TABLE 220-1 National Institute of Health Stroke Scale: A Rapid, Reproducible Neurologic Evaluation of Patients with Stroke

Category	Patient Response	Score
1a. Level of consciousness (LOC)	Alert	0
	Drowsy	1
	Stuporous	2
	Coma	3
1b. LOC questions	Answers both correctly	0
	Answers one correctly	1
	Answers none correctly	2
1c. LOC commands	Obeys both correctly	0
	Obeys one correctly	1
	Obeys none correctly	2
2. Best gaze	Normal	0
	Partial gaze palsy	1
	Forced deviation	2
3. Best visual	No visual loss	0
	Partial hemianopsia	1
	Complete hemianopsia	2
4. Facial palsy	Normal	0
	Minor facial weakness	1
	Partial facial weakness	2
	No facial movement	3
5. Best motor arm	No drift after 10 s	0
	Drift	1
	Cannot resist gravity	2
	No effort against gravity	3
6. Best motor leg	No drift after 5 s	0
	Drift	1
	Cannot resist gravity	2
	No effort against gravity	3
7. Limb ataxia	Absent	0
	Present in upper or lower extremities	1
	Present in both upper and lower extremities	2
8. Sensory	Normal	0
	Partial loss	1
	Dense loss	2
9. Neglect	No neglect	0
	Partial neglect	1
	Complete neglect	2
10. Dysarthria	Normal articulation	0
	Mild to moderate dysarthria	1
	Near unintelligible or worse	2
11. Best language	No aphasia	0
	Mild to moderate aphasia	1
	Severe aphasia	2
	Mute	3

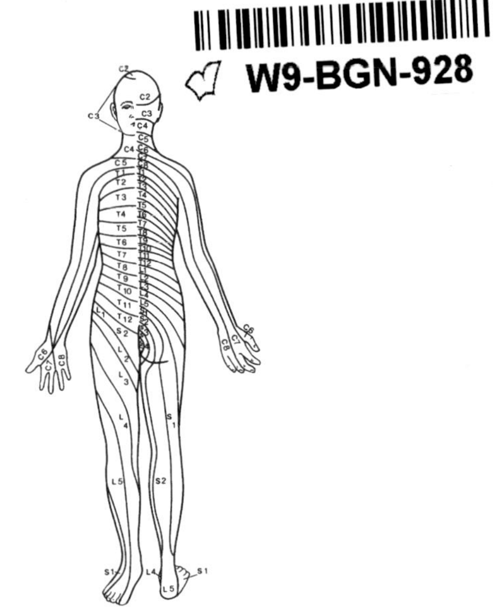

FIG. 264-1. Dermatomes.

TABLE 244-2B Revised Trauma Score

Number	Glasgow Coma Score	Systolic Blood Pressure	Respiratory Rate
4	13–15	>89	10–29
3	9–12	76–89	>29
2	6–8	50–75	6–9
1	4–5	1–49	1–5
0	3	0	0

TABLE 244-2A Pediatric Trauma Score

	−1	+1	+2
Size (kg)	<10	10–20	>20
Airway	Unmaintained	Maintained	Normal
Systolic blood pressure (mmHg)	<50	50–90	>90
Level of consciousness	Comatose	Altered	Awake
Wounds	Major open	Minor open	None
Skeletal trauma	Open/multiple	Closed	None

TABLE 226-1 Drugs That Should Be Used With Caution in Myasthenia Gravis

Steroids
- ACTH*
- Methylprednisolone*
- Prednisone*

Anticonvulsants
- Dilantin
- Ethosuximide
- Trimethadione
- Paraldehyde
- Magnesium sulfate
- Barbiturates

Antimalarials
- Chloroquine*
- Quinine*

IV Fluids
- Na lactate solution

Antibiotics
- Aminoglycosides
  - Neomycin*
  - Streptomycin*
  - Kanamycin*
  - Gentamicin
  - Tobramycin
  - Dihydrostreptomycin*
  - Amikacin
- Polymyxin A
- Polymyxin B
- Bacitracin
- Sulfonamides
- Viomycin
- Colistin
- Colistimethate*
- Lincomycin
- Clindamycin
- Tetracycline
  - Oxytetracycline
  - Rolitetracycline

Psychotropics
- Chlorpromazine*
- Lithium carbonate*
- Amitriptyline
- Droperidol
- Haloperidol
- Imipramine
- Paraldehyde
- Trichlorethanol

Antirheumatics
- D-Penicillamine
- Colchicine
- Chloroquine

Cardiovascular
- Quinidine*
- Procainamide*
- Beta blockers
  - Propranolol
  - Oxprenolol
  - Practolol
  - Pindolol
  - Sotalol
- Lidocaine
- Dilantin
- Trimethaphan

Local Anesthetic
- Lidocaine*
- Procaine*

Analgesics
- Narcotics
  - Morphine
  - Dilaudid
  - Codeine
  - Pantopon
  - Meperidine

Endocrine
- Thyroid replacement*

Eyedrops
- Timolol*
- Ecothiopate

Others
- Amantadine
- Diphenhydramine
- Emetine
- Diuretics
- Muscle relaxants
- CNS depressants
- Respiratory depressants
- Sedatives
- Procaine*
- Tranquilizers

Neuromuscular blocking agents
- Tubocurarine
- Pancuronium
- Gallamine
- Dimethyl tubocurarine
- Succinylcholine
- Decamethonium

*Case reports implicate drugs in exacerbations of MG.

Source: This table is a modified version of the table from Adams SL, Matthews J, Grammer LC: Drugs that may exacerbate myasthenia gravis. *Ann Emerg Med* 13:532, 1984. Used with permission.

EMERGENCY MEDICINE

A COMPREHENSIVE STUDY GUIDE

NOTICE

FIFTH EDITION

EMERGENCY MEDICINE

A COMPREHENSIVE STUDY GUIDE

Editor-in-Chief

Judith E. Tintinalli, M.D., M.S.

Professor and Chair
Department of Emergency Medicine
University of North Carolina at Chapel Hill
Chapel Hill, North Carolina

Co-Editors

Gabor D. Kelen, M.D.

Professor and Chair
Department of Emergency Medicine
Johns Hopkins University
Baltimore, Maryland

J. Stephan Stapczynski, M.D.

Professor and Chair
Department of Emergency Medicine
University of Kentucky
Lexington, Kentucky

American College of Emergency Physicians®

New illustrations by Holly R. Fischer, MFA
Ann Arbor, Michigan, and
Cinnamon Larson
Carrboro, North Carolina

McGraw-Hill
Health Professions Division
New York St. Louis San Francisco Auckland Bogatá Caracas Lisbon Madrid Mexico City Milan Montreal New Delhi San Juan Singapore Sydney Tokyo Toronto

McGraw-Hill
A Division of The McGraw-Hill Companies

EMERGENCY MEDICINE A Comprehensive Study Guide

1234567890 DOWDOW 09876543210

ISBN 0-07-065351-8

This book was set in Times New Roman by The PRD Group, Inc.
The editors were John J. Dolan, Mariapaz Ramos Englis,
Pamela T. Hanley, and Lester A. Sheinis.
The production supervisor was Richard C. Ruzycka.
The text and cover designer was Joan O'Connor.
The indexer was Irving Condé Tullar.
R. R. Donnelley & Sons Company was printer and binder.
This book is printed on acid-free paper.

LIBRARY OF CONGRESS CATALOGING-IN-PUBLICATION DATA
Tintinalli, Judith E.
Emergency medicine : a comprehensive study guide / Judith E. Tintinalli, Gabor D. Kelen, J. Stephan Stapczynski ; American College of Emergency Physicians.—5th ed.
p. cm.
Rev. ed. of: Emergency medicine / American College of Emergency Physicians ; Judith E. Tintinalli. 4th ed. c1996.
Includes bibliographical references and index.
ISBN 0-07-065351-8
1. Emergency medicine. I. Kelen, Gabor D. II. Stapczynski, J. Stephan. III. American College of Emergency Physicians.
IV. Emergency medicine. V. Title.
[DNLM: 1. Emergency Medicine. 2. Emergencies. WB 105 T593e 1999]
RC86.7.E586 1999
616.02′5—dc21
DNLM/DLC
for Library of Congress 99-10685
CIP

To the physicians, nurses, paramedics, students, and administrative staff of the Emergency Department at the University of North Carolina Hospitals, who make sure I never have a dull moment in the practice of emergency medicine. JET

To my parents, Andrew and Susan Kelen, who instilled in me the ethic and love of discovery. GDK

To my wife, to my sons, and to my parents. The challenges of being a husband, a father, and a son have made me a better person. My love and appreciation. JSS

CONTENTS

Section Twelve Infectious Diseases 943

Section Thirteen Toxicology 1057

CONTRIBUTORS*

STEPHANIE B ABBUHL, M.D. [296]
Associate Professor and Medical Director
Department of Emergency Medicine
Hospital of the University of Pennsylvania
Philadelphia, Pennsylvania

RIYAD B. ABU-LABAN, M.D., M.H.Sc., F.C.R.P.C. [83]
Assistant Clinical Professor of Surgery
University of British Columbia
Attending Physician and Associate Research Director
Department of Emergency Medicine
Vancouver General Hospital
Vancouver, BC, Canada

WILLIAM R. AHRENS, M.D. [128]
Director of Emergency Medicine for Pediatrics
Department of Emergency Medicine
University of Illinois at Chicago College of Medicine
Chicago, Illinois

MICHAEL F. ALTIERI, M.D., F.A.A.P. [136]
Pediatric Section Chief
Department of Emergency Medicine
Inova Fairfax Hospital
Falls Church, Virginia
Associate Clinical Professor of Emergency Medicine and Pediatrics
Georgetown University School of Medicine
Washington, DC
George Washington University School of Medicine
Washington, DC
Associate Clinical Professor of Pediatrics
University of Virginia School of Medicine
Charlotte, Virginia

DAVID C. ANDERSON, M.D. [227]
Department of Neurology
Hennepin County Medical Center
Minneapolis, Minnesota

ERIC ANDERSON, M.D., F.A.C.E.P. [60]
Clinical Faculty
Department of Emergency Medicine
Case Western Reserve University
MetroHealth Emergency Medicine
Cleveland Clinic Foundation
Cleveland, Ohio

WILLIAM T. ANDERSON, M.D., F.A.C.E.P. [144]
Department of Emergency Medicine
William Beaumont Hospital
Troy, Michigan

PAUL S. AUERBACH, M.D., M.S., F.A.C.E.P. [190]
Clinical Professor of Emergency Medicine
Department of Surgery
Stanford University School of Medicine
Stanford, California
Life Sciences Advisor
Palo Alto, California

TOM P. AUFDERHEIDE, M.D. [81]
Associate Professor
Research Director
Department of Emergency Medicine
Medical College of Wisconsin
Milwaukee, Wisconsin

CHENICHERI BALAKRISHNAN, M.D. [194]
Assistant Professor
Department of Surgery
Wayne State University School of Medicine
Detroit, Michigan

J. MICHAEL BALLESTER, M.D. [195]
Clinical Instructor
Department of Emergency Medicine
Southern Illinois University School of Medicine
St. Johns Hospital
Springfield, Illinois

JEFFREY D. BAND, M.D. [142]
Division of Infectious Diseases
William Beaumont Hospital
Royal Oak, Michigan

ROBERT A. BARISH, M.D., F.A.C.E.P., F.A.C.P. [72]
Professor of Surgery and Medicine
Associate Dean of Clinical Affairs
University of Maryland School of Medicine
Baltimore, Maryland

STEVEN BRENT BARNES, M.D. [187]
Assistant Professor of Emergency Medicine
Associate Residency Program Director
Department of Emergency Medicine
University of Oklahoma Health Sciences Center
Oklahoma City, Oklahoma

L. JARRETT BARNHILL, M.D. [302]
Associate Professor
Department of Psychiatry
University of North Carolina Chapel Hill School of Medicine
Chapel Hill, North Carolina

BONNY J. BARON, M.D. [248, 250]
Assistant Professor
Department of Emergency Medicine
State University of New York Health Science Center at Brooklyn
Attending Physician
Department of Emergency Medicine
Kings County Hospital Center
Brooklyn, New York

WILLIAM G. BARSAN, M.D. [220]
Professor and Chair
Department of Emergency Medicine
University of Michigan Health System
Ann Arbor, Michigan

*The numbers in brackets following the contributors' names indicate the chapters written or cowritten by that contributor.

CHRISTOPHER W. BARTON, M.D., F.A.C.E.P. [20]
Associate Professor
Head, Division of Informatics
Department of Emergency Medicine
University of North Carolina Chapel Hill School of Medicine
Chapel Hill, North Carolina

DANIEL G. BATTON, M.D. [113]
Chief, Neonatology
Department of Pediatrics
William Beaumont Hospital
Royal Oak, Michigan

NORMAN J. BEAUCHAMP, Jr., M.D. [229]
Assistant Professor
Division of Neuroradiology
Department of Radiology
The Johns Hopkins Hospital
Baltimore, Maryland

RONALD W. BEAUDREAU, D.M.D., M.D., F.A.C.E.P. [234]
Assistant Director
Department of Emergency Medicine
Columbia Augusta Medical Center
Augusta, Georgia

AMY J. BEHRMAN, M.D. [105]
Assistant Professor
Director of Occupational Medicine
Hospital of the University of Pennsylvania
Department of Emergency Medicine
Philadelphia, Pennsylvania

WILLIAM A. BERK, M.D., F.A.C.E.P. [17, 160, 299]
Associate Professor
Department of Emergency Medicine
Wayne State University
Detroit, Michigan

CAROL D. BERKOWITZ, M.D., F.A.A.E.M. [110, 114, 289]
Acting Chair and Professor
Department of Pediatrics
Harbor–UCLA Medical Center
Torrance, California

EDWARD BERNSTEIN, M.D., F.A.C.E.P. [287]
Professor of Emergency Medicine
Boston University School of Medicine and Boston Medical Center
Professor of Social and Behavioral Sciences
Boston University School of Public Health
Vice Chairperson for Academic Affairs
Boston University School of Medicine
Boston, Massachusetts

JUDITH A. BERNSTEIN, R.N.C., Ph.D. [287]
Assistant Professor
Department of Maternal and Child Health
Boston University School of Public Health
Assistant Professor
Department of Emergency Medicine
Boston University School of Medicine
Boston, Massachusetts

HOWARD A. BESSEN, M.D. [186]
Director
Emergency Medicine Residency Program
Harbor–UCLA Medical Center
Torrance, California

EDWARD S. BESSMAN, M.D., F.A.C.E.P., F.A.A.E.M. [18]
Chairman
Department of Emergency Medicine
Johns Hopkins Bayview Medical Center
Assistant Professor
Associate Residency Director
Department of Emergency Medicine
Johns Hopkins University School of Medicine
Baltimore, Maryland

JESSICA L. BIENSTOCK, M.D., M.P.H. [102]
Assistant Professor
Department of Gynecology and Obstetrics
Johns Hopkins University School of Medicine
Johns Hopkins Hospitals
Baltimore, Maryland

ROBERT BILKOVSKI, M.D. [26]
Assistant Professor
Department of Emergency Medicine
Virginia Commonwealth University School of Medicine
Richmond, Virginia

JIM BLAKE, M.D. [43]
Resident
Department of Emergency Medicine
University of Kentucky
Lexington, Kentucky

BARBARA K. BLOK, M.D. [46]
Instructor
Department of Emergency Medicine
Johns Hopkins University
Baltimore, Maryland

DAVID M. BLUEMKE, M.D., Ph.D. [57]
Clinical Director, MRI
Department of Radiology
Johns Hopkins Hospital
Baltimore, Maryland

EILEEN M. K. BOBEK, M.D. [27]
Resident Physician
Section of Emergency Medicine
University of Michigan Medical Center
University of Michigan School of Medicine
Ann Arbor, Michigan

MARK P. BOGNER, M.D. [93]
Assistant Professor of Medicine
University of Wisconsin
Madison, Wisconsin

EDMUND BOLTON, M.D. [24]
Emergency Medicine HealthCare Physicians
Westmont, Illinois

MICHAEL J. BONO, M.D., F.A.C.E.P. [87]
Associate Professor
Associate Director
Emergency Medicine Residency Program
Department of Emergency Medicine
Eastern Virginia Medical School
Norfolk, Virginia

MARC BORENSTEIN, M.D., F.A.C.E.P., F.A.C.P. [217]
Vice-Chair and Residency Program Director Department of Emergency Medicine
St. Luke's-Roosevelt Hospital Center
Associate Professor of Clinical Medicine
Columbia University College of Physicians and Surgeons
New York, New York

CARL L. BOSE, M.D. [4]
Department of Pediatrics
Chief, Division of Neonatal-Perinatal Medicine
University of North Carolina
Chapel Hill, North Carolina

GEORGE M. BOSSE, M.D. [158]
Associate Professor
Department of Emergency Medicine
University of Louisville
Louisville, Kentucky

SHARON A. BOSWELL, R.N., C.E.N. [252]
Research Nurse
R. Adams Crowley Shock Trauma Center
University of Maryland Medical Center
Baltimore, Maryland

JAMES K. BOUZOUKIS, M.D., F.A.C.E.P. [78]
Medical Center of Delaware
Wilmington, Delaware

WILLIAM M. BOWLING, M.D. [251]
Resident Physician
Department of Surgery
Washington University School of Medicine
St. Louis, Missouri

WILLIAM J. BRADY, M.D. [81, 155, 202, 237, 241]
Assistant Professor of Emergency Medicine and Internal Medicine
Program Director, Emergency Medicine Residency
Associate Director, Chest Pain Unit
University of Virginia School of Medicine
Department of Emergency Medicine
University of Virginia Health System
Charlottesville, Virginia

G. RICHARD BRAEN, M.D., F.A.C.E.P. [179]
Professor and Chair
Department of Emergency Medicine
State University of New York, Buffalo
Buffalo, New York

ANNE F. BRAYER, M.D., F.A.A.P. [200]
Assistant Professor of Emergency Medicine and Pediatrics
Department of Emergency Medicine
University of Rochester Medical Center
Strong Memorial Hospital
Rochester, New York

JANE H. BRICE, M.D., M.P.H. [147]
Assistant Professor
Department of Emergency Medicine
University of North Carolina Chapel Hill School of Medicine
Chapel Hill, North Carolina

JAMES E. BROWN, M.D. [286]
Assistant Professor
Department of Emergency Medicine
Wright State University School of Medicine
Dayton, Ohio

KATHLEEN M. BROWN, M.D. [119]
Assistant Professor of Pediatric Emergency Medicine
Department of Emergency Medicine
State University of New York Health Science Center at Syracuse
Syracuse, New York

BRIAN J. BROWNE, M.D., F.A.C.E.P. [79]
Head, Division of Emergency Medicine
Director of Emergency Medical Services
University of Maryland Medical System
University of Maryland School of Medicine Baltimore
Baltimore, Maryland

ROBERT A. BROWNSTEIN, M.D. [150]
Attending Physician
Department of Emergency Medicine
Rex Hospital
Raleigh, North Carolina

G. RICHARD BRUNO, M.D. [166, 175, 180]
Assistant Professor
Department of Emergency Medicine
Assistant Director
Emergency Medicine Residency Program
State University of New York–Brooklyn
New York, New York

JAMES H. BRYAN, M.D., Ph.D., F.A.C.E.P. [149]
Assistant Professor of Emergency Medicine
Department of Emergency Medicine
Oregon Health Sciences University
Portland Veterans Affairs Medical Center
Portland, Oregon

TIMOTHY G. BUCHMAN, M.D., Ph.D. [251]
Professor of Surgery, Anesthesiology, and Medicine
Chief Section of Burn, Trauma, Surgical Critical Care
Department of Surgery
Barnes-Jewish Hospital
Washington University School of Medicine
St. Louis, Missouri

JOHN H. BURTON, M.D., F.A.C.E.P. [278]
Research Director
EMS Director
Department of Emergency Medicine
Maine Medical Center
Portland, Maine
Assistant Professor
Department of Surgery
University of Vermont School of Medicine
Burlington, Vermont

CHARLES B. CAIRNS, M.D., F.A.C.E.P. [49]
Associate Professor; Director, Colorado Emergency Medicine Research Center
Division of Emergency Medicine
University of Colorado Health Sciences Center
Denver, Colorado

MARY CAMARCA, M.D. [136]
Department of Emergency Medicine
Inova Fairfax Hospital
Falls Church, Virginia

DONNA L. CARDEN, M.D., F.A.C.E.P. [140]
Associate Professor of Internal Medicine, Emergency Medicine, and Molecular and Cellular Physiology
Louisiana Chapter of ACEP
Louisiana State University Medical Center
Shreveport, Louisiana

TERESA M. CARLIN, M.D. [25]
Fellow
St. Christopher's Hospital for Children
Pediatric Emergency Medicine
Philadelphia, Pennsylvania
Instructor
Department of Emergency Medicine
Johns Hopkins University School of Medicine
Baltimore, Maryland

CHRISTINE M. CARR, M.D., F.A.C.E.P. [23]
Clinical Instructor
Department of Emergency Services
Medical University of South Carolina
Charleston, South Carolina

WALLACE A. CARTER, M.D. [36, 39, 166, 175, 180]
Director, Emergency Medicine Residency
New York University/Bellevue Medical Center
Assistant Professor
Clinical Surgery/Emergency Medicine
New York University School of Medicine
New York, New York

MICHAEL S. CATAPANO, M.D., F.A.C.E.P. [131]
Department of Emergency Medicine
Southampton Hospital
Southampton, New York

EUGENE E. CEPEDA, M.D. [9]
Pediatrician
Department of Pediatrics
The Detroit Medical Center
Hutzel Hospital
Detroit, Michigan

ROBERT S. CHANG, M.D. [39]
Clinical Instructor
Department of Emergency Medicine
Boston Medical Center
Boston, Massachusetts

ARJUN S. CHANMUGAM, M.D., F.A.C.E.P. [53, 171]
Assistant Professor
Department of Emergency Medicine
Johns Hopkins Hospital
Baltimore, Maryland

MICHAEL E. CHANSKY, M.D. [203]
Associate Professor and Acting Chairman
Department of Emergency Medicine
UMDNJ–Robert Wood Johnson Medical School at Camden
The Cooper Health System
Camden, New Jersey

BENNETT CHIN, M.D. [57]

HAROLD W. CHIN, M.D., F.A.C.E.P. [261, 262]
Medical Director
Occupational Health
Lake Forest Hospital
Lake Forest, Illinois

ANN S. CHINNIS, M.D., M.S.H.A., F.A.C.E.P. [196, 197]
Associate Professor of Emergency Medicine
Interim Chair of Emergency Medicine
Emergency Department Medical Director
West Virginia University School of Medicine
Morgantown, West Virginia

ANIL CHOPRA, M.D. [55]
Assistant Professor of Medicine
Division of Emergency Medicine
The Toronto Hospital
University of Toronto
Toronto, Canada

RICHARD A. CHRISTOPH, M.D. [132, 135]
Associate Professor of Emergency Medicine and Pediatrics
Director, Pediatric Emergency Medicine
Department of Emergency Medicine
University of Virginia
Charlottesville, Virginia

RICHARD F. CLARK, M.D., F.A.C.E.P., F.A.C.M.T. [188]
Associate Professor of Medicine and Director
Division of Medical Toxicology
Department of Emergency Medicine
UCSD Medical Center
San Diego, California

DAVID M. CLINE, M.D., F.A.C.E.P. [34, 50]
Clinical Associate Professor and Assistant Residency Director
Department of Emergency Medicine, University of North Carolina at Chapel Hill
Chapel Hill, North Carolina
Education Director, Department of Emergency Medicine
WakeMed
Raleigh, North Carolina

WENDY C. COATES, M.D., F.A.C.E.P. [38, 40]
Associate Professor of Medicine
UCLA School of Medicine
Los Angeles, California
Director, Medical Education
Department of Emergency Medicine
Harbor–UCLA Medical Center
Torrance, California

DANIEL J. COBAUGH, Pharm.D. [156]
Managing Director
Finger Lakes Regional Poison and Drug Information Center
Assistant Professor of Emergency Medicine
Department of Emergency Medicine
University of Rochester Medical Center
Rochester, New York

STEPHEN A. COLUCCIELLO, M.D. [249]
Assistant Chair
Director of Clinical Services and Trauma Coordinator
Department of Emergency Medicine
Carolinas Medical Center
Assistant Clinical Professor
Department of Emergency Medicine
University of North Carolina
Chapel Hill, North Carolina

ALASDAIR K. T. CONN, M.D., F.A.C.S., F.A.C.E.P. [253]
Chief of Emergency Services
Department of Emergency Services
Massachusetts General Hospital
Assistant Professor of Surgery
Harvard Medical School
Boston, Massachusetts

JOHN R. COOKE, M.D., J.D. [216]
St. Luke's–Roosevelt Hospital Center
Columbia College of Physicians and Surgeons
New York, New York

RANDOLPH J. CORDLE, M.D., F.A.A.P., D.A.B.E.M. [125, 129]
Director Pediatric Emergency Medicine
Department of Emergency Medicine
St. Luke's Hospital
Boise, Idaho

EDWARD E. CORNWELL III, M.D., F.A.C.S., F.C.C.M. [243]
Associate Professor of Surgery
Chief, Adult Trauma Service
Department of Surgery
The Johns Hopkins Medical Institutions
Baltimore, Maryland

C. JAMES CORRALL, M.D., M.P.H, F.A.A.P, F.A.C.E.P. [115]
Clinical Associate Professor of Emergency Medicine
and Pediatrics
Adjunct Associate Professor of Clinical Pharmacology
Department of Emergency Medicine
Emergency Medicine and Trauma Center
Methodist Hospital of Indiana
Indiana University School of Medicine
Indianapolis, Indiana

FRANCIS L. COUNSELMAN, M.D., F.A.C.E.P. [271]
Professor, Chairman, and Program Director
Department of Emergency Medicine
Eastern Virginia Medical School
Staff Physician
Emergency Physicians of Tidewater
Norfolk, Virginia

NATALIE M. CULLEN, M.D. [126]
Assistant Professor
Department of Emergency Medicine
Wright State University School of Medicine
Dayton, Ohio

RITA K. CYDULKA, M.D., F.A.C.E.P. [64, 65]
Associate Professor and Residency Director
Department of Emergency Medicine
MetroHealth Medical Center
Case Western Reserve University
Cleveland, Ohio

FRANK F. S. DALY, M.B.B.S. [189]
Fellow
Medical Toxicology
Rocky Mountain Poison and Drug Center
University of Colorado Health Sciences Center
Denver, Colorado

DANIEL F. DANZL, M.D., F.A.C.E.P. [15]
Professor and Chair
Department of Emergency Medicine
University of Louisville
Louisville, Kentucky

RICHARD C. DART, M.D., Ph.D. [164, 189]
Director
Rocky Mountain Poison and Drug Center
Associate Professor of Surgery,
Medicine, and Pharmacy
University of Colorado Health Sciences Center
Denver, Colorado

ELIZABETH M. DATNER, M.D. [12]
Assistant Professor of Emergency Medicine
Department of Emergency Medicine
University of Pennsylvania School of Medicine
Hospital of the University of Pennsylvania
Presbyterian Medical Center
Philadelphia, Pennsylvania

DANIEL J. DEBEHNKE, M.D., F.A.C.E.P. [241]
Associate Professor of Emergency Medicine
Department of Emergency Medicine
Medical College of Wisconsin
Milwaukee, Wisconsin
Director of Clinical Operations
Department of Emergency Medicine
Froedtert Memorial Lutheran Hospital
Milwaukee, Wisconsin

KATHLEEN A. DELANEY, M.D. [182]
Clinical Professor in Medicine and Surgery
Division of Emergency Medicine
Department of Surgery
Southwestern Medical School
Dallas, Texas

KENNETH C. DIRK, M.D. [149]
Resident Physician
Department of Emergency Medicine
Oregon Health Sciences University
Portland, Oregon

GAIL D'ONOFRIO, M.D. [287]
Associate Professor
Yale University School of Medicine
Director of Research
Department of Surgery, Section of Emergency Medicine
Yale University School of Medicine
Yale New Haven Hospital
New Haven, Connecticut

SUZANNE DOYON, M.D. [161]
Assistant Professor
Division of Emergency Medicine, Department of Surgery
University of Maryland Medical System
Baltimore, Maryland

WILLIAM H. DRIBBEN, M.D. [168]
Medical Toxicology Fellow
Indiana Poison Center and Emergency Medicine and Trauma Center at Methodist Hospital
Indiana University School of Medicine
Indianapolis, Indiana

STEVEN C. DRONEN, M.D. [27]
Associate Professor
Associate Section Head and Residency Director
Section of Emergency Medicine
University of Michigan Medical Center
University of Michigan School of Medicine
Ann Arbor, Michigan

MARY E. EBERST, M.D. [210–215]
Assistant Professor
Departments of Emergency Medicine and Medicine
University of North Carolina at Chapel Hill
Chapel Hill, North Carolina

CHARLES A. ECKERLINE JR., M.D., F.A.C.E.P. [43]
Associate Professor and Associate Chief of Service
Department of Emergency Medicine
University of Kentucky
Lexington, Kentucky

COL. EDWARD M. EITZEN, JR., M.D., M.P.H. [181]
Chief
Division of Operational Medicine
USAMRIID
Ft. Detrick, MD
Associate Clinical Professor
Uniformed Services
University of the Health Sciences
Bethesda, Maryland

CHARLES L. EMERMAN, M.D. [59, 167]
Associate Professor of Emergency Medicine
Case Western Reserve University
Chairman of Emergency Medicine
MetroHealth Medical Center
Cleveland Clinic Foundation
Cleveland, Ohio

STEPHEN D. EMOND, M.D., F.A.C.E.P. [216]
Assistant Professor of Medicine
Department of Emergency Medicine
Weill Medical College of Cornell University
Director of Clinical Research
Department of Emergency Medicine
New York-Presbyterian Hospital
New York, New York

JOHN ENG, M.D. [294]
Assistant Professor of Radiology
Department of Radiology and Radiological Science
Johns Hopkins University
Baltimore, Maryland

BRIAN D. EUERLE, M.D. [31]
Assistant Professor
Division of Emergency Medicine
Emergency Department
University of Maryland Medical Center
Baltimore, Maryland

RAWDEN W. EVANS, M.D., Ph.D. [82]
Assistant Professor
Department of Emergency Medicine
University of Michigan Medical Center
Ann Arbor, Michigan

MARTIN L. FACKLER, MD
President
International Wound Ballistics Association
Hawthorne, Florida

KIM M. FELDHAUS, M.D., F.A.C.E.P. [290]
Associate Residency Director
Denver Health Medical Center
Denver, Colorado
Assistant Professor
Division of Emergency Medicine
Department of Surgery
University of Colorado Health Sciences Center
Denver, Colorado

MADONNA FERNÁNDEZ, M.D. [40]
Chief Resident and Clinical Teaching Fellow
Harbor–UCLA Department of Emergency Medicine
Torrance, California

DENIS J. FITZGERALD, M.D. [74]
Department of Emergency Medicine
University of Cincinnati Medical Center
University of Cincinnati School of Medicine
Cincinnati, Ohio

STEVEN G. FOLSTAD, M.D., F.A.C.E.P. [146]
Mid-Atlantic Emergency Medicine Associates
Charlotte, North Carolina

MARSHA D. FORD, M.D., F.A.C.E.P., F.A.C.M.T. [178]
Director
Carolinas Poison Center
Assistant Chairman
Director, Division of Toxicology
Department of Emergency Medicine
Carolinas Medical Center
Charlotte, North Carolina

MARK W. FOURRE, M.D. [277]
Associate Clinical Professor of Surgery
University of Vermont
Burlington, Vermont
Program Director
Department of Emergency Medicine
Maine Medical Center
Portland, Maine

HAROLD E. FOX, M.D., M.S. [102]
Professor and Chair
Residency Program Director
Obstetrician/Gynecologist-in-Chief
Department of Gynecology and Obstetrics
Johns Hopkins University School of Medicine
Johns Hopkins Hospital
Baltimore, Maryland

SUSAN FUCHS, M.D. [116]
Associate Director
Division of Pediatric Emergency Medicine
Children's Memorial Hospital
Chicago, Illinois
Associate Professor of Pediatrics
Northwestern University Medical School
Chicago, Illinois

WADE R. GAASCH, M.D., F.A.C.E.P. [72]
Assistant Professor of Surgery
Clinical Director
Adult Emergency Services and Medical Director
Maryland ExpressCare
Division of Emergency Medicine
University of Maryland School of Medicine
Baltimore, Maryland

E. JOHN GALLAGHER, M.D. [68]
University Chair
Department of Emergency Medicine
Professor of Emergency Medicine, Medicine, Epidemiology, and Social Medicine
Albert Einstein College of Medicine
Bronx, New York

DAVID R. GENS, M.D., F.A.C.S. [16]
Assistant Professor
Department of Surgery and Program in Trauma
University of Maryland School of Medicine
R. Adams Cowley Shock Trauma Center
University of Maryland Medical Center
Baltimore, Maryland

MAXIME ALIX GILLES, M.D. [60]
Clinical Faculty
Co-Director, Medical Students
Department of Emergency Medicine
Case Western Reserve University
MetroHealth Emergency Medicine
Cleveland, Ohio

LEWIS R. GOLDFRANK, M.D. [303]
Associate Professor of Clinical Medicine
New York University School of Medicine
Director of Emergency Medicine
Bellevue Hospital Center and New York University Medical Center
New York, New York

BRIAN GOLDMAN, M.D., F.A.C.E.P. [223]
Assistant Professor
Department of Family and Community Medicine
University of Toronto
Staff Emergency Physician
Mount Sinai Hospital
Toronto, Ontario, Canada

ANTHONY GOMEZ, M.D. [94]
Attending Physician
Department of Emergency Medicine
St. Luke's–Roosevelt Hospital Center
New York, New York

HERMAN F. GOMEZ, M.D. [189]
Clinical Instructor
Division of Emergency Medicine
University of Michigan Medical Center
Ann Arbor, Michigan

PHILLIP V. GORDON, M.D., Ph.D. [4]
Fellow in Neonatal-Perinatal Medicine
Department of Pediatrics
University of North Carolina
Chapel Hill, North Carolina

SUSAN J. GOTTLIEB, M.D. [283]
Department of Psychiatry
William Beaumont Hospital
Royal Oak, Michigan

MICHELLE S. GRADY, R.N., B.S.N. [56]
Heart and Heart-Lung Transplant Coordinator
Heart and Heart-Lung Transplantation Program
University of North Carolina Hospitals
Chapel Hill, North Carolina

CHARLES S. GRAFFEO, M.D. [205]
Associate Professor and Assistant Residency Director
Department of Emergency Medicine
Eastern Virginia Medical School
Norfolk, Virginia

MATTHEW C. GRATTON, M.D. [73]
Associate Professor/EMS Medical Director
Department of Emergency Medicine
University of Missouri at Kansas City School of Medicine
Truman Medical Center
Kansas City, Missouri

GARY B. GREEN, M.D., M.P.H., F.A.C.E.P. [45]
Assistant Professor
Director
Cardiac Evaluation Unit
Department of Emergency Medicine
Johns Hopkins University
Baltimore, Maryland

RACHELLE A. GREENMAN, M.D. [106]
Assistant Professor of Emergency Medicine
Department of Emergency Medicine
Cooper Hospital University Medical Center
UMDNJ–Robert Wood Johnson Medical School at Camden
Camden, New Jersey

CHERYL H. HACK, M.D. [134]
Assistant Clinical Professor
Wayne State University School of Medicine
Medical Director, Myelomeningocele Care Center
Medical Director, Comprehensive Multi-Handicapped Team
Children's Hospital of Michigan
Detroit, Michigan

JASON B. HACK, M.D. [151]

THERESA A. HACKELING, M.D. [235, 236]
Attending Physician
Department of Emergency Medicine
WakeMed Center
Raleigh, North Carolina

PETER H. HACKETT, M.D., F.A.C.E.P. [191]
Affiliate Associate Professor
Department of Medicine
University of Washington School of Medicine
Seattle, Washington
Attending Physician
Emergency Department
St Mary's Hospital and Medical Center
Grand Junction, Colorado

PAUL R. HALLER, M.D. [267]
Assistant Professor
Emergency Medicine Program
University of Minnesota
Minneapolis, Minnesota

GLENN C. HAMILTON, M.D., M.S.M. [286]
Professor and Chair
Department of Emergency Medicine
Wright State University School of Medicine
Dayton, Ohio

MARK P. HAMLIN, M.D., M.S. [22]
Fellow
Critical Care Medicine
Department of Anesthesiology and Critical Care Medicine
Johns Hopkins University School of Medicine
Baltimore, Maryland

DANIEL G. HANKINS, M.D., F.A.C.E.P. [6]
Assistant Professor
Department of Emergency Medicine
Mayo Clinic
Medical Director
Mayo Medical Transport and Communications
Rochester, Minnesota

KAREN N. HANSEN, M.D. [163]
Assistant Professor
Department of Emergency Medicine
Johns Hopkins University
Baltimore, Maryland

CHRISTINA E. HANTSCH, M.D. [99]
Medical Toxicology Fellow
Middle Tennessee Poison Center
Center for Clinical Toxicology
Vanderbilt University Medical Center
Nashville, Tennessee

FRED P. HARCHELROAD, JR., M.D. [195]
Director
Medical Toxicology Treatment Center
Associate Professor
Department of Emergency Medicine
MCP–Hahneman School of Medicine
Allegheny General Hospital
Pittsburgh, Pennsylvania

KAREN J. MORRILL HARDART, M.D. [108]
Attending Physician
Department of Obstetrics and Gynecology
Anne Arundel Medical Center
Annapolis, Maryland

RICHARD A. HARRIGAN, M.D., F.A.C.E.P. [155, 202]
Associate Professor of Medicine
Temple University School of Medicine
Acting Chief and Associate Research Director
Division of Emergency Medicine
Temple University Hospital
Philadelphia, Pennsylvania

ANN L. HARWOOD-NUSS, M.D., F.A.C.E.P. [138]
Professor and Assistant Dean for Educational Affairs
Department of Emergency Medicine
University of Florida Health Science Center–Jacksonville
Jacksonville, Florida

M. YOUSUF HASAN, M.D., F.A.A.P. [112]
Fellow
Critical Care Medicine
Department of Pediatrics
University of Florida Health Science Center–Jacksonville
The Nemours Children's Clinic and Wolfson Children's Hospital
Jacksonville, Florida

WILLIAM E. HAUDA II, M.D. [10, 127, 224]
Assistant Clinical Professor of Emergency Medicine
George Washington University School of Medicine
Washington, DC
Clinical Instructor of Pediatrics
University of Virginia School of Medicine
Charlottesville, Virginia
Co-Director
Pediatric Emergency Medicine Fellowship
Inova Fairfax Hospital
Falls Church, Virginia

BRUCE E. HAYNES, M.D. [193]
Medical Director
Emergency Medical Services
County of Imperial
El Centro, California
County of Orange
Santa Ana, California

MICHAEL B. HELLER, M.D., F.A.C.E.P. [295]
Director
Emergency Medicine Residency
St. Luke's Hospital
Bethlehem, Pennsylvania
Clinical Professor
Temple University School of Medicine
Philadelphia, Pennsylvania

WILMA V. HENDERSON, M.D., F.A.C.E.P. [160]
Assistant Professor
Medical Student Coordinator
Department of Emergency Medicine
Wayne State University
Detroit, Michigan

LEE U. HERFEL, M.D. [30]
Resident
Department of Emergency Medicine
University of Kentucky
Lexington, Kentucky

ROB HERFEL, M.D. [37]
Resident
Department of Emergency Medicine
University of Kentucky
Lexington, Kentucky

PATTI J. HERLING, M.D. [296]
Assistant Professor
Department of Radiology
Section of Emergency Radiology
University of Pennsylvania Health System
Philadelphia, Pennsylvania

PETER M. HILL, M.D., M.Sc. [45]
Instructor
Assistant Chief of Service
Department of Emergency Medicine
Johns Hopkins Bayview Medical Center
Johns Hopkins University
Baltimore, Maryland

JON MARK HIRSHON, M.D., M.P.H., F.A.C.E.P., F.A.A.E.M. [8]
Assistant Professor
Department of Emergency Medicine
Johns Hopkins University
Baltimore, Maryland

ROBERT S. HOFFMAN, M.D, F.A.C.E.P., F.A.A.C.T., F.A.C.M.T. [151, 162]
Assistant Professor of Clinical Surgery and Emergency Medicine
New York University School of Medicine
Director
New York City Poison Center
New York, New York

TERESITA M. HOGAN, M.D., F.A.C.E.P. [247]
Associate Professor
Department of Emergency Medicine
University of Illinois
Program Director
Resurrection Emergency Medicine Residency Program
Resurrection Medical Center
Chicago, Illinois

JUDD E. HOLLANDER, M.D. [47, 48]
Associate Professor
Clinical Research Director
Department of Emergency Medicine
Hospital of the University of Pennsylvania
Philadelphia, Pennsylvania

JEREMY J. HOLLERMAN, M.D. [256]
Assistant Chief
Department of Medical Imaging
Hennepin County Medical Center
Minneapolis, Minnesota
Assistant Professor
Department of Radiology
University of Minnesota School of Medicine
Minneapolis, Minnesota

CHRISTOPHER M. HOLMES, M.D. [122]
Department of Pediatrics
University of Michigan Medical Center
Ann Arbor, Michigan

RONALD D. HOLMES, M.D. [122]
Clinical Professor
Division of Pediatric Gastroenterology
Department of Pediatrics and Communicable Diseases
University of Michigan Medical Center
Ann Arbor, Michigan

EDMOND A. HOOKER, M.D. [84, 85]
Assistant Clinical Instructor
Department of Emergency Medicine
University of Louisville
Louisville, Kentucky

MARK A. HOSTETLER, M.D., F.A.C.E.P. [201]
Assistant Professor
Associate Director
Pediatric Emergency Medicine
Departments of Emergency Medicine and Pediatrics
Vanderbilt University
Nashville, Tennessee

DAVID S. HOWES, M.D., F.A.C.E.P. [90, 93]
Program Director
University of Chicago Emergency Medicine Residency
Associate Professor of Clinical Medicine
University of Chicago
Chicago, Illinois

J. STEPHEN HUFF, M.D., F.A.C.E.P. [221, 222]
Associate Professor of Emergency Medicine and Neurology
Department of Emergency Medicine
University of Virginia
Charlottesville, Virginia

ROGER LOYD HUMPHRIES, M.D. [62]
Assistant Professor
Department of Emergency Medicine
University of Kentucky
Lexington, Kentucky

OLIVER L. HUNG, M.D. [165]
Assistant Professor of Clinical Surgery and Emergency Medicine
Department of Emergency Medicine
Bellevue Hospital Center and New York University Medical Center
New York, New York

D. MONTE HUNTER, M.D. [275]
Clinical Instructor
Section of Sports Medicine
Department of Orthopaedics
UCLA Medical Center
Los Angeles, California

JEFFERY C. HUTZLER, M.D. [281]

KENNETH G. JACKIMCZYK, M.D., F.A.C.E.P. [285]
Associate Chairman
Director of Academic Affairs
Department of Emergency Medicine
Maricopa Medical Center
Phoenix, Arizona

RAYMOND E. JACKSON, M.D., M.S. [29]
Clinical Associate Professor
Wayne State University School of Medicine
Department of Emergency Medicine
William Beaumont Hospital
Royal Oak, Michigan

DAVID M. JAFFE, M.D., F.A.A.P., F.A.C.E.P. [116]
Professor of Pediatrics
Director
Division of Emergency Medicine
Washington University School of Medicine
Director
Emergency Services
St. Louis Children's Hospital
St. Louis, Missouri

DAVID M. JANICKE, M.D. [100]
Associate Research Director
Clinical Assistant Professor
Department of Emergency Medicine
State University of New York–Buffalo
Millard Fillmore Hospital
Buffalo, New York

DIETRICH VON KUENSSBERG JEHLE, M.D., F.A.C.E.P. [109]
Director of Emergency Services
Erie County Medical Center
Associate Professor and Vice Chairman
Department of Emergency Medicine
State University of New York at Buffalo
Buffalo, New York

GARY A. JOHNSON, M.D., F.A.C.E.P. [54]
Associate Professor
Residency Program Director
Department of Emergency Medicine
State University of New York Health Sciences Center at Syracuse
Syracuse, New York

ELAINE B. JOSEPHSON, M.D., F.A.C.E.P. [94]
Attending Physician
Department of Emergency Medicine
St. Luke's–Roosevelt Hospital Center
New York, New York

JONATHAN JUI, M.D., M.P.H. [28, 149]
Associate Professor
EMS Medical Director, Multnomah County
Department of Emergency Medicine
Oregon Health Sciences University
Portland, Oregon

LAWRENCE M. KATZ, M.D., F.A.C.E.P. [20]
Assistant Professor
Department of Emergency Medicine
University of North Carolina Chapel Hill School of Medicine
Chapel Hill, North Carolina

GABOR D. KELEN, M.D. [21, 23, 139, 251, 254]
Professor and Chair
Department of Emergency Medicine
Johns Hopkins University
Baltimore, Maryland

ARTHUR L. KELLERMANN, M.D., M.P.H., F.A.C.E.P. [258]
Professor and Chair
Department of Emergency Medicine
Emory University School of Medicine
Director
Center for Injury Control
Rollins School of Public Health
Emory University
Atlanta, Georgia

SCOTT S. KELLEY M.D. [272]
Vice-Chairman and Associate Professor
Department of Orthopaedic Surgery
University of North Carolina at Chapel Hill
Chapel Hill, North Carolina

WILLIAM P. KERNS II, M.D., F.A.C.E.P., A.C.M.T. [169]
Clinical Instructor
Department of Emergency Medicine
Carolinas Medical Center
Charlotte, North Carolina

SORABH KHANDELWAL, M.D. [64, 65]
Attending Physician
Department of Emergency Medicine
Assistant Professor
The Ohio State University College of Medicine
Columbus, Ohio

MARK A. KIRK, M.D. [168]
Medical Toxicology Fellowship Director
Indiana Poison Center and Emergency Medicine and Trauma Center at Methodist Hospital
Indiana University School of Medicine
Indianapolis, Indiana

THOMAS D. KIRSCH, M.D., M.P.H., F.A.C.E.P. [247]
Chairman
Department of Emergency Medicine
Resurrection Medical Center
Chicago, Illinois

NIRANJAN KISSOON, M.B.B.S., F.A.A.P., F.C.C.M., F.R.C.P.(C.) [112]
Professor and Chief
Division of Critical Care Medicine
Department of Pediatrics
University of Florida Health Science Center–Jacksonville
The Nemours Children's Clinic and Wolfson Children's Hospital
Jacksonville, Florida

KENNETH W. KIZER, M.D., M.P.H. [192]
Department of Veterans Affairs
Under Secretary for Health
Washington, DC

JEFFREY A. KLINE, M.D. [170]
Assistant Director of Research
Department of Emergency Medicine
Carolinas Medical Center
Charlotte, North Carolina

SANFORD H. KOLTONOW, M.D., Psy.S., F.A.C.E.P. [288]
Attending Physician
Residency Faculty
Director of Physician Wellness Programs
Department of Emergency Medicine
William Beaumont Hospital
Royal Oak, Michigan

MAYBELLE KOU, M.D. [120, 133]

RONALD F. KOURY, D.O. [43]
Resident
Department of Emergency Medicine
University of Kentucky
Lexington, Kentucky

SHAHEED I. KOURY, M.D., F.A.C.E.P. [30]
Assistant Professor
Department of Emergency Medicine
University of Kentucky
Lexington, Kentucky

ALAN J. KOZAK, M.D. [227]
Attending Physician
Division of Infectious Disease
Department of Medicine
Mary Imogene Bassett Hospital
Cooperstown, New York

DANIEL J. KRANITZ, D.O. [167]
Attending Staff
Department of Emergency Medicine
Cleveland Clinic Foundation
Cleveland, Ohio

GARY S. KRAUSE, M.D., M.S., F.A.C.E.P. [19]
Professor
Department of Emergency Medicine
Wayne State University School of Medicine
Detroit, Michigan

RICHARD S. KRAUSE, M.D. [100]
Clinical Assistant Professor
Department of Emergency Medicine
Buffalo General Hospital
State University of New York at Buffalo
Buffalo, New York

STEVEN KRONICK, M.D., M.S. [86]
Lecturer
Department of Emergency Medicine
University of Michigan
Ann Arbor, Michigan

LOUIS J. KROOT, M.D., F.A.C.E.P. [35, 44]
Associate Professor
Department of Emergency Medicine
University of Kentucky
Chandler Medical Center
Lexington, Kentucky

GLORIA J. KUHN, D.O., Ph.D, F.A.C.E.P.
Associate Professor
Virginia Commonwealth University
Medical College of Virginia
Director of Faculty Development
Department of Emergency Medicine
Richmond, Virginia

ALLAN KUMAR, M.D. [255]

MYRON M. LABAN, M.D. [273, 274]
Director
Physical Medicine and Rehabilitation
William Beaumont Hospital
Royal Oak, Michigan

RICHARD L. LAMMERS, M.D., F.A.C.E.P. [42]
Research Director
Michigan State University and Kalamazoo Center for Medical Studies
Associate Professor of Emergency Medicine
Michigan State University
Kalamazoo, Michigan

JAMES L. LARSON, JR., M.D. [264]
Assistant Professor
Department of Emergency Medicine
University of North Carolina Chapel Hill School of Medicine
Chapel Hill, North Carolina

HARRISON A. LATIMER, M.D. [272]
Kinston Clinics
Kinston, North Carolina

FRANK W. LAVOIE, M.D. [76]
Chief
Department of Emergency Medicine
Southern Maine Medical Center
Biddeford, Maine

EDWARD LEE, M.D. [95]
Attending Physician
Department of Emergency Medicine
St. Luke's–Roosevelt Hospital Center
New York City, New York

NADINE LEVICK, M.D. [32, 130]
Assistant Professor
Division of Pediatric Emergency Medicine
Department of Pediatrics
Johns Hopkins University School of Medicine
Baltimore, Maryland

HORACE K. LIANG, M.D., M.A., F.A.C.E.P., F.A.A.E.M. [206, 207]
Assistant Professor of Emergency Medicine
Residency Director
Department of Emergency Medicine
Johns Hopkins University School of Medicine
Baltimore, Maryland

ERICA L. LIEBELT, M.D. [32, 130]
Assistant Professor
Division of Pediatric Emergency Medicine
Department of Pediatrics
Johns Hopkins University School of Medicine
Baltimore, Maryland

G. PATRICK LILJA, M.D. [1]
Clinical Professor
Department of Emergency Medicine
University of Minnesota School of Medicine
North Memorial Medical Center
Minneapolis, Minnesota

JOÃO A. C. LIMA, M.D. [57]

MICHAEL LONDNER, M.D. [23, 107]
Instructor
Department of Emergency Medicine
Johns Hopkins University School of Medicine
Baltimore, Maryland

KEITH E. LORING, M.D., M.P.H., F.A.C.E.P. [227]
Assistant Clinical Professor of Surgery
Department of Surgery
Division of Emergency Services
University of California, San Francisco
San Francisco General Hospital
Director of Graduate Medical Education
Department of Emergency Medicine
St. Mary's Medical Center
San Francisco, California

CARY L. LUBKIN, M.D. [203]
Assistant Director
Assistant Professor of Emergency Medicine
Department of Emergency Medicine
UMDNJ–Robert Wood Johnson Medical School at Camden
The Cooper Health System
Camden, New Jersey

MICHAEL LUCCHESI, M.D. [231]
Associate Professor and Chairman
Residency Director
Department of Emergency Medicine
State University of New York
Health Sciences Center at Brooklyn
Kings County Hospital Center
Brooklyn, New York

O. JOHN MA, M.D. [245]
Assistant Professor and Research Director
Department of Emergency Medicine
Truman Medical Center
Kansas City, Missouri

RICHARD MALLEY, M.D. [117]
Instructor
Division of Emergency Medicine
Children's Hospital
Boston, Massachusetts

JAMES E. MANNING, M.D., F.A.C.E.P. [20]
Associate Professor of Emergency Medicine, Surgery, and Anesthesiology
Department of Emergency Medicine
University of North Carolina Chapel Hill School of Medicine
Chapel Hill, North Carolina

CATHERINE A. MARCO, M.D. [13]
Assistant Professor
Department of Emergency Medicine
Johns Hopkins Bayview Medical Center
Johns Hopkins University
Baltimore, Maryland

JENNIFER MARRAST-HOST, M.D. [97]
Attending Physician
Roosevelt Emergency Department
St. Luke's–Roosevelt Hospital Center
New York, New York

JULIA E. MARTIN, M.D., F.A.C.E.P. [37]
Assistant Professor
Department of Emergency Medicine
University of Kentucky
Lexington, Kentucky

MARCUS L. MARTIN, M.D. [237]
Professor and Chair
Department of Emergency Medicine
University of Virginia Health Sciences Center
Charlottesville, Virginia

LISA MAY, M.D. [238–240, 242]
Assistant Professor
Department of Dermatology
University of North Carolina Chapel Hill School of Medicine
Chapel Hill, North Carolina

THOM A. MAYER, M.D., F.A.C.E.P., F.A.A.P. [120, 124, 127, 133, 136]
Chairman
Department of Emergency Medicine
Medical Director
Flight Services
Inova Fairfax Hospital
Falls Church, Virginia
Professor of Emergency Medicine
Georgetown University School of Medicine
George Washington University School of Medicine
Washington, DC
Associate Clinical Professor of Pediatrics
University of Virginia School of Medicine
Charlottesville, Virginia

MARSHALL C. McCOY, M.D., F.A.C.E.P. [293]
Associate Professor
Head
Carolina Air Care
Department of Emergency Medicine
University of North Carolina Chapel Hill School of Medicine
Chapel Hill, North Carolina

ROBERT McNAMARA, M.D., F.A.A.E.M. [69]
Professor and Chief of Emergency Medicine
Department of Medicine
Temple University Hospital
Philadelphia, Pennsylvania

GREGORY D. MEARS, M.D., F.A.C.E.P. [6]
Associate Professor
Head
Division of EMS
Department of Emergency Medicine
University of North Carolina at Chapel Hill
Chapel Hill, North Carolina

WILLIAM J. MEGGS, M.D., Ph.D. [176]
Professor of Emergency Medicine
Vice-Chair for Clinical Affairs
Chief
Division of Toxicology
East Carolina University School of Medicine
Greenville, North Carolina

HAGOP S. MEKHJIAN, M.D. [77]
Professor of Internal Medicine
Division of Gastroenterology
Medical Director
The Ohio State University Hospitals
Assistant Vice President for Health Services
Associate Dean of Clinical Affairs
Ohio State University Medical Center
Columbus, Ohio

SCOTT W. MELANSON, M.D., F.A.C.E.P. [295]
Associate Director
Emergency Medicine Residency
St. Luke's Hospital
Bethlehem, Pennsylvania
Assistant Clinical Professor
Temple University School of Medicine
Philadelphia, Pennsylvania

FRANTZ R. MELIO, M.D., F.A.C.E.P. [279]
Associate Clinical Professor of Emergency Medicine
University of North Carolina at Chapel Hill
Chapel Hill, North Carolina
Chairman and Medical Director
Department of Emergency Medicine
WakeMed
Raleigh, North Carolina

PETER T. MELLIS, M.D., F.A.A.P. [111, 118]
Director
Department of Pediatric Emergency Medicine
Chippenham Medical Center and Henrico Doctors' Hospital
Richmond, Virginia

MOSS H. MENDELSON, M.D., F.A.C.E.P. [71]
Assistant Professor
Department of Emergency Medicine
Eastern Virginia Medical School
Norfolk, Virginia

JEFFREY S. MENKES, M.D. [259]
Attending Physician
Department of Traumatology and Emergency Medicine
Hartford Hospital
Hartford, Connecticut
Assistant Professor of Emergency Medicine
University of Connecticut School of Medicine
Farmington, Connecticut

JOHN T. MEREDITH, M.D., F.A.C.E.P. [145]
Assistant Professor
Department of Emergency Medicine
East Carolina University School of Medicine
Greenville, North Carolina

JOHN A. MICHAEL, M.D., F.R.C.P.C., F.A.A.E.M. [268, 269]
Attending Physician
The North Shore Medical Center
Salem, Massachusetts

HUBERT S. MICKEL, M.D., F.A.C.E.P. [218]
Assistant Professor
Department of Emergency Medicine
Johns Hopkins Bayview Medical Center
Johns Hopkins University
Baltimore, Maryland

SALVATORE A. MIGLIORE, M.D. [247]
Resident Physician
Resurrection Emergency Medicine Residency Program
Resurrection Medical Center
Chicago, Illinois

MICHAEL R. MILL, M.D., F.A.C.S., F.A.C.C., F.C.C.P. [56]
Professor and Interim Chief
Division of Cardiothoracic Surgery
Director
Heart and Heart-Lung Transplantation Program
Director
University of North Carolina Comprehensive Transplantation Center
University of North Carolina at Chapel Hill School of Medicine
University of North Carolina Hospitals
Chapel Hill, North Carolina

KIRK C. MILLS, M.D., F.A.C.E.P. [152–154]
Medical Toxicologist
Assistant Clinical Professor
Department of Emergency Medicine
Detroit Receiving Hospital
Detroit, Michigan

JOHN D. MITCHELL, M.D. [230]
Program Director
Ophthalmology Residency
Washington National Eye Center/Washington Hospital Center
Washington, DC
Attending Physician, Emergency Medicine
Fair Oaks Hospital
Fairfax, Virginia

DONALD A. MOFFA, JR., M.D. [59]
Clinical Faculty
Department of Emergency Medicine
Case Western Reserve University
MetroHealth Emergency Medicine
Cleveland Clinic Foundation
Cleveland, Ohio

JOEL MOLL, M.D. [61, 92]
Senior Instructor
Case Western Reserve University
Department of Emergency Medicine
MetroHealth Medical Center
Cleveland, Ohio

GREGORY P. MOORE, M.D., F.A.C.E.P. [285]
Clinical Associate Professor
Department of Emergency Medicine
Indiana University School of Medicine
Attending Faculty
Methodist Hospital
Indianapolis, Indiana

DEXTER L. MORRIS, Ph.D., M.D., F.A.C.E.P. [137]
Vice-Chair
Associate Professor
Department of Emergency Medicine
University of North Carolina Chapel Hill School of Medicine
Chapel Hill, North Carolina

LAURIE MORRISON, M.D., F.R.C.P.C., A.B.E.M. [98]
Director
Division of Emergency Medicine
Assistant Professor
Department of Medicine
University of Toronto
Department of Emergency Services
Sunnybrook and Women's Health Sciences Center
Toronto, Ontario, Canada

ROBERT L. MUELLEMAN, M.D., F.A.C.E.P. [260]
Section Chief
Department of Emergency Medicine
University of Nebraska Medical Center
Medical Director
Emergency Services
Nebraska Health System
Omaha, Nebraska

LEWIS S. NELSON, M.D., F.A.C.E.P. [165, 173, 183, 184]
Assistant Professor of Clinical Surgery and Emergency Medicine
New York University School of Medicine
Director
Fellowship in Medical Toxicology
New York City Poison Control Center
New York, New York

LINDA MEREDITH NICHOLAS, M.D., M.S. [284]
Assistant Professor
Director of Outpatient Clinics
Director of Crisis Emergency Service
Department of Psychiatry
University of North Carolina Chapel Hill School of Medicine
Chapel Hill, North Carolina

DAVID D. NICOLAOU, M.D., F.A.C.E.P. [21, 33]
Assistant Professor
Department of Emergency Medicine
Johns Hopkins University School of Medicine
Baltimore, Maryland

JAMES T. NIEMANN, M.D., F.A.C.E.P. [51]
Professor of Medicine
UCLA School of Medicine
Senior Faculty
Department of Emergency Medicine
Harbor–UCLA Medical Center
Torrance, California

MICHAEL A. NIGRO, D.O., F.A.C.N. [121]
Professor of Neurology and Pediatrics
Chief
Division of Pediatric Neurology
Children's Hospital of Michigan
Wayne State University School of Medicine
Detroit, Michigan

RICHARD A. NOCKOWITZ, M.D. [282]
Department of Psychiatry
The Ohio State University College of Medicine
Columbus, Ohio

THOMAS P. NOELLER, M.D. [66]
Assistant Professor–Clinical
Ohio State University
Department of Emergency Medicine
Cleveland Clinic Foundation
Cleveland, Ohio

ERIC K. NOJI, M.D., M.P.H. [5]
Senior Medical Officer
Department of Emergency and Humanitarian Action
World Health Organization
Geneva, Switzerland

JOSEPH P. ORNATO, M.D., F.A.C.C., F.A.C.E.P. [7]
Professor and Chairman
Department of Emergency Medicine
Virginia Commonwealth University's Medical College of Virginia
Richmond, Virginia

HAROLD H. OSBORN, M.D., F.A.C.E.P. [143, 172]
Professor and Chair
Department of Emergency Medicine
Long Island College Hospital
Brooklyn, New York

DAVID T. OVERTON, M.D., M.B.A., F.A.C.E.P., F.A.C.P. [70]
Emergency Medicine Program Director
Michigan State University Kalamazoo Center for Medical Studies
Professor and Chairman of Emergency Medicine
Michigan State University College of Human Medicine
Kalamazoo, Michigan

JOSEPH PAGANE, M.D. [228]
Attending Physician
Department of Emergency Medicine
Orlando Regional Healthcare System
Orlando, Florida

PETER J. PAGANUSSI, M.D., F.A.C.E.P. [133]
Department of Emergency Medicine
Inova Fairfax Hospital
Falls Church, Virginia

ARTHUR M. PANCIOLI, M.D., F.A.C.E.P. [74]
Assistant Professor
Associate Residency Director
Department of Emergency Medicine
University of Cincinnati College of Medicine
Cincinnati, Ohio

WILLIAM FRANKLIN PEACOCK IV, M.D., F.A.C.E.P. [92, 232, 233]
Director of Clinical Operations
Department of Emergency Medicine
The Cleveland Clinic
Associate Professor
Department of Emergency Medicine
Ohio State University
Cleveland, Ohio

DEBRA G. PERINA, M.D. [204]
Associate Professor
Director
Prehospital Care Division
Medical Director
Pegasus Flight Operations
Department of Emergency Medicine
University of Virginia Health Sciences Center
Charlottesville, Virginia

JEANMARIE PERRONE, M.D. [162]
Co-Director, Division of Toxicology
Assistant Professor
Department of Emergency Medicine
University of Pennsylvania School of Medicine
Attending Physician
Emergency Department
Hospital of the University of Pennsylvania
Philadelphia, Pennsylvania

SHAWNA J. PERRY, M.D. [138]
Department of Emergency Medicine
University of Florida Health Science Center–Jacksonville
Jacksonville, Florida

PAMELA L. PIGGOTT, M.D. [199]
Resident Physician
Department of Emergency Medicine
Pitt County Memorial Hospital
East Carolina University School of Medicine
Greenville, North Carolina

NANCY A. POOK, M.D. [126]
Assistant Clinical Professor
Department of Emergency Medicine
Kettering Medical Center
Dayton, Ohio

JANET M. POPONICK, M.D. [61, 67]
Clinical Faculty
Department of Emergency Medicine
Case Western Reserve University
MetroHealth Emergency Medicine
Cleveland, Ohio

TIMOTHY G. PRICE, M.D. [75]
Assistant Professor
Department of Emergency Medicine
University of Louisville
Louisville, Kentucky

SUSAN B. PROMES, M.D. [12]
Associate Residency Director
Department of Emergency Medicine
Alameda County Medical Center–Highland General Hospital
Oakland, California

PETER J. PRONOVOST, M.D., Ph.D. [22]
Assistant Professor of Anesthesiology and Critical Care Medicine, Surgery, and Health Policy and Management
Johns Hopkins University School of Medicine
Baltimore, Maryland

KIMBERLY S. QUAYLE, M.D. [116]
Professor of Pediatrics
Medical Director
Pediatric Transport Team
Division of Emergency Medicine
Department of Pediatrics
St. Louis Children's Hospital
Washington University School of Medicine
St. Louis, Missouri

MARK B. RABOLD, M.D., F.A.C.E.P. [185, 191]
Saint Peter's Hospital
Department of Emergency Medicine
Helena, Montana

MOHAMED Y. RADY, M.D. [26]
Mayo Clinic Scottsdale
Scottsdale, Arizona

KATHLEEN A. RAFTERY, M.D. [304]
Department of Emergency Medicine
Brigham and Women's Hospital
Boston, Massachusetts

GENE RAGLAND, M.D., F.A.C.E.P. [208]
Associate Director
Emergency Services
St. Joseph Mercy Hospital
Ann Arbor, Michigan
Clinical Assistant Professor
University of Michigan Medical School
Ann Arbor, Michigan

RAMA B. RAO, M.D. [303]
Department of Emergency Medicine
Bellevue Hospital Center and New York University Medical Center
New York, New York

ROBERT F. REARDON, M.D. [109]
Assistant Professor of Clinical Emergency Medicine
University of Minnesota
Department of Emergency Medicine
Hennepin County Medical Center
Minneapolis, Minnesota

SEAN M. REES, M.D. [183]
Attending Physician
Bethesda and Good Samaritan Hospitals
Cincinnati, Ohio

EARL J. REISDORFF, M.D. [41]
Program Director
Department of Emergency Medicine
Inghram Regional Medical Center
Lansing, Michigan

NICHOLAS C. RELICH, M.D. [129]
Co-Director
Neonatal Intensive Care Unit
Department of Emergency Medicine
St. John Hospital and Medical Center
Detroit, Michigan

JOSEPH G. RELLA, M.D. [173, 184]
Clinical Instructor Surgery and Emergency Medicine
New York University School of Medicine
Fellowship in Medical Toxicology
New York City Poison Control Center
New York, New York

KATHY J. RINNERT, M.D., M.P.H. [148]
Instructor in Emergency Medicine
EMS Fellowship Director
Department of Surgery
Division of Emergency Medicine
University of Texas Southwestern Medical Center at Dallas
Parkland Health and Hospital Systems
Dallas, Texas

EMANUEL P. RIVERS, M.D., M.P.H. [26]
Assistant Professor of Emergency Medicine and Surgery
Director of Research
Department of Emergency Medicine
Associate Director of Hyperbaric Therapy
Department of Emergency Medicine
Henry Ford Health Systems
Case Western Reserve University
Detroit, Michigan

WALTER C. ROBEY III, M.D. [176]
Clinical Associate Professor of Emergency Medicine
Associate Director
Emergency Medicine Residency Program
East Carolina University School of Medicine
Greenville, North Carolina

MARIBEL RODRIGUEZ, M.D., F.A.C.E.P. [124]
Department of Emergency Medicine
Inova Fairfax Hospital
Falls Church, Virginia

A. MICHAEL ROMAN, M.D., F.A.C.E.P. [14]
Assistant Professor
Department of Emergency Medicine
University of Arkansas Medical Sciences
Little Rock, Arkansas

C. RICHARD ROSS, M.D., Ph.D. [95]
Attending Physician
Department of Emergency Medicine
St. Luke's–Roosevelt Hospital Center
New York, New York

RICHARD E. ROTHMAN, M.D., Ph.D. [139]
Assistant Professor
Department of Emergency Medicine
Johns Hopkins University
Baltimore, Maryland

MARCIE RUBIN, M.D., F.A.C.E.P. [11]
Department of Emergency Medicine
Brigham and Women's Hospital
Boston, Massachusetts

JOHN P. RUDZINSKI, M.D. [263]
Department of Emergency Medicine
Rockford Memorial Hospital
Rockford, Illinois

ERNEST RUIZ, M.D. [267, 270]
Professor and Director
Emergency Medicine Program
University of Minnesota
Minneapolis, Minnesota

DOUGLAS A. RUND, M.D., F.A.C.E.P. [77, 280–282]
Professor and Chairman
Department of Emergency Medicine
Ohio State University
University Medical Center
Columbus, Ohio

MICHEAL D. RUSH, M.D. [209]
Assistant Program Director
Department of Emergency Medicine
University of Missouri–Kansas City School of Medicine
Truman Medical Center
Kansas City, Missouri

WILLIAM A. RUTALA, Ph.D., M.P.H. [141]
Professor of Medicine
Director, Occupational Health, Hospital Epidemiology, and Environmental Health and Safety
University of North Carolina at Chapel Hill
University of North Carolina Hospitals
Chapel Hill, North Carolina

ALEXANDER H. SACKEYFIO, M.D. [283]
Department of Psychiatry
William Beaumont Hospital
Royal Oak, Michigan

ANNIE TEWEL SADOSTY, M.D. [79]
Department of Emergency Medicine
University of Maryland Medical System
University of Maryland School of Medicine
Baltimore, Maryland

NICHOLAS SADOVNIKOFF, M.D. [11]
Department of Anesthesiology
Critical Care Medicine
Brigham and Women's Hospital
Boston, Massachusetts

PATRICIA R. SALBER, M.D., F.A.C.E.P., F.A.C.P. [291, 292]
Medical Director
Managed Care
Health Care Initiatives
General Motors in Conjunction with The Permanente Company
Emergency Physician
The Permanente Medical Group
Oakland, California

ARTHUR B. SANDERS, M.D., M.H.A. [300]
Professor
Section of Emergency Medicine
Department of Surgery
University of Arizona Health Sciences Center
Tucson, Arizona

THOMAS M. SCALEA, M.D., F.A.C.S. [31, 248, 252]
Director, Program in Trauma
Professor of Surgery, Section Chief, Critical Care Medicine
Section Chief, Trauma Surgery
R. Adams Cowley Shock Trauma Center
University of Maryland Medical System
Baltimore, Maryland

ROBERT W. SCHAFERMEYER, M.D. [123]
Clinical Professor of Emergency Medicine and Pediatrics,
University of North Carolina Chapel Hill School of Medicine
Chapel Hill, North Carolina
Associate Chairman
Department of Emergency Medicine
Carolinas Medical Center
Charlotte, North Carolina

RAQUEL M. SCHEARS, M.D., M.P.H. [157, 159]
Assistant Professor
Department of Emergency Medicine
Hospital of the University of Pennsylvania
Philadelphia, Pennsylvania

ROBERT E. SCHNEIDER, M.D., F.A.C.E.P. [91]
Clinical Assistant Professor
Department of Emergency Medicine
Carolinas Medical Center
Charlotte, North Carolina

SANDRA M. SCHNEIDER, M.D., F.A.C.E.P. [156, 200, 201]
Professor and Chair
Department of Emergency Medicine
University of Rochester
Rochester, New York

CHARLES N. SCHOENFELD, M.D., F.A.C.E.P., F.A.A.E.M. [52]
Vice-Chair
Assistant Professor
Department of Emergency Medicine
Johns Hopkins School of Medicine
Johns Hopkins Bayview Medical Center
Baltimore, Maryland

MICHAEL SCHULL, M.D., M.Sc., F.R.C.P.C. [219]
Clinical Epidemiology Unit and Emergency Department
Sunnybrook Health Science Center
University of Toronto
Toronto, Ontario, Canada

LAWRENCE R. SCHWARTZ, M.D., F.A.C.E.P. [194]
Assistant Professor
Department of Emergency Medicine
Wayne State University School of Medicine
Detroit Receiving Hospital
Detroit, Michigan

PHILLIP A. SCOTT, M.D., F.A.A.E.M. [220]
Assistant Professor
Director
Emergency Stroke Team
Department of Emergency Medicine
University of Michigan Health System
Ann Arbor, Michigan

DONNA L. SEGER, M.D. [99]
Assistant Professor of Medicine
Medical Director
Middle Tennessee Poison Center
Center for Clinical Toxicology
Vanderbilt University Medical Center
Nashville, Tennessee

SEETHA SHANKARAN, M.D. [9]
Neonatal Resuscitation and Emergencies
Director
Neonatal-Perinatal Medicine Professor of Pediatrics
Department of Pediatrics
Detroit Medical Center
Wayne State University School of Medicine
Detroit, Michigan

SUZANNE MOORE SHEPHERD, M.D., F.A.C.E.P. [105, 298]
Associate Professor and Program Director
Department of Emergency Medicine
Hospital of the University of Pennsylvania
Philadelphia, Pennsylvania

RICHARD O. SHIELDS JR., M.D., F.A.C.E.P. [80]
Department of Emergency Medicine
St. Joseph's—Candler Health System
Savannah, Georgia 31405

CARA B. SIEGEL, M.D. [274, 301]
Assistant Professor
Department of Physical Medicine and Rehabilitation
University of North Carolina Chapel Hill School of Medicine
Chapel Hill, North Carolina

SUSAN L. SIEGFRIED, M.D. [284]
Resident Physician
Department of Psychiatry
University of North Carolina Chapel Hill School of Medicine
Chapel Hill, North Carolina

LINMARIE SIKICH, M.D. [302]
Assistant Professor
Department of Psychiatry
University of North Carolina Chapel Hill School of Medicine
Chapel Hill, North Carolina

MICHAEL A. SILVERMAN, M.D. [108]
Operations Director
Department of Emergency Medicine
Saint Agnes Healthcare
Instructor of Emergency Medicine
Johns Hopkins University School of Medicine
Baltimore, Maryland

RICHARD SINERT, D.O. [88, 89, 96]
Research Director
Assistant Professor
Department of Emergency Medicine
State University of New York–Health Science
Center at Brooklyn
Brooklyn, New York

JONATHAN I. SINGER, M.D. [126]
Professor of Emergency Medicine and Pediatrics
Vice-Chair and Residency Program Director
Department of Emergency Medicine
Wright State University School of Medicine
Dayton, Ohio

EDWARD P. SLOAN, M.D., M.P.H., F.A.C.E.P. [226]
Associate Professor and Research Development Director
Department of Emergency Medicine
University of Illinois
Attending Physician
Emergency Services
University of Illinois Hospital
Chicago, Illinois

JOHN E. SMIALEK, M.D. [257]
Head
Division of Forensic Pathology
Associate Professor
Department of Pathology
University of Maryland School of Medicine
Baltimore, Maryland

JULIE SPENCE, M.D. F.R.C.P.C. [98]
Director
Residency Program
Division of Emergency Medicine
Assistant Professor
Department of Medicine
University of Toronto
Department of Emergency Services
St. Michael's Hospital
Toronto, Ontario, Canada

SARAH A. STAHMER, M.D., F.A.C.E.P. [298]
Associate Professor
Division of Emergency Medicine
Cooper Hospital
Robert Wood Johnson Medical School
Camden, New Jersey

J. STEPHAN STAPCZYNSKI, M.D., F.A.C.E.P. [58, 216]
Professor and Chair
Department of Emergency Medicine
University of Kentucky
Lexington, Kentucky

MICHAEL W. STAVA, M.D. [63]
Department of Emergency Medicine
University of Kentucky College of Medicine
Lexington, Kentucky

MARK T. STEELE, M.D. [265, 266]
Associate Professor and Chairman
Department of Emergency Medicine
University of Missouri–Kansas City School of Medicine
and Truman Medical Center
Kansas City, Missouri

IAN G. STIELL, M.D., M.Sc., F.R.C.P.C. [268, 269]
Senior Principal Investigator
Clinical Epidemiology Unit
Ottawa Hospital Loeb Research Institute
Associate Professor
Division of Emergency Medicine
Faculty of Medicine
University of Ottawa
Ottawa, Ontario, Canada

C. KEITH STONE, M.D., F.A.C.E.P. [3]
Residency Director and Associate Professor
Department of Emergency Medicine
University of Kentucky
Lexington, Kentucky

SUSAN C. STONE, M.D., M.P.H. [36]
Clinical Instructor
Department of Surgery
Division of Emergency Medicine
University of Colorado Health Sciences Center
Denver, Colorado

BHARAT B. SUTARIYA, M.D. [17]
Assistant Professor
Department of Emergency Medicine
Wayne State University
Detroit, Michigan

JOHN J. SVERHA, M.D. [217]
Clinical Instructor
Department of Emergency Medicine
University of North Carolina Chapel Hill School of Medicine
Chapel Hill, North Carolina

ROBERT A. SWOR, D.O., F.A.C.E.P. [1]
Director, EMS Programs
William Beaumont Hospital
Royal Oak, Michigan
Clinical Associate Professor
Department of Emergency Medicine
Wayne State University
Detroit, Michigan

ELLEN H. TALIAFERRO, M.D. [291, 292]
Associate Professor
Department of Surgery
Division of Emergency Medicine
University of Texas Southwestern Medical Center
Dallas, Texas

NELSON TANG, M.D. [246]
Assistant Professor
Department of Emergency Medicine
Johns Hopkins University
EMS Medical Director
Johns Hopkins Hospital
Baltimore, Maryland

PAUL J. W. TAWNEY, M.D. [274, 301]
Assistant Professor
Department of Physical Medicine and Rehabilitation
University of North Carolina Chapel Hill School of Medicine
Chapel Hill, North Carolina

THOMAS E. TERNDRUP, M.D., F.A.C.E.P. [119]
Professor and Chair
Department of Emergency Medicine
University of Alabama at Birmingham
Birmingham, Alabama

CAROL A. TERREGINO, M.D. [106]
Associate Professor of Emergency Medicine
Department of Emergency Medicine
Cooper Hospital University Medical Center
UMDNJ–Robert Wood Johnson Medical School at Camden
Camden, New Jersey

STEPHEN H. THOMAS, M.D., M.P.H., F.A.C.E.P. [3]
Assistant in Emergency Medicine
Instructor in Medicine
Harvard Medical School
Assistant in Emergency Medicine and Director of Undergraduate Emergency Medicine Education
Massachusetts General Hospital
Associate Medical Director
Boston MedFlight
Boston, Massachusetts

JUDITH E. TINTINALLI, M.D., M.S., F.A.C.E.P. [81, 281]
Professor and Chair
Department of Emergency Medicine
University of North Carolina Chapel Hill School of Medicine
Chapel Hill, North Carolina

KNOX H. TODD, M.D., M.P.H., F.A.C.E.P. [258]
Associate Professor and Vice Chair for Academic Affairs
Department of Emergency Medicine
Emory University School of Medicine
Atlanta, Georgia

KIMBERLY N. TREAT, M.D. [196, 197]
Resident in Emergency Medicine
West Virginia University
Morgantown, West Virginia

RUDOLPH J. TRIANA, JR. [235, 236]
Attending Physician
Department of ENT Surgery
WakeMed Center
Raleigh, North Carolina

DENNIS T. UEHARA, M.D., M.S.A.M. [261–263]
Clinical Associate Professor of Surgery
University of Illinois College of Medicine
Rockford, Illinois
Chairman
Department of Emergency Medicine
Medical Director
Emergency Services
Rockford Health System
Rockford, Illinois

ANNE T. URDANETA, M.D. [231]
Clinical Assistant Instructor
Department of Emergency Medicine
State University of New York
Health Sciences Center at Brooklyn
Kings County Hospital Center
Brooklyn, New York

KEITH W. VAN METER M.D., F.A.C.E.P. [198]
Clinical Associate Professor
Department of Medicine
Louisiana State University School of Medicine
Clinical Associate Professor
Department of Surgery
Tulane School of Medicine
Louisiana State University Section Head
Department of Emergency Medicine
Charity Hospital
New Orleans, Louisiana

JULIA B. VANROOYEN, M.D. [103, 107]
Clinical Instructor
Department of Obstetrics and Gynecology
Johns Hopkins University
Baltimore, Maryland

MICHAEL J. VANROOYEN, M.D., M.P.H., F.A.C.E.P. [103]
Associate Professor
Department of Emergency Medicine
Johns Hopkins University
Baltimore, Maryland

SALVATOR J. VICARIO, M.D. F.A.C.E.P. [75]
Associate Professor
Vice Chair
Department of Emergency Medicine
Director
Emergency Department
Director
Residency Program
University Medical Center
University of Louisville
Louisville, Kentucky

CHRISTINA CATLETT VIOLA, M.D. [224]
Assistant Chief of Service
Department of Emergency Medicine
Johns Hopkins University
Baltimore, Maryland

ROBERT J. VISSERS, M.D., F.R.C.P.C., F.A.C.E.P. [83, 304]
Residency Program Director
Assistant Professor
Department of Emergency Medicine
University of North Carolina at Chapel Hill
Chapel Hill, North Carolina

JAMES S. WALKER, D.O., F.A.C.E.P. [187]
Associate Professor of Emergency Medicine
Medical Student Coordinator
Department of Emergency Medicine
University of Oklahoma Health Sciences Center
Oklahoma City, Oklahoma

MICHAEL M. WANG, M.D., Ph.D. [225]
Research Fellow
Department of Neurology
Johns Hopkins Hospital
Baltimore, Maryland

MARY CHESTER WASKO, M.D., M.Sc. [276]
Department of Medicine
Division of Rheumatology and Clinical Immunology
University of Pittsburgh
Pittsburgh, Pennsylvania

THOMAS A. WATERS, M.D. [233]

PAUL M. WAX, M.D., F.A.C.M.T., F.A.C.E.P. [174]
Associate Professor
Emergency Medicine
University of Rochester School of Medicine
Assistant Medical Director
Finger Lakes Regional Poison and Drug Information Center
Rochester, New York

DAVID J. WEBER, M.D., M.P.H. [141]
Associate Professor of Medicine, Pediatrics, and Epidemiology
University of North Carolina Hospitals
Assistant Dean
University of North Carolina Chapel Hill School of Medicine
Medical Director, Occupational Health
Medical Director, Hospital Epidemiology
Medical Director, Environmental Health and Safety
University of North Carolina at Chapel Hill
University of North Carolina Hospitals
Chapel Hill, North Carolina

MICHAEL S. WEINSTOCK, M.D., F.A.A.P., F.A.C.E.P. [131]
Professor Clinical Medicine
Penn State University College of Medicine
Chair
Department of Emergency Medicine
Lehigh Valley Hospital and Health Care Network
Allentown, Pennsylvania

IRWIN D. WEISMAN, M.D., Ph.D. [297]
Assistant Professor
Department of Radiology
Hennepin County Medical Center
University of Minnesota Medical School
Minneapolis, Minnesota

HOWARD A. WERMAN, M.D., F.A.C.E.P. [77]
Associate Professor of Clinical Emergency Medicine
Medical Director
MedFlight
Department of Emergency Medicine
Ohio State University Medical Center
Columbus, Ohio

BLAINE C. WHITE, M.D. [19]
Professor
Department of Emergency Medicine
Wayne State University School of Medicine
Detroit, Michigan

SUZANNE R. WHITE, M.D., F.A.C.E.P. [181]
Assistant Professor
Departments of Emergency Medicine and Pediatrics
Wayne State University School of Medicine
Detroit, Michigan

DAN E. WIENER, M.D. [97]
Assistant Professor of Clinical Medicine
Columbia College of Physicians and Surgeons
Director
Roosevelt Emergency Department
St. Luke's Roosevelt Hospital Center
New York, New York

JANET M. WILLIAMS, M.D., F.A.C.E.P. [196, 197]
Director
Center for Rural Emergency Medicine
Department of Emergency Medicine
West Virginia University
Morgantown, West Virginia

ROBERT F. WILSON, M.D. [251]
Professor
Department of Surgery
Detroit Receiving Hospital
Wayne State University School of Medicine
Detroit, Michigan

SONIA WINSLETT [209]
Senior Staff Physician
Department of Emergency Medicine
Henry Ford Health System
Detroit, Michigan

KIMBERLEY DAWN WISDOM, M.D. [209]
Assistant Professor
Department of Medical Education
University of Michigan Medical School
Ann Arbor, Michigan

DAVID ALAIN WOHL, M.D. [141]
Clinical Assistant Professor
Division of Infectious Diseases
Department of Medicine
University of North Carolina
Chapel Hill, North Carolina

LESLIE R. WOLF, M.D., A.C.M.T. [177]
Associate Professor and Toxicology Coordinator
Wright State University School of Medicine
Department of Emergency Medicine
Dayton, Ohio

WILLIAM A. WOODS, M.D., F.A.A.P. [204]
Assistant Professor of Emergency Medicine and Pediatrics
Department of Emergency Medicine
University of Virginia Health System
Charlottesville, Virginia

MELISSA M. WU, M.D. [53]
Administrative Fellow
Department of Emergency Medicine
Johns Hopkins University
Baltimore, Maryland

ARTHUR H. YANCEY II, M.D., M.P.H., F.A.C.E.P. [6]
Assistant Professor
Department of Surgery
Emory University School of Medicine
Atlanta, Georgia

LUKE YIP, M.D. [164]
Rocky Mountain Poison and Drug Center
Denver, Colorado

WILLIAM FRANKLIN YOUNG, JR., M.D., F.A.C.E.P. [62, 63, 90]
Assistant Professor
Department of Emergency Medicine
University of Kentucky
Lexington, Kentucky

RICHARD D. ZANE, M.D. [255]
Instructor
Department of Emergency Medicine
Johns Hopkins University School of Medicine
Baltimore, Maryland

REVIEWERS

WILLIAM R. AHRENS, M.D.
Illinois Masonic Medical Center
Chicago, Illinois

HOWARD A. BESSEN, M.D.
Harbor–UCLA Hospitals
Torrance, California

EDWARD BESSMAN, M.D.
Johns Hopkins University
Baltimore, Maryland

HERBERT G. BIVINS, M.D.
Fresno Medical Center
Fresno, California

MARC A. BORENSTEIN, M.D.
St. Luke's–Roosevelt Hospital Center
New York, New York

JANE H. BRICE, M.D., M.P.H.
University of North Carolina Hospitals
Chapel Hill, North Carolina

ROBERT BROWNSTEIN, M.D.
Rex Hospital
Raleigh, North Carolina

MICHAEL L. CALLAHAN, M.D.
University of California, San Francisco
San Francisco, California

TERESA CARLIN, M.D.
Johns Hopkins University
Baltimore, Maryland

CAROL L. CLARK, M.D.
Crittenton Hospital
Troy, Michigan

DAVID M. CLINE, M.D.
WakeMed Hospital
Raleigh, North Carolina

RANDOLPH JAY CORDLE, M.D.
St. Luke's Hospital
Boise, Idaho

RITA K. CYDULKA, M.D.
MetroHealth Medical Center
Cleveland, Ohio

SUSAN M. DUNMIRE, M.D.
Presbyterian Hospital
Pittsburgh, Pennsylvania

STUART R. FRITZ, M.D.
Emergency Physicians Professional Association
Bloomington, Minnesota

GARY B. GREEN, M.D., M.P.H.
Johns Hopkins University
Baltimore, Maryland

STEPHEN W. HARGARTEN, M.D.
Froedtert Memorial Lutheran Hospital
Milwaukee, Wisconsin

WILLIAM E. HAUDA II, M.D.
University of Virginia Health Sciences Center
Charlottesville, Virginia

ROBERT D. HERR, M.D.
Health Clinics of Utah
Salt Lake City, Utah

MARILYN P. HICKS, M.D.
WakeMed Hospital
Raleigh, North Carolina

JAY HOHENHAUS, R.N., E.M.T.-P.
University of North Carolina Hospitals
Chapel Hill, North Carolina

STEPHEN G. HOLTZCLAW, M.D.
Johns Hopkins University
Baltimore, Maryland

YING C. HUANG, M.D.
Kaohsiung Medical College
Kaohsiung, Taiwan

J. STEPHEN HUFF, M.D.
University of Virginia Health Science Center
Charlottesville, Virginia

SHELDON JACOBSON, M.D.
Mount Sinai Medical Center
New York, New York

SAMUEL M. KEIM, M.D.
University of Arizona Health Sciences Center
Tucson, Arizona

KIMBERLY D. KEITH, M.D.
Outer Banks Medical Center
Nags Head, North Carolina

THOMAS D. KIRSCH, M.D., M.P.H.
Resurrection Medical Center
Chicago, Illinois

KRISTI L. KOENIG, M.D.
Highland General Hospital
Oakland, CA

ERIK LETOVSKY, M.D.
University of Toronto
Toronto, Ontario, Canada

KEITH E. LORING, M.D., M.P.H.
San Francisco General Hospital
San Francisco, California

CATHERINE A. MARCO, M.D.
Johns Hopkins University Hospitals
Baltimore, Maryland

JULIA E. MARTIN, M.D.
University of Kentucky Hospitals
Lexington, Kentucky

ANDREW McCALLUM, M.D.
Sunnybrook Health Science Center
Toronto, Ontario, Canada

MARA ANN McERLEAN, M.D.
Albany Medical Center
Albany, New York

HURBERT S. MICKEL, M.D.
Johns Hopkins University
Baltimore, Maryland

GREGORY J. MORAN, M.D.
Olive View/UCLA Medical Center
Los Angeles, California

DAVID D. NICOLAOU, M.D.
Johns Hopkins University Hospitals
Baltimore, Maryland

KRISTEN NORDENHOLZ, M.D.
Tuba City Indian Medical Center
Tuba City, Arizona

BERNADETTE R. PAGE, M.D.
Duke University Medical Center
Durham, North Carolina

JACK R. PAGE, M.D.
Durham, North Carolina

ARTHUR M. PANCIOLI, M.D., F.A.C.E.P.
University of Cincinnati Hospitals
Cincinnati, Ohio

WILLIAM FRANKLIN PEACOCK IV, M.D.
The Cleveland Clinic
Cleveland, Ohio

MARK B. RABOLD, M.D.
Saint Peter's Hospital
Helena, Montana

KAREN M. RESTIFO, M.D.
Yale–New Haven Medical Center
Madison, Connecticut

JAMES R. ROBERTS, M.D.
Mercy Hospital of Philadelphia
Philadelphia, Pennsylvania

CARLOS GARCIA ROSAS, M.D.
Puerto Vallarta, Jalisco, Mexico

MARCIE A. RUBIN, M.D.
Johns Hopkins University
Baltimore, Maryland

TIM RUTLEDGE, M.D.
North York General Hospital
North York, Ontario, Canada

JOSEPH A. SALOMONE III, M.D.
Truman Medical Center
Kansas City, Missouri

SANDRA M. SCHNEIDER, M.D.
University of Rochester Medical Center
Rochester, New York

CHARLES N. SCHOENFELD, M.D.
Johns Hopkins University
Baltimore, Maryland

WALTER A. SCHRADING, M.D.
York Hospital
York, Pennsylvania

SUZANNE MOORE SHEPHERD, M.D.
Hospital of the University of Pennsylvania
Philadelphia, Pennsylvania

C. KEITH STONE, M.D., F.A.C.E.P.
University of Kentucky Medical Center
Lexington, Kentucky

NELSON TANG, M.D.
Johns Hopkins University
Baltimore, Maryland

ANNE T. URDANETA, M.D.
Kings County Hospital Center
Brooklyn, New York

VINCENT P. VERDILE, M.D.
Albany Medical Center
Albany, New York

JOHN VINEN, M.D.
Royal North Shore Hospital
New South Wales, Australia

YEHEZKEL WAISMAN, M.D.
Schneider Children's Medical Center of Israel
Petab Tikva, Israel

STEVEN J. WHITE, M.D., F.A.C.E.P.
Vanderbilt University Medical Center
Nashville, Tennessee

KIMBERLY D. WILLIAMS, M.D.
St. Claire Medical Center
Morehead, Kentucky

WILLIAM F. YOUNG, M.D., F.A.C.E.P.
University of Kentucky Medical Center
Lexington, Kentucky

RICHARD ZANE, M.D.
Johns Hopkins University
Baltimore, Maryland

PREFACE

The Study Guide is the fifth edition to follow the first one published by the American College of Emergency Physicians in 1979. The increasing complexity of each edition has reflected the maturation of our practices over twenty years.

To prepare for this edition, we solicited written reviews of the fourth edition from emergency medicine residents, clinical practitioners, and academicians. We expanded the format of the Study Guide to incorporate evidence from the medical literature to support clinical practice. Chapter structure was improved, several new sections have been added, and many new emergency medicine authors were recruited. It is surprising how little of the practice of medicine is founded on the results of clinical investigation. We hope that our readers and users will be stimulated to design their own clinical investigations to help us improve our future practices.

We have incorporated the EMRA Antibiotic Handbook into the body of the Study Guide, to make this excellent resource more widely available.

The list of reviewers and authors for the Study Guide is impressive. We are especially proud of the many contributions by young emergency medicine faculty and practitioners. Their knowledge, clinical expertise, and commitment to emergency medicine reflect positively on our specialty.

Of the skills important for an emergency physician—knowledge, technical proficiency, compassion, and wisdom—this book can only provide the first, knowledge, to help us practice. Technical ability is learned at the bedside under the watchful eyes and hands of a teacher—a book cannot guide your hands through a difficult procedure. Compassion comes from the values and beliefs that we bring to our profession—a book cannot infuse us with compassion and advocacy for the patients we treat. And wisdom comes from awareness of your own strengths, weaknesses, abilities, and limitations. Our hope is that this text, containing the experience of hundreds of emergency physicians, will stimulate your own development as an emergency physician.

EMERGENCY MEDICINE

A COMPREHENSIVE STUDY GUIDE

EMERGENCY MEDICAL SERVICES

G. Patrick Lilja

Robert A. Swor

Emergency medical services (EMS) constitute the extension of emergency medical care into the community. Strong emergency department leadership is absolutely essential to a safe and effective EMS system.

The 1966 National Highway Safety Act authorized the US Department of Transportation (DOT) to fund ambulances, communications, and training programs for prehospital medical services.[1] Coincidentally, in 1967 J. Frank Pantridge began using a mobile coronary care unit in Belfast, Northern Ireland, to extend coronary care into the prehospital setting.

In 1973, public law 93-154 defined a goal of improving emergency medical care and EMS on a national scale. Although much has changed in EMS since passage of that initial act, the original definition of EMS systems is useful for understanding their functions. This law identified 15 elements of an EMS system: (1) personnel, (2) training, (3) communications, (4) transportation, (5) facilities, (6) critical care units, (7) public safety agencies, (8) consumer participation, (9) access to care, (10) transfer of care, (11) standardization of patients' records, (12) public information and education, (13) independent review and evaluation, (14) disaster linkage, and (15) mutual aid agreements. Thus, an EMS system is the entire system in place to provide care to emergency patients, from the initial 911 call until definitive care is rendered.

State laws broadly outline what is safe and prudent for the public good. State EMS laws and regulations typically define levels of ambulance service capability, training requirements, equipment requirements, and requirements for physician leadership and accountability. In addition, the state health department may be the lead agency in promoting and funding EMS activity.

LOCAL ROLE IN EMERGENCY MEDICAL SERVICES

To be effective, an EMS system must be planned, organized, and operated at the local level. Any community contemplating an EMS system must identify its resources and needs and determine how much service its citizens are willing or able to afford. The 15 elements of an EMS system defined by public law 93-154 can provide guidance in this process. Each element is discussed below.

Personnel

In urban areas, public safety and ambulance personnel provide prehospital medical care, but in rural or wilderness areas, volunteers, park rangers, or ski patrols are commonly employed. Citizen volunteers should not be overlooked, especially in rural communities. Public interest and participation are key ingredients in any EMS system.

Training

Training begins with the education of the private citizen. Courses in EMS system access, cardiopulmonary resuscitation (CPR), and other forms of first aid are essential. Communications media can be utilized to reach large populations with the minimum information necessary to educate citizens to respond to emergencies.

Some communities use a dual-response system consisting of first responders (FRs) followed by ambulance personnel. The FRs may be firefighters, police, park rangers, or citizen volunteers. The DOT National Highway Traffic Safety Administration (NHTSA) was initially given the responsibility of developing training curricula for EMS providers. The use of these curricula was tied to receipt of federal EMS grants, and the training programs were widely accepted and utilized nationally. Although their use is no longer required, DOT training standards are the de facto national standard for EMS education. Training for FRs may include the DOT FR course (which encompasses 60 h of classroom training) or similar courses developed by the American Red Cross or American Heart Association. The training for ambulance personnel usually requires completion of an emergency medical technician (EMT) course. Although various levels of EMT training have evolved in various states, there are three nationally recognized levels of EMTs: EMT basic (EMT-B), EMT intermediate (EMT-I), and EMT paramedic (EMT-P). The EMT-Bs have the necessary first aid skills to take care of immediately life-threatening prehospital emergency conditions. These skills include CPR, use of an automated external defibrillator (AED), and safe extrication, immobilization, and transportation of emergency victims. EMT-Bs are now being trained to assist patients in using their own nitroglycerin, epinephrine, and inhalers. There is an optional module in the DOT EMT-B curriculum on advanced airway techniques; it teaches EMT-Bs to perform endotracheal intubation or to use an advanced airway adjunct, such as a Combitube (Sheridan Corp, Argyle, NY). The decision to teach the optional airway module is generally made by the state EMS agency. EMT-I training includes the additional skills of intravenous access, pneumatic antishock garment use, and advanced airway techniques. EMT-P training adds drug therapy for selected prehospital conditions, interpretation of electrocardiogram (ECG) rhythms, synchronized cardioversion, and manual defibrillation. Clearly, physicians need to be deeply involved in EMT training to ensure that knowledge and skills are being taught appropriately and safely.

Communications

The universal 911 emergency telephone number, available in most locations, has greatly facilitated citizens' access to emergency medical care. In many systems, 911 answering centers have enhanced 911 (E-911) equipment that provides automatic number and location identification as well as additional information to assist the responding personnel. However, the advent of cellular telephones has complicated this process. In some urban areas, up to 25 percent of all 911 calls are made from cellular phones. Technology is being developed to address this issue.

The call to 911 is the essential front door of the EMS system. The EMS system must assure that those answering the calls have the knowledge and training to properly obtain initial medical information, dispatch appropriate personnel, and offer first aid information to the caller when appropriate. A variety of courses have been developed to train 911 dispatchers, those who answer calls and dispatch appropriate personnel and equipment. The 911 center must have adequate staff and equipment to ensure that calls are answered and responded to in a timely manner. The public should be encouraged to use the 911 number rather than call a hospital or physician when certain symptoms (e.g., acute chest pain, dyspnea, loss of consciousness, or focal weakness) occur.

Information can be collected and ambulances dispatched by the 911 center in many ways. The process known as priority dispatch utilizes structured information gathering by the 911 dispatcher, followed by direction concerning the most appropriate EMS response.

Use of this procedure is on the rise. Many of the 911 dispatch protocols also contain first aid information that the dispatcher can give to the caller so that the caller can provide care until EMS arrives. Ambulance personnel must be able directly or indirectly to communicate with the hospital of destination. Most EMTs operate in the field under ''off-line'' medical control, according to standing orders and patient care protocols developed by physicians. However, there are times when EMS personnel may require ''on-line'' medical control, in which they talk directly with a physician for specific direction or orders. The communications system functions to provide public access, prompt dispatch of the appropriate vehicles and personnel, timely hospital notification, and on-line medical control.

Transportation

Ground ambulances have evolved from transport vehicles into sophisticated and efficient mobile patient care areas where lifesaving maneuvers can be performed. Federal standards provide specifications for ambulance construction, and vehicles that meet these specifications can display the ''star of life'' emblem. Nontransporting vehicles, such as rescue response units, carry personnel and equipment to the scene but cannot transport patients. Type I ambulances have a conventional cab and chassis fitted with a modular patient care compartment; there is no passageway between the driver's and the patient's compartments.Type II ambulances are van-type vehicles; the body and the cab form a single unit, and most models have a raised roof for extra stand-up space. Type III ambulances are larger units with a forward cab connected by a walk-through passage to the patient care compartment. The most important aspect of ambulance design is that the attendants must be able to provide airway and ventilatory support while safely transporting the patient. Basic life support (BLS) ambulances carry equipment appropriate for attendants trained at the EMT-B level. Advanced life support (ALS) ambulances are equipped for EMT-Ps or other health care personnel capable of providing drug therapy and performing other advanced medical procedures. Ground transportation is appropriate for the majority of ill or injured patients, especially in urban and suburban areas. Air transport should be considered if the time elapsed before definitive care is important and air transport would shorten that interval.

Facilities

In general, emergency patients should be transported to the closest appropriate hospital or, if there are multiple hospitals within the same transport time, to the hospital of the patient's choice. However, if the EMS system has identified a specific hospital with better resources to treat seriously ill or injured patients (e.g., a trauma center), the patient should be transported to that institution, bypassing closer hospitals. Several systems of categorizing hospitals exist, and this process should precede or coincide with the development of the EMS system. In a number of regions, the state has the statutory authority to designate certain specialty hospitals to receive a subset of patients (most commonly trauma patients), based on an objective review of the hospitals' capabilities. Some states and the American College of Surgeons have also developed a process to provide external verification of trauma centers. This process requires a review of hospital facilities, treatment processes, and patients' outcomes to confirm that quality trauma care is in place. Many EMS systems are now also identifying hospitals as specialized receiving facilities that can provide 24-h emergency angioplasty for patients with acute myocardial infarction (AMI) or that have special expertise with thrombolytic therapy for acute stroke patients.

Decisions to divert patients to specialty centers have substantial health care and commercial implications. These decisions should be made in a collaborative manner for the EMS region based on clearly defined criteria.

Critical Care Units

Tertiary care facilities should be identified by every EMS system to provide specialty care that is not available in typical community hospitals. These facilities may be either within the EMS service area or, more commonly, outside the area. Usually, patients are initially transported to a local hospital for assessment and treatment and then transferred to a tertiary center. In some EMS regions, it may be possible to develop criteria for the transport of patients requiring tertiary specialty care directly from the scene to these centers. The most common reasons for tertiary care emergency transfer are trauma, neonatal intensive care, high-risk obstetrics, burns, spinal cord injury, and neurosurgical and cardiac care. It is not cost effective or feasible for every community to support all of these specialty services.

Public Safety Agencies

The EMS system must have strong ties with police and fire departments. Public safety officials must have input into the decisions of EMS councils, and, conversely, EMS providers must have input into public safety decisions that affect emergency medical care. Public safety agencies provide first-response services because their personnel are often the first on the scene of an emergency, and they are vital links in the delivery of emergency care. For example, police in some municipalities have begun carrying automatic defibrillators in order to improve outcomes for patients suffering cardiac arrest.[2]

Consumer Participation

The public must have input into the governance of its EMS system. Laypersons should be represented on EMS councils. If the public does not understand what a good EMS system offers, public support for the system, including financial support, will dwindle. Two important components of a successful EMS system are lay public first aid training and the implementation of a 911 system.

Access to Care

A successful EMS system ensures that all individuals have access to emergency care regardless of their ability to pay or type of insurance coverage. Often the EMS system is a patient's only point of entry into the health care system. As pressure increases to control health care costs, patients may be discouraged by a variety of sources from accessing the EMS system for perceived emergencies. Emergency physicians must serve as patients' advocates on this issue to ensure that patients access the system in a timely fashion.

A more difficult problem exists when population densities or terrain dictate longer response times for some citizens than others. EMS councils must be able to handle such inequities, which are, both politically and economically, difficult to adjust. Typically, EMS councils are advisory bodies to county boards or other political entities. An informed, representative governing body ultimately makes the best decisions.

Transfer of Care

Patients must sometimes be transferred from one medical care facility to another either within or outside of the EMS service area. These transfers must be made with maximum safety for the patient. Many problems can be avoided if both the transferring and the receiving medical facilities develop transfer agreements in advance. For example, the prospective agreement to accept a trauma patient decreases the time spent arranging for the transfer of a critical patient when necessary. The referring physician should be assured of receiving follow-up information about the patient, and the receiving physician should be assured of receiving all important information about the patient on arrival. Proper medical support en route should be ensured by establishing contact with the receiving center as soon as possible and having appropriate medical personnel accompany the patient.

Standardization of Patients' Records

A patient's care depends on good medical records, and prehospital records are no exception. All ambulance services within a specific region should use a similar reporting form that can be quickly and easily interpreted by receiving nurses and physicians. It is more difficult to standardize emergency department records. However, flow sheets that are easily interpretable by receiving physicians and nurses can be used. Uniform data elements for EMS care have been developed by the NHTSA and are coming into common use.[3] Uniform data elements for emergency department care have also been developed by a cooperative effort among the NHTSA, the Centers for Disease Control, and many emergency medical organizations. It is wise to design record systems that facilitate data extraction for trauma registries, severity scoring, and cardiac arrest outcome studies.

Public Information and Education

The public should be well informed on how to deal with medical emergencies. In designing a public information program, the EMS council should consider the following:

1. The public should understand how the community stands to benefit from an excellent EMS system.
2. The public should be prepared to render first aid care.
3. The public must know how to access the EMS system quickly.
4. The public should understand that patients may not be delivered to the hospital of their choice under life-threatening conditions.

Independent Review and Evaluation

Governing agencies should be assured that there is ongoing review of the EMS system. Monitoring of radio communications, review of response times, and review of patients' care records are relatively mechanical methods of quality control that are easily implemented. Outcome studies of such entities as cardiac arrest and multiple trauma require considerable physician input and cooperation. The system medical director should require that mechanisms be in place to ensure and improve the quality of EMS care. EMS system access to hospital charts should be a requirement for participating hospitals, with proper controls to ensure patients' confidentiality.

Disaster Linkage

The EMS system is an integral part of disaster preparedness and should be involved in planning and practice drills along with public safety agencies and others. Public safety agencies should keep the EMS system informed of potential disaster situations or hazards that may temporarily be present. Also, hospitals must be prepared to keep the EMS system informed of their capacity to receive certain kinds of patients under disaster conditions.

Mutual Aid Agreements

EMS services should develop mutual aid agreements with neighboring jurisdictions so that uninterrupted emergency care is available when local agencies are overwhelmed or unable to provide services.

MEDICAL CONTROL

A safe and effective EMS system requires considerable physician input and surveillance to provide the best possible care for patients.[4] Medical control can be either on line (immediate and direct) or off line (indirect).

On-line medical control is the provision of direct medical communication to personnel in the field either in person or by radio or phone communication. The EMS medical director delegates this authority to other physicians who understand the protocols under which paramedics administer care. Also, the medical director may allow ambulance personnel to carry out certain standing orders when timely contact with the controlling physician is not feasible.

Off-line medical control is the responsibility of the service medical director. Three main components of off-line medical control are (1) development of protocols, (2) development of medical accountability (quality assurance), and (3) development of ongoing education. Protocol development determines those treatment procedures that prehospital personnel may perform under the medical license of the medical director. Protocols should not only address care but should also specify the utilization of medical devices and equipment. It is the medical director's responsibility to approve the medical devices utilized by EMS personnel. The protocols must be reviewed and rewritten on a regular basis to keep pace with current medical knowledge. Quality assurance requires ongoing surveillance and study of the system. The medical director should enlist other physicians to review existing protocols and suggest improvement where deficiencies are noted. Finally, the medical director is responsible for the ongoing educational needs of the prehospital care providers under his or her direction. The medical director should direct the quality and content of the training. Physicians must remember that they have the ultimate responsibility for the overall quality of prehospital medical care.

MEDICAL BASIS FOR EMERGENCY MEDICAL SERVICES

While a relatively small number of emergency physicians are involved in the direction and control of an EMS system, virtually every emergency physician deals with prehospital care in day-to-day practice. This section reviews the medical basis for EMS care as well as common problems in medical practice in a prehospital setting.

Emergency Cardiac Care

While it is clear that ALS saves lives after sudden cardiac arrest, the number of lives saved and the cost are often debated.[5,6] Since sudden cardiac death (SCD) is the number one cause of out-of-hospital death in the United States, the potential benefit of treatment is enormous. Some have argued that the successful treatment of out-of-hospital cardiac arrest alone by EMS systems justifies their existence.[6] Population studies with an age distribution of the entire US population find that the annual incidence of out-of-hospital cardiac arrest is about 1 per 1000.[6] In regions with a higher concentration of elderly persons, the annual incidence is higher.

Without treatment at the scene, the survival rate of out-of-hospital cardiac arrest is virtually zero. Early studies by groups in Seattle and King County, Washington, have demonstrated that as many as 26 percent of patients may be successfully resuscitated from out-of-hospital cardiac arrest.[5] Resuscitation rates in other communities are not as high. The overwhelming majority of survivors of out-of-hospital sudden cardiac arrest were those whose cardiac arrests were witnessed and who had an initial cardiac rhythm of ventricular fibrillation (VF). Multiple studies have shown that survival is clearly related to the time from the collapse of the patient to the delivery of defibrillation and that survival rates decline dramatically with delays of only a few minutes.[7]

These findings have lead a number of physicians to train FRs or EMT-Bs, who usually arrive first at the scene of an emergency, to recognize and treat VF. Systems in King County, Washington, and in Iowa have documented that this approach improves survival from cardiac arrest if the interval between collapse and defibrillation is short. That observation has lead to the wide proliferation of automated external defibrillators (AEDs). The American Heart Association has identified AED defibrillation as the standard of care for vehicles that respond to emergencies and transport patients. However, there is conflicting evidence concerning whether equipping FRs or EMT-Bs with AEDs incrementally improves survival in an existing EMS system with paramedics.[2] Clearly, a cost-benefit analysis should be undertaken in individual systems, and, if implementation of AEDs by police or fire FRs can significantly decrease the time to defibrillation in a system, this modality should be part of the system. Automatic defibrillation is clearly efficacious, but for maximum benefit (more survivors in the community) the local system must optimize the ''chain of survival'': early access, early CPR, early defibrillation, and early ALS.[7] Citizen awareness of the signs of cardiac arrest, quick access to the system, and rapid and appropriate dispatch of units are all critical links to maximizing survival. Pilot programs are being conducted to test whether laypersons, or targeted FRs, such as casino security guards, can effectively utilize AEDs to treat SCD patients.

Despite the emphasis on cardiac arrest during the development of EMS systems, such cases make up less than 5 percent of the volume of an EMS system. The most common clinical entities seen in EMS systems are the manifestations of cardiac disease, usually ischemic chest pain and its complications. Common treatment includes relief of ischemic chest pain with nitrates and narcotic analgesics, control of cardiac arrhythmias with antiarrhythmics, treatment of symptomatic bradyarrhythmias with external pacemakers, and treatment of congestive failure with diuretics and, if necessary, endotracheal intubation. While most EMS authorities agree that such treatment to prevent a cardiac arrest is the true benefit of an ALS system, there is a lack of research to document this assertion.

Many EMS systems are now also facilitating emergency department care through the field use of 12-lead electrocardiography (ECG). Either paramedics interpret the initial rhythm or a computer-generated algorithm is used to diagnose an AMI and contact an intended receiving facility. Limited studies have found that field ECG decreases the time to initiate thrombolysis or to perform angioplasty in patients with AMI. Some EMS systems have used field 12-lead ECG to triage AMI patients to ''cardiac centers'' that have been prospectively identified to provide emergency angioplasty.

Early administration of thrombolytics has been shown to significantly reduce mortality and morbidity. Logistical obstacles to field thrombolytic therapy include the difficulty in diagnosing myocardial infarction in the field, identification of contraindications by paramedics, and management of complications by the limited resources available in the field. Studies of field administration of thrombolytics by paramedics have identified that this therapeutic approach is feasible, but it does not improve outcome when compared to patients who are diagnosed in the field (by 12-lead ECG) and are treated promptly on arrival in the emergency department.[8]

Trauma Care

While the care of trauma patients is more controversial than cardiac care for EMS systems, there is widespread agreement that delivery of critically injured trauma patients to trauma centers saves lives.[9] Systems are designed to bypass certain hospitals under predetermined protocols based on the mechanism of injury or the patient's physiologic status.

There is less agreement on what therapy should be given by EMS providers to trauma victims in the field and en route.[10,11] Some early literature documented a decreased survival rate if patients received ALS (intravenous fluid administration and intubation) at the scene instead of immediate transport to the hospital; presumably this occurred because of the delay to definitive care. More recent studies have found that paramedics may secure an airway, establish an intravenous line, and infuse significant volumes of fluid rapidly without delaying transport of the patient. While the value of providing a secure airway is unarguable, the value of prehospital intravenous fluid administration has been challenged. Thought-provoking work from Houston found that, for hypotensive victims of penetrating truncal trauma who required surgical repair, withholding fluid and blood in both the prehospital and emergency department phases until arrival in the operating room improved survival rates, reduced the amount of blood loss, and shortened the overall hospital stay compared to patients who received fluid and blood in the field and emergency department.[12] Many questions concerning the value of prehospital fluid therapy for trauma victims remain. Until further studies are done, emphasis remains on rapid transport and airway support of the trauma victim, with intravenous fluid administration an unproven but commonly performed treatment.

Adult Medical Care

While much of the initial research in EMS has centered on cardiac and traumatic emergencies, interest has evolved in management of other emergencies by EMS providers as they have broadened their scope of practice. There is evidence that prehospital ALS care improves a patient's condition during transport.[13] However, it is not known whether the ultimate outcome is improved by such care.

The management of airway obstruction and respiratory arrest is an important function of the EMS system. Airway control by endotracheal and nasotracheal intubation is readily achieved by paramedics with a high success rate and an acceptable complication rate. Early advanced airway measures for upper airway obstruction from burns, trauma, foreign body, or allergic causes may be lifesaving. Some EMS systems have shown that neuromuscular paralytic agents, such as succinylcholine, may be safely used by paramedics in the field with appropriate instruction and close medical oversight.

Respiratory distress in patients with chronic obstructive pulmonary disease and asthma is a common clinical entity treated in EMS systems. β_2 agonists have been shown to be safe and effective bronchodilators for field use. Pulse oximetric studies for the evaluation of occult hypoxemia have become widely utilized.

Paramedics are commonly called to evaluate patients with altered mental status. Glucose is frequently given to hypoglycemic patients and naloxone to patients with suspected narcotic overdose. Similarly, control of seizures with diazepam and airway support for status epilepticus are important EMS functions.

Pediatric Care

With the development of pediatric emergency care as an area of interest, experts and organizations have started to review the care of children in EMS systems.[14] It is estimated that 5 to 10 percent of a system's volume consists of pediatric cases, and the most common pediatric emergencies are trauma, respiratory emergencies, and seizures.[15] Cardiac arrest in children is rare (approximately 1 per 10,000 children per year in the United States) usually with a dismal outcome. The ability of paramedics to perform procedures to treat pediatric cardiac arrest, respiratory emergencies, and trauma is extremely variable and age dependent. For most age groups, endotracheal intubation success rates are comparable to those for adults. As would be expected, endotracheal intubation and intravenous access are performed with poor success in infants. In a large regional study of pediatric intubation, Gausche and others have shown no change in patient outcome after field endotracheal intubation.[16] The Los Angeles County EMS system has withdrawn the use of pediatric intubation by paramedics, although it has greatly increased clinical education regarding field bag-valve-mask ventilation.

RURAL EMERGENCY MEDICAL SERVICES

Most EMS literature has been developed by urban and suburban systems, with little emphasis on rural EMS care. However, rural EMS systems are an integral part of health care for the ill and injured rural patient. The rural environment provides a number of unique challenges to providers of emergency care.[17] Long distances over which to reach and transport patients are a central issue. Specialized search and rescue capabilities may be needed for off-road and wilderness emergencies. Because of the low population density of rural areas, there is a decreased likelihood that an emergency will be witnessed and emergency aid summoned. Compared to urban and suburban populations, the population in rural areas tends to be less affluent, older, and less likely to request emergency aid unless it is truly needed.

The implementation of a 911 system has not occurred in many rural communities. Enhanced 911 services, which provide automatic location identifiers, may not be as useful in rural as in urban locations because there may not be addresses to guide emergency providers. The infrastructure for basic radio communications may not be as well developed or supported. The contraction of the health care system in the United States has caused the closure of a number of hospitals, most of them in rural areas. If an emergency facility exists, it may not have specialty or critical care services. Therefore, patients must have access to air or ground interfacility transport service. Fortunately, large tertiary care facilities can facilitate these transfers, and most rural facilities are able to prospectively develop the necessary relationships and transfer agreements.

The key component of any EMS system is its personnel. Rural EMS systems face particular challenges in maintaining a cadre of EMS personnel. The volume of EMS responses in most rural communities is too low to allow for the employment of full-time EMS providers; thus, rural EMS services often use volunteers or on-call part-time personnel who are paid only when called out. Volunteer and part-time personnel have limited time for initial training and continuing education and limited experience necessary for skill maintenance. Most, but not all, rural EMS services are provided at the EMT-B level. The recent revision of the model DOT EMT curriculum allows for an increased level of service by EMT-Bs that would be useful in rural areas. They can now assist patients with self-administration of some medications (e.g., nitroglycerin for angina or bronchodilators for asthma), use AEDs for cardiac arrest, and, with the optional 10-h training module, utilize advanced airway techniques. These modifications allow a higher level of basic EMT service without having to commit rural providers to the much longer time required to obtain a higher level of certification. Innovative approaches to continuing education are also needed, particularly in isolated areas. Distance learning approaches, often in collaboration with local schools, are invaluable. Videotape conferences, satellite transmission of lectures, and computer- and Internet-based education programs are all valuable adjuncts to rural EMS continuing education.

The provision of lifesaving services on a volunteer basis entails particular obstacles. Daytime coverage for service is a challenge because most volunteers or part-time personnel have other full-time employment. As a result, many services hire a cadre of full-time providers to respond during business hours. Dispatching volunteers from home or work directly to the scene may be one method of providing daytime coverage and reducing response times.[18] Recruitment and retention of providers is an ongoing problem. To address it, volunteer services may be able to provide incentives, such as retirement benefits, death benefits, and scholarships for volunteers and their children. Undoubtedly, the most powerful incentive for EMS volunteers is the fellowship bonds that develop within volunteer EMS agencies.

Medical leadership of any EMS system is crucial. Identification of a physician who is knowledgeable and experienced in emergency care and willing to take time away from his or her family and practice is a difficult problem for rural systems. Many systems depend on nonemergency physicians, such as family physicians with an interest in community health or general surgeons with an interest in acute surgical care, to provide medical leadership.

EMERGENCY MEDICAL SERVICES AGENDA FOR THE FUTURE

With wide input from the EMS community, NHTSA sponsored the development of a visionary planning document, ''The EMS Agenda for the Future.''[19] This document defines EMS as the ''intersection of public safety, public health, and health care systems'' and as an essential component of the emergency care safety net. It proposes that EMS systems and providers play a role in illness and injury prevention. As a result, EMS systems have become involved in drowning prevention for children, social service referral and fall prevention for the elderly, and immunization of adults and children for infectious disease.[20] This concept will evolve significantly in the years ahead.

REFERENCES

1. Mustalish AC, Post C: History, in Kuehl AE (ed): *Prehospital Systems and Medical Oversight.* St. Louis, National Association of EMS Physicians, Mosby Lifeline, 1994, pp 3–27.
2. Auble TE, Menegazzi JJ, Paris PM: Effect of out of hospital defibrillation by basic life support providers on cardiac arrest mortality: A metaanalysis. *Ann Emerg Med* 25:642, 1995.
3. Spaite D, Benoit R, Brown D, et al: Uniform prehospital data elements and definitions: A report from the uniform prehospital emergency medical services data conference. *Ann Emerg Med* 25:525, 1995.
4. Alonso-Serra H, Blanton D, O'Connor RE: Physician medical direction in EMS. *J Prehosp Care* 2:153, 1998.
5. Eisenberg MS, Horwood BT, Cummins RO, et al: Cardiac arrest and resuscitation: A tale of 29 cities. *Ann Emerg Med* 19:179, 1990.
6. Eisenberg MS, Pantridge JF, Cobb LA, Geddes JS: The revolution and evolution of prehospital cardiac care. *Arch Intern Med* 156:1611, 1996.
7. Becker LB, Pepe PE: Ensuring the effectiveness of community-wide emergency cardiac care. *Ann Emerg Med* 22(part 2):354, 1993.
8. Weaver DW, Cerqueira M, Hallstrom AP, et al: Prehospital-initiated vs hospital-initiated thrombolytic therapy: The MITI trial. *JAMA* 270:1211, 1993.
9. Smith JS, Martin LF, Young WW, Macioce DP: Do trauma centers improve outcome over non-trauma centers: The evaluation of regional trauma care using discharge abstract data and patient management categories. *J Trauma* 30:1533, 1990.
10. Sampalis JS, Lavoie A, Williams JI, et al: Impact of on-site care, prehospital time, and level of in-hospital care on survival in severely injured patients. *J Trauma* 34:252, 1993.
11. Cayten CG, Murphy JG, Stahl WM: Basic life support versus advanced life support for injured patients with an injury severity score of 10 or more. *J Trauma* 35:460, 1993.
12. Bickell WH, Wall MJ, Pepe PE, et al: Immediate vs delayed fluid resuscitation for hypotensive patients with penetrating torso injuries. *N Engl J Med* 331:1105, 1994.
13. Shuster M, Shannon HS: Differential prehospital benefit from paramedic care. *Ann Emerg Med* 23:1014, 1994.
14. Pediatric Education Task Force, Gausche M, Henderson DP, et al: Education of out-of-hospital emergency medical personnel in pediatrics: Report of a national task force. *Ann Emerg Med* 31:58, 1998.
15. Joyce SM, Brown DE, Nelson EA: Epidemiology of pediatric EMS practice: A multistate analysis. *Prehosp and Disas Med* 11:180, 1996.
16. Gausche M, Lewis RJ, Stratton SJ, et al: A prospective, randomized study of the effect of out-of-hospital pediatric intubation on patient outcome. *Acad Emerg Med* 5:428, 1998.
17. Thompson AM: Rural emergency medical volunteers and their communities: A demographic comparison. *J Community Health* 18:379, 1993.
18. Johnson DR, Maggiore WA, Davis DR: A method to reduce rural EMS response times. *Prehosp and Disas Med* 6:143, 1991.

19. EMS Agenda for the Future Steering Committee, Delbridge TR, Bailey B, et al: EMS agenda for the future: Where we are . . . where we want to be. *Prehosp Emerg Care* 2:1, 1998.
20. Garrison HG, Foltin GL, Becker LR, et al: The role of EMS in primary injury prevention. *Prehosp Emerg Care* 1:156, 1997.

PREHOSPITAL EQUIPMENT AND ADJUNCTS

Daniel G. Hankins

Early emergency medical services (EMS) equipment began as hospital equipment that was extrapolated to the field. It soon became apparent that hospital equipment did not always perform under the more rigorous conditions of out-of-hospital care. Over the last 25 years, equipment has evolved specifically for EMS that is better adapted to field use in terms of size, weight, and durability. This equipment is designed for resuscitating and packaging the patient for transport to the hospital and for maintenance of stability during emergency or interfacility transport.

Much EMS equipment has been placed in vehicles without clear-cut proof of efficacy. More and more equipment will be scrutinized for effectiveness, with good equipment being kept and useless equipment being discarded.[1] Reimbursement for out-of-hospital transports is changing, and the cost-benefit ratio becomes important in the face of ever-tightening EMS budgets. The EMS medical director should be actively involved in evaluating and choosing equipment for use in the field. The nature of EMS equipment is changing due to the expanded scope of practice by paramedics and the blurring of care levels between basic and advanced life support personnel. Equipment once considered only for advanced level care (e.g., defibrillators) is now being carried routinely on basic life support ambulances. There are still differences in the equipment carried by providers of the two levels of care, primarily due to differences in the demographics of prehospital care. Advanced life support (ALS) services tend to be paid, full-time, and urban, while basic life support (BLS) services tend to be volunteer, part-time, and rural.

There are four basic questions that must be answered about EMS equipment: (1) Does it do the job?, (2) Is it safe?, (3) Does it do the job and is it safe in the field environment?, and (4) Does it do the job and is it safe in the field environment in the hands of field personnel?[2]

VEHICLES

The equipment used in out-of-hospital care includes the vehicles and everything on them. The two most common EMS vehicles are first-response units (fire engines, police cruisers, and rescue vehicles), which do not transport patients, and ground ambulances, which do transport patients. Ground ambulances come in three common varieties: type I, a standard pick-up chassis with a modular box to carry personnel, patient, and equipment; type II, an enlarged van-type vehicle; and type III, a van chassis with a modular box on the back.

Ground vehicles have warning devices (lights and siren) as part of their equipment. Unwarranted use of red lights and sirens is dangerous for the EMS crew, any patient on board, and the general public on the streets. Ambulance transport with lights and sirens does not save significant amounts of time in most urban and suburban transports.[3] Every EMS system must have protocols or guidelines written by the medical director to use these devices only at times when medically indicated when the crew is responding to the scene, transporting the patient back to the hospital, and during interfacility transports.[4]

UNIVERSAL PRECAUTIONS

Every EMS provider must be protected against exposure to blood and other body fluids from patients. This protection includes masks, goggles, and gloves for routine use. On occasion, more extensive protection may be needed, such as gowns or perhaps heavier gloves. This equipment must be carried on any EMS vehicle.

RESUSCITATION EQUIPMENT AND THERAPEUTIC MODALITIES

Defibrillators

Defibrillators have been an essential part of out-of-hospital care since Pantridge showed that defibrillation could be done in the field on the streets of Belfast in 1965. Early defibrillation is the most important factor in surviving an out-of-hospital cardiac arrest. To meet this need, defibrillators have become smaller, less expensive, and easier to use. Many BLS services carry automated external defibrillators (AEDs) (Fig. 2-1). These devices are more precisely called shock advisory defibrillators because they analyze the patient's rhythm, determine whether a defibrillatory shock is indicated, charge the capacitors, and then inform the operator that a shock is advised. The operator can press the appropriate button to deliver the defibrillatory shock. The arrhythmia recognition algorithm of the AED is designed to advise defibrillation only for ventricular fibrillation and very fast wide QRS complex tachycardias (usually over 180 beats per minute). Rhythm monitoring and defibrillation are performed with combination pads, one placed over the cardiac apex and the other placed over the left paraspinal area at approximately the T6 level. Automated external defibrillators are designed to be used only on pulseless and apneic patients. Because AEDs have become so easy to use and function almost always as designed, a debate is ongoing whether these devices should be available for public access defibrillation by laypersons. While layperson defibrillation is beyond the scope of this discussion, there is developing evidence that rapid first-response defibrillation before the ambulance arrives, (e.g., by law enforcement officers using an AED) results in improved survival rates.[5]

Automated external defibrillators are priced at about $2500 to $3500 for a basic version without a rhythm monitor display, $5000 to $7000 for versions with monitor display screens, and $9000 to $10,000 for versions with full-function defibrillation, synchronized cardioversion, and external pacing capabilities. The AEDs without rhythm display monitors may actually function better because a displayed rhythm may only serve to distract a non-ALS operator. The event-recording capabilities of AEDs facilitate later review of the cardiac arrest for medical oversight and quality assurance reasons. The medical director must be involved in the selection of these devices, the training of EMS personnel, and subsequent review of their use.

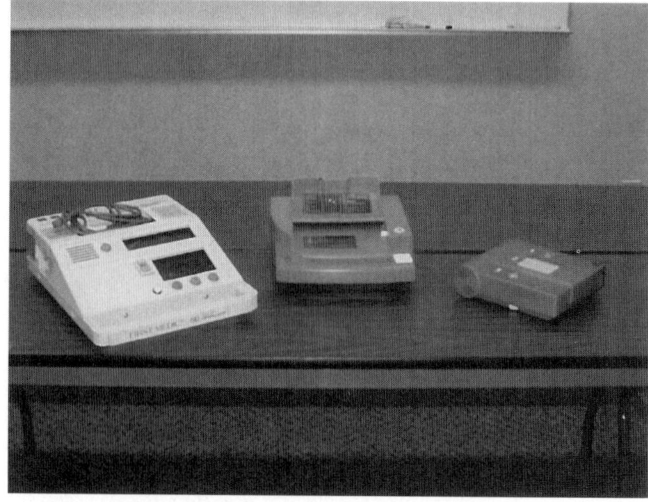

FIG. 2-1. Automated external defibrillators (AEDs).

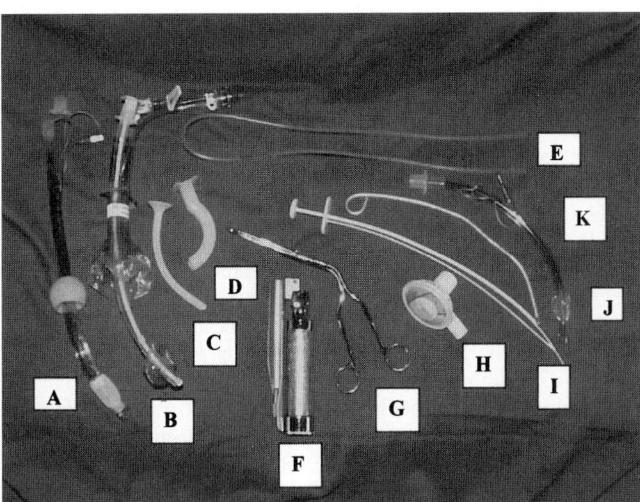

FIG. 2-2. Airway devices and adjuncts. A. Combitude. B. Pharyngeal tracheal lumen airway. C. Nasopharyngeal airway. D. Oropharyngeal airway. E. Tube exchanger. F. Laryngoscope. G. Magill forceps. H. Qualitative end expiratory CO_2 detector. I and J. Stylets for endotracheal intubation. K. Endotracheal tube.

Defibrillators used by ALS personnel are more sophisticated, with monitoring screens, printout units, manual defibrillation ability, and synchronized cardioversion capability. Defibrillation is often done with combination pads (as with the AED) rather than with paddles. These pads provide better contact with the skin, resulting in decreased resistance and allowing for more current to be delivered with a higher success rate for conversion. Such pads are also safer for the operator, who does not have direct contact with the patient when the shock is delivered. The monitor screen is used by the paramedics for initial interpretation of rhythms, ongoing monitoring of patients' rhythms, synchronizing a countershock for rhythms other than ventricular fibrillation, and pacing bradycardiac rhythms. The ALS defibrillators will soon be equipped with the technology to monitor blood pressures, pulse oximetry, and end tidal CO_2. The ALS personnel will use these machines for monitoring very ill patients from emergent calls or interfacility transfers.

Airway and Ventilation Adjuncts

For patients with acute respiratory failure or arrest, airway and ventilation adjuncts are useful to maintain an airway that would otherwise require continuous bag-valve-mask (BVM) ventilation. In addition, some airway adjuncts aid in preventing gastric distention or aspiration (Fig. 2-2).

The simplest devices for airway management used with BVM ventilation are the oropharyngeal and nasopharyngeal airways. These devices prevent obstruction of the upper airway so that externally applied positive-pressure ventilation can reach the trachea. Effective portable suction devices are available that can be carried to the patient's side to help clear the airway (Fig. 2-3).

More advanced airway devices are required if the patient needs more prolonged airway management or is at risk for aspiration. At the BLS level, available options include the pharyngeal tracheal lumen (PTL) airway, the esophagotracheal double lumen tube (or, simply, Combitube), and the laryngeal mask airway (LMA). Each of these is used in conjunction with a bag-valve for ventilation. These devices are great improvement over the old esophageal obturator airway and esophageal gastric airway, both of which had unacceptably high complication rates and are no longer recommended for use. Both the PTL and the Combitube (Sheridan Corp.) are only for adult patients in full cardiac arrest. The PTL and Combitube provide a seal in the upper airway—to promote better ventilation than the BVM with oral airway—and a seal in the esophagus—to prevent gastric regurgitation and aspiration. Both devices are passed blindly, and the tube usually passes into the esophagus. A small percentage of the time, the device goes into the trachea, where it can function as an endotracheal tube. There is some evidence that the Combitube is an easier device to use than the PTL because the large PTL mouth balloon is more easily broken than the Combitube balloon.[6] The Combitube may be easier for basic emergency medical technicians (EMTs) to ventilate through. There are few data on usage of the LMA for out-of-hospital care. While the LMA provides a seal for ventilation, it does not prevent aspiration. One possible advantage of the LMA is that it is less expensive than the Combitube or the PTL. The PTL and/or Combitube is mostly used by BLS ambulance personnel but may be used by ALS personnel (or even by hospital personnel) for a patient with a difficult airway who cannot be intubated with an endotracheal tube. The disadvantages of the PTL, Combitube, or LMA is that it cannot be used in small adults, children, or patients who are somewhat responsive with a gag reflex.

Endotracheal intubation is the "gold standard" for airway management; it provides the best access for ventilation and the greatest protection against aspiration. The majority of ALS systems use endotracheal intubation as the airway of choice for the patient in respiratory failure or with an unprotected airway. Therefore, a number of different-sized endotracheal tubes, laryngoscope blades with handles, stylets, lubricants, and Magill forceps must be carried in the airway kit. Tube exchanger catheters or gum bougies can also aid with establishing a difficult endotracheal tube. Directors of EMS must ensure that ALS personnel maintain their intubation skills through field experience and practice.

The new basic EMT model curriculum has made endotracheal intubation an optional module. Therefore, intubation training may be provided to basic EMTs and intubation equipment may be placed on some BLS ambulances. Increasing the number of ambulance personnel in need of endotracheal intubation training in an EMS system may cause logistical problems for the medical director. It is sometimes difficult to obtain adequate live intubation opportunities for the personnel in an EMS system in order to develop and maintain skills. Some studies have found that basic EMTs do not maintain endotracheal intubation skills and have low rates of successful field intubations.[7,8] This would suggest that intubation will generally remain an ALS skill.[9]

Another intubation-related modality that has bearing on the equipment carried on the ambulance is rapid sequence intubation (RSI)

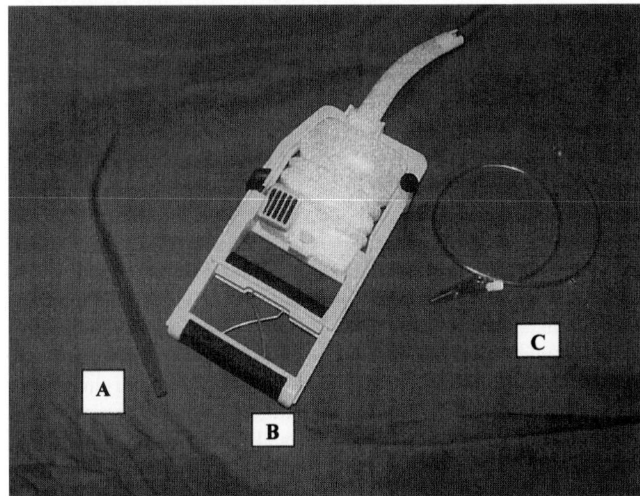

FIG. 2-3. Suction devices. A. Yankauer rigid suction catheter. B. V-Vac (Laerdal Medical Corp., Wappingers Falls, NY) portable suction device. C Flexible suction catheter.

using intravenous (IV) hypnotics and neuromuscular paralytic drugs.[10] Critical care transport services have been using RSI for more than a decade, but now a number of ALS systems are doing so, also with good success. The use of RSI raises the level of psychomotor and judgment skills required of the paramedic. While the use of RSI increases the amount of training needed, it enables paramedics to secure more difficult airways. In addition to the usual equipment required for intubation, these ALS services must carry the drugs needed for sedation and paralysis.

Vascular Access Equipment

The equipment used to establish IV access in the field is the same as at the hospital: tourniquets, cleaning agent, IV catheters, IV fluid bags, and IV tubing. In ALS ambulances, IV access is used for fluid resuscitation and administration of drugs. In general, vascular access is obtained for drug administration as soon as possible after the patient is assessed and it is determined that pharmacologic intervention is required. Paramedics are very adept at rapid IV placement.[11] For fluid resuscitation, usually in trauma patients, vascular access is usually started en route to the hospital after the patient is immobilized, unless there is prolonged scene time due to extrication difficulties. Obtaining IV access should not prolong scene times in a trauma patient, especially when ''LOAD AND GO'' criteria are present. Prehospital fluid administration may make little difference in the patient's outcome.[12] First, the amount of fluid that can be administered during transport in most urban and suburban EMS systems is modest and may not be physiologically significant. Second, there is evidence that prehospital (and emergency department) fluid administration to hypotensive victims of penetrating truncal trauma does not improve survival and may even decrease survival in those patients who require surgery.[13] The medical director is responsible for developing protocols for prehospital IV access and monitoring their use in an ongoing manner.

Vascular access is also utilized by some BLS services, not for drug administration, but for fluid resuscitation. Since BLS services usually serve rural areas and have longer transport times, fluid resuscitation may be more beneficial (although this is unproven) for the hypovolemic trauma patient.

Pneumatic Antishock Garment

The military antishock trousers (MAST) garment is a one-piece layered device made of polyvinyl fabric that encircles the legs and lower abdomen and can be inflated to apply external pressure to enclosed body parts. The legs are enclosed separately from the inguinal crease to the ankle; the feet are exposed. The abdominal component encloses the body from the lower rib cage to the pelvis, with the perineal area exposed. Three compartments are fastened with Velcro (Velcro USA, Inc.). Most versions of the garment allow separate inflation and deflation of the three compartments. The MAST is inflated with a foot pump, and some units are equipped with inflation pressure monitoring gauges. Internal pressures of the suit are limited by pressure relief valves (set at 104 mmHg) and the ability of the Velcro fasteners to withstand stress.

The MAST is a old concept but was rediscovered in Vietnam when a commercially available ''G-suit'' inflated to a pressure of 30 to 40 cmH_2O was used during the transport of seriously injured soldiers from combat areas to the hospital.[14] The authors of this study felt that the device was beneficial because four soldiers survived while using it who otherwise would have died, a judgment based on the physician's previous experience with similar casualties. Since then, considerable study, thought, and opinion have been published concerning the utility of the MAST in civilian EMS.[15,16] Currently, the MAST has fallen into disfavor because there is little evidence that it improves survival rates for the condition for which it is most commonly used: hemorrhagic shock after trauma. In fact, there is evidence from the Houston EMS system that the MAST may be detrimental in cases of cardiac and thoracic trauma with short transport times.[17] It is not clear whether MAST may be useful in other situations or in disease entities other than trauma. For instance, there is theoretical and anecdotal evidence that the MAST may be useful in bluntly traumatized patients with long transport times, in ruptured abdominal aortic aneurysms (AAAs), or in pelvic fractures. A position paper from the National Association of EMS physicians attempts to bring a reasoned approach to the use of MAST by categorizing the possible indications into classes I, II-A, II-B, and III, based on possible efficacy or lack thereof.[15] Incidentally, the only class I intervention (usually indicated, useful, and effective) for MAST in that paper is ruptured AAA. It may be reasonable to keep MAST on ambulances for now, especially for rural services, to use it primarily for blunt trauma with long transport times and to avoid its use with penetrating thoracic injury.

The physiologic effects of the MAST are often misunderstood.[16] The MAST increases blood pressure primarily by increasing peripheral vascular resistance (afterload). The MAST does not reliably mobilize pooled blood (autotransfuse) from the legs or abdomen, especially in hypovolemic trauma patients. The MAST does decrease bleeding from vessels under the compartments by applying external pressure that decreases the pressure gradient for continued hemorrhage.

In practice, the MAST is applied as the patient is being immobilized on the long spine board. After physical assessment of the abdomen, pelvis, and legs, the three compartments are closed over the patient. If the patient is hypotensive, the garment is inflated sequentially, first the legs and then the abdomen. Inflation is done in stages until the desired response by the patient is seen—usually a systolic blood pressure greater than 90 mmHg—and the MAST is not inflated further. While the compartments have pressure relief valves set at 104 mmHg, the Velcro fasteners usually give way at pressures far less, usually around 60 mmHg; thus, it is difficult to achieve high MAST compartment pressures.

Once a patient has been placed in a MAST and the compartments have been inflated, their cardiovascular system responds and adapts to the increased afterload. If that external pressure is suddenly relieved, systolic blood pressure can fall precipitously, especially in a hypovolemic patient. Therefore, MAST deflation in the emergency department should be done slowly, with blood pressure monitoring and IV fluid administration in case of sudden hypotension.

Since the MAST increases afterload, pulmonary edema is the one absolute contraindication to its use. Contraindications for use of the abdominal compartment of the MAST (and relative contraindications to the use of the MAST in general) are pregnancy, the presence of impaled objects, evisceration of the abdominal contents, and thoracic and diaphragmatic injuries.

SPINAL IMMOBILIZATION

The preservation of integrity of the spinal column and the enclosed spinal cord is of paramount importance in the field. Cervical spine stabilization and airway assessment are performed simultaneously. Manual stabilization of the neck is not released until the patient has been transferred and securely strapped to a board. The length of boards used (whether short, long, or both) depends on the initial position in which the patient is found by the first responder or EMT.

Carrying boarded patients takes a heavy toll on the backs of EMTs and paramedics. Evaluation of the boarded patient is expensive and time-consuming in the emergency department because of the need to ''clear the spine.'' Not all trauma victims require spinal immobilization for transport. The medical director should develop protocols or guidelines to avoid unnecessary field immobilization.[18] For example, a patient with no neck pain or tenderness (neck pain must be defined liberally and includes stiffness or ''feels funny''), not in the extremes of age (below 10 or above 65), with no altered sensorium (no drugs or alcohol present and no head injury), and with no distracting injuries (e.g., long bone fracture or abdominal or chest injury) does not routinely require immobilization because there is an extraordinarily low probability of neck injury. Ideal guidelines for prehospital personnel necessarily would have virtually 100 percent sensitivity with acceptable specificity for cervical spine injuries.

Spinal Boards and Cervical Collars

Spine boards, either short or long, are made from plastic or wood to provide a rigid surface on which to bind the patient to ensure that no movement occurs in the cervical, thoracic, or lumbar spine during transportation. Straps with buckles or Velcro fasteners are used to secure the patient to the board. Some boards have attached firm head blocks for either side of the head and straps to go across these blocks to keep the head steady between them. Rolled up blankets (''blanket rolls'') secured to the board with tape are also effective head blocks. A popular and effective variation of the short board is the Kendrick extrication device (KED) (Ferno, Wilmington, OH), which consists of slats of rigid material bound together by heavy cloth. The KED immobilizes the cervical spine, wraps partly around the patient, and is then strapped the rest of the way around the thorax and around the thighs for secure immobilization. The patient can be lifted using the KED straps, allowing for easier and safer extrication from a vehicle.

Rigid cervical collars are more accurately called cervical extrication devices. Multiple types are commercially available for use in the field: Philadelphia collar (Philadelphia Cervical Collar Co., Westville, NJ), the StifNeck (Laerdal Medical Corp., Wappingers Falls, NY), and the Neck-Loc (Un-I-Med, Louisville, KY). These collars come either as two asymmetric pieces, which are used and marked for back and front, or as a single piece that is folded into the correct shape. By themselves, collars are not adequate for complete cervical immobilization; additional lateral support is required to avoid lateral movement. For complete immobilization, the patient needs to be strapped on the backboard and secured with head blocks and head straps. Once the patient is well secured to the board, the collar does not add a significant amount of stabilization and can actually be removed without compromise of the spine. However, the collar is often left in place for added protection. Patients with mandible or soft tissue neck injuries should probably not have a collar applied because of the potential for airway compromise that could be masked by the collar. More recent designs have openings in the front to allow observation of the trachea and jugular veins, but this may not be adequate for observing other neck areas. Soft cervical collars are not adequate or appropriate for out-of-hospital care.

Sequence of Spinal Immobilization

Prehospital personnel are taught to have a high index of suspicion for spine trauma. If the patient is sitting in a car after an accident and is stable from respiratory and circulatory standpoints, the short spine board and rigid cervical collar or KED are first used to safely get the patient onto a long spine board and out of the vehicle in a orderly manner. If time is critical because of the patient's condition or the threat of hazards such as chemicals, fire, or water, the patient can be extricated more rapidly without the short board or KED. The risk of rapid extrication must be weighed carefully but quickly against the benefit of getting out of the vehicle promptly.

At a noncritical scene, when the patient is still sitting in the vehicle upon EMS arrival, one EMT secures the neck with his or her hands and applies the necessary airway maneuvers while the second EMT secures the rigid cervical collar. The short board is then slid in behind the patient and the patient is strapped to the board while still seated (short boards are not used if the patient is not seated in a vehicle). The first EMT maintains manual stabilization of the neck until the patient is secured to the short board. The patient can then be rotated around and slid directly onto the long board positioned on the car seat or directly onto the ambulance stretcher. The MAST garment, if needed, is often already placed on the long board underneath the patient. The patient is then strapped to the long board. A properly secured patient can be turned on the board or even stood on end if necessary to move the patient to the ambulance. If the patient vomits, for instance, the board can be partly turned (''logrolled'') to prevent aspiration.

Because of the difference in relative size and positions of head and body, adults and children need slightly different positioning on a backboard. An adult needs more padding under the head, while a child needs more padding under the body, to maintain neutral neck position.

In more dangerous situations where rapid extrication is required, the short board is omitted, but the rigid cervical collar should still be used. The patient is carefully rotated out and slid onto the waiting long board.

If a patient is walking at the scene when EMS personnel arrive but complains of neck pain, the patient should be boarded from a standing position. If the patient is lying on the ground when the EMTs arrive, the patient should be carefully logrolled by several attendants onto a long backboard.

Radiographs can be obtained without difficulty through short and long boards. In general, patients should not be removed from these devices until the spine has been ''cleared'' clinically or radiographically. If removal off the spine board is necessary before clearing, the patient should be logrolled or lifted off carefully.

EXTREMITY IMMOBILIZATION

Most fractures encountered in the field are splinted for the patient's comfort and ease of transport. Air splints, or circumferential bladders that are inflated by mouth, are adequate for most distal fractures of the upper and lower extremities. In hot weather, air splints can be difficult to remove when they stick to the skin. An air splint with a zipper and powder on the inside is easier to remove. The MAST garment can function as an air splint for one or both lower extremities. Other splinting possibilities include simple sling and swathe, tying the legs together with cravats to splint one injured leg with the other normal one, or using a pillow wrapped around an extremity and secured with tape. A pillow splint is comfortable and secure for the patient either out-of-hospital or in the emergency department. Other splints are available on the market, such as vacuum splints, but add cost with perhaps no clear-cut advantages over older cheaper splinting methods.

Traction Splints

Pelvic fractures and fractures of the femoral shaft are potentially life- and limb-threatening. Stabilization of pelvic fractures is difficult. Indeed, the only effective method in the field or in the emergency department is using the MAST garment with all compartments inflated. Radiographs can be performed through the garment.

Fractures of the femur can damage vessels and nerves from movement of bony fragments. Stabilization of femur fractures in the field is imperative to minimize blood loss and soft tissue damage. While MAST garments are often used to immobilize femur fractures, they do limit the assessment of the patient and cannot reduce the fracture. The femoral traction splint is the preferred device for femur fractures.

Several leg traction splint variations are commercially available. The two most commonly used types are the Hare splint (Dyna Med, Carlsbad, CA) and the Sager splint (Minto Research and Development, Inc.) (Figs. 2-4 and 2-5). Other traction splints (Thomas Ring, Donway, and Klippel) are less commonly used. The underlying principle is the application of traction by a hitch on the ankle against resistance when the splint impinges proximally on the pelvis. The padded proximal end of the Hare splint abuts the ischial tuberosity (Fig. 2-4). The proximal end of the Sager splint rests against the ischial tuberosity medial to the shaft of the femur (Fig. 2-5). These splints cannot be used if a pelvic fracture is suspected, since the pressure on the pelvis may further displace a fracture and cause more bleeding. Another

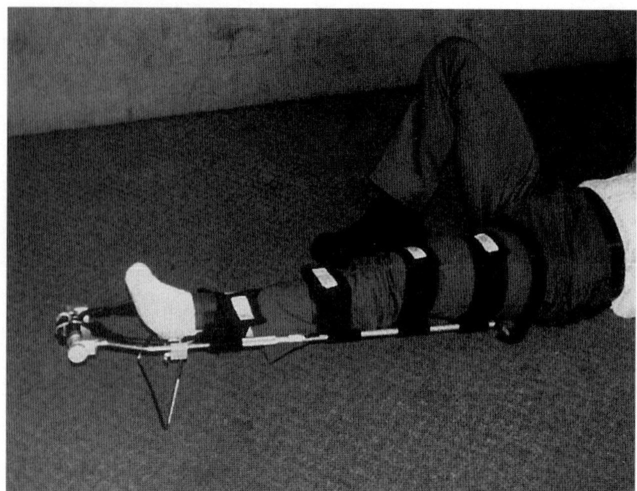

FIG. 2-4. Hare traction splint.

contraindication to the use of femoral traction splints is a hip dislocation.

Leg traction splints may also be used for tibial shaft fractures. Traction splints should not be used for fractures near the knee; since longitudinal traction may damage the neurovascular structures in the popliteal area. Traction splints for the tibia should be reserved for angulated or displaced fractures; otherwise, an air splint or the MAST would suffice.

Before applying a femoral traction splint at the scene, enough clothing must be cut or removed so that the extremity can be assessed for injury and distal neurovascular function. If the Hare splint (Fig. 2-4) is used, the proximal half ring is placed in the crease of the buttocks against the ischial tuberosity. Traction is placed on the ankle with the padded ankle strap by one rescuer while the splint is strapped to the leg. The ankle strap is then attached to a ratcheting mechanism, and traction is applied. If a Sager splint (Fig. 2-5) is used, the splint is placed on the medial side of the limb up against the groin. The padded ankle hitch is applied, and traction-applied elastic straps are then secured to hold the splint to the leg. With both splints, traction is applied until malalignment is reduced and pain is relieved. Overtraction can be harmful.

The Hare splint can be longer than an ambulance stretcher when fully extended, and care needs to be taken when closing the rear door of the ambulance. The Sager splint is shorter than the Hare splint, and one Sager splint can be used to splint both legs simultaneously. The Sager device is less bulky and therefore takes up less room in an ambulance or a helicopter, which can be very important in the latter.

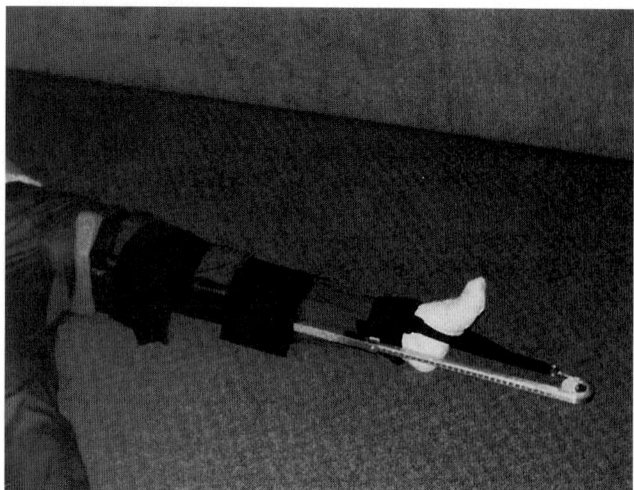

FIG. 2-5. Sager traction splint.

PHARMACEUTICAL EQUIPMENT

Another area where practice is becoming blurred between BLS and ALS is in the realm of medications. The new basic EMT model curriculum has a module on certain classes of pharmaceuticals to prepare basic EMTs for helping the patient administer his or her medication in a limited fashion. This module includes nitroglycerin for chest pain, inhaled beta-adrenergic agonists for bronchospasm, glucagon for hypoglycemia, and epinephrine preloaded injections for anaphylaxis. The curriculum assumes that the patient already has the medication and the EMT is simply assisting; the drugs are not carried on the ambulance. Some states have gone beyond that and allowed limited carrying of medications on BLS ambulances.

Drugs carried by ALS services are more extensive, but it must be emphasized that out-of-hospital pharmaceutical interventions are limited to a few that will make a real difference before the patient gets to the hospital. The drugs that can make a real difference when administered by a paramedic include oxygen for hypoxia; glucose for hypoglycemia; nitroglycerin for chest pain and pulmonary edema; inhaled beta-adrenergic agonists for bronchospasm; naloxone for suspected narcotic overdose; morphine for pain; benzodiazepines for seizures, delirium, or intubation; furosemide for fluid overload; epinephrine for cardiac arrest and anaphylaxis; and lidocaine, magnesium, bretylium, and perhaps amiodarone for cardiac arrest. Adenosine and diltiazem are useful for rate control of tachycardia, but most patients would be able to wait until arrival in the emergency department for treatment. Sodium bicarbonate is helpful for suspected or known hyperkalemia but probably not for cardiac arrest. Calcium may also be of use in cardiac arrest, especially if hyperkalemia is suspected. In some systems, paralytic drugs (e.g., succinylcholine and vecuronium) are used along with the sedating agents for RSI. Out-of hospital care providers do not need the whole spectrum of drugs found in the emergency department; drugs carried by ALS services should be restricted to those that improve patients' outcomes.

REFERENCES

1. Callaham M: Quantifying the scanty science of prehospital emergency care. *Ann Emerg Med* 30:785–790, 1997.
2. Stewart RD: The search for the better mousetrap . . . are the mice winning? *Prehosp Emerg Med* 1:58–59, 1997
3. Hunt RC, Brown LH, Cabinum ES, et al: Is ambulance transport time with lights and siren faster than that without? *Ann Emerg Med* 25:507–511, 1995.
4. National Association of EMS Physicians, National Association of State EMS Directors: Position paper: Use of warning lights and siren in emergency medical vehicle response and patient transport. *Prehosp and Disas Med* 9:133–136, 1994.
5. White RD, Asplin BR, Bugliosi TF, Hankins DG: High discharge survival rate after out-of-hospital ventricular fibrillation with rapid defibrillation by police and paramedics. *Ann Emerg Med* 28:480–485, 1996.
6. Rumball CJ, MacDonald D: The PTL, combitube, laryngeal mask, and oral airway: A randomized prehospital comparative study of ventilatory device effectiveness and cost-effectiveness in 470 cases of cardiorespiratory arrest. *Prehosp Emerg Care* 1:1–10, 1997.
7. Bradley JS, Billows GL, Olinger ML, et al: Prehospital oral endotracheal intubation by rural basic emergency medical technicians. *Ann Emerg Med* 32:26–32, 1998.
8. Sayre MR, Sakles JC, Mistler AF, et al: Field trial of endotracheal intubation by basic EMTs. *Ann Emerg Med* 31:228–233, 1998.
9. Spaite DW: Intubation by basic EMTs: Lifesaving advance or catastrophic complication? *Ann Emerg Med* 31:276–277, 1998.
10. McDonald CC, Bailey B: Out of hospital use of neuromuscular-blocking agents in the United States. *Prehosp Emerg Care* 2:29–32, 1998.

11. Sapite DW, Valenzuela TD, Criss EA, et al: A prospective in-field comparison of intravenous line placement by urban and nonurban emergency medical services personnel. *Ann Emerg Med* 24:209–214, 1994.
12. Kaweski SM, Sise MJ, Virgilio RW: The effect of prehospital fluid on survival in trauma patients. *J Trauma* 30:1215–1219, 1990.
13. Bickell WH, Wall MJ, Pepe PE, et al: Immediate versus delayed fluid resuscitation for hypotensive patients with penetrating torso injuries. *N Engl J Med* 331:1105–1109, 1994.
14. Cutler BS, Daggett WM: Application of the ''G-suit'' to the control of hemorrhage in massive trauma. *Ann Surg* 173:511–514, 1971.
15. Domeier RM, O'Connor RE, Delbridge TR, Hunt RC: National Association of EMS Physicians: Position paper: Use of pneumatic anti-shock garment (PASG). *Prehosp Emerg Care* 1:32–35, 1997.
16. O'Connor RE, Domeier RM: Collective review: An evaluation of the pneumatic anti-shock garment (PASG) in various clinical settings. *Prehosp Emerg Care* 1:36–44, 1997.
17. Mattox KL, Bickell W, Pepe PE, et al: Prospective MAST study in 911 patients. *J Trauma* 29:1104–1112, 1989.
18. Brown LH, Gough JE, Simonds WB: Can EMS providers adequately assess trauma patients for cervical spine injury? *Prehosp Emerg Care* 2:33–36, 1998.

AIR MEDICAL TRANSPORT

C. Keith Stone
Stephen H. Thomas

Air medical transport is part of an integrated emergency medical services (EMS) system. Field EMS personnel or physicians transferring patients between hospitals should be able to select the proper mode of transportation for an individual patient, depending on the particular circumstances (Fig. 3-1). Effective implementation of all these EMS tools requires well-trained communications and dispatch personnel who can quickly assess the situation at hand and then institute the right EMS response. In addition, the entire out-of-hospital care system must be designed with and medically supervised by physicians well versed in EMS care.

The terms *aeromedical* and *air medical* are not interchangeable: *air medical* refers to the use of aircraft for evacuation of patients, whereas *aeromedical* refers to the study of the medical effects of flight and altitude on humans.

HELICOPTER TRANSPORT

The history of air evacuation is closely connected to the history of warfare. Igor Sikorsky's invention, the helicopter, first flown on September 14, 1939, was used for the first rotor-wing medical evacuation in Burma in 1945. From this small start in World War II, helicopter usage blossomed extensively in the Korean war, when more aircraft of sturdier construction were available. About 20,000 patients were transported by helicopter in the Korean war. During the Vietnamese war, about 370,000 patients were carried by helicopter from 1965 to 1969.

The first hospital-based civilian program began in 1972 in Denver. Currently, there are 385 air medical service providers identified by the Association of Air Medical Services (AAMS), 362 domestic and 23 international.[1] Most of these programs are run by hospitals or groups of hospitals. Helicopters are expensive, ranging from $750,000 to $5 million. Because of the high cost of purchase, maintenance, and pilot training, most programs lease their helicopters from aircraft vendors. In this arrangement, the air medical program provides the medical personnel (paramedics, nurses, physicians, and dispatchers) and medical supplies, while the aircraft vendor supplies the helicopters, pilots, and maintenance personnel. The annual cost of operating a rotor-wing service typically exceeds $2 million.

For safety reasons, air medical services have increasingly moved toward using two-engine helicopters with instrument flight rating (IFR), rather than single-engine helicopters with visual flight rating (VFR).[2] Twin-engine helicopters have greater lifting capacity, range, and speed. They are also safer if one engine fails in flight; the helicopter can make a more controlled landing on the remaining engine. Under similar conditions, a single-engine helicopter must make an autorotation landing with a dead engine. A VFR aircraft can only fly with good visibility, whereas an IFR craft can fly under conditions of poorer visibility. Both VFR and IFR helicopters have strict visibility limitations imposed by the Federal Aviation Administration (FAA), but the IFR helicopter has fewer restrictions. If the pilot unexpectedly encounters bad weather during a flight, an IFR helicopter has a better chance of successfully (and safely) completing the mission than does a VFR helicopter.[3] In areas with frequent bad weather periods, some programs have elected to use two-pilot IFR.[2] The addition of more sophisticated equipment, a second pilot, and a second engine increases both initial and ongoing costs for a helicopter air medical program.

As technology becomes increasingly available to civilian aviation, air medical services often incorporate the newer avionics. A survey from 115 domestic air medical services found that 78 percent of services were using the gobal positioning system (GPS) in 1997.[2]

A survey of 126 United States air medical programs found that the mean number of patients transported in 1997 was 827 per program; this figure has been generally stable since 1992.[1] Programs that responded to this survey were generally the larger programs. Total estimates of annual air medical transports are in the range of 150,000 to 300,000 patients.

Crew Configuration and Training

The medical crew on a rotor-wing craft can be configured in multiple ways: nurse-paramedic, nurse-nurse, nurse-physician, or nurse-respiratory therapist. The literature suggests that the addition of a physician to the crew does not add a significantly higher level of care to that already rendered by a flight nurse or flight medic, although there is a minority view that on-board physicians do improve patient care.[4,5] The most frequently used crew is nurse-paramedic because of their complementary skills. Since rotor-wing missions vary on the spectrum between scene flights and interfacility transports, a broad skill basis is essential in the medical crew. A comprehensive curriculum guide developed by a number of national air medical organizations under contract from the U.S. Department of Transportation is available to use for training medical flight crews.[6] This curriculum covers all aspects of air medical care and is intended for use by paramedics, nurses, and physicians.

The medical flight crew needs to know how the environment on board an aircraft will affect the patient's illness and how to transport the patient safely in the relatively hostile environment of that aircraft.[7] Since helicopters generally transport patients at about 1000 to 3500 ft, low barometric pressure with barotrauma is usually not a factor; but it could become a consideration if transportation were to occur over mountains. The noise, close quarters, vibration, and temperature changes of the cabin of a rotor-wing craft can have a marked effect on the patient's condition. Likewise, these factors make assessment of the patient more difficult. For example, measurement of blood pressure or ausculation of the lungs with a stethoscope is generally impossible during flight due to the noise and vibration.

Clinical Use of Helicopters

Helicopters are fast ambulances, cruising at 125 to 175 mph, depending on the aircraft. They are not limited by traffic or road quality. The usual flight range for a helicopter is 150 to 200 mi. Helicopters bring sophisticated medical care to areas that otherwise might have only basic life support (BLS) ground ambulance service. The air medical

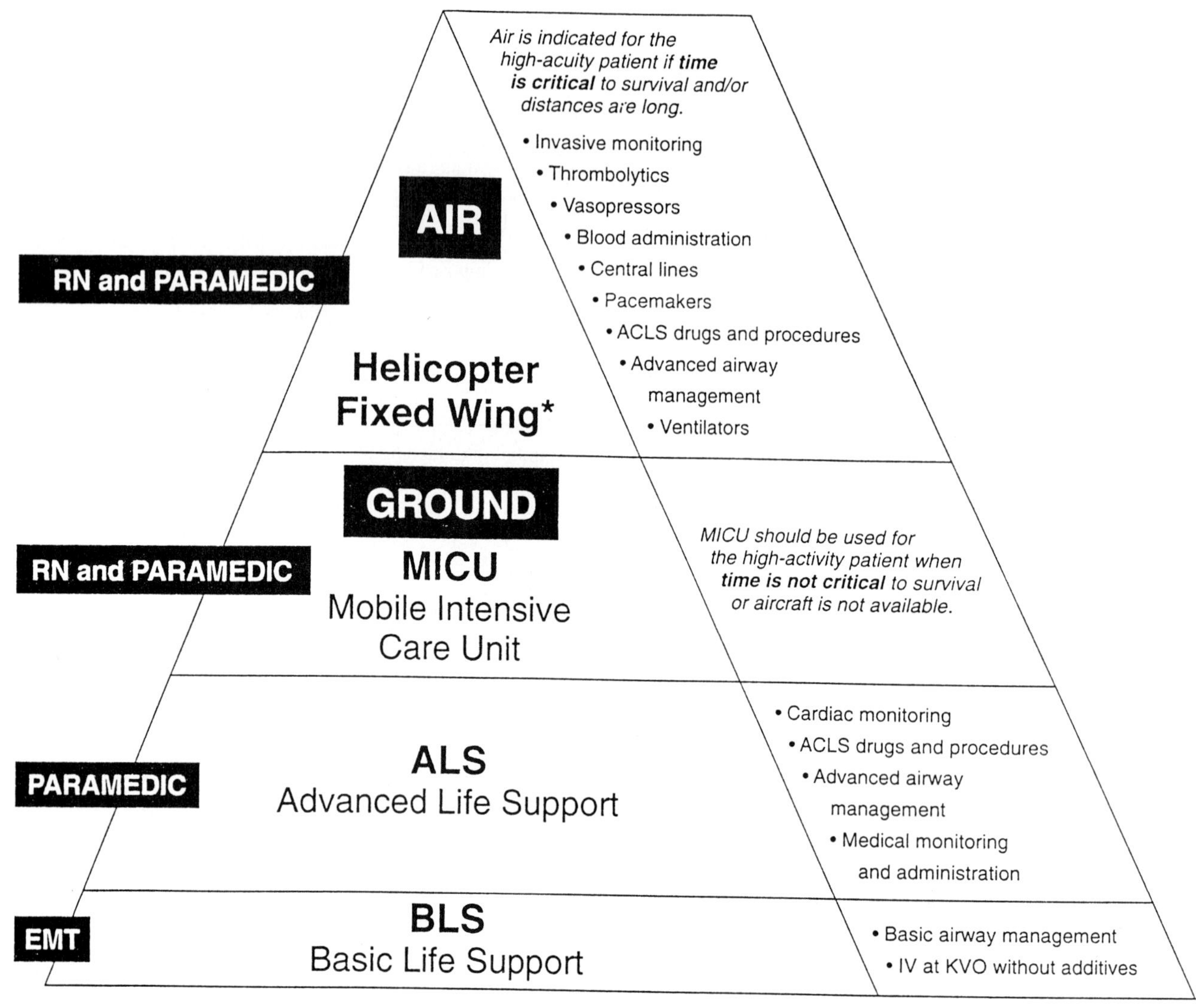

FIG. 3-1. The patient transport guidelines pyramid. (From North Flight EMS: *J Emerg Med Serv,* 18:50, 1993. Used by permission.)

crews bring tertiary critical care and transfer patients back to the tertiary center at two to three times the speed of a ground ambulance. The two major types of helicopter missions are trauma/medical scene responses and interfacility transfers. Mission patterns vary widely among flight programs, with the national average in 1997 for scene and interfacility flights being 30 and 70 percent, respectively.[1]

Scene Helicopter Response

There is evidence that helicopter scene response for victims of trauma decreases morbidity and mortality rates for critically ill and injured patients.[8–12] In spite of this, there is still a concern that air medical services are inappropriately overutilized for trauma scene responses. The appropriate use of helicopters at trauma scenes involves a complex interplay of factors: How far away is the scene from the helicopter base? What resources are already responding to the patient or patients? What is the distance from the scene to the local hospital or the trauma center? How many victims are there, and what is the severity of their injuries? Is there a significant amount of extrication needed before a patient can be moved to definitive care?

National guidelines (Table 3-1) have been developed to assist in making decisions for trauma scene responses.[13] Clinical information such as mechanism of injury, severity of injury, vital signs, and level of consciousness are one part of the equation. Emergency medical technicians on the scene are very accurate at defining which patients are critical and need air medical transport to the trauma center.[14]

There are also logistical and operational factors to be considered. If the patient is not accessible because of location (e.g., off-road or wilderness), traffic, road conditions, or weather, a helicopter dispatch may be appropriate. However, helicopters are much more weather-sensitive than ground ambulances; if the weather is bad for ambulances, it is probably worse for helicopters.

Time and distance play key roles in electing to send a helicopter. A severe trauma or medical situation in an urban area close to a trauma center does not have the implications for the patient that the same situation would in a rural area 100 mi from a major medical center. If the time for transport to the trauma center is greater than 15 min by ground ambulance, if the transport time to the local hospital by ground is greater than the time required for the helicopter to reach the trauma center, or if patient extrication will take longer than 20 min, then dispatch of the helicopter should be considered. In general, scene responses occur within 25 mi of the helicopter base, although this varies with local conditions and protocols. It is likely that at distances greater than 25 mi the patient will be transported to the local hospital first for stabilization and then a helicopter will transfer the patient to the trauma center. Sometimes, if the patient is extricated faster than initially thought, the ground EMS personnel communicate to the helicopter to divert to the local hospital rather than go to the scene.

There is one group of trauma patients for whom air medical scene response has a very low rate of resuscitation and essentially zero survival: traumatic cardiac arrest.[15] Some services have developed protocols that patients in traumatic cardiac arrest are not flown back to the trauma center, but instead the air medical crew assists the ground EMS service and transports the patient to the local hospital.

TABLE 3-1 Air Medical Dispatch: Guidelines for Trauma Scene Response

I. Clinical situations
  A. General
    1. Trauma victims need to be delivered as soon as possible to a regional trauma center.
    2. Stable patients who are accessible to ground vehicles probably are best transported by ground.
  B. Specific patients with critical injuries resulting in unstable vital signs require the fastest, most direct route of transport to a regional trauma center in a vehicle staffed with a team capable of offering critical care en route. Often this is the case in the following situations:
    1. Trauma score <12
    2. Glasgow coma score <10
    3. Penetrating trauma to the abdomen, pelvis, chest, neck, or head
    4. Spinal cord or spinal column injury, or any injury producing paralysis of any extremity if any lateralizing signs
    5. Partial or total amputation of an extremity (excluding digits)
    6. Two or more long-bone fractures or a major pelvic fracture
    7. Crushing injuries to the abdomen, chest, or head
    8. Major burns of the body surface area, or burns involving the face, hands, feet, or perineum, or burns with significant respiratory involvement, or major electrical or chemical burns
    9. Patients involved in a serious traumatic event who are <12 or >55 years of age
    10. Patients with near-drowning injuries, with or without existing hypothermia
    11. Adult patients with any of the following vital sign abnormalities:
      a. Systolic blood pressure <90 mmHg
      b. Respiratory rate <10 or >35 per min
      c. Heart rate <60 or >120 per min
      d. Unresponsive to verbal stimuli

II. Operational situations in which helicopter use should be considered
  A. Mechanism of injury
    1. Vehicle roll-over with unbelted passengers
    2. Vehicle striking pedestrian at >10 mph
    3. Falls from >15 ft
    4. Motorcycle victim ejected at >20 mph
    5. Multiple victims
  B. Difficult access situations
    1. Wilderness rescue
    2. Ambulance egress or access impeded at the scene by road conditions, weather, or traffic
  C. Time/distance factors
    1. Transportation time to the trauma center >15 min by ground ambulance
    2. Transport time to the local hospital by ground greater than transport time to trauma center by helicopter
    3. Patient extrication time >20 min
    4. Utilization of local ground ambulance leaves local community without ground ambulance coverage.

Source: From National Association of EMS Physicians.[13] Used by permission.

Scene responses for patients with medical conditions (as opposed to traumatic conditions) vary from program to program.[16,17] Especially in rural areas, it is common for helicopters to intercept BLS ambulances that are transporting deteriorating or unstable patients. Basic life support technicians may call for a helicopter if the patient could be transported faster to the tertiary center by air than the ground ambulance could get the patient to the local hospital. Medical scene responses have not received as much attention in the literature as have trauma scene responses, although criteria for medical scene responses have been developed.[18] The small number of medical scene responses reported in the literature makes it difficult to judge the utility of this mode of response and transport. However, if a patient is in cardiac arrest and the ground ambulance crew has a defibrillator and has secured the airway, it is unlikely that the arrival of the helicopter crew will result in any more successful resuscitation.[19] Such intercept situations must be dealt with on a local or regional level by guidelines and protocols, and they reinforce the importance of an integrated EMS system in which air and ground units work smoothly together under medical direction.

One important factor to be considered in initiating helicopter transport of a patient is whether ground transport of the patient by the local ambulance will deprive that community of vital EMS services. If the local ambulance is out of service for 5 to 6 h and emergency ambulance coverage in that area is compromised, then use of the helicopter should be strongly considered.

Another other important use for helicopters is in disaster situations. Rotor-wing craft can not only bring in sophisticated triage and treatment personnel for better medical care at the scene, but they can also give the incident commander a bird's-eye view of the events, which can assist in best distributing the available resources. These functions can be served in addition to the usual role of the helicopter in evacuating the most seriously ill and injured to the trauma center.

Interfacility Helicopter Transports

The majority of air medical transports are interfacility. It is surprising to note that there have been few studies on the benefit of interfacility air medical transports. A recent study from Norway on 370 interfacility helicopter transfers found that positive benefit could be judged in only 11 percent of patients, and almost all of the total additional life-years gained from such transport was confined to only 9 patients.[20] Benefits were most often seen in neonates, children with infection, and adults with cardiovascular disease. While some adults with trauma benefited from the interfacility helicopter transfer, the total additional life-years gained was very small. Published studies in the United States have usually focused on acute myocardial infarction and unstable angina.[21,22] These studies have not found a positive benefit of interfacility helicopter transfer over ground ambulance.

The Federal Emergency Medical Treatment and Active Labor Act (EMTALA), originally passed in 1985 as part of the Consolidated Omnibus Budget Reconciliation Act (COBRA) and strengthened through amendment in 1989, directed the Health Care Financing Administration (HCFA) to develop regulations concerning the examination, treatment, and transfer of individuals with emergency medical conditions. The final interim rule issued by the HCFA in 1994 contains a prohibition against the transferring physician's having a patient transported to a medical facility with a lesser or inadequate level of care en route. Thus, if the patient is unstable or requires intensive care during transport, then it is not appropriate to use a BLS ambulance. The position paper from the Air Medical Committee of the National Association of EMS Physicians states: "Reducing out-of-hospital time for these patients seems to be in their best interest. Ground-based out-of-hospital care providers, faced with a patient whose needs obviously exceed their abilities, may wish to access a rotor-wing air medical transport service, especially if they are distant from an appropriate medical facility."[18] This position is strengthened by the literature, which suggests that a tertiary center can extend its care out to several hundred miles via rotor- or fixed-wing aircraft with no change in mortality compared with patients transported locally to the same trauma center.[23] However, air medical services may violate certain EMTALA sections by transporting "unstable" patients (as defined by the regulations) and bypassing closer "appropriate" hospitals in order to return to their base hospital.[24] The issue is complex, the regulations are vague, and case law is limited to date.

In this regard, then, air medical care and transport protocols should operate to ensure that the patient is transported with the highest appropriate level of service and to the closest appropriate hospital.

Safety

Flight programs are exceedingly safety conscious. While it is true that EMS helicopters have a crash rate exceeding that of non-EMS helicopters, it is probably true that, per patient-mile, EMS helicopters are safer than ground ambulances.[3,25] Air medical programs must follow FAA rules. The industry itself has set forth additional stringent standards under the auspices of the AAMS and, more recently, the Commission on Accreditation of Air Medical Services (CAAMS).[26] On request, CAAMS performs site visits of air medical programs to certify that they comply with strict safety and operational standards.

On a mission, safety is the chief responsibility of the pilot. Because weather and collisions against ground obstacles are the leading hazards, in most programs, the pilot is not told the nature of the mission until a weather check is done and it is decided that the flight can be made safely. The pilot does not then feel pressured into flying a mission under borderline weather conditions because of the patient's condition. For helicopters, visibility, wind, and icing conditions are major limiting conditions.

The use of fire-resistant flight clothing, helmets, and emergency absorbing seats are felt to be effective in reducing preventable injuries to the medical crew in survivable crashes.[27]

Safety training must involve everybody in contact with the aircraft, including the communicators and dispatchers, aircraft mechanics, and especially on-scene EMS personnel. The latter must be taught to function around the helicopter at the scene.

Scene flights are inherently more dangerous than landing at a regular hospital landing zone. The unfamiliar landing area at a scene has more obstacles, such as wires and trees. More material may be scattered on the ground and blown around by the rotor wash from the helicopter. Scenes to which EMS has been called tend to be uncontrolled, with more bystanders who have the potential of walking into a tail or main rotor. A small helicopter needs a minimum of 60 ft by 60 ft for a landing zone, and a medium-sized or larger aircraft requires at least 100 ft by 100 ft. A landing zone of this size may be difficult to secure on a rural highway or at other accident scenes.

Several points are important for scene helicopter safety. First, the craft should always be approached from the front, where the pilot can see approaching personnel and can then acknowledge their presence and motion them into the helicopter. In general, a flight team member will guide ground personnel into the aircraft. Second, a rotor-wing aircraft should never be approached from the rear, since the tail rotor is going very fast and is virtually invisible. The tail rotor is the most dangerous area of a helicopter. Third, landings and takeoffs are the most likely times for adverse incidents to occur. Ground personnel need to stand well away as the helicopter lifts off.

Cost and Reimbursement

Helicopter transport is more expensive than ground transport, with an average helicopter transport charge in 1997 of $3882 for a medium-sized twin-engine helicopter and a 50-mi one-way patient transport.[1] The fees charged by almost all programs include a base fee for liftoff plus a fee for loaded (one-way) mileage.[1] Some programs charge for professional services and drugs or medical supplies used in flight.

Reimbursement issues are complex and vary between government (Medicare and Medicaid), private insurance, and managed care health insurance plans. One program found that, with an average flight charge of $2298 in 1991 through 1992, mean reimbursement was $991, or 43 percent of charges.[28] Reimbursement rates varied from nearly zero for Medicaid to 90 percent for commercial insurance.

The cost-versus-benefit analysis of air medical transport is not easy. It is not easy to predict how a patient might deteriorate if sent by ground rather than by air. It is not enough to ask the simple question: "Would the patient have died if not transported by helicopter?" Other medical factors, such as the number of days in intensive care, duration of rehabilitation, and quality of future life may be positively affected by air medical transport. Models have been developed to analyze the cost-effectiveness of using a helicopter to provide advanced life support (ALS) to local BLS ambulance services instead of placing additional ground ALS vehicles. A recent analysis found that a single helicopter could provide ALS backup over a 50 km radius replacing six ground ALS units at less annual operating cost.[29]

In summary, the determinants of helicopter usage must be medical and driven by national standards, as described above. Currently, there is inherent conflict between the requirements of EMTALA/COBRA for adequate transport and the frequent unwillingness of other federal programs (Medicare) and third parties to pay for the service rendered.

FIXED-WING AIR MEDICAL TRANSPORT

Fixed-wing aircraft can serve a wide variety of missions, from urgent to routine, over great distances. Since airplanes land only at airports, they cannot make scene flights, and they need ground ambulance connections at both ends of the flight to transport the patient between the hospital and airport. Because of this need, fixed-wing flights generally take longer to arrange and are not used for truly emergent patients.

In the United States, more fixed-wing than rotor-wing aircraft are used for air medical transport. Rotor craft are usually dedicated as air medical transport units, while planes are often multifunctional, used for charter flights or business. Unfortunately, this may sometimes lead to inadequate equipping and staffing of airplanes when used for air medical work. Medical fixed-wing craft need to have an adequate cargo-type door to allow access to a patient on a stretcher. Removeable medical equipment modules have been developed for airplanes to ensure the presence of adequate medical equipment when required.

Fixed-wing transports are less expensive per mile and usually more practical than helicopters at distances over 150 mi. On average, helicopter transport costs about three to four times more than fixed-wing transport per patient-loaded mile.[1] This estimate is rough because of the large number of variables involved in determining charges: distance, aircraft type and speed, crew configuration, and the nature of the patient's condition.

Airplanes vary in size and speed. Jet aircraft typically cruise at 400 to 500 mph, turboprop airplanes at 200 to 300 mph, and piston-driven airplanes at 120 to 150 mph. The appropriate aircraft to use for any one mission depends on many factors: distance, the nature of the airport at the patient's pick-up point, the condition of the patient, the amount of equipment, and the crew required in transport. The more critically ill the patient, the more equipment and crew may be needed and the larger the aircraft required. The choice of aircraft must also take into account the comfort of the crew and the patient for a trip of that distance. The cabins of fixed-wing aircraft are more spacious than those of rotor-wing craft. A larger plane that is able to be pressurized can fly above 10,000 ft, which means the plane can go faster, farther, and more comfortably.

Since airplanes can fly above bad weather and are less susceptible to icing conditions, fixed-wing craft can often fly when helicopters cannot. Fixed-wing planes can also fly under more difficult visibility circumstances than rotor craft because of on-board instrumentation and ground control from an airport.

All fixed-wing services must comply with FAA rules for airplanes. Standards have been developed for air medical fixed-wing aircraft by the Association of Air Medical Services and CAAMS, just as they have been developed for helicopters.[26] These standards deal with aircraft configuration, medical equipment requirements, medical crew configuration and training, and medical director qualifications.

MEDICAL DIRECTION OF AIR MEDICAL SERVICES

Medical direction may be even more important with rotor- and fixed-wing services than with ground services; it is certainly more complicated. Guidelines for the medical director of air medical transport programs has been developed by the National Association of EMS Physicians.[30] The medical director should be familiar with the physiology and stress of flight on the patient. A flight crew requires more initial training and more ongoing education than do ground EMS personnel because patients transported by air are generally sicker and require more advanced interventions than those transported by ground. Because flight crews are often far from their base of operations and out of voice contact, they must act independently. Standing orders or protocols for complex procedures such as chest tube insertion or cricothyrotomy are needed. More intense review of transport records is needed for quality control.

REFERENCES

1. Rau W, Lathrop G: 1998 transport statistics and fees survey. *Air Med* 4:19, 1998.
2. Rau W: 1998 helicopter avionics and operations survey. *Air Med* 4:20, 1998.
3. Low RB, Dunne MJ, Blumen IJ, Tagney G: Factors associated with the safety of EMS helicopters. *Am J Emerg Med* 9:103, 1991.
4. Hamman BL, Cue JI, Miller FB, et al: Helicopter transport of trauma victims: Does a physician make a difference? *J Trauma* 31:490, 1991.
5. Baxt W, Moody PG: The impact of a physician as part of the areomedical prehospital team in patients with blunt trauma. *JAMA* 257:3246, 1987.
6. US Dept of Transportation: *Air-Medical Crew National Standard Curriculum, Advanced Student Manual.* Washington, DC, 1988.
7. Blumen IJ, Rinnert KJ: Altitude physiology and the stresses of flight. *Air Med J* 14:87, 1995.
8. Baxt WG, Moody P, Cleveland HC, et al: Hospital-based rotorcraft aeromedical emergency care service and trauma mortality: A multicenter study. *Ann Emerg Med* 14:859, 1985.
9. Moylan JA, Fitzpatrick KT, Beyer AJ, Georgiade GS: Factors improving survival in multisystem trauma patients. *Ann Surg* 207:670, 1988.
10. Boyd CR, Corse KM, Campbell RC: Emergency interhospital transport of the major trauma patient: Air versus ground. *J Trauma* 29:789, 1989.
11. Moront ML, Gotschall CS, Eichelberger MR: Helicopter transport of injured children: System effectiveness and triage criteria. *J Pediatr Surg* 31:1183, 1996.
12. Nicholl JP, Brazier JE, Snooks HA: Effects of London helicopter emergency medical service on survival after trauma. *Br Med J* 311:217, 1995.
13. National Association of EMS Physicians: Air medical dispatch: Guidelines for scene response. *Prehosp Disas Med* 7:75, 1992.
14. Emerman CL, Shade B, Kubincanek J: A comparison of EMT judgement and prehospital trauma triage instruments. *J Trauma* 31:1369, 1991.
15. Wright SW, Dronen SC, Combs TJ, Storer D: Aeromedical transport of patients with post-traumatic cardiac arrest. *Ann Emerg Med* 18:721, 1989.
16. Savitsky E, Rodenberg H: Demographics of prehospital helicopter EMS responses in rural Florida. *Prehosp Disas Med* 7:279, 1992.
17. Jones JB, Leicht M, Dula DJ: A 10-year experience in the use of air medical transport for medical scene calls. *Air Med J* 17:7, 1998.
18. National Association of EMS Physicians: Criteria for prehospital air medical transport: Non-trauma and pediatric considerations. *Prehosp Disas Med* 9:140, 1994.
19. Lindbeck GH, Groopman DS, Powers RD: Aeromedical evacuation of rural victims of nontraumatic cardiac arrest. *Ann Emerg Med* 22:1258, 1993.
20. Hotvedt R, Kristiansen IS, Forde OH, et al: Which group of patients benefit from helicopter evacuation? *Lancet* 347:1362, 1996.
21. Schneider S, Borok Z, Heller M, et al: Critical cardiac transport: Air versus ground? *Am J Emerg Med* 6:449, 1988.
22. Stone CK, Hunt RC, Sossa JA, et al: Interhospital transport of cardiac patients: Does air transport make a difference? *J Air Med Trans* 11:54, 1992.
23. Valenzuela TD, Criss EA, Copass MK, et al: Critical care air transportation of the severely injured: Does long distance transport adversely affect survival? *Ann Emerg Med* 19:169, 1990.
24. McCleary N: Air medical transfers: Are you COBRA compliant? *Air Med J* 16:113, 1997.
25. Boyd CR, Hungerpiller JC: Patient risk in prehospital transport: Air versus ground. *Emerg Care Q* 5:48, 1990.
26. Association of Air Medical Services: *Standards and Safety Guidelines.* Pasadena, CA, AAMS, 1992.
27. Dodd RS: The cost-effectiveness of air medical helicopter crash survival enhancements: An evaluation of the costs, benefits and effectiveness of injury prevention interventions. *Air Med J* 13:281, 1994.
28. Lindbeck G: Hospital and flight program reimbursement for patients transferred by helicopter. *Am J Emerg Med* 13:405, 1995.
29. Lechleuthner A, Koestler W, Voigt M, Laufenberg P: Helicopters as part of a regional EMS system: Cost-effectiveness analysis for three EMS regions in Germany. *Eur J Emerg Med* 1:159, 1994.
30. National Association of EMS Physicians: Medical director for air medical transport programs. *Prehosp Disas Med* 10:283, 1995.

NEONATAL AND PEDIATRIC TRANSPORT

Carl L. Bose
Phillip V. Gordon

Regionalized intensive care is a concept that has gained wide acceptance in many fields of medicine, including neonatology, pediatric intensive care, and emergency medicine. This concept mandates that expensive, high-technology, labor-intensive therapies be limited to a few regional centers. Because patients in need of these services may initially present to other hospitals, interfacility transport has developed as a complement to regionalized intensive care.[1]

Either the referring hospital or the regional center may assume the responsibility for the transport of a patient to a regional center. Because regional neonatal and pediatric intensive care centers often provide transport services and because community emergency medical services (EMS) systems are often not equipped to transport critically ill children, the interfacility transport of pediatric patients is often conducted by regional centers. Under these circumstances, the referring hospital still has important responsibilities related to transport. Emergency department personnel must often assume these responsibilities because the emergency department is the site of initial care. This chapter focuses on the stabilization and preparation of critically ill children for transport. Since some emergency departments are also responsible for operating transport services, a brief discussion of the organization and administration of a pediatric transport program is also included.

THE TRANSPORT ENVIRONMENT

Moving critically ill patients between hospitals or even within a hospital invariably adds to the risks of the illness or injury because of the hazards associated with the transport environment. Patient care can be influenced dramatically by the unique features of this environment and is particularly affected during the transport of neonatal and pediatric patients.[2] For this reason, an understanding of the transport environment is essential for individuals who participate in the preparation or transport of children.

Features

The features of the transport environment that may distinguish this environment from the inpatient setting and the effects of these features on patients and caretakers include the following:

1. *Excessive noise.* The acute effects of excessive noise on older pediatric and adult patients are probably minimal. By contrast, persistent sound in excess of 80 dB appears to dramatically increase the frequency of arterial oxygen desaturation in premature infants. In addition, excessive noise makes it virtually impossible to use the sense of hearing to evaluate patients during transport.
2. *Vibration.* The effects of vibration on patients are uncertain but are probably not of great significance. However, vibration may limit the reliability of transport equipment. Monitor artifact must be recognized, and alternative techniques for monitoring should be employed as needed.
3. *Inadequate lighting.* Inadequate lighting is rarely a problem during the transport of adult patients because EMS vehicles generally have lighting designed for adult patients on stretchers. However, task lighting for illuminating small areas and small patients is usually not available.
4. *Variable ambient temperature.* Although the range of ambient temperature encountered during transport rarely influences the body temperature of adult patients, environmental conditions can have a dramatic influence on the body temperature of neonates and small children.
5. *Changes in barometric pressure.* Changes in barometric pressure during ascent in nonpressurized aircraft cause expansion of gases in closed spaces (e.g., with endotracheal tube cuffs or pulmonary interstitial emphysema) and a fall in the partial pressure of oxygen. These changes are rarely of sufficient magnitude to influence physiologic characteristics unless the change in altitude is greater than approximately 1500 m.
6. *Confined space.* The confined space in transport vehicles is an obvious handicap because it limits the number of caretakers and the amount of support equipment.
7. *Limited support services and personnel.* Similarly, the extent and precision of care is limited during transport by the lack of support services (e.g., radiographic and laboratory services) and specialty personnel.
8. *Equipment failure.* Equipment failure during transport is common and is particularly problematic because replacement equipment is less likely to be available in the vehicle than in an inpatient setting. The most common problem is the unexpected exhaustion of an oxygen tank.
9. *Motion-induced illness.* Many medical personnel develop motion-induced illnesses during transport. Symptoms are often categorized into one of two syndromes: the sopite syndrome, which is characterized by drowsiness and inability to concentrate, and the nausea syndrome. Either syndrome may impair the ability of personnel to provide skilled care.

Precautions

Plans to minimize the impact of the handicaps inherent in a transport environment are essential. Suggested guidelines include the following:

1. *Stabilize the patient carefully prior to transport.* Unless the immediate needs of the patient can only be met in the receiving hospital (e.g., severe trauma), ample time should be devoted to stabilizing the patient in the referring hospital.
2. *Anticipate deterioration.* Preparation of the patient should include not only care for the identified problems but also anticipation of problems that may arise during transport.
3. *Monitor as many physiologic parameters as possible electronically.* Because physical examination is nearly impossible during transport and because pediatric patients are often transported during dynamic changes in their physiologic condition, electronic monitoring is essential.
4. *Prepare the transport vehicle.* If repeated transport of pediatric patients is anticipated, one or more vehicles should be prepared to meet the special needs of these patients (e.g., accessory lighting and a more precisely controlled thermal environment).

PREPARATION OF A PATIENT FOR TRANSPORT

Decision to Transport

The decision to transport should be based on a patient's needs at the time of presentation and anticipated needs during the evolution or treatment of the disease or injury. If the patient's needs will exceed the resources of the hospital at any time, then the patient should be transported as soon as possible.

Basic Preparation

When a critically ill child arrives in the emergency department and the decision is made to transport that child to another institution, extensive preparation of the child should occur. This preparation should be completed by the referring hospital personnel to the limits of their abilities and resources, regardless of whether they or a receiving hospital will perform the transport. Two aspects of care to which referring hospitals should direct immediate attention are airway management and vascular access.

AIRWAY MANAGEMENT The decision to intubate and mechanically ventilate a patient is usually based on objective evidence of respiratory failure. This principle applies to both inpatients and those being prepared for transport. However, the threshold for intervention should be lowered for most patients requiring transport. For example, an infant with an arterial partial pressure of carbon dioxide ($Paco_2$) of 50 mmHg might be observed without ventilatory support in the inpatient setting but probably should be intubated and ventilated in preparation for transport. In addition, children without respiratory failure but in whom deterioration is anticipated should be intubated in preparation for transport. This more aggressive approach to airway management is justified because the ability to identify respiratory failure and to intubate is often impaired during transport.[3]

All emergency departments should be supplied with equipment to intubate and ventilate patients of all sizes (Table 4-1). All nonneonatal patients should be medicated prior to intubation unless they are unconscious or in extreme distress. Neonatal patients should be premedicated only if they are alert and vigorous. An opiate analgesic (morphine or fentanyl) should be administered intravenously to patients less than approximately 3 months of age. Older children should be intubated following rapid-sequence anesthesia and paralysis.

Neonatal intubation may be challenging for personnel not experienced in airway management in this population.[4] Attention to the following problems may increase the likelihood of success:

1. A common mistake made during neonatal intubation is to insert the blade into the esophagus and then fail to withdraw it far enough to visualize the glottis.
2. The glottis is in a more ventral position in infants than in older children; therefore, it is more difficult to visualize. This problem can be minimized by avoiding overextension of the neck and by applying gentle pressure to the cricoid. Too much pressure should be avoided because it can occlude the airway and prevent intubation.
3. Premature infants have very small mouths and upper airways, making insertion of the endotracheal tube difficult. Gentle traction on the infant's right cheek by an assistant can usually provide sufficient

TABLE 4-1 Intubation Guide for Pediatric Patients

Age, Weight	Laryngoscope Blade	Tube Size, mm*	Insertion Distance, cm†
<1 kg	Straight 0	2.5	6.0–7.0
<1 kg	Straight 0	2.5	6.0–7.0
1–2 kg	Straight 0	3.0	7.0–8.0
2–3 kg	Straight 0 or 1	3.0–3.5	8.0–9.0
2–3 kg	Straight 0 or 1	3.0–3.5	8.0–9.0
3–4 kg	Straight 1	3.5–4.0	9.0–9.5
0.5–3 years	Straight 1	4.0–4.5	‡
3–5 years	Straight or curved 2	4.5–5.5	‡
5–8 years	Straight or curved 2	5.5–6.5	‡
>8 years	Straight or curved 2 or 3	6.5–7.5	‡

*Cuffed endotracheal tubes should not be used in children <7 years of age.
†Insertion distance is the distance from the tip of the tube to the lip.
‡See Chap. 11 for more details.

opening to allow insertion of the endotracheal tube just to the right of the blade. This maneuver also helps preserve the intubator's field of view.

4. Because the skin of newborns is usually moist, extra care must be taken during taping of the endotracheal tube.

Because the distance between the thoracic inlet and the carina is extremely short in small children, the position of the tip of the endotracheal tube should be confirmed with a chest radiograph as soon after insertion as possible. A radiograph should be obtained even when reassuring signs of a successful intubation are present (condensation on the wall of the tube, symmetrical chest rise and breath sounds, and positive CO_2 detection). Right main-stem intubation is common in neonates. Prolonged right main-stem intubation increases the likelihood of pneumothorax and is particularly hazardous in premature infants. Soon after the initiation of mechanical ventilation, arterial blood gas analysis should be performed to ensure appropriate ventilator settings. Overventilation is a common error that may have serious consequences.

VASCULAR ACCESS All patients should have intravascular access during transport. Critically ill children should have at least two lines in case one becomes dislodged or several drugs must be administered simultaneously. Access should be through a device that includes a nonmetallic intravascular component. The metal butterfly needles often used in pediatric inpatient units are not satisfactory during transport because they frequently perforate the vessel as a result of vibration and movement. Intraosseous cannulation is an alternative technique for fluid and drug administration when intravascular lines cannot be placed and the severity of illness demands immediate access.

In small children, intravenous lines should be infused with the use of pumps. Open "drips" should not be used, even with volumetric drip chambers, because of the risk of fluid intoxication from inadvertent administration of large boluses. The amount of fluid administered should be carefully monitored and recorded.

SPECIAL PROBLEMS OF THE NEONATE

The stabilization and transport of critically ill neonates is complicated by their dependence on extrinsic factors to maintain homeostasis. This is particularly true when birth occurs prior to term. In fact, the complexity of care is often inversely related to birth weight and gestational age. The following aspects of care deserve special consideration: thermal regulation, mechanical ventilation, glucose homeostasis, vascular access, risk of infection, and determining viability.

Thermal Regulation

Humans conserve body temperature by several mechanisms, including (1) shunting blood from the skin and periphery to the core, (2) increasing basal metabolic rate, (3) voluntary muscle activity, (4) shivering, and (5) nonshivering thermogenesis. With the exception of nonshivering thermogenesis, all of these mechanisms are less effective in the neonate. Although older children and adults can maintain normal core body temperature when subjected to a wide range of environmental conditions, neonates, particularly premature infants, are very limited in this regard. In addition, even under conditions in which a neonate can maintain normal body temperature, this is often accomplished at the expense of increased oxygen consumption and carbon dioxide production. These consequences are particularly onerous in infants with respiratory failure.

Neonates should be cared for in a neutral thermal environment in which core temperature remains normal and oxygen consumption is minimized. Such an environment is best provided by treating a neonate on or within a thermo-controlled bed specially designed for neonates. Thermo-controlled beds come in two varieties: an open platform heated with an overhead radiant heat source and a closed plastic incubator heated with a convection heater. Although not satisfactory for transport, open incubators with radiant heaters are ideal for the care of critically ill neonates in the emergency department because they permit access by several caretakers. An alternative is the use of a portable overhead heat lamp and a standard crib. These devices should be used with extreme caution because they do not usually include a servo-control mechanism. The patient's body temperature should be monitored frequently to avoid hyperthermia. The neutral thermal environment is presumed when the infant's body temperature is normal and there is a minimal gradient between the core and the skin temperature.

Humans lose body heat in four ways: (1) evaporation, (2) conduction, (3) convection, and (4) radiation. Neonates, especially preterm infants, are particularly susceptible to heat loss because they have a relatively large surface–to–body mass ratio when compared to older patients. Also, their skin is more permeable to water vapor, and they

TABLE 4-2 Initial Ventilator Settings for Neonates

Disease Severity	Mild	Moderate	Severe
PIP (cmH_2O)	18	24	28
PEEP (cmH_2O)	4	4	5
T_i, s	0.5	0.4	0.4
Rate, breaths/min	20	24	30

may have a paucity of subcutaneous tissue. In addition to providing a heat source, attempts to create a neutral thermal environment should include provisions to minimize heat loss:

1. Infants should be thoroughly dried to avoid evaporative heat loss. This is critical after an emergent delivery. Drying should not be delayed under any circumstances. If emergent procedures are necessary, such as intubation, another caretaker should simultaneously dry the infant.
2. Whenever possible, infants should be placed on a pre-warmed surface to avoid conductive heat loss. The temperature of these surfaces or auxiliary heat sources (e.g., hot water bottles) should not exceed 104°F (40°C) because of the risk of thermal injury.
3. When treating an infant in an open crib or platform warmer, the room temperature should be increased to avoid convective heat loss. The infant should be located away from drafts (e.g., heat and/or air conditioning vents).
4. An infant should be clothed to the extent that it does not interfere with patient care and should not be placed near cold surfaces (e.g., exterior windows) to avoid radiant heat loss. At a minimum, a hat should be placed on the infant's head.[5]

Mechanical Ventilation

Most neonates are ventilated with time-cycled, pressure-limited ventilators using intermittent mandatory ventilation. As with volume ventilation, the clinician must determine the fraction of inspired oxygen (Fio_2) and ventilator rate. In contrast to volume ventilation, the tidal volume is not set, and in fact is not known with most infant ventilators. The volume of each breath is determined by setting a peak inspiratory pressure (PIP), a positive end-expiratory pressure (PEEP), and an inspiratory time (T_i) with suggested initial ventilator settings for infants that vary according to the severity of lung disease (Table 4-2).

The adequacy of oxygenation and ventilation should be assessed immediately after initiation of ventilation by observing the degree of chest expansion and the change in the color of mucous membranes. Arterial blood is the most accurate source for blood gas analysis, but capillary or venous blood is acceptable for measurement of the partial pressure of carbon dioxide (Pco_2) and pH in the absence of access to arterial blood. Adequacy of oxygenation can be assessed using pulse oximetric measurements. The target ranges for oxygenation and ventilation of neonates are somewhat different than those for older patients (Table 4-3). The blending of oxygen and air to deliver the minimum Fio_2 required to achieve adequate oxygenation is highly desirable, particularly in premature infants, in whom hyperoxia may result in retinal damage.

Glucose Homeostasis

During fetal life, the placenta and the maternal circulation closely regulate metabolic homeostasis. In healthy full-term neonates, homeostasis is maintained by the infant's autoregulatory mechanisms. Unfortunately, these mechanisms often fail during acute illness or after preterm birth. The result is increasing dependence on caretakers for normal metabolic function.

The most common metabolic abnormality in newborns is hypoglycemia. At birth, blood glucose in the neonate is approximately 60 to 70 percent of the maternal level. Within 1 to 2 h, the level falls to approximately 40 mg/dL. This decline may be accentuated in premature infants, acutely ill infants of any gestational age, and certain other high-risk infants (e.g., infants of diabetic mothers).

Because of the risk of hypoglycemia, all neonates should receive glucose containing fluids in preparation for and during transport. Ten-percent dextrose infused at a rate of 80 mL/kg/d should be used in infants with birth weight greater than 1000 g. Five-percent dextrose should be used in smaller infants because they are likely to develop hyperglycemia with high glucose intake. In these infants, the infusion rate should be increased to approximately 100 mL/kg/d because of excessive insensible water loss. In all infants at risk for hypoglycemia, measurement of blood sugar should be repeated at frequent intervals, at least every 2 h.[6]

Vascular Access

Peripheral venous access in the neonate may be technically challenging and is usually performed successfully only by caretakers skilled in this technique. Femoral line placement is difficult in neonates and should rarely be considered. Intravascular lines placed through the umbilicus are a simple and desirable alternative for both arterial and venous access in infants less than 1 week of age. The most rapid way to obtain vascular access is to temporarily place an umbilical venous catheter (UVC) 2 to 3 cm below the level of the skin. A UVC located in this position can be used to administer fluid, medications, and pressors in emergency situations, but it is not a sufficiently stable form of access during transport. By contrast, UVCs with the tip located near the junction of the inferior vena cava and the right atrium are ideal for all infusions, both during stabilization and transport. The position of the tip of the catheter should be determined radiographically prior to use to ensure that medications are not being infused into the liver. An umbilical artery catheter is desirable when frequent blood gas analysis is anticipated or central blood pressure monitoring is crucial. However, umbilical artery catheters should not generally be used for the administration of pressors.

Risk of Infection

Signs and symptoms of infection in a neonate are often nonspecific and may be indistinguishable from those associated with other diseases. Therefore, infection should be presumed as a cause of illness in any sick neonate. Broad-spectrum antibiotics should be administered unless the signs and symptoms can be attributed with reasonable certainty to a cause other than infection. Antibiotics should also be administered to premature infants because uterine and placental infection is a common cause of preterm labor.

Antibiotics should be administered as soon as possible because early treatment decreases mortality and morbidity rates. It is preferable to collect a blood culture prior to the initiation of antibiotic therapy,

TABLE 4-3 Target Ranges for Oxygenation and Ventilation of Neonates

OXYGENATION		
Premature infant	Pao_2 50–70 mmHg	Sao_2 93–98%
Term infant	Pao_2 60–100 mmHg	Sao_2 96–100%
VENTILATION		
All infants	$Paco_2$ 35–50 mmHg	

Note: Pao_2 = partial pressure of arterial oxygen; Sao_2 = percent saturation of oxygen.

but therapy should not be withheld because of difficulties in collecting a blood culture.

Determining Viability

Delivery of premature infants who are at the limits of viability is not an uncommon occurrence in the emergency department. Under these circumstances, the first priority of the physician caring for the infant is to determine whether resuscitation is justified. An infant born at a gestational age of less than 24 weeks, weighing less than 500 g, who has gelatinous skin and fused eyes should not, except under unusual circumstances, be resuscitated. By contrast, infants born at greater than 24 weeks are likely to have a relatively good outcome and should be supported aggressively after birth. The decision to initiate support must be made immediately. If the decision is not clear, proceed with resuscitation.

Death of an infant judged to be nonviable might not occur rapidly even in the absence of respiratory support. After a decision has been made to withhold aggressive care, it is important that the staff remain supportive and available to the parents. If the parents desire, the child can be held in a quiet place with a physician checking periodically to determine the time of death. This period, around the time of death, may be emotionally difficult for the staff as well as the family. However, families often recall these irreplaceable moments with fondness. Futile efforts at resuscitation or interfacility transport should not be a substitute for compassionate support without medical intervention.

MONITORING DURING TRANSPORT

One of the critical aspects of care during transport is electronic monitoring. At a minimum, the following monitors should be considered:

1. *Heart rate and respiratory monitor.* All transported patients should be monitored with impedance electrocardiogram (ECG) and respiratory monitoring. The selection of a monitor should be based on its size, weight, battery life, and resistance to motion artifact. The monitor should include a screen with a graphic display of ECG and respiratory tracings. Ideally, the monitor should display pressure waveforms and digital readings of systolic, diastolic, and mean blood pressures from transduced intravascular catheters. It is not essential that the monitoring system include the capability of electrical cardioversion or pacing. The need for such a device in the care of pediatric patients is extremely rare. However, this capability should be available during the transport of patients with known arrhythmias or patients at risk for such problems (e.g., tricyclic poisoning).
2. *Pulse oximetry.* Continuous pulse oximetry is essential in patients with cardiorespiratory illness. Devices that display a plethysmographic waveform are ideal because they assist in identifying motion artifact.
3. *Body temperature monitor.* Continuous temperature monitoring is helpful in neonates and small infants because of their predisposition to hypothermia.
4. *Carbon dioxide monitor.* Continuous estimation of $Paco_2$ is helpful in patients with respiratory failure. Transcutaneous carbon dioxide monitors may be useful in young infants, but their value in transport is limited because of the need for frequent calibration using special calibration gases. In addition, they cannot be relied on to provide accurate absolute measurements. Rather, they are valuable only for identifying trends. Capnography, utilizing continuous in-line infrared analysis to measure end-tidal carbon dioxide, is becoming increasingly popular as an alternative to transcutaneous carbon dioxide monitoring. As yet, capnography has not been widely used during transport.
5. *Blood pressure monitor.* Noninvasive blood pressure monitoring is advisable in children without indwelling arterial catheters. The cuff should cycle frequently enough to provide meaningful information about changes in hemodynamics. Arterial pressure can be monitored directly in patients with indwelling arterial catheters. Direct monitoring is preferable because it is more accurate and provides an alarm system in the event that arterial pressure suddenly falls (e.g., if the line becomes disconnected and the neonate suddenly has unimpeded arterial hemorrhage). Noninvasive blood pressure monitoring may also be useful in patients with direct monitoring to differentiate abnormal findings from technical artifacts.
6. *Portable blood analyzer.* Small, battery-powered devices are now available for the performance of blood gas analysis and measurement of selected blood chemistries (e.g., electrolytes and blood glucose). These devices may be valuable for monitoring patients with dynamic diseases, particularly when the transit time between hospitals is long.

CONDUCT OF A TRANSPORT

The transport of a critically ill child from the emergency department in a community hospital to a regional center is rarely a scheduled event. Nevertheless, the transfer should proceed in an orderly fashion if protocols exist within the emergency department for referral of critically ill children. These protocols should provide information about each regional center to which a patient might be referred, including (1) special services available; (2) criteria for referral; (3) telephone numbers for consultation, referral, and transport; (4) distance and usual response time; (5) type of transport personnel and their capabilities; (6) type of transport vehicles; and (7) protocols for preparation of patients. It is also advisable to establish formal agreements with regional centers that outline the circumstances under which patients can be transported without prior administrative approval.

Once the decision has been made to transport a child, the referring hospital has certain obligations in addition to medical care.[7] The Consolidated Omnibus Budget Reconciliation Acts of 1985 and 1989 mandate some of these responsibilities. The referring physician must contact the receiving hospital and secure a receiving physician. The choice of receiving institution is critical because the referring physician is liable for the adequacy of that facility.

In preparation for transport, the referring hospital should assemble all available information pertinent to the current illness. This generally includes a copy of the emergency department record, laboratory data, radiographs, and old medical records if available. The referring physician should inform the parents of the need for transfer and discuss the mechanism by which the child will be transferred. Consent to transport should be obtained from a parent or other responsible individual.

Receiving physicians often make recommendations regarding stabilization of the patient. This information should be requested if necessary. However, referring physicians are not obligated to follow these recommendations if they are considered to be medically inappropriate or beyond the capabilities of the referring hospital. Under these circumstances, it is advisable for the referring and receiving physicians to develop an alternative plan.

A collaborative decision must also be made regarding who will assume the responsibility for transporting the patient. There are usually four options: private automobile, local ambulance service, local ambulance with personnel from the referring hospital, or service provided by the receiving hospital. The selection should be based on the appropriate balance between the needs of the patient and the resources of each type of provider. Cost should be a consideration only when more than one provider can satisfy the patient's needs.

For most critically ill pediatric patients, ideal care is provided when the emergency department of the referring hospital devotes its energy to providing emergent short-term care and the responsibility for transport is left to the regional center. This is particularly true for neonatal patients because of the special equipment and expertise required for transport. It is rarely in the best interest of critically ill children to "pick them up and run." When transport services are not provided by the regional center or when time is critical, it may be appropriate for the referring hospital to provide transport. In these circumstances, it is the referring hospital's responsibility to ensure the adequacy of care during transport. The converse is true if transport is conducted by the receiving hospital.

In many areas, physicians also have a choice between air and ground transportation. Again, this decision should be made collaboratively.[8] Air transport should be reserved for situations in which reduction of a critical period of time during transport is likely to reduce morbidity or mortality. In some emergencies, the critical period ends with the arrival of the receiving hospital's transport team because the team is able to administer a definitive intervention. Under these circumstances, the advantage of air compared to ground transport is directly related to the reduction in time between the referral and the arrival of the team at the referring hospital. Air transport may offer the greatest advantage when the definitive therapy is available only in the receiving hospital (e.g., a surgical procedure) because the patient benefits from the reduction in transit time for the round trip between the receiving and referring hospitals.

When the transport team arrives, the referring physician should be present to coordinate the transition of care. Under most circumstances, a transport team originating from a hospital other than the referring hospital does not receive a detailed history of the patient's illness prior to arrival. It is essential that the referring physician be available to provide this history and a brief review of recent events. In addition to the referring physician, one or two support personnel should also be available to aid the transport team with further stabilization.

TABLE 4-4 Training for Pediatric Critical Care Transport Team

CERTIFICATION
Basic life support (BLS) (provider class type C)
Pediatric advanced life support (PALS)
Neonatal resuscitation program (NRP)
DIDACTIC TRAINING
Respiratory failure
Airway obstruction
Respiratory therapies
Congestive heart failure
Shock
Sepsis and other infections
Status epilepticus
Near drowning
Drug overdose
Comatose child
Mutiple trauma
Pharmacotherapy
X-ray interpretation
Aviation physiology
Radio communications
Vehicle safety
TECHNICAL SKILLS TRAINING
Endotracheal intubation
Arterial puncture
Central line placement
Intraosseous needle placement
Thoracentesis
Thoracostomy tube placement

ORGANIZATION OF A PEDIATRIC TRANSPORT PROGRAM

The administration and staffing of a neonatal transport program is rarely the responsibility of emergency department personnel, and therefore is not discussed in this chapter. However, programs responsible for transporting older pediatric patients often originate in the emergency department. While a detailed discussion of the conduct of a pediatric transport program is beyond the scope of this book, this section outlines the principles of the organization of a transport program with emphasis on pediatric transport. The focus is on interhospital transport, although many of the principles also apply to prehospital and intrahospital transport.

Administration

Components of a transport program can be divided into two general categories: medical and nonmedical components.[9] The medical components include medical personnel, equipment, and supplies. The nonmedical components include transportation, communications, billing, and marketing. A physician with training and expertise in pediatric intensive care or pediatric emergency medicine should supervise the medical components of a pediatric transport program. While this individual assumes overall responsibility for the program, many management decisions may be shared with or delegated to a nurse manager or other professional. Because of the time constraints on medical professionals and their usual lack of administrative expertise, the responsibility for direction of the nonmedical components of the program is often best assumed by a member of the hospital administration.

Transport Team Personnel

A variety of personnel might serve as attendants during pediatric transport including physicians, nurses, nurse practitioners, respiratory therapists, physician assistants, and paramedic-emergency medical technicians.[10] Practical issues such as availability, salary costs, and the requirement for training most often govern the selection of a particular professional group. Although it would be desirable to have a physician with expertise in pediatric emergency medicine in attendance during each transport, this is rarely practical. Utilizing physicians in training is an alternative, but the competition between transport activities and other aspects of their training often makes this an unattractive alternative. An increasing number of programs now utilize specially trained nonphysician personnel exclusively.

Ideally, pediatric transport personnel would have responsibility for pediatric patients only. Unfortunately, few centers have the volume of pediatric transports or the resources to support a stand-alone team for pediatric patients. More often, the responsibility for transporting infants and small children falls to teams who also transport neonatal patients, while another team transports older children and adults. The latter model of care can result in competent patient care if special effort is devoted to preparing personnel to manage pediatric emergencies.

Training requirements for team members may vary and depend on their designated responsibilities during transport. For example, programs that utilize physicians may not need to train nonphysicians

TABLE 4-5 Content of Equipment Packs for Pediatric Critical Care Transport

PEDIATRIC NURSING PACK	
Procedure tray, sterile	Masks
IV catheters	Suction catheters
Lancets, sterile	Buretrol
Blood culture bottle	Disposable transducer
Blood collection tubes	Heimlich valves
IV limb boards	Thoracostomy tubes
Tape	Foley catheters
Dextrostix bottle	Blood component filter
Intraosseous needles	Scissors
Rubber bands	Hemostat
Safety pins	Tape measure
Tourniquets	Pacifier
Syringes	K-Y jelly
IV fluids	Butterfly needles
Transilluminator	Sterile gauze
Stethoscope	Stopcock
Sphygmomanometer (pediatric cuffs)	Extension IV tubing
Cotton balls	Thermometer, digital
Stockinette for caps	Alcohol and betadine swabs
Silver thermal cap and blanket	IV extension T connectors
Ear plugs	Needles
Sterile gloves	ECG leads or pads
Yankauer suction tube	Feeding tubes
Replogle tube	Bulb syringe

PEDIATRIC RESPIRATORY THERAPY PACK	
Airway Supplies	
Laerdal masks	Oral airways
Oxygen tubing	Pediatric MVB with PEEP valve
Non-rebreathing mask	Face tent
Nasal cannula	Blood gas syringes
Venturi mask	Laryngoscope
Aerosol mask	Endotracheal tubes
Pediatric tracheotomy collar	McGill forceps
Other Equipment	
Benzoin applicators	Normal saline vials
Tape	Blood gas syringes
Cable ties	Oxygen connectors
Septisol	O_2 flowmeter nipple
Chemical hot packs	Suction catheters
Stethoscope	Tape measure
Pulse oximeter sensors	

MEDICATION PACK	
Acyclovir	Gentamicin
Adenosine	Heparin
Albumin 25%	Heparin lock flush
Aminophylline	Hydralazine
Ampicillin	Isotonic saline vials
Atropine	Isoproterenol
Bretylium tosylate	Lacrilube
Calcium chloride	Lidocaine 1%
Calcium gluconate	Lidocaine 2%
Cefotaxime	Mannitol
Ceftriaxone	Naloxone
Clindamycin	Vecuronium
Dexamethasone	Pancuronium
Dextrose 50%	Potassium chloride
Digoxin	Phentolamine
Phenytoin/fosphenytoin	Flumazenil
Dobutamine	Sodium bicarbonate
Dopamine	Sodium chloride, concentrated
Epinephrine 1 : 1000	Methylprednisolone
Epinephrine: 1 : 10,000	Sterile water vials
Furosemide	Vitamin K
Controlled Substances	
Lorazepam	Phenobarbital
Chloral hydrate suppositories	Diazepam
Fentanyl	Midazolam
Morphine	

Note: MVB = manual ventilation bag.

in skills related to airway management. At least one member of the team attending every patient should include an individual who is experienced in diagnosing and managing virtually all life-threatening pediatric emergencies. It is helpful to cross-train if more than one discipline (e.g., respiratory therapy and nursing) is represented on the team. In addition, all team members should have a thorough understanding of the transport environment and should be familiar with all communication devices.

Many different training strategies have been utilized to prepare transport personnel. Common to most are didactic sessions during which cognitive knowledge is attained, laboratory sessions during which technical skills are taught, and supervised patient care (Table 4-4). This training is generally followed by participation in transport accompanied by an experienced team member.

Vehicles

Three types of vehicles are used during interhospital transport: ground ambulances, helicopters, and fixed-wing aircraft. The choice of a vehicle for a program is often dictated by the features of the anticipated population and the relative advantages and disadvantages of each mode of transportation.

AMBULANCES Ground ambulances are available at most medical centers but may require modification for optimal transport of pediatric patients. Their disadvantage is excessive travel time between hospitals when distances are great or when terrain, road conditions, or traffic congestion require slow travel. Their advantage is relatively low operating costs compared to other forms of transportation.

HELICOPTERS Helicopters provide the most rapid service when distances between hospitals are within approximately 150 mi. When landing facilities are available at both hospitals, helicopter transportation reduces transit time by at least two-thirds compared to ground ambulance. Noise and vibration levels are high, and it is rarely practical to stop the vehicle for the management of an emergency requiring a more stable environment. They also have a more confined patient care compartment compared to other vehicles. The impact of these problems can be minimized by extensive preparation of the patient prior to transport and sophisticated electronic monitoring. Because of their speed, helicopters are the vehicle of choice for programs transporting a high proportion of trauma patients for whom time to the receiving hospital is much more important than in-transit care. The major disadvantage of helicopters is the extremely high cost of operation. The purchase cost of a helicopter is usually in excess of $2,500,000; lease/operation contracts usually exceed $100,000 per month.

FIXED-WING AIRCRAFT Fixed-wing aircraft also offer the advantage of speed, which is five to six times that of ground ambulances. This advantage is only appreciated when distances exceed approximately

120 mi because of the additional time needed to transfer the patient and medical personnel between airports and hospitals. Fixed-wing aircraft are also much less costly to operate than helicopters.

Equipment and Supplies

Equipment used to care for pediatric patients during transport is similar to that found in most emergency departments except that it is portable and reduced in size and weight. This is in contrast to equipment used during neonatal transport, which is usually specially designed for its unique function. The basic equipment required for pediatric transport includes a ventilator, a cardiorespiratory monitor with invasive pressure monitoring capability, a pulse oximeter, intravenous pumps, and a noninvasive blood pressure monitor. This equipment should be mounted to a stretcher or fitted with devices that can be secured to the vehicle or stretcher during transport.

Supplies and small equipment should be preassembled in equipment packs. These supplies can be divided into separate packs based on those required for airway management and all other care. Suggested inventories for these packs are included in Table 4-5.

Communications

Reliable and rapid communication is essential for the efficient operation of a transport program. Communication systems that support transport programs are of three varieties: 911 emergency dispatch centers, communication centers within emergency departments, and communication centers dedicated solely to transport programs. Centers that support EMS as well as transport programs are generally more economical. This combined function also helps facilitate the integration of EMS and the transport program. However, 911 dispatch centers are usually governed by agencies other than hospitals and therefore may not be responsive to the needs of the transport program.

The dispatch center should have equipment capable of coordinating communications among referring and receiving medical personnel, transport attendants, vehicle operators, local EMS providers, and area air traffic controllers. Coordinating communications may require the integration of local and long-distance telephone lines, cellular telephones, UHF and VHF band radios, and radio pagers. Ideally, the dispatch center should also have a device for recording all communications.

Transport vehicles should be equipped to provide the same range of communications as the dispatch center. At a minimum, both UHF and VHF band radios are required. Cellular telephones should also be considered in regions where cellular coverage is extensive. Telephones offer the advantage of user friendliness and a style of communication with which more medical personnel are familiar.

Patient Care Protocols and Quality Assurance

The medical director of the program should develop patient care protocols. They should reflect the institutional standards of care for the full range of emergencies likely to be encountered. The program should also document the techniques for training personnel and certifying competency.

During the conduct of a transport, the team should be supervised by a physician with expertise in the care of pediatric emergencies. If such an individual is not in attendance, phone or radio communication with an appropriate physician is advisable at some point during the transport.

To ensure quality of care, the program should also have a systematic plan to review transports. This plan should involve all disciplines represented by the team.

REFERENCES

1. McCloskey KA, Orr RA: Pediatric transport issues in emergency medicine. *Emerg Med Clin North Am* 9:475, 1991.
2. Bose CL: The transport environment, in MacDonald MG, Miller MK (eds): *Emergency Transport of the Perinatal Patient.* Boston, Little, Brown, 1989, pp 194–211.
3. Berens R, Day S: Airway management, in Jaimovich DG, Vidyasagar D (eds): *Handbook of Pediatric and Neonatal Transport Medicine.* Philadelphia, Hanley and Belfus, 1996, pp 157–178.
4. Fletcher MA: Tracheal intubation, in Fletcher MA, MacDonald MG (eds): *Atlas of Procedures in Neonatology.* Philadelphia, Lippincott, 1993, pp 253–269.
5. Klaus MH, Martin RJ, Fanaroff AA: The physical environment, in Klaus MH, Fanaroff AA (eds): *Care of the High Risk Neonate,* 4th ed. Philadelphia, Saunders, 1993, pp 114–129.
6. Kliegman RM: Problems in metabolic adaptation: glucose, calcium, and magnesium, in Klaus MH, Fanaroff AA (eds): *Care of the High Risk Neonate,* 4th ed. Philadelphia, Saunders, 1993, pp 282–301.
7. Bolte R: Responsibilities of the referring physician and hospital, in McCloskey KAL, Orr RA (eds): *Pediatric Transport Medicine.* St Louis, Mosby, 1995, pp 33–42.
8. Schneider C, Gomez M, Lee R: Evaluation of ground ambulance, rotor-wing, and fixed-wing aircraft services. *Crit Care Clin* 8:533, 1992.
9. Bose CL: An overview of the organization and administration of a perinatal transport service, in MacDonald MG, Miller MK (eds): *Emergency Transport of the Perinatal Patient.* Boston, Little, Brown, 1989, pp 34–75.
10. AAP Task Force on Interhospital Transport: *Guidelines for Air and Ground Transport of Neonatal and Pediatric Patients.* Elk Grove, IL, American Academy of Pediatrics, 1993.

DISASTER MEDICAL SERVICES

Eric K. Noji

Natural disasters, such as earthquakes, tornadoes, floods, and hurricanes, have claimed about 3 million lives worldwide during the past 25 years, adversely affecting the lives of at least 800 million more people, and have resulted in property damages exceeding $23 billion. While past disasters have produced their share of mass-casualty situations, the future appears to be even bleaker.[1] Increasing population density in flood plains and earthquake- and hurricane-prone areas, the development of thousands of toxic and hazardous materials and their transportation on public roads, the potential risks from incidents at fixed-site industrial facilities, and the catastrophic possibilities of nuclear, biological, and chemical terrorism all suggest the probability of major emergencies in the future. Recent significant disasters include massive summer flooding in the Midwest (1993); earthquakes in Northridge, California (1994), and Kobe, Japan (1995); the bombing of a federal office building in Oklahoma City (1995); a sarin chemical weapon attack on a Tokyo subway (1995); a bombing during the Olympic Games in Atlanta (1996); severe El Nino-related flooding in California (1997); and Hurricane Mitch (1998).[2–4]

This chapter discusses disaster planning and operations with particular emphasis on the emergency department and the role of the emergency physician. Emergency physicians have extensive responsibilities for community disaster preparedness and other disaster medical services. In several position papers, the American College of Emergency Physicians (ACEP) has outlined the scope of emergency physicians' involvement in disaster medical services and stated its belief that "emergency physicians should assume a primary role in the medical aspects of disaster planning, management, and patient care . . . [and that] emergency physicians should pursue training that will enable them to fulfill this responsibility."[5–7] Despite efficient field management of disaster victims, a rapid flow of victims from a disaster scene can quickly overwhelm a hospital emergency department. Emergency departments must have a specific set of protocols that direct the mobilization of personnel and equipment outside of the emergency department and permit rapid assessment, stabilization, and triage to definitive care of victims of a mass-casualty incident.[8]

DEFINITION OF DISASTER

According to the World Health Organization, a disaster is a sudden ecological phenomenon of sufficient magnitude to require external assistance.[9] From the perspective of the emergency department, however, a disaster exists when the number of patients and/or the severity of illness or injury are such that normal daily emergency department operations are no longer possible. In other words, the number of patients presenting in a given time period are such that the emergency department cannot provide care for them without external assistance.[10] Disasters that cause large numbers of deaths and injuries are referred to as mass-casualty incidents.[11] However, disasters cannot be defined simply by a given number of victims. Large university hospitals with house staff may not have the facilities to manage even two chemically contaminated patients.[12,13] The arrival of one important political person or celebrity with severe injuries (e.g., the President of the United States, the Pope, or a rock star) completely disrupts the normal operations of even the most efficient emergency department.[14]

Regardless how a disaster is defined numerically or situationally for a given institution, it is imperative that the hospital and, more specifically, the emergency department institute preestablished protocols for effectively dealing with such extraordinary situations. These protocols (e.g., for chemically contaminated patients or for the mobilization of appropriate outside assistance) must be instituted rapidly in order to prevent death or severe complications.

In many hospitals in the United States, disasters are often divided into external and internal events. External disasters are events that occur physically outside the hospital (e.g., transportation accidents, terrorist actions, etc.). As a result of such an external event, patients are brought to the hospital from the outside, usually to the emergency department. Unless the outside disaster is a chemical accident with contaminated patients, the hospital and its staff, patients, and visitors are in no immediate physical danger.

Internal disasters are events that occur within the physical plant of the hospital itself (e.g., a fire or laboratory accident involving radioactive material) that severely compromise the ability of the hospital to function.[15] A disaster may be both internal and external, for example, an earthquake that severely damages the hospital.[16] Such an event may damage the structural integrity of the hospital, cause dangerous equipment or supplies to fall over, and injure or kill hospital staff, patients, and visitors.

EFFECT OF MASS-CASUALTY EVENTS ON AN EMERGENCY DEPARTMENT

Extensive social and organizational research on the management of mass-casualty events has shown that emergency departments experience great difficulty coping with even moderate numbers of patients following a disaster.[17] The reasons for this difficulty include confusion, lack of planning, and lack of training in the principles of disaster management. Hospitals are often not well integrated into the surrounding community's disaster planning efforts.[18] Hospital disaster plans often exist only on paper and are rarely referred to, let alone carried out, during a real disaster. Shortcomings of hospital disaster plans include (1) delayed or improper notification of hospital staff, (2) poor delineation of the command structure, (3) overloaded or broken communications networks, (4) improper or incomplete identification of patients and the dead, (5) lack of supplies, and (6) lack of public relations.[19]

When a disaster occurs, transportation of patients to emergency departments is usually uncoordinated, with no thought given to equitable distribution of patients among potential receiving medical facilities.[20] As a result, nearby hospitals are usually overwhelmed with the majority of severely injured patients, while those farther away see very few patients.[21] Most casualties are transported to a hospital over a relatively short period of time, with most patients arriving at an emergency department within $1\frac{1}{2}$ h after the disaster has occurred.[22] Most patients presenting to an emergency department in a disaster have minor injuries and do not require advanced trauma services.[21]

Victims of mass-casualty events may arrive at hospitals by a variety of means, including ambulances, private automobiles, police vehicles, taxis, and on foot.[23] Since hospitals may receive patients in all sorts of unplanned ways, the flow of patients is not under the control of the official or formal emergency medical services (EMS) system.[22] In addition, ambulatory patients and those with relatively minor injuries may arrive at the emergency department before patients with more serious injuries because they are able to leave the disaster site by their own devices, using taxis, buses, private cars, vans, and police vehicles. The more severely injured, who often need extrication (e.g., from collapsed buildings following earthquakes), arrive at a later stage. The result is that less severely injured patients often tend to be treated before the more seriously injured. The early arrival of a large number of ambulatory patients can create serious problems because the emergency department may become badly overcrowded early, resulting in confusion in the efforts to provide treatment.[24] Similarly, when attention is being paid to early arrivals at a hospital, it is easy for the more seriously injured patients brought in later not to be noticed immediately or to be given delayed treatment.

Rescuers, emergency medical technicians, and representatives of the media may rapidly converge on the emergency department and contribute to chaos.

DISASTER PLANNING

Overview

Roles, responsibilities, and working relationships among those responsible for disaster operations should be clarified in the planning process to lessen the confusion that invariably occurs during a disaster.[25] Selected protocols should require personnel to perform functions that are relatively similar to their day-to-day activities.

The disaster planning process should begin by answering the following questions:

1. What types of disasters are most likely to occur in the community (hazard analysis)?
2. What are the disaster planning requirements of the Joint Commission on the Accreditation of Healthcare Organizations (JCAHO), as well as local and state health agencies?[26]
3. What are the capabilities and responsibilities of the hospital?

Hazard Analysis

Hospital disaster planners must plan for those disasters most likely to occur in their community.[27] Hospitals in Hawaii and along the Gulf coast of the United States should plan for hurricanes,[28,29] those in California should plan for earthquakes,[30–34] and those near chemical industries should have facilities for decontamination. Hospitals located near facilities using large amounts of hazardous materials are required by Title III of the Superfund Amendments and Reauthorization Act to participate in local emergency planning committees.[35] Accidents at large transportation facilities, such as airports and harbors, and at festivals, stadiums, and amusement parks can generate large numbers of casualties.[36–39] Various types of disasters are characterized by specific morbidity and mortality rate patterns, and thus health care requirements.[40] Earthquakes cause many deaths and severe injuries.[41–43] Hurricanes cause primarily property damage, with low numbers of deaths and predominantly minor injuries.[28] Pulmonary irritation from fires or hazardous chemicals requires large supplies of oxygen, as the 1984 industrial accident in Bhopal, India, demonstrated.[44] The Tokyo sarin chemical weapon attack in 1995 required large quantities of the antidote atropine.[45] Fortunately, some disasters, such as hurricanes, may afford several days' lead time, and preparations for management can begin early.

JCAHO Requirements

JCAHO requires that member hospitals have a written plan for the timely care of casualties arising from both external and internal disasters, and the hospital must document the rehearsal of these plans.[26]

Hospital-Community Cooperation in Disaster Planning

Every hospital should integrate its own disaster plan with those of community disaster management agencies.[10,27] Such integration is especially important in the areas of disaster notification and communications, transportation of casualties, and provisions for dispatch of hospital medical teams to a disaster site. Strong relationships with community agencies, such as the fire department, the regional EMS system, the local emergency management agency, and the civil defense agency, are important to ensure a coordinated disaster response. Table 5-1 lists key members of the community disaster team.

The hospital may also interact with utility companies, the military, the local American Red Cross, the Salvation Army, the Federal Emergency Management Agency (FEMA), the National Disaster Medical System, and the Centers for Disease Control and Prevention during a disaster.

Medical planning for disasters in the community is usually the responsibility of local EMS councils.[46] Such councils include representatives from the local ambulance services, the fire department, and other nonmedical and government agencies as well as the physician EMS director. Physicians involved in community disaster planning must be familiar with the local EMS communications and treatment protocols.[5]

The hospital must develop its external disaster plan in conjunction with other emergency facilities in the community. For example, prearranged mutual aid agreements with hospitals outside the immediate area ensure that patients are cared for when hospital capacities are exceeded. Plans should also be made for referral to area tertiary centers and special units (e.g., burn, spinal cord, and pediatric trauma centers).

Hospital disaster planners should anticipate that information about specific hazards (e.g., chemicals and radiation), expert personnel (e.g., poison control), and special supplies (e.g., antidotes) not readily available may be needed in a particular disaster situation. Plans should consider how to rapidly access these resources and how to obtain additional shelter, food, and water if necessary.

TABLE 5-1 Community Disaster Team

Community Agency	Responsibilities
EMS service	Patient triage in the field, stabilization, transfer to definitive care facility
Fire service Police service	Overall scene command, victim rescue, hazard control, traffic management, scene security
Emergency manager	Communications, personnel and equipment support, liaison with state and federal agencies
Public works	Support equipment and personnel, structural safety expertise
Chief executive officer	Management of overall operation, assurance of public safety, communication with public, direction of requests for outside assistance to appropriate state and federal authorities

TABLE 5-2 Key Functions of the Hospital Disaster Plan

Activation of the plan
Assessment of the hospital's capacity
Establishment of a disaster command
Communications
Supplies
Hospital disaster administrative and treatment areas
Training and drills

THE HOSPITAL DISASTER PLAN

Basic Requirements of Hospital Planning

Hospital disaster planning is the responsibility of the administration, the nursing staff, and the medical staff. A good hospital disaster plan should be coordinated with community organizations and should provide an organized response for the management of casualties transported to the hospital from the disaster site. Finally, it should take into account disasters arising within or near the hospital that require hospital evacuation.

Staff members perform most efficiently when they are performing relatively familiar tasks. The disaster plan should therefore rely on standard operating procedures as much as possible. Key functions of the hospital plan are listed in Table 5-2.

Activating the Disaster Plan

The plan must designate an individual and alternate who have the responsibility of putting the hospital's disaster plan into effect. Situations that warrant activation of the plan should also be defined (see "Definition of Disaster," above). For example, the emergency department disaster manual must define how the on-duty physician and nurse determine when to mobilize staff from other departments and when to involve the hospital administrator and nursing supervisor.

Following activation of the plan, there must be immediate mobilization of anticipated disaster resources: personnel, supplies, equipment, communications, and transportation.

Assessment of the Hospital's Capacity

Before the hospital can receive casualties, it must be determined whether the hospital itself has sustained any structural damage or loss of utility as a result of a disaster. Such damage may include blocked passageways; inoperable elevators; potential for fire, explosion, or building collapse; failure of any utility; loss of equipment and/or supplies, including oxygen; contamination of water; and outside access problems. Damage assessment is usually the responsibility of the plant safety officer or hospital engineer. If the structural integrity of the hospital has been compromised, it may be necessary to evacuate staff and patients.[16]

Once it is ascertained that the hospital itself is safe, the hospital must determine how many casualties from the disaster site it can safely manage. This capacity may be limited by available personnel, beds, and supplies as well as by the type of disaster and the availability of other community resources. At the time of disaster notification, it is necessary to know the status of many of the hospital's capabilities, including how many beds are available, how much blood is available, how many personnel are on duty, what damage has been done, how many operating rooms are in use, and which doctors are present. Either someone must tour the hospital to accumulate this information or a form for reporting it must be available in each department ahead of time.

Establishment of Disaster Command

A predesignated command site within the hospital should be established. The command site should be able to communicate with the emergency department receiving and triage area, with patient care areas, and with regional EMS, police, fire, and governmental authorities. Provisions for multiple modes of communication should be made. The command personnel should include at least a physician, a nurse, and an administrator.[10]

Communication

Establishment of good communications is critical in any disaster or mass-casualty situation. Past experience, however, has shown that this essential function is difficult to achieve for a variety of reasons. Telephones frequently become inoperative due to switchboard overload and damage to telephone lines and other equipment. A major goal should be full utilization of all possible communications resources, including citizens' band groups, cellular phones, blackboards, E mail, intercoms, closed-circuit television, short-wave radio and radio-equipped individuals of all kinds, runners, and even messenger and courier services.

Interhospital communication may be necessary because of shortages of supplies, such as blood or intravenous fluids; certain equipment, such as incubators or surgical instruments; or personnel, such as nurses, x-ray technicians, respiratory therapists, or physicians. When a hospital is overloaded, it may be desirable to transfer patients to a prearranged receiving hospital. Unfortunately, interhospital communications may present a weak link in the community's disaster response. After one Los Angeles earthquake in 1971, 67 percent of hospitals had difficulty with interhospital communications.[46a]

Supplies

During a disaster, necessary supplies and equipment must be ready for immediate distribution to appropriate locations in the hospital (e.g., stretchers and wheelchairs to the receiving area). Each hospital must estimate the amount of disaster supplies that will be needed in addition to its regular stock. The trend toward last-minute inventories may exacerbate problems in this area.

Hospital Disaster Administrative and Treatment Areas

Specific areas of the hospital must be designated for specific functions (Table 5-3). Staffing requirements and basic supplies for each area should be defined.

DISASTER COMMAND Disaster command provides overall direction and coordination of the hospital disaster response activities. These activities include activation of the plan, coordination of hospital activities with those at the disaster site, opening up additional hospital wards or clinics, obtaining outside assistance, evacuation of endangered patients, assignment of staff to treatment areas, and adjustment of the plan as necessary. Good, reliable communication is essential.

TRIAGE Entry of all patients should be restricted to one location: the triage area. The primary function of a disaster triage area is rapid assessment of all incoming casualties, assignment of priorities for management, and distribution of patients to various patient care areas in the hospital. A senior emergency physician or resident should be responsible for triage.

PATIENT IDENTIFICATION, REGISTRATION, AND DOCUMENTATION Emergency department registration personnel are key components of the emergency department disaster response. Ideally, they should be part of the triage team. Prepared documents assigned to each patient should include a unique disaster number for each patient, the patient's name and key information if available, the triage designation, the patient's wristband identification and charting materials, and copies for postevent analysis. A system should be in place to quickly obtain more patient documents when the supply is depleted. A separate triage log should be maintained. Individuals must also be assigned to transfer registration information to the hospital computer system so that laboratory requests, admissions, blood for type and cross-match, and dispositions can be systematically recorded. Finally, if unique disaster numbers are used, a system for transferring to the hospital medical record number system should be in place.

PATIENT CARE STATIONS One suggested method of organizing patient care stations includes division into resuscitation, major illness and injury, and minor trauma/primary care.

A resuscitation area should handle all life-threatening problems. Seriously injured patients who do not require immediate airway management or resuscitation are sent to the major illness or injury area, located in the emergency department.

In most disaster situations, the majority of patients are not seriously injured. Such patients can be sent to the minor trauma/primary care area for splinting of fractures, primary closure of lacerations, and tetanus prophylaxis. This area can be established in the hospital's outpatient clinics.

PRESURGICAL HOLDING Most trauma patients stabilized in the major illness or injury area (emergency department) will be sent to the admission presurgical holding area.

SURGERY The number of operating rooms that can be staffed is the main limiting factor in the provision of definitive care for a large

TABLE 5-3 Hospital Disaster Areas

Disaster command
Triage
Patient identification, registration, and documentation
Patient care stations
Presurgical holding
Surgery
Morgue
Decontamination
Psychiatry
Family waiting and discharge area
Public relations

number of severely injured casualties.[47] The most senior surgeon available must take the responsibility for prioritizing cases and assigning surgeons to them as rapidly as possible.

MORGUE Many disasters can result in a large number of fatalities. Morgue capacities may need to be expanded or outside facilities, such as a church or stadium, temporarily utilized.[48]

DECONTAMINATION JCAHO requires hospitals to have provisions for emergency treatment and decontamination of individuals who are radioactively or chemically contaminated.[13,49] Some basic requirements for hospitals are (1) a safe area for decontamination, (2) a means of washing external contamination from patients, (3) a method of containing contaminated materials, (4) adequate protection for persons handling patients and for other hospital personnel, and (5) disposable and/or cleanable medical equipment.

The goals are to reduce external contamination, contain the contamination that remains, and prevent further spread of potentially dangerous substances.[12,50] After being decontaminated, the patient can be treated as a ''normal'' accident victim. To accomplish this, three things must be achieved: (1) termination of exposure to toxic material, (2) stabilization of the patient, and (3) initiation of proper definitive care.

PSYCHIATRY In the event of a disaster involving mass casualties and extensive property damage, it is common for patients to present with episodes of anxiety, depression, and psychosis. Hysterical persons, whether patients, visitors, or staff, can be extremely disruptive to hospital disaster operations. A separate, isolated area must be predesignated to receive individuals in need of psychological intervention.

FAMILY WAITING AND DISCHARGE AREA Families and friends will converge on the hospital seeking information about victims. A separate area must be predesignated for family members seeking information. This area may also be utilized to discharge in-hospital patients and victims of the disaster. It may be staffed by volunteers, chaplains, and members of the public relations staff.

PUBLIC RELATIONS COMMAND The medical disaster plan should include a section on the proper relationship with the media. Representatives of the media are present at all medical disasters. They may be a valuable resource for announcing hazards or the need for evacuation. In addition, they may be used to make a general announcement that hospital or rescue personnel should report to work. The plan should include a means of providing the media with adequate information both at the site and in the hospital. At the disaster site, regular briefings help prevent representatives of the media from becoming victims as they search for more information. At the hospital, regular briefings and a room with adequate telephone access will prevent members of the media from invading patient care areas. A hospital public relations officer should act as liaison to the media. His or her duties are to prepare the pressroom, hold regular briefings, and arrange appropriate photographic opportunities. These functions must be carried out while balancing the public's right to know with individual victims' rights to privacy.

Training and Drills

Regular training and drills help to familiarize staff with their disaster roles and responsibilities. They also serve to point out weaknesses or omissions in the plan that require additions or revisions. Drills can range from full-scale community-wide simulations with moulage victims to tabletop triage games to minidrills that test only certain components of the disaster plan, such as call-up of personnel and testing of communications. JCAHO requires two drills a year; the scenarios should reflect incidents that are likely to occur in the community.

FIELD DISASTER OPERATIONS

On-Site Medical Care

In the field, rescue personnel often use a simple triage and rapid treatment (START) technique that depends on a quick assessment of respiration, perfusion, and mental status.[51] Subsequently, determining how much and what type of care to administer at the disaster site depends on several factors. If the number of patients is small and sufficient prehospital personnel and transportation resources are available, on-site medical care can proceed in a fairly normal manner, with rapid stabilization and transportation to nearby hospitals. When extrication will be prolonged, potentially lifesaving interventions, such as crystalloid infusion for hypovolemic shock, should be instituted in the field.[52,53] On the other hand, early, rapid transportation with a minimum of treatment should be practiced when there is danger to rescuers and casualties from fire, explosion, falling buildings, hazardous materials, or extreme weather conditions.

When there is an overwhelming number of casualties that exceed transportation capacities, advanced field medical and surgical treatment may be beneficial, since it may be hours before seriously injured patients can be evacuated.[54] This may necessitate the establishment of field hospitals with operating-theater capabilities. Casualties are brought there from the disaster site for further assessment and initial treatment of their injuries. After a period of observation and stabilization, they are either sent home or transported to a hospital.

If evacuation of ambulatory victims and those with minor injuries rapidly overwhelm local hospitals prior to the arrival of the more severely injured, it may be better to treat them locally. To address these considerations, the secondary assessment of victim endpoint (SAVE) system of triage has been proposed.[55] The SAVE triage system is designed to identify patients who are most likely to benefit from the care available under austere field conditions. When combined with the START protocol, the SAVE triage is useful for any scenario where multiple patients experience a prolonged delay to definitive care (Fig. 5-1). The SAVE triage method divides patients into three categories: (1) those who will die regardless of how much care they receive, (2) those who will survive whether or not they receive care, and (3) those who will benefit significantly from austere field interventions.

Incident Command System

The incident command system (ICS) is a standard emergency management system used throughout the United States to provide a flexible command and control structure upon which to organize a response.[56] The ICS is generally used when there is an identifiable single scene for a disaster event, such as the site of a plane crash. By standardizing an organizational structure and using common terminology, the ICS provides a management system that is adaptable to incidents involving a multiagency or multijurisdictional response. At the most basic level, the organizational structure has five main components: (1) incident command, (2) operations, (3) planning, (4) logistics, and (5) finance. The principles of a prehospital ICS can also be applied to the hospital setting. With this type of organizational infrastructure and the flexibility to expand and collapse as needed, an orderly and efficient response to any incident can theoretically be implemented.

Communication from Disaster Site to Hospital

The local emergency communications or disaster operations center should alert hospitals in the affected area of a possible mass- or multiple-casualty situation. Ideally, this report should include the number of injured divided into categories: serious injuries, minor injuries, and special patients (e.g., pregnant women). Hospitals should report to the local emergency communications center the following informa-

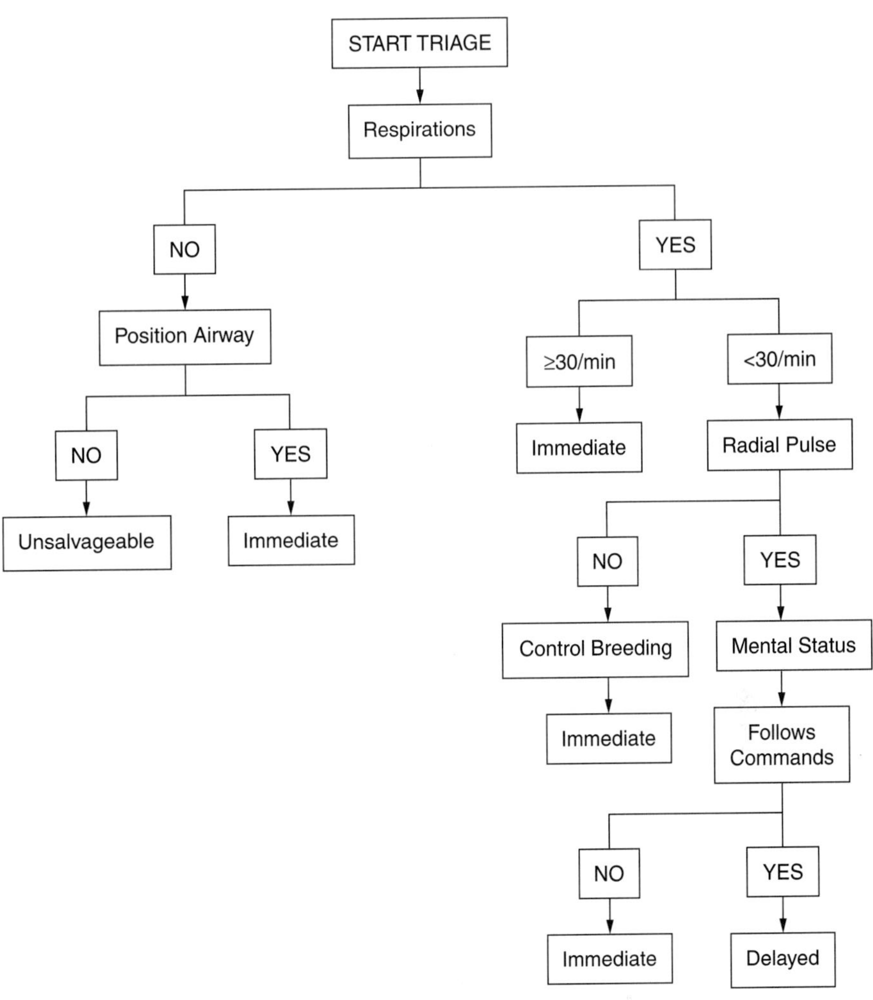

FIG. 5-1. Medical disaster response modified simple triage and rapid treatment (START). There are three SAVE triage categories: unsalvageable, immediate care, and delayed care. (Used with permission, copyright Medical Disaster Response Inc., Dana Point, CA, 1990.)

tion: (1) bed availability, (2) number of casualties received thus far, (3) number of additional casualties that the hospital is prepared to accept, and (4) specific items in short supply.

Distribution of Casualties to Receiving Hospitals

Typically, in the past, the hospital closest to the disaster site received an inordinately large number of disaster victims as well as the most critically injured. It is important that the casualty load be distributed among available hospitals so that the injured receive prompt and appropriate treatment and individual hospitals do not become overwhelmed.

However, such a situation may be unavoidable due to large numbers of critically injured patients, blocked transportation routes, or weather conditions. Nevertheless, such problems can be minimized by maintaining good communications between hospitals and on-site EMS command. The on-scene incident commander should be alerted immediately by a potentially overloaded hospital so that less injured and more stable patients can be sent to other hospitals. Secondary triage from one hospital to another may also be necessary if the hospital's capability to handle victims has been exceeded.

Casualties with special problems, such as major burns, carbon monoxide poisoning, and spinal cord injuries, may need to be transferred directly to specialized units, although it may not be possible for these units to accept a large number of injured.

On-Site Disaster Medical Teams from Hospitals

On-site disaster medical teams dispatched from local hospitals may be of value if victims require prolonged extrication; transportation routes are blocked, preventing easy evacuation to hospitals; or the number of casualties exceeds transportation capacities. Such a team should be dispatched with great caution. Most physicians and nurses function well in an in-hospital setting, but few are prepared, either by training or experience, to work under austere field conditions. Such hospital-based teams should probably not come from the emergency department staff until backup staff has arrived to care for patients expected from the disaster site and those already in the emergency department. The resources for such teams should be carefully planned on a regional basis. The capability to send hospital teams to a disaster site can be developed in a number of ways. For example, an on-site triage team of physicians and nurses can come from teaching hospitals or be created from a pool of volunteer medical staff in office practice. Ideally, at least one institution from each region should maintain such a capability. The designated hospital should store disaster triage kits containing essential resuscitation and stabilization equipment in the emergency department for such circumstances.

EMERGENCY DEPARTMENT

The emergency department is the most critical part of a hospital's initial response to virtually any type of external disaster. It is the department of the hospital that usually receives first notification that a disaster has occurred, and it is usually the entry point for incoming victims.

Initial Response

When a call is made to a hospital about a disaster or a potentially mass-casualty-producing event, the recipient of the call must have a procedure to follow for verification of the incident. A disaster notification form is used by some facilities to remind the staff of the questions they are to ask the caller.

The appropriate hospital official or administrator on duty is then given this information. When the emergency department is notified by hospital administration (now Disaster Command) that the external disaster plan is in effect, it sets in motion a series of activities. The information obtained from the call is given to the charge nurse; the clerical, registration, nursing, and medical personnel in the department are notified of the impending arrival of casualties; and the emergency department plan for calling additional staff is activated.

An initial needs assessment is conducted by the nurse and physician in charge, given the information available. They must evaluate and prioritize the patients currently in the department and admit, discharge, or transfer them. All stable and nonurgent patients should be given plans for follow-up care and discharged from the emergency department with responsible individuals.

Based on this initial assessment, the number of patients that the department can receive is determined and communicated to the prehospital disaster communications center. The nurse and the physician in charge then determine whether more physician and nursing coverage is required in the emergency department and assign staff to those areas in the department to be used during the disaster. As patients begin to arrive, the charge nurse must be alert to signs of staff stress and work overload before the problem gets out of hand. Family members and representatives of the media should be directed away from the emergency department.

Personnel Notification

The director of the emergency department or a designee should have a phone list of appropriate personnel to be called in to work during a disaster. Lists of addresses and phone numbers of these individuals should be distributed to all key personnel. This information should be regularly updated.

If hospital telephone communications have been completely disrupted, emergency department personnel may have to be reached by cellular phone, E mail, or radio or television announcement. Alternatively, a telephone remote from the hospital, even at a personal residence, may be able to handle this extensive calling job.

Security and Traffic Control

Hospital security personnel play a key role in the emergency department by diverting nonessential vehicles and ensuring a smooth, one-way flow of traffic to the ambulance entrance.

Reception of Patients

Since many patients will arrive independently of the official or formal EMS system, reports from the field may greatly underestimate the total number of patients.

All available litters and wheelchairs should be taken to the ambulance ramp immediately on announcement of the disaster status. Patients from the disaster site are met at the receiving area by hospital escorts, who assist the emergency medical technicians in transferring patients to wheelchairs or stretchers.

Essential equipment, such as endotracheal tubes, intravenous solutions, cervical collars, splints, and bandages should be placed near the ambulance entrance to permit convenient restocking of the ambulance and rapid return to the disaster site.

Medical Care during Disaster Situations

PATIENT IDENTIFICATION, REGISTRATION, AND CHARTING

Documentation is limited to patient identification and charting of critical findings and treatments. Some plans call for the use of the prehospital disaster tag to record this limited information. Other plans include the preparation of kits containing the emergency department records, x-ray requests, laboratory slips and tubes, and wristbands, all prelabeled with a discrete disaster number. Medical records and laboratory computers accept these numbers, which are used for patient identification until full normal registration is possible. At that point the computer will search previous medical records to match disaster numbers with the records of victims who have been patients previously. Such a prelabeled kit system can be used during normal operations on unidentified critically ill or injured patients, so that all hospital departments are familiar with the concept. Admissions personnel are needed to log key information rapidly. Hours or days later they will be able to complete the registration process.

TRIAGE Triage is the prioritization of care based on severity of injury or illness, prognosis, and availability of resources. The triage personnel determine to which predesignated patient care area a patient should be sent based on priorities for care. For example, patients needing immediate decontamination or resuscitation are taken to decontamination and resuscitation areas. The dead are moved directly to the morgue. The severely but less critically injured are taken to the major illness/injury area. The walking injured are directed to the minor injury/primary care treatment area, often located in outpatient clinic areas.

A team consisting of an emergency physician or a surgeon skilled in triage, an emergency department nurse, and a medical records or admitting clerk should assess every patient. In extraordinary situations, several triage teams may be required to handle the casualty load. The physician performing hospital triage should be acknowledged as being in command in the triage area, should be clearly identified by a specially colored vest or other garment, and must understand all triage options.

Even though patients may have been triaged at the scene, they should undergo a second triage upon arrival at the hospital at the ambulance/triage entrance to the emergency department. Triage teams must remain at triage and cannot be diverted for patient care. Another team should be called to triage if immediate life support is needed. Only the most basic steps, such as opening the airway and applying pressure to active bleeding, should be done.

The triage team may need to communicate information on the number of casualties, severity of injuries, and need for additional resources to both the emergency department and the hospital Disaster Command center. Likewise, triage personnel need to be informed about the capability of the various treatment areas (e.g., major and minor injury) to handle additional casualties or special problems, such as eye injuries or burns. They also need to know about the establishment and location of patient overflow areas.

The admitting clerk's role as part of the triage team is to complete triage tags, attach them to victims, retrieve valuables and clothing for bagging, and maintain the triage area casualty log.

The approach to patient evaluation and treatment is quite different under disaster situations resulting in large numbers of casualties. While some principles of medical care are unchanged in a mass-casualty incident, other principles must be altered to achieve the best outcome for the largest number of patients rather than concentrating resources on a single patient. There is no role for advanced life support resuscita-

TABLE 5-4 Triage Categories

Red	Yellow	Green	Black
First priority Most urgent Life-threatening shock or hypoxia is present or imminent, but patient can be stabilized and, if given immediate care, will probably survive.	Second priority Urgent Injuries have systemic implications or effects, but patient is not yet in life-threatening shock or hypoxia; although systemic decline will ensue, given appropriate care, patient seems able to withstand a 45- to 60-min wait without immediate risk.	Third priority Nonurgent Injuries are localized and without immediate systemic implications; with a minimum of care, patient generally does not deteriorate for up to several hours.	Dead No distinction can be made between clinical and biologic death in a mass-casualty incident, and any unresponsive patient who has no spontaneous ventilation or circulation is classified as dead; some classify in this category catastrophically injured patients who have a poor chance for survival regardless of care.

tion at triage; care should be limited to manual opening of airways and control of external hemorrhage. Routine emergency department care is also modified: patients in cardiac arrest do not usually receive advanced life support and cardiopulmonary resuscitation in order that other seriously injured patients with a better chance of survival can be treated with available resources; radiologic and laboratory studies are used only if they will provide critical information; patients are hospitalized only when necessary; nurses have increased autonomy; and paramedics operate under standing orders without the need for on-line medical control.

The most common triage classification involves assigning patients to one of four color-coded categories (red, yellow, green, or black) depending on injury severity and prognosis (Table 5-4). In addition to taking into account the nature and urgency of the patient's condition, triage decisions should be sensitive to such factors affecting prognosis as age, general health, and prior physical condition of the patient.

WOUND CARE AND CRUSH SYNDROME This section addresses some concepts of care that are not found in the routine management of emergency patients.

Wound infections may occur in virtually all types of disasters. Infected wounds and gangrene were major problems following an earthquake in Armenia (1988) and tornadoes in Illinois (1991).[57,58] In hurricanes or tornadoes, persons may be cut by flying glass and other, potentially highly contaminated material. Because of this, all wounds should be copiously irrigated. Primary closure of heavily contaminated wounds may result in major complications, as was the case following the Armero volcanic eruption in Colombia in 1985.[59] If lacerations are more than 6 to 12 h old or appear contaminated, they should be treated by debridement and left open for primary delayed closure. Tetanus prophylaxis and tetanus immunoglobulin should be administered if indicated.

Victims who have been trapped by rubble for several hours or days should be watched very closely for signs and symptoms of crush syndrome, such as cardiac arrhythmias, hyperkalemia, and renal failure.[60,61] Fulminant pulmonary edema or pneumonia from dust inhalation may also be a delayed cause of death for victims of building collapse.

RADIOGRAPHIC AND LABORATORY STUDIES Radiographic and laboratory studies should be used only if test results will change therapeutic intervention. For example, x-rays of closed, nonangulated potential fractures can be safely delayed for 24 to 48 h, during which time effective splinting, elevation, and ice can be utilized. On the other hand, cervical spine, pelvic, and femur x-rays may be indicated, considering their potential complications. A chest radiograph is needed in patients complaining of chest pain, dyspnea, or abnormal chest wall motion.

Indications for clinical laboratory studies are minimal. In cases of hemorrhagic shock, a baseline hematocrit and type and cross-matching for blood should be obtained. A urine dipstick test for blood may be useful in detecting renal or urinary tract injuries. All other laboratory studies should be considered accessory and ordered only in specific circumstances (e.g., determination of serum carboxyhemoglobin levels in cases of smoke inhalation).

BLOOD BANK In a disaster situation involving many casualties, it is recommended that the blood bank have as many as 50 units of blood available.[62] It is also important that the bank have ready access to a source of volunteer donors who can be rapidly mobilized. Other potential sources of blood include friends and family members of patients as well as those with minor injuries.

PATIENT IDENTIFICATION AND RECORD KEEPING Emergency department records of disaster victims have usually been poor or nonexistent in past disasters.[63] The general absence of detailed and systematic record keeping in disasters, except for serious cases in which patients were admitted to hospitals for surgery or to intensive care units, has implications for reimbursement and quality improvement.

Documentation of the patient's hospital course starts in the triage area. Proper tagging with a triage tag is essential for patient identification, documentation of medical care rendered, and supplying information for relatives and the news media. Unfortunately, triage tags are frequently underutilized in actual disasters because they are a departure from normal emergency department routine.

One member of the triage team (admitting or medical records clerk) should be assigned to record the patient's name and triage destination. If identification of the patient is not available, race, gender, and approximate age should be noted on the tag. An initial diagnostic impression should also be registered on the tag. This information is entered in the triage area log.

MEDIA RELATIONS AND FAMILY The hospital may become inundated by more members of the media than disaster victims.[64] Members of the news media should be directed to an area away from patient care. The pressroom should be closely supervised by a hospital administrator or public relations specialist who is in direct contact with the disaster command center. To ensure that consistent information is released by the hospital, the staff must leave all communications with the media to the public relations team.

Family members should not be allowed into patient care areas. Special policies should be developed for handling family members whose relatives are critically ill or who have died. The hospital operator will also be inundated with calls of inquiry. Such calls should be directed to a single predesignated desk or office.

Aftermath of Disaster

As soon as possible, efforts should be directed toward returning the hospital to normal operations. Besides restocking and cleaning, consideration must be given to the emotional stress experienced by both prehospital and hospital staff. Short- and long-term emotional problems, including posttraumatic stress disorder, particularly among rescuers, have been reported on numerous occasions.[65] A technique known as critical incident stress debriefing (CISD) was introduced in 1983,[66,67] and such an intervention can assist providers in maintaining job performance and satisfaction, resulting in improved patient care.[68]

Deficiencies in a hospital's disaster plan that are revealed during a disaster should be carefully recorded, reviewed, and criticized. Immediate steps should then be taken to correct these flaws in the plan.

MAJOR DISASTER RESPONSE ORGANIZATIONS IN THE UNITED STATES

Federal Emergency Management Agency

In the United States, the Federal Emergency Management Agency (FEMA) is the federal government agency responsible for emergency preparedness and response. FEMA helps state and local organizations prepare for, respond to, and recover from emergencies. Under the Robert T. Stafford Disaster Relief and Emergency Assistance Act, public law 93-288 (the Stafford Act, 1988), the President is authorized to direct federal agencies to provide emergency assistance to save lives and protect property, public health, and safety in emergencies. "The Federal Response Plan" developed by FEMA in the early 1990s is the operational blueprint for the implementation of the Stafford Act in responding to all disasters and emergencies. The plan is a cooperative agreement signed by all 26 federal agencies and the American Red Cross for providing services when there is a need for federal response assistance following any type of disaster or emergency. The plan outlines a problem-oriented or functional approach to identifying the types of federal assistance that a state is most likely to need following a major disaster. Emergency support functions are grouped into 12 categories, such as food, health and medical services, transportation, and communications. For each emergency support function, one agency is charged with being the major provider of the service, with several other agencies responsible for supporting the primary agency. For health and medical services, the primary agency is the US Department of Health and Human Services.

Disaster Medical Assistance Teams

The National Disaster Medical System (NDMS) is a federally coordinated initiative designed to augment the emergency medical response capability of the United States in the event of a catastrophic disaster.[69] This system is a cooperative program of four federal government agencies: the Department of Defense, the Department of Health and Human Services, FEMA, and the Department of Veterans Affairs. The NDMS provides an interstate medical mutual-aid system linking federal, state, and local agencies and private-sector institutions to address medical care needs in a catastrophic disaster. The program was designed to supplement the activities of state and local governments during a massive civil disaster and to supplement the military medical care system in the event of an overseas conventional conflict. The NDMS contains a medical response element to provide organized aid to a disaster-affected area, an evacuation system, and a network of precommitted hospital beds throughout the United States. Its medical response element includes dozens of volunteer civilian disaster medical assistance teams (DMATs), which (1) operate supplemental casualty clearing facilities for triage, stabilization, and holding care for disaster victims; and (2) operate evacuation facilities for patients in excess of local hospital capacity. DMATs have also been developed for specialized needs, such as quick response, preventive medicine, burn care, renal dialysis, mental health, intensive care, and mortuary services.

In a disaster, NDMS will be activated only when state resources have been overwhelmed and the governor has requested federal assistance.[70] The DMATs are designated by the Department of Health and Human Services and must meet specific NDMS standards. Although DMAT members are volunteers, they become temporary federal employees if they are activated and are paid a per diem rate.

Throughout the NDMS, emergency physicians play key roles in the definition of training standards, the deployment of clinical services, the administration of field operations, and the further development of the civilian-federal disaster response capacity during times of national emergency.

DISASTER MEDICINE

The field of disaster medicine has become an area of major interest within the specialty of emergency medicine.[71,72] A section for disaster medicine has been organized within the American College of Emergency Physicians. Several national and international forums present the results of disaster medical research (e.g., annual conferences sponsored by the Florida chapter of ACEP, World Congresses on Disaster and Emergency Medicine, and meetings of the International Society for Disaster Medicine).[73] Since ACEP first defined a disaster medicine curriculum for residencies and fellowships, a number of disaster medicine fellowships have been established in the United States.[74] Disaster medicine continues to develop as a professional discipline in the United States, and emergency physicians are becoming increasingly involved in the areas of disaster response and humanitarian medical relief.[56]

REFERENCES

1. Noji EK: Progress in disaster management. *Lancet* 343:1239, 1994.
2. Tanaka K: The Kobe earthquake: The system response, a disaster report from Japan. *Eur J Emerg Med* 3:263, 1996.
3. Chartoff SE, Gren JM: Survey of Iowa emergency medical services on the effects of the 1993 floods. *J Prehosp Disaster Med* 12:210, 1997.
4. Noji EK, Miller GL: Emergency department response to a disaster from an emerging pathogen [editorial]. *Ann Emerg Med* 24:512,1994.
5. American College of Emergency Physicians: The role of the emergency physician in mass casualty/disaster management. *JACEP* 5:901, 1976.
6. ACEP Practice Management Committee: Definition of emergency medicine and the emergency physician. *Ann Emerg Med* 15:1240, 1986.
7. ACEP Disaster Committee: Disaster medical services. *Ann Emerg Med* 14:1026, 1985.
8. Chaff L: Emergency preparedness, in: *Safety Guide for Health Care Institutions,* 5th ed. Chicago, American Hospital Publishing, 1994.
9. Noji EK: *The Public Health Consequences of Disasters.* New York, Oxford University Press, 1997.
10. Callum JR, Dinerman NM: Disaster preparedness, in Sheehy S (ed): *Emergency Nursing: Principles and Practice,* 3d ed. St. Louis, Mosby, 1992.
11. Cowley RA: *Proceedings of "Mass Casualties: A Lessons Learned Approach," 13–17 June, 1982.* Baltimore, Maryland Institute for Emergency Medical Services Systems, 1982.
12. Currance PL, Bronstein AC: *Emergency Care for Hazardous Materials Exposure.* St. Louis, Mosby, 1988.
13. Agency for Toxic Substances and Disease Registry: *Managing Hazardous Materials Incidents: Hospital Emergency Departments, a Planning Guide for the Management of Contaminated Patients.* Atlanta, Agency for Toxic Substances and Disease Registry, 1992.
14. Edelstein S, Giordano J: Presidential assassination attempt, in Cowley RA (ed): *Proceedings of "Mass Casualties: A Lessons Learned Approach," 13–17 June, 1982.* Baltimore, Maryland Institute for Emergency Medical Services Systems, 1982, pp 17–28.
15. Aghababian R, Lewis CP, Gans L, et al: Disasters within hospitals. *Ann Emerg Med* 23:771, 1994.
16. Noji EK, Jones NP: Hospital preparedness for earthquakes. *J Comm Accredit Health Care Organ Plant Technol Saf Ser* 2:13, 1990.
17. Dynes RR: Emergency medical services delivery in disasters, in: *Collected Papers in Emergency Medical Services and Traumatology.* Baltimore, University of Maryland, 1979, pp 56–58.

18. Quarentelli EL: The delivery of disaster emergency medical services: Recommendations from systematic field studies. *Disaster Med* 1:41, 1983.
19. Auf der Heide E: *Disaster Response: Principles of Preparation and Coordination.* St. Louis, Mosby, 1989.
20. Tierney K: Emergency medical preparedness and responses in disasters: The need for interorganizational coordination. *Public Adm Rev* 45:77, 1985.
21. Tierney KJ, Taylor VA: EMS delivery in mass emergencies: Preliminary research findings. *Mass Emerg* 2:151, 1977.
22. Quarantelli EL: *Delivery of Emergency Medical Services in Disasters: Assumptions and Realities.* New York, Irvington, 1983.
23. Orr M, Robinson A: The Hyatt Regency skywalk collapse: An EMS-based disaster response. *Ann Emerg Med* 12:601, 1983.
24. Taylor VA: *Hospital Emergency Facilities in a Disaster: An Analysis of Organizational Adaptation to Stress.* Disaster Research Center preliminary paper 11. Columbus, OH, Ohio State University, 1974.
25. Waeckerle JF: Disaster planning and response. *N Engl J Med* 324:815, 1991.
26. *Accreditation Manual for Hospitals, 1998.* Oak Brook Terrace, IL, Joint Commission on the Accreditation of Healthcare Organizations, 1998.
27. Auf der Heide E: Community hospital and medical disaster planning guidelines, in *ACEP Handbook: Disaster Preparedness.* Dallas, American College of Emergency Physicians, 1993.
28. Henderson AK, Lillibridge SR, Salinas C, et al: Disaster medical assistance teams: Providing health care to a community struck by Hurricane Iniki. *Ann Emerg Med* 23:726, 1994.
29. Noji EK: Analysis of medical needs in disasters caused by tropical cyclones: The need for a uniform injury reporting scheme. *J Trop Med Hyg* 96:370, 1993.
30. Schultz CH, Koenig KL, Noji EK: A medical disaster response to reduce immediate mortality after an earthquake. *N Engl J Med* 334:438, 1996.
31. Pointer JE, Michaelis J, Saunders C, et al: The 1989 Loma Prieta earthquake: Impact on hospital care. *Ann Emerg Med* 21:1228, 1992.
32. Haynes BE, Freeman C, Rubin JL, et al: Medical response to catastrophic events: California's planning and the Loma Prieta earthquake. *Ann Emerg Med* 21:368, 1992.
33. Martchenke R, Pointer JE: Hospital disaster operations during the 1989 Loma Prieta earthquake. *Prehosp Disaster Med* 9:146, 1994.
34. Palafox J, Pointer JE, Martchenke J, et al: The 1989 Loma Prieta earthquake: Issues in medical control. *Prehosp Disaster Med* 8:291, 1993.
35. Leonard RB, Calabro JJ, Noji EK, et al: SARA (Superfund Amendments and Reauthorization Act): Implications for Emergency Medicine. *Ann Emerg Med* 18:1212, 1989.
36. Leonard RB, Petrilli R, Calabro J, Noji EK: *Provision of Emergency Medical Care for Crowds.* Monograph. Dallas, American College of Emergency Physicians, 1990.
37. Federman JH, Giordano LM: How to cope with a visit from the Pope. *Prehosp Disaster Med* 12:86, 1997.
38. Lorenzo RA: Mass gathering medicine: A review. *Prehosp Disaster Med* 12:68, 1997.
39. Michael JA, Barbera JA: Mass gathering medical care: A twenty-five year review. *Prehosp Disaster Med* 12:305, 1997.
40. Noji EK, Sivertson KT: Injury prevention in natural disasters: A theoretical framework. *Disasters* 11:290, 1987.
41. Noji EK, Kelen GD, Armenian HK, et al: The 1988 earthquake in Soviet Armenia: A case study. *Ann Emerg Med* 19:891, 1990.
42. Durkin ME, Thiel CC, Schneider JE: Casualties and emergency medical response, in Tubbesing SK (ed): *The Loma Prieta, California, Earthquake of October 17, 1989: Loss Estimation and Procedures.* USGS professional paper 1553-A. Washington DC, US Government Printing Office, 1993, pp A9–A38.
43. Durkin ME, Thiel CC, Schneider JE, et al: Injuries and emergency medical response in the Loma Prieta earthquake. *Bull Seismol Soc Am* 81:2143, 1991.
44. Dhara RV: Health effects of the Bhopal gas leak: A review. *Arch Environ Health* 47:385, 1992.
45. Okumura T, Takasu N, Ishimatsu S, et al: Report on 640 victims of the Tokyo subway sarin attack. *Ann Emerg Med* 28:129, 1996.
46. Leonard RB: Planning EMS disaster response, in Roush WR (ed): *Principles of EMS Systems,* 2d ed. Dallas, American College of Emergency Physicians, 1994.
46a. Arnold C, Durkin M: *Hospitals and the San Fernando Earthquake of 1971: The Operational Experience.* San Mateo, CA: Building Systems Development, 1983.
47. Burkle FM, Sanner PH, Wolcott BW (eds): *Disaster Medicine.* New York, Medical Examination Publishing, 1984.
48. Hooft PJ, Noji EK, Van de Voorde HP: Fatality management in mass-casualty incidents. *Forensic Sci Int* 40:3, 1989.
49. Borak J, Callan M, Abbott W: *Hazardous Materials Exposure.* Englewood Cliffs, NJ, Brady, 1991.
50. Cashman JR: *Hazardous Materials Emergencies: Response and Control.* Lancaster, PA, Technomic Publishing, 1988.
51. Super G, Groth S, Hook R, et al: *START: Simple Triage and Rapid Treatment Plan.* Newport Beach, CA, Hoag Memorial Hospital Presbyterian, 1994.
52. Noji EK: Medical consequences of building collapse, in: *Proceedings of the International Symposium on the Forensic Aspects of Mass Disasters and Crime Scene Reconstruction, 23–29 June, 1990, FBI Academy, Quantico, Virginia.* Washington, DC, Federal Bureau of Investigation, Department of Justice, 1993, pp 97–108.
53. Barbera JA, Lozano M: Urban search and rescue medical teams: FEMA task force system. *Prehosp Disaster Med* 8:349, 1993.
54. Baskett P, Weller R: *Medicine for Disasters.* London, Wright, 1988.
55. Medical Disaster Response: Triage: START and SAVE, in Bade R (ed): *Medical Disaster Response Syllabus.* Dana Point, CA, Medical Disaster Response, 1995.
56. Koenig KL, Schultz CH: Disaster medicine: Advances in local catastrophic disaster response. *Acad Emerg Med* 1:133, 1994.
57. Noji EK: Medical and healthcare aspects of the 1988 earthquake in Soviet Armenia. *Earthquake Spectra special suppl:*101, 1989.
58. Brenner SA, Noji EK: Wound infections after tornadoes [letter]. *J Trauma* 33:643, 1992.
59. Oxtoby MJ, Broome CV, Pinzon MR: Late mortality in Nevado del Ruiz victims, in: *Disaster Chronicles No. 4: The Volcanic Eruption in Colombia, November 13, 1985.* Washington, DC, Pan American Health Organization, 1986, pp 144–160.
60. Noji EK: Prophylaxis of acute renal failure in traumatic rhabdomyolysis [letter]. *N Engl J Med* 323:550, 1990.
61. Oda Y, Shindoh M, Yukioka H, et al: Crush syndrome sustained in the 1995 Kobe, Japan, earthquake: Treatment and outcome. *Ann Emerg Med* 30:507, 1997.
62. Sandler SG: Strategies for blood management in mass casualty incidents, in Cowley RA (ed): *Proceedings of "Mass Casualties: A Lessons Learned Approach," 13–17 June, 1982.* Baltimore, Maryland Institute for Emergency Medical Services Systems, pp 229–234.
63. Lillibridge SA, Noji EK: The importance of medical records in disaster epidemiology research. *J Am Health Inf Manage Assoc* 63:137, 1992.
64. Churchill RE: Effective media relations, in Noji EK (ed): *The Public Health Consequences of Disasters.* New York, Oxford University Press, 1997, pp 122–132.
65. Waeckerle JF: The skywalk collapse: A personal response. *Ann Emerg Med* 12:651, 1983.
66. Mitchell J, Everly GS: *Critical Incident Stress Debriefing: An Operations Manual for the Prevention of Traumatic Stress among Emergency and Disaster Workers.* Ellicott City, MD, Chevron Publishing, 1993.
67. Linton JC, Kommor MJ, Webb CH: Helping the helpers: The development of a critical incident stress management team through university/community cooperation. *Ann Emerg Med* 22:663, 1993.
68. Gerrity ET: Critical incident stress debriefing (CISD): Value and limitations in disaster response. *Nat Cent PTSD Clin Q* 4:17, 1994.
69. Roth PB: Status of a national disaster medical response. *J Am Med Assoc* 266:1266, 1991.
70. Roth PB, Vogel A, Key G, et al: The St. Croix disaster and the National Disaster Medical System. *Ann Emerg Med* 20:391, 1991.
71. Waeckerle JF, Lillibridge SR, Burkle FM, Noji EK: Disaster medicine: Challenges for today. *Ann Emerg Med* 23:715, 1994.
72. SAEM Disaster Medicine White Paper Subcommittee: Disaster medicine: Current assessment and blueprint for the future. *Acad Emerg Med* 2:1068, 1995.
73. Scientific Committee of the International Society of Disaster Medicine: *Education and Training in Disaster Medicine: Curriculum.* Rijswijk, The Netherlands, Ministry of Health, 1992.
74. Noji EK: Core content development project. *ACEP Disaster Medicine Section News* 1:5, 1990.

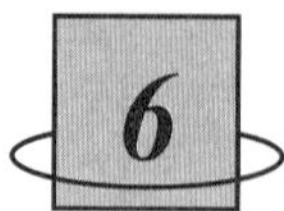

MASS GATHERINGS

Gregory D. Mears
Arthur H. Yancey II

Medical care for mass gatherings represents an intersection of emergency medicine with public health and public safety requiring working talents in business, logistics, disaster preparedness, telecommunications, and public relations. The ingredients for success lie in understanding the health and medical care of populations through systems.

Each year over 200,000,000 people show their support for their favorite sports team by attending an event affiliated with the National Basketball Association, the National Football League, major league baseball, the National Hockey League, National Collegiate Athletic Association division I college football and basketball, or National Association for Stock Car Auto Racing (NASCAR) (Table 6-1). Not included in these figures are the millions who attend high school athletics events, Olympic festivals, local and state fairs, music concerts, and religious, political, or professional gatherings.

A mass gathering is any collection of greater than 1000 people at one site or location. Although this definition specifies an exact number of people, many unique smaller gatherings have many of the same characteristics. Such gatherings include groups of people on commercial airliners, passenger trains, and offshore transportation modes, such as ferries or hydrofoils, and groups at other events that may be smaller but that create a situation where a large number of people are crowded into a limited area somewhat isolated from routine emergency medical services (EMS). The same treatment principles can often be applied in each of these settings. It is important for emergency physicians to understand the structure and organization of mass gatherings. It has been shown that these events are characterized by higher injury and illness rates than for the general population and create unique treatment and transportation dilemmas.

HISTORY

In 1965, two spectators collapsed and died in the University of Nebraska football stadium. Cardiopulmonary resuscitation (CPR) was not available. Based on the need to address this problem and the expanding philosophy at that time involving CPR, airway management and defibrillation were included in the emergency medical care provided for the stadium. In the 8 years that followed, 18 spectators developed a cardiac or pulmonary emergency. Of these, 9 experienced cardiac arrest. Eight of the 9 were successfully resuscitated and discharged from the hospital. Other specific experiences with medical care provided at mass gatherings have been reported by the Denver Mile High Stadium; the University of Arizona, Tucson; the 1984 Los Angeles and 1996 Atlanta Summer Olympic Games; the 1986 World's Exposition In Vancouver, British Columbia; the XV Winter Olympic Games in Calgary, Canada; the Indianapolis 500, the Carrier Dome at Syracuse University; and the 1982 US Rock Music Festival in Devore, California. Statistics generated from these events have shown an incidence of medical problems ranging from 0.12 to 6.00 per 1000 spectators and cardiac arrests ranging from 0.3 to 4.0 per 1,000,000 spectators. These numbers reflect the unique medical setting and indicate a need for a medical care plan and program in any mass gathering.

TABLE 6-1 Attendance at Major Sporting Events, 1997–1998 Season

Sport	No. of Events	Average Attendance per Event	Season Total Attendance
Major league baseball	2,430	28,000	68,040,000
National Basketball Association	1,189	17,135	20,373,079
National Football League	316	60,284	19,049,886
National Hockey League	1,066	16,196	17,264,678
National Association for Stock Car Auto Racing			
Winston Cup	32	190,335	6,091,356
All other series	233	46,223	10,769,935
National Collegiate Athletic Association			
Men's football division I	1,297	25,272	32,778,007
Men's basketball division I	4,265	5,459	23,282,774
Women's basketball division I	3,890	1,384	5,382,042
Totals	14,718		203,031,757

Source: Verbal communication with the individual organizations.

EVENT RECONNAISSANCE

Physical Setting

Preparation should begin with repeated reconnaissance of the event setting with respect to the event type and expected population. Will the participants be seated at a sports event in a stadium or a political rally at a convention center or arena, or will they be ambulatory at a golf or racecourse, an aviation exhibit, or a cross-country running, biking, or equestrian event? The mobility of the attendees has important implications for the population density and expected morbidity rate. At events where spectators are predominantly ambulatory, especially on irregular terrain, lower extremity trauma should be anticipated. Reports from both the 1984 Los Angeles and 1996 Atlanta Summer Olympics revealed the highest medical care use in venues where spectators moved about during the events.

Within the venue, the medical director must investigate the total geographic area of medical responsibility as well as the physical barriers to accessing potential patients. These factors can affect the ability to discover, locate, and extricate victims from a crowd as well as the ability to transport them to the most appropriate treatment site. Are there dedicated public safety ingress and egress routes adequate to handle anticipated medical needs? What is the estimated transport time to the nearest hospital for noncritical patients and the nearest appropriate facility for critical patients? These factors hold profound implications for both the number and expertise of medical care providers needed for the event as well as their mode of transportation within the venue.

Will the event be held indoors? Adequate ventilation and access to exits are important issues indoors and are usually specified by jurisdictional fire codes. If the event is outdoors, climatic exposure, access to shelter, and protection from indigenous species must be evaluated. In both settings, access to potable water, adequate numbers and distribution of restrooms, and the geographic range of the public address system must be investigated. The history of severe weather conditions during the time of the event should be researched in anticipation of resultant illness or injury, such as heat syndromes or hypothermia and frostbite.

Expected Populations and Hazardous Exposures

The event attendance bears some relationship to the expected volume of patients and has implications for the numbers and type of medical personnel needed. However, retrospective research has not yielded any universally acceptable mathematical relationship, and the exposure of the crowd to hazards at an event bears a much greater relationship to the volume of patients than does crowd size. In studying Syracuse University's rock concert, basketball, and football events for 7 years,

De Lorenzo found a correlation between crowd size and volume of patients only for the concerts. The duration of the event also correlates with the volume of patients through the duration of exposure to the event and population health risk factors. The 1982 US Rock Music Festival experienced a significant increase in the daily volume of patients on the second day of the 3-day event.

Therefore, investigating expected population characteristics and hazardous exposures is crucial to planning for their medical care. The expected density and range of ambulatory movement within a venue may foretell the risk of heat exhaustion. Will this event attract an older population at risk for sudden cerebrovascular and cardiovascular events or one in which a younger population will likely be exposed to street drugs? Children presenting the danger of separation from responsible adults can be tagged with identification upon entry to the event. Will alcohol be allowed and/or served, and, if so, what is the history of its effect on participants' behavior and health at previous and similar events? Will food be offered at the event, and, if so, what public health officials have responsibility for monitoring and enforcing its sanitation and disposal? Will VIPs (e.g., politicians, heads of state, diplomats, media personalities, corporate executives, etc.) participate, and, if so, what special health and medical care measures are planned? Who are the officials responsible for these measures?

INTERACTIONS

Plans for medical care must proceed simultaneously along interdisciplinary and intradisciplinary lines. Coordination with fire, rescue, and hazardous materials teams; public health departments; and law enforcement agencies and/or security providers is essential. What law enforcement agency and officials are responsible for precautions against terrorism and the coordinated response to it? What agency and officials are responsible for the jurisdictional disaster or multicasualty incident (MCI) plan? What is the communications path to officials responsible for initiating execution of the plan and what intravenue officials are in the decision tree to trigger the request?

Planning for mass gatherings must also consider the EMS services responsible for responding to 911 calls within the jurisdiction surrounding the venue. The patient transport capacity at which the service becomes saturated and needs to shift into an MCI mode of operation must be known or determined. The extra patient transport capacity afforded by any existing mutual aid agreements with other services should be examined. What potential patient capacities do the surrounding hospitals possess? Limited external medical facilities (e.g., in a rural setting) may force more advanced care to be performed on site, requiring more medical personnel at a higher level of expertise, more supplies, and intravenue facilities. Both the medical and administrative directors of potentially affected EMS and hospital emergency services should be repeatedly updated on medical care plans for the event.

RESPONSIBILITY FOR COVERAGE

The producer or promoter of any mass gathering has an obligation to provide for the safety and security of its participants, spectators, and workers. Few venues have enough regularly scheduled events to be able to provide medical care without assistance. This assistance is typically provided through an affiliation or contractual arrangement with an EMS system and/or a health care provider, such as a hospital. The goal of any venue should be to provide the same quality of health care and security one could reasonably expect as a normal citizen outside the venue.

The medical director plays a key role in the planning of the medical facility and the care it is to provide during a mass gathering. The medical director should be involved in the plan, setup, and maintenance of the medical facility and the selection, training, and function of each medical team member. This requires involvement not only in the event planning but, if possible, in the design and construction of the facility. The medical director's goal is to provide the best possible care within the constraints of the available resources. Early involvement of the medical director can only improve the amount and quality of the resources available at the event.

The licensing of all medical personnel is extremely important. Large events may be able to benefit from a "Good Samaritan law" permitting health care workers to practice outside their licensed state or jurisdiction. Such laws are typically useful only when the worker is practicing in a voluntary capacity. Any such legal ramifications should be investigated prior to the event. Unless a Good Samaritan law is in effect, all health care providers must be licensed to function as such during the event. Liability insurance is also extremely important to the medical director as well as the health care providers. The producer or promoter of an event may be able to obtain coverage for the medical care, or coverage may have to provided by the health care providers or their employers.

Several legal issues should be addressed in a contract with the producer of the event. A contract should allow the medical director to have the authority to obtain whatever supplies or resources are needed prior to and during the event. The contract should spell out who pays for the equipment, resources, and personnel. At a minimum, the contract should include start and end dates, fee structures, health department and medical license structures, equipment and personnel requirements, minimum medical care requirements, medical direction authority level, and emergency provisions for disasters or MCIs. As much detail as possible should be listed with respect to the size, location, and physical construction of the medical treatment facility; the transportation of patients and personnel; the lodging, parking, food, and hygiene provisions for personnel; and the communications system and devices.

ANATOMY OF A MEDICAL CARE SYSTEM

Planning

The first step in designing any medical care system is to determine the level of medical care that is needed or desired. Levels of care may be (1) transportation only, (2) basic life support (BLS) only, (3) treatment without transportation, (4) advanced life support (ALS), or (5) aggressive ALS care targeting cardiac arrest victims. The patient population must also be established; it may be participants or performers, spectators, or employees. As mentioned above, the goal of any medical care system should be the same as that of any EMS system: to provide the maximum care possible with the resources available. Spectators should receive the same quality of care that they would have received if they had not attended the event. This goal requires the system to be cooperative, adjustable, organized, intelligent, and prepared.

If possible, the design of a medical care system should be based on factors known to positively affect patients' outcomes. For instance, a response time of 3 to 5 min can positively influence the ability to successfully resuscitate a cardiac arrest victim. Rapid CPR (optimally, performed by a bystander) is the cornerstone of BLS care, and airway management and early defibrillation are the cornerstones of ALS care. These skills must be applied if positive outcomes are to be realized. Therefore, responders who are trained at least at a BLS level should be stationed within 5 min of anyone in the venue.

Medical personnel and supplies should be allocated based on the anticipated number of patients and the seriousness of the anticipated medical problems. As stated, a general estimate of patient volume is from 0.12 to 6.00 patients per 1000 spectators and 0.3 to 4.0 cardiac arrests per 1,000,000 spectators. The medical problems encountered at mass gatherings are often similar (Table 6-2). The volume of patients and the nature of their complaints can depend to a large degree on

TABLE 6-2 Common Presenting Complaints at Mass Gatherings

Complaint	Relative Frequency, %
TRAUMA	
Dermal injury	13.0–40.9
Eye injury	0.6–2.8
Foreign body	1.0–5.9
Head injury	0.6–2.0
Insect bites	0.3–3.8
Musculoskeletal	5.4–20.5
Other trauma	0.3–2.0
MEDICAL	
Abdominal pain	1.8–8.8
Alcohol or drug ingestion	0.4–4.0
Cardiac arrest	0.7–1.2
Chest pain	0.6–4.0
Dehydration	1.1
Diabetes	0.6–0.7
Dizziness	0.6–6.8
Epistaxis	0.6–4.0
Gastrointestinal	1.6–17.5
Headache	2.5–36.2
Heat- or cold-related	1.2–11.9
Hyper- or hypotension	0.3–1.7
Obstetrical or gynecologic	0.3–1.2
Other medical	1.8–44.9
Respiratory distress	0.4–13.7
Seizure	0.1–0.8
Syncope	0.2–9.7

the variables previously discussed. If possible, it is helpful to obtain preevent medical intelligence from the records of previous and/or similar events or from law enforcement agencies with experience with the particular event. This investigation may give insight to the potential for violence, alcohol, and drug use.

Patient Care Path

The medical care plan should address the entire flow of patients' care from the occurrence of the medical problem to definitive care. Ushers, volunteers, and security personnel should be equipped with adequate communications devices and trained to relay information concerning any individual in need of medical care. Those without communications devices should be informed of the location of the nearest security officer or device for contacting the command center. Training should include the ability to communicate the appropriate information in a clear, concise format. These individuals must also act as first responders in providing a path to the patient and, when necessary, providing bystander CPR.

The command center or dispatch center is responsible for coordinating the response to a medical incident. Provision of a clear, concise chief complaint to the center is vital to coordinating an appropriate response. The command center should provide all the necessary medical and security resources, including maintenance personnel to address plumbing and electrical mishaps. The command center is also responsible for the flexibility of personnel duties and the positioning of the response teams within the facility to provide the best response time.

Once a response team has been dispatched, they should respond and initiate patient care. This is best accomplished by the rapid extrication of the patient from the crowd to the nearest space (e.g., a tunnel or open entryway) isolated by security personnel. At this point, treatment can be initiated by protocol or with on-line medical direction. The amount of treatment provided at this time depends on the medical condition of the patient and the layout of the facility. Transport to a designated treatment site or ambulance should occur as soon as possible so that a specialist can provide care at the highest level appropriate to definitive treatment. Ideally, direct supervision by the medical director should be available. Staffing of the treatment facility can be variable, including nurses, physician assistants, emergency medical technicians, paramedics, Red Cross volunteers, medical students, or first responders.

Transportation from the event should be by the most efficient mode possible considering all factors. If no access roads are available, helicopter transport may be the most appropriate option. A medical care plan should integrate the local EMS system to allow for increased transport capabilities to external hospitals if needed. EMS units, in normal service within the community, can be dispatched to the designated sites of medical incidents at the facility or can replace a unit that is already transporting a patient to the hospital.

MEDICAL CARE RESOURCES

Personnel

Often events are staffed by a combination of paid personnel and volunteers. The number of personnel is based on the layout of the facility and the size and characteristics of the crowd, adequacy of EMS coverage, and proximity to adequate hospital facilities. These factors determine the level of intravenue care needed. Response teams should be located throughout the facility to keep response times within a 3- to 5-min time period. It is often very beneficial to couple security officers with medical personnel in order to provide a safer environment and quicker response. In special situations, it may be necessary to add others, such as firefighters or water rescuers, to the response team. Each response team should be efficiently staffed and equipped to easily transport a nonambulatory patient.

Treatment facilities should be staffed with personnel capable of delivering definitive emergency care. The number of patients and the medical complaint categories can be estimated based on the attributes previously discussed. It is the function of the medical director to determine how to best meet the demands of patient care within the budget of the facility. The expertise level of nonphysician personnel varies greatly. Their availability can have a direct impact on the number of physicians required. The number of physicians recommended for on-site care ranges from 1 for every 5000 to 1 for every 50,000 people. These staffing requirements should be part of a formal contract with the facility management.

Equipment

It is the responsibility of the medical director to determine the supply level and type of equipment to be used within the facility and to incorporate these specifications into both the contract and the medical care plan. Often this is dictated by the local EMS system, which provides equipment for the facility. Response teams should be equipped with basic airway and first aid equipment. The teams must also have adequate extrication and transportation devices based on the layout of the facility. In the event of a cardiac arrest, a defibrillator should be available to be sent to the location of the patient along with ALS personnel with advanced airway equipment. This may not be necessary if an intravenue treatment facility is within 3 to 5 min transport time under actual event conditions. The medical care system should have enough defibrillators to allow access to one from any location within the facility in 5 min or less.

Equipment within the treatment sites should be based on the level of care provided, the number of patients anticipated, and the length of time each patient would be required to stay at the site awaiting disposition or transportation. If not on-site, transportation should be established in the plan to have the capabilities of transporting the patient to a hospital within 30 min of the request.

Communications

Audio and visual communications represent the glue that joins not only the myriad medical care and surveillance components into an efficiently functioning system but also the venue health care system to the other systems vital to managing a mass gathering.

The spectator level presents the greatest challenge. The first "first responders" are always fellow performers or spectators. Upon entry to an event, they should be educated in how to communicate knowledge of an illness or injury to the venue's medical care system so that rapid assistance can be rendered. In preparation for the 1996 Olympics, health promotion brochures were mailed with ticket information. Concise information on ticket stubs accompanied by periodic public service announcements can serve the same purpose.

At the medical care system personnel level, every event official, from ushers, volunteers, security guards, and public relations personnel to the top rung of management, must be educated in and updated on the most expedient manner in which to obtain medical assistance. Because radios are expensive, for the most numerous event workers, usually ushers, alternatives such as flag systems have been devised. At the US Open tennis tournament, in New York, a flare system has been organized. All event personnel should know the venue location of the nearest official who has a radio.

Among those officials with radios, frequencies and/or "talk groups" (800 MHz trunking) can be organized to minimize interruptions and maximize effective radio traffic from incident discovery through responders to definitive care givers. At the most highly evolved events, discovery of a victim by the system usually proceeds from bystanders, ushers, or vendors to in-field security personnel to a central communications or command center where the event medical director is based. Venue surveillance cameras can augment verbal reports on the victim's location and can show the scope of the incident. The medical director can then select and radio-dispatch the nearest most appropriate responders with adequate security and/or public relations assistance. Event field providers must be able to communicate with dedicated event ambulance crews, venue medical facilities, and the medical director to coordinate the transportation of the patient from the incident site to the next most appropriate level of care. Fixed facility providers must be on line with field providers, event ambulance crews, and the medical director. The medical director must be able to communicate with all venue-dedicated ambulances, the jurisdictional 911 public safety answering point for access to the public EMS system, and those officials responsible for the jurisdictional disaster plan. In addition, medical command should have voice access to all area hospital emergency departments.

RELATIONSHIP OF FUNCTIONAL AREAS

Optimally, a central location should be designated for stationing the directors of the following functions: medical emergencies, event management, logistics, facility maintenance, public relations, security and law enforcement, ushers, and event performers or athletes. If not within the immediate area, the fire-rescue, public health, and public transportation and parking directors must be easily and reliably accessible by telephone and/or radio. From the medical care perspective, the leadership's close physical proximity is especially important if on-site care is provided, since such an arrangement allows for efficient information exchange and problem solving among the directors whose functional areas are integral to medical care delivery. A less reliable alternative involves intravenue radio links among the directors of these functional areas.

Internally, event management has to mediate issues at the interface of one functional area with another. Externally, event management represents the window with a view to outside resources, a vital function in the management of MCIs. Whenever depletion of operational resources is threatened, logistics personnel must immediately access and deliver additional equipment and supplies as patient demand dictates. The medical director and logistics supervisor must prospectively determine a threshold level for each essential supply item below which resupply is undertaken. The facility maintenance department has a major public health role in providing and maintaining an adequate potable water supply, sanitary facilities, and the venue electrical system vital to operating the public address system, air conditioning and ventilation, and lighting. Public relations plays a crucial role in directing crowd control and informing the event population of preventive public health measures as well as the location of medical care. Security and/or law enforcement personnel serve the entire spectrum of illness and injury prevention. Their primary preventative role includes pedestrian safety through the regulation of the interface of vehicular and pedestrian traffic, clearance of emergency vehicle access routes and pedestrian entrances and exits of the venue, and surveillance for and investigation of terrorist threats. The discovery of the ill or injured by direct sight or television surveillance, subsequent dispatch of medical care providers, and clearance of the path through crowds to patients represents the secondary preventative role of security and law enforcement personnel. They play a part in definitive care (tertiary prevention) when administering CPR or using automatic external defibrillators (AEDs). Similarly, ushers play a crucial role in the direct-sight discovery of victims and must know how to inform the predesignated personnel responsible for dispatching medical response teams. As with security and law enforcement personnel, their ubiquitous positioning makes ushers invaluable in the delivery of response-time-sensitive CPR. Finally, the event performers, whether they are athletes, politicians, musicians, or animals, represent a separate and distinct population requiring medical care specifically geared to their performance. The care of event performers is best provided by personnel most familiar with the performers' specific health care needs. When affordable, a separate medical care system and separate resources should be provided to ensure that care for performers does not interfere with care for spectators and vice versa.

QUALITY MANAGEMENT

Documentation

A medical record should be generated for each medical encounter, with the type of record based on the severity of the complaint. An officially sanctioned event form should be used to record the encounter date and time, patient's name, sex, age, race, medical complaint, drug allergies, and relevant medical history and examination findings. The tentative diagnosis and treatment plan should be documented, complete with discharge instructions. Because all patients provided ALS care will be transported to a hospital, the transporting EMS patient care report form can conveniently document the continuum of care provided at the scene and in transit.

As with every quality medical care system, treatment at mass gatherings should be evaluated systematically to improve care at subsequent events. The medical director should review all medical records. If the patient volume was large or included a MCI, a multidisciplinary audit committee should perform the review.

Event Training

Event training represents prospective quality management and puts into operation the aforementioned planned relationship of functional areas. Optimally, a representative of each of the personnel functions described under ''Relationship of Functional Areas'' should be represented at event training sessions held on site. However, especially with public safety, health, and medical care personnel, their regularly scheduled duties can be an obstacle to training participation. Possible alternatives for addressing this problem include videoconferencing and virtual reality applications. However, both of these modes preclude a realistic grasp of time-space relationships (e.g., patient access obstacles) that are facilitated by drills at the venue.

A central goal of event briefings must include instruction in the following venue locations: the command-center, medical care facilities, ambulance and radio-equipped security postings, and emergency ingress and egress routes. All personnel must know their geographic postings and coverage areas, receive instruction in communications equipment use, and practice the appropriate communications pathways to be used for medical care. Instruction in filling out a standardized medical care report form must be included. Practice scenarios should include a mock MCI requiring designation of ambulance staging and contingent triage zones and a request for outside intervention. Contingency plans for critical incident stress debriefing should be made and explained. Difficult access extrication, hyper- and/or hypothermia prevention and treatment, cardiac arrest, event player or performer injury, and dignitary or VIP care must also be rehearsed. Within each of these scenarios, communication (radio and cell phone) and physical routes to optimal care (ambulance evacuation to venue facility care) should be tested. Event briefings and training sessions should translate into efficient medical care. The retrospective aspect of the quality management process should detect this through instruments that document the quality of care (patient care report forms) and gauge the public image of care rendered at the event (patient-targeted surveys) and through management's degree of satisfaction with the results.

SPECIAL CONSIDERATIONS

Cardiac Arrests

As mentioned previously, the incidence of cardiac arrests in mass gatherings is higher than that in the normal population. It has been postulated that, due to the natural excitement generated by competitive sports, individuals who have cardiac disease are more likely to become symptomatic. However, medical systems at mass gatherings have demonstrated much higher success rates than even the most advanced EMS systems, primarily due to the ability to provide early bystander CPR, airway control, defibrillation, and ALS care. Survival rates for hospital discharge have varied from 20 to 100 percent survival from documented cardiac arrest. This evidence also supports the use of AEDs in mass gatherings where ALS support is not available in less than 5 min.

Commercial Airline In-Flight Emergencies

All US-commercial airlines are classified by federal law as ''common carriers,'' and, as such, the airlines are not required to provide passengers with emergency care that meets jurisdictional EMS standards. Because of the population density on airliners, many of the principles of mass gathering medical care apply.

The medical problems encountered on airlines occur with a frequency and in an organ system category type resembling those of populations at ground-level mass gatherings. For the calendar year 1996, an average of three in-flight medical emergencies per day occurred on one major US airline. An average of one life-threatening (i.e., asthma, choking, cardiac arrest, heart attack, loss of consciousness, or stroke) emergency occurred every 2.5 days. Nationally, data covering nine major US air carriers from 1991 to 1993 revealed that the most frequent (in decreasing order) complaints were neurologic, syncopal, cardiac, psychiatric, and respiratory. Intentional injury of crews by unruly passengers increased each year from 1993 to 1995, when 174 incidents were reported. The emergency rate (incidents per million enplanements) has increased each year from 1990 to 1993.

The airplane environment presents several unique aspects of medical emergencies and their treatment. Following discovery of a medical incident, the response time to on-board care is minimal. Care givers' access to victims is compromised by their seated position in a setting similar to that in a crowded stadium. The victim's safe, timely extraction to a secured space allowing the supine (left lateral decubitus for pregnant patients) position is a foremost priority but is a great challenge in such a confined environment not dedicated to even provisional medical care. Oxygen sources are plentiful, but their location is not configured for optimal care of patients. At cruising altitude, despite cabin pressurization, ambient air oxygen availability is below that at sea level (Po_2 118 mmHg in flight versus 159 mmHg at sea level) and has the potential of causing respiratory problems in the marginally compensated. Flight attendants receive basic first aid training to a degree that varies among airlines.

The uneven training of flight attendants leads to requests for emergency assistance from ''educated bystanders.'' National survey data reveal that from 1986 to1988, when all medical kit usage on the major air carriers was monitored, physicians responded in 85 percent of the 2322 cases. The US Department of Transportation mandated the study at the inauguration of its medical kit placement on board all commercial aircraft (Table 6-3). This kit places priority on airway, breathing, and circulation problems. Noticeably absent are aerosolized bronchodilators, anticonvulsants, and AEDs, the latter currently being placed and studied on some airlines.

When addressing the most frequent types of medical emergencies referred to above, as well as any involving vital functions, the issue of plane diversion arises. The desire to divert the aircraft stems from either the recognition that a patient is in immediate need of care and that expertise is not available on board or by radio, or the need for further evaluation of that condition. The decision to divert a commer-

TABLE 6-3 Medical Equipment on US Commercial Aircraft

Sphygmomanometer
Stethoscope
Oropharyngeal airways (3 sizes)
Syringes and needles
Dextrose (50%, 50 mL)
Diphenhydramine (2 ampules)
Epinephrine (1:1000, 2 ampules)
Nitroglycerin tablets (10)
Standard industry-type first aid kit

cial aircraft rests ultimately with the pilot. However, in 2321 cases representing 10.7 percent of all US domestic air carrier activity between 1990 and 1993, the crews complied with a physician's recommendation to divert 97 percent of the time. In addition to the time sensitivity of the patient's condition, this strategic decision involves issues of proximity to an airport suitable for the aircraft versus the original destination port, availability of adequate EMS resources (ALS versus BLS) to meet the diverted craft, and proximity of appropriate hospital resources to the diversion airport. Many US air carriers contract with in-flight medical consultation companies to assist crews and on-board medical personnel in making an appropriate diversion decision.

If the incidence of medical emergencies continues to increase, as it has from 1991 to 1993, on-board medical personnel will be called upon more frequently to become involved in patient care in this unique environment. On a more global scale, emergency physicians, by virtue of their expertise, should collaborate with the airlines to ensure optimal in-flight patient care.

BIBLIOGRAPHY

Baker WM, Simone BM, Niemann JT, et al: Special event medical care: The 1984 Los Angeles summer Olympics experience. *Ann Emerg Med* 15:185, 1986.

Bock HC, Cordell WH, Hawk AC, Bowdish GE: Demographics of emergency medical care at the Indianapolis 500 mile race (1983–1990). *Ann Emerg Med* 21:1204, 1992.

Carveth SW: Eight-year experience with a stadium-based mobile coronary-care unit. *Heart Lung* 3:770, 1974.

DeJohn CA, Veronneau SJH, Hordinsky JR: *In-Flight Medical Care: An Update.* Washington, US Dept of Transportation, Federal Aviation Administration, document DOT/FAA/AM-97/2, 1997.

De Lorenzo RA, Gray BC, Bennett PC, Lamparells VJ: Effect of crowd size on patient volume at a large multipurpose, indoor stadium. *J Emerg Med* 7:379, 1989.

Dubin GH: *Medical Care at Large Gatherings: A Manual Based on Experiences in Rock Concert Medicine.* Rockville MD, US Dept. of Health, Education, and Welfare Public Health Service, Alcohol, Drug Abuse, and Mental Health Admin., 1976.

Hordinsky JR, George MH: Response capability during civil air carrier in-flight medical emergencies. *Aviat Space Environ Med* 60:1211, 1989.

Illinois State Medical Society: *Guidelines for the Provision of Medical Care at Large-Scale Events. Chicago,* 1984.

Meehan P, Toomey KE, Drinnon J, et al: Public health response for the 1996 Olympic games. *JAMA* 279:1469, 1998.

Ounanian LL, Salinas C, Shear CL, Rodney WM: Medical care at the 1982 US Festival. *Ann Emerg Med* 15:520, 1986.

Pons PT, Holland B, Alfrey E, et al: An advanced emergency medical care system at National Football League games. *Ann Emerg Med* 9:203, 1980.

Sanders AB, Criss E, Steckl P, et al: An analysis of medical care at mass gatherings. *Ann Emerg Med* 15:515, 1986.

Spaite DW, Criss EA, Valenzuela TD, et al: A new model for providing prehospital medical care in large stadiums. *Ann Emerg Med* 17:825, 1988.

Speizer C, Rennie CJ, Brenton H: Prevalence of in-flight medical emergencies on commercial airlines. *Ann Emerg Med* 18:26, 1989.

Thompson JM, Savoia G, Powell G, et al: Level of medical care required for mass gatherings: The XV winter Olympic games in Calgary, Canada. *Ann Emerg Med* 20:385, 1991.

US Dept of Transportation, Federal Aviation Administration: Emergency Medical Equipment Final Rule 14CFR, parts 11 and 121. *Fed Regist* January 9, 1986.

Weaver WD, Sutherland K, Wirkus MJ, et al: Emergency medical care requirements for large public assemblies and a new strategy for managing cardiac arrest in this setting. *Ann Emerg Med* 18:155, 1989.

Wetterhall SF, Coulombier DM, Herndon JM, et al: Medical care delivery at the 1996 Olympic games. *JAMA* 279:1463, 1998.

RESUSCITATIVE PROBLEMS AND TECHNIQUES

SUDDEN CARDIAC DEATH

Joseph P. Ornato

Sudden cardiac death (SCD) due to unexpected cardiac arrest claims the lives of an estimated 250,000 adult Americans each year. Despite advances in resuscitation and emergency medical services (EMS), only about 3 to 8 percent of all cardiac arrest victims survive to leave the hospital neurologically intact. However, there is substantial variability in the odds for survival among various geographic locations, with published survival to hospital discharge for patients with all initial rhythms ranging from 1 to 25 percent.[1–3] This chapter reviews the epidemiology and pathophysiology of SCD in adults and the strategies to prevent and treat the problem. Sudden infant death syndrome and cardiac arrest in children are discussed in Chaps. 9 and 10, respectively.

EPIDEMIOLOGY

Most episodes of unexpected SCD in adults occur in the home.[4] The most common victim is a male who is 50 to 75 years of age. The majority of SCD victims have underlying structural heart disease, usually in the form of coronary atherosclerosis and/or cardiomegaly. Although 75 percent of SCD victims have significant atherosclerotic narrowing (greater than 75 percent) in one or more major coronary arteries, fewer than half of all sudden deaths occur *during* an acute myocardial infarction (AMI).

Epidemiologic studies have identified both a circadian and a seasonal pattern of SCD and AMI, suggesting the presence of underlying biological triggers of the onset of both disease processes.[5] Both SCD and AMI are most likely to occur within the first few hours after awakening from sleep, at a time when there is increased sympathetic stimulation. Beta blockade appears to protect against SCD, particularly in patients with known coronary artery disease who have had an AMI. In addition, both SCD and AMI are much more likely to occur during climatic winter rather than summer.[5,6] These and other epidemiologic and experimental findings suggest that neurophysiologic factors, such as autonomic tone, may alter the heart's propensity to develop and sustain a serious ventricular dysrhythmia. An alternative possibility is that there are factors external to the atherosclerotic plaque, such as triggers of plaque rupture or thrombus formation, which may affect the onset of ischemic cardiac events.

PATHOPHYSIOLOGY

Ventricular Tachyarrhythmias

Sudden cardiac death is usually caused by chance arrhythmic events that are triggered by an interaction between structural heart abnormalities and transient, functional electrophysiologic disturbances. In the majority of cases the initiating event is a ventricular tachyarrhythmia, either pulseless ventricular tachycardia (VT) that degenerates rapidly to ventricular fibrillation (VF) or "primary" VF.[7,8] From a public health standpoint, strategies for preventing and treating SCD in the community can be targeted primarily at VT and VF because these rhythms are not only the most frequent, but also the most potentially treatable, currently identified initiating event.

The mechanisms responsible for triggering fatal ventricular dysrhythmias are only partially understood. Frequent ventricular ectopy alone, in the absence of significant underlying structural heart disease, does not generally result in cardiac arrest. However, ventricular extrasystoles in the presence of transient myocardial ischemia, left ventricular dysfunction, and/or cardiomegaly often trigger runs of VT that may degenerate into pulseless VT or VF.

Many types of structural heart disease can predispose to SCD. One common denominator is dispersion of ventricular depolarization and/or repolarization, allowing "islands" of ventricular tissue to depolarize and repolarize at different rates. This lack of homogeneity in electrical activation and recovery fosters the development of circus movement reentry, which can initiate and sustain ventricular tachyarrhythmias. Myocardial ischemia and/or infarction can also transiently diminish the homogeniety of left ventricular depolarization and repolarization.

Left ventricular hypertrophy (often due to hypertension and/or valvular heart disease) or conduction disturbances (left or right bundle branch block or a nonspecific intraventricular conduction disturbance) can create similar functional disturbances on a more chronic basis. An example of this SCD mechanism is the mysterious illness that causes death during sleep in young Asian (especially Thai) men who have no evidence of structural heart disease.[9] Many of these men have an abnormal cardiac conduction system that can be diagnosed by electrophysiologic testing. It is interesting to note that many of these Asian men who are at risk of SCD can be identified from a standard electrocardiogram (ECG), which shows a characteristic pattern of right bundle branch block with ST-segment elevation in $V_{1\text{-}3}$.

The long QT syndrome, in which the corrected QT interval is pathologically prolonged, is also associated with SCD.[10] Prolongation of the corrected QT interval probably represents dispersion in ventricular repolarization and can be congenital (with or without nerve deafness) or acquired (due to hypokalemia, hypomagnesemia, hypocalcemia, anorexia, ischemia, central nervous system pathology, terfenadine-ketoconazole combinations, or certain antipsychotic or antiarrhythmic drugs). The "corrected QT interval" can be calculated easily by the following formula:

$$QT_c = \frac{QT_m}{\sqrt{R\text{–}R}}$$

where QT_c is the corrected QT interval in seconds, QT_m is the measured QT interval in seconds, and R–R is the interval between any two consecutive R waves on the ECG in seconds. This formula, known as Bazett's equation, while seeming to be complex, is actually quite simple and easy to remember. Since the QT interval is heart rate dependent, the formula "corrects" the measured QT interval to a heart rate of 60 beats per minute (at which the R–R interval is 1.0 s). Since the square root of 1 = 1, the QT_c equals the QT_m at a heart rate of 60 beats per minute (at which the normal QT interval limits are 0.35 to 0.44 s).

Most SCD victims have cardiac abnormalities on postmortem examination. The most common autopsy findings in SCD victims are evidence of coronary atherosclerosis and its complications, cardiomegaly with left ventricular hypertrophy and contraction band necrosis. The latter appears to be a marker for catecholamine stimulation and occurs with high frequency regardless of whether cardiopulmonary resuscitation (CPR) was performed.[11]

Factors affecting survival of out-of-hospital VF include witnessed collapse, prompt initiation of CPR, early defibrillation, younger age, and arrest occurring away from home.[12] Comorbid illnesses, such as a history of congestive heart failure, contribute to hospital mortality following successful resuscitation but only account for one-fourth of the variation in survival from SCD. Cardiac arrest during AMI is associated with a significantly *improved* outcome compared to cases not occuring in the setting of AMI.[13] Although the reason for improved long-term survival of AMI patients is not fully known, it is probably due to the fact that such patients have *transient* electrical instability, unlike patients with chronic cardiomyopathy, in whom there is a persistent vulnerability to VT or VF.

The outcome of resuscitation is strongly influenced by the patient's initial cardiac rhythm. The likelihood of survival is relatively high (up to 40 to 60 percent) if the initial rhythm is VT or VF (particularly if the VF is "coarse," the arrest was witnessed, and prompt CPR and defibrillation are provided). If the initial rhythm is not VT or VF, survival is typically less than 5 percent in most reported series. Asystolic patients whose cardiac arrest was unwitnessed rarely survive neurologically intact to hospital discharge. The only common exceptions are witnessed cardiac arrest patients whose initial asystole is due to increased vagal tone or other relatively easily correctible factors, such as hypoxia of brief duration.

Bradyasystole

Although this chapter emphasizes VT and VF, an important minority of SCD events begin with a bradyarrhythmia[14] or an organized rhythm without a pulse (e.g., pulseless electrical activity, or PEA). Bradyasystole refers to a cardiac rhythm that has a ventricular rate below 60 beats per minute in adults and/or periods of absent heart rhythm (asystole). Bradyasystolic states are clinical situations during which bradyasystole is the dominant heart rhythm.

Bradyasystolic rhythms other than asystole can either be accompanied by a pulse or there can be no discernible pulse with each QRS (PEA). Bradyasystole with a pulse is often accompanied by a significant decrease in cardiac output, leading to hypotension and/or syncope. Bradycardia with or without a pulse occurs frequently during cardiac arrest, either as the initial rhythm, during the course of resuscitation, or following electrical defibrillation. Obviously, asystole occurs eventually in all dying patients.

Ewy et al.[15] have shown that electrically induced coarse VF in dogs can have a direction or vector. When recordings are made using an ECG lead perpendicular to the main axis of the coarse fibrillation in experimental models, tracings show what appears to be asystole or fine VF. To ensure that VF is not masquerading as asystole, the American Heart Association recommends confirmation of asystole by switching to another lead whenever a "flat line" is recorded on the ECG during resuscitation. Although there are anecdotal case reports in the literature suggesting that this phenomenon can occur in humans, "masquerading" VF probably occurs rarely during clinical resuscitation and is not responsible for the misdiagnosis of large numbers of cases of asystole.[16]

Bradyasystole can be either primary or secondary. Primary bradyasystole occurs when the heart's electrical system intrinsically fails to generate and/or propagate an adequate number of ventricular depolarizations per minute to sustain consciousness and other vital functions. Secondary bradyasystole is present when factors external to the heart's electrical system cause it to fail (e.g., hypoxia). It is unclear why conventional treatment of bradyasystolic cardiac arrest with atropine, epinephrine, or electrical pacemakers rarely results in survival to hospital discharge.

Cellular metabolic functions must be intact for normal electrical impulse generation and propagation to occur. Severe ischemia of the sinoatrial (SA) node can disable cellular metabolism, preventing pacemaker cells from actively transporting the ions necessary to control the transmembrane action potential. Proximal occlusion of the right coronary artery (RCA) can cause ischemia and/or infarction of both the SA and atrioventricular (AV) nodes, since the SA node is supplied by a branch from the proximal RCA 55 percent of the time and the AV node receives its nourishment from a branch of the distal RCA 90 percent of the time. Ischemia or infarction of the AV node can disrupt normal conduction, causing bradycardia due to AV block. Because the bundle branches receive their blood supply from multiple coronary arteries, bradyasystole caused by ischemic bilateral bundle branch block is rare and generally only occurs when there is extensive myocardial infarction due to severe, multivessel coronary artery disease.

The spectrum of disorders affecting the heart's primary pacemaker, known as the sick sinus syndrome, can cause intermittent lightheadedness, syncope, or SCD. The disorder affects both men and women. Although it is more common with advancing age, primary electrical failure of the heart can even occur in infants and children. The precise cause of sick sinus syndrome is unknown. Pathologic studies usually reveal histologic degeneration of the SA node. In addition, the disorder often involves the AV node and the conduction tissue between the SA and AV nodes. Thus, sick sinus syndrome should be thought of as a diffuse degenerative disease of the heart's electrical generation and conduction system. Idiopathic sclerodegeneration of the AV node and the bundle branches (Lenegre's disease) or invasion of the conduction system by fibrosis or calcification spreading from adjacent cardiac structures (Lev's disease) can lead to bradyasystolic heart block with or without cardiac arrest. In rare cases, a clinical presentation resembling the sick sinus syndrome can occur when the heart's electrical system is affected by systemic disease, vascular compromise, or tumor (e.g., melanoma metastatic to the AV node).

Atropine, transcutaneous pacing, dopamine, or epinephrine can be used to treat acute, symptomatic bradyasystole (including cardiac arrest) that is due to the sick sinus syndrome. Permanent ventricular or AV sequential pacing is usually necessary for patients with persistent symptomatic bradycardia. Patients who manifest the tachycardia-bradycardia variant (periods of supraventricular tachycardia followed by prolonged sinus arrest or bradycardia) may also require antiarrhythmic therapy or radiofrequency ablation.

Pacemaker cells and conducting tissue can be affected by a variety of endogenous chemical, hormonal, pharmacologic, toxicologic, and neurogenic influences. Hypoxia and hypercarbia due to respiratory arrest cause bradyasystole frequently, due to both a direct depressant effect on cardiac pacemaker cells and increased parasympathetic discharge. Common clinical conditions that often cause bradyasystole include suffocation, near drowning, stroke, and opiate overdose. Beta-adrenergic blocking agents, calcium channel blockers, digitalis glycosides, parasympathomimetic agents (e.g., edrophonium), hypoxia, hypercarbia, adenosine, and adenosine triphosphate can also cause bradyasystole.

Endogenous adenosine that is released when there is myocardial hypoxia and ischemia relaxes vascular smooth muscle, decreases atrial and ventricular contractility, depresses pacemaker automaticity, and impairs AV conduction. During normal aerobic metabolism, adenosine is formed primarily by intracellular degradation of S-adenosylhomocysteine (SAH), catalyzed by the enzyme SAH hydrolase (SAH pathway). During myocardial ischemia, adenosine is formed primarily by dephosphorylation of adenosine monophosphate (AMP), catalyzed by the enzyme 5′ nucleotidase (adenosine triphosphate [ATP] pathway).

The cellular electrophysiologic effects of adenosine can be antagonized competitively by methylxanthines but not by atropine. A specific adenosine antagonist (BW-A1433U) has been shown to reverse and prevent postdefibrillation bradyasystole and hemodynamic depression in a domestic pig model. In small pilot studies, aminophylline, a competitive nonspecific adenosine antagonist, restored cardiac electrical activity within 30 s in more than half of the bradyasystolic cardiac arrest patients who were refractory to atropine and epinephrine.[17,18]

Myocardial ischemia excites cardiac vagal and sympathetic afferents, leading to vagally mediated depressor reflexes and/or sympathetic reflex cardioexcitation. In addition, myocardial infarction can interrupt afferent and efferent neural transmission, potentially triggering dysrhythmias. Autonomic disturbances have been documented in the majority of AMI patients, especially during the first 30 to 60 min after coronary artery occlusion. Stimulation of afferent vagal cardiac receptors, particularly those located in the posterior left ventricle, during ischemia or infarction can trigger sympathetic inhibition, vasodilation, bradycardia, and hypotension (the Bezold-Jarisch reflex). Activation of this reflex may explain the higher incidence of nausea and vomiting in patients with inferior (69 percent) compared to anterior (29 percent) infarction. Bradyasystole triggered by the Bezold-Jarisch reflex is usually short-lived and often responds to atropine.

One of the most baffling mysteries of bradyasystolic cardiac arrest relates to myocardial mechanics. Bradyasystole, unlike ventricular fibrillation, is accompanied by very little myocardial oxygen consumption in animal models. Because of this, myocardial high-energy phosphate stores should decay relatively slowly during bradyasystole. This should theoretically result in a high incidence of return of spontaneous circulation following restoration of a more normal rhythm (e.g., with the early use of electrical pacing). However, return of spontaneous circulation is infrequent, and long-term neurologically intact survival is rare in bradyasystolic cardiac arrest.

These findings strongly suggest that other factors must play a determining role in the pathophysiology and subsequent outcome of bradyasystolic cardiac arrest. Bradyasystolic arrest is not just a disorder of rhythm generation or propagation: it is a perplexing syndrome characterized by such rhythm disturbances accompanied, in many cases, by profound depression of myocardial and vascular function. The causes of the latter derangements have yet to be elucidated. Suspected causes include endogenous myocardial depressants (including downregulation of catecholamine receptors and/or toxic influences of intense sympathetic stimulation), neurogenic influences, postischemic myocardial stunning, and/or free radical injury.

Pulseless Electrical Activity

Pulseless electrical activity can be caused by a variety of pathophysiologic conditions. The sine qua non of this syndrome is the presence of an organized rhythm without the presence of a detectable pulse in an individual who is clinically in cardiac arrest. The latter is important to differentiate conditions in which the rescuer is unable to detect a pulse but there is unmistakable evidence that there is adequate blood pressure and cardiac output to maintain vital organ perfusion (e.g., a conscious patient with profound vasoconstriction due to hypothermia). There is evidence that PEA encompasses a spectrum of pathophysiologic effects ranging from good LV function with an empty ventrical or widely dilated arterial bed, to a stiff ventrical.

The underlying physiologic cause of PEA is a marked reduction in cardiac output that is due to either profound myocardial depression or mechanical factors that reduce venous return or impede the flow of blood through the cardiovascular system. Common conditions that can cause PEA are shown in Table 7-1. In one recent analysis, PEA was present initially during resuscitation in 22 percent of cardiac arrest cases.[19] Compared to other patients, individuals with PEA were more likely to be women whose cardiac arrest was unwitnessed, at night, and without bystander-initiated CPR. Only 2 percent of these patients survived to hospital discharge. The management of patients with PEA is directed at identifying and treating the underlying cause or causes.

TABLE 7-1 Common Causes of Pulseless Electrical Activity

Hypovolemia
Tension pneumothorax
Pericardial tamponade
Pulmonary embolism
Massive myocardial dysfunction due to infarction, ischemia, myocarditis, toxic myocardial depressants
Profound shock of any cause
Hypoxia
Acidosis
Severe hypercarbia

SCD PREVENTION

Prediction of SCD

It is necessary to accurately predict who is at risk for SCD for any prevention strategy to be of value. Unfortunately, the majority of future SCD victims cannot be identified in advance. Prodromal symptoms in the days to weeks preceding cardiac arrest are common but usually too nonspecific to be of important predictive value. In one of the largest series in which survivors of SCD were questioned about events preceding their collapse, Goldstein et al.[20] found that 71 percent of SCD survivors reported no prodromal symptoms or symptoms of 1 h or less in duration. Prodromal symptoms were present for more than 1 h in only 29 percent of patients. The most common symptoms reported by SCD survivors or family members of SCD victims are chest pain, dyspnea, and palpitations.

Even aggressive attempts to predict SCD in high-risk patients, such as those who have suffered a prior AMI or those with a chronic cardiomyopathy, have been of limited value. Various diagnostic techniques have been used to try to ''risk-stratify'' these patients, including invasive and noninvasive assessment of left ventricular ejection fraction, coronary angiography, ambulatory ECG (Holter) monitoring, exercise testing, detection of ventricular late potentials using signal averaging, programmed ventricular stimulation of the heart to test the inducibility of ventricular tachydysrhythmias, and assessment of heart rate variability.[21] None of these tests, alone or in combination, has sufficient sensitivity and specificity to identify more than a small fraction of those who will develop SCD. For example, only 15 to 30 percent of even ''high-risk'' post-AMI patients identified by a variety of these screening tests will experience a sustained ventricular tachydysrhythmia over the next several years of follow-up.[22]

Antidysrhythmic Drug Therapy

Although both an underlying substrate (cardiac pathology) and a trigger (a ventricular extrasystole) are commonly needed to initiate VT or VF, recent results of large randomized, controlled, clinical trials of antidysrhythmic agents for primary and secondary prevention of VT and VF are changing traditional beliefs regarding the actions, efficacy, and risk of antidysrhythmic agents. For example, it once seemed reasonable to expect that class I sodium channel blocking drugs (e.g., quinidine, procainamide, encainide, flecainide, and moricizine) that effectively suppress premature ventricular beats should reduce the risk of SCD. To test this theory, the Cardiac Arrhythmia Suppression Trial (CAST) was conducted to determine whether potent class I sodium channel blocking antidysrhythmic drugs are effective in preventing SCD in post-AMI patients compared to placebo. The trial had to be terminated prematurely because each of the antidysrhythmic agents tested (encainide, flecainide, and moricizine) paradoxically *increased* the odds of developing SCD, compared to placebo, in patients at relatively low risk for death in the long term.[23] The excess mortality in this trial was due to proarrhythmic effects of the type I drugs, resulting in a *facilitation* of reentry, especially during acute ischemia.

Antidysrhythmic drugs with class III and/or beta-blocking activity may be of some value in protecting patients at high risk of SCD. In the randomized, double-blind, placebo-controlled European Myocardial Infarct Amiodarone Trial (EMIAT), the type III antidysrhythmic drug amiodarone reduced all-cause mortality (primary endpoint) and cardiac mortality/dysrhythmic death (secondary endpoints) in survivors of myocardial infarction who had a left ventricular ejection fraction of less than 40 percent.[24] The Cardiac Arrest in Seattle: Conventional Versus Amiodarone Drug Evaluation (CASCADE) study evaluated antidysrhythmic drug therapy in VT and VF survivors who were thought to be at high risk for VT or VF recurrence. Therapy with empirical amiodarone was compared to therapy with other antidysrhythmic agents as guided by electrophysiologic testing and/or Holter recording. Survival was better in patients treated with amiodarone than in patients treated with other antidysrhythmic agents. Patients treated with amiodarone were less likely to receive a shock from an implanted defibrillator, and syncope followed by a shock from a defibrillator was less common in patients treated with amiodarone. However, overall mortality was high, and side effects of therapy were common. Patients treated with amiodarone, even at the low doses used in the study, were still at risk for thyroid dysfunction (both hyperthyroidism and hypothyroidism) and for pulmonary toxicity. The combined class II/III agent sotalol has also been shown to be better at reducing VT and VF recurrence than are conventional class I antidysrhythmic agents.[25]

Class II (beta-blocking drugs) also appear to offer some protection against SCD, particularly in patients with myocardial ischemia or prior AMI.[26] These agents probably exert their protective effects by reducing the risk of VT and VF during myocardial ischemia and following AMI by direct suppression of adrenergic myocardial stimulation, decreasing the rate of atheroma formation, directly suppressing the influence of the central nervous system on ventricular tachydysrhythmias, and preventing or attenuating fracture of vulnerable atherosclerotic plaques. In addition, beta blockers reduce morbidity and may even lower mortality in patients suffering from moderate to severe heart failure.[27] In these patients, careful titration of the drug dosage may be necessary.

Implantable Cardioverter Defibrillator Therapy

The benefits of beta blockade, sotalol, and amiodarone in decreasing mortality from SCD pale in comparison to the protective effects of the implantable cardioverter defibrillator (ICD) on high-risk patients.[28] The results of recent studies indicate that treatment with an ICD is more effective than electrophysiologically guided treatment with antidysrhythmic agents.[29] Although these devices are expensive to insert, their effectiveness over conventional therapy results in a cost of less than $30,000 per year of life saved, which is highly cost-effective.[30] At present, these devices are indicated for preventing SCD in high-risk patients, particularly those with clinically significant coronary artery disease, depressed left ventricular function, and spontaneous life-threatening and/or inducible ventricular dysrhythmias. Further research is necessary to determine the value of ICD therapy in patients with nonischemic cardiomyopathy accompanied by reduced left ventricular function.

RESCUE FROM SCD

Emergency medical services and in-hospital resuscitation (also known as code blue or code 99) systems are the most effective means currently known to rescue patients from SCD. Survival from pulseless VT or VF is inversely related to the time interval between its onset and its termination. Each minute that a patient remains in VF, the odds of survival decrease by 7 to 10 percent. Survival is optimal when both CPR and advanced cardiac life support (ACLS), including defibrillation and drug therapy, are provided early.

The American Heart Association has introduced the ''chain of survival'' concept to represent a sequence of events that ideally should occur to maximize the odds of successful resuscitation from cardiac arrest.[8] The links in the chain include early access (recognition of the problem and activation of the EMS system by a bystander), early CPR, early defibrillation for patients who need it, and early advanced cardiac life support.

Early Access

Because most SCDs occur suddenly and without warning, the victim cannot activate the emergency response system prior to collapse. Bystanders who witness the event can improve a victim's chances for survival significantly by alerting the emergency response system promptly. All too often, the untrained citizen only further delays treatment by attempting to inform relatives, call the neighbors, or contact the patient's personal physician instead of calling the local community emergency telephone number (in most places, it is 911).

Early CPR

Public CPR education can improve the behavior of bystanders significantly when a cardiac emergency occurs in the community. Availability of the simple three-digit 911 emergency number in the United States can reduce confusion and decrease delay in activating the EMS system. There are a number of problems associated with training the public to perform CPR. For example, it can be argued that the wrong rescuers have been trained. The typical cardiac arrest victim is male, is 50 to 75 years old, and usually arrests at home, often in the presence of a spouse of similar age. Most citizens who have taken CPR training are under 30 years of age; typically, fewer than 10 percent live with family members known to have heart disease. Most citizens who have received CPR training never actually witness or participate in managing a cardiac arrest; conversely, bystanders who witness a cardiac arrest usually do not know how to perform CPR. The majority of laypersons who attempt to perform CPR out of hospital are actually employed or volunteer their services as health professionals. The best solution to the problem is to target CPR training to ''high-risk'' individuals, such as middle-aged persons, senior center residents and staff, and family members (particularly the spouse) of patients who are survivors of AMI or cardiac arrest or who have other risk factors for SCD.

Skill retention is also a problem because CPR is a psychomotor technique that deteriorates rapidly over time unless practiced or used. In Belgium, 46 percent of bystanders who performed CPR forgot to perform mouth-to-mouth breathing; chest compressions were not done 17 percent of the time.[31] It is important for laypersons or health care professionals who perform CPR infrequently to receive at least annual reinforcement. However, only about 20 percent of trainees return for annual training in the United States. Irrational fear of communicable disease, particularly infection with the human immunodeficiency virus (HIV), that is disproportionate to the known minimal risk of disease transmission may decrease the likelihood that trained rescuers will actually perform mouth-to-mouth ventilation on strangers.[32]

Although the value of bystander CPR was once debatable, virtually all recent studies have shown that early initiation of CPR by a bystander improves survival from cardiac arrest significantly, and it also results in improved neurologic outcome of survivors.[8] The presumed mechanism by which CPR by a bystander improves outcome is the preservation of flow to the heart, brain, and other vital organs, providing a ''holding action'' until other therapies (e.g., defibrillation) can result in restoration of spontaneous circulation.

Early Defibrillation

The rationale for the use of early defibrillation stems from four observations: (1) ventricular tachydysrhythmias are the most common cause of SCD in adults; (2) defibrillation is the most effective treatment for VT and VF; (3) the effectiveness of defibrillation diminishes rapidly over time; and (4) unless treated promptly, VF becomes less coarse and eventually converts to the less treatable rhythm of fine VF or asystole.

The best outcomes from VT and VF in adults occur regularly in the electrophysiology laboratories, where prompt defibrillation (typically within 20 to 30 s of dysrhythmia onset) from pulseless VT or VF results in virtually 100 percent survival. The next best outcomes have been noted in cardiac rehabilitation programs, where defibrillation can be performed within the first minute or two. In such "ideal" settings, as many as 85 to 90 percent of patients are resuscitated and return to their prearrest neurologic status. Survival from out-of-hospital VT and VF treated by police officers equipped with automatic external defibrillators (AEDs) in Rochester, Minnesota, has averaged 50 percent, with a median time from collapse to defibrillation of about 5 min. Outcomes in many locations with EMS systems that cannot provide defibrillation until 10 min or more after a patient's collapse typically yield survival rates of less than 10 percent.[8]

The best survival is attained in EMS systems that can provide early defibrillation to a large percentage of patients. In most cases, this is most cost-effectively accomplished by a tiered response system, in which large numbers of rapid first-response firefighters or emergency medical technicians (EMTs) are trained and equipped to provide first aid, CPR, and early defibrillation using an AED. Unfortunately, not all communities in the United States have yet implemented a comprehensive, tiered EMS system. Many systems, particularly in suburban or rural areas, have EMTs who are neither trained nor equipped to defibrillate. For such areas, adding rapid defibrillation capability offers a cost-effective alternative that can significantly improve survival from out-of-hospital VF or pulseless VT.

The American Heart Association advocates the widespread implementation of rapid defibrillation programs throughout the nation in its belief that "all emergency personnel should be trained and permitted to operate an appropriately maintained defibrillator if their professional activities require that they respond to persons experiencing cardiac arrest. This includes all first responding emergency personnel, both hospital and nonhospital (e.g., emergency medical technicians (EMTs), non-EMT first responders, fire fighters, volunteer emergency personnel, physicians, nurses, and paramedics). To further facilitate early defibrillation, it is essential that a defibrillator be immediately available to emergency personnel responding to a cardiac arrest. Therefore, all emergency ambulances and other emergency vehicles that respond to or transport cardiac patients should be equipped with a defibrillator."[33]

More novel strategies have also been tried to increase the availability of rapid defibrillation in the community. There are many densely populated public areas in which conventional EMS systems *cannot* respond within an acceptable response time interval. The most innovative idea is termed *public access defibrillation* (PAD), so named because the intent is to have citizens from outside the health care fields perform early defibrillation using AEDs.

There are four "levels" of PAD based on the type of potential first responder expected to use the AED (Table 7-2). There has been considerable experience demonstrating benefit with minimal risk for level I (firefighters) and level II (police officers and airline flight attendants) first responders.[34–36] Other experimental approaches to rapid defibrillation in the workplace include use in British rail stations, oil platforms in the North sea, electricity plants, passenger cruise ships, and merchant marine vessels.[8] There has been little experience thus far with level III PAD, and the few studies that have been reported have been somewhat disappointing. For example, Eisenberg et al. trained family members of 59 patients who had survived out-of-hospital cardiac arrest in King County, Washington.[37] Only 6 of the 10 cardiac arrests that occurred in these patients were defibrillated successfully, and only 1 patient survived for a few months and sustained new neurologic impairment. Since AEDs are currently approved for marketing in United States under prescription only, there has been no experience thus far with level IV PAD.

TABLE 7-2 Levels of Public Access Defibrillation

Level	Personnel
1	Traditional first responders who have a duty to respond (firefighters)
2	Nontraditional first responders who have a secondary duty to respond (police, lifeguards, security officers, flight attendants)
3	Trained citizen CPR providers who volunteer to be trained to respond (building supervisors, family members of high-risk individuals)
4	Minimally trained or untrained lay witnesses who may try to respond (laypersons in the right place at the right time)

Early ACLS

Physicians provide prehospital ACLS by staffing specially equipped ambulances in many countries (e.g., western Europe, Scandinavia, and Canada). In the United States, "intermediate"-level EMTs or paramedics provide most prehospital ACLS intervention (e.g., defibrillation or synchronized cardioversion, endotracheal intubation, intravenous fluid therapy, or drug administration). Intermediate EMTs (often called cardiac technicians) typically receive several hundred hours of training; paramedics usually receive 1000 or more hours. Adding field ACLS capability appears to affect survival from out-of-hospital cardiac arrest favorably, although the degree of benefit is relatively minimal compared to the powerful effect of early defibrillation.[8]

REFERENCES

1. Lombardi G, Gallagher J, Gennis P: Outcome of out of hospital cardiac arrest in New York City: The Pre-Hospital Arrest Survival Evaluation (PHASE) Study. *JAMA* 271:678–683, 1994.
2. Becker LB, Ostrander MP, Barrett J, et al: Outcome of CPR in a large metropolitan area: Where are the survivors? *Ann Emerg Med* 20:355–361, 1991.
3. Eisenberg MS, Howard BT, Cummins RO, et al: Cardiac arrest and resuscitation: A tale of 29 cities. *Ann Emerg Med* 19:179–186, 1990.
4. Becker L, Eisenberg M, Fahrenbruck C, Cobb L: Public locations of cardiac arrest: Implications for public access defibrillation. *Circulation* 97:2106–2109, 1998.
5. Ornato JP, Peberdy MA, Chondra NC, Bush DE: Seasonal pattern of acute myocardial infarction in the National Registry of Myocardial Infarction. *J Am Coll Cardiol* 28:1684–1688, 1996.
6. Hohnloser SH, Klingenheben T: Insights into the pathogenesis of sudden cardiac death from analysis of circadian fluctuations of potential triggering factors. *Pacing Clin Electrophysiol* 17:428–433, 1994.
7. Bayes de Luna A, Coumel P, Leclercq JF: Ambulatory sudden cardiac death: Mechanisms of production of fatal arrhythmia on the basis of data from 157 cases. *Am Heart J* 117:151–159, 1989.
8. Cummins RO, Ornato JP, Thies WH, Pepe PE: Improving survival from sudden cardiac arrest: The "chain of survival" concept: A statement for health professionals from the Advanced Cardiac Life Support Subcommittee and the Emergency Cardiac Care Committee, American Heart Association. *Circulation* 83:1832–1847, 1991.
9. Nademanee K, Nimmanit S, Chaowakul V, et al: Arrhythmogenic marker for the sudden unexplained death syndrome in Thai men. *Circulation* 96:2595–2600, 1997.
10. Brugada P, Geelen P: Some electrocardiographic patterns predicting sudden cardiac death that every doctor should recognize. *Acta Cardiol* 52:473–484, 1997.
11. Davies MJ: Anatomic features in victims of sudden coronary death: Coronary artery pathology. *Circulation* 85(suppl 1):119–124, 1992.
12. Hallstrom AP, Cobb LA, Ben Hui Y: Influence of comorbidity on the outcome of patients treated for out-of-hospital ventricular fibrillation. *Circulation* 93:2019–2022, 1996.
13. Beuret P, Feihl F, Vogt P, et al: Cardiac arrest: Prognostic factors and outcome at one year. *Resuscitation* 25:171–179, 1993.
14. Ornato JP, Peberdy MA: The mystery of bradyasystole during cardiac arrest. *Ann Emerg Med* 27:576–587, 1996.
15. Ewy GA, Dahl CF, Zimmerman MEA: Ventricular fibrillation masquerading as ventricular standstill. *Crit Care Med* 9:841–844, 1981.
16. Cummins RO, Austin D Jr: The frequency of "occult" ventricular fibrillation masquerading as a flat line in prehospital cardiac arrest. *Ann Emerg Med* 17:813–817, 1988.

17. Viskin S, Belhassen B, Roth A, et al: Aminophylline for bradyasystolic cardiac arrest refractory to atropine and epinephrine. *Ann Intern Med* 118:279–281, 1993.
18. Mader TJ, Gibson P: Adenosine receptor antagonism in refractory asystolic cardiac arrest: Results of a human pilot study. *Resuscitation* 35:3–7, 1997.
19. Herlitz J, Estrom L, Wennerblom B, et al: Survival among patients with out-of-hospital cardiac arrest found in electromechanical dissociation. *Resuscitation* 29:97–106, 1995.
20. Goldstein S, Mendendorp SV, Landis JR, et al: Analysis of cardiac symptoms preceding cardiac arrest. *Am J Cardiol* 58:1195–1198, 1986.
21. Breithardt G, Borggrefe M, Fetsch T, et al: Prognosis and risk stratification after myocardial infarction. *Eur Heart J* 16(suppl G):10–19, 1995.
22. Gilman JK, Jalal S, Naccarelli GV: Predicting and preventing sudden death from cardiac causes. *Circulation* 90:1083–1092, 1994.
23. Pratt CM, Moye LA: The Cardiac Arrhythmia Suppression Trial: Background, interim results and implications. *Am J Cardiol* 65:20B–29B, 1990.
24. Kennedy HL: Beta-blocker prevention of proarrhythmia and proischemia: Clues from CAST, CAMIAT, and EMIAT (Cardiac Arrhythmia Suppression Trial, Canadian Amiodarone Myocardial Infarction Arrhythmia Trial, and European Myocardial Infarct Amiodarone Trial) (editorial). *Am J Cardiol* 80:1208–1211, 1997.
25. Klein RC: Comparative efficacy of sotalol and class I antiarrhythmic agents in patients with ventricular tachycardia or fibrillation: Results of the Electrophysiology Study Versus Electrocardiographic Monitoring (ESVEM) Trial. *Eur Heart J* 14(suppl H): 78–84, 1993.
26. Kendall MJ, Lynch KP, Hjalmarson A, Kjekshus J: Beta blockers and sudden cardiac death. *Ann Intern Med* 123:358–368, 1995.
27. Van Gelder IC, Brugemann J, Crijns HJ: Current treatment recommendations in antiarrhythmic therapy. *Drugs* 55:331–346, 1998.
28. Haverkamp W, Eckardt L, Borggrefe M, Breithardt G: Drugs versus devices in controlling ventricular tachycardia, ventricular fibrillation, and recurrent cardiac arrest. *Am J Cardiol* 80:67G–73G, 1997.
29. Cannom DS: A review of the implantable cardioverter defibrillator trials. *Curr Opin Cardiol* 13:3–8, 1998.
30. Mushlin AI, Hall WJ, Zwanziger J, et al: The cost-effectiveness of automatic implantable cardiac defibrillators: Results from MADIT (Multicenter Automatic Defibrillator Implantation Trial). *Circulation* 97:2129–2135, 1998.
31. Bossaert L, Van Hoeyweghen R, Cerebral Resuscitation Study Group: Evaluation of cardiopulmonary resuscitation (CPR) techniques. *Resuscitation* 17:S99–S109, 1989.
32. Ornato JP, Hallagan LF, McMahan SB, et al: Attitudes of BCLS instructors about mouth-to-mouth resuscitation during the AIDS epidemic. *Ann Emerg Med* 19:151–156, 1990.
33. Kerber RE: Statement on early defibrillation from the Emergency Cardiac Care Committee, American Heart Association. *Circulation* 83:2233, 1991.
34. Nichol G, Hullstrom RP, Kerbner R, et al: American Heart Association report on the second public access defibrillation conference, April 17–19, 1997. *Circulation* 97:1309–1314, 1998.
35. Weisfeldt ML, Kerber RE, McGoldrick RP, et al: Public access to defibrillation: The Automatic Defibrillation Task Force. *Am J Emerg Med* 14:684–692, 1996.
36. O'Rourke MF, Donaldson E, Geddes JS: An airline cardiac arrest program. *Circulation* 96:2849–2853, 1997.
37. Eisenberg MS, Moore J, Cummins RO, et al: Use of the automatic external defibrillator in homes of survivors of out-of-hospital ventricular fibrillation. *Am J Cardiol* 63:443–446, 1989.

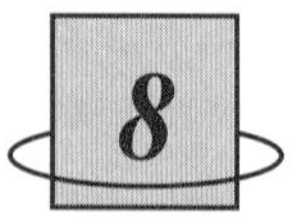

CARDIOPULMONARY RESUSCITATION IN ADULTS

Jon Mark Hirshon

Cardiopulmonary resuscitation (CPR) is a key part of emergency medical care designed to resuscitate individuals in cardiac arrest. The purpose of cardiopulmonary resuscitation is to temporarily provide effective oxygenation of vital organs, especially the brain and heart, through artificial circulation of oxygenated blood until the restoration of normal cardiac and respiratory activity occurs. This is to stop the degenerative processes of ischemia and anoxia caused by inadequate circulation and inadequate oxygenation. Time to initiation of cardiopulmonary resuscitation is critical to improve likelihood of recovery; ideally, it should be started within 4 min of arrest, and advanced cardiac life support should be initiated within 8 min of arrest. While basic life support alone may be lifesaving in some instances, in most cases, advanced interventions such as the delivery of electric current for defibrillation and the addition of various pharmacologic therapies are required to maximize the likelihood of patient recovery. Without rhythm-specific interventions, recovery from cardiac arrest is highly unlikely.

This chapter reviews basic CPR for adults, including approach to an unresponsive patient, basic airway opening procedures including initial management of an obstructed airway, and the physiology and mechanics of closed-chest compression techniques.

BASIC CARDIOPULMONARY RESUSCITATION

Overview

As with all aspects of emergency medicine, it is important to approach basic CPR systematically. When someone is found unresponsive, the following should be performed rapidly and in sequence:

1. Assess responsiveness. If unresponsive, then
2. Obtain assistance/activate the local emergency medical service system.
3. Call for a defibrillator (if available).
4. Position the patient and open the airway (maintain cervical spine immobilization if trauma is potentially involved).
5. Assess breathing. If no breathing is noted, then
6. Give two slow breaths.
7. Assess circulation. If no pulse noted, then
8. Begin closed-chest compressions and continue ventilations. Use the defibrillator if available.

Initial Actions

Upon discovery of a collapsed individual, the first medical action should be to assess the victim and determine whether the person is in fact unresponsive. However, prior to approaching a collapsed individual, the scene needs to be fully assessed for dangers to providers. Potential risks, whether from hazardous materials, unstable physical environment, or violence, should be considered. Becoming an additional victim will not aid patients and only add to the work load of other care providers. Once the patient is reached, level of responsiveness can be determined quickly through the administration of various stimuli from mild through noxious. If the individual is not responding, this is the time to obtain help prior to starting ventilations and chest compressions. Within a hospital, this may mean calling for the arrest team and requesting the arrest cart; outside the hospital, this is likely to be activation of the local emergency medical services system. Additionally, efforts should be made to obtain a defibrillator. Time to rhythm-specific therapy, especially defibrillation for unstable ventricular tachycardia or ventricular fibrillation, is critical for the recovery of patients in cardiac arrest.

Open the Airway

Once unresponsiveness has been determined, assistance obtained, and a defibrillator requested, the next step is to assess the upper airway of the victim. This usually requires positioning the individual supine on a flat, firm surface with arms along the sides of the body, followed by opening the person's airway. Unless trauma can be definitely excluded, any movement of the victim must take into account the potential of a spine injury; as the patient is placed supine, stabilize the cervical spine by maintaining the head, neck, and trunk in a straight line. If for some reason the patient cannot be placed supine, consider using the jaw-thrust maneuver (see below) from a lateral position to open the airway. Properly opening the airway is a critical and potentially lifesaving step. Common causes for airway obstruction in an unconscious patient are occlusion of the oropharynx by the tongue and laxity of the epiglottis. With loss of muscle tone, the tongue or the epiglottis can be forced back into the oropharynx on inspiration. This can create the effect of a one-way valve at the entrance to the trachea, leading to airway obstruction manifesting as inspiratory stridor. After positioning the patient, the mouth and oropharynx should be inspected for secretions or foreign objects. If secretions are present, they can be removed with the use of oropharyngeal suction; a foreign body may be dislodged by use of a finger sweep and then manually removed (see below).

Once the oropharynx has been cleared, two basic maneuvers for opening the airway may be tried to relieve upper airway obstruction. These are the head tilt–chin lift and the jaw thrust. These maneuvers help to open the airway by mechanically displacing the mandible and the attached tongue out of the oropharynx.

HEAD TILT–CHIN LIFT MANEUVER The head tilt–chin lift is usually the first maneuver attempted if there is no concern for cervical spine injury. The head tilt is performed by gently extending the neck. This is done by placing one hand under the patient's neck and the other on the forehead and extending the head in relation to the neck. This should place the patient's head in the "sniffing position" with the nose pointing up. In conjunction with the head tilt, the chin lift is performed. This is done by carefully placing the hand, which had been supporting the neck for the head tilt, under the symphysis of the mandible so as not to compress the soft tissues of the submental triangle and the base of the tongue. The mandible is then lifted forward and up until the teeth barely touch. This supports the jaw and helps tilt the head back.

JAW-THRUST MANEUVER The jaw thrust is the safest method for opening the airway if there is the possibility of cervical spine injury. It helps to maintain the cervical spine in a neutral position during resuscitation. The rescuer, who is positioned at the head of the patient, places the hands at the sides of the victim's face, grasps the mandible at its angle, and lifts the mandible forward (Fig. 8-1). The rescuer's elbows may rest on the surface on which the victim lies. This lifts the jaw and opens the airway with minimal head movement.

Assess Breathing and Initiate Ventilation

Once the airway has been opened, assessment of respiratory effort and air movement should occur. The care provider should look for chest expansions and listen and feel for airflow. The simple act of opening the airway may be adequate for the return of spontaneous respirations. However, if the victim remains without adequate respiratory effort, then further intervention is required. Two slow breaths of $1\frac{1}{2}$ to 2 s each should be given. At this point, a foreign body obstruction, as indicated by lack of chest rise or airflow on ventilation, may be noted, which would require efforts to relieve the obstruction (Fig. 8-2). Agonal respirations in an individual who has just suffered a cardiac arrest are not considered adequate. Intermittent positive-pressure ventilation, if possible with oxygen-enriched air, should be initiated.

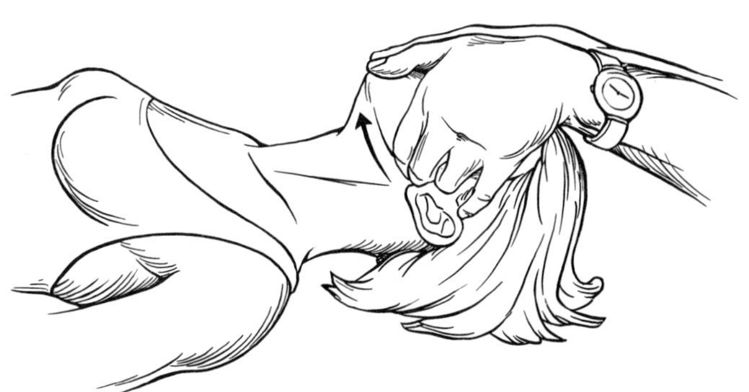

FIG. 8-1. Jaw-thrust maneuver.

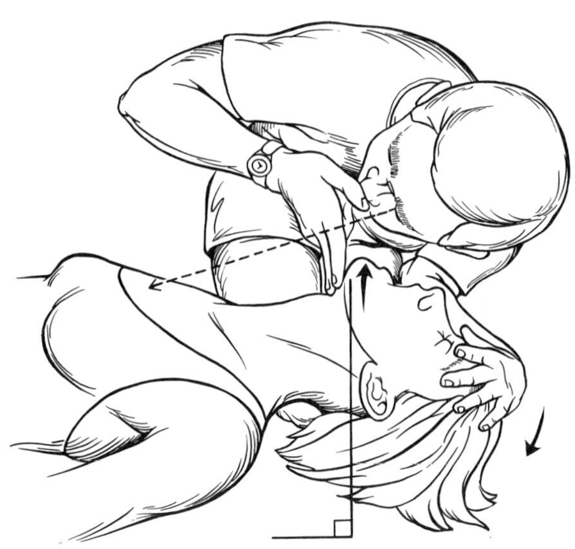

FIG. 8-2. Determine breathlessness.

VENTILATION TECHNIQUES There are a number of techniques for ventilating an individual, including mouth to mouth, mouth to nose, mouth to stoma, mouth to mask. Rescue breaths of an inspiratory time of $1\frac{1}{2}$ to 2 s each should be given at a rate of 10 to 12 per minute, with a volume adequate to make the chest rise—800 to 1200 mL in most adults. Too large a volume or too rapid an inspiratory flow rate will likely cause gastric distention, which can lead to regurgitation and aspiration. Expired air has an $F_{I}O_2$ of 16 to 17 percent. Supplemental oxygen should be delivered as soon as possible.

Mouth to Mouth With the airway open, the patient's nose should be gently pinched shut with the rescuer's thumb and index finger (Fig. 8-3). This prevents air escape. After a deep breath, the rescuer places his or her lips around the patient's mouth, forming an airtight seal. The rescuer slowly exhales. Release the seal and allow adequate time for passive exhalation by the victim, and then repeat the procedure.

Mouth to Nose At times, as with severe maxillofacial trauma, mouth-to-nose ventilation may be more effective. With the airway open, the rescuer lifts the patient's jaw, closing the mouth. After a deep breath, the rescuer places his or her lips around the patient's nose, forming an airtight seal. The rescuer slowly exhales.

Mouth to Stoma or Tracheostomy After laryngectomy or tracheotomy, the stoma or tracheostomy becomes the patient's airway. As with the previous techniques, a seal is made around the stoma or tracheostomy tube, and the rescuer slowly exhales.

Mouth to Mask Placement of the mask properly and securely on a victim's face is important when using a mask for ventilation, either with a bag or via mouth to mask. The mask should be placed over the bridge of the patient's nose and around the mouth. The rescuer

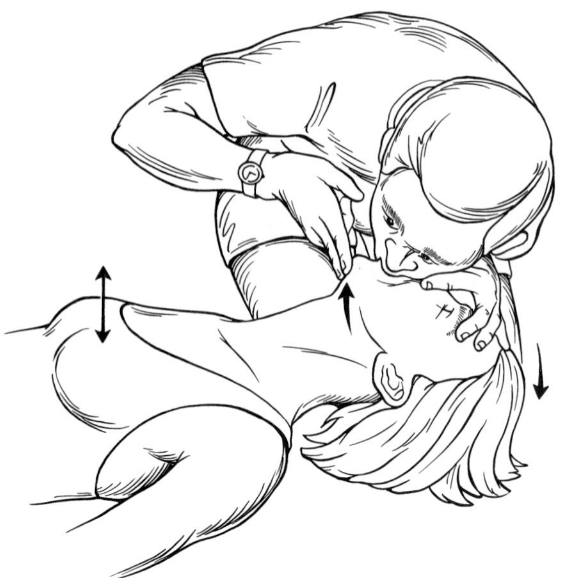

FIG. 8-3. Mouth-to-mouth rescue breathing.

places the thumb on the part of the mask that is sitting on the patient's nose and places the index finger of the same hand on the part of the mask sitting on the patient's chin (Fig. 8-4). The three other fingers of the same hand are then placed along the bony margin of the jaw. The mask can then be firmly sealed to the patient's face. Two hands may be used for this technique if a second rescuer is available. Ventilations are then performed through the mask; some masks also allow for supplemental oxygenation.

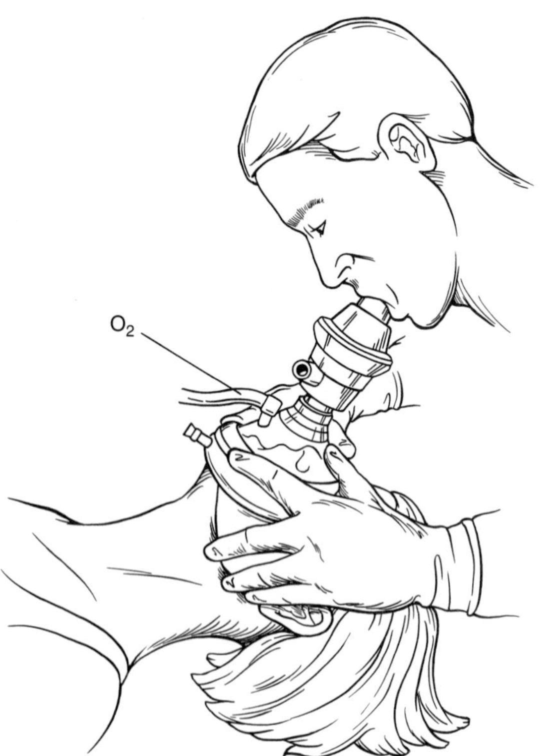

FIG. 8-4. Mouth-to-mask rescue breathing with proper mask placement.

Foreign Body Obstruction

It is important to recognize and be able to assist someone with an airway obstruction from a foreign body. The National Safety Council reported that approximately 2900 deaths from foreign body airway obstruction occurred in 1993.[1] An individual in distress from a compromised airway is likely to use the universal sign for an airway obstruction, which is for the individual to grab his or her neck with both hands. Foreign bodies can cause partial or complete obstruction. With a partial airway obstruction, air exchange may be adequate or inadequate. If the victim is able to speak, cough, and exchange air, then he or she should be encouraged to continue spontaneous efforts. Assistance, such as activation of the local emergency medical services system, should be obtained. No interference should be made with the patient's attempts to cough or expel the foreign body. If air exchange becomes inadequate, indicated by increased difficulty breathing, weak and ineffective cough, worsening inspiratory stridor, or cyanosis, direct medical intervention should occur. Inadequate air exchange from either a severe partial or a complete airway obstruction should be managed the same. In an unconscious person, airway obstruction may be noted through inadequate airflow and poor chest rise on efforts to ventilate.

OBSTRUCTION-RELIEVING MANEUVERS Maneuvers used to relieve foreign body obstructions include the Heimlich maneuver (subdiaphragmatic abdominal thrusts), chest thrusts, and the finger sweep. As a single method, back blows are no longer recommended to relieve obstructions in adults. In a conscious individual, the Heimlich maneuver is the recommended maneuver in most adults for relieving airway obstruction from a solid object. It is not useful for liquids. In an unconscious individual suspected of having an aspirated foreign body, the recommended first step is the finger sweep. Otherwise, in an unconscious patient the recommended sequence is the Heimlich maneuver up to five times, open mouth and perform a finger sweep, and then attempt to ventilate. This sequence may be repeated as long as needed until the patient recovers or additional assistance arrives.

Heimlich Maneuver (Fig. 8-5) Described by Dr. Heimlich in 1975, this maneuver creates an artificial cough through elevating the diaphragm and forcing air from the lungs.[2] It may be repeated multiple times; each individual thrust should be performed with the intent to relieve the obstruction. It can be performed with the victim standing, sitting, or lying down, or it can be self-administered. To perform with the patient standing or sitting, the rescuer stands behind the patient and places the thumb side of a fist against the victim's abdomen midline just above the navel and well below the xiphoid process. Grasping the fist with the other hand, the rescuer presses the fist into the victim's abdomen with a quick upward thrust. This is repeated until the item is dislodged or the patient becomes unconscious. For an unconscious patient, the individual is placed supine on a firm surface with the rescuer sitting astride the victim's thighs (Fig. 8-6). The heel of a hand is positioned midline just above the patient's umbilicus, and the second hand is placed directly on top of the first. The rescuer then delivers quick upward thrusts. To self-administer thrusts, the individual can either use his or her own fist to delivery the thrusts or lean against a firm object, such as a porch rail or back of a chair. Potential complications of the Heimlich maneuver include injury or rupture of abdominal or thoracic viscera or regurgitation of stomach contents.

Chest Thrusts This maneuver is used primarily if someone is morbidly obese or in the late stages of pregnancy and the rescuer cannot reach around the patient's abdomen to perform abdominal thrusts (Fig. 8-7). To perform chest thrusts with the patient standing or sitting, the rescuer stands behind the patient and places the thumb side of a fist against the victim's sternum, avoiding the costal margins and the xiphoid process. Grasping the fist with the other hand, the rescuer

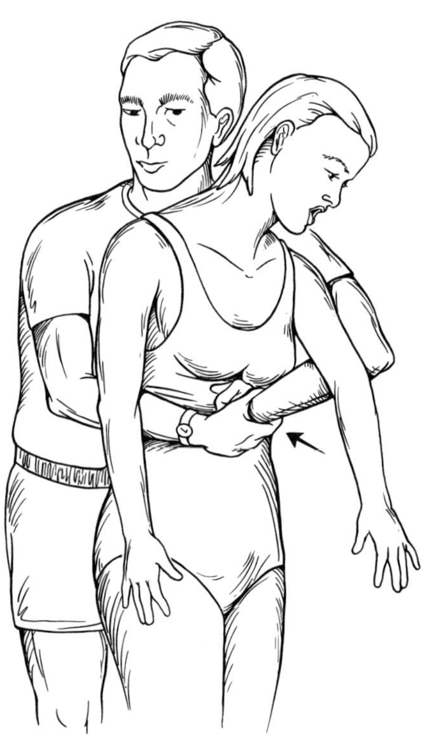

FIG. 8-5. Standing Heimlich maneuver administered to conscious victim of foreign body airway obstruction.

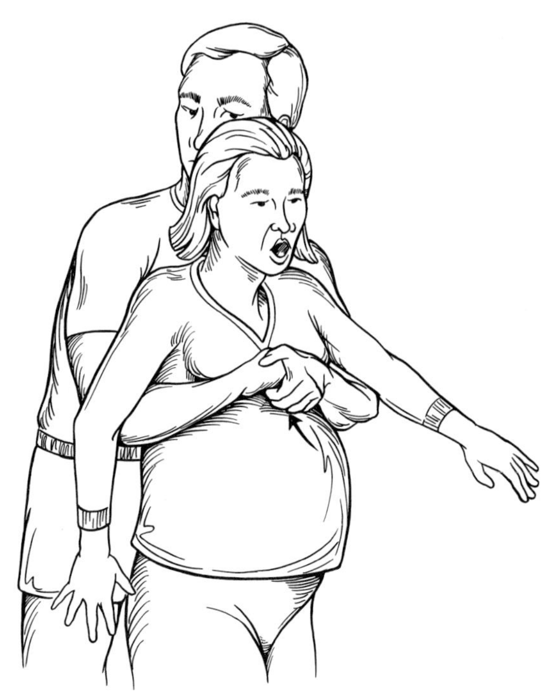

FIG. 8-7. Standing chest-thrust maneuver administered to conscious victim of foreign body airway obstruction.

presses the fist into the victim's chest with a quick backward thrust. This is repeated until the item is dislodged or the patient becomes unconscious. For an unconscious patient, the individual is placed supine on a firm surface with the rescuer kneeling close to the victim's side. The hands are placed in the same position as for chest compression, i.e., the lower sternum, and quick thrusts are delivered.

Finger Sweep This maneuver is used only in unconscious patients (Fig. 8-8). Using the thumb and fingers of one hand, the rescuer grasps both the tongue and the mandible and lifts. This may partially relieve the obstruction by lifting the tongue away from the back of the throat. With the other hand, the rescuer then inserts his or her index finger into the back of the throat and uses a hooking action in an attempt to dislodge the foreign body to move it into the mouth for manual removal. Care must be used so as to not push the foreign object deeper into the throat.

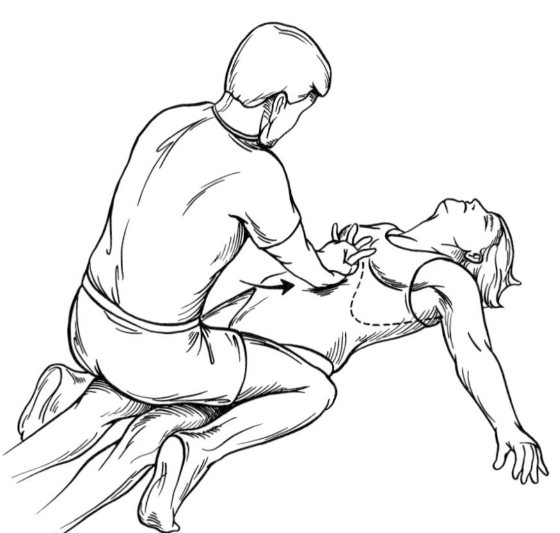

FIG. 8-6. Prone Heimlich maneuver administered to unconscious victim of foreign body airway obstruction.

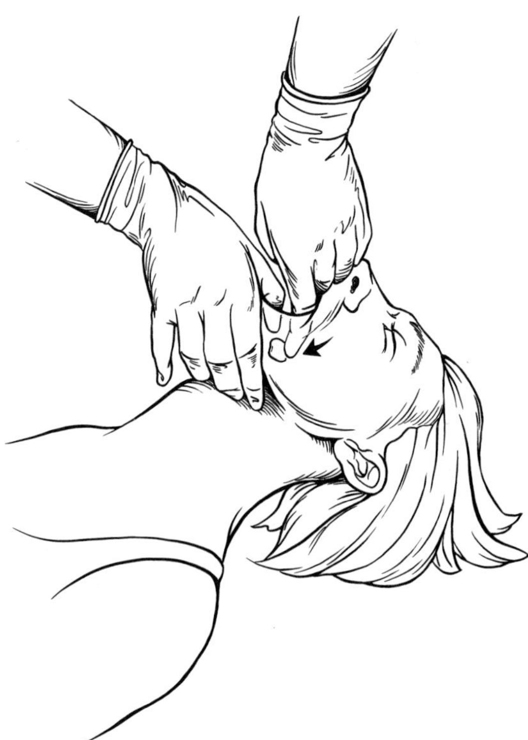

FIG. 8-8. Finger-sweep maneuver administered to unconscious victim of foreign body airway obstruction.

Assess Circulation and Initiate Compressions

The carotid artery is generally the most reliable and accessible location to palpate a pulse. The artery can be located by placing two fingers on the trachea and then sliding them down to the groove between the trachea and the sternocleidomastoid muscle. Simultaneous palpation of both carotid arteries should not be performed because this could obstruct cerebral blood flow. In low-pressure states, forceful palpation may interfere with the ability to detect a pulse. The femoral artery may be used as an alternative site to palpate a pulse. This can be found just below the inguinal ligament approximately halfway between the anterosuperior iliac spine and the pubic tubercle. If no pulse is felt after 5 to 10 s, chest compressions should begin.

PHYSIOLOGY OF CLOSED-CHEST COMPRESSIONS Since the technique of closed-chest compressions was put forth initially by Kouwenhoven and colleagues in the 1960s, there has been an active debate as to the mechanism of blood flow.[3,4] In a closed system, liquid flows when pressure gradients develop. There are two basic theories for how pressure gradients and flow are produced during closed-chest cardiac massage.[5] The conventional theory of blood flow during compressions is called the *cardiac pump theory*. This postulates that direct compression of the heart between the spine and the sternum leads to increased pressure in the ventricles. This causes closure of the mitral and tricuspid valves, leading to blood flow into the aorta and the pulmonary arteries. The *thoracic pump theory* postulates that compressions lead to an increase in pressure throughout the thoracic cavity, leading to a pressure gradient from intrathoracic to extrathoracic arteries. It is possible that both mechanisms produce blood flow to varying degrees during closed-chest cardiac massage in humans. However, regardless of mechanism, conventional chest compressions generate one-fourth to one-third of physiologic cardiac output. Lower ratios can be expected with delays in initiating compressions.

TECHNIQUE OF CLOSED-CHEST COMPRESSIONS Upon confirmation that an individual is without a pulse, serial rhythmic closed-chest compressions should be initiated. The victim is placed supine on a firm surface with the rescuer at the side. The care provider places the heel of one hand midline on the lower half of the sternum, approximately 2 in cephalad of the xiphoid process (Fig. 8-9). The heel of the hand should be parallel with the long axis of the patient's body. The second hand is then placed on top of the first hand so that the hands are parallel with each other. The fingers of the two hands may be interlaced if desired. The arms should be straight and the elbows preferably locked. The vector of the compression force should start from the rescuer's shoulders and be directed downward; lateral forces will decrease efficiency of the compressions and increase the likelihood of complications. The sternum should be depressed $1\frac{1}{2}$ to 2 in (3.8 to 5.1 cm) in an adult at a minimum rate of 80 to 100 compressions per minute. Rates less than this are inadequate. The compression-release phases should be roughly equal. With a single rescuer, 2 ventilations should be given after every 15 compressions; with two rescuers, a ventilation should be given after every fifth compression.

There are currently several experimental techniques for closed-chest cardiac massage. In one method, circumferential chest compressions are performed by a pneumatic vest CPR to more effectively increase intrathoracic pressure during chest compressions.[6] In interposed abdominal compression CPR, abdominal compression occurs during the relaxation phase of chest compression, causing increased aortic diastolic pressure and leading to improved blood flow to organs above the diaphragm.[7] In active compression-decompression CPR, a hand-held suction device is used to decrease intrathoracic pressure during the relaxation phase of chest compression and to improve ventricular filling.[8] Additionally, self-initiated cardiopulmonary resuscitation can be performed by forceful coughing. This increases intrathoracic pressure, leading to blood flow to the brain for as long as the patient remains conscious and able to cough.[9]

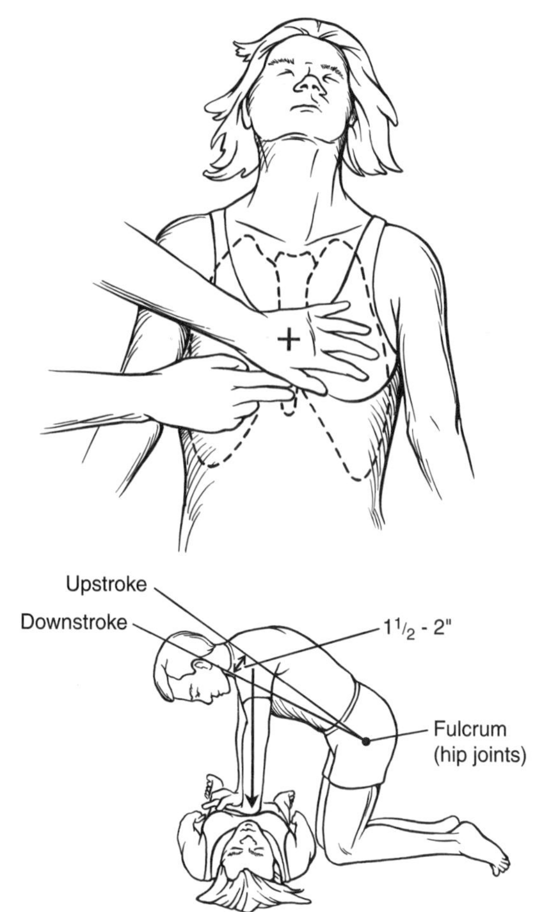

FIG. 8-9. Proper hand and rescuer positioning for chest compression.

Complications of Cardiopulmonary Resuscitation

Ventilations can cause insufflation of the stomach, leading to regurgitation and possible aspiration or possibly to gastric rupture. Closed-chest compressions can lead to fractures of the sternum or the ribs, separation of the ribs from the sternum, pulmonary contusion, pneumothorax, myocardial contusion, hemorrhagic pericardial effusions, splenic laceration, or liver laceration. Proper techniques can minimize these complications but not totally prevent them. Late complications include pulmonary edema, gastrointestinal hemorrhage, pneumonia, and recurrent cardiopulmonary arrest. Anoxic brain injury can occur in a resuscitated individual who had suffered prolonged hypoxia; it is the most common cause of death in resuscitated patients.

Terminating Resuscitation

Efforts at resuscitation should be continued until the patient recovers spontaneous respirations and cardiac output, the rescuer becomes exhausted, or the patient is pronounced dead. Atraumatic individuals who recover spontaneous respirations and circulation should be placed on their sides—the *recovery position*. Recovery from cardiac arrest depends on time to CPR and rhythm-specific intervention. Resuscitation and long-term outcome in normothermic patients with arrest times of 20 min or more are very poor.

FUTURE DIRECTIONS

It should be noted that many of the current basic CPR guidelines are based on expert consensus derived from limited scientific studies and clinical experience, and much active research is currently occurring.[10] Well-designed and executed outcome-directed scientific research will help to further develop the quality and efficacy of basic CPR.

REFERENCES

1. National Safety Council: *Accident Facts 1994*. Chicago: National Safety Council, 1994.
2. Heimlich HJ: A life-saving maneuver to prevent food-choking. *JAMA* 234:398, 1975.
3. Kouwenhoven WB, Jude JR, Knickerbocker GG: Closed-chest cardiac massage. *JAMA* 173:1064, 1960.
4. Jude JR, Kouwenhoven WB, Knickerbocker GG: Cardiac arrest: Report of application of external cardiac massage on 118 patients. *JAMA* 178:1063, 1961.
5. Halperin HR: Mechanisms of forward flow during CPR, in Paradis N, Nowak R, Halperin H (eds): *Cardiac Arrest: The Science and Practice of Resuscitation Medicine,* Baltimore: Williams & Wilkins, 1996.
6. Sack JB, Kasselbremmer MB, Bregman D, et al: Survival from in-hospital cardiac arrest with interposed abdominal counter pulsation during cardiopulmonary resuscitation. *JAMA* 267:379, 1992.
7. Cohen TJ, Goldner BG, Maccaro PC, et al: A comparison of active compression-decompression cardiopulmonary resuscitation with standard cardiopulmonary resuscitation for cardiac arrests occurring in the hospital. *N Engl J Med* 329:1918, 1993.
8. Halperin HR, Tsitlik JE, Gelfand M, et al: A preliminary study of cardiopulmonary resuscitation by circumferential compression of the chest with use of a pneumatic vest. *N Engl J Med* 329:762, 1993.
9. Criley JM, Blaufuss AH, Kissel GL: Cough-induced cardiac compression: Self-administered form of cardiopulmonary resuscitation. *JAMA* 236:1246, 1976.
10. Gazmuri RJ, Becker J: Cardiac resuscitation: The search for hemodynamically more effective methods. *Chest* 111:712, 1997.

9 NEONATAL RESUSCITATION AND EMERGENCIES

Eugene E. Cepeda
Seetha Shankaran

NEONATAL RESUSCITATION

Approximately 6 percent of all newborns require life support in the delivery room or nursery, and in those neonates whose birth weights are less than 1500 g, the need for resuscitation rises to 60 percent. Personnel skilled in neonatal resuscitation should be available at every delivery. It is important to anticipate the delivery of high-risk neonates so that delivery room personnel may be alerted to the possible need for resuscitation.

There are no guidelines available to assist in making the decision to resuscitate extremely premature infants in the emergency department. When in doubt, resuscitate. At the present time, survival at 22 weeks of gestation or less is rare. However, a 20 to 30 percent survival rate is reported at 24 weeks' gestation, although often with severe resultant morbidity.

The following factors are associated with an increased risk for neonatal resuscitation:

Maternal factors
- Inadequate prenatal care
- Age <16 and >35 years
- History of previous perinatal morbidity or mortality
- Toxemia, hypertension
- Diabetes
- Chronic renal disease
- Anemia
- Drug therapy (e.g., reserpine, lithium, carbonate, magnesium, adrenergic-blocking agents)
- Substance abuse
- Blood type or group isoimmunization
- Oligohydramnios

Intrapartum factors
- Abnormal presentation
- Caesarean section
- Prolonged labor or precipitous delivery
- Prolonged rupture of membranes, chorioamnionitis
- Cephalopelvic disproportion
- Forceps delivery other than outlet or vacuum extraction
- Prolapsed cord
- Cord compression
- Maternal hypotension, shock
- Analgesic or sedative drugs given within 2 h of delivery

Fetal factors
- Prematurity
- Postmaturity
- Intrauterine growth failure
- Multiple gestation
- Acidosis per fetal scalp capillary monitoring
- Abnormal fetal heart rate per monitor
- Thick meconium in amniotic fluid
- Congenital infection
- Fetal malformation or edema diagnosed by ultrasound

The following conditions should alert nursery personnel to the possibility of apnea: previous need for resuscitation, prematurity, sepsis and/or meningitis, congenital abnormalities, respiratory distress, or seizures.

Normal newborns are equipped with physiologic, pharmacologic, and metabolic responses to enable them to survive the hypoxia that develops as a consequence of asphyxia. Generally, brain injury occurs only when the asphyxia is severe enough to impair cerebral blood flow. Initially the injury is reversible, and only longer periods of ischemia lead to permanent damage. The pattern of injury is strongly influenced by the distribution of blood flow. During asphyxia, blood flow is redirected to the heart, brain, and adrenals at the expense of other organs, such as the kidneys and the gastrointestinal tract. Within the brain, flow is directed to the brainstem at the expense of the high cerebral structures, such as the cortex. In the preterm neonate, the periventricular white matter is susceptible to injury. In the full-term or postterm neonate, the gray-matter regions, such as the overlying parasagittal "watershed" cortex, are more vulnerable to ischemic injury. When the asphyxial insult is severe or prolonged, hypoxic multiorgan dysfunction occurs because of the redistribution of organ blood flow and results in cardiopulmonary distress, renal failure, impaired hepatic function, seizures and encephalopathy, gastrotintestinal dysfunction, and coagulopathies.

Principles of Resuscitation

The Apgar score (Table 9-1) is assessed at 1 and 5 min of age for every newly delivered infant. Although the scoring system has been useful in evaluating the condition of the newborn, 1 min is too long to wait to make the decision to initiate resuscitation. If the 5-min score is less than 7, additional scores are obtained every 5 min for a total of 20 min.

Perinatal asphyxia is currently defined as the presence of the following: umbilical artery acidemia (pH <7.00), 5-min Apgar score of 0 to 3, neonatal neurologic sequelae, and multiorgan dysfunction. Certain conditions require specific measures during resuscitation in addition

TABLE 9-1 Apgar Score

Sign	0	1	2
Heart rate	Absent	<100/min	>100/min
Respiratory effort	Absent	Weak cry	Strong cry
Muscle tone	Limp	Some flexion	Good flexion
Reflex irritability (when feet stimulated)	No response	Some motion	Cry
Color	Blue, pale	Body pink, extremities blue	Pink

to those outlined below. These conditions are discussed following the general principles.

Resuscitation should be continued for a maximum of 30 min. Neonatal morbidity and mortality rates are high after 20 to 30 min of cardiac asystole and resulting encephalopathy in term infants. Infants who were successfully resuscitated at birth should have continuous monitoring of vital signs, blood gases, hematocrit, dextrose levels, blood pressure, fluid status, and clinical condition. Complications associated with severe asphyxia are seizures, hypoxic-ischemic encephalopathy, intracranial hemorrhage, inappropriate antidiuretic hormone (ADH) secretion, hypocalcemia, persistent pulmonary hypertension, ischemic cardiomyopathy, hypovolemia or shock, necrotizing enterocolitis, renal failure, and coagulopathy.

EQUIPMENT The following is a list of the equipment necessary for resuscitation.

1. Bag and mask with manometer attached, connected to a source of 100 percent oxygen (oxygen should be heated and humidified; bag should be a rubber anesthesia bag, a rebreathing bag of 500-mL capacity, or a self-inflating bag designed for newborns)
2. Rubber face masks of varying sizes, 1, 2, 3, and 4
3. Wall suction, sterile catheters, and bulb syringes
4. DeLee suction catheter with mucus trap
5. Laryngoscope with 0 and 1 blades
6. Oral endotracheal tubes with stylet, sizes 2.5, 3.0, 3.5, and 4.0 mm
7. Radiant heater with servomechanism
8. Sterile umbilical vessel catheterization tray
9. Glucose oxidase blood test strips
10. Heart rate monitor with easily applicable leads
11. Intravenous infusion equipment
12. Transcutaneous oxygen monitor or saturation pulse oximeter
13. Appropriate light
14. Infant stethoscope
15. Nasogastric tubes, 5F and 8F
16. Clock with sweep second hand

Resuscitation Steps

MAINTAIN BODY TEMPERATURE Maintain the infant below the level of the placenta prior to clamping the cord. When the cord is clamped, blot the infant dry with a sterile towel and place the infant under a preheated radiant warmer on a sterile table. Neonates should be placed either on the back or the left side somewhat in the Trendelenburg position, with the neck in a neutral position.

CLEAR THE AIRWAY Gently suction the nose and mouth with a bulb syringe, DeLee trap, or mechanical suction apparatus with an 8F suction catheter. A 5- to 10-s examination should be performed to determine the need for resuscitation. This examination should include an assessment of heart rate, respiratory effort, color, and muscular activity. If the infant has a lusty cry, is pink, has spontaneous respirations, and has a heart rate above 120 beats per minute (Apgar > 8), no further therapy is needed.

INITIATE BREATHING If the infant is apneic or the heart rate is slow and irregular (<100 beats per minute) and the color is cyanotic (Apgar 4 to 7), administer positive-pressure ventilation with the mask over the infant's face and 100% oxygen. The respiratory rate should be maintained at 40 breaths per minute, with pressure applied to gently move the chest wall. In an infant who has not yet taken a breath, over 40 cmH_2O pressure may be necessary to expand the lungs. In mildly depressed infants, this will produce a prompt increase in heart rate and the onset of regular spontaneous respirations. If no improvement is noted in 15 to 30 s and the condition deteriorates (Apgar ≤ 4), the trachea should be intubated and assisted ventilation continued.

MECONIUM STAINING Meconium staining of the amniotic fluid occurs in from 0.5 to 20 percent of all births. Aspiration of thick meconium carries a 20 to 50 percent mortality rate; however, with proper management it is almost entirely preventable. When gross meconium is noted at the time of delivery, the following procedure should be followed. After delivery of the infant's head (but before delivery of the shoulders), the nose, mouth, and pharynx should be thoroughly suctioned with a DeLee suction catheter. Repeat suctioning of the upper airway should be performed as the infant is placed under the radiant warmer. The trachea should then be visualized with a laryngoscope and meconium aspirated by direct suctioning through an endotracheal tube. Suctioning should be repeated until no more meconium is present in the trachea. The infant may then be ventilated with positive pressure as indicated. Failure to clear the trachea before assisted or spontaneous ventilation may result in dissemination of the meconium through the airways.

ENDOTRACHEAL INTUBATION

Indications

1. Mechanical ventilation
2. To clear the trachea of meconium

Equipment

Pediatric laryngoscope handle
Laryngoscope blade no 0 for infants < 2000 g
Laryngoscope blade no 1 for infants > 2000 g
Self-inflating bag and mask apparatus
Adapter
Scissors
Stylet
Tape
Suction apparatus
Tincture of benzoin

Procedure

1. Check that the light source on the laryngoscope blade is working. Place the infant supine and suction the mouth and oropharynx. Monitor the heart rate and color.
2. Hold the laryngoscope in the left hand and open the infant's mouth by sliding your right index finger between the infant's right upper and lower gums. Insert the laryngoscope into the infant's mouth by sliding the blade down against your right index finger. Push the tongue with the blade to the left.
3. Advance the blade and lift. You should be able to see the epiglottis. Remove your right index finger, holding the blade with left hand.
4. Pass the endotracheal tube along the right side of the mouth and advance it past the vocal cords. If a stylet is used, it should be

gently removed while the tube is held firmly in place. The tip of the tube should not go past 2.5 cm beyond the cords.

5. Attach the resuscitation bag to the tube and listen for breath sounds, which should be equal on both the right and left chest. The infant's oxygen saturation should improve. A chest x-ray will confirm proper placement.
6. Paint the skin with tincture of benzoin and tape the tube securely.

CARDIAC MASSAGE If the heart rate is below 50 beats per minute with assisted ventilation, cardiac massage should be initiated by placing both hands around the infant's chest with two thumbs over the midsternum so that the sternum will be depressed two-thirds of the distance to the vertebral column at 120 compressions per minute. Cardiac massage may be stopped periodically to assess improvement, and ventilation and cardiac massage should be synchronized (1:3 ratio). The chest should expand, bilateral breath sounds should be heard in the axilla, and heart rate should increase if the resuscitation is effective and the endotracheal tube is in good position. *In most instances* it is possible to obtain an adequate response with the use of external cardiac massage and assisted ventilation. If there is no response to these measures, drug therapy should be considered. Any route of access to the circulatory system is acceptable, including a peripheral vein, the umbilical vein, or an umbilical artery.

UMBILICAL ARTERY CATHETERIZATION

Indications

1. To measure arterial blood gases
2. To monitor continuous blood pressure
3. To infuse fluids

Equipment

2 × 2 sponges, 5
Curved hemostat
Medicine glasses, 2
Scalpel blade, no 11
Iris forceps, curved, serrated end, no teeth, 2
Lacrimal probe
Needle holder
Debriding scissors
Umbilical tape, 6 in
Knife handle
4-0 silk suture with needle
Three-way stopcock
10-mL syringes, 2
Iodine solution
3.5F catheter for infant < 1200 g
5.0F catheter for infant > 1200 g

Procedure

1. Immobilize the patient. Measure the distance between the umbilicus and the right shoulder.
2. Clean the umbilical stump and surrounding area with iodine solution. Drape the umbilical area, but leave the head and feet uncovered.
3. Tie the base of the cord with the umbilical tape to minimize blood loss.
4. Cut the cord cleanly across its length to 1 cm with the scalpel. The arteries are small and have pinpoint openings. The vein is larger and has thinner walls and a larger opening.
5. Grasp the edge of the cord with the forceps. Using the iris forceps, enlarge the opening of the umbilical artery first with the tip of one arm of the forceps.
6. Insert both arms of the forceps to dilate the artery so that it will accept the catheter.
7. The length of the catheter inserted for the low position is two-thirds of the distance from the umbilicus to the right shoulder and for the high position, the full measurement from the right shoulder to the umbilicus.
8. Attach the three-way stopcock and aspirate blood with a syringe. Clear the catheter with normal saline.
9. Anchor the catheter with silk suture to the umbilical stump.
10. Check the position of the catheter tip with an x-ray. It should be at the level of L4 for the low position, or between T6 and T9, which is above the diaphragm, for the high position.

Patency of the umbilical arterial line can be maintained by a continuous infusion of fluid. The catheter should be removed when the need for arterial blood gas monitoring is no longer necessary (oxygen requirement $\leq 80\%$) or complications occur.

Complications Possible complications of umbilical artery catheterization are infection, thrombosis and vasospasm, and hemorrhage. Renal hypertension is a delayed complication.

UMBILICAL VEIN CATHETERIZATION The most expedient procedure for obtaining vascular access is to insert the venous catheter through the umbilicus via the umbilical vein, and the ductus venosus into the inferior vena cava. The venous catheter should be inserted 10 to 12 cm and anchored to the abdominal wall. Obtain radiographs of chest and abdomen to rule out other abnormalities and evaluate the position of the catheters.

Drug Therapy in Resuscitation

There is a very minor role for drug therapy in resuscitation. Most resuscitative efforts in the delivery room respond to adequate support of ventilation and circulation without drug therapy (see Table 9-2).

DEXTROSE To provide metabolic substrate and expansion of plasma volume, 10 percent dextrose in water ($D_{10}W$) at 100 (mL/kg)/day or 6 to 8 (mg/kg)/min should be infused. If the Dextrostix is less than 45 mg/dL, 5 mL/kg of 10 or 15% glucose solution should be infused; 25% dextrose infusions should be avoided because of the risk of rebound hypoglycemia.

EPINEPHRINE To stimulate heart rate if it is under 120 beats per minute, 0.1 mL/kg of a 1:10,000 solution may be given through the endotracheal tube or intravenously. Cardiac massage should continue following epinephrine administration.

NALOXONE Use naloxone only to reverse narcotic respiratory depression, 0.01 mg/kg of a neonatal solution (0.2 mg/mL) may be administered intravenously, subcutaneously, or through the endotracheal tube. The time for peak concentration of transplacentally acquired narcotics in the fetus is 2 h following administration of medication to the mother; thus, delivery of the fetus at that time would predispose the fetus to maximal depression. Naloxone may precipitate withdrawal in infants whose mothers are addicted to narcotics.

ISOPROTERENOL If epinephrine has failed to raise the heart rate to at least 120 beats per minute, 1:10,000 solution or 0.05 to 0.1 μg/min may be infused.

A delay in onset of spontaneous regular respiration of more than 30 min following birth has been associated with a poor prognosis. Attempts at resuscitation after 30 min of no response do not appear to be warranted.

BICARBONATE In the presence of metabolic acidosis, 2 to 3 meq/kg of sodium bicarbonate should be administered as an intravenous infusion. A continuous infusion may be necessary [not to exceed 8 meq/kg/day] if acidosis is protracted.

TABLE 9-2 Neonatal Resuscitation Drug Chart

Drug and Concentration	Syringe Size, mL	Dose by Weight	PATIENT DOSE Weight, kg	VOLUME, mL IV	VOLUME, mL ET	Administration
Epinephrine 1:10,000 (0.1 mg/mL) for bradycardia	1	0.01–0.03 mg/kg	1 2 3 4	0.2 0.4 0.6 0.8	0.5 1 1.5 2	IV push or endotracheally followed by 1 mL normal saline solution. Repeat q 5 min as needed. *Do not mix with sodium bicarbonate. Never inject into an artery.*
Sodium bicarbonate 4.2% (0.5 meq/mL) for metabolic acidosis	6, 10, or 12	2 meq/kg	1 2 3 4	4 8 12 16		IV over at least 2 min. *Do not mix with epinephrine.* Ensure adequate ventilation.
Whole blood, albumin 5%, normal saline solution, or Ringer's lactate for volume expansion	20 or 35	10 mL/kg	1 2 3 4	10 20 30 40		IV over at least 10 min.
Naloxone (Narcan) 0.4 mg/mL for narcotic respiratory depression	1	0.1 mg/kg	1 2 3 4	0.25 0.50 0.75 1		IV push, intermuscularly, or endotracheally. May repeat 2 to 3 times. *Use cautiously if maternal narcotic addiction is suspected.*

Source: Adapted from Bloom RS, Cropley C: *Textbook of Neonatal Resuscitation*. Chicago, American Heart Association, 1994.

DOPAMINE Dopamine should be initiated to raise the blood pressure after adequate fluids have been administered. At low doses (2 to 5 μg/kg/min) dopamine preserves renal and mesenteric perfusion; at higher doses (10 to 20 mg/kg/min) it has both inotropic and vasoactive properties through α- and β-adrenergic effects.

NEONATAL EMERGENCIES

Neonatal Shock

The risk factors for shock and hypotension in newborn infants are low birth weight, maternal sepsis, prolapsed cord, and acute onset of maternal vaginal bleeding. Clinical signs of hypovolemia are pallor, tachycardia, grunting respirations in the absence of pulmonary disease, mottling of skin, poor capillary filling, thready pulse and hypotension (systolic < 45 mmHg in a 1000-g premature neonate or < 60 mmHg in a term infant), and persistent metabolic acidosis. A hematocrit should be obtained, and if anemia (hematocrit < 45 vol%) or hypotension is diagnosed, immediate plasma expansion in the form of packed red blood cells 5 mL/kg or whole blood, fresh-frozen plasma, Plasmanate, or 5% salt-poor albumin 10 to 20 mL/kg should be given intravenously over 10 min.

Seizures

Seizures in neonates are common, with an incidence of 1 in 200 live births, and may represent primary central nervous system (CNS) disease or a systemic or metabolic disorder. Recent data suggest that seizure activity itself may adversely affect the growing brain. It is important to distinguish seizures from tremors or jitteriness, which may be seen in infants who have hypocalcemia, hypoglycemia, drug withdrawal, or no identifiable disease. Tremors are uniform, fine movements that respond to sensory stimuli, stop with manual stabilization, and do not occur spontaneously. They are not accompanied by eye, oral, or lingual movements. The types of neonatal seizures include subtle seizures, tonic seizures, multifocal clonic seizures, focal clonic seizures, and myoclonic seizures.

Subtle seizures occur in both preterm and term neonates. These seizures consist of ocular, facial, oral, or lingual movements and respiratory manifestations, such as apnea or stertorous breathing.

Tonic seizures are characteristic of premature infants. The seizures appear as decerebrate or decorticate posturing. There are sustained deviation of the eyes and assymetric posturing of the limbs and trunk.

Multifocal clonic seizures are seen in term infants. These are initially noted in one limb and migrate to another part of the body. There are rhythmic and slow movements at one to six times per second.

Focal clonic seizures are well localized and are accompanied by specific sharp activity on the electroencephalogram (EEG). These seizures occur more commonly in full-term infants.

Myoclonic seizures are expressed as single or multiple jerks of flexion of the upper or lower extremities. They are rare and occur in both premature and full-term infants.

CLINICAL FEATURES There are numerous causes of neonatal seizures. Hypoxic-ischemic encephalopathy is the most common cause of seizures. The seizures occur between 6 and 18 h of life. In full-term neonates, the hypoxic injury may result in a cerebral hemorrhage, watershed infarct, posterior fossa hematoma, or subarachnoid or subdural hemorrhage. In premature infants, hypoxic injury often results in periventricular-intraventricular hemorrhage. This type of seizure has a poor prognosis.

The metabolic disturbances associated with neonatal seizures include hypoglycemia, hypocalcemia, hypomagnesemia, hyperammonemia, hypernatremia, and hyponatremia. Hypoglycemia, hypocalcemia, and hypomagnesemia are often found in premature infants with perinatal asphyxia. Hypernatremia occurs in neonates with dehydration secondary to excessive fluid losses or treatment with large doses of sodium bicarbonate. Hyponatremia may be seen secondary to inappropriate ADH secretion or acute volume overload. Inborn errors of amino acid metabolism also may present as seizures.

Seizures can result from bacterial meningitis, and encephalitis associated with TORCH complex (toxoplasmosis, rubella, cytomegalovirus infection, and herpes simplex infection) or coxsackie B encephalitis. Developmental abnormalities including congenital hydrocephalus, microcephaly, and other congenital brain anomalies can cause seizures. Drug withdrawal from maternal use of methadone, barbiturates, alcohol, pentazocine (Talwin), and tripelannamine (Pyribenzamine) rarely presents as seizures. Pyridoxine dependence occurs rarely but must be considered in neonatal seizures unresponsive to standard therapy. A rare cause of neonatal seizures is inadvertent fetal scalp injection of maternal local anesthetic agents. Finally, neonatal stroke diagnosed by computed tomography (CT) has recently been described in term infants with focal motor seizures. Neonatal stroke may occur in the setting of diverse cerebrovascular disorders, such as hypoxic-ischemic encephalopathy, polycythemia, acute severe hypertension, and cocaine use.

A careful history, including intrapartum monitoring data and physical examination, is essential when considering drug withdrawal, birth asphyxia, or metabolic disorders as a cause of the seizures. A lumbar puncture with analysis of cell count, culture, and Gram stain along with blood specimens for culture and determinations of sugar, calcium, magnesium, and blood urea nitrogen (BUN) levels should be obtained. The skull x-ray, echoencephalogram, and EEG can be obtained after the seizures have been controlled. In a full-term infant, a CT scan of the head to look for ischemic injury may be necessary, since an echoencephalogram may not provide adequate visualization of the subarachnoid space or posterior fossa. Recently, positron emission tomography of the head has been utilized to evaluate the effects of asphyxia and seizures on cerebral blood flow.

TREATMENT Repeated seizures in neonates may be accompanied by hypoventilation and apnea, resulting in hypercapnia and hypoxemia. Increases in cerebral blood flow and arterial hypertension occur with neonatal seizures. Treatment of seizures should be initiated while awaiting results of laboratory data. An intravenous access route should be established immediately and the airway maintained; assisted ventilation should be initiated if apnea persists. Hypoglycemia and hypocalcemia should be treated as stated above. Hypomagnesemia is often associated with hypocalcemia and should be treated by intravenous administration of 2 to 4 mL of a 2 percent magnesium sulfate solution.

The anticonvulsant drugs used most frequently include phenobarbital and diphenylhydantoin. The loading dosage of phenobarbital is 20 mg/kg intravenously given slowly over 10 min, and the maintenance dose is 5 (mg/kg)/day intramuscularly or orally in two divided doses. If the initial 20 mg/kg dose of phenobarbital is not effective in controlling the seizures, additional doses of 5 mg/kg may be administered every 5 min until the seizures have ceased or the total dose of 40 mg/kg has been reached. In unresponsive cases, diphenylhydantoin may be administered with a similar loading dose followed by maintenance dose of 3 to 5 (mg/kg)/day by the intravenous route in only two divided doses 20 min apart to avoid disturbance of cardiac function. Lorazepam is recommended for status epilepticus as long as ventilation and blood pressure are supported. The dose of lorazepam is 0.01 mg/kg administered intravenously. Infants with pyridoxine dependence respond immediately to an intravenous injection of 50 to 100 mg of pyridoxine.

Diaphragmatic Hernia

A failure of development of the posterolateral parts of the diaphragm at the Bochdalek foramen or retrosternally at the Morgagni foramen allows herniation of the gut into the chest cavity. Left-sided Bochdalek hernias are more common than those on the right. The defect occurs in one out of 2200 births. Associated anomalies with diaphragmatic hernias include congenital heart diseases, genitourinary anomalies, gastrointestinal anomalies, hydronephrosis, and cystic kidneys. Frequently the lungs are hypoplastic bilaterally and have abdominal pulmonary vasculature, predisposing the infant to pulmonary hypertension.

Fifty percent of fetuses with diaphragmatic hernia have difficulty swallowing, and the condition is therefore associated with polyhydramnios. The diagnosis can often be made by prenatal ultrasonography.

CLINICAL FEATURES The clinical findings are localized to the respiratory and digestive tracts. The chest is large, while the abdomen is scaphoid. Bowel sounds are heard in the left chest, and the heart is displaced to the right. Dyspnea, cyanosis, retractions, and vomiting are proportional to the amount of abdominal viscera herniated into the thorax. Radiologic study reveals air-filled loops of bowel in the chest cavity and an absent diaphragmatic margin. The heart is often displaced and the lungs are small in size.

TREATMENT Immediate surgical repair is a method of treatment, and the neonate should be stabilized as much as possible prior to surgery. Alternatively, the neonate can be placed on extracorporeal membrane oxygenation (ECMO) prior to repair. The infant should be intubated immediately, and little or no attempt should be made to ventilate with a mask. The endotracheal tube should be positioned above the carina. Rapid ventilatory rates and low peak inspirator pressures are used to ventilate the infant and prevent reactive respiratory acidosis and hypercarbia, which are potentially conducive to the development of pulmonary hypertension. A large-caliber 10F tube should be placed in the stomach with low continuous suction applied. An umbilical artery catheter is useful to monitor blood gases and pH. Any acidemia should be corrected and the pH maintained in the alkalotic range (pH $>$ 7.45) if possible. Intravenous fluids should be given and the patient kept warm.

The outcome of management of diaphragmatic hernia is dependent on pulmonary parenchymal and vascular hypoplasia, as well as the complex syndrome of persistent fetal circulation. The morbidity is higher when the symptoms present at birth and when the diaphragmatic hernia is detected prenatally. Morgagni hernias, if they do not affect cardiac output, generally have a better prognosis than do Bochdalek hernias. Common complications that occur pre- and postoperatively are pneumothorax, persistent fetal circulation, overdistension of hypoplastic lungs, and chylothorax. The recent introduction of the use of ECMO for infants with persistent pulmonary hypertension after hernia repair has made a minimal impact on prognosis.

Tracheoesophageal Fistula

A defect in the separation of the trachea from the esophagus results in a persistent channel connecting the trachea and the esophagus. There are five types of tracheoesophageal fistulas (TEFs) which are descriptive of the malformations possible: (1) esophageal atresia with a distal communication between the trachea and the esophagus, the most common presentation (85 percent), (2) isolated esophageal atresia occurs, less common, (3) isolated TEF or H type, (4) esophageal atresia with a proximal TEF, and (5) esophageal atresia with a double TEF.

Tracheoesophageal fistulas occur in one out of every 4500 births. One-third of the affected infants weigh less than 2500 g. The incidence of associated anomalies with TEF ranges from 40 to 55 percent. The smaller the infant with TEF, the greater the number of other associated anomalies. Congenital heart malformation, vertebral anomalies, imperforate anus, and radial aplasia are common associated anomalies.

The inability to pass a catheter more than 20 cm through the gastrointestinal tract is the hallmark of esophageal atresia. An x-ray may show the air-filled proximal pouch, and if the catheter is left in place, it may coil in the proximal esophagus. Recurrent pneumonias occur in infants with an H-type fistula.

It is important to provide respiratory support by assisted ventilation if needed to correct acidosis before any surgical repair can be undertaken. A plastic sump catheter should be left in the pouch and connected to constant, low-pressure suction. The patient should be maintained in the reverse Trendelenburg or semi-Fowler position to prevent further reflux of gastric secretions through the fistula into the trachea. Intravenous fluids and antibiotics are indicated. Other coexistent problems, such as a heart defect, should be evaluated. Primary anastomosis is done in cases of esophageal atresia with a distal tracheoesophageal fistula.

The majority (80 percent) of infants with TEF survive. Operative mortality is low. Complications of surgery are pneumonia, atelectasis, anastomotic leak, anastomotic strictures, and (rarely) recurrent fistulas.

Pulmonary Air Leaks

Pulmonary air leaks are a common occurrence in the neonatal intensive care unit. The air may present as pneumothorax, pulmonary interstitial emphysema, pneumomediastinum, pneumopericardium, or pneumoperitoneum.

CLINICAL FEATURES Spontaneous pneumothorax can occur in term and postterm infants following intrapartum asphyxia and meconium aspiration. Currently, however, pneumothorax has increased in incidence with the use of continuous positive airway pressure, positive end-expiratory pressure, mechanical ventilation, and cardiopulmonary resuscitation. Uneven ventilation caused by aspirated blood, mucus, meconium, and amniotic fluid debris can also result in an air leak. Atelectasis, poor ventilation, and air trapping are common predisposing factors. Premature, low-birth-weight infants with surfactant deficiency have a high incidence of air leaks (30 percent), as do newborns with meconium aspiration syndrome (10 percent).

The signs and symptoms of an air leak are those of respiratory distress and often present as an acute clinical deterioration. Grunting respirations and intercostal, sternal, and subcostal retractions may be seen. Cyanosis, elevated respiratory rate, and elevated heart rate are common. Auscultation of the chest reveals decreased breath sounds on the affected side of a pneumothorax, distant heart sounds, and a shift of the mediastinum. Transillumination of the chest with a high-intensity lamp may aid in the diagnosis. A chest x-ray is diagnostic. The accuracy can be improved with a cross-table lateral film of the chest taken along with the anteroposterior and lateral views.

TREATMENT An asymptomatic pneumothorax that is less than 20 percent of the volume of the affected side may be followed clinically with no therapy and with serial radiographic studies every 4 h. Any pneumothorax with severe respiratory distress and clinical deterioration needs emergency treatment. When there are mediastinal shift and cardiovascular collapse, rapid decompression at the fourth intercostal space with a 21-gauge needle attached to a three-way stopcock and a large syringe can be lifesaving.

THORACOSTOMY

Indications

1. To decompress tension pneumothorax, which results in decreased venous return, decreased cardiac output, and low blood pressure
2. To relieve respiratory compromise, in which there is decreased ventilation, increased work of breathing, as well as hypoxia and hypercarbia
3. To drain pleural fluid

Equipment

Sterile towels, 4
4 × 4 Sterile gauze pads, 6
Curved hemostat
Scalpel
Scalpel blade, no 15
Needle holder
000 silk suture
5-mL syringe
10F chest tube for infant <1500 g
12F chest tube for infant >1500 g
Stopcock
Chest tube drainage system
6 ft connecting tubing
Wall suction gauge
Iodine solution
Lidocaine, 1%

Procedure

1. Restrain the patient in the supine position and extend the arm to 90° on the affected side. Monitor heart rate, respiratory rate, and oxygen saturation if possible.
2. Mark the site for placement of the tube. Placement of the tube is at the second or third intercostal space on the midclavicular line. Posterior placement of the chest tube is at the fifth or sixth intercostal space on the anterior axillary line.
3. Clean the area with iodine solution. Infiltrate the site of insertion with lidocaine, and then infiltrate the intercostal muscles and parietal pleura. Incise the skin over the rib, 1 to 1.5 cm.
4. Take the curved hemostat, and, with the tip in the incision, enter the chest cavity just above the rib. Avoid the intercostal nerve, artery, and vein, which run on the lower edge of the rib.
5. Spread the hemostat open and slide the chest tube between the blades of the hemostat to the point where the side holes on the tube are within the pleural cavity. Connect the tube to a water-sealed vacuum system and apply 5 to 10 cm of negative pressure.
6. Increase the pressure to reduce the pneumothorax, if necessary.
7. Close the skin wound and secure the chest tube with silk suture. Verify the position of the chest tube with a chest x-ray. The lung should reexpand promptly following evacuation of the air in the pleural space.

Gastroschisis and Omphalocele

An omphalocele is a defect in the umbilical ring that allows the intestines to protrude out of the abdominal cavity in a sac. A gastroschisis is a defect in the abdominal wall that allows the antenatal evisceration of abdominal structures without a sac being present. There is some controversy as to the exact embryology of the two conditions.

Omphaloceles are found in one out of 6000 to 10,000 births, while gastroschisis occurs twice as frequently in the newborn population. Omphaloceles have a higher (37 percent) incidence of associated anomalies, including chromosomal abnormalities. Three specific syndromes are associated with omphalocele: the upper midline pentalogy of Cantrell, Haller, and Ravitch (sternal, ventral, diaphragmatic, pericardial, and cardiac defects); the lower midline syndrome (vesicointestinal fissure); and the Beckwith-Wiedemann syndrome (macroglossia, visceromegaly, and hypoglycemia).

The emergency management of the two conditions is not different, especially when the sac in an omphalocele is ruptured. The eviscerated bowel should be wrapped in saline-soaked gauze and placed in a plastic bag to protect it from hypothermia and evaporative losses. A nasogastric tube should be inserted to decompress the intestines. Rapid infusion of 20 mL/kg of 5% Ringer's lactate may be necessary to restore vital signs, after which the infusion should be adjusted to maintain a urine output of at least 2 (mL/kg)/h. Intravenous antibiotics should be administered.

Primary fascial closure is the treatment of choice and is often accomplished within hours after birth. When the defect is large, a

Silastic silo may be used, but survival nonetheless correlates with rapid closure and removal of the prosthesis.

Complications include gastroesophageal reflux, malabsorption, diarrhea, dehydration, and failure to thrive. The mortality of omphalocele is 25 to 30 percent, largely as a result of congenital heart disease and sepsis, while death in patients with gastroschisis is associated with intestinal atresia.

Necrotizing Enterocolitis

Necrotizing enterocolitis is a disease entity that affects the asphyxiated or stressed premature infant of less than 2000-g weight. Full-term newborns with polycythemia or congenital heart disease and those who have had umbilical arterial or venous catheters in situ have been reported to also be at risk for necrotizing enterocolitis.

The exact cause of necrotizing enterocolitis remains unknown, and it is likely that there are multiple factors that ultimately lead to stasis, ischemia, and infection of the bowel wall. The risk factors include hypertonic feeding solutions producing damage to mucosal epithelium of the intestine, patent ductus arteriosus and episodes of apnea diverting blood flow away from the gastrointestinal tract, ischemia following exchange transfusions, and infections with *Escherichia coli, Klebsiella pseudomonas, Clostridium* species, coronavirus, rotavirus, and other enteroviruses.

The signs and symptoms, seen in decreasing frequency, are abdominal distention, gastric distention, retention of gastric feeds, apnea, gastrointestinal bleeding, and lethargy. Other signs are abdominal tenderness, redness of abdominal wall, and the presence of reducing substances in the stool.

A supine anteroposterior and cross-table lateral and upright view will aid in the radiographic diagnosis. Nonspecific findings are distention, air-fluid levels, and separation of intestinal loops, suggesting mural edema. Pneumatosis intestinalis is the radiographic hallmark, and its presence indicates gas in the bowel wall. Portal venous gas is an ominous sign, and pneumoperitoneum indicates perforation of the bowel.

The medical management consists of bowel rest, with the infant receiving nothing by mouth, and gastric decompression with a nasogastric tube. Cultures of blood, urine, and cerebrospinal fluid should be obtained. Ampicillin and cefotaxime 100 mg/kg q 8 to 12 h should be administered. The blood pressure and hydration status should be maintained with liberal use of crystalloids and Plasmanate. Fluid intake may have to be increased to 200 (mL/kg)/24 h and inotropic agents used if needed. Thrombocytopenia, neutropenia, and disseminated intravascular coagulopathy are often seen in neonates who are deteriorating, and platelet transfusions should be administered if there is evidence of systemic or gastrointestinal bleeding. Respiratory support may be required, and any acidosis should be corrected. Patients with early necrotizing enterocolitis should have close clinical observations and serial x-rays to look for signs of gangrene or intestinal perforation. The medical treatment includes bowel rest for 2 weeks and nutritional support with parenteral alimentation. The complications of necrotizing enterocolitis are bowel stricture, fistula, abscess, malabsorption, and failure to thrive.

Pneumoperitoneum related to signs of necrotizing enterocolitis is an absolute indication for surgical repair. Recent data indicate that paracentesis indicative of intestinal gangrene prior to intestinal perforation may be an indication for surgery. Persistent acidosis, oliguria, abdominal wall erythema, and portal vein air are associated with advanced disease. The surgical repair consists of removal of the segment of involved bowel and an enterostomy. Reanastomosis is usually performed after 4 to 6 weeks of bowel rest.

Rectal Bleeding

The conditions most often associated with rectal blood or blood in the diaper are polyps (24 to 25 percent), swallowed maternal blood (12 percent), anal fissures (1 to 36 percent), intussusception (7 to 26 percent), Meckel diverticulum (6 percent), and unexplained causes (31 to 48 percent). In unstable patients, management requires volume replacement followed by evaluation, identification, and control of the bleeding. Swallowed maternal blood from the delivery or from nursing on a nipple with a fissure appears in the second or third day of life. The Apt test can identify blood that is maternal in origin. Anal fissures are readily diagnosed as hairline breaks in the epithelium of the anus. In both swallowed blood and anal fissures, small amounts of blood are passed. Diaper blood stains are rarely larger than the size of a 50-cent piece. Patients present with no other signs and are stable and well hydrated. Meckel diverticulum, colonic polyps, and rectal varices are rare in newborns. The history is that of painless, fresh bleeding but no loose and no hard stools. Meckel diverticulum is seen in infants less than 1 year old, while polyps and varices are seen in infants older than 1 year. Intussusception presents with intermittent cramping, abdominal pain, and vomiting. Blood in the stools ("currant-jelly stools") is a late sign. Radiographic studies with contrast confirm the diagnosis.

Sepsis

Sepsis occurs at a rate of about one case per 1000 live births, and one-third of septic newborn babies develop meningitis. Factors associated with perinatal infection are either maternal or perinatal. Premature rupture of membranes, prolonged rupture of membranes, and maternal infection presenting as chorioamnionitis or urinary tract infection increase the likelihood of newborn disease. Low birth weight is the single most important risk factor for the infant. Group B β-hemolytic *Streptococcus* most frequently causes newborn sepsis and meningitis. *E. coli* is second in prevalence, and *Lysteria monocytogenes* and *Haemophilus influenzae* are other pathogens.

Infants often present with subtle and nonspecific findings. Ninety percent of sepsis infants have respiratory distress in the form of apnea, rapid respirations, grunting, nasal flaring, and cyanosis. Temperature instability, decreased activity, metabolic acidosis, low blood pressure, bruising, abdominal distention, ileus, diarrhea, lethargy, and seizures alone or in combination are manifestations of newborn sepsis.

Blood and cerebrospinal fluid samples should be cultured and evaluated for total and differential white blood cell counts, serum glucose level, and cerebrospinal fluid protein. Urinalysis has not been helpful in the management of neonatal sepsis. All infants suspected of being septic should be admitted to the hospital. Ampicillin and cefotaxime concomitantly and each at a dose of 50 to 100 mg/kg q 8 to 12 h will provide the broadest coverage until the organism and antibiotic susceptibility have been determined.

Apnea

Apnea is the absence of respirations for a period of 20 s or if it is associated with a decrease in heart rate of 80 beats per minute and/or accompanied by cyanosis or pallor. Apnea is categorized as *central apnea* when it is of CNS origin. There are no respiratory efforts and no gas flow in central apnea. In *obstructive apnea,* there is impaired gas flow in the presence of respiratory effort. In *mixed apnea,* there are components of both of the above. *Periodic breathing* is apnea of a few seconds' duration in a 20-s span of otherwise normal breathing. In term infants, apnea is never physiologic and is usually secondary to a serious disorder.

PATHOPHYSIOLOGY Apnea and periodic breathing are thought to arise from an immature respiratory center. There is an abnormal biphasic response to hypoxia with a period of tachypnea of several seconds followed by apnea. In premature babies, there is a shift in the carbon dioxide curve so that higher levels of CO_2 are required for respiration. Airway muscle weakness, as well as skeletal muscle weakness, probably contribute to the problem. Finally, the preterm infant may have problems during the sleep-waking states in much the same way as shifts from one sleep state to another are accompanied by respiratory instability in adults.

CLINICAL FEATURES Apnea may occur during any time in the neonatal period. It is always abnormal in the first day of life. After the age of 3 days in a preterm neonate, if it is not associated with any pathologic condition, it may be called benign apnea of prematurity. Apnea is always abnormal in a term newborn. Siblings of children who have died of sudden infant death syndrome have periods of apnea. The pathologic conditions associated with apnea are as follows:

1. Central nervous system: asphyxia, cerebral infarction, hydrocephalus, intracranial hemorrhage, meningitis, and seizures
2. Cardiovascular: congestive heart failure, and patent ductus arteriosus
3. Respiratory: chronic lung disease, hypoxia, pneumonia, and obstruction
4. Digestive system: necrotizing enterocolitis, overfeeding, and vagal response to a nasogastric tube
5. Other causes: anemia, polycythemia, sepsis, temperature instability, hyponatremia, hyperkalemia, hypocalcemia, hypermagnesemia, and high serum levels of phenobarbital, diazepam, opiates, and chloral hydrate

A complete blood count, electrolytes, calcium, glucose, blood gases, drug screen, chest x-ray, electrocardiogram, lumbar puncture, EEG, and an abdominal flat-plate film may be indicated on admission. Further workup may be necessary.

TREATMENT All infants who have benign apnea of prematurity respond to tactile stimulation. When apnea is recurrent and sustained, specific treatment is indicated. The infant who presents in the emergency department should be admitted for evaluation.

Theophylline, 5 to 6 mg/kg should be administered as an oral or intravenous loading dose, followed by 2 mg/kg q 2 h as maintenance. An alternative drug is oral or intravenous caffeine citrate, 20 to 40 mg/kg as loading dose, with 2.5 to 5 mg/kg as maintenance dose.

Continuous positive airway pressure at 2 to 4 cmH_2O may be applied if the above drugs do not resolve the problem.

Mechanical ventilation with endotracheal intubation should be initiated if there is prolonged apnea or repeated episodes are not responsive to the above medications.

Cyanotic Newborns

Cyanosis in neonates may be central or peripheral. Central cyanosis is defined as cyanosis of the tongue, mucous membranes, and peripheral skin and indicates the presence of 5 g or more of reduced hemoglobin. Peripheral cyanosis is defined as blue discoloration confined to the skin of the extremities; the arterial saturation is greater than 94 percent. Peripheral cyanosis is common in neonates and may persist for 2 to 3 days. It is usually due to vasomotor instability secondary to a cold environment.

Normal newborn infants have a Po_2 above 50 mmHg by 5 to 10 min of age; hence, it is pathologic for central cyanosis to persist beyond 20 min after birth. Diagnostic considerations in central cyanosis include right-to-left shunts, pulmonary disorders, CNS disorders, polycythemia, or shock or sepsis.

Congenital heart disease presenting with cyanosis secondary to intracardiac right-to-left shunt includes transposition of the great vessels, tricuspid atresia, truncus arteriosus, tetralogy of Fallot and total anomalous pulmonary venous return with obstruction, pulmonary atresia, and preductal coarctation.

These lung disorders associated with cyanosis include hyaline membrane disease, pneumonia, meconium aspiration syndrome, and persistent fetal circulation due to pneumonia or asphyxia. Mechanical interference with lung function by air leaks (pneumothorax), diaphragmatic hernia, lobar emphysema, or mucous plugs also causes cyanosis.

Intracerebral hemorrhage, when severe, may be associated with shock and cyanosis. The increased viscosity and stagnation of blood in polycythemia may produce cyanosis. Shock and sepsis result in alveolar hypoventilation, causing central cyanosis.

DIAGNOSTIC APPROACH TO CENTRAL CYANOSIS Neonates with cyanosis secondary to cyanotic heart disease rarely have respiratory symptoms other than tachypnea. A murmur may be present. Neonates with lung disease producing cyanosis have respiratory distress, grunting, tachypnea, and sternal and intercostal retractions. Cyanotic infants with CNS disturbances or sepsis have apnea, bradycardia, lethargy, and seizures. Neonates with methemoglobinemia have minimal distress despite their cyanotic appearance.

The "hyperoxia test" (the Pao_2 in response to breathing 100% oxygen) may be of use in distinguishing heart disease from other causes of cyanosis. Neonates with cyanotic heart disease do not demonstrate any increase in Pao_2 over 20 mmHg because of the right-to-left shunting of the circulation. Most neonates with lung disease, however, demonstrate an increase in Pao_2 after breathing 100% oxygen for 20 min. The neonate with persistent fetal circulation, CNS disorders, polycythemia, sepsis, and shock also demonstrates an increase in Pao_2. There is no response elicited in the neonate with methemoglobinemia. When a blood specimen is exposed to air, it turns pink in all the conditions described above except in methemoglobinemia, where the blood remains chocolate colored.

The chest radiograph may demonstrate pulmonary oligemia with normal heart size in tetralogy of Fallot and pulmonary or tricuspid atresia, while pulmonary vascularity is increased in transposition of great vessels, truncus arteriosus, anomalous pulmonary venous return, and hypoplastic left heart. Neonates with lung disease have radiographs that are characteristic of the underlying disease. The electrocardiogram and echocardiogram are useful in diagnosing cyanotic heart disease. Right ventricular hypertrophy may be seen in lung disease with associated pulmonary hypertension.

TREATMENT Most of the cyanotic heart diseases are amenable to palliative or corrective surgery. Infants with severe or complete right ventricular outflow obstruction are dependent on the postnatal patency of the ductus arteriosus for maintenance of adequate pulmonary blood flow and systemic oxygenation. Short-term infusions of prostaglandin E_1 0.05 to 0.1 (μg/kg)/min in these infants have allowed stabilization prior to surgery.

Congestive Cardiac Failure

Heart failure in newborn infants is caused not only by structural heart disease but also by other systemic disorders. Causes of congestive heart failure include (1) structural heart disease (most commonly transposition of the great vessels and hypoplastic left heart syndromes), (2) heart disease without structural abnormalities (myocarditis, cardiac dysrhythmias, glycogen storage disease, and endocardial fibroelastosis), (3) respiratory disease with patent ductus arteriosus with left-to-right shunt, (4) anemia (hemoglobin < 3.5 g/dL), (5) polycythemia, (6) cerebral or other arteriovenous malformation, and (7) sepsis.

The most frequent symptoms are feeding difficulties, tachypnea, increased sweating, tachycardia, rales and rhonchi, liver enlargement, and cardiomegaly. Less common signs and symptoms are ascites, gallop rhythm, pulsus alternans, and increase in central venous pressure. Peripheral edema is exceedingly rare. A clear distinction between right heart failure (characterized by liver enlargement, tachycardia, and dependent edema) and left heart failure (cardiomegaly, rales, tachypnea, and tachycardia) is not as obvious in the neonate as in the older child or adult.

TREATMENT It is essential to monitor the heart and respiratory rates and blood pressure closely. Blood gas levels should be determined frequently to identify and treat hypoxemia or acidosis. Fluid intake should be restricted to 100 (mL/kg)/day and adjusted according to the weight, liver size, and urine output. Electrolyte levels should be monitored closely. Anemia should be corrected with packed red blood cell transfusions. The neonate should be on a 10 to 30° incline with the head elevated inside the incubator.

Infants with heart failure should receive digoxin unless the heart rate is below 100 beats per minute. The digitalizing oral dose of digoxin is 0.03 mg/kg for term neonates. For digitalization, half the calculated digitalizing dose should be given initially, a fourth in 8 h, and another fourth in 8 h, with maintenance started 12 h after the last digitalizing dose. The maintenance dose is one-fourth of the total digitalizing dose in two divided doses. Serum K^+ levels should be checked and monitored.

Furosemide (Lasix) is the drug of choice for a rapid response and should be used intravenously (1 to 3 mg/kg). Maintenance therapy with hydrochlorothiazide (Diuril) and spironolactone (Aldactone) to help conserve potassium may be necessary.

Neonates with severe heart failure from left-to-right shunts with cardiogenic shock and bradycardia may require β-adrenergic drugs for inotropic action. Isoproterenol (Isuprel) may be infused at 0.1 (μg/kg)/min, increased to 0.4 (μg/kg)/min until the heart rate is 140 beats per min. Dopamine is useful in hypotensive shock and should be infused at 5 to 15 (μg/kg)/min. Both medications should be discontinued slowly while heart rate and blood pressure are monitored.

BIBLIOGRAPHY

Avery GB, Fletcher MA, MacDonald MG (eds): *Neonatology: Pathophysiology and Management of the Newborn,* 4th ed. Philadelphia, Lippincott, 1994.

PEDIATRIC CARDIOPULMONARY RESUSCITATION

William E. Hauda II

This chapter reviews cardiopulmonary resuscitation (CPR) in children and notes pertinent differences compared with adults. Perhaps the greatest difference between adult and pediatric arrest is etiology. The most common cause of primary cardiac arrest in adults is coronary artery disease. Children usually develop cardiac arrest secondary to respiratory arrest and shock syndromes. Children have very poor survival rates from cardiac arrest, because it is often associated with prolonged hypoxia or shock.[1,2] Following a cardiac arrest, the survival rate without devastating neurologic sequelae in children is only 2 percent.[3] The best chance for a good outcome is to recognize impending respiratory failure or shock and intervene to prevent the development of cardiopulmonary arrest.

Age-related differences must still be considered with the pediatric population.[4] An appropriate drug dose for a 6-month-old may be excessive for a 1-month-old and yet inadequate for a 5-year-old. Other aspects of resuscitation, such as endotracheal tube size, tidal volumes, cardiac compression rates, and respiratory rates, also vary with a child's age. All emergency medicine practitioners who treat children must be familiar with appropriate size of equipment and rapidly determine the correct dosage of medication for any given child.

The priorities of resuscitation are airway, oxygenation, ventilation, and shock management. These factors are easily compromised in children, but, with prompt intervention, cardiopulmonary arrest may be prevented.[4] International consensus guidelines for basic life support procedures[5] are listed in Table 10-1.

AIRWAY

Anatomy

A child's airway is much smaller than an adult's, and the size varies depending on age. The anatomic and functional differences are more pronounced in infants and young children. The airway is higher and more anterior in a child's neck than in the adult's. The tongue and epiglottis are relatively larger and, thus, more likely to be an obstructing element in a child's airway. Infants younger than 6 months of age are primarily nasal breathers. Thus, keeping the nasal passages clear is vital in a young, spontaneously breathing infant. When a child is supine, the prominent occiput causes flexion of the neck on the chest, occluding the airway. This can be corrected by mild extension of the neck to the sniffing position. Overextension or hyperextension, acceptable for adults, causes obstruction and may kink the trachea, since the cartilaginous support is poor.

Positioning

The sniffing position can be maintained by placing a towel or other object beneath the shoulders. Despite good head position, a child's hypotonic mandibular tissues may still allow the relatively large tongue to occlude the airway posteriorly. This can be relieved by a chin lift or jaw thrust that elevates the mandible anteriorly and separates the tongue from the posterior pharyngeal wall. The jaw-thrust technique is preferred in a child with a possible cervical spine injury, because it minimizes the movement of the neck while allowing maintenance of a neutral position of the cervical spine. If these maneuvers are unsuccessful, an oral airway or endotracheal tube should be considered.

NASOPHARYNGEAL AIRWAY Nasopharyngeal airways tend to be less useful in children because of the small nasal passages and the presence of hypertrophic adenoid tissue in the posterior nasopharynx, which is easily traumatized when inserting a nasopharyngeal airway.

ORAL AIRWAY Oral airways, which should be used only in unconscious children, are most useful in patients who require a continuous jaw thrust or chin lift to maintain airway patency. Oral airways are inserted with a tongue depressor to push the tongue into the mandible so that the airway can be inserted under direct vision.

Intubation

Endotracheal intubation of infants and children is felt by many to be easier than the same procedure in adults. There are, however, some differences related to a child's anatomy and proper sizing of equipment. Pediatric airway management is discussed in detail in Chap. 11. A brief overview is provided here for perspective.

POSITIONING Hyperextension of the neck must be avoided by placing the child in the sniffing position prior to intubation. Also, the stretcher should be raised so that the child's head is at least at the level of the intubator's waist. All equipment should be located within easy reach of the team, including the bag-valve mask, oxygen source, monitoring equipment, and, perhaps most importantly, the suction device.

LARYNGOSCOPE BLADES For two reasons, the curved (MacIntosh) blade is rarely used in children who are younger than age 4. The relatively large and flaccid epiglottis is not effectively displaced by pulling on it indirectly from the vallecular space. Second, an exact-

TABLE 10-1 Guidelines for Pediatric Basic Life Support

Maneuver	Newborn	Infant <1 Year	Child 1–8 Years	Adult >8 Years
Airway	Head tilt/chin lift	Head tilt/chin lift	Head tilt/chin lift	Head tilt/chin lift
If trauma	Jaw thrust	Jaw thrust	Jaw thrust	Jaw thrust
If foreign body	Suction	Back blows and chest thrusts	Abdominal thrusts	Abdominal thrusts
Breathing rate	30–60/min (every 1–2 s)	20/min (every 3 s)	20/min (every 3 s)	12/min (every 5 s)
Circulation				
Pulse check	Umbilical	Brachial	Carotid	Carotid
Compression				
Location	1 finger below intramammary line	1 finger below intramammary line	Lower half of sternum	Lower half of sternum
Method	2 fingers or 2 thumbs	2 fingers	Heel of 1 hand	2 hands
Depth	$\frac{1}{3}$ of chest	$\frac{1}{3}$ of chest	$\frac{1}{3}$ of chest	$\frac{1}{3}$ of chest
Rate	120/min	100/min	100/min	100/min
Ventilation ratio	3:1	5:1	5:1	5:1 (15:2 for 1 rescuer)

sized blade must be used to fit the curvature of the tongue. For these reasons, a straight (Miller) blade is preferred. The straight blade is inserted in the midline with the tip underneath the epiglottis such that the epiglottis is directly lifted up to allow tracheal visualization.

ENDOTRACHEAL TUBE Tracheal tube sizes vary with a patient's age. An often-quoted rule is that the correct internal diameter tube size is approximately the same size as the end of the patient's little finger. However, this tenet has been shown to not hold true.[6,7] The age-based formula (age + 16)/4 is a good predictor of correct endotracheal tube size for children. Uncuffed tubes are used for children up to 7 or 8 years old (tube size, 2.5 to 5.5 mm). The subglottic trachea (unlike in adults) is the narrowest spot of the tracheal apparatus and forms an adequate seal around the endotracheal tube in this age group. After this age, the vocal cords become the narrowest part to the airway and a cuff is needed to provide an adequate seal for positive pressure ventilation. One can almost always intubate with a laryngoscope blade that is too large and with a tube that is too small, but not vice versa.

SECURING THE AIRWAY Once a child has been intubated, one person should be assigned to hold the endotracheal tube in place until it is securely fastened. Confirmation of endotracheal intubation is similar to that in adults: adequate chest rise, symmetric breath sounds, capnographic or capnometric readings,[8] improved oxygenation, and clinical improvement.[4] Because a young child has a small chest, listening to breath sounds in each axilla as well as over the stomach will minimize the chance of hearing sounds transmitted from the other lung.[4] The tube should be taped to the upper lip and jaw, ideally from both sides of the face. Especially in small infants, small movements can easily displace the tube from the trachea into the esophagus. Tape or ties should not be wrapped around the head of a young child, because these can slide off the occiput and easily allow displacement of the tube. Mechanical ventilation is discussed in *Breathing,* which follows.

Foreign Body Management

Controversy exists as to the safest and most effective emergency maneuvers to use with a choking child. The American Heart Association specifically discourages two common maneuvers used with adult patients: (1) the Heimlich maneuver for patients younger than age 1, because of the potential for injury to abdominal organs, and (2) blind finger sweeps, because of the possibility of pushing the foreign body further into the airway.[4] Serious differences of opinion exist, but current recommendations rely on the back blow and chest thrust to clear an infant's airway.

CONSCIOUS CHILDREN A child who is choking but is able to maintain some ventilation or vocalization should be allowed to clear her or his own airway by coughing. Once a child cannot cough, vocalize, or breathe, a sequence of steps must be immediately instituted. Choking infants are treated with an alternating sequence of five back blows and five chest thrusts. With the infant's torso positioned prone and head down along the rescuer's arm, or the older child draped prone and head down across the rescuer's knees, five blows are delivered to the interscapular area. The infant is then repositioned supinely along the rescuer's arm, or the larger infant can be placed on the floor as for external cardiac compression, and five chest thrusts (cardiac compressions) are delivered. These are continued until the child's airway obstruction is relieved or the child becomes unconscious. In older children, the Heimlich maneuver is used, with the rescuer kneeling or standing behind the child. The clenched fist is placed at the level of the umbilicus, and firm upward thrusts are continued until the obstruction is cleared or the child becomes unconscious.

UNCONSCIOUS CHILDREN In all cases where a child becomes unconscious with the rescuer present, the rescuer should first attempt ventilation because the object may have become dislodged. If an obstruction is still present, then airway clearance maneuvers must be continued. For infants, the same sequence is used, but between each cycle of back blows and chest thrusts (the same technique as for CPR) an attempt at ventilation should be made. Before attempting a ventilation, the airway should be inspected to see whether an object is present. Only remove a visualized object, do not use blind finger sweeps. If the obstruction persists, the sequence is repeated. For children older than age 1, the Heimlich maneuver is performed with the child lying down and the rescuer straddling the child's thighs. Future investigation may well lead to revised recommendations.

The foregoing recommendations are directed primarily at a first responder who has neither access to, nor the skills to use, airway management equipment. For unconscious children in emergency departments, direct laryngoscopy, visualization, and removal of the foreign body with McGill forceps should be attempted rapidly. Until this equipment is ready, however, use the basic life support techniques.

BREATHING

Mouth to Mouth

Whether to employ mouth-to-mouth or mouth-to-mouth-and-nose ventilation depends on the size of the patient. The rate of ventilation is shown in Table 10-1. Ventilations are done slowly to avoid the generation of high airway pressures, which can overcome esophageal resistance and result in gastric distention.

Bag-Valve Mask

The self-inflating bag-valve mask system is most commonly used for ventilation. Ventilation bags used for infants and children should have a minimum volume of 450 mL. There is a common misconception that children are more susceptible to pneumothoraces at high inspiratory pressures. In fact, pediatric lung compliance is very good, and children can tolerate relatively high pressures. Pneumothoraces more commonly result from the administration of excessive tidal volume. The tidal volume necessary to ventilate children is the same as that for adults: 10 to 15 mL/kg. Since it is impractical to calculate the tidal volume in emergency situations, start ventilating with the smallest volume that causes adequate chest rise. Careful monitoring of the rate of ventilation is crucial to avoid excessive hyperventilation, a very common mistake.

Mechanical Ventilation

If an endotracheal tube is placed, then mechanical ventilation should soon be instituted. Determining appropriate initial settings for the mechanical ventilation of children can be difficult. For children weighing less than 10 kg, time-flow or pressure preset ventilators should be used. For time-flow ventilators, inspiratory and expiratory times are needed. Typical inspiratory times are $\frac{1}{2}$ to 1 s, depending on ventilation frequency. For pressure ventilators, inflating pressures are determined by using pressures necessary to inflate the lungs and cause the chest to rise. Pressures usually range from 15 to 40 mmHg. Excess pressures can cause barotrauma. For older children, volume ventilators can be used, starting with a tidal volume of 10 mL/kg, as for adults. If the lungs have normal compliance and the child does not require hyperventilation, then the respiratory rate should be started at $\frac{1}{2}$ the normal rate for age (20 breaths/min for infants, 15 breaths/min for young children, and 10 breaths/min for older children and adolescents). Children should be adequately sedated and paralyzed during mechanical ventilation until definitive care is started in a pediatric intensive care unit.

CIRCULATION

External Cardiac Compression

The brachial pulse is recommended for monitoring purposes for infants younger than age 1. Above this age, the femoral pulse is most easily accessible, but most guidelines recommend assessment of the carotid pulse by laypersons. Absence of pulse, or poor perfusion with a heart rate of 60 bpm or less, mandates external cardiac compression. Most patients should be placed on a hard surface. With smaller infants, the wraparound two-thumb technique can be used.

Current standards advocate compressions over the lower sternum as opposed to midsternum.[5] Whether to use two fingers, two thumbs, three fingers, or the heel of the hand depends on the size of the child. Whichever method comfortably produces a compression depth of approximately one-third the anteroposterior diameter should be used. The rate of compressions is at least 100/min in infants and older children. The ratio of ventilations to compressions is 1:5 for both one-person CPR and two-person CPR. A pause of 1 to 1.5 s between ventilations should be allowed for adequate exhalation. To assess the adequacy of the compression depth and rate, the femoral or carotid artery should be palpated during compressions.

TABLE 10-2 Body Weight Estimation Guidelines

Age	Weight, kg	
Term infant	3.5	Birth weight (BW)
6 Months	7	2 × BW
1 Year	10	3 × BW
4 Years	16	$\frac{1}{4}$ Adult weight of 70 kg
10 Years	35	$\frac{1}{2}$ Adult weight

TABLE 10-3 Essential Drugs

Drug	Concentration	Dose
Epinephrine		
First dose	1:10,000 (0.1 mg/mL)	0.01–0.02 mg/kg
High dose	1:1000 (1 mg/mL)	0.1–0.2 mg/kg
Atropine	1:10,000 (0.1 mg/mL)	0.02 mg/kg*
Sodium bicarbonate	1 meq/mL	1.0 meq/kg

*Minimum dose is 0.1 mg regardless of weight.

VASCULAR ACCESS

Difficulty in obtaining rapid intravenous (IV) access is certainly one of the major differences between adult and pediatric resuscitation (see Chap. 17, "Vascular Access"). Two important facts should be kept in mind. First, a significant portion of children respond to airway management alone, since most cardiac arrests in children are secondary to hypoxic respiratory arrest. Time spent securing vascular access at

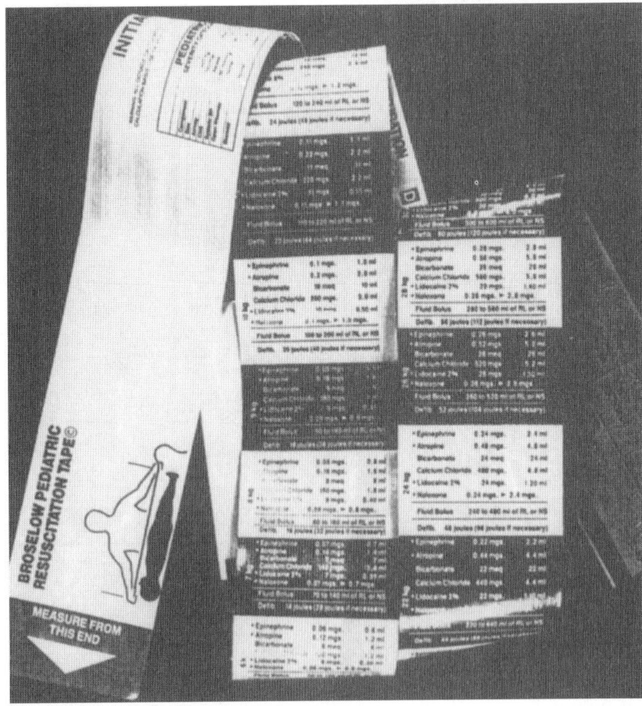

FIG. 10-1. The Broselow Resuscitation Tape.

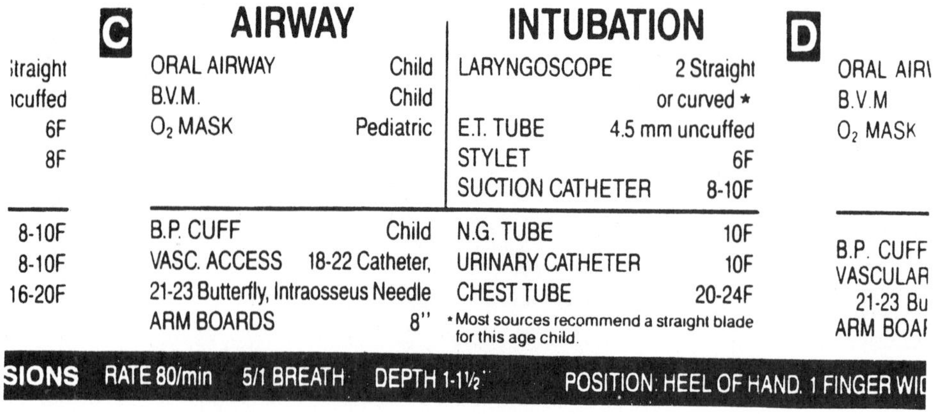

	C AIRWAY		INTUBATION		D
;traight	ORAL AIRWAY	Child	LARYNGOSCOPE	2 Straight or curved *	ORAL AIR\
ıcuffed	B.V.M.	Child			B.V.M
6F	O_2 MASK	Pediatric	E.T. TUBE	4.5 mm uncuffed	O_2 MASK
8F			STYLET	6F	
			SUCTION CATHETER	8-10F	
8-10F	B.P. CUFF	Child	N.G. TUBE	10F	B.P. CUFF
8-10F	VASC. ACCESS	18-22 Catheter,	URINARY CATHETER	10F	VASCULAR
16-20F	21-23 Butterfly, Intraosseus Needle		CHEST TUBE	20-24F	21-23 Bu
	ARM BOARDS	8"	* Most sources recommend a straight blade for this age child.		ARM BOAI

SIONS RATE 80/min 5/1 BREATH DEPTH 1-1½" POSITION: HEEL OF HAND. 1 FINGER WI

FIG. 10-2. Equipment side of the Broselow Resuscitation Tape. One of seven color equipment zones.

the expense of adequate airway management is a common mistake in dealing with children. Second, once a patient has been intubated, the tracheal route may be used to administer drugs such as lidocaine, epinephrine, atropine, and naloxone (mnemonic: LEAN). The dose of endotracheal epinephrine for symptomatic bradycardia or pulseless cardiac arrest is 0.1 mg/kg, 1:1000 concentration q 3 to 5 min. Although the ideal doses for other drugs have never been studied in children, current recommendations support the use of two to three times the IV dose.[4]

Although central access would be ideal for administration of drugs during CPR, many emergency medicine practitioners are not highly skilled in placing central lines in children. Therefore, the most frequently used sites are peripheral: scalp, arm, hand, or antecubital veins; the external jugular vein; femoral vein; or distal saphenous vein via cutdown. Intraosseous infusion is a quick, safe route for resuscitation drugs as well as fluid administration. This is discussed in Chap. 17, "Vascular Access." The general order of attempts during a resuscitation should be antecubital, hand, or foot and then intraosseous.

FLUIDS

In the face of hypotension due to volume depletion, isotonic fluid boluses of 20 mL/kg should be given as rapidly as possible and repeated, depending on response.[4] A syringe attached to a three-way stopcock and extension tubing can be used to deliver aliquots of fluid rapidly, until the entire bolus is administered. Do not depend on gravity or pressure bags. The bolus should be delivered in a maximum of 20 min, and then the child's condition should be reassessed. If volume depletion has been corrected (at most, three to four boluses) and hypotension persists, a pressor agent should be strongly considered, preferably with the aid of a central venous pressure catheter. In normotensive patients or when the IV line is being used for drug administration only, it should be maintained at the minimum rate that will keep the vein open (KVO). Fine fluid and electrolyte calculations and adjustments can be made after the emergency treatment has been completed. Overhydration, even when IV lines are set at KVO, is common when adult equipment is used in pediatric resuscitations. To enable easy monitoring of the total volume given, preventing accidental overhydration, a pediatric microdrip should always be used when resuscitating children.

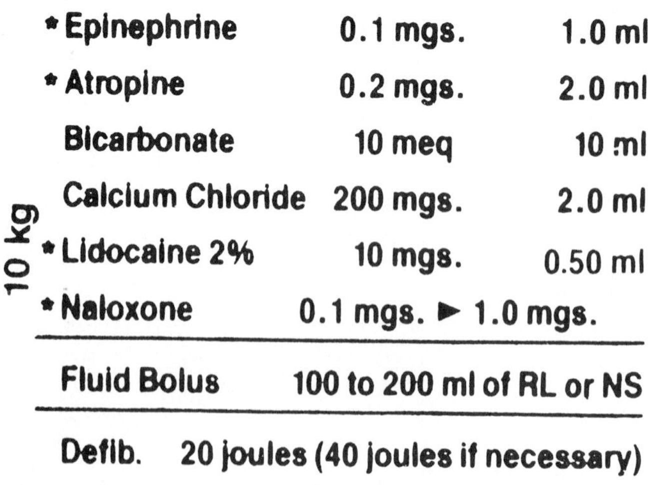

10 kg			
	* Epinephrine	0.1 mgs.	1.0 ml
	* Atropine	0.2 mgs.	2.0 ml
	Bicarbonate	10 meq	10 ml
	Calcium Chloride	200 mgs.	2.0 ml
	* Lidocaine 2%	10 mgs.	0.50 ml
	* Naloxone	0.1 mgs. ► 1.0 mgs.	
	Fluid Bolus	100 to 200 ml of RL or NS	
	Defib.	20 joules (40 joules if necessary)	

FIG. 10-3. Drug side of the Broselow Resuscitation Tape. One of 25 precalculated weight zones for resuscitation drugs.

PHARMACOLOGIC AGENTS

The indications for the use of specific drugs are essentially the same for children as for adults. Particular to pediatrics, however, is the problem of drug dosage. Proper dosage in children requires knowledge of the patient's weight (Table 10-2), knowledge of the dose (usually given in milligrams per kilogram), and error-free calculation and delivery. Problems may arise in remembering the correct dose, performing calculations in the crisis situation (a common error involves the misplacement of a decimal point and results in 10 times or one-tenth the correct dosage), and delivery of the correct dosage (because of an error in drawing up the correctly calculated amount). Use of a chart with precalculated drug doses can help reduce dosage errors (Table 10-3). However, estimating a child's weight accurately so that the proper dosage can be determined from the table is not easy, especially in a crisis situation. Choosing the proper sized equipment for pediatric patients is similarly difficult. Valuable time can be lost in weight estimation, dosage calculations, and equipment selection.

Recently, systems based on a direct measurement of a patient's length have been developed for estimating dosages and selecting equipment in pediatric emergencies (see Table 10-3).[9] In children, length has a direct correlation with weight. It has also been shown to be one of the most accurate predictors of correct equipment sizes for pediatric patients, especially endotracheal tube sizes. The use of a length-based system is currently included in the American Heart Association's Pediatric Advanced Life Support Course (PALS). These systems use a tape to assist making appropriate selections. Most tapes are two sided and display emergency resuscitation drug dosage and equipment selection based on length (see Figs. 10-1 to 10-3). Fluid volumes for resuscitation as well as appropriate basic life support techniques are often also displayed. To make optimal use of these systems, emergency personnel must be able to find the proper equipment rapidly. Equipment can be stored in shelves or drawers labeled by age and weight, or a

TABLE 10-4 Calculation for Dosage of Medications Delivered by Constant Infusion Using the Rule of 6

Drug	Continuous Infusion Dose, μg/kg/min	Conversion Factor, mg × wt (kg)	Delivery
Epinephrine dose	0.1–1.0 μg/kg/min	0.6 mg × wt (kg)	1 mL/h = 0.1 μg/kg/min
Dobutamine dose	5–10 μg/kg/min	6 mg × wt (kg)	1 mL/h = 1.0 μg/kg/min
Dopamine	5–20 μg/kg/min	6 mg × wt (kg)	1 mL/h = 1.0 μg/kg/min
Isoproterenol	0.1–1.0 μg/kg/min	.6 mg × wt (kg)	1 mL/h = 0.1 μg/kg/min
Lidocaine	20–50 μg/kg/min	60 mg × wt (kg)	1 mL/h = 10 μg/kg/min

Dosage of medications delivered by constant infusions is calculated in terms of micrograms per kilogram per minute. Actual calculation can be confusing and a source of lethal decimal errors. The *rule of 6* can be used for *dopamine* and *lidocaine* to simplify dosage calculation:

6 mg × wt (kg), *fill* to 100 mL with D_5W

The medication is mixed in an intravenous set with a measured chamber and a microdrip (1 drop/min = 1 mL/h). Rate of administration is best set by an electric pump.

Example: For a 10-kg infant requiring dopamine:

6 mg × 10 = 60 mg dopamine

In a measured chamber *fill* to 100 mL with D_5W. Weight is now factored in so that

1 mL/h = 1 μg/kg per min
5 mL/h = 5 μg/kg per min
10 mL/h = 10 μg/kg per min

For *isoproterenol* the rule of 6:

0.6 mg × wt (kg), *fill* to 100 mL with D_5W
1 mL/h = 0.1 μg/kg per min
5 mL/h = 0.5 μg/kg per min

system of color codes can be used in which color-coded shelves, carts, or equipment organizers correspond to specific length categories.

The pharmacology of resuscitation drugs has been well described in other chapters (see Chap. 25), but a few peculiarities pertain to pediatric resuscitation drug use.

Epinephrine

Epinephrine is the one drug proven beneficial in cases of cardiac arrest. It is specifically indicated for hypoxia- or ischemia-induced slow rates that fail to respond to adequate oxygenation and ventilation and to pulseless arrest situations (i.e., asystole, pulseless electrical activity, and ventricular fibrillation). If the initial dose of epinephrine is not effective, 10 to 20 times that dose should be given subsequently. However, the use of high-dose epinephrine (0.1 mg/kg of the 1:1000 concentration) for resuscitation in infants and children has not been associated with increased survival rate in any controlled prospective studies. PALS has recommended,[4] and at the time of this writing continues to recommend, that high-dose epinephrine be used if there is no response to the initial standard dose. Studies addressing this issue that are currently concluding are not expected to show an increase in neurologically intact survival. Adverse effects associated with the use of high-dose epinephrine in the clinical setting include intracranial hypertension, myocardial hemorrhage, and myocardial necrosis.[5] Epinephrine, rather than dopamine, is the vasopressor infusion of choice in children, because dopamine requires release of endogenous norepinephrine. In children with cardiac arrest, norepinephrine stores may be low.

Atropine

Primary cardiac causes of slow rates are rare with the pediatric population and may also be treated with atropine. The recommended dose of atropine is 0.02 mg/kg IV. The minimum dose is 0.1 mg, with a maximum single dose of 0.5 mg for children and 1.0 mg for adolescents. The dose may be repeated once, with a maximum total dose of 1.0 mg for children and 2.0 mg for adolescents. There is no particular proscription against further doses, but the maximum dose is considered to be fully vagolytic. If no response to atropine is seen, then dosing beyond the vagolytic amount is unlikely to be effective. If an effect is seen, but not maintained, further doses may be tried.

Sodium Bicarbonate

Sodium bicarbonate is no longer a first-line drug, because it worsens acidosis when administered in the presence of inadequate ventilation and perfusion. It is administered only after epinephrine administration has not improved a clinical situation. An initial dose of 1 meq/kg IV is given only after the airway has been secured, the patient hyperventilated, and CPR initiated. An exception may be a situation where hyperkalemia is a factor, and where metabolic acidosis is severe. Resuscitation drugs are ineffective in the face of severe acidosis and severe alkalosis. In neonates or premature infants, sodium bicarbonate should be diluted 1:1 with sterile water, not saline. Indications for bicarbonate use are the same as for adults.

Calcium

Because of lack of proven efficacy and because of possible deleterious effects, calcium administration is no longer routinely recommended during resuscitation. Calcium should be used for documented hyperkalemia, hypocalcemia, and calcium-channel blocker overdose.

The Rule of 6

Often there is great confusion when attempting to calculate the dose of a medication to be delivered by constant infusion. The *rule of 6* can

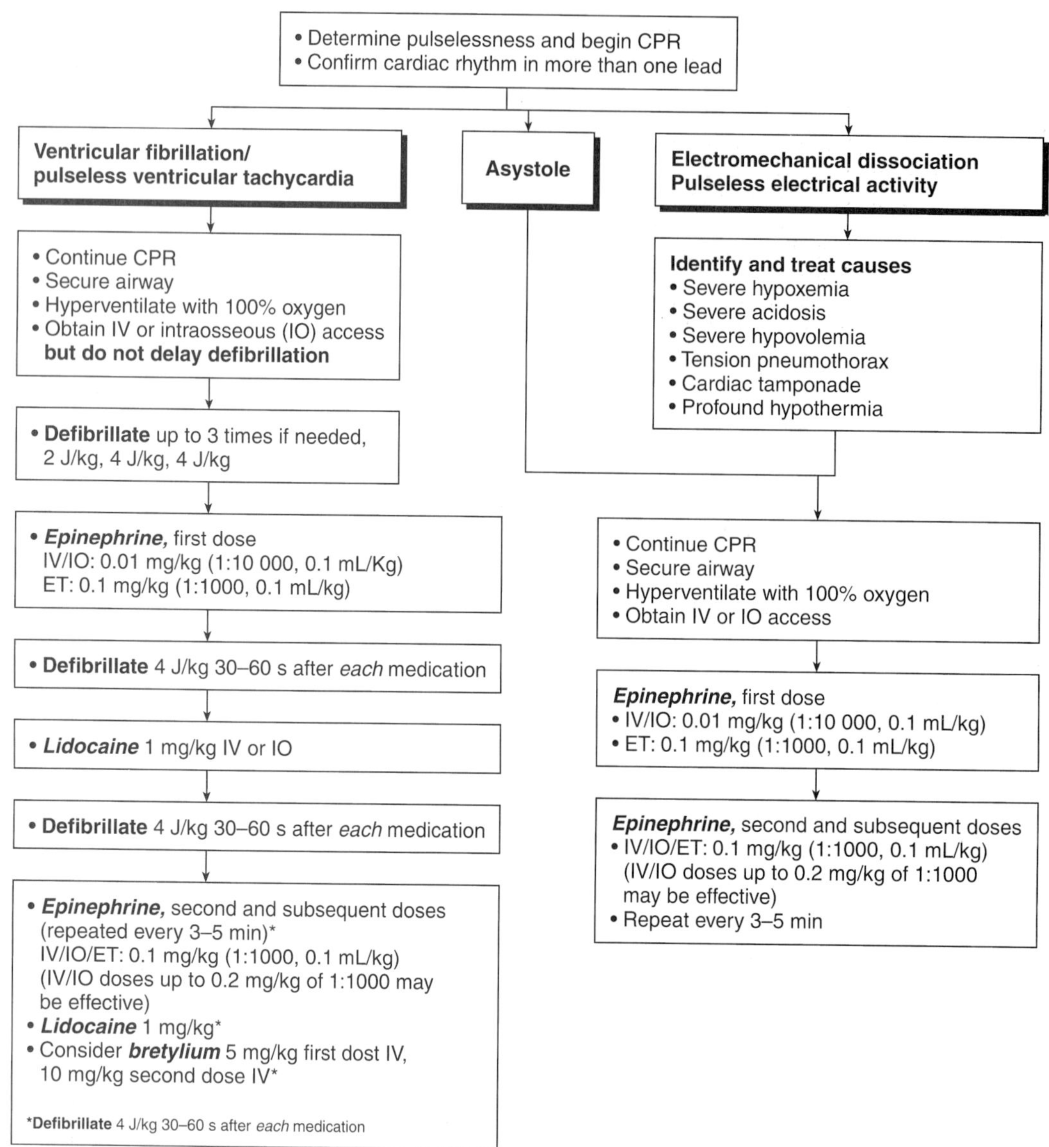

FIG. 10-4. Asystole and pulseless arrest decision tree. IV, intravenous/IO, intraosseous; ET, endotracheal.

be used to avoid mistakes (Table 10-4). The Broselow tape (Armstrong Medical Industries) can be used to assist.

DYSRHYTHMIAS

Dysrhythmia management plays only a small role in the resuscitation of children. Since rhythm disturbances are usually secondary to hypoxia and not primary cardiac events, careful attention must be given to the correction of hypoxia, acidosis, and fluid balance. Ventilation and oxygenation must be accomplished first. Pulse oximetry, or arterial blood-gas analysis, should be performed to assess oxygen and blood-gas status. An IV of 0.9% NaCl or lactated Ringer solution should be established and the child placed on a cardiac monitor.

A patient with an abnormal cardiac rhythm or rate, coupled with evidence of poor end-organ perfusion (cyanosis, mottled skin, lethargy, etc.), has an unstable cardiac rhythm and requires immediate intervention. The parameters of clinical assessment and expression of instability vary with a child's age. In neonates, blood pressure measurement is difficult, and a heart rate of 80 bpm or less, coupled with evidence of poor end-organ perfusion, requires immediate intervention. In infants and children, variations in heart rate may be well tolerated clinically, and a blood pressure of 70 mmHg or less, coupled with evidence of poor end-organ perfusion, is used to define instability. Figures 10-4 and 10-5 summarize electrical and drug therapy of unstable cardiac rhythms in children.

The most common rhythms seen in pediatric arrest are the bradycardias, which lead to asystole if untreated. Treatment consists of maximizing oxygenation and ventilation. Chest compression should be started in children with a heart rate of less than 60 bpm and signs of poor perfusion.

Paroxysmal atrial tachycardia (supraventricular tachycardia, or SVT) is most commonly seen in infants and most often presents as a narrow complex tachycardia with rates usually between 250 and 350 bpm. Treatment of unstable patients consists of rapid synchronized cardioversion. Treatment of stable patients varies. Adenosine, vagal maneuvers, or cardioversion are used to treat stable SVT. Adenosine (0.1 mg/kg) is the current recommended drug for SVT in children. This dose can be doubled if the first dose is unsuccessful.

Differentiating a rapid secondary sinus tachycardia from a rapid primary cardiac tachycardia can be difficult. Although heart rates of 150 to 200 bpm in adults are usually cardiac in origin, young children not uncommonly have compensatory sinus tachycardias as fast as

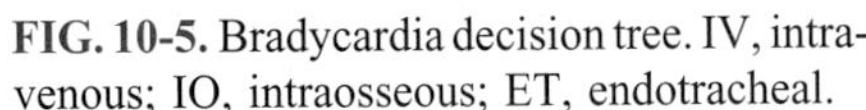

FIG. 10-5. Bradycardia decision tree. IV, intravenous; IO, intraosseous; ET, endotracheal.

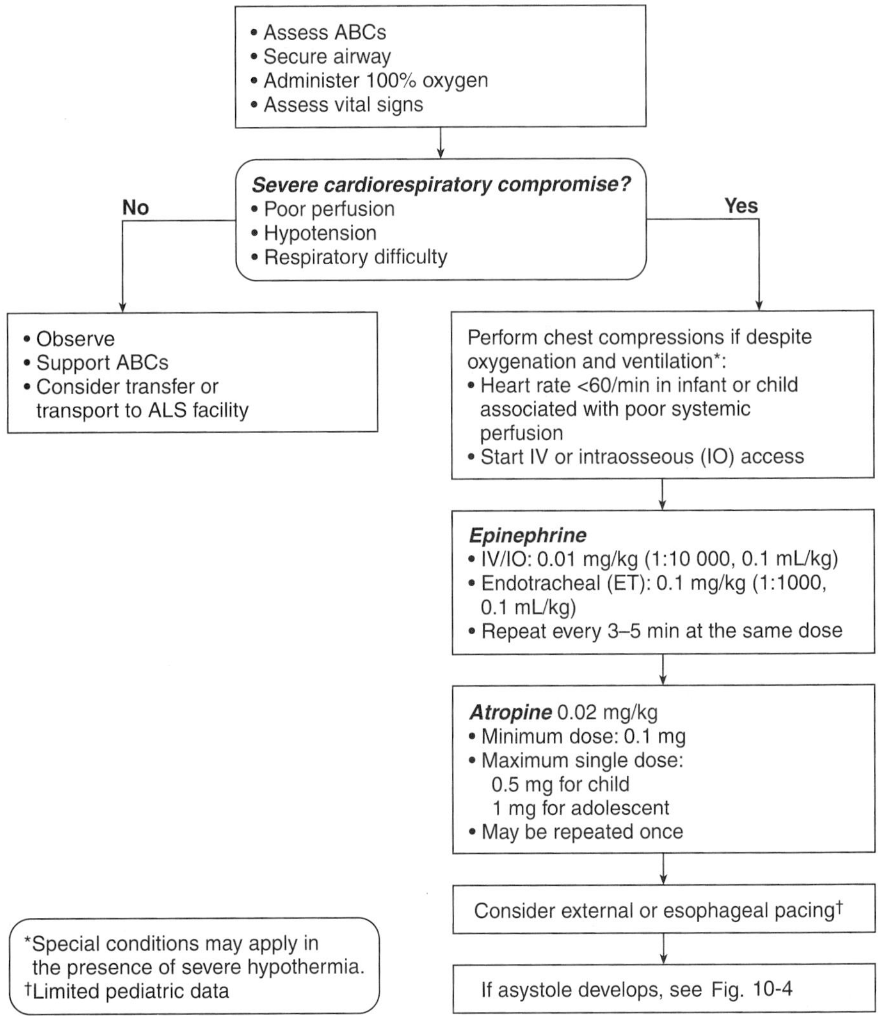

200 to 220 bpm, especially small infants. Children can tolerate rapid primary cardiac heart rates for long periods before congestive heart failure or lethal dysrhythmias develop. Differentiating primary from secondary tachycardia is critical to patient management. However, an ECG may not be very helpful because, at very fast rates, in either sinus tachycardia or SVT, identifiable P waves may not be readily apparent. Historical features pointing to volume loss likely suggest sinus tachycardia. Evidence of congestive heart failure is more likely associated with a pathologic rhythm.

CARDIOVERSION, DEFIBRILLATION, AND PACING

Electric conversion is used on an emergency basis to treat ventricular fibrillation (defibrillation) and symptomatic tachydysrhythmias (cardioversion). Ventricular fibrillation as a cause of cardiac arrest is rare in children and even more rare in infants.[10]

Paddle Size

Paddle size is usually 4.5 cm for infants (who weigh less than 10 kg) and 8 cm for children. The paddle should be in contact with the chest wall over its entire surface area. The larger 8-cm paddles can be used for infants in the anteroposterior position.

Interface

Electrode cream, electrode paste, and saline-soaked gauze pads are all acceptable. Alcohol pads are to be discouraged, because serious burns may be produced. Care must be taken so that the interface substance from one paddle does not come in contact with the substance from the other paddle. This creates a short circuit, and insufficient energy may be delivered to the heart.

Electrode Position

One paddle is placed on the right of the sternum at the second intercostal space. The other is placed in the left midclavicular line at the level of the xyphoid. The anteroposterior approach can be used as well.[4]

Defibrillation

Initially, 2 J/kg should be used. If that is unsuccessful, the amount should be doubled and performed twice at the higher energy level, if necessary. If the three attempts are unsuccessful, epinephrine should be given at the standard dose. The oxygenation and ventilation of the child should be maximized for 1 to 2 min before repeating a defibrillation attempt at the higher setting.

Cardioversion

Tachydysrhythmias are generally very sensitive to electric conversion. Initial dose is $\frac{1}{2}$ J/kg. The energy level is doubled if the first attempt is unsuccessful. If the device only has a few energy settings available, choose the one that is closest to the desired energy setting. All tachydysrhythmias should be treated with synchronized cardioversion. If

TABLE 10-5 Length-Based Equipment Chart (Length, cm)

Item	54–70	70–85	85–95	95–107	107–124	124–138	138–155
Endotracheal tube size (mm)	3.5	4.0	4.5	5.0	5.5	6.0	6.5
Lip-tip length (mm)	10.5	12.0	13.5	15.0	16.5	18.0	19.5
Laryngoscope	1 Straight	1 Straight	2 Straight	2 Straight or curved	2 Straight or curved	2–3 Straight or curved	3 Straight or curved
Suction catheter	8F	8–10F	10F	10F	10F	10F	12F
Stylet	6F	6F	6F	6F	14F	14F	14F
Oral airway	Infant/small child	Small child	Child	Child	Child/small adult	Child/adult	Medium adult
Bag-valve mask	Infant	Child	Child	Child	Child	Child/adult	Adult
Oxygen mask	Newborn	Pediatric	Pediatric	Pediatric	Pediatric	Adult	Adult
Vascular access	22–24/23–25	20–22/ 23–25	18–22/ 21–23	18–22/ 21–23	18–20/ 21–23	18–20/ 21–22	16–20/ 18–21
Catheter/butterfly	Intraosseous		Intraosseous		Intraosseous		Intraosseous
Nasogastric tube	5–8F	8–10F	10F	10–12F	12–14F	14–18F	18F
Urinary catheter	5–8F	8–10F	10F	10–12F	10–12F	12F	12F
Chest tube	10–12F	16–20F	20–24F	20–24F	24–32F	28–32F	32–40F
Blood pressure cuff	Newborn/infant	Infant/child	Child	Child	Child	Child/adult	Adult

Directions for use:
1. Measure patient length with centimeter tape.
2. Using measured length in centimeters, access appropriate equipment column.
Source: Adapted from Luten et al,[9] with permission.

synchronization in not possible (i.e., if the device cannot identify the QRS), then use the defibrillator in the unsynchronized mode.

Transcutaneous Pacing

Children with a severe bradycardia or asystole may respond to pacing. Because transvenous pacing requires central venous access with large tubing and proficient skill in placing the pacing electrodes, most emergency practitioners and prehospital providers should only attempt transcutaneous pacing. Adult patches should be used in children who weigh over 15 kg.[11] The negative electrode patch should be placed on the anterior chest at V_3, and the positive electrode patch is placed on the posterior chest between the shoulder blades at the T4 vertebral level.[12] Ventricular capture is determined by the palpation of a pulse or the appearance of an arterial waveform if an arterial pressure catheter is present. Begin with the maximal energy output.[12] If ventricular capture occurs, then decrease the energy setting progressively until the lowest setting is found that allows ventricular capture. The pacing rate should be set at a rate slightly higher than the normal rate for age. Transcutaneous pacing has not been associated with greatly improved survival rates, but it can be life-saving if applied quickly in a child with sudden asystole or bradycardia.

SUMMARY OF MANAGEMENT GUIDELINES

The age-related differences are difficult to remember and cause major problems in pediatric resuscitation. One should not have to memorize numbers such as drug doses, tube sizes, or cardiac compression ratios. The proper organization of equipment, the posting of pediatric CPR data and equipment sheets, and the use of a length-based system (Table 10-5) can eliminate the need to commit many variables to memory and can reduce the possibility of errors. This eliminates much of the general anxiety connected with pediatric resuscitation and leaves clinicians free to apply the principles of resuscitation to the children as presented.

TERMINATION OF EFFORTS

Pediatric cardiopulmonary arrest of longer than 20 min or with no response to two doses of epinephrine has been associated with a dismal outcome.[1] Resuscitation should be continued until a core temperature of 30°C is reached if cardiac electrical activity is present in a child with hypothermia.

COPING WITH THE DEATH OF A CHILD

Both family members and the resuscitation team members will mourn the death of a child. Little attention has been focused on this issue for either the family or the emergency department staff. Several *tasks of mourning* have been described that must occur for successful resolution of grieving (Table 10-6).[13] Whether a child dies in the emergency

TABLE 10-6 Tasks of Family Mourning a Lost Child

1. Accept the reality of the loss
2. Work through painful grieving
3. Adjust to the life without the child
4. Emotional resolution and return to normal activities

TABLE 10-7 Giving Bad News Effectively

1. Utilize support staff such as chaplains and social workers
2. Early in your delivery of the news, let the family know the child died
3. Use simple, direct, understandable language
4. Speak with compassion and caring
5. Answer questions from any family members honestly

department or after several days of hospitalization does not seem to affect the grieving process.[14] Pathologic grief reactions are often the result of fear that the child will be forgotten. Excessive focus of time, energy, and effort is spent on remembering the child without resolving the grief. Sharing feelings and memories about the child is crucial; persons who do not allow parents to express their feelings may mar the grieving process.[14]

Physician and other health care providers can shape the way families remember the death of a child. Guidelines for communicating with parents are listed in Table 10-7.[14] Parents remember how compassionately the bad news is given, but most families still want the "bottom line" when they are first told of their child's death. They are waiting for it. Saying "I am very sorry, we did everything we could, but Sally died" is compassionate and direct. Most families do not want all the technical details about the resuscitation efforts. After delivering the bad news, have a chaplain or social worker stay with the family to allow the family time to deal initially with the shocking news. The physician should remain quietly in the room or return after a few minutes (or later, if other duties require) to answer questions. This is also the time to ask whether the family would like to see the child and to prepare them for what they will see. This is also the time to inquire about organ or tissue donation, if a regional transplant consortium does not provide this service already. Although parents do not regret organ donation, donation is not associated with a higher likelihood of successful grieving.[14]

Many hospitals have policies requiring that family wait outside the area where resuscitation efforts are being conducted, but family presence during resuscitation efforts is increasing in popularity. Both positive and negative family responses can occur during resuscitation.[15] Family presence during an attempted resuscitation may enable family members to begin appropriate grieving earlier. No studies have shown that the long-term effects on family grieving are beneficial, however. Some family members may become distressed or exceedingly emotional while care is being given to a loved one. Worries by emergency department staff members about the family's critiques of the resuscitation, or the family's unwillingness to terminate efforts, also contribute to the desire not to have the family present during resuscitation. However, the desire to have family members present during a resuscitation is a holistic approach to patient care with both the family's and the patient's needs addressed simultaneously. In general, the resistance of emergency department staff members to the presence of family members during a resuscitation has been diminishing. Policies are being created to train emergency department staff on how to assist family members and what to expect when families are present during a resuscitation.

REFERENCES

1. Schindler MB, Bohn D, Cox PN, et al: Outcome of out-of-hospital cardiac and respiratory arrest in children. *N Engl J Med* 335:1473, 1996.
2. Teach SJ, Moore PE, Fleisher GR: Death and resuscitation in the pediatric emergency department. *Ann Emerg Med* 25:799, 1995.
3. Ronco R, King W, Donley DK, et al: Outcome and cost at a children's hospital following resuscitation for out-of-hospital cardiopulmonary arrest. *Arch Pediatr Adolesc Med* 149:210, 1995.
4. Chameides L, Hazinski MF: *Textbook of Pediatric Advanced Life Support*. Dallas, American Heart Association, 1994.
5. Nadkarni V, Hazinski MF, Zideman D, et al: Pediatric resuscitation: An advisory statement from the Pediatric Working Group of the International Liaison Committee on Resuscitation. *Circulation* 95:2185, 1997.
6. King BR, Baker MD, Braitman LE, et al: Endotracheal tube selection in children: A comparison of four methods. *Ann Emerg Med* 22:530, 1993.
7. Van den Berg AA, Mphanza T: Choice of tracheal tube size for children: Finger size or age-related formula. *Anaesthesia* 52:695, 1997.
8. Bhende MS, Thompson AE: Evaluation of an end-tidal CO_2 detector during pediatric cardiopulmonary resuscitation. *Pediatrics* 95:395, 1995.
9. Luten RC, Wears RL, Broselow J, et al: Length-based endotracheal tube sizing and emergency equipment for pediatric resuscitation. *Ann Emerg Med* 21:900, 1992.
10. Schoenfeld PS, Baker MD: Management of cardiopulmonary and trauma resuscitation in the pediatric emergency department. *Pediatrics* 91:726, 1993.
11. Beland MJ, Hesslein PS, Finlay CD, et al: Non-invasive transcutaneous cardiac pacing in children. *PACE* 10:1262, 1987.
12. Rosenthal E, Thomas N, Quinn E, et al: Transcutaneous pacing for cardiac emergencies. *PACE* 11:2160, 1988.
13. Worden JW: Attachment, loss, and the tasks of mourning, in *Grief Counselling and Grief Therapy: A Handbook for the Mental Health Practitioner*, 2d ed. New York, Springer-Verlag, 1991.
14. Oliver RC, Fallat ME: Traumatic childhood death: How well do parents cope? *J Trauma* 39:303, 1995.
15. Van der Woning M: Should relatives be invited to witness the resuscitation attempt? A review of the literature. *Accid Emerg Nurse* 5:215, 1997.

PEDIATRIC AIRWAY MANAGEMENT

Marcie Rubin
Nicholas Sadovnikoff

As in all resuscitative efforts, the airway in pediatric patients has the highest priority. Skillful management of the pediatric airway requires a thorough familiarity with airway anatomy, an organized approach to the assessment of a compromised airway, and availability of the necessary tools for securing and maintaining a patent airway.

This chapter discusses the differences between adult and pediatric airways as well as causes for abnormal pediatric airways. It reviews the tools and techniques required for establishing and maintaining an airway and ventilation. It also addresses specific pathologic conditions leading to pediatric airway compromise and the appropriate interventions for such situations.

NORMAL PEDIATRIC AIRWAY ANATOMY

The normal airway of a pediatric patient has important anatomic differences from that of the adult. These differences are most apparent in infants and become relatively insignificant by age 8. They include the size of the occiput and the tongue in the infant, the high position of the larynx, the configuration of the larynx, and the position of the vocal cords.

The infant has a large occiput. Positioning of the head to obtain the optimum orientation for laryngoscopy, or the "sniffing position," is accomplished simply by rotating the head so that it rests on the occiput. Elevating the head with padding can lead to excessive flexion of the neck and may contribute to upper airway obstruction and difficulty during intubation. The infant's tongue is also relatively large, and this can impair laryngoscopy as well as contribute to upper airway obstruction. An infant's larynx is higher in the neck, located at the C3 level, than that of an adult, which is found at the C4 to C5 level. The larynx is also funnel-shaped in infants, with the narrowest portion at the subglottic area, rather than at the level of the vocal cords, as in an adult. Hence, in infants and small children, an endotracheal tube that passes easily through the vocal cords may encounter resistance more distally. Finally, infants' vocal cords are slanted anteriorly rather than being perpendicular to the trachea, as in an adult, and this characteristic, too, can result in more difficult visualization and intubation in the pediatric population.[1]

ABNORMAL PEDIATRIC AIRWAYS

Congenital

Numerous airway anomalies may be present at birth or develop over the first several months of life. While they rarely of themselves lead to the need for emergent airway control, their presence will complicate management of other emergencies requiring intubation.

Choanal atresia is the most common congenital anomaly of the nose. It may be unilateral or bilateral. Infants with this condition may not have difficulty breathing at birth if they can breathe orally, but they often present several months after birth when there is a concurrent problem, such as an upper respiratory infection. Maintaining an oral or tracheal airway overcomes the obstruction. Emergency department treatment is placement of oral airway, tube feedings, and admission for surgical repair.

Cystic hygroma is a benign congenital tumor of lymphatic origin. About 60 percent appear within the first year of life, and 80 to 90 percent occur before the second year. Cystic hygroma usually occurs in the neck or tongue but may also be found in the mediastinum. Progressive growth can lead to compromise of the structures of the pharynx and trachea, leading to airway obstruction and impairing or preventing laryngoscopy. The treatment is surgical resection.[2]

There are five types of tracheoesophageal fistulas, the most common defect consisting of a blind upper esophageal pouch and a fistula between the lower esophagus and the trachea. The diagnosis is usually made soon after birth when an infant becomes cyanotic and starts coughing after feeding or when a catheter cannot be passed into the stomach. Although most patients present soon after birth, a few with tracheoesophageal fistula with esophageal atresia present some time after discharge with pneumonia, and cyanosis with feeding. Placement of the endotracheal tube in patients with tracheoesophageal fistula is crucial to avoid gastric insufflation and resultant aspiration. The tube should be above the carina but below the fistula. This is often achieved by intubation of the right mainstem bronchus, then pulling back until breath sounds are heard bilaterally.

The common congenital syndrome of trisomy 21 (Down syndrome) may present significant difficulties in airway management. Characteristic of these patients are a short neck, small mouth, narrow nasopharynx, and large tongue; moreover, approximately 20 percent have asymptomatic dislocation of the atlas on the axis.[3] All of the potential difficulties must be considered prior to initiating intubation. Many congenital syndromes include airway abnormalities (Table 11-1). In controlled settings, management is preceded by careful evaluation and planning. Unfortunately, in the emergency department, this is rarely possible, and thus the approach to airway management must be mastered in all facets by those whose practice, even infrequently, involves pediatrics.

TABLE 11-1 Pediatric Syndromes and Associated Airway Abnormalities

Prominent Airway Abnormality	Syndromes
Mandibular hypoplasia	Hallermann-Steiff-François Pierre-Robin Goldenhaber's Nager's Treacher Collins
Maxillary hypoplasia	Apert's Pfeiffer's Crouzon's
Macroglossia	Trisomy 21 Beckwith-Wiedemann Hurler's
Tracheomalacia	Apert's Crouzon's

Note: If patient has history of significant airway obstruction or apnea, premedication is best avoided or used with extreme caution.

Acquired

Acquired abnormalities in pediatric airways can be subdivided into acute and chronic. Acute obstruction can result from foreign-body aspiration, infection such as laryngotracheobronchitis or epiglottitis, subglottic edema secondary to previous intubation or allergy, or internal or external airway trauma. Chronic obstruction can result from subglottic stenosis (posttraumatic or postsurgical), tumor, or abscess formation.

The management of an infant or child with airway obstruction depends on utilization of a safe, calculated approach to securing the airway. Such an approach requires a systematic evaluation of the pediatric airway, familiarity with pediatric airway equipment and pharmacologic agents, and recognition of a difficult airway and its appropriate management.

EVALUATION OF A PEDIATRIC AIRWAY

The first step in evaluating a pediatric airway is a directed history and physical examination. The time course of the present episode should be determined, as should a history of any recent fever, cough, or sore throat. Any history of previous airway problems should be elicited. If time permits, the history should include a review of the antenatal and perinatal periods, with an emphasis on feeding or sleeping difficulties. Any history of snoring or noisy breathing, recurrent croup or upper respiratory infections, or cyanosis or coughing during feedings should alert the clinician to the possibility of an abnormal airway.

The physical examination of a pediatric patient may be hindered by lack of cooperation, and care should be taken not to frighten the child. Visual signs of possible airway compromise include tachypnea, cyanosis, drooling, nasal flaring, and intercostal retractions. The child may assume a ''tripod'' position to enhance the use of accessory respiratory muscles. Auscultation may reveal stridor, wheezing, or grunting. Any change in the child's mental status, including agitation or somnolence, may further indicate airway difficulties. As in adults, features suggesting potentially difficult intubation include a small or recessed mandible, a prominent tongue, prominent upper incisors, and impairment of neck mobility.

Pediatric patients often have a period of compensated respiratory compromise prior to an arrest.[4] Pulse oximetric measurements should be continuously monitored, but adequate oxygen saturation should not be considered assurance of respiratory stability, since this measurement may not reflect declining ventilatory performance. All patients with potential airway compromise require attentive observation and frequent examination.

PEDIATRIC AIRWAY EQUIPMENT

Oropharyngeal and Nasopharyngeal Airways

Oropharyngeal airways are easy to use and available for pediatric patients of all ages. An oral airway should extend from the corner of the mouth to just cephalad to the angle of the mandible. To estimate the correct size, the airway can be placed next to the face. The oral airway should not be used in a conscious child because it may induce vomiting. The nasopharyngeal airway can be used in awake or semicomatose patients. The proper length is estimated by measuring the distance from the tip of the nose to the tragus of the ear. Complications include damage to adenoid tissue, epistaxis, and laryngospasm. Because the diameter of the nasal airways are so small in the pediatric population, they easily may become obstructed with blood, mucus, or vomitus and thus require frequent suctioning.

Bag-Valve-Mask Devices

The ideal pediatric mask should provide an airtight seal between the mask and the patient's face. A poor mask fit results in gas leaks, inability to maintain positive pressure, and potential compromise to ventilation and oxygenation. It has been found that child-size and adult-size self-inflating (Ambu, Inc., Linthicum, MD) bags may be utilized for the entire range of infants and children. Maximum oxygen delivery occurs at an oxygen flow of 15 L/min.[1]

Laryngoscope Blades

Two types of blades are most commonly available in emergency departments for pediatric intubation: curved (Macintosh) and straight (Miller). The tip of the Macintosh blade is inserted into the vallecula anterior to the epiglottis, and, as the blade is lifted, the epiglottis is elevated passively beneath the blade tip to expose the glottic opening. The tip of the Miller blade is placed beneath the epiglottis, which is directly elevated as the blade is lifted. A straight blade is superior to a curved blade in children under 2 years of age. Table 11-2 is a guide for laryngoscope selection in pediatric patients.

Endotracheal Tubes

There are numerous methods for selecting the correct endotracheal tube size for a given pediatric patient, including age, height, weight, and diameter of the fifth digit. Endotracheal tube size for premature and full-term infants is usually selected by weight, since, given the rapid growth during this period, age formulas become invalid. The rule usually employed is a 2.5-mm tube below 1.5 kg body weight, a 3.0-mm tube between 1.5 and 2.5 kg, and a 3.5-mm tube above 2.5 kg. The most commonly used formula for age determination of endotracheal tube size in children over 1 year of age is tube size (in millimeters) = 4 + age (in years)/4.[5] However, single-formula methods based on age have been shown to lead frequently to inappropriate tube selection.[6] Resuscitation measuring tapes have been found to be more accurate than age-based formulas, which in turn are superior to the diameter of the fifth digit.[7,8] The tube should fit sufficiently snugly to prevent any leakage at pressures up to 10 cmH_2O but should leak at a pressure lower than 30 cmH_2O. An insufficiently snug fit will result in difficulty ventilating, compromised airway protection, and leakage of inhalational agents if the patient undergoes anesthesia. An overly tight-fitting tube risks endotracheal injury with the potential for development of subglottic stenosis due to the anatomic reasons noted above. For the same reason, cuffed tubes are generally avoided in patients 8 years old and under. Clearly, in the care of an unstable patient in the emergency department, a suboptimal tube that provides adequate ventilation is preferable to no airway at all, and exchange for a more appropriate tube can be deferred until the patient has been stabilized. The ideal depth of placement is midway between the glottis and the carina. Because of substantial variability in tracheal length, especially before the age of 1 year, formulas predicting the distance to the lips are unreliable. Since most pediatric tubes have a series of marks at the distal end, one technique is to simply advance the tube so that the second mark is just past the vocal cords. This results in a conservatively high tube that will not risk bronchial intubation. However, inadvertent dislodgement of the tube with head and neck manipulation may occur. A second technique is to initially deliberately perform a bronchial intubation, advancing the tube until breath sounds are heard only unilaterally, and then to back the tube up to a point 1 cm above where the breath sounds are again heard bilaterally. This method results in a conservatively low tube, but with little risk of inadvertent displacement out of the airway.

TABLE 11-2 Laryngoscope Blade Selection for Pediatric Patients

	SIZE	
Age	Miller	Macintosh
Premature	0	
Neonate	0 or 1	
1 month to 2 years	1	
2–6 years	*	2
6–12 years	2	2 or 3
12 or older	2 or 3	3

* If a straight blade is desired in this age group, a Wis-Hipple 1.5 may be used.

TABLE 11-3 Laryngeal Mask Airway Size Selection

Weight, kg	LMA Size
<5	1
5–10	1.5
10–20	2
20–30	2.5
30–50	3
50–70	4
>70	5

Laryngeal Mask Airway

The laryngeal mask airway (LMA) has been widely used in the pediatric population.[9] It has been found to be extremely useful in the management of difficult airways. It consists of a large-bore tube terminating in an ovoid, fenestrated cup with an inflatable rim that, when properly placed, forms a seal over the laryngeal orifice (Fig. 14-6). The result is an airway that is superior to a face mask in that it prevents supraglottic obstruction and greatly reduces the likelihood of gastric insufflation, but is less reliable at preventing aspiration than an endotracheal tube. Since it is placed blindly, it avoids the complications of endotracheal intubation that arise from the need to visualize and penetrate the glottic opening. It provides a useful rescue device in the event of a failed endotracheal intubation. Once in place, it can be used as a conduit for fiberoptically guided endotracheal intubation. Its applications and experience with its use continue to expand, and emergency physicians should be familiar with its insertion. LMAs can be sized from neonates to adults. Table 11-3 is a guideline of sizes according to weight.

RAPID-SEQUENCE INTUBATION OF THE PEDIATRIC PATIENT

Rapid-sequence intubation (RSI) is the nearly simultaneous administration of a potent intravenous anesthetic agent and a neuromuscular blocking agent to facilitate endotracheal intubation. The process involves preparation, preoxygenation, application of cricoid pressure (Sellick maneuver), induction of anesthesia, neuromuscular blockade, and intubation without attempting mask ventilation. While there remain advocates of other airway management methods, this technique provides unsurpassed airway access while minimizing complications. Its use in critically ill children is well described, and it is regarded as the first choice in the absence of contraindications (see below).[10,11]

Preparation

Prior to undertaking a RSI, all necessary tools and materials should be prepared. A well-functioning intravenous line must be in place, and all drugs to be used for the RSI should be predrawn in syringes and labeled. Laryngoscopes with blades of the appropriate sizes, with lights checked and working, should be within reach, as should suction equipment and a bag-mask-ventilation apparatus connected to oxygen. Any materials for rescue maneuvers following failed intubation, such as LMAs, jet ventilation devices, and cricothyrotomy trays, should be immediately available. An endotracheal tube of the estimated size should be styletted, with tubes a size larger and a size smaller present. At least one additional experienced provider should be present to apply cricoid pressure and provide assistance as needed. Continuous pulse oximetric monitoring is mandatory.

Preoxygenation

Due to their relatively high oxygen consumption, smaller children, and especially infants, undergo rapid desaturation with cessation of ventilation, even with normal lungs. Once drugs have been administered in RSI, patients rapidly become apneic. Positive-pressure mask ventilation is not performed at this point due to the risk of gastric insufflation and resultant regurgitation. Therefore, it is important to maximize the length of time that adequate saturation is maintained by maximizing the reservoir of oxygen in the lungs. The lung volume remaining at end-expiration, or functional residual capacity (FRC), contains less than 20% oxygen in a patient breathing room air, with nearly 80% occupied by nitrogen. Preoxygenation is effectively denitrogenation of FRC, and it increases by roughly fivefold the oxygen reservoir in the lungs once apnea occurs. Effective denitrogenation is ideally accomplished by having a patient breathe 100% oxygen from a tight-fitting mask for 2 min or for four vital capacity breaths. This is often not possible with a critically ill prediatric patient, but as long a period of preoxygenation as circumstances permit should be provided prior to RSI.

Cricoid Pressure

Application of cricoid pressure entails the manual application of firm pressure at the level of the cricoid cartilage anteroposteriorly to occlude the esophagus and minimize the risk of aspiration. It should not be applied over the thyroid cartilage or over the entire larynx. It should be initiated immediately prior to the administration of the RSI drugs and not released until correct endotracheal tube position is confirmed. The amount of pressure should be graded according to the size of the patient. In smaller patients, the person applying cricoid pressure may wish to use the other hand under the neck to avoid altering the neck position.

Induction of Anesthesia

Laryngoscopy and endotracheal intubation are extremely stimulating events that are powerfully resisted by the unanesthetized patient. The goal of RSI is to overcome this resistance while preserving hemodynamic stability. The term *induction of anesthesia* is used here rather than *sedation* because, while the distinction between the two is somewhat indistinct, performance of laryngoscopy and intubation without causing major hemodynamic perturbations requires a deep state of anesthesia, for which the term *sedation* is inappropriate. The drugs commonly used for induction of anesthesia and their pediatric doses are listed in Table 11-4. Note the absence of opioid agents, which do not reliably induce rapid hypnosis. These doses are appropriate for healthy, well-hydrated patients. The dose for critically ill patients, as well as for those who have received other agents, such as opioid analgesics, should be adjusted downward accordingly. All of these drugs are appropriate for this indication; however, the profiles and side effects of each differ somewhat, as discussed below.

SODIUM THIOPENTAL Sodium thiopental is the most commonly employed drug for induction of anesthesia and has been in use for some five decades. It is very inexpensive and provides reliable induction of anesthesia within 1 min. It causes significant venodilation and moderate direct myocardial suppression, which result in decreases in blood pressure and cardiac output in spite of an increase in heart rate mediated by a minimally suppressed baroreceptor reflex. It lowers intracranial and intraocular pressures and has long been the drug of choice where elevations of these pressures are a concern. Only barbiturates, of all the pharmacologic interventions studied, have been shown to provide cerebroprotection in acute brain injury, leading to the preference for this drug in the setting of intracranial mass lesions or head trauma. Its side effects include histamine release, which may manifest as flushing, exaggerated hypotension, and wheezing in patients with reactive airways. Neuroexcitatory effects during induction, such as twitching, cough, and hiccups, are relatively common. It can cause extensive tissue necrosis if extravasated.

PROPOFOL Since its release in the United States in 1989, this drug has enjoyed increasing popularity, particularly in elective settings. Its onset of action is similar to that of thiopental, and it produces comparable decreases in blood pressure and cardiac output. Unlike thiopental, there is no reflex increase in heart rate. Propofol appears to be superior to thiopental at suppressing pharyngeal and laryngeal reflexes and for this reason is usually chosen for insertion of an LMA without paralysis. Like thiopental, it lowers intracranial and intraocular pressures, and, while experience with propofol is less extensive, it is probably as good a choice as thiopental in similar settings. It does not cause histamine release or stimulate bronchospasm, and extravasation has not been reported to cause significant tissue injury. It is notorious for causing pain on injection, which may be markedly attenuated by preadministration of a small dose of lidocaine. It is significantly more expensive than thiopental, and, given the overall similarity of their profiles, propofol has not been widely adopted for use in RSI due to this factor. Because it is prepared as an emulsion that readily supports bacterial growth, propofol must either be administered on discarded within 6 h of opening its container.

KETAMINE Unlike any of the other induction agents, ketamine tends to increase heart rate, blood pressure, and cardiac output. These effects appear to be mediated through central sympathetic stimulation, since ketamine appears to be a weak myocardial depressant in isolated heart preparations. Such effects enhance its attractiveness in settings such as trauma with hypovolemia. It is also a bronchodilator with no suppression of ventilatory drive, making it an excellent choice for patients with known reactive airway disease. In addition, it has significant analgesic and amnestic properties. It can be given intramuscularly in a dose of 4 to 6 mg/kg with onset of anesthesia within 5 min. This may be desirable in the combative patient in whom intravenous access has not been secured. Unfortunately, it also carries a number of undesirable side effects. Despite the bronchodilatation, there are marked in-

TABLE 11-4 Drugs Used for Induction of Anesthesia

Drug	Usual Dilution	IV Induction Dose	Duration of Action After an Induction Dose	Advantages	Disadvantages
Sodium thiopental	25 mg/mL	5–6 mg/kg	5–10 min	Safe with ICP Possibly cerebroprotective Inexpensive	Hypotension Extravasation Histamine release
Propofol	10 mg/mL	2–3 mg/kg	4–8 min	Safe with ICP Possibly cerebroprotective Not tissue toxic	Pain on injection Expensive Short life when opened
Ketamine	50 or 100 mg/mL	2–3 mg/kg	10–15 min	Supports blood pressure, heart rate Can be given IM Bronchodilator Inexpensive Potent analgesic	Raises ICP Emergence hallucinations Increases respiratory tract secretions
Midazolam	1 mg/mL	0.2–0.3 mg/kg	20–30 min	Cardiostable Reversible	Slow onset Long recovery time Expensive
Etomidate	2 mg/mL	0.2–0.3 mg/kg	5–10 min	Cardiostable Safe with ICP Minimal histamine release	No analgesic effect Pain on injection

Abbreviations: ICP, intracranial pressure; IM, intramuscular; IV, intravenous.

creases in upper airway secretions, which can occur briskly and complicate airway management. It increases cerebral blood flow, intracranial pressure, and intraocular pressure and should not be used in patients in whom these effects are a concern. Finally, it is associated with a significant incidence of emergence hallucinations, particularly in patients with a known history of psychosis, although this reaction is less common in children than in adults. This response can be attenuated by coadministration of benzodiazepines.

MIDAZOLAM Of the benzodiazepines, midazolam is the most popular for induction of anesthesia due to its rapid onset time and lack of venous irritation. The doses required for induction are much larger than those used for sedation. The onset of action is still somewhat slower than with the other induction agents discussed here. As a consequence of the large dose, the time to recovery is prolonged compared to that for the other induction agents. Unlike the other induction agents, however, midazolam can be reversed by the benzodiazepine antagonist flumazenil, although this should be done with caution due to the risk of seizures. Remarkably little hemodynamic perturbation occurs with an induction dose, although significant hypotension may occur in a hypovolemic or critically ill patient. Apnea is common, and coadministration of opioids markedly potentiates respiratory suppression. Amnesia is most reliably accomplished with this induction agent. While expensive compared to thiopental, it is commonly used in the emergency department due to its stable hemodynamic profile.

ETOMIDATE Etomidate is worthy of discussion due to its stable hemodynamic profile. An induction dose results in almost no change in heart rate, blood pressure, or cardiac output, since it appears to affect neither vascular tone nor baroreceptor reflex. It has little effect on ventilatory drive and none on airway smooth muscle. It lowers cerebral blood flow, intracranial pressure, and intraocular pressure much to the same degree as do thiopental and propofol. It completely lacks any analgesic properties and may require a low (2- to 4-μg/kg) dose of fentanyl to fully suppress the response to intubation. Side effects include pain on injection, myoclonic movements on induction, and a high incidence of subsequent nausea and vomiting. Reports suggesting adrenal suppression occurring with only an induction dose of the drug decreased its popularity, but evidence of the clinical significance of this observation has not been reported.

CHOICE OF AGENTS The choice of agent should be dictated by the specifics of the patient's physiologic status as well as by the experience of the emergency physician. Factors such as cost and convenience of storage and administration affect a department's choice of options. Specific scenarios for which pharmacologic management may be tailored are discussed below.

Neuromuscular Blockade

The goal of neuromuscular blockade in RSI is to obtain the optimal conditions for laryngoscopy as quickly as possible. The neuromuscular-blocking drug (NMB) is thus injected immediately after the injection of the induction agent. Complete neuromuscular blockade enables maximal laryngoscopic displacement of the tongue and mandible to optimize the view of the glottic aperture. In most children without anatomic deformities, glottic visualization is relatively simple once neuromuscular blockade is accomplished. Neuromuscular blockade also ensures that the vocal cords will be open, facilitating atraumatic passage of the endotracheal tube. There are many NMBs available, but only those with the most rapid times of onset can be recommended for RSI. These include the depolarizing NMB succinylcholine and two nondepolarizing NMBs, vecuronium and rocuronium.

While many practitioners may be more familiar with pancuronium which is inexpensive and has a long history of use in the emergency department, its long time of onset and very long duration of action make it a suboptimal choice for RSI.

SUCCINYLCHOLINE Succinylcholine, the only depolarizing NMB available in the United States, remains the drug of choice for RSI. While the US Food and Drug Administration has issued an advisory against its elective use in children, it continues to be approved for emergency airway management. The reason for the limitation of its use is that it has been associated with hyperkalemic arrest in children subsequently found to have underlying but undiagnosed myopathies (see below).

The advantages of succinylcholine include its extremely reliable and rapid time to onset of action; intubating conditions are obtained generally within 45 s. As noted, children become hypoxemic with apnea more rapidly than do adults, and even a 15-s advantage can be meaningful. Unlike nondepolarizing NMBs, duration of action is short. Spontaneous ventilation usually returns within 3 to 5 min. This is particularly important when ongoing neurologic assessment is desired, or when a difficult airway is anticipated or encountered, as options are preserved in the case of a failed intubation.

Unfortunately, the disadvantages of the drug are relatively numerous:

1. Hyperkalemia, with resultant cardiac arrest, is the most severe disadvantage. All patients experience a small rise, on the order of 0.5 meq/L, in their serum potassium following administration of succinylcholine. However, in certain subsets of patients, this rise is greatly exaggerated. Most of these are not likely to be a factor in an emergency department setting given the short time proximity of the injury or illness event to the need for intervention. In addition to myopathies, as mentioned above, other conditions that predispose to this occurrence include chronic immobilization, denervation lesions, spinal cord injuries, burns, crush injuries, and extensive necrotic soft tissue infections. The exaggerated response is due to unregulated proliferation of acetylcholine receptors on the muscle membrane. This response takes 2 to 3 days to occur after burns and neurologic injuries; thus, succinylcholine is safe to use in the immediate postinjury period in such patients.
2. Malignant hyperthermia can be triggered by succinylcholine in susceptible individuals. Since the lesion causing this disease is hereditary, patients known to have a history *or a family history* of malignant hyperthermia should not receive this agent.
3. Fasciculations precede the onset of neuromuscular blockade as the depolarization of the muscle membranes occurs. These uncontrolled muscle contractions are not inherently dangerous as long as the patient is protected from involuntary physical injury. Thought to increase the occurrence of myalgias, they can be prevented by preadministration of a small "defasciculating" dose (10 percent of an intubating dose) of a nondepolarizing NMB 2 min before succinylcholine is given.
4. Elevations in intracranial, intraocular, and intragastric pressures have been documented. Such rises are not reliably prevented by defasciculating premedication. However, they are transient, and their clinical importance is largely theoretical. In a patient in whom elevated intracranial pressure is a concern, securing the airway and providing ventilation (and thus controlling P_{CO_2}) are of primary importance.
5. Bradycardia occurs unpredictably in some patients receiving succinylcholine and is more common after a second dose. When it does occur, hypoxia, rather than drug effect, should be the first consideration. This is of particular concern in small children and neonates, whose cardiac output is directly dependent on heart rate. Premedication with atropine 0.15 to 0.20 mg/kg is advisable in children under five years old or in any child with a heart rate less than 120 bpm.
6. Prolonged blockade, lasting hours instead of minutes, occurs in a small subset of patients who have decreased activity of plasma cholinesterase, the enzyme responsible for the inactivation of succinylcholine. This may be due either to a defective enzyme or to diminished levels of normal enzyme. The frequency of clinically significant prolongation in the population is roughly 1:3000. This condition is not inherently dangerous in and of itself. The implication is that occasionally a patient has a prolonged apparent absence of neurologic function that could be mistaken for central nervous system injury. Train-of-four monitoring, the elicitation of muscular response following a standardized series of four electrical pulses stimulating a particular nerve, is used primarily in the operating room and intensive care unit settings. Absence of any twitch response to train-of-four muscular stimulation 10 min after a dose of succinylcholine reflects prolonged neuromuscular blockade.
7. A small subset of patients develop masseter spasm on receiving succinylcholine, making intubation more difficult. These patients are at increased risk of developing myoglobinuria and have a higher propensity for developing malignant hyperthermia. Fewer than 1 percent of patients manifest this complication.

In the event that succinylcholine is contraindicated, a fast-acting nondepolarizing NMB may be chosen with the knowledge that the onset will be slightly slower and the duration of action substantially longer.

VECURONIUM Vecuronium was the first nondepolarizing NMB to be recommended for use in RSI. In order to obtain intubating conditions in 60 to 90 s, a dose of 0.3 to 0.4 mg/kg is given. This results in a duration of action of 90 to 150 min. Alternatively, if time permits, a "priming" dose of 0.01 mg/kg should be given 2 to 3 min before an intubating dose of 0.15 to 0.2 mg/kg. The priming technique entails no clinically significant issues, but it speeds the onset of intubating conditions after the intubating dose and shortens the duration of action to 60 to 75 min. Vecuronium is essentially devoid of hemodynamic effects and does not cause histamine release. It is stored as a powder that is easily diluted for use.

ROCURONIUM Rocuronium is similar to vecuronium in its lack of hemodynamic effects. It is somewhat less potent, giving it a more rapid time to onset of intubating conditions, sufficiently so that priming is not considered necessary. Doses of 0.9 and 1.2 mg/kg have been shown in adults to result in times to intubating conditions of 75 and 55 s, respectively, approaching the 45 s typical of succinylcholine.[12] The duration of action is comparable to that of vecuronium 0.1 mg/kg at the 0.9 mg/kg dose and somewhat longer at the 1.2 mg/kg dose. Rocuronium is supplied as a solution that requires refrigeration, making it slightly less convenient to stock and store than vecuronium.

Contraindications

There are few contraindications to RSI. A known difficult airway requires an alternative approach. A variety of other approaches may be considered in a patient known to have experienced failed laryngoscopic intubation in the past or whose anatomy or injuries preclude direct laryngoscopy. These approaches include blind techniques, fiberoptically assisted techniques, and techniques employing an LMA. (These are detailed in Chap. 15.) Invasive emergency airway management approaches are discussed below. Patients who are judged to be too ill to receive anesthetic drugs, such as those comatose, profoundly hypotensive, or without circulation, may be intubated without pharmacologic assistance. Cricoid pressure should nonetheless be applied, since regurgitation and aspiration may still occur in these patients.

INVASIVE AIRWAY TECHNIQUES

Needle Cricothyroidotomy

Emergency surgical airways are often difficult to establish in children and have high complication rates. Hence, needle cricothyroidotomy has been advocated as the preferred airway access technique in the pediatric population. Needle cricothyroidotomy is performed by first identifying the cricothyroid membrane. A large-bore (14-gauge) intravenous catheter is passed through the membrane into the airway at a 45-degree caudad angle. The needle is removed, and an adapter is placed on the catheter so a standard bag-valve mask can be connected for oxygenation. This system has been shown to provide adequate oxygenation for prolonged periods of time. It cannot, however, provide adequate ventilation.[13]

Transtracheal jet ventilation allows ventilation and oxygenation through a catheter. Ventilation is provided with short, intermittent bursts of oxygen. This requires high-pressure (50 psi) oxygen-delivery systems. The system of choice is a jet injector regulated by a flow meter attached to a wall or tank unit. The less optimal choice is an unregulated wall or tank system. A 1-s jet of oxygen followed by a 4-s expiratory phase achieves satisfactory ventilation.[14]

Complications of needle cricothyroidotomy include bleeding, infection, esophageal perforation, breakage or bending of the needle, subcutaneous emphysema, pneumothorax, pneumomediastinum, and pneumopericardium.

Surgical Cricothyroidotomy and Tracheostomy

Emergency surgical cricothyroidotomy and tracheostomy in pediatric patients is much more difficult than in adults due to the smaller dimensions of the structures and the relatively higher position of the larynx in the neck. Sufficient literature documenting the true complication rates of these procedures in the pediatric population is not available, but the procedures should be undertaken only as measures of last resort.

SPECIAL CONSIDERATIONS

Head Trauma or Intracranial Mass Lesion

Securing the airway in a pediatric patient with head trauma or an intracranial mass lesion plays an important role by correcting or preventing hypercarbia and hypoxemia, factors that can cause increases in intracranial pressure. Since endotracheal intubation itself is inherently stimulating to intracranial pressure, as noted above, all possible precautions should be taken to suppress this response. In addition, in the setting of head trauma, RSI should be undertaken with strict head and neck immobilization due to the potential for concomitant cervical spine injuries.

RSI is the preferred method of intubation in pediatric patients with suspected or known intracranial hypertension. In addition to the agents previously discussed, lidocaine at a dose of 1.5 mg/kg intravenously should be given prior to laryngoscopy.[15] This intervention blocks the rise in intracranial pressure that commonly accompanies endotracheal intubation. It is important to remember that in pediatric patients, as in adults, head injuries can also be associated with intraoral and intratracheal injuries. When managing the airway of a head-injured patient, one must always be prepared for invasive airway management.

Epiglottis and Croup

For a detailed discussion of pediatric upper airway obstruction, see Chap. 129. Optimal airway management for pediatric patients with epiglottitis is in the operating room. If the patient is stable, he or she should be transported to the operating room accompanied by a skilled airway manager and the proper equipment. A patient with complete airway obstruction can often be ventilated until an airway can be established. If this is unsuccessful, emergent orotracheal intubation should be attempted. If this fails, invasive airway techniques should be utilized.

Uncommonly, a child with croup may be unresponsive to medical management and may require an artificial airway. An endotracheal tube is optimally placed in the operating room allowing for inhalation induction of anesthesia. Intubation, however, may have to be performed in the emergency department if the patient is in extremis.

Airway Foreign Bodies

Management of an unstable patient with acute airway obstruction requires immediate attention to the airway. In the prehospital setting, the American Heart Association recommends a series of five back blows and five chest thrusts in a child under the age of 1 (see Chap. 10). The child should have the oropharynx examined between each series. In a child older than 1, the recommendation is a series of abdominal thrusts in either the upright or the supine position.

In the emergency department, the child with a partially obstructed airway should be rapidly assessed. If the child will tolerate it, a visual inspection of the hypopharyngeal and laryngeal areas should be attempted. Commonly, a child will tolerate this procedure poorly and thus should be taken to the operating room for general anesthesia and removal of the foreign body. In an unstable or completely obstructed patient, orotracheal intubation may dislodge the foreign body, and this should be attempted prior to needle cricothyroidotomy.

REFERENCES

1. Todres D: Pediatric airway control and ventilation. *Ann Emerg Med* 22:440, 1993.
2. Macdonald DJF: Cystic hygroma: An anesthetic and surgical problem. *Anaesthesia* 49:433, 1978.
3. Williams JP, Somerville GM, Miner ME, Reilly D: Atlanto-axial subluxation and trisomy 21: Another perioperative complication. *Anesthesiology* 67:253, 1987.
4. Guidelines for cardiopulmonary resuscitation and emergency cardiac care. Emergency Cardiac Care Committee and Subcommittees, American Heart Association. Part VI. Pediatric advanced life support. *JAMA* 268:2262, 1992.
5. Ferrari LR, Cunningham MJ: Determination of endotracheal tube size in pediatric patients. *Arch Otolaryngol Head Neck Surg* 118:448, 1992.
6. Mostafa SM: Variation in subglottic size in children. *Proc R Soc Med* 29:494, 1976.
7. Luten RC, Wears RL, Broselow J, et al: Length-based endotracheal tube and emergency equipment in pediatrics. *Ann Emerg Med* 21:900, 1992.
8. King BR, Baker MD, Braitman LE: Endotracheal tube selection in children: A comparison of four methods. *Ann Emerg Med* 22:530, 1993.
9. Lopez-Gil M, Brimacombe J, Alvarez M: Safety and efficacy of the laryngeal mask airway: A prospective survey of 1400 paediatric patients. *Anesthesia* 51:969, 1996.
10. Gerardi MJ, Sacchetti AD, Cantor RM, et al: Rapid-sequence intubation of the pediatric patient. *Ann Emerg Med* 28:55, 1996.
11. Walls RM: Rapid-sequence intubation comes of age. *Ann Emerg Med* 28:79, 1996.
12. Magorian T, Flannery KB, Miller RD: Comparison of rocuronium, succinylcholine and vecuronium for rapid-sequence induction of anesthesia in adult patients. *Anesthesiology* 79:913, 1993.
13. Cote CJ, Eavey RD, Todres ID, et al: Crycoid membrane puncture: Oxygenation and ventilation in a dog model using an intravenous catheter. *Crit Care Med* 16:615, 1988.
14. Benumof JC, Scheller MS: The importance of transtracheal jet ventilation in the management of the difficult airway. *Anesthesiology* 71:769, 1989.
15. Walls RM: Rapid-sequence intubation in head trauma. *Ann Emerg Med* 22:1008, 1993.

RESUSCITATION ISSUES IN PREGNANCY

Elizabeth M. Datner
Susan B. Promes

ETIOLOGY OF MATERNAL DEATH

Although cardiac arrest in pregnant patients is rare—it is estimated to occur once in every 30,000 deliveries—the incidence of maternal death has been increasing recently. From 1987 to 1990, the overall pregnancy-related mortality ratio was 9.2 deaths per 100,000 live births. However, the National Health Promotion and Disease Preven-

TABLE 12-1 Common Etiologies of Maternal Cardiopulmonary Arrest

Preexisting medical conditions
- Congenital heart disease
- Acquired valvular disease
- Dysrhythmia
- Myocardial infarction
- Traumatic myocardial contusion
- Cerebral pathology
  - Intracranial hemorrhage
  - Aneurysm
- Pulmonary pathology
  - Asthma
- Malignant hyperthermia
- Illicit drug use

Obstetric complications
- Hemorrhage
  - Uterine atony
  - Placental abruption
  - Placenta previa, accreta, increta, or percreta
  - Disseminated intravascular coagulopathy
- Severe pregnancy-induced hypertension
- Amniotic fluid embolism
- Idiopathic peripartum cardiomyopathy

Iatrogenic events
- Failed intubation
- Pulmonary aspiration
- Intravascular local anesthetic overdose
- Drug error, overdose, or allergy
- Hypermagnesemia

Pulmonary embolism
- Thrombus
- Air
- Fat

Trauma
- Homicide
- Suicide
- Motor vehicle accident
- Electrical injury

Infection or sepsis

Source: Adapted with permission from Johnson MD, Luppi CJ, Over D: Cardiopulmonary resuscitation in pregnancy, in Gambling DR, Douglas MJ (eds): *Obstetric Anesthesia and Uncommon Disorders.* Philadelphia, WB Saunders, 1997, and Doan-Wiggins L in Benrubi GI (ed): *Obstetric and Gynecologic Emergencies,* Philadelphia, Lippincott, 1994.

tion Objectives of Healthy People 2000 identifies a rate of no more than 3.3 maternal deaths per 100,000 live births as a national goal. Because critically ill obstetric patients are uncommon, optimal care is sometimes jeopardized. Many maternal deaths may be preventable if managed appropriately. Some of the factors associated with a higher risk of pregnancy-related death include increasing maternal age, race, increasing live birth order, lack of prenatal care, and unwed mothers.[1]

The leading causes of maternal death are pulmonary embolism, trauma, hemorrhage, and maternal cardiac disease (Table 12-1). While pulmonary embolism is considered the most common medical cause of death in pregnant women, several studies indicate that injury is the most common etiology of maternal death and homicide the most common form of injury.[2,3] Domestic violence and its relationship to pregnancy and homicide is poorly understood, but domestic violence indicators should be examined in all newly diagnosed pregnancies as a preventive measure.

MATERNAL AND FETAL PHYSIOLOGIC CHANGES THAT AFFECT CARDIAC ARREST

Uteroplacental blood flow is directly related to maternal blood volume and arterial pressure. Support of maternal blood volume and oxygenation is the best way to prevent fetal hypoxia. With this principle in mind, a detailed understanding of cardiac arrest physiology is important. A full discussion of fetomaternal physiology can be found in Chap. 99, but several points are discussed and put in perspective here.

The maternal cardiovascular system undergoes dramatic changes. Cardiac output increases to 30 to 45 percent above baseline levels by the twentieth week of gestation and remains at that level until delivery. In addition, the mean arterial blood pressure gradually falls throughout the first two trimesters of pregnancy and returns to baseline levels by term. This change is a result of decreased resistance in the pulmonary and uteroplacental circulations. The uteroplacental mass increases and requires 10 percent of systemic blood volume by term, compared to a baseline 2 percent. By the second half of pregnancy, the uteroplacental vascular bed functions as a passive low-resistance system, with flow determined by maternal perfusion pressure. Thus, in a state of cardiac compromise, uterine blood flow is greatly diminished. The addition of vasopressors with α- and β-adrenergic effects can cause significant vasoconstriction, decreasing uterine blood flow even further.

By the twentieth week of pregnancy, the enlarged uterus mechanically compresses the great vessels in the pelvis, particularly when the patient is in the supine position. As a result of decreased venous return from compression of the inferior vena cava, cardiac output is reduced 10 to 30 percent during spontaneous circulation (Fig. 12-1). Administration of medications through intravenous sites in the infradiaphragmatic vessels, such as the femoral or saphenous veins, is also compromised because of poor venous flow. These vascular sites are therefore

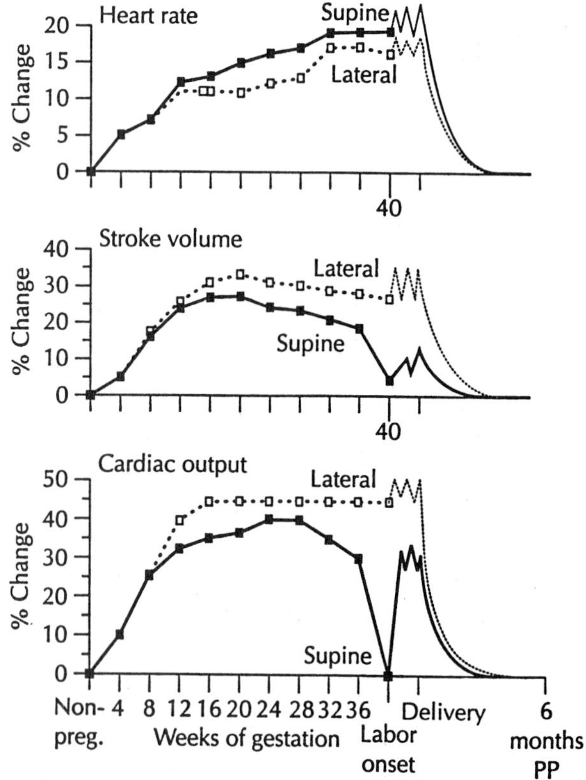

FIG. 12-1. Changes in maternal heart rate, stroke volume, and cardiac output during pregnancy with the gravida in the supine and lateral positions. (From Barclay ML, in Pearlman MD, Tintinalli JE (eds): *Emergency Care of the Woman,* McGraw-Hill, 1998.)

not recommended for intravenous access in the resuscitation of a pregnant patient greater than 20 weeks' gestation. Aortal compression also occurs, causing diminished distal blood flow. The untoward effects of great vessel compression are worsened in the setting of maternal hypotension and uterine contractions, leading to an even more pronounced decrease in uteroplacental blood flow.

Pregnancy also alters the respiratory system. A state of partially compensated respiratory acidosis develops during the first trimester of pregnancy due to progesterone-stimulated hyperventilation. The resulting decrease in serum bicarbonate levels and Pco_2 makes the woman less able to buffer a state of acidosis from hypotension or cardiac arrest. In addition, the decreased functional residual capacity (FRC) and increased maternal oxygen consumption and basal metabolic rate during pregnancy, results in more rapid onset of anoxia with respiratory arrest. Arterial oxygen content drops three times more quickly in pregnant than in nonpregnant patients.[4] Rapid resumption of respiration, whether mechanical or spontaneous, is essential to minimize hypoxic damage. Progesterone also increases gastric emptying time and decreases lower esophageal sphincter tone, making the gravid patient prone to aspiration. This is another reason to initiate endotracheal intubation early.

Fetal physiology appears to be protective of severe hypoxia. There are several reports of fetal survival when delivery occurred more than 20 min after maternal cardiac arrest in patients receiving cardiopulmonary resuscitation (CPR). The trauma literature indicates that absence of maternal vital signs for greater than 20 min renders emergency cesarean section futile. It is unclear whether CPR plays a role in potential fetal survival beyond 20 min. The fetal oxyhemoglobin dissociation curve is shifted to the left relative to the maternal oxyhemoglobin dissociation curve because of the greater affinity of hemoglobin F for oxygen. Thus, at any partial pressure of oxygen, fetal hemoglobin will bind oxygen more strongly, resulting in greater saturation. Fetal Po_2 does not fall significantly unless maternal Po_2 falls below 60 mmHg.[5] Below this level, only slight decreases in maternal Po_2 will result in significant decreases in fetal Po_2. In addition, there is a higher concentration of fetal hemoglobin in fetal erythrocytes than maternal hemoglobin in maternal erythrocytes, and the fetus exists in a physiologically acidemic state relative to the mother, which allows preferential oxygen transfer at the fetal tissue level. Acidemia favors a rightward shift of the oxyhemoglobin dissociation curve. Thus, a greater amount of oxygen is supplied to fetal tissues.

Fetal cardiac output protects against hypoxia with increases in umbilical blood flow and placental gas exchange. Fetal blood flow is then preferentially redistributed to vital tissues. As a result, fetuses exposed to short periods of maternal hypoxia may not suffer neurologic damage.

Resuscitation of a pregnant patient can become a chaotic event. Particularly in major centers, there may be other specialists involved, including pediatricians, neonatologists, anesthesiologists, obstetricians, and possibly others. These specialists have unique skills and experience that will help in the resuscitation. However, many of the specialists are poorly versed in emergency medicine and advanced cardiac life support (ACLS) protocols. It is particularly important that the team leader of the resuscitation take strict control of the events and the order in which they occur. The other specialists involved should not be allowed to deviate from the proper process. The team leader for such resuscitations may be decided by hospital policy. If such a policy does not exist, then typically the emergency physician must be the director of the resuscitation and take firm control.

AIRWAY ISSUES

The airway presents special concerns in obstetric patients. Attention to a few details, particularly in the setting of maternal cardiac arrest, may reduce morbidity and mortality. Airway management and its associated problems represent the greatest risk factor for anesthetic-related maternal deaths, the majority of which occur in the setting of an emergent cesarean section. Maternal death related to anesthesia most commonly results from aspiration of gastric contents or failure to intubate the trachea, resulting in hypoxia, which ultimately can result in cardiac arrest.[6] Mask ventilation can be difficult and ineffectual in obstetric patients because of low FRC, elevated diaphragms, and raised intraabdominal pressure. The incidence of failed intubations in pregnant patients is approximately 1 in 300 to 500 patients undergoing general anesthesia.[7] Complicating the fact that pregnant patients develop hypoxia more quickly and are less tolerant of apneic periods, the airway poses more difficulties than in the general population. The potential factors accounting for these difficulties should be assessed prior to attempting an intubation.

Parturients in general are in an edematous state, which effects the tongue and supraglottic soft tissues.[8] The edema may compromise the airway lumen, making mask ventilation, laryngoscopy, and endotracheal intubation more challenging. Smaller endotracheal tubes may be needed to achieve a successful intubation and should be readily available. Mucosal engorgement and increased friability make the airway more likely to bleed and swell. This in itself can cause rapid deterioration. Decreased gastric emptying and diminished lower esophageal sphincter tone allow for increased gastric insufflation and result in a higher risk of aspiration during intubation. The intubating physician should make as few attempts as possible, to avoid making a difficult airway worse. Blind nasotracheal intubation is relatively contraindicated, and nasogastric tubes should generally be avoided, given the engorgement and friability of the mucosa in pregnant patients. Orogastric tubes may be used with caution in pregnant patients in cardiac arrest.

Several other physical conditions should be considered prior to intubating a parturient. Pregnant patients are likely to have full and intact dentition, and there may be little interdental distance in which to maneuver a laryngoscope. Obesity is relatively common in pregnant patients, causing relative neck extension when patients are supine, which results in greater anterior placement of the larynx. The neck is foreshortened, and there are often redundant pharyngeal and palatal folds in the airways of obese gravid women. In addition, enlarged and engorged breasts may obstruct placement of the laryngoscope in the mouth and the hand of an assistant attempting to maintain cricoid pressure.

The technique for intubating pregnant patients may require several modifications. As in any intubation, adjunctive equipment, including small endotracheal tubes, short laryngoscope handles, and stylets, should be readily available and familiar to the physician managing the airway. The patient should be placed in the supine position with the right hip elevated 10 to 12 cm to minimize aortocaval compression. The head and shoulders can be elevated with a pillow or folded sheets to achieve the sniffing position. This maneuver is particularly important in obese patients.

Use of rapid-sequence induction with cricoid pressure has become the standard of care for intubating pregnant women, particularly unstable patients with airway compromise. Administration of an induction agent, such as thiopental or etomidate, is followed by administration of succinylcholine, the muscle relaxant of choice, unless there is a contraindication to its use. It is helpful to allow a sufficient amount of time for muscle relaxants to take effect and for adequate preoxygenation prior to attempting laryngoscopy, given its potential hazards in pregnant patients. Preoxygenation prior to intubation is important because of the parturient's decreased FRC. However, hyperventilation may lead to respiratory alkalosis, which, in addition to shifting the oxyhemoglobin dissociation curve to the left, causes decreased uterine blood flow. Cricoid pressure must be carefully applied throughout the intubation procedure. In the case of failed intubation, more invasive maneuvers, such as percutaneous transtracheal jet ventilation or cricothyrotomy, may need to be performed in order to maintain oxygenation and prevent hypercarbia. Ventilator settings for pregnant patients are

TABLE 12-2 Algorithm for Cardiopulmonary Resuscitation in Pregnant Patients

Effect early intubation, protecting the vulnerable airway and supplying oxygen.
Tilt the patient, limiting aortocaval compression.
Obtain rapid intravenous access, avoiding the femoral and saphenous veins.
Follow current ACLS recommendations.
Perform perimortem cesarean section within 5 min of maternal arrest if fetus >20 weeks.
Consider open-chest CPR within 15 min of maternal arrest.
Explore differential diagnosis, including iatrogenic causes, e.g., spinal analgesia.
Consider cardiopulmonary bypass if indicated.

similar to those for nonpregnant patients, with minor modifications. Minute ventilation should aim to maintain a P_{CO_2} of approximately 30 mmHg. Significant respiratory alkalosis must be avoided to prevent decreased uterine blood flow.

MODIFICATIONS OF CARDIOPULMONARY RESUSCITATION

The etiology of cardiac arrest in pregnant patients is different from that in nonpregnant patients and includes pulmonary embolism, amniotic fluid embolism, eclampsia, drug toxicity (e.g., magnesium sulfate or epidural anesthetics), cardiomyopathy, aortic dissection, trauma, and hemorrhage. As always, one should address the potential underlying etiology as well as the cardiovascular collapse.

Cardiopulmonary arrest in a pregnant patient must be considered under two scenarios: prior to fetal viability and after fetal viability. The accepted age of fetal viability may vary among institutions, but 24 to 26 weeks is generally considered the age of viability. The uterine fundus is palpable at the umbilicus at 20 weeks. After 20 weeks, the gestational age of the fetus can be estimated by measuring the fundus from the pubic symphysis to the top of the fundus. The fundal height in centimeters corresponds roughly to the gestational age in weeks. Prior to 24 weeks' gestation, all efforts should focus on the mother, with no modifications to CPR. However, early intubation and resumption of respirations and circulation is essential in all gravid arrests for the reasons mentioned earlier. Beyond 20 weeks or if the gravid uterus can be palpated above the umbilicus, several modifications of CPR should be instituted: (1) the patient should be positioned to minimize aortocaval compression, and (2) an emergency cesarean section should be considered.

Aortocaval compression must be limited in all patients beyond the twentieth week of gestation. This can be achieved by (1) having someone manually displace the uterus to the left, (2) tilting the patient 15 to 30° on a tiltable table, or (3) placement of a roll or a Cardiff wedge, if available, under the patient's right hip and flank. The Cardiff wedge provides a tilt of 27 percent, allowing 80 pecent of perfusion compared with CPR in the supine position.[9] Even this is minimal blood flow, considering that correctly performed CPR maintains 30 percent or less of normal cardiac output in nonpregnant adults.[10,11] The "human wedge" has been advocated for bystander CPR. In this technique, the patient lies across the thighs of the rescuer, who is in a kneeling position. Despite relatively clear current recommendations regarding resuscitation in pregnancy, summarized in Table 12-2, there remains a paucity of research in this area.[6]

Five factors have been suggested as important to improving the chance of fetal survival when the mother suffers cardiac arrest: gestational age greater than 28 weeks or fetal weight greater than 1 kg, short interval between maternal death and delivery, a cause of maternal death not related to chronic hypoxia, fetal status before maternal death, availability of neonatal intensive care facilities, and quality of maternal resuscitation.[12,13]

The role of open chest cardiopulmonary resuscitation (OCCPR) remains unclear. There is some evidence that early thoracotomy and open chest cardiac massage may improve both maternal and fetal outcome. If, after several minutes of external CPR (15 min has been suggested), a pregnant woman has failed to achieve return of spontaneous circulation, OCCPR should be considered.

DEFIBRILLATION AND MEDICATIONS

Pregnant patients who experience cardiac arrest should be treated using current ACLS guidelines. Defibrillation has never been found to have adverse effects on the fetus and thus is not contraindicated. The patient should be placed in the left lateral tilt position if possible prior to defibrillation or cardioversion. Large-bore intravenous lines should be placed, preferably above the diaphragm, and lactated Ringer's or normal saline solution infused. Supplemental oxygen should be given. APGAR scores and fetal outcome are positively affected by greater fetal oxygen reserves.[14] In limited published reports, the standard medications used in ACLS have not been demonstrated to have adverse effects on the fetus and thus are recommended in the setting of cardiac arrest.[15] See Table 12-3 for details regarding ACLS medications. Vasopressors, such as epinephrine and dopamine, may be detrimental in the setting of maternal hypotension, since they cause uteroplacental vasoconstriction, but should be used as needed during cardiac arrest. In the setting of hypotension alone without cardiac arrest, ephedrine, in standard doses, is the preferred pressor when fluids fail to restore adequate blood pressure. (The dose is 5 mg IV q 5 min until a response is seen.) The use of sodium bicarbonate is not well studied. Sodium bicarbonate crosses the placenta slowly and can potentially be problematic for the fetus for the following reason. Rapid correction of maternal metabolic acidosis will decrease maternal respiratory compensation and lead to a rise in or normalization of maternal P_{CO_2}. As maternal P_{CO_2} increases, the concomitant rise in fetal P_{CO_2} occurs at a faster rate than does the rise in HCO_3^-, causing the fetus to become more acidotic.

COMPLICATIONS FROM CARDIOPULMONARY RESUSCITATION

Complications may occur from standard resuscitation. Maternal problems secondary to CPR include liver lacerations, uterine rupture, hemothorax, and hemopericardium. Fetal complications include cardiac dysrhythmias from maternal defibrillation and ACLS drugs, central nervous system toxicity from ACLS drugs, and altered uteroplacental blood flow from maternal hypoxia, acidosis, and vasoconstriction. Despite all of the aforementioned problems, standard ACLS protocols, with the addition of a pelvic tilt, are still the standard of care in resuscitating pregnant patients. The ultimate goal is to oxygenate the mother, and in turn the fetus, and achieve return of spontaneous circulation as soon as possible.

CARDIAC ISCHEMIA

Pregnant women thought to be experiencing cardiac ischemia are treated the same as nonpregnant patients, with the exception of thrombolytic therapy. Pregnancy is considered a relative contraindication to thrombolytic therapy by the American College of Cardiology/American Heart Association.[16] No controlled trials using thrombolytic agents, such as streptokinase, urokinase, or tissue plasminogen activator, have been performed on pregnant women or are currently feasible.

TABLE 12-3 Medications Used During Cardiopulmonary Resuscitation—Considerations in Pregnancy*

Drug	Indications	Considerations in Pregancy
Epinephrine	Potentially beneficial in all forms of cardiac arrest	Category C. Has been shown to be teratogenic in animals in large doses; may induce uteroplacental vasoconstriction.
Lidocaine	Ventricular ectopy, tachycardia, and fibrillation	Category C. Use during pregnancy is not well studied; crosses the placenta but in therapeutic doses has no teratogenic effect on the fetus; may cause fetal bradycardia.
Bretylium	Ventricular fibrillation and tachycardia unresponsive to other therapy	Category C. Safety has not been established in human pregnancy; use only if clearly indicated.
Atropine	Symptomatic bradycardia, asystole	Category B. Crosses placenta but results in no fetal abnormalities; can cause fetal tachycardia.
Sodium bicarbonate	Cardiac arrest unresponsive to other measures; documented preexisting metabolic acidosis	Category C. Studies to define risk of hypertonic sodium bicarbonate therapy in pregnancy have not been done.
Dopamine	Hemodynamically significant hypotension in the absence of hypovolemia	Category C. No teratogenic effects have been observed in laboratory animals but sufficient studies in humans are lacking. Use only when clearly indicated.
Dobutamine	Short term inotropic support of patients with depressed myocardial contractility	Category C. Not found to be teratogenic in animal studies but its effects in pregnant humans are unknown. Use only if clearly indicated.

*Tamari I, Eldar M, Rabinowitz B, Neufeld HN: Medical treatment of cardiovascular disorders during pregnancy, *Am Heart J* 104:1357, 1982.
Gibler WB: Antiarrhythmics, in Barsan WG, Jastremski MS, Syverud SA (eds): *Emergency Drug Therapy,* Philadelphia, WB Saunders, 1991, p 147.
Saunders CF: Vasoactive agents, in Barsan WG, Jastremski MS, Syverud SA (eds): *Emergency Drug Therapy,* Philadelphia, WB Saunders, 1991, p 281.
Singal B: Acidifying and alkalizing agents, in Barsan WG, Jastremski MS, Syverud SA (eds): *Emergency Drug Therapy,* Philadelphia, WB Saunders, 1991, p 281.

Patients with suspected myocardial infarction should be evaluated for emergent percutaneous interventional therapy or medical management.

PULMONARY EMBOLISM

Thromboembolic disease is increased in pregnancy. Anticoagulation with heparin is currently the treatment of choice for a pulmonary embolism, along with ensuring adequate oxygenation and treating hypotension. Both unfractionated and low-molecular-weight heparin are acceptable treatment regimens. When a pulmonary embolism is suspected, empiric treatment with heparin should be started immediately, especially if the patient is hypoxic or hemodynamically unstable. Once treatment has begun, a Doppler ultrasound or ventilation-perfusion scan should be obtained to confirm the diagnosis. Traditionally, thrombolytic therapy for pulmonary embolism has been considered relatively contraindicated in pregnant patients. However, pregnant women have been treated successfully with thrombolytics with no untoward complications.[17] The use of thrombolytics should be reserved for patients in extremis.

AMNIOTIC FLUID EMBOLISM

The classic presentation of amniotic fluid embolism is the development of dyspnea and hypotension in association with labor or an abortion. Milder forms can present with sudden onset of shortness of breath and air hunger along with a decreased oxygen saturation that resolves spontaneously. Amniotic fluid embolism can be difficult to distinguish from pulmonary embolism. Patients can develop cardiac arrest within minutes, and if they survive they will go on to develop disseminated intravascular coagulation. Treatment is primarily supportive care along with invasive cardiac monitoring and correction of the coagulopathy. The use of cardiopulmonary bypass and open pulmonary artery thromboembolectomy has been used with success in a moribund patient with AFE.[18]

PERIMORTEM CESAREAN SECTION

Perimortem cesarean section must be considered as part of any resuscitation in the case of maternal cardiac arrest and a viable fetus. Prognosis for intact survival of the infant is excellent if delivery occurs within 5 min of maternal arrest and initiation of CPR. If the 5-min time frame has been exceeded, it is still recommended to perform a perimortem cesarean section. One case has been reported of a perimortem cesarean section performed 22 min after maternal cardiac arrest that resulted in a normal living infant.[19] No cases have been reported of live births by perimortem cesarean section beyond 25 min after maternal arrest. Ideally, an obstetrician and a pediatrician or neonatologist are present at the time of a perimortem cesarean section. In the absence of these specialists, the emergency physician must be prepared to perform the procedure. It is not necessary and only delays a potentially lifesaving procedure to evaluate fetal viability prior to initiation of the cesarean section. For the same reasons, the patient should not be moved to an operating suite, since this only wastes time. The decision to perform a perimortem cesarean section should be made by 4 min after cardiac arrest, with delivery of the fetus by 5 min postarrest.

Maternal CPR should be continued throughout the procedure and for a brief time afterward, since a few cases of successful resuscitation following such a procedure have been reported. Necessary equipment includes a scalpel, bandage scissors, Mayo scissors, toothed forceps, Richardson retractors, needle drivers, and suture material (Table 12-4). The goal of this procedure is to remove and resuscitate the fetus.

Abdominal preparation and insertion of a Foley catheter to decompress the bladder may be performed prior to initial incision if time allows but should not delay the procedure. No anesthesia is required, since the mother is in cardiac arrest. A vertical midline (classical) incision is made from 4 to 5 cm below the xiphoid process to the pubic symphysis through the abdominal wall. The rectus muscles may be separated with blunt dissection, and the peritoneum is entered with a midline incision that is continued superiorly and inferiorly to allow visualization of the uterus. A vertical uterine incision is made from

TABLE 12-4 Equipment Required for Emergency Cesarean Section

Scalpel
Mayo scissors
Bandage scissors
Toothed forceps
Needle holders
0 chromic sutures on a CT 1 needle
Richardson retractors
10 U/mL oxytocin vials
10 mL normal saline solution vials
10 mL syringe with intramuscular needles

the fundus to the point at which the opaque bladder is adherent to the uterus. An initial small inferior incision may be made until amniotic fluid is obtained and then extended with scissors using the free hand to elevate the uterus, avoiding injury to the fetus. An anterior placenta should be incised in order to reach the fetus. The fetus is then delivered and resuscitated. The placenta is then manually removed from the uterus, and the uterus is wiped clean of membranes with a sponge or towel. The uterus is closed with one or two layers with a locked running stitch using number 0 or number 1 semipermanent suture and a large needle. The fascia and peritoneum may be closed with a permanent or semipermanent number 0 or number 1 suture with a running stitch. Finally the skin is closed. Closure of the abdomen may be delayed until maternal pulse and blood pressure are restored, to allow direct observation of the uterus for ongoing bleeding. Uterine atony after perimortem cesarean section is common and may lead to significant blood loss when the uterus fails to contract after delivery. Because maternal blood circulation may not be sufficient to deliver intravenously administered medication, dilute oxytocin (10 U in 9 mL normal saline solution) may be injected directly into the myometrium in divided doses until contraction occurs. Other possible therapeutic medications include ergometrine (intravenous or intramuscular) or prostaglandin $F_{2\alpha}$ into the uterus.

Informed consent for perimortem cesarean section is not necessary. The procedure needs to be performed expediently and should be considered part of the resuscitation. The performance of a non-life-threatening operation in the setting of cardiac arrest abides by the ethics of absence of malfeasance and beneficence for both the mother and the fetus. The question of when emergent cesarean section should be performed in critically ill, prearrest patients has not been adequately addressed in the literature. In addition, the recommendations for perimortem cesarean section are based on multiple case reports. No experimental studies have been done to evaluate this procedure.

DISPOSITION

The presence of experienced obstetricians, anesthesiologists, and pediatricians or neonatologists will facilitate the care of pregnant patients with cardiac arrest. However, none of the required care and procedures should be delayed if these specialists are not available. When trained staff are available to perform external fetal tococardiography without diverting care from the mother, it should be provided for pregnancies beyond 20 weeks' gestation. If this technology is not available or personnel are limited, the often-quoted maxim "Maternal resuscitation is the best fetal resuscitation" should be kept in mind. The closest center providing neonatal services should be contacted as soon as possible to facilitate rapid transport of the newly delivered infant.

REFERENCES

1. Berg CJ, Atrash HK, Koonin LM, Tucker M: Pregnancy-related mortality in the United States, 1987–1990. *Obstet Gynecol* 88:161, 1996.
2. Harper M, Parsons L: Maternal deaths due to homicide and other injuries in North Carolina: 1992–1994. *Obstet Gynecol* 90:920, 1997.
3. Dannenberg AL, Carter DM, Lawson HW, et al: Homicide and other injuries as causes of maternal death in New York City, 1987 through 1991. *Am J Obstet Gynecol* 172:1557, 1995.
4. Archer GW Jr, Marx GF: Arterial oxygen tension during apnoea in parturient women. *Br J Anaesth* 46:358, 1974.
5. Sobrevilla LA, Cassinelli MT, Carcelen A, et al: Human fetal and maternal oxygen tension and acid-base status during delivery at high altitude. *Am J Obstet Gynecol* 111:1111, 1971.
6. Crosby ET: The difficult airway in obstetric anesthesia, in Benumof JL (ed): *Airway Management: Principles and Practice.* St. Louis, Mosby-Year Book, 1996.
7. Davies JM, Weets S, Crone LA, Paulin E: Difficult intubation in the parturient. *Can J Anaesth* 36:668, 1989.
8. Cheek TG, Gutsche BB: Maternal physiologic alterations during pregnancy, in Shnider SM, Levinson G (eds): *Anesthesia for Obstetrics,* 3d ed, Baltimore, Williams & Wilkins, 1993.
9. Rees GAD, Willis BA: Resuscitation in late pregnancy. *Anaesthesia* 43:347, 1988.
10. Ornato JP, Paradis N, Bircher N, et al: Future directions for resuscitation research: III. External cardiopulmonary resuscitation advanced life support. *Resuscitation* 32:139, 1996.
11. Chandra NC, et al: *Textbook of Basic Life Support for Healthcare Providers.* New York, American Heart Association, 1994.
12. Strong TH, Lowe RV: Perimortem cesarean section. *J Emerg Med* 7:489, 1989.
13. Dillon WD, Lee RV, Tronolone MJ, et al: Life support during maternal brain death during pregnancy. *JAMA* 248:1089, 1982.
14. Marx GF, Mateo CV: Effects of different oxygen concentrations during general anaesthesia for elective caesarean sections. *Can Anaesth Soc J* 18:587,1971.
15. Selden BS, Burke TJ: Complete maternal and fetal recovery after prolonged cardiac arrest. *Ann Emerg Med* 17:346,1988.
16. Ryan TJ, Anderson JL, Antman EM, et al: ACC/AHA guidelines for the management of patients with acute myocardial infarction: A report of the American College of Cardiology/American Heart Association Task Force on Practice Guidelines (Committee on Management of Acute Myocardial Infarction). *J Am Coll Cardiol* 28:1328, 1996.
17. Turrentine MA, Braems G, Ramirez MM: Use of thrombolytics for the treatment of thromboembolic disease during pregnancy. *Obstet Gynecol Surv* 50:534, 1995.
18. Esposito RA, Grossi EA, Coppa G, et al: Successful treatment of postpartum shock caused by amniotic fluid embolism with cardiopulmonary bypass and pulmonary artery thromboembolectomy. *Am J Obstet Gynecol* 163:572, 1990.
19. Oates S, Williams GL, Rees GGAD: Cardiopulmonary resuscitation in late pregnancy. *Br Med J* 297:404, 1988.

ETHICAL ISSUES OF RESUSCITATION

Catherine A. Marco

GENERAL PRINCIPLES OF MEDICAL ETHICS

The study of ethics has been defined as the way of *understanding and examining the moral life* (Beauchamp and Childress, *Principles of Biomedical Ethics*, 4th ed., 1994), and as the study of standards of conduct and moral judgment (*Webster's Dictionary*). The Hippocratic Oath has been revered as one of the oldest codes of medical ethics. More recently, the American Medical Association (AMA) Code of

Ethics (earliest version from 1847) and American College of Emergency Physicians (ACEP) Code of Ethics (1997) have provided guidance to emergency physicians in application of ethical principles to clinical practice. Most ethical codes address common features, such as beneficence (doing good), nonmalfeasance (primum non nocere, or "do no harm"), respect for patient autonomy, confidentiality, honesty, distributive justice, and respect for the law. Ethical dilemmas may arise when there is a seeming conflict between two ethical principles or values. Ethical dilemmas may be resolved by various means, including individual physician judgment, additional information gathering, meetings with health care professionals, patients, and families. In some circumstances, the involvement of the institutional ethics committee or the judicial system may be sought. Several ethical situations related to emergency medicine are explored in this chapter.

CARDIAC RESUSCITATION AND OUTCOMES

There are an estimated 750,000 sudden deaths in the United States annually. The outcome of resuscitative efforts for victims of cardiac arrest is uniformly poor, but varies, dependent on a variety of factors. The most important factor determining outcome is the time elapsed since arrest ("downtime"). One study showed a 27 percent resuscitation rate for patients who received advanced cardiac life support (ACLS) within 8 min of arrest, and a dismal outcome if more than 20 min elapses.[1] Improved outcomes have been demonstrated for witnessed arrests, who received early cardiopulmonary resuscitation (CPR) and advanced life support (ALS). Another important prognostic factor is the presenting rhythm. Previous studies have demonstrated improved survival rates for patients with presenting rhythms of ventricular fibrillation or ventricular tachycardia, and reduced survival rates for patients with asystole or pulseless electrical activity. The underlying medical condition of the patient is another important factor affecting outcome.

A potentially poor response to resuscitation can be expected for patients with metastatic disease, acute cerebrovascular accident, sepsis, renal failure, or pneumonia. Failure to respond to prehospital ALS protocols leads to a survival rate of less than 2 percent. The age of the patient also affects predicted survival rate, with a 0 percent survival rate for unwitnessed arrests of elderly patients[2] and for long-term care patients.[3] Overall survival of victims of cardiac arrests, to hospital discharge, has been estimated to be between 0 and 16 percent.

Based on such data, several authors have suggested proposed criteria for withholding resuscitative efforts for patients in certain clinical settings with low likelihood of successful resuscitation (e.g., apneic, pulseless for longer than 10 min prior to Emergency Medical Service arrival, no response to ACLS, and preexisting terminal disease).[4,5] Knowledge of data regarding resuscitation outcomes in various clinical settings is crucial when making evidence-based decisions regarding the risks and benefits of attempting cardiopulmonary resuscitation and the duration of the resuscitation attempt.

RISKS AND BENEFITS OF RESUSCITATIVE EFFORTS

When considering offering or withholding resuscitative efforts, risks and benefits of resuscitative efforts should be carefully considered. The goal of resuscitative efforts is to restore circulation, and life to the patient. Other less tangible benefits may include such entities as resolution of guilt of the survivors, and the additional time for acceptance of bad news for survivors.

However, often resuscitative measures are undertaken in clinical situations in which physiologic survival is very unlikely. In some situations, there is a substantial risk that, if circulation is restored, significant anoxic brain injury will result, possibly resulting in impairment of quality of life (dementia, persistent vegetative state, or other cognitive impairments). Additionally, substantial resources (supply costs, as well as personnel) are often invested in this clinical setting of low likelihood of benefit, while the care of many other patients is delayed (distributive justice). Another consideration for limiting resuscitative efforts is the potentially increased human resources that could be available for family counseling, rather than investing such resources in resuscitative efforts unlikely to be successful.

"FUTILITY" AND NONBENEFICIAL INTERVENTIONS

The term *futility* is fraught with difficulties in definition and interpretation. Health care professionals may interpret futile interventions as those that carry an absolute impossibility of successful outcome, a low likelihood of success, a low likelihood of survival to discharge from the hospital, or a low likelihood of restoration of meaningful quality of life. Schneiderman and colleagues defined "futility" as "any effort to achieve a result that is possible but that reasoning or experience suggests is highly improbable and that cannot be systematically produced."[6] Several authors have demonstrated that there is no consensus among physicians about the meaning of futility.[7,8] Because of these difficulties, it is probably more accurate to use the appropriate terminology, such as "nonbeneficial," "ineffectual," or "low likelihood of success."

The withholding or limitation of medical interventions that have a predicted low likelihood of producing a successful outcome can be a difficult and far-reaching decision. Many emergency physicians continue to attempt resuscitation on patients in cardiac arrest, in situations considered nonbeneficial, often because of fears of litigation or criticism.[9] Medical ethicists have stated widely variable opinions regarding rendering treatments considered futile or of low likelihood of benefit. The AMA Council on Ethical and Judicial Affairs stated that "the social commitment of the physician is to sustain life and relieve suffering. Where the performance of one duty conflicts with the other, the choice of the patient should prevail."[10] One extreme viewpoint is that even the irrational choices of a competent patient must be respected if the patient cannot be persuaded to change them.[11] However, most ethicists agree that physicians are under no obligation to render treatments that they deem of little or no benefit to the patient. ACEP has a policy which states that "physicians are under no ethical obligation to render treatments that they judge have no realistic likelihood of medical benefit to the patient."[12]

There have been numerous ethical opinions supportive of the position of offering only those treatments judged to be of likely medical benefit. The Hastings Center concluded, "if a treatment is clearly futile . . . there is no obligation to provide the treatment."[13] The AMA Council on Ethical and Judicial Affairs holds that CPR may be withheld, even if requested by the patient, "when efforts to resuscitate a patient are judged by the treating physician to be futile."[14] Blackhall stated that in cases of low likelihood of successful resuscitation, "the issue of patient autonomy is irrelevant."[15] Tomlinson and Brody stated that "physicians have no obligation to provide, and patients and families have no right to demand, medical treatment that is of no demonstrable benefit."[16] Hackler and Hiller believe that "respect for patient autonomy does not require that the physician initiate decisions of medically pointless procedures."[17] Schneiderman and colleagues wrote that "futility is a professional judgement that takes precedence over patient autonomy and permits physicians to withhold or withdraw care deemed to be inappropriate without subjecting such a decision to patient approval."[6] Jecker and Schneiderman also stated that physicians have no ordinary ethical obligation to offer futile interventions.[18] Paris and Reardon wrote that "physicians as moral agents should exercise professional judgment in assessing patient requests. If the request goes beyond well-established criteria of reasonableness, the physician ought not feel obliged to provide it."[19]

Ultimately, the decision regarding CPR, its likelihood of benefit to the patient, and decisions to provide, limit, or withhold resuscitative efforts are to be made by the emergency physician in the context of well-established research results, patient and family wishes, and professional judgment. Individual bias regarding quality of life or other related issues should be avoided. There are many cases where dying should be accepted as a natural process, even in an emergency setting. Perhaps palliative care, communication, and counseling with the patient, family, and friends may be of greater benefit then technology of unlikely benefit.

ADVANCE DIRECTIVES

The *living will,* which was adopted by many states in 1990. The treating physician abides by the providions when an ill individual can no longer make competent decisions regarding their medical care. Many living wills are created to ensure that no high-technology life support be used in cases where meaningful recovery will not occur. *Durable power of attorney* specifies a surrogate decision maker in the event the patient no longer has the capacity to make medical decisions. An *advance directive* refers to any document stating the patient's wishes in various situations, should the patient be unable to state them in an actual clinical encounter. In 1991, the Federal Patient Self-Determination Act mandated the opportunity to sign an advance directive, for all patients admitted to a hospital. In many cases, the existence of an advance directive can facilitate the implementation of the patient's specific wishes. However, there still exist numerous problems with the widespread implementation of advance directives in the emergency setting, including the fact that very few patients compose them, the designated decision maker may be unavailable, or the advance directive may not reflect a changed opinion. State law often limits advance directives, and patients may lack understanding of decisions and ramifications of the advance directive. Even when an advance directive exists, compliance may be variable, dependent on the clinical circumstances.[20] When an advance directive exists, but is unavailable, the emergency physician must make a decision regarding the reliability of the information available and make every attempt to offer treatment congruent with the patient's previously stated wishes. In the absence of an advance directive, a surrogate may be consulted to aid in the determination of the most appropriate course of action. Decision-making authorities may be a court-appointed guardian, patient-designated decision maker, spouse, adult child (or majority of children available), parents, or the nearest living relative.

PROCEDURES ON RECENTLY DECEASED PATIENTS

The practices of teaching and performing procedures on recently deceased patients are controversial. The most important benefit of these practices is the fulfillment of the recognized need for hands-on practice for students and housestaff, as well as experienced physicians.[21] The setting of the recently deceased patient provides a unique clinical setting with literally *no* tangible risk to the patient. Following this rationale, physicians so inclined are able to perform these procedures competently on future, living patients, resulting in overall benefit to society. However, informed consent is rarely obtained or available in these settings. Some consider performing procedures without informed consent to be disrespectful, deceptive, or unethical.[22]

Until formal policies are developed by governing organizations in emergency medicine, emergency physicians must make the choices they judge most appropriate in the specific clinical situations encountered. Factors to be considered, when making such decisions, include the teaching benefit, to the student and his/her future patients, the overall benefit to society, invasiveness and disfigurement produced by the procedure(s), availability of the family and feasibility of informed consent, potential distress to the family, other potential avenues for teaching procedures, and any institutional policies on this issue.

RESUSCITATION RESEARCH

Research on resuscitation techniques and pharmaceuticals has been problematic, due to the frequent inability to obtain informed consent and the constraints of the decision-making process. Ordinarily, the process of obtaining informed consent for human subject research is designed to assure protection and autonomy of the subject. However, the process of obtaining informed consent is time consuming and requires competence of the subject. Because of these difficulties, the Food and Drug Administration recently issued guidelines under which resuscitation research may be performed, with a waiver of informed consent, under certain conditions.[23] When designing such research protocols, factors to be considered include the patient's wishes (if known), expected safety of the study protocol, expected benefit of the therapeutic intervention, overall expected benefit to society by improved knowledge regarding resuscitation, related animal data, feasibility of surrogate consent, local Institutional Review Board opinion, and local general public opinion, if available.

COMMUNICATION AND COUNSELING FOR SURVIVORS

In many cases, the communication, care, and counseling provided for survivors (family, friends, and the like) of victims of cardiac arrest will have more impact than the actual resuscitative efforts. A majority of emergency physicians find the notification of death to survivors emotionally difficult.[24] Optimum care should be provided for families and friends of victims of cardiac arrest, regardless of the level of treatment rendered and outcome. Some general guidelines for such support might include the following:[25,26]

1. Give advance warning, if possible. During the resuscitative efforts, a member of the health care team should communicate the gravity of the patient's condition.
2. Provide a private, quiet location for communications.
3. Spend adequate time in counseling and in answering questions.
4. Use clear and succinct language. Often medical jargon is not accurately understood. It is generally appropriate to use straightforward language, such as "died" and "death," rather than "didn't make it," "passed on," and the like.
5. Use proper names of the deceased and family members.
6. Accept any reaction as normal. Even unexpected reactions, such as apathy, anger, and hysteria may not be inappropriate.
7. Don't hesitate to show emotion. Families may benefit from sharing emotions.
8. Reassure loved ones that the patient likely did not suffer.
9. Attempt to absolve any guilt feelings. It is generally inappropriate to suggest that a different course of action (calling 911 sooner, different actions by prehospital personnel, and so on) may have changed the outcome.
10. When appropriate, discuss organ donation. Many families find organ donation a positive experience.
11. Allow the family to view the body. This may provide some closure and aid in their acceptance of the death.
12. Utilize additional resources when appropriate. These may include social work, nursing, psychiatry, clergy, or other ancillary and support staff.
13. Invite further questioning. The emergency physician may serve as an important resource for future concerns or questions that may arise.

Recently, some facilities have allowed family members to be present during the resuscitative phase of a dying child or adult. The practice is growing but remains controversial.

REFERENCES

1. Eisenberg MS, Bergner L, Hallstrom A: Cardiac resuscitation in the community. Importance of rapid provision and implications for program planning. *JAMA* 241:1905, 1979.
2. Murphy DJ, Murray AM, Robinson BE, et al: Outcomes of cardiopulmonary resuscitation in the elderly. *Ann Intern Med* 111:199, 1989.
3. Awoke S, Mouton CP, Parrott M: Outcomes of skilled cardiopulmonary resuscitation in a long-term-care facility: Futile therapy? *J Am Geriatr Soc* 40:593, 1992.
4. Bonnin MJ, Pepe PE, Kimball KT, et al: Distinct criteria for termination of resuscitation in the out-of-hospital setting. *JAMA* 270:1457, 1993.
5. Kellerman AL, Hackman BB, Somes G: Predicting the outcome of unsuccessful prehospital advanced cardiac life support. *JAMA* 270:1433, 1993.
6. Schneiderman LJ, Jecker NS, Jonsen AR: Medical futility: Its meaning and ethical implications. *Ann Intern Med* 112:949, 1990.
7. Lantos JD, Singer PA, Walker RM, et al: The illusion of futility in clinical practice. *Am J Med* 87:81, 1989.
8. Brody BA, Halevy A: Is futility a futile concept? *J Med Philos* 20:123, 1995.
9. Marco CA, Bessman ES, Schoenfeld CN, et al: Ethical issues of cardiopulmonary resuscitation: Current practice among emergency physicians. *Acad Emerg Med* 4:898, 1997.
10. AMA Council on Ethical and Judicial Affairs: *Current Opinions of the CEJA-AMA*, Chicago, American Medical Assoc., 1989, pp 12–13.
11. Brock DW, Wartman SA: When competent patients make irrational choices. *N Engl J Med* 322:1595, 1990.
12. ACEP: Policy statement: Nonbeneficial (''futile'') emergency medical interventions. Irving, TX, American College of Emergency Physicians, 1998.
13. Hastings Center: *Guidelines on the Termination of Life-Sustaining Treatment and the Care of the Dying*. Briarcliff Manor, NY, The Hastings Center, 1987, p 19.
14. AMA Council on Ethical and Judicial Affairs: Guidelines for the appropriate use of do-not-resuscitate orders. *JAMA* 265:1868, 1991.
15. Blackhall LJ: Must we always use CPR? *N Engl J Med* 317:1281, 1987.
16. Tomlinson T, Brody H: Ethics and communication in do-not-resuscitate orders. *N Engl J Med* 318:43, 1988.
17. Hackler JC, Hiller FC: Family consent to orders not to resuscitate: reconsidering hospital policy. *JAMA* 264:1281, 1990.
18. Jecker NS, Schneiderman LJ: Futility and rationing. *Am J Med* 92:189, 1992.
19. Paris JJ, Reardon FE: Physician refusal of requests for futile or ineffective interventions. *Cambridge Quarterly of Healthcare Ethics* 2:127, 1992.
20. Davidson KW, Hackler C, Caradine DR, et al: Physicians' attitudes on advance directives. *JAMA* 266:402, 1991.
21. Iserson KV: Law versus life: The ethical imperative to practice and teach using the newly dead emergency department patient. *Ann Emerg Med* 25:91, 1995.
22. Goldblatt AD: Don't ask, don't tell: Practicing minimally invasive resuscitative techniques on the newly dead. *Ann Emerg Med* 25:86, 1995.
23. Department of Health and Human Services, Food and Drug Administration: Protection of human subjects; informed consent and waiver of informed consent requirements in certain emergency research; final rules. *Federal Register* FR 96-24968, 9/26/96.
24. Schmidt TA, Tolle SW: Emergency physicians' responses to families following patient death. *Ann Emerg Med* 19:125, 1990.
25. Marco CA: Coping with unexpected death. *J Coll Aesculapium* Spring: 29, 1993.
26. Olsen JC, Buenese ML, Falso W: Death in the emergency department. *Ann Emerg Med* 31:758, 1998.

NONINVASIVE AIRWAY MANAGEMENT

A. Michael Roman

The principal goal of this chapter is to familiarize the physician with upper airway control by presenting alternatives to tracheal intubation. Reviewed is a brief anatomic and pathophysiologic description of the upper airway, the (oral, nasal) airway management, bag-valve mask, esophageal airway devices, and noninvasive pressure support ventilation techniques.

ANATOMY AND PATHOPHYSIOLOGY

Prior to airway management procedures, when there is sufficient time, the physician should:

1. Inspect the patient's mouth for size of teeth and size and mobility of the jaw.
2. Open the patient's mouth and observe the palate, tongue, and oropharynx.
3. Flex the stable neck (in the absence of trauma), and assess mobility, and place in the sniffing position.
4. Examine the size and alignment of the neck.
5. Inspect the nasal openings for patency.
6. Ask the patient's history, if possible.
7. Listen for abnormal airway sounds like stridor, hoarseness, or gurgling.
8. Be sure to have suction available at all times, especially during any procedures.

The anatomic airway (Fig. 14-1) begins at the oral/nasal cavities and continues posteriorly to the tongue/turbinates; the tonsils/adenoids; past the palate; through the oropharynx; across the epiglottis, which protects the glottis (the narrowest portion of the airway); past the false and true vocal cords; and into the larynx. Surrounding the larynx is the thyroid cartilage, cricoid cartilage, and thyroid gland. The upper airway ends here; the lower airway then continues to the trachea and into the lungs. Potential obstruction may develop anywhere along this route. In infants and small children, the anatomy is somewhat different than in the adult. The tongue is relatively larger in relation to the mandible. The glottis is higher and more anterior and the vocal cords are angled more anteriorly and inferiorly. The epiglottis is large and floppy and may lie against the posterior wall of the pharynx.

AIRWAY OBSTRUCTION

Potential causes of upper airway obstruction are shown in Table 14-1. Basic management of the obstructed airway is discussed in Chap. 8. Most of these entities cause soft tissue swelling or themselves are soft tissue masses that compromise the upper airway, but a few need mentioning. Certain medical diseases like respiratory syncytial virus (RSV) and cystic fibrosis produce copious secretions in the upper airway that can lead to partial or complete occlusion. Angioedema may present with soft tissue swelling sufficient to preclude an oral airway, requiring a nasal pharyngeal airway, nasotracheal intubation, or surgical intervention to reestablish patency. Laryngospasm, the feared complication of any invasive airway technique, needs to be considered in any patient with a compromised airway, especially in children. It is defined as closure of the glottis by the constriction of intrinsic/extrinsic laryngeal muscles, which can completely restrict ventilation. This pathophysiologic state often persists long after the stimulus has ceased. Laryngospasm may occur secondary to contact with the upper airway receptors on the tongue, palate, and oropharynx. Light touch to the upper airway, anal stretch, traction on the pelvic/abdominal viscera, chemical irritation, secretions, blood, water, and vomitus may all cause laryngospasm. Hypoxia and hypercapnea depress the activity of laryngeal adductor neurons, so laryngospasm is somewhat self-limited. Laryngospasm and bronchospasm occur more frequently in children and particularly following a recent respiratory tract infection.

Altered mental status, somnolence, or even sleep can depress the intrinsic and extrinsic muscle tone of the airway and produce obstruction. Some authors question the long-standing belief that the tongue falling back and occluding the lower pharynx is the major cause of airway obstruction in the somnolent or comatose patient. In a supine individual, the degree of extension of the head required to open the airway depends on elevation of the occiput above the horizontal plane.

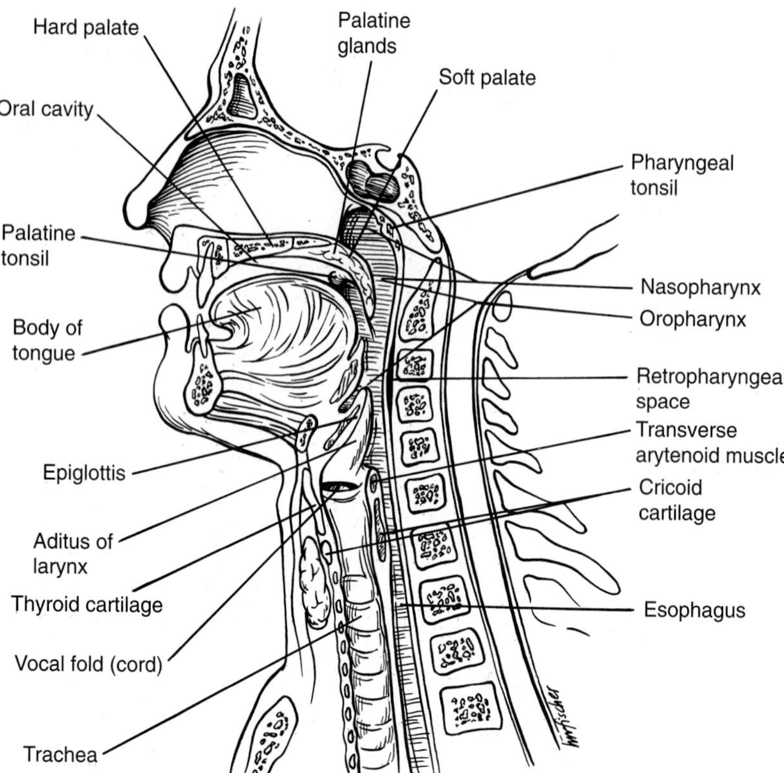

FIG. 14-1. The anatomic airway.

Relative to the neck, the more the occiput is elevated, the less extension is required to open the airway, which explains why patients with airway compromise need to have their heads in the "sniffing" position. One can place a folded towel or foam rubber device behind the patient's occiput (not neck) to create this position. Flexion of the neck has a marked effect of closing the airway, specifically the oropharynx. Recently, it has been shown that during anesthesia in the supine patient, the tongue does in fact displace posteriorly, but it does not appear to occlude the pharynx. Upper airway obstruction in the unconscious patient occurs primarily because the epiglottis occludes the laryngeal inlet due to intrinsic muscle relaxation, which can be relieved simply by extending the neck. Extension of the neck and anterior displacement of the mandible moves the hyoid bone anteriorly and, in turn, lifts the epiglottis away from the laryngeal inlet. Recent magnetic resonance imaging (MRI) studies show that the soft palate also relaxes significantly during sedation, partially occluding the nasopharynx and causing complete obstruction when the patient is fully anesthetized. Moreover, retraction of the anterior tongue does not appear to relieve this obstruction.[1]

TABLE 14-1 Causes of Upper Airway Obstruction

Congenital/ Genetic	Infectious	Medical	Trauma/ Tumor
Large tonsils	Tonsillitis	Cystic fibrosis	Laryngeal trauma
Macroglossia	Peritonsilar abscess	Angioedema	Hematoma/ masses
Micrognathia	Retropharyngeal abscess	Laryngospasm	Smoke inhalation
Neck masses	Pretracheal abscess	Airway muscle relaxation	Thermal injuries
Large adenoids	Epiglottitis	Inflammatory	Foreign body
	Laryngitis/RSV*	Asthma	
	Ludwig angina		

*Respiratory syncytial virus.

Esophageal foreign bodies can also obstruct the airway. They can impinge upon the larynx or trachea, causing either acute or subacute obstruction. Some foreign bodies, such as large fruit pits, may have been present for some time; thus there may not be a history of swallowing an object.

ORAL/NASAL AIRWAYS

The oral airway (Fig. 14-2) is an "S"-shaped, rigid instrument used to prevent the base of the tongue from occluding the hypopharynx. It should be used to maintain the airway only in a patient with an absent gag reflex. It can also be used as a bite block during orotracheal intubation. The operator places the oral airway over the tongue, being careful not to push it further into the hypopharynx. A tongue blade can be used to aid insertion. The concave portion is placed cephalad, rotated 180°, or aimed toward the ear and rotated 90° inferiorly to hold the tongue away from the pharyngeal wall.

A nasal airway (nasopharyngeal tube) (Fig. 14-3) is made of a pliable (latex) material that allows it to be placed into the nostril of a somnolent patient with an intact gag reflex. The nasal airway is a wonderful tool that can be quickly placed in a sonorous patient who may have decreased pharyngeal muscle tone and an obstructing soft palate and tongue. It allows air to bypass such obstructions, and if topical anesthesia was used as a lubricant, may ease subsequent passage of a nasogastric tube. The nasopharyngeal tube should be inserted into the most patent nostril (with the tip lubricated, ideally with a topical anesthetic such as lidocaine jelly) horizontal to the palate, and advanced until maximal airflow is heard. It is important to use the correct size tube and to avoid inserting it far enough to stimulate the gag reflex.

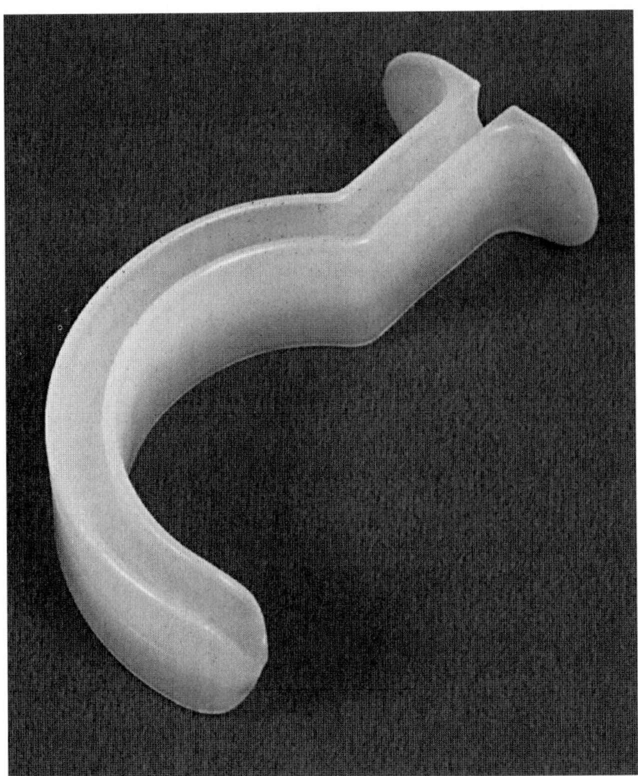

FIG. 14-2. An oral airway.

THE BAG-VALVE-MASK UNIT

The bag-valve-mask (BVM) unit (Fig. 14-4) is a self-inflating bag with a nonrebreathing valve that can be attached to a face mask. This design allows room air or oxygenated air to be manually delivered into the victim's lungs after any obstruction has been eliminated. This apparatus can be used initially while preparing for definitive airway maintenance. After the mask is placed, the handler clamps it snugly to the face. The thumb and index finger grasp the mask while the other fingers grasp the chin and pull it forward to hyperextend the stable neck. The other hand compresses the bag, expelling air into the patient's respiratory tree. This procedure can be used to manage respiratory failure temporarily, to assist poor inspiratory effort, or to temporize respiratory fatigue. The most common problem with a one-person operation is air leaks around the mask. A two-person operation employs two hands to hold the mask flush and has been shown to result in more effective ventilation.[2] After an intubation, the BVM unit can be attached to the proximal end of the endotracheal tube. Placement of an oral or nasal airway further facilitates airflow. The BVM unit may also be used prior to rapid-sequence intubation (RSI) to quickly assess the ease of BVM ventilation in cases where oral intubation fails.

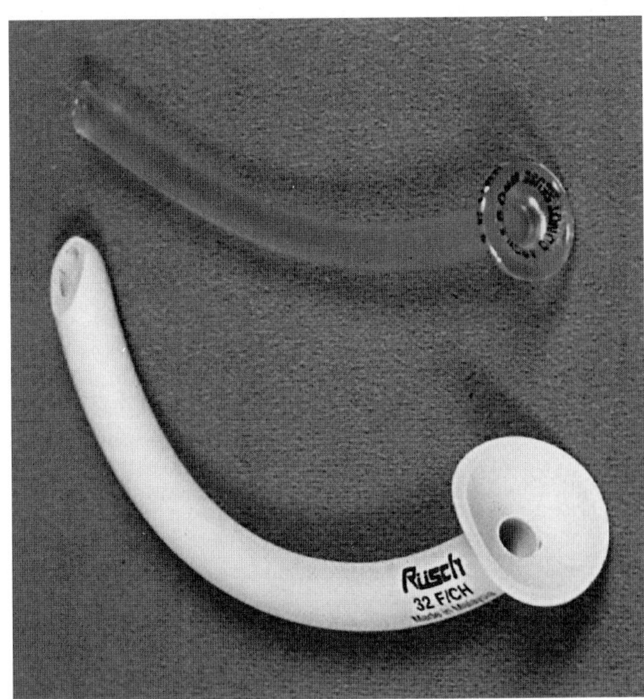

FIG. 14-3. Nasal airways.

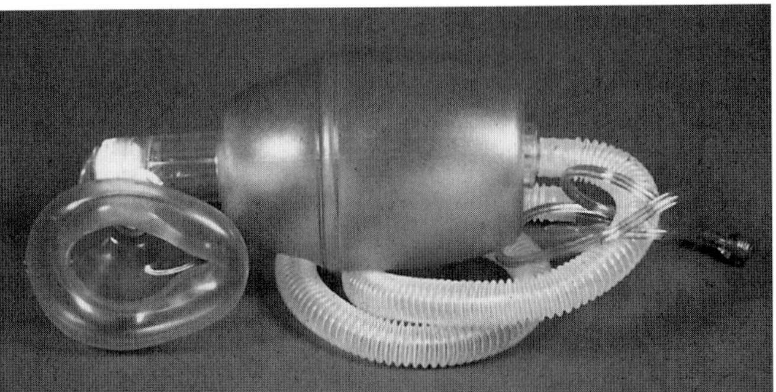

FIG. 14-4. Bag-valve-mask unit.

To deliver 100% oxygen, there must be a reservoir with the same volume as the bag and an oxygen flow rate equal to the respiratory minute volume of the patient. By using a 2.5-L reservoir bag with an oxygen flow of 15 L/min, 100% oxygen can be delivered. Similarly, a demand valve attached to the reservoir port of the ventilation bag will deliver a high concentration of oxygen.

ESOPHAGEAL AIRWAYS

Esophageal obturator airways (EOAs) (Fig. 14-5)—the pharyngotracheal lumen airway, and the esophageal tracheal Combitube—are all devices used in the prehospital setting when oral endotracheal intubation is not a viable option. These devices are designed to be placed in apneic, unconscious adults only.

Esophageal Obturator Airway/Esophageal Gastric Tube Airway (EOA/EGTA)

The EOA, a 34-cm tube (Fig. 14-5*A*), is placed by flexing the neck and blindly inserting the device into the esophagus. The closed-tube distal cuff is inflated and the more proximal holes allow pressurized air to enter the hypopharyngeal area for ventilation. The EOA has a proximal face mask that requires a good seal to ensure adequate ventilation. The primary benefit is placement without direct laryngeal visualization. The secondary benefits are prevention of gastric distention, regurgitation, and aspiration. The esophageal gastric tube airway (EGTA) (Fig. 14-5*B*), a modification of the EOA, has an open distal tube containing a valve that allows passage of a nasogastric tube.

Once placed, the EOA is left alone until definitive oral endotracheal intubation is performed, at which point the EOA tube is pulled. EOAs have been shown to be more effective in oxygenation than mask ventilation, but the potential complications are the main reason this tool is used only when endotracheal intubation is not an option. Inadvertent tracheal intubation occurs in approximately 4 to 10 percent of cases. Esophageal injury, including laceration, occurs in up to 10 percent

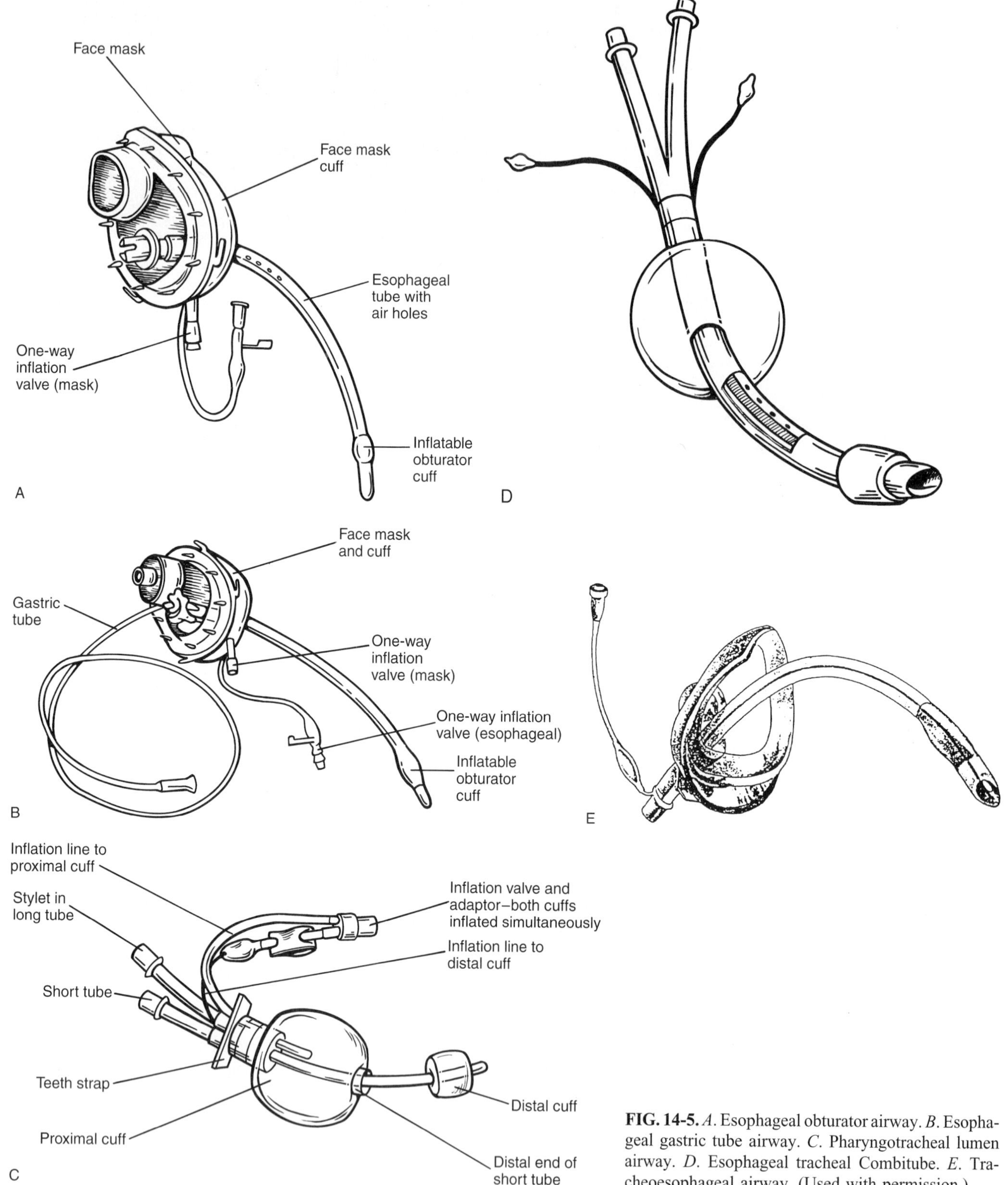

FIG. 14-5. *A*. Esophageal obturator airway. *B*. Esophageal gastric tube airway. *C*. Pharyngotracheal lumen airway. *D*. Esophageal tracheal Combitube. *E*. Tracheoesophageal airway. (Used with permission.)

and perforation in approximately 2 percent. Related mortality is 10 to 15 percent. Other considerations include the possibility of vomitus with aspiration and difficulty in maintaining a good seal with the face mask.

Since airway management in the prehospital setting is now more sophisticated in most jurisdictions than it was in the past, the use of EOAs has become quite uncommon. One study showed that some physicians had never seen an EOA, and unfamiliarity is reason enough to avoid using this tool.

Pharyngotracheal Lumen Airway

The pharyngotracheal lumen airway (PTLA) (Fig. 14-5*C*) is another two-tubed, cuffed airway that seals the oropharynx proximally and allows ventilation below the cuff. If the trachea is intubated, no complication arises because the open lumen allows ventilation to occur. This design was the first to offer an esophageal airway without the need for a face-to-mask seal.

Esophageal Tracheal Combitube

The esophageal tracheal Combitube (ETC) (Sheridan Catheter Corp.) (Fig. 14-5*D*) is a plastic twin-lumen tube with a proximal low-pressure cuff that seals the pharyngeal area and a distal cuff that seals the esophagus, allowing ventilation between the cuffs. The proximal seal also removes the need for a facemask and, as compared with the PTLA, minimizes dental damage to the cuff. The distal cuff is similar to an ETT and serves to seal either the esophagus or the trachea when inflated. If the distal tube enters the esophagus, perforations in the esophageal lumen serve to ventilate the patient. If the trachea is intubated, the patient is ventilated directly, as with the cuffed ETT.

Studies show that by comparison to the simple oral airway, the EOAs are superior in preventing regurgitation and thus aspiration. Compared with the ETT, ventilation and oxygenation studies reveal varying results but suggest that the EOAs are adequate during cardiac arrest.[3] However, the method of choice for airway management for both hospital and prehospital therapy remains direct oral endotracheal intubation.

Tracheoesophageal Airway

Another modification of the EOA is the tracheoesophageal airway (TEA) (Fig. 14-5*E*). It has a standard endotracheal tube (ETT) with two openings, one for the ETT and the other for oropharyngeal ventilation. It is designed to function equally well if inserted into the trachea or the esophagus. Tracheal intubation is facilitated by using cricoid pressure and extending the neck. While the tube is in the trachea, the cuff is inflated and the patient is ventilated normally. While the tube is in the esophagus, the patient is ventilated through the mask and the ETT allows for gastric venting or decompression.

Laryngeal Mask Airway

The laryngeal mask airway (LMA) (Intavent, Ltd.) (Fig. 14-6) was developed by Brain in 1983 as another artificial airway that can be placed blindly yet can provide a positive-pressure airway. The LMA consists of a tubular oropharyngeal airway similar to the ETT, but it is shorter and has a distal silicone laryngeal mask (balloon-type bulb) that inflates and provides a seal around the larynx. The LMA, when placed, is similar to other esophageal airways in that it can be inserted without manipulation of the patient's head. Because of its large diameter and short length, intubation of the bronchi or esophagus is circumvented. The hypopharynx, which is adapted to the passage of food, is less sensitive to a foreign body than the larynx and vocal cords, which have sensitive, protective reflexes. Many published cases show the LMA to be an effective alternative when the ETT fails because of nonvisualization of the cords secondary to ETT difficulty, airway masses, or cervical pathology.[4] Studies of LMA use by nonphysician emergency personnel in fasting patients found it easier to place than the ETT. The LMA never failed, versus 21 percent of failures for the ETT, required only half as many attempts and one-fifth the time to perform, and was rated equal to the ETT as an airway by anesthesiologists.[5] Some of the complications included partial or complete respiratory obstruction (3 percent). In general, failure to protect against aspiration of gastric contents was noted. The LMA was also inadequate in severe chronic obstructive pulmonary disease (COPD) because of the high pressure requirement.[6] Applying cricoid pressure in the acute setting almost always impedes insertion of the LMA and therefore reduces the chance of successful ventilation of the patient.[7] Therefore the LMA seems an effective alternative to the ETT when endotracheal intubation fails or when cervical pathology exists.

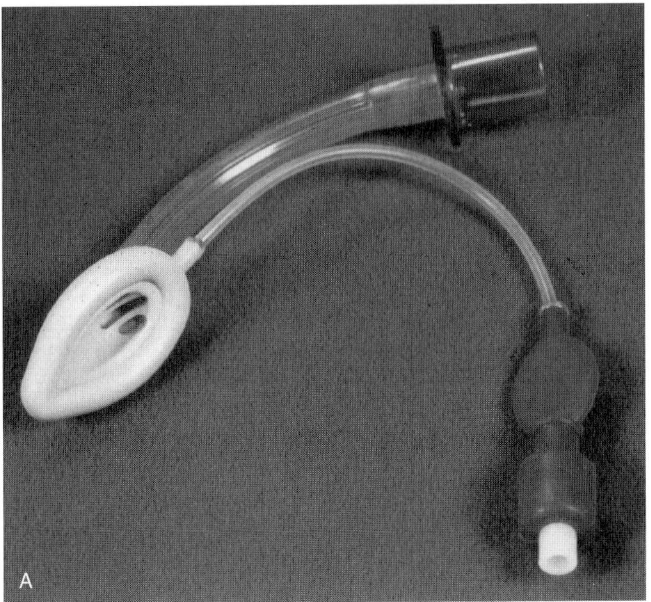

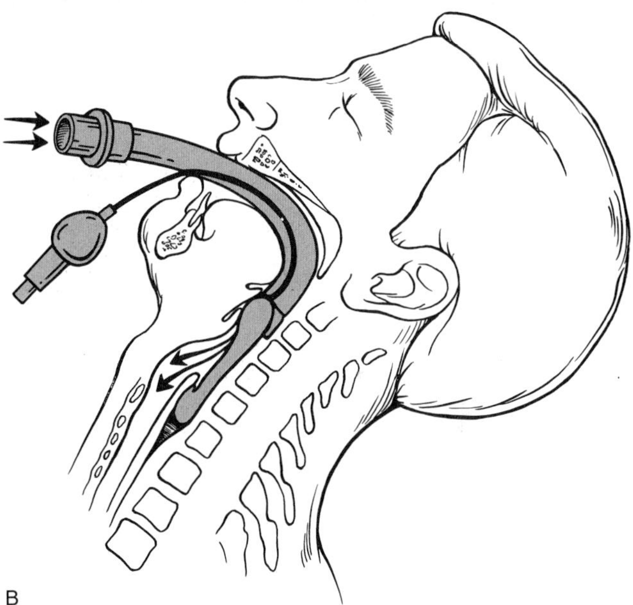

FIG. 14-6. *A*. Laryngeal mask airway (LMA). *B*. LMA diagram showing placement at the larynx. (Used with permission.)

NONINVASIVE POSITIVE-PRESSURE VENTILATION

The widespread use of noninvasive positive-pressure ventilation (NIPPV) for chronic sleep apnea in the 1980s has prompted investigators to look at NIPPV in the acute setting today. NIPPV can be described as an application of a preset volume/pressure of inspiratory air through a face or nasal mask.

Inspiratory muscle fatigue is the final phase of ventilatory failure in patients with severe reactive airway disease, COPD, and end-state pulmonary edema/pneumonia. The airway resistance overcomes the patient's muscular ability to ventilate. Another noninvasive technique used as an effective alternative to the traditional ETT, with its potential complications, is noninvasive, mechanically assisted ventilation with continuous positive pressure (CPAP) or bilevel positive pressure (BiPAP). CPAP applied through a face or nasal mask has recently received renewed application in the treatment of patients with *acute* hypoxemic respiratory failure.[8] NIPPV has been used to support patients with acute respiratory failure but has been primarily studied in the intensive care setting. Patient diagnostic categories individually studied in the emergency department (ED) include those with COPD, status asthmaticus, adult respiratory distress syndrome (ARDS), those who have been intubated, and those with pulmonary edema, pneumonia, or traumatic respiratory insufficiency. In early published and unpublished studies, CPAP used in the hospital and prehospital settings showed potential improvement of vital signs (heart rate, respiratory rate, and blood pressure) and oxygen saturation. In the pediatric patient population, BiPAP appears to improve respiratory rate, heart rate, Pa_{CO_2}, and O_2 saturation; it also decreases the need for intubation in obstructive apnea. The use of face-mask positive-pressure ventilation with acute exacerbation of COPD has been shown to avoid intubation up to 76 percent of the time.[9] It has been proven to decrease the requirement for mechanical support and to lower the average stay in the intensive care unit.[10] The patients studied all had impending respiratory failure but were hemodynamically stable. Studies showed arterial blood gas improvement (85 percent), intubation avoidance (72 to 76 percent), decreased respiratory rates (31 percent), with low complication risk.[8,11] In the elderly, where the decision to intubate is more complex (because of age, illness, or cancer), nasal-mask ventilation yielded improvements in Pa_{O_2} similar to those of other studies (60 percent), but hypercarbia improved more slowly.[12]

Trauma patients frequently have a significant loss of functional residual capacity (FRC) that often leads to mild to moderate respiratory insufficiency. In such instances, CPAP has been used to improve respiratory function and reduce hypoxemia.[13] CPAP is helpful in decreasing the work of breathing and improving FRC, thus preventing hypoxemia, hypocarbia, and tachypnea. Criteria for NIPPV have included spontaneous respirations, absence of respiratory acidemia/hypercarbia, intact mental status, a Pa_{O_2} above 65 torr, presence of a functioning nasogastric tube, and absence of severe maxillofacial injury. Improvement may be seen starting at 5 cm of H_2O. Studies have shown a mean CPAP of 8.6 cmH_2O meets therapeutic goals. Duration of therapy may range from a few hours to 2 days. Trauma conditions that have been studied include pulmonary contusion, flail chest, pneumothorax, hemopneumothorax, and multiple chest and abdominal gunshot/stab wounds. In this setting, a functioning nasogastric tube and respective chest tube placement, when indicated, are extremely important. Patients suffering high esophageal or tracheal injuries should not be supported with a CPAP mask. Maxillofacial and basilar skull fractures are also contraindications to CPAP ventilation by face mask. Since many traumatized patients exhibit a remarkable capacity to breathe spontaneously and improvements in hemodynamics have been shown to be one of the benefits of using spontaneous ventilation versus mechanical ventilation, CPAP is an appropriate adjunct for managing the airway in the trauma patient.

Technique

Nasal-mask or facial-mask ventilation employs a tight-fitting mask that allows for a CPAP or BiPAP support system. The patient with impending respiratory failure receives either continuous pressure or inspiratory/expiratory (bilevel) support, thus allowing a decrease in inspiratory effort, rest for respiratory and accessory muscles, improvement of gas exchange, avoidance of intubation, and improved comfort.[9,14] A nasal-mask protocol with BiPAP appears to be the most advanced protocol and appears to allow more sensitive changes during the course of treatment (Fig. 14-7). The nasal mask allows the patient to eat, drink, and converse with the emergency staff. However, the nasal positive-pressure ventilation (NPPV) does allow for air leaks through the mouth.

The ventilatory support system frequently preferred is the BiPAP ventilator (Respironics, Murraysville, PA). It is small, relatively inexpensive, very mobile, and tolerates leaks better than other systems. It is possible to set the inspiratory positive airway pressure (IPAP) and the expiratory positive airway pressure (EPAP/PEEP) independently. Three modes of ventilatory triggering are available: spontaneous, combined spontaneous/timed, and timed. The proper-size mask should be chosen (allowing no mouth coverage) and tight enough to allow a good, comfortable seal. Settings should include spontaneous mode, IPAP set at 10, EPAP set at 3 cmH_2O initially and increasing IPAP by 3-cm increments and EPAP slowly. Continuing hypercarbic failure is treated by increasing IPAP alone by 3-cm increments.[15]

Complications

Some of the complications described include difficulty with mask seal requiring multiple readjustments, gastric distention, aspiration (rare),

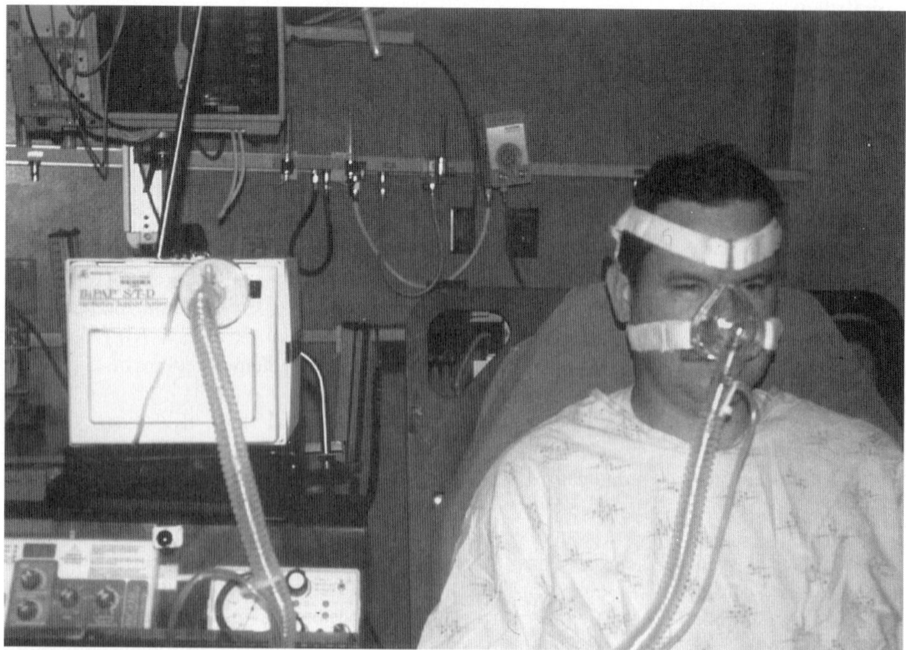

FIG. 14-7. A patient with severe COPD on nasal BiPAP. (Used with permission.)

intolerance of the positive pressure, and facial skin breakdown (with long-term use). These complications appear to occur infrequently, but the most common intolerance was excessive respiratory secretions, which, in fact, may be a relative contraindication to NPPV. Other contraindications to NPPV are severe maxillofacial trauma and potential basilar skull fracture where pneumocephalus may occur. Another problem with *mask* ventilation is that using a conventional ventilator can be difficult or even counterproductive because of the inadvertent triggering of alarms in systems that are not designed for this use. The BiPAP ventilatory system, which has been used with success, may not be readily available in the ED, and respiratory services may have to be contacted for this setup.

Application of NPPV provides ventilatory support for impending respiratory failure and has been shown to decrease the workload of the respiratory muscles. Oxygen saturation, Pa_{CO_2}, and pH remain stable or improve as compared with unassisted ventilation. Therefore this technique may prove useful in respiratory failure when intubation is questionable. Facial/nasal-mask–assisted ventilation is a simple, noninvasive method that has few complications, and is shown to be well tolerated over long periods of time. It also decreases negative intrathoracic pressure but needs to be studied more fully for situations where suppression of inspiratory effort is desired, as in flail chest.

This modality may decrease long-term hospital admissions, prevent unwanted intubations in the elderly or severely ill, and circumvent borderline respiratory failure intubations. Each patient must be closely monitored for tolerance of upper airway positive pressure. Multiple mask/ventilator adjustments may be required. Finally, any instability in ventilation or oxygenation requires close monitoring in case a more invasive intervention is required.

Patients who receive NIPPV need to be cooperative and should not have life-threatening cardiac ischemia, dysrhythmias, or hypotension. NIPPV is inappropriate in patients who have absent respiratory effort, who are agonal, or who produce excessive airway secretions. Airway management and apparatus associated with NIPPV can be distracting. However, medical treatment, such as in-line nebulized updrafts, anticholinergics, steroids, and respiratory hygiene must proceed as appropriate simultaneous with NIPPV.

REFERENCES

1. Nandi PR, Charlesworth CH, Taylor SJ, et al: Effects of general anesthesia on the pharynx. *Br J Anesth* 66:157, 1990.
2. Jesudian MCS, Harrison BA, Keenan RL, et al: Bag-valve mask ventilation: Two rescuers are better than one. Preliminary report. *Crit Care* 13:122, 1985.
3. Hammargren Y, Clinton JE, Ruiz E: A standard comparison of esophageal obturator airway and endotracheal tube ventilation in cardiac arrest. *Ann Emerg Med* 14:953, 1985.
4. Calder I, Ordman AJ, Jackowski A, Crockard HA: The Brain laryngeal mask airway—An alternative to emergency tracheal intubation. *Anaesthesia* 45:137, 1990.
5. Reinhart DJ, Simmons G: Comparison of placement of laryngeal mask airway with endotracheal tube by paramedics and respiratory therapists. *Ann Emerg Med* 24:260, 1994.
6. Maltby JR, Loken RG, Watson NC: The laryngeal mask airway: Clinical appraisal in 250 patients. *Can J Anesth* 37:509, 1990.
7. Gabbott DA, Sasada MP: Laryngeal mask airway insertion using cricoid pressure and manual in-line neck stabilization. *Anaesthesia* 50:674, 1995.
8. Meduri GU, Abou-Shala N, Fox RC: Noninvasive face mask mechanical ventilation in patients with acute hypercapnic respiratory failure. *Chest* 100:445, 1991.
9. Brochard L, Isabey D, Piquet J, et al: Reversal of acute exacerbations of chronic obstructive lung disease by inspiratory assistance with a face mask. *N Engl J Med* 323:1523, 1990.
10. Bersten AD, Holt AW, Vedig AE, et al: Treatment of severe cardiogenic pulmonary edema with continuous positive airway pressure delivered by face mask. *N Engl J Med* 325:1825, 1991.
11. Pennock BE, Kaplan PD, Carlin BW, et al: Pressure support ventilation with a simplified ventilatory support system administered with a nasal mask in patients with respiratory failure. *Chest* 100:1371, 1991.
12. Benhamou D, Girault C, Raure C, et al: Nasal mark ventilation in acute respiratory failure. *Chest* 102:912, 1992.
13. Hurst JM, DeHaven CB, Branson RD: Use of CPAP mask as the sole mode of ventilatory support in trauma patients with mild to moderate respiratory insufficiency. *J Trauma* 25:1065, 1985.
14. Carrey Z, Stewart BG, Levy RD: Ventilatory muscle support in respiratory failure with nasal positive pressure ventilation. *Chest* 97:150, 1990.
15. Pennock BE, Crawshaw L, Kaplan PD: Noninvasive nasal mark ventilation for acute respiratory failure. *Chest* 105:441, 1994.

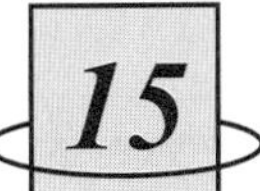

TRACHEAL INTUBATION AND MECHANICAL VENTILATION

Daniel F. Danzl

Airway integrity, assurance of oxygenation, ventilation, and prevention of aspiration are the mainstays of emergency airway management. The indications for tracheal intubation in the emergency setting most commonly include correction of hypoxia or hypercarbia, prevention of impending hypoventilation, and assuring maintenance of a patent airway. Secondary indications include provision of a route for resuscitative medication administration and to permit temporizing paralysis during diagnostic testing. This chapter reviews tracheal intubation techniques to establish an airway and ventilate a patient after basic maneuvers have been utilized.

OROTRACHEAL INTUBATION

The most reliable means to ensure a patent airway, provide oxygenation and ventilation, and prevent aspiration is endotracheal intubation. Many unconscious and even conscious patients may be unable to spontaneously clear the airway of secretions, may require mechanical ventilation, may have aspirated, or may lack protective airway reflexes.

The clinical assessment of oxygenation and ventilation is often unreliable in a chaotic ED. Continuous noninvasive bedside monitoring of arterial oxygen saturation by oximetry is helpful. Isolated oximetry, however, does not assess the status of alveolar ventilation. Capnography does allow estimation of the Pa_{CO_2} based on the waveform display of the end-tidal Pa_{CO_2}. *Capnometry* refers to the numerical display. In combination, both of these noninvasive modalities affect decisions regarding tracheal intubation.

One should take the time to evaluate the upper airway anatomy. Examination of the teeth, size of the oral cavity, thyromental distance, mobility and posterior depth of the mandible, and neck mobility may point to a difficult airway. The normal adult mouth opening measures three finger breadths. The alert, sober patient may be asked to open the mouth as widely as possible and point the tongue in the examiner's direction. The ease of laryngoscopy correlates well with the examiner's ability to visualize the soft palate, uvula, and faucial pillars (see "Difficult Airway," below).

While calling for an assistant, check and arrange the necessary equipment. The appropriate-size tube and an additional tube (0.5 to 1 mm in size smaller) should be selected and the cuff checked for air leaks with a 10-mL syringe. Selecting a tube of the proper diameter is essential (Table 15-1). The second hole at the end of the tube above

TABLE 15-1 Approximate Adult Sizes for Endotracheal Tubes and Suction Catheters

Patient	Endotracheal Tube Inner Diameter, mm*	Suction Catheter Size (French) Outer Diameter
Adult Female	7.5–8.0	12–14
Adult Male	8.0–8.5	14

*Tubes of 0.5 to 1 mm smaller inner diameter are used for nasotracheal intubation.

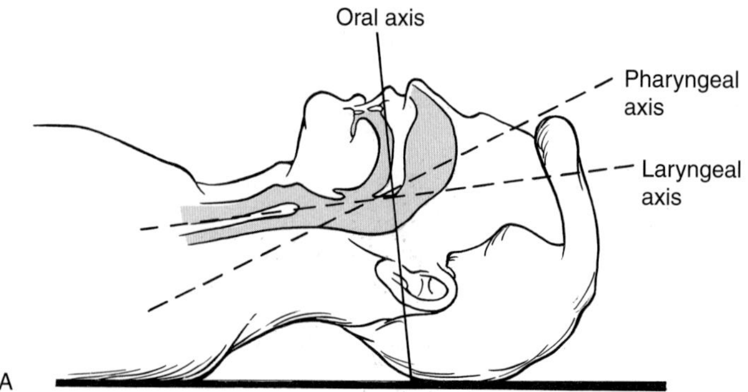

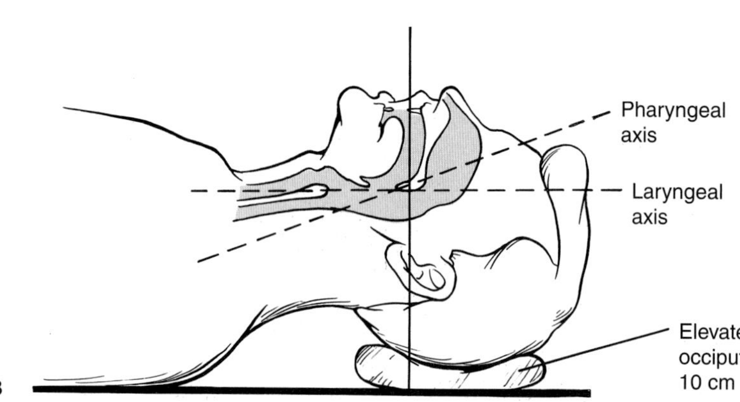

FIG. 15-1. *A.* Oral pharyngeal laryngeal axes. *B.* Sniffing position.

the bevel is called Murphy's eye. This permits some uninterrupted airflow if the tip is occluded.

Endotracheal tubes (ET) tubes with high-volume, low-pressure cuffs are the best design for adults. When properly inflated, thin-walled cuffs prevent aspiration better than medium-walled cuffs. The operator should test the light on the laryngoscope and then pick an appropriate sized blade. The straight Magill blade physically lifts the epiglottis. The curved Macintosh blade rests in the vallecula above the epiglottis and indirectly lifts the epiglottis off the larynx owing to the traction on the frenulum.

The development of expertise with both blades is desirable, since they offer differing advantages, depending on the clinical setting and the patient's body habitus. The curved blade may cause less trauma and be less likely to stimulate an airway reflex since it does not directly touch the larynx. It also allows more room for adequate visualization during tube placement and is helpful in the obese patient. The straight blade is mechanically easier to insert in many patients who do not have large central incisors. Simply point the tip of the blade directly at the epiglottis and aim for it. Selecting the proper-size blade greatly facilitates intubation. In adults, the curved Macintosh no. 3 is the most popular, or no. 4 for large patients. The straight Miller no. 2 or 3 is similarly most often ideal.

When all equipment is in order, the patient should be placed in the sniffing position. Flexion of the lower neck with extension at the atlantooccipital joint (sniffing position) aligns the oropharyngeolaryngeal axis, allowing a direct view of the larynx. Placing a folded towel or small pillow under the occiput is often helpful (Fig. 15-1). The inexperienced laryngoscopist's most common reasons for failure—inadequate equipment preparation and poor patient positioning—arise prior to the use of the laryngoscope.

The patient should be thoroughly preoxygenated prior to intubation if time permits. Begin with the laryngoscope in the left hand and an ET tube or suction apparatus in the right hand. After dentures and any obscuring blood, secretions, or vomitus are removed, the suction is exchanged for the ET tube and inserted during the same laryngoscopy.

The blade is inserted into the right corner of the patient's mouth. If a curved Macintosh blade is used, the flange will push the tongue toward the left side of the oropharynx. If the blade is inserted directly down the middle, the tongue can force the line of sight posteriorly—which is a common reason for the putative ''anterior larynx.'' After visualization of the arytenoids, lift the epiglottis directly with the straight blade or indirectly with the curved blade. The larynx is exposed by pulling the handle in the direction that it points, that is, 90° to the blade. Cocking the handle back, especially with the straight blade, risks fracturing central incisors and is ineffective at revealing the cords.

There are a variety of other straight and curved blades available. To mention a few, the Guedel blade is a straight blade with an acute 72° angle to the handle. The Schapira straight blade has a side concavity that helps cradle the large tongue and push it toward the left side of the mouth. The CLM curved laryngoscope blade has a hinged tip. This permits elevation of the epiglottis with minimal force, since the fulcrum is repositioned down within the pharynx.

One technique to avoid the most common error, overly deep insertion of the blade, is to look for the arytenoid cartilages. If only the posterior commissure is visible, have an assistant apply more pressure on the cricoid (Sellick maneuver) or perform the laryngeal lift. Another option is the ''BURP'' technique.[1] The larynx is manually displaced posteriorly (backward) against the cervical vertebrae, superiorly (upward), and laterally to the right (rightward pressure). To avoid error, the cuff must be seen passing completely through the cords. Last-ditch attempts at blind passage will only invite anoxia. The intubator should never be reluctant to abort the attempt if visualization of the larynx is not successful. Whenever feasible, have an assistant apply steady cricoid pressure with the thumb and index finger during the intubation to help prevent aspiration.

With proper technique and practice, semirigid, malleable, blunt-tipped metal or plastic stylets are not usually necessary for most patients. Should the patient's anatomy call for them, a selection of proper-sized stylets must be available. The tip of the stylet should not extend beyond the end of the ET tube or exit Murphy's eye.

One aid to intubation with direct vision is the use of a thin, flexible intubation stylet. This type of stylet can be inserted blindly around the epiglottis into the trachea. The ET tube is then threaded over it into the trachea and the stylet is removed. The Eschmann tracheal tube introducer or stylet, also known as the "gum elastic bougie," is a valuable aid for difficult oral intubations. Another option is to use the tip on the laryngeal tracheal anesthesia kit. With either stylet, orient the tube so that Murphy's eye is at 12 o'clock.

The tube should never be forced through the vocal cords. Forced insertion can result in avulsion of the arytenoid cartilages or laceration of the vocal cords. Usually, any difficulty in passing the tube is a result of either the tube being too large or too soft and flexible. Directed transoral or translaryngeal anesthesia with lidocaine can help relax the cords. If this fails, sometimes lining up the bevel with the glottic opening will also be successful.

The tube should be advanced until the cuff disappears below the cords. Correct tube placement is about 2 cm above the carina. From the corner of the mouth, this is approximately 23 cm in men and 21 cm in women. The base of the pilot tube is usually at teeth level. The tube is also positioned by palpating its tip at the suprasternal notch and advancing it 2 to 3 cm. To avoid ischemia of the tracheal mucosa, keep the cuff pressure below 40 cmH_2O. The minimal intracuff pressure to prevent aspiration is 25 cmH_2O.[2]

After cuff inflation, auscultate to verify bilateral lung expansion and if satisfied insert an oropharyngeal airway or bite block. Some advocate first listening over the stomach, since the early detection of errant esophageal intubation is desirable to minimize insufflation of the stomach with subsequent regurgitation. Inadvertent endobronchial intubation is usually on the right side. The operator should secure the tube, being careful not to impede cervical venous return with the umbilical tape or fixator. The use of a modified clove-hitch knot or a commercial fixator is ideal and also helps avoid kinking the pilot tube. Ventilation should be initiated using 100% oxygen with a tidal volume of 10 to 15 mL/kg at a rate of 10 to 15 breaths per minute.

Confirmation and Complications of Intubation

Endobronchial or esophageal intubation will result in hypoxia or hypercarbia. There is no clinically reliable substitute for direct visualization of the tube passing through the vocal cords. Hence the adage, "when in doubt, take it out." Nevertheless, there are a number of options to help confirm intratracheal tube positioning. Clinical assessments—including chest and epigastric auscultation, tube condensation, and symmetrical chest wall expansion—are not infallible in the ED. "Breath sounds" from the stomach can be transmitted through the chest following gastric insufflation.

The two basic categories of adjuncts include end-tidal CO_2 detectors or monitors and esophageal detection devices (EDDs). Both have advantages provided that the operator remains cognizant of the sources of interpretation error. Capnometers are the devices that measure CO_2 in the expired air. The most commonly used capnometric devices used in the ED are colorimetric, with a pH-sensitive purple-colored filter paper. When in contact with CO_2, hydrogen ions are formed resulting in color changes depending upon the concentration of CO_2. For example, with the Nellcor Easy Cap II, a yellow color develops on exposure to 2 to 5% $ETco_2$, equivalent to 15 to 38 mmHg CO_2. There is no color change, that is the filter paper remains purple, with an $ETco_2$ of <0.5%, equivalent to <4 mmHg CO_2. An intermediate color results with an $ETco_2$ of 0.5% to 2%, corresponding to 4 to 15 mmHg CO_2. Generally these readings are accurate within +/− 3 mmHg. While capnometers are useful for general readings, as in assessing proper ETT placement, they are not accurate enough when precise determinations are necessary. Capnography is the real-time display of characteristic CO_2 waveforms.

The use of end-tidal CO_2 pressure ($Petco_2$) monitoring can help confirm endotracheal intubation.[3] A color change to yellow indicates endotracheal placement. Colorimetric or infrared detection of $Petco_2$, however, may not occur even with proper ETT placement, during states of low pulmonary perfusion such as during cardiac arrest, inadequate chest compressions during CPR, or massive pulmonary embolism. Other causes of false-negative interpretations include massive obesity. Severe pulmonary edema may obstruct the $ETco_2$ monitor with secretions. On the other hand, there may be an initial false-positive detection of CO_2 following esophageal intubation if carbonated beverages have been ingested by the patient, or for a few minutes after bolus sodium bicarbonate administration. Another cause is gastric distention resulting from bag-valve-mask ventilation. A heated humidifier or nebulizer or epinephrine instilled via the ET tube can also cause false-positive interpretations.

Correct technique is essential for accurate interpretation. After intubation and cuff inflation, attach the capnometer to the ET tube. Then attach a bag-valve-mask unit to the detector and ventilate the patient with about six ventilations to wash out residual CO_2. Then check for the $Petco_2$-induced color changes. If capnography is also available, a persistent positive capnograph formation after clear and direct visualization of tube placement approaches certainty. On rare occasion, misplacement of the hypopharyngeal glottic tube tip may result in misleadingly normal oximetry and capnography. This error can be recognized by the inadequate depth of tube insertion, ventilatory volumes, or on chest x-ray.

Esophageal detection devices also offer the potential to accurately determine tube location. The various designs all depend on their proper function as in-line aspirators of the ET tube. The device adaptors fit over the 15-mm ET tube connector. One of the advantages of the EDD is that accuracy does not depend on adequate cardiac output and pulmonary perfusion. Instead, proper functioning is predicated on the anatomic differences between the esophagus and the trachea. When the ET tube is in the esophagus, the soft, noncartilagenous walls will collapse and air cannot be aspirated easily.[4]

To perform the syringe aspiration technique, attach the device after intubation but before ventilation. Then attempt to retract the syringe plunger. Resistance to aspiration reflects occlusion from esophageal collapse. If there is no resistance during aspiration, one assumes that the tube is in the trachea. If a self-inflating bulb is used, first compress the bulb and then attach it to the ET tube. One advantage of the bulb is that it requires only a single hand.

As expected, these devices are also not infallible. When the seal with the device leaks, there may be an erroneous assumption of intratracheal tube placement. In the prehospital setting, some studies report that the EDDs demonstrate poor sensitivity for esophageal intubations. On the other hand, the EDDs have a potential advantage over $Petco_2$ in cardiac arrest patients.[4]

The emergency physician should never assume that continued airway patency is assured after ET tube insertion. Repeated suctioning is necessary to prevent thrombotic or inspissated secretions from obstructing the tube. Endobronchial ball-valve obstruction can also occur with a clot. This will impair ventilation and produce hyperinflation of individual lobes.

Cuff displacement or overinflation can result in ball-valve obstruction of the airway. Cuffs inflated in the field during frigid conditions will expand with warming. Deflate the cuff when tracheal ball-valve obstruction is suspected. If the tube is blocked, deflation will allow exhalation.

There are a variety of other correctable intubation complications that should be kept in mind. If the ET tube cuff leaks after the intubation, first check for a defective inflation valve. One simple fix is to attach a three-way stopcock to the valve and reinflate the cuff. Then turn the stopcock off. If the cuff itself seems to be leaking slowly, it may be sealable. An option is to instill an aspirable mixture of normal saline and 2% lidocaine jelly into the cuff in a 3:1 ratio.

If the ET tube needs to be replaced, consider the use of a tube changer. A classic technique is to use nasogastric tubing at least three times longer than the ET tube. Standard room-temperature tubing, however, may not be a sufficiently rigid guide. There are a number of commercially available semirigid catheters that include 15-mm adaptors or connectors to permit ventilation during the tube exchange. These devices have quick-connect adapters that incorporate through-lumen designs to ensure adequate airflow during the procedure.

If the ET tube is inserted too deeply, carinal stimulation can cause bronchospasm. Unilateral pulmonary edema is also reported. The ET tube may be obstructed by a bulging cuff, secretions, kinking, or biting. The cuff may simply be overinflated. If the cuff was inflated with frigid air in the field, it may expand and compress the tube after warming.

Although uncommon, morbidity related to emergent endotracheal intubation does occur and may be quite debilitating. Arytenoid cartilage avulsion or displacement, usually on the right, prevents the patient from phonating properly. Intubation of the pyriform sinus and pharyngeal-esophageal perforation has been reported. Chordal synechiae may develop anteriorly or commissural stenosis posteriorly.

Subglottic stenosis is the most disastrous sequela. The physician should avoid cuff overinflation and attempt to minimize tube motion in the larynx and trachea. This usually occurs in patients with poorly secured tubes who are combative or on ventilators. Gastric rupture with tension pneumoperitoneum can occur after a difficult intubation.

NASOTRACHEAL INTUBATION

Nasotracheal intubation (NTI) is an essential psychomotor skill that may be useful in many difficult situations. Operators adept at both NTI and rapid-sequence intubation (RSI) are in the best position to assess and act on the following two prime considerations. What are the potential risk-benefits to having spontaneous respirations preserved versus ablated? Is there a safe alternative in this patient that may avoid precipitating the need for a potentially unnecessary surgical airway?[5]

Nasal intubation is helpful in situations where laryngoscopy or cricothyrotomy may be difficult and neuromuscular blockade hazardous. Severely dyspneic patients with congestive heart failure (CHF), chronic obstructive pulmonary disease (COPD), or asthma who are awake often cannot remain supine but do tolerate nasotracheal intubation in the sitting position. Nasotracheal tubes are better tolerated by some patients than oral tubes. There is often less intratracheal tube movement against the tracheal muscosa with head motion.

It may be impossible to align the oropharyngeolaryngeal axis in patients with arthritis, masseter spasm, temporomandibular dislocation, or recent oral surgical procedures. Patients with a peculiar body habitus may be difficult to intubate orally. Other considerations for NTI include trismus from seizures, facial trauma, infection, tetanus, or decorticate-decerebrate rigidity.

To minimize epistaxis, spray both nares with a topical vasoconstrictor anesthetic. While waiting briefly, select a cuffed ET tube 0.5 to 1 mm smaller than optimal for oral intubation. Check the integrity of the cuff and ensure snug fitting of the tube adapter. Since secretions and blood may be expelled into the air and onto the intubator's face, observe universal precautions. An option in addition to a face shield includes the use of a protective filtering adapter such as the Humid-Vent 1, which can be attached to the proximal end of the ET tube (Gibeck Respiration, Sweden).

Advance the tube, lubricated with a water-soluble (2% lidocaine or K-Y) jelly along the nasal floor on the more patent side. If the nares appear equal, initially try the right side. It helps to prevent abrasions of the Kiesselbach plexus by having the bevel face the septum. Steady, gentle pressure or slow rotation of the tube usually bypasses small obstructions. Passage of the tube is straight back toward the occiput. If the right side is not passable, try the other side before resorting to a smaller tube.

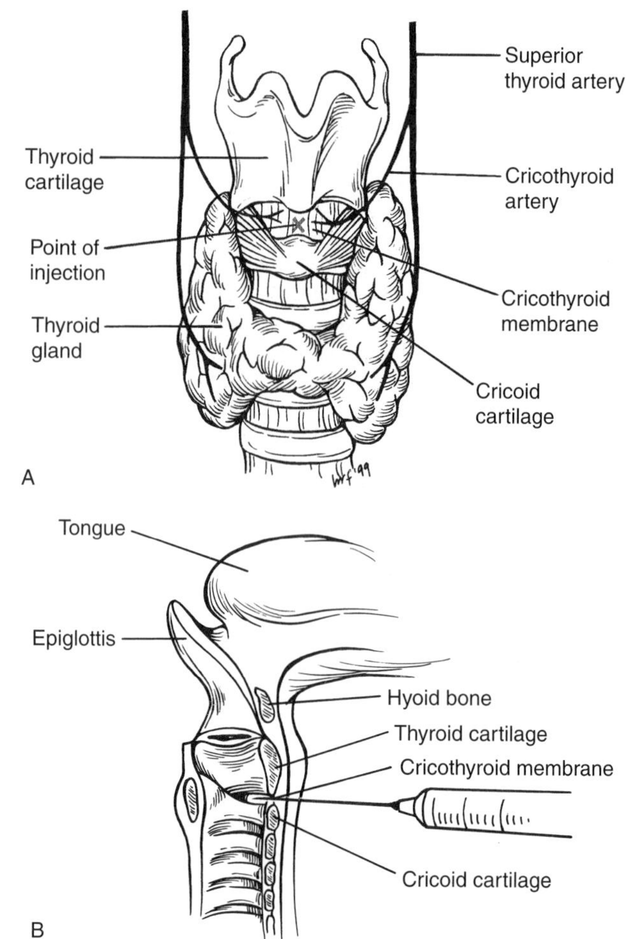

FIG. 15-2. Translaryngeal anesthesia via cricothyroid puncture. *A.* Anatomy—anterior view. *B.* Anatomy—cross-sectional view.

In patients with intact protective airway reflexes, directed transoral or translaryngeal anesthesia often facilitates intubation. Translaryngeal anesthesia, although not widely utilized in the ED, should be considered when the initial intubation attempt is unsuccessful. After palpating the superior border of the cricoid cartilage in the midline, puncture the cricothyroid membrane with a 22- to 25-gauge 0.5- to 1-in. needle (Fig. 15-2). The needle should be perpendicular to the membrane in the midline, with the point of injection just cephalad to the cricoid cartilage. Aspirate air, then swiftly inject 1.5 to 2.0 mL of 4% lidocaine (sterile for injection) and press the site firmly with a finger for a few seconds. This prevents small degrees of subcutaneous emphysema that would erroneously suggest a laryngeal injury.

The literature would suggest a complication rate of less than 0.5 per 1000 procedures. Translaryngeal anesthesia is contraindicated if the landmarks are obscured by thyroid or tumor impingement on the cricothyroid membrane and in obese or combative patients.

An assistant should immobilize the patient's head and initially maintain it in a neutral or slightly extended position ("sniffing position"). Stand to the side of the patient, with one hand on the tube and with the thumb and index finger of the other hand straddling the larynx. Advance the tube while rotating it medially 15 to 30° until you hear maximal airflow through the tube. Then gently but swiftly advance the tube. The best time for advancement is at the initiation of inspiration. Entrance into the larynx may initiate a cough, and most expired air should exit through the tube even though the cuff is uninflated. "Fogging" of the tube, while not foolproof, is usually a good sign. The presence of any vocal sounds indicates a failed attempt.

The advancement of the tube toward the carina can be observed externally. The normal distance from the external nares to the carina is 32 cm in the adult male and 27 to 28 cm in the adult female. Therefore, prior to obtaining a chest x-ray, the optimal initial depth of tube placement in NTI of adults, measured at the naris, is 28 cm in men and 26 cm in women.[6] Preformed nasal tracheal tubes are also available, with an acute angle bent at the 29-cm mark. Auscultate to verify bilateral lung expansion and cuff inflation and perform tube confirmation techniques. Secretions or blood in the tube should be removed prior to initiating positive-pressure ventilation.

If intubation is unsuccessful, carefully inspect the neck to determine malposition of the tube. Most commonly, the tube is in the pyriform fossa on the same side as the nostril used. A bulge will be seen and can be palpated laterally. Withdraw the tube into the retropharynx until breath sounds are again heard. Then redirect while manually displacing the larynx toward the bulge. If there is no contraindication, flexion and rotation of the neck to the ipsilateral side while the tube is rotated medially will often help.

The other most common tube misplacement is posteriorly in the esophagus. There will be no breath sounds through the tube, and the trachea will be slightly elevated. The intubator should attempt redirection after extending the patient's head and performing a Sellick maneuver. When cervical spine pathology is suspected, consider the use of a directional tip control tube (Endotrol) or a fiberoptic laryngoscope. Endotrol tubes smaller than 7.5 mm(ID) tend to soften and obstruct and can be difficult to suction. The use of these directional-tip tubes may improve the success rate of the first attempt at NTI.[7]

When the tube hangs up on the vocal cords, shrill, turbulent air noises will be heard. Rotate the tube slightly to realign the bevel with the cords or squirt 2 mL of 4% lidocaine (80 mg) down the tube onto the cords if transoral or translaryngeal anesthesia was omitted. There have been anecdotal reports that if NTI is unsuccessful with passage of the tube into the esophagus, leaving the original tube in place may facilitate passage of the tube using the other nostril. This technique may also afford some protection from aspiration.

Nasal intubation with a fiberoptic laryngoscope may be required when neoplastic lesions, lymphoid tissue, Ludwig angina, peritonsillar abscess, or epiglottitis obstructs the pharynx.

The presence of facial trauma does not appear to be a contraindication to NTI intubation.[8] Complex nasal and massive midfacial fractures as well as bleeding disorders are relative contraindications to NTI. Oral intubation, on the other hand, can impede prompt reduction and stabilization of some maxillary fractures. Since a LeFort I fracture does not extend to the cribriform plate, this is not a contraindication. Fiberoptic guidance or RSI is preferable for LeFort II and III fractures.

The risk of inadvertent intracranial passage of a nasotracheal tube is extremely low, unlike nasogastric tube insertion. Very poor technique in the setting of obvious massive head trauma would be required. Severe traumatic nasal or pharyngeal hemorrhage may necessitate orotracheal intubation or cricothyrotomy. Contamination of the spinal fluid is a hazard with some basilar skull fractures.

Serious complications of nasotracheal intubation are rare. In a number of large series, there was no permanent laryngeal damage. Epistaxis will occur with inadequate topical vasoconstriction, excessive tube size, poor technique, or anatomic defects. Excessive force can damage the nasal septum or turbinates.

Frequent suctioning, especially if epistaxis or other upper airway hemorrhage is present, will help to prevent thrombotic occlusion of the tube or a mainstem bronchus. Retropharyngeal lacerations, abscesses, and nasal necrosis are reported.

Paranasal sinusitis, especially occurring with prolonged nasotracheal intubation or severe cranial trauma, can be an unrecognized source of sepsis. The risk of postintubation sinusitis correlates with the duration of intubation, which often reflects the neurologic insult. In the setting of craniofacial trauma, any subsequent computed tomography (CT) scans should include views of the paranasal sinuses. Other factors causing sinusitis include presence of a nasogastric tube, sinus hemorrhage or fracture, and administration of glucocorticoids.

DIGITAL INTUBATION

Digital intubation is an underutilized noninvasive technique for ET tube insertion. The performance of this maneuver requires tactile recognition of the epiglottis. Visual landmarks may be impossible to identify with a laryngoscope because of patient positioning, anatomic disruption, or significant hemorrhage. Tactile digital intubation can avert cricothyrotomy when direct laryngoscopy has failed following neuromuscular blockade. Patients with micrognathia or temporomandibular immobility are poor candidates for the technique.

The patient must be deeply comatose, in cardiac arrest, or in a state of adequate neuromuscular blockade. Prior to insertion, shape the well-lubricated ET tube with a stylet into a J configuration. Then, unless the operator is quite confident, a bite block should be inserted in the opposite side of the mouth. Lift the tongue and pull the mandible forward with your gloved dominant hand. Then insert the lubricated middle and index fingers of the gloved nondominant hand down the middle of the tongue and palpate the cartilaginous epiglottis with the middle finger.

While palpating the epiglottis, insert the well-lubricated J-shaped tube with stylet and slide it along your middle finger. The path from the corner of the mouth opposite the bite block to the epiglottis is the shortest distance. The index finger can help guide the tube from behind. As the larynx is entered, resistance will be encountered. At this point, it is essential to partially withdraw the stylet. Otherwise, the tube will lodge against the anterior wall of the trachea and be difficult to advance. Left mainstem intubation is the unusual complication reported with this technique.

Transillumination

Transillumination with a lighted stylet can facilitate oral or nasal intubation and help to confirm ET tube placement and positioning. This technique is of particular assistance when direct laryngoscopy is anatomically impossible. Oral intubation is easiest with a semirigid stylet. Prior to insertion, transilluminate the patient's cheek. This serves as a check of the ambient light and will predict the laryngeal light intensity. It may be necessary to dim or shield bright ambient light from the neck. Obese patients who do not transilluminate buccally may not do so laryngeally.

For oral insertion, insert the lubricated ET tube with lighted stylet after pulling the tongue forward with a 4- by 4-in. gauze pad. The tube should initially be directed into the ipsilateral pyriform fossa, thus establishing the depth of the epiglottis. Then the tube is slightly withdrawn, and the tip directed toward the midline. The intubator must discriminate between the light emanating from the larynx and the much dimmer light transmitted from the esophagus. Usually the "jack-o-lantern" glow arising from the larynx or trachea is not appreciated when the light source is misplaced in the esophagus. Some manufacturers incorporate timed blinking lights that suggest when it is time for reoxygenation.

For nasal intubation, the flexible stylet or wand instrument is inserted into a directional tip ET tube (Endotrol). After positioning the tube in the retropharynx, very gentle traction is applied on the ring to achieve slight flexion of the tip of the ET tube. Standard training programs for transillumination-guided ET intubation may require didactic, video, and repeated demonstration and practice sessions.[9]

FIBEROPTIC ASSISTANCE

The flexible fiberoptic laryngoscope or bronchoscope can be a valuable adjunct when there are anatomic or traumatic limitations that prevent

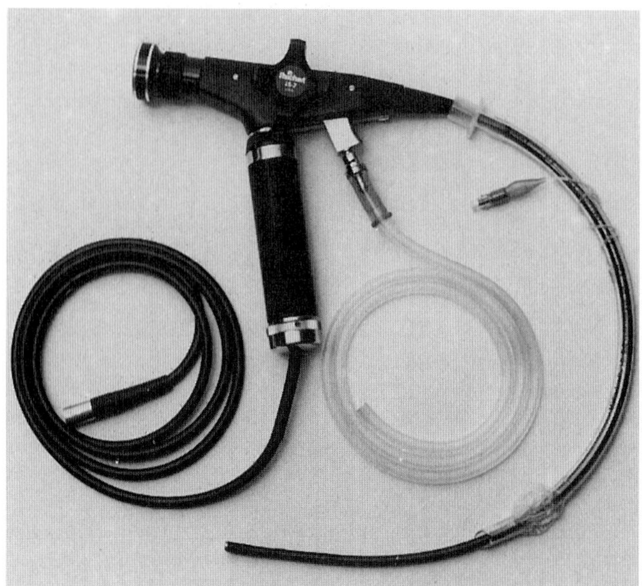

FIG. 15-3. Fiberoptic laryngoscope. An ET tube covers the shaft; suction or oxygen tubing is attached.

visualization of the vocal cords. Clinical examples include conditions that prevent opening or movement of the mandible, congenital anatomic abnormalities, and cervical spine immobility. These instruments allow visualization of laryngeal structures and can enable difficult intubations, including those around expanding hematomas (Fig. 15-3). Patients in need of an immediate airway or those with ongoing hemorrhage or copious secretions are poor candidates.

Directed transoral or transnasal and translaryngeal topical anesthesia is essential. The nasal mucosa should be sprayed with a vasoconstrictor. Dual suctioning capability is needed; a suction port should be attached to a suction apparatus for oral blood and secretions. Tongue extrusion and anterior mandibular displacement will be helpful if the oral route is chosen. Fragile equipment is more frequently damaged transorally. The nasal route is better also because the optic tip can enter the glottis at a less acute angle.

Begin by focusing the eyepiece and lubricating the flexible shaft. Then immerse the lens at the tip of the laryngoscope in warm water to prevent fogging. The intubator should continuously monitor pulse oximetry and assure that the gag reflex is not present. After attachment of oxygen tubing to the suction port, intermittent insufflation of oxygen at 10 to 15 L/min to keep the optic tip clear should be considered. Insufflation is usually superior to suction for clearing secretions.

Initially remove the adapter from an ET tube that is at least 7.0 mm (ID) in size. To prevent barotrauma when high-flow oxygen is insufflated, use at least a 7.5-mm (ID) tube. Then slip the lubricated ET tube over the shaft up to the handle. The distal end of the laryngoscope must extend beyond the end of the ET tube. The laryngoscope is held with your left hand, and tip deflection is controlled while advancing it through the cords. The laryngoscope will function as a stylet for the tube. After the laryngoscope is in the trachea, advance the ET tube and remove the laryngoscope.

Another option is to insert a nasotracheal tube blindly into the posterior pharynx and stop about 1 to 2 cm proximal to the epiglottis. The scope is then inserted through this hollow conduit and the fiberoptic tip can be directed into the glottis. Be careful not to pass the lubricated scope through Murphy's eye. If this occurs, it will be impossible to advance the ET tube.

The fiberoptic scope cannot be used as a stylet to guide the ET tube into the trachea. The stiffer ET tube will often deflect the thin scope tip posteriorly into the esophagus. In addition, this keeps the concavity of the ET tube anterior toward 12 o'clock and places the tube tip and Murphy's eye at 3 o'clock (90° to the right). The tip will then often hit the right arytenoid cartilage. Rotating the tube 90° counterclockwise lines up the tip with the upper triangular entrance into the trachea.

Fiberoptic ET tubes are also commercially available. Direct line of sight can improve visualization in many difficult intubations. The advantages of direct vision include verification of tube positioning, identification of the right- or left-sided source of pulmonary hemorrhage, and inspection of tracheal injury.

RETROGRADE TRACHEAL INTUBATION

Retrograde tracheal intubation (RTI) is another viable option when conventional airway approaches fail. This skill can be taught in a variety of ways, including the use of a mannequin.[10] The landmarks are the same as for cricothyroid puncture (Fig. 15-2). Severe maxillofacial trauma, cervical or mandibular ankylosis, and upper airway masses are some of the potential conditions in which RTI may help. Another advantage of RTI is that it is not impeded by the blood that obscures fiberoptically guided intubation.

The insertion of a retrograde translaryngeal catheter is a less invasive option than cricothyrotomy. This technique can be time-consuming and will not be quick enough for apneic patients. Before beginning the procedure the patient should be preoxygenated. Bag-valve-mask ventilation can continue to be performed without interrupting this technique. Then consider administering translaryngeal anesthesia via an 18-gauge needle through the caudal aspect of the membrane.

Alignment of the needle bevel with the syringe markings will help determine the bevel direction after puncture of the cricothyroid membrane. The initial angle of the needle should be 30 to 45° cephalad, and a 70- to 75-cm flexible-tip guidewire is advanced through the needle. The wire is then grasped in the oropharynx or nares with Magill forceps. Occasionally the wire will exit spontaneously.

Another option when hemorrhage is present is to insert a 75-cm CVP catheter and insufflate. To locate the tip, observe for bubbles and use forceps. J wire, which can be slowly twisted once it arrives at the oropharynx, can also be easier to locate than a straight guidewire. Most central line kits will have 60- to 80-cm wires. Use of a multilumen catheter is yet another option.

The next step is to clasp the guidewire securely with a hemostat at the neck. Then the proximal end of the guidewire is threaded through the Murphy's eye on the ET tube. This allows more of the ET tube to enter the trachea before the guidewire is removed. With both hands, tighten the wire like a tightrope and advance the tube. When the ET tube will pass no further, cut the guidewire or catheter flush with the cricothyroid membrane to minimize soft tissue contamination.

If the tube will not pass through the cords, try a 90° counterclockwise tube rotation to bring the Murphy's eye anterior; this realigns the bevel. Another technique is to insert the guidewire end that exits the mouth into the suction port of a fiberoptic scope. The scope is then inserted over the retrograde guidewire and functions as an antegrade guide.

RAPID-SEQUENCE INTUBATION

The term *induction* refers to the production of a deep level of unconsciousness. *Rapid-sequence induction* is the classic anesthesia term pertaining to the induction of anesthesia. In emergency medicine parlance, rapid sequence intubation (RSI) most commonly involves the combined administration of a sedative and a neuromuscular blocking agent to facilitate tracheal intubation (Table 15-2). This technique is a component of standard airway management in the emergency department.[11] Tracheal intubation follows laryngoscopy, while cricoid pressure is maintained to prevent aspiration. The principal contraindication is any condition preventing mask ventilation or intubation, since this may be the only way to ventilate a patient once the patient is paralyzed.

TABLE 15-2 Rapid-Sequence Intubation

1. Set up IV × 2; cardiac monitor; oximetry, and capnography.
2. Check equipment: suction, airway devices: translaryngeal ventilation and cricothyrotomy tray.
3. Explain procedure; document neurologic status.
4. Preoxygenate (100% F_iO_2); *no* positive-pressure ventilation.
5. Consider sedation, analgesia, adjunctive lidocaine and/or atropine.
6. Defasciculation agent if necessary.
7. Induce with sedative agent.
8. Do Sellick maneuver.
9. Give neuromuscular blocking agent.
10. Intubate trachea and release Sellick maneuver.

Patient care is optimized if emergency physicians are adept with all methods for managing standard and difficult airways in nonfasting patients. Otherwise, the incidence of cricothyrotomy will exceed the current 1 to 2 percent of patients when RSI is selected and fails.[12] The prime goal is to avoid placing the breathing patient in the "can't ventilate, can't intubate" predicament.

Topical laryngeal and intravenous lidocaine (1.5 mg/kg) is a useful adjunct during RSI. Lidocaine suppresses coughing, and adverse airway reflexes. The efficacy of pretreatment with intravenous lidocaine during tracheal intubation of patients with reactive airway disease is unclear. Lidocaine levels achieved through an ET tube side port designed to administer medication may not be therapeutic, and will be lower than than those achievable intravenously or via the ET tube's main lumen.

There is no single initial agent of choice for achieving hypnosis and sedation during rapid-sequence induction in the ED. Pharmacotherapy must be tailored to the patient's unique circumstances. All of the commonly used agents offer distinct advantages in specific clinical conditions. Each agent, however, also has signifcant potential side effects, and specific contraindications (Table 15-3).

Thiopental (Pentothal) is a short-acting barbiturate sedative. An intravenous dose of 3.0 to 5.0 mg/kg will induce unconsciousness in 30 to 60 s and last 10 to 30 min. It is a widely used induction agent. Hypotension is commonly observed because of myocardial depression and venous dilatation. An ultra-short-acting barbiturate option is methohexital (Brevital). It is twice as potent as thiopental with onset of action in 60 s, and a duration of action of 5 to 7 min. These cerebroprotective agents should be avoided if systemic hypotension is a problem. This is a major consideration in the multiple trauma patient. Thiopental and methohexital can cause laryngospasm. A more feared but very rare complication is trismus, or masseter muscle spasm, which has also been reported with fentanyl and propofol, often with rapid bolus administration. Methohexital reduces the seizure threshold.

Another pharmacologic alternative is a short-acting benzodiazepine, such as midazolam (Versed) at a dose of 0.1 mg/kg. This drug has valuable amnesic and anticonvulsant properties and is reversible with the antagonist flumazenil. One disadvantage is that it has a wide therapeutic index.

Some agitated and combative patients can be reasoned with only by using rapid-acting major tranquilization. The combative multiple trauma patient is the most common example. Repeated intravenous

TABLE 15-3 Sedative Induction Agents

Agent	Dose	Onset	Duration	Benefits	Caveats
Thiopental	3–5 mg/kg	30–40 s	10–30 min	↓ ICP	↓ BP Laryngospasm
Methohexital	1 mg/kg	<1 min	5–7 min	↓ ICP Short duration	↓ BP Seizures Laryngospasm
Midazolam	0.1 mg/kg	1–2 min	20–30 min	Reversible Amnesic Anticonvulsant	Apnea No analgesia Highly variable dose
Ketamine	1–2 mg/kg	1 min	5 min	Bronchodilator "Dissociative" amnesia	↑ Secretions ↑ ICP Emergence phenomenon
Etomidate	0.3 mg/kg	<1 min	10–20 min	↓ ICP ↓ IOP Rare ↓ BP	Myoclonic excitation Vomiting No analgesia
Propofol	0.5–1.5 mg/kg	20–40 s	8–15 min	Antiemetic Anticonvulsant ↓ ICP	Apnea ↓ BP No analgesia
Haloperidol	5-mg aliquots	5–10 min	Variable	Rare ↓ BP	Titrate Dystonia
Droperidol	2.5-mg aliquots	5–10 min	Variable	Rare ↓ BP Antiemetic	Titrate Dystonia ↓ BP
Fentanyl	3–8 μg/kg	1–2 min	30–40 min	Reversible analgesia	Highly variable dose ICP—variable effects Chest wall rigidity

Key: BP, blood pressure; ICP, intracranial pressure; IOP, intraocular pressure.

aliquots of haloperidol (Haldol) 5 to 10 mg will eventually control severe agitation. Another butyrophenone, droperidol (Inapsine), titrated with aliquots of 2.5 to 5.0 mg IV, is a more potent and rapid-onset agent. Droperidol can blunt the cardiovascular response to intubation. Hypotension is rare, and there are fewer dystonic reactions than with haloperidol. Since it is a potent antiemetic, it is an ideal option as a premedication or for neuroleptanalgesia.

Ketamine, a phencyclidine derivative, is a potent bronchodilator to be considered particularly in difficult hypotensive or bronchospastic patients. This agent is indicated for refractory status asthmaticus. Since ketamine increases the blood pressure, it is an appropriate choice in hypovolemic patients. It can, however, increase the intracranial pressure (ICP) in patients with head injuries. Owing to its inotropic and chronotropic cardiac effects, it should be used with caution in the elderly. As ketamine wears off and consciousness returns, the patient may experience "emergence phenomenon" in the form of nightmares, visual hallucinations, and dissociative sensations. Benzodiazepines (e.g., midazolam 0.5 mg aliquots limited to a maximum of 4 mg) may attenuate this phenomenon.

Etomidate is a nonbarbiturate nonreceptor hypnotic. It significantly inhibits adrenocortical function with continuous infusion. For single administration as an induction agent, however, this is not a major concern. The advantages of etomidate in the ED include protection from myocardial and cerebral ischemia, minimal histamine release, a stable hemodynamic profile, and short duration of action. This is another drug to consider if patients are hypovolemic or with closed head injury. Myoclonus, nausea, and vomiting do occur, and seizure foci may be stimulated. The incidence of severe etomidate-induced myoclonus can be decreased by pretreatment with diazepam or fentanyl. Etomidate lacks analgesic efficacy and does not blunt the sympathetic response to intubation.

Another option is propofol, a highly lipophilic, rapid-acting sedative. During RSI, this agent provides effective hypnosis. Propofol has a more rapid onset of action than etomidate and a shorter duration of action. Some of the pharmacologic advantages include its anticonvulsant and antiemetic properties and its ability to lower intracranial pressure.

While not first-line selections, opioids are also potent reversible induction agents. Fentanyl has an onset of action of less than 2 min. The ideal dose is highly variable (Table 15-3). Fentanyl is popular because of its sedative and analgesic properties. This agent provided the most neutral hemodynamic profile during RSI in a randomized double-blind study on sedatives and hemodynamics in the ED.[13] Rapid injection of high doses may cause chest wall rigidity. A related compound, alfentanil, is more potent and has a more immediate onset of action.

NEUROMUSCULAR BLOCKADE

Neuromuscular blocking agents facilitate airway management of selected patients in the emergency department. There are two major classes of drugs, depolarizing and nondepolarizing. Depolarizing neuromuscular blocking agents have high affinity for cholinergic receptors of the motor end plate, and are resistant to acetylcholinesterase. Initially they produce transient muscle fasciculations, followed by paralysis. This type of blockade is not antagonized, and may be enhanced, by anticholinesterase agents. Nondepolarizing neuromuscular blocking agents compete with acetylcholine for the cholinergic receptors, and can usually be antagonized by anticholinesterase agents. Succinylcholine, a depolarizing agent, inhibits neuromuscular transmission as long as an adequate concentration remains at one receptor site. However, succinylcholine is rapidly hydrolyzed by plasma cholinesterase. Potential adverse effects are listed in Table 15-4. In contrast, pancuronium, vecuronium, atracurium, cisatracurium, rocuronium, and mivacurium are nondepolarizing agents (Table 15-5).

In the ED, neuromuscular blockade can facilitate tracheal intubation, improve mechanical ventilation, and help control intracranial hypertension. Paralysis improves oxygenation and decreases peak airway pressures in a variety of disorders, including refractory pulmonary edema and the respiratory distress syndrome. Patients with refractory status asthmaticus, status epilepticus, or tetanic spasms resulting from clostridial infections or a variety of toxins, including strychnine, may improve with blockade.

In addition, extremely violent, agitated patients who jeopardize aeromedical personnel or their own airway security, spinal cord integrity, or fracture stability may require the ultimate pharmacologic restraint.

For the conditions mentioned above, nondepolarizing agents are preferable to succinylcholine. Although the onset of action is delayed, nondepolarizing agents have fewer adverse cardiovascular and histaminic effects coupled with a longer duration of paralysis. The delayed onset (1 to 5 min) and prolonged duration of action (25 to 120 min) require that the patient be ventilated with a bag-mask unit or other alternative, should intubation fail.

After documentation of the neurologic examination, including pupil size, presedation with an induction agent is advised unless there are other mitigating circumstances such as significant head injury or overdose. Neuromuscular blockers (NMBs) are neither anxiolytics nor analgesics. Omission of sedation is a common error in patients who remain aware of their paralysis. The resultant increased sympathetic tone can also exacerbate dysrhythmias.

The normal sequence in RSI is to induce sedation prior to administration of the depolarizing NMB agent. If a nondepolarizing agent is selected, some physicians reverse the sequence of administration, giving the nondepolarizing agent first because of its longer onset of action. Giving a rapid-acting hypnotic agent seconds later results in both medications having a synchronized peak effect.

Succinylcholine

When the indication for neuromuscular blockade is tracheal intubation, succinylcholine is the most commonly used agent. It has a more rapid onset (30 to 60 s) and shorter duration of action (average 5 to 6 min) than do the nondepolarizing agents. After a brief fasciculation, complete relaxation occurs at 60 s, with maximal paralysis at 2 to 3 min.

The dosage of succinylcholine is 1.0 to 1.5 mg/kg IV for adults. Succinylcholine can result in excellent intubation conditions in the ED. There are some significant potential complications.

Before injection of succinylcholine, atropine 0.01 mg/kg IV may attenuate the muscarinic vagal effects, especially in vagotonic adults and adolescents. An additional pretreatment to consider is a subparalytic dose of 0.01 mg/kg vecuronium or another nondepolarizing agent of similar duration to prevent the initial muscle fasciculations, which may cause long bone fractures to become displaced. Such fasiculations are most pronounced in muscular adolescents.

Succinylcholine increases intraocular pressure. In addition, the increased intragastric pressure will predispose to aspiration, hence the importance of cricoid pressure. Another concern with succinylcholine

TABLE 15-4 Succinylcholine

Adult Dose	Onset	Duration	Benefits
1.0–1.5 mg/kg	30–60 s	3–8 min	Rapid onset Short duration

Complications

Bradyarrhythmias	Masseter spasm
Increased intragastric, intraocular, and intracranial pressure	Malignant hyperthermia
Hyperkalemia	Prolonged apnea with pseudocholinesterase deficiency
Fasciculation-induced musculoskeletal trauma	Histamine release
	Cardiac arrest

TABLE 15-5 Nondepolarizing Neuromuscular Relaxants

Agent	Adult Intubating Dose IV	Onset	Duration	Complications
Vecuronium (intermediate/long)	0.8–0.15 mg/kg 0.15–0.28 mg/kg (high-dose protocol)	2–4 min	25–40 min 60–120 min	Prolonged recovery time in obese or elderly, or if there is hepatorenal dysfunction
Pancuronium (long)	0.1–0.15 mg/kg	3–5 min	80–100 min	Vagolytic tachyarrhythmias Prolonged recovery in elderly or if there is hepatorenal dysfunction
Doxacurium (long)	0.05–0.08 mg/kg	3–5 min	80–100 min	Prolonged block
Atracurium (intermediate)	0.4–0.6 mg/kg	2–3 min	25–45 min	Histamine release Hypotension Bronchospasm
Cisatracurium (intermediate)	0.15–0.20 mg/kg	2–3 min	50–60 min	Cardiovascular
Rocuronium (intermediate)	0.6–1.0 mg/kg	1–3 min	30–45 min	Tachycardia
Mivacurium (short)	0.15–0.20 mg/kg	2–3 min	10–20 min	Histamine release

is its potential to increase the ICP. This increase in ICP is greater in patients with central nervous system (CNS) neoplasms and may not be clinically significant in those with acute CNS hemorrhage or trauma.

There are other, less preventable side effects of succinylcholine. The serum potassium will transiently rise an average of 0.5 meq/L with succinylcholine. A clinically significant hyperkalemic response following succinylcholine administration in prescreened ED patients is uncommon.[14] Nevertheless, hyperkalemia may be pronounced hours after muscle trauma or burns. It should not be a factor in the immediate aftermath of such injury. Still, it is advisable to avoid depolarizing agents in patients with burns, muscle trauma, crush injuries, myopathies, rhabdomyolysis, narrow-angle glaucoma, renal failure, or neurologic disorders. Any patient with ''denervated musculature'' (e.g., Guillain-Barré syndrome or spinal cord injury) is particularly at risk. Genetically susceptible individuals may develop acute malignant hyperthermia.

Dantrolene sodium should always be available. Patients with an atypical pseudocholinesterase will require prolonged ventilatory support, as will those with burns, cirrhosis, or carcinomas who have low plasma pseudocholinesterase levels.

Also, patients recently abusing cocaine may have a prolonged duration of neuromuscular blockade, since cocaine is metabolized by plasma cholinesterase, reducing the amount of enzyme available for succinylcholine metabolism.

Nondepolarizing Agents

Pancuronium is a nondepolarizing agent which is less likely than most others to cause histamine release. However, it more commonly results in tachycardia, so should be avoided in patients with underlying cardiac disease. While still commonly used, agents with a shorter duration of action and fewer cardiac effects have supplanted its use in some institutions.

Vecuronium bromide is an intermediate- to long-acting nondepolarizing agent. This drug is approximately one-third more potent than pancuronium. The duration of action is one-third to one-half as long. The usual dose of vecuronium is 0.08 to 0.15 mg/kg IV. Maximal paralysis occurs within 2 to 4 min, with full blockade lasting for 25 to 40 min. Vecuronium does not cause the degree of tachycardia commonly seen after pancuronium, since it has one-twentieth of the vagolytic effect. This simplifies interpretation of a tachycardia developing in the trauma patient.

A major advantage is the lack of hemodynamic alterations. Hypersensitivity reactions are rare, doses are only minimally cumulative, and excretion is biliary. Despite the lack of histamine release, hypotension may occur through two other mechanisms. Blockage of sympathetic ganglia occurs, and venous return is decreased from both absent muscle tone and the positive-pressure ventilation.

Doxacurium chloride is a long-acting nondepolarizing NMB used to facilitate prolonged mechanical ventilation after tracheal intubation. It provides skeletal muscle relaxation with no dose-related cardiovascular effects.

Atracurium is an agent well suited for patients with hepatic or renal failure. Elimination is via ester hydrolysis and Hoffman degradation, a nonenzymatic process. This nondepolarizing agent's elimination half-life is approximately 20 min, versus 65 to 75 min for vecuronium. Recovery time is consistent and unaffected by anticonvulsants. Consider this agent for intubated patients requiring brief diagnostic or therapeutic procedures.

Atracurium also offers advantages when continuous infusion is essential to maintain a precise, required level of neuromuscular blockade. A disadvantage is that histamine release can cause bronchospasm and hypotension. The risk with prolonged infusion is accumulation of laudanosine, a neuroexcitatory metabolic by-product.

Other nondepolarizing options include cisatracurium, rocuronium, and mivacurium. Cisatracurium is an intermediate-duration NMB agent. None of the metabolites have NMB activity, and excretion is independent of hepatorenal function. Rocuronium also has an intermediate duration of action, but the onset of action is much faster. Excretion is predominantly hepatic. Mivacurium is the nondepolarizing agent with the shortest duration of action. Histamine release can be minimized by slow infusion.

The reversal of nondepolarizing muscle relaxants is rarely necessary in the ED. Reversal should not be attempted prior to some sign of motion or spontaneous recovery. Reversal requires atropine 0.01 mg/kg IV to prevent muscarinic side effects, followed by edrophonium 0.5 to 1.0 mg/kg IV. The onset of action is 30 to 60 s, with a duration of 10 to 30 min. This reversal may be shorter than the duration of the muscle relaxant. Edrophonium is an acetylcholinesterase inhibitor with a faster onset and fewer muscarinic side effects than the longer-acting neostigmine.

Strategies

DIFFICULT AIRWAY The management of the difficult airway in the ED is, in many regards, more challenging than in the controlled setting of the operating room. The patient generally has not been fasting and

TABLE 15-6 "Difficult Airway" Kit

ET tubes: assorted sizes, designs, tip control, fiberoptic
Laryngoscope blades: alternate sizes and designs, fiberoptic
Stylets: Eschmann bougie, semirigid, hollow, light wand
Syringes, fixators, and Magill forceps
4% lidocaine and laryngotracheal anesthesia kit
1% phenylephrine (Neo-Synephrine)-lidocaine jelly
Tube changers
Emergency ventilation option: Laryngeal-mask airway Translaryngeal ventilation equipment Esophageal tracheal Combitube
Retrograde tracheal intubation equipment
Cricothyrotomy equipment: dilators, #4 Shiley

is not premedicated. There is rarely time for a leisurely evaluation of the "airway history" and "airway physical examination." The difficult airway constitutes the clinical scenario in which mask ventilation or tracheal intubation is challenging. Approximately 2 to 3 percent of tracheal intubations prove impossible with standard techniques. Difficult mask ventilation is defined as the inability to maintain the Sa_{O_2} above 90 percent. Intubation is defined as difficult if more than three attempts are necessary or if conventional laryngoscopy requires more than 10 min. Many emergency physicians prefer to assure the availability of the appropriate airway equipment by customizing the contents of a portable airway kit (Table 15-6).

In some stable ED patients, it may be feasible to screen for those physical findings that might suggest a difficult laryngoscopy. The three most predictive tests include assessments of atlantooccipital extension, thyromental distance, and the Mallampati criteria[15] (Fig. 15-4).

Proper visualization of the larynx requires flexion of the lower cervical vertebrae coupled with extension at the atlantooccipital joint (the "sniffing position"). In addition, the mandibular opening in a normal adult should be at least 4 cm or two to three finger breadths. A thyromental distance less than 6 cm or a mandibular length less than 9 cm correlates with difficulties. Finally, the size of the tongue relative to the oral cavity affects visualization of the glottis. The Mallampati criteria (Fig. 15-4) help predict the degree of difficulty in visualizing the vocal cords.[15] The ability to visualize the faucial pillars, base of the uvula, and the soft palate predicts the degree of difficulty in laryngeal exposure.

These clinical findings should affect the judgment of the emergency physician who is considering the feasibility of the various approaches to airway management. The decision is basically centered on two initial considerations: will a nonsurgical approach succeed, and is preservation versus ablation of spontaneous ventilation wise (Fig. 15-5).

CEREBRAL RESUSCITATION Patients with suspected acute intracranial hypertension require aggressive airway management. Direct laryngoscopy can elevate the ICP. Prior to oral or nasal intubation, pretreatment with intravenous lidocaine may help blunt this deleterious cardiovascular response. Fentanyl will also blunt the hemodynamic changes.

Since in certain situations succinylcholine may also increase ICP, the intubator should consider prior use of a defasciculating dose of a nondepolarizing NMB agent. If one is selected, the use of a priming dose will shorten the onset of action. However, a significantly prolonged duration of action may be the result, extending the risks if a difficult airway is encountered. Another consideration is the use of a short-acting sedative induction agent. Several of these drugs, including thiopental, fentanyl, and etomidate, directly decrease the ICP.

Effective oxygenation and ventilation during cerebral resuscitation often requires prolonged neuromuscular blockade. Autoregulation of cerebral blood flow (CBF) over a range of perfusion pressures may be impaired. As a result, CBF becomes pressure-dependent ($CBF = CPP/CVR$, where *CPP* is cerebral perfusion pressure and *CVR* is cerebral vascular resistance). Autoregulation is usually intact when the CPP ranges between 50 and 130 mmHg. The CPP equals the mean arterial pressure minus the ICP.

In traumatic brain injury, the goal is therefore to maintain the mean arterial pressures over 90 mmHg throughout the patient's course; this will usually maintain the CPP over 70 mmHg. Other treatment modalities, such as mannitol administration and hyperventilation, do have the potential for exacerbation of intracranial ischemia. Therefore, prophylactic hyperventilation therapy (P_{CO_2} less than 35 mmHg) should be avoided during the first 24 h after injury.[16]

On the other hand, brief hyperventilation therapy should rapidly be initiated in the ED in patients with definite acute signs of intracranial hypertension. If the intracranial hypertension does not respond to adjunctive osmotic diuretics, sedation, neuromuscular blockade, and neurosurgical drainage of cerebrospinal fluid, protracted hyperventilation may be necessary.

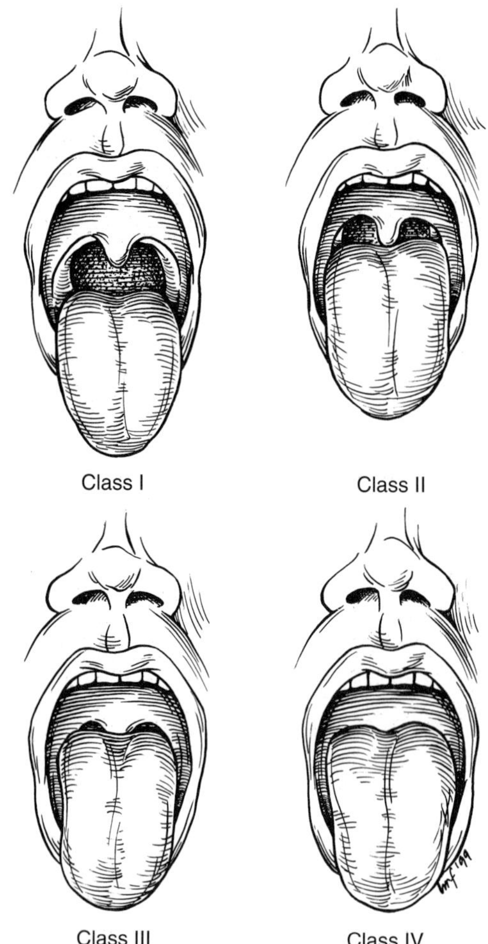

FIG. 15-4. The classification of tongue size relative to the size of the oral cavity as described by Mallampati and colleagues.[15] Class I: faucial pillars, soft palate, and uvula can be visualized. Class II: faucial pillars and soft palate can be visualized, but the uvula is masked by the base of the tongue. Class III: only the base of the uvula can be visualized. Class IV: none of the three structures can be visualized.

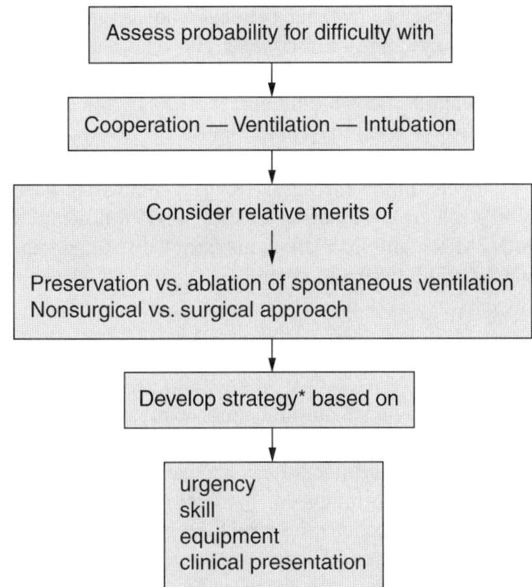

FIG. 15-5. Difficult airway algorithm.
* Options include bag-valve-mask intubation, endotracheal intubation, nasotracheal intubation, rapid-sequence intubation, digital intubation, fiberoptic transillumination, laryngeal mask airway, Combitube, retrograde tracheal intubation, translaryngeal ventilation, and cricothyrotomy. (Adapted from American Society of Anesthesiologists,[5] with permission.)

After blockade, select the Fio_2 sufficient to maintain an arterial Po_2 of 100 mmHg, fully saturating hemoglobin. Positive end-expiratory pressure (PEEP) of up to 5 cmH_2O may help prevent atelectasis. Higher levels will impair cerebral venous drainage because of the elevated intrathoracic pressure. Avoid other modalities that also increase the ICP, including excessively tight ET tube straps, tight cervical collars, or Trendelenburg positioning.

CARDIOPULMONARY DISEASE Tracheal intubation and mechanical ventilation can also have other significant physiologic consequences. In a prospective investigation of 297 tracheal intubations in an intensive care unit setting, there were 7 deaths.[17] These occurred predominantly among those requiring emergent tracheal intubation. Mortality risk, however, was greatest among those receiving prior vasopressor therapy. Any conditions that result in the cardiovascular system's reliance on preload to maintain perfusion will predispose to hypotension and cardiac decompensation. Particular caution is needed when intubating previously hypotensive patients who require vasopressor support. In addition, patients with hypercarbia and chronic obstructive pulmonary disease (COPD) require special consideration. As mentioned, mechanical ventilation increases the positive intrathoracic pressure. This decreases the preload by decreasing venous return. Hypotension may be anticipated. Additional physiologic considerations include the decreased left ventricular compliance and the fact that most of the medications useful in RSI decrease the sympathetic tone.

INTUBATION IN CERVICAL SPINE INJURY

Airway management of patients with the potential to have an unstable injury of the cervical spine challenges clinical judgment. There is no single best algorithm. Cervical spine radiography without a thorough and reliable neurologic examination does not "clear the neck." From 20 to 30 percent of cervical spine injuries are not appreciated on a single cross-table lateral view. In addition, patients with blunt major trauma requiring tracheal intubation have associated unstable cervical spine injuries that range from 1 to 12 percent. Spinal cord injury without radiographic abnormality (SCIWORA), is an important consideration, especially in adolescents and children.

The initial decision is to determine whether immediate airway intervention is really needed. Patients not in urgent need of an airway should be neurologically and radiographically evaluated as thoroughly as is practical given their condition. The need for in-line cervical stabilization should not be considered a license for axial in-line traction. For example, attempting to visualize C7 radiographically by countertracting on the head and shoulders of the near-hanging patient is counterintuitive.

There is a large selection of airway options to consider while attempting to maintain cervical spine immobilization. The selection is far less critical than the timing. Nasotracheal intubation, transillumination, fiberoptic laryngoscopy, and RTI are commonly selected options. Oral intubation appears safe when achieved without hyperdistraction, flexion, or extension of the neck. Maintenance of cervical spine immobilization is the paramount issue—not the approach to secure the airway. Careful endotracheal intubation (ETI) causes less cervical spine motion than bag-valve-mask (BVM) ventilation.

Visualization of the larynx prior to cervical spine clearance is difficult, since alignment of the oropharyngeolaryngeal axis is not possible. One method to move the tip of the tube anteriorly is to use a slightly flexed directional-tip tube (Endotrol) coupled with the Sellick maneuver. Another is to use a flexible stylet, such as the Flexiguide, which passes through the tube and has a trigger similar to the Endotrol. Another option is to aim the tip of the tube anteriorly with Magill forceps while an assistant advances the tube.

There are several new commercially available laryngoscope blade designs that allow vocal cord visualization without manipulation of the neck. Most designs have fiberoptic attachments to the blade. This allows elevation of the tongue to avoid the blood or secretions. Technically, these blades may prove simpler to use than conventional fiberoptic laryngoscopes.

The Bullard blade incorporates a fiberoptic bundle along the posterior aspect of the straight blade. After visualization, a stylet carries the ET tube, which is advanced through the vocal cords. The Direct View blade incorporates fiberoptics with a curved MacIntosh-style blade. A nonfiberoptic design is the Bainton blade; this has a tubular, square design to facilitate visualization when there is significant soft tissue swelling. This design helps displace tissue circumferentially.

SUCTIONING

A variety of conditions render patients unable to clear their own secretions. Aspiration usually occurs when the tone of the lower esophageal sphincter is insufficient to deal with the increased intragastric pressure and the protective laryngeal airway reflexes are depressed. The common iatrogenic causes include BVM ventilation, the presence of nasogastric tubes, and pharmacologic neuromuscular paralysis. Some common predisposing conditions include trauma, bowel obstruction, obesity, overdose, pregnancy, hiatus hernia and seizures.

Aspiration after urgent ET intubation occurs infrequently in ED patients if there is inattention to technique.[18] The intubator should consider using large-diameter suction systems or tubing for the removal of particulate matter or clots that are larger than the standard Yankauer tip can handle.[19] The rigid-tip plastic tonsil suction catheter can remove large quantities of oropharyngeal secretions.

When necessary, place the patient in a left lateral Trendelenburg position. This helps get the tongue out of the laryngoscopist's way and will facilitate immediate endotracheal suctioning.

To suction the nasopharynx and tracheobronchial tree, use a well-lubricated, soft, curved-tip catheter. Straight catheters will usually pass into the right mainstem bronchus. If a curved-tip catheter is available, turning the head to the right in addition to catheter rotation will often facilitate passage into the left bronchus.

A suction catheter of a size no larger than half the diameter of the tube to be suctioned should be selected. This will prevent pulmonic collapse from insufficient ventilation during suctioning. Then oxygenate the patient before and after suctioning to avoid transient desaturation. The catheter is inserted without suctioning and then slowly removed, suctioning with rotation over 10 to 15 s.

Some of the complications of suctioning include hypoxia, cardiac dysrhythmias, hypotension, pulmonic collapse, and direct mucosal injury. The magnitude of the ICP increase during endotracheal suctioning may be related to the increase in intrathoracic pressure with coughing if lidocaine has been omitted.

MECHANICAL VENTILATORY SUPPORT

The knowledge of the pathophysiology of acute respiratory failure and the changes in lung physiology during positive-pressure ventilation will aid in the selection of an appropriate ventilatory modality and in the selection of the initial settings.[20] Ventilators are pressure- or volume-cycled. Volume-cycled ventilators are used routinely in EDs. Other decisions regarding mechanical ventilatory support in the ED include the rate, mode, F_iO_2, minute ventilation, and use of positive end-expiratory pressure (PEEP) or continuous positive airway pressure (CPAP).

There are three common ventilator modes or methods for providing the tidal volume: controlled mechanical ventilation (CMV), assist-control (A/C), and intermittent mandatory ventilation (IMV). Use the control mode for apneic patients. The A/C mode allows the patient to trigger a cycle by inhaling and lowering the air pressure, which can be adjusted by the ventilator's trigger "sensitivity" (1 to 3 cmH_2O). The ventilator will provide an untriggered "controlled" breath unless one is triggered during the selected time cycle. Finally, a predetermined number of ventilator-generated tidal volumes can be assured either unsynchronized (IMV) or more commonly synchronized (to patient effort) intermittent mandatory ventilation (SIMV). In the ED, the A/C or SIMV is the preferred initial mode except with an apneic patient.

The initial FiO_2 should be guided by the oximetry. Set the tidal volume at 10 to 15 mL/kg ideal body weight and adjust the rate accordingly. Allow sufficient time for expiration. Maintain the *peak* airway pressure (PAP) below 35 to 45 cmH_2O to prevent barotrauma. The PAP appears to be related to barotrauma more than the level of CPAP. The tidal volume can be increased up to 15 mL/kg to adjust the $PaCO_2$ unless it elevates the PAP excessively.

To reclaim lung volumes, PEEP or CPAP should be considered if the decreased pulmonary compliance prevents delivery of an adequate tidal volume or if hypoxemia persists despite 100% FiO_2. Even low levels (3 to 5 cmH_2O) of PEEP/CPAP usually render ventilator "sighs" (1.5 × tidal volume) unnecessary. If hypotension develops, adjust the respiratory rate and PEEP to lower the *mean* airway pressure.

Some alert patients with mild respiratory insufficiency who do not meet intubation criteria can be temporarily managed with continuous positive airway pressure (CPAP) through a snug-fitting face mask. This reduces the functional residual capacity and the work of breathing. Mask CPAP may thus delay or reduce the need for intubation. In patients with severe maxillofacial trauma and potential basilar skull fractures, pneumocephalus is a hazard. Noninvasive positive-pressure ventilation delivered through a face mask has been compared to conventional mechanical ventilation and is an effective option for many types of acute respiratory failure.[21]

Face-mask CPAP may also prove to be a valuable initial adjunct in some patients with pulmonary edema. The pressure can be maintained below 18 cmH_2O if it is intermittently released. This decreases the potential for gastric insufflation and subsequent aspiration.

Patients who require prolonged CPAP to maintain oxygenation and adequate alveolar ventilation may subsequently benefit from airway pressure release ventilation (APRV). APRV is basically a CPAP system for spontaneously breathing patients who cannot maintain adequate alveolar ventilation on their own and who also require an increased functional residual capacity. This technique attempts to ventilate the lungs while avoiding higher PAPs by releasing the level of CPAP to a lower pressure. These ventilators incorporate a second relief valve that allows for the cyclical release of CPAP to the desired lower level. Inverse ratio ventilation (IRV), in contrast, is the technique to completely control ventilation and the PAP following NMB. In other words, APRV and IMV allow unrestricted spontaneous ventilation, while IRV and CMV do not.

EXTUBATION

Inherently more relaxing than intubation, extubation is nevertheless potentially hazardous. It should rarely occur in the ED. Patients who are recovering their protective airway reflexes may "fight" the tube yet still need to remain intubated. Instillation of 1 to 2 mL of 4% lidocaine (sterile for injection) down the ET tube will decrease bucking. The absorption of lidocaine via the airway yields a maximum serum level that is only slightly lower than that from an equivalent intravenous dose.

Prior to extubation, consider the impact of metabolic or circulatory abnormalities. The patient should be checked for respiratory insufficiency, and nasogastric decompression is advised. On command, the patient should have an inspiratory capacity of at least 15 mL/kg. Ideally there should be no intercostal or suprasternal reactions, and the patient's grip should be firm.

After suctioning secretions, assure adequate oxygenation and explain the procedure to the patient. Positive-pressure ventilation using a mask will help to exsufflate secretions while the cuff is deflated. At the end of a deep inspiration, to prevent secretory reaccumulation, remove the tube and oxygenate by mask.

Closely observe the patient for stridor. Postextubation laryngospasm is initially treated with oxygen by positive pressure. If necessary, nebulized racemic epinephrine (0.5 mL of 2.25% epinephrine in 4-mL saline) often helps.

REFERENCES

1. Takahata O, Kubota M, Mamiya K, et al: The efficacy of the "BURP" maneuver during a difficult laryngoscopy. *Anesth Analg* 84:419, 1997.
2. Barnhard WN, Cottrell JE, Sirakumarana C, et al: Adjustment of intracuff pressure to prevent aspiration. *Anesthesiology* 50:313, 1979.
3. Ward KR, Yealy DM: End-tidal carbon dioxide monitoring in emergency medicine, Part 2: clinical applications. *Acad Emerg Med* 5:637, 1998.
4. Bozeman WP, Hexter D, Liang HK, Kelen GD: Esophageal detector device versus detection of end-tidal carbon dioxide level in emergency intubation. *Ann Emerg Med* 27:595, 1996.
5. American Society of Anesthesiologists Task Force on Management of the Difficult Airway: Practice Guidelines for Management of the Difficult Airway. *Anesthesiology* 78:597, 1993.
6. Reed DB, Clinton JE: Proper depth of placement of nasotracheal tubes in adults prior to radiographic confirmation. *Acad Emerg Med* 4:1111, 1997.
7. Hooker EA, Hagan S, Coleman R, et al: Directional-tip endotracheal tubes for blind nasotracheal intubation. *Acad Emerg Med* 3:586, 1996.
8. Rosen CL, Wolfe RE, Chew SE, et al: Blind nasotracheal intubation in the presence of facial trauma. *J Emerg Med* 15:141, 1997.
9. Margolis GS, Menegazzi J, Abdlehak M, et al: The efficacy of a standard training program for transillumination-guided endotracheal intubation. *Acad Emerg Med* 3:371, 1996.
10. van Stralen DW, Rogers M, Perkin RM, et al: Retrograde intubation training using a mannequin. *Am J Emerg Med* 13:50, 1995.
11. Ma OJ, Bentley B II, Debehnke DJ: Airway management practices in emergency medicine residencies. *Am J Emerg Med* 13:501, 1995.
12. Sakles JC, Laurin EG, Rantapaa AA, et al: Airway management in the emergency department: A one-year study of 610 tracheal intubations. *Ann Emerg Med* 31:325, 1998.

13. Sivilotti MLA, Ducharme J: Randomized, double-blind study on sedatives and hemodynamics during rapid-sequence intubation in the emergency department: The SHRED Study. *Ann Emerg Med* 31:313, 1998.
14. Zink BJ, Snyder HS, Raccio-Robak N: Lack of a hyperkalemic response in emergency department patients receiving succinylcholine. *Acad Emerg Med* 2:974, 1995.
15. Mallampati SR, Gatt SP, Gugino LD, et al: A clinical sign to predict difficult tracheal intubation: A prospective study. *Can Anaesth Soc J* 32:429, 1985.
16. Brain Trauma Foundation: The use of hyperventilation in the acute management of severe traumatic brain injury. *J Neurotrauma* 13:699, 1996.
17. Schwartz DE, Matthay MA, Cohen NH: Death and other complications of emergency airway management in critically ill adults: A prospective investigation of 297 tracheal intubations. *Anesthesiology* 82:367, 1995.
18. Thibodeau LG, Verdile VP, Bartfield JM: Incidence of aspiration after urgent intubation. *Am J Emerg Med* 15:562, 1997.
19. Vandenberg JT, Rudman NT, Burke TF, et al: Large-diameter suction tubing significantly reduces evacuation time of simulated vomitus. *Am J Emerg Med* 16:242, 1998.
20. Orebaugh SL: Initiation of mechanical ventilation in the emergency department. *Am J Emerg Med* 14:59, 1996.
21. Antonelli M, Conti G, Rocco M, et al: A comparison of noninvasive positive-pressure ventilation and conventional mechanical ventilation in patients with acute respiratory failure. *N Engl J Med* 339:429, 1998.

BIBLIOGRAPHY

USPDI, vol I. 19th ed, 1999, Micromedia and the US Pharmacopeia Connection.

SURGICAL AIRWAY MANAGEMENT

David R. Gens

Surgical airway management is an important skill for all medical personnel treating patients with potentially life-threatening airway emergencies. Up to 2 percent of emergency department intubations have been reported to result in a cricothyroidotomy, but the actual rate is certainly considerably lower.[1] It is probably underutilized as a technique.

The term *cricothyroidotomy* technically means vertically incising (splitting) both the cricoid and thyroid cartilages, and *coniotomy* means incising the cricothyroid (conic) ligament, which runs from the cricoid to the thyroid cartilage. Although *coniotomy* is the correct term for incising between these two cartilages, the term *cricothyroidotomy* is now commonly used to denote this procedure and is used throughout this chapter.

CLINICAL FEATURES

The indications for an emergency surgical airway are several; however, the majority are due to an inability to establish an orotracheal or nasopharyngeal airway. This may be due to anatomy (short, obese neck), a disease state (epiglottis, laryngeal edema, paralyzed vocal cords, or retropharyngeal abscess), trauma from distortion of the neck by hematoma (cervical fracture or major vessel injury), aspiration of blood (facial trauma), or loss of supporting structures (mandibular fractures). Clinical manifestations of acute airway obstruction are stridor (in a patient who is still able to breath) or cyanosis. Clinical signs and symptoms are listed in Table 16-1.

TABLE 16-1 Clinical Manifestations Associated with Acute Airway Obstruction

Etiology	Manifestation
Vascular	Hematoma External hemorrhage Hypotension Hemoptysis
Laryngotracheal	Stridor Subcutaneous air (massive) Hoarseness Dysphonia Hemoptysis
Pharyngeal and/or hypopharyngeal	Subcutaneous air Hematemesis Dysphagia Sucking wound

SPECIFIC ISSUES THAT AFFECT EVALUATION AND TREATMENT

Age

Needle cricothyroidotomy is the preferred emergency surgical airway in children under the age of approximately 12 years who cannot be intubated orotracheally or nasotracheally. A 12- or 14-gauge catheter over a needle will support ventilation and oxygenation in a child until a tracheostomy can be performed in the operating room by a surgeon familiar with the anatomy of a child's neck. Surgical cricothyroidotomy should not be considered. The larynx is easily damaged by surgical cricothyroidotomy, and younger individuals have a higher incidence of late airway complications.[2]

Associated Injuries

The standard indications for an airway in emergency patients are mentioned below; however, some specific types of trauma usually have a greater need for a surgical airway.

Penetrating trauma to the neck (gunshot or stab wound) that injures a major artery (carotid, vertebral, or thyroid) demonstrates an expanding hematoma around the injured artery and may cause obstruction of the airway by pressure. The need for a surgical airway should be anticipated. Infrequently, free blood from concomitant vascular and pharyngeal or tracheal injuries spills into the oro- or hypopharynx and causes severe aspiration of blood; in such cases a cuffed tube (surgical cricothyroidotomy, not needle cricothyroidotomy) is needed. Difficulty in establishing an airway occurs in approximately 10 percent of penetrating cervical trauma cases.[3]

Blunt trauma to the neck or face may cause hemorrhage of the soft tissues or injury to the trachea or larynx itself. The trachea may become detached from the larynx at the level of the first tracheal ring, and the larynx or the trachea itself may become ruptured. In either of these rare circumstances, an emergency tracheostomy is required. This procedure should be performed by someone with experience in surgery of the neck. It is difficult to perform as an emergency tracheostomy, especially with an awake patient who is becoming hypoxic and combative. Severe edema of the larynx or, rarely, fracture of the cartilages of the larynx may obstruct the airway.

In blunt facial trauma, the principal cause of death is obstruction of the airway. This occurs for several reasons. In patients with mandibular fractures, the loss of supporting structure for the tongue allows the base of the tongue to fall back into the hypopharynx and obstruct the airway. Also, these patients, placed supine and with major facial bleeding, will aspirate blood continuously.

Type of Emergency Airway and Tube Selection

Surgical cricothyroidotomy is always preferred over needle cricothyroidotomy (except for children under 12 years of age, as noted above) simply because of the larger diameter of the 6-mm (internal diameter)

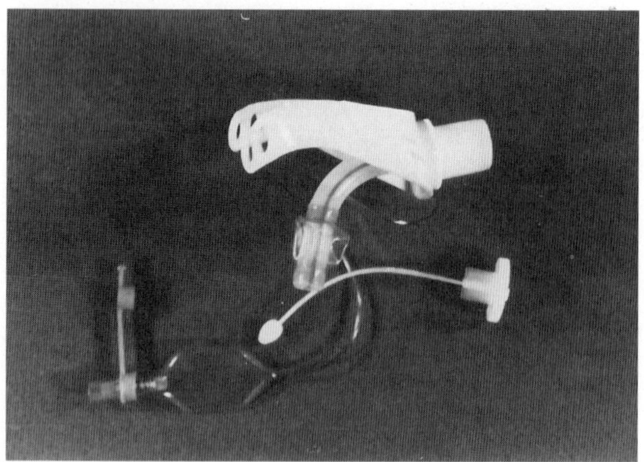

FIG. 16-1. Tracheostomy tube with obturator.

endotracheal or tracheostomy tube compared to the needle cricothyroidotomy catheter. Adequate ventilation is crucial in the early prevention of cerebral edema after brain injury. Ventilation is practically impossible through a 14- or 12-gauge catheter. Emergency tracheostomy is rarely indicated and extremely difficult to perform. This procedure should be performed only by physicians who are familiar with surgical anatomy and skilled with the procedure.

A tracheostomy tube is preferred to an endotracheal tube for several reasons. A tracheostomy tube has an obturator, which makes entry through the narrow cricothyroid membrane easier. The tracheostomy tube is shorter and therefore easier to suction through. Most important, it has phalanges on each side that allow it to be sutured to the neck and secured with a cloth ribbon around the neck (Fig. 16-1). The endotracheal tube (when used for cricothyroidotomy) is very difficult to affix to the neck and moves easily no matter how well secured with adhesive tape. Unfortunately, many emergency departments are not stocked with tracheostomy tubes because of their infrequent need, or when they are stocked, they may not be readily available. Therefore, an endotracheal tube is most commonly used and is readily available. When a tracheostomy tube becomes available, a tube change can be made using the Seldinger technique; a suction catheter with the suction vent cut off at one end is readily available and easy to use.

The diameter of the tube inserted is crucial. A 6-mm tracheostomy or 6-mm endotracheal tube is preferred (never larger than 7 mm in either case). Tubes with diameters larger than 7 mm are difficult to insert in the narrow space between the cricoid and thyroid cartilages. If airway pressures are high with the small-diameter tube, the cricothyroidotomy tube may be changed to a tracheostomy or endotracheal tube with a larger diameter at a later, convenient time.

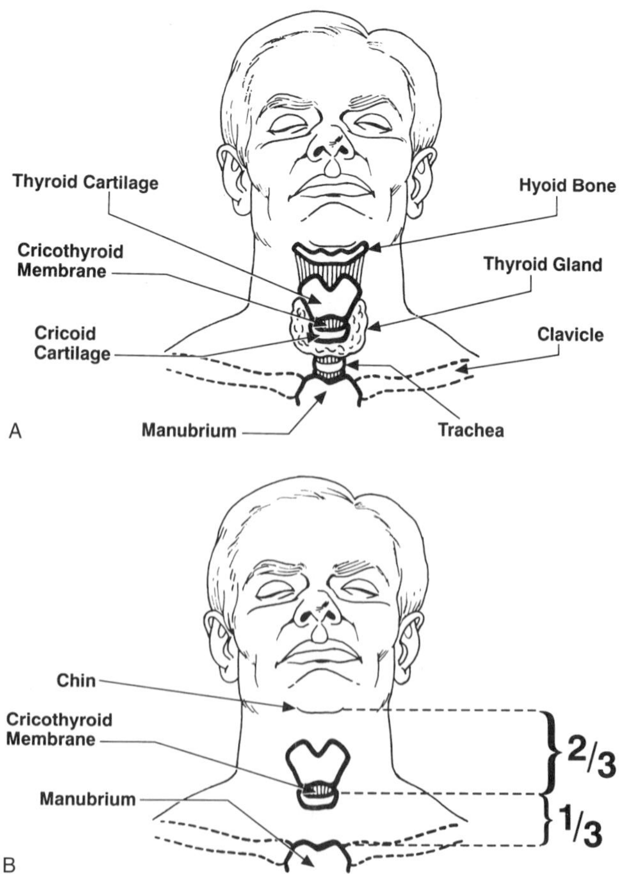

FIG. 16-2. A. Anatomy of the neck. **B.** Location of the cricothyroid membrane.

Conversion from Cricothyroidotomy to Tracheostomy

The question frequently arises as to how long to leave a cricothyroidotomy tube in place in the larynx. A tube left in the narrow space between the cricoid and thyroid cartilages can erode both cartilages, and a bacterial chondritis may occur. The cartilages will be destroyed and eventually scar, leading to stenosis and loss of the function of the larynx. Because cricothyroidotomy has a higher incidence of airway stenosis, a cricothyroidotomy should be converted to a tracheostomy.[4] As a rule of thumb, if the airway will be needed for more than 2 to 3 days, the cricothyroidotomy should be changed to a tracheostomy. Otherwise, the cricothyroid tube may stay in place.

PROCEDURE

Surgical Cricothyroidotomy

ANATOMY The cricothyroid membrane is located between the thyroid and cricoid cartilages (Fig. 16-2A). Both of these structures are easily palpated. The cricothyroid membrane can be found approximately one-third the distance from the manubrium to the chin in the midline in patients with normal habitus (Fig. 16-2B). In a patient with a short, obese neck, the membrane may be hidden at the level of the manubrium, while in a patient with a thin, long neck, it may be midway between the chin and the manubrium. The thyroid gland overlies the trachea; both of these structures are difficult to palpate.

The only vascular structure that may be injured during the course of a properly performed cricothyroidotomy is the thyroid ima artery, a branch of the aorta that runs up to the thyroid gland in the midline and infrequently reaches the level of the cricothyroid membrane. When injured, it needs to be surgically ligated to control the hemorrhage.

INDICATIONS AND CONTRAINDICATIONS Inability to orotracheally intubate an emergency patient is the prime indication for surgical or needle cricothyroidotomy. Orotracheal (or nasotracheal) intubation should be attempted first. In-line cervical stabilization must be maintained in trauma patients. If orotracheal intubation is unsuccessful, then cricothyroidotomy should be performed.

As mentioned earlier, surgical cricothyroidotomy is reserved for patients over the age of 12 years and is contraindicated in patients under the age of 12. Needle cricothyroidotomy is the procedure of choice in this age group.

COMPLICATIONS Acute complications following emergency cricothyroidotomy occur in up to approximately 10 percent of cases.[5] Such complications include

1. *Bleeding from the insertion site.* Venous bleeding is almost always from small veins and usually stops (using a vertical neck incision decreases the chance of bleeding). Arterial bleeding can be from the thyroid ima artery or from a small artery at the base of the cricothyroid membrane. Apply gentle pressure to stop the bleeding. If bleeding persists, surgical control may be necessary in the operating room.
2. *Misplacement of the tube.* In an obese neck, it is possible to place the tube anterior to the larynx and trachea into the mediastinum. Ventilation is not possible. Manifestations of an incorrectly positioned tube are high airway pressures, absent breath sounds, and massive subcutaneous emphysema. The tube should be removed and a second attempt should be made.
3. *Laceration of the structures of the neck.* Laceration of the trachea, esophagus, or recurrent laryngeal nerves is extremely rare and is due to inadequate knowledge of the anatomy of the neck.
4. *Pneumothorax.* This complication is probably secondary to barotrauma caused by ventilation initiated immediately after tube placement.

Late airway complications may occur in up to 52 percent of cases. These complications include voice changes and laryngeal and/or tracheal stenosis.[6–8]

EQUIPMENT NEEDED

1. Personal protective equipment
2. Scalpel with number-10 blade (preferable due to its greater width) or a number-11 blade
3. A 6-mm endotracheal tube or 6-mm tracheostomy tube (preferred) (Do not use a tube that is larger than 6 mm. A larger size is difficult to place through the cricothyroid membrane.)
4. Tape to secure the endotracheal tube in place; cloth ribbon and sutures to secure tracheostomy tube in place
5. Bag-valve-mask device and oxygen source

PATIENT PREPARATION AND POSITIONING The patient should be placed supine with the neck positioned in the midline. Povidone iodine solution should be quickly applied to the skin if time permits. If the patient still has a patent airway (albeit minimal), oxygen should be administered by mask.

STEPS OF PROCEDURE

1. Stand to one side of the patient at the level of the neck. A right-handed practitioner should stand on the right side, and a left-handed practitioner on the left side.
2. Locate the cricoid ring. Place the index finger at the sternal notch and palpate cephalad until the first rigid structure is felt (cricoid ring). Roll the index finger one finger breadth above to locate the ''hollow'' between the cricoid and thyroid cartilages. This is the cricothyroid membrane (Fig. 16-3).

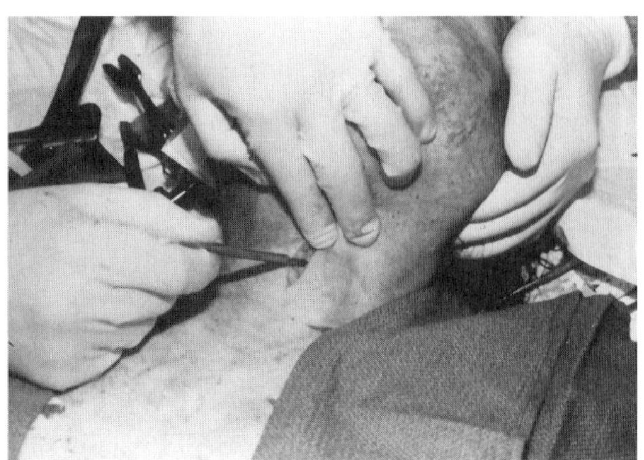

FIG. 16-4. Surgical cricothyroidotomy: puncturing the cricothyroid membrane with a scalpel blade.

3. Using the thumb and middle finger of the nondominant hand, stabilize the two cartilages.
4. Use the scalpel to make a vertical incision in the midline between the two cartilages. The incision should go through the skin and subcutaneous tissues. The structures are superficial, and care should be taken not to incise deeper, since this may result in damage to the cricoid or thyroid cartilage or vascular structures.
5. With the scalpel blade positioned horizontally, perforate the cricothyroid membrane so that the blade goes in approximately half its length (Fig. 16-4).
6. Place the back end of the scalpel handle into the incision in the cricothyroid membrane to widen the opening (Fig. 16-5).
7. Place the endotracheal tube (or tracheostomy tube) in the opening (Fig. 16-6).
8. Secure the tube carefully with a ribbon and/or adhesive tape. If using an endotracheal tube, take special care that the tube is in no more than 2 to 3 cm; otherwise, the tube will slip down the right main-stem bronchus with even minimal movement.
9. Connect to a bag-valve-mask device for ventilation. Check for breath sounds for ventilation. If no ventilation is heard bilaterally, then pull the tube out and reinsert it. Constantly recheck for breath sounds to ensure that the endotracheal tube is correctly positioned. If breath sounds are absent only on the left side, then the tube has been inserted down the right main-stem bronchus and needs to be pulled back a few centimeters. This usually occurs with the use of an endotracheal tube.

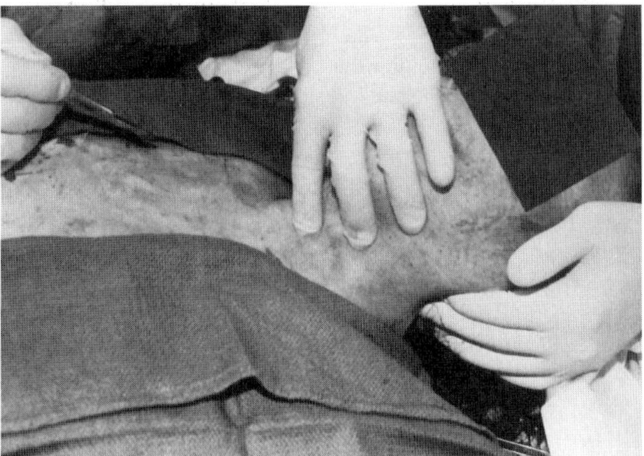

FIG. 16-3. Surgical cricothyroidotomy: palpating the cricothyroid membrane.

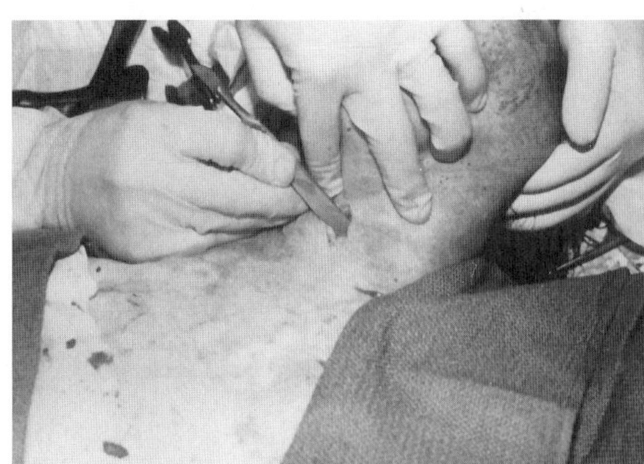

FIG. 16-5. Surgical cricothyroidotomy: placing the scalpel handle to widen the hole in cricothyroid membrane.

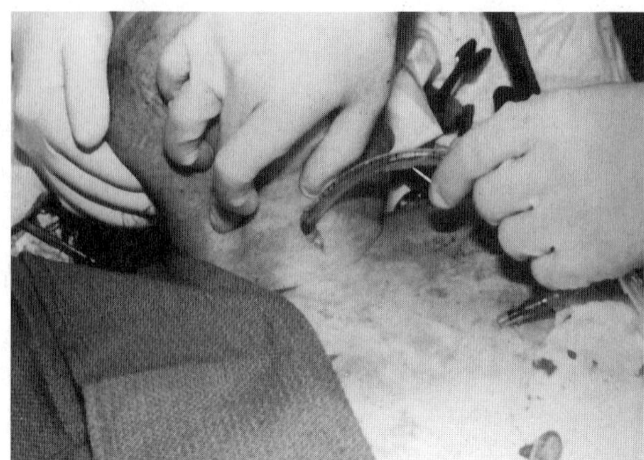

FIG. 16-6. Surgical cricothyroidotomy: endotracheal tube in place.

DRESSING AND STABILIZATION If a tracheostomy tube has been used, a simple dressing may be fashioned by cutting a slit half-way down the middle of a 4-by-4 cm dressing and placing it under the tracheostomy tube. This tube may be secured with a ribbon placed through the phalanges of the tracheostomy tube. For added security, 2-0 nylon sutures may be used to fix the tube to the skin. Endotracheal tubes are extremely difficult to secure properly to the neck and should be changed to tracheostomy tubes whenever possible.

DEVICE REMOVAL The cricothyroidotomy tube may be removed once the patient has a patent airway, or has been changed to a tracheostomy tube, as mentioned above. Patency may be evaluated by deflating the cuff of the tube and assessing airflow by breathing or by speech.

Needle Cricothyroidotomy

Needle cricothyroidotomy entails insertion of a catheter (generally an intravenous catheter) through the cricothyroid membrane. Although this procedure is easier to perform than surgical cricothyroidotomy, it is greatly inferior in providing adequate ventilation. The diameter of the catheter used is the limiting factor for airflow.

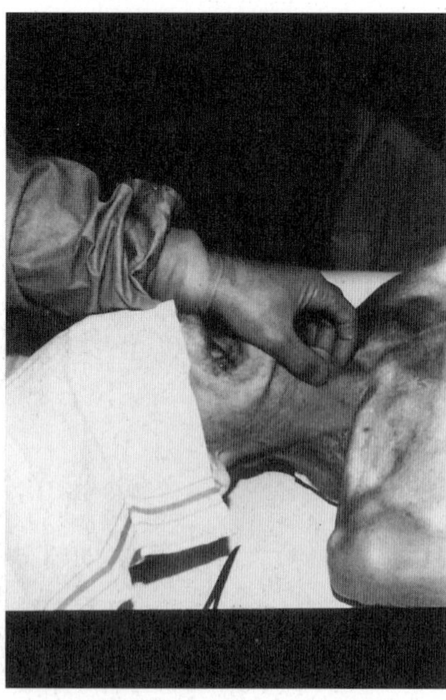

FIG. 16-7. Needle cricothyroidotomy: palpating the cricothyroid membrane.

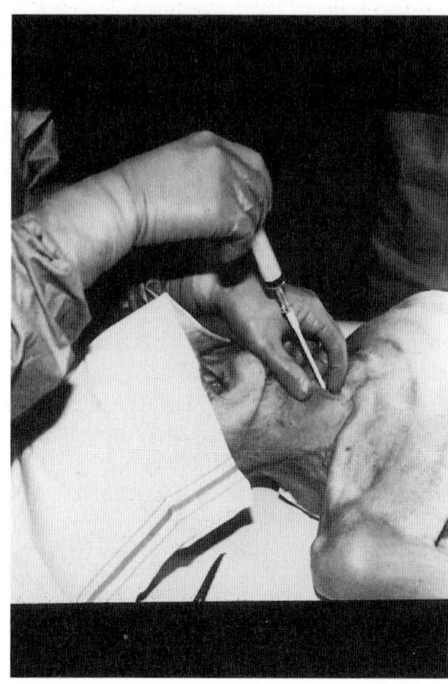

FIG. 16-8. Needle cricothyroidotomy: puncturing the skin with the needle and catheter.

ANATOMY See the discussion under ''Surgical Cricothyroidotomy.''

INDICATIONS AND CONTRAINDICATIONS The general indications are listed under ''Surgical Cricothyroidotomy.'' However, needle cricothyroidotomy is usually deemed the only type of emergency surgical airway that is indicated in children under the age of 12 years. Although generally there are no contraindications to needle cricothyroidotomy, adult patients can be ventilated for only approximately 15 to 20 min and should have an alternative airway secured immediately (by surgical cricothyroidotomy, endotracheal intubation, or tracheostomy).

COMPLICATIONS Complications after needle cricothyroidotomy are less frequent than after surgical cricothyroidotomy. Bleeding at the puncture site and infection may occur. Inadvertent perforation of the esophagus or back wall of the trachea or larynx is infrequent. Massive subcutaneous emphysema will develop during ventilation. The catheter may also be misplaced in the soft tissues of the neck.

EQUIPMENT NEEDED

1. Personal protective equipment
2. A 14- or 12-gauge sheathed needle catheter
3. A 3-mL syringe
4. Adapter from the end of a 7-mm endotracheal tube
5. Wall oxygen source at 15 L/min (40 to 50 lb/in^2) connected by tubing with a Y connector or fashioned with a side hole (a bag-valve-mask device can be substituted but is not optimal)

PATIENT PREPARATION AND POSITIONING See the discussion under ''Surgical Cricothyroidotomy.''

STEPS OF PROCEDURE

1. The operator should be positioned above the head of the patient.
2. Locate the cricoid ring. Place the index finger at the sternal notch and palpate cephalad until the first rigid structure is felt (cricoid

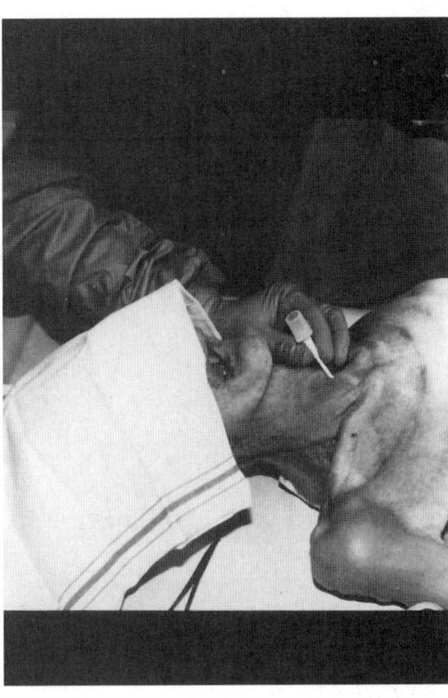

FIG. 16-9. Needle cricothyroidotomy: holding the catheter in place.

ring). Roll the finger one finger breadth above to locate the "hollow" between the cricoid and thyroid cartilages. This is the cricothyroid membrane (Fig. 16-7).

3. Attach a 3-mL syringe to the catheter (12- or 14-gauge).
4. Introduce the catheter into the subcutaneous tissue at a 90° angle to the skin. Aspirate gently while advancing the catheter over the needle. When air suddenly returns (indicating entry into the airway), change the angle to 45°, and advance the catheter over the needle into the larynx. Withdraw the needle and syringe (Figs. 16-8).
5. Disconnect the 3-mL syringe from the bare needle.
6. Withdraw the plunger from the syringe and attach the plungerless 3-mL syringe barrel to the catheter in the neck.
7. Attach the adapter (from the end of a 7-mm endotracheal tube) to the end of the inserted catheter or the open end of the 3-mL syringe (Figs. 16-9 and 16-10), or place a 7-mm endotracheal tube into the empty syringe barrel and inflate the balloon (Fig. 16-11).
8. Attach the oxygen source to the adapter and start ventilation using 100% oxygen. Intermittent jet insuflation (50 lb/in^2) can be achieved by occluding the Y connector or side hole in the connecting tubing. Insuflate 1 s; then release the occlusion for 4 s. To achieve the required high pressures, it is best to use a jet injector regulated by a flowmeter attached to a wall unit on a tank. An unregulated wall unit or tank is a less optimal choice.
9. The operator must hold the catheter in place at all times until a definitive airway is obtained. The catheter is easily displaced with minimal movement. (The inspiration-to-expiration ratio may be as high as 1:10 or 1:15 due to the high resistance to flow. Ventilation will be inadequate, and a definitive airway must be obtained. This is only a temporary airway.)

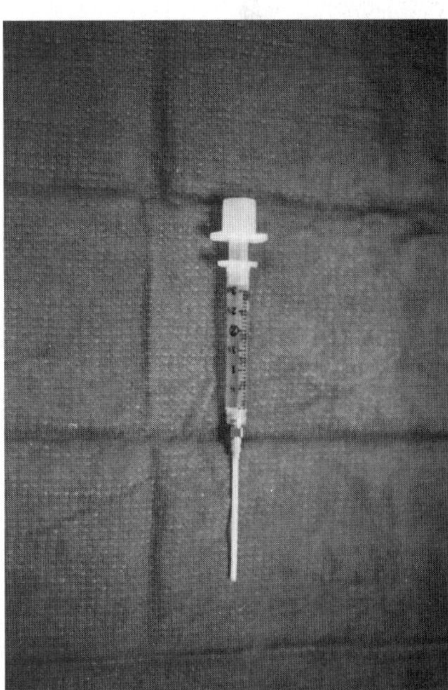

FIG. 16-10. Needle cricothyroidotomy: adapter-syringe-catheter setup.

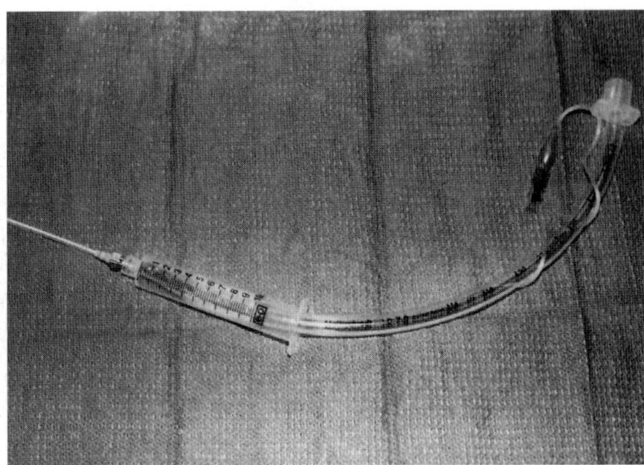

FIG. 16-11. Needle cricothyroidotomy: endotracheal tube-syringe-catheter setup.

DRESSING AND STABILIZATION Stabilization is achieved by the operator until another choice of airway is established, either tracheostomy or oro- or nasotracheal intubation (if possible). Dressings are not necessary.

DEVICE REMOVAL A needle cricothyroidotomy catheter should be removed as expediently as possible. The catheter almost always becomes inadvertently dislodged from the airway, and the ability to ventilate is poor.

REFERENCES

1. Erlandson MJ, Clinton JE, Ruiz E, Cohen J: Cricothyroidotomy in the emergency department revisited. *J Emerg Med* 7:115, 1989.
2. Sise MJ, Shackford SR, Cruickshank JC, et al: Cricothyroidotomy for long-term tracheal access: A prospective analysis of morbidity and mortality in 76 patients. *Am Surg* 200:13, 1984.
3. Grewal H, Rao PM, Mukerji S, Ivantury RR: Management of penetrating laryngotracheal injuries. *Head Neck* 17(6):494, 1995.
4. Esses BA, Jafek BW: Cricothyroidotomy: A decade of experience in Denver. *Ann Otol Rhino Laryngol* 96:519, 1987.
5. Isaacs JH Jr, Pedersen AD: Emergency cricothyroidotomy. *Am Surg* 63:346, 1997.
6. Gleeson MJ, Pearson RC, Armistead S, Yates AK: Voice changes following cricothyroidotomy. *J Laryngol Otol* 98:1015, 1984.
7. Kuriloff DB, Setzen M, Portnoy W, Gadaleta D: Laryngotracheal injury following cricothyroidotomy. *Laryngoscope* 99:125, 1989.
8. Holst M, Hertegard S, Persson A: Vocal dysfunction following cricothyroidotomy: A prospective study. *Laryngoscope* 100:749, 1990.

VASCULAR ACCESS

Bharat B. Sutariya
William A. Berk

Obtaining access to the venous and arterial circulation enables the administration of drug, crystalloid, and blood products and measurement of central venous and arterial pressures. About one-third—or more than 32 million emergency department (ED) patients each year—require vascular access. This chapter discusses indications, techniques, and potential complications of vascular access.

During resuscitation, venous access should be obtained at the site of the largest vein that is accessible without disrupting resuscitation. When peripheral sites are not available, central veins should be accessed for monitoring of central venous pressure or the administration of drugs directly into the central circulation.

VASCULAR ACCESS BY ENDOTRACHEAL TUBE

A number of medications may be administered by endotracheal tube in the critical minutes of resuscitation before intravenous (IV) access is obtained. These include atropine, diazepam, epinephrine, isoproterenol, lidocaine, and naloxone but *not* sodium bicarbonate, calcium chloride, or bretylium. The American Heart Association Advanced Cardiac Life Support (ACLS) and Pediatric Advanced Life Support (PALS) guidelines recommend increasing IV dosages of resuscitation medications by a factor of 2 to 3 with dilution of 3 to 5 mL before administration via endotracheal tube. Epinephrine as a preparation of 1 mg/mL (1:1000) should be given in a dosage of 0.1 mg/kg (standard dosage). Drug administration is followed by several positive-pressure ventilations using a bag-to-tube device.[1]

ISSUES OF FLOW DYNAMICS

Infusion rate is crucial in resuscitation for severe hypovolemia or hemorrhage. Fluid in a medical catheter behaves for practical purposes according to the Poiseuille law:

$$\text{Rate of flow} = \frac{\pi \times (\text{catheter radius})^4 \times \text{pressure gradient}}{8 \times \text{dynamic fluid viscosity}}$$

The fact that flow is a function of the fourth power of the radius of the tube lumen means that the internal catheter diameter is a major limiting factor.[2] A fluid delivery system is only as effective as its slowest component, whether this is intravenous tubing, in-line filters, or the catheter itself. Flow rates may also be affected by pressure and viscosity, the latter being an especially important consideration in relation to red blood cell transfusion. Rate of infusion is also directly proportional to catheter length, which is why a long central catheter will have a slower infusion rate than a shorter catheter of the same caliber in a peripheral vein.[3]

Placement of two large-bore 16-gauge or greater catheters is indicated in stable adult trauma patients whose injuries could cause potentially life-threatening hemorrhage or for initial therapy of medical patients with hypovolemic shock. In the management of exsanguination, an 8.5-Fr catheter with a manually operated pressure bag or a wall-mounted external pneumatic device delivers crystalloid at the rate of almost 1 L/min. A second catheter may be needed for drug infusion. Rapid infusion of larger volumes of fluid should be accompanied by careful monitoring for volume overload, especially in older patients and those with cardiovascular disease.

Volume repletion and measurement of central venous pressure can be accomplished by a Y-arm catheter sheath passed percutaneously into the femoral vein. An 8.5-Fr catheter can then be used for volume repletion, while a smaller catheter can simultaneously be inserted through the other arm of the Y and directed into the right atrium for the measurement of central venous pressure. Femoral catheters should generally be left in place no longer than 48 h, since iliofemoral thrombophlebitis can result. However, with sterile technique and the use of Silastic catheters, the deep femoral system may safely be employed for a longer duration.

Pressure infusion increases flow two to three times above that achieved by gravity alone and is superior to the use of on-line hand-pumped bulbs. Pressure devices are available for the administration of packed red blood cells. Use of a standard urologic Y irrigation set augments flow rates by reducing resistance in the tubing leading to the catheter site. For maximum infusion rates of either blood or crystalloid, use of blood administration tubing eliminates on-line micropore filters, stopcocks, and one-way valves, which increase resistance. Addition of saline to packed red blood cell infusions decreases viscosity, increasing the speed of transfusion.[2]

Volume repletion is effective through IV catheters placed distal to an inflated military antishock trouser (MAST) suit. In patients with abdominal hemorrhage, lines in the legs as well as those in the arms augment volume.

Warming of crystalloid and blood before infusion is essential when volume resuscitation is massive. Crystalloid may be stored in a heating bath or oven, safely microwaved, or warmed with a heating coil or heat packs. Blood warming coils that allow transfusion rates of up to 500 mL/min are now available. Alternatively, cold-packed red blood cells may be warmed by diluting them with an equal amount of warmed saline (up to 60°C); this will also decrease viscosity and thus enhance flow.[2] An in-line microwave blood warmer may be used to heat blood safely to 49°C without any significant increase in hemolysis.[2,4]

VENOUS ACCESS SITES

Peripheral venous catheterization is a routine everyday component of emergency medical practice. The normal human anatomy offers many potential sites for catheterization (Figs. 17-1 and 17-2). The arm veins are associated with an increased risk of phlebitis and are often technically more difficult to access than leg veins. The cephalic vein, in both the forearm and the upper arm, is large, constant, and straight; easily catheterized, it is the time-honored choice for peripheral access in both adults and children. The superficial radial vein at the wrist is well developed in adults, though it is difficult to locate in a small child. Veins of the hand are usually accessible even in obese persons but are short, tortuous, and difficult to stabilize. Veins in the antecubital fossa are excellent in emergency situations, but an armboard is necessary to prevent catheter kinking or dislodgement with movement. This is a relatively uncomfortable position for patients if access is required beyond a few hours. The large basilic vein in the upper arm is usually not visible, but with practice it can be catheterized by palpating the brachial artery and searching ''blindly'' for the medially placed vein. Puncture of the brachial artery is common but rarely of clinical significance if care is taken to prevent hemorrhage or hematoma formation; transitory paresthesias may also occur.

Veins in the legs often require cutdown for catheter placement. The superficial saphenous vein at the ankle is large, constant, and easy to isolate and cannulate. The proximal great saphenous vein in the thigh may be found reliably 5 cm below the inguinal ligament at the junction of the medial and middle third of the thigh in the supine patient. The deep femoral vein is accessible percutaneously, just medial to the femoral artery (Fig. 17-2). In the pulseless patient, the landmark is the junction of the medial and middle third of the inguinal ligament. From the great saphenous and deep femoral veins, advancement of catheters into the right atrium for the measurement of central venous pressure is possible.

Peripheral venous catheterization should not be attempted distally in an extremity involved by cellulitis, burns, or serious injury or when drainage occurs to an area that has sustained an acute serious injury (e.g., the right arm in the presence of a gunshot wound to the right chest). In such situations, the proximal veins may not be patent. Catheterization of arms in the presence of an indwelling fistula or serious neck trauma should also be avoided. Hyperosmolar fluids and agents known to cause chemical phlebitis or sclerosis of peripheral veins should not be infused through such veins.

Internal jugular, subclavian, or femoral vein catheterization is performed when peripheral access is impossible or when the measurement of central venous pressure is desired. The external jugular vein can provide reliable access in both adults and children. Although this vein is readily distended by the Valsalva or Trendelenburg maneuvers, scant subcutaneous support can make it difficult to catheterize. Access to central veins without the risk that attends direct internal jugular and subclavian puncture is a major advantage. In young children, intraosseous infusion provides rapid and reliable access in emergencies. A bone marrow or intraosseous infusion needle placed in the proximal, distal tibial, or distal femoral bone marrow can provide emergency access.

TECHNIQUE FOR PERIPHERAL VENOUS ACCESS

Care must be taken to minimize the risk of local infectious complications, which occur in up to one-third of patients undergoing venous catheterization and may rarely result in septicemia. Insertion of peripheral venous catheters should be preceded by a surgical prep and followed routinely by placement of a sterile dressing. Consideration of the indications for venous access and what constitutes appropriate and adequate access in individual patients will minimize risk and facilitate management of emergencies when they occur. If peripheral veins are small, size and visibility can be enhanced by application of hot, moist compresses for 5 min, by tapping gently on the vein before attempting puncture, or by application of nitroglycerin ointment (0.4% for children less than 1 year old; 2% for others) over an area 1 in. in diameter for 2 min and then wiping off. Once access has been obtained, gentle circumferential occlusive taping may be necessary if stability of the site is tenuous, with the IV line looped and secondarily secured to prevent traction at the point at which the line penetrates the skin. The size of the catheter can usually be determined by the color of the hub; otherwise, it should be written on the tape dressing. When venous access is required primarily for drug administration, consideration should be given to placing a saline or heparin lock. By comparison with adults, obtaining IV access in children is often a challenge. Children tend to be more anxious and thus uncooperative. Generous subcutaneous fat may prevent vessel palpation and direct visualization. Finally, a child's vessels are smaller, and children readily lose body heat, which promotes vasoconstriction.

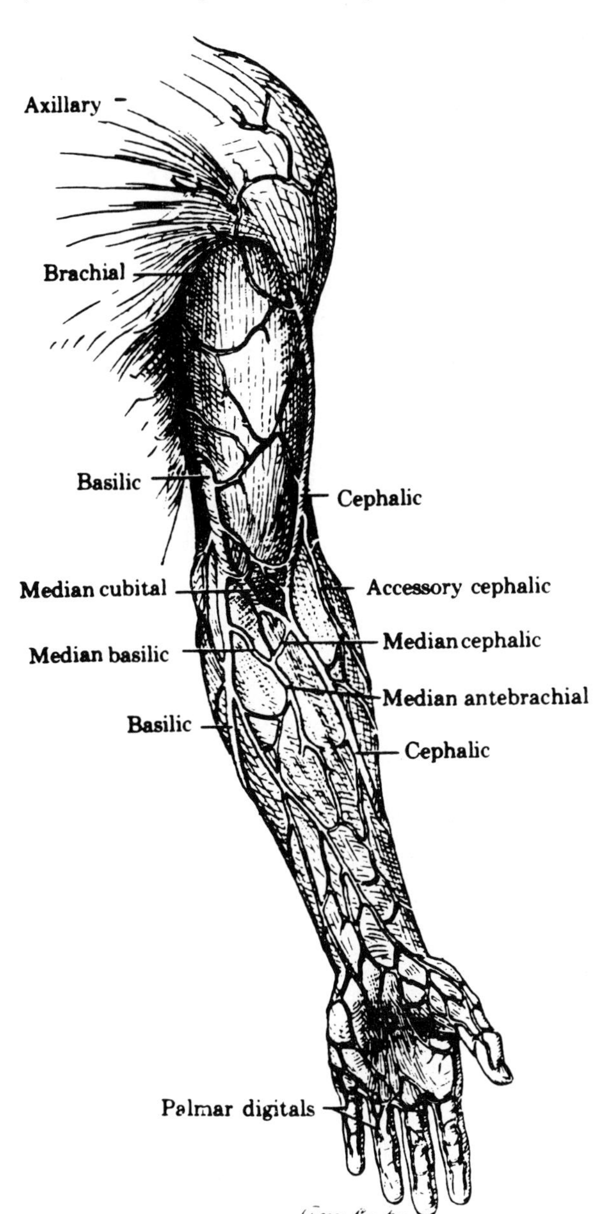

FIG. 17-1. Veins of the upper extremity.

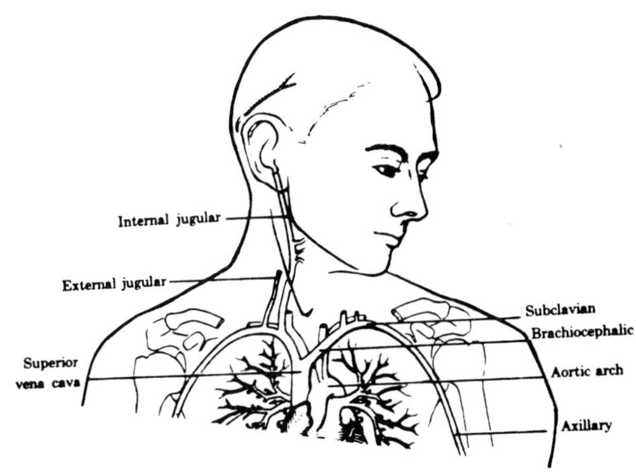

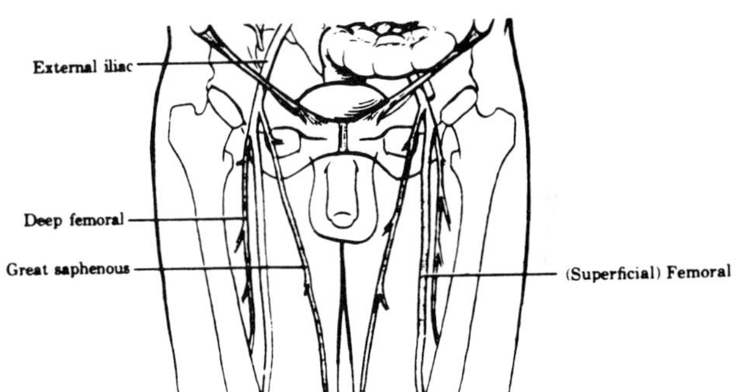

FIG. 17-2. Veins of the torso and lower extremities.

Complications

Complications from placement of peripheral IV lines include hematoma formation, phlebitis, and cellulitis. Phlebitis may occur in up to 75% of hospitalized patients. There is general agreement that catheters should not be left in place for longer than 3 days before replacement. Nerve and tendon damage, deep venous thrombosis, suppurative thrombophlebitis, and septicemia are rare. The unusual event of extravasation of irritative, vasoconstricting, or tissue-toxic substances such as 50% dextrose, epinephrine, phenytoin, and some drugs used for chemotherapy of malignancies may cause problems ranging from minor pain and inflammation to full-thickness sloughing of skin, necessitating skin grafting. In rare situations, reactive arterial vasospasm has led to ischemia and ultimately tissue necrosis in extremities with very distally placed IV lines that may have infiltrated. Catheter-over-needle assemblies are now in common use and provide more stable, reliable access than the steel needles they replaced. Microparticulate matter in IV solutions is removed by in-line micropore filters.

CENTRAL VENOUS PRESSURE CATHETERIZATION AND MONITORING

Central venous catheterization should be performed (1) when rapid delivery of cardiac medications to the coronary circulation is required during cardiopulmonary resuscitation (CPR);[1,5] (2) for access when peripheral veins are inadequate; and (3) when measurement of central venous pressure is desired. Hypovolemic shock by itself is not, however, an indication for central venous catheterization. Many patients who require large-volume infusions or transfusion with multiple units of blood can be managed with large-bore peripheral IVs. Determination of central venous pressure is indicated when (1) massive volume repletion is administered to elderly patients or those with heart disease, (2) fluid administration is being monitored in patients with visceral trauma and severe head injuries, and (3) pericardial tamponade is suspected.

A variety of sites and techniques are available to access the central circulation. Most commonly, a catheter is placed in the upper vena cava via the internal jugular or subclavian vein; less commonly, via the external jugular vein. The femoral vein may also be used, but it requires subsequent immobilization of the leg and the procedure is accompanied by a higher rate of infection and thrombosis. Emergency physicians should become skilled in at least two approaches for central venous catheterization, using one as primary while reserving the other as a backup.

Use of peripheral veins to access the central circulation and measure central venous pressure has the indisputable advantage of avoiding the risk associated with direct puncture of the subclavian and internal jugular veins. However, low flow is inevitable due to the long course of the catheter from the extremity to the superior vena cava. Peripheral sites also fail frequently due to catheter malposition and kinking. In the arm the brachial-basilic system must be used, since catheters in the cephalic system often become kinked in the plexus of veins at the shoulder. Smooth passage and correct tip positioning are more likely if the patient is sitting with his or her head angulated sharply toward the catheterized arm, the arm is held abducted, and the catheter is wire-guided. In emergency situations, however, this time-consuming approach to the central circulation is often impractical. The femoral and axillary veins are safe and reliable alternatives. However, in the presence of cardiac arrest, internal jugular or subclavian lines are highly desirable for drug administration.

Anatomy

A brief review of anatomy is warranted (Figs. 17-1 and 17-3). The major veins of the upper thorax are deeply and centrally placed and well protected by the clavicles, sternum, and strap muscles. The internal jugular veins join the subclavian veins to form the brachiocephalics (innominates), which, in turn, join to become the superior vena cava. The sternocleidomastoid muscle attaches separately by two heads to the sternum and clavicle; the triangle formed by these two heads and the clavicle is just above the internal jugular vein. The right internal

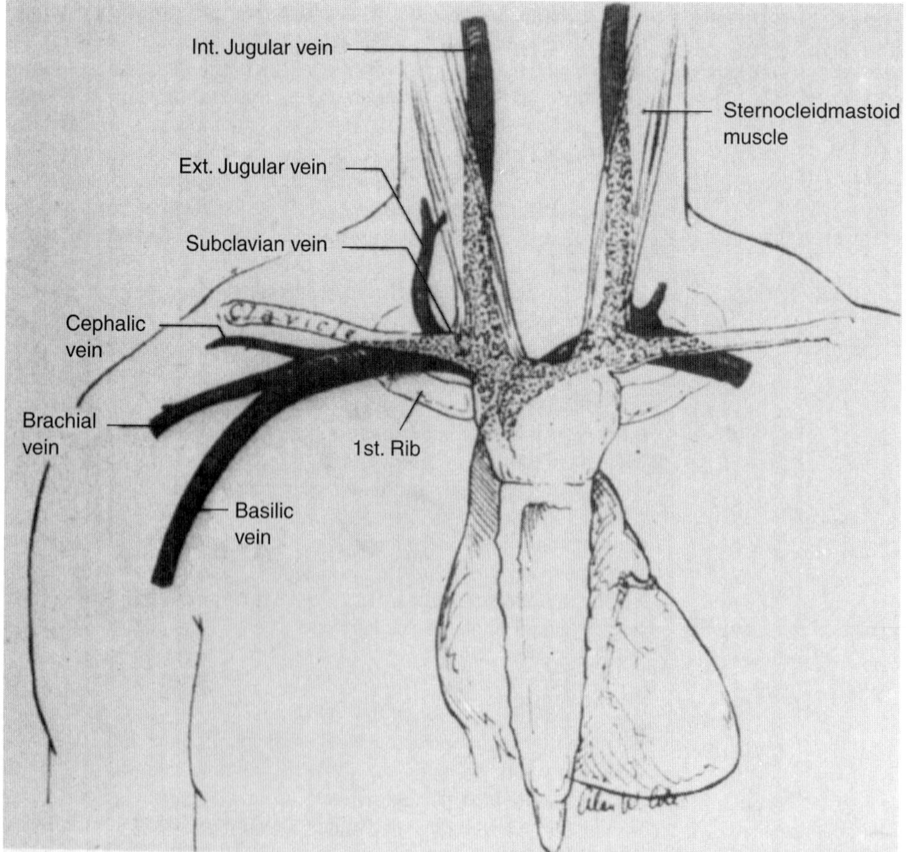

FIG. 17-3. Relationship of major torso veins to other anatomy.

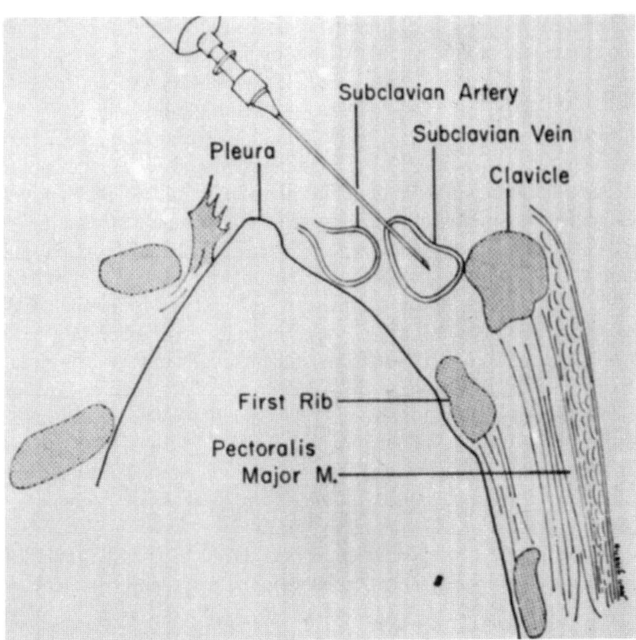

FIG. 17-4. Coronal section through the midclavicle.

jugular has a straight path into the superior vena cava, whereas all the other major tributaries curve. Both external jugular veins enter the subclavian veins at close to right angles. The subclavian veins lie immediately posterior to the junction of the medial and middle thirds of the clavicle and are anterior and inferior to the artery; the pleura are immediately posterior and inferior to the subclavian vessels (Fig. 17-4). The internal jugular vein usually lies anterolateral to the carotid. The basilic and brachial veins join to form the axillary vein. The cephalic vein joins the axillary vein more superiorly, just before it becomes the subclavian vein. The axillary vein continues the distal subclavian vein and runs medial to the axillary artery from the distal arm. The femoral vein is medial to the femoral artery. The relative locations of components of the neurovascular-lymphatic bundle in the groin from lateral to medial can be recalled by the mnemonic NAVEL (nerve, artery, vein, empty space, lymphatic).

Equipment and General Technique for Central Venous Catheterization

All equipment should be at the bedside, including a central venous (CV) pressure manometer if CV pressure monitoring is desired. Catheter-through-needle devices, whose large 14-gauge insertion needles are prone to complications and whose 16-gauge catheters allow maximum gravity-assisted flow of 100 to 150 mL/min, have been largely supplanted by wire-guided (Seldinger) catheters.[6] Their use allows use of a small needle to place any size catheter into a vessel.

The patient should be placed in a neutral to maximum of 30° head rotation and 15° Trendelenburg's position, and the entire route of the neck should be prepped so that all three approaches are possible in case the primary approach fails. The right side is preferred over the left, since (1) the lung apex is slightly lower, (2) there is a straight relationship between the right internal jugular vein and the superior vena cava, and (3) the left-sided thoracic duct cannot be injured. With unilateral chest trauma in the absence of suspected vessel injury, the attempt should be on the injured side in order to protect the uninjured hemithorax in the event of complications from the procedure.

When the procedure is performed electively, preceding the approach for catheter placement with a 22-gauge needle attached to a 5- or 10-mL syringe filled with lidocaine facilitates local anesthesia and allows the operator to "locate" the vein. After landmarks are identified, an 18-gauge needle is then inserted into the vein (Fig. 17-5*A*). Gentle, continuous negative pressure on the syringe should be maintained until free flow of blood is obtained. The syringe is removed and a fingertip is used to occlude the hub before wire insertion (Fig. 17-5*B*). This often forgotten or ignored maneuver is important to prevent aspiration of air, particularly in internal jugular or subclavian vein catheterizations. The needle is then removed (Fig. 17-5*C*), leaving just the wire in the vein. A small skin incision (1 to 2 mm) is often made over the wire (Fig. 17-5*D*) to facilitate smooth entry of the catheter, which is threaded over the wire and into the vein with a twisting motion (Fig. 17-5*E*). The wire is then removed, leaving only the catheter in place (Fig.17- 5*F*). If a large-bore catheter is necessary, the apparatus is used with a venodilator. In this situation, the venodilator is removed with the wire, leaving the large-bore 8.5-Fr catheter sheath in place.

The principal advantages of wire-guided catheters are (1) use of a small (and thus safer) needle for insertion; (2) the step-up capability with a venodilator, allowing for the higher flow rates often required in trauma resuscitation; (3) the flexibility of exchanging standard intravenous catheters, central venous catheters, and Swan-Ganz catheters without repeated stabs; and (4) the use of J wires to access the central circulation from the external jugular vein.

Ultrasound visualization of the central vein while puncture is attempted reduces the number of punctures necessary for cannulation and the time required to establish central access while also reducing the incidence of complications. The technique is particularly helpful when the traditional landmark-based techniques fail or are impractical due to vascular anomalies or body habitus, or when patients with a coagulopathy require central venous access.[7,8]

Complications

The three most common serious complications of direct puncture of a central vein are pneumothorax, arterial puncture, and local infection. With subclavian puncture, the incidence of pneumothorax is 2 to 4

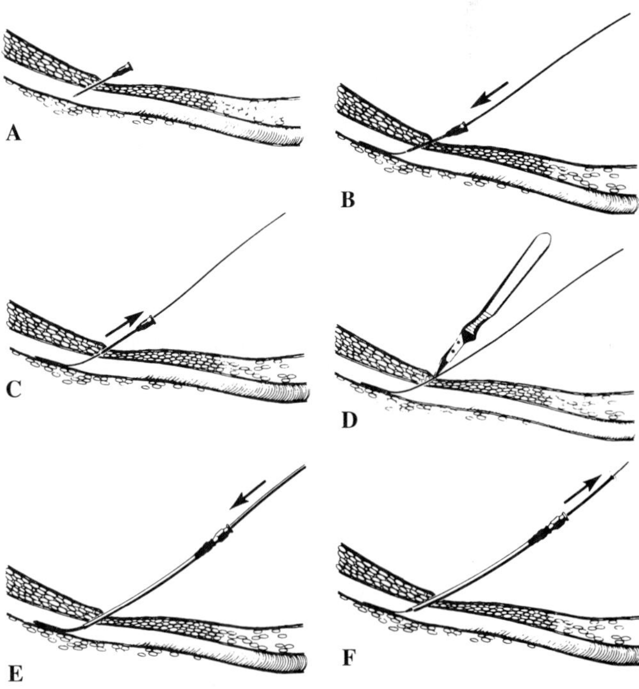

FIG. 17-5. Seldinger technique of catheter insertion (wire-guided). (From Conahan TJ III, Schwartz AJ, Geer RT: Percutaneous catheter introduction: The Seldinger technique. *JAMA* 237:446, 1977. With permission.)

percent, significantly greater than with either internal jugular approach. The incidence of arterial puncture, 3 to 7 percent, is similar for all approaches. In children, success rates for subclavian venous catheterization are higher than for internal jugular venous catheterization and the complication rate is lower. Other, less common complications include hydrothorax, chylothorax (left side), hydromediastinum, air or catheter embolism, thrombosis, dysrhythmia, nerve injuries, osteomyelitis of the clavicle, catheter tip perforation of the superior vena cava (causing hydromediastinum or hydrothorax) or right atrium (causing hydropericardium), knotting with other catheters, and puncture of endotracheal tube cuffs.[9] Care in executing the procedure and in the selection of patients who will benefit from central venous catheterization will minimize the occurrence of complications.

Technique of Commonly Used Approaches

EXTERNAL JUGULAR VEIN The external jugular vein is a superficial, readily accessible vessel that lies in the subcutaneous tissue over the sternocleidomastoid muscle. The vein courses inferior and joins the subclavian vein under the clavicle (Fig. 17-3). Central venous access via this route has an increased success rate (57 to 95%) if a J wire-guided catheter assembly is used. Success is enhanced by introducing the wire through a 16-gauge catheter rather than through a needle, using a J tip with no more than a 3-mm radius, exaggerating head tilt with marked traction on the skin of the neck, and—when initial attempts with wire through needle techniques are met with resistance at the level of the clavicle—twisting the tip of the J wire 180° before making a second attempt. It is also recommended that a small syringe (insulin or TB syringe) be attached to the introducing needle-catheter assembly for both stabilization and to maintain negative pressure. The external jugular vein is very pliable and collapses easily during initial skin puncture. Gently withdrawing the needle back while maintaining suction improves chances of catheterization.

The main disadvantage of the external jugular catheterization is difficulty in securing the catheter in the neck. The venous valves within its course may impede catheter placement as well. The constant movement of the patient makes most external jugular lines short-lived. Also, turning of the neck impedes flow of the infusion, making the line unreliable for fluid or medications unless it is constantly watched.

INTERNAL JUGULAR VEIN There are three traditional approaches to catheterization of the internal jugular vein. The central approach may be the most popular. After the patient is placed in Trendelenburg position, the needle should puncture the skin 1 cm below the apex of a triangle at the midpoint formed by the tendinous and muscular heads of the sternocleidomastoid muscle. The palpation and definition of the margin of the carotid artery is not as important as in the anterior approach but is helpful in locating the vein and to avoid puncture of the artery. Held at a 60° angle with the plane of the skin, the needle is directed slightly lateral to the axis of the body (lateral to the pulsation of carotid artery). Common helpful landmarks for needle direction include the ipsilateral nipple and a plane parallel to the medial border of the lateral head of the sternocleidomastoid muscle. Blood return should be obtained within 3 cm, since the vein is very superficial here. If the attempt fails, the needle should be withdrawn completely before the next attempt.

In the lateral or posterior approach, the head is turned slightly away from the selected side; after the patient is placed in Trendelenburg

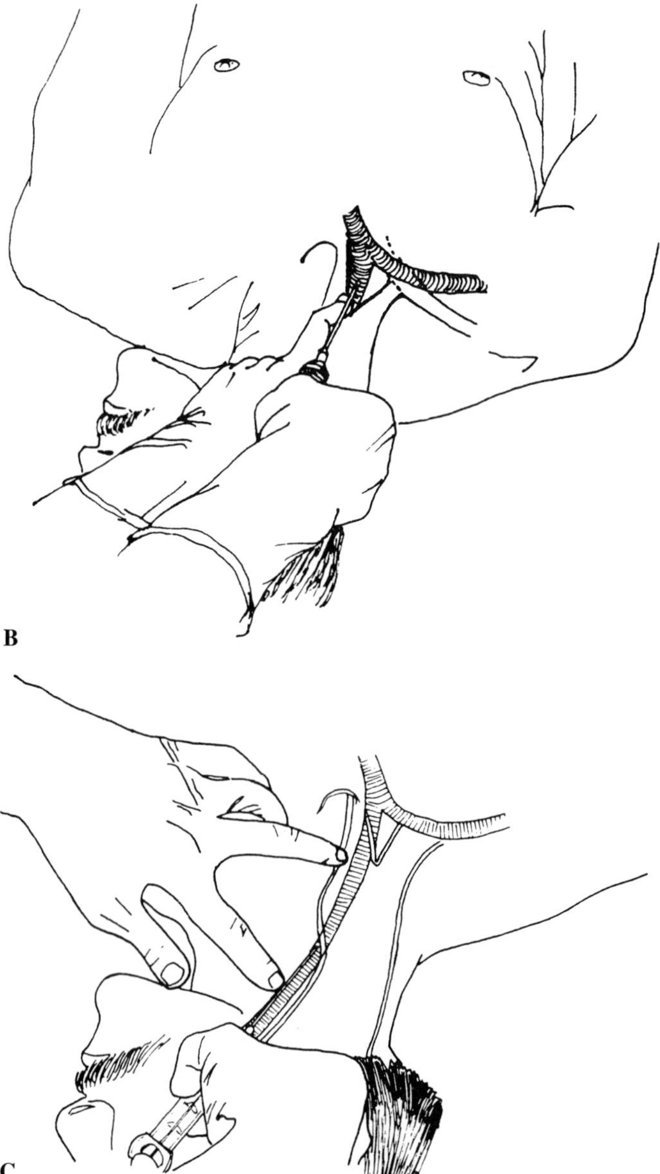

A

FIG. 17-6. **A.** Posterior approach for internal jugular venipuncture. **B.** Central approach. **C.** Anterior approach. (From *Textbook of Advanced Life Support,* 2d ed. Dallas, American Heart Association, 1990, pp 149–150. With permission.)

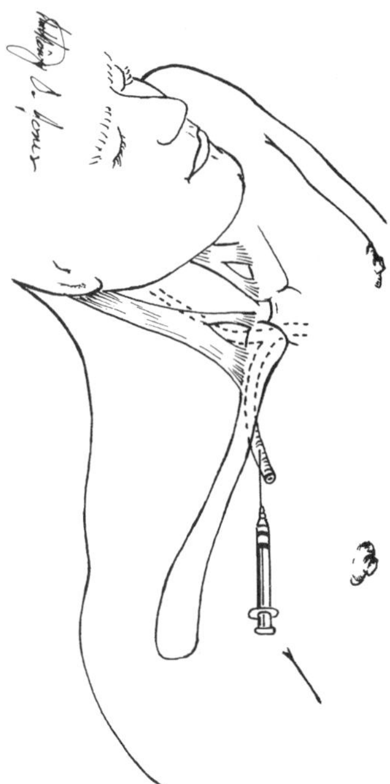

FIG. 17-7. Infraclavicular subclavian venipuncture.

postion, the needle is inserted at the posterior margin and deep to the sternocleidomastoid muscle two to three fingerbreadths above the clavicle and directed toward the suprasternal notch (Fig. 17-6). Frequently, the external jugular vein crosses the lateral wall of the sternocleiomastoid muscle at this point. If it does, the needle should be inserted at the junction of the crossing at a 90° angle to the external jugular vein. Blood should be aspirated within 4 to 5 cm. The carotid artery is just behind this path, albeit slightly posterior, and may be at increased risk for puncture.

The anterior approach and its variants may well be the most technically difficult. After the carotid is identified, the needle is entered at the midpart of the medial border of the sternocleidomastoid. With the fingers over the carotid, the needle is directed 30 to 45° from the midline plane toward the ipsilateral nipple. This approach has the greatest likelihood of carotid puncture and appears to be the least favored of the IV cannulation approaches.

SUBCLAVIAN VEIN The subclavian vein is still the most commonly used site for central venous access. The right side is preferred because the pleural dome is lower on that side. The fact that the point of insertion is in a broad, flat area of the chest makes it ideal for use when central venous access will be required for a prolonged period. The patient is placed in the Trendelenburg position. If the patient is a child, a towel is placed under the thoracic spine. This may also be helpful in some adults.

The *infraclavicular* subclavian approach is the most commonly taught technique. There is no universal agreement on exactly where the needle should enter (Fig. 17-7). The bisection of the middle and medial thirds of the clavicle is an appropriate landmark. Another is a point just lateral and inferior to the junction of the clavicle and first rib. For this latter approach the needle is aimed at the bisection of the junction. Using the former landmark, the skin is penetrated about 1 cm inferior to the clavicle and directed inferomedially. With the index or middle finger of the other hand in the suprasternal notch, the needle is aimed at the superior and most posterior portion of the ipsilateral clavicular head (Fig. 17-7). Inferomedial orientation of the needle bevel facilitates entry of the wire or catheter into the brachiocephalic vein. Vessel entry occurs at a depth of 3 to 4 cm.

For the *supraclavicular* subclavian approach, the patient's head is turned slightly away from the involved side. The needle enters just above the clavicle, 1 cm lateral to the insertion of the clavicular head of the sternocleidomastoid muscle and 1 cm posterior to the clavicle. It is then directed to bisect the angle formed between the sternocleidomastoid and the clavicle, at an angle of 10° above the horizontal, with the tip pointing just caudad to the contralateral nipple. Keeping the bevel up prevents trapping of the wire or catheter against the inferior wall of the vessel. Vessel puncture occurs at a depth of 2 to 3 cm.

FEMORAL VEIN Femoral vein catheterization is used when the vessels of the upper body are not suitable, and when access is required above and below an injury. Although femoral vein catheterization is somewhat easier than subclavian or internal jugular catheterization, the insertion site is difficult to sterilize and keep clean, and patient movement may make it difficult to keep the line secured.

The patient should be supine with the ipsilateral hip in a neutral to slightly externally rotated position. The approximate position of the femoral vein can be determined by dividing the distance between the anterior superior iliac spine and the pubic tubercle into three equal segments (Fig. 17-2). The femoral artery usually lies at the junction of middle and distal thirds. If the femoral pulse is palpable, the needle puncture site should be 1.5 cm medial and 1.5 cm inferior to the inguinal ligament. Once venous blood is obtained, the guide wire is inserted though the needle, the needle is removed, and the catheter is inserted over the wire.

This access can be used for the measurement of central venous pressure, for intravenous pacing, for Swan-Ganz pulmonary artery catheterization, and to administer large volumes of fluids rapidly; the increased risk of infection and thrombosis make it less than ideal as a route for hyperalimentation. It is not an ideal central access site for administration of ACLS medications.

AXILLARY VEIN The axillary vein (Fig. 17-2) is used for central venous access when the femoral, subclavian, and jugular veins are unavailable. This useful technique is unfortunately rarely used by emergency physicians. With practice, the success rate for central access via the axillary vein is similar to that for puncture of the internal jugular or subclavian vein. There is no risk of pneumothorax and the method has the advantage that, when arterial puncture occurs, direct pressure can be applied.

Patients are placed supine with head-down tilt and the arm abducted to 45°. In this position the axillary vein follows a straight course from the arm to the subclavian vein. An insertion point is chosen approximately 2.5 cm inferior to the axillary pulse and lateral to the midclavicular line. The introducer needle is then inserted along a line formed by the insertion point and suprasternal notch, at an angle of 30° to the skin, and directed parallel to the course of the artery toward the chest wall. In children and thin adults, the artery is easily palpable.

VENOUS CUTDOWN

The basilic vein in the antecubital fossa and the saphenous vein in the leg are the most commonly utilized vessels for cutdowns. The basilic vein is located two fingerbreadths above and two fingerbreadths medial to the olecranon. The saphenous vein is just anterior to the malleolus at the ankle and is also accessible in the proximal thigh three fingerbreadths below the midpoint of the inguinal ligament (Fig. 17-8). Although experienced operators may be able to complete the procedure in less than a minute, for most operators 5 or 6 min will be required. In many situations, this implies that cutdown should be resorted to only when percutaneous access has failed or is deemed likely to be unsuccessful.

The operator begins by prepping and anesthetizing the skin. A transverse skin incision is made, and by blunt dissection the subcutaneous tissue is separated until the vein is exposed. Any accompanying

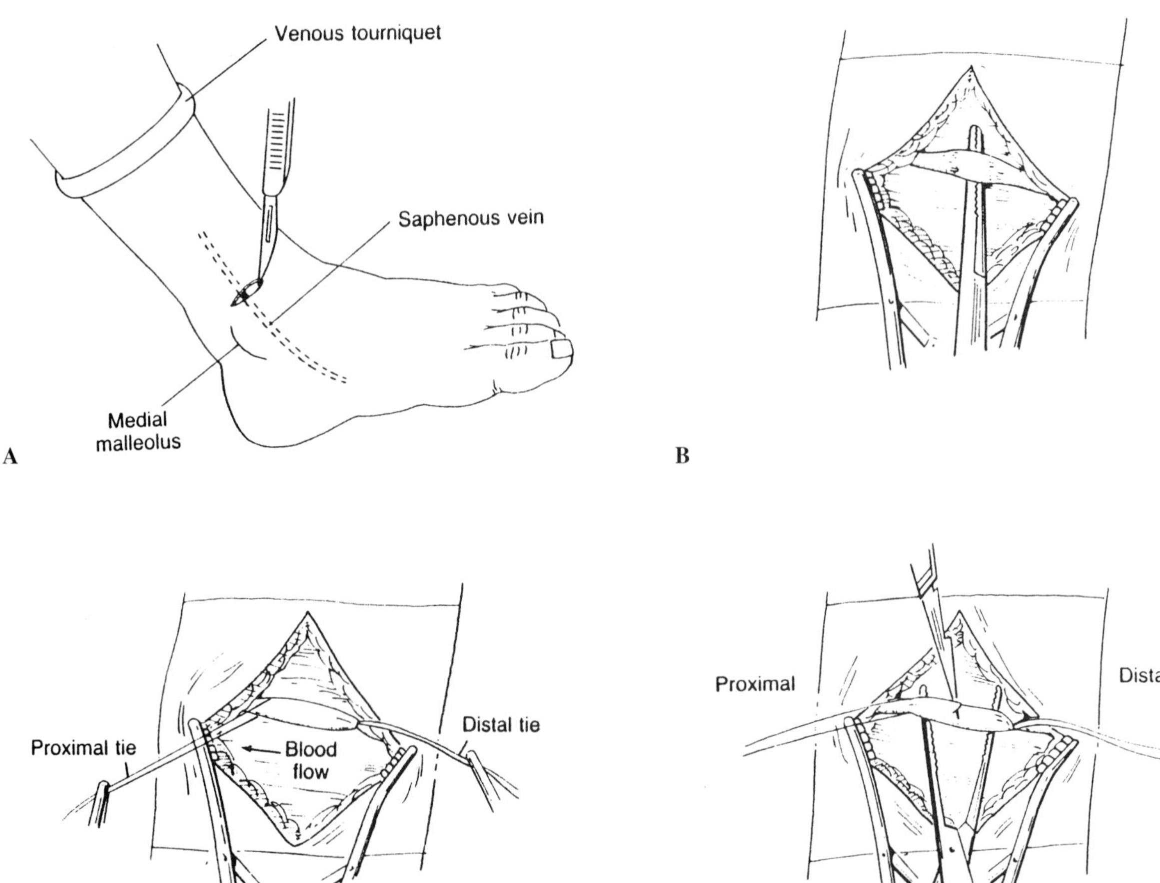

FIG. 17-8. Venous cutdown. **A.** A skin incision is made perpendicular to the course of the vein. **B.** Skin retracted and vein exposed. **C.** Proximal and distal ties are passed under the vein. If the vein is to be sacrificed, the distal suture is tied to prevent bleeding, and the ends are left long to help stabilize the vein during cannulation. The proximal tie is not tied at this point, but traction on it will control back bleeding. **D.** The vein is stretched flat and incised at a 45° angle. Approximately one-third of the lumen must be exposed. Traction on the proximal tie will control back bleeding. (From Roberts JR, Hedges JR: *Clinical Procedures in Emergency Medicine,* 2d ed. Philadelphia, Saunders, 1991, p 321. With permission. Parts B and C first appeared in Vander Salm TJ et al: Atlas of Bedside Procedures. Boston, Little, Brown, 1979.)

artery is identified by slipping a forceps or hemostat under the vessels and applying pressure; pulsatile flow will be evident in the artery. (However, with patients who are in shock, this maneuver may be unsuccessful.) After freeing the vein from the surrounding tissues, two separate sutures are passed beneath the vein, one proximally and one distally. The proximal sutures are left untied, while the distal suture is tied to occlude the vein. The ends of the sutures are kept long so that they can be used for applying traction to the vein. A small incision is made in the vein between the proximal and the distal sutures. (It should not be cut through and through). While applying traction on the vein, the operator inserts the catheter into the vein. Some cutdown kits contain a vein "holder," which may help to prepare the vein to accept a catheter. The proximal suture is tied to secure the catheter in the vein and the skin is closed. Care must be exercised throughout the procedure, since poor technique can result in injury to a tendon or nerve or extensive hemorrhage from soft tissue.

An alternate method of cannulating the vessel is to perform a "mini-cutdown" (Fig. 17-9). In this technique, the vein is fully exposed and an over-the-needle catheter is inserted into the vein under direct visualization. Great care must be taken to avoid through-and-through puncture. The advantage of this technique is that it is easier to perform, especially in young children; and the vessel does not have to be sacrificed. Extensive tissue dissection and complete isolation of the vein are avoided, there is no need to place proximal and distal suture ties, and the catheter can be discontinued with simple pressure at the site.

The potential complications of venous cutdown include infection, phlebitis, and laceration of a nerve or artery.

INTRAOSSEOUS VASCULAR ACCESS

When vascular access cannot be obtained through other sites, intraosseous infusion may be life- or limb-saving. This method of vascular access, usually considered for children, may be used in adults as well. After 5 years of age, however, red marrow is steadily replaced by yellow marrow in the limbs, making infusion more difficult, and decreasing the infusion rate.

For pediatric patients up to 5 years of age, the tibia is the preferred site (Fig. 17-10). In adults, the most commonly used site is the medial malleolus. Although the sternum offers higher infusion rates for adults, this approach is attended by the potentially disastrous complication of puncture into the thoracic cavity. The tibia is technically more difficult in adults than in children because the adult bone is thicker and the needle tends to slip off the bone. Other potential insertion sites include the distal femur, clavicle, humerus, and ileum.

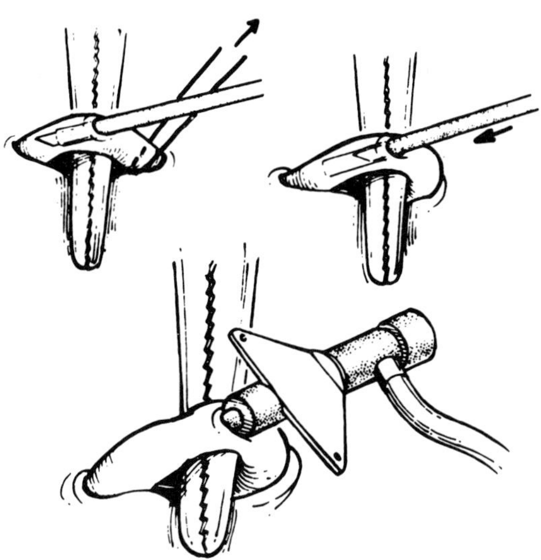

FIG. 17-9. The vessel is elevated with a hemostat and occluded with gentle traction from a distal tie. The needle is inserted and the sheath is advanced into the vessel. The vessel should not be tied off with this techinque.

A word about skeletal vascular anatomy is in order. Arterial supply to bones is by a nutrient artery that pierces the cortex and bifurcates into ascending and descending branches; these further divide into arterioles that pierce the endosteal surface to become capillaries. The capillaries drain into medullary venous sinusoids within the medullary space; these then drain into a central venous channel. Catheter placement in the sinusoids provides ready access to the venous circulation.

Technique

Either standard bone marrow aspiration needles or specialized intraosseous infusion needles must be used because standard intravenous stylets and spinal needles are likely to bend during the procedure. For the proximal tibia, the puncture site is 1 to 2 cm distal to the midpoint between the tibial tuberosity and the medial aspect of the tibia; for the distal tibia, it is the medial surface of the ankle just proximal to the medial malleolus; and for the distal femur, it is the dorsal surface at the point where the condyles join the shaft of the bone. After prepping and anesthetizing skin and periosteum, the operator inserts the needle with the point directed away from the joint space (distally if the site is the proximal tibia, proximally at the other two sites). The needle is grasped in the palm of the hand and directed into the bone using a twisting motion to break through the cortex. Once this has occurred, resistance decreases and crepitus is encountered as the needle enters the marrow cavity. The stylet is then removed and aspiration with a syringe is performed to obtain blood and marrow for confirmation of positioning. If shock is present, aspiration may be unsuccessful; if this is the case, cautious infusion of several milliliters of saline should be attempted with careful observation for extravasation. If there is none, then the needle may be assumed to be positioned in the marrow cavity. A postprocedure x-ray should be performed to rule out the complication of iatrogenic fracture.

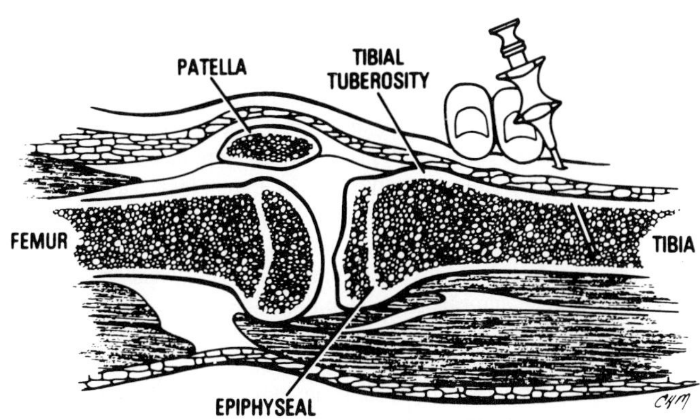

FIG. 17-10. The needle is inserted 2-cm distal to the tibial tuberosity on the medial aspect of the tibia. It is inserted in a caudal direction, away from the joint space.

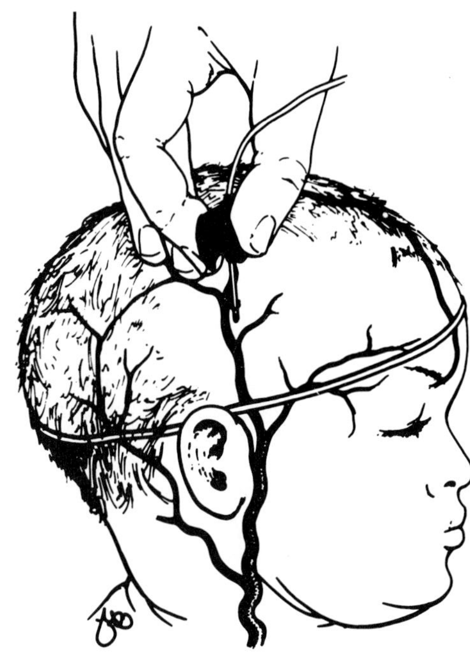

FIG. 17-11. A tourniquet is placed around the infant's head and the needle inserted 0.5 cm from the intended puncture site in the direction of blood flow.

Complications

The incidence of infection, including both cellulitis and osteomyelitis, is less than 1 percent, similar to that for other techniques. The potential for infection can be minimized by limiting the duration of intraosseous infusion and avoiding hypertonic solutions. Fractures of the tibia have been reported. Fat embolism is rare and has been reported only in adult patients. Injury to the growth plate has also been mentioned as a potential complication, but there are no reports of serious morbidity arising from an injury to developing bone.

VASCULAR ACCESS IN CHILDREN

Scalp Vein Access

Scalp veins are easily accessible in children less than 1 year of age and provide a good route for maintenance fluid and drug administration (Fig. 17-11). The superficial temporal, posterior auricular, and supratrochlear veins are the most easily catheterized scalp veins. In all cases, the vein must be differentiated from its respective artery. Arteries are generally more tortuous; they pulsate, and they fill from below, whereas veins fill from above.

The operator begins by shaving and prepping an area large enough to secure butterfly needle wings. A rubber-band tourniquet is placed around the head proximal to the venipuncture site and a butterfly needle—usually 23 to 27 gauge—is advanced into the vein. The needle is then taped at the skin entry point and at the butterfly with cotton support under the wings. A cover (medicine cup) may be used to protect the area. Complications from this procedure include infection, bleeding, extravasation of fluid or medications, and inadvertent arterial puncture.

Umbilical Vein Access

In the first 1 to 2 weeks after birth, the umbilical vessels offer easy central venous access. Even a severely dehydrated umbilical stump may yield good vessels with adequate preparation. In a normal infant, there are two small umbilical arteries and a single larger vein. The arteries arise from the internal iliac artery while the vein is continuous with the portal vein.

The operator begins by cleansing the cord. A transverse cut is made 1 cm above the junction of skin and cord, at which point a purse-string suture is placed. The single large vein and two smaller arteries are identified. A 3.5- to 5.0-Fr catheter is inserted into the vein and advanced to 4 to 5 cm in a term infant; further advancement may cause liver damage. The catheter should be filled with saline solution and flushed properly prior to placement to ensure an air-free system.

The most common complications relate to vascular insufficiency induced by the catheter. Evidence of ischemia—such necrotic enterocolitis, liver necrosis, poor peripheral circulation, or abdominal distention—is an indication for immediate removal of the catheter. The potential for infectious complications is equivalent to that for other indwelling catheters.

ARTERIAL ACCESS

Arterial cannulation should be performed when emergency physicians are managing patients with conditions requiring arterial pressure monitoring or repeated arterial blood sampling—for example, hypertensive crisis, cardiogenic shock, and respiratory failure. Although the radial artery is the most frequently employed site, extensive experience using the brachial, femoral, and dorsalis pedis arteries has shown them to be equally satisfactory. In infants and neonates, the temporal or umbilical and dorsalis pedis arteries are most often accessed, although radial artery cannulation is also acceptable. While many operators are most familiar with the radial artery site, use of the femoral artery leaves the arm clear for other procedures and, in the presence of shock, the femoral artery is less difficult to cannulate percutaneously.

Assessment and Complications

Although catheterization of the radial artery is associated with up to a 20 percent incidence of temporary flow obstruction by Doppler study, permanent ischemic complications requiring surgical reanastomosis or amputation are quite rare. Confirmation of collateral flow through a patent ulnar artery can be obtained by performing the Allen test: while the patient clenches the wrist for 1 min the examiner compresses the radial and ulnar vessels with thumb and forefinger.[10] On release of ulnar compression, the patient partially extends the fingers, which are observed for rubor accentuated in comparison to the untested side. Patent ulnar circulation is indicated by return of rubor within 7 s; an equivocal result is 7 to 14 s. Greater than 14 s is considered definitely abnormal. If ulnar cannulation is contemplated, patency of the radial artery can be tested by the same test, with release of that vessel following compression. Percutaneous cannulation of the brachial or femoral arteries may be possible when the radial pulse is absent in a hypotensive patient. The technique is similar to radial artery cannulation, although a careful groin prep, preceded by removal of hair at that site to minimize the risk of infection, is necessary. With profound hypotension, cutdown to the radial artery may be required to cannulate the artery. This is performed through a transverse incision, with the artery punctured by utilizing a technique identical to the percutaneous approach, only under direct vision. The wound should be sutured and the catheter affixed with a silk suture. Serious complications—infection and occlusion—are most closely related to duration of cannulation and are much more common among critically ill patients than among those undergoing monitoring as an adjunct to a surgical procedure. During a typical stay in an intensive care unit, the incidence of local infection can be expected to approach 20 percent, while that of generalized sepsis from primary catheter infection is 4 percent, with little site-dependent variation. Other complications include hematoma formation and hemorrhage requiring transfusion.

Technique

The patient's nondominant extremity should be selected for radial artery cannulation. The wrist is placed in mild extension by placing a roll of gauze behind it and taping it to a splint. A sterile prep is applied and the operative area draped. Local infiltration should be performed with a small amount of lidocaine so that the pulse is not obscured. While a 20- or 22-gauge 1.25-in. Teflon catheter over a needle is held in one hand, the radial pulse is palpated with the other. The skin over the radial aspect of the wrist is punctured with the needle pointing proximally and at a 45° angle with the plane of the skin. The needle is advanced into the artery until pulsations appear. The catheter is then slid off the needle into the artery. If pulsatile flow ceases, the catheter may be withdrawn until arterial flow again appears, and a second attempt may be made to advance the catheter. If this is unsuccessful, the procedure must be repeated. After each attempt, care should be taken to apply pressure to the site long enough to prevent hematoma formation. Once in the artery, the catheter is connected to the monitoring system and flushed through a three-way stopcock with a sterile cap. The catheter should then be secured to the skin at its hub using silk or nylon suture. Kits are available for wire-guided arterial catheterization.

If cutdown is necessary to achieve arterial puncture, exposure of the artery is performed in a manner similar to that outlined for venous cutdown above. When 1 cm of artery is visible, the vessel is isolated by passing two lengths of silk suture beneath it, using a hemostat. A catheter through needle device is passed through the skin distal to the area of exposure and advanced into the site. The artery may then be punctured and the catheter advanced. The suture, which is used only to control the artery, may then be removed and the skin incision closed.

SPECIAL PROBLEMS RELATED TO VENOUS ACCESS

Complications of Total Parenteral Nutrition

Central venous catheter placement for total parenteral nutrition (TPN) may be done short-term as a part of hospital care or long-term at home or in extended-care facilities. TPN is usually administered through a catheter placed into either the subclavian or jugular vein. The incidence of mechanical and septic complications depends upon the skill, experience, and commitment of both the patient and the nutrition support team.[11] Suspicion of line sepsis demands immediate consultation. Most patients should be admitted, although the catheter may not need to be removed in selected cases.

Catheter occlusions occur in approximately 5 percent of patients receiving long-term TPN. If the first-line remedy of flushing the catheter with normal saline or heparin solution fails, thrombolytic agents, such as urokinase, may be used to lyse clots that obstruct the lumen of catheter without obstructing the vessel. The recommended dose of urokinase ranges from 5000 to 15,000 IU, depending on the type of intravascular device and its filling volume. A syringe with 1 to 2 mL of urokinase solution is instilled into the catheter, which is then clamped for 30 min. If no blood return is achieved, the maneuver may be repeated, with urokinase left in the catheter for 60 min. If there is still no return, then a third attempt may be made, this time leaving the urokinase solution in place for 12 h. Failure to clear the catheter after 12 h suggests either organized thrombus or anatomic abnormality; further diagnostic study such as angiography and ultrasound-Doppler duplex scanning may be indicated. Some authors have reported high success rates infusing ethanol (up to 3 mL of 70% solution) for presumed lipid occlusions or hydrochloric acid (HCl, 0.1N, up to 3 mL) to clear presumed mineral oil or other precipitates.

Catheter-related sepsis in patients receiving TPN is usually a result of catheter contamination by organisms colonizing the skin. Gram-negative bacteremia, sepsis syndrome, and fungemia are treated by removal of catheter in association with appropriate antimicrobial therapy. Gram-positive infections can often be managed with the catheter left in place while antibiotic therapy is administered. The delivery of TPN through peripherally inserted central catheters (PICCs) is associated with slightly lower infection rates but a higher rate of mechanical failure. Because there is a considerably increased risk of both infection and thrombosis when femoral lines are used for TPN, this mode of access is less than optimal for patients requiring parenteral nutrition. Other reported complications include pulmonary embolism, line fracture, embolized catheter fragment, mediastinitis, superior vena cava syndrome, pneumothorax, air embolism, and lymphatic duct injury.

Accessing Indwelling Catheters

It is increasingly common for patients to present to EDs with specialized devices, such as Hickman catheters, which have been placed to provide long-term IV access. Such devices facilitate outpatient treatment in an era of increasing cost-consciousness. Emergency physicians can access these devices to obtain specimens for laboratory study as well as to administer IV fluids and medications.

When indwelling catheters are accessed, meticulous care should be taken to maintain sterility at the site. Depending on the type of device (implanted versus externalized), specialized equipment may be required to obtain access. Five milliliters of either normal saline or heparin flush (100 U/mL) is injected and then withdrawn gently to ensure catheter patency. Blood for laboratory study is collected only after a dead-space volume (5 to 10 mL) has been collected and discarded. Since these devices are heparinized, coagulation studies performed on such samples are unreliable; blood for these studies should be obtained from other sites. After access has been terminated, implanted devices should be flushed with heparin solution of 1000 U/mL strength. Other externalized devices should be flushed using a solution of 100 U/mL strength.

Arteriovenous fistulas and shunts should be used only for access in the most extreme of emergency situations, since complications, including loss of the access site, are common. The smallest needle appropriate to the task at hand should be inserted. Afterward, local pressure should be applied for 5 min or more, and these arterialized sites should be carefully monitored for hemorrhage for 12 h.

REFERENCES

1. Gonzalez ER: Pharmacologic controversies in CPR. *Ann Emerg Med* 22:317, 1993.
2. Floccore DJ, Kelen GD, Altman NJ, et al: Rapid infusion of additive red blood cells: Alternative techniques for massive hemorrhage. *Ann Emerg Med* 19:129, 1990.
3. Dutky PA, Stevens SL, Maull KI: Factors affecting rapid fluid resuscitation with large bore intravenous catheters. *J Trauma* 29:856, 1989.
4. Herron DM, Grabowy R, et al: The limits of bloodwarming: maximally heating blood with an inline microwave bloodwarmer. *J Trauma* 43:219, 1997.
5. Hedges JR, Barsan WB, Doan LA, et al: Central versus peripheral intravenous routes in cardiopulmonary resuscitation. *Ann J Emerg Med* 2:385, 1984.
6. Conahan TJ, Schwartz AJ, Geer RT: Percutaneous catheter introduction: The Seldinger technique. *JAMA* 237:446, 1977.
7. Gilbert TB, Seneff MG, Becker RB: Facilitation of internal jugular venous cannulation using an audio-guided Doppler ultrasound vascular access device: Results from a prospective, dual-center, randomized, crossover clinical study. *Crit Care Med* 23:60, 1995.
8. Slama M, Novara A, Safavian A, et al: Improvement of internal jugular vein cannulation using an ultrasound-guided technique. *Intens Care Med* 23:916, 1997.
9. Snazajder JI, Zveibil FR, Bitterman H, et al: Central vein catheterization: Failure and complication rates by three percutaneous approaches. *Arch Intern Med* 146:259, 1986.
10. Allen EV: Thromboangiitis obliterans: Methods of diagnosis of chronic occlusive arterial lesions distal to the wrist with illustrative cases. *Am J Med Sci* 178:237, 1929.
11. Savage AP, Picard M, Hopkins CC, Malt RA: Complications and survival of multilumen central venous catheters used for total parenteral nutrition. *Br J Surg* 80:1287, 1993.

18 INVASIVE MONITORING, PACING TECHNIQUES, AND AUTOMATIC AND IMPLANTABLE DEFIBRILLATORS

Edward S. Bessman

During critical resuscitations the emergency physician may be called upon to institute invasive pressure monitoring or to use emergency pacing techniques. Emergency physicians must also be familiar with the relevant aspects of automatic external defibrillators and implantable cardioverter defibrillators. This chapter reviews these technologies as applied to emergency cardiac care.

INVASIVE MONITORING TECHNIQUES

General Considerations

Invasive pressure monitoring should never be the initial step in resuscitation. When clinically indicated, arterial line or pulmonary artery catheter (PAC) placement may be considered after initial stabilization is completed. If possible, these procedures should be deferred until the patient reaches the more controlled environment of the intensive care unit, unless there will be a significant delay.

The two essential components of any pressure monitoring system are a properly placed and secured catheter and a functioning pressure transducer-monitor. Ideally, the transducer and line for pressure monitoring should be set up and ready for use prior to the patient's arrival in the emergency department. Examples of transducer systems are illustrated in Fig. 18-1.

Arterial Cannulation

Arterial lines offer several advantages over monitoring blood pressure with an arm cuff. The arterial line provides continuous measurement of blood pressure and can be used for easy sequential sampling of blood gases. In the setting of marked vasoconstriction or hypotension, the arterial line usually gives more accurate pressure readings than a blood pressure cuff. The American College of Cardiology/American Heart Association practice guidelines for patients with acute myocar-

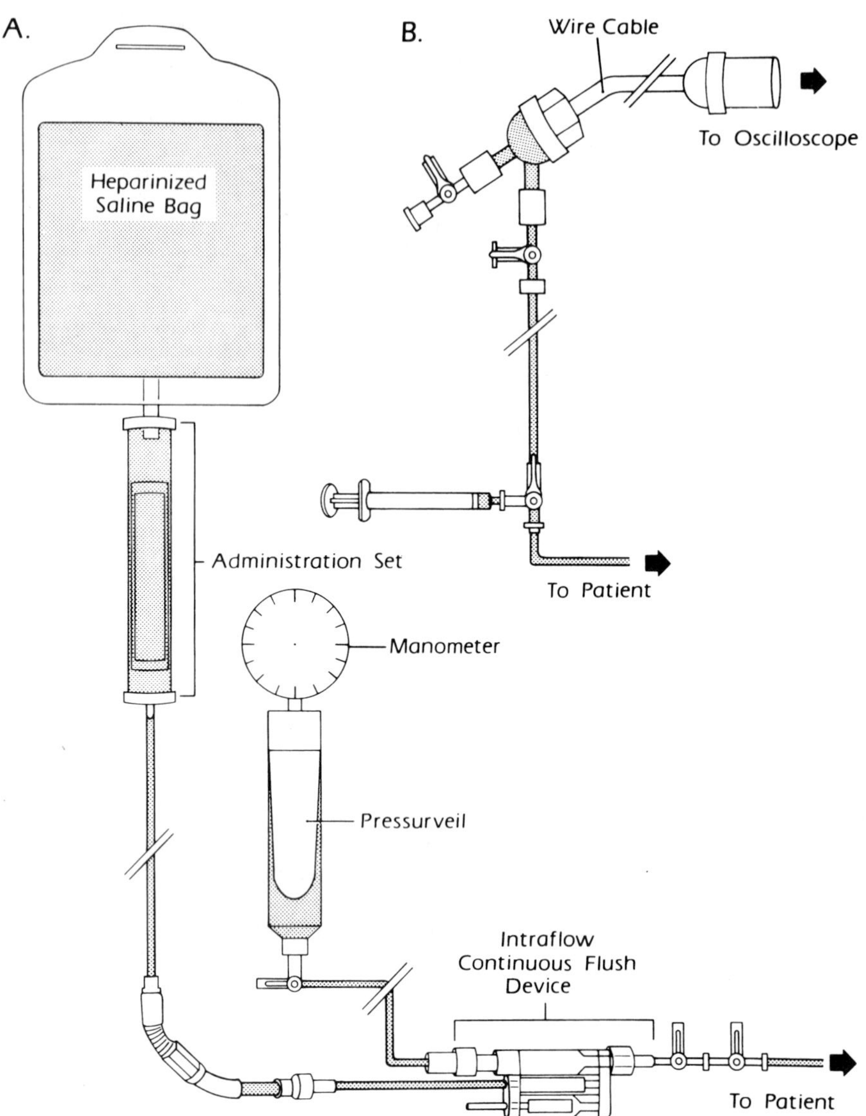

FIG. 18-1. Arterial pressure monitoring systems. **A.** Systems for continuous flush with heparinized saline solution connected to a mechanical pressure transducer. **B.** System for manual flush. Either system can be used with an electronic pressure transducer, shown in **B.** The pressure done should be maintained at the level of the patient's heart. [From Beal JM (ed): *Critical Care for Surgical Patients.* New York, Macmillan, 1982. Used by permission.]

dial infarction recommend intraarterial pressure monitoring for patients with severe hypotension or cardiogenic shock or who are receiving potent vasoactive infusions.[1] Other appropriate scenarios include hypertensive crisis, hypothermic cardiac arrest, and prolonged emergency department resuscitation.

The radial and femoral arteries are readily accessible for rapid cannulation. Percutaneous puncture is preferred. In hypotensive patients it may be easier to cannulate the femoral artery (because it is a larger vessel with constant landmarks) than the radial artery. Cutdown on the radial artery is an alternative in such patients. It is prudent to document the result of Allen's test for ulnar artery patency prior to radial arterial line placement, although its accuracy is questionable.[2] If the test result is positive, another site should be considered, but if that is not practical, then the clinician may have to proceed with radial artery cannulation.[3]

Landmarks for radial and femoral artery cannulation are shown in Fig. 18-2. The catheter (usually 20 gauge, 2 in long for radial cannulation and 18 gauge, 4 in long for femoral cannulation) can be introduced by direct puncture threaded over the needle or by Seldinger technique threaded over a guidewire. Freely flowing, pulsatile, bright-red blood indicates proper placement. With marked hypotension or hypoxia, arterial blood flow may be mistaken for venous (nonpulsatile, dark blood returned). In all cases, connection to the transducer should reveal an arterial waveform if the catheter is in the proper position. Failure to visualize a waveform can be due to venous placement, air in the line, a closed stopcock, or a malfunction in the transducer or monitor.

The complication rate for either radial or femoral artery cannulation is about 7 percent.[4] These include local hematoma and hemorrhage; both can usually be controlled with a pressure dressing. Arterial occlusion, thrombosis, or embolization with distal ischemia may occur; they are associated with placement in smaller vessels or in atherosclerotic vessels, with prolonged catheterization, and with use of end arteries that supply areas with poor collateral circulation. Sepsis may result from local infection at the insertion site. Using the femoral or radial site can minimize these complications, along with proper attention to sterile technique and removal of the line as soon as feasible after the patient is stabilized.[1]

Pulmonary Artery Cannulation

A PAC is helpful in the measurement of critically ill patients with hemodynamic instability, particularly in the setting of acute myocardial infarction. Most important, the PAC can help to differentiate between shock due to intravascular volume depletion and that due to extensive left ventricular (LV) dysfunction. When the balloon tip of a PAC is properly wedged in a branch of the pulmonary artery, the pressure sensed by the catheter corresponds approximately to that in the left atrium. Left atrial pressure (which equals LV filling pressure) is an

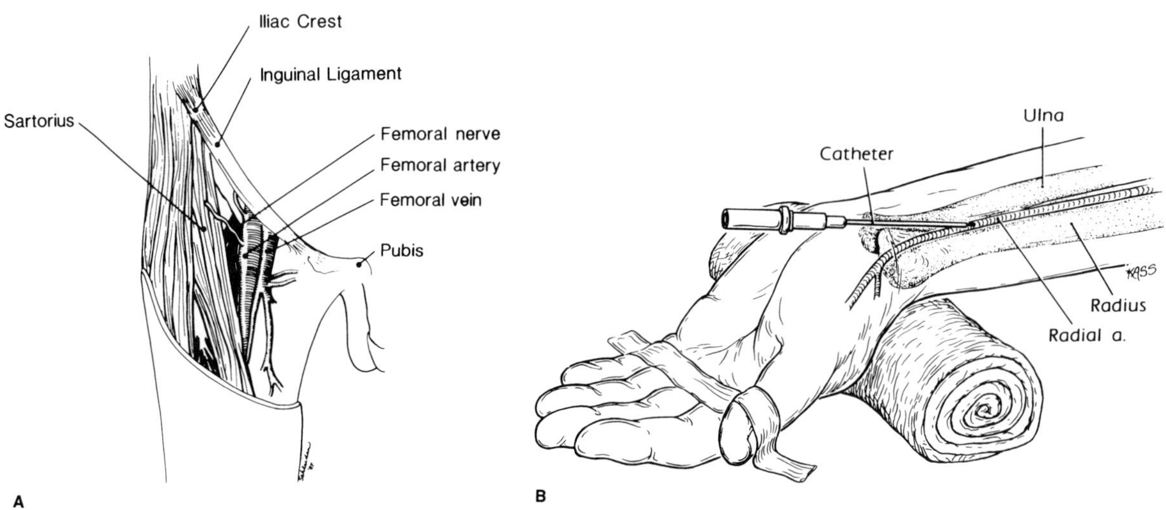

FIG. 18-2. Anatomic landmarks for arterial line placement. **A.** Femoral triangle. Note that the femoral artery lies lateral to the vein and midway between the pubis and the iliac crest. **B.** Radial aspect of the wrist. Note that mild extension of the wrist aids in successful placement. [From Beal JM (ed): *Critical Care for Surgical Patients.* New York, Macmillan, 1982. Used by permission.]

excellent indication of the adequacy of fluid resuscitation. If this pressure is low (<12 mmHg), additional fluid resuscitation is indicated. If this pressure is high (>20 mmHg), additional fluids are unlikely to improve cardiac performance; instead diuresis, afterload reduction, inotropic support, or vasopressors should be considered. Although the PAC can yield useful diagnostic information (Tables 18-1 and 18-2), the distinction between the need for more fluids and the need for more LV support is its most useful application during resuscitation.[1] Volume assessment via central venous pressure monitoring is less reliable than PAC, especially in the presence of valvular or pulmonary disease.

A standard PAC is shown in Fig 18-3. The catheter has two fluid paths, one that terminates at the tip (the distal port) and a second that opens 10 to 15 cm from the tip (the proximal port). A third lumen connects to a 1.5-mL balloon located at the tip of the catheter. When inflated during insertion, the balloon surrounds the tip of the PAC to prevent it from causing injury to the heart or great vessels as well as to help float the catheter through the heart as it is advanced. A temperature sensor is located about 5 cm proximal to the catheter tip and can be used to measure cardiac output via the thermodilution technique.

The procedure for insertion is described in detail elsewhere[5] but briefly is as follows. After central venous access is secured (see Chap. 17, "Vascular Access") the PAC, which has already been attached to a monitor and a pressure transducer, is slowly advanced through the introducer sheath. Once the tip of the catheter enters the vein, the balloon is inflated. By observing the pressure waveform transmitted via the distal port, the operator can follow the progress of the catheter through the heart and, ultimately, into a branch of the pulmonary artery (Fig. 18-4). Fluoroscopy is helpful to ensure quick and proper placement but rarely is available in the emergency department.

With the PAC in position, the clinician can occlude the branch pulmonary artery by inflating the balloon and wedging it in the artery. This gives the pulmonary artery occlusion pressure, or, as it is more commonly known, the pulmonary capillary wedge pressure, which best reflects the pressure in the pulmonary capillary bed and the left atrium. The clinician can also rapidly measure pulmonary artery pressure, cardiac output, and central venous pressure. These measurements, when combined with arterial pressure measurement, enable the clinician to calculate systemic vascular resistance. These parameters are useful in the diagnosis and treatment of various shock states and in guiding therapy in acute myocardial infarction (Tables 18-1 and 18-2).

As with arterial cannulation, therapeutic procedures or definitive care should not be delayed solely to allow PAC placement. Complications include all the complications of central venous line placement (Chap. 17). In addition, cardiac dysrhythmias and right bundle branch block may occur as the catheter traverses the heart. Other potential complications include pulmonary embolism or infarction, knotting of the catheter, infection, and rupture of a small branch of the pulmonary artery.

The safety of PACs in the critical care environment has been questioned recently because of an association between its use and

TABLE 18-1 Hemodynamic Diagnosis of Shock States

Type of Shock	CO	PCWP	SVR
Cardiogenic	↓	↑	↑
Hypovolemic	↓	↓	↑
Septic	↓ or ↑	↓	↓
Neurogenic	↑	↓	↓
Anaphylactic	↓	↓	↓

Abbreviations: CO, cardiac output; PCWP, pulmonary capillary wedge pressure; SVR, systemic vascular resistance; ↑, increased; ↓, decreased.

TABLE 18-2 Hemodynamic Subsets in Acute Myocardial Infarction

Cardiac index, (L/min)/m²		<18 PCWP	>18 PCWP
	>2	I	II
	<2	III	IV

Note: Initial therapy and prognosis can be determined by class. Mortality rates by class are 1%, 11%, 18%, and 60% for classes I–IV, respectively. Patients in class I require supportive care only. Patients in class II require treatment for pulmonary edema due to lower pulmonary capillary wedge pressure. Patients in class III may improve with fluid administration. Patients in class IV require maximal circulatory support for cardiogenic shock.
Abbreviation: PCWP, pulmonary capillary wedge pressure.

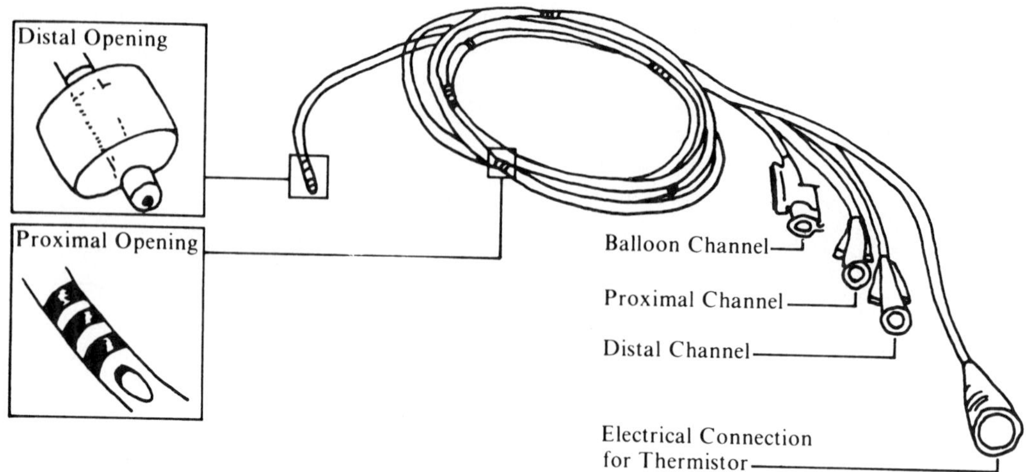

FIG. 18-3. Pulmonary artery thermodilution catheter. [From Beal JM (ed): *Critical Care for Surgical Patients.* New York, Macmillan, 1982. Used by permission.]

increased mortality rates.[6] Current consensus favors the continued use of PACs[1] but underscores the need for definitive investigation.[7] Thus, the appropriateness of PAC insertion in the emergency department setting for a given patient must be weighed carefully. The advent of newer techniques, such as transesophageal echocardiography,[8,9] transthoracic impedance cardiography,[10] and magnetic resonance velocimetry[11] may further reduce the role of PACs in the emergency department.

EMERGENCY PACING TECHNIQUES

General Considerations

Emergency cardiac pacing may be instituted either prophylactically or therapeutically. Prophylactic indications include those situations where there is high risk of atrioventricular block. Therapeutic indications include symptomatic bradyarrhythmias, asystole, and overdrive

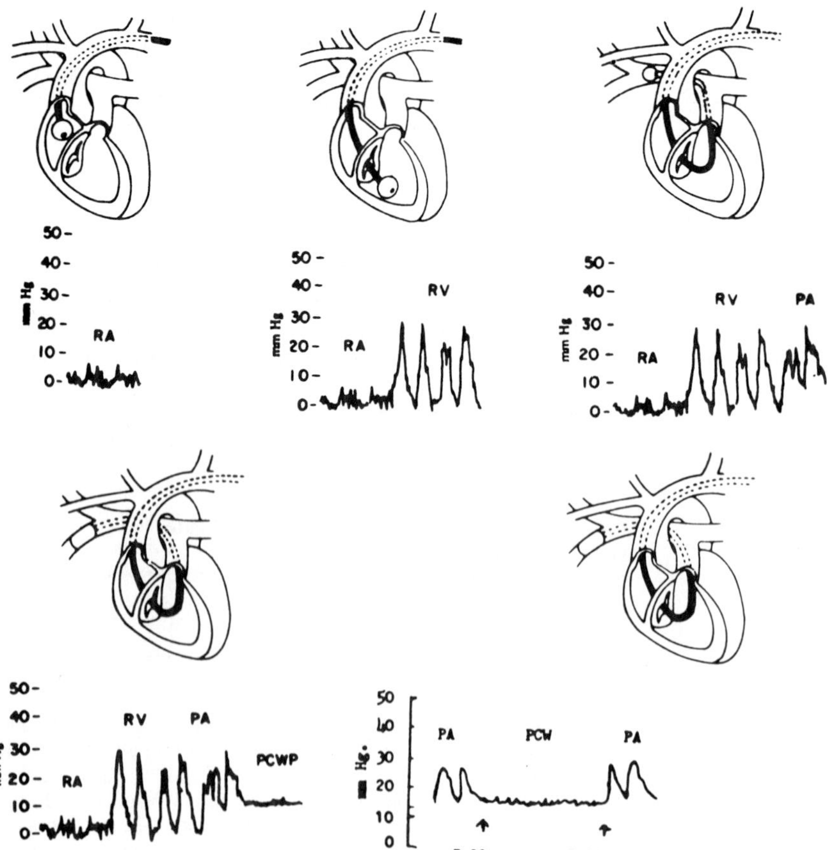

FIG. 18-4. Hemodynamic aspects of balloon catheter insertion into the pulmonary artery. [From Gottlieb AJ (ed): *The Whole Internist Catalog.* Philadelphia, Saunders, 1980. Used by permission.]

pacing. Since it can be instituted quickly and noninvasively, transcutaneous pacing is the technique of choice in the emergency department. Transvenous pacing should be used in patients who require prolonged pacing or who have a very high (>30 percent) risk of heart block. Detailed guidelines are available in Chaps. 24 and 48.

Transcutaneous Pacing

Transcutaneous pacing has become the emergency technique of choice because of its easy application. It uses externally applied electrodes to deliver an electric impulse directly across the intact chest wall to stimulate the myocardium. Transcutaneous pacers differ from standard pulse generators in several important ways. The pulse duration of the stimulating impulse is longer and the current output higher than for standard internal leads. Muscle contraction (usually the chest wall or diaphragm) is notable during pacing, especially at higher outputs. This results in a twitching or bucking activity that can make assessment of cardiac output by palpation of the radial, carotid, or femoral pulse unreliable during transcutaneous pacing. The higher current outputs used make cardiac monitoring with standard electrocardiogram (ECG) monitors problematic due to interference from the large-amplitude pacing spike. Most transcutaneous pacing units come equipped with a monitor that automatically filters the pacing spike so that simultaneous monitoring is possible.

The external pacing electrodes are quickly and easily applied to the chest and back. If separate defibrillator pads or paddles are used, they should be placed at least 2 to 3 cm away from the pacing pads. There is little risk of electrical injury to health care providers during transcutaneous pacing. The electrodes are insulated, and chest compressions [cardiopulmonary resuscitation (CPR)] can be administered directly over them while pacing, although it is recommended that pacing be discontinued during CPR to minimize inappropriate stimulation of the patient due to electrical artifacts. Inadvertent contact with the active pacing surface results only in a mild shock. In the setting of bradyasystolic arrest, it is reasonable to turn the stimulating current to maximum output and then decrease the output if capture is achieved. In a patient with a hemodynamically compromising bradycardia (but not in cardiac arrest), the operator should slowly increase the output from the minimum setting until capture is achieved. Capture is assessed by following the ECG on the filtered monitor of the pacing unit and palpation of peripheral pulses. The hemodynamic response to pacing must also be assessed, either by blood pressure cuff or arterial catheter. Ideally, pacing should be continued at 1.25 times the threshold of initial electrical capture.

As with other pacing systems, transcutaneous pacing may be fixed rate (asynchronous) or demand (synchronous). Asynchronous pacing delivers an electrical impulse at a regular interval without regard to intrinsic cardiac pacemaker activity. This creates the risk of precipitating dysrhythmias if a pacing stimulus is given during the vulnerable period of ventricular repolarization. Synchronous pacing is therefore safer, since the pacing impulse is delivered only if an intrinsic electrical complex is not sensed within a preset interval. An increasing number of defibrillators include a built-in transcutaneous pacemaker. These units are equipped with multifunctional electrodes that allow defibrillation, pacing, and ECG monitoring through one set of pads. This development ensures that pacing will be available as soon as the defibrillator reaches the patient in cardiac arrest.

Failure to capture with transcutaneous pacing may be related to electrode placement or the patient's size. Patients who are conscious or who regain consciousness during transcutaneous pacing may experience discomfort due to muscle contraction. Analgesia with incremental doses of morphine or sedation with a benzodiazepine makes this discomfort tolerable. There is no evidence of clinically significant myocardial damage from properly performed transcutaneous pacing.[12] Nonetheless, transcutaneous pacing should be used for temporary stabilization only and should always be followed as soon as feasible by an internal pacing technique if there is a prolonged need for pacing.

Transvenous Pacing

Transvenous pacing consists of endocardial stimulation of the right ventricle by an electrode introduced into a central vein. The most commonly encountered difficulties with transvenous pacing are securing venous access and obtaining proper placement of the stimulating electrode, both of which can be time consuming. Venous access routes most commonly used include the subclavian, internal or external jugular, femoral, and brachial. Transvenous pacing catheters can be inserted through a variety of venous introducers. A soft, flexible, semifloating bipolar catheter is preferred. This type of pacer is safest to use and takes advantage of any forward blood flow that may be present.

Placement of the catheter tip into the apex of the right ventricle is the key to successful transvenous pacing. Several techniques can aid successful placement. Fluoroscopic guidance is the surest method of right ventricular placement but is rarely available in the emergency department. Electrocardiographic guidance is useful in patients with narrow complexes and/or P waves when fluoroscopy is unavailable. Balloon-tipped floating catheters may aid placement when used in conjunction with ECG and fluoroscopic guidance or when used alone. The balloon is inflated after catheter insertion into a central vein. Forward blood flow then directs the catheter tip toward the ventricle as the operator slowly advances the catheter. As with all balloon-tipped catheters, the balloon should always be deflated prior to withdrawal; the catheter should never be pulled back with the balloon inflated.

When patients have decreased or no forward blood flow (including many circumstances in which transvenous pacing would be used in the emergency department), positioning of the pacer tip within the right ventricle is difficult. Balloon-tipped catheters are not much of an aid in placement during low- or no-flow states. In a true emergency, the pacemaker electrodes are connected to the power source and the catheter advanced blindly in hopes that the tip will encounter the endocardium of the right ventricle and that capture will result. In this setting a right internal jugular venous access route should be used. From this approach, the catheter traverses a straight line into the right ventricle and rarely curls in the atrium or deflects into the inferior vena cava.

Pacer settings vary with the clinical situation. An initial rate of 80 to 100 impulses/min is appropriate for most patients. Asynchronous mode (sensitivity off) is used initially in patients requiring emergency pacing for hemodynamically unstable bradycardias. The ECG should be followed to determine the presence or absence of capture (Fig. 18-5). Output should initially be set at maximum (usually 20 mA) and then decreased after capture is achieved. With optimal tip position, capture should occur at less than 2 mA. Pacing should be continued at 1.5 to 2 times the threshold output required for capture. Subsequent rate and sensitivity settings should be adjusted as clinically indicated by the patient's hemodynamic status and underlying rhythm disturbance.

Chest radiographs should be obtained after the patient is stabilized to ensure proper tip placement and to evaluate the possibility of pneumothorax from the preceding central venous line placement. Finally, care should be taken to firmly affix the pacing catheter to the insertion site prior to transferring the patient. Transvenous pacing is best used in urgent rather than emergent situations, particularly when there is adequate time to utilize fluoroscopy. In the setting of cardiac arrest, transcutaneous pacing is preferred.

Transthoracic pacing is mentioned here largely for historic reasons, since external pacing techniques have largely replaced its use. However, whenever transvenous pacing is tried but unsuccessful, transthoracic pacing may still be attempted. When the latter technique is performed blindly, the likelihood of successful placement is low, with risk of liver, pulmonary artery, diaphragm, lung, or coronary artery

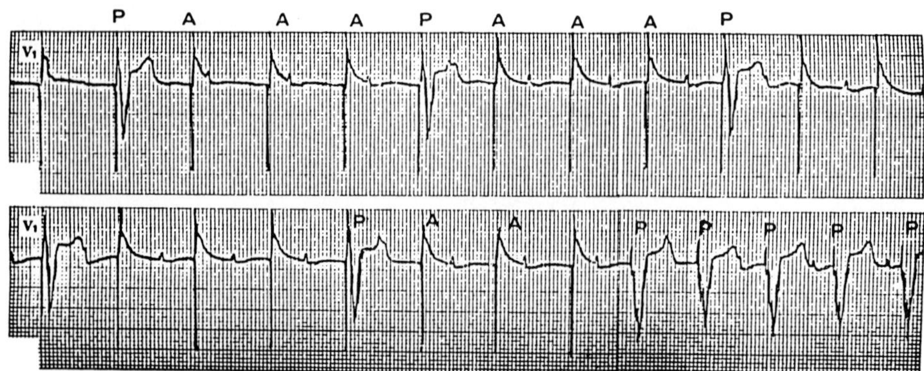

FIG. 18-5. Pacing with intermittent capture. "P" indicates paced beats and "A," pacer artifact without capture.

puncture.[13] Although it has not been studied, use of ultrasound-guided placement may improve placement.

AUTOMATIC AND IMPLANTABLE DEFIBRILLATORS

In 1933, William Kouwenhoven observed in dogs that closed-chest electrical shocks delivered within 30 s of inducing ventricular fibrillation (VF) were 98 percent effective in terminating the dysrhythmia. After 2 min of VF, the rate of resuscitation fell to 27 percent. He reported similar results in human subjects.[14] Modern research indicates that the likelihood for successful resuscitation decreases roughly 10 percent/min after the onset of VF. Thus, the goal of emergency cardiac care is to deliver defibrillation as quickly as possible.

Two recent technological developments have led to the more rapid application of defibrillation. Automatic external defibrillators allow first responders to rapidly institute defibrillation. Even laypersons, such as family members or bystanders, can learn to use these devices. In addition, implanted defibrillators allow patients with frequent malignant ventricular dysrhythmias to carry their own defibrillators with them at all times. Emergency physicians need to be familiar with these devices and the special considerations associated with their use.

Automatic External Defibrillators

Automatic external defibrillators (AEDs) have relatively simple controls and can be used by minimally trained providers to initiate defibrillation. At the patient's right sternal border and cardiac apex, the operator places electrode pads, which are used both for monitoring and defibrillating. Once attached, the AED analyzes the cardiac rhythm and initiates its treatment algorithm. A fully automatic device will deliver a countershock once ventricular tachycardia or VF has been sensed. The AED gives an audible announcement that defibrillation will commence, and the only way the operator can prevent discharge is to turn off the device. A semiautomatic AED analyzes the rhythm and then advises whether a shock is indicated. The operator must press the control button in order to initiate defibrillation; the operator may also override the AED and administer a countershock even if the device has not sensed a shockable rhythm.

AEDs shock patients in VF several times sequentially until an organized cardiac rhythm results or until the maximum number of shocks allowed by the programmed algorithm is reached. Many devices also provide a record of rhythms and events during their use, which allows the emergency physician to subsequently reconstruct the sequence of events during resuscitation.

An AED may be placed on an unstable patient in anticipation of subsequent deterioration, but the device should not be activated until or unless the patient is pulseless. Since motion artifacts may confuse the rhythm-analysis circuitry, the AED should not be in the sensing mode during CPR, during transport, or if the patient has a seizure. Unlike transcutaneous pacemakers, AEDs can deliver a debilitating shock to the operator or other personnel, and the same precautions regarding contact with the patient during defibrillation should be followed with AEDs as with standard defibrillators. The failure of an AED to restore a perfusing rhythm is a poor prognostic sign often associated with long arrest times or arrest rhythms other than VF. When an AED fails to resuscitate a patient in arrest, the cardiac rhythm should be identified and treated. If the rhythm is refractory VF, drug therapy should be instituted while continuing further defibrillation attempts.

AEDs are most effective in tiered emergency medical services systems where AED-equipped first responders reach the patient rapidly and are backed up by the later arrival of paramedics with full advanced life-support capabilities.[15] There is ongoing interest in making AEDs available for widespread use by nonmedical personnel and the lay public.[16,17]

Implantable Cardioverter-Defibrillators

The first human placement of an implantable cardioverter-defibrillator (ICD) took place in 1980 at the Johns Hopkins Hospital.[18] Since that time it has become the treatment of choice for sudden cardiac death, reducing mortality from about 30 to 45 percent/year to less than 2 percent/year.[19] This remarkable efficacy, coupled with the failure (and potentially proarrhythmic effects) of pharmacologic therapy and the increasing sophistication and miniaturization of the devices, has led to an explosion in ICD use. Through 1994 there had been over 50,000 ICDs implanted worldwide; in 1995 there were more than 20,000 implantations in the United States alone.

An ICD consists of a pulse generator, a lead system with both sensing and shocking electrodes, circuitry to analyze the cardiac rhythm and trigger defibrillation, and a power supply. There are currently three generations of ICDs. In each successive generation, the devices have become smaller, more sophisticated, more reliable, and easier to implant. Second-generation ICDs are still quite common. These devices generally were placed by thoracotomy or sternotomy, and defibrillation occurred through electrodes positioned inside or outside the pericardium. Rate-sensing electrodes were placed epicardially or transvenously (Fig. 18-6). The sensing algorithms for second-generation ICDs were relatively unsophisticated; they reliably detected ventricular tachycardia and VF but would cause the devices to inappropriately shock supraventricular rhythms as well. Roughly one-third of patients with second-generation ICDs receive at least one shock triggered by a supraventricular tachycardia during the working life of the device.

Third-generation ICDs have a volume of about 60 mL, or roughly one-quarter that of second-generation devices. The sensing-pacing-defibrillation electrodes are placed transvenously, and the device itself is generally implanted subcutaneously in the subpectoral region or in an abdominal pocket. A subcutaneous patch electrode may be used to help lower the defibrillation threshold. On a chest radiograph, at first glance these devices can easily be mistaken for conventional

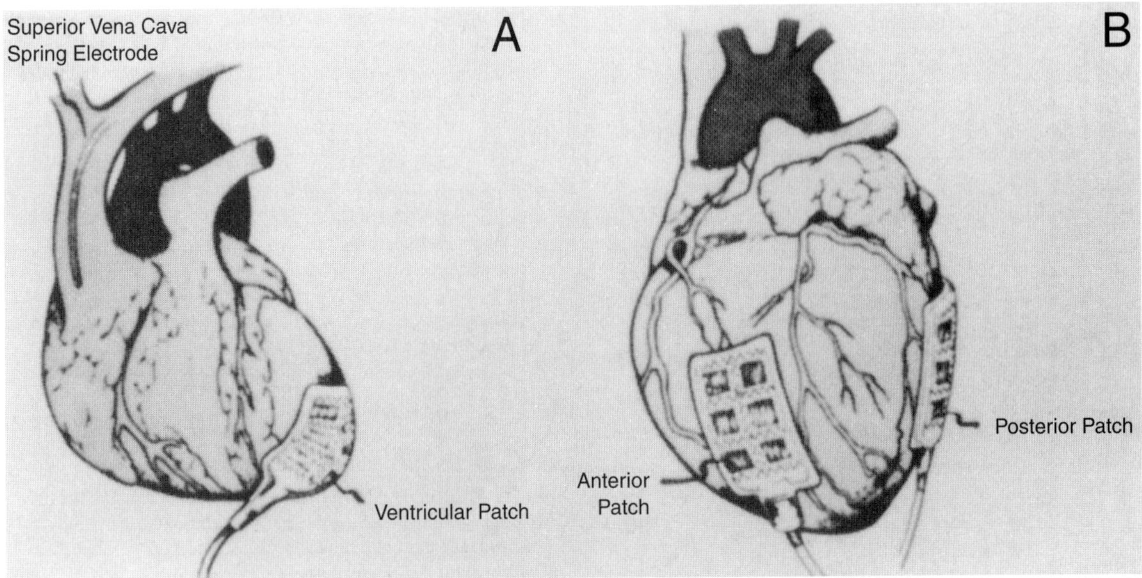

FIG. 18-6. Typical second generation ICD electrode arrangements. **A.** Spring-patch pathway. **B.** Patch-patch pathway. (From Chapman PD, Veseth-Rogers JL, Duquette SE: The implantable defibrillator and the emergency physician. *Ann Emerg Med* 18:579, 1989. Used by permission.)

pacemakers. Careful examination of the electrodes will reveal their true nature (Fig. 18-7). Newer ICDs are better at discriminating supraventricular tachycardia and are capable of a variety of responses to ventricular tachycardia and VF. Most are programmed to follow a tiered approach to ventricular dysrhythmias: antitachycardia pacing, low-energy cardioversion, and finally defibrillation. Depending on the frequency of discharge and whether the pacemaker function is used, the latest ICDs have a projected life span of about 8 years.

EMERGENCY DEPARTMENT EVALUATION AND THERAPY ICDs are remarkably effective in preventing sudden cardiac death. The most common cause of death in patients with ICDs is congestive heart failure, which should be managed in standard fashion in the emergency department. However, the most common reason an ICD patient comes to the emergency department is to be evaluated for the appropriateness of a previously delivered shock. Causes of inappropriate shock delivery are summarized in Table 18-3. In evaluating a patient complaining of one or more ICD shocks, it is important to determine the number of shocks delivered, the activity of the patient at the time, and any prodromal symptoms or postshock trauma. Recent changes in antiarrhythmic drug dosage should be noted. The physical examination should focus on the vital signs, the cardiovascular status, the generator pocket, and evidence of incidental trauma. The patient should be monitored during the evaluation. An ECG should be obtained and interpreted with the knowledge that ST-segment elevations or depressions due exclusively to the shock will resolve within 15 min. A chest radiograph may reveal electrode migration, displacement, or fracture. Drug levels of antiarrhythmics should be determined and electrolyte disturbances explored.

Since admission criteria are often institution- and cardiologist-specific, consultation with the patient's cardiologist is essential. General admission guidelines include all unstable patients, patients with two or more shocks in a 1-week period, the presence of correctable causes of dysrhythmia (e.g., electrolyte imbalances, drug toxicity, or

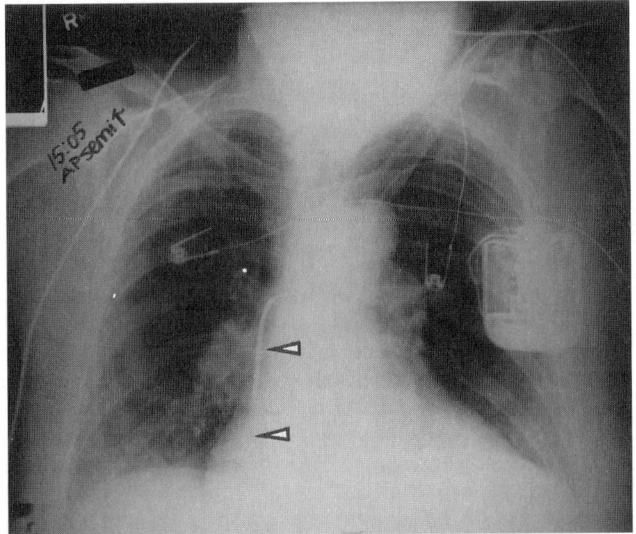

FIG. 18-7. Chest radiograph of a patient with a nonthoracotomy implanted third generation defibrillator. The ICD is in the left subpectoral area. The electrodes (arrows) have been placed transvenously. The proximal spring electrode is positioned at the junction of the superior vena cava and the right atrium. The distal electrode is in the right ventricle; only a portion of its lead is visible.

TABLE 18-3 Potential Causes of Inappropriate ICD Shock Delivery

False sensing Supraventricular tachycardia with rapid ventricular response Muscular activity (shivering, diaphragmatic contraction) Extraneous source (tapping of chest wall, vibrations, pacer spikes) Sensing T waves as QRS complex (double counting) Sensing lead fracture or migration
Unsustained tachyarrhythmia
ICD-pacemaker interactions
Component failure

Source: Adapted from Munter WM, DeLacey WA: Automatic implantable cardioverter defibrillators. *Emerg Med Clin North Am* 12:579, 1994. Used by permission.

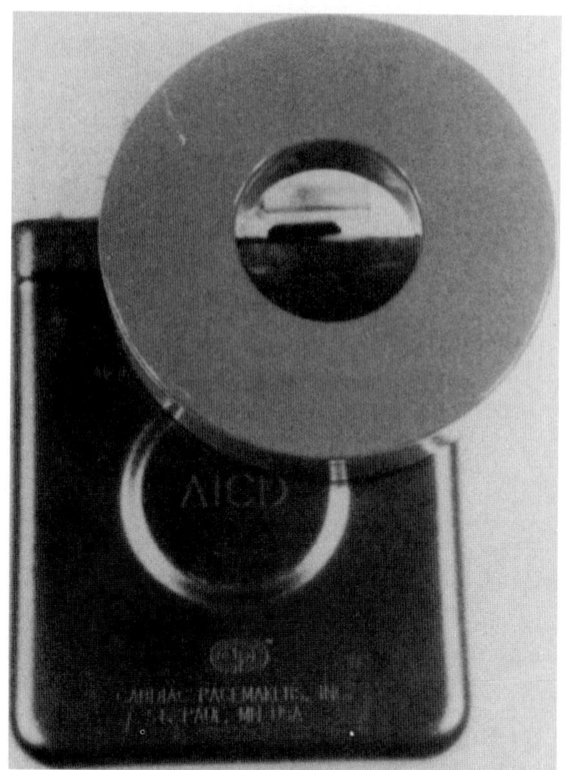

FIG. 18-8. Correct magnet placement to deactivate second generation ICD. (From Chapman PD, Veseth-Rogers JL, Duquette SE: The implantable defibrillator and the emergency physician. *Ann Emerg Med* 18:579, 1989. Used by permission.)

ischemia), any sign of infection, mechanical disruption of the ICD or leads, and patients who need additional cardiologic investigation for possible malfunction of the device.

For an ICD patient in cardiac arrest, normal basic and advanced resuscitation measures are indicated. If defibrillation is necessary, the operator should avoid placing either paddle directly over the ICD. The presence of epicardial patch electrodes may shield the myocardium from the countershock and may therefore necessitate repositioning of the paddles. CPR may be performed in the usual fashion. If the ICD should discharge during CPR, the provider may perceive a small electrical shock, but it is neither uncomfortable nor dangerous.

Occasionally it may become necessary to temporarily deactivate the ICD, as in the case of inappropriate shock for a stable rhythm. Second-generation devices may be deactivated by placing a donut-shaped magnet over the right upper quadrant (Fig. 18-8) of the pulse generator for 30 s until the intermittent beeping ceases and a solid tone is heard. The magnet is then removed. If this does not succeed, then deactivation is attempted by placing the magnet over the opposite corner of the pulse generator (some are surgically positioned upside down). The response of third-generation devices to a magnet can be complex, but generally defibrillation is deactivated only when the magnet is present. This requires taping the magnet to the skin overlying the ICD. Defibrillation can be reenabled by removing the magnet. Some third-generation devices are programmed so that they cannot be deactivated by a magnetic field. All ICDs should be evaluated by a cardiologist after exposure to a magnet.

REFERENCES

1. Ryan TJ, Anderson JL, Antman EM, et al: ACC/AHA guidelines for the management of patients with acute myocardial infarction: A report of the American College of Cardiology/American Heart Association Task Force on Practice Guidelines (Committee on Management of Acute Myocardial Infarction). *J Am Coll Cardiol* 28:1328, 1996.
2. Fuhrman TM, McSweeney E: Noninvasive evaluation of the collateral circulation to the hand. *Acad Emerg Med* 2:195, 1995.
3. Slogoff S, Keats AS, Arlund C: On the safety of radial artery cannulation. *Anesthesiology* 59:42, 1983.
4. Russell JA, Joel M, Hudson RJ, et al: Prospective evaluation of radial and femoral artery catheterization sites in critically ill adults. *Crit Care Med* 11:936,1983.
5. Kong R, Singer M: Insertion of a pulmonary artery flotation catheter: How to do it. *Br J Hosp Med* 57:432, 1997.
6. Connors AF, Speroff T, Dawson NV, et al: The effectiveness of right heart catheterization in the initial care of critically ill patients. *JAMA* 276:889, 1996.
7. Pulmonary Artery Catheter Consensus Conference: Consensus Statement. *Crit Care Med* 25:910, 1997.
8. Kuecherer HF, Foster E: Hemodynamics by transesophageal echocardiography. *Cardiol Clin* 11:475, 1993.
9. Nomura M, Hillel Z, Shih H, et al: The association between Doppler transmitral flow variables measured by transesophageal echocardiography and pulmonary capillary wedge pressure. *Anesth Analg* 84:491, 1997.
10. Woltjer HH, Bogaard HJ, Bronzwaer JG, et al: Prediction of pulmonary capillary wedge pressure and assessment of stroke volume by noninvasive impedance cardiography. *Am Heart J* 134:450, 1997.
11. Mohiaddin RH, Gatehouse PD, Henien M, Firmin DN: Cine MR fourier velocimetry of blood flow through cardiac valves: Comparison with Doppler echocardiography. *J Magn Reson Imaging* 7:657, 1997.
12. Hedges JR, Syverud S, Dalsey WC, et al: Threshold, enzymatic, and pathologic changes associated with prolonged transcutaneous pacing in a chronic heart block model. *J Emerg Med* 7:1, 1989.
13. Brown CG: Injuries associated with percutaneous placement of transthoracic pacemakers. *Ann Emerg Med* 14:223, 1985.
14. Kouwenhoven WB: Closed chest defibrillation of the heart. *Surgery* 42:550, 1952.
15. Eisenberg MS, Pantridge JF, Cobb LA, et al: The revolution and evolution of prehospital cardiac care. *Arch Intern Med* 156:1611, 1996.
16. Mosesso VN, Davis EA, Auble TE, et al: Use of automated external defibrillators by police officers for treatment of out-of-hospital cardiac arrest. *Ann Emerg Med* 32:200, 1998.
17. Kerber RE, Becker LB, Bourland JD, et al: Automatic external defibrillators for public access defibrillation: Recommendations for specifying and reporting arrhythmia analysis algorithm performance, incorporating new waveforms, and enhancing safety. A statement for health professionals from the American Heart Association Task Force on Automatic External Defibrillation, Subcommittee on AED Safety and Efficacy. *Circulation* 95:1677, 1997.
18. Mirowski M, Morton MM, Staewen WS, et al: The development of the transvenous automatic defibrillator. *Arch Intern Med* 129:773, 1972.
19. Fogoros RN: Impact of the implantable defibrillator on mortality: The axiom of overall implantable cardioverter-defibrillator survival. *Am J Cardiol* 78:57, 1996.

CEREBRAL RESUSCITATION

Gary S. Krause
Blaine C. White

Cerebral resuscitation continues to affect a substantial portion of the population of the United States. Data from the ARIC (Atherosclerotic Risk in Communities), CHS (Cardiovascular Health Study), and the NHLBI (National Heart, Lung, and Blood Institute) show that about 600,000 people suffer a new or recurrent stroke each year. Furthermore, stroke is the leading cause of serious, long-term disability in the United States. Three million Americans are currently permanently disabled because of stroke, and 31 percent of stroke survivors need help caring for themselves, 20 percent need help walking, 71 percent have an impaired vocational capacity when examined an average of 7 years later, and 16 percent have to be institutionalized. The direct and indirect cost of stroke in 1998 was estimated at over $40 billion. In addition, cardiopulmonary resuscitation for victims of cardiac arrest, both within and outside of the hospital, succeeds in restoring spontaneous circulation in about 70,000 patients a year in the United States. At least 60 percent of these patients subsequently die in the hospital as a result of extensive brain damage; only 3 to 10 percent of resuscitated patients are finally able to resume their former lifestyles. Clearly, the development of effective interventions to prevent these sequela of brain ischemia and reperfusion would enormously enhance the value of the investment already made and would return thousands of now lost patients to renewed vigorous and productive time with their families and in our society.

There are two important issues involved in the ongoing effort to reduce this neurologic morbidity. One is discovery of the mechanisms involved in tissue injury and repair, and the other is the identification of clinically effective therapy. Clinical trials conducted more than a decade ago utilizing postresuscitation treatment with barbiturates[1] or calcium antagonists[2] were disappointing. More recently, clinical treatment of stroke with the radical scavenger tirilazad was found ineffective,[3] and laboratory investigations of treatment with glutamate receptor antagonists after resuscitation from cardiac arrest produced disappointing results.[4] The wide variety of therapeutic agents now in single-drug clinical trials (e.g., involving thrombolysis, glutamate release inhibition, *N*-methyl-D-aspartate receptor antagonism, opioid antagonism, calcium channel blockade, free radical scavenging, membrane stabilization, intercellular adhesion molecule-1 antagonism, ganglioside administration, and growth factor administration) suggests that understanding of the mechanisms involved in damage and repair in neurons remains incomplete.

Four major observations have provided the foundation for investigation of brain injury by ischemia and reperfusion:[5] (1) rapid loss of high-energy phosphate compounds during ischemia followed by their recovery within the first 15 min of reperfusion, (2) morphologic evidence that most structural damage occurs during reperfusion, especially in selectively vulnerable zones, (3) progressive brain hypoperfusion during postischemic reperfusion, and (4) prolonged suppression of protein synthesis in selectively vulnerable neurons.

Cardiac arrest resulting in ischemic-anoxic brain injury is characterized by three phases: ischemia, early reperfusion, and late reperfusion. We have published extensive reviews of our theoretical model of the causal interactions of neuronal injury and repair mechanisms during ischemia and reperfusion.[5,6] Briefly, primary injury mechanisms include, at a minimum, activation of phospholipases and proteolytic enzymes (calpain) during ischemia and generation of radicals accompanied by lipid peroxidation during reperfusion. This chapter outlines the crucial role of calcium and iron in these injury mechanisms and suggests possible therapies to ameliorate brain injury following an ischemic insult.

ISCHEMIC PHASE

Morphologic studies have shown that the extent of tissue injury observed following ischemia largely reflects damage incurred during reperfusion and have identified specific populations of brain neurons that are exceptionally susceptible to damage and death. These selectively vulnerable neurons include the pyramidal neurons in layers 3 and 5 of the cortex and those found in the CA1 and hilus of the hippocampus. Minimal ultrastructural injury is seen in the brain during complete ischemia. Some margination and clumping of nuclear chromatin is seen by 10 to 15 min of complete ischemia. Mitochondria may be slightly swollen, but their structure does not show major degenerative alterations for up to 30 min of complete ischemia. Similarly, some swelling of the endoplasmic reticulum (ER) may be seen during ischemia, but the polyribosomes remain appropriately associated with the ER, and disaggregation of polyribosomes does not occur during complete ischemia. Nuclear and plasma membranes show a normal, well-defined bilaminar structure without evidence of holes or general structural disintegration.

In contrast to the paucity of morphologic findings, there are severe biochemical alterations. With the onset of cardiac arrest there is precipitous decline in brain oxygen content, which approaches zero within 6 to 12 s. The brain has very limited reserves of glucose, glycogen, or phosphocreatine; therefore, oxygen depletion leads to a sharp decline in tissue adenosine triphosphate (ATP) levels, which approach zero within 4 min. Anaerobic glycolysis and ATP depletion lead to lactic acidosis and hypoxanthine accumulation, respectively, during the ischemic phase. Since about 80 percent of the brain's ATP is used to maintain transmembrane ionic gradients for potassium, sodium, and calcium, these ionic gradients also decay rapidly. During complete ischemic anoxia, these ions equilibrate between the extra- and intracellular fluid within 5 to 10 min of the insult.

The high cytosolic calcium level, thought to be a major initiating event leading to cell death,[7] causes four key events: the activation of membrane phospholipase A_2, proteolytic cleavage of xanthine dehydrogenase, activation of the proteolytic enzyme calpain, and release of excitatory neurotransmitters such as glutamate. Phospholipase A_2 cleaves a fatty acid, primarily arachidonate, from the cell membrane lipids, yielding a free fatty acid and in the process damaging the membrane's structure. The proteolysis of xanthine dehydrogenase in brain endothelial cells produces xanthine oxidase, which will react with hypoxanthine to produce the superoxide radical (O_2^-) upon reperfusion. Proteins that are degraded by calpain during either ischemia or reperfusion include microtubule-associated 2, tubulin, neurofilament protein, spectrin, protein kinase C, calcium/calmodulin kinase II, and the translation initiation factors eIF4E and eIF4G.

EARLY REPERFUSION

During early reperfusion, ATP levels and total adenylate charge recover rapidly. If the ischemic insult has been less than 20 min, the membrane ionic gradients also recover quickly. After much longer insults of 1 to 3 h, total tissue calcium loads actually increase during reperfusion. It is felt that this reflects extensive and irreversible cell membrane injury during these very prolonged periods of ischemia.

Arachidonate is rapidly oxidized by both cyclooxygenase and lipoxygenase, and returns to preischemic levels within 30 min of reperfusion. Several vasoactive substances are produced by the metabolism of arachidonate. The prostaglandins are the products of cyclooxygenase, and the leukotrienes are the products of lipoxygenase. The production of the vasodilatory prostaglandin prostacyclin is severely inhibited during early reperfusion. Thus, vasospastic compounds predominate in the leukotriene and prostaglandin products. While the free arachidonic acid levels rapidly return to baseline during reperfusion, leukotrienes remain markedly elevated for at least 24 h. The time course of leukotriene elevation may explain the alterations in blood flow seen in the postischemic brain (the "no-reflow" phenomenon). Restoration of normal or mildly hypertensive systemic arterial pressure produces an initial brain hyperperfusion. However, within 1 h, global brain perfusion has dropped to levels of 20 to 40 percent of normal, where it remains for up to 1 to 2 days. This phenomenon occurs without a change in intracranial pressure and was originally thought to lead to failure of high-energy metabolism and neuronal death during reperfusion. However, therapy that inhibited postischemic brain hypoperfusion had little effect on neurologic outcome.

Membrane lipids are extensively peroxidized by iron-dependent radical reactions during reperfusion. Within the first 30 s of reperfusion, there is a brief burst of oxygen-based free radical production, although the precise identity of the radical species remains unknown. Xanthine oxidase and cyclooxygenase, whose substrates are hypoxanthine and arachidonate respectively, produce O_2^- as a side product. Availability of a transition metal, such as iron, is required for reaction of oxygen radicals with tissue macromolecules, including lipids (lipid peroxidation). The brain glia have abundant stores of oxidized (ferric) iron, mostly in ferritin and transferrin, forms in which the iron is unable to act as a catalyst for oxygen radical reactions. However, O_2^-, which is present in excessive amounts during early reperfusion, promotes reduction of ferric iron and release of ferrous iron from ferritin, and lipid peroxidation in the reperfused brain has been demonstrated by many laboratories and maps to selectively vulnerable neurons. These reactions also appear to be involved in the genesis of the postischemic hypoperfusion phenomenon, which is inhibited by superoxide dismutase and deferoxamine or U74006F, a lipid peroxidation chain terminator.

Excitatory amino acid neurotransmitters appear to play a role in the injury produced by focal brain ischemia such as stroke; it is unclear whether the same holds true in global brain ischemia. However, excitatory neurotransmitter uptake is inhibited by arachidonate and products of lipid peroxidation, and thus continued stimulation of receptors may contribute to neuronal damage by as yet unidentified mechanisms.

Protein synthesis is suppressed during ischemia by lack of ATP.[8] However, even with the rapid restoration of ATP levels that accompanies reperfusion, there is a severe suppression of protein synthesis that varies with duration of ischemia, brain region, and individual proteins. Whereas most regions of the brain recover their ability to synthesize protein following a short ischemic period, protein synthesis in the selectively vulnerable regions is depressed by about 90 percent early in reperfusion and does not recover significantly. Failure of protein synthesis is due to a disruption in the formation of new ribosomal translation complexes. Initiation, the rate-limiting step in translation, requires the coordinated assembly of the ribosomal subunits, the mRNA to be translated, and the amino-acyl tRNA for the first amino acid (always methionine in eukaryotes). This process is orchestrated by a family of proteins named eukaryotic initiation factors (eIFs). The eIF4 and eIF2 complexes are the major regulatory points for translation initiation. Cellular mRNAs vary greatly in their binding efficiency to eIF4E, and under normal physiologic situations message selection for translation initiation is modulated by altering the phosphorylation of Ser^{209} on eIF4E. However, under conditions of cellular stress (e.g., heat shock, viral infection, or starvation), rates of global protein synthesis are downregulated by phosphorylating Ser^{51} on the α subunit of eIF2 [eIF2α(P)].

Studies have now identified three important changes in eIFs that occur during brain ischemia and reperfusion: (1) a modest degree of proteolytic degradation of eIF4E occurs during ischemia, but without change in its phosphorylation state during either ischemia or reperfusion;[9,10] (2) there is substantial proteolytic degradation of eIF4G mediated by calpain during both ischemia and reperfusion;[11,12] and (3) probably most important, there is an approximately twentyfold increase in eIF2α(P) during early reperfusion. In nonischemic tissue, phosphorylated eIF2α is found exclusively in astrocytes.[13] After only 10 min postischemic reperfusion, there is prominent eIF2α(P) immunostaining in the cytoplasm of neurons in both the hippocampus and cortex. After 1 h of reperfusion, eIF2α(P) is prominent in both the nuclei and cytoplasm of selectively vulnerable neurons in both the hippocampus and cortex; nuclear eIF2α(P) is never seen in ischemia-resistant neurons. By 4 h reperfusion, the pattern of nuclear eIF2α(P) immunostaining in vulnerable neurons suggests nuclear condensation consistent with the early stages of apoptosis. These results provide a mechanism for the inhibition of protein synthesis in vulnerable neurons during reperfusion and, together with other evidence suggesting a role for eIF2α(P) in causing apoptosis, may represent a fundamental phenomenon in the causal pathway leading to the death of vulnerable neurons. It is interesting to note that animals treated with 20 U/kg insulin at resuscitation are able to dephosphorylate eIF2α(P) and recover protein synthesis in vulnerable hippocampal neurons by 90 min reperfusion. Thus, growth factors, including fibroblast growth factor, nerve growth factor, insulin-like growth factor 1, and insulin, all of which have been shown to improve neuronal survival in the laboratory, may have a role in limiting and repairing neuronal damage.[6]

LATE EVENTS DURING REPERFUSION

Brain tissue ionic concentrations are indistinguishable from normal after 4 h of reperfusion following a 15-min cardiac arrest. The tissue iron has been recovered into high-molecular-weight species by 8 h of reperfusion. However, after 8 h large shifts of the concentrations of calcium, potassium, and sodium are observed. These shifts most likely reflect equilibration between the cytosol and the interstitial fluid for these ions. Electron microscopic examination of brains fixed in situ after 8 h reperfusion reveals in the vulnerable neurons an obvious general degradation of membrane structure with large holes in the plasmalemma. Nuclear chromatin is densely clumped, with grossly abnormal nuclear architecture. Mitochondrial architecture is well preserved. The ER is dilated and ragged, and normally arranged polyribosomes are virtually nonexistent. Histochemical evidence of lipid peroxidation can be seen by as early as 90 min following a 10-min arrest and involves approximately 30 percent of the neurons in the cortex and most neurons in CA1 and the hilus.[14] Membrane injury by lipid peroxidation produces degradation of membrane structure to the point that the membrane becomes freely permeable to ions and the cell is irreversibly injured.

THERAPY

Clearly, the first priority in the treatment of cerebral ischemia is the reestablishment of blood flow. Trials of thrombolytics have shown tissue plasminogen activator to be of some benefit in select subgroups of stroke patients, but it must be administered within a 3-h window.[15] Methods of restoring spontaneous circulation in cardiac arrest are described in Chaps. 8, 10, and 20.

Because the ultimate extent of injury observed following ischemia largely reflects damage incurred during reperfusion (reperfusion injury), effective therapy must not only limit ongoing mechanisms of damage but also facilitate repair of the damage that has already occurred. Optimum therapy to obviate continuing injury and salvage viable brain tissue is unknown.[16] Most therapeutic studies use animal models, use pretreatment, or contain small numbers of patients. However, a few general principles can be stated. Perfusion should be maintained at normal levels. It does not appear that intracranial pressure is increased in the postresuscitation period, and therefore therapies directed at increased intracranial pressure (hyperventilation and osmotic agents) are unnecessary. Hypotension should be avoided for obvious reasons. Oxygenation should be maintained at or near normal levels. Hyperoxia should be avoided, since it is toxic to the lungs and may increase brain damage. Prearrest hyperglycemia is associated with poor neurologic outcome, and although glucose administered postinsult has not been adequately studied, hyperglycemia should probably be avoided.[17] As mentioned above, several other therapies have been advocated, but human studies have failed to show efficacy. These therapies include pentobarbital coma, calcium antagonists, and glucocorticoids.[18,19]

Ischemic injury of the brain is complex, and this complexity indicates that single-drug therapeutic approaches will continue to fail. The pattern of ATP and ionic recovery and DNA transcription during reperfusion shows that several cellular systems are intact following prolonged ischemia and reperfusion. Future investigation of therapeutic approaches may combine calpain antagonists, iron chelators, lipid peroxidation chain reaction terminators, and growth factors to forestall further lipid peroxidation and to stimulate repair mechanisms. Effective therapeutic protocols will be identified only by continued studies.

REFERENCES

1. Brain Resuscitation Clinical Trial I Study Group: Study of thiopental loading in comatose survivors of cardiac arrest. *N Engl J Med* 314:397–401, 1986.

2. Brain Resuscitation Clinical Trial II Study Group: A randomized clinical study of a calcium-entry blocker (lidoflazine) in the treatment of comatose survivors of cardiac arrest. *N Engl J Med* 324:1225–1231, 1991.
3. RANITAS investigators: A randomized trial of trilazad mesylate in patients with acute stroke. *Stroke* 27:1453–1458, 1996.
4. Nellgard B, Gustafson I, Wieloch T: Lack of protection by the *N*-methyl-D-aspartate receptor blocker dizocilpine (MK-801) after transient cerebral ischemia in the rat. *Anesthesiology* 75:279–287, 1991.
5. O'Neil BJ, Krause GS, Grossman LI, et al: Global brain ischemia and reperfusion by cardiac arrest and resuscitation: Mechanisms leading to death of vulnerable neurons and a fundamental basis for therapeutic approaches, in Paradis NA, Halperin HR, Nowak RM (eds): *Cardiac Arrest: The Science and Practice of Resuscitation Medicine.* Baltimore, Williams & Wilkins, 1996, pp 84–112.
6. White B, Grossman L, Krause G: Membrane damage and repair in brain injury by ischemia and reperfusion. *Neurology* 43:1656–1665, 1993.
7. Siesjo BK, Bengtsson F, Grampp W, et al: Calcium, excitotoxins, and neuronal death in the brain. *Ann N Y Acad Sci* 568:234–251, 1989.
8. Krause GS, Tiffany BR: Protein synthesis in the reperfused brain. *Stroke* 24:747–756, 1993.
9. Krause GS, DeGracia DJ, Neumar RW, et al: eIF4E degradation during brain ischemia. *J Neurochem* 63:1391–1394, 1995.
10. Neumar RW, DeGracia DJ, Konkoly LL, et al: Calpain I mediates eukaryotic initiation factor 4G degradation during global brain ischemia. *J Cereb Blood Flow Metab* 18:876–881, 1998.
11. DeGracia DJ, Neumar RW, White BC, Krause GS: Global brain ischemia and reperfusion: Modifications in eukaryotic initiation factors are associated with inhibition of translation initiation. *J Neurochem* 67:2005–2012, 1996.
12. Neumar RW, Hagle SM, DeGracia DJ, et al: Brain calpain autolysis during global cerebral ischemia. *J Neurochem* 66:421–424, 1996.
13. DeGracia DJ, Sullivan JM, Neumar RW, et al: Effect of brain ischemia and reperfusion on the localization of phosphorylated eukaryotic initiation factor 2α. *J Cereb Blood Flow Metab* 17:1291–1302, 1997.
14. White BC, Daya A, DeGracia DJ, et al: Flourescent histochemical localization of lipid peroxidation during brain reperfusion following cardiac arrest. *Acta Neuropathol (Berlin)* 86:1–9, 1993.
15. National Institute of Neurological Disorders and Stroke rt-PA Stroke Study Group: Tissue plasminogen activator for acute ischemic stroke. *N Engl J Med* 333:1581–1587, 1995.
16. del Zoppo GJ, Wagner S, Tagaya M: Trends and future developments in the pharmacological treatment of acute ischemic stroke. *Drugs* 54:9–38, 1997.
17. Wass CT, Lanier WL: Glucose modulation of ischemic brain injury: Review and clinical recommendations. *Mayo Clin Proc* 71:801–812, 1996.
18. Grafton ST, Longstreth WT Jr: Steroids after cardiac arrest: A retrospective study with concurrent, nonrandomized controls. *Neurology* 38:1315–1316, 1988.
19. Jastremski M, Sutton-Tyrrell K, Vaagenes P, et al: Glucocorticoid treatment does not improve neurological recovery following cardiac arrest: Brain Resuscitation Clinical Trial I Study Group. *JAMA* 262:3427–3430, 1989.

20 NEWER RESUSCITATIVE TECHNIQUES

James E. Manning
Christopher W. Barton
Laurence M. Katz

Despite advances in the science of cardiopulmonary-cerebral resuscitation, the prospects for long-term survival with good neurologic recovery remain exceedingly poor. A major limitation of present therapy is the marginal blood flow generated by closed-chest cardiopulmonary resuscitation (CPR). Cardiac output has been reported to be 25 to 33 percent of normal at best and decreases with time delays to initiation of CPR. With increasing duration of arrest and progressive loss of peripheral arterial resistance, even optimally performed closed-chest CPR is unlikely to result in return of spontaneous circulation (ROSC).

Successful resuscitation of the patient in cardiac arrest requires at least some minimal amount of blood flow to the heart. Myocardial perfusion during closed-chest CPR has been shown to be directly related to the pressure gradient across the coronary vasculature. This gradient is equal to the aortic pressure minus the right atrial pressure and is termed the *coronary perfusion pressure* (CPP). Aortic pressure largely determines the CPP gradient and is dependent upon the level of residual peripheral arterial vasomotor tone. Research has shown that the CPP gradient is greatest during the relaxation phase of CPR chest compressions (CPR diastole). Both laboratory and clinical data indicate that a CPP of at least 15 mmHg is almost always required to achieve ROSC. Yet human studies indicate that CPP gradients attained with standard CPR are usually in the ineffective range of 1 to 8 mmHg.

TABLE 20-1 Alternative Methods of Closed-Chest CPR

Mechanical piston CPR
Simultaneous compression and ventilation (SCV CPR)
Interposed abdominal compression (IAC CPR)
CPR with abdominal binding
CPR with medical antishock trousers (MAST)
High-impulse CPR
Circumferential thoracic vest CPR
Active compression-decompression (ACD CPR)
Phased chest and abdominal compression-decompression (Lifestick)

Much of the research into cardiopulmonary resuscitation has focused on methods to improve artificial perfusion during cardiac arrest. In addition to the originally described "conventional" CPR technique, several alternative methods of performing closed-chest CPR have been investigated (Table 20-1). Vasoconstrictor agents have long been used as the pharmacologic adjunct to improve vital organ perfusion by increasing aortic pressure and coronary perfusion pressure. Adrenergic-mediated vasoconstriction remains the major pharmacologic intervention in all forms of cardiac arrest. Although epinephrine has been the principal drug used, other adrenergic agents have been studied and, more recently, nonadrenergic vasoconstrictors as well.

Noninvasive and invasive monitoring techniques have been examined in an effort to identify clinically useful and reliable parameters to guide resuscitative efforts (Table 20-2).

Invasive perfusion techniques capable of providing near-normal artificial vital organ perfusion have also been described (Table 20-3). Direct mechanical ventricular assistance (or actuation) and cardiopulmonary bypass have been reported in laboratory models and a few clinical reports. Methods of artificial perfusion using aortic balloon catheters have recently been described in laboratory investigations. These newer invasive techniques have attempted to address the issue of clinical feasibility during sudden cardiac death.

TABLE 20-2 Monitoring Techniques for Assessing CPR Effectiveness

Noninvasive
Ventricular fibrillation amplitude
End-tidal carbon dioxide ($ETco_2$)
Median frequency of ventricular fibrillation
Invasive
Arterial pressure
Coronary perfusion pressure (CPP)
Central venous oxygen saturation

TABLE 20-3 Invasive Perfusion Techniques

Open-chest manual cardiac compression
Minimally invasive direct cardiac massage (MID CM)
Direct mechanical ventricular assistance (DMVA)
Cardiopulmonary bypass (CPB)
Hemopump
Aortic catheter perfusion techniques —Intra-aortic balloon pump (IABP) —Selective aortic arch perfusion (SAAP)/selective aortic perfusion and oxygenation (SAPO) —Intermittent ascending aortic occlusion

Reperfusion-induced injury is a major focus of research in many fields of medicine and for numerous ischemic diseases states, including cardiac arrest, and is discussed in detail elsewhere (see Chap. 19). Cerebral resuscitation with favorable neurologic outcome after prolonged global ischemia will be the ultimate obstacle to overcome in cardiac arrest therapy. Brain-oriented therapies, such as hypothermia, may substantially improve postresuscitation neuronal survival and functional neurologic recovery. Pharmacologic agents capable of limiting ischemia-induced cellular damage and reperfusion-induced injury from reactive oxygen species will likely be an important form of therapy for cardiac arrest patients in the resuscitation and postresuscitation phases.

This chapter briefly discusses some of the alternative methods of closed-chest CPR, pharmacologic agents, monitoring methods, and invasive perfusion techniques that are presently undergoing investigation and hold promise for the future clinical management of cardiac arrest.

ALTERNATIVE METHODS OF CLOSED-CHEST CPR

The rationale for most of the alternative methods of closed-chest CPR that have been decribed are based on one of two proposed mechanisms of blood flow during CPR chest compression. The *cardiac pump theory* proposes that compression of the heart between the sternum and the spine squeezes blood out of the ventricles in a forward flow direction in a manner generally similar to normal myocardial contraction. The *thoracic pump theory* proposes that pressurization of the entire thorax, not just the heart, is responsible for blood flow and that the heart serves only as a passive or partially compressed conduit for blood flow. Net forward blood flow occurs due to competent closure of venous valves during diastole at the thoracic inlet during chest compression. The evidence for and against each theory is beyond the scope of this chapter, but it is accurate to state that the precise mechanism of blood flow during closed-chest CPR remains controversial and may vary based on individual anatomic features. Alternative methods of performing closed-chest CPR have largely been based on efforts to exploit one or both of the two proposed mechanisms.

High-Impulse CPR

In 1984, Maier et al reported a laboratory study comparing compression rates of 100 per minute and 150 per minute with the conventional rate of 60 per minute advocated prior to 1986.[1] They observed increases in cardiac output that were roughly linear to the increase in compression rate, while stroke volume remained relatively constant. The compression force and velocity of impact used with these rapid CPR compression rates led to the term ''high-impulse'' CPR. This work was partially responsible for the increase in the recommended CPR compression rate from 60 min^{-1} to 80 to 100 per minute.

Interposed Abdominal Compression CPR (IAC CPR)

Compression of the abdomen during cardiac arrest generates aortic pressures similar to chest compressions. The hypothesis that CPR diastolic aortic pressure and venous return from the abdomen might be augmented by abdominal compressions led to the idea of IAC CPR. One person performs the chest compressions of standard CPR while another person applies a similar compression over the central abdomen during the relaxation phase of chest compression. The hemodynamic effects of IAC CPR in laboratory investigations have not been consistent, but most have shown increases in CPR diastolic aortic pressure, coronary perfusion pressure, and cardiac output. Results of clinical studies of IAC CPR have been highly variable. Some studies have shown no evidence of improved resuscitation outcome, whereas others have demonstrated significant improvements in ROSC and survival to hospital discharge.[2] Differences in study populations and the technical performance of IAC CPR may be the reasons for the variable results obtained. At present, the data supporting the use of IAC CPR are not sufficient to recommend its routine application. It could also be argued that IAC CPR is physiologically very similar to high-impulse CPR with the compressions performed by two persons rather than one. However, if perfusion with standard CPR is judged to be inadequate, attempting IAC CPR is a reasonable alternative intervention.

Active Compression-Decompression CPR (ACD CPR)

Standard CPR involves a forceful or ''active'' chest compression phase with elastic recoil of the chest wall during the relaxation phase (''passive'' decompression). The ACD CPR device consists of a circular suction cup connected to a handle with a force gauge (Fig. 20-1). With the suction cup securely attached at the midsternal chest, CPR is performed with force applied both downward (active compression) and upward (active decompression) during CPR.[3] One advantage of the ACD CPR device is that it tends to decrease the venous system

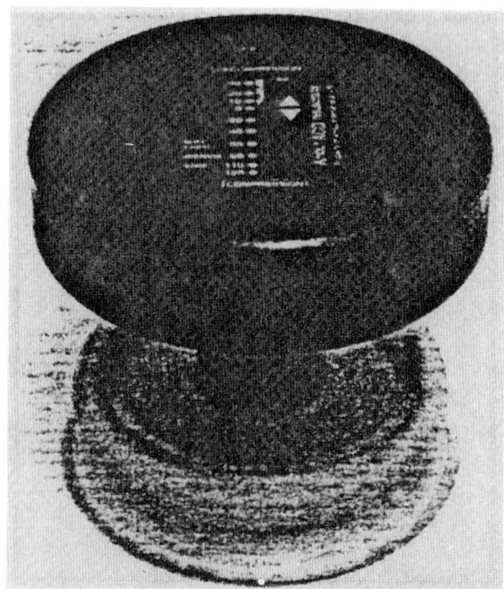

FIG. 20-1. The Ambu CardioPump (Ambu International Inc., Copenhagen, Denmark) is used for active compression-decompression cardiopulmonary resuscitation (ACD-CPR). The silicone rubber suction cup is positioned mid-chest at the level of the nipples. Using the circular plastic handle, the device is pushed downward during the compression phase followed by active withdrawal during the decompression phase. Force of compression and decompression is measured by the gauge located within the handle and is easily viewed by the operator during CPR. (From Lurie KG, Shultz JJ, Callaham ML, et al: Evaluation of active compression-decompression CPR in victims of out-of-hospital cardiac arrest. *JAMA* 271:1405, 1994, with permission.)

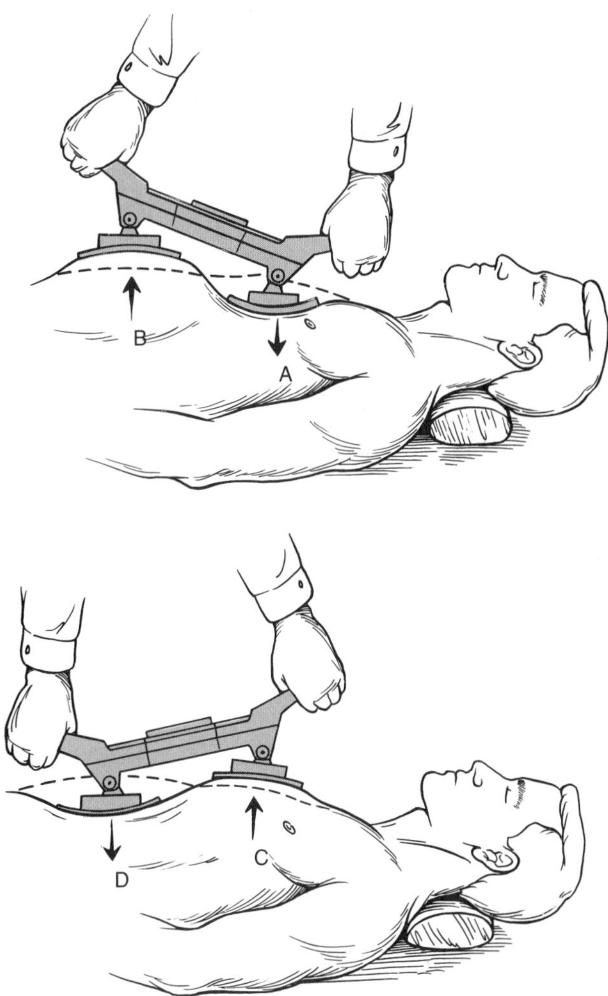

FIG. 20-2. Sequencing compression-decompression with the Lifestick resuscitator. The subject's head is on the right. Chest compression (**A**) is coincident with abdominal decompression (**B**). This is followed by chest decompression (**C**) and abdominal compression (**D**). (From Tang et al,[4] with permission.)

pressure to a greater extent than the arterial pressures during the active decompression phase. This may increase venous return and increase the coronary perfusion pressure gradient during CPR diastole. Although initial clinical reports have indicated some improvement in ROSC and survival, a large randomized clinical trial in in-hospital cardiac arrest (773 patients) and out-of-hospital cardiac arrest (1011 patients) showed no improvement in survival for the ACD CPR device as compared with standard CPR.[3] There is presently insufficient evidence to support the routine use of ACD CPR. However, as noted for other alternative CPR techniques, if standard CPR is judged to be ineffective, ACD CPR is another option. Unlike some of the other alternative techniques, ACD CPR requires a special device, and this limits its applicability.

Phased Chest and Abdominal Compression-Decompression

Tang et al have described the use of a device that combines the concepts of IAC CPR and active compression-decompression.[4] This technique involves the use of a device called the Lifestick resuscitator. This device has chest and abdominal pads connected to an adjustable rigid frame with a handle at each end (Fig. 20-2). The pads are attached to the sternum and the upper abdomen by an adhesive. Using a seesaw motion, the chest and abdomen are compressed in an alternating pattern. The preliminary report of this technique by Tang et al in a survival model of swine cardiac arrest showed improved CPP, ROSC, and 48-h survival. At present, there have been no reports of the use of this device in human cardiac arrests.

Circumferential Thoracic Vest CPR

As noted above, the thoracic pump theory proposes that cyclic fluctuations in intrathoracic pressure created by CPR chest compressions are responsible for blood flow. Thus, efforts to maximize the intrathoracic pressure generated while limiting trauma to the chest would be advantageous. This led to the conception of the circumferential thoracic vest CPR device. This involves the placement of a vest around the thorax and pressurizing the thorax from all directions as opposed to localized pressure over the lower sternum (Fig. 20-3). Halperin et al have reported their preliminary experience in humans with a refined circumferential vest CPR device and found significant improvements in coronary perfusion pressure and initial ROSC.[5] In patients failing prolonged resuscitative efforts, peak CPR–systolic aortic pressure increased from an average of 78 mmHg with manual CPR to an average of 138 mmHg with vest CPR. In 34 patients randomized to receive manual CPR versus vest CPR after an average of 11 min of unsuccessful manual CPR, 8 of 17 vest CPR patients had ROSC compared with only 3 of 17 manual CPR patients. Although this appears to be a promising alternative method of CPR, a substantial amount of clinical investigation is still needed to clarify its potential benefit. Such clinical investigations have been hampered by issues of informed consent.

PHARMACOLOGIC INTERVENTIONS

Adrenergic Therapy

Adrenergic drugs have been the primary agents studied and utilized in all types of cardiac arrest. Epinephrine is the predominant adrenergic drug and remains the recommended agent. The mechanism of action of adrenergic therapy in cardiac resuscitation has been convincingly shown to be primarily alpha adrenergic receptor–mediated vasoconstriction in the peripheral arterial system resulting in increased aortic pressure and thus increased coronary perfusion pressure. In addition to epinephrine, several other pure alpha-adrenergic or mixed alpha- and beta-adrenergic agents have been studied. However, none of these agents has been shown to increase ROSC or long-term survival as compared with epinephrine.

The appropriate dosage of adrenergic drugs during cardiac arrest is the subject of ongoing controversy. Although based on early animal studies and on very limited anecdotal clinical evidence, an epinephrine dose of 1 mg was the standard recommendation for many years. Laboratory investigations and clinical reports in the 1980s suggest that substantially higher doses were required for optimal beneficial effect. These studies led to large, randomized, controlled clinical trials in the early 1990s that showed variable effects on the rate of ROSC but failed to show improvement in survival to hospital discharge or neurologic outcome.[6] Although no benefit was demonstrated, no adverse results were identified with the use of higher doses of epinephrine. Still, there have been anecdotal complaints from intensivists that the temporary ROSC achieved unnecessarily diverts intensive care resources for futile situations. The American Heart Association has left the option of using higher doses of epinephrine open to the clinician's discretion in the clinical arena.[6]

Nonadrenergic Vasoconstriction

Although adrenergic therapy has been the pharmacologic cornerstone of vasoconstrictor therapy, there are nonadrenergic agents capable

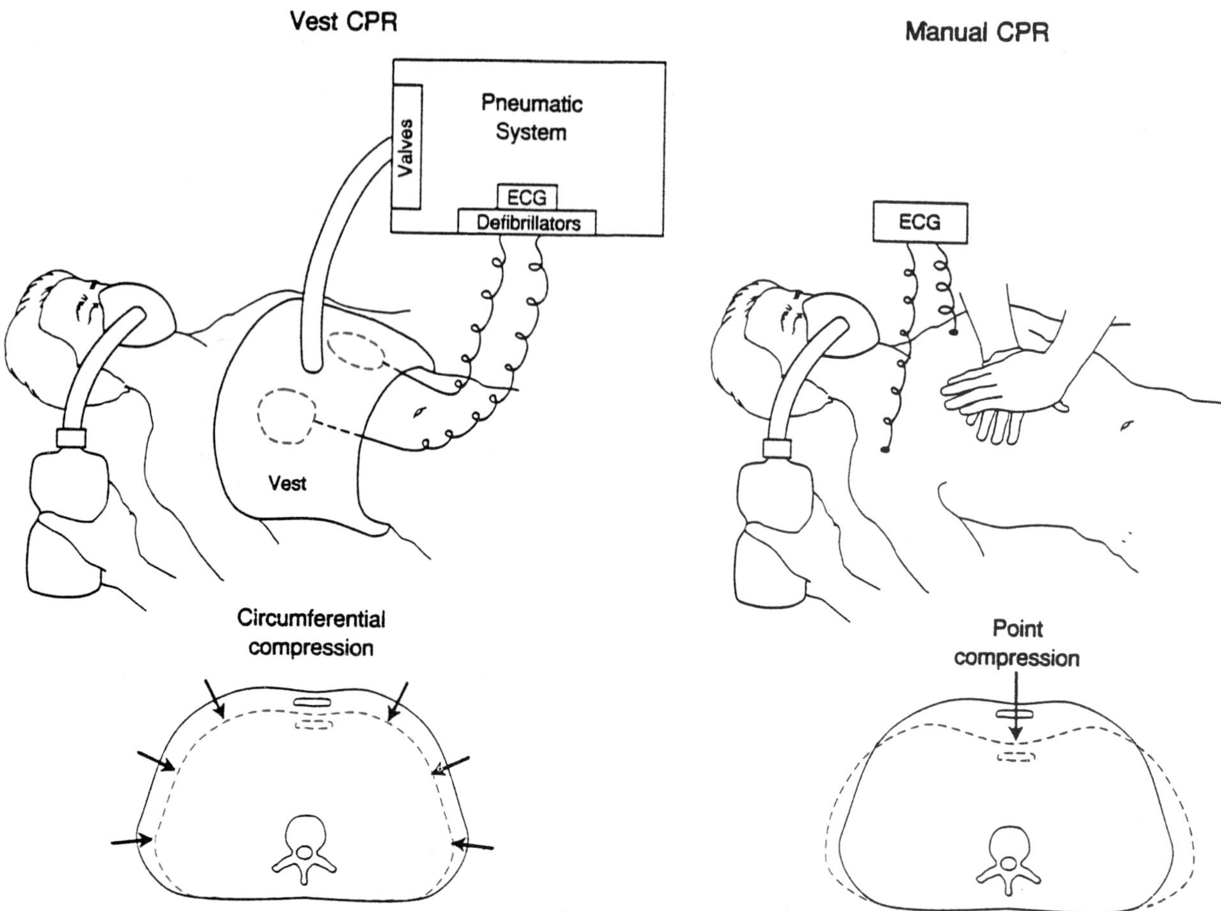

FIG. 20-3. A comparison of the thoracic vest system for cardiopulmonary resuscitation (vest CPR) with the standard manual CPR. The vest contains a bladder that is inflated and deflated by the pneumatic system. Defibrillation can be accomplished during chest compression through the flat defibrillator electrodes (*dashed circles*) under the vest. The ECG can be recorded through the same electrodes. The lower panels show schematic representations of transverse sections of the midthorax during vest CPR and manual CPR. The thoracic size during chest relaxation is shown by the solid lines. The arrows indicate force applied to the thorax during chest compression. With vest inflation, there is a relatively uniform decrease in the dimensions of the thorax. With manual CPR, the sternum is displaced during compression (*arrow*) and the lateral thorax can bulge, thereby increasing thoracic volume and reducing the intrathoracic pressure generated during compression. (From Halperin et al,[5] with permission.)

of producing significant arterial vasoconstriction; these could prove beneficial in the treatment of cardiac arrest. The most promising nonadrenergic agent is vasopressin. Laboratory studies and early clincial reports have shown favorable effects as compared with epinephrine. Linder et al reported a small randomized clinical study comparing intravenous vasopressin (40 U) with intravenous epinephrine (1 mg) and showed a significant increase in initial ROSC, hospital admission, and 24-h survival.[7] There was also a trend toward improved survival to hospital discharge. Another nonadrenergic agent that has undergone only limited laboratory investigation is angiotensin II. The use of nonadrenergic vasoconstrictor agents either alone or in conjunction with adrenergic vasoconstrictor agents may prove to be more effective than adrenergic therapy alone.

Adenosine Antagonism

Release and accumulation of adenosine in ischemic tissues and adenosine's role as a depressant of cardiac pacemaker automaticity has been more clearly defined in recent years. There is limited clinical evidence to suggest that aminophylline can reverse these effects (by acting as an adenosine antagonist) and may be useful in the treatment of bradydysrhythmias associated with myocardial ischemia. Clinical studies have shown favorable initial response to aminophylline bolus, but long-term survival does not appear to be affected.[8,9] Laboratory studies have shown no apparent benefit of aminophylline in cardiac arrest. Thus, adenosine antagonism remains an unproven therapy. However, given the dismal prospects for survival associated with bradyasystolic arrest, a clinician could not be faulted for administering aminophylline in such a setting, especially if there was no response to standard therapy. However the caveat noted earlier for high-dose epinephrine would apply here also.

Amiodarone

Amiodarone is an antiarrhythmic agent with a complex electropharmacologic profile that has been used for long-term control of a variety of atrial and ventricular dysrhythmias. Despite its reportedly limited effect on ventricular effective refractory period after acute intravenous administration, it has been shown to be effective in the treatment of acute unstable ventricular dysrhythmias refractory to lidocaine and procainamide. In a randomized, double-blind, multicenter clinical trial, two amiodarone regimens (low-dose and high-dose) were compared to a standard bretylium regimen in 302 patients with refractory, hemodynamically unstable ventricular tachycardia and ventricular fibrillation.[10] The high-dose amiodarone regimen (an initial rapid infusion of 150 mg over 10 min, followed by 1 mg/min for 6 h and 0.52 mg/h thereafter to 48 h) was equivalent to bretylium in terms of suppression of subsequent unstable ventricular dysrhythmias and showed a better side-effect profile. Amiodarone is, therefore, an emerging antiarrhythmic agent in the treatment of acute ventricular dysrhythmia, especially those cases that are refractory to more traditional antiarrhythmic therapy.

Magnesium

Clinical studies have shown improved survival with magnesium supplementation in the setting of acute myocardial infarction. The cardioprotective effects of magnesium are thought to be related to suppression of automaticity, coronary vasodilation, platelet inhibition, and inhibition of calcium influx. Although an association between hypomagnesemia and cardiac dysrhythmias has been recognized, the value of magnesium in the treatment of acute, life-threatening ventricular dysrhythmias has not been established. Thel et al reported a randomized, double-blind, placebo-controlled clinical trial of magnesium administration in 156 in-hosptial cardiac arrest patients.[11] Administration of magnesium (initial 2 g bolus during cardiac arrest followed by an infusion of 8 g over 24 h) showed no difference in ROSC, survival to 24 h, survival to hospital discharge, or Glasgow Coma Scale score on discharge as compared with placebo. However, among survivors to hospital discharge (21 percent in each group), quality of life assessed by Karnofsky performance status was better in the magnesium group, and no adverse effects of magnesium administration were noted. Thus, the use of magnesium in cardiac arrest remains incompletely defined. Magnesium administration during cardiac arrest seems acceptable based on clinical judgment, especially in cases of suspected hypomagnesemia or refractory cardiac arrest.

Routes for Medication Delivery

Recommended routes for the administration of resuscitation drugs include intravenous, endotracheal, and intraosseous routes. Intravenous administration is considered optimal, with central venous delivery preferred over peripheral venous delivery provided that there is no delay in gaining central venous access. Intracardiac drug injection has largely been discouraged. Central arterial administration of medications has received little attention but may be a useful alternative, especially for delivery of vasoconstrictor agents, which have their effector sites in the peripheral arterial system.

Catheterization to measure arterial pressure during cardiac arrest is becoming a more accepted intervention to help guide resuscitative efforts. Thoracic aortic catheterization via a femoral artery approach allows for both pressure monitoring and homogeneous arterial drug administration. When aortic arch and central venous routes of epinephrine administration were compared in a laboratory model, aortic arch delivery resulted in a more rapid increase in CPR diastolic aortic pressure, a greater magnitude of aortic pressure increase, and a maximal response consistently seen within 30 to 50 s of injection.[12] The rapidity of initial and maximal aortic pressure response suggests that adrenergic therapy could be rapidly adjusted based on a parameter reflecting vital organ perfusion. Thus, thoracic aortic catheterization allows for both rapid delivery of vasoconstrictor agents to effector sites and rapid assessment of therapeutic effect, such that therapy can be rapidly titrated on an individual basis. The major limitation of this route is the need to establish central arterial access.

TECHNIQUES FOR ASSESSMENT OF RESUSCITATIVE EFFORTS

The lack of an accurate and readily measurable parameter to guide resuscitative efforts has long frustrated clinicians and clinical investigators. Pulse quality, pupillary reactivity, serial blood gases, and the coarseness of ventricular fibrillation were the only parameters available until relatively recently. None of these was sufficiently accurate to allow for therapeutic adjustments on an individual case basis. Fortunately, recent technological advances have led to monitoring techniques which allow for much more accurate assessment and guidance of therapy.

Capnometry or End-Tidal Carbon Dioxide

Capnometry (the measurement of exhaled end-tidal carbon dioxide levels) has become a valuable and standard monitoring tool in the emergency department. Although used primarily to assess endotracheal tube placement and monitor ventilation, end-tidal carbon dioxide ($ETCO_2$) can also be used to assess blood flow. $ETCO_2$ is proportional to pulmonary perfusion, which, in turn, reflects systemic perfusion. It is this principle that makes $ETCO_2$ monitoring of value in the assessment of perfusion during CPR.

The use of quantitative or semiquantitative $ETCO_2$ as an indicator of the effectiveness of artificial perfusion has received considerable attention over the past decade or so. Laboratory models or cardiac arrest demonstrated a statistically significant correlation between $ETCO_2$ and coronary perfusion pressure, suggesting that $ETCO_2$ could serve as a useful noninvasive method to monitor the effectiveness of resuscitative efforts and to guide therapy. In one clinical study, the initial $ETCO_2$ served to predict which patients would regain a pulse during the resuscitation. Those patients with an $ETCO_2$ of at least 15 mmHg on arrival in the emergency department (ED) had a greater than 90 percent probability of regaining a pulse, while those patients with an $ETCO_2$ of less than 15 mmHg almost never regained a pulse.[13] In many of these patients, a sudden, dramatic increase in the $ETCO_2$ was noticed well before a pulse could be detected. Unfortunately, $ETCO_2$ does not always correlate precisely with coronary perfusion pressure, and the relationship between the two can be affected by therapeutic interventions such as adrenergic therapy. While these studies cannot be used as an endorsement for deciding when to quit or continue CPR, they do lend support to the validity of $ETCO_2$ as a reflection of cardiac output. $ETCO_2$ is the most accurate noninvasive method of monitoring CPR effectiveness currently available, and its use is encouraged. The most appropriate way to use $ETCO_2$ is to maintain minute ventilation relatively constant while adjusting the mechanics of CPR chest compression and titrating adrenergic therapy in an effort to maximize the $ETCO_2$.

Ventricular Fibrillation Waveform Analysis

It has long been recognized that the coarseness of the ventricular fibrillation (VF) waveform has a rough correlation with the duration of cardiac arrest and the prospects for successful defibrillation with ROSC. With the onset of VF, thcrc is a gradually progressive decrease in the peak-to-trough amplitude of the VF waveform in the absence of resuscitative interventions. The recorded amplitude of the VF waveform, however, is subject to such factors as body habitus, electrode location, and contact, and instrumentation. Using mathematical formulas (the fast Fourier transform) and high-speed computers, a digital characterization of the VF waveform can be derived. This method provides a discreet digital number with which to describe the distribution of frequencies present in the waveform. One measure, the median or centroid frequency, has been found to correlate with defibrillation success and to predict the duration of VF. As VF continues without resuscitation, the median frequency gradually deteriorates over time. When effective resuscitation measures are instituted, the median frequency promptly increases.[14] Such interventions as invasive perfusion support or pharmacologic therapy with epinephrine or vasopressin have successfully raised the median frequency of VF and have been associated with enhanced resuscitation success in animal models. The median frequency (or other measures derived from the fast Fourier transform) may eventually find their way to the bedside in the form of a monitor used by the clinician to guide therapy during resuscitation attempts.

Invasive Hemodynamic Pressure Monitoring

Laboratory and clinical studies have demonstrated that both aortic pressure and CPP correlate strongly with coronary blood flow and ROSC. Although placement of arterial pressure catheters is a common occurrence in critical care medicine, arterial catheterization is not routinely performed in cardiac arrest patients. This is partially because of the technical difficulties associated with performing this during CPR. However, arterial pressure monitoring provides a very useful parameter to guide resuscitative efforts. The CPR-diastolic arterial pressure is the major predictor of the actual CPP. Thus, adjusting therapeutic interventions to maximize CPR-diastolic arterial pressure will result in greater CPP and improved chances of survival.

Central venous catheterization in addition to arterial and aortic catheterization allows for the accurate measurement of the aortic-to-right atrial pressure gradient or CPP. Although clearly one of the most useful measurable parameters in human resuscitation, it has been studied by only a few investigators and only as an in-hospital procedure. Thus, out-of-hospital cardiac arrest patients undergoing CPP monitoring have generally been in arrest for an extended period of time. Paradis et al reported that ROSC in the ED correlated with achieving a CPP greater than 15 mmHg among patients with prolonged cardiac arrest.[15] None of the patients with ROSC survived, suggesting that CPP monitoring after prolonged cardiac arrest is likely to be of limited benefit. Thus, efforts to perform invasive monitoring more rapidly upon hospital arrival or even in the prehospital setting should be pursued. The feasibility of performing prehospital invasive hemodynamic monitoring has been demonstrated with the use of a commercially available, lightweight, and portable monitoring system that can be easily transported to the scene of out-of-hospital cardiac arrest.

Central Venous Oxygen Saturation Monitoring

Rivers et al have reported the use of central venous oximetry in evaluation of cardiac arrest patients.[16] Central venous oxygen saturation yields important information about tissue oxygen delivery/consumption balance and was predictive of ROSC. A central venous oxygen saturation of less than 30% resulted in a zero percent ROSC rate, whereas a value greater than 72% resulted in a 100 percent ROSC rate. Impending ROSC was foreshadowed by an abrupt or gradual increase in central venous oxygen saturation. Interestingly, a supranormal central venous oxygen saturation, termed *venous hyperoxia,* was frequently seen during the early phase of ROSC, followed by a return to normal levels.

INVASIVE PERFUSION TECHNIQUES

Direct Mechanical Ventricular Assistance

Direct mechanical ventricular assistance (DMVA) was first described by Anstadt et al in 1965 and several laboratory studies have investigated this technique in cardiac arrest models. DMVA utilizes a cup-shaped device that fits around the ventricles and is held in place by a vacuum at the apex of the heart (Fig. 20-4). Cyclic positive and negative pressures are transmitted to a flexible diaphragm on the inner surface of the cup, resulting in compression and reexpansion of the ventricles, respectively. The major difference between DMVA and open-chest manual compression of the heart is the active ventricular dilatation, which enhances ventricular filling for the next compression phase. DMVA has been shown to generate higher arterial pressures and greater cardiac output than open-chest manual compression. The clinical utility of this technique in the treatment of cardiac arrest has not been established. The major advantage of DMVA is that it can be sustained for an extended period of time. The major limitation of DMVA is the requirement of a thoracotomy, which largely precludes its use within an effective time frame for most victims of out-of-hospital cardiac arrest.

Cardiopulmonary Bypass

Cardiopulmonary bypass (CPB) (Fig. 20-5) is an effective means of providing sustained global perfusion and has been advocated in the treatment of cardiac arrest. Several laboratory studies have demonstrated improved ROSC and neurologic recovery with CPB compared with standard advanced cardiac life support (ACLS) interventions. There are also several case series describing the successful use of femorofemoral CPB in the treatment of cardiac arrest. The major advantages of CPB are that it can be performed with only a femoral vessel cutdown, artificial perfusion can be sustained for an extended period of time, and perfusion support can be gradually withdrawn. The major disadvantage is the equipment, skill, and time required to

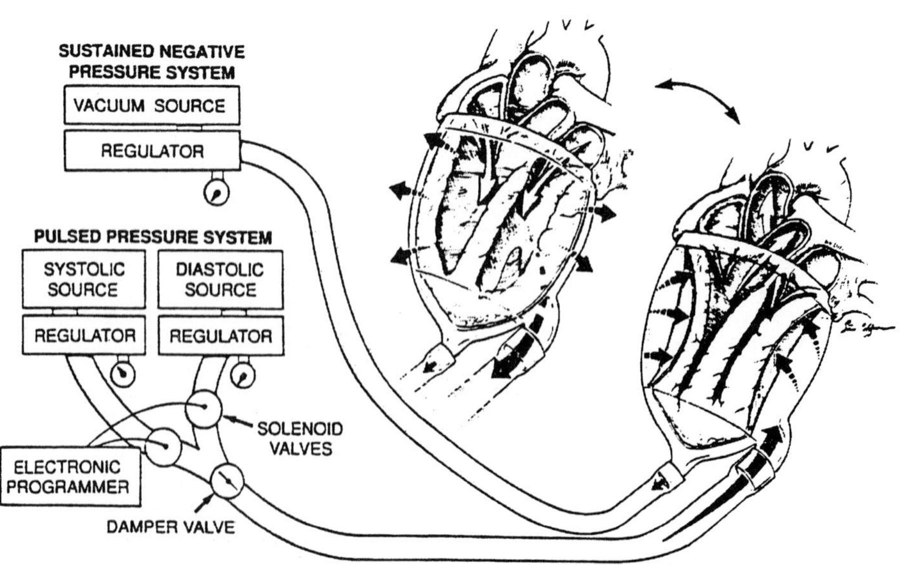

FIG. 20-4. Direct mechanical ventricular assistance (DMVA). Schematic diagram of DMVA drive system and cup. Note the device actuates the ventricular myocardium into systolic (*right*) and diastolic (*left*) configurations. (From Anstadt MP, Anstad GL, Lowe JE: Direct mechanical ventricular actuation: A review. *Resuscitation* 21:7, 1991, with permission.)

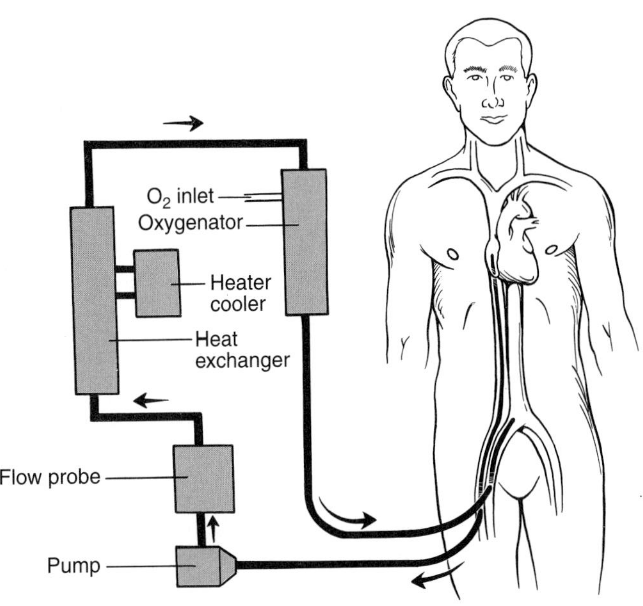

FIG. 20-5. Schematic diagram of CPB system used.

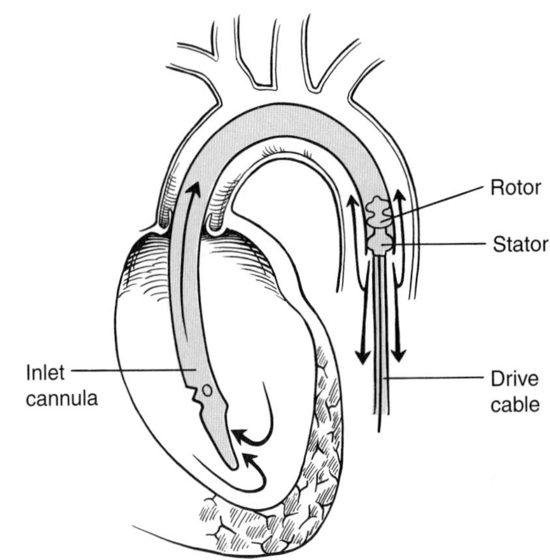

FIG. 20-6. Schematic diagram of the Hemopump positioned in the left ventricle.

perform CPB. A recent report of 10 cardiac arrest victims in whom CPB was initiated in the ED showed that ROSC was achieved in all 10, but there were no long-term survivors.[17] The average-time from onset of arrest to onset of CPB support was 32 min. In order to achieve long-term survival, the time interval to CPB support must be much shorter. Unless the technique can be extended to the prehospital setting, it will be of very limited value in the treatment of victims of out-of-hospital cardiac arrest. However, technological advances offer the prospect of developing CPB devices that can be used in the prehospital setting.

Hemopump

The Hemopump is a catheter-based temporary ventricular assist device consisting of an axial flow pump component at the distal end of the catheter powered by an external motor via a flexible drive cable that runs the length of the catheter. The distal tip of the axial flow pump component is advanced from a femoral artery into the left ventricle (Fig. 20-6). When it is in operation, forward blood flow is generated by blood entering the axial flow pump component in the left ventricle and exiting in the aortic arch. Laboratory investigation in a cardiac arrest model has demonstrated sustained mean arterial pressures of approximately 60 mmHg and cardiac output averaging 2.3 L/min.[18] The major drawback with the use of this device in the setting of cardiac arrest is that one must be able to insert the catheter from a femoral artery to the left ventricle.

Aortic Catheter Perfusion Techniques

During the past decade, there has been an interest in the use of aortic balloon occlusion catheters to enhance vital organ perfusion during cardiac arrest. The use of standard intraaortic balloon pumping has been shown to increase CPP during closed-chest CPR, but the effect is not dramatic. However, the use of aortic balloon catheters for the infusion of resuscitation solutions during cardiac arrest holds greater promise for improving resuscitation outcome.

Selective aortic arch perfusion (SAAP) as described by Manning et al[19] or selective aortic perfusion and oxygenation (SAPO) as described by Paradis et al[20] uses a large-lumen balloon occlusion catheter positioned in the descending aortic arch to provide selective perfusion of the heart and brain during cardiac arrest (Fig. 20-7). The catheter

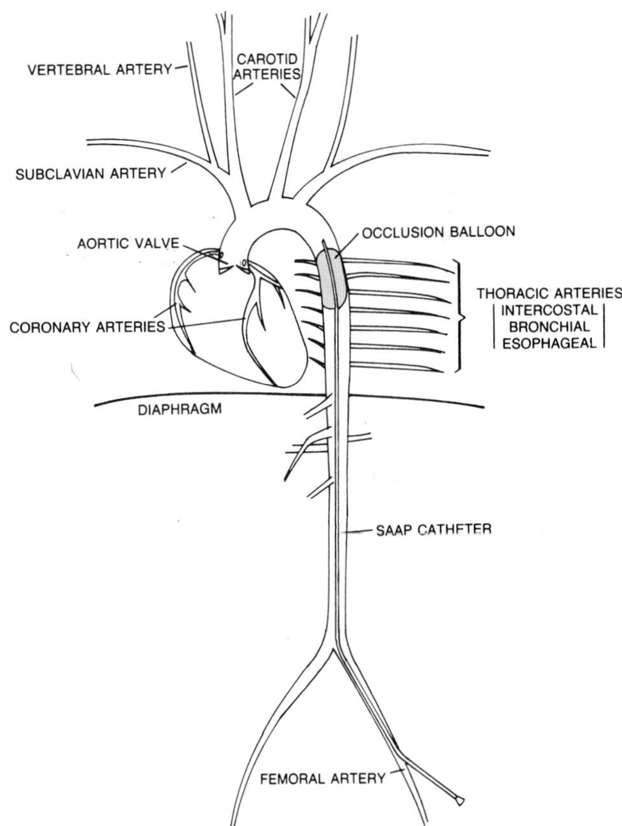

FIG. 20-7. Selective aortic arch perfusion (SAAP). Positioning of the SAAP balloon occlusion catheter at the end of the descending aortic arch through a femoral artery. Placement of the balloon at this level restricts flow to aortic arch vessels including coronary arteries. (From Manning et al,[19] with permission).

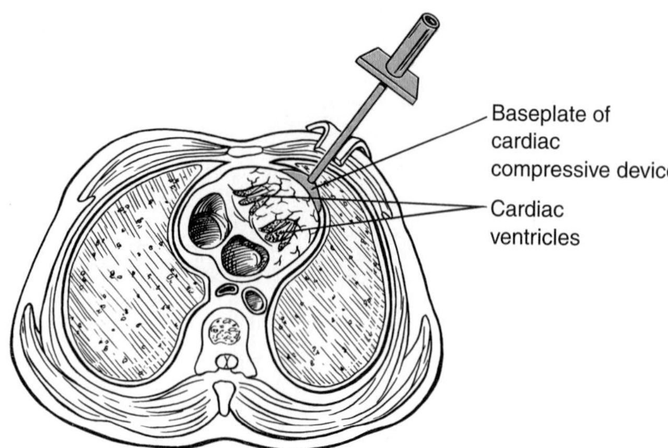

FIG. 20-8. The heart-contacting baseplate and a portion of the stem of the cardiac compressive device are inserted into the thorax through a small, parasternal incision. The manually-operated handle remains outside the chest. The base plate is positioned directly on the cardiac ventricles, lying within an intact pericardium. Manual depression of the device compresses the heart and produces an artificial systole.

is inserted into a femoral artery (percutaneously or via a cutdown) and blindly advanced into the thoracic aorta. With the balloon inflated and pressure cuffs applied to the upper arms, the coronary and cerebral circulations are relatively isolated for brief perfusion. The resuscitation solution infused consists of an oxygenated blood substitute, such as a perfluorocarbon emulsion or polymerized hemoglobin solution, that might contain various agents to enhance restoration of spontaneous cardiac contraction, maintain neuronal viability, and limit both myocardial and neuronal reperfusion injury. One of the major advantages of SAAP is the ability to administer agents to combat reperfusion injury at the moment of reperfusion or just prior to it. SAAP was designed for use in the prehospital as well as the in-hospital setting. Although laboratory results have been very favorable, the efficacy of this invasive perfusion technique in human cardiac arrest has not been studied.

Tang et al have described the use of a balloon occlusion catheter positioned in the ascending aortic arch.[21] Laboratory investigations of this technique have shown marked increases in coronary perfusion with intermittent balloon occlusion. Infusion of fluid via the catheter results in isolated coronary artery perfusion. The technical feasibility of rapidly and reliably positioning the tip of this catheter in the ascending aortic arch may prove to be a significant challenge in the clinical setting.

Minimally Invasive Direct Cardiac Massage

In 1995, Buckman et al reported the use of a relatively simple device for the rapid initiation of internal cardiac compression through a small thoracic incision.[22] The technique, called minimally invasive direct cardiac massage, uses a rectangular, curved, padded plate connected to a handle to compress the heart through an intercostal incision at the anterolateral left chest at the level of the lower sternum (Fig. 20-8). In a swine cardiac arrest model, the device generated CPP and cardiac output similar to that produced by manual open-chest cardiac massage. It has been suggested that a modified device could potentially be inserted via a smaller (2 to 3-cm) intercostal incision.

REFERENCES

1. Maier GW, Tyson GS, Olsen CO, et al: The physiology of external cardiac massage: High-impulse cardiopulmonary resuscitation. *Circulation* 70:86, 1984.
2. Sack JB, Kesselbrenner MB: Hemodynamics, survival benefits, and complications of interposed abdominal compression during cardiopulmonary resuscitation. *Acad Emerg Med* 1:490, 1994.
3. Stiell IG, Hebert PC, Wells GA, et al: The Ontario trial of active compression-decompression cardiopulmonary resuscitation for in-hospital and prehospital cardiac arrest. *JAMA* 267:2916, 1992.
4. Tang W, Weil MH, Schock RB, et al: Phased chest and abdominal compression-decompression: A new option for cardiopulmonary resuscitation. *Circulation* 95:1335, 1997.
5. Halperin HR, Tsitlik JE, Gefand M, et al: A preliminary study of cardiopulmonary resuscitation by circumferential compression of the chest with use of a pneumatic vest. *N Engl J Med* 329:762, 1993.
6. Emergency Cardiac Care Committee and Subcommittees, American Heart Association: Guidelines for cardiopulmonary resuscitation and emergency cardiac care: III. Adult advanced cardiac life support. *JAMA* 268:2199, 1992.
7. Lindner KH, Dirks B, Strohmenger HU, et al: Randomised comparison of epinephrine and vasopressin in patients with out-of-hospital ventricular fibrillation. *Lancet* 349:535, 1997.
8. Viskin S, Belhassen B, Roth A, et al: Aminophylline for bradyasystolic cardiac arrest refractory to atropine and epinephrine. *Ann Intern Med* 118:279, 1993.
9. Mader TJ, Gibson P: Adenosine receptor antagonism in refractory asystolic cardiac arrest: Results of a human pilot study. *Resuscitation* 35:3, 1997.
10. Kowey PR, Levine JH, Herre JM, et al for the Intravenous Amiodarone Multicenter Investigators Group: Randomized, double-blinded comparison of intravenous amiodarone and bretylium in the treatment of patients with recurrent hemodynamically destabilizing ventricular tachycardia and fibrillation. *Circulation* 92:3255, 1995.
11. Thel MC, Armstrong AL, McNulty SE, et al: Randomised trial of magnesium in in-hospital cardiac arrest. *Lancet* 350:1272, 1997.
12. Manning JE, Murphy CA, Batson DN, et al: Aortic arch versus central venous epinephrine during CPR. *Ann Emerg Med* 22:703, 1993.
13. Callaham ML, Barton CW: Prediction of outcome of cardiopulmonary resuscitation from end-tidal carbon dioxide concentration. *Crit Care Med* 18:358, 1990.
14. Brown CG, Dzwonczyk R: Signal analysis of the human electrocardiogram during ventricular fibrillation: Frequency and amplitude parameters as predictors of successful countershock. *Ann Emerg Med* 27:184, 1996.
15. Paradis NA, Martin GB, Rivers EP, et al: Coronary perfusion pressure and the return of spontaneous circulation in human cardiopulmonary resuscitation. *JAMA* 263:1106, 1990.
16. Rivers EP, Martin GB, Smithline H, et al: The clinical implications of continuous central venous oxygen saturation during human CPR. *Ann Emerg Med* 21:1094, 1992.
17. Martin GB, Rivers EP, Paradis NA, et al: Emergency department cardiopulmonary bypass in the treatment of human cardiac arrest. *Chest* 113:743, 1998.
18. Schroder T, Hering JP, Uhlig P, et al: Efficiency of the left ventricle assist device Hemopump in cardiac fibrillation. *Br J Anaesth* 68:536, 1992.
19. Manning JE, Murphy CA, Hertz CM, et al: Selective aortic arch perfusion during cardiac arrest: A new resuscitation technique. *Ann Emerg Med* 21:1058, 1992.
20. Paradis NA, Rose MI, Gawryl MS: Selective aortic perfusion and oxygenation: An effective adjunct to external chest compression–based cardiopulmonary resuscitation. *J Am Coll Cardiol* 23:497, 1994.
21. Tang W, Weil MH, Noc M, et al: Augmented efficacy of external CPR by intermittent occlusion of the ascending aorta. *Circulation* 88:1916, 1993.
22. Buckman RF Jr, Badellino MM, Mauro LH, et al: Direct cardiac massage without major thoracotomy: Feasibility and systemic blood flow. *Resuscitation* 29:237, 1995.

ACID-BASE DISORDERS

David D. Nicolaou
Gabor D. Kelen

The homeostasis of the human organism is critically dependent upon the function of its proteins. Protein function is optimal at specific levels of acidity. Thus, plasma acidity is closely regulated.

Many diseases including those presenting an imminent life threat produce acid-base disturbances that provide important clues concerning the nature of the underlying illness and suggest immediate therapeutic interventions. The following is a practical approach to the clinical evaluation of acid-base disorders.

MEASUREMENT OF PLASMA ACIDITY

Plasma hydrogen ion concentration ($[H^+]$) is normally 40 meq (40 mmol) per liter and corresponds to a pH of 7.4. It is inconvenient to work with such small concentrations, and the negative base 10 logarithm of the hydrogen ion concentration (pH) is therefore often used to express plasma acidity. Because pH is a logarithmic transformation of $[H^+]$, the relationship of $[H^+]$ to pH is not linear for all pH values (Table 21-1). However, for pH values from 7.20 to 7.50, the relationship between hydrogen ion concentration and pH is nearly linear; pH changes of 0.01 unit correspond to approximately 1 mmol/L change in $[H^+]$.

Plasma Acid Homeostasis

Plasma hydrogen ion concentration is influenced by rate of endogenous production, rate of excretion, and buffering capacity of the body. Buffers mitigate the impact on plasma pH of large changes in available hydrogen ion. A buffer pair consists of a weak acid and its conjugate base, which are in equilibrium, as seen in Eq. (1), below:

$$[HA] \Leftrightarrow [H^+] + [A^-] \qquad (1)$$

Addition or removal of hydrogen ion causes a shift in the equilibrium, resulting in a reduction or increase in $[H^+]$, respectively. The effectiveness of a buffer system is optimal when the concentrations of its base and conjugate acid are equal; that is, the system is equally able to buffer excess protons or to release them. This point is the dissociation constant, or K_A.

Equation (1) can now be written quantitatively to describe the hydrogen ion concentration, as shown in Eq. 2.

$$[H^+] = K_A \frac{[HA]}{[A^-]} \qquad (2)$$

Equation (2) demonstrates that a buffer system's efficiency is determined by how close its pK_A is to physiologic pH. Buffer systems that are effective at physiologic pH include hemoglobin, phosphate, proteins, and bicarbonate (Fig. 21-1).[1] One can consider the hydrogen ion concentration to be the result of all physiologic buffers acting on the common pool of hydrogen ions.

TABLE 21-1 pH and Hydrogen Ion Concentrations

pH	$[H^+]$
6.8	158
6.9	126
7.0	100
7.1	79
7.2	63
7.3	50
7.4	40
7.5	32
7.6	25
7.7	20

Source: From Narins and Emmett,[1] with permission.

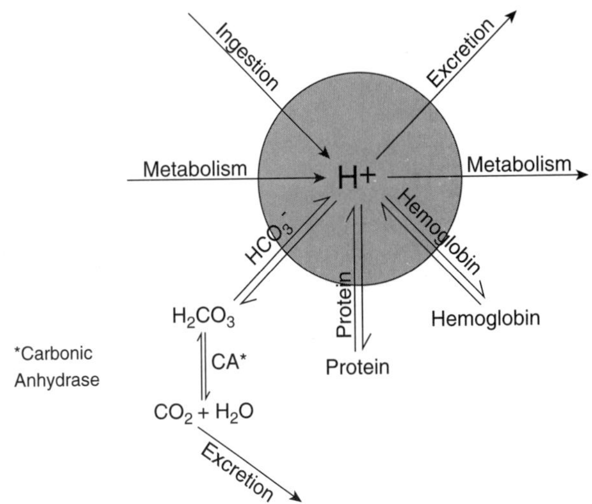

FIG. 21-1. Schematic representation of hydrogen ion homeostasis.

If the base 10 logarithm of each term in Eq. (2) is taken and the resulting equation is applied to the bicarbonate/carbonic acid buffer system, the familiar Henderson-Hasselbalch equation—Eq. (3)—results.

$$pH = pK + \log \frac{[HCO_3^-]}{[H_2CO_3]} \qquad (3)$$

This equation demonstrates the interrelationship between carbonic acid, bicarbonate, and pH; any two of these determine the third.

The clinical utility of the Henderson-Hasselbalch equation, however, is limited. The values of each term in Eq. (3) except pH are not convenient to measure. The bicarbonate concentration is approximated by the total CO_2,* but carbonic acid must be calculated from the P_{CO_2} and the solubility constant of CO_2 in blood. This requires substitution of the pK_A with a modified value. Finally, the logarithm of all terms must be calculated.

However, if all constants are inserted into the Henderson-Hasselbalch equation and the antilog of all its terms is taken, the resulting simplified equation—Eq. (4)—is of great clinical utility.[2]

$$[H^+] = 24 \times \frac{P_{CO_2}}{[HCO_3^-]} \qquad (4)$$

The Kassirer-Bleich equation may be used to calculate the concentration of any component of the bicarbonate buffer system provided that the concentrations of the other two components are known. It therefore allows clinicians to determine, for example, what the pH *must be* when the P_{CO_2} and the bicarbonate concentration are known. Performing such a calculation using values reported by the laboratory permits the clinician to check the internal consistency of the reported data. (In fact, hospital laboratories do not measure $[HCO_3^-]$ but calculate the number based on pH and P_{CO_2} measurements.)

*The "bicarbonate concentration" measured by the clinical laboratory is actually the total CO_2, a figure that is the sum of bicarbonate and dissolved CO_2 plus H_2CO_3. The latter term is the P_{CO_2} multiplied by the solubility coefficient of CO_2 in blood (α), 0.03. Thus, total CO_2 = $[HCO_3^-]$ + (0.03) (P_{CO_2}). Most clinicians simply neglect the second term when the P_{CO_2} is normal; when hypercapnia is present, however, the second term contributes significantly to total CO_2.[1]

PHYSIOLOGY OF ACID PRODUCTION AND EXCRETION

The bicarbonate/carbonic acid buffer system is an open system; that is, the quantity of buffer present in the system is not fixed but varies according to physiologic need. This flexibility is largely provided by pulmonary excretion of P_{CO_2}, which can vary significantly and rapidly according to the exigencies of the acid-base milieu. The kidney regulates both bicarbonate excretion and the formation of new bicarbonate and is able to change the rate of these processes when demanded by the acid-base milieu, while pulmonary response to immediate renal compensation requires hours to days to complete.

Hepatic Influence on Acid-Base Balance

Although the lungs and kidney are traditionally considered the cornerstone organs of acid-base balance, increasing attention is being given to the role of the liver in acid-base homeostasis. Approximately 1 mol each of bicarbonate and ammonium is generated every day by protein catabolism. The irreversible synthesis of urea by the liver results in consumption of virtually all of this bicarbonate. The rate of this reaction is closely tied to both extracellular pH and bicarbonate concentration. This control, mediated by glutaminase and carbonic anhydrase, can result in significant retention and neutralization of bicarbonate during acidosis. The fixation of ammonium ions into urea slows, but the kidney increases ammonia synthesis and excretion. This process not only prevents ammonia accumulation but also allows hydrogen ion trapping in the distal tubule. Furthermore, hepatic cells without the cellular machinery to fix ammonia into urea avidly use excess ammonia to synthesize glutamine.[3] Thus, the liver is the ''third organ'' of acid-base balance.

Renal Influence on Acid-Base Balance

The maintenance of bicarbonate homeostasis by the kidney requires reclamation of the daily filtered load of bicarbonate, 85 percent of which occurs in the proximal convoluted tubule. The Na^+,K^+-ATPase system extrudes sodium into plasma and draws potassium into the tubule cell. The filtrate in the tubule lumen, however, has a sodium concentration equal to that of plasma. An antiporter of sodium and hydrogen ion is driven by this gradient, transporting sodium from the tubule lumen into the tubule cell in exchange for hydrogen ion. The hydrogen ion combines with filtered bicarbonate in the tubule lumen, producing carbonic acid. Carbonic anhydrase, resident in the luminal cell membrane, catalyzes the conversion of carbonic acid to water and CO_2. CO_2, which is soluble, diffuses down a concentration gradient into the tubule cell, where cytoplasmic carbonic anhydrase regenerates carbonic acid (and thereby creates the CO_2 concentration gradient). The carbonic acid dissociates, providing hydrogen ion for extrusion and bicarbonate, which enters the plasma. If the rate of proton extrusion is reduced by tubular disease, bicarbonate will be lost until the serum concentration has fallen to a level that can be reclaimed by the limited hydrogen ion extrusion available. This is the pathophysiology underlying proximal renal tubular acidosis (RTA).

The kidney reclaims the balance (approximately 15 percent) of filtered bicarbonate in the distal tubule. Carbonic anhydrase in the cytoplasm of distal tubule cells generates carbonic acid, which dissociates. An electrogenic H^+-ATPase on the luminal cell membrane secretes the resulting hydrogen ion into the tubule lumen, where it is titrated by inorganic phosphate or binds to ammonia and is ''trapped'' in the tubule lumen. The bicarbonate resulting from dissociation of intracellular carbonic acid diffuses into plasma. The loss of H^+ and HCO_3^- from the cell maintains electroneutrality, so the process of bicarbonate reclamation in the distal tubule is *sodium-independent.* Thus, the process of proton secretion in the distal tubule functions not only to reclaim filtered bicarbonate but also to excrete protons generated by metabolism. The failure of proton secretion is the mechanism underlying distal renal tubular acidosis.

The kidney also generates new bicarbonate in the distal tubule in a *sodium-dependent* process. A Na^+,K^+-ATPase on the antiluminal cell membrane creates a low intracellular sodium concentration. At the same time, intracellular glutamine is metabolized to bicarbonate and ammonium. Sodium then moves from the tubule lumen into the tubule cell down its concentration gradient, and ammonium moves from the tubule cell into the tubule lumen. (Impairment of ammonium excretion results in its incorporation into urea in the liver, a process that *consumes* bicarbonate.) Bicarbonate formation by this process may increase 6 to 10 times over 4 to 5 days when acidosis so demands. However, drugs that alter uptake or delivery of sodium to the distal tubule significantly affect this process.

The effect of the kidney on acid-base balance is to prevent bicarbonaturia and to excrete the daily metabolic load of acid. The process of acid excretion allows the kidney to regenerate bicarbonate in proportion to the quantity consumed by buffering of the daily acid load. The result is that urine, especially under conditions of acidosis, can be made almost entirely free of bicarbonate.

FUNDAMENTAL ACID-BASE DISORDERS

Any condition that disturbs acid-base balance by increasing $[H^+]$—whether through endogenous production, decreased buffering capacity, decreased excretion, or exogenous addition—is termed *acidosis.* Similarly, any condition that decreases $[H^+]$ is termed *alkalosis.* The terms *acidemia* and *alkalemia* refer to the net imbalance of $[H^+]$ in the blood. The difference between acidosis and acidemia is not merely semantic but of great clinical importance. For example, a patient with an acidosis and an alkalosis of equal magnitude will have a normal pH. A patient with these disturbances, then, has neither acidemia nor alkalemia but has both an acidosis and an alkalosis. It is therefore important to appreciate that while acidemia is diagnostic of acidosis and alkalemia of alkalosis, a normal or high pH does not exclude acidosis and a normal or low pH does not exclude the presence of an alkalosis.

Acid-base disturbances are further classified as either respiratory or metabolic. Respiratory acid-base disorders first affect P_{CO_2}, while metabolic disorders first alter bicarbonate concentration. If there were no compensatory mechanism, the Kassirer-Bleich equation states that the magnitude of change in either P_{CO_2} or $[HCO_2^-]$ would directly determine the magnitude of change in the pH. However, physiologic mechanisms tend to mitigate pH changes by effecting offsetting changes in bicarbonate and CO_2 levels. For example, the P_{CO_2} (and thus $[H^+]$) is elevated in respiratory acidosis, but the corresponding fall in pH is attenuated over time by renal retention of bicarbonate.

Compensatory mechanisms are, by definition, not ''disorders.'' Such mechanisms constitute normal physiologic responses to acid-base derangements, and such terms as a *compensatory respiratory alkalosis* are therefore not only confusing but also misleading. The clinician is concerned with the adequacy of compensation, however, because failure of adequate compensation implies the presence of another primary acid-base disturbance. For example, a patient with metabolic acidosis who does not exhibit adequate respiratory compensation has a superimposed respiratory acidosis. Normal compensatory responses to each primary acid-base disturbance have been established through careful study and are presented later in this chapter.

It is important to note that compensatory mechanisms return the pH toward but not to normal.† The fact that compensatory mechanisms cannot become complete is evident when one considers that complete

†The sole exception is in chronic respiratory alkalosis, where bicarbonate levels may decline to a level that nearly normalizes the pH such that differentiating the actual pH from normal falls within the range of lab error.

compensation would necessarily remove the (physiologic) stimulus driving the compensation.[1]

The "normal" values of pH, P_{CO_2}, and $[HCO_3^-]$ for a given laboratory are ranges, intended to include 95 percent of patients without an acid-base disorder. The normal pH range is 7.35 to 7.45, the normal P_{CO_2} range is 35 to 45 mmHg, and the normal $[HCO_3^-]$ is usually 21 to 28 meq/L. However, a patient may have no value outside the "normal range" and still have significant acid-base disturbances. As detailed further below, a patient with a wide anion gap acidosis and a concomitant metabolic alkalosis of near-equal magnitude will have a normal pH, P_{CO_2}, and $[HCO_3^-]$. On the other hand, abnormal-appearing values may, in fact, be appropriate for a given simple acid-base disturbance. For example, in the presence of a metabolic acidosis ($[HCO_3^-] = 15$; pH $= 7.3$), an appropriate respiratory compensation should result in a P_{CO_2} of about 30 mmHg. The P_{CO_2} is below the "normal" range but at the expected level for the degree of (metabolic) acidosis. In this example, the finding of 40 mmHg for P_{CO_2}, a "normal"-appearing value, actually implies the presence of a respiratory acidosis, since the expected physiologic respiratory response is inadequate.

The Anion Gap

The principle of electroneutrality requires that plasma have no net charge. The charge of the predominant plasma cation, sodium, must therefore be "balanced" by the charge of plasma anions. Although bicarbonate and chloride constitute a significant fraction of plasma anions, the sum of their concentrations does not equal that of sodium. There must therefore be other anions present in the serum that preserve electroneutrality. These anions are mostly serum proteins, phosphate, sulfate, and organic anions such as lactate and the conjugate bases of ketoacids. Because these substances are not commonly measured, they are termed *unmeasured anions* (UA). Unmeasured cations (UC) also exist largely in the form of Ca^{2+} and Mg^{2+}. Since all cations, both measured and unmeasured, must equal all anions (both measured and unmeasured),

$$MC + UC = MA + UA$$

it follows that

$$MC - MA = UA - UC = \text{anion gap (AG)}$$

Thus substituting measured ions

$$[Na^+] - ([HCO_3^-] + [Cl^-]) = AG$$

The difference between the serum sodium (the contribution of potassium, largely an intracellular ion, is usually neglected) and the sum of serum chloride and bicarbonate, then, equals the concentration of the unmeasured anions. Correction of serum sodium for hyperglycemia is unnecessary because this condition similarly reduces chloride concentrations.[4]

The unmeasured anion concentration is commonly called the *anion gap* (AG), and in the past its normal value had been considered to be 12 ± 4 meq/L. Recent reports have suggested that a normal anion gap value of 7 ± 4 meq/L may be more appropriate to electrolyte measurements made with ion-specific electrodes.[5] However, the value used by the clinician should reflect institutional practice.[6] As with other acid-base concepts, the accepted "normal" range for the AG is less important than whether it has changed in relation to the patient's steady-state (baseline) value. Thus, a relative change in AG is more important than the actual value. However, virtually all values above 15 meq/L can be considered abnormal even when there is no previous comparison value available.

The anion gap may change even in the absence of acid-base disturbances. It may rise when (unmeasured) cations are decreased, as in severe states of hypomagnesemia, hypokalemia, and hypocalcemia. A reduced or even negative anion gap may result from an increase in unmeasured *cations,* such as lithium and unmeasured positively charged proteins resulting from myeloma and polyclonal gammopathies, or a decrease in unmeasured anions such as albumin and gamma globulin. A narrow or negative anion gap may also be the result of confounders of chloride measurement. Bromide is measured as chloride on an equimolar basis by chloride-specific electrodes. Other techniques of chloride measurement may produce even more inaccurate results in the presence of bromide.[7] Triglyceride levels greater than 600 mg/dL produce overestimation of chloride levels measured by colorimetric techniques and may also result in underestimation of serum sodium, resulting in an apparently negative anion gap.[4]

While increases in the AG are traditionally considered in the context of metabolic acidosis, elevation of the anion gap may be seen with any acid-base disturbance. Metabolic and respiratory alkalosis, for example, may elevate the AG by 2 to 3 meq/L because of elevations in lactate produced by enhancement of glycolysis. Penicillin and carbenicillin, as anions, produce elevations in the AG. Their charges must be balanced by sodium, which is retained by renal tubules at the cost of enhancing secretion of potassium and hydrogen ion. This effect is enhanced by the presence of the poorly reabsorbed penicillin and carbenicillin ions in the tubule lumen, the negative charges of which serve as an electrical gradient for hydrogen and potassium ion secretion. The result is an elevated AG with a hypokalemic alkalosis, illustrating the principle that anions principally cleared by the kidney may elevate the AG, particularly when aldosterone activity is high.

However, elevation of the AG is most commonly associated with metabolic acidosis. The unmeasured anions associated with an elevated AG and metabolic acidosis are listed in Table 21-2. Traditional mnemonics for the differential diagnosis of an elevated AG acidosis unfortunately suggest that iron, theophylline, cyanide, biguanides, and other compounds *are* unmeasured anions. These substances actually elevate the anion gap by producing lactic acidosis, discussed later in this chapter. The result of using traditional mnemonics in evaluating elevated AG acidosis may be a satisfaction-of-search error, where the discovery of lactic acidosis provides a ready explanation for the elevated AG and thereby inhibits pursuit of the causes of lactic acidosis. We suggest that the differential diagnosis of metabolic acidosis with an elevated AG should emphasize distinctions between endogenous and exogenous unmeasured anion sources and avoid mixing the differential diagnosis of lactic acidosis with that of increased unmeasured anions.

Clinical use of the AG requires an appreciation of its limitations. While an AG greater than 30 meq/L is usually caused by lactic acidosis or ketoacidosis, these conditions may exist even when the AG is normal. An AG value less than 25 meq/L has been found to be an insensitive indicator of elevated lactate levels in critically ill patients,[8] and in trauma patients the postresuscitation AG does not predict lactate levels.[9] Thus, the "normal" AG does not exclude the presence of increased concentrations of unmeasured anions. As noted previously, an AG increased from baseline but still within the "normal" range may be a clue. Direct measurements of lactate, formate, ketoacids, methanol (parent of formic acid), ethylene glycol (parent of oxalic acid and numerous other organic acids), and salicylate should be ordered when the AG is "normal" but the presence of any these substances is suspected.

A common clinical problem is the diagnosis of mixed acid-base disturbances in the presence of an elevated AG. Simple acid-base disturbances that produce elevated AGs are referred to as *wide*-AG *metabolic acidoses.* If a wide-AG metabolic acidosis is the only disturbance, then the change (elevation from baseline) in value of the AG (sometimes referred to as the *delta gap*)[10] should exactly equal the change (decrease) in the $[HCO_3^-]$. This is a one-to-one relationship. This concept is represented mathematically in Eq. (5).

$$\Delta \uparrow AG = \Delta \downarrow [HCO_3^-] \quad (5)$$

TABLE 21-2 Unmeasured Anions Associated with an Elevated Anion Gap and Metabolic Acidosis

Diagnostic Category	Species	Origin	Diagnostic Adjuncts
Renal failure (uremia)	PO_4, SO_4	Protein metabolism	BUN/Creatinine
Ketoacidosis Diabetic (DKA) Alcoholic (SKA) Starvation (SKA)	Ketoacids β-hydroxybutyrate Acetoacetate	Fatty acid metabolism	Serum/urine ketones
Lactic acidosis	Lactate	Metabolism	Lactate level
Exogenous poisoning			
Methanol	Formate	Methanol metabolism	Osmolal gap
Ethylene glycol	Oxylate and organic anions	EG metabolism, also results in high NAD/NADH ratio, favoring pyruvate conversion to lactate	Osmolal gap Oxylate crystals (urine)
Salicylate	Salicylate	Salicylate, lactate, ketoacids	Concomitant respiratory alkalosis, and metabolic alkalosis

This simple relationship can be used to great advantage in determining the presence of other metabolic acid-base disturbances. If the $[HCO_3^-]$ is even lower than predicted by the delta AG, then there must be a concomitant hyperchloremic (i.e., non-AG type) metabolic acidosis (Fig. 21-2*A*). Similarly, if the decrease in $[HCO_3^-]$ is less than expected based on the delta AG, there must be a concomitant metabolic alkalosis present. Note that acute respiratory conditions (respiratory acidosis or alkalosis) do not affect these determinations. Potential acid-base disturbances related to respiratory status must be further determined, as discussed below (Fig. 21-2*A–C*).

Parameters Required for Clinical Acid-Base Evaluation

Clinical evaluation of acid-base disorders is an art requiring the synthesis of information gleaned from the clinical encounter and the laboratory. The history should emphasize events that may result in the gain or loss of acid or base, such as vomiting, diarrhea, or ingestion of acids or bases. There may also be evidence of diseases of the organs of acid-base homeostasis: the liver, kidneys, and lungs.

Laboratory evaluation requires blood samples for determination of electrolyte concentrations (potassium, sodium, chloride, and bicarbonate) and blood gases (pH, P_{CO_2}, and bicarbonate concentration). Most clinical laboratories measure two of the parameters reported in blood gas results, most commonly the pH and P_{CO_2}, and use the Henderson-Hasselbalch equation to calculate the third.

Blood samples for acid-base evaluation are traditionally obtained by arterial puncture, but there is some evidence that venous blood may be used instead. Arterial and capillary values of pH and CO_2 content in normal patients and those with diabetic ketoacidosis correlate well (correlation coefficient 0.9 and 0.98, respectively). Recent work has demonstrated high correlations between arterial and venous pH (r = 0.9689) and arterial and venous bicarbonate concentrations (r = 0.9543) in emergency department (ED) patients with diabetic ketoacidosis.[11] The correlation between venous and arterial blood gas values in patients with severe shock remains uncertain, but in other circumstances, the use of venous values seems reasonable. Inexperienced clinicians frequently resort to arterial blood gas (ABG) determination as a means to "know" the pH. However, the pH per se is often the least important value for diagnosis and management. When respiratory status is not compromised, the pH can be calculated from knowing the venous $[HCO_3^-]$ alone, as described below.

METABOLIC ACIDOSIS

Metabolic acidosis may result from bicarbonate loss per se, administration of acid, or endogenous production and accumulation of acid. Loss of bicarbonate occurs in externalization of intestinal contents (e.g., vomiting, enterocutaneous fistulae) and renal wasting of bicarbonate (e.g., renal tubular acidosis, carbonic anhydrase inhibitor therapy). Administration of acid occurs primarily in total parenteral nutrition, where patients receive hydrochloric salts of basic amino acids. Finally, endogenous acids accumulate in renal tubular acidosis, ketoacidosis, and lactic acidosis.

Metabolic acidosis results in a decreased serum bicarbonate concentration, and its development causes respiratory compensation through increases in alveolar ventilation, resulting in a reduction in P_{CO_2}. The steady-state relationship between the P_{CO_2} and the bicarbonate concentration, determined from a study of 60 patients who had only metabolic acidosis of more than 24-h duration is shown in Eq. (6)[12]‡

$$P_{CO_2} = (1.5 * [HCO_3^-] + 8) \pm 2 \tag{6}$$

When the bicarbonate concentration is greater than about 8 meq/dL, the relationship between P_{CO_2} and bicarbonate is simpler: *P_{CO_2} falls by 1 mmHg for every 1 meq/dL fall in bicarbonate.* Use of these relationships allows the clinician to calculate the expected P_{CO_2} from the measured bicarbonate concentration. If the expected P_{CO_2} value differs from the measured value in uncomplicated steady-state metabolic acidosis, a respiratory disorder also exists. For example, if the $[HCO_3^-]$ is 15, the expected P_{CO_2} is about 30 mmHg. If it is higher than this value (say 35 mmHg), then by definition there is also concomitant primary respiratory acidosis (see Fig. 21-2*A*). If the value is lower than expected (say 25 mmHg), then there is a concomitant respiratory alkalosis. This latter case is not an "overcompensation" but rather a second primary disturbance occurring simultaneously. These are important concepts. The body cannot tolerate both a metabolic and respiratory mechanism for acidosis simultaneously, as one cannot buffer or compensate for the other.

The ED patient's illness can, unfortunately, rarely be assumed to be in steady state. Pierce and colleagues, in physiologic studies of otherwise healthy persons with acute metabolic acidosis caused by diarrhea, discovered that the completeness of the respiratory response to metabolic acidosis depends upon the duration of the acidosis, the time course of its development, and its severity.[13] If acidosis develops quickly, the P_{CO_2} is often higher than that observed in steady state; the more rapid and severe the acidosis, the larger the difference between the observed P_{CO_2} and the predicted steady-state P_{CO_2}. When bicarbonate concentration is then held constant, steady-state P_{CO_2} is reached in 11 to 24 h. When acidosis develops or is corrected more slowly, there is no lag in respiratory compensation.

‡The constants in this equation (orginally $P_{CO_2} = 1.54 * [HCO_3^-] + 8.36 \pm 2$) have been rounded for ease of use.

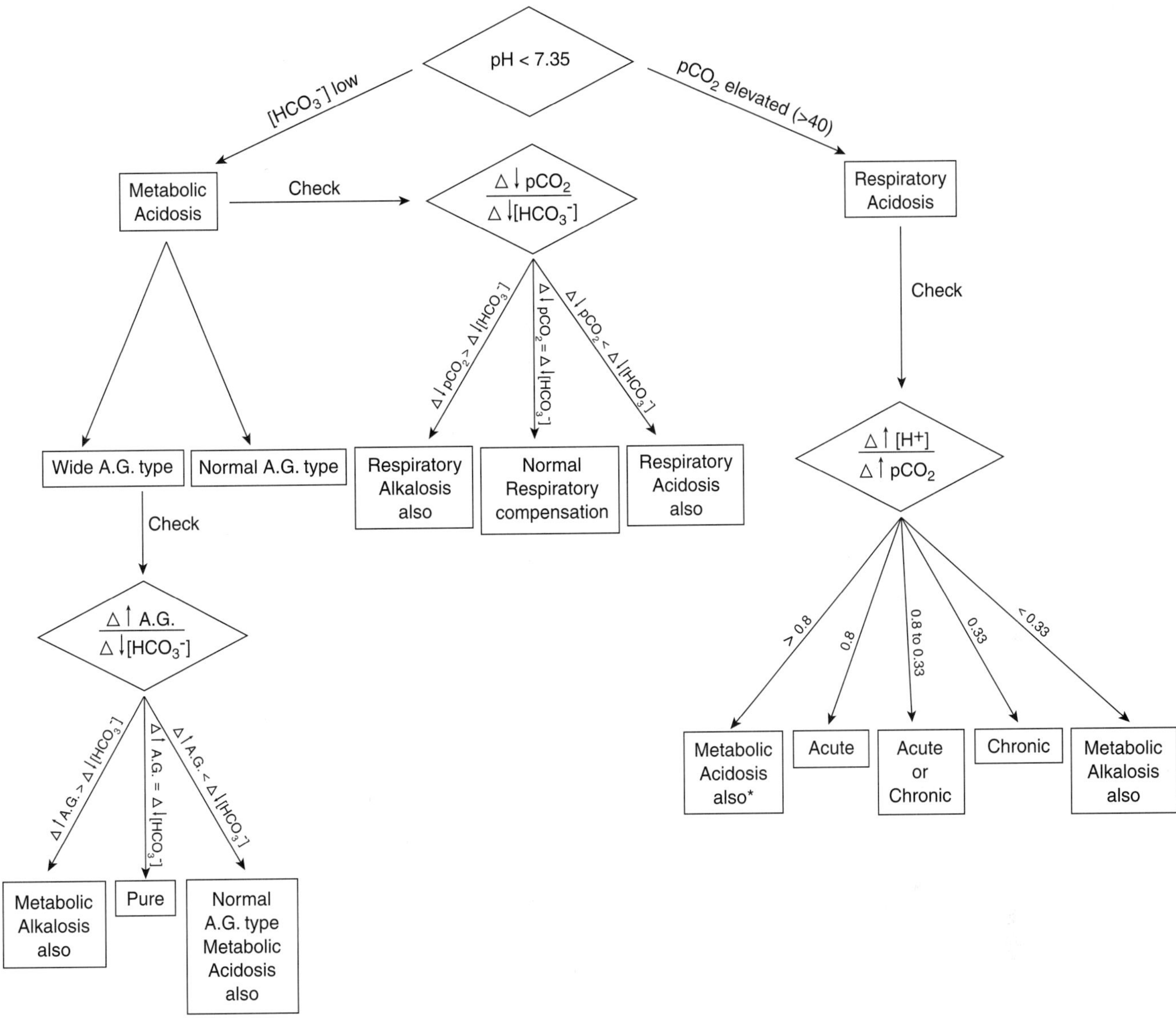

Key: *It is likely that $[HCO_3^-]$ is < 25 in this scenario and the tree could have been started on the left.
A.G., anion gap.

FIG. 21-2A. Algorithm for determination of type of acidosis and mixed acid-base disturbances when pH indicates acidemia.

There are limits to the adequacy of respiratory compensation during metabolic acidosis. A study early in the twentieth century of diabetic ketoacidosis by Kety and colleagues found that respiratory minute volume actually declined when pH fell below 7.10.[14] This finding led both Albert et al.[12] and Pierce et al.[13] to initiate bicarbonate therapy if their subjects' pH fell below 7.10. The nature of respiratory compensation in untreated severe metabolic acidosis is therefore unknown. Furthermore, these studies appear to have ensconced 7.10 as the definition of "severe" metabolic acidosis. It is particularly important to appreciate any contribution to the acidosis from inadequate respiratory response. Simply initiating bicarbonate therapy when a pH of less than 7.1 is encountered may miss the respiratory insufficiency, which, if addressed, may obviate the need to use solutions containing HCO_3^-. Further, administration of HCO_3^- in the face of inadequate ventilatory response actually exacerbates the respiratory acidosis, as the HCO_3^- is converted to CO_2 and H_2O. The development of metabolic acidosis in which the pH is below 7.10 is probably associated with a very high risk of ventilatory insufficiency. There is another limit to respiratory compensation. The lowest level that P_{CO_2} can attain is about 12 mmHg. The restriction of air movement and the CO_2 generated by the exertion required for rapid ventilation limits the attainable nadir for P_{CO_2}. The superimposition of respiratory acidosis upon a patient in such straits will result in a rapid decline of pH to levels at which organ function and pharmacotherapy will fail. Mechanical ventilation should usually be instituted in such situations.

The serum potassium level is affected by metabolic acidosis. The movement of hydrogen ion into cells is associated with extrusion of potassium. Changes in potassium concentration are more substantial in inorganic acidosis, though elevated serum potassium values are typically seen in diabetic ketoacidosis. Generally, for each 0.10 change in the pH, serum $[K^+]$ will increase by approximately 0.5 meq/L. Whatever the mechanism of the acidosis, it is important to remember that low-normal or low serum potassium values probably reflect severe intracellular potassium depletion. The reversal of the acidosis in such circumstances may result in severe hypokalemia, with attendant cardiovascular effects.

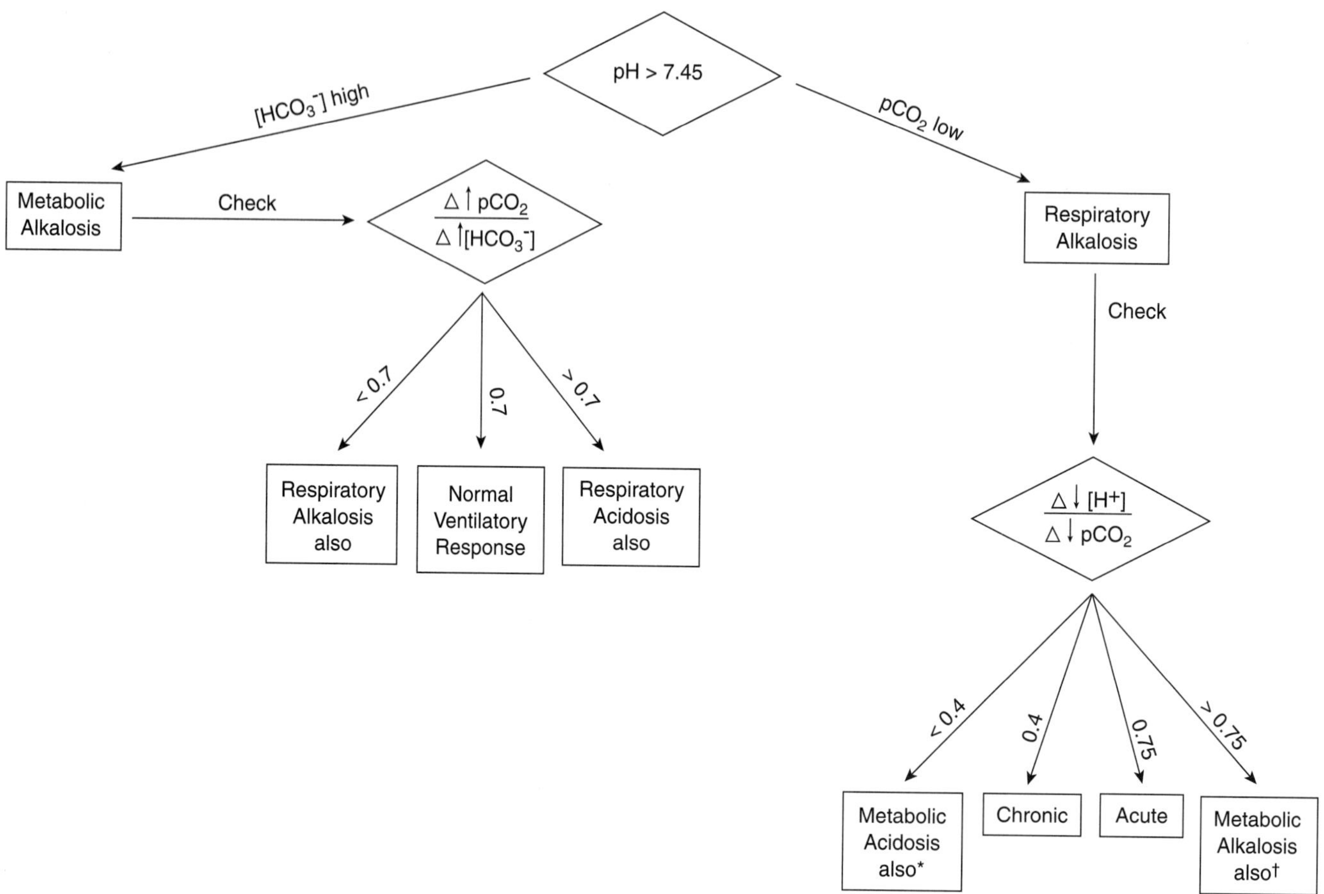

FIG. 21-2B. Algorithm for determination of type of alkalosis and mixed acid-base disturbances when pH indicates alkalemia.

Causes of Metabolic Acidosis

Metabolic acidosis results in a depression of serum bicarbonate, whose negative charge must be replaced. The negatively charged species are either unmeasured anions (elevated-AG acidosis) or chloride (normal-AG acidosis, also referred to as hyperchloremic metabolic acidosis).

The causes of elevated-AG metabolic acidosis are listed in Table 21-2. We reemphasize that the anion gap may be within the normal range even when a metabolic acidosis associated with increased concentrations of unmeasured anions is present. A comparison with the patient's steady-state AG is warranted or measurement of specific anions in such cases is indicated. However, caution is necessary when serum ketone testing is performed, as the chemical reaction used to measure serum ketones has an important limitation: the nitroprusside reaction for ketones is positive only for species whose carbonyl moiety has an α-methyl group. The major ketone present in the serum of patients with diabetic ketoacidosis may be β-hydroxybutyrate, which has no α-methyl group and is not detected by the nitroprusside reaction. The result may be a paradox: initial serum ketone assays in a patient with clinically severe diabetic ketoacidosis are only weakly positive yet rise in spite of clear clinical improvement. This occurs because appropriate resuscitation alters the hepatic NAD/$NADH_2$ ratio and the restoration of NAD concentrations allows oxidation of β-hydroxybutyrate to acetoacetate. The addition of several drops of hydrogen peroxide to serum will also oxidize β-hydroxybutyrate to acetoacetate in cases where this distinction is clinically important. See Chap. 203 for a detailed discussion.

Lactic acidosis occurs whenever lactate production exceeds lactate utilization or metabolism and is classically of two types. The first, in which tissue hypoxia is present and lactate production is elevated, is referred to as type A. Normal tissue oxygenation and impairment of lactate utilization define the second, called type B. Type B lactic acidosis is further subdivided. B_1 lactic acidosis is associated with systemic disorders such as diabetes, renal insufficiency, sepsis, and leukemia; type B_2 is associated with various substances, especially biguanides (phenformin, metformin), salicylates, methanol, iron and isoniazid; and type B_3 is associated with hereditary metabolic diseases.

The pyruvate produced by glycolysis may be transported across mitochondrial membranes and metabolized in the Krebs cycle under aerobic conditions. However, under anaerobic conditions, it is oxidized to lactate by lactate dehydrogenase. This reaction is reversible, but the conversion of lactate to pyruvate in the liver requires NAD. Thus, it is not surprising that many patients with type B lactic acidosis have underlying liver disease. For example, an alcoholic may develop lactic acidosis after giving up heavy drinking because impaired gluconeogenesis prevents pyruvate fixation into glucose, while the metabolism of ethanol has left little NAD available to convert lactate to pyruvate. The distinction between type A and type B lactic acidosis is useful in conceptualizing the therapeutic approach. However, there is some

FIG. 21-2C. Algorithm to check for acid-base disturbances when pH is in "normal" range.

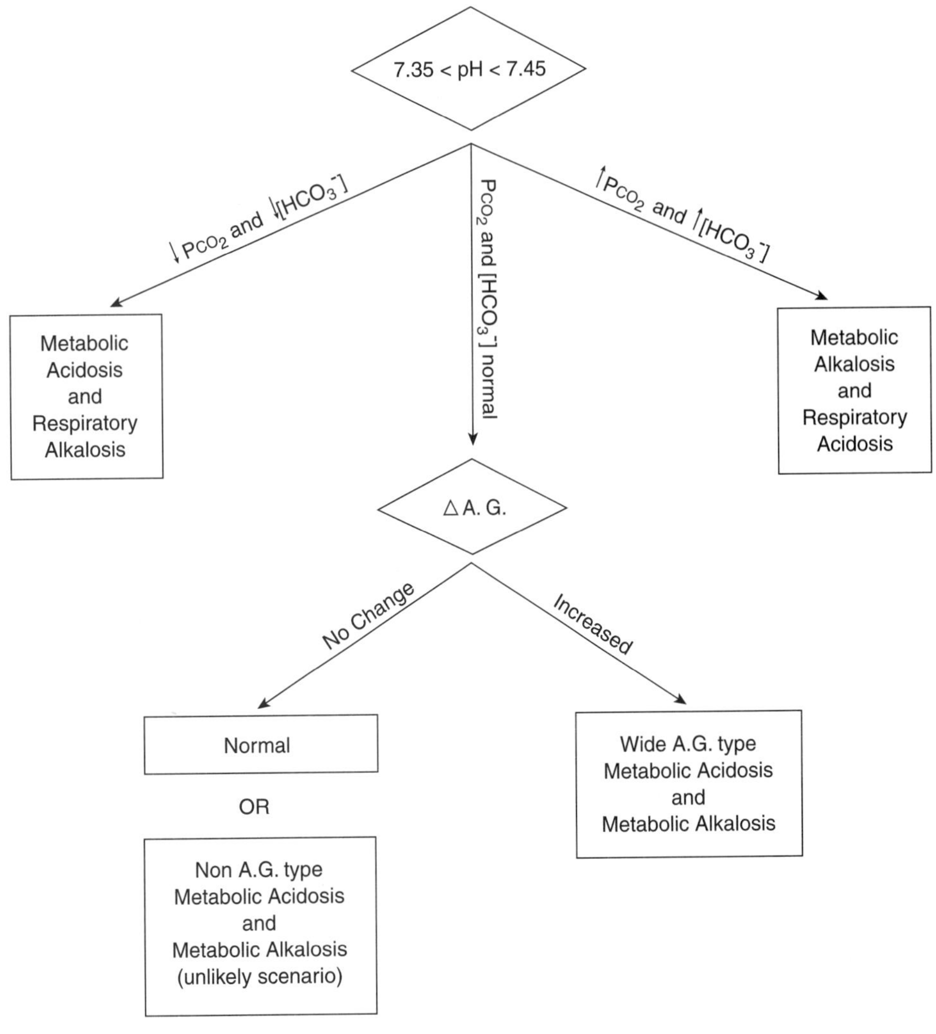

impairment of lactate utilization in both types, usually because of impaired hepatic oxygenation or perfusion in the case of type A and because of underlying liver disease in type B.

Differential Diagnoses of Wide-AG Acidosis

Note that an ABG is completely immaterial in determining whether a wide-AG metabolic acidosis exists. The determination is made with simple venous electrolytes. The differential diagnosis falls into four broad categories: renal failure (uremia), lactic acidosis, ketoacidosis (DKA, AKA, SKA), and ingestions (methanol, ethylene glycol, salicylates).

Renal failure should be evident from the serum chemistries. Positive serum ketones point to one of the ketoacidoses. In known insulin-dependent diabetes mellitus (IDDM), DKA is likely, although there is usually a small component of lactic acidosis also. In alcoholics who have recently stopped binge drinking, AKA should be considered. Starvation ketosis will be found in patients with inadequate recent oral intake (fasting, dieting, or protracted vomiting).

Determination of the osmolal gap will help differentiate two of the ingestants from other etiologies. Elevated gaps are seen in methanol and ethylene glycol poisoning. Although methanol is measured in most hospital laboratories, determination of ethylene glycol levels is still performed off-site in many institutions. A widened osmolal gap without evidence of methanol ingestion may determine the diagnosis long before confirmatory laboratory evidence is available. Calculation adjustments to the osmolal gap may need to be made if ethanol is a coingestant (see Chap. 23 for detailed discussion).

When the diagnosis remains in doubt or poor tissue perfusion is a diagnostic possibility, lactate levels should be specifically sent. It should be noted that several poisonings may result in lactic acidosis, including isoniazid (INH), iron, carbon monoxide (CO), methemoglobin, and cyanide. This is but one reason why the authors shun the overtaught mnemonic of *MUDPILES.* For example, this mnemonic does not clearly reflect the fact that INH and iron exert their effects on the AG through lactic acidosis. Also, ethanol is frequently taught as a cause of wide-AG acidosis. *Ethanol should never be considered the etiologic source of any significant metabolic acidosis.* While ethanol alcohol metabolism may lead to very mild lactic acidosis, usually in association with AKA, its effect is very mild and all but clinically immaterial.

Severe acidosis that is resistant to treatment is seen in various B1 lactic acidoses and ingestions. AKA and SKA tend to be mild. Acidosis seen in initial stages of renal failure may be severe but is stable ($[HCO_3^-]$ about 15 meq/L) in chronic renal failure. Concomitant acid-base disturbance may further assist in determining the etiology. The triple acid-base disturbance of wide-AG metabolic acidosis, metabolic alkalosis, and respiratory alkalosis is seen with sepsis (lactic acidosis), and salicylate poisoning. The latter may be associated with a mild temperature elevation also.

TABLE 21-3 Causes of Normal Anion Gap Metabolic Acidosis

With a tendency to hyperkalemia	With a tendency to hypokalemia
Subsiding DKA	Renal tubular acidosis—type I (classical distal acidosis)
Early uremic acidosis	Renal tubular acidosis—type II (proximal acidosis)
Early obstructive uropathy	Acetazolamide
Renal tubular acidosis—type IV	Acute diarrhea with losses of HCO_3^- and K^+
Hypoaldosteronism (Addison's disease)	Ureterosigmoidostomy with increased resorption of H^+ and Cl^- and losses of HCO_3^- and K^+
Infusion or ingestion of HCl, NH_4Cl, lysine-HCl, or arginine-HCl	Obstruction of artificial ileal bladder
Potassium-sparing diuretics	Dilution acidosis

Finally, the relationship of [HCO_3^-] to the anion gap and expected P_{CO_2} compensation must be examined in every patient with wide anion gap acidosis to determine if other (respiratory) acid-base disturbances exist (see Fig. 21-2*A*).

Differential Diagnosis of Unchanged (Normal) AG Acidosis

The non-AG type of acidosis is often referred to as ''normal'' anion gap acidosis. As discussed above, issues related to the AG are relative, so the term *unchanged* or *non-AG type* is preferred. Some texts refer to this as hyperchloremic metabolic acidosis.

Non-AG acidosis results from loss of bicarbonate, failure to excrete hydrogen ion, or administration of hydrogen ion. Bicarbonate may be lost from either the urine or gastrointestinal tract and is usually accompanied by potassium. However, potassium-sparing diuretics, hypoaldosteronism, urinary tract obstruction, and type IV renal tubular acidosis all result in loss of bicarbonate with retention of potassium (Table 21-3).

One should be wary of the traditional classification based on K^+, as serum [K^+] itself is dependent on the actual pH. Thus, in severe acidosis, a normal range [K^+] may be deceiving unless the clinician corrects for the degree of acidosis.

Since all diuretics have a tendency to result in mild contraction alkalosis, the metabolic acidosis that occurs simultaneously with potassium-sparing diuretics may not be evident, as the two distinct physiologic processes may simply cancel each other out (see Fig. 21-2*C*). Since the AG is unchanged, there is no clue that two opposed processes may be occurring.

Acetazolamide exerts its effect through carbonic anhydrase inhibition, inducing a functional RTA.

Treatment of Acidosis

Acidemia has numerous negative physiologic consequences, impairing the function of many different organs through mechanisms not yet well understood. Cardiac contractile function is reduced, probably due to impaired oxidative phosphorylation as well as intracellular acidosis. The threshold for ventricular fibrillation falls while the defibrillation threshold rises. Hepatic and renal perfusion decline, along with systemic blood pressure, while pulmonary vascular resistance increases. The physiologic effects of catecholamines are attenuated, and when acidosis is sufficiently severe, vascular collapse may result. A catabolic state develops, including a generalized increase in metabolism, resistance to insulin, and inhibition of anaerobic glycolysis. Finally, the effect of hypoxia on all organs is aggravated.[15]

The treatment of acidosis reflects that of the underlying disorder but particularly emphasizes restoration of normal tissue perfusion and oxygenation. As noted above, the most important step is to determine whether there is a respiratory component to the acidosis (i.e., a primary respiratory acidosis), because the treatment approach differs. If there is inadequate respiratory compensation, the most appropriate treatment will be to first correct the respiratory problem.

The adverse effects of acidemia make the concept of buffer therapy teleologically appealing, but the role of buffer therapy in both cardiac arrest and severe metabolic acidosis is uncertain. The traditional therapeutic buffer, sodium bicarbonate, may have negative effects in the treatment of acidosis. Bicarbonate therapy results in the generation of significant quantities of CO_2, which diffuses readily into cells—particularly those of the central nervous system—and may therefore cause paradoxical worsening of intracellular acidosis. An abrupt CO_2 load may also exceed the ventilatory capacity of a maximally ventilating patient, producing respiratory failure. After successful treatment with bicarbonate, ''overshoot'' alkalosis may result; this problem occurs most commonly in organic acidosis, when reversal of the acidosis results in reformation of bicarbonate. Finally, bicarbonate therapy imposes an osmotic and sodium load (1000 meq/L of typical 1N solution). These concerns suggest that bicarbonate therapy should not be used in the ED treatment of mild to moderate metabolic acidosis. Bicarbonate therapy is reasonable, however, in situations where the effects of acidosis are so severe that they preclude or jeopardize therapy for the underlying disease (Table 21-4).

When bicarbonate is used, Adrogue and Madias[15] recommend administering 0.5 meq/kg bicarbonate for each meq/dL desired rise in [HCO_3^-]. The goal is to restore adequate buffer capacity ([HCO_3^-] > 8 meq/dL) or achieve clinical improvement in shock or dysrhythmias. Bicarbonate should be given as slowly as the clinical situation permits; 1.5 ampules of sodium bicarbonate in 500 mL D_5W produces a nearly isotonic solution for infusion. Adequate time should be allowed for the desired effect to be achieved, and close monitoring of acid-base balance, especially in patients with organic acidosis, is critical.

Newer buffers appear to show promise in the treatment of metabolic acidosis. Carbicarb, an equimolar solution of sodium bicarbonate and sodium carbonate (CO_3^{2-}), produces significantly less CO_2 than an equimolar dose of bicarbonate. The carbonate ion, a strong base, combines avidly with protons to form bicarbonate, resulting in increased pH, an increased bicarbonate concentration, and limited CO_2 production. Clinical studies of Carbicarb use in lactic acidosis models have shown improvements in pH with little or no change in P_{CO_2}.[16,17] However, large-scale studies in ED patients do not yet exist, and Carbicarb, while promising, remains experimental.

TABLE 21-4 Indications for Bicarbonate Therapy in Metabolic Acidosis

Indication	Rationale
Severe hypobicarbonatemia (<4 meq/L)	Insufficient buffer concentrations may lead to extreme increases in acidemia with small increases in acidosis
Severe acidemia (pH <7.20) with signs of shock or myocardial irritability that is not rapidly responsive to supportive measures	Therapy for the underlying cause of acidosis depends upon adequate organ perfusion
Severe hyperchloremic acidemia*	Lost bicarbonate must be regenerated by kidneys and liver, which may require days

*No specific definition by pH exists. The presence of serious hemodynamic insufficiency despite supportive care should guide the use of bicarbonate therapy for this indication.

METABOLIC ALKALOSIS

Metabolic alkalosis is typically classified as chloride-sensitive and chloride-insensitive, indicating the treatment approach itself. Metabolic alkalosis results from either gain of bicarbonate or loss of acid. The relationship of metabolic alkalosis to chloride balance defines both pathophysiologic features of the disease and its therapy. Bicarbonate and chloride represent the major serum anions whose concentration may be readily altered, and their homeostasis is therefore closely intertwined.

Conditions that produce chloride loss, such as vomiting (which also produces acid loss), diarrhea, diuretic therapy, and chloride-wasting diseases (e.g., cystic fibrosis and chloride-wasting enteropathy) all tend to reduce both serum chloride concentration and extracellular volume. The reduction in extracellular volume produces increased mineralocorticoid activity, which enhances sodium reabsorption and potassium and hydrogen ion secretion in the distal tubule, which, in turn, enhance bicarbonate generation. The resulting increase in serum bicarbonate concentration eventually exceeds the tubule's maximum ability to reabsorb filtered bicarbonate. The resulting alkaline urine, because its anionic content is mostly bicarbonate, is largely free of chloride ($<$10 meq/L), though when diuretics have been administered, the urine chloride may be normal. The result is hypokalemic, hypochloremic alkalosis that responds to normal (chloride-responsive alkalosis).

Other diseases that cause metabolic alkalosis are usually associated with normovolemia or hypervolemia and often hypertension. These diseases usually cause excess mineralocorticoid activity, resulting in the same pathophysiologic cascade described above. However, the excess mineralocorticoid activity is not associated with hypovolemia, so the urine chloride is generally normal or elevated ($>$10 meq/L) and the alkalosis cannot be reversed with normal saline. Diseases producing "chloride-unresponsive alkalosis" and hypertension include renal artery stenosis, renin-secreting tumors, adrenal hyperplasia, hyperaldosteronism, Cushing syndrome, Liddle syndrome, and exogenous mineralocorticoids (e.g., licorice, Florinef). Chloride-unresponsive alkalosis caused by Bartter syndrome and Gitelman syndrome is usually associated with normotension.

The compensation for metabolic alkalosis involves reduction in alveolar ventilation, but the exact relationship between P_{CO_2} and hydrogen ion concentration is not well established. Most studies to date have been conducted either in dialysis patients or patients with conditions that predispose to alveolar hyperventilation (e.g., sepsis, pneumonia). As a guideline, P_{CO_2} in patients with significant metabolic alkalosis should rise 0.7 mmHg for each milliequivalent increase in $[HCO_3^-]$. The P_{CO_2} also rarely rises above 55 mmHg in compensation for metabolic alkalosis.

The physiologic effects of alkalemia are substantial. Neurologic abnormalities—especially tetany, neuromuscular instability, and seizures—are common. Reduction in hydrogen ion concentration results in reductions in ionized calcium, potassium, magnesium, and phosphate levels. Constriction of arterioles occurs, resulting in reduced coronary and cerebral blood flow. Finally, refractory dysrhythmias may develop.[15] Alkalemia may be of particular concern in patients with chronic obstructive pulmonary disease (COPD) because of the shift of the oxygen-hemoglobin to the left, making O_2 less available to the tissues. Many such patients are taking diuretics, which lead to a contraction alkalosis. Also, the alkalotic environment tends to depress ventilatory drive further.

Therapy of alkalemia, as with all acid-base disorders, emphasizes treatment of the underlying cause and careful supportive care. Acetazolamide produces significant bicarbonaturia and is effective in the treatment of metabolic alkalosis, but its use requires very careful monitoring of potassium, magnesium, and phosphate concentrations. If alkalemia is severe ($[HCO_3^-] > 45$ mmol/L) and associated with serious signs or symptoms not responsive to supportive care, the use of intravenous hydrochloric acid should be considered. A 0.1 normal solution (100 mmol/L), infused at no more than 0.2 mmol/kg/h through a central venous catheter is used; higher concentrations may produce degradation of catheter material.[18] The dose is calculated as shown in Eq. (7), with the result in millimoles of bicarbonate.

$$\text{Dose} = (\Delta[HCO_3^-])(\text{weight})(0.5) \tag{7}$$

RESPIRATORY ACIDOSIS

Respiratory acidosis is defined by alveolar hypoventilation and is diagnosed when the P_{CO_2} is greater then the expected value. Acute respiratory acidosis may have origins such as increased CO_2 production (high-glucose diet) and abnormal gas exchange (e.g., pneumonia). Final common path is inadequate ventilation.

Inadequate minute ventilation is most frequently due to head trauma, chest trauma, or disease or excess sedation. The chronic hypoventilation seen in extremely obese patients is often referred to as the *pickwickian syndrome,* after an obese character in Charles Dickens' *Pickwick Papers.* Patients with severe COPD have increased dead space and frequently also have a decreased minute ventilation.

In general, a rise in the P_{CO_2} stimulates the respiratory center to increase respiratory rate and minute ventilation. However, if the arterial P_{CO_2} chronically exceeds 60 to 70 mmHg, as may occur in 5 to 10 percent of patients with severe emphysema, the respiratory acidosis may depress the respiratory center. Under such circumstances, the stimulus for ventilation is provided primarily by hypoxemia acting on chemoreceptors in the carotid and aortic bodies. Giving oxygen could take away the main stimulus to breathe, causing the P_{CO_2} to rise abruptly to extremely dangerous levels. Consequently, one should not administer oxygen to patients with COPD without carefully watching for the development of apnea or hypoventilation.

Evaluation of ventilation requires attention to several important clinical issues. First, the ventilation that would be expected based on assessment of the respiratory rate and depth should be compared to the actual ventilation of the patient (i.e., P_{CO_2}). A "normal" P_{CO_2} of 40 mmHg in a tachypneic, dyspneic patient probably reflects significant ventilatory insufficiency. Second, the impact of respiratory acidosis on PA_{O_2} in such a patient may be considerable. The alveolar gas equation suggests that if inspired oxygen concentration and respiratory quotient do not vary, increases in P_{CO_2} will result in reductions in PA_{O_2}.

The relationship of P_{CO_2} to hydrogen ion concentration in acute respiratory acidosis is suggested by the Kassirer-Bleich equation:

$$\Delta[H^+] = 0.8(\Delta P_{CO_2}) \tag{8}$$

Each 1-mmHg increase in P_{CO_2} results in a 1-mmol increase in $[H^+]$. Across the linear portion of the pH–hydrogen ion concentration relationship, then, each 1-mmHg increase in P_{CO_2} should theoretically produce a 0.01-unit decrease in pH. The actual relationship between changes in P_{CO_2} (up to values of 90 mmHg) and changes in $[H^+]$ determined in normal humans is about 8:10, as shown in Eq. (7). Thus, a 10-mmHg increment in P_{CO_2} produces an 8-mmol increase in hydrogen ion concentration, with little change in bicarbonate concentration (usually 1 meq/dL) or urinary acid excretion.[19] If the $[H^+]$ is higher or lower than that suggested by the change in the P_{CO_2}, a mixed disorder is present.

The adaptation to chronic respiratory acidosis is complex. Over time, chronic elevation of P_{CO_2} results in a reduction in the sensitivity of carotid sinus sensitivity to hypercapnia; ventilatory drive is then controlled by Pa_{O_2}. The acidosis results in significant increases in renal bicarbonate generation and avid reclamation of filtered bicarbonate. The relationship between $[H^+]$ and $[HCO_3^-]$ in chronic respiratory acidosis at steady state, derived from studies in humans, is shown in Eq. (9).

$$\Delta[H^+] = 0.3(\Delta P_{CO_2}) \tag{9}$$

TABLE 21-5 Evaluation of Acid-Base Status in Respiratory Acidosis

Ratio = $\Delta[H^+]/\Delta P_{CO_2}$				
Ratio < 0.3	Ratio = 0.3	0.3 < Ratio < 0.8	Ratio = 0.8	Ratio > 0.8
Change in hydrogen ion concentration is less than accounted for by chronic change in P_{CO_2}. Metabolic alkalosis is also present.	Change in hydrogen ion concentration matches chronic change in P_{CO_2}. Chronic respiratory acidosis is present.	Change in hydrogen ion concentration is larger than accounted for by chronic change in P_{CO_2}. Chronic respiratory acidosis plus either acute respiratory alkalosis or metabolic acidosis is present; examine pH.	Change in hydrogen ion concentration matches acute change in P_{CO_2}. Acute respiratory acidosis is present.	Change in hydrogen ion concentration is larger than accounted for by acute or chronic change in P_{CO_2}. Metabolic acidosis is also present.

It is rarely certain during a given clinical encounter whether a patient has an acute respiratory acidosis, a chronic respiratory acidosis, or an acute exacerbation of chronic COPD. Evaluation of the acid-base status in such circumstances does not require "baseline" arterial blood gas values. Instead, the change in hydrogen ion concentration is compared with the change in P_{CO_2}. If this ratio is 0.3, the patient has a chronic respiratory acidosis; if it is 0.8, the patient has an acute respiratory acidosis. States resulting in other ratios suggest a mixed acid-base disturbance, as shown in Table 21-5.

Treatment of respiratory acidosis is primarily designed to improve alveolar ventilation. In general, if the minute ventilation is doubled, the P_{CO_2} will be reduced by 50 percent. In patients with COPD, bronchodilators such as aminophylline or various sympathomimetic agents such as isoproterenol or adrenalin, together with careful administration of small amounts of oxygen, may substantially improve ventilation. However, ventilating assistance may be required in some patients who do not respond adequately to lesser measures, particularly if the pH falls below 7.25 to 7.30. Unfortunately, it may be extremely difficult to extubate such patients later.

In patients with a chronic respiratory acidosis, reduction of the P_{CO_2} should generally proceed slowly. The minute ventilation for a 70-kg person is normally about 6 L/min, and in COPD patients it may be less than 4 L/min. In a patient with COPD and severe hypercarbia, it may be wise to start treatment with a minute ventilation of about 5 L/min and then gradually increase it according to the clinical response and changes in P_{CO_2}.

Rapid correction of a chronic respiratory acidosis can cause sudden development of a severe combined metabolic and respiratory alkalosis with resulting dysrhythmias. A rapid rise in pH can cause an abrupt fall in ionized calcium. The resulting ionic hypocalcemia can then cause dangerous dysrhythmias or seizures. In patients with a chronic respiratory acidosis, the arterial P_{CO_2} should not be reduced by more than 5.0 meq/h.

RESPIRATORY ALKALOSIS

Respiratory alkalosis is defined by alveolar hyperventilation and exists when P_{CO_2} is less then expected. It is caused by conditions that stimulate respiratory centers, including central nervous system tumors or stroke, infections, pregnancy, hypoxia, and toxins (e.g., salicylates). Anxiety, pain, and overventilation of patients on mechanical ventilators also cause respiratory alkalosis.

Whatever the etiology, the clinical symptoms of acute respiratory alkalosis are predictable from its physiologic effects. Acute reduction in P_{CO_2} produces a reduction in hydrogen ion concentration, resulting in an increase in negative charge on anionic buffers. The now relatively negatively charged proteins instead bind calcium, and this reduction in ionized calcium produces carpopedal spasm and paresthesias.[15] Hypocapnia also produces substantial reductions in cerebral blood flow, and results in reduced tissue oxygen delivery because of increased hemoglobin oxygen binding.

The theoretical relationship of hydrogen ion concentration and P_{CO_2} predicted by the Kassirer-Bleich equation is that a 1-mmol decrease in $[H^+]$ results from each 1-mmHg reduction in P_{CO_2}. The actual observed relationship is very close to that predicted by the Kassirer-Bleich equation.[20] Each mmHg reduction in P_{CO_2} results in a 0.75-mmol reduction in $[H^+]$ (Eq. 10).[20]

$$\Delta[H^+] = 0.75(\Delta P_{CO_2}) \qquad (10)$$

Chronic respiratory alkalosis is unique among the acid-base disorders in that its compensation may be complete. Compensatory events include bicarbonaturia and a reduction in acid excretion, requiring 6 to 72 h to develop fully and at least 1 week to normalize pH. The steady-state relationship between hydrogen ion concentration and P_{CO_2} in chronic respiratory alkalosis observed in normal human subjects at high altitude is shown in Eq. (10).[21]

$$\Delta[H^+] = 0.4(\Delta P_{CO_2}) \qquad (11)$$

Therapy for acute respiratory alkalosis emphasizes identification and treatment of the underlying cause. The use of paper-bag rebreathing in the treatment of respiratory alkalosis should be avoided. Callaham evaluated paper-bag rebreathing in voluntarily hyperventilating volunteers and found that while the inspired P_{CO_2} increased by 20 mmHg in 30 s, it never increased above 40 mmHg. However, inspired oxygen concentration fell by an average of 27 mmHg in 180 s, and in 5 percent of subjects the fall was greater than or equal to 42 mmHg.[22] If the cause of hyperventilation is actually cellular hypoxia, such a fall could be catastrophic.[23] Furthermore, there is evidence that expectation of efficacy and suggestion, rather than elevations of inspired CO_2 tension, are responsible for relief of symptoms in hyperventilation.[24] An oxygen mask might provide benefits similar to those of paper-bag rebreathing with less risk of hypoxia.

Chronic respiratory alkalosis is seen at high altitudes, particularly among mountaineers climbing over 12,000 ft (where the partial pressure of O_2 is significantly diminished). Acetazolamide is frequently prescribed to counter the physiologic respiratory effects of such ascents.

CLINICAL APPROACH TO ACID-BASE PROBLEMS AND MIXED ACID-BASE DISTURBANCES

The evaluation of an acid-base problem begins with a history and physical examination, with particular attention to sources of acid or alkali gain or loss and to diseases that affect renal, hepatic, or pulmonary function. Blood should be obtained for gas analysis and electrolyte determination, and the anion gap should be calculated. Finally, blood gas results should be checked for internal consistency using the Henderson-Hasselbalch or Kassirer-Bleich equation—Eq. (3) or Eq. (4).

Note that in metabolic acidosis, where the respiratory response appears clinically appropriate, both the P_{CO_2} and pH can be predicted.

Thus, a single ABG to prove there is no abnormal respiratory component may be all that is necessary and further evaluation can be determined from serum (venous) [HCO_3^-] alone. For example when, the [HCO_3^-] is 15, the expected physiologic respiratory compensatory response is expected to be a decline in P_{CO_2} equal to the decline in [HCO_3^-]—i.e., in this scenario, 30 mmHg. The values for both known [HCO_3^-] and predicted P_{CO_2} can then be inserted in the Kassirer-Bleich equation–Eq. (4)—to determine the [H^+], which in this case is calculated to be about 48. The [H^+] can then be related to the corresponding pH, which, as noted earlier, is close to linear for values from 22 to 55 nmol/L, in this case about 7.32.

Methodical interpretation of laboratory results followed by correlation with the clinical scenario is necessary to prevent erroneous acid-base evaluation. While we suggest one method that has worked well for us, the particular method used matters less than the consistency of its application. However, we do frown on reliance on ''acid-base disturbance maps.'' First, they may be misleading, particularly where there is more than one primary disturbance. Second, they offer no understanding of the processes. Without an understanding of the complex but not difficult to master concepts of interrelationships in acid-base balance, the clinician misses diagnoses and has little understanding of the appropriate approach to therapy. As long as the method selected reflects the acid-base relationships presented in this chapter, the result should be the same. One suggested method follows:

1. Look at the pH. If it is decreased, the primary or predominant disturbance is acidosis. If the pH is increased, the predominant disturbance is alkalosis.
2. If the pH indicates acidosis, the primary (or predominant) mechanism can be ascertained by examining the [HCO_3^-] and P_{CO_2} (see Fig. 21-2*A*).
   a. If the [HCO_3^-] is low (implying a primary metabolic acidosis) then the AG should be examined and, if possible, compared with a known steady-state value.
      i. If the AG is increased compared to the known previous value, or is greater than 15, then by definition a wide-AG metabolic acidosis is present and the absolute change in the AG should be compared with the absolute change in the [HCO_3^-] from normal.
      ii. If the AG is unchanged, then the disturbance is a nonwidened (sometimes termed *unchanged AG* or *hyperchloremic*) metabolic acidosis.
      iii. If the change in the AG is equal to the change in the [HCO_3^-], then the wide AG-acidosis is termed *pure.* If the AG has risen more than the [HCO_3^-] has decreased, then there is also likely to be a concomitant metabolic alkalosis. If the change in the AG is less than the change in the [HCO_3^-], then a non-AG acidosis is also present. (This is a difficult concept, but two separate physiologic mechanisms both resulting in increased [H^+] can occur simultaneously.)
      iv. Next examine whether the ventilatory response is appropriate.
         1. If the decrease in the P_{CO_2} equals the decrease in the [HCO_3^-], there is appropriate respiratory compensation. Note that the pH will not return to normal.
         2. If the decrease in the P_{CO_2} is greater than the decrease in the [HCO_3^-], there is a concomitant respiratory alkalosis. (Although there are other formulas for this comparison, this is the simplest, as explained earlier in the text.)
         3. If the decrease in the P_{CO_2} is less than the decrease in [HCO_3^-], there is also a concomitant respiratory acidosis.
   b. If the P_{CO_2} is elevated (rather than the [HCO_3^-] decreased), the primary disturbance is respiratory acidosis (see Fig. 21-2*A*). The next step is to figure out which type it is by examining the ratio of (the change in) [H^+] to (the upward change in) the P_{CO_2}.
      i. If the ratio is 0.8, it is considered acute.
      ii. If the ratio is 0.33, it is considered chronic.
      iii. If the ratio is between 0.8 and 0.33, it is probably an acute exacerbation of the chronic condition.
      iv. If the ratio is greater than 0.8, there must be a metabolic explanation for the excess [H^+].
      v. If the ratio is less than 0.33, a metabolic alkalosis must also be present.
3. If the pH is greater than 7.45, the primary or predominant disturbance is a metabolic alkalosis (see Fig. 21-2*B*).
   a. It is best to look at the [HCO_3^-] first. If it is elevated, there is a primary metabolic alkalosis. There is an expected ventilatory response, although it is quite varied. The ratio of the change upward in P_{CO_2} to the change upward in [HCO_3^-] can be examined.
      i. If the ratio is much less than 0.7, there is also a respiratory alkalosis (in addition to the metabolic alkalosis). If the ratio is more or less 0.7, this is likely to be a compensatory ventilatory response. If the ratio is well above 0.7, respiratory acidosis is concomitantly present.
   b. If the P_{CO_2} is low, there is a primary respiratory alkalosis and the ratio of the change in [H^+] to the change in P_{CO_2} should be examined. Acute respiratory alkalosis has a ratio of about 0.75. If the ratio is well above 0.75, there is probably also a concomitant metabolic alkalosis to explain the greater than expected decline in [H^+]. If the ratio is smaller, the condition is either chronic or there may also be a metabolic acidosis component.
4. Every ABG that shows no or minimal pH derangement should still call for examination of the P_{CO_2} and [HCO_3^-], as there may well be a mixed acid-base disturbance (see Fig. 2*C*). As noted earlier, it is quite possible for the pH, [HCO_3^-], and P_{CO_2} all to be normal and yet for there to be significant acid-base disturbances. The only clue will be the anion gap. Take the example of a [Na^+] of 145, [Cl^-] 97, [K^+] 4.5, and [HCO_3^-] of 25 and a normal ABG. All the numbers look reasonably normal. However, the AG is 23, so by definition there must be a wide-AG metabolic acidosis. The only explanation for the normal numbers is that there must be a concomitant metabolic alkalosis.

REFERENCES

1. Narins RG, Emmett M: Simple and mixed acid-base disorders: A practical approach. *Medicine* 59:161, 1980.
2. Kassirer JP, Bleich HL: Rapid estimation of plasma carbon dioxide from pH and total carbon dioxide content. *N Engl J Med* 272:1067, 1965.
3. Häussinger D: Liver and kidney in acid-base regulation. *Nephrol Dial Transplant* 10:1536, 1995.
4. Graber ML, Quigg RJ, Stempsey WE, Weis S: Spurious hyperchloremia and decreased anion gap in hyperlipidemia. *Ann Intern Med* 98(pt 1):607, 1983.
5. Winter SD, Pearson JR, Gabow PA, et al: The fall of the serum anion gap. *Arch Intern Med* 150:311, 1990.
6. Roberts W, Johnson R: The serum anion gap: Has the reference interval really fallen? *Arch Pathol Lab Med* 121:568, 1997.
7. Elin R, Robertson E, Johnson E: Bromide interferes with determination of chloride by each of four methods. *Clin Chem* 27:778, 1981.
8. Levraut J, Bounatirou T, Ichai C, et al: Reliability of anion gap as an indicator of blood lactate in critically ill patients. *Intens Care Med* 23:417, 1997.
9. Mikulaschek A, Henry SM, Donovan R, Scalea TM: Serum lactate is not predicted by anion gap or base excess after trauma resuscitation. *J Trauma* 40:218, 1996.
10. Wrenn K: The delta (Δ) gap: An approach to mixed acid-base disorders. *Ann Emerg Med* 19:1310, 1990.
11. Brandenburg MA, Dire DJ: Comparison of arterial and venous blood gas values in the initial emergency department evaluation of patients with diabetic ketoacidosis. *Ann Emerg Med* 31:459, 1998.
12. Albert MS, Dell RB, Winters RW: Quantitative displacement of acid-base equilibrium in metabolic acidosis. *Ann Intern Med* 66:312, 1967.
13. Pierce NF, Fedson DS, Brigham KL, et al: The ventilatory response to acute base deficit in humans: Time course during development and correction of metabolic acidosis. *Ann Intern Med* 72:633, 1970.

14. Kety SS, Polis BD, Nadler CS, Schmidt CF: The blood flow and the oxygen consumption of the human brain in diabetic acidosis and coma. *J Clin Invest* 27:500, 1948.
15. Adrogue HJ, Madias NE: Management of life-threatening acid-base disorders: Second of two parts. *N Engl J Med* 338:107, 1998.
16. Kucera RR, Shapiro JI, Whalen MA, et al: Brain pH effects of $NaHCO_3$ and Carbicarb in lactic acidosis. *Crit Care Med* 17:1320, 1989.
17. Bersin RM, Arieff AI: Improved hemodynamic function during hypoxia with Carbicarb, a new agent for the management of acidosis. *Circulation* 77:227, 1988.
18. Kopel RF, Durbin CG Jr: Pulmonary artery catheter deterioration during hydrochloric acid infusion for the treatment of metabolic alkalosis. *Crit Care Med* 17:688, 1989.
19. Brackett NC, Cohen JJ, Schwartz WB: Carbon dioxide titration curve of normal man: Effect of increasing degrees of acute hypercapnia on acid-base equilibrium. *N Engl J Med* 272:6, 1965.
20. Arbus GS, Herbert LA, Levesque PR et al: Characterization and clinical application of the ''significance band'' for acute respiratory alkalosis. *N Engl J Med* 280:117, 1969.
21. Krapf R, Beeler I, Hertner D, Hulter HN: Chronic respiratory alkalosis: The effect of sustained hyperventilation on renal regulation of acid-base equilibrium. *N Engl J Med* 324:1394, 1991.
22. Callaham M: Hypoxic hazards of traditional paper bag rebreathing in hyperventilating patients. *Ann Emerg Med* 18:622, 1989.
23. Callaham M: Panic disorders, hyperventilation, and the dreaded brown paper bag. *Ann Emerg Med* 30:838, 1997.
24. van der Hout MA, Boek C, van der Molen GM, et al: Rebreathing to cope with hyperventilation: Experimental tests of the paper bag method. *J Behav Med* 11:303, 1989.

BLOOD GASES: PATHOPHYSIOLOGY AND INTERPRETATION

Mark P. Hamlin
Peter J. Pronovost

Human lungs serve two distinct functions: ventilation and oxygenation. Ventilation, which determines the clearance of carbon dioxide from the body, is a function of the rate and depth of breathing. Oxygenation is the diffusion of oxygen from the lungs to the bloodstream for subsequent delivery to the tissues. The separation between oxygenation and ventilation is dramatically demonstrated by the apnea test for determining brain death. During this test, 100% oxygen is insufflated via a thin catheter placed near the carina in an apneic, unventilated patient. The peripheral oxygen saturation is 90 to 100% despite no clearance of carbon dioxide with severe acidosis. This dramatic example clearly distinguishes the two functions.

VENTILATION

Minute Ventilation

Minute ventilation (VM), the total amount of new air moved in and out of the airways and lungs each minute, is equal to the tidal volume (VT) multiplied by the respiratory rate (f). The normal VT is about 7 mL/kg, or 500 mL in an adult, and the normal f is 12 breaths per minute. Therefore, the normal minute ventilatory volume required to maintain a partial pressure of carbon dioxide (P_{CO_2}) of 40 mmHg averages about 6 L/min. However, the VM required to maintain a normal P_{CO_2} depends on the amount of CO_2 being produced and the amount of dead space in the lung. People who are exercising or patients who are febrile or hypermetabolic have increased CO_2 production and thus a VM greater than 10 to 20 L/min, while patients who are severely hypothermic may have decreased CO_2 production and thus VM equals 2 L/min. A VM less than 2 L/min, even in a hypothermic patient, leads to respiratory acidosis. The f occasionally rises to as high as 40 to 50 breaths per minute, and the VT can become almost as great as the forced vital capacity, which is about 4500 to 5000 mL, or 65 to 70 mL/kg in a young adult male. However, at rapid rates a person usually cannot sustain a VT greater than 40 percent of the vital capacity for more than a few hours.

Dead Space

Approximately 30% of the air that a person breathes does not participate in the alveolar gas exchange process and is thus called dead space ventilation (VDS). Dead space ventilation is made up of anatomic dead space and alveolar dead space. Anatomic dead space is the volume of air that fills the conducting airways (trachea, bronchi, and bronchioles), while alveolar dead space is the volume of air in alveoli that are not perfused. The combination of alveolar and anatomic dead space is called the physiologic dead space, which in a young male adult with a VT of 500 mL is about 150 mL (about 2 mL/kg of body weight), or about 30% of the VT.

Dead space can be increased by certain disease states, such as adult respiratory distress syndrome (ARDS), where the physiologic dead space can exceed 60% of the VT. The increased dead space requires a tremendous increase in the VM (usually by an increase in the respiratory rate) to prevent the development of respiratory acidosis.

Alveolar Ventilation

The main function of the pulmonary ventilatory system is to continually renew the air in the alveoli, where it is brought in close proximity to the pulmonary capillary blood. The rate at which new air reaches these areas is called alveolar ventilation (VA), or VM − VDS. Consider a patient with myasthenia gravis who is developing progressive respiratory failure. The patient's baseline VA is [VM(500 × 12 = 6 L/min) − VDS(150 × 12 = 1.8 L/min) = VA(4.2 L/min)]. If the patient's VT is decreased to 250 due to weakness, the patient cannot simply double f but must increase it almost 4 times, to 42 breaths per minute [(250 × 42 = 10.5 L/min) − (150 × 42 = 6.3 L/min) = 4.2 L/min], to maintain the same alveolar ventilation. An increased f increases the patient's work of breathing and may lead to respiratory failure.

GAS PRESSURES

Pressure is caused by the constant impact of moving molecules against a surface. Therefore, the pressure of a gas acting on the surfaces of the respiratory passages and alveoli is proportional to the sum of the impaction forces of all the molecules striking the surface at any given instant. The important gases to consider in the lung are oxygen, nitrogen, and carbon dioxide. The rate of diffusion of each gas is directly proportional to its partial pressure.

The concentration of a gas in solution (e.g., blood) is determined not only by its partial pressure but also by the solubility coefficient of the gas. The solubility coefficients for the important respiratory gases at body temperature are oxygen, 0.024; carbon dioxide, 0.57; carbon monoxide, 0.018; and nitrogen, 0.012. Thus, carbon dioxide is more than 20 times as soluble as oxygen, and oxygen is twice as soluble as nitrogen. The solubilities help determine the quantity of gas dissolved in the fluids of the body, which is a major factor in determining the rate at which the gas can diffuse through tissues.

Diffusion of Gases

Major factors that affect the rate of gas diffusion in a fluid include (1) the partial pressure of the gas, (2) the solubility of the gas in the fluid, (3) the surface area available for diffusion, (4) the distance through which the gas must diffuse, (5) the molecular weight of the gas, and (6) the temperature of the fluid.

The greater the solubility of the gas and the greater the surface area for diffusion, the greater the number of molecules available to diffuse for any given pressure difference. On the other hand, the greater the distance the molecules must diffuse, the longer it takes for the diffusion to occur. Finally, the greater the velocity of the molecules, which at any given temperature is inversely proportional to the square root of the molecular weight, the greater the rate of diffusion of the gas. All these factors can be expressed in a single formula:

$$D = \frac{PAS}{d\sqrt{\text{MW}}}$$

where D = diffusion rate
P = pressure difference between the two ends of the diffusion pathway
A = cross-section area of the pathway
S = solubility of the gas
d = distance of diffusion
MW = molecular weight of the gas

The characteristics of a gas determine its solubility and molecular weight, which determine the diffusion coefficient of the gas. The diffusion coefficient, which equals $S\sqrt{\text{MW}}$, determines the relative rates at which different gases at the same pressure will diffuse. If the diffusion coefficient of oxygen is 1.0, the relative diffusion coefficients of other gases of respiratory importance are carbon dioxide, 20.3; carbon monoxide, 0.81; nitrogen, 0.53; and helium, 0.95.

Oxygen, carbon dioxide, and nitrogen are all highly soluble in lipids and consequently are also highly soluble in cell membranes. The major limitation to the movement of these gases in tissues is the rate at which the gases can diffuse through the tissue water, an important consideration in pulmonary edema.

The respiratory unit is composed of a respiratory bronchiole, alveolar ducts, atria, and alveoli. The alveolar walls are extremely thin and closely applied to an almost continuous network of interconnecting capillaries. The membrane through which gaseous exchange between the alveolar air and the pulmonary blood occurs is known as the respiratory (pulmonary) membrane. For oxygen to get from the alveolus into the pulmonary capillary bed, it must pass through four separate layers, referred to collectively as the alveolar-capillary, or respiratory, membrane. These layers include (1) a layer of fluid, called alveolar fluid, lining the alveolus and containing surfactant that reduces its surface tension; (2) the alveolar epithelium, composed of very thin epithelial cells and a basement membrane; (3) a very thin interstitial space between the alveolar epithelium and the capillary membrane; and (4) the capillary endothelial membrane and its basement membrane, which fuses with the alveolar basement membrane in many places.

The average diameter of the pulmonary capillaries is less than 8 mm, which means that red blood cells must actually squeeze through them. Therefore, at least part of the red blood cell membrane touches the capillary wall. Where this occurs, oxygen does not have to pass through significant amounts of plasma as it diffuses from the alveolus to the red blood cell. This reduces the diffusion distance and thus increases the rapidity of diffusion of gases between the alveolus and the hemoglobin molecules.

Gas Diffusion Through the Respiratory Membrane

The total diffusing surface area of the lung is enormous (160 m^2) and very thin (averaging 0.63 mm). These characteristics, combined with the solubility of CO_2 and O_2, make the lungs very efficient for maximizing gas exchange. The factors that determine how rapidly a gas passes through the respiratory membrane are (1) the thickness of the membrane, (2) the surface area of the membrane, (3) the diffusion coefficient of the gas in the water of the membrane, and (4) the pressure difference between the two sides of the membrane.

TABLE 22-1 Partial Pressure of Gases while Breathing Room Air, (mmHg)

Value	Air	Inspired Air in Trachea	Average Alveolar Gas	Average Expired Gas
P_{O_2}	159.0	149.3	104.0	120.0
P_{CO_2}	0.3	0.3	40.0	28.0
P_{N_2}	597.0	563.4	569.0	565.0
P_{H_2O}	3.7	47.0	47.0	47.0
Total	760.0	760.0	760.0	760.0

Thickness of the membrane is rarely a significant impediment to the transfer of CO_2, but O_2, being 20 times less soluble than CO_2, can be effected by processes that increase the diffusion distance. Two common clinical entities that increase the diffusion distance are pulmonary edema and pulmonary fibrosis, which explains the common finding of hypoxemia in patients with congestive heart failure. Another example of how the factors that determine gas diffusion can be applied clinically is the treatment of carbon monoxide poisoning with 100% oxygen, or hyperbaric oxygen, to increase the pressure difference between the two sides of the alveolar capillary membrane and thus facilitate oxygen loading.

The surface area of the respiratory membrane may be greatly decreased by a variety of conditions, such as atelectasis, resection of lung tissue, or emphysema. In emphysema, many of the alveoli coalesce, with dissolution of alveolar walls. The new alveolar chambers are much larger than the original alveoli, but the total surface area of the respiratory membrane available for gas diffusion is considerably decreased. When the total surface area of the lung is decreased to approximately one-third to one-fourth normal, exchange of gases through the membrane is impeded significantly, even under resting conditions. During strenuous exercise, even the slightest increase in dead space in patients with severe emphysema can seriously interfere with the exchange of gases.

The pressure difference across the respiratory membrane is the difference between the partial pressure of the gas in the alveoli and the partial pressure of the gas in the blood. In room air, the normal difference between the partial pressure of alveolar oxygen (P_{AO_2}) and the partial pressure of arterial oxygen (P_{aO_2}), ($P_{AO_2} - P_{aO_2}$), or $[P(A - a)O_2]$, is 2 to 10 mmHg. The normal difference between the partial pressure of alveolar carbon dioxide (P_{ACO_2}) and the partial pressure of arterial carbon dioxide (P_{aCO_2}), ($P_{ACO_2} - P_{aCO_2}$), or $[P(A - a)CO_2]$, is zero. An increase in the $P(A - a)CO_2$ is due to an increase in dead space. The dead-space air does not participate in gas exchange and thus dilutes the alveolar CO_2.

ALVEOLAR GASES

Inspired Gases

Air at sea level has an average barometric pressure of 760 mmHg and contains approximately 21% oxygen and 0.04% carbon dioxide, with nitrogen making up most of the remainder. Thus, the partial pressures of oxygen and carbon dioxide in the air at sea level are 159 and 0.3 mmHg, respectively (Table 22-1).

Alveolar air does not have the same concentration of gases as atmospheric air. The reasons for the difference include the following: (1) dry atmospheric air that enters the respiratory passages is humidified before it reaches the alveoli, (2) alveolar air is only partially replaced by atmospheric air with each breath, (3) oxygen is constantly being absorbed from the alveolar air, and (4) carbon dioxide is constantly diffusing from the pulmonary blood into the alveoli.

Humidification of Inspired Air

When air enters the respiratory passageways, water immediately evaporates from the surfaces of these passages and humidifies the inhaled air. At 37°C (98.6°F), water has a vapor pressure of 47 mmHg. Therefore, once the gas mixture is fully humidified, the partial pressure of the water vapor in the gas mixture is 47 mmHg (regardless of barometric pressure). This partial pressure is designated P_{H_2O} and must be subtracted from atmospheric pressure (760 mmHg) prior to calculation of the partial pressures of the dry gases in the alveolus (760 − 47 = 713). The remaining gases are predominantly nitrogen (79%, or 563 mmHg), oxygen (21%, or 149 mmHg), and CO_2 (0.04%, or 0.3 mmHg) (Table 22-1). If the patient is breathing 60% oxygen (fraction of inspired oxygen [F_{IO_2}]) = 0.6, the inspired oxygen pressure (P_{IO_2}) in the trachea or bronchi is determined as follows:

$$
\begin{aligned}
P_{IO_2} &= (P_B - P_{H_2O})F_{IO_2} \\
&= (760 - 47)(0.6) \\
&= 427.8 \text{ mmHg}
\end{aligned}
$$

where PB is barometric pressure (assumed to be 760 mmHg at sea level).

Rate at Which Alveolar Air Is Renewed by Atmospheric Air

The functional residual capacity of the lungs, which is the amount of air remaining in the lungs at the end of normal expiration, is approximately 2500 to 3000 mL (35 to 45 mL/kg). Only 350 mL of new air is brought into the alveoli with each new V_T and the same amount of old alveolar air is expired.

The slow replacement of alveolar air helps prevent sudden changes in gas concentrations in the blood. This helps to prevent excessive changes in tissue oxygenation, tissue carbon dioxide concentration, and tissue pH when ventilation is temporarily interrupted. This is also the basis of preoxygenation of patients prior to elective intubation, which could be more accurately described as denitrogenation, or replacing the alveolar nitrogen with oxygen.

Oxygen Concentration and Partial Pressure in the Alveoli

Oxygen is continually being absorbed into the blood in the alveolar capillaries, and new oxygen is continually entering the alveoli from the atmosphere. The more rapidly oxygen is absorbed, the lower its concentration in the alveoli. The more rapidly new oxygen is brought into the alveoli from the atmosphere, the higher its concentration becomes. Therefore, oxygen concentration in the alveoli is controlled by the rate of absorption of oxygen into the blood and the rate of entry of new oxygen into the lung.

Carbon Dioxide Concentration in the Alveoli

Carbon dioxide is continually formed and discharged into the alveoli and continually removed from the alveoli by ventilation. Therefore, the two factors that determine the P_{ACO_2} are (1) the rate of excretion of carbon dioxide from the blood into the alveoli and (2) the rate at which carbon dioxide is removed from the alveoli by V_A.

At a normal rate of V_A of 4.2 L/min, the P_{ACO_2} is usually 40 mmHg. If V_A is doubled, the P_{ACO_2} is reduced to 20 mmHg. If V_A is decreased to 2.1 L/min, the P_{ACO_2} rises to 80 mmHg. These estimations change with metabolic activity, nutritional state, temperature, and so on.

Alveolar Gas Equation

Inspired gas in the trachea has a partial pressure of oxygen (P_{O_2}) of about 149 mmHg and a P_{CO_2} of about 0.3 mmHg. As the warm, water-saturated air enters the alveoli, oxygen diffuses through the alveolar capillary membranes into the plasma and carbon dioxide diffuses from the blood into the alveoli. The mixed venous blood brought to the pulmonary capillaries normally has a P_{O_2} of about 40 mmHg and a P_{CO_2} of 46 mmHg. On the average, for each milliliter of oxygen that leaves the alveolus, 0.8 to 1.0 mL of carbon dioxide enters it. This relationship is defined as the respiratory quotient (RQ), which can be expressed as

$$RQ = \frac{\text{rate of } CO_2 \text{ production}}{\text{rate of } O_2 \text{ consumption}}$$

In order to determine how well the lungs are functioning at oxygenation, the difference between P_{AO_2} and P_{aO_2} is often estimated. To estimate P_{AO_2} from the P_{IO_2} and P_{aCO_2}, one needs a correction factor to determine how much oxygen is consumed for each 1.0 mmHg of P_{aCO_2} resulting from carbon dioxide that enters the alveoli. Thus, for the usual circumstances, in which the RQ is 0.8, the alveolar gas equation is

$$P_{AO_2} = (P_B - P_{H_2O})(F_{IO_2}) - (P_{aCO_2})/RQ$$

In room air (F_{IO_2} = 0.21) at sea level with a P_{aCO_2} of 40 mmHg, the P_{AO_2} is expected to be

$$P_{AO_2} = (760 - 47)(0.21) - (40)/0.8 = 150 - 50 = 100$$

The normal difference between P_{AO_2} and P_{aO_2} is 2 to 10 mmHg.

End-Tidal Gases

Expired air is a combination of dead space air and alveolar air, and its overall composition is determined by the proportion of each in expired air. Dead space air is expired first. Then progressively more alveolar air becomes mixed with the dead space air until all the dead space air has finally been washed out. At the end of normal exhalation nothing but alveolar air is expired. Therefore, to collect alveolar air for study, one simply collects end-tidal gas. Determination of end-tidal carbon dioxide (ET_{CO_2}) levels is a useful measure of the adequacy of ventilation. In patients with normal lungs, ET_{CO_2} is approximately 3 mmHg lower than P_{ACO_2}, but in patients with obstructive airways disease, typically asthma, there can be a large difference between ET_{CO_2} and P_{ACO_2}, since dead space air is never fully exhaled and thus neither is pure alveolar air. The use of ET_{CO_2} monitors is responsible for the reduction in undetected esophageal intubations.

ARTERIAL BLOOD GASES

Partial Pressure of Arterial Carbon Dioxide

ALVEOLAR VENTILATION Carbon dioxide diffuses so rapidly that the P_{aCO_2} usually provides an excellent index of the adequacy of ventilation. If the P_{aCO_2} is greater than normal in a patient with a normal or low arterial pH, one can assume that V_A is inadequate. The patient may have a low respiratory rate or tidal volume or may also have increased dead space due to emphysema, pulmonary emboli, or increased carbon dioxide production as in thyroid storm or sepsis. An elevated P_{aCO_2} in the presence of metabolic alkalosis usually reflects compensatory effort to restore arterial pH to normal while an increased P_{aCO_2} in a patient with metabolic acidosis generally indicates impending respiratory failure.

DEAD SPACE When the ventilation of an alveolar-capillary unit is normal but perfusion of the alveolar capillary is absent, the ventilation of these alveoli and their associated airways is referred to as dead space, or high ventilation-perfusion (V/Q) mismatching. V_{DS} and the tidal volume (V_T) are often expressed as a ratio (V_{DS}/V_T). This is determined in a pulmonary function laboratory (or a bedside metabolic cart) by measuring the Pa_{CO_2}, measuring the *average* expired gas (PE_{CO_2}) (not to be confused with ET_{CO_2}), and using the Bohr equation:

$$\frac{V_{DS}}{V_T} = \frac{Pa_{CO_2} - PE_{CO_2}}{Pa_{CO_2}}$$

The normal values are

$$\frac{V_{DS}}{V_T} = \frac{40 - 28}{40} = \frac{12}{40} = 0.3$$

When the physiologic dead space is increased, some of the work of ventilation is wasted because a greater fraction of ventilated air never reaches the functioning alveolar-capillary units. A patient with a dead space greater than 0.6 generally requires mechanical ventilation to maintain normal Pa_{CO_2}.

TRANSPORT OF CARBON DIOXIDE IN THE BLOOD Under resting conditions, each 100 mL of blood transports an average of 4 mL of carbon dioxide from the tissues to the lungs. Transport of carbon dioxide is not as great a problem as is transport of oxygen because, even under the most abnormal conditions, carbon dioxide can usually be transported in far greater quantities than can oxygen. However, carbon dioxide in the blood does affect acid-base balance.

The carbon dioxide formed in cells diffuses out in the form of carbon dioxide rather than bicarbonate because the cell membrane is almost impermeable to bicarbonate ions. As the carbon dioxide enters the capillary, it initiates a number of almost instantaneous reactions essential for carbon dioxide transport.

First, a small portion of the carbon dioxide is transported to the lungs dissolved in plasma. The dissolved portion is approximately 0.36 mL of carbon dioxide in each 100 mL of blood. This is about 9% of all carbon dioxide transported.

Much of the dissolved carbon dioxide in the blood reacts with water to form carbonic acid; a reaction facilitated by carbonic anhydrase inside the red blood cells speeds up the reaction about 500-fold. The reaction occurs so rapidly that it reaches almost complete equilibrium within a fraction of a second. This allows tremendous amounts of carbon dioxide to react with red blood cell water even before the blood leaves the tissue capillaries.

In another fraction of a second, the carbonic acid formed in the red blood cells dissociates into hydrogen and bicarbonate ions. Most of the hydrogen ions then combine with the hemoglobin in the red blood cells because hemoglobin is a powerful acid-base buffer. At the same time, many of the bicarbonate ions diffuse into the plasma; to offset this ionic shift, chloride ions diffuse into the red blood cells. This diffusion is made possible by the presence of a special bicarbonate-chloride carrier protein in the red blood cell membrane that rapidly shuttles these two ions in opposite directions. Thus, the chloride content of venous red blood cells is greater than that of arterial red blood cells. This phenomenon is called the chloride shift.

The reversible combination of carbon dioxide with water in the red blood cells, under the influence of carbonic anhydrase, accounts for at least 60 to 70% of all the carbon dioxide transported from the tissues. Indeed, when a carbonic anhydrase inhibitor (acetazolamide) is administered to block the action of carbonic anhydrase in the red blood cells, carbon dioxide transport from the tissues becomes very poor and the tissue P_{CO_2} rises abruptly.

CARBAMINOHEMOGLOBIN AND CARBAMINOPROTEINS Carbon dioxide also reacts directly with hemoglobin to form carbaminohemoglobin ($Hb-CO_2$). Since this reversible reaction occurs with a very loose bond, the carbon dioxide is easily released into the alveoli, where the P_{CO_2} is lower than that in the tissue capillaries. A small amount of carbon dioxide (usually equivalent to about 0.5 to 1.0 meq/L of bicarbonate) also reacts in this way with the plasma proteins, forming carbaminoproteins. This reaction is much less significant because the quantity of these proteins is only about one-fourth to one-half the quantity of hemoglobin.

The theoretical quantity of carbon dioxide that can be carried to the lungs in combination with hemoglobin and plasma proteins is approximately 20 to 30% of the total quantity transported—that is, about 1.5 mL of carbon dioxide in each 100 mL of blood. However, this reaction is much slower than the reaction of carbon dioxide with water, and it is doubtful that more than 15 to 25% of the total quantity of carbon dioxide is transported this way.

CARBON DIOXIDE DISSOCIATION CURVE Carbon dioxide can exist in the blood as free carbon dioxide and in chemical combinations with water, hemoglobin, and plasma proteins. The total quantity of carbon dioxide combined with the blood in all forms depends on the Pa_{CO_2}.

The normal blood Pa_{CO_2} averages about 40 mmHg in arterial blood and 46 mmHg in mixed venous blood. Although the normal total concentration of carbon dioxide in the blood is about 50 mL/dL (vol%), only 4 mL/dL of this is actually exchanged during normal transport of carbon dioxide. Thus, the concentration of carbon dioxide rises to about 52 mL/dL after the blood passes through the tissues and falls to about 48 mL/dL after the blood passes through the lungs.

EFFECT OF THE OXYGEN-HEMOGLOBIN REACTION ON CARBON DIOXIDE TRANSPORT: THE HALDANE EFFECT An increase in the carbon dioxide level in the blood causes oxygen to be displaced from the hemoglobin, and this promotes oxygen release to tissues at the capillary level. The reverse is also true; binding of oxygen with hemoglobin tends to displace carbon dioxide as blood moves through the pulmonary capillaries. Indeed, this so-called Haldane effect is quantitatively far more important in promoting carbon dioxide transport than the Bohr effect (see the section on "Oxyhemoglobin Saturation") is in promoting oxygen transport.

CHANGE IN BLOOD ACIDITY DURING CARBON DIOXIDE TRANSPORT The carbonic acid formed when carbon dioxide enters the blood in the tissue capillaries decreases the pH. However, the buffers of the blood prevent the hydrogen ion concentration from rising greatly. Ordinarily, arterial blood has a pH of approximately 7.40, and as the blood acquires carbon dioxide in the tissue capillaries, the pH falls to approximately 7.35. The reverse occurs when carbon dioxide is released from the blood in the lungs. Under conditions of high metabolic activity or when blood flow through the tissues is extremely sluggish, the decrease in pH in the blood as it leaves the tissues can be 0.50 or more.

CHANGES IN RESPIRATORY QUOTIENT As stated above, the RQ is the ratio of CO_2 produced to O_2 consumed. The RQ for the standard patient metabolizing a mixed diet of carbohydrates, fats, and protein is approximately 0.8. The RQs of the individual components are listed below:

Nutritional source	*RQ*
Carbohydrates	1.00
Protein	0.83
Fats	0.7

Thus, the RQ can change in patients who eat (or are fed) diets containing predominantly fat or carbohydrates. Relying heavily on carbohydrates for a patient with little respiratory reserve can lead to respiratory acidosis due to an increase in required V_M. However, the effect

TABLE 22-2 Expected Pa_{O_2} in Patients Inhaling Various Concentrations of Oxygen, mmHg

F_{IO_2}	0.21 (room air)	0.4	0.6	0.8	1.0
Expected Pa_{O_2}*	100	227	370	512	655

*Assuming a $PA_{O_2} - Pa_{O_2}$ of 10 mmHg and a P_{CO_2} of 40 mmHg.

of diet on RQ is usually only an issue in the intensive care unit in a minority of patients with severe lung disease who are attempting to wean from mechanical ventilation.

MONITORING OXYGENATION AND VENTILATION A patient who is awake, alert, comfortable, and cooperative and has normal vital signs is generally oxygenating and ventilating adequately. However, if a patient is tachypneic and/or tachycardic and appears to be anxious and/or confused, hypercarbia or hypoxemia should be suspected. In comatose patients, it is sometimes very difficult to judge how well the patient is oxygenating or ventilating without serial blood gas determinations.

Cyanosis as a sign of inadequate oxygenation is almost worthless when the hemoglobin is less than 10 g/dL. Under such circumstances, the arterial oxygen saturation (Sa_{O_2}) must be less than 65%, corresponding to a Pa_{O_2} of about 30 to 35 mmHg, before the patient looks cyanotic. It must be remembered that oxygenation and ventilation are two separate systems. A frequent clinical misconception is that a patient with an adequate Sa_{O_2} must be ventilating adequately. This assumption is incorrect and dangerous, particularly with patients who are receiving supplemental oxygen. This is discussed below under ''Noninvasive Monitoring, Pulse Oximetry.''

Partial Pressure of Arterial Oxygen

The Pa_{O_2} in normal, healthy young adults breathing room air at sea level is considered to be 90 to 100 mmHg. The Pa_{O_2} is extremely important because it not only reflects the functional capabilities of the lungs but also determines the rate at which oxygen enters the tissue cells.

Factors that affect the Pa_{O_2} include the V_A, the F_{IO_2}, the functional capabilities of the lungs, the mean airway pressure in mechanically ventilated patients, and the oxyhemoglobin dissociation curve.

ALVEOLAR VENTILATION If the patient hyperventilates, the Pa_{CO_2} tends to fall and the Pa_{O_2} tends to rise. If the Pa_{CO_2} falls by 1 mmHg, the Pa_{O_2} rises by about 1.0 to 1.2 mmHg; in accordance with the law of additive partial pressures. The lungs can make up for some pulmonary dysfunction by hyperventilating. This is seen in pregnant patients who have normal arterial blood gas values at term showing normal pH, a Pa_{CO_2} of 30 to 32, a Pa_{O_2} of 110 to 115, and a serum bicarbonate level of 20 to 22 meq/L. This is due to an increase in V_M (predominantly due to increased V_T), with resultant respiratory alkalosis with increased urinary excretion of bicarbonate to compensate.

FRACTION OF INSPIRED OXYGEN Unfortunately, the F_{IO_2} is often not considered adequately in evaluating the Pa_{O_2}. If a patient is receiving oxygen by nasal cannula, the actual delivered F_{IO_2} is usually only 25 to 30 percent. With a properly fitting face mask, the inhaled F_{IO_2} is usually less than half that delivered to the mask. The approximate Pa_{O_2} values that might be expected in normal persons who are inhaling various concentrations of oxygen are listed in Table 22-2.

The expected PA_{O_2} when the patient is given oxygen can be estimated by multiplying the actual delivered percentage of oxygen by 6. Thus, a patient getting 60% oxygen would be expected to have a PA_{O_2} of about 60 × 6, or 360 mmHg.

TABLE 22-3 Changes in P_{O_2} at Various Altitudes

Altitude Above Sea Level, ft	Atmospheric Pressure, mmHg	P_{O_2} in Air, mmHg	PA_{O_2}, mmHg	Pa_{O_2}, mmHg*
0	760	159	105	100
2,000	707	148	97	92
4,000	656	137	90	85
6,000	609	127	84	79
8,000	564	118	79	74
10,000	523	109	74	69
20,000	349	73	40	35
30,000	226	47	21	19

*Assuming ideal circumstances with a $PA_{O_2} - Pa_{O_2}$ of 5 mmHg or less.

ALTITUDE The Pa_{O_2} expected when a patient is breathing room air varies with height above sea level. The greater the altitude, the lower the P_{O_2} in the air and the greater the tendency for the patient to hyperventilate (Table 22-3).

The Pa_{O_2} drops about 3 to 4 mmHg for each 1000-foot rise above sea level. Up to an altitude of approximately 10,000 ft, the Sa_{O_2} remains about 90 percent. However, above 10,000 ft, the Sa_{O_2} progressively falls about 1 percent for each 1 mmHg drop in P_{O_2} until at 20,000 ft altitude the Pa_{O_2} is about 35 mmHg and the Sa_{O_2} is only about 65 percent.

When a person breathes air at 30,000 ft, where the barometric pressure is about 226 mmHg, the Pa_{O_2} is only 21 mmHg. At this height above sea level, almost three-fourths of the alveolar air is nitrogen. However, if the person breathes pure oxygen instead of air, most of the space in the alveoli formerly occupied by nitrogen becomes occupied by oxygen. Nevertheless, even if the person is breathing 100% oxygen at 30,000 ft, the Pa_{O_2} is only 139 mmHg (Table 22-4).

AGE Even in healthy individuals, pulmonary changes that cause a fall in the Pa_{O_2} occur with advancing age. On the average, the Pa_{O_2} falls about 3 to 4 mmHg per decade after the patient reaches 20 to 30 years of age. Thus, an otherwise normal 20-year-old patient with

TABLE 22-4 Effects of Acute Exposure to Low Atmospheric Pressure on Alveolar Gas Concentrations and on Sa_{O_2}

		WHILE BREATHING AIR		WHILE BREATHING 100% O_2	
Altitude, ft	Barometric Pressure, mmHg	PA_{O_2}, mmHg	PA_{CO_2}, mmHg	PA_{O_2}, mmHg	Oxygen Saturation, %
0	760	159	40	673	100
10,000	523	110	40	436	100
20,000	349	73	40	262	100
30,000	226	47	40	139	99
40,000	141	29	36	58	87
50,000	87	18	24	16	22

TABLE 22-5 Relation Between Oxyhemoglobin Saturation and Plasma Po_2

Oxygen saturation, %	100.0	98.4	95	90	80	73	60	50	40	35	30
Po_2, mmHg	677	100	80	59	48	40	30	26	23	21	18

TABLE 22-6 Changes in Pao_2 Related to pH

PH	7.60	7.50	7.40	7.30	7.20	7.10	7.00
PAO_2, MMHG*	80	90	100	111	122	134	148

*Assuming a temperature of 37°C (98.6°F) and a hemoglobin saturation of 98.4%.

a Pao_2 of about 90 to 100 mmHg (breathing room air at sea level) might be expected to have a Pao_2 of only about 75 to 80 mmHg at 80 years of age.

Alveolar-Arterial Oxygen Differences

One method of determining the degree to which lung function is impaired is to determine the alveolar-arterial oxygen gradient $[P(A - a)o_2]$. The Pao_2 can be determined from arterial blood samples and the PAo_2 and be determined from the alveolar air equation previously discussed. One can also estimate the PAo_2 in patients with a normal cardiac output breathing room air by subtracting the $Paco_2$ from 145. This is possible because PAo_2 and $PAco_2$ add up to about 145 mmHg when a patient breathes room air at sea level. Since the $PAco_2$ is usually the same as the $Paco_2$, the PAo_2 can be estimated from the arterial gas pressure by the following formula:

$$PAo_2 = 145 - Paco_2$$

If the patient has a $Paco_2$ of 40 mmHg,

$$PAo_2 = 145 - 40 = 105 \text{ mmHg}$$

This equation can be used to determine the $P(A - a)o_2$. The PAo_2 is estimated from the above formula, and the Pao_2 is determined from arterial blood gas analysis. If the Pao_2 were 90 mmHg, the $P(A - a)o_2$ would be 15 mmHg, which is relatively normal. A $P(A - a)o_2$ of 20 to 30 mmHg on room air usually indicates mild pulmonary dysfunction, and a $P(A - a)o_2$ greater than 50 mmHg on room air usually indicates severe pulmonary dysfunction. The causes of an increased A-a gradient include intrapulmonary shunt (relatively less ventilation than perfusion, or a low V/Q ratio), intracardiac shunt, and diffusion abnormalities.

Oxyhemoglobin Saturation

NORMAL RELATIONSHIPS When arterial blood gas study results are obtained, clinicians are often concerned by PaO_2 levels in the 60 to 90-mmHg range. A Pao_2 of 60 mmHg correlates to an Sao_2 of 90%. Furthermore, if the hemoglobin level is 15.0 g/dL and the tissue removes 5.0 mL of oxygen from each 100 mL of blood, the Po_2 of the venous blood falls to about 36 mmHg, which is only 4 mmHg below the normal value. Thus, the tissue Po_2 often changes minimally despite a marked fall in Pao_2.

On the other hand, if the Pao_2 rises far above the upper limit of normal (90 to 100 mmHg), the oxygen saturation of hemoglobin cannot rise above 100%. Therefore, even if the Pao_2 rose to 600 mmHg or more, the saturation of hemoglobin would increase only 1 to 2% because, at Pao_2 of 100 mmHg, the Sao_2 is only 98 to 99%. This, combined with some evidence (predominantly in animals) that an Fio_2 greater than 50 can be associated with pulmonary toxicity, should guide the clinician to supply only the amount of oxygen required to produce a Pao_2 between 70 and 100 mmHg.

Under circumstances of normal body temperature [37°C (98.6°F)] and blood pH 7.40, certain standard relationships exist between the oxyhemoglobin saturation and the plasma Po_2 (Table 22-5). Thus, the relationship between Sao_2 and plasma Po_2 is almost linear when the Sao_2 is 60 to 90%. However, as the Sao_2 rises above 90%, the Po_2 begins to rise much faster than the saturation. A simplification to remember for clinical practice is that a Pao_2 of 30, 40, 50, and 60 correspond approximately to an Sao_2 of 60, 70, 80, and 90 percent, respectively.

FACTORS AFFECTING OXYHEMOGLOBIN DISSOCIATION The best known of the factors affecting the oxyhemoglobin dissociation curve are pH, temperature, and the amount of 2,3-diphosphoglycerate (2,3-DPG) in the red blood cells. Other related factors include Pco_2 and exercise.

pH The more acidic the blood, the more readily hemoglobin gives up its oxygen and the higher the Pao_2 (the partial pressure of oxygen dissolved in blood) is for a particular oxyhemoglobin saturation. In contrast, alkalosis makes hemoglobin hold on to its oxygen more tightly, lowering the Pao_2 present at a particular oxyhemoglobin saturation. In general, a rise or fall in pH of 0.10 causes a fall or rise (i.e., an opposite change) in the Pao_2 of about 10% (Table 22-6).

Partial Pressure of Carbon Dioxide A shift of the oxyhemoglobin dissociation curve, as a result of changes in the blood levels of carbon dioxide (Haldane effect) and hydrogen ions (Bohr effect), enhances oxygenation of the blood in the lungs and promotes release of oxygen from the blood in the tissues. As the blood passes through the lungs, carbon dioxide diffuses from the blood into the alveoli. This reduces the blood Pco_2 and decreases the hydrogen ion concentration because of the resulting decrease in the blood carbonic acid level. Both changes shift the oxyhemoglobin dissociation curve to the left. With a shift to the left, the quantity of oxygen binding to hemoglobin at any given Pao_2 is increased, allowing greater oxygen transport to the tissues. Then, when the blood reaches the tissue capillaries, the opposite effect occurs. Carbon dioxide entering the blood from the tissues shifts the curve to the right. This displaces oxygen from the hemoglobin and delivers oxygen to the tissues at a higher Po_2 than would otherwise occur.

Temperature As blood temperature increases, hemoglobin gives up oxygen more readily, raising the Po_2 in the plasma. The opposite occurs during cooling. For each 1°C rise in temperature, the Pao_2 rises about 5% (Table 22-7). With hypothermia, the Pco_2 falls by about the same amount.

Exercise During strenuous exercise, several factors can shift the oxyhemoglobin dissociation curve to the right. Exercising muscles release large quantities of carbon dioxide and other acids, increasing

TABLE 22-7 Po_2 Levels at Various Temperatures

Temperature, °F	104.0	102.2	100.4	98.6	95.0	86.6
Temperature, °C	40	39	38	37	35	32
Pao_2, mmHg*	117	111	105	100	90	76

*Assuming a pH of 7.40 and a hemoglobin saturation of 98.4%.

TABLE 22-8 Interpretation of Pao_2/Fio_2 Ratio

Pao_2, mmHg	Fio_2, mmHg	Ratio	QS/QT, %	Abnormality
240	0.4	600	5	None
120	0.4	300	10	Minimal
100	0.4	250	15	Mild
80	0.4	200	20	Moderate
60	0.4	150	30	Severe*
40	0.4	100	40	Very severe*

*In trauma or septic patients, ventilatory assistance and PEEP to reduce the QS/QT to 15 percent should be considered. The higher the QS/QT, the greater the need for ventilatory assistance and PEEP.

the hydrogen ion concentration in muscle capillary blood. In addition, the temperature of the muscle often rises as much as 3 to 4°C, and phosphate compounds are also released. All these factors acting together shift the oxyhemoglobin dissociation curve of the blood in the muscle capillaries considerably to the right. This allows oxygen to be released to the muscle at a Po_2 as high as 40 mmHg even though as much as 75% of the oxygen has been removed from the hemoglobin. In the lungs, the shift occurs in the opposite direction, allowing pickup of extra amounts of oxygen from the alveoli.

2,3-Diphosphoglycerate Except for hemoglobin, the compound present in greatest quantity in red blood cells is 2,3-DPG. A normal concentration of 2,3-DPG in a red blood cell keeps the oxyhemoglobin dissociation curve shifted slightly to the right all the time. In addition, under hypoxic conditions lasting longer than a few hours, the quantity of 2,3-DPG increases considerably, shifting the oxyhemoglobin dissociation curve even farther to the right. This can cause the Po_2 in the plasma to be as much as 10 mmHg higher than it would have been otherwise. However, the presence of increased 2,3-DPG makes it more difficult for the hemoglobin to combine with oxygen in the lungs.

If the concentration of 2,3-DPG falls, as it does in stored blood or during sepsis, the hemoglobin holds on to its oxygen more tightly and the Pao_2 tends to fall. This is an important consideration during large-volume resuscitations with banked blood.

Other Methods of Evaluating Oxygenation

Pao_2/Fio_2 RATIO A quick way to estimate the impairment of oxygenation is to calculate the Pao_2/Fio_2 ratio. Normally, the ratio is about 500 to 600, which usually correlates to a pulmonary shunt (QS/QT) of about 3 to 5%. However, if a patient has a Pao_2 of 80 mmHg on 40% oxygen, the Pao_2/Fio_2 ratio is 80/0.4, or 200. A Pao_2/Fio_2 ratio of less than 200 corresponds with a QS/QT of about 20%. The usual relationship between Pao_2/Fio_2 ratios and the QS/QT in patients with a normal cardiac output is shown in Table 22-8. Pao_2/Fio_2 ratios are also used as criteria for the diagnosis of ARDS/acute lung injury (ALI). In a patient with alveolar infiltrates in at least 3 of 4 quadrants on chest x-ray, a normal pulmonary capillary wedge pressure, and a mechanism known to cause ARDS/ALI, a Pao_2/Fio_2 of less than 300 indicates ALI, while a ratio less than 200 indicates ARDS. However, some researchers no longer distinguish between ARDS and ALI and classify all patients with a Pao_2/Fio_2 ratio less than 300 as having ARDS.

Physiologic Shunting in the Lung (Venous-Arterial Admixture)

Although abnormal gas diffusion or distribution in the lungs can cause abnormal blood gas values, the most important cause is usually V/Q mismatching. When considering ventilation and perfusion, there can be four types of alveolar capillary units: (1) if ventilation and perfusion are normal, the unit is normal; (2) if there is ventilation without perfusion, the unit is considered to be dead space (or high V/Q); (3) if there is perfusion without ventilation, the unit is considered to be a (right-to-left) shunt (or low V/Q); and (4) if there is neither ventilation nor perfusion, the unit is silent.

The amount of physiologic shunting in the lung, or venous-arterial admixture (QS/QT), is probably the most sensitive guide to the onset and progression of acute respiratory failure. The shunt is that fraction of blood passing through the lungs without being oxygenated. Normally, the amount for venous-arterial admixture is about 3 to 5 percent of the cardiac output. This small amount of shunting is largely due to the drainage of deoxygenated blood in bronchial veins into oxygenated blood in pulmonary veins.

Physiologic shunting is harder to determine than alveolar-arterial oxygen differences because it requires drawing both arterial and mixed venous (pulmonary artery) blood samples and determining their oxygen contents. Mixed venous samples from the pulmonary artery are preferable to those obtained from central venous pressure catheters. However, central venous blood does give a reasonable estimate of the amount of shunting present if cardiac output is relatively normal.

Although an Fio_2 of 1.0 was generally used in the past to determine the amount of physiologic shunting in the lung, the high Fio_2 in itself may cause increased shunting. Now the shunt with an Fio_2 of 0.4 is considered to be a better indicator of lung function.

The QS/QT can be calculated from a modification of Berggren's formula:

$$\frac{QS}{QT} = \frac{Cco_2 - Cao_2}{Cco_2 - Cvo_2}$$

where Cco_2 is the pulmonary capillary oxygen content, Cao_2 is the arterial content, and Svo_2 is the mixed venous oxygen content. Thus, if Cco_2 is 20 mL/dL, Cao_2 is 19 mL/dL, and Svo_2 is 14 mL/dL, the shunt is

$$\frac{QS}{QT} = \frac{20 - 19}{20 - 14} = \frac{1}{6} = 17\%$$

The amount of shunting in the lung can also be estimated from arterial blood alone, using an assumption that the arteriovenous oxygen difference is approximately 5 mL/dL.

In general, if cardiac output doubles, the amount of shunt associated with a particular $P(A - a)o_2$ increases by about 50 percent (Table 22-9). This is partly related to the fact that, if only a small amount of blood is going through the lung, the blood flow tends to go to well-ventilated alveoli. If cardiac output increases, there is increasing likelihood that some of the blood will go through less well-ventilated tissue.

Thus, if cardiac output is high, relatively mild hypoxemia can result from a high shunt. For example, at a Pao_2 of 300 mmHg, if the cardiac output is 2.5 L/min, the shunt might be 11 percent, but at a cardiac output of 10.0 L/min, the shunt would be 32 percent. To factor in the changes due to an increased or decreased cardiac output, one uses the shunt index (SI). The SI is the percent shunt divided by the cardiac index. For example, at a normal cardiac index of 3.5 $(L/min)/m^2$ and a shunt of 5.0 percent, the SI is 5.0/3.5 = 1.4. If a patient has a shunt of 20 percent with a cardiac index of 2.5 $(L/min)/m^2$, the SI is 8.0. Patients with an SI above 5.0 usually require oxygenation support.

If the cardiac index is not known, the critical QS/QT is about 20 to 25 percent. Above these values, the patient usually has enough of

TABLE 22-9 Relation Between the Physiologic Shunt in the Lung(Q_S/Q_T) and $P(A - a)O_2$ while Breathing 100% O_2

		Qs/QT, %		
Pa_{O_2}	$P(A - a)O_2$ on 100% O_2	CO = 2.5 L/min	CO = 5 L/min	CO = 10 L/min
600	70	2	4	8
500	170	5	10	17
400	270	8	16	25
300	370	11	19	32
200	470	13	24	38
150	520	14	26	42
100	570	18	31	47
90	580	20	34	50
80	590	22	36	53
70	600	24	39	56
60	610	28	44	61
50	620	33	50	67

Abbreviation: CO, cardiac output.

a V/Q abnormality to warrant oxygenation support and positive end-expiratory pressure (PEEP).

Oxygen Availability

Oxygen availability is determined by the amount of oxygen brought to the capillaries, or oxygen delivery (D_{O_2}), and the dissociation of oxygen from hemoglobin at the tissues. To a certain extent, a good heart, which can increase cardiac output appropriately, can make up for bad lungs and a low hemoglobin level. The reverse is also true. However, a combination of poor oxygenation, low hemoglobin level, and low cardiac output may be rapidly fatal.

OXYGEN CONTENT The oxygen content of blood is determined primarily by the hemoglobin level and the oxyhemoglobin saturation. When fully saturated, each gram of hemoglobin measured clinically can carry 1.34 mL of oxygen. Thus, a patient with a hemoglobin concentration of 15.0 g/dL can carry about 20.1 mL of oxygen per 100 mL in the red blood cells when the hemoglobin is fully saturated. Although the Pa_{O_2} determines the rate at which oxygen enters the tissues, it contributes very little to the total oxygen content of blood. Each millimeter of mercury of Pa_{O_2} represents only 0.0031 mL of oxygen in 100 mL of blood. Thus, a patient with a normal Pa_{O_2} of 100 mmHg has only 0.31 mL of oxygen dissolved in the plasma.

The oxygen content of arterial blood (Ca_{O_2}) can be calculated from the following formula:

$$Ca_{O_2} = [Hb](1.34)(Sa_{O_2}/100) + (Pa_{O_2})(0.003)$$

Thus, in a patient with a hemoglobin concentration of 15.0 g/dL, an Sa_{O_2} of 98%, and a Pa_{O_2} of 100 mmHg,

$$\begin{aligned} Ca_{O_2} &= (15)(1.34)(98/100) + (100)(0.003) \\ &= 20.0 \text{ mL } O_2 \text{ per deciliter of blood} \end{aligned}$$

If the hemoglobin concentration falls to 10.0 g/dL, even if Sa_{O_2} and Pa_{O_2} remain the same, Ca_{O_2} falls by about a third. For example,

$$\begin{aligned} Ca_{O_2} &= (10)(1.34)(98/100) + (100)(0.003) \\ &= 13.132 + 0.30 \\ &= 13.4 \text{ mL } O_2 \text{ per deciliter of blood} \end{aligned}$$

Even with only 10 g of hemoglobin, the red blood cells are carrying over 40 times as much oxygen as is the plasma.

CARDIAC OUTPUT Oxygen content (in milliliters per liter of blood) multiplied by cardiac output (in liters per minute) is equal to D_{O_2}. Thus, the D_{O_2} in a patient with 15.0 g of 98% saturated hemoglobin, a Pa_{O_2} of 100 mmHg, and a cardiac output of 5 L/min is

$$\begin{aligned} D_{O_2} &= (Ca_{O_2} \text{ per dL})(10)(\text{cardiac output}) \\ &= \{[\text{hemoglobin}](1.34)(Sa_{O_2}/100) \\ &\quad + (Pa_{O_2})(0.003)\}(10)(\text{cardiac output}) \\ &= [(15)(1.34)(98/100) + (100)(0.003)](10)(5) \\ &= [(19.698 + 0.3)](50) \\ &= (19.998)(50) = (20)(50) \\ &= 1000 \text{ mL/min} \end{aligned}$$

The factor 10 is used to convert oxygen content from milliliters per 100 mL of blood to milliliters per liter of blood.

Since the normal oxygen consumption of an average resting adult male is about 250 to 300 mL/min [approximately 3 (mL/kg)/min], the tissue on average takes up about 25% of the oxygen brought to it, although the percent oxygen extraction varies by organ. Thus, the Sa_{O_2} falls from about 98% in arterial blood to about 73% in mixed venous blood. If there is no change in oxygen consumption but cardiac output doubles to 10 L/min, the amount of oxygen removed from each liter of blood is halved, and the venous oxyhemoglobin saturation will be about 85%. On the other hand, if cardiac output falls to 2.5 L/min, venous oxyhemoglobin saturation will fall to about 48 percent.

OXYGEN DISSOCIATION IN THE TISSUES The ability of blood to give up more oxygen (increasing the arteriovenous oxygen difference) as cardiac output falls and thus maintain oxygen delivery is an important defense mechanism sometimes referred to as oxygen reserve. Unfortunately, there is a limit to this so-called oxygen reserve because the P_{O_2} in most tissues seldom falls below 26 mmHg, which is the P_{50} for hemoglobin (P_{O_2} at which hemoglobin is 50% saturated).

The lowest value to which the P_{O_2} in capillaries can fall is about 18 to 20 mmHg because this is the usual capillary-mitochondrial gradient for oxygen. The saturation at a P_{O_2} of 20 mmHg is referred to as the S_{20}, and this is normally about 33%. The only places where the P_{O_2} in venous blood is normally as low as 20 mmHg are the coronary sinus, renal medulla, and perhaps the jugular venous bulb at the base of the brain. A relatively mild degree of alkalosis can raise the S_{20} by 4 to 5%, thereby greatly reducing oxygen availability to the myocardium. Thus, alkalosis (e.g., when metabolic acidosis is treated with bicarbonate) in low-flow states can be deleterious.

COMBINATION OF HEMOGLOBIN WITH CARBON MONOXIDE Carbon monoxide combines with hemoglobin at the same point on the hemoglobin molecule that oxygen does. Furthermore, it binds about 230 times more strongly than oxygen does. Therefore, an alveolar carbon monoxide level of 0.4 mmHg, which is $\frac{1}{230}$ that of the Pa_{O_2}, allows the carbon monoxide to compete equally with oxygen for combination with hemoglobin, causing half the hemoglobin in the blood to bind with carbon monoxide instead of oxygen. An alveolar carbon monoxide level of 0.7 mmHg (about 0.1% in air) can be lethal. Oxygen at high alveolar pressures displaces carbon monoxide from hemoglobin much more rapidly than atmospheric oxygen does. Patients with carbon monoxide poisoning can also benefit from simultaneous administration of 4 to 5% carbon dioxide, which strongly stimulates the respiratory center, increasing V_A, reducing the alveolar carbon monoxide concentration and allowing increased carbon monoxide to be released from the blood. A 96% oxygen and 4% carbon dioxide therapy removes carbon monoxide from the blood 10 to 20 times more rapidly than would be removed by breathing room air. The half-life of Hb—CO in a patient breathing room air is 2 to 3 h; if the patient is breathing 100% O_2, the half-life is about 20 to 30 min. The most effective way to clear Hb—CO is by increasing the Pa_{O_2} above that attainable by breathing 100% oxygen—that is, in a hyperbaric oxygen chamber.

OTHER METHODS OF EVALUATING BLOOD GASES

Pulmonary Artery Catheters

A number of pulmonary artery catheters have been developed to continuously monitor mixed venous oxygen saturation (Sv_{O_2}). The normal Sv_{O_2} is about 70 to 75%. A change in Sv_{O_2} could serve as an early warning of inadequacy of perfusion and oxygenation. A rise in Sv_{O_2} can signal an increase in cardiac output and D_{O_2} beyond that required for metabolism, shunting of blood from tissues (sepsis), or an inability of the peripheral tissues to extract and utilize O_2 (cyanide poisoning). It can also be simply a reflection of the location of the catheter tip in a persistently wedged position so that pulmonary capillary (oxygenated) blood is being analyzed. A fall in Sv_{O_2} below 50 to 60% is usually due to a significant decrease in cardiac output or lung function and requires urgent investigation. It is important to remember that, while a change in Sv_{O_2} may indicate important physiologic change, there can be major changes in the patient's condition without corresponding changes in the Sv_{O_2}. A major criticism of the usage of Sv_{O_2} to guide therapy is that it is a measure of all of the blood returning to the lungs and can give no information about the adequacy of perfusion of individual organ systems, such as the kidneys, brain, heart, or liver.

Noninvasive Monitoring

PULSE OXIMETRY The use of pulse oximetry for monitoring Sa_{O_2} and pulse amplitude in the fingers, nose, or toes can provide early warning of pulmonary or cardiovascular deterioration before it is clinically apparent. This technique employs a microprocessor that continuously measures pulse rate and oxyhemoglobin saturation. The photosensor is not heated and does not require calibration. Oxyhemoglobin is red and reduced hemoglobin is blue, and each has a different absorption of light at their given wavelengths. Because the ratio of transmittance at each of the two wavelengths (660 nm, red, and 940 nm, infrared) varies according to the percentage of oxyhemoglobin, pulse oximeters can be programmed to calculate and display the percentage of oxyhemoglobin saturation at each pulse.

There is a predictable correlation between noninvasive Sa_{O_2} monitoring and measured arterial oxygen saturation from arterial blood gas over a wide range of values. Pulse oximetry has only a minimal error, of 1 to 2 percent, above 60% saturation. However, a number of factors can limit the effectiveness and accuracy of pulse oximetry, including impaired local perfusion (e.g., in patients who are hypothermic or on vasopressors); ambient light, particularly flourescent (easily eliminated by placing a towel over the pulse oximeter); nail polish (particularly blue, which absorbs near 660 nm); abnormal hemoglobin; and very high P_{O_2}. Carboxyhemoglobin falsely raises oxyhemoglobin saturation readings because bedside pulse oximeters read carboxyhemoglobin as oxyhemoglobin, while methemoglobin lowers them (at high levels of methemoglobin the pulseoximeter will read 85% regardless of the actual blood oxygenation, as may be seen after the treatment of cyanide poisoning). Fetal hemoglobin has nearly the same absorption spectrum as hemoglobin A and thus has little effect on the readings.

It is important to remember that a pulse oximeter does not provide a good measure of the adequacy of ventilation of patients on supplemental oxygen. A quick calculation using the alveolar gas equation shows that a person on 50% oxygen would be able to increase the Pa_{CO_2} to greater than 230 mm Hg before that saturation would drop below 90 [$Pa_{O_2} = 0.5(713) - 230/0.8 = 356 - 287 = 69$].

CAPNOGRAPHY By providing a real-time estimate of Pa_{CO_2}, capnography is a useful and accurate means of assessing ventilation, respiratory gas exchange, and carbon dioxide production, and it can give some indication of cardiovascular status (primarily cardiac output). Although the measurement of end-tidal carbon dioxide partial pressure (PET_{CO_2}) usually underestimates Pa_{CO_2} by about 3 mmHg, it may be greater if the patient has a high dead space. However, the difference between PET_{CO_2} and Pa_{CO_2} is constant for a given patient, provided that the V_{DS}/V_T ratio and airway resistance are not changing.

Mainstream and side-stream infrared capnometers are commercially available. A mainstream capnometer connects directly to the endotracheal tube, thus providing real-time breath-by-breath analysis. The major disadvantages of this system are its size and bulk and the fact that it cannot be used in nonintubated patients. Side-stream capnometers aspirate gas at the sample site. The principal advantages of this system are that it reduces mechanical dead space and can be used in nonintubated patients; however, many mechanical factors related to gas sampling require much expert attention and time, and can affect the results.

Because carbon dioxide production is directly dependent on metabolic rate, there are a large number of conditions that can lower PET_{CO_2}. However, sudden decreases in PET_{CO_2} suggest mechanical problems in the airway, hypoventilation, or increased dead space. A gradual decrease in the PET_{CO_2} is usually due to changes in the lung itself. Increases in the PET_{CO_2} are generally due to hypermetabolic states or unrecognized inadequate ventilation. If a simultaneous Pa_{CO_2} value is available, one can estimate the $P(A - a)_{CO_2}$ (using PET_{CO_2} as a proxy for PA_{CO_2}). Normally, this is less than 3 mmHg, and if it suddenly increases, one should suspect a pulmonary embolus or drastic reduction in cardiac output.

The most frequent use of PET_{CO_2} is to evaluate the adequacy of ventilation. Inadvertent esophageal intubation, tracheal extubation, and endotracheal tube obstruction can be readily detected. These monitors can reduce the number of arterial blood gas determinations obtained and can be very useful in weaning patients from mechanical ventilatory support. They can also be useful in determining the adequacy of circulation during cardiopulmonary resuscitation.

Pulse oximetry and, to some extent, capnography have become standard monitors in most locations that provide for the acute care of unstable patients. While understanding that they have limitations, the clinician can use them for second-to-second indications of the adequacy of ventilation and oxygenation.

CLINICAL APPROACH TO THE VENTILATOR AND RESPIRATORY FAILURE

As mentioned earlier, it is best to think of blood gases as participating in two separate systems: oxygenation and ventilation. When interpreting blood gas values, the clinician can evaluate the oxygenation system with the Pa_{O_2} and the ventilation system with the Pa_{CO_2} and pH. The therapies can also be separated into oxygenation and ventilation.

Oxygenation

There are generally five causes of hypoxemia (low Pa_{O_2} in the blood). They include hypoventilation, low Fi_{O_2}, V/Q mismatch, shunt, and diffusion.

HYPOVENTILATION As seen from the alveolar air equation, hypoventilation causes hypoxemia by having a high carbon dioxide. This is usually corrected with increased V_A, which reduces the P_{CO_2}. If a patient is on supplemental oxygen, hypoventilation is rarely a cause of hypoxemia, since the F_{IO_2} would be significantly elevated.

LOW INSPIRED OXYGEN This causes hypoxemia in two clinical situations. The first is at altitudes where the atmospheric pressure is reduced and thus P_{IO_2} is reduced. The second, more common cause is inadvertent administration of hypoxic gases to a patient. This most commonly occurs when an E cylinder (green oxygen canister) becomes empty. A full E cylinder contains 2200 lb/in^2 of pressure and 660 L of oxygen. Since oxygen is stored as a gas, the amount of oxygen in an E cylinder is directly proportional to the pressure. Thus, a canister with 1100 lb/in^2 contains approximately 330 L of oxygen. If one knows how much oxygen, in liters, is contained in an E cylinder and the flow rate of oxygen, one can determine when the E cylinder will become empty. This calculation should be performed for all patients receiving supplemental oxygen from an E cylinder.

VENTILATION-PERFUSION MISMATCH V/Q mismatch is the most common cause of hypoxemia. Atelectasis, pneumonia, congestive heart failure, pulmonary embolus, and ARDS all cause V/Q mismatch. V/Q mismatch causes hypoxemia because areas of low V/Q ratios (low ventilation and high perfusion) act like a shunt. However, these disorders respond to supplemental oxygen.

SHUNT Shunt occurs when areas of the lung are perfused but not ventilated. Hypoxemia due to shunt does not respond to supplemental oxygen. Severe ARDS and cardiac anomalies, such as tetralogy of Fallot, are examples of shunt.

DIFFUSION As discussed previously, oxygen diffuses rapidly across the alveolus. This factor does not generally cause hypoxemia at rest. Rather, it usually causes hypoxemia during exercise.

Treatment

Treatment for hypoxemia is supplemental oxygen. There are three levels of therapy for hypoxemia: (1) supplemental oxygen via nasal canula or face mask; (2) noninvasive ventilation, such as a continuous positive airway pressure (CPAP) or bilevel positive pressure ventilation (BiPAP) mask, in which a patient is given positive-pressure ventilation via a face mask; and (3) mechanical ventilation via an endotrachial tube. Due to entrainment of air around a face mask, the maximum amount of supplemental oxygen that can be administered is 60% but varies with the tightness of the seal. If a patient is still hypoxemic, the clinician needs to administer one of the positive-pressure modes of ventilation. For invasive and noninvasive mechanical ventilation, it is helpful to think of oxygenation separately from ventilation. Specifically, F_{IO_2} and PEEP or CPAP should be used to control oxygenation. Both F_{IO_2} and PEEP or CPAP should be titrated upward until hypoxemia is resolved.

Ventilation

Ventilatory failure is often diagnosed by a P_{CO_2} that is greater than expected for a given bicarboninate level. However, the diagnosis can also be made clinically with a high sensitivity by evaluating the respiratory rate, (f), the use of accessory muscles, and the degree of distress. Ventilatory failure can be broken into two broad categories: (1) neuromuscular disorders, including stroke, Guillain-Barré syndrome, and drugs, such as narcotics, that alter the drive to breath; and (2) increased work of breathing, which can be due to asthma, chronic obstructive pulmonary disease, ARDS, and sepsis, which increase CO_2 production.

Ventilatory failure is usually treated with mechanical ventilation either invasively or noninvasively. Like oxygenation, ventilation can be thought of as a separate system and is controlled by f and V_T, the components of V_M (Table 22-10). When the P_{CO_2} is elevated, f and V_T can be changed to increase the V_M and reduce the P_{CO_2}.

TABLE 22-10 An Approach to the Ventilator Management of Hypoxic and Hypercarbic Patients*

	P_{aO_2}	P_{CO_2}
Ventilator variables	F_{IO_2}	V_T
	PEEP	f

*f, respiratory rate.

AutoPEEP When placing patients who may have obstructive airway disease on mechanical ventilation, it is important to evaluate for auto-PEEP. AutoPEEP, or dynamic hyperinflation, occurs when a patient receives a breath from the ventilator prior to fully exhaling the previous breath. Dynamic hyperinflation is usually caused by a limitation to airflow, such as asthma. Such limitation results in a buildup of intrathoracic pressure and has the same physiologic consequences as does PEEP: decreased right heart preload, increased right heart afterload, and decreased left heart afterload). Indeed, autoPEEP is an unfortunate cause of pulseless electrical activity in ventilated patients, and the physiologic characteristics are similar to those of a tension pneumothorax and result in decreased preload. While one may suspect a diagnosis of autoPEEP in a wheezing patient with increased airway pressures, autoPEEP can be directly measured from the ventilator by blocking the exhalation port (usually found under the ventilator) just prior to inhalation (end exhalation). The pressure that the manometer reads is the measure of autoPEEP. Like regular PEEP, autoPEEP of 5 mmHg or greater can decrease preload.

If autoPEEP is detected, the treatment is to change the ventilator settings to allow a longer time for exhalation or to have a smaller breath to exhale. This is best accomplished by decreasing f, decreasing V_T, and increasing the inspiratory-to-expiratory ratio. In patients with obstructive airway disease and elevated P_{CO_2}, one must be cautious about attempting to normalize the P_{CO_2}, since this may result in significant autoPEEP. Rather, an elevated P_{CO_2} may have to be accepted until the obstructive airway disease is reversed.

BIBLIOGRAPHY

Berne RM, Levy MN: *Physiology,* 2d ed. St. Louis, MO, Mosby, 1988, pp 605–620.

Bhavani-Shankar K, Kumar AY, Moseley HS, et al: Terminology and the current limitations of time capnography: A brief review. *J Clin Monitoring* 11:175, 1995.

Bhende MS: Colorimetric end-tidal carbon dioxide detector. *Pediat Emerg Care* 11:58, 1995.

Braman SS: The regulation of normal lung function. *Allergy Proc* 16:223, 1995.

Clanton TL, Diaz PT: Clinical assessment of the respiratory muscle. *Phys Ther* 75:983, 1995.

Conrad SA: Advances in the management of respiratory failure: Advanced strategies for mechanical ventilation in severe acute respiratory failure. *ASAIO J* 42:204, 1996.

Hess D, Maxwell C: Which is the best index of oxygenation: $P(A - a)O_2'$ P_{aO_2}/P_{AO_2} or P_{aO_2}/F_{IO_2}? *Respir Care* 30:961, 1985.

Hillberg RE, Johnson DC: Noninvasive ventilation. *N Engl J Med* 337: 1746, 1997.

Hlastala MP: Ventilation/perfusion: From the bench to the patient. *Cardiologia* 41:405, 1996.

Kram HB, Shoemaker WC: Transcutaneous, conjunctival, and organ P_{O_2} and P_{CO_2} monitoring in the adult, in Shoemaker WC, Ayres S, Grenvik A, et al (eds): *Textbook in Critical Care*. Philadelphia, Saunders, 1989, pp 283–291.

Make BJ, Hill NS, Goldberg AI, et al: Mechanical ventilation beyond the intensive care unit: Report of a consensus conference of the American College of Chest Physicians. *Chest* 113(suppl 5):289S, 1998.

Orebaugh SL: Initiation of mechanical ventilation in the emergency department. *Am J Emerg Med* 14:59, 1996.
Pinsky MR: The hemodynamic consequences of mechanical ventilation: An evolving story. *Intens Care Med* 23:493, 1997.
Plant JCD: Functional anatomy of the respiratory tract and lungs, in Wilson RF, Wilson JA (eds): *Pulmonary Function and Respiratory Failure in Critically Ill and Injured Patients.* Detroit, Wayne State University, 1974.
Samaja M: Blood gas transport at high altitude. *Respiration* 64:422, 1997.
Shapiro BA, Cane RD: Blood gas monitoring: Yesterday, today and tomorrow. *Crit Care Med* 17:966, 1989.
Shneerson JM: Techniques in mechanical ventilation: Principles and practice. *Thorax* 51:756, 1996.
Stock MC: Capnography for adults. *Crit Care Clin* 11:219, 1995.
Syabbalo N: Measurement and interpretation of arterial blood gases. *Br J Clin Pract* 51:173, 1997.
Tung A: Indications for mechanical ventilation. *Int Anesthesiol Clin* 35:1, 1997.
West JB: Ventilation perfusion relationships. *Am Rev Respir Dis* 116:919, 1977.
Wiklund L: Carbon dioxide formation and elimination in man: Recent theories and possible consequences. *Upsala J Med Sci* 101:35, 1996.

23 FLUID AND ELECTROLYTE PROBLEMS

Michael Londner
Christine M. Carr
Gabor D. Kelen

Fluid and electrolyte disturbances encompass a broad spectrum of acute and chronic disease. The body deals with abnormalities under a specific stratification. Its first concern is oxygenation and ventilation, the second is circulation, and then equilibrium of acid-base status. Although derangements in any of these are often interrelated, abnormalities in any of these often lead to fluid and electrolyte derangement that may correct once the underlying abnormality itself is addressed. There are some general principles to follow in the initial evaluation of patients with fluid and electrolyte disturbances:

1. Treat the patient, not the laboratory value, particularly if the abnormality was unexpected. An aberrant laboratory value may simply be spurious. Errors occur obtaining, labeling, performing, and reporting laboratory tests. The patient's history and physical examination should be reviewed to determine whether the abnormality is congruous with the patient's presentation. When results remain seemingly inexplicable, the test should be repeated.

2. Often the rate of change defines the severity of an ailment, not the absolute value. In the same light, the rate of correction should generally mirror the rate of derangement. The rapid correction of disorders that developed slowly may lead to worse iatrogenic outcome or possible overcorrection. The body often can help itself once the underlying disorder is corrected. Full deficit correction of electrolytes is rarely appropriate during the initial period. As a rule of thumb, approximately half the deficit is replaced during the initial period (8 to 12 h), and the situation is then further addressed.

3. When fluids and electrolytes are altered, they should be corrected in the following orderly fashion:

1. Volume
2. pH
3. Potassium, calcium, and magnesium
4. Sodium and chloride

Equilibrium of fluid, electrolytes, and pH depends on adequate tissue perfusion and often corrects spontaneously with resolution of the underperfused state.

4. Lastly, fluids, electrolytes, and pH status are all intertwined. Correction of any one facet must be undertaken with deference to the overall effect. For example, correction of the pH will have a significant effect on the serum potassium, ionized calcium, and ionized magnesium. Rapid replacement of volume may result in a dilutional non-anion-gap acidosis that, in turn, will decrease serum potassium.

FLUIDS

Compartments

A prerequisite to the anatomy of body fluids and the physiologic principles that maintain normal fluid and electrolyte balance is a firm understanding of the extent and composition of the various body fluid compartments. Homeostasis is the maintenance of the composition of the internal environment that is essential for health. This includes consideration of the distribution of water in the body, along with appropriate maintenance of pH and electrolyte balance.

Water is the major constituent of the body and accounts for between 50 and 70 percent of total body weight (Fig. 23-1). The proportion of total body water (TBW) varies with age, gender, and lean body mass. For example, fat contains very *little* water; therefore, the more lean body mass there is, the larger is the proportionate TBW. In the healthy average male, TBW approximates up to 60 percent of weight.[1] Since females have relatively more subcutaneous adipose tissue and less muscle, they have less water or about 50 percent TBW. Similarly, muscle mass decreases with age and sometimes is replaced by fat, leading to a lower percentage of TBW.

The water of the body is divided into two basic functional compartments. The intracellular fluid (ICF) compartment accounts for approximately two-thirds of TBW, and the extracellular fluid (ECF) compartment accounts for approximately one-third of TBW. Most cell membranes are freely permeable to water, and thus, at steady state, the osmolality (discussed below) of these two compartments is equal. A change in osmolality of one compartment results in the passive movement of water from the area of lower osmolality to the area of higher osmolality.

The electrolyte concentration of ICF varies greatly from tissue to tissue. Skeletal muscle accounts for a large proportion of the intracellular component, and thus it is customary to use its electrolyte concentration as representative of the total body intracellular electrolyte concentration. Electrolytes are further classified according to electronic charge, cations (positively charged ions) and anions (negatively charged ions). The principal cations in the intracellular compartment are K^+ and Mg^{2+}, whereas the principal anions are PO_4^- and proteins (Table 23-1).

The ECF is partitioned by vascular epithelium into an intravascular compartment and the interstitial (sometimes referred to as extravascular) compartment. The intravascular compartment contains circulating plasma and accounts for approximately 20 to 25 percent of extracellular water. The interstitial compartment bathes all cells and accounts for approximately 75 to 80 percent of extracellular water. The interstitial compartment is much more complicated in that it has a rapidly equilibrating functional component and several slowly equilibrating nonfunctioning components. The nonfunctioning components account only for a small percentage of extracellular water, which includes the connective tissue water and the ''transcellular'' water, made up of the cerebrospinal and joint fluids. A dynamic equilibrium exists between the intravascular and interstitial compartments. There is a constant movement of fluid back and forth across the capillary bed between the intravascular and interstitial spaces. This movement is determined by the permeability of the membrane, the net difference between the hydrostatic pressure gradient (which drives fluid out of the intravascular space), the oncotic pressure gradient (which holds fluid within the intravascular space), and tissue turgor pressure countering the hydrostatic pressure. At the arteriolar end, there is a net efflux. At the venule end, there is a net influx. This simple system known as the Starling hypothesis[2] is insufficient to account for the large volume of

As a function of	TBW	ICF	ECF	IF	IVF
Total Weight	60%	40%	20%	15%	5%
TBW		67%	33%	25%	8%
ECF compartment				75%	25%

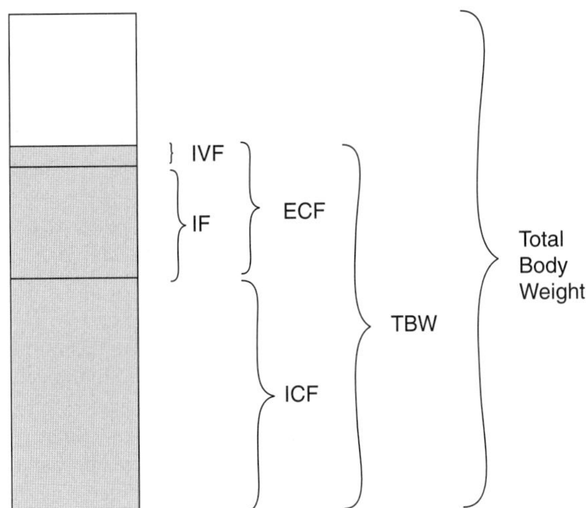

FIG. 23-1. Relationship of fluid compartment to body weight and each other. *Abbreviations:* IVF, intravascular fluid; IF, interstitial fluid, ECF, extracellular fluid; ICF, intracellular fluid; TBW, total body water.

fluid exchange that actually occurs and for the transport of nutrients and materials to and from tissues. It has been calculated that capillaries exchange water with interstitial fluid up to 300 times/min in the forearm capillary beds. NaCl, urea, and glucose exchange 40 to 120 times/min.[3] Vasomotion of the capillaries (rhythmic contraction and relaxation) determines rate of flow. During the dilator phase, hydrostatic pressure is high, and fluid filters out readily. During the constrictor phase, flow is diminished, and fluid readily enters the capillaries throughout their length. Vasomotion depends on vasomotor nerve outflow, hormones, and local concentrations of tissue metabolites.

One can readily appreciate how a malfunction or imbalance in this system can be buffered to some extent but will ultimately lead to edema (high hydrostatic pressures, loss of vasomotion, decreased oncotic pressure, and decreased tissue turgor).

TABLE 23-1 The Electrolyte Concentration of Body Fluids (meq/L)

Solution	Plasma Fluid	Interstitial Fluid	Intracellular Fluid
Cations			
Sodium	**142**	**144**	10
Potassium	4	4.5	**150**
Magnesium	2	1.0	**40**
Calcium	5	2.5	
Total	153	152	200
Anions			
Chloride	**104**	**113**	
Phosphates	2	2	**120**
Sulfates	1	1	30
Bicarbonate	**27**	**30**	10
Protein	13	1	**40**
Organic acids	6	5	
Total	153	152	200

Note: The major components of each compartment are in bold.

The proportionate relationship of the fluid compartment to body weight and TBW can be quite confusing, depending on whether the compartment is spoken in terms of body weight or TBW (see Fig. 23-1). For example, the ECF is 20 percent of total body weight but 33 percent of TBW.

Solutes

The other difficulty in understanding fluid and electrolytes is in the understanding of the various terms that are used and commonly misused to describe them. In considering the effects of various physiologically important substances and the interactions between them, the number of molecules, electrical charges, or particles of a substance per unit volume of a particular body fluid are more meaningful than simply the weight of a substance per unit volume. Therefore, concentrations are often expressed in moles, equivalents, or osmoles per liter. The use of grams per 100 mL expresses the weight of electrolytes per unit volume but does not enable a physiologic comparison of the solutes in solution.

The term *mole* describes the chemical basis for quantifying substances. It represents the molecular weight of a substance in grams (g) and is the standard unit of expressing the amount of a substance in the Systeme International d'Unites (SI) unit system. However, this quantification gives no direct information as to the number of osmotically active ions in a solution or to the electrical charges they carry. For example,

$$1 \text{ mol (mole) of NaCl} = 23 \text{ g (Na)} + 35.5 \text{ g (Cl)} = 58.5 \text{ g}$$

thus

$$1 \text{ mmol (millimole)} = 58.5 \text{ mg}$$

Equivalents represent the chemical combining activity of electrolytes. An equivalent (eq) of an ionized (charged) substance is 1 mol divided by its valence, whereas a milliequivalent (meq) is that figure expressed in milligrams (mg). In any given solution, the number of milliequivalents of cations is balanced precisely to the same number of milliequivalents of anions. This is referred to as electroneutrality. For example,

$$1 \text{ mol of NaCl dissociates to 1 eq of } Na^+ \text{ and 1 eq of } Cl^-$$

$$1 \text{ eq of } Na^+ = 23 \text{ g/L} = 23 \text{ g, but } 1 \text{ eq of } Ca^{2+} = 40 \text{ g}/2 = 20 \text{ g}$$

When considering the osmotic pressure of a solution, it is more descriptive to discuss this in terms of osmoles and milliosmoles. The osmolal concentration of a substance in a fluid is measured by the degree to which it depresses the freezing point, 1 mol/L of ideal solute depressing the freezing point 1.86°C. Osmoles refer to the actual number of osmotically active particles present in a solution. One osmole (osm) equals the molecular weight of the substance (in grams) divided by the number of freely moving particles each molecule liberates in solution. This is not dependent on the equivalents (electrochemical combining activity) each substance possesses.

Osmolarity is the number of osmoles per liter of solution, whereas osmolality is the number of osmoles per kilogram of solvent. Thus, the volume of the various solutes in the solution and the temperature affect osmolarity but not osmolality. The density of water is 1, so 1 L = 1 kg. Therefore, in water-based systems (such as the human body) where osmotically active substances are dissolved in plasma that is 91 to 93 percent H_2O, osmolal concentrations can be expressed as osmoles per liter (osm/L). This more closely approximates osmotic pressure, since osmolarity will be 7 to 9 percent lower than osmolality.

The serum osmolality can be measured directly by determining the freezing point of the serum, or it can be estimated by adding the measured $[Na^+]$, $[Cl^-]$, and bicarbonate to the glucose and blood urea nitrogen (BUN) divided by their respective molecular weights divided by 10 (to yield mg/dL):

$$\text{mosm/L} = 2 \times [Na^+] + \frac{\text{glu}}{18} + \frac{\text{BUN}}{2.8}$$

Since the sum of the measured $[Cl^-]$ and bicarbonate approximate the measured $[Na^+]$, twice the measured $[Na^+]$ is generally used in this calculation.

The normal serum osmolality ranges from 275 to 295 mosm/L. The urine and serum osmolality are much more accurate to use to diagnose the state of hydration than hematocrit, serum proteins, or BUN, since these are dependent on factors other than hydration. The presence of other osmotically active agents must be taken into account, since they influence serum osmolality. The presence of these osmotically active agents should be suspected when the measured osmolality differs from the calculated osmolality by greater than 10. This is termed an osmotic gap. If an *osmotic gap* is encountered, the following should be considered:

1. Laboratory analytic error
2. Decreased serum water content
   - Hyperlipidemia
   - Hyperproteinemia
3. Additional low-molecular-weight substances in the serum
   - Ethanol, methanol, isopropyl alcohol, ethylene glycol, acetone, ethyl ether, paraldehyde, lactate, or mannitol

The osmolal gap can be used to estimate the blood alcohol level (BAL), since osmolality increases 22 mg/dL for every 100 mg/dL of ethanol. Other substances can be similarly estimated (Table 23-2).

$$\text{BAL (estimated)} = \text{osmolal} \times (100/22)$$

The differences in ionic concentrations between the ICF and ECF are maintained by a semipermeable cell membrane. A semipermeable membrane is one that allows the free passage of solvent (H_2O) but not solute (crystalloid such as cations and anions, or colloids such as plasma proteins). At equilibrium, the concentration of molecules in the fluid of one compartment is equal to that in all the others. If free water is lost from one compartment, its concentration of molecules increases. This attracts water into that compartment until the concentration equalizes. The solutes (particles) that can not freely pass from one compartment to the next through the semipermeable membrane create the osmotic gradient (i.e., exert a force on water) and are termed

TABLE 23-2 Contribution to Osmolal Gap of Osmotic Substances

Substance	Factor
Ethanol	4.6
Methanol	3.2
Ethylene glycol	6.3
Isopropyl alcohol	5.9
Mannitol	18
Glycerol	9

Note: The osmolal gap is multiplied by the factor to arrive at an estimated level of mg/dL.

effective osmoles. These include the electrolytes and, in most tissues, glucose. Glucose readily enters red blood cells, hepatocytes, and osmoreceptors in the brain and thus exerts no force on water in relation to these cellular compartments. The solutes (particles) that distribute across the semipermeable membrane freely and therefore don't contribute to the osmotic gradient are termed "ineffective" osmoles.

Tonicity is used to describe the osmolality of a solution relative to plasma. Solutions with the same osmolality are said to be *isotonic,* those with comparatively higher osmolality are *hypertonic,* and those with lower osmolality are *hypotonic.* Tonicity is created by *effective* osmoles. Effective osmoles exert a force on water. The *ineffective* osmoles (urea, ethanol, methanol, or ethylene glycol) contribute to serum osmolality but not to tonicity. They do not exert a force on water across a semipermeable membrane as they freely diffuse.

Homeostasis

Fluid balance is exceedingly important to maintain homeostasis. To maintain balance, an average normal adult requires approximately 2000 to 3000 mL intake of water per day. This accounts for the volume of water lost in a day due to insensible and urinary losses. The insensible losses include the respiratory tract (500 to 700 mL/day), the skin (250 to 350 mL/day), and the feces (100 mL/day). This insensible loss can accelerate dramatically in the setting of fever (500 mL per 1°C fever), sweating (up to 1500 mL), and gastrointestinal losses.

The disorders of fluid balance may be classified into three categories: volume, concentration, and composition. Although all of these are interrelated, they are each separate entities.

1. Disturbances of volume occur when an isotonic solution is added or lost from a fluid compartment. Solute will not transfer from an adjacent compartment; only the volume of that compartment will change as long as the osmolality remains the same in the different compartments.
2. Disturbances of concentration occur when water alone is added or lost from a fluid compartment. The concentration of osmotically active particles will change, exerting an osmotic force into the compartment with the higher osmolality. This will continue until osmolality balances between the two compartments.
3. Disturbances of composition occur when the concentration of ions changes within a compartment without significantly altering the total number of osmotically active particles.

It is important to note that the volume lost is relative to the overall volume. A child who loses fluid is much more susceptible to its effects since this absolute quantity is a greater percentage of its overall volume. Signs of volume loss are related to not only volume but also to rate of loss. The faster the loss, the less time the body has to counterregulate and the greater the deleterious effects will be. They include weight loss, thirst, tachycardia, oliguria, and dry mucous membranes.

Flexibility in the body's ability to control water volume is provided by two mechanisms: antidiuretic hormone (ADH) and aldosterone. In the setting of volume depletion with increased serum osmolality and/or decreased plasma volume, the posterior pituitary is stimulated to release ADH and renin (from the kidney), stimulating the adrenal gland to release aldosterone. The ADH leads to retention of free water in the collecting ducts of the kidneys while aldosterone stimulates retention of Na^+ in the renal tubules, leading to further retention of water. In the setting of extra body water, there is a decrease in serum osmolality and/or an increase in plasma volume. This leads to a suppression of ADH secretion from the posterior pituitary and suppression of aldosterone release from the adrenal gland. The suppression of ADH leads to free water diuresis.

Overall, volume status is a much more potent stimulator of ADH than is osmolality. Therefore, change in volume alone will have a greater influence on ADH. For example, hypovolemia is a stronger stimulus for ADH secretion than hypo-osmolality is an inhibitor. Nausea and pain are considered to be of even greater potency for ADH stimulation.

CLINICAL ASSESSMENT OF VOLUME STATUS

Volume Loss

Volume loss can often be suspected from the history. Poor oral intake or history of vomiting, diarrhea, poorly controlled diabetes, renal disease, or adrenal disease are suggestive. With moderate volume loss, there may be postural hypotension and possibly a resting tachycardia. There may be narrowing of the pulse pressure. Jugular venous pressure will be difficult to appreciate clinically (assuming no right heart disease). Patients with moderate to severe volume loss may be weak and often have altered sensorium. They may be hypotensive even when recumbent. Mucous membranes will be dry, tissue turgor decreased, and eyes sunken (usually a finding in the pediatric population, along with sunken fontanelles). Oliguria is frequently in accompaniment. Volume loss may be sufficient to induce shock.

Laboratory findings include hemoconcentration (interpretable only if baseline values are known) and, usually, increased creatinine and urea nitrogen levels. In an acute setting, the ratio of urea nitrogen to creatinine will be 20:1 or even greater. Serum [Na^+], as explained, in and of itself, reveals nothing about volume status. If the volume loss is extrarenal, then urine [Na^+] will be less than 10 meq/L.

Treatment depends on the underlying disorder, but the cornerstone is volume repletion. Treatment is detailed elsewhere in this chapter and, for shock states, in the relevant chapters in this volume.

Volume Overload

Volume overload is most often encountered in disease states where excretion of free water is impaired. Most of these conditions are related to renal disease, diseases that impair blood flow to the kidneys (resulting in Na^+ retention), diseases that diminish intravascular osmolality (liver failure and low-protein states), or diseases that cause undesirable Na^+ retention by various mechanisms. Decreased intravascular osmolality results in a functional intravascular contraction, with expanded interstitial and cellular volume. These are discussed elsewhere in this chapter.

Volume overload clinically manifests as edema, whether peripheral or central (e.g., pulmonary). Early findings are weight gain, resting tachycardia, and peripheral edema. Jugular venous pressure is elevated. If severe, volume overload eventually results in severe right heart failure with resultant anasarca and ascites, and ultimately severe left heart failure, with pulmonary edema and pump failure manifesting as hypotension. Unfortunately, the contracted intervascular volume from hypotension causes the kidney to conserve Na^+, exacerbating the problem.

Specific treatments are discussed in this chapter and elsewhere in this volume.

ELECTROLYTES

Electrolyte abnormalities are often challenging to diagnose and treat. Overall, each disorder can be assessed with the same general approach. Increased concentration (hyper-) is a result of (1) excess total body amount, (2) shift among compartments, and (3) a relative fluid loss. Decreased concentrations (hypo-) are a result of (1) depleted total body amount, (2) shift among compartments, and (3) relative fluid gain.

SODIUM (Na^+)

The total body Na^+ content is between 40 and 50 meq/kg, which is approximately 2800 meq in a normal 70-kg man. It is found predominantly in the ECF space (98 percent) with a concentration of approximately 140 meq/L. One-third of this is fixed in bone while two-thirds is readily exchangeable. The intracellular concentration is usually less than 10 to 12 meq/L. Na^+, which is primarily responsible for the osmolality of the ECF space, moves passively into cells along its concentration gradient and then is actively "pumped" back out against its concentration gradient. When physiologic alterations cause intracellular-extracellular osmotic disequilibrium, movement of solute across the cell membrane is not the predominant corrective action but, rather, movement of water. The water travels to the fluid space with the higher osmolal concentration in an attempt to restore osmotic equilibrium.

Disorders of Na^+ often accompany disorders of water regulation where either *too little* or *too much* water is present in the body relative to solute. Therefore, hyponatremia and hypernatremia can occur with normal, low, or high total body Na^+ content, and with hypovolemic, euvolemic, and increased TBW states. This point cannot be overemphasized. The serum [NA^+] reveals nothing by itself of the patient's volume status. Determination of the serum [Na^+] is generally indicative of body fluid tonicity. The regulation of Na^+ and regulation of water are closely coupled. Together they are regulated by two controls: by ADH (vasopressin) and by the renin-angiotensin-aldosterone system. ADH release is stimulated by increases in serum osmolality, but a much more potent response is to volume depletion. ADH stimulation increases renal water absorption and decreases urine output by increasing tubular water permeability and by increasing water reabsorption in the collecting ducts of the kidney. Renin is synthesized by the kidney in response to decreased intravascular volume or pressure and stimulates the production of aldosterone in the adrenal gland. Aldosterone acts on the distal tubules to increase Na^+ reabsorption, and water passively follows.

Aberrant levels of Na^+ should be diagnosed on clinical grounds through history and physical examination findings and confirmed with laboratory evaluation. Clinical signs of increase or decrease tend to occur early and are greater in severity if the rate of Na^+ change in the extracellular space is rapid. Diagnosis should be suspected and confirmed early in patient management and corrected within the appropriate time frame to prevent the dangerous sequelae associated with these abnormalities.

Hyponatremia

Hyponatremia is strictly defined as a measured serum [Na^+] less than 135 meq/L. This can result from primary water gain and/or greater Na^+ loss (than water), alteration in the distribution of body water, or aberrant laboratory measurement. The development of symptoms is more related to the rate of change of the serum [Na^+] than the absolute value. Values less than 120 meq/L are more likely to lead to symptoms, even when slowly developing. Common presenting symptoms include, but are not limited to, confusion, lethargy, nausea, vomiting, anorexia, muscle cramps, and hypothermia, and culminate ultimately in seizures and coma. Seizures are quite likely at [Na^+] of 113 meq/L or less.

PATHOPHYSIOLOGY The pathophysiologic changes of hyponatremia are most obvious when serum [Na^+] levels fall below 120 meq/L in less than 12 to 24 h. The central nervous system (CNS) effects are usually the most obvious, but cardiovascular and musculoskeletal dysfunction may also occur.

Central Nervous System As serum [Na^+] fall, the osmotic gradient that develops across the blood-brain barrier causes water to move into the brain, causing apathy, agitation, headache, altered consciousness, seizures, and even coma. The severity of symptoms is dependent not only on the rapidity but also the magnitude of the fall in the serum [Na^+]. Acute hyponatremia occurring in 24 h or less and resulting in a serum [Na^+] of less than 120 meq/L, or a rate of fall of 0.5 meq/L or more per hour, can cause muscular twitching, seizures, and coma. The mortality rate with acute severe hyponatremia with CNS changes has been reported to be as high as 50 percent in adults. In animals in which serum [Na^+] is reduced to 110 mmol/L in 2 h, the mortality rate is 88 percent, and there is gross evidence of brain edema. When plasma Na^+ is lowered slowly during several days or weeks by a combination of Na^+ depletion and water ingestion, patients are usually less symptomatic, but even patients with chronic hyponatremia may experience focal weakness, hemiparesis, ataxia, and a positive Babinski sign.

As hyponatremia develops, the osmotic equilibrium between brain and plasma allows movement of increased amounts of water into the brain. However, brain swelling is less than would be predicted on the basis of the osmotic shifts alone. The brain's adaptation to hyponatremia is accomplished by two mechanisms: (1) movement of interstitial fluid into the cerebrospinal fluid and (2) loss of cellular potassium and organic osmolytes. With acute hyponatremia, water moves into the brain from the plasma, causing an increase in the hydrostatic pressure of the cerebral interstitial fluid. The increased interstitial pressure accelerates the clearance of interstitial fluid into the cerebrospinal fluid, which is returned to the systemic circulation via the arachnoid villi. The movement of Na^+-rich interstitial fluid out of the brain reduces brain Na^+, which in turn reduces the osmotic gradient for water moving into the brain.

The loss of sodium, potassium, and chloride from the brain provides most of the protection against cerebral edema in the first hours of hyponatremia; however, when hyponatremia is sustained, the brain slowly loses other intracellular osmolytes, mainly amino acids. Losses of organic osmolytes during prolonged or severe hyponatremia are especially important in defending the brain against swelling.

The adaptive changes that protect the brain from excessive swelling also render it susceptible to dehydration during correction of the fluid and electrolyte problem. Indeed, there is often more risk of brain damage during treatment than from the hyponatremia itself. The rate of rise of brain intracellular potassium and organic osmolytes during correction of the hyponatremia is much slower than the rate of loss of these substances during the development of the problem. If correction of hyponatremia occurs more rapidly than the brain can recover solute, the higher plasma osmolality may dehydrate and injure the brain, producing what is now called the *osmotic demyelination syndrome,* or *central pontine myelinolysis* (CPM). (See section on ''Complications of Therapy.'')

Cardiovascular System The cardiovascular response to hyponatremia depends primarily on the effective arterial blood volume, which may be increased, decreased, or normal depending on the underlying disorder. Intravascular volume is determined in part by the distribution of water between the ICF and ECF compartments. Thus, in volume-depleted patients, hyponatremia can cause a further decrease in the intravascular volume by allowing movement of water out of the ECF compartment into the ICF space. Accordingly, shock occurs at lesser degrees of TBW depletion in hyponatremia than similar fluid deficits when the plasma is hypertonic or isotonic.

ADH is one of the main factors opposing the hypovolemic effect of fluid shifts induced by hyponatremia. The ADH is released primarily as a response to the decreased effective arterial blood volume that often accompanies hyponatremic edematous disorders. Nonosmotic stimulation of ADH release overrides the hypo-osmotic suppressive effect of hyponatremia, and increased ADH is present in almost all hyponatremic conditions. The function of ADH in this setting initially may seem paradoxical, because it potentiates the hyponatremic state by increasing water reabsorption by the renal tubules. ADH is also a potent vasoconstrictor, however, and even at the low ADH concentrations that are characteristic of clinical hyponatremia, it increases peripheral vascular resistance, thereby increasing blood flow to the liver and kidneys at the expense of the skin and muscle.

Musculoskeletal System Most patients with hyponatremia have normal muscle tone and function. However, muscle cramps and weakness can occur during strenuous exercise, especially if excess sweating is replaced with water. These symptoms usually resolve rapidly when the serum [Na^+] is corrected back toward normal.

Renal System The usual renal response to hyponatremia is production of dilute urine; however, this process is abrogated to some extent by the presence of increased concentrations of ADH. The amount of ADH present depends on the primary disease process and the effective arterial blood volume.

A urine [Na^+] less than 10 meq/L usually indicates that the renal handling of Na^+ is intact and that the effective arterial blood volume is contracted. In contrast, a urine [Na^+] greater than 20 meq/L often indicates intrinsic renal tubular damage or a natriuretic response to hypervolemia. The urine [Na^+] will also vary somewhat according to the ongoing gains and losses of salt and water. Urine [Na^+] will tend to increase if the underlying disease significantly impairs renal function.

DIAGNOSIS The diagnosis and ultimate etiology of hyponatremia are determined via a staged algorithm (Fig. 23-2). Since Na^+ and its attendant anions are the primary determinants of ECF osmolality,

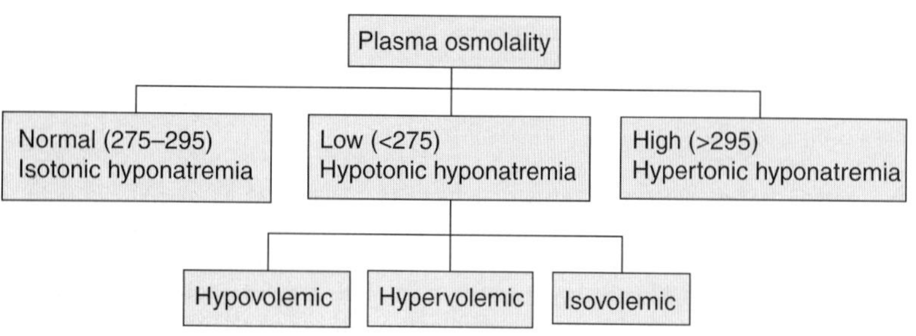

FIG. 23-2. Algorithm for diagnosis of hyponatremia.

TABLE 23-3 Etiology of Hyponatremia

I. Hypertonic hyponatremia ($P_{osm} > 295$)
   Hyperglycemia
   Mannitol excess
   Glycerol therapy

II. Isotonic (pseudo)hyponatremia (P_{osm} 275–295)
   Hyperlipidemia
   Hyperproteinemia (e.g., multiple myeloma, Waldenstrom macroglobulinemia)

III. Hypotonic hyponatremia ($P_{osm} < 275$)
   a. Hypovolemic (usually associated with volume replacement with hypotonic fluids)
      i. Renal
         Diuretic use
         Salt-wasting nephropathy (renal tubular acidosis, chronic renal failure, interstitial nephritis)
         Osmotic diuresis (glucose, urea, mannitol, hyperproteinemia)
         Mineralocorticoid (aldosterone) deficiency
      ii. Extrarenal
         Volume replacement with hypotonic fluids
         Gastrointestinal loss (vomiting, diarrhea, fistula, tube suction)
         Third-space loss (e.g., burns, hemorrhagic pancreatitis, peritonitis)
         Sweating (e.g., cystic fibrosis)
   b. Hypervolemic
      i. Urinary [Na^+] >20 meq/L
         Renal failure (inability to excrete free water)
      ii. Urinary [Na^+] <20 meq/L
         Congestive heart failure (perceived as low-flow state by kidneys, stimulates ADH)
         Nephrotic syndrome (low serum protein secondary to urinary loss)
         Cirrhosis (low intravascular oncotic pressure secondary to decreased protein production)
   c. Euvolemic (urine [Na^+] usually >20 meq/L)
      i. SIADH (see Table 23-4)
      ii. Hypothyroidism (possible increased ADH or decreased GFR)
      iii. Pain, stress, nausea, psychosis (stimulates ADH)
      iv. Drugs: ADH, nicotine, sulfonylureas, morphine, barbiturates, NSAIDs, acetaminophen, carbamazepine, phenothiazines, TCAs, colchicine, clofibrate, cyclophosphamide, isoproterenol, tolbutamide, vincristine, MAOI
      v. Water intoxication (psychogenic polydipsia, lesion in thirst center)
      vi. Glucocorticoid deficiency (glucocorticoids required to suppress ADH)
      vii. Positive-pressure ventilation
      viii. Porphyria
      ix. Essential (reset osmostat or sick cell syndrome—usually in the elderly)

Abbreviations: ADH, antidiuretic hormone; GFR, glomerular filtration rate; MAOI, monoamine oxidase inhibitor; NSAIDs, nonsteroidal anti-inflammatory drugs; TCAs, tricyclic antidepressants.

hyponatremia is usually accompanied by hypo-osmolality. However, hyponatremia may be associated with a normal or even elevated plasma osmolality. Therefore, the first step in the evaluation of a patient with a low measured [Na^+] should include a clinical evaluation of ECF volume status and both measured and calculated plasma osmolality. This provides a means for the first tier in categorizing hyponatremic disorders. In *true* hyponatremia, the plasma osmolality is reduced, whereas in *factitious* hyponatremic states, the plasma osmolality is either normal or increased.

HYPERTONIC HYPONATREMIA ($P_{osm} > 295$) Hyponatremia with an increase in osmotically active solutes occurs when there is an accumulation of large quantities of solutes restricted primarily to the ECF space. In this setting, there is a net movement of water from the ICF to the ECF, thereby effectively diluting the ECF [Na^+]. The most common cause of this is hyperglycemia. Each 100-mg/dL increase in plasma glucose decreases the serum [Na^+] by 1.6 to 1.8 meq/L. The differential diagnosis of hypertonic hyponatremia is shown in Table 23-3. Treatment of hyponatremia in this class includes reduction of the ECF hypertonicity by correction of the underlying disorder with close observation. Unless detected during the very acute phase, or in the face of renal failure, an osmotic diuresis is likely, resulting in total body Na^+ deficit. Volume depletion is often associated, and, thus, volume repletion with Na^+-containing fluids is required.

ISOTONIC HYPONATREMIA (P_{osm} 275–295) Hyponatremia associated with normal plasma osmolality is often termed *pseudohyponatremia.* High levels of plasma proteins and lipids increase the nonaqueous, non-Na^+-containing fraction of plasma. This represents an artifact in serum [Na^+] measurement. Na^+ usually is distributed within 910 and 930 mL in each liter of plasma. Since traditional methods of Na^+ measurement employ a ''mass per volume'' of serum method (such as flame emission spectrophotometry, or FES), the laboratory analysis reports a factitious lower value of [Na^+] than the serum truly contains. The true [Na^+] and osmolality of plasma water are normal. The differential diagnosis of isotonic hyponatremia is shown in Table 23-3. Treatment of hyponatremia itself in this class is not required.

HYPOTONIC HYPONATREMIA ($P_{osm} < 275$) This category of hyponatremia results in intracellular volume expansion with consequent derangement of cellular functions. This category can be further subdivided into classifications based on functional ECF volume (Fig. 23-2) and urinary [Na^+] (accounting for possible recent use of diuretics). The assessment of ECF should focus on predisposing factors once volume status is ascertained. In addition to the electrolytes and plasma osmolality already obtained, urine electrolytes and osmolality should be added. This will help facilitate classification into hypovolemic, hypervolemic, and euvolemic categories.

TABLE 23-4 Etiology of Syndrome of Inappropriate Antidiuretic Hormone (SIADH)

Central Nervous System Disease	Pulmonary Disease	Carcinoma
Tumor	Tumor	Lung
Trauma	Pneumonia	Pancreas
Infection	Chronic obstructive pulmonary disease	Thymoma
Cerebral vascular accident, subarachnoid hemorrhage	Lung abscess	Ovarian
Guillain-Barré syndrome	Tuberculosis	Lymphoma
Delerium tremens	Cystic fibrosis	
Multiple sclerosis		

Hypovolemic hyponatremia is associated with a loss of both Na^+ and water, often with disproportionate water replacement through oral intake or the administration of hypotonic fluids. Losses of Na^+ may be either renal or extrarenal.

Patients with extrarenal losses of Na^+ and water will demonstrate a urinary $[Na^+]$ of less than 20 meq/L. The unequal balance of electrolyte and water loss produces a contracted ECF and hyponatremia. This is maintained by the physiologic effect of volume depletion on the kidneys inhibiting the excretion of free water. The impairment of water excretion to defend ECF volume at the expense of tonicity is accomplished by four mechanisms:

1. Decreased glomerular filtration
2. Increased proximal tubular reabsorption of solute and water
3. Decreased delivery of fluid to the diluting segment of the nephron
4. ADH released by nonosmotic stimuli

The differential diagnosis of hypovolemic hyponatremia from extrarenal losses is shown in Table 23-3.

The decreased ECF volume may also be due to renal losses (see Table 23-3). In this setting, the urinary $[Na^+]$ will be greater than 20 meq/L. The clinical manifestations are usually due to the volume deficit rather than the hyponatremia itself. Treatment of hypovolemic hyponatremia includes reexpansion of the ECF volume with isotonic saline and appropriate correction of any underlying disorder.

Euvolemic hyponatremia is described as having a combination of normal volume status and hyponatremia. Although these patients may have a slightly increased ECF volume, they are not clinically edematous and have near-normal total body Na^+ content despite the presence of hyponatremia. When symptoms are present, they usually relate to CNS hypotonicity. Urinary $[Na^+]$ is usually greater than 20 meq/L and may be much higher in instances of ADH excess. The most notable cause of euvolemic hyponatremia is the syndrome of inappropriate ADH (SIADH) secretion. This is characterized by six criteria:

1. Hypotonic hyponatremia
2. Inappropriately elevated urinary osmolality (usually greater than 200 mosm/kg)
3. Elevated urinary $[Na^+]$ (typically greater than 20 meq/L)
4. Clinical euvolemia
5. Normal adrenal, renal, cardiac, hepatic, and thyroid function
6. Correctable with water restriction

The diagnosis of SIADH is primarily made by exclusion (Table 23-4). The other causes of euvolemic hyponatremia are listed in Table 23-3. Some of these may stimulate ADH secretion. Treatment for patients with euvolemic hyponatremia requires fluid restriction and appropriate workup and management of the underlying disorder. Admission is usually warranted.

Hypervolemic hyponatremia is described as TBW in great excess. These patients present with manifestations of volume overload, such as peripheral and/or pulmonary edema. They usually have impaired ability to excrete a water load. This allows for water retention in excess of Na^+ retention. These patients can be further categorized into two groups (Table 23-3): The first of these is generalized edematous states without advanced renal insufficiency. These patients have urinary $[Na^+]$ of less than 20 meq/L. They include patients with cirrhosis and/or ascites, congestive heart failure, and nephrotic syndrome. The second category is advanced acute or chronic renal insufficiency. These patients have urinary $[Na^+]$ in excess of 20 meq/L.

Management of patients with hypervolemic hyponatremia includes optimizing treatment for the underlying disorder coupled with judicious salt and water restriction. Often diuretics are required to aid in management. Dialysis may be necessary.

EMERGENCY TREATMENT OF SEVERE HYPONATREMIA While specific or general treatment of hyponatremia for the condition discussed may be initiated in the ED, there is little urgency to address the hyponatremia itself immediately when $[Na^+]$ is above 120 meq/L. In cases where hyponatremia is severe (less than 120 meq/L), develops rapidly (a greater than 0.5-meq/L decrease in serum $[Na^+]$ per hour), or is associated with a patient in extremis (i.e., coma or seizures), administration of 3% saline solution (513 meq/L) is usually indicated. This can be administered at 25 to 100 mL/h, with careful observation for fluid overload and the rise in serum $[Na^+]$. The rise in $[Na^+]$ should be no greater than 0.5 to 1.0 meq/L per hour. In the face of seizures, this can be increased to 1 to 2 meq/L per hour. It is sometimes necessary to administer concomitant furosemide to reduce the amount of water present in the body, allowing more rapid correction of plasma $[Na^+]$.[4]

CALCULATION OF SODIUM DEFICIT In hypovolemic patients, the Na^+ deficit should be calculated and replaced with normal saline solution. The formula is

$$(\text{desired plasma } [Na^+] - \text{actual plasma } [Na^+]) * (\text{TBW}) = \text{total body } Na^+ \text{ deficit (in meq/L)}$$

COMPLICATIONS OF THERAPY Complications with the treatment of acute hyponatremia, especially when there is no underlying CNS, hepatic, or renal disorder, are uncommon and occur in fewer than 2 percent of patients. In chronic hyponatremia, brain edema is usually not severe, and little evidence exists that chronic hyponatremia itself causes brain damage. Nevertheless, these patients appear to be at greater risk for brain injury (CPM) during the correction process. The injury reportedly occurs after the hyponatremia has been corrected and progresses in a predictable manner. These neurologic changes are believed to be due to correction of the serum $[Na^+]$ at a rate faster than the brain can adapt to the higher osmolality. In patients with chronic hyponatremia, other factors contributing to the CPM may include alcoholism, malnutrition, toxins, and metabolic imbalance.

Brain histology in fatal cases shows myelinolysis and demyelination of central pontine and extrapontine myelin-bearing neurons. In typical cases, the neurologic findings include fluctuating levels of consciousness, behavioral disturbances, dysarthria, dysphagia, or convulsions progressing to pseudobulbar palsy and quadriparesis. Improvement may occur after several weeks of severe debilitation, but some patients are permanently impaired.

In patients with chronic severe hyponatremia, the threshold for the production of CPM is a rate of correction of Na^+ levels faster than 0.5 meq/L per hour (12 meq/L per day). In patients with acute severe hyponatremia, correction at rates exceeding 0.5 to 1.0 meq/L per hour, with or without diuretics, does not usually cause any problems. Severe neurologic complications have occurred almost exclusively in clinically hypernatremic patients treated with hypertonic or isotonic saline without the addition of furosemide or an osmotic diuretic. Similar patients treated with the same fluids but with furosemide almost uniformly have done well. Patients with chronic hyponatremia corrected at a rate less than 0.5 meq/L per hour have also done well.

Hypernatremia

Hypernatremia is strictly defined as serum [Na^+] greater than 150 meq/L. The most frequent cause of hypernatremia is a decrease in TBW secondary to either reduced intake or excessive loss. The main defense against hypernatremia is likely thirst. A 2 percent increase in plasma osmolality should stimulate thirst and thereby increase free water intake. The problem arises when patients, such as those in a coma or those who are bedridden, are unable to obtain adequate fluid. All hypernatremic states are hyperosmolar (Table 23-5).

Clinical manifestations are much more severe with acute rapidly developing hypernatremia than with chronic hypernatremia. In the elderly and in infants (two groups at great risk), the morbidity and mortality rates are high when [Na^+] is greater than 160 meq/L. Symptoms usually occur when plasma osmolality exceeds 350 mosm/kg of water. Neurologic dysfunction predominates (Table 23-6).

Virtually all hypernatremia encountered in the ED is related to volume loss, usually severe. There are two potential mechanisms seemingly opposed but having the same result. The first is the ADH response

TABLE 23-5 Etiologic Classification of Hypernatremia

I. Pure water loss
  A. Inability to obtain or swallow water; examples include
    Infancy, coma, dementia, bed confined
  B. Impaired thirst drive; examples include
    Hypothalamic lesion
  C. Increased insensible loss

II. Excessive sodium
  A. Iatrogenic sodium administration
    1. Sodium bicarbonate
      Cardiac arrest, treatment of lactic acidosis
    2. Hypertonic saline
  B. Accidental/deliberate ingestion of large quantities of sodium
    Substitution of salt for sugar in infant formula or tube feedings
  C. Seawater ingestion or drowning
  D. Mineralocorticoid or glucocorticoid excess
    1. Primary aldosteronism
    2. Cushing's syndrome
    3. Ectopic adrenocorticotropic hormone production

III. Loss of water in excess of sodium (without simultaneous water intake)
  A. Gastrointestinal
    Vomiting, diarrhea, intestinal fistula
  B. Renal loss
    1. Central diabetes insipidus
      a. Head trauma
      b. Granulomatous disease
        Sarcoidosis, tuberculosis, Wegener granulomatosis, syphilis, hystiocytosis
      a. Posthypophysectomy
      b. Tumor
      c. Central nervous system infection
      d. Congenital
      e. Vascular lesion
        CVA, aneurysm, sickle cell disease, Sheehan syndrome
    2. Impaired renal concentrating ability
      a. Osmotic diuresis
        Diabetic ketoacidosis, chronic renal failure (i.e., polycystic or medullary cystic disease), partial urinary tract obstruction, postobstruction diuresis, diuretic phase of acute renal failure, mannitol, tube feedings/infant formula (especially cow's milk), excessive diuretic use, hypokalemia
      b. Hypercalcemia
      c. Decreased protein intake
      d. Prolonged, excessive water intake
      e. Sickle cell disease
      f. Multiple myeloma
      g. Amyloidosis
      h. Sarcoidosis
      i. Sjögren syndrome
      j. Nephrogenic diabetes insipidus
      k. Congenital
  C. Drugs, including
    Alcohol, lithium, phenytoin, propoxyphene, sulfonylurea hypoglycemic agents, amphotericin B, colchicine
  D. Skin loss
    Burns, sweating
  E. Peritoneal dialysis

IV. Essential hypernatremia

TABLE 23-6 Clinical Manifestations of Hypernatremic States Related to Serum Osmolality

Manifestations	Osmolality, mosm/kg
Restlessness, irritability	350–375
Tremulousness, ataxia	375–400
Hyperreflexia, twitching, spasticity	400–430
Seizures and death	>430

to low volume and hypertonicity. The renal response to ADH, conservation of free water, results in low urine output (less than 20 mL/h) that has a high osmolality (usually greater than 1000 mosm/kg H_2O). The second mechanism is failure of ADH response, either central or peripheral (vide infra). In essence, the patient cannot excrete Na^+ properly. Urine osmolality is low (200 to 300 mosm/kg with urinary $[Na^+]$ of 60 to 100 meq/kg).

Finally, one mechanism of hypernatremia may result in hypervolemia. This is excessive intake of Na^+. Usually, the kidney is able to regulate Na^+ at a very constant level. However, if the kidneys are impaired, then serum $[Na^+]$ will increase and a dangerous ECF volume expansion will occur. Note that even large volumes of normal saline administration by itself cannot result in hypernatremia, because the $[Na^+]$ is only 154 meq. However, administration of concentrated Na^+ solutions (e.g., hypertonic saline, addition of $NaHCO_3$ to normal solution) can result in euvolemic or hypervolemic hypernatremia.

DIABETES INSIPIDUS A particularly interesting cause of hypernatremia is diabetes insipidus (DI), which results in excessive loss of hypotonic urine. Diabetes insipidus may be central in origin (due to a failure of secretion of ADH) or nephrogenic (due to renal unresponsiveness to ADH). About 30 percent of central DI is idiopathic and about 70 percent is secondary to neoplasms (25 percent), pituitary surgery (20 percent), or trauma (15 percent). Most of the remaining 10 percent is due to various granulomas (tuberculosis, sarcoidosis, or eosinophilic granuloma) or local vascular problems (aneurysms, thrombosis, or Sheehan syndrome). Nephrogenic DI may be primary (familial) or secondary to a wide variety of causes, including hypercalcemia, hypokalemia, renal disorders, various drugs (including lithium, demeclocycline, amphotericin B, aminoglycosides, and cisplatin), hematologic disorders (sickle cell disease and myeloma), malnutrition, or amyloidosis.

Traumatic DI is typically triphasic. After an initial polyuria from insufficient ADH secretion by hypothalamic cells, there is a transient second phase lasting 1 to 7 days characterized by release of previously formed hormone from the posterior pituitary and resolution of the polyuria. In the third phase, central DI returns after the released hormone has been utilized. Regeneration of cells that secrete ADH may occur weeks to months after injury. The ADH-secreting cells have their cell bodies in the hypothalamus, and these are not usually completely destroyed by trauma.

Differentiation between central and nephrogenic DI is best achieved by noting (1) the response of serum and urine osmolarity to water deprivation (trying to reach a serum osmolarity greater than 295 mosm/L) and (2) the response to 5 units of subcutaneous aqueous vasopressin. Patients with central DI show little or no response to dehydration but respond well to vasopressin (urine osmolarity of 800 mosm/L or greater). Nephrogenic DI shows little or no response to dehydration or vasopressin.

PATHOPHYSIOLOGY Because Na^+ does not freely penetrate tissue cell membranes, ECF and plasma volume tend to be maintained in hypernatremic dehydration until the water loss is greater than 10 percent of body weight. Although there may be rather profound dehydration in some patients with severe hypernatremia, shock is an infrequent occurrence. When the dehydration results in loss of 10 percent of body weight, skin turgor becomes reduced and the skin of the abdomen has a characteristic ''doughy'' feel when it is pinched between the fingers.

Acute symptomatology is seen in many patients once serum $[Na^+]$ exceeds 158 meq/L. Patients tend to become irritable, and infants may also have a high-pitched cry or wail alternating with periods of severe lethargy. As dehydration and hypernatremia become more severe, one may see increased muscle tone or even coma with eventual seizures. Fever can be both a contributing cause and a result of hypernatremic dehydration.

Restlessness and irritability occur when serum osmolality increases to between 350 and 375 mosm/kg, while ataxia and tremulousness tend to occur when osmolality is between 375 and 400 mosm/kg. When serum osmolality rises above 400 mosm/kg, asynchronous jerks and tonic spasms are apt to occur. Death usually occurs at an osmolality above 430 mosm/kg.

Permanent sequelae are not uncommon in children when serum $[Na^+]$ exceeds 160 to 165 meq/L. Up to 16 percent of children with hypernatremia develop chronic neurologic deficits as a consequence. The overall mortality rate of hypernatremia is above 10 percent. If the plasma osmolality exceeds 350 mosm/kg, the incidence of severe morbidity or mortality may exceed 25 to 50 percent.

Hypocalcemia, which is frequently seen in patients with hypernatremia, may contribute to the CNS symptomatology. However, the mechanism of the hypocalcemia is unclear.

Massive brain hemorrhage or multiple small hemorrhages and thromboses may occur when hypernatremia causes enough cellular dehydration and resultant brain shrinkage to cause tearing of cerebral blood vessels. This has been observed most frequently in neonates following acute administration of a large Na^+ load. As a consequence, the amount of sodium bicarbonate administered to acidotic infants must be limited.

If the hypernatremia persists for more than a few days, the brain dehydration may resolve, and brain water content may return to normal or near-normal levels due to accumulation in the brain cells of amino acids known as *idiogenic osmoles,* particularly taurine. The formation of these idiogenic osmoles increases intracellular osmolality, attracts water back into the brain cells, and restores their cellular volume. If the hypertonicity develops gradually, this protective mechanism tends to prevent severe brain cell shrinkage.

TREATMENT The cornerstone of treatment is volume replacement. There are many opinions regarding appropriate initial fluid and subsequent therapy. Where volume is the issue, we believe volume should be replaced first with either normal saline or Ringer's lactate. Either of these will have, by definition, a lower $[Na^+]$ than the patient's serum. Plasma-expanding fluids should continue until tissue perfusion is restored. Once perfusion has been established, the solution should be converted to 0.45% saline or other isotonic solution. This should continue until the urine output is at least 0.5 mL/kg per hour. The reduction in $[Na^+]$ should not exceed 10 to 15 meq/L per day. A calculation to estimate free water deficit is

$$\text{water deficit (in liters)} = \text{TBW} * (1 - \text{actual } [Na^+]/\text{desired } [Na^+])$$

As a general rule, each liter of water deficit results in a rise of serum $[Na^+]$ of 3 to 5 meq/L.

Rapid correction of hypernatremia, especially if it is chronic, can cause seizures and severe neurologic sequelae. Unless the hypernatremia is of short duration, idiogenic osmoles are presumably present in brain cells. Consequently, too rapid rehydration and lowering of serum $[Na^+]$ can cause brain cells to swell, resulting in cerebral edema and an increased likelihood of seizures, permanent neurologic sequelae, or even death. Serum electrolyte levels should be monitored frequently to ensure that the appropriate rate of decline of serum [Na^+] occurs.

In the case of acute hypernatremia, serum [Na^+] levels can be corrected rather rapidly with little fear of cerebral edema because idiogenic osmoles will not yet be present in brain cells. However, rapid fluid administration in patients with hypernatremia due to excessive Na^+ administration may result in hypervolemia and pulmonary edema.

In children with acute severe Na^+ excess and a serum [Na^+] of more than 180 to 200 meq/L, peritoneal dialysis using a high-glucose (7.5%), low-Na^+ dialysate may be lifesaving, but must be done with frequent monitoring of serum electrolyte levels.

In the case of central DI, administration of either vasopressin or 1-deamino-8-D-arginine vasopressin (dDAVP) must be undertaken carefully, and fluid intake should be regulated so that the serum [Na^+] does not drop too rapidly.

POTASSIUM (K^+)

Elemental K^+ is the major intracellular cation of the body. The normal intracellular concentration is 100 to 150 meq/L, while the normal extracellular concentration is 3.5 to 5.0 meq/L. The total body K^+ store ranges from 35 to 55 meq/kg or 3500 meq in a healthy 70-kg man. Approximately 70 to 75 percent of total body K^+ is found in muscle tissue; therefore, in patients with severe muscle wasting, total body stores may be as low as 20 to 30 meq/kg. Daily intake of K^+ ranges from 50 to 150 meq. Foods high in K^+ include oranges, grapefruit, tomatoes, bananas, avocados, and raisins. K^+ is excreted predominantly by the kidneys (90 percent) and with some loss in the stool and by sweating. K^+ is filtered freely through the glomerulus and then reabsorbed in the proximal and ascending tubules. It is secreted in the distal tubule in exchange for Na^+. In healthy individuals, the kidneys are able to excrete up to 6 meq/kg per day. Even in severe K^+ deficit, 5 to 15 meq/L may be excreted.

In the absence of an acid-base disturbance, measuring extracellular [K^+] is a reasonably accurate way to assess total body K^+ in relatively healthy patients. A decrease in measured serum [K^+] from 4 to 3 meq/L represents a total body deficit of approximately 200 to 400 meq. An increase in measured serum [K^+] from 4 to 5 meq/L represents a total body K^+ increase of approximately 100 to 200 meq/L. Extracellular K^+ represents about 2 percent of total body K^+, or 70 meq, and is influenced by two important variables: total body K^+ stores, and distribution between the ICF and ECF spaces. Significant and rapid intracellular to extracellular shifting occurs in response to severe injury (i.e., surgical stress, trauma, or burns), acid-base imbalance, catabolic states, increased extracellular osmolality, or insulin deficiency. These shifts are important when viewed in light of the role of K^+ in maintaining the resting membrane potential. The normally balanced intracellular-extracellular gradient facilitates propagation of electrical impulses. This is particularly important in the functioning of the heart.

Hypokalemia

Hypokalemia is defined as a serum [K^+] of less than 3.5 meq/L. The most frequent causes of hypokalemia are intracellular shifts and increased losses (Table 23-7). K^+ tends to shift into cells as the pH of the ECF rises in exchange for hydrogen ions. A rise in the pH of 0.10 generally causes a 0.5 ± 0.2-meq/L decrease in serum [K^+] levels. This relationship applies to metabolic acid-base derangements. Although the reasons are unclear, respirator alkalosis and acidosis have minimum effect on K^+ shift. K^+ losses usually involve either the gastrointestinal tract or the kidneys. It is important to note that the hypokalemia associated with vomiting has very little to do with the actual K^+ lost in the vomitus and much more to do with the metabolic alkalosis that follows. The hypovolemia from volume loss leads to increases in aldosterone secretion, which acts on the kidney to preserve Na^+ and bicarbonate in exchange for K^+. The resultant alkalosis also causes K^+ to shift into cells in exchange for H^+.

TABLE 23-7 Etiology of Hypokalemia

Extra → intracellular potassium shifts
Alkalosis
Increase plasma insulin (treatment of diabetic ketoacidosis)
β Adrenergics
Hypokalemic periodic paralysis
Decreased intake
Poor dietary intake, geophagia
Gastrointestinal loss
Vomiting, nasogastric suction, diarrhea (laxative, enema abuse), malabsorption, ureterosigmoidostomy, enteric fistula, villous adenoma
Renal loss
Diuretic therapy
Primary aldosteronism
Secondary aldosteronism
Malignant hypertension, renal artery stenosis, congestive heart failure, cirrhosis and ascites, ACTH or glucocorticoid excess, Bartter syndrome, Liddle syndrome, renin-secreting tumor
Licorice ingestion
Excessive use of chewing tobacco
Renal tubular acidosis
Postobstructive diuresis
Osmotic diuresis
Drugs and toxins
Carbenicillin, penicillin, amphotericin B, L-dopa, lithium, thalium, theophylline, dopamine
Sweat loss
Heavy exercise, heatstroke, febrile illness
Other
Hypomagnesemia, acute leukemia, state of rapid cellular synthesis, intravenous hyperalimentation, recovery from megaloblastic anemia

The clinical manifestations of hypokalemia usually start when serum concentrations reach 2.5 meq/L, although they may appear sooner with rapid decreases in concentration. The symptoms result from abnormalities in membrane polarization and affect almost every system. Manifestation by system includes

Neuromuscular: Generalized malaise, weakness, fatigue, hyporeflexia, cramps, and paresthesias all begin as early signs. Paralysis (even of the respiratory muscles) and rhabdomyolysis are seen at levels below 1.5 meq/L.

Gastrointestinal: The gastrointestinal tract demonstrates an increased tendency to intestinal ileus.

Renal: Hypokalemia increases renal tubular production of ammonia, which may aggravate hepatic encephalopathy. Its direct effect on the kidney results in urinary-concentrating defects and decreased glomerular filtration and tends to cause a metabolic alkalemia with increased acid excretion in the urine (paradoxical aciduria). Severe hypokalemia can lead to nephrogenic DI with volume loss.

Endocrine: Hypokalemia leads to glucose intolerance.

Cardiovascular: Perhaps the most important effects are those on the cardiovascular system. These include worsening hypertension, orthostatic hypotension, potentiation of digitalis, and dysrhythmias. The classic electrocardiographic (ECG) abnormalities associated with hypokalemia include T-wave flattening, prominent U waves, and ST-segment depression. Tachyarrhythmias predominate.

TREATMENT The treatment of hypokalemia is quite simple: replacement of K^+. This can be done orally in stable patients who are able to tolerate oral intake. Either foods rich in K^+, salt substitutes, or K^+ supplements will work. Intravenous replacement is appropriate for patients with severe hypokalemia. It can also be given as 10 to 20 meq/L in 100 mL of 0.9% saline. The ECG should be continually monitored for any patient receiving intravenous K^+. As a rule, no more than 40 meq of K^+ should be in a single liter of intravenous fluid and no more than 40 meq should be given in 1 h. Concentrations greater than 20 meq/L should be infused through a central line. A 20-meq infusion will raise serum [K^+] by approximately 0.25 meq/L.[5]

Hyperkalemia

Hyperkalemia is defined as measured serum [K^+] of greater than 5.5 meq/L. If hyperkalemia is noted, oliguric renal failure, severe hemolysis, or excessive tissue breakdown should be suspected. However, the most common cause of hyperkalemia is pseudohyperkalemia. This may be due to hemolysis during blood draw or from breakdown of cells if blood is not analyzed within 30 min of phlebotomy. Other causes of hyperkalemia are listed in Table 23-8.

Clinical manifestations of hyperkalemia usually result from derangement in membrane polarization. Cardiac manifestations are the most serious. They include ECG changes ranging from

6.5 to 7.5 meq/L: tall peaked T waves, short QT interval, and prolonged PR interval
7.5 to 8.0 meq/L: QRS widening, and flattening of the P wave
10 to 12 meq/L: the QRS complex may degrade into a "sine wave" pattern

Ventricular fibrillation, complete heart block, and asystole may occur. Death from hyperkalemia is usually the result of diastolic arrest or ventricular fibrillation. Neuromuscular manifestations include weakness, paresthesias, areflexia, and ascending paralysis. The gastrointestinal symptoms include nausea, vomiting, intermittent intestinal colic, and diarrhea. Patients with slowly developing hyperkalemia often tolerate serum [K^+] of 7 to 8 meq/L, whereas, with acute elevations, significant problems, including cardiac arrest, can occur at most lower levels.

TREATMENT If there are no cardiac derangements, the initial step in the treatment of hyperkalemia is to confirm the presence of "true" hyperkalemia. Immediate cessation of further K^+ administration as well as clinical determination of severity will drive management. Asymptomatic patients with relatively small elevation of K^+ (5.0 to 6.0 meq/L) require determination and treatment of the underlying cause. As patients become symptomatic, management must become more aggressive. It is divided into three phases:

1. Membrane stabilization (especially cardiac tissue)
2. Shift K^+ from ECF to ICF
3. Removal of K^+ from the body

Membrane stabilization can be achieved with calcium gluconate or calcium chloride. This is usually indicated in any patient with evidence of cardiac irritability or acutely elevated levels of greater than 7.5 meq/L. It acts to antagonize the effect of K^+ on the cardiac conduction system. It is administered in a dose of 10 to 20 mL of 10% calcium gluconate (4.6 meq/10 mL) or as 5 mL of 10% calcium chloride (13.6 meq/10 mL) intravenously over 2 to 5 min. The effect of calcium occurs within 1 to 3 min of administration and remains pharmacologically active for up to 1 h.

If calcium is to be given to a patient on digitalis, great caution must be exercised, as hypercalcemia potentiates the toxic cardiac effects of digitalis. If it is to be given in this setting, it is best added to 100 mL of D_5W and infused slowly over at least 20 to 30 min, allowing a more even distribution throughout the extracellular space.

Patients without evidence of cardiac irritability or instability may be approached more slowly. The shifting of K^+ to the ICF can be achieved in various ways. The administration of 50 g of glucose with 5 to 10 units of regular insulin intravenously will help to redistribute K^+. Onset of action is approximately 30 min, with duration of action from 4 to 6 h. Some authorities believe that in patients with normal pancreatic function, glucose administration alone suffices, as the patient's own physiologic mechanism will result in insulin secretion. After the initial glucose has been administered, 1 L of 20% glucose with 20 to 40 units of regular insulin may be infused over the next 2 to 4 h, if necessary. Sodium bicarbonate acts through both antagonism and redistribution. It should be administered as 50 to 100 meq (1 to 2 ampules) intravenously over 2 min. Its onset of action is 5 to 10 min, with duration of 1 to 2 h. Lastly, β agonists help to redistribute K^+ into cells. The most practical route of administration is nebulized albuterol.

The removal of K^+ from the body can be achieved in three ways: via the urine, via stool, or through dialysis. Diuretics block the reabsorption of K^+, leading to increased excretion. Furosemide is the drug of choice, administered at 40 mg intravenously. Other diuretic options include ethacrynic acid or other loop diuretics. For obvious reasons, avoid K^+-sparing diuretics. Cation-exchange resins such as sodium polystyrene (Kayexalate) can be taken either orally or rectally. Each gram of sodium resin exchanges and thus eliminates about 1 meq of

TABLE 23-8 Etiology of Hyperkalemia

Pseudohyperkalemia	Intra to Extra Cellular Potassium Shift	Potassium Load	Decreased Potassium Excretion
Tourniquet use	Acidosis	Potassium supplements	Renal failure
Hemolysis (in vitro)	Heavy exercise	Potassium-rich foods	Drugs Potassium-sparing diuretics, β blockade, NSAIDs, ACE inhibitors
Leukocytosis	β Blockade	Intravenous potassium	Aldosterone deficiency
Thrombocytosis	Insulin deficiency Digitalis intoxication Hyperkalemic periodic paralysis	Potassium-containing drugs Transfusion of aged blood Hemolysis (in vivo) Gastrointestinal bleeding Cell destruction after chemotherapy Rhabdomyolysis/crush injury Extensive tissue necrosis	Selective defect in renal potassium excretion Pseudohypoaldosteronism, SLE, sickle cell disease, obstructive uropathy, renal transplantation, congenital

Abbreviations: ACE, angiotensin-converting enzyme; NSAIDs, nonsteroidal anti-inflammatory drugs.

TABLE 23-9 Emergency Therapy of Hyperkalemia

Therapy	Mechanism	Dose	Onset of Action	Duration of Hypokalemic Effect
Ca gluconate (10%)	Antagonism	10–20 mL IV	1–3 min	30–50 min
Na bicarbonate	Antagonism and redistribution	50–100 meq IV	5–10 min	1–2 h
Insulin plus glucose	Redistribution	20 U regular insulin with 50 g glucose IV over 1 h	30 min	4–6 h
Diuretics Furosemide Ethacrynic acid	Excretion	 40 mg IV 50 mg IV	With diuresis	With diuresis
Cation-exchange resin (sodium polystyrene)	Excretion	15–50 g PO or rectally with sorbitol	1–2 h	4–6 h
Peritoneal dialysis or hemodialysis	Excretion		Within minutes	During dialysis

K^+. Orally, 15 to 50 g of sodium polystyrene is given with 50 mL of a 20% sorbitol solution every 4 to 6 h. The sorbitol helps overcome the constipating effect of the resin and speeds bowel transit. Rectal administration is 20 g in 200 mL of a 20% sorbitol solution every 4 h, with the enema retained for at least 30 min. Care must be taken in patients with fluid overload or those sensitive to Na^+. Congestive heart failure may be precipitated. Dialysis is reserved for severely ill patients or those already on dialysis. Peritoneal dialysis or hemodialysis may be instituted depending on the situation.

If a dangerous tachyarrhythmia develops, all of the foregoing steps may have to be undertaken nearly simultaneously (Table 23-9). In patients with oliguric renal failure, hemodialysis (or peritoneal dialysis) stat consultation for dialysis should also be undertaken.

CALCIUM (Ca^{2+})

Calcium is the most abundant mineral in the body. The total body calcium is between 1.0 and 1.5 kg or 10 and 20 g/kg of body weight in an average-sized adult. Calcium, also the most abundant cation in the body, is 99 percent bound in bone as phosphate and carbonate (mineral apatite), with the remainder in the ECF compartment. The normal daily intake of calcium is 800 to 3000 mg, one-third of which is absorbed primarily in the small bowel via both active (vitamin D–dependent) and passive (concentration-dependent) absorption. Most of the calcium we ingest is found in milk and milk products. Most of this calcium is excreted through the gastrointestinal tract via the stool, with 200 mg or less in the urine.

The gradient between the intravascular and extravascular compartments is highly regulated to maintain a ratio of 10,000:1. The measured serum concentration of calcium ranges from 8.5 to 10.5 mg/dL and is maintained by the function of parathyroid hormone, vitamin D metabolites (1α,25-dihydroxyvitamin D_3, or calcitriol), and calcitonin.

Parathormone (parathyroid hormone, or PTH) is secreted by the parathyroid gland in response to low ionized calcium or magnesium levels. It raises serum calcium primarily by stimulating osteoclasts to increase bone resorption. It secondarily increases serum calcium by both indirect action in the kidney (increases calcium resorption and phosphorus excretion) and in conjunction with calcitriol to increase intestinal absorption. Calcitonin is influenced by elevations in serum calcium, epinephrine, glucagon, and gastrin. Its primary effect is to inhibit the activity of osteoclasts, with a limited secondary effect to potentiate calcium loss through the kidney. Vitamin D can be produced nonenzymatically by ultraviolet irradiation of skin or can be absorbed directly from the gastrointestinal tract. It is hydroxylated first in the liver and again in the kidney to create its more potent form. Upregulation of this process occurs with hypocalcemia or hypophosphatemia.

The intravascular calcium exists as 50 percent bound to plasma proteins, i.e., albumin (4.0 to 4.5 mg/dL), 45 percent free active ions (4.2 to 4.8 mg/dL), and 5 percent nonionized (bound to other substances in plasma and interstitial fluids). A laboratory value reported in meq/L is equal to half the amount in mg/dL; therefore, a value of 4.2 mg/dL = 2.1 meq/L (= 1.05 mosm/L).

Changes in hydrogen concentration result in changes to the ionized calcium concentration. This occurs because calcium binds to the protein in place of hydrogen ions. For example, hyperventilation leads to respiratory alkalosis and an attendant decrease in $[H^+]$. The decreased $[H^+]$ causes an increase in protein-bound calcium and a decrease in serum ionized calcium (relative hypocalcemia).

It is the ionized fraction that is physiologic activity. Signs and symptoms of hypocalcemia usually occur when the ionized fraction drops below 3.0 mg/dL, while those associated with hypercalcemia occur with total serum calcium greater than 11 mg/dL.

Various factors affect serum calcium:

1. Serum protein, of which albumin is the major component. On average, 0.8 mg of calcium binds to 1 g of protein. Therefore, total serum $[Ca^{2+}]$ = ionized $[Ca^{2+}]$ + (0.8 * total protein). A 1-g decrease in albumin results in a 0.8 mg/dL decrease in calcium with no change in ionized fraction.
2. Alkalosis: decrease in ionized fraction with no change in the total serum calcium. Each 0.1 rise in pH lowers ionized $[Ca^{2+}]$ by about 3 to 8 percent.
3. Acidosis: increase in ionized fraction with no change in the total serum calcium.

Hypocalcemia

Hypocalcemia is defined by an ionized calcium level of below 2.0 meq/L. In the presence of hypoalbuminemia, total calcium may be very low, yet ionized calcium remains normal. Some more common causes of hypocalcemia include shock, sepsis, renal failure, and pancreatitis. It is quite uncommon in ambulatory patients, except those with hypoparathyroidism (secondary to surgery) or in chronic renal disease.

TABLE 23-10 Etiology of Hypocalcemia

Hypoalbuminemia
Vitamin D deficiency Sunlight deficiency Dietary deficiency Malabsorption Postgastrectomy, sprue, pancreatic insufficiency, hepatobiliary disease with bile salt disease, laxative abuse Abnormal metabolism of vitamin D Renal failure (acute or chronic), liver failure, vitamin D–dependent rickets, anticonvulsants, microsomal enzyme inducers Hypoparathyroidism Congenital, idiopathic, acquired (surgical, iron overload, irradiation, neoplasm) Pseudohypoparathyroidism (types I and II) Hyperphosphatemia Phosphate administration Enemas, laxatives, intravenous administration, cow's milk in infant formula Renal failure Rhabdomyolysis Cytotoxic therapy for leukemia or lymphoma Malignancy Osteoblastic metastases Malignancy with increased thyrocalcitonin levels (medullary thyroid cancer)
Magnesium depletion
Drugs (see Table 23-11)
Massive transfusions or plasma exchange
Acute pancreatitis
Shock or sepsis
Fat embolism syndrome
Healing phase of rickets
Hyperkalemic periodic paralysis (acute)
Neonatal tetany

ETIOLOGY (TABLE 23-10) **Movement into "Sick" Cells** The concentration of ionized calcium in the ECF is about 1.0 mmol/L or 10^{-3} *M*. The concentration of ionized calcium in the cytoplasm of most cells is about 10^{-7} *M*. This gradient of 10^4, or 10,000, to 1 is maintained by active metabolic processes. Any process that interferes with cell metabolism, such as shock or sepsis, will tend to reduce ionized calcium levels by allowing increased net movement of calcium across the cell membrane into the cytoplasm of the poorly functioning cells. Following trauma, serum calcium levels may be low, especially with the fat embolism syndrome, not only because of cell dysfunction and binding of calcium to free fatty acids, but also because of fatty inhibition of cell membrane calcium pumps.

Pancreatitis Acute pancreatitis is an important cause of hypocalcemia. Pancreatic lipase breaks down fat into fatty acids and glycerol. The fatty acids combine with calcium to form insoluble calcium soaps and reduce serum calcium levels. The combination of necrotic fat cells plus calcium soaps makes up much of what is recognized as the fat necrosis of pancreatitis. In addition, as protein moves into the inflammatory exudate, the resultant hypoproteinemia may cause total calcium levels to fall. Pancreatitis can also reduce PTH secretion and the response of tissues to it. If total calcium levels fall below 7.0 or 8.0 mg/dL, there is an increased chance of severe complications from pancreatitis.

Drugs A large number of drugs can cause hypocalcemia (Table 23-11). One of the most frequently used of these is cimetidine. This histamine receptor–blocking agent apparently lowers serum calcium levels by decreasing the synthesis or secretion of parathyroid hormone.

Postoperative Hypocalcemia HYPOPARATHYROIDISM Currently, more than 10 percent of postparathyroidectomy patients may have hypoparathyroidism as defined by a fasting calcium level of less than 8.5 mg/dL and a simultaneous inorganic phosphorus level of greater than 4.5 mg/dL. Postoperative hypocalcemia can be due to hypoparathyroidism from the permanent surgical removal of parathyroid tissue, from transient ischemia of the parathyroid glands in patients who have extensive bilateral neck surgery, or because of long-term hypercalcemic suppression of the nonadenomatous parathyroid glands.

HUNGRY-BONE SYNDROME The term *hungry-bone syndrome* was coined by Albright and now indicates postparathyroidectomy hypocalcemia due to rapid remineralization of the skeleton. During this accelerated remineralization, a persistent hypocalcemia and hypophosphatemia may be severe enough to cause tetany. These patients may require vigorous calcium and vitamin D supplementation for prolonged periods of time.

The hungry-bone syndrome may be found in over 10 percent of patients after parathyroid surgery. Patients are at risk if they have a fasting calcium level of less than 8.5 mg/dL and a simultaneous inorganic serum phosphorus of less than 3.0 mg/dL on postoperative day 3 or later.

Renal Failure Hypocalcemia is a frequent finding in renal failure. This may be partially due to the resulting hyperphosphatemia, but there is also decreased production of 1α,25-$(OH)_2$-vitamin D in the kidney, which, in turn, causes decreased intestinal absorption of calcium. Secondary hyperparathyroidism with increased PTH levels often results from the chronic hypocalcemia. If PTH levels remain elevated and hypercalcemia develops in spite of cure of the renal failure by renal transplantation, the patient is said to have tertiary hyperparathyroidism.

TABLE 23-11 Drugs that Can Cause Hypocalcemia

Cimetidine
Phosphates (e.g., enemas, laxatives)
Dilantin, phenobarbital
Gentamicin, tobramycin, actinomycin
Cisplatin
Heparin
Theophylline
Protamine
Glucagon
Norepinephrine
Citrate (blood)
Loop diuretics
Glucocorticoids
Magnesium sulfate
Sodium nitroprusside

TABLE 23-12 Symptoms and Signs of Hypocalcemia

General	Muscular
Weakness, fatigue	Spasms, cramps
Neurologic	Weakness
Tetany	Skeletal
Chvostek sign, Trousseau sign	Osteodystrophy
Circumoral and digital paresthesias	Rickets
Impaired memory, confusion	Osteomalacia
Hallucinations, dementia, seizures	Miscellaneous
Extrapyramidal disorders	Dental hypoplasia
Dermatologic	Cataracts
Hyperpigmentation	Decreased insulin secretion
Coarse, brittle hair	
Dry, scaly skin	
Cardiovascular	
Heart failure	
Vasoconstriction	

Phosphate Overload Phosphate overload from nonrenal causes may also lead to hypocalcemia. This is the presumed mechanism in the acute rhabdomyolysis of hyperpyrexia and major trauma. Excessive use of phosphate cathartics and sodium phosphate enemas can cause significant hyperphosphatemia in patients with renal disease, in children with Hirschsprung disease, and in small infants.

Hypomagnesemia Hypomagnesemia in association with hypocalcemia may be seen in alcoholism, diuretic use, epilepsy, and renal failure. Neonatal hypomagnesemia leads to low PTH secretion, decreased responsiveness of bone cells to PTH, and decreased calcium mobilization from bone.

Idiopathic Hypoparathyroidism Idiopathic hypoparathyroidism is probably an autoimmune disorder in which pernicious anemia, exostoses, moniliasis, Hashimoto disease, sterility, and Addison disease may be seen. This syndrome may also be associated with cataracts, mental retardation, intracranial calcifications, and papilledema due to increased intracranial pressure.

Nonsurgical Primary Hypoparathyroidism Hypocalcemia with primary hypoparathyroidism has been reported from parathyroid infarction, metastases to the parathyroids, and hemochromatosis of the parathyroids.

Pseudohypoparathyroidism Pseudohypoparathyroidism is a familial disorder characterized by decreased end-organ responsiveness to PTH resulting in hypocalcemia, hyperphosphatemia, parathyroid hyperplasia, and excessive serum PTH concentrations. These patients usually have a very low urinary cyclic AMP excretion that only slightly increases with infusion of parathormone. This condition may be inherited as an X-linked dominant trait with variable penetrance; the male to female ratio is 2 to 1. Patients are short and have round faces; brachycephaly; a short, thick neck; short, pudgy fingers and toes; and growth failure of the fourth and fifth metacarpals. Mental retardation, seizures, and subcutaneous soft tissue calcification may be seen. The skin can be dry and coarse, and the hair is often brittle.

Vitamin D Deficiency Hypocalcemia due to vitamin D deficiency is rare in the United States. Infants born to vitamin D–deficient mothers who lack sunlight exposure and receive no vitamin D supplementation may have rickets. Breast milk has low vitamin D content, and breast milk feeding without sunshine exposure in unsupplemented infants may result in infantile rickets.

PHYSIOLOGIC EFFECTS Although normal ionized calcium levels are 2.1 to 2.6 meq/L (1.05 to 1.3 mmol/L), serious physiologic changes do not usually occur until ionized levels in serum are less than 1.4 to 1.6 meq/L (0.7 to 0.8 mmol/L). Below those levels, hypocalcemia can cause a wide variety of signs and symptoms (Table 23-12).

The severity of signs and symptoms depends greatly on the rapidity of the fall in calcium. The more acute the drop in the serum calcium, the more likely are significant pathophysiologic changes. As serum calcium levels fall, neuronal membranes become increasingly more permeable to sodium, enhancing excitation. Potassium and magnesium have an antagonizing effect on this excitation.

Decreased ionized calcium levels reduce the strength of myocardial contraction primarily by inhibiting relaxation. They also decrease the sensitivity of the heart to digitalis. Hypocalcemia should be considered in patients with refractory heart failure.

Low ionized calcium levels increase PTH secretion, which mobilizes calcium from bone and decreases renal tubular absorption of phosphate and bicarbonate. This, in turn, may cause an increased absorption of chloride, producing a tendency to hyperchloremic hypophosphatemic renal tubular acidosis. A ratio of chloride to phosphate greater than 35 to 1 in meq/mg in the plasma is sometimes considered to be highly suggestive of hyperparathyroidism.

Increased cytoplasmic calcium activates phospholipase, which increases prostaglandin production and alters cell lipids. Increased cytoplasmic calcium also interferes with cell metabolism. Efforts by mitochondria to pump the excess calcium from the cytoplasm into the mitochondrial matrix greatly reduce adenosine triphosphate (ATP) formation. Consequently, giving calcium during shock or sepsis may transiently improve hemodynamics, but if cell metabolism does not also improve, some of the additional calcium moves into the cytoplasm within 30 to 40 min and further impairs cell metabolism.

Movement of calcium into ischemic cerebrovascular smooth muscle cells may cause persistent cerebral vasoconstriction with resultant failure of cerebral reperfusion after strokes or cardiac arrest. This may be a major cause of the poor results in management of these problems. Consequently, there has been some interest in the use of calcium blockers for cerebral resuscitation.

DIAGNOSIS **Symptoms** The most characteristic initial symptom of hypocalcemia following thyroid or parathyroid surgery is paresthesias around the mouth or in the fingertips. Hypocalcemia should be suspected in any patient who is irritable and has hyperactive deep tendon reflexes following neck surgery. It should also be suspected in patients who have seizures particularly if they have ever had thyroid surgery, even if many years previously.

Signs A positive Chvostek or Trousseau sign is generally considered to be good clinical evidence of hypocalcemia. A positive Chvostek sign is a twitch at the corner of the mouth when the examiner taps over the facial nerve just in front of the ear. However, it is present in about 10 to 30 percent of normal individuals. Nevertheless, eyelid muscle contraction with the Chvostek maneuver is said to be almost diagnostic of hypocalcemia.

Trousseau sign, which is generally a more reliable indicator of hypocalcemia, is positive if carpal spasm is produced when the examiner applies a blood pressure cuff to the upper arm and maintains a pressure above systolic for 3 min. The fingers are spastically extended at the interphalangeal joints and flexed at the metacarpophalangeal joints. The wrist is flexed and the forearm is pronated.

Laboratory Findings Signs of hypocalcemia may be found with normal total serum calcium levels if a patient is very alkalotic. Each 0.1 rise in pH lowers ionized calcium levels by about 3 to 8 percent. Consequently, a very alkalotic patient may have normal total serum calcium levels with ionic hypocalcemia. Similar signs and symptoms may be caused by hypomagnesemia, strychnine, or tetanus toxin.

Decreased plasma levels of ionized calcium are diagnostic, but one should also suspect ionic hypocalcemia if a patient has decreased levels of total calcium in the presence of normal plasma proteins. Primary hypoparathyroidism is characterized by a low serum PTH concentration, hyperphosphatemia, and hypocalcemia.

TABLE 23-13 Causes of Hypercalcemia

Malignancy	Granulomatous disease
Lung (squamous cell cancer)	Sarcoidoses
Breast	Tuberculosis
Kidney	Histoplasmosis
Myeloma	Coccidioidomycosis
Leukemia	Immobilization
Endocrinopathies	Miscellaneous
Primary hyperparathyroidism	Paget's disease of bone
Hyperthyroidism	Postrenal transplantation
Pheochromocytoma	Recovery from acute renal failure
Adrenal insufficiency	Phosphate depletion syndrome
Acromegaly	
Drugs	
Hypervitaminosis D and A	
Thiazides	
Lithium	
Hormonal therapy for breast cancer	

ECG The most characteristic ECG finding in hypocalcemia is prolonged QT intervals. However, the T wave is of normal width, and it is the ST segment that is really prolonged. This finding is usually seen with total serum calcium levels less than 6.0 mg/dL.

X-rays Radiologically, rickets is characterized by craniotabes, frontal skull bossing, rachitic rosary ribs, widened rib cage (Harrison groove), bowed legs, and, often, fractures. Other radiographic changes include cupping and splaying of the metaphyseal ends of long bones, widening between the metaphyses and epiphysis, bone demineralization, and thinning of cortical bone.

TREATMENT Treatment of hypocalcemia is tailored to the individual and directed toward the underlying cause. If a patient is asymptomatic, oral calcium therapy with or without vitamin D may be all that is required. Calcium lactate, calcium glubionate, calcium ascorbate, calcium carbonate, and calcium gluconate are available in oral preparations. Milk, because of the large amount of phosphate present, is not really a very good source of calcium, except in normal growing children who also need the phosphate.

Symptomatic patients following thyroid or parathyroid surgery are often treated with parenteral calcium. With severe acute hypocalcemia, 10 mL of 10% $CaCl_2$ (or 10 to 30 mL of 10% calcium gluconate) may be given intravenously (IV) over 10 to 20 min followed by a continuous IV drip providing 1 g of $CaCl_2$ over a period of 6 to 12 h. If the patient is not asymptomatic or if the hypocalcemia is not severe and prolonged for more than 10 to 14 days, treatment with calcium may not be required. One should not administer calcium rapidly IV to asymptomatic patients with mild to moderate hypocalcemia because it can cause severe unnecessary cardiovascular, neuromuscular, and renal complications.

During massive transfusions, if the blood is being given faster than 1 unit every 5 min, 10 mL of 10% calcium chloride can be given after every 4 to 6 units of blood if a patient is in shock or heart failure in spite of adequate volume replacement therapy. Calcium is seldom required during transfusions for elective surgery.

Hypercalcemia

Hypercalcemia is a relatively common entity. It is defined as a total calcium level exceeding 10.5 mg/dL or an ionized calcium level exceeding 2.7 meq/L. Over 90 percent of occurrences are associated with hyperparathyroid or malignancy. Various mnemonics exist to help recall the long list of potential etiologies for hypercalcemia (Table 23-13).

PATHOPHYSIOLOGIC EFFECTS The effects of hypercalcemia can be neuromuscular, cardiovascular, gastrointestinal, renal, and skeletal. Neuromuscular changes include decreased sensitivity, responsiveness, and strength of muscular contraction and nerve conduction. This causes increasing weakness and fatigue that may progress to ataxia and altered mental status.

In mild hypercalcemic states, the heart's conduction is slowed and automaticity is decreased with a shortening of the refractory period. There is also increased sensitivity to digitalis preparations.

Loss of renal concentrating ability, as might be expected with nephrogenic DI, is the most frequent renal effect of hypercalcemia. This is a reversible tubular defect, which results in polyuria and dehydration in spite of polydipsia. Potassium wasting results in hypokalemia in up to one-third of patients. Nephrocalcinosis and nephrolithiasis are caused by the hypercalcemia and aggravated by volume depletion. As the hypercalcemia persists, increasing microscopic calcium deposits in the kidney may result in progressive renal insufficiency.

Hypertension is seen with increased frequency in hypercalcemic patients, probably as a result of arteriolar vasoconstriction.

DIAGNOSIS Hypercalcemic patients with plasma total calcium levels below 12.0 mg/dL are usually asymptomatic, but higher levels can cause a wide variety of symptoms and signs (Table 23-14).

Patients with total calcium levels above 14 to 16 mg/dL are usually very weak, lethargic, and confused. Coma is uncommon, but calcium levels should probably be determined in any patient with coma of unknown etiology. Polyuria, in spite of polydipsia, tends to cause increasing volume depletion. Weariness and weakness are common with hypercalcemia. Polyuria and polydipsia are due to impaired renal tubular reabsorption of water. Total calcium levels above 15.0 mg/dL may cause somnolence, stupor, and even coma.

A mnemonic sometimes used for the signs and symptoms of hypercalcemia is *stones* (renal calculi), *bones* (osteolysis), *moans* (psychiatric disorders), and *groans* (peptic ulcer disease and pancreatitis). The most common gastrointestinal symptoms are anorexia and constipation, but these are very nonspecific.

Hypercalcemia should be suspected in patients with extensive metastatic bone disease, particularly if the primary site involves the breast, lungs, or kidneys, and in individuals with combinations of clinical problems such as renal calculi, pancreatitis, or ulcer disease. As with hypocalcemia, ionized calcium levels should be measured and/or total

TABLE 23-14 Symptoms and Signs of Hypercalcemia

General	Cardiovascular
Malaise, weakness	Hypertension
Polydipsia, dehydration	Dysrhythmias
Neurologic	Vascular calcifications
Confusion	ECG abnormalities
Apathy, depression, stupor	QT shortening
Decreased memory	Coving of ST-T wave
Irritability	Widening of T wave
Hallucinations	Digitalis sensitivity
Headache	Gastrointestinal
Ataxia	Anorexia, weight loss
Hyporeflexia, hypotonia	Nausea, vomiting
Mental retardation (infants)	Constipation
Metastatic calcification	Abdominal pain
Band keratopathy	Peptic ulcer disease
Conjunctivitis	Pancreatitis
Pruritus	Urologic
Skeletal	Polyuria, nocturia
Fractures	Renal insufficiency
Bone pain	Nephrolithiasis
Deformities	

TABLE 23-15 Treatment of Hypercalcemia

Drug	Dose	Cautions
	TO TREAT DEHYDRATION	
Saline	Until ECF is restored	Watch for hypokalemia
Furosemide	40–100 mg IV q 2–4 h	Digitalis, renal failure
	TO DECREASE BONE ABSORPTION	
Calcitonin	4 IU/kg sq or IM q12h	
Mithramycin	25 μg/kg IV	Bone marrow and renal toxicity
Hydrocortisone	3 mg/kg per day IV in divided doses q6h	May take 3 weeks to lower Ca^{2+}
Indomethacin	25 PO q6h	Peptic ulcer disease, GI bleeding

Abbreviations: ECF, extracellular fluid; GI, gastrointestinal.

calcium levels should be correlated with serum proteins. If a patient is hypoproteinemic, total calcium levels may be normal or low in spite of increased ionized calcium levels.

On ECG, hypercalcemia may be associated with depressed ST segments, widened T waves, and shortened ST segments and QT intervals. Bradyarrhythmias may occur, and bundle branch patterns may progress to second-degree block and then complete heart block. Levels above 20 mg/dL may cause cardiac arrest.

TREATMENT Up to one-third of patients with hypercalcemia have hypokalemia, and in those with malignant disease, more than half the patients may have hypokalemia. Some patients also have hypomagnesemia. The tendency toward hypokalemia and hypomagnesemia will be aggravated by diuresis and should be monitored carefully. A number of modalities are available to treat hypercalcemia (Table 23-15). Mithramycin, calcitonin, and hydrocortisone should be used in severe cases. Mithramycin is a cytotoxic drug that suppresses bone resorption and calcium release from bone. It is infused over 3 h. It is particularly useful in patients with metastatic bone disease. Calcitonin is also an osteoclast inhibitor but less toxic than mithramycin. When used in conjunction with corticosteroids, resistance to calcitonin may be delayed. Glucocorticoids are useful in patients with sarcoidosis, vitamin A or D intoxication, multiple myeloma, leukemia, or breast cancer. They work by inhibiting bone resorption and gastrointestinal absorption of calcium. It is also postulated that they cause Ca^{2+} to shift inside cells where it may become bound to mitochondria. Gallium nitrate has been approved for use in the United States.[6] It acts by decreasing the solubility of base crystals. It is administered in a dose of 200 mg/m^2 added to 1 L of fluid in 24 h. It potentiates nephropathy and its use should be avoided in renal disease. Intravenous phosphates are no longer used.

MAGNESIUM (Mg^{2+})

Mg^{2+} is a vital element in all biologic systems and is the key element in chlorophyll, the first link in the world's food chain. The total body content of Mg^{2+} is 24 g, or 2000 meq. Of this, 50 to 70 percent is fixed in bone and is only slowly exchangeable. Most of the remaining Mg^{2+} (approximately 40 percent) is found in the ICF space, with a concentration of approximately 40 meq/L. The distribution of Mg^{2+} is similar to that of potassium, with the major portion intracellular. It is the second most abundant intracellular cation. Serum [Mg^{2+}] ranges between 1.5 and 2.5 meq/L. Mg^{2+} present in blood is 25 to 35 percent protein-bound, 10 to 15 percent complexed, and 50 to 60 percent ionized. The normal dietary intake of Mg^{2+} is approximately 20 to 28 meq/day, or 240 to 336 mg/day, and is found in vegetables such as dry beans and leafy greens, meat, and cereals. The majority of Mg^{2+} is excreted through the gastrointestinal tract in the stool (60 percent) with the remainder (40 percent) in the urine. The kidney is very capable of conserving Mg^{2+}. A person on an Mg^{2+}-free diet will excrete less than 1 meq/day through the urine. Mg^{2+} promotes enzyme reactions within the cell during metabolism, helps in the production of ATP, participates in protein synthesis, and plays a role in coagulation, platelet aggregation, and neuromuscular activity.

Hypomagnesemia

The three major intracellular components—Mg^{2+}, K^+, and PO_4^-—usually travel together; therefore, the loss and deficiency of one constituent usually leads to the loss and deficiency of the others. As with most intracellular components, loss of total body Mg^{2+} may occur when serum levels are normal.

ETIOLOGY A wide variety of problems can cause hypomagnesemia (Table 23-16). In adults, magnesium deficiencies are most frequently seen in alcoholics, in malnourished patients, and in patients with cirrhosis, pancreatitis, or excessive gastrointestinal fluid losses. Diarrhea is usually more of a problem (Mg^{2+} content of 10 to 14 meq/L) than upper gastrointestinal loss (1 to 2 meq/L).

Intravenous hyperalimentation or treatment of diabetic ketoacidosis without providing adequate magnesium, especially in a previously malnourished patient, can cause an abrupt fall in plasma magnesium levels. This is largely due to magnesium being ''pulled'' into cells with glucose or as new lean body mass is synthesized. Hypophosphatemia, which can also develop with IV hyperalimentation, can contribute to the hypomagnesemia.

Renal wasting of magnesium can be seen with loop diuretics, hypophosphatemia, ketoacidosis, aminoglycosides, and nephrotoxic chemotherapeutic agents.

The normal renal threshold for magnesium (1.5 to 2.0 meq/L) is significantly decreased by cisplatin, diuretics, hypercalcemia, growth hormone, thyroid hormone, and calcitonin. Cisplatin causes dose-dependent, cumulative, reversible renal tubular injury. Even when the glomerular filtration rate is not diminished by cisplatin, renal magnesium wasting along with a secondary hypocalcemia and hypokalemia may develop. Potassium wasting is thought to occur as a result of impaired ATP production when magnesium is low. This in turn impairs the function of the membrane Na^+/K^+ transport system and causes loss of the normal Na^+/K^+ gradient. The accompanying hypocalcemia may be due to (1) impaired PTH release by the parathyroid gland, (2) decreased peripheral sensitivity to PTH, or (3) abnormal blood-bone calcium balance independent of PTH.

PHYSIOLOGIC EFFECTS Magnesium is essential to a large number of vital enzymes, including membrane-bound ATPase. Consequently hypomagnesemia may result in a wide variety of neuromuscular, gastrointestinal, and cardiovascular changes (Table 23-17).

Hypomagnesemia may cause increased muscular irritability similar to that seen with hypocalcemia. It can also cause many CNS signs and symptoms, including depression, vertigo, ataxia, and seizures. In severe chronic alcoholics, delirium tremens is often associated with moderate to severe magnesium deficiencies. Cardiac dysrhythmia, particularly in patients on digitalis, is often due to both potassium and magnesium deficiencies.

Some metabolic manifestations of magnesium deficiency include difficulties in treating hypokalemia, impaired PTH secretion, decreased response to thiamine, and vitamin D–resistant hypocalcemia. Other manifestations include hypothermia, hypotension, nephropathy, incomplete distal renal tubular acidosis, dysphagia, and anemia due to shortened red blood cell survival.

It has been noted that patients with severe acute pancreatitis and hypocalcemia usually have normal serum magnesium levels; however,

TABLE 23-16 Causes of Hypomagnesemia

Redistribution	Extrarenal Loss	Decreased Intake	Increased Renal Loss
Postparathyroidectomy	Nasogastric suction (infrequent)	Alcoholism (cirrhosis)	Ketoacidosis
Correction of diabetic ketoacidosis	Lactation	Malnutrition, poor intake	Drugs: loop diuretics Aminoglycosides Amphotericin B Vitamin D intoxication Alcohol Cisplatin
Intravenous glucose	Profuse sweating, burns, sepsis	Small bowel resection	SIADH
Intravenous hyperalimentation	Intestinal or biliary fistula	Malabsorption	Hyperthyroidism
Refeeding after starvation	Diarrhea		Hyperparathyroidism
Acute pancreatitis			Hypercalcemic states Diabetic ketoacidosis Primary or secondary aldosteronism Tubulointerstitial renal disease Postobstructive or postacute renal failure diuresis Saline or osmotic diuresis Potassium depletion Familial Hypophosphatemia

Abbreviation: SIADH, syndrome of inappropriate antidiuretic hormone.

there is an intracellular and total body magnesium deficiency. This may contribute to the severity of the pancreatitis and the pathogenesis of the hypocalcemia.

DIAGNOSIS One cannot rely on plasma levels to diagnose magnesium deficiencies because it is not unusual to have severe total body magnesium depletion before plasma levels are lowered. The diagnosis of hypomagnesemia in the presence of normal serum calcium levels is suggested by increased neuromuscular irritability (hyperreflexia, positive Chvostek or Trousseau signs, tremor, tetany, or even convulsions). Hypomagnesemia should be suspected in alcoholics, cirrhotics, and patients on IV fluids for prolonged periods. Hypomagnesemia may also develop rapidly during IV hyperalimentation, especially when anabolism begins.

The ECG changes seen with magnesium deficiencies include prolonged PR and QT intervals, widened QRS complexes, depression of ST segments, and inversion of T waves, especially in the precordial leads. The changes may be somewhat similar to those caused by hypokalemia and/or hypocalcemia, and many of these changes may be related to Mg^{2+} deficiency altering cardiac intracellular potassium content.

TABLE 23-17 Symptoms and Signs of Hypomagnesemia

Neuromuscular	Gastrointestinal
Tetany	Dysphagia
Muscle weakness	Anorexia, nausea
Cerebellar (ataxia, nystagmus, vertigo)	Cardiovascular
Confusion, obtundation, coma	Heart failure
Seizures	Dysrhythmias
Apathy, depression	Hypotension
Irritability	Miscellaneous
Paresthesias	Hypokalemia
	Hypocalcemia
	Anemia

TREATMENT Hypokalemia, hypocalcemia, and hypophosphatemia are often present with hypomagnesemia and must be monitored carefully. Hypocalcemia does not develop until [Mg^{2+}] falls below 1.2 mg/dL.

Patients with magnesium deficiency may require more than 50 meq of oral magnesium (6 g $MgSO_4$) per day. In chronic alcoholics with delirium tremens and in patients with severe proven hypomagnesemia, up to 8 to 12 g of $MgSO_4$ may be given intramuscularly or intravenously the first day. The first 10 to 15 meq (1.5 to 2.0 g) of IV $MgSO_4$ can be given over 1 to 2 h. This may be followed by up to 4 to 6 g/day thereafter.

If magnesium is being given rapidly, as in the treatment of eclampsia, the deep tendon reflexes (which disappear at about 3 to 4 meq/L) should be checked frequently, and blood levels should be measured once or twice daily. If deep tendon reflexes decrease or disappear, magnesium administration should stop, at least temporarily.

Hypermagnesemia

Hypermagnesemia is rarely encountered in emergency practice. A small elevation in serum concentration has little clinical significance. The most common etiology for hypermagnesemia can be found in patients with renal insufficiency or renal failure who ingest Mg^{2+}-containing drugs. Hypermagnesemia may be seen in the perinatal setting in both a mother and her neonate secondary to the treatment of preeclampsia/eclampsia. Other etiologies of hypermagnesemia include lithium ingestion, volume depletion, or familial hypocalciuric hypercalcemia (Table 23-18).

PHYSIOLOGIC EFFECTS Hypermagnesemia only rarely produces symptoms. Mg^{2+} significantly decreases the transmission of neuromuscular messages and thus acts as a CNS depressant and decreases neuromuscular activity. An initial finding in hypermagnesemic patients is nausea that appears with serum levels greater than 2.0 meq/L. Somnolence may develop as levels approach 3.0 meq/L. Deep tendon reflexes tend to disappear at serum concentrations of 4.0 to 8.0 meq/L, and respiratory compromise or apnea is seen at higher levels, approxi-

TABLE 23-18 Causes of Hypermagnesemia

Renal failure (acute or chronic)
Increased magnesium load
Magnesium-containing laxatives, antacids, or enemas
Treatment of preeclampsia/eclampsia (mothers and neonates)
Diabetic ketoacidosis (untreated)
Tumor lysis
Rhabdomyolysis
Increased renal magnesium absorption
Hyperparathyroidism
Familial hypocalciuric hypercalcemia
Hypothyroidism
Mineralocorticoid deficiency, adrenal insufficiency

mately 8.0 to 12.0 meq/L. Hypotension, heart block, or cardiac arrest may be seen with levels approaching 15.0 meq/L. ECG abnormalities such as prolonged PR and QT intervals and increased QRS duration may be seen at any level above 5.0 meq/L.

DIAGNOSIS Serum magnesium levels are usually diagnostic. The possibility of hypermagnesemia should be considered in patients with hyperkalemia or hypercalcemia. Hypermagnesemia should also be suspected in patients with renal failure, particularly in those who are taking magnesium-containing antacids, such as Maalox (see Table 23-18).

TREATMENT The only treatment available is the immediate cessation of Mg^{2+} administration. If renal failure is not evident, dilution by IV fluids followed by furosemide (40 to 80 mg IV) may be helpful. In symptomatic patients, 1 ampule (10 mL of 10%) calcium gluconate or 5 mL of 10% IV $CaCl_2$ (given over 5 to 10 min is appropriate). Patients with renal failure may benefit from dialysis against a decreased Mg^{2+} bath that lowers serum Mg^{2+} levels.

CHLORIDE (Cl^-)

Alteration in serum chloride is seldom a primary disturbance. Chloride is a major extracellular anion that has the reciprocal power of increasing or decreasing in concentration whenever changes occur in the concentration of other anions. For example in non-anion-gap metabolic acidosis, the decrease in serum $[HCO_3^-]$ is replaced by Cl^-. Cl^- plays a major role in the maintenance of urinary output, ECF, acid-base, potassium balance, and normal anion gap. Cl^- concentration is approximately 70 percent that of Na^+ and is diffusable and active. $[Cl^-]$ should be between 95 and 105 meq/L. Cl^- is easily absorbed in the intestine by active and passive transport coexistent with Na^+ and HCO_3^-. Hydrogen and chloride ions are secreted into the gastric fluid while HCO_3^- is transported into the bloodstream. Therefore, significant gastric loss of H^+ and Cl^- from vomiting results in metabolic alkalosis. A total of 90 percent of Cl^- is excreted through the kidney, with a small percentage (10 percent) secreted in sweat and stool.

Hypochloremia

Hypochloremia usually manifests when levels are less than 95 meq/L. It is usually caused by excessive diuresis, vomiting, or nasogastric tube drainage. Volume loss results in alkalosis. When Cl^- is lost via the urine or gastrointestinal fluids, there is an increase in both Na^+ and HCO_3^- resorption secondary to the volume contraction. Na^+ may be resorbed in the kidney with either Cl^- or HCO_3^- acid. When Cl^- levels become low, the Na^+ is exchanged for H^+, and HCO_3^- is accentuated in the renal tubules. This loss of H^+ in the urine further worsens the alkalosis. There is also an increased delivery of Na^+ to the distal nephron for H^+ and K^+ exchange. This exchange potentiates the loss of H^+ and K^+ in the urine, exaggerating the alkalosis further. Secondary skin losses from severe sweating or burns, along with states in which sweat has excessive Cl^- (cystic fibrosis), often lead to a metabolic alkalosis also.

APPROACH There are no signs or symptoms specific for hypochloremia. However, the clinical approach may be based on the findings of the secondary effects. For example, if a metabolic alkalosis is diagnosed and is judged to be due to volume contraction, the approach is to address the metabolic alkalosis. In fact, $[Cl^-]$ can largely be ignored. Vomiting, nasogastric tube drainage, diuretics, or volume depletion may lead to hypochloremia but virtually never without an associated metabolic alkalosis. The symptoms of metabolic alkalosis include muscle weakness, irritability, and hypoventilation. Patients usually present with symptoms of volume depletion from the aforementioned etiologies, and electrolyte levels demonstrate a low $[Cl^-]$ and $[Na^+]$.

It is important then to determine the urinary $[Cl^-]$ because low urinary $[Cl^-]$ (less than 10 meq/L) in the setting of metabolic alkalosis implies chloride-responsive alkalosis (see Chap. 21, "Acid-Base Disorders"). If the urinary Cl^- levels are higher (greater than 40 meq/L), the hypochloremia may be secondary to volume overload or dilution. Increased urinary Cl^- may also result from increased mineralocorticoid activity, which leads to the retention of HCO_3^- and Na^+ at the expense of H^+, K^+, and Cl^-. This results in further positive feedback derangement. The Na^+ retention leads to volume expansion that increases the Na^+ delivery to the distal tubule. This ultimately leads to a greater exchange with K^+ and H^+, resulting in more H^+ and K^+ urinary losses. This acts to further the metabolic alkalosis.

The treatment of Cl^--responsive metabolic alkalosis (urinary $[Cl^-]$ 10 meq/L) is IV NaCl administration. Generally speaking, emergency practice concerns itself with addressing the acute issues associated with the underlying condition. Chloride deficit per se rarely needs separate or specific consideration in the ED setting. However, as emergency practice extends to the realm of acute extended care, it is worthwhile to note that total body deficit can be determined by:

serum Cl^- deficit * 20% of the body weight = total body Cl^- deficit

The total body Cl^- should be repleted by giving 25 percent of the calculated Cl^- deficit as KCl and 75 percent as NaCl. In the setting of renal insufficiency or failure, treatment options are more complicated in that NaCl administration may lead to volume problems and KCl may lead to hyperkalemia. The replacement method of choice, amino acid hydrochlorides or 0.1 *N* HCl, will lead to a non-anion-gap acidosis, worsening the underlying wide-anion-gap acidosis associated with renal failure.

Hyperchloremia

Excessive amounts of Cl^- are usually the result of administration of NaCl, volume depletion, or entities causing metabolic acidosis without a widened anion gap (see Chap. 21, "Acid-Base Disorders").

NaCl, KCl, or amino acid hydrochlorides readily dissociate and bind with bicarbonate, leading to metabolic acidosis. The effects of hyperchloremia are a result of volume depletion or acidosis. Since Na^+ and Cl^- travel together, high levels of serum Na^+ are associated with high levels of serum Cl^-. Bicarbonate is inversely proportional to Cl^-, so hyperchloremia is associated with non-widened-anion-gap metabolic acidosis. If Na^+ levels are normal in the face of elevated Cl^-, one must think of KCl or amino acid hydrochloride administration (again leading to non-anion-gap acidosis). Finally, bromism, rarely seen today, may present with hyperchloremia, as Br^- is factitiously measured as Cl^- in hospital laboratories. A narrow anion gap will be an important clue in this latter diagnosis.

APPROACH Similar to hypochloremia, clinical conditions associated with hyperchloremia, are rarely considered from the perspective of the serum [Cl^-]. Rather, the [Cl^-] is used as a diagnostic adjunct. For example, in the setting of metabolic acidosis, an elevated [Cl^-] will merely help confirm the acidosis type when it is also noted that the anion gap is not widened. Thus, rather than seeking the cause of the hyperchloremia, clinicians can approach the differential diagnosis from the perspective of the nonwidened metabolic acidosis (see Chap. 21, "Acid-Base Disorders"). Similarly, when [Cl^-] is elevated in hypernatremic states, the differential diagnosis can be considered from the perspective of elevated [Na^+] and the volume status of the patient (vide supra).

TREATMENT If there is excess administration of chloride or excessive losses of bicarbonate, this should be corrected. Hyperchloremia due to dehydration is best treated by slowly administering increased isotonic fluids with little or no chloride. However, if too much isotonic fluid is given too rapidly, seizures due to cerebral edema may develop.

PHOSPHORUS

Phosphorus is an essential mineral that exists mainly as hydroxyapatite (85 percent) or as an intracellular constituent (10 to 15 percent). Only about 1 percent is in the ECF, and therefore serum measurements may not accurately reflect total body stores. Serum phosphate levels decrease with age from a high of 4.0 to 7.0 mg/dL in newborns to 3.0 to 5.0 mg/dL in adults. The total body phosphorus in a normal man is approximately 700 g (10 to 15 g/kg). This is predominantly in bone (80 percent), where phosphorus plays a major role in structural integrity. Serum Ca^{2+} and phosphate are inversely proportional, and the product of their two concentrations is approximately 30 to 40 mg/dL. When phosphorus is not in the form of hydroxyapatite, it may be extracellular where it is in the form of inorganic ions. Intracellular phosphorus is bound to protein or exists as organic esters. Levels of inorganic phosphates are normally between 2.3 and 4.5 mg/dL.

Phosphorus, unlike the other elements, is 85 percent free and only 15 percent bound to proteins. Phosphate may be present in different forms such as $H_2PO_4^-$ or HPO_4^{2-}, and levels change with pH. The 85 percent of phosphorus that is free can be bound to Na^+, Ca^{2+}, or Mg^{2+}. Plasma phosphorus levels, unlike Ca^{2+} or Mg^{2+}, demonstrate diurnal variation with a morning nadir and are affected by age, hormones (insulin and growth hormone), and the amount of carbohydrate ingestion. Therefore, fasting levels should be measured, since glucose infusion as well as carbohydrate and phosphorus ingestion lower serum levels.

Normal daily intake is between 10 and 12 mmol. Phosphorus absorption is proportional to dietary intake. Approximately 70 percent is absorbed via passive transport, with the remainder via active transport, which is dependent on 1,25-$(OH)_2$-vitamin D. phosphate deficiency is rarely caused by a decrease in phosphorus oral intake unless absorption is affected. Phosphate excretion is proportional to oral intake. Excretion is predominantly in the urine by the glomerulus, with the majority resorbed in the proximal tubules. This is regulated by PTH, which acts to lower serum phosphate by increasing renal excretion. Proximal tubule absorption increases when serum phosphate levels drop, as well as with hypoparathyroidism, volume depletion, hypocalcemia, or the presence of growth hormone. Excretion increases in the presence of volume expansion, hypercalcemia, acidosis, hypomagnesemia, hypokalemia, glucocorticoids, diuretics, calcitonin, or PTH. Phosphate is essential to a wide variety of biochemical reactions, especially energy metabolism in the form of high-energy phosphate and phosphocreatine.

Hypophosphatemia

Since phosphorus is abundant in many foods and readily absorbed, hypophosphatemia is relatively unusual. Mechanisms leading to hypophosphatemia are reduced oral intake, excessive loss, or shift from the ECF into cells. Significant hypophosphatemia is unlikely to be encountered in the ED, because it is most often associated with hyperalimentation. There may be a shift into cells seen with alkalosis (respiratory or metabolic). Alcoholics may be in a sufficiently poor nutritional state that hypophosphatemia becomes an issue. Other conditions that may on occasion present to the ED with complications related to phosphate depletion include hyperparathyroidism, malignancy with hypercalcemia (phosphaturia), renal tubular defects, and use of phosphate-binding antacids. As explained earlier, hypokalemia and hypomagnesemia are likely to be associated with hypophosphatemia. Conditions unlikely to be seen in ED practice but associated with hypophosphatemia include rapid healing, prolonged anabolic states, recovery from starvation or severe burns, and partial hepatectomy.

Redistribution phenomena also can occur with glucose infusion. Phosphorus is consumed during phosphorylation as glucose moves into cells. This is one of the theoretical reasons why potassium phosphate is advocated as part of K^+ replacement regimens in the treatment for diabetic ketoacidosis. However, it should not be the initial form of K^+ replacement in the ED, as significant hypophosphatemia is unlikely to occur for 12 to 24 h, and parenteral administration may cause precipitous falls in serum [Ca^{2+}]. (Also see Chap. 203, "Diabetic Ketoacidosis.")

DIAGNOSIS Symptoms of hypophosphatemia are unlikely to appear until levels are quite low, usually less than 1 mg/dL. Patients with diabetic or alcoholic ketoacidosis or severe malnutrition may develop complications of hypophosphatemia. It should be particularly sought as a potential complication 12 to 24 h after initiating treatment for diabetic ketoacidosis and 24 to 96 h after treatment for alcoholic ketoacidosis. Detecting total body depletion cannot reliably be ascertained from blood phosphorus levels, as the ratio of intracellular to extracellular phosphorus is approximately 100:1.

PHYSIOLOGIC EFFECTS The most frequent consequences of hypophosphatemia are hematologic and neuromuscular. Hypophosphatemia may be associated with depletion of ATP in platelets, red blood cells, and white blood cells, reducing their survival time and function. Platelet membrane changes may result in a bleeding tendency due to impaired aggregation. Phosphate deficiency also causes a tendency for red blood cells to become rigid spherocytes, thereby impairing capillary perfusion. In addition, decreased 2,3-diphosphoglycerate (2,3-DPG) increases the affinity of hemoglobin for oxygen, thereby reducing the arterial P_{O_2} and oxygen availability to tissues. Phosphate depletion in macrophages may impair chemotaxis, phagocytosis, and intracellular killing, resulting in decreased resistance to infection.

Progressive weakness and tremors may be noted as blood phosphate levels fall below 0.5 to 1.0 mg/dL. Circumoral and fingertip paresthesias may be present along with absent deep tendon reflexes. Mental obtundation, anorexia, and hyperventilation may also occur. Myocardial function, as measured by left ventricular stroke work, may also be impaired.

TREATMENT Fortunately, phosphate deficiency is easily reversible by correcting the underlying disorder and replacing phosphorus. Milk is an excellent source of phosphorus and contains 1000 mg/L. Tablets come in the form of sodium or potassium phosphate and must be given in divided doses.

For severe hypophosphatemia with blood levels less than 1.0 mg/dL (0.32 mmol/L) or symptoms, immediate IV replacement is required. Otherwise, oral preparations can be often used.

If the hypophosphatemia is recent and uncomplicated, the initial recommended daily dose is 2.5 mg/kg. Prolonged or multifactorial hypophosphatemia may require 5 mg/kg. Up to 25 to 50 percent more phosphorus is needed if a patient is symptomatic; however, less is required in the presence of hypercalcemia. Each dose is administered

IV over 6 h, and serum phosphorus is checked after each dose. To minimize the risks of hyperphosphatemia, a total dose of no more than 7.5 mg/kg should be administered.

Risks of phosphate therapy include hypocalcemia, metastatic calcification, hypotension, and hyperkalemia from the potassium salts. One should switch to oral therapy as soon as possible.

Hyperphosphatemia

ETIOLOGY Hyperphosphatemia may be due to reduced renal excretion, increased phosphate movement out of cells into the ECF, or increased phosphorus or vitamin D intake. Hyperphosphatemia is most apt to be seen with renal dysfunction. It may also be seen with hypoparathyroidism or any problem associated with hypocalcemia or hypomagnesemia.

PHYSIOLOGIC EFFECTS Problems due to hyperphosphatemia are usually those due to associated renal failure, hypocalcemia, or the hypomagnesemia that is usually present.

THERAPY Therapy is aimed at treating the underlying cause and restricting calcium phosphate intake to less than 200 mg/day. With normal renal function, phosphate excretion can be increased with saline (1 to 2 L every 4 to 6 h) and acetazolamide (500 mg every 6 h). Phosphorus absorption from the gastrointestinal tract is decreased with oral phosphate binders (i.e., aluminum carbonate or hydroxide 30 to 45 mL qid). These binders also absorb phosphate secreted into the gut lumen and are of benefit even if no oral phosphorus is given. If clinically significant hypocalcemia exists, calcium should be cautiously administered. If renal failure is present, calcium carbonate is the treatment of choice to avoid aluminum toxicity. Hemodialysis may be required.

It may take years to correct the structural changes in bone that occur secondarily to long-term hypophosphatemia.

REFERENCES

1. Schlaerb PR, Friis-Hansen BJ, Edelman IS, et al: The measurement of total body water in the human subject by deuterium oxide dilution with consideration of the dynamics of deuterium distribution. *J Clin Invest* 29:1296, 1950.
2. Starling EH: Physiological factors involved in the causation of dropsy. *Lancet* 1:1405, 1896.
3. Pappenheimer JR: Passage of molecules through capillary walls. *Physiol Rev* 33:387, 1953.
4. Schrier RW: Treatment of hyponatremia. *N Engl J Med* 312:1121, 1985.
5. Krause JA, Carlson RW: Rapid correction of hypokalemia using concentrated intravenous potassium chloride infusion. *Arch Intern Med* 150:613, 1990.
6. Warrell PR Jr, Bachmon RJ, Coonley CJ, et al: Gallium nitrate inhibits calcium resorption and is effective treatment for cancer-related hypercalcemia. *J Clin Invest* 73:1487, 1984.

24 DISTURBANCES OF CARDIAC RHYTHM AND CONDUCTION

Edmund Bolton

The interpretation and treatment of cardiac dysrhythmias is basic to the practice of emergency medicine. This chapter reviews the important cardiac rhythm and conduction disturbances, their clinical significance, and their emergency treatment. Discussions of defibrillation, cardioversion, and artificial cardiac pacemakers are also included.

Although emphasis is appropriately placed on drug treatment of these dysrhythmias, it is also important that underlying and reversible causes of rhythm and conduction disturbance—such as hypoxia, alkalosis, electrolyte abnormalities, and drug toxicity—be recognized and treated.

THE NORMAL CARDIAC CONDUCTING SYSTEM

The heart consists of three types of specialized tissue: (1) pacemaker cells that undergo spontaneous depolarization and can initiate an electric impulse (this property is called *automaticity*); (2) cells that conduct electrical waves more rapidly than other cardiac cells, causing a very rapid propagation of the electric impulse throughout the heart, and (3) contractile cells, which contract when electrically depolarized.

The sinus [sinoatrial (SA)] node is normally the dominant cardiac pacemaker unless disease or drugs depress its activity. The SA node is located near the junction of the superior vena cava and right atrium. Blood supply is from the sinus node artery, which arises from either the proximal few centimeters of the right coronary artery (in about 55 percent of individuals) or from the proximal few millimeters of the left circumflex artery (in the other 45 percent). Both sympathetic and parasympathetic nerves, which are the primary controls of the heart rate, innervate the SA node. The normal sinus discharge rate is 60 to 100 beats per minute.

The electric impulse generated by the SA node spreads in waves through the cardiac muscles of the atria, activating atrial contraction. Additionally, specialized atrial conduction tracts (anterior, middle, and posterior internodal tracts) serve to propagate the electric impulse through the atria and between the sinus node and the atrioventricular (AV) node.

The atria and ventricles are insulated electrically from each other by the fibrous connective tissue of the AV ring (annulus fibrosus). Normally, electric impulses from the atria can reach the ventricles only by passing through the AV node and infranodal conducting system.

The AV node is under the surface of the right atrial endocardium and directly above the insertion of the septal leaflet of the tricuspid valve. The AV node receives its blood supply from the right coronary artery as it turns to form the posterior descending artery in 90 percent of individuals and, in the other 10 percent, as it comes off the left circumflex artery. This accounts for the common occurrence of AV conduction disturbances with acute inferior myocardial infarctions. The AV node is innervated by both sympathetic and parasympathetic fibers. It has two important electrophysiologic characteristics: a slow conduction velocity and a long refractory period. The slow conduction velocity through the AV node allows time for atrial contraction to give an extra 10 percent ventricular filling, which increases stroke volume according to the Frank-Starling principle. This "atrial kick" is most important for patients with ventricular failure. The long refractory period of the AV node protects the ventricles from excessively rapid stimulation; very rapid heart rates decrease the diastolic filling period and thereby reduce cardiac output, which may cause deterioration into ventricular fibrillation or cardiac failure. Cells near the AV node have automaticity and will escape from the control of the SA node if its rate becomes too low, normally below 60 beats per minute.

Electric impulses leave the inferior pole of the AV node along the bundle of His, which travels downward along the posterior margin of the membranous portion of the intraventricular septum to reach the top of the muscular portion. The bundle of His consists of Purkinje cells, which are the most rapidly conducting cells of the heart. The common bundle is only 1 to 2 cm in length before it divides at the crest of the muscular intraventricular septum into the right and left bundle branches (RBB and LBB). The RBB is a compact group of fibers that travels down to the apex of the right ventricle before separating into smaller branches. The LBB travels 2 to 3 cm before fanning out into a virtual sheet of fibers to cover the left ventricle. There are two relatively distinct pathways to the base of the papillary muscles, the left anterior superior fascicle (LASF) and the left posterior inferior fascicle (LPIF). These fascicles are distinguished more readily by

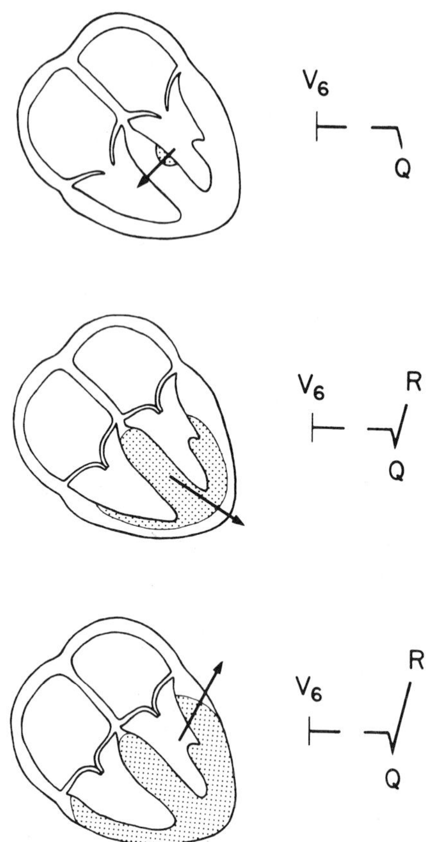

FIG. 24-1. Ventricular depolarization recorded in lead V_6.

electrical means in humans than by anatomy, but they can be seen clearly in animals.

The blood supply to the RBB and LASF is from the same sources: about half the time from both the AV nodal artery and branches from the left anterior descending coronary artery and the other half from the left anterior descending artery alone. The LPIF is supplied about half the time from the AV nodal artery and the other half by both the AV nodal artery and left anterior descending artery. Infarction in the region supplied by the left anterior descending artery is capable of affecting the RBB and LASF but very rarely the LPIF.

Accessory tracts are embryologic remnants of myocardium found in the AV annulus that can transmit electric impulses between the atria and ventricles, bypassing all or part of the AV node and infranodal system. These bypass tracts conduct at different rates and are the anatomic basis for the preexcitation syndrome.

THE NORMAL ELECTROCARDIOGRAM (ECG)

The clinical surface ECG records the potential (voltage) differences between "neutral" ground and recording electrodes. The ECG is generated by the electrical activity of the heart and depicts the net sum of this activity recorded over time. By convention, a potential difference that points toward a recording electrode is assigned a positive deflection on the ECG, and a potential that points away from the recording electrode is assigned a negative deflection. Also by convention, routine ECG recordings are obtained with paper speed at 25 mm/s (2.5 cm/s) and signal calibration of 1.0 mV/10 mm (1.0 cm).

In Fig. 24-1, depolarization starts on the left side of the ventricular septum and initially proceeds to the right; this is recorded as a small negative deflection in the recording electrode. Subsequent depolarization involves the free walls of both ventricles, and since the left side has a much larger mass, the net sum of electrical activity is directed toward the recording electrode and a tall, positive deflection is recorded.

The P-QRS-T complex of the normal ECG represents electrical activity over one cardiac cycle (Fig. 24-2).

The P wave is caused by atrial depolarization. The QRS complex usually obscures atrial repolarization. The normal P wave duration is less than 0.10 s (2.5 mm), and normal amplitude is less than 0.3 mV (3 mm). A P wave originating from the SA node is directed inferiorly and to the left on the frontal plane.

The PR interval is the time between the onset of depolarization in the atria and the onset of depolarization in the ventricles. It is commonly used as an estimation of AV nodal conduction time because the AV node is the most likely site for delay in conduction. For adults in sinus rhythm, the PR interval is 0.12 to 0.20 s (3 to 5 mm) at 25 mm/s.

The QRS complex indicates ventricular depolarization. In general, depolarization starts on the endocardium and spreads outward to the epicardium. Despite the large amount of myocardium that must be depolarized, the specialized conducting system makes this a rapid process and the normal QRS duration is 0.06 to 0.10 s (1.5 to 2.5 mm). Any delay in intraventricular conduction results in a wide QRS. Ectopic impulses that originate below the bundle of His or that arrive prior to repolarization of the bundle branches also result in a widened QRS because they do not use the Purkinje network.

While small negative initial deflections (Q waves) are normal, large Q waves can be due to an electrically unexcitable area just under the recording electrode. An abnormal Q wave has a width of 0.04 s or greater and a height one-third that of the QRS complex.

The ST segment represents the plateau phase of ventricular depolarization. While the ST segment is usually isoelectric, a small deviation, less than 0.1 mV (1 mm), is not always pathologic.

The T wave is caused by ventricular repolarization. Depolarization is a rapid, near-simultaneous release of stored energy (like the release of a compressed spring); repolarization is a slow, asynchronous event where the metabolic machinery of each individual cell restores the transmembrane potential. Therefore, the T-wave duration is much longer and the amplitude much lower than those of the QRS complex. In general, repolarization starts on the epicardium and spreads to the endocardium. Many factors can influence this normal repolarization sequence: (1) metabolic factors (hypoxia, fever, drugs), (2) autonomic stimuli (abdominal pain, hyperventilation), (3) myocardial hypertrophy, (4) myocardial ischemia or inflammation, and (5) abnormal depolarization (Bundle branch block).

The QT interval represents ventricular depolarization and repolarization. While QT duration is commonly between 0.33 and 0.42 s, it does vary inversely with heart rate. The corrected interval is obtained by dividing the measured QT interval (in seconds) by the square root of the R-R interval (in seconds). The normal corrected QT interval is less than 0.47 s. This corrected QT should be checked prior to giving drugs such as ibutilide (Corvert), a recently released drug for the conversion of new onset atrial fibrillation. If Corvert is given in face of a prolonged correct QT, it may cause torsades de pointes.

The U wave may be seen as a normal component of the surface ECG. It is best seen in leads V_1 and V_2. There is still some dispute as to the origin of the U wave. The classic explanation is that the U wave represents the delayed repolarization of the Purkinje network. More recent research has shown that the U wave can be seen at the same time as early afterdepolarizations (EADs) in patients with a prolonged QT interval and torsades de pointes.

CARDIAC DYSRHYTHMIAS

There are many protocols for the classification of dysrhythmias and conduction disturbances. Dysrhythmias are basically classified in rela-

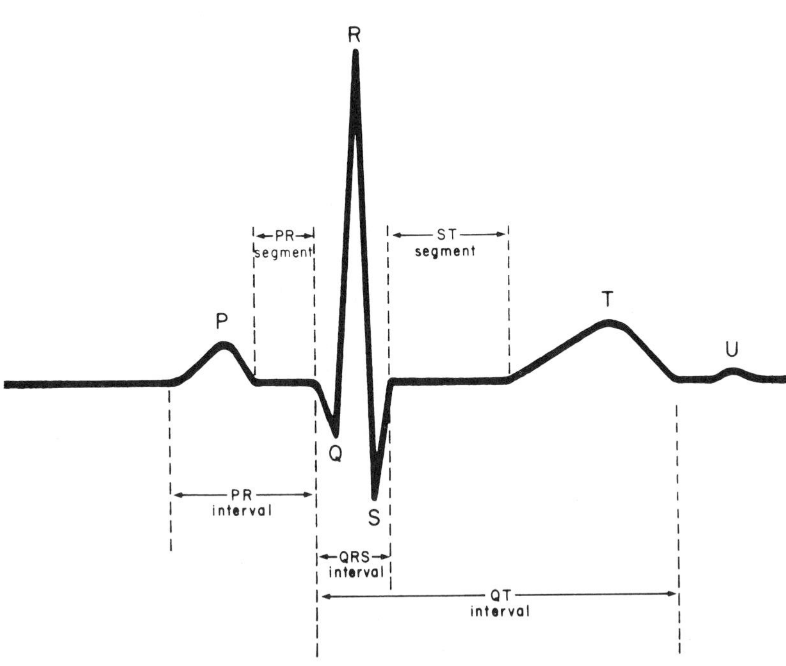

FIG. 24-2. Normal P-QRS-T ECG pattern.

tion to the rate and site of abnormality. Conduction disturbances are usually classified as to the site and degree of block.

Cardiac dysrhythmias may decrease cardiac output if the ventricular rate is too fast or slow. In an adult without cardiac disease, heart rates between 40 and 160 are usually well tolerated because physiologic adaptations are able to maintain an adequate cardiac output and blood pressure. In adults with significant heart disease, rates below 50 or above 120 may produce decreased cardiac output based on a poorly functioning ventricle because of basic myocardial cell damage, ischemic cells, valvular disease, or a combination of these.

Mechanisms of Tachydysrhythmias

There are three accepted mechanisms for dysrhythmias: (1) increased automaticity in a normal or ectopic site, (2) reentry in a normal or accessory pathway, and (3) afterdepolarizations causing triggered rhythms. While treatment is best directed by an understanding of the underlying process, uncertainty still exists over the precise mechanism of many dysrhythmias, and therapy is still often empiric.

An ectopic focus is an area of the heart, away from the normal sinus node pacemaker, that acquires independent pacemaker activity and usurps the pacemaking role. The result can be a single extrasystole or multiple extra depolarizations. These ectopic pacemakers can be the result of (1) enhanced automaticity of subsidiary pacemaker cells (i.e., in the AV node or infranodal conduting system) or (2) abnormal automaticity of myocardial cells, which seldom possess pacemaking activity (i.e., Purkinje cells). Dysrhythmias due to an ectopic focus usually have a gradual onset ("warmup period"). The termination is also gradual, as opposed to the abrupt onset and termination seen with reentry or triggered mechanisms.

Reentry was initially described when researchers took myocardial tissue and increased the K^+ concentration in a part of the tissue. They found that when stimulated, a rhythm was sustained without further stimulation at certain K^+ concentrations. Reentry requires a temporary or permanent unidirectional block in one limb of a circuit and slower-than-normal conduction around the entire circuit. These conditions are secondary to disease, drugs, accessory pathways, or when tissue is stimulated during the partial refractory period (before full repolarization), as with premature depolarizations.

As indicated in Fig. 24-3, the inciting impulse traveling in the normal downward direction encounters the two limbs, finds limb *a* blocked, and travels down limb *b*. Upon reaching the bottom portion of the circuit where the two limbs rejoin, the impulse can then travel retrograde up limb *a* and reach the upper connection of the circuit. Normally, conduction is so rapid that the impulse would encounter limb *b* still refractory to stimulation, and no further propagation would occur. However, if conduction around the circuit were slow enough, limb *b* would be able to conduct the impulse again in the antegrade direction. With the right size circuit and conduction velocity, an electric impulse can be maintained traveling around the circuit in a cyclic manner. Each time the impulse passes the upper and lower limb connections, a depolarization occurs.

Reentry can occur around anatomically defined circuits, resulting in a regular rapid rhythm such as paroxysmal supraventricular tachycardia. Conversely, reentry can also occur in a disorganized and chaotic fashion through a syncytium of myocardial tissue—as seen, for example, in atrial or ventricular fibrillation.

Triggered dysrhythmias are due to the oscillations of the transmembrane potential during or after repolarization (afterpotentials). Under

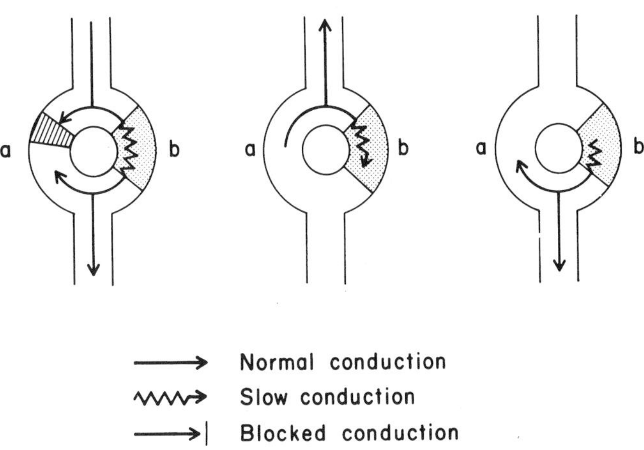

FIG. 24-3. Reentry circuit.

ideal conditions of rate, afterpotentials reach threshold and trigger a complete depolarization (afterdepolarization). Once triggered, this process may be self-sustaining. Triggered dysrhythmias associated with early afterpotentials are enhanced by slow heart rates and usually treated by accelerating the ventricular rate with positive chronotropic drugs or electrical pacing. Triggered dysrhythmias associated with delayed afterpotentials are enhanced by fast heart rates. Treatment with agents that have a negative chronotropic action is usually effective.

The urgency with which tachydysrhythmias require treatment is guided by two considerations: (1) evidence of hypoperfusion (shock, altered mental status, anginal chest pain, or pulmonary edema) and (2) the potential to degenerate into a more serious dysrhythmia or cardiac arrest. The two treatment methods most commonly used are intravenous drugs for the clinically stable patient and synchronized cardioversion or defibrillation for the unstable patient. Some tachydysrhythmias are amenable to overdrive electrical pacing but frequently require rates over 200 in order to capture the ventricle.

Mechanisms of Bradydysrhythmias

Bradydysrhythmias can be caused by two mechanisms: depression of sinus nodal activity or conduction system blocks. In both situations, subsidiary pacemakers take over and pace the heart; and provided the pacemaker is located above the bifurcation of the bundle of His, the rate is generally adequate to maintain cardiac output.

The need for emergent treatment of bradycardias is guided by two considerations: (1) evidence of hypoperfusion and (2) the potential to degenerate into a more profound bradycardia or ventricular asystole. In general, emergent treatment is not required, unless (1) the heart rate is below 50 and there is clinical evidence of hypoperfusion or (2) the bradycardia is due to structural disease of the infranodal conducting system (either transient or permanent) that has a risk of progressing to complete AV block. The first group of patients requires immediate treatment during assessment of the etiology of the bradycardia and consideration of whether internal pacing will be required. The second group of patients does not always require immediate treatment but should be monitored closely, with therapy readily available, while arrangements are made for further evaluation and possible internal cardiac pacing.

Three methods are currently available for emergent treatment of bradycardias: atropine, isoproterenol, and transcutaneous cardiac pacing.

Atropine should be the initial agent, at doses of 0.5 mg IV every 5 min until the desired response is achieved or a total vagolytic dose (about 0.05 mg/kg in humans) is given. Usually, if no response is seen by a dose of 2.0 mg, further doses are not effective. The vast majority of bradycardias due to problems of either the sinus or AV node respond to atropine. Even some patients with infranodal blocks may respond, so atropine deserves consideration in most bradycardias when emergent treatment is desired. Atropine can increase rate and myocardial oxygen consumption; therefore it has no place in an otherwise stable patient with bradycardia.

Isoproterenol can be used when atropine is ineffective, generally as a result of disease of the infranodal conducting system. Isoproterenol is given as a constant infusion, starting at a rate of around 0.5 μg/min and increasing as required to maintain a heart rate of 60. Isoproterenol increases myocardial oxygen demand, stimulates ventricular ectopy, and produces peripheral vasodilation, making it a less attractive agent than atropine. The reported response to isoproterenol is less than that observed with atropine, although isoproterenol is usually used only in patients who fail while receiving atropine. It is difficult to say how effective isoproterenol would be if used initially, and we do not suggest that.

External cardiac pacing represents a reemergence of an old concept with new electronics that make the technique more sensitive and likely to capture rhythm. This should be available in every emergency facility.

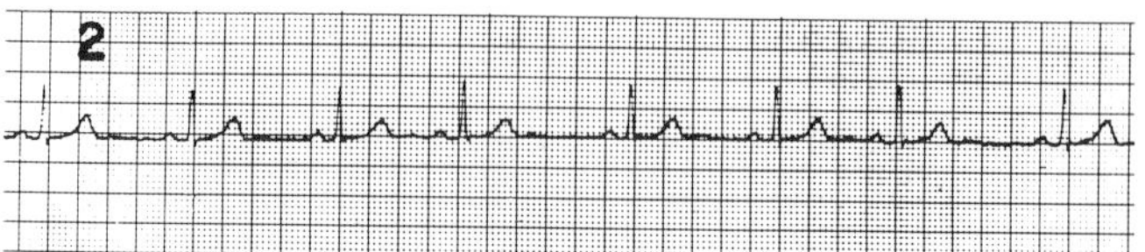

FIG. 24-4. Sinus dysrhythmia.

The emergency physician must become familiar with the technique of applying the transcutaneous pacemaker so that it will sense and pace appropriately.

Internal pacing is the definitive treatment for progressive or persistent bradycardias. Emergent internal pacing is possible with the use of balloon-tipped flotation catheters, although, without fluoroscopic guidance, it is often technically difficult to achieve stable placement in a patient with low cardiac output.

Supraventricular Dysrhythmias

SINUS DYSRHYTHMIA Some variation in the sinus node discharge rate is common, but if the variation exceeds 0.12 s between the longest and shortest intervals, sinus dysrhythmia is present. The ECG characteristics of sinus dysrhythmia are (1) normal sinus P waves and PR intervals, (2) 1 : 1 AV conduction, and (3) variation of at least 0.12 s between the shortest and longest P-P interval (Fig. 24-4).

Clinical Significance Sinus dysrhythmia is frequently a normal finding in children and young adults; it tends to disappear with advancing age. Sinus dysrhythmia is most commonly a phasic (respiratory variation) variety and less commonly a nonphasic variety. In the phasic variety, the sinus node rate accelerates during inspiration and decelerates during expiration because of changes in vagal tone occurring with respiration (Bainbridge reflex). The irregularity in either the phasic or nonphasic varieties can be exaggerated by conditions that increase vagal tone. During long intervals of sinus dysrhythmia, junctional escape beats may occur.

Treatment None is required.

SINUS BRADYCARDIA Sinus bradycardia occurs when the sinus node rate falls below 60. The ECG characteristics of sinus bradycardia are (1) normal sinus P waves and PR intervals, (2) 1 : 1 AV conduction, and (3) atrial rate below 60 (Fig. 24-5).

Clinical Significance Sinus bradycardia represents a suppression of the sinus node discharge rate. Sinus bradycardia can be (1) physiologic (in well-conditioned athletes, during sleep, or with vagal stimulation), (2) pharmacologic (digoxin, narcotics, reserpine, β-adrenergic antagonists, calcium channel blockers, quinidine), or (3) pathologic (acute inferior myocardial infarction, increased intracranial pressure, carotid sinus hypersensitivity, hypothyroidism).

Treatment

1. Sinus bradycardia usually does not require specific treatment unless the heart rate is below 50 and there is evidence of hypoperfusion.

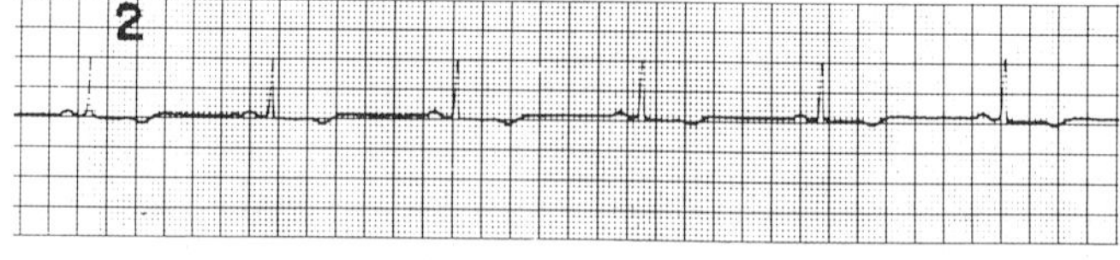

FIG. 24-5. Sinus bradycardia, rate 44.

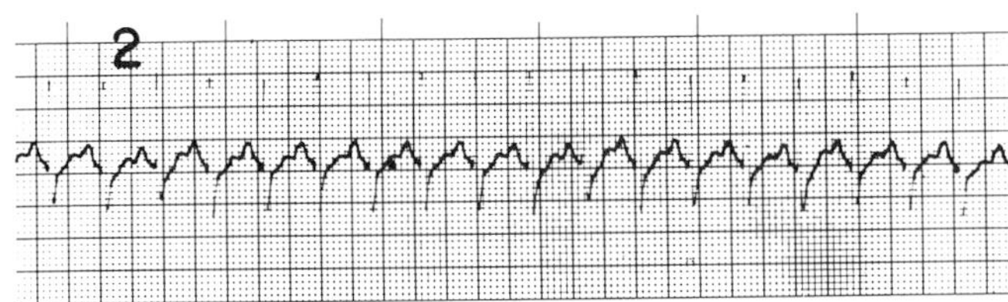

FIG. 24-6. Sinus tachycardia, rate 176.

2. Therapy should begin with atropine as previously described. Most patients will respond to one or two doses.
3. Isoproterenol can be used if atropine is ineffective.
4. External cardiac pacing can be used in the patient refractory to atropine or isoproterenol.
5. Internal pacing is required in the patient with symptomatic recurrent or persistent sinus bradycardia.

SINUS TACHYCARDIA Sinus tachycardia originates from acceleration of the sinus node discharge rate. The ECG characteristics of sinus tachycardia are (1) normal sinus P waves and PR intervals and (2) an atrial rate usually between 100 and 160 (Fig. 24-6).

Clinical Significance Sinus tachycardia represents an acceleration of the sinus node discharge rate, usually in response to three categories of stimuli: (1) physiologic (infants and children, exertion, anxiety, emotions), (2) pharmacologic (atropine, epinephrine and other sympathomimetics, alcohol, nicotine, caffeine), or (3) pathologic (fever, hypoxia, anemia, hypovolemia, pulmonary embolism). In many of these conditions, the increased heart rate is due to an effort to increase cardiac output to match increased circulatory needs.

Treatment

1. No specific treatment is usually required, but any underlying conditions should be investigated and treated.
2. Some patients with acute myocardial infarction have an "inappropriate" tachycardia and may benefit from slowing heart rate with β-adrenergic antagonists.

PREMATURE ATRIAL CONTRACTIONS (PACs) PACs originate from ectopic pacemakers anywhere in the atrium other than the sinus node. The ECG characteristics of PACs are that (1) an ectopic P′ wave appears sooner (prematurely) than the next expected sinus beat, (2) the ectopic P′ wave has a different shape and axis, and (3) the ectopic P′ wave may or may not be conducted through the AV node (Fig. 24-7). A PAC is not conducted through the AV node if it reaches the AV node during the absolute refractory period and is conducted with a delay (longer P′R interval) during the relative refractory period. Most PACs are conducted with typical QRS complexes, but some may be conducted aberrantly through the infranodal system if they reach a bundle branch during the refractory period. The sinus node is often depolarized and "reset," so that while the interval following the PAC is often slightly longer than the previous cycle length, the pause is less than fully compensatory.

Clinical Significance PACs are common at all ages and often seen in the absence of heart disease. It is generally assumed, although it remains unproven, that stress, fatigue, alcohol, tobacco, and coffee may precipitate PACs. Frequent PACs may also be seen in chronic lung disease, ischemic heart disease, or digitalis toxicity. PACs may precipitate sustained atrial tachycardia, flutter, or fibrillation under the right circumstances.

Treatment

1. Any precipitating drugs or toxins should be discontinued.
2. Underlying disorders should be treated.
3. PACs that produce symptoms or initiate sustained tachycardias can be suppressed with quinidine, procainamide, or β-adrenergic antagonists.

MULTIFOCAL ATRIAL TACHYCARDIA (MFAT) MFAT (also known as "chaotic atrial rhythm" or "wandering atrial pacemaker") is an irregular rhythm caused by at least three different sites of atrial ectopy. The ECG characteristics of MFAT are (1) three or more differently shaped P waves; (2) varying PP, PR, and RR intervals; and (3) atrial rhythm usually between 100 and 180 (Fig. 24-8). MFAT is frequently confused with atrial flutter or fibrillation.

Clinical Significance MFAT is most often found in elderly patients with decompensated chronic lung disease, but it may also complicate congestive heart failure or sepsis or be caused by methylxanthine toxicity. Digoxin toxicity is an unlikely cause of MFAT.

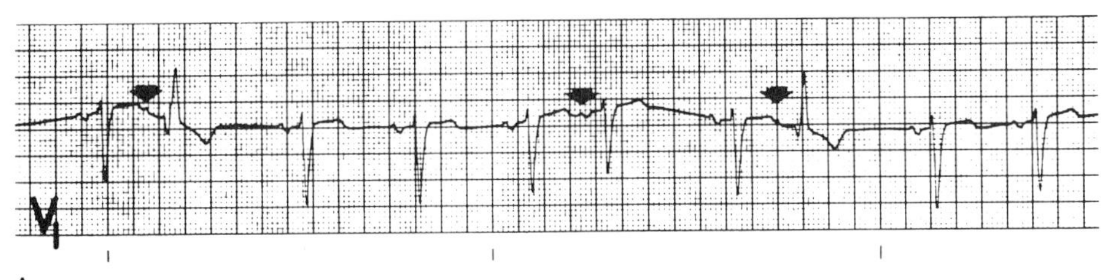

A

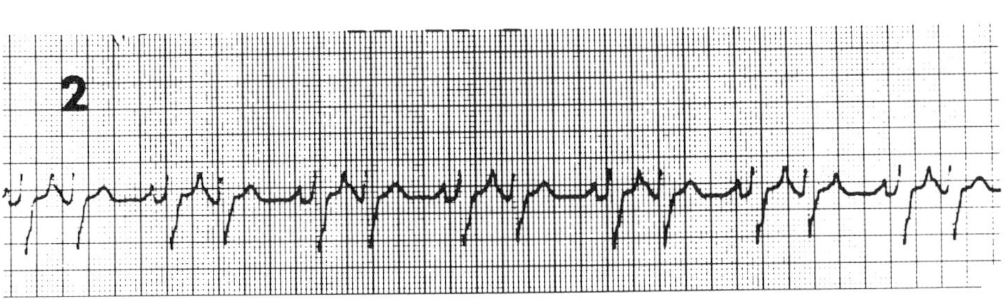

B

FIG. 24-7. Premature atrial contractions (PACs). Top: ectopic P′ waves (arrows). Bottom: atrial bigeminy.

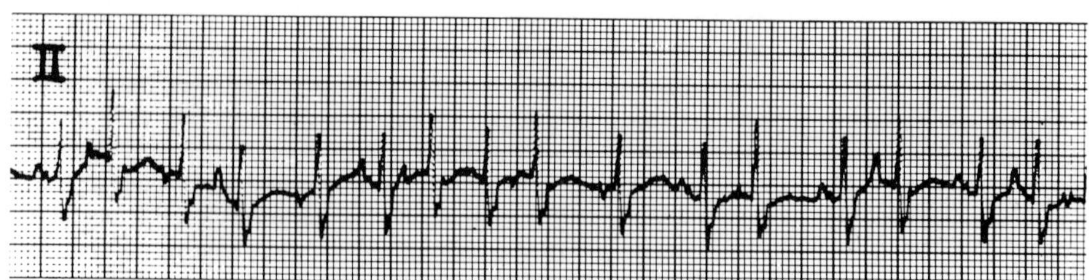

FIG. 24-8. Multifocal atrial tachycardia (MFAT).

Treatment

1. Treatment is directed toward the underlying disorder. With decompensated lung disease, oxygen and bronchodilators improve pulmonary function and arterial oxygenation and decrease atrial ectopy. Theophylline agents have been associated with the production or exacerbation of this dysrhythmia.
2. Specific antiarrhythmic treatment is rarely indicated. Standard antiarrhythmics appear to be ineffective in suppressing these multiple sites of atrial ectopy, and toxic side effects from these agents have been reported. Likewise, attempts to slow the ventricular rate by depressing AV nodal conduction with digoxin is also difficult without producing toxic side effects. Recently, three modes of therapy have been described that may be helpful in some patients. Magnesium sulfate 2 g IV over 60 s followed by a constant infusion of 1 to 2 g/h has been shown to reduce atrial ectopy in these patients and is sometimes associated with conversion to sinus rhythm. The full antiarrhythmic effect of magnesium requires supplemental potassium to maintain serum potassium levels above 4 meq/L. Intravenous verapamil (5 to 10 mg) slows the ventricular response in most patients, decreases atrial ectopy in some patients, and is associated with conversion to sinus rhythm in many patients. The β-adrenergic antagonists esmolol, acebutolol, and metoprolol all decrease the ventricular rate in MFAT, and metoprolol is associated with conversion to sinus rhythm in a majority of patients. However, theoretically, β-adrenergic therapy may worsen bronchospasm. The value of such specific antiarrhythmic treatment in MFAT is unproven.
3. Cardioversion has no effect on these multiple sites of atrial ectopy.

ATRIAL FLUTTER Atrial flutter usually originates from a localized area within the atria. The exact mechanism—whether reentry, automatic focus, or triggered dysrhythmia—is not yet known. Intracardiac studies demonstrate electrical activity usually originating in the inferior right atrium and propagating upward and to the left. ECG characteristics of atrial flutter are (1) regular atrial rate between 250 and 350 (most commonly 280 and 320); (2) sawtooth flutter waves directed superiorly and most visible in leads II, III, aV_F; and (3) AV block, usually 2 : 1, but occasionally greater, causing an irregular ventricular response (Fig. 24-9). One-to-one AV conduction may occur in the presence of bypass tracts or if drugs are used to slow the atrial rate to the level that the junction will be able to conduct one-to-one. If the ventricular rate is greater than 300, this should definitely be investigated with EP studies. Carotid sinus massage is a useful technique to slow the ventricular response, increase the AV block, and unmask flutter waves.

Clinical Significance Atrial flutter is usually associated with heart disease. It is most commonly found in patients with ischemic heart disease or acute myocardial infarction. Less common causes include congestive cardiomyopathy, pulmonary embolus, myocarditis, blunt chest trauma, and, rarely, digoxin toxicity. Atrial flutter may be a transitional dysrhythmia between sinus rhythm and atrial fibrillation.

Treatment

1. Low-energy cardioversion (25 to 50 J) is very successful in converting more than 90 percent of cases of atrial flutter into sinus rhythm. Energies less than 10 J should be avoided, as they are more likely to convert atrial flutter into atrial fibrillation than into sinus rhythm.
2. If cardioversion is contraindicated, control of ventricular rate can be achieved with digoxin, verapamil, diltiazem, esmolol, or propranolol. If there is 1 : 1 conduction and the rate is 300 and above, preexcitation should be considered and procainamide may be the drug of first choice.
3. Quinidine or procainamide can be used for 1 : 2 conduction after ventricular rate control is achieved to chemically slow or convert atrial flutter or prevent recurrence of the dysrhythmia.
4. Intravenous esmolol will convert up to 60 percent of patients with new-onset atrial flutter to sinus rhythm.
5. Intravenous verapamil will occasionally convert atrial flutter into sinus rhythm (up to 30 percent) or atrial fibrillation (up to 20 percent).
6. Some of the newer antiarrhythmics may also have a role in the chemical conversion of atrial flutter. Ibutilide (Corvert), mentioned earlier, can convert both atrial flutter and fibrillation to normal sinus rhythm. This drug should be used in new-onset atrial flutter (AF) because of the chance of emboli if used in long-term AF. Ibutilide is very effective in the conversion of atrial flutter or atrial fibrillation; however, there is a significant chance of torsades de pointes (TdP). To reduce the chance of TdP, it is suggested that the K^+ and the corrected QT (QTc) interval be checked prior to administration of the agent. This agent should not be given in the presence of

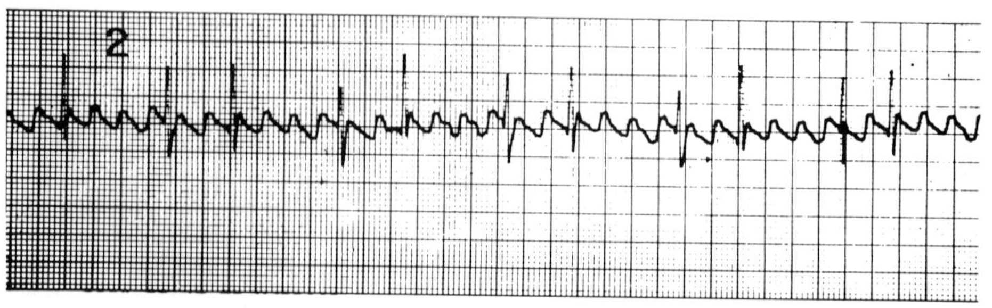

FIG. 24-9. Atrial flutter.

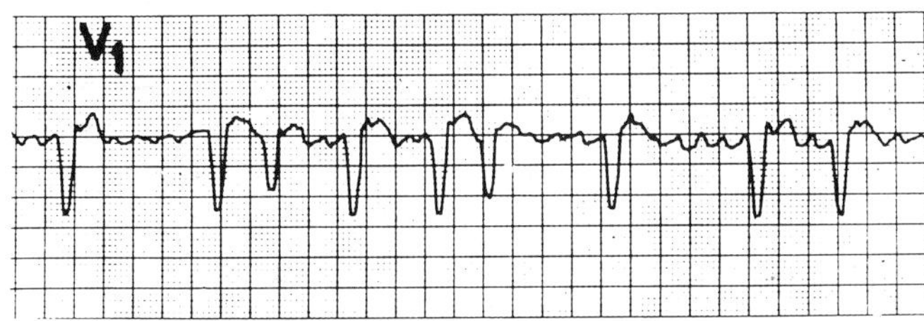

FIG. 24-10. Atrial fibrillation.

hypokalemia, prolonged QTc, or history of congestive heart failure (CHF). The chance of TdP can extend 4 to 6 h after the drug is given.

ATRIAL FIBRILLATION Atrial fibrillation occurs when there are multiple small areas of atrial myocardium continuously discharging and contracting. There is no uniform atrial depolarization and contraction—instead, only a quivering of the atrial wall. While the atrial rate is usually above 400, the ventricular rate is limited by the refractory period of the AV node or an accessory pathway. The ECG characteristics of atrial fibrillation are (1) fibrillatory waves of atrial activity, best seen in leads V_1, V_2, V_3, and aV_F; and (2) irregular ventricular response, usually around 170 to 180 in patients with a healthy AV node (Fig. 24-10). Disease or drugs (especially digoxin) may reduce AV node conduction and markedly slow ventricular response. A more rapid ventricular response may be seen in patients with bypass tracts, and the rate in these patients has been suggested as a way of estimating the refractory period of the accessory path. Rates above 300 are possible and dangerous. In this case, since ventricular activation occurs by way of the bypass tract, the QRS complex is usually wide. The configuration of the aberrancy may vary with the site of the one or more accessory pathways.

Clinical Significance Atrial fibrillation can occur in a paroxysmal or in a sustained manner. Predisposing factors for atrial fibrillation are increased atrial size and mass, increased vagal tone, and variation in refractory periods between different parts of atrial myocardium. Atrial fibrillation is usually found in association with four disorders: rheumatic heart disease, hypertension, ischemic heart disease, and thyrotoxicosis. Less common causes are chronic lung disease, pericarditis, acute alcoholic intoxication, or atrial septal defect.

In patients with left ventricular failure, left atrial contraction contributes significantly to cardiac output. The loss of effective atrial contraction, as in atrial fibrillation, may produce heart failure in these patients. Atrial fibrillation also predisposes to peripheral venous and atrial emboli, with the risk of pulmonary and systemic arterial embolism. Up to 15 percent of patients per year in chronic atrial fibrillation have at least one embolic episode. Conversion from chronic atrial fibrillation to sinus rhythm also carries up to a 1 to 2 percent risk of arterial embolism. Patients with chronic atrial fibrillation are frequently anticoagulated.

Treatment

1. Atrial fibrillation with a rapid ventricular response and acute hemodynamic deterioration should be treated with synchronized cardioversion. Over 60 percent of patients can be converted with 100 J and over 80 percent with 200 J. Conversion to and retention in sinus rhythm is more likely when atrial fibrillation is of short duration and the atria are not greatly dilated. If initial cardioversion is unsuccessful, procainamide should be given intravenously to facilitate further cardioversion attempts. Oral quinidine or low-dose amiodarone can enhance maintenance of sinus rhythm. Metanalysis and decision analysis of postconversion antiarrhythmic treatment has found that the benefits of maintaining sinus rhythm with antiarrhythmics is partially offset by an increase in sudden death, presumably due to the proarrhythmic properties of these drugs. In the emergency department (ED) setting, all other causes of hypotension, such as acute blood loss, must be ruled out before concluding that the rate is causing the hemodynamic deterioration.
2. In the more stable patient, the first priority is to achieve ventricular rate control. Diltiazem 10 to 20 mg (0.125 to 0.25 mg/kg) given intravenously over 2 min is extremely effective in achieving ventricular rate control, with the peak response seen in 2 to 7 min. An infusion of 10 mg/h is usually started after the initial dose to maintain control and a second dose of 25 mg (0.35 mg/kg) can be given at 15 min if rate control is not achieved. Verapamil 5 to 10 mg IV is effective in slowing the ventricular response in 60 to 70 percent of patients with atrial fibrillation and converts 10 to 15 percent into sinus rhythm. Intravenous β-adrenergic blockers (e.g., esmolol and propranolol) are effective, especially in patients with thyrotoxicosis or rheumatic mitral stenosis, but the depressive effects on myocardial contractility make them poor agents to use in patients with ventricular failure. Intravenous digoxin is an effective agent for this purpose, although the onset of action is slow, with a mean time of over 11 h to achieve ventricular rate control.
3. Once ventricular rate control has been achieved, chemical conversion can be considered with procainamide, quinidine, or verapamil. Intravenous procainamide has also been used as a single agent to chemically convert atrial fibrillation of short duration into sinus rhythm; however, ibutilide is being touted as a better agent. Because of the risk of intraatrial thrombi and arterial embolization, patients with atrial fibrillation of more than 2 days' duration should be anticoagulated systemically for 1 to 3 weeks prior to attempts at either chemical or electrical conversion. More recent work indicates that there may be some increased risk of embolism even with AF of less than 2 days' duration. An alternative to anticoagulation is to exclude atrial thrombi by transesophageal echocardiography. Those without visible thrombi can be safely cardioverted without the need for preconversion oral anticoagulation.
4. Patients with a slow ventricular response not due to digitalis have AV node disease and probably a more generalized disorder of cardiac conduction (second- or third-degree AV block is seen in these patients when in sinus rhythm). These patients are at increased risk for profound bradycardias or asystole following cardioversion or antiarrhythmic drug therapy.
5. In some patients with a rapid ventricular response, conversion will reveal a very slow rate (tachy-brady syndrome) because of underlying disease of the pacemaker tissue (sick sinus syndrome).

SUPRAVENTRICULAR TACHYCARDIA (SVT) Supraventricular tachycardia is a regular, rapid rhythm that arises from either reentry or an ectopic pacemaker in areas above the bifurcation of the bundle of His. The reentrant variety is clinically the most common. These patients often present with acute, symptomatic episodes termed *paroxysmal supraventricular tachycardia* (PSVT).

Ectopic SVT usually originates in the atria with an atrial rate of 100 to 250 (most commonly 140 to 200) (Fig. 24-11). The regular P waves can be mistaken for atrial flutter, or, if there is a 2 : 1 AV block, sinus rhythm.

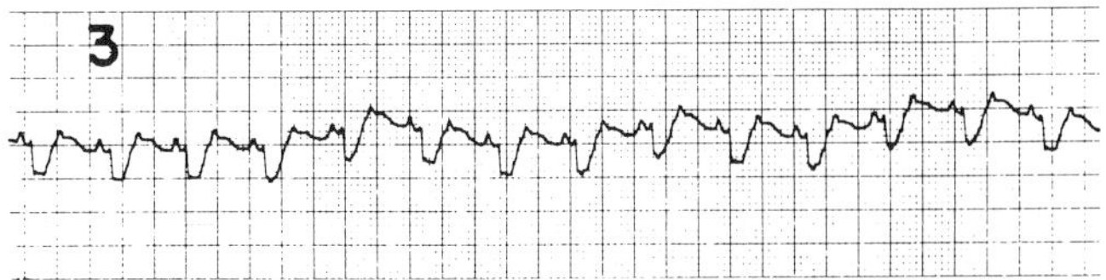

FIG. 24-11. Ectopic supraventricular, tachycardia (STV) with 2 : 1 AV conduction.

Reentrant SVT is seen in the majority of patients with SVT: about 60 percent of these patients have reentry within the AV node and 20 percent have reentry involving a bypass tract. The remainder have reentry in other sites. In the normal heart, reentrant SVT at the typical rates of 160 to 200 is often tolerated for hours or days. However, cardiac output is usually depressed—regardless of the blood pressure—and rapid rates may produce heart failure depending upon the health of the myocardium.

Reentrant SVT within the AV node usually is initiated when an ectopic atrial impulse encounters the AV node during the partially refractory period (Fig. 24-12). There are two functionally different parallel conducting limbs within the AV node that are connected above at the atrial end and below at the ventricular end of the node. This circuit is capable of sustained reentry when properly stimulated. In AV nodal reentry, the P wave is usually buried in the QRS complex and not visible, there is 1 : 1 conduction, and the QRS complex is normal.

Patients with bypass tracts have two parallel limbs of the reentry circuit, the AV node and the bypass tract, with connections at the atrial and ventricular ends by myocardial cells. While reentry can occur in either direction, it usually occurs in a direction that goes down the AV node and up the bypass tract, producing a narrow QRS complex (orthodromic conduction). In the Wolff-Parkinson-White syndrome, about 85 percent of the reentrant SVTs have narrow QRS complexes. If the conduction is down the accessory bundle and up the AV node (antidromic conduction), the complexes are wide and are difficult to differentiate from ventricular tachycardia.

Clinical Significance Ectopic SVT may be seen in patients with acute myocardial infarction, chronic lung disease, pneumonia, alcohol intoxication, and digoxin toxicity [where it is often associated with AV block and termed *paroxysmal atrial tachycardia* (PAT) with block]. It is commonly held that a high percentage of SVT with block, as much as 75 percent, is due to digoxin toxicity. However, not all studies have found this to be the case. In the test situation, PAT with block is still pathognomonic for digitalis toxicity. The common dysrhythmias of digoxin toxicity are listed in Table 24-1.

Reentrant SVT can occur in a normal heart or in association with rheumatic heart disease, acute pericarditis, myocardial infarction, mitral valve prolapse, or one of the preexcitation syndromes.

SVT often causes a sensation of palpitations and light-headedness. In patients with coronary artery disease, anginal chest pain and dyspnea may occur from the rapid heart rate. Frank heart failure and pulmonary edema may occur in patients with poor left ventricular function. The decrease in diastolic filling period and subsequent decrease in cardiac output cannot be tolerated in the patient with left ventricular failure.

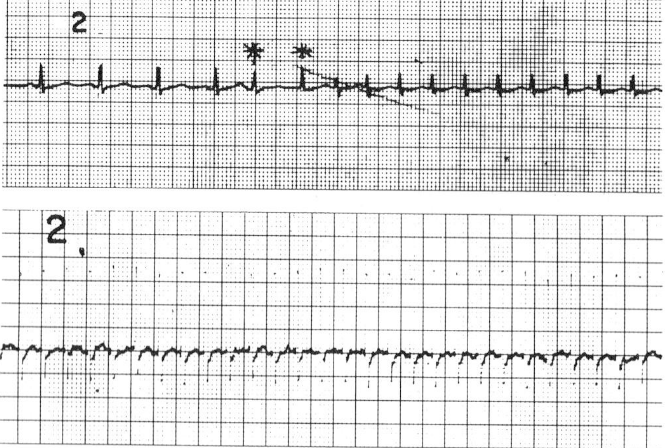

FIG. 24-12. Reentrant supraventricular tachycardia (SVT). Top: 2d (*) initiates run of PAT. Bottom: SVT, rate 286.

TABLE 24-1 Common Dysrhythmias of Digoxin Toxicity (Approximate Incidence)

PVCs (60%)
Unifocal, multifocal, bigeminy, or trigeminy
AV block (20%)
Second degree
Mobitz I, Mobitz II
Third degree
Ectopic SVT (20–30%)
Rate 70–130
Gradual appearance and disappearance
AV dissociation and or block
Junctional escape beats (10%)
Ventricular tachycardia (10%)
Bidirectional ventricular tachycardia associated with high mortality
Sinus bradycardia, SA block, and sinus pause (1–10%)

Treatment Ectopic SVT due to digoxin toxicity is treated as follows:

1. Discontinuation of the digoxin.
2. As long as there is not a high-grade AV block, correction of any existing hypokalemia to bring serum potassium into the high-normal range in an effort to reduce atrial ectopy is indicated.
3. Digoxin-specific antibody fragments (Fab) should be considered for patients with hemodynamic deterioration or serious ventricular dysrhythmias due to digoxin toxicity.
4. Either phenytoin, lidocaine, or magnesium given intravenously can reduce atrial ectopy. Published reports are not methodologically adequate for determination of the response rate, risks, and benefits of each agent, so the choice is often guided by personal preference. Historically, phenytoin has been the most commonly used drug, but its response rate has not been impressive and toxic side effects are common with full loading doses (15 to 18 mg/kg IV). Lidocaine has not been considered a useful agent for this dysrhythmia, but a recent report indicates some benefit. Recent studies indicate that magnesium sulfate 1 g IV impressively reduces atrial ectopy due to digoxin toxicity, and perhaps this agent has a greater effect than phenytoin or lidocaine.
5. Cardioversion is not effective and is potentially hazardous.

Reentrant SVT can be converted by impeding conduction through one limb of the reentry circuit; sustained reentry is then impossible and extinguishes, allowing sinus rhythm to resume ventricular pacing. Since it is usually impossible to differentiate ectopic from reentrant SVT clinically, treatment should be the same.

1. Maneuvers that increase vagal tone have been shown to slow conduction and prolong the refractory period in the AV node. These maneuvers can be done by themselves or after administration of drugs.
   a. Carotid sinus massage. This attempts to massage the carotid sinus and its baroreceptors against the transverse process of C6. Massage should be done for 10 s at a time, first attempted on the side of the nondominant cerebral hemisphere, and should never be done simultaneously on both sides. In addition, bruits should be discovered prior to the procedure. Prolonged AV block during carotid massage may occur in patients with AV node disease or who are on digoxin. Patients with carotid artery stenosis may develop cerebral ischemia or infarction from overvigorous carotid massage.

b. Facial immersion in cold water for 6 to 7 s with the nostrils held closed (''diving reflex''). This maneuver is particularly effective in infants. The parents usually have more vagal tone than the infant so this must be approached carefully.

c. The Valsalva maneuver. Done in the supine position, it appears to be the most effective vagal maneuver for the conversion of reentrant SVT. For maximal effectiveness, the strain phase must be adequate (usually at least 10 s) with slowing or conversion seen during the release phase.

2. Administration of adenosine. An ultra-short-acting (20 s) agent, adenosine produces AV block and has been observed to convert over 90 percent of reentrant SVT. The initial dose is a 6-mg rapid IV bolus. This must be given in a large vein, preferably in the antecubital space. If no effect is seen within 2 min, a second dose of 12 mg can be given. There is no proven benefit to repeated doses or administration of more than 20 mg. Half or more of patients experience distressing albeit transient side effects of facial flushing or chest pain. This should obviously be discussed with the patient when possible. Because adenosine possesses no sustained antiarrhythmic effect, subsequent ectopic beats are able to initial the dysrhythmia again, and early recurrences of SVT are seen in up to 25 percent of patients. The major advantage of adenosine is its ultrashort effect and its lack of hypotensive or myocardial depressive activity. Adenosine is also safe and effective in unstable patients (chest pain and/or hypotension) with reentrant SVT. It is safer in pregnancy. In addition, it is not contraindicated in the presence of Wolff-Parkinson-White syndrome.

3. Verapamil, 0.075 to 0.15 mg/kg (3 to 10 mg) IV over 15 to 60 s, with a repeat dose in 30 min if necessary. Studies have found that more than 90 percent of adults with reentrant SVT will respond within 1 to 2 min to verapamil. In patients with a normal blood pressure, intravenous verapamil is almost always associated with a decrease in blood pressure, even following successful conversion of SVT. The falls in systolic and mean arterial pressures are around 20 and 10 mmHg, respectively. The drop in blood pressure due to verapamil can be prevented and/or treated with intravenous calcium without reducing the antiarrhythmic action of verapamil. While the use of different calcium doses and salts has been reported, 90 mg of elemental calcium given intravenously over 3 to 6 min appears safe and effective (90 mg elemental calcium = 10 mL calcium gluconate 10% solution = 3.3 mL calcium chloride 10% solution). Whenever verapamil is used intravenously, calcium should be readily available. Intravenous verapamil is generally considered to be contraindicated in the hypotensive patient. Studies of intravenous verapamil in hypotensive patients with SVT report an excellent conversion rate (80 percent or better), the ventricular rate almost always slows, and rarely does the systolic blood pressure decrease without a change in ventricular rate. I would consider cardioversion a better approach to the hypotensive patient with SVT.

4. Diltiazem 20 mg (0.25 mg/kg) IV over 2 min. This is reported to be 75 to 100 percent effective in converting reentrant SVT.

5. Parasympathetic tone can be increased with edrophonium. A standard treatment protocol is a 1-mg IV test dose, a wait of 3 to 5 min, followed by 5 to 10 mg IV over 60 s. Historically, edrophonium does not have the 90 percent response rate seen with verapamil. I have not used this drug for the last 12 years but have noted that, most likely, it was the profound vomiting that caused the conversion rather than the direct effect of the drug.

6. Vagal tone can be enhanced by pharmacologically evaluating blood pressure with a pure peripheral vasoconstrictor; do not use agents with β-adrenergic activity. This method should be combined with carotid sinus massage. Blood pressure should be monitored frequently, and diastolic pressure should not be allowed to exceed 130 mmHg. This method should not be used if hypertension is already present.

a. Metaraminol 200 mg/500 mL D_5W or norepinephrine 4 mg/500 mL D_5W can be infused at rates of 1 to 2 mL/min and titrated until the rhythm converts.

b. Methoxamine or phenylephrine 0.5 to 1.0 mg IV over 2 to 3 min, with repeat doses as required.

7. Esmolol is an intravenous β-adrenergic blocker with an ultrashort duration of activity that can be titrated to effect. This agent can be used to control the ventricular rate in most tachycardias of supraventricular origin and is capable of converting about half of reentrant SVT. Esmolol is given as a bolus dose of 300 μg/kg over 60 s, followed by an infusion starting at 50 μg/kg per min. If there is an inadequate response after 2 to 5 min, a repeat bolus of 300 μg/kg should be given and increases in the infusion rate in increments of 50 μg/kg per min. should be made. The maximal recommended infusion rate is 300 μg/kg per min., although most patients respond to rates of 200 μg/kg per min. or less. With aggressive dosing regimens, hypotension occurs in about half of patients but can be quickly reversed by halting the infusion.

8. Propranolol 0.5 to 1.0 mg IV slowly over 60 s, repeated every 5 min, until the rhythm converts or the total dose reaches 0.1 mg/kg. Overall, propranolol has about a 50 percent success rate in converting reentrant SVT: about 80 percent with AV nodal reentry and 15 to 20 percent with accessory tract retrograde reentry.

9. Digoxin 0.5 mg IV with repeat doses of 0.25 mg in 30 to 60 min until a response occurs or the total dose reaches 0.02 mg/kg. The chief drawback of digoxin has been its long onset of action and potential hazard in patients with accessory (bypass) tracts who develop either atrial fibrillation or flutter.

10. External noninvasive pacing has been used in a limited number of patients to terminate reentrant SVT. Asynchronous pacing with 2 to 10 external pulses at a rate 240 to 280 (typically 40 faster than the SVT rate) with an impulse amplitude of 120 mA is effective in young, hemodynamically stable adults. Most pacing units in the ED do not pace at 240 to 280 beats per min. Some automatic internal cardiac defibrillators (AICDs) have overdrive pacing capability.

11. Synchronized cardioversion should be done in any unstable patient with hypotension, pulmonary edema, or severe chest pain. The dose required is usually small, less than 50 J.

Junctional Dysrhythmias

Traditionally, a junctional impulse is considered to be one that arises from the AV node or bundle of His above the bifurcation. Pacemaker tissue cannot be found in the AV node of experimental animals. The question is not settled in humans. From its source, probably in the junction, the impulse spreads retrograde toward the atria and antegrade toward the ventricles. Depending on the site of origin, conduction velocity, and refractory periods, the atria may be activated before, during, or after ventricular depolarization. Atrial depolarization may not be visible if retrograde conduction is blocked or atrial activation occurs simultaneously with ventricular activation and the QRS complex obscures the P waves. AV dissociation may occur if the rate of discharge from the junctional pacemaker is faster than the sinus node rate and the junctional impulse is blocked from retrograde conduction toward the atria.

JUNCTIONAL PREMATURE CONTRACTIONS (JPCs) JPCs are due to an ectopic pacemaker within the AV node or common AV bundle. The ECG characteristics of JPCs are as follows:

1. The ectopic QRS complex is premature.
2. The ectopic P′ wave has a different shape and direction (usually inverted in leads II, III, and aV_F).
3. The ectopic P′ wave may occur before or after the QRS complex.
4. The PR interval of the ectopic beat is shorter than normal.

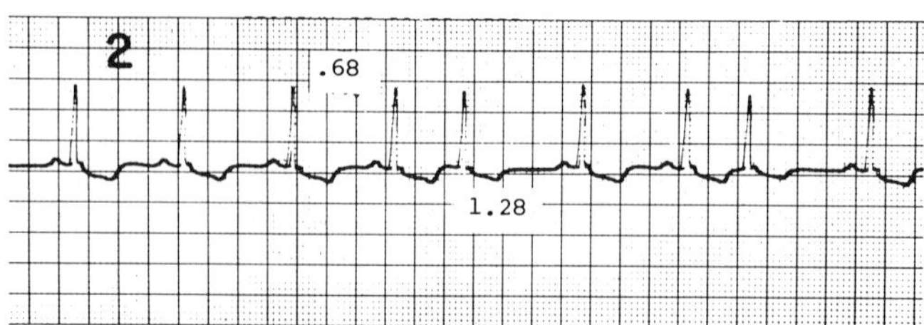

FIG. 24-13. Junctional premature contractions (JPCs).

5. The QRS complex is usually of normal shape unless there is aberrant conduction.
6. The sinus node is usually affected and the postectopic pause is not fully compensatory (Fig. 24-13). Some JPCs do not conduct retrograde; therefore a compensatory pause may be seen.

JPCs may be isolated, multiple (as in bigeminy or trigeminy), or multifocal.

Clinical Significance JPCs are uncommon in healthy hearts. They occur in congestive heart failure, digoxin toxicity, ischemic heart disease, and acute myocardial infarction (especially of the inferior wall).

Treatment

1. No specific treatment is usually required.
2. Treat the underlying disorder.
3. Antiarrhythmic therapy with quinidine or procainamide may be useful if JPCs are frequent, symptomatic, or initiate more serious dysrhythmias.

JUNCTIONAL RHYTHMS Under normal circumstances, the sinus node discharges at a faster rate than the AV junction, so the pacemaker function of the AV junction and all other slower pacemakers is suppressed (overdrive suppression). If sinus node discharges slow or fail to reach the AV junction, then junctional escape beats may occur, usually at a rate between 40 and 60, depending on the level of the pacemaker. Generally, junctional escape beats do not conduct retrograde into the atria, so a QRS complex without a P′ wave is usually seen (Fig. 24-14).

Under other circumstances, enhanced junctional automaticity may override the sinus node and produce either an accelerated junctional rhythm (rate 60 to 100) or junctional tachycardia (rate greater than 100). Usually, the enhanced junctional pacemaker (Fig. 24-15) captures both the atria and ventricles.

Clinical Significance Junctional escape beats may occur whenever there is a long enough pause in the impulses reaching the AV junction: sinus bradycardia, slow phase of sinus dysrhythmia, AV block, or during the pause following premature beats. Sustained junctional escape rhythms may be seen with congestive heart failure, myocarditis, hypokalemia, or digoxin toxicity. If the ventricular rate is too slow, myocardial or cerebral ischemia may develop.

Accelerated junctional rhythm and junctional tachycardia may occur from digoxin toxicity, acute rheumatic fever, or inferior myocardial infarction. With digoxin toxicity, the rate is usually between 70 and 130. If this rhythm develops in a patient being treated with digoxin for atrial fibrillation, the ECG is characterized by regular QRS complexes superimposed on atrial fibrillatory waves. Regulation of ventricular response during digoxin therapy in a patient with atrial fibrillation should therefore raise the suspicion of digoxin toxicity.

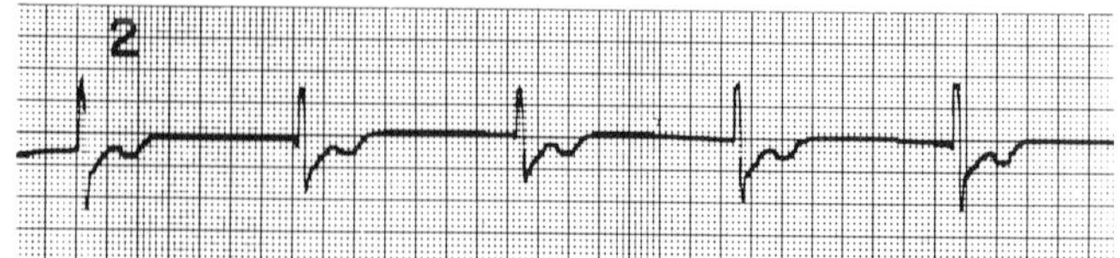

FIG. 24-14. Junctional escape rhythm, rate 42.

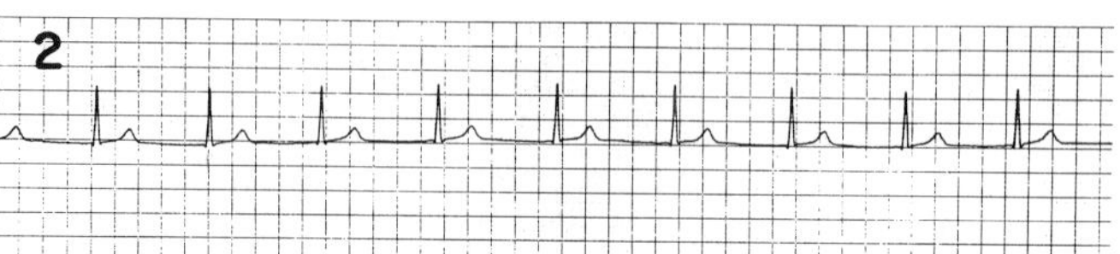

FIG. 24-15. Accelerated junctiional rhythm, rate 61.

Treatment

1. Isolated, infrequent junctional escape beats usually do not require specific treatment.
2. If sustained junctional escape rhythms are producing symptoms, the underlying cause should be treated. Atropine can be used to accelerate the sinus node discharge rate temporarily and enhance AV nodal conduction.
3. Accelerated junctional rhythm and junctional tachycardia usually do not produce significant symptoms. If the cause is digoxin toxicity, the drug should be discontinued. If the rate is fast and producing symptoms, giving supplemental potassium to increase the serum level into the high-normal range may decrease it.

Ventricular Dysrhythmias

PREMATURE VENTRICULAR CONTRACTIONS (PVCs) PVCs are due to impulses originating from single or multiple areas in the ventricles. The ECG characteristics of PVCs are as follows:

1. There is a premature and wide QRS complex.
2. There is no preceding P wave.
3. The ST segment and T wave of the PVC are directed opposite the major QRS deflection.
4. Most PVCs do not affect the sinus node, so there is usually a fully compensatory postectopic pause or the PVC may be interpolated between two sinus beats.
5. Many PVCs have a fixed coupling interval (within 0.04 s) from the preceding sinus beat.
6. Some PVCs are conducted into the atria, producing a retrograde P wave (Fig. 24-16).

Occasionally, a ventricular fusion beat occurs when supraventricular and ventricular impulses depolarize the ventricles almost simultaneously. The QRS configuration of a fusion beat contains features of the individual components.

A PVC may be confused with an aberrantly conducted supraventricular beat. Several clinical and ECG criteria can be used to help distinguish aberrantly conducted supraventricular beats from PVCs; this is discussed later in this section.

Clinical Significance PVCs are very common, even in patients without evidence of heart disease. They occur in most patients with ischemic heart disease and are universally found in patients with acute myocardial infarction (MI). Other common causes of PVCs include digoxin toxicity, congestive heart failure, hypokalemia, alkalosis, hypoxia, and sympathomimetic drugs.

While there is a correlation between the severity of underlying coronary artery disease and the degree of ventricular ectopy, there is disagreement as to whether ventricular ectopy itself is an independent risk factor for future morbidity or mortality. Most studies indicate that

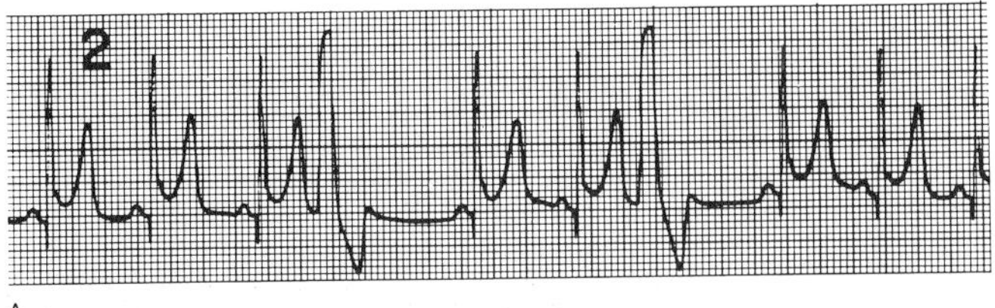

A

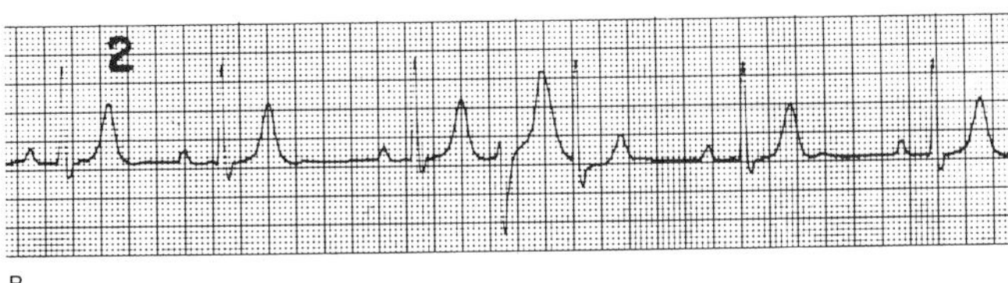

B

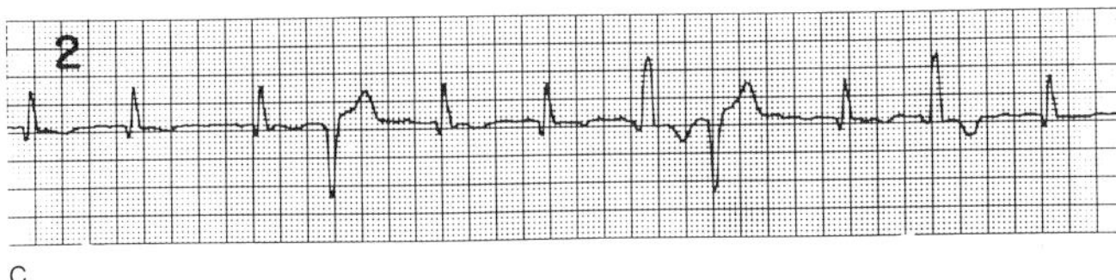

C

FIG. 24-16. Premature ventricular contractions (PVCs). Top: unifocal PVC. Center: interpolated PVC. Bottom: multifocal PVCs.

repetitive PVCs (two or more in a row) do have some associated independent risk in patients with coronary artery disease, but the evidence for other forms of ventricular ectopy is less convincing. Lown has made an attempt with his classification to quantitate the risks associated with chronic ventricular ectopy, but his classification is not universally accepted (Table 24-2). It must be remembered that his classification was made using patients with recent acute MIs.

In the setting of an acute MI, PVCs indicate the underlying electrical instability of the heart. The patients are at increased risk for the development of primary ventricular fibrillation. Current work indicates that various degrees of PVCs (''warning dysrhythmias'') are not reliable predictors of subsequent ventricular fibrillation.

Although it is experimentally established that electric impulses, such as PVCs, that occur during or soon after repolarization (the so-called vulnerable period) can initiate ventricular tachycardia or fibrillation, clinical studies have found that late-coupled PVCs initiate more paroxysms of ventricular tachycardia than early-coupled PVCs (R-on-T phenomenon).

Treatment

1. Most patients with acute myocardial disease and PVCs will respond to intravenous lidocaine, although some patients may require procainamide. In the setting of acute myocardial ischemia (unstable angina or acute MI), many physicians would treat frequent or multiform PVCs with the goal of reducing deaths due to sudden ventricular tachycardia or fibrillation. While single studies have suggested benefit, pooled data and metanalyses find no reduction in mortality from either suppressive or prophylactic treatment of PVCs.
2. In patients with chronic PVCs, there is no evidence that oral antiarrthymics enhance survival. To the contrary, large, randomized studies of postinfarction patients found that treatment with encainide, flecainide, or moricizine increased the incidence of cardiac arrest or arrhythmic death, probably related to their proarrthymic effects. Before treating chronic PVCs, the physician should consider several factors:
   a. Underlying heart disease
   b. The nature of the ectopy
   c. The presence or absence of symptoms
   d. The potential side effects of oral antiarrhythmic therapy
   e. Which technique will be used to judge efficacy of therapy (continuous monitoring versus EP studies)? Oral antiarrhythmic therapy requires careful monitoring. In some patients at risk of sudden cardiac death, automatic internal cardiac defibrillators (AICDs) are used in conjunction with antiarrthymics.

TABLE 24-2 Lown Grading System for Ventricular Ectopy

Grade	ECG Characteristics
1	Uniform PVCs < 30/h
2	Uniform PVCs > 30/h
3	Multiform PVCs
4A	Couplets (2 consecutive PVCs)
4B	Triplets (3 or more consecutive PVCs)
5	R-on-T PVCs

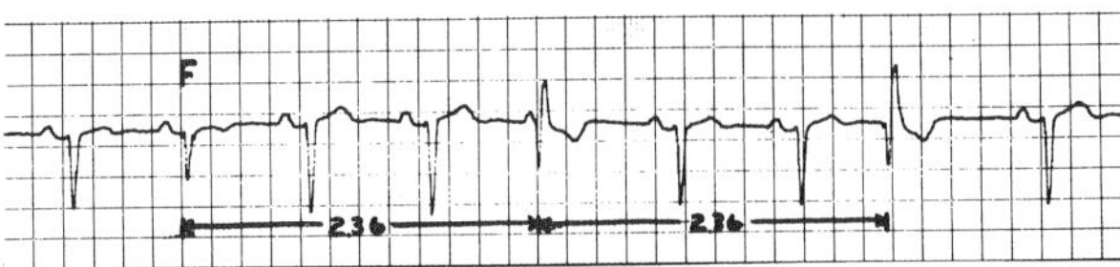

FIG. 24-17. The fifth and eighth ventricular complexes are premature and of similar morphology but have different coupling intervals. The second complex (marked ''F'') represents a fusion beat. The interectopic interval is 2.36 s. (From Heger JW, Niemann JT, Boman KG, et al: *Cardiology for the House Officer.* Baltimore, Williams & Wilkins, 1982. Used by permission.)

VENTRICULAR PARASYSTOLE Parasystole occurs when an independent ectopic pacemaker is protected from the influence of outside impulses (entrance block) and competes with the dominant pacemaker to produce myocardial depolarizations. A parasystolic pacemaker can arise anywhere in the heart but is most often located in the ventricles, where it produces a rhythm that operates in competition with the sinus node. This ectopic pacemaker has an innate rate; however, not all beats depolarize the ventricle (exit block).

The ECG characteristics of ventricular parasystole are (1) variation in the coupling interval between the preceding sinus beat and the ectopic beat, (2) common relation between the interectopic beat intervals, and (3) occurrence of fusion beats (Fig. 24-17). Usually, long rhythm strips are necessary to establish that the interectopic intervals are multiples of a common parasystolic pacemaker. Because of the difference in response to antiarrthymics, it is important to recognize and differentiate parasystolic beats from PVCs.

Clinical Significance Ventricular parasystole is most often associated with severe ischemic heart disease, acute MI, hypertensive heart disease, or electrolyte imbalance. Parasystole is often self-limited and benign but infrequently may lead to ventricular tachycardia or fibrillation.

Treatment

1. The underlying disease should be treated.
2. Antiarrhythmics are indicated in patients with symptomatic episodes or beats that initiate ventricular tachycardia.

ACCELERATED IDIOVENTRICULAR RHYTHM (AIVR) AIVR is an ectopic rhythm of ventricular origin occurring at a rate of 40 to 100.

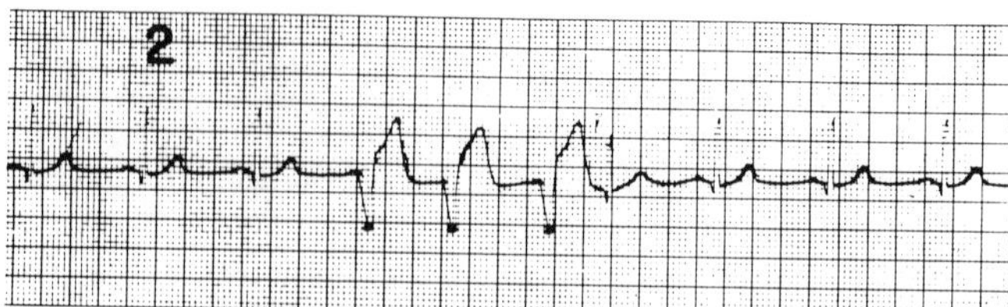

FIG. 24-18. Accelerated idioventricular rhythms (AIVR).

Even though AIVR is not a tachycardia, such terms as *idioventricular tachycardia, nonparoxysmal ventricular tachycardia,* or *slow ventricular tachycardia* are sometimes used to describe this rhythm.

The ECG characteristics of AIVR are (1) wide and regular QRS complexes, (2) a rate between 40 and 100 that is often close to the preceding sinus rate, (3) most runs of short duration (3 to 30 beats), and (4) an AIVR often beginning with a fusion beat (Fig. 24-18).

Clinical Significance This condition is found most commonly in the setting of an acute MI. Reports indicate that AIVR sometimes appears during successful thrombolysis of an occluded coronary artery. AIVR and other ventricular dysrhythmias seen during this time are termed *reperfusion dysrhythmias.* AIVR may be seen infrequently in patients without organic heart disease. While there is some variable association with ventricular tachycardia, there is no apparent association with ventricular fibrillation. AIVR usually produces no symptoms itself. Sometimes the loss of atrial contraction and subsequent fall in cardiac output may produce hemodynamic deterioration.

Treatment

1. Treatment is not necessary. On occasion, AIVR may be the only functioning pacemaker, and suppression with lidocaine can lead to cardiac asystole.
2. If sustained AIVR produces symptoms secondary to a decrease in cardiac output, treatment with atrial pacing may be required.

VENTRICULAR TACHYCARDIA Ventricular tachycardia is the occurrence of three or more depoplarizations from a ventricular ectopic pacemaker at a rate greater than 100. The ECG characteristics of ventricular tachycardia are (1) wide QRS complexes; (2) rate greater than 100 (most commonly 150 to 200); (3) rhythm usually regular, although there may be some beat-to-beat variation; and (4) QRS axis usually constant (Fig. 24-19). Uncommonly (about 5 percent of episodes), ventricular tachycardia may have a narrow (<120 ms) QRS complex. In these cases, ECG criteria usually suggest a ventricular origin (see ''Aberrant versus Ventricular Tachyarrhythmias,'' below). Ventricular tachycardia can occur in a nonsustained manner—usually short episodes, lasting seconds, with spontaneous termination—or in a sustained fashion—longer episodes that typically require treatment.

There are several variants of ventricular tachycardia. *Ventricular flutter* is the phrase used for a regular zigzag pattern without distinguishable QRS complexes or T waves. In *bidirectional ventricular tachycardia,* the QRS complexes alternate polarity as recorded in a single lead. In *alternating ventricular tachycardia,* the QRS complexes alternate in height (but not polarity) in a single lead. (Both bidirectional and alternating ventricular tachycardia indicate serious myocardial disease and are often due to digitalis toxicity.) In *polymorphous ventricular tachycardia,* the QRS complexes have many different shapes in one lead. *Atypical ventricular tachycardia* [torsade de pointes (TdP), or ''twisting of the points''] is where the QRS axis swings from a positive to negative direction in a single lead (Fig. 24-20). This rhythm results from a triggered arrhythmic mechanism. TdP usually occurs in short runs of 5 to 15 s at a rate of 200 to 240. This form of ventricular tachycardia generally occurs in patients with serious myocardial disease who have a prolonged and uneven ventricular repolarization (prolonged QT interval) (Table 24-3).

Drugs that further prolong repolarization—quinidine, disopyramide, procainamide, phenothiazines, and tricyclic antidepressants—

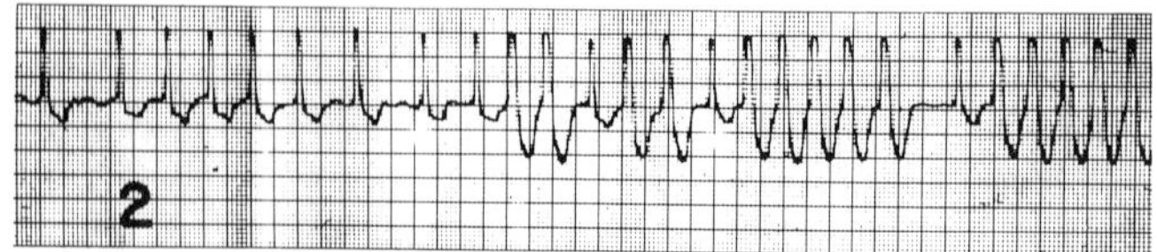

FIG. 24-19. Ventricular tachycardia.

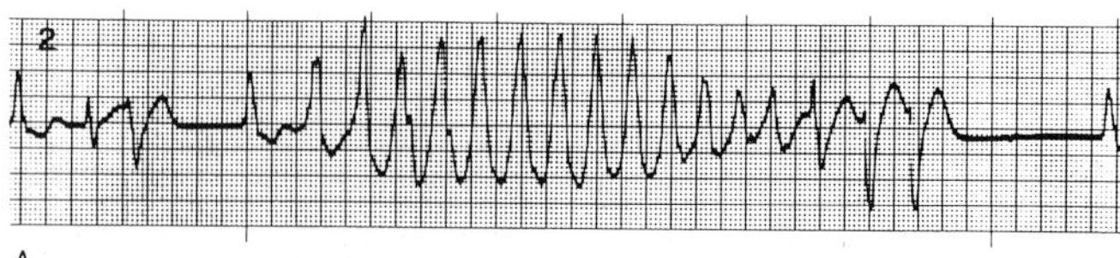

A

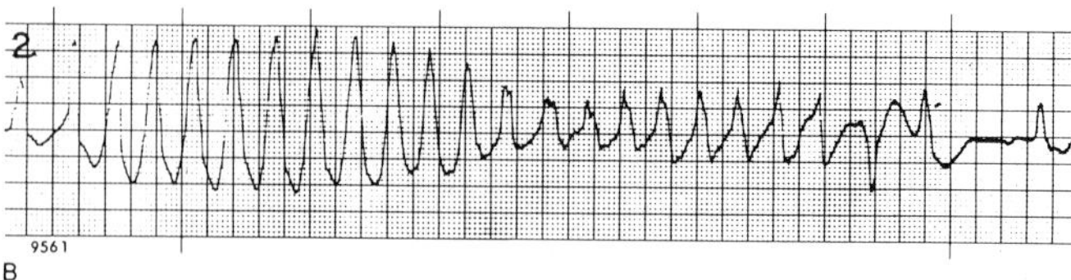

B

FIG. 24-20. Two examples of short runs of atypical ventricular tachycardia showing sinusoidal variation in amplitude and direction of the QRS complexes: ''Le torsade de pointes'' (twisting of the points). Note that the top example is initiated by a late-occurring PVC (lead II).

TABLE 24-3 Etiologies and Associated Conditions in Torsades de Pointes

Familial
Jervell-Lange-Nielson syndrome (congenital deafness)
Romano-Ward syndrome (without deafness)
Toxins and drugs
Antiarrhythmics: most common with classes IA, IC, and III
Psychotropics: tricyclic antidepressants, some phenothiazines (thioridazine), tetracyclics (maprotiline)
Organophosphate insecticides
Liquid protein diets
Cerebrovascular disease
Cerebrovascular accidents, intracranial hemorrhage, carotid endarterectomy
Electrolyte disorders
Hypokalemia, hypomagnesemia, hypocalcemia
Endocrine disorders
Hypothyroidism
Cardiac disease
Acute rheumatic carditis, mitral valve prolapse syndrome, inflammatory myocarditis
Coronary artery disease
Myocardial ischemia or infarction, left ventricular failure
Pacemaker malfunction
Postoperative complication

exacerbate this dysrhythmia. Conventional treatment with lidocaine often is ineffective. To date, treatment for TdP consisted of accelerating the heart rate (thereby shortening ventricular repolarization) with isoproterenol (2 to 8 μg/min) while making arrangements for a ventricular pacemaker to overdrive the heart at rates of 90 to 120. Temporary pacing is the most effective and safest method to treat TdP and prevent its recurrence in the emergency setting. Recent reports have revealed that magnesium sulfate 1 to 2 g IV over 60 to 90 s followed by an infusion of 1 to 2 g/h is effective in abolishing these runs of TdP, although recurrences are seen despite continued infusion. A wide variety of other agents and antiarrhythmics have reported anecdotal success, but overall efficacy has been inconsistent.

Clinical Significance Ventricular tachycardia is very rare in patients without underlying heart disease. The most common causes of ventricular tachycardia are ischemic heart disease and acute MI. Less common causes include hypertrophic cardiomyopathy, mitral valve prolapse, and toxicity from many drugs (digoxin, quinidine, procainamide, and sympathomimetics). Hypoxia, alkalosis, and electrolyte abnormalities exacerbate the tendency toward ventricular ectopy and tachycardia.

It is a common misconception that patients with ventricular tachycardia appear clinically unstable; this is the basis for the mistaken assumption that patients who appear stable with a wide complex tachycardia have SVT with aberrancy rather than ventricular tachycardia. This is definitely wrong. Ventricular tachycardia cannot be differentiated from SVT with aberrancy on the basis of clinical symptoms, blood pressure, or heart rate. Patients who are unstable should be cardioverted; this is effective for both dysrhythmias. In patients who are stable, a 12-lead ECG should be obtained first and examined for evidence favoring one dysrhythmia over another; but even then, it is often difficult to decide. Therefore, in general, it is best to treat all wide complex tachycardias as ventricular tachycardia with lidocaine or procainamide. These drugs are obviously effective in ventricular tachycardia and often surprisingly effective in SVT with aberrancy, and they carry little risk of harming the patient. Conversely, verapamil is harmful in most patients with ventricular tachycardia, accelerating the heart rate and the decreasing blood pressure without converting the rhythm. Adenosine appears to do little harm in patients with ventricular tachycardia and has potential merit for the treatment for wide QRS complex tachycardias. However, until further experience is gained with this agent, it cannot be recommended for routine use in this setting.

Treatment

1. Unstable patients or those in cardiac arrest should be treated with synchronized cardioversion. Ventricular tachycardia can be converted with energies as low as 1 J, and over 90 percent can be converted with less than 10 J. Rarely is more than 100 J needed. Current advanced cardiac life support (ACLS) guidelines recommend that pulseless ventricular tachycardia be *defibrillated* (unsynchronized cardioversion) with 200 J.
2. Clinically stable patients should be treated with intravenous antiarrhythmics.
   a. Lidocaine 75 mg (1.0 to 1.5 mg/kg) IV over 60 to 90 s, followed by a constant infusion at 1 to 4 mg/min (10 to 40 μg/kg per minute). A repeat bolus dose of 50 mg lidocaine may be required during the first 20 min to avoid a subtherapeutic dip in serum level due to the early distribution phase.
   b. Bretylium 500 mg (5 to 10 mg/kg) IV over 10 min, followed by a constant infusion at 1 to 2 mg/min.
   c. Procainamide at a rate of less than 50 mg/min IV until the dysrhythmia converts, the total dose reaches 15 to 17 mg/kg in normals (12 mg/kg in patients with congestive heart failure), or early signs of toxicity develop with hypotension or QRS prolongation. The loading dose should be followed by a maintenance infusion of 2.8 mg/kg per hour in normal subjects (1.4 mg/kg per hour in patients with renal insufficiency).
   d. A variety of other antiarrhythmics have been studied for the treatment of ventricular tachycardia. Most class I and III agents are effective for the acute termination of ventricular tachycardia when given intravenously. Recommendations concerning their routine use will have to await further studies.

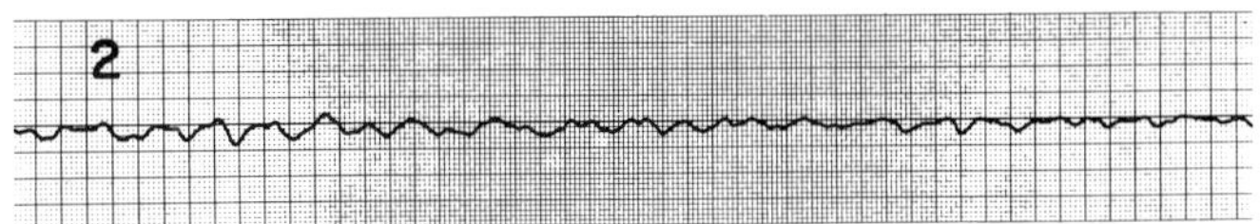

FIG. 24-21. Ventricular fibrillation.

VENTRICULAR FIBRILLATION Ventricular fibrillation is the totally disorganized depolarization and contraction of small areas of ventricular myocardium—there is no effective ventricular pumping activity. The ECG of ventricular fibrillation shows a fine to coarse zigzag pattern without discernible P waves or QRS complexes (Fig. 24-21).

A pulse or blood pressure never accompanies ventricular fibrillation. In patients who are awake and responsive, the ECG pattern of ventricular fibrillation is caused by a loose lead artifact or electrical interference.

Clinical Significance Ventricular fibrillation is most commonly seen in patients with severe ischemic heart disease, with or without an acute MI. Primary ventricular fibrillation occurs suddenly, without preceding hemodynamic deterioration, while secondary ventricular fibrillation occurs after a prolonged period of left ventricular failure and/or circulatory shock. Ventricular fibrillation may also occur from digoxin toxicity, quinidine toxicity, hypothermia, blunt chest trauma, severe electrolyte abnormality, or myocardial irritation caused by an intracardiac catheter or pacemaker electrode.

Treatment

1. Current ACLS guidelines recommend immediate electrical defibrillation with 200 J. If ventricular fibrillation persists, defibrillation should be repeated immediately with 200 to 300 J for the second attempt and increased to 360 J for the third attempt.
2. If the initial three attempts at defibrillation are unsuccessful, CPR should be initiated and, according to ACLS guidelines, further electrical defibrillations done after the administration of various intravenous drugs.

ABERRANT VERSUS VENTRICULAR TACHYDYSRHYTHMIAS

Differentiation between ectopic beats of ventricular origin and those of supraventricular origin but conducted aberrantly can be difficult, especially in sustained tachycardias with wide QRS complexes [wide complex tachycardia (WCT)]. In general, the majority of patients with WCT have ventricular tachycardia and should be approached as having ventricular tachycardia until proved otherwise. Several guidelines might help in the distinction.

1. A preceding ectopic P′ wave is good evidence favoring aberrancy, although coincidental atrial and ventricular ectopic beats or retrograde conduction can occur. During a sustained run of tachycardia, AV dissociation greatly favors a ventricular origin of the dysrhythmia.
2. Postectopic pause. A fully compensatory pause is more likely after a ventricular beat, but exceptions do occur.
3. Fusion beats are good evidence for ventricular origin, but exceptions do occur.

TABLE 24-4 Aberrancy versus Ventricular Ectopy

QRS Pattern in V_1	Favors	QRS Pattern in V_6	Favors
rSR′(RBBB pattern)	Aberrancy	qRS	Aberrancy
rR′			
R		rS	
qR		S	
RS	Ventricular	qR or QR	Ventricular
Slurred downslope R		R qQ′	
Slurred upstroke R	Either	RS Slurred R	Either

Source: Wellens HJJ, Frits WHMB, Lie KI: *Am J Med* 64:27, 1978, with permission.

4. A varying bundle branch block pattern suggests aberrancy.
5. Coupling intervals are usually constant with ventricular ectopic beats unless parasystole is present. Varying coupling intervals suggest aberrancy.
6. Response to carotid sinus massage or other vagal maneuvers will slow conduction through the AV node and may abolish reentrant SVT and slow the ventricular response in other supraventricular tachyarrhythmias. These maneuvers have essentially no effect on ventricular dysrhythmias.
7. A QRS duration of longer than 0.14 s is usually only found in ventricular ectopy or tachycardia.
8. QRS morphology: Wellens et al have studied patients with both ventricular tachycardia and SVT with aberrancy using His bundle electrocardiography. Several morphologic ECG criteria were found useful in differentiating between the two (Table 24-4). In the ED, these morphologic criteria are not helpful.
9. Historical criteria have also been found to be useful: age of the patient over 35 and/or history of MI, congestive heart failure, or coronary artery bypass graft strongly suggest ventricular tachycardia in patients with WCT.

CONDUCTION DISTURBANCES

Sinoatrial (SA) Block

The sinus node discharge must be conducted into the atria to pace the heart during sinus rhythm. If sinus node discharges are delayed or blocked in their outward propagation (exit block), then sinoatrial block is present. Sinoatrial block is divided into first-, second-, and third-degree varieties.

First-degree SA block means that the impulse is delayed in its conduction out of the sinus node into the atria—a condition that cannot be recognized on the clinical ECG.

Second-degree SA block means that some impulses get through and some are blocked. Second-degree SA block can be suspected whenever an expected P wave and the corresponding QRS complex are absent. In the variable (Wenckebach) type of second-degree SA block, the missing P wave would come after a period of progressive prolongation of the conduction time from the sinus node to the atrium, something undetectable on the clinical ECG. However, another ECG finding common to the Wenckebach phenomenon can be seen—progressive shortening of the P-P intervals prior to the missing P wave (Fig. 24-22). In the constant type of second-degree SA block, the sinoatrial conduction time remains constant before and after the

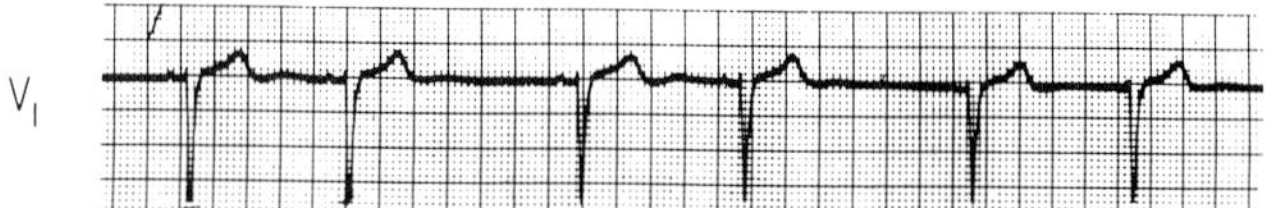

FIG. 24-22. Second-degree SA block type I (Wenckebach). (From Braunwald E: Heart Disease. *A Textbook of Cardiovascular Medicine* Philadelphia, Saunders, 1980. Used by permission.)

blocked impulses. In this situation, the interval encompassing the missing beat is an exact or near-exact multiple of the cycle length (Fig. 24-23).

Third-degree SA block occurs when the sinus node discharge is completely blocked and no P wave originating from the sinus seen. There are three other causes of absent sinus P waves in addition to third-degree SA block: (1) sinus node failure, (2) a sinus node stimulus inadequate to activate the atria, and (3) atrial unresponsiveness.

CLINICAL SIGNIFICANCE Sinoatrial block usually arises from myocardial disease (acute rheumatic fever, acute inferior MI, other causes of myocarditis) or drug toxicity (digoxin, quinidine, salicylates, β-adrenergic blockers, or calcium channel blockers). In rare individuals, vagal stimulation can produce SA block.

TREATMENT

1. Treatment depends on the underlying cause, associated dysrhythmias, and whether symptoms of hypoperfusion are present.
2. Sinus node discharge rate and sinoatrial conduction can be facilitated by atropine or isoproterenol when clinically required; however, ischemia may result from a rhythm that is accelerated.
3. Cardiac pacing is indicated for recurrent or persistent symptomatic bradycardia.

Sinus Arrest (Pause)

Sinus pause is a failure of impulse formation within the sinus node. In sinus arrest, the P-P interval has no mathematical relation to the basic sinus node discharge rate (Fig. 24-24).

CLINICAL SIGNIFICANCE The same conditions that produce SA block can also produce sinus arrest, especially digoxin toxicity and aging disease of the SA node, as in sick sinus syndrome, discussed below. The combination of digoxin and carotid sinus massage is well known to be able to produce prolonged sinus arrest. Brief periods of sinus arrest may occur in healthy individuals from increased vagal tone. If sinus arrest is prolonged, AV junctional escape beats often occur.

TREATMENT

1. Treatment depends on the underlying cause, associated dysrhythmias, and whether symptoms of hypoperfusion are present.
2. If sinus arrest is symptomatic, atropine will usually increase the sinus node discharge rate.
3. Cardiac pacing is indicated for recurrent or persistent symptomatic bradycardia.

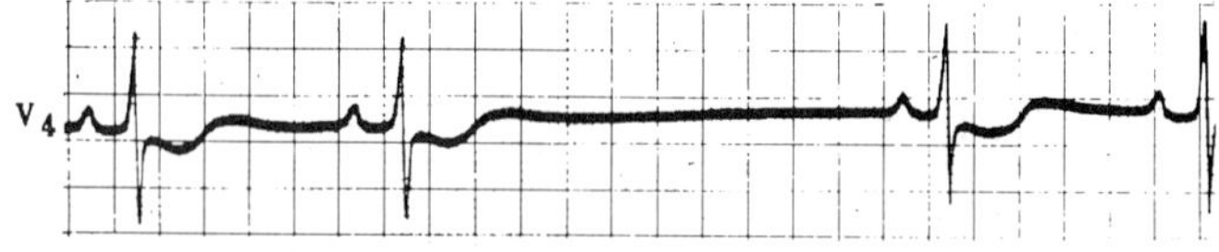

FIG. 24-23. Second-degree constant SA block type II (lead V_4).

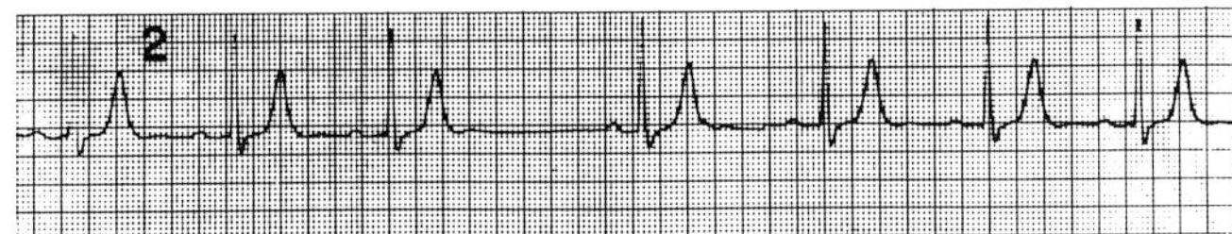

FIG. 24-24. Sinus pause.

Atrioventricular (AV) Dissociation

AV is a condition in which separate and independent pacemakers drive the atria and ventricles. It is not a primary rhythm disturbance but is secondary to another conduction or rhythm abnormality. There are two varieties of AV dissociation: passive (default or "escape") and active (usurpation).

Passive AV dissociation occurs when an impulse fails to reach the AV node because of sinus node failure or block. Usually an escape rhythm takes over and paces the ventricles. When the sinus node recovers, atrial activity resumes, but there may be a period during which the ventricles are still driven by the escape pacemaker and the P waves and QRS complexes occur independently of each other (Fig. 24-25).

Active AV dissociation occurs when a lower pacemaker accelerates to usurp the sinus node and captures the ventricles but the atria are still paced as before (Fig. 24-26).

In both varieties of AV dissociation, fusion beats are common. It is also common for the two pacemakers to operate with nearly identical rates, possibly as a result of mechanical or electrical influences that tend to keep them in phase with each other—a condition termed *isorhythmic dissociation*.

CLINICAL SIGNIFICANCE Passive AV dissociation occurs when the sinus node discharge rate is slowed by sinus bradycardia, sinus dysrhythmia, SA block, or sinus pause. Common causes of this include (1) ischemic heart disease (especially acute inferior myocardial infarction), (2) myocarditis (especially acute rheumatic fever), (3) drug toxicity (especially digoxin), and (4) vagal reflexes. It may also be seen in well-conditioned athletes.

Active AV dissociation occurs when the automaticity of lower pacemakers is enhanced. Common causes include myocardial ischemia and drug toxicity (especially digoxin). This form of AV dissociation is seen only when the lower tachycardiac rhythm is not conducted to the sinus node with capture of the SA node. Ventricular tachycardia is the classic example of an active AV dissociation.

TREATMENT

1. Most occurrences of AV dissociation have an acceptable heart rate and are well tolerated.
2. Therapy, if any, is directed toward the underlying cause.

Atrioventricular (AV) Block

Clinical classification of AV block was done before the sites and mechanisms involved in impairing conduction between the atria and ventricles were understood. As a matter of fact, Wenkebach described

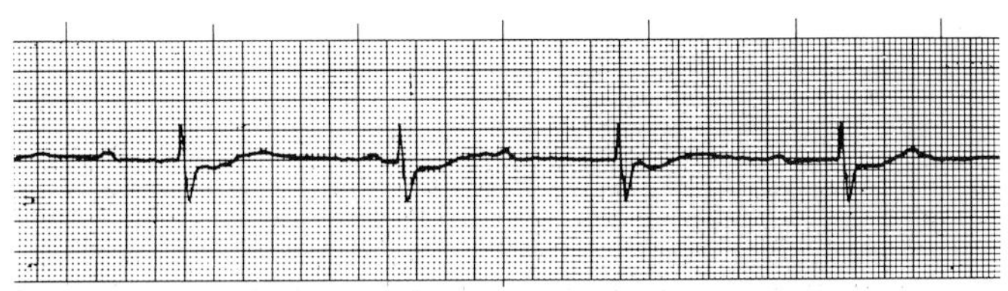

FIG. 24-25. Passive AV dissociation, secondary to third-degree AV block.

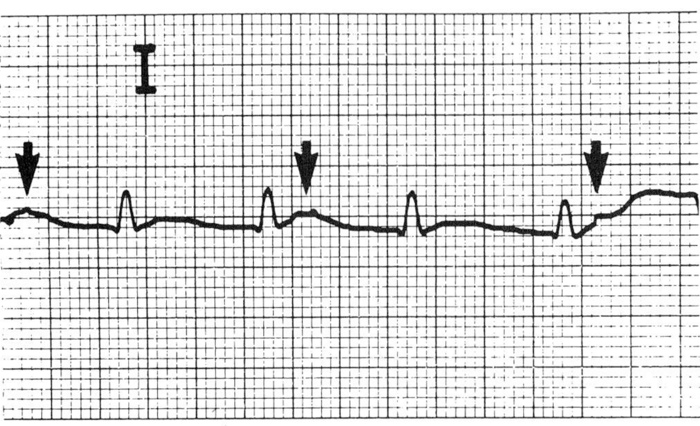

FIG. 24-26. Active AV dissociation. (Arrows indicate P waves.)

his block prior to the development of ECGs by looking at the A and V waves in the jugular veins. Mobitz described his classification after the invention of the ECG but before His bundle recordings. This classification is too simple to categorize all the problems that may occur with AV conduction. However, this system is almost universally used in respect to their observations.

First-degree AV block is characterized by a delay in AV conduction manifest by a prolonged PR interval. Second-degree AV block is characterized by intermittent AV conduction—some atrial impulses reach the ventricles and others are blocked. Third-degree AV block is characterized by the complete interruption of AV conduction.

Precise localization of AV conduction blocks can be made with His bundle electrocardiography. Although this method is not available for use in the ED, correlations can be made between the clinical ECG, approximate location of the block, and risk of future progression.

AV blocks can also be divided into nodal and infranodal blocks. This is an important distinction because the clinical significance and prognosis vary with the site. AV nodal blocks (block at the AH area by the His bundle) are usually due to reversible depression of conduction, are often self-limited, and generally have a stable infranodal escape pacemaker pacing the ventricles. AV nodal blocks therefore do not usually have a serious prognosis. Infranodal blocks (block at the HV area by the His bundle) are usually due to organic disease of the His bundle or bundle branches; often the damage is irreversible. They generally have a slow and unstable ventricular escape rhythm pacing the ventricles, and they may have a serious prognosis depending on the clinical circumstance.

FIRST-DEGREE AV BLOCK In first-degree AV block, each atrial impulse is conducted into the ventricles, but more slowly than normal. This is recognized by a PR interval of greater than 0.20 s (Fig. 24-27). The AV node is usually the site of conduction delay, although this may occur at any infranodal level.

Clinical Significance First-degree AV block is occasionally found in normal hearts. Other common causes include increased vagal tone (whatever the cause), digoxin toxicity, acute inferior MI, and myocar-

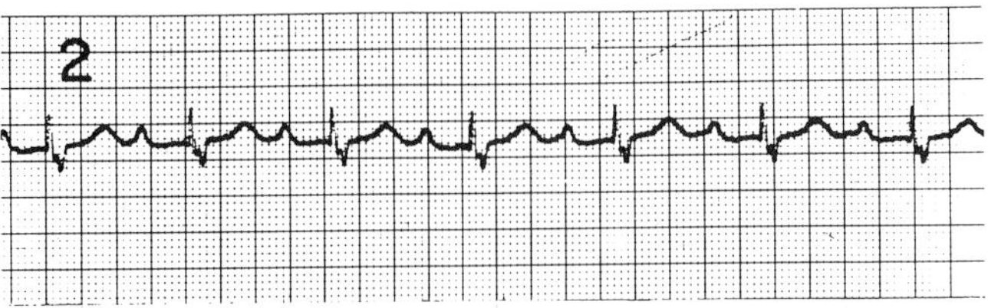

FIG. 24-27. First-degree AV block (PR interval = 0.3 s).

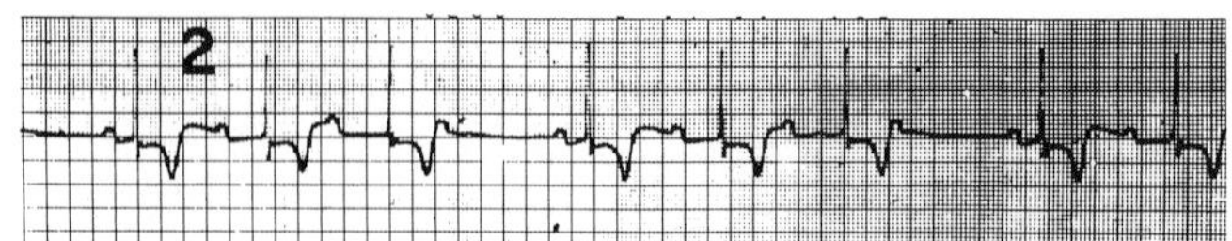

FIG. 24-28. Second-degree Mobitz I (Wenckebach) AV block 4 : 3 AV conduction.

ditis. Patients with first-degree AV block without evidence of organic heart disease appear to have no significant difference in mortality compared with matched controls.

Treatment

1. None is usually required.
2. Prophylactic pacing in acute myocardial infarction is not indicated unless more serious infranodal conduction disturbances are present.

Second-Degree Mobitz I (Wenckebach) AV Block

In this block there is progressive prolongation of AV conduction (and the PR interval) until an atrial impulse is completely blocked (Fig. 24-28). This property of gradually increasing block until complete block is a normal property of cardiac tissue. In the face of disease, this property occurs at a much slower rate. In the electrophysiology laboratory (EP), a Wenkebach type of block is frequently seen when atrial pacing occurs at fast rates to uncover an accessory pathway. Conduction ratios are used to indicate the ratio of atrial to ventricular depolarizations: 3 : 2 indicates that two out of three atrial impulses are conducted into the ventricles. Usually, only a single atrial impulse is blocked. After the dropped beat, the AV conduction returns to normal and the cycle usually repeats itself with either the same conduction ratio (fixed ratio) or a different conduction ratio (variable ratio). This type of block almost always occurs at the level of the AV node and is often due to reversible depression of AV nodal conduction.

The Wenckebach phenomenon involves a seeming paradox. Even though the PR intervals progressively lengthen prior to the dropped beat, the increments by which they lengthen decrease with successive beats; this produces a progressive shortening of the R-R interval prior to the dropped beat (Fig. 24-28). This sign can be used to indicate that a Wenckebach phenomenon is occurring even when the conduction delay cannot be seen, as in SA Wenckebach block.

Wenckebach block is believed to occur because each successive depolarization produces prolongation of the refractory period of the AV node. When the next atrial impulse comes upon the node, it is earlier in the relative refractory period and conduction occurs more slowly relative to the previous stimulus. This process is progressive until an atrial impulse reaches the AV node during the absolute refractory period and conduction is blocked altogether. The pause allows the AV node to recover and the process can resume.

CLINICAL SIGNIFICANCE This block is often transient and usually associated with an acute inferior MI, digoxin toxicity, or myocarditis, or it is seen after cardiac surgery. As mentioned, Wenckebach block may also occur when a normal AV node is exposed to very rapid atrial rates.

TREATMENT

1. Specific treatment is not necessary unless slow ventricular rates produce signs of hypoperfusion.
2. 0.5 mg IV of atropine is given, repeated every 5 min as necessary, titrated to the desired effect, or until the total dose reaches 2.0 mg. Almost all patients will respond to atropine. The need for an increased rate and hopefully increased perfusion must be consistently balanced with the increased myocardial O_2 consumption in the ischemic patient.
3. Isoproterenol is hazardous in the setting of acute myocardial infarction or digoxin toxicity and its use should be avoided.
4. Transcutaneous or transvenous ventricular demand pacing should be initiated if atropine is unsuccessful. It must be confirmed that the hypoperfusion is due to the rate and not to decreased preload, as in some patients with an inferior MI.

Second-Degree Mobitz II AV Block

In this block, the PR interval remains constant before and after the nonconducted atrial beats (Fig. 24-29). One or more beats may be nonconducted at a single time.

Mobitz II blocks usually occur in the infranodal conducting system, often with coexistent fascicular or bundle branch blocks, and the QRS complexes are therefore usually wide. Even if the QRS complexes are narrow, the block is generally in the infranodal system.

When second-degree AV block occurs with a fixed conduction ratio of 2 : 1, it is not possible to differentiate between a Mobitz type I (Wenckebach) or Mobitz type II block. If the QRS complex is narrow, then the block is in the AV node or infranodal system with about equal incidence. If the QRS complex is wide, the block is more likely to be in the infranodal system.

CLINICAL SIGNIFICANCE Type II blocks imply structural damage to the infranodal conducting system, are usually permanent, and may progress suddenly to complete heart block—especially in the setting of an acute MI.

TREATMENT

1. Emergent treatment is required when slow ventricular rates produce symptoms of hypoperfusion. Atropine should be the first drug used, and up to 60 percent of patients will respond. Isoproterenol is effective in up to 50 percent of cases but is potentially hazardous in the setting of acute myocardial infarction or digoxin toxicity, and its use should be avoided. Transcutaneous cardiac pacing is a useful modality in patients unresponsive to atropine.
2. Most patients, especially in the setting of acute MI, will require permanent transvenous cardiac pacing.

Third-Degree (Complete) AV Block

In third-degree AV block, there is no atrioventricular conduction. The ventricles are paced by an escape pacemaker at a rate slower than the

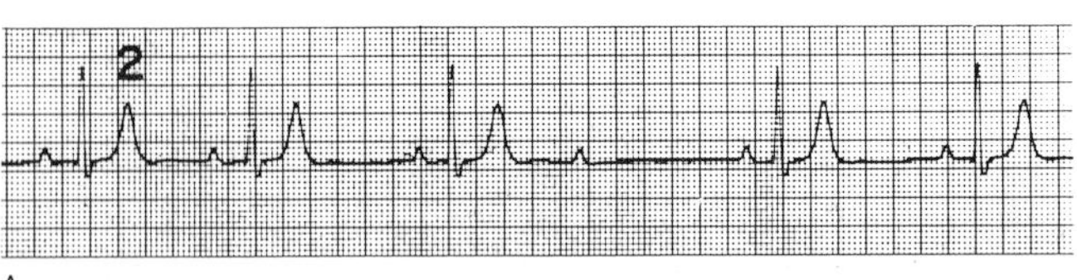

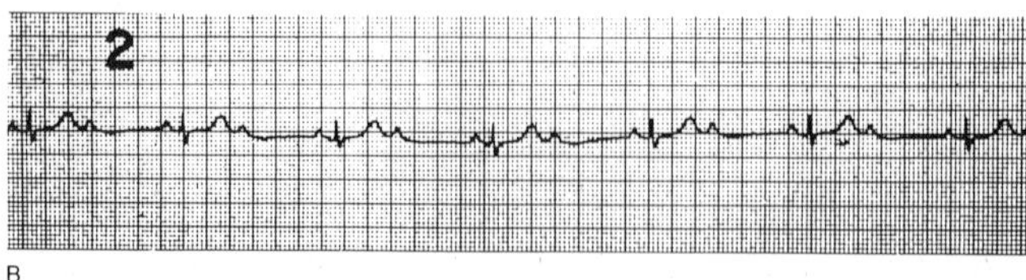

FIG. 24-29. Top: second-degree Mobitz II AV block. Bottom: second-degree AV block with 2 : 1 AV conduction.

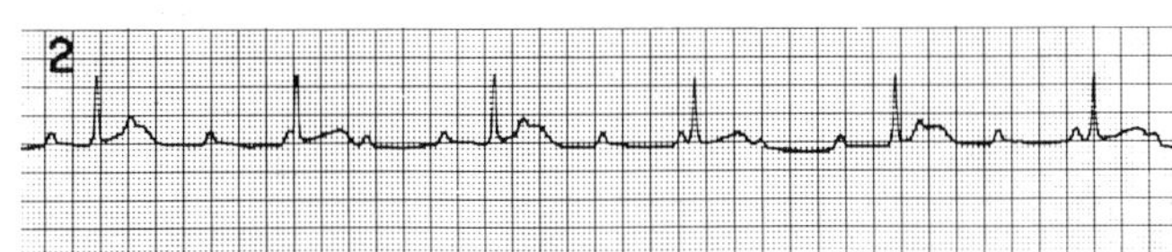

FIG. 24-30. Third-degree AV block.

atrial rate (Fig. 24-30). Third-degree AV block can occur either at nodal or infranodal levels.

When third-degree AV block occurs at the AV node, a junctional escape pacemaker takes over with a ventricular rate of 40 to 60, and—since the rhythm originates above the bifurcation of the bundle of His—the QRS complexes are narrow.

When third-degree AV block occurs at the infranodal level, the ventricles are driven by a ventricular escape rhythm at a rate of less than 40. In third-degree AV block located at the His bundle level, the escape rhythm has narrow QRS complexes about half of the time. Presumably in these cases, the escape pacemaker resides above the bifurcation of the conducting system into the separate bundle branches. Third-degree AV block located in the bundle branch or elsewhere in the Purkinje system invariably have escape rhythms with wide QRS complexes.

CLINICAL SIGNIFICANCE Nodal third-degree AV block may develop in up to 8 percent of acute inferior MIs, where it is usually transient, although it may last for several days.

Infranodal third-degree AV blocks indicate structural damage to the infranodal conducting system, as seen with an extensive acute anterior myocardial infarction (AMI). The ventricular escape pacemaker is usually inadequate to maintain cardiac output and is unstable, with periods of ventricular asystole. When third-degree block is seen in acute AMI, mortality is increased even when rhythm is controlled with pacing.

TREATMENT

1. Nodal third-degree AV blocks should be treated like second-degree Mobitz I AV blocks with atropine or ventricular demand pacemaker as required.
2. Infranodal third-degree AV blocks require a ventricular demand pacemaker. Isoproterenol can be used temporarily to accelerate the ventricular escape rhythm, or external cardiac pacing can be performed before transvenous pacemaker placement.

FASCICULAR BLOCKS

Unifascicular Block

Unifascicular block is a conduction block that affects one of the three major infranodal conduction pathways: right bundle branch (RBB), left anterior superior fascicle (LASF), or left posterior inferior fascicle (LPIF). A wide variety of disease processes can produce conduction block in the fascicles: ischemia, cardiomyopathies, valvular (especially aortic), myocarditis, cardiac surgery, congenital conditions, and degenerative processes affecting the conduction tissue (Lenegre or Lev diseases). The RBB and the LASF are relatively small and easily affected parts of the conduction system. The LPIF is very broad and is caused by disease affecting a large area of myocardium.

In LASF block, left ventricular activation is by way of the LPIF and proceeds in an inferior-to-superior and right-to-left direction. The ECG characteristics of LASF block are (1) normal QRS duration, (2) frontal plane mean QRS axis of less than −45°, (3) R wave in lead I greater than the R waves in leads II or III, (4) a qR complex in lead AVL, and (5) deep S wave in leads II, III, and AVF (Fig. 24-31). The LASF is small and easily affected by focal lesions. Other causes of left axis deviation should be excluded—inferior MI, hyperkalemia, preexcitation syndromes, or body habitus. Left ventricular hypertrophy can cause left axis deviation as seen with LASF block; however, the axis is infrequently less than −30.

In LPIF block, left ventricular activation is by way of the LASF and proceeds in a superior-to-inferior and left-to-right direction. The ECG characteristics of LPIF block are (1) normal QRS duration, (2) frontal plane mean QRS axis greater than 110°, (3) small r and deep S waves in lead I, (4) an R wave in lead III larger than the R wave in lead II, and (5) a qR complex in lead III (Fig. 24-32). The LPIF is broad and not affected by focal lesions; its presence indicates widespread organic heart disease. Other causes of right axis deviation are chronic cor pulmonale, right ventricular hypertrophy, and lateral MI.

In RBB block, ventricular activation is by way of the left bundle branch, proceeding from the left to the right ventricle. The ECG characteristics of RBB block are (1) prolonged QRS duration (greater than 0.12 s); (2) triphasic QRS complexes (RSR′) in lead V_1; (3) wide

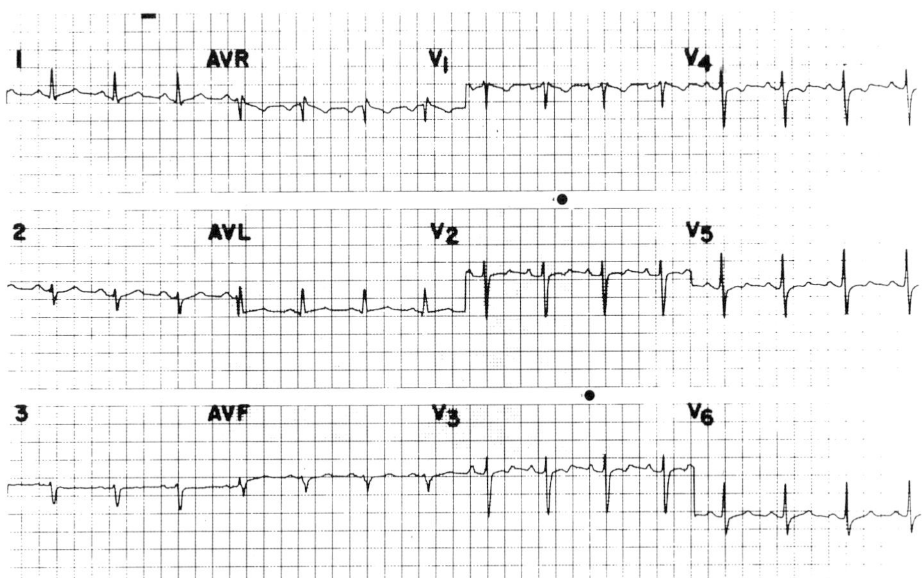

FIG. 24-31. Left anterior superior fascicular block (LASF block).

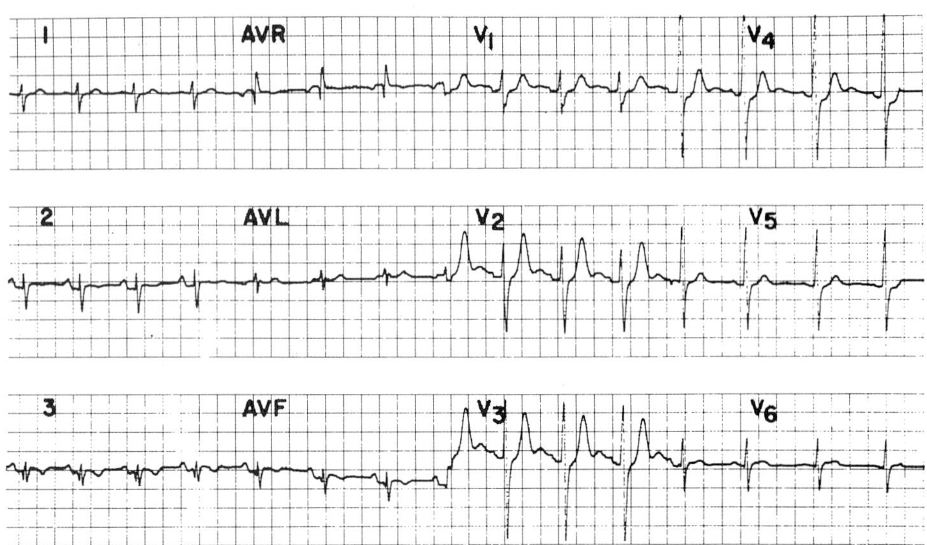

FIG. 24-32. Left posterior inferior fascicular block (LPIF block).

S waves in the lateral leads I, V_5, and V_6; and (4) normal onset of ventricular activation in lead V_6 (Fig. 24-33). The frontal plane mean QRS axis is usually not deviated to the right unless there is associated right ventricular hypertrophy or LPIF block.

Bifascicular Block

The term *bifascicular block* refers to conduction blocks over two fascicles: (1) RBB and LASF, (2) RBB and LPIF, or (3) left bundle branch (LBB) block.

In LBB block, ventricular activation is by way of the RBB and proceeds from right to left and inferior to superior. The ECG characteristics of LBB block are (1) prolonged QRS duration (greater than 0.12 s); (2) large and wide R waves in leads I, aV_L, V_5, and V_6; (3) small r wave followed by deep S wave in leads II, III, aV_F, and V_1 to V_3; and (4) no q waves in leads I, aV_F, V_5, and V_6 (Fig. 24-34).

Trifascicular Block

The term *trifascicular block* refers to a combination of conduction blocks in all three fascicles, either permanent or transient: (1) RBB and LASF with first-degree AV block, (2) RBB and LPIF with first-degree AV block, (3) LBB with first-degree AV block, or (4) alternating RBB and LBB block.

While bi- and trifascicular conduction blocks indicate advanced organic heart disease, long-term follow-up studies of ambulatory patients indicate that the risk of sudden progression to complete heart block and sudden death due to ventricular asystole is not high. Placement of a ventricular demand pacemaker is indicated only for symptoms due to documented bradyarrhythmias.

In the face of an acute myocardial infarction, the risks of complete heart block are much greater when new or preexistent bi- or trifascicular conduction blocks are present. In this setting, prophylactic placement of a ventricular demand pacemaker is indicated.

PRETERMINAL RHYTHMS

Several dysrhythmias may be seen during cardiac resuscitation. Ventricular tachycardia and fibrillation potentially are treatable and resuscitation may result in a functional survivor. The four other dysrhythmias included here have a low rate of successful resuscitation and are much less likely to yield a functional survivor.

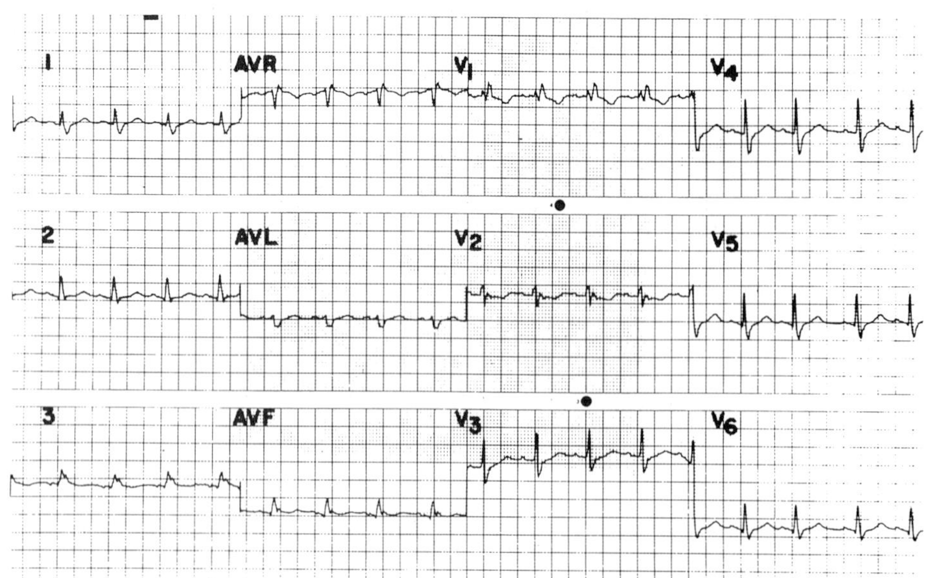

FIG. 24-33. Right bundle branch block (RBB block).

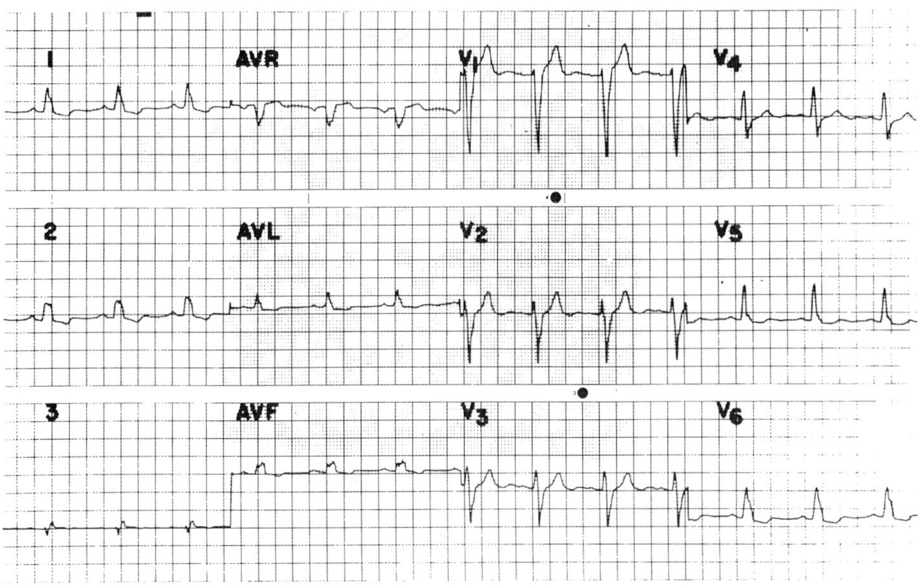

FIG. 24-34. Left bundle branch block (LBB block).

Pulseless Electrical Activity (PEA)

PEA is the presence of electrical complexes without accompanying mechanical contraction of the heart (Fig. 24-35). In the setting of a cardiac arrest, PEA is due to a profound metabolic abnormality of the myocardium, rendering it noncontractile. At this time, there is no clearly beneficial therapy; the best that can be recommended currently is continued cardiopulmonary resuscitation and α-adrenergic agents. Although calcium has been advocated traditionally, most studies have found no consistent benefit, and there are serious biophysiologic reasons to question the use of calcium in the setting of cardiac arrest. Electrical pacing is, of course, not effective.

Other conditions that may mimic PEA are (1) severe hypovolemia, (2) cardiac tamponade, (3) tension pneumothorax, (4) massive pulmonary embolus, and (5) rupture of the ventricular wall. The first three conditions are potentially treatable if recognized early.

Idioventricular Rhythm (IVR)

An IVR is an escape rhythm of ventricular origin with very wide QRS complexes (more than 0.16 s) and a rate less than 40 (Fig. 24-36). Effective cardiac contractions and pulses may or may not be present. Idioventricular rhythm may occur as the result of complete infranodal AV block, AMI, cardiac tamponade, or exsanguinating hemorrhage. Treatment consists of attempting to accelerate the heart rate and enhance mechanical contractility using cardiopulmonary resuscitation and α-adrenergic agents. There is no proven benefit to the use of atropine or isoproterenol to treat IVR during cardiac resuscitation.

Agonal Ventricular Rhythm

Agonal rhythm is the occurrence of very broad and irregular ventricular complexes at a slow rate, usually without associated ventricular contractions (Fig. 24-37).

Cardiac Asystole (Cardiac Standstill)

Asystole is complete absence of any cardiac electrical activity. Treatment consists of attempting to stimulate electrical activity and mechanical contractions with continued cardiopulmonary resuscitation and α-adrenergic agents. Transthoracic or transvenous ventricular pacing may occasionally produce electrical capture but rarely yields effective pumping action if prior agents were unsuccessful.

TACHYCARDIA-BRADYCARDIA SYNDROME (SICK SINUS SYNDROME)

Sick sinus syndrome (SSS) is a heterogeneous disorder consisting of abnormalities of supraventricular impulse generation and conduction that produce a wide variety of intermittent supraventricular tachy- and bradydysrhythmias. The tachydysrhythmias are usually atrial fibrillation, junctional tachycardia, reentrant SVT, and atrial flutter. The bradydysrhythmias are marked sinus bradycardia, prolonged sinus arrest, and sinoatrial block, usually associated with AV nodal conduction abnormalities and inadequate AV junctional escape rhythms.

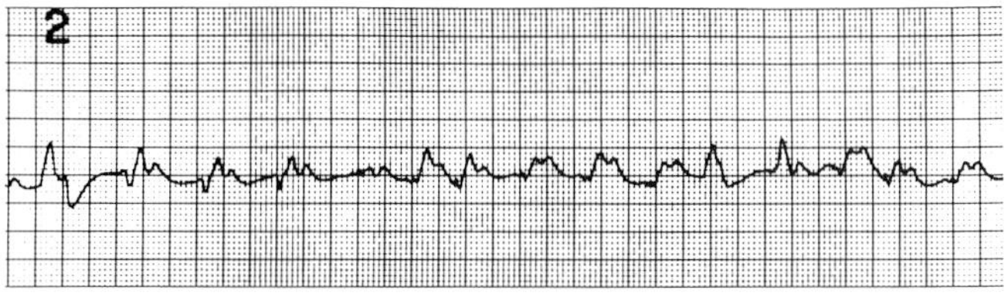

FIG. 24-35. Pulseless electrical activity (PEA).

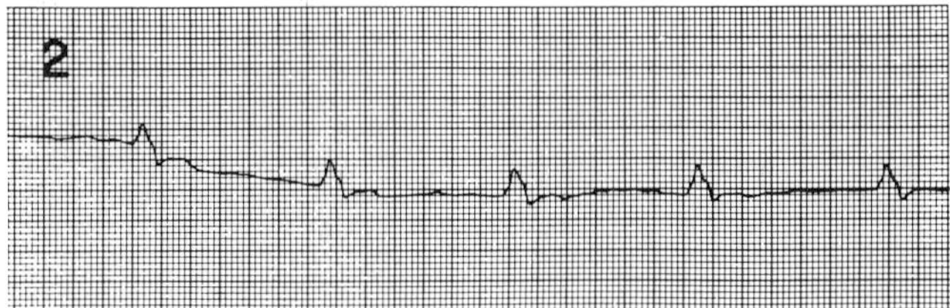

FIG. 24-36. Idioventricular rhythm (IVR).

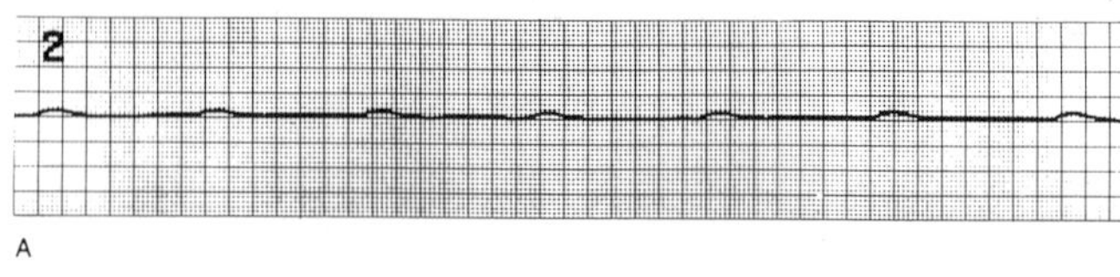

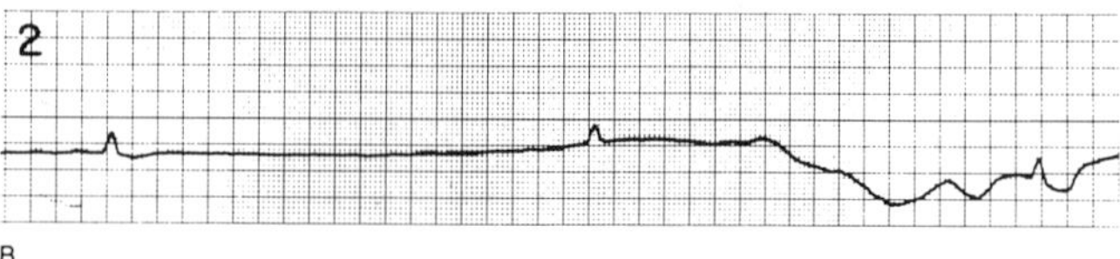

FIG. 24-37. Agonal ventricular rhythm. Top: regular. Bottom: irregular.

Clinical Significance

Symptoms of SSS are due to the effects of either fast or slow heart rate. Common symptoms include syncope or near-syncope, palpitations, dyspnea, chest pain, and cerebrovascular accidents.

A wide variety of cardiac diseases can affect the sinus and AV nodes, producing the dysrhythmias of SSS: ischemic and rheumatic disorders, myocarditis and pericarditis, rheumatologic disease, metastatic tumors, surgical damage, or cardiomyopathies.

Conditions such as abdominal pain, increased intracranial pressure, thyrotoxicosis, and hyperkalemia, which increase vagal tone, may exacerbate the abnormalities of SSS and cause increased symptoms. Drugs such as digoxin, quinidine, procainamide, disopyramide, nicotine, β-adrenergic antagonists, or calcium channel blockers also cause increased symptoms.

Ambulatory ECG monitoring or EP studies are usually necessary for the diagnosis of SSS, since a routine ECG will not normally demonstrate the intermittent dysrhythmias common in this syndrome. The demonstration of increased sensitivity of the sinus node to carotid sinus massage, the Valsalva maneuver, or atropine suggests sinus node dysfunction but is not conclusive proof for the diagnosis of SSS.

Treatment

1. SSS is the most common indication for a permanent pacemaker. This disease of the SA and AV nodes accounts for 48 percent of primary pacemaker implants. Retrospective analysis indicates that a reduction in mortality and in the incidence of CHF, AF, and thromboembolism occurs in patients with atrial pacing (AAI or DDD) compared to ventricular pacing (VVI).
2. Treatment of atrial tachyarrhythmias with digoxin, quinidine, disopyramide, procainamide, propranolol, or verapamil carries the risk of aggravating preexisting AV block or sinus arrest. Therefore, most patients should have pacemaker implantation before drug therapy is begun.

PREEXCITATION SYNDROMES

Preexcitation occurs when the ventricles are activated by an impulse from the atria sooner than would be expected if the impulse were transmitted down the normal conducting pathway (the AV node). Several different forms of preexcitation have been described, based on anatomic, clinical, electrocardiographic, and electrophysiologic abnormalities. All forms of preexcitation are felt to be due to accessory tracts that bypass all or part of the normal conducting system. These bypass tracts have specific names (Fig. 24-38).

James fibers (atriohisian connection) are a continuation of the posterior internodal tract and connect the atrium and proximal His bundle. Atrial impulses can therefore completely bypass the AV node to activate the ventricles. On ECG, this appears as (1) a short PR interval because the usual delay in the AV node is bypassed and (2) a normal QRS because James fibers insert directly into the infranodal conducting system and the ventricles are activated normally. When this is associated with reentrant SVT, the clinical condition is termed the Lown-Ganong-Levine (LGL) syndrome.

Mahaim bundles are composed of myogenic tissue; they originate from either the AV node, His bundle, or bundle branches and insert into the ventricles in the septal region. Atrial impulses pass through the AV node but then bypass all or part of the infranodal conducting system to activate the ventricles. Ventricular activation then occurs from two sources, the bypass tract and the normal conducting system, and the QRS complex represents a fusion of the two. The initial depolarization starts at the ventricular insertion of the bypass tract and is spread slowly by cell-to-cell transmission of the impulse. Subsequent depolarization by way of the faster normal conducting system then overtakes the initial depolarization and activates the bulk of ventricular myocardium. The QRS complex is basically normal with a slurred and distorted initial portion termed a *delta wave.* On ECG, this appears as a normal PR interval, and an initial distortion of ventricular depolarization (delta wave).

Kent bundles are composed of myogenic tissue and directly link the atria to the ventricles, completely bypassing the AV node and infranodal system. This is the most common form of preexcitation and is the anatomic basis for the Wolff-Parkinson-White (WPW) syndrome. On ECG, this appears as a shortened PR interval and with an initial distortion of ventricular activation (delta wave). Sometimes the bypass tract does not conduct an atrial impulse in the antegrade direction and the QRS complex is entirely normal. However, these concealed bypass tracts may conduct retrograde and be able to sustain reentrant SVT.

The WPW syndrome has been divided into types, depending on the direction of the initial delta wave on the surface ECG. This, in turn, is determined by where the bypass tract (bundle of Kent) inserts into the ventricles and which portion of the ventricles is activated first. In reality, accessory tracts can insert anywhere around the AV annulus; the three types are just the most common locations.

In type A WPW, ventricular activation first occurs in the inferior-posterior region of the left ventricle and the delta wave is directed anteriorly. A positive initial deflection with a dominant R wave is seen in lead V_1. Q waves in leads II, III, and aV_F are common (Fig. 24-39).

In type B WPW, ventricular activation first occurs in the inferior-posterior region of the right ventricle and the delta wave is directed posteriorly and to the left. A negative initial deflection and rS or QS pattern are seen in lead V_1 (Fig. 24-40).

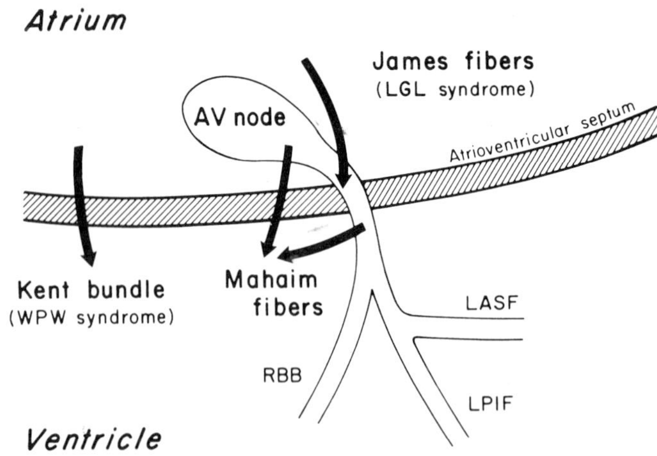

FIG. 24-38. Anatomic sites of bypass tracts.

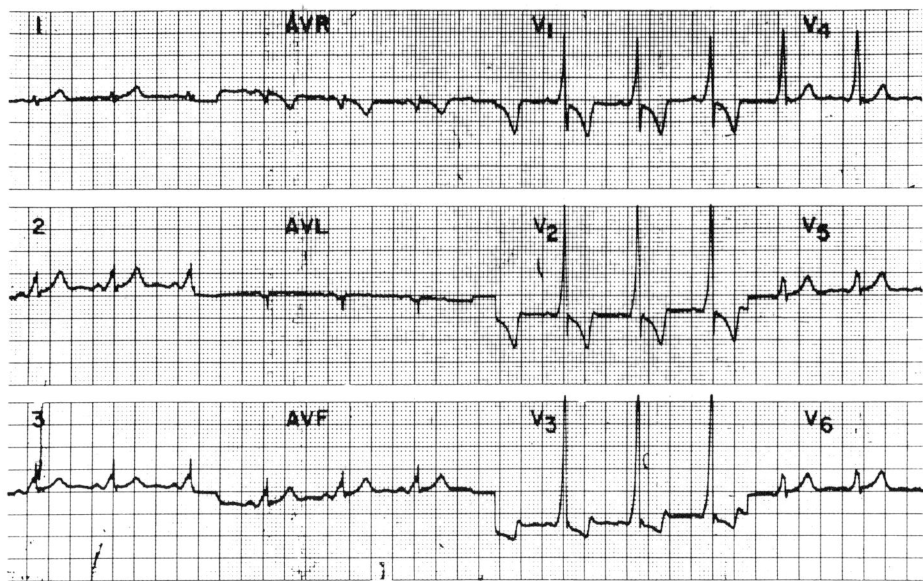

FIG. 24-39. Type A Wolff-Parkinson-White syndrome.

In type C WPW, ventricular activation first occurs in the posterior-lateral region of the left ventricle and the delta wave is directed to the right, superiorly, and anteriorly. A positive delta wave is seen in lead V_1, with a negative or isoelectric delta wave in leads V_5 and V_6.

Because there is altered depolarization, repolarization is often abnormal, with changes in the ST segments and T waves. The ECG changes of WPW may mimic changes seen with myocardial ischemia, infarction, or ventricular hypertrophy. Type A WPW may imitate as a posterior MI, and type B WPW may imitate an inferior MI.

Clinical Significance

There is a high incidence of tachyarrhythmias in patients with WPW. Atrial flutter occurs in about 5 percent, atrial fibrillation in 10 to 20 percent, and paroxysmal reentrant SVT in 40 to 80 percent.

Reentrant SVT occurs when an impulse is sustained around a loop composed of the bypass tract and the AV conducting system, the impulse traveling down one and up the other. Whether the QRS complex is wide or narrow depends on which limb of the circuit is used as the downward pathway to activate the ventricles. About 80 to 95 percent of the time, reentrant SVT occurs with the impulse being conducted down the normal AV conducting system and up the bypass tract [orthodromic AV reciprocating tachycardia (OAVRT)]. In this situation, ventricular activation occurs entirely over the normal system, the QRS complex is normal, and no delta wave is seen. Because the entire heart is used as the reentrant pathway, these arrythmias are easily converted. Conversely, 5 to 10 percent of the time, the impulse is conducted down the bypass tract and retrograde up the AV node [antidromic AV reciprocating tachycardia (AAVRT)]. In this case, the QRS complex is wide, and in the ED setting, this arrythmia is treated as ventricular tachycardia. Reentry is usually initiated by a premature atrial contraction that encounters a bypass tract which still is refractory from the previous sinus beat, but the AV node has recovered partially and conducts the impulse more slowly than normal (Fig. 24-41). In some patients, the bypass tract does not conduct antegrade during sinus rhythm and so no delta wave is seen, but it does conduct retrograde so reentrant SVT occurs. Patients with concealed bypass tracts account for about 20 percent of all patients with reentrant SVT.

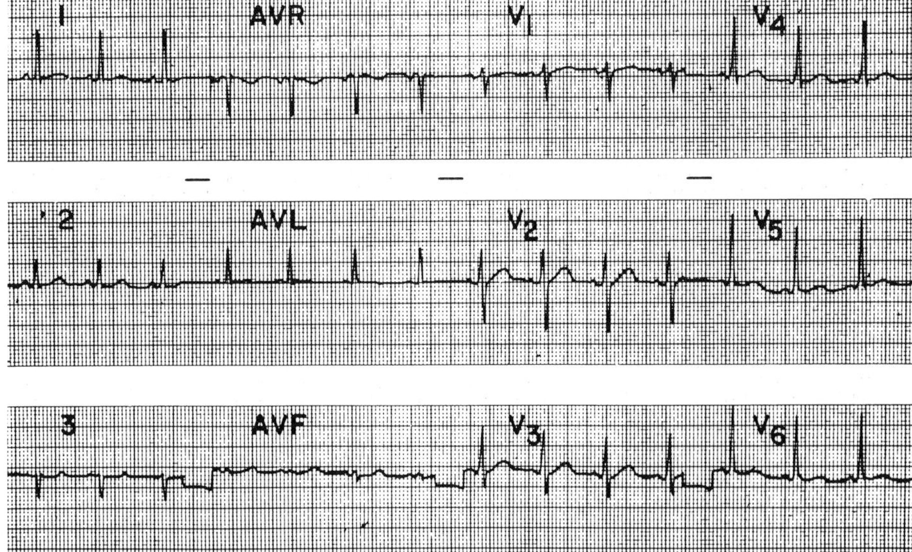

FIG. 24-40. Type B Wolff-Parkinson-White syndrome.

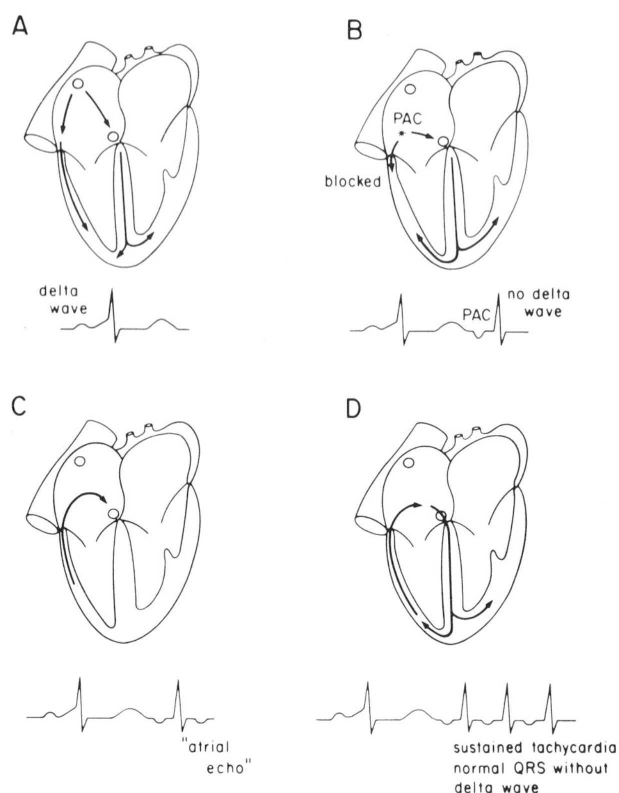

FIG. 24-41. Onset of reentrant SVT in Wolff-Parkinson-White syndrome.

If patients with WPW develop atrial flutter or fibrillation, impulses can reach the ventricles via the accessory tract, the normal conducting system, or both. Which pathway is used depends on the refractory period of each. Most patients with WPW have longer refractory periods in their accessory tracts than in the AV node, but a minority have the opposite. In patients with short refractory periods in their accessory tracts, more atrial impulses can be conducted through the accessory tract than the AV node, so most of the QRS complexes will be wide. In atrial flutter, 1 : 1 AV conduction is possible with ventricular rates of 300 (Fig. 24-42). In atrial fibrillation, very rapid and irregular ventricular rates are possible. These rapid rhythms may resemble ventricular tachycardia, and excessive stimulation of the ventricles may precipitate ventricular fibrillation. Any patient with a ventricular rate of over 300 should raise the suspicion of preexcitation syndrome.

Treatment

1. Reentrant SVT (OAVRT, narrow QRS complex) in the WPW syndrome can be treated like other cases of reentrant SVT. Since the AV node is involved in the reentry circuit, any maneuver or drug that slows conduction through the AV node is usually effective. Verapamil in the patient who is not hypotensive or in CHF is by some accounts the optimal drug. Adenosine is very successful at terminating this dysrhythmia in patients with WPW; however, there is some proclivity to increase atrial vulnerability to AF and to ectopic atrial activity, which may reinitiate the dysrhythmia.
2. Antidromic tachycardia (AAVRT, wide QRS complex) is usually associated with a short refractory period in the bypass tract, and such patients are at risk for rapid ventricular rates and degeneration into ventricular fibrillation. Stable patients should be treated with intravenous procainamide and unstable patients should be cardioverted. β-adrenergic agents, adenosine, and calcium channel blockers should be avoided.
3. Atrial flutter or fibrillation with a rapid ventricular response is best treated with cardioversion. As an alternative, agents that prolong the refractory period of the accessory tract—such as intravenous procainamide—can be used. Lidocaine may have some utility, and experimental studies with intravenous flecainide have shown promise. In general, phenytoin, esmolol, propranolol, or verapamil should not be used because of their variable effect on accessory conduction. Digoxin is contraindicated, as it may shorten the refractory period and enhance conduction over the bypass tract.

DEFIBRILLATION AND SYNCHRONIZED CARDIOVERSION

Defibrillation and cardioversion is the technique of passing a short burst (about 5 ms) of direct electric current across the thorax to terminate tachyarrhythmias. The electric current simultaneously depolarizes all excitable cardiac tissue and terminates any areas of reentry by halting further propagation of the impulse around the reentry loop. This places all cardiac cells in the same depolarized state, and a dominant pacemaker (usually the sinus node) paces the heart in a regular manner.

Defibrillation or cardioversion uses the same type of equipment. A device stores a known quantity of electrical energy in a storage

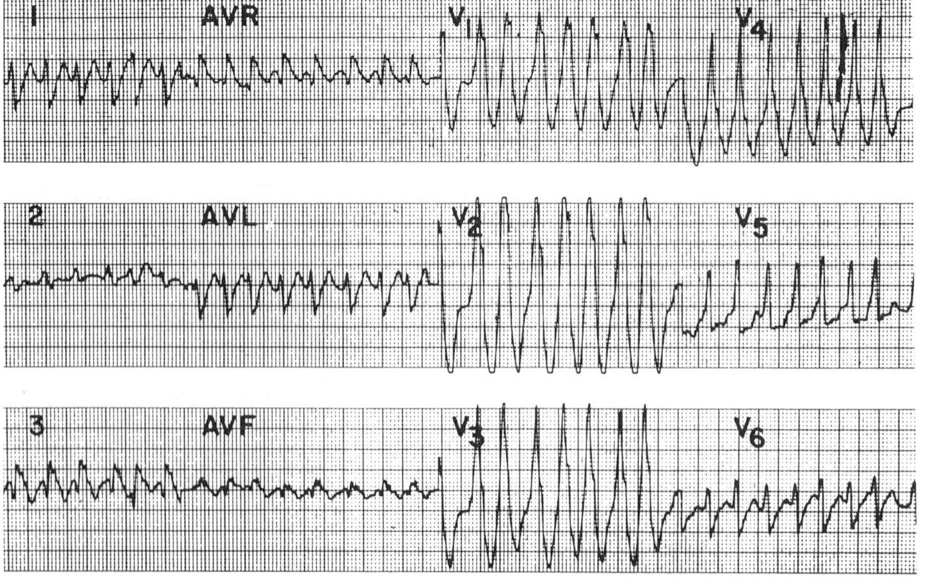

FIG. 24-42. Atrial fibrillation in Wolff-Parkinson-White syndrome.

capacitor and, on command, discharges it through two paddles placed on the chest wall. Usually, a rhythm monitor and a synchronizer circuit are built into the device. Paddle placement can be either anterior-posterior or apex–right parasternal. While some authors found a lower energy requirement for conversion using anterior-posterior paddles, others have not. For emergencies, paddle placement probably does not matter.

To reduce transthorax electrical impedance and increase the amount of current passing through the heart, certain techniques are important at the paddle–chest wall interface. Electrode paste, gel, or saline pads are applied to the surface of the paddles. Firm pressure of 10 to 12.5 kg/cm^2 (20 to 25 lb/in.^{2}) is used to achieve good electrical contact. Larger paddles or defibrillator pads, within reason, have a reduced impedance, but this does not appear to significantly influence the energy required for conversion.

Older devices had significant internal energy losses and delivered as little as 40 percent of the stored energy to the patient. This is not a problem with modern defibrillators, as they deliver very close to the stored amount.

Defibrillation should be done as soon as ventricular fibrillation is diagnosed. The longer ventricular fibrillation persists, the less likely it is that resuscitation will be successful. Current ACLS guidelines recommend 200 J for the first attempt, 200 to 300 J for the second attempt, and 360 J for subsequent defibrillations. Several studies have found that most patients can be defibrillated with 160 to 200 J. Recommendations for children are 2 J/kg (1 J/lb) in the initial attempt and 4 J/kg on subsequent attempts.

Synchronized cardioversion applies the electric current at a time during the cardiac cycle well away from the vulnerable period when there is little chance of inducing ventricular fibrillation—usually about 10 ms after the peak of the R wave. On most machines, the synchronizer circuit must be turned on each time an impulse is desired. Many devices also display by the monitor screen or a flashing light that the synchronizer circuit is detecting properly the QRS complex. Cable leads, rather than the paddles, should be used to monitor the cardiac rhythm to avoid any movement artifact that could be misinterpreted by the synchronizer circuit as the QRS complex.

Complications of defibrillation or cardioversion include the following:

1. Direct myocardial damage: unusual unless there are repeated shocks at high energy (more than 325 J).
2. Ventricular fibrillation: incidence is less than 5 percent with a synchronized discharge but probably greater in the presence of digoxin or quinidine toxicity, hypokalemia, or AMI. However, patients on maintenance digoxin therapy can be safely cardioverted using low energies (less than 50 J).
3. Systemic emboli: about 1.2 to 1.5 percent in patients with chronic atrial fibrillation.
4. ST segment changes: transient elevations or depressions, usually resolving within 5 min.
5. Bradycardias: more common in patients with inferior MIs and those requiring multiple defibrillations-cardioversions. Bradycardias are usually evident during the first 5 s after shock and may occasionally persist for longer than 20 s and require external or internal pacing.
6. Tachycardias: usually sinus tachycardia, occasionally atrial flutter or fibrillation, and usually resolving spontaneously within 5 min.
7. Atrial, junctional, or ventricular ectopy: usually transient and benign.
8. Pulmonary edema: uncommon but may occur in patients with mitral or aortic valvular disease or left ventricular failure.
9. Hypotension: rare, inexplicable, and may last for several hours before spontaneously resolving.
10. Muscle damage: elevated levels of creatine phosphokinase and lactate dehydrogenase are common, but other more specific indicators (CPK-MB and troponin) are rarely abnormal.

CARDIAC PACEMAKERS

Artificial cardiac pacemakers have two components: a power source (battery with pulse generator) and an electrode that delivers current to the heart (transvenous, epicardial, transthoracic, and transcutaneous). In permanent pacemaker placement, the power source is implanted subcutaneously, and the electrodes are run through the veins to inside the heart or through the subcutaneous tissue to the epicardial surface. In temporary pacemaker placement, the power source is external to the body, and electrodes are placed in one of two ways: (1) transvenously to an intracardiac location or (2) transcutaneously with electrodes placed on the thoracic skin. The pulse generator can be designated to operate in either a fixed-rate mode (asynchronous or competitive) or a demand mode (synchronous or noncompetitive). In the fixed-rate mode, the pulse generator produces an electrical signal at the preset rate regardless of the patient's own intrinsic cardiac rhythm. Serious dysrhythmias or ventricular fibrillation may occur if the pacemaker discharges during the vulnerable period (T wave); for this reason, fixed-rate pacing is rarely done.

In the demand mode, the pulse generator has a sensing circuit that detects spontaneous cardiac activity and will discharge only if no cardiac depolarization is detected for a preset interval. Demand pacemakers may have two response modes, either inhibited or triggered. Pacemakers set to be inhibited have a pulse generator that is inhibited by the sensed cardiac activity and do not generate an impulse. In the triggered response mode, the pacemaker detects the patient's intrinsic cardiac activity and then discharges during the absolute refractory period. On ECG, this appears as pacing spikes following each intrinsic QRS complex.

The latest five-letter code system is shown in Table 24-5. This coding system has added antitachyarrhythmic and shocking capabilities of the latest pacemakers. Many patients carry cards indicating the type of pacemaker they have. The simplest type of pacemaker used—the ventricular-demand inhibited-response pacemaker—would be designated as VVI.

The modern permanent pacemaker is powered by a lithium battery that has an approximate lifetime of 8 to 12 years. Most units are preset for rates around 70, with a pacing interval of 0.84 s. The demand pacemaker has a built-in refractory period (0.2 to 0.4 s) during which it will not sense. This prevents it from being inhibited by its own stimulus. Most demand pacemakers have a magnetic switch, which temporarily converts the pulse generator from the demand mode to the fixed-rate mode when a magnet is held over the unit. In this way, the pacing rate can be quickly determined, but the magnet should be applied for only short periods to avoid initiating tachyarrhythmias. The rate and stimulus strength can be reset by noninvasive means in programmable pacemakers. Some of the more sophisticated pacemakers can be interrogated to indicate events such as tachyarrhythmias and conversions. Since pacemaker complexity varies, the manufacturer supplies an identification card with each unit that patients should carry.

Temporary pacemakers are powered by 9-V radio-type batteries. On these pacemakers, there are settings for the mode (fixed or demand), rate (40 to 140), and stimulus strength (0.2 to 20 mA). During emergency pacing, initial settings should be in the demand mode with a rate around 70 and stimulus strength around 3.0 mA. The negative terminal should be connected to the distal electrode.

The transvenous intracardiac electrode may be either unipolar or bipolar. The unipolar setup has the negative electrode within the heart and the positive electrode in the chest wall. Permanent pacemakers using the unipolar setup have the positive electrode in their surface covering. Temporary pacemakers using the unipolar setup have their positive electrode connected to a needle implanted in the skin of the anterior thorax. With the bipolar setup, both electrodes are within a few millimeters of each other and both lie within the heart. Transvenous electrodes are placed most commonly into the apex of the right ventricle. This causes an LBBB pattern when pacing. Different catheters are used depending on the clinical situation. Semirigid catheters (6 or

TABLE 24-5 NASPE/BPEG Generic (NBG) Pacemaker Code*

Letter Position	I	II	III	IV	V
Category	Chamber(s) Paced	Chamber(s) Sensed	Response to Sensing	Programmability, Rate	Antitachyarrhythmis Function(s)
	O, none	O, none	O, none	O, none	O, none
	A, atrium	A, atrium	T, triggered	P, simple programmable	P, pacing
	V, ventricle	V, ventricle	I, inhibited	M, multiprogrammable	S, shock
	D, dual (A + V)†	D, dual (A + V)†	D, dual (D + I)‡	C, Communicating (telemetry)	D, dual (P + S)§
	S, single chamber	S, single chamber		R, rate modulation	

*NASEP/BEPEG, North American Society for Pacing and Electrophysiology/British Pacing and Electrophysiology Group.
†Atrial and ventricular.
‡Dual (atrial and ventricular) and inhibited.
§Pacing and shock.

7 Fr) are inserted through a venous puncture or cutdown. They usually require fluoroscopy for correct placement. Semifloating (3 or 4 Fr) or flexible balloon-tipped catheters (3 or 5 Fr) can be introduced and directed into the right ventricle without fluoroscopy, using blood flow. Flexible catheters can become dislodged by patient or cardiac movement and are usually replaced with semirigid catheters within 24 h.

Transthoracic cardiac pacing has been largely replaced by transcutaneous pacing. Transthoracic pacing is fraught with many complications, including coronary artery laceration and cardiac tamponade in addition to pneumothorax (Fig. 24-43).

Transcutaneous electrodes are self-adhesive pads that are usually placed with the negative electrode over the left anterior precordium and the positive electrode over the left infrascapular area. Transcutaneous pacing is then initiated by using the lowest current setting, which is increased until electrical capture is achieved. Most patients can be paced with 100 mA, but some may require up to 200 mA. The newer pacemakers cause much less discomfort, can be applied faster, and combine defibrillator and pacing functions from the same pads.

Indications for Emergency Pacing

Emergency cardiac pacing is indicated either therapeutically (for symptomatic bradyarrhythmias) or prophylactically (for conduction defects that pose a high risk of sudden complete heart block or asystole).

As noted before, symptomatic bradyarrhythmias should be treated with atropine and/or isoproterenol as a temporary measure to support cardiac rhythm prior to pacemaker placement. Some patients may respond adequately to atropine alone and do not require pacemaker insertion.

Most authors would recommend prophylactic placement of a pacemaker in any patient with acute myocardial infarction who has a new or age-indeterminant bi- or trifascicular block. In addition, second-degree Mobitz II and, of course, third-degree AV blocks are also indications for pacemaker insertion or transcutaneous pacer pads. Despite successful pacing, many patients with acute myocardial infarction and these serious conduction blocks have extensive left ventricular damage and a high mortality from pump failure.

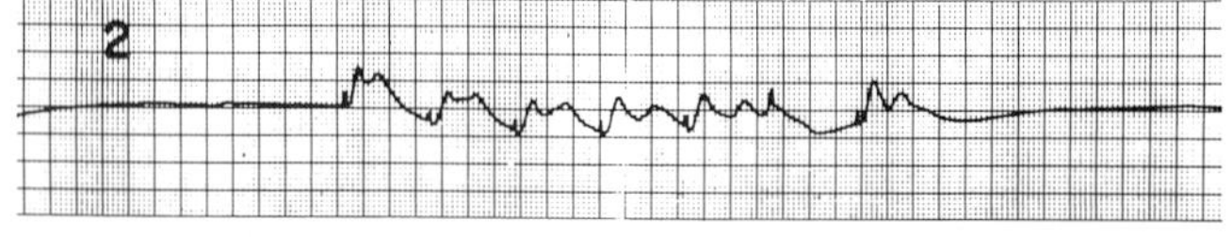

FIG. 24-43. Ventricular capture with transthoracic pacing.

Pacemaker Malfunction

Malfunction of a permanent pacemaker can be categorized as either (1) failure to sense, (2) failure to pace, (3) oversensing, or (4) combinations of the first three. With current lithium batteries and reliable circuitry, most pacemaker malfunctions are due to problems with the electrodes and not the result of battery exhaustion or pulse-generator failure.

Failure to sense may occur when the voltages of the patient's own intrinsic QRS complex is too low to be detected by the sensing circuit of the pacemaker. Changing from a bipolar to a unipolar setup (if possible) may help the pacemaker sense the intrinsic cardiac activity. Failure to sense may cause the pacemaker to become a fixed-rate pacemaker, discharge during the T wave, and trigger serious dysrhythmias.

Failure to pace may occur when tissue reaction around the electrode makes the myocardium insensitive to the electric discharge that is generated by the pacemaker. It is common for the pacing threshold to increase during the first few weeks after insertion, but further rises are infrequent.

Failure to both sense and pace may be due to battery exhaustion, fracture of the wires in the catheter, or displacement of the electrodes. Battery exhaustion is indicated when the pacing rate slowly decreases. With lithium batteries, such decreases usually occur years before actual battery exhaustion. Greater than a 10 percent change from the initial rate is an urgent indication for replacement. Catheter wire fracture may cause either sustained or intermittent interruption in electrical conductivity. Sudden onset of symptoms and/or bradyarrhythmias suggests catheter fracture. Catheter fractures are rarely seen on routine chest radiographs. The transvenous electrode is usually positioned in the right ventricular apex, with a characteristic appearance on the chest radiograph and ECG. Displacement can be suggested when changes on radiographs or ECG occur.

Oversensing is used to describe the situation where the pacemaker senses electrical activity not associated with atrial or ventricular depolarizations; it is thus inhibited and generation of the pacemaker impulse is suppressed. Causes of oversensing include physiologic electrical activity (T waves, muscle potentials), external electromagnetic interference, and signals generated by the interaction of different portions of the pacing system. Unipolar electrodes are more sensitive to physiologic electrical activity and electromagnetic interference than bipolar electrodes.

Under certain conditions, pacemakers may initiate tachyarrhythmias despite functioning as designed; this usually results from an intrinsic depolarization occurring during the pacemaker refractory period, therefore not being sensed, and the pacemaker firing soon thereafter and initiating a reentrant tachycardia. In this setting, maintenance of the dysrhythmia does not require further participation of the pacemaker. Dual-chamber pacemakers can also induce and sustain dysrhythmias. In this situation, emergent treatment requires reprogramming the pacemaker, if possible, or converting to synchronous mode by placing a magnet over the pulse generator.

EVALUATION OF PALPITATIONS

Palpitations are common symptoms that may be due to an dysrhythmia. Frequently, palpitations are no longer present when the patient presents to the emergency department. The term is nonspecific, but certain descriptions may be helpful in pointing toward certain types of rhythm disturbances. Premature atrial or ventricular contractions followed by a compensatory pause are often described as a flip-flopping in the chest. Atrial or ventricular dysrhythmias can cause a fluttering feeling. Pounding in the neck can be felt when atrial and ventricular contractions are dissociated as in supraventricular or junctional tachycardias. Inappropriate sinus tachycardia is also in the differential diagnosis.

History taking should include questions regarding prescribed medications, including herbals; recreational drugs, and use of caffeine-containing beverages. History suggestive of endocrine disorders such as hyperthyroidism should also be sought. If the clinical presentation suggests potassium abnormality, electrolytes can be checked.

Palpitations associated with dizziness, syncope, or presyncope should be assumed to be associated with ventricular tachycardia until proven otherwise. While panic attack is often assumed to be associated with palpitations; this diagnosis cannot be established in the ED.

The ECG should be examined for evidence of dysrhythmia, bypass tracts, and QT-interval prolongation. Patients with a family history of sudden death, syncope, or dysrhythmia, those with any evidence of organic heart disease, and those with presyncope, syncope, or dizziness can be admitted or placed in an observation unit for monitoring and electrophysiologic testing. Patients felt to be at lower risk can be discharged and ambulatory monitoring arranged by the continuing care physician.

BIBLIOGRAPHY

Brugada P, Brugada J, Mont L, et al: A new approach to the differential diagnosis of regular tachycardia with a wide QRS complex. *Circulation* 83:1649, 1991.

Dreifus LS, Hessen SE: Supraventricular tachycardia: diagnosis and treatment. *Cardiology* 77:259, 1990.

Epstein AE, Hallstrom AP, Rogers WJ, et al: Mortality following ventricular dysrhythmia suppression by encainide, flecainide, and moricizine after myocardial infarction: The original design concept of the cardiac dysrhythmia suppression trial (CAST). *JAMA* 270:2451, 1993.

Rankin AC, Brooks R, Ruskin JN, et al: Adenosine and the treatment of supraventricular tachycardia. *Am J Med* 92:655, 1992.

Teo KK, Yusuf S, Furberg CD: Effects of prophylactic antiarrhythmic drug therapy in acute myocardial infarction. An overview of results from randomized controlled trials. *JAMA* 270:1589, 1993.

Zimetbaum P, Josephson ME: Evaluation of patients with palpitations. *N. Engl J Med* 338:1369, 1998.

PHARMACOLOGY OF ANTIDYSRHYTHMIC AND VASOACTIVE MEDICATIONS

Teresa M. Carlin

To understand antidysrhythmic therapy, one must be familiar with the cardiac cycle. The action potential is made up of four phases, with phase 4 representing diastole. During diastole, pacemaker cells slowly depolarize (automaticity) while all other myocytes are electrically quiescent. Once the pacemaker reaches threshold, through propagation of an action potential, myocardial cells rapidly depolarize in coordinated fashion because of influx of sodium through voltage-dependent sodium channels (phase 0). The efflux of potassium down its concentration gradient initiates repolarization (phase 1). The phase 2 plateau occurs when ion fluxes across membranes are in equilibrium—namely, calcium influx via slow calcium channels and potassium efflux. The influx of calcium allows the heart to contract. During phase 3, the calcium channels close and potassium permeability increases, which permits rapid repolarization. The beginning of phase 0 (rapid depolarization) until midway through phase 3 (rapid repolarization) represents the absolute refractory period. During the effective refractory period (ERP), a second action potential cannot be elicited. (Fig. 25-1).

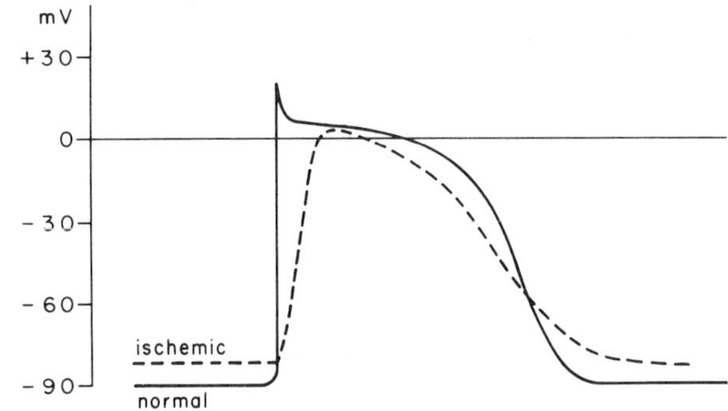

FIG. 25-1. Ventricular myocardial cell transmembrane action potential.

The Vaughan Williams classification of antidysrhythmics groups drugs based on their ability to block sodium channels (class I), block calcium channels (class IV), block beta-adrenergic receptors (class II), or prolong the refractory period (class III) (Table 25-1). Digoxin and adenosine do not fit into this scheme.

ANTIDYSRHYTHMIC AGENTS

Class I Antidysrhythmic Agents

PROCAINAMIDE Procainamide is useful as an antidysrhythmic agent in the treatment of various ventricular and supraventricular dysrrhythmias. Procainamide was developed after the antidysrhythmic effects of the local anesthetic agent procaine were realized. However, procaine's short duration of action and its prominent central nervous system (CNS) effects rule it out for its clinical use.

Like all class I agents, procainamide blocks sodium channels and depresses the speed of impulse conduction (phase 0) of the cardiac action potential. It prolongs the duration of the action potential and the effective refractory period. This is reflected on the electrocardiogram (ECG) as QRS, QT, and PR interval prolongation. These effects directly depress myocardial conduction, suppress fibrillatory activity in the atria and ventricles, and prevent ectopic or reentrant dysrhythmias. These electrophysic effects of procainamide are more pronounced at faster heart rates.

Procainamide suppresses automaticity (phase 4), especially of ectopic pacemakers, secondary to its anticholinergic properties. The effects on AV node conduction are variable. Sodium channel blockade slows AV node conduction time. However, anticholinergic stimulation tends to speed AV node conduction. The antimuscarinic effects are dose dependent. Large doses of procainamide will provide extensive anticholinergic effects and may even increase automaticity (inducing a prodysrhythmic effect). Unlike quinidine, procainamide produces more local anesthetic effects but less vagolytic effects. Procainamide

TABLE 25-1 Electrophysiologic Actions of Antidysrhythmic Agents

	Agent	Action
CLASS I AGENTS		
Sodium (post) channel blockers		
IA:	Quinidine Procainamide	Depress phase 0 (conduction), moderate depression, especially depolarized tissue
		Depress phase 4 (automaticity), especially ectopic sites
		Prolong refractoriness—APD lengthened, ERP lengthened
IB:	Lidocaine Phenytoin	Depress phase 0 (conduction), slight
		Depress phase 4 (automaticity), affects depolarized tissue, not normal tissue
		Refractoriness essentially unchanged—APD shortened, ERP lengthened
IC:	Encainide Flecainide	Depress phase 0 (conduction), marked depression; no place in ED setting.
		Depress phase 4 (automaticity)
		Refractoriness unchanged—APD, ERP unchanged
CLASS II AGENTS		
β blockers		
	Propranolol (prototype)	Depress phase 4 (automaticity), especially in high catecholamine states
		Depress phase 0 (conduction)
		Prolong refractoriness, specifically of the AVN
CLASS III AGENTS		
Antifibrillatory agents		
	Amiodarone	Prolong refractoriness
	Bretylium	Potassium channel modulation
	Sotalol	Each agent has a unique pharmacodynamic profile
CLASS IV AGENTS		
Calcium channel blockers		
	Verapamil (prototype)	Depress phase 4 (automaticity)
		Depress phase 0 (conduction)
		Prolong refractoriness
UNCLASSIFIED AGENTS:		
	Digoxin	Increase phase 4 (automaticity), specifically of ectopic pacemakers at toxic levels
		Depress phase 0 (conduction), particularly through the AVN
		Prolong refractoriness, particularly through the AVN
	Adenosine	Decrease phase 4 (automaticity)
		Depress phase 0 (conduction), especially in the AVN; effects not blocked by atropine

Key: APD, action potential duration; ERP, effective refractory periods; AVN, atroventricular node.

is less depressing to cardiac contractility than quinidine; negative inotropy is most pronounced in ischemic tissue.

Pharmacokinetics The onset of action of procainamide is 5 to 10 min following intravenous administration and 15 to 60 min following intramuscular injection. Procainamide has an elimination half-life of 2.5 to 4.7 h (in normal renal function) and an apparent volume of distribution (Vd) of 2 L/kg. However, in patients with congestive heart failure (CHF) and renal dysfunction, the elimination half-life may increase and the Vd may decrease (i.e., requiring smaller doses). Procainamide is metabolized to an active compound, *N*-acetyl procainamide (NAPA), in the liver via *N*-acetyltransferase. This active metabolite has an average half-life of 7 h in patients with normal renal function. Rapid acetylators convert greater amounts of procainamide to NAPA than do slow acetylators. Plasma procainamide levels of approximately 4 to 10 mg/mL are usually required to suppress ventricular dysrhythmias. Refractory dysrhythmias may require levels up to 20 mg/mL (usually 10 to 15 mg/mL). Adverse effects often appear with levels greater than 12 mg/mL.

Common Emergency Department (ED) Indications Procainamide is a second-line agent generally used to treat and prevent recurrence of ventricular dysrhythmias, specifically stable ventricular tachycardia (VT) and premature ventricular contractions (PVCs) that are unresponsive to lidocaine. It is infrequently used in ventricular fibrillation (VF) or pulseless VT because it takes so long to achieve therapeutic concentrations. Procainamide may also be used for slowing or converting supraventricular tachycardias (SVT) including atrial flutter and fibrillation [especially in Wolff-Parkinson-White (WPW) syndrome], paroxysmal supraventricular tachycardia (PSVT), paroxysmal atrial tachycardia (PAT), and paroxysmal atrioventricular (AV) junctional rhythm. Contraindications include complete AV heart block, second- or third-degree heart block (without an electrical pacemaker present), long QT intervals, and torsades de pointes. The drug should be used cautiously in patients with systemic lupus erythematosus, CHF, and hepatic or renal disease and avoided in those with allergies to procaine or amide-type drugs.

Dosing and Administration In the past, the recommendation for intravenous loading of procainamide for treating ventricular dysrhythmias was as a bolus injection. However, a continuous infusion has been shown to be safer (fewer adverse effects) than a bolus injection until the dysrhythmia is controlled, hypotension develops, the QRS complex widens more than 50 percent, prolongation of the QT interval develops, or a total of 17 mg/kg (1.2 g for a 70-kg patient) has been given. The recommended infusion rate is 20 mg/min; in urgent situations, however, 30 mg/min may be given cautiously. Blood pressure and QRS complex must be monitored during intravenous administration. If procainamide suppresses the VT, initiate a continuous infusion at 1 to 4 mg/min to maintain the suppression. Lower doses are generally necessary for patients with CHF, hypotensive states, and hepatic or renal failure. Measurement of daily serum levels of procainamide or NAPA should be considered in patients with risk factors for impaired clearance.

Alternatively, oral therapy may be started after intravenous loading with procainamide (375 to 500 mg PO q3–4h) or a sustained-release preparation may be used (Procan SR or Pronestyl-SR in a dose of between 500 and 1000 mg q6–8h).

Adverse-Effects Profile The most serious adverse effects of procainamide are from myocardial depression. ECG changes may include prolongation of the QRS and QT intervals, impairment of AV conduction, VF, and torsades de pointes. High doses or rapid infusion can cause severe hypotension. It should be initiated cautiously in patients with acute myocardial infarction (AMI) owing to its potential proarrhythmic effect. Procainamide and NAPA levels should be monitored in the following patients: (1) those on procainamide longer than 24 h, (2) those on a maintenance infusion of 3 mg/min or higher, and (3) those with acute CHF or renal failure. Symptoms of systemic lupus erythematosus (SLE) have been reported with chronic administration. Hypersensitivity reactions—characterized by angioedema, acute bronchoconstriction, vascular collapse, febrile episodes, and respiratory arrest—may occur. In addition, idiosyncratic reactions—including agranulocytosis, hepatomegaly, confusion, nausea, vomiting, urticaria, fever, maculopapular eruptions, and thrombocytopenia—may develop with procainamide.

QUINIDINE (GLUCONATE OR SULFATE) **Actions** Quinidine is a class IA antidysrhythmic agent with essentially the same mechanism of action as procainamide. However, anticholinergic effects are more pronounced with quinidine. These anticholinergic effects may facilitate conduction across the AV node.

Pharmacokinetics Onset of action following intravenous administration is within minutes, whereas the onset for the intramuscular and oral routes usually occurs in 1 to 3 h. Therapeutic cardiovascular effects last for the half-life of the drug, 6 to 8 h. The oral sustained-release gluconate preparation, however, can last up to 12 h. Therapeutic serum levels range between 2 and 7 mg/mL. Quinidine has an average Vd of 2 L/kg in healthy adults. It is metabolized in the liver to two active metabolites. Approximately 10 to 50 percent of a dose is excreted as unchanged drug in the urine within 24 h.

Common ED Indications Quinidine is effective in the treatment of atrial and ventricular dysrhythmias and thus has the same indications as procainamide. It is not commonly used parentally in the ED, since other agents such as procainamide are safer alternatives.

Dosing and Administration The oral route is preferred in administering quinidine. Oral quinidine is available in three salts: sulfate (83 percent active drug), gluconate (62 percent active drug), and polygalacturonate (60 percent active drug). Only the gluconate and sulfate salts are available for parenteral use. Intramuscular administration is effective in acute but not in critical dysrhythmias. Intravenous administration is now rarely used. The dosage of quinidine varies, depending on the indication and salt used. For example, the adult dosage for suppressing atrial, AV junctional, and ventricular complexes is 324 to 600 mg PO of extended-release quinidine gluconate q8–12h, while the dosage for quinidine sulfate to maintain sinus rhythm after conversion is 200 to 400 mg three or four times daily. The initial IM dose is 600 mg PO of quinidine gluconate, then 400 mg PO as often as q2h until desired effects are seen. Generally, the intravenous dosage required to abolish ventricular dysrhythmias is 300 mg or less; however, 500 to 750 mg may be needed. The rate of infusion should not exceed 16 mg/min, and the ECG and blood pressure should be continuously monitored to gauge the efficacy and safety of treatment.

Adverse-Effects Profile The adverse-effect profile of quinidine is similar to that of procainamide (including a prodysrhythmic effect) and includes QT prolongation, torsades de pointes, SLE, and hypersensitivity reactions. Toxicity usually impairs therapeutic effectiveness. High serum levels of quinidine may result in cinchonism, which includes tinnitus, blurred vision, headache, nausea, and deafness. Severe cases may lead to delirium and psychosis. Quinidine may also cause SA or AV nodal block and decrease cardiac contractility. It is also associated with acute hemolytic hemolysis, thrombocytopenia, and hepatitis. Hypotension, heart failure, and hepatic disease decrease clearance. Quinidine has also been implicated in raising serum digoxin levels two- to threefold.

Class IB Agents

LIDOCAINE **Actions** Lidocaine is the prototype of a class IB agent. It is a first-line agent in the treatment of serious ventricular dysrhythmias. It preferentially depresses the automaticity (phase 4) of the distal conduction system of depolarized and ischemic tissue; it does not affect normal myocardium. It has greater activity at faster heart rates. Lidocaine is not effective against atrial dysrhythmias because it preferentially acts on the His-Purkinje and more distal conduction system. Unlike class IA and IC agents, lidocaine only minimally depresses phase 0 (conduction). The refractory period is essentially unchanged, since the shortening of the action potential duration is offset by the relative lengthening of the effective refractory period.

Lidocaine has local anesthetic effects that stabilize membranes, elevate the ventricular fibrillation threshold, and suppress ventricular ectopy in tissues during acute myocardial ischemia. However, lidocaine is no longer routinely recommended for prophylaxis after myocardial infarction (MI). Although it reduces the incidence of ventricular ectopy and fibrillation after MI, it may increase mortality secondary to asystole, which may occur if ventricular escape rhythms are abolished.

The benefits of lidocaine include its rapid onset of action, its short time to recovery from sodium channel blockade, and its relative lack of adverse hemodynamic effects. It is protein bound and undergoes hepatic metabolism. Given the extensive first-pass effect, it is not available as an oral medication.

Pharmacokinetics The onset of action is 30 to 90 s following intravenous administration and 10 min following an intramuscular dose. Subsequent bolus doses are generally required to attain therapeutic plasma levels early in treatment; maintenance infusions started without an initial bolus dose will not attain therapeutic levels for up to 30 min to several hours (based on disease state). Lidocaine has an approximate Vd of 1.3 L/kg in normal patients and 0.9 L/kg in patients with liver disease or CHF or in those who are hypotensive. The drug is available for intravenous use only because of its lack of gastrointestinal (GI) absorption and its high first-pass metabolism. Less than 10 percent is excreted unchanged in the urine. The major metabolites, monoethylglycinexylidide (MEGX) and glycinexylidide (GX), possess antidysrhythmic and neurotoxic actions and are excreted renally.

Lidocaine has a short distribution half-life of 7 to 8 min following an intravenous bolus and 12 to 28 min following intramuscular administration. This short distribution half-life accounts for the short duration of action after a bolus injection. The elimination half-life in healthy patients ranges from 80 to 108 min, but this may increase up to 7 h in patients with CHF or liver disease and is also greatly prolonged in cardiac arrest. Renal dysfunction does not alter kinectics. Therapeutic serum levels range from 1.5 to 6 mg/mL; serum levels greater than 5 mg/mL may cause CNS toxicity. It readily crosses the blood brain barrier, which accounts for its CNS effects. Not all patients require maximum serum levels.

Common ED Indications Lidocaine is the drug of choice for the suppression of ventricular dysrhythmias and ventricular ectopy (frequent multifocal PVCs, couplets, salvos, and especially long runs of VT) in suspected acute myocardial ischemia or unstable angina.[1] Although once popular, the prophylactic routine use of lidocaine during acute MI is generally not recommended. Such therapy has not been shown to reduce mortality following AMI. In addition, lidocaine should not be used to treat chronic PVC that occur in an asymptomatic patient, as it does not prevent VF. The drug is indicated for control of VT and VF refractory to defibrillation and epinephrine. Lidocaine should be given following successful conversion of ventricular tachydysrhythmias to normal sinus rhythm. It is also indicated for ventricular dysrhythmias associated with cardiac arrest, myocardial infarction, and unstable angina. Lidocaine can be an adjunct to procainamide for the treatment of wide-complex supraventricular dysrhythmias of uncertain type (e.g., WPW syndrome).

Dosing and Administration Lidocaine is given as an initial bolus dose of 1.0 to 1.5 mg/kg followed by additional bolus doses of 0.5 to 0.75 mg/kg q5–10 min as needed up to a cumulative dose of 3 mg/kg. An alternative method is to give 1.5 mg/kg initially followed by 50-mg bolus doses every 5 min up to a total dose of 225 mg or 3 mg/kg. When VF is present and defibrillation and epinephrine have failed, an initial bolus of 1.5 mg/kg is recommended for all patients. Conscious patients should receive lidocaine at a rate not exceeding 50 mg/min to minimize adverse CNS effects (< 25 mg/min if infused through a central line). However, in pulseless VT or VF, lidocaine can be given by rapid intravenous push. When intravenous lines are not available, the drug may be instilled endotracheally, in which case 2 to $2\frac{1}{2}$ times the intravenous dose diluted with normal saline solution to a total volume of 10 mL is recommended for optimal drug absorption.

TABLE 25-2 Summary of Dosing and Administration of Common Antidysrhythmic Agents*

Agent	Indication	Dose
Procainamide (pronestyl)	Treatment of ventricular dysrhythmias and recurrent ventricular tachycardias refractory to lidocaine. Second-line therapy for pulseless VT/VF. Convert supraventricular dysrhythmias, particularly those associated with WPW.	20-mg/min IV infusion. Stop when: total dose of 17 mg/kg reached, QRS complex widens more than 50 percent, QT interval prolongation, dysrhythmia is controlled, or hypotension develops.
Lidocaine (Xylocaine)	VF/pulseless VT	1.5-mg/kg IV bolus, then 0.5-mg/kg bolus q5 min as needed until 3 mg/kg total given. Follow with continuous infusion at 2 to 4 mg/min. Increase to 2 to 2.5 times the IV dose for ET administration. Mix with saline or sterile water for a total drug volume of 10 mL. Decrease the loading dose and maintenance by 50 percent in patients more than 70 years of age, those with CHF, liver disease, or impaired hepatic blood flow.
Atenolol (Tenormin)	Hypertension Angina AMI	5 mg IV over 5 min. Repeat in 10 min, then convert to PO medication.
Metoprolol (Lopressor)	Hypertension Angina AMI	5 mg IV over 5 min for three doses, then convert to 50 mg PO q12h.
Esmolol (Brevibloc)	Ventricular rate control of SVT	500-μg/kg bolus over 1 min, with a maintenance infusion of 50 μ/kg per min over 4 min. If inadequate clinical response, reload with 500-μg/kg bolus over 1 min followed by a maintenance infusion of 100 μg/kg per min. Continue the cycle of reloading with 500 μg/kg followed by an incremental increase of the maintenance infusion by 50 μg/kg per min until the desired heart rate is obtained. If hypotension occurs, hold the bolus and decrease the infusion by 50 μg/kg per min.
Propranolol (Inderal)	Life-threatening tachydysrhythmias.	The dose is 0.5 mg to 1.0 mg IV up to 3 mg at a rate not exceeding 1.0 mg/min. Repeat dose in 2 min if necessary. Of note, esmolol is as effective in reducing heart rate; it has the advantage of a more rapid reversal of β blockade and less β_2 effects as compared with propranolol.
Labetalol (Normodyne, Trandate)	Hypertensive crisis Dissecting aneurysm Pregnancy-induced hypertension Pheochromocytoma	20 mg IV (0.25 mg/kg in an 80-kg patient) over 2 min. Double the dose until desired supine BP achieved or 300 mg cumulative dose is given. Or, 0.5 mg/min to 2 mg/min IV as a continuous infusion until desired response or 300 mg cumulative dose is given.

**Key:* AMI, acute myocardial infarction; SVT, supraventricular tachycardia.

VF and pulseless VT should be managed only with intravenous bolus doses. Maintenance infusions should be started at 2 mg/min and titrated up to 4 mg/min as needed (30 to 50 mg/kg per minute) only upon return of perfusion (poor perfusion will hamper the drug's elimination).

Patients more than 70 years of age as well as those with CHF, liver disease, or impaired hepatic blood flow should have their loading dose and maintenance infusion rate lowered by 50 percent. Drug interactions that can prolong the half-life of lidocaine or increase toxicity include those that potentiate neurologic effects (e.g., procainamide, tubocurarine), drugs that undergo metabolism in the liver and increase lidocaine levels (e.g., cimetidine, propranolol), and drugs that can produce excessive cardiac depression (e.g., phenytoin). Septic shock will also produce increased cardiac depression. Since the half-life of lidocaine can be increased after 24 to 48 h in any of the above, serum levels should be obtained and infusions adjusted if therapy is used for longer than 24 h. Lidocaine toxicity may also develop in patients with renal dysfunction because of accumulation of the metabolites. Patients should be switched over to oral antidysrhythmics within the first 24 h.

Adverse-Effects Profile Adverse effects from lidocaine usually occur when the drug is administered too rapidly in a conscious patient, when excessive doses are administered, or when a drug interaction potentiates toxicity. Symptoms of mild lidocaine toxicity that correlate with levels greater than 5 mg/mL include slurred speech, drowsiness, confusion, nausea, vertigo, ataxia, tinnitus, paresthesias, muscle twitching and tremor. An abrupt change in mental status is classic for lidocaine toxicity and may indicate that an excessive dose was administered or that the rate of administration was excessive. Serious symptoms occurring at plasma levels greater than 9 mg/mL may include psychosis, seizures, and respiratory depression. Lidocaine is contraindicated in patients with known sensitivities to amide-type local anesthetics and those with high degrees of sinoatrial (SA) or AV block. Lidocaine should be used cautiously in sulfite-allergic patients.

PHENYTOIN Phenytoin also a class IB agent, is used to treat ventricular and supraventricular dysrhythmias associated with digitalis intoxication because of its ability to increase AV nodal conduction time. Unlike lidocaine, phenytoin increases AV nodal conduction. Additionally, it has central sympatholytic activity which is responsible for some of its antidysrhythmic effects. The dose for digoxin-induced dysrhythmias is 100 mg IV q5 min to a total of 1000 to 1500 mg. With parental administration, hypotension can occur secondary to the phenol carrier. Toxic serum levels can result in CNS changes. A further general discussion of phenytoin appears in Chap. 172.

TABLE 25-2 Summary of Dosing and Administration of Common Antidysrhythmic Agents* (*continued*)

Agent	Indication	Dose
Amiodarone	Life-threatening ventricular tachydysrhythmias refractory to first line agents.	150 mg IV over 10 min, then, 1 mg/min for 6 hr, then 0.5 mg/min as maintenance. Re-bolus with 150 mg over 10 min for breakthrough VT or VF.
Bretylium	VF/pulseless VT Recurrent VT with a pulse resistant to first-line agents.	1. Give 5 mg/kg by IV push followed by a 20-mL flush. 2. Defibrillate. Re-bolus with 10 mg/kg by IV push followed by a 20-mL flush. 3. Repeat step 2 q15 min until a maximal cumulative dose of 35 mg/kg is given.
Diltiazem (Cardizem)	Ventricular rate control of SVT Conversion of NSR of PSVT.	1. Give 0.25 mg/kg of actual body weight (average adult dose is 20 mg) IV bolus over 2 min. 2. If inadequate response, then re-bolus with 0.35 mg/kg (average adult dose is 25 mg) over 2 min. 3. Give a continuous infusion at 5 to 15 mg/h to maintain reduced heart rate in patients with atrial fibrillation and/or flutter.
Verapamil (Isoptin, Calan)	Ventricular rate control of SVT. Conversion of NSR of PSVT.	Adults: 5 to 10 mg (0.075 to 0.15 mg/kg) IV over 2 to 3 min. A second dose may be given 15 to 30 min later as needed. Children 1 to 15 y: 0.1 to 0.3 mg/kg IV (usual dose range, 2 to 5 mg) over 2 to 3 min. A second dose may be given 15 to 30 min later as needed. Infants below 1 y: Do not use. There is an association with severe bradycardia, hypotension, and asystole.
Adenosine (Adenocard)	Convert PSVT into NSR. Uncover atrial rhythm of a narrow complex tachycardia of unknown etiology.	1. Give 6-mg IV bolus over 1 to 3 s followed by a 20-mL IV flush. 2. If no response, re-bolus with 12 mg IV push followed by a 20-mL IV flush. 3. If no response, a third 12 mg IV bolus may be given followed by a 20-mL IV flush.
Magnesium ($MgSO_4$)	Torsades de pointes AMI and cardiac arrest with suspected hypomagnesemia.	1 to 2 g IV in 100 mL D_5W over 1 to 2 min.
	Preeclampsia, eclampsia, and preterm labor.	1 to 2 g IV in 100 mL D_5W over 20 min

Class IC Antidysrhythmic Agents

Encainide and flecainide are prototypical class IC agents. They have no effect on the duration of the action potential or the refractory period. They cause marked depression of automaticity (phase 4) of pacemaker cells and slow conduction velocity (phase 0). These agents are not used in the ED setting because of associated prodysrhythmic effects. They were earlier thought helpful for the treatment of atrial fibrillation and refractory VT. However, the Cardiac Arrhythmia Suppression Trial (CAST) demonstrated an increased mortality associated with class IC agents when used to suppress ventricular ectopy in patients with a history of a recent MI and LV dysfunction.[2] In fact, encainide was voluntarily taken off the market because of its prodysrhythmic tendencies. It is available only on a limited basis.

Class II Antidysrhythmic Agents: β Blockers

There are numerous β blockers, each being an effective antidysrhythmic because it prevents circulating catecholamines from binding to beta receptors. However, specific to each drug is its degree of cardioselectivity, intrinsic sympathomimetic activity, α-adrenergic blockade, and quinidine-like membrane stabilization. The metabolic effects (such as alterations in glycogen metabolism) and pharmacokinetics (relative potency, route of elimination, distribution in fat and brain, and duration of action) of each agent are also unique.

Two types of beta receptors exist in the body. β_1 receptors are chiefly found in the heart (also kidney and eye), whereas β_2 receptors are primarily extracardiac. The cardiovascular response to β_1 stimulation includes increased inotropy, increased chronotropy, and increased dromotropy. Therefore β_1 blockade reduces cardiac contractility and myocardial oxygen consumption, decreases heart rate and blood pressure, and slows cardiac conduction velocity.

β_2 receptors are primarily in respiratory, uterine, and vascular smooth muscles as well as in the human liver. β_2 stimulation promotes smooth muscle relaxation and glycogenolysis while β_2 blockade is associated with bronchoconstriction and alterations in glucose metabolism, namely hypoglycemia.

Metoprolol, atenolol, and esmolol are β_1-cardioselective drugs. They are better choices for use in patients with a history of asthma, chronic obstructive pulmonary disease (COPD), and diabetes, since the blockade of β_2 receptors may result in adverse outcomes. At high doses, some agents lose their cardioselectivity; the exact dose at which this occurs, however, has not been clearly established.

Propranolol is a noncardioselective β-blocker prototype since it inhibits both the β_1- and β_2-receptor response. It reduces the incidence of sudden cardiac death after MI. Labetalol is a noncardioselective β blocker with α_1-adrenergic blocking effects. The β-blocking effects of intravenous labetalol are approximately seven times more potent than the α-blocking effects. Sotalol is a class III antidysrhythmic that has β-antagonistic properties. It is discussed later in the chapter.

Cardioselective β blockers with intrinsic sympathomimetic activity (Table 25-2), such as acebutol, occupy the β receptor and produce low-level stimulation. Despite this stimulation, the receptor is functionally blocked to high sympathetic tone. Theoretically, these drugs would be safer to use in patients with low cardiac output states because of their intrinsic ability to stimulate the heart. This ability may prevent acute drug-induced heart failure, but this has not been proven in clinical trials.

β antagonists have a wide spectrum of clinical usefulness. This discussion is limited to acute cardiovascular indications. β blockers slow conduction through the AV node and are therefore useful in slowing the ventricular response in SVT, atrial fibrillation, and atrial flutter. They are particularly useful when these dysrhythmias are dependent on catecholamine stimulation or occur in the setting of an acute myocardial infarction. They are used for rate control but not chemical cardioversion.

β blockers are negative inotropic agents that decrease myocardial oxygen tension. They are therefore useful adjuncts to the treatment of angina and acute myocardial infarction. β blockers limit infarct size, decrease the risk of reinfarction, and reduce mortality in the setting of an AMI. Specifically, propranolol, metoprolol, and atenolol can decrease mortality in AMI patients. This is particularly true if administered early in the course of an AMI (within 6 h of onset), or during an acute anterior infarct. In low-risk patients receiving thrombolytics, β blockade may reduce mortality and recurrent MI if administered within 2 h of symptom onset and it can lower the rate of nonfatal reinfarction and recurrent ischemia if used within 4 h.

Patients with hypertrophic cardiomyopathy develop diastolic dysfunction. β blockers are first-line therapy for ischemic chest pain associated with diastolic dysfunction and may be used very cautiously in CHF associated with this condition. β blockers help reduce shearing forces in patients with dissecting thoracoabdominal aneurysms. Catecholamine excess such as thyroid storm and hypertensive crisis are successfully treated with β antagonist. Symptoms associated with alcohol withdrawal and with mitral valve prolapse are also ameliorated with β blockers.

Mechanism of Action Some β-receptor antagonists have quinidine-like membrane stabilization properties. They depress all phases of the cardiac action potential. Specifically, they depress automaticity (phase 4) and conduction velocity (phase 3) and prolong the refractory period (phase 0). Sinus node discharge and AV conduction velocity are both slowed. Heart rate, blood pressure, and contractility are reduced because of the negative inotropic and negative chromotropic effects. The net result is decreased myocardial oxygen consumption.

Adverse-Effects Profiles The adverse-effects profiles of all β blockers are remarkedly similar. Bronchospasm secondary to β_2 blockade is particularly exaggerated in individuals with asthma or COPD. Therefore, these agents are avoided in the severe COPD/asthma population. However, if a clear indication for β blockade exists in the mild COPD/asthma patient, a cardioselective drug may be used. Cardioselective β agonists are less likely to cause bronchoconstriction than are noncardioselective agents. Bradycardia, hypotension, and heart block can occur. Therefore, patients receiving parental medication should be placed on a cardiac monitor with frequent blood pressure assessments. β blockers may precipitate CHF in patients with LV dysfunction secondary to negative inotropic effects. Hypoglycemia and hyperglycemia may occur. Hypoglycemia needs to be considered, since β blockers may mask signs and symptoms of low blood sugar. Other general side effects include nausea, vomiting, diarrhea, dizziness, lassitude, weakness, and sexual dysfunction.

These drugs are generally contraindicated in patients with heart block greater than first degree, CHF, and cardiogenic shock. However, β blockers may provide some relief when CHF is secondary to diastolic dysfunction or tachycardia. They must be used cautiously in patients with asthma, COPD, and diabetes. Cardioselective drugs cause less bronchospasm and glucose abnormalities than nonselective agents. β blockers are pregnancy class C drugs but can be given when benefits outweigh the risks.

PROPRANOLOL **Actions** In therapeutic doses, the major effect of propranolol is its β-adrenergic blocking activity. The drug blocks the effects of catecholamines on β receptors, inhibiting chronotropic, inotropic, and vasodilator responses to β-adrenergic stimulation. Propranolol slows the sinus rate, depresses AV conduction, decreases cardiac output, reduces blood pressure on exercise, and reduces both supine and standing blood pressures. In addition, propranolol decreases renin release and myocardial oxygen demand and protects against sudden cardiac death.

Pharmacokinetics The onset of action of propranolol following intravenous administration is within 1 min, with a half-life of elimination that varies with duration of therapy. In short-term treatment, the elimination half-life approximates 2 to 3 h; in chronic treatment, however, the elimination half-life is 4 h. Propranolol is widely distributed throughout the body, undergoes extensive first-pass metabolism by the liver, and is also significantly bound to sites within the liver. For these reasons, propranolol has a low bioavailability when taken orally as compared to intravenous administration, requiring the intravenous dose to be approximately 10 times smaller than the oral dose. Several metabolites have been discovered; they are primarily excreted in the urine and feces. In significant renal impairment, the proportion of metabolites excreted by the feces will increase. No dosage adjustments are required in patients with kidney disease. Propranolol has the highest lipid solubility of all β blockers as well as the highest protein binding (93 percent).

Common ED Indications Propranolol is indicated for a wide variety of supraventricular dysrhythmias. These include paroxysmal atrial tachycardia, particularly those dysrhythmias induced by digoxin or catecholamines or associated with the WPW syndrome; refractory sinus tachycardia; atrial flutter or fibrillation refractory to digoxin; persistent atrial extrasystoles that do not respond to conventional therapy; and tachydysrhythmias associated with thyrotoxicosis.[1] Propranolol is less effective for ventricular than for supraventricular dysrhythmias, but it can be used for ventricular tachycardias or ectopic beats due to digoxin or catecholamine toxicity.

Other indications for propranolol include the management of angina and acute myocardial ischemia or infarction because it decreases myocardial oxygen demands; management of all chronic types of hypertension, either alone or in combination with other antihypertensive agents (propranolol is not indicated for hypertensive emergencies); the treatment of idiopathic hypertrophic subaortic stenosis; prophylaxis for common migraine headaches; management of familial or hereditary essential tremor; and as an adjunctive drug following an α-adrenergic blocker in controlling tachycardia due to pheochromocytoma.

Dosing and Administration For life-threatening dysrhythmias, the intravenous dose of propranolol is 0.5 to 1 mg given as an intravenous bolus up to 5 mg at a rate not exceeding 1 mg/min. The dose may be repeated in 2 min. Since significant myocardial depression can occur when doses greater than 3 mg are given, caution should be used if additional doses are necessary. Intravenous esmolol infusion has been as effective as intravenous propranolol in reducing heart rate and has resulted in a more rapid reversal of β blockade as compared with propranolol.

Adverse-Effects Profile The adverse-effects profile of propranolol is similar to that of other nonselective β blockers. The drug is generally not given to patients with asthma or allergic rhinitis and is contraindicated in those with sinus bradycardia or advanced SA or AV block. Propranolol should also not be used in CHF or cardiogenic shock unless these conditions are due to tachydysrhythmias. Following an AMI with the presence of heart failure, ''cardiac asthma'' can be aggravated with propranolol, but less so with cardioselective agents (e.g., esmolol, metoprolol, and atenolol).

ESMOLOL **Actions** Esmolol possesses cardioselective β-adrenergic blocking properties. It selectively blocks the β_1 receptor. As with other β blockers, this drug exhibits both negative inotropic and negative chronotropic effects. Esmolol prevents excessive adrenergic stimulation on the myocardium by blocking the β_1 receptors, thus producing an increase in sinus cycle length, prolongation of SA nodal recovery time, and a prolongation in conduction through the AV node. Esmolol is effective for treating SVT and also possesses antihypertensive effects. These may be due to its ability to decrease cardiac output, sympathetic outflow, and renin release from the kidneys, or perhaps from the direct vasodilatory action of the drug.

Pharmacokinetics Within 1 to 4 min of intravenous loading with esmolol, both the heart rate and blood pressure decline and the PR interval becomes prolonged on the ECG. Of all the available β-blocking agents, esmolol has the shortest duration of action. The elimination half-life is approximately 9 min, and effects of the drug completely reverse within 30 min after cessation of intravenous therapy. This feature makes intravenous esmolol a useful agent for the treatment of acute and unstable SVT, since the adverse or toxic effects disappear quickly upon discontinuation of the drug. The short duration of action also allows the drug to be titrated to effect. Although 90 percent of an administered dose is excreted renally as metabolites, the metabolites possess minimal if any β-blocking effects. Dosing adjustments are thus not required in patients suffering from hepatic or renal insufficiency. At high doses, esmolol loses its cardioselectivity.

Common ED Indications Esmolol is currently indicated to control ventricular rate for the short term when the termination of SVT is desired. It prevents and treats SVT resulting from increased sympathetic tone during or following surgical procedures. Intravenous esmolol may also be used during surgery as replacement β-blocker therapy to prevent rebound hypertension in patients who have been receiving long-term β-blocker treatment. Esmolol can also be used to maintain normal sinus rhythm (NSR) in post-AMI patients who cannot tolerate oral medications. Esmolol is not indicated for long-term management of SVT.

Dosing and Administration A loading dose of esmolol is given as an IV bolus of 500 μg/kg over 1 min, followed by IV infusion starting at 50 μg/kg per min infused over 4 min. Assess for therapeutic and adverse effects immediately following the infusion. If there is no response, give another loading dose over 1 min and increase the infusion rate to 100 μg/kg per min for 4 min. If there is still no response, repeat this procedure, using the same bolus dose each time and increasing the infusion rate by increments of 50 μg/kg per min until the rate of infusion reaches 200 μg/kg per min, the desired response is achieved, or adverse effects appear. The majority of patients will respond within this dosage range. A dose-dependent action is noticed, however, and doses above 200 μg/kg per min are usually of no greater benefit. Once adequate therapeutic response is obtained, it is advisable to change infusion rates by no more than 25 μg/kg per min and not use a bolus dose. Also, avoid concentrations greater than 10 μg/mL. The use of esmolol infusions up to 24 h has been well documented. Limited data indicate that esmolol is well tolerated up to 48 h. After achieving a desired hemodynamic response, transition to alternative antidysrhythmic agents should be considered. Wean the patient off esmolol gradually.

The majority of patients will respond within this dosage range. A dose-dependent action is noticed, however, and doses above 200 μg/kg per min are usually of no greater benefit. Once adequate therapeutic response is obtained, it is advisable to change infusion rates by no more than 25 μg/kg per min and not use a bolus dose. Also, avoid concentrations greater than 10 μg/mL. The use of esmolol infusions up to 24 h has been well documented. Limited data indicate that esmolol is well tolerated up to 48 h. After a desired hemodynamic response is achieved, transition to alternative antidysrhythmic agents should be considered. Wean the patient off esmolol gradually.

Adverse-Effects Profile Esmolol shares the same toxic potential and adverse effect profile as the other β-blocking agents. The most common adverse effect associated with esmolol use is hypotension, which occurs in approximately 20 to 50 percent of patients being treated for SVT. This usually occurs within 30 min of the initiation of therapy. Other common adverse effects include dizziness, somnolence, and nausea.

LABETALOL **Actions** Labetalol possesses membrane-stabilizing effects and thus has some antidysrhythmic action; however, the drug is often used as an antihypertensive agent because it blocks both α- and β-adrenergic receptors. The β-adrenergic blocking effects are nonselective, while the α-blocking effects are selective for the α_1 receptor. The β-blocking effects of labetalol are much greater than its α-blocking effects, in a ratio between 3:1 for oral and 7:1 for intravenous administration. Labetalol possesses some ability to stimulate rather than block the β_2 receptors.

The mechanisms by which labetalol elicits its antihypertensive effects may include any or all of the following: (1) synergistic effects resulting in hypotension when both α_1 and β_1 receptors are blocked, (2) β_2-receptor stimulation, and (3) direct vasodilatory action. Labetalol decreases heart rate, contractility, cardiac output, cardiac work, and total peripheral resistance.

Pharmacokinetics Labetalol is primarily eliminated by the liver and undergoes extensive first-pass metabolism, with approximately 30 percent of the drug reaching circulation following oral administration. It is excreted in the urine and feces. Very little crosses the blood-brain barrier. Geriatric patients and those with liver disease, however, may have a greater bioavailability. The onset of action of intravenous labetalol is within 2 to 5 min; it peaks in 10 to 15 min and lasts 2 to 4 h. Oral labetalol acts within 20 min to 2 h, peaks within 1 to 4 h, and lasts 8 to 24 h. The elimination half-life is approximately 3 to 8 h in normal individuals. Only 5 percent of the drug is excreted unchanged.

Common ED Indications Labetalol is used in emergency medicine primarily for its antihypertensive actions. Intravenous labetalol rapidly and effectively reduces elevated pressures, causing only minimal alterations in heart rate and cardiac output. It is a good alternative for treating the hypertensive patient with myocardial ischemia. Oral labetalol may be substituted once control of blood pressure has been established. Intravenous labetalol can be used in pregnancy as long as benefits outweigh risks. It is a class C drug in pregnancy.

Dosing and Administration Labetalol can be administered intravenously via multiple intravenous boluses or a continuous infusion. When initiating an intravenous bolus, the clinician should start with 20 mg (0.25 mg/kg in an 80-kg patient) and repeat with 40 mg to 160 mg every 10 min until the desired effect is reached or until a total cumulative dose of 300 mg has been given. It is best to double the previous dose every 10 min, thus allowing a gradual dosage increase. A smaller alternative dosage would be 10 to 15 mg given every 15 min. Alternatively, labetalol may be given via continuous infusion at a rate of 0.5 to 2 mg/min until the desired response or a total cumulative dose of 300 mg has been reached. There are reports where labetalol has been used as a continuous drip over a 24-h period in severe and refractory cases. Patients receiving labetalol via the intravenous route should be placed in a supine position and remain supine for approximately 3 h after receiving any intravenous doses, since symptomatic orthostatic hypotension may occur. Following patient stabilization, labetalol may be given orally up to 2400 mg per day in two to four divided doses. Acute dosing of intravenous labetalol can lead to a "cumulative effect," as each dose will persist for 2 to 4 h. These patients must be under diligent observation to avoid hypotensive episodes.

Adverse-Effects Profile Labetalol has the same adverse-effects profile as the other β- and α_1-blocking agents. The most common adverse effect is orthostatic hypotension, which occurs most frequently upon initial therapy. Syncope has been reported following both intravenous and oral administration. Symptomatic heart failure may also occur. Adverse CNS effects that may occur include light-headedness, drowsiness, dizziness, fatigue, lethargy, and vivid nightmares. Tingling of the scalp and skin may occur with the initiation of therapy. Occasionally, reversible elevation of the hepatic enzymes may lead to jaundice and hepatitis. Other effects include lupus-like complaints, elevated renal function tests, blood dyscrasias, and allergic reactions. There is synergism between labetalol and halothane anesthesia.

Class III Antidysrhythmic Agents

The Cardiac Arrhythmia Suppression Trial illustrated the prodysrhythmic effects and increased mortality of certain Class I sodium channel blocking agents. Class III antidysrhythmics serve as an alternative to the sodium channel blocking drugs.[3] They are a heterogenous group of antifibrillatory agents that lack negative hemodynamic effects. Class III drugs are characterized by prolongation of the effective refractory period by a mechanism other than or in addition to sodium blockade. Amiodarone, bretylium, and sotalol are discussed below.

AMIODARONE The parental formulation of amiodarone was recently approved by the FDA for the treatment of life-threatening ventricular dysrhythmia refractory to standard first-line therapy. Amiodarone lacks significant hemodynamic effects, making it useful in patients with severe LV dysfunction.

Action Amiodarone is classified as a class III antidysrhythmic; it has a complex pharmacodynamic profile that also includes class I, class II, and class IV properties. It is a noncompetitive α- and β-receptor blocking agent, which is responsible for its negative inotropic and chronotropic effects. The negative inotropic response is countered by the decreased SVR; therefore cardiac output and ejection fraction are unchanged. Calcium channel blockade contributes to the peripheral vasodilatory response and decreased SVR. Amiodarone also weakly inhibits sodium channels, which depresses the myocardial conduction velocity by slowing the upstroke of phase 0. It is therefore a negative dromotropic agent. Last, amiodarone directly depresses the automaticity of the SA and AV nodes. It modifies the automaticity of spontaneously firing fibers in the Purkinje system and prolongs the refractory period in accessory pathways (e.g., WPW syndrome).

The hallmark of class III antifibrillatory drugs is prolongation of the action potential duration and the refractory period. The antifibrillatory effect of amiodarone is caused by inhibition of potassium ion fluxes that normally occur during phases 2 and 3 of the cardiac cycle. Amiodarone interferes with thyroid metabolism, which may also contribute to its antidysrhythmic properties. Repolarization time is lengthened as reflected by the prolonged QT interval on ECG. Although amiodarone prolongs the QT interval, torsades de pointes rarely occurs.

Hypotension can occur with the intravenous formulation secondary to its rapid vasodilatory effects. The ECG may show sinus bradycardia, PR and QT interval prolongation, and U waves.

Pharmacokinetics Amiodarone hydrochloride is slowly and variably absorbed following oral administration. Systemic absorption ranges from 22 to 86 percent (average, 50 percent). The drug is approximately 96 percent plasma protein–bound. The effect of food on absorption has not been determined. The Vd is 1.3 to 12 L/kg allowing the drug to be extensively distributed. Peak serum concentrations may occur from 2 to 12 h (average, 3 to 7 h) after oral administration. The half-life appears to be substantially prolonged following multiple rather than single doses. The terminal elimination half-life is 28 to 107 days. Because of the drug's slow elimination, discontinuance of the drug will still allow therapeutic levels to be maintained for weeks.

After parenteral administration, amiodarone has rapid distribution to various sites, particularly adipose tissue and highly perfused organs such as the liver, spleen, and lungs. Serum levels correlate poorly with clinical efficacy. Each individual responds differently to the initial intravenous infusion; thus supplemental dosages are frequently needed for breakthrough dysrhythmias.

Amiodarone is metabolized in the liver by cytochrome P-450 enzyme and is eliminated by biliary excretion. Enterohepatic recirculation occurs. Negligible amounts are found in the urine, and it is not dialyzable.

Common ED Indications Labeled uses for parenteral and oral therapy include treatment and suppression of VF/pulseless VT refractory to other medications. Unlabeled uses include the treatment and suppression of refractory PSVT, paroxysmal atrial fibrillation, symptomatic atrial flutter, and suppression of ventricular dysrhythmias in patients with cardiomyopathy.

Oral amiodarone appears to be effective in the management of a wide variety of ventricular and supraventricular dysrhythmias. However, due to the severe potential adverse effects, it is used only if alternative drug and electrical therapy is ineffective or contraindicated.

Dosing and Administration The initial parenteral dose of amiodarone is 150 mg over 10 min. This is followed by an infusion of 1 mg/min for 6 h, after which 0.5 mg/min is infused as maintenance. Rebolus of 150 mg over 10 min is given for breakthrough VT or VF. The recommended dose for supraventricular dysrhythmias is the same.

Amiodarone is a highly toxic drug; therefore the lowest effective dosage should be used to minimize the risk and occurrence of adverse effects. The dosage of amiodarone must be carefully adjusted according to individual requirements and response, patient tolerance, and the general condition and cardiovascular status of the patient. The oral loading-dose phase of therapy should be performed only where close monitoring is available, especially until the risk of recurrent VT or VF has abated. All other antidysrhythmic agents should be gradually discontinued, if possible, before oral amiodarone therapy is initiated. In addition, ophthalmologic and pulmonary tests should be performed to obtain a baseline before amiodarone is started.

In adults, oral daily loading dosages of 800 to 1600 mg are generally required for 1 to 3 weeks (occasionally longer) until an initial therapeutic response is seen. Recommended oral doses of amiodarone to treat ventricular dysrhythmias are administered once daily. However, when doses of 1 g or more are administered (e.g., during the loading-dose phase of therapy) or when intolerable adverse effects (usually GI effects) occur, a twice-daily regimen with meals is suggested. Dosage reduction is essential when there is adequate control of the ventricular dysrhythmias or if adverse effects become a problem. Dosages can be gradually titrated down to 600 to 800 mg daily for about 1 month and then again to the lowest effective maintenance dose. Typically, 400 to 600 mg/day is an adequate maintenance dose.

Adverse-Effects Profile With parenteral use, hypotension is the most common side effect; it usually presents within the first few hours of therapy. Bradycardia may also occur. Hypotension and bradycardia should be treated by slowing or stopping the intravenous infusion. Refractory bradycardia may require pacemaker placement.

The most serious noncardiac side effects of amiodarone is pulmonary toxicity. Pneumonitis should be suspected in any patient who presents with fever, cough, and progressive shortness of breath. Steroids and dose reduction or discontinuation of amiodarone may prove beneficial. Asymptomatic rise in liver function tests may occur, but cirrhosis is rare. QT prolongation occurs hours after initiation of therapy, but dysrhythmias do not occur for a few days.

Oral therapy is associated with several serious and potentially fatal toxicities, including pulmonary toxicity, prodysrhythmic effects, and, rarely, hepatic toxicity. The likelihood of most adverse reactions appears to increase after the first 6 months of therapy and remains relatively constant beyond 1 year of therapy. With chronic administration, corneal microdeposits are reported in all patients. Additional adverse effects may include rash, skin discoloration, photosensitivity, serious neurologic effects, constipation and other GI symptoms, and others. These effects may persist for weeks or months after discontinuance. Also, thyroid function tests may appear falsely elevated or decreased.

For a variety of medications, concomitant administration of amiodarone may result in either increased levels and/or potential toxicities; such medications include digoxin, procainamide, quinidine, calcium channel blockers, β-adrenergic blocking agents, other antidysrhythmics, anticoagulants, theophylline, and thyroid medications. Amiodarone should not be used in patients with marked sinus bradycardia or second- and third-degree AV block unless emerging pacing is available.

BRETYLIUM **Actions** Bretylium is a class III drug with a biphasic cardiovascular response. There is an appreciable increase in heart rate, blood pressure, and cardiac output after intravenous infusion. This effect lasts approximately 20 min. Next, there is a sympatholytic response with subsequent reduction in heart rate, blood pressure, and systemic vascular resistance. The biphasic response is due to the initial release of norepinephrine from the sympathetic ganglia and the postganglionic nerve terminals, results in increased adrenergic tone. Subsequently bretylium blocks further release of norepinephrine by depressing the excitability of adrenergic nerve terminals after sympathetic stimulation. This results in a sympatholytic effect that can cause orthostatic hypotension.

Like all class III agents, bretylium prolongs the action potential duration and the effective refractory period in the ventricular myocardium. Modulation of fluxes across potassium channels is responsible for this action. Additionally, bretylium reduces the disparity of the length of the action potential duration and the effective refractory period between ischemic and normal myocardium. It is also likely that bretylium increases the fibrillatory threshold. These additive effects contribute to bretylium's antifibrillatory action. Lidocaine is still considered first-line treatment of VF/unstable VT since bretylium is associated with more adverse hemodynamic outcomes during cardiopulmonary resuscitation (CPR). However, some studies suggest a synergistic response when lidocaine is used with bretylium.

In ischemic myocardium, the resting membrane potential (phase 4) is depressed. Bretylium transiently restores the phase 4 membrane potential toward normal. Curiously, bretylium has no effect on the resting membrane potential in normal myocardium.

Pharmacokinetics The onset of action for intravenous bretylium in VF is within minutes, but it may take from 20 min up to 2 h when used for other ventricular dysrhythmias. Peak effects occur in 1.5 to 6 h and last 6 to 12 h following a single dose. Bretylium is well absorbed following intramuscular injection, but this should be avoided in cardiac arrest and shock. Bretylium is eliminated primarily as unchanged drug via the kidney (70 to 85 percent) and thus may have a prolonged duration of action in patients with renal dysfunction.

Common ED Indications Bretylium is indicated for the treatment of refractory VF/pulseless VT unresponsive to repeated countershocks, epinephrine, and lidocaine. It is also indicated for the treatment of sustained VT with a pulse resistant to lidocaine and procainamide.[1] Last, bretylium may convert a wide complex tachycardia of uncertain origin unresponsive to adenosine and lidocaine. Bretylium is considered first-line therapy when lidocaine and procainamide are contraindicated (i.e., hypersensitivity reactions).

Dosing and Administration The initial dose of bretylium for VF or pulseless VT is 5 mg/kg (500 mg = 1 ampule) administered by rapid intravenous push. If VF persists, the dose can be increased to 10 mg/kg and repeated at 15- to 30-min intervals up to a maximum dose of 35 mg/kg. Undiluted drug may be given for life-threatening emergencies, otherwise diluted drug should be used. If a peripheral line is used, the bolus is followed with a 20-mL flush. For recurrent or refractory ventricular tachydysrhythmias with a pulse, 5 to 10 mg/kg of drug should be infused over a period of 8 to 10 min. Nausea, vomiting, and hypotension can occur with a more rapid infusion. If these dysrhythmias persist, repeated boluses of 5 to 10 mg/kg can be given q1–2h as necessary.

For maintenance, give 1 to 2 mg/min by continuous intravenous infusion. Alternatively, give 5 to 10 mg/kg over 10 min every 6–8 h. If the intramuscular route is used, no more than 5 mL should be injected at any one site, and injection sites should be rotated. Consider short-term use when possible (e.g., <24 h).

Adverse-Effects Profile Transient hypertension, tachycardia, and increased frequency of dysrhythmias secondary to ventricular irritability may follow drug injection secondary to the initial release of catecholamine. Nonspecific symptoms such as nausea, vomiting, vertigo, and light-headedness can occur following rapid injection. Bretylium should be avoided, if possible, in the setting of digoxin toxicity, since catecholamines are believed to exacerbate the toxic effects of digoxin.

Postural hypotension is the most common adverse reaction and may occur within 15 to 30 min in as many as 60 percent of patients. If this occurs, the patient should be placed in a supine or Trendelenburg position and be resuscitated with crystalloid fluids. If hypotension persists, vasopressors may be employed, but note that these agents will increase automaticity and may negate bretylium's effects.

Avoid bretylium in patients with renal failure, since the drug is excreted principally unchanged in the urine. Use cautiously in patients with fixed cardiac output, such as aortic stenosis, since severe hypotension may occur.

SOTALOL **Actions** Sotalol (Betapace) is a class III antidysrhythmic with noncardioselective β-blocking activity (class II) without intrinsic sympathomimetic or local anesthetic activity. It prolongs repolarization, like other class III drugs, through modulation of potassium currents. As a result, the action potential duration and the effective refractory period are prolonged. This is reflected on the ECG as QT prolongation, which is more pronounced at lower heart rates. Sotalol is approved for use in life-threatening ventricular dysrhythmias only.

Pharmacokinetics Sotalol is rapidly and completely absorbed from the GI tract. Food reduces its bioavailability. It is hydrophilic and does not accumulate in the brain. Sotalol does not bind to plasma proteins, forms no metabolites, and is eliminated mainly in the urine. The elimination half-life of the drug is about 12 h. Peak concentrations are reached at 2.5 to 4 h after oral dosing. Unlike many other drugs, sotalol does not interact with the pharmacokinetics of other cardiac drugs (e.g., digoxin, warfarin).

Common ED Indications Sotalol effectively suppresses life-threatening ventricular dysrhythmias refractory to other conventional antidysrhythmic agents but is associated with a 2 percent incidence of torsades de pointes, VT, or VF. While sotalol can suppress SVT and atrial fibrillation, it is not approved for this use.

Dosing and Administration Only the oral formula is approved for usage in the United States. The usual initial oral dosage is 80 mg bid, which can be increased to 240 or 320 mg/day; a therapeutic response is usually obtained at a total daily dose of 160 to 320 mg/day. There should be 2 to 3 days with QT monitoring allowed between increments. The maximum dosage is 480 to 640 mg/day; however, this should be used only when the potential benefit outweighs the increased risk of adverse effects. The dosing interval should be extended for renal insufficiency. Dose escalations in these patients should be done after administration of at least five to six doses and be based on the creatinine clearance. If the creatinine clearance is 30 to 60 mL/min, the dosing interval should be q24h; at 10 to 30 mL/min, adjust the dosing interval to 36 to 48 h; and when the clearance is $<$10 mL/min, the dose should be individualized.

Adverse-Effects Profile Sotalol is well tolerated and many adverse effects are dose-related; the most common are related to nonselective β blockade. Sotalol can also have prodysrhythmic effects, particularly in those who are taking high doses of the drug or those with torsades de pointes, prolonged QTc intervals, hypokalemia, or bradycardia. Torsades de pointes, secondary to prolonged QT interval, is the most common dysrhythmia.

Class IV Antidysrhythmic Agents

By blocking the calcium-dependent slow channel response, calcium channel blockers slow myocardial conduction velocity, relax vascular smooth muscle, and depress cardiac contractility. They are indicated for the treatment of cardiac dysrrhythmias, hypertension, Prinzmetal angina, migraine headache, and recent subarachnoid hemorrhage (SAH). The use of calcium channel blockers (CCBs) in AMI is controversial. Some studies suggest an increased risk of adverse cardiovascular events, particularly in the presence of left ventricular dysfunction;[4] other studies dispute these findings.[5] Currently, the American College of Cardiology/American Heart Association (ACC/AHA) Guidelines for the Management of Acute Myocardial Infarction do not recommend calcium channel blockers for routine use in AMI since β-adrenergic blocking agents are generally a more appropriate choice. However, if β blockers are ineffective or contraindicated, verapamil or diltiazen may be given in patients with AMI without evidence of congestive heart failure, left ventricular dysfunction, or AV block. Nifedipine is generally contraindicated.

Class IV antidysrhythmics block calcium-dependent slow channels in vascular smooth muscle, contractile cells, and the conduction system. Specifically, they prevent the influx of calcium through the suprahisian (SA and AV nodes) conduction tissue, which is involved in the propagation of the action potential. Therefore, the conduction velocity is slowed, particularly in the AV node.

Calcium is responsible for myocardial excitation-contraction coupling. Class 4 agents block slow calcium channels in cardiac muscle, which depress excitation-contraction coupling and myocardial contractile function. As a result, CCBs exert a negative inotropic effect. Slow channels also exist in smooth muscle. By interfering with the excitation-contraction coupling in vascular smooth muscle, CCBs promote vasodilatation.

Each agent has variable effects on AVN conduction, SVR, and contractile function. For example, verapamil causes moderate prolongation of atrioventricular conduction and moderate negative inotropic effects, while nifedipine has negligible effects on each. Conversely, nifedipine causes a moderate reduction of systemic vascular resistance, while the effects of verapamil on SVR are much less pronounced. The spectrum of action of diltiazem is midway between those of verapamil and nifedipine. Only diltiazem and verapamil are used as antidysrhythmic drugs.

VERAPAMIL **Actions** Verapamil (Isoptin, Calan), a calcium channel blocking agent, is a class IV antidysrhythmic agent. In diseased tissue, verapamil decreases conduction velocity, prolongs the refractory period in the AV node, and decreases the discharge rate in the SA node. It interrupts the AV node reentrant pathway associated with PSVT, thus causing the myocardium to return to normal sinus rhythm (NSR). In addition, verapamil can slow ventricular response in patients with atrial fibrillation and/or flutter by its action on the AV node. A decrease in heart rate and/or SA nodal block may occur in patients with SA nodal disease. Verapamil has minimal effects on normal conduction tissue.

Although verapamil has negative inotropic effects, they are often offset by the decrease in afterload. Thus, the hemodynamic effects are negligible in normal myocardium. Those with severe heart failure, however, may experience a decrease in ejection fraction.

Most patients with PSVT and WPW syndrome demonstrate narrow QRS complexes of tachycardias. This indicates antegrade conduction through the AV node, with retrograde conduction over the bypass tract completing the circuit. Verapamil is safe and effective in patients with narrow-complex PSVT, even in the presence of WPW syndrome, because of the pronounced negative dromotropic effects of verapamil on the AV node. If antegrade conduction occurs over the accessory pathway, the QRS complex widens. Verapamil may decrease the refractory period of an accessory tract. Therefore, verapamil is contraindicated for atrial fibrillation or flutter due to WPW syndrome and in any type of wide-complex tachycardia, since it can increase rather than decrease the ventricular rate. In addition, in many cases, wide complex tachycardia can represent VT. In this case, verapamil could worsen hemodynamics because of vasodilatory and negative inotropic effects.

By inhibiting the influx of calcium, verapamil impairs the contractile processes that calcium normally activates, thereby causing dilatation of coronary and systemic arteries. Dilatation of coronary arteries improves oxygen delivery, while dilatation of the systemic arteries decreases oxygen consumption by decreasing afterload. These effects provide the myocardium with a beneficial oxygen balance in patients with vasospastic, unstable, and chronic stable angina.

Pharmacokinetics Verapamil elicits its hemodynamic effects within 3 to 5 min following intravenous administration, with effects lasting approximately 30 min. Effects on conduction begin within 1 to 2 min, peak in 10 to 15 min, and persist for 1 to 6 h. The Vd of verapamil is 4.5 to 7.1 L/kg. Verapamil undergoes first-pass metabolism in the liver and is metabolized to several metabolites. Norverapamil, an active metabolite, appears in the greatest amount. The elimination half-life of verapamil is 2 to 8 h, increasing to 4 to 12 h after 1 to 2 days of therapy.

Common ED Indications Verapamil is as effective as adenosine and diltiazem for terminating narrow-complex PSVT and for controlling the ventricular rate in atrial fibrillation/flutter. Avoid verapamil in patients with WPW syndrome who present in atrial fibrillation/flutter since ventricular fibrillation may occur.[6–8] Similarly, it is best avoided in patients with wide complex PSVT. It should also be avoided in patients with wide complex tachycardias. Diagnosis of PSVT should be confirmed by 12-lead ECG and managed with vasovagal maneuvers prior to administering verapamil whenever possible. Oral verapamil can be used for the management of vasospastic, chronic stable, and unstable angina and may also be used for the prophylaxis of PSVT. It is also used for essential hypertension.

Dosing and Administration For PSVT, many recommend an initial intravenous dose of 2.5 mg given over 2 to 3 min and repeated in 15 to 30 min if the response is inadequate. Others are more aggressive, particularly if the blood pressure is elevated and the patient is known to respond to a higher dose. In such cases, 5 mg may be slowly infused and repeated every 5 min. The blood pressure should be checked immediately before and after the drug has been given. Lower initial doses of verapamil and slower administration techniques should be considered in older patients and those with hepatic dysfunction. Pretreatment with calcium chloride, gluconate, or gluceptate (500 to 1000 mg) can be given before or after verapamil infusion to prevent or reverse hypotension. Reports using calcium with verapamil have been largely anecdotal, but such use may be most efficacious in patients whose hemodynamic status is borderline (i.e., systolic blood pressure <90 mmHg). Administration of calcium may also be considered for intentional overdose or accidentally poisoned patients who demonstrate severe bradydysrhythmias.

For the prevention of recurrent PSVT, oral administration of verapamil, 240 to 480 mg daily, should be given in three to four divided doses. Control of ventricular rate in digitalized adults with chronic atrial fibrillation and/or flutter is 240 to 320 mg daily in three or four divided doses. Maximum antidysrhythmic effects are generally seen within 48 h after initiating a verapamil dose. For the treatment of vasospastic, unstable, or chronic stable angina, oral doses of verapamil can be given (80 mg q6–8h), with doses titrated up or down to desired clinical response. In patients with hypertension, verapamil is initiated with 80 mg three times daily and titrated to blood pressure response. Patients who are elderly or of small stature can be started on 40 mg three times daily. Although doses of 480 mg/day have been used, efficacy with doses greater than 360 mg/day has not conclusively been proven.

The only current recommended use for Verapamil SR is for hypertension. When switching from immediate-release tablets, the total daily dose (in milligrams) may remain the same. Breaking the sustained-release (SR) tablet does not affect the therapeutic effect of verapamil SR. The SR tablets, as an initial dose of 240 mg every morning, may be used for hypertension. Titration may be accomplished with 120-mg (one-half SR tablet) increments added in the evening. Antihypertensive effects are evident within the first week.

Adverse-Effects Profile The majority of adverse effects secondary to verapamil are related to its pharmacologic action. The incidence is increased in patients with severe heart failure, hypertrophic cardiomyopathy, and conduction disturbances. The incidence of hypotension is 5 to 10 percent with intravenous administration and may rarely require treatment with intravenous calcium salts or vasopressors. Conduction disturbances such as bradycardia, AV block, and bundle branch block occur in approximately 2 percent or fewer of patients and usually respond to a dosage reduction or discontinuation of the drug; rarely, use of atropine, cautious use of isoproterenol, or cardiac pacing may be necessary. In addition, approximately 2 percent may develop acute pulmonary edema secondary to the negative inotropic effects of verapamil. Verapamil may increase serum digoxin concentrations. Avoid the concomitant use of intravenous β blockers.

Noncardiac side effects with verapamil include constipation, dizziness, headache, and nausea. Other side effects, occurring in fewer than 1 percent of patients, include sleep disturbances, blurred vision, shakiness, drowsiness, confusion, dry mouth, rash, urticaria, bruising, flushing, polyuria, sexual difficulties, apnea, and muscle cramps. Several cases of hepatocellular injury accompanied by clinical signs of hepatotoxicity have also been reported. Verapamil should be given with caution to patients who are receiving agents such as β blockers, digoxin, antihypertensives, and antidysrhythmics, since their effects may be additive. Cimetidine may reduce hepatic metabolism. Do not use verapamil in children younger than 1 year old, since its use is associated with sudden circulatory collapse.

DILTIAZEM **Actions** The actions of diltiazem (Cardizem) on the coronary and systemic arteries resemble those of verapamil. Diltiazem, also a calcium antagonist, is a less potent vasodilator than nifedipine. Vasodilation is predominant in the coronary arteries, allowing improved oxygen delivery and thus benefiting patients with vasospastic angina. Systemic arterial dilation also reduces afterload, resulting in decreased oxygen consumption and improvement in oxygen balance in those with chronic stable angina. Diltiazem slows AV nodal conduction time and prolongs AV nodal refractoriness. It may selectively reduce the heart rate during tachycardias involving the AV node with little or no effect on normal AV nodal conduction at normal heart rates. The ventricular rate is slowed in patients with a rapid ventricular response during atrial fibrillation or atrial flutter. PSVT is converted to NSR by interrupting the reentry circuit in AV nodal reentrant tachycardias and reciprocating tachycardias (e.g., WPW syndrome). Diltiazem has no effects on sinus node recovery or the sinoatrial conduction time in patients without SA nodal dysfunction.

Pharmacokinetics An intravenous bolus dose appears to follow linear pharmacokinetics over a dosage range of 10.5 to 21.0 mg. The apparent Vd is 305 L. The plasma elimination of diltiazem is approximately 3 to 7 h. The drug is extensively metabolized in the liver with a systemic clearance of 65 L/h. After a continuous intravenous infusion, one study cited development of nonlinear pharmacokinetics over an infusion range of 4.8 to 13.2 mg/h for 24 h. As the dose is increased over this infusion range, systemic clearance decreases from 64 to 48 L/h and the apparent Vd remains unchanged (360 to 391 L). Generally, systemic clearance averaged 42 and 31 L/h in patients given continuous infusions of diltiazem at 10 to 15 mg/h, respectively, for 24 h. However, in comparison with healthy volunteers, patients with atrial fibrillation or atrial flutter had decreased systemic clearance.

Oral doses also have a 40 percent bioavailability due to first-pass effect. Oral bioavailability does increase as doses increase. The onset of action of conventional tablets is 30 to 60 min, with the peak effect occurring in 2 to 4 h. SR tablets, however, have a gradual onset of action, with a peak effect occurring in 6 to 11 h. Comparable products, with a 24-h controlled drug delivery system (Cardizem-CD; Dilacor-XR), have similar absorption throughout the dosing intervals, and peak serum levels occur generally between 10 and 14 h.

Diltiazem is 70 to 80 percent protein-bound; 35 to 40 percent is bound to albumin and is metabolized in the liver to one active and several inactive metabolites. Approximately one-third of diltiazem is metabolized to desacetyldiltiazem, a metabolite with 25 to 50 percent of the coronary vasodilating activity of diltiazem. Diltiazem and its metabolites are excreted via glucuronide and/or sulfate conjugation.

Common ED Indications Intravenous diltiazem is as effective as verapamil and adenosine for rapid conversion of PSVT to NSR and to slow ventricular rate in atrial fibrillation or atrial flutter. It should not be used in patients with a wide complex tachydysrhythmia suggesting an accessory bypass tract (e.g., WPW syndrome).

Oral diltiazem is indicated for the treatment of vasospastic and chronic stable angina and is considered one of the drugs of choice for vasospastic angina. In patients with chronic stable angina, diltiazem is thought to be as effective as β-blocking agents and/or nitrates but is usually reserved for those who fail therapy with these agents.

Oral diltiazem is also approved for the treatment of hypertension either alone or in combination with other agents. An additive effect is commonly seen when thiazide diuretics are added to diltiazem therapy. Like other calcium channel blockers, diltiazem may be especially useful in hypertensive patients with low renin levels, those who have angina, or in African Americans.

Dosing and Administration The intravenous bolus dose for control of PSVT, atrial fibrillation, or atrial flutter is 0.25 mg/kg using actual body weight (average adult dose is 20 mg) over a 2-min period. If a further response is desired, a second intravenous bolus of 0.35 mg/kg actual body weight can be given at the same rate (average adult dose, 35 mg). Subsequent bolus dosing should be individualized on a milligram-per-kilogram basis. It should be noted that some patients may not need an initial dose greater than 0.15 mg/kg, yet duration of action may be shorter. For continued reduction of the heart rate (up to 24 h) in atrial fibrillation or atrial flutter, a diltiazem maintenance infusion may be started immediately following the bolus dose(s). The recommended initial rate is 10 mg/h, yet some patients may respond to a 5-mg/h dose. If needed, subsequent increases can be in 5-mg/h increments up to 15 mg/h. The infusion may be maintained for up to 24 h. Patients should have continuous ECG monitoring and frequent blood pressure checks. For patients being converted from intravenous to oral diltiazem, the following suggestions are based on oral steady state: 5 mg/h or approximately 180 mg/day; 7 mg/h or approximately 240 mg/day; 11 mg/h or approximately 360 mg/day. The oral doses and dosing intervals are variable, based on the indication and the product selected. For the treatment of vasospastic or chronic stable angina, the usual initial diltiazem dose is 30 mg before meals and at bedtime (four times daily). Most patients can be controlled with 180 to 360 mg/day in divided doses. Sustained release tablets are indicated for the control of hypertension and chronic stable angina. Angina episodes and weekly nitroglycerin consumption decreases with the use of extended release diltiazem. SR products start at 60 to 120 mg/day, with optimum dosage 240 to 360 mg/day.

For patients with hypertension, diltiazem is usually given as the extended-release tablet in 60- or 120-mg doses twice daily. Maintenance doses are usually 240 to 360 mg/day. Doses should be titrated to clinical response in each of the above situations. Additionally, patients with hepatic and/or renal dysfunction should be dosed cautiously and may require dosage adjustments. The Cardizem-CD and the Dilacor-XR products offer 180 and 240 mg with once-daily dosing. Cardizem-CD is also available in a 300-mg strength. SR products use 60- to 120-mg strengths and are started with 120 or 180 mg daily. Some patients may respond to higher doses of up to 480 mg/day. As necessary, the optimum dose for hypertension can be titrated over a 7- to 14-day period.

Adverse-Effects Profile Many of the adverse effects associated with diltiazem are an extension of its pharmacologic profile. Cardiovascular effects may include angina, bradycardia, asystole, CHF, AV block (first, second, or third degree), bundle-branch block, PVC, flushing, decreased blood pressure, palpitations, and peripheral edema.

Noncardiac side effects include headache (2 to 10 percent), dizziness (1 to 7 percent), asthenia (2 to 5 percent), nausea (1 to 3 percent), constipation (1 to 2 percent), rash (1 to 2 percent), vomiting, diarrhea, dry mouth, pruritus, nervousness, somnolence, insomnia, tinnitus, abnormal dreams, depression, sexual difficulties, bruising, polyuria, hyperglycemia, epistaxis, alopecia, and photosensitivity.

Diltiazem may cause a transient increase in liver function test values (e.g., AST, ALT, LDH), which may resolve despite continued therapy. However, hepatocellular toxicity has been reported in some patients. Patients receiving digoxin or β blockers may experience additive conduction disturbances. Cimetidine may increase diltiazem levels secondary to inhibition of metabolism.

OTHER CALCIUM CHANNEL BLOCKERS *Nifedipine* and the other dihydropyridines (e.g., amlodipine, felodipine, nicardipine, nimodipine, and nisoldipine) lower blood pressure by blocking calcium influx into vascular smooth muscle. This prohibits excitation-contraction coupling, which lowers systemic vascular resistance and dilates the coronary arteries. The coronary artery dilatation results in improved oxygen delivery, benefiting patients with vasospastic angina. Systemic arterial dilatation results in decreased afterload, leading to decreased oxygen consumption in patients with chronic stable angina. A reflex increase in heart rate and an increase in cardiac output may be seen with nifedipine. Unlike verapamil and diltiazem, nifedipine has little effect on the SA and AV nodal conduction clinically. Nifedipine may, however, result in a decrease in left ventricular end diastolic pressure (LVEDP) or left ventricular end diastolic volume (LVEDV) in patients with moderate to severely impaired LV function, thereby worsening their condition.

Approved indications for nifedipine include management of vasospastic and chronic stable angina. Nifedipine, either alone or in combination with other antihypertensives, is indicated for the management of essential hypertension. In comparison to other classes of antihypertensives (i.e., angiotensin-converting enzyme inhibitors and β blockers), nifedipine may benefit patients with low-renin hypertension, coexisting angina, or peripheral vascular disease. Nifedipine is also used for hypertensive urgencies. Sublingual administration and chewing should be avoided as this may result in a precipitous fall in blood pressure.

Nimodipine (Nimotop) is a calcium channel blocker structurally similar to nifedipine. Like other calcium channel blockers, it inhibits the influx of calcium across the transmembrane channels, thereby inhibiting the contractile activity in the cell. The inhibition of calcium influx is seen in myocardial muscle, vascular smooth muscle, and neuronal cells. Nimodipine has a relative selectivity for vascular smooth muscle—as opposed to the myocardium—and therefore has minimal effects on the conduction and inotropy of the myocardium. Its greatest affinity is for the CNS vasculature. It increases cerebral blood flow and may shunt blood to ischemic areas. Although inhibition of cerebral vasospasm (which often occurs following SAH) was initially thought to be responsible for the beneficial effects of nimodipine in SAH, angiography has not proven this. Improved collateral blood flow and prevention of large calcium influxes into neurons (causing cell destruction) may be of greater importance.

Nimodipine is indicated for the treatment of recent (within 96 h) SAH from ruptured congenital intracranial aneurysm in patients whose postictal neurologic condition is good (e.g., Hunt and Hess grades I to III), where it can decrease the degree of morbidity and mortality. Patients with more severe disability (Hunt and Hess grades IV to V) do not seem to benefit and may become worse with nimodipine.

Nicardipine (Cardene) is a dihydropyridine calcium channel blocker structurally related to nifedine. Like nifedipine, nicardipine inhibits the transmembrane flux of calcium into cardiac and vascular smooth muscle. The inhibition results in a decrease in the contractile activity within the myocardium and vascular smooth muscle. This agent provides selective activity on the vasculature as opposed to the myocardium. Nicardipine possesses both systemic and peripheral vasodilatory action primarily through a decrease in peripheral vascular resistance. Increases in cardiac output and cardiac index can be seen in a dose-dependent manner with nicardipine. It does not have demonstrable effects on renal blood flow or glomerular filtration rate.

Intravenous nicardipine decreases systemic vascular resistance, improves coronary artery perfusion, and increases cardiac index without raising myocardial oxygen demand or left ventricular filling pressure. Despite systemic and hemodynamic effects (hypotension and tachycardia), intravenous nicardipine does not have a depressant effect on the myocardium or a negative action on right or left ventricular filling pressure in patients with uncomplicated MI. However, it has been shown to produce a decrease in contractility in patients with severe heart failure.

Intravenous nicardipine is indicated for the short-term treatment of hypertension when oral therapy is not feasible or desirable. Oral nicardipine (Cardene) is indicated for chronic stable angina and essential hypertension. It is as effective as nifedipine in treating chronic stable angina and hypertension.

Other Antidysrhythmic Agents

ADENOSINE Adenosine (Adenocard) is an endogenous nucleoside produced by the dephosphorylation of adenosine triphosphate (ATP) and is contained in every cell of the body. Cardiac adenosine receptors are concentrated in the coronary arteries, the SA node, the AV node, and the atrial myocytes.[9] A1 adenosine receptor stimulation alters potassium channels. The increase in K^+ conductance hyperpolarizes the cell membrane and shortens the action potential of supraventricular cells. Therefore, the threshold of the SA and AV nodes to trigger another action potential is increased. This results in the long sinus pause on the rhythm strip following adenosine administration.

The positive inotropic, chronotropic, and dromotropic response of catecholamines depends on cAMP. Adenosine exerts antiadrenergic effects by inhibiting the adenyl cyclase/cAMP pathway. Therefore, adenosine antagonizes the effect of catecholamines on supraventricular and ventricular myocardium. This may explain why some wide complex tachycardias of ventricular origin are terminated with adenosine.

In summary, the modulation of K^+ currents and the blunting of catecholamine response are responsible for the antidysrhythmic properties of adenosine.

Action Adenosine exerts negative chronotropic and negative dromotropic actions on the SA and AV nodal tissue secondary to its influence on potassium conductance. Adenosine terminates PSVT primarily via blockade of the AV node without altering conduction through accessory pathways, as is seen with the WPW syndrome. Reentrant SVTs not involving the AV node are not terminated by adenosine. Adenosine is a potent vasodilator; however, there is no change in systemic blood pressure following its administration because it is rapidly metabolized by circulating adenosine deaminase and undergoes rapid sequestration by vascular endothelial cells.

Pharmacokinetics Onset of action is within approximately 30 s, with a duration of 60 to 90 s. The drug is rapidly metabolized in the blood, with a half-life less than 7 s. The primary routes of elimination are cellular uptake and simple or facilitated diffusion by a nucleoside transport system, metabolism to various by-products, and renal excretion of these metabolic products. The predominant final metabolite of adenosine is uric acid. Specific pharmacokinetic parameters—such as Vd, therapeutic plasma concentrations, and clearance—are difficult to assess due to the extremely short half-life of the drug.

Common ED Indications Adenosine is the drug of first choice to convert PSVT involving the AV node into sinus rhythm. It is as efficacious as intravenous verapamil and diltiazem in terminating the dysrhythmia. Its ultrashort action and its lack of serious side effects make it the preferred drug. While it is extremely effective in the initial conversion of reentrant PSVTs, recurrence of the dysrhythmia (within minutes after the initial conversion) may occur. Although repeat doses of adenosine are effective, consideration of a longer-acting antidysrhythmic agent will often be necessary.

Adenosine causes transient AV block in narrow complex tachycardias of unknown origin. Adenosine will not convert atrial fibrillation or atrial flutter to normal sinus rhythm. However, it may expose the underlying atrial rhythm (atrial fibrillation, atrial flutter, or some other atrial tachycardias), so that therapy may be appropriately initiated. Adenosine may also detect a previously latent accessory pathway.

It is often difficult to differentiate between SVT with aberrancy and ventricular tachycardia in the ED setting. Adenosine will convert SVT with aberrancy to normal sinus rhythm or reveal the underlying atrial mechanism. Adenosine will not terminate VT (unless the dysrhythmia is dependent on adrenergic drive), nor does it block conduction over accessory pathways.

This drug is the preferred agent for treatment of PSVT in infants, children, and pregnant women. Because adenosine shortens the action potential duration and slows the heart rate, it is contraindicated in second- or third-degree AV heart block or sick sinus syndrome. Adenosine is not effective in converting atrial tachydysrhythmias (e.g., atrial fibrillation or flutter) or VT to NSR. However, it has been shown to be safe to administer in situations where VT and SVT cannot be differentiated.[10]

Dosing and Administration The initial dose for the treatment of acute PSVT is 6 mg (6 mg/2 mL) given as a *rapid* intravenous bolus over 1 to 2 s directly into the vein or into the most proximal port of the intravenous tubing on the peripheral intravenous site. When the latter method is used, the bolus should be followed by a 20-mL saline flush and the arm immediately elevated. This method will expedite travel of the drug to the heart and lessen the amount of drug getting caught in the intravenous tubing, where it rapidly breaks down. If the heart rate does not decrease within 2 min, a second bolus injection of 12 mg should be given in the same manner. A final, third bolus dose may be given in 1 to 2 min if the dysrhythmia persists. It is imperative that adenosine be administered *fast;* if it is infused too slowly, systemic vasodilation may occur, which can result in reflex tachycardia.

Adverse-Effects Profile When adverse effects due to adenosine occur, they are minor and well tolerated because they last less than 1 min, owing to the drug's short half-life. The most common are dyspnea, cough, syncope, vertigo, paresthesias, numbness, nausea, and metallic taste. Cardiovascular adverse effects may include facial flushing, headache, diaphoresis, palpitations, retrosternal chest pain, sinus bradyarrhythmias (i.e., bradycardia, sinus arrest, AV block), atrial tachyarrhythmias (i.e., atrial fibrillation or flutter), PVCs, and hypotension. These adverse effects rarely require specific management. Dipyridamole and carbamazepine have been shown to enhance the negative chronotropic and dromotropic effects of adenosine and may increase the degree of toxicity. Methylxanthines and caffeine, on the other hand, compete for adenosine receptors. Therefore, asthmatics or those who drink large amounts of coffee may require a higher dose of adenosine to achieve a therapeutic effect. The induction of atrial fibrillation and/or flutter is problematic in patients with an accessory pathway as in WPW syndrome, since adenosine does not block conduction over accessory pathways. For reentrant pathways, adenosine will only block conduction of the antegrade AV loop. Adenosine has been shown to be safe in the setting of hypotension and CHF.[10]

DIGOXIN Intravenous digoxin is an effective inotropic agent with weak AV blocking effects. It exerts ventricular rate control through vagal tonic effects, which may take several hours to become clinically apparent.

Actions Digoxin has three basic actions: (1) it increases the force, strength, and velocity of cardiac contractions (positive inotropic effects); (2) it slows the heart rate (negative chronotropic effects); and (3) it slows conduction velocity through the AV node.

Digoxin exerts its direct inotropic and electrophysiologic effects by binding to and inhibiting the sodium and potassium ATPase pump in the cell membrane. This action results in higher intracellular levels of sodium and causes calcium to move intracellularly in exchange for sodium. The elevated intracellular calcium concentration allows more calcium to be available to increase the rate and force of cardiac contractions.

Digoxin increases the refractory period and decreases the conduction velocity of both the SA and AV nodes but shortens the refractory period and increases conduction velocity in the atrial muscles (including atrial bypass tracts, as present in WPW syndrome). The primary effect on SA and AV nodal conduction is secondary to direct enhancement of parasympathomimetic tone. ECG changes include PR interval prolongation and QT interval shortening. High doses of digoxin enhance ventricular automaticity.

Slowing of the heart results in a prolonged diastolic period, allowing a greater period for improving coronary blood and myocardial perfusion. A decrease in oxygen demand may also occur secondary to the decrease in heart rate.

Pharmacokinetics The onset of action is about 5 to 30 min following intravenous administration and 30 to 120 min for oral tablets, while peak effects occur in 1 to 4 h and 2 to 6 h, respectively. The onset of action following parenteral therapy varies based upon the rate at which digoxin is administered. In oral dosing, however, patient variability is the primary cause of variation. The large variation in peak effect can be explained by the fact that digoxin has a large Vd of 5.6 L/kg. Digoxin crosses the blood-brain barrier and the placenta, and high concentrations are found in the liver, heart, kidney, and intestines. Digoxin may also be given by oral tablets, elixir, and capsules, the bioavailability being approximately 70, 80, and 90 percent, respectively. Digoxin is inactivated by hepatic degradation and excreted unchanged in the urine. The half-life of digoxin in patients with normal renal function is 30 to 40 h and can extend to 4 to 6 days in anuric patients. Because digoxin concentrates in the tissues, serum levels of digoxin may not accurately reflect the amount of drug in the body, making procedures such as dialysis or exchange transfusion ineffective.

Common ED Indications Digoxin is indicated to improve cardiac output in CHF and to control heart rate in atrial fibrillation, atrial flutter, and paroxysmal atrial tachycardia (PAT). Use of digoxin in the treatment of CHF should be considered only when diuretics and vasodilators fail to improve cardiac output. Digoxin may be particularly effective in providing beneficial hemodynamic and symptomatic improvement in heart failure patients presenting with an S_3 gallop or ''low-output'' heart failure associated with depressed ventricular function. Digoxin is less effective with ''high-output'' heart failure, which occurs in patients with bronchopulmonary insufficiency, anemia, infection, hyperthyroidism, or arteriovenous fistulas.

Dosing and Administration Digoxin can be administered by the oral or intravenous route. The latter is preferred when a more rapid onset of action and peak effect is desired. The intravenous dose is 20 to 30 percent less than an oral dose. Digoxin should not be administered by intramuscular injection, since this route offers no advantages and can cause severe pain at the injection site.

For control of SVT, digoxin should be administered intravenously in a dose of 10 to 15 mg/kg (up to a total of 0.75 to 1.5 mg given over the first 24 h). This dose should be divided, with 0.25 to 0.5 mg given as the initial dose and 0.125 to 0.25 mg q2–6h as subsequent doses until the entire dose is administered or the heart rate is sufficiently lowered. The dose for patients with CHF without atrial fibrillation is generally lower (8 to 12 mg/kg) but can be given in a similar fashion as above until an appropriate response has been achieved. Higher doses are often required to control the ventricular response to atrial fibrillation or flutter, but higher doses have more adverse effects. Loading doses should be calculated using lean body weight, since this method generally provides therapeutic effects with minimal risk of toxicity. Intravenous loading doses should be administered slowly over a 5-min period or longer, undiluted or diluted, to a fourfold or greater volume. Serum digoxin levels should not be obtained earlier than 6 to 8 h after loading because of the slow distribution of the drug. Dosing in infants and children must be extremely careful. The small amounts given to children can easily be miscalculated.

Maintenance therapy should be adjusted according to clinical response or to maintain a serum digoxin concentration between 0.8 to 2.0 ng/mL. Dosage adjustments are necessary in renal failure, dehydration, hypokalemia, hypercalcemia, hypomagnesemia, and hypothyroidism. Drugs that interact with digoxin to cause increases in serum digoxin levels include amiodarone, verapamil, nifedipine, hydroxychloroquine, propafenone, quinidine, erythromycin, tetracycline, and anticholinergic agents. In contrast, the use of cholestyramine, metoclopramide, kaolin-pectin, penicillamine, and dietary fiber has resulted in lower serum digoxin concentrations.

Adverse-Effects Profile When digoxin toxicity is suspected, the drug should be stopped and a serum level obtained. Toxicity may actually occur in some patients with low serum levels, since it is often the myocardial tissue level rather than the serum level that determines the degree of toxicity. Symptoms of digoxin toxicity include mental depression, confusion, headache, drowsiness, anorexia, nausea, vomiting, weakness, visual disturbances (green or yellow vision and/or halo effects), delirium, electroencephalographic (EEG) abnormalities, and seizures. Patients may also present with diarrhea and abdominal discomfort. Almost any type of dysrhythmia may manifest in digoxin toxicity. The most common dysrhythmias include an increased number of unifocal or multiform PVCs, VT, junctional tachycardia, high-degree AV block, PSVT with block, and sinus arrest. Atrial fibrillation, bradycardia, and ventricular fibrillation may also occur. Other adverse effects may include gynecomastia, skin rash, eosinophilia, and thrombocytopenia. See Chap. 168 for a detailed discussion of digitalis toxicity.

While hypokalemia increases the risk of digoxin toxicity, significant digoxin toxicity itself may produce hyperkalemia due to paralysis of the transmembrane sodium-potassium pump. However, when hypokalemia develops in less severe cases of toxicity, potassium can be replaced by intravenous infusion provided that there is no evidence of high-degree AV conduction block. When digoxin toxicity is associated with hyperkalemia, a corresponding intracellular deficiency of potassium exists, which may be the causative factor of subsequent dysrhythmias. Treatment in this circumstance is controversial. It is not clear whether measures should be taken to decrease the total body supply of potassium (at the risk of increasing intracellular hypokalemia), to increase the total body potassium in the face of extracellular hyperkalemia, or to use measures that would ordinarily encourage movement of potassium back into cells (e.g., use of bicarbonate, glucose, and insulin). These methods may all prove useless in the absence of a functioning transmembrane sodium-potassium pump.

Lidocaine and phenytoin are antidysrhythmics that have classically been used in digoxin toxicity, but their efficacy has not been proven. Atropine and electrical pacing have been tried in cases of bradydysrhythmias, but these too have had limited success. Hemodialysis and resin hemoperfusion have been attempted in some cases of severe digoxin poisoning but have generally been unsuccessful because of the large volume of distribution of digoxin. Digoxin antibody fragments, otherwise known as digoxin immune FAB (fragmented antibodies) or Digibind (Burroughs-Wellcome), is available for use in treating life-threatening digoxin toxicity. This antidote is indicated for life-threatening ventricular tachydysrhythmias, sinus bradydysrhythmias, or severe AV blocks resulting from overdose or accidental pediatric ingestion of digoxin and digitalis-like glycosides that are unresponsive to conventional therapy. An additional indication for FAB, by the manufacturer, is in patients experiencing severe digoxin toxicity who have serum potassium levels greater than 5 meq/mL. See Chap. 168 for more information.

MAGNESIUM **Actions** Magnesium affects skeletal and smooth muscle contractility, vasomotor tone, and neuronal transmission directly via the Na^+, K^+-ATPase pump and indirectly via calcium blocking activity. It increases membrane potential, prolongs AV conduction, and increases the absolute refractory period. Hypomagnesemia can precipitate life-threatening cardiac dysrhythmias, symptoms of cardiac insufficiency, and sudden cardiac death after an AMI. Resupplementation of magnesium helps to replenish intracellular potassium in hypomagnesemic, hypokalemic patients, blocks calcium to cause vasodilation, and reduces platelet aggregation. Magnesium also decreases myocardial sensitivity to catecholamines as well as their release, which can lead to an excessive adrenergic surge. This surge can lead to dysrhythmias, hypertension, and increased myocardial oxygen consumption.

Common ED Indications The national council on CPR classified magnesium as usually indicated, always acceptable, and considered useful and effective in each of the following situations: treatment of torsades de pointes, cardiac arrest with suspected magnesium deficiency, and AMI with suspected magnesium deficiency. Suspect magnesium deficiency if a patient has a history of diuretic use, chronic illness, or malnutrition (including chronic alcoholism).

Some studies have suggested that magnesium therapy reduces the incidence of serious dysrhythmia as well as mortality in AMI. However, routine use of magnesium in AMI is not currently advocated by the ACC/AHA Task Force on Practice Guidelines.[11] Conflicting data exists for its usefulness. The second Leicester Intravenous Magnesium Infusion Trial (LIMIT-2) showed decreased mortality post-MI at 28 days.[12] However, the Fourth International Study of Infarct Survival (ISIS-4) did not demonstrate any benefit to magnesium therapy.[13] In fact, it was associated with an increased incidence of heart failure. Timing of administration of magnesium therapy may account for the conflicting results. Magnesium is recommended if there is a documented or suspected magnesium deficiency or if thrombolytics are contraindicated. If magnesium is used, it should be given as soon as possible.

Magnesium is indicated for ventricular fibrillation and sustained ventricular tachycardia refractory to standard therapy regardless of serum magnesium levels.[14] Polymorphic ventricular tachycardia will probably not respond to magnesium therapy if the QT interval is normal. Magnesium may reduce the frequency of PVCs, since this dysrhythmia is associated with low serum levels. Several studies indicate the usefulness of magnesium for the treatment of multifocal atrial tachycardia.[14] Its mechanism of action may be inhibition of afterdepolarizations. Magnesium also proves helpful in digoxin toxic dysrhythmias, which often occur in hypomagnesemic states. Magnesium may also terminate PSVT by prolonging atrioventricular nodal conduction. Other uses for parenteral magnesium sulfate include seizures associated with toxemia/eclampsia/nephritis, hypomagnesemia (mild to severe), and hyperalimentation. Unlabelled uses include the termination of preterm labor and bronchodilation in a subset of asthma patients.

Pharmacokinetics When magnesium sulfate is given intravenously, its onset of action is immediate and the duration of action is about 30 min. Following intramuscular administration, the time to onset of action is about 1 h and the duration is 3 to 4 h. Magnesium is excreted by the kidney at a variable rate directly proportional to the serum concentration and the glomerular filtration rate.

Dosing and Administration An intravenous loading dose of magnesium sulfate is administered as 1 to 2 g (8 to 16 meq), mixed in 50 or 100 mL D_5W, using either the 10% (100 mg/mL) or 50% (500 mg/mL) solutions. In cardiac arrest scenarios, the intravenous dose can be injected over 1 to 2 min. However, if time permits, a safer method is to administer 2 to 4 g as an intravenous infusion over 20 to 60 min. The rate of infusion should be slowed or stopped if hypotension develops. Several trials recommend the routine use of magnesium at doses of 8 to 12 g/24 h for AMI or suspected MI in the face of magnesium deficiency. While most recommendations suggest that an intravenous maintenance infusion at 0.5 to 1 g/h (4 to 8 meq) should follow for up to 24 h, the rate and duration of infusion should be based on the clinical situation and the degree of hypomagnesemia.

Adverse-Effects Profile Hypotension is the predominant adverse effect, yet it is surprisingly uncommon, even when a 1- to 2-g IV push is given over a few minutes. Other signs of hypermagnesemia, which may begin at serum concentrations of 4 meq/mL, include flushing, sweating, CNS depression, depression of reflexes, flaccid paralysis, hypotension, circulatory collapse, hypothermia, and fatal respiratory paralysis. Depression of reflexes usually precedes respiratory collapse.

VASOACTIVE DRUGS

Vasoactive drugs have two functions: (1) to improve cardiac perfusion pressure during cardiac arrest and (2) to support the circulation during hemodynamic compromise. During cardiac arrest, the myocardium needs to be perfused with adequately oxygenated blood before the return of spontaneous circulation can occur. Since α-adrenergic stimulation is responsible for improved coronary perfusion pressure, for this reason as well as others, adrenergic agents are used. Epinephrine is the agent most frequently employed. Currently, no evidence exists to support the superiority of an alternative agent although many have been tested in animal models.

Adrenergic agents are divided into pure α agents (phenylephrine), mixed α and β agents (epinephrine, norepinephrine, dopamine), and pure β or primarily β agonists (isoproterenol, dobutamine). The α receptors are found primarily in blood vessels, where α stimulation causes vasoconstriction. The β agonists work primarily on the heart and promote increased heart rate, increased contractility, and increased myocardial oxygen consumption. The β_2 receptors are found in smooth muscle of the bronchi, blood vessels, and uterus; stimulation causes bronchodilatation, vasodilatation, and uterine relaxation. If the etiology of the hemodynamic compromise is identified (e.g., cardiogenic, vasogenic, hypovolemic, or septic shock, etc.), then the judicious selection of a sympathomimetic agent can be achieved. See Tables 25-3, 25-4, and 25-5 for details.

TABLE 25-3 Cardiovascular Actions and Signal Transduction Pathways Initiated by Adrenergic Receptor Activation

Receptor Type	Cardiovascular Actions	Signal Pathway
α_1	Vasoconstriction	Activation of phospholipase C
α_2	Decreased central sympathetic outflow; feedback inhibition of norepinephrine release; vasoconstriction	Inhibition of adenyl cyclase
β_1	Increased heart rate, contractility, and conduction velocity	Activation of adenyl cyclase
β_2	Vasodilation	Activation of adenyl cyclase
Dopamine	Vasodilation	Activation of adenyl cyclase

EPINEPHRINE **Actions** Epinephrine is a potent, nonselective α- and β-adrenergic agonist. It is first-line therapy for cardiac arrest. The myocardium needs to be perfused before return of spontaneous

TABLE 25-4 Ability of Commonly Used Sympathomimetic Agents to Stimulate Adrenergic Receptors

	Receptor Type			
	α	β_1	β_2	Dopamine
Phenylephrine	++/+++	–	–	
Norepinephrine	++++	++++	+/++	
Epinephrine	+++	++++	+++	
Dopamine	++/+++	++++	++	++++
Dopexamine			++	+++
Dobutamine	+	++++	++	
Isoproterenol	–	++++	++++	

TABLE 25-5 Vasopressor Agents

Agent	Indications and Dosage	Remarks
Epinephrine	Cardiac arrest (asystole, VF/pulseless VT), symptomatic bradycardia, PEA: IV: 1 mg (1:10,000) q3 min ET: 2–2.5 mg (1:10,000) diluted with NSS to a volume of 10 mL Anaphylaxis, bronchospasm: SQ: 0.3 mg (1:1000) q20 min Pressor and chronotropic agent IV: 1 μg/min titrated to desired effect (2 to 10 μg/min)	The use of high-dose epinephrine in cardiac arrest is neither recommended nor supported by the AHA. Alpha effects are responsible for increased coronary artery perfusion pressure, which may promote return of spontaneous circulation. β effects may precipitate myocardial ischemia.
Dopamine	Renal dose (dopaminergic effects): IV: 1–5 μg/kg per minute infusion Cardiac dose (β_1 effects): IV: 5–10 μg/kg per minute infusion Vasopressor dose (α effects): IV: 10–20 μg/kg per minute infusion	Renal dose improves renal blood flow. Cardiac doses exert positive inotropic and chronotropic effects. Indicated for the treatment for cardiogenic shock. Vasopressor doses cause vasoconstriction and cardiac stimulation. If shock is refractory to 20 μg/kg per minute, add norepinephrine.
Dobutamine	Inotropic agent with little effect on SVR: IV: 2–20 μg/kg per minute infusion	Good inotropy, weak chronotropy. Little α effects. Useful adjunct to dopamine for treating cardiogenic shock. May use alone for cardiac decompensation associated with normal or slightly low blood pressure.
Isoproterenol	Inotropy without any alpha effects: IV: 2–10 μg per minute infusion	Used for bradycardia and heart block associated with a denervated heart (e.g. a transplanted heart) until pacing capabilities available. Increases myocardial oxygen consumption, which limits clinical usefulness in the adult population. Pediatric asthma.
Amrinone	Inotropy for CHF therapy: IV: 0.75 mg/kg over 3–5 min, then maintenance infusion at 5–10 μg/kg per minute	Positive inotropy with potent vasodilatation and increased stroke volume. Associated with thrombocytopenia. Cardiac dysrhythmias more pronounced with milrinone therapy.
Phenylephrine	Vasopressor: IV: 40 to 60 μg/min, titrate until clinical response or maximum infusion of 180 μg/min reached	Pure alpha agonist, no β effects. α effects of epinephrine and norepinephrine are more potent. Avoid in cardiogenic shock.
Norepinephrine	Vasopressor: (septic shock, sympathectomy) IV: 0.5–1 μg/min initial infusion. Increase infusion until clinical response or infusion rate reaches 30 μg/min Standard adult dose is 2 to 12 μg/min	Powerful vasoconstrictor with some β_1 cardiac stimulatory effects. Unlike epinephrine, it lacks β_2 effects. Useful for dopamine-refractory septic shock. Associated with reflex bradycardia. High doses associated with cardiac irritability.

circulation can occur. The α-adrenergic properties of epinephrine increase coronary artery perfusion pressure, which improves myocardial blood flow. Epinephrine is also a potent vasoconstrictor and increases mean arterial pressure by stimulating α-adrenergic receptors. This effect causes vasoconstriction of arterioles in the skin, mucosa, and mesenteric vasculature, redistributing blood to the heart and brain, and in turn results in improved cardiac and cerebral perfusion during resuscitation. However, its β-adrenergic qualities can have deleterious effects in the patient with myocardial ischemic or coronary artery disease. The β agonists increase heart rate, improve myocardial contractility, and therefore increase myocardial oxygen demand.

The β_2 adrenergic effects of epinephrine cause bronchodilation and antagonize the effects of histamine. Therefore, epinephrine is a useful adjunct for the treatment of severe bronchospasm and severe hypersensitivity reaction.

Pharmacokinetics Both the onset and the duration of action of epinephrine are relatively short: 1 to 2 min and 2 to 10 min, respectively. The drug quickly becomes fixed in the tissues and is rapidly inactivated via oxidation by monoamine oxidase (MAO) and via methylation by catechol-O-methyltransferase (COMT). Subsequent metabolites are excreted in the urine as sulfates and glucuronides.

Common ED Indications Epinephrine is considered a first-line agent in the treatment of cardiac arrest and may be used in pulseless VT/VF that has not responded to electrical countershock, asystole, and pulseless electrical activity (PEA). The drug has also been purported to "coarsen" fine ventricular fibrillation, but there is no documented evidence that this is true. Epinephrine does, however, increase the likelihood of continued hemodynamic stability in animals that have been successfully defibrillated. This has been attributed to the effect of epinephrine on systemic vascular resistance. Historically, the standard 1-mg dose came from the operating room practice of intracardiac injections, which were effective in restarting the arrested heart. But when studies showed that 1 to 3 mg of intracardiac epinephrine seemed to be more effective, higher dosages were adopted. Further animal studies were performed, and their dose-response curves demonstrated that vasoactive effects of epinephrine were dose-dependent. The lower doses favored β-adrenergic effects (cardiac stimulation), while higher doses revealed α-agonist effects (vasoconstriction). Over the years, it was assumed that 1 mg of epinephrine administered intravenously was equivalent and would be useful for all body weights. The dose-response curve was studied in the 1980s and early 1990s, revealing that higher doses of epinephrine (ranging from 0.045 to 0.2 mg/kg) were required to improve hemodynamics and demonstrate increased rates of return of spontaneous circulation (ROSC). However, trials failed to demonstrate significant improvement in survival rates to hospital discharge compared with the standard epinephrine doses (see "Dosing and Administration," below). Experience with "high-dose" epinephrine resulted in increased numbers of patients with ROSC admitted to intensive care settings, who previously would likely have failed resuscitation. While these results were initially exciting, the routine practice of administering high-dose epinephrine has waned as clinicians have come to appreciate the poor outcomes and needless consumption of precious medical resources.

Epinephrine is also used as an antidote to reverse bronchospasm due to anaphylactic and hypersensitivity reactions. It can be used as a vasopressor to increase blood pressure in septic shock. It should be employed as second-line therapy after norepinephrine. Be aware of its β-agonist properties, namely cardiac stimulation, which can increase the risk of dysrhythmias.

Dosing and Administration Current AHA guidelines recommend that epinephrine in a 1-mg (1:10,000) IV bolus continue to be the initial dose in cardiac arrest. It is now recommended that the dosing frequency be increased to 3 to 5 min from a 5-min interval. The AHA recognizes that higher doses of epinephrine are acceptable but can neither recommend nor discourage their use; however, they do say higher doses should be used only after the 1-mg dose has failed. The intermediate epinephrine dose suggestion is 2 to 5 mg IV push, also given every 3 to 5 min; the escalating regimen is 1 mg to 3 mg to 5 mg IV push, 3 min apart; the high dose reflects use of a bolus of 0.1 mg/kg every 3 to 5 min.

Epinephrine may be given by peripheral vein, central line, or endotracheally. The optimal dose for endotracheal drug delivery is unknown; however, a dose that is at least 2 to $2\frac{1}{2}$ times the peripheral intravenous dose may be needed. Endotracheal (ET) administration is performed by placing 10 mL of a 1:10,000 solution (preload syringe) down the ET tube and then performing several rapid ventilations to disperse the drug throughout the airways for maximal absorption. If the more concentrated epinephrine vial is used (30 mg/30 mL, 1:1000), the dose should be diluted to 10 mL.

Intracardiac administration should be used only during open cardiac massage so as to avoid the risk of pneumothorax, coronary artery laceration, and cardiac tamponade. Transthoracic intracardiac injections will interrupt ventilations and closed chest compressions and are thus no longer recommended.

Although ephinephrine is not the first choice, a continuous epinephrine infusion can be used to elicit the vasopressor response in patients who are not in cardiac arrest. The initial dose should begin at 1 mg/min (range 2 to 10 mg/min) and be titrated to a desired hemodynamic response. Continuous intravenous infusions of epinephrine should be administered by central venous access to ensure prompt transport to the heart and reduce the risk of extravasation.

Adverse-Effects Profile Adverse effects are of minimal importance in the setting of cardiac arrest. Epinephrine does increase myocardial oxygen consumption significantly and thus can exacerbate ventricular irritability in the setting of myocardial ischemia. The α-adrenergic activity of epinephrine produces an increase in systemic vascular resistance, which could conceivably be detrimental to a failing myocardium in that increased afterload can significantly decrease cardiac output. Also, if the patient is resuscitated, hypertension, tachycardia, and dysrhythmias should be anticipated. Because epinephrine causes renal artery vasoconstriction, it may cause a detrimental decrease in the glomerular filtration rate (GFR). Epinephrine is not compatible with alkaline solutions (e.g., sodium bicarbonate) in the same intravenous line, as some studies show slow inactivation of catecholamine.

DOPAMINE **Actions** Dopamine (Intropin), an endogenous catecholamine and the precursor of endogenous norepinephrine, acts on dopaminergic, β_1 and α receptors. In low doses (1 to 3 μg/kg per min), dopamine acts on dopaminergic receptors, causing vasodilation of the renal, mesenteric, coronary, and intracerebral vascular beds. This effect improves organ perfusion and increases urine output. At moderate doses (3 to 10 μg/kg per min), dopamine acts on its β_1-adrenergic receptors, exerting inotropic and chronotropic effects and increasing cardiac output without marked increases in pulmonary wedge pressure. Stimulation of α receptors increases peripheral resistance, increases pulmonary wedge pressure, and decreases blood flow to the kidney. The α effects begin at 10 μg/kg per min and predominate above 15 μg/kg per min.

Pharmacokinetics Dopamine has an onset of action within 2 to 4 min and a duration of action of less than 10 min. It is used only as an intravenous infusion. Renal response may take 20 to 30 min. Dopamine is metabolized primarily (75 percent) to homovanillic acid and other metabolites (including norepinephrine) by MAO and COMT and is subsequently excreted in the urine. Only a fraction of the dose eliminated by the kidneys is unchanged dopamine.

Common ED Indications Dopamine is used to treat hemodynamic compromise associated with MI, heart failure, septic shock, and renal failure. It is indicated for reversing hemodynamically significant hypotension due to MI, overt heart failure, renal failure, and chronic CHF when fluid resuscitation is unsuccessful (using the appropriate crystalloid or colloid solution) or not appropriate. It is also used to improve renal blood flow and to increase urine output, especially in the patient with septic shock. It is a preferred agent for treatment of cardiogenic shock.

Dopamine can be used in septic shock, especially if the primary goal is improvement in myocardial contractility. At high α-adrenergic doses (>10 μg/kg per min), dopamine can effectively raise the blood pressure in the fluid-resuscitated patient with septic shock. However, cardiac stimulation also occurs at high doses, which increases the risk of dysrhythmias. Often low-dose dopamine is used in combination with a more pure α vasoconstrictor to treat septic shock. Dopamine should be avoided in trauma until the patient has been adequately fluid-resuscitated.

Dosing and Administration The range for low-dose dopamine is 1 to 3 μg/kg per min, while the moderate dose is 3 to 10 μg/kg per min. High-dose dopamine begins at 10 μg/kg per min and should be titrated to adequate blood pressure response. These three levels of dosage are also referred to as "renal," "cardiac," and "vasopressor," respectively, in recognition of the different physiologic effects at different doses. Renal dose dopamine improves renal blood flow and urine output. Cardiac dose dopamine improves myocardial contractility and increases heart rate secondary to β_1-adrenergic effects. Peripheral arterial and venous vasoconstriction caused by α adrenergic stimulation occurs with vasopressor dose dopamine. As with all vasoactive infusions, dopamine should be discontinued by tapering the dosage. Most patients can be managed on 20 μg/kg per min or less. If higher doses are needed for septic shock, an intravenous norepinephrine infusion should be added. The combination of dopamine and dobutamine improves cardiac performance during cardiogenic shock.

Adverse-Effects Profile Dopamine may produce dose-dependent adverse effects, including hypotension at low infusion rates, hypertension at high infusion rates, ectopic beats, headache, nausea, vomiting, angina pectoris, and tachycardia. Necrosis may occur if the infusion extravasates. Gangrene of the extremities has occurred in patients with occlusive vascular disease or diabetes as well as in those who received prolonged high-dose infusions. Monoamine oxidase inhibitors, halogen anesthetics, sympathomimetics, and phosphodiesterase inhibitors will prolong and intensify the effects of dopamine, possibly causing hypertensive and dysrhythmogenic activity. Phenytoin may interact with dopamine and cause hypotension, seizures, and bradycardia. Dopamine is contraindicated in pheochromocytoma. Like epinephrine, dopamine should not be mixed with alkaline solutions in the same line.

DOBUTAMINE **Actions** Dobutamine (Dobutrex) is a synthetic sympathomimetic agent that exerts potent inotropic and mild chronotropic activity by directly stimulating β-adrenergic receptors. Dobutamine also has mild α_1-agonist activity, but the effects are balanced by the more potent β_2-agonist effects, cumulatively resulting in mild vasodilation. Dobutamine has potent β_1 effects, which make it an excellent inotrope, but it lacks the α vasoconstricting activity of dopamine. Doses of 2 to 20 μg/kg per min increase cardiac output, induce peripheral vasodilation, and decrease pulmonary occlusive pressures, causing minimal increase in heart rate. However, higher doses of dobutamine will accelerate the heart rate and induce dysrhythmogenic effects. An increased cardiac output usually results in increased renal and mesenteric blood flow.

Pharmacokinetics Dobutamine has an onset of action of 1 to 2 min, but peak plasma levels may not be reached for 10 min. Its duration of action is 10 to 15 min. The plasma half-life is 2 min. Dobutamine is metabolized in the liver and other tissues by COMT and glucuronic acid, and over two-thirds of a dose is excreted as metabolites in the urine within 48 h.

Common ED Indications Dobutamine is used to increase inotropic activity in the short-term management of cardiac decompensation due to depressed contractility resulting either from organic heart disease or from cardiac surgical procedures. The drug should be used to increase cardiac output in patients with chronic CHF when standard therapy (diuretics, vasodilators, and digoxin) fails to improve symptoms and/or in the patient with pulmonary congestion and low cardiac output.

Dosing and Administration Dobutamine is administered only by intravenous infusion. The dosage range is 2 to 20 μg/kg per min; however, most patients can be maintained on 10 μg/kg per min or less. In some cases, very low doses (0.5 μg/kg per min) may be effective. Conversely, infusions up to 40 μg/kg per min have been used, but doses greater than 20 μg/kg per min should be used with caution because of increased risks of tachydysrhythmias. To assess the effectiveness of the drug correctly, patients should be monitored with a Swan-Ganz catheter.

Adverse-Effects Profile The primary adverse effects of dobutamine are increased heart rate (increases greater than 5 to 15 beats per minute are uncommon), blood pressure (increases greater than 10 to 20 mmHg are uncommon), and ectopic dysrhythmias (escape beats, unifocal and multifocal ventricular ectopic beats, and ventricular bigeminy). Less common effects include headache, paresthesias, tremors, nausea, angina, and dyspnea. Increases in heart rate greater than 10 percent may induce or exacerbate myocardial ischemia.

NOREPINEPHRINE **Actions** Norepinephrine bitartrate (Levophed) is identical to the endogenous catecholamine synthesized in the adrenal medulla and sympathetic nervous tissue. Norepinephrine acts primarily on α receptors, inducing powerful vasoconstrictor actions on arterial and venous beds (i.e., renal and mesenteric vasoconstriction). It is particularly useful in patients with dopamine refractory septic shock. The drug also has direct action on β_1 receptors, thus inducing inotropic and chronotropic effects. Paradoxical decreases in heart rate may result from reflex increases in parasympathetic tone. Norepinephrine therefore produces less tachycardia than dopamine. It differs from epinephrine in that it has little effect on β_2 receptors.

Pharmacokinetics Norepinephrine is administered only as intravenous infusion. The pressor effect has an onset of action within 1 to 3 min and stops within 5 to 10 min of discontinuation of the infusion. The primary elimination of norepinephrine is via uptake by adrenergic neurons and metabolism in the liver and other tissues, mainly by COMT and to a lesser extent by MAO. Norepinephrine metabolites are excreted in the urine as sulfate and glucuronate conjugates.

Common ED Indications Norepinephrine is used primarily as a vasopressor for the treatment of severe hypotension refractory to fluids and other pressor agents, specifically dopamine. Norepinephrine may be particularly effective when endogenous norepinephrine stores are low. This scenario may arise in patients who have been on prolonged infusions of dopamine. To a certain degree, norepinephrine increases inotropic activity and may be indicated in severe hypotension occurring during an AMI. However, norepinephrine is a potent vasoconstrictor that increases afterload and may impede cardiac output. Therefore norepinephrine should be employed in cardiogenic shock only after more traditional therapy has failed. Other specific uses for norepinephrine include controlling hypotensive states during poliomyelitis, treating drug overdose (various phenothiazines and tricyclic antidepressants), and for spinal anesthesia, pheochromocytomectomy, and sympathectomy. Its potent α effects make it a good choice to treat septic shock.

Dosing and Administration Norepinephrine should be used only as an intravenous infusion. The initial adult dose is 0.5 to 1 μg/min. Rates must be titrated carefully, increasing by 1 to 2 μg/min q3–5 min until a systolic blood pressure of 80 to 100 mmHg is attained. The drug should be infused at the lowest effective dose for the shortest period of time possible. Occasionally, high doses of norepinephrine may be necessary to reverse hypotension (e.g., 8 to 30 mg/min). Usually, the maintenance dose is 2 to 4 μg/min. Adjust the rate of flow q3–5 min to maintain blood pressure. Once the blood pressure is adequate, the infusion may be gradually titrated down. Abrupt withdrawal may result in acute hypotension.

Adverse-Effects Profile Large doses of norepinephrine may result in ventricular irritability, cardiac depression, decreased renal blood flow, and a reflex bradycardia. Acute hypertension may result in patients on MAO inhibitors or tricyclic antidepressants. Use norepinephrine with extreme caution in these patients. Use as large a vein as possible to minimize the risk of extravasation. If extravasation occurs, phentolamine, 5 to 10 mg in 10 to 15 mL of normal saline solution, should be infiltrated as soon as possible to prevent necrosis and sloughing. Check frequently for intravenous extravasation if a small vein is used. Norepinephrine is contraindicated in patients with hypotension resulting from cyclopropane or halogenated hydrocarbon anesthesia or uncorrected blood volume deficits as well as in mesenteric or peripheral vascular thrombosis. Norepinephrine must be used with caution in patients with known or suspected pulmonary hypertension, since norepinephrine is a potent vasoconstrictor of the pulmonary vasculature.

PHENYLEPHRINE **Actions** Phenylephrine is an α-adrenergic agent that possesses few β-adrenergic effects. It is useful for the treatment of septic shock, particularly if further cardiac stimulation is to be avoided. However, phenylephrine lacks the vasoconstrictor potency of epinephrine and norepinephrine.

Pharmacokinetics The vasoconstrictor activity of phenylephrine lasts approximately 20 min after intravenous infusion, 1 to 2 h after an intramuscular dose, and 50 min after subcutaneous administration. It is associated with reflex bradycardia, which is blocked by atropine. The sympathomimetic effects are potentiated by MAO inhibitors.

Common ED Indications Phenylephrine is a powerful α-receptor stimulant. It causes peripheral vasoconstriction, which causes an elevation of the systolic and diastolic blood pressure and reflex bradycardia. Unlike epinephrine and norepinephrine, phenylephrine lacks cardiac stimulant β effects. Therefore cardiac complications are rarely seen. It is useful in shock states caused by sepsis and by some drug toxicities. Patients with cardiogenic shock and left ventricular dysfunction require more β-inotropic support. Phenylephrine should be avoided in this patient population.

Dosing and Administration Phenylephrine can be administered intravenously or as a continuous infusion. In shock, the initial dose is 100 to 180 μg/kg as an intravenous infusion. Once the blood pressure is stable, the infusion can be decreased to 40 to 60 μg/kg. An alternate regimen is 0.1 to 0.5 mg intravenously q15 min. Do not exceed an individual dose of 0.5 mg IV. This should elevate the blood pressure for at least 15 min. Clinical response to the continuous infusion occurs between 40 to 180 μg/min. Blood pressure should be monitored continuously for both routes and hypertension avoided.

Adverse-Effects Profile Phenylephrine is associated with headache and restlessness. Reflex bradycardia commonly occurs. Since phenylephrine is pure α stimulant, cardiac dysrhythmias are rare. The α receptors are located in large coronary arteries but not commonly found in the small coronary arteries. Vasoconstriction of the large coronary arteries is particularly dangerous in the elderly, in those with severe atherosclerosis, and in patients with a history of MI. Extravasation of the drug is associated with sloughing and tissue necrosis, often requiring surgical debridement. Phentolamine, an α-adrenergic blocking agent, may prevent necrosis. (Dilute 10 mg of phentolamine in normal saline solution to a volume of 15 mL. Infiltrate the "at risk" area.)

ISOPROTERENOL **Actions** Isoproterenol is a synthetic sympathomimetic with strong β_1 and β_2-adrenergic-agonist properties; it increases the myocardial oxygen consumption. β_1 actions increase the inotropic and chronotropic activity of cardiac muscle, resulting in increased cardiac output despite a reduction in the mean blood pressure. The drop in blood pressure can be attributed to the β_2-adrenergic relaxation of smooth muscle in the splanchnic vascular bed and alimentary tract, the lungs, and skeletal muscle, which causes peripheral vasodilation and venous pooling. Therefore, isoproterenol is not a vasopressor agent and should not be used in shock.

Pharmacokinetics After intravenous administration, isoproterenol has an onset of action within 1 to 5 min and a duration of action lasting 1 to 2 h. Some 50 percent of the drug is eliminated unchanged in the urine, while 25 to 35 percent is metabolized primarily to 3-O-methylisoproterenol (which has been reported to have weak β-adrenergic blocking activity) by COMT in the lung, liver, and other body tissues and then excreted unchanged or as a sulfate conjugate.

Common ED Indications Isoproterenol is now indicated only for refractory torsades de pointes and immediate temporary management of hemodynamically significant bradycardias in the denervated heart of patients at or and after heart transplantation. Isoproterenol is not considered the drug of choice for either of these conditions; it should be considered only as a temporary measure until pacemaker therapy is instituted. For hemodynamically unstable bradydysrhythmias transcutaneous pacing (TCP) is the definitive treatment, since it provides better control and is a safer mode of therapy. Other agents that should be considered before isoproterenol are intravenous fluid challenge, atropine, and a dopamine or epinephrine infusion. The vasodilator effects of isoproterenol have been shown to lower coronary perfusion pressure during cardiac arrest and to increase the mortality rate in experimental animals; the drug has not been shown to be efficacious in cardiac arrest or for use in hypotension.

Dosing and Administration Isoproterenol should be administered only via intravenous infusion. The initial infusion rate, 2 to 10 μg/min, should be titrated to the desired heart rate. The drug has been shown to be more helpful at low doses rather than high doses.

Adverse-Effects Profile It must be emphasized that the β_1-agonist action of isoproterenol will cause an increase in chronotropic effect. This effect raises myocardial oxygen requirements and can possibly precipitate or exacerbate myocardial ischemia, inducing serious dysrhythmias (e.g., VT and VF). Other adverse effects include anxiety, mild tremors, and anginal pain in patients with previously reported angina pectoris. Therefore, the drug should be avoided in patients with preexisting ischemic heart disease. Isoproterenol may also induce tachydysrhythmias in hypokalemic and digoxin-toxic patients. The primary adverse effects from β_2-adrenergic actions are facial flushing, headache, and hypotension.

AMRINONE **Actions** Amrinone is thought to be a positive inotropic agent not related to digitalis glycosides, catecholamines (e.g., epinephrine, dopamine, and norepinephrine), or synthetic β_1-adrenergic agonists (e.g., dobutamine and isoproterenol); it possesses potent vasodilator activity. While its true mechanism is not known, amrinone is believed to act by inhibiting cyclic adenosine monophosphate (cAMP) phosphodiesterase activity, which results in increased levels of cellular cAMP. Increased levels of cAMP are thought to increase calcium availability to the myocardial contractile components. These actions increase myocardial contractility and force of contractions (i.e., positive inotropic effect) without significant increases in heart rate and blood pressure. Some believe that the vasodilator action is the primary mechanism responsible for increasing myocardial performance. Vasodilation with amrinone may be the result of direct action by the drug on the vessels or may be caused by a reflex withdrawal of sympathetic tone following the improvement of myocardial function. Nonetheless, the primary effect of amrinone is an increase in myocardial contractility and stroke volume with a reduction in preload and afterload.

Pharmacokinetics Cardiovascular effects usually begin within 2 to 5 min and generally peak within 10 min at all doses. The duration of effect is dose-related. Following a 0.75-mg/kg bolus dose, the duration is about 30 min, while a 3-mg/kg dose will last approximately 2 h. Amrinone is metabolized in the liver, excreted in the urine, and has a Vd of 1.2 L/kg. In patients with normal renal function, amrinone has an elimination half-life of 3.6 h. In patients with CHF and/or hepatic or renal dysfunction, amrinone has a prolonged elimination half-life (average 5.8 h).

Common ED Indications Amrinone is indicated for increasing myocardial performance in the short-term management of CHF. Because of its adverse-effects profile, the drug should be used only when other therapies, such as diuretics, digoxin, and vasodilators, have failed. Amrinone has been studied in class III and IV CHF. It may serve as an alternative or adjunctive agent to dobutamine in the treatment of cardiogenic shock.

Dosing and Administration The initial dose is 0.75 mg/kg followed by a maintenance infusion at 5 to 10 μg/kg per min. Amrinone should be administered as a slow direct intravenous injection (undiluted) over 2 to 3 min or as a continuous infusion diluted in 0.9 or 0.45% saline. Dextrose-containing solutions may result in a loss of the drug's activity. The total daily dose should not exceed 10 mg/kg. A second intravenous bolus injection may be given 30 min following the first dose if desired effects have not been achieved. Adjustments in the maintenance infusion should be titrated to clinical response.

Adverse-Effects Profile The most common adverse effects are thrombocytopenia (<100,000/mm^3, in 2.4 percent), ventricular and supraventricular dysrhythmias (3 percent), hypotension (1.3 percent), and nausea (1.7 percent). Other adverse effects, which occur in fewer than 1 percent of patients, include vomiting, anorexia, fever, chest pain, and burning at the site of injection. Although rare, hepatotoxicity with amrinone has been reported. Acute marked elevations of hepatic enzymes along with clinical symptoms may suggest a hypersensitivity reaction, which would require prompt discontinuation of the drug.

MILRINONE Milrinone is a phosphodiesterase inhibitor with positive inotropic and vasodilator effects. It is similar to amrinone in its spectrum of action. Milrinone has a lower incidence of thrombocytopenia but a higher risk of cardiac dysrhythmias as compared with amrinone. Milrinone minimally slows AV node conduction time, which may speed the ventricular response in patients with atrial fibrillation or atrial flutter. Ventricular ectopy, ventricular dysrhythmias, and supraventricular dysrhythmias may also occur with milrinone, especially in high-risk patients.

Milrinone inhibits cAMP phosphodiesterase activity. Like amrinone, cAMP mediated increases in intracellular calcium permit the cardiac muscle to contract with increased force. Milrinone promotes improved diastolic function and vascular muscle relaxation. It is indicated for the treatment of CHF. The loading dose is 50 μg/kg administered over 10 min, then a maintenance infusion at 0.375 to 0.75 μg/kg per min (standard is 0.5 μg/kg per min).

ATROPINE **Actions** Atropine sulfate, an antimuscarinic agent, enhances sinus node automaticity and AV conduction by blocking vagal activity; thus it has been termed a parasympatholytic drug. It has anticholinergic properties.

Pharmacokinetics The onset of action of atropine following intravenous, intramuscular, and endotracheal administration is rapid, with peak increases in heart rate occurring within 5 min. The half-life of atropine is 2 to 4 h or longer. Well absorbed and distributed throughout the body, atropine is metabolized in the liver and excreted in the urine.

Common ED Indications Atropine is the treatment of choice for increasing heart rate in hemodynamically unstable bradycardias (e.g., decreased heart rate with hypotension, altered mental status, "escape beats," and chest pain). Higher doses have been used in asystolic cardiac arrest, specifically if it is associated with increased vagal tone. It improves AV node conduction time in first degree and type I second degree AV block. Caution should be exercised with type II second degree and third degree AV block, since atropine may be associated with paradoxical slowing of the heart rate. The drug reverses cholinergic medications and toxins that cause a decrease in systemic vascular resistance, heart rate, and blood pressure. Additionally, atropine may reduce nausea and vomiting that occur as a result of morphine administration.

Dosing and Administration The dose of atropine for hemodynamically unstable bradycardia is 0.5–1.0 mg by rapid IV push, repealed q3–5 min until a desired heart rate is achieved or symptoms resolve. Do not administer less than 0.5 mg since lower doses are associated with paradoxical bradycardia. Bolus doses of 1 mg can be given for asystole and repeated once if necessary. A total dose of 3 mg (0.04 mg/kg) results in full vagolytic blockade in humans. It has been conventional practice to stop atropine administration when the total "vagolytic dose" has been given as outlined in standard ACLS teaching. This practice is appropriate when there is no response to atropine; further doses are unlikely to be effective. However, if a response is seen, there is no proscription to exceeding the "vagolytic" dose, if further dosing maintains the desired effect.

Atropine can be administered by intravenous push, intramuscularly, and via endotracheal tube. If given via the endotracheal tube, recommendations include a bolus of at least 1 mg at a time. No dilution is necessary when a preload syringe (1 mg/10 mL) is used. However, if the 1-mg/mL ampules are used, dilution with up to 10 mL of normal saline is recommended. It appears that absorption across tracheobronchial structure is good and substantial atropine levels are achieved within 10 min of dosing. The pediatric dose is 0.02 mg/kg with a minimum dose of 0.1 mg. Do not administer less than 0.1 mg since lower doses are associated with paradoxical bradycardia.

Adverse-Effects Profile Atropine is not indicated for bradycardia in hemodynamically stable patients. If it is administered, marked increases in heart rate can increase myocardial oxygen consumption, possibly inducing ischemia and precipitating ventricular tachydysrhythmias (including VT and VF). This is particularly true with doses greater than 0.5 mg. Doses less than 0.5 mg along with a therapeutic dose administered slowly can cause paradoxical bradycardia. This may be due to a central reflex stimulation of the vagus or a peripheral parasympathomimetic effect on the heart. There is concern by some about using atropine in AV block at the His-Purkinje level (type II AV block and third-degree block with new wide QRS complexes). Other effects that may occur include anticholinergic symptoms (e.g.,

TABLE 25-6 Nitroglycerin Chart

Sublingual:
- Dissolve 1 tablet under tongue q5 min until pain relief or hypotension occurs
- Onset: 1–3 min
- DOA: 1–3 min

Translingual spray:
- 1–2 metered-dose sprays into oral mucosa q3–5 min
- Onset: 2 min
- DOA: 30–60 min

Topical ointment:
- Apply 1 to 2 in. to chest wall q4–8 hr
- Onset: 20–60 min
- DOA: 2–12 h

Intravenous infusion:
- Give 5–10 μg/min, titrate in increments of 5–10 μg/min q3–5 min until desired results (standard dose 50–200 μg/min)
- Onset: 1–2 min
- DOA: 3–5 min

Sustained-release pill:
- Starting dose is 2.5 mg PO tid
- Onset: 20–45 min
- DOA: 4 h

Transmucosal tablets:
- Place 1-mg pill between lip and gum above incisors or between cheek and gum q3–5 h while awake
- Onset: 1–2 min
- DOA: 3–5 h

Transdermal patch
- Apply to hair-free area and rotate sites. 2.5–15-mg patches are available; start with low dose and titrate upward
- Onset: 30–60 min
- DOA: up to 24 h

*DOA, duration of action.

TABLE 25-7 Drugs Commonly Used in Pediatric Resuscitation

Drug	Pediatric Dosage	Remarks
Adenosine	IV: 0.1–0.2 mg/kg, followed by 2–5 mL NSS bolus. Double dose and repeat × 1	Maximum single dose is 12 mg.
Atropine	IV: 0.02 mg/kg, repeat in 5 minutes (minimum single dose is 0.1 mg) ET: double IV dose and dilute with NSS to 3–5 mL	Maximum single dose: 0.5 mg (child) and 1.0 mg (adolescent). Maximum cumulative dose: 1.0 mg (child) and 2.0 mg (adolescent).
Bretylium	5 mg/kg, may be increased to 10% mg/kg	Rapid IV
Calcium chloride (10%)	20 mg/kg	Slow push
Dopamine infusion	IV: 2.0–20 μg/kg per minute titrate to desired effect renal dose (dopaminergic effects): IV: 2–5 μg/kg per minute infusion cardiac dose (B1 effects) IV: 5–10 μg/kg per minute infusion vasopressor dose (alpha effects): IV: 10–20 μg/kg per minute infusion	6 × weight in kg = mg of drug to add to a diluent to make a final volume of 100 mL. 1 mL/h = 1 μg/kg per minute.
Dobutamine infusion	IV: 2.0–20 μg/kg per minute, titrate to desired effect	6 × weight in kg = mg of drug to add to a diluent to make a final volume of 100 mL. 1 mL/h = 1 μg/kg per minute.
Epinephrine	bradycardia: IV/IO: 0.01 mg/kg (0.1 mL/kg) of 1:10,000 ET: 0.1 mg/kg (0.1 mL/kg) of 1:1000 pulseless arrest: First dose: IV/IO: 0.01 mg/kg (0.1 mL/kg) of 1:10,000 ET: 0.1 mg/kg (0.1 mL/kg) of 1:1000 Second dose: IV/IO/ET: 0.1 mg/kg (0.1 mL/kg) of 1:1000 q3 min	Unlike other agents, epinephrine per ET tube is 10 times the IV dose. Follow ET dose with several positive pressure ventilations.
Epinephrine infusion	IV: 0.1–1.0 μg/kg per minute	0.6 × weight in kg = mg of drug to add to a diluent to make a final volume of 100 mL. 0.1 mL/h = 0.1 μg/kg per minute.
Lidocaine	IV: 1.0 mg/kg bolus, then 20–50 μg/kg per min ET: double IV dose and dilute with NSS to 3–5 mL	
Lidocaine infusion	IV: 20–50 μg/kg per minute	60 × weight in kg = mg of drug to add to a diluent to make a final volume of 100 mL. 1 mL/h = 10 μg/kg per minute.
Naloxone	If < 5 yrs or ≤ 20 kg: 0.1 mg/kg If > 5 yrs and > 20 kg: 2.0 mg	Titrate to desired effect
Nitroprusside infusion	IV: 0.5–5.0 μg/kg per minute	6 × weight in kg = mg of drug to add to a diluent to make a final volume of 100 mL. 1 mL/h = 1 μg/kg per minute.
Norepinephrine infusion	IV: 0.1–1.0 μg/kg per minute	0.6 × weight in kg = mg of drug to add to a diluent to make a final volume of 100 mL. 1 mL/h = 0.1 μg/kg per minute.
Sodium bicarbonate	1 meq/kg	Infuse slowly and use only if ventilation is adequate.

Source: Chameides L, Hazinski MF (eds): *Textbook of Pediatric Advanced Life Support*. Dallas: American Heart Association, 1997.

blurred vision, dry mouth, CNS stimulation, hallucinations, mydriasis, tachycardia).

Vasodilator Agents

NITROGLYCERIN **Actions** Although the mechanism of action of nitroglycerin is not fully understood, its therapeutic benefit appears to be due to its actions on the peripheral circulation and the coronary blood flow. Nitroglycerin is a direct vasodilator that induces venodilation at low doses (<100 mg/min) and arteriolar vasodilation at high doses (>200 mg/min). Coronary artery dilation occurs throughout the dosage range.

Pharmacokinetics Table 25-6 describes the onset and duration of action of various nitroglycerin products. Nitroglycerin has a plasma half-life of 1 to 4 min and is metabolized in the liver. Oral doses undergo an extensive first-pass metabolism.

Common ED Indications Nitroglycerin is approved for the prophylaxis, treatment, and management of angina pectoris. Intravenous nitroglycerin is used to control hypertension associated with surgery and also in CHF associated with AMI.

Dosing and Administration Refer to Table 25-6 for dosing details of specific nitrates used in clinical practice. Nitroglycerin can be administered sublingually, lingually, intrabuccally, orally, topically, or by intravenous infusion. The sublingual and intrabuccal tablets should not be swallowed, and the extended-release buccal tablets (transmucosal) should not be chewed or swallowed. Patients should be in a sitting or supine position immediately following sublingual, lingual, or intrabuccal administration.

An intravenous infusion of nitroglycerin (Tridil) should be administered by a controlled-infusion device. Since data on the incompatibility of nitroglycerin with other parenteral agents are unclear, a separate intravenous site for a nitroglycerin infusion should be used. Infusions should not be suddenly discontinued, since abrupt withdrawal reactions (including angina pectoris or MI) may result. Attempts should be made to gradually wean down the infusion. Specific dosing regimens are shown in Table 25-6. There is no specific upper limit to the dose. Although most patients will be managed well below 200 μg/min or even 100 μg/min, a few patients may require a dose several fold higher. The dose of nitroglycerin for each patient should be titrated to individual response, using the smallest effective dose.

Adverse-Effects Profile Most adverse effects are related to the cardiovascular actions induced by nitroglycerin. These effects include headache, dizziness, weakness, syncope, flushing, hypotension, reflex tachycardia, and occasionally bradycardia. Use in patients concomitantly using alcohol may potentiate hypotension. Nitroglycerin has been shown to decrease the anticoagulant effects of heparin. Also, rash has been reported with topical nitroglycerin use.

Caution is advised when nitroglycerin is used in patients who are hemodynamically unstable (including those who are volume-depleted) or who have increased intracranial pressure or severe anemia. The drug should also be used cautiously in cases of constrictive pericarditis, pericardial tamponade, and hypertrophic cardiomyopathy. Also, there have been reports of associated brief increases in intraocular pressure in patients with glaucoma. Extended-release preparations of nitroglycerin should be avoided in patients with GI hypermotility or malabsorption syndromes.

Transdermal patches and topical ointment must be removed prior to attempting defibrillation or synchronized cardioversion. Topical nitroglycerin products alter electrical conductivity and enhance the potential for electrical arcing. To avoid excessive dosing, topical products should also be removed if additional nitroglycerin is given for acute symptoms.

NITROPRUSSIDE Sodium nitroprusside (Nipride) is another potent arterial and venous dilator used to treat the full spectrum of hypertensive emergencies. A full discussion of nitroprusside is found in Chap. 53.

Pediatric Considerations

Children, unlike adults, seldom have primary ventricular dysrhythmias in the absence of congenital heart disease. Rather, pediatric arrest is usually secondary to severe respiratory insufficiency. Bradydysrhythmias are the most common rhythms seen in pediatric arrest. Table 25-7 shows the drugs most commonly used in pediatric advanced life support. Pediatric resuscitation is discussed in depth in Chap. 10.

REFERENCES

1. Guidelines for Cardiopulmonary Resuscitation and Emergency Care: Recommendation of the 1992 National Conference: Part III. Adult cardiac life support. *JAMA* 268:2205, 1992.
2. Echt D, Leibson P, Mitchell L, et al: Mortality and morbidity in patients receiving encainide, flecainide, or placebo: The Cardiac Arrhythmia Suppression Trial. *N Engl J Med* 324:781, 1991.
3. Kowey P, Marinchak R, Rial S, et al: Pharmacologic and pharmacokinetics profile of class III antiarrhythmic drugs. *Am J Cardiol* 80:8A, 16G.
4. Kostis J, Lacy B, Cosgrove N, et al: Association of calcium channel blocker use with increased rate of acute myocardial infarction in patients with left ventricular dysfunction. *Am Heart J* 133:550, 1997.
5. Hagar WD, Davis B, Riba A, et al: Absence of a deleterious effect of calcium channel blockers in patients with left ventricular dysfunction after myocardial infarction: The SAVE study experience. *Am Heart J* 135:406, 1998.
6. Gulamhusein S, Ko P, Klein GJ: Ventricular fibrillation following verapamil. A Wolff-Parkinson-White syndrome. *Am Heart J* 106:145, 1983.
7. Strasberg B, Sagie A, Rechavia E, et al: Deleterious effects of intravenous verapamil in Wolff-Parkinson-White patients and atrial fibrillation. *Cardiovasc Drugs Ther,* 2(6):801, 1989.
8. McGovern B, Garan H, Ruskin JN: Precipitation of cardiac arrest by verapamil in patients with Wolff-Parkinson-White syndrome. *Ann Intern Med* 104:791, 1986.
9. Shryock J, Belardinelli L: Adenosine and adenosine receptors in the cardiovascular system: Biochemistry, physiology, and pharmacology. *Am J Cardiol* 79(12A):2, 1997.
10. Marco CA, Cardinale JF: Adenosine for the treatment of supraventricular tachycardia in the ED. *Am J Emerg Med* 12:485, 1994.
11. Ryan T, Anderson J, Antonan E, et al: ACC/AHA Guidelines for the Management of Patients with Acute Myocardial Infarction: executive summary. *J Am Coll Cardiol* 28(5):1372, 1996.
12. Woods K, Fletcher S, Roffe C, et al: Intravenous magnesium sulfate in suspected myocardial infarction: The Second Leicester Intravenous Magnesium Trial (LIMIT-2). *Lancet* 339:1553, 1992.
13. ISIS-4 (Fourth International Study of Infarct Survival) Collaborative Group. ISIS-4: A randomized factorial trial assessing oral captopril, oral mononitrate, and intravenous magnesium sulfate in 58,050 patients with suspected myocardial infarction. *Lancet* 345:669, 1995.
14. Frakes M, Richardson L: Magnesium sulfate therapy in certain emergency conditions. *Am J Emerg Med* 15:182, 1997.

APPROACH TO THE PATIENT IN SHOCK

Emanuel P. Rivers
Mohamed Y. Rady
Robert Bilkovski

EPIDEMIOLOGY

Over 1 million cases of shock present to the emergency department (ED) each year; the presentation may be cryptic or obvious as in the ultimate shock state of cardiac arrest. The definition and treatment of shock continue to evolve because of new understanding and technologies, some of which are now available for ED use. With a contemporary understanding of shock, the emergency physician can initiate expert and timely intervention. Regardless of the specific precipitating events, modifying circumstances, and variable presentations, common principles apply concerning the general approach to a patient in the initial stages of shock.

THE RATIONALE FOR EARLY INTERVENTION

The ''golden hour'' is the tenet of early intervention in surgical resuscitation. Due to inpatient crowding, this ''golden hour'' can frequently be *hours* in hospitals, requiring the provision of critical care in the ED.[1,2] The benefit of ED care in nontraumatic critical illness has not been adequately studied. Using a measure of illness severity that also predicts mortality (APACHE II), a study of critically ill patients admitted to the medical critical care unit demonstrated that ED intervention significantly decreased the incidence of organ failure by 25 percent and predicted mortality by 12.5 percent.[3] This study, and others like it, provide evidence that expert and timely ED care reduces morbidity and mortality in patients with nontraumatic critical illness.

PATHOPHYSIOLOGY

Shock is now defined as circulatory insufficiency that creates an imbalance between tissue oxygen supply and oxygen demand. Global tissue hypoperfusion is associated with a decreased venous oxygen content and metabolic acidosis (lactic acidosis). Shock is classified into four categories by etiology: (1) hypovolemic (due to inadequate circulating volume), (2) cardiogenic (due to inadequate cardiac pump function), (3) distributive (maldistribution of blood flow), and (4) obstructive (extracardiac obstruction to blood flow). Clinically, shock may have a predominant cause, but as the shock state persists or progresses, other pathophysiologic mechanisms become operative.

Knowledge of the principles of oxygen transport and consumption is important to the understanding of shock. A maximum of four molecules of oxygen is loaded onto each molecule of hemoglobin as it passes through the lungs. If all available oxygen sites are occupied (four per molecule of hemoglobin), $Sa{O_2}$ is 100 percent (see Table 26-1 for abbreviation definitions). The $Ca{O_2}$ is the amount of oxygen bound to hemoglobin plus a small amount dissolved in plasma (Table 26-2). Oxygen is delivered to the tissues by the pumping function of the heart. The $D{O_2}$ is the product of the $Ca{O_2}$ and CO.

$D{O_2}$ and $V{O_2}$ comprise a sensitive balance of supply and demand. Normally, 25 percent of the oxygen carried on hemoglobin is consumed by the tissues, and venous blood returning to the right heart is normally 75 percent saturated. When oxygen supply is insufficient to meet demands, the first compensatory mechanism is an increase in CO. If the increase in CO is insufficient, the amount of oxygen extracted from hemoglobin by the tissues increases, which decreases $Smv{O_2}$.

When compensatory mechanisms have failed to correct the imbalance between tissue supply and demand, anaerobic metabolism occurs, resulting in the formation of lactic acid. Elevated lactic acid levels are associated with an $Smv{O_2}$ of less than 50 percent. Most cases of lactic acidosis are due to inadequate oxygen delivery, as in cardiogenic shock, but lactic acidosis occasionally can develop from an excessively high oxygen demand (abnormally elevated $V{O_2}$), for example, status epilepticus. Sometimes, lactic acidosis can occur because of an impairment of tissue oxygen utilization, as in septic shock and postresuscitation from cardiac arrest.[4] Elevated lactic acid and normal $Smv{O_2}$ in the presence of adequate delivery indicate an impairment of tissue oxygen utilization. Lactic acid levels are markers of the severity of the tissue oxygen supply-to-demand imbalance and can be used in the triage, diagnosis, therapy, and prognosis of critically ill patients.

In addition to lactic acid, $Smv{O_2}$ can be used as a measure of tissue oxygen supply and demand imbalance. $Smv{O_2}$ is usually obtained from the pulmonary artery catheter, but similar information can be obtained by sampling the central venous blood through an internal jugular or subclavian catheter ($Scv{O_2}$), which has been shown to correlate with $Smv{O_2}$ and can be more easily obtained in the ED.

Shock is usually, but not always, associated with arterial hypotension: systolic blood pressure less than 80 or 90 mmHg. Since the product of flow and resistance determines pressure, blood pressure may not fall if, along with a marked reduction in flow, there is a corresponding increase in peripheral vascular resistance. MAP, CO, and SVR are related by the equation: $\text{MAP} = \text{CO} \times \text{SVR}$. A marked reduction in CO may not be reflected by a decrease in MAP if SVR increases as a compensatory response. In this situation, the result will be global tissue hypoperfusion. The insensitivity of blood pressure to detect global tissue hypoperfusion has been repeatedly confirmed.[5] Thus, shock may occur with a normal blood pressure, and hypotension may occur without shock.

The onset of shock induces autonomic responses, many which serve to maintain perfusion pressure to vital organs. Stimulation of the carotid baroreceptor stretch reflex activates the sympathetic nervous system leading to (1) arteriolar vasoconstriction, which overcomes local autoregulation and redistributes blood volume from the skin, skeletal muscle, kidneys, and splanchnic viscera; (2) an increase in heart rate and contractility that increases cardiac output; (3) constriction of venous capacitance vessels, which augments venous return; (4) release of the vasoactive hormones epinephrine, norepinephrine, dopamine, and cortisol to maintain arteriolar and venoconstriction; and (5) release of antidiuretic hormone and activation of the renin-angiotensin axis to enhance water and sodium conservation to maintain intravascular volume. These compensatory mechanisms attempt to maintain $D{O_2}$ to the most critical organs: the coronary and cerebral circulation. In this process, blood flow to other organs such as the kidney and gastrointestinal tract may be compromised.

The cellular response to decreased $D{O_2}$ is adenosine triphosphate depletion leading to ion-pump dysfunction, an influx of sodium, an efflux of potassium, and a reduction in membrane resting potential. Cellular edema occurs secondary to increased intracellular sodium while cellular membrane receptors become poorly responsive to the stress hormones insulin, glucagon, cortisol, and catecholamines. As shock progresses, lysosomal enzymes are released into the cells with

TABLE 26-1 Definitions of Abbreviations

$(a\text{-}v)CO_2$	arterial-central venous carbon dioxide difference
Cao_2	arterial oxygen content
$Cmvo_2$	mixed venous oxygen content
CI	cardiac index (cardiac output/body surface area)
CO	cardiac output
CPP	coronary perfusion pressure
CT	computed tomography
CVP	central venous pressure
Do_2	systemic oxygen delivery
DBP	diastolic blood pressure
ED	emergency department
Hb	hemoglobin
MAP	mean arterial pressure
MODS	multiorgan dysfunction syndrome
OER	oxygen extraction ratio
$Paco_2$	arterial carbon dioxide pressure
PAOP	pulmonary artery occlusion pressure
Sao_2	arterial oxygen saturation
$Scvo_2$	central venous oxygen saturation
$Smvo_2$	mixed venous oxygen saturation (pulmonary artery)
$Srao_2$	retinal venous oxygen saturation
SIRS	systemic inflammatory response syndrome
SVR	systemic vascular resistance
Vo_2	systemic oxygen consumption

subsequent hydrolysis of membranes, deoxyribonucleic acid, ribonucleic acid, and phosphate esters. As the cascade of shock continues, the loss of cellular integrity and the breakdown in cellular homeostasis result in cellular death. These pathologic events give rise to the clinical features of hyperkalemia, hyponatremia, metabolic acidosis, hyperglycemia, and lactic acidosis.

In the early phases of shock, these physiologic changes produce SIRS, defined as the presence of two or more of the following features: (1) temperature greater than 38°C or less than 36°C; (2) heart rate faster than 90 beats per minute; (3) respiratory rate faster than 20 breaths per minute; and (4) white blood cell count greater than 12.0×10^9/L, less than 4.0×10^9/L, or with greater than 10 percent immature forms or bands.[6] If shock progresses, SIRS may be accompanied by MODS manifested by myocardial depression, adult respiratory distress syndrome, disseminated intravascular coagulation, hepatic failure, or renal failure. Inflammatory mediators or cytokines, which arise from endothelial cell disruption, have a significant pathogenic role in the progression from SIRS to MODS. How fulminant the progression is from SIRS to MODS is determined by the balance of these anti-inflammatory and proinflammatory mediators (Fig. 26-1).[7]

Global tissue hypoperfusion alone can independently activate SIRS or serve as a comorbid variable in the pathogenesis of other forms of shock. The progression from SIRS to MODS is frequently accompanied by cardiovascular insufficiency.[8] The failure to diagnose and treat global tissue hypoperfusion in a timely manner leads to an accumulation of an oxygen debt; the magnitude of which correlates with increased mortality.[9]

CLINICAL FEATURES

History

Often the presence of shock will be instantly apparent along with the underlying cause, such as acute myocardial infarction, anaphylaxis, or hemorrhage. Some patients may be in shock with few symptoms other than generalized weakness, lethargy, or altered mental status. Symptoms that suggest volume depletion include bleeding, vomiting, diarrhea, excessive urination, insensible losses due to fever, or orthostatic light-headedness. A history of cardiovascular disease is important, particularly episodes of chest pain or symptoms of congestive heart failure. Prior neurologic diseases can render patients more susceptible to complications from hypovolemia. Drug use, both prescribed and nonprescribed, is important. Some drugs will cause volume depletion (e.g., diuretics) whereas others depress myocardial contractility (e.g., β blockers). The possibility of an anaphylactic reaction to a new medication or cardiovascular depression due to drug toxicity should be considered.[10]

Physical Examination

The clinical presentation of shock can be dramatic, as in profound hypotension caused by hemorrhage from a gunshot wound. Or shock can be subtle, as in heart failure or, even paradoxically, hypertensive crisis.[11,12] No single vital sign or value is diagnostic of shock; all vital signs are insensitive in detecting and assessing the severity of shock. Measurement of blood pressure can be particularly difficult due to peripheral vascular disease, tachycardia with a small pulse pressure, and irregular rhythms such as atrial fibrillation. Although not specific, physical findings taken as a composite are useful in the assessment of patients in shock (Table 26-3).

DIAGNOSIS

Ancillary Studies

The clinical presentation and the presumptive etiology of shock will dictate the use of ancillary studies. A battery of standard hematologic, coagulation, and biochemical tests usually provides an assessment of a patient's general physiologic condition and occasionally detects an abnormality that requires specific treatment (Table 26-4). A wide range of laboratory abnormalities may be encountered in shock, but most abnormal values merely point to the particular organ system that is either contributing to or being affected by the shock state. No single laboratory value is sensitive or specific for shock.

Hemodynamic monitoring is important in the assessment of patients in shock and following response to treatment. Monitoring capabilities will vary from institution to institution, but basic capabilities should include electrocardiographic monitoring, continuous noninvasive but preferably intraarterial blood pressure monitoring, pulse oximetry, end-tidal CO_2 monitoring, and CVP monitoring.

A variety of tubes and catheters are used to monitor patients or prevent complications: nasogastric tube, continuous rectal or esophageal temperature, and bladder catheterization. A pulmonary artery catheter, although impractical in the ED, is useful in monitoring mixed venous oxygen saturation, cardiac output, and left ventricular filling pressure. The benefit of monitoring patients with a pulmonary artery catheter is subject to debate.[13] Because hemodynamic measurements are physiologic values, they should be used to answer specific physiologic questions rather than to serve as end points themselves.

TABLE 26-2 Oxygen Transport and Utilization Components

Arterial oxygen content	$CaO_2 = 0.0031 \times PaO_2 + 1.38 \times Hb \times SaO_2$
	CaO_2 is the amount of O_2 within 100 mL blood. Oxygen is contained within blood in two forms: dissolved in plasma and chemically combined with hemoglobin. Assuming 15 g hemoglobin per 100 mL blood and an oxygen saturation of 97%, the representative normal value of CaO_2 is 20.1 mL/100 mL blood (vol%).
Central venous/mixed venous oxygen saturation	$ScvO_2$ or $SmvO_2$
	$SmvO_2$ reflects physiologic efforts to meet tissue O_2 demands. Normal $SmvO_2$ is 65 to 75%. When the $SmvO_2$ falls below 50%, the body's limits to compensate have been reached and O_2 availability for tissue metabolism will be compromised, leading to lactic acidosis.
Central venous/mixed venous oxygen content	$CmvO_2 = 0.0031 \times PmvO_2 + 1.38 \times Hb \times SmvO_2$
	$CmvO_2$ is the amount of oxygen content returning to the heart. Normal $CmvO_2$ is 15 mL/100 mL blood (vol%).
Systemic oxygen extraction ratio	$OER = C(a - v)O_2/CaO_2$
	The amount of O_2 taken out of the blood by the tissues is the systemic OER. It is described as a percentage. Normal OER is about 25%. Lactic acid production, an indicator of anaerobic metabolism, usually accompanies an OER of greater than 60%.
Oxygen delivery	$DO_2 = CO \times CaO_2 \times 10$
	DO_2 is the amount of O_2 delivered to the tissues per minute. Assuming a normal cardiac output of 5 L/min and a CaO_2 of 20.1 vol%; a normal value for O_2 delivery would be 1000 mL O_2/min.
Oxygen consumption	$VO_2 = CO \times Hb \times 1.38 \times (SaO_2 - SmvO_2) \times 10$
	The amount of O_2 consumed by tissues each minute and is equal to the difference in O_2 delivered to tissues and the O_2 returning from tissues. The normal value is about 250 mL O_2/min. Note that this formula ignores the small contribution from dissolved oxygen.
Oxygen affinity	
	Shifts in the oxyhemoglobin dissociation curve affect the release of O_2 in the peripheral circulation. Increased pH, decreased temperature, decreased carbon dioxide concentration (PCO_2) and decreases in 2,3-DPG levels all result in a shift of the oxyhemoglobin curve to the left. Thus, for any particular value of PaO_2, the O_2 saturation will be higher. This increased affinity of hemoglobin for O_2 makes O_2 loading easier, but release of O_2 in the peripheral tissues is impaired. The reverse is true with a decreased pH, increased temperature, increased PCO_2, and increased 2,3-DPG: there is a shift of the oxyhemoglobin dissociation curve to the right resulting in a decreased affinity of hemoglobin for O_2.

Note: See Table 26-1 for abbreviation definitions.

TREATMENT

Initial Treatment

The tenets of shock resuscitation are *A*irway establishment, control the work of *B*reathing, optimization of the *C*irculation, preventing inappropriate oxygen *C*onsumption, assuring adequate oxygen *D*elivery and tissue oxygen *E*xtraction.

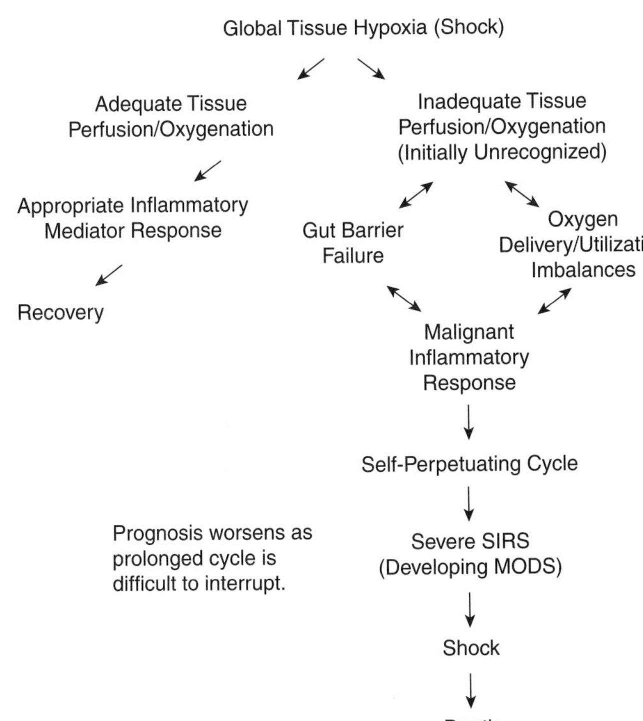

FIG. 26-1. The pathophysiology of shock, SIRS, and MODS.

Airway Control

Airway control is best obtained through endotracheal intubation for airway *p*rotection, *p*ositive *p*ressure ventilation (oxygenation), *p*atency, and *p*ulmonary toilet. Sedatives, which are frequently used to facilitate intubation, can exacerbate hypotension through arterial vasodilatation, venodilation, and myocardial suppression. Furthermore, positive pressure ventilation reduces preload and cardiac output. The combination of these interventions can lead to hemodynamic collapse. Volume resuscitation or application of vasoactive agents may be required prior to intubation.

Control of the Work of Breathing

Control of breathing is required when tachypnea accompanies shock. Respiratory muscles are significant consumers of precious DO_2 during shock and contribute to lactic acid production. Mechanical ventilation and sedation and decrease the work of breathing in shock and have been shown to improve survival. In the absence of a full shock picture, arterial blood-gas analysis can assist in the decision to perform intubation and mechanical ventilation. SaO_2 should be restored to greater than 93 percent and ventilation controlled to maintain a $PaCO_2$ of 35 to 40 mmHg. Attempts to normalize pH above 7.3 by hyperventilation are not beneficial. Mechanical ventilation not only provides oxygenation and corrects hypercapnia, but assists, controls, and synchronizes ventilation, which ultimately decreases the work of breathing.

Circulatory Stabilization

Circulatory or hemodynamic stabilization begins with adequate intravenous access. For fluid resuscitation, large-bore peripheral lines are

TABLE 26-3 Physical Examination

Temperature	Hyperthermia or hypothermia may be present. It is important to distinguish endogenous hypothermia (hypometabolic shock) from exogenous hypothermia secondary to environmental exposure. The treatment is obviously aggressive resuscitation in the former and exogenous heat application in the latter.
Heart rate	Usually elevated. However, paradoxical bradycardia can be seen in shock states such as hemorrhagic shock (up to 30%), hypoglycemia, β-blocker use, and preexisting cardiac disease.
Systolic blood pressure	May actually increase slightly when cardiac contractility increases in early shock and then fall as shock advances.
Diastolic blood pressure	Correlates with arteriolar vasoconstriction and may rise early in shock and then fall when cardiovascular compensation fails.
Pulse pressure	Systolic minus diastolic pressure and related to stroke volume and rigidity of the aorta. Increases early in shock and decreases before systolic pressure.
Pulsus paradoxus	The change in systolic blood pressure with respiration. The rise and fall in intrathoracic pressure affects cardiac output. This can be seen in asthma, cardiac tamponade, and severe cardiac decompensation.
Mean arterial blood pressure	Diastolic blood pressure + (pulse pressure)/3. The relationship between cardiac output and vascular resistance determines the capability of systemic blood pressure to provide adequate tissue perfusion.
Shock index	Shock index = heart rate/systolic blood pressure. Normal = 0.5 to 0.7. The shock index is related to left ventricular stroke work in acute circulatory failure. A persistent elevation of the shock index (>1.0) indicates an impaired left ventricular function (due to blood loss and/or cardiac depression) and carries a high mortality rate.[26]
Central nervous system	Acute delirium or brain failure; restlessness, disorientation, confusion, and coma secondary to decrease in cerebral perfusion pressure (mean arterial pressure − intracranial pressure). Patients with chronic hypertension may be symptomatic at normal blood pressures.
Skin	Pallor, pale, dusky, clammy, cyanosis, sweating, altered temperature, and decreased capillary refill.
Cardiovascular	Neck vein distention or flattening, tachycardia, and arrhythmias. An S3 may result from high-output states. Decreased coronary perfusion pressures can lead to ischemia, decreased ventricular compliance, increased left ventricular diastolic pressure, and pulmonary edema.
Respiratory	Tachypnea, increased minute ventilation, increased dead space, bronchospasm, hypocapnia with progression to respiratory failure, and adult respiratory distress syndrome.
Splanchnic organs	Ileus, gastrointestinal bleeding, pancreatitis, acalculous cholecystitis, and mesenteric ischemia can occur from low flow states.
Renal	Reduced glomerular filtration rate, renal blood flow redistributes from the renal cortex toward the renal medulla leading to oliguria. Paradoxical polyuria can occur in sepsis, which may be confused with adequate hydration status.
Metabolic	Respiratory alkalosis is the first acid-base abnormality, as shock progresses metabolic acidosis occurs. Hyperglycemia, hypoglycemia, and hyperkalemia.

equally as effective as central venous access, thus peripheral venous access should be the procedure of choice if peripheral veins are available. Trendelenburg positioning does not significantly improve cardiopulmonary performance compared with the supine position. Trendelenburg positioning may also worsen pulmonary gas exchange and enhance aspiration of vomitus. If a volume challenge is felt to be urgent, rather than using the Trendelenburg position, a compromise would be to raise the patient's legs above the level of the heart with the patient supine. Central venous access will aid in assessing volume status (CVP) and monitoring $Scvo_2$. It is a preferred route for the long-term administration of vasopressor therapy, and provides rapid access to the heart if pacemaker placement is required.

Fluid resuscitation begins with isotonic crystalloid: the amount and rate are determined by an estimate of the hemodynamic abnormalities. Most patients in shock have either an absolute or relative volume deficit. The one exception is cardiogenic shock with pulmonary edema. Fluid is given rapidly, in set quantities (e.g., 500 to 1000 mL), with reassessment of the patient after each amount. Patients with modest degrees of hypovolemia usually require about 20 mL/kg of isotonic crystalloid; much more may be required with profound volume deficits.

The colloid-versus-crystalloid resuscitation controversy remains despite evidence that there is a slight increase in mortality when colloids are used for volume replacement in critically ill patients.[14] Some studies have found a lower incidence of pulmonary edema and possibly greater benefit in elderly patients with colloid resuscitation, although survival is not statistically improved.

Without invasive hemodynamic monitoring, noncardiogenic pulmonary edema may be difficult to differentiate from cardiogenic pulmonary edema in the ED. Even though the former may respond to fluids, fluids should be minimized until appropriate monitoring can be placed.

Vasopressor agents are usually used when there has been an inadequate response to volume resuscitation or when a patient has contraindications to volume infusion. Vasopressors are most effective when the vascular space is "full" and least effective when the vascular space is depleted. However, vasopressors may be necessary early in the treatment of shock, before volume resuscitation is complete, in order to prevent potentially lethal consequences of prolonged systemic arterial hypotension. This is especially important in elderly patients with significant coronary and cerebrovascular disease. Rapidly restoring the MAP to 60 mmHg or systolic pressure to 90 mmHg may avoid the coronary and cerebral complications of

TABLE 26-4 Ancillary Studies

Basic evaluation
Hemogram: white blood cell and differential, hemoglobin and hematocrit, platelet count
Electrolytes, glucose, calcium, magnesium, phosphorus
Blood urea nitrogen, creatinine
Prothrombin, partial thromboplastin time
Urinalysis
Chest radiograph
Electrocardiograph
Moderate physiologic assessment
Arterial blood gas (measured saturation)
Lactic acid (serum lactate)
Fibrinogen, fibrin split products, D dimer
Hepatic function panel
Noninvasive hemodynamic assessment
End-tidal carbon dioxide
Noninvasive cardiac output measurement
Echocardiogram
Invasive hemodynamic assessment
Filling pressures: CVP or PAOP
Cardiac output
Central venous oxygen saturation: $Smvo_2$
Calculation of hemodynamic values: SVR, CO, Do_2, Vo_2
As clinically indicated to define etiology or detect complications
Blood, sputum, urine, and pelvic cultures
CT of head and sinuses
Lumbar puncture
Culture suspicious wounds
Cortisol level
Pregnancy test
Acute abdominal series
Abdominal or pelvic ultrasound
Abdominal or pelvic CT

Note: See Table 26-1 for abbreviation definitions.

decreased blood flow. Vasopressor agents are based on the catecholamine molecule and have variable effects on the α- and β-adrenergic receptors (Table 26-5).

The use of vasopressors is a double-edged sword. While improving perfusion pressure in the large vessels, they may decrease capillary blood flow in certain tissue beds. Vasopressors also may alter the relationship between volume and pressure measurements through their effect on the pulmonary and peripheral vascular beds. In other words, vasopressors will falsely elevate CVP and pulmonary artery occlusion pressure. They should be used judiciously, generally only after volume resuscitation. When multiple vasopressors are used, they should be simplified as soon as the most therapeutic vasopressor is identified. Volume resuscitation and intravascular volume assessment should be a dynamic process. This will increase the opportunity for the earliest possible discontinuation of vasopressor.

Control of Oxygen Consumption

The control of Vo_2 is important in restoring the balance of oxygen supply and demand to tissues. A hyperadrenergic state results from the compensatory response to shock, physiologic stress, pain, and anxiety. Shivering frequently results when a patient is unclothed for examination and then left inadequately covered in a cold resuscitation room. The combination of these variables increases systemic oxygen consumption. Pain further suppresses myocardial function, thus impairing Do_2 and Vo_2.[15] Providing analgesia, muscle relaxation, warm covering, anxiolytics, and even paralytic agents, when appropriate, decreases this inappropriate Vo_2. It is also important to provide appropriate anesthesia/analgesia for invasive procedures, since this is many times inappropriately forgotten in the haste of expedient intervention.

Oxygen Delivery

Once blood pressure is stabilized through optimization of preload and afterload, Do_2 can be assessed and further manipulated. Arterial saturation should be returned to physiologic levels (93 to 95 percent) and hemoglobin maintained above 10 g/dL.[16] If cardiac output can be assessed, it should be increased using volume infusion and inotropic agents in incremental amounts until the $Smvo_2$ and lactic acid are normalized.

Oxygen Extraction

Tissue oxygen extraction assesses adequacy of the resuscitation in meeting the oxygen needs of the tissues. Sequential examination of lactic acid and $Scvo_2$ or $Smvo_2$ is a method to assess adequacy of tissue oxygen extraction. Continuous measurement of $Scvo_2$ through fiberoptic technology can be used in the ED.[17] Other technologies have potential to assess Do_2 during the resuscitation of shock in the ED (Table 26-6).

Resuscitation End Points

Traditional end points have been normalization of blood pressure, heart rate, and urine output. Since these underestimate the degree of remaining hypoperfusion and oxygen debt, more physiologic end points have been investigated[18] (Tables 26-7 and 26-8). No therapeutic end point is universally effective, and only a few have been tested in prospective trials, with mixed results.[18,19] The goal of resuscitation is to maximize survival and minimize morbidity using objective hemodynamic and physiologic values to guide therapy.

Troubleshooting a Persistently Hypotensive Patient

Treatment of a persistently hypotensive patient after maximal therapy can be a harrowing experience in the ED. The patient who has obvious trauma with ongoing hemorrhage, the reason is usually apparent, and the outcome is dismal if uncorrected. In medical cases of shock or in cases without ongoing hemorrhage, potential pitfalls should be rapidly reviewed. Is the patient appropriately monitored? Is there malfunctioning arterial blood pressure monitoring, such as dampening of the arterial line or disconnection from the transducer? Is the patient adequately volume resuscitated? The early use of vasopressor will falsely elevate CVP and disguise hypovolemia. Is the intravenous tubing into which the vasopressors are running connected appropriately? Are the vasopressor infusion pumps working? Are the vasopressors mixed adequately? Does the patient have a pneumothorax after that CVP placement? Has the patient been adequately assessed for an occult penetrating injury (a bullet hole or stab wound)? Is there hidden bleeding from a ruptured spleen or ectopic pregnancy? Does the patient have adrenal insufficiency? The incidence of adrenal dysfunction can be as high as 30 percent in this subset of patients.[20] Is the patient allergic to the medication just given (e.g., penicillin) or taken before arrival? Is the renal failure or cancer patient in cardiac tamponade?

Bicarbonate Use in Shock

The primary treatment of acidosis in shock is to reverse the underlying cause. Because this goal is not rapidly attainable, intravenous bicarbonate is often administered. The rationale for giving bicarbonate is that

TABLE 26-5 Commonly Used Vasoactive Agents

			EFFECTS				
Drug	Dose	Actions	Cardiac Stimulation	Vasoconstriction	Vasodilation	Cardiac Output	Side Effects and Comments
Dopamine	0.5–25 μg/kg/min	α, β, and dopaminergic	++ at 2–10 μg/kg/min	++ at 7 μg/kg/min	+ at 0.5–5.0 μg/kg/min	Usually increases	Tachydysrythmias, increases myocardial O_2 consumption. A cerebral, mesenteric, coronary, and renal vasodilator.
Norepinephrine	0.01–0.5 μg/kg/min	Primarily α_1 some β_1	++	++++	0	Slight decrease	Dose related, reflex bradycardia. Useful when loss of venous tone predominates, spares the coronary circulation.
Phenylephrine	0.15–0.75 μg/kg/min	Pure α	0	++++	0	Decrease	Reflex bradycardia, headache, restlessness, excitability, rarely dysrhythmias. Ideal for patients in shock with tachycardia or supraventricular dysrhythmias.
Ephedrine	5–25 mg bolus	α and β	+++	++	+	Increases	Causes palpitations, hypertension, cardiac arrhythmias. An indirect-acting central nervous system stimulant; limited long-term value as therapy for shock.
Epinephrine	0.01–0.75 μg/kg/min	α and β	++++ at 0.03–0.15 μg/kg/min	++++ at 0.15–0.30 μg/kg/min	+++	Increases	Causes tachydysrythmias, leukocytosis. Increases myocardial oxygen consumption.
Dobutamine	2.0–20 μg/kg/min	β_1, some β_2, and α_1 in large dosages	++++	+	++	Increase	Causes tachydysrythmias, occasional gastrointestinal distress. Increases myocardial oxygen consumption, hypotension in volume depleted patient. Has less peripheral vasoconstriction than dopamine. Can cause fewer arrhythmias than isoproterenol.
Isoproterenol	0.01–0.02 μg/kg/min	β_1 and some β_2	++++	0	++++	Increases	Causes tachydysrythmias, facial flushing, hypotension in hypovolemic patients. Increases myocardial oxygen consumption. Never use alone in shock.

Note: 0, no effect; +, mild effect; ++, moderate effect; +++, marked effect; ++++, very marked effect.

it will diminish myocardial depression and counteract the insensitivity to endogenous catecholamines attributed to acidosis, but experimental data indicate that exogenous bicarbonate can actually worsen intracellular acidosis, and prospective studies have not shown benefit.[21] Bicarbonate also shifts the oxygen-hemoglobin dissociation curve to the left and impairs tissue unloading of hemoglobin-bound oxygen. However, many clinicians remain uncomfortable withholding bicarbonate, which has created disparate opinions in the medical literature.[22] A middle ground to correct the metabolic acidosis partially over time is as follows: calculate the bicarbonate deficit, which is equal to (normal HCO_3^- minus the patient's HCO_3^-) × 0.4 × body weight (kilograms), with one-half of this amount infused slowly and the remainder over 6 to 8 h to a pH of no greater than 7.25.

DISPOSITION

Transition to the Intensive Care Unit

Documentation and communication are important. Resuscitation in the ED is commonly performed in ''ordered chaos'' and, even though resuscitation is systematic and thoughtful, miscommunication with the intensivist or subspecialist accepting the patient can undo the benefits of initial treatment. A system-oriented problem list with an assessment and plan, including all procedures and complications, should be verbally communicated, written, or dictated prior to transfer. For prolonged ED stays, notations regarding patient status, diagnostic and therapeutic intervention, and sentinel events should be provided frequently, if possible.

Prognosis

Outcome prediction at ED disposition has not been fully studied, however, some clinical variables are associated with poor outcome: severity of shock, temporal duration, underlying cause, preexisting vital organ dysfunction, and reversibility. Direct noninvasive measurement of V_{O_2} has been shown to be predictive of outcome in patients who developed cardiogenic shock secondary to myocardial infarction and after cardiac arrest.[4,23] Serial elevated lactic acid levels have been shown to be predictive in trauma, septic shock, and after cardiac arrest.[4,24] Base-deficit correction has also been correlated with the development of multisystem organ failure in trauma.[25] Outcome predictions using physiologic scoring systems in the ED are currently being studied.[3]

TABLE 26-6 Adjuncts in Assessing Tissue Perfusion

Base deficit	Base deficit is an indicator of metabolic acidosis and an index of hemodynamic and tissue perfusion changes in shock. Predicts illness severity in intraabdominal hemorrhage and blunt trauma.[25]
Invasive blood pressure monitoring	Intense vasoconstriction caused by sympathetic activity or vasopressors given will cause the cuff pressure to underestimate true blood pressure. A Doppler used in conjunction with a sphygmomanometer may enable more accurate measure of systolic blood pressure once Korotkoff sounds are no longer audible. Intraarterial pressure measurement is preferable because vasoactive drugs may cause rapid swings in blood pressure and multiple blood samplings will typically be required.
Central venous pressure	Aid in assessing volume status. May not reliably reflect the left ventricular filling pressure in clinical states such as pulmonary embolus, obstructive airway disease, right ventricular infarction, and pericardial effusion. Common iliac venous pressure can approximate CVP.[27]
Central venous oximetry ($Scvo_2$)	$Scvo_2$ closely approximates traditionally used mixed venous oxygen saturation ($Smvo_2$) and can be monitored by continuous infrared oximetry. This technology enables clinicians to detect clinically unrecognized global tissue hypoperfusion in the treatment of myocardial infarction, general medical shock, trauma hemorrhage, septic shock, hypovolemic shock, end-stage heart failure, and cardiogenic shock during and after cardiopulmonary arrest.[11,17,28–31]
Arterial-central venous CO_2 difference	Increased arterial-mixed venous carbon dioxide gradients or (a-v)CO_2 are seen in acute circulatory failure and inversely correlate with the CI.[32]
Noninvasive cardiac output	CO can be measured by transesophageal Doppler, cutaneous bioimpedence, and lithium dilution (through an injection of lithium through the CVP line and by using the radial artery catheter to measure clearance).[33,34]
Gastric tonometry	Serial measurements of gastric mucosal blood flow are based on hydrogen ion diffusion and equilibration with normal saline in a balloon-tipped gastric tonometry catheter. Inadequate visceral perfusion as evidenced by persistently low intramucosal pH after resuscitation is associated with subsequent organ dysfunction and death.[18]
Retinal venous O_2 saturation	Retinal venous oxygen saturation ($Srao_2$) correlates with blood volume and central venous oxygen saturation. The $Srao_2$ correlates with Sao_2 during graded hypoxia.[35]
Pulmonary artery catheterization	The standard of care for assessing cardiac status. Valuable in determining left-sided heart filling pressure and pulmonary artery pressure and in assessing the risk of pulmonary edema. Can obtain CO and mixed venous oxygen saturation. Will be able to calculate hemodynamic (i.e., SVR) and oxygen transport variables (Vo_2 and Do_2). The effectiveness of this modality on improving outcome is now being challenged.[13]
Metabolic cart	Directly measures Vo_2 without a pulmonary artery catheter. A reduction in Vo_2 predicts the development of cardiogenic shock after acute infarction and survival after cardiac arrest.[5,23]

Note: See Table 26-1 for abbreviation definitions.

TABLE 26-7 End Points of Resuscitation

Traditional: normalization of blood pressure, pulse, and urine output
Restoration of circulating volume
Restoration of all fluid compartments
Vascular space is "full"
Hemodynamic parameters are "normalized"
Tissue oxygen delivery is maximized
Restoration of aerobic metabolism, elimination of tissue acidosis, and repayment of oxygen debt

TABLE 26-8 Hemodynamic Resuscitation End Points

	Modality	Goals
Preload	CVP PAOP	10–12 mmHg 12–18 mmHg
Afterload	MAP SVR = (MAP − CVP/CO)(80)	90–100 mmHg 800–1400 dyne·s/cm^5
Contractility	CO CI SV = CO/heart rate	5.0 L/min 2.5–4.5 L/min/m^2 50–60 mL/min
Heart rate	60–100 bpm	Avoid >100 bpm; this will decrease SV and increase myocardial oxygen consumption
Coronary perfusion pressure	CPP = DBP − CVP (or PAOP)	>60 mmHg
Tissue oxygenation	$Scvo_2$ or $Smvo_2$ Lactic acid	>70% <2 mM/L

Note: See Table 26-1 for abbreviation definitions.

REFERENCES

1. Varon J, Fromm RE, Levine RL: Emergency department procedures and length of stay for critically ill medical patients. *Ann Emerg Med* 23:546, 1994.
2. Svenson J, Besinger B, Stapczynski JS: Critical care of medical and surgical patients in the ED: Length of stay and initiation of intensive care procedures. *Am J Emerg Med* 15:654, 1997.
3. Rivers EP, Doyle D Nguyen HB, et al: Physiologic assessment of the critically ill: An outcome evaluation of emergency department intervention. *Acad Emerg Med* 5:530, 1998.
4. Rivers EP, Rady MY, Martin GB, et al: Venous hyperoxia after cardiac arrest: Characterization of a defect in systemic oxygen utilization. *Chest* 102:1787, 1992.
5. Wo CC, Shoemaker WC, Appel PL, et al: Unreliability of blood pressure and heart rate to evaluate cardiac output in emergency resuscitation and critical illness. *Crit Care Med* 21:218, 1993.
6. American College of Chest Physicians–Society of Critical Care Medicine Consensus Conference. Definitions for sepsis and organ failure and guidelines for the use of innovative therapies in sepsis. *Crit Care Med* 20: 864, 1992.
7. Bone RC: Sir Isaac Newton, sepsis, SIRS, and CARS. *Crit Care Med* 24:1125, 1996.
8. Rangel-Frausto MS, Pittet D, Costigan M, et al: The natural history of the systemic inflammatory response syndrome (SIRS): A prospective study [see comments]. *JAMA* 273:117, 1995.
9. Meade P, Shoemaker WC, Donnelly TJ, et al: Temporal patterns of hemodynamics, oxygen transport, cytokine activity, and complement activity in the development of adult respiratory distress syndrome after severe injury. *J Trauma* 36:651, 1994.
10. Fink M: Shock: An overview, in *Intensive Care Medicine,* Boston, Little Brown, 1991, pp 1417–1435.
11. Rady M, Jafry S, Rivers E, Alexander M: Characterization of systemic oxygen transport in end-stage chronic congestive heart failure. *Am Heart J* 128:774, 1994.
12. Quezado ZN, Keiser HR, Parker MM: Reversible myocardial depression after massive catecholamine release from a pheochromocytoma. *Crit Care Med* 20:549, 1992.
13. Connors AF Jr, Speroff T, Dawson NV, et al: The effectiveness of right heart catheterization in the initial care of critically ill patients: SUPPORT Investigators [see comments]. *JAMA* 276:889, 1996.
14. Schierhout G, Roberts I: Fluid resuscitation with colloid or crystalloid solutions in critically ill patients: A systematic review of randomized trials. *BMJ* 316:961, 1998.
15. Rady MY, Kirkman E, Cranley J, Little RA: Nociceptive somatic nerve stimulation and skeletal muscle injury modify systemic hemodynamics and oxygen transport and utilization after resuscitation from hemorrhage. *Crit Care Med* 24:623, 1996.
16. Greenburg AG: A physiologic basis for red blood cell transfusion decisions. *Am J Surg* 170(suppl 6A):44S, 1995.
17. Rady MY, Rivers EP, Martin GD, et al: Continuous central venous oximetry and shock index in the emergency department: Use in the evaluation of clinical shock. *Am J Emerg Med* 10:538, 1992.
18. Porter JM, Ivatury RR: In search of the optimal end points of resuscitation in trauma patients: A review. *J Trauma* 44:908, 1998.
19. Gattinoni L, Brazzi L, Pelosi P, et al: A trail of goal-oriented hemodyanmic therapy in critically ill patients. *N Engl J Med* 333:1025, 1995.
20. Blake HC, Rivers EP, Dereczyk B, et al: Adrenal insufficiency in high-risk emergency department patients. *Acad Emerg Med* 3:438, 1996.
21. Cooper DJ, Walley KR, Wiggs BR, Russell JA: Bicarbonate does not improve hemodynamics in critically ill patients who have lactic acidosis. A prospective, controlled clinical study [see comments]. *Ann Intern Med* 112:492, 1990.
22. Arieff AI: Current concepts in acid-base balance: Use of bicarbonate in patients with metabolic acidosis. *Anaesth Crit Care* 7:182, 1996.
23. Rady MY, Edwards JD, Rivers EP, Alexander M: Measurement of oxygen consumption after uncomplicated acute myocardial infarction. *Chest* 104: 930, 1993.
24. Bakker J, Gris P, Coffernils M, et al: Serial blood lactate levels can predict the development of multiple organ failure following septic shock. *Am J Surg* 171:221, 1996.
25. Rutherford EJ, Morris JA, Reed CW, Hall KS: Base deficit stratifies mortality and determines therapy. *J Trauma* 33:417, 1992.
26. Rady MY: The role of central venous oximetry, lactic acid concentration and shock index in the evaluation of clinical shock: A review. *Resuscitation* 24:55, 1992.
27. Ho KM, Joynt GM, Tan P: A comparison of central venous pressure and common iliac venous pressure in critically ill mechanically ventilated patients. *Crit Care Med* 26:461, 1998.
28. Scalea TM, Hartnett RW, Duncan AO, et al: Central venous oxygen saturation: A useful clinical tool in trauma patients. *J Trauma* 30:1539, 1990.
29. Krafft P, Steltzer H, Hiesmayr M, et al: Mixed venous oxygen saturation in critically ill septic shock patients: The role of defined events. *Chest* 103:900, 1993.
30. Creamer JE, Edwards JD, Nightingale P: Hemodynamic and oxygen transport variables in cardiogenic shock secondary to acute myocardial infarction, and response to treatment. *Am J Cardiol* 65:1297, 1990.
31. Rivers EP, Martin GB, Smithline H, et al: The clinical implications of continuous central venous oxygen saturation during human CPR. *Ann Emerg Med* 21:1094, 1992.
32. Cuscheri J, Hays G, Rivers EP, et al: Arterial-venous carbon dioxide gradients as an indicator of cardiac index: A comparison between the mixed and central venous circulation. *Crit Care Med* 26(abstract):A62, 1998.
33. Cuscheri J, Rivers EP, Caruso J, et al: A Comparison of transesophageal Doppler, thermodilution and Fick cardiac output measurements in critically ill patients. *Crit Care Med* 26(abstract):A56, 1998.
34. Shoemaker WC, Wo CC, Bishop MH, et al: Noninvasive hemodynamic monitoring of critical patients in the emergency department. *Acad Emerg Med* 3:675, 1996.
35. Denninghoff KR, Smith MH, Hillman LW, et al: Retinal venous oxygen saturation correlates with blood volume. *Acad Emerg Med* 5:577, 1998.

27 FLUID AND BLOOD RESUSCITATION

Steven C. Dronen
Eileen M. K. Bobek

Fluid resuscitation is the mainstay of therapy of hemorrhagic shock in the emergency department (ED) setting, with the goal of restoring or maintaining tissue oxygenation despite ongoing blood loss. Considerable research has been devoted to identifying the optimal resuscitation fluid, as well as its rate of delivery. Despite significant advances, questions regarding the ideal resuscitation agent and the timing and endpoints of resuscitation remain unanswered. Recently, the standard practice of rapidly infusing crystalloid during resuscitation of hypotensive trauma victims has been called into question. Ultimately, the ability to answer these questions and optimize the care of the shock victim will require a better understanding of the physiologic and biochemical events that characterize acute hemorrhage.

PATHOPHYSIOLOGY

Acute hemorrhage is defined as a rapid blood loss that may accompany a wide variety of medical and surgical conditions. The most common causes of significant hemorrhage include trauma, disorders of the gastrointestinal and reproductive tracts, and vascular disease (Table 27-1). Hemorrhagic shock occurs when blood loss is of sufficient magnitude to overcome normal physiologic compensatory responses and compromise tissue perfusion and oxygenation.

Acute hemorrhage triggers a series of physiologic responses involving the cardiovascular, respiratory, renal, hematologic, and neuroendocrine systems. The net effect of these responses is an increase in cardiac rate and contractility, a redistribution of blood flow to preserve vital organ function, conservation of water and sodium, and control of blood loss at the site of injury.

TABLE 27-1 Etiologic Classification of Acute Hemorrhage

Trauma
Solid organ injury
Pulmonary parenchymal injury
Myocardial laceration/rupture
Vascular injury
Retroperitoneal hemorrhage
Pelvic fracture
Ruptured duodenum
Ruptured kidney
Fractures, especially bones and pelvis
Lacerations, especially scalp
Epistaxis
Gastrointestinal tract
Esophageal varices
Ulcer disease
Gastritis/esophagitis
Mallory-Weiss tear
Malignancies
Vascular lesions (arteriovenous malformations, rare congenital anomalies)
Inflammatory bowel disease
Ischemic bowel disease
Reproductive tract
Vaginal bleeding
Malignancies
Miscarriage
Metrorrhagia
Retained products of conception
Placenta previa
Ectopic pregnancy
Ruptured ovarian cyst
Vascular
Aneurysms
Dissections
Arteriovenous malformations

Cardiovascular

One of the very first responses observed in animal studies of acute hemorrhage is a fall in blood pressure that cannot be accounted for simply by the initial reduction in intravascular volume.[1] It is likely that the fall in blood pressure is caused by a sudden reduction in systemic vascular resistance, although the mechanism has not been explained. The fall in blood pressure is sensed by both high-pressure baroreceptors in the carotid artery sinus and the aortic arch as well as low-pressure baroreceptors in the left atrium and pulmonary veins. Stimulation of these baroreceptors, in turn, causes disinhibition of the medullary vasomotor center, a subsequent decrease in vagal tone, and an increase in the secretion of norepinephrine (NE). Decreased vagal tone increases heart rate and cardiac output. NE increases heart rate and myocardial contractility, stimulates renin secretion, and causes intense vasoconstriction, especially of splanchnic and musculoskeletal blood vessels. Such vasoconstriction provides a functional reservoir that can be used to compensate for acute blood loss, since 20 to 30 percent of the circulating blood volume resides in the splanchnic bed.

Cardiac output typically falls during hemorrhage, due to a decrease in atrial filling or preload, despite increases in myocardial rate and contractility. It is commonly taught that afterload rises during acute hemorrhage in order to maintain blood pressure. In fact, there is little evidence to support this claim. It is more likely that, early in the course of hemorrhage, total systemic vascular resistance falls or remains at near-normal levels in order to facilitate flow to vital organs. There are, however, increases in regional resistance that cause redistribution of blood flow away from skin, muscle, and gut to favor the brain, heart, and kidneys.

Endocrine and Humoral

Conservation of sodium and water during hemorrhage is mediated by an increase in the levels of aldosterone and antidiuretic hormone. Stretch receptors in the afferent arterial walls of the juxtaglomerular apparatus (JGA) respond to a drop in blood pressure by stimulating an increase in renin secretion. Renin converts angiotensinogen to angiotensin I, which is then converted in the lung and liver to angiotensin II. The effects of angiotensin II include intense vasoconstriction of arteriolar smooth muscle and stimulation of aldosterone secretion by the adrenal cortex. Aldosterone is also secreted in response to elevation of potassium and adrenocorticotropic hormone (ACTH) levels, both of which occur during acute hemorrhage. Aldosterone increases the reabsorption of sodium and the excretion of potassium in the distal convoluted tubule. Water passively follows sodium and is therefore reabsorbed and conserved. Aldosterone also stimulates the secretion of hydrogen ions, thus decreasing acidosis.

Osmo- and baroreceptors also regulate the release of arginine vasopressin or antidiuretic hormone (ADH), which is synthesized in the hypothalamus and stored in the posterior pituitary. Release of ADH occurs in response to both a fall in blood pressure and a decrease in sodium concentration. ADH increases the permeability of the renal distal tubule collecting ducts, and loop of Henle to NaCl and water, with the net result being fluid and salt retention. In higher concentrations, ADH also acts as a vasoconstrictor.

Acute hemorrhage causes local activation of the coagulation system. In response to injury, affected blood vessels contract, and activated platelets rapidly adhere to the edges of the damaged vessels. Platelets release thromboxane A_2, which is a potent local vasoconstrictor and further platelet activator. Platelets form an unstable jelly-like plug during the first 20 min after injury. Control of hemorrhage during this period depends upon a regional reduction in flow caused by systemic hypotension and local vasoconstriction. Vessel injury exposes collagen and releases tissue thromboplastin, causing fibrin deposition in the platelet plug and gradual formation of a stable clot. The entire process for complete fibrinous transformation takes approximately 24 h.

Compensatory Limitations

The compensatory mechanisms described above are quite effective at maintaining critical organ perfusion even in the face of severe hemorrhage. Animal studies demonstrate complete recovery without intervention in animals bled as much as 40 percent of their estimated blood volumes. However, if the hemorrhage is not controlled, a vicious cycle of increased myocardial work and decreased perfusion eventually develops. Progressive increases in heart rate shorten diastole, with a resultant decrease in myocardial perfusion and oxygenation as well as cardiac filling and output. The low perfusion state increases acidemia, which in turn decreases myocardial contractility.

Eventually, cardiac output becomes inadequate to maintain cellular oxygen delivery, and characteristic changes occur. The first cellular response to hypoperfusion is an attenuation of the cell membrane and an increase in sodium influx. Adenosine triphosphate (ATP) is utilized to maintain function of the sodium-potassium pump; during periods of low flow, however, it cannot be regenerated in sufficient quantities through the normal oxygen-dependent pathways. As the supply of oxygen and high-energy substrates diminishes, the cells revert to anaerobic metabolism to generate ATP, resulting in the accumulation of lactic acid. As ATP availability decreases, sodium continues to enter the cells, causing progressive swelling first of the cytoplasm, then the endoplasmic reticulum, and finally the mitochondria. Eventually the cells undergo clumping of mitochondria, loss of membrane integrity, and death.

There appears to be a point of no return for individual cells as well as for the overall organism in shock. Although this point is well defined for the cell, the clinician caring for patients in shock is less able to identify this landmark. It has been suggested that a sudden and substantial decrease in oxygen consumption may be a reliable marker of irreversible shock.

CLINICAL FEATURES

Factors that affect the clinical presentation of acute hemorrhage include the etiology, duration, and severity of hemorrhage and the patient's age and underlying medical condition. Acute hemorrhage most often accompanies blunt or penetrating trauma and is generally the presumed cause of shock in the trauma patient. Hemorrhage must be differentiated from other causes of shock associated with trauma, including cardiac tamponade (distinguished by elevated central venous pressure), tension pneumothorax (distinguished by unilaterally diminished breath sounds), and spinal cord injury (distinguished by the presence of neurologic deficits, warm skin, and a lower than expected pulse rate).

Hemorrhage not associated with trauma may present with a myriad of complaints depending upon the primary organ system involved. Nausea and vomiting; dizziness; syncope; pain in the chest, abdomen, or back; and rectal or vaginal bleeding are some common chief complaints associated with bleeding from those organ systems.

The classic clinical features of acute hemorrhage include tachycardia; tachypnea; a narrow pulse pressure; decreased urine output; cool, clammy skin; poor capillary refill; low central venous pressure; and, in the later stages, hypotension and altered mentation. Elderly patients and those with preexisting cardiac disease may show more severe signs and symptoms with less blood loss. Medications such as β blockers can mask some of the early signs and symptoms of hemorrhage. On the other hand, young, athletic patients can lose considerable amounts of blood before they appear ill. Up to a third of patients who sustain intraabdominal hemorrhage severe enough to develop hypotension [systolic blood pressure (BP) <90 mmHg] will not develop a tachycardia (heart rate >100), presumably due to vagal simulation from blood in the peritoneal cavity.

In general, however, there is a somewhat predictable and orderly progression of pathophysiologic events through which the patient passes as organ and cellular perfusion deteriorate and shock develops. Blood loss of less than 20 percent of circulating blood volume causes cool, clammy skin, delayed capillary refill, and decreased pulse pressure. Tachycardia may be present, and generally the blood pressure is normal, although the pulse pressure may be narrow. As hemorrhage progresses, with blood loss of 20 to 40 percent, patients are tachycardic and tachypneic, have postural changes in blood pressure, and may be confused or agitated. If the patient is not resuscitated and the bleeding continues, hypotension and oliguria develop, respirations quicken and become deeper, tachycardia worsens, and the skin becomes mottled. With hemorrhage exceeding 40 percent of the circulating blood volume, patients commonly demonstrate tachycardia, profound hypotension, either tachypnea or irregular respirations, markedly decreased urine output, decreased or absent peripheral pulses, pallor, and lethargy and obtundation. Death from severe hemorrhage is generally marked by respiratory arrest prior to circulatory arrest due to fatigue of the respiratory musculature and, sometimes, bradyasystolic rhythms.

MANAGEMENT

There are two goals in the treatment of hemorrhagic shock: control of hemorrhage and maintenance of oxygen delivery. The definitive therapy of hemorrhage is control of the source of bleeding; this often requires operative intervention. Thus, for most patients with hemodynamic instability secondary to hemorrhage, prompt surgical consultation and intervention are mandatory.

TABLE 27-2 Approximate Maximal Infusion Rates of Normal Saline or Ringer's Lactate

IV Catheter Size	Gravity 80 cm height	Pressure 300 mmHg
18 g IV	50–60 mL/min	120–180 mL/min
16 g IV	90–125 mL/min	200–250 mL/min
14 g IV	125–160 mL/min	250–300 mL/min
8.5 Fr introducer	200 mL/min	400–500 mL/min

Oxygenation and Ventilation

Maintenance of tissue oxygen delivery requires, first and foremost, an assessment of the adequacy of oxygenation and ventilation. Items requiring immediate evaluation include airway patency, skin color, depth and rate of respiration, as well as the presence of any mechanical obstruction to ventilation including pneumothorax, hemothorax, or flail chest. Supplemental oxygen should be administered to all patients in shock and to most patients who are bleeding acutely. Many patients will require endotracheal intubation and ventilatory support. Respiratory arrest caused by fatigue of the intercostal muscles and diaphragm commonly precedes cardiac arrest as a terminal event in hemorrhagic shock; therefore it is essential that liberal guidelines for ventilatory support be used.

Intravenous Access

Tissue oxygenation also requires restoration of circulating blood volume, and it is routine to place at least two large-bore intravenous lines for infusion of crystalloid and potentially blood. A practical limitation during fluid resuscitation is sometimes the size of the intravenous access, which limits the rate of infusion (Table 27-2). The largest-bore catheter possible should be used in patients who may require aggressive fluid administration. All patients should be placed on a continuous cardiac monitor and pulse oximeter. As the intravenous lines are placed, initial blood samples should be drawn for type and cross matching, coagulation studies [prothrombin time (PT), partial thromboplastin time (PTT), platelet count] and a baseline complete blood count (CBC). All women of childbearing age need a pregnancy test. An immediate serum glucose assessment is critical in the patient with a depressed level of consciousness. A baseline metabolic assessment requires more extensive laboratory study, including serum electrolytes, blood urea nitrogen (BUN), creatinine, and liver function tests. An arterial blood gas (ABG) provides crucial information about the patient's acid-base, oxygenation, and ventilatory status and, if available on the blood gas analyzer, data regarding the patient's hematocrit and bicarbonate level. An initial electrocardiogram (ECG) is also indicated in adult patients. All patients should have a Foley catheter placed, as urine output is believed to reflect underlying renal perfusion.

Standard Monitoring

Parameters that should be routinely monitored during resuscitation of acute hemorrhage include vital signs, mentation, skin temperature, capillary refill, oxygen saturation of arterial blood, and urine output.

There is a tendency to follow BP quite closely and to gauge the adequacy of therapy by the extent to which BP returns to normal levels. It is important to recognize, however, that BP is not precisely correlated with cardiac output and provides a poor assessment of the state of cellular metabolism.[2] Also, as noted below, restoration of normotension in the presence of a vascular injury may merely increase the severity of hemorrhage. Central venous pressure (CVP) monitoring may be of some value in confirming the diagnosis of hypovolemia and judging the response to therapy. A low CVP (<5 cmH_2O) supports the diagnosis of hypovolemia; probably more useful, a failure of the CVP to increase after fluid infusion suggests persistent hypovolemia and indicates the need for further fluid. Swan-Ganz catheterization is usually not necessary in the acute setting except in elderly patients or those with respiratory or cardiac disease.

TABLE 27-3 Representative Volume Properties of 1 L of Intravenous Fluid

	VOLUME EXPANSION		
Fluid Space	Intracellular	Interstitial	Plasma
D5W	660 mL	255 mL	85 mL
NS or RL	−100 mL	825 mL	275 mL
7.5% NaCl	−2950 mL	2960 mL	990 mL
5% Albumin	0	500 mL	500 mL
Whole blood	0	0	1000 mL

Prehospital Treatment

There have been many debates in recent years over the extent to which patients should be resuscitated prior to operative intervention, both in the prehospital setting and the ED. The concept of field stabilization of trauma victims has been discredited for those with hemorrhagic shock. The prehospital interventions that improve survival include attention to the airway, ventilation, immobilization, and rapid transport; not fluid resuscitation.[3] Standard prehospital interventions directed at restoring blood pressure, such as application of a pneumatic antishock garment (PASG) and infusion of intravenous fluids, have not been shown to improve survival.[4,5]

The PASG became standard prehospital treatment in the late 1970s based on anecdotal reports of efficacy and its extensive use during the Vietnam War. While there is no doubt that application of the PASG often raises blood pressure, most likely through a rise in systemic vascular resistance, there is no evidence that use of the PASG to achieve such a result actually improves outcome. Several controlled trials have failed to prove that any significant benefit is derived from its use in trauma victims.[4,6,7] In fact, in the presence of shock and chest trauma, PASG use may actually increase the severity of hemorrhage and also mortality.[8] Thus, enthusiasm for the PASG has begun to wane except for patients with unstable pelvic fractures, for whom it may stabilize the fractures and potentially tamponade retroperitoneal hemorrhage. The PASG may also prove useful for splinting of multiple lower extremity fractures and control of soft tissue bleeding from lower extremities.

There has also been debate over the efficacy of prehospital line placement and fluid resuscitation. Proponents of field resuscitation state that skilled paramedics are able to place intravenous lines with little or no delays in transport.[9] Opponents state that since blood loss cannot be controlled in the field, any delay in definitive treatment is excessive. Clinical studies have shown that the amount of fluid infused en route is usually minimal as compared with the total fluid requirement, and one randomized study of victims of penetrating trauma has failed to show any benefit associated with preoperative fluid therapy.[10] Prehospital fluid therapy probably does not affect outcome in the vast majority of cases, but it may be valuable given a specific combination of hemorrhage severity and distance from the hospital. Until conclusive data for a particular position can be obtained, it is reasonable to place intravenous lines once en route to the hospital whenever possible. This practice avoids potentially lethal delays in the field and grants patients the potential benefits of prehospital fluid therapy.

Fluid Resuscitation

It should be noted, however, that the benefits of early and aggressive fluid replacement in victims with ongoing hemorrhage, whether given in the prehospital setting or the ED, remain unproven. Many animal studies have shown that raising the blood pressure with either vasopressors or fluid also worsens mortality, sometimes dramatically.[11] Such findings were recently validated in a prospective clinical study of hypotensive patients with penetrating torso injuries in which improved outcome was demonstrated for those whose fluid resuscitation was delayed until the start of operative intervention.[10] These studies indicate that resuscitation to normotension is harmful because it exacerbates continued hemorrhage and that some degree of "underresuscitation" may be beneficial.[12] Conversely, to purposefully withhold resuscitation as the patient exsanguinates is also wrong.

Both animal and human studies continue in an attempt to determine the ideal rate and volume of fluid administration as well as the appropriate therapeutic end point of resuscitation.[13] The traditional end point of isotonic fluid resuscitation has been clinical assessment of the adequacy of tissue perfusion. In addition, the use of red cells was generally identified as a hemoglobin of 10 g/dL or a hematocrit of 30 percent as the "transfusion trigger." However, such a guideline is not reliable in an actively hemorrhaging patient, particularly in the setting of trauma. At the present time, the amount and type of volume expander used depends primarily on the clinical status of the patient and to a lesser extent on individual institutional preference. In most hospitals, isotonic crystalloid—either 0.9% NaCl [normal saline (NS)] or Ringer's lactate (RL)—is the agent of choice for the initial management of acute hemorrhage. Standard therapy of the hemodynamically unstable patient is rapid infusion of 20 to 40 mL/kg as fast as possible, typically over 10 to 20 min. Since, at best, only about 30% of infused isotonic crystalloid stays intravascular, blood volume restoration with NS or RL requires a volume approximately three times that of the lost blood (Table 27-3).[14] An isotonic infusion of 30 mL/kg can be expected to expand blood volume by about 10 mL/kg, roughly one-seventh of the estimated blood volume of 70 mL/kg. Thus, if an adult patient continues to show signs of impaired perfusion after a total of 30 mL/kg (roughly 2 L), it is likely that blood loss exceeds 15 percent of the total blood volume.

Blood Transfusion

At this point, it is appropriate to begin red cell transfusions, particularly if blood loss has not been controlled. If the patient appears to be stable, it usually is possible to wait for fully cross-matched blood, but that decision must be individualized, based on the assessment of ongoing blood loss and the efficiency of the local blood bank. When in doubt, it is advisable to use type-specific blood. Several studies have shown this to be a very safe practice, and delays in providing needed oxygen-carrying capacity are potentially more harmful to the patient. Early blood therapy is particularly important in the elderly and in those with significant respiratory and cardiac disease, as their ability to tolerate a decrease in oxygen-carrying capacity is significantly reduced.

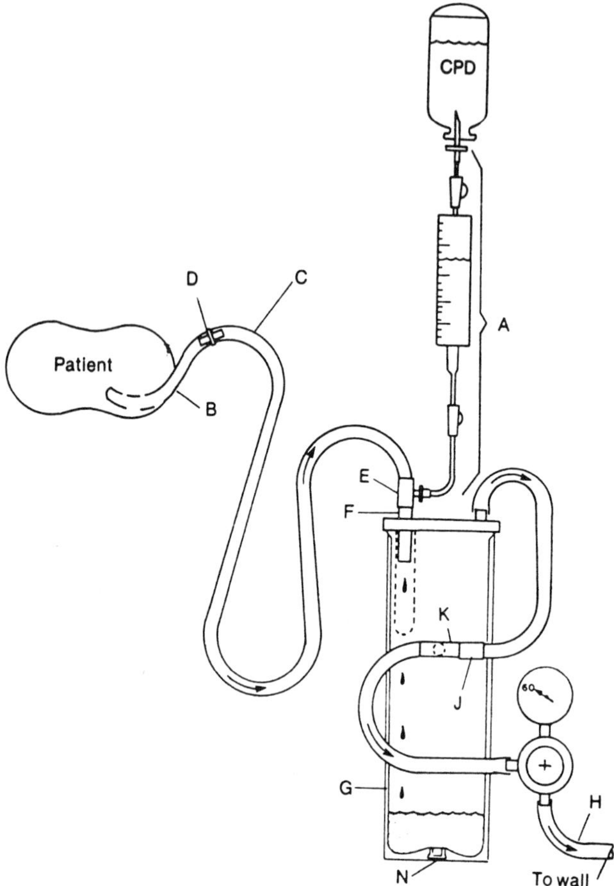

FIG. 27-1. Collection apparatus. **A**, anticoagulant volume control burette; **B**, chest tube; **C**, latex drainage tubing; **D**, male-to-male connector; **E**, end of drainage tubing with side port; **F**, inlet port of red liner cap attached to collection canister; **G**, collection liner bag; **H**, downstream suction hose; **J**, liner lid tubing connector; **K**, canister tee; and **N**, liner stem with protective cap. *Abbreviation:* CPD, citrate phosphate dextrose. [From Roberts JR, Hedges JR (eds): *Clinical Procedures in Emergency Medicine,* 2d ed. Philadelphia, Saunders, 1991, p 412, with permission.]

More aggressive therapy is mandated in the hemorrhaging patient exhibiting any degree of hemodynamic instability or signs of end-organ hypoperfusion. These patients almost always require blood transfusions, and it is appropriate to begin type-specific blood early unless there is a prompt and persistent improvement in perfusion with saline solution alone. Type-specific blood is indicated in patients who are profoundly hypotensive on initial presentation, those who remain in shock after crystalloid infusion, and those who demonstrate rapid ongoing hemorrhage. Continued administration of crystalloid without blood may result in profound dilution of the remaining red blood cell mass, platelets, and coagulation factors. It may also disrupt clot formation in the injured vessels. Volume restored at the expense of oxygen-carrying capacity and hemostasis is of questionable therapeutic value.

The moribund patient requires even more prompt restoration of circulating red blood cell mass. In this case, type O blood should be used immediately if it is available. Type O Rh-negative blood should be given to females of childbearing age. In most other situations Type O Rh-positive blood is preferred because of its greater availability. A sample for type and cross match should always be drawn and sent before administration of type O blood.

Autologous whole blood may be given if the hemorrhage is intrathoracic and the capabilities for autotransfusion exist (Fig. 27-1). Autotransfusion decreases the risk of transmission of diseases such as acquired immunodeficiency syndrome (AIDS) and hepatitis, and it also decreases the demand on the blood bank. There has been some discussion concerning autotransfusion in patients with intraabdominal injuries. It can be difficult to determine, especially in the ED, if there is fecal contamination of intraabdominal blood. Transfusion of contaminated blood has not been shown to be safe, and it may be prudent to autotransfuse blood from intraabdominal injuries only in the operating suite, after the source of blood has been discovered and the risk of transfusing contaminated blood is known.

Colloid Resuscitation

Although isotonic saline solution is most commonly used in the initial management of hemorrhagic shock, debate continues over the value of adding colloid to the resuscitation regimen. Albumin has fallen into disfavor, but purified protein fraction (PPF) and fresh frozen plasma (FFP) continue to be recommended and used. Central to the issue are the effects of fluid resuscitation on the pulmonary interstitium.[15] Proponents of protein replacement argue that saline resuscitation of hemorrhage results in a fall in intravascular oncotic pressure and a reversal of the normal gradient favoring intravascular fluid retention. Theoretically, this may lead to pulmonary edema and impaired tissue oxygenation. Colloid administration is advocated because it raises oncotic pressure in the pulmonary capillary bed. This argument ignores the fact that the pulmonary capillary endothelium permits considerable flow of fluids, including plasma proteins, between the capillaries and the interstitium. A fall in intravascular oncotic pressure is compensated for by a fall in pulmonary interstitial oncotic pressure, thereby minimizing changes in the pressure gradient. It appears likely that pulmonary capillary hydrostatic pressure [measured as pulmonary artery (occlusion) wedge pressure] is far more important than pulmonary capillary oncotic pressure in determining the amount of fluid flowing to the interstitium. Maintenance of the pulmonary artery occlusion pressure below 15 mmHg is probably the most important factor in preventing pulmonary edema. Systematic reviews of clinical studies have found no clear benefit to colloid resuscitation compared with crystalloid resuscitation.[16] Clinicians inclined to use albumin, PPF, or FFP in the resuscitation of hemorrhagic shock should question whether the undocumented benefits of this therapy are worth the substantial increase in cost or, in the case of FFP, the risk of disease transmission.

Alternatives to the use of naturally occurring colloid preparations include synthetic colloid solutions such as hydroxyethyl starch (HES) and dextran 70. The volume-expanding properties of HES are equivalent to those of 5% albumin. These agents differ significantly from albumin, however, in that they remain predominantly in the intravascular space because of their high molecular weight and branched structure. Their plasma-expanding effects are more prolonged than those of albumin, and interstitial edema is not a significant concern. Their inability to restore oxygen-carrying capacity, however, is a significant disadvantage shared by all crystalloid and colloid solutions with the exception of blood.

Oxygen-Carrying Resuscitation Fluids

Blood remains, from a physiologic perspective, the ideal resuscitation agent, but there are substantial practical limitations to its routine use. Although the potential for disease transmission has been significantly reduced by modern donor screening techniques, it has not been completely eliminated.[17] Other concerns include the limited availability of blood products; the cost of collection, storage and transfusion; a limited shelf-life; and the existence of religious prohibitions against the transfusion of blood products. These issues have led researchers to search for alternative agents that can safely and effectively deliver oxygen to the cells.[18] To date the use of stoma-free hemoglobin as well as pyridoxalated-hemoglobin-polyoxyethylene (PHP) conjugate represent examples of hemoglobin-based substitutes under investigation. Hemoglobin solutions became of interest during World War II owing to practical difficulties of blood storage and compatibility testing on the battlefield. Their use was ultimately rejected due to their short half-lives and the frequent occurrence of significant hypotension. Subsequent research was directed at the modification of these solutions to eliminate side effects such as renal failure and bleeding abnormalities. Currently, although some modified hemoglobin solutions may be effective at restoring blood pressure and cardiac index, their clinical efficacy remains limited by their short half-lives and potential toxic effects.[19] Hemoglobin has been identified as a neurotoxin and has been shown to promote vasoconstriction, platelet adhesion, and free radical damage.

Perfluorocarbons (PFCs) have also been investigated as possible blood substitute candidates because of their high oxygen solubility. Unfortunately, new PFC emulsions produce toxic effects on the lung in a dose-dependent fashion, thereby severely limiting their ability to improve oxygen-carrying capacity. Because of these problems, blood substitutes are not currently recommended as an alternative to blood transfusion in the treatment of hemorrhagic shock. The importance of developing a safe and effective blood substitute is not diminished, however, and this remains a fertile area for future research.

Hypertonic Resuscitation Fluids

Hypertonic saline (HS) has been recommended as a possible alternative fluid resuscitation therapy based upon impressive hemodynamic effects in numerous animal studies of acute hemorrhage. Given in small amounts and often in combination with 6% dextran 70, HS caused a prompt and sustained shift of fluid from the interstitial to the intravascular compartment. Based upon these studies, HS was once promoted as an ideal agent for the prehospital resuscitation of hemorrhage. Thus far, clinical studies have not demonstrated overall improvement in survival in victims of hypotensive trauma given HS.[20,21] However, there was a trend toward improved outcome in some subpopulations of hypotensive trauma victims given HS. There may be particular injury patterns (such as combined hypovolemia and head injury) in which a benefit exists. Given the absence of a demonstrated benefit in the general population of hemorrhage patients, the widespread use of HS cannot be recommended because of uncommon but potentially significant complications. These include confusion, seizures, and central pontine myelinolysis. The addition of dextran also presents disadvantages, as it may induce anaphylactic reactions and coagulopathies.

End Points to Resuscitation

Perhaps one of the greatest challenges in shock management facing both clinicians and researchers today is the identification of valid and reliable shock parameters to assess the severity of hemorrhage and the adequacy of resuscitation.[2,13] In the past, gross physiologic indices such as heart rate, blood pressure, capillary refill, urine output, and central venous pressure have been used to assess the severity of hemorrhage. Despite a long history of frequent clinical use, these parameters have repeatedly been shown to be unreliable. More reliable indicators include mixed venous oxygen saturation and serum lactate concentrations, both of which may reflect the presence of hypoperfusion, even in the face of normal vital signs.[13,22]

Several different parameters have been introduced as potential markers for the end point of resuscitation, including supernormal oxygen transport variables, mixed venous oxygen saturation ($Smvo_2$), central venous oxygen saturation ($Scvo_2$), gastric intramucosal pH, end-tidal CO_2, serum lactate, and base deficit.[13] Oxygen transport variables of particular interest include cardiac index (CI), oxygen delivery (Do_2), and oxygen consumption(Vo_2). It has been proposed that the measurement of such indices would supply an accurate reflection of oxygen debt and therefore tissue perfusion. Adjusting therapeutic interventions in an effort to achieve supernormal values would therefore presumably be indicative of an adequate level of resuscitation. Studies have demonstrated, however, that although attainment of supernormal oxygen transport variables may have some prognostic significance, it is not an appropriate resuscitation end point.[13] This may also be true for $Smvo_2$. Although it also provides a measure of tissue oxygen extraction, it does not provide information about regional hypoperfusion, and normal or elevated values do not necessarily imply the absence of shock, particularly in the face of sepsis.

The measurement of oxygen transport variables and mixed venous oxygen saturation requires the placement of a pulmonary artery catheter, a procedure that is both time-consuming and has inherent risks. Central venous oxygen saturation monitoring has therefore been proposed as an alternative, since $Scvo_2$ measurements have been shown to correlate with $Smvo_2$. Although it still requires invasive monitoring and its use is limited by similar factors as $Smvo_2$ measurements, placement is certainly less time-consuming. Until prospective studies demonstrate its validity as a potential guide for resuscitation though, its use cannot be unequivocally advocated.

Gastric intramucosal pH (pHi) has been investigated as a potential minimally invasive marker of regional perfusion. The splanchnic bed is particularly sensitive to hypoperfusion states because blood is shunted from its mucosa to preserve flow to the brain, heart, and kidneys. Theoretically, restoration of splanchnic perfusion should indicate adequacy of resuscitation. To date though, studies evaluating gastric intramucosal pH have been limited and do not demonstrate a reliable correlation with indices of global hypoperfusion, such as serum lactate and base deficit.

End-tidal CO_2 monitoring has also been recommended as a noninvasive monitoring tool during shock.[23] The reduction in cardiac output and pulmonary blood flow should be accompanied by reduced production of CO_2 and reflected in low end-tidal CO_2 measurements. Similarly, restoration of normal flow should be accompanied by increased end-tidal CO_2 measurements. Preliminary studies have shown that persistently low end-tidal CO_2 measurements are associated with poor outcome, but no prospective trials exist evaluating its contribution to clinical decision making.

Serum lactate concentrations have gained prominence as an indirect measure of tissue perfusion and oxygenation, because shock ultimately results in a shift from aerobic to anaerobic metabolism and increased production of lactate. Elevated serum lactate levels have been shown to correlate with both the severity of shock and the adequacy of resuscitative measures. In addition, changes in serial lactate values during resuscitation have provided prognostic information about patients in shock.[22] Although the use of lactate has been limited by its lack of real-time availability, the development of accurate bedside lactate analyzers may eliminate this disadvantage in the future.

Base deficit has also been utilized as a measure of global tissue acidosis due to inadequate tissue perfusion. Base deficit is defined as the amount of base, in millimoles, required to titrate 1 L of whole arterial blood to a pH of 7.40, with the sample fully saturated with O_2 at 37° and a Pco_2 of 40 mmHg. Although some studies have found a correlation between serum lactate and base excess, the relationship is not always predictable.[24]

One element that is certainly common to all potential markers for the end points of resuscitation is that isolated values in time have significantly less importance than the identification of a trend. It is clear that both the development and resuscitation of a shock state are dynamic processes and in many respects remain elusive ones to monitor.

COMPLICATIONS

The overwhelming bulk of clinical and scientific data indicate that the infusion of resuscitation fluids is an extraordinarily safe procedure but still with risk for complications. The overall percentage of interventions that lead to complications is quite low, but given the frequency with which fluid resuscitation occurs, complications arise regularly. This is particularly true when blood products are infused and especially when they are infused in massive quantities. Although there is no strict criteria, massive transfusion is generally defined as the transfusion of the equivalent of one blood volume (70 to 80 mL/kg in an adult) within 24 h. Clotting abnormalities are commonly noted after massive transfusion owing to dilutional thrombocytopenia and the effects of storage on coagulation factors and platelet number and function. Previous guidelines recommended the routine transfusion of FFP and platelets based upon the number of units of red cells transfused. It has been demonstrated, however, that the occurrence of bleeding diathesis in trauma correlates not just with the number of red cell transfusions, but also with the duration of the shock state and the type and severity of injury sustained. Therefore it is recommended that transfusion of FFP and platelets be based on clinical evidence of impaired hemostasis and frequent monitoring of coagulation parameters.[25] Platelets are indicated in the actively bleeding trauma patient with a platelet count of 50,000 or less. FFP is indicated if the PT is prolonged more than 1.5 times normal (usually 18). When an underlying coagulation disorder is suspected, as in patients taking warfarin or with evidence of severe liver disease, it may be appropriate to administer FFP without waiting for laboratory confirmation.

Other potential complications of massive transfusion include electrolyte abnormalities. Hypocalcemia and hypomagnesemia may occur due to citrate toxicity, particularly in neonates, patients transfused with whole blood and those with preexisting liver disease. Reductions in these electrolytes may precipitate cardiac dysrhythmias; therefore careful monitoring of their levels is essential. Empiric therapy with calcium and magnesium is not recommended. Treatment, when indicated, includes administration of calcium or magnesium solutions as the chloride salts.

Potassium levels also require close monitoring, because massive transfusion may precipitate both hyperkalemia, due to leakage of potassium from stored cells, and hypokalemia, due to hepatic conversion of transfused citrate and lactate to bicarbonate, with resultant metabolic alkalosis. Theoretically, massive transfusion of banked blood may also precipitate the development of a metabolic acidosis, as banked blood is relatively acidic owing to its citrate and lactate content. It cannot be overstated however, that the presence of ongoing acidosis in the patient in shock should not be attributed to massive transfusion but to ongoing hemorrhage. Although persistent acidosis is ominous, bicarbonate administration is not routinely recommended unless pH remains persistently at or below 7.1 despite aggressive resuscitative measures.

Many trauma patients arrive in the ED with a lower than normal temperature, possibly due to prolonged exposure as well as the shock state. In the face of massive transfusion, hypothermia may contribute to the development of platelet dysfunction and cardiac dysrhythmias. Whenever possible, therefore, blood warmers should be utilized throughout the course of resuscitation.

At the extremes of age, trauma patients have limited cardiovascular reserve to tolerate the large shifts of fluid that occur during massive transfusion. One potential consequence of such physiologic restrictions is the development of signs and symptoms of congestive heart failure and potentially adult respiratory distress syndrome (ARDS). At such times, aggressive fluid administration may paradoxically defeat efforts to improve a patient's oxygenation status.

Perhaps the most feared consequences of transfusion are hemolytic transfusion mediated reactions and transfusion-transmitted disease. The most common cause of hemolytic transfusion reactions is ABO incompatibility, accounting for a mortality of 1/100,000 units transfused. The viruses of most concern are hepatitis B virus (HBV), hepatitis C virus (HCV), human immunodeficiency virus (HIV), and human T-cell lymphotrophic virus (HTLV).[17] Recently, the risk of donating blood during an infectious window period were estimated as 1 in 63,000 for HBV; 1 in 103,000 for HCV; 1 in 493,000 for HIV; and 1 in 641,000 for HTLV.[17] Although modern screening techniques have substantially reduced the risk of blood-borne infection, the potential risk must always be considered when transfusion is contemplated.

REFERENCES

1. Bellamy RF, Maningas PA, Wenger BA: Current shock models and clinical correlations. *Ann Emerg Med* 15:1392, 1986.
2. Wo CC, Shoemaker WC, Appel PL, et al: Unreliability of blood pressure and heart rate to evaluate cardiac output in emergency resuscitation and critical illness. *Crit Care Med* 21:218, 1993.
3. Cayten CG, Murphy JG, Stahl WM: Basic life support versus advanced life support for injured patients with an injury severity score of 10 or more. *J Trauma* 35:460, 1993.
4. Maddox KL, Bickell WH, Pepe PE, et al: Prospective randomized evaluation of antishock MAST in posttraumatic hypotension. *J Trauma* 26:779, 1986.
5. Kaweski SM, Sise MJ, Virgilio RW: The effect of prehospital fluid on survival in trauma patients. *J Trauma* 30:1215, 1990.
6. Domeier RM, O'Connor RE, Delbridge TR, Hunt RC: National Association of EMS Physicians Position Paper: Use of pneumatic anti-shock garment (PASG). *Prehosp Emerg Care* 1:32, 1997.
7. O'Connor RE, Domeier RM: Collective Review: An evaluation of the pneumatic anti-shock garment (PASG) in various clinical settings. *Prehosp Emerg Care* 1:36, 1997.
8. Honigman B, Lowenstein FR, Moore EE, et al: The role of the pneumatic shock garment in penetrating cardiac wounds. *JAMA* 266:2398, 1991.
9. Spaite DW, Valenzuela TC, Criss EA, et al: A prospective in-field comparison of intravenous line placement by urban and nonurban emergency medical personnel. *Ann Emerg Med* 24:209, 1994.
10. Bickell WM, Wall MJ, Pepe PE, et al: Immediate versus delayed fluid resuscitation for hypotensive patients with penetrating torso injuries. *N Engl J Med* 331:1105, 1994.
11. Stern SA, Dronen SC, Birrer P, Wang X: Effect of blood pressure on hemorrhage volume and survival in a near-fatal hemorrhage model incorporating a vascular injury. *Ann Emerg Med* 22:155, 1993.
12. Dries DJ: Hypotensive resuscitation. *Shock* 6:311, 1996.
13. Porter JM, Ivatury RR: In search of the optimal end points of resuscitation in trauma patients: A review. *J Trauma* 44:908, 1998.
14. Wagner BKJ, D'Amelio LT: Pharmacologic and clinical consideration in selecting crystalloid, colloid, and oxygen carrying resuscitation fluids. *Clin Pharm* 12:335, 1993.
15. Peter RM, Hargens AR: Protein vs electrolytes and all of the Starling forces. *Arch Surg* 116:1293, 1981.
16. Schierhout G, Roberts I: Fluid resuscitation with colloid or crystalloid solutions in critically ill patients: A systematic review of randomized trials. *Br Med J* 316:961, 1998.
17. Schreiber GB, Busch MP, Kleinman SH, et al: The risk of transfusion-transmitted viral infections. *N Engl J Med* 334:1685, 1996.
18. Hess J: Blood substitutes. *Semin Hematol* 33:369, 1996.
19. Sprung J, Mackenzie CF, Barnas GM, et al: Oxygen transport and cardiovascular effects of resuscitation from severe hemorrhagic shock using hemoglobin solutions. *Crit Care Med* 23:1540, 1995.
20. Mattox KL, Maningas PA, Moore EE, et al: Prehospital hypertonic saline/dextran infusion for post-traumatic hypotension: The USA multicenter trial. *Ann Surg* 213:482, 1991.
21. Vassar MJ: A multicenter trail for resuscitation of injured patients with 7.5% sodium chloride. *Arch Surg* 128:1003, 1993.
22. Manikis P, Jankowski S, Zhang H, et al: Correlation of serial blood lactate levels to organ failure and mortality after trauma. *Am J Emerg Med* 13:699, 1995.
23. Domsky M, Wilson RF, Heins J: Intraoperative end-tidal carbon dioxide values and derived calculations correlated with outcome: Prognosis and capnography. *Crit Care Med* 23:1497,1995.
24. Mikulaschek AS, Henry SM, Donovan R, et al: Serum lactate is not predicted by anion gap or base excess after trauma resuscitation. *J Trauma* 40:218, 1996.
25. Development Task Force of the College of American Pathologists: Practice parameters for the use of fresh-frozen plasma, cryoprecipitate, and platelets. *JAMA* 271:777, 1994.

SEPTIC SHOCK

Jonathan Jui

Sepsis is a heterogenous clinical syndrome that can be caused by any class of microorganism. Although both gram-negative and gram-positive bacteria account for the majority of sepsis cases, fungi, mycobacteria, rickettsia, viruses, or protozoans can cause similar presentations. Microbial blood invasion is not essential to the development of sepsis.

EPIDEMIOLOGY

It is commonly believed that the incidence of sepsis has continued to rise over the last 3 decades, but most figures, including the often quoted 300,000 to 500,000 patients developing sepsis every year in the U.S., are largely estimations. A study from 8 academic medical centers reported an incidence of 2 cases of sepsis per 100 hospital admissions. Of these cases, 55 percent occurred in the ICU, 12 percent in the emergency department, and 33 percent in a non-ICU patient care unit. Up to half of sepsis patients develop shock with an overall mortality rate of about 45 percent, but with a wide range of 20 to 80 percent depending on the host. In 1991, sepsis was the thirteenth leading cause of death in the United States with approximately two-thirds of the cases occurring in hospitalized patients. Recent clinical studies in patients with bacteremia indicate that gram-positive and gram-negative bacteria are the etiology of the sepsis in 35 to 40 percent and 55 to 60 percent of the episodes, respectively. The most frequent sites of infection are the lungs, abdomen, and the urinary tract. Factors that predispose to gram-negative bacteremia include diabetes mellitus, lymphoproliferative diseases, cirrhosis of the liver, burns, invasive procedures or devices, and chemotherapy. Major gram-positive bacteremia risk factors include vascular catheters, indwelling mechanical devices, burns, and intravenous drug injection. Fungemia most often occurs in immunocompromised patients.

While there is no reason to suspect that the occurrence of septic shock would vary according to the patient's sex, two large-scale prospective studies have found a slightly higher incidence of systemic inflammatory response syndrome (SIRS) and sepsis syndrome in men; 60 percent and 56 percent, respectively. This slight difference may reflect a higher rate of preceding surgical procedures in men as opposed to women. Sepsis is more common in older adults; the mean age reported is 55 to 60 years. Older patients are more likely to have conditions that predispose to bacterial infection, such as diabetes, surgical procedures, and cancer.

DEFINITIONS AND RISK CATEGORIZATION

In 1991, the American College of Chest Physicians and the Society of Critical Care proposed a set of definitions that could be applied to patients with sepsis and its sequelae. These definitions are contained in Table 28-1. The primary goals of this classification were to provide a conceptual and practical framework of the systemic inflammatory response to infection; to improve the ability of clinicians to make early bedside detection of sepsis, thus allowing early therapeutic intervention; and to standardize the definition which would allow better comparison and analysis of research protocols.

The identification of SIRS does not confirm a diagnosis of infection or sepsis because the features of SIRS can be seen in many other conditions such as trauma, pancreatitis, burns, or infection (Fig. 28-1). SIRS is not a diagnosis nor is it a good indicator of outcome. Its presence, however, must be explained adequately.

The SIRS criteria may be seen as a crude stratification for patients with systemic inflammation. In a recent prospective study of the epide-

TABLE 28-1 Definitions

Infection = microbial phenomenon characterized by an inflammatory response to the presence of microorganisms or the invasion of normally sterile host tissue by those organisms.

Bacteremia = the presence of viable bacteria in the blood.

Systemic inflammatory response syndrome (SIRS) = the systemic inflammatory response to a variety of severe clinical insults. The response is manifested by two or more of the following conditions: (1) temperature >38°C or <36°C; (2) heart rate >90 beats per minute; (3) respiratory rate >20 breaths per minute or Pa_{CO_2} <32 mmHg; and (4) white blood cell count >12,000/μL, <4,000/cu mm, or >10% immature (band) forms.

Sepsis = the systemic response to infection, manifested by two or more of the following conditions as a result of infection: (1) temperature >38°C or <36°C; (2) heart rate >90 beats per minute; (3) respiratory rate >20 breaths per minute or Pa_{CO_2} <32 mmHg; and (4) white blood cell count >12,000/cu mm, <4,000 μL, or >10% immature (band) forms.

Severe sepsis = sepsis associated with organ dysfunction, hypoperfusion, or hypotension. Hypoperfusion and perfusion abnormalities may include, but are not limited to lactic acidosis, oliguria, or an acute alteration in mental status.

Septic shock = sepsis-induced with hypotension despite adequate fluid resuscitation along with the presence of perfusion abnormalities that may include, but are not limited to, lactic acidosis, oliguria, or an acute alteration in mental status. Patients who are receiving inotropic or vasopressor agents may not be hypotensive at the time that perfusion abnormalities are measured.

Sepsis-induced hypotension = a systolic blood pressure <90 mmHg or a reduction of ≥40 mmHg from baseline in the absence of other causes for hypotension.

Multiple organ dysfunction syndrome (MODS) = presence of altered organ function in an acutely ill patient such that homeostasis cannot be maintained without intervention.

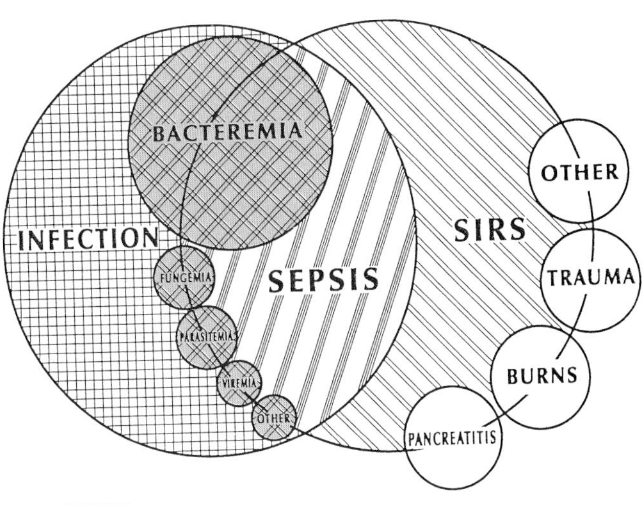

FIG. 28-1. The interrelationship between systemic inflammatory response syndrome (SIRS), sepsis, and infection. (From *Chest* 101:6, 1992.)

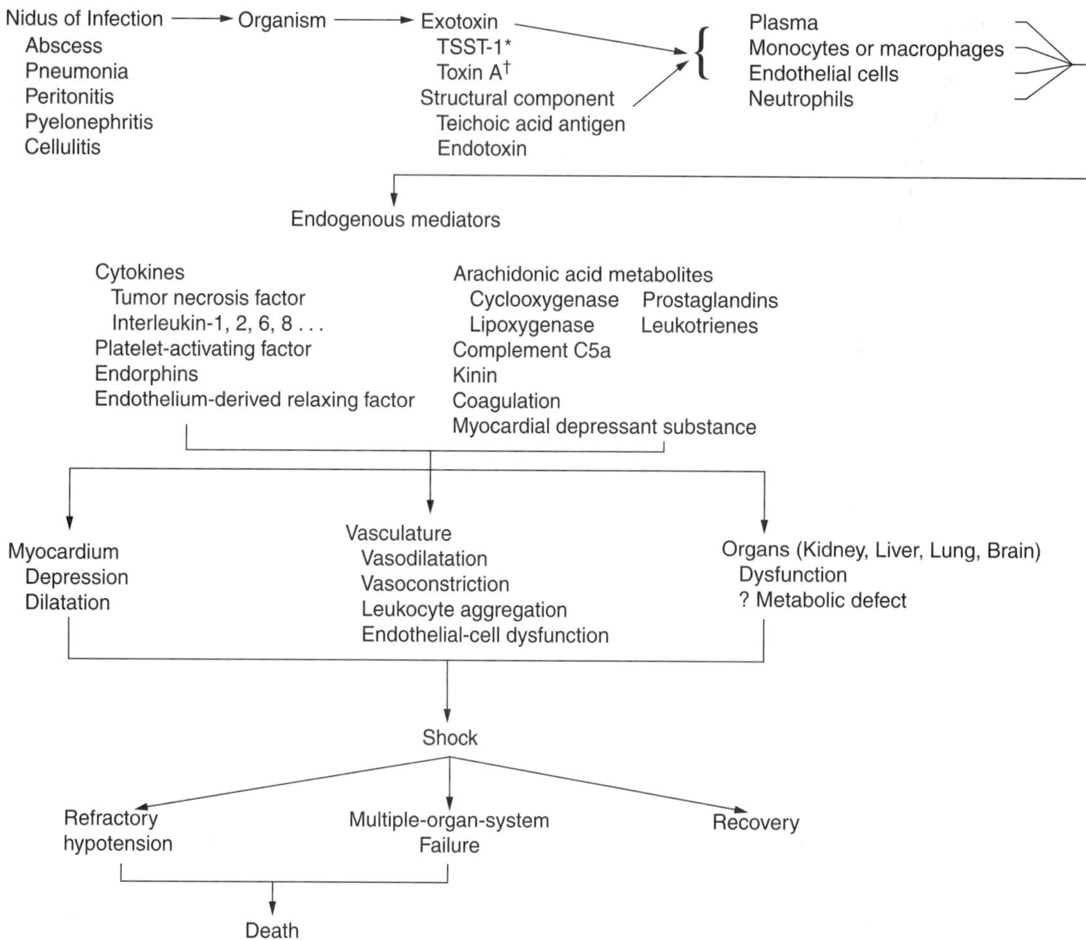

FIG. 28-2. Pathogenic sequence of the events in septic shock.
*TSST-1 denotes toxic shock syndrome toxin 1.
†Toxin A is *Pseudomonas aeruginosa* toxin A.

miology of SIRS in medical and surgical patients, mortality was 3 percent in patients without SIRS, 6 percent in those with two criteria, 10 percent in those with three positive criteria, and 17 percent in those meeting all four criteria. Death rates were similar for patients with culture-negative SIRS and those with culture-positive SIRS. Other investigators propose a complementary method of classification of sepsis based primarily on physiologic abnormalities such as the APACHE III acuity system. These investigators found that multivariate analysis using initial APACHE score, etiology of sepsis (urosepsis or other), and treatment location prior to ICU admission provided the greatest degree of discrimination of patients by risk of hospital death.

PATHOPHYSIOLOGY

Sepsis starts as a focus of infection (urinary tract infection, pneumonia, cellulitis, abscess, or indwelling prosthetic device) resulting in either blood stream invasion or a proliferation of organisms at the infected site (Fig. 28-2). These growing organisms release a large amount of exogenous toxins consisting of endotoxins, exotoxins, and other components of the organism's structural components. The host's reaction to these toxins results in the release of endogenous mediators and other humoral defense mechanisms including complement, kinins, and coagulation factors. Among the most prominent of the endogenous mediators are the cytokines (tumor necrosis factor, interleukins), platelet activating factor (PAF), arachidonic acid metabolites, and myocardial depressant substances (MDS). Release of MDS results in the depression of myocardial function, dilation of the ventricles, and vasodilation. These vascular and myocardial abnormalities combine to result in generalized cardiovascular insufficiency leading to refractory hypotension and multiple organ system failure, and death.

One of the most important of the vasoactive mediators is nitric oxide. Nitric oxide is a low-molecular weight membrane-permeable gas with both harmful and beneficial effects in shock. Under normal conditions, this gas is produced in the endothelium by a calcium and calmodulin-dependent nitric oxide synthase (NOS) which converts L-arginine and O_2 to L-citrulline and nitric oxide. This pathway is normally well regulated by signal transduction pathways linked to cell-surface receptors for vasodilators such as acetylcholine and histamine. However, inflammatory mediators induce a calcium-independent form of nitric oxide synthase that is not controlled by this mechanism. This form may rise to abnormal amounts of nitric oxide in septic patients and patients given IL-2 for cancer treatment.

Three distinct NOS enzyme complexes have been described. The first, neuronal nitric oxide synthase (nNOS) is found in central nervous system cells and is thought to support a neurotransmitter function. The second, constitutive NOS (cNOS) is found in endothelial cells and is thought to play a role in the maintenance of normal vascular tone. The third, a high output inducible enzyme called inducible NOS (iNOS) is found in many cell types including, endothelial cells, vascular smooth muscle cells and macrophages.

Nitric oxide actions include functioning as a neurotransmitter; regulating vascular tone; and inhibiting platelet aggregation and leukocyte adhesion. At higher doses, nitric oxide has antitumor and antimicrobial activity. Nitric oxide is thought to have a beneficial role in sepsis. It is important in maintaining visceral and microvascular blood flow acting as a counter-regulatory mechanism to the vasoconstriction mediators (thromboxane and endothelin-1) released in inflammation. It is thought to be an important free radical scavenger that prevents microvascular stasis and thrombosis by blocking platelet aggregation and leukocyte adhesion.

Nitric oxide may have several harmful effects in sepsis. Nitric oxide has been implicated as a major mediator for vasodilation and hypotension in septic shock. The inducible form of nitric oxide synthase is stimulated by inflammatory mediators (including TNFα and interleukin-1), which leads to increased release of nitric oxide from endothelial cells, vascular smooth muscle cells, and macrophages. Once induced, iNOS is likely to persist for many hours to days. Peroxynitrite, which is formed from the reaction between superoxide radicals and nitric oxide, may cause direct cellular injury. Nitric oxide may also contribute to the myocardial depression and increased permeability seen in septic shock.

Anti-inflammatory substances are also released. These include endogenous steroids and catecholamines, interleukin-10 (IL-10), interleukin-4 (IL-4), prostaglandin E_2, interleukin-1 receptor antagonists, and tumor necrosis factor receptors. All of these substances alter immune function, which leads to a period of immune depression after the initial shock episode.

Molecular Pathophysiology of Sepsis

There is now compelling evidence that septic shock and its morbid consequences are the direct result of endogenous proteins and phospholipid mediators secreted by the infected individual. Molecular pathophysiology of sepsis can be divided into 3 phases: induction of cytokine synthesis, cytokine synthesis and secretion, and cascade phase of sepsis.

The induction of cytokine synthesis involves the interaction of certain microbial molecules that, when recognized by the host, results in the production of mediators that amplify and transmit the microbial signal to other cells and tissues.

Of currently available models, the pathophysiology of gram-negative infection is best understood. An individual suffering from a gram-negative infection is not only exposed to membrane bound lipopolysaccharides (LPS) at the site of infection, but is also systemically exposed to the free endotoxin on fragments of bacterial outer membrane commonly shed during bacterial growth and replication. LPS binds to LPS-binding protein forming an LPS-LPS-binding protein complex. This complex is 1000-fold more potent than LPS alone in inducing TNF production by macrophages. The receptor for this complex is known to be the CD14 molecule that is found on monocytes, macrophages, and neutrophils. The peptidoglycan and lipoteichoic acids of gram-positive bacteria, certain polysaccharides, extracellular enzymes, and toxins induce cytokine synthesis in animals similar to those of LPS.

The phase of cytokine synthesis and secretion involves several regulated steps. These steps include transcription (synthesis of messenger RNA from the DNA template), translation of mRNA into protein, post-translational processing, and secretion of protein. An example is when LPS-LPS-binding protein complex interacts with the CD14, transcription of TNF gene in vitro increases threefold with levels of TNF mRNA increasing 100-fold. Biosynthesis and secretion of TNF, however, increase over 10,000-fold; this is primarily due to increased translational efficiency of preformed TNF mRNA as well as efficient translation of newly transcribed TNF mRNA.

The cascade portion of sepsis results from the activation and release of a central mediator (TNF, IL-1), which results in the secretion of various secondary mediators (IL-1, IL-6, IL-8, PAF, prostaglandins, leukotrienes); the activation of neutrophils, the complement system, and vascular endothelial cells; and synthesis of acute phase reactants. LPS and TNF probably promote intravascular coagulation initially by inducing blood monocytes to express tissue factor, by initiating the release of plasminogen activator inhibitor-1 (PAI-1) and inhibiting the expression of thrombomodulin and plasminogen activator by vascular endothelial cells. TNF, IL-1, and IL-6 are cytokines that have been detected in increased concentrations in the serum of patients with septic shock. The physiologic outcome of this complex cascade comprises the SIRS.

Parallel to SIRS is the body's intrinsic anti-inflammatory response. This response "compensatory anti-inflammatory response syndrome (CARS)" attempts to downregulate the SIRS response. Agents identified as participating in CARS include interleukins (IL-4, -10, -11, -13), transforming growth factor-β (TGF-β), colony-stimulating factor (CSF), soluble receptors to tumor necrosis factor (sTNFR), and antagonists to tumor necrosis factor (TNFra) and IL-1 (IL-1ra) receptors. These mediators inhibit T and B lymphocyte activity, as well as decrease antigen-presenting activity on the monocyte. The body normally maintains a delicate balance between SIRS and CARS. Uncontrolled sepsis and SIRS lead to profound hypotension, inadequate perfusion, and death. If the CARS reaction is severe, it will manifest clinically as anergy and increase susceptibility to infection.

CLINICAL FEATURES

Constitutional

Hyperthermia or hypothermia, tachycardia, wide pulse pressure, tachypnea, and mental status changes are early systemic signs of infection and septic shock. Endotoxin, TNF, IL-1, and interferon-α have all been shown to elicit febrile responses in humans. Acute hyperventilation with respiratory alkalosis ($Paco_2$ $\leq$30 mmHg) is common in sepsis. The etiological mechanism of this tachypnea is thought to be due either to the direct effects of endotoxins or secondary to kallikreins, bradykinin, prostaglandins, or complement activation.

The most frequent mental status change in sepsis is mental obtundation. The neurological findings are nonfocal and range from mild disorientation to confusion, lethargy, agitation, and coma. The pathophysiology is still unknown; an altered state of amino acid metabolism producing a state similar to portosystemic encephalopathy or decreased cerebral blood flow with secondary disruption of the blood-brain barrier are proposed mechanisms.

Cardiovascular

In the early stages of septic shock, the vasodilatory mediators predominate, and patients present with warm extremities. Cardiac output and stroke volume are usually well maintained. Frequently, cardiac output is increased concomitantly with tachycardia. Hemodynamic measurements during the first 24 hours show that the characteristic pattern of septic shock consists of an initial decrease in left and right ventricular ejection fractions (RVEF, LVEF) with an increase in both end-diastolic and end-systolic volume indices, normal stroke volume and decreased peripheral vascular resistance. In survivors, the changes are reversible, and the ventricular function and size return to normal by 7 to 10 days after septic shock onset. Patients with septic shock have been shown to have markedly diminished cardiac response to volume administration with only minor increments in both end-diastolic volume index (EDVI) and left ventricular stroke work index (LVSWI). Hemodynamic factors that are significant predictors of survival are an initial heart rate of $<$106 beats per minute, a 24-h heart rate of $<$95 beats per minute, or a systemic vascular resistance of $>$1529 dyne/s/cm^{-5}), and a change over the initial 24-h heart rate with a decrease in heart rate $>$18 beats per minute or a decrease in cardiac index by $>$0.5 L/min/m^2.

Myocardial depression is present in early septic shock. Studies show that the perfusion of the coronary arteries in patients with septic shock are equal to or greater than controls. This data strongly argues against the hypothesis that coronary hypoperfusion with secondary ischemic myocardial dysfunction is the cause of the myocardial depression. Significant evidence points towards the existence of several active circulating myocardial depressant substances.

Substances that have demonstrated myocardial depressant activity include TNFα (when IL-1β is present), nitric oxide, and IL-1β (when TNF is present), PAF, oxygen free radicals, interferon-γ, and arachidonic acid metabolites. The compounds that have received the most scrutiny are the combination of TNFα and IL-1β as well as nitric oxide. TNFα, in the presence of IL-1β, has been shown to produce significant myocardial depression in vitro. Another major contributor to the prolonged myocardial depression is cytokine-mediated nitric oxide. Nitric oxide can be produced in cardiac tissue, as in the vasculature, by two distinct pathways. Constitutive NOS (cNOS) appears to be involved in the physiologic regulation of myocardial contractility through the interaction between endothelial cells and cardiac myocytes. cNOS is stimulated by cytokines such as TNF, IL-1, and possibly IL-2, and activated macrophages. This inflammatory stimulus of sepsis is sustained at higher capacity through iNOS, which is responsible for the larger portion of the prolonged myocardial depression in sepsis.

Pulmonary

Sepsis remains the most common condition associated with adult respiratory distress syndrome (ARDS). ARDS is a physiologic syndrome characterized acutely by lung edema resulting from increased alveolar-capillary permeability. Recently, the concept of global microcirculatory injury has won favor with many investigators. In the setting of trauma and sepsis, ARDS affects capillary beds throughout the body concurrently. The lung is a conspicuous organ because when increased microvascular permeability develops in the lung, alveolar flooding occurs, causing dyspnea, hypoxemia, and abnormal opacities on chest x-ray. The appearance of ARDS varies from minutes to hours after the onset of sepsis. Although there are no specific and sensitive markers for ARDS, diagnostic criteria for ARDS include bilateral pulmonary infiltrates, pulmonary capillary wedge pressure (PCWP) $<$18 mmHg, Pa_{O_2}/PA_{O_2} ratio $<$0.2, and static compliance $<$40 mL/cm H_2O. Clinically, severe refractory hypoxemia, noncompliant "heavy" lungs, and a chest radiograph showing bilateral pulmonary alveolar infiltrates should suggest the presence of ARDS. The hypoxemia is due to perfusion of the underventilated alveoli; right-to-left shunting has been reported as high as 30 to 50 percent in this syndrome. Pathogenic factors implicated in the global microcirculatory injury are endotoxin, TNFα, IL-1, IL-6, IL-8, and bacterial permeability increasing protein.

Renal

Renal manifestations of septic shock include acute renal failure (ARF) with azotemia, oliguria, and active urinary sediment. Factors associated with the development of ARF in septic shock include hypotension, dehydration, aminoglycoside administration, and pigmenturia. Within the kidney, both vasoconstrictive and vasodilator mediators are generated and their balance dictates renal hemodynamics. If renal hypoperfusion predominates, renal ischemic injury occurs. Renal hypoperfusion is considered to be a major factor in the pathogenesis of ARF in sepsis. Toxic products resulting from neutrophil-endothelial interactions, endothelial damage by various mediators, reperfusion injury, and microvascular thrombosis in the kidney also contribute to renal dysfunction. In patients without septic shock, renal insufficiency may occur as a consequence of glomerulonephritis or interstitial nephritis. Glomerular disease in the setting of sepsis has been reported in subacute bacterial endocarditis, pyogenic visceral abscesses, and infections at other sites. Urine sediment in glomerular disease contains red blood cells, casts (red, white, or pigmented), and protein. Renal biopsy usually shows proliferative changes. Immune complex deposition with glomerular deposits of IgG, IgM, C3, bacterial antigens, and antibodies to these antigens has been reported. Tubulointerstitial disease has been associated with *Streptococcus pneumoniae, Staphylococcus pyogenes, Legionella pneumophila,* salmonellosis, brucellosis, and diphtheria infections. Acute interstitial nephritis secondary to allergic reaction to antibiotics (most commonly, methicillin) has also been reported; eosinophilia and eosinophiluria are usually present in this setting.

Hepatic

Liver dysfunction is frequently seen in patients with sepsis. The most frequent presentation is cholestatic jaundice. Increases in transaminase, alkaline phosphatase (one to three times normal) and bilirubin concentrations (usually not $>$10 mg/dL) are frequently noted. The proposed mechanism for bilirubin elevation involves hemolysis of red blood cells and hepatocellular dysfunction due to endotoxin, cytokines, or immune complex disease. Prolonged or severe hypotension may induce acute hepatic injury or ischemic bowel necrosis.

Hematologic

Major blood loss secondary to upper gastrointestinal bleeding occurs in only a small percentage of patients with sepsis. However, minor blood loss within 24 h of developing a severe infection is common as patients develop painless 1- to 2-mm erosions in the mucosal layer of the stomach and/or duodenum. Proposed mechanisms for these ulcerations include decrease in the blood flow, hypoxia of the mucosal cells, interruption of the gastric mucosal barrier, and release of mucosal lysozyme.

The most frequent hematologic changes in the septic patient are neutropenia or neutrophilia, thrombocytopenia, and disseminated intravascular coagulation (DIC). Sepsis most frequently produces a neutrophilic leukocytosis with a "left shift." These early changes result from demargination and release of less-mature granulocytes from the marrow storage pools. One proposed mechanism for demargination and bone marrow release is the presence of endotoxin or other similar substances and activation by complement (C3a) causing the release of a neutrophil-releasing substance. The sustained neutrophilia that accompanies chronic infection is thought to be secondary to colony stimulating factors. These glycoproteins increase granulocyte production by activating committed stem cells. Infection increases the colony-stimulating factor elaboration by macrophages, lymphocytes, and other tissues. In certain cases of sepsis, leukemoid reactions with leukocyte counts of 50,000 to 100,000 cells/μL have been reported.

Neutropenia, occurring rarely, is associated with an increase in mortality. The etiology of this neutropenia includes increased peripheral utilization of neutrophils, damage to neutrophils by bacterial byproducts, or depression of marrow granulocyte production by inflammatory mediators. Both morphologic and functional changes to neutrophils have been reported in sepsis. The most commonly reported morphologic changes include the presence of toxic granulations, Dohle bodies, and vacuolization. Functional changes reported in sepsis include increased phagocytic and cytotoxic activities. Eosinophilia occurring in the presence of sepsis has been attributed to the effect of margination or migration of these cells from the vascular space, inhibition of bone marrow release, and a decrease in marrow production. Activated complement C5a has been implicated.

Red cell number and morphologic characteristics are not usually affected by sepsis. However, red cell production and survival are decreased during sepsis. Decreased production and survival do not usually cause anemia unless the infection is prolonged. Septic patients generally possess low serum iron concentrations. Sepsis and its intermediaries cause a rapid iron flux into the liver and other parts of the reticuloendothelial cells, with the serum iron concentration decreasing by 50 percent or more within a period of hours. This effect may last days. An attractive hypothesis is that this represents a host defense mechanism. The addition of iron to normal human serum enhances the growth of organisms. Also, iron in the reticuloendothelial system may be beneficial to the host cells in detoxifying bacterial activity.

Thrombocytopenia most frequently arises as a consequence of DIC, although isolated thrombocytopenia is present in over 30 percent of cases of sepsis. Thrombocytopenia may be an early clue to bacteremia and may also be useful in observing patient's response to therapy. The proposed mechanisms for the thrombocytopenia include inhibition of thrombopoiesis, increased platelet turnover, increased endothelial adherence, and increased destruction secondary to immunologic mechanisms.

DIC is a condition in which the clotting and/or fibrinolytic system are systemically activated, leading to the consumption of many coagulation factors and platelets. DIC, with disseminated fibrin depositions in the microcirculation of various organ systems, is a frequent finding in patients with septic shock. The activation of the hemostatic (clotting) system is due primarily to the activation of the extrinsic pathway of clotting. This cascade is triggered by multiple sources including bacteria (gram-negative and gram-positive), viruses, fungi, endotoxins, and exotoxins (see Fig. 28-2). Gram-negative infections precipitate DIC more readily than does gram-positive bacteremia. The fibrinolytic system is also activated in sepsis and plays an important role in the regulation of fibrin deposition in the microcirculation. Several studies of septic patients have demonstrated the release of tissue type plasminogen activator, which activates the fibrinolytic system, at least initially in sepsis. As sepsis progresses, there is an increased release of plasminogen activator inhibitor type 1 (PAI-1), which blocks plasmin generation and thus contributes to fibrin deposition in the microcirculation and subsequent multiple-organ failure.

DIC can be categorized into two forms. The compensated form of DIC is characterized by a "slower" generalized activation of the hemostatic system. Although platelets and coagulation factors are consumed more rapidly than normal, bleeding is prevented by increasing coagulation factor production in the liver, by the release of the platelets from reserve storage sites, and by the synthesis of inhibitors at an accelerated rate. Patients with decompensated DIC will have clinical bleeding and/or thrombosis. Laboratory studies suggesting the presence of DIC include thrombocytopenia, prolonged prothrombin and activated partial thromboplastin values, decreased fibrinogen and antithrombin III levels, and increased fibrin monomer, fibrin split products, and D-dimer values.

Endocrine

Hyperglycemia may suggest the presence of sepsis in diabetic patients. Proposed pathogeneses include increased amounts of catecholamines, increased cortisol and glucagon in the circulation, peripheral insulin resistance, impaired glucose utilization, and decreased insulin secretion. Hypoglycemia with glucose levels as low as 10 to 20 mg/dL has been reported but is a relatively uncommon manifestation of sepsis. Bacterial infections associated with hypoglycemia include *S. aureus, S. pyogenes, S. pneumoniae, Listeria monocytogenes, Haemophilus influenzae, Neisseria meningitidis,* and *Enterobacteriaceae*. The proposed pathogenesis of hypoglycemia includes the depletion of hepatitic glycogen and inhibition of gluconeogeneses.

Acid-Base

Blood gas analysis performed early in the course of septic shock usually finds respiratory alkalosis. Relative or absolute hypoxemia is often present due to ventilation perfusion mismatches. The development of metabolic acidosis reflects inadequate tissue perfusion and increased glycolysis in peripheral tissues, along with impaired hepatic clearance of lactate and pyruvate. As perfusion worsens and continues, tissue hypoxia generates more lactic acid and metabolic acidosis worsens.

Cutaneous

Cutaneous lesions that occur as a result of sepsis can be divided into three categories: direct bacterial involvement of the skin and underlying soft tissues (cellulitis, erysipelas, and fasciitis); lesions that occur as a consequence of sepsis, hypotension, and/or DIC (acrocyanosis and necrosis of peripheral tissues); and lesions secondary to infective endocarditis (microemboli and/or immune complex vasculitis).

DIAGNOSIS

Septic shock should be suspected in any individual with temperature >38°C or <36°C and a systolic blood pressure of <90 mmHg with evidence of inadequate organ perfusion. The hypotension should not reverse with rapid volume replacement of at least 1 L of isotonic crystalloid. Frequently, the diagnosis is straightforward with the patient presenting with hypotension or inadequate perfusion and complaints attributable to a serious infection such as pneumonia, acute pyelonephritis, or an acute abdomen. Other early clinical features of sepsis include mental obtundation; hyperventilation; hot, flushed skin; and a widened pulse pressure. In the elderly, very young, or immunocompromised patient, the clinical presentation may be atypical with no fever or localizable source of infection.

The differential diagnosis of septic shock includes the other nonseptic causes of shock such as cardiogenic, hypovolemic, anaphylactic, neurogenic, obstructive (pulmonary embolism, tamponade), and endocrinal (adrenal insufficiency, thyroid storm) causes.

History and physical examination with some basic laboratory or radiologic investigations are usually successful in the initial assessment and identification of a presumptive source of sepsis. Particular attention should be focused on infections in these organ systems: central nervous system; pulmonary; intra-abdominal; skin and soft tissue.

Acute bacterial meningitis is the CNS infection that is most commonly associated with shock. Community-acquired meningitis with shock is usually due to *S. pneumoniae* or *N. meningitidis*. The majority of patients present with nuchal rigidity and a depressed level of consciousness. Chest radiographs may show a pneumonia with secondary bacteremia due to *S. pneumoniae*. Disseminated meningococcemia may present only with shock without meningismus. Frequently, these patients possess a "new petechial rash," which is the major clue to the etiology of shock. Brain abscesses, subdural or epidural empyemas, and viral CNS infections are seldom associated with shock on the initial presentation. Shock is also unusual in neurosurgical patients with *S. aureus* or enteric gram-negative meningitis secondary to neurosurgical procedure or skull fracture.

The major pulmonary entity commonly leading to septic shock is acute bacterial pneumonia. The most frequent organisms are *S. pneumoniae, S. aureus,* gram-negative bacilli, and *L. pneumophila.* The physical examination and chest radiograph almost always suggest the presence of pneumonia.

Intraabdominal processes are the source of infection leading to septic shock in the largest proportion of patients. Acute pancreatitis with or without infection can result in a presentation identical to septic shock. Suppurative cholangitis and empyema of the gallbladder are the primary considerations for the biliary tree. In women of childbearing age, septic abortion and postpartum endometritis/myometritis are the dominating presenting infections leading to septic shock. Acute pyelonephritis secondary to gram-negative enteric bacteria or enterococci can occasionally present with shock. Ureteric obstruction is often present in these syndromes.

The most common skin and soft tissue infection associated with septic shock is cellulitis due to *S. aureus* or *S. pyogenes.* Soft tissue infections secondary to gram-negative organisms are indistinguishable from those due to primary infection by staphylococci or streptococci. Shock associated with soft tissue infections is clinically obvious and frequently associated with bacteremia. Shock associated with a generalized erythematous macular rash may represent toxic shock syndrome. Necrotizing soft tissue infections are suspect in infections in immunocompromised patients or in patients with history of poor vascular circulation. Populations at risk for necrotizing infections are diabetics and individuals with peripheral vascular disease.

Individuals without obvious source of septic shock may have a primary bacteremia, or endocarditis. The most prevalent etiologies of primary bacteremias in outpatients are *S. aureus, S. pneumoniae*, and *N. meningitidis.* Encapsulated species such as *Salmonella* or *H. influenzae* are important pathogens in individuals who are asplenic. *Pseudomonas aeruginosa* and other gram-negative bacteria are occasionally etiologies of bacteremia and endocarditis in intravenous drug users.

Ancillary Studies

While there is no specific laboratory test for the diagnosis of septic shock, tests are useful because they (1) assess the general hematologic and metabolic state of the patient, (2) provide results that suggest the potential for occult bacterial infection, and (3) detect a specific microbial etiology for infection. Basic laboratory studies should include a complete blood count including platelet count; DIC panel (prothrombin time, activated partial thromboplastin time, fibrinogen, D-dimer, antithrombin III concentration); serum electrolytes (including magnesium, calcium, phosphate, and serum glucose); liver function panel (bilirubin, alkaline phosphate, and ALT); renal function panel (blood urea nitrogen and creatinine); arterial blood gas analysis; and urinalysis. Blood should be typed and crossed if low hematocrit is suspected. A chest radiograph should also be a part of the basic evaluation. Flat and upright abdominal films are helpful in patients in which there is a potential abdominal source of infection and should be considered in every patient except individuals with a completely benign abdomen or an obvious alternate source. Any patient with a clinical presentation compatible with a CNS source of infection should undergo a lumbar puncture with CSF collected for analysis. This should be performed without delay in the emergency department. In individuals with papilledema, focal neurologic deficits, or with potential for brain abscess or epidural or subdural empyema, the LP should be deferred until an imaging study is performed. However, if meningitis is an important consideration, empiric antimicrobial therapy should be initiated prior to the study.

Bacterial cultures of blood and urine should be obtained on all septic patients. At least two separate sets of blood cultures from different venipuncture sites should be obtained. Gram's stain and culture of secretions from any potential site of infection should be performed. A Gram's stain or other means of rapid identification of microbial etiologies are generally the only immediately available tests useful in selection of antimicrobial therapy.

TREATMENT

Airway and Respiratory Management

Immediate assessment of oxygenation and ventilation status is the first priority in the management. Oxygen by mask and consideration of endotracheal intubation should be done immediately if the patient's airway is not secure or if respirations are inadequate. In addition, patients with hypotension not responding acutely to rapid fluid resuscitation should be intubated to avoid respiratory arrest from fatigue of the respiratory muscles due to inadequate perfusion of these muscles. There is no consensus as to acceptable levels of oxygen saturation or tensions; however, most experts recommend maintaining oxygen saturations above 90 percent in a septic patient.

Hemodynamic Stabilization

FLUID ADMINISTRATION Correction or stabilization of hypotension and inadequate perfusion is the second goal of resuscitation. Rapid fluid administration at a rate of 0.5 L (20 mL/kg in children) of normal saline or similar isotonic crystalloid should be administered every 5 to 10 min as needed; it is not unusual for the patient to require 4 to 6 L (60 mL/kg in children) or more of crystalloid in the initial phase of resuscitation. Stabilization of the patient's mentation, blood pressure, respiration, pulse rate, skin perfusion, and central venous pressure, with urine output greater than 30 mL/h (1 mL/kg/h in pediatric patients) are useful clinical parameters in monitoring the response to fluid administration.

INOTROPIC SUPPORT If no response to the fluid infusion is noted after 3 to 4 L of fluid, or if there are signs of fluid overload (elevated central venous pressure or pulmonary edema), an infusion of dopamine can be started. If the patient has a pulmonary artery catheter in place during this resuscitation, dopamine should be added in the setting of a PCWP of 15 to 18 mmHg or if there are marked increases of the PCWP with additional fluids. Doses of dopamine often required are 5 to 20 μg/kg/min resulting in both β-adrenergic inotropic and α-adrenergic vasopressor activity. If the patient is still unresponsive above a rate of 20 μg/kg/min of dopamine infusion, norepinephrine should be started with the goal of keeping the mean blood pressure at least 60 mmHg. Although previous investigations have raised doubts concerning the efficacy of norepinephrine in these cases, recent studies have demonstrated that norepinephrine can reverse septic shock in patients unresponsive to fluid administration and dopamine. Once the blood pressure and perfusion have been stabilized by norepinephrine, the lowest dosage that maintains blood pressure should be utilized to minimize the complications of vasoconstriction. Additionally, data from the canine model has suggested the use of low-dose dopamine (1 to 4 μg/kg/min) in patients on norepinephrine results in significantly higher renal blood flow and reduced renal vascular resistance. In one series, the norepinephrine survival group approached 40 percent. Vasodilators are rarely used in the emergency department, but they have been used in the intensive care units in situations of severe myocardial depression, increased system vascular resistance, and adequate blood pressure.

HEMODYNAMIC ENDPOINTS Most authorities recommend that the optimal hematocrit should be maintained between 30 and 35 percent to maximize oxygen transport capacity. A number of studies have suggested that increased global oxygen delivery has improved survival in critically ill patients. However, a recent multicenter trial involving more than 10,000 patients in 56 intensive care units suggested that hemodynamic therapy aimed at achieving supranormal values for cardiac index, with normal values of mixed venous oxygenation, failed to reduce morbidity or mortality in critically ill patients when compared to a control group that was supported to normal cardiac index levels.

Empiric Antimicrobial Therapy

All patients with septic shock should receive empiric antimicrobial therapy as soon as possible. Whenever possible, samples of blood or fluids from potential sites of infection should be obtained prior to the initiation of antimicrobial therapy. Selection of antibiotics should be based upon the adequate coverage of all potential pathogens of the potential infection sites as well as the anticipated antimicrobial susceptibility patterns of the bacterial isolate(s).

Empiric therapy should be effective against gram-positive organisms (*Streptococcus spp.* and *Staphylococcus spp.*) and gram-negative bacteria. The route of administration should be intravenous in the maximum doses allowed. In neonates, a regimen of ampicillin plus cefotaxime is recommended. For infants one to three months of age, the combination of ampicillin with cefotaxime or ceftriaxone is recommended. In nonimmunocompromised children three months or older, cefotaxime or ceftriaxone is the drug of choice. In adults (non-neutropenic) without an obvious source of infection, a third-generation cephalosporin or an antipseudomonal β-lactamase-susceptible penicillin is recommended. Some experts advise the addition of an aminoglycoside (tobramycin, gentamicin, or amikacin) to this regimen. Alternatively, imipenem or meropenem alone is acceptable. In neutropenic children and adults, ceftazidime, imipenem, or meropenem alone is acceptable. Alternatively, the combination of an antipseudomonal aminoglycoside plus ceftazidime or antipseudomonal β-lactamase-susceptible penicillin is acceptable. In patients with high probability of a gram-positive etiology (history of illicit drug abuse), nafcillin or vancomycin should be added to the regimen. If an anaerobic source is suspected (intraabdominal, biliary, female genital tract, necrotizing cellulitis, aspiration pneumonia, odontogenic infection, or an anaerobic soft tissue infection) metronidazole or clindamycin should be added to the regimen. In patients with potential for *Legionella* species infection, the addition of erythromycin to the regimen is recommended. In patients with indwelling vascular devices, vancomycin should be added to the regimen.

Removal of Source of Infection

If a focal source of sepsis is identified, removal of the nidus of infection is absolutely mandatory for successful treatment. Indwelling intravenous catheters should be removed and replaced. The tip should be sent for quantitative culture. Foley catheters should be replaced if obstructed. Intraabdominal or soft tissue sites of pus require urgent drainage.

Initial Baseline Assessment

Hemodynamic and laboratory monitoring is critical to the resuscitation of a patient in septic shock. Some clinicians advocate following the serum lactate as a monitor of response to therapy. Arterial blood gas should be repeated to monitor adequacy of ventilation and perfusion. Septic shock patients should have at least two large-bore intravenous catheters for administration of fluids and vasoactive drugs. Early placement of a central venous catheter (ideally with a 8.5-Fr catheter introducer) may help in the monitoring of fluid resuscitation. Placement of a flow-directed thermal-dilution pulmonary artery wedge-pressure catheter should be considered in patients requiring vasoactive therapy, where there is difficulty in assessing volume status, or ongoing hemodynamic instability is present. Generally, the placement of this catheter can wait until the patient is in the intensive care unit.

New noninvasive methods of patient monitoring are currently under investigation. Clinical studies have shown that only the measurement of gastric pH has a significant impact on the treatment and prognosis of patients with sepsis. Among the most promising of the newer techniques being investigated are near-infrared spectroscopy and transcranial Doppler measurements. Near-infrared spectroscopy (NIRS) enables the assessment of intracerebral oxygenation and may be suitable for monitoring critically ill patients. Investigations in patients with sepsis have suggested that NIRS detected evidence of impaired vasoregulation. Its clinical use is limited by its only giving relative values and no critical values of tissue perfusion can be given. Currently, NIRS is used for the cerebral monitoring of newborn infants and patients undergoing cardiopulmonary bypass or operations involving the carotid artery.

Transcranial Doppler measurements enable the noninvasive evaluation of blood flow velocities of some cerebral arteries. Investigations have suggested that the monitoring cerebral blood flow is vital in critically ill patients. In particular, the risks of cerebral vasoconstriction induced by hyperventilation, and the sepsis-induced nonhomogenous cerebral blood flow seen in some patients with sepsis, may place certain patients at risk for cerebral ischemia.

Other Therapies

BICARBONATE Some investigators advocate the administration of bicarbonate for individuals with severe acidosis (pH <7.2). The efficacy of this intervention is not established.

THERAPY OF DIC The management of the patient in DIC has three basic approaches: elimination of the underlying disorder or source of infection; substitution of coagulation constituents lost in the clotting process; and arrest of the intravascular clotting process. If the patient is actively bleeding and decompensated DIC is present, urgent replacement of the components of the coagulation and fibrinolytic systems is indicated with the rapid infusion of fresh-frozen plasma and/or platelets. Reasonable guidelines in the actively bleeding patient with DIC include the transfusion of platelets to maintain a concentration of 50 to $100 \times 10^3/\mu L$ and fresh-frozen plasma to keep the coagulation parameters (prothrombin time and activated prothrombin time) less than twice normal.

Interruption of the activated hemostatic system has been attempted by a number of investigators. Heparin has been used (primarily outside the United States) with mixed results. Currently, no conclusive evidence is available to suggest that heparin therapy reduces morbidity or mortality in septic patients with DIC. Administration of a natural anticoagulant, such as antithrombin III (ATIII) may arrest clotting without concomitant risk of bleeding. ATIII is a single-chain glycopeptide that is produced by the liver. ATIII is an important regulator of hemostasis by inhibiting several serine proteases of the coagulation system, predominately thrombin and factor Xa. Plasma ATIII levels decrease in septic patients with DIC. In healthy individuals, the half-life of ATIII is approximately 60 h. In patients with sepsis and septic shock, this may be reduced to as little as 4 to 6 h. The possibility that replacement of ATIII neutralizes excess thrombin and dampens the intravascular coagulation process has prompted several experimental and clinical studies. In several animal models of DIC, infusion of ATIII concentrates shortened the duration of DIC and reduced multiple organ failure and mortality. Results of human clinical studies have been mixed. These investigations have suggested either a trend towards efficacy or no significant difference between patients who received ATIII and controls. Until a definitive study is available, some experts recommend that patients with DIC secondary to a septic process should receive replacement of ATIII to a level of 70 to 80 percent of normal. Other investigators suggest that a much higher level of ATIII (140 to 150 percent) is required for efficacy.

ANTI-INFLAMMATORIES Although some animal models have shown that high-dose corticosteroid therapy was effective, large clinical trials have shown no differences in mortality between corticosteroid treated patients and control patients. These studies also have documented the occurrence of superinfection in corticosteroid treated patients. Thus the primary role of steroids is in patients with suspected or documented adrenal insufficiency. Adrenal insufficiency should be considered in septic patients with fulminant *N. meningitidis* bacteremia, disseminated tuberculosis, AIDS, prior glucocorticoid use, or with refractory hypotension. The use of inhibitors to metabolites elaborated in sepsis (inhibitors include ibuprofen, naloxone, eicosanoids, or antihistamines) has not proven to be effective in the management of septic shock.

NEW AGENTS IN THE TREATMENT OF SEPSIS

Recent advances in molecular biology and immunology suggest that the host's inflammatory response to infection contributes substantially to the development of septic shock. Standard sepsis treatment strategies include the use of life support procedures, antibiotics to kill invading bacteria, and surgical procedures to eradicate the nidus of infection. Despite these aggressive measures, the mortality rate of septic shock remains high. The development of new interventions is based on the premise that neutralizing bacterial toxins and the potentially harmful host mediators could stop or slow this syndrome. Researchers have targeted interventions at all three phases of the host's inflammatory responses. Interventions targeting the induction phase include all those against the endotoxin's lipopolysaccharide molecule. This category includes E5 and HA-1A therapy monoclonal antibodies. Therapies targeting cytokine synthesis include pentoxifylline, β-agonists (amrinone and dobutamine), and corticosteroids. Therapies directed against the cascade phase of sepsis include monoclonal antibodies to TNF- and IL-1-receptor antagonist, monoclonal antibodies against the neutrophil CD11/18 adhesion complex, nitric oxide synthase inhibitors, and cyclooxygenase inhibitors.

Currently, none of the therapies aimed at single targets in the inflammatory cascade has been proven to be effective in the treatment of septic shock in humans. In the cases of interventions that are directed at endogenous inflammatory mediators, none of the studies has produced unequivocal benefit in the treatment of sepsis. Great potential danger exists in altering the natural balance of inflammatory mediators. These mediators perform important functions, such as clearing bacterial toxins and the mobilization of the host defenses that control the infection. Attempting to block the harmful effect of inflammatory mediators may compromise host defenses and ultimately worsen the outcome. Successful therapeutic approaches may depend on determining which inflammatory mediators should be inhibited or augmented and when to do so. In almost all the animal models, anti-LPS therapy is only effective if given before or simultaneously with LPS challenge. Thus, it is very unlikely that anti-LPS treatment alone will change outcome in patients in shock and with organ failure. The situations in which these agents may be the most effective are those in which the patients are in early gram-negative sepsis or as a prophylaxis for high-risk patients.

Anti-Endotoxin Antibodies

The most studied exogenous mediator is endotoxin. This macromolecule is found in gram-negative bacteria as one of the integral components of the outer bacterial lipopolysaccharide cell wall. The molecule can be functionally divided into 3 parts: a highly variable O-polysaccharide side-chain that provides the heat-stable serologic specificity of gram-negative bacteria and is the basis for the O (somatic) antigen type scheme; an oligosaccharide or R-core region composed of approximately 10 monosaccharides; and a lipid backbone referred to as lipid A. The lipid A portion of endotoxin is responsible for the majority of the molecule's toxicity; this portion is also highly conserved and is essentially invariable and ubiquitous.

Experimental studies of the administration of endotoxin have produced physiologic changes paralleling those of septic shock. Administration of endotoxin in dogs results in severe hypotension. Administration of endotoxin in humans produces an increase in heart rate and cardiac index, and a decrease in peripheral vascular resistance. Later hemodynamic changes include a depressed cardiac state with a dilated left ventricle. Endotoxin administration in rabbits produces DIC and bilateral renal cortical necrosis. Endotoxin administration in both animals and humans results in fever.

Endotoxin (otherwise known as lipopolysaccharide) alone can induce septic shock. Recently, scientists have discovered a major cellular basis for the pathophysiologic response to LPS. Endotoxin (LPS), lipopolysaccharide-binding protein (LBP), and CD14 (a protein found on the surface of monocytes and macrophages) form a complex that is critical for macrophage and neutrophil activation by LPS. LBP is present in the circulation and concentrations are increased in the response to inflammatory stimuli. LBP binds LPS and this LPS-LBP complex then interacts with CD14. CD14 is thought to act as a carrier molecule presenting LPS to a signaling receptor. It is the LPS-sCD14 complex that is thought to be the major module that binds to endothelial cells and triggers the cascade of events leading to septic shock.

Many strategies have been developed to manipulate this complex, including enhanced LPS clearance (anti-LPS antibodies, direct removal of LPS via filtration and use of hemoglobin); direct neutralization of circulating LPS (anti-LPS antibodies, LPS neutralizing proteins); inhibition of LPS-LBP; and removal of both endotoxin and cytokines by hemofiltration, hemadsorption, or hemodialysis. Limited information from using continuous veno-venous hemofiltration (CVVH) on patients with sepsis and oliguric renal failure has suggested that CVVH may increase the predominance of circulating anti-inflammatory cytokines over pro-inflammatory cytokines. This change is thought to be beneficial. However, there are no randomized trial data to support the routine use of plasma filtration or hemodialysis in sepsis. Other interventions include the use of LPS-sCD14 complex modifiers (lipid A analogues, anti-LBP antibodies, anti-CD14 antibodies); blocking cellular LPS receptors (lipid A analogues, anti-CD14 antibodies); and inhibition of cell signal transduction via tryosine kinase or protein kinase C inhibitors.

J5 (POLYCLONAL ANTI-ENDOTOXIN ANTIBODY) Despite initial promise, five subsequent clinical trials using either J5 antiserum, immune plasma, or intravenous immunoglobulin have not improved survival in sepsis or septic shock.

E5 (MONOCLONAL ANTI-ENDOTOXIN ANTIBODY) Monoclonal antibodies were developed to produce a more specific anti-endotoxin therapy with less risk for transmission of infection. E5 is an IgM antiendotoxin monoclonal antibody produced by immunizing mice with the core lipopolysaccharide antigen of the E5 mutant of *E. coli.* E5 is manufactured by an antibody-producing hybridoma created by the fusion of mouse spleen cells with a murine myeloma cell line. Preliminary animal studies suggested potential efficacy in septic shock. Double-blind, placebo-controlled investigations of patients in sepsis and septic shock have produced mixed results. Overall mortality has not been consistently reduced in either sepsis or septic shock. The only consistent benefit appears to be a more rapid resolution of organ failure in patients with gram-negative sepsis without hypotension or shock. Allergic reactions to the murine antibody were minimal, and adverse effects were minimal. Overall, the benefits of E5 are too limited to justify the expense of routine use.

HA-1A (HUMAN-HYBRID MONOCLONAL ANTI-ENDOTOXIN ANTIBODY) While the hybridoma that produces HA-1A is about 80% murine, the antibody itself is predominately human. Studies of HA-

1A in animals have met with varied results; some models showing benefit and others showing harm. The first human study with HA-1A originally reported a decrease in mortality and a more rapid resolution of organ system failure in patients with gram-negative bacteremia. HA-1A treatment did not improve survival in patients who had non-bacteremic gram-negative infections and in patients without gram-negative infections. Despite these favorable results, significant concerns were raised, and when the data were analyzed using the original analytic plan, HA-1A did not show a significant effect on survival. In the second placebo-controlled study with HA-1A, mortality in patients with gram-negative bacteremia was unaffected and mortality in patients without gram-negative bacteremia was actually worsened. Further development of HA-1A for the treatment of septic shock was halted.

T88 (MONOCLONAL ANTIBODY) This is an antibody to a common enterobacterial antigen that has shown promise in animal studies. A phase III trial of patients with sepsis has recently been completed and preliminary data suggest that no overall benefit resulted from the administration of this medication.

LPS-NEUTRALIZING PROTEIN A number of lipopolysaccharide-neutralizing proteins has been described of which BPI has been most extensively studied and is currently in clinical trials for gram-negative sepsis. BPI is a 55 to 60 kDa neutrophil primary granule protein with 45 percent sequence homology to LBP. BPI has a higher affinity for LPS than LBP and therefore displaces LPS from the LPS-LBP complex. In addition, BPI is cytotoxic for many gram-negative bacteria. Phase II and phase III clinical studies of BPI_{23} are in progress including a multicenter trial of patients with meningococcemia.

LIPID A ANALOGUES Inhibition of the LPS-LBP interaction is an attractive and potential method of intervention. Analogues based upon the structure of lipid A display reduced or absent cellular toxicity. The most attractive of these compounds is E5331. This compound has been shown to block endotoxin binding to cells, to inhibit LPS-induced TNFα release, and to protect mice from *E. coli* challenge. E5331 inhibits endotoxin-induced cytokine release in human volunteers in response to low-dose endotoxin infusion and phase I/II studies are in progress.

A number of conclusions can be made. Antiendotoxin core-directed antibodies have not shown a reproducible survival benefit for patients with sepsis in 10 clinical trials. However, both E5 and HA1A may have beneficial roles in a subgroup of patients presenting with sepsis. Further investigations are needed to determine if monoclonal antibody to endotoxin is an appropriate therapeutic modality for treatment of septic shock.

The setting where antiendotoxin antibody therapy is therapeutic and cost-effective remains to be defined. Neither E5 nor HA-1A benefited the approximately 30 percent of individuals who did not have a gram-negative infection. Separating patients with gram-positive sepsis from those with gram-negative sepsis based upon clinical symptoms and presenting signs alone is difficult. Early laboratory diagnosis of gram-negative bacteremia or endotoxemia is not currently available. The rapid identification of the presence of gram-negative organisms from potential sites of infection (UTI; pneumonia; abdominal infection; CNS infections; soft tissue infections; decubitus or cellulitis in the setting of diabetes or peripheral vascular disease) is critical for interventions and antiendotoxin antibody therapy. Gram's stain and other rapid assays remain the most valuable tests for rapid identification of gram-negative organisms in clinical specimens.

Anticytokine Therapy

Cytokines are peptides that function as cellular signals to regulate the amplitude and duration the host's inflammatory response. TNF, IL-1, and other cytokines play protective roles in the host's immune response to infection. The host's response to these cytokines consists of recruited and activated neutrophils, macrophages and lymphocytes, increased gene expression, and release of granulocyte colony-stimulating factors. Two cytokines, TNF and IL-1, have been studied extensively in patients with sepsis.

TUMOR NECROSIS FACTOR Tumor necrosis factor is a polypeptide hormone that can stimulate the release of other mediators including IL-1, IL-6, and PAF. TNF also promotes the metabolism of arachidonic acid, leading to eicosanoid formation. TNF is directly toxic to endothelial cells, increases the adhesion of polymorphonuclear leukocytes to the endothelial cells, and enhances the phagocytic activity of these cells. Finally, TNF reduces the transmembrane potential of muscle cells, depresses myocardial function, and activates coagulation.

Administration of TNF to experimental animals and healthy human subjects duplicates many of the signs and symptoms of sepsis. Injection of TNF into animals results in hemodynamic collapse, multiple-organ injury, and a life-threatening vascular leak syndrome. In humans, injection of TNF produces hypotension, chills, fever, headache, and malaise synchronously with the time of the peak serum TNF level. In addition, rapid and sustained activation of the common pathway of the coagulation system occurs.

Numerous studies have reported a positive correlation between level of serum concentrations of TNF and clinical outcome in patients with sepsis. Significantly higher levels of TNF were found in nonsurvivors of meningococcemia, sepsis, children with infectious purpura, and adult respiratory distress syndrome. Close association of the presence of TNF and septic shock has been demonstrated. Absolute TNF levels were a significant predictive factor for morbidity and mortality in patients with septic shock.

The most compelling evidence that TNF is a causal rather than an associative factor are animal studies demonstrating that antibodies to TNF enhance survival and reduce physiologic derangements after challenge with endotoxin or live bacteria.

Human studies on the feasibility of monoclonal antibodies are currently underway. Two phase I and one phase II trials have reported that administration of monoclonal anti-TNF antibodies was well tolerated and that the serum half-life ranged from 40 to 54 h in septic patients. Unfortunately, the multicenter North American trial of 478 patients with septic shock and the multicenter European trial of 420 patients with sepsis found no reduction in either the 3-day or 28-day mortality. Further analysis suggested significantly more rapid reversal of shock and a decreased incidence of multiorgan failure with anti-TNF antibody administration.

Investigators have attempted to "trap and eliminate" TNF. There are two major types of TNFα receptors that exist in surface-bound and circulating forms. Researchers have developed a recombinant human TNF receptor termed p75. Hypothetically, this receptor should act as a matrix for removal of TNF from the circulation but preliminary human study found the 28-day mortality was unchanged.

INTERLEUKIN-1 Interleukin-1β is also present in the blood of patients with septic shock. Both TNF and IL-1β induce hypotension, and a combination of the two cytokines is a more potent inducer of shock than either cytokine alone. Both cytokines induce IL-6, a nonlethal cytokine, that serves as an excellent marker of cytokine activity in patients with sepsis. An interleukin-1 receptor antagonist (IL-1ra) has been shown to block the hemodynamic consequences of *E. coli* endotoxin and heat-killed *S. epidermidis* in experimental animals. Human recombinant IL-1ra decreased the mortality rate of endotoxin-induced shock in rabbits and lethal *E. coli*-induced septic shock in primates. In addition, IL-1ra attenuated the decrease in mean artery blood pressure and cardiac output in the primate model.

Results are available from three human studies on the efficacy of IL-1ra in patients with septic syndrome. Reduction in 28-day mortality has been in the two smaller studies but not the largest study with 696 patients.

In summary, most investigators believe that TNF is a key and perhaps central mediator in sepsis. To date, anti-TNF and anti-IL-1 agents have not been shown to consistently improve outcome in the treatment of septic patients.

The Neutrophil

Evidence suggests that the neutrophil has both beneficial and harmful effects in sepsis and septic shock. The neutrophil is a key component of the host defense. Data from neutropenic animals and humans suggest that augmented neutrophil count and function reduce the risk of infection. Conversely, studies have also shown that the neutrophil and its toxic byproducts produce tissue injury and organ dysfunction in sepsis and septic shock.

One area of intense interest is the leukocyte endothelium interaction. This interaction appears to be a crucial step in the inflammatory cascade during sepsis. A membrane glycoprotein complex termed CD11/18 has been suggested as the primary adhesion receptor site on endothelial cells and leukocytes for this interaction, and has been the target of many investigators. This complex is a cell-surface receptor that regulates neutrophil-endothelial cell adhesion, the first step in the neutrophil migration to sites of infection or inflammation.

Researchers have developed monoclonal antibodies against the CD11/18 complex. These antibodies, both in vitro and in vivo, prevent endotoxin, TNF, and complement-induced neutrophil adhesion; injury to endothelial cells; and neutrophil extravascular migration. In some animal models of sepsis and meningitis, monoclonal anti-CD 11/18 antibodies improved mortality rates, decreased adverse hemodynamic parameters, and decreased meningeal inflammation. In a study of dogs pretreated with CD11/18 monoclonal antibody and challenged with TNF, animals treated with CD11/18 had a reduced mortality rate and better arterial oxygenation in the first 24 hours; but this effect was not sustained and the overall survival between the two groups was not significantly different. In a subsequent study in dogs using a similar design but challenged with *E. coli,* investigators found that the CD11/18 monoclonal antibody worsened cardiovascular instability and decreased tissue perfusion during sepsis. In conclusion, studies to date suggest that efforts to inhibit neutrophil function may lead to more tissue injury and more adverse outcomes.

Nitric Oxide

There is good evidence from a large number of studies that humans suffering from sepsis syndrome also have increased systemic nitric oxide production. The higher the nitric oxide level, the more pronounced the septic hypotension seems to be.

Animal studies using nitric oxide synthase inhibitors have mixed results. Researchers have reported that nitric oxide synthase inhibitors restored the responsiveness of septic vasculature to catecholamines and improved survival in endotoxin-challenged animals. Other investigators have reported opposite and harmful effects. These investigators found that the administration of a nitric oxide synthase inhibitor increased systemic and renal vascular resistance, decreased renal blood flow, increased capillary leak, decreased cardiac output, and increased mortality.

Only a handful of studies using an iNOS antagonist, such as arginine analogues, in septic patients has been published. In a small placebo-controlled study with 12 individuals, an arginine analogue was shown to be an effective pressor but was associated with diminished cardiac output and continued high mortality rates. Other limited, uncontrolled studies have shown that the septic patients treated with nitric oxide inhibitors demonstrated transient improvements in blood pressure but no effect on overall mortality. The role of nitric oxide in septic shock warrants further investigation. To date, only nonselective nitric oxide synthetase inhibitors that block both forms of nitric oxide synthase inhibitors have been extensively studied. Future research is most likely to be performed with highly selective inhibitors.

Other Agents

PENTOXIFYLLINE Pentoxifylline, a methylxanthine derivative, inhibits cytokine activation of neutrophils and the production of TNF by endotoxin-exposed monocytes. This prevents the adherence of neutrophils to endothelium and the release of toxic degranulation products. The mechanism of this action is believed to be via increasing cyclic adenosine monophosphate concentrations. Animal experiments suggest that treatment with pentoxifylline decreases mortality rate and prevents lung injury by inhibiting migration of neutrophils through the pulmonary capillary endothelium. Also, better survival rates and lower meningeal inflammation have been observed in animals with experimental bacterial meningitis. In healthy human volunteers, pentoxifylline inhibits the rise in TNF induced by endotoxin.

CYCLOOXYGENASE INHIBITORS Two principal pathways of arachidonic acid metabolism exist. The lipoxygenase pathway leads to the production of leukotrienes. Leukotrienes are potent leukocyte chemoattractants. The cyclooxygenase pathway results in the release of thromboxanes and prostaglandins that are important regulators of vascular tone.

Ibuprofen is a cyclooxygenase inhibitor. In animal models of endotoxin shock and shock from peritoneal implantation or intravenous infusion of bacteria, ibuprofen decreases mortality, reverses hemodynamic, metabolic, and blood coagulation abnormalities, improves pulmonary gas exchange, and attenuates the development of increase in microvascular permeability. These results are seen with ibuprofen when administered before and after the septic insult. In preliminary human studies, treatment with ibuprofen attenuates flu-like symptoms and reduces fever, tachycardia, and metabolic rate in volunteers exposed to endotoxin. Recently, the Ibuprofen Sepsis Study Group published its findings of a randomized, double-blind, placebo-controlled trial of intravenous ibuprofen (10 mg/kg per body weight given every 6 h for a total of 8 doses) in 455 patients who had sepsis. It found that the ibuprofen-treated group had significant declines in temperature, heart rate, oxygen consumption, lactic acidosis, and urinary levels of prostacyclin and thromboxane. However, ibuprofen did not reduce the incidence or duration of shock or ARDS, and did not significantly improve the rate of survival at 30 days (mortality, 37 percent with ibuprofen versus 40 percent with placebo). No increase in adverse events (renal dysfunction, gastrointestinal bleeding) was noted in the ibuprofen group. No definitive conclusions can be made from any of the studies regarding the efficacy of ibuprofen in sepsis. However, both human and animal studies to date have suggested that ibuprofen results in decreased metabolic demand on patients with sepsis.

BIBLIOGRAPHY

General

Astiz ME, Rackow EC: Septic shock. *Lancet* 351:1501, 1998.

Definitions

Bone RC: The sepsis syndrome: Definition and general approach to management. *Clin Chest Med* 17:175, 1996.

Bone RC, Balk RA, Cerra FB, et al: Definitions for sepsis and organ failure and guidelines for the use of innovative therapies in sepsis. The ACCP/SCCM Consensus Conference Committee. *Chest* 101:1644, 1992.

Epidemiology

Brun-Buisson C, Doyon F, Carlet J, et al: Incidence, risk factors, and outcome of severe sepsis and septic shock in adults. *JAMA* 274:968, 1995.

Lundberg JS, Perl TM, Wiblin T: Septic shock: An analysis of outcomes for patients with onset on hospital wards versus intensive care units. *Crit Care Med* 26:1020, 1998.

Rangel-Frausto NS, Pittet D, Costigan M: The natural history of the systemic inflammatory response syndrome (SIRS): A prospective study. *JAMA* 273:117, 1995.

Sands KE, Bates DW, Lanken PN: Epidemiology of sepsis syndrome in 8 academic medical centers. *JAMA* 278:234, 1997.

Pathophysiology

Glauser MP, Heumann D, Baumgartner JD, Cohen J: Pathogenesis and potential strategies for prevention and treatment of septic shock: An update. *Clin Infect Dis* 18(supp 2):S205, 1994.

Ognibene FP: Pathogenesis and innovative treatment of septic shock. *Adv Intern Med* 42:313, 1997.

Parrillo JE: Pathogenetic mechanisms of septic shock. *N Engl J Med* 328:1471, 1993.

Saez-Llorens X, McCracken GH Jr: Sepsis syndrome and septic shock in pediatrics: Current concepts of terminology, pathophysiology, and management. *J Pediatr* 123:497, 1993.

Clinical Features

Bock HA: Pathophysiology of acute renal failure in septic shock: From prerenal to renal failure. *Kidney Int* 64(suppl):S15, 1998.

Carleton SC: The cardiovascular effects of sepsis. *Cardiol Clin* 13:249, 1995.

Mammen EF: The haematological manifestations of sepsis. *J Antimicrob Chemother* 41(supp A):17, 1998.

Parrillo JE: The cardiovascular pathophysiology of sepsis. *Ann Rev Med* 40:469, 1989.

Parrillo JE, Parker MM, Natanson C, et al: Septic shock in humans: Advances in the understanding of pathogenesis, cardiovascular dysfunction, and therapy. *Ann Intern Med* 113:227, 1990.

Snell RJ, Parrillo JE: Cardiovascular dysfunction in septic shock. *Chest* 99:1000, 1991.

Singer M: Management of multiple organ failure: Guidelines but no hard-and-fast rules. *J Antimicrob Chemother* 41(supp A):103, 1998.

Treatment

Abraham E, Wunderink R, Silverman H: Efficacy and safety of monoclonal antibody to human tumor necrosis factor-alpha in patients with sepsis syndrome. A randomized, controlled, double-blind, multicenter clinical trial. *JAMA* 273:934, 1995.

Cronin L, Cook DJ, Carlet J: Corticosteroid treatment for sepsis: A critical appraisal and meta-analysis of the literature. *Crit Care Med* 23:470, 1995.

Kuhl SJ, Rosen H: Nitric oxide and septic shock: From bench to bedside. *West J Med* 168:176, 1998.

Lefering R, Neugebauer EAM: Steroid controversy in sepsis and septic shock: A meta-analysis. *Crit Care Med* 23:1294, 1995.

Lynn WA, Cohen J: Adjunctive therapy for septic shock: A review of experimental approaches. *Clin Infect Dis* 20:143, 1995.

Task Force of the American College of Critical Care Medicine, Society of Critical Care Medicine: Practice parameters for hemodynamic support of sepsis in adult patients in sepsis. *Crit Care Med* 27(3):639–660, 1999.

Zeni F, Freeman B, Natanson C: Anti-inflammatory therapies to treat sepsis and septic shock: A reassessment. [editorial; comment] *Crit Care Med* 25:1095, 1997.

Ziegler EJ, Fisher CJ Jr, Sprung CL, et al: Treatment of gram-negative bacteremia and septic shock with HA-1A human monoclonal antibody against endotoxin. A randomized, double-blind, placebo-controlled trial. *N Engl J Med* 324:429, 1991.

CARDIOGENIC SHOCK

Raymond E. Jackson

The syndrome of cardiogenic shock results from an impairment of the heart's pumping action to the degree that there is insufficient blood flow to the tissues to meet resting metabolic demands. Cardiogenic shock is usually caused by contractile failure of the myocardium, although other processes may impair cardiac output enough to produce shock (Table 29-1). Cardiogenic shock is a true emergency requiring rapid recognition and aggressive interventions to avert the extremely high mortality.[1–6]

EPIDEMIOLOGY

Cardiogenic shock is the most frequent cause of in-hospital death from acute myocardial infarction (AMI), resulting in 50,000 to 70,000 deaths per year in the United States alone. The reported incidence in recent studies of cardiogenic shock after AMI is about 5 to 7 percent. Since the mid-1980s, the incidence seems to be decreasing, possibly secondary to early reperfusion, invasive monitoring, and rapid correction of hypovolemia. Cardiogenic shock typically occurs early in the course of an AMI, with a median time of about 7 h from the onset after symptoms to the recognition of shock. Although a small minority may present to the emergency department in shock, it is more likely that a patient may develop signs of shock while in the department. Some factors have been identified as independent predictors of the risk for developing cardiogenic shock after AMI: advanced age, female gender, large myocardial infarction as indicated by marked increases in creatinine kinase (CK), an anterior wall infarction, previous MI, previous congestive heart failure (CHF), multivessel disease, proximal occlusion of the left anterior descending coronary artery, and diabetes mellitus.[7] Increased numbers of risk factors convey greater risk and indirectly reflect a unifying principle: The greater the amount of myocardium at risk, the greater is the probability of developing shock. Early identification of patients at increased risk may reduce the incidence of shock with aggressive strategies for reperfusion. Despite recent major advances in the treatment of acute cardiac conditions and heart failure,

TABLE 29-1 Etiology of Cardiogenic Shock

I. Loss of effective contractility
  A. Acute myocardial infarction
    Loss of critical mass of LV myocardium
    RV pump failure
  B. LV aneurysm
  C. End-stage cardiomyopathy
  D. Myocardial contusion
  E. Acute myocarditis
  F. Global LV dysfunction secondary to toxins/drugs
  G. Dysrhythmia/heart block
II. Mechanical impairments to systemic blood flow
  A. Impairment to LV outflow
    Acute mitral regurgitation due to papillary muscle dysfunction or rupture
    Aortic stenosis
    Hypertrophic obstructive cardiomyopathy
    Aortic dissection with acute aortic insufficiency
    Ventricular septal wall rupture
  B. Impairment to LV inflow
    Mitral stenosis
    Atrial myxoma
    Massive pulmonary embolus
    Ventricular septal wall rupture
    Free-wall rupture leading with tamponade
    Aortic root dissection with tamponade
    Pericardial tamponade

the mortality from cardiogenic shock remains 70 to 90 percent with medical treatment alone.

PATHOPHYSIOLOGY

Although there are many etiologies for cardiogenic shock, most occur from acute left ventricular (LV) infarction (see Table 29-1). While some degree of LV dysfunction occurs with most acute infarcts, once 40 percent of the LV mass is akinetic, clinical evidence of shock is likely to ensue. This amount of LV mass loss need not have occurred with the current AMI, since there may be preexisting impairment from previous infarcts. Therefore, a patient with a past history of infarction may develop cardiogenic shock with a relatively small new MI.

In cases of cardiogenic shock after AMI, the infarct border zone appears irregular with evidence of marginal infarct extension. Myocytes in this border zone demonstrate evidence of various stages of cell death, probably due to inadequate collateral blood flow, which is exacerbated further by hypotension. Areas of focal necrosis develop throughout the right and left ventricles, suggesting widespread coronary vascular pathology and perfusion insufficiency. Resulting hypotension leads to further reduction in coronary perfusion pressure, exacerbating already compromised myocardial oxygen delivery and leading to additional loss of myocardium, additional loss of contractility, additional hypotension, and so on. This process leads to a progressive and rapid cycle of deterioration into irreversible shock. If the patient develops pulmonary edema, the hypoxia and acidosis further diminish contractility.

The severe reduction in cardiac output and the subsequent compensatory mechanisms result in acute oliguria, hepatic failure, gastrointestinal ischemia, anaerobic metabolism, lactic acidosis, and hypoxia. All these further impair myocardial contractility. Salvage of myocardium by preventing infarct extension into the border zone can prevent development of shock. Although loss of LV mass is the major predictor of shock, disease in other coronary arteries, diastolic dysfunction, and arrhythmias can amplify the negative effects of loss of LV mass and produce shock with a loss of myocardium of less than 40 percent.

Many compensatory mechanisms are recruited in the face of an AMI in an effort to maintain cardiac output and tissue perfusion. Initially, the sympathetic nervous system is activated, leading to an increased heart rate and arterial and venoconstriction. The sympathetic activity increases myocardial contractility, which can be visualized as compensatory hyperkinesis in the uninvolved myocardium by echocardiography. When the uninvolved myocardium is fibrotic or blood flow is compromised due to diffuse coronary disease, this compensatory hyperkinesis does not occur. Lack of compensatory hyperkinesis results in increased end-systolic LV volume, increasing the probability of cardiogenic shock. The renin-angiotensin system is activated by the sympathetic stimulation of renal nerves and the inadequate perfusion pressure. Increased angiotensin II activity leads to peripheral vasoconstriction and aldosterone synthesis, causing sodium and water retention and increasing blood volume. When these compensatory actions are inadequate or overwhelmed, shock may ensue.

Right ventricular (RV) infarction can occur in up to 50 percent of inferior wall infarctions. Although hypotension is not uncommon with RV infarction, shock is much less common, accounting for only 3 to 4 percent of the cases of cardiogenic shock. The major determinate of shock with RV infarction is the presence of concomitant LV dysfunction. With decreased LV contractility, the normal systolic septal function of aiding the RV to perfuse the pulmonary bed is impaired. This leads to loss of LV preload, hypotension, and a further decrease in coronary perfusion pressure.

Hemodynamic assessment of patients with AMI has disclosed four profiles based on measurement of cardiac output (either decreased or not) and LV preload (either elevated or not):

Class I: Normal cardiac output and LV preload. Infarction is tolerated without significant hemodynamic impairment; the prognosis is very good, with about a 3 percent mortality rate.

Class II: Normal cardiac output but elevated LV preload. Pulmonary edema is usually evident on clinical examination. Vasodilation and diuresis result in clinical improvement. Overall mortality is approximately 9 percent.

Class III: Decreased cardiac output but normal LV preload. There is relative or absolute volume deficiency. Cardiac output can be improved by volume infusions that increase stroke volume utilizing the Frank-Starling relationship. Overall mortality is about 23 percent.

Class IV: Decreased cardiac output and an elevated LV preload. Clinical shock is present. Overall mortality is 50 percent or greater.

Patients with occult cardiogenic shock may be clinically indistinguishable from those with stable end-stage CHF.[8] Patients at risk appear to be those with CHF duration greater than 3 months and known decreased ejection fraction of less than 30 percent.

CLINICAL FEATURES

The patient with evolving cardiogenic shock often will exhibit a rapid progression of findings indicating poor perfusion. Clinical evaluation, diagnostic testing, and treatment are initiated simultaneously. History from the patient is often blunted by the severity of the patient's condition, so family, EMS personnel, and medical records should supplement the patient's history. Key information includes current medications, allergies, and past history of MI, CHF, diabetes mellitus, and renal failure. Although the patient may experience chest pain, ischemic equivalents include profound weakness, shortness of breath, or a feeling of impending doom.

The hallmark of shock is hypoperfusion, often, but not always, accompanied by hypotension. The systolic blood pressure is typically less than 90 mmHg, although it may be within a "normal" range, especially if the patient has preexisting hypertension. Another blood pressure parameter that may be more sensitive is a 30 mmHg decrease in mean blood pressure or a pulse pressure (systolic-diastolic) of less than 20 mmHg. Although a compensatory sinus tachycardia is common and does not require specific treatment, excessively high or low heart rates do require immediate therapy. Compensatory sympathetic stimulation leads to cool and clammy skin. Oliguria reflects development of poor renal perfusion. Diminishing cerebral perfusion and hypoxemia lead to anxiety and confusion.

Signs of acute LV failure accompanied by pulmonary edema are tachypnea, rales, wheezing, and frothy sputum. The presence of jugular venous distension in the face of hypotension without signs of pulmonary edema suggest acute RV failure, from either RV infarction, tamponade, or pulmonary embolus. Careful cardiac examination is needed to identify an S_3 or S_4. Mitral regurgitation due to chordae tendinae rupture will exhibit a soft holosystolic murmur at the apex radiating to the axilla, although the murmur is often obscured by rales. Mitral regurgitation due to papillary muscle dysfunction usually will not be completely holosystolic. It starts with the first heart sound but terminates before the second. Acute septal rupture (acute ventricular septal defect) initially will have a loud parasternal ejection murmur, often with a palpable thrill, that decreases in intensity as the intraventricular pressures equalize.

DIAGNOSIS

Although the diagnosis of cardiogenic shock can be suspected from the initial history and physical examination, ancillary tests are essential for confirmation, to define the specific causes, and to direct therapy. Findings of an AMI on the standard 12-lead electrocardiograph (ECG) support the diagnosis of cardiogenic shock. In cases of an inferior wall infarction, patients at risk to develop cardiogenic shock will have ST-segment elevation in the right-sided precordial leads, ST-segment depression in the left precordial leads, or third-degree heart block. Diffuse ST-T changes can be seen with acute myocarditis. The absence of ECG changes consistent with AMI suggests alternate causes of shock, such as aortic dissection, pulmonary embolus, pericardial tamponade, acute valvular insufficiency, hemorrhage, or sepsis.

The chest radiograph (usually an anteroposterior view obtained with a portable machine) should be inspected for evidence of pulmonary vascular congestion: Kerley-B lines, cephalization, interstitial edema, or frank pulmonary edema. A large heart size suggests prior CHF, and a globular cardiac shape provides a clue for chronic pericardial effusion. A wide mediastinum may indicate aortic dissection.

Baseline laboratory studies are of little immediate diagnostic value but provide a hematologic and metabolic assessment of the patient. The severity of tissue hypoperfusion is reflected in the degree of metabolic acidosis, as measured by arterial blood gases, serum bicarbonate, or serum lactate. Serum markers of myocardial injury support the clinical and ECG evidence: CK-MB, troponin I, and troponin T.

The best bedside diagnostic tool available for differentiating the causes of cardiogenic shock is the two-dimensional transthoracic echocardiogram (TTE). This imaging modality can reveal signs of myocardial pump failure by detecting regional hypokinetic, akinetic, or dyskinetic abnormalities. The TTE can detect early signs of distress by visualizing lack of compensatory hyperkinesis in uninvolved segments, which can alert the clinician to take steps to prevent further loss of myocardium, initiate inotropic support, and consult the invasive cardiologist. The TTE also can evaluate other causes of decreased cardiac output. The presence of acute RV dilatation, tricuspid insufficiency, paradoxical systolic septal motion, and high estimated pulmonary artery and right ventricular pressures suggest pulmonary hypertension, often seen with acute pulmonary embolus. Loss of RV contractility, RV dilatation, and normal estimated pulmonary pressures are observed more commonly with RV infarction. Use of the color flow Doppler can easily diagnose acute valvular stenosis or insufficiency, as well as septal and free wall rupture. Pericardial effusion with collapse of the right atrium or diastolic right ventricle collapse indicates cardiac tamponade. Although not the best imaging modality for aortic dissection, TTE sometimes can visualize dissection of the aortic root.

Although more often done in the intensive care unit than in the emergency department, invasive hemodynamic monitoring with a pulmonary artery catheter can provide confirmatory information and guide treatment. As noted earlier, patients with cardiogenic shock have decreased cardiac output (defined as a cardiac index <2.2 L/min/m^2) and elevated LV preload (defined as a pulmonary artery occlusion or wedge pressure >18 mmHg). Because of impaired tissue oxygen delivery with continued metabolic need, there is an elevated oxygen extraction (arterial-venous oxygen content difference >5.5 mL/dL), and blood returning back to the heart is low in oxygen (pulmonary artery oxygen saturation <60 percent or partial pressure less than 30 mmHg). Continuous hemodynamic monitoring and treatment are facilitated by using both (1) a balloon-tipped pulmonary artery catheter with continuous oximetry and cardiac output monitoring and (2) an arterial catheter for pressure measurements. There is a fair correlation between clinical and hemodynamic assessments of cardiac output and LV preload during an AMI, but the overlaps between the different classes limit therapy based solely on clinical criteria.

Noninvasive hemodynamic monitoring by a variety of techniques shows promise, but the currently available devices lack sufficient accuracy for clinical use where important therapeutic decisions require precise measurement.

TREATMENT

In the prehospital setting, the medical control physician should consider directing the patient suspected to be in cardiogenic shock to a facility that has an intraaortic balloon pump, 24-h emergency percutaneous transluminal coronary angioplasty (PTCA), and emergent coronary artery bypass graft (CABG) capabilities.

In both the prehospital and emergency department setting, monitoring should begin immediately: oxygen, intravenous access, cardiac monitor, and continuous pulse oximetry. When detected, hypoxia, hypovolemia, rhythm disturbances, electrolyte abnormalities, and acid-base alterations should be corrected. In the setting of an AMI, aspirin should be given unless the patient is allergic or has an absolute contraindication. Pain control can be attempted judiciously using intravenous nitroglycerin or morphine sulfate with attentive concern for maintaining the systemic blood pressure. In the absence of evidence for pulmonary edema, careful boluses of normal saline (100–250 mL) should be administered. As noted earlier, some patients with AMI and hypotension have a degree of relative or absolute volume deficiency and benefit from fluid administration. In a RV infarct with hypotension, fluid support is the first action. Oral tracheal intubation is often necessary to maintain oxygenation and ventilation, but the change to positive-pressure ventilation may further decrease preload and cardiac output. Alternatively, continuous positive airway pressure can be used in selected patients with a reduction in the need for intubation and a trend toward decreased mortality.[9]

In the absence of profound hypotension, dobutamine is a mainstay of initial pharmacologic treatment.[10,11] This sympathomimetic agent improves myocardial contractility and augments diastolic coronary blood flow without inducing excessive tachycardia. Usually, cardiac output increases and LV filling pressures decrease. Infusions should be started at 2.5 to 5.0 μg/kg per minute, titrating at 2.5 μg/kg per minute increments to achieve the desired effect. Increases should be stopped at 15 μg/kg per minute. With profound hypotension (systolic pressure <70 mmHg), dopamine is preferred, either as a single agent or in combination with dobutamine. Dopamine is started at 2.5 to 5.0 μg/kg per minute and titrated to desired effect. The lowest possible dose of dopamine should be used because this agent can produce excessive tachycardia, increase myocardial oxygen demands, and induce arrhythmias. When shock persists despite use of these agents, mechanical inotropic support with an intraaortic balloon pump is required.[12,13]

The intraaortic balloon pump can temporarily stabilize the hemodynamics in cardiogenic shock.[12,13] It decreases afterload and augments diastolic pressure and coronary perfusion, resulting in decreased myocardial work. It is only temporizing and does not improve survival without successful revascularization of the culprit coronary artery or surgical correction of an acute mechanical catastrophe.[13,14] If a patient requires transfer for surgical therapy, the balloon pump can be used to support the patient during transport.

Limiting infarction size with reperfusion is the key to successful therapy of cardiogenic shock. Although early use of fibrinolytic therapy in AMI has been shown to markedly decrease morbidity and mortality, once cardiogenic shock has developed, the mortality rate remains high, at about 75 percent. One reason for the high mortality despite the use of fibrinolytics is that documented clot lysis in the infarct-related artery and reperfusion in cases of cardiogenic shock is only 40 to 50 percent with these agents. Another reason is that shock combined with the existence of multivessel disease limits the effectiveness of these agents. Thus, while fibrinolytic agents are successful in preventing cardiogenic shock in AMI, they have much less benefit once shock has developed.

A number of nonrandomized trials have reported relatively good mortality rates as low as 30 percent with primary PTCA in conjunction with balloon pump support for patients in cardiogenic shock. Although these results await confirmation by randomized trials, PTCA, if available within 60 minutes, appears to be the reperfusion modality of choice for patients who present with or develop cardiogenic shock in the emergency department.[5,13] Conversely, in hospitals without PCTA immediately available, fibrinolytics should be administered as soon as possible.

Emergent CABG also has been reported to decrease mortality in cardiogenic shock. However, the extensive surgical and medical resources required, as well as the operative risk for these seriously ill patients, have limited its use. For patients who develop a mechanical complication of infarction (e.g., ventricular septal rupture or acute mitral insufficiency) with cardiogenic shock, temporary inotropic support with the intraaortic balloon pump followed by early surgical repair produces the best outcome.

Acute RV failure leading to cardiogenic shock may occur with RV infarction. Although attempts to reverse hypotension should begin with rapid infusion of normal saline, dobutamine should be started if no improvement is observed after 1 L. As with LV infarction, early reperfusion is essential.

Acute mitral valve insufficiency accounts for about 8 percent of cases of cardiogenic shock and can be suspected at the bedside in the face of sudden hypotension, pulmonary edema, and a holosystolic apical murmur. Hemodynamic support can be initiated with dobutamine and nitroprusside to support contractility and provide afterload reduction to promote forward systemic blood flow. The intraaortic balloon pump is also beneficial for temporary support. Acute septal rupture accounts for about 4 percent of cases of cardiogenic shock and is treated with dobutamine, nitroprusside, and the intraaortic balloon pump. Confirmatory evidence for these emergent conditions with two-dimensional echocardiography should be sought concomitant with emergency notification of the cardiac surgical team.

Clearly, not all patients may benefit from aggressive care. The decision to perform or withhold therapies should be made in light of the patient's desires and wishes. Factors that may influence the decision to pursue aggressive therapy include advanced age, diminished functional status, and comorbid conditions.

REFERENCES

1. Alpert JS, Becker RC: Cardiogenic shock: Elements of etiology, diagnosis and therapy. *Clin Cardiol* 16:182, 1993.
2. Barry WI, Sarembock IJ: Cardiogenic shock: Therapy and prevention. *Clin Cardiol* 21:72, 1998.
3. Califf RM, Bengtson JR: Cardiogenic shock. *N Engl J Med* 330:1724, 1994.
4. Grella RD, Becker RC: Cardiogenic shock complicating coronary artery disease: Diagnosis, treatment, and management. *Curr Probl Cardiol* 19:693, 1994.
5. Moscucci M, Bates ER: Cardiogenic shock. *Cardiol Clin* 13:391, 1995.
6. Rodgers KG: Cardiovascular shock. *Emerg Med Clinics North Am* 13:793, 1995.
7. Peterson ED, Shaw LJ, Califf RM: Risk stratification after myocardial infarction. *Ann Intern Med* 126:561, 1997.
8. Ander DS, Jaggi M, Rivers E, et al: Undetected cardiogenic shock in patients with congestive heart failure presenting to the emergency department. *Am J Cardiol* 82:888, 1998.
9. Pang D, Keenan SP, Cook DJ, Sibbald WJ: The effect of positive pressure airway support on mortality and the need for intubation in cardiogenic pulmonary edema: A systematic review. *Chest* 114:1185, 1998.
10. Chernow B: New advances in the pharmacologic approach to circulatory shock. *J Clin Anesth* 8:67S, 1996.
11. McGhie AI, Goldstein RA: Pathogenesis and management of acute heart failure and cardiogenic shock: Role of inotropic therapy. *Chest* 102(suppl 2):671S, 1992.
12. Anderson RD, Ohman EM, Holmes DR, et al: Use of intra-aortic balloon counterpulsation in patients presenting with cardiogenic shock: Observations from the GUSTO-1 study. *J Am Coll Cardiol* 30:708, 1997.
13. Webb JG: Interventional management of cardiogenic shock. *Can J Cardiol* 14:233, 1998.
14. Berger PB, Holmes DR, Stebbins AL, et al: Impact of aggressive invasive catheterization and revascularization strategy on mortality in patients with cardiogenic shock in the Global Utilization of Streptokinase and Tissue Plasminogen Activator for Occluded Coronary Arteries (GUSTO-1) trial: An observational study. *Circulation* 96:122, 1997.

30 ANAPHYLAXIS AND ACUTE ALLERGIC REACTIONS

Shaheed I. Koury
Lee U. Herfel

Anaphylaxis, a term used inconsistently in the literature, is a severe systemic hypersensitivity reaction characterized by either hypotension or airway compromise that is potentially life threatening in nature and that is caused by chemical and IgE mediators released from mast cells. *Anaphylactoid* was coined to describe responses clinically identical to anaphylaxis that were found to be non-IgE mediated and that did not require a sensitizing exposure.[1] Recent work has shown that the final pathway in "classic" anaphylactic and anaphylactoid reactions is identical, and *anaphylaxis* is now used to refer to both IgE and non-IgE reactions.[2] Hypersensitivity is an exaggerated immune system response to presented antigens. Anaphylaxis lies at one end of a gradient of hypersensitivity reactions, and it is important to keep in mind that even apparently mild allergic reactions may progress to severe anaphylaxis.

EPIDEMIOLOGY

Neither age, occupation, race, gender, nor geographic factors have been shown to increase the risk of anaphylaxis.[3] Most studies indicate that atopic individuals (sufferers of asthma, allergic rhinitis, atopic dermatitis, etc.) are at no greater risk for anaphylaxis from insect stings or drugs reactions than are nonatopic individuals.[1] Atopy is a risk factor, however, for idiopathic anaphylaxis.[4] The only other factors known to increase the risk of anaphylaxis are a previous exposure to a sensitizing antigen and a previous anaphylactic reaction. Notably, anaphylaxis recurrence risks are not 100 percent for reexposure. The reoccurrence rate is 40 to 60 percent for insect stings, 20 to 40 percent for radiocontrast agents, and 10 to 20 percent for penicillin.[1]

Limited data are available on the incidence and prevalence of anaphylaxis. The rate of fatal anaphylaxis is approximately 4 deaths per 10 million people per year.[5] The incidence of allergic reactions and anaphylaxis in one study at a university hospital emergency department was 0.5 percent (5 per 1000) and 0.02 percent (2 per 10,000) of the total emergency department population, respectively.[6] The most common causes of serious anaphylaxis are antibiotics, such as penicillin, and radiocontrast agents.[1] Penicillin is estimated to cause 100 to 500 deaths in the United States annually, with a systemic allergic reaction occurring in 1 per 10,000 exposures.[3] *Hymenoptera* stings constitute the next most common cause of anaphylaxis, with fewer than 100 deaths in the United States annually.[1] Table 30-1 contains a partial list of some of the more common causative agents.

PATHOPHYSIOLOGY

Allergic or hypersensitivity reactions vary from localized pruritus to anaphylactic shock and death. The basic mechanism underlying allergic reactions is mast cell degranulation and mediator release.[7] The causes of mast cell degranulation include IgE cross-linking, complement activation, nonimmunologic or direct activation, modulation of arachadonic acid metabolism, exercise, catamenial effects, and idiopathic causes.[7,8]

Hypersensitivity has traditionally been divided into four types by Coombs and Gell. Type I hypersensitivity is mediated by IgE and IgG and involves cross-linking of two adjacent IgE molecules on a mast cell or basophil. Type II hypersensitivity is the reaction of IgG and IgM to cell-surface antigens, resulting in complement activation and killer-cell phagocytosis. Type III involves soluble antigen-antibody complexes that activate the complement system. Type IV is mediated

TABLE 30-1 Common Causes of Anaphylaxis and Anaphylactoid and Allergic Reactions

DRUGS
Penicillin and related antibiotics
Aspirin
Trimethoprim-sulfamethoxazole
Vancomycin
Nonsteroidal anti-inflammatory agents
FOODS AND ADDITIVES
Shellfish
Soybeans
Nuts
Wheat
Milk
Eggs
Monosodium glutamate
Nitrates and nitrites
Tartrazine dyes
OTHER
Hymenoptera stings
Insect parts and molds
Radiographic contrast material

by activated T lymphocytes and has not been mentioned in the literature in relation to anaphylaxis.[9] Research has shown that there is much overlapping among the types and has identified mechanisms that do not fit into the system. Therefore, the classification is for the most part not used in the current literature.

The "classic" anaphylaxis (type I hypersensitivity) pathway involves the production of IgE and requires two separate exposures to either an antigen or a hapten-protein antigenic complex. An antigen is a molecule, usually a protein, that can stimulate the immune system. Haptens are molecules, such as penicillin, that are too small to stimulate the immune system unless they are bound to endogenous proteins (e.g., albumin), resulting in an antigenic complex large enough to be recognized.[9]

Antigens are internalized by antigen-presenting (macrophages and dendritic cells), processed, and then presented externally on the cell surface bound to the major histocompatibility (MHC) 2 complex. T-helper cells recognize the antigen-MHC 2 complex and subsequently induce specific B lymphocytes to undergo proliferation and differentiation to plasma cells. These plasma cells produce and release IgE antibody into the bloodstream. The IgE antibody (like all antibodies) has a variable and a constant region. The variable region is specific for the antigen that initiated the immune response, and the constant region binds to IgE receptors present in vast quantities on mast cells (and basophils), resulting in mast cells covered with antigen-specific IgE molecules. This sensitizing process takes days to weeks, resulting in a latent period during which no clinical response to antigen occurs. After the latent period, on antigen reexposure the variable regions on the IgE bind the antigen, resulting in bridging of adjacent IgE molecules on the mast cell surface. This IgE-antigen-IgE bridging results in activation of serine proteases, a rise in intracellular cyclic AMP and calcium levels, new mediator synthesis, and mast cell degranulation with release of preformed chemical mediators.[3] Examples of IgE-mediated reaction triggers include antibiotics, foods, and *Hymenoptera* stings.

Complement-mediated anaphylactic reactions occur after the administration of blood products secondary to the formation of immune complexes. Immune complex formation results in activation of the complement pathway and formation of the anaphylatoxins C3a and C5a, which cause mast-cell and basophil degranulation.[7,8] Immune complexes include IgG aggregates and IgA-IgG from human immunoglobin therapy, and IgE-IgA complexes formed in selective IgA-deficient patients (1 : 600 people) who have been given blood products repeatedly.[7] Administration of mismatched blood also causes complement activation secondary to the production of IgG and IgM antibodies against transfused red blood cells, resulting in cell lysis, agglutination, anaphylatoxin generation, and subsequent anaphylaxis. This is an example of a cytotoxic type II reaction.[7]

Nonimmunologic anaphylaxis occurs when an exogenous substance results in mast-cell degranulation either by direct stimulation of the mast cell or by unknown mechanisms. These reactions have been referred to as anaphylactoid reactions.[1,7] Substances that cause anaphylactoid reactions include radiocontrast dyes, muscular depolarizing drugs, narcotics, and dextrans. The mechanism of radiocontrast reactions is uncertain but is believed to be caused by the activation of the complement, contact, and coagulation systems. Since the advent of nonionic contrast dyes, the incidence of reactions has decreased. Narcotics and neuromuscular depolarizing drugs cause direct release of mediators from mast cells, although there is little documentation of generalized reactions.[7]

Aspirin and other nonsteroidal drugs cause anaphylactic symptoms by a non-mast-cell process. The mechanism is not precisely known but is thought to involve modulation of the cyclooxygenase-arachidonic acid metabolism pathway. Five to 10 percent of asthmatics have these reactions, which include bronchospasm, bronchorrhea, rhinorrhea, and, rarely, hypotension. Nonasthmatics may experience urticaria, angioedema, and hypotension.[7]

Idiopathic anaphylaxis is by definition of unknown cause. Patients suffer recurrent attacks, with no trigger identified after extensive evaluation by an allergist. They often need prolonged treatment with alternate-day prednisone to maintain remission from attacks.[4] A rare subset of anaphylaxis is catamenial, or menstrual, anaphylaxis. The patient has repeated attacks, often coinciding with the luteal phase of menstruation due to hypersensitivity to endogenous progesterone. Treatment is with medical ovarian suppression by either luteinizing-hormone-releasing-hormone agonists or oophorectomy.

Concurrent use of β-blocking drugs by the patient is a risk factor for severe prolonged anaphylaxis. In one study, three out of five patients who had severe protracted reactions were being treated with β-blocking drugs. Furthermore, they were the only patients in the study who were taking β blockers out of the 67 anaphylactic patients in the study.[6] Use of epinephrine in patients taking β blockers may result in severe hypertension secondary to unopposed α-adrenergic stimulation.[1] β blockers should be discontinued in any patient with new-onset anaphylaxis and should not be prescribed for any patient with a history of anaphylaxis.[3] As would be expected, asthmatics are often more refractory to the treatment of allergic bronchospasm.[1]

CLINICAL FEATURES

Anaphylaxis is the most severe life-threatening form of a systemic allergic reaction involving respiratory or cardiovascular compromise. The clinician must keep in mind that even mild, localized urticaria can progress to full anaphylaxis and death. The clinical signs of systemic allergic reactions include urticaria, angioedema, abdominal pain or cramping, nausea, vomiting, diarrhea, bronchospasm, rhinorrhea, conjunctivitis, dysrhythmias, and/or hypotension.[3] Anaphylaxis can include any combination of these signs along with hypotension or airway compromise. Dermatologic manifestations of pruritus and urticaria are the most common initial symptoms. The "classic" presentation of anaphylaxis begins with pruritus, cutaneous flushing, and urticaria. These symptoms are followed by a sense of fullness in the throat, anxiety, a sensation of chest tightness, shortness of breath, lightheadedness, and finally loss of consciousness.[5] A complaint of a "lump in the throat" and hoarseness heralds life-threatening laryngeal edema in a patient with symptoms of anaphylaxis.

In the vast majority of patients, signs and symptoms begin within 60 min after exposure. In general, the faster the onset of symptoms, the more severe the reaction, as evidenced by the fact that one-half of anaphylactic fatalities occur within the first hour.[10] After the initial signs and symptoms have abated, patients are at risk for a recurrence of symptoms. This biphasic phenomenon occurs in 3 to 20 percent of patients.[6] The effect is caused by a second phase of mediator release, peaking 4 to 8 h after the initial exposure and exhibiting itself clinically 3 to 4 h after the initial clinical manifestations have cleared. The pathophysiology of this phenomenon is poorly understood.[6]

DIAGNOSIS

The diagnosis of anaphylaxis is by history and physical examination, and is easily made with a clear history of exposure, such as a bee sting, shortly followed by the multisystemic signs and symptoms described above. Unfortunately, diagnosis is not always so evident. Symptom onset is delayed over an hour in a small percentage of cases.[3] Often, such as in food allergy, the inciting substance may not be known. The differential diagnosis of anaphylactic reactions is extensive, including vasovagal reactions, myocardial ischemia, arrhythmias, status asthmaticus, seizure, epiglottitis, hereditary angioedema, foreign-body airway obstruction, carcinoid, mastocytosis, and drug reactions.[1] The most common anaphylaxis imitator is a vasovagal reaction, which is characterized by hypotension, pallor, bradycardia, diaphoresis, weakness, and sometimes syncope.[3]

Laboratory values have essentially no role in making the diagnosis. Histamine levels are elevated for 5 to 30 min postreaction and thus are usually in decline by presentation to the emergency department.[3] Tryptase is a neutral protease of unknown function in anaphylaxis that is found only in mast-cell granules and is released with degranulation. Serum tryptase levels are elevated for several hours and are useful for research purposes for later confirmation of an anaphylactic episode.[1]

TREATMENT

Emergency Treatment

The patient having an anaphylactic reaction, as defined by airway compromise or hypotension, is a true medical emergency and must be rapidly assessed and treated. Exposure to the causative agent, if identified, must be terminated if ongoing. Vital signs, intravenous (IV) access, oxygen, cardiac monitoring, and pulse oximetry measurements should be ordered immediately. Securing the airway is the first priority. The airway should be examined for angioedema. If angioedema is producing respiratory distress, the patient should be intubated immediately, since delay may result in complete airway obstruction secondary to progression of angioedema. An endotracheal tube one or more sizes smaller than normal may be needed.[10] The patient should be given sufficient oxygen to maintain a pulse oximetry value greater than 92%. Intubation is indicated if hypoxemia is refractory to 100% oxygen therapy.

Epinephrine is the cornerstone of treatment for anaphylactic reactions. If the patient has severe bronchospasm, laryngeal edema, signs of upper airway obstruction, respiratory arrest, or signs of shock, IV epinephrine is indicated.[10] Initially, 100 μg of IV epinephrine should be given in a 1:100,000 dilution. This can be done by placing 0.1 mL of 1:1000 epinephrine in 10 mL of normal saline solution (NS) and infusing it over 5 to 10 min (a rate of 1 to 2 mL/min).[2,11] If the patient is refractory to the initial bolus, then an epinephrine infusion can be started, according to the 1997 Advanced Cardiac Life Support (ACLS) guidelines, by placing 1 mg of 1:1000 epinephrine in 500 mL of dextrose in water (D_5W) or NS and running at a rate of 1 to 4 μg/min (0.5 to 2 mL/min), titrating to effect. The pediatric epinephrine infusion rate starts at 0.1 μg/kg/min and can be increased up to 1.5 μg/kg/min.[11] If hypotension is present, the patient should receive a NS bolus of 1 to 2 L concurrently with the epinephrine infusion. For hypotension refractory to 2 L NS infusion and epinephrine, colloid infusion should be considered. Physicians are often hesitant to give IV epinephrine due to its side effects. It should be stressed that the initial adult dose is 100 μg (0.1 mg) IV of 1:100,000 dilution given over 5 to 10 min and that the dose can be stopped immediately if arrhythmias or chest pain occurs.

For less severe signs, such as decreasing blood pressure without hypotension [systolic blood pressure (SBP) $>$ 90 mmHg], symptomatic dyspnea, abdominal cramps, and urticaria, subcutaneous (SC) epinephrine can be given.[10] The dose is 0.3 to 0.5 mL of 1:000 epinephrine (pediatric dose 0.01 mL/kg 1:1000) SC, repeated every 5 to 10 min according to response. If the patient is refractory to treatment despite repeated SC epinephrine, then IV epinephrine infusion should be instituted.

The first-line therapies for anaphylaxis are epinephrine, IV fluids, and oxygen, which have immediate effect during the acute stage of anaphylaxis. The second-line drugs are antihistamines, corticosteroids, glucagon, albuterol, and aminophylline. These drugs are used to prevent recurrences and treat anaphylaxis refractory to the first-line treatments. All patients with anaphylaxis should receive corticosteroids and antihistamines. Methylprednisolone 125 mg IV and a histamine$_1$ (H_1) blocker, such as diphenhydramine 25 to 50 mg IV, should be given.[2] Since the histamine$_2$ (H_2) blockers have been shown to be effective in shock refractory to epinephrine, fluids, steroids, and H_1 blockers, it is recommended that H_2 antihistamines be given as well.[2,7] It is the authors' opinion that an H_2 blocker other than cimetidine should be used in anaphylaxis. Cimetidine prolongs metabolism of β blockers, resulting in a possible prolongation of the anaphylactic state in patients who take β blockers. Cimetidine likewise interferes with the metabolism of many other drugs, including aminophylline, which may be used in refractory bronchospasm. After the initial IV dose of steroids and antihistamines, the patient may be switched to oral medication (Table 30-2).

If wheezing or tightness is part of the patient's presentation, a bronchodilator, such as a continuous albuterol nebulizer, should be instituted. For severe bronchospasm refractory to the above-mentioned treatments, aminophylline can be added. The dose should be 5 mg/kg IV over 30 min, with a lower rate for elderly patients, patients taking cimetidine or erythromycin, and patients with cardiac or liver failure.[2]

For patients taking β blockers with hypotension refractory to fluids and epinephrine, glucagon should be used in a dose of 1 mg IV every 5 min until hypotension resolves, followed by an infusion of 5 to 15 μg/min.[2] The side effects of glucagon include nausea, vomiting, hypokalemia, dizziness, and hyperglycemia.

For minor allergic reactions that do not involve hypotension or respiratory symptoms, epinephrine is not needed. The causative agent should be identified and discontinued. The patient may be given oral (PO), intramuscular (IM), or IV diphenhydramine 25 to 50 mg and observed for a response for at least 1 h.[10] If the patient is stable, he or she can be discharged on an antihistamine and prednisone 20 mg bid or 40 mg qd for 4 days.[2]

TABLE 30-2 Anaphylaxis and Allergic Reactions Drug Dosing

Drug	Adult Dose	Pediatric Dose
Epinephrine	IV single dose: 100 μg of 1:100,000 IV over 5–10 min IV infusion: 1–4 μg/min SC: 0.3–0.5 mL 1:1000	IV infusion: 0.1–0.3 μg/kg/min maximum 1.5 μg/kg/min SC: 0.01 mL/kg of 1:1000
IV fluids: NS or LR	1–2 L	20 mL/kg
Diphenhydramine (Benadryl)	25–50 mg q6h IV, IM, or PO	1 mg/kg q6h IV, IM, or PO
Ranitidine (Zantac)	50 mg IV over 5 min	0.5 mg/kg IV over 5 min
Methylprednisolone (Solumedrol)	125 mg IV	1–2 mg/kg IV
Albuterol	Single treatment: 2.5 mg nebulized (0.5 mL 0.5% solution) Continuous nebulization: 5–10 mg/h	Single treatment: 1.25 mg nebulized (0.25 mL 0.5% solution) Continuous nebulization: 3–5 mg/h
Glucagon	1 mg IV q5min until hypotension resolves, followed by 5–15 μg/min infusion	50 μg/kg IV q5min
Aminophylline	5–6 mg/kg IV	5–6 mg/kg IV
Prednisone	40–60 mg/d divided bid or qd	1–2 mg/d divided bid or qd

Abbreviations: LR, lactated Ringer's solution.

DISPOSITION

Admission

An unstable patient with anaphylaxis refractory to treatment should be admitted to the intensive care unit. All patients who receive epinephrine should be observed for a minimum of 6 h. If the patient remains symptom free during this time, he or she may be discharged home.[2] Factors to consider in discharge planning include distance from medical care, whether the patient lives alone, significant comorbidity, age, past history of severe reaction, and the use of β-blocking agents.[6]

Outpatient Care

For all allergic reactions, the patient should be instructed on how to eliminate exposure to the causative agent. This may be difficult, especially in the case of food allergy. An adult or pediatric Epi-Pen prescription should be given with clear instructions for serious allergic reactions or anaphylaxis when the risk of another reaction is judged to be substantial. The patient should be referred to an allergist for in-depth preventive management and attempts at allergen identification.[12] Patients with anaphylactic reactions should be encouraged to wear Medic-Alert bracelets. Any anaphylactic patient on a β blocker should be switched to another antihypertensive drug.[1] The patient should be instructed to return immediately if there is any recurrence of symptoms.

URTICARIA AND ANGIOEDEMA

Urticaria, or hives, is a cutaneous IgE-mediated reaction marked by the development of pruritic, erythemic wheals of varying size that generally disappear quickly. Erythema multiforme is a more pronounced urticarial variant, characterized by typical target lesions. Angioedema is believed to be an IgE-mediated reaction characterized by edema formation in the dermis, most generally involving the face and neck. These manifestations may accompany many allergic reactions. As with all allergic manifestations, a detailed history of exposures, ingestions, medications, and infections and a family history should be obtained. If an etiologic agent can be identified, future reactions may be avoided. Treatment of these reactions is generally supportive and symptomatic, with attempts to identify and remove the offending agent. Epinephrine, antihistamines, and steroids are most often tried. Oral antihistamines and steroids for several days may be beneficial. The addition of an H_2 receptor blocker, such as ranitidine, may also be useful in more severe cases. Cold compresses may be soothing to affected areas. Referral to an allergy specialist is indicated.[13]

Angioedema of the tongue, lips, and face occurs in 0.1 to 0.2 percent of patients taking angiotensin-converting enzyme (ACE) inhibitor antihypertensives. Fortunately, most cases are mild and transient. Management is supportive, with special attention to the airway, which can become occluded rapidly and unpredictably. One must anticipate and be prepared for airway problems in any patient who presents with angioedema. Typical allergic-reaction drugs, such as antihistamines and steroids, are not proven to be beneficial due to the pathophysiology of ACE-inhibitor angioedema. Normally, ACE inactivates bradykinin, a potent vasodilator, and converts angiotensin I to angiotensin II, a potent vasoconstrictor. ACE inhibitors therefore allow accumulation of bradykinin and angiotensin I, which leads to vasodilation, hypotension, and angioedema. Also, ACE inhibitor angioedema is not associated with an increase in IgE. For this reason, angioedema is usually refractory to standard medical therapy. Epinephrine, antihistamines, and steroids are still used; however, their benefits have not been clearly demonstrated in the literature. Immediate withdrawal from the ACE inhibitor is indicated, and another antihypertensive should be prescribed as needed. Patients with mild swelling and no evidence of airway obstruction can be observed in the emergency department and discharged if swelling diminishes. Rebound or recurrent swelling will not occur unless the patient takes an ACE inhibitor again. Patients with moderate-to-severe swelling, dysphagia, or respiratory distress are best admitted for close observation.[14,15]

Hereditary angioedema is an autosomal dominant disorder with a characteristic complement pathway deficiency: low levels of C1 esterase inhibitor or elevated levels of dysfunctional C1 esterase inhibitor with low levels of C4 between acute attacks. Reactions often involve the upper respiratory tract and gastrointestinal tract. Attacks can last from a few hours to 1 to 2 days. Minor trauma often precipitates a reaction. Many of the typical treatments of allergic problems, such as epinephrine, steroids, and antihistamines, have been tried, but their effectiveness is not clearly demonstrated.[13] Prophylaxis of acute attacks is possible with attenuated adrogens, such as stanozolol 2 mg/d or danazol 200 mg/d.[16] Acute attacks can be shortened by C1 esterase inhibitor replacement, either by a concentrate or fresh-frozen plasma infusion.[17] Treatment of patients is complex and best done in coordination with the appropriate specialist.

OTHER COMMON ALLERGIC PROBLEMS

Food Allergy

Hypersensitivity reactions to ingested foods are generally due to IgE-mediated reactions to food components or additives. IgE-coated mast cells lining the gastrointestinal tract react to presented allergens in ingested foods and produce clinical findings associated with the release of biologic mediators, as previously described. Non-IgE-mediated food allergy reactions have also been described. Dairy products, eggs, and nuts are some of the most commonly implicated foods.

A detailed history will provide the best clues to food allergy, with particular attention to other allergic history and prior reactions. Diagnosis is often difficult, since the offending food or foods may only occasionally produce symptoms, depending on the amount ingested and other foods present.

Symptoms of food allergy include swelling and itching of the lips, mouth, and pharynx; nausea; abdominal cramps; vomiting; and diarrhea. Cutaneous manifestations, such as angioedema and urticaria, as well as anaphylaxis, can occur. Treatment for mild reactions is supportive, with the administration of antihistamines to lessen symptoms. More severe reactions or anaphylaxis are managed as previously described. Referral to an allergy specialist is indicated.[3,7,13]

Insect Sting Allergy

Insect stings can produce significant and sometimes fatal reactions, particularly in sensitized patients. Approximately 100 patients die annually from insect sting reactions, making insect sting the second most common cause of fatal anaphylaxis. True stinging insects belong to the order *Hymenoptera,* which includes three families: *Apoidea* (honeybee), *Formicoidea* (fire ants), and *Vespidae* (wasps, yellow jackets, and hornets). The venoms of each family are unique, although all have similar types of components, mostly proteins. This difference accounts for the limited cross-reactivity seen. The usual reaction to these stings includes localized pain, pruritus, swelling, and redness. Sensitized individuals may have exaggerated local reactions with or without systemic manifestations. Systemic reactions run from mild nausea and malaise to urticaria, angioedema, or anaphylaxis.

Diagnosis depends on clinical history, with particular attention to past reactions, and an examination to locate the site of the sting. Occasionally, the site of envenomization is overlooked, and predominance of reaction in one organ system can lead to misdiagnosis.

Treatment is symptomatic and supportive. Mild local reactions can be managed with application of ice and oral antihistamines. More generalized reactions or local reactions of the head and neck may benefit from a short steroid course. Severe reactions are managed as outlined under ''Treatment'' above. Patients with severe reactions should be advised to carry self-administered epinephrine and antihistamines. A referral to an allergy specialist is indicated.[1,3,7,13]

Drug Allergy

Although adverse reactions to drugs are a common clinical problem, true immunologically mediated hypersensitivity reactions probably account for less than 10 percent of these problems. Since most drugs are small organic molecules, they are generally unable to stimulate the immune system alone. However, when a drug or metabolite becomes protein bound, either in serum or on cell surfaces, the drug-protein complex can become an allergen and stimulate immune system responses. Thus, the ability of a drug or its metabolites to sensitize the immune system depends on the ability to be bound to tissue proteins. Approximately 100 to 500 patients die yearly of anaphylactic drug reactions. Penicillin is the drug most commonly implicated in eliciting true allergic reactions and accounts for approximately 90 percent of all allergic drug reactions. Of those patients who had fatal anaphylactic drug reactions, over 95 percent reacted to penicillin. Only about 25 percent of patients who die of penicillin anaphylaxis had exhibited allergic reactions during previous courses of the drug. Parenterally administered penicillin was more than twice as likely to produce fatal allergic reactions as orally administered penicillin.[3,13]

The clinical manifestations of drug allergy are widely varied and can involve all four types of hypersensitivity reactions. A generalized reaction similar to immune-complex or serum-sickness reactions is very common. Beginning usually in the first or second week after the administration of the drug, this reaction may take many weeks to subside after drug withdrawal. Generalized malaise, arthralgias, pruritus, urticarial eruptions, and fever are common. Drug fever may occur without other associated clinical findings and may also occur without an immunologic basis. Circulating immune complexes are probably responsible for the lupus-like reactions caused by some drugs. Cytotoxic reactions, such as penicillin-induced hemolytic anemia, can occur. Skin eruptions may include erythema, pruritus, urticaria, angioedema, erythema multiforme, and photosensitivity, and severe reactions, such as those seen in Stevens-Johnson syndrome and toxic epidermal necrolysis, may also occur. Pulmonary complications, including bronchospasm and airway obstruction, can occur. Delayed hypersensitivity reactions may be manifested as a contact dermatitis from drugs applied topically.

Diagnosis is best determined by a careful and thorough history. Treatment is supportive, with oral or parenteral antihistamines, glucocorticoids, and β-adrenergic agents, as discussed above. Immediate drug withdrawal is important; however, reactions can continue or recur after a period of abstinence. Referral to an allergy specialist may be indicated.[13]

REFERENCES

1. Bochner BS, Lichtenstein LM: Anaphylaxis. *N Engl J Med* 324:1785, 1991.
2. Brown AFT: Therapeutic controversies in the management of acute anaphylaxis. *J Accid Emerg Med* 15:89, 1998.
3. Yunginger JW: Anaphylaxis. *Ann Allergy* 69:87, 1992.
4. Ditto AM, Harris KE, Krasnick J, et al: Idiopathic anaphylaxis: A series of 335 cases. *Ann Allergy Asthma Immunol* 77:285, 1996.
5. Friday GA, Fireman P: Anaphylaxis. *ENTJ* 75:21, 1996.
6. Brady WJ, Luber S, Carter CT, et al: Multiphasic anaphylaxis: An uncommon event in the emergency department. *Acad Emerg Med* 4:193, 1997.
7. Atkinson TP, Kaliner MA: Anaphylaxis. *Med Clin North Am* 76:841, 1992.
8. Galli SJ: New concepts about the mast cell. *N Engl J Med* 328:257, 1993.
9. Coombs RRA, Gell PGH: Classification of allergic reactions responsible for clinical hypersensitivity and disease, in Gell PGH, Coombs RRA, Lachmann PJ (eds): *Clinical Aspects of Immunology*, 3d ed. Oxford, Blackwell Scientific, 1975.
10. Gavalas M, Sadana A, Metcalf S: Guidelines for the management of anaphylaxis in the emergency department. *J Accid Emerg Med* 15:96, 1998.
11. Barach EM, Nowak RM, Lee TG, et al: Epinephrine for treatment of anaphylactic shock. *JAMA* 251:2118, 1984.
12. AAAI Board of Directors: Position Statement: The use of epinephrine in the treatment of anaphylaxis. *J Allergy Clin Immuno* 94:666, 1994.
13. Beer DJ, Rocklin RE, David JR: Immunology VII, in *Scientific American Medicine*. New York, Scientific American, 1996.
14. Slater EE, Merrill DD, Guess HA: Clinical profile of angioedema associated with ACE inhibition. *JAMA* 260:967, 1988.
15. Roberts JR, Wuerz RC: Clinical characteristics of angiotensin converting enzyme inhibitor-induced angioedema. *Ann Emerg Med* 20:555, 1991.

16. Cicardi M, Bergamaschini L, Cugno M, et al: Long-term treatment of hereditary angioedema with attenuated adrogens: A survey of a 13-year experience. *J Allergy Clin Immunol* 87:768, 1991.

17. Waytes AT, Rosen FS, Frank MM: Treatment of hereditary angioedema with a vapor-heated C1 inhibitor concentrate. *N Engl J Med* 334:1630, 1996.

NEUROGENIC SHOCK

Brian Euerle
Thomas M. Scalea

Neurogenic shock, characterized by hypotension and bradycardia, occurs after an acute spinal cord injury that disrupts sympathetic outflow, leaving unopposed vagal tone.[1] The term neurogenic shock must be carefully differentiated from another that has a very different meaning—namely, *spinal shock*. Spinal shock refers to the temporary loss of spinal reflex activity that occurs below a total or near total spinal cord injury.[2] These terms are not interchangeable. This chapter focuses on neurogenic shock.

The vast majority of patients who sustain a spinal cord injury are initially evaluated in an emergency department (ED). Although the definitive care of these patients is provided by a variety of specialists, the emergency physician usually performs the initial evaluation, resuscitation, stabilization, and transfer. The patient's prognosis and eventual outcome depend on initial ED care. Early recognition of the potential injury, along with early spinal immobilization, will help prevent any possible worsening of an injury. For high-dose methylprednisolone therapy to be effective, it should be given within 8 h of injury.[3] The search for associated injuries must be done early, often by the emergency physician.

EPIDEMIOLOGY

Acute spinal cord injury is usually due to blunt trauma; penetrating trauma causes only 10 to 15 percent of cases.[1,4] Focusing only on penetrating injuries, the majority are caused by gunshot wounds, with a small minority due to stab wounds.[1] Of the blunt trauma causes, automobile accidents are the most frequent, followed by falls and sports.[4–6] The cervical region is the most commonly injured, followed by the thoracolumbar junction, the thoracic region, and the lumbar segments.[6] The area of the spinal cord injured has important implications for the incidence and severity of neurogenic shock. Approximately 10,000 people sustain spinal cord injury in the United States each year.[6] Because of the long-term care involved with many of these patients, the economic costs are staggering.

PATHOPHYSIOLOGY

The spinal column is composed of 33 bony vertebrae with interspersed cartilaginous intervertebral disks. The typical vertebra consists of an anterior vertebral body and a posterior vertebral arch. These elements form the borders of the vertebral foramen, which contains and protects the spinal cord. The superior and inferior articular processes arising from most vertebrae allow the spine to be a strong yet flexible structure. The pedicles and laminae form the sides of the vertebral arch and are notched to allow for the passage of nerves and blood vessels.

The spinal cord is a cylindrical structure arising at the base of the brain and passing through the skull at the foramen magnum. It is surrounded and protected by three layers of meninges as well as cerebrospinal fluid. Thirty-one pairs of spinal nerves exit the spinal column via the intervertebral foramen. The spinal nerves are formed by the junction of the anterior and posterior nerve roots as they exit from the spinal cord.

The spinal cord consists of both white and gray matter. In general, the white matter is the outer covering of the cord. It contains the nerve fibers running up and down the spinal cord in tracts. The gray matter is made up of nerve cells and is formed in the shape of an H when viewed on cross section (Fig. 31-1).

The autonomic nervous system, which maintains the internal balance of the body's many systems, has two main divisions: the sympathetic and parasympathetic. The sympathetic nervous system activates the "fight or flight" response, increasing the heart rate and blood pressure and constricting arterioles of the skin and intestines in order to redistribute blood flow, preferentially to the brain, heart, and skeletal muscle. The parasympathetic nervous system has the opposite effect, slowing the heart rate, decreasing blood pressure, and increasing the peristaltic activity of the gastrointestinal tract.

The anatomy of the autonomic nervous system is quite complex (Fig. 31-1). The outflow portion of the sympathetic system starts with neuron cell bodies located in the lateral gray horns of the first thoracic to the second lumbar segments. In some cases they may extend to the third lumbar segment. These cells are controlled by the hypothalamus via descending tracts of the reticular formation. The axons from the sympathetic nerve cells in the lateral gray horns leave the spinal cord in the anterior nerve roots and connect to the ganglia of the paraspinal sympathetic trunk. The sympathetic trunk is located along each side of the spinal column and extends along the entire length of the vertebral column. Axons arising from neurons in the sympathetic ganglia then travel throughout the body. The sympathetic fibers that innervate the heart arise primarily from the second to fourth thoracic segments.

The anatomy of the parasympathetic system is very different. The majority of the parasympathetic system is carried along the cranial nerves, although there is a portion that involves the second to fourth sacral segments of the spinal cord. The parasympathetic axons synapse with the cranial nerves in peripheral ganglia close to or within the target organ. The parasympathetic axons from the sacral segments form the pelvic splanchnic nerves. The portion of the parasympathetic system that innervates the heart originates in the dorsal nucleus of the vagus nerve and travels to the heart via the vagus nerves.

In evaluating patients with spinal cord injuries, the concepts of primary and secondary cord injury are important. When the spinal cord is initially injured, the pathologic picture may be relatively benign, showing some scattered hemorrhages and edema.[7] Several weeks later, the appearance is much worse, with large cavities surrounded by gliosis and fibrosis.[7]

These primary or initial changes are caused by the traumatic event, which can cause compression, laceration, or stretching of the cord.[8] Over several days to weeks, the initial injury evolves to what is termed *secondary cord injury*. Spinal cord ischemia has been suggested as the principal etiology of secondary changes, although other mechanisms may exist.[3,8] Ischemia of the spinal cord can be caused by a variety of events. The blood supply to the spinal cord is, in general, not very substantial, and can be easily disrupted by either local trauma to the small anterior and posterior spinal arteries or injury and thrombosis to a large regional vessel, such as the great radicular artery of Adamkiewicz. General systemic hypotension and shock, if severe enough, can cause a low-flow state such that blood flow to the cord is compromised, even with an intact arterial supply.

The clinical relevance of secondary injury is that a patient's presentation can change in the period following the traumatic event. An incomplete lesion can evolve to a complete injury, or the level of injury can become higher because of the cord changes that occur during secondary cord injury.

CLINICAL FEATURES

The initial cardiovascular response after spinal cord injury may include hypertension, widened pulse pressure, and tachycardia.[1] This acute response has been shown experimentally to last from 2 to 3 min.[9] In animal experiments, the hypotension that is characteristic of neuro-

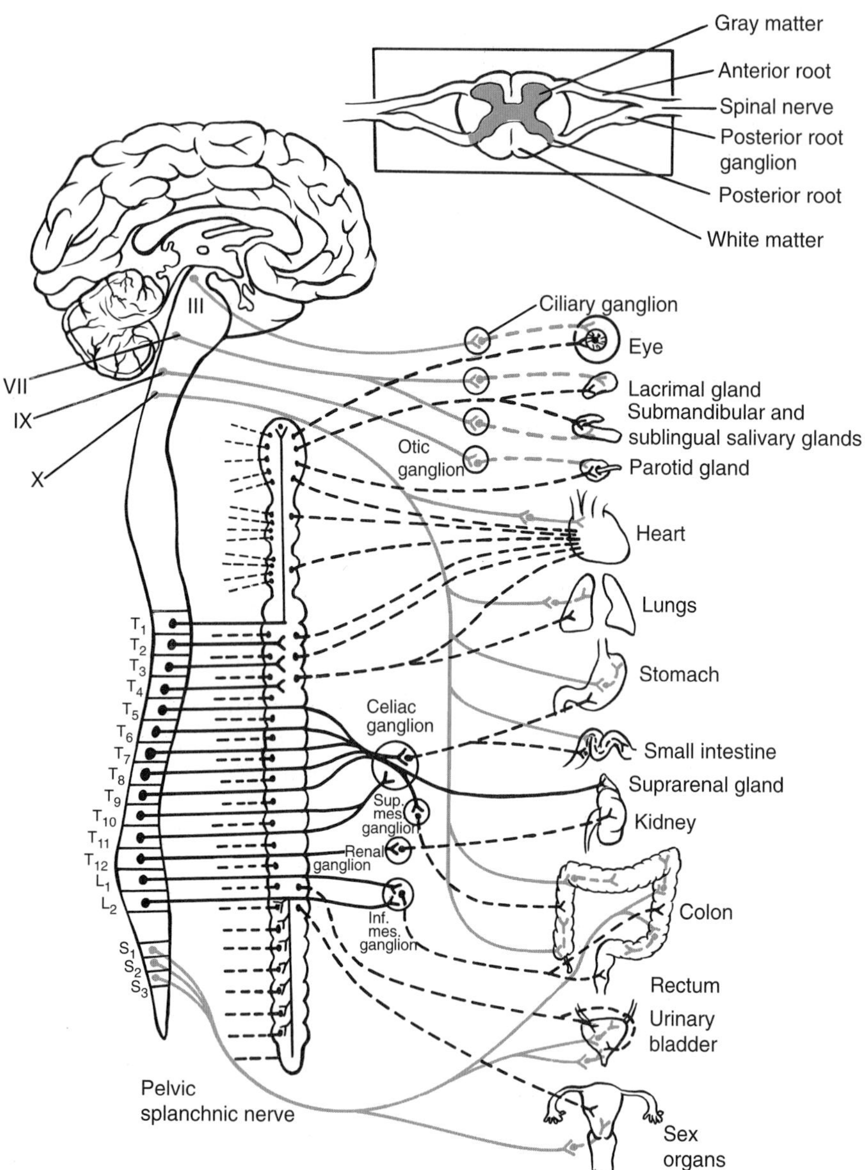

FIG. 31-1. Section of the spinal cord, showing the white and gray matter, spinal roots, and spinal nerve (Adapted with permission from Snell RS: *Clinical Anatomy for Medical Students.* Philadelphia, Lippincott-Raven, 1973, p. 828.), as well as the efferent portion of the autonomic nervous system. (Used with permission from Snell RS: *Clinical Neuroanatomy for Medical Students.* 4th ed. Philadelphia, Lippincott-Raven, 1997, p. 463.)

genic shock generally begins within 5 min of the acute spinal cord injury.[9]

Patients with neurogenic shock are hypotensive and usually have warm, dry skin.[10] Bradycardia is characteristic but not universal. The patient may lose the ability to redirect blood from the periphery to the core because of the loss of sympathetic tone.[10] This can result in excessive loss of heat from the skin, with subsequent hypothermia.[10]

These symptoms of neurogenic shock can be expected to last from 1 to 3 weeks.[10] In some cases, significant rehabilitation using elastic stockings, an abdominal binder, and a tilt table may be required to prevent an orthostatic drop in blood pressure when the patient is placed upright.[11]

The anatomic level of the spinal cord injury influences the likelihood and severity of neurogenic shock. Any injury above T1 should be capable of disrupting the spinal tracts that control the entire sympathetic system. Any injury from T1 to L3 has the potential to partially disrupt the sympathetic outflow; intuitively, the higher the injury in this zone, the more likely or more severe the resulting neurogenic shock.[1] In one of the few studies to quantify this relationship, Zipnick and colleagues described this relationship in five patients with true neurogenic shock resulting from penetrating injuries: two in the cervical region, one in the lumbar region, and one each in the upper and lower thoracic regions.[1]

The question of an incomplete versus a complete spinal cord lesion causing neurogenic shock has also been considered. In a large study of 408 patients with cervical cord/column injuries, Soderstrom and Ducker reported a near equal incidence of neurogenic shock in patients with incomplete versus complete lesions.[12] The explanation for this is not entirely clear. Guha and Tator, working with an acute spinal cord injury model in rats, have suggested that the decline in cardiac output following acute cord injury is not due to decreased sympathetic tone alone but may also be caused by direct myocardial injury, similar to that seen after head injury or subarachnoid hemorrhage.[9]

An interesting difference has been found with regard to incidence of neurogenic shock between patients with blunt versus penetrating spinal cord injuries.[1] In a study of patients with blunt cervical spine/cord injury, neurogenic shock alone was believed to be responsible in 69 percent of all patients in shock.[5] In Zipnick's study of patients with penetrating spinal injury at various anatomic levels, neurogenic shock was thought to be responsible in only 22 percent of patients in shock.[1] The reason for the difference is unclear but probably related to the fact that the two groups were not equivalent: blunt trauma patients had only cervical injuries, while the penetrating injury patients had injuries at all levels of the spinal cord. Also, part of the difference may stem from the fact that patients with penetrating trauma are more likely to have associated injuries.

TREATMENT

Evaluation and treatment of patients with spinal injury and neurogenic shock starts with the ''ABCDEs'' of trauma assessment: the ''A'' is not only for airway but also includes cervical spine protection, and the ''D'' represents disability, or neurologic evaluation[13] (Table 31-1). Cervical spine protection and neurologic evaluation are not discussed further here except to say that they form the cornerstone of all further management of patients with neurogenic shock.

It is impossible to separate the initial evaluation and management of the patient with neurogenic shock from that of the general trauma patient. In essence, the diagnosis of neurogenic shock should be one of exclusion. Certain clues—such as bradycardia and warm, dry skin—may be evident, but hypotension in the trauma patient can never be presumed to be due to neurogenic shock until all other possible sources of hypotension have been eliminated.[1] Again, a difference has been noted between blunt and penetrating spinal injuries, but a large percentage of these patients will have significant concomitant injuries, causing blood loss, which will explain their hypotension.[1,5] It is only after these other injuries have been excluded that neurogenic shock can be said to be present.

Once the ABCDEs have been attended to and all other possible sources of hypotension have been investigated and treated, the treatment will focus on the hypotension and bradycardia of neurogenic shock.

Hypotension is treated by rapid infusion of crystalloid; this is usually effective in treating neurogenic shock.[14] During neurogenic shock, blood pools in the distal circulation because of the loss of sympathetic innervation. Infusion of intravenous crystalloid will correct this relative hypovolemia. Adequate fluid resuscitation should be undertaken with the aim of keeping the mean arterial blood pressure above 70 mmHg.[14] This level of blood pressure is a bit arbitrary and has been arrived at by clinical experience. It is thought that this level of pressure provides adequate perfusion and minimizes the effects of secondary cord injury.

The use of fluids in neurogenic shock must, however, be judicious. There is a danger of excessive fluid replacement, with resultant heart failure and pulmonary edema.[15] The placement of a pulmonary artery catheter and its resultant pressure measurements can be of tremendous benefit and help prevent excess fluid administration.[16] If intravenous fluids are not adequate to maintain organ perfusion, the use of positive inotropic pressor agents such as dopamine or dobutamine may be beneficial.[10] These agents will improve cardiac output and raise perfusion pressure.[10] The doses required are variable and should be titrated to the patient's hemodynamic response.

Bradycardia, when present, usually occurs within the first few hours or days of spinal cord injury[9] because of a predominance of vagal tone to the heart. In severe cases and when the patient's hemodynamics warrant, atropine can be used for treatment. In some patients who may present with heart block or asystole, a pacemaker may be required.[9]

One topic that deserves discussion is the physiologic significance of the hypotension associated with neurogenic shock. For most patients treated in the ED, an adequate blood pressure is important to ensure perfusion and normal functioning of end organs. This can be especially important in the patient with a spinal cord injury, in whom optimal perfusion and oxygenation of the spinal cord may maximize nervous system recovery.[15] On the other hand, the authors' clinical experience has shown that moderate hypotension may be tolerated by some of these patients without any evident sequelae. In these patients, more harm than good may be done by trying to normalize the blood pressure, as evidenced by the pulmonary edema that can result from overvigorous fluid resuscitation. Perhaps, in these patients, careful monitoring and the tincture of time, allowing the sympathetic nervous system to recover its function, might be the best course of action. This group of patients might more accurately be labeled as having ''neurogenic hypotension'' rather than ''neurogenic shock.'' This is because these patients, though hypotensive, have no problems with peripheral perfusion. They maintain clear mentation and adequate urine output, and do not develop the typical laboratory abnormalities of patients that are in shock.

TABLE 31-1 Treatment of Neurogenic Shock

ABCDE: Airway with cervical spine protection Breathing Circulation Disability (neurologic evaluation) Exposure
Fluid resuscitation with crystalloid—consider pulmonary artery catheter to avoid over hydration.
Administer methylprednisolone 30 mg/kg over 15 min in the first hour; then 5.4 mg/kg/hr × 23 hours.
Carefully search for and treat any possible causes of hypotension and blood loss.
Consider vasopressor support with dopamine or dobutamine.
Transfer patient, after resuscitation, to regional spine or trauma center.

DISPOSITION

Any patient with neurogenic shock has suffered a severe traumatic injury and obviously will be admitted to the hospital. In general, the patient with a spinal cord injury is best cared for at a trauma or spine center. Most areas have a regional spine care center, centralizing the extensive resources needed for the care of these patients and standardizing patient care.

While in the ED, the patient with a spinal cord injury and neurogenic shock can benefit from early consultation and involvement of the appropriate specialty services, namely neurosurgery, trauma surgery, and orthopedics. Early consultation and the consideration of transfer is most important for the patient with continuing or worsening hypotension, an evolving deficit, or a progressing level of injury.

REFERENCES

1. Zipnick RI, Scalea TM, Trooskin SZ, et al: Hemodynamic responses to penetrating spinal cord injuries. *J Trauma* 35:578, 1993.
2. Atkinson PP, Atkinson JLD: Spinal shock. *Mayo Clin Proc* 71:384, 1996.
3. Bracken MB, Shepard MJ, Hellenbrand KG, et al: A randomized, controlled trial of methylprednisolone or naloxone in the treatment of acute spinal-cord injury. *N Engl J Med* 322:1405, 1990.
4. Savitsky E, Votey S: Emergency department approach to acute thoracolumbar spine injury. *J Emerg Med* 15:49, 1997.
5. Soderstrom CA, McArdle DQ, Ducker TB, Militello PR: The diagnosis of intraabdominal injury in patients with cervical cord trauma. *J Trauma* 23:1061, 1983.
6. Meyer PR, Cybulski GR, Rusin JJ, Haak MH: Spinal cord injury. *Neurol Clin* 9:625, 1991.
7. Tator CH: Acute spinal cord injury: A review of recent studies of treatment and pathophysiology. *Can Med Assoc J* 107:143, 1972.
8. Tator CH, Rowed DW: Current concepts in the immediate management of acute spinal cord injuries. *Can Med Assoc J* 121:1453, 1979.
9. Guha AB, Tator CH: Acute cardiovascular effects of experimental spinal cord injury. *J Trauma* 28:481, 1988.

10. Gilson GJ, Miller AC, Clevenger FW, Curet LB: Acute spinal cord injury and neurogenic shock in pregnancy. *Obstet Gynecol Surv* 50:556, 1995.

11. McCagg C: Postoperative management and acute rehabilitation of patients with spinal cord injuries. *Orthop Clin North Am* 17:171, 1986.

12. Soderstrom CA, Ducker TB: Increased susceptibility of patients with cervical cord lesions to peptic gastrointestinal complications. *J Trauma* 25:1030, 1985.

13. Committee on Trauma, American College of Surgeons: *Advanced Trauma Life Support for Doctors: Student Course Manual.* Chicago: American College of Surgeons, 1997.

14. Fehlings MG, Louw D: Initial stabilization and medical management of acute spinal cord injury. *Am Fam Physician* 54:155, 1996.

15. Wilson RH, Whiteside MCR, Moorehead RJ: Problems in diagnosis and management of hypovolaemia in spinal injury. *Br J Clin Pract* 47:224, 1993.

16. Soderstrom CA, Brumback RJ: Early care of the patient with cervical spine injury.*Orthop Clin North Am* 17:3, 1986.

ANALGESIA, ANESTHESIA, AND SEDATION

ACUTE PAIN MANAGEMENT, ANALGESIA, AND ANXIOLYSIS IN THE ADULT PATIENT

Erica Liebelt
Nadine Levick

In both the United States and the United Kingdom, in excess of 60 percent of all emergency department (ED) patients present with conditions associated with pain. However, inadequate analgesia continues to be documented in the ED setting. Acute pain management consists of pain relief and anxiolysis with preservation of airway reflexes and consciousness. The Agency for Health Care Policy and Research (AHCPR) guidelines for acute pain management[1] are a useful guide but should be supplemented with more detailed and current information.[2]

The experience of pain is determined by many factors, including medical condition, developmental level, emotional and cognitive state, personal concerns, meaning of pain, family issues and attitudes, culture, and environment. Fear and anxiety accentuate physical pain. Effective pain management should address psychological and physical aspects by using both nonpharmacologic and pharmacologic modalities.

The utility of oral medications in the ED is limited because emergent operative or investigational procedures often mandate NPO status, and gastrointestinal absorption may be poor because of the patient's underlying condition. Repeated intramuscular doses of narcotic analgesia no longer represent an approach of choice except in patients where vascular access must be preserved (sickle cell patients). A multifaceted approach combining titrated intravenous medications, regional and topical medications, adequate anxiolysis, and incorporation of nonpharmacologic techniques to enhance patient care and comfort is preferred.

PATHOPHYSIOLOGY

Pain involves release of potent mediators of inflammation, and is modulated by neurocognitive factors resulting in an unpleasant sensory and emotional experience. The peripheral pain system (e.g., nociceptors, C fibers, A-δ fibers, free nerve endings) registers the original noxious stimulus and conducts it to the central nervous system (CNS). The primary afferent peripheral nociceptors have poorly differentiated nerve fiber terminals and slow conduction velocities (ranging from C fibers at 2.5 ms^{-1} to A-δ fibers at 2.5 to 20.0 ms^{-1}) and are normally activated by stimuli of strong to noxious intensity. They release several neurotransmitters. Glutamate, an excitatory amino acid (EAA) released from these nociceptors, elicits fast synaptic responses in second-order neurons that are mediated by at least two EAA receptor subtypes. Some primary afferent nerve fibers also express and synthesize neuropeptides (substance P, neurokinin A, and calcitonin gene–related peptide) that are coreleased with glutamate within the spinal cord.[3] The dorsal horn of the spinal cord (e.g., dorsal root ganglion, inhibitory interneurons, ascending pain tracts) integrates and modulates pain and other sensory stimuli. Supraspinal centers (e.g., hypothalamic centers, thalamic nuclei, the limbic and reticular activating systems) integrate and process pain information, allowing detection and perception of pain. Cognitive interpretation, localization, and identification of pain and triggering of emotional and physiologic reactions also occur at this site. Parietal pain pathways are more complex and differ in structure from visceral pain pathways, which may explain the poor localization of visceral pain as opposed to parietal pain.

Assessment and Reassessment of Pain

Pain assessment in the ED involves determining its location, quality, and severity. Since pain is dynamic and changes with time, its severity requires assessment and reassessment, ideally involving the use of validated objective and subjective pain assessment instruments.

The awake, cooperative, competent patient can describe and locate pain and be assessed easily and reliably.[1] Patients who have difficulty communicating are at risk of inadequate pain management. Patients who are cognitively impaired, psychotic, or severely emotionally disturbed as well as children, the elderly, patients who do not speak the language of their health care team, and patients whose level of education or cultural background differs significantly from that of their health care team are at particular risk.[4] These scenarios require a more objective than subjective approach. Involvement of family members is often valuable.

For comprehensive assessment of pediatric pain, age-appropriate, developmentally specific techniques are essential, and assessment is enhanced by the involvement of the parents or caregiver. (See Chap. 130.)

The elderly often report pain very differently from younger patients because of physiologic as well as psychological and cultural changes associated with aging. The high prevalence of visual, hearing, motor, and cognitive impairments among the elderly can be barriers to effective pain assessment, affecting the reliability of traditional pain assessment instruments.

Ethnicity has bearing on different cultural concepts of pain and on the characteristics of culturally appropriate pain-related behaviors. There is also interplay between the ethnicity of patient and physician. Most pain instruments are to some extent language-dependent. In practical consideration of language difficulties and cross-cultural measurement, visual analogue scales have been preferred. Confounding issues are the interplay of socioeconomic status and also the degree of accommodation to the dominant culture.[5]

Gender-related differences in reporting of pain intensity are equivocal, but women are more likely to express pain and to actively seek treatment. Physicians have a tendency to underestimate and undertreat pain in female patients.[6]

Approaches to Pain Assessment

NON-SELF-REPORT MEASUREMENT Respiratory and cardiovascular changes as well as changes in patient expression and movement can all occur due to pain. However, factors other than pain can cause or inhibit the same changes, making interpretation difficult. Physiologic parameters may be more useful to confirm a clinical impression than as a primary assessment tool. The more developed non-self-report tools are used in the pediatric setting. (See Chap. 130.)

SELF-REPORT MEASUREMENT Self-report measurement scales include numerical or adjective ratings and visual analogue scales. These tools may also be used simply by asking the patient for a verbal response. Small changes in pain severity may not have clinical importance. For example, with a 100-mm visual analogue scale, a change in severity of less than 13 mm has statistical but minimal clinical significance.

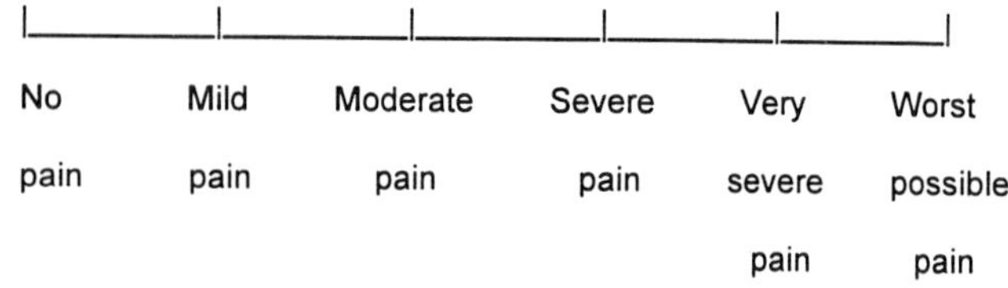

FIG. 32-1. Adjective rating scale.

Pain Assessment Tools

Self-report tools are the mainstay of pain assessment. These tools should be reliable, valid, and easy for the patient and health care provider to use in the ED environment. The ideal tool should be applicable to any individual regardless of psychological, emotional, cultural, cognitive, or developmental status.

The adjective rating scale (ARS) is a simple, descriptive pain-intensity scale presented graphically or verbally as a linear list of pain descriptors (Fig. 32-1). A 10-cm baseline is recommended.[1]

A numerical rating scale (NRS) can be presented as a verbal or graphic scale to describe pain intensity (Fig. 32-2). The patient is asked to self-report pain on a scale of zero to ten (0 = no pain, 10 = worst possible pain) and mark it off graphically, self-report verbally, or—where language or speech is difficult—indicate the numerical value with upheld fingers. While not as precise as the visual analogue scale (VAS), (see below), the NRS requires no visual or manual skill and is easy to use.[1]

The VAS is a 10-cm linear scale marked at one end with a term like *no pain* and at the other with *worst imaginable pain* (Fig. 32-3). The patient places a mark on the line at the point that best represents the pain. The VAS scale is scored by measuring the distance of the patient's mark from either end. The VAS has been validated,[7] but debate continues over the clinical relevance of statistically significant differences in VAS scores.[8] A disadvantage of the VAS is that it requires visual, manual, and some conceptual skill.

MODALITIES OF PAIN MANAGEMENT

Effective management of acute pain includes nonpharmacologic cognitive-behavioral and physical techniques combined with the pharmacologic agents—administered systemically, regionally, locally or sometimes via novel delivery systems.

Pharmacologic Modalities

The pharmacologic management of acute pain includes systemic agents such as opioid and nonopioid analgesics and adjunct medications (anxiolytics and antiemetics) in addition to the nonsystemic local and regional agents (Table 32-1). Agents such as nonsteroidal anti-inflammatory drugs (NSAIDs) should be considered for mild pain, and systemic opioids and/or NSAIDs should be considered for moderate to severe pain. Local or regional neural blockade is a useful technique to minimize the use of narcotic agents (Table 32-2).

Analgesics are the drugs most often associated with adverse drug events, with similar rates for overmedication as for undermedication

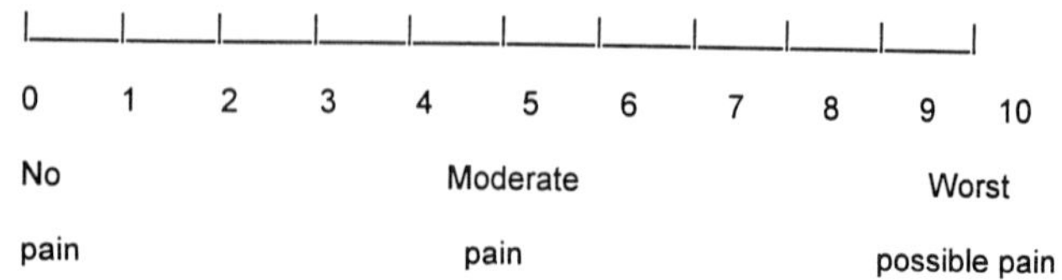

FIG. 32-2. Numeric rating scale.

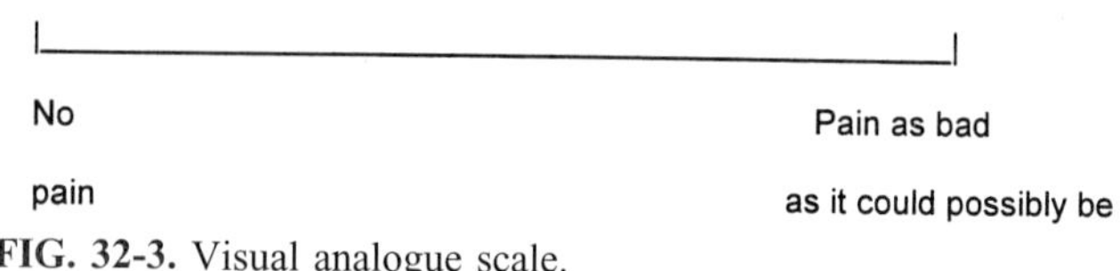

FIG. 32-3. Visual analogue scale.

despite the likely reporting bias for overmedication. Sedatives are the next most likely category of medication to cause adverse reactions.[9]

NONOPIOID AGENTS *Acetaminophen* (*paracetamol* in some countries) is an effective analgesic, adequate for mild to moderate pain. Its efficacy is significantly enhanced when it is combined with codeine. Acetaminophen does not affect platelet aggregation, nor is it anti-inflammatory. Acetaminophen may be hepatotoxic above 140 mg/kg per day in the setting of normal hepatorenal function.

NSAIDs are a class of drugs including aspirin, naproxen, indomethacin, ibuprofen, and ketorolac (standard doses are shown in Table 32-3). In therapeutic doses these agents decrease levels of inflammatory mediators generated at the site of tissue injury. They do not cause sedation or respiratory depression or interfere with bowel or bladder function.[10] Even when insufficient alone, NSAIDs have significant opioid dose-sparing effects. There are oral, rectal, intravenous, and topical preparations. The NSAID ketorolac is approved by the U.S. Food and Drug Administration for parenteral use. Topical NSAIDs, effective in acute musculoskeletal injuries, are associated with the lowest side-effect profile.[11] They are available in Australia and the United Kingdom but currently not in the United States. Adverse effects of NSAIDs include platelet dysfunction, impaired coagulation, and gastrointestinal irritation and bleeding; hence they should be used with care in patients with thrombocytopenia or coagulopathies and in those at risk for bleeding or gastric ulceration. Acute renal failure has been reported and may be precipitated in patients who are volume depleted or have lost more than 10 percent of their blood volume, have preex-

TABLE 32-1 Pharmacologic Agents for Analgesia and Anxiolysis

Systemic
Nonopioid
Acetaminophen
NSAIDs
Nitrous oxide
Ketamine
Opioid
Morphine
Meperidine
Hydromorphone
Oxycodone
Fentanyl
Codeine
Adjuncts
Anxiolytics: benzodiazepines
Antiemetics: hydroxyzine, metaclopromide, promethazine
Nonsystemic
Local Anesthetics
Lidocaine
Bupivacaine
Prilocaine
Tetracaine
Procaine
Other
Topical NSAIDs
Ethyl Chloride spray
Capsaicin
Alternative/allopathic

TABLE 32-2 Comparison of Pharmacologic Agents

Drug	Route	Advantages	Disadvantages
NSAIDs	Oral alone or adjunct to opioid	Effective for mild to moderate pain Potentiates effect of opioids	Relatively contraindicated in patients with renal disease and risk of gastric ulceration coagulopathy May mask fever
	Parenteral	Effective in moderate to severe pain Useful where opioids are contraindicated, especially to avoid respiratory depression and sedation	As above Expensive
Opioids	Oral	Can be as effective as parenteral in appropriate doses	Variable absorption
	Intramuscular	No IV access required	Injections painful and absorption unreliable Avoid this route when possible
	IV	Suitable for titrated bolus or continuous administration	Requires monitoring Significant risk of respiratory depression with inappropriate dosing
Local anesthetics	Infiltration Peripheral nerve block IV regional	Technical ease Opioid sparing Opioid and general anesthetic sparing	Limited duration of action Requires specific skill and knowledge Requires full monitoring and resuscitation facilities Risk of hypotension, cardiac dysrhythmias, and convulsions
Nitrous oxide	Inhalational	Painless delivery system	Need patient compliance Scavenger system necessary Nausea and vomiting frequent

isting renal or cardiac disease, or are taking loop diuretics. Ibuprofen is safer than ketorolac in this respect.[12]

OPIOID AGENTS Opioid analgesics are the cornerstone of pharmacologic management of moderate to severe acute pain (standard doses are shown in Table 32-4). Proper use of opioids involves selecting a particular drug, and considering (1) route of administration, (2) suitable initial dose, (3) frequency of administration titrated against analgesic response, (4) optimal use of nonopioid analgesics and adjunct agents, (5) incidence and severity of side effects, and (6) whether the analgesic will be continued in an inpatient or ambulatory setting. Patients vary greatly in their responses to opioid analgesics; these variations are related to age, body mass, and previous or chronic exposure to opioids. Relative potency estimates provide a rational basis for selecting the appropriate starting dose to initiate analgesic therapy, changing the route of administration (e.g., from parenteral to oral), or switching to another opioid (Table 32-5). An oral opioid such as a codeine-acetaminophen combination, or a stronger compound such as oxycodone with acetaminophen is useful for ED pain patients able to take oral medications.

The opioids include the phenanthrene derivatives (e.g., morphine, codeine, and hydromorphone), the phenylpiperidine derivatives (e.g., meperidine and fentanyl), and the diphenylheptane derivative (methadone). When they are used in equianalgesic doses, there is no compelling evidence to recommend one opioid over another. Accumulation of the toxic metabolite of meperidine (normeperidine) has been shown to cause CNS toxicity in patients with compromised renal function or those taking monoamine oxidase inhibitors (MAOIs).[13] Morphine, in contrast to meperidine, has an active rather than a toxic metabolite. Adverse effects of opioids include nausea, vomiting, constipation, pruritus, urinary retention, and respiratory depression.

Codeine, hydromorphone (Dilaudid), oxycodone, morphine, and meperidine can be administered orally (Table 32-4), hydromorphone and codeine being readily absorbed from the gastrointestinal tract.

TABLE 32-3 Nonopioid Analgesics

Drugs	Adult Dose	Pediatric Dose	Toxicity/Adverse Reactions
Oral/rectal			
Acetaminophen (paracetamol)	Oral: 650–1000 mg q4h Rectal: 1–2000 mg q12h	Oral: 10–15 mg/kg q4h Rectal: as above	Toxic dose: 140 mg/kg in 24 h Toxic dose: 150 mg/kg in 24 h
Aspirin	Oral: 650–1000 mg q4h	Oral: 10–15 mg/kg q4h	Reye's syndrome in children; tinnitus
Ibuprofen	Oral: 400 mg q4–6h	Oral: 10 mg/kg q6–8h	GI irritation, platelet dysfunction, renal dysfunction, bronchospasm
Naproxen	Oral: 250 mg q6–8h Rectal: 500–1000 mg q12h	Oral: 5–7 mg/kg q12h Rectal: as above	GI irritation, platelet dysfunction, renal dysfunction, hepatic impairment, interacts with protein bound drugs
Indomethacin	Oral: 25–50 mg q12h Rectal: 100 mg q24h	N/A	As for naproxen
Parenteral			
Ketorolac	IV: 30 mg/dose IM: 60 mg/dose	IV: 0.5 mg/kg q6h Max. dose: 120 mg/day	GI irritation, platelet dysfunction (24–48 h), renal dysfunction (volume-depleted patient)

TABLE 32-4 Opioid Analgesics

Drugs	Adult Dose	Pediatric Dose	Duration of Action, min	Toxicity/Adverse Reactions
Opioids				
Morphine	IV: 2–5 mg IM: 10 mg Oral: 60 mg	Oral: 0.3–0.5 mg/kg IV or IM: 0.05–0.15 mg/kg	2–4 h	Histamine release may result in hypotension
Hydromorphone	IV: 1 mg IM: 1.5 mg	Oral: 0.02 mg/kg IV: 0.015 mg/kg	3–4 h	Less pruritus and nausea than morphine
Meperidine	IV: 50 mg IM: 75–100 mg	IV/IM: 1–2 mg/kg	2–3 h	Toxic metabolite
Codeine	Oral: 10–60 mg IM: 30–100 mg	Oral: 1–3 mg/kg/day in 4–6 divided doses IM: 0.5–1.2 mg/kg	4 h	Causes nausea Caution in renal failure Not recommended for IV use
Oxycodone	Oral: 5 mg Rectal: 30 mg	Oral: 0.1 mg/kg	3–6 h	See codeine Less nauseating than codeine
Fentanyl	IV: 50–100 μg IM: 50–100 μg	IV or IM: 0.5–3 μg/kg Transmucosal: 10–15 μg/kg	30–45 min	Chest wall rigidity (see text for ℞) Use ⅓ dose in children < 6 months Avoid in children < 4 months Emesis with transmucosal prep.
Other				
Ketamine	IM: 0.5–1.0 mg/kg IV: 0.5–1.0 mg/kg over 60 sec	IV: 0.25–0.5 mg/kg IM: 2–4 mg/kg Oral/rectal: 4–6 mg/kg	IV: 5–15 min IM: 10–20 min	Causes increased intracranial and intraocular pressure, nystagmus Emergence reactions

Fentanyl is now available as a raspberry-flavored fentanyl-impregnated lozenge preparation (Oralet).

Codeine can be given both orally and intramuscularly; intravenous administration is not recommended due to a higher side-effect profile via this route. Codeine is a very useful agent in the ED for adjunct oral pain therapy with acetaminophen for discharge analgesia. At therapeutic doses, the analgesic effect reaches a peak within 2 h and persists between 4 and 6 h. The plasma concentration does not correlate with brain concentration or relief of pain. Codeine crosses the blood-brain barrier and is found in fetal tissue and breast milk, but it is not bound to plasma proteins. The plasma half-life is about 2.9 h. The elimination of codeine is primarily via the kidneys, and about 90 percent of an oral dose is excreted by the kidneys within 24 h of dosing. Patients who report allergy to codeine or morphine (phenanthrine) can usually be offered meperidine or fentanyl (phenylpiperidine) unless they describe allergies to both classes of agents.

TABLE 32-5 Equianalgesic Opioid Doses

Opioid	Equipotent IV Dose, mg/kg	Equipotent PO Dose, mg/kg	Parenteral/Oral Ratio
Morphine	0.1	0.3–0.5	20–33%
Meperidine	1.0	1.5–2.0	50–60%
Fentanyl	0.001	0.01–0.015 (transmucosal)*	25–50% (of transmucosal dose)
Alfentanil	0.05	—	—
Hydromorphone	0.015	0.02–0.1	20–70%
Codeine	1.2	2.0	66%
Oxycodone	—	0.1	—

*Less than 25–50% of a transmucosal dose in absorbed systemically.
Source: Adapted from Yaster M, Krane E, Kaplan R, et al: *Pediatric Pain Management and Sedation Handbook,* St. Louis, Mosby, 1997, p 40.

Opioids are frequently combined with an anxiolytic as an adjunct (hydroxyzine or benzodiazepines), which may provide pain relief at a lower opiate dose than using an opiate alone. However, hydroxyzine can only be given intramuscularly. Use of antiemetics (such as metoclopramide, prochlorperazine, or promethazine) is useful to control the side effects of nausea and vomiting. When a benzodiazepine or promethazine is given with an opioid, the sedative effects will be additive.

Concerns have been raised about delayed-release transdermal formulations, because of delayed onset and prolonged duration of action. Transdermal fentanyl preparations are used in the chronic pain and oncology setting. Generally, transdermal fentanyl should be avoided for acute pain management.

Side effects (e.g., confusion, respiratory depression, hypotension, urinary retention, or pruritus) associated with opioids are greater with intravenous, transmucosal, and epidural administration than oral administration and require frequent assessment and monitoring. Opioids should generally be withheld whenever there is respiratory depression (usually fewer than 10 breaths per minute).

OTHER AGENTS Ketamine and nitrous oxide are two agents that have been used widely for brief analgesic therapy; these agents also have sedative properties.

Ketamine, a phenylcyclidine derivative, produces analgesia and dissociative anesthesia and has the advantage of causing minimal respiratory depression. The ability of ketamine to produce amnesia makes it a good agent for brief minor procedures and for wound dressing. Adverse effects include increased intracranial pressure (ICP) and intraocular pressure, hypersalivation, and reemergence phenomena (disagreeable dreams or hallucinations upon awakening). It should be avoided in patients with closed head injuries or other conditions associated with increased intracranial pressure. It is a useful agent in the pediatric ED (see chapter 130).

Nitrous oxide is a fast-onset, short-acting analgesic and sedative inhalational agent useful for wound dressing, and brief minor procedures. The primary adverse effects are nausea and vomiting. Barriers to ED use of nitrous oxide include the need for patient cooperation and an effective scavenging system. Adverse effects are nausea and vomiting. In addition, it cannot be used in patients with altered mental status, head injury, suspected pneumothorax, or perforated abdominal viscus. Severe pulmonary disease may also alter the respiratory elimination of nitrous oxide.

Choosing a Route to Administer a Pharmacologic Agent

Systemic pain medications can be given orally, rectally, intravenously, intramuscularly, transmucosally, transdermally, by inhalation, or by epidural administration (Table 32-6). Intravenous opioids are suitable for bolus administration or continuous infusion and are preferred to intermittent intramuscular injections. Patient controlled intravenous analgesic systems do have a role in the ED for the stabilized patient who is to be admitted. Repeated intramuscular injections can themselves cause pain and trauma and may deter patients from requesting pain medication. Oral administration is convenient and inexpensive and is appropriate once the patient can tolerate oral intake; it is a mainstay of pain management in the ambulatory ED population. Nonsystemic agents can be delivered transdermally or transmucosally or by infiltrative local and regional injection, or intravenously for specific regional blocks. Alternative delivery techniques such as iontophoresis and single-dose jet injectors, which are now available for topical local anesthetic drug delivery, warrant consideration and further investigation.

Analgesic Dosage, Precautions, and Comorbidity

The key principle for safe and effective use of opioids is to titrate the dose against the desired effect—pain relief—and minimize unwanted effects. Opioids in larger doses than necessary to control pain, or when given to patients who are not in pain, can result in respiratory depression and hypotension. Relative potency estimates provide a rational basis for selecting the appropriate dose (see Table 32-5). In the setting of comorbid conditions that include underlying neurologic deficits, altered mental status, hemodynamic instability, respiratory dysfunction, or multisystem trauma, systemic narcotics should be used cautiously.

TABLE 32-6 Comparison of Delivery Routes for Systemic Pharmacologic Agents

Method	Advantages	Disadvantages
Systemic		
Oral	Ease Painless Minimal cost, inexpensive No technical skill required Patient acceptability	Unreliable GI absorption Requires effective gastric absorption Nil by mouth status Slow onset Titration less reliable
IV (it is preferable to secure IV access than intraosseous access for analgesia administration)	Rapid onset Titratable Usually easier to reverse Can use medications with short half-life.	Venous access required Potential for overdose
IM or subcutaneous	Convenient More rapid analgesia onset than oral	Titration difficult and necessitates repeated painful injections Absorption depends on effective peripheral circulation More expensive than oral route
Rectal (transmucosal)	No first-pass effect No reliance on gastric motility	Patient cooperation/acceptability Variable absorption
Buccal/nasal (transmucosal)	Ease Painless	Difficult to control dosage Can cause irritation to nasal mucosa
Transdermal	Ease Painless	Variable dosage and duration Difficult to titrate Slow onset Prolonged action after removal
Inhalational	Rapid onset and offset Painless	Patient cooperation required Scavenger facilities necessary
Nonsystemic		
Regional		
Peripheral nerve block	Minimizes total dose of agent used Minimizes need for systemic sedation/analgesia	Technical skill required
Hematoma block	Minimizes need for systemic sedation/analgesia	Potential for infection Distressing to patient
IV regional block (Biers block)	Minimizes need for systemic sedation/analgesia	Requires specific equipment and technical skill Potential for overdose
Local		
Infiltration	Simple and convenient	Painful injection and tissue distortion
Transdermal Novel transdermal: Local anesthetic jet injector "guns"* Iontophoresis†	Painless Shorter onset than routine transdermal	Slow onset Specific equipment required May cause skin irritation or pain
Topical	Painless No tissue distortion	Slower onset than filtration

*Potential for cross infection.
†Reliability dependent on skin type.

Patients at the extremes of age are at risk for both inadequate analgesia and pharmacotherapy complications. For the comprehensive management of pediatric pain, age-appropriate assessment techniques and medication dosages and developmentally specific nonpharmacologic adjuncts are essential (see chapter 130). Elderly patients may have more than one source of pain and comorbidity and are at increased risk for drug-drug as well as drug-disease interactions. The elderly, especially opioid-naive patients, are more sensitive to the analgesic effects of opioid drugs as they experience a higher peak and longer duration of pain relief. Moreover, they are more sensitive to sedation and respiratory depression and cognitive and neuropsychiatric dysfunction. Some patients may have concerns about physiologic or psychological dependence and should be informed that this is extremely unlikely after short-term use for acute pain.[1,14,15]

As most analgesics are metabolized by the liver or kidney, caution is essential when using opioids in patients with altered hepatic or renal function. Renal excretion is a major route of elimination for such pharmacologically active opioid metabolites as norpropoxyphene, normeperidine, morphine-6-glucuronide, and dihydrocodeine. Mild renal failure can impede excretion of the metabolites of many opioids, resulting in clinically significant narcosis and respiratory depression.

Patients with respiratory insufficiency and those with chronic obstructive pulmonary disease, cystic fibrosis, and neuromuscular disorders affecting respiratory effort (e.g., muscular dystrophy, myasthenia gravis) are particularly vulnerable to the respiratory depressant effects of opioids and nitrous oxide. Appropriate monitoring of respiratory rate and effort and adequacy of gas exchange is necessary.

Opioids may have adverse synergistic sedative effects in patients with psychiatric illnesses taking anxiolytics or other psychoactive drugs. The use of MAOIs with meperidine has been associated with severe adverse reactions, including death through mechanisms that mimic malignant hyperthermia. The tricyclic antidepressants clomipramine and amitriptyline may increase morphine levels.

Patients in shock, as well as those with trauma and burns, and hemodynamic or respiratory instability mandate judicious use of narcotics. Cautious titration, in consideration of cardiovascular and respiratory stability, of an intravenous short-acting opioid analgesic such as fentanyl[16] and maximal use of regional analgesia are recommended.[1] The intramuscular route has poor and variable absorption and bioavailability in this setting and should be avoided. Additionally, in the trauma patient there is potential for masking occult trauma with excessive use of systemic narcotics. Use of analgesic therapy also must allow for continuous monitoring of neurologic status after a head injury and neurovascular status after limb injury. In the setting of closed head injury or multiple injuries, maximal use of regional and nonpharmacologic modalities minimizes the use of systemic analgesics. While of value in the patient with minor trauma, the use of NSAIDs in the major trauma patient remains controversial. The risk of excessive bleeding from platelet dysfunction, gastric stress ulcers, and potential for acute renal failure in the volume-depleted patient minimize their utility for this patient group.

Nonpharmacologic Modalities (Cognitive-Behavioral and Physical Therapies for Analgesia and Anxiolysis)

Traditionally, nonpharmacologic techniques of pain management in the ED are limited to application of heat or cold, and immobilization and elevation of injured extremities. Other techniques may prove to have a role in the ED and post-ED setting. Among these are cognitive-behavioral techniques, which are effective in reducing pain and anxiety, may control mild pain when used alone, and also enhance patient satisfaction. These techniques include reassurance, explanation, relaxation, music, psychoprophylaxis, biofeedback, guided imagery, hypnosis, and distraction. They are a useful adjunct to pharmacologic management of moderate to severe pain.[1] Successful application of these therapies requires a cognitively intact patient and skilled personnel, but many of the techniques require only a few minutes to teach the patient.

Physical nonpharmacologic agents are becoming increasingly relevant to ED pain management. In addition to the traditional techniques noted above, the less commonly used physical modalities such as transcutaneous electrical nerve stimulation (TENS) and acupuncture, particularly the newer electroacupressure techniques,[17] may have some potential role in the ED environment in the future. Although specific technical skills and equipment are required, there is no need for intravenous access, and there is no systemic effect or depression of respirations or mental status.

Specific Situations

There are a number of situations where the ideal ED analgesic management approach is complex or somewhat controversial. Acute abdominal pain and migraine are two such situations.

ABDOMINAL PAIN Unfortunately, withholding of analgesics in the setting of abdominal pain remains widespread practice that is not evidence based.[18] Early administration of intravenous opiate has been shown to be a safe[19] and effective analgesic in patients with acute abdominal pain in the ED and does not have adverse effects on the accuracy of the evaluation,[20] the diagnosis, and management.[18] Some studies have shown that narcotic administration not only does not mask the diagnosis but actually enhances diagnostic accuracy.[21]

MIGRAINE The choice of the best analgesic agent for use in the ED to manage a migraine headache remains broad. There have been reported success rates as high as 95 percent for the phenothiazines, chlorpromazine (Thorazine) and prochlorperazine (Compazine).[22] Both drugs were associated with decreasing pain scores, but the effect of prochlorperazine was greater. Headache recurrence has been reported to be as high as 50 percent with 5-hydroxytryptamine agonist (Sumatriptan) or dihydroergotamine (DHE). Headache rate at 24 h was significantly higher for patients who left the ED with persisting headache compared to those who left with no pain. More aggressive ED treatment may result in higher successful treatment rates but may also be associated with more adverse effects from the therapy. Dopamine antagonist, antiemetics, metoclopramide, phenothiazines, haloperidol, Sumatriptan, DHE, NSAIDs, acetaminophen, codeine, and narcotics have all been studied.[23] The relative benefit of these agents or combinations of therapies remains unclear. Ketorolac, meperidine, and saline each produced significant pain reduction in a recent study.[24] Opioid use has lost favor due to poor performance in clinical trials as well as the potential to be associated with drug-seeking behavior.[25]

Management of pain related to other conditions is discussed in their respective chapters and is outlined in Table 32-7.

DISPOSITION

Inpatient or outpatient management determination of certain conditions may be affected by pain intensity alone. However, acute pain significant enough to warrant inpatient management is often associated with an underlying condition that is the primary reason for the admission. Safety of discharging patients home on narcotics with conditions necessitating acute pain management is dependent on two main precautions: a disease process that could be masked by analgesic medications and the likelihood of serious complications with the use of these medications in an unmonitored environment. Knowledge of the underlying pathologic diagnosis and an awareness of the home environment, support system, and the ability of the patient to manage home medications safely all impact on the determination for admission. Awareness of the duration of action of analgesic medications and the time of offset with respect to discharge planning and disposition is essential. Where the cause of the pain is determined and under control, long-

TABLE 32-7 Painful Conditions and Suggested Analgesic Management Approaches (a Conjunction to Definitive Care)

	Suggested Systemic Analgesic Options	Adjuncts
Injury		
Acute back pain	Oral/rectal NSAIDs, acetaminophen, oral benzodiazepines, codeine oral	Regional techniques Physical therapies: TENS, acupuncture, massage
Burns/Crush injury/Fractures	Acutely: narcotic IV ± NSAIDS IV/PR For discharge: acetaminophen oral/PR, codeine oral	Elevate Burns: saline dressings (caution re: hypothermia over large areas) Fractures/crush: splint
Concussion	Acetaminophen oral/PR ± codeine oral	Elevate head
Soft tissue contusion strain	NSAIDs oral/PR Acetaminophen oral/PR ± codeine oral	Topical NSAIDs Splint, elevate
Illness		
Medical		
Chest pain		
ischemic	Narcotic IV	Oxygen, correct ischemia
pleuritic	NSAIDs oral/PR	
myocarditis/pericarditis	Acetaminophen oral/PR	
Migraine headache	NSAIDs oral/IV/PR + acetaminophen oral/PR ± codeine oral/IM Consider prochlorperazine *or* chlorpromazine *or* dihydroergotamine *or* sumatriptan (see text)	IV fluid
Dyspepsia	H_2 antagonists	Antacids + lidocaine viscous
Surgical		
Abdominal pain		
Parietal	Narcotic IV	
Visceral, hollow (renal, biliary)	NSAIDs IV/PR Narcotic IV Acetaminophen PR	Antispasmodics
Neurosurgical		
Subarachnoid	Narcotic IV	Antivasospastic agents Antiemetics
Other		
Sickle cell crisis	Narcotic IV or IM NSAIDs oral/IV/PR Acetaminophen oral/PR Hydromorphone Codeine, oxycodone oral	Regional techniques

acting medications minimize the frequency of analgesic medication. However, where there is less diagnostic clarity, these agents could be problematic in delaying symptom recognition by the patient until after discharge home. Longer acting pain medications are likely to result in longer ED stays, to monitor the patient's baseline pain and also to ensure the safety of discharge.

Written discharge instructions detailing specific medication procedures will help patients to take their medications correctly and also enhance patients' awareness of side effects. This information should include names of medications, dosages and frequencies, and adverse effects.

LOCAL ANESTHESIA

Local and regional anesthesia are essential tools in the ED for procedural- and trauma-related pain management, such as for wound repair, lumbar puncture, insertion of intravenous catheters, arterial lines, chest tubes, arthrocentesis, fracture pain, and fracture manipulation and reduction. Local anesthetic (LA) techniques provide short-term pain relief by (1) infiltration or application of LA directly into the area to be anesthetized, (2) infiltration of local anesthetic into the environment of nerve fibers supplying the area, or (3) intravenous regional block. Knowledge of the dosages, actions, and toxicity of the LA medications is required for safe use of these agents. In addition, specific skills and anatomic knowledge for regional anesthesia techniques are necessary for the effectiveness of these procedures.

Local Anesthetic Agents

LAs are all synthetic drugs derived from cocaine. The chemical structure includes a hydrophillic and hydrophobic region and a linkage (amide or ester) region. LAs are weak bases supplied as a salt (usually HCl), with an acidic pH to increase stability, solubility, and shelf life. The most commonly used pharmacologic agents for local infiltrative as well as regional anesthesia are the amide agents, lidocaine and bupivacaine. Lidocaine has a shorter duration of action compared to bupivicaine but has a lower toxicity profile. Tetracaine, an ester LA, is frequently used in topical anesthetic preparations. Esters are metabolized via hydrolysis by cholinesterase enzymes in plasma. Amide LAs are metabolized by hepatic microsomal enzymes. The metabolism rates of amide LAs (prilocaine > lidocaine > bupivacaine) are slower overall than those of ester LAs, creating the potential for sustained plasma levels and cumulative effects of amide LAs. Maximum doses, volumes, and duration of action of various anesthetics are shown in Table 32-8.

The mechanism of action of LAs is to decrease the rate and degree of depolarization and repolarization, decrease conduction velocity, and prolong the refractory period of the neural action potential. LAs bind to receptor sites on the voltage-gated sodium channels (a four-subunit transmembrane protein) in the neuronal membrane and impair or block sodium influx, thereby blocking or slowing nerve conduction. Potency is related to lipid solubility and pK_a; the higher the lipid solubility and the lower the pK_a, the more un-ionized drug present at tissue pH. The un-ionized form traverses lipid layers to the axoplasm. However, the drug must return to the cationic state to bind to the channel receptors. Buffering, by the addition of sodium bicarbonate ($NaHCO_3$), increases the amount of uncharged drug available and decreases pain of infiltration. Duration of action is related to protein binding: the longer the LA binds to the sodium channel, the longer the duration of the blockade.

Addition of epinephrine (usually 1:200,000 or 5 μg/mL) provides a longer duration of anesthesia, provides wound hemostasis, and slows systemic absorption, thereby decreasing the potential for toxicity and allowing a greater volume of agent to be used for extensive laceration repair. Epinephrine may actually increase the pain of infiltration because it lowers the overall pH of the solution. *Epinephrine should never be used in an end-arterial field,* e.g., digits, pinna, nose, penis. Inadvertent intraarterial injection of LA with epinephrine or infiltration into an end-arteriole region can cause prolonged vasospasm and ischemia. This may be reversed with local or intravascular injection of 1.5 to 5 mg phentolamine. Phentolamine, 2 mg, has been used successfully as a "digital block" for digital ischemia. Use of 10 mg has been reported for local infiltration in the extremities. The side effect of phentolamine, hypotension, is less likely in this setting.

Toxicity

Toxicity is determined by the total dose and mode of LA delivered, modulated by factors influencing systemic uptake. The relative absorp-

TABLE 32-8 Local Anesthetic Dosages for Infiltration

				MAXIMUM DOSE†							
				WITHOUT EPINEPHRINE				WITH EPINEPHRINE			
Drug	Concentration for Infiltration*	Onset, min	Duration, min	mg/kg	Total mg	mL/kg	Total mL	mg/kg	Total mg	mL/kg	Total mL
Lidocaine‡	1%	2–5	30–60	4.5	300	0.45	30	7	500	0.7	50
Bupivacaine§	0.25%	3–7	90–360	2	175	0.8	40	3	225	1.2	60
Procaine	1%	2–5	15–45	7.0	500	0.7	50	8	600	0.8	60
Prilocaine	4%	2–5	30–60	5	400	0.13	10	7	600	0.18	15

*Percent (%) solution defines the number of grams of substance per 100 mL. To determine mg/mL from a % solution, multiply the drug's % solution by 10, i.e., 2% lidocaine = 20 mg/mL, 0.25% bupivicaine = 2.5 mg/mL.
†Maximum total mg is based on 70-kg patient; maximum volumes cited are for the % solutions listed in the table.
‡Lidocaine dose may be repeated in 2–4 h.
§Bupivacaine dose may be repeated once every 4–6 h to a maximum of 400 mg/day.

tion of LA is site dependent. The absorption, from highest to lowest, is: intercostal/intratracheal > epidural/caudal > brachial plexus > mucosal > distal peripheral nerve > subcutaneous. Caution should be exercised with intercostal blocks: the recommended LA dose for intercostal blocks is one-tenth of maximum for peripheral blocks. Serious adverse reactions including systemic toxic reactions are more frequently encountered with the use of amide rather than ester LAs, due in part to the slower amide metabolism. However, patients with atypical plasma cholinesterase may be prone to systemic toxicity from ester LAs. The systemic toxicity of LAs is enhanced by hypercarbia, hypoxemia, and acidosis. Systemic toxicity is usually the result of rapid inadvertent intravenous injection or delivery of an excessive total dose of LA.

Serious toxicity primarily involves the CNS and cardiovascular system. CNS toxicity results from a combination of central excitatory and depressant activity of the LA, ranging from perioral tingling and numbness to confusion, seizure, and coma (see Table 32-9). Cardiovascular toxicity relates to the Na+ channel blockade and results in myocardial depression and dysrhythmias. Bupivacaine, due in part to its prolonged binding to the receptor site and slow metabolism, is particularly cardiotoxic and for this reason contraindicated for intravenous regional anesthesia. Methemoglobinemia has also been reported from excessive dosage.

TABLE 32-9 Toxicity of Local Anesthetics

	Toxic Effects
CNS	Mild: visual disturbance, tongue numbness, lightheadedness, apprehension, restlessness Moderate: perioral paresthesia, muscle twitching, slurred speech, excitability, drowsiness Severe: seizures, cardiorespiratory depression, coma, death
Cardiovascular system	Palpitations, vasodilation, hypertension, ventricular dysrhythmias (partic. bupivacaine), myocardial depression, hypotension, bradycardia, cardiovascular collapse
Respiratory system	Hypoventilation, respiratory arrest
Allergy	Amides (uncommon) Esters (more common) associated with PABA allergy
Methemoglobinemia specific to prilocaine	Manifestations: cyanosis, dyspnea, dizziness, lethargy; coma occurs if dose in adults > 600 mg prilocaine (8 mg/kg); newborns more susceptible

True allergic reactions to local anesthetics are rare. They are usually due to the metabolite para-aminobenzoic acid (PABA) in the case of ester anesthetics and the preservative methylparaben (MPB), structurally similar to PABA, in the case of amide anesthetics. Esters are more commonly associated with allergic reactions than amides. If a true allergy is suspected based on history or documentation, the optimal approach is to use a preservative-free agent from the other class.

Diphenhydramine (0.5 to 1.0 percent) is an alternative anesthetic choice in patients allergic to the amides and/or ester-type anesthetics. Although it is effective in reducing local infiltrative pain, it has been demonstrated to be more painful than lidocaine and can cause tissue irritation and even skin necrosis. Thus, its role for local anesthesia is extremely specific and limited to those patients who have true allergies to ester or amide anesthetics, which are quite rare.

Management of systemic LA toxicity should follow standard advanced life-support protocols (ensure a patent airway, 100 percent oxygen, ventilatory and circulatory support), and there should be immediate discontinuation of administration of LA and prompt treatment of the CNS and cardiovascular complications. Correcting hypoxia, hypercarbia, and metabolic acidosis is paramount as all of these conditions enhance the toxicity of LAs. Incremental doses of intravenous benzodiazepines are usually effective to control seizures.

Specific Agents

Lidocaine is an amide anesthetic available in 0.5 percent, 1.0 percent, and 2 percent concentrations and is the most commonly used anesthetic in the ED because of its excellent efficacy and low toxicity profile. Decreased metabolism occurs with hepatic failure and decreased hepatic blood flow (e.g., congestive cardiac failure) and in these circumstances can lead to high plasma levels. Its onset of action is within 2 to 5 min and its duration of action is 1 to 2 h. Lidocaine can be combined with epinephrine and bicarbonate.

Bupivacaine (0.25 percent) is an amide anesthetic and is highly protein bound. It has a longer duration of action than lidocaine, 4 to 6 h, and is more cardiotoxic. Bupivacaine is preferred for prolonged procedures (such as ingrown toenail removal), when longer postprocedural analgesia is desired, and for non-IV regional blocks. Bupivacaine is contraindicated for IV regional blocks due to its cardiac toxicity, from which fatalities have been reported. Similar caution regarding conditions affecting hepatic metabolism should be followed as for lidocaine. The onset of action of bupivacaine is similar to that of lidocaine, but some studies suggest its injection is more painful.

Prilocaine, an amide LA with a lower cardiac toxicity profile than lidocaine or bupivacaine, has similar anesthetic potency, milligram for milligram. After intravenous injection, its CNS toxicity is less than lidocaine due to a lower blood level because of differences in its distribution and peripheral uptake. It is also broken down by amidases in the liver more rapidly than lidocaine, resulting in a shorter duration of toxic effects. Prilocaine and tetracaine are the active agents in EMLA cream (eutectic mixture of local anesthetics) for topical use on intact skin. Prilocaine may lead to methemoglobinemia after a large intravenous bolus (or total dose > 600 mg). Due to its lower toxicity, it is commonly used in Australia for intravenous regional arm blocks.

Procaine is an ester LA and can be used for patients who are allergic to the amide anesthetics (e.g., lidocaine). It has a rapid onset but short duration of action. *Tetracaine* is an ester LA and is more lipid soluble and longer acting than other LAs in its class. It is commonly used for topical LA preparations.

Additives and Adjuncts to Minimize Pain of Infiltration

Many variables influence the degree of pain experienced with local anesthetic infiltration. Slow infiltration of the anesthetic (30 s per mL) with a 27- or 30-gauge needle will decrease the pain compared to rapid injection with a larger needle, probably because of less rapid distension of local tissue. Numerous clinical studies have demonstrated attenuation of pain on infiltration with buffered lidocaine. It is prepared by mixing 9 mL of 1 percent lidocaine (with or without epinephrine) with 1 mL of 8.4 percent (1 meq/mL) sodium bicarbonate solution. Bicarbonate can cause precipitation of bupivacaine and should not be used with this anesthetic unless it can be used immediately. It is prepared by mixing 29 mL bupivacaine (0.25 percent) with 1 mL (1 meq/mL) $NaHCO_3$ solution.

The exact mechanisms by which buffering of lidocaine reduces pain is not clear. Buffering to a higher pH may reduce direct tissue irritation by reducing the acidity of the agent. Additionally, buffering increases the concentration of lidocaine in the uncharged form, which theoretically may allow more rapid tissue dispersion resulting in more rapid sensory nerve blockade. Because buffered lidocaine undergoes biodegradation at room temperature, its shelf life is limited. One study suggests 7 days, while another suggests that efficacy is maintained up to 30 days. Each ED must compare the cost and utilization of premixed solution with single dose preparation.

Studies evaluating the efficacy of warm lidocaine (anywhere from 37 to 42°C) to decrease injection pain have yielded equivocal results. It is postulated that heating the anesthetic causes faster diffusion into tissues and reduces or avoids stimulation of cold receptors, increasing the rate of onset of neuronal block. Lidocaine can be warmed either in dry heat (blanket warmers) or in temperature-regulated water baths at 37°C. From a practical standpoint, anesthetics should at least be administered at room temperature. Unlike buffered lidocaine, heated lidocaine undergoes no chemical denaturation, placing no limitations on shelf life.

Local Anesthetic Infiltration

The most common usage of LA in the ED is local infiltration for wound repair and invasive painful procedures. It is a rapid-onset technique. Infiltration can be into the wound margins or as a field block in a ''diamond-shaped wheal'' of LA surrounding the wound. Lidocaine is the drug of choice for local anesthetic infiltration for brief procedures. Bupivacaine is preferable for longer procedures due to its longer duration of action, but with due caution regarding the increased toxicity. Epinephrine can be added to enhance safety and efficacy, and bicarbonate to minimize pain of infiltration. The maximal dosages commonly cited (see Table 32-8) apply to infiltration of local anesthetic, in contrast to the lower maximal dosages for most regional procedures.

TOPICAL ANESTHETICS

Topical anesthetics such as tetracaine (0.5 percent), adrenaline (0.05 percent, 1:2000), and cocaine (4 percent to 11.8 percent) (TAC); lidocaine (4 percent), epinephrine (0.1 percent, 1:1000), and tetracaine (0.5 percent) (LET); and EMLA can be used for a number of different painful procedures and may eliminate or decrease the need for painful infiltrative injection. Compared to infiltrative anesthesia, TAC and LET provide good hemostasis, do not distort wound edges, and can be applied painlessly. Until recently, TAC was the most frequently used topical anesthetic in the United States. Concerns over the safety of TAC stem from the reported cases of seizures, respiratory arrest, and even death in children from the inadvertent systemic absorption of cocaine from its improper application. TAC is a controlled substance, making it less readily available and creating the potential for abuse. In addition, TAC has been estimated to cost from 10 to 17 times more than LET, depending on the concentration of cocaine. LET has been found to be just as effective as TAC in providing local anesthesia for laceration repair. For these reasons, LET is a safer, more practical, and more cost-effective choice.

LET should be made available in single-dose individual vials with a maximum volume of 5 mL. Several drops of the solution can be dripped into the wound with a syringe. Alternatively, a gel can be made by adding methylcellulose powder to each vial, allowing the LET to be ''painted'' in the wound with a sterile, cotton-tipped swab, with less chance for dripping the solution into mucous membranes. The remainder of the solution/gel should be placed on a cotton ball or sterile gauze roughly the size of the wound and either taped to the wound or held by the patient or caregiver wearing a glove. It should be left in place at least 20 min for the maximum anesthetic effect. LET should be avoided on mucous membranes, the pinna of the ear, the nose, penis, and fingers and toes. The gel form may be used cautiously near the eyes, nose, or mouth.

Lidocaine may be used as a topical anesthetic for a variety of painful conditions and procedures. It is marketed in solution, jelly, and ointment forms in concetrations from 2 percent to 10 percent. Viscous lidocaine solutions (2 percent) can be used for temporary relief of inflamed or irritated mucous membranes of the mouth and pharynx (viral stomatitis). A sterile preparation of the viscous solution can be used for insertion of Foley catheters and gastrostomy tubes. Strict instructions to the patient and caregivers about sparing use of the viscous oral solution must be given. Only a limited amount (about 2 ml) of the solution should be applied. Topical benzocaine anesthetic solutions such as Auralgan (antipyrene/benzocaine) may be effective in temporarily alleviating pain due to acute otitis media or external otitis media.

EMLA is an emulsion in which the oil phase is a eutectic (melting point below room temperature) mixture of lidocaine and prilocaine in a ratio of 1:1 by weight (lidocaine 2.5 percent and prilocaine 2.5 percent). Each gram of cream contains 25 mg lidocaine and 25 mg prilocaine, carboxypolymethylene (thickening agent), sodium hydroxide to adjust to a pH of 9, and purified water to 1 gram. EMLA is for use on intact skin. It contains no preservative, is not sterile, and is not recommended for anesthesia of open wounds, although this is being further investigated. Onset, depth, and duration of dermal analgesia depend primarily on the duration of the application. EMLA cream should be applied under an occlusive dressing. There are also new EMLA prepackaged transdermal adhesive disks available. Satisfactory analgesia is achieved after 1 h, peaks at 2 h, and persists for 1 h after removal; both delivery systems have similar pharmacokinetics. The indications are to provide topical anesthesia for venipuncture, arterial puncture, vascular cannulation, drug reservoir or port access, lumbar puncture, sites for needle insertion for regional blocks, and superficial minor skin procedures. However, the time required for adequate anesthesia limits its use for emergent procedures in the ED. Higher effectiveness observed in children over 7 years and adults suggests the importance of emotional and psychological support of younger children undergoing procedures.

Absorption is more rapid on diseased, facial, or Caucasian skin, when compared with nondiseased intact skin, the extremities, or African American skin. Although the incidence of systemic adverse reactions is very low, caution should be exercised, particularly with application to large areas or for longer than 2 h (Table 32-10). Local reactions of blanching or erythema are common. In infants <3 mos there is a theoretical risk of methemoglobinemia because of the low levels of methemoglobin reductase at this age. Toxicity as for lidocaine and prilocaine may be encountered, but is unlikely when EMLA is used as recommended; it is not contraindicated in labor and delivery.[26,27]

Refrigerant Anesthetic Sprays

Refrigerant anesthetic sprays such as Ethyl Chloride (chloroethane) and Fluori-Methane (dichlorodifluoromethane, trichloromonofluoromethane) offer another effective and convenient alternative for topical anesthesia. Ethyl Chloride has been used as a local anesthetic for over 100 years. Vaporization of the liquid spray on the skin lowers its temperature to −20°C, thereby temporarily freezing it. Anesthesia is almost immediate, providing a distinct advantage in a busy outpatient clinic or ED over EMLA cream.

Refrigerant anesthetic sprays have been used to reduce pain associated with minor surgical procedures on the skin, abscess incision, deep intramuscular injections (immunizations), lumbar punctures, venous cannulation, bone marrow aspiration, digital blocks, and port access in children. In addition, these vapocoolants have been used to reduce pain associated with athletic injuries, muscle pain, and myofascial pain. This needle-less form of anesthesia offers a clear psychological advantage to a child's perception and anxiety about pain, compared to a needle injection.

Ethyl Chloride can be applied by inverting the bottle and directing a stream of spray about 30 cm from the skin until the area turns white, while protecting the adjacent skin with petrolatum. Alternatively, apply the spray to a sterile cotton ball for 10 s and then apply it to the skin for 10 s. The liquid maintains its sterility and the cost is minimal. Disadvantages includes its short duration of only 30 seconds to 1 minute, superficial level of anesthesia only, possible pain on thawing, possible lowered resistance to infection, and delayed skin healing. Prolonged spraying causes chemical ''frostbite'' and skin ulceration. These sprays cannot be used on the mucosa. Inhalation should be avoided because it can produce opioid and general anesthetic effects. Ethyl Chloride is flammable and must be used in a well-ventilated room, never in the presence of open flames or electric cautery.

TABLE 32-10 EMLA Contraindications and Precautions

Do not use in infants <1 month (or infants <12 months at risk of methemoglobinemia)
Limit the area and duration of application with children <20 kg
Avoid ingestion (potential for toxicity); ensure the dressing is well secured
Not for ophthalmic use
Not recommended for use on open wounds
Caution with nursing mother, milk:plasma ratio for lidocaine is 0.4 and is not determined for prilocaine
Caution in patients on class I antiarrhythmics (as for injectable local anesthetics)

Novel Topical Techniques and Agents

JET INJECTOR Compressed air high-pressure jet injectors are available to deliver LA agents both in liquid and powder form through the epidermis in a needle-less fashion. This is a delivery method suitable for most skin types and has been used extensively by blood banks to minimize pain during blood donation. There is concern about potential cross infection due to ''splash back'' when these devices are used on multiple patients without sterilization occurring between each use. However, single dose systems are now available.

IONTOPHORESIS Iontophoresis is a recently developed, single-use delivery system to enhance the speed and depth of delivery of topical LA agents. It also is a needle-less system. However, its effect is variable depending on skin type, thickness, and degree of skin moisture. This system requires specific equipment, is more expensive than the routine topical preparations, and can only be used on intact skin. The anesthetic effect is not immediate and may take up to 15 minutes. The patient may experience a burning sensation under the adhesive electrical pad used for this delivery system.

OTHER PHARMACOLOGIC AGENTS Topical preparations of NSAIDs are being introduced. These preparations are analgesics, not anesthetics. Topical NSAIDs have relatively lower efficacy than oral NSAIDs but also have lower systemic side effects. Another topical agent currently used for chronic pain management that may also have a role in local acute pain management is capsaicin cream, which blocks substance P. There are a number of allopathic preparations available without prescription for topical analgesia, such as aloe and tea-tree oil. Scientific evidence supporting the effectiveness of these preparations is limited. Tea tree oil is toxic if ingested.

REGIONAL PROCEDURES

Regional procedures include peripheral nerve blocks, hematoma blocks, intravenous arm blocks (Biers block), neural plexus blocks, and epidural anesthesia. Although the latter two techniques may be performed in the ED, they usually require anesthesiology participation and oversight in most institutions. The scope of ED practice encompasses the remaining regional blocks. These procedures can shorten ED patient stays, minimize narcotic requirements, and decrease the need for general anesthesia and admissions. The safety and effectiveness of LAs for regional blocks depend on proper dosage, correct technique, adequate precautions, and readiness for emergencies. Regional procedures with LA should be employed only by clinicians who are well versed in diagnosis and management of LA dose-related toxicity and other acute emergencies that might result from inadvertent systemic absorption of the LA or intraarterial injection of an epinephrine-containing LA solution. The setting should be such that resuscitative measures can be initiated immediately if necessary. For major regional blocks (Biers block, brachial plexus blocks) IV access must be established. LA should be administered in the lowest dosage that results in an effective block. Epinephrine is often added to enhance the duration, quality, efficacy, reliability, and safety of a block. Epinephrine is contraindicated in nerve blocks in end-arterial areas. There have been reports of cardiac arrest and death with the use of bupivacaine for intravenous regional anesthesia, and thus its use is contraindicated.

Nerve Blocks

Peripheral nerve blocks are advantageous in the ED environment, particularly for procedures on the digits or penis. They require less

TABLE 32-11 Suggested Dosages for Regional Blocks for Adults (and Children >40 kg)

	WITH EPINEPHRINE 1% LIDOCAINE OR 0.25% BUPIVACAINE	
Nerve Blocks	Volume, mL	Total Dose, mg
Femoral	10–25	100–250
Intercostal	2–10	20–100
Pudendal	3	30
	WITHOUT EPINEPHRINE 1% LIDOCAINE OR 0.25% BUPIVACAINE	
	Volume, mL	Total Dose, mg
Digital	1–3	10–40
Web space	2–5	20–50
Penile	10	100

total LA medication, and the site of drug delivery is often less painful than for local infiltration. It is important to document neurovascular status prior to application of the block, to prevent masking a primary traumatic neurovascular injury. The onset of anesthesia is more delayed than by direct infiltration and may be up to 15 min. The duration depends on the agent used and the amount of drug injected. Complications of nerve blocks include nerve injury. During a block, severe pain suggests that contact has been made with the nerve. In this circumstance, the needle must be withdrawn and repositioned before anesthetic is injected. Intravascular injection can result in limb and systemic toxicity. LA dose exceeding the maximum may result in systemic toxicity (primarily cardiac and CNS), as discussed above. In order to minimize the likelihood of intravascular injection, the plunger on the needle syringe apparatus should be drawn back in all nerve block procedures prior to infiltration. If blood is withdrawn, the procedure is halted. The suggested dosages for regional blocks are shown in Table 32-11.

HAND BLOCKS/ANATOMY **Median Nerve** The median nerve provides sensation to the lateral two-thirds of the palm of the hand, palmar surfaces of the lateral three and one-half digits and their finger tips. The palmar branches of the median digital nerves extend dorsally over the digit to supply the dorsum of the thumb, the index, the middle finger and lateral half of the ring finger distal to the interphalangeal joint and including the nail and the nail bed. The median nerve enters the hand through the carpal tunnel, deep to the flexor retinaculum, between the tendons of the flexor digitorum superficialis and the tendon of the flexor carpi radialis. The median nerve sends cutaneous sensory fibers to the entire palmar surface and sides of the thumb, index finger, middle and lateral half of the ring finger, and the dorsum of these digits distal to their proximal interphalangeal joints (Fig. 32-4).

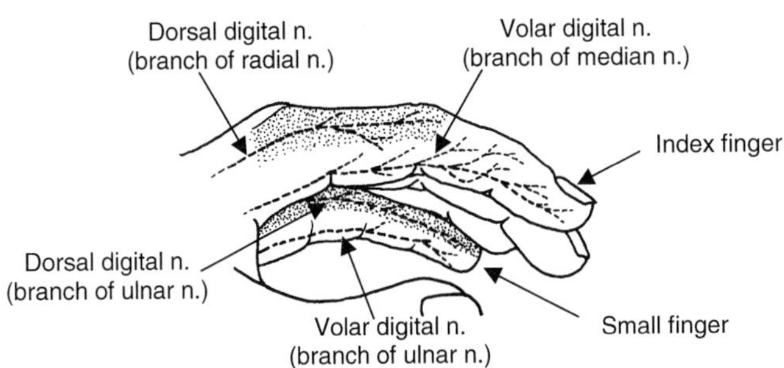

FIG. 32-5. The dorsal digital nerve extends to the tip of the digit in the small finger. In areas of the median nerve distribution (i.e., the ring finger), the volar nerve supplies the dorsum of the digit distal to the interphalangeal joint.

Ulnar Nerve The ulnar nerve can be blocked at the elbow or the wrist to provide anesthesia to the medial aspect of the hand and the small finger, including its nail and nail bed. Just proximal to the wrist, the ulnar nerve gives off a palmar cutaneous branch, which passes superficially to the flexor retinaculum and palmar aponeurosis to supply the skin of the ulnar side of the palm (see Fig. 32-4). It also gives off a dorsal cutaneous branch that supplies the ulnar half of the dorsum of the hand, the small finger, and the ulnar half of the ring finger. The ulnar nerve ends by dividing into a superficial and a deep branch. The superficial branch supplies cutaneous fibers to the anterior surfaces of the small finger and the ulnar half of the ring finger. In the small finger, the dorsal digital nerve extends to the tip of the digit. In the median nerve distribution, the volar nerve supplies the dorsum of the digit distal to the proximal interphalangeal joint (Fig. 32-5).

Radial Nerve The radial nerve provides sensation to the lateral two-thirds of the dorsum of the hand, the proximal aspect of the dorsum

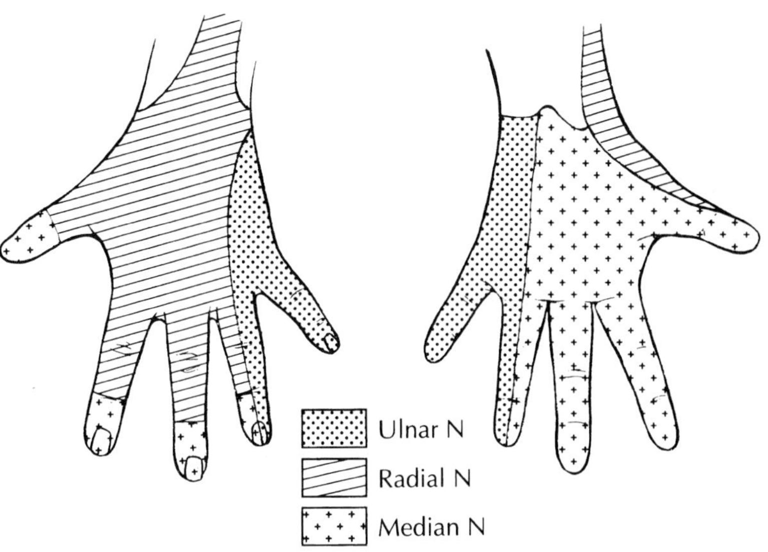

FIG. 32-4. The cutaneous distribution of anesthesia with block of major nerves of the wrist.

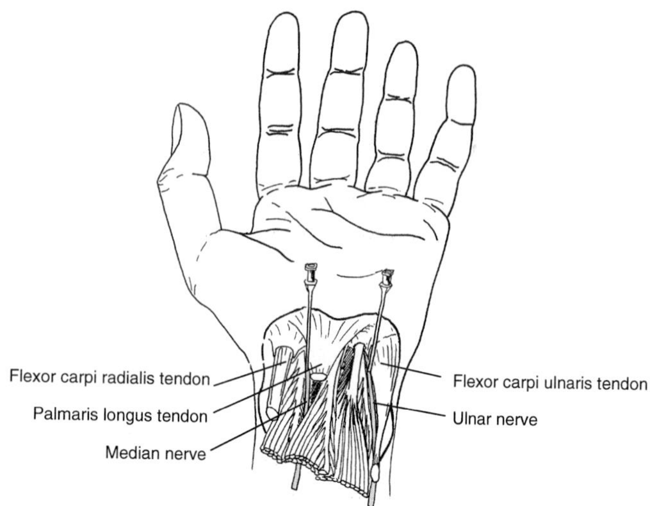

FIG. 32-6. Regional blocks of the ulnar and median nerves.

of the thumb and index finger and lateral aspect of the dorsum of the middle finger, excluding the nails and nailbeds of these digits. The superficial branch of the radial nerve is the direct continuation of the radial nerve along the anterolateral side of the forearm and is entirely sensory. It pierces the deep fascia near the dorsum of the wrist to supply skin and fascia over the lateral two thirds of the dorsum of the hand, the dorsum of the thumb, and proximal parts of the lateral one and one-half fingers (see Fig. 32-4).

HAND BLOCKS/TECHNIQUE For lacerations of the hand, regional blocks at the wrist are performed at the level of proximal volar skin crease (Fig. 32-6). The median nerve is anesthetized by inserting a 27-gauge needle perpendicular to the skin between the tendons of the palmaris longus and flexor carpi radialis muscles at the midpoint of the distal volar crease. A regional block of the ulnar nerve is accomplished by passing the needle between the ulnar artery and the flexor carpi ulnaris. Once inserted, the needle is moved fanwise transversely until paresthesia is elicited. When paresthesia occurs, the needle is held in place and 5 to 10 mL of 1 percent lidocaine with epinephrine (1:100,000) is injected slowly.

The superficial rami of the radial nerve can be blocked by raising the subcutaneous ring with 5 to 10 mL of 1 percent lidocaine with epinephrine (1:100,000) beginning at the level of the tendon of the extensor carpi radialis and extending around the radial border of the wrist dorsal to the styloid process (Fig. 32-7).

FINGER BLOCKS **Digital Nerve Block** The digital nerve block provides excellent anesthesia for fingers and toes and has a more rapid onset although it is as painful a block as the metacarpal block. It is

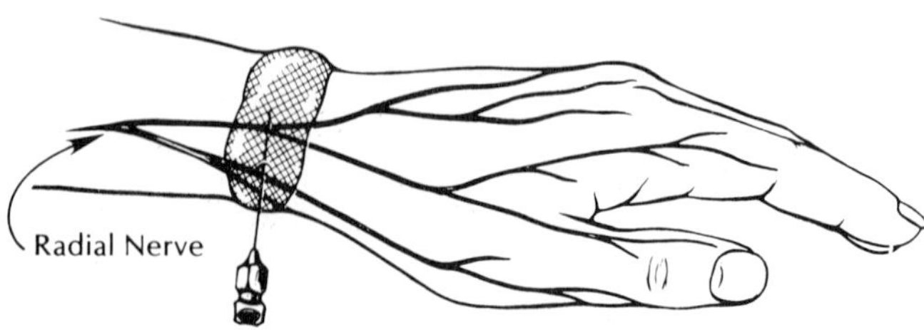

FIG. 32-7. Regional block of several rami of the radial nerve.

commonly used for laceration repair, incision and drainage of paronychia, finger or toenail removal or repair. Preparation with EMLA or Ethyl Chloride can minimize the pain of injection for these blocks. Epinephrine is contraindicated for this block. Contraindications to performing this block are any compromise to the digits' blood supply. Complications are few, however, large volumes of anesthetic can result in a 'compartment' syndrome. Each digit is supplied by a palmar (volar) and dorsal digital nerve on each side of the digit, superficial to the digital arteries (Fig. 32-8*A*).

TECHNIQUE A 27- or 30-gauge needle is inserted through the skin into one side of the extensor tendon of the affected finger just proximal to the web (Fig. 32-8*B*,1). After aspirating, approximately 1 mL of 1 percent lidocaine or 0.25% bupivacaine is injected superficially into the subcutaneous tissue lying on the dorsal surface of the extensor tendon to block the dorsal digital nerve. The needle is then advanced toward the palm until its tip is palpable beneath the volar skin at the base of the finger, just distal to the web (Fig. 32-8*B*). After aspirating, another 1 mL of the anesthetic solution is injected to block the volar digital nerve.

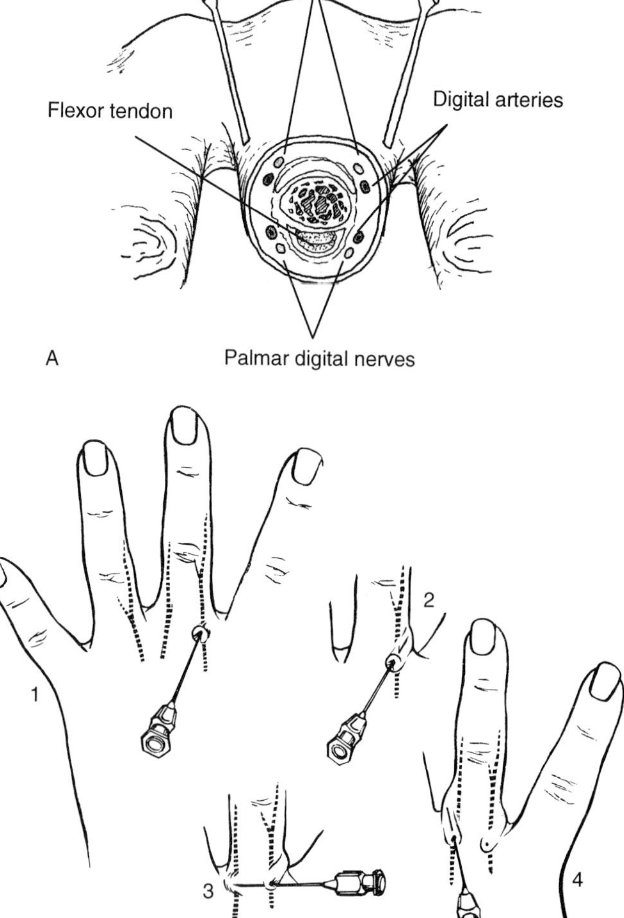

FIG. 32-8. Digital nerve block. **A.** Cross section. (From Yaster M et al: *Pediatric Pain Management and Sedation Handbook.* St. Louis, Mosby, 1997, p 183. Used by permission.) **B.** Positions for needle (see text).

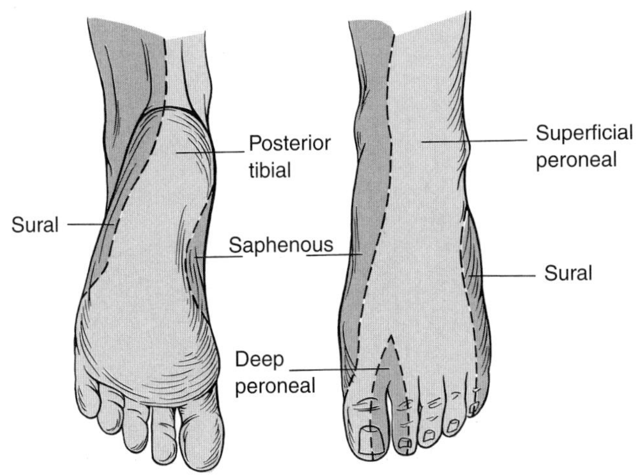

FIG. 32-9. Sensory innervation of the foot and ankle.

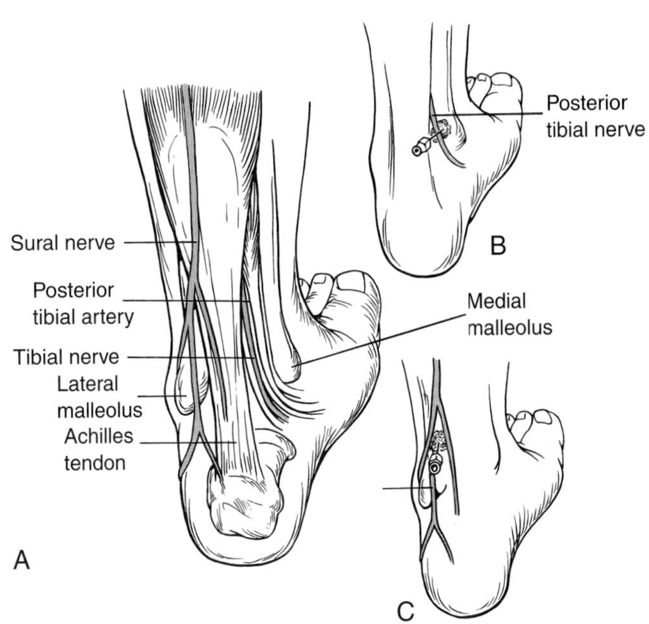

FIG. 32-10. Posterior view of the left foot demonstrating the sites for tibial and sural nerve blocks.

Before removing the needle, it is redirected across the extensor tendon to the opposite side of the finger and approximately 1 mL of the anesthetic solution is injected into the tissue overlying the other dorsal digital nerve (Fig. 32-8*C*). Five minutes later, the needle is reintroduced in the anesthetized skin on the opposite side of the finger and the same technique is repeated (Fig. 32-8*D*). The total volume of the anesthetic agent should not exceed 4 mL. Epinephrine must *not* be used as an adjunct to lidocaine because it may result in irreversible ischemic injury to the finger.

Metacarpal Block Metacarpal blocks can be used to anesthetize either the index, long, ring, or small finger although digital blocks are preferred. The block is performed on each side of the affected finger by inserting a 27-gauge needle at a 90° angle to the dorsum of hand approximately 1 cm proximal to the metacarpophalangeal joint midway between each metacarpal bone. The needle is then advanced at a 90° angle to the skin until its tip is at the level of the lateral volar surface of the metacarpal head or until resistance of the palmar aponeurosis is detected. After aspirating, 3 mL of 1 percent lidocaine is injected slowly.

ANKLE BLOCKS/ANATOMY These regional nerve blocks are used for anesthesia of surgical procedures of the foot. There are 5 nerves which supply sensation to the foot. Most foot blocks involve a block of at least two nerves. It is unusual in the ED setting to have need to block the whole foot. The sole of the foot is a commonly injured area. Regional nerve blocks are the preferred LA technique. Local infiltration directly into the sole is extremely painful and difficult to perform effectively and is not recommended. Buffered lidocaine 1%, or bupivacaine 0.25% are the LA agents of choice. Epinephrine is contraindicated, and these blocks should not be used in patients with peripheral vascular disease, or traumatic circulatory compromise.

The peripheral nerves involved in blocks of the foot are all branches of the sciatic nerve, except for the saphenous nerve (a branch of the femoral nerve) (Fig. 32-9). The sensory innervation of the plantar surface of the foot is primarily the two main branches of the tibial nerve (posterior tibial and sural nerves) which lie posteriorly, and a small contribution from the saphenous nerve medially over the arch. The sensory innervation of the dorsum of the foot is predominantly from the two main branches of the common peroneal nerve (the superficial and deep peroneal nerves), with contribution from the sural nerve laterally and the saphenous nerve medially.

The saphenous nerve is the only branch of the femoral nerve below the knee. It becomes subcutaneous at the medial side of the knee joint and then follows the saphenous vein to a site anterior to the medial malleolus. It provides sensory innervation to the skin over the medial malleolus extending to the skin over the medial side of the foot to the base of the great toe.

The superficial peroneal nerve becomes the dorsal digital nerves. It descends toward the ankle in the lateral compartment, entering the ankle just lateral to the extensor digitorum longus, and provides the cutaneous supply to the dorsum of the foot and all five toes, except for the adjacent sides of the first and second toes (deep peroneal nerve) and lateral side of the fifth toe (sural nerve) (see Fig. 32-9). It is most commonly located lateral to the extensor digitorum longus at the level of the lateral malleolus superficially. It also supplies the peroneus longus and brevis. The sensory supply of the deep peroneal nerve is limited to the 1 cm area of web space between the first and second toes. Thus, blocks of the deep peroneal nerve are not reasonable or practical to perform.

SOLE OF FOOT BLOCK (SURAL NERVE, POSTERIOR TIBIAL NERVE AND SAPHENOUS NERVE) The three nerves which supply the sole of the foot are the posterior tibial nerve via its medial and lateral plantar branches (medial and lateral sole) and medial calcaneal branch (the heel), the sural nerve (posterolateral sole) and the saphenous nerve (small area, medially over the arch) (Fig. 32-9).

The posterior tibial nerve is located along the medial aspect of the ankle, lying between the medial malleolus and the Achilles tendon, just posterior and slightly deeper than the posterior tibial artery (Fig. 32-10) and gives off the three terminal branches, medial calcaneal branch, and medial and lateral plantar nerves. The sural nerve travels with the short saphenous vein (Fig. 32-10), posterior and inferior to the lateral malleolus, it terminates as the dorsal lateral cutaneous nerve. The saphenous nerve follows the great saphenous vein to the medial malleolus.

Technique This block is best performed with the patient in the prone position. The posterior tibial nerve is blocked as it passes posterior to the medial malleolus, the tibial artery is palpated just posterior to the medial malleolus (Fig. 32-10). Buffered lidocaine 1% (or bupivacaine 0.25%) is injected with a 30-gauge needle lateral to the tibial artery and just anterior to the medial border of the Achilles tendon, at the level of the upper border of the medial malleolus. A syringe with a 25-gauge needle is then introduced at 90° to the skin, just lateral and posterior to the tibial artery (Fig. 32-10). Once paresthesia is elicited and after careful aspiration to ensure no inadvertent intravascular access, 3 to 5 mLs of LA is injected. If no paresthesia is encountered, then 5 to 7 mLs of LA should be injected as the needle is withdrawn. Onset of anesthesia should occur within about 5 to 10 minutes if paresthesia has been elicited and in about 30 minutes if it is not elicited. The sural nerve is blocked between the lateral malleolus and the Achilles tendon (Fig. 32-10). It is superficial, lying just anterior to the short saphenous vein. Buffered lidocaine 1% (or bupivacaine 0.25%) is injected with a 30-gauge needle just lateral to the Achilles tendon 1 cm above the lateral malleolus. A 25-gauge needle is then introduced into this area and 3 to 5 mLs of LA is injected subcutaneously as the needle is withdrawn. The saphenous nerve lies superficially between the medial malleolus and the anterior tibial tendon (Fig. 32-11) and is blocked anteriorly by infiltration of 3 to 5 mLs of LA between these landmarks as the needle is withdrawn.

DORSUM OF FOOT BLOCK Regional block of the dorsum of the foot has fewer ED applications than blocks for the sole of the foot, as direct infiltration of the dorsum is more easily performed. The sensory innervation of the dorsum of the foot is primarily supplied by the superficial peroneal nerve, with contribution from the deep peroneal nerve over the first web space, the sural nerve laterally extending to the lateral malleolus, and the saphenous nerve medially over the arch and the medial malleolus (Fig. 32-11).

TECHNIQUE This block is best performed with the patient in the supine position. With a 30-gauge needle a small wheal of LA is raised just above the level of the talocrural joint in the midline anteriorly, between the extensor digitorum longus and the extensor hallucis longus. The superficial peroneal nerve is then blocked by infiltration of 5 mLs of buffered lidocaine 1% (or bupivacaine 0.25%) in a large wheal extending from this point just superior to the talocrural joint at the anterior border of the tibia to the lateral malleolus (Fig. 32-11).

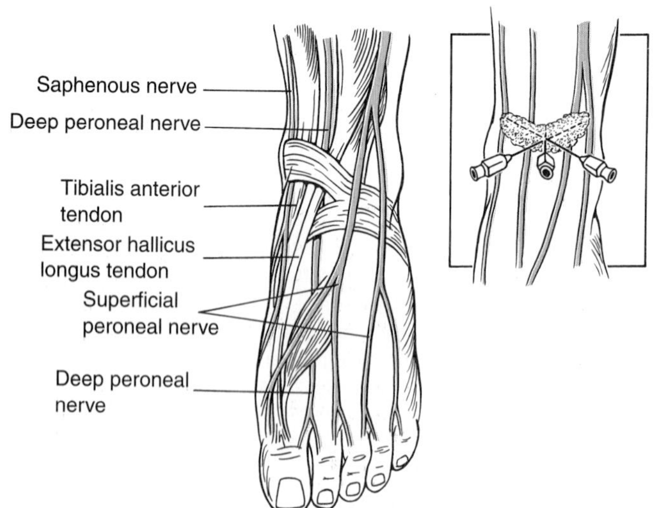

FIG. 32-11. Deep peroneal, saphenous, and superficial peroneal nerve blocks.

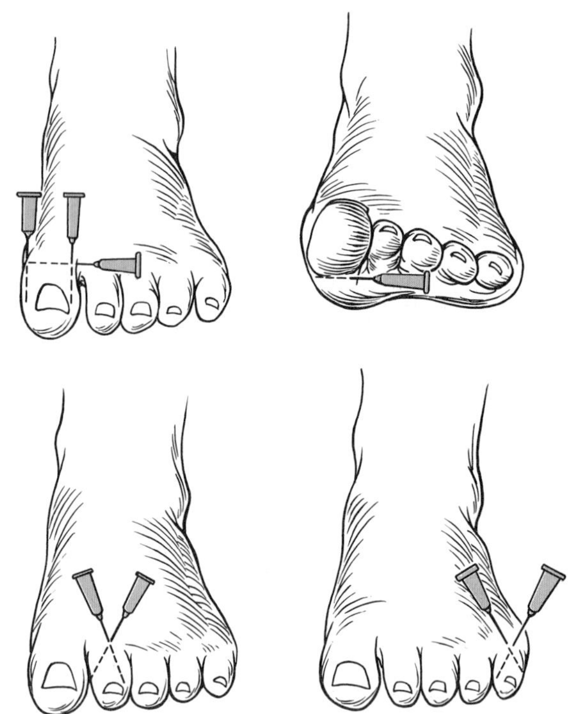

FIG. 32-12. (*Top*) Regional block of great toe. (*Bottom*) Regional block of other toes.

The deep peroneal nerve can be blocked by infiltrating 5 mLs of buffered lidocaine 1% (or bupivacaine 0.25%) between the tendons of the tibialis anterior and the extensor hallucis longus also just above the talocrural joint. However, the area supplied by the deep peroneal nerve is so small a digital block or local infiltration would achieve the same effect. Saphenous and sural nerves are described above.

TOE BLOCKS Digital nerve blocks of the toe are used for laceration repair and minor surgical procedures of the toe. Epinephrine must not be used as an adjunct to lidocaine because it may result in irreversible ischemic injury. A 27- or 30-gauge needle should be introduced through the skin on the dorsal aspect of the base of the midpoint of the involved toe (Fig. 32-12). The needle should be angled around the bone until it induces blanching of the skin on the plantar surface. As the needle is withdrawn, approximately 1.5 mL of 1% lidocaine is injected. Before the needle is withdrawn completely from the skin, it should be redirected to the opposite side of the injured toe to inject the local anesthetic agent in a similar manner. The total volume of the injected local anesthetic agent should not exceed 3 mL.

For the hallux (great toe), a modified collar (ring) block is used (see Fig. 32-12). The 27-gauge needle is inserted through the skin on the dorsolateral aspect of the base of the toe until it blanches the plantar skin. As the needle is withdrawn, 1.5 mL of 1% lidocaine is injected into the tissues. Before the needle is removed completely from the skin, the needle is passed under the skin on the dorsal aspect of the toe and 1.5 mL of 1% lidocaine is injected as the needle is withdrawn from the skin. The needle is then introduced through the anesthetized skin on the dorsomedial aspect of the toe and advanced until it produces blanching of the plantar skin, at which time the needle is withdrawn and 1.5 mL of 1% lidocaine is injected. Usually, approximately 4.5 mL of 1% lidocaine is needed to anesthetize the hallux.

FACIAL AND ORAL BLOCKS Facial blocks are ideal anesthesia techniques for commonly injured areas such as the forehead, chin, lips, nose, tongue and ear, where local infiltration is often either not possible, extremely painful or results in tissue distortion or potential tissue necrosis. These blocks, as for foot blocks, often require blockade of more than one nerve to provide for adequate regional anesthesia. For all intraoral routes of infiltration, a small amount of 2% viscous lidocaine should be applied to the mucosa prior to injection. For percutaneous routes of infiltration, topical EMLA cream or refrigerant sprays should be applied prior to injection.

Forehead (Trigeminal Nerve, Ophthalmic Branch, Frontal and Supratrochlear Nerves) The sensory innervation of the forehead (anterior aspect from eyebrows extending posteriorly to the lambdoid suture) is supplied by the lateral and medial branches of the frontal (or supraorbital) nerve and the supratrochlear nerve, branches of the ophthalmic branch of the trigeminal nerve (Fig. 32-13). Regional nerve block can be easily achieved by infiltration of 3 to 6 mLs of lidocaine 1% (or bupivacaine 0.25%) with a 27-gauge needle into the skin immediately above the full length of the eyebrow.

Lower Lip, Chin (Trigeminal Nerve, Mandibular Branch, Inferior Alveolar and Mental Nerve) Direct infiltration to the lip is very painful and causes tissue distortion which can interfere with the quality of the repair of lacerations. The skin of the chin and lower lip are supplied by the mental nerve (branch of the inferior alveolar nerve). A block of the inferior alveolar nerve as it enters the mandibular foramen, medial and just below the anterior border of the ramus of the mandible is performed by the intraoral route (Fig. 32-14). Regional block of the mental nerve can be performed by an intraoral (Fig. 32-15) or extraoral route. The mental foramen is located at the mucosal reflection of the lower lip and the lower gum, just posterior to the first premolar tooth.

TECHNIQUE The landmarks for the inferior alveolar nerve block are the inferior aspect of the vertical ridge of the anterior border of the ramus of the mandible (oblique line), and the oral mucosa 1 cm above the occlusal surface of the third molar tooth. After the mucosal injection site is anesthetized, the oblique line is identified by palpation. A 27-guage needle is inserted just medial to this ridge and 1 cm above the third molar tooth, and slowly advanced along the medial side of the ramus of the mandible to a depth of 2 cm, keeping the syringe in parallel position with the body of the mandible and the occlusal surfaces of the teeth of the lower jaw. While the needle remains in proximity to the medial aspect of the ramus of the mandible, 2 to 4 mLs of lidocaine 1% (with or without epinephrine) is infiltrated after the syringe is rotated over to the premolar region of the opposite side of the mandible, maintaining the same horizontal plane.

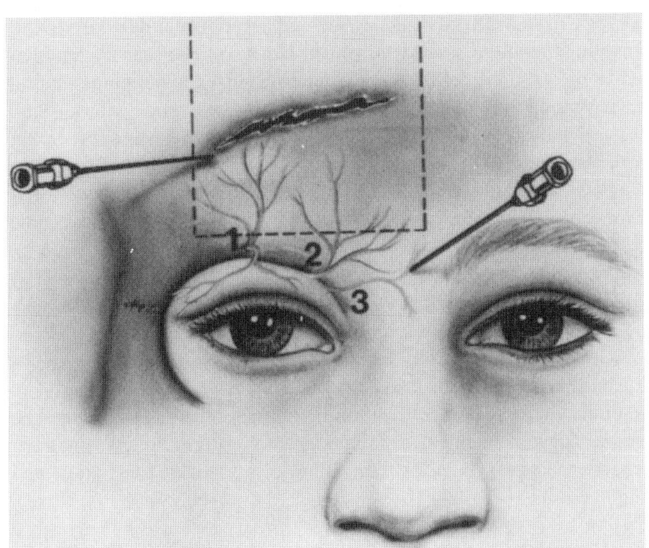

FIG. 32-13. Regional blocks of (1) the lateral branch of the frontal nerve, (2) the medial branch of the frontal nerve, and (3) the supratrochlear nerve. Infiltration anesthesia is an alternative approach to anesthetizing lacerations of the forehead.

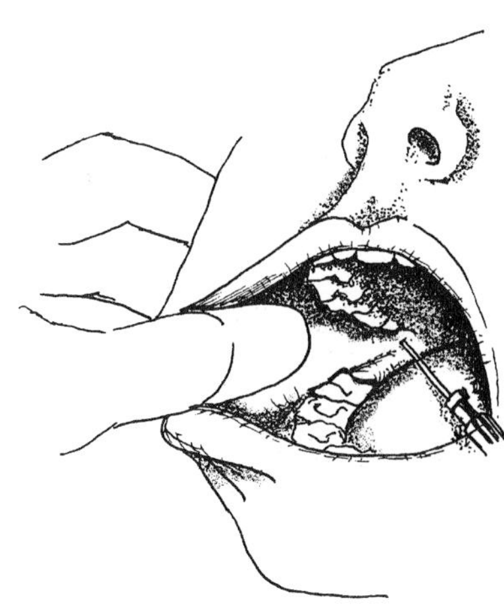

FIG. 32-14. Regional intraoral block of the lingual and inferior alveolar nerves.

For the oral approach to the mental nerve the lip is retracted with the thumb and index finger (see Fig. 32-15). A 27-gauge needle is inserted at the mucosal junction of the lower lip and gum near the mental foramen. 2 ml of lidocaine 1% with epinephrine (1:100,000) is infiltrated taking care that the needle is not introduced into the mental foramen to avoid neural injury. Similarly for the extraoral approach, identification of landmarks, and percutaneous infiltration of 2 mL of LA close to the mental foramen.

Tongue (Trigeminal Nerve, Mandibular Branch, Lingual Nerve) Direct infiltration into the sensate and moving of the tongue is very painful and poorly effective, and a regional block is preferred. The lingual nerve provides sensory innervation to the anterior two-thirds of the tongue, the floor of the mouth and gums. It lies in close proximity to the inferior alveolar nerve at the entrance to the mandibular foramen. The lingual nerve can be blocked by the intraoral route similarly to the inferior alveolar nerve (see Fig. 32-14).

TECHNIQUE From an intraoral approach the vertical ridge of anterior border of the ramus of the mandible is identified by palpation with the index finger (Fig. 32-15). After the mucosal injection site is anesthe-

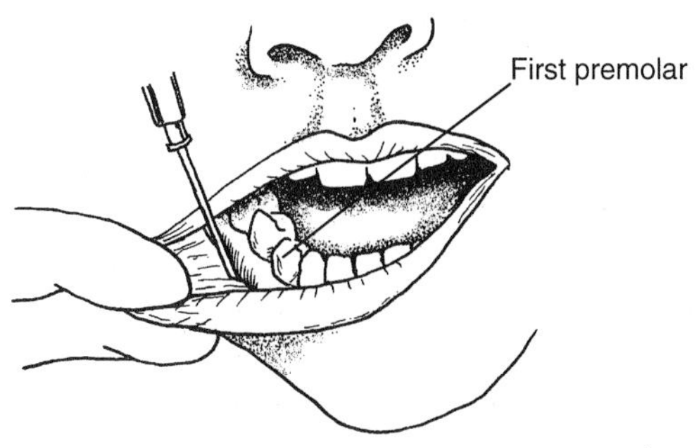

FIG. 32-15. Regional intraoral block of the mental nerve.

tized topically, the procedure for an inferior alveolar nerve block (same as above) is followed. Infiltration of the LA as the needle is withdrawn will anesthetize the lingual nerve. Alternatively the lingual nerve can be anesthetized by injecting 2 to 3 mLs of LA into the lateral floor of the mouth adjacent to the premolar teeth.

Cheek, Lower Eyelid, Upper Lip and Lateral Aspect of Nose (Trigeminal Nerve, Maxillary Branch, Infraorbital Nerve) The infraorbital nerve supplies sensory innervation to the cheek, lower eyelid, upper lip and lateral aspect of the side of the nose. A regional block of the infraorbital nerve can be performed by an intraoral approach (Fig. 32-16) or extraoral transcutaneous approach. The duration of action is more prolonged with the intraoral approach.

TECHNIQUE To identify the infraorbital foramen, the midpoint of the lower margin of the orbit is palpated, approximately 1 cm inferior to this point the infraorbital nerve exits the infraorbital foramen. For the intraoral approach, a palpating finger is positioned over the infraorbital foramen (Fig. 32-16). The cheek is retracted cephalad with the thumb and index finger and a 27-gauge needle with syringe, held in the other hand directed through the mucosa at the reflection of the upper gum opposite and parallel to the long axis of the upper premolar tooth. The needle is then advanced until it is palpated near the infraorbital foramen, approximately a depth of 2.5 cm. Use caution not to introduce the needle directly into the infraorbital foramen to avoid neural injury and subsequent numbness of the cheek, also use caution not to direct the needle too far superiorly or posteriorly to avoid inadverntently entering the orbit. Aspirate to ensure facial artery and vein are avoided. Instil 2 to 3 mLs of lidocaine 1% (or bupivacaine 0.25%) adjacent to the foramen. The extraoral approach uses the same landmarks for identification of the infraorbital foramen, but with a percutaneous approach. Epinephrine is best avoided due to the proximity of the facial artery.

Nose (Trigeminal Nerve, Ophthalmic Branch, Infratrochlear and External Nasal Nerves; Maxillary Branch, Infraorbital Nerve, Posterior Nasal and Nasopalatine Nerves) The sensory supply of the nose is supplied by both the ophthalmic and maxillary branches of the trigeminal nerve. It is important to note that block of the infraorbital nerve alone will not provide adequate anesthesia of the nose. The mucosal surface of the nose can be anesthetized by topical application of LA spray or gel. The ophthalmic branch of the trigeminal nerve (infratrochlear and external nasal nerves) provides sensation to the majority of the external nose in the midline. These nerves can be blocked by percutaneous infiltration of LA at the sites of their emergence from bony foraminae. The remaining aspects of the nose are supplied by the maxillary branch of the trigeminal nerve, the infraorbital nerve for the lateral aspect (see above for intraoral and extraoral block technique) and the posterior nasal and nasopalatine nerves for the septum and inferior midline. The posterior nasal and nasopalatine nerves are best approached intraorally in the midline from the mucosal surface of the reflection of the upper lip.

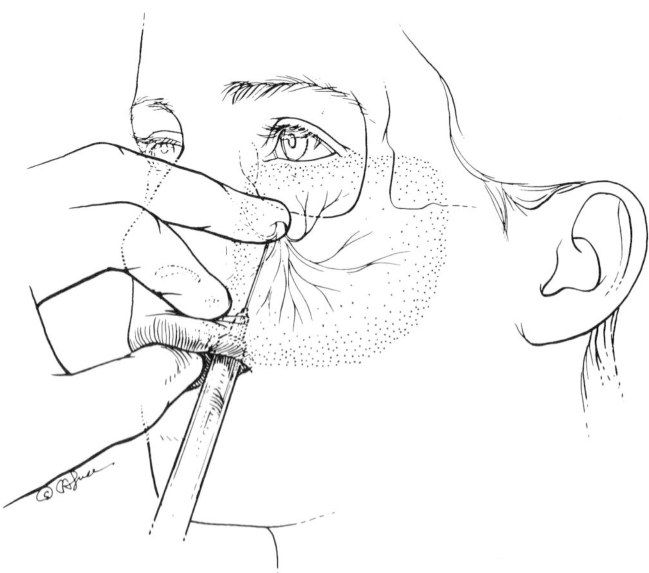

FIG. 32-16. Intraoral approach to regional nerve block of the infraorbital nerve.

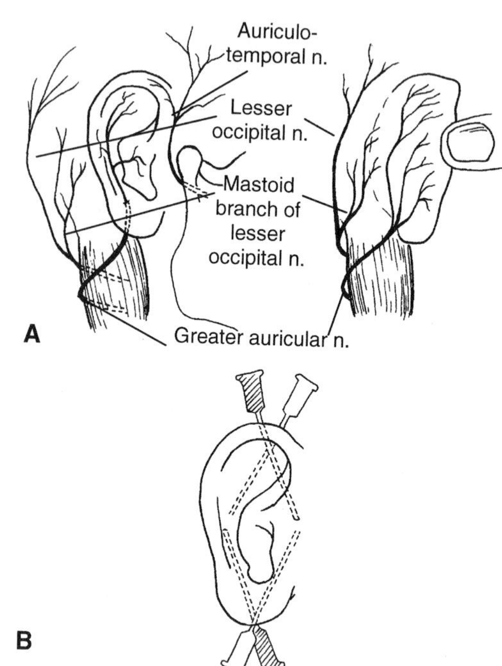

FIG. 32-17. A. Sensory nerve supply of the auricle. **B.** Technique of regional anesthesia of the auricle.

Ear (Trigeminal Nerve, Mandibular Branch, Auriculotemporal Nerve; Cervical Plexus C2 and C3; Greater Auricular Nerve and Mastoid Branch of Lesser Occipital Nerve) The sensory innervation to the external ear is supplied anteriorly by the auriculotemporal nerve (mandibular branch of the trigeminal nerve), and posteriorly by the greater auricular nerve and the mastoid branch of the lesser occipital nerve (branches of the cervical plexus). Direct infiltration of the pinna should be avoided due to the risk of tissue necrosis. Regional block of the ear is achieved by infiltration of lidocaine 1% (or bupivacaine 0.25%) via a 27- or 30-gauge needle at the base of the ear from an inferior and superior direction both anteriorly and posteriorly (Fig. 32-17, *A* and *B*)

FEMORAL NERVE BLOCK Femoral nerve block is an effective technique for relieving pain of a femoral shaft fracture and is useful in the multitrauma patient when minimizing narcotics is important. The femoral nerve is lateral to the femoral artery at the inguinal ligament and innervates the anterior thigh, the periosteum of the femur, and the knee joint (Fig. 32-18).

Technique Bupivacaine, 0.5 mL/kg (maximum 1 mL/kg, or 25 mL) of a 0.25 percent solution, is suggested as the preferred LA agent because of its longer duration of action. The usual adult dose is 10 to 20 mL. A sterile field is prepared over and surrounding the femoral triangle. The femoral artery is located midway between the anterior superior iliac crest and the pubic tubercle. The femoral artery is compressed 1 to 2 cm below the inguinal ligament with the nondominant hand. A weal of local anesthetic is raised in the skin and subcutaneous tissues lateral to the artery; the needle is then introduced 60° to the skin lateral and parallel to the femoral artery. A double loss of resistance or ''pop'' is felt as the needle traverses the fascia overlying the femoral nerve. Onset of anesthesia is 10 to 20 min, and the duration is 3 to 8 h.

INTERCOSTAL BLOCK Intercostal block is valuable for the management of pain after chest trauma (typically rib fracture) or discomfort from a chest tube. It is a simple block; however, caution should be exercised due to the rapid and high systemic absorption of local anesthetic at this site. Contraindications are local soft tissue disease and contralateral pneumothorax. Complications include pneumothorax and systemic toxicity. The intercostal nerves run anteriorly within the neurovascular bundle along the inferior portion of the rib. Addition of epinephrine enhances the safety of this block. The dosage range for an adult is 3 to 5 mL per segment (child, 1 to 3 mL) 1% lidocaine or 0.25% bupivacaine. To perform this procedure, the landmarks are the palpable intercostal spaces and the midaxillary line. The intercostal space is identified by palpation. On the upper margin of this space the inferior border of the upper rib is palpated. At the mid or posterior axillary line the needle is inserted and advanced at a 90° angle until the rib is reached. The needle is withdrawn slightly and redirected caudally to the inferior aspect of this upper rib (Fig. 32-19).

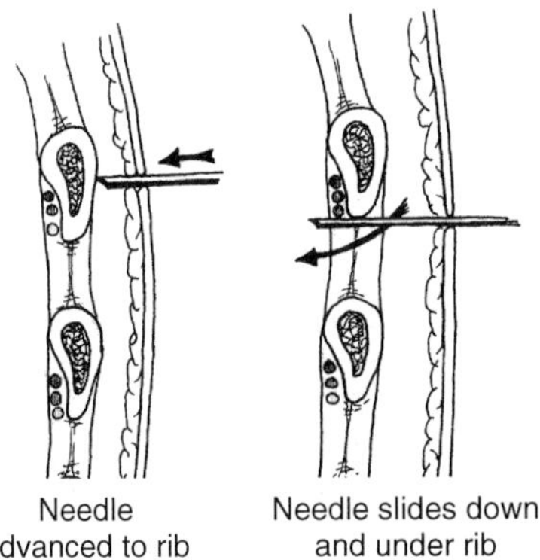

FIG. 32-19. Intercostal nerve block. (From Nichols DG et al: *Golden Hour: The Handbook of Advanced Pediatric Life Support,* 2d ed. St. Louis, Mosby Yearbook, 1996, p 336. Used by permission.)

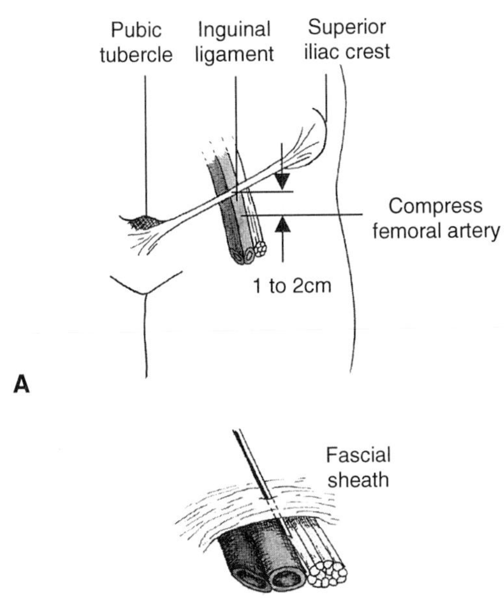

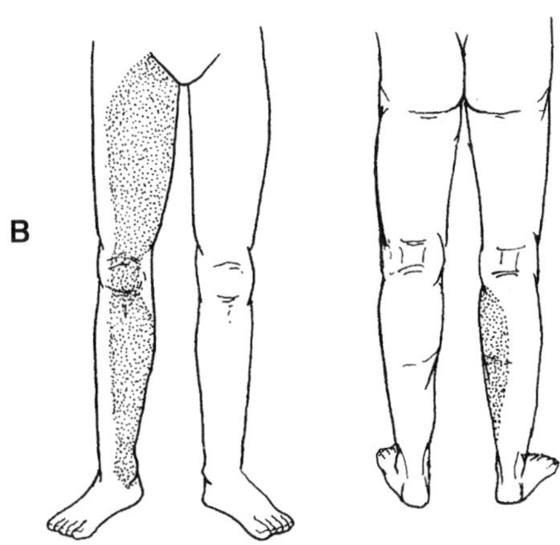

FIG. 32-18. A. Regional block of the femoral nerve. (Adapted from Nichols DG et al: *Golden Hour: The Handbook of Advanced Pediatric Life Support,* 2d ed. St. Louis, Mosby Yearbook, 1996, p 335. Used by permission.) **B.** Sensory innervation of the skin and femur by the femoral nerve is depicted in the shaded area. (From Yaster M et al: *Pediatric Pain Management and Sedation Handbook.* St. Louis, Mosby, 1997, p 176. Used by permission.)

Hematoma Blocks

Hematoma blocks are a simple, quick, and effective mode of regional anesthesia for isolated closed fracture reduction. Although hematoma blocks are safe the anesthesia that they provide is not as efficacious as the intravenous regional Bier block (see below). The hematoma block is a useful alternative when the Bier block is contraindicated.[28]

Technique Superficial anesthesia is obtained with local infiltration or other technique such as EMLA applied to the skin over the fracture site. An analgesic dose of narcotic can also be given if deemed appropriate. The fracture site is identified and using sterile technique, the hematoma is aspirated using a 10-mL syringe and 20- to 22-gauge needle. Lidocaine 1% without epinephrine is infiltrated (3 to 10 mL, maximum of 0.5 mL/kg) into the fracture cavity and around the periosteum. The block is effective within 5 to 10 min, with several hours duration.

Intravenous Regional Block (Bier Block)

A Bier block is a reliable regional anesthetic procedure involving intravenous administration of local anesthetic distal to an inflated pneumatic tourniquet. It is useful for fracture reductions, large laceration repairs, and foreign body removal. Duration of regional anesthesia is 30 to 60 min. In addition to routine monitoring and resuscitation equipment, the procedure requires a double-cuff tourniquet with a constant pressure gas source (Table 32-12). A standard blood pressure cuff is not acceptable and can result in catastrophic systemic leakage

TABLE 32-12 Equipment and Medications for Bier Block

Equipment
Double pneumatic cuff with constant-pressure gas source
ECG and BP monitoring
Oxygen
IV access ×2 (24 gauge in the injured limb)
Resuscitation equipment
Medication
Lidocaine 0.5%, 3 mg/kg (1.5 mg/kg minidose)
*Prilocaine 0.5%, 3 mg/kg
Availability of diazepam and resuscitation meds.

*Only in Australia and the United Kingdom.

of local anesthetic. Contraindications are listed in Table 32-13. The need for patients to have nothing by mouth for 4 h prior to the procedure may limit the usefulness of the technique. Use of this technique has also been applied to the lower limb in children, but it is less frequently used for the lower limb with larger children or adults.

Technique Lidocaine (0.6 mL/kg of 0.5 percent solution) without epinephrine is used. In Australia and the United Kingdom, prilocaine (0.6 mL/kg of 0.5 percent solution) is used. Increased efficacy has been shown with the addition of 60 mg of intravenous ketorolac or fentanyl (1 μg/kg) to the lidocaine. Bupivacaine is absolutely contraindicated due to cardiac toxicity. A "minidose" of 1 to 1.5 mg/kg 0.5 percent lidocaine without epinephrine has been used effectively in children.[29]

The patient should have nothing by mouth for at least 4 h. Vital signs and limb neurologic status and perfusion should be recorded and monitored. Intravenous access should be established in both upper limbs, distal to the fracture site on the affected limb. Standard resuscitation equipment and medications should be available. A small dose of narcotic may allay apprehension and the pain of the cuff, which usually occurs after 15 to 30 min.

The injured extremity is elevated and an Esmarch bandage may be applied (distal to proximal) to exsanguinate the limb. Protective padding is then applied to the upper arm to minimize cuff discomfort. Pneumatic double cuffs are then positioned over the padding on the upper arm. The proximal cuff is inflated to 50 to 100 mmHg above systolic pressure. A venous tourniquet may be positioned just proximal to the fracture site to contain the intravenous local anesthetic to this site. The lidocaine (or 0.5 percent prilocaine) is injected slowly over 2 min into the intravenous cannula in the affected limb. Mottling of the affected limb should occur within 2 to 5 min, followed by anesthesia and paresis of the limb. After 10 min, the distal cuff should be inflated (the area under this cuff should now be anesthetized); once the distal cuff is securely inflated, the proximal cuff can be deflated to minimize cuff pain. The distal cuff should not be de-inflated until at least 20 min has elapsed from the time of LA injection for tissue binding of the LA agent to occur, and thus to minimize the potential for toxicity. Loss of tourniquet pressure prior to this time will result in a systemic bolus of local anesthetic and potential systemic cardiac and CNS toxicity.

TABLE 32-13 Contraindications to Bier Block

Peripheral vascular disease
Raynaud's syndrome
Sickle cell disease
Cardiac conduction abnormalities
Hypertension, BP > 200 mmHg systolic
Cellulitis/infected extremity
Uncooperative patients
Young children (<5 years)
Local anesthetic allergy

REFERENCES

1. Acute Pain Management Guideline Panel: *Acute Pain Management: Operative or Medical Procedures and Trauma.* Guideline Report. AHCPR Pub. No. 92-002. Rockville, MD: Agency for Health Care Policy and Research, Public Health Service, U.S. Department of Health and Human Services, 1993.
2. Follin SL, Charland SL: Acute pain management: Operative or medical procedures and trauma. *Ann Pharmacother* 31:1068, 1997.
3. Grubb BD: Peripheral and central mechanisms of pain. *Br J Anaesth* 81:8, 1998.
4. Todd KH, Samaroo N, Hoffman JR: Ethnicity as a risk factor for inadequate emergency department analgesia. *JAMA* 269:1537, 1993.
5. Todd KH: Pain assessment and ethnicity. *Ann Emerg Med* 27:421, 1996.
6. Nevin K: Influence of sex on pain assessment and management. *Ann Emerg Med* 27:427, 1996.
7. McCormack HM, Home DJ, Sheather S: Clinical applications of visual analog scales: A critical review. *Psychol Med* 10:1007, 1988.
8. Todd KH: Clinical versus statistical significance in the assessment of pain relief. *Ann Emerg Med* 27:439, 1996.
9. Bates DW, Cullen DJ, Laird N, et al: Incidence of adverse drug events and potential adverse drug events: Implications for prevention. *JAMA* 274:29, 1995.
10. Brooks PM, Day RO: Nonsteroidal anti-inflammatory drugs: Differences and similarities. *N Engl J Med* 324:1716, 1991.
11. Moore RA, Tramer MR, Carroll D, et al: Quantitative systematic review of topically applied nonsteroidal inti-inflammatory drugs. *Br J Med* 316:333, 1998.
12. Neighbor ML, Puntillo KA: Intramuscular ketorolac vs oral ibuprofen in emergency department patients with acute pain. *Acad Emerg Med* 5:118, 1998.
13. Szeto HH, Inturrisi CE, Houde R, et al: Accumulation of normeperidine, an active metabolite of meperidine, in patients with renal failure of cancer. *Ann Intern Med* 86:738, 1977.
14. Jones JS, Johnson K, McNinch M: Age as a risk factor for inadequate emergency department analgesia. *Am J Emerg Med* 14:157, 1996.
15. Portenoy RK, Dole V, Joseph H, et al: Pain management and chemical dependency: Evolving perspectives. *JAMA* 278:592, 1997.
16. Wagner BE, O'Hare DA: Pharmacokinetics and pharmacodynamics of sedatives and analgesics in the treatment of agitated critically ill patients. *Clin Pharmacokinet* 33:426, 1997.
17. Ulett GA, Han S, Han JS: Electroacupuncture: Mechanisms and clinical application. *Biol Psychiatry* 44:129, 1998.
18. LoVecchio F, Oster N, Sturmann K, et al: The use of analgesics in patients with acute abdominal pain. *J Emerg Med* 15:775, 1997.
19. Attard AR, Corlett MJ, Kidner NJ, et al: Safety of early pain relief for acute abdominal pain. *Br Med J* 305:554, 1992.
20. Pace S, Burke TF: Intravenous morphine for early pain relief in patients with acute abdominal pain. *Acad Emerg Med* 3:1081, 1996.
21. Zoltie N, Cust MP: Analgesia in the acute abdomen. *Ann R Coll Surg* 68:209, 1986.
22. Seim MB, March JA, Dunn KA: Intravenous ketorolac versus intravenous prochlorperazine for the treatment of migraine headaches. *Acad Emerg Med* 5:573, 1998.
23. Capobianco DJ, Cheshire WP, Campbell JK: An overview of the diagnosis and pharmacologic treatment of migraine. *Mayo Clin Proc* 71:1055, 1996.
24. Harden RN, Gracely RH, Carter T, Warner G: The placebo effect in acute headache management: Ketorolac, meperidine, and saline in the emergency department. *Headache* 1996; 36:352, 1996.
25. Ducharme J, Beveridge RC, Lee J, Beaulieu S: Emergency management of migraine: Is the headache really over? *Acad Emerg Med* 5:899, 1998.

26. Buckley MM, Benfield P: Eutectic lidocaine/prilocaine cream: A review of the topical anaesthetic/analgesic efficacy of a eutectic mixture of local anaesthetics (EMLA). *Drugs* 46:126, 1993.
27. Robieux I, Kumar R, Radhakrishnan S, Koren G: Assessing pain and analgesia with a lidocaine-prilocaine emulsion in infants and toddlers during venipuncture. *J Pediatr* 971, 1991.
28. Furia JP, Alioto RJ, Marquardt JD: The efficacy and safety of the hematoma block for fracture reduction in closed, isolated fractures. *Orthopedics* 20:423, 1997.
29. Reuben SS, Steinberg RB, Kreitzer JM, Duprat KM: Intravenous regional anesthesia using lidocaine and ketorolac. *Anesth Analg* 81:110, 1995.

SYSTEMIC ANALGESIA AND SEDATION FOR PAINFUL PROCEDURES

David D. Nicolaou

Pain is either the chief complaint or is implicit in the chief complaint of many patients who seek care in the emergency department (ED). The recognition of its significance is sufficiently widespread that it has been included in the list of symptoms comprising the "prudent layperson" statutory definition of a medical emergency. The treatment of pain is therefore the essence of emergency medicine practice.

The provision of analgesia by physicians has historically been inadequate, and this has been shown to be true in the ED. A study of 198 patients admitted with acutely painful conditions found that only 89 (44 percent) received analgesics in the ED. Of these, 69 percent waited more than 1 h and 42 percent waited more than 2 h for opioid analgesia.[1] Similar findings have been demonstrated in other ED studies of pain treatment, both in the United States and abroad.[2,3] "Oligoanalgesia," the term coined by Wilson and Pendleton to describe the inadequate use of opioids to treat pain, unfortunately is often still present in EDs. Patients likely to receive inadequate analgesia include those over 70 years of age[4] and members of certain ethnic groups.[5] There is conflicting evidence, though, as to whether age is a factor.[6]

The reasons for inadequate analgesia are numerous. Minimal attention to pain management in medical school and residency, concern about narcotic diversion, abuse or addiction, and a limited understanding of analgesic pharmacology have all been hypothesized to contribute to "oligoanalgesia" in the ED. Physical evidence of distress, such as facial expressions and pulse rate, correlates poorly with the patient's perception of pain.[7]

DEFINITIONS

Pain is a noxious sensation transmitted by specialized nervous structures to the brain, where its perception is modified by cognition and emotion.[7] Analgesic and anesthetic techniques may modulate pain at the level of the peripheral nerves, spinal cord, thalamus, or cortex.

Analgesia is "relief of perception of pain without intentional production of a sedated state. Altered mental status may be a secondary effect of medications administered for this purpose."[8] Agents for pain relief interrupt axonal action potential propagation (i.e., "local anesthetics"), modulate the inflammatory cascade (e.g., ibuprofen), or modulate central nervous system (CNS) responses to pain (e.g., enkephalins and opioids).[7,9]

Anxiolysis is the reduction of apprehension without alterations in the level of consciousness.[8] A kind approach to the patient, a realistic and unhurried explanation of what may be expected, distracting conversation, and music have anxiolytic properties.

Neurolepsis is quiescence, indifference to surroundings, and reduced motor activity. Agents used for this purpose include haloperidol and droperidol.

Dissociation is characterized by amnesia, analgesia, sedation, and maintenance of muscle tone. Ketamine is the only commonly used dissociative agent.

Sedation is controlled reduction of environmental awareness.[8] It is not so much a specific level of consciousness as it is a continuum, incorporating anxiolysis or light sedation at one extreme and general anesthesia at the other. The agent or agents chosen, the rate of delivery, the pharmacokinetics of CNS uptake and redistribution, the kinetics of metabolic and elimination pathways, and the degree of patient stimulation may result in varying degrees of sedation over time. The level of sedation is dynamic within a given patient and must be continually assessed to detect changes in its depth. *Light* or *conscious sedation* (CS) produces minimal depression in the level of consciousness and enables the patient to maintain a patent airway and respond appropriately to stimulation or commands.[8] *Deep sedation* produces marked depression of consciousness or unconsciousness and frequently results in loss of independent airway maintenance, protective reflexes, adequate respirations, and satisfactory hemodynamics.[8]

General anesthesia is the presence of "sensory, mental, reflex, and motor blockade and concurrent loss of all protective reflexes."[10]

PRINCIPLES OF CONSCIOUS SEDATION

The indications for CS include the treatment of severe pain, attenuation of the pain and anxiety associated with procedures, rapid tranquilization, and the need to perform a diagnostic procedure (Table 33-1). No single regimen fits all patients and their clinical problems, so doses and agents should be individualized. The physician must integrate the nature of the planned procedure with an assessment of the patient's wishes and physical status, the physician's skills, the patient's intended disposition, the available resources, and a sound knowledge of the pharmacology of the available drugs to formulate a management plan.

The agents used for CS often have a relatively narrow therapeutic index. *They should therefore be given in small incremental intravenous doses, allowing adequate time for the development and assessment of peak effect.* If the desired effect seems unusually difficult or easy to achieve, no additional medication should be administered and the patient should be carefully monitored until the cause is determined (Table 33-2). Monitoring of patients and medication administration should be performed by a second provider who understands the pharmacology of the agents used, possesses sound advanced airway-management skills, and will not be distracted by other tasks during the period when the patients' ability to independently maintain their airway is in doubt.

TABLE 33-1 Selected Indications for Systemic Analgesia and Sedation

Indication
Abscess incision and drainage
Wound debridement
Tube thoracostomy
Laceration repair
Fracture manipulation
Joint reduction
Cardioversion
Diagnostic interview
Diagnostic study
Rapid tranquilization

TABLE 33-2 Differential Diagnoses of Unexpected Drug Effects by Phase of Drug Disposition

	CLINICAL EFFECT	
Phase of Dispositon	Less Than Expected	More Than Expected
Delivery	Blood pressure cuff/tourniquet up IV catheter dislodged IV line clamped/kinked IV bag empty Syringe contents incorrect	Syringe contents incorrect
Uptake and distribution	Hypovolemia Acidosis (for opioids) Elevated acute-phase reactants (fentanyl)	Alkalosis (for opioids) Hypoproteinemia (for bound drugs) Pregnancy (fentanyl)
Redistribution	Obesity (fentanyl)	Reperfusion of muscle (after large doses of fentanyl)
Clearance	Alcohol use	P-450 oxidase inhibitors (e.g., cimetidine) Use of drugs which compete for P-450 metabolism (e.g., erythromycin, lidocaine, midazolam) (opioids) Liver disease (morphine) Renal disease Hypovolemia (especially fentanyl) Advanced age (especially fentanyl)
Other	Tolerance	Use of other drugs Delirium Metabolic encephalopathy

Table 33-3 lists equipment for CS. A dedicated area for CS should ideally be established, with well-labeled supplies and equipment always in a consistent location. It can easily be stocked with drugs and labels, resuscitation and monitoring equipment, and equipment for common procedures. Drug dosages and documentation tools may be kept in a single location, improving risk management and quality-improvement efforts.

The use of pulse oximetry during CS is important. By 1990, more than 80 deaths had been reported following the use of midazolam, commonly in conjunction with an opioid, for sedation.[11] Coadministration of midazolam (0.05 mg/kg) and fentanyl (2.0 μg/kg) to 12 healthy volunteers produced hypoxemia (Sa_{O_2} <90 percent for longer than 10 s) in 11 and apnea in 6.[11] A study of pulse oximetry and nasal end-tidal CO_2 values in 27 ED patients who were sedated with benzodiazepines and/or opiates for a painful procedure noted that one patient developed clinically significant apnea and eight developed clinically silent hypoxemia.[12] The American Medical Association's (AMA) Council on Scientific Affairs subsequently called for the development of standards by specialty societies for the use of pulse oximetry during conscious sedation.[13] Several authors have noted that when oxygen supplementation is given, extreme ventilatory insufficiency may develop in the absence of hypoxemia. The clinical significance of hypoxemia during sedation is still uncertain, but abnormal pulse oximetry certainly counsels providers to evaluate the patient carefully.

TABLE 33-3 Equipment for Intravenous Analgesia and Sedation

High-flow oxygen source*
Suction source with large-bore catheters*
Vascular access equipment*
Airway-management equipment*
Monitoring equipment Electrocardiography Pulse oximeter* Blood pressure* Capnograph (if available)
Resuscitation drugs*
Reversal agents (appropriate to drugs being used*)
Adequate staff for monitoring and documentation*

Note: Not all equipment is required for all patients, procedures, and regimens. Suggested minimum equipment is marked with an asterisk.

ASSESSMENT OF PATIENTS

A patient's general physical status can be conveniently described by using the American Society of Anesthesiologists' (ASA) classification (Table 33-4). Any medications or intoxicants should be solicited and their effects considered when selecting medications. The patient's airway should be systematically evaluated by the provider who will be responsible for its management during CS (see Chap. 15, "Tracheal Intubation and Mechanical Ventilation"). Depending on clinical circumstances, a patient with an anticipated difficult airway or an ASA classification of 3 or 4 may require consultation with an anesthesiologist. Patients with underlying neurologic diseases such as cerebral palsy, myasthenia gravis, or mental retardation may be much more sensitive to sedatives and consultation is suggested in such cases.

CS requires careful assessment of its risks and benefits based on the clinical scenario and the agents to be used. Patients should be fully informed of the risks of the procedure and the alternatives available. The patient's expectations should be carefully explored and should be corrected when they are not reasonable. Clarify that CS is not general anesthesia and that no surety of complete amnesia and analgesia can be offered. Written informed consent documents may

TABLE 33-4 American Society of Anesthesiologists Physical Status Classification

Class	Description	Examples
I	Normal, healthy patient	—
II	Mild systemic disease	Asthma, controlled diabetes
III	Moderate systemic disease	Stable angina, diabetes with hyperglycemia, moderate chronic obstructive pulmonary disease
IV	Severe systemic disease	Unstable angina, diabetic ketoacidosis
V	Moribund	—
+E	Modifier added to any classification indicating "emergency" status	All emergency department patients

TABLE 33-5 Dose Equivalents and Pharmacokinetics of Analgesics

Generic Name/ Products	Dose	Approximately Equivalent to	Peak Effect	Duration of Effect	Plasma Half-life	Notes
Opioids						
Morphine sulfate	5 mg IV 10 mg IM 60 mg PO	Morphine 5 mg IV	15–30 min 1 h 2 h	2–4 h 4–5 h 4–5 h	2.5–3 h	Releases histamine
Fentanyl citrate	50 μg IV	Morphine ~4 mg IV*	~2.5–10 min	30–90 min	3–4 h	Does not release histamine May cause chest wall rigidity Higher doses prolong clinical effects
Meperidine	50 mg IV 75 mg IM	Morphine 5 mg IV	5–15 min 30–60 min	3–4 h	3–6 h	Normeperidine is epileptogenic Normeperidine half-life: 15–20 h; up to 30–40 h in renal failure
Hydromorphone	1 mg IV 1.5 mg IM	Morphine 5 mg IV	15 min 30–60 min	2–3 h 3–4 h	2–3 h	
Oxycodone	5 mg PO	Morphine 3 mg IV Morphine 10 mg IM	1 h	2–3 h		Tylox: 5 mg oxycodone + 500 mg APAP Percocet: 5 mg oxycodone +325 mg APAP; liquid: 5 mg oxycodone +325 mg APAP per 5 mL (1 tsp)
Codeine	200 mg PO	Morphine 5 mg IV Codeine 130 mg IM				
Nonopioids						
Ibuprofen	400 mg PO	Morphine 5–10 mg IM				
Ketorolac	30 mg IV	Morphine 12 mg IM				
Acetaminophen (APAP)	650 mg PO	Morphine 1 mg IV				
Acetylsalicylic acid (ASA)	650 mg PO	Morphine 1 mg IV				

Note: *Fentanyl is highly lipophilic and is therefore difficult to compare directly with morphine.
Abbreviation: APAP, *N*-acetyl-*p*-aminophenol.

be required at certain hospitals, but are not a substitute for the physician's note documenting patient discussion.

PHARMACOLOGY

Analgesics

Opioids are the most common analgesics used in CS. Classes of opioid analgesics include opium (morphine and codeine) and phenylpiperidine (meperidine, fentanyl, sufentanil, and alfentanil) derivatives. The analgesic activity of a drug is traditionally referenced to morphine (Table 33-5). Following systemic administration, morphine analgesia is mediated through supraspinal μ_1 receptors (possibly by activating descending inhibitory pathways to the dorsal horn cells, and possibly by activating more rostral mechanisms in the brainstem). Spinal cord analgesia is mediated by μ_2 receptors. All opioids have analgesic, sedative, and antitussive effects; they do not reliably produce amnesia when given in doses commonly used for CS. Opioids may also produce muscle rigidity, pruritis, nausea, vomiting, and constipation, and impair ventilation. Respiratory depression is potentiated in the presence of other CNS depressants.

Agents in common use for ED CS include morphine, fentanyl, and meperidine.

Meperidine may be a poor choice for ED analgesia in general. It causes more histamine release than either morphine or fentanyl. Its primary metabolite, normeperidine, is bioactive and toxic. Normeperidine causes CNS excitation, including tremors, myoclonus, and seizures, effects that are not antagonized by naloxone. Because normeperidine is excreted by the kidneys, it accumulates in renal insufficiency and with repeated doses.[14] Meperidine may also cause a fatal reaction when coadministered with monoamine oxidase inhibitors. This reaction may be excitatory (agitation, rigidity, hyperpyrexia, seizures, and coma) or depressive (respiratory depression, hypotension, and coma). For these reasons, meperidine is considered a second-line agent in the treatment of pain when opioid analgesics are considered.

MORPHINE Morphine is a naturally occurring opioid that is approximately 35 percent protein bound, 77 percent ionized at pH 7.4, and poorly lipid soluble. It therefore is slow to penetrate the blood-brain barrier and, after small bolus injections, 10 to 30 min are required before its peak effects are seen. Doses of 0.2 mg/kg result in peak effects in less than 1 h that may last for 4 to 6 h. It releases histamine and therefore may produce hypotension, especially in preload-dependent patients. Its analgesic effects, and its respiratory depression, have been shown to be potentiated by coadministration of hydroxyzine in postoperative patients;[15] the significance of this finding for ED CS is uncertain, especially since hydroxyzine is not recommended for intravenous (IV) use. Morphine undergoes hepatic glucuronidation to morphine-3-glucuronide and morphine-6-glucuronide; the latter is four times as potent as morphine and has a duration of action approximately double that of its parent. The daughter compounds are renally excreted and accumulate in renal insufficiency.

FENTANYL Fentanyl is a synthetic phenylpiperidine derivative that is approximately 80 to 85 percent protein bound and 92 percent ionized at pH 7.4. However, it is highly lipid soluble, resulting in rapid CNS uptake and an effect onset half-time of 6.4 min. Fentanyl is also distributed into adipose tissue, though, creating a ''reservoir'' of fentanyl. The size of this reservoir is dose dependent, with higher doses resulting in a progressively increasing duration of effect as the drug is released from tissue stores and then eliminated. Furthermore, distribution from plasma may not result in drug levels below those associated with clinical effects and respiratory depression. Thus, the use of relatively high doses of fentanyl (i.e., in the range of 10 μg/kg) results in greatly prolonged clinical effects and elimination half-times. Fentanyl is metabolized in the liver to inactive compounds.

Fentanyl has been shown to have a low complication rate when used for CS in the ED. Chudnofsky and colleagues noted six cases of respiratory depression (largely in patients who were intoxicated or had received other drugs) and three cases of hypotension among 841 ED patients receiving fentanyl.[16] Respiratory depression occurs at significantly lower fentanyl doses when another respiratory depressant, such as alcohol or midazolam, is present. Chest wall rigidity may occur in a dose-dependent fashion following fentanyl administration; approximately half of healthy volunteers develop chest wall rigidity in response to 15 μg/kg, a dose not usually used in CS in the ED. Rigidity and apnea, however, may occur with even small doses of fentanyl, resulting in respiratory insufficiency. The rigidity is not reliably antagonized by naloxone and may require neuromuscular blockade and intubation to enable adequate ventilation. Fentanyl does not release histamine, which mediates most of the peripheral vascular effects of narcotics, so it rarely produces hypotension.[17]

Anxiolytics

The prototypical anxiolytics in common use for CS in the ED are the benzodiazepines, which potentiate the inhibitory activity of γ-aminobutyric acid (GABA) in the CNS by binding to benzodiazepine-specific receptors on the $GABA_A$-benzodiazepine receptor complex, which induces a conformational change that potentiates GABA-mediated chloride influx. This activity results in sedation, amnesia, anxiolysis, and anticonvulsant effects, as well as respiratory depression. The benzodiazepine most commonly used for CS in the ED is midazolam, which produces earlier sedation, more frequent amnesia, less pain on injection, and improved 90-min alertness and readiness for discharge when compared with diazepam.[18]

Midazolam has a number of characteristics favorable for use in ED CS. Its diazepine ring opens at pH values of less than 4, in which form it is quite water soluble. At physiologic pH, the ring closes, rendering midazolam highly lipid soluble, with associated rapid CNS uptake producing peak effects within a few minutes of IV administration. Midazolam's relatively high volume of distribution compared with other benzodiazepines derives from its lipophilicity. This characteristic is greatly amplified in obese patients, resulting in an increase in plasma half-life from 2.7 to 8.4 h. Midazolam is cleared by hepatic hydroxylation to 1-hydroxymidazolam (which is pharmacologically active) and to 4-hydroxymidazolam and 1,4-dihydroxymidazolam, which are conjugated and excreted in the urine.

The combination of midazolam with alcohol or opioids greatly increases sedative and respiratory-depressant effects, and increases the risk of cardiovascular depression. Midazolam should be used cautiously in such cases, with careful monitoring of respiratory and hemodynamic status.

The dose of midazolam should be individualized. Midazolam should be given in small incremental doses until the desired effect is achieved. Aliquots of 0.25 to 0.5 mg given every 3 to 5 min in healthy adults, or 0.1 to 0.25 mg every 5 to 10 min in the intoxicated or elderly patient, is a reasonable starting point. Chronic alcohol users who do not have cirrhosis may require relatively high doses of midazolam to achieve the clinical effects desired.

Anesthetics

PROPOFOL Propofol (2,6-diisopropylphenol) is a lipid-soluble anesthetic agent that is supplied in an emulsion of soybean oil and purified egg phosphatide, which most egg-allergic patients should tolerate, since it contains no protein. The emulsion is responsible for frequent burning on injection and contains no preservatives, resulting in the risk of bacterial growth in improperly handled solutions. When given by infusion, the onset of sedation is rapid (5 to 10 min), and it resolves rapidly (5 to 10 min) upon discontinuation of the infusion.[19] Amnesia, however, is not reliably produced in doses used for sedation. The drug possesses antiemetic properties. Propofol produces significant cardiovascular depression, with dose-related declines in systolic blood pressure of up to 25 to 40 percent when given in induction doses. This effect is more pronounced in those with hemodynamic compromise and in the elderly.

The use of propofol for ED CS is controversial, and its use outside the operating room by nonanesthesia personnel may be restricted by hospital policy. However, Swanson and colleagues employed a regimen of 2 μg/kg fentanyl and a propofol infusion at a loading rate of 0.21 (mg/kg)/min, followed by a maintenance rate of 3 to 6 (mg/kg)/h in 20 ED patients who required CS. This provided rapid onset of sedation (mean, 6.6 min) and rapid recovery (mean, 6.1 min), with high patient and physician satisfaction scores. Three patients had pain on injection, one had pain and brief hypotension, and two had brief episodes of apnea; 75 percent had amnesia for the procedure at 24 h.[19]

Propofol is a promising agent for CS in the ED because it rapidly produces sedation that quickly abates when the infusion is discontinued. In doses usually used for CS, however, both analgesic and amnestic agents may be required, which may result in hypoventilation and potentiate the already significant hemodynamic effects of propofol. Further study is required before the routine use of propofol in the ED can be recommended.

KETAMINE Ketamine is a phencyclidine derivative that has analgesic and anesthetic properties. Ketamine anesthesia is often called ''dissociative,'' reflecting electroencephalographically demonstrable discontinuity of the corticothalamic and limbic systems. The patient's eyes often remain open, with spontaneous horizontal and vertical nystagmus. Muscle tone may be increased, and corneal reflexes and spontaneous swallowing are preserved; occasional purposeful movements unrelated to the environment occur. Emergence reactions, characterized by disturbing dreams and vivid, sometimes frightening hallucinations, occur in 5 to 30 percent of patients. Patients at greatest risk for emergence reactions are over 16, female, normally dream, have personality disorders, or receive droperidol or atropine. These phenomena may be attenuated with benzodiazepines given before or at the completion of the procedure.

Ketamine is highly lipid soluble and has a pKa of 7.5, accounting for the rapid (within 1 min) onset of hypnosis following IV injection.

Peak brain and plasma concentrations develop within 1 min; rapid redistribution to peripheral tissues results in a mean hypnosis time of 6 min (1.0 mg/kg) to 10 min (2.0 mg/kg). Ketamine is metabolized by the hepatic P-450 system to several active metabolites, the chief among which is norketamine. Norketamine appears within 2 min of a bolus injection and is one-tenth to one-third less potent than the parent drug, but does not appear to penetrate the CNS in quantities sufficient to produce hypnosis. Subsequent metabolites are conjugated and renally excreted, but, because they are much less active, the dose appears not to require adjustment in patients with renal insufficiency. Drugs which induce the P-450 system increase the metabolism of ketamine, whereas inhibitors prolong the duration of effect.

The hemodynamic response to ketamine is complex. It is a direct myocardial depressant and vasodilator, but these effects are typically overshadowed by stimulation of significant CNS sympathetic outflow, resulting in tachycardia and vasoconstriction. (The author's experience is that fentanyl, 1 to 2 μg/kg given 3 to 5 min prior to the procedure, attenuates this effect but increases the frequency of hypoxemia, especially when ketamine is given rapidly.) However, profoundly hypovolemic patients or those with little sympathetic reserve (e.g., cocaine users) may develop hypotension, particularly at rapid rates of injection.

The pulmonary effects of ketamine make it an appealing agent. Although it produces bronchodilation and bronchorrhea, it rarely causes significant respiratory depression unless given by rapid injection (over less than 60 s) or coadministered with other agents. Patients usually retain protective airway reflexes, but this is not a certainty, and careful monitoring is necessary when ketamine is used.

Before giving ketamine, it is important to consider the drug's likely nontherapeutic effects. If a hyperdynamic state or bronchorrhea may not be well tolerated, then appropriate premedication (opioids or glycopyrrolate) should be given or another agent chosen. A specific discussion of the emergence phenomenon with the patient, family, and friends will reduce the impact of this occasionally dramatic event.

The dose of ketamine commonly used for analgesia is 0.5 to 1.0 mg/kg over 60 s. Anesthesia is produced by doses of 1 to 2 mg/kg. When anesthetic doses are administered, midazolam should be given during the emergence phase to attenuate emergence phenomena.

Adjunctive Agents

Antiemetic agents are useful in the treatment of nausea and vomiting accompanying opioid therapy. Their value as "potentiators" of opioids is not clear, and they should not be routinely employed for this purpose.

Antidotal agents

NALOXONE Naloxone, which is a competitive antagonist of opioids at μ receptors, is indicated for reversal of unwanted respiratory depression following opioid administration. Patients who are opioid dependent may develop withdrawal following the administration of naloxone. Naloxone may not reverse chest wall rigidity caused by fentanyl. It should be given in small increments (0.1 to 0.2 mg every 1 to 2 min) until the desired effect is achieved. Because patients who receive long-acting opioids or who clear opioids slowly may redevelop respiratory depression after clearing all or part of an effective dose of naloxone, continual patient reassessment is required after naloxone administration.

FLUMAZENIL Flumazenil, which is a competitive antagonist of benzodiazepines, is given in IV aliquots of 0.1 to 0.2 mg every 1 to 2 min until the desired effect is achieved. It has a half-life of 45 to 104 min, rendering resedation a possibility if the effects of a long-acting benzodiazepine are reversed with flumazenil. It should be used with caution in benzodiazepine-dependent patients. Flumazenil was shown in a study of 133 ED patients to reverse midazolam-induced sedation safely and effectively. However, the time from completion of the procedure to discharge from the ED was no shorter in the group treated with flumazenil than in the control group.[20] Flumazenil is indicated for reversal of respiratory depression caused by benzodiazepine during CS, but its routine use to "awaken" patients cannot be recommended.

TABLE 33-6 Discharge Criteria for Patients Receiving Conscious Sedation

Vital signs stable for at least a half hour
No evidence of respiratory distress
Minimal or no nausea, vomiting, or dizziness
Alert, oriented, and able to retain information
Able to take fluids and medications by mouth
Ambulation consistent with preprocedure status
Receives, comprehends, and retains discharge instructions
Responsible person present to accompany patient

DISCHARGE

Discharge criteria for CS are outlined in Table 33-6. These guidelines may require modification based on patient age, clinical circumstances, the agents used, and the patient's social situation. Patients must not be permitted to drive or operate heavy machinery for at least 24 h after CS. The agents used for CS often produce anterograde amnesia, which may be present even when consciousness appears otherwise normal. It is therefore vital to evaluate the patient's ability to retain information prior to discharge.

Discharge planning is an important component of CS and should be part of the preprocedure evaluation process. A patient who is likely to require prolonged postprocedure monitoring or treatment should be considered for hospital admission. If a companion is required for discharge, he or she should be identified prior to beginning CS.

POLICY ISSUES

Clinical Standards and Documentation

The increasingly widespread use of IV sedation and analgesia outside the operating room has garnered the attention of various organizations. The clinician's decisions regarding CS are increasingly subject to

TABLE 33-7 Cost* of Drugs Used During Conscious Sedation

Drug	Formulation	Cost
Morphine sulfate	10 mg/mL	$0.60
Fentanyl	100 μg/2 mL	$2.06
Midazolam	5 mg/mL	$10.90
Ketamine	500 mg/5 mL	$19.44
Propofol	200 mg/20 mL	$14.48
Naloxone	0.4 mg/1 mL	$5.25
Flumazenil	0.5 mg/5 mL	$36.88

Note: *Cost to pharmacist per unit of use (1 vial) based on case prices.

regulations and standards, and these in turn are evolving in parallel with local and national CS experience. The development of guidelines concerning ED CS has been hampered by the lack of high-quality clinical evidence, such as clinical trials, supporting particular practices. As a result, few evidence-based standards exist.

The Joint Commission on Accreditation of Healthcare Organizations (JCAHO) standard specifies that a uniform standard of care must be provided throughout an accredited institution. This means that situations in which protective airway reflexes are typically expected to be lost might be held to the standard of care provided in the operating room.[21] The American College of Emergency Physicians[22] and the American Society of Anesthesiologists[23] have also begun to promulgate guidelines. Each ED should develop standards for CS, and then strive to provide and document care consistent with that standard.

Costs

The true costs and benefits of CS are presently difficult to judge. The current costs of individual drugs are presented in Table 33-7. The costs of a properly equipped CS room, staff to monitor patients, drugs, and risk management have not been rigorously studied. The impact of CS on the length of stay, patient satisfaction, and referral patterns is difficult to assess. Although outcome and cost issues are not yet well defined, CS is nonetheless fundamental to the effective and humane performance of painful procedures in the ED.

REFERENCES

1. Wilson JE, Pendleton JM: Oligoanalgesia in the emergency department. *Am J Emerg Med* 7:620, 1989.
2. Jantos TJ, Paris PM, Menegazzi JJ, Yealy DM: Analgesic practice for acute orthopedic trauma pain in Costa Rican emergency departments. *Ann Emerg Med* 28:145, 1996.
3. Reichl M, Bodiwala GG: Use of analgesia in severe pain in the accident and emergency department. *Arch Emerg Med* 4:25, 1987.
4. Jones JS, Johnson K, McNinch M: Age as a risk factor for inadequate emergency department analgesia. *Am J Emerg Med* 14:157, 1996.
5. Todd KH, Samaroo N, Hoffman JR: Ethnicity as a risk for inadequate emergency department analgesia. *JAMA* 269:1537, 1993.
6. Lewis LM, Lasater LC, Brooks CB: Are emergency physicians too stingy with analgesics? *South Med J* 87:7, 1994.
7. Paris PM: No pain, no pain. *Am J Emerg Med* 7:660, 1989.
8. Sacchetti A, Schafermeyer R, Gerardi M, et al: Pediatric analgesia and sedation. *Ann Emerg Med* 23:237, 1994.
9. Menegazzi JJ, Paris PM, Kersteen CH, et al: A randomized, controlled trial of the use of music during laceration repair. *Ann Emerg Med* 20:348, 1991.
10. Ward KR, Yealy DM: Systemic analgesia and sedation for procedures, in Roberts JR, Hedges JR (eds): *Clinical Procedures in Emergency Medicine.* Philadelphia, WB Saunders, 1998, pp 516–531.
11. Bailey PL, Pace NL, Ashburn MA, et al: Frequent hypoxemia and apnea after sedation with midazolam and fentanyl. *Anesthesiology* 73:826, 1990.
12. Wright SW: Conscious sedation in the emergency department: The value of capnography and pulse oximetry. *Ann Emerg Med* 21:551, 1992.
13. Council on Scientific Affairs AMA: The use of pulse oximetry during conscious sedation. *JAMA* 270:1463, 1993.
14. Szeto HH, Inturrisi CE, Houde R, et al: Accumulation of normeperidine, an active metabolite of meperidine, in patients with renal failure of cancer. *Ann Intern Med* 86:738, 1977.
15. Hupert CP, Yacoub M, Turgeon LR: Effect of hydroxyzine on morphine analgesia for the treatment of postoperative pain. *Anesth Analg* 59:690, 1980.
16. Chudnofsky CR, Wright SW, Dronen SC, et al: The safety of fentanyl use in the emergency department. *Ann Emerg Med* 18:635, 1989.
17. Rosow CE, Moss J, Philbin DM, Savarese JJ: Histamine release during morphine and fentanyl anesthesia. *Anesthesiology* 56:93, 1982.
18. Wright SW, Chudnofsky CR, Dronen SC, et al: Comparison of midazolam and diazepam for conscious sedation in the emergency department. *Ann Emerg Med* 22:201, 1993.
19. Swanson ER, Seaberg DC, Mathias S: The use of propofol for sedation in the emergency department. *Academic Emergency Medicine* 3:234, 19
20. Chudnofsky CR: Group TEMCSS: Safety and efficacy of flumazenil in reversing conscious sedation in the emergency department. *Acad Emerg Med* 4:944, 1997.
21. Sklar DP: Joint commission on accreditation of healthcare organizations requirements for sedation. *Ann Emerg Med* 27:412, 1996.
22. American College of Emergency Physicians: Clinical policy for procedural sedation and analgesia in the emergency department. *Ann Emerg Med* 31:663, 1998.
23. Task Force on Sedation and Analgesia by Non-Anesthesiologists: A report by the American Society of Anesthesiologists task force on sedation and analgesia by non-anesthesiologists. *Anesthesiology* 84:459, 1996.

MANAGEMENT OF PATIENTS WITH CHRONIC PAIN

David M. Cline

Chronic pain is defined as a painful condition that lasts longer than 3 months.[1] Chronic pain can also be defined as pain that persists beyond the reasonable time for an injury to heal or a month beyond the usual course of an acute disease. There are four basic types of chronic pain: (1) pain persisting beyond the normal healing time for a disease or injury, (2) pain related to a chronic degenerative disease or persistent neurologic condition, (3) cancer-related pain, (4) pain that emerges or persists without an identifiable cause. Chronic pain differs from acute pain in its function. Acute pain is an essential biologic signal to warn the individual to stop a potentially injurious activity or to prompt one to seek medical care. Chronic pain serves no obvious biologic function. Chronic pain patients presenting to the emergency department (ED) have not been well studied, despite their apparent numbers.

Complete eradication of pain is not a reasonable end point in most cases. Rather, the goal of therapy is pain reduction and return to functional status. Chronic pain syndromes discussed in this chapter include myofascial headaches, ''transformed'' migraine headaches, fibromyalgia, myofascial chest pain, back pain, complex regional pain types I and II, postherpetic neuralgia, and phantom limb pain. Drug-seeking patients are also covered.

EPIDEMIOLOGY

Chronic pain affects about a third of the population at least once during a patient's lifetime, at a cost of—80 to 90 billion dollars in health care payments and lawsuit settlements annually. Chronic pain is also common in those who do not seek medical attention. Despite similar subjective pain, those who seek medical attention are less physically active, experience more social alienation and more psychologic distress than those who do not seek medical attention.

The causes of chronic pain are more complex than the causes of acute pain. Chronic pain may be caused by (1) a chronic pathologic process in the musculoskeletal or vascular system, (2) a chronic pathologic process in one of the organ systems, (3) a prolonged dysfunction in the peripheral or central nervous system, or (4) a psychological or environmental disorder. In contrast, acute pain may be influenced by, but is not primarily caused by, a psychological or continuous environmental disorder. A detailed listing of all the epidemiologic factors of the various chronic pain syndromes is beyond the scope of this chapter. However, in general, patients who attribute their pain to a specific traumatic event experience more emotional distress, more life interference, and more severe pain than those with other causes.[2]

PATHOPHYSIOLOGY

The pathophysiology of chronic pain can be divided into three basic types. Nociceptive pain is associated with ongoing tissue damage.

Neuropathic pain is associated with nervous system dysfunction in the absence of ongoing tissue damage. Finally, psychogenic pain has no identifiable cause.[3] Many chronic pain states begin with an episode of nociceptive pain and then continue with neuropathic or psychogenic pain. For example, an acute injury with fracture involves nociceptive pain, but an associated nerve injury may lead to neuropathic pain. Chronic disability may lead to psychogenic pain. Nociceptive pain results from the stimulation of nociceptors in tissues or organs by noxious mechanical, thermal, or chemical stimuli. Chemical mediators of inflammation such as bradykinins and prostaglandins are essential elements in the pathophysiology of nociceptive pain. Examples of chronic nociceptive pain include cancer pain and pain due to chronic pancreatitis. Patients with nociceptive pain usually respond well to centrally acting analgesics. Neuropathic pain is caused by disease of the central or peripheral nervous system. Examples of neuropathic pain include complex regional pain type II (causalgia), postherpetic neuralgia, and phantom limb pain. Neuropathic pain responds poorly to common analgesics, including narcotics. Psychogenic pain is a diagnosis of exclusion and can be difficult to establish in the ED. Patients with psychogenic pain believe their pain is physical and tend to strongly reject the concept that it is psychological.

CLINICAL FEATURES

To better define the psychology of chronic pain, psychiatrists have divided patients' characteristics into two groups.[4] The first group has normal psychologic function at baseline. However, continued pain and its effects, such as inability to work or altered body image, result in psychological dysfunction. The second group has primary psychopathology that predates the onset of chronic pain. Hypochondriacal, hysterical, pain-prone, and depressive personalities are included in this group. The ''seven D's'' (Table 34-1) summarize the clinical features of these groups.[5]

The following set of historical inquiries may prove helpful in the ED. The patients should be asked to describe the nature of the current pain, initiating and exacerbating or relieving factors. Other useful information includes determination of the chronic nature of their pain, quantification of similar episodes, and sources and modes of treatment, including medications and dosages for physician-prescribed, over-the-counter, or alternative medications. Outcomes of previous therapeutic efforts and the effect of the condition on the patient's functional status are also important. Addiction to drugs or alcohol or experience with detoxification programs should also be noted. Finally, a review of systems should be done to rule out any other conditions.

TABLE 34-1 Psychological Characteristics of Chronic Pain Patients

Characteristic	Features
Drugs	Misuse of narcotics or other medications
Doctors	Tendency to ''doctor shop'' and play one physician against another
Dysfunction	Bodily impairment related to the physical and emotional factors
Disability	Inability to work or hold a job
Dependance	Loss of self-reliance and helplessness
Dramatization	Exaggeration, acting out by verbalization or by body language
Depression	Despair and negative attitudes

Source: From Brena and Chapman.[5]

Substance abuse is a frequent problem in chronic pain patients. Patients referred to chronic pain clinics meet *Diagnostic and Statistical Manual of Mental Disorders,* third revised edition (DSM III-R) criteria for active substance abuse disorders in 12 to 24 percent of cases, while 9 percent meet criteria for remission diagnosis.[6,7] Drug detoxification is often the first step of the therapeutic plan for new patients referred to a pain clinic.

Objective findings of acute pain include tachycardia, hypertension, diaphoresis, and muscle spasms on stimulation. Objective evidence of chronic pain includes muscle atrophy in the distribution of pain due to disuse, skin temperature changes due to the effects of the sympathetic nervous system after disuse or secondary to nerve injury, and trigger points, which are focal points of muscle tenderness and tension. However, these findings do not have to be present for the pain to be factual.

Signs and symptoms of chronic pain syndromes are summarized in Table 34-2.

MYOFASCIAL HEADACHES AND TRANSFORMED MIGRAINE

Myofascial headache is a variant of tension headache and is characterized by the presence of trigger points on the scalp; constant, squeezing pain; and occasionally shooting pain. Nausea, vomiting, neck pain, and neck tenderness may be present. It is important to differentiate this disorder from common tension headache because myofascial headache may benefit from referral for injection of trigger points. ''Transformed migraine'' is a syndrome in which classic migraine headaches change over time and develop into a chronic pain syndrome. One cause of this change is frequent treatment with narcotics.[8] In this regard, patients who initially have ''vascular symptoms'' eventually have predominantly muscular symptoms: nonthrobbing, squeezing, bandlike pain associated with muscle tenderness and tension. Nausea and vomiting or failure of oral antimigraine medications often prompts an ED visit.

FIBROMYALGIA AND CHRONIC MYOFASCIAL CHEST PAIN Fibromyalgia is classified by the American College of Rheumatology as the presence of 11 of 18 specific tender points, nonrestorative sleep, muscle stiffness, and generalized aching pain, with symptoms present longer than 3 months.[9] Chronic myofascial chest pain is classically a dull, constant pain associated with trigger points on the chest wall. Symptoms may mimic ischemic myocardial-type chest pain but usually is not provoked by exercise (unless the movement involves the use of chest or arm muscles) and is not completely relieved by rest.

BACK PAIN Risk factors for chronic back pain following an acute episode include male gender, advanced age, evidence of nonorganic disease, leg pain, prolonged initial episode, and significant disability at onset.[10] Chronic back pain symptoms and causes can be divided into myofascial or muscular, articular, and neurogenic types. Myofascial back pain is characterized by constant dull and occasional shooting pain that does not follow a classic nerve distribution. Pain may or may not be exacerbated by movement. Usually trigger points can be found at the site of greatest pain, and muscle atrophy is not found. Range of motion of the involved muscle is reduced, but there is no actual muscle weakness. Previous recommendations for bed rest in the treatment of back pain have proven counterproductive.[11] Exercise programs have been found to be helpful in chronic low back pain.[12] Articular back pain is characterized by constant or sharp pain that is exacerbated by movement and associated with local muscle spasm. Myofascial and articular back pain may be indistinguishable from each other except by advanced imaging techniques beyond the usual scope of practice in the ED. Neurogenic back pain is classically characterized by constant or intermittent pain that is burning, shooting, or aching. The pain is usually more severe in the leg than in the back and follows a dermatome. Muscle atrophy as well as reflex changes can be seen over time.

TABLE 34-2 Signs and Symptoms of Chronic Pain Syndromes

Disorder	Pain Symptoms	Signs
Myofascial headache	Constant dull pain, occasional shooting pain	Trigger points on scalp, muscle tenderness and tension
Transformed migraine	Initially migraine-like, becomes constant, dull; nausea, vomiting	Muscle tenderness and tension, normal neurologic examination
Fibromyalgia	Diffuse muscle pain, stiffness, fatigue, sleep disturbance	Diffuse muscle tenderness, >11 trigger points
Myofascial chest pain	Constant dull pain, occasional shooting pain	Trigger points in area of pain
Myofascial back pain syndrome	Constant dull pain, occasional shooting pain, does not follow nerve distribution	Trigger points in area of pain, usually no muscle atrophy, poor ROM in involved muscle
Articular back pain	Constant or sharp pain exacerbated by movement	Local muscle spasm
Neurogenic back pain	Constant or intermittent, burning or aching, shooting or electric shock-like; may follow dermatome; leg pain > back pain	Possible muscle atrophy in area of pain, possible reflex changes
Complex regional pain type I (RSD)	Burning persistent pain, allodynia, associated with immobilization or disuse	Early: edema, warmth, local sweating Late: above alternates with cold; pale, cyanosis, eventually atrophic changes
Complex regional pain type II (causalgia)	Burning persistent pain, allodynia, associated with peripheral nerve injury	Early: edema, warmth, local sweating Late: above alternates with cold; pale, cyanosis, eventually atrophic changes
Postherpetic neuralgia	Allodynia; shooting, lancinating pain	Sensory changes in the involved dermatome
Phantom limb pain	Variable: aching, cramping, burning, squeezing or tearing sensation	None

Abbreviations: ROM, range of motion; RSD, reflex sympathetic dystrophy.

COMPLEX REGIONAL PAIN Complex regional pain type I, also known as reflex sympathetic dystrophy, and complex regional pain type II, also known as causalgia, may be seen in the ED 2 weeks or more after an acute injury.[13] These disorders cannot be differentiated from one another on the basis of signs and symptoms. Type I occurs because of prolonged immobilization or disuse, and type II occurs because of a peripheral nerve injury. These disorders should be suspected when a patient presents with classic symptoms: allodynia (pain provoked with gentle touch of the skin), and a persistent burning or shooting pain. Associated signs early in the course of the disease include edema, warmth, and localized sweating. Therefore, it may be difficult to distinguish this disorder from an underlying wound infection or osteomyelitis. Later signs include periods of edema and warmth that alternate with cold, pale, cyanotic skin and eventually atrophic changes. Complex regional pain is an important diagnosis to make, since early steroid treatment may prevent ongoing symptoms.

POSTHERPETIC NEURALGIA The classic pain of postherpetic neuralgia may follow the course of an acute episode of herpes zoster. Pain is characterized by allodynia (defined above) and shooting, lancinating (tearing or sharply cutting) pain. Often, patients have hyperesthesia in the involved dermatome. Occasionally there are pigmentation changes in the distribution of the involved dermatome, but this is not unique to postherpetic neuralgia.

PHANTOM LIMB PAIN Phantom limb pain is quite variable in presentation but is more frequent in patients who had pain in the extremity before amputation. Pain may be aching, cramping, burning, tearing, or squeezing. Failure to respond to any treatment, including narcotics, is common.

DIAGNOSIS

The most important task of the emergency physician is to distinguish chronic pain from an exacerbation that heralds a life- or limb-threatening condition. A complete history and physical examination should either confirm the chronic condition or point to the need for further evaluation when unexpected signs or symptoms are elicited. An electrocardiogram (ECG) may be needed in some cases of chronic myofascial chest pain to help differentiate it from acute ischemic chest pain. Because chronic pain patients may be frequent visitors to the ED, the entire staff may prejudge their complaint as chronic or factitious. Physicians should insist that routine procedures be followed, including a full triage assessment and a complete set of vital signs.

Rarely is a provisional diagnosis of a chronic pain condition made for the first time in the ED. The exception is a form of post–nerve-injury pain, complex regional pain. The sharp pain from acute injuries, including fractures, rarely continues beyond 2 weeks' duration. Pain in an injured body part beyond this period should alert the clinician to the possibility of nerve injury, and proper treatment, discussed below, should be instituted.

Definitive diagnostic testing of chronic pain conditions is difficult, requires expert opinion, and often expensive procedures such as magnetic resonance imaging (MRI), computed tomography (CT), and thermography. Therefore, referral back to the primary source of care and eventual specialist referral are warranted to confirm the diagnosis.

TREATMENT

Emergency physicians must avoid labeling patients with pain as either drug seekers or legitimate patients deserving narcotics for pain relief.

With these labels, emergency physicians may exacerbate the problem and promote the learned pain response, where patients believe that they must come to the ED for pain relief. Chronic pain patients often request narcotics, although the lure of going to the ED can be just as strong without receiving narcotics. Any drug that alters sensorium can exacerbate the learned pain response. The external rewards of visiting the ED for medication or evaluation are many: attention and comforting from family and nursing staff, status as a special patient who must go the ED for pain control, avoiding responsibilities at work and at home, potential money if litigation is involved, and potential income if a disability claim is pending.

Treatment with opiates frequently contributes to the psychopathologic aspects of the disease. Chronic pain and disability lead to distress and increased stress in the life of the patient. The potentiated psychological stress heightens physiologic arousal, which increases pain sensations. Elevated pain sensations exacerbate the patient's disability. Opiate use only temporarily relieves the pain sensations, but the side effects frequently increase the disability associated with chronic pain, therefore exacerbating the psychological stress and the syndrome. Furthermore, a new problem is created as the patient becomes preoccupied with seeking pain relief from opiates. Another essential consideration is that many types of chronic pain are poorly controlled by opiates, and yet the side effects remain. It is interesting to note that the presence of objective evidence of pain does little to influence a physician's administration of narcotics. Physicians' opiate-prescribing habits are most commonly prompted by observed pain behaviors, such as facial grimacing, audible expressions of distress, or patients' avoidance of activity regardless of the physical findings.[15]

With the exception of cancer-related pain, the use of opioids in the treatment of chronic pain is controversial. Many pain specialists feel that they should not be used. There are two essential points that affect the use of opioids in the ED on which there is agreement: (1) opioids should only be used in chronic pain if they enhance function at home and at work, and (2) a single practitioner should be the sole prescriber of narcotics or should be aware of their administration by others. Finally, a previous narcotic addiction is a relative contraindication to the use of opioids in chronic pain. In contrast to the concerns listed above, narcotics are both recommended and effective treatment for cancer pain. Long-acting narcotics such as methadone or transdermal fentanyl may be more effective than the short-acting agents.

The management of chronic pain conditions is listed in Table 34-3. The medications listed under "Primary ED Treatment" are familiar to emergency physicians. While NSAIDs are most helpful in conditions where there is ongoing tissue injury, such as chronic inflammatory arthritis or cancer-related nerve or bone damage, they are also helpful in many cases of chronic pain where no evidence of tissue damage or inflammation is evident. Nonsteroidal anti-inflammatory drugs have been shown to be more helpful in acute than in chronic pain.[16] However, the need for long-standing treatment of chronic pain conditions may limit the safety of the NSAIDs. Standard dosing procedures may be followed except in the elderly (see following section).

Antidepressants and, most commonly, the tricyclic antidepressant drugs, are the most frequently used drugs for the management of chronic pain. Often, effective pain control can be achieved at doses lower than typically required for relief of depression.[3] Tricyclic antidepressants appear to enhance endogenous pain inhibitory mechanisms.[17] When antidepressants are prescribed in the ED, a follow-up plan should be in place. Discussion with a pain specialist is often beneficial. The most common drug and dose is amitriptyline 10 to 25 mg, 2 h prior to bedtime.

Anticonvulsants are used for several pain disorders, especially neuropathic pain. Anticonvulsants prevent bursts of action potentials, which may prevent the severe lancinating pain of certain neuropathic syndromes. Carbamazepine (start 100 to 200 mg bid), valproic acid (start 15 mg/kg/d divided bid), and clonazepam (start 0.5 mg tid) are the most frequently used.

Muscle relaxants, such as cyclobenzaprine 10 mg every 8 h, have been useful for chronic pain patients. Their sedating effects may limit their success.

Tramadol is an atypical centrally active analgesic. It has less respiratory depression, less tolerance, and less abuse potential than do opiates. Tramadol has been used with success in patients with fibromyalgia, migraine headaches, low back pain, and neuropathic pain. The dose of tramadol is 50 to 100 mg every 4 to 6 h by mouth.

Chronic Pain in the Elderly

Elderly patients frequently complain of chronic pain. Unfortunately, many of the commonly used medications for pain have higher complication rates in the elderly. In particular, the nonsteroidal anti-inflammatory drugs (NSAIDs) are associated with higher rates of gastrointestinal bleeding and renal disease in the elderly. Opioids also may cause debilitating sedation and/or constipation in the elderly; however, opioids may have less debilitating side effects than NSAIDs. Doses of many agents should be reduced when treating the elderly, to avoid side effects, and it is essential that a follow-up plan be in place at the time of discharge. There is a perception that the elderly are undermedicated for pain control. While this may be true, the elderly do not seem to be undermedicated more than other age groups.[14]

DISPOSITION

Referral to an appropriate specialist is one of the most productive means of aiding in the care of chronic pain patients who present to the ED. Chronic pain clinics have been successful at changing the lives of patients by eliminating opioid use, decreasing medication use by two-thirds, and pain levels by one-third, and increasing work hours twofold.[18] Patients' compliance with pain clinics may improve if the benefits are explained. The Canadian health system has initiated a chronic pain registry.[19] Patients are referred to the registry if they have had ten or more pain-related visits to the ED in a 12-month period or by the discretion of an emergency physician. An independent third-party consultation with a chronic pain specialist is provided. The success of the system is being assessed.

Admission to the hospital is rarely indicated for chronic pain patients. However, occasionally patients may be admitted for pain control, possibly using self-controlled analgesic administration.

MANAGEMENT OF PATIENTS WITH DRUG-SEEKING BEHAVIOR

There are few controlled studies on "drug-seeking behavior." Although it is known that approximately 10 percent of patients seeking treatment for drug addiction identify a prescription drug as the principal drug of abuse,[20] there is no statistical documentation of the problem in the ED. The spectrum of drug-seeking patients includes those who have chronic pain and have been advised to avoid taking narcotics, the drug addict who is trying to supplement his or her habit, and the "hustler" who is obtaining prescription drugs to sell on the street. Patients may move from chronic pain patient to addict to hustler as their social and financial support deteriorates.

Epidemiology

It is impossible to separate prescription drug abuse from other forms of substance abuse. Narcotics, stimulants, depressants, and unexpected drugs of abuse, such as antibiotics (used to treat patients with suspected intravenous drug abuse infections) and β blockers (used to limit debilitating subjective anxiety), are examples of abused agents. The magnitude of this problem has been cited as being huge, but the accuracy of the statistics has been called into question.[21] Physicians have been well implicated in this process. The "four D's" have been used

TABLE 34-3 Management of Chronic Pain Syndromes

Disorder	Primary ED Treatment	Secondary Treatment*	Possible Referral Outcome
Cancer pain	NSAIDs, opiates	Long-acting opiates	Optimization of medical therapy
Myofascial headache	NSAIDs, cyclobenzaprine	Antidepressants, phenothiazines	Trigger-point injections, optimization of medical therapy
Transformed migraine	NSAIDs, cyclobenzaprine	Antidepressants	Optimization of medical therapy, narcotic withdrawal
Fibromyalgia	NSAIDs	Antidepressants, exercise program	Optimization of medical therapy, dedicated exercise program
Myofascial chest pain	NSAIDs	Antidepressants	Trigger-point injections, optimization of medical therapy
Myofascial back pain syndrome	NSAIDs, stay active	Antidepressants	Trigger-point injections, optimization of medical therapy
Articular back pain	NSAIDs		Surgery, physical therapy
Neurogenic back pain	Acute: tapered solumedrol or prednisone	NSAIDs, muscle relaxants	Epidural steroids, surgery, exercise program
Complex regional pain types I and II (RSD and causalgia)	Acute: prednisone 60 mg/d × 4 days and taper to include 3 weeks of therapy	Chronic: antidepressants, anticonvulsants	Sympathetic nerve blocks, TENS, spinal analgesia
Postherpetic neuralgia	Acute: simple analgesics	Chronic: antidepressants, capsaicin	Regional nerve blockade
Phantom limb pain	Simple analgesics	Antidepressants, anticonvulsants	TENS, sympathectomy

*If started in the ED, consultation and/or follow-up with pain specialist or personal physician recommended.
Abbreviations: NSAIDs, nonsteroidal anti-inflammatory drugs; RSD, reflex sympathetic dystrophy; TENS, transcutaneous electrical nerve stimulation.

by the American Medical Association to describe physicians who contribute to prescription drug abuse: (1) the disabled (impaired) doctor; (2) the dishonest (''script'') doctor, who illegally sells drugs; (3) the duped doctor, who unwittingly prescribes drugs of abuse to drug-seeking patients; and (4) the dated doctor, whose obsolete prescribing practices may lend themselves to drug dependency or abuse.[22] Drug-seeking patients are very persistent and successful. A study conducted in Portland found that drug-seeking patients presented to the ED 12.6 times per year, visited 4.1 different hospitals, and used 2.2 different aliases. Patients who were refused narcotics at one facility were successful in obtaining narcotics at another facility 93 percent of the time and were later successful at obtaining narcotics from the same facility 71 percent of the time.[23]

Clinical Features

Because of the spectrum of drug-seeking patients, the history given may be factual or fraudulent. Drug seekers may be demanding, intimidating, or flattering. In one ED study, the most common complaints of patients who were drug seeking were (in decreasing order): back pain, headache, extremity pain, and dental pain.[23] Patients may complain of panic disorder or drug withdrawal symptoms and request benzodiazepines. Additional fraudulent techniques are listed in Table 34-4. In some cases, observations of vital signs and physical examination findings will help the physician identify factitious illness, but even experienced clinicians are frequently misled.[23]

Patients should be examined for signs of intravenous drug addiction, including needle marks and healed or active superficial cutaneous abscesses, and the heart should be examined for evidence of a new murmur and other signs of endocarditis. Patients attempting to simulate nephrolithiasis can falsify hematuria by biting their buccal mucosa and spitting into the urine sample or by pricking their finger and dipping it into the urine sample. Patients who are suspected of factitious hematuria should be examined for these findings. Patients with factitious acute injury may massage old deformities to create the appearance of erythema and swelling, but this will dissipate over time if the clinician stops the patient from holding the extremity. Patients may self-mutilate, usually with the dominant hand, and seek narcotics. Patients may have evidence of chronic pain or, most commonly, have completely normal physical examination findings. Finally, it is widespread anecdotal experience that such patients will relate ''allergy'' to alternative pharmacotherapy, insisting that only one or two specific narcotics are effective.

Diagnosis

The diagnosis of drug-seeking behavior may not be possible in the ED. The medical record can provide a wealth of information regarding the patient, including documentation proving the patient is supplying false information. Often the diagnosis is suspected in the ED but cannot be confirmed. In such cases, a notation should be made in the chart listing the physician's concerns, but physicians should be careful when using diagnoses such as ''drug-seeking behavior'' without solid evidence. A listing or card file at the nurses' desk of ''drug seekers'' violates patient-physician confidentiality unless it is part of the patient's permanent medical record and subject to the same controls restricting access. Drug-seeking behaviors can be divided into two groups: ''predictive'' and ''less predictive'' of drug-seeking behavior (Table 34-5). The behaviors listed under ''predictive'' are illegal in many states and form a solid basis to refuse narcotics to the patient. However, the possibility still exists that the patient could have pain

TABLE 34-4 Common Fraudulent Techniques Used by Drug Seekers and Their Management

Technique	Characteristics	Management
Lost prescription	Calls or returns stating that narcotic prescription was lost prior to being filled	Establish a policy: no narcotic prescriptions refilled. Notify all patients at discharge as they receive prescriptions.
Impending surgery	Wants temporizing narcotics, doctor "unavailable," previous surgery, patient from out of town	Call physician. Check medical records. Offer substitute for narcotics.
Carries own records and x-rays	Suspicious or forged records, doctor's written permission to receive narcotics, patient from out of town	Make phone calls. Check records. Offer substitute for narcotics.
Factitious hematuria with complaint of kidney stones	Appears comfortable or overacting, pricked finger dipped in urine, lip/cheek bitten and blood spit into urine	Examine fingers and mouth. Obtain witnessed UA urinalysis. Use ketorolac IV. Obtain confirmatory test prior to giving narcotics.
Self-mutilation	Done with dominant hand, requests narcotics for pain	Use bupivacaine for local block. Do not prescribe narcotics without indications. Offer substitute for narcotics.
Dental pain	Dental caries only	Give local nerve block with bupivacaine. Refer to dentist.
Factitious injury	Old injury, old deformity, self-massaged to produce erythema, patient from out of town	X-ray prior to treatment. Check records. Check for erythema that dissipates over time.
Partner waiting near telephone at home	"Call my doctor," handwritten number offered, partner answers: "Doctor so-and-so."	Question respondent for medical knowledge. Verify number with telephone company.
Partner in ED	Confirms history, urges narcotics	Check records. Send to waiting room if verbally abusive.

and should be evaluated for a medical or surgical illness and possibly treated with a nonnarcotic drug.

Specific Issues: Legal Implications

The Drug Enforcement Agency licenses physicians (along with state agencies) to administer or dispense controlled substances. However, it is state law that determines most prescribing regulations. All physicians should be aware of state laws regulating controlled substances prescribed in their practice setting. For example, some states mandate reporting the use of schedule II agents, and some states limit monthly dosing. Prescribing narcotics to a known drug addict could result in restriction of the physician's medical license in some states. However, if a patient refuses to acknowledge his or her addiction, the physician cannot be held accountable unless medical records at the facility where the patient presents document the addiction. In all states it is illegal for patients to forge or alter prescriptions. In some states it is illegal for patients to use aliases or factitious illness to obtain narcotics. Further, in some states, concealing previous or recent prescriptions for narcotics when requesting narcotics from a new practitioner is illegal. Physicians should ask patients about previous addiction and recent treatment with narcotics.

TABLE 34-5 Characteristics of Drug-Seeking Behavior

Behaviors Predictive of Drug-Seeking Behavior*
Sells prescription drugs
Forges/alters prescriptions
Factitious illness, requests narcotics
Uses aliases to receive narcotics
Admits to illicit drug addiction
Conceals multiple physicians prescribing narcotics
Conceals multiple ED visits receiving narcotics
Less Predictive of Drug-Seeking Behavior
Admits to multiple doctors prescribing narcotics
Admits to multiple prescriptions for narcotics
Abusive when refused
Multiple drug allergies
Uses excessive flattery
From out of town
Asks for drugs by name

*Behaviors in this category are unlawful in many states.

Treatment and Disposition

The treatment of drug-seeking behavior is to refuse the controlled substance, consider the need for alternative medication or treatment, and consider referral for drug counseling. Unfortunately, successful management has been documented only by anecdote and case report.[24]

The patient who complains of multiple drug allergies can be difficult. Occasionally the medical record will show previous administration of the drug in question (usually a narcotic substitute) with no adverse reaction other than no pain relief. When confronted with a physician's discovery of their fraudulent behavior, many drug-seeking patients become verbally abusive, and hospital security may be required to escort the patient out of the department. Alternatives to narcotics can be offered, and patients should understand that refusal to prescribe narcotics is not a refusal of care.

When drug-seeking behavior is confirmed or suspected in ED, it should be documented in the chart with careful attention to the facts. When physicians are notified by a pharmacist of forged or altered prescriptions, law enforcement authorities should be called, and physicians should cooperate with the legal investigation. The prosecution of many fraudulent behaviors, such as using aliases to obtain narcotics, requires the involvement of the state bureau of investigation or a similar agency of the state. Physicians may inquire about the legal proceedings with either the hospital attorney or the police. Finally, the primary care provider or pain specialist can be contacted to establish a contract with the patient. Such contracts may include specific directions for ED treatment and usually stipulate that prescriptions will only be given by the primary care provider. Such contracts ease the burden for emergency physicians and set realistic expectations for the patient.

REFERENCES

1. Merskey HM: Classification of chronic pain: Descriptions of chronic pain syndromes and definitions of pain terms. *Pain* 3(suppl):S217, 1986.
2. Turk D, Okifuji A: Perception of traumatic onset, compensation status, and physical findings: Impact on pain severity, emotional distress, and disability in chronic pain patients. *J Behav Med* 14:435, 1996.
3. Garcia J, Altman RD: Chronic pain states: Pathophysiology and medical therapy. *Semin Arthritis Rheum* 27:1, 1997.
4. Kinney SS, Brin EN: Diagnostic evaluation and management of the patient with chronic pain, in Aronoff GM (ed): *Evaluation and Treatment of Chronic Pain.* Baltimore, Williams & Wilkins, 1992, pp 26–55.
5. Brena SF, Chapman SL: The "learned pain syndrome:" Decoding a patient's pain signals. *Postgrad Med* 69:53, 1981.
6. Hoffman NG, Olofsson O, et al: Prevalence of abuse and dependency in chronic pain patients. *Int J Addiction* 30:919, 1995.
7. Kouyanou K, Pither CE, Wessely S: Medication misuse: Abuse and dependence in chronic pain patients. *J Psychosomat Res* 43:497, 1997.
8. Mathew NT, Stubitis E, Nigam M: Transformation of migraine headache into daily headache: Analysis of factors. *Headache* 22:66, 1982.
9. Wolfe F, Smythe HA, et al: The American College of Rheumatology 1990 criteria for the classification of fibromyalgia. *Arthritis Rheum* 33:160, 1990.
10. Valat JP, Goupille P, Vedere V: Low back pain: Risk factors for chronicity. *Rev Rhum Engl Ed* 64:189, 1997.
11. Waddell G, Feder G, Lewis M: Systemic reviews of bed rest and advice to stay active for acute low back pain. *Br J Gen Pract* 47:647, 1997.
12. Faas A: Exercises: Which ones are worth trying, for which patients, and when. *Spine* 21:2874, 1996.
13. Cooney WP: Somatic versus sympathetic mediated chronic limb pain: Experiences and treatment options. *Hand Clin* 13:355, 1997.
14. Lewis LM, Lasler LC, Brooks CB: Are emergency physicians too stingy with analgesics? *South Med J* 87:7, 1994.
15. Turk DC, Okifuji A: What factors affect physicians' decisions to prescribe opioids for chronic non-cancer pain patients? *Clin J Pain* 13:330, 1997.
16. Deyo RA: Drug therapy for back pain: Which drugs help which patients. *Spine* 21:2840, 1996.
17. Satterthwaite JR, Tollison CD, Kriegel ML: The use of tricyclic antidepressants for the treatment of intractable pain. *Compr Ther* 16:10, 1990.
18. Hubbard JE, Tracy J, et al: Outcome measures of a chronic pain program: A prospective statistical study. *Clin J Pain* 12:330, 1996.
19. MacLeod DB, Swanson R: A new approach to chronic pain in the ED. *Am J Emerg Med* 14:323, 1996.
20. Batten HL, Horgan CM, et al: *Drug Services Research Survey: Phase I Final Report: Non-correctional Facilities,* contract 271. Rockville, MD, National Institute of Drug Abuse, 1990, pp 90–91.
21. Cooper JR, Czechowicz DJ, et al: Prescription drug diversion control and medical practice. *JAMA* 268:1306, 1992.
22. American Medical Association Council on Scientific Affairs: Drug abuse related to prescribing practices. *JAMA* 247:864, 1982.
23. Zechnich AD, Hedges JR: Community-wide emergency department visits by patients suspected of drug seeking behavior. *Acad Emerg Med* 3:312, 1996.
24. Sousa JA, Cline DM, Stout R, et al.: Extortion in the emergency department. *J Emerg Med* 15:537, 1997.

EMERGENCY WOUND MANAGEMENT

EVALUATION OF WOUNDS

Louis J. Kroot

Acute traumatic wounds are routinely evaluated in emergency departments. The most common include isolated lacerations, abrasions, and avulsions, along with those wounds associated with multiple trauma. This chapter discusses the basic principles of acute wound assessment.

EPIDEMIOLOGY

Approximately 12 million traumatic wounds are treated annually in US emergency departments, accounting for more than 10 percent of all visits.[1] The two groups most frequently treated are males, aged 15 to 44, and women over age 75. The most frequently involved body locations are the face, scalp, fingers, and hands.[2–5] Approximately half of traumatic lacerations seen in the emergency department are sustained from blunt objects. Children have different wound epidemiologic characteristics: wounds are more likely to be located on the head, linear, shorter, less contaminated, and more often caused by blunt trauma, compared with wounds of adults.[6]

PATHOPHYSIOLOGY

Acute traumatic wounds are caused either by shear, compressive, or tensile forces, which vertically separate the epithelium and dermis.[7] Shear forces are produced by sharp objects that cut through the skin. The amount of energy required to cut through the skin with a sharp object is relatively low and directed to a very small area. Thus, little energy is deposited into the surrounding tissue and there is minimal cell damage. Typically, the resultant wound has straight edges, little contamination, and heals with a good result. Compressive and tensile forces are produced when a blunt object impacts the skin at right and oblique angles, respectively. In contrast to shear forces, the amount of energy deposited from compressive and tensile injuries is larger, with significant amounts applied to the area around the wound causing disruption of the microvasculature. The amount of force required to produce a cutaneous laceration is in the range of 2.5 J/cm^2. The devitalized tissue creates an anaerobic environment, which impairs the ability of leukocytes to function and supports bacterial proliferation. Experimentally, wound infections have been produced in compressive injuries with inoculums of about 100,000 organisms per gram of tissue compared with the requirement for about 10,000,000 organisms per gram in shear injuries. Compressive wounds tend to be stellate or complex, with ragged or shredded edges. Tensile wounds tend to be triangular or produce a flap. In cross section, tensile wounds tend to be "skived," that is, cut oblique through the skin with a thin edge on one side and a thick edge on the other.

The body responds to the injury by initiating a series of restorative stages to recover tissue continuity and strength. In general, tensile strength of the wounded area recovers approximately 50 percent by 40 days and nearly 100 percent by 150 days after injury. These stages of wound healing are described as hemostasis, inflammation, epithelialization, angiogenesis, fibroplasia, contraction, and scar maturation. All these stages are stimulated by various tissue growth factors (Table 35-1).

Hemostasis is initiated at the time of injury. Tissue and vascular smooth muscle contraction compresses small bleeding vessels. Activation of platelets and the coagulation cascade produce a fibrin clot within the lumens of the severed vessels and within the exposed wound.

Inflammation is stimulated by chemotactic factors released by activated platelets and the complement cascade, which initially attract neutrophils followed by macrophages. Neutrophils and macrophages phagocytose dead tissue, foreign material, and bacteria, providing physiologic debridement and preventing infection. Neutrophils perform this function for the first 72 h after injury, and macrophages perform this task for up to 30 days after a traumatic wound.

Epithelialization reaches a peak about 24 h after the injury as the inflammatory response stimulates cell division in the stratum germinativum. Epithelial cells migrate across a closed traumatic wound during the first 24 to 48 h, making the wound impervious to water. Eschar and surface debris impede this process.

Angiogenesis is vital to wound repair. New vessel growth is detectable at 72 h and reaches its peak at 7 to 10 days, accounting for the often-marked erythema seen at this time. As the wound matures, vascularity decreases nearly back to baseline at 30 days.

Fibroplasia, with collagen synthesis, reaches a peak by 7 days and essentially replaces the inflammatory mass in the wound by 3 weeks. At the same time as increasing collagen synthesis, hydrolysis and breakdown of old and damaged collagen are also taking place. The period between 7 and 10 days is the vulnerable time when the balance between collagen synthesis and breakdown is most tenuous and unwanted wound separation occurs.

Wound contraction and scar remodeling occur over the next several months. Contraction significantly modifies the cosmetic appearance of treated wounds. An important principle of wound repair is to take this expected contraction into account and repair lacerations with everted edges. Remodeling is such a powerful process that, at the time of suture removal, it is impossible to predict the ultimate appearance of wounds.[8]

During wound healing, excess fibroblastic activity can create excess tissue, developing either a hypertrophic scar or a keloid. Hypertrophic scars are excess collagen confined to the original boundaries of the wound and are more common in areas of increased tissue tension. Keloids have excess scar tissue from the wound extending beyond the original borders. Keloids are most often seen in African Americans but can occur in any dark-pigmented skin area.

PRIORITIES

Unless airway and breathing are compromised or there is active bleeding from the wound edge, acute traumatic wounds are evaluated and treated after other life- or limb-threatening conditions have been evaluated and managed. To maximize patient safety and comfort, it is generally best to evaluate patients supine on a stretcher. Hemostasis may be required and is best done by local pressure. Sometimes, wound repair must be delayed to address other issues. In this case, fresh wounds should be covered by saline-moistened gauze to prevent drying. Most wounds can be assessed without analgesia and anesthesia, provided the physician proceeds slowly and carefully. Encircling clothing, rings, and jewelry should be removed as soon as possible to reduce the potential for damaging edema and contamination.

Wound repair has been traditionally divided into three categories. *Primary closure* (healing by primary intention) is performed with sutures, staples, or adhesives at the time of initial evaluation. *Secondary closure* (healing by secondary intention) is where the wound is allowed to granulate and fill in with eventual epithelialization with only cleaning and minimal debridement. *Tertiary closure* (delayed primary clo-

TABLE 35-1 Tissue Growth Factors and Their Effects

Platelet derived
- Transforming growth factors (TGFs): TGF-α and TGF-β
  - Stimulate fibroblasts and epithelial and vascular endothelial cells
  - Promote epithelialization and neovascularization
- Platelet-derived growth factor (PDGF)
  - Stimulates fibroblasts and smooth muscle cells to migrate toward the wound
  - Facilitates formation of procollagen and collagen fibrils

Macrophage derived
- Acidic fibroblast growth factor (aFGF)
- Basic fibroblast growth factor (bFGF)
- Macrophage-derived growth factor (MDGF)
- Interleukin 1 (IL-1)
  - Stimulates procollagen production to form collagen fibrils
  - Smooth muscle cells help collagen fibrils contract and increase tensile strength

Epithelial cell derived
- Epidermal cell-derived growth factor (EDF)
  - Stimulates epithelial cells mitosis and accelerates healing

sure) is where the wound is initially cleaned, debrided, and observed for a period of time (typically 4 or 5 days) before closure.

MEDICAL HISTORY

The existence of the wound is often so obvious that the importance of a proper medical history is sometimes forgotten[9] (Table 35-2). The patient's symptoms should be noted, including pain, swelling, paresthesias, and loss of function. It is important to elicit information about the specific mechanism of injury that will either influence treatment or affect outcome. Blunt-force wounds with compressive or tensile forces are more prone to infection. Wounds sustained from contaminated objects or occurring in contaminated environments have increased risk of infection. The most common foreign body in wounds is soil, and the particular composition greatly affects the risk of infection. Clay-containing soils and soils with large amounts of organic material (e.g., swamps) have a high potential for wound infection, whereas sand and black dirt from the highway surface have a low potential. Some body locations have a higher concentration of normal flora and are more prone to infection. For example, most of the surface area of the human body has only a few thousand bacteria per square centimeter, but the perineum, axilla, toe webs, fingernail edges, and intertriginous areas can have over a 1 million/cm^2. Animal bite wounds are prone to infection with organisms different than those, which produce infection in nonbite wounds.

A patient should be asked whether the wound was sustained from an intentional act (e.g., assault or self-inflected) or unintentional event. Most states have regulations that require the reporting of intentional injuries, and self-inflicted injuries are grounds for involuntary holding and psychiatric evaluation. Occupational injuries are reportable to the appropriate agency.

The time of the injury and delay in seeking care will influence the decision for primary closure. In experimental models, a delay of more than 3 to 5 h allows the bacterial population to increase to greater than 1 million bacteria per gram of tissue and significantly increases the chances of infection. Treatment performed by a patient before seeking care, or lack thereof, may influence wound appearance. The possibility of a retained foreign body should be assessed by asking about the wounding object and any sensation of an object still in the wound. The presence of a foreign body dramatically increases the potential for infection; experimentally, infection can be initiated with as little as 100 bacteria per gram of tissue.

TABLE 35-2 Medical History

Symptoms
- Pain
- Swelling
- Paresthesias
- Loss of function

Type of force
- Shear
- Compressive
- Tensile

Contamination
- Time since injury
- Prior wound care
- Object
- Environment
- Body location
- Animal bite

Event
- Intentional versus unintentional
- Assault or self-inflicted
- Occupational

Potential for foreign body
- Friable wounding object
- Incomplete removal
- Residual foreign-body sensation

Function
- Handedness
- Occupation

Tetanus immunization status

Allergies
- Analgesics, anesthetics, antibiotics
- Latex

Medications

Chronic medical conditions
- Comorbid diseases: diabetes, chronic renal failure, immunosuppression
- Internal prosthetic device: prosthetic heart valves

Previous scar formation
- Keloid
- Hypertrophic scars

The impact of the wound on the patient's daily function will vary according to handedness and occupation. Tetanus immunization status should be assessed for every traumatic wound. Allergies will influence treatment with analgesics, anesthetics, antibiotics, and dressings. Patients with a latex allergy must be examined with latex-free gloves.[10] Current medications, including those purchased without prescription, should be noted. Patients who are taking warfarin or aspirin may not be able to spontaneously stop bleeding. Lastly, chronic medical conditions that may influence the incidence of wound infection or be associated with poor outcome should be noted. Patients with severe peripheral vascular diseases may not have an adequate blood supply to an injured part of the body for proper healing. Old age can affect healing through debility of a patient's physiology.

PHYSICAL EXAMINATION

Wound examination is greatly facilitated by a calm and cooperative patient, appropriate positioning, adequate lighting, and, sometimes, magnification.[11] Sterile technique would seem to be important, but studies using clean, but nonsterile, gloves found no increase in the

TABLE 35-3 Physical Examination

Location Scalp and face Neck and trunk Extremity Perineum Hand Foot Over joint
Size Length Width
Shape Linear Flap Stellate Complex Avulsion
Margins Smooth Jagged
Depth Layers involved
Aligned with skin tension lines
Neurologic function Sensory Motor
Vascular function Pulses Capillary refill
Tendon function
Underlying and adjacent structures Bone Joint capsule
Wound contamination Visible debris
Foreign body

incidence of wound infections. However, it is important to practice universal precautions and protect the patient and physician from cross infection.

Several factors should be noted and documented during wound examination (Table 35-3). Areas with excellent vascular supply and a low incidence of infection include the scalp, face, neck, and trunk. Lacerations on the extremities are at increased risk for infection, and those on the feet and hands are at greatest risk. Lacerations on the hands can damage tendons, nerves, and joints important for normal function. Lacerations over joints may penetrate into the joint capsule and are at risk for hypertrophic scar formation. Any laceration over the metacarpophalangeal joint is suspicious for a clenched-fist injury. Lacerations in the perineum have a high likelihood for contamination.

Wound characteristics are important to note. Large wounds, both in length and width (gaping), are at increased risk of infection. Likewise, wounds with flaps, stellate shape, complex arrangement, avulsed tissue, jagged edges, or deep penetration are at increased risk of infection.

The skin has static and dynamic forces that normally create tension within the tissue and vary depending on anatomic site. Lacerations heal with the best results when the long axis of a laceration is in the direction of the maximal skin tension. When static skin tension is perpendicular to the wound edges, tissue retracts and the wound edges gap. Although Langer more than a century ago published his text on the orientation of these forces on the human body, it is now realized that the majority of his findings were incorrect and have almost no application in the care of acute traumatic wounds. The degree of skin tension depends more on the length and configuration of the wound: there is less tension on a jagged wound compared with a straight wound because of the increased length of the laceration in a jagged wound. Therefore, the meticulous repair of a jagged wound, rather than converting it into a straight wound, results in a more cosmetically satisfactory outcome.

TABLE 35-4 Wounds That Usually Require Consultation

Wounds involving the tarsal plate of the eyelid or lacrimal duct
Wounds involving an open fracture or joint space
Wounds associated with multiple trauma that need surgical admission
Wounds of the face that require extensive plastic reconstruction
Wounds associated with amputation
Wounds associated with loss of function
Wounds that involve tendons, nerves, or vessels
Wounds that involve a significant loss of epidermis

Neurologic function should be assessed by evaluating distal sensory and motor function. Absent distal pulses and capillary refill indicate a vascular injury, but their presence does not exclude one. Tendon function should be performed for each one in isolation, where possible. The underlying and adjacent structures should be carefully inspected. The wound should be inspected to its full extent and depth for visible contamination and foreign bodies.

Although most traumatic wounds can be treated by an emergency physician, a prudent physician knows when to call for a consultant (Table 35-4).

ANCILLARY STUDIES

In general, there is very little need for ancillary tests in most patients with traumatic wounds, with the exception of possible imaging studies to detect and locate retained foreign bodies. Foreign bodies are suggested by either the mechanism of injury, persistent foreign-body sensation reported by the patient, or palpation of a hard object by the examining physician. Fortunately, pieces of metal, glass, gravel, teeth, and bone larger than 1 mm are readily visible on plain radiographs when taken using the soft tissue technique and with multiple views to avoid overlapping bone (see Chap. 42, ''Soft Tissue Foreign Bodies''). Unfortunately, some foreign bodies (plastic, wood, and other organic material) are radiolucent and not visible on plain radiographs. For these objects, computed tomography is the best imaging modality for detection and localization. Ultrasound, though attractive, does not have the required sensitivity to exclude a retained foreign body under clinical circumstances.

REFERENCES

1. Stussman BJ: *National Hospital Ambulatory Medical Care Survey: 1994 Emergency Department Summary.* Hyattsville, MD: National Center for Health Statistics, 1996; DHHS publication (PHS) 96-1250. (Advance Data from Vital and Health Statistics, no. 275.)
2. Hollander JE, Singer AJ, Valentine S, Henry MC: Wound registry: Development and validation. *Ann Emerg Med* 25:675, 1995.

3. Harker C, Matheson AB, Ross JA, Seaton A: Occupational accidents presenting to the accident and emergency department. *Arch Emerg Med* 9:185, 1992.
4. Layne LA, Castillo DN, Stout N, Cutlip P: Adolescent occupational injuries requiring hospital emergency department treatment: A nationally representative sample. *Am J Public Health* 84:657, 1994.
5. Lillis KA, Jaffe DM: Playground injuries in children. *Pediatr Emerg Care* 13:149, 1997.
6. Hollander JE, Singer AJ, Valentine S: Comparison of wound care practices in pediatric and adult lacerations repaired in the emergency department. *Pediatr Emerg Care* 14:15, 1998.
7. Edlich RF, Rodeheaver GT, Morgan RF, et al: Principles of emergency wound management. *Ann Emerg Med* 17:1284, 1988.
8. Hollander JE, Blasko B, Singer AJ, et al: Poor correlation of short- and long-term cosmetic appearance of repaired lacerations. *Acad Emerg Med* 2:983, 1995.
9. American College of Emergency Physicians: Clinical policy for the initial approach to patients presenting with penetrating extremity trauma. *Ann Emerg Med* 23:1147, 1994.
10. Warshaw EM: Latex allergy. *J Am Acad Dermatol* 39:1, 1998.
11. Howell JM, Chisholm CD: Wound care. *Emerg Med Clin North Am* 15:417, 1997.

WOUND PREPARATION

Susan Stone
Wallace A. Carter

Wound preparation is a vital step in emergency department wound care for restoring the integrity and function of the injured tissue while minimizing the risk of infection and maximizing the cosmetic result. While the vast majority of wounds treated in emergency departments heal with a good outcome, careful preparation is particularly important when underlying medical conditions or wound factors may alter wound healing and increase the chance of infection (Table 36-1). Many traditional methods of wound preparation have surprisingly little scientific validation.[1,2] This chapter reviews the basic principles of wound preparation, using available experimental models and prospective clinical studies, where available, to justify these techniques.

TABLE 36-1 Risk Factors for Poor Wound Repair Outcome

Immunosuppression
Diabetes
Chemotherapeutic agents
Steroids
Chronic renal failure
Hematologic malignancies
Congenital immunodeficiencies
Tissue ischemia
Peripheral vascular disease
Anemia
Vasculitis
Poor wound repair
Elderly
Malnourished
Connective tissue disorder
Wound factors
Crush injury
Tissue loss
Contamination
Foreign bodies
Location

ANESTHESIA

In general, pain control should be provided before extensive wound preparation. Not only more humane, anesthesia and analgesia will enable better preparation and treatment if patients are relaxed and able to cooperate without undue anxiety and pain. Prior to the administration of local or regional anesthetic, the sensory, motor, and vascular examination should be performed.

HEMOSTASIS

Control of bleeding is necessary for both hemodynamic stability and for proper evaluation of a wound. Bleeding most often occurs from the subdermal plexus and superficial veins. Direct pressure with saline-soaked sponges or gauze is usually effective in stopping this type of bleeding.

Bleeding from an exposed lacerated vessel is best controlled by direct pressure with a gloved fingertip directly onto the vessel. Once bleeding is halted, persistent control can be achieved by clamping the involved vessel, isolating a short length, and ligating with absorbable synthetic suture (typically 5-0). This approach is most useful for rapidly bleeding minor vessels in the extremities, but major arteries of an extremity should not be ligated. Extreme caution must be exercised in the face because of the proximity of important facial structures. Scalp lacerations can bleed extensively from the wound edges due to the highly vascular subcutaneous layer. This bleeding can be controlled by the use of specially designed clips applied along the wound edges. For bleeding wounds where the involved vessel is not visible, a figure-of eight or horizontal mattress suture applied adjacent to the wound edge near the site of bleeding will sometimes achieve control. However, this technique may obstruct significant blood flow and leave nonviable tissue in the wound.

Chemical means of hemostasis include epinephrine, Gelfoam, Oxycel, Actifoam, and cyanoacrylates. Topical epinephrine is not very effective. More commonly, epinephrine is mixed with local anesthetics in concentrations of 1:100,000 or 1:200,000 and injected into the wound area. This will induce local vasoconstriction that will allow a longer duration of anesthesia and a larger total dose due to the depot effect of the vasoconstriction. Epinephrine should never be used in end organs such as fingers, toes, and tip of nose, ears, and penis. Although there is a theoretical risk of increased infection with the addition of epinephrine to local anesthetics, observational studies on emergency department wound repair have not found a significant increase in the incidence of wound infection after suturing. Gelfoam, made from denatured gelatin, has no intrinsic homeostatic properties and works by the pressure it exerts as it becomes a fluid-filled sponge. Oxycel, a cellulose derivative, and Actifoam, a collagen sponge, react with blood, forming an artificial clot. These products are not particularly effective for actively bleeding wounds, as the blood can wash them out. Cyanoacrylates form a gluelike substance, bringing wound edges together when applied to the skin surface. Cyanoacrylates should never be applied into the depth of a wound.

Bipolar electrocautery can achieve hemostasis from blood vessels smaller than 2 mm in diameter but, if improperly or too extensively applied, results in tissue necrosis. Electrocautery units are not routinely available in many emergency departments. Battery-powered hand-held cautery units are more readily available but do not generate sufficient heat to produce coagulation in vessels larger than capillaries.

Extremity wounds that are refractory to direct pressure, ligation, or cautery may require a tourniquet. Although helpful in stopping exsanguination, tourniquets may compress and damage underlying blood vessels and nerves, reducing tissue viability. The simplest tourniquet to use in an emergency department is a blood pressure cuff placed proximal to the wound and inflated above the patient's systolic pressure. Elevating the extremity to reduce venous blood volume prior to cuff inflation is useful. If an extremity tourniquet is needed to control bleeding, the patient is best explored and repaired in the operating room and a surgeon should be immediately consulted.

FOREIGN-BODY REMOVAL

Obvious foreign debris should be carefully removed from the wound, with care to avoid injury to the physician from sharp edges or points. Retained foreign bodies can cause wound infections. Some diagnostic clues to the presence of a foreign body may include point tenderness or increased pain on range of motion, in conjunction with clinical suspicion. Visual wound inspection, down to the full depth and along the full course of the wound, is the most important method of detecting foreign bodies. Imaging modalities—plain radiology, ultrasound, computed tomography (CT), and magnetic resonance imaging—have a role in selected patients (see Chap. 42, "Soft Tissue Foreign Bodies"). In general, glass, metal, and gravel fragments larger than 1 mm should be readily visible on plain radiographs taken with soft tissue technique and with multiple views to avoiding overlapping bone. Painted plastic and wood may be radiopaque and visible on plain radiographs. However, unpainted plastic or wood and other organic material is radiolucent and not routinely visible on plain radiographs. If these potential foreign bodies are suggested by the history and not detected during wound exploration, CT is the imaging modality most successful in detecting and locating such objects. Ultrasound, an attractive modality because of the lack of radiation exposure and the ability to image and assist during foreign-body removal, lacks sufficient sensitivity for soft tissue foreign-body detection and cannot be recommended as the sole imaging modality.

HAIR REMOVAL

Because it can act as a foreign body, increasing the risk of wound infection, hair should be removed as completely as possible with clipping 1 to 2 mm above the skin with scissors.[1,2] Shaving the area with a razor damages the hair follicle, allowing bacterial invasion, and is associated with a tenfold increase in infection rates when compared with clipping. An alternative method to clipping is to use ointment or saline to clear hair away from wound edges. Hair should never be taken from the eyebrows, because of the potential failure of that hair to regenerate. Likewise, hair may provide good landmarks for alignment of wound edges during suturing, and removal at the skin-hair interface (eyebrows or scalp) should be avoided when possible.

IRRIGATION

Effective high-pressure irrigation decreases bacterial count and helps to remove foreign bodies, thereby reducing the risk of wound infection.[1,2] Because of the discomfort involved, local anesthetic should be given prior to irrigation. Irrigation pressures of 5 to 8 psi are recommended, which is easily achieved using a 19-gauge needle with either a 35-mL or 65-mL syringe.[3] Sufficient pressures will not be generated using a bulb syringe or fluid directly from the intravenous fluid bags. Although the exact volume of irrigant required is not known, some authors have found 60 mL/cm of wound length as a useful guideline.[2] The other approach is to use 1 L of saline as a standard volume, although a large prospective observational study found little correlation between the incidence of infection and the volume of irrigation, provided at least 200 mL was used.[4]

Wound soaking is not effective in cleansing contaminated wounds and may actually increase wound bacterial counts.[5] Scrubbing traumatic wounds with a sponge is also ineffective and inflicts trauma and impairs resistance to infection.

Saline, the least expensive irrigant, also has the lowest toxicity. There is no added benefit to the addition of an antiseptic (such as povidone-iodine or hydrogen peroxide) to the irrigant.[6] These agents are actually toxic to open wounds and impair resistance. Povidone-iodine, hydrogen peroxide, chlorhexidine, and detergents all cause tissue and fibroblast toxicity. Therefore, although these agents are bactericidal, they are not beneficial in wound care.

Universal Precautions should be observed while participating in wound care. Irrigation is often a time when contaminated fluid can be splashed onto the health care workers. Barrier protection should be used. Irrigation wet shields attached to the irrigation system may prevent some of the splashing associated with irrigation but are still not a substitute for Universal Precautions.

Recently, the need for routine irrigation of traumatic wounds has been questioned, particularly for simple nonbite, noncontaminated wounds in highly vascular areas, such as the scalp and face.[7,8] Although irrigation produced a slight trend toward a better outcome (less wound infection and optimal cosmetic appearance), the results were not statistically significant.[7] However, this was a nonrandomized observational study and therefore routine irrigation is still recommended at this time.

DEBRIDEMENT

The next step in wound preparation is debridement of nonviable tissue.[1,2] Devitalized tissue may increase the risk of infection and delay healing by acting as a culture medium and inhibiting leukocyte phagocytosis. Debridement not only removes foreign matter, bacteria, and devitalized tissue, but also creates a sharp wound edge that is easier to repair. After debridement is completed, wounds should be reirrigated.

The most effective type of debridement is excision, because it converts a contaminated wound into a clean surgical wound. A standard surgical blade and scissors are used. Tissue that has a narrow base or lacks capillary refill will require excision. Heavily contaminated wounds require more extensive debridement, whereas adequate debridement of soft tissue, which includes specialized tissue such as tendons and nerves, may require consultation.

The goal of debridement is to reestablish a margin of normal tissue at wound edges. The easiest technique for excisional debridement is to mark an elliptical area around the sides of the wound and then, using a no. 15 surgical blade, cut only through epidermis. Skin lines should be respected, and extensive excision should be avoided.

Wounds with an extensive amount of nonviable tissue are more problematic. They may require a large amount of tissue removal (e.g., crush injuries) and will need more delayed wound closure or grafting. In general, a surgeon should be consulted to manage these wounds.

Debridement has become such a standard in wound care, it is difficult to conceive of a situation where this technique should not be applied. However, a recent study of low-velocity civilian gunshot wounds to the extremities found that conservative wound care had the same incidence of wound infection as routine wound debridement.[9]

ANTIBIOTICS

Infections occur in approximately 3 to 5 percent of traumatic wounds repaired in emergency departments, although this rate varies widely according to mechanism, location, and patient factors.[1,7,8,10–12] Delays of over 3 h in seeking care, wound location, extremes of age, crush injuries, puncture or avulsion wounds, retained foreign bodies, and contamination with saliva, feces, and soil are all risk factors for infection. Delays of over 3 h in seeking care allow bacterial proliferation to increase exponentially. Less vascular areas, moist areas (axilla and perineum), and exposed areas (feet and hands) also tend to be at higher risk for infection. Crush or puncture wounds are more prone to infection due to the tensile and compressive forces generated that increase the potential for devitalized tissue. Additionally, wounds contaminated with saliva or feces are at risk. Soil may increase infection by direct interference with leukocyte function.

To reduce the incidence of wound infections, antibiotics have been commonly used for years, although there is no clear evidence that

TABLE 36-2 Guidelines for Tetanus Prophylaxis

Wound Type	Incomplete Immunization (Unknown or <3 Doses)	<5 Years from Last Immunization	5–10 Years from Last Immunization	>10 Years from Last Immunization
Clean/minor	Begin immunization with tetanus toxoid	None	None	Tetanus toxoid
All other wounds	Tetanus immune globulin 250 units *and* Tetanus toxoid	None	Tetanus toxoid	Tetanus toxoid

Tetanus toxoid:
<7 years old Diphtheria tetanus (DT) toxoid 0.5 mL
>7 years old Tetanus-diphtheria (Td) toxoid 0.5 mL

antibiotic prophylaxis prevents wound infections in most patients whose wounds are closed in the ED.[1,2] Antibiotic prophylaxis has been studied and well accepted in some surgical procedures. The principles learned from these studies are that effectiveness requires the achievement of antimicrobial blood levels prior to or rapidly after wound contamination, and there is no benefit for continuing antibiotics past 24 h in most cases.[13–15] The common practice of giving a patient a prescription for an oral cephalosporin for 7 days upon discharge, which the patient may not fill for hours, clearly fails to meet these principles. If used, antibiotic prophylaxis for traumatic wounds in an emergency department should be (1) started rapidly, ideally within 1 h and before significant tissue manipulation; (2) performed with agents that are effective against predicted pathogens; and (3) administered by routes that rapidly achieve desired blood levels. For most circumstances, this will require intravenous broad-spectrum or combination antibiotic regimens. Oral administration, though theoretically less effective, may also work if done in the emergency department before manipulation and by using an agent with appropriate spectrum and rapid oral absorption.

The most important step in prevention of a wound infection is adequate irrigation and debridement.

Current literature does not support the routine use of antibiotics for most wounds encountered in emergency departments.[12] However, in wounds contaminated by debris or feces, or caused by punctures or bites, in wounds with tissue destruction or in avascular areas, and in neglected wounds, sufficient bacteria may be present to cause infection, and antibiotics are often administered. If antibiotics are chosen, and since most wound infections are due to staphylococci or streptococci, a penicillinase-resistant penicillin (e.g., dicloxacillin) or a first-generation cephalosporin (e.g., cephalexin) provides reasonable coverage. For dog, cat, and human bites, penicillin should be added to cover both *Pasteurella* and *Eikenella,* respectively. Alternatively, amoxicillin-clavulanate alone can be used for therapy in bite wounds but is a more expensive alternative. There is no proven benefit, though, for antibiotic prophylaxis of low-risk dog-bite wounds.[11,16] Full-thickness oral lacerations also warrant antibiotics and should be treated with penicillin.[17] Wounds contaminated by freshwater, and plantar puncture wounds through athletic shoes, should include *Pseudomonas* coverage, preferably with a fluoroquinolone.

The duration for antibiotic prophylaxis is unknown; most physicians use 5 to 7 days. Patients with established wound infections usually require longer treatment. A wound warranting antibiotics can be reevaluated at 24 to 48 h, or patients should be given clear instructions to return at the earliest sign of infection. Contaminated wounds, or those with undetected foreign bodies, may still develop infection despite antibiotic prophylaxis.

TETANUS PROPHYLAXIS

Tetanus is a devastating disease with significant morbidity and mortality rates, and all patients must be asked about their immunization status, even those with clean, ''minor'' wounds. Of the 124 cases of tetanus reported in the United States during 1995 through 1997, a total of 93 were related to acute injury.[18] Importantly, the most common injury type that preceded tetanus infection was a puncture wound in 46 cases (49 percent). Since the incubation period is from 7 to 21 days, it is acceptable to give the adsorbed tetanus toxoid days after injury. The concept of ''tetanus-prone wounds'' is still cited, although the incidence of tetanus occurring in minor wounds makes this distinction suspect. Tetanus-prone wounds are considered to be those that are older than 6 h; stellate or avulsion; over 1 cm deep; due to a missile, crush, or frostbite; or have visible contamination with dirt or saliva.

Guidelines for tetanus prophylaxis in wound management have been developed by several public and professional organizations. Most clinicians refer to the recommendations developed by the Centers for Disease Control (CDC) Advisory Committee on Immunization Practice (ACIP)[19] (Table 36-2). Tetanus immune globulin (TIG) will provide passive protection for several weeks and can be given days after an injury, particularly in patients presenting with high-risk wounds and not up to date on vaccination. TIG and toxoid should be given at separate sites. Due to the large number of inadequately immunized adults, a liberal policy should be used with regard to prophylaxis. Immunization and immune globulin administration are safe during pregnancy.

WOUND COVERAGE

Wounds should be covered after irrigation and cleaning. Allowing a wound to stay open during time in the emergency department increases the risk of continued contamination and interferes with healing. After discharge, coverage with a topical antibiotic reduces the incidence of wound infection.[20] Wounds closed with tissue adhesives should not have topical ointments applied as they may remove the adhesive.

REFERENCES

1. Singer A, Hollander JE, Quinn JV: Evaluation and management of traumatic lacerations. *N Engl J Med* 337:1142, 1997.
2. Howell JM, Chisholm CD: Wound care. *Emerg Med Clin North Am* 15:417, 1997.
3. Singer AJ, Hollander JE, Subramanian S, et al: Pressure dynamics of various irrigation techniques commonly used in the emergency department. *Ann Emerg Med* 24:36, 1994.
4. Singer AJ, Hollander JE, Cassara G, et al: Level of training, wound care practices, and infection rates. *Am J Emerg Med* 13:265, 1995.
5. Lammers RL, Fourre M, Callaham ML, Boone T: Effect of povidone-iodine and saline soaking on bacterial counts in acute traumatic contaminated wounds. *Ann Emerg Med* 19:709, 1990.
6. Dire DJ, Welch AP: A comparison of wound irrigation solutions used in the emergency department. *Ann Emerg Med* 19:704, 1990.
7. Hollander JE, Richman PB, Werblud M, et al: Irrigation in facial and scalp lacerations: Does it alter outcome? *Ann Emerg Med* 31:73, 1998.

8. Hollander JE, Singer AJ, Valentine S: Comparison of wound care practice in pediatric and adult lacerations repaired in the emergency department. *Pediatr Emerg Care* 14:15, 1998.
9. Brunner RG, Fallon WF: A prospective, randomized clinical trial of wound debridement versus conservative wound care in soft-tissue injury from civilian gunshot wounds. *Am Surg* 56:104, 1990.
10. Hollander JE, Singer AJ, Valentine S, Henry MC: Wound registry: Development and validation. *Ann Emerg Med* 25:675, 1995.
11. Dire DJ, Hogan DE, Walker JS: Prophylactic oral antibiotic for low risk dog bite wounds. *Pediatr Emerg Care* 8:194, 1992.
12. Cumming P, Del Beccaro MA: Antibiotics to prevent infection of simple wounds: A meta-analysis of randomized studies. *Am J Emerg Med* 13:396, 1995.
13. McDonald M, Grabsch E, Marshall C, Forbes A: Single- versus multiple-dose antimicrobial prophylaxis for major surgery: A systematic review. *Aust NZ J Surg* 68:388, 1998.
14. Song F, Glenny AM: Antimicrobial prophylaxis in colorectal surgery: A systematic review of randomized controlled trials. *Br J Surg* 85:1232, 1998.
15. Committee on Antimicrobial Agents, Canadian Infectious Disease Society: Antimicrobial prophylaxis in surgery. *Can Med Assoc J* 151:925, 1994.
16. Dire DJ, Hogan RE, Riggs MW: A prospective evaluation of risk factors for infections from dog-bite wounds. *Acad Emerg Med* 1:258, 1994.
17. Steele MT, Sainsbury CR, Robinson WA, et al: Prophylactic penicillin for intraoral wounds. *Ann Emerg Med* 18:847, 1989.
18. Centers for Disease Control and Prevention (CDC): Tetanus surveillance: United States, 1995–1997. *MMWR* 47(SS-2):1, 1998.
19. Centers for Disease Control (CDC) Advisory Committee on Immunization Practices: Diphtheria, tetanus, and pertussis: Recommendations for vaccine use and other preventive measures. *MMWR* 40(RR-10):1, 1991.
20. Dire DJ, Coppola M, Fwyer DA, et al: Prospective evaluation of topical antibiotics for preventing infections in uncomplicated soft-tissue wounds repaired in the ED. *Acad Emerg Med* 2:4, 1995.

METHODS FOR WOUND CLOSURE

Julia Martin
Rob Herfel

The ideal wound closure is one that will repair tissue, recover function, reduce the risk of infection, and restore appearance. In order to obtain a cosmetic closure, it is important to understand the principles of wound healing, have a knowledge of the different techniques, and practice these approaches to become efficient. This chapter addresses the general concepts of closure techniques useful in the emergency department (ED).

After wound preparation, the physical integrity and function of the injured tissue must be restored. Most wounds seen in the ED require some form of closure, and the method chosen depends on the type of wound. There are three categories of wound closure: primary, delayed primary, and secondary.

Primary wound closure is the closing of the wound near the time of injury. Primary closure without tissue loss is almost always possible with clean wounds seen within 4 h after injury. The incidence of bacterial contamination and the risk of infection increase with injuries more than 4 h old. However, with clean wounds in highly vascular areas (scalp, face, and neck), the incidence of infection is so low that primary closure may be possible even up to 24 h after injury.[1] Primary closure of wounds in areas with poor blood supply (e.g., distal extremities) and contamination (e.g., debris) can generally be attempted if they are seen within 4 to 8 h and should be avoided if they present after 12 h from the time of the injury. Wounds with associated tissue loss usually require grafts or flaps to close the defect; these procedures are usually performed by specialists, often in the operating room.

Delayed primary closure is the approach of cleaning the wound, leaving the wound open under a moist dressing for approximately 4 to 5 days, and then suturing the wound if there is no evidence of infection. Heavily contaminated wounds, wounds resulting from high-energy missile injuries, or large wounds due to animal bites are ideal for delayed primary closure. Wounds contaminated by pus, vaginal discharge, feces, or saliva as well as those where treatment is delayed longer than 12 h should also be considered for open wound management. The first step in delayed primary closure is through cleaning and removal of debris and devitalized tissue. Prophylactic antibiotics should be started in the ED. The wound is packed open with moist, sterile, fine-meshed gauze and then covered by a dry sterile dressing. The wound should not be disturbed for the first 4 to 5 days after injury unless the patient develops an unexplained fever; unnecessary inspection during this period increases the risk of contamination and subsequent infection. On the fourth or fifth day, the wound can be undressed and inspected. In the absence of infection (no purulence or erythema beyond the edges of the wound) and devitalized tissue, the wound edges can be approximated with minimal risk of infection.[2]

Closure by secondary intention is allowing the wound to heal without mechanical closure. Over a period of time the tissue slowly granulates, forming a slightly larger scar than that would be seen with primary wound closure yet less of a scar than would be seen if a sutured wound became infected.

Once it is decided to close the wound, a closure technique must be selected that allows the most accurate and secure approximation of the skin edges. Suturing is the oldest and most commonly used method. However, alternative techniques—including skin staples, skin-closure tapes, and tissue adhesives—can be used in selected patients. The short-term goal of any closure method is to hold tissue in apposition until the tensile strength of the wound is sufficient to withstand stress. The long-term goal of wound closure is to accurately reapproximate wound edges with the most esthetically pleasing results.

CLOSURE METHODS

Sutures

The placement of sutures is the oldest and most common method of wound closure. An ideal suture material would have the following characteristics:

1. A low friction coefficient, so it will not stick to tissue as it is drawn through and not bind to itself as knots are being tied.
2. High pliability, so the suture will not deform tissue when it attempts to straighten itself after being tied.
3. Knot security, so that the ties will not unravel. Sutures with a low friction coefficient will slip more easily and the knots will spontaneously unravel, as opposed to materials with a high friction coefficient.
4. Tensile strength to hold the wound closed.
5. Low tissue reaction to reduce inflammation and the risk of infection.

No suture material possesses all these characteristics; different suture materials are chosen as acceptable compromises for specific types of wounds (Table 37-1). Sutures are generally divided into two general classes based on their rate of degradation:

1. Sutures that undergo rapid degradation in tissues, losing essentially all their tensile strength within 60 days, are considered ''absorbable'' sutures.
2. Sutures that maintain their tensile strength for longer than 60 days are ''nonabsorbable'' sutures.

This terminology is somewhat misleading, because most absorbable sutures lose half their tensile strength within 4 weeks and some nonabsorbable sutures (e.g., silk and nylon) lose some tensile strength during this 60-day interval. Silk loses approximately half of its tensile strength in 1 year and has no strength at the end of 2 years. Nylon preserves its strength the longest, losing only about 25 percent of its original strength over 2 years.

TABLE 37-1 Sutures Commonly Used for ED Wound Repair

		Low Friction	Pliability	Knot Security	Tensile Strength	Tissue Non-Reactivity	Tensile Strength Half-Life	Comments
Nonabsorbable								
Silk	Natural multifilament	2+	3+	4+	2+	1+	12 months	Easiest to handle but poses greatest risk of infection
Nylon (Ethilon and Dermalon)	Synthetic monofilament or multifilament	3+ 2+	1+ 2+	2+ 3+	3+ 3+	3+ 3+	>2 years	Low tissue reactivity and most often used for cutaneous closure
Polypropylene (Prolene)	Synthetic monofilament	3+	1+	1+	4+	4+		Stiffest suture, requires multiple throws for knot security
Polyester (Mersilene)	Synthetic multifilament	3+	3+	4+	2+	2+		Easy to handle with excellent security, often used for vascular sutures
Polybutester (Novafil)	Synthetic monofilament	3+	2+	4+	4+	4+		Excellent characteristics, can stretch with wound edema and then contract back to original size
Absorbable								
Gut	Natural	1+	1+	2+	2+	1+	5–7 days	Stiff, rapidly absorbed, used for mucosal closures only
Chronic gut	Natural	1+	1+	2+	2+	1+	10–14 days	Used in situations where suture removal may be difficult
Polyglycolic acid (Dexon)	Synthetic multifilament	2+	3+	3+	3+	3+	10–15 days	Subcutaneous sutures, coated variety easier to use
Polyglactin 910 (Vicryl)	Synthetic multifilament	2+	3+	2+	4+	3+	14–21 days	Use clear variety on face
Polyglyconate (Maxon)	Synthetic monofilament	3+	2+	3+	4+	4+	28–36 days	Very strong and low reactivity
Polydioxanone (PDS II)	Synthetic monofilament	3+	1+	2+	4+	4+	28 days	Very strong and low reactivity

4+ highest and most desirable; 1+ lowest and least desirable.

Sutures are sized according to their diameter. The smallest in general use is designated 6-0 and is used for percutaneous closure on the face and other cosmetically important areas. Suture sizes 5-0 and 4-0 are progressively larger and used on the trunk and extremities. Very thick skin, like that on the scalp and sole of the foot, may require percutaneous closure with size 3-0 sutures.

NONABSORBABLE SUTURES Nonabsorbable sutures can be of either natural or synthetic origin. Natural nonabsorbable sutures include fibers (silk) and metal (stainless steel). Natural materials like silk are easy to handle but incite moderate tissue reaction. Synthetic nonabsorbable fibers include polyamides (nylon), polyesters (Dacron, Dupont), polypropylene, and polybutester. Synthetic suture materials are useful for wound closure because they cause the least tissue reaction. Sutures may be classified according to their physical configuration. Sutures made of one filament are called *monofilament sutures* (nylon, polypropylene, polybutester, and stainless steel). Knot security with monofilaments is low; therefore at least two square knots (four throws) are required to achieve an adequate hold with 4-0 suture.[3] Sutures composed of multiple fibers braided together are called *multifilament sutures* (silk, nylon, polyester, and stainless steel). Multifilament sutures have greater pliability and increased knot security; they are less likely to unravel than monofilament sutures.[4] The disadvantage of multifilament sutures is that bacteria can migrate down the gaps between the individual filaments into the wound, increasing the likelihood of infection. Nylon and stainless steel are available as both monofilament and multifilament sutures.

ABSORBABLE SUTURES Absorbable sutures are made from either collagen or synthetic polymers. Collagen sutures are derived either from the submucosa of ovine or bovine small intestine (gut suture) or from reconstituted collagen manufactured from bovine tendon collagen (collagen suture). This collagenous tissue is treated in an aldehyde solution, which cross-links and strengthens the suture, making it more resistant to enzymatic degradation. Suture materials treated in this way are called *plain gut* or *plain collagen*. If the suture is additionally treated in chromium trioxide, it becomes *chromic gut* or *chromic collagen*, which is more highly cross-linked and more resistant to absorption than plain gut or collagen. The shortcomings of collagen and gut sutures include variable strength, unpredictable absorption, and marked inflammation during absorption by proteolytic enzymatic digestion. Gut sutures should be avoided in areas close to surface. Other disadvantages of gut sutures are less tensile and knot strength, a higher infection rate, and more dehiscence than with synthetic sutures. Gut sutures are primarily used to close oral mucosal lacerations, as these wounds heal rapidly and do not require prolonged suture support. Chromium-treated sutures are absorbed less rapidly than plain gut but more rapidly than synthetic sutures. Because of its coating, chromic gut causes less inflammation than plain gut. Chromic gut can also be used in the oral mucosa and for closure of scalp lacerations in children; these sutures typically fall out in 1 to 2 weeks with little or no complication and no need for a return visit for suture removal.

Synthetic substitutes commonly used instead of gut sutures are produced from polyglycolic acid (Dexon, Sherwood Davis & Geck)

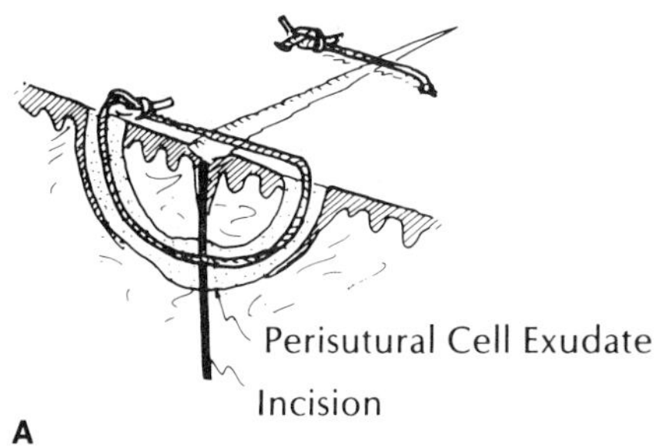

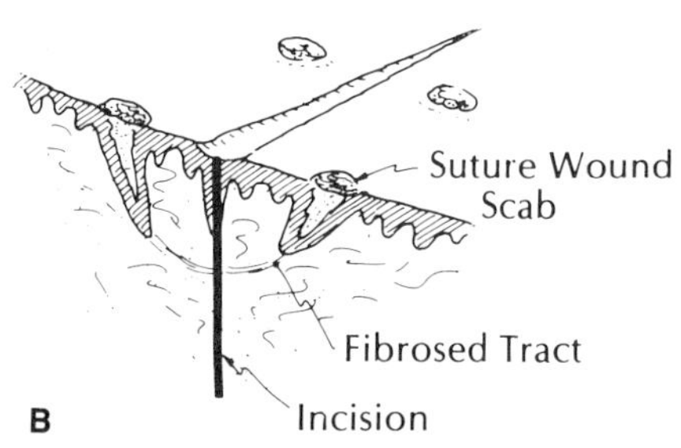

FIG. 37-1. A. Epithelial cells migrate along the suture track, forming a perisutural cuff. **B.** If percutaneous sutures are not removed before 8 days, needle puncture scars develop.

or polyglactin 910 (Vicryl, Ethicon, Inc.). These braided sutures lose half their strength in tissues approximately 2 weeks after implantation, with absorption essentially complete by 2 months. Two other synthetic absorbable monofilament sutures, polyglyconate (Maxon, Sherwood Davis & Geck) and polydioxanone (PDSII, Ethicon, Inc.), retain their tensile strength longer. The chemical degradation of all these synthetic absorbable sutures is by hydrolysis of their ester bonds and opposed to the proteolytic inflammatory reaction required to degrade gut sutures. Absorbable suture materials are useful when working just below skin surface and in special circumstances when later suture removal is awkward (in children and inaccessible sites). Synthetic braided polymers are less reactive and more resistant to infection from contaminating bacteria than plain or chromic catgut. Polyglycolic acid has excellent knot security and will hold tight with a single square knot (two throws). The main drawback is that its high friction coefficient makes it "bind and snag" when wet. Major uses of polyglycolic acid are for single deep (dermal) closures or superficial fascial closure as well as ligature of small bleeding vessels. Dexon Plus (Sherwood Davis & Geck) is coated with polaxamer 188, which reduces friction and drag through tissues; it is easier to handle but more throws (four to six) are required to prevent knot slippage than with plain polyglycolic acid. Polyglactin 910 (Vicryl, Ethicon, Inc.), mentioned above, is used for deep closures. It has less knot security, similar dry tensile strength, and longer in vivo strength as compared with polyglycolic acid.

INFECTION All sutures compromise local tissue defenses and increase the potential for infection for the following reasons:

1. The trauma of inserting a needle is sufficient to incite an inflammatory response.
2. Sutures that are tied too tightly impair blood flow and cause tissue necrosis of the wound edges.
3. Sutures that penetrate the intact skin provide an avenue for wound contamination through the perisutural cuff (Fig. 37-1).
4. The quantity of suture and the chemical reactivity of the material increase the susceptibility to infection.

Sutures made of natural fiber potentate infection more than other nonabsorbable sutures and should be avoided in contaminated wounds. The incidence of infection from monofilament sutures is less than that from multifilament sutures made of comparable materials. Therefore synthetic monofilament sutures should be used for wounds at risk for infection.

NEEDLES The ideal surgical needle should guide the suture through the tissue and provide for meticulous approximation of the wound edges with the least damage.[5] All surgical needles are produced from stainless steel alloys, which have excellent resistance to corrosion. High nickel maraging adds resistance to bending and breakage compared with plain stainless steel surgical needles. Every surgical needle has three basic components: swage, body, and point.

The swage is the point of attachment of the suture to the needle. The swaging process provides a smooth junction between the needle and suture as opposed to the rough junction of a thread being attached to the needle by insertion through an eye. Almost all sutures used today have laser-drilled swages down the center of the needle for about 2 mm for the attachment of sutures. Channel needles have a channel cut into one side of the needle for about 6-mm for attachment of the suture. The needle is attached to the suture by uniformly compressing the walls of the swage against the suture. In most uses, this attachment strength is so great that separation of the needle from the suture is most easily accomplished by cutting the suture. A swage requiring lower uniform forces to detach its suture, sometimes called *pop-off* or *control release*, is also available. The control release was originally developed for abdominal wound closure, bolus dressings for skin grafts, and hysterectomies in which large numbers of interrupted sutures are used; eliminating the need to cut the suture considerably reduces the length of the operation. For ED wound closure, where a single length of suture is used for multiple loops, the control-release attachment is rarely used.

Both laser-drilled and channel swaged needles are more susceptible to bending and breakage by the needle-holder jaws when grasped over the swage than the body of the needle. To prevent this, the needle should be grasped with the needle holder on the body of the needle, not over the swage. Conversely, suturing is easier when as much of the needle as possible is available for passage through the tissue in one stroke, therefore the needle holder should be close to the swage end but not over it. Since laser-drilled swages are shorter than channel swages, the needle can be grasped with more available for passage through the tissue (Fig. 37-2).

The body of the needle is the portion that is grasped by the needle holder. The security with which needle-holder jaws grasp the needle is influenced primarily by the presence of teeth in the needle-holder jaws and the ratchet setting of the needle-holder handle and less so by the cross-sectional shape of the needle body.

The overall biomechanical performance of the surgical needle and holder combination is determined by (1) needle sharpness, (2) needle resistance to bending, (3) needle ductility, and (4) needle-holder clamping moment. Sharpness measures the force needed to pass a needle through a membrane that simulates the density of human tissue, and needle resistance to bending is measured by recording the force required to bend the needle 90°. But the more critical measurement to the emergency physician is the force required to deform the needle irreversibly—the yield moment. Ductility is a measure of the needle's resistance to complete breakage. The needle-holder clamping moment is a measure of the force exerted by the needle-holder jaws on a curved surgical needle.

The body of a suture needle can be defined according to (1) the cross-sectional shape and (2) the geometric configuration. The cross-sectional shape will determine the resistance of the needle to bending as well as the security with which the needle-holder jaws grasp the needle. The cross-sectional shapes in common use are round, triangular, trapezoidal, rectangular with rounded sides, and side-flattened.

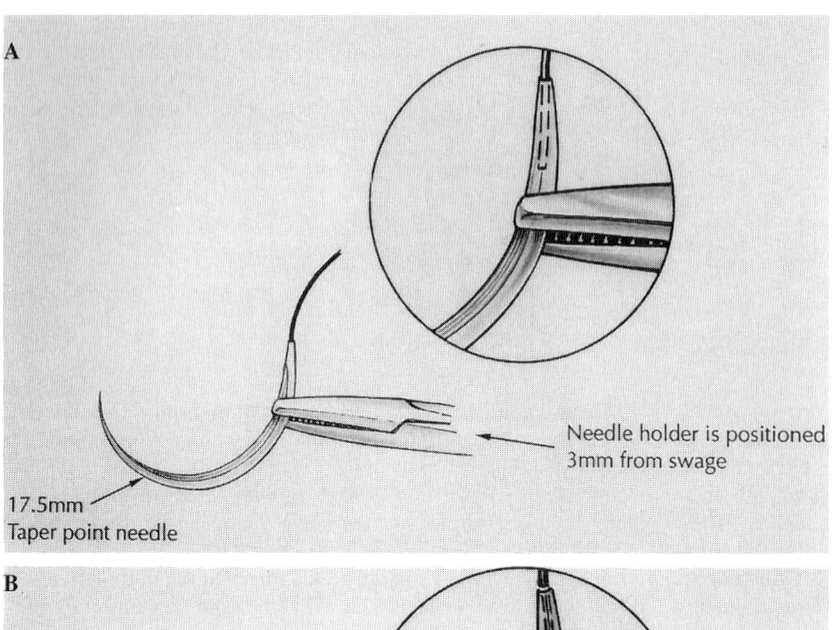

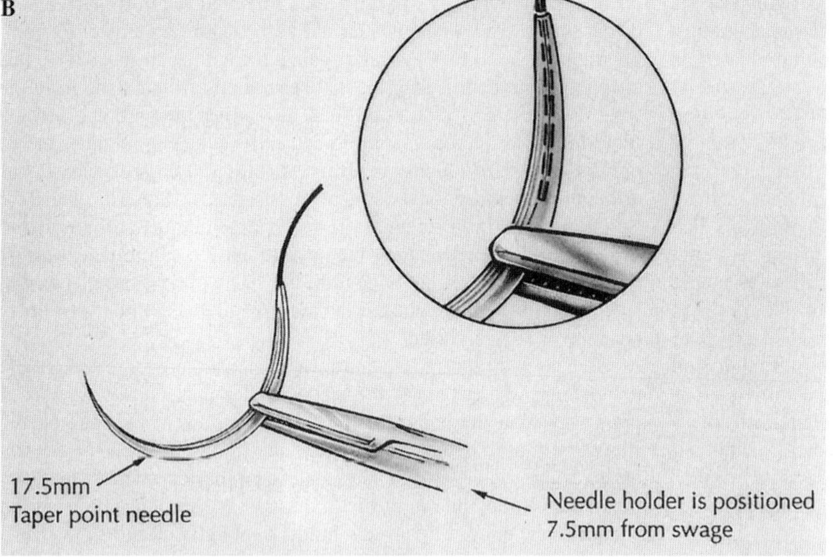

FIG. 37-2. A. The laser-drilled swage is only 1.5 mm long and the needle holder can grip close to the end of the needle, leaving more length available for passage through tissue on the initial movement. **B.** The channel swage is 6 mm long and the needle holder must grip further along the needle, leaving less needle available for passage through tissue on the initial movement.

Rectangular cross sections are created by flattening the inner and outer surfaces of the circular wire during the manufacturing process. Needle holders are able to hold the body more securely when it has flat surfaces parallel to the grasping face of the jaws. With rectangular and trapezoidal shapes, the needle-holding security against twisting and rotation is greater than with any other cross-sectional configuration. Unfortunately, flattening the inner surface reduces resistance to bending, partially reducing the benefit of enhanced needle holding security. For suturing of tough tissues, side-flattened needle bodies are preferred because they exhibit greater resistance to bending than any other cross-sectional shape.

The geometry of the suture needle can be described by its radius, curvature, diameter, length, and chord length. The radius of the needle is the distance from the center of the circle to the body of the needle if the curvature of the needle is continued to make a full circle. The curvature at the needle is measured in degrees of the subtended arc and may vary from 90° ($\frac{1}{4}$) to 225° ($\frac{5}{8}$) (Fig. 37-3). Needles with a curvature of 135° are ideal to approximate divided edges of thin planar structures that are readily accessible (e.g., skin), requiring a limited arc of wrist rotation to pass the needle. It is difficult to use the 135° needle in deeper tissues (e.g., muscle, fascia) because the limited arc of the wrist rotation involved in passing this needle is usually not sufficient to expose the needle point, which will remain buried in the tissue. The 180° needle is ideally suited for use in deeper tissues because a limited arc of wrist rotation will successfully pass the entire needle through the tissue, allowing adequate exposure of the needle point for easy retrieval of the needle. Curved needles are ideally suited for closure of thin layers, such as epidermis and fascia. The compound curved needle is most often used to alter the 135° needle; the straight point readily facilitates initial entrance through the tissue and controls the depth, while the tight curvature beyond the point permits accurate exiting at a selected level. This design offers a mechanical advantage over the standard needle with one radius of curvature. The compound needle is useful for closure of the dermis.

Needle diameter is the width of the original circular wire utilized in the manufacturing process for the production of the needle. Cord length is the linear distance measured from the central point of the needle swage to the point of the needle. Needle length is the length of the needle measured at the center of the wire's cross section.

The point of the needle extends from the tip of the needle to the maximum cross section of the body. A variety of needle-point configurations have been designed to penetrate specific types of tissue.

The simplest configuration is the taperpoint, where the needle tapers to a sharp tip (Fig. 37-4). The taperpoint spreads the tissue without

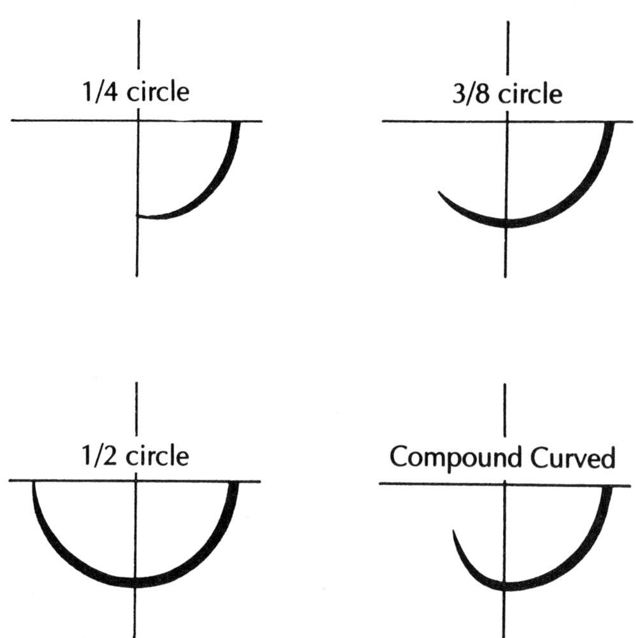

FIG. 37-3. Geometry of length of needle.

cutting and is used for soft tissue that does not resist needle penetration, such as vessels, fascia, and muscle. The taperpoint makes the smallest hole in tissue and does not cut small incisions at the periphery of the hole.

For suturing cutaneous wounds in the ED, needles with cutting edges are useful to penetrate the relatively tough skin. Cutting-edge needles have at least two opposing edges that are designed to separate tough tissue. Usually, a third cutting edge is added, and the position of this third cutting edge categorizes the needle as either a conventional cutting-edge needle or a reverse cutting-edge needle.

A conventional cutting-edge needle has the third edge located on the inner or concave surface, which produces two effects during suturing: (1) cutting action directed toward the center of the wound and (2) pressure that directs the needle point toward the skin as it passes through tissue (surface-seeking) (Fig. 37-5). The central cutting action has a tendency to divide tissues that ultimately will be encircled by the suture. As the needle passes through the skin, it produces a triangular defect, the apex of which is directed toward the incision. If it is positioned in this apex, the suture may cut through when tied.

In contrast, the reverse cutting-edge needle has the third cutting edge located on the outer, convex curvature of the needle (Fig. 37-6). This configuration has the flat surface of the needle closest to the edges of the incision or wound and directs the point of the needle toward the depth of the wound (depth-seeking). The skin hole left by the reverse cutting-edge needle leaves a flattened wall of tissue for the suture to be tied against, which should resist suture cut-through.

Sharpness of cutting needles can be enhanced by narrowing the point configuration, reducing the angles of the cutting edges, and coating the point with silicone. For conventional and reverse cutting-edge needles, the shape of the needle point is triangular, with two lateral cutting edges and a cutting edge at the apex. The bevel-edge

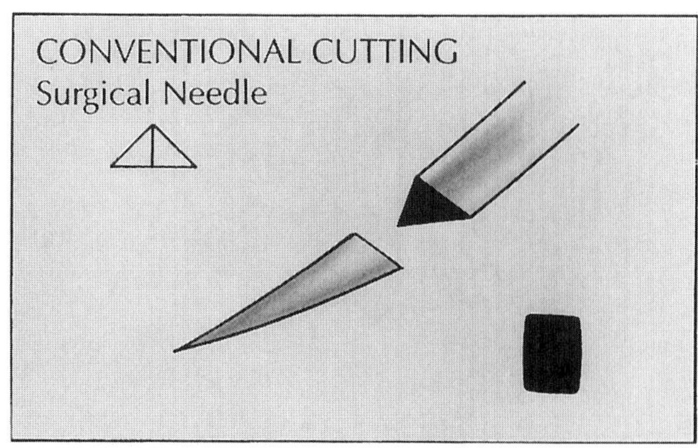

FIG. 37-5. Conventional cutting edge surgical needle. **Top left**. Front view of point. The point of the needle has three cutting edges, with its apical cutting edge on the inside, concave surface of the needle. **Side view**. Its apical cutting edge is positioned on the inside, concave surface of the needle. **Bottom right**. The body of the needle has a side-flattened cross-sectional configuration.

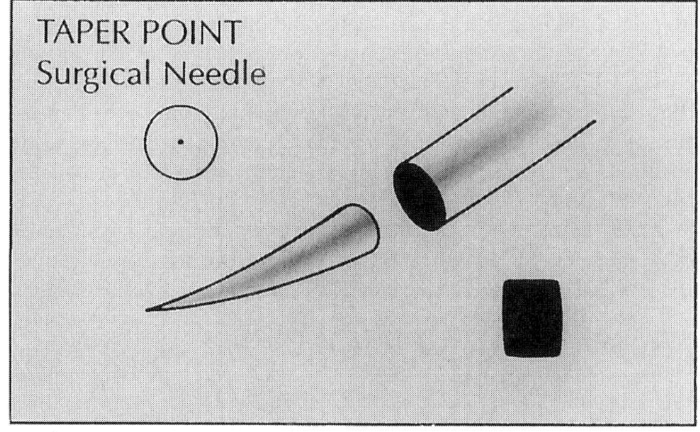

FIG. 37-4. Taperpoint surgical needle. **Top left**. Front view of point. The geometry of this needle tapers to a point and has no cutting edges. **Side view**. The point of this needle has a narrow taperpoint geometry. **Bottom right**. The body of the needle has a side-flattened cross-sectional configuration.

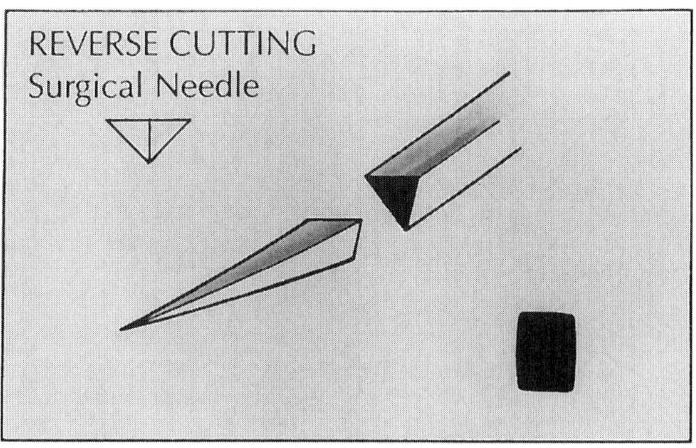

FIG. 37-6. Reverse cutting edge surgical needle. **Top left**. Front view of point. The point of the needle has three cutting edges, with its apical cutting edge on the outer, convex surface of the needle. **Side view**. Its apical cutting edge is located on the outer, convex side of the needle. **Bottom right**. The body of the needle has a side-flattened cross-sectional configuration.

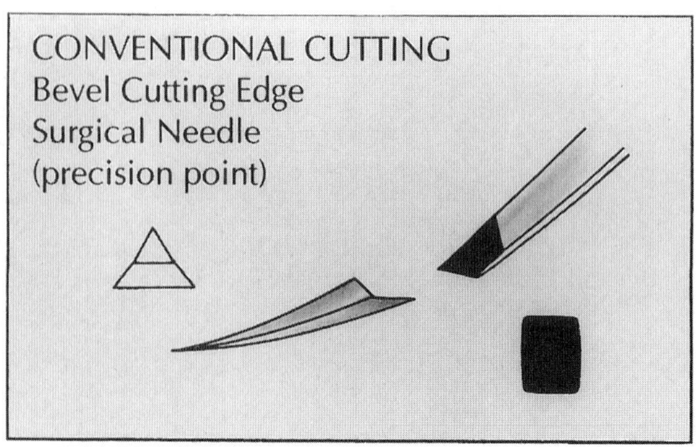

FIG. 37-7. Bevel conventional cutting edge surgical needle. **Top left**. Front view of point. The opposing sides of the point of the needle have a concave geometry that reduces the angle of its cutting edges. **Side view**. The sides of the point of this bevel conventional cutting edge needle are beveled to reduce the angle of its cutting edges. **Bottom right**. The body of the needle has a side-flattened cross-sectional configuration.

needle has opposing concave surfaces rather than the straight planar surfaces encountered in the standard cutting-edge needles (Fig. 37-7). The angles of the cutting edges at the apex and sides of the bevel cutting edges are 45° and 52.5°, respectively, rather than the 60° for the standard cutting-edge needles, which enhances the sharpness. Coating the cutting-edge surfaces with silicone increases their initial sharpness in tissues and maintains the sharpness after repeated passage (durability).

Tapercut needles combine the unique features of taperpoint and cutting-edge needles (Fig. 37-8). The cutting edges of the tapercut needle extend only a very short distance from the needle tip and blend into a round taper body. This needle provides smooth passage through oral mucous membrane, yet its round shaft without cutting edges will not cut through the deeper tissues.

Surgical sutures currently in use have a needle-to-suture diameter ratio of approximately 2:1; the hole left by the needle will not be completely filled by the suture and the unfilled space at each suture hole may invite infection to pass through. To resolve this problem,

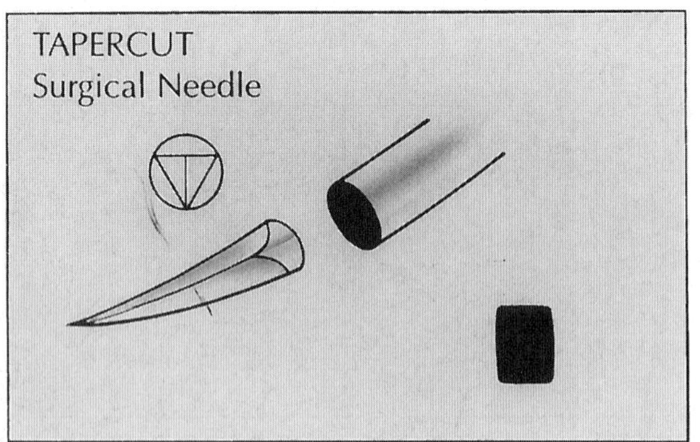

FIG. 37-8. Tapercut surgical needle. **Top left**. Front view of point. This tapercut needle has a short reverse cutting edge that blends into a taperpoint geometry. **Side view**. The reverse cutting edges are confined to a small portion of the tip of this needle. **Bottom right**. The body of the needle has a side-flattened cross-sectional configuration.

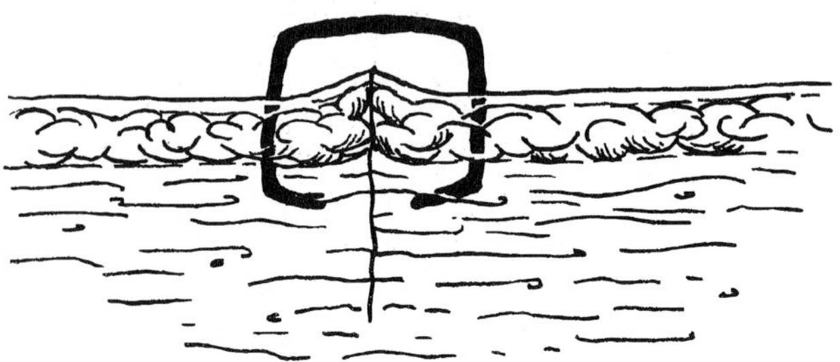

FIG. 37-9. A cutaneous staple properly placed will evert the skin edges and not be in contact with the skin surface.

two new sutures attached to taperpoint needles have been developed. A polytetrafluoroethylene monofilament suture can be produced with a porous microstructure that is approximately 50 percent air by volume. This porous nature allows it to be swaged to a needle that closely approximates its suture diameter; a needle-to-suture ratio of 1:1. Alternatively a monofilament polypropylene suture can be made with a tapered end that is significantly smaller than that of the remainder of the suture, and swaged to a needle with a needle-to-suture diameter ratio approaching 1:1.

Staples

Skin closure by metal staples is quick (at least four times faster than closure with sutures) and economical (slightly less total cost than suturing).[6–8] An additional advantage of staples is their low level of tissue reactivity; wounds with staple closure exhibit resistance to infection superior even to that of the least reactive suture.[9] These advantages of skin staples must be weighed against one notable drawback—the skin staple does not provide the same meticulous coaptation of lacerations with irregular skin edges that can be achieved with sutures. For staples to achieve accurate closure, the skin edges must be aligned before the staples are placed. Because accurate prepositioning of the wound edges is very difficult in many lacerations, staple implantation will often result in malapposition of wound edges, which is an invitation to the development of scar deformity. Consequently, skin staples are usually reserved for lacerations in anatomic sites where the healing scar is not readily apparent (e.g., scalp).

The basic shape of an applied cutaneous staple is an incomplete rectangle; the top bridges the laceration off the skin surface and the points are directed 90° inward off the side legs (Fig. 37-9). As staples are placed, the stapling device pushes the points toward each other; they impinge the skin and evert the wound edges. When placing staples, the wound edges should be held together with tissue forceps. The stapling device should be placed gently (not firmly or with pressure) against the skin surface before the trigger is slowly (not rapidly) squeezed. A properly placed staple should have its top side off the skin surface.

A variety of stapling devices that implant stainless steel staples are commercially available for use in the ED. There are several features of a stapling device to be considered in choosing a particular product:

1. The stapler should be designed so that it does not obstruct the physician's view of the wound edge.
2. The stapler should have a mechanism that holds the staple securely during its formation.
3. The stapler should have an ejection spring that automatically releases the staple.
4. The handling characteristics of the stapler should be such that the physician can easily implant a large number of staples without becoming fatigued.

Other features to be considered in choosing stapling devices include size (smaller ones are better for lacerations in tight areas) and quantity of staples (more are required when closing large lacerations).

Staples were originally developed to close surgical incisions, and there was initially a reluctance to use them for traumatic lacerations.[6] Clinical studies have found that for the scalp, neck, trunk, and extremities, staples produce a cosmetic result that is identical to that from sutures.[6–8] Staple removal requires a special instrument that deforms the top and spreads open the points. Staple removal is slightly more painful than suture removal.

Skin-Closure Tapes

Skin-closure tapes are used as an alternative to sutures and staples for wound closure and for additional support after suture and staple removal.[9] Tapes do not require anesthesia and the patient does not need to return for their removal. Skin-closure tapes work best on flat, dry, nonmobile surfaces where the wound edges fit together without tension. Conversely, oily or wet surfaces, movable areas, or wounds that stay open with tension are not appropriate for surgical tape closure. Taped wounds are more resistant to infection than sutured wounds; therefore tapes are useful for wounds at increased risk of infection. Tapes can be used for skin flaps, where sutures may compromise perfusion, and for lacerations with thin, friable skin that will not hold sutures.

The ease with which wounds can be closed by tape varies according to the anatomic and biomechanical properties of the wound site. Linear cutaneous wounds subjected to minimal static and dynamic tensions are easily approximated by tape. The relatively lax skin of the face and abdomen makes it amenable to wound closure by tapes. Contrary to expectation, tape closure without sutures is more easily accomplished in obese patients, and the thick cut edges of adipose tissue tend to evert the skin. The taut skin of the extremities, which is subjected to frequent dynamic joint movements, requires dermal sutures before taping. The copious secretions from the skin of the axillae, palms, and soles discourage tape adherence.

A variety of skin-closure tapes are commercially available, with differing biomechanical characteristics. The ideal tape should primarily possess excellent adhesion and strength; porosity, flexibility, and elasticity are less important. In the United States, tapes sold for ED use come in widths of $\frac{1}{4}$ and $\frac{1}{2}$ in., in varying lengths, in sterile, single-use packages. The $\frac{1}{4}$-in. width is appropriate for wounds less than 3 to 4 cm in length; longer wounds should use the $\frac{1}{2}$-in. width. The individual tapes are applied to nonadherent backing that can be bent at a scored perforation to free up one end of the tape without deforming it. The tapes should be removed from the backing by grasping the free end with forceps.

Adherence of tapes is enhanced by the use of benzoin or mastic to the skin surface 2 to 3 cm beyond the wound edges. These agents are best applied with applicator sticks or applicator-tipped single-use vials. Care should be taken not to allow any benzoin or mastic to enter the wound. The agent should be allowed to dry and become tacky before the tape is applied.

Tapes should be long enough to stretch 2 to 3 cm on either side of the wound. Using forceps, the tape is attached to the skin on one side, then pulled across the wound to coadapt the wound edges and applied to the opposite side. Coadaption of the wound edges can be facilitated by using a finger to push the wound together as the tape is being pulled across. Longitudinal alignment of the wound edges is facilitated when taping starts in the middle and progresses toward each end. Individual tapes are applied with some space between them but not so much that the wound edges gap open between the individual tapes (Fig. 37-10).

When skin-closure tapes are properly employed to close linear wounds subjected to weak tensions, cosmetic results are excellent. Additionally, the discomfort of anesthetic infiltration, the need for suture removal, and the development of suture puncture scars is avoided. Wounds closed with tape cannot get wet or be washed. Dressing over a taped wound is problematic; on the one hand, the dressing may protect the tape ends from becoming lifted, but, on the other, a dressing may promote the collection of moisture and premature tape separation. Tapes should stay in place about as long as an equivalent suture and will spontaneously detach as the underlying epithelium exfoliates.

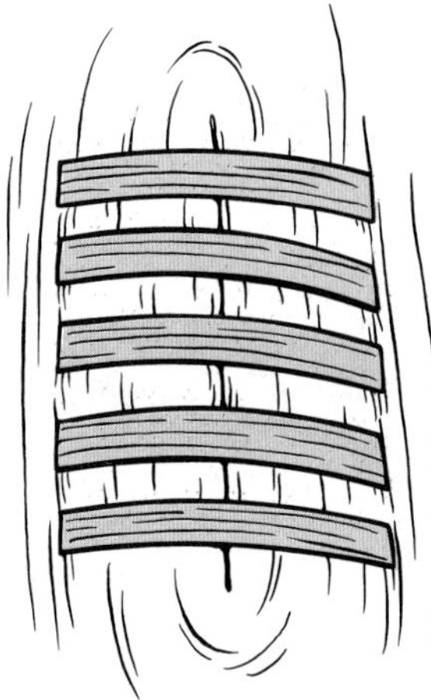

FIG. 37-10. Skin-closure tapes should be applied perpendicular to the wound edges and spaced so that the edges do not gape.

Tissue Adhesives

Cyanoacrylate tissue adhesives have been available in Canada and Europe for years, and one product, 2-octylcyanoacrylate, is now available in the United States (Dermabond, Ethicon, Inc.).[10] Cyanoacrylate adhesives polymerize rapidly when applied to tissues through an exothermic reaction catalyzed by a small amount of moisture. These adhesives close wounds by forming an adhesive layer on top of intact epithelium, which holds the edges together. Cyanoacrylate adhesives cause an intense inflammatory reaction within subcutaneous tissues and should never be applied within wounds. Adhesives cannot be used near the eye, on mucous membranes or mucosal surfaces, on infected areas, on wounds that are wet or exposed to body fluids, or in areas with dense hair (e.g., scalp). When used on appropriately selected wounds, tissue adhesives can be applied in less than half the time required for sutures and without the need for anesthesia or return for removal.[11–13]

Adhesives are most useful when they are used on wounds that close spontaneously, have clean or sharp edges, and are located on clean, nonmobile areas. Wounds where the edges are separated more than 5 mm by the underlying skin tension are unlikely to stay closed with tissue adhesives alone. In this case, subcutaneous sutures can be inserted to relieve this tension and approximate the edges. Also, lacerations longer than 5 cm are prone to shear forces and unlikely to remain closed with tissue adhesives alone.

Two-octylcyanoacrylate is commercially available in a single-use vial with an applicator tip. A violet colorant is added to make it visible during application. Wounds should be cleaned and bleeding controlled before the tissue adhesive is applied, but absolute dryness is not required. The wound should be held together and the edges slightly everted with tissue forceps. Adhesive is applied by lightly wiping the applicator tip over the area (at least 5 mm beyond the skin edges) in the direction of the long axis of the wound (Fig. 37-11). Three to four thin layers should be applied successively; droplets or a single thick layer is to be avoided. The wound edges should be held together for

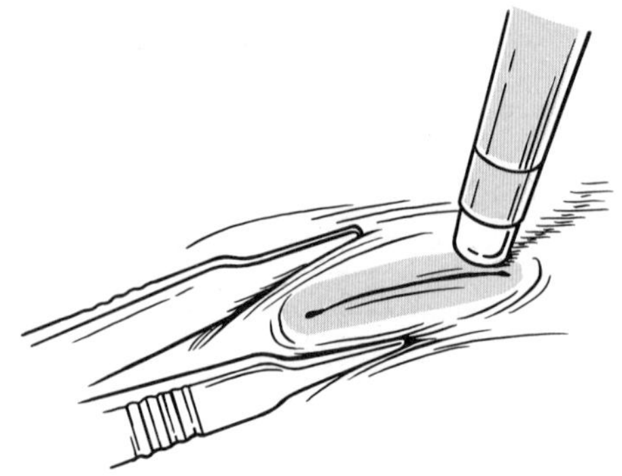

FIG. 37-11. Tissue adhesives are applied in several light coats over the wound, carefully avoiding entry of the adhesive into the wound.

about 60 s after the last adhesive application to ensure that the adhesive has time to set fully. Some articles have described the application of tissue adhesives as "spots" along the laceration or as intermittent "stripes" applied perpendicular to the laceration. These techniques might be less useful, since cyanoacrylates are only slightly more viscous than water and subcutaneous penetration is possible from dabs applied to the skin or from unintentional opening of the edges by wiping the applicator tip across the wound. Adhesive applied to unwanted areas can be removed by using petroleum jelly or acetone. Once applied, cyanoacrylates should not be covered with ointment, bandage, or dressing.

Patients should be instructed not to use ointments, apply bandages, or pick at edges of the adhesive. After 24 h, the area can be gently washed with plain water but should not be scrubbed, soaked, or exposed to moisture for any length of time. The adhesive will spontaneously slough off in 5 to 10 days. Should a wound open, the patient should immediately return for closure.

As compared with suturing, wounds closed with tissue adhesives initially have less tensile strength; after 7 days, however this difference disappears.[10] The manufacturer of 2-octylcyanoacrylate notes that the incidence of wound infection with this product is 3.6 percent and the incidence of dehiscence requiring retreatment is 2.2 percent; neither was statistically different by comparison with equivalent wounds closed with sutures. An animal model has found that 2-octylcyanoacrylate can be used to close contaminated wounds with a lower infection rate, although this use has not been validated in humans.[14] The ultimate cosmetic appearance of wounds closed with tissue adhesives is identical to that of closure with sutures.[13,15]

SUTURING TECHNIQUES

General Principles

Suturing continues to be the most common method for laceration repair in the ED and percutaneous sutures that pass through both the epidermal and dermal layers are the type most frequently used. Dermal, or subcuticular, sutures reapproximate the divided edges of the dermis without penetrating the epidermis. Occasionally, dermal and percutaneous sutures are used together in a layered closure. As noted above, dermal sutures can be used with either surgical tapes or tissue adhesives for epidermal closure. Sutures can be applied in a continuous manner ("running," with knots at each end of a long closure) or as interrupted sutures (each loop being individually tied).

Monofilament nylon or polypropylene sutures are most commonly used for skin closure because these materials have acceptable mechanical properties and low tissue reaction. Polybutester sutures have unique performance characteristics that may be advantageous for the closure of wounds that might expand from edema and then contract as the swelling resolves. Polybutester can elongate in response to low forces and has elasticity, enabling it to return to its original length once the load is removed. Sutures with less extensibility under low forces—like nylon, polypropylene, polyester, or silk—will frequently lacerate or necrose encircled tissue in edematous wounds, thereby increasing the susceptibility to infection.

Percutaneous sutures are recommended for closure of stellate lacerations resulting from crush injuries. In these wounds, meticulous closure with percutaneous sutures approximates the skin edges more exactly than does tape. Closing these wounds is often like putting together a jigsaw puzzle, and tapes have little practical value. The more accurate approximation of skin edges by skillfully applied sutures leads to a more pleasing cosmetic result. Damage to the local tissue defenses is related to the quantity of the suture within the wound (diameter and length); therefore, the suture with the narrowest diameter and sufficient strength to resist disruption of the closure should be used.

Straight, shallow lacerations can be closed with percutaneous sutures only, sewing from one end toward the other and aligning edges with each individual suture bite. Deep, irregular wounds with uneven, unaligned, or gaping edges are more difficult to suture. Certain principles have been identified by years of clinical experience:

1. The uneven edges can be aligned by first approximating the midportion of the wound with the initial suture. Subsequent sutures are placed in the middle of each half, and so on, until the wound edges are aligned and closed.
2. Wounds where the edges cannot be brought together without excessive tension should have dermal sutures placed to close the gap partially and reduce the force on the epidermal closure.
3. Adipose tissue beneath the skin should not be sutured; obliteration of this potential dead space between the cut edge of adipose tissue by even the least reactive suture increases the incidence of infection.
4. When wounds of different thickness are to be reunited, the needle should be passed through one side of the wound and then drawn out before reentry through the other side. This maneuver ensures that the needle is inserted at comparable levels on each side of the wound. Unless appropriate adjustment of the bite is made on the thinner side, uneven coaptation of the skin will occur, resulting in a step-off scar.

Dermal sutures can be used alone or as adjuncts to percutaneous sutures in wounds subjected to strong skin tensions, to serve as an added precaution against disruption of the wound. Some physicians prefer a synthetic absorbable suture for dermal closure, while others favor a synthetic nonabsorbable suture. The nonabsorbable suture is applied in a continuous manner with the ends brought out the skin and secured at both ends of the wound. This suture can then be removed before the eighth day after wound closure to prevent the development of needle puncture scars. When dermal closure alone is used, it is advisable to close the skin with surgical tapes or tissue adhesive for more accurate approximation of the epidermis.

In clean wounds (e.g., elective surgical incisions), subcutaneous sutures do not significantly increase the incidence of wound infection. However, in traumatic wounds, particularly with contamination, dermal sutures potentate wound infection.[16] Once an infection develops, the collecting purulent exudate spreads preferentially between the divided edges of fat rather than penetrating the closed dermis. By the time the infection becomes clinically apparent, it has usually involved the entire extent of the wound. One value of dermal closure is thought to be that by reducing tension across the wound, scar width will be lessened. However, despite the immediate, esthetically pleasing appearance of dermal skin closure, it does not improve the ultimate cosmetic appearance of the healing wound; scar width after dermal skin closure is comparable to the scar width of wounds healing in the absence of dermal sutures. Another effective method of reducing tension during closure is to undermine the skin edges. However, this benefit must be weighed against the potential damage to the skin blood supply, which may compromise the host's defenses and invite infection. Consequently, undermining of the wound edges of lacerations should be done in carefully selected situations in the ED.

Suturing Instruments

The surgical needle holder used in suturing lacerations should have several features.[5] First, it should hold the needle securely to direct it through the tissue. Second, it should release the needle easily to allow the suture to be tied. And third, it should have a design that can readily grasp the suture end to be used for the instrument tie.

The appropriate needle holder should hold the needle firmly without crushing it. The jaws of the needle holder may be flat or scored ("teeth"). Teeth may limit twisting and rotation of the needle, allowing it to be directed through tissue more accurately. However, teeth may damage needles and monofilament synthetic sutures, reducing their breaking strength. Smooth-face needle-holder jaws with rounded edges do not cause structural damage to either monofilament suture or needles. However, their smooth jaw surfaces provide limited resistance to twisting or rotation of the needle. Needle-holder jaw faces can be textured with tungsten carbide particles to create a fine granular surface, making them an attractive alternative to either smooth jaws or those with teeth. The textured face provides more needle-holding security than smooth jaws but significantly less than jaws with teeth. The needle-holder jaw should grasp only the needle body; clamping the needle point damages the cutting edge and dulls the needle. The suture needle should be aligned perpendicularly to the long axis of the needle holder and grasped between the jaws about 2 mm from the their tips. As noted above, the needle should be grasped 1.5 mm beyond the depth of the channel or swage hole, a site that provides optimal resistance to bending.

The finger holes of the needle holder are used for directing the needle and latching and unlatching the jaws. The needle holder can be grasped by either the thenar grip or the thumb-ring finger grip; each has its advantages. Both grips, however, do not place the index or middle finger through the ringlet holes; instead, the index finger is placed along the side of the needle-holder arms and the middle finger is pressed against the outside curve of the bottom ringlet for more control as the suture is placed. When placing a suture, the hypothenar side of the hand holding the needle holder can be placed against the patient's skin in order to brace the hand against sudden movement. This is particularly useful when placing a suture in a child or a moving patient.

With the thenar grip, the thenar eminence and skin overlying the first metacarpophalangeal joint are pressed against one ringlet, while the long, ring, and small fingers encircle the other ringlet. This position aligns the needle holder in the same direction as the longitudinal axis of the wrist and forearm, allowing the hand and needle holder to be positioned comfortably into recessed cavities (e.g., the oral cavity). In addition, the needle can be released and regrasped by the needle holder without changing positions. The needle can be redirected in preparation for the next stitch by spinning the needle holder clockwise in the palm. The disadvantage of this grip is the lack of precision when releasing the needle; when the thenar eminence applies pressure to the ringlet, it disengages the ratchet mechanism uncontrollably, causing inadvertent movement of the needle.

In the thumb-ring finger grip, the tip of the thumb is positioned in one ringlet, while the tip of the ring finger is placed in the other ringlet. The greatest advantage of this grip is its controlled disengagement of the ratchet mechanism, permitting precise manipulation of the needle. This advantage must be weighed against the relatively larger size of the physician's hand and needle holder; the palm is separated from the needle holder, making it more difficult to position the needle holder in recessed cavities (e.g., the mouth).

To align skin edges, a skin hook is preferred over forceps with teeth; hooks do not crush tissue, as do forceps. When forceps are used, they should pick up and elevate the skin as opposed to grasping the epidermis between the teeth. Conversely, the dermis can be grasped with the forceps, again, avoiding grasping the epidermis.

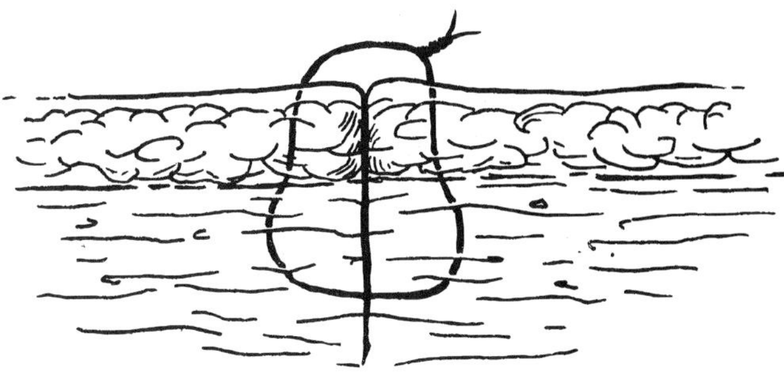

FIG. 37-12. A single interrupted percutaneous suture with everted edges.

Because the ratchet mechanism of most needle holders is designed for right-handed individuals, most physicians prefer to hold the needle holder with the right hand, allowing them to hold skin hook or tissue forceps with the left hand. Before passing the needle through tissue, lay the free end of the suture away from the wound. The curved suture needle is passed through the tissue by starting with the hand prone and then twisting the wrist to a supine alignment, driving the needle through in one motion. For small lacerations being closed with only percutaneous sutures, this one motion can drive the needle from one side, across the wound, and out the other side without the need to release the needle. For larger lacerations, those with gaps, or those where approximating the layers is important, the needle is released after the point comes out in the wound, regrasped, and repositioned for placement through the other side.

Percutaneous sutures should be placed to achieve eversion of the edges. To accomplish this, the needle should enter the skin at a 90° angle. The curving motion of the needle and wrist movement then drives the needle first downward and then across the wound. The needle point should also exit the opposite side at 90°. It is desirable for the depth of the suture to be wider than the width (from entry to exit). Sutures placed in this manner (similar to the shape of an Erlenmeyer flask) will encompass a portion of tissue that will evert when the knot is tied (Fig. 37-12). Percutaneous sutures should also match opposing layers; the exit at one side of the wound should be at the same level as the entrance on the opposite side.

An adequate number of sutures should be placed so that the wound edges are closed without gaping. The general rule that the space between individual sutures should be roughly equal to the length of each bite (distance from needle entry point to the wound edge) can really be used only in straight wounds with sharp edges (e.g., surgical incisions). Experience and practice are the most useful guides to placement and spacing of percutaneous sutures in traumatic wounds.

Bleeding should be controlled before wound closure. Most bleeding stops after gentle compression with gauze sponges applied to the wound surface, using aseptic technique. Persistent bleeding should be controlled as noted in Chap. 36.

Knot Construction

Sutures are secured by tying the free ends into a series of square knots, often beginning with the surgeon's knot, where the initial double throw offers better knot security with less slipping of the suture material as the wound is pulled together during tying. The initial double throw is followed by subsequent single throws to create the series of square knots. The square knot is used because it is the strongest knot that can be tied while still keeping the knot small. Knot tying can be accomplished by either instrument or hand tying technique. The instru-

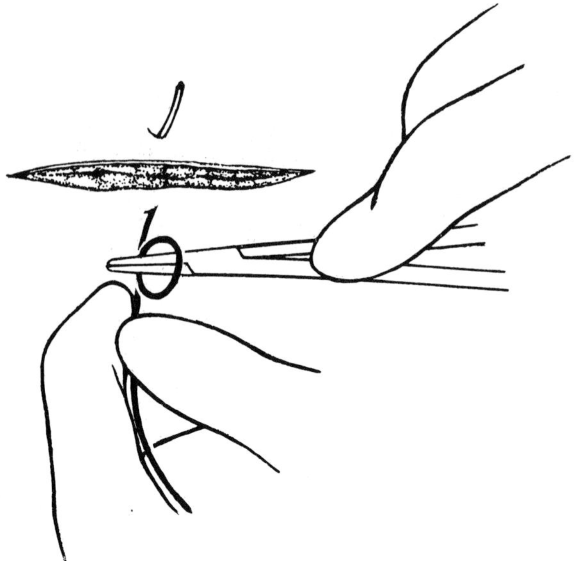

FIG. 37-13. Formation of the first suture loop. The fixed suture end held by the left hand is wrapped counter-clockwise over and around the needle holder jaws to form the first suture loop. (If the suture is wrapped twice around the needle holder jaws, the first, double-wrap throw of the surgeon's knot square will be formed. A double-wrap, first throw displays a greater resistance to slippage than a single-wrap throw, accounting for its frequent use in instrument ties in wounds subjected to strong, static skin tensions.)

ment tie is useful for both deep and superficial closures. Because the needle holder does not have to be moved on and off the hand, the instrument tie is also faster than hand tying for placing a series of percutaneous sutures during wound closure.

Formation of each throw is accomplished in three steps. The first step is the formation of a suture loop. In the second step, the free suture end is passed through the suture loop to create a throw. The final step is to advance the throw to the wound surface as tension is applied to the suture ends in opposite directions. The initial throw should approximate the wound edges as it is advanced down to the wound surface. Once this throw contacts the wound, the physician will have a preview of the ultimate apposition of the wound edges. Additional throws are placed in succession, reversing the direction of the suture ends as tension is applied. The knot should be constructed by carefully snuggling each throw tightly against the preceding one. The rate of applying tension to each throw should be relatively slow. Ideally, the knotted suture should reapproximate the wound edges without strangulating the tissue encircled by the suture loop.

With the instrument tie, knots can be tied rapidly in the following steps:

1. The suture is placed through the tissue leaving a short free end, usually 2 cm.
2. The initial throw is started by looping the portion of suture attached to the needle around the instrument in a counterclockwise manner.
3. A complete loop is then formed around the tip of the needle holder with the long end directed away from the wound (Fig. 37-13).
4. The needle holder then grasps the free end of the suture and pulls it through the suture loop while the left hand slides the loop off the needle holder down and around the free end of the suture.
5. Tension is applied to both the fixed and free ends in opposite directions to form half of the square knot.
6. The second throw is created by passing the suture around the needle holder tip in a clockwise direction, opposite that of the first throw.
7. The loop created again has the long end directed away from the wound.
8. The free end is grasped and pulled through the suture loop.
9. The suture loop is slipped off the needle holder to form the second half of the square knot, this time with tension applied in a direction opposite the first throw.
10. Additional square knots are placed down over the first knot. For monofilament and multifilament nylon sutures of 2-0 to 4-0 size, two square knots (four throws) placed snugly against each other are adequate for knot security. Finer sutures, 5-0 and 6-0, should have three square knots (six throws).

The direction of the suture loops will determine the type of knot created. When successive throws are in opposite directions, a square-type is created. In contrast, a granny-type knot will result when the suture loops are in the same direction for two successive throws.

The major disadvantage of an instrument tie is that it is difficult to apply continuous tension to the suture ends and maintain wound edge coaptation during the process of tying. Consequently, widening of the suture loop and separation of wound edges due to slippage is frequently encountered in wounds subjected to strong tensions. Instrument ties are ideally suited for closing a wound that is subjected to weak tensions. Instrument ties can be accomplished more rapidly and accurately than hand ties while conserving considerably more suture; the parsimonious physician can complete 10 interrupted suture loops from one length of suture measuring 18 in. (46 cm), a feat that would be impossible if the knots were tied by hand. Instrument ties are invaluable in special situations where hand ties are impractical or impossible, such as body recesses or cavities (e.g., the mouth); there, instruments can form knots where hands could never gain access.

Failure of the knotted suture loop may be the result of either knot slippage or breakage, suture cutting through tissue, or mechanical crushing of the suture by surgical instruments. All knots slip to some degree, regardless of the type of suture material, and the cut ends of the knot must provide the additional material to compensate. If the amount of knot slippage exceeds the length of the cut ends, the throws of the knot become untied. In general, leaving the free ends approximately 3 mm in length will accommodate most knot slippage. To facilitate removal in some locations (e.g., scalp or eyebrow), it may be useful to leave longer suture ends so that they can be easily located and grasped with forceps. Dermal sutures are, however, an exception to this rule. Because the ends of dermal suture knots may protrude through the wound, it is best to cut the dermal suture ends close to the knot. It must be emphasized that knot security is enhanced by additional throws and not by longer ends.

Suture Patterns

Simple interrupted sutures represent the most versatile suture technique and are good for realigning irregular wound edges and stellate lacerations with more meticulous approximation of the wound edges (Fig. 37-14). An advantage of interrupted sutures is that only the involved sutures need to be removed in the case of wound infections. Wound integrity is greater and the risk of premature separation (dehiscence) is less because the wound is held together with multiple individual suture loops.

Continuous running sutures are quick, easy, and may save time in the ED because only two knots need to be tied at each end of the laceration as opposed to individual knots for each interrupted suture loop (Fig. 37-15). Continuous sutures are best when repairing linear wounds. However, a break in suture may ruin the entire repair and may cause permanent marks if placed too tightly. This type of suture is often used where hemostasis is important, such as the vagina and scalp, where locking the running suture aids in hemostasis (Fig. 37-16). Another advantage of the continuous suture is that it accommodates to the developing edema of the wound edges during healing. In contrast,

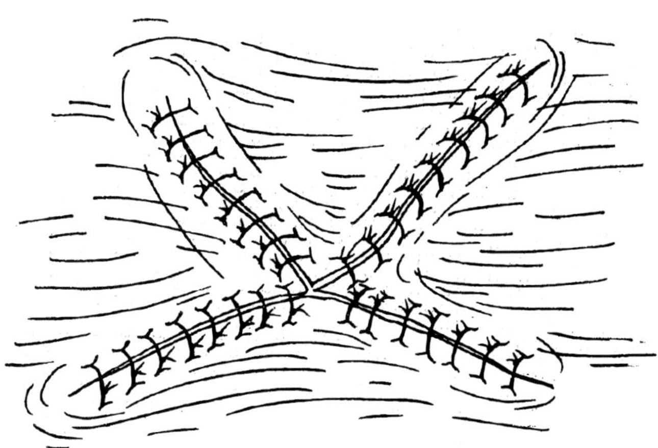

FIG. 37-14. Stellate laceration closed with interrupted sutures.

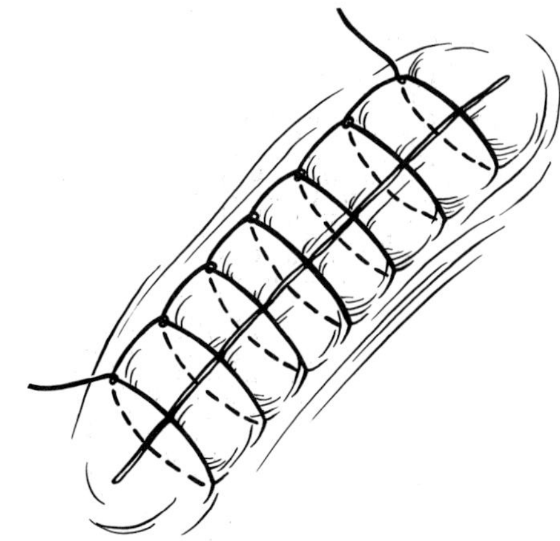

FIG. 37-16. Running locked suture.

the dimensions of the interrupted suture remain unchanged, constricting the edematous tissue within each suture loop. For either interrupted or continuous percutaneous suture closure, a monofilament synthetic nonabsorbable suture is used.

Continuous suture closure of a laceration can be accomplished by two different patterns. In the first pattern, the needle pathway is at a 90° angle to the wound edges and results in a visible suture that crosses the wound edges at a 45° angle (Fig. 37-17*A*). In the other pattern, the needle pathway is at a 45° angle to the wound edges, so that the visible suture is at a 90° angle to the wound edges (Fig. 37-17*B*). In either case, the physician starts the continuous suture closure at the corner of the wound that is farthest away, and suturing progresses toward the physician, rather than away.

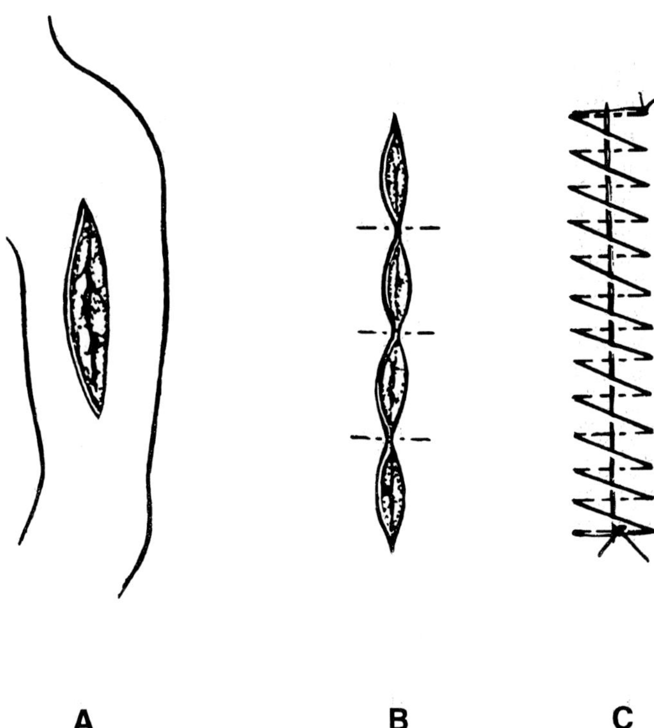

FIG. 37-15. **A.** Linear laceration of the arm subjected to strong skin tensions, with marked retraction of wound edges. **B.** Three interrupted dermal sutures markedly reduce the retraction of the skin edges. **C.** Continuous percutaneous suture.

Dermal (subcuticular) sutures, either interrupted or continuous, may be necessary prior to skin closure to reduce tension and gaping. Interrupted dermal sutures are started by entering the skin near the base and exiting just beneath the dermal-epidermal junction. Entry into and exit from the opposite side is at corresponding levels. Tying the ends with an instrument tie ''buries'' the knot in the wound depth; starting the suture at the dermal-epidermal junction would leave the knot close to surface (Fig. 37-18). The compound curved needle is ideal for this type of suture because the suture loop is smaller than that achieved with a simple curved needle.

Continuous dermal (or subcuticular) sutures are useful in wounds subjected to strong skin tensions, patients prone to keloid formation, children frightened by suture removal, and those individuals who are unable to contact a health professional for suture removal. Absorbable synthetic braided or monofilament sutures (4-0 and 5-0 size) are ideally suited for continuous dermal sutures because they do not have to be removed. In contrast, nonabsorbable continuous dermal sutures have to exit percutaneously from the ends of the wound as well as surfacing every 3 cm through the skin, to facilitate removal. Continuous dermal sutures are begun as an interrupted dermal suture with its knot buried in the subcutaneous tissue (Fig. 37-19). After the physician cuts the

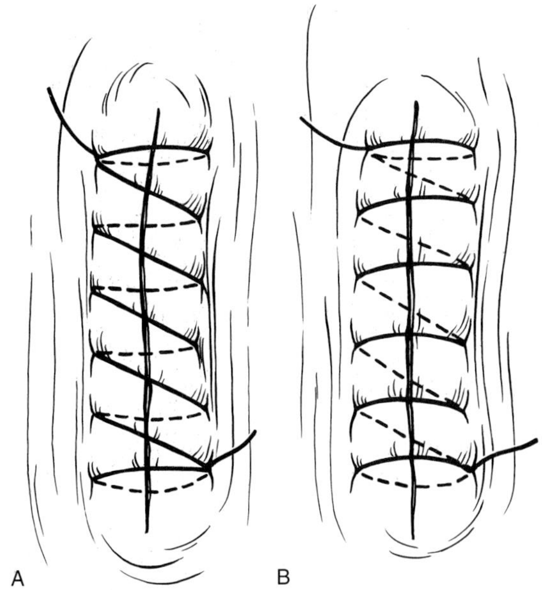

FIG. 37-17. **A.** Running suture crossing wound at 45°. **B.** Running suture crossing wound at 90°.

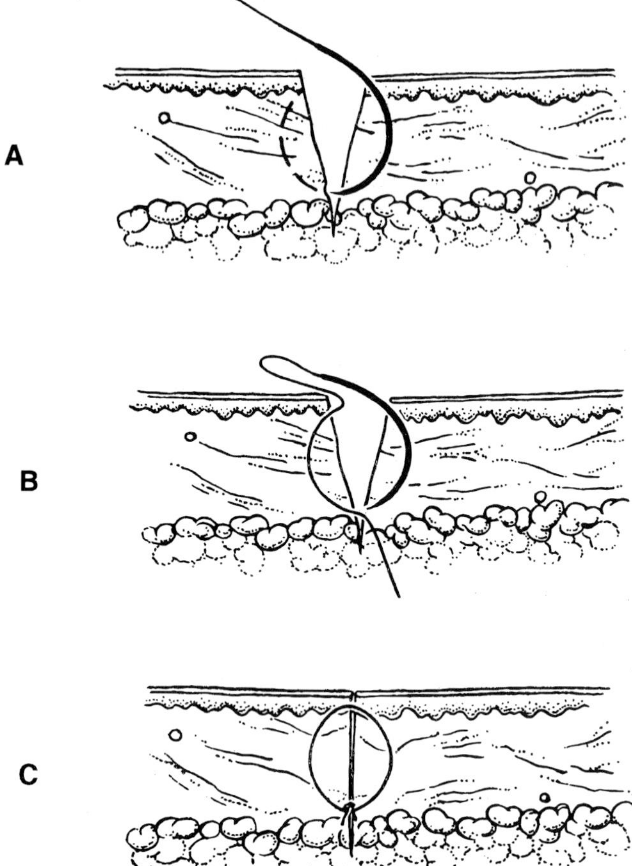

FIG. 37-18. Dermal suture. **A.** Entry is at base of wound on one side and exit at the dermal-epidermal junction. **B.** Entry on the opposite side is at the dermal-epidermal junction with exit at the base. **C.** The tied loop has the knot buried in the wound away from the skin surface.

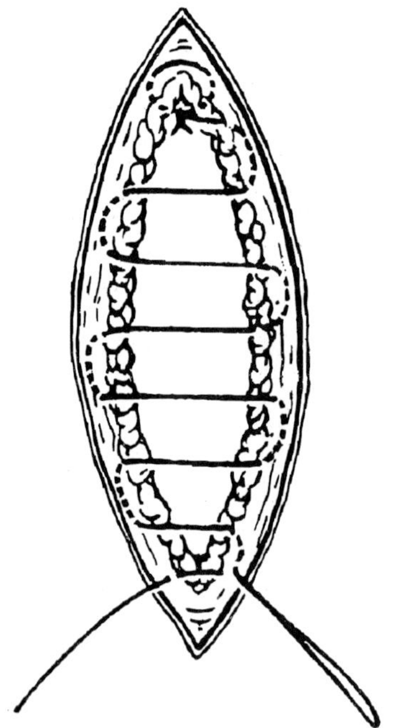

FIG. 37-19. Continuous subcuticular suture.

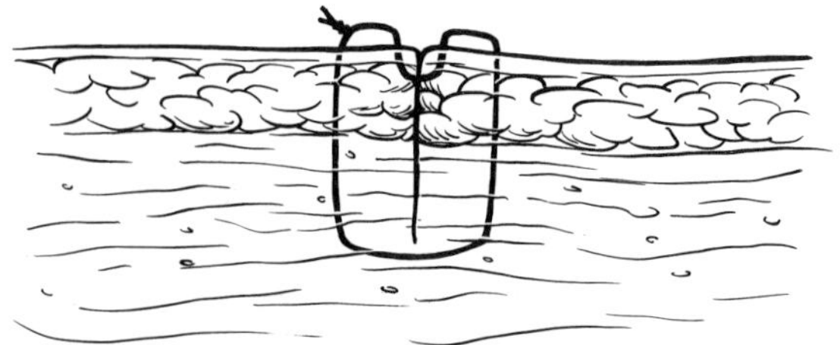

FIG. 37-20. Vertical mattress suture.

free end close to the knot, the suture attached to the needle is used for the continuous closure. The next stitch is passed horizontally along the length of the wound through the superficial dermis (Fig. 37-19). After the dermis is exited, the position of the next bite is identified by pulling the suture across at right angles to the wound. Accurate positioning is assured by slight backtracking of each bite. During passage of the needle, the skin is stabilized by one arm of the toothed forceps. As the horizontal bites are taken, gentle constant traction on the fixed suture brings the wound edges together. At a point one bite from the end of the wound, a smaller horizontal bite is passed toward the end of the wound. The suture from this corner stitch is withheld, forming a loop that will be used in constructing the knot. After passing the suture horizontally through a small bite of dermis in the opposite wound edge, the fixed suture end and the long loop of the free suture are used to construct the terminal square knots. The skin edges can be approximated with either percutaneous sutures, skin staples, skin-closure tapes, or tissue adhesives.

Continuous dermal sutures can be used by themselves when percutaneous sutures might cause cosmetic problems. They are ideal for linear facial lacerations, where sutures placed completely below the surface of the skin minimize scaring. One disadvantage is that complete suture removal may be required if local infection demands wound reopening. Wound integrity is dependent on only one piece of suture as opposed to multiple loops if interrupted sutures were used. For the best cosmetic results, a compound-curved, reverse cutting-edge precision-point needle is recommended.

Vertical mattress sutures allow for precise edge to edge alignment and are especially good to match thick to thin skin (Fig. 37-20). This suture enhances skin edge eversion and avoids the tendency for inversion common with deep nonlinear lacerations. When placing the sutures, care must be taken not to make them too tight, which might strangulate the tissues. The resulting scar may be inferior to that from some of the other suturing techniques; therefore this approach should be used for areas that are not cosmetically important. For conventional vertical mattress sutures, the first bite is a large one starting approximately 1 to 1.5 cm away from the wound edge and crossing through the wound to an equal distance on the opposite side. The needle is then reversed and a very small, shallow bite (1 to 2 mm) at the epidermal/dermal edge is placed in order to closely approximate the epidermal layer. The ends are tied with the knot falling on one side of the wound. The vertical mattress suture is useful in areas of lax skin (elbow, dorsum of hand), where the wound edges tend to fall or fold into the wound and eversion of the skin is harder to obtain. The vertical mattress suture can also act as a deep as well as superficial suture—an "all in one" suture; avoiding the need for a layered closure. The modified vertical mattress suture places the small bite first and then uses elevation on the suture ends to raise the wound edges, to make placing the larger and deeper second bite easier. This modification allows faster placement of individual stitches.[17]

Horizontal mattress sutures are faster and better at eversion than vertical mattress (Fig. 37-21). The repair may look poor early on, but with good eversion, the scar will have a better cosmetic effect in 2 to 3 months. This suturing technique may be faster because it covers more linear distance. It is especially useful in areas of increased tension

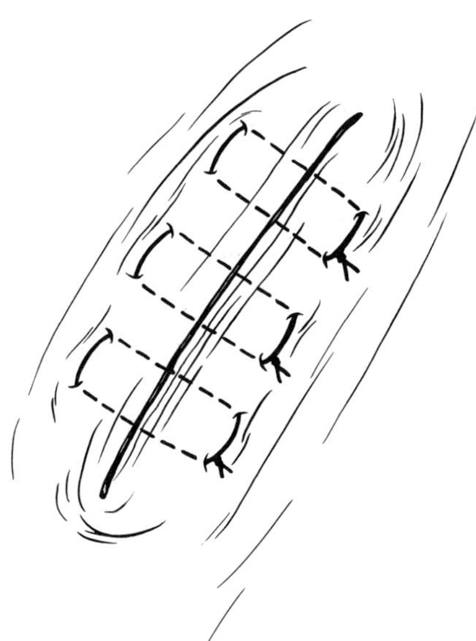

FIG. 37-21. Horizontal mattress suture.

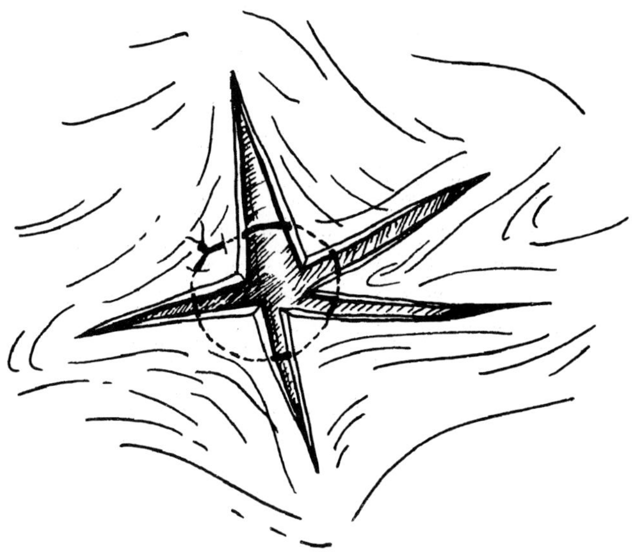

FIG. 37-23. Purse-string suture.

such as fascia, joints, and callused skin. Individual sutures must be tied loosely to avoid tissue strangulation. The first throw is similar to a simple interrupted suture but instead of tying the suture a second bite is taken approximately 5 mm adjacent to the first exit on the same side and directed back to the initial side. This second bite exits approximately 5 mm from the initial entry point. The knot is tied leaving an everted edge.

Horizontal half buried sutures are good for repairing flaps and triangular wounds (Fig. 37-22). It minimizes tissue tension so it doesn't strangulate the interposed tissue. Similar to vertical mattress sutures, horizontal half buried sutures are also useful to approximate thick to thin edges. To accomplish this, it is important to bury the suture in the thicker edge and tie the suture on the thinner side to allow eversion and reapproximation of the skin edges.

Purse-string suture is very useful at reapproximating multiple flap tips and corner wounds back together (Fig. 37-23). This technique is used in these areas in order to preserve the blood supply and minimize tissue destruction at the tips of the skin edges.

The dog-ear maneuver is a technique used to handle excess tissue at one end of the wound (Fig. 37-24). Basically the wound is extended from the apex toward the long side in the form of a hockey stick. Then the triangular piece of excess skin is removed and the skin edges are sewn together. Undermining may be necessary to help remove the excess tissue and suture the edges closed.

PROBLEM WOUNDS

Several factors should be considered in choosing the best approach for wound closure. For example, deep wounds produce potential spaces, which, when the overlying skin is closed, can be susceptible to infection. Closure of deep space is controversial, as absorbable sutures placed to close this potential space increase the risk of infection due to the presence of the suture foreign body. Parallel lacerations may have compromised perfusion to the ''island'' of skin between the lacerations that could be further impaired by percutaneous sutures. To minimize damage to subcutaneous blood vessels and reduce skin tension on the intervening strips of skin, horizontal mattress sutures or

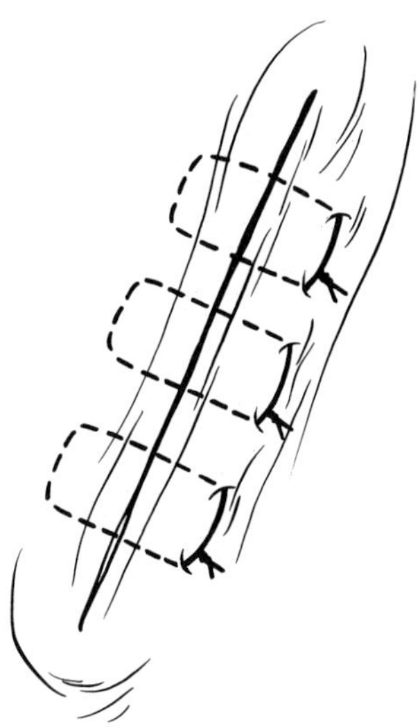

FIG. 37-22. Horizontal half-buried suture.

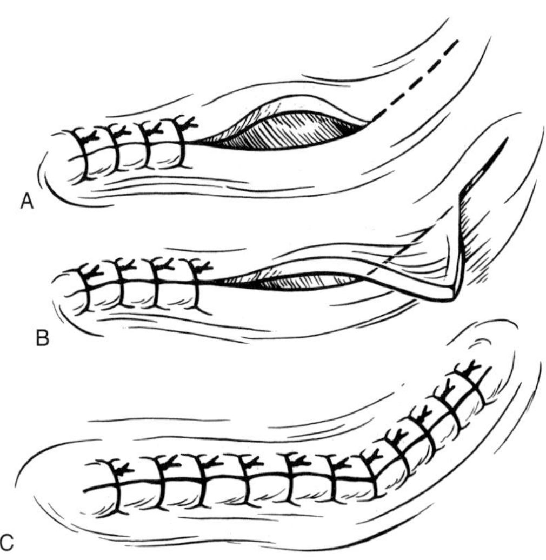

FIG. 37-24. Dog-ear maneuver. **A.** Incision is carried off one end of the wound at 45° toward the side with excess tissue. **B.** The excess tissue is pulled over the incision and cut away. **C.** The sutured laceration now has a ''hockey stick'' angulation.

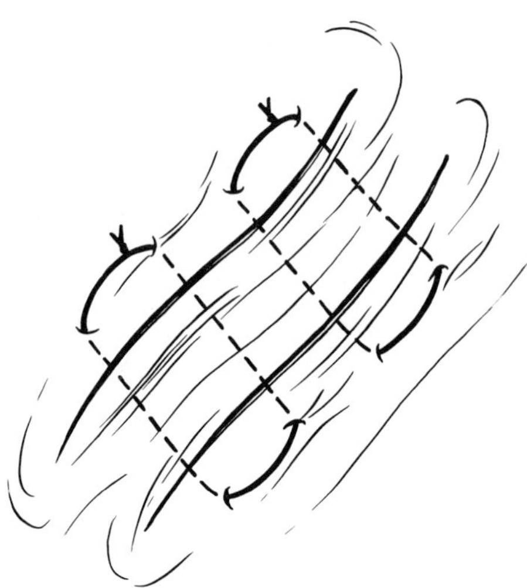

FIG. 37-25. Parallel lacerations can be closed with horizontal mattress sutures.

closure with skin-closure tapes or tissue adhesives alone should be considered (Fig. 37-25).

Elderly Skin

With aging, there is a decrease in the cellular growth rate and a degeneration of collagen and elastic fibers, resulting in a loss of both dermal and subcutaneous tissues and a thinning of the epidermis. Consequently, the skin loses its elasticity and appears transparent, wrinkled, thin, dry, fragile, and lacking in tensile strength. Normally, the epidermis attaches firmly to the dermis by projecting extensions of epidermis into the dermis in a tongue-in-groove fashion (rete pegs). With aging, this dermal-epidermal junction flattens owing to loss of capillaries, collagen fibers, and glycoproteins. There is also an increase in the fragility of the capillaries in the basement membrane zone, making the skin prone to subcutaneous hemorrhage or senile purpura. Because of all of these changes, aging skin tears with minor friction or shearing forces. These tears become an invitation to bacterial invasion and subsequent infection.

In the elderly, skin tears usually present as epidermal flaps. If the flap remains attached to its pedicle, it should be replaced on the dermis and approximated to adjacent tissue by skin-closure tapes or tissue adhesives (not sutures or skin staples). When the epidermal flap becomes separated from the skin, healing of the wound will be considerably delayed. With complete loss of the epidermal flap and exposure of 500 mm^2 or more of the dermis, coverage with a split-thickness skin graft may be necessary.

U-Shaped Flaps and Jagged Lacerations

A U-shaped skin flap is often caused by compressive forces on skin overlying bone. The flap usually has abraded skin and extends deep with attached subcutaneous tissues. The edges of the flap are usually irregular and fit together with adjacent wound edges, like a jigsaw puzzle. The survival of a rectangular-shaped flap is dependent on the blood supply from vessels that enter the flap at its base. Survival of a flap is more dependent on its length and not the width of the base; wide and narrow-based flaps survive equally if they are of the same length. Other factors that favor survival include the following: (1) the presence of direct cutaneous arteries or veins coursing the longitudinal axis of the flap (axial-pattern flap); (2) location of the flap in the head or neck, where the vascularity is excellent; (3) younger patients and those without diabetes mellitus or arteriosclerosis; (4) location above the knee and not in areas of scar or previous exposure to radiation, which, especially in the elderly, have diminished vascularity; and (5) absence of excessive tension, kinking, pressure, hematoma, or infection, which may interfere with circulation.

The most reliable way to determine tissue viability in a flap is reexamination 24 h after injury, at which time the viability is well demarcated and can be clearly ascertained. For fresh skin wounds, active bleeding from the distal and dermal margins indicates viability. U-, C-, or V-shaped flaps usually heal with a trapdoor or pincushion effect that results in an elevated bulging of the tissues. Various theories to explain this phenomenon are lymphatic and venous obstruction, hypertrophy of the scar, excessive fatty and redundant tissues, beveled wound edges, and contracture of the scar. Because the traumatic wound is susceptible to the development of infection, it is best to reapproximate the edges of a vascularized flap with the least reactive synthetic monofilament suture using interrupted percutaneous sutures. Approximation of the irregular wound edges is like putting together a jigsaw puzzle (Fig. 37-26). The wound edges of these lacerations often have

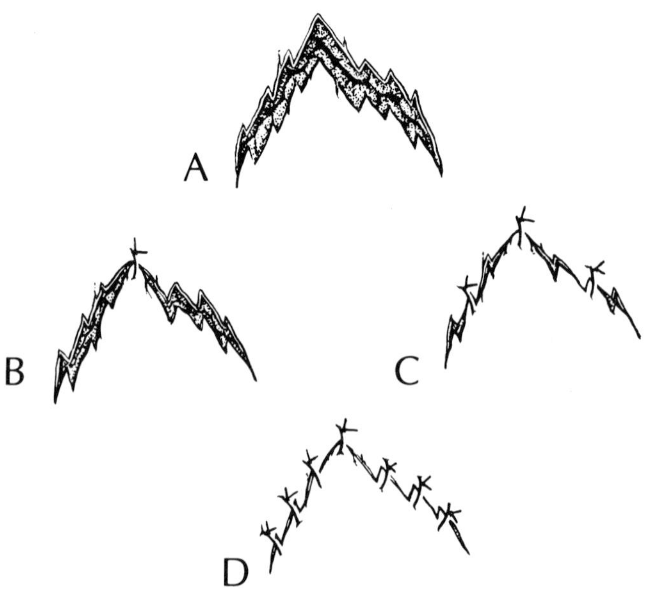

FIG. 37-26. **A.** V-shaped laceration with irregular wound edges. **B.** An interrupted percutaneous suture approximates the midportion of the wound. **C.** Two additional percutaneous sutures are used to approximate the lateral sides of the wound. **D.** Additional percutaneous sutures are positioned between the previously placed percutaneous sutures. **E.** The interrupted percutaneous sutures allow the wound to be reconstructed like a jigsaw puzzle.

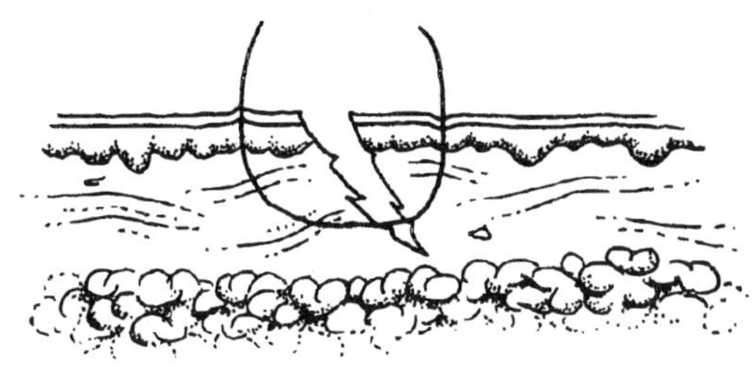

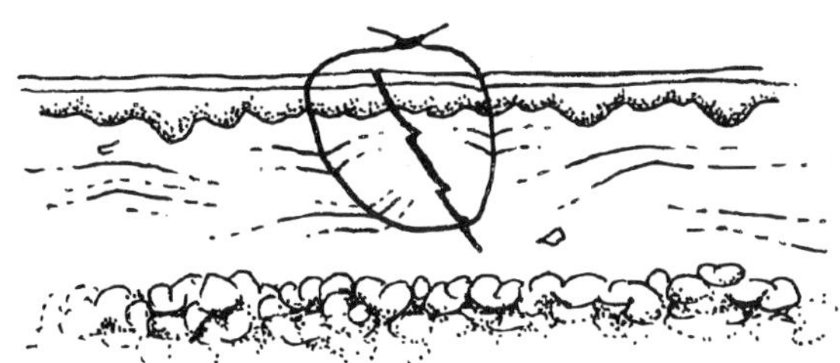

FIG. 37-27. Closure of beveled edges requires careful approximation of the wound edges. This is facilitated by removing the needle from the needle holder after passage through one side, regrasping the needle, and passing it through the opposite side.

a beveled edge rather than a perpendicular configuration (Fig. 37-27). It can be argued that this beveled edge may have a favorable influence on healing by providing a large interface between the divided edges, thereby enhancing repair. Consequently, repair of the beveled edges is advocated rather than revising the edges to create perpendicular edges. Suturing beveled edges may be time-consuming because the needle must be passed separately through one edge before it is passed through the other to ensure that the suture passes through the same depth on each side of the wound to align equivalent layers. This time-consuming maneuver is worthwhile because it prevents malapposition of the wound edges and an unattractive scar deformity.

When a portion of the flap is devascularized, this segment should be excised. The excised flap should then be defatted, converting the flap into a skin graft that is applied to the defect and secured by a tie-over bolus dressing. After the skin graft heals without infection, the patient should be referred to a plastic surgeon for follow-up evaluation. Six months after wound closure, the plastic surgeon can correct the trapdoor deformity by performing Z- and W-plasties accompanied by peripheral undermining of the wound. For small trapdoor deformities, simple excision of the deformity resulting in a lenticular defect that can be primarily closed is an excellent alternative.

Corners

Irregular lacerations often have corners or sharp angles; from a simple corner to V-shaped, Y-shaped, or stellate lacerations. Corners have less blood supply than edges, and closure should be done carefully to prevent further impairment of perfusion and minimize tension. The horizontal half buried suture is designed to accomplish both purposes (Fig. 37-22).

Lacerations Subjected to Strong Skin Tensions

Lacerations subjected to strong skin tensions are prone to wound dehiscence and healing with wide, hypertrophic scars. These lacerations can be identified by retraction of their wound edges more than 5 mm and the alignment of the long axis of the wound with the wrinkle lines or transverse axis of the joint. Undermining the wound edges is one method to reduce tension, but this technique can diminish the blood supply to the wound, thereby damaging wound defenses and inviting the development of infection. Attempting to reduce tension by closure of adipose tissue is to be avoided because it enhances infection without strengthening the wound.

Dermal skin closure is recommended in these wounds to maintain their strength and prevent the development of wound dehiscence after removal of the skin sutures or the exfoliation of skin-closure tapes or tissue adhesives. Because dermal sutures allow early removal of the percutaneous suture, needle puncture scars and tracts do not develop, but there is no reduction in scar width. Dermal repair should be accomplished with the least number of interrupted sutures and with buried knots using braided synthetic absorbable sutures. The suture ends are cut flush with the knot. Interrupted percutaneous synthetic monofilament sutures positioned between the dermal sutures are then used to close the skin edges (Fig. 37-28). Alternatively, if the skin edges are close together after dermal suturing, the epidermis can be closed with skin-closure tapes or tissue adhesives.

Wound undermining reduces wound tension by releasing the dermis and superficial fascia from their deeper attachments, allowing the wound edges to be brought together with less force. Undermining is

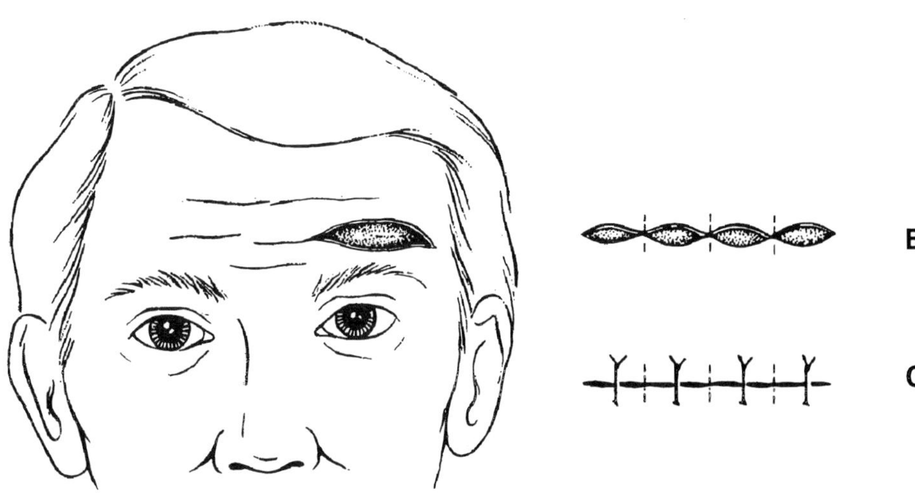

FIG. 37-28. A. Linear laceration of left forehead subjected to strong static skin tensions. **B.** Three interrupted dermal skin sutures bring the retracted wound edges together. **C.** Four interrupted percutaneous sutures positioned between the dermal sutures provide meticulous approximation of the wound edges.

potentially useful in the scalp, forehead, and lower legs, particularly in the tibia area, where the skin is under a great deal of natural tension. Caution must be taken because this procedure can spread bacteria into deeper tissues as well as creating a deeper and larger dead space. Undermining is performed by using scissors placed underneath the dermis and gently spreading them to bluntly dissect in a parallel fashion, releasing the dermis from deeper attachments. Cutting is kept to a minimum to minimize bleeding.

Crushed Tissue

As a general rule, crushed tissue should be excised. Crushed tissue leads to additional edema, fibroplasia, and more scarring. The extent of crushed tissue may not be easily visible. One way to demonstrate the extent of crushed tissue is to use hydrogen peroxide, which will produce a white patch wherever the wound edges were crushed. However, full excision of all crushed tissue may create more problems in the long run, particularly if excision will leave defects that cannot be covered with available skin. During the repair of traumatic lacerations in the ED, excision should be limited and completely avoided on the nose, vermilion-cutaneous junction, or eyelid. Wounds in these areas should be closed while preserving as much tissue as possible. The most important principle in repairing crushed tissue is to do most of the work at the subcutaneous level and use very few percutaneous sutures. Another principle is to position the pieces so that they heal in proper relation to each other so that scar revision, if necessary, will be easier. With all crush injuries, the patient should be warned about the possibility of a residual scar but also informed that plastic surgery revision is an option.

TIPS FOR A PLASTIC CLOSURE

There are several general principles to cosmetic closure. All wounds heal with some scarring, the goal is to use techniques that make the scar as small and invisible as possible. Scars become visible when they cast a shadow, have a rough surface, are wide, or develop permanent secondary color change.

Scars most often cast a shadow when they become concave from wound contraction during healing. Wound-edge eversion during the initial repair will therefore gradually flatten with healing and have a final appearance that is cosmetically acceptable. Wounds that are not everted will contract into linear depressions that will become noticeable cosmetic defects because of the tendency to cast shadows under incident light.

In closing a laceration, it is important to match each layer of a wound edge to its counterpart. The epithelium-to-epithelium interface should match perfectly to create a hairline smooth scar. Care must be taken to avoid having one wound edge rolled inward, so that the cut edge of the epithelium on one side is opposed against the dermis on the other side. The skin edges may look matched up but actually are not. The rolled-in edge occludes the capillaries, promoting wound infection. The dermal side will not heal to the rolled epidermal side, causing wound dehiscence when the sutures are removed. Everting the edges helps prevent skin rolling. Likewise, overeverting the edges causes problems; the exposed dermal surfaces promote granulation tissue and a rough scar.

The relationship between the wound tension and the distance between sutures is also important for a cosmetic repair. The more tension on the wound, the closer the sutures need to be to each other to minimize the tension on the wound edge. Further spaced sutures have more tension that is distributed to each loop leading to cut-over marks, stitch marks, and stitch holes. Another technique to reduce tension on the wound is to close the wound in layers. However, deep stitches can cause an inflammatory response, leading to increased scarring as well as an increased risk of infection. Sutures placed through the epidermis can cause stitch-mark scars. Therefore, the minimum number of sutures necessary to accomplish closure should be placed just far enough from each other that no gap appears between the wound edges. The knots should be placed away from the wound edges to prevent an inflammatory response.

To prevent the development of needle-puncture scars, percutaneous sutures must be removed as soon as possible and the wound edges reinforced with skin-closure tape to prevent wound dehiscence.

Topical agents (antibiotics, vitamin E, and aloe vera) have been found to reduce the incidence of wound infection, accelerate healing, and increase wound tensile strength after suturing. Dressings are usually necessary for only the first 12 to 24 h, after which gentle periodic cleaning with mild soap and water can commence. The area should be gently patted dry and re-dressed with a sterile dressing. Wounds closed with skin-closure tapes or tissue adhesives should not be covered with a dressing or washed. Pressure dressings are useful in minimizing intercellular fluid collection and limiting the dead space, both useful in achieving cosmetic closure. Abraded wound areas may develop an exudate that dries on the surface, forming a scab during the first 24 h. This dry scab resists epidermal cell migration and interferes with wound healing. If abraded areas are covered with a dressing to maintain moisture during the first 24 h, epidermal cell migration is encouraged and healing promoted. If sutures are placed in and around abraded areas, small amounts of water-soluble ointment may be beneficial in preventing scab formation. Gently cleaning the wound with half-strength hydrogen peroxide every 6 h until the wound edge is free of blood prevents scarring due to clot formation around the wound edge.

Exposure of abraded skin and healed lacerations to sunlight during the first 6 months after injury may cause permanent hyperpigmentation. Hyperpigmentation can be prevented by protecting the injured skin area from sunlight with a sun-blocking agent with sun protection factor of 15 to 30 for 6 to 12 months.

REFERENCES

1. Berk WA, Osbourne DD, Taylor DD: Evaluation of the ''golden period'' for wound repair: 204 cases from a third world emergency department. *Ann Emerg Med* 17:496, 1988.
2. Smilanich RP, Bonnet I, Kirkpatrick JR: Contaminated wounds: The effect of initial management on outcome. *Am Surg* 61:427, 1995.
3. Zimmer CA, Thacker JG, Powell DM, et al: Influence of knot configuration and tying technique on the mechanical performance of suture. *J Emerg Med* 9:107, 1991.
4. Batra EK, Franz DA, Towler MA, et al: Influence of emergency physician's tying technique on knot security. *J Emerg Med* 10:309, 1992.
5. Edlich RF, Thacker JG, McGregor W, et al: Past, present, and future for surgical needles and needle holders. *Am J Surg* 166:522, 1993.
6. Bickman KR, Lambert RW: Evaluation of skin stapling for wound closure in the emergency department. *Ann Emerg Med* 18:1122, 1989.
7. Orlinksy M, Goldberg RM, Chan L, et al: Cost analysis of stapling versus suturing for skin closure. *Am J Emerg Med* 13:77, 1995.
8. Kanegaye JT, Vance CW, Chan L, Schonfeld N: Comparison of skin stapling devices and standard sutures for pediatric scalp lacerations: A randomized study of cost and time benefits. *J Pediatr* 130:808, 1997.
9. Edlich RF, Becker DG, Thacker JG, et al: Scientific basis for selecting staple and tape skin closures. *Clin Plast Surg* 17:571, 1990.
10. Noordzij JP, Foresman PA, Rodeheaver GT, et al: Tissue adhesive wound repair revisited. *J Emerg Med* 12:645, 1994.
11. Quinn J, Wells G, Sutcliffe T, et al: A randomized trial comparing octylcyanoacrylate tissue adhesive and sutures in the management of lacerations. *JAMA* 277:1527, 1997.
12. Bruns TB, Robinson BS, Smith RJ, et al: A new tissue adhesive for laceration repair in children. *J Pediatr* 132:1067, 1998.
13. Singer AJ, Hollander JE, Valentime SM, et al: Prospective, randomized, controlled trial of tissue adhesive (2-octylcyanoacrylate) vs standard wound closure techniques for laceration repair. *Acad Emerg Med* 5:94, 1998.
14. Quinn J, Maw J, Ramotar KM, et al: Octylcyanoacrylate tissue adhesive versus suture wound repair in a contaminated wound model. *Surgery* 122:69, 1997.

15. Quinn J, Wells G, Sutcliffe T, et al: Tissue adhesive versus suture wound repair at 1 year: Randomized clinical trial correlating early, 3-month, and 1-year cosmetic appearance. *Ann Emerg Med* 32:645, 1998.
16. Mehta PH, Dunn KA, Bradfield JF, Austin PE: Contaminated wounds: Infection rates with subcutaneous sutures. *Ann Emerg Med* 27:43, 1996.
17. Jones JS, Gartner M, Drew G, Pack S: The shorthand vertical mattress stitch: Evaluation of a new suture technique. *Am J Emerg Med* 11:483, 1993.

38 LACERATIONS TO THE FACE AND SCALP

Wendy C. Coates

EPIDEMIOLOGY

Each year, more than 12 million wounds are treated in emergency departments (EDs) across the United States.[1] The most cosmetically devastating are those that appear on the face; therefore careful evaluation and meticulous repair technique are important for excellent results. The emergency physician can repair the majority of facial lacerations; however, because of the cosmetic impact of these wounds, consultation with specialists is encouraged when the technical aspects of closure exceed the physician's ability. In addition, the patient may insist on a specialist to repair such wounds as are readily visible. Wounds to the face that involve areas of tissue avulsion may best be repaired primarily in the operating room so that flaps or grafts can be applied. When the emergency physician initially evaluates the wound, it should be cleaned and properly irrigated even if a delayed repair by a specialist is anticipated.

In today's society, a growing number of victims of domestic violence are being identified in the ED. Anyone with facial trauma should be questioned about the possibility of domestic violence; if this is strongly suspected, appropriate authorities should be notified. Prompt identification and intervention are critical in preventing future injury.[2,3]

PATHOPHYSIOLOGY

Facial and scalp wounds are most often caused by a combination of sharp and blunt mechanisms. For example, a victim of a motor vehicle accident may bluntly strike the windshield and be cut by the glass as it shatters. People involved in interpersonal trauma or falls may have a similar pattern of injury. Lacerations caused by sharp objects are likely to have more discrete edges but may be deeper and involve underlying structures such as the muscles of facial expression, nerves, and/or arteries. Wounds caused by blunt forces burst the skin open, damage cells, and produce tissue edema, which slows down the wound-healing process. As a result, it takes an average of ten times fewer bacteria to cause an infection as in a blunt wound as opposed to a sharp wound. Blunt forces are more likely to cause diffuse underlying damage, such as fractures of the facial bones or skull. The presence of foreign bodies such as soil, glass, or wood fragments further complicates the potential for good healing.[1,4–6]

SCALP AND FOREHEAD

Anatomy

The scalp and forehead have similar structure (Fig. 38-1). The skin is thick, and over the scalp has abundant hair follicles and sebaceous glands. There is a rich network of blood vessels: the arterial supply to each side of the scalp involves three branches off the external carotid artery (occipital, superficial temporal, and posterior auricular arteries) and two branches from the internal carotid artery (supraorbital and supratrochlear arteries).[7] Since the dermal tissue is so fibrous,

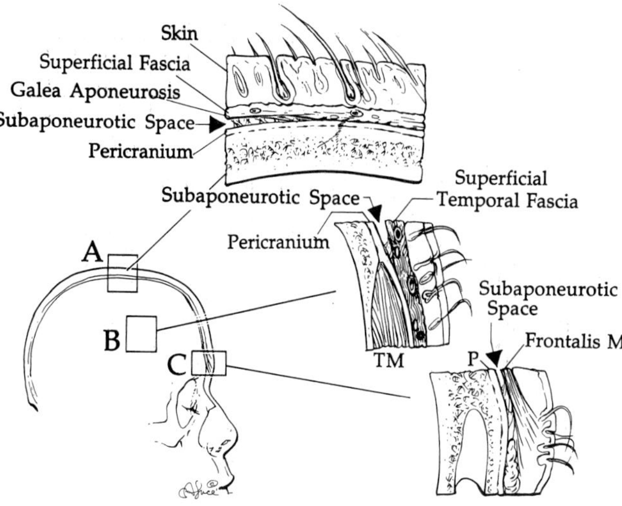

FIG. 38-1. The layers of the **A.** scalp, **B.** forehead, **C.** and eyebrow.

vessel retraction is limited following injury, and significant hemorrhage can result. The potential space between the periosteum and the galea aponeurosis allows for easy movement of the scalp over the cranium. However, hematoma and infection can collect and spread within this space to involve the entire forehead and scalp. This high degree of mobility sometimes leads to a scalping injury, in which a large segment of the scalp is torn off in one piece.

Evaluation

For many patients with scalp and forehead lacerations, the wound may be a minor part of the overall injury; prior to definitive wound care, airway, breathing, circulation, hemorrhage control, and spinal and neurologic injury should be addressed. In some cases, it may be necessary to control scalp hemorrhage urgently by applying direct pressure or clamping the involved vessel(s) at the wound edges (e.g., using Raney clips).

Routine lacerations should be inspected and gently palpated to their depth, noting whether the galea is lacerated or if there is an underlying depressed skull fracture. Palpable depressions in the outer table of the skull should be evaluated further by computed tomography. The orientation of forehead lacerations has important cosmetic implications. In general, wounds that fall along the lines of skin tension have better cosmetic results. Skin tension lines are always perpendicular to the underlying muscles. As an obvious example, the horizontal lines seen on the forehead when the brow is raised are perpendicular to the frontalis muscle underneath (Fig. 38-2). Forehead lacerations that

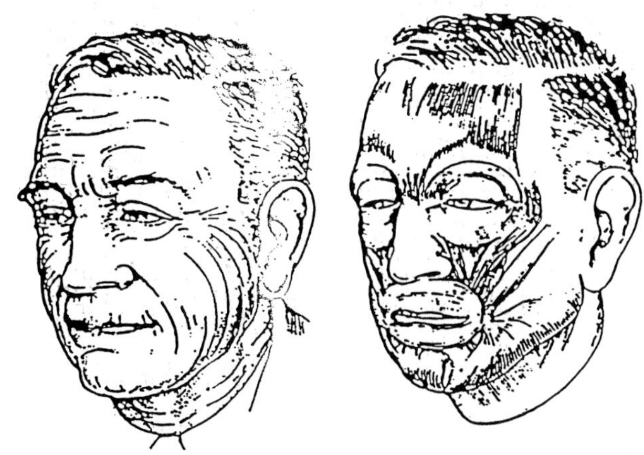

FIG. 38-2. Skin tension lines are perpendicular to underlying muscles.

extend to other structures, such as the eyebrow, nose, or ear must be evaluated and managed with the cosmetic result of these structures in mind.

Wound Preparation

Routine wound care should be undertaken. Sedation may be required to ensure that the patient is safe and relaxed during the procedure.[8] Anesthesia can be provided by topical, local, or regional infiltration. A supraorbital block can be used to anesthetize one side of the forehead and anterior third of the scalp. The advantage of a regional block in the face is that the volume of locally instilled anesthetic does not distort the wound.[9] Local anesthetics containing epinephrine are often used in these highly vascular wounds to help control hemorrhage from small vessels. While many clinicians describe this effect, there are few data to support the belief that epinephrine reduces bleeding during wound repair. Conversely, the theoretical adverse effects of added epinephrine (increased risk of infection, ischemia of portions of the wound with poor circulation, and cardiovascular effects of epinephrine) are rarely an issue with facial and scalp lacerations. Thus, the use of a local anesthetic with or without epinephrine is a matter of personal preference. Topical agents such as TAC (tetracaine-adrenaline-cocaine) or LET (lidocaine-epinephrine-tetracaine) may be useful in this area.[10,11] LET has several practical advantages and is recommended over TAC.

All traumatic wounds are commonly irrigated to reduce contamination and lessen the risk of wound infection. However, in nonbite, noncontaminated facial and scalp wounds presenting within 6 h, routine irrigation does not alter the rate of infection or subsequent cosmetic appearance after suture repair.[12] Regardless of irrigation, the overall incidence of wound infection in sutured scalp and facial wounds is about 1 percent.

Repair of Scalp Lacerations

It is not necessary to shave the scalp prior to closure; shaving actually increases the likelihood of a wound infection and produces a less desirable cosmetic result in the short term. In most cases, the hair can be brushed aside. One can also apply an ointment such as bacitracin zinc or petrolatum to mat down the hair adjacent to the laceration. Hair braiding has been described as an alternate closure technique.[13] Large galeal defects should be repaired if possible to prevent a wide, depressed appearance of the final scar and to minimize the development of a subgaleal hematoma. Buried 4-0 nonabsorbable monofilament nylon [e.g., Ethilon (Ethicon, Inc.)], coated nylon [e.g., Surgilene (Sherwood Davis & Geck)], or polypropylene [e.g., Prolene (Ethicon, Inc.)] interrupted or horizontal mattress sutures may be used (Table 38-1). In large wounds, the muscle layer may be approximated with 4-0 absorbable monofilament [e.g., Monocryl (Ethicon, Inc.)] or multifilament [e.g., Dexon (Sherwood Davis & Geck) or Vicryl (Ethicon, Inc.)] in a simple interrupted fashion. This also serves to reduce the apparent width and depth of the final scar. Conversely, the skin and muscle layers can be closed with a single suture layer through both structures. The skin can be closed with surgical staples or by simple interrupted nylon or rapidly absorbable braided [e.g., Vicryl rapide (Ethicon, Inc.)] sutures.[14] It is helpful to leave the tails long and use sutures of a color different than the hair to facilitate removal. Tissue adhesive is not recommended for the scalp. A pressure dressing should be considered for the first 24 h on a deep laceration to prevent the formation of a hematoma. Patients who have sustained a significant scalping injury should be sent to the operating room for definitive repair.

Repair of Forehead Lacerations

The deep layers may be approximated in a similar fashion to the scalp. In this area, unrepaired muscle layers are more likely to produce noticeable scars, especially when the facial muscles of expression are involved. The superficial layers may be closed with 6-0 nonabsorbable interrupted suture (nylon, coated nylon, or polypropylene) or tissue adhesive. For deep wound under tension, a buried 5-0 intradermal, absorbable monofilament (e.g., Monocryl) or multifilament (e.g., Dexon or Vicryl) can be used. The epidermal layer can be closed with 6-0 nonabsorbable nylon in a simple, interrupted fashion; with wound closure strips [e.g., Steri-strips (3M Company) or Dermaseal (Personna Medical)] over tincture of benzoin; or with tissue adhesive.[15,16] These

TABLE 38-1 Suturing Guidelines for the Face and Scalp

Area	Suture	Size	Anesthetic	Removal
Scalp and face				
Galea	Nylon	4–0	Local or supraorbital	Not removed
Muscle	Monofilament or braided absorbable	4–0	Local or supraorbital	Not removed
Skin	Staples	Standard	Local or supraorbital	10–14 days
	Nylon	4–0		
	Rapidly absorbing	4–0		
Forehead	Coated or plain nylon	6–0	Local or supraorbital	5 days
	Tissue adhesive	May need deep layer		
Face	Coated or plain nylon	6–0	Local, infraorbital, or mandibular	5 days
	Tissue adhesive	May need deep layer		
Eyelids	Coated or plain nylon	6–0 or 7–0	Supra- or infraorbital	3 days
Nose				
Cartilage	Braided absorbable	5–0	Intranasal pack (no epinephrine)	Do not remove
Skin	Coated or plain nylon	6–0	Intranasal pack (no epinephrine)	3–5 days
Ears				
Cartilage	Coated nylon	6–0	Auricular block (no epinephrine)	Do not remove
Skin	Coated nylon	6–0	Auricular block (no epinephrine)	5 days
Lips				
Mucosa	Rapidly absorbing	5–0	Local, infraorbital, or mandibular	Do not remove
Muscle	Monofilament or braided absorbable	4–0 or 5–0	Local, infraorbital, or mandibular	Do not remove
Skin	Plain or coated nylon	6–0	Local, infraorbital, or mandibular	3–5 days

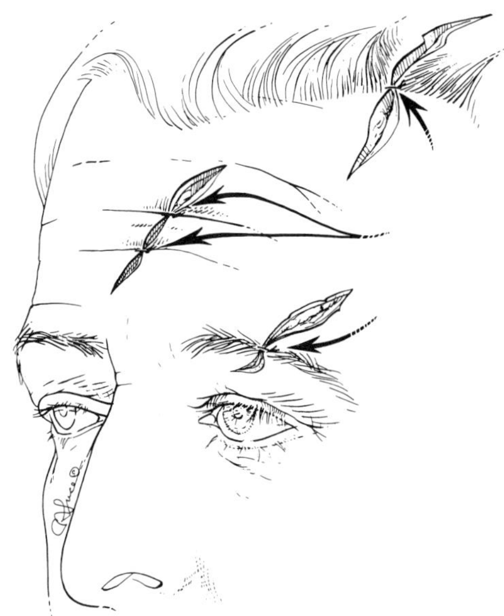

FIG. 38-3. Key stitches in the forehead.

alternate methods of closure are especially attractive if the patient is at risk to develop keloids or hypertrophic scars (e.g., people with darkly pigmented skin). Care should be taken in the forehead to approximate the skin tension lines and hairline precisely (Fig. 38-3).

Repair of Eyebrow Lacerations

The eyebrow marks the lowest portion of the forehead. The eyebrows should never be clipped or shaved because their delicate contour and form are valuable landmarks for the meticulous reapproximation of the wound edges. Furthermore, it is unlikely that they will grow back in exactly the same fashion as they had been prior to the injury. If debridement in any hairy area must take place, the scalpel should cut in an angle parallel to the hair follicles to minimize the area of subsequent alopecia.

Disposition

Patients whose overall medical condition does not warrant surgery or admission to the hospital can be discharged safely with routine wound-care instructions. If their injury resulted from a major blunt impact, a companion should be instructed to bring the patient back for altered level of consciousness, nausea or vomiting, or persistent bleeding or headache. Removal of scalp sutures or staples should take place in 10 to 14 days, while nonabsorbable sutures in the face should be removed in 3 to 5 days.

EYELIDS

Anatomy

The eyelid is a thin tissue that covers the globe and is composed of five layers: skin, subcutaneous tissue, orbicularis oculi muscle, tarsal plate, and conjunctiva. The muscular layer controls lid closure and forms both the medial and lateral canthus; fibers of the orbicularis oculi wrap around the lacrimal system. Nerve supply to the eyelid arises from the temporal and zygomatic branches of the facial nerve. The tarsal plate forms the main body of the lower half of the lid and consists of elastic tissue in a dense matrix of connective tissue. Embedded in the tarsal plate are the meibomian glands, which open into the white line just in front of the conjunctival edge of the lid margin. In the lid margin, the eyelashes are arranged in three irregular rows with their follicles extending obliquely into the tarsal plate.

The lacrimal system begins at the upper and lower puncta as they form the canaliculi. The nasolacrimal duct extends 3 to 5 mm above the level of the medial canthus. It is responsible for tear drainage.[7]

Evaluation

The structures surrounding the eye and eyelids are very delicate; they are cosmetically and functionally important. Depending on the mechanism of injury, a high degree of suspicion for injury to these structures must be maintained. The emergency physician should have a low threshold for referring lacerations in this area to an ophthalmologist or oculoplastic specialist for definitive treatment.

The eyelids are very thin and do not offer any protection from penetrating injuries to the globe. A complete exam of the eye's structure and function and a search for the presence of foreign bodies must be completed before local wound care can be attempted. Once the integrity of the globe and muscular structures is verified, the lid should be examined for involvement of the canthi, the lacrimal system, or penetration through the tarsal plate or lid margin. The following wounds should be referred to an ophthalmologist or oculoplastic specialist: (1) those involving the inner surface of the lid, (2) those involving the lid margins, (3) those involving the lacrimal duct, (4) those associated with ptosis, and (5) those that extend into the tarsal plate. Poor approximation of the lid margins leads to a notched appearance (ectropion). Failure to recognize and properly repair the lacrimal system can result in chronic tearing (epiphora) or dacrocystitis. In general, wounds that are superficial and especially those parallel to the lid margins may be carefully repaired by the emergency physician (Fig. 38-4).[17]

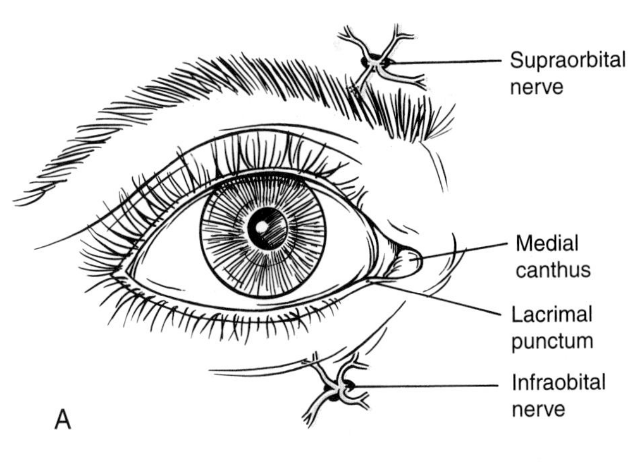

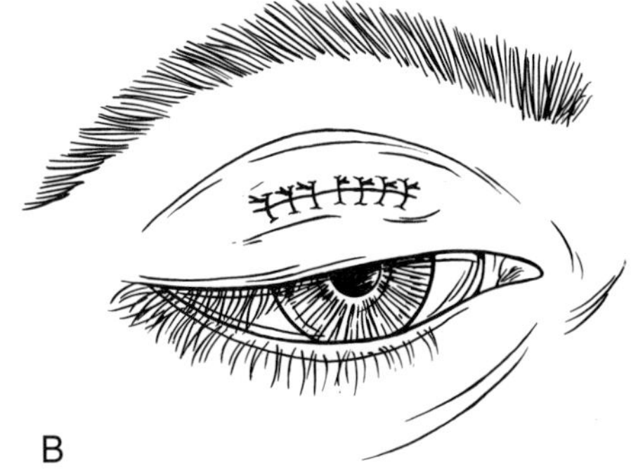

FIG. 38-4. Eyelid anatomy. **A.** External landmark. **B.** Simple closure of a superficial laceration of the upper lid.

Treatment and Disposition

Gentle irrigation to prevent lid edema should be performed after anesthesia. Caustic substances should be avoided. Closure with 6-0 or 7-0 nonabsorbable simple interrupted nylon suture (e.g., Ethilon, Dermalon) or polypropylene (e.g., Surgilene, Prolene) is preferred. Extreme care should be taken to avoid deep penetration of the needle into the globe as it is passed through the skin. Small bites only through the skin layer should be taken. Tissue adhesive is contraindicated near the eye. In the event of inadvertent contact with the eye, copious irrigation and/or application of a petrolatum ointment is indicated. Routine evaluation and treatment of the subsequent corneal abrasion should be followed. Sutures should be removed in 3 to 5 days. A thin layer of antibiotic ointment may be applied in place of a dressing.

NOSE

Anatomy

Being a protuberant structure, the nose is especially vulnerable to blunt trauma. It is composed of cartilaginous and osseous structures that support the overlying skin and musculature and the underlying mucosa. It is separated into halves by the septum. The tip of the nose is formed by two C-shaped alar cartilages that are covered directly by skin. The interior of the nose is covered by specialized skin with mucus-producing cells and thick, long hairs near the end, while the proximal portion of the nasal lining is made up of ciliated pseudostratified columnar epithelial cells.[7]

Evaluation

The most important assessment of nasal lacerations is to determine their depth and the involvement of the deeper tissue layers. Exposed cartilage or penetration through all tissue layers increases the risk of infection. When there is septal trauma, the presence of a hematoma underneath the cartilage and its protective mucoperichondrial layer may eventually lead to permanent thickening of the septum, causing partial airway obstruction of the nasal passage. Alternatively, the pressure exerted by a large, untreated septal hematoma may cause necrosis and subsequent erosion of the septum, enabling communication between the nasal passageways. Besides the annoyance to the patient, it may lead to a cosmetic saddle-nose deformity. If the mechanism of injury included a blunt force delivered to the nose, the presence of cerebrospinal fluid rhinorrhea should be sought to diagnose a possible injury to the cribriform plate.

Treatment and Disposition

Local anesthesia of the nose may be attempted but is difficult because of the tightly adhering skin. Injection of epinephrine-containing anesthetics should be avoided on the nose. Regional anesthetic injection is difficult, but topical application of lidocaine mixed with epinephrine may provide sufficient anesthesia. Insertion of multiple cotton-tipped swabs or plain nasal packing gauze soaked in the mixture is usually sufficient (Fig. 38-5). After several minutes and prior to repair, the swabs or gauze should be removed.

Superficial lacerations to the skin layer may be closed with 6-0 nonabsorbable monofilament simple interrupted sutures, which may be removed in 3 to 5 days. Lacerations in which the cartilage is exposed should be closed promptly. Small pieces of cartilage that may be present should be preserved under the skin to provide the optimal cosmetic result. Future revision by a plastic surgeon will be easier if there is abundant tissue available for reconstruction.

If the laceration extends through all tissue layers, closure should begin with a 5-0 monofilament synthetic suture that aligns the skin surrounding the entrance to the nasal canals at the alar rim (Fig. 38-5). Initially, the ends can be left untied and long to facilitate the closure of the deeper structures. *Gentle* traction on this suture provides alignment of the mucosa and cartilage layers. The mucosal layer is closed with a 5-0 rapidly absorbable interrupted suture (e.g., Vicryl rapide) and the area is reirrigated gently from the outside. The cartilage may rarely need to be approximated with a minimal number of 5-0 absorbable sutures. In sharply demarcated linear lacerations, closure of the overlying skin is usually sufficient. Finally, the initial stitch at the alar margin should be reevaluated for precise alignment and tied; then the remainder of the skin should be sutured with 6-0 monofilament nonabsorbable material. Removal of the external sutures may take place in 3 to 5 days.

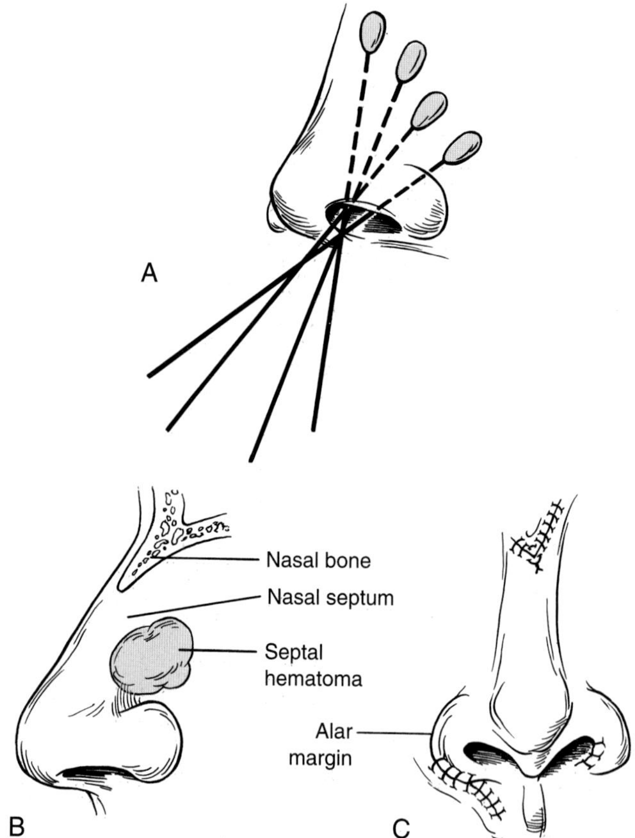

FIG. 38-5. The nose. **A.** Nasal anesthetic technique using cotton-tipped applicators. **B.** Septal hematoma and lateral anatomy. **C.** Frontal view showing closure of skin edges.

Septal hematomas should be drained. For a small, unilateral hematoma, the clot can often be aspirated through an 18-gauge needle. Larger hematomas require a horizontal incision at the base (Fig. 38-5). Following the procedure, nasal packing prevents the reaccumulation of blood. A brief course of prophylactic antibiotics is recommended to prevent infection of the cartilage. The packing may be removed in 2 to 3 days. Bilateral hematomas should probably be drained in the operating room.

LIPS

Anatomy

The external surfaces of the lips have three distinct regions: the skin, the vermilion, and the oral mucosa. The cosmetically important junction of the skin and the red portion of the lip is called the *vermilion border.* The orbicularis oris muscle surrounds the mouth. Its integrity is respon-

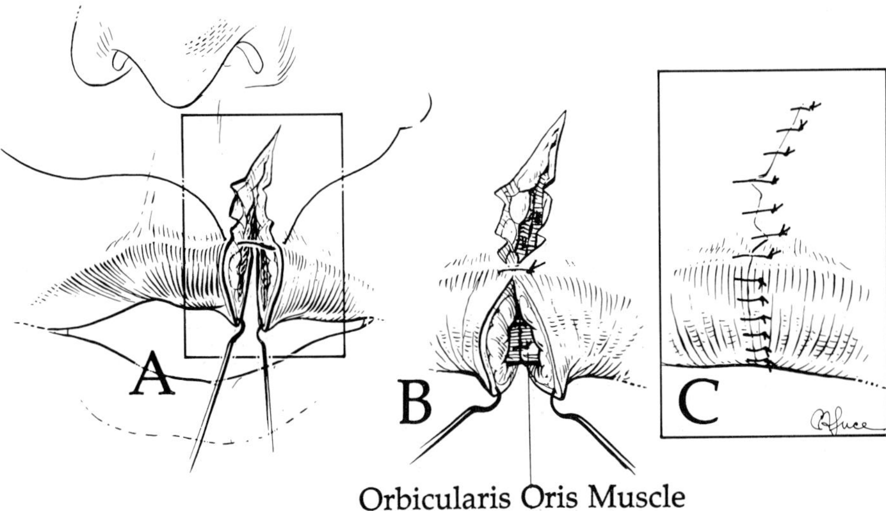

FIG. 38-6. Irregular-edged vertical laceration of the upper lip. **A.** Traction is applied to the lips and closure of the wound is begun first at the vermilion-skin junction. **B.** The orbicularis oris muscle is then repaired with interrupted, absorbable 4-0 synthetic sutures. **C.** The irregular edges of the skin are then approximated.

sible for retaining the saliva inside the mouth, producing the bilabial sounds of speech, and providing important facial expressions. The infraorbital nerve supplies the upper lip and the mental nerve supplies the lower lip. Both are branches of the trigeminal nerve and can easily be blocked by regional anesthetic techniques. The lips are richly supplied by the labial arteries.[7]

Evaluation

External as well as intraoral examination must take place to appreciate the complete injury, and lacerations should be fully explored. Missing, impacted, or fractured teeth; involvement of the parotid (Stensen's) duct; or exposed bone of the maxilla or mandible should be noted. Lacerations that cross the vermilion border are of the utmost cosmetic importance.

Treatment and Disposition

Isolated intraoral mucosal lacerations may not need to be sutured. Through-and-through lacerations that do not include the vermilion border can be closed in layers. The mucosal layer is closed with a 5-0 rapidly absorbable suture (e.g., plain gut, Vicryl rapide). Gentle re-irrigation from the outside is recommended to prevent wound infection from intraoral organisms. Next, the orbicularis oris muscle is approximated with 5-0 absorbable suture material (e.g., Vicryl, Dexon, Monocryl) with a simple interrupted or horizontal mattress technique. Finally, the skin is sutured with 6-0 nonabsorbable monofilament material in a simple interrupted fashion. The sutures should be removed in 5 days. Alternatively, the skin can be approximated with tissue adhesive. The use of tissue adhesive on mucosal surfaces is contraindicated.

Wounds that cross the vermilion border should be repaired by placing the first stitch to approximate the edges of the vermilion border precisely (Fig. 38-6). Even 1 mm of step-off will be cosmetically unpleasing. Following this first stitch, the repair can proceed as previously described. In some cases, it is helpful to place this crucial suture and leave it untied until the remainder of the skin is sutured. Gentle traction on the ends can help approximate underlying tissue to provide optimal cosmesis. Care should be taken to avoid pulling the suture through the skin in this cosmetically delicate area.

If an underlying fracture of the maxilla or mandible is suspected, radiographic evaluation is required. Patients with open fractures should receive prophylactic antibiotics that provide coverage against oral flora, and a maxillofacial specialist should be consulted.

EARS

Anatomy

The external ear begins with the external auditory canal and extends to the fibrocartilaginous framework and finally the earlobe. The blood supply arises from the superficial temporal and posterior auricular arteries. The majority of the sensory innervation is from the anterior and posterior branches of the greater auricular nerve. The posterior wall of the external auditory canal is supplied by the auricular branches of the vagus nerve, so lacerations that involve this area must be anesthetized separately.[7]

Evaluation

It is crucial to identify lacerations caused by blunt forces to the ear, as a ruptured tympanic membrane or the formation of a subchondral hematoma can have devastating consequences. Hematomas must be identified and treated even in the absence of a laceration. The presence of cerebrospinal fluid otorrhea may signal a basilar skull fracture. Lacerations caused by blunt or shear forces may involve the cartilage.

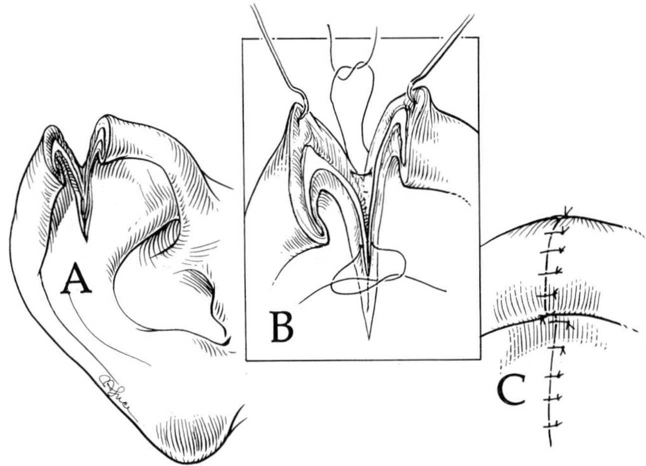

FIG. 38-7. **A.** Laceration through auricle. **B.** One or two interrupted, 6-0 coated nylon sutures will approximate divided edges of cartilage. **C.** Interrupted nonabsorbable 6-0 synthetic sutures approximate the skin edges.

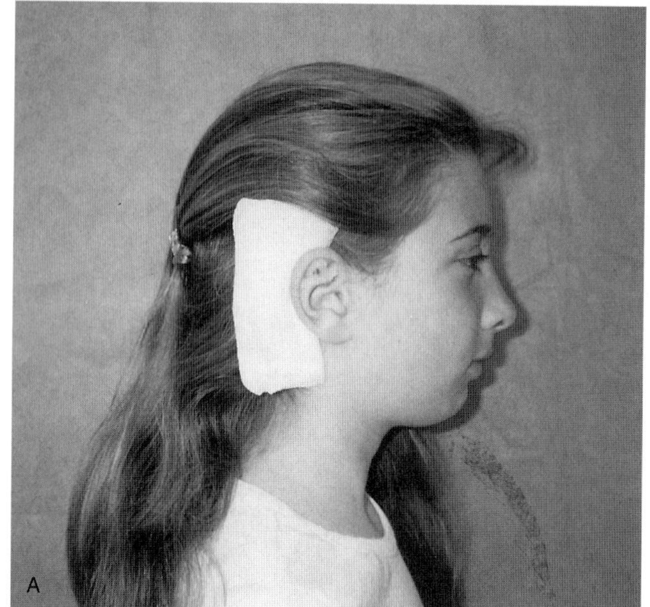

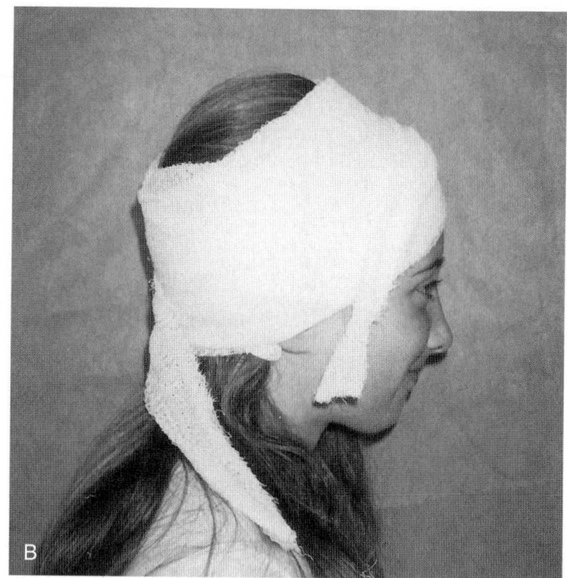

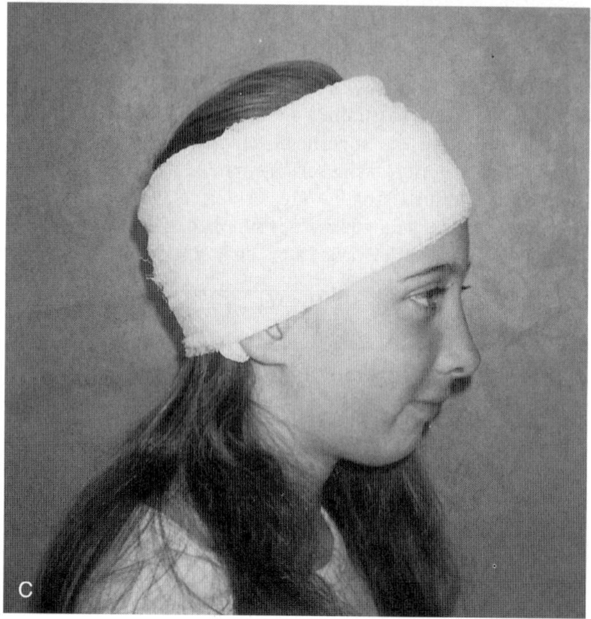

FIG. 38-8. Pressure dressing for ear lacerations. **A.** Gauze placed behind auricle. **B.** Bandage wrapped around head with two ends cut for tying. **C.** Ends tied.

Treatment and Disposition

Routine wound preparation is appropriate for ear lacerations. For patient comfort, a cotton plug can be inserted into the ear canal during irrigation. If a wound extends deep into the canal, the integrity of the tympanic membrane should be verified. Regional anesthesia by auricular block is ideal. Epinephrine should be avoided in lacerations involving the ear. Impeccable hemostasis prior to repair is required to prevent the formation of a hematoma.

Superficial lacerations to the skin can be closed with 6-0 monofilament interrupted sutures (Fig. 38-7). Any exposed cartilage should be covered to prevent subsequent infection. If an injury produces several crushed pieces of cartilage under the skin, they should not be removed; remaining cartilage will be beneficial if reconstructive surgery is necessary. Debridement of skin is not advisable, since there is very little excess skin available to cover the existing cartilage. In most through-and-through lacerations of the auricle, the skin can be approximated and the underlying cartilage will be supported adequately. In a large, gaping wound, one or two 6-0 nonabsorbable coated nylon stitches can be used to approximate the edges of cartilage. The knots should be tied so they will not cause an obvious deformity through the skin. If the overlying skin is avulsed, referral to a plastic surgeon for repair using a flap is recommended. Following repair of the simple ear laceration, a small piece of nonadherent gauze may be applied over the laceration only and a pressure dressing applied. Gauze squares are placed behind the ear to apply pressure and the head is wrapped circumferentially with gauze [e.g., Kerlix (Kendall Healthcare Products, Inc.)]. The dressing may be tied into place by cutting the last portion of the gauze longitudinally (Fig. 38-8). Sutures should be removed in 5 days. Complete avulsion of the ear must be urgently referred to a plastic surgeon.

If an auricular hematoma is suspected, consultation with a plastic surgeon or otolaryngologist is recommended. Proper treatment requires the complete and permanent evacuation of the hematoma and definitive control of the bleeding that caused it. Neglecting to treat an auricular hematoma may produce a ''cauliflower'' ear type of cosmetic defect of the cartilage.

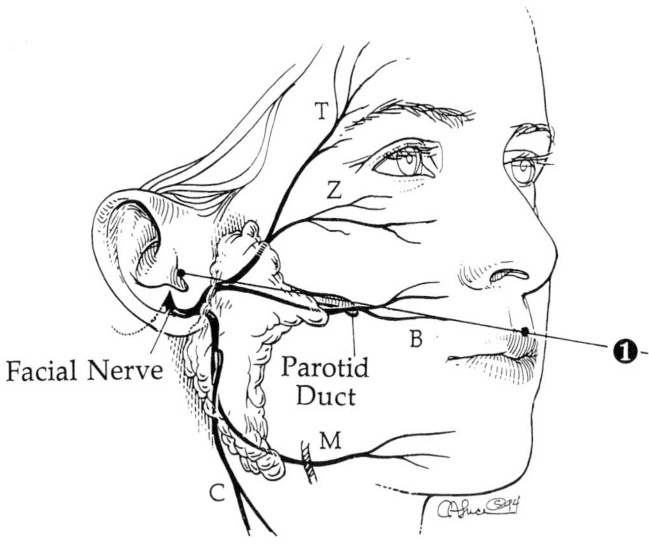

FIG. 38-9. Anatomic structures of the cheek. The course of the parotid duct is deep to a line drawn from the tragus of the ear to the midportion of the upper lip. Branches of the facial nerve: temporal (T), zygomatic (Z), bucial (B), mental (M), and cervical (C).

THE CHEEKS AND FACE

Lacerations that involve the surface of the face may be repaired carefully using standard wound-care techniques. In general, facial lacerations are closed with 6-0 monofilament nylon simple interrupted sutures that are removed in 5 days. Tissue adhesive may be used in superficial wounds after proper irrigation. If there is significant tension, an underlying layer of 4-0 absorbable suture closure is indicated. Attention to underlying anatomic structures including the facial nerve and parotid gland is necessary[7] (Fig. 38-9). If these structures are involved, operative repair is indicated.

REFERENCES

1. Singer AJ, Hollander JE, Quinn JV: Evaluation and management of traumatic lacerations. *N Engl J Med* 337:1142, 1997.
2. Salber PR, Talieferro E: *The Physician's Guide to Domestic Violence: How to Ask the Right Questions and Recognize Abuse—Another Way to Save a Life.* Volcano, CA, Volcano Press, 1995.
3. Ochs HA, Neuenschwander MC, Dodson TB: Are head, neck and facial injuries markers of domestic violence? *J Am Dent Assoc* 127:757, 1996.
4. Edlich RF, Rodeheaver GT, Morgan RF, et al: Principles of emergency wound management. *Ann Emerg Med* 17:1284, 1988.
5. Berk WA, Welch RD, Bock BF: Controversial issues in clinical management of the simple wound. *Ann Emerg Med* 21:72, 1992.
6. Howell JM, Chisholm CD: Wound care. *Emerg Med Clin North Am* 15:417, 1997.
7. Moore KL: *Clinically Oriented Anatomy,* 3d ed., Philadelphia: Williams & Wilkins, 1992.
8. Algren JT, Algren CL: Sedation and analgesia for minor pediatric procedures. *Pediatr Emerg Care* 12:435, 1996.
9. Ferrera PC, Chandler R: Anesthesia in the emergency setting: Part II. Head and neck, eye and rib injuries. *Am Fam Physician* 50:797, 1994.
10. Blackburn PA, Butler KH, Hughes MJ, et al: Comparison of tetracaine-adrenaline-cocaine (TAC) with topical lidocaine-epinephrine (TLE): Efficacy and cost. *Am J Emerg Med* 13:315, 1995.
11. Ernst AA, Marvez-Valls E, Nick TG, Weiss SJ: LAT (lidocaine-adrenaline-tetracaine) versus TAC (tetracaine-adrenaline-cocaine) for topical anesthesia in face and scalp lacerations. *Am J Emerg Med* 13:151, 1995.
12. Hollander JE, Richman PB, Werblud M, et al: Irrigation in facial and scalp lacerations: Does it alter outcome? *Ann Emerg Med* 31:73, 1998.
13. Aoki N, Oikawa A, Sakai T: Hair braiding closure for superficial wounds. *Surg Neurol* 46:150, 1996.
14. Orlinsky M, Goldberg RM, Chan L, et al: Cost analysis of stapling versus suturing for skin closure. *Am J Emerg Med* 13:77, 1995.
15. Quinn JV, Drzewiecki A, Li MM, et al: A randomized, controlled trial comparing tissue adhesive with suturing in the repair of pediatric facial lacerations. *Ann Emerg Med* 22:1130, 1993.
16. Bresnahan KA, Howell JM, Wizorek J: Comparison of tensile strength of cyanoacrylate tissue adhesive closure of lacerations versus suture closure. *Ann Emerg Med* 26:575, 1995.
17. Janda AM: Ocular trauma: triage and treatment. *Postgrad Med* 90:51, 1991.

FINGERTIP AND NAIL INJURIES

Robert S. Chang
Wallace A. Carter

Fingertip injuries are those that occur distal to the insertion of the flexor and extensor tendons at the level of the lunula. This is among the most frequently injured parts of the hand and such injuries may involve the skin, pulp tissue, distal phalanx, and perionychium, made up of the nail, nail bed, and surrounding structures (Fig. 39-1). Injuries may be classified as closed crush, simple lacerations, open crush with partial amputation, and complete amputation.[1] The approach to treatment depends on the number versus other factors, including the specific digit involved (thumb or index finger); patient's age, sex, handedness, and occupation; as well as the size and angle of the wound, presence or absence of exposed bone, mechanism of injury, concurrent medical problems, and anticipated future use of the hand. The goals are to maintain length and cosmetic appearance, have the fingertip approach normal sensation and function, and have as short and uncomplicated a healing period as possible. This chapter is organized to separate distal fingertip injuries with and without bone exposure from those directly involving the perionychium.

MANAGEMENT—GENERAL PRINCIPLES

History and Examination

The majority of fingertip injuries are isolated injuries and can be managed in the emergency department (ED). Complex or extensive injuries calling for skin grafting or technically demanding skills will require consultation with a specialist, as will those associated with other bodily injuries. Before evaluating the injury, an adequate history must be taken. Specific considerations must be taken into account if the digit involved is the thumb or index finger. In the thumb, it is crucial to establish a functional, sensate tip with preservation of as much length as possible. The second most important digit to consider is the index finger, where the goal is to preserve pinch.[2] The mechanism of injury (crush versus clean cut), age, hand dominance, occupation, and future hand use will influence the method of repair. Where the function of the fingers is vital to the patient's occupation (e.g., that of a concert pianist), early consultation with a hand or plastic surgeon is necessary.

In all cases, however, one is dealing with contaminated wounds in the hand; therefore examination and care of the involved digit must begin with meticulous attention to wound care. In addition to active tetanus toxoid immunization, a severely contaminated wound—one that has been in contact with soil, feces, or organic material—may require passive immunization using tetanus immune globulin (TIG) at the time of presentation. Further examination of the involved digit includes assessment of the extent of damage to the soft tissue, the nail, and nail bed; the level and angle of amputation; the presence or absence of exposed bone; and vascular status (e.g., capillary refill). A sterile needle applied along either side of the involved digit can easily test for sensation. Similarly, the ability to flex and extend at

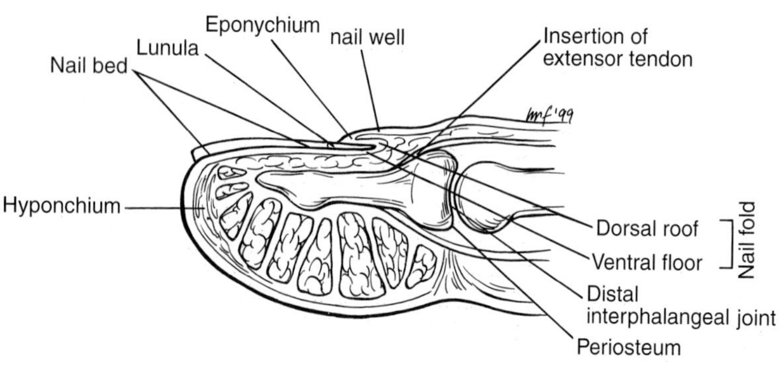

FIG. 39-1. Anatomy of the perionychium. [From Zook, EG: The perionychium, in Green, DP (ed): *Operative Hand Surgery*, 2d ed. New York: Churchill Livingstone, 1988, p 1332, with permission.]

the distal interphalangeal (DIP) joint suggests that the integrity of the flexor and extensor tendons is at least partially intact.

Radiographic evaluation with anteroposterior (AP), lateral, and oblique views of the involved finger is necessary to assess for bone injuries and retained radiopaque foreign bodies.

Anesthesia and Irrigation

Adequate anesthesia is then administered to further delineate the extent of injury as well as allow for copious saline irrigation and débridement of necrotic tissue, as needed. There are several different types of nerve blocks that can be used, such as the digital, metacarpal, carpal, and axillary blocks. The choice of which to use is based on various factors, such as the number of digits involved, the size and location of the wound, as well as the personal preference of the physician. In the ED, the digital nerve block is a simple yet usually effective means of achieving digital anesthesia.

Following adequate anesthesia, the wound should be irrigated to remove foreign debris, reduce bacterial contamination, and lessen the risk of wound infection. Animal studies suggest that irrigation under pressure with adequate total volume lowers the infection rate in contaminated wounds; however, the required pressure and amount of irrigant is subject to debate. Irrigation through an 18- to 20-gauge needle attached to a 30- to 60-mL syringe generates a peak pressure of about 30 psi; this is usually adequate to dislodge foreign material from wounds. As to the irrigation amount, many clinicians have adopted the rule of thumb of 60 mL/cm of wound length. However, the total amount must be adjusted according to the condition and location of the wound. Unless there is extraordinary contamination, irrigation of fingertip wounds can usually be accomplished with a total amount of 250 to 500 mL of normal saline.

Adequate Visualization

A bloodless field provides the optimal setting for the performance of a digital repair. Several types of tourniquets have been described in the literature, including the pneumatic tourniquet placed around the upper arm, the digital tourniquet using a 1-in. Penrose drain, and a surgical glove. In the last of these techniques, the patient wears a glove that has a cut fingertip corresponding to the injured digit. As the glove is rolled from distal to proximal, a tight band acting as a tourniquet is created around the base of the digit.[3] The disadvantage of this technique is that different glove sizes, the varying thickness of the glove material, and the varying number of rolls produced may generate a wide range of pressures, making this technique less desirable in the ED setting. In the ED, a simple yet safe means of achieving hemostasis is with the digital Penrose tourniquet. With a 1-in. Penrose drain, the finger is carefully wrapped from distal to proximal, thereby exsanguinating the digit. The drain is then carefully removed from distal to proximal and placed around the base of the finger, secured with a hemostat, to serve as a ''tourniquet.'' Excessively high pressures, which can cause neurovascular damage, may be avoided by limiting the stretch of the drain to no more than 50 percent of the original length.[4]

A magnification loupe can be extremely useful in the surgical repair of an injured finger. However, not many EDs are equipped with this tool. If a repair cannot be achieved without a loupe, the hand or plastic surgery specialist must be consulted.

Wound Dressing and Postrepair Care

Once the fingertip injury is repaired, it should be dressed in nonadherent gauze, such as Adaptic (Johnson & Johnson Medical, Inc.) or an antibiotic-impregnated petrolatum gauze, such as Xeroform (Kendall Healthcare Products) and wrapped with sterile gauze dressings. If possible, it is desirable to observe capillary refill after the dressing has been placed. The fingertip should always be wrapped loosely to allow for adequate circulation. A metal or plastic-cap splint should be incorporated into the last layer of dressing for protection and avoidance of painful stimulation. The hand should be kept elevated. These injuries tend to be very painful, so adequate analgesia with oxycodone or hydrocodone should be offered to all patients. A follow-up wound check by the hand or plastic surgeon is recommended after 2 days. Sutures are usually removed 2 weeks after the injury. Exercises to prevent joint stiffness are begun 10 to 14 days following soft-tissue injuries and after 3 weeks if a distal phalangeal fracture is involved.[5]

Broad-spectrum antibiotics are not routinely recommended. They may be considered in wounds that are contaminated, for injuries that are more than 12 h old, in the presence of exposed bone, or in patients with concurrent medical problems that may affect wound healing (i.e., those with diabetes, renal, or peripheral vascular disease).[5] Antibiotics should be chosen to cover suspected contaminants and pathogens: *Staphylococcus aureus*, streptococci, gram-negative bacilli, and/or anaerobes, depending on the circumstances. Antibiotics should be given early and by a route to achieve high blood and tissue levels, often intravenously.

Indications for admission to the hospital include injuries that require repair in the operating room, those that require a course of intravenous antibiotics, as well as social issues such as homelessness or the patient's inability to follow basic aftercare instructions.

SPECIAL CONSIDERATIONS

In a child, identifying a fracture with plain radiographs may be difficult owing to an open epiphysis. It is often necessary to obtain radiographs of the uninvolved hand for comparison. If a surgical procedure is indicated and the child is unable to tolerate the procedure after a digital nerve block alone, conscious sedation may be required. Medications commonly used for conscious sedation include the sedatives/anxiolytics, such as benzodiazepines and barbiturates; pain relief is achieved using opioids such as fentanyl and morphine. In children, a commonly used agent is ketamine, a nonopiate phencyclidine derivative that produces both analgesia and sedation. Before performing conscious sedation, specific attention should be paid to allergies (including those to latex), current medications, and last oral intake of solids and liquids.

Keeping dressings intact on children poses a problem because of their continuous activity, rendering a routine hand dressing and protective finger splint ineffective. If the dressing is deemed essential to wound healing, the child should be placed in a long arm cast.[6] Consultation with the hand or plastic surgeon is recommended for proper follow-up and neurovascular evaluation.

SPECIFIC TREATMENT STRATEGIES

Digital Tip Injuries with Skin and Pulp Tissue Loss Only

Distal fingertip amputations that are 1 cm^2 or less in size without exposed bone can usually be treated conservatively in the ED with serial dressing changes alone. This is a desirable option, because healing occurs by secondary intention and results in very little scarring. Follow-up is arranged in 2 days for wound check and the patient is made aware that wound care is vital to the success of this technique. The patient is instructed to soak the injured fingertip in warm water to which an antibacterial soap has been added once a day for 10 min, followed by tap-water irrigation and application of a sterile nonadherent dressing. This procedure is performed daily for the first 10 to 15 days and every other day thereafter. On average, complete healing may take 4 to 8 weeks, and both the cosmetic appearance and sensibility of the fingertip are quite satisfactory with this technique. Conservative management is advocated in children less than 12 years of age, since they have greater regenerative potential than do adults.[6] Loss of volume, lack of pulp firmness, and increased sensibility (particularly to cold) have been reported in approximately 30 percent of patients.[7]

In cases where the severed skin tip is available, an alternative means of treatment is to use the amputated portion as a full-thickness skin graft. The amputated tissue is cleaned and debrided of nonviable tissue, the undersurface of the skin is then defatted with sharp scissors and sutured to the defect using nylon sutures. Sutures are left long and tied over a 2- by 2-cm gauze stent dressing to compress the graft firmly against the fingertip. Appropriate follow-up is made and unless obvious purulence ensues, the stented dressing is left undisturbed for 7 to 12 days.

A split- or full-thickness skin graft harvested from a distant site is another means of wound closure. This procedure may be indicated in situations where the severed skin tip is either not available or nonviable, significant pulp tissue loss is greater than 1 cm^2, or the patient's desire to have full use of the hand precludes waiting the 4 to 8 weeks necessary for healing by secondary intention. In these cases, consultation with a specialist is appropriate. Most surgeons recommend using the hypothenar eminence of the injured hand as the donor site, since the skin from this region is the same type of glabrous skin as is present on the fingertips.[1] The graft is left in place for 7 to 12 days and allows for rapid wound closure and healing. Complications with skin grafts include decreased sensibility of the fingertip, scar tenderness both at donor and graft sites, cosmetically poor quality of coverage, and hyperpigmentation in patients with dark skin.[7]

Many authors agree that conservative management of fingertip injuries without bone exposure, as opposed to the above techniques, is superior in terms of cosmetic appearance, improved function, and sensibility of the involved digit.[1,6,8]

Digital Tip Injuries with Exposed Bone

If a significant loss of tissue to the fingertip causes exposure of the tuft of the distal phalanx, skin grafting will be unsuccessful since bone does not provide adequate vascularity to support the donor tissue. Several treatment options exist, always keeping in mind the important goals of preserving digit length, especially with regard to the thumb and index finger, as well as sensitivity and functionality of the fingertip. The size and geometry of the injury, the angle of tip amputation, and the availability of the amputated tip will determine the options available for wound closure.

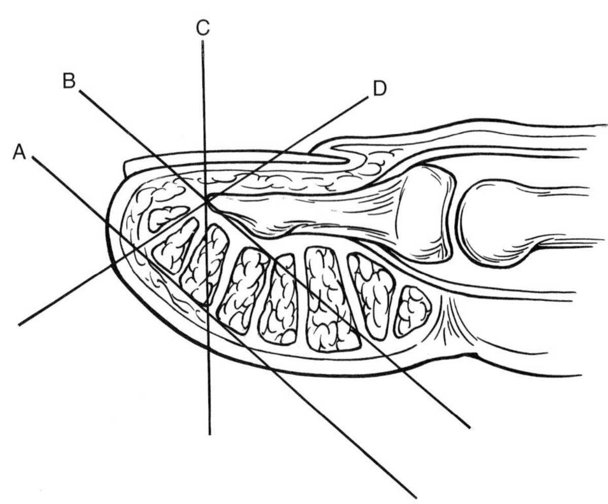

FIG. 39-2. Fingertip amputations. **A.** Volar angulation without bone exposure. **B.** Volar angulation with bone exposure. **C.** Transverse or perpendicular angulation with bone exposure. **D.** Dorsal angulation with bone exposure. [From Russell RC: Fingertip injuries, in McCarthy J (ed): *Plastic Surgery*. Philadelphia: Saunders, 1990, p 4479, with permission.]

If the bony protuberance is less than 0.5 cm in length and the soft tissue defect is less than 1 cm^2, the bone may be trimmed back using a rongeuer and the wound left to heal by secondary intention as previously described. A dorsal obliquely angulated wound (Fig. 39-2*D*) may be treated in the ED with bone shortening followed by primary closure of the wound using the adjacent volar tissue. An injury of this type has a favorable prognosis because the sensate volar skin is intact. Fat from the local tissue may need to be trimmed to allow wound closure without tension. The nail should be removed and attention paid to associated injuries to the nail bed and surrounding structures. Although results are comparable to those following conservative management, shortcomings include loss of length as well as tenderness of the fingertip and some degree of functional disability.

Amputations that are angled either in a transverse or volar direction (Fig. 39-2*B* and *C*) have less favorable outcomes because they do not always have adequate soft tissue and skin coverage to allow for primary closure and preservation of length. Consultation with a plastic or hand surgeon is necessary, as these injuries often require the use of sophisticated local V-Y advancement or adjacent pedicle flaps to maintain length and provide tissue coverage, a technique beyond the scope of practice by most emergency physicians.

Incomplete digital tip amputations, defined by the retention of the neurovascular bundle as well as portions of the underlying bone, may be replaced as a composite graft. However, as reported in the literature, these are among the most difficult injuries to reconstruct and require consultation with a specialist. If adequate circulation is retained in the tip, the injury is treated with fracture reduction, internal pin fixation, and repair of the soft tissue injury. This procedure is optimally performed in the operating room.

In all patients with a complete amputation that occurs proximal to the lunula, consultation with the hand or plastic surgeon is recommended for possible replantation in the operating room. Conversely, in the adult patient, replantation of a complete amputation distal to the lunula is not usually advocated. This is because the procedure is technically demanding owing to the arborization of the neurovascular bundle at this location, and it carries a poor prognosis. However, consultation with the surgical specialist is clearly indicated in all patients with specific occupational concerns and when the injured digit is the thumb or index finger.

Although fingertip injuries are quite common in children, most require only conservative management because of the rapid healing process. Repairs should be done using absorbable sutures. Surgical procedures such as grafts and advancement flaps should be avoided where possible. A completely amputated composite tip may be reattached to serve solely as a biological dressing, and parents should be informed that the tip might necrose, dry up, and turn black as the underlying wound continues to heal. However, in children less than 6 years of age, replantation and revascularization of the composite tip may be a viable treatment option performed by the surgical specialist.

Injuries Involving the Perionychium

The nail, nail bed, and surrounding soft tissue make up the perionychium (see Fig. 39-1). The nail bed is made up of the germinal and sterile matrix. The germinal matrix begins 3 to 5 mm proximal and deep to the eponychium and extends distally to the lunula. From there, the sterile matrix (responsible for producing the majority of the nail) extends distally to the hyponychium. Injury to the perionychium is most commonly due to closure of the fingertip in a door and often occurs in the distal portion of the nail bed; it may occur as an isolated injury or in combination with any of the injuries previously discussed. Injuries can be described as simple nail bed laceration, stellate laceration, severe crush, and complete avulsion. The mechanism of injury is a force directed to the dorsum of the nail, causing it to bend or break and crushing the nail bed against the unyielding tuft of the distal phalanx. There is an associated distal tuft fracture in approximately 50 percent of nail bed injuries; thus all patients require the standard three radiographic views of the involved digit(s). Nail plate deformity affecting permanent nail growth is the most common complication resulting from lack of treatment. Therefore it is important to recognize when these injuries have occurred and to treat them appropriately.

Subungual Hematoma

These are injuries due to the disruption of the blood vessels of the nail bed. The area of the hematoma is directly proportional to the degree of vascular damage. If the hematoma covers less than 50 percent of the area beneath the nail, treatment can be accomplished with trephination of the nail plate to allow for adequate decompression and drainage of the hematoma. Various tools have been used effectively for this purpose, including a heated paper clip, electric nail drill, electrocautery, 18-gauge needle, and scalpel. The disadvantages with the heated paper clip include coagulation of the hematoma and introduction of carbon particles called "lampblack" into the nail bed, which may delay healing.[8] Use of a needle, scalpel, or nail drill can be painful and may necessitate local anesthesia. A handheld electrocautery device permits rapid and painless trephination and is sterile and disposable.[8] However, not every ED will be equipped with such a tool, and emergency physicians will likely perform nail trephination using tools they are familiar with. Patients are discharged with local wound care instructions to soak the affected finger in warm water containing antibacterial soap two to three times a day for 7 days.

It is commonly recommended that for a subungual hematoma occupying more than 50 percent of the nail bed area, the nail be removed in order to evaluate the nail bed and repair any associated laceration.[2,5,8] However, there are two prospective studies which found that simple trephining produces a good to excellent outcome in about 85 percent of patients with subungual hematoma regardless of its size, the presence of fracture, or infection.[9,10] Therefore, simple trephination is an adequate treatment for most simple subungual hematomas, with nail removal recommended if there is associated nail avulsion or surrounding nail fold disruption.

Nail removal can be accomplished with adequate anesthesia, digit exsanguination, nail elevation using a small hemostat, elevation of the eponychium off the nail, and then removal by gentle longitudinal traction with a hemostat. Lacerations of the nail bed are carefully repaired using 7-0 absorbable sutures. Crush injuries often result in stellate lacerations, which may require extensive meticulous repair with a magnification loupe. The nail is gently cleaned with saline, taking care not to damage the germinal matrix; it is then trephinated and secured in its anatomic position. This is accomplished by placing a 5-0 nylon suture through the distal end of the nail plate and then passing it underneath and through the center of the eponychial fold. Once the nail plate is returned to its anatomic position, the suture is tied down over the nail. The replaced nail acts as a natural splint to the terminal phalanx, prevents formation of synechiae, and protects the sensitive nail bed. If the nail is not available, nonbiological stents made of Silastic (Dow Corning) or silicone may be used to elevate the eponychium and protect the nail bed. Similarly, a sterile piece of aluminum foil used to wrap suture materials may be fashioned into the dimension of the avulsed nail and inserted under the eponychium. The fingertip is then dressed in nonadherent gauze and placed in a volar splint to limit movement at the DIP joint. Patients are given postoperative wound care instructions (e.g., as to hand elevation) as well as neurovascular checks and given adequate pain relief. Unless obvious purulence is noted, the dressing is left undisturbed for 5 to 7 days after which the site is examined for new hematoma formation. The suture attached to the nail is removed after 3 weeks; the existing nail will be dislodged by the new ingrowing nail after 1 to 3 months.

If an associated distal phalanx fracture coexists with a nail bed laceration, it usually manifests as an avulsion of the nail out of the proximal eponychial fold. If this happens, the nail is removed, the fracture is stabilized by manual reduction, and the nail bed is repaired as previously described. The nail replaced in its anatomic position serves as a biological splint to maintain fracture reduction, owing to its proximity to the underlying bone. Unstable reductions require consultation with a plastic or hand surgeon for internal fixation using Kirschner wires to prevent deformity of the nail bed.

Nail Bed Avulsion Injuries

An avulsion or crush injury may tear the nail completely away from the digit or raise a flap of nail bed matrix. Often fragments of matrix tissue may be left on the underside of the avulsed nail; these should be preserved for use as free grafts and, when possible, attached to the nail bed using fine 7-0 absorbable sutures. When the nail or avulsed nail bed fragments are not available, or in the case of a large defect, a full-thickness nail bed graft can be harvested from the patient's toe and sutured into the nail bed of the affected finger. As these injuries are complex and their repair is technically challenging, consultation with a hand or plastic surgeon is appropriate. In addition, avulsion injuries to the nail bed have the poorest prognosis of any fingertip injury.

Avulsion injuries may also incompletely tear the proximal portion of the nail bed or the germinal matrix, normally located under the eponychium. When this happens, the germinal matrix may lie on top of the eponychium. Management entails replacement of the matrix into its anatomic position using a series of three horizontal mattress sutures (Fig. 39-3). One suture is placed through the center and one in each corner of the eponychial fold. The sutures are then passed through the proximal portion of the corresponding segment of avulsed germinal matrix and then back out through the nail fold, pulling the matrix back to its anatomic position.[8]

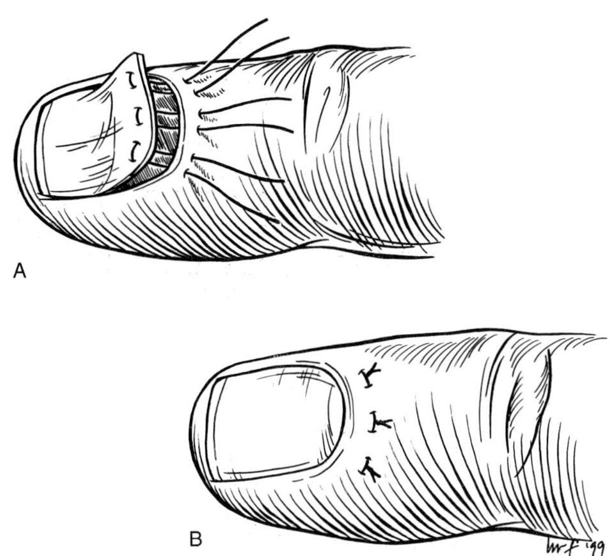

FIG. 39-3. Technique for repair of an avulsion of the germinal matrix using three horizontal mattress sutures. (From Chudnofsky CR, Sebastian S: Special wounds—Nail bed, plantar puncture, and cartilage. *Emerg Med Clinics North Am* 10:808, 1992, with permission.)

RING TOURNIQUET SYNDROME

A tight ring encircling the proximal phalanx may become entrapped because of distal swelling. Such swelling may be the result of trauma, infections, skin disorders, allergic reactions, or the tight ring alone. As the digit expands, venous outflow is restricted by the tight ring, producing more swelling. This vicious cycle may lead to nerve damage, ischemia, and digital gangrene.

The finger should be assessed for lacerations, sensory function (two-point discrimination), and perfusion (color and capillary refill). Digital artery pulsations can be detected with a Doppler flow meter, although this is usually not required. The presence of impaired sensation or diminished perfusion indicates significant constriction; rapid ring removal is then warranted. Rapid removal usually requires cutting the ring. If sensation and perfusion are intact, removal can be attempted with slower techniques that preserve the ring. The exception to ring preservation methods arises when there is an underlying phalangeal fracture; it is then prudent to cut the ring off.

In all methods, the hand should be elevated to encourage venous and lymphatic drainage, thus reducing swelling. Alternatively, the finger can be circumferentially wrapped with a 1/2- to 1-in. elastic band (e.g., Penrose drain), starting from the distal tip and winding the band tightly around the finger, progressing toward the proximal phalanx to reduce swelling. The wrap is left in place for several minutes before it is unwrapped and the ring is removed by one of the methods described below. Regional anesthesia is often required, particularly in patients who cannot tolerate the pain of circumferential compression. The metacarpal block is ideal because it produces less swelling of the finger than a digital block.

The simplest technique is lubrication. A variety of water-soluble lubricants can be applied to the digit and the ring removed with circular motion and traction.

The string technique uses a length of string wound circumferentially around the finger. When string is unwrapped, the ring is advanced toward and off the distal tip of the finger. Either string, umbilical tape, or 0-gauge silk sutures can be used. Synthetic monofilament sutures should not be used because they tend to cut the skin. The required length depends on the diameter of the string and the size of the finger; up to 100 in. of string may be required. The method starts by passing one end of the string under the ring and then wrapping the finger, starting next to the ring and winding clockwise, with each loop snug against the previous one, from proximal to distal. With each loop, the tissue underneath is compressed. When it is completely wrapped, the finger should be entirely covered by the string with no tissue showing between the loops (Fig. 39-4*A*). Wrapping and compression is a painful process and usually requires regional anesthesia. To remove the ring, the proximal end of the string is slowly unwrapped in a counterclockwise manner, advancing the ring toward the distal end as the string unwinds (Fig. 39-4*B*). The proximal interphalangeal region is the widest portion of the finger and is the most difficult site over which to maneuver the ring. Abrasions are commonly produced with the string method.

A variety of modifications to the string technique have been described. One involves wrapping from distal to proximal so as to reduce distal edema. Elastic band compression to reduce digital edema can be combined with a blood pressure cuff inflated above systolic pressure to prevent reaccumulation of edema once the elastic band is removed.[11] Another method uses a self-adherent compression bandage.[12]

The rubber band technique uses a 3- to 4-mm rubber band that is passed between the ring and skin; the two ends of the rubber band are then picked up by a clamp and used to place distal traction on the ring. The finger and ring are then lubricated. Traction is applied to the rubber band as it is moved circumferentially around the ring, slowly pulling it distal.[13]

Ring cutters are available in both manual and power models. The cutter has a small guard that fits underneath the ring and contains a channel allowing the circular blade to cut down through the ring without coming in contact with the skin. Sometimes, the swelling is so tight that the guard cannot slip under the ring. In these cases, reducing edema by using an elastic band, as noted above, may be successful. Alternatively, the circular ring may be deformed into an oval, creating a gap on the long axis of the ring. Rings should be cut in the thinnest and most accessible site. Thin and flexible rings may require only one cut; the ring is then removed by bending the two ends and pulling the ring open. Thick rings cannot easily be bent; such rings may need to be cut in two locations, opposite each other, separating the ring into two halves.

Very thick or tempered industrial objects (nuts or machine parts) may occasionally be placed on fingers and become stuck. Removal

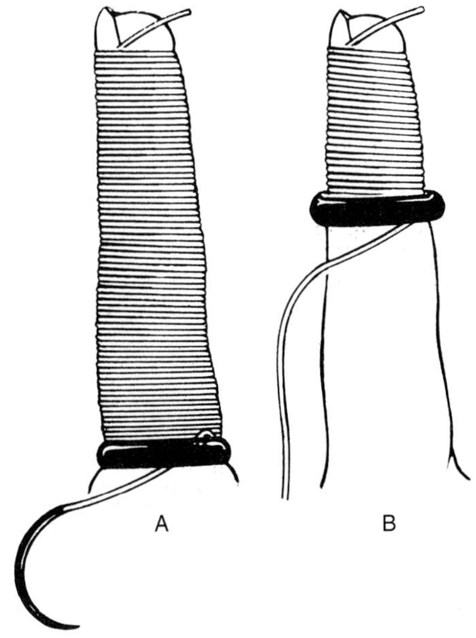

FIG. 39-4. String technique for ring removal. **A.** Completely wrapped. **B.** Unwrapping with ring advancing off with the string.

of these objects may require bolt cutters or motorized hand-held cutters. When these devices are used, the underlying skin should be protected from injury by a Silastic band or similar material. To prevent thermal burn from motorized cutters, water should be used for cooling during the cutting process.

After removal, sensation and perfusion should be reassessed. Tetanus prophylaxis may be required.

REFERENCES

1. Burkhalter WE: Fingertip injuries. *Emerg Med Clin North Am* 3:245, 1985.
2. Hart RG, Kleinert HE: Fingertip and nail bed injuries. *Emerg Med Clin North Am* 11:755, 1993.
3. Karev A: A simple fingertip tourniquet. *Br J Plastic Surg* 32:136, 1979.
4. Shaw JA, DeMuth WW, Gillespy AW: Guidelines for the use of digital tourniquets based on physiologic pressure measurements. *J Bone Joint Surg* 67A:1086, 1985.
5. Abbase EA, Tadjalli HE, Shenaq SM: Fingertip and nail bed injuries: Repair techniques for optimum outcome. *Postgrad Med* 98:217, 1995.
6. Herndon JH: Hand injuries—Special considerations in children. *Emerg Med Clin North Am* 3:405, 1985.
7. Browne EZ: Complications of fingertip injuries. *Hand Clin* 10:125, 1994.
8. Chudnofsky CR, Sebastian S: Special wounds: Nail bed, plantar puncture, and cartilage. *Emerg Med Clin North Am* 10:801, 1992.
9. Seaberg DC, Angelos WJ, Paris PM: Treatment of subungual hematomas with nail trephination: A prospective study. *Am J Emerg Med* 9:209, 1991.
10. Meek S, White M: Subungual hematomas: is simple trephining enough? *J Accid Emerg Med* 15:269, 1998.
11. Cresap CR: Removal of hardened steel ring from an extremely swollen finger. *Am J Emerg Med* 13:318, 1995.
12. Mullett ST: Ring removal from the oedematous finger: An alternative method. *J Hand Surg (Br)* 20:496, 1995.
13. McElfresch EC, Peterson-Elijah RC: Removal of a tight ring by the rubber band. *J Hand Surg (Br)* 16:225, 1991.

40 LACERATIONS OF THE EXTREMITIES AND JOINTS

Madonna Fernández
Wendy C. Coates

Greater than 12 million traumatic lacerations are treated every year in emergency departments (EDs) across the United States.[1] Extremities provide most of the interaction with the environment and are therefore particularly prone to injury.

Wounds may be caused by sharp or blunt mechanisms; each has different implications for evaluation and treatment (Table 40-1). Blunt-force wounds often have edges that are irregular and difficult to close; they are also more likely to contain an underlying fracture and are more susceptible to infection than wounds caused by sharp forces.[2] Contamination by soil, chemicals, and foreign bodies can adversely affect the outcome of any laceration, increasing the risks of infection and scarring and slowing the healing process. A more detailed discussion of hand and digit injuries can be found in Chapter 260.

TABLE 40-1 Sharp versus Blunt Trauma Wounds

	Sharp	Blunt
Edges	Straight	Irregular
Edema	Less	More
Underlying structures likely to be damaged	Tendons, nerves, vessels	Bones (fractures)
Susceptibility to infection	Less	More

TABLE 40-2 Relevant History—Questions to Ask the Patient

When did the injury occur?
What object caused the injury?
Are there possible contaminants?
Is there a foreign body sensation?
Is there numbness or decreased sensation distal to the wound?
In what position was the extremity at the time of injury?
Which is the dominant hand?
What is the patient's occupation?
When was the patient's last tetanus immunization?
Was the injury self-inflicted?
Was the injury the result of an assault?

CLINICAL AND DIAGNOSTIC FEATURES

History

The history required to evaluate lacerations to the extremities is the same as that required to evaluate lacerations elsewhere, with two important additions (Table 40-2). First, because of the mobility of the extremities, the position of the limb at the time of injury may influence the potential for damage to underlying tendons, nerves, blood vessels, and joints. Second, injuries to the dominant hand or limb are potentially more devastating than injuries to the nondominant limb.

Physical Examination

The diagnosis of an extremity laceration is straightforward, but damage to underlying structures must be excluded. Prior to administering anesthesia, the wound should be grossly inspected and the extremity assessed for injury to underlying tendons, nerves, and blood vessels. Pulses and capillary refill distal to the wound should be present and symmetrical when compared to the contralateral extremity. Distal peripheral nerve sensation should be tested separately for light touch (Figs. 40-1 and 40-2). Two-point discrimination at 5 mm should be

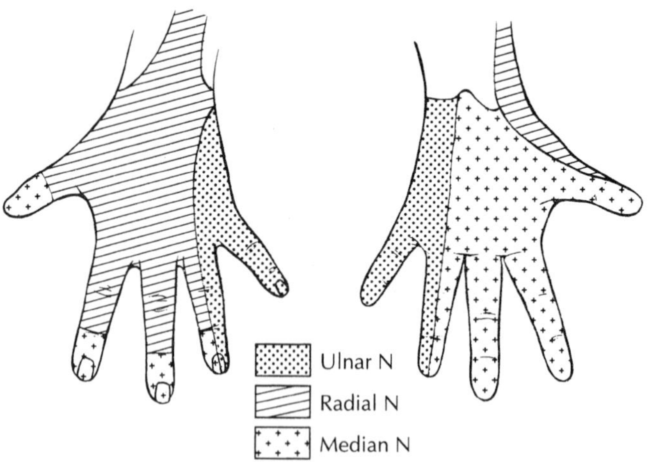

FIG. 40-1. Sensory innervation to the hand.

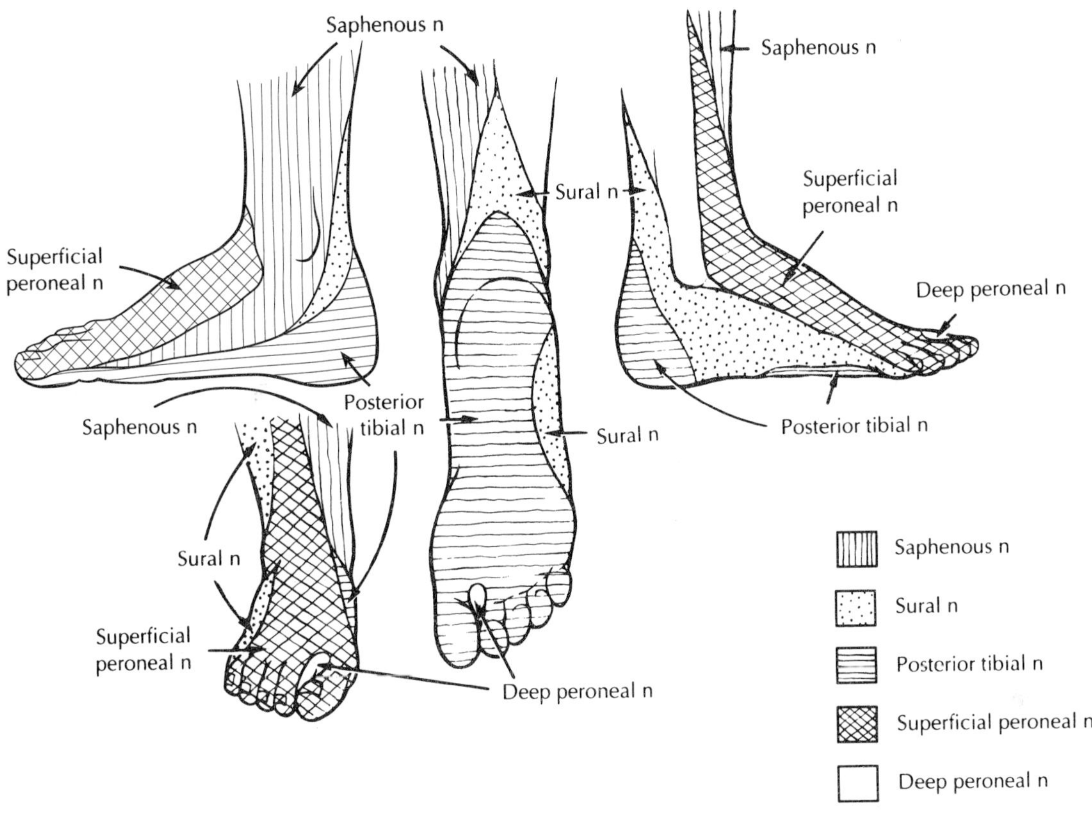

FIG. 40-2. Sensory innervation to the foot.

assessed on both sides of each involved finger to evaluate individual digital nerves. Motor function may be assessed more easily after the wound is anesthetized, since the patient's effort will be less affected by pain. After administering a local or regional anesthetic, examine the wound for depth and size. The involved extremity or joint should be placed through its complete range of motion, both actively and passively.[3] Motor nerve function should be treated individually (Table 40-3). Particular attention to underlying structures in the position of injury is essential, since this is where damage is most likely to be seen. Each tendon function should be tested separately (Fig. 40-3 and Table 40-4). A partially lacerated tendon will still function, and the injury may be overlooked if visual inspection is not performed. Care should be taken to avoid excessive countertraction during physical examination because this could completely disrupt a partial tendon laceration.

TABLE 40-3 Motor Function of Peripheral Nerves

Nerve	Motor Function
Radial	Wrist extension Digit extension
Ulnar	Finger abduction Finger adduction Thumb adduction
Median	Thumb flexion Thumb opposition Thumb abduction
Superficial peroneal	Foot eversion
Deep peroneal	Foot inversion Ankle dorsiflexion
Tibial	Ankle plantar flexion

Ancillary Studies

Soft tissue radiographs are required for all lacerations involving glass and any wound suspected of having a retained foreign body. Radiographs can detect glass fragments greater than 2 mm in diameter and gravel greater than 1 mm in diameter with greater than 95 percent sensitivity.[3] Wood, plastic, and most organic material is radiolucent. If a radiolucent foreign body is strongly suspected, computed tomography (CT) or magnetic resonance imaging (MRI) is recommended.[4] Although ultrasound has been advocated as a method to detect radiolucent foreign bodies, this technique has not been validated in prospective clinical studies. Plain radiographs of the involved extremity should be performed when an underlying fracture is suspected.

Lacerations over joints should be examined for joint capsule integrity. Unfortunately, prediction of joint penetration on physical examination alone is incorrect up to 43 percent of the time when compared with diagnosis by injecting the joint.[5] If joints are penetrated, management may change in up to 40 percent of these patients. If the depth of a wound suggests that the joint capsule could be violated, further evaluation is recommended. Plain radiographs may demonstrate air within the joint space, a clear sign of joint penetration. One also may consider injecting the joint. The skin should be cleaned with antiseptic and the joint injected with sterile normal saline (NS) through one of the standard arthrocentesis approaches at a site separate from the

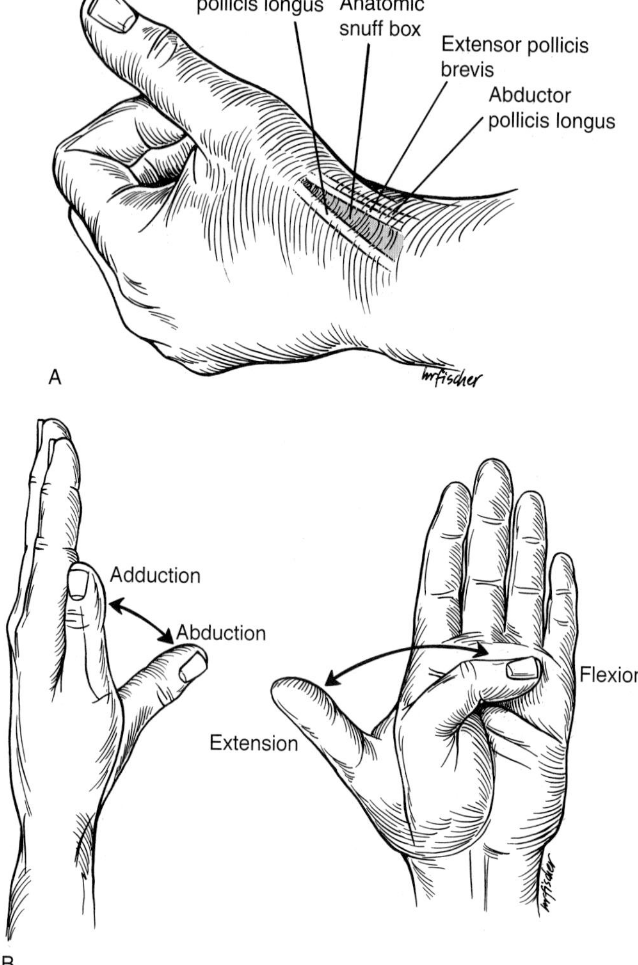

FIG. 40-3. A. Tendons of the thumb. **B.** Thumb movements.

TABLE 40-4 Tendon Function of the Upper and Lower Extremities

Tendon	Motor Function
Flexor digitorum profundus	DIP* joint flexion
Flexor digitorum superficialis	PIP† joint flexion
Flexor carpi ulnaris	Flexion at wrist with ulnar deviation
Flexor carpi radialis	Flexion at wrist with radial deviation
Extensor carpi ulnaris	Extension at wrist with ulnar deviation
Extensor carpi radialis	Extension at wrist with radial deviation
Extensor digitorum communis	Extension of digits 2–5
Flexor pollicis longus	Thumb flexion
Extensor pollicis longus	Thumb extension at DIP*
Extensor pollicis brevis	Thumb extension at MCP‡
Abductor pollicis longus	Thumb abduction
Extensor hallicus longus	Great toe extension with ankle inversion
Tibialis anterior	Ankle dorsiflexion and inversion
Achilles tendon	Ankle plantar flexion and inversion

*Distal interphalangeal.
†Proximal interphalangeal.
‡Metacarpophalangeal.

laceration (Table 40-5). Fluid leaking from the wound indicates joint penetration. For smaller joints or lacerations, a few drops of sterile fluorescein can be added to the NS and the wound inspected under a Wood's lamp after injection.

SPECIFIC ISSUES THAT IMPACT EVALUATION AND TREATMENT

Several factors can have an impact on wound healing in the extremities and over joints. These include intrinsic patient characteristics and chronic diseases that may hinder the normal healing process, such as age, comorbidities, keloids, and suspected abuse or assault.

Extremes of age have clinical relevance to wound healing. Elderly patients tend to have thin skin and decreased subcutaneous fat, especially over the dorsum of the hand or the anterior shin, making wound edges more difficult to oppose. This also results in decreased tissue viability when under the tension of sutures. Elderly patients are more likely than others to have underlying systemic medical conditions that may contribute to delayed wound healing. In addition, they are less likely to be adequately immunized against tetanus. Only 28 percent of people over age 70 in the United States have detectable serum antibody to tetanus.[6]

Extremely young patients are also at high risk for poor wound healing. They may have difficulty limiting movement of the injured extremity, and they are more likely to contaminate their wounds. The general rule to follow is "the smaller the child, the larger the dressing."

Many comorbid medical conditions may adversely affect wound healing in the extremities. Patients with diabetes mellitus are more prone to wound infection as a result of peripheral vascular disease and hyperglycemia. Other medical conditions that can hamper wound healing include chronic renal insufficiency, end-stage liver disease, anemia, chronic corticosteroid use, obesity, and connective tissue diseases such as Ehlers-Danlos and Marfan syndromes and osteogenesis imperfecta.

Keloid formation can be a problem for many patients. It is more common in patients of African and Asian descent but can occur in patients of any ethnic origin. The most common sites are the ears, lower abdomen, sternum, and upper extremity. Previous keloid formation in a given patient should alert the physician to the risk of subsequent keloids.

Injuries over the midshafts of long bones should alert the emergency physician to the possibility of assault. The patient should be questioned as to the mechanism of injury and examined thoroughly for ecchymoses and lacerations in various stages of healing. It is the physician's duty

TABLE 40-5 Recommended Volumes of NS and Needle Size for Joint Injection

Joint	Needle (gauge)	Volume of NS
Knee	18–20 G	60 mL
Elbow	18–20 G	20 mL
Ankle	20–22 G	20 mL
Wrist	20–22 G	5 mL
Digits	22–25 G	1–2 mL

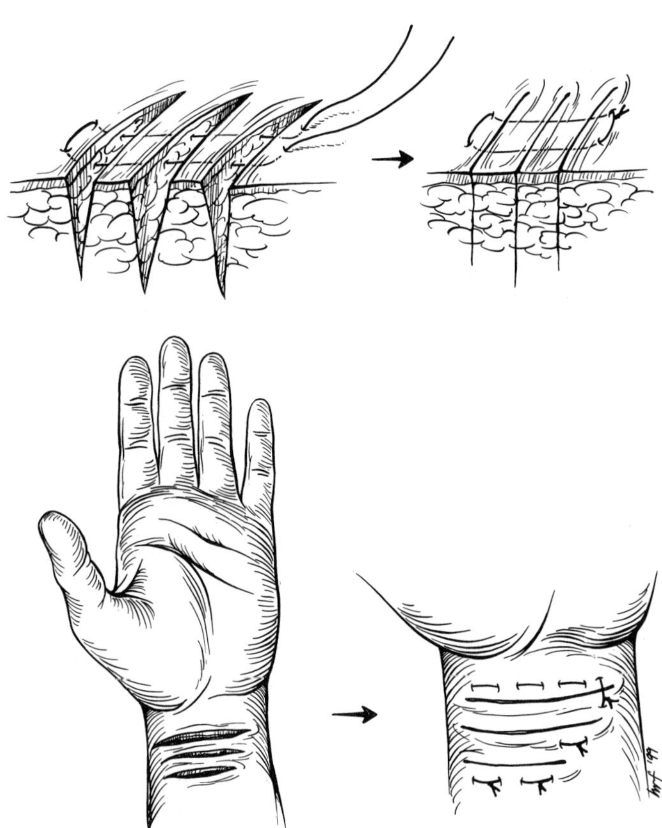

FIG. 40-4. Horizontal mattress sutures for multiple parallel lacerations.

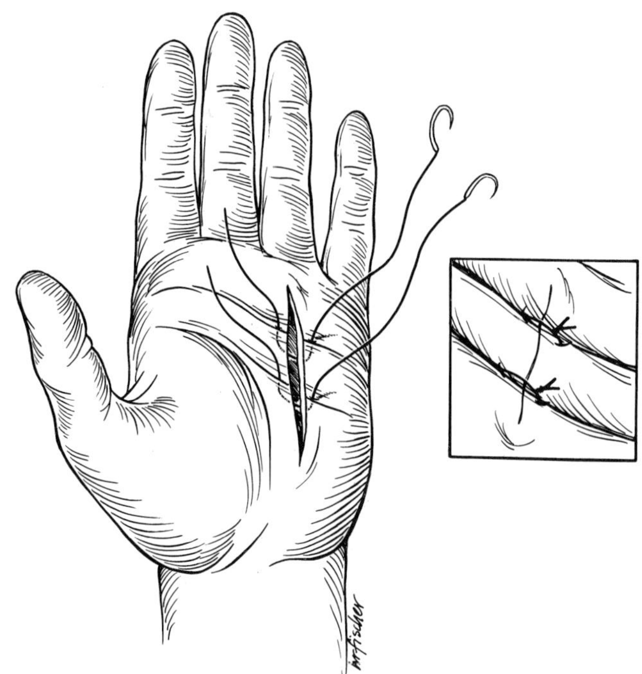

FIG. 40-5. Approximating palmar creases.

to report suspected abuse to the local law enforcement agency in accordance with individual state laws.

TREATMENT

The Forearm and Wrist

Any patient with a laceration to the wrist or forearm must be questioned about suicide. If the laceration is the result of a suicide attempt or gesture, the patient should be placed in a secure environment with adequate supervision.

The function of all tendons and neurovascular structures, especially the abductor pollicis longus and extensor pollicis brevis functions, should be checked in lacerations of the radial aspect of the distal forearm. Most of these wounds can be closed with simple 4-0 nonabsorbable interrupted sutures (nylon or polypropylene). If the wound is gaping or under high tension, absorbable deep buried sutures or nonabsorbable horizontal mattress suture are recommended. The multiple parallel lacerations that are classic for a suicide attempt often preclude closure with simple interrupted sutures, and the horizontal mattress suture method, running through all lacerations with one suture is ideal (Fig. 40-4). The depth of this suture should be uniform throughout the entire stitch. This reduces wound tension, prevents ischemia, and approximates the edges with fewer sutures.

The Palm

Anesthesia of the palm by local infiltration may be cumbersome, and a regional wrist block is often more effective. Lacerations of the palm should be examined carefully through range of motion to exclude flexor tendon or tendon sheath involvement (Table 40-4). Two-point discrimination should be carefully checked since the digital nerves are very superficial in the palm. Deeper lacerations between the metacarpophalangeal joints and distal wrist crease are judged to be in ''no man's land,'' and specialty consultation for exploration often is needed. All flexor tendon lacerations require consultation by a hand surgeon, but primary repair of flexor tendon lacerations can be delayed. In this case, the emergency physician should close the skin, splint the extremity in the position of function, and have the patient evaluated by the hand surgeon within the next few days. The closure method of choice in the palm is horizontal mattress sutures with 5-0 nylon or polypropylene. This reduces the chance that the suture material will pull through the skin edges. Every attempt should be made to reapproximate palmar creases by placing a suture directly through the crease on either side of the laceration (Fig. 40-5). It is important to observe the placement of the needle with each pass to avoid catching underlying tendons or tendon sheaths.

The Dorsum of the Hand

A radial nerve block is an excellent alternative to local infiltration for anesthesia on the dorsum of the hand. The skin on the dorsum of the hand is quite thin and can be difficult to approximate. Simple interrupted sutures using 5-0 nonabsorbable material are usually adequate. Since the dorsum of the hand is a cosmetically important area, alternatives include a dermal pull-through using 5-0 polypropylene or subcuticular sutures using 5-0 absorbable material (Fig. 40-6).

Lacerations over the metacarpophalangeal (MCP) joints suggest a potential clenched-fist injury (CFI) or ''fight bite,'' a laceration sustained with a closed fist to the mouth of another person during a fight. Patients may be reluctant to admit to the mechanism but should be warned of the serious risk of infection. These wounds should be inspected carefully with the digits flexed, reproducing the position at the time of injury. Any visible laceration of the extensor tendon or the joint capsule overlying the MCP joint indicates possible joint penetration, and a hand surgeon should be consulted. Radiographs should be obtained to evaluate for underlying foreign bodies, fracture, and air in the MCP joint. Even if the evaluation finds no evidence of joint penetration or deeper injury, it is probably best to assume that all lacerations over the MCP joints sustained in fights are too contami-

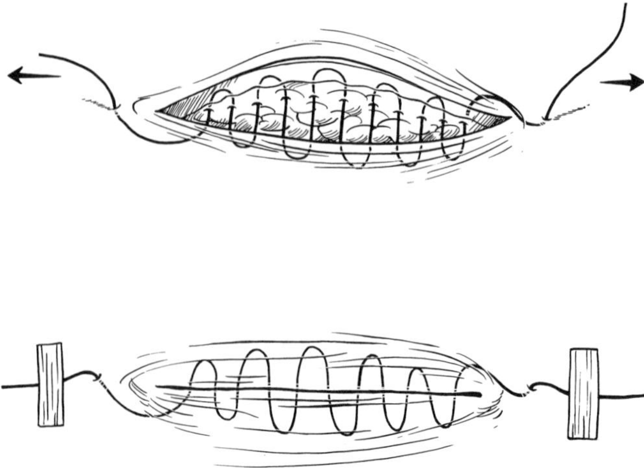

FIG. 40-6. Dermal pull through suture.

nated for primary closure, and such wounds should be allowed to heal by secondary intention. The wound should be irrigated and dressed and the hand splinted. The patient should be placed on a 5-day course of an oral antibiotic to cover mouth flora. The patient should be reevaluated in 2 to 3 days, or sooner if signs of infection develop.

Extensor Tendon Lacerations

Wounds over the dorsum of the hand and fingers may involve extensor tendons. These lacerations must be examined through complete range of motion, paying particular attention to reconstructing the position of injury. Extensor tendon lacerations that are proximal to the MCP joint in some cases can be repaired by an emergency physician who is experienced and comfortable with the procedure.[7] Many methods are used for extensor tendon laceration repair. One simple and effective method is a figure-of-eight suture (Fig. 40-7). This method places the knot on the side of the tendon, making it less obvious under the skin after repair. Nonabsorbable 4-0 suture should be used. Consultation and follow-up with a hand surgeon are recommended. Extensor tendon lacerations over the distal interphalangeal joint result in mallet finger (Fig. 40-8A), and those over the proximal interphalangeal joint result in a boutonniere deformity (Fig. 40-8B). These are treated with splinting for 6 weeks when closed, but when they are open, they require surgical repair.[8] Tendon lacerations of the thumb should be repaired by a hand surgeon.

Lower Extremity Lacerations

Lacerations of the lower extremity are under greater tension than those of the upper extremity. Fascia may be loosely approximated with buried sutures of 4-0 absorbable material. Any lower extremity laceration under significant tension should be repaired with a multiple-layered closure first using buried deep 4-0 absorbable sutures followed by simple interrupted 4-0 nonabsorbable sutures. Simple interrupted sutures of 4-0 nonabsorbable suture material may be used for skin closure in lacerations under minimal tension, and horizontal mattress sutures are ideal for wounds under moderate tension in the lower extremity. Wounds proximal to the knee and in areas that are usually covered (i.e., where cosmesis is not an issue) can be closed with skin staples. In patients with diabetes or those with stasis changes, deep sutures should be avoided because they markedly increase the risk of wound infection. Skin staples or horizontal mattress sutures are an excellent alternative in these patients.

The Knee

Lacerations to the knee are under marked active tension. The wound should be examined through range of motion, checking for the integrity of all ligamentous structures (Fig. 40-9). If joint capsule involvement is suspected, approximately 60 ml NS should be injected in a sterile fashion at a site separate from the wound to assess for leakage. The common peroneal nerve is prone to injury as it runs over the head of the fibula laterally, and distal function should be assessed. Deep popliteal wounds can injure the popliteal artery and tibial nerve. Distal pulses and nerve function should be documented prior to anesthetic administration and closure. Popliteal artery injury requires emergent angiography and vascular surgery consultation because the leg has minimal collateral circulation distal to the knee. Skin can be closed with 4-0 nonabsorbable material, using simple interrupted or horizontal mattress sutures. Skin staples are an alternative in patients subject to poor wound healing. The knee should be splinted or placed in a knee

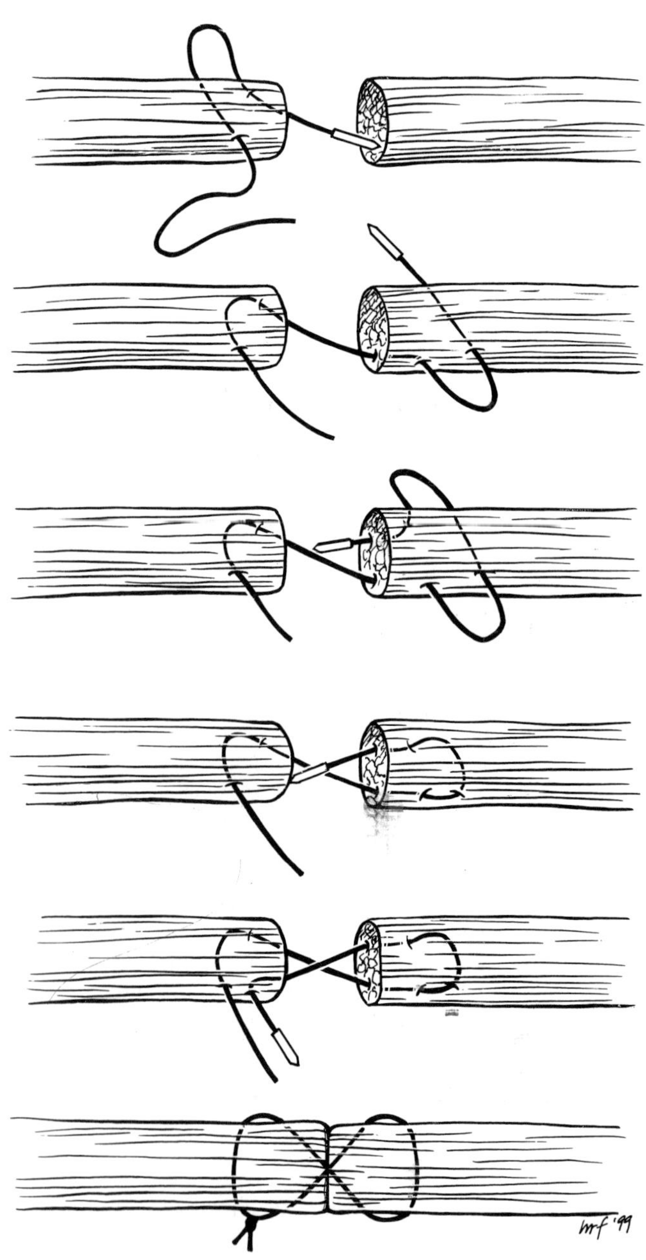

FIG. 40-7. Extensor tendon laceration repair with a figure-of-eight stitch.

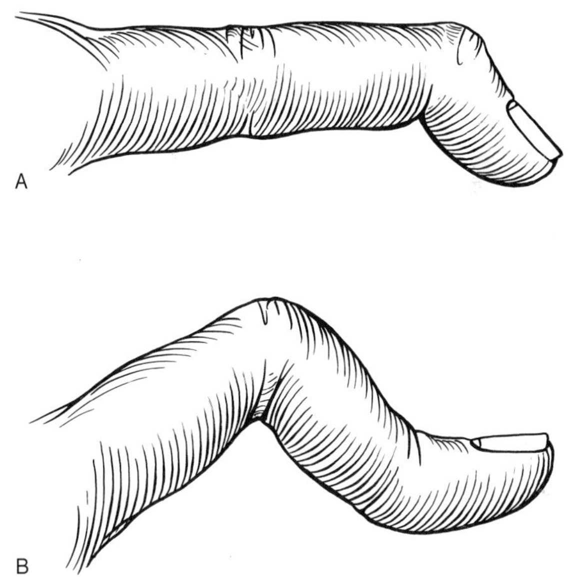

FIG. 40-8. **A.** Mallet finger. **B.** Boutonniere deformity.

immobilizer to decrease active tension and promote better wound healing.

Anterior Tibial Surface

Wounds over the anterior tibial surface are under considerable tension. Whenever possible, they should be approximated with a multiple-layered closure, first using buried deep 4-0 absorbable sutures followed by simple interrupted 4-0 nonabsorbable sutures. Horizontal mattress sutures using 4-0 nonabsorbable material are an alternative, especially in patients who are prone to wound infection.

The Ankle and Foot

Lacerations to the ankle and foot may involve the underlying tendons and neurovascular structures (Fig. 40-10). Sensory function should be assessed before anesthesia (see Fig. 40-2). After administering local or regional anesthesia, the ankle should be examined through complete range of motion, paying particular attention in the position of injury. The function of the extensor hallucis longus (EHL), tibialis anterior (TA), and Achilles tendons should be assessed (see Fig. 40-2). Partial tendon lacerations may be missed if the wound is not inspected visually through the range of motion, since some tendon function will remain unless the tendon is completely lacerated. The Achilles tendon is not the only tendon responsible for plantar flexion of the foot, and its individual function may be difficult to assess. The Achilles tendon can be palpated for defects; if it is completely lacerated, there should be a conspicuous absence of the tendon at the posterior ankle. The patient also can lie prone on the examination table with the foot dangling over the edge of the bed for the Thompson test (Fig. 40-11). The bellies of the gastrocnemius and soleus muscles are squeezed by the examiner. This should produce plantar flexion of the foot if the Achilles tendon is at least partially intact. Lacerations of the EHL, TA, and Achilles tendons require surgical consultation for repair because damage to these tendons can result in foot drop. The skin should be closed with simple interrupted or horizontal mattress sutures using 4-0 nonabsorbable material, and the ankle should be splinted.

Lacerations to the sole of the foot should be inspected for a foreign body because they often result from stepping on a sharp object. Regional anesthesia is ideal for the sole of the foot (see Fig. 40-2). Horizontal mattress sutures using 4-0 nonabsorbable material are recommended. The patient should be given crutches or a walking boot for comfort and to minimize trauma to the laceration while it heals.

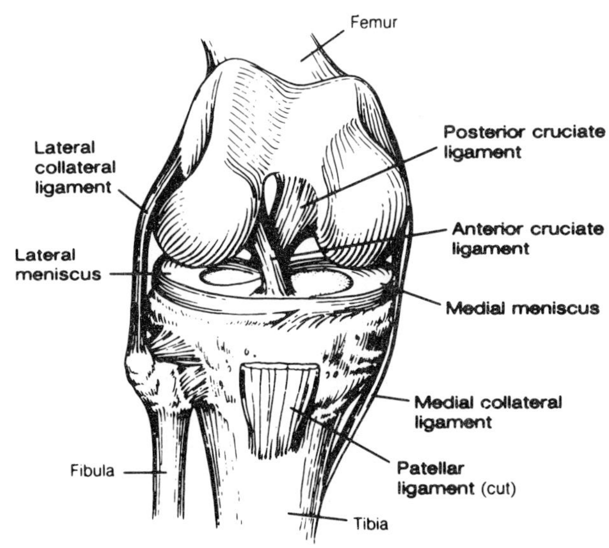

FIG. 40-9. Ligaments of the knee.

DISPOSITION

Admission Criteria

The majority of patients with extremity lacerations can be discharged after repair. Indications for admission include associated injuries that would otherwise require admission, joint contamination requiring irrigation in the operating room, compartment syndrome, severe infection, or significant infection in an immunocompromised individual.

Consultation

Orthopedic consultation is required for joint capsule penetration, open fractures, nerve lacerations, lacerations of the EHL, TA, or Achilles tendon, and for suspected compartment syndrome. Hand surgery consultation must be obtained for all flexor tendon lacerations, as well as for extensor tendon lacerations distal to the MCP joint, and should be considered for extensor tendon lacerations proximal to the MCP joint. With peripheral nerve and tendon injuries, it is appropriate for the emergency physician to close the skin and have the patient followed in the consultant's office within the next few days. Injury to the large, named arteries requires vascular surgical consultation.

After-Care Instructions

Wounds should be kept clean and dry for 24 h after suturing. Thereafter, they may be cleaned with running water and covered with a clean, dry dressing. Discharged patients should return for suture or staple removal in 7 to 10 days for upper extremity lacerations, 10 to 14 days for lower extremity lacerations, and 14 days for lacerations over joints. This time can be extended a few days in patients over age 65 years because epithelialization and noncollagenous protein accumulation are delayed.[8] Routine antibiotic prophylaxis is not recommended.[1,9] Prophylactic antibiotics are recommended for joint penetration, bite wounds, and in delayed primary closure. For markedly contaminated

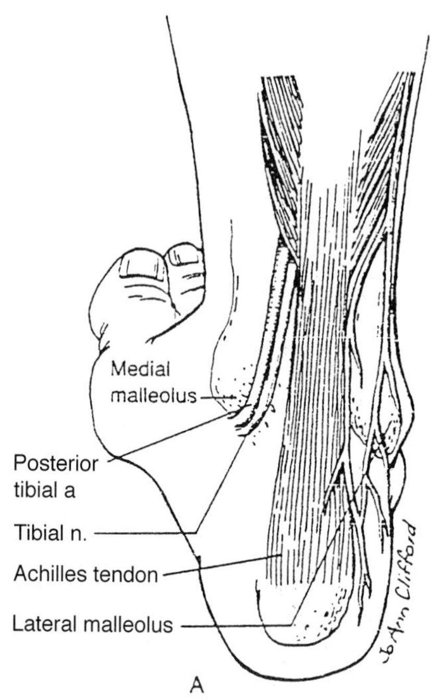

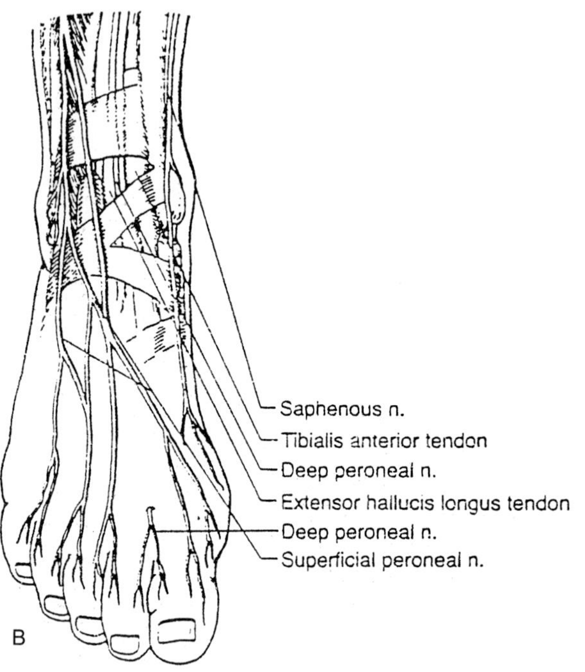

FIG. 40-10. Anatomy of the ankle and foot.

wounds, which required extensive debridement and irrigation, it is appropriate to reexamine the patient in 48 h for signs of infection and then begin antibiotics if necessary. Patients should be instructed to return for severe pain, erythema, purulent discharge, fever greater than 38.6°C (101.5°F), ascending lymphangitis, paresthesias, or weakness. Acetaminophen or nonsteroidal anti-inflammatories are usually sufficient for pain control. Elevation of the injured extremity will decrease tissue edema and expedite healing.

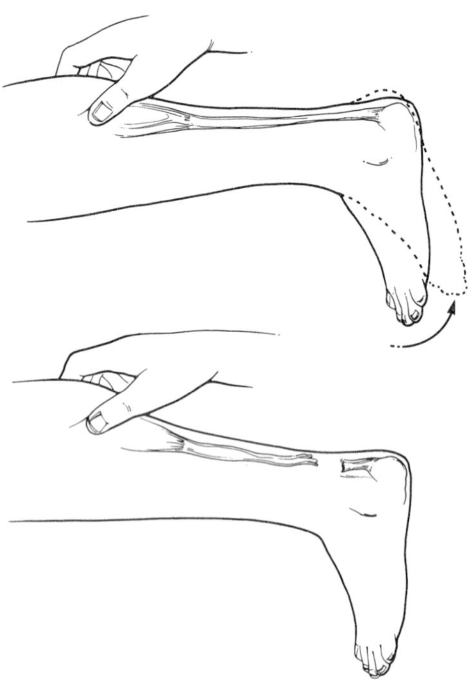

FIG. 40-11. The Thompson test.

REFERENCES

1. Singer AJ, Hollander JE, Quinn JV: Evaluation and management of traumatic lacerations. *N Engl J Med* 337:1142, 1997.
2. Edlich RF, Rodeheaver GT, Morgan RF, et al: Principles of emergency wound management. *Ann Emerg Med* 17:1284, 1988.
3. Howell JM, Chisholm CD: Wound care. *Emerg Med Clinic North Am* 15:417, 1997.
4. Russell RC, Williamson DA, Sullivan JW, et al: Detection of foreign bodies in the hand. *J Hand Surg* 16:2, 1991.
5. Voit G, Irvine G, Beals RK: Saline load test for penetration of periarticular laceration. *J Bone Joint Surg* 78:732, 1996.
6. Gergen PJ, McQuillan GM, Kiely M, et al: A population-based serologic survey of immunity to tetanus in the United States. *N Engl J Med* 332:761, 1995.
7. Ingari JV, Pederson WC: Update on tendon repair. *Clin Plast Surg* 24:161, 1997.
8. Noeller T, Cydulka RK: Laceration repair techniques. *Emerg Med Rep* 17:207, 1996.
9. Cummings P, DelBeccaro MA: Antibiotics to prevent infection of simple wounds: A meta-analysis of randomized studies. *Am J Emerg Med* 13:396, 1995.

41 FOOT LACERATIONS

Earl J. Reisdorff

EPIDEMIOLOGY

The human walks upright. Therefore, any injury to the foot jeopardizes the ability to function fully. Penetrating trauma involving the foot is sustained in a variety of novel manners from simple plantar puncture wounds to castastrophic lawnmower injuries. Urban children are at risk for sustaining foot lacerations while playing in water from fire hydrants.[1] These most commonly result from stepping on broken glass. Bicycle-spoke injuries result in complex lacerations with marked surrounding abrasions and even tissue loss.[2] Skin loss from bicycle-spoke injuries often occurs over the lateral malleolus and the base of the fifth metatarsal. Disastrous lawnmower injuries are usually sustained by push mowers, often when being pulled backwards.[3] Lawnmower-induced lacerations are heavily contaminated, averaging 3.1 organisms at the time of intraoperative culture. Lawnmower-induced foot lacerations are also sustained from debris flying out from the under carriage. Footwear does not usually prevent injury from mowers. High-pressure water-spray cleaning systems cause complex laceration-injection injuries. Due to the biomechanical importance of the foot and the enhanced risk of infection with wounds to the foot, lacerations must be treated properly to avoid complications.

PATHOPHYSIOLOGY

During standing and walking, the soles of the feet are in contact with the ground. This relatively small area of contact surface tells the body about its position, as well as detailed information about the terrain being traversed. The tough plantar epidermis and dermis are thick and able to withstand the numerous forces that a moving body produces. The primary "shock absorber" of the sole of the foot is a modified layer of fat. The blood and lymphatic vessels of the foot are under high hydrostatic pressure. As a consequence, edema easily results from injury and can retard healing. Except for the arch area, the epidermis and dermis of the soles are quite thick. Despite this, the foot is quite sensitive to two-point discrimination and pressure. The heel has an 18-mm-thick modified pad of fat separated into chambers by fibrous septae. There is an additional broad internal fibrous arch, called the inner cup ligament, aiding to maintain the shape of the heel. The skin of the sole readily hypertrophies and can become quite thickened, especially in people who walk barefooted.

The dorsal aspect of the foot provides little protection to underlying tendons, nerves, and blood vessels. The dorsum of the foot is particularly vulnerable to work-related injuries such as when heavy objects are dropped on the foot.

The pattern of pedal tendons roughly approximates that of the hand. One important location is just posterior to the lateral malleolus, where the peroneus longus tendon runs.

The structural design of the foot severely limits exploration of wounds to the plantar surface. The dense fibrous fatty tissue of the ball and heel makes exploration and visualization nearly impossible in the emergency department (ED), and the underlying structures are easily damaged. However, lacerations to the arch, although more uncommon, are more readily explored.

CLINICAL FEATURES

History

A limited, injury-specific history should determine when the trauma occurred. The mechanism of the injury helps determine the degree of injury, as well as the likelihood of injury to underlying tissue. High-energy injuries (e.g., a lawnmower injury) and crush injuries have a greater complication rate. The risk of a retained foreign-body and contamination risk should be determined. For example, was the laceration sustained by a farming accident (*Clostridium perfringens* contamination) or when wading in a freshwater stream (*Aeromonas hydrophila* infection)? High-pressure water systems used for cleaning surfaces cause severe laceration-injection injuries that are at risk for *Acinetobacter calcoaceticus* infection. Animal bites require consideration of infection by the rabies virus or bacterial pathogens such as *Pasteurella multocida* and *Capnocytophaga canimorsus* (formerly called DF-2 bacillus). The circumstances surrounding the injury are usually of limited concern unless dangerous activities are involved (e.g., knife-throwing contests among adolescents). Finally, the complaint of any new paresthesia, anesthesia, weakness, or the loss of function suggests a neurovascular or tendon injury, prompting a rigorous examination of the affected site.

The past medical history should include questions concerning tetanus immunization status and conditions that increase the risk for infection or delayed wound healing (diabetes mellitus, immunosuppression, valvular heart disease, and asplenia). The patient with diabetic neuropathy is at risk for recurrent trauma. Asplenic patients with a dog bite require prophylactic antibiotic treatment against *C. canimorsus*.[4]

Physical Examination

The physical examination determines the location, length, depth, and shape of the wound. Any wound on the weight-bearing surface is noted, because the wound care plan should consider avoiding weight bearing. As with all lacerations, the distal nerve function, motor function, and vascular integrity (pallor, capillary refill) should be checked. A foreign body is sought on general examination as well as during sterile inspection of the laceration just prior to wound closure. When possible, the wound is explored using a dry field. The loose thin skin over the dorsum of the foot allows for adequate visual, digital, and instrument exploration for tendon lacerations, as well as for foreign-body discovery. The dense tissue of the plantar surface of the foot severely limits wound visualization and exploration. The risk of creating new or further injury limits the exploration of wounds to the sole of the foot, especially at weight-bearing sites. The exception to this general policy is if a retained foreign body is suspected, such as an infected puncture wound presenting 48 h after the initial injury.

DIAGNOSIS

Laboratory studies are not indicated during the initial evaluation of an uncomplicated wound. If the wound becomes infected, a complete blood cell count may assist in determining the degree of cellulitis and the effectiveness of antibiotic therapy. Obviously, the most important parameter to monitor is the clinical appearance of the infection. Some clinicians also follow an erythrocyte sedimentation rate. Blood cultures and a wound culture are obtained if bacteremia is anticipated in immunocompromised patients. A wound culture of the laceration site immediately obtained in the ED for an open fracture or a grossly contaminated wound may be useful.

Radiographic imaging is required when an open fracture is suspected. The ideal form of radiographic imaging for foreign-body detection is debated. In cases of inert materials, standard plain-film radiographs and adequate wound exploration suffice. On the radiograph, the wound site is indicated with a radiodense marker. Though the retained material may be radiographically "invisible," there can be distortion of soft tissue shadows indicating the foreign body. When retained organic material is highly suspected, computed tomography is required. Retained foreign bodies can be visualized on ultrasound, although experience using this modality on the foot is limited.

TREATMENT

Wound Anesthesia

Certain areas of the foot, especially the plantar surface, are particularly sensitive to the infiltration of a local anesthetic. Lacerations involving the toes are anesthetized using standard digital blocks. Likewise, the lacerations to the dorsum of the foot are sufficiently prepared by local infiltration of lidocaine. Use of epinephrine-containing lidocaine is avoided in toe lacerations. Conscious sedation should be considered for plantar surface lacerations in children. For extensive lacerations, regional nerve blocks are used. Local infiltration of an anesthetic to supplement a regional block is frequently required. The two most commonly used foot nerve blocks are the sural nerve block and the posterior tibial nerve block. The posterolateral aspect of the sole is anesthetized using a sural nerve block, by depositing a generous band-like deposit of lidocaine 1 cm posterior to the distal aspect of the lateral malleolus. The tibial nerve block numbs the anteromedial aspect of the sole. A posterior tibial nerve block is performed by infiltrating the area just next to the posterior tibial artery just posterior to the distal aspect of the medial malleolus. (See Chap. 279.)

Topical anesthetic preparations use lidocaine mixed with any combination of tetracaine, cocaine, and epinephrine. These preparations are poorly effective on the dense epidermis of the sole, especially at the contact areas. Adequate anesthesia with topical preparations can usually be achieved on a dorsal laceration. If topical preparations are used, the blood coagulum is first removed and the solution-soaked cotton pledget is placed firmly into the wound.

Wound Preparation and Repair

The repair of foot lacerations, and especially plantar surface lacerations, has been poorly studied.[5] Few clinical practices regarding foot lacerations have been scientifically evaluated. Due to the inherent risk of infection with foot lacerations, excellent wound irrigation with copious amounts of saline irrigation is essential. The ideal time to perform a thorough dry-field exploration to determine tendon integrity and to detect foreign bodies is when the wound is completely anesthetized.

Debridement removes devitalized tissue, reducing the risk of wound complication. Nonetheless, debridement should be limited on the plantar surface because the thick, dense, fibrous tissue is not pliable. On the sole, any defect resulting from debridement is, therefore, closed under tension across the laceration.

Lacerations associated with nail injuries require close attention. On the dorsum of the phalanx, the skin is attached directly to the periosteum with no intervening layer of subcutaneous tissue. Therefore, a laceration to the nailbed places the underlying bone at risk for bacterial contamination.

The timing of closure must be considered. The foot is a body area with a high concentration of bacteria. Therefore, the risk of foot infection increases significantly 4 to 6 h after the injury.[6] A delayed presentation should prompt consideration of a delayed primary closure. Most foot wounds should not be closed after 6 h. If heavily contaminated, the laceration should not be repaired using a primary closure technique, especially if it presents to the ED beyond 3 h from the time of injury. For delayed primary closure, the wound is packed with saline-soaked gauze and the patient is placed on an antistaphylococcal antibiotic. At 96 h after injury, the wound is closed by using interrupted nonabsorbable monofilament sutures.

PLANTAR LACERATIONS When repairing a laceration on the plantar surface, the patient is placed in a prone position. The foot should overhang the cart or be elevated by placing a pillow beneath the ankle. Heavy, large suture needles are required to penetrate the hypertrophied epidermis and dermis of the sole of the foot. Heavy nonabsorbable monofilament suture is used; absorbable suture material is typically avoided in the foot. The plantar surface is approximated without tension usually using 3-0 and sometimes 4-0 suture with a large curved cutting needle. On the plantar surface, simple interrupted sutures usually suffice. The advantage of interrupted sutures is that if the foot becomes infected, individual sutures can be selectively removed. If there is tissue loss or a site is under tension, a vertical mattress suture may be required. In the arch area, achieving tissue eversion can be difficult. Tapes and adhesives are avoided on the plantar surface. Likewise, staples provide an irregular surface for weight bearing.

DORSAL LACERATIONS Dorsal surface lacerations are repaired almost exclusively with nonabsorbable monofilament suture material. Most commonly, 4-0 is used; for small simple lacerations, 5-0 suture can be used. Though running sutures are avoided on the sole, they are acceptable on the dorsal surface. Under select circumstances, tapes and staples can be used.

INTERDIGITAL LACERATIONS Lacerations between the toes are difficult to repair. The interdigital space is confined with a deep-set web space. Having an assistant gently separate the toes enhances the exploration and repair of interdigital lacerations. The use of simple interrupted sutures often leads to skin inversion and risk of failure of the initial wound repair. The most effective closure technique, albeit somewhat more difficult, is to place horizontal or vertical mattress sutures. This is best accomplished with 5-0 monofilament nonabsorbable suture on a small cutting needle. In young children, monofilament absorbable suture can be used, thus avoiding suture removal. When a web space laceration involves the neurovascular bundle, the skin is usually closed without any subsequent consideration to repairing the neurovascular injury.

TENDON LACERATIONS Similar to hand lacerations, flexor tendons are more aggressively repaired than are extensor tendons. Extensor tendon lacerations are sometimes treated with skin closure and splinting. Moreover, extensor tendon lacerations involving the midfoot and forefoot can often go unrepaired without sacrificing any necessary foot function. Regarding tendon lacerations across the toes (excluding the great toe), both extensor and flexor tendon injuries can be ignored without significant functional sequelae. Occasionally, a hammer toe or claw toe deformity results from the failure to repair a tendon (usually flexor tendon) laceration.[7] Although 80 to 93 percent of surgeons recommend repair of the flexor hallucis longus, no long-term evaluation has determined that this is essential.[5] In fact, there is limited information that unrepaired flexor hallucis longus tendon lacerations do not result in a functional deficit, even among athletes.[8] Nonetheless, adhesion formation is a common complaint. Lacerations to the flexor tendons of the other toes are usually unrepaired.

RETAINED FOREIGN BODIES Retained (nonreactive) foreign bodies such as glass can pose a problem. Chronic pain, especially during walking, can occur if the material is not removed. In the absence of chronic discomfort, inert foreign bodies can remain in the foot. The material typically becomes encapsulated, as is sometimes seen with insulin needles retained in the foot of patients with diabetic neuropathy. Obviously, organic material must be aggressively sought. Deep foreign bodies in the foot can be extremely difficult to remove in the ED. Surgical consultation and removal under fluoroscopy can be required.

HAIR STRANGULATION Hair strangulation-amputation is an unusual type of toe injury that is seen during infancy. A long strand of hair becomes wrapped around a toe and can involve several loops of the hair strand, all of which must be removed. This can be an occult source of irritability for infants. Removal must be complete so that the neurovascular bundle is not transected. Moreover, complete removal eliminates any further circumferential laceration of the skin around the toe. A novel approach to removal involves the use of hair-dissolving compounds. This approach has not been studied sufficiently to recommend it. The most certain approach to salvage the compromised digit is to make a midline longitudinal incision along the extensor surface of the toe. The incision should be deep enough to split the fibers of the extensor ligament without transecting the fibers. The multiple strands of hair are then removed using fine forceps without teeth. Unfortunately, the toe often retains the initial appearance, making one uncertain whether all of the strands have been removed or cut.

DISPOSITION

A bulky dressing is applied to the plantar surface to cushion any plantar laceration. For large lacerations on the plantar surface, weight bearing is avoided for at least 5 days. However, infants will naturally step on the injured site. Crutches are too difficult to use in children younger than age 7 years. Therefore, younger children may need to be carried. Elevation of the extremity decreases swelling and infection risk. Sutures are removed in 10 to 14 days.

Antibiotic prophylaxis should be considered in foot lacerations. Infection occurs in 18[9] to 34[1] percent of foot lacerations. In small lacerations to the dorsum of the foot, antibiotic prophylaxis is unnecessary. Animal bites require coverage against *Staphylococcus, Streptococcus,* and *Pasteurella*. Asplenic or immunocompromised patients who sustain a dog bite to the foot should receive coverage against *C. canimorsus*. Amoxicillin-clavulanate will cover all four organisms. A foot laceration caused from wading in freshwater streams should receive antibiotic prophylaxis for *Aeromonas hydrophila* (a gram-negative bacillus) with a fluoroquinolone. An *Aeromonas* infection should be suspected for rapidly developing infections involving foot lacerations. *Aeromonas* infections occur 8 to 48 h after inoculation and are rapidly progressive. There is a tendency for deeper structures to become involved: fascia, tendon, muscle, bone, or joint involvement occurs in 39 percent of cases.[10] Compartment syndrome, myonecrosis, and foot amputation can result. Effective antibiotic coverage against *Aeromonas* includes aminoglycosides, trimethoprim-sulfamethoxazole, and fluoroquinolones. Though fluoroquinolones are routinely used in the adult for *A. hydrophila*, their use is avoided in children. Open fractures are most commonly infected by *S. aureus*, so patients should receive a first-generation cephalosporin and an aminoglycoside in the ED. For other lacerations, antistaphylococcal antibiotics are sufficient.

REFERENCES

1. Joffe M, Torrey SB, Baker D: Fire hydrant play: Injuries and their prevention. *Pediatrics* 87:900, 1991.
2. D'Souza LG, Hynes DE, et al: The bicycle spoke injury: An avoidable accident? *Foot Ankle Int* 17:170, 1996.
3. Anger DM, Ledbetter BR, Stasikelis PJ, Calhoun JH: Injuries of the foot related to the use of lawn mowers. *J Bone Joint Surg [Am]* 77:719, 1995.
4. American College of Emergency Physicians: Clinical policy for the initial approach to patients presenting with penetrating extremity trauma. *Ann Emerg Med* 3:1147, 1994.
5. Yancey HA Jr: Lacerations of the plantar aspect of the foot. *Clin Orthop* 122:46, 1977.
6. Trott AT: *Wounds and Lacerations: Emergency Care and Closure*, 2d ed. St. Louis: Mosby, 1997, p 33.
7. Floyd DW, Heckman JD, Rockwood CA: Tendon lacerations in the foot. *Foot Ankle* 4:8, 1983.
8. Frenette JP, Jackson DW: Lacerations of the flexor hallucis longus in the young athlete. *J Bone Joint Surg [Am]* 59:673, 1977.
9. Baker MD: Lacerations in urban children. *Am J Dis Child* 144:87, 1990.
10. Semel JD, Trenholme G: *Aeromonas hydrophila* water-associated traumatic wound infections: A review. *J Trauma* 30:324, 1990.

SOFT TISSUE FOREIGN BODIES

Richard L. Lammers

Soft tissue foreign bodies may be encountered when managing new wounds or evaluating complications of old wounds.[1] When evaluating fresh injuries, the physician is responsible for detecting foreign bodies and for deciding if removal is urgent, can be delayed, or is even necessary. Many foreign bodies should be removed in the emergency department (ED); for example, all foreign material within the cavities of fresh lacerations should be irrigated away, debrided, or extracted with instruments. The decision to remove foreign bodies embedded below the dermal layer of skin depends on the size, location, composition, accessibility, and anticipated mechanical and inflammatory effects of the object. Occasionally, patients with subcutaneous foreign bodies should be referred to appropriate physicians for delayed removal.

Many foreign bodies are detectable during clinical examination, but some will not be apparent to the sight or touch of the examining physician. Various imaging studies can be used to evaluate wounds when nothing is found during exploration but the probability of a concealed object remains high; some foreign bodies, however, may not be visible with any type of radiographic or sonographic study. Consequently, malpractice actions for missed foreign bodies will continue to plague emergency physicians.

PATHOPHYSIOLOGY

Transient inflammation is an integral part of normal wound healing. A small amount of foreign debris in a wound provokes an inflammatory response in an effort to eliminate or contain the invader. When large quantities of devitalized tissue, foreign debris, bacteria, or other irritants are present within a wound, this protective response intensifies. Excessive or prolonged inflammation may delay wound healing or destroy surrounding soft tissue and bone, producing periosteal reactions, osteolytic lesions, synovitis, and arthritis. If the body fails to dissolve or extrude foreign material, it will encapsulate it within a fibrous capsule. Many granulomas result from chronic inflammation caused by foreign bodies that inflammation could not eliminate. Once a retained foreign body is encapsulated, inflammation subsides.[1]

The type and intensity of an inflammatory reaction is determined primarily by the chemical composition and physical form of the foreign object. Material that is inert—such as glass, metal, or plastic—may not elicit any abnormal tissue response. Objects with smooth, nonporous surfaces produce less inflammation and fibrosis than those with rough surfaces. Most metals are inert, but those which oxidize will cause mild to moderate inflammation. Earrings with studs dipped in gold paint cause earlobe swelling and inflammation when the paint flakes off. Vegetative foreign bodies, such as wood, thorns, and spines, trigger the most severe inflammatory reactions. Sea urchin spines, other marine foreign bodies, and hair may cause chronic inflammation with granuloma formation.

In some cases, inflammation is caused by a local toxic reaction. For example, blackthorns contain an alkaloid that produces intense inflammation. The oils and resins in redwood and cedar splinters also cause considerable inflammation. Sea urchin spines and catfish spines contain venoms that cause severe burning pain at the puncture site and a variety of systemic symptoms.[2] A sudden, local inflammatory reaction from a rose thorn or cactus spine may be an allergic response to fungi on the plant. Some cacti cause a delayed hypersensitivity reaction. Systemic toxic and allergic reactions are unusual but serious complications of foreign bodies. Foreign bodies containing lead have the potential to produce systemic lead poisoning, particularly if they are in contact with pleural, peritoneal, cerebrospinal, or joint fluid.[3]

Infections are the most common complication of retained foreign bodies. Infection may result even when the foreign material itself is not contaminated.[4] Foreign bodies may incite a variety of soft tissue infections, including local wound infection, cellulitis, abscess formation, lymphangitis, tenosynovitis, bursitis, and osteomyelitis. These infections are characteristically resistant to therapy; antibiotics, anti-inflammatory drugs, and steroids may produce a partial regression of symptoms but seldom eradicate the infection. Some infections will resolve spontaneously once the foreign bodies are removed. Vegetative foreign bodies may cause fungal infections, particularly in immunosuppressed patients.

Foreign objects also can cause mechanical damage by compressing or lacerating anatomic structures or occluding vessels. Repeated movement of tissue containing a foreign object increases the fibrous reaction.

CLINICAL FEATURES

History

Every wound has the potential for concealing a foreign body, but only a small percentage of the lacerations and puncture wounds actually contain them.[1,5] Certain historical events are associated with a higher risk for a retained foreign body: the mechanism of injury, composition and shape of the wounding object, and the shape and location of the resulting wound. Objects that shatter, splinter, or break in the process of causing a wound often leave remnants behind. For example, a wound caused by glass that broke on the skin is more likely to contain shards than a wound caused by previously broken glass. Dental fractures following a blow to the mouth serve as a warning that fragments of teeth may be embedded in the lip or tongue of the patient or in the hand of the assailant. Thorns, spines, and sharp wooden branches are usually brittle and tend to penetrate deeply into puncture wounds before breaking. Wood splinters are notorious for fragmenting when they are pulled out of a puncture wound. Patients impaled by long, thin metallic objects such as hypodermic or sewing needles may remove them without realizing that a portion of the object broke off beneath the skin surface. Both remnants of a needle and impurities in street drugs can cause persistent pain or abscess formation at the site of intravenous drug use. Nails that penetrate socks and shoes may drive leather, rubber, or cloth into the plantar surface of a patient's foot. Blunt objects with a diameter greater than 4.5 mm may push a plug of skin deep into a wound, resulting in an epidermal inclusion cyst. If any object pulled from a wound does not appear intact, the wound should be explored for further contaminants.

Patients with retained foreign bodies may present to the ED after a wound heals, complaining of sharp pain with movement or with pressure over the site. Failure to heal a wound also may be evidence of a retained irritant. Chronic, delayed, and recurrent infections also can be associated with retained foreign bodies. New puncture wounds that become infected and infections that are resistant to antibiotic therapy suggest that a foreign body has been missed. Arthritis in a joint near an old puncture wound may be a thorn-induced synovitis. Delayed nerve, vessel, or tendon injuries also require further investigation.

Physical Examination

Physicians are occasionally surprised by foreign bodies that can be embedded in small or seemingly superficial wounds.[5] Several physical findings indicate the presence of a foreign body. A discoloration or visible mass under the epidermis makes the diagnosis obvious. Sometimes a mass cannot be seen but can be palpated. Sharp, well-localized pain with palpation over a puncture wound is a useful sign. Patients who report the sensation of ''something in the wound'' should be taken seriously because their perceptions are often correct. If passive range of motion of a joint near a wound is limited, a foreign body may be responsible.

Old wounds with retained foreign bodies may have a persistent purulent drainage, a chronic draining sinus, or a chronic granulomatous reaction. A sterile abscess that complicates wound healing may be the result of a foreign body.

Some foreign bodies are discovered in wounds unexpectedly, but most are found during a deliberate and careful exploration of wounds considered to be at risk. Adequate lighting, good hemostasis, complete local anesthesia, and patient cooperation are essential. Every effort should be made to visually inspect all recesses of a wound. Wounds deeper than 5 mm and wounds whose depth cannot be visualized have a higher association with foreign bodies.[5] If punctures and other narrow wounds make direct visualization difficult and the physician is concerned about the possibility of a foreign body below the surface, the wound margins should be extended with a scalpel (Fig. 42-1). However, wounds that penetrate deeply into adipose tissue are difficult to explore and easily hide foreign material. Blind probing with a hemostat is a less effective but sometimes acceptable alternative to wound exploration when the wound is narrow and deep and extending the wound is not desirable. This method is used frequently to evaluate plantar puncture wounds caused by nails and to search for clear glass, which is difficult to see in a wound. A closed hemostat should be introduced into the wound and either used as a probe or spread open and then withdrawn. If an instrument strikes a metallic or glass foreign

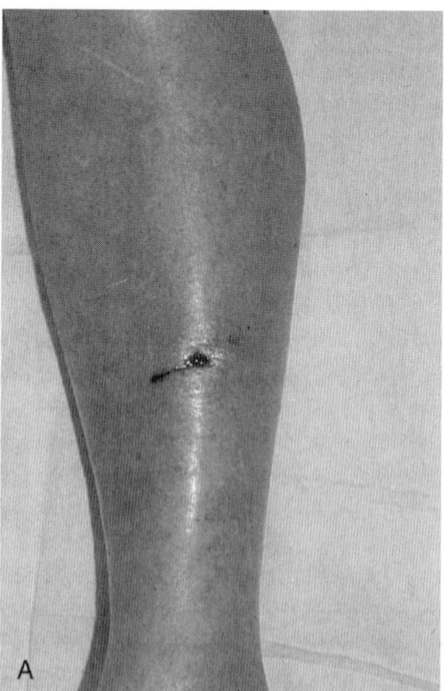

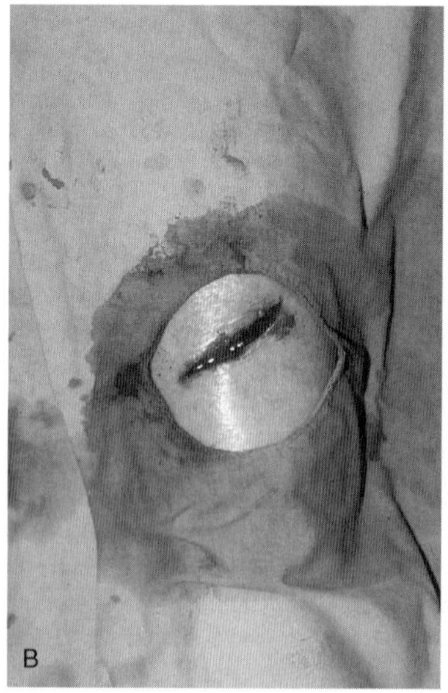

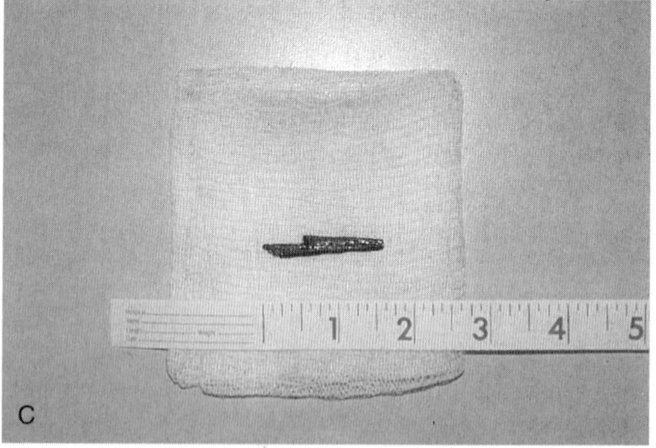

FIG. 42-1. A. (Plate 1) This patient's leg was punctured by a wooden stake 2 days prior to presentation. Surrounding cellulitis and point tenderness lateral to the wound increased the probability of a retained foreign body. **B.** (Plate 2) The entrance to the wound was extended. **C.** (Plate 3) A 1.5-cm piece of wood was removed from a 3.5-cm-deep wound.

TABLE 42-1 Experimental Studies on Foreign Body Imaging

Material, Author (Ref.)	Object Size (approximate)	N (No. of Observations)	Plain Radiography Sensitivity (95% CI)	Ultrasound Sensitivity (95% CI)
Aluminum:				
Ellis[8]	0.5 mm	1	100% (50–100%)	NS*
Glass:				
Courter[7]	0.5 mm	150	61% (53–69%)	NS
Courter[7]	1 mm	150	83% (76–88%)	NS
Courter[7]	2 mm	150	99% (95–100%)	NS
Manthey[17]	2 mm	20	95% (75–100%)	50% (27–73%)
Schlager[16]	5 mm	NS	NS	90% (56–99%)
Gravel:				
Chisholm[11]	0.5 mm	120	72% (63–80%)	NS
Chisholm[11]	1 mm	120	99% (95–100%)	NS
Chisholm[11]	2 mm	120	94% (88–97%)	NS
Schlager[16]	4 mm	10	NS	100% (92–100%)
Manthey[17]	5 mm	20	100% (96–100%)	40% (19–64%)
Plastic:				
Schlager[16]	1 × 2 mm	10	NS	100% (92–100%)
Manthey[17]	10 mm length	20	0% (0–17%)	40% (19–64%)
Wood:				
Jacobson[15]	1.0 × 2.5 mm	30	NS	87% (69–96%)
Jacobson[15]	1.0 × 5.0 mm	30	NS	93% (78–99%)
Manthey[17]	10 mm length	20	0% (0–17%)	50% (27–73%)
Schlager[16]	15 mm length	10	NS	100% (92–100%)
Cactus spine:				
Manthey[17]	10 mm	20	0% (0–17%)	30% (12–54%)
Schlager[16]	Agave spine	10	NS	100% (92–100%)

*NS = not studied.

body, it will produce a grating sensation. The instrument should not be used to grasp blindly in hopes of clamping an unseen object. This technique is especially dangerous in hands, feet, or faces, where direct visualization is the preferred method of exploration.

DIAGNOSIS

Soft tissue foreign bodies must be identified and located before treatment decisions can be made. Imaging studies should be ordered in most cases where a retained foreign body is suspected but not found during wound exploration or when thorough wound exploration is technically impossible. They are also useful after initial removal of multiple foreign bodies to determine if all the pieces were found.

A number of imaging modalities are available. The ability of any of these modalities to find a foreign body depends on the characteristics of the study as well as the object's size, shape, density, and orientation relative to the imaging beam. Materials that are the same density as surrounding soft tissue are difficult to see with any type of radiographic or sonographic technique.

Plain Radiography

It is fortunate that many foreign bodies are radiopaque; most foreign bodies that can be missed during the initial clinical evaluation can be seen on plain films.[6] Plain films are readily available but must be obtained with appropriate technique and inspected carefully to detect small and faint foreign bodies. Metal, mammalian bone, some types of fish bones, teeth, pencil graphite, certain plastics, glass, gravel, sand, and aluminum are visible on plain radiographs[1,7–12] (Table 42-1). Almost all glass is visible on radiographs if it is 2 mm or larger, and contrary to myth, glass does not have to contain lead to be visible on plain films.[1,5,7] A radiopaque fragment is more easily seen if it is positioned parallel to the central ray of the x-ray beam, which increases its apparent thickness.

Radiographs should be obtained with an underpenetrated "soft tissue technique," producing a lighter film that increases the contrast between the foreign body and surrounding tissue.[1] Plain films should be taken in multiple projections to separate the shadow of the foreign body from underlying bone and to help gauge the depth of the object in the tissue. Chronic inflammatory changes may create secondary bony changes such as osteolytic and osteoblastic lesions, pseudotumor formation, and periosteal reaction, revealing the object's location.

Many common or highly reactive materials such as wood, thorns, cactus spines, fish bones, most plastics, and other organic matter are not visible on plain films.[1] Sometimes there is indirect evidence of their presence; a radiolucent filling defect may occur when the object is less dense than surrounding tissue. Even radiopaque foreign bodies may be invisible on plain films if they are projected over bone or impacted in bone.

Computed Tomography (CT)

CT is capable of detecting more types of foreign materials than plain-film radiography because it is 100 times more sensitive in differentiating densities.[6,10] Subtle density differences can be distinguished with a narrow radiographic density window adjustment, particularly if a computer workstation is used to vary the gain and contrast settings.[10] Thorns, spines, wood toothpicks, and plastic foreign bodies have been identified with this method. CT may detect objects embedded in bone, and isodense objects may be outlined by surrounding air within the wound. Digital edge enhancement can further improve the visibility of these objects.[9] CT images can be created in multiple planes and can demonstrate the relationship of a foreign object to important anatomic structures. The principal disadvantages of CT are its cost and higher radiation dose. However, even CT may not demonstrate thorns, spines, and some types of wood. Wood may have a CT pattern that is similar to a gas bubble or bone fragment.[9] As wood absorbs fluid from tissue, it becomes isodense and difficult to distinguish from surrounding tissue.

Ultrasonography

Sonography has been described in clinical case reports to identify soft tissue foreign bodies such as wood, fish bones, sea urchin spines, and other vegetative materials.[13–15] However, this method has had a wide variation in sensitivity, specificity, and overall accuracy for the detection of soft tissue foreign bodies in experimental studies (see Table 42-1). Depending on the experimental model, the sensitivity for foreign body detection with ultrasound is 30 to 100 percent with a specificity of 70 to 90 percent.[15–17] In clinical practice, variation may be due to the size and sonographic nature of the foreign body, the presence of confounding objects (e.g., bone, blood, air, purulence, scars, old sutures) near or about the foreign body, and operator skill and experience. Areas with many echogenic structures such as calcifications, sesamoid bones, and tendons may hide foreign bodies within their acoustic shadows, so these areas must be scanned slowly to detect foreign bodies that are small or oriented perpendicular to the skin surface. Some areas of the body that are prone to foreign body penetration, such as the web spaces of the hands or toes, may not accommodate an ultrasound probe.

Once a foreign body is confirmed by plain films or CT studies, sonography can be used in place of fluoroscopy to guide an instrument to the object during retrieval.[18] The scanning beam should be oriented parallel to the long axis of a hemostat, which can be directed toward the long axis of the foreign body. Transverse and longitudinal scans provide views in multiple planes. A 7.5-MHz linear-array transducer can be used to find objects that are up to 3 cm deep.

The primary advantage of ultrasonography is that this imaging modality avoids radiation exposure. In addition, portable ultrasound machines are becoming increasingly available in EDs. The principal disadvantage of this modality is the variable sensitivity for foreign body detection for the reasons noted earlier.

Xeroradiography

Xeroradiographs enhance soft tissue images, improving images already visible on plain films. However, this modality fails to detect radiolucent foreign bodies and has been supplanted by other imaging techniques.[1,6,13]

Magnetic Resonance Imaging (MRI)

MRI can detect nonmetallic radiolucent foreign bodies and in limited comparison studies is more accurate than any other modality in identifying wood, plastic, spines, and thorns.[6] MRI should not be used with gravel or metal-containing foreign bodies because ferromagnetic streaks obscure visualization. MRI may prove more effective than CT in visualizing organic foreign bodies, but comparison studies are needed.

Selecting an Imaging Study

If a foreign body is suspected but not found during exploration of a wound, a plain film should be ordered first, since plain radiography will detect as many as 80 to 90 percent of all foreign bodies. It is prudent to order films if a patient believes there is a retained object. If the wound was caused by metal, glass, or gravel and no foreign body was found on plain films or wound exploration, the physician can end the search. For objects not routinely visible on plain radiography, CT scans are the modality of choice. Both plain films and CT scans are useful for identifying the composition, size, shape, and approximate location of an object in tissue. Ultrasound is not as reliable as CT in confirming the presence or absence of nonradiopaque foreign bodies. However, ultrasonography and fluoroscopy are effective methods for guiding an instrument toward a soft tissue foreign body.[18,19]

TABLE 42-2 Indications for Foreign Body Removal

Potential for inflammation or infection:
Vegetative or chemically reactive material
Heavy bacterial contamination (e.g., teeth, soil)
Proximity to fractured bone
Established infection
Allergic reaction
Toxicity:
Spines with venom
Heavy metals
Functional and cosmetic problems:
Impingement on nerves, vessels, or tendons
Restriction of joint mobility
Proximity to tendons
Impairment of gait
Persistent pain
Cosmetic deformity (e.g., tattooing)
Psychological distress
Potential for later injury:
Intraarticular location
Intravascular location
Migration toward important structures

TREATMENT

General Principles

Once a soft tissue foreign body is discovered, the physician must weigh the risk of leaving the foreign body in place against the potential harm of attempting to remove it. Not all foreign bodies must be removed, and not all that require removal must be extracted in the ED. However, every effort should be made to identify their presence during the initial visit. General indications for foreign body removal include potential for later infection, toxicity, injury, and functional problems (Table 42-2). Usually, objects that are small, inert, deeply embedded, and causing no symptoms can be left in place. A common question concerns bullets that come to rest deep within a muscle belly; they are usually not removed because the procedure can cause more damage than leaving the foreign object in place. Projectiles may drag bits of clothing or skin into the wound, so the entrance wound deserves cleaning and debridement. Bullet migration and embolization are rare but possible complications. Bullets near vessels can enter the systemic circulation. Bullets that cause distal ischemia, thrombus formation, or wall erosion or that lie within the lumen of a blood vessel require immediate removal in the operating room.

Thorns, spines, wood splinters, and other vegetative materials require immediate removal because they cause intense and excessive inflammation.[20] Foreign objects that are heavily contaminated, such as fractured teeth and soil-covered objects, should be removed as soon as possible; antibiotic treatment will not take the place of foreign body removal. Glass, metal, and plastic are relatively inert, and removal can be postponed, if necessary. Glass foreign bodies in hands or feet can cause persistent pain with gripping or walking, and they can sever nerves or tendons years after the initial injury. Patients with deep, sharp foreign bodies in these locations should be referred to appropriate specialists for eventual removal.

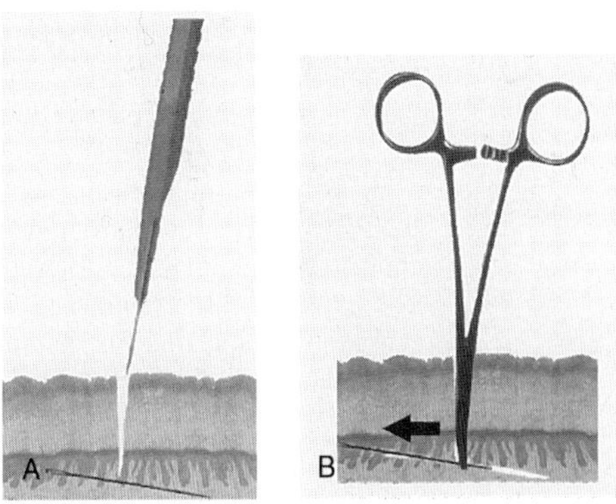

FIG. 42-2. **A.** (Plate 4) An incision is made perpendicular to the needle at its midpoint. **B.** The needle is grasped through the incision with a hemostat and backed out of the puncture wound.

Sometimes harmless foreign bodies are psychologically distressing to patients, particularly when they are visible under the skin surface or produce a lump. Patient concern may be a justification for elective removal.

Successful removal of foreign bodies requires adequate local or regional anesthesia and good lighting. Depending on location and depth, tourniquet control of bleeding and assistance may be needed. Depth and accessibility of the object and physician time are the limiting factors for removal of foreign bodies by the emergency physician. Foreign bodies buried deeply in adipose tissue or muscle are difficult to locate. Most foreign bodies in hands should be removed because the hand is mobile and sensitive. Deep exploration of hands by the emergency physician is not recommended because magnification and experience are needed to avoid injury to numerous closely spaced vital structures.

The emergency physician may not be able to devote more than about 15 to 30 min to the removal procedure, particularly when other seriously ill or injured patients demand attention. This amount of time is sufficient for locating most foreign bodies. The patient should be informed before the procedure that the duration of the exploration will be limited. If more time is required, the patient should be referred to a surgeon.

Methods of Localization

Accurate localization of a foreign body prior to removal is important because blind searching is time-consuming and can cause further injury. However, it is usually easier to detect the presence of a foreign body than to locate its exact position. If a foreign body is radiopaque, one can estimate its location and depth by taping radiopaque skin markers such as lead circles or paper clips on the skin at the wound entrance or directly over the object. With multiple projections, the object can be seen in relation to the markers. Hypodermic needles can be used as skin markers. Two or three needles are inserted into the skin near the object at approximately 90° to each other to provide a frame of reference around the object. Plain films taken in multiple projections allow the physician to gauge the distance of the object from the closest needle or its distance between two needles.

FIG. 42-4. To remove a friable foreign body such as a wood splinter that is parallel to the skin surface, an incision is made along its long axis. The object can be lifted out and the entire length of the wound inspected for remnants.

The limitations of this technique are that it does not provide a true three-dimensional image and that images on radiographs are distorted by divergence and parallax. Tendons and other structures may block the most accessible path to the foreign body. Alternatively, the site of injury can be rotated under fluoroscopy to visualize the object between the markers.[19] Radiation exposure should be minimized by brief, intermittent imaging and appropriate shielding. An incision is made between needles or markers, or dissection is carried along the path of the closest needle.

Specific Foreign Bodies and Removal Procedures

METALLIC NEEDLES Long, thin foreign bodies such as sewing and hypodermic needles may be difficult to locate in soft tissue. Two techniques are available for removing needles that are parallel to the surface of the skin. If the needle is superficial enough to be palpable, an incision is made at one end to expose and grasp it with a hemostat. If the needle is deep, an incision is made perpendicular to the needle at its midpoint, where it can be clamped with a hemostat and pushed out of the entrance of the original wound (Fig. 42-2).

Long, thin foreign bodies that are oriented perpendicular to the skin surface can be elusive. If a needle can be reached with an alligator forceps or hemostat, it can be pulled straight out. If a needle lies beyond the reach of a hemostat, the entrance wound must be enlarged with a skin incision (Fig. 42-3). However, the incision can easily pass to the side of the object, so the skin edges should be undermined, and

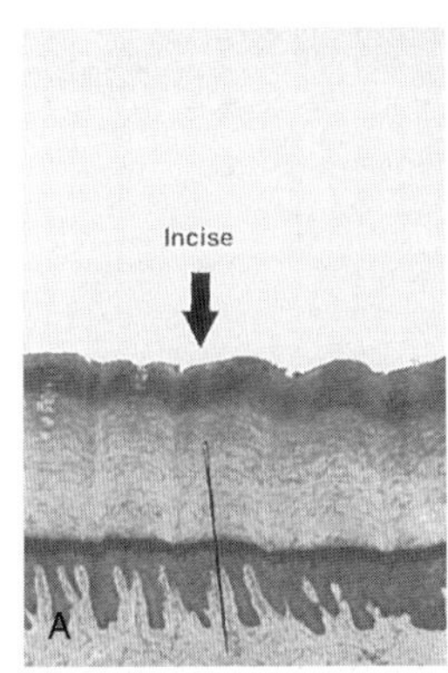

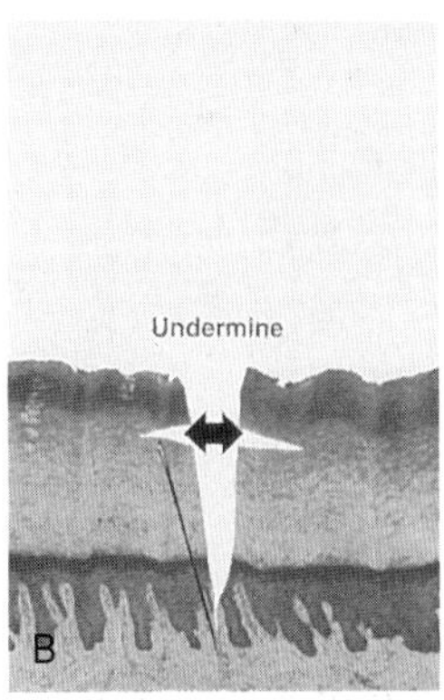

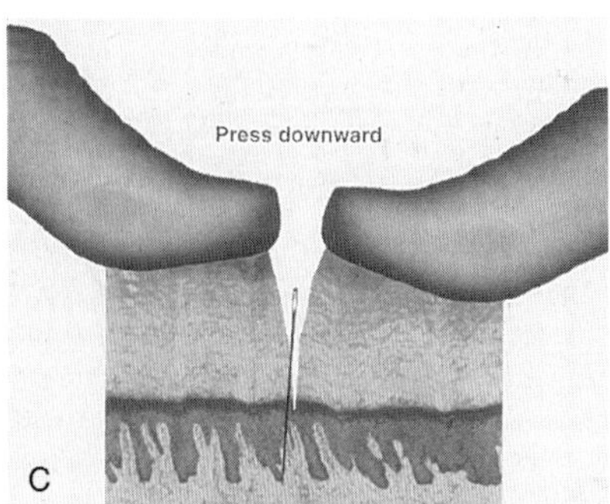

FIG. 42-3. **A.** The entrance site is enlarged with a skin incision. **B.** If the incision passes to the side of the object, the skin is undermined. **C.** (Plate 5) Pressure on the skin edges displaces the foreign body into the center of the wound.

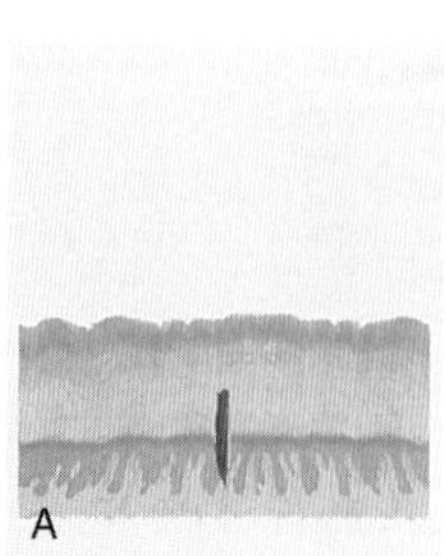

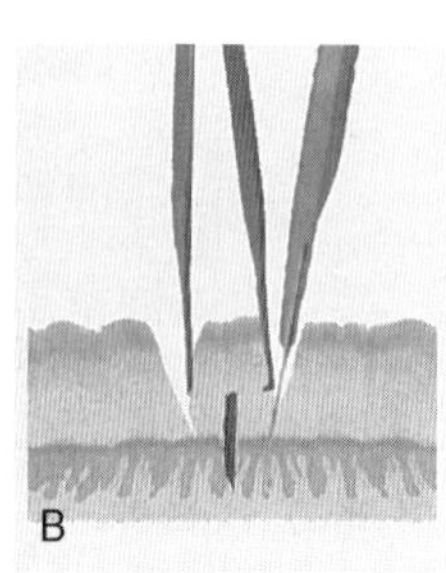

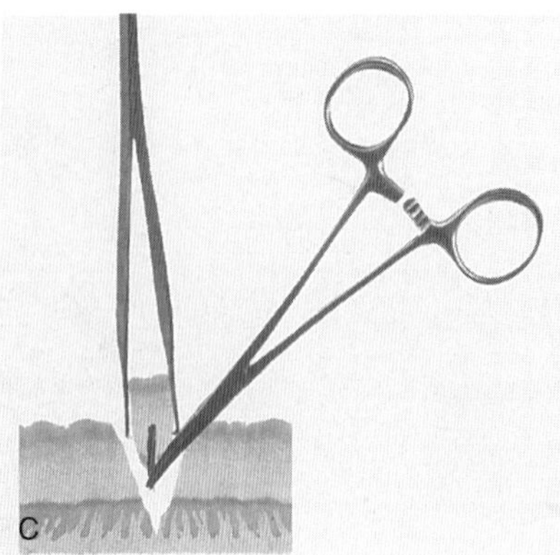

FIG. 42-5. Block excision is effective for foreign bodies that are friable, difficult to find, buried in fatty tissue, or stain surrounding tissue. **A.** A small, elliptical incision is made around the original wound. **B.** (Plate 6) The incision is undercut until contact is made with the foreign body. **C.** The block of tissue is grasped with a forceps, the foreign body is clamped with a hemostat, and both are removed.

pressure applied on the skin edges may displace the foreign body into the center of the wound, where it can be seen and grasped. Once removed, the needle and the wound should be inspected to ensure that the object was removed in its entirety.

WOOD SPLINTERS AND ORGANIC SPINES Solid foreign bodies can be pulled out of puncture wounds with forceps, but wood splinters and organic spines (e.g., cactus, sea urchin, and fish) may disintegrate with this technique. Only superficial splinters that are a few millimeters long can be grasped and removed with a fine-point splinter forceps. A splinter parallel to the skin surface should be lifted out of the wound after incising the skin along the long axis of the object (Fig. 42-4). If the splinter is lodged in the subcutaneous tissue, the entrance wound must be enlarged with a skin incision so that the foreign body can be grasped under direct visualization. Wood fragments may be impossible to locate precisely. One solution is to create an elliptical incision around the puncture wound and extract the fragment in a block of tissue (Fig. 42-5). The physician should avoid incorporating nerves, vessels, or tendons within the excised block. Either technique creates a larger wound but allows a better inspection and more thorough cleaning after removal.

Subungual splinters must be removed because subsequent infection is almost inevitable, and the distal phalanx is at risk for osteomyelitis. If the splinter is underneath the distal end of the nail, it can be grasped by a splinter forceps or hooked by a hypodermic needle bent at its tip. More proximal splinters can be reached by anesthetizing the finger and removing a wedge of the nail overlying part of the foreign body (Fig. 42-6). If pieces of the splinter remain, the entire nail can be removed.

Numerous, tiny cactus spines in the dermis can be plucked out individually with forceps or extracted together with depilatory wax, professional-quality facial gel, rubber cement, or household glue.[20,21] Larger spines and thorns should be removed with incision or excision techniques.

FISHHOOKS Fishhooks have a variety of sizes and shapes based on a common pattern (Fig. 42-7). The barb, which is a projection extending backward from the point of the hook, keeps the point embedded in the fish's mouth and makes removal from skin a challenging task. Most injuries with fishhooks involve the hand, head, or face.

Several methods for removing fishhooks in skin have been reported. The best strategy depends primarily on the depth of the hook. If the hook has multiple barbs, precautions should be taken to avoid impaling the treating physician, bystanders, or the patient (a second time) during removal by taping or cutting off the exposed barbs. With any technique, the skin should be prepared and anesthetized at the entry site. If the hook is superficial, gentle downward pressure is placed on the shank while the hook is simply pulled in a retrograde direction along the path of entry (Fig. 42-8).

The *string-pull method* is a variation on the retrograde technique. String is wrapped around the bend of the hook where it enters the skin. The end of the shank is depressed with one hand to disengage the barb from deeper tissue. The other hand then gives a quick pull on the string, extracting the hook (Fig. 42-9). The disadvantages of

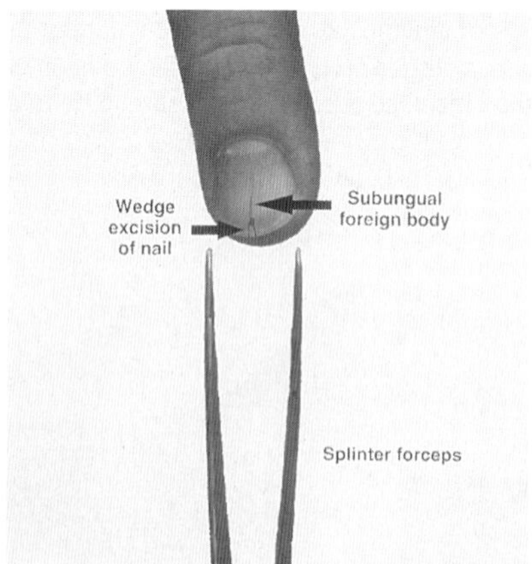

FIG. 42-6. Subungual foreign bodies that are beyond the reach of a splinter forceps can be exposed by excising a wedge of the overlying nail.

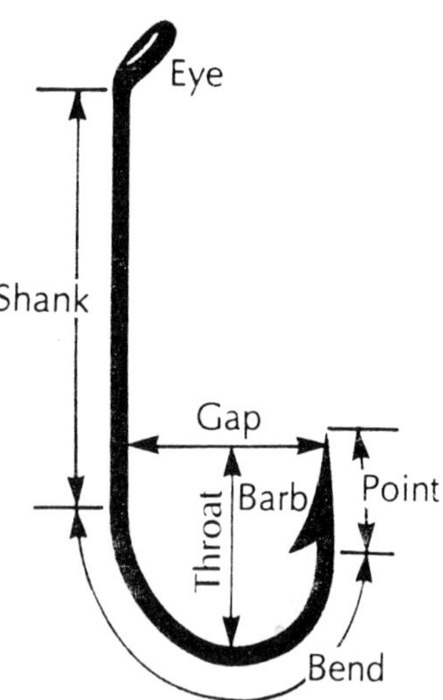

FIG. 42-7. Anatomy of a fishhook.

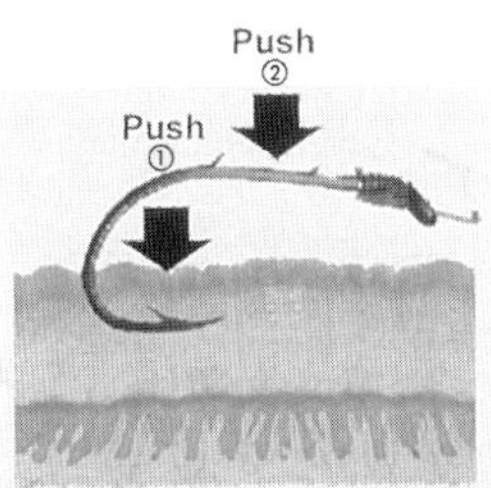

FIG. 42-8. Simple retrograde technique. While pressing the skin over the tip of the hook to disengage the barb and applying gentle downward pressure on the shank, the physician backs the hook out of the skin. If the barb catches on skin fibers, other techniques must be used.

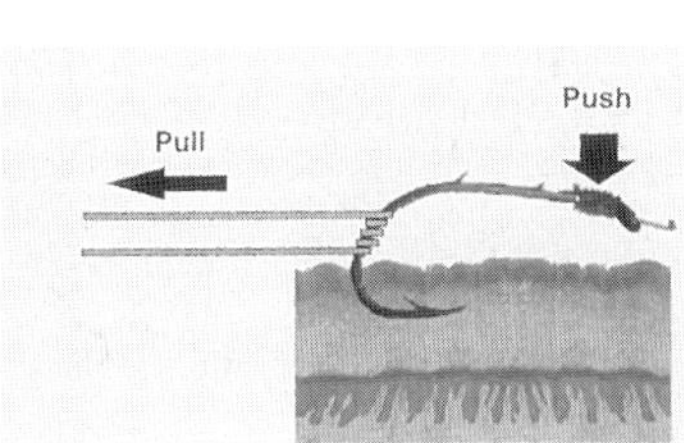

FIG. 42-9. String-pull technique. String or suture material is tied to the curve of the hook. The hook is positioned as described in the simple retrograde technique, and a quick pull on the string will dislodge the hook.

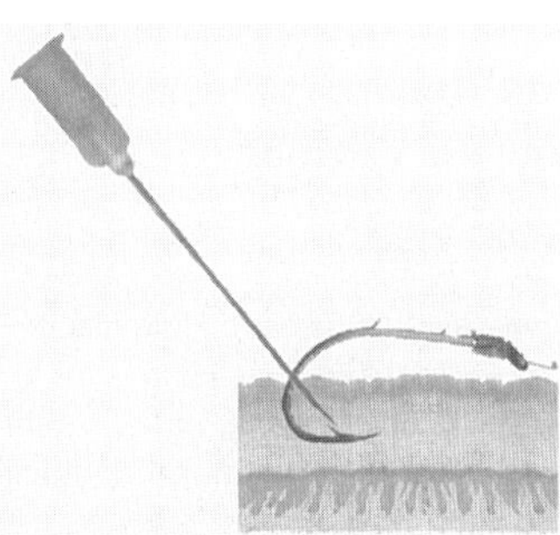

FIG. 42-10. Needle-cover technique. The area is anesthetized, and an 18-gauge needle is inserted into the entrance wound along the hook. The lumen of the needle is placed over the barb to cover it, and both the hook and needle are backed out of the wound.

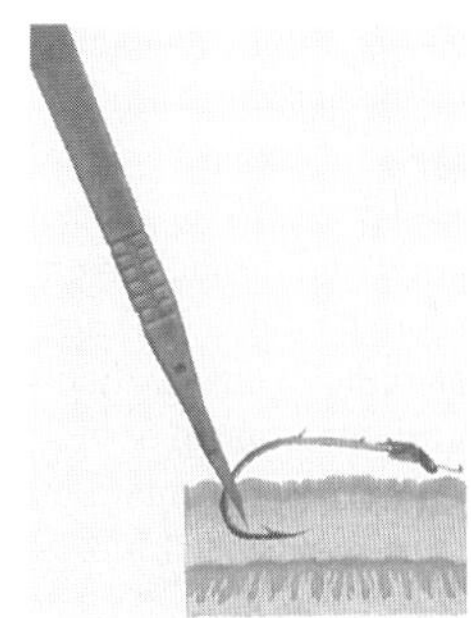

FIG. 42-12. Incision technique. The area is anesthetized, and a small incision is made along the shaft of the hook to the barb. The hook is withdrawn through the incision.

this technique are that failure can cause further pain to the patient and success can result in ripped tissue or a sharp, blood-contaminated object flying uncontrollably across the room.

The *needle-cover technique* requires physician dexterity. An 18-gauge needle is inserted into the entrance wound alongside the shank of the hook. The needle follows the bend of the hook until the lumen of the needle can be placed over the barb to sheathe it. The hook and needle are then withdrawn from the wound as a unit (Fig. 42-10).

The *advance-and-cut technique* is another alternative (Fig. 42-11). The tip of the hook is advanced through the skin surface. Once exposed, the point and barb are cut with wire cutters, and the remaining part of the hook is rotated out of the original wound. If barbs along the shank are embedded beneath the dermis, the shank can be clipped near the hook's eye. The remaining part of the hook is then passed antegrade through the skin. Since the advance-and-cut method further traumatizes and contaminates tissue, it probably should be reserved for wilderness situations. However, this may be an effective method in the ED if the barb has nearly or already penetrated the surface of the skin or is embedded within a joint, cartilage, or tendon.

A fifth technique requires the services of a physician but has important advantages over other methods. When the barb penetrates into the dermis, it usually cannot be backed out or pulled out of the wound. In these cases, the entrance wound should be enlarged 2 to 3 mm with a No. 11 scalpel blade. A small incision is carried along the bend of the hook to the barb until the barb is disengaged from the soft tissue. The hook can then be withdrawn easily through the larger entrance (Fig. 42-12). If necessary, the barb can be grasped with a hemostat to prevent it from snagging tissue on the way out. There are two major benefits to enlarging puncture wounds containing foreign bodies. First, the wound is more easily inspected for additional foreign bodies. In the case of fishhook impalement, the wound may be harboring the bait that was on the hook. Second, the wound tract is more easily

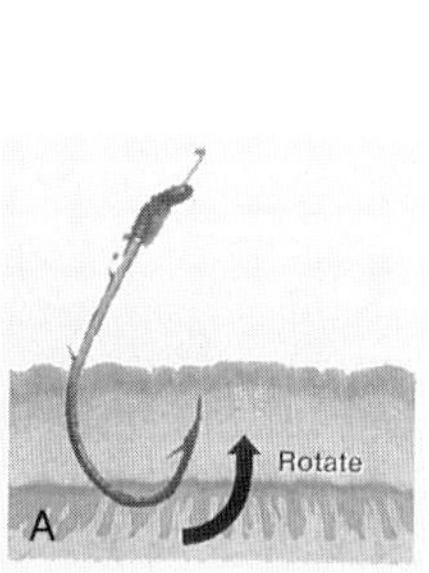

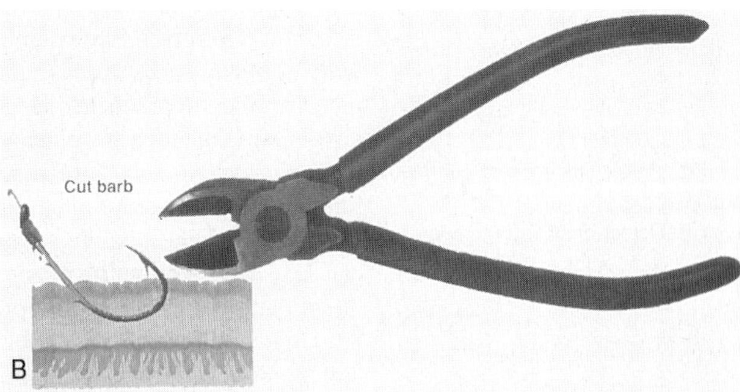

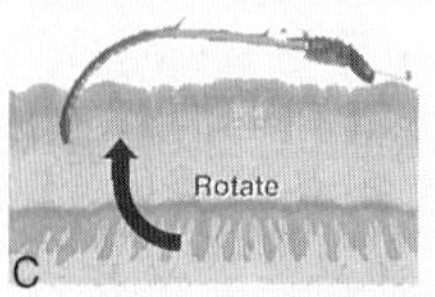

FIG. 42-11. Advance-and-cut technique. The area is anesthetized, and the tip of the hook is advanced through the skin surface **(A)**, the barb is cut **(B)**, and the hook is rotated back out of the original wound **(C)**.

irrigated through a larger opening. However, the physician must avoid injuring tendons, nerves, or vessels with the scalpel.

TRAUMATIC DERMAL TATTOOING Foreign particulates may be embedded in the epidermal and dermal layers of skin by an abrasion, which permanently stains or "tattoos" the surrounding tissue. If vigorous scrubbing does not remove the particulates, the patient can be referred to specialists for dermabrasion or block excision. The graphite from pencil lead can produce a pigmentation that will never dissolve, and graphite tattoos should be excised in cosmetic areas.

DISPOSITION

Postremoval Treatment

After removal of a foreign body, the wound should be irrigated thoroughly. A puncture wound is difficult to clean adequately because either the small wound diameter prevents the irrigation fluid from reaching the wounded tissue or the fluid enters the wound but does not completely drain. If the puncture is contaminated, the entrance wound can be enlarged to allow more effective cleaning. If foreign debris is impregnated in tissue, the contaminated area can be debrided or excised. If multiple radiopaque objects were removed, a postprocedure plain film should be obtained. The decision to close lacerations, incisions, and block excisions depends on the potential for infection; wounds where all foreign contaminants can be removed and those in locations with good blood supply can be closed primarily. Otherwise, delayed primary closure is preferred to immediate closure. Necessary tetanus immunization (TIG and/or Td) should be provided. If a foreign body is deliberately left in place, the patient should be informed. If foreign material was removed, the patient should be warned that there is always a possibility that not all pieces were found.

Delayed Removal

Many patients must be referred to surgical specialists for delayed removal of foreign bodies. It is important to inform the patient that the object is present but unlikely to cause harm before it is removed. The benefit of prophylactic antibiotics for uninfected wounds containing foreign bodies has not been studied. Antibiotics are justified for infected wounds, particularly when removal must be postponed, even though removal allows infections to clear rapidly. If a foreign body is near a joint or highly mobile region, the affected area should be splinted prior to removal to prevent further injury or migration of the object.

REFERENCES

1. Lammers RL: Soft tissue foreign bodies. *Ann Emerg Med* 17:1336, 1988.
2. Auerbach P: Marine envenomation, in Auerbach PS (ed): *Wilderness Medicine,* 3d ed. St. Louis: Mosby, 1995, pp 1327–1374.
3. Farrell SE, Vandevander P, Lee D, et al: Elevated serum lead levels in ED patients with retained lead foreign bodies [abstr]. *Acad Emerg Med* 3:418, 1996.
4. Zimmerli W, Zak O, Vosbeck K: Experimental hematogenous infection of subcutaneously implanted foreign bodies. *Scand J Infect Dis* 17:303, 1985.
5. Avner JR, Baker MD: Lacerations involving glass: The role of routine roentgenograms. *Am J Dis Child* 146:600, 1992.
6. Russell RC, Williamson DA, Sullivan JW, et al: Detection of foreign bodies in the hand. *J Hand Surg* 16A:2, 1991.
7. Courter BJ: Radiographic screening for glass foreign bodies: What does a "negative" foreign body series really mean? *Ann Emerg Med* 19:997, 1990.
8. Ellis G: Are aluminum foreign bodies detectable radiographically? *Am J Emerg Med* 11:12, 1993.
9. Roobottom CA, Weston MJ: The detection of foreign bodies in soft tissue: Comparison of conventional and digital radiography. *Clin Radiol* 49:330, 1994.
10. Reiner B, Siegel E, McLaurin T, et al: Evaluation of soft-tissue foreign bodies: Comparing conventional plain film radiography, computed radiography printed on film, and computed tomography displayed on a computer workstation. *AJR* 167:141, 1996.
11. Chisholm CD, Wood CO, Chua G, et al: Radiographic detection of gravel in soft tissue. *Ann Emerg Med* 29:725, 1997.
12. Ell SR, Sprigg A, Parker AJ: A multi-observer study examining the radiographic visibility of fishbone foreign bodies. *J R Soc Med* 89:31, 1996.
13. De Flaviis L, Scaglione P, Del Bo P, et al: Detection of foreign bodies in soft tissues: Experimental comparison of ultrasonography and xeroradiography. *J Trauma* 28:400, 1988.
14. Gilbert FJ, Campbell RSD, Bayliss AP: The role of ultrasound in the detection of non-radiopaque foreign bodies. *Clin Radiol* 41:109, 1990.
15. Jacobson JA, Powell A, Craig JG, et al: Wooden foreign bodies in soft tissue: Detection at ultrasound. *Radiology* 206:45, 1998.
16. Schlager D, Sanders AB, Wiggins D, et al: Ultrasound for the detection of foreign bodies. *Ann Emerg Med* 20:189, 1991.
17. Manthey DE, Storrow AB, Milbourn JM, et al: Ultrasound versus radiography in the detection of soft-tissue foreign bodies. *Ann Emerg Med* 28:7, 1996.
18. Turner J, Wilde CH, Hughes KC, et al: Ultrasound-guided retrieval of small foreign objects in subcutaneous tissue. *Ann Emerg Med* 29:731, 1997.
19. Cohen DM, Garcia CT, Dietrich AM, Hickey RW: Miniature C-arm imaging: An in vitro study of detecting foreign bodies in the emergency department. *Pediatr Emerg Care* 13:247, 1997.
20. Lindsey D, Lindsey WE: Cactus spine injuries. *Am J Emerg Med* 6:362, 1988.
21. Martinez TT, Jerome M, Barry RC, et al: Removal of cactus spines from the skin: A comparative evaluation of several methods. *Am J Dis Child* 141:1291, 1987.

PUNCTURE WOUNDS AND BITES

Charles A. Eckerline, Jr
Jim Blake
Ronald F. Koury

PUNCTURE WOUNDS

Puncture wounds are usually accidental and usually involve the hands and soles of the feet.[1] Sharp, elongated objects that pierce the skin may penetrate into the deeper tissues, injuring underlying structures, introducing foreign bodies, and planting the inoculum for infection. Organized evaluation and management is necessary to minimize complications.

Pathophysiology

The most common sequela of puncture wounds is infection, which, depending on the location and puncturing instrument, is reported to occur from 6 to 11 percent of the time.[2,3] Infection is more common in puncture wounds than in open lacerations because of inoculation of organisms into the deep tissues, followed by skin closure. Most infections from puncture wounds are due to gram-positive organisms, with *Staphylococcus aureus* predominating, followed by other staphylococcal and streptococcal species. Many other microorganisms have also been isolated from puncture wound infections, including *Aerobacter aerogenes* and *Mycobacterium fortuitum*. Puncture wounds over joints can penetrate through the joint capsule, producing septic arthritis. Penetration to the relatively vascular cartilage, periosteum, and bone can lead to osteomyelitis. *Pseudomonas aeruginosa* is the most frequent pathogen isolated post-puncture wound osteomyelitis, particularly when foreign-body penetration occurs through the sole of an athletic shoe.[4,5] Because this organism is not detected in new shoes, it has been postulated that the foam rubber material becomes colonized in the warm, humid summer months. Post–puncture wound infections are accentuated by the presence of a foreign body, and failure of an

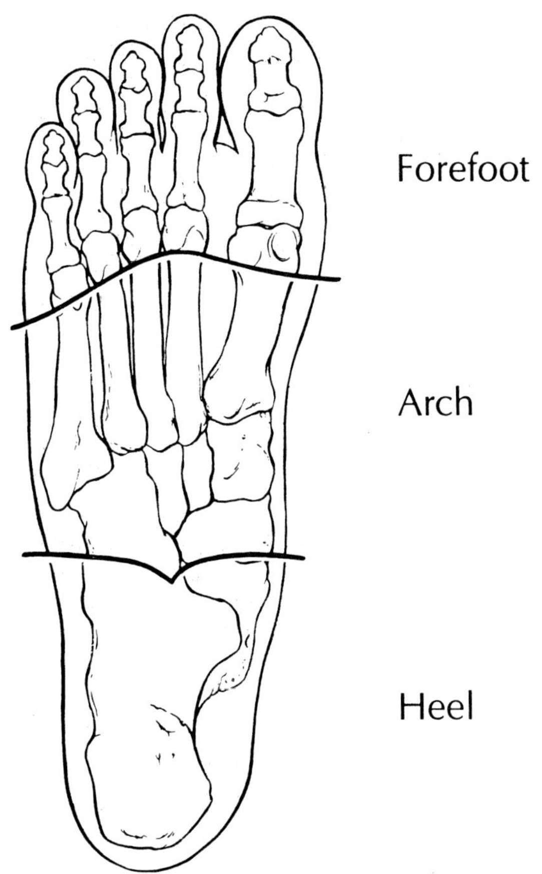

FIG. 43-1. The bony and cartilaginous structures in the forefoot region of the sole of the foot are the most prone to development of osteomyelitis after plantar puncture wounds.

infection to respond to antibiotics suggests the presence of a retained foreign body.

Puncture wounds that present soon after injury generally appear simple and innocuous. Appropriate history should be obtained and documented: (1) the time interval since the injury (discomfort at >6 h increases the probability of infection), (2) type and condition of the penetrating object, (3) complete or partial removal of the object, (4) residual foreign-body sensation in the wound, (5) whether footwear was worn (plantar punctures), (6) an estimation of the depth of penetration, (7) whether the injury occurred indoors or outdoors, and (8) potential contamination (rust, dirt, cloth contaminants). A retained foreign body is suggested if the patient reports either the sensation of a retained object or incomplete removal of the penetrating instrument. The incidence of post–puncture wound infection is increased if the patient has decreased resistance to infection from diabetes mellitus, peripheral vascular disease, or immunosuppression.[6] As in the case of any wound, tetanus immunization status should be determined and appropriate prophylaxis performed.

Puncture wounds associated with an increased incidence of infection are those involving (1) more than 6 h from injury to presentation, (2) larger lesions with deeper penetration, (3) obvious contamination with foreign matter and debris, (4) occurrence outdoors, (5) penetration through footwear, (6) puncture of the forefoot, and (7) patients with poor resistance to infection (Fig. 43-1).[7]

Clinical Features

Physical examination of puncture wounds should evaluate and document the wounds as well as the function of underlying structures. In puncture wounds of the hand, distal function of tendons (flexor and extensor), nerves (motor and sensory), and vessels (perfusion) should be assessed. Puncture wounds should be carefully inspected for their location, the condition of the surrounding skin, and the presence of foreign matter, debris, or devitalized tissue. Wound infection is suggested by increased pain, swelling, erythema, warmth, fluctuance, decreased range of motion at joints, or drainage from a wound site.

Because puncture wounds are potentially deep and cannot be easily inspected to their depth, there remains the possibility of a foreign body. Some materials are prone to break, leaving retained fragments behind: these include wood, glass, and plastic and thin objects such as pins and needles. Probing of the wound with a sterile, thin, blunt instrument is common practice to determine the depth of the wound and the presence of foreign body. However, this practice has not been validated in prospective studies. Wound probing is usually harmless and generally useless.

Plain-film radiographs should be obtained in all infected puncture wounds and in any wound suspicious for a retained radiopaque (metal, gravel, and glass) foreign body. Radiopaque foreign bodies greater than 0.5 to 1.0 mm in size will be identifiable in 80 to 90 percent of plain films. Radiographs should be obtained with multiple views and the ''soft tissue'' technique to maximize detection. Most organic substances—such as wood splinters, cactus spines, thorns, and vegetable matter—have radiodensities close to that of soft tissue and cannot be identified with plain-film radiographs. Ultrasound has been successfully used to identify substances invisible on plain films, although the reported sensitivity, specificity, and accuracy varies widely in experimental studies of this modality. Computed tomography (CT) is the method of choice for the detection of retained foreign bodies not seen with other techniques, especially wood and plastic. The ability of CT to differentiate densities permits detection of substances previously ''invisible'' by other imaging modalities. Magnetic resonance imaging (MRI) has excellent ability to differentiate contrast between soft tissues and may be superior to other imaging modalities in the detection of plastics. However, MRI cannot be used to image metallic objects or gravel because of the production of significant ferromagnetic artifacts. CT or MRI should be used if the penetrating object was radiolucent and there is historical or clinical evidence of a retained foreign body.

Treatment

Many aspects of the treatment of puncture wounds remain controversial.[4,8] Uncomplicated, clean punctures presenting less than 6 h after injury require only wound cleansing and tetanus prophylaxis as indicated. Soaking of the wound has no proven benefit. Low-pressure irrigation (e.g., 0.5 psi) of wounds is recommended to assist in cleansing of the wound for better visualization of the entrance site as well as removal of visible foreign matter. The injection of irrigation fluid under high (e.g., 7 psi) pressure into a closed wound tract may lead to displacement of foreign matter secondary to hydrodissection along tissue planes and disseminate bacteria deeper into the surrounding tissue.

Debridement or ''coring'' of the wound tract in clean wounds is sometimes recommended, but there is no evidence that this procedure reduces the risk of infection, even for plantar puncture wounds. Large objects may produce lacerations that should be anesthetized, explored, irrigated, and debrided. The expertise, time required for the procedure, and postprocedure management may dictate referral to a surgical specialist.

There is no proven benefit to routine prophylactic antimicrobial therapy in the management of clean, nonplantar puncture wounds. In fact, it has been suggested that this practice may actually contribute to the development of secondary infections with gram-negative organisms by altering the normal flora. Puncture wounds in patients with peripheral vascular disease, diabetes mellitus, and immunocompromising disorders are associated with an increased incidence of infection and *may* benefit from antibiotics.[6] Plantar puncture wounds, especially those in high-risk patients, those located in the forefoot, or those through athletic shoes should be treated with antibiotics.[9] The ability of antibiotics to reduce the incidence of wound infections is correlated with the early achievement of antimicrobial blood levels. In the past, this required parenteral (intravenous or intramuscular) administration of both a cephalosporin and an aminoglycoside in the emergency department (ED). The development of fluoroquinolones now provides the physician with a broad-spectrum antibiotic that rapidly achieves high blood levels following an oral dose.[10] Either route is acceptable in plantar puncture wounds; the choice is up to the physician's judgment. Following the initial dose in the ED, the patient should be discharged with an oral regimen. The ideal duration of treatment is not known. A dilemma is posed by plantar puncture wounds through athletic shoes, where infection with *Pseudomonas* has been reported to occur in up to 25 percent. The only oral agents consistently effective against *Pseudomonas* are the fluoroquinolones ciprofloxacin and levofloxacin, and these agents are not approved by the FDA for use in children. The alternative would be hospital admission for intravenous antibiotics. Experience with ciprofloxacin in children with cystic fibrosis indicates a low rate of complications, particularly with short courses. A tentative recommendation can be made for the prophylactic use of ciprofloxacin in children with plantar puncture wounds either in the forefoot or through athletic shoes.

Complications

Infections that develop after puncture wounds can be differentiated into (1) local cellulitis, (2) local abscess, (3) deeper spreading soft tissue infections, and (4) infections of bone or cartilage.

CELLULITIS A localized inflammation of the dermis surrounding the puncture wound, usually without significant drainage, developing within 1 to 4 days. Distal swelling or swelling opposite the puncture site (e.g., dorsum of the foot when the puncture site is the plantar surface) is not encountered. Pain is generally noted around the puncture site, causing the patient to limit weight bearing on the affected foot.

A local abscess may develop at the puncture site, especially if a foreign body remains. Swelling, fluctuance, and local drainage may be present.

Deeper soft tissue infections also present with painful cellulitis around the puncture site that limits weight bearing on the affected foot; in addition, most patients also have pain and swelling distal to or opposite the puncture site. Serious infections may involve gram-negative and anaerobic bacteria, generating crepitus and a foul order from the site.

Cellulitis from a puncture wound can occur at any site in the foot, as contrasted with bone infections, which are limited to specific regions of the foot. Puncture wounds involving the forefoot pose the highest risk of osteomyelitis. The forefoot is a major weight-bearing region and the underlying bones, as compared with the heel and the arch, have very little overlying soft tissue. Therefore, a puncture wound is more prone to penetrate bone and cartilage in forefoot injuries, predisposing to osteomyelitis.

Patients who present with infections developing after puncture should have plain radiographs taken to detect the possibility of a radiopaque foreign body, soft tissue gas indicating a deeper infection, or the bone changes of osteomyelitis. If the wounding object was radiolucent, a CT scan may be necessary.

With simple cellulitis developing after puncture wounds in otherwise healthy patients, there is no need for routine cultures, and antimicrobial coverage should be directed at gram-positive organisms, especially *S. aureus*. Effective agents include penicillinase-resistant penicillin (e.g., dicloxacillin), first-generation cephalosporins (e.g., cephalexin, cefadroxil), or ciprofloxacin. Local abscesses are treated with incision, drainage, and careful exploration for a retained foreign body. Serious, deep soft tissue infections require surgical exploration and debridement in the operating room.

OSTEOMYELITIS Bone and joint infections are the most disastrous sequelae of puncture wounds, often resulting in significant long-term morbidity. The overall incidence following plantar puncture wounds is about 4 percent, but this figure increases to nearly 25 percent in patients with forefoot puncture wounds through athletic shoes. Patients with post–puncture wound osteomyelitis or septic arthritis have typically received initial management of their puncture wound and tetanus immunization. Often, antimicrobial agents may have been given prophylactically or for early cellulitis, with a short period of symptomatic improvement that is typically followed by increasing pain, swelling, redness, drainage, or a combination of these. Radiographs, if taken at this time, are usually normal and a second course of antibiotics may be administered. Partial resolution or persistence of symptoms prompts patients to seek further evaluation. It is not until an average of 3 weeks after the initial injury, or even longer for diabetics, that radiographs are repeated and the diagnosis of osteomyelitis is made. Any patient who relapses or fails to improve after initial therapy for a puncture wound should be suspected of having osteomyelitis. Radiographs should be obtained and blood sent for a white blood cell (WBC) count and an erythrocyte sedimentation rate (ESR). While an elevated WBC and ESR may alert the physician to the presence of a deep infection, normal values cannot be relied upon to exclude one.[11] A bone scan will show changes consistent with osteomyelitis 48 to 72 h after the onset of symptoms. There is a poor correlation between cultures of overlying wounds and those obtained from the involved bone in osteomyelitis. For that reason, culture of wounds and drainage should not be relied upon for antibiotic selection. In general, initiation of antibiotics should wait until cultures have been obtained from the involved bone, usually in the operating room. Pending cultures results, antibiotics are started that cover *Staphylococcus* and *Pseudomonas* species. An acceptable regimen would consist of parenteral nafcillin and ceftazidime. Definitive management frequently necessitates operative intervention for debridement.

The majority of those who develop local infections after puncture wounds can be managed as outpatients. These patients should be provided with instructions on rest, with avoidance of weight bearing for plantar puncture wounds, elevation, warm soaks, and information detailing events that should prompt immediate return. Close follow-up with a routine recheck within 48 h is recommended.

Needle-Stick Injuries

Needle-stick injuries are common among health care professionals. Like other puncture wounds, these injuries carry the risk of bacterial infection in addition to the risk of infection with hepatitis and human immunodeficiency virus (HIV). The risk of infection after an inadvertent needle stick from an infectious source has been estimated to be negligible for hepatitis A virus (HAV), 9 percent (range 5 to 27 percent) for hepatitis B virus (HBV), 1.8 percent (range 0 to 7 percent) for hepatitis C virus (HCV), and 0.3 percent (range 0.2 to 0.5 percent) for HIV.[12–14]

Preexposure prophylaxis is currently possible for HAV and HBV with appropriate vaccines.[12] Postexposure prophylaxis is possible for HAV with immune serum globulin (ISG), for HBV with hepatitis B immune globulin (HBIG), and for HIV with combination antiviral therapy.[12–14] There is no proven postexposure prophylaxis for HCV.[13] Many factors enter into the decision process concerning the risks and benefits of treatment: (1) location of the needle stick, (2) ability to test the source, (3) immune status of the recipient, and (4) time from injury until treatment. Recommendations in this area are complex and changing. Each hospital should have a predesigned protocol developed by infectious disease specialists for the expeditious evaluation, testing, and possible treatment of needle-stick injuries.

High-Pressure-Injection Injuries

A high-pressure injection injury may present as a puncture wound, usually to the hand or foot.[15] High-pressure equipment is designed to force liquids such as paint, paint thinner, grease, oil, or diesel fuel through a small nozzle under high pressure—sometimes up to several thousand psi. If held against or close to the skin, the liquid stream coming out of the nozzle will be injected through the skin and deposited in the subcutaneous tissues. Pressure required to penetrate the skin is approximately 100 psi, which is easily achieved by this type of equipment. These injuries are severe owing to the intense inflammation incited by the injected liquid and the vascular compromise that develops from edema within these tight tissue compartments. The type, amount, and velocity of material injected will determine the degree of tissue inflammatory response, and this material often spreads widely along fascial planes.

Patients who present soon after injury typically have pain out of proportion to the appearance of the injection wound, and swelling is minimal.[15] Despite this innocuous appearance, potentially serious damage can develop. Neurovascular function should be carefully assessed. Pain control should be achieved with parenteral analgesics; digital blocks are contraindicated so as to avoid increases in tissue pressure with resultant further compromise in perfusion. The extremity should be elevated in order to reduce swelling. Parenteral antibiotics against the gram-positive skin flora (*Staphylococcus* and *Streptococcus*) should be administered. Radiographs should be taken because some material may be radiopaque and may demonstrate the extent of subcutaneous spread from the injection site. An appropriate hand specialist should be consulted and early surgical debridement implemented for an optimal outcome.[16]

HUMAN BITES

Human bites are most often reported on the hands and upper extremities (60 to 75 percent), head and neck (15 to 20 percent), trunk (10 to 20 percent), and lower extremities (5 percent) as the result of fighting.[17] Passionate sexual activity can lead to bites on the penis, scrotum, and vulva. Self-inflicted bites are usually on the fingers, hands, and forearms. An occlusional bite, when human teeth bite through the body part, commonly occurs at the distal portion of a digit during an altercation and may result in complete amputation. The ''clenched-fist'' injury (CFI) occurs on the dorsum of the metacarpophalangeal region of the fist as it strikes the mouth and teeth of another individual.[18] Human bites to the hands have serious sequelae, including infection, loss of function, and potential amputation if untreated or misdiagnosed. In the ED, patients may try to conceal or even deny the true etiology of human bite wounds. The ED physician should be suspicious, especially when confronted by any small laceration over the dorsum of the metacarpophalangeal joint, that such an injury should be considered a CFI until proven otherwise.

Pathophysiology

Human bites produce a crushing or tearing mechanism with tissue destruction and devitalization. Underlying structures, particularly in the hand, are at risk of injury; these include the tendons, vessels, nerves, deep spaces, joints, and bone. Inoculation into these wounds with the normal human aerobic and anaerobic oral flora predisposes to infection; 1 ml of human saliva can contain up to 10^8 organisms. Many infected human bite wounds are polymicrobial, with studies reporting up to 43 percent mixed gram-positive and gram-negative organisms, and 26 to 83 percent yielding both aerobic and anaerobic bacteria.[17] The most frequent aerobic organism isolated is *Streptococcus viridans*, followed by *S. epidermidis*, *Corynebacterium* sp., *S. aureus*, *Eikenella* sp., and *Haemophilus* sp. Common anaerobic isolates include *Bacteroides* sp., *Fusobacterium* sp., and anaerobic cocci (e.g., *Peptostreptococcus* sp.). *Eikenella corrodens*, a slow-growing opportunistic aerobic gram-negative bacillus, has been isolated in up to 15 percent of CFI wounds and is a common cause of osteomyelitis, septic arthritis, and abscesses in the hand. *Eikenella corrodens* is susceptible to penicillin but resistant to penicillinase-resistant penicillin, clindamycin, and metronidazole; it has variable resistance to cephalosporins.

Complications from human bites occur most frequently in hand wounds, particularly CFI. These infections include localized cellulitis, lymphangiitis, abscess formation, tenosynovitis, septic arthritis, and osteomyelitis. Human bites in locations other than the hand appear to have similar rates of infection as nonbite lacerations. It is noteworthy that human bites in children and bites in the face have low rates of infection, often less than 5 percent. Paronychia is frequent in children who suck their thumbs and may inoculate oral flora to the region of the nail bed. In addition, two viral diseases are commonly transmitted by human bites. Herpetic whitlow results from contact or bites to the finger by a person infected with herpes simplex virus. Hepatitis B virus has also been transmitted after human bites from infected individuals. The potential risk of HIV infection through human bites appears to be negligible, likely due to the low levels of HIV present in saliva.

Clinical Features

The evaluation of human bites should identify the time interval since the injury, mechanism (i.e., occlusion versus closed fist), location, estimated depth of penetration, tetanus immunization status, medications, allergies, and underlying medical conditions predisposing to poor wound healing. As mentioned, human bites in the hands have an increased predilection for infection, but clinical signs of infection may not be present even after 24 h postinjury. Documentation of the vascular, motor, and sensory examination is essential. Following appropriate anesthesia, careful wound exploration is necessary to examine underlying structures for injury and possible foreign bodies. Examination of a CFI wound must take into account the flexed position at the interphalangeal and metacarpophalangeal joints at the time of injury; the injured segment of tendon will retract proximally in the unclenched, open hand and be missed if the physician evaluates the wound only in this position. The wound must be examined with the hand taken through a full range of motion at the metacarpophalangeal joint to detect extensor tendon injury. The joint capsule should be inspected to detect potential joint-space penetration. Radiographs should be taken of human bites to the hand, particularly CFI. Radiographs may disclose radiopaque foreign bodies (e.g., fragments of teeth), fractures, and air within the joint space (indicating joint-space penetration).

Treatment

Patients presenting more than 24 h after injury may already exhibit evidence of infection, with swelling, erythema, warmth, and a purulent, often malodorous discharge. Aerobic and anaerobic cultures should be obtained from the wound prior to any irrigation or cleansing of the wound. Careful examination of the wound following irrigation and cleansing is required to inspect the tendons and joint capsules. Radiographs should be taken.

Patients who present with a fresh CFI should have careful inspection under anesthesia, as noted above, and radiographs taken. If no laceration of the extensor tendon or joint capsule is seen, the wound should be copiously irrigated; it should be left open with an appropriate dressing, the hand immobilized in a bulky dressing and elevated for 24 h, followed by reevaluation in 1 to 2 days.[18,19] If there is a laceration to either the extensor tendon or the joint capsule or radiographic findings (foreign bodies, fractures, or joint-space air), a hand specialist should be consulted; these patients usually require exploration in the operating room.[20] In general, non-CFI human bite wounds of the hand should also be left open after examination and irrigation.

Wounds in other locations—such as the face, head, and neck—can be successfully repaired with primary closure after copious irrigation and judicious limited debridement.[21,22]

Prophylactic antibiotics should be considered in all human bites of the hands and in bites to other locations in high-risk patients (asplenia, diabetes mellitus, and immune deficiency).[17,19] Antibiotics should cover the expected mouth flora. Acceptable agents include amoxicillin/clavulanate, dicloxacillin plus penicillin, a first-generation cephalosporin plus penicillin, or a fluoroquinolone. Patients allergic to penicillin can be treated with clindamycin plus trimethoprim-sulfamethoxazole. Three to 5 days of therapy is appropriate. All patients with human bite wounds should be provided with tetanus immunization according to standard guidelines.

Patients with human bite hand wounds, particularly CFI, presenting more than 24 h after injury usually have clinical evidence of infection. Mildly infected wounds, such as those showing a localized cellulitis, in otherwise healthy and reliable patients may be managed on an outpatient basis with oral antibiotics, immobilization, and close follow-up. The wound should be explored and irrigated, left open with a dressing, and immobilized in a bulky dressing. Initial antibiotics should be administered in the ED with prescriptions for an additional 7 days given to the patient on discharge. These wounds should be reexamined in 24 h.

Moderate to severe infections manifest by fever, tachycardia, spreading cellulitis, or lymphangitis or possible involvement of deep tissue require admission for parenteral antibiotic therapy. Appropriate coverage can be provided by ampicillin/sulbactam, cefoxitin, ticarcillin/clavulanate, or piperacillin/tazobactam. Penicillin-allergic patients can be treated with clindamycin plus ciprofloxacin. Additional management includes copious irrigation and drainage (usually in the operating room), bulky dressings with daily changes, elevation, and immobilization. Delayed primary closure or healing by secondary intention is the preferred approach for the closure of hand wounds.

ANIMAL BITES

It is generally recognized that estimates of the number of animal bites are inaccurate and previous figures of 1 to 2 million people bitten per year in the United States are far too low. A survey of 5238 households in 1994 produced an estimated number of almost 4.5 million for dog bites alone (18 per 1000 population), with 756,000 requiring medical attention.[23] A review of the National Hospital Ambulatory Medical Care Survey for 1992 through 1994 yielded an estimated 333,000 annual emergency department visits for dog bites alone.[24] School-age children (5 to 14 years) sustain the majority of reported animal bites. The most frequently reported sites of animal bites include the hands (48 to 59 percent), arms (16 to 26 percent), legs (15 percent), and face (8 to 30 percent). Animal bite wounds comprise punctures, lacerations, avulsions, and abrasions. Patients seek medical attention with concerns about infection, tetanus and rabies prophylaxis in addition to treatment for the wound. Wound infection is the most frequent complication; other complications seen less frequently include sepsis, septic arthritis, tenosynovitis, osteomyelitis, meningitis, and disfiguring wounds.

The risk of infection from animal bite wounds depends on several factors: (1) the type of injury (puncture, laceration, avulsion, or abrasion), (2) presence of foreign bodies, (3) anatomic location, (4) time delay to treatment, (5) wound care techniques, (6) patient's age, and (7) underlying medical conditions.[25,26] Factors that predict a probability of infection greater than 5 to 10 percent include (1) full-thickness skin puncture; (2) wounds of the hands or feet; (3) wounds requiring debridement; (4) wounds involving joints, ligaments, or tendons; (5) wounds associated with fractures; and (6) wounds in patients who are high-risk hosts. Treatment with antibiotics in such circumstances is recommended.

Animal bites should be considered tetanus-prone wounds; guidelines for tetanus immunization should be followed. The need for postexposure rabies immunoprophylaxis must also be considered in cases of animal bite wounds. Factors to consider concern the animal type, nature of the attack, and evaluation and disposition of the animal. In general, skunks, raccoons, bats, foxes, and most carnivores should be considered as posing a high risk for rabies and postexposure immunoprophylaxis should be initiated. It is generally best to consult local public health officials for the most current recommendations.

The physician should evaluate and document the number, type, location, and depth of all bite wounds as well as the presence of any clinical evidence of infection. Lacerations and avulsions should be explored to evaluate potential involvement of any underlying structures, including vessels, nerves, tendons, soft tissue, and joint spaces. In general, fresh bite wounds do not require extension and exploration. Radiographs should be obtained if there is evidence of infection or any suspicion of foreign-body or bone involvement. Bites from animals known to have strong jaws, such as pit bulls, mastiffs, tigers, and cougars, should be assumed to produce fractures until proven otherwise by x-ray. All animal bite wounds require appropriate local wound care with copious irrigation and debridement of compromised or necrotic tissue. Primary closure following appropriate wound care has been successful in wounds to the head and neck, torso, and proximal extremities, but in general bites without cosmetic implications should be allowed to heal by secondary intention. Hand wounds are best managed open initially, followed by delayed primary wound closure in 3 to 5 days. Antibiotics should not be used as a substitute for proper local wound care.

Dog Bites

Dogs account for 80 to 90 percent of reported animal bites in the United States.[23] Boys are victims of dog bites twice as often as girls, and the dog is known to the victim in about 90 percent of cases. Dog bite injuries occur most frequently on the extremities (upper slightly more often than lower), followed by the head and neck, and least frequently on the trunk. Head and neck bites are more common in children. Infection occurs in dog bites in approximately 5 percent of cases. Factors that increase the rate of infection include (1) victim age greater than 50 years, (2) delay in seeking treatment greater than 24 h, (3) hand wounds, and (4) deep puncture wounds. Dog bites are rarely lethal, but they may produce significant damage secondary to the force delivered—approximately 150 to 450 psi.[27,28]

Infection of dog bite wounds usually results from the organisms inoculated into the depth of the wound by the animal's teeth, not from the bacterial flora normally found on the patient's skin. Infections from dog bite wounds are often polymicrobial; aerobic bacteria are present in most wounds and anaerobic bacteria are found in up to 40 percent.[25] Aerobic isolates are usually alpha-hemolytic streptococci, followed by *S. aureus*, *Pasteurella multocida*, and *S. intermedius*. Other pathogenic aerobes include β-hemolytic streptococci, γ-hemolytic streptococci, *E. corrodens*, *Capnocytophaga canimorsus*, other *Pasteurella* sp., and *Haemophilus aphrophilus*. Anaerobic bacteria isolated from dog bite wounds include *Actinomyces* sp., *Bacteroides* sp., *Fusobacterium* sp., and *Peptostreptococcus* sp.

Capnocytophaga canimorsus, formerly known by the Centers for Disease Control and Prevention as "dysgonic fermenter-2" (DF-2), is a fastidious, thin, gram-negative bacillus that has been associated with severe infection in immunocompromised patients (asplenia, alcoholism, chronic lung disease, or other immunosuppression). It was first recognized as a human pathogen in 1976. Infection with this organism may produce severe sepsis with disseminated intravascular coagulation, acute renal failure, endocarditis, peripheral gangrene, and cardiopulmonary failure. Fatalities are seen in up to 25 percent of cases. Penicillin is the drug of choice when infection with this organism is suspected and should be used prophylactically in high-risk individuals. This bacterium is also usually sensitive to cephalosporins, tetracyclines, erythromycin, and clindamycin.

Lacerations of the scalp, face, and trunk from dog bites can be irrigated, debrided, and sutured in the ED with a low risk of infection.[29,30] Lacerations of the distal extremities, especially the feet and hands, should not be sutured. Lacerations of the proximal extremities—the upper arm and the thigh—can probably be closed after irrigation and exploration. Large, extensive lacerations, especially in small children, are best explored and repaired in the operating room.[27]

Discharge instructions should include information about signs and symptoms of infection and assurance of follow-up within 24 to 48 h. Bites to the hand, and wounds in high-risk individuals should receive prophylactic treatment with amoxicillin/clavulanate, clindamycin plus ciprofloxacin, or clindamycin plus trimethoprim-sulfamethoxazole for 3 to 5 days. Antibiotics should be initiated in the ED. There is no evidence that antibiotic therapy for dog bite wounds in other anatomic locations is beneficial.

Wounds obviously infected at the time of presentation need to be cultured and antibiotic therapy must be initiated. Infection developing within 24 h after injury suggests *P. multocida* and treatment with penicillin, ciprofloxacin, or trimethoprim-sulfamethoxazole is recommended. Wound infection developing beyond 24 h after the dog bite implicates *Staphylococcus* and *Streptococcus*; treatment with a penicillinase-resistant penicillin or first-generation cephalosporin is indicated. Low-risk patients with local cellulitis only and no involvement of underlying structures can be treated and observed closely as outpatients. Admission and parenteral antibiotic therapy are indicated in patients with infected wounds and evidence of lymphangitis, lymphadenitis, tenosynovitis, septic arthritis, or osteomyelitis; systemic signs such as fever; or injury to underlying structures such as tendons, joints, or bone. Aerobic and anaerobic cultures should be obtained from the deep structures, preferably during exploration in the operating room. Initial antibiotic therapy should begin with ampicillin/sulbactam or clindamycin plus ciprofloxacin. If the Gram stain shows gram-negative bacilli, a third- or fourth-generation cephalosporin or aminoglycoside should be added. When sepsis is present, broad-spectrum coverage with imipenem/cilastatin is warranted pending culture results.

Cat-Scratch Disease (CSD)

CSD most often occurs in young (80 percent less than 21 years of age) immunocompetent hosts.[31] The initial site develops a transient erythematous papule or pustule for which the patients do not often seek medical attention. They usually come after the development of persistent regional lymphadenopathy in an area of the body draining lymph from the scratch or bite, usually 7 to 12 days after the injury. Symptomatic lymphadenopathy usually resolves in 2 to 4 months. Systemic complications—with involvement of the central nervous system, eye, liver, spleen, and bone—can be seen in up to 2 percent of cases. It has been estimated that CSD affects about 22,000 individuals annually in the United States (9.3 per 100,000 population) and results in about 2000 hospitalizations. There is a male as well as a fall/winter seasonal predominance.

The precise etiologic agent has been difficult to determine. Most investigations implicate *Bartonella henselae*, a small gram-negative rod. Diagnosis is made by (1) history of cat exposure, (2) typical lymphadenopathy, (3) no other cause of lymph gland swelling, and (4) a positive serologic test for *B. henselae*. Serologic assay using the polymerase chain reaction (PCR) is the most accurate method (86 percent sensitive and 96 percent specific) and more sensitive than either the IgG indirect fluorescence assay (IgG IFA) (41 percent sensitive) or the IgM enzyme-linked immunoassay (IgM EIA) (71 to 80 percent sensitive).[32] Serologic testing can be improved by using PCR to assay pus and lymph node specimens, with sensitivities approaching 100 percent.[33]

Most patients with CSD are not seriously ill, spontaneous resolution is common, and antibiotic therapy has not been studied in large controlled clinical trials. As a result, most reviews do not recommend antibiotic therapy for uncomplicated cases. A recent controlled study of 29 patients with typical CSD found that a 5-day course of azithromycin led to more rapid resolution in lymph node volume during the first 30 days.[34] After that, there was no difference in rate or degree of resolution. Antimicrobial susceptibility testing has shown favorable minimum inhibitory concentration (MIC) values to a number of antibiotics, but since the bacterium resides intraceullularly, agents that achieve high concentrations inside human cells would probably be the most effective—rifampin, gentamicin, doxycycline, and the macrolides. Severely ill patients, those with systemic complications, and those who are immunocompromised should be treated with either rifampin or trimethoprim-sulfamethoxazole.

Cat Bites

Cat bites account for 5 to 18 percent of reported animal bites in the United States.[26] The majority of wounds are inflicted on the arm, forearm, and hand and with decreasing frequency to the head and neck, lower extremity, and trunk. Owing to the long, slender fangs of cats, most bites result in puncture wounds (57 to 86 percent); the remainder are superficial abrasions (9 to 25 percent) and lacerations (5 to 17 percent). Up to 80 percent of cat bites become infected, due to such factors as (1) older age of the patient, (2) attempting wound care at home with longer treatment delays, (3) higher percentage of puncture wounds, and (4) a higher likelihood of *P. multocida* in feline oral flora.

Pasteurella multocida is the major pathogen found in infected cat bite wounds; it is isolated in 53 to 80 percent.[25,26] These infections are characterized by a rapidly developing, intense inflammatory response, often within a few hours and rarely more than 24 h after the bite. Pain and swelling are prominent. *Pasteurella multocida* may cause serious bone and joint infections. Septic arthritis usually involves a single joint, with predilection for joints previously damaged by arthritis or prosthetic joints, and more than half the patients also have altered host defenses from glucocorticoids or alcoholism. Bacteremia may occur in serious infections with *P. multocida*.

Treatment for cat bite wounds is essentially the same as for dog bite wounds. Larger lacerations (>2 cm) can be primarily closed after cleaning without an increased risk of infection.[29] Puncture wounds and lacerations smaller than 1 to 2 cm in length cannot be adequately cleaned and should not be primarily closed. Delayed primary closure can be employed for wounds smaller than 1 to 2 cm in length located in cosmetically important areas. Prophylactic antibiotics should be administered to high-risk patients including those with punctures of the hand; immunocompromised patients; and patients with arthritis or prosthetic joints. The case can be made that all cat bites should receive prophylactic antibiotics because of the high risk of infection. Three to five days of penicillin, amoxicillin/clavulanate, cefuroxime, or doxcycline are appropriate for prophylactic treatment following cat bites. For cat bites that develop infection, evaluation and treatment is similar to dog bite infections.

Exotic Animal Bites

Extensive clinical data and treatment recommendations pertaining to bite wounds made by exotic animals and resulting infection are based on anecdotal case reports. In general, it is best to adhere to the dictum that the bacteriology of the bite wound will reflect the normal oral flora of the inflicting animal as opposed to the normal skin flora of the patient. General principles of local wound care—including irrigation and surgical debridement, wound cultures as appropriate, and tetanus and rabies prophylaxis—should be followed.

Nonhuman primate (monkey) bites are likely to be seen in animal handlers and researchers. The organisms most often encountered in the mouths of rhesus monkeys (*Macaca mulatta*) are *Neisseria* sp., α-hemolytic streptococci, and *Haemophilus parainfluenza*. Also, *E. corrodens* is a pathogen from primate bite infections. The combination of penicillin and cefoperazone has been recommended as an initial antibiotic regimen for monkey bite injuries. In addition, the potential for transmission of *Herpesvirus simiae* (B virus) must be considered, from bites, scratches, or needle sticks. The potential consequences of inoculation with B virus are grave and include local neurologic symptoms, encephalitis (91 percent), and death (68 percent). The affected area must be scrubbed with povidine-iodine for 15 min, and then copiously rinsed with water. Ocular or mucous membrane exposure requires a 15-min irrigation with saline or water. Treatment with acyclovir 800 mg PO five times a day beginning immediately after injury should be considered when a wound from a rhesus monkey is sustained. The monkey should be quarantined and carefully examined for oral mucosal lesions. Questions can be directed to the NIH B virus Research Laboratory (404-651-0808).

The large feline carnivores, such as lions and tigers, like domestic cats, also carry *Pasteurella* among their normal oral flora. Wound care should be the same as for other species, with awareness for the potential for major skeletal and internal injuries.

Alligator bites (*Alligator mississippiensis*) may be frequently encountered in the southeastern United States. Bite wounds can be polymicrobial, but the aerobic organism *Aeromonas hydrophila* has been a consistent isolate. Trimethoprim-sulfamethoxazole is considered a front-line agent for treatment, with an aminoglycoside, imipenem, meropenem, or tetracycline as an alternative. *Bacteroides* and *Clostridium* species have also been isolated from alligator bites.

Bites from the common or green iguana (*Iguana iguana*), readily available in the United States as a pet, are generally innocuous. These animals do not harbor the rabies virus. Local topical antiseptic wound care and verification of tetanus status is all that is needed for the emergency treatment of an iguana bite.

Rat bites may be complicated by leptospirosis, a zoonosis transmitted primarily through the direct or indirect exposure of mucous membranes or abraded skin to the urine of an infected animal. The domestic rat may serve as the primary reservoir of leptospirosis in urban areas. Subclinical infections are common and most clinical infections are self-limiting. Oral doxycycline for 7 days is effective when initiated within 4 days of symptom onset. Parenteral penicillin G for 7 days is indicated for the more severe icteric disease. In addition, rat-bite fever may be transmitted by several small rodents, including the rat, mouse, and gerbil. The causative organisms are *Streptobacillus moniliformis* and *Spirillum minor*. Prophylactic therapy with penicillin, amoxicillin/clavulanate, or doxcycline for 5 days is recommended.

Camels can inflict serious bites as well as other associated injuries due to their enlarged canine teeth and long necks, which allow them to reach around and bite the rider violently, lift the rider into the air, and throw him or her to the ground. The bacteriology of camel bite wounds has not been well studied; however, an anecdotal report of successful treatment with high-dose penicillin G, gentamicin, and clindamycin has been published.

REFERENCES

1. Laughlin TJ, Armstrong DG, Caporusso J, Lavery LA: Soft tissue and bone infections from puncture wounds in children. *West J Med* 166:126, 1997.
2. Weber EJ: Plantar puncture wounds: A survey to determine the incidence of infection. *J Accid Emerg Med* 13:274, 1996.
3. Schwab RA, Powers RD: Conservative therapy of plantar puncture wounds. *J Emerg Med* 13:291, 1995.
4. Chisholm CD, Schlesser JF: Plantar puncture wounds: Controversies and treatment recommendations. *Ann Emerg Med* 18:1352, 1989.
5. Inaba AS, Zukin DD, Perro M: An update on the evaluation and management of plantar puncture wounds and *Pseudomonas* osteomyelitis. *Pediatr Emerg Care* 8:38, 1992.
6. Armstrong DG, Lavery LA, Quebedeaux TL, Walker SC: Surgical morbidity and the risk of amputation due to infected puncture wound in diabetics and nondiabetic adults. *J Am Podiatr Med Assoc* 87:321, 1997.
7. Patzakis MJ, Wilkins J, Brien WW, Carter VS: Wound site as a predictor of complications following deep nail punctures to the foot. *West J Med* 150:545, 1989.
8. Book JW: Management of pedal puncture wounds. *J Foot Ankle Surg* 33:463, 1994.
9. Pennycock A, Makower R, O'Donnell AM: Puncture wounds of the foot: Can infectious complications be avoided? *J R Soc Med* 87:581, 1994.
10. Raz R, Miron D: Oral ciprofloxacin for treatment of infection following nail puncture wounds of the foot. *Clin Infect Dis* 21:194, 1995.
11. Lavery LA, Armstrong DG, Quebedeaux TL, Walker SC: Puncture wounds: Normal laboratory values in the face of severe infection in diabetics and non-diabetics. *Am J Med* 101:521, 1996.
12. Centers for Disease Control and Prevention: Prevention of hepatitis A through active and passive immunization. *MMWR* 45(RR-15):1, 1996.
13. Centers for Disease Control and Prevention: Recommendations for prevention and control of hepatitis C virus (HCV) infection and HCV-related chronic disease. *MMWR* 47(RR-19):1, 1998.
14. Centers for Disease Control and Prevention: Public Health Service guidelines for the management of health-care worker exposures to HIV and recommendations for postexposure prophylaxis. *MMWR* 47(RR-7):1, 1998.
15. Fialkov JA, Freiberg A: High-pressure injection injuries: An overview. *J Emerg Med* 9:367, 1991.
16. Pinto MR, Turkula-Pinto LD, Cooney WP, et al: High-pressure injection injuries of the hand: Review of 25 patients managed by open technique. *J Hand Surg [Am]* 18:125, 1993.
17. Bunzli WF, Wright DH, Hoang AT, et al: Current management of human bites. *Pharmacotherapy* 18:227, 1998.
18. Kelly IP, Cunney RJ, Smyth EG, Colville J: The management of human bite injuries of the hand. *Injury* 27:481, 1996.
19. Zubowicz VN, Gravier M: Management of early human bites of the hand: A prospective randomized study. *Plast Reconstr Surg* 88:111, 1991.
20. Chadaev AP, Jukhtin VI, Butkevich AT, Emkuzhev VM: Treatment of infected clench-fist human bite wounds in the area of the metacarpophalangeal joints. *J Hand Surg [Am]* 21:299, 1996.
21. Donkor P, Bankas DO: A study of primary closure of human bite injuries to the face. *J Oral Maxillofac Surg* 55:479, 1997.
22. Uchendu BO: Primary closure of human bite losses of the lip. *Plast Reconstr Surg* 90:841, 1992.
23. Sachs JJ, Kresnow M, Houston B: Dog bites: How big a problem? *Inj Prev* 2:52, 1996.
24. Weiss HB, Friedman DI, Coben JH: Incidence of dog bite injuries treated in emergency departments. *JAMA* 279:51, 1998.
25. Weber DJ, Hansen AR: Infections resulting from animal bites. *Infect Dis Clin North Am* 5:663, 1991.
26. Griego RD, Rosen T, Orengo IF, Wolf JE: Dog, cat, and human bites: A review. *J Am Acad Dermatol* 33:1019, 1995.
27. Brogan TV, Bratton SL, Dowd MD, Hegenbarth MA: Severe dog bites in children. *Pediatrics* 96:947, 1995.
28. Centers for Disease Control and Prevention: Dog-bite-related fatalities—United States, 1995–1996. *MMWR* 30:463, 1997.
29. Dire DJ: Management of animal bites. *Acad Emerg Med* 1:178, 1994.
30. Wolff KD: Management of animal bite injuries of the face: Experience with 94 patients. *J Oral Maxillofac Surg* 56:838, 1998.
31. Bass JW, Vincent JM, Person DA: The expanding spectrum of *Bartonella* infections: II. Cat-scratch disease. *Pediatr Infect Dis J* 16:163, 1997.
32. Bergmans AM, Peeters MF, Schellekens JF, et al: Pitfalls and fallacies of cat scratch disease serology: Evaluation of *Bartonella henselae*–based indirect fluorescence assay and enzyme-linked immunoassay. *J Clin Microbiol* 35:1931, 1997.
33. Avidor B, Kletter Y, Abulafia S, et al: Molecular diagnosis of cat scratch disease: A two step approach. *J Clin Microbiol* 35:1924, 1997.
34. Bass JW, Freitas BC, Freitas AD, et al: Prospective randomized double blind placebo controlled evaluation of azithromycin for treatment of cat-scratch disease. *Pediatr Infect Dis J* 17:447, 1998.

POSTREPAIR WOUND CARE

Louis J. Kroot

Following repair in the emergency department (ED), continued care and instructions should be provided to minimize complications and optimize outcome. This chapter discusses the principles of postrepair wound care as commonly practiced in the United States. These steps may not be necessary with every patient; in fact, while many of them are based on common sense, scientific validation is lacking.[1,2]

DRESSING

The value of wound dressings has been debated for years. Studies indicate that an important component of wound repair is reepithelialization as the regenerating epithelial cells migrate across the moist exudate of a wound.[1] A moist environment is crucial for this process, and epithelial repair is significantly impaired in desiccated wounds. Wound dressings that follow this basic principle of maintaining a moist environment for the first 24 to 48 h facilitate healing.

The simplest wound dressing is a layer of petrolatum-based ointment applied directly over the sutures. This approach is most useful to treat simple, uncontaminated lacerations of the face and scalp but should not be implemented when tissue adhesives are applied. These areas have an excellent vascular supply; they heal with little risk of infection and a good cosmetic result. The addition of an antibiotic to the petrolatum-based ointment reduces the risk of infection, particularly in extremity wounds.[3] Available agents include bacitracin zinc, neomycin, and polymixin B, usually in combination. The ointment should be gently washed off and reapplied two or three times per day for the first 2 to 3 days and once a day thereafter until suture removal.[3] This approach has been criticized as being unnecessary, time-consuming, and uncomfortable.[4] Instead, the use of a topical antibiotic in a water-soluble base (such as mupirocin in polyethylene glycol) has been advocated, for abraded skin surrounding stellate lacerations. Topical antibiotic ointments, which contain povidone-iodine, should be avoided, since this antiseptic impairs wound healing. Application of ointment facilitates suture removal by preventing the exposed tails from becoming encrusted in a dried wound exudate.

Small lacerations can be dressed with self-adhesive elastic strips. These strips almost always have a nonadherent center that goes directly over the wound. Petrolatum-based antibiotic ointment can be placed either on the elastic strip or on the wound.

Most other wounds are commonly dressed; although there is little evidence that dressing reduces the risk of infection or improves ultimate cosmetic appearance. The less ''scientific'' but highly practical reasons for wound dressing include the following:

1. General cleanliness as the dressing absorbs exudate
2. Protection from external contamination when the patient returns home or work
3. Camouflage, so that the patient or others do not have to see the wound
4. Prevention of premature suture removal from spontaneous unraveling or the patient's curiosity
5. Prevention from excessive movement by providing a ''soft'' splint
6. Satisfying the patient's expectation that the repaired wound will be dressed

The basic wound dressing has four layers: (1) a nonadherent layer adjacent to the wound, (2) gauze sponges to absorb any exudate, (3) wrapping to hold the first two layers in place, and (4) tape or elastic bandage to secure the entire package (Table 44-1).

The simplest nonadherent dressing is a ribbon of petrolatum-based ointment applied to the wound with a small gauze pad over it. When wrapped with gauze and secured with tape, such a dressing will remain moist for the first 24 h. This simple approach is appropriate for clean, closed wounds with minimal exudate. Several nonadherent dressing materials have been developed for use on open, larger, and more exudative wounds and burns. These materials can be occlusive, semipermeable, or porous. While wounds treated with the newer semipermeable materials may tend to heal faster and with less pain, there is no clear benefit over the older and less expensive porous materials. The nonadherent material should be cut to extend beyond the wound area.

TABLE 44-1 Wound Dressing Materials—Representative Examples

Petrolatum-based ointment
Plain
Bacitracin zinc
Neomycin/polymyxin B/bacitracin zinc (Neosporin)
Polymyxin B/bacitracin zinc (Polysporin)
Polyethylene glycol–based ointment
Mupirocin (Bactroban)
Nonadherent layer
Adaptic (Johnson & Johnson Medical)
Epi-Lock (Lock Laboratories)
Tegaderm (3M Health Care)
Telfa (Kendall Healthcare Products)
Xeroform (Kendall Healthcare Products)
Absorbent layer
Gauze squares
Alginate dressing
Wrapping layer
Gauze wrap
Securing layer
Tape
Elastic bandages

A layer of gauze squares is placed over the nonadherent layer to absorb any exudate. While it is possible to tape the gauze squares directly to the adjacent skin, this is uncomfortable for the patient; moreover, as the sweat loosens the tape, such a dressing usually does not last for more than a few days. In general, the first two layers are held in place by a wrap, usually of gauze. Wrapping is easy over tubular body portions (e.g., the forearm) and more difficult over irregular areas (e.g., the shoulder).

Either tape or elastic bandages secures the wrapping layer. Tape should be applied in a spiral manner to allow for edema and swelling; it should never be wrapped circumferentially around an extremity or digit. Elastic bandages must likewise be applied with allowance for expansion during the following 24 h.

DRESSING CHANGES

The general principle is that wound dressings should be changed as often as needed for removal of exudate, inspection, and general cleaning. That said, there is great variety in the need for dressing changes. A routine change in 24 h serves several purposes: removal of most of the exudate and inspection for bleeding and early signs of infection. The wound should be dressed again, often with a simpler bandage than was initially required. Thereafter, dressing changes depend on the rate of wound healing, the continued presence of exudate, and the patient's ability to keep the area clean.

PAIN CONTROL

Wounds, particularly burns and abrasions, can be painful. Patients should be instructed about the potential for pain and measures to help control it. The need for analgesics should also be considered for every wound patient. Narcotic analgesics, particularly hydrocodone and oxycodone, may be necessary. Studies have consistently found that ED patients are often untreated with analgesics for acute, painful injuries while in the ED and upon discharge. Patients who do receive appropriate analgesics upon discharge report greater satisfaction with overall care.[5] The pain from wounds decreases during the first 48 h and narcotic analgesics are not usually required beyond that time.

ANTIBIOTIC PROPHYLAXIS

As discussed in other chapters, antibiotic prophylaxis is effective when a wound has more than baseline bacterial contamination, antibiotics effective against expected pathogens are chosen, and such antibiotics are given as soon as possible to achieve antimicrobial blood levels before repair. However, as commonly practiced, antibiotic prophylaxis from the ED is suspect for the following reasons: (1) the use of antibiotics for simple, uncomplicated lacerations fails to satisfy the first requirement; (2) the use of cephalexin for cat bites fails to meet the second requirement; and (3) handing the patient a prescription on discharge fails the third.[6] Antibiotic prophylaxis should be initiated in the ED, before significant wound manipulation, and with agents that rapidly achieve antibacterial blood levels.

The following types of wounds have shown evidence to support the use of continued antibiotic prophylaxis upon discharge from the ED:

1. Intraoral lacerations: penicillin
2. Complicated human bites: amoxicillin/clavulanate or penicillin plus a first-generation cephalosporin
3. Complicated dog bites: amoxicillin/clavulanate or penicillin plus a first-generation cephalosporin
4. Cat bites: penicillin or amoxicillin/clavulanate
5. Plantar puncture wounds, particularly through athletic shoes: ciprofloxacin

Although antibiotic prophylaxis is commonly employed for patients with comorbid conditions predisposing to wound infection (diabetes, cirrhosis, advanced age, and immunosuppression), there is little supporting evidence for this practice in all circumstances except for the types of wounds described above.

ROUTINE RECHECKS

The routine recheck policy serves two purposes: (1) professional cleaning and redressing of the wound and (2) early identification of bleeding or wound infection. Routine rechecks have been criticized because: (1) most wounds are uncomplicated and do not require professional cleaning and redressing; (2) the routine recheck is usually performed at 48 h, slightly before the 3- to 5-day peak incidence for wound infection; and (3) the vast majority of wounds heal without complication and do not benefit from a recheck.

A more appropriate approach would be to implement selective rechecks on patients with complicated wounds at risk for infection. Comorbidity status and social situation may also be used to select patients for recheck. Patients may not have a clear understanding of the symptoms and signs of wound infection. Those at significant risk should be told to return on a specific day. Practically speaking, rechecks are easier when they are scheduled in the morning, when the ED is less busy and these patients can be seen expeditiously. Since the bulk of ED wound care is provided in the late afternoon and evening, having the patient return on the second and fourth day corresponds to rechecks at approximately 36 and 84 h. The first recheck would be appropriate for redressing and the second would occur when signs of wound infection usually become manifest.

CLOSURE REMOVAL

Sutures and staples are generally removed when the wound closure has become strong enough to withstand normal activity. The major exception to this principle is the face, where cosmetic outcome is important. Percutaneous sutures incite the development of small epithelial plugs at the suture puncture sites, leaving behind a "railroad track" if sutures are left in place for 7 days or more. Therefore, facial sutures are removed at 4 to 5 days, before tensile strength is adequately recovered. Such wounds may require adhesive closure strips for an additional 3 to 4 days. Sutures and staples in other areas can be removed in 7 to 14 days (Table 44-2). Sutures and staples applied over highly mobile areas, particularly the extensor surfaces of large joints, are best left in place for 3 to 4 days longer.

TABLE 44-2 Timing for Removal of Cutaneous Sutures and Staples

Face	4–5 days
Scalp	7–10 days
Trunk	10 days
Arm (surface)	10 days
Arm (joint)	10–14 days
Hand	10–14 days
Leg (surface)	10 days
Leg (joint)	10–14 days
Foot	14 days

Wounds closed with adhesive tape or tissue adhesives do not require specific removal; the tape or adhesive will slough off by itself by epithelial exfoliation. In general, such adhesives should be expected to remain on the skin for about the same time as sutures would.

WASHING AND GROOMING

Within 8 to 24 h after closure, wounds in highly vascular areas (scalp, face, and neck) can be washed without any impairment to healing or an increase in infection; shampooing of the scalp or washing of the face and neck is allowable the day after suture repair. Likewise, wounds in other areas can be washed after 12 to 24 h without increased risk of an adverse outcome. However, immersion or soaking should be avoided, as this tends to track moisture down the percutaneous sutures and macerate the wound; showering is allowable, but bathing is to be discouraged. Following cleaning, the wound should be dried with a clean towel and redressed as directed. While shaving is rarely a danger, patients may have to be told not to shave around or over a wound.

Stapled wounds can be washed and groomed in the same way as sutured wounds. However, wounds that have been closed by adhesive tape should not be moistened or washed. Wounds closed with tissue adhesive may be very gently cleaned after 24 h, but immersion should be prohibited.

DISCHARGE INSTRUCTIONS

For the majority of lacerations sutured in the ED, patients should be instructed that a small amount of bloody discharge is to be expected; enough only to form a small surface clot or to stain the dressing. More than that is unexpected, and if such is found, the patients should return for recheck. Deep, complex lacerations that require drains or remain open may bleed more, and the patient should receive appropriate instructions to this potential.

Patients should be instructed about early symptoms and signs of infection: increasing pain, redness that extends more than $\frac{1}{4}$ in. (5 mm) beyond the wound edges, red streaks that extend from the wound, purulent drainage, and fever. As noted above, many patients unfortunately do not recognize these signs of infection; in a study of 433 patients with 21 physician-diagnosed wound infections, only 11 (52 percent) were able to self-diagnose their infection.[7] Instructions must be clear, simple, and specific.

Wounds may open spontaneously, especially during the vulnerable period: 7 to 10 days after injury. Infection, fluid, and blood collections within the wound facilitate dehiscence. Patients should be instructed to return if a wound opens, particularly if blood or pus is expressed.

Patients discharged with a planned delayed primary closure require additional instructions:

1. They will generally be given antibiotics to take after they are sent home
2. They should leave the dressing intact until they return for a recheck
3. A recheck is generally done within 4 to 5 days

In carefully selected patients, delayed primary closure is associated with a low incidence of wound infection.[8]

Patients may inquire about the long-term outcome of the wound; in such instances, the physician should respond with a candid prognosis explaining that wound outcome is primarily determined by factors beyond the physician's control, including:

1. Wounding mechanism
2. Type of wound
3. Location of wound
4. Comorbid diseases

Patients should be told that the wound's appearance will change during the healing process and that the ultimate cosmetic outcome cannot be predicted at the time of suture removal.[9,10] If necessary, wound revision should wait about 6 to 9 months from the initial injury. Some wounds on sun-exposed areas may be less pigmented than the surrounding skin and more sensitive to ultraviolet radiation. Color generally fills in over the next 12 months and sunscreens may be required for several months.

REFERENCES

1. Edlich RF, Rodeheaver GT, Morgan RF, et al: Principles of emergency wound management. *Ann Emerg Med* 17:1284, 1988.
2. Berk WA, Welch RD, Bock BF: Controversial issues in clinical management of the simple wound. *Ann Emerg Med* 21:72, 1992.
3. Dire DJ, Coppola M, Dwyer DA, et al: Prospective evaluation of topical antibiotics for preventing infections in uncomplicated soft-tissue wounds repaired in the ED. *Acad Emerg Med* 2:4, 1995.
4. Edlich RF, Sutton ST: Postrepair wound care revisited. *Acad Emerg Med* 2:2, 1995.
5. Chan L, Verdile VP: Do patients receive adequate pain control after discharge from the ED? *Am J Emerg Med* 16:705, 1998.
6. Cummings P, Del Beccaro MA: Antibiotics to prevent infections of simple wounds: A meta-analysis of randomized studies. *Am J Emerg Med* 13:396, 1995.
7. Seaman M, Lammers R: Inability of patients to self-diagnose wound infections. *J Emerg Med* 9:215, 1991.
8. Smilanich RP, Bonnet I, Kirkpatrick JR: Contaminated wounds: The effect of initial management on outcome. *Am Surg* 61:427, 1995.
9. Hollander JE, Blasko B, Singer AJ, et al: Poor correlation of short- and long-term cosmetic appearance of repaired lacerations. *Acad Emerg Med* 2:983, 1995.
10. Hollander JE, Valentine SM, McCluskey CF, et al: Long-term evaluation of cosmetic appearance of repaired lacerations: Validation of telephone assessment. *Ann Emerg Med* 31:92, 1998.

CARDIOVASCULAR DISEASES

APPROACH TO CHEST PAIN AND POSSIBLE MYOCARDIAL ISCHEMIA

Gary B. Green
Peter M. Hill

OVERVIEW

Approximately 5 percent of all emergency department (ED) visits, or about 5 million visits a year, are for chest pain, yet accurate diagnosis remains a challenge. Owing to a complex interplay of anatomic, physiologic, and psychological factors, serious illness often mimics benign conditions. Symptoms are often intermittent, so the patient may appear well on evaluation. This chapter outlines an approach to patients presenting with chest pain and other symptoms of possible ischemia. Detailed discussion of patients with findings diagnostic of acute coronary syndromes (ACS) can be found in other chapters of this text.

Pathophysiology of Chest Pain

Afferent pain fibers are classified into two broad categories, visceral and somatic, with their stimulation resulting in distinct pain syndromes. The dermis and parietal pleura are innervated by somatic pain fibers. They enter the spinal cord at specific levels, are arranged in dermatomal patterns, and map to specific areas on the parietal cortex. Visceral pain fibers are found in internal organs such as blood vessels, the esophagus, and the visceral pleura. These fibers enter the spinal cord at multiple levels, along with somatic pain fibers, and map to areas on the parietal cortex corresponding to the cord levels shared with the somatic fibers. Therefore, pain from somatic fibers is usually easily described, precisely located, and experienced as a sharp sensation. Pain from visceral fibers is more difficult to describe and is imprecisely localized. Those experiencing visceral pain are more likely to use terms such as *discomfort, heaviness,* or *aching.* Further, patients frequently misinterpret the origin of visceral pain because it is often referred to a different area of the body corresponding to an adjacent somatic nerve. For example, diaphragmatic irritation can present as shoulder pain, and arm pain may actually represent myocardial ischemia.

Many physiologic, psychological, and cultural factors further influence how patients perceive, interpret, and communicate their symptoms. Gender, age, comorbidities, polypharmacy, drugs, and alcohol can all affect perception of pain.

Pathophysiology of Anginal Pain

For a detailed discussion of the pathophysiology of ischemia, see Chap. 47. In brief, angina pectoris can be defined as any pain syndrome that is caused by lack of oxygen supply to the heart. Anginal symptoms are typically caused by obstructive coronary artery disease or coronary spasm, or both. Atherosclerotic plaques lining the walls of coronary arteries cause luminal stenosis in patients with coronary artery disease. During periods of low myocardial oxygen demand, blood flow through the stenosed vessels may be adequate to meet demand. However, during times of increased oxygen demand, flow through the fixed lesion is limited and the region of myocardium supplied by the affected vessel may become ischemic. Cardiac myocytes respond to oxygen deprivation by switching from aerobic to anaerobic metabolism, during which sufficient ATP cannot be produced to meet the metabolic demands of the cell. The lack of ATP causes dysfunction of all intracellular ATP-dependent processes, including ion channels in the sarcoplasmic and cell membranes, causing diminished contractility and cell integrity. Chemical mediators are subsequently released, stimulating visceral afferent nerve fibers in sympathetic nerves of coronary vessels. These nerves travel through deep and superficial cardiac plexuses and the sympathetic ganglia and enter the spinal cord through the lower cervical and upper five thoracic spinal nerve roots. Because of this wide spinal cord distribution of the cardiac pain fibers, the cerebral cortex often misinterprets the location and origin of the pain, therefore confusing myocardial ischemia with pain from any of the other structures in the chest.

INITIAL APPROACH TO THE PATIENT

All chest pain patients, like trauma patients, should receive a high triage priority and be evaluated without delay. The patient care team—nurses, electrocardiography (ECG) technicians, and physicians—should be mobilized around the patient simultaneously. During this time, the patient should be placed on a cardiac monitor, have intravenous access established, oxygen administered, vital signs measured, and a 12-lead ECG obtained.

The initial moments with the patient must be considered similar to a primary survey for trauma, with the focus on identifying an immediate life threat. First, there is a rapid assessment of the patient's airway, breathing, and circulation, general appearance, and vital signs. The initial history should include only a few directed questions—e.g., as to the presence and character of any ongoing symptoms and the presence of significant underlying cardiovascular or pulmonary pathology, such as a history of pulmonary embolism, acute myocardial infarction (AMI), or coronary revascularization. A focused pulmonary and vascular exam is performed next.

If immediate life threats have not been detected or have already been addressed, a more extensive evaluation can then be performed. The secondary survey consists of a more comprehensive history and physical examination and appropriate laboratory and diagnostic testing. This evaluation should focus on those variables that will aid in establishing a tentative diagnosis.

Every patient in whom ACS is entertained, particularly those that present with CP, must have concurrent consideration of several entities that may have similar presentation. Missing any of these diagnoses carries the same order of risk of morbidity and even mortality as missed ACS. These include PE, pneumothorax, pericarditis, pneumonia, aortic dissection, perforated peptic ulcer, and under certain circumstances esophageal rupture. These represent a minimum differential diagnosis of consequence. Some authorities would add such entities as aortic stenosis (CP, syncope, DOE) and possibly acute cholecystitis and pancreatitis within the list of conditions to be simultaneously considered. It is important to emphasize that this differential must be pursued simultaneous, and the evaluation should be concerned with ruling in, or ruling out, each entity. While important history that may point to an ACS is detailed below, the history and physical exam should also include consideration of the above conditions (Table 45-1). Fortunately, the evaluation of the patient with possible ACS readily includes ancillary investigations that also appropriately consider most of the above noted entities. For example, a chest x-ray and an EKG readily consider PE, pneumothorax, pericarditis, pneumonia, dissection, and even perforated viscus. Among these, PE requires more evaluation if other evidence suggests further investigation. Cholecystitis, pancreatitis, and aortic stenosis may require additional avenues of investigation,

TABLE 45-1 Life-Threatening and Serious Causes of Chest Pain and Their Clinical Characteristics

Diagnosis	Presentation	Physical Exam	Ancillary Tests
Pulmonary embolism	Sudden onset, pleuritic pain, and dyspnea	Tachypnea, tachycardia Deep vein thrombosis	ABG, CXR, V/Q scan, Angiogram
Aortic dissection	Tearing pain with radiation to back Neurologic symptoms	New murmer, bruits Unequal BP in upper extremities	CXR Angiogram
Pericarditis	Positional ache, dyspnea	Rub, distended neck veins	ECG, CXR, sonogram
Pneumothorax	Pleuritic pain and dyspnea	Decreased breath sounds	CXR
ACS	Vague, pressure-like pain Radiation to arm, neck, jaw Associated diaphoresis, dyspnea, nausea	Diaphoresis, rales	ECG, Myocardial markers
Esophageal rupture	Constant retrosternal, epigastric pain History of inciting event	Variable	CXR
Pneumonia	Pleuritic pain, cough, dyspnea, chills	Fever, rhonchi, Decreased breath sounds	CXR, WBC

although routine chemistries may assist in establishing or refuting the diagnosis of the first two.

Other important diagnoses such as mitral valve prolapse (covered later in this chapter) may yet be the underlying etiology, but there is little risk of morbidity in the short term if missed during the ED evaluation. Diagnoses such as musculoskeletal chest pain, hiatal hernia, or gastritis may be a source of both concern and discomfort to the patient, but there is minimal to no consequence if such diagnoses were in fact the underlying cause but not seriously pursued in the ED.

CLINICAL FEATURES

History

Routine questions should determine the quality, location, radiation, intensity. frequency, associated symptoms, and precipitating factors of chest pain. For patients who have difficulty explaining symptoms in a narrative fashion, directed questions should be asked. Patients without previously diagnosed ischemic heart disease may have difficulty describing the quality of pain and may resort to textbook terms. Specific questioning is needed about radiation to the jaw, neck, arms, back, or epigastrium. However, lack of such specific pain location is not differentiating. Pain intensity is commonly graded on a scale of 1 to 10, with 10 representing the worst pain the patient can imagine. The frequency of pain episodes should be assessed over a continuum of the past weeks to better determine whether the condition is stable or unstable angina. Patients can be asked about episodes relative to a past holiday or event and should compare frequency to the current time frame. They should identify precipitating factors such as changes with inspiration, movement, palpation, or exertion and during sleep or at rest. The presence of associated symptoms such as diaphoresis, near syncope, nausea, or vomiting raises concern about ischemic disease. Family members, friends, or emergency medical technicians (EMTs) who may have witnessed the episode can be questioned about the patient's general appearance while in pain. If the patient is described as appearing ill, suspicion for ischemia is heightened.

The classic description of angina pectoris is that of a retrosternal left anterior chest or epigastric discomfort consisting of crushing, tightening, squeezing, or pressure. The presence of certain associated symptoms during chest pain—including dyspnea, diaphoresis, nausea, and/or vomiting—is common and indicates a twofold higher risk of ischemia. Many patients also complain of discomfort radiating from the chest to the left shoulder, arm, hand, or jaw, a finding whose presence is also associated with a significantly greater risk of ischemia.[4,5] However, atypical characteristics are the rule rather than the exception. For example, up to 22 percent of patients with AMI describe their symptoms as being sharp or stabbing in character and up to 6 percent describe a pleuritic component of their pain.[6]

Anginal pain (or other anginal symptoms) is typically described as lasting from 2 to 20 min and pain from an uncomplicated AMI lasting up to 2 h. In contrast, chest pain that is described as lasting a ''split second'' or only a few seconds is more likely to be due to another cause, as is constant, unremitting pain lasting 12 to 24 h or more. Anginal pain is often brought on by exertion and relieved by rest, while pain worsened by body movement or body position is suggestive (but certainly not diagnostic) of another etiology. Angina may also occur at rest and is often attributed to coronary artery spasm with or without underlying atherosclerotic lesions.

All patients should also be questioned regarding the presence of cardiac risk factors, although ''risks'' are valid only for predicting the presence of coronary artery disease within a given population and not in an individual patient. Major risk factors identified by the American Heart Association include age above 40, male or postmenopausal female, hypertension, cigarette smoking, hypercholesterolemia, diabetes, truncal obesity, family history, and sedentary lifestyle. Cocaine use is associated with AMI even in young people with minimal or no coronary artery disease. Chronic cocaine use has also been associated with accelerated atherosclerosis and severe coronary artery disease.

The patient's medical record should always be reviewed when analyzing chest pain. Previous ECGs should always be compared with the current tracing. Results of prior stress testing, echocardiograms, catherizations, or radionuclide scans should be reviewed, if available, and the present symptoms interpreted in light of those results. The ''gold standard'' for determining the presence or absence of coronary artery disease is angiography. In general, catherization reports from within the previous 2 years are considered to be generally reflective of the current extent of disease.

Ischemic Equivalents

Because of the visceral afferent innervation of the myocardium as well as the many confounding factors affecting the perception of ischemia, many patients with ACS will not experience chest discomfort. Up to one-third of AMIs may be silent, occurring without any reports of symptoms from the patient and discovered incidentally on routine ECG.[1] Many other patients present with ischemic-equivalent symptoms, which may include one or any combination of the following: dyspnea at rest or exertion; shoulder, arm, or jaw discomfort; epigastric discomfort; nausea; light-headedness; generalized weakness; acute changes in mental status; or diaphoresis. Other atypical features associated with ischemia, particularly in women, include repetitive chest pain, pain relieved by antacids, pain unrelated to exercise, pain not relieved with rest or nitoglycerin, or palpitations without chest pain.[2] Upper abdominal discomfort, despite relief with antacids, can also be a symptom of myocardial ischemia; for patients over 50 and those with known CAO, the evaluation of abdominal pain should include an ECG. Patients predisposed to sensory impairment due to diabetes, advanced age, or altered mental status are especially likely to present in atypical ways.[3]

Atypical chest pain is more common in women than in men,[2] and disorders such as vasospastic and microvascular angina and mitral valve prolapse are more common in women. In women, typical angina is strongly suggestive of cardiac ischemia, and nonischemic pain is associated with a lower though not well defined likelihood of disease.

Ischemia produces different patterns of pain in women with known coronary artery disease. Chest pain at rest but not during exercise does not decrease the likelihood of disease in women as it does in men. Women with stable angina are more likely than men to have pain during rest, sleep, or stress. Risk factors for coronary artery disease in women are listed below:[2]

Typical angina
Postmenopausal, no hormone replacement
Diabetes
Peripheral vascular disease
Hypertension
Smoking
Hyperlipidemia
Truncal obesity
Sedentary lifestyle

Palpitations are common symptoms that raise concern about myocardial ischemia. Palpitation may indicate dysrhythmia induced by ischemia, or the inducement of ischemia by a primary tachyarrhythmia. Palpitations are usually intermittent, and symptoms may have disappeared by the time ED evaluation occurs. The patient may describe palpitations in association with nonspecific chest discomfort or dyspnea, making evaluation difficult. The history should include questions about prescribed or over-the-counter medications or herbals; use of caffeine-containing beverages, symptoms of metabolic disorders such as hyperthroidism; and any prior individual or familial heart disease. If the clinic setting suggests hypokalemia or hypomagnesemia, electrolytes can be checked.

Physical Examination

The physical examination is often normal. Abnormalities in vital signs include hyper- or hypotension, sinus tachycardia, or bradycardia. Tachycardia often results from increased sympathetic tone and decreased left ventricular stroke volume, while bradycardia is often present among patients with inferior wall ischemia.

Patients with acute ischemia have a higher incidence of abnormal heart sounds such as a diminished S_1, a paradoxically split S_2, and/or an S_3 or S_4 due to changes in ventricular function or compliance. Auscultation of the lungs may reveal the presence of ischemia-induced congestive heart failure. However, none of these findings are uniformly present, nor are they diagnostic. Chest wall tenderness reproducing the patient's pain is somewhat suggestive of a musculoskeletal etiology. However, reproducible chest wall tenderness has also been reported in up to 15 percent of patients with confirmed MI; therefore, this finding should never be used to exclude the diagnosis of myocardial ischemia.[6] Despite a lack of specific diagnostic findings, a thorough physical examination remains essential, as it may provide clues to a nonischemic origin of the patient's symptoms and is often helpful in identifying or excluding other life-threatening causes of chest pain.

Electrocardiography

The ECG may help to identify nonischemic causes of chest pain such as dysrhythmias, acute pericarditis, or pulmonary embolism.

Because of the importance of early diagnosis of MI (and hence reduced delay of thrombolytic treatment), specific recommendations have been made concerning the procurement of the initial ECG in the ED. That is, under standing orders, patients with ischemic-type pain should have a 12-lead ECG performed within 10 min of arrival in the ED and the ECG should be handed directly to the treating physician for immediate interpretation. Considering the difficulty of defining ''ischemic type'' pain and the frequency of atypical presentations, it would be prudent to extend this protocol to all adult patients with chest pain.

Although the ECG is a critical guide to therapy when positive, a normal or nonspecific ECG is not reassuring. Among patients presenting to the ED with AMI, only about half will present with diagnostic changes on the initial ECG. Serial ECGs, even over several hours during the patient's ED stay, will increase the sensitivity of the ECG for the detection of AMI and should therefore be encouraged.[7] The inclusion of right-sided, posterior, or 22-lead ECGs can also improve the diagnostic yield and should be considered in all patients with known or suspected ischemia of the inferior, lateral, or posterior walls or of the right ventricle.[8] The use of continuous 12-lead ST-segment monitoring in the ED may also aid in the detection of patients with transient and/or silent ischemia.

Risk stratification based on the initial ED ECG has also been suggested as a way of improving ED decision making. Although the initial ECG cannot exclude AMI, stable ED patients whose initial ECG is without ischemic changes are at low risk of subsequent life threatening complications and can usually be managed in a non-intensive-care setting.[9]

ANCILLARY TESTING

Computerized Decision Aids

In an effort to facilitate more accurate disposition decisions and thereby reduce mounting health care costs, several investigators have developed computerized decision aids or computer-based triage protocols for ED patients with chest pain. One well-known computer-derived decision aid, developed by Goldman et al., applied recursive partitioning to clinical and ECG data to derive and prospectively validate an algorithm that could stratify ED patients into groups at variable risk of infarction (Fig. 45-1).[10] Although hypothetical testing predicted improved specificity of coronary care unit (CCU) triage decisions, a prospective study did not result in a significant decrease in the rates of CCU admission from the ED. Other methods, such as multivariate analysis and artificial neural networks, have also been used to develop predictive instruments for the detection of acute ischemic heart disease. In a large multicenter prospective trial (as yet unpublished), one of these decision aids, the time-insensitive predictive instrument (TIPI), was shown to decrease CCU admissions by 26 percent and increase ED discharges to home by 48 percent, but this approach has not yet been validated.

Myocardial Markers

CREATINE KINASE (CK), CK ISOENZYMES, AND ISOFORMS CK (adenosine triphosphate creatine *N*-phosphotransferase) is an intracellular enzyme involved in the transfer of high-energy phosphate groups

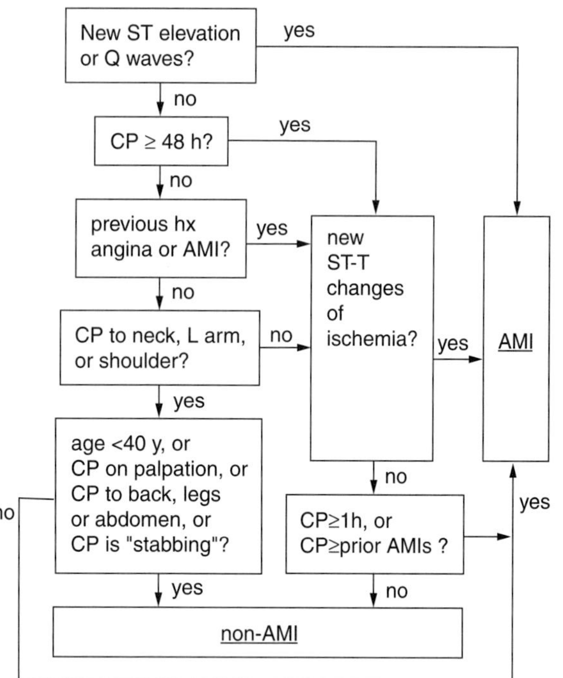

FIG. 45-1. Goldman algorithm. (An abridged version. Modified from Ref. 10.)

from ATP to creatine. Although found in small quantities in many tissues, CK is present in large concentrations in cardiac and skeletal muscle as well as brain. The enzyme is a dimer composed of two subunits, each of which may be either the M (muscle) type or the B (brain) type, thus creating three distinct dimers, or isoenzymes: CK-BB, predominantly found in brain tissue; CK-MM, the predominant isoenzyme in skeletal muscle (although CK-MB is also found there in small amounts); and CK-MB, accounting for 14 to 42 percent of the total enzyme activity present in cardiac muscle (the predominant enzyme remaining CK-MM).

The quantitative and temporal patterns of appearance and disappearance of CK and its isoenzymes in the blood occur in a reproducible manner but can vary considerably depending on the amount of CK released from cells, the amount of perfusion of damaged tissues, and the rate of clearance by the reticuloendothelial system. CK levels usually become abnormally high within 4 to 8 h after coronary artery occlusion (onset of symptoms), peak between 12 and 24 h, and return to normal between 3 and 4 days (Fig. 45-2). Reports of the sensitivity

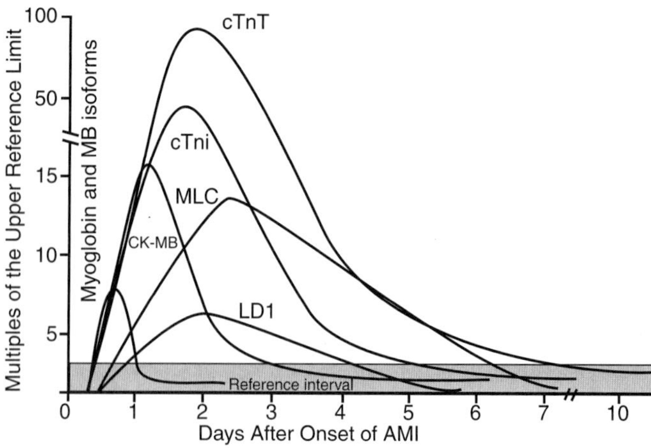

FIG. 45-2. Multiple marker curve.

of total CK vary from 93 to 100 percent, whereas the specificity is lower, ranging from 57 to 86 percent. Owing to the presence of CK in other tissues, many conditions other than AMI may cause an elevated total CK level, thus limiting this marker's usefulness.

Soon after MI, the CK-MB isoenzyme curve parallels the total CK curve, with levels detectable 4 to 8 h after onset of symptoms (Fig. 45-2). CK-MB may peak slightly earlier than total CK, and it is cleared more rapidly, usually within 48 h (versus 72 to 96 h). Using CK-MB and the ratio of MB to total CK, most studies report both sensitivity and specificity to be greater than 95 percent. Cutoff values vary between techniques, laboratories and populations, but CK-MB values in healthy controls may be up to 5 U/L and up to 5 percent of total CK. Until recently, CK-MB had been almost universally adopted as the ''gold standard'' for diagnosis of MI. Although specificity is generally improved over total CK, 37 conditions other than MI have been associated with elevated CK-MB levels (Table 45-2). Fortunately, most of these conditions can be easily differentiated from MI on clinical grounds. The relatively rapid return of elevated MB levels to normal is another potential disadvantage because of the possibility of missing the diagnosis in patients presenting later in the course of MI. However, this rapid clearance may be used to a different advantage because it enables the identification of infarct extension and reinfarction.

One major limitation of CK-MB use is that in MI, abnormal levels of the isoenzyme cannot be detected until 4 to 8 h after onset of symptoms, regardless of the assay used. This problem has been partially overcome with the development of rapid assays for CK-MB isoforms (subforms). The isoenzymes CK-MM, CK-MB, and CK-BB are dimeric molecules consisting of three different combinations of two monomers, M and B. On its release from damaged cells, the M-monomer found in tissue CK (M_t) is acted on by an enzyme present in serum, carboxypeptidase-N, which cleaves off the C-terminal lysine. This action results in its conversion into the M-monomer found in serum CK (M_s). Because lysine is a positively charged amino acid, its cleavage results in the M_s-monomer being more negatively charged than M_t. Because the rate of this conversion is limited, newly released, unmodified tissue CK-M_tM_t dimers (referred to as CK-MM_3) undergo sequential C-terminal cleavage of its two M_t-monomers to create CK-M_tM_s (CK-MM_2) and, subsequently, CK-M_sM_s (CK-MM_1). Although the clinical utility of CK-MM isoform measurement is limited by its lack of specificity, the same modification also occurs to the M_t-monomer of CK-MB (CK-MB_2), resulting in the formation of CK-MB_1. By measuring MB_2 activity and the MB_2/MB_1 ratio, evidence of infarction can be detected before the total level of CK-MB exceeds the normal range. Using this method, one multicenter study has reported a sensitivity of 95.7 percent and specificity of 93.9 percent for AMI among 1110 patients within 1.2 h of ED presentation (6 h from symptom onset).[11]

Myoglobin is a small (17,500-Da), heme-containing protein found in striated (skeletal) and cardiac muscle cells. When disrupted, these cells rapidly release myoglobin into the serum. Myoglobin serum levels increase rapidly after significant muscle damage and return to baseline values relatively quickly in the presence of normal kidney function. This property makes myoglobin potentially valuable as a serum marker for myocardial necrosis. After MI, serum myoglobin levels begin to rise within 3 h of onset of symptoms and are abnormally elevated in 80 to 100 percent of patients after 6 to 8 h, peak from 4 to 9 h after symptom onset (Fig. 45-2), and return to baseline within 24 h. Because of this rapid rise and fall, serum myoglobin is very sensitive as a marker of MI when determined early in the course of infarction. However, a false-negative result may occur if the test is performed after myoglobin has already been cleared from the serum. Also, because the myoglobin found in myocardium is indistinguishable from that found in skeletal muscle, it is a nonspecific marker. Aside from MI, all conditions that cause significant skeletal muscle injury must be considered as possible causes of an elevated myoglobin level. Fortunately, these conditions can usually be detected clinically in patients with symptoms related to infarction.

TABLE 45-2 Conditions Associated with Elevated CK-MB Levels

Patient's Condition or Preceding Event	Frequency Reported
Unstable angina (intermediate coronary syndrome), acute coronary ischemia	Common
Inflammatory heart diseases	Common
Cardiomyopathies	Common
Circulatory failure and shock	Common
Cardiac surgery	Common
Cardiac trauma	Common
Skeletal muscle trauma (severe)	Common
Dermatomyositis, polymyositis	Common
Myopathic disorders	Common
Muscular dystrophy, especially Duchenne	Common
Extreme exercise	Common
Malignant hyperthermia	Common
Reye's syndrome	Common
Rhabdomyolysis of any cause	Common
Delirium tremens	Common
Ethanol poisoning (chronic)	Common
Congestive heart failure	Uncommon
Coronary artery disease after stress test	Uncommon
Angina pectoris	Uncommon
Valvular defects	Uncommon
Tachycardia	Uncommon
Cardiac catheterization	Uncommon
Electrical countershock	Uncommon
Noncardiac surgery	Uncommon
Brain and head trauma	Uncommon
Peripartum period	Uncommon
Miscellaneous drug overdoses	Uncommon
CO poisoning	Uncommon
Prostatic cancer	Uncommon
Isolated case in normal person	Rare
Acromegaly	Unclear
Hypothermia	Unclear
Rocky Mountain spotted fever	Unclear
Typhoid fever	Unclear
Chronic bronchitis	Unclear
Lumbago	Unclear
Febrile disorder	Unclear

Evaluation of the myoglobin/carbonic anhydrase III ratio can enhance the specificity of myoglobin. The enzyme carbonic anhydrase III is released from skeletal muscle in a fixed ratio with myoglobin. Combined assays can therefore help determine whether myoglobin is of skeletal or cardiac origin. When these dual assays are used, the high early sensitivity of myoglobin is maintained and specificity is improved. However, these assays are not yet commercially available and the use of dual assays for risk stratification has not yet been evaluated.

Troponin I and T

The troponin complex is the main regulatory protein of the thin filament of the myofibrils that regulate the Ca^{2+}-dependent ATP hydrolysis of actomyosin. The troponin complex consists of three subunits: an inhibitory subunit (troponin I), a tropomyosin binding subunit (troponin T), and a calcium-binding subunit (troponin C). Because each subunit has cardiac, slow-twitch, and fast-twitch skeletal isoforms, immunoassays based upon the significant heterogeneity in amino acid sequences can detect the specific isoforms. The cardiac isoform of troponin I is not found in skeletal muscle during any stage of development. As a result, elevations of cardiac troponin I do not occur in the setting of acute or chronic skeletal muscle damage in the absence of myocardial necrosis.

Following AMI, both cardiac troponin I and troponin T become elevated after approximately 6 h, peak at 12 h, and remain elevated for 7 to10 days. Both have a higher specificity for myocardial necrosis than CK-MB in selected subsets of patients, such as those presenting late in the course of MI, those with recent surgery, a cocaine habit, or skeletal muscle disease. Either troponin may be elevated in patients with renal failure. In ED patients with symptoms of possible ischemia, both troponins have been shown to have high sensitivity and specificity for AMI. Elevation of either cardiac troponin also predicts subsequent cardiovascular complications independent of CK-MB and the ECG.[12,13]

Clinical Applications of Myocardial Marker Measurements

The current literature supports the inclusion of myocardial marker measurements in protocols governing the ED evaluation of patients with chest pain for four distinct purposes (Table 45-3). First, for the ability of myocardial markers to confirm or ''rule in'' suspected MI within the first hours after presentation in patients with nondiagnostic ECGs. Second, for the ability of markers to identify some patients with otherwise unrecognized MI from among the many patients with atypical presentations and non-diagnostic ECGs. Third, to risk-stratify patients early in their ED course—i.e., to identify those patients at particularly high risk for subsequent adverse events. Fourth, to definitively exclude the diagnosis of AMI using an accelerated myocardial marker curve during an extended observation and monitoring period in the ED. The first three applications are discussed here, while the fourth is discussed in the following section.

EARLY DIAGNOSIS OF AMI In those patients whose initial ECG is diagnostic for MI, no further testing is required and appropriate

TABLE 45-3 Uses of Markers of Myocardial Injury in the ED

Early confirmation of AMI (*rule in*)
Identification of otherwise unrecognized AMI in patients with atypical presentations
Early risk stratification
Accelerated exclusion of AMI in an ED-based observation unit (*rule out*)

interventions can be initiated. As stated previously, approximately 50 percent of MI patients will have an initially nondiagnostic ECG. The release kinetics of currently available markers generally require 6 h or more after coronary occlusion to exclude infarction; therefore MI cannot be definitively ruled out within the first few hours of the ED visit. However, some MI patients with nondiagnostic initial ECGs will have positive marker tests upon ED arrival, and many more will develop positive tests soon after presentation. Therefore, early, rapid serial sampling of myocardial markers may identify many MI patients with nondiagnostic ECGs (rule in MI) and thus allow earlier utilization of time-dependent treatments.

Studies of single CK-MB measurement upon ED presentation have demonstrated a sensitivity for MI of less than 60 percent. However, by using serial CK-MB measurements, several authors have demonstrated sensitivities ranging from 80 to 96 percent.[14–16]

Owing to its earlier release into serum after coronary artery occlusion, the heme-containing protein myoglobin has a potential advantage over CK-MB for early diagnosis of MI. In one study, samples taken at presentation yielded a sensitivity of 62 percent for myoglobin as compared with 14 percent for CK-MB. At 3 h, the sensitivity for MI increased to 90 percent for CK-MB and to 100 percent for myoglobin.[17] A subsequent, similar study reported sensitivities at 2 h of 82.1 percent for CK-MB and 100 percent for myoglobin.[18]

IDENTIFYING "MISSED MI" PATIENTS Single-sample myocardial marker measurements cannot be used to exclude the diagnosis of MI in the ED. However, results of several investigations suggest that the incorporation of markers into patient care algorithms for low-risk patients prior to discharge may help to identify those with unsuspected MI.

In the first such study (1987), three of 482 chest pain patients discharged from the ED were found to have had a positive CK-MB. In another investigation (1991) among 271 ED patients, 5 discharged patients and 2 admitted to unmonitored beds with noncardiac diagnoses were identified by a single positive CK-MB value and later determined to have had a clinically unsuspected MI. All 7 of these patients had nondiagnostic initial ECGs and 3 had presented with symptoms other than chest pain.[19] In a later multicenter study that prospectively assessed the effect on ED physician decision making of two CK-MB measurements drawn 3 h apart, 3 of 265 patients selected for discharge by the ED physician were identified and admitted solely on the basis of a positive CK-MB. These results suggest that ED patients to be sent home or admitted to unmonitored beds after presenting with chest pain as well as with other presentations of possible ischemia may benefit from prerelease "screening" for MI using CK-MB.[20] Although these results are promising, there is not yet sufficient data concerning either cost or clinical effectiveness of this practice to advocate it's widespread use.

EARLY RISK STRATIFICATION As use of newer anti-ischemic therapies, such as early angiographic interventions and anti-platelet and antithrombotic drugs, become more common, the morbidity and mortality associated with ACS are likely to decline further. However, the greater risk of therapy related complications and the higher costs associated with these newer interventions necessitate a selective approach to their use. Several investigations suggest that markers of myocardial injury can successfully be used in the ED to rapidly identify those patients most likely to benefit from a more aggressive approach.

Positive CK-MB tests obtained upon presentation and 2 h later have been shown to predict up to a fivefold increased likelihood of subsequent ischemic complication, regardless of the final diagnosis. A subsequent similar study of 5120 patients from 53 EDs confirmed the prognostic significance of a positive CK-MB value, regardless of final diagnosis. Other investigations have shown that early ED testing of either troponin-T or troponin-I also yields clinically useful prognostic data and suggest that simultaneous testing of both troponin and CK-MB may identify additional high-risk patients.[12,21,22]

APPROACH TO LOW PROBABILITY OF ISCHEMIA

After initial evaluation, early data collection, and interpretation, a high potential for the presence of an ACS will be recognized in many patients. The approach to further risk stratification and treatment of these patients is detailed in Chap. 47. Many others can be classified as having a low probability of acute ischemia based on clinical information available at the time of their ED visit. However, there is currently no consensus in the literature on their optimal management or even a widely accepted definition of who belongs to this group. There is consensus on two issues: that history alone is inadequate to exclude the presence of acute ischemia and that the goal must be "zero tolerance" for missed AMI.[23] A systematic approach based on objective data is required to identify these lower-risk patients early in their course (Table 45-4) while also resulting in lower costs and, perhaps, improved outcomes (Fig. 45-3).

Diagnostic tools now available for this group of patients include myocardial marker measurements (see above), stress testing, nuclear or ultrasound imaging, and advanced monitoring techniques. A description of the commonly used approaches for low-risk patients follows.

TABLE 45-4 Proposed Prognosis-Based Classification System for ED Chest Pain Patients*

I. Acute myocardial infarction: candidate for immediate revascularization

II. Probable acute ischemia: high risk for adverse events
Any of the following:
- Evidence of clinical instability (i.e., pulmonary edema, hypotension, dysrhythmia)
- Ongoing pain thought to be ischemic
- Pain at rest associated with ischemic ECG changes
- One or more positive myocardial marker measurements
- Positive myocardial imaging study

III. Probable acute ischemia: intermediate risk for adverse events
History suggestive of ischemia with any of the following:
- Rest pain, now resolved
- New onset of pain
- Crescendo pattern of pain
- Ischemic pattern on ECG not associated with pain

IV. A. Stable angina pectoris: low risk for adverse events
Requires all of the following:
- More than 2 weeks of unchanged symptom pattern or long-standing symptoms with only mild change in exertional pain threshold
- ECG normal, unchanged from previous or nonspecific changes
- Negative myocardial marker measurement

IV. B. Probably not ischemia: low risk for adverse events
Requires all of the following:
- History not strongly suggestive of ischemia
- ECG normal, unchanged from previous or nonspecific changes
- Negative myocardial marker measurement

V. Definitely not ischemia: very low risk for adverse events
Requires all of the following:
- Clear objective evidence of nonischemic symptom etiology
- ECG normal, unchanged from previous or nonspecific changes
- Negative myocardial marker measurement

*This system has not been prospectively investigated.

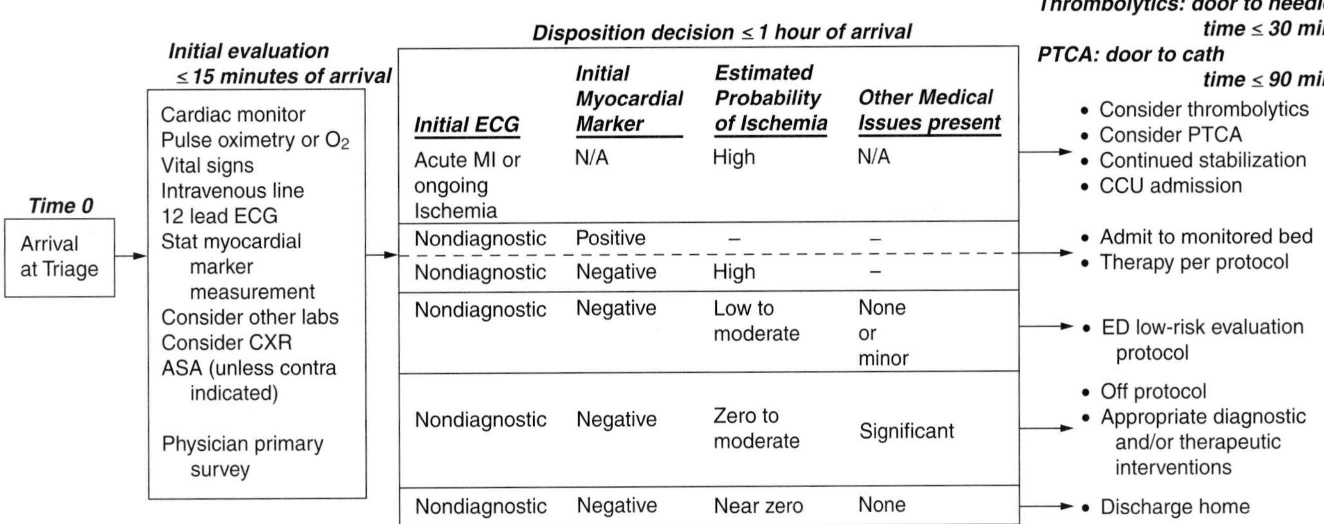

FIG. 45-3. Algorithm for risk-based decision making.

Characteristics of Common Diagnostic Tests Used in Emergency Cardiac Care

ECG BASED (STANDARD) EXERCISE STRESS TESTING In the ED setting, exercise testing has been recommended for patients applied either as the final component of a chest pain observation protocol after the exclusion of AMI or, in selected low-risk patients, soon after presentation as an alternative to an extended observation period.

Many variations exist in the equipment, procedures, and interpretive algorithms used. Both treadmill and cycle ergometer devices are acceptable and commercially available. Cycle devices are smaller and less expensive, offering reduced motion artifact. However, treadmills are still more commonly used in the United States because many patients are unable to reach the desired point of maximum oxygen uptake on the cycle owing to quadriceps muscle fatigue. Other mandatory equipment includes a nearby crash cart with defibrillator and rhythm monitoring capability. Testing may be reliably performed by a trained technician or other allied health professional, although an experienced physician must be readily available. Dysrhythmia, AMI and death have been reported and can be expected to occur at rates of 4.8, 3.6 and 0.5 per 10,000 tests, respectively.[24]

Several exercise and monitoring protocols are in use, differing in duration and level of exercise reached as well as testing end points. No consensus exists on the preferred protocol, although the Bruce protocol is the most common and best studied. At the time of testing, informed consent is obtained and the procedure is explained to the patient in detail. The patient's skin is prepared for electrode placement by trimming hair, use of a defatting agent, e.g., alcohol, and abrading the superficial skin layer. After electrode placement, baseline measures of heart rate, blood pressure, and 12-lead ECG are obtained at rest in both supine and standing positions. Exercise is then initiated, with exertion increased in a step-wise fashion predetermined by protocol with the desired endpoint ideally reached within 8 to 12 min of test initiation. Throughout the test and during recovery, ECG rhythm is monitored continuously and 12 lead ECGs are recorded at least once each min. Heart rate, blood pressure, patient symptoms, and perceived exertion (via a visual analog scale) is also recorded at each workload level. Depending on the protocol followed, exercise is terminated when the subject reaches a predetermined percentage of predicted maximum heart rate (i.e., 85 percent) or when another defined end point is reached (Table 45-5). The most commonly used definition of a positive exercise test result from an ECG standpoint is greater than or equal to 1 mm of horizontal or downsloping ST-segment depression or elevation for at least 60 to 80 ms after the end of the QRS complex.

Exercise stress testing may be contraindicated for various reasons (Table 45-6).[25] If the patient has physical limitations preventing exercise but no other contraindications, a pharmacologic stress test using

TABLE 45-5 Indications for Terminating Exercise Testing

Absolute indications
Drop in systolic blood pressure of >10 mmHg from baseline blood pressure despite an increase in workload when accompanied by other evidence of ischemia
Moderate to severe angina
Increasing nervous system symptoms (e.g., ataxia, dizziness, or near-syncope)
Signs of poor perfusion (cyanosis or pallor)
Technical difficulties in monitoring ECG or systolic blood pressure
Subject's desire to stop
Sustained ventricular tachycardia
ST elevation (≥1.0 mm) in leads without diagnostic Q waves (other than V_1 or aVR)
Relative indications
Drop in systolic blood pressure of ≥10 mmHg from baseline blood pressure despite an increase in workload in the absence of other evidence of ischemia
ST or QRS changes such as excessive ST depression (>2 mm of horizontal or downsloping ST-segment depression) or marked axis shift
Dysrhythmias other than sustained ventricular tachycardia, including multifocal PVCs, triplets of PVCs, supraventricular tachycardia, heart block, or bradydysrhythmias
Fatigue, shortness of breath, wheezing, leg cramps, or claudication
Development of bundle branch block or IVCD that cannot be distinguished from ventricular tachycardia
Increasing chest pain
Hypertensive response*

*In the absence of definitive evidence, the committee suggests systolic blood pressure of >200 mmHg and/or a diastolic blood pressure of >115 mmHg.
Key: ECG, electrocardiogram; PVCs, premature ventricular contractions; ICD, implantable cardioverter-defibrillator discharge; IVCD, intraventricular conduction delay.
Source: Fletcher GF, Balady G, Froelicher VF, et al.: Exercise standards: A statement for healthcare professionals from the American Heart Association Writing Group. Special Report. *Circulation.* 91:580, 1995.

TABLE 45-6 Contraindications to Exercise Testing

Absolute
- Acute myocardial infarction (within 2 d)
- Unstable angina not previously stabilized by medical therapy*
- Uncontrolled cardiac dysrhythmias causing symptoms or hemodynamic compromise
- Symptomatic severe aortic stenosis
- Uncontrolled symptomatic heart failure
- Acute pulmonary embolus or pulmonary infarction
- Acute myocarditis or pericarditis
- Acute aortic dissection

Relative†
- Left main coronary stenosis
- Moderate stenotic valvular heart disease
- Electrolyte abnormalities
- Severe arterial hypertension‡
- Tachydysrhythmias or bradydysrhythmias
- Hypertrophic cardiomyopathy and other forms of outflow tract obstruction
- Mental or physical impairment leading to inability to exercise adequately
- High-degree atrioventricular block

*Appropriate timing of testing depends on level of risk of unstable angina as defined by AHCPR Unstable Angina Guidelines.
†Relative contraindications can be superseded if the benefits of exercise outweigh the risks.
‡In the absence of definitive evidence, the committee suggests systolic blood pressure of >200 mmHg and/or diastolic blood pressure of >110 mmHg.
Source: Fletcher GF, Balady G, Froelicher VF, et al.: Exercise standards: A statement for healthcare professionals from the American Heart Association Writing Group. Special Report. *Circulation.* 91:580, 1995.

a chronotropic drug (i.e., dobutamine) may be appropriate. Exercise testing may not be safe for patients at high risk for acute ischemia or those with other uncontrolled cardiovascular or pulmonary pathology. Further, patients with an abnormal baseline ECG—such as those with left ventricular hypertrophy, bundle branch block, or digoxin effect—are less likely to benefit from standard exercise testing owing to difficulties in interpretation of exercise-induced ECG changes.

The clinical utility of ED stress testing depends upon the test result's ability to modify the pretest probability of the diagnosis and to change treatment and disposition. ED stress testing is particularly difficult to quantify because test sensitivity and specificity are greatly influenced by the population being tested. As the pretest probability of significant coronary artery disease increases, the likelihood of a false-negative test also increases. Conversely, when a population with a very low pretest probability of disease is tested, the likelihood of a false-positive result increases. Therefore, based on current data, *diagnostic* stress testing is recommended for patients with a low pretest probability of coronary artery disease and is unlikely to be helpful in those at either very low risk (<5 percent) or those at moderate to high risk (>30 percent).[25,26] The pretest probability of disease can be determined semiquantitatively based on demographic, historical, and ECG data using a number of validated decision aids. ED stress testing may be of further value when applied to a broader range of patients if the goal of testing is to predict prognosis rather than diagnosis. Stress-test performance of post-AMI patients is a valid and commonly used predictor of post-event prognosis, and several recent studies suggest that ED stress testing of selected patients can reliably predict short-term prognosis.

Myocardial Imaging

Advantages of *echocardiography* include its noninvasive nature, that it does not utilize radioactive materials, and that it can be performed in the ED. Further, it is a dynamic technique, allowing time-related observations of anatomy and function at rest and/or under stress (exercise- or pharmacology-induced). Additionally, it has potential value in assessing other sources of chest pain, including aortic dissection, pericardial pathology, valvular disease, and pulmonary embolism.

The value of echocardiography in evaluating ischemic heart disease is largely based upon the experimental finding, in both animal and human studies, that acute myocardial ischemia reliably and rapidly results in observable wall motion abnormalities. Thus, theoretically, a normal echocardiogram during chest pain should exclude the presence of ischemia. Unfortunately, this finding is limited by several factors. Since the effects of adjacent wall segments commonly lead to false-positive and false-negative interpretations of wall motion abnormalities, systolic wall thickening is used as a more specific indicator of ischemia. However, detection of wall-thickening abnormalities is highly dependent on imaging technique and interpretative skills, with up to 10 percent of tests being technically inadequate. Further, the echocardiogram cannot distinguish between myocardial ischemia and acute infaction, cannot reliably detect subendocardial ischemia, and may be falsely interpreted as positive in the presence of several conditions (conduction disturbances, volume overload, heart surgery, trauma). Finally, timing of the test relative to the onset of symptoms is critical, as transient wall motion abnormalities may resolve within minutes of an ischemic episode.

Contrast echocardiography using physiologically safe microbubbles is a newer technique that holds future promise. Studies suggest that this technique significantly improves the detection of regional wall motion abnormalities and wall thickening. In one study, 28 percent of standard stress echos performed were inconclusive due to difficulties in interpretation but were decisively normal or abnormal with the use of contrast. Further, contrast echocardiography may potentially be used to assess coronary vessel patency directly, even at the microvascular level, with sensitivity similar to or greater than that of nuclear perfusion imaging.

Myocardial perfusion imaging utilizes an intravenously injected radioactive tracer that is distributed throughout the coronary circulation. The tracer is actively transported across the sarcolemma membrane into myocardial cells. Local myocardial uptake and subsequently, myocardial imaging, is therefore dependent on both adequate regional coronary flow and myocardial cell integrity, with tracer uptake occurring in direct proportion to regional myocardial blood flow.

Thallium 201 is the oldest and most studied tracer in common use today. Thallium, a cation, behaves similarly to potassium in tissues and is rapidly redistributed after initial uptake, making it particularly well suited for the detection of stress induced ischemia. When imaging occurs within 20 min after thallium injection (immediately after exercise or pharmacologic stress testing), areas of positive uptake reflect both adequate coronary flow and viable myocardium, while areas without uptake represent either infarcted or ischemic myocardium. On repeat imaging several hours later, continued lack of perfusion (''irreversible defect'') indicates an area of infarction, while areas with tracer uptake only on delayed images (''reversible defect'') represent formerly ischemic myocardium. Combined with conventional ECG-based stress testing, thallium imaging offers improved sensitivity and specificity for detection of significant coronary artery disease over ECG-based testing alone. Further, thallium testing (or other perfusion imaging) is likely to be of value in patients who would not otherwise benefit from stress testing due to a confounding or potentially masking abnormal baseline ECG. There are several limitations of thallium testing. Imaging must be performed immediately after injection, making it impractical for use in patients with ongoing chest pain. Moreover, because of a long half life, the injected dose of thallium must be kept low to avoid excessive radiation exposure. This and other properties of the tracer result in a relatively poor image quality and the frequent occurrence of artifactual perfusion defects (false positives) due to overlying tissue attenuation. This is particularly common in women and obese patients. Based on these limitations and the lack of ED-based efficacy studies, a 1997 National Heart Attack Alert Program

Working Group concluded that "thallium-201 does not appear to be an ideal agent for use in ED management of patients with chest pain."[27]

Owing to several technical factors, myocardial perfusion imaging using *technetium 99m* (^{99m}Tc)-labeled agents such as sestamibi offers advantages over thallium for ED use. Since the half-life of ^{99m}Tc is much shorter than that of thallium (6 versus 73 h), a larger dosage can be injected without harm to the patient. This results in the superior image quality, decreased tissue attenuation–related artifacts, and higher specificity of sestamibi imaging. Newer ^{99m}Tc agents currently under investigation are likely to further improve image quality. Additionally, in contrast to thallium, the initial distribution of ^{99m}Tc agents is stable for several hours. Therefore, accurate imaging can occur up to 3 h after injection. As with thallium, resting and stress (exercise or pharmacologic) images can be compared to yield additional data.

Low-Risk Patient Protocols

INPATIENT ADMISSION In settings where extended observation and definitive diagnostic testing is not available in the ED, all patients whose presentation suggests any reasonable plausibility of an acute ischemic event must be admitted to an inpatient bed. Even in the presence of an ED-based cardiac evaluation protocol, inpatient admission is often prudent for patients whose presentation suggests a low probability of ischemia but who also have other acute medical, surgical, or psychiatric diseases requiring a prolonged or intensive level of attention, which cannot be optimally given in the ED. Once the need for inpatient admission has been determined, further stratification based on assessment of the patient's short-term risk of morbidity or mortality can be made based on the patient's history and physical exam, initial ECG,[9] and early myocardial marker measurement.[12,21,22] Patients with a prior history of coronary artery disease, evidence of congestive heart failure on physical exam, recurrent chest pain in the ED, or new or presumed new ischemic ECG changes are at higher short-term risk and may be more appropriately managed in an intermediate-care (step-down) unit.[6] Conversely, patients whose initial ED ECG is normal or unchanged from a previous ECG have a very low risk of adverse events and can safely be evaluated on a monitored floor or telemetry bed. Those with nonspecific changes on the initial ECG represent an intermediate risk group. A single myocardial marker measurement soon after ED presentation can also identify those patients at greater risk from among those with atypical presentations.[22]

ED OBSERVATION/MONITORING In 1984, the Multicenter Chest Pain Study Group was formed to develop new lower-cost strategies for managing "ROMI" (rule out MI) patients. In 1991, this group published the results of a seven-center investigation of 2684 patients admitted for chest pain and reported that the diagnosis of infarction could have been safely excluded within a 12-h observation period among a subgroup identifiable at presentation as having a low probability of AMI.[28] The authors also suggest routine predischarge stress testing of these patients in order to reduce the risk of discharging patients with unstable coronary syndromes prematurely.

This approach was further refined by Gibler et al. in a study of 1010 patients admitted to an ED-based chest pain evaluation and treatment unit ("Heart ER") over 32 months. Patients with symptoms consistent but not highly suggestive of acute ischemia were observed for 9 h with continuous 12-lead ST-segment ECG monitoring and serial CK-MB testing at 0, 3, 6, and 9 h after presentation. Those who completed a negative 9-h evaluation subsequently underwent echocardiography followed by graded exercise stress testing in the ED prior to discharge. Utilizing this approach, 82.1 percent of patients were released home from the cardiac evaluation unit (CEU).[29]

The ideal length of observation (12, 9, or 8 h), the best choice and timing of myocardial marker measurements, and the value of continuous ST-segment monitoring are among the many questions that have not yet been answered definitively. Additionally, while several studies have documented cost savings associated with use of an ED-based CEU compared with traditional inpatient admission, the cost effectiveness of their widespread use is still not uniformly accepted.

Although AMI can be reliably excluded by this type of observation protocol (Fig. 45-4), normal serial ECGs and myocardial marker measurements do not preclude the presence of other ACSs (i.e., unstable angina), which may still put the patient at high risk for a subsequent adverse event. Therefore, further evaluation is usually indicated prior to discharge. The various forms of stress testing (with or without myocardial imaging) currently offer the best noninvasive method to both predict the presence of coronary artery disease as well as assess prognosis. In the Cincinnati study previously mentioned,[29] 791 patients underwent treadmill exercise stress testing after a negative observation period with no adverse events reported during testing. Among these, 9 of the patients had positive tests and 4 of these subsequently confirmed to have significant coronary artery disease not otherwise identified (positive predictive value = 44.4 percent). Of the 782 negative results, 10 were false negatives, yielding a negative predictive value of 98.7 percent. The authors concluded that although a negative observation period and stress test still does not completely rule out the possibility of coronary artery disease, they do identify a large group of patients who could be safely released from the ED with subsequent follow-up.[29] In a subsequent study, 86 percent of 502 patients who underwent a similar observation protocol and ECG stress testing were discharged after a negative evaluation, with no deaths or AMIs reported after 5 months of follow-up. In this investigation, 24 patients with subsequently confirmed ischemic heart disease were identified only through positive ED stress tests. However, the effectiveness of this technology is still not uniformly accepted. A recent consensus panel report from the National Heart Attack Alert Program cited the need for additional investigation and concluded that "ECG exercise stress testing in the ED cannot be recommended in the absence of additional data demonstrating safety and effectiveness."[26]

IMMEDIATE SCREENING In addition to admission or ED-based observation, immediate myocardial perfusion imaging, echocardiography, or stress testing without prior observation have been suggested as rapid, safe, and cost-effective alternatives among selected patients. However, few ED-based studies have been published concerning these approaches and many questions remain unanswered concerning their limitations and relative value.

Because of its minimal redistribution, myocardial perfusion imaging using ^{99m}Tc sestamibi (sestamibi scanning) is particularly suited for the early ED assessment of both diagnosis and prognosis among patients with *ongoing chest pain.* The agent can be injected in the ED upon presentation without interfering with other therapeutic or diagnostic interventions. Imaging can then be delayed for up to 3 h without significant degradation of the resulting image. With this technique, the image acquired will represent the state of myocardial perfusion at the time of injection, and a normal perfusion scan should therefore reliably exclude myocardial ischemia as a cause of the patient's chest pain. Indeed, multiple investigations have confirmed that an abnormal study has a high sensitivity (94 to 100 percent) for the prediction of AMI when injection occurred during active pain.

The value of resting sestamibi scanning in patients who present after the resolution of chest pain is less clear. Some investigators have reported a substantial decrease in diagnostic accuracy related to increasing delay from symptom resolution to tracer injection. However, in another study among those with greater than 30 min of chest pain within the 12 h prior to presentation, sensitivity for AMI remained 100 percent.[30] In the largest published series to date, 100 percent sensitivity for AMI was also reported among 438 low-risk patients enrolled and scanned without regard to the presence or absence of chest pain at the time of injection.[31] In this study, among the 338 "low-risk" patients with normal perfusion scans in the ED, there were

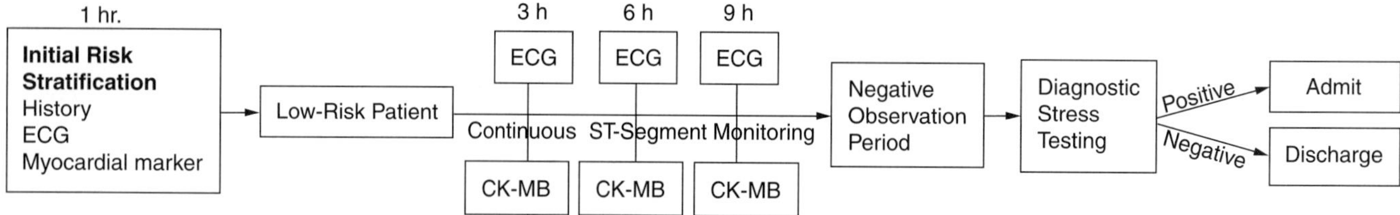

FIG. 45-4. Algorithm for the evaluation of low-risk patients.

no AMIs or deaths within the 1-year follow-up period. However, seven (2.1 percent) low-risk patients with normal scans did require a coronary revascularization procedure within 1 month of their ED visit. Taken as a whole, the current literature suggests that low-risk patients with negative sestamibi scans may be safely discharged from the ED without an extended observation period. Pharmacologic or exercise stress imaging using sestamibi may subsequently be performed either after an observation period or during a follow-up visit to assess for the presence of stress-induced ischemia.

Several small studies have been published in which chest pain patients were assessed with standard *echocardiography* soon after ED presentation. Among these, the sensitivity for the detection of acute ischemia or AMI among all patients ranged from 88 to 96 percent, significantly higher than that of the 12-lead ECG. However, even among selected patients with adequate studies who are evaluated during ongoing chest pain, false-negative echocardiograms may occur in up to 8 percent of AMI patients, thus precluding the possibility of discharging a patient on the basis of a negative study. Primarily due to this limitation, the National Heart Attack Alert Program Working Group on echocardiography has concluded that this tool cannot currently be recommended for ED use.[32]

A few reports have advocated *immediate exercise testing* of low-risk chest pain patients presenting to the ED without prior observation or ruling out of AMI. One small series of 32 patients who presented with "chest pain suggestive of cardiac origin but not typical of angina," normal or nondiagnostic ECG, and less than two cardiac risk factors reported that all stress tests were negative and no adverse events occurred. Another investigation of 212 ED patients with similar inclusion criteria found that 13 percent had a positive stress test, 59 percent a negative test, and 2 percent a nondiagnostic result with no adverse events in any group.[33] The limited amount of available data concerning both clinical effectiveness and safety preclude routine application of this approach at the present time.

DIFFERENTIAL DIAGNOSIS

During the initial assessment of patients with chest pain, it is important that the diagnosis of ACS be considered in concert with other life-threatening conditions. These include aortic dissection, pulmonary embolism, pneumothorax, pericarditis, pericardial tamponade, pneumonia, and esophageal rupture (Table 45-1). Other significant causes of chest pain include mitral valve prolapse, aortic stenosis, and gastrointestinal conditions, such as perforated ulcer and cholecystitis.

Risk factors for *aortic dissection* include atherosclerosis, uncontrolled hypertension, coarctation of the aorta, bicuspid aortic valves, aortic stenosis, Marfan syndrome, Ehlers-Danlos syndrome, and pregnancy. The pain of aortic dissection—midline substernal chest pain—is classically described as tearing, ripping, or searing and radiating to the interscapular area of the back. Typically, the pain is at its worst at symptom onset and is often felt both above and below the diaphragm. Symptoms of "secondary" pathologies resulting from arterial branch occlusions—such as stroke, AMI, or limb ischemia—may overshadow the clinical presentation of the dissection and make an accurate diagnosis difficult. Aortic dissection should be considered in the patient with continuing chest pain but without ECG evidence of evolving myocardial infarction.

The most common radiographic finding is mediastinal widening (>75 percent of cases). While aortography remains the "gold standard" in evaluating aortic dissection, both transesophageal echocardiography and high-resolution contrast spiral computed tomography are less invasive techniques that are now widely accepted for this evaluation. Acute dissection is discussed in detail in Chap. 54.

Pulmonary embolism (PE) can manifest in a multitude of presentations including chest pain, syncope, shock, hypoxia, and dyspnea. The pain associated with a PE occurs when inflammation of the parietal pleura overlying the infarction causes chest pain that is generally sharp and related to respiration. Dyspnea, fever, cough, and/or hemoptysis may also be present and the chest wall may be tender to palpation. Patients with massive pulmonary emboli often present with unstable vital signs and the classic presentation of sharp, pleuritic chest pain and dyspnea associated with tachypnea, tachycardia, and hypoxemia.

Spontaneous pneumothorax may occur due to sudden changes in barometric pressure, in smokers or patients with chronic obstructive pulmonary disease, idiopathic pleural bleb disease, in AIDS patients on pentamidine, or in those with other pulmonary pathology. Patients usually complain of a sudden, sharp, lancinating, pleuritic chest pain and dyspnea. If not recognized early, the condition can progress to tension pneumothorax, which is characterized by severe dyspnea, jugular venous distention, tracheal deviation to the contralateral side, and hypotension. Auscultation of the lungs may reveal absence of breath sounds on the ipsilateral side and hyperresonance to percussion but clinical impression alone is unreliable. Diagnosis of a simple pneumothorax is made by chest x-ray.

The pain of *acute pericarditis* is typically acute, sharp, severe, and constant. It is usually described as substernal, with radiation to the back, neck, or shoulders, and is exacerbated by lying down and by inspiration. It is relieved by leaning forward. The presence of a pericardial friction rub is suggestive of the diagnosis, but absence of a rub does not exclude the diagnosis. The ECG may show diffuse ST-segment elevation and T-wave inversion. Additionally, depression of the PR segment is a highly specific ECG finding for pericarditis. The etiologies of pericarditis are many and must be pursued prior to determining a final disposition and treatment plan.

Mitral valve prolapse (MVP) is the most frequently diagnosed cardiac valvular abnormality and is more commonly diagnosed in women than in men.[34] The discomfort of mitral valve prolapse often occurs at rest, is atypical for myocardial ischemia, and can be associated with dizziness, hyperventilation, anxiety, depression, palpitations, and fatigue. The discomfort may be related to papillary muscle tension, and many patients benefit from the administration of beta-adrenergic blocking agents.[35] The more serious complications of MVP are syncope, stroke, infective endocarditis, congestive heart failure, and dysrhythmia. MVP is characterized by a midsystolic click and late systolic murmur detected on cardiac auscultation. Two-dimensional echocardiography is the diagnostic tool of choice and, together with physical exam findings, helps to stratify patients into high- and low-risk categories for developing serious complications. Patients with MVP who do not have a murmur or mitral regurgitation on Doppler have a lower rate of serious complications than those with the following abnormalities on echocardiogram: severe mitral regurgitation, left ventricular enlargement, redundant or thickened mitral valve leaflets, and left atrial enlargement.[35] Palpitations and every type of supraventricular or ventricular dysrhythmia have been associated with MVP.

Any patient who may be in the high-risk category, presenting with concerning signs and symptoms, should be considered for either inpatient evaluation or cardiology consultation and close follow-up as an outpatient.

Pneumonia can produce chest pain or discomfort that is usually sharp and pleuritic. It is usually associated with fever, cough, and hypoxia. Physical exam may reveal rales over the affected lobes, decreased breath sounds, and signs of consolidation, (i.e., bronchial breath sounds). A chest radiograph confirms the diagnosis.

Esophageal rupture (Boerhaave syndrome) is a rare but potentially life-threatening cause of chest pain. Patients classically present with a history of substernal, sharp chest pain of sudden onset that occurs immediately following an episode of forceful vomiting. The patient is usually ill-appearing, dyspneic, and diaphoretic. The physical exam is often normal but may reveal evidence of pneumothorax or subcutaneous air. Chest radiography may be normal or may demonstrate pleural effusion (left more common than right), pneumothorax, pneumomediastinum, pneumoperitoneum and/or subcutaneous air. The diagnosis can be confirmed by a study with water-soluble contrast.

Musculoskeletal or chest wall pain syndromes are diagnoses of exclusion. These syndromes are often characterized by highly localized, sharp, pleuritic and positional chest pain. Pain that is completely reproducible by light to moderate palpation of a discrete area of the chest wall often represents pain of musculoskeletal origin, although musculoskeletal pain commonly accompanies coronary artery disease. Costochondritis is an inflamation of the costal cartilages and/or their sternal articulations and causes chest pain that is variably sharp, dull, and/or increased with respirations. Tietze syndrome is a particular cause of costochondral pain related to fusiform swelling in one or more upper costal cartilages and has a pain pattern similar to that of other costochondral syndromes. Xiphodynia is another inflammatory process that causes sharp, pleuritic chest pain reproduced by light palpation over the xiphoid process. Texidor twinge or precordial catch syndrome is described as a short, lancinating chest discomfort located near the cardiac apex associated with breathing as well as with poor posture and inactivity.

GASTROINTESTINAL DISORDERS It is very difficult to discriminate gastrointestinal disorders from myocardial ischemia. Dyspepsia syndromes, including gastroesophageal reflux disease (GERD), often produce pain described as burning or gnawing, usually in the lower half of the chest and often accompanied by a brackish or acidic taste in the back of the mouth. The recumbent position usually exacerbates the symptoms, and although the pain is usually relieved with antacids, this therapeutic response is also common with myocardial ischemia. Esophageal spasm is often associated with reflux disease and is characterized by a sudden onset of dull, tight, or gripping substernal chest pain, frequently precipitated by the consumption of hot or cold liquids or a large food bolus and often lasting for hours. The pain also responds to sublingual nitroglycerin. Thus, nitroglycerin does not differentiate esophageal spasm from myocardial ischemia.

Peptic ulcer disease is classically characterized as postprandial, dull, boring pain located in the midepigastric region. Patients often describe being awakened from sleep by it. Duodenal ulcer pain is usually relieved after eating food, in contrast to gastric ulcer symptoms, which are often exacerbated by eating. Symptomatic relief is usually achieved by antacid medications. Acute pancreatitis and biliary tract disease present with right-upper-quadrant or epigastric pain and tenderness but can also present with chest pain.

There are no data to support the practice of a therapeutic intervention as diagnostic challenge. The episodic nature of the pain in many of these symdromes, the very strong potential for placebo effect, and the substantial impact of ''negative tests'' and reassurance in alleviating anxiety and pain cannot be underestimated. There are no data to prove that chest discomfort relieved by antacids is more likely to be noncardiac in origin than pain that is not so relieved. Conversely, nitroglycerin is a smooth muscle dilator that may afford relief in cases of lower esophageal spasm or biliary colic. As a rule, diagnostic decisions should not be influenced by response to a therapeutic trial. When the history, physical examination, and diagnostic workup point to a gastrointestinal etiology of the pain, the patient may be treated with antacids and H_2 blockers, with follow-up referral to an internist or gastroenterologist.

REFERENCES

1. Sigurdsson E, Thorgeirsson G, Sigvaldason H, et al: Unrecognized myocardial infarction: Epidemiology, clinical characteristics, and the prognostic role of angina pectoris: The Reykjavik Study. *Ann Intern Med* 122:96, 1995.
2. Douglas PS, Ginsburg GS: The evaluation of chest pain in women. *N Engl J Med* 334:1311, 1996.
3. Lumley MA, Torosian T, Rowland LL, et al: Correlates of unrecognized acute myocardial infarction detected via perfusion imaging. *Am J Cardiol* 79:1170, 1997.
4. Panju AA, Hemmelgarn BR, Guyatt GH, Simel DL: Is this patient having a myocardial infarction? *JAMA* 280:1256, 1998.
5. Jonsbu J, Rollag A, Aase O, et al: Rapid and correct diagnosis of myocardial infarction: standardized case history and clinical examination provide important information for correct referral to monitored beds. *JAMA* 229:143, 1991.
6. Lee TH, Cook EF, Weisberg M, et al: Acute chest pain in the emergency room: Identification and examination of low-risk patients. *Arch Intern Med* 145:65, 1985.
7. Silber SH, Leo PJ, Katapadi M: Serial electrocardiograms for chest pain patients with initial nondiagnostic electrocardiograms: Implications for thrombolytic therapy. *Acad Emerg Med* 3:147, 1996.
8. Justis DL, Hession WT: Accuracy of 22-lead ECG analysis for diagnosis of acute myocardial infarction and coronary artery disease in the emergency department: A comparison with 12-lead ECG. *Ann Emerg Med* 21:1, 1992.
9. Brush JE, Brand DA, Acampora D, Chalmer B, Wackers F: Use of the initial electrocardiogram to predict in-hospital complications of acute myocardial infarction. *N Engl J Med* 312:1137, 1985.
10. Goldman L, Cook EF, Brand DA, et al: A computer protocol to predict myocardial infarction in emergency department patients with chest pain. *N Engl J Med* 318:797, 1988.
11. Puleo PR, Meyer D, Wathen C, et al: Use of a rapid assay of subforms of creatine kinase- MB to diagnose or rule out acute myocardial infarction. *N Engl J Med* 331:561, 1994.
12. Green GB, Li DJ, Bessman ES, et al: The prognostic significance of troponin I and troponin T. *Acad Emerg Med* 5:758, 1998.
13. Antman EM, Tanasijevic MJ, Thompson B, et al: Cardiac specific troponin I levels predict the risk of mortality in patients with acute coronary syndromes. *N Engl J Med* 335:1342, 1996.
14. Gibler WB, Lewis LM, Erb RE, et al: Early detection of acute myocardial infarction in patients presenting with chest pain and nondiagnostice ECGs: Serial CK-MB sampling in the emergency department. *Ann Emerg Med* 19:1359, 1990.
15. Marin MM, Teichman SL: Use of rapid serial sampling of creatine kinase MB for very early detection of myocardial infarction in patients with acute chest pain. *Am Heart J* 123:354, 1992.
16. Gibler WB, Young GP, Hedges JR, et al: The Emergency Medicine Cardiac Research Group: Acute myocardial infarction in chest pain patients with nondiagnostic ECGs: Serial CK-MB sampling in the emergency department. *Ann Emerg Med* 21:504, 1992.
17. Gibler WB, Gibler CD, Weinshenker E, et al: Myoglobin as an early indicator of acute myocardial infarction. *Ann Emerg Med* 16:851, 1987.
18. Tucker JF, Collins RA, Anderson RA, et al: Value of serial myoglobin levels in the early diagnosis of patients admitted for acute myocardial infarction. *Ann Emerg Med* 24:704, 1994.
19. Green GB, Hansen KW, Chan DW, et al: Potential utility of a rapid CK-MB assay in evaluating emergency department patients with possible myocardial infarction. *Ann Emerg Med* 20:954, 1991.

20. Hedges JR, Gibler WB, Young GP, et al: Multicenter study of creatine kinase MB use: Effect on chest pain clinical decision making. *Acad Emerg Med* 3:7, 1996.
21. Green GB, Beaudreau R, Chan DW, et al: Troponin T for risk stratification of ED patients with possible myocardial ischemia. *Ann Emerg Med* 31:19, 1998.
22. Pettijohn TL, Doyle T, Spiekerman AM, et al: Usefulness of positive troponin-T and negative creatine kinase levels in identifying high-risk patients with unstable angina pectoris. *Am J Cardiol* 80:510, 1997.
23. Ryan TJ, Anderson JL, Antman EM, et al: ACC/AHA guidelines for the management of patients with acute myocardial infarction: a report of the American College of Cardiology/American Heart Association Task Force on Practice Guidelines (Committee on Management of Acute Myocardial Infarction). *J Am Coll Cardiol* 28:1328, 1996.
24. Stuart RJ Jr, Ellestad MH: National survey of exercise stress testing facilities. *Chest* 77:94, 1980.
25. Gibbons RJ, Balady GJ, Beasley JW, et al: ACC/AHA guidelines for exercise testing: A report of the American College of Cardiology/American Heart Association task force on practice guidelines (Committee on Exercise Testing). *J Am Coll Cardiol* 30:260, 1997.
26. Selker HP, Zalenski RJ, Antman EM, et al: ECG exercise stress test. In an evaluation of technologies for identifying acute cardiac ischemia in the emergency department: A report from a national heart attack alert program working group. *Ann Emerg Med* 29:33, 1997.
27. Selker HP, Zalenski RJ, Antman EM, et al: Thallium scanning in an evaluation of technologies for identifying acute cardiac ischemia in the emergency department: A report from a national heart attack alert program working group. *Ann Emerg Med* 29:74, 1997.
28. Lee TH, Juarez G, Cook F, et al: Ruling out acute myocardial infarction: A prospective multicenter validation of a 12-hour strategy for patients at low risk. *N Engl J Med* 324:1239, 1991.
29. Gibler WB, Runyon JP, Levy RC, et al: A rapid diagnostic and treatment center for patients with chest pain in the emergency department. *Ann Emerg Med* 25:1, 1995.
30. Varetto T, Cantalupi D, Altieri A, Orlandi C: Emergency room technetium-99m sestamibi imaging to rule out acute myocardial ischemic events in patients with nondiagnostic electrocardiograms. *J Am Coll Cardiol* 22:1804, 1993.
31. Tatum JL, Jesse RL, Kantos MC, et al: Comprehensive strategy for the evaluation and triage of the chest pain patient. *Ann Emerg Med* 29:166, 1997.
32. Selker HP, Zalenski RJ, Antman EM, et al: Echocardiogram: In an evaluation of technologies for identifying acute cardiac ischemia in the emergency department: A report from a national heart alert program working group. *Ann Emerg Med* 29:69, 1997.
33. Kirk JD, Turnipseed S, Lewis WR, Amsterdam EA: Evaluation of chest pain in low-risk patients presenting to the emergency department: the role of immediate exercise testing. *Ann Emerg Med* 32:1, 1998.
34. McLachlan J, Reddy PC, Ratts TE: Mitral valve prolapse: A common cardiac diagnosis in women. *J LA State Med Soc* 150:29, 1998.
35. Devereaux RB: Recent developments in the diagnosis and management of mitral valve prolapse. *Curr Opin Cardiol* 10:107, 1995.

46 SYNCOPE

Barbara K. Blok

Syncope is a sudden, transient loss of consciousness associated with inability to maintain postural tone. Syncope accounts for approximately 3 percent of ED visits each year. The elderly population has the highest incidence and is at increased risk for morbidity from syncopal episodes.[1] Near-syncope, a premonition of syncope without loss of consciousness, shares the same basic pathophysiologic processes as syncope.

PATHOPHYSIOLOGY

The final common pathway of syncope is a lack of vital nutrient delivery to the brainstem reticular activating system, leading to loss of consciousness and postural tone. Most commonly, an inciting event causes a drop in cardiac output, which, unless corrected rapidly, decreases oxygen and substrate delivery to the brain. Less commonly, vasospasm or other alterations in flow singularly reduce central nervous system blood flow. The reclined posture of syncope and the response of autonomic autoregulatory centers reestablish cerebral perfusion, leading to a spontaneous return of consciousness.

TABLE 46-1 Etiology of Syncope

Reflex-mediated	**Cardiac**
Vasovagal	Structural cardiopulmonary disease
Situational	Valvular heart disease
Cough	Aortic stenosis, tricuspid stenosis
Micturition	Mitral stenosis
Defecation	Cardiomyopathy
Swallow	Pulmonary hypertension
Neuralgia	Congenital heart disease
Carotid sinus syndrome	Myxoma
	Pericardial disease
Orthostatic hypotension	Aortic dissection
	Pulmonary embolism
Psychiatric	Myocardial ischemia
	Myocardial infarction
Neurologic	Dysrhythmias
Transient ischemic attacks	Bradydysrhythmias
Subclavian steal	Sinus node disease
Migraines	2nd- or 3rd-degree heart block
	Pacemaker malfunction
Medications (Table 46-2)	Tachydysrhythmias
	Ventricular tachycardia
	Torsades de pointes
	Supraventricular tachycardia

ETIOLOGY

The differential diagnosis of syncope is vast and includes everything from common benign disorders to life-threatening processes (Table 46-1). The most common causes of syncope are cardiac dysrhythmia and vasovagal reflex and orthostatic hypotension.[2,3]

Reflex-Mediated Syncope

Under normal circumstances a physical or emotional stress leads to increased sympathetic outflow and a subsequent increase in heart rate, blood pressure, and cardiac output. In patients with reflex-mediated syncope, the stimulus produces an abnormal autonomic nervous system reflex. Most commonly, an initial increase in sympathetic outflow is inappropriately withdrawn and replaced by increased vagal tone. Hypotension with or without bradycardia follows, leading to decreased cerebral perfusion and syncope. Less commonly, the stimulus leads directly to vagal hyperactivity and symptoms. Prodromal symptoms are varied, but include blurring of vision, dizziness, pallor, nausea, and diaphoresis.

The classic example of reflex-mediated syncope is the vasovagal faint incited by a noxious stimulus (pain, fear) or a characteristic setting. Vasovagal syncope rarely occurs without warning symptoms, which may last several minutes. A clinical diagnosis of vasovagal syncope should not be made without the typical prodromal symptoms described above. The individual is usually in the vertical position at the time of the event, and attacks are aborted or resolved after assuming a reclined position, which allows an increase in central circulation and thus increases cerebral perfusion. Whereas in the past, vasovagal syncope was diagnosed by history alone, upright tilt-table testing serves as an objective measure for vasovagal syncope and has led to the diagnosis in a number of patients with previously unclear etiology.[4]

Carotid sinus hypersensitivity is another type of reflex-mediated syncope. The carotid body, located at the carotid bifurcation, is a pressure-sensitive organ. The stimulation of an abnormally sensitive carotid body by external pressure may lead to two autonomic responses. Most commonly, there is an abnormal vagal response leading to bradycardia and asystole of greater than 3 s. Less commonly, there is a vasodepressor response leading to a decrease in blood pressure of more than 50 mmHg without a significant change in heart rate. Both responses may occur simultaneously. Carotid sinus hypersensitivity is more common in men, the elderly and among those with ischemic heart disease, hypertension, and certain head and neck malignancies. Although a number of patients may have a hypersensitive carotid sinus response on testing, unless this response culminates in syncope or recurrence of prodromal symptoms and can be associated with an inciting event, such as shaving or turning of the head, it cannot be diagnosed as the cause of a syncopal event. Only 5 to 20 percent of patients with carotid sinus hypersensitivity have a true carotid sinus syndrome with spontaneous symptoms. Carotid sinus hypersensitivity should be considered in all older patients with recurrent syncope and negative cardiac evaluations.

In situational syncope, there is an abnormal or hypersensitive autonomic reflex response to a specific physical stimulus (Table 46-1). Additionally, there may be a component of raised intracranial pressure or increased intrathoracic pressure leading to decreased cerebral perfusion. The physical stimulus may be associated with another underlying disease process: esophageal stricture in swallow syncope, prostatic hypertrophy or bladder neck obstruction with micturition syncope, and constipation with defecation syncope.

Orthostatic Syncope

When a person assumes an upright posture, blood is shifted to the lower part of the body and cardiac output drops. When a drop in cardiac output or blood pressure occurs in a healthy individual, the autonomic nervous system responds with an increase in sympathetic output and a decrease in parasympathetic output. This autonomic nervous system reflex produces an increase in heart rate and peripheral vascular resistance, leading to an increase in both cardiac output and blood pressure, thereby allowing the individual to maintain an upright posture. If the autonomic response is insufficient to counter the drop in cardiac output, decreased cerebral perfusion and syncope may follow if the person remains upright. Symptom onset is usually within the first 3 min after assuming the upright posture, but may be more delayed in some patients. Symptoms are characteristic of decreased cerebral perfusion, with blurred vision, dizziness, and tunnel vision. Orthostatic hypotension is defined as a fall in systolic blood pressure of greater than 20 mmHg upon assuming the upright posture. Caution must be taken in diagnosing a patient with orthostatic syncope based on orthostatic blood pressure measurements alone, because 5 to 55 percent of patients with other causes of syncope have orthostatic hypotension on physical examination.[5] To establish orthostasis as the cause of syncope, the patient should have recurrence of syncopal symptoms on orthostatic testing.

Serious orthostatic symptoms may be due to autonomic dysfunction, with failure of vasoconstriction during orthostatic stress. This may be a primary disease process or secondary to peripheral neuropathy, certain medications such as ganglionic blockers, spinal cord injury, and a variety of other neurologic diseases. More commonly, orthostatic symptoms are due to other conditions that lead to volume depletion, including gastrointestinal losses, bleeding, and diuresis. Medications commonly contribute to orthostatic syncope by blunting the chronotropic response of the heart to orthostatic stress or by leading to relative or absolute volume depletion. The elderly are more susceptible to orthostatic hypotension for many reasons, including use of diuretics and β-blocking agents, varying degrees of autonomic dysfunction, and other changes related to aging.

Cardiac Syncope

Cardiac syncope can be divided into two basic pathophysiologic categories: dysrhythmias and structural cardiopulmonary lesions. In both settings, the heart is unable to provide adequate cardiac output to maintain cerebral perfusion.

Although both brady- and tachydysrythmias may lead to transient cerebral hypoperfusion, there is no absolute high or low heart rate that will produce syncope. Symptoms depend on both the autonomic nervous system's ability to compensate for a decrease in cardiac output and the degree of cerebrovascular atherosclerotic disease. A variety of dysrythmias may lead to syncope (Table 46-1). A bradydysrhythmia is more likely to be an incidental finding on EKG rather than the actual cause of syncope.[6] Dysrhythmias are most likely to occur in the setting of ischemic heart disease but also may occur in other disease processes, such as in prolonged QT syndrome (torsades de pointes) and Lyme disease (heart blocks). Syncope from dysrhythmias is typically sudden, with prodromal symptoms lasting less than 3 s. Many patients report lack of any warning or premonition when questioned.

A wide variety of structural cardiopulmonary lesions may lead to an obstruction to flow and syncope. Syncope due to underlying structural cardiopulmonary disease often occurs in the setting of physical exertion but also may be seen in response to an acute vasodilation from medication or a hot environment. The resultant decrease in systemic vascular resistance is normally compensated by an increase in cardiac output to maintain arterial perfusion. In the presence of obstruction to flow, the upper limit of cardiac output is relatively fixed, limiting the compensation for decreased systemic vascular resistance and leading to a decrease in arterial perfusion and possible syncope. Aortic stenosis, a disease primarily of the elderly, is the most common structural cardiac abnormality causing syncope. In aortic stenosis there may be an additional component of abnormal reflex response, with increased ventricular pressures leading to inappropriate vasodilatation. Hypertrophic cardiomyopathy also leads to outflow obstruction and high ventricular pressures. It is characterized by asymmetric left ventricular hypertrophy and occurs most commonly in the young, although this entity is frequently present in persons over the age of 60. Pulmonary outflow obstruction may also lead to syncope. Up to 13 percent of patients diagnosed with pulmonary embolism have an initial syncopal episode that is likely secondary to the acute obstruction to flow by a large embolus.[7]

Medications

Medications frequently contribute to syncope (Table 46-2), particulary among the elderly. The most commonly implicated medications include antihypertensives and antidepressants.[8] Medications may contribute to syncope by a variety of means. Antihypertensive medications such as β blockers or calcium channel blockers commonly lead to a blunted heart rate response after an orthostatic or vasodilatory stress and may lead to bradycardia and conduction disturbances. Diuretics may produce volume depletion and subsequent orthostatic hypotension. Other medications may have proarrhythmic properties, increasing the concern for dysrhythmia as the cause of syncope. To entertain a medication as a cause of syncope, the untoward effects of the medications such as bradycardia or symptomatic orthostatic hypotension must be documented or demonstrable.

Psychiatric Illness

Studies have reported a high incidence of syncope in patients with psychiatric illness. The most frequent psychiatric diagnoses among these patients were generalized anxiety disorder, panic disorder, and major depressive disorder.[9,10] Syncope in these patients may have a variety of causes. Hyperventilation has been used as a provocative

TABLE 46-2 Drugs Commonly Implicated in Syncope

Antihypertensives
β Blockers
Cardiac glycosides
Diuretics
Antidysrhythmics
Antipsychotics
Antiparkinsonism drugs
Antidepressants
Phenothiazines
Nitrates
Alcohol
Cocaine

maneuver in diagnosing panic disorders and generalized anxiety disorders and can lead to hypocarbia, cerebral vasoconstriction, and subsequent syncope.[11,12] The hyperventilation may not be obvious to the observer but has been documented by end-tidal CO_2 monitoring.[11] Additionally, patients with psychiatric disorders may not have adequate coping skills and therefore may be more likely to have a vasovagal response culminate in syncope after an acute stress. Uncommonly, syncope may be psychogenic in nature with no measurable physical basis. In general, a patient with syncope and a psychiatric disorder is likely to be young, with repeated episodes of syncope, multiple prodromal symptoms, and a universally positive review of symptoms.[9,13]

Neurologic Syncope

Cerebrovascular disorders are rarely the primary cause of syncope, but must be considered in any patient with syncope and signs or symptoms indicating central nervous system pathology.

Brain stem ischemia may cause a decrease in blood flow to the reticular activating system, leading to sudden brief episodes of loss of consciousness, called *drop attacks.* These episodes of loss of consciousness are typically associated with other signs and symptoms of posterior circulation ischemia, including diplopia, vertigo, and nausea and possibly vertebrobasilar bruits. Subclavian steal is a rare cause of brain stem ischemia. It is characterized by an abnormal narrowing of the subclavian artery proximal to the origin of the vertebral artery (more commonly on the left) such that with exercise of the ipsilateral arm, blood is shunted, or "stolen," from the vertebrobasilar system to the subclavian artery supplying the arm muscles. Because of anatomy, it is more common on the left. Physical examination may reveal decreased pulse volume and diminished blood pressure in the affected arm. Other causes of brainstem ischemia include vertebrobasilar atherosclerotic disease and basilar artery migraines.

Subarachnoid hemorrhage (SAH) is a devastating disease process that may present with syncope. Accurate data regarding frequency of syncopal presentation of SAH is not readily available, but it does not seem to be particularly common. As the intracranial pressure increases there is a decrease in cerebral perfusion pressure, which may cause syncope. The patient typically complains of sudden severe headache and may have focal neurologic findings.

Syncope in Special Populations

The majority of hospital admissions for syncope are for patients aged 55 and older. Because of both normal physiologic changes with aging and age-related disease processes, the elderly are at increased risk of syncope. They are susceptible to increased morbidity from either the trauma of a syncopal episode or from iatrogenic events during subsequent hospital admission. Additionally, syncope in the elderly is frequently recurrent.

As a person ages, the blood vessels become calcified and less compliant, leading to diminished flow rates. The left ventricle also becomes less compliant, resulting in increased diastolic filling pressures and an increased dependence on the "atrial kick." There is a general decrease in adrenergic receptor responsiveness of both the heart and the peripheral blood vessels. This decreased adrenergic responsiveness contributes to the diminished chronotropic response seen after orthostatic stresses in the elderly. The incidence of vasovagal syncope actually decreases with age, in part due to this decreased responsiveness of the autonomic nervous system. The elderly also have a less-sensitive thirst mechanism and a decreased endocrine response after volume depletion. In addition to these normal changes with aging, the elderly may have a number of pathophysiologic processes that may contribute to diminished cerebral perfusion. Cardiac disease is prevalent in the elderly population. Chronic hypertension shifts the cerebral autoregulation mechanism to higher pressures. Additionally, orthostatic hypotension and postprandial hypotension are more common among the hypertensive elderly. Atherosclerotic disease leads to ischemia and myocardial infarction and subsequent congestive heart failure and dysrhythmias. Aortic stenosis is the most common obstructive cardiac lesion in the elderly, producing a fixed cardiac output and thus a risk of syncope when increased demand for cardiac output cannot be met.[14] Diabetes is another disease process common in the elderly and may lead to autonomic dysfunction and peripheral neuropathy. Finally, medication usage is much more common in the elderly population, again increasing the risk of orthostasis and decreasing autonomic responsiveness to orthostatic stress. It is important to note that syncope in the elderly population is most often multifactorial and the etiology may, therefore, be difficult to establish, particularly in the ED.

Pregnancy is associated with numerous physiologic changes including increased heart rate, decreased peripheral resistance, and increased stroke volume. In late pregnancy, the enlarged uterus may compress the inferior vena cava, decreasing venous return. The incidence of cardiac dysrhythmias, especially premature ventricular contractions, increases during normal pregnancy in young healthy women. However, a positive correlation has not been shown between symptoms of presyncope or syncope and cardiac dysrhythmia.[15] Vasovagal syncope is the most common cause of syncope during normal pregnancy and may be the presenting cause for an ED visit.

Syncope in the pediatric population is discussed elsewhere in this text (Chap. 127).

DIFFERENTIAL DIAGNOSIS

Seizure disorders are frequently listed as a cause of syncope, and although they often cause a brief loss of consciousness, they do not share the same pathophysiologic mechanisms as syncope. Seizure is the most common event mistaken as syncope. History is very important in differentiating seizure from syncope.[16] Brief tonic movements of extremities may accompany syncope but do not represent true seizure activity. Urinary incontinence, which is often seen with seizures, may also occur with syncope. The most reliable differentiating factor is the postictal confusion period, which is commonly seen after a generalized seizure but is rarely associated with syncope. However, syncope itself may trigger a seizure, so that a seizure presentation does not exclude a syncopal origin.

EMERGENCY DEPARTMENT EVALUATION

The core components of the ED evaluation of syncope are a careful history, a thorough physical examination, and the electrocardiogram.

The history and physical examination are essential in determining a patient who is at risk of serious morbidity from subsequent syncope, and will identify the cause of syncope up to 85 percent of patients in whom a diagnosis can be established.[2] It should be obtained from the patient and any witness of the event. Emphasis should be placed on the events leading up to the loss of consciousness, the characteristics of the loss of consciousness, and symptoms occurring after regaining consciousness. The history should begin with a detailed description of the events preceding the loss of consciousness, including position, environmental stimuli, and the involvement of strenuous activity or arm exercise. All premonitory symptoms should be recorded, looking for neurologic symptoms, such as vertigo or focal weakness, and cardiac symptoms, such as palpitations. Duration of loss of consciousness and symptoms occurring after regaining consciousness should also be documented. Symptoms associated with syncope that should raise concern of an immediately life-threatening diagnosis include chest pain (acute myocardial infarction, aortic dissection, pulmonary embolism, aortic stenosis), headache (subarachnoid hemorrhage), and abdominal or back pain (leaking abdominal aortic aneurysm, ruptured ectopic pregnancy). A sudden event without warning and events associated with exertion should increase suspicion of a cardiac dysrhythmia or structural cardiopulmonary lesion. Antecedent illness or substance use should be documented. The past medical history must include details about prior cardiopulmonary events, including prior myocardial infarction, ventricular dysrhythmias, and congestive heart failure. All medications should be recorded, including over-the-counter medications such as laxatives. Patients aggressively dieting to lose weight may have electrolyte disturbances or be taking amphetamine-like medications. The family history is important in regards to history of prolonged QT syndrome, dysrhythmias, or other cardiac risks.

Particular attention should be paid to patients presenting with single-car motor vehicle crashes (especially driving off the road), particularly if the patients are elderly. Clinicians may become preoccupied by the trauma evaluation and miss the possibility of syncopal event.

Physical examination may also give important information. For example, evidence of trauma without defensive injuries to the hands or knees should raise suspicion of a sudden event without warning, such as a dysrhythmia. The physical examination should focus on both the cardiovascular and neurologic systems. Blood pressure measurements should be taken in both arms. Unequal blood pressures should increase suspicion of aortic dissection or subclavian steal. The presence of orthostatic hypotension and symptoms should be recorded. To appropriately evaluate orthostasis, the patient should be supine for a period of 5 to 10 min and then should arise to the standing position. After standing, blood pressure measurements should be taken two to three times over the next few minutes. A detailed cardiac examination may reveal the murmur of hypertrophic cardiomyopathy or aortic stenosis. The neurologic examination may uncover findings of focal neurologic disease or peripheral neuropathy. Rectal examination must be performed on all patients to evaluate for gastrointestinal bleeding.

A 12-lead ECG should be obtained, even though the electrocardiogram and rhythm strip lead to a diagnosis in only a small number of patients.[3] The ECG should be evaluated for evidence of prior cardiopulmonary disease, acute ischemia, dysrhythmia, and heart block. Patients should be monitored for abnormal cardiac activity until a cardiac origin has been reasonably excluded.

Other ED testing should be done on selected patients based on the above initial evaluation. Laboratory testing should not be performed unless the history and physical examination suggest an abnormality. For example, a patient with orthostatic symptoms and heme-positive guaiac test warrants at least a CBC. A reproductive-age female should have a urine pregnancy test. Although electrolyte abnormalities may be implicated as a cause of seizures, they are rarely the cause of syncope and therefore routine testing in the evaluation of syncope is not warranted.[3] Evidence of an irritable myocardium, profound weakness, dehydration, or diuretic use merits serum electrolyte determination.

Carotid massage is used to diagnose carotid sinus hypersensitivity. It can be done at the bedside with continuous electrocardiographic and blood pressure monitoring. Each carotid body is separately massaged for 5 to 10 s. Carotid massage should not be done if bruits are present, if there is history of recent stroke or myocardial infarction, or if there is a history of ventricular tachycardia. Only a small number of patients with carotid hypersensitivity will have the true carotid sinus syndrome.

A hyperventilation maneuver (open-mouthed, slow, deep breaths at a rate of 20 to 30 breaths per minute for 2 to 3 min) can be very useful in the young patient with undiagnosed syncope. A recurrence of prodromal symptoms or syncope significantly correlates with psychiatric (anxiety-provoking) causes of syncope.[11]

Studies fail to show any benefit of routine CT scanning, EEG, or lumbar puncture for patients who lack a history or physical examination that supports a neurologic cause of syncope.[3] An echocardiogram should be reserved for patients with a history or physical findings consistent with structural heart disease.

Patients with an unknown etiology of syncope after this initial evaluation need a further inpatient or outpatient medical evaluation that focuses on dysrhythmia detection and identification of vasovagal syncope or psychiatric illness (Fig. 46-1).

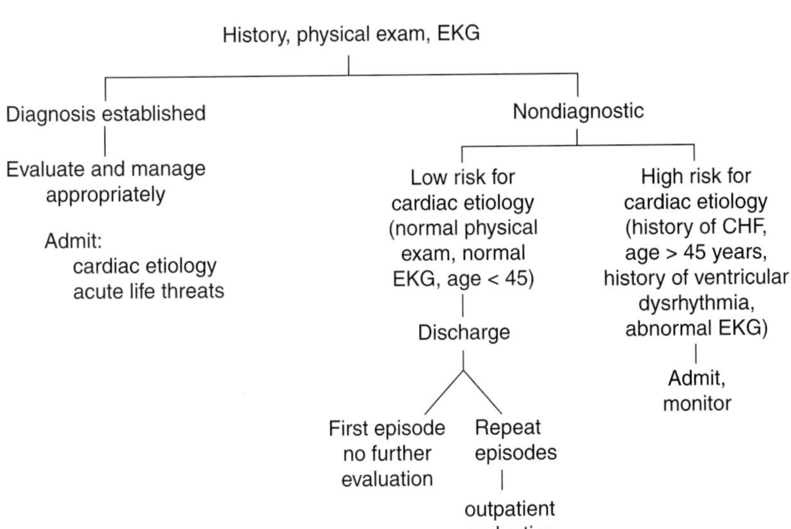

FIG. 46-1. Approach to the ED management of syncope.

PROGNOSIS

If a cause of syncope can be determined on ED evaluation, identification of high-risk patients is simple. Those patients with acute neurologic deficits or life-threatening disorders are at immediate risk of morbidity. Additionally, patients with cardiac causes of syncope represent a high-risk group for major morbidity or death. On evaluation in the emergency department, however, a cause of syncope is not identifiable in up to half of patients.[3] Efforts must then be focused to identify those patients at high risk for a cardiac cause of syncope. A recent prospective study focused on risk stratification based on clinical and electrocardiographic characteristics.[17] The study found four significant predictors of sudden cardiac death or significant dysrhythmia within one year of a syncopal event: abnormal electrocardiogram (anything other than nonspecific ST-T changes), age greater than 45 years, history of ventricular dysrhythmia, and history of congestive heart failure. The risk went up with increased numbers of these predictors. This supports prior studies that show that the prognosis of syncope in patients without heart disease is very good.[18,19] The young patient with syncope, a normal physical examination, and a normal electrocardiogram has a very low risk of morbidity. Additionally, patients who have recurrent syncope with more than five episodes in 1 year are more likely to have vasovagal syncope or a psychiatric diagnosis than dysrhythmia as the cause.[2]

Indications for hospital admission, therefore, include patients with acute neurologic or life-threatening disorders and patients at risk for a cardiac etiology of syncope (Fig. 46-1). Patients with more than one episode, who are discharged from the ED should be accompanied by a responsible adult and be advised not to drive, work at heights, or operate machinery until further outpatient evaluation.

REFERENCES

1. Kapoor WN: Syncope in older persons. *J Am Geriatr Soc* 42:426, 1994.
2. Kapoor WN: Evaluation and management of the patient with syncope. *JAMA* 268(18):2553, 1992.
3. Linzer M, Yang EH, Estes NA III, et al: Diagnosing syncope. Part 1: Value of history, physical examination and electrocardiography. The clinical efficacy assessment project of the American College of Physicians. *Ann Intern Med* 126:989, 1997.
4. Strasberg B, Rechavia E, Sagie A, et al: The head up tilt-table test in patients with syncope of unknown origin. *Am Heart J* 118(5 part 1):923, 1989.
5. Atkins D, Hanusa B, Sefcik T, et al: Syncope and orthostatic hypotension. *Am J Med* 91:179, 1991.
6. McAnulty JH, Rahimtoola SH, Murphy E, et al: Natural history of "high risk" bundle-branch block: Final report of a prospective study. *N Engl J Med* 307:137, 1987.
7. Thames MD, Alpert JS, Dalen JE: Syncope in patients with pulmonary embolism. *JAMA* 238:2509, 1977.
8. Hanlon JH, Linzer M, MacMillan JP, et al: Syncope and presyncope associated with probable adverse drug reaction. *Arch Intern Med* 150:2309, 1990.
9. Kapoor WN, Fortunato M, Hanusa BH, et al: Psychiatric illness in patients with syncope, *Am J Med* 99:505, 1995.
10. Linzer M, Felder A, Hackel A, et al: Psychiatric syncope: A new look at an old disease. *Psychosomatics* 31:181, 1990.
11. Koenig M, Pontinen M, Divine GW: Syncope in young adults: Evidence for a combined medical and psychiatric approach. *J Intern Med* 232:169, 1992.
12. Naschitz JE, Gaitini L, Mazov I, et al: The capnography-tilt test for the diagnosis of hyperventilation syncope. *QJMed* 90:139, 1997.
13. Linzer M, Varia I, Pontinen M, et al: Medically unexplained syncope: Relationship to psychiatric illness. *Am J Med* 92:185, 1992.
14. Lindroos K, Kupari M, Keikkila M, et al: Prevalence of aortic valve abnormalities in the elderly: An echocardiographic study of a random population. *J Am Coll Cardiol* 21:1220, 1993.
15. Shotan A, Ostrzega E, Mehra A, et al: Incidence of arrhythmias in normal pregnancy and relation to palpitations, dizziness, and syncope. *Am J Cardiol.* 79:1061, 1997.
16. Hoefnagels WAJ, Padberg GW, Overweg J, et al: Transient loss of consciousness: The value of the history for distinguishing seizure from syncope. *J Neurol* 238:39, 1991.
17. Martin TP, Hanusa BH, Kapoor WN: Risk stratification of patients with syncope. *Ann Emerg Med* 29:4, 1997.
18. Eagle KA, Black HR, Cook EF, et al: Evaluation of prognostic classifications for patients with syncope. *Am J Med* 79:455, 1985.
19. Martin GJ, Adams SL, Martin HG, et al: Prospective evaluation of syncope, *Ann Emerg Med* 13(7):499, 1984.

ACUTE CORONARY SYNDROMES: UNSTABLE ANGINA, MYOCARDIAL ISCHEMIA, AND INFARCTION

Judd E. Hollander

PATHOPHYSIOLOGY

Knowledge of the anatomy of the coronary arteries is essential to understand the effects of myocardial ischemia and why some complications are more common with anterior or inferior wall myocardial infarction. (Fig. 47-1). The left coronary artery arises from the ascending aorta in the left sinus of the aortic valve. It courses through the atrioventricular sulcus on the left side and divides into the left circumflex and the left anterior descending branch. The left anterior descending branch courses down the anterior aspect of the heart around the inferior margin and anastomoses with the posterior diagonal branch of the right coronary artery. It is the main blood supply to the anterior and septal regions of the heart. The circumflex branch continues around the atrioventricular sulcus, where it anastomoses with the right coronary artery. It supplies blood to some of the anterior wall and a large portion of the lateral wall of the heart. The right coronary artery arises from the right sinus of the aortic valve and runs in the atrioventricular sulcus between the right atrium and right ventricle. It gives off a marginal branch near the lower aspect of the heart and terminates as the right posterior descending artery. The right coronary artery supplies the right side of the heart with blood and it provides some perfusion to the inferior aspect of the left ventricle through the posterior descending artery.

The atrioventricular (AV) conduction system receives blood supply from both the AV branch of the right coronary artery and septal perforating branch of the left anterior descending coronary artery. Similarly, both the right bundle branch and the left posterior division obtain a dual blood flow from the left anterior descending and right coronary arteries. The posteromedial papillary muscle receives blood

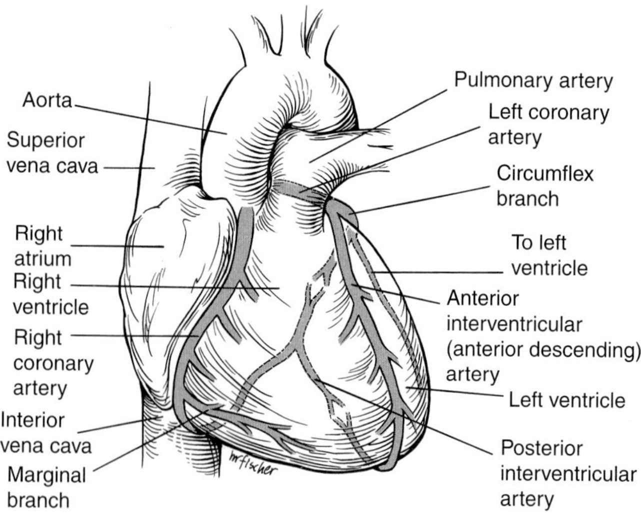

FIG. 47-1. Schematic diagram of the coronary arteries.

TABLE 47-1 Canadian Cardiovascular Society Classification of Angina

Class I	Angina occurs only with strenuous, rapid or prolonged exertion. Ordinary physical activity does not cause angina.
Class II	Slight limitation of ordinary activity. Angina occurs with climbing stairs rapidly, walking uphill, walking after meals, in cold, in wind, or under emotional stress.
Class III	Marked limitations of ordinary physical activity. Angina occurs on walking 1–2 blocks on level or climbing one flight of stairs at usual pace.
Class IV	Inability to carry on physical activity without discomfort; anginal symptoms may be present at rest.

Source: Braunwald et al.[1]

supply from only a single coronary artery, usually the right coronary artery.

EPIDEMIOLOGY AND DEFINITIONS

Ischemic heart disease is the leading cause of death among adults in the United States. Over 6 million U.S. citizens have coronary artery disease. There are 4 to 5 million emergency department (ED) visits for acute chest pain syndromes annually. Coronary artery disease results in approximately 500,000 deaths annually in the United States. The total economic burden is over $100 billion per year.

Acute coronary syndromes (ACS) represent a spectrum of disease from chronic stable angina to acute myocardial infarction.[1] The Canadian Cardiovascular Society divides angina into four classes (Table 47-1). Class I represents those patients in whom ordinary physical activity does not cause angina and class IV is reserved for those patients who develop anginal symptoms at rest. Unstable angina has been divided into three principal presentations by the Agency for Health Care Policy and Research (AHCPR) Clinical Practice Guidelines.[1] These three presentations are rest angina, new-onset angina, and increasing angina (Table 47-2).

The use of these classifications and definitions in the ED is problematic. When patients present with acute chest pain syndromes, it is often not clear whether the chest pain is cardiac or noncardiac in origin. The proper application of both the Canadian Cardiovascular Society Classification and the AHCPR guidelines assumes a diagnosis of ischemic chest pain. These guidelines can be difficult to incorporate into emergency practice, where the diagnosis is often uncertain. They are not as useful as other methods to assess risk of an acute cardiac event or adverse events (Table 47-3).

TABLE 47-2 Main Presentations of Unstable Angina

Rest angina	Angina occurring at rest and usually prolonged >20 min, occurring within a week of presentation
New onset angina	Angina of at least CCSC* III severity with onset within 2 months of presentation
Increasing angina	Previously diagnosed angina that is distinctly more frequent, longer in duration, or lower in threshold (increased by at least one CCSC class to at least CCSC III severity)

*CCSC, Canadian Cardiovascular Society Classification.
Source: Braunwald et al.[1]

TABLE 47-3 Short-Term Risk of Death or Nonfatal Myocardial Infarction in Patients with Unstable Angina

High Risk—At Least One of the Following Features Must Be Present:	Intermediate Risk—No High Risk Feature But Must Have One of the Following:	Low Risk—No High or Intermediate Risk Feature But May Have Any of the Following Features:
Prolonged ongoing (>20 min) rest pain	Prolonged (20 min) rest angina, now resolved, with moderate or high likelihood of CAD	Increased angina frequency, severity, or duration
Pulmonary edema, most likely related to ischemia	Rest angina (>20 min or relieved with rest or sublingual nitroglycerin)	Angina provoked at a lower threshold (e.g. with less exertion than before)
Angina at rest with dynamic ST changes ≥1 mm	Nocturnal angina	Isolated new-onset angina with onset 2 weeks to 2 months prior to presentation
Angina with new or worsening MR murmur	Angina with dynamic T-wave changes	Normal or unchanged ECG
Angina with S_3 or new/worsening rales	New onset CCSC III or IV angina in the past 2 weeks with moderate or high likelihood of CAD	
Angina with hypotension	Pathologic Q waves or resting ST depression ≤1 mm in multiple lead groups (anterior, inferior, lateral)	
	Age >65 years	

Key: CAD, coronary artery disease; CCSC, Canadian Cardiovascular Society Classification; ECG, electrocardiogram.
Source: Braunwald et al.[1]

Hypoxia is a reduction in oxygen supply to tissue despite adequate perfusion. Ischemia is oxygen deprivation accompanied by inadequate removal of metabolites due to reduced perfusion. Both ischemia and hypoxia must be discussed in relative terms, since conditions that result in ischemia in one patient may not result in ischemia in another. Ischemia occurs when there is an imbalance between oxygen demand and oxygen supply. Oxygen supply is influenced by the oxygen-carrying capacity of the blood and the coronary arterial blood flow. The oxygen-carrying capacity of the blood is determined by the amount of hemoglobin present. Coronary arterial blood flow is determined by diastolic relaxation of the heart and the vascular resistance. Humoral, neural, metabolic, and extravascular compressive forces and local autoregulation mechanisms determine the coronary vascular resistance.

Myocardial ischemia and its sequelae usually occur as a result of fixed atheroscerotic lesions or secondary reduction in myocardial blood flow due to coronary arterial spasm, disruption of atherosclerotic plaques, and platelet aggregation or thrombus formation. Nonatherosclerotic etiologies of acute myocardial infarction are considerably less common (Table 47-4).

TABLE 47-4 Some Nonatherosclerotic Etiologies of Acute Myocardial Ischemia

Other causes of coronary artery disease
- Trauma
  - Laceration
  - Thrombosis
  - Radiation
  - Myocardial contusion
- Connective tissue diseases
  - Takayasu arteritis
  - Polyarteritis nodosa
  - Systemic lupus erythematosus
  - Rheumatoid arthritis
  - Ankylosing spondylitis
- Long-term sequelae of infectious diseases
  - Syphilis
  - Kawasaki disease
- Metabolic diseases leading to thickening of intima or media
  - Homocystinuria
  - Amyloid
  - Fabry disease
  - Mucopolysaccharidosis

Congenital anomalies of the coronary arteries
- Anomalous origin of the left coronary artery from pulmonary artery or anterior sinus of Valsalva
- Coronary artery aneurysms
- Coronary artery fistulas

In situ thrombosis
- Disseminated intravascular coagulation
- Thrombotic thromboytopenic purpura
- Polycythemia vera
- Thrombocytosis

Emboli
- Endocarditis
  - Bacterial
  - Nonbacterial
- Thrombotic emboli from left atrium or ventricle

Dissection of aorta or coronary arteries
- Idiopathic
- Iatrogenic (postcatheterization)

Drug use
- Cocaine
- Amphetamines
- Other

Plaque formation occurs through repetitive injury to the vessel wall. Macrophages and smooth muscle cells are the main cellular elements in plaque development, whereas lipids are the predominant in the extracellular milieu. Plaque fissuring and rupture is affected by features inherent to the plaque, such as its composition and shape, as well as local factors such as shear forces, coronary arterial tone, coronary arterial perfusion pressure, and movements of the artery in response to myocardial contractions. When plaque rupture occurs, potent thrombogenic substances are exposed to circulating platelets.

The platelet response involves adhesion, activation, and aggregation. Platelet adhesion occurs through the weak platelet interactions with subendothelial adhesion molecules such as collagen, fibronectin, and laminin and the binding of the glycoprotein 1b receptor to the subendothelial form of Von Willebrand factor. Adherent platelets are strongly thrombogenic. Subendothelial collagen is a potent inducer of platelet activation. Lipid-laden macrophages in the plaque core and adventitia of the vessel wall release tissue factor, which stimulates the conversion of prothrombin to thrombin. Thrombin, collagen, and the local shear forces are all potent platelet activators. Platelet secretion of adenosine diphosphate, thromboxane A_2, and serotonin are autostimulatory agonists of platelet activation. Activated platelet glycoprotein IIb/IIIa receptors become cross-linked by fibrinogen or Von Willebrand factor in the final common pathway of platelet aggregation.

The extent of oxygen deprivation and thus clinical presentation of acute coronary syndromes, depends upon the limitation of O_2 delivery imposed by thrombus adhering to fixed, fissured, or eroded atherosclerotic plaque. Myocardial ischemia can be manifest by chest discomfort, dyspnea, characteristic or nonspecific electrocardiographic changes, depressed myocardial function, reduced central and peripheral perfusion, or any combination. In stable angina, ischemia occurs only when activity induces O_2 demands beyond the supply restrictions imposed by a partially occluded coronary vessel. This occurs at a relatively fixed and predictable point and changes slowly over time. Atherosclerotic plaque has not ruptured and there is little if any superimposed thrombus. In unstable angina and acute myocardial infarction, atherosclerotic plaque rupture and platelet-rich thrombus develops. Coronary blood flow is reduced and myocardial ischemia occurs. The degree and duration of the oxygen supply–demand mismatch determines whether the patient develops reversible myocardial ischemia without injury (unstable angina) or myocardial ischemia with injury (myocardial infarction). More severe obstruction and prolonged obstruction is related to an increased likelihood of myocardial injury.

Acute myocardial ischemia may inhibit myocardial contractability, affecting both central and peripheral perfusion. In acute myocardial infarction, the fundamental alteration is loss of functioning myocardium. When an area of the myocardium does not receive adequate O_2, the functional deterioration is progressive through four sequentially abnormal contraction patterns. Dyssynchrony, the dissociation in time course of contraction of adjacent segments of myocardium, occurs first. Hypokinesis, the reduction in the extent of shortening with contraction, occurs next. Akinesis, the cessation of shortening with systolic contraction follows. Finally dyskinesis, the paradoxical expansion of infarcted tissue, occurs during systole. With increasing size of the infarcted myocardium, left ventricular pump function decreases. Left ventricular end-diastolic pressure increases and left ventricular end-systolic volume increases. Cardiac output, stroke volume, and blood pressure may decrease. When left atrial and pulmonary capillary wedge pressures increase, congestive heart failure may develop. Poor perfusion to the brain and kidneys can result in altered mental status and impaired renal function, respectively.

CLINICAL FEATURES

Clinical History

The symptoms of ischemic heart disease that should be sought and characterized include chest discomfort, severity, location, radiation, duration, and quality. In addition, the presence of associated symptoms such as nausea, vomiting, diaphoresis, dyspnea, light-headedness, syncope, and palpitations may be helpful. A detailed history regarding the onset and duration of symptoms, activities that precipitate symptoms, and prior evaluations for similar symptoms should be ascertained. Cardiac risk-factor assessment should be performed.

Symptoms of chest discomfort or pain may be cardiac or noncardiac in origin. Diseases of the esophagus, lungs, stomach, mediastinum, pleura, and viscera may all simulate cardiac discomfort. In addition, many patients may have concurrent diseases.

Symptoms of acute myocardial ischemia will often be described as discomfort rather than pain. Anginal symptoms include chest pressure, heaviness, tightness, fullness, or squeezing. Less commonly but not infrequently, patients will describe their symptoms as knifelike, sharp, or stabbing. The classic location is substernal or in the left chest. Radiation to the arm, neck, or jaw may occur. Reproducible chest wall tenderness is not uncommon, since the pericardium may become inflamed and it sits beneath the chest wall. A complete discussion of the differential diagnosis of chest pain syndromes can be found in Chap. 45.

Exercise, stress, or a cold environment classically precipitates angina pectoris. Angina usually has a duration of symptoms of up to 15 to 20 min and usually improves within 2 to 5 min after rest or nitroglycerin. However, early classic descriptions of angina describe episodes as short as 2 min. On the other hand, acute myocardial infarction is usually accompanied by more prolonged and severe chest discomfort, more prominent associated symptoms (nausea, diaphoresis, shortness of breath, etc.), and little if any response to sublingual nitroglycerin. Easy fatigability may be a prominent symptom of ACS.

It is important to know the frequency of anginal episodes and any change in frequency of episodes over the past months. The patient should be questioned to determine any increase in severity or duration of symptoms or whether less effort is required to precipitate them.

Atypical presentations or silent myocardial ischemia are common. Up to 30 percent of patients with acute myocardial infarction identified in large longitudinal studies are clinically unrecognized. Some of these patients have had atypical symptoms for which they did not pursue medical advice. Others cannot recall any symptoms. The prognosis for patients who have atypical symptoms at the time of their infarction is worse than that of patients who had more typical symptoms. Women and the elderly are more likely to have atypical presentations.[2]

Cardiac risk factors are modestly predictive of coronary artery disease in asymptomatic patients. In the ED, cardiac risk factors are poor predictors of cardiac risk for myocardial infarction or other acute coronary syndromes.[1,2] Traditional cardiac risk factors—such as hypertension, diabetes mellitus, tobacco use, family history of coronary artery disease at an early age, and hypercholesterolemia—are not predictive of the cardiac risk in female ED chest pain patients. In male patients, only diabetes and family history were weakly predictive.[2] The distinction between the utility of cardiac risk factors in the asymptomatic patient and the ED chest pain patient is easy to understand. The cardiac risk factors were derived from population-based longitudinal cohort studies of asymptomatic patients. In contrast, ED chest pain patients have already been identified as being at increased risk by the very fact that they have symptoms. The mere presence of symptoms outweighs the predictive value of cardiac risk factors. A lack of cardiac risk factors does not sufficiently decrease cardiac risk in ED patients such that triage and disposition strategies should be altered.[2]

Physical Examination

The physical examination is not helpful in distinguishing patients with acute coronary syndromes from those with noncardiac chest pain syndromes unless an alternate diagnosis is clear. Patients with acute coronary syndromes may appear deceptively well without any clinical signs of distress or may be uncomfortable, pale, cyanotic, and in respiratory distress. Vital signs may reveal bradycardia, tachycardia, or irregular pulses. Bradycardic rhythms are more common with inferior wall myocardial ischemia. In the setting of an anterior wall infarction, bradycardic rhythms or heart block is an extremely poor prognostic sign. Blood pressure can be normal, elevated (due to baseline hypertension, sympathetic stimulation, and anxiety) or decreased (due to pump failure or inadequate preload). Extremes of blood pressure are associated with a worse prognosis.

The first and second heart sounds are often diminished due to poor myocardial contractility. An S_3 is present in 15 to 20 percent of patients with acute myocardial infarction. An S_4 is common in patients with long-standing hypertension or myocardial dysfunction. The presence or absence of the noted heart sounds is not usually helpful in the ED, although an S_3, if truly detected, may imply a failing myocardium. However, the presence of a new systolic murmur is an ominous sign, as it may signify papillary muscle dysfunction, a flail leaflet of the mitral valve with resultant mitral regurgitation, or a ventricular septal defect.

The presence of rales, with or without an S_3 gallop is associated with left ventricular dysfunction and left-sided congestive heart failure. Jugular venous distention, hepatojugular reflex, and peripheral edema suggest right-sided congestive heart failure. It is important to determine the patient's baseline condition from medical records or from the patient's physician to establish the presence of new findings that may help guide management.

Electrocardiography

The normal myocardium depolarizes from endocardium to epicardium and repolarizes in the opposite direction. When injured, the myocardium remains electrically more positive than the uninjured area at the end of depolarization. The relatively positive potential in this area will result in ST elevation of electrocardiogram leads over this area. Conversely, if the electrode is located over uninjured myocardium opposite the injured area, ST depression will be noted (reciprocal changes). If the injury is limited to the subendocardial area, the electrode will be separated from the injured area by the normal epicardial layer. The epicardial layer becomes more electrically negative than the injured subendocardial layer at the end of depolarization, resulting in ST-segment depressions.

Transmural myocardial ischemia also delays the repolarization process. The ischemic area is electrically more negative than the uninjured area. The T-wave recording over the ischemic area will be negative or downward. In subendocardial ischemia, the delay in repolarization does not alter the direction of the recovery period because the normal repolarization process is from the epicardium to the endocardium. T-wave inversions will not be seen. Since the electrical potential generated by the delayed repolarization in the subendocardium is not opposed, the T wave will be larger than normal (hyperacute T waves).

After acute myocardial infarction (AMI), the area of necrosis is electrically silent. The resultant forces generated from the myocardium during repolarization (the QRS complex) will be affected by this electrically silent area. Electrodes facing the infarcted area will record an abnormal negative deflection during depolarization (pathologic Q waves).

The standard 12-lead electrocardiogram (ECG), is the single best test to identify patients with acute myocardial infarction upon ED presentation.[3] National guidelines require that it be obtained and interpreted within 10 min of presentation.[4] Although it is the best immediately available test in the ED, it still has relatively low sensitivity for detection of acute myocardial infarction. The ST-segment is elevated during an AMI in approximately 50 percent,[1,3] i.e., half of the patients who present to the ED with AMI would not be detected solely on the basis of the electrocardiogram. Most patients with AMI will have some nondiagnostic abnormalities on the ECG.[3] Some 1 to 5 percent of patients with AMI have an entirely normal ECG.[3–6] These figures refer to myocardial infarction, not angina.

Standard diagnostic ECG criteria for AMI are shown in Table 47-5. ST-segment elevations in the distributions shown suggest acute transmural injury. ST-segment depressions in these distributions suggest subendocardial ischemia. All inferior wall acute myocardial infarctions should have a right-sided lead V_4 (rV_4) obtained because ST-segment elevation in rV_4 is highly suggestive of right ventricular infarction. There is no proven role for other right-sided leads.

Reciprocal ST-segment changes (such as ST-segment depressions in the anterior precordial leads in the setting of an inferior wall AMI) predict a larger infarct distribution, an increased severity of underlying coronary artery disease, more severe pump failure, a higher likelihood of cardiovascular complications, and increased mortality. In general, the more elevated the ST segments and the more ST segments that are elevated, the more extensive the injury.

TABLE 47-5 Electrocardiographic Criteria for Acute Myocardial Infarction

Location	ECG Findings
Anteroseptal	QS deflections in V_1, V_2, V_3, and possibly V_4
Anterior	rS deflection in V_1 with Q waves in V_2–V_4 or Decrease in amplitude of initial R waves from V_1 through V_4
Anterolateral	Q waves in V_4 through V_6, I, and aVL
Lateral	Q waves in I and aVL
Inferior	Q waves in II, III, and aVF
Inferolateral	Q waves in II, III, aVF, V_5, and V_6
True posterior	Initial R waves in V_1 and V_2 >0.04 s and R/S ratio ≥1
Right ventricular	Q waves in II, III, and aVF and ST-segment elevation in V_{4R}

The ECG can also be used to predict the infarct-related vessel. Inferior wall myocardial infarctions can result from occlusion of the left circumflex artery or the right coronary artery. In the setting of an inferior wall AMI, ST-segment elevation in at least one lateral lead (V_5, V_6, or aVL) with an isoelectric or elevated ST segment in lead I is strongly suggestive of a left circumflex lesion. The presence of ST-segment elevation in lead III greater than that in lead II predicts a right coronary artery occlusion. When accompanied by either ST-segment elevation in V_1 or aVR, it predicts a proximal right coronary artery lesion with accompanying right ventricular infarction. Reciprocal anterior ST-segment depressions in V_1 through V_4 are equally prevalent in both right coronary and left circumflex inferior wall AMI.

The main utility of the ECG is to detect AMI. The standard 12-lead ECG is less helpful in the detection of other acute coronary syndromes (stable angina or unstable angina). One widely used classification breaks down the ECG into six categories:

- Normal;
- nonspecific ST-segment or T-segment wave changes;
- abnormal but not diagnostic of ischemia or infarction;
- ischemia, strain, or infarction known to be old;
- ischemia, strain or infarction not known to be old;
- probable myocardial infarction.

This classification and others like it have been used to show that patients with more significant ECG abnormalities are more likely to have AMI, unstable angina, and serious cardiovascular complications. On the other hand, even the patients with normal or nonspecific ECGs have a 1 to 3 percent incidence of AMI and a 4 to 23 percent incidence of unstable angina. Patients with nondiagnostic ECGs or with ischemia that is not known to be old have a 4 to 7 percent incidence of AMI and a 21 to 48 percent incidence of unstable angina. Demonstration of new ischemia increases the risk of AMI 25 to 73 percent and the unstable angina risk to 14 to 43 percent.[3] The standard 12-lead ECG is useful for cardiovascular risk stratification of patients with acute coronary syndromes. It can be used in conjunction with clinical history and cardiac markers to determine admission location for such patients.

Novel approaches to electrocardiography have been proposed in the last decade. A continuous 12-lead ECG monitor has been developed that records a new 12-lead ECG every 20 s. When the ST-segment baseline is altered, an alarm is raised and a copy of the new ECG is automatically shared or printed. This type of technology might be useful for monitoring patients who present with non-AMI acute coronary syndromes for ECG evidence of injury.[4] Because of costs, concerns regarding labile ST-segment and T-wave changes from hyperventilation or patient movement and a lack of ED-based prospective studies, continuous-12 lead ECG monitoring has not been recommended for routine use.[4]

ECGs with 15, 18, and 22 leads have been studied.[4,7] The addition of V_{4R}, V_8, and V_9, increased the sensitivity without a loss of specificity for the detection of ST-segment elevation.[7] The addition of V_{4R} through V_{6R} and V_7 through V_9 as posterior leads led to increased sensitivity, but at the cost of decreased specificity. ECGs with 22 leads and body-surface mapping have not been sufficiently studied. The report from the National Heart Attack Alert Program recommends the use of standard ECGs with right-sided leads in the setting of inferior wall infarction.[4]

There are several clinical conditions where ECG interpretation is difficult (Table 47-6). It has been shown that in the setting of paced rhythms and left bundle branch blocks, acute myocardial ischemia can be identified. In the setting of a left bundle branch block, the presence of ST-segment elevation ≥1 mm and concordant with the QRS complex or ST segment depression ≥1 mm in leads V_1, V_2, or V_3 suggests acute myocardial infarction.[8] ST-segment elevation ≥5 mm and discordant with the QRS complex increases the likelihood of AMI but has poor specificity.

Right ventricular pacing causes secondary repolarization changes of opposing polarity to that of the predominant QRS complex. Most leads have predominant negative QRS complexes followed by ST-segment elevation and positive T waves. ST-segment elevation ≥5 mm was most indicative of AMI in leads with predominantly negative QRS complexes. Any ST-segment elevation concordant to the QRS

TABLE 47-6 Some Clinical Conditions Where the Electrocardiogram Interpretation Can Be Difficult

May have ST-segment elevation in the absence of acute myocardial infarction
- Early repolarization
- Left ventricular hypertrophy
- Pericarditis
- Myocarditis
- Left ventricular aneurysms
- Idiopathic hypertrophic subaortic stenosis
- Hypothermia
- Paced rhythms
- Left bundle branch block

May have ST-segment depressions in the absence of ischemia
- Hypokalemia
- Digoxin effect
- Cor pulmonale and right heart strain
- Early repolarization
- Left ventricular hypertrophy
- Paced rhythms
- Left bundle branch block

May have T-wave inversions in the absence of ischemia
- Persistent juvenile pattern
- Stokes-Adams syncope or seizures
- Post-tachycardia T-wave inversion
- Post-pacemaker T-wave inversion
- Intracranial pathology (CNS bleeds)
- Mitral valve prolapse
- Pericarditis
- Primary or secondary myocardial diseases
- Pulmonary embolism or cor pulmonale from other causes
- Spontaneous pneumothorax
- Myocardial contusion
- Left ventricular hypertrophy
- Paced rhythms
- Left bundle branch block

TABLE 47-7 Characteristics of Cardiac Markers

Marker	Molecular Mass (kDa)	Elevation	Peak	Duration
Myoglobin	17,800	1–4 h	6 h	24 h
Myosin light chains	25,000	6–12 h	2–4 days	6–12 days
Cardiac troponin I	23,500	3–12 h	18 h	5–10 days
Cardiac troponin T	33,000	3–12 h	12 h	5–14 days
CK-MB	86,000	3–12 h	18–24 h	2 days
MB subforms	86,000	3–12 h	18 h	2 days
LDH	135,000	10 h	1–2 days	10–14 days
Glycogen phosphorylase BB	188,000	2–4 h	8 h	1–2 days
Myosin heavy chain	400,000	48 h	5–6 days	14 days

Source: Adams et al,[14] with permission.

complex in a predominantly positive QRS complex was highly specific for AMI. The QRS complex is predominantly negative in leads V_1 to V_3. ST-segment depression in these leads had 80 percent specificity for AMI.[9]

Markers of Myocardial Injury

A detailed discussion on the physiology and value of myocardial markers can be found in Chap. 45. Only contextual material is presented here.

The utility of cardiac markers (Table 47-7) depends upon their ability to detect and risk-stratify patients with acute coronary syndromes. Markers vary in terms of their molecular weight, cellular localization, solubility, plasma concentration, clearance, and ability to be accurately detected in serum with rapid immunochemical techniques (see Chap. 45).

CK-MB is the ''gold standard'' and most commonly used marker for the diagnosis of AMI. In the setting of AMI, CK-MB levels rise to twice normal at 6 h and peak within approximately 24 h. Serial CK-MB measurement has a sensitivity of over 90 percent 3 h after ED presentation (approximately 5 to 6 h after symptom onset); it is only 50 percent sensitive when utilized at or shortly after presentation.[10–12] Patients with skeletal muscle disease, acute muscle exertion, chronic renal failure, and cocaine use often have elevated levels of CK-MB in the absence of infarction.

$CK\text{-}MB_2$ is the subform that is released from the myocardium. Following release, it is cleaved by lysine carboxypeptidase, producing a more negatively charged molecule, $CK\text{-}MB_1$. Normally both subforms are in equilibrium. When $CK\text{-}MB_2$ is greater than 1.0 U/L or the MB_2:MB_1 ratio is >1.5, the sensitivity and specificity for the diagnosis of AMI is improved. When serial sampling every 30–60 min is used, CK-MB subforms have a sensitivity for detection of AMI of 96 percent and a specificity of 93 to 96 percent within 6 h of ED arrival. Less frequent sampling has resulted in less impressive results.[13] The value of CK-MB subforms for the risk stratification of patients with acute coronary syndromes is unknown. The main advantage of CK-MB subform analysis is that it can identify patients with AMI earlier than CK-MB.

The troponin complex is the main regulatory protein of the thin filament of the myofibrils that regulate the Ca^{2+}-dependent ATP hydrolysis of actomyosin. The troponin complex consists of three subunits: an inhibitory subunit (troponin I), a tropomyosin binding subunit (troponin T), and a calcium-binding subunit (troponin C). Because each subunit has cardiac, slow-twitch, and fast-twitch skeletal isoforms, immunoassays based upon the significant heterogeneity in amino acid sequences can detect the specific isoforms. The cardiac isoform of troponin I is not found in skeletal muscle during any stage of development. As a result, elevations of cardiac troponin I do not occur in the setting of acute or chronic skeletal muscle damage unless concurrent myocardial necrosis is present.

Following AMI, cardiac troponin I becomes elevated after approximately 6 h, peaks at 12 h, and remains elevated for 7 to 10 days. Troponin I has a higher specificity for myocardial necrosis than CK-MB in selected subsets of patients with acute coronary syndromes such as those with recent surgery, cocaine use, chronic renal failure, and skeletal muscle disease.[14] In ED patients with symptoms of acute coronary syndromes, cardiac troponin I has been shown to have similar sensitivity and specificity for detection of acute myocardial infarction as CK-MB.[15–17] In patients with acute coronary syndromes, elevations in cardiac troponin I values predict cardiovascular complications independent of CK-MB and the ECG.[16,17] The cardiac specificity of troponin I is clearly an advantage, especially when CK-MB elevations are suspected to be false.

The cytosolic component of cardiac troponin T is released from the cell within 2 to 6 h following symptom onset. Its diagnostic sensitivity for AMI approaches 100 percent 10 h after symptom onset and it remains elevated for 7 to 10 days after injury. This extended period of elevation results from disintegration of the contractile apparatus and the continued release of cardiac troponin T. It is not as specific for myocardial injury as cardiac troponin I. It may be elevated in patients with renal disease who do not have acute coronary syndromes. Cardiac troponin T is an independent marker of cardiovascular risk in patients with acute coronary syndromes.[16,18] Risk can be further stratified when cardiac troponin T is combined with the ECG and CK-MB. However, the lower specificity of troponin T compared with cardiac troponin I is a disadvantage.

Myoglobin has a lower molecular weight and is released more rapidly than CK-MB during AMI. As a result, serum myoglobin levels rise faster than CK-MB, reaching twice normal values within 2 h and peaking within 4 h of AMI symptom onset. The sensitivity of older assays was poor. The newer monoclonal immunoassay techniques demonstrate higher sensitivity and specificity of myoglobin for AMI than older assays in patients presenting within 3 h of symptom onset. Serial quantitative testing with an immunochemical assay for myoglobin has 91 percent sensitivity and up to a 99 percent negative predictive value for AMI within 1 h of ED presentation (approximately 3 to 4 h after symptom onset).[19] The advantage of myoglobin is early detection of patients with acute myocardial infarction. The disadvantage is that it has poor specificity for AMI in patients with concurrent trauma renal failure, rhabdomyolysis, and various hemolytic syndromes.

Evaluation of the myoglobin/carbonic anhydrase III ratio can enhance the specificity of myoglobin.[20] Carbonic anhydrase III is released from skeletal muscle in a fixed ratio with myoglobin. Combined assays can therefore help determine whether myoglobin is of skeletal or cardiac origin. With use of these dual assays, the high early sensitivity of myoglobin is maintained and specificity is improved. These assays are not yet commercially available. The use of dual assays for risk stratification has not yet been evaluated.

Other cardiac markers, such as glycogen phosphorylase BB and myosin light chains, are currently being evaluated. In addition, markers of platelet activation such as P-selectin and other integrins are theoretically attractive as indicators of acute coronary syndrome. They might detect platelet activation prior to myocardial injury. Their role in the diagnosis and triage of patients with acute coronary syndromes remains to be determined.

Cardiac Imaging

The use of echocardiography and nuclear imaging for risk stratification of chest pain patients was discussed in Chap. 45. Echocardiography can identify myocardial wall motion abnormalities. It has sensitivity for detection of AMI of approximately 93 percent but a specificity of only 53 to 57 percent.[4] Despite the high sensitivity, it cannot distinguish old from new infarcts. As a result, it is more useful in patients without prior coronary artery disease. Larger areas of infarction and more depressed left ventricular function predict a higher likelihood of cardiovascular complications and increased mortality.[21] Early echocardiography can be used for risk stratification and should be considered to help determine the need for transfer from smaller community to larger tertiary-care hospitals.

Sestamibi imaging may be useful for ED risk stratification of patients experiencing chest pain at the time of study. Technetium sestamibi is a radioisotope that is taken up by the myocardium in proportion to myocardial blood flow. It has prolonged retention in the myocardium and redistributes minimally after injection. This allows injection during symptomatic episodes but enables imaging after patient stabilization. This imaging modality is highly sensitive and specific for coronary artery disease. Sestamibi has higher independent predictive value in detecting acute coronary syndromes than the clinical history or ECG.[22] In one study, an abnormal sestamibi scan in the ED during pain predicted a 50-fold relative risk of AMI, 15-fold risk of revascularization, and 30-fold increased risk of death at 1 year. Disadvantages of sestamibi scanning include the need for 24 h availability of nuclear radiology technicians and time needed to prepare the isotope.

Exercise stress testing has become commonplace in EDs with chest pain observation units. Exercise treadmill testing with or without nuclear imaging, as well as stress echocardiography, can assist in cardiovascular risk stratification in the ED. Current studies demonstrate that patients with an uneventful observation period, negative cardiac markers, and a normal stress test can be safely discharged with a referral for follow-up in 24–48 hours. Stress testing is usually used on patients at very low risk for acute coronary syndromes or patients who have been "ruled out" for AMI. It is not routinely used for patients with acute coronary syndromes while in the ED. Further details on various forms of stress testing can be found in Chap. 45.

COMPLICATIONS OF MYOCARDIAL INFARCTION AND ISCHEMIA

Myocardial perfusion and cardiac function affect blood flow to the entire body. As a result, any end organ can be damaged when cardiac pump function is decreased. In this section, discussion of the complications of acute coronary syndromes is limited to the direct effects on the heart. The systemic effects of cardiac function are discussed in organ-appropriate chapters of this book. The treatment of these complications is discussed in the following chapter.

TABLE 47-8 Frequency of Occurrence of Dysrhythmias during Acute Myocardial Infarction

Dysrhythmia	Frequency of Occurrence
Bradydysrhythmias	
Sinus bradycardia	15–40%
First-degree AV block	4–14%
Second-degree AV block—type I	4–10%
Second-degree AV block—type II	<1%
Third-degree AV block	5–8%
Asystole	1–14%
Tachydysrhythmias	
Sinus tachycardia	33%
Atrial premature contractions	50%
Supraventricular tachycardia	2–11%
Atrial fibrillation	10–15%
Atrial flutter	1–3%
Ventricular premature beats	>90%
Accelerated idioventricular rhythm	8–20%
Ventricular tachycardia	10–40%
Ventricular fibrillation	4–18%

Source: Pasternak et al,[23] with permission.

Dysrhythmias

The genesis, diagnosis, and treatment of dysrhythmias are presented in Chap. 24. The effect dysrhythmias have in complicating the course of patients with acute coronary syndromes is the subject of this section.

Dysrhythmias occur in 72 to 100 percent of AMI patients treated in the coronary care unit. Table 47-8 shows the approximate frequency of the various dysrhythmias observed in patients with AMI. Many of these dysrhythmias occur in the prehospital and ED setting. The main consequence of these dysrhythmias is that they may impair hemodynamic performance, compromise myocardial viability by increasing myocardial oxygen requirements, and predispose to even more serious rhythm disturbances by diminishing the ventricular fibrillation threshold.

Early in the course of AMI, patients frequently exhibit evidence of increased autonomic nervous system activity. Sinus bradycardia, atrioventricular block, and hypotension may occur from increased vagal tone. Activation of atrial and ventricular receptors in the myocardium may result in enhanced efferent sympathetic activity, increased circulating catecholamines, and increased local catecholamine release. These increased catecholamines in the setting of a sensitive myocardium form the substrate for the generation of tachyarrhythmias. Electrical instability during acute myocardial infarction results in ventricular premature beats, ventricular tachycardia, ventricular fibrillation, accelerated idioventricular rhythms, and some AV junctional tachycardias.

The hemodynamic consequences of dysrhythmias are dependent on ventricular function. Patients with left ventricular dysfunction have a relatively fixed stroke volume. They depend upon changes in heart rate to alter cardiac output. The range of heart rate that is optimal becomes narrowed with increasing dysfunction. Slower or faster heart rates may further depress cardiac output.

Additionally, maintenance of the atrial kick is important for patients with AMI. Patients with normal hearts have a loss of 15 to 20 percent of left ventricular output when the atrial kick is eliminated. Patients with reduced left ventricular compliance, as occurs from AMI, have a 35 percent reduction in stroke volume when the atrial systole is eliminated.

''Pump'' failure with resultant increased sympathetic stimulation results in sinus tachycardia, atrial fibrillation/flutter, and supraventricular tachycardias. Conduction disturbances result in bradydysrhythmias such as sinus bradycardia, junctional escape rhythms, and atrioventricular and idioventricular blocks.

The significance of cardiac dysrhythmias during acute myocardial infarction is the subject of some debate. Sinus bradycardia during the early phases of AMI may predispose to hypotension and repetitive ventricular dysrhythmias. On the other hand, it appears to be protective because it reduces the myocardial oxygen requirement. The net effect is that the presence of sinus bradycardia does not appear to increase mortality during AMI.

Almost all patients with first-degree AV block have infranodal disturbances above the His bundle and will not progress to higher degrees of AV block. Mobitz I (Wenckebach) accounts for 90 percent of second-degree AV block. It generally occurs within the AV node, is associated with narrow QRS complexes, and results from ischemic injury. It is more common with inferior than anterior AMI, is intermittent usually during the first 72 h after infarction, and rarely progresses to complete heart block or other pathologic rhythm. Conversely, Mobitz 2 second-degree heart block originates from conduction lesions below the His bundle, is associated with a wide QRS complex, is usually associated with anterior AMI, and does progress to complete heart block.

Complete heart block can occur in patients with both anterior and inferior AMI. This is because the atrioventricular conduction system receives blood supply from both the AV branch of the right coronary artery and the septal perforating branch of the left anterior descending coronary artery. Complete heart block occurs in the setting of inferior myocardial infarction; it usually progresses from lesser forms of AV block. This form of third degree block is usually stable and should resolve. In the absence of right ventricular involvement, the mortality is approximately 15 percent. It rises to greater than 30 percent when right ventricular involvement is present. In contrast, complete heart block in the setting of an anterior MI is seldom benign and portends a grave prognosis. Junctional rhythms are usually transient and occur within 48 h of infarction. Whether they affect long-term prognosis is not clear.

Sinus tachycardia is quite prominent in patients with anterior wall AMI. Because of increased myocardial oxygen utilization, persistent sinus tachycardia is associated with a poor prognosis. The etiology of the sinus tachycardia should be determined. It may include anxiety, pain, left ventricular failure, fever, pericarditis, hypovolemia, atrial infarction, pulmonary emboli, or use of medications that accelerate heart rate. Similarly, paroxysmal supraventricular tachycardia, atrial fibrillation, and atrial flutter are associated with an increased mortality. Atrial premature contractions are common. They occur in up to 50 percent of AMI patients, and are not associated with an increased mortality related to the acute event.

Ventricular premature contractions are common in patients with AMI. They do not appear to have much prognostic ability. Accelerated idioventricular rhythms in patients with AMI have not been shown to have an effect on prognosis. Ventricular tachycardia shortly after AMI is often transient and does not portend a poor prognosis. When ventricular tachycardia occurs late in the course of AMI, it is usually associated with transmural Q-wave infarction and left ventricular dysfunction, induces hemodynamic deterioration, and is associated with a mortality rate approaching 50 percent. Primary ventricular fibrillation, occurring shortly after symptom onset does not appear to have a large effect on mortality and prognosis. Delayed or secondary ventricular fibrillation during hospitalization is associated with severe ventricular dysfunction and a 75 percent in-hospital mortality.

Intraventricular conduction disturbances occur in 10 to 20 percent of patients with AMI. Approximately half of these disturbances are already present at the time of ED presentation and may not represent a new finding. Blood supply to the left anterior division comes from septal perforators of the left anterior descending coronary artery. Both the right bundle branch and the left posterior division obtain a dual blood flow from both the left anterior descending and right coronary arteries. For this reason, left anterior hemiblock is more common.

TABLE 47-9 Forrester-Diamond-Swan Hemodynamic Classification

Class	Cardiac Index, L/min per m^2	Pulmonary Artery Wedge Pressure, mmHg	Approximate Mortality
I. No pulmonary congestion or hypoperfusion	>2	<18	2–3%
II. Isolated pulmonary congestion	>2	>18	10%
III. Isolated peripheral hypoperfusion	<2	<18	20–25%
IV. Both pulmonary congestion and peripheral hypoperfusion	<2	>18	50–55%

New right bundle branch block occur in approximately 2 percent of AMI patients, most commonly anteroseptal AMI, and is associated with an increased mortality because it often leads to complete AV block. New left bundle branch block occurs in 5 percent of patients with AMI and is associated with a high mortality. The left posterior fascicle is larger than the left anterior fascicle. Thus, left posterior hemiblock is associated with a higher mortality than isolated left anterior hemiblock because it represents a larger area of infarction. Bifascicular block (right bundle branch block and a left hemiblock) is associated with an increased likelihood of progression to complete heart block; it represents a large infarction and is associated with an increased likelihood of pump failure and mortality. Other combinations of heart block and their treatment are discussed in Chap. 48.

Cardiac Failure

Some 15 to 20 percent of patients with AMI present in some degree of congestive heart failure. One-third of these patients have circulatory shock. In the setting of AMI, congestive heart failure can occur through either diastolic dysfunction alone or a combination of systolic and diastolic dysfunction. Left ventricular diastolic dysfunction leads to pulmonary congestion. Systolic dysfunction is responsible for decreased forward flow, reduced cardiac output, and reduced ejection fraction. In general, the more severe the degree of left ventricular dysfunction, the higher the mortality. The degree of left ventricular dysfunction in any single patient is dependent upon the net effect of prior myocardial dysfunction (prior AMI), baseline myocardial hypertrophy, acute myocardial necrosis, and acute reversible myocardial dysfunction (''stunned myocardium'').

Patients with AMI can be classified into four subsets based upon hemodynamic status (Forrester-Diamond classification) and clinical status (Killip classification), shown in Tables 47-9 and 47-10. These classifications are useful to guide therapy and predict response to treatment. Patients with decreasing cardiac outputs or increasing pulmonary congestion have an increasingly higher mortality in the setting of AMI. Class I patients have a mortality of 2 to 5 percent. Class IV patients, (i.e., those with cardiogenic shock), are at very high risk of mortality (50 to 80 percent).

TABLE 47-10 Killip Clinical Classification

Class	Approximate Mortality
I. No congestive heart failure	5%
II. Mild congestive heart failure (bibasilar rales and an S_3)	15–20%
III. Frank pulmonary edema	40%
IV. Cardiogenic shock	80%

The presence of shock in AMI results in a complex spiral relationship. Coronary obstruction leads to myocardial ischemia, which, in turn, impairs myocardial contractility and ventricular outflow. The resulting reduction in arterial blood pressure leads to further decreases in coronary arterial perfusion, resulting in worsening myocardial ischemia and more severe myocardial necrosis. Interruption of this downward spiral requires careful attention to fluid management, preload, afterload, and the Frank-Starling relationships. Resolution of ischemia and preventing or minimizing the area of stunned myocardum that progresses to infarction is imperative.

Mechanical Complications of AMI

Sudden decompensation of previously stable patients should always raise concern of the ''mechanical'' complications of AMI. As a group, these complications usually involve the tearing or rupture of infarcted tissue. Therefore, they are unlikely to occur in patients with non-AMI acute coronary syndromes. The clinical presentation of these entities depends upon the site of rupture (papillary muscles, interventricular septum, or ventricular free wall).

Free wall rupture occurs in 10 percent of AMI fatalities, usually 1 to 5 days after infarction. Rupture of the left ventricular free wall usually leads to pericardial tamponade and death (in more than 90 percent). Patients may complain of tearing pain or sudden onset of severe pain. They will be hypotensive and tachycardic and may have onset of confusion and agitation. Increased neck veins, decreased heart sounds, and pulsus paradoxus may be present. Echocardiography is the diagnostic test of choice, although near equalization of right atrial, right ventricular middiastolic, and right ventricular systolic pressures on pulmonary artery catheterization may also be useful. Treatment is surgical.

Rupture has been attributed to intense necrosis at the distal end of blood supply along with poor collateral blood flow and a thin apical left ventricular wall in conjunction with the shearing effects of muscle contraction. Anti-inflammatory medications, steroids, and late administration of thrombolytic agents have all been linked to an increased likelihood of cardiac rupture. However, studies remain contradictory. The elderly appear to be more prone to cardiac rupture. Left ventricular hypertrophy appears to be protective.

Rupture of the interventricular septum is more often detected clinically than rupture of the ventricular free wall, despite the fact that rupture of the ventricular free wall is more commonly detected in autopsy studies. The size of the defect determines the degree of left-to-right shunt and the ultimate prognosis. Clinically, interventricular septal rupture presents with chest pain, dyspnea, and sudden appearance of a new holosystolic murmur. The murmur is usually accompanied by a palpable thrill and is heard best at the lower left sternal border. Doppler echocardiography is the diagnostic procedure of choice. Demonstration of left-to-right shunt by pulmonary catheter blood sampling may be useful. An oxygen step up of more than 10 percent from right atrial to right ventricular samples is diagnostic. Rupture of the interventricular septum is more common in patients with anterior wall myocardial infarction and patients with extensive (three vessel) coronary artery disease.

Papillary muscle rupture occurs in approximately 1 percent of patients with AMI, is more common with inferior myocardial infarction, and usually occurs 3 to 5 days after AMI. In contrast to rupture of the interventricular septum, papillary muscle rupture often occurs with a small to modest-sized AMI. Patients may have relatively limited coronary artery disease. Patients present with acute onset of dyspnea, increasing degree of congestive heart failure, and a new holosystolic murmur consistent with mitral regurgitation. The posteromedial papillary muscle is most commonly ruptured because it receives blood supply from only a single coronary artery, usually the right coronary artery. Echocardiography can often distinguish rupture of a portion of the papillary muscle from other etiologies of mitral regurgitation. Treatment is surgical.

Pericarditis

Post-AMI pericarditis occurs in 10 to 20 percent of patients. It is more common in patients with transmural AMI. It results from inflammation adjacent to the pericardium on the epicardial surface of a transmural infarction. It generally occurs 2 to 4 days after AMI. Pericardial friction rubs are more often detected with inferior wall and right ventricular infarction because the right ventricle lies immediately beneath the chest wall. The pain of pericarditis can be confused with that of infarct extension or post-AMI angina. Classically the discomfort of pericarditis becomes worse with a deep inspiration and may be somewhat relieved by sitting forward. Echocardiography may demonstrate a pericardial effusion, but pericardial effusions are much more common than pericarditis and are often present in the absence of pericarditis. Similarly, pericarditis can be present in the absence of a pericardial effusion. The resorption rate of post-AMI pericardial effusions are slow, often taking several months. Dressler syndrome (post-AMI syndrome) occurs 2 to 10 weeks after AMI and presents as chest pain, fever, and pleuropericarditis.

Right Ventricular Infarction

Isolated right ventricular infarction is extremely rare and it is usually seen as a complication or other infarction. The right ventricle most commonly receives its blood supply from the right coronary artery. In patients with left dominant systems, the blood supply may come from the left circumflex. The anterior portion of the right ventricle is supplied by branches of the left anterior diagonal artery. Approximately 30 percent of inferior wall myocardial infarctions involve the right ventricle. The presence of right ventricular infarction is associated with a significant increase in mortality and cardiovascular complications. Right ventricular infarction can be diagnosed by the presence of ST-segment elevation in the right precordial lead V_4 (rV_4), in the setting of an inferior wall myocardial infarction. The presence of elevated neck veins or hypotension in response to nitroglycerin is also suggestive. Echocardiography or nuclear imaging can be diagnostic, but they are less readily available in the ED.

The most serious complication of right ventricular infarction is shock.[24] The severity of the hemodynamic derangement in the setting of right ventricular infarction is related to the extent of right ventricular dysfunction, the interaction between the ventricles (the right and left ventricle share the interventricular septum), and the interaction between the pericardium and the right ventricle. Right ventricular infarction results in a reduction in right ventricular end-systolic pressure, left ventricular end-diastolic size, cardiac output, and aortic pressure as the right ventricle becomes more of a passive conduit to blood flow. Left ventricular contraction causes bulging of the interventricular septum into the right ventricle, with resultant ejection of blood into the pulmonary circulation. As a result, right ventricular infarction with concurrent left ventricular infarction has a particularly devastating effect on hemodynamic function. Fluid balance and maintenance of adequate preload is critical in the treatment of right ventricular infarction. Treatment of right ventricular infarction is discussed in Chap. 48.

Other Complications

Other complications of AMI that occur but are not usually seen in the ED include left ventricular thombus formation, arterial embolization, venous thrombosis, pulmonary embolism, postinfarction angina, and infarct extension. With the more rapid discharge of uncomplicated AMI patients, the emergency physician should keep these possibilities in mind for patients who return to the ED shortly after hospital discharge.

SPECIFIC ISSUES

Age and Gender

Age and gender play a role in the presentation of patients with acute coronary syndromes. Both increased age and female gender are associated with more atypical presentations. There is no evidence that AMI patients should be evaluated differently in the ED as a result of age or gender.

Postprocedure Chest Pain

Patients who present with symptoms of an acute coronary syndrome shortly after percutaneous coronary interventions such as angioplasty or stent placement should be assumed to have had abrupt vessel closure until proven otherwise. Subacute thrombotic occlusion following stent placement occurs in approximately 4 percent of patients 2 to 14 days postprocedure. Although less common than closure following percutaneous transluminal coronary angioplasty (PTCA), it is associated with a high likelihood of major ischemic complications. Patients should be treated aggressively for an acute coronary syndrome, and cardiology or interventional cardiology consultation should be obtained. Patients with chest pain syndromes following coronary artery bypass grafting may also have abrupt vessel closure; however, symptoms of recurrent ischemia must be distinguished from post-AMI pericarditis or Dressler syndrome, as discussed above.

Cocaine Use

Myocardial ischemia and infarction can occur secondary to cocaine insufflation, smoking, intravenous use, and possibly withdrawal. Serum levels or route of administration does not play a role in the likelihood of developing ischemia.

Patients with cocaine-associated acute coronary syndromes frequently have atypical chest pain or chest pain delayed for hours to days after their most recent use of cocaine. AMI can occur after use of only small amounts of cocaine. Approximately 6 percent of patients with cocaine associated chest pain syndromes sustain AMI.[25] An additional 20 to 60 percent suffer from transient myocardial ischemia. Most infarctions occur within 24 h of cocaine use; however, reports of cocaine use leading to AMI several weeks after last use exist.

Cocaine causes myocardial ischemia through a complex pathophysiology resulting from its acute and chronic effects.[24] Acutely, cocaine results in coronary artery vasoconstriction, tachycardia, systemic arterial hypertension, increased myocardial oxygen demand, platelet aggregation, and in situ thrombus formation. Chronic cocaine users develop accelerated atherosclerosis and left ventricular hypertrophy, which can further exacerbate the O_2 supply–demand mismatch. Myocardial ischemia and infarction have occurred in patients without any underlying atherosclerotic disease or other evidence of preexisting heart disease. Q-wave and non-Q-wave infarctions occurred with equal frequency. Although cocaine can cause myocardial ischemia in patients without coronary artery disease, the majority of patients with cocaine-associated AMI have atherosclerotic coronary artery disease. Patients with cocaine-associated myocardial infarction should receive an evaluation for underlying coronary artery disease.

Risk stratification of patients with cocaine-associated acute coronary syndromes has been difficult. Clinical criteria have not been useful. ECGs reveal abnormalities consisting of ST-segment elevation and T-wave inversions that often persist during hospitalization; however, the ECG is less sensitive and less specific for myocardial infarction in patients who have recently used cocaine. CK-MB assays have diminished specificity for AMI in cocaine users. Cardiac troponin I appears to be more useful. On the other hand, risk stratification of patients with cocaine-associated acute coronary syndromes may be less important, since even patients with cocaine-associated myocardial infarction have a favorable short-term prognosis. The 1-year mortality in patients with cocaine-associated acute coronary syndromes is largely related to comorbid conditions and continued cocaine use.

DISPOSITION

All patients with acute chest pain syndromes need to be evaluated for the possibility of acute coronary syndromes. Based upon the initial history, physical examination, and ECG, patients can be subdivided into those with and without known coronary artery disease. Patients with known coronary artery disease should be further subdivided into those who meet criteria for AMI (and may or may not meet criteria for reperfusion therapy), those with a stable anginal pattern that do not require acute intervention, and those with unstable angina. Patients with unstable angina should be treated according to their risk for acute myocardial infarction and death (Table 47-1).

Patients without known coronary artery disease who do not have an obvious myocardial infarction should be evaluated for their likelihood of coronary artery disease (Table 47-11) and the possibility of an alternative diagnosis (not ischemic heart disease). Those with a clear alternative diagnosis should be treated accordingly.

Patients at high risk of coronary artery disease, AMI, or death should be admitted to an intensive care unit (ICU). Moderate risk patients should be admitted to a non-ICU monitored setting. Patients at low risk can be treated in a non-ICU monitored setting or can be observed in an ED observation unit. Both ED observation units and non-ICU monitored settings are safe and cost-effective for patients with normal ECGs and other low-risk clinical features. Prior invasive and noninvasive assessments of cardiac function should be taken into account in making disposition decisions. Patients known to have severe coronary artery disease or depressed left ventricular function might be triaged to a more intensive setting than patients with a similar presentation without such dysfunction.

Results of prior cardiac catheterization are very useful for risk stratification. Patients who have previously been documented to have minimal (less than 25 percent) stenosis or normal coronary arteriograms have an excellent long-term prognosis. More than 98 percent of patients with this profile are free from myocardial infarction 10 years later.[26] Repeat cardiac catheterizations an average of 9 years later found that approximately 90 percent of patients did not develop even single-vessel coronary artery disease. Thus, a recent (in the past 2 years) cardiac catheterization with normal or minimally diseased vessels almost eliminates the possibility of an acute coronary syndrome, due to atherosclerosis. It would not eliminate the possibility of vasospasm. Without other complicating circumstances, even observation protocols are unnecessary.

Stress tests are less useful because the precise results of such tests may not be available. When patients complete all stages of the emergency protocol, have no ECG changes, and have normal imaging studies, exercise testing can rule out acute ischemic syndromes with sensitivities in the range of 80 to 90 percent. When patients do not meet their target heart rates, exercise testing has poor sensitivity (less

TABLE 47-11 Likelihood of Significant Coronary Artery Disease in Patients with Symptoms Suggesting Unstable Angina

High Likelihood—85–99%—Any of the Following Features:	Intermediate Likelihood—15–84%—Absence of High Likelihood Features and Any of the Following:	Low Likelihood—1–14%—Absence of High or Intermediate Likelihood Features But May Have Any of the Following:
History of prior AMI or sudden death or other known history of CAD	Definite angina: males <60 or females <70 years of age	Chest pain classified as probably not angina
Definite angina: males ≥60 or females ≥70 years of age	Probable angina: males ≥60 or females ≥70 years of age	One risk factor other than diabetes
Transient hemodynamic or ECG changes during pain	Chest pain probably not angina in patients with diabetes	T-wave flattening or inversion <1 mm in leads with dominant R waves
Variant angina (pain with reversible ST-segment elevation)	Chest pain probably not angina and two or three risk factors other than diabetes	Normal ECG
ST-segment elevation or depression ≥1 mm	Extracardiac vascular disease	
Marked symmetrical T-wave inversion in multiple precordial leads	ST-segment depression 0.05–1 mm	
	T-wave inversion ≥1 mm in leads with dominant R waves	

Key: AMI, acute myocardial infarction; CAD, coronary artery disease; ECG, electrocardiogram.
Source: Braunwald et al.[1]

than 80 percent) leading to false-negative results. Unless the patient reached the maximal heart rate (220 beats per minute minus the patient's age), had no ECG changes, and had normal imaging (when done), one cannot rely heavily on the results of prior exercise testing in making disposition decisions. However, a negative maximal exercise stress predicts a favorable 1-year survival free of cardiac events.

REFERENCES

1. Braunwald E, Mark DB, Jones RH, et al: *Unstable Angina: Diagnosis and Management.* Clinical Practice Guideline No. 10 (amended). AHCPR Publication No. 94-0602. Rockville, MD: Agency for Health Care Policy and Research and the National Health, Lung and Blood Institute, Public Health Service, U.S. Department of Health and Human Services, 1994.
2. Jayes RL, Beshansky JR, D'Agostino RB, Selker HP: Do patients' coronary risk factor reports predict acute cardiac ischemia in the emergency department? A multicenter study. *J Clin Epidemiol* 45:621, 1992.
3. Lee T, Cook F, Weisberg M, et al: Acute chest pain in the emergency room: identification and examination of low risk patients. *Arch Intern Med* 145:65, 1985.
4. Selker HP, Zalenski RJ, Antman EM, et al: An evaluation of technologies for identification of acute cardiac ischemia in the emergency department: A report from a National Heart Attack Alert Program Working Group. *Ann Emerg Med* 29:13, 1997.
5. Slater DK, Hlatky MA, Mark DB, et al: Outcome in suspected acute myocardial infarction with normal or minimally abnormal admission electrocardiographic findings. *Am J Cardiol* 60:766, 1987.
6. Brush JE, Brand DA, Acampora D, et al: Use of the initial electrocardiogram to predict in-hospital complications of acute myocardial infarction. *N Engl J Med* 312:1137, 1985.
7. Zalenski RJ, Cooke D, Rydman R, et al: Assessing the diagnostic value of an ECG containing leads V4R, V8 and V9: The 15 lead ECG. *Ann Emerg Med* 22:786, 1993.
8. Sgarbossa EB, Pinski SL, Barbagelata A, et al: Electrocardiographic diagnosis of evolving acute myocardial infarction in the presence of left bundle branch block. *N Engl J Med* 334:481, 1996.
9. Sgarbossa EB, Pinski SL, Gates KB, Wagner GS, for GUSTO-1 Investigators. Early electrocardiographic diagnosis of acute myocardial infarction in the presence of ventricular paced rhythm. *Am J Cardiol* 77:423, 1996.
10. Gibler WB, Lewis LM, Erb RE, et al: Early detection of acute myocardial infarction in patients presenting with chest pain and nondiagnostic ECGs: Serial CK-MB sampling in the emergency department. *Ann Emerg Med* 19:1359, 1990.
11. Hedges JR, Young GP, Henkel GF, et al: Early CK-MB elevations predict ischemic events in stable chest pain patients. *Acad Emerg Med* 1:9–16, 1994.
12. Hoekstra JW, Hedges JR, Gibler WB, et al: Emergency department CK-MB: A predictor of ischemic complications. *Acad Emerg Med* 1:17, 1994.
13. Puleo PR, Meyer D, Wathen C, et al: Use of a rapid assay of subforms of creatine kinase MB to diagnose or rule out acute myocardial infarction. *N Engl J Med* 331:561, 1994.
14. Adams JE III, Bodor GS, Davila-Roman VG, et al: Cardiac troponin I: A marker with high specificity for cardiac injury. *Circulation* 88:101, 1993.
15. Brogan GX, Hollander JE, McCuskey CF, et al: Evaluation of a new assay for cardiac troponin I versus CK-MB for the diagnosis of acute myocardial infarction. *Acad Emerg Med* 4:6, 1997.
16. Green GB, Li DJ, Bessman ES, Cox JL, et al: The prognostic significance of troponin I and troponin T. *Acad Emerg Med* 5:758, 1998.
17. Antman EM, Tanasijevic MJ, Thompson B, et al: Cardiac specific troponin I levels predict the risk of mortality in patients with acute coronary syndromes. *N Engl J Med* 335:1342, 1996.
18. Ohman EM, Armstrong PW, Christenson RH, et al: Cardiac troponin-T levels for risk stratification in acute myocardial ischemia. *N Engl J Med* 335:1333, 1996.
19. Brogan GX Jr, Friedman S, McCuskey C, et al: Evaluation of a new rapid quantitative immunoassay for serum myoglobin versus CK-MB for ruling out acute myocardial infarction in the emergency department. *Ann Emerg Med* 24:665, 1994.
20. Brogan GX, Vuori J, Freidman S, et al: Improved specificity of myoglobin plus carbonic anhydrase versus that of creatine kinase-MB for the early diagnosis of acute myocardial infarction. *Ann Emerg Med* 27:22, 1996.
21. Fleischmann KE, Lee TH, Come PC, et al: Echocardiographic prediction of complications in patients with chest pain. *Am J Cardiol* 79:292, 1997.
22. Tatum JL, Jesse RL, Kontos MC, et al: Comprehensive strategy for the evaluation and triage of the chest pain patient. *Ann Emerg Med* 29:116, 1997.
23. Pasternack RC, Braunwald E, Sobel BE: Acute myocardial infarction, in Braunwald E (ed): *Heart Disease: A Textbook of Cardiovascular Medicine,* 4th ed. Philadelphia, Saunders, 1992, pp 1239–1245.
24. Kinch JW, Ryan TJ: Right ventricular infarction. *N Engl J Med* 330:1211, 1994.
25. Hollander JE: Management of cocaine associated myocardial ischemia. *N Engl J Med* 333:1267, 1995.
26. Pitts WR, Lange RA, Cigarroa JE, Hillis LD: Repeat coronary angiography in patients with chest pain and previously normal coronary angiogram. *Am J Cardiol* 80:1086, 1997.

INTERVENTION STRATEGIES FOR ACUTE CORONARY SYNDROMES

Judd E. Hollander

Acute coronary care syndromes (ACS) can be inhibited or reversed with a wide variety of interventions. In this chapter, major therapeutic treatment trials are summarized. Where available, evidence-based consensus panel treatment recommendations are provided. Some dosage recommendations are intentionally not provided because ongoing clinical trials are likely to result in changed dosing strategies.

Treatment of ACS is individualized based on duration and persistence of symptoms, cardiac history, and findings on physical examination and initial electrocardiogram. Generally speaking, patients with persistent symptoms and ST-segment elevation should receive therapy or mechanical reperfusion (angioplasty). Treatment with heparin, β antagonists, nitrates, and angiotensin-converting enzyme inhibitors should be considered, based on symptoms, vital signs, and the presence or absence of heart failure. Patients with unstable angina or non-Q-wave infarctions without ST-segment elevation should be treated with aspirin and heparin, and possibly β antagonists and nitrates. Patients refractory to these therapies or patients scheduled to undergo percutaneous interventional procedures also benefit from the use of glycoprotein IIb/IIIa antagonists.

GENERAL MEASURES

Intravenous access and continued electrocardiographic monitoring should be established in all patients with ACS. Supplemental oxygen may reduce ST-segment elevation in patients with acute myocardial infarction. It is therefore reasonable to provide 2 to 4 L of oxygen routinely by nasal cannula, but higher doses can lead to arterial vasoconstriction and increased afterload. Treatment strategies are those that achieve immediate reperfusion and those that limit infarct size (Table 48-1).

TABLE 48-1 Recommended Doses of Drugs Used in the Treatment of Coronary Care Syndromes

Drug	Dose
Nitroglycerin (sl)	0.4 mg q5 min × 3
Nitroglycerin IV	Start at 10 μg/min, titrate to 10% reduction in mean arterial pressure (map) if normotensive, 80% reduction in map if hypertensive
Morphine	2–5 mg q 5–15 min
Aspirin	160 mg
Ticlopidine*	250 mg po bid
Metoprolol	5 mg IV over 2 min; repeat q5 min for total dose 15 mg; follow with 50 mg po q6h 15 min after last IV
Atenolol	5 mg IV over 5 min, repeat once 10 min later, follow with 50 mg po
Streptokinase	1.5 million U over 60 min
Alteplase (accelerated infusion)	*>67 kg:* 100 mg: 15 mg initial IV bolus, 50 mg infused over next 30 min, 35 mg infused over next 60 min *<67 kg:* 15 mg initial IV bolus, 0.75 mg/kg infused over next 30 min, 0.50 mg/kg infused over next 60 min Maximum dose 100 mg
Heparin† (unfractionated)	80-U/kg bolus, then 18-U/kg/h infusion, monitor PTT
Enoxaparin (LMWH)†	1 mg/kg q12h sq†

*Alternative for aspirin allergy.
†Need dose adjustment when used in conjunction with glycoprotein IIb/IIIa inhibitors.
Abbreviations: LMWH, low-molecular-weight heparin; PTT, partial thromboplastin time; sl, sublingual.

TABLE 48-2 Contraindications to Fibrinolytic Therapy in Acute Myocardial Infarction

Absolute contraindications
- Previous hemorrhagic stroke at any time
- Bland strokes or cardiovascular accident in past year
- Known intracranial neoplasm
- Active internal bleeding (excluding menses)
- Suspected aortic dissection
- Diabetic retinopathy

Relative contraindications
- Severe uncontrolled blood pressure (>180/100 mmHg)
- History of prior cerebrovascular accident or known intracranial pathology not covered in contraindications
- Current use of anticoagulants with international normalized ratio >2 to 3
- Known bleeding diathesis
- Recent trauma (past 2 weeks)
- Prolonged cardiopulmonary resuscitation > 10 min
- Major surgery < 3 weeks
- Noncompressible vascular punctures
- Recent internal bleeding (2–4 weeks)
- Prior allergic reaction to streptokinase (should not receive streptokinase)
- Pregnancy
- Active peptic ulcer disease
- History of chronic severe hypertension

REPERFUSION

Reperfusion therapies can be mechanical or pharmacologic. Angioplasty, coronary stent placement, and atherectomy are the major methods of mechanical reperfusion. Pharmacologic interventions include fibrinolytic and antiplatelet therapy.

Fibrinolytics

Fibrinolytic agents act on the acute coronary thrombosis directly or indirectly as plasminogen activators. Plasminogen, an inactive proteolytic enzyme, binds directly to fibrin during thrombus formation, forming a plasminogen-fibrin complex. This plasminogen-fibrin complex is more susceptible to activation than plasma plasminogen, and this promotes fibrin proteolysis.

Randomized controlled clinical trials comparing streptokinase to placebo for treatment of acute myocardial infarction demonstrated that fibrinolytic therapy improved left ventricular function and short-term and long-term mortality rate.[1–3] A meta-analysis of all nine clinical trials that randomized more than 1000 patients to fibrinolytic therapy or control treatments found that the net benefit of treatment in the first 3 h was more than 30 lives saved per thousand patients. The loss of benefit per hour delay in thrombolytic administration was 1.6 lives per 1000 patients per hour.

Fibrinolytic therapy is indicated for patients with symptoms compatible with acute myocardial infarction, a time to treatment of less than 6 to 12 h, and an electrocardiogram that has at least 1-mm ST-segment elevation in two or more contiguous leads.[4] Therapy is most beneficial if given early and is more beneficial for larger infarctions and anterior infarctions than it is for smaller or inferior wall infarctions.

In the elderly, the overall risk of mortality from acute myocardial infarction (AMI) is high with and without therapy. The proportionate reduction in mortality rate appears to be less in patients older than age 75, but the absolute number of patients who may be saved is still large.

Contraindications to thrombolytic therapy are those that increase the risk of hemorrhage (Table 48-2). The most catastrophic complication is intracranial bleeding. Clinical variables that can be assessed in the emergency department and predict an increased risk of intracranial hemorrhage are age (older than 65 years, odds ratio of 2.2), low body weight (less than 70 kg, odds ratio 2.1), and hypertension on presentation (odds ratio, 2.0).[4] Intracranial hemorrhage is also more common with tissue plasminogen activator (tPA) than with streptokinase (odds ratio, 1.6). Patients with relative contraindications may still receive fibrinolytic therapy when the benefits of therapy outweigh the risks of the complications, but institutions with direct percutaneous intervention availability might consider direct angioplasty over fibrinolytic therapy in the presence of relative contraindications. Reperfusion therapy with fibrinolysis is the standard of care for patients with ST-segment elevation AMI. However, this treatment has limitations. First, even the most potent fibrinolytic agents do not achieve early and complete restoration of coronary blood flow in 40 to 50 percent of patients. Fibrinolytics are plasminogen activators. When fibrin is lysed, thrombin is exposed. The exposed thrombin is one of the most potent biologic platelet activators known. As a result, the more fibrin that is lysed, the more thrombin is exposed and more prothrombotic substrate is engendered. The second limitation of fibrinolytic therapy is that approximately 1 percent of patients have intracranial hemorrhage, which usually results in death or disabling stroke.

Controversy continues to surround the choice of fibrinolytic agent. There have been three large trials comparing streptokinase to tPA and one large trial comparing reteplase to alteplase.

STREPTOKINASE Streptokinase is a polypeptide derived from β-hemolytic *Streptococcus* cultures. It binds 1:1 to plasminogen, causing a conformational change that activates the plasminogen-streptokinase complex. This complex cleaves peptide bonds on other plasminogen molecules to activate them. This activated complex does not have fibrin specificity.

Initial trials demonstrated a reduction in mortality rate and improvement in left ventricular function with streptokinase relative to placebo.[1–3] Other fibrinolytic agents have not been evaluated in large randomized placebo-controlled clinical trials.

Antibodies may develop after treatment, so retreatment should be avoided. Streptokinase allergy can be seen in approximately 5 percent of patients treated for the first time, especially those with a recent *Streptococcus* infection. Self-limited allergic reactions usually respond to antihistamines. Fewer than 0.2 percent of patients experience a serious anaphylactic reaction. During intravenous administration, approximately 15 percent of patients will experience hypotension, which usually responds to decreasing the rate of infusion and volume expansion. The 1998 recommended dose of streptokinase is 1.5 million units over 60 min, which produces a fibrinolytic state for up to 24 h. Streptokinase is less costly than other fibrinolytic agents.

TISSUE PLASMINOGEN ACTIVATOR tPA is a naturally occurring enzyme produced by the vascular endothelium and other tissues. It has a binding site for fibrin that allows it to attach to a formed thrombus and trigger fibrinolysis (fibrin specificity). Small trials (28 to 144 patients) compared infarct-related patency rates of tPA to placebo and found that tPA achieved higher patency rates than was seen with placebo or in trials of streptokinase. Three large randomized controlled clinical trials have compared streptokinase to tPA. Using the composite end point of stroke or death at 30 to 35 days, GISSI-2 (more than 20,000 patients) found that tPA resulted in an increased rate of stroke/death of 5 per 1000 patients relative to streptokinase.[5] ISIS-3 (27,000 patients) found a 1 per 1000 patient benefit in favor of tPA.[6] GUSTO-1 found a 5.4 per 1000 patient benefit in favor of tPA, which increased to 9 patients per 1000 when the accelerated tPA regimen was given.[7] As a result, most cardiologists recommend the use of the accelerated tPA regimen.

When these trials are taken together, these three megatrials found no statistical difference between streptokinase and tPA with respect to the composite end point of stroke and death. A meta-analysis of the data from these three trials found that tPA offered a nonstatistical benefit of 1.6 ± 1.9 per 1000 patients ($p = 0.4$). Using only death as the end point, tPA rather than streptokinase use results in a nonstatistical difference of 2.0 ± 1.9 lives saved per thousand patients ($p > 0.1$). Based on this analysis, the choice of which thrombolytic agent to use is probably less relevant than the speed of thrombolytic administration (which results in saving an additional 1.6 per 1000 lives per hour earlier that treatment is provided). In addition, it is probably better to choose streptokinase over tPA when the risk for intracranial hemorrhage is highest (elderly, etc.) since tPA has an increased likelihood of resulting in hemorrhagic stroke.[4]

The mechanism of improved benefit of tPA in the GUSTO angiographic substudy is early patency of the infarct-related vessel.[8] For tPA, streptokinase-subcutaneous heparin, streptokinase-intravenous heparin, and streptokinase-tPA, the patency rates at 90 min were 81, 56, 61, and 73 percent, respectively.[8] These patency rates were predictive of survival outcomes.

The accelerated regimen of tPA, as used in the GUSTO trial, is an initial bolus of 15 mg, followed by 0.75 mg/kg (up to 50 mg) in the first 30 min and 0.5 mg/kg (up to 35 mg) in the next hour.[7]

RETEPLASE rPA is a genetically engineered modification of tPA with a prolonged half-life (18 min vs 3 min) and reduced fibrin binding. GUSTO-3 compared rPA to tPA in 15,000 patients and found similar mortality and stroke rates between the two agents.[9] Smaller studies suggest that reteplase has a faster time to reperfusion. Reteplase can be given as a double bolus, 10 mg each, 30 min apart.

Other genetically engineered molecules are currently in the developmental stages, and results of clinical trials are not yet available. TNK-tPA is another tPA mutant with prolonged half-life, that is resistant to endogenous plasminogen activator inhibitor-1 (PIA-1) inactivation, and has high fibrin specificity and binding. In animal models, it produces more active and complete fibrinolysis with less risk of intracranial bleeding. Results of clinical trials are pending. n-PA is a deletion and point mutant of tPA that has a more extended half-life (30 to 45 min) with improved lytic activity in animal models and reduced fibrin affinity.

Mechanical Reperfusion

Coronary angioplasty is the most common percutaneous intervention. Alternatives include coronary stent placement, atherectomy, and laser angioplasty. Balloon angioplasty increases the size of the arterial lumen through endothelial denudation; cracking, splitting, and disruption of atherosclerotic plaque; dehiscence of intima and plaque from underlying media; and stretching or tearing of underlying media and adventitia.[10] With successful dilation, small amounts of arterial wall dissection and aneurysmal expansion may be seen. The greater the increase in luminal size, the lower is the risk of restenosis. On the other hand, more aggressive balloon inflation can be associated with excessive dissection, platelet deposition, thrombus formation, and plaque hemorrhage.[10]

Alternative percutaneous interventional procedures have been developed in an attempt to limit complications. Directional and rotational coronary atherectomy extract atherosclerotic tissue from the coronary artery. Excimer laser atherectomy vaporizes atheromatous tissue. Their use results in larger luminal diameters but has not reduced rates of restenosis or other complications associated with percutaneous angioplasty procedures.

Coronary stents are fenestrated stainless-steel tubes that are expanded by a balloon to provide scaffolding within the coronary arteries. The addition of antiplatelet therapies (in particular, glycoprotein IIb/IIIa inhibitors) has been associated with reduced rates of abrupt vessel closure and improved outcomes up to 3 years following the procedure.

Direct coronary angioplasty has compared favorably with fibrinolytic therapy for the treatment of patients with AMI. In centers with significant expertise in direct angioplasty, primary angioplasty reduces the cardiovascular complication rate in patients with AMI relative to fibrinolytic therapy. The PAMI trial compared the efficacy of intravenous tPA with immediate percutaneous coronary angioplasty (PTCA) in 395 patients with AMI. The in-hospital mortality rate in the tPA group was 6.5 percent and in the PTCA group was 2.6 percent. In-hospital reinfarction rates, 6-month rates of reinfarction or death, and rates of intracranial hemorrhage were all lower in the PTCA group.[11] In GUSTO IIb, 1138 patients who presented within 12 h of AMI were randomized to accelerated tPA or to primary angioplasty. The incidence of death, nonfatal reinfarction, and nonfatal disabling stroke was 33 percent lower in patients who received primary angioplasty.[12] A large study of patients presenting to community hospitals did not show a benefit of direct angioplasty over fibrinolysis.[13]

Primary angioplasty may offer benefits in highly specialized centers with ready availability of cardiac catheterization and skilled operators that are not apparent with longer delays or less skilled operators. The decision to use primary interventional procedures rather than fibrinolysis should be individualized based on the institutional expertise and availability and risk of complications from fibrinolysis.

Antiplatelet Agents

Platelets are at the core of coronary artery thrombosis.[14] Platelet activation and adhesion to subendothelial matrix elements occur as a result of plaque rupture. Platelet aggregation may be initiated by shearing forces, fibrinolytics, thrombin, thromboxane A_2, ADP, epinephrine, serotonin, or plasmin. These trigger the arachidonic acid pathway, the protein kinase C pathway, or other pathways that result in platelet aggregation. The final common pathway of platelet activation is exposure of glycoprotein IIb/IIIa receptors on the surface of the platelet. Bivalent fibrinogen molecules cross-link activated platelets together by using these receptors. The glycoprotein IIb/IIIa antagonists are considerably stronger antiplatelet agents than aspirin, because they interrupt platelet activation regardless of agonist. In contrast, aspirin only inhibits platelet aggregation stimulated through thromboxane A_2 and mediated through the arachidonic acid pathway.

GLYCOPROTEIN IIb/IIIa INHIBITORS Several different forms of glycoprotein IIb/IIIa antagonists are available. Abciximab (ReoPro) is a chimeric antibody that binds irreversibly to the glycoprotein IIb/IIIa antagonists. The duration of action is longer than that of the smaller peptide molecules. As a result, benefits may be realized with a shorter duration of infusion. Eptifibatide (Integrelin) is a synthetic heptapeptide that binds reversibly to the glycoprotein IIb/IIIa receptor. Lamifiban and tirofiban (Aggrastat) are synthetic small molecules with reversible binding to the glycoprotein IIb/IIIa receptor. All require a 48- to 72-h infusion to demonstrate sustained benefits. Reversal of platelet inhibition following cessation of infusion is more rapid with the polypeptide or small molecules, offering an advantage when bleeding complications occur.

The glycoprotein IIb/IIIa inhibitors have been evaluated for use in three clinical areas: percutaneous interventional procedures (PCI), in combination with low-dose fibrinolysis, and for medical stabilization of patients with ACS. In EPIC, 2099 high-risk patients receiving PTCA or atherectomy were randomized to abciximab bolus alone, abciximab bolus plus 12-h infusion, or placebo, in conjunction with aspirin and heparin.[15] Patients who received abciximab bolus plus infusion had a 35 percent reduction in the composite end point of death, AMI, or urgent reintervention. Some of this benefit was sustained for up to 3 years (13 percent reduction). Of note, the rate of bleeding was increased twofold in the patients treated with abciximab. The EPILOG trial randomized 2792 patients undergoing PCI to abciximab plus low-dose weight-adjusted heparin, abciximab plus standard-dose heparin, or placebo plus standard-dose heparin. This trial, using lower doses of heparin, retained the reduction in the risk of death, AMI, or urgent revascularization (56 percent at 30 days and 43 percent at 6 months), without an increased risk of bleeding complications.[16] As a result of these trials, glycoprotein IIb/IIIa inhibitors are often used in high-risk patients undergoing percutaneous interventions in the cardiac catheterization laboratory.

A variety of glycoprotein IIb/IIIa antagonists have been shown to be efficacious for patients with ACS. In the CAPTURE trial,[17] 1265 patients who had failed medical stabilization with heparin and nitroglycerin were randomized to abciximab or placebo bolus and infusion in addition to aspirin, standard-dose heparin, and intravenous nitroglycerin while waiting 24 h for percutaneous intervention. Medical therapy with abciximab resulted in a 71 percent decrease in AMI and 29 percent decrease in composite end point of death, AMI, or urgent reintervention. This reduction in adverse cardiovascular events occurred prior to the percutaneous intervention, suggesting a role for glycoprotein IIb/IIIa antagonists in medical stabilization of refractory unstable angina patients.

Four large trials (PURSUIT, PRISM, PRISM-PLUS, and PARAGON) evaluated glycoprotein IIb/IIIa antagonists for the medical stabilization of patients with unstable angina or non-Q-wave AMI.[18–21] In the PRISM study,[18] 3232 patients who were already receiving aspirin were randomized to additional treatment with intravenous tirofiban or heparin for 48 h. The composite end point (death, AMI, or refractory ischemia at 48 h) was 32 percent lower in the glycoprotein IIb/IIIa antagonist group. The reduction in mortality rate persisted to 30 days. In PRISM-PLUS,[19] 1915 patients were randomized to tirofiban, heparin, or both for 3 days. Patients treated with tirofiban and heparin had a reduction in the composite end point of death, AMI, or refractory ischemia at 7 days. Reduction in rates of death and AMI persisted for up to 6 months. Notably, in contrast to the PRISM results, patients who received tirofiban alone had an increased rate of adverse cardiovascular events. PURSUIT randomized 10,948 patients to bolus and infusion treatment with eptifibatide or placebo for up to 72 h.[20] The glycoprotein IIb/IIIa antagonist resulted in 1.5 percent absolute reduction (10 percent relative reduction) in death and nonfatal AMI that was evident by 96 h and persisted to 30 days. The PARAGON trial randomized patients to various doses of lamifiban with or without heparin and did not find that lamifiban reduced clinical events at 30 days; however, there was a 40 percent reduction in death and AMI at 6-month follow-up.[21]

Taken together, these trials strongly suggest a role for the glycoprotein IIb/IIIa antagonists in the treatment of patients with refractory unstable angina. The various glycoprotein IIb/IIIa antagonists have not been compared with one another in any trial. Long-term benefits have been documented with abciximab and tirofiban. Abciximab differs from the other glycoprotein IIb/IIIa antagonist in terms of duration of infusion (12 h vs 48 to 72 h) and duration of sustained benefit (up to 3 years in the EPIC study). In contrast, the intracranial hemorrhage rate of the glycoprotein IIb/IIIa antagonists is considerably lower (0.1 percent) than with fibrinolysis, although severe catheter site bleeding and transfusion needs are approximately 6 percent.

COMBINATION FIBRINOLYTIC AND GLYCOPROTEIN IIb/IIIa INHIBITORS Although most of the coronary thrombosis is red clot (fibrin and erythrocytes), the central platelet thrombus (white clot) is fully resistant to fibrinolytic therapy. These platelets secrete PAI-1, which is a potent inhibitor of fibrinolysis. In theory, combination therapy with antiplatelet agents and fibrinolytics will attack both components of coronary thrombosis. This is one explanation why even a weak antiplatelet agent reduces mortality rate as much as treatment with streptokinase alone.[3]

Preclinical studies of low-dose fibrinolytic therapy with glycoprotein IIb/IIIa antagonists that have utilized a reduction in the standard fibrinolytic dose to 50 percent of the standard dose have found that fibrinolysis occurs more rapidly and is more stable. TIMI-14 evaluated abciximab plus either tPA or streptokinase in patients who also received aspirin and low-dose heparin.[22] Abciximab was able to increase the rate of TIMI grade 3 flow by 20 to 25 percent (a 10 percent absolute improvement). The SPEED trial is a dose finding trial to determine the optimal doses of abciximab and reteplase to be used together. GUSTO-IV will compare low dose fibrinolysis in combination with abciximab versus standard dose fibrinolysis alone to determine if the theoretical benefits of low dose fibrinolytics in conjunction with glycoprotein IIb/IIIa antagonists can be realized.

ASPIRIN Aspirin should be given as soon as possible to all patients with ACS. In platelets, aspirin prevents formation of thromboxane A_2, an agonist of platelet aggregation. This inhibition persists for the 9 to 10 life of the platelet, since platelets are unable to generate new cyclooxygenase.[23] Aspirin alone has been shown to be efficacious as streptokinase alone.[3] Aspirin alone reduces mortality rate by 23 percent. In conjunction with streptokinase, mortality rate is reduced 43 percent. Aspirin used in conjunction with fibrinolytic therapy further reduces ischemic events and coronary artery reocclusion. Doses greater than 160 mg cause immediate near complete inhibition of thromboxane A_2. Lower doses may be effective for long-term prophylaxis but may not be effective for acute use. Aspirin reduces vascular events in patients with AMI and patients with unstable angina.[4,24] In patients with prior myocardial infarction or stroke, it reduces vascular events by up to 40 events per 1000 patients.[23]

The side effects of aspirin are mainly gastrointestinal and dose related. They can be reduced by using diluted or buffered aspirin solutions, lowest possible doses, or concurrent antacid or H_2 antagonist administration. In the setting of acute ischemia, the delay in absorption of enteric-coated aspirin may be best avoided. Due to the substantial benefits of aspirin therapy during AMI, it should not be withheld from patients with minor contraindications (vague allergy, history of remote peptic ulcer, or gastrointestinal bleeding).[4] Other antiplatelet agents, such as ticlopidine, can be substituted if true aspirin allergy or active peptic ulcer disease exists.[4] The aspirin dose should be at least 160 mg.

TICLOPIDINE This is an antiplatelet agent that inhibits platelet aggregation induced by a wide range of agonists. The inhibitory effect of ticlopidine is delayed 24 to 48 h after its administration.[4] It is effective in reducing 6-month vascular death and AMI rate in patients with unstable angina.[25] Side effects include neutropenia, which is more common in patients treated for more than 2 weeks. The dose is 250 mg twice per day.

Antithrombins

HEPARIN Heparin is a specific antithrombin agent.[23] As already discussed, thrombin generation plays an intricate role in the pathogenesis of coronary artery thrombosis. Thrombin converts soluble fibrinogen to insoluble fibrin; activates coagulation factors V and VIII, which exert positive feedback on coagulation through the prothrombinase complex; and activates factor XIII, which stabilizes thrombus formation by promoting fibrin cross-linking. In addition, thrombin serves as a platelet agonist.

Unfractionated heparin consists of a mixture of molecules with molecular weights varying between 2000 and 20,000. The different-sized molecules have different effects on the coagulation system. Heparin complexes with antithrombin III, and this complex inactivates both thrombin and activated factor X. The heparin-antithrombin III complex is not effective against clot-bound thrombin. Heparin reduces the risk of AMI and death during the acute phase of unstable angina.[26] The combination therapy of aspirin and heparin reduces the short-term risk of death or myocardial infarction by 56 percent, compared with aspirin alone.[26] When heparin is used in combination with aspirin, reactivation of ischemia is prevented after cessation of the heparin infusion.[27] Thus, combination therapy with aspirin and heparin is indicated for patients with ACS not treated with fibrinolytic agents.

For patients who have been treated with aspirin and fibrinolytic therapy, the incremental value of the addition of heparin is small. The 35-day mortality rate is not improved, and the rate of major or severe bleeding is slightly increased.

Unfractionated heparin has some limitations. It has an unpredictable anticoagulant response because the bioavailability of heparin is variable. It requires careful laboratory monitoring and dose adjustment.

LOW-MOLECULAR-WEIGHT HEPARINS The low-molecular-weight heparins (LMWHs) have greater bioavailability, lower protein binding, a longer half-life, and achieve a more reliable anticoagulant effect. As a result, they can be administered in a fixed dose subcutaneously once or twice a day and achieve a stable therapeutic response without the need for monitoring anticoagulation.

Several clinical trials have compared LMWH to standard heparin regimens for treatment of ACS. The ESSENCE trial randomized 3171 patients with unstable angina and non-Q-wave myocardial infarction to treatment with aspirin and either subcutaneous enoxaparin (LMWH) or intravenous unfractionated heparin.[28] At 14 and 30 days, the risk of death, AMI, or recurrent angina was more than 15 percent lower in patients who received LMWH, without an increase in major bleeding complications.[28] The dose of enoxaparin for treatment of ACS is 1 mg/kg body weight. The dose may change depending upon results of ongoing trials.

Direct Thrombin Inhibitors

These bind to the catalytic site of thrombin, bind to thrombin in clot, and are resistant to agents that degrade heparin. Hirudin, a 65-amino-acid peptide, is derived from the medicinal leech and is one of the most potent naturally occurring anticoagulants. A recent large clinical trial was terminated because hirudin resulted in an increased incidence of intracranial bleeding relative to heparin (1.3 vs 0.7 percent).[29] Bivalirudin (Hirulog) reduced the short-term risk of postischemic complications relative to high-dose unfractionated heparin in patients who underwent percutaneous interventions for unstable or postinfarction angina, but benefits did not persist long term.[30] Also, a low-molecular-weight thrombin inhibitor, inogatran, does not appear to offer benefits over unfractionated heparin for the treatment of patients with ACS.[31] Thus, at this time, there is no clearly defined role for direct thrombin inhibitors in the treatment of ACS.

LIMITING INFARCT SIZE

Nitrates

Nitrates relax vascular smooth muscle in arteries, arterioles, and veins through the metabolic conversion of organic nitrates to nitric oxide. The pulmonary capillary wedge pressure, systemic arterial pressure, and left ventricular end-systolic and end-diastolic volumes all decrease. Reduction in right and left ventricular filling pressures that result from peripheral dilatation combined with afterload reduction that results from arterial dilatation decrease cardiac work and myocardial oxygen requirements. Nitroglycerin has direct vasodilator effects on the coronary vascular bed, increasing global and regional myocardial blood flow. When obstructing atherosclerotic lesions contain intact vascular smooth muscle, nitrates may dilate these vessels, improving blood flow. Platelet aggregation is also inhibited by nitroglycerin.

When nitroglycerin is used in AMI patients who are not treated with thrombolytics, several clinical trials have demonstrated a reduction in infarct size, improved regional function, and decreased rate of cardiovascular complications.[32–34] The mortality rate appears to be reduced by 35 percent with the use of nitrates.[34] It is important to note that, in most studies, intravenous nitroglycerin was titrated to 10 percent reduction in mean arterial pressure for normotensive patients and 30 percent reduction in mean arterial pressure for hypertensive patients. It was not titrated to symptom resolution. Thus, when intravenous nitroglycerin is used for patients with AMI, the dose should be titrated to blood pressure reduction rather than to symptom (chest pain) resolution.

Studies in patients who have received fibrinolytic agents have not found a benefit to the use of nitroglycerin. Unfortunately, large numbers of the control (non-nitroglycerin) patients were prescribed nitroglycerin by their physician, precluding optimal data interpretation.

The American College of Cardiology/American Heart Association (ACC/AHA) guidelines recommend the use of intravenous nitroglycerin for the first 24 to 48 h for patients with AMI and recurrent ischemia, congestive heart failure, or hypertension.[4] Benefits are likely to be greatest in the patients not receiving concurrent fibrinolytic therapy. The Agency for Health Care Policy and Research (AHCPR) unstable angina guidelines recommend that intravenous nitroglycerin be used in patients with unstable angina who are not responsive to an initial three sublingual nitroglycerin tablets and initiation of β-antagonist therapy.[24]

The most serious side effect of nitroglycerin is hypotension, which may result in reflex tachycardia and worsening ischemia. Nitrates should not be used for patients with right ventricular infarction.[35] Nitroglycerin should be used very cautiously for patients with inferior wall ischemia, because one-third of such patients might have right ventricular involvement. Patients with right ventricular infarction are volume dependent. Administration of nitrates reduces preload and commonly results in hypotension in these patients. The development of hypotension is associated with an increased infarct size.

When nitroglycerin results in hypotension and bradycardia, the drug should be discontinued, legs elevated, and fluid administered. Atropine may be necessary in some cases.[4]

β Blockers

β-Adrenergic antagonists have antiarrhythmic, anti-ischemic, and antihypertensive properties. During AMI, they diminish myocardial oxygen demand by decreasing heart rate, systemic arterial pressure, and myocardial contractility. Prolongation of diastole may augment perfusion to ischemic myocardium.[32]

Immediate β-antagonist administration in AMI reduces chest pain, wall stress, infarct size, incidence of cardiovascular complications, and mortality rate for patients not treated with fibrinolytics. The International Collaborative Study Group randomized 144 patients with AMI to treatment with timolol or placebo.[36] The timolol group had a reduction in pain, analgesic use, and infarct size. The Metoprolol in Acute Myocardial Infarction (MIAMI) trial randomized 5778 patients to metoprolol or placebo. Metoprolol reduced mortality rate in high-risk patients, and infarct size was reduced in patients treated within 7 h of symptom onset.[37] ISIS-1 randomized 16,027 patients to atenolol or placebo and found a 14 percent sustained reduction in mortality rate equating to 6 lives saved per 1000 patients.[38]

For patients treated with fibrinolytics, the TIMI-II trial showed that β antagonists decrease the risk of nonfatal reinfarction and recurrent ischemia if given within 2 h after symptom onset. Mortality rate and ventricular function were not affected.[39]

The ACC/AHA guidelines recommend that all patients with Q-wave AMI who do not have a contraindication to β antagonists be treated with these agents within 12 h of onset of infarction, regardless of whether they have received fibrinolytic therapy.[4] Patients with recurrent ischemia and tachyarrhythmias should receive β-antagonist therapy. The role of β antagonists in non-Q-wave infarctions is less clear. The AHCPR guidelines do recommend that patients with unstable angina receive treatment with β antagonists, when possible.[24]

Relative contraindications to β-adrenergic antagonists are heart rate less than 60 beats per minute, systolic blood pressure less than 100 mmHg, moderate to severe left ventricular failure, signs of peripheral hypoperfusion, PR interval more than 0.24 s, second-degree or third-degree atrioventricular block, severe chronic obstructive pulmonary disease, history of asthma, severe peripheral vascular disease, and insulin-dependent diabetes mellitus.[4] Use of β antagonists should be individualized for patients with these conditions.

Angiotensin-Converting Enzyme Inhibitors

Angiotensin-converting enzyme (ACE) inhibitors reduce left ventricular dysfunction and left ventricular dilatation and slow the development of congestive heart failure during AMI. Studies have consistently shown a reduction in mortality rate for patients treated with oral ACE inhibitors during and soon after AMI.[32] A meta-analysis of 15 trials including over 100,000 patients supports a 6.5 percent reduction in short-term mortality rate, with an absolute benefit of 4.6 fewer deaths per 1000 patients treated with early ACE inhibitor therapy.[40] Intravenous enalaprilat was associated with increased hypotension and is not recommended for use during AMI.

The ACC/AHA guidelines recommend that patients with AMI and ST-segment elevation in two or more anterior precordial leads or with clinical heart failure in the absence of contraindications receive treatment with ACE inhibitors.[4] Contraindications to ACE inhibitors include hypotension, bilateral renal artery stenosis, renal failure, or history of cough or angioedema due to prior ACE inhibitor use. The efficacy of ACE inhibitors in unstable angina has not been well evaluated.

Magnesium

Magnesium produces systemic and coronary vasodilatation, possesses antiplatelet activity, suppresses automaticity, and protects myocytes from calcium influx during reperfusion. One meta-analysis of seven randomized trials found a significant mortality-rate benefit in patients with AMI.[41] In the 2316 patients in the Leicaster Intravenous Magnesium Intervention Trial (LIMIT-2), magnesium-treated patients had a 21 to 25 percent reduction in short-term mortality rate and the incidence of congestive heart failure and 4-year cardiovascular mortality rate was also reduced.[42] Studies, however, are conflicting: some have found mortality rate reduced by about 75 percent, whereas others have showed no benefit at all. The disparity in findings may be related to the interval between symptom onset and magnesium administration, and various concurrent therapies (including fibrinolysis). In light of these conflicting data, the ACC/AHA guidelines support correction of documented hypomagnesemia during AMI and treatment of torsades-type ventricular tachycardia with a prolonged QT interval.[4] Magnesium bolus and infusion in high-risk patients, such as the elderly and those in whom reperfusion therapy is not suitable, is considered possibly beneficial.[4]

Calcium-Channel Antagonists

Calcium-channel blockers have antianginal, vasodilatory, and antihypertensive properties.[32] Calcium antagonists have not been shown to reduce mortality rate after AMI. In fact, they may be harmful to some patients with cardiovascular disease.[4] Nifedipine is the most studied of the calcium-channel blockers for the treatment of AMI. This short-acting dihydropyridine has been associated with a nonsignificant increase in mortality rate when given during or shortly after AMI in several clinical trials.[43] Immediate-release nifedipine may be harmful as a result of a coronary "steal" syndrome in which coronary perfusion pressure is reduced through disproportionate dilatation of the coronary arteries adjacent to the ischemic zone and/or reflex activation of the sympathetic nervous system with a resultant increase in myocardial oxygen demand.

Diltiazem has also been found to be associated with increased mortality rate, particularly for patients with congestive heart failure.[44] Similarly, studies evaluating verapamil have not found mortality-rate benefits.[32] Verapamil is detrimental for patients with congestive heart failure or bradydysrhythmias. There are no data supporting the use of second-generation dihydropyridines (amlodipine and felodipine) for treatment of AMI.

The ACC/AHA guidelines state that "these agents are still used too frequently in patients with acute MI and that beta-adrenoreceptor blocking agents are a more appropriate choice.''[4] Verapamil and diltiazem are considered potentially beneficial for use in patients with ongoing ischemia or atrial fibrillation with rapid ventricular response who do not have congestive heart failure, left ventricular dysfunction, or atrioventricular block, and β-adrenergic antagonists are contraindicated.[4,24]

SPECIAL ISSUES IN TREATMENT OF AMI COMPLICATIONS

Recurrent or Refractory Ischemia

Patients unresponsive to medical management with continued ischemia should be treated on an individual basis. Depending on the infarct distribution and coronary anatomy, decisions could be made regarding continued medical management, rescue angioplasty, or coronary artery bypass grafting. Emergency cardiology referral should be considered. Refractory ischemia is often investigated with coronary catheterization.

Intraaortic balloon counterpulsation delivers phased pulsations synchronized to the electrocardiograph so that balloon inflation will occur at the time of aortic valve closure and deflation occurs just prior to onset of systole. The augmented coronary perfusion pressure during diastole enhances coronary blood flow. Balloon deflation during systole allows the left ventricle to eject blood against a lower resistance. The net effect of intra-aortic balloon counterpulsation is an increase in cardiac output, reduction in systolic arterial pressure, increase in diastolic arterial pressure, little change in mean arterial pressure, and reduction in heart rate. The reduction in left ventricular afterload leads to reduced myocardial oxygen consumption, decreasing the amount of myocardial ischemia. Intraaortic balloon counterpulsation is recommended for patients with ACS who are refractory to aggressive medical management or are hemodynamically unstable, as a means to bridge a patient's stability en route to the cardiac catheterization laboratory or the operating room.[24]

Cardiogenic Shock

This is discussed in Chap. 29.

Right Ventricular Infarction

One-third of patients with inferior wall myocardial infarction have right ventricular involvement. The most serious complication of right ventricular infarction is shock. Right ventricular infarction results in a reduction in right ventricular end-systolic pressure, left ventricular end-diastolic size, cardiac output, and aortic pressure as the right ventricle becomes more of a passive conduit to blood flow. Left ventricular contraction causes bulging of the interventricular septum into the right ventricle, with resultant ejection of blood into the pulmonary circulation. As a result, right ventricular infarction in the setting of a large left ventricular infarction has a particularly devastating effect on hemodynamic function. Factors that reduce preload (volume depletion, diuretics, and nitrates) or decrease right atrial contraction (atrial infarction and loss of atrioventricular synchrony) and factors that increase right ventricular afterload (left ventricular failure) can lead to significant hemodynamic derangements.

Treatment of right ventricular infarction includes maintenance of preload, reduction of right ventricular afterload, and inotropic support of an ischemic right ventricle, in addition to early reperfusion.[45] Patients with right ventricular infarction should not be treated with drugs, such as nitrates, that reduce preload. In the setting of right ventricular infarction, nitrates will often reduce cardiac output and produce hypotension. Instead, patients with marginal preload or hypotension should be treated with volume loading (normal saline). The increased preload will improve right ventricular cardiac output. If cardiac output is not improved after 1 to 2 L of normal saline, inotropic support with dobutamine should be initiated.

High-degree heart block is very common in patients with right ventricular infarction. The loss of right atrial kick can greatly compromise right ventricular cardiac output. Restitution of atrioventricular synchrony is important. For patients who require pacing in the setting of right ventricular infarction, it may be necessary to establish atrioventricular sequential pacing leads. Patients who do not attain hemodynamic improvement after placement of a ventricular pacer may still improve with atrioventricular sequential pacing reestablishing a right atrial kick.

When right ventricular infarction is accompanied by left ventricular dysfunction, the use of nitroprusside to reduce afterload, or intraaortic balloon counterpulsation, may be of benefit. Reduction in left ventricular afterload may help passive movement of blood through the right ventricle.

Selected Dysrhythmias in AMI

ATRIAL FIBRILLATION Atrial fibrillation associated with AMI most typically occurs in the first 24 hours and is usually transient. It more often occurs in patients with excess catecholamine release, hypokalemia, hypomagnesemia, hypoxia, chronic lung disease, and sinus node or left circumflex ischemia. Patients with supraventricular tachycardia, atrial fibrillation, and atrial flutter who have hemodynamic compromise should receive cardioversion with 100 J, then 200 to 300 J, then 360 J if lower energies fail. Patients without hemodynamic compromise, clinical left ventricular dysfunction, reactive airway disease, or heart block can be treated with beta-adrenergic antagonists, such as atenolol (2.5–5 mg over 2 min to a total of 10 mg) or metopropol (2.5–5 mg every 2–5 min to a total of 15 mg). Patients with contraindications to beta-adrenergic antagonists can be treated with digitalis (0.3 mg–0.5 mg initial bolus with a repeat in 4 h) or a calcium antagonist such as verapamil or dilitiazem. Digitalis will take longer to work but is still preferred by the ACC/AHA guidelines because of the potential negative inotropic effects of calcium antagonists, their lack of efficacy in reducing mortality during AMI, and potentially harmful effects in some subsets of AMI patients.[2] The etiology of the tachydysrhythmia should also be addressed. Heparin should be given since atrial fibrillation during AMI is associated with a 3-fold risk in systemic embolization.

BRADYDYSRHYTHMIAS The increased mortality in patients with heart block during AMI is related to more extensive myocardial damage and not the heart block itself. As a result, pacing has not been shown to reduce mortality in patients with AV block or intraventricular conduction delay. Nonetheless, pacing is still recommended to protect against sudden hypotension, acute ischemia, and precipitation of ventricular dysrhythmias in certain patients.

The risk of developing third degree heart block during AMI is increased in the setting of first degree AV block, both types of second degree AV block (more likely with Mobitz II), left anterior hemiblock, left posterior hemiblock, right bundle branch block, and left bundle branch block. The prognosis is related to the site of infarction, site of the block (intranodal vs. infranodal), the type of escape rhythm, and the hemodynamic response to the rhythm.

Atropine is recommended for sinus bradycardia when it results in hypotension, ischemia, or ventricular escape rhythms and for treatment of symptomatic AV block occurring at the AV nodal level (second degree type 1 or third degree AV block). Atropine will reverse decreases in heart rate, systemic vascular resistance, and blood pressure that are mediated by parasympathetic activity. It should be used cautiously in the setting of AMI because the parasympathetic tone is protective against infarct extension and ventricular fibrillation.

Temporary *transcutaneous* pacers are recommended for patients at moderate to high risk of progression to AV block, e.g: unresponsive symptomatic bradycardia, Mobitz-II, or higher AV blocks, new LBBB and bifascicular blocks, RBBB, or LBBB with 1 degree block. It can also be considered for some cases with stable bradycardia and new or indeterminate age RBBB. *Transvenous* pacing should be considered in patients who require permanent pacing and in patients with a very high likelihood (>30%) of requiring permanent pacing, e.g. asystole, unresponsive symptomatic bradycardia, Mobitz-II, 3 degree block, alternating BBB, or RBBB or LBBB with 1 degree block. It can also be considered in some cases of RBBB with left anterior or posterior hemiblocks, new or indeterminate age LBBB, for atrial or ventricular overdrive pacing in unresponsive V_T, and unresponsive recurrent sinus pauses (>3 s). Patients with right ventricular infarction who are very dependent on atrial systole may require atrioventricular sequential pacing to maintain cardiac output.

Cocaine Associated Myocardial Ischemia

Management of patients with cocaine associated myocardial ischemia focuses on reversal of coronary vasoconstriction, hypertension, tachycardia, and predisposition to thrombus formation.[31] Central nervous system protection and decreased sympathetic outflow should be accomplished with the administration of benzodiazepines. Multiple animal experiments and widespread anecdotal experience in humans support the use of diazepam as the initial agent for the management of cocaine intoxicated patients. Diazepam alone will often calm the agitated patient and return abnormal vital signs to the normal range. Reduction in hypertension and/or tachycardia will decrease the myocardial oxygen demand.

Aspirin and/or heparin should be used as they would be in patients with myocardial ischemia unrelated to cocaine, despite the lack of any clinical or experimental data. The success with platelet inhibitors and anticoagulants in traditional myocardial infarction patients and the propensity of cocaine to induce platelet aggregation supports their use.

Specific anti-ischemic therapy begins with nitroglycerin. Nitroglycerin reverses cocaine induced coronary artery vasoconstriction and relieves cocaine associated chest pain. Although infarct size reduction or mortality benefits have not been assessed, based on direct vasodilatory effects of nitroglycerin, experimental reversal of coronary vasoconstriction, and clinical relief of chest pain, it should be used.[31]

Patients with continued myocardial ischemia, after the use of nitroglycerin should be treated with either phentolamine, calcium channel blockers, or thrombolytic agents depending on the clinical circumstances.[31] Phentolamine blocks the alpha adrenergic effects of cocaine and reverses the coronary vasoconstrictive effects of cocaine. Phentolamine should be used with caution, as it is generally considered contraindicated after benzodiazepine use, and may result in marked hypotension. Low doses (1 mg every 2.5 min) have been used multiple times without any adverse consequences.

Verapamil, a calcium channel antagonist, reverses cocaine induced coronary artery vasoconstriction. Unfortunately, animal studies demonstrate enhanced central nervous system toxicity from concurrent administration of cocaine and any one of several calcium antagonists (verapamil, diltiazem, and nifedipine). The potentiation of cocaine associated central nervous system toxicity, combined with the limited success of calcium antagonists in traditional myocardial infarction patients makes them less attractive for use in patients with cocaine associated myocardial infarction.[31]

Thrombolytic therapy has become the standard of care for patients with myocardial infarction unrelated to cocaine, however, the use of these agents in cocaine associated myocardial ischemia must proceed with great caution. Although initial concerns regarding safety have been tempered, there has been no demonstrated efficacy in this patient population. Up to 43% of patients with cocaine associated chest pain without myocardial infarction meet TIMI criteria for the administration of thrombolytic agents despite the fact they did not infarct. The potential administration to patients who are not infarcting coupled with a very low mortality from cocaine associated myocardial infarction limits the utility of thrombolytic agents. Patients who have new ST segment elevations (based on comparison with prior electrocardiograms), or echocardiographic wall motion abnormalities may be suitable candidates since "false positive" ST elevations should be less of a concern.

Beta adrenergic antagonists should be avoided in patients who have recently used cocaine.[31] They have been shown to increase central nervous system toxicity and exacerbate coronary artery vasospasm in several animal models of cocaine toxicity. Clinical series have demonstrated that they fail to reverse the hpertensive and tachycardic effects of cocaine. The alpha-adrenergic agonist effects of cocaine on the coronary vasculature are enhanced by beta adrenergic antagonists which worsen the severity of cocaine induced coronary vasoconstriction. Thus, despite the overwhelming success of beta adrenergic antagonists in patients with myocardial infarction unrelated to cocaine, they are to be avoided in patients who have recently used cocaine. Labetalol does not appear to offer any advantage over the use of pure beta adrenergic antagonists.

The treatment of post infarction dysrhythmias secondary to cocaine has not been well studied. The local anesthetic and sodium channel blocking effects of cocaine were hypothesized to be worsened by concomitant lidocaine administration, however, several animal models have yielded conflicting results. One clinical series, in which patients received lidocaine more than 4 hours after cocaine use, did not find serious dysrhythmias or central nervous system toxicity after lidocaine administration. Sodium bicarbonate narrows the QRS complex in cocaine induced dysrhythmias through its effects of the sodium channels. Sodium bicarbonate is recommended for the early treatment of cocaine induced dysrhythmias.[31] Lidocaine can also be used for treatment of patients with later development dysrhymias.[31]

REFERENCES

1. Kennedy JW, Ritchie JL, Davis KB, et al: The Western Washington randomized trial of intracoronary streptokinase in acute myocardial infarction. *N Engl J Med* 312:1073, 1985.
2. ISAM Study Group: A prospective trial of intravenous streptokinase in acute myocardial infarction (ISAM): Mortality, morbidity, and infarct size at 21 days. *N Engl J Med* 314:1465, 1986.
3. ISIS-2 Collaborative Group: Randomized trial of intravenous streptokinase, oral aspirin, or neither among 17,187 cases of suspected AMI. *Lancet* 2:349, 1988.
4. Ryan TJ, Anderson JL, Antman EM, et al: ACC/AHA guidelines for the management of patients with acute myocardial infarction: A report of the American College of Cardiology/American Heart Association Task Force on Practice Guidelines (Committee on Management of Acute Myocardial Infarction). *J Am Coll Cardiol* 28:1328, 1996.
5. International Study Group: In-hospital mortality and clinical course of 20,891 patients with suspected acute myocardial infarction randomized between alteplase and streptokinase with or without heparin. *Lancet* 336:71, 1990.
6. ISIS-3 Collaborative Group: A randomized comparison of streptokinase vs tissue plasminogen activator vs anistreplase and of aspirin plus heparin vs aspirin alone among 41,299 cases of suspected acute myocardial infarction: ISIS-3. *Lancet* 339:753, 1992.
7. GUSTO Investigators: An international randomized trial comparing four thrombolytic strategies for acute myocardial infarction. *N Engl J Med* 329:673, 1993.
8. GUSTO Angiographic Investigators: The effects of tissue plasminogen activator, streptokinase, or both on coronary-artery patency, ventricular function, and survival after acute myocardial infarction. *N Engl J Med* 329:1615, 1993.
9. GUSTO III Investigators: A comparison of reteplase with alteplase for acute myocardial infarction. *N Engl J Med* 337:1118, 1997.
10. Bittl JA: Advances in coronary angioplasty. *N Engl J Med* 335:1290, 1996.
11. Grines CL, Browne KF, Marco J, et al: A comparison of immediate angioplasty with thrombolytic therapy for acute myocardial infarction. *N Engl J Med* 328:673, 1993.
12. GUSTO IIB Angioplasty Substudy Investigators: A clinical trial comparing primary coronary angioplasty with tissue plasminogen activator for acute myocardial infarction. *N Engl J Med* 336:1621, 1997.
13. Every NR, Parsons LS, Hlatky M, et al</AU>, for MITI Investigators: A comparison of thrombolytic therapy with primary coronary angioplasty for acute myocardial infarction. *N Engl J Med* 335:1253, 1996.

14. Topol EJ: Toward a new frontier in myocardial reperfusion therapy: Emerging platelet preeminance. *Circulation* 97:211, 1998.
15. EPIC Investigators: Use of a monoclonal antibody directed against the platelet glycoprotein IIb/IIIa receptor in high risk coronary angioplasty. *N Engl J Med* 330:956, 1994.
16. EPILOG Investigators: Platelet glycoprotein IIb/IIIa receptor blockade and low dose heparin during percutaneous coronary revascularization. *N Engl J Med* 336:1689, 1997.
17. CAPTURE Investigators. Randomized placebo-controlled trial of abciximab before and during acute coronary intervention in refractory unstable angina. *Lancet* 349:1429, 1997.
18. Platelet Receptor Inhibition in Ischemic Syndrome Management (PRISM) Study Investigators: A comparison of aspirin plus tirofiban with aspirin plus heparin for unstable angina. *N Engl J Med* 338:1498, 1998.
19. Platelet Receptor Inhibition in Ischemic Syndrome Management in Patients Limited by Unstable Signs and Symptoms (PRISM-PLUS) Study Investigators: Inhibition of the platelet glycoprotein IIb/IIIa receptor with tirofiban in unstable angina and non-Q-wave myocardial infarction. *N Engl J Med* 338:1488, 1998.
20. PURSUIT Investigators: Inhibition of platelet glycoprotein IIb/IIIa with eptifibatide in patients with acute coronary syndromes. *N Engl J Med* 339:436, 1998.
21. PARAGON Investigators: A randomized trial of potent platelet IIb/IIIa antagonism, heparin, or both in patients with unstable angina: The PARAGON study [abst]. *Circulation* 94(suppl I):I-553, 1996.
22. Antman EM: TIMI-14: Abciximab plus thrombolytic therapy, in *George Washington University 13th International Workshop: Thrombolysis and Interventional Therapy in Acute Myocardial Infarction, Orlando, Florida, November 1997.*
23. Collins R, Peto R, Baigent C, Sleight P: Aspirin, heparin, and fibrinolytic therapy in suspected acute myocardial infarction. *N Engl J Med* 336:847, 1997.
24. Braunwald E, Mark DB, Jones RH, et al: *Unstable Angina: Diagnosis and Management—Clinical Practice Guideline 10 (Amended).* Rockville, MD, Agency for Health Care Policy and Research and the National Health, Lung and Blood Institute, Public Health Service, US Department of Health and Human Services, May 1994; AHCPR publication 94-0602.
25. Balsano F, Rizzon P, Violoi F, et al: Antiplatelet treatment with ticlopidine in unstable angina: A controlled multicenter clinical trial—The Studio della Ticlopidina nell'Angina Instabile Group. *Circulation* 82:17, 1990.
26. Theroux P, Ouimet H, McCans J, et al: Aspirin, heparin or both to treat acute unstable angina. *N Engl J Med* 319:1105, 1988.
27. Theroux P, Waters D, Qiu S, et al: Aspirin versus heparin to prevent myocardial infarction during the acute phase of unstable angina. *Circulation* 88:2045, 1993.
28. Cohen M, Demers C, Gurfinkel EP, et al: A comparison of low molecular weight heparin with unfractionated heparin for unstable coronary artery disease. *N Engl J Med* 337:447, 1997.
29. GUSTO IIA Investigators: Randomized trial of intravenous heparin versus recombinant hirudin for acute coronary syndromes. *Circulation* 90:1631, 1994.
30. Bittl JA, Strony J, Brinker JA: Treatment with bivalirudin (Hirulog) as compared with heparin during coronary angioplasty for unstable angina or postinfarction angina. *N Engl J Med* 333:764, 1995.
31. Anderson K, Dellborg M, for the TRIM Study Group: Heparin is more effective than inogatran, a low molecular weight thrombin inhibitor, in suppressing ischemia and recurrent angina in unstable coronary disease. *Am J Cardiol* 81:939, 1998.
32. Hennekins CH, Albert CM, Godfried SL, et al: Adjunctive drug therapy of acute myocardial infarction: Evidence from clinical trials. *N Engl J Med* 335:1660, 1996.
33. Judgutt BI, Warnica JW: Intravenous nitroglycerin therapy to limit myocardial infarct size, expansion, and complications: Effect of timing, dosage, and infarct location. *Circulation* 78:906, 1988.
34. Yusuf S, Collins R, McMahon S, Peto R: Effect of intravenous nitrates on mortality in acute myocardial infarction: An overview of randomized trials. *Lancet* 1:1088, 1988.
35. Fergusen JJ, Diver DJ, Boldt M, Pasternak RC: Significance of nitroglycerin-induced hypotension with inferior wall acute myocardial infarction. *Am J Cardiol* 64:311, 1989.
36. International Collaborative Study Group: Reduction of infarct size with the early use of timolol in acute myocardial infarction. *N Engl J Med* 310:9, 1984.
37. MIAMI Trial Research Group: Metoprolol in acute myocardial infarction (MIAMI): A randomised placebo controlled international trial. *Eur Heart J* 6:199, 1985.
38. ISIS-1 Collaborative Group: Randomised trial of intravenous atenolol among 16,027 cases of suspected myocardial infarction: ISIS-1. *Lancet* 2:57, 1986.
39. TIMI Study Group. Comparison of invasive and conservative strategies after treatment with intravenous tissue plasminogen activator in acute myocardial infarction: Results of the TIMI phase II trial. *N Engl J Med* 320:618, 1989.
40. Latini R, Maggioni AP, Flather M, et al: ACE inhibitor use in patients with acute myocardial infarction: Summary of evidence from clinical trials. *Circulation* 92:3132, 1995.
41. Antman EM, Lau J, Kupelnick B, et al: A comparison of results of meta-analyses of randomized control trials and recommendations of clinical experts: Treatments for myocardial infarction. *JAMA* 268:240, 1992.
42. Woods KL, Fletcher S: Long term outcome after intravenous magnesium sulphate in suspected acute myocardial infarction: The second Leicaster Intravenous Magnesium Intervention Trial (LIMIT-2). *Lancet* 343:816, 1994.
43. Furberg CD, Patsy BM, Meyer JV: Nifedipine: Dose-related increase in mortality in patients with coronary heart disease. *Circulation* 92:1326, 1995.
44. Multicenter Diltiazem Postinfarction Trial Research Group: The effect of diltiazem on mortality and reinfarction after myocardial infarction. *N Engl J Med* 319:385, 1988.
45. Kinch JW, Ryan TJ: Right ventricular infarction. *N Engl J Med* 330:1211, 1994.

HEART FAILURE AND PULMONARY EDEMA

Charles B. Cairns

HEART FAILURE

The principal functions of the heart are to receive blood from the veins, send it to the lungs for oxygenation, and pump the oxygenated blood to the body. *Heart failure* occurs when there is a substantial disruption of these functions secondary to a loss of normal contractile ability.[1] Heart failure that results in abnormal fluid retention is commonly referred to as *congestive heart failure* (CHF). The major clinical manifestation of heart failure is shortness of breath, especially with exercise. The heart may fail when it performs excessive work for a prolonged period, such as in patients with hypertension and valvular heart disease. Heart failure is also seen in a variety of infectious, inflammatory, and infiltrative conditions that affect heart muscle. In the acute setting, heart failure is commonly due to a loss of heart muscle via infarction or to a loss of nourishment via ischemia.[1,2] The common causes of heart failure are summarized in Table 49-1.[1–9]

Over 2 million people in the United States have heart failure.[3] The incidence of heart failure appears to be increasing, and over 500,000 new cases are detected each year.[4] In addition, the mortality rate from heart failure is also increasing,[5] and one-half of patients with severe heart failure (left ventricular ejection fraction less than 35 percent) die within 1 year of diagnosis.[6]

Pathophysiology of Heart Failure

The three factors of contractility, preload, and afterload determine ventricular stroke volume.[1] Coupled with heart rate, stroke volume determines cardiac output. Cardiac *contractility* is related to the amount of myocardial stretch, known as *preload.* Clinical measurements of cardiac stretch include the ventricular end-diastolic pressure and volume. *Afterload* is defined as the ventricular wall tension that develops during systole and reflects the resistance to outward blood flow. It is clinically estimated by the systolic arterial pressure. Many sorts of heart failure are associated with decreased contractility. The Frank-

TABLE 49-1 Common Causes of Heart Failure and Pulmonary Edema

Myocardial ischemia: Acute and chronic
Valvular dysfunction
Aortic valve disease
Aortic stenosis
Aortic insufficiency
Aortic dissection
Infectious endocarditis
Mitral valve disease
Mitral stenosis
Mitral regurgitation
Papillary muscle dysfunction or rupture
Ruptured chordae tendineae
Infectious endocarditis
Prosthetic valve malfunction
Other causes of left ventricular outflow obstruction
Supravalvular aortic stenosis
Membranous subvalvular aortic stenosis
Idiopathic cardiomyopathy
Hypertrophic cardiomyopathy
Dilated
Restrictive
Acquired cardiomyopathy
Toxic: Alcohol, cocaine, adriamycin
Metabolic: Thyrotoxicosis, myxedema
Myocarditis: Radiation, infection
Constrictive pericarditis
Cardiac tamponade
Systemic hypertension
Miscellaneous
Anemia
Cardiac dysrhythmias

Starling relationships between stroke volume, preload, and contractility in both normal hearts and failing hearts are illustrated in Fig. 49-1.[1]

Heart failure can be further classified into three categories related to physiology and functional anatomy: high versus low cardiac output, right versus left heart failure, and systolic versus diastolic dysfunction.[1,2,7–12]

Heart failure can produce either low or high cardiac output states.[1] Whereas *low-output failure* is due to an inherent problem in myocardial contraction, *high-output failure* is due to an inability of functionally intact myocardium to keep up with excess functional demands. The causes of high-output failure are relatively few and include anemia, thyrotoxicosis, large arteriovenous shunts, beriberi, and Paget disease of the bone.

In congestive heart failure, excess fluid accumulates behind the affected chamber of the heart. In patients with left ventricular dysfunction due to either mechanical overload or infarction, excess fluid develops in the lungs. This resulting *pulmonary edema,* or congestion, is the cardinal manifestation of *left-sided heart failure.* In patients where the right ventricle is compromised (pulmonary embolus, right ventricular infarction), jugular venous distention and other signs of *right-sided heart failure* occur. Long-standing heart failure, however, usually results in compromise of both ventricles.[11]

Systolic heart failure is characterized by an impairment of myocardial contraction, and diastolic failure by an impairment in myocardial relaxation. *Systolic failure* can occur from excessive afterload (systemic hypertension) or from damaged myocytes (infarction).[11] *Diastolic failure* can be seen in both acute and chronic heart failure. Inhibited early diastolic relaxation as seen in myocardial ischemia is due to altered energy availability.[10] Chronic processes such as hypertrophic cardiomyopathy increase ventricular stiffness and inhibit relaxation. Many etiologies, such as transient myocardial ischemia, can result in either systolic or diastolic failure.

Once heart failure has developed, several neurohormonal compensatory mechanisms occur.[12] Alterations in adrenergic tone redistribute blood flow to the brain and myocardium, reducing blood flow to the skin, kidneys, gastrointestinal tract, and skeletal muscle. The reduction in blood flow to the kidneys results in increased stimulation of the renin-angiotensin-aldosterone axis and secretion of antidiuretic hormone. The end result of these processes is enhanced sodium and water retention by the kidneys, which leads to fluid overload and the clinical manifestations of CHF. Additionally, the increased adrenergic tone leads to arteriolar vasoconstriction, a significant raise in afterload, and finally, to increased cardiac work.

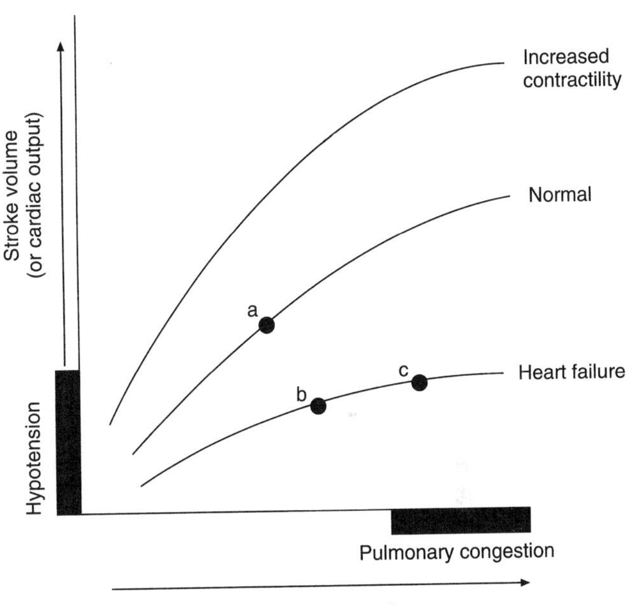

FIG. 49-1. Left ventricular (LV) performance (Frank-Starling) curves relate preload, measured as LV end-diastolic volume (EDV) or pressure (EDP), to cardiac performance, measured as ventricular stroke volume or cardiac output. On the curve of normal individuals (*middle line*), cardiac performance continuously increases as a function of the preload. States of increased contractility (e.g., dobutamine infusion) are characterized by an augmented stroke volume at any level of preload (*top line*). Conversely, decreased LV contractility (commonly associated with heart failure) is characterized by a curve that is shifted downward (*bottom line*). Point *a* is an example of a normal individual at rest. Point *b* represents the same individual after developing systolic dysfunction and heart failure (e.g., after a large myocardial infarction): stroke volume has fallen, and the decreased LV emptying results in elevation of the EDV. Because point *b* is on the ascending portion of the curve, the increased EDV serves a compensatory role because it results in an increase in subsequent stroke volume, albeit much less so than if operating on the normal curve. Further augmentation of LV filling (e.g., increased circulating volume) in the heart failure patient is represented by point *c*, which resides on the relatively flat part of the curve: stroke volume is only slightly augmented, but the markedly increased EDP results in pulmonary congestion.

TABLE 49-2 Common Symptoms and Physical Findings in Heart Failure

Symptoms	Physical Findings
Left sided	
Fatigue	Tachycardia, tachypnea
Dyspnea	S_3 gallop
Paroxysmal nocturnal dyspnea	Diaphoresis
Orthopnea	Pulmonary rales, wheezes
Right sided	
Dependent edema	Jugular venous distention
Right upper quadrant pain	Peripheral edema
	Hepatomegaly
	Hepatojugular reflux

Source: Adapted from Coday et al,[21] with permission.

Clinical Features of Heart Failure

The clinical features of heart failure may be due to impaired perfusion or elevated venous pressures and relate to which ventricle is primarily affected (Table 49-2). Patients may present with either the chronic progressive symptoms of heart failure or with acute pulmonary edema due to sudden left-sided decompensation.[1,2,7,8]

The manifestations of heart failure depend on which ventricle is primarily affected (Table 49-2). Left ventricular failure can result from either diastolic or systolic dysfunction and can lead to increased pulmonary venous pressures, interstitial lung fluid, and pulmonary edema. Right ventricular failure leads to jugular venous distention, peripheral edema, hepatic congestion, and ascites.

The most common symptom of left-sided heart failure is breathlessness, or *dyspnea,* particularly with exertion.[1,7] When pulmonary venous pressure reaches a critical level (20 mmHg), there is movement of fluid into the pulmonary interstitium, compressing airways and alveoli.[1] The increased resistance to airflow intensifies the work of breathing. In addition, stimulation of the juxtacapillary receptors (J receptors) causes rapid shallow breathing. Other manifestations of pulmonary congestion include orthopnea and paroxysmal nocturnal dyspnea (PND).[1,8,9–11] Orthopnea is the sensation of breathlessness while lying flat and is relieved by sitting upright. Orthopnea results from the redistribution of intravascular blood from the gravity-dependent portions of the body to the lungs. The degree of orthopnea is usually assessed by the number of pillows a patient uses at night to avoid breathlessness. PND is severe breathlessness that awakens a patient from sleep 2 to 3 h after lying down. PND is due to the gradual reabsorption of interstitial lower extremity edema after lying down, with subsequent greater venous return to the heart and lungs.[1]

Clinical manifestations of left-sided heart failure due to alterations in blood flow include fatigue, altered mental status, and reduced urine output (especially during the day). At night, urine output may increase due to increases in venous return. The increased urinary frequency at night is termed nocturia.[1]

Right-sided heart failure causes increased systemic venous pressures and peripheral edema.[1,8] Additional edema of the gastrointestinal tract causes anorexia and nausea, and right upper quadrant abdominal pain occurs as the liver becomes engorged.

Physical findings of left-sided heart failure include dusky or pale skin, diaphoresis, and cool extremities due to poor perfusion and peripheral arterial vasoconstriction.[1,8] Pulmonary congestion commonly results in tachypnea and bilateral inspiratory crackles on auscultation. Additional auscultatory findings include rhonchi and wheezing (''cardiac asthma'') due to airway edema. Pleural effusions may develop, detected by dullness to percussion at the lung bases. In advanced heart failure, Cheyne-Stokes respiration can occur and is a respiratory pattern characterized by periods of hyperventilation separated by periods of apnea.[1]

Frequently, sinus tachycardia secondary to sympathetic nervous system activity is present in heart failure patients.[1,8] Cardiac auscultation may reveal a third heart sound (S_3), an early diastolic sound resulting from abnormal filling into the dilated ventricle. Also present may be a fourth heart sound (S_4), which results from forceful atrial contraction into a stiffened ventricle. Finally, *pulsus alternans* (alternating strong and weak contractions detected in the peripheral pulse) may occur in advanced heart failure.[1]

Right-sided heart failure may result in additional physical findings due to elevated systemic venous pressures. Jugular venous distention (JVD) is common.[1,8] Engorgement of the liver results in hepatomegaly, right upper quadrant tenderness, and the presence of the hepatojugular reflux (JVD with liver palpation). Peripheral edema accumulates in the dependent areas of the body, including the ankles and legs of ambulatory patients and the presacral region of bedridden patients.[1,8]

Radiographic manifestations of left-sided CHF generally relate to the increases in pulmonary venous pressures.[1] When the pulmonary pressures exceed 15 mmHg, hydrostatic pressure increases in the gravity-dependent edematous lower zones of the lung. Because of the higher resistance to flow in the lower regions, blood flow is selectively shunted to the upper regions, and the chest radiograph shows upper-zone vascular redistribution. As pulmonary pressures exceed 20 mmHg, interstitial edema occurs with loss of distinct vascular margins on chest x-ray. Interlobular edema results in Kerley B lines, which are short linear markings at the periphery of the lower lung fields on the chest x-ray.[1] When pulmonary pressures reach 25 mmHg, alveolar pulmonary edema develops with opacification of the airspaces on x-ray. However, in patients with long-standing CHF, enhanced lymphatic drainage may minimize these radiographic findings.[1]

Depending on the cause of the CHF, additional radiographic findings include cardiomegaly and pleural effusions.[1] Cardiomegaly is defined as a cardiothoracic ratio greater than 0.5 on a posteroanterior film.[1] Pleural effusions may occur in either left-sided or right-sided failure but are usually the result of bilateral heart failure. High right atrial pressure may cause azygos vein enlargement on chest x-ray.

The electrocardiogram (ECG) may reveal evidence of acute myocardial infarction or ischemia as a cause of acute decompensation of CHF. In chronic CHF, the ECG usually reveals evidence of ventricular hypertrophy, atrial enlargement, or conduction abnormalities.[1]

In patients with dyspnea or evidence of pulmonary edema, arterial blood gases will help define the acid-base status and are necessary to quantitate the level of respiratory effort. Hypoxia is a frequent finding with pulmonary edema and, when associated with hypercarbia and acidosis, can portend impending respiratory failure.[1,8]

Treatment of Chronic Congestive Heart Failure

The treatment of heart failure involves either correction of the underlying cause of the heart failure or elimination of the symptoms.[1,7] Treatment of the underlying condition may be curative in patients with readily correctable conditions such as valvular disorders, acute infections, or dysrhythmias. For the remaining patients with CHF, treatment is geared toward reduction of cardiac work, control of fluid retention, and enhancement of myocardial contractility.

The reduction of cardiac work is accomplished by restriction of both physical and emotional activity coupled with pharmacologic afterload reduction. Vasodilators help to reduce the increase in afterload that occurs with the neurohormonal compensatory response to CHF. Even a modest reduction in afterload may elevate the stroke volume of the heart and reduce ventricular end-diastolic pressures.

Vasodilators can be classified by their effects—primarily on the venous bed, arterial bed, or both beds—or by their route of administration.[4,7,13,14] Venodilators tend to shunt blood away from the chest to the peripheral circulation, reducing preload. Venodilators include nitroglycerin and isosorbide dinitrate. Arteriolar dilators reduce afterload and enhance stroke volume. Arteriolar dilators include hydralazine, minoxidil, and calcium-channel blockers. Agents with mixed venous and arterial effects include prazosin and the angiotensin-converting enzyme (ACE) inhibitors. Intravenous agents with mixed venous and arterial dilatory effects include sodium nitroprusside and phentolamine.

The control of excess fluid retention in patients with CHF is accomplished mainly by dietary restriction of sodium intake and the use of diuretics. Diuretics reduce intravascular volume and preload by promoting the elimination of sodium and water via the kidney. However, overly vigorous reduction of preload with diuresis can result in a marked reduction of cardiac contractility.[4] Therefore, the use of diuretics in CHF is usually restricted to those patients with evidence of pulmonary or peripheral edema.[4]

Diuretics acting on the loop of Henle are the most potent and include furosemide, bumetanide, and ethacrynic acid.[7] Thiazide diuretics are useful in mild CHF when renal perfusion is preserved.[8] The most important adverse effects of these drugs are overdiuresis, with impairment of cardiac output, and electrolyte abnormalities, including hypokalemia and hypomagnesemia. Potassium-sparing diuretics, such as spironolactone and triamterene, can potentiate the action of thiazides and loop diuretics. Such combinations are useful in severe CHF, although they should not be used in patients with impaired renal fucntion or hyperkalemia.[4,8]

Enhancement of myocardial contraction with inotropic agents can be useful in patients with systolic dysfunction.[1,4,7,8,10] Inotropic drugs increase cardiac output by shifting the Frank-Starling curve upward. Thus, for any given preload, stroke volume and contraction are augmented. The inotropic therapy of chronic CHF is mainly through the use of digitalis glycosides. In addition to enhancing contractility, digitalis reduces afterload by blunting the cardiac sympathetic response. Digitalis prolongs the refractory period of the atrioventricular node and is effective in controlling the ventricular response to atrial fibrillation. Digitalis intoxication, however, can be a life-threatening disorder characterized by atrial and ventricular dysrhythmias and hyperkalemia, as well as central nervous system and gastrointestinal complaints.[1,8]

The long-term use of other inotropic agents, such as sympathomimetic amines, is limited by a lack of oral forms and the development of drug tolerance.

In patients with diastolic dysfunction, the use of inotropic drugs is contraindicated.[4,7] Diuretics may reduce pulmonary congestion and peripheral edema, and calcium-channel blockers may be useful in cases of hypertension and hypertrophic cardiomyopathy.

While the use of β-adrenergic blockers is usually contraindicated in patients with significant systolic dysfunction, β blockade may be useful in counteracting the effects of excessive sympathetic stimulation. Recent studies have demonstrated a functional benefit with the use of β-adrenergic blockers, although a benefit in survival has not yet been found.[7]

Prognosis

The prognosis of patients with heart failure secondary to acute myocardial infarction has been related to their hemodynamic status. The Killip-Scheidt classification[15] is based on the physical examination findings: class I (no evidence of pulmonary edema or shock), class II (rales in less than one-half of lung fields), class III (rales in greater than one-half of lung fields; and class IV (cardiogenic shock with arterial systolic pressure greater than 90 mmHg). These hemodynamic classifications were modified by Forrester and colleagues[16] to include pulmonary capillary wedge pressure (PCWP) measurements: class I, no pulmonary edema (normal vital signs; PCWP, <18 mmHg), class II, isolated pulmonary edema (normal vital signs; PCWP, >18 mmHg), class III, isolated cardiogenic shock (hypotension; PCWP, <18 mmHg), and class IV, both pulmonary edema and cardiogenic shock (hypotension; PCWP, >18 mmHg).

TABLE 49-3 Treatment of Cardiogenic Pulmonary Edema[7]

- Oxygen
- Nitroglycerin, 0.4–0.6 mg sublingually q 5–10 min up to 4 times or 0.3–0.5 μg/kg/min IV infusion
- Furosemide 20–80 mg IV
- Morphine sulfate 1–5 mg IV, with caution in pulmonary insufficiency
- Cardiovascular supportive drugs: nitroprusside, dobutamine, dopamine
- Thrombolytic therapy or urgent revascularization if due to acute myocardial infarction
- CPAP, BiPAP, or intubation and mechanical ventilation if refractory
- Definitive repair of underlying anatomic cause if indicated and feasible

Unfortunately, heart failure is a progressive, fatal condition. In the absence of a correctable underlying cause, the prognosis of patients with CHF is poor, with a 5-year mortality rate of 50 percent.[1,4,5,11] Most of these deaths are due to development of refractory failure, although a large number of patients die suddenly, presumably of ventricular dysrhythmias. There is no evidence, however, that these fatal dysrhythmias can be prevented by the use of antiarrhythmic medications.

Recent studies have found that ACE inhibitors prolong survival in patients with heart failure and delay the onset of death in patients with impaired heart function.[1,8] Combined with β-adrenergic receptor blockers, these drugs may be helpful in prolonging the life of patients with heart disease at risk for developing heart failure.

PULMONARY EDEMA

Cardiogenic pulmonary edema is an acute, life-threatening form of left-sided heart failure.[1,4,7,8] Severe hypoxia can result in this condition due to the shunting of pulmonary blood flow to hypoventilated alveoli.

Treatment of Acute Pulmonary Edema

While attention must be given to potential precipitating causes, acute pulmonary edema is a life-threatening emergency that requires immediate improvement of systemic oxygenation. (See Table 49-3.)

OXYGENATION AND VENTILATION Oxygen (100%) should be given by mask and arterial blood gases obtained. The patient should be seated upright to pool systemic blood and reduce venous return. If hypoxia persists with supplemental oxygen, then positive pressure ventilation is required. Positive end-expiratory pressure (PEEP) applied via face mask as continuous positive airway pressure (CPAP) or bilevel continuous positive airway pressure (BiPAP) or via endotracheal tube can be used to prevent alveolar collapse.[8] Although impedance of venous return with PEEP via the endotracheal tube can be beneficial in reducing preload, care must be taken in using the lowest possible pressure in order to avoid compromising cardiac output. Noninvasive pressure support decreases the work of breathing, enhances oxygen and carbon dioxide exchange, and increases cardiac output. If hypercarbia and acidosis are also present, then endotracheal tube ventilation is warranted.[4,7]

VASODILATORS Nitrates are effective preload reducers. Nitroglycerin can be given by the sublingual, oral, topical, or intravenous routes.[4,7] For acute pulmonary edema, higher doses of sublingual nitroglycerin than those used in angina may be required (0.4 to 0.8 mg sublingually, 5 to 10 min × 4).[4] Intravenous administration of either nitroglycerin or sodium nitroprusside can rapidly reduce preload and afterload. Because nitroprusside has the potential to induce ischemia, intravenous nitroglycerin is preferred in the treatment of pulmonary edema in patients with coronary artery disease.[4] Infusion of nitroglycerin is safer with close hemodynamic monitoring. Dosing should begin at 0.3 to 0.5 (μg/kg)/min and titrated to relief of symptoms or until mean blood pressure falls 30 percent or systolic blood pressure below 90 mmHg.[1]

DIURETICS Intravenous furosemide (20 to 80 mg IV) can rapidly induce a potent diuresis.[7] These doses may be repeated in 10 to 15 min, and higher doses may be required in patients with renal failure.[8] Although furosemide can have a venodilatory effect, use of intravenous furosemide alone may not significantly lower preload until 30 min after administration.[17] In contrast, the combination of intravenous furosemide and nitrates can rapidly reduce preload.[13,17] In a recent randomized trial, the combination of intravenous high-dose isosorbide dinitrate with low-dose furosemide was more efficacious in the treatment of pulmonary edema than was low-dose isosorbide dinitrate with high-dose furosemide.[13]

The effects of furosemide may be augmented by pretreatment with metolazone (2.5 to 5 mg PO) or chlorothiazide (250 to 500 mg PO).[8] An alternative diuretic for patients with acute pulmonary edema is bumetanide (0.5 to 1.0 mg IV initially; double the dosage every 2 h to a total daily dose of 10 mg).[8]

INOTROPIC AGENTS In patients refractory to oxygen, nitrates, and diuretics, intravenously administered β-adrenergic agonists can be used to augment myocardial contractility.[4,7] *Dopamine* is particularly useful in the setting of pulmonary edema and hypotension.[4,7] At low doses (1 to 2 μg/kg/min), dopamine increases renal and mesenteric blood flow by stimulation of dopaminergic receptors. At moderate doses (2 to 10 μg/kg/min), dopamine increases myocardial contractility via β_1-adrenergic stimulation, and at high doses (more than 20 μg/kg/min), arterial pressure is elevated due to α-adrenergic stimulation.[4] *Dobutamine* at a dose of 2 to 20 μg/kg/min may produce a more favorable balance between myocardial oxygen supply and demand and is the choice for treatment of pulmonary edema in normotensive patients.[4] The administration of these drugs should be accompanied by close ECG and arterial pressure monitoring and may be optimized with pulmonary artery pressure recording. There is a minimal role for digitalis in the management of acute congestive heart failure.[4]

MORPHINE Morphine in doses of 1 to 5 mg IV decreases afterload and produces a sedative effect, thereby reducing cardiac work.[4,7] It should be given with caution to those with respiratory insufficiency and sustained respiratory acidosis.[4,18] The use of nitrates has supplanted the use of morphine in many instances.[19] Morphine's vasodilatory effects are in part due to histamine release, and it can cause potenthypotension.

PHLEBOTOMY Phlebotomy is a rapid, effective method of reducing circulating volume and may be particularly useful in the renal failure patient with acute pulmonary edema.[1] The practice of rotating tourniquets has not been found to be clinically beneficial.[20]

REFERENCES

1. Braunwald E: Heart failure, in Isselbacher KJ, Braunwald, K, Wilson TD, et al (eds): *Harrison's Principles of Internal Medicine,* 13th ed. New York, McGraw-Hill, 1994, pp 998–1009.
2. Cummings RO (ed): *Textbook of Advanced Cardiac Life Support.* Dallas, American Heart Association, 1997.
3. Kannel WB, Ho K, Thom T: Changing epidemiologic features of cardiac failure. *Br Heart J* 72(suppl):S3, 1994.
4. Cowie MR, Mosterd A, Wood DA, et al: The epidemiology of heart failure. *Eur Heart J* 18:208, 1997.
5. Centers for Disease Control and Prevention: Mortality from congestive heart failure: United States, 1980–1990. *MMWR* 43:77, 1994.
6. Carson P, Johnson G, Fletcher R, et al: Mild systolic dysfunction in heart failure: Baseline characteristics and response to therapy in the Vasodilator in Heart Failure Trials (V-HeFT). *J Am Coll Cardiol* 27:642, 1996.
7. ACC/AHA Task Force: Guidelines for the evaluation and management of heart failure: A report of the American College of Cardiology/American Heart Association Task Force on Practice Guidelines (Committee on Evaluation and Management of Heart Failure). *Circulation* 92:2764, 1995.
8. Pennington J, Jouriles N: *Clinical review: Heart failure.* Denver, Micromedex, 1998. (Micromedex Health Care Series, vol 98.)
9. Konstam M, Dracup K, Baker D, et al: *Heart Failure: Management of Patients with Left Ventricular Systolic Dysfunction.* Rockville, MD, Agency for Health Care Policy and Management Public Health Service, United States Department of Health and Human Services, June 1994. (Quick Reference Guide for Clinicians, 11, AHCPR Publication 94-0613.)
10. Bonow RO, Udelson JE: Left ventricular diastolic dysfunction as a cause of congestive heart failure: Mechanisms and management. *Ann Intern Med* 117:502, 1992.
11. Katz AM: Cardiomyopathy of overload: A major determinant of prognosis in congestive heart failure. *N Engl J Med* 322:100, 1992.
12. Packer M: The neurohormonal hypothesis: A theory to explain the mechanism of disease progression in heart failure. *J Am Coll Cardiol* 20:248, 1992.
13. Cotter G, Metzkor E, Kaluski E, et al: Randomized trial of high-dose isosorbide dinitrate plus low-dose isosorbide dinitrate in severe pulmonary oedema. *Lancet* 351:389, 1998.
14. Northridge D: Furosemide or nitrates for acute heart failure? *Lancet* 347:667, 1998.
15. Scheidt S, Wilner G, Fillmore S, et al: Objective haemodynamic assessment after acute myocardial infarction. *Br Heart J* 35:908, 1973.
16. Forrester JS, Diamond GA, Swan HJC: Correlative classification of clinical and hemodynamic function after acute myocardial infarction. *Am J Cardiol* 39:137, 1977.
17. Kraus PA, Lipman J, Becker PJ: Acute preload effects of furosemide. *Chest* 98:124, 1990.
18. Hoffman JR, Reynolds S: Comparison of nitroglycerin, morphine and furosemide in treatment of presumed prehospital pulmonary edema. *Chest* 92:586, 1987.
19. Beltrame JF, Zeitz CJ, Unger SA, et al: Nitrate therapy is an alternative to furosemide/morphine therapy in the management of acute pulmonary edema. *J Card Fail* 4:271–279, 1998.
20. Francis GS: Rotating tourniquets for acute cardiogenic pulmonary edema. *JAMA* 274:1192, 1995.
21. Coday A, Vikram J, Fifer MA: Heart failure, in Lilly LS (ed): *Pathophysiology of Heart Disease: A Collaborative Project of Students and Faculty.* Malvern, PA, Lea and Febiger, 1993, p 159.

VALVULAR EMERGENCIES AND ENDOCARDITIS

David M. Cline

Ninety percent of valvular disease is chronic, with decades between the onset of the structural abnormality and symptoms. The emergency physician most commonly encounters patients with valvular disease after the diagnosis has been made but is occasionally the first to suspect valvular dysfunction based on the patient's symptoms and examination. Through chronic adaptation by dilation and hypertrophy, cardiac function can be preserved for years, which may delay the diagnosis for one to two decades until a murmur is detected on auscultation. In contrast to the more common chronic presentations, acute rupture of a cardiac valve presents with dramatic symptoms.

The four heart valves prevent retrograde flow of blood during the cardiac cycle, allowing efficient ejection of blood with each contraction of the ventricles. The mitral valve has two cusps, while the other three heart valves normally have three cusps. The right and left papillary muscles promote effective closure of the tricuspid and mitral valves, respectively. The papillary muscles are attached to the cusps of the atrioventricular valves by tendinous cords, the chordae tendineae. Abnormalities of the valvular cusps, the papillary muscles, the chordae tendineae, or the cardiac chambers themselves can cause valvular dysfunction.

The pathophysiology of and clinical findings for each of the classic valvular disorders are presented below. Following these descriptions, the treatment of the disorders is presented collectively. When important differences occur in the indicated management, these recommendations are contrasted and explained.

MITRAL STENOSIS

Pathophysiology

Despite its declining frequency, rheumatic heart disease is still the most common cause of mitral valve stenosis. Scarring from rheumatic endocarditis causes fusion of the commissures and matting of the chordae tendineae, which interfere with valve closure. Calcification over time makes the valve less mobile. Progressive stenosis may lead to pulmonary hypertension, which may signal the need for surgery. The majority of patients eventually develop atrial fibrillation because of progressive dilation of the atria. Pulmonary hypertension may lead to pulmonary and tricuspid valve incompetence.

Clinical Features

Even though mitral stenosis is a chronic condition, increased demands on cardiac output may precipitate acute symptoms. Conditions that prompt symptoms in mitral stenosis include exertion, tachycardia, anemia, pregnancy, infection, emotional upset, and atrial fibrillation. As with all valvular diseases, exertional dyspnea is the most common presenting symptom (80 percent of patients with mitral stenosis). Paroxysmal nocturnal dyspnea may occur with more severe disease. Hemoptysis is the second most common presenting symptom and may be massive if a bronchial vein ruptures. Other common symptoms and signs include orthopnea, premature atrial contractions, and atrial fibrillation, which is almost inevitable with the passage of time. Systemic emboli may occur and result in myocardial, kidney, central nervous system, or peripheral infarction. Embolic stroke is more frequent in the presence of atrial fibrillation. As the disease progresses, symptoms of right heart failure may develop.

Signs of mitral stenosis include middiastolic rumbling murmur, with crescendo toward the S_2. With the onset of atrial fibrillation the presystolic accentuation of the murmur disappears. Typically the S_1 is loud and is followed by a loud opening "snap" that is high-pitched and heard best at the right of the apex. A prominent *a* wave in the neck may be seen, as may an early systolic parasternal lift, which is due to right heart pressure overload. The apical impulse is small and tapping, representing an underfilled left ventricle. Systemic blood pressure is typically normal or low. Rales may be heard at the lung bases as the disease progresses. If pulmonary hypertension is present, signs may include a thin body habitus, peripheral cyanosis, and cool extremities because of low cardiac output. With pulmonary hypertension the auscultatory findings are less evident.

The electrocardiogram (ECG) may demonstrate notched or diphasic P waves and right axis deviation. On the chest radiograph, straightening of the left heart border, indicating left atrial enlargement, is a typical early radiographic finding. Eventually, findings of pulmonary congestion are noted: redistribution of flow to the upper lung fields, Kerley B lines, and an increase in vascular markings. The chest radiograph is useful in assessing the degree of pulmonary congestion.

MITRAL INCOMPETENCE

Pathophysiology

Infective endocarditis or myocardial infarction can cause acute rupture of the chordae tendineae or papillary muscles or cause perforation of the valve leaflets. Inferior myocardial infarction due to right coronary occlusion is the most common cause of ischemic mitral valve incompetence. Rarely, trauma may cause acute mitral incompetence. Patients with acute mitral valve rupture deteriorate rapidly. Intermittent mitral incompetence can be due to ischemia, which causes papillary muscle dysfunction. Rheumatic heart disease is the most common cause of chronic mitral incompetence. Recently, an association has been found between the use of appetite suppressant drugs (fenfluramine and phentermine, or dexfenfluramine) and cardiac valve incompetence,[1] although this has been questioned.[2]

Acute regurgitation into a noncompliant left atrium quickly elevates pressures and causes pulmonary edema. In contrast, in the chronic state the left atrium dilates so that left atrial pressure rises little, even with a large regurgitant flow. As an adaptation, the total stroke volume of the left ventricle increases so that effective forward flow into the aorta is maintained despite the large regurgitant volume across the mitral valve.

Clinical Features

Acute mitral incompetence presents with dyspnea, tachycardia, and pulmonary edema. Usually an S_3 and S_4 will be heard. Acutely, the harsh apical systolic murmur starts with S_1 and may end before S_2. Patients may quickly deteriorate to cardiogenic shock or cardiac arrest. Intermittent mitral incompetence usually presents with acute episodes of respiratory distress due to pulmonary edema and can be asymptomatic between attacks. The pronounced dyspnea may mask angina that accompanies the ischemia. Patients may have an active apical impulse, systolic thrust, and thrill at the apex. Jugular venous distention may be seen, with a prominent *a* wave and a left parasternal lift. The ECG may show evidence of acute inferior wall infarction (more common than anterior wall infarction in this setting). On the chest radiograph, acute mitral incompetence from papillary muscle rupture may result in a minimally enlarged left atrium and pulmonary edema, with less cardiac enlargement than expected.

Chronic mitral incompetence may be tolerated for years or even decades. The first symptom is usually exertional dyspnea, sometimes prompted by atrial fibrillation. If patients are not anticoagulated, systemic emboli occur in 20 percent and are often asymptomatic. Endocarditis is still a feared complication. Signs of chronic mitral incompetence include a late systolic left parasternal lift. There is a high-pitched holosystolic murmur that is best heard in the fifth intercostal space, mid left thorax, which radiates to the axilla. The first heart sound is soft and often obscured by the murmur. An S_3 is usually heard and is followed by a short diastolic rumble, indicating increased flow into the left ventricle. The ECG may demonstrate findings of left atrial and left ventricular hypertrophy (LVH). On the chest radiograph, chronic mitral incompetence produces left ventricular and atrial enlargement that is proportional to the severity of the regurgitant volume.

MITRAL VALVE PROLAPSE

Pathophysiology

The etiology of mitral valve prolapse (MVP), or the click-murmur syndrome, is not known but may be congenital. MVP is the most common valvular heart disease in industrialized countries, affecting about 3 percent of the population.[3] One or both of the mitral valve leaflets prolapse into the atrium during systole, and this may or may not be accompanied by regurgitant flow. Male sex, age over 45, and the presence of regurgitation, recognized clinically by a short diastolic murmur, places the patient in a higher risk group for complications.[4] Click-murmur syndrome has unique symptoms that differentiate it from other forms of mitral regurgitation.

Clinical Features

Most patients are asymptomatic. Symptoms include atypical chest pain, palpitations, fatigue, and dyspnea unrelated to exertion. Symptoms are more common in those who know they have the syndrome. However, there is an increased incidence of sudden death and dysrhythmias in patients with MVP. There is also an increased incidence of transient ischemic attacks under the age of 45. In patients with MVP without mitral regurgitation at rest, exercise provokes mitral regurgitation in 32 percent of patients and predicts a higher risk for morbid events.[5] The classic cardiac finding is a midsystolic click. The second heart sound may be diminished by the late systolic murmur, with crescendos into S_2 (not present in all patients). Some patients may have pectus excavatum, a straight thoracic spine, or scoliosis. The ECG is usually normal, as is the chest radiograph unless the thoracic cage abnormalities described above are seen.

AORTIC STENOSIS

Pathophysiology

Congenital heart disease is the most common cause of aortic stenosis, with the presence of a bicuspid valve accounting for 50 percent of cases. Rheumatic heart disease is the second most common cause, followed by degenerative heart disease or calcific aortic stenosis, which is the most common cause in patients over age 70. Blood flow into the aorta is obstructed, producing progressive LVH and low cardiac output. This produces a marked reduction in coronary blood flow.

Clinical Features

The classic triad is dyspnea, chest pain, and syncope. Exercise may induce acute symptoms. Symptoms appear late in the course of the disease. In active persons, the symptoms appear more rapidly. Dyspnea is usually the first symptom, followed by paroxysmal nocturnal dyspnea, syncope on exertion, angina, and myocardial infarction. Atrial fibrillation is less common than in mitral disease, but 10 percent of patients have atrial fibrillation at time of surgery. With isolated aortic stenosis, endocarditis occurs in only 2 percent of patients.

The most common signs include a pulse of small amplitude. The carotid pulse can be most accurately assessed and is found to have a slow rate of increase. Blood pressure is normal or low, with a narrow pulse pressure. LVH is common. There is paradoxic splitting of S_2, and S_3 and S_4 are commonly present. Classically, there is a harsh systolic ejection murmur that is best heard in the second right intercostal space and that radiates to the right carotid artery. Brachioradial delay is an important finding in aortic stenosis. The examiner palpates simultaneously the right brochial artery of the patient with the thumb and the right radial artery of the patient with the middle or index finger. Any palpable delay between the brachial artery and radial artery is considered abnormal.[6] Sudden death, usually from an dysrhythmia, occurs in 25 percent of patients. The ECG usually demonstrates criteria for LVH and, in 10 percent of patients, left or right bundle branch block. The chest radiograph is normal early, but eventually LVH and findings of congestive heart failure are evident if the patient does not have valve replacement.

AORTIC INCOMPETENCE

Pathophysiology

In 20 percent of patients, the cause of aortic incompetence is acute in nature. Infective endocarditis accounts for the majority of acute cases; aortic dissection at the aortic root causes the remainder. In acute cases, a sudden increase in backflow of blood into the ventricle raises left ventricular end-diastolic pressure, which may cause acute heart failure. Increased ventricular pressure elevates pressure in the left atrium, and pulmonary congestion results. Rheumatic heart disease and congenital disease cause the majority of chronic cases. Syphilis, ankylosing spondylitis, and Reiter syndrome are less frequent causes. An association between the appetite-suppressant drugs (fenfluramine and phentermine or dexfenfluramine) has also been found for aortic incompetence.[2] Chronic disease is more common in males than in females, with a ratio of 3:2. In chronic disease, the ventricle progressively dilates to accommodate the regurgitant blood volume. Wide pulse pressures result from the fall in diastolic pressure, and marked peripheral vasodilation is seen. During exercise and tachycardia, the diastolic filling period shortens, thus decreasing the number of times per minute that regurgitation can occur. Cardiac function is therefore close to normal with exercise early in the course of the disease. In contrast, isometric exercise or stress may precipitate symptoms.

Clinical Features

In acute disease, dyspnea is the most common presenting symptom, seen in 50 percent of patients. Many patients have acute pulmonary edema with pink frothy sputum. Patients may complain of fever and chills if endocarditis is the cause. Patients may present with systemic emboli or a persistent sinus tachycardia. Dissection of the ascending aorta typically produces a ''tearing'' chest pain that may radiate between the shoulder blades. Sudden death is common in patients with both acute and chronic aortic incompetence.

The two major causes of acute aortic incompetence present with different signs. Elevated temperature is common with acute endocarditis. ECG changes may be seen with aortic dissection, including ischemia or findings of acute inferior myocardial infarction, suggesting involvement of the right coronary artery. Patients commonly have signs of peripheral circulatory collapse, such as sweating, marked tachycardia, tachypnea, and rales. Classically there is a high-pitched blowing diastolic murmur heard immediately after S_2, best heard in the right second or third intercostal parasternal area. There may be an S_3 with long diastolic murmurs, and there may be a systolic flow murmur. In the acute state, the chest radiograph demonstrates acute pulmonary edema with less cardiac enlargement than expected.

In the chronic state, about one-third of patients have palpitations associated with a large stroke volume and/or premature ventricular contractions. Frequently these sensations are noticed in bed. Patients may complain of stabbing chest pain, fatigue, or dyspnea. Two-thirds of patients have no symptoms for up to 20 years despite a hemodynamically significant lesion, defined as a diastolic blood pressure under 70 mmHg. Symptoms of left ventricular failure may occur late in the course of the disease and include dyspnea, pulmonary edema, ischemic chest pain, and sweating.

In the chronic state, signs include a wide pulse pressure with a prominent ventricular impulse, which may be manifested as head bobbing. ''Water hammer pulse'' may be noted; this is a peripheral pulse that has a quick rise in upstroke followed by a peripheral collapse. Other classic findings may include accentuated precordial apical thrust, pulsus biferiens, Duroziez sign (a to-and-fro femoral murmur), and Quincke pulse (capillary pulsations visible at the proximal nailbed, while pressure is applied at the tip). In chronic aortic incompetence, the ECG demonstrates LVH, and the chest radiograph shows LVH, aortic dilation, and possibly evidence of congestive heart failure.

HYPERTROPHIC CARDIOMYOPATHY (IDIOPATHIC HYPERTROPHIC SUBAORTIC STENOSIS)

Hypertrophic cardiomyopathy (HCM) is known by other terms, including idiopathic hypertrophic subaortic stenosis and asymmetrical septal hypertrophy. This disorder is best described as *hypertrophic cardiomyopathy* and is defined by a hypertrophied, nondilated left ventricle. In 95 percent of cases, the septum is asymmetrically enlarged, but the free wall of the ventricle is also hypertrophied. The atrium is typically enlarged, and the mitral valve is thickened. Only one-fourth of patients with this disorder have a ventricular outflow obstruction sufficient to cause symptoms; therefore, *idiopathic hypertrophic subaortic stenosis* incompletely describes this disorder. This disease is discussed in Chapter 51, ''Cardiomyopathies, Myocarditis, and Pericardial Disease," and is mentioned here only to aid in its differentiation from valvular aortic stenosis.

Clinical Features

Patients with HCM may become symptomatic at any age, but most present between age 30 and 40 years, approximately 10 years earlier than the average of onset of symptomatic valvular aortic stenosis. Symptoms are similar to those of aortic stenosis, except that the patient with HCM may report that symptoms are relieved with squatting.

Signs may be absent in this disease. The classic auscultatory finding is a crescendo-decrescendo harsh systolic murmur heard best at the fifth left intercostal space, mid left thorax, which radiates to the lower left sternal border. The Valsalva maneuver intensifies the murmur by decreasing venous return, which contracts the left ventricle and increases the obstruction. Squatting and passive leg elevation diminish the murmur. Listening at the apex, one can hear an increased murmur as the patient goes from a squatting to a standing postion, due to decreased venous return from pooling. There is no opening snap, as is commonly heard in valvular aortic stenosis. The apical impulse may be double secondary to an abrupt interruption of early systolic ejection by the asymmetrical septum, which blocks outflow, as the ventricle contracts. The pulse has a brisk rise and a double peak, unlike valvular aortic stenosis, in which the pulse has a slow rise and a sustained single peak.

HCM is one cause of sudden death among athletes, and all patients are at significant risk. The mechanism of sudden death is not well understood and is probably due to several mechanisms, including dysrhythmias and massive myocardial infarction. Patients with HCM are at risk for endocarditis, usually involving the thickened mitral valve. Antibiotic prophylaxis is recommended for certain procedures performed in the emergency department (Table 50-1).

RIGHT-SIDED VALVULAR HEART DISEASE

Pathophysiology

Right-sided valvular heart disease is much less common than left-sided valvular disease. Drug users with endocarditis due to aggressive organisms, such as *Staphylococcus aureus,* are the largest group of patients with isolated tricuspid disease. Right ventricular failure with dilation may lead to tricuspid incompetence. Rheumatic heart disease may affect more than one valve, and tricuspid disease is frequently seen in conjunction with left-sided valvular disease. Rarely, blunt trauma can lead to tricuspid incompetence.

Pulmonary incompetence is most commonly due to pulmonary hypertension, and symptoms of pulmonary hypertension dominate the clinical picture. The most common cause of pulmonary stenosis is congenital tetralogy of Fallot, which is usually corrected surgically in infancy.

Clinical Features

The most common presenting symptoms of right-sided valvular disease are dyspnea and orthopnea. Because of the organisms involved, patients presenting with tricuspid incompetence in association with endocarditis are acutely ill with sepsis. As the disease progresses, signs of right-sided heart failure are evident: jugular venous distention with a prominent *a* wave, peripheral edema, hepatomegaly, splenomegaly, and ascites.

In tricuspid incompetence, the murmur is soft blowing, holosystolic, and best heard along the lower left sternal border. In tricuspid stenosis, the rumbling crescendo- decrescendo diastolic murmur occurs

TABLE 50–1 Prophylaxis for Infective Endocarditis

Procedure	Standard Regimen*	Alternative Regimen
Dental procedure known to cause bleeding	Amoxicillin 2.0 g PO 1 h before procedure or Ampicillin 2.0 g IV or IM 30 min before procedure	Clindamycin 600 mg PO 1 h before procedure or Cephalexin 2.0 g PO 1 h before procedure or Cefadroxil 2.0 g PO 1 h before procedure or Azithromycin 500 mg PO 1 h before procedure or Clarithromycin 500 mg PO 1 before procedure
Urethral catheterization if infection is present Urethral dilation	Ampicillin 2.0 g IV or IM plus gentamicin 1.5 mg/kg IV or IM (not to exceed 120 mg) 30 min before procedure followed by half the original dose of ampicillin	Vancomycin 1.0 g IV over 1 h plus gentamicin 1.5 mg/kg IV or IM (not to exceed 120 mg), complete infusion within 30 min of starting procedure; for moderate-risk patients, amoxicillin 2 g PO 1 h before procedure
Incision and drainage of infected tissue	Cefazolin 1.0 g IV or IM 30 min before procedure or Cephalexin 2.0 g PO 1 h before procedure or Cefadroxil 2.0 g PO 1 h before procedure	Vancomycin 1.0 g IV over 1 h plus gentamicin 1.5 mg/kg IV or IM (not to exceed 120 mg), complete infusion within 30 min of starting procedure

*Includes patients with prosthetic heart valves and others at high risk. Initial pediatric doses are as follows: amoxicillin 50 mg/kg, ampicillin 50 mg/kg, cephalixin 50 mg/kg, cefadroxil 50 mg/kg, azithromycin 15 mg/kg, clarithromycin 15 mg/kg, clindamycin 20 mg/kg, gentamicin 2 mg/kg, and vancomycin 20 mg/kg. Pediatric dose should not exceed listed adult dose.

Abbreviations: IM, intramuscularly; IV, intravenously; PO, per os (by mouth, orally).

just prior to S_1. This murmur is best heard along the lower left sternal border.

MULTIVALVULAR DISEASE

Multivalvular disease is common, but the presence of more than one abnormal valve makes the diagnosis of others more difficult. In addition, there may be coexisting stenosis and incompetence of diseased valves. Multivalvular and combined stenotic-incompetent valvular disease present with slightly different symptoms from the classic symptoms of single-valve disease.

Pathophysiology

Rheumatic heart disease remains an important cause of combined aortic and mitral disease. Between 32 and 50 percent of patients with cardiac manifestations of rheumatic fever have both aortic and mitral disease. In aged patients, calcification can lead to both aortic stenosis and mitral incompetence. Infective endocarditis can extend from either the mitral or aortic valve to the adjacent valve though the inflammatory process. Intravenous drug users may have multivalvular disease. Tricuspid regurgitation often occurs with right ventricular dilation secondary to pulmonary hypertension that may be due to mitral disease or combined aortic and mitral disease.

Clinical Features

Patients with combined valvular disease generally present at a younger age than those with a single chronic lesion. The most common symptom of combined valvular disease is dyspnea. Symptoms of multivalvular disease may resemble those of single-valve disease when advanced disease of one valve dominates the clinical picture. Although both syncope and angina pectoris are infrequent in patients with mitral regurgitation alone, chest pain and syncope are more common with incompetence of both the aortic and mitral valves. The presence of a chronic lesion of one valve exaggerates the effects of an acute lesion of another valve.

Physical signs are more difficult to interpret in mixed lesions. With combined aortic and mitral stenosis, the aortic systolic murmur is reduced. The mitral opening snap is infrequently audible in this setting. In regurgitant lesions of both aortic and mitral valves, the usual fall in diastolic blood pressure commonly seen with aortic incompetence may be absent. As many as 40 percent of patients with this combined valvular disease have diastolic blood pressures above 70 mmHg.

DIAGNOSIS OF VALVULAR HEART DISEASE

The loud background noise in the emergency department makes the accurate auscultation of subtle murmurs difficult. Despite this, the emergency physician may suspect undiagnosed valvular dysfunction on incidental cardiac auscultation. The ECG and chest radiograph may be of help, but neither is confirmatory. The suspected diagnosis should be confirmed by echocardiography and/or consultation with a cardiologist. Transesophageal echocardiography yields a more complete analysis of valvular dysfunction, especially for the mitral valve. However, transthoracic echocardiography is generally performed first.[7] The urgency for an accurate diagnosis and appropriate referral depends on the severity of symptoms and the suspected diagnosis. For example, a patient presenting with syncope and auscultatory findings of aortic stenosis should be admitted to the hospital for observation and further evaluation.

DIAGNOSING A NEWLY DISCOVERED MURMUR The first step in diagnosing a newly discovered murmur is to consider it in the context of the patient's medical condition. Patients with normal cardiac anatomy may have murmurs associated with anemia, thyrotoxicosis, sepsis, fever, renal failure with volume overload, pregnancy, and other clinical conditions. A diastolic murmur or a new murmur associated with symptoms at rest should always be considered abnormal and warrants referral for a workup and possible echocardiographic study and admission. Figure 50-1 presents an algorithm for the clinical assessment of a newly discovered systolic murmur. The algorithm, based on the work of Etchells and colleagues,[8] presents a step-by-step method of assessment to uncover an abnormal murmur. Each murmur category lists characteristics or maneuvers that have been shown to predict the presence of the named abnormal murmurs. The studies referred to by Etchells and colleagues have used cardiologists as examiners, and these issues have not been tested in the emergency department setting. However, the algorithm can be expected to prompt the clinician to perform the appropriate examinations and maneuvers to help uncover an abnormal murmur. Whenever the clinician is uncertain of the diagnosis of a newly discovered murmur, referral should be made to a cardiologist or back to the primary care physician for an appropriate workup.

A truly innocent (physiologic) murmur is associated with no abnormal symptoms or signs. The soft systolic ejection murmur begins after S_1 and ends before S_2, and the heart sounds are completely normal. The review of systems should elicit no symptoms compatible with cardiovascular disease, and findings upon complete physical examination are normal with the exception of the flow murmur.

Acute mitral and aortic incompetence are important and urgent diagnoses. Due to the severity of symptoms, it is unlikely that such a patient would go unnoticed in the emergency department, but the patient may be admitted with the murmur unrecognized. Acute mitral or aortic incompetence should always be suspected in patients with acute pulmonary edema, especially when the heart is smaller than expected on the chest radiograph or when the patient does not respond to conventional therapy. When aortic dissection is suspected as the cause of acute aortic incompetence and the patient is sufficiently stable, transesophageal echocardiography or computed tomographic (CT) scanning of the chest is useful. Angiography may still be required after CT scanning.

In infants, a newly diagnosed murmur demands the consideration of congenital heart disease, such as ventricular septal defect, atrial septal defect, and pulmonic stenosis in association with tetralogy of Fallot. See Chapter 115, ''Heart Disease,'' for a more detailed discussion of congenital heart disease in children.

EMERGENCY DEPARTMENT CARE OF SYMPTOMATIC VALVULAR HEART DISEASE

There is little that the emergency physician can do to change the structural abnormality of the diseased cardiac valve. The exception to this rule is acute mitral incompetence due to myocardial infarction. The infusion of thrombolytic therapy may reestablish blood flow to the papillary muscle, with restoration of function.[9] The alternative to thrombolytic therapy is coronary angioplasty.[10] The majority of treatments are directed toward symptomatic relief of the manifestations of valvular disease. However, there are certain medical treatments that can reduce the consequences of the mechanical defect. The regurgitation of aortic and mitral incompetence may be lessened by reducing afterload. When the cause of mitral incompetence is myocardial ischemia, regurgitation can be lessened by treatment with nitrates.

Pulmonary edema should be treated with oxygen, intubation for failing respiratory effort, diuretics, and nitrates if tolerated. Patients with aortic stenosis usually have normal-to-low blood pressure and do not tolerate afterload reducers. In contrast, patients with mitral incompetence or aortic incompetence can benefit from intravenous nitroprusside or nitroglycerin even with normal blood pressures.[11] Reducing afterload helps to reduce regurgitation and relieve pulmonary edema. Tachycardia reduces the regurgitant volume by reducing the time during the cardiac cycle during which backflow may occur.

FIG. 50-1. Algorithm for workup of newly discovered systolic murmur.

Listen for a murmur in the second right intercostal space that radiates to the right carotid artery and determine:

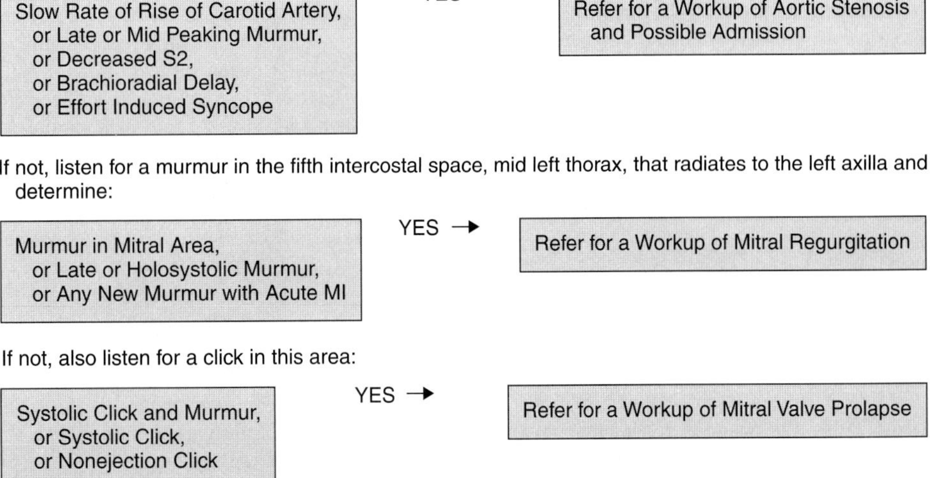
Slow Rate of Rise of Carotid Artery,
or Late or Mid Peaking Murmur,
or Decreased S2,
or Brachioradial Delay,
or Effort Induced Syncope
YES →
Refer for a Workup of Aortic Stenosis and Possible Admission
If not, listen for a murmur in the fifth intercostal space, mid left thorax, that radiates to the left axilla and determine:
Murmur in Mitral Area,
or Late or Holosystolic Murmur,
or Any New Murmur with Acute MI
YES →
Refer for a Workup of Mitral Regurgitation
If not, also listen for a click in this area:
Systolic Click and Murmur,
or Systolic Click,
or Nonejection Click
YES →
Refer for a Workup of Mitral Valve Prolapse

If not, listen for a murmur in the fifth intercostal space, mid left thorax that radiates to the lower left sternal border and determine:

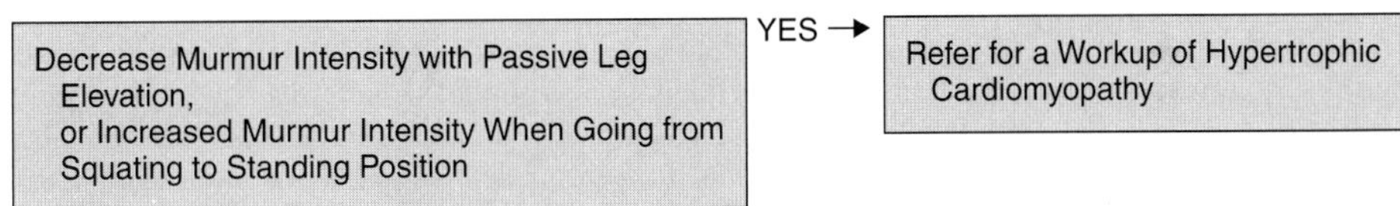
Decrease Murmur Intensity with Passive Leg Elevation,
or Increased Murmur Intensity When Going from Squating to Standing Position
YES →
Refer for a Workup of Hypertrophic Cardiomyopathy

If not, listen for a murmur in the lower left sternal border that radiates to the lower right sternal border and determine:

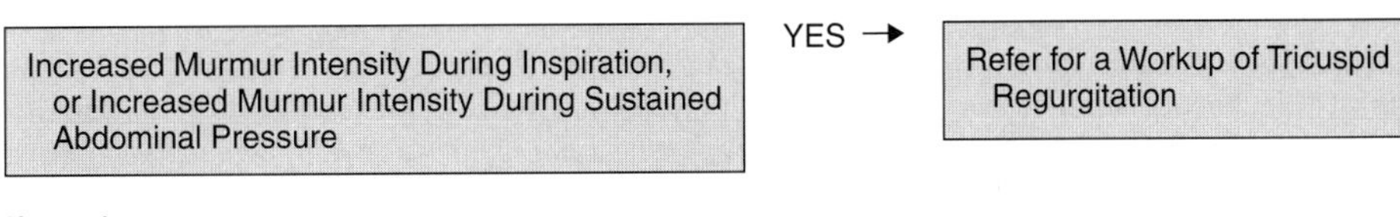
Increased Murmur Intensity During Inspiration,
or Increased Murmur Intensity During Sustained Abdominal Pressure
YES →
Refer for a Workup of Tricuspid Regurgitation

If not, then:

Refer to a Family Physician to Follow Murmur

Therefore, artificially lowering the pulse with a β-blocking agent may worsen symptoms.

The hypertension associated with aortic dissection should be controlled with intravenous nitroprusside and β blockade. Labetalol has been used with success in this setting. Patients with valvular heart disease and acute pulmonary edema should be considered for Swan-Ganz catheter insertion. The presence of valvular disease, especially stenosis, may complicate the procedure of catheter insertion. In patients who do not respond to medical management, intraaortic balloon counterpulsation should be considered. However, this is contraindicated in wide-open aortic regurgitation.

Rapid atrial fibrillation, which may precipitate symptoms in patients with silent valvular disease, should be rate-controlled with intravenous diltiazem or digoxin. Intravenous propranolol or verapamil may be considered, but their negative inotropic action may cause more problems. Emergency cardioversion may be needed in severely compromised patients, but dysrhythmia recurrence is common. The most common cause of the dysrhythmia in valvular heart disease, a dilated atrium, remains unchanged by cardioversion. The danger of embolization is greater in patients with atrial fibrillation.

Hemoptysis associated with valvular heart disease most frequently accompanies pulmonary edema and is frothy pink. This form of hemoptysis does not in and of itself require treatment. However, if pulmonary hypertension is present, gross hemoptysis may occur from the rupture of distended bronchial veins. Mitral stenosis is the most frequent valvular heart disease associated with hemoptysis, which can be severe enough to require blood transfusion and emergency surgery.

In the event of embolization, anticoagulation should be undertaken with intravenous heparin as long as there is no evidence of central nervous system bleeding. Anticoagulation is especially needed in the setting of atrial fibrillation.

Emergency surgery should be considered in all cases of acute symptomatic valvular disease.[12] Because stenotic lesions are slowly progressive, emergency surgery is rarely needed for stenotic defects. However, a patient with new onset of syncope in association with aortic stenosis should be considered for urgent repair. The need for emergency surgery most commonly accompanies acute regurgitant lesions of the mitral or aortic valves. Patients are acutely ill and present considerable surgical risks. The urgency of these two acute regurgitant lesions leaves little time for intubation, intravenous afterload reducers, echocardiography, and assembling the surgical team for emergency valve replacement.

Patients with acute fevers should be suspected of having infective endocarditis. The evaluation and management of endocarditis are discussed below, under ''Infective Endocarditis.'' Antibiotic prophylaxis for infective endocarditis is recommended during procedures that may produce bacteremia in patients at risk for developing endocarditis, and the American Heart Association guidelines, which were revised in

1997, should be followed.[13] Patients considered at risk include those with a prosthetic heart valve, a history of endocarditis, rheumatic heart disease, acquired and congenital valvular disease, idiopathic hypertrophic subaortic stenosis, mitral valve prolapse with a murmur, or surgically constructed pulmonary shunts or conduits. The common procedures performed by emergency physicians that require prophylaxis are listed in Table 50-1. Endotracheal intubation does not require antibiotic prophylaxis. When a febrile patient is being evaluated for urinary tract infection, emergency physicians should consider the need for prophylaxis before using a catheter to obtain a urine specimen. However, recent data from an epidemiologic study suggest that medical and dental procedures cause only 5 percent of endocarditis cases and prophylaxis does not prevent all cases.[13]

Admission Considerations

The presence of persistent symptoms in patients with valvular heart disease determines the indications for admission to the hospital. Patients with acute onset of valvular incompetence are acutely ill and require admission. This should be clinically obvious. Patients with aortic stenosis presenting with syncope on exertion should be considered for admission because of the critical limitation of blood flow that syncope usually heralds. Patients with valvular heart disease and a new symptomatic dysrhythmia should also be considered for admission. Considerations for admission of patients with suspected infective endocarditis are discussed later in this chapter. Patients with intermittent symptoms from valvular heart disease can be management dilemmas. Consultation with a cardiologist may be required to determine the need for hospital admission.

Discharge Instructions

Stable patients suspected of having valvular heart disease not previously diagnosed should be referred to a cardiologist or back to their private physician for an evaluation and possible echocardiographic study. Patients should be instructed to avoid strenuous exercise and work, and psychologically stress-provoking activity until they have been cleared for such activity by the referral physician.

PROSTHETIC VALVE DISEASE

Prosthetic valves are implanted in 40,000 patients per year in the United States. There are approximately 80 types of artificial valves, each with advantages and disadvantages. Patients who receive prosthetic valves are instructed to carry a descriptive card in their wallet. The prosthetic valves can be divided into two basic groups: mechanical, nontissue models and bioprostheses using porcine, bovine, or human valves. Complications of prosthetic valves are more common in patients who have advanced heart disease, including cardiac dilation, LVH congestive heart failure, or dysrhythmias, at the time of their original operation.

Pathophysiology

Prosthetic valves tend to be slightly stenotic, and a very small amount of regurgitation is common because of incomplete closure. Patients with mechanical valves require continuous anticoagulation. Some bioprostheses do not require anticoagulation. Several complications can lead to dysfunction of artificial valves. Thrombi can form on a prosthetic valve and become large enough to obstruct flow or prevent closure. The dysfunction due to thrombi can be acute or slowly progressive. Bioprostheses may gradually degenerate, undergoing gradual thinning, stiffening, and possibly tearing, which result in valvular incompetence. The sutures that secure the prosthetic valve may become disrupted, leading to paravalvular regurgitation as a fistula forms at the periphery of the valve. Mechanical models may suddenly fracture or fail. These failures usually bring sudden symptoms and often are fatal before corrective surgery can be accomplished.

Bleeding and systemic embolism originating from a thrombus on the prosthetic valve are the most important complications of mechanical heart valves, occurring at a rate of 1.4 percent and 1 percent per year, respectively, for patients on warfarin. Life-long anticoagulation is required to reduce the risk of thromboembolism and valve thrombosis. The optimal anticoagulation regimen is controversial, with disagreement concerning the intensity of warfarin therapy as well as the need for an antiplatelet agent. Embolism is more common after mitral valve replacement. Embolism occurs less frequently with bioprostheses, and bleeding complications depend on the therapy given.

Patients with artificial valves develop endocarditis at a rate of 0.5 percent per year. Infections occur more frequently during the first 2 months after operation. The most common organisms during this period are *Staphylococcus epidermidis* and *S. aureus*. Gram-negative organisms and fungi are also frequent causes of endocarditis during this early period. Late cases of endocarditis are similar to those affecting native valves. The most frequent organism is *Streptococcus viridans,* but *Serratia* and *Pseudomonas* also occur. Patients with prosthetic valves and endocarditis may develop a ring abscess around the valve, which requires valve replacement. Patients with mechanical prostheses have an increased rate of intravascular destruction of red blood cells. Usually the red blood cell loss is easily corrected by the bone marrow, but hemolytic anemia may be severe and indicate a paravalvular leak. Finally, patients with prosthetic valves may be particularly susceptible to hemodynamic compromise from a new arrhythmia, such as atrial fibrillation.

Clinical Features

Many patients have persistent dyspnea and reduced effort tolerance after successful valve replacement. This is more common in the presence of preexisting heart dysfunction or atrial fibrillation. Many symptoms of valvular dysfunction described in the preceding sections on specific valvular disease may occur in the setting of prosthetic valves. However, in addition to those symptoms, patients with prosthetic valves experience symptoms specific to the presence of the artificial valve.

Large paravalvular leaks usually present with congestive heart failure or hemolytic anemia. Patients with new neurologic symptoms may have thromboembolism associated with the valve thrombi or endocarditis. Minor embolic episodes, such as transient neurologic symptoms, amaurosis fugax, or self-limited ischemic episodes in the extremities or organs in the absence of endocarditis, are common. Patients may present with major embolic events, including stroke, mesenteric infarction, or sudden death. Major bleeding due to anticoagulant therapy can also occur, with hemorrhagic stroke the most common lethal bleeding complication.

Patients with prosthetic valves usually have abnormal cardiac sounds. Mechanical valves have loud, metallic closing sounds. Systolic murmurs are commonly present with mechanical models. Loud diastolic murmurs are generally not present with mechanical valves. Patients with bioprostheses usually have normal S_1 and S_2, with no abnormal opening sounds. The aortic bioprostheses is usually associated with a short midsystolic murmur. Only the mitral bioprostheses is normally associated with a diastolic rumble.

Diagnosis of Prosthetic Valve Dysfunction

New or progressive symptoms referable to the heart suggest a prosthetic valve disorder. Therefore, new or progressive dyspnea of any form, new onset or worsening of congestive heart failure, decreased exercise tolerance, or a change in chest pain compatible with ischemia all suggest valvular dysfunction.[14] Severe hemolytic anemia may indicate a paravalvular leak. Persistent fever in patients with prosthetic valves should be evaluated for possible endocarditis. Changes in valve position may be noted on chest radiographs if comparison views are available. Blood studies that may be helpful include a blood count with red blood cell indices and coagulation studies if the patient is on warfarin. Emergency echocardiographic studies should be requested if there is any question about valve dysfunction. Ultimately, echocardiography and/or cardiac catheterization may be required for diagnosis.

Emergency Department Management and Admission Indications

The medical management of patients with valvular dysfunction is the same as that described under "Emergency Department Care of Symptomatic Valvular Heart Disease," above. The evaluation and management of endocarditis is described in the following section. Acute prosthetic valvular dysfunction due to thrombotic obstruction has been successfully treated with thrombolytic therapy, but the diagnosis requires angiography and therefore is not be done by an emergency physician without consultation with a cardiologist.

Patients suspected of having acute prosthetic valvular dysfunction or endocarditis require admission to the hospital and evaluation for possible valve replacement. Disposition of patients with worsening of symptoms can be problematic, and consultation with the patient's regular physician is needed.

INFECTIVE ENDOCARDITIS

The preferred term, *infective endocarditis*, encompasses all types of endocarditis caused by infectious organisms and represents an infection of the endocardium occurring on the valve leaflets, the walls of the heart cavities, or the tissue surrounding prosthetic heart valves. The infection may be subacute or acute, depending on the virulence of the organism, the susceptibility of the host, and the presence of intravenous drug use. Because of the declining frequency of rheumatic heart disease, the increasing number of cardiac surgical procedures, and the increasing numbers of intravenous drug users, the nature of this disease has changed dramatically in the last 20 years.[15]

Pathophysiology

The cardiac valve leaflets are the portion of the heart most susceptible to infection because of their limited blood supply. Endocarditis can occur with normal valves but is more common with congenital and acquired valve disease and prosthetic valves. Bacteria and fungi gain entry to the circulation through various routes and settle on valvular tissue. A platelet-fibrin matrix forms, and further growth of the organisms forms a vegetation on the valve that makes the organisms inaccessible to normal cellular host defenses. Risk factors for infective endocarditis include congenital or acquired valvular heart disease, intravenous drug abuse, prosthetic valves, hemodialysis or peritoneal dialysis, indwelling venous catheters, postcardiac surgery, and calcific valve degeneration that occurs with increasing age. Rheumatic heart disease, although still important, is declining in frequency.

Infective endocarditis can be divided into acute and subacute forms, depending on the virulence of the infecting organism. Subacute disease more commonly infects abnormal valves, while acute disease more commonly infects previously normal valves. In the acute form, devastating complications are more common, including rapid disruption of the valve, leading to incompetence and heart failure. Embolism of the vegetations is responsible for many of the clinical features of the disease in both forms. Younger patients are more likely to have acute endocarditis, while older individuals are more likely to have subacute disease. In the subacute form, anemia is common and is probably a reflection of the chronicity of the disease. Antibodies form in reaction to foreign antigen, and immune-complex injury to basement membranes of the kidney may result in glomerulonephritis, which can occur in both acute and subacute disease.

Endocarditis can be further divided into left and right heart disease. Left-sided disease (aortic and mitral involvement) is the most common, except in injecting drug users. The most common organisms include *S. viridans* (declining in frequency), *S. aureus* (increasing in frequency), *Enterococcus*, and fungal organisms. *Pseudomonas* and *Serratia* are important etiologic agents in intravenous drug users in certain areas of the United States, especially Detroit and San Francisco, respectively. Cardiac failure is the most common cause of death in left-sided disease, but deaths due to neurologic complications are increasing. Patients with aortic involvement are more prone to ring abscess and atrioventricular block. Vegetations may embolize from the left heart, causing neurologic complications, systemic infarction, or metastatic infection.

Right-sided disease is usually seen in intravenous drug abusers (60 percent) and is caused by *S. aureus* (75 percent) and *Streptococcus pneumonia* (20 percent), gram-negative organisms (4 percent), and fungal organisms.[16] Vegetations may embolize from the right heart, causing pulmonary infection or infarction. The fatality rate for right-sided endocarditis is lower than that for left-sided disease because the incidence of cardiac failure is less than that for left-sided disease.

Children with endocarditis most commonly have complex congenital heart disease (35 percent) or unrepaired ventricular septal defect (14 percent).[17] Echocardiography may fail to uncover vegetations despite the presence of acute infection. *Staphylococcus aureus* is the most common organism isolated.

Clinical Features

Acute left-sided disease presents with a picture of sepsis with or without cardiac failure. Typically, patients appear ill with fever, chills, and tachycardia and may have significant congestive failure symptoms, such as dyspnea, frothy sputum, and chest pain. Patients may quickly deteriorate, with acute rupture of mitral or aortic valves. Murmurs are typically the sounds of aortic or mitral regurgitation; however, the murmur is often absent or unable to be heard over lung sounds in acute cases. Neurologic symptoms secondary to aseptic meningoencephalitis and embolization of vegetations account for about one-third of emergency department presentations. These complications most commonly are mental status changes, hemiplegia, aphasia, ataxia, or severe headache. Monocular blindness may also occur.

Patients with subacute left-sided disease present with recurrent intermittent fever and constitutional symptoms such as malaise, anorexia, or weight loss. The diagnosis is frequently missed. Patients may give a history of recurrent "flu" or report several courses of antibiotics for presumed bacterial infections, such as bronchitis. The majority of patients with left-sided subacute disease have a murmur of aortic or mitral regurgitation or a change in their previous murmur at the time of their admission to the hospital. However, many admitted patients have been examined previously by a physician who did not detect the murmur. Patients may have Roth spots, which are retinal hemorrhages with central clearing. Peripheral evidence of endocarditis includes Osler nodes, tender nodules on the tips of the toes and fingers, and Janeway lesions, nontender plaques on the soles of the feet and palms of the hands, and clubbing. Petechiae may be seen on the conjunctiva, hard palate, neck, and upper trunk. Splinter hemorrhages may be seen in the nails of the fingers or toes. Splenomegaly is noted in 25 percent of patients. Patients may present with back pain as their only complaint. New criteria for diagnosis that include echocardiographic findings have been suggested.[18,19]

Right-sided disease is usually acute and presents with fever and respiratory symptoms: cough, chest pain, hemoptysis, and dyspnea. Subacute presentations are unusual with right-sided disease. Murmurs are detectable in fewer than 50 percent of patients with right-sided disease. The chest radiograph may reveal pulmonary effusions and multiple pulmonary infiltrates of variable size and shape. Although meningitis coexists in only 5 percent of patients with left-sided disease, bacterial meningitis is seen in up to 30 percent of patients with right-sided disease.

Diagnosis

The diagnosis of endocarditis is based on positive blood culture results and echocardiographic evidence of valvular injury or vegetations. Three separate cultures from different veins should be obtained. Aerobic, anaerobic, and fungal cultures should be obtained before antibiotics are started. Echocardiography is helpful but should not delay appropriate stabilizing treatments. Transesophageal echocardiography is preferred, but in experienced centers transthoracic echocardiography may suffice. Evidence of vasculitis or embolic events contributes to the clinical diagnosis. Nonspecific laboratory findings that support the diagnosis of endocarditis include leukocytosis, elevated C-reactive proteins, positive rheumatoid factor, normocytic anemia, hematuria (25 to 50 percent), and pyuria.

Emergency Department Care

The first priority in the care of patients with acute infective endocarditis is stabilization of respiratory and cardiac symptoms. For patients with mental status changes and hypoxia or a compromised airway, intubation may be required. Cardiac decompensation is usually due to left-sided valvular incompetence and/or rupture. Acute rupture of the mitral or aortic valve should be stabilized with afterload reducers such as sodium nitroprusside, with insertion of a Swan-Ganz catheter for monitoring therapy as soon as possible. Preparation for emergency surgery should be made for patients suspected of acute valvular rupture.[20] Aortic balloon counterpulsation may be helpful for mitral valve rupture but is contraindicated for wide-open aortic valve rupture.

The second priority is drawing three blood cultures from different sites and then starting empiric antibiotic therapy.[21] For acute infective endocarditis, a penicillinase-resistant penicillin, such as oxicillin 2 g q4h, should be given with an aminoglycoside, such as gentamicin 1 mg/kg up to 80 mg q8h, chosen on the basis of local patterns of susceptibility. In areas where there is a high incidence of methicillin-resistant *Staphylococcus* or in the case of a patient taking oral antibiotics already, vancomycin 1 g intravenously should be used in addition to an aminoglycoside. Patients with prosthetic valve endocarditis should be treated with antibiotics that cover *S. epidermidis,* usually vancomycin, 1 g intravenously, in addition to an aminoglycoside and rifampin. Although subacute cases are frequently caused by *S. viridans* and this bacteria is covered by penicillin G, patients with subacute presentations that require admission should be started on a newer cephalosporin, such as ceftriaxone, 1 g intravenously, in addition to an aminoglycoside until cultures and sensitivities are known. For patients with subacute disease who were taking oral antibiotics for another presumed infection, consideration should be given to collecting at least seven cultures or waiting until culture results turn positive before giving intravenous antibiotics.

Admission Indications

In general, patients with suspected endocarditis should be admitted to the hospital. Currently, injecting drug users who present to the emergency department with fever are admitted routinely at many centers regardless of whether there are other findings or potential explanations for the fever. Since only 10 percent prove to have evidence of endocarditis, studies are currently under way to determine whether emergency department "rules" can be developed for risk categorization.

Ambulatory Treatment

The ambulatory treatment of culture-proven *S. viridans* endocarditis has been advocated.[22] Patients treated with intramuscular injections of ceftriaxone, 2 g daily for 4 weeks, did well. This finding should not affect emergency medicine practice, however, since cultures are not usually available until some time after admission to the hospital. For patients for whom blood cultures are drawn and who are then sent home, a referral should be made to a cardiologist for evaluation and follow-up.

NONVALVULAR INFECTIONS OF THE HEART

Nonvalvular infections of the heart involve the endocardium, the myocardium, and the pericardium.[23] In addition, pacemakers; automatic, implantable cardioverter-defibrillators; and other cardiac devices may become infected in the subcutaneous device pocket or along the vascular tracks leading to and including the heart. Most commonly these devices become infected at the device pocket, where they are more readily diagnosed because of tenderness and erythema easily noted on physical examination. Myocardial abscesses and mural endocarditis are discussed here because of their similarities to valvular endocarditis. These two conditions are difficult to diagnose because their signs and symptoms are subtle.

Pathophysiology

Risk factors for the development of myocardial abscesses or mural endocarditis include chronic debilitating illness, immunosuppression, indwelling catheters, prolonged antibiotic therapy, and valvular endocarditis. The source of infection may be from hematogenous seeding or contiguous extension from valvular endocarditis. These two infections may coexist, or one may lead to the development of the other. In the case of mural endocarditis, bacteria may seed damaged endocardium or aneurysms in the ventricular wall. In the case of myocardial abscesses, multiple areas of the myocardium may be involved, but when valvular endocarditis is the source of bacterial seeding, the paravalvular areas are usually involved. The most common organisms in these nonvalvular infections of the heart are *S. aureus, S. viridans,* and other organisms associated with valvular endocarditis.

Clinical Features

The symptoms and signs may be completely nonspecific, especially with myocardial abscesses. Patients usually experience vague fevers and chills but may present with more obvious sepsis. Frequently patients are given antibiotics on an outpatient basis for some presumed bacterial infection, such as bronchitis. Patients may be suspected of having valvular endocarditis and may be admitted to the hospital for intravenous antibiotics, and yet the correct diagnosis is not made and symptoms recur after discharge. Many symptoms, including positive blood culture results, peripheral embolization, and splenomegaly, are found in both valvular and nonvalvular infections of the heart. Frequently patients have sudden fatal complications, such as myocardial rupture, tamponade, or severe peripheral embolization, diagnoses made only at autopsy.

Diagnosis

The diagnosis of myocardial abscess and mural endocarditis is difficult. Blood culture results are positive in 75 percent of patients with myocardial abscess, but this finding is nonspecific. In cases of mural endocarditis, patients frequently have peripheral embolization and splenomegaly, but these findings do not distinguish mural from valvular endocarditis. When these conditions are found at autopsy in a previously undiagnosed patient, endocarditis is frequently the misdiagnosis. Whenever patients present with findings compatible with endocarditis and yet both physical examination and echocardiographic study fail to demonstrate valvular lesions, myocardial abscess and mural endocarditis should be considered. Unfortunately, diagnosis with echocardiography or even cardiac angiography is difficult. Transesophageal echocardiography may offer the best results.

Emergency Department Management

When nonvalvular infections of the heart are suspected by the emergency physician, the patient should be admitted to the hospital. Accurate structural and microbiologic diagnosis is essential to proper management, which may include surgical drainage and repair. Therefore, antibiotics should be withheld until the plan for diagnostic evaluation can be initiated.

REFERENCES

1. Jick H, Vasilakis C, Weinrauch LA, et al: A population-based study of appetite-suppressant drugs and the risk of cardiac valve regurgitation. *N Engl J Med* 339:719, 1998.
2. Weissman NJ, Tighe JF, Gottdiener JS, Guynne JT: An assessment of heart-valve abnormalities in obese patients taking dexfenfluramine, sustained release dexfenfluramine, or placebo. *N Engl J Med* 339:725, 1998.
3. Devereux RB, Kramer-Fox R, Kligfield P: Mitral valve prolapse: Causes, clinical manifestations, and management. *Ann Intern Med* 111:305, 1989.
4. Zuppiroli A, Rinaldi M, Kramer-Fox R, et al: Natural history of mitral valve prolapse. *J Am Cardiol* 75:1028, 1995.
5. Stoddard MF, Prince CR, Dillon S, et al: Exercise-induced mitral regurgitation is a predictor of morbid events in subjects with mitral valve prolapse. *J Am Coll Cardiol* 25:693, 1995.
6. Leach RM, McBrian DJ: Brachioradial delay : A new clinical indicator of the severity of aortic stenosis. *Lancet* 335:1199, 1990.
7. Cheitlin MD, Alpert JS, Armstrong WF, et al: ACC/AHA guidelines for the clinical application of echocardiography: A report of the American College of Cardiology/American Heart Association Task Force on Practice Guidelines (Committee on Clinical Application of Echocardiography). *Circulation* 95:1686, 1997.
8. Etchells E, Bell C, Robb K: Does this patient have an abnormal systolic murmur? *JAMA* 277:564, 1997.
9. Hickey M, Smith R, Muhlbaier LH, et al: Current prognosis of ischemic mitral regurgitation. *Circulation* 78:151, 1988.
10. Heuser RR, Maddoux GL, Goss JE, et al: Coronary angioplasty for acute mitral regurgitation due to myocardial infarction. *Ann Intern Med* 107:852, 1987.
11. Carabello BA: Management of valvular regurgitation. *Curr Opin Cardiol* 10:124, 1995.
12. Antunes MJ, Franco CG: Advances in surgical treatment of acquired valve disease. *Curr Opin Cardiol* 11:139, 1996.
13. Dajani AS, Taubert KA, Wilson W, et al: Prevention of bacterial endocarditis. *JAMA* 277:1794, 1997.
14. Binder T, Baumgartner H, Maurer G: Diagnosis and management of prosthetic valve dysfunction. *Curr Opin Cardiol* 11:131, 1996.
15. Child JS: Risks for and prevention of infective endocarditis. *Cardiol Clin* 14:327, 1996.
16. Watonakunakorn C, Burlart T: Infective endocarditis at a large community teaching hospital, 1980–1990: A review of 210 episodes. *Medicine* 72:90, 1993.
17. Saiman L, Prince A, Gersony WM: Pediatric infective endocarditis in the modern era. *J Pediatr* 122:847, 1993.
18. Durack DT, Lukes AS, Bright DK: New criteria for diagnosis of infective endocarditis: Utilization of specific echocardiographic findings. *Am J Med* 96:200, 1994.
19. Lamas CC, Eykyn SJ: Suggested modifications to the Duke criteria for the clinical diagnosis of native valve and prosthetic valve endocarditis: Analysis of 118 pathological proven cases. *Clin Infect Dis* 25:713, 1997.
20. Moon MR, Stinson EB, Miller DC: Surgical treatment of endocarditis. *Prog Cardiovasc Dis* 40:239, 1997.
21. Kubak BM, Nimmagadda AP, Holt CD: Advances in medical and antibiotic management of infective endocarditis. *Cardiol Clin* 14:405, 1996.
22. Francioli P, Etienne J, Hoigne R, et al: Treatment of streptococcal endocarditis with a single daily dose of ceftriaxone sodium for 4 weeks. *JAMA* 267:264, 1992.
23. Kearney RA, Eisen HJ, Wolf JE: Nonvalvular infections of the cardiovascular system. *Ann Intern Med* 121:219, 1994.

THE CARDIOMYOPATHIES, MYOCARDITIS, AND PERICARDIAL DISEASE

James T. Niemann

THE CARDIOMYOPATHIES

The term *cardiomyopathy* is used to describe a group of diseases that directly alter cardiac structure and impair myocardial function. Four types of cardiomyopathy are currently recognized: (1) dilated cardiomyopathy (DCM), (2) hypertrophic cardiomyopathy (HCM), (3) restrictive cardiomyopathy, and (4) arrhythmogenic right ventricular cardiomyopathy.[1] It is acknowledged that there are some primary heart muscle disorders that do not fit readily into one of these four groups, and these conditions have been termed unclassified cardiomyopathies. Finally, the term *specific cardiomyopathies* is now used to describe heart muscle diseases that are associated with specific cardiac or systemic disorders. They often present with hemodynamic findings similar to those of the idiopathic dilated or restrictive form of cardiomyopathy. Some specific cardiomyopathies are listed in Table 51-1. The cardiomyopathies, as a group, are the third most common form of cardiac disease encountered in the United States, following coronary (ischemic) heart disease and hypertensive heart disease. HCM is the second most common cause of sudden cardiac death in the adolescent population and the leading cause of sudden death in competitive athletes.[2]

Dilated Cardiomyopathy

Hemodynamically, DCM is characterized by depressed myocardial systolic function and systolic pump failure. Left ventricular (LV), and often right ventricular (RV), contractile force is diminished, resulting in a low cardiac output and increased end-systolic and end-diastolic ventricular volumes and intracavitary pressures. LV, and often RV,

TABLE 51-1 Common Causes of Specific Cardiomyopathies

Toxins
Ethanol
Chemotherapeutic agents (doxorubicin)
Antiretroviral drugs (zidovudine, didanosine)
Phenothiazines
Cocaine
Infections
Viruses (coxsackievirus, echovirus, cytomegalovirus, HIV)
Rickettsia
Bacteria (diphtheria, rheumatic fever)
Mycobacteria
Fungal
Parasitic (toxoplasmosis, Chagas disease)
Collagen vascular disorders
Scleroderma
Systemic lupus erythematosus
Dermatomyositis
Hypersensitivity myocarditis
Peripartum cardiomyopathy
Metabolic
Nutritional deficiency (thiamine)
Endocrine (hypothyroidism, Cushing disease, hyperthyroidism)
Electrolyte distrubances (hypophosphatemia, hypocalcemia)
Neuromuscular disorders (muscular dystrophy, Friedreich ataxia)
Familial cardiomyopathy

dilatation accompanied by compensatory hypertrophy are the hallmarks of DCM. Histologic findings are nonspecific.

Approximately 80 percent of cases of DCM are of unknown etiology; that is, they are not associated with specific cardiac or systemic disorders (Table 51-1) and are considered idiopathic.[3] The idiopathic form of DCM is the cause in approximately 25 percent of all cases of congestive heart failure (CHF) and the primary indication for cardiac transplantation in the United States. The prevalence of idiopathic DCM is estimated to be approximately 36 cases per 100,000 population. Blacks and males have a 2.5-fold increase in risk compared to whites and females. Most patients are diagnosed between the ages of 20 and 50 years, and the majority have advanced symptoms of CHF at the time of initial presentation.[3]

CLINICAL FEATURES AND DIAGNOSIS As a result of systolic pump failure, the patient presents with signs and symptoms of CHF: dyspnea on exertion, orthopnea, and paroxysmal nocturnal dyspnea. Depressed ventricular contractile function and dilatation may result in the formation of mural thrombi, and the patient may present with manifestations of peripheral embolization (e.g., an acute neurologic deficit, flank pain, and hematuria or a pulseless, cyanotic extremity). Chest pain with features of typical angina pectoris occurs in approximately one-third of patients. Chest pain in these patients is felt to be due to limited coronary vascular reserve rather than atherosclerotic coronary artery disease.

Murmurs are frequently heard during cardiac auscultation and are not necessarily indicative of primary valvular disease. Ventricular dilatation and the resultant annular dilatation and displacement of the papillary muscles of the atrioventricular valves inhibit leaflet coaptation and complete valve closure. Holosystolic regurgitant murmurs of mitral and tricuspid valve origin are frequently heard at the apex or lower left sternal border in the patient with biventricular failure. On occasion an apical diastolic rumble may be heard and is due either to accentuated, early-diastolic atrial-to-ventricular flow (the result of mitral regurgitation and left atrial overload) or to a loud summation gallop. An enlarged, pulsatile liver may be found if tricuspid insufficiency is significant. Bibasilar rales and dependent edema are common additional findings.

The chest x-ray invariably shows an enlarged cardiac silhouette and increased cardiothoracic ratio; biventricular enlargement is common. Evidence of pulmonary venous hypertension (''cephalization'' of flow and enlarged hila) is also frequent and may serve to differentiate cardiac enlargement due to myocardial failure from that due to a large pericardial effusion.

The electrocardiogram (ECG) is almost always abnormal. Left ventricular hypertrophy and left atrial enlargement are the most common findings. Q or QS waves and poor R-wave progression across the anterior precordium may produce a pseudoinfarction pattern. Atrial fibrillation and ventricular ectopy are frequently encountered rhythm disturbances.

Echocardiographic studies in a symptomatic patient demonstrate a decreased ejection fraction, increased systolic and diastolic volumes, and ventricular and atrial enlargement.

TREATMENT AND DISPOSITION A timely workup is indicated in patients who present with newly diagnosed symptomatic CHF, and evaluation typically requires hospitalization. Echocardiography is indicated to exclude known causes of heart failure that may be correctable (e.g., precordial effusion or valvular disease), to estimate ejection fraction, and to rule out other potential complications (e.g., mural thrombi) that may be amenable to therapy. Symptom-directed therapy is best initiated in the in-patient setting in order to minimize adverse drug effects. Almost all patients will benefit symptomatically from digitalis glycoside therapy and diuretics, but these drugs have not been shown to improve survival rates. The use of angiotensin-converting enzyme inhibitors and β blockers, specifically carvedilol, have been shown to improve survival rates in patients with DCM and CHF.[4,5] Patients with complex ventricular ectopy may benefit from amiodarone therapy.[6]

TABLE 51-2 Cause of Acute Exacerbation of Chronic Congestive Heart Failure

Anemia
Infection
Noncompliance (diet, medications)
Paroxysmal atrial fibrillation
Bradyarrhythmias or heart block
Acute valvular insufficiency
Renal dysfunction (overdiuresis, angiotensin-converting enzyme inhibitor induced)
Myocardial ischemia or infarction
Pulmonary thromboembolism
Thyroid dysfunction

Patients with a known DCM and chronic CHF may present to the emergency department with a mild-to-moderate worsening of symptoms. In most instances, the cause is noncompliance with medical therapy or dietary indiscretion. Such patients can often be managed in the emergency department with intravenous diuretics, reinstitution of prescribed medications, counseling of the patient, and timely referral to the primary care physician.[7] However, other causes of an acute exacerbation of symptoms in a disease characterized by a slow and progressive history must be considered (Table 51-2) and, if present or suspected, require hospitalization for definitive management.

Hypertrophic Cardiomyopathy

Hypertrophic cardiomyopathy is characterized by LV and/or RV hypertrophy that is usually asymmetrical and involves primarily the interventricular septum. The diagnostic hallmarks of the disease are echocardiographic asymmetical septal hypertrophy and histologic hypertrophy associated with myocardial fiber disarray surrounding areas of increased loose connective tissue.[8] In approximately 50 percent of cases, it is a familial disease with autosomal dominant inheritance. In the rest, it is sporadic. There is no apparent sex or ethnic predilection. Molecular genetics has demonstrated that HCM is a heterogeneous disease of the sarcomere with many mutations. The most common mutation involves the β-myosin heavy chain. There is evidence that particular genotypes have more rapidly progressive courses. The prevalence in the general population is approximately 1 in 500. The annual mortality rate the unselected population is about 1 percent per annum but 4 to 6 percent in childhood and adolescence.

Hemodynamically, HCM is characterized by abnormal LV diastolic function due to reduced compliance of the hypertrophied left ventricle. This decreased compliance is reflected by an increase in LV filling pressure. Cardiac output, ejection fraction, and end-systolic and end-diastolic volumes are usually normal. During cardiac catheterization and hemodynamic monitoring, a systolic pressure gradient between the body of the left ventricle and the subvalvular outflow tract can be recorded in some patients at rest or after provocation (e.g., exercise or isoproterenol infusion). The majority of clinical symptoms in this heart muscle disease are the result of impaired diastolic relaxation and restricted LV filling.

CLINICAL FEATURES AND DIAGNOSIS Severity of symptoms in most instances is related to the patient's age; the older the patient, the more severe the symptoms. Dyspnea on exertion is the most frequent initial complaint and is due to exercised-induced sinus tachycardia, which results in an abrupt elevated LV diastolic pressure and pulmonary venous hypertension. Additional symptoms include chest pain, palpitations, and syncope. A family history of death due to cardiac disease, frequently described as "massive heart attack" or "heart failure," is not uncommon. Complaints of paroxysmal nocturnal dyspnea and pedal edema are infrequent.

Chest pain in HCM patients is due to an imbalance between the oxygen demand of the hypertrophied left ventricle and the available myocardial blood flow. In older patients, associated atherosclerotic coronary artery disease may further limit myocardial perfusion. Precordial or retrosternal chest discomfort in HCM may mimic angina pectoris or may be "atypical." Response to nitroglycerin administration is poor and highly variable.

The HCM patient may be aware of forceful ventricular contraction and complain of an abnormal heartbeat or "palpitations." Atrial and ventricular dysrhythmias are not uncommon in these patients; rapid atrial dysrhythmias, especially atrial fibrillation, and particularly poorly tolerated because of the increased importance of the atrial contribution to LV filling in the poorly compliant heart and require aggressive management in hemodynamically unstable patients.

Jugular venous pressure is usually not elevated; however, a prominent *a* wave may be noted on close inspection of the neck veins. The upstroke of the carotid arterial pulse is rapid and frequently biphasic or bifid (pulsus bisferiens). The apical impulse is sustained and hyperdynamic, and a presystolic lift is common.

The first and second heart sounds are usually normal, and a fourth sound (S_4) will be heard in most patients. The characteristic systolic ejection-type murmur of HCM is heard best at the lower left sternal border or at the apex and rarely radiates to the carotid arteries. Easily performed bedside maneuvers can be used to increase the intensity and duration of the murmur (Table 51-3). Interventions that decrease LV filling and the distending pressure in the LV outflow tract or that increase the force of myocardial contraction accentuate the murmur of HCM. Such interventions include standing and the Valsalva maneuver. The murmur is also louder with the first sinus beat following a premature ventricular contraction. Maneuvers that increase LV filling (squatting, passive leg elevation, and hand grip) have an opposite effect on murmur characteristics. The murmurs of HCM and mitral valve prolapse are similar and are compared in Table 51-3.

ECG findings of LV hypertrophy and left atrial enlargement are found in 30 percent and 25 to 50 percent, respectively, of HCM patients. Evidence of chamber enlargement is most common in patients with large gradients across the LV outflow tract. Q waves of considerable amplitude (more than 0.3 mV), termed septal Q waves, are seen in about 25 percent of patients and may be encountered in the anterior, lateral, or inferior leads. These Q waves may mimic those seen following myocardial infarction (pseudoinfarction pattern). The polarity of the T wave may serve as a diagnostic clue in the separation of HCM septal Q waves from Q waves due to myocardial infarction. Upright T waves in those leads with QS or QR complexes are usually found in HCM; T-wave inversion in such leads is highly suggestive of ischemic heart disease.

TABLE 51-3 Effect of Bedside Interventions on the Murmur of Hypertrophic Cardiomyopathy Compared to Mitral Valve Prolapse

	Hypertrophic Cardiomyopathy	Mitral Valve Prolapse
Valsalva maneuver	Murmur increased	Click closer to S_1, murmur increased
Standing after squatting	Murmur increased	Click closer to S_1, murmur increased
Passive leg elevation by supine patient	Murmur decreased	Click closer to S_2, murmur decreased
Hand grip	Murmur decreased	Click closer to S_1, murmur increased
Squatting	Murmur decreased	Click closer to S_2, murmur decreased

The chest x-ray is frequently normal, and identifiable abnormalities are largely nonspecific. Many patients do not show radiographic evidence of LV or left atrial enlargement. Evidence of pulmonary venous congestion is unusual but has been reported.

Echocardiography has played a substantial role in the diagnosis of HCM, in the correlation of the auscultatory and hemodynamic events with LV anatomic changes, and in defining inheritance patterns. The characteristic echocardiographic finding is disproportionate septal hypertrophy. Additional described echocardiographic abnormalities include normal or reduced LV end-diastolic dimensions, systolic anterior motion of the mitral valve, and midsystolic closure of the aortic valve.

TREATMENT AND DISPOSITION The majority of patients with HCM who seek medical care typically do so because of declining exercise tolerance, chest pain, or syncope.[9] Symptoms may mimic those of ischemic heart disease, or in the young patient, symptoms may be ascribed to a noncardiac cause. The patient who presents complaining of exercise intolerance or chest pain in whom the typical murmur of HCM is heard should be referred for echocardiographic evaluation. Syncope in patients with HCM typically occurs during or immediately after exercise. If HCM is suspected in a patient with syncope, hospitalization is indicated. The workup in such cases is extensive and includes echocardiographic studies as well as extended ambulatory (Holter) monitoring, exercise stress testing to assess blood pressure response, and tilt testing. Syncope in patients with HCM may be due to one or more factors and may presage sudden cardiac death.[9] Vigorous exercise is discouraged for such patients, and preparticipation screening guidelines have been developed for competitive athletes to minimize the risk of sudden death due to HCM.[10] β blockers are the mainstay of therapy for patients with chest pain.

Restrictive Cardiomyopathy

The restrictive forms are among the least common of the described cardiomyopathies. *Restrictive cardiomyopathy* is defined as heart muscle disease that results in "restricted" ventricular filling, with normal or decreased diastolic volume of either or both ventricles. Systolic function is usually normal, and ventricular wall thickness may be normal or increased, depending on the underlying cause. The hemodynamic hallmarks include (1) elevated LV and RV end-diastolic pressure, (2) normal LV systolic function (ejection fraction greater than 50 percent), and (3) an abrupt and rapid rise in early-diastolic ventricular pressure following a marked decline at the onset of diastole. The rapid rise and abrupt plateau in the early-diastolic ventricular pressure trace produce a characteristic "square-root sign" or "dip-and-plateau" filling pattern due to increased myocardial stiffness. This pattern is not diagnostic, however, and may be seen in constrictive pericarditis, with which restrictive cardiomyopathy is commonly confused. Differentiation between the two is critical because constrictive pericarditis can be cured surgically. The diagnosis of restrictive cardiomyopathy should be considered in a patient presenting with CHF but no evidence of cardiomegaly or systolic dysfunction.[11]

Restrictive cardiomyopathy may result from systemic disorders (Table 51-4), but most cases are idiopathic. The idiopathic form is sometimes familial, with autosomal dominant transmission. There has been no clearly demonstrated predilection for gender or ethnicity.

TABLE 51-4 Common Causes of Restrictive Cardiomyopathy

Idiopathic
Amyloidosis
Sarcoidosis
Hemochromatosis
Progressive systemic sclerosis (scleroderma)
Carcinoid heart disease
Endomyocardial fibrosis
Hypereosinophilic syndrome

CLINICAL FEATURES AND DIAGNOSIS Symptoms are typical of CHF and include dyspnea, orthopnea, and pedal edema. Right-sided manifestations may predominate and result in hepatomegaly, right upper quadrant pain, and ascites. Chest pain is uncommon, except in amyloidosis.

Findings on physical examination depend on the stage or severity of myocardial involvement. An S_3 is almost always present, and an S_4 is often heard if the patient is in sinus rhythm. Pulmonary rales, jugular venous distention, Kussmaul sign (jugular venous pulse rises during inspiration rather than falling), hepatomegaly, pedal edema, and ascites are also typical findings.

The chest x-ray may reveal signs of CHF in the absence of cardiomegaly. Chamber enlargement due to wall thickening, but not dilatation, and nonspecific ST-T-wave changes are usually noted on the ECG. Cardiac conduction disturbances are common in amyloidosis and sarcoidosis. Atrial fibrillation may occur in the setting of atrial enlargement. Low-voltage QRS complexes (QRS amplitude less than 0.7 mV) have been frequently described in patients with restrictive cardiomyopathy secondary to amyloidosis and hemochromatosis.[12]

TREATMENT AND DISPOSITION Symptoms and signs of CHF, particularly right-sided failure, with a normal-size cardiac silhouette on chest x-ray should prompt a suspicion of underlying restrictive cardiomyopathy, constrictive pericarditis, or diastolic LV dysfunction (most commonly due to ischemic heart disease, hypertension, or age-related changes in ventricular diastolic compliance). Doppler echocardiographic studies and cardiac catheterization with hemodynamic assessment are often required to differentiate between the above-mentioned entities. Computed tomography and magnetic resonance imaging of the heart have also been shown to be of value in differentiating constrictive pericarditis and restrictive cardiomyopathy.[11] Timely diagnosis is important because constrictive pericarditis can be surgically corrected and diastolic LV dysfunction not due to restrictive cardiomyopathy usually responds well to drug therapy (β blockers or calcium-channel blockers). The medical management of restrictive cardiomyopathy is less effective and symptom directed (diuretics and angiotensin-converting enzyme inhibitors) unless due to sarcoidosis (corticosteroid therapy) or hemachromatosis (chelation therapy). The need for admission is usually determined by the severity of symptoms and the availability of a timely and usually invasive workup.

Arrhythmogenic Right Ventricular Cardiomyopathy

Arrhythmogenic cardiomyopathy, or dysplasia, is the rarest of the cardiomyopathies. Familial disease is common in an autosomal dominant inheritance pattern with incomplete penetrance. This cardiomyopathy is characterized by progressive replacement of the RV myocardium with fibrofatty tissue in an eventual global distribution. The left ventricle and septum are usually spared.[13]

CLINICAL FEATURES AND DIAGNOSIS The typical presentation is that of sudden death or ventricular dysrhythmia in a young or middle-aged patient. The findings upon physical examination are normal. The chest x-ray shows no specific findings, and the heart size is not enlarged. The ECG may show a right bundle branch pattern and precordial T-wave inversion. Echocardiographic studies, radionuclide angiography, and cardiac catheterization are routinely required to confirm the diagnosis. The echocardiogram has the highest sensitivity and positive predictive value for the diagnosis of RV abnormalities and typically shows RV contraction abnormalities and RV enlargement.[13] Magnetic resonance imaging has been shown to detect fatty infiltration of the myocardium and may become the preferred diagnostic test.

TREATMENT AND DISPOSITION The majority of patients present after aborted sudden cardiac death, with syncope, or with complex ventricular ectopy. Due to the nature of these complaints, hospitalization is indicated. Ventricular tachycardia can be suppressed with antiarrhythmic drugs, but ablative procedures or implantation of an antiarrhythmic device may be necessary.

MYOCARDITIS

Definition

Myocarditis is broadly but nonspecifically defined as inflammation of the heart muscle and is most frequently characterized pathologically by focal infiltration of the myocardium by lymphocytes, plasma cells, and histiocytes. Varying amounts of myocytolysis and destruction of the interstitial reticulin network are also seen.[14] The pathologic changes have been ascribed to a number of infectious agents (Table 51-5), some of which involve the myocardium secondarily as part of a systemic disease process. Myocarditis is frequently accompanied by pericarditis.

Clinical Features and Diagnosis

Fever is common, as is sinus tachycardia, which is usually ''out of proportion'' with respect to the extent of temperature elevation. Signs and symptoms depend on the extent of myocardial involvement and resultant depression of myocardial systolic function. In severe cases, progressive heart failure, with its associated symptoms, may be seen. With less extensive myocardial involvement, pericarditis and the clinical manifestations of systemic illness (fever, myalgias, headache, and rigors) may overshadow clinical signs of myocardial dysfunction, and myocarditis may not be suspected. Retrosternal or precordial chest pain is a frequent presenting complaint and is most commonly secondary to associated pericardial inflammation (myopericarditis). This chest pain may mimic angina in its character. A pericardial friction rub is commonly heard in patients with myopericarditis.[15]

The chest roentgenogram is usually normal, and reported abnormalities (cardiomegaly and pulmonary venous hypertension and/or pulmonary edema) vary with disease severity and are nondiagnostic.

TABLE 51-5 Common Infectious Causes of Myocarditis

Viral Agents	Bacteria
Coxsackie B virus	*Corynebacterium diphtheriae*
Echovirus	*Neisseria meningitides*
Influenzavirus	*Mycoplasma pneumoniae*
Parainfluenzavirus	β-Hemolytic streptococci (rheumatic fever)
Epstein-Barr virus	Lyme disease
Hepatitis B virus	
HIV	

Reported ECG changes include nonspecific ST-T-wave changes, ST-segment elevation (due to associated pericarditis), atrioventricular block, and prolonged QRS duration. Levels of cardiac enzymes (creatine kinase and CK-MB) and troponin may be elevated.[16] Echocardiographic studies may reveal depressed systolic function in severe cases.

Treatment and Disposition

Current therapy in cases of idiopathic or viral myocarditis is largely supportive and symptom directed. Myocarditis in rheumatic fever and complicating diphtheria or meningococcemia necessitates directed antibiotic therapy. Immunosuppressive therapy is of unproven value. Because most patients present with rapidly progressive CHF, admission is usually indicated.[17]

UNEXPLAINED HEART FAILURE AND CARDIOMEGALY: DIFFERENTIAL DIAGNOSIS AND EVALUATION

Symptoms of CHF and associated cardiomegaly or evidence of cardiomegaly in an asymptomatic patient necessitates a directed evaluation. In the vast majority of instances, one of the following five disease entities will eventually be diagnosed. Where appropriate, recognized diagnostic clues are noted.

1. *Hypertensive heart disease.* Systemic arterial hypertension affects 10 to 20 percent of the adult population. This is a disease with a high prevalence that may be diagnosed at a number of stages. Patients with a dilated cardiomyopathy and untreated cardiac failure frequently present with an elevated blood pressure due to autonomically mediated compensatory reflexes. Isolated involvement of the myocardium as the major manifestation of systemic arterial hypertension is rare. A careful search for evidence of other end-organ damage due to arterial hypertension should be undertaken (examination of fundi, assessment of renal function, evaluation for focal neurologic changes, or history of such entities).
2. *Ischemic heart disease (ischemic cardiomyopathy).* Most patients with clinical signs of biventricular heart failure and cardiomegaly due to obstructive coronary arterial disease relate a history of typical anginal pain or documented myocardial infarction. A few do not, and clinical presentation and physical findings in these cases mimics those of an idiopathic dilated cardiomyopathy.
3. *Valvular heart disease.* Although the incidence of rheumatic heart disease in the United States is low, it remains prevalent in underdeveloped countries and is frequently first diagnosed in recent immigrants. The growing geriatric population is prone to calcific aortic stenosis and mitral annular calcification. In addition, bicuspid or unicuspid aortic valve abnormalities remain the most common congenital heart disease. All valvular diseases may present with CHF or incidental cardiac enlargement, and systolic and diastolic murmurs may be noted. Echocardiographic studies are the diagnostic tests of choice in patients with suspected valvular heart disease. Hemodynamic and angiographic studies may be confirmatory.
4. *Myocarditis.* Patients with severe myocarditis may present with signs and symptoms of cardiac insufficiency. Such patients are usually young, have no significant past cardiac history, have few risk factors for atherosclerotic coronary arterial disease, and present with a recent, abrupt onset of symptoms during or immediately following a systemic or viral illness.
5. *Idiopathic cardiomyopathy.* This diagnosis should be considered only if the first four entities have been excluded. A careful search for potential causes should then be undertaken.

PERICARDIAL DISEASE

The pericardium consists of a serous or loose fibrous membrane (visceral pericardium) overlying the epicardium and a dense collagenous sac (parietal pericardium) surrounding the heart. The space between the visceral and parietal pericardium may contain up to 50 mL of fluid under normal conditions, and intrapericardial pressure is normally subatmospheric. Because its layers are serosal surfaces and because of its proximity and attachments to other structures, the pericardium may be involved in a number of systemic or localized disease processes (Table 51-6). The clinical presentation of pericardial heart disease is variable and dependent on the pericardium's response to injury and how this response affects cardiac function. In this section the clinical manifestations and evaluation of acute and constrictive pericarditis and nontraumatic cardiac tamponade are discussed.[18]

TABLE 51-6 Common Causes of Acute Pericarditis

Idiopathic
Infectious Viral (coxsackievirus, echovirus, HIV) Bacterial [especially Staphylococcus, *Streptococcus pneumoniae*, β-hemolytic streptococci (acute rheumatic fever), *Mycobacterium tuberculosis*] Fungal (especially *Histoplasma capsulatum*)
Malignancy (leukemia, lymphoma, metastatic breast and lung carcinoma, melanoma)
Drug-induced (procainamide, hydralazine)
Connective tissue disease
Radiation-induced
Postmyocardial infarction (Dressler syndrome)
Uremia
Myxedema

Acute Pericarditis

CLINICAL FEATURES The most common symptom is precordial or retrosternal chest pain, which is most frequently described as sharp or stabbing. It may be of sudden or gradual onset and radiate to the back, neck, left shoulder, or arm; referral to the left trapezial ridge (due to inflammation of the joining diaphragmatic pleura) is a particular distinguishing feature. Chest pain due to acute pericarditis may be aggravated by inspiration or movement. It may be most severe when the patient is supine and is often relieved when the patient sits up and leans forward. In most instances, these characteristics allow the pain of acute pericarditis to be distinguished from the ischemic pain of angina or acute myocardial infarction.

Associated symptoms include (1) low-grade, intermittent fever, particularly if pericarditis is infectious in origin or of the idiopathic type; (2) dyspnea, due to accentuated pain with inspiration; and (3) dysphagia, ascribed to irritation of the esophagus by the posterior pericardium.

A pericardial friction rub is the most common and important physical finding in pericarditis. A pericardial rub most closely resembles a superficial grating or scratching sound. It is best heard with the diaphragm of the stethoscope at the lower left sternal border or apex when the patient is sitting and leaning forward or in the hands-and-knees position. It may be audible only during a certain phase of respiration and characteristically is transient (e.g., heard one hour and not the next). No inference as to the amount of pericardial fluid should be drawn from the presence or absence of a pericardial friction rub.

A pericardial rub is most often triphasic in character, consisting of a systolic component, an early diastolic component occurring during the early phase of ventricular filling, and a presystolic component synchronous with atrial systole. It is less commonly biphasic, with a systolic component with either an early diastolic or presystolic compo-

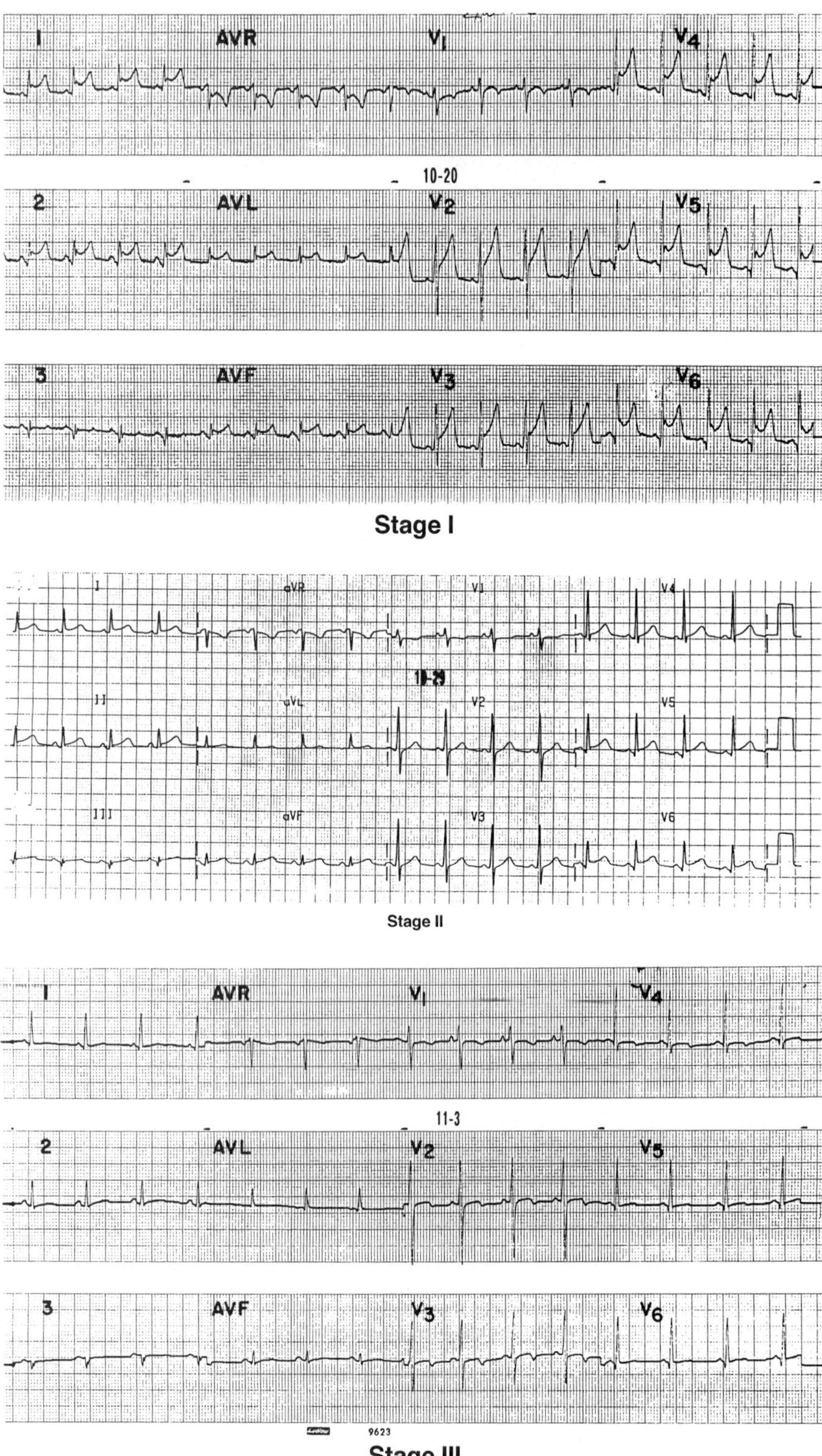

FIG. 51-1. This series of ECGs was recorded in a 28-year-old male who presented complaining of pleuritic retrosternal pain, cough, and fever. The initial ECG (dated 10-20) demonstrates diffuse ST-segment elevation (stage I). The ST-segment to T-wave amplitude ratio measured in V_6 is 5 mm/10 mm, or 0.50, thus meeting criteria for pericarditis rather than early repolarization (see the text). The ECG dated 10-29 demonstrates a return of the ST segment to the isoelectric point in most leads in which they had been elevated (stage II). The third tracing (dated 11-3) demonstrates resolution of ST changes and the appearance of T-wave inversion in the anterior precordial leads (stage III). These evolutionary changes are typical of and diagnostic for pericarditis and usually occur over several weeks.

nent. A monophasic rub is unusual (18 percent of cases) but is most often systolic.

DIAGNOSIS **Electrocardiogram** Serial ECGs recorded over a number of days may be diagnostic in acute pericarditis. The evolutionary ECG changes during acute pericarditis and convalescence have been divided into four stages. During stage 1, or the acute phase, ST-segment elevation (reflecting associated subepicardial inflammation and/or injury) is prominent in the precordial leads, especially V_5 and V_6, and in standard lead I. PR-segment depression may be noted in leads II, aV_f, and V_4 to V_6 (Fig. 51-1). In stage 2, the ST segment begins returning to the isoelectric line, and T-wave amplitude decreases. T-wave inversion is rarely seen until stage 3. Stage 3 is characterized by an isoelectric ST segment and T-wave inversion in those leads previously showing ST-segment elevation. Resolution of repolarization abnormalities is the hallmark of stage 4.

If a large pericardial effusion develops during the course of acute pericarditis, additional ECG abnormalities may be noted, including low-voltage QRS complexes and electrical alternans. These phenomena are due to the "insulating" effect of pericardial fluid, which attenuates electrical signals of myocardial origin, and the pendular motion of the heart within the fluid-filled pericardial space.

Although serial ECG tracings are of diagnostic value in acute pericarditis, sequential ECG assessment is not a diagnostic luxury afforded the emergency physician. Differentiating pericarditis from the normal variant with "early repolarization" is a common problem and can be difficult when only a single 12-lead ECG is available. Acute pericarditis is a common cause of chest pain and abnormal ECGs in young adults. The ST-T-wave changes present in the early repolarization or normal variant ECG mimic those of pericarditis and have been reported in 2 percent of healthy young adults. Investigations attempting to distinguish these two conditions have yielded conflicting results. However, a simple criterion offers considerable diagnostic utility, namely, the ST-segment/T-wave amplitude ratio in leads V_5, V_6, or I.[19] Using the end of the PR segment as baseline, or 0 mV, the amplitude or height of the ST segment at its onset is measured in one of the aforementioned leads and recorded in millivolts. The height of the T wave in the same lead is measured from the baseline to the T-wave peak. If the ratio of ST amplitude (in millivolts) to T-wave amplitude (in millivolts) is below 0.25, a normal variant or early repolarization is most probable. If the ratio is above 0.25, acute pericarditis is likely. This criterion may allow differentiation of acute pericarditis (stage 1) from early repolarization during emergency department evaluation (Fig. 51-1). Pericarditis alone does not cause significant cardiac rhythm disturbances.

Radiographic Assessment Conventional posteroanterior and lateral chest x-rays are of limited value. The cardiac silhouette may be of normal size and contour in acute pericarditis and, in some instances, the setting of cardiac tamponade. If previous chest x-rays are available for comparison, a recent increase in the size of the cardiac silhouette or an increase in the cardiothoracic ratio without radiographic evidence of pulmonary venous hypertension aids in distinguishing an expanding pericardial effusion from left heart failure. The epicardial "fat-pad sign" is rarely seen on the lateral chest x-ray and has been reported in only 15 percent of cases of acute pericarditis during fluoroscopy with image intensification. If acute pericarditis is suspected on the basis of history, physical examination, or ECG, posteroanterior and lateral chest x-rays, which may demonstrate a pleuropulmonary or mediastinal abnormality, may assist in establishing a cause (e.g., neoplastic or infectious).

Echocardiographic Studies Echocardiography has become the procedure of choice for the detection, confirmation, and serial follow-up of patients with acute pericarditis and a pericardial effusion.[18]

Normally, the pericardial sac is only a "potential" space, and the myocardium is echocardiographically in direct contact with surrounding thoracic structures. The anterior RV wall is in contact with the chest wall, and the posterior LV wall is in contact with the posterior pericardium and adjacent pleura. When a pericardial effusion is present, the pericardial space fills with echo-free fluid. Echocardiographically, a separation is seen between the right ventricle and the chest wall and between the left ventricle and the posterior pericardium. Quantitation of the size of the effusion is arbitrary and is determined by where the echo-free space is seen (anterior or posterior) and when in the cardiac cycle it occurs. For example, when an echo-free space is seen only posteriorly and only during systole, a small effusion is said to present.

Ancillary Laboratory Evaluation The laboratory studies listed in Table 51-7 may be of value in establishing an etiologic diagnosis.

TABLE 51-7 Ancillary Diagnostic Studies in Acute Pericarditis

Complete blood count and differential white blood cell count: may suggest infection or leukemia
Blood urea nitrogen/creatinine: may suggest a diagnosis of uremic pericarditis
Streptococcal serologic testing (antistreptolysin O, anti-DNAse, antihyaluronidase), particularly in patients with a history of rheumatic heart disease or pharyngitis
Blood cultures if bacterial infection suspected
Acute and convalescent viral titers
Serologic studies: antinuclear antibodies, anti-DNA titers, or right atrial latex fixation in patients with systemic symptoms
Thyroid function studies
Erythrocyte sedimentation rate: will not facilitate an etiologic diagnosis but can be followed serially to assess response to therapy

Creatine kinase and CK-MB may be elevated in acute pericarditis due to associated myocarditis.

TREATMENT AND DISPOSITION Most patients with idiopathic or presumed viral pericarditis will respond to nonsteroidal anti-inflammatory agents administered for 7 days to 3 weeks. If a specific cause is identified, therapy should be directed toward the underlying disease.[20] Patients with an enlarged cardiac silhouette on chest x-ray should be admitted for early Doppler echocardiography to assess the extent of the effusion and degree of hemodynamic compromise.

Nontraumatic Cardiac Tamponade

PATHOPHYSIOLOGY An increase in the amount of fluid within the pericardial sac results in an increase in intrapericardial pressure. The normal fibrocollagenous parietal pericardium has elastic properties and stretches to accommodate increases in intrapericardial fluid. The initial portion of the pericardial volume-pressure curve is flat: relatively large increases in volume result in comparatively small changes in intrapericardial pressure. The curve becomes steeper as the parietal pericardium reaches the limits of its distensibility. If fluid continues to accumulate, intrapericardial pressure rises to a level greater than that of the normal filling pressures of the right heart chambers. When this occurs, ventricular filling is restricted and results in cardiac tamponade. The point at which this occurs is determined by the slope of the pericardial volume-pressure curve, which is dependent on the rate of fluid accumulation, pericardial compliance (a thickened parietal pericardium is less distensible), and intravascular volume (hypovolemia lowers ventricular filling pressure).[18] Common causes of cardiac tamponade in nontrauma patients are listed in Table 51-8.[21–23]

CLINICAL FEATURES AND DIAGNOSIS Symptoms are nonspecific, and patients most commonly complain of dyspnea and profound exertional intolerance. Additional complaints may be present due to the underlying disease (e.g., uremia) or if the pericardial effusion has developed gradually (e.g., tuberculous pericarditis). Such symptoms may include weight loss, pedal edema, ascites, and so on.

Physical examination most commonly reveals tachycardia and low systolic arterial blood pressure with a narrow pulse pressure. Pulsus paradoxus may also be present. A paradoxical arterial pulse is said to be present when the cardiac rhythm is regular and there are apparent

TABLE 51-8 Cardiac Tamponade in Medical (Nontrauma) Patients

Cause	Approximate Frequency, %
Metastatic malignancy	40
Acute idiopathic pericarditis	15
Uremia	10
Bacterial or tubercular pericarditis	10
Chronic idiopathic pericarditis	10
Hemorrhage (anticoagulant)	5
Other (systemic lupus erythematosus, postradiation, myxedema, etc.)	10

TABLE 51-9 Echocardiographic Findings in Cardiac Tamponade

Right atrial compression
Right ventricular diastolic collapse
Abnormal respiratory variation in tricuspid and mitral flow velocities (Doppler)
Dilated inferior vena cava with lack of inspiratory collapse

dropped beats in peripheral pulse during inspiration. There is usually a greater than 10-mmHg decrease in systolic blood pressure during inspiration in the supine position. A value greater than 25 mmHg usually separates true tamponade from lesser degrees of restricted cardiac filling.[24] Pulsus paradoxus occurs because there is an inspiratory decrease in LV filling secondary to the dominance of inspiratory right heart filling within the confined intrapericardial space. Pulsus paradoxus is not diagnostic of cardiac tamponade and may be noted in other cardiopulmonary processes, as listed in Table 51-6. The neck veins are usually distended with an absent *y* descent. The apical impulse is indistinct or tapping in quality. Cardiac auscultation may reveal "distant" or soft heart sounds. Pulmonary rales are usually absent, and there may be right upper quadrant tenderness due to hepatic venous congestion.

The chest x-ray may or may not reveal an enlarged cardiac silhouette, and this finding is dependent on the amount of intrapericardial fluid accumulation. The pulmonary vasculature typically appears normal. An epicardial fat-pad line, or sign, may occasionally be seen within the cardiac silhouette.

The ECG usually shows low-voltage QRS complexes (less than 0.7 mV) and ST-segment elevation (due to the inflammation of the epicardium) with PR-segment depression, as in pericarditis. Electrical alternans (beat-to-beat variation in the amplitude of the P and R waves unrelated to the respiratory cycles) is a classic but uncommon finding (about 20 percent of cases). Electrical alternans is demonstrated in Fig. 51-2.

The diagnosis should be suspected based on the clinical examination and chest x-ray findings. Echocardiographic assessment is the diagnostic test of choice. In addition to a large pericardial fluid volume, typical echocardiographic findings described in cardiac tamponade are listed in Table 51-9.[25]

TREATMENT AND DISPOSITION Volume expansion with a bolus of normal saline solution (500 to 1000 mL) will increase intravascular volume, facilitate right heart filling, and increase cardiac output and arterial pressure. However, it is a temporary measure, and patients will require pericardiocentesis as initial definitive therapy and for diagnostic evaluation.

Pericardiocentesis should be performed under optimal circumstances, usually within the cardiac catheterization laboratory using echocardiographic guidance. The major potential complications, namely, cardiac perforation and coronary artery laceration, can be minimized. In addition, a pigtail catheter can be inserted to allow continuous fluid drainage and prevention of fluid accumulation.

Pericardiocentesis must be performed within the emergency department if dictated by hemodynamic instability. The subxiphoid approach with the patient sitting at a 45° angle is the preferred technique. A 16- to 18-gauge spinal needle is inserted between the xiphoid process and the left costal margin at a 30 to 40° angle to the skin. The needle is directed toward the right shoulder and continuous negative pressure applied to the syringe until fluid is withdrawn. Due to the shape of the pericardial volume-pressure curve, removal of only a small volume of fluid (e.g., 50 mL) can result in dramatic hemodynamic improvement. If time permits and the equipment is available, the V lead of an ECG monitor electrode can be attached to the needle using an alligator clip or Harrison adapter to detect epicardial contact (ST-segment elevation) as the needle is advanced beneath the skin.

If the equipment is available, echocardiographically guided emergency pericardiocentesis can be performed in the emergency department. Definitive management (insertion of an intrapericardial pigtail catheter through a pericardial window) is best undertaken following admission. After pericardiocentesis, patients require admission in a monitored setting.

Constrictive Pericarditis

PATHOPHYSIOLOGY Constrictive pericarditis is pathologically distinct from acute pericarditis.[18] Following pericardial injury and the

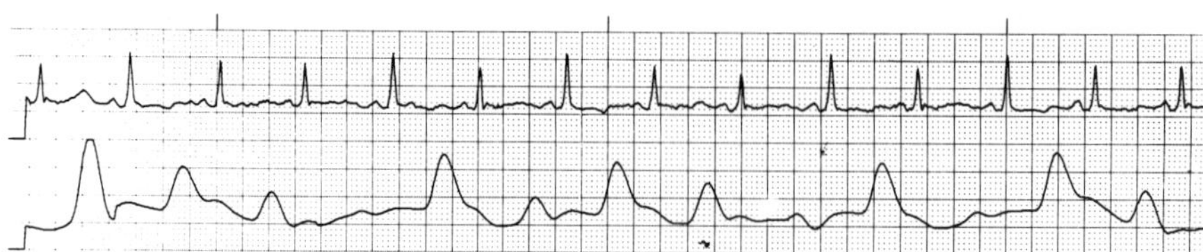

FIG. 51-2. This rhythm strip *(lead II, top tracing)* and plethysmograph *(bottom tracing)* were recorded in a patient who presented with dyspnea, hypotension, and clinical and echocardiographic evidence of cardiac tamponade. A paradoxical pulse was noted on palpation of the radial artery. The amplitude of the R waves varies from beat to beat (electrical alternans). Similar changes are seen in P-wave amplitude. These ECG changes are not related to the respiratory cycle.

resultant inflammatory and reparative process, fibrous thickening of the layers of the pericardium may occur. This fibrous reparative process is most commonly encountered after cardiac trauma with intrapericardial hemorrhage, after pericardiotomy (open-heart surgery, including coronary revascularization), in fungal or tuberculous pericarditis, and in chronic renal failure (uremic pericarditis). When the fibrous and/or collagenous response prevents passive diastolic filling of the normally distensible cardiac chambers, constriction is said to be present. Intrapericardial fluid is not required to produce such a hemodynamic effect. By its nature, constrictive pericarditis is most commonly a clinically chronic process. However, clinical manifestations may occur early if fluid also accumulates within the thickened, noncompliant pericardial sac (so-called effusive constrictive pericarditis). In the vast majority of cases of constrictive pericarditis, proved by hemodynamic assessment (see below), a specific cause is never determined.

CLINICAL FEATURES The symptoms of constrictive pericarditis usually develop gradually and may mimic those of CHF and restrictive cardiomyopathy.[11] If symptoms develop within months of a pericardial injury, a combination of pericardial effusion and constriction should be suspected. Exertional dyspnea and decreased exercise tolerance are common complaints; however, orthopnea, paroxysmal nocturnal dyspnea, and chest pain are unusual. Lower-extremity swelling (pedal edema) and increasing abdominal girth (ascites) are also common complaints and are the result of decreased RV diastolic compliance and the resultant increase in systemic venous pressure.

In most instances, physical findings and their correct interpretation will lead the clinician to suspect constrictive pericarditis.[18] Examination of the neck veins with the torso of the patient at a 45° angle from horizontal will reveal jugular venous distention and a rapid *y* descent of the cervical venous pulse. Elevated venous pressure is also seen in CHF, but a rapid *y* descent is infrequently encountered. The Kussmaul sign (inspiratory neck vein distention) is frequently but not invariably noted in constrictive pericarditis but rarely noted in uncompensated CHF. A paradoxical pulse is found in a minority of patients, and thus its absence does not exclude a diagnosis of constrictive pericarditis. On cardiac auscultation, an early diastolic sound, a pericardial "knock," may be heard at the apex 60 to 120 ms after the second heart sound. The pericardial knock sounds like a ventricular gallop but occurs earlier than the S_3 of CHF, which it may mimic. The knock is due to accelerated RV inflow in early diastole and early myocardial distention, followed by an abrupt slowing of further ventricular expansion. There is usually no pericardial friction rub. Hepatomegaly, ascites, and dependent edema of varying severities are usually found.

DIAGNOSIS **Electrocardiogram** Diagnostic ECG changes have not been described in constrictive pericarditis. However, low-voltage QRS complexes and inverted T waves are common.

Radiographic Assessment Conventional posteroanterior and lateral chest x-rays most commonly demonstrate a normal or slightly enlarged cardiac silhouette, clear lung fields, and little or no evidence of pulmonary venous congestion. Pericardial calcification, which may be evident in up to 50 percent of patients with constrictive pericarditis, is seen best on the lateral chest x-ray but is not diagnostic of constrictive pericarditis.

Echocardiographic Studies On occasion, two-dimensional echocardiography may demonstrate pericardial thickening and abnormal ventricular septal motion in a patient with suspected constrictive pericarditis. However, its diagnostic utility is much less than in a patient with acute pericarditis. Doppler echocardiography is preferred, and cardiac computed tomography and magnetic resonance imaging may also be useful.

TREATMENT AND DISPOSITION In cases of significant constriction and impaired ventricular filling, pericardiectomy is the treatment of choice.

REFERENCES

1. Richardson P, McKenna W, Bristow M, et al: Report of the 1995 World Health Organization/International Society and Federation of Cardiology Task Force on the definition and classification of cardiomyopathies. *Circulation* 93:841, 1996.
2. Liberthson RR: Sudden death from cardiac causes in children and young adults. *N Engl J Med* 334:1039, 1996.
3. Dec GW, Fuster V: Idiopathic dilated cardiomyopathy. *N Engl J Med* 331:1564, 1994.
4. Williams JF, Bristow MR, Fowler MB, et al: Guidelines for the evaluation and management of heart failure: Report of the American College of Cardiology/American Heart Association Task Force on Practice Guidelines (Committee on Evaluation and Management of Heart Failure). *Circulation* 92:2764, 1995.
5. Packer M, Bristow MR, Cohn JN, et al: The effect of carvedilol on morbidity and mortality in patients with chronic heart failure. *N Engl J Med* 334:134 1996.
6. Singh SN, Fletcher RD, Fisher SG, et al: Amiodarone in patients with congestive heart failure and asymptomatic ventricular arrhythmia. *N Engl J Med* 333:77, 1995.
7. Karon BL: Diagnosis and outpatient management of congestive heart failure. *Mayo Clin Proc* 70:1018, 1995.
8. Wigle ED, Rakowski H, Kimball BP, et al: Hypertrophic cardiomyopathy: Clinical spectrum and treatment. *Circulation* 92:1680, 1995.
9. Spirito P, Seidman CE, McKenna WJ, et al: The management of hypertrophic cardiomyopathy. *N Engl J Med* 336:775, 1997.
10. Maron BJ, Thompson PD, Puffer JC, et al: Cardiovascular preparticipation screening of competitive athletes: A statement for health professionals from the Sudden Death Committee (Clinical Cardiology) and Congenital Cardiac Defects Committee (Cardiovascular Disease in the Young), American Heart Association. *Circulation* 94:850, 1996.
11. Kushwaha SS, Fallon JT, Fuster V: Restrictive cardiomyopathy. *N Engl J Med* 336:267, 1997.
12. Falk RH, Comenzo RL, Skinner M: The systemic amyloidoses. *N Engl J Med* 337:898, 1997.
13. Fontaine G, Fountaliran F, Frank R: Arrhythmogenic right ventricular cardiomyopathies: Clinical forms and main differential diagnoses. *Circulation* 97:1532, 1998.
14. Lange LG, Schreiner GF: Immune mechanisms of cardiac disease. *N Engl J Med* 330:1129, 1994.
15. Lieberman EB, Hutchins GM, Herskowitz A, et al: Clinicopathologic description of myocarditis. *J Am Coll Cardiol* 18:1617, 1991.
16. Smith SC, Ladenson JH, Mason JW, et al: Elevations of cardiac troponin I associated with myocarditis: Experimental and clinical correlates. *Circulation* 95:163, 1997.
17. Mason JW, O'Connell JB, Herskowitz A, et al: A clinical trial of immunosuppressive therapy for myocarditis. *N Engl J Med* 333:269, 1995.
18. Spodick DH: Pathophysiology of cardiac tamponade. *Chest* 113:1372, 1998.
19. Ginzton LE, Laks MM: The differential diagnosis of acute pericarditis from the normal variant: New electrocardiographic criteria. *Circulation* 65:1004, 1982.
20. Maisch B: Pericardial diseases, with a focus on etiology, pathogenesis, pathophysiology, new diagnostic imaging methods, and treatment. *Curr Opin Cardiol* 9:379, 1994.
21. Corey GR, Campbell PT, Van Trigt P, et al</NM>: Etiology of large pericardial effusions. *Am J Med* 95:209, 1993.
22. Markiewicz W, Borovik R, Ecker S: Cardiac tamponade in medical patients: Treatment and prognosis in the echocardiographic era. *Am Heart J* 111:1138, 1986.
23. Guberman BA, Fowler NO, Engel PJ, et al: Cardiac tamponade in medical patients. *Circulation* 64:633, 1981.
24. Curtiss EI, Reddy S, Uretsky BF, et al: Pulsus paradoxus: definition and relation to the severity of cardiac tamponade. *Am Heart J* 115:391, 1988.
25. Fowler NO: Cardiac tamponade: A clinical or an echocardiographic diagnosis? *Circulation* 87:1738, 1993.

Pulmonary Embolism

Charles N. Schoenfeld

Pulmonary embolism (PE) is difficult to diagnose. It has a significant mortality, especially if not recognized in a timely fashion, but lacks a typical presentation. Only with a high index of suspicion and knowledge of predisposing risk factors, coupled with an understanding of the limitations of the diagnostic tests used, can the clinician reliably confirm or exclude the disease and initiate timely and appropriate therapy.

EPIDEMIOLOGY

The incidence of PE in the United States is estimated to be 650,000 cases per year; with over 200,000 patients dying each year, PE is the third leading cause of death. Approximately one-third of these deaths occur within the first hour and over 16,000 patients die despite treatment. Overall mortality ranges from 2 to 10 percent in patients treated for PE and from 20 to 30 percent in those with unrecognized PE. More than 50 percent of fatal PE is diagnosed at autopsy.[1] PE is more common in males than females before the age of 50; this gender difference disappears in older age groups. PE is the most common cause of nonsurgical maternal death in the peripartum period. Pregnant women over the age of 40 and those of African-American descent are at highest risk.[2]

The overwhelming majority of PEs are caused by thromboemboli. In situ pulmonary artery thrombosis is rare. When sought, deep venous thrombosis (DVT) of the lower extremities proves to be the source of 80 to 90 percent of cases.[3] DVT of the upper extremity has been reported to cause 10 to 15 percent of PE, especially if associated with indwelling central venous catheters.[4] Other sources of PE include pelvic vein thrombosis, right heart thrombosis, and amniotic or fat emboli. Septic emboli—associated with valvular vegetations in right-sided endocarditis, infected central venous catheters, and septic thrombphlebitis from intravenous drug use (IDU)—present unique diagnostic and therapeutic challenges.

PATHOPHYSIOLOGY

In the presence of predisposing factors (Table 52-1), clot forms in the deep venous system. Thrombosis usually begins at venous valve sinuses and propagates proximally over minutes to hours. Lysis of the clot generally occurs over 1 to 2 weeks. The risk of embolization is highest in the first week of thrombus formation.

The pathophysiologic effects of PE are caused both by mechanical obstruction of the pulmonary arterial system and by the release of vaso- and bronchoactive mediators. Mechanical obstruction produces the clinical picture of acute cor pulmonale. The trigger for the release of chemical mediators is platelet degranulation in the lung. These mediators—prostaglandins, catecholamines, serotonin, and histamine—cause bronchoconstriction as well as pulmonary artery vasoconstriction. This results in an overall reduction in lung compliance. Vasoconstriction is the predominant effect, leading to a ventilation/perfusion ($\dot{V}/\dot{Q}$) mismatch. Vasoconstriction may be severe enough to cause pulmonary hemorrhage or infarct, producing an infiltrate on the chest radiograph. The infiltrate of pulmonary hemorrhage usually resolves in 1 to 2 weeks, while that of infarct may take months to disappear.[5]

PE tend to be multiple and bilateral, with the right lower lobe of the lung being the most commonly involved lung segment. Angiographic evidence of PE generally resolves in 1 to 4 weeks and pulmonary artery (PA) pressure usually normalizes within a month. If the PE fails to resolve, chronic cor pulmonale may occur.

TABLE 52-1 Predisposing Factors for Thromboembolic Disease

Immobilization	Burns
Hospitalization/bed rest	History of DVT or PE
Stroke/spinal cord injury	Hypercoagulable states
Prolonged travel	Pregnancy
Recent surgery	Protein C deficiency
Trauma (especially lower extremity, pelvis)	Protein S deficiency
	Antithrombin III deficiency
Obesity	Malignancy
Cardiac disease	Estrogen therapy

CLINICAL FEATURES

Predisposing Factors

PE usually results from DVT, and DVT occurs because of predisposing risk. Thus, patients at risk for DVT are at risk for PE. Venous stasis, hypercoagulability, and endothelial damage—Virchow's triad—are well-recognized factors favoring the development of DVT. Table 52-1 lists the commonly recognized risk factors for DVT and PE. The majority of patients with PE will have at least one risk factor, with immobilization being the most prevalent.[6] While a minority of patients may not have clinically evident risk factors at presentation, they will generally be found to have abnormalities of coagulation or occult cancer on further evaluation. IDU may cause septic or aseptic thrombophlebitis by extension from superficial phlebitis, external compression by and septic extension from a perivascular abscess, or direct injection into the deep venous system. In addition, agents contaminating illicit drugs, such as talc and bacteria, have direct thrombogenic properties.

Clinical Presentation

There is no typical presentation of PE. The classic triad of dyspnea, hemoptysis, and pleuritic chest pain occurs in less than 20 percent of patients. Table 52-2 lists the frequency of symptoms and signs found in patients with angiographically proven PE.[5] Chest pain (usually pleuritic) and dyspnea were the only symptoms and tachypnea (respirations >16/min) was the only sign occurring with sufficient frequency to be clinically useful. The absence of any of these three findings is strong though inconclusive clinical evidence in excluding the diagnosis of PE. The presence of any of these, especially in association with predisposing risks for DVT, must raise the index of suspicion for PE if no other cause is found.

PE may present as syncope or near-syncope in 10 to 15 percent of cases and should be considered in the differential diagnosis of this presenting complaint.[5,7] Altered mental status, especially in the elderly, may be the presenting complaint, as may be generalized seizures. Anxiety, a diagnosis of exclusion in all emergency department (ED) patients, occurs in more than 50 percent of patients with PE.[5]

Physical Examination

The physical findings in patients with PE are as varied and nonspecific as the clinical presentations. Vital signs reveal tachypnea (RR > 16/min) in over 90 percent of cases, while tachycardia (PR > 100/min) and fever (>37.8°C) occur in less than 50 percent.[5] Blood pressure may be elevated, normal, or low.

Depending on the extent of the PE and preexisting cardiopulmonary disease, the patient may appear to be in no apparent distress or be found to be anxious, diaphoretic, or dyspneic. Cyanosis is uncommon, generally signifying massive PE or underlying cardiopulmonary disease.

TABLE 52-2 Symptoms and Signs of 327 Patients With Angiographically Proven PE

Symptoms and Signs	Total Series, %
Symptom	
Chest pain	88
Pleuritic	74
Nonpleuritic	14
Dyspnea	84
Apprehension	59
Cough	53
Hemoptysis	30
Sweats	27
Syncope	13
Sign	
Respirations >16/min	92
Rales	58
P2 > S2	53
Pulse >100/min	44
Temperature >37.8°C	43
Phlebitis	32
Gallop	34
Diaphoresis	36
Edema	24
Murmur	23
Cyanosis	19

Source: Adapted from Bell WR, Simon TL, DeMets DL: The clinical features of submassive and massive pulmonary emboli. *Am J Med* 62:355, 1977. With permission.

Findings of acute right heart dysfunction—neck vein distention, accentuation of the pulmonic heart sound, and right parasternal heave—may occur in massive and submassive PE. Chest exam reveals a pleural friction rub in less than 20 percent of cases. Rales are a more common but less specific finding. Localized wheezes are suggestive of PE but uncommon. Clinical evidence of DVT occurs in less than 50 percent of patients. However, up to 80 percent of patients with PE have positive venography.[3]

CLASSIFICATION OF PE

Patients with PE are characterized as having massive or submassive PE. Massive PE presents in dramatic form, including hypotension and hypoxemia, which may be refractory to therapy. In general, 40 to 50 percent of the pulmonary arterial circuit must be occluded to produce these effects. Patients with preexisting cardiac or pulmonary disease may show the signs of massive PE with lesser degrees of occlusion. Massive PE accounts for approximately 5 percent of all PE but has a mortality of about 40 percent.

Submassive PE presents with normal systemic hemodynamics and hypoxemia, which is correctable with supplemental oxygen. Mortality is low (about 2 percent) if the diagnosis is made and therapy initiated. Failure to make the diagnosis and treat accordingly increases the mortality 10-fold.

A subset of patients with submassive PE warrants special mention. These patients, while having normal systemic pressures on presentation, have evidence of moderate to severe right ventricular dysfunction by physical exam or echocardiography. If not treated, this dysfunction may progress to right ventricular infarction, leading to hypotension and death. Lungs scans reveal perfusion defects of more than 30 percent of the pulmonary circuit. More aggressive therapy than simple anticoagulation may be warranted in this set of patients.[8,9]

DIAGNOSIS

Establishing or excluding the diagnosis of PE is a challenge requiring the synthesis of clinical suspicion, awareness of predisposing risk factors, and the interpretation of diagnostic studies utilizing pretest probability of PE. While only a negative pulmonary angiogram excludes the diagnosis of PE,[10] this test is required only when sufficient doubt about the diagnosis or contraindications to empiric therapy exist.[11]

Unexplained chest pain, dyspnea, or tachypnea should always raise the question of PE as the cause. If these findings occur in a patient at risk for thromboembolic disease the diagnosis of PE must be strongly considered. All patients with chest pain, dyspnea, or tachypnea not explained by the history or physical exam should undergo screening tests, including an electrocardiogram (ECG), chest x-ray (CXR), and arterial blood gas (ABG) analysis.

Electrocardiography

The most common ECG abnormality in PE is nonspecific ST-T wave changes, seen in more than 40 percent of patients. T-wave inversions in the precordial leads mimicking subendocardial infarction may be seen in massive PE. Other ECG changes include new right bundle branch block, p-pulmonale, S1Q3T3 pattern, and clockwise axis rotation.

Sinus tachycardia is the most common rhythm disturbance, although atrial fibrillation or flutter may occur.[7] There is no diagnostic pattern of PE on the ECG. The greatest utility of the ECG is to exclude disorders such as pericarditis or myocardial infarction.

Chest X-ray

The initial CXR is normal in nearly one-third of patients with PE.[7] A normal CXR in the setting of dyspnea and hypoxemia without evidence of reactive airway disease is strongly suggestive of PE.[12] The overwhelming majority of patients will develop some CXR abnormality during the course of their disease.[13] Infiltrate or atelectasis will appear in nearly 50 percent, while an elevated hemi-diaphragm occurs in about 40 percent, often in association with a pleural effusion.[7]

The classically described Hampton hump, a pleural-based wedge-shaped infiltrate, is uncommon. The Westermark sign, relative oligemia distal to engorged pulmonary arteries, may be seen in patients with massive PE (Fig. 52-1). The CXR is of greatest utility in ruling in other causes of the patient's complaints, such as pneumothorax or

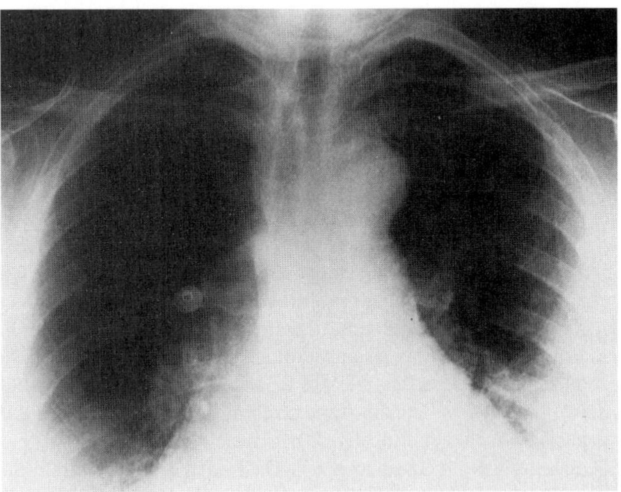

FIG. 52-1. Westermark sign: AP CXR demonstrating relative oligemia in right upper lobe and dilated proximal pulmonary artery.

pneumonia. It is essential for the subsequent interpretation of lung scans and pulmonary arteriograms.

Arterial Blood Gas

Hypoxemia occurs in about 90 percent of patients with PE, but the Pa_{O_2} may be normal. While a Pa_{O_2} of 80 to 90 mmHg is 90 to 95 percent sensitive in identifying patients with PE, it is less than 50 percent specific.[5] Further, the degree of hypoxemia fails to accurately predict the size of the PE.[5] However, a Pa_{O_2} of less than 70 mmHg not explained by findings on the CXR strongly suggests PE. The calculation of the alveolar-arterial (A-a) oxygen gradient may be useful in reducing the suspicion of PE if it and the Pa_{CO_2} are both normal.[14]

$$\text{A-a gradient} = [(F_iO_2) \times (\text{barometric pressure} - 47)] - [(1.2) \times (Pa_{CO_2})] - (Pa_{O_2})$$

However, the A-a gradient has been shown to be normal in nearly 25 percent of patients with PE[15] and should never be used alone to exclude the diagnosis. The A-a gradient has been shown to be even less useful in the elderly.[16] These screening tests (ECG, CXR, and ABG) are most useful in defining the patient's complaints to be caused by diseases other than PE. A normal ECG, presenting CXR, Pa_{O_2}, Pa_{CO_2}, and A-a gradient cannot be used to exclude the diagnosis of PE in patients at risk for thromboembolic events. In this subset of patients, a number of additional tests are used to increase or decrease the clinical suspicion of PE.

Biochemical Tests

A variety of biochemical tests have been studied as aids in the confirmation or exclusion of the diagnosis of PE. The combination of elevated lactate dehydrogenase (LDH) and bilirubin in association with a normal serum glutamic oxaloacetic transaminase has long been recognized as insufficiently sensitive or specific. The absence of fibrinopeptide A in the urine combined with a low-probability lung scan may be useful in excluding PE but needs further study.[17] Plasma DNA measurements have received variable acceptance in the diagnosis of PE.

Measurement of serum levels of dimerized plasmin fragment D (D-dimer) is considered by many to have utility in excluding the diagnosis of PE. D-dimer is a sensitive but nonspecific indicator of thromboembolic disorders, and a level less than 500 U/mL is strong evidence against thrombosis (negative predictive value of about 90 percent). Recent reviews question the utility of this test in excluding PE, since results are highly dependent on the assay used and have a high incidence of false positives. At the present time there is no biochemical test, alone or in combination, that possesses sufficient sensitivity and specificity to allow the confirmation or exclusion of the diagnosis of PE.

Imaging Studies

Echocardiography, either transthoracic or transesophageal, may demonstrate right atrial, right ventricular, or proximal pulmonary arterial emboli. If right ventricular dysfunction is present in combination with normal systemic hemodynamics the need for careful monitoring and consideration of more aggressive therapy is suggested.[18] Transesophageal echocardiography is also useful in excluding thoracic aortic dissection as well as detecting massive PE in transit in hemodynamically unstable patients.[18,19] The ability to perform these tests at the bedside is especially useful in critically ill patients.

Other studies are used to detect DVT in the lower extremities, since the treatment of DVT and hemodynamically stable PE is the same. Noninvasive studies such as duplex ultrasonography (DUS) and impedance plethysmography (IPG) have largely replaced invasive contrast venography, although this last test remains the "gold standard." Using the criteria of vein compressibility, DUS is 95 to100 percent sensitive and more than 95 percent specific in diagnosing proximal DVT. Both IPG and DUS are insensitive in detecting DVT below the knee, but PE from this site is rare without proximal propagation. If DVT is strongly suspected and DUS or IPG are negative, serial exams are needed to detect extension of thrombus into the ileofemoral system.

TABLE 52-3 Definition of $\dot{V}/\dot{Q}$ Scan Probabilities

$\dot{V}/\dot{Q}$ Scan Category	Definition
High probability (>80%)	Two or more large mismatched segments or the equivalent
Intermediate probability (20–79%)	One moderate to two large mismatched segments
Low probability (<20%)	Nonsegmental perfusion defects, matched defects
Normal	No perfusion defects

Source: Adapted from Sostman HD, Coleman RE, DeLong DM, et al: Evaluation of revised criteria for ventilation-perfusion scintigraphy in patients with suspected pulmonary embolism. *Radiology* 193:103, 1994. With permission.

$\dot{V}/\dot{Q}$ scans of the lung often raise more questions than they answer. Although they are commonly used to diagnose or exclude PE, they have been shown to be reliable only at the extremes of interpretation—normal or high probability. All other results require further investigations to confirm or exclude PE, depending on the à priori probability.

One of the difficulties in interpreting $\dot{V}/\dot{Q}$ scans is that they are reported as "probabilities" rather than normal or abnormal. This probability must then be judged based on the clinical suspicion for PE. Table 52-3 shows an interpretation of $\dot{V}/\dot{Q}$ probabilities based on PIOPED data.[20] This demonstrates that a high-probability scan (Fig. 52-2*A* and *B*) is only 80 percent accurate in diagnosing PE, while a low-probability result is only 20 percent accurate in excluding the diagnosis. Overall, $\dot{V}/\dot{Q}$ scans are 98 percent sensitive but only 10 percent specific in the diagnosis of PE.[10] Infiltrate on CXR, preexisting cardiopulmonary disease, and previous PE all increase the rate of false-positive results.

Combining $\dot{V}/\dot{Q}$ results with the degree of clinical suspicion for PE has been shown to increase the accuracy of the test.[10] The combination of a low-probability scan with a low clinical suspicion has a 96 percent predictive value for the exclusion of PE, while a high-probability scan in the setting of high clinical suspicion has a 96 percent positive predictive value. The presence or absence of PE in this study was confirmed by pulmonary arteriography. Unfortunately, only a minority of patients (174 out of 887) in the PIOPED study were found to have the diagnosis of PE confirmed or excluded by the combination of pretest probability and $\dot{V}/\dot{Q}$ results.[10]

Further difficulty arises in defining "clinical suspicion." While most authors use the terms *high, moderate,* or *low* suspicion and some studies even assign a percent probability, no universally accepted diagnostic algorithm is available. The presence or absence of risk factors predisposing to the development of DVT is of prime importance, although unrecognized risk factors (e.g., occult cancer, deficiency of protein C or S) may exist in a given patient. The existence of unexplained symptoms of chest pain and dyspnea or signs such as tachypnea should raise the index of suspicion for PE. Findings of DVT, an elevated A-a gradient unexplained by exam or CXR, and the presence of a Westermark sign are all strong predictors of PE.

Spiral computed tomography (CT) compared favorably to pulmonary arteriography in one study, with an overall sensitivity of 82 to 90 percent and specificity of 93 to 96 percent. Accuracy was lowest in

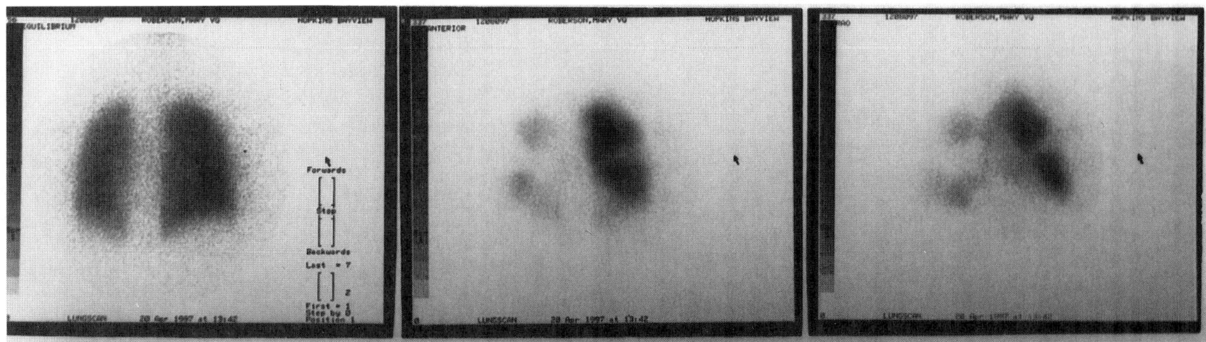

A. Ventilation - Equilibrium phase B. Perfusion - Anterior View C. Perfusion - RAO view

FIG. 52-2. High-probability $\dot{V}/\dot{Q}$ scan of patient whose CXR is shown in Fig. 52-1. **A.** Ventilation, equilibrium phase, demonstrates no ventilation defect. Washout phase demonstrated no air trapping. **B.** Perfusion, anterior. **C.** Right anterior oblique projections show multiple segmental defects. Note absence of flow to right upper lobe.

the setting of subsegmental PE.[21] Magnetic resonance imaging (MRI) angiography has reported sensitivity of 75 to 100 percent and specificity of 95 to 100 percent in PE proven by pulmonary arteriography.[22] It is of limited utility in unstable patients, however.

Pulmonary arteriography remains the standard by which all other studies are judged. A negative study reliably excludes the diagnosis of PE.[7,10] It should be obtained when clinical suspicion for PE is high and other studies ($\dot{V}/\dot{Q}$ scans, tests for leg DVT) are inconclusive or likely to produce false-positive results. It is often used prior to the initiation of thrombolytic therapy but is not necessary. Indeed, it increases the risk of bleeding complications in these patients.[18] Pulmonary arteriography has a mortality rate up to 0.5 percent and morbidity of 4 percent. These complications may be reduced by the use of selective angiography.

Diagnostic Approach

Suspect PE in a patient presenting with unexplained chest pain, dyspnea, tachypnea, syncope, or shock. Figure 52-3 is an algorithm for the approach to patients with suspected PE.

Historical evidence of risk for DVT, physical findings suggestive of DVT or PE and findings from ECG, CXR, and ABG are used to determine a pretest probability of PE.

Patients whose signs and symptoms remain unexplained should undergo further diagnostic evaluation, taking into account their clinical stability (Fig. 52-3). Stable patients should be studied for leg DVT (DUS, IPG, or venography) or PE ($\dot{V}/\dot{Q}$ scan). If DVT is confirmed, the patient should be admitted for anticoagulation therapy.

If a $\dot{V}/\dot{Q}$ scan is of high probability and clinical suspicion for PE is high, admission for anticoagulation is warranted. If the $\dot{V}/\dot{Q}$ scan is of low probability and the pretest suspicion also low, another diagnosis should be sought. A normal $\dot{V}/\dot{Q}$ scan reliably excludes PE regardless of clinical suspicion. All other combinations of $\dot{V}/\dot{Q}$ probabilities and clinical suspicion require further evaluation, whether pulmonary angiography, spiral CT, or MRI angiography.

For unstable patients suspected of having PE, transthoracic or transesophageal echocardiography is especially useful. Evidence of proximal pulmonary artery emboli or right ventricular embolus in transit is sufficient evidence to justify thrombolytic therapy without pulmonary angiography.[18] Echocardiography has the additional benefit of identifying patients with acute right ventricular dysfunction and normal systemic hemodynamics—a group at risk for catastrophic clinical deterioration. Sending an unstable patient to the nuclear medicine or angiography suite is potentially hazardous, requires intensive nursing and physician support, and should be done only as a last resort.

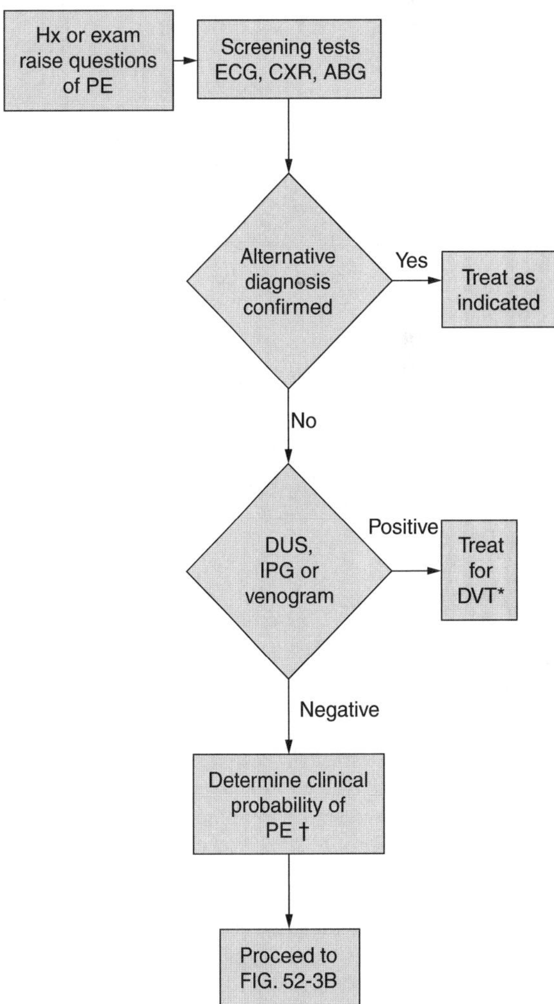

A

FIG. 52-3. A. Evaluation of stable patients with suspected PE. *Refer to text and Chap. 55. †Refer to text.

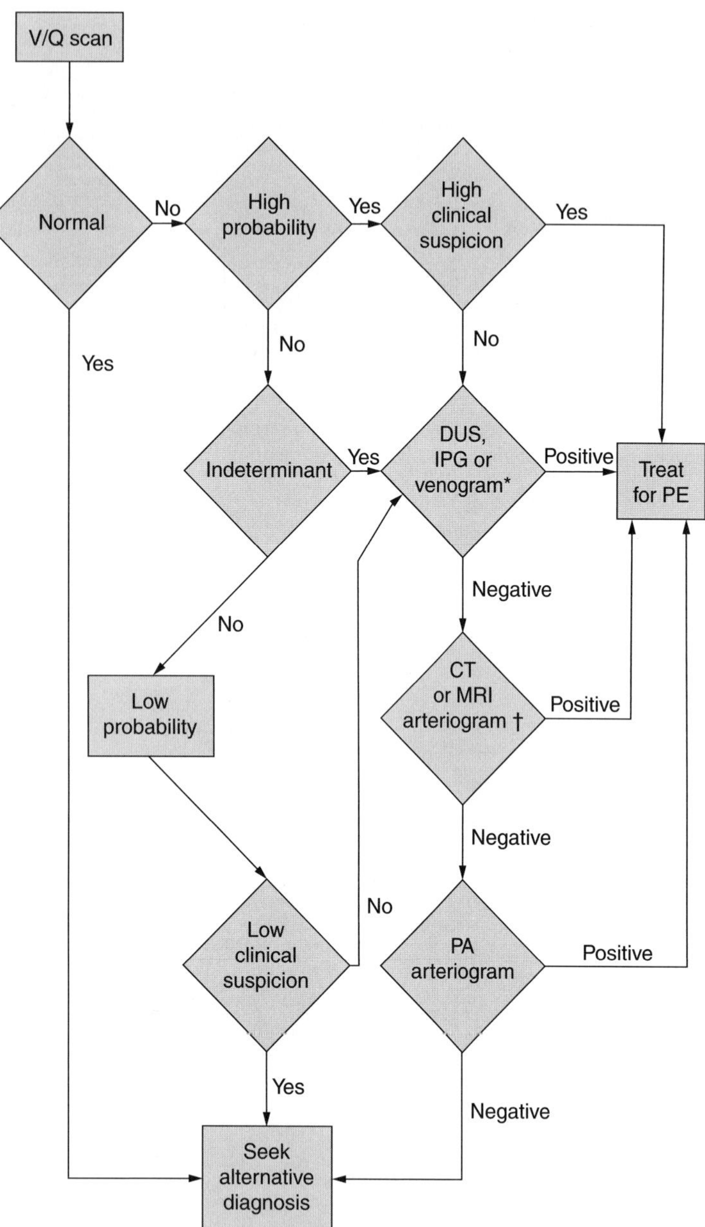

FIG. 52-3. B. Further evaluation of patients with suspected PE whose earlier tests have been negative.
*Perform these studies only if not previously obtained.
†The clinician may proceed directly to pulmonary arteriography depending on local availability and practice.

TREATMENT

All patients with significant chest pain, dyspnea, or tachypnea should receive cardiac monitoring, intravenous access, and supplemental oxygen while their evaluation proceeds. Failure to correct hypoxemia with supplemental oxygen may necessitate endotracheal intubation in order to provide a higher F_iO_2 directly. Shock in the absence of pulmonary edema should be treated with aggressive intravenous administration of crystalloid. If vasopressors are required, dopamine is considered the drug of choice in PE.

Stable patients with PE are treated with anticoagulant (AC) therapy. After obtaining baseline coagulation studies, intravenous heparin is administered first as a bolus (either 5000 U or 80 U/kg) and then as a constant infusion (1280 U/h or 18 U/kg per hour). Dosing of heparin based on the patient's weight is preferred, as it is less likely to produce subtherapeutic levels. The activated partial thromboplastin time (aPTT) is measured every 6 h, altering the heparin infusion, until a stable aPTT of 50 to 90 s is achieved; it is then checked daily. After 24 h of heparin, oral warfarin is begun at 5 to 10 mg/day and the prothrombin time (PT) is checked daily. Warfarin administration is best delayed owing to an initial hypercoagulability effect of reducing protein before reduced prothrombin levels are achieved. The dose is adjusted until PT measurements show a stable International Normalized Ratio (INR) of between 2 and 3 (or PT of 1.5 to 2.5 times control). Heparin and warfarin therapy should overlap for at least 4 days. Patients should continue warfarin therapy for at least 3 months, with monitoring of the PT. Low-molecular-weight heparin (LMWH) has been shown to be as safe and effective as unfractionated heparin,[23] allows for twice daily subcutaneous administration, and precludes the need for aPTT measurements. For these reasons many consider LMWH preferable in the treatment of DVT and PE. Chapter 216 discusses the major complication of AC therapy and their treatment.

Thrombolytic therapy is used in patients with massive PE associated with refractory hypoxemia or circulatory collapse. It should also be considered for patients with moderate to severe right ventricular dysfunction, since they may progress to circulatory collapse. Urokinase (4400 U/kg load followed by 4400 U/kg per hour by infusion for 12 to 24 h), streptokinase (250,000 U load followed by 100,000 U/h infusion for 24 h) and recombinant tissue plasminogen activator (r-tPA) at 100 mg over 2 h have all been shown to be effective in normalizing pulmonary artery pressures, improving right ventricular function, correcting hypoxemia, and improving systemic hemodynamics. However, r-tPA has been shown to be fastest in improving these parameters. Beneficial effects may be seen with thrombolytic therapy up to 2 weeks after the PE is activated, although the effects are greatest early in the course of the disease.[24] Therapy with heparin and warfarin is begun after the thrombolytic infusion is completed. Intrapulmonary artery infusion is no more effective than peripheral intravenous administration, and the risk of bleeding at the site of pulmonary artery catheter placement is high. The use of thrombolytics has largely replaced embolectomy in unstable patients.

Septic emboli, whether from indwelling central venous catheters or associated with IDU, represent a diagnostic and therapeutic challenge. Septic DVT requires not only appropriate AC therapy but also antibacterial or antifungal treatment. Removal or drainage of septic foci, whether due to an intravenous catheter or an abscess cavity, must be accomplished. In some circumstances surgical removal of an infected vein segment is required. AC therapy of septic PE from right-sided endocarditis is controversial, since heparin administration in endocarditis is associated with a higher incidence of intracranial hemorrhage.

Patients with recurrent PE despite adequate AC therapy or those with contraindications to AC therapy may require interruption of the inferior vena cava. Transvenous placement of a Greenfield (umbrella) filter is most commonly used for this.

DISPOSITION

All patients with known PE should be admitted for close monitoring and AC or thrombolytic therapy. Patients strongly suspected of having PE should be admitted if the diagnosis cannot be rapidly confirmed. Generally, the patient should be admitted to the service of an internist, pulmonologist, or cardiologist. A radiologist must be consulted to arrange and interpret invasive and noninvasive leg studies for DVT, $\dot{V}/\dot{Q}$ scans, spiral CT, MRI, and pulmonary arteriograms. Consultation with a thoracic surgeon is necessary if pulmonary embolectomy is contemplated.

The decision to initiate AC therapy prior to establishing the diagnosis of PE should be made in consultation with the admitting physician. The clinical situation and degree of suspicion for PE dictate this decision. AC therapy should be continued for at least 3 months in patients with first-time PE. Recurrent PE may dictate the need for chronic AC therapy.

REFERENCES

1. Morgenthaler TI, Ryu JH: Clinical characteristics of fatal pulmonary embolism in a referral hospital. *Mayo Clin Proc* 70:417, 1995.
2. Franks AL, Atrash HK, Lawson HW, et al: Obstetrical pulmonary embolism mortality, United States, 1970–85. *Am J Publ Health* 80:720, 1990.
3. Hirsch J: Diagnosis of venous thrombosis and pulmonary embolism. *Am J Cardiol* 65:45C, 1990.
4. Montreal M, Lafoz E, Ruiz J, et al: Upper-extremity deep venous thrombosis and pulmonary embolism: A prospective study. *Chest* 99:280, 1991.
5. Bell WR, Simon TL, DeMets DL: The clinical features of submassive and massive pulmonary emboli. *Am J Med* 62:355, 1977.
6. Stein PD, Terrin ML, Hales CA, et al: Clinical, laboratory, roentgenographic and electrocardiographic finding in patients with acute pulmonary embolism and no pre-existing cardiac or pulmonary disease. *Chest* 100:598, 1991.
7. Leeper KV Jr, Popovich J Jr, Adams D, et al: Clinical manifestations of acute pulmonary embolism: Henry Ford Hospital experience, a five-year review. *Henry Ford Hosp Med J* 36:29, 1988.
8. Cannon CP, Goldhaber SZ: Cardiovascular risk stratification of pulmonary embolism. *Am J Cardiol* 78:1149, 1996.
9. Lualdi JC, Goldhaber SZ: Right ventricular dysfunction after acute pulmonary embolism: Pathophysiologic factors, detection, and therapeutic implications. *Am Heart J* 130:1276, 1995.
10. PIOPED: Value of the ventilation/perfusion scan in acute pulmonary embolism: Results of the Prospective Investigation of Pulmonary Embolism Diagnosis (PIOPED). *JAMA* 263:2753, 1990.
11. Stein PD, Athanasoulis C, Alavi A, et al: Complications and validity of pulmonary angiography in acute pulmonary embolism. *Circulation* 85:462, 1992.
12. Stein PD, Alavi A, Gottschalk A, et al: Usefulness of noninvasive diagnostic tools for diagnosis of acute pulmonary embolism in patients with a normal chest radiograph. *Am J Cardiol* 67:1117, 1991.
13. Buckner CB, Walker CW, Purnell GL: Pulmonary embolism: Chest radiographic abnormalities. *J Thorac Imaging* 4:23, 1989.
14. Cvitanic O, Marino PL: Improved use of arterial blood gas analysis in suspected pulmonary embolism. *Chest* 95:48, 1989.
15. Stein PD, Goldhaber SZ, Henry JW: Alveolar-arterial oxygen gradient in the assessment of acute pulmonary embolism. *Chest* 107:139, 1995.
16. Jones JS, VanDeelen N, White L, et al: Alveolar-arterial oxygen gradients in elderly patients with suspected pulmonary embolism. *Ann Emerg Med* 22:1177, 1993.
17. Tulchinsky M, Zeller JA, Reba RC: Urinary fibrinopeptide A in the evaluation of patients with suspected acute pulmonary embolism. *Chest* 100:394, 1991.
18. Goldhaber SZ, Morpurgo M: Diagnosis, treatment, and prevention of pulmonary embolism: Report of the WHO/International Society and Federation of Cardiology Task Force. *JAMA* 268:1727, 1992.
19. Krivec B, Voga G, Zuran I, et al: Diagnosis and treatment of shock due to massive pulmonary embolism: Approach with transesophageal echocardiography and intrapulmonary thrombolysis. *Chest* 112:1310, 1997.
20. Sostman HD, Coleman RE, DeLong DM, et al: Evaluation of revised criteria for ventilation-perfusion scintigraphy in patients with suspected pulmonary embolism. *Radiology* 193:103, 1994.
21. van Rossum AB, Pattynama PMT, Ton ER, et al: Pulmonary embolism: Validation of spiral CT angiography in 149 patients. *Radiology* 201:467, 1996.
22. Meaney JFM, Weg JG, Chenevert TL, et al: Diagnosis of pulmonary embolism with magnetic resonance angiography. *N Engl J Med* 336:1422, 1997.
23. The Columbus Investigators: Low-molecular-weight heparin in the treatment of patients with venous thromboembolism. *N Engl J Med* 337:657, 1997.
24. Daniels LB, Parker A, Patel SR, et al: Relation of duration of symptoms with response to thrombolytic therapy in pulmonary embolism. *Am J Cardiol* 80:184, 1997.

HYPERTENSION

Melissa M. Wu
Arjun Chanmugam

Hypertension is considered one of the most important modifiable risk factors for cardiovascular disease and is the fourth most prevalent chronic medical condition in the United States.[1,2] Up to 24 percent of the United States general adult population and 32 percent of African Americans may be affected by hypertension.[3]

Overall morbidity and mortality rates, and, in particular, the risk of developing serious cardiovascular, renal, or cerebrovascular disease increase with poorly controlled blood pressure. Although the public has become more knowledgeable, only two-thirds of Americans with high blood pressure are aware of their diagnosis. Of greater concern is that nearly 75 percent of adult Americans with hypertension are not controlling their blood pressure to below 140/90 mmHg, and only half are taking their prescription medications as directed.[1,3] Accordingly, elevated blood pressure is frequently encountered in many emergency department (ED) patients.

The primary responsibilities of emergency physicians in the approach to hypertensive patients are to recognize and treat true emergencies, to manage the complications of chronic disease, and to arrange the most appropriate follow-up for nonemergent cases. To fulfill these responsibilities, emergency physicians need to have an understanding

TABLE 53-1 Classification of Blood Pressure for Adults Aged 18 Years and Older

Category	Systolic Blood Pressure (mmHg)	Diastolic Blood Pressure (mmHg)
Optimal	< 120	<80
Normal	<130	<85
High-normal	130–139	85–89
Hypertension		
Stage 1	140–159	90–99
Stage 2	160–179	100–109
Stage 3	≥180	≥110

Note: When systolic and diastolic pressures fall into different categories, the higher category should be used to classify the individual's blood pressure status.
Source: From JNC,[1] with permission.

of the definitions, pathophysiology, and pharmacotherapy of hypertension.

CLASSIFICATION

Among individuals, a wide variation in blood pressures occurs along a continuum from normotensive to hypertensive. In an effort to standardize terminology, the Joint National Committee on Prevention, Detection, Evaluation, and Treatment of High Blood Pressure developed a consensus regarding the definition of hypertension, which includes a graded classification dependent on risk factors and clinical condition (Table 53-1).[1] In general, either a systolic blood pressure (SBP) greater than 140 mmHg or a diastolic blood pressure (DBP) greater than 90 mmHg constitutes hypertension. However, management of hypertension depends more on the individual's clinical condition rather than the absolute systolic or diastolic values. In the ED, it is helpful to consider four general categories for the management of high blood pressure.

Hypertensive emergencies are those situations that require immediate blood pressure reduction to prevent or limit damage to target organs (i.e., brain, eyes, heart, or kidneys). The terms *malignant hypertension* or *hypertensive crisis* may also be used to refer to this category. Target-organ damage occurs in syndromes such as hypertensive encephalopathy, intracranial hemorrhage, acute left ventricular failure with pulmonary edema, unstable angina pectoris, acute myocardial infarction, dissecting aortic aneurysm, and eclampsia.[1] A hypertensive emergency is not defined by any absolute pressure measurements but, instead, is contingent on the presence of relative blood pressure increases combined with injury to any of the so-called target organs. In fact, a patient with a low baseline pressure can present with ''normal'' or mildly elevated pressure and be considered to have a true hypertensive emergency, if there is evidence of concurrent related central nervous system (CNS), cardiovascular, or renal dysfunction.

The treatment goal in hypertensive emergency is the immediate reduction of mean arterial pressure (MAP = [1/3(SBP-DBP) + DBP]) in a controlled, graded manner, using improvement in the patient's condition as a guide. Blood pressures should not exceed a 20 to 25 percent reduction within the first 30 to 60 min. Although hypertensive emergencies are the most serious complications of hypertension, they occur in only 1 percent of all hypertensive patients.

Hypertensive urgency is less clearly defined in the literature. Most sources concur that hypertensive urgency occurs when the blood pressure elevation presents a risk for imminent target-organ damage. Although acute organ injury has not yet occurred in hypertensive urgency, the risk of injury is high if the elevated blood pressure is allowed to persist. In many cases of hypertensive urgency, elevated blood pressure in the presence of preexisting conditions (e.g., renal insufficiency, congestive heart failure, coronary artery disease, or CNS disorders) increases the likelihood of target-organ damage. As with hypertensive emergencies, in hypertensive urgencies, relative increases in blood pressure are more important than absolute values. The main challenge for the clinician is determining whether the asymptomatic hypertensive patient is experiencing a hypertensive urgency. The first priority in recognizing this condition is to determine whether target-organ dysfunction exists. If dysfunction does not exist, the clinician must determine whether damage to the CNS, cardiovascular, or renal system is impending, given the elevated blood pressure and relevant past medical history. If target-organ dysfunction exists, the emergency physician must identify whether the end-organ dysfunction is chronic and at risk of acute further impairment, or whether the dysfunction is acute and related to the hypertension (i.e., then to be considered an emergency rather than an urgency). This may be difficult without knowledge of the patient's past medical history, including prior laboratory values and clinical findings. In many cases, the clinician may be obligated to initiate antihypertensive treatment without being certain of the diagnostic classification.

The treatment goal in hypertensive urgencies is the gradual reduction of blood pressure within 24 h by using oral antihypertensive agents, although the recommended duration to reduce the blood pressure varies in the literature from a few hours to 48 h. Because a common cause of hypertensive urgency is noncompliance with medications, restarting a patient on a previously established regime is an acceptable strategy. Any patient with a diagnosis of hypertensive urgency should be started on an antihypertensive medication with follow-up in 24 h. Admission decisions depend on the patient's comorbid conditions, and the clinician's impression of the patient's anticipated response to therapy.

Acute hypertensive (nonemergency/nonurgency) episode occurs when a patient is found to have stage 3 hypertension (Table 53-1; systolic pressure of 180 mmHg or more, and diastolic pressure of 110 mmHg or more) with no signs or symptoms of evolving or impending target-organ damage.[1] Although many of these patients receive treatment in an effort to prevent target-organ damage, there is some controversy regarding the need for immediate treatment. There is evidence to show that in some cases acute interventions may actually be harmful.[4] In chronically hypertensive individuals, complications of acute blood pressure reduction can include altered sensorium, seizures, transient ischemic attacks, and amaurosis and other visual changes. In addition, there is no evidence of a beneficial effect of acute blood pressure reduction on long-term control or on the chronic effects of hypertension. In general, these patients require no acute intervention but should be referred to a primary care physician for follow-up and initiation of therapy. If these patients have previously been diagnosed as hypertensive but have been noncompliant with medications, a reasonable strategy would be to restart the patients on their previous treatment regimen and then refer for appropriate follow-up care within 24 to 48 h.

Transient hypertension occurs in association with other conditions such as anxiety, alcohol-withdrawal syndromes, and some toxicologic substances. One specific type of transient hypertension is *white-coat hypertension,*[5] a phenomenon that occurs when a patient has an elevated blood pressure in a clinical setting but has a normal pressure at other times. White-coat hypertensive patients have elevated pressures only in a medical setting but are normotensive when followed over a 24-hour period with ambulatory blood pressure monitoring. A number of studies have shown that at least 20 percent of newly diagnosed hypertensive individuals are actually normotensive in their normal environment.[5] The cardiovascular morbidity and mortality rates of individuals with white-coat hypertension correlate with their ambulatory blood pressure as opposed to their pressure measurements in the medical setting. Therefore, a single encounter in the ED setting should not be the basis for diagnosis of new-onset hypertension, nor does it constitute an indication to initiate antihypertensive therapy. However, patients do require prompt and close follow-up care for repeat blood pressure testing.

PATHOPHYSIOLOGY

Systemic blood pressure is related to vascular smooth muscle tone. At the cellular level, postsynaptic α_1 and α_2 receptors are stimulated by norepinephrine released from the presynaptic sympathetic nerve ending, ultimately leading to the release of intracellular calcium stores. Calcium release results in smooth muscle contraction via activation of actin and myosin. The increase in smooth muscle tone results in increased peripheral vascular resistance thereby causing increased blood pressure. The presynaptic α_2 receptors, when stimulated by norepinephrine, help to limit this response by preventing further release of norepinephrine through a negative-feedback loop.

There are two major theories to explain how hypertension develops: (1) as a result of alterations in the contractile properties of smooth muscle in arterial walls, or (2) as a response to failure of normal autoregulatory mechanisms. Most individuals with hypertension have elevated peripheral vascular resistance with normal cardiac output. However, some patients may also have elevated cardiac output as a result of increased α-adrenergic and β-adrenergic tone.

The concept of autoregulation is important in the vascular beds of the vital organs, including the heart, kidneys, and brain, but has been most extensively studied in the latter.[6] In the brain, as blood pressure falls, cerebral vasodilation occurs. When blood pressure rises, the autoregulatory response is vasoconstriction, ensuring a stable cerebral blood flow rate among a range of blood pressures. However, autoregulation is effective only within a specific range of blood pressures. Most authorities specify a range of 50 to 150 mmHg for MAP, within which there is effective autoregulation in an uninjured brain. At pressures beyond this narrow range, the limits of autoregulation are breached, and hypoperfusion or hyperperfusion results. In patients with chronically elevated blood pressure, the narrow range at which autoregulation functions is shifted higher. Thus, chronically hypertensive patients can develop symptoms of brain hypoperfusion if their blood pressure is lowered to "normal" levels, because normal levels may be below the limits of the individual's adjusted autoregulation. The lower limit of cerebral autoregulation is based on a patient's baseline MAP and is generally about 25 percent below this baseline.[6]

When poorly controlled blood pressure is allowed to persist long enough, it can cause damage to specific organs and vascular beds. The pathologic change responsible for target-organ damage is fibrinoid necrosis of small arterioles. At a microscopic level, this process begins when vessels in capillary beds dilate in response to an elevated blood pressure that overwhelms the autoregulatory mechanism. The persistently elevated pressures cause injury to the endothelium, leading to increased vascular permeability and vascular wall injury. Eventually, endothelial damage leads to deposition of fibrin within the vessel walls and causes activation of mediators of coagulation and cell proliferation.[7] A recurrent cycle of vascular reactivity develops, with an increased release of vasoconstrictors, endothelial damage, platelet aggregation, myointimal proliferation, and progressive narrowing of arterioles.

Hypertensive retinopathy is traditionally graded into four categories. In grade I, there is minimal diffuse or focal narrowing of arterioles. In grade II, "copper" and "silver" wiring (increased light reflex) is evidence of long-standing uncontrolled hypertension. These are considered relatively mild target-organ effects. In grade III and IV retinopathy, cotton-wool spots (focal ischemia), hard exudates and hemorrhages (vessel leakage), and extensive microvascular changes are seen. Grade IV retinopathy is distinguished by disk edema and defines malignant hypertension or hypertensive crisis. (The term *papilledema* is frequently used, but the disk edema is due to infarction and hypoxia of the optic disk. Thus, the term papilledema is best reserved for disk edema associated with elevated cerebrospinal fluid pressure.) Grade I and grade II retinopathy are evidence of chronic hypertension. Grades III and IV are evidence of accelerated retinopathy particularly in the young. Also grade III and IV changes might not be seen in the elderly. The mechanism of underlying pathology—arteriolar spasm—ultimately leads to degeneration of the muscle of the blood vessel, with subsequent degeneration of the endothelial cells of the vessel lumen. The elderly, who are likely to have arteriosclerotic vessels, are paradoxically protected by the presence of this other pathology.

In the brain, an abrupt, sustained rise in blood pressure exceeding the limits of cerebral autoregulation may be associated with stroke, intracerebral hemorrhage, or hypertensive encephalopathy.[6] Vascular injury caused by an abrupt or persistent elevation in blood pressure may result in ischemia or infarction in vulnerable regions of the brain. Intracerebral bleeding from dilated vessels may result in cerebral or subarachnoid hemorrhage. Hypertensive encephalopathy is characterized by marked vasospasm with ischemia, punctate hemorrhages, and increased vascular permeability all leading to cerebral edema (a mechanism similar to retinopathy). This mechanism is different from localized cerebral edema in the area of ischemic stroke caused by emboli or thrombi. An increase in blood pressure may be a physiologic response to maintain adequate cerebral perfusion to areas distal to the occlusion and may not justify classification as a hypertensive emergency.

In the heart, increased afterload occurring after an acute rise in blood pressure results in increased left ventricular wall tension that, in turn, increases myocardial oxygen demand. Angina or myocardial infarction occurs when hypertension causes a decrease in coronary blood flow relative to an increased demand. Pulmonary edema occurs when the sudden increase in MAP results in elevated end-diastolic pressure and decreased end-diastolic filling volume precipitating acute left ventricular failure.

In the kidneys, impaired autoregulation due to elevated blood pressure results in decreased renal perfusion. Decreased renal perfusion stimulates the renin-angiotensin (I and II) cascade, leading to increased vasoconstriction. If this cycle continues, arteriolar necrosis occurs, ultimately leading to renal impairment. Angiotensin II can exacerbate hypertension not only by causing vasoconstriction but also by stimulating aldosterone secretion to promote sodium retention. Sodium retention induces hypertension in susceptible individuals by a variety of mechanisms, including (1) increased sympathetic nervous system activity; (2) decreased response to dopamine; (3) change in calcium and potassium metabolism; (4) resistance to insulin; and (5) inappropriate response of renal vasculature and adrenals to angiotensin II.[8]

Hypertension is associated with major cardiovascular risk factors such as smoking, hyperlipidemia, diabetes mellitus, age older than 60 years, gender (men and postmenopausal women), obesity, and a family history of cardiovascular disease.[1] In addition, dietary sodium excess in salt-sensitive individuals (50 percent of hypertensive patients) can induce hypertension. Although no single cause of hypertension has been identified, a combination of factors such as these are believed to contribute to elevated blood pressure.

Although most cases of hypertension are considered to be essential with no known cause, several specific causes do exist. Of the known causes, renal disease is the most prevalent and includes renal arteriostenosis, fibromuscular disease of the renal arteries, chronic pyelonephritis, and nonspecific glomerulonephritis. Coarctation of the aorta, although uncommon, is also an important cause of secondary hypertension and should be suspected in any patient with the triad of upper extremity hypertension, a systolic murmur best heard over the back, and delayed femoral pulses. Another cause of hypertension is excessive glucocorticoids, seen in Cushing syndrome, but usually due to exogenous steroid therapy. Endogenous overproduction is less common but results from excessive adrenocorticotropic hormone (ACTH) production by a pituitary tumor, ectopic ACTH production by a nonpituitary tumor, or glucocorticoid production by tumors of the adrenal cortex. Pheochromocytomas are tumors that produce catecholamines arising from cells of the sympathetic nervous system (most commonly from the adrenal medulla) and account for fewer than 1 percent of cases of hypertension. The characteristic feature of pheochromocytomas is paroxysms of hypertension associated with palpitations, tachycardia, malaise, apprehension, and sweating.[9] Finally, ingestion of foods containing large amounts of tyramine can raise blood pressure by causing release of norepinephrine stored in nerve endings. This normally transient response may become prolonged in patients taking monoamine oxidase (MAO) inhibitors, since these agents block the enzyme that destroys tyramine.

CLINICAL EVALUATION AND MANAGEMENT

Overview

The clinical evaluation of hypertensive patients is aimed at determining the underlying reason for the hypertensive episode and ascertaining the effects on end organs. Management is determined by this assessment. Although patients with hypertension present to the ED relatively frequently, the number of individuals who actually require emergent intervention is small.[10] ED management should begin with an accurate blood pressure measurement, confirmed by repeat assessment in both arms if the initial value is elevated. The challenge is to determine whether the presenting blood pressure reading is only a transient circumstantial elevation or is representative of the patient's baseline. The approach to hypertensive patients in the ED is summarized in the flow diagram in Fig. 53-1.

Medical History

Any prior diagnosis of hypertension, including treatment regimens, compliance patterns, and baseline recordings of past blood pressures, are important to determine. Elevated blood pressure in the context of several months of noncompliance with antihypertensive medications likely represents a patient's baseline, whereas hypertension after several days of noncompliance could be a more serious abrupt cessation syndrome. A history of all medication use, including over-the-counter and illicit drugs, should be obtained, since many commonly used

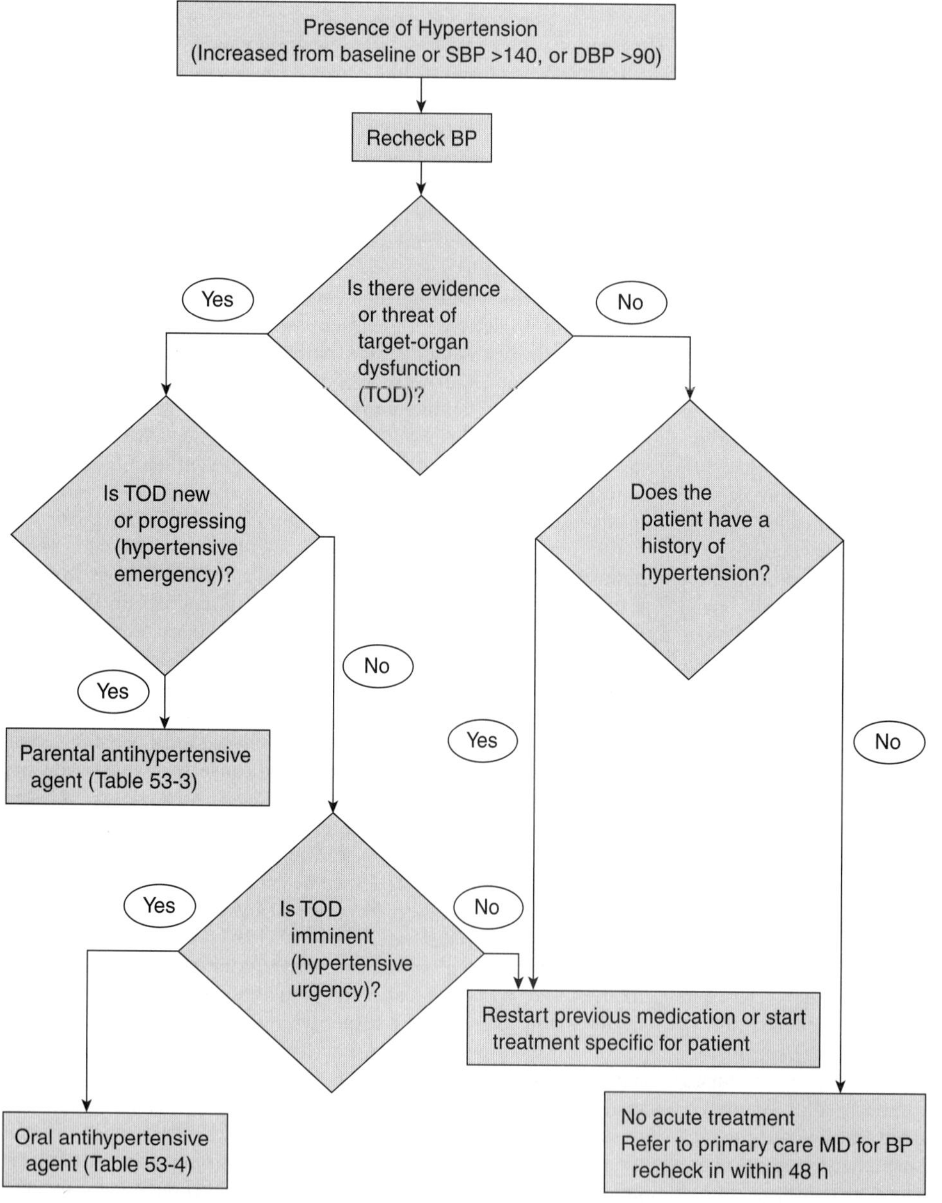

FIG. 53-1. Algorithm for approach to hypertensive patients.

agents—including cocaine, amphetamines, decongestants, stimulants, oral contraceptives, and nonsteroidal anti-inflammatory drugs (NSAIDs)—may elevate blood pressure. MAO inhibitors in combination with tyramine-containing foods (e.g., beer and aged cheese) or certain drugs (e.g., amphetamines and tricyclic antidepressants) can also precipitate acute blood pressure elevation. Any past medical history of cardiovascular, cerebrovascular, or renal disease; diabetes; hyperlipidemia; chronic obstructive pulmonary disease (COPD); asthma; or gout; or a family history of hypertension or premature heart disease should also be elicited.[1] Patients with elevated pressures should be asked specifically about CNS symptoms (e.g., headache, diplopia, blurred vision, confusion, hemiparesis, and seizures), cardiac symptoms (e.g., chest pain, dyspnea, tachycardia, and palpitations), and renal symptoms (e.g., hematuria and anuria) that may be indicative of progressive end-organ damage.[1]

Physical Examination

The blood pressure should be measured with a cuff of the appropriate size for the patient. The width of the inflatable portion of the cuff should be about 40 percent of the circumference of the limb and the length of the inflatable portion should equal 80 percent of the limb's circumference. Using a cuff that is too short or narrow or too loose may cause falsely high readings. The blood pressure should be measured at least twice if the first value is elevated (SBP of more than 140 mmHg or DBP of more than 90 mmHg). For severe elevation, measure pressure in both arms and legs, and palpate pulses in all extremities. In adults, a differential in brachial systolic pressures of more than 20 mmHg may indicate the presence of aortic coarctation, aneurysm, or dissection.

Focus the physical examination on the detection of target-organ damage and determine the acuity. Neurologic examinations that reveal focal findings or mental status changes may indicate hypertensive encephalopathy, subarachnoid hemorrhage, or stroke. A careful funduscopic examination may reveal acute changes such as hemorrhages, cotton-wool exudates, or disk or retinal edema (grade III or IV retinopathy). Alternatively, grade II retinopathy suggests chronic uncontrolled hypertension. Hyperreflexia with peripheral edema in a pregnant woman is suggestive of preeclampsia. This physical finding may also be found in elderly patients with multiple small ischemic strokes (lacunes).

On cardiovascular examination, auscultate for carotid bruits, murmurs, third and fourth heart sounds (S_3 and S_4), and a pericardial rub. An S_3 occurs in association with ventricular failure (either right or left), whereas an S_4 occurs when there is left ventricular hypertrophy and a noncompliant left ventricle. A right-sided S_4 may be heard with coexisting pulmonary hypertension. Left-sided congestive heart failure is associated with unexplained tachycardia as an early finding and pulmonary rales as a late finding. Diminished extremity pulses may be found in patients with coarctation of the aorta or aortic dissection. The abdomen should be examined for a bruit and a palpable pulsatile mass that may indicate the presence of an abdominal aortic aneurysm.[1]

Diagnostic Studies

Blood urea nitrogen (BUN), creatinine, electrolyte, and glucose levels should be determined, and complete blood count (CBC), electrocardiography (ECG), urinalysis, and chest x-ray should be obtained in cases of suspected hypertensive emergencies to look for evidence of target-organ damage.[1] Renal impairment may present as hematuria, proteinuria, or elevations in BUN, creatinine, and potassium levels. Red cell casts suggest glomerulonephritis. The blood glucose level is important because hypoglycemia can elevate blood pressure and also simulate hypertensive encephalopathy or stroke. The CBC may reveal microangiopathic hemolytic anemia that may occur as a result of vascular damage after an acute, severe rise in blood pressure. The ECG should be compared with previous tracings. ST-T wave changes may be evidence of ischemia, electrolyte abnormalities, or left ventricular hypertrophy. The chest x-ray may be helpful in showing evidence of left-sided congestive heart failure or aortic dissection. In patients with neurologic symptoms, computed tomography (CT) of the head should be performed to look for evidence of stroke or hemorrhage.

TYPES OF HYPERTENSIVE EMERGENCIES

Hypertensive Encephalopathy

Although no specific blood pressure is pathognomic, the elevated pressure must exceed the limits of cerebral autoregulation of the small-resistance arteries, resulting in cerebral hyperperfusion with loss of integrity of the blood-brain barrier. In most cases, autoregulation usually cannot accommodate a constant cerebral blood flow above a MAP of 150 to 200 mmHg. Immediate reduction of blood pressure by 20 to 25 percent will help reverse the vasospasm that occurs at these pressures; however, excessive reduction in blood pressure must be avoided in order to prevent hypoperfusion and further cerebral ischemia.[11,12]

Hypertensive encephalopathy is usually acute in onset and reversible. It is characterized by severe headaches, nausea, and vomiting, and may also include altered mental status. Neurologic symptoms can range from confusion and drowsiness to seizures, decreased visual acuity, focal deficits, or even coma. Since the pathologic mechanisms are the same, accelerated hypertensive retinopathy is often seen. The differential diagnosis is wide and includes intracranial hemorrhage, stroke, meningoencephalitis, brain tumors, toxidromes, and metabolic coma. If hypertensive encephalopathy is suspected, antihypertensive therapy should be initiated while awaiting the results of certain key studies such as chemistry tests and CT scan.

Hypertensive encephalopathy is a true medical emergency and, if left untreated, can progress over hours and lead to coma and death. The treatment of choice is sodium nitroprusside infused at an initial dose of 0.5 (μg/kg)/min and titrated up to a maximum of 10 (μg/kg)/min. Intravenous nitroglycerin and labetalol have been successfully used, but they have not replaced nitroprusside as first-line therapy for hypertensive encephalopathy.

Stroke Syndromes (see Chap. 220)

Elevated blood pressure is commonly associated with stroke syndromes and is often the result of a physiologic response to the stroke itself (to maintain adequate cerebral perfusion to the viable but edematous tissue surrounding the ischemic area) and not its immediate cause. In the area of the stroke, cerebral autoregulation is lost, causing tissue blood flow to become directly pressure dependent. Most patients suffering from embolic or thrombotic strokes without associated hemorrhage do not have substantial elevations in blood pressure and do not need aggressive antihypertensive treatment. Furthermore, if the patient has a long-standing history of hypertension, any rapid reduction in blood pressure may further reduce cerebral blood flow to watershed areas and cause increased ischemia.[11,12] In the rare case of a stroke patient with extreme blood pressure elevation or sustained diastolic pressure greater than 140 mmHg, the blood pressure may be reduced in a controlled manner by no more than 20 percent with intravenous labetalol in small doses beginning with 5-mg increments.

In contrast to the relatively minor blood pressure elevations with most strokes, intracranial hemorrhage commonly results in profound reactive rise in blood pressure. Causes of intracranial hemorrhage include hypertensive vascular disease, arteriovenous anomalies, arterial aneurysms, bleeding associated with tumors, and trauma. Hypertension associated with hemorrhagic stroke is usually transitory and the result of increased intracranial pressure and irritation of the autonomic nervous system. The acute management of blood pressure associated with intracranial hemorrhage is controversial. In the case of subarachnoid hemorrhage, oral nimodipine (60 mg every 4 h) has been used to reverse the vasospasm associated with subarachnoid blood. Intravenous nicardipine (2-mg boluses followed by a 4- to 15-mg/h infusion) is also beginning to have a role in the management of hypertension during this type of hemorrhage.

Acute Pulmonary Edema

The hypertension associated with acute pulmonary edema is usually a result of increased peripheral vascular resistance caused by elevated catecholamines. In some cases, pulmonary edema occurs because an abrupt rise in blood pressure precipitates acute left ventricular failure. The blood pressure must be lowered to reverse this process, and nitroprusside and intravenous nitroglycerin are the agents of choice, although the latter does not reduce blood pressure as much as nitroprusside. Additional standard therapy for pulmonary edema includes nitrates (to reduce preload and afterload), oxygen, diuretics, and morphine sulfate.

Acute Coronary Syndromes

Increased left ventricular end-diastolic pressure increases the workload of the heart. Wall tension is one of the greatest determinants of myocardial oxygen needs. Increases in oxygen demand secondary to hypertension may result in angina. Myocardial infarction may also develop particularly among those with fixed lesions in coronary arteries, preventing appropriate delivery of required oxygen. Acute left ventricular failure with pulmonary edema may also develop. Treatment of left-sided heart failure should include agents that decrease both preload and afterload. Other agents that have been used as adjuvant therapy include oxygen, morphine sulfate, and diuretics. The use of agents that increase myocardial oxygen demand, such as diazoxide, hydralazine, and minoxidil, should be avoided.

In cases of hypertension and angina, immediate blood pressure reduction is indicated to prevent myocardial damage, and therapy should be initiated with nitroglycerin, either sublingually or parenterally. For a greater degree of pressure reduction, sodium nitroprusside may be started.

Aortic Dissection (see Chap. 54)

Because aortic dissection is associated with hypertension in about 90 percent of cases, medical therapy aimed at reducing blood pressure can limit the extent of the dissection. The process begins as a tear in the aortic intima, allowing blood to dissect into the media and then to reenter the lumen of the aorta via a second intimal tear, resulting in a double-barreled aorta. Approximately half of all nontraumatic dissections begin in the ascending aorta, a third in the arch, and the rest in the descending aorta. The dissection may extend proximally to involve the carotid arteries, coronary arteries, or pericardium, or it may extend distally to include the spinal artery or renal arteries.

The classic description is the abrupt onset of severe, tearing chest pain, radiating to the back or the abdomen. The location of the pain, the signs and symptoms, and the findings on physical examination vary with the site of the dissection and the direction in which it extends. The blood pressure is generally elevated but may be normal or even low. There may be differences in the pulses and blood pressure in different extremities. Because of the variety of presentations, the diagnosis of aortic dissection is often a difficult one and may require the aid of imaging studies. In 80 to 90 percent of cases, the chest x-ray may show a widening of the cardiac silhouette or, less often, a widened superior mediastinum may be evident. The chest x-ray may also show a separation of calcified intima from the aortic wall, but other more definitive studies, including transesophageal ultrasound, CT, magnetic resonance imaging, and aortography, may be needed to confirm the diagnosis and identify the level of dissection (see Chap. 54 for details).

The initial medical therapy for a suspected dissection is the use of an antihypertensive agent to lower the blood pressure and reduce the ventricular ejection force (rate of change in pressure with time, dp/dt) of the heart. Treatment of choice includes either a combination of a β-adrenergic antagonist (such as esmolol) and sodium nitroprusside, or labetalol alone. Emergency surgical consultation should be obtained for all suspected aortic dissections, although dissections involving the descending aorta are often medically managed. Surgical intervention is indicated in dissections involving the ascending aorta or aortic arch and in cases in which pain and blood pressure cannot be adequately controlled.

Renal Failure

Blood pressure and renal function are intrinsically related. Hypertension may cause acute renal failure or exacerbate chronic renal failure, whereas renal disease may result in hypertension. In patients with renal disease, the control of hypertension can delay the progression of further injury. Worsening renal function in the setting of elevated pressure, with elevation of BUN and creatinine levels, proteinuria, or the presence of red cells and red cell casts in the urine, is considered a hypertensive emergency that requires immediate reduction of blood pressure. Nitroprusside is the preferred agent in these cases. Patients who have known renal failure and are dialysis dependent and have volume overload may require emergent dialysis if they present with uncontrolled hypertension with other evidence of end-organ dysfunction.

Preeclampsia and Eclampsia

These are discussed in Chapter 101.

Childhood Hypertensive Emergencies

Hypertension is an uncommon problem in children, occurring in less than 5 percent,[13] and is defined as SBP or DBP equal to or greater than the 95th percentile for age and sex. Blood pressure should be measured with a cuff of the appropriate size as noted earlier. In the majority of confirmed cases of hypertension, renal/renovascular disease and pheochromocytoma are the most common etiologies.

Children often will have nonspecific complaints such as throbbing frontal headache or blurred vision. Physical findings associated with hypertension are similar to those found in adults.

The decision to treat is based on the combination of blood pressure and symptoms, but a guideline for urgent treatment is blood pressure that exceeds previous measurements by 30 percent. The goal of treatment, as in adults, is to reduce pressure within 1 h by 25 percent. Nitroprusside [0.5 to 8 (μg/kg)/min] and labetalol [1 to 3 (mg/kg)/h] are the agents of choice to treat hypertensive emergencies of childhood. Pediatric hypertension that may require intervention in the ED probably mandates consultation and likely admission.

SELECTION OF AN ANTIHYPERTENSIVE AGENT

The following section outlines therapies for hypertensive emergency and urgency. For those patients in an ambulatory setting, Table 53-2 summarizes guidelines for the selection of an antihypertensive agent for patients with various coexisting conditions.[14] Diuretics should be one of the agents of first choice in patients with renal disease and congestive heart failure who are judged to be volume overloaded. Because of their greater prevalence of stage 3 hypertension (systolic pressure of 180 mmHg or more, and diastolic pressure of 110 mmHg or more), African American patients may require multidrug therapy. For treatment of patients with angina pectoris or postmyocardial infarc-

TABLE 53-2 Antihypertensive Treatment Regimens for Specific Populations

Coexisting Condition	Diuretic	β Blocker	Antiotensin-Converting Enzyme Inhibitor	α_1 Blocker	Ca^{2+}-Channel Blocker
Older age	++	+/−	+	+	+
Black race	++	+/−	+/−	+	++
Angina pectoris	+	++	+	+	++
Postmyocardial infarction	+	++	+	+	−
Congestive heart failure with systolic dysfunction	++	−	++	+	−
Cerebrovascular disease	+	+	+	+/−	+
Renal disease (Cr > 200 μmol/L)	++	+/−	−	+	+
Diabetes mellitus with nephropathy	+	+/−	+	+	+
Migraine	+	++	+	+	+
Atrial fibrillation (with rapid ventricular response)	+	++	+	+	+
Paroxysmal supraventricular tachycardia	+	++	+	+	+
Senile tremor	+	++	+	+	+

Symbols: ++, preferred; +, suitable; +/−, usually not preferred; −, usually contraindicated.
Source: From Kaplan and Gifford,[14] with permission.

tion, β blockers are indicated. They are also indicated for those patients with a history of migraines, atrial fibrillation with rapid ventricular response, paroxysmal supraventricular tachycardia, and senile tremor. The use of β blockers is safe in the latter part of pregnancy, but their use should be avoided in early pregnancy because of an association with fetal growth retardation. Angiotensin-converting enzyme (ACE) inhibitors should be used in patients with congestive heart failure and can also be used in patients with a history of diabetes mellitus, especially those with diabetic nephropathy. The use of ACE inhibitors should be avoided in pregnant women. In the elderly, diuretics are the first choice for antihypertensive therapy because the pathophysiology of their hypertension is usually related to total peripheral resistance rather than cardiac output. β blockers are also recommended as alternative therapy. Use of agents that cause significant orthostatic changes (e.g., calcium-channel blockers, peripheral adrenergic blockers, and α blockers), as well as drugs that cause cognitive dysfunction (e.g., central α_2 agonist), should be avoided in the elderly.

AGENTS FOR TREATMENT OF HYPERTENSIVE EMERGENCIES

Agents used in hypertensive emergencies are shown in Table 53-3.

Sodium Nitroprusside (Nipride)

ACTIONS AND PHARMACOLOGY This rapidly acting arteriolar dilator and venodilator is the drug of choice for hypertensive emergencies and is the standard against which all other agents are compared. It acts by reacting with cysteine to form nitrosocysteine, a potent activator of guanylate cyclase, which in turn stimulates the formation of cyclic GMP to relax smooth muscle in both arteries and veins. This decreases preload and afterload, resulting in decreased myocardial oxygen demand. The heart rate may increase slightly secondary to a baroreceptor-mediated reflex, but there is no change in cardiac output or myocardial blood flow unless there is preexisting coronary artery disease which can result in a significant reduction in regional blood flow ("coronary steal") (see below). Cerebral blood flow may be affected, decreasing in a dose-dependent manner. Renal blood flow remains unchanged, but plasma renin activity is increased. Pulmonary shunting may occur with nitroprusside use.

The rate of onset is extremely rapid, with a duration of action of 1 to 2 min and a plasma half-life of 3 to 4 min. Nitroprusside is metabolized to thiocyanate in the liver and is excreted slowly by the kidneys. Cyanide is an intermediate metabolite, but cyanide toxicity is rare.[15]

INDICATIONS Sodium nitroprusside is an excellent agent for all hypertensive emergencies except eclampsia prior to delivery (because it crosses the placenta). It is only indicated for postpartum eclampsia or in eclampsia resistant to other interventions.

USE The MAP should not be reduced by more than 20 to 25 percent within 30 to 60 min.[15] The solution is made by mixing 50 mg of sodium nitroprusside in 500 mL of 5% dextrose in water (D_5W) (10 mg/mL). The infusion is usually started at 0.5 (μg/kg)/min, titrating up to a maximum of 10 (μg/kg)/min until the desired blood pressure has been achieved. The blood pressure needs to be closely monitored; therefore, an arterial line should be placed once the infusion is initiated. Because of rapid degradation and sensitivity to light, sodium nitroprusside solution should be used within 24 h of mixing and be protected from the light by wrapping the solution and tubing in aluminum foil.

SIDE EFFECTS AND CONTRAINDICATIONS The most common complication is hypotension. Prolonged infusions may lead to the rare complications of cyanide toxicity, which may occur in patients with hepatic dysfunction, and thiocyanate toxicity, which is associated with renal failure.[15] This rarely occurs in the ED. Because nitroprusside inhibits hypoxia-induced vasoconstriction in the pulmonary vasculature, there may be increased perfusion to nonventilated areas of the lung. Myocardial ischemia may be worsened by a coronary steal syndrome because of dilation of coronary arteries or by the combina-

TABLE 53-3 Parenteral Agents for Hypertensive Emergencies

Drug	Mechanism of Action	Dose	Onset of Action	Duration	Contra-indications	Adverse Effects
Nitroprusside	Vascular smooth muscle dilator	0.3 (μg/kg)/min IV	Seconds	3–5 min	Hepatic dysfunction	Cyanide toxicity
Labetalol	α_1,β-Adrenergic blocker	20–80 mg/10 min or 1–2 mg/min IV max 300 mg	5 min	4–8 h	Asthma, COPD, 2nd- or 3rd-degree heart block	Bronchoconstriction, heart block
Esmolol	β_1-Adrenergic blocker	0.05–0.3 (mg/kg)/min	5–30 min	30 min	Asthma, COPD	Bronchoconstriction
Nitroglycerin	Vascular smooth muscle dilator	5–100 μg/min IV	2–5 min	5–10 min		Headache
Hydralazine	Arteriolar dilator	10–20 mg IV or 10–50 mg IM	10 min 20 min	4–6 h	Aortic dissection, CAD	Tachycardia, increases catecholamines
Trimethaphan	Ganglionic blocker	0.3–3.0 mg/min IV	1–5 min	10 min		Autonomic effects, tachycardia
Enalaprilat	ACE inhibitor	0.625–1.25 mg IV	15 min	6 h	Renal artery stenosis	Acute renal failure, angioedema
Fenoldopam	Dopaminergic receptor agonist	0.05–1.5 (mg/kg)/min IV	4 min	8–10 min		Headache, flushing
Nicardipine	Calcium-channel blocker	4–15 mg/h IV	15–30 min	40 min	Aortic stenosis	Headache tachycardia

Abbreviations: ACE, angiotensin-converting enzyme; CAD, coronary artery disease; COPD, chronic obstructive pulmonary disease; IM, intramuscularly; IV, intravenously.

tion of nitroprusside and clonidine. Another consequence of the vasodilatory effect of nitroprusside is increased intracranial pressure.

Labetalol

ACTIONS AND PHARMACOLOGY This antihypertensive agent is a competitive, selective α_1 blocker and a competitive, nonselective β blocker, with the β-blocking action being 4 to 8 times the α-blocking action. It can be given either orally or intravenously. It lowers blood pressure by blocking α_1 adrenoreceptors in vascular smooth muscle but, because of the simultaneous β blockade, causes no reflex tachycardia.

When given intravenously, the distribution to peripheral tissues is rapid, with a large volume of distribution (15.7 L/kg). Onset of action is 5 to 10 min, and the duration of action is 8 h. The elimination half-life is 5.5 h. When taken orally, it is rapidly absorbed, with an absorption half-life of about 12 min and peak plasma concentrations at about 50 min. Labetalol is safe for use in patients with renal insufficiency, because it is predominantly (95 percent) hepatically metabolized; however, oral dosing may need to be reduced in patients with hepatic disease, because of significant first-pass hepatic metabolism. Oral bioavailability is only 25 percent but increases in the elderly or when taken with food or cimetidine. The elimination half-life after an oral dose is 8 h.

Labetalol reduces systolic arterial pressure and total peripheral vascular resistance. Cardiac output may be slightly decreased or unchanged, pulmonary artery and wedge pressures decrease, and angiotensin II activity decreases, while cerebral blood flow, renal blood flow, and glomerular filtration rates are unchanged. With prolonged use, fluid retention may occur. Labetalol should be used with caution in patients with asthma and COPD, because of its nonselective β-blocking activity, which decreases the forced expiratory volume in 1 s (FEV_1) by causing bronchospasm. The use of labetalol should also be avoided in patients with bradycardia and second- or third-degree heart block.

INDICATIONS Labetalol can be used intravenously for hypertensive emergencies and be easily converted to the oral formulation as the first-line agent for hypertensive urgencies. It offers the advantages of providing a steady, consistent drop in blood pressure without decreasing cerebral blood flow or producing reflex tachycardia. It can be safely used in patients with cerebral vascular disease and coronary artery disease. Labetalol is ideal for use in syndromes associated with excessive catecholamine stimulation, such as from pheochromocytoma, MAO inhibitor-induced emergencies, and abrupt clonidine withdrawal. It has also been used in pregnancy-induced hypertension. It is a class C drug in pregnancy.

USE Labetalol can be given for hypertensive emergencies with repeated, incremental boluses starting with 20 to 40 mg IV, until the target blood pressure is achieved or a total dose of 300 mg is reached. After an intravenous bolus, the blood pressure falls in 5 min, with a maximum response in 10 min, and antihypertensive effect lasting for up to 6 h. After a 20-mg loading dose, labetalol may also be given as a continuous infusion by mixing 200 mg in 200 mL of D_5W and running this at 2 mg/min (2 mL/min). The infusion should be stopped when the target pressure has been achieved.

The initial oral dose in hypertensive urgencies is 200 mg. Patients can experience the onset of effects within 1 to 3 h.[16]

SIDE EFFECTS AND CONTRAINDICATIONS Labetalol has a prolonged action because of its large volume of distribution and long elimination half-life. In 5 percent of patients, orthostatic hypotension is a complication of therapy. The nonselective β-blocking action can exacerbate heart failure and induce bronchospasm. A paradoxical hypertensive effect may occur when the drug is used in low doses in catecholamine-induced crisis, because of the predominant β blockade, leaving relatively unblocked α receptors for the circulating catecholamines.[17] In addition, patients with ischemic heart disease may experience exacerbation of angina and, in some cases, myocardial infarction after abrupt discontinuation of oral therapy.

Esmolol

ACTIONS AND PHARMACOLOGY This is an ultra-short-acting β_1-selective adrenergic blocker, which has rapid distribution and elimination half-lives of 2 and 9 min, respectively. When given as an intravenous bolus, followed by an infusion, 90 percent of β blockade is achieved within 5 min; however, when given as an infusion without a bolus, steady-state blood levels are reached within 30 min. Within 2 min of discontinuing an infusion, there is a significant decrease in the β-antagonist activity, and, generally, all blockade will resolve within 30 min. Because of its rapid onset of action, short duration of action, and easy reversibility—properties not found in other β blockers—esmolol is very useful in acute settings.[18] When compared with sodium nitroprusside, esmolol provides similar rapid control of hypertension without producing the excessive reduction in DBP and reflex tachycardia that are seen with sodium nitroprusside.

INDICATIONS Esmolol has been used in the treatment of supraventricular tachycardias; to lower pulse and blood pressure in perioperative patients and in patients with myocardial infarction, unstable angina, and thyrotoxicosis; and to blunt rises in blood pressure associated with intubation. It has also been used for severe hypertension but is not particularly efficacious as monotherapy.

USE A loading dose of 0.5 (mg/kg)/min may be given over 1 min prior to the initiation of an infusion of 0.05 to 0.3 (mg/kg)/min. Esmolol may also be given without a loading dose but then takes longer to reach a steady state. It is usually used in combination with other agents such as nitroprusside or phentolamine for hypertensive emergencies.

SIDE EFFECTS AND CONTRAINDICATIONS Because of its β-antagonist activity, the use of esmolol should be avoided in patients with asthma or COPD. It also should not be used to treat patients with cocaine-induced cardiovascular complications, because of the predominant β blockade, leaving relatively unblocked α receptors.

Intravenous Nitroglycerin

ACTIONS AND PHARMACOLOGY This agent acts by causing both arteriolar dilation and venodilation, with a greater effect on the venous system than on the arterial vasculature. Onset of action is almost immediate when nitroglycerin is given intravenously, and the half-life is 4 min. The mechanism of action is thought to involve the reduction of sulfhydryl groups at a smooth muscle nitrate receptor, resulting in an increase in cyclic GMP. Nitroglycerin is hepatically metabolized. Cardiac output usually remains unchanged but may decrease slightly.

INDICATIONS The main indication for nitroglycerin is in the setting of myocardial ischemia, because it is a better vasodilator of the coronary vessels than is nitroprusside; therefore, it is the agent of choice for moderate hypertension complicating unstable angina, myocardial infarction, or pulmonary edema. It also has a less harmful effect on pulmonary gas exchange than does nitroprusside.

USE The initial infusion rate should be 5 to 20 μg/min, with 5-μg/min incremental increases every 5 min until symptoms are improved or adverse effects necessitate stopping the infusion.

SIDE EFFECTS AND CONTRAINDICATIONS The most common side effects include headache, tachycardia, nausea, vomiting, hypoxia, and hypotension.

Hydralazine

ACTIONS AND PHARMACOLOGY This agent acts as a direct arteriolar dilator, with onset of action within 10 min when given intravenously and a duration of action of 4 to 6 h. The onset of action increases to 20 min when hydralazine is given intramuscularly and to 30 min after an oral dose. The plasma half-life is 2 to 4 h, but the antihypertensive affect may outlast this time interval. Its mechanisms of action are not well understood, but it is known to directly relax vascular smooth muscle, resulting in vasodilation. Hydralazine is metabolized by acetylation in the liver and gut walls by ring hydroxylation and conjugation. In patients who are ''slow acetylators'' (50 percent of the US population), there is a higher incidence of hypotension and toxic complications. Within 24 h, 80 percent of hydralazine and its metabolites are excreted in the urine. Doses need to be decreased in patients with renal insufficiency.

INDICATIONS The main indication for use of intravenous hydralazine is pregnancy-induced hypertension.[19] The drug can be used orally and in combination with other drugs.

USE In cases of eclampsia, hydralazine can be given as either a 10- to 20-mg intravenous dose or a 10- to 50-mg intramuscular dose. This dose can be repeated in 30 min.

SIDE EFFECTS AND CONTRAINDICATIONS Hydralazine should not be used in patients with aortic dissection or a history of coronary artery disease, because it causes reflex tachycardia and increases plasma renin and catecholamines. It also causes sodium and water retention and can cause headaches, nausea, tachycardia, lethargy, and postural hypotension. A lupuslike syndrome can result from chronic oral use.

Trimethaphan

ACTIONS AND PHARMACOLOGY This is a ganglionic blocking agent that inhibits both sympathetic and parasympathetic discharge by occupying receptor sites, thus stabilizing postsynaptic membranes from the effects of acetylcholine. This blockade results in vasodilation, improved blood flow to some vascular beds, and a decrease in blood pressure. The heart rate may rise in response to the decrease in peripheral vascular resistance. Cardiac output, stroke volume, and left ventricular work decrease. It has a rapid onset of action, and its effects are of short duration.

INDICATIONS Historically, trimethaphan had been the drug of choice for acute aortic dissection, especially of the descending type. However, because it causes a number of serious side effects, it has been replaced by the combination of nitroprusside and β blockade as the therapy of choice. It continues as a second-line agent in this setting.

USE Trimethaphan is given by intravenous infusion at a rate of 0.3 to 3.0 mg/min. It is sometimes used in combination with propranolol (1 to 3 mg IV or 10 to 40 mg orally qid) to reduce the velocity and force of left ventricular ejection.

SIDE EFFECTS AND CONTRAINDICATIONS A number of serious side effects can occur including bladder atony with urinary retention, ileus, gastric atony, cycloplegia, severe postural hypotension from blockade of circulatory reflex pathways, and even respiratory arrest. Tolerance develops with continued use; therefore, it is mainly useful

TABLE 53-4 Oral Agents for Hypertensive Urgencies

Drug	Mechanism of Action	Dose	Onset of Action	Duration	Contra-indications	Adverse Effects
Nitroglycerin	Vascular smooth muscle dilator	0.3–0.6 mg SL	5 min	5–10 min	Aortic stenosis	Headache
Labetalol	α_1,β-Adrenergic blocker	200–400 mg PO, repeat every 2–3 h	30–120 min	6–12 h	Asthma, COPD, 2nd- or 3rd-degree heart block	Bronchoconstriction, heart block
Clonidine	Central α agonist	0.1–0.2 mg PO, repeat every hour	30–60 min	6–8 h	CHF, 2nd- or 3rd-degree heart block	Drowsiness, sedation, tachycardia, dry mouth
Captopril	ACE inhibitor	6.5–25 mg PO	15–30 min	4–6 h	Renal artery stenosis	Acute renal failure, angioedema
Nifedipine (extended release)	Calcium-channel blocker	10 mg/30 min PO	5–15 min	3–6 h	Angina, acute hypertension	MI, CVA, syncope, heart block, CHF
Losartan	Angiotensin II receptor antagonist	10–50 mg PO	60 min	12–24 h	2nd and 3rd trimesters of pregnancy	Allergic (rare)

Abbreviations: ACE, angiotensin-converting enzyme; CHF, congestive heart failure; COPD, chronic obstructive pulmonary disease; CVA, cerebrovascular accident; MI, myocardial infarction; PO, per os (orally); SL, sublingual.

for short-term administration such as in patients awaiting surgery or in inoperable patients until oral therapy with another agent can be started.

AGENTS FOR TREATMENT OF HYPERTENSIVE URGENCIES

See Table 53-4.

Sublingual Nitroglycerin

INDICATIONS It is the agent of choice for unstable angina, for immediate treatment of pain in acute myocardial infarction, and for the treatment of left ventricular insufficiency and pulmonary edema.[20]

USE Nitroglycerin is absorbed very quickly through the oral mucosa. It is given as a 0.3- to 0.6-mg tablet or spray under the tongue. The onset of hypotensive effect is in 5 min and can last several hours.

SIDE EFFECTS AND CONTRAINDICATIONS The most common side effects include headache, tachycardia, nausea, vomiting, hypoxia, and hypotension. It should be used with caution in patients with aortic stenosis.

Clonidine

ACTIONS AND PHARMACOLOGY This agent is a centrally acting, α_2-adrenergic agonist that decreases central sympathetic activity, lowering plasma catecholamine levels. Clonidine causes little postural hypotension, because vasomotor reflexes are unchanged. It also does not increase heart rate or cardiac output and does not change renal blood flow or glomerular filtration rates. Overall, the effect of clonidine is to lower blood pressure, slow the heart rate, and cause sedation.

The onset of action is 30 to 60 min after an oral dose, with peak effect in 2 to 4 h. The duration of action is 6 to 8 h. Clonidine crosses the blood-brain barrier. Because approximately 50 percent is excreted unchanged in the urine in the first 24 h, it can accumulate in patients with renal insufficiency and is not dialyzable; however, in cases of renal failure, it is excreted in the feces.

INDICATIONS This is considered to be a second-line agent for the treatment of hypertensive urgencies. It can be used safely in the elderly and in renal failure. However, because it sometimes requires up to 6 h for an adequate response, it is not ideal for ED use.

USE The initial dose is 0.1 mg, with additional doses of 0.1 mg every hour until the diastolic pressure is below 115 mmHg or a maximum dose of 0.7 mg has been given. A patient who is given clonidine in the ED setting does not need to be discharged on this specific agent long term.

SIDE EFFECTS AND CONTRAINDICATIONS The most common side effects include dry mouth, drowsiness, and constipation. Rarely, bradycardia can occur in patients with sick sinus syndrome. Clonidine may interact with other drugs, causing adverse effects such as orthostatic hypotension in patients taking diuretics, decreased antihypertensive effects with cyclic antidepressants, increased sedation with alcohol, and bradyarrhythmias or other dysrhythmias with negative inotropic agents. When high doses of clonidine are abruptly stopped, the well-documented phenomenon of clonidine withdrawal with severe rebound hypertension, tachycardia, flushing, and abdominal symptoms may be seen. If this syndrome occurs, the patient should be given clonidine therapy promptly. The use of β blockers should be avoided because they may worsen the withdrawal symptoms.

Captopril

ACTIONS AND PHARMACOLOGY This is an angiotensin-I-converting enzyme inhibitor that is rapidly absorbed orally, with an onset of action within 15 to 30 min, peak effects of blood pressure reduction between 50 and 90 min, and duration of antihypertensive effect of 4 to 6 h. It causes no change in cardiac output, heart rate, or cerebral blood flow. Since captopril is renally metabolized, its dosing must be decreased in patients with renal insufficiency. Postural hypotension is a rare problem, because it has no effect on baroreceptor reflexes.

INDICATIONS Captopril is effective in cases of refractory acute congestive heart failure and is also useful in treating hypertensive urgencies with known renovascular hypertension.

USE The usual oral dose is 25 mg. The dose-response curve for captopril is flat; therefore, increasing doses generally do not cause greater reductions in blood pressure.

SIDE EFFECTS AND CONTRAINDICATIONS Several common side effects include skin rash, cough, and loss of taste. Laboratory abnormalities that can occur include leukopenia, proteinuria, and hyperkalemia. Captopril should not be used in combination with potassium-sparing diuretics. It also should not be given to patients with bilateral renal artery stenosis or unilateral stenosis with one kidney, because of the risk of acute renal failure. In patients with chronic renal failure or collagen-vascular disease, there is an increased risk of side effects. A potentially life-threatening complication of this therapeutic agent is angioneurotic edema, which can result in airway compromise.[18] This condition presents as a pale and sometimes severe swelling of the face and upper airway, and should be treated with epinephrine, antihistamines, and glucocorticoids.

Nifedipine

ACTIONS AND PHARMACOLOGY This dihydropyridine calcium-channel antagonist has been one of the most extensively studied agents for rapid control of blood pressure. Until the last few years when awareness of serious side effects became more widespread, it had been the most frequently used agent for acute blood pressure lowering in hospitalized patients. It is a coronary and peripheral arterial dilator, which causes a slight increase in heart rate but rarely causes postural hypotension. It can be given orally, sublingually, or rectally and has been shown to lower blood pressure quickly and in a rapid dose-dependent manner. After sublingual administration, the onset of action is 1 to 5 min, with a maximal effect at 20 to 60 min. The duration of action is 3 to 5 h. The clearance half-life is 2 to 4 h and the time to peak level remains constant with all doses. It undergoes extensive hepatic metabolism.

With an oral dose, peripheral vascular resistance falls, cardiac output increases, and pulmonary capillary wedge pressures decrease. There is a slight increase or no change in the glomerular filtration rate and renal blood flow. Nifedipine may improve cardiac performance in patients with impaired ventricular function but, because of its negative inotropic effect, should be used with caution in patients with severe congestive heart failure.

INDICATIONS The US Food and Drug Administration (FDA) has never specifically approved the use of short-acting nifedipine for the treatment of hypertension of any kind. Because of the risks of serious adverse reactions, such as acute coronary events or an ischemic stroke, the US National Heart, Lung, and Blood Institute issued a warning in 1995 stating that this agent should not be used in the treatment of hypertension, angina, and myocardial infarction.[21] The extended-release form of nifedipine appears to have less adverse effects than the short-acting formulations.

SIDE EFFECTS AND CONTRAINDICATIONS The common side effects of flushing, headache, pedal and periorbital edema formation, and palpitations are relatively well tolerated. The less common, but more serious, complications that have occurred include cerebral ischemia, syncope, complete heart block, symptomatic hypotension, sinus arrest, retinal ischemia, congestive heart failure, and myocardial ischemia/infarction. Rebound hypertension can also occur when nifedipine therapy is stopped abruptly.

Although nifedipine has been used widely for hypertensive urgencies, some patients are predisposed to unfavorable outcomes with the use of this drug. Five effects have been identified that can cause complications when nifedipine is used to treat acute hypertension in some vulnerable patient populations.[22] These are (1) proischemic effects—the potential to worsen ischemia unpredictably, especially in areas of the myocardium with good collaterals, (2) prohemorrhagic effects—antiplatelet activity combined with vasodilation, (3) negative inotropy—especially in patients with a history of congestive heart failure, (4) hypotension—with resultant hypoperfusion of the subendocardium, and (5) arrhythmogenic effects—predisposition to ventricular tachyarrhythmias in some populations.

PROMISING NEW ANTIHYPERTENSIVE AGENTS

Enalaprilat

ACTIONS AND PHARMACOLOGY This agent, which is the first intravenous ACE inhibitor approved for clinical use, is the biologically active form of the oral ACE inhibitor enalapril that occurs after deesterification in the liver. It is effective in patients with chronic heart failure with left ventricular ejection fractions of 20 to 44 percent, because it causes coronary vasodilation and significant reduction in mean arterial blood pressure and pulmonary capillary wedge pressure. It also improves cardiac index and stroke volume without affecting the heart rate or stroke work index.[18]

The onset of antihypertensive effect is within minutes of an intravenous bolus injection, with the maximal decrease in DBP in 30 min and duration of action up to 6 h. The degree of blood pressure reduction seems to be associated with the degree of pretreatment plasma renin activity, thus suggesting that the mechanism of antihypertensive effect may be renin-angiotensin inhibition.[18] Enalaprilat is excreted primarily by the kidney; therefore, its dosage should be decreased in patients with severe renal insufficiency.

INDICATIONS Enalaprilat is an effective intravenous antihypertensive agent in hypertensive emergencies that can be easily replaced by oral enalapril for long-term maintenance therapy.

USE An initial dose of 0.625 to 1.25 mg by intravenous bolus has been found to be effective in reducing blood pressure and heart rate. Doses of 2.5, 5, and 10 mg, up to a maximum of 40 mg, have been tried in different studies but have not been found to show appreciable difference in the magnitude of blood pressure reduction with increasing dose.[23] A bolus can be given every 6 h. The onset of hypotensive effects is variable.

SIDE EFFECTS AND CONTRAINDICATIONS This agent produces complications and effects that are similar to those of other ACE inhibitors, most notably angioneurotic edema and deterioration of renal function.

Fenoldopam

ACTIONS AND PHARMACOLOGY This antihypertensive agent is a selective postsynaptic dopaminergic receptor (DA_1) agonist that has potent vasodilative and natriuretic properties.[18] Recent clinical trials have shown this intravenous agent to be effective in the treatment of severe hypertension without causing a change in heart rate. The onset of action is 4 min, with duration of antihypertensive effect of 8 to 10 min.

INDICATIONS Fenoldopam shows promise for use in treating hypertensive emergencies but is not yet FDA approved for this purpose.

USE The initial dose is 0.05 to 0.1 (mg/kg)/min and can be increased at increments of 0.1 (mg/kg)/min to a maximum infusion rate of 1.6 (mg/kg)/min or to a diastolic pressure of less than 110 mmHg.

SIDE EFFECTS AND CONTRAINDICATIONS Mild side effects of headache and flushing occur in about 25 percent of patients.

Nicardipine

ACTIONS AND PHARMACOLOGY This is a dihydropyridine calcium-channel blocker that decreases afterload by reducing total peripheral resistance without reducing cardiac output and without apparent negative inotropic effect on the heart. It improves left ventricular pumping activity in patients with mild to moderate heart failure.[18] Nicardipine also displays a greater vasodilator effect on coronary than on systemic vessels and produces a clinically significant decrease in cerebral vasospasm after subarachnoid hemorrhage.[24] The onset of action is 15 to 30 min, with a duration of action of 40 min.

INDICATIONS It has been used for the treatment of postoperative hypertension, stable angina, and congestive heart failure, and shows promise for use in patients with subarachnoid hemorrhage.

USE Nicardipine can be given initially as a 2-mg intravenous bolus, followed by a 4- to 15-mg/h infusion.

SIDE EFFECTS AND CONTRAINDICATIONS Nicardipine does not produce the negative inotropic effects seen with other calcium-channel blockers such as nifedipine. Headache occurs as a side effect in 20 to 50 percent of patients. Other less common effects include hypotension, tachycardia, nausea, and vomiting. The use of nicardipine is contraindicated in patients with severe aortic stenosis.

Losartan

ACTIONS AND PHARMACOLOGY This is a highly selective angiotensin II receptor antagonist that blocks the vasoconstrictor and aldosterone-secreting effects of angiotensin II. It selectively blocks the binding of angiotensin II to specific receptors found in vascular smooth muscle and the adrenal gland.[18] It undergoes substantial first-pass metabolism by cytochrome P-450 enzymes and is converted to an active metabolite. The half-life of losartan is about 2 h and of the metabolite is about 6 to 9 h. Peak concentrations of losartan and its active metabolite are reached in 1 h and in 3 to 4 h, respectively.

INDICATIONS Losartan has been used in clinical trials in the treatment of hypertensive urgency.

USE It is available as 10-, 25-, or 50-mg tablets. The 50-mg dose has been found in studies to produce better results than the lower doses, but higher doses do not produce a more significant blood pressure reduction.

SIDE EFFECTS AND CONTRAINDICATIONS Because of potential fetal injury, the use of losartan should be avoided in the second and third trimesters of pregnancy. Dosing should be decreased in patients with hepatic insufficiency.

REFERENCES

1. Joint National Committee (JNC) on Prevention, Detection, Evaluation, and Treatment of High Blood Pressure: The sixth report of the Joint National Committee on Prevention, Detection, Evaluation, and Treatment of High Blood Pressure. *Arch Intern Med* 157:2413, 1997.
2. US Department of Health and Human Services. Prevalence of selected chronic conditions: United States, 1986–1988. *Vital Health Stat* 182:10, 1993.
3. Burt VL, Whelton P, Roccella EJ, et al: Prevalence of hypertension in the U.S. adult population: Results from the Third Health and Nutrition Examination Survey, 1988–1991. *Hypertension* 25:305, 1995.
4. Fagan TC: Acute reduction of blood pressure in asymptomatic patients with severe hypertension: An idea whose time had come and gone. *Arch Intern Med* 149:2169, 1989.
5. Pierdomenico SD, Mezzetti A: White coat hypertension in patients with newly diagnosed hypertension: Evaluation of prevalence by ambulatory monitoring and impact on cost of health care. *Eur Heart J* 16:692, 1995.
6. Strandgaard S: Autoregulation of cerebral blood flow in hypertensive patients: The modifying influence of prolonged anti-hypertensive treatment on the tolerance of acute, drug-induced hypotension. *Circulation* 53:720, 1976.
7. Kitiyakara C: Malignant hypertension and hypertensive emergencies. *J Am Soc Nephrol* 9:133, 1998.
8. Grossman E, Messerli FH: High blood pressure: A side effect of drugs, poisons, and food. *Arch Intern Med* 155:450, 1995.
9. Sheps SG, Jiang NS, Klee GG, van Heerden JA: Recent developments in the diagnosis and treatment of pheochromocytoma. *Mayo Clin Proc* 65:88, 1990.
10. Zampaglione B, Pascale C: Hypertensive urgencies and emergencies: Prevalence and clinical presentation. *Hypertension* 27:144, 1996.
11. Barry DI: Cerebrovascular aspects of antihypertensive treatment. *Am J Cardiol* 63:14C, 1989.
12. Graham DI: Ischaemic brain following emergency blood pressure lowering in hypertensive patients, *Acta Med Scand* 678(suppl):61, 1983.
13. Sinaiko AR: Hypertension in children. *N Engl J Med* 335:1968, 1996.
14. Kaplan NM, Gifford RW: Choice of initial therapy for hypertension. *JAMA* 275:1577, 1996.
15. Vesey CJ, Cole PV, Simpson PJ: Cyanide and thiocyanide concentrations following sodium nitroprusside infusion in man. *Br J Anaesth* 48:651, 1976.
16. McDonald AJ, Yealy DM, Jacobson S: Oral labetalol versus oral nifedipine in hypertensive urgencies in the ED. *Am J Emerg Med* 11:460, 1993.
17. Reach G, Thibonnier M, Chevillard C, et al: Effect of labetalol on blood pressure and plasma catecholamine concentrations in patients with pheochromocytoma. *BMJ* 280:1300, 1980.
18. Abdelwahab W, Frishman W, Landau A: Management of hypertensive urgencies and emergencies. *J Clin Pharmacol* 35:747, 1995.
19. Lowe SA, Rubin PC: The pharmacologic management of hypertension in pregnancy. *J Hypertens* 10:201, 1992.
20. Bussman WD, Kenedi P, von Mengden HJ, et al: Comparison of nitroglycerin with nifedipine in patients with hypertensive crisis or severe hypertension. *Clin Invest* 70:1085, 1992.
21. McCarthy M: US NIH issues warning on nifedipine. *Lancet* 346:689, 1995.
22. Furberg CD, Psaty BM: Should dihydropyridines be used as first-line drugs in the treatment of hypertension? The con side. *Arch Intern Med* 155:2157, 1995.
23. Hirschl MM, Binder M, Bur A, et al: Clinical evaluation of different doses of intravenous enalaprilat in patients with hypertensive crisis. *Arch Intern Med* 155:2217, 1995.
24. Haley EC Jr, Kassell NF, Torner JC: A randomized controlled trial of high-dose intravenous nicardipine in aneurysmal subarachnoid hemorrhage. *J Neurosurg* 78:537, 1993.

54 AORTIC DISSECTION AND ANEURYSMS

Gary A. Johnson

Thoracic and abdominal aneurysmal disease comprises a significant subset of emergencies. A ruptured aneurysm or dissecting aneurysm is a prominent cause of sudden death as well as severe abdominal, chest, or back pain. These diseases disproportionately affect the elderly. As our patient population becomes older, the incidence of presentations for aneurysms will continue to increase.[1–3]

Abdominal aortic aneurysms (AAA) have a clear familial trend. Eighteen percent of patients with AAA have a family history of aneurysm (a first-degree relative) compared with less than 3 percent of controls. Patients with Marfan syndrome have been found to have mutations in the FBN1 gene on chromosome 15.[2] Other genetic abnormalities have been investigated as well.[2,3]

The incidence of AAA increases with age and rarely presents before age 50. Most patients are older than 60 and males have an increased risk of disease. Patients with other aneurysms and peripheral arterial disease are at an increased risk as well.

PATHOGENESIS

Risk factors for aneurysms include connective tissue disorders, familial history of aneurysm, and atherosclerotic risk factors (age, smoking, hypertension, hyperlipidemia, and diabetes). These risk factors combine to increase the expansile force on the aortic wall or to impair the patient's ability to withstand these forces. The Laplace law [wall tension = (pressure × radius)/tensile force] dictates that as the aorta dilates, the force on the aortic wall increases, therefore causing further aortic dilation.

The destruction of the media of the aorta is a prominent feature in aneurysm pathogenesis. Elastin and collagen are markedly reduced in the aneurysmal aorta and fibrolamellar units are dramatically decreased. In addition, the normal abdominal aorta has a decreasing number of elastic lamellae as the aorta becomes more distal. This may help account for the prominent infrarenal location of aneurysm in many patients.

Histologic examination of an aneurysmal wall will show an intima that is infiltrated by atherosclerosis and a thinned media. There may be intraluminal thrombus, and the adventitia has often been infiltrated by inflammatory cells. Patients with saccular outpouchings (blisters) may have an increased risk of rupture. Such blisters have been shown to increase the incidence of rupture of small (less than 5-cm) aneurysms.[4]

Rate of aneurysmal dilation is variable. As a consequence of the LaPlace law, larger aneurysms will expand more quickly than smaller ones. An average rate may be 0.25 to 0.5 cm per year.[4] Patients with known aneurysms must be followed closely for unpredictably fast expansion.

Dissecting Aneurysms

Aortic dissections occur from a violation of the intima, which allows blood to enter the media and dissect between the intimal and the adventitial layers. Common sites for tear include the ascending aorta and the region of the ligamentum arteriosum. The dissecting column of blood ruptures the intima and thus maintains a true and false lumen. The dissection may extend proximally, distally, or both. The patient's symptoms may cease abruptly when the dissection extends back through the intima; this may suggest a spontaneous cure. Alternatively blood may dissect through the adventitia and will nearly always be fatal.

Aortic dissection presents in a bimodal fashion. One group consists of younger patients with specific predisposing conditions. The predominant group is patients above age 50 with hypertension. Atherosclerosis is only a minor contributor to the pathogenesis of dissection.

Predisposing conditions for dissection include multiple forms of congenital heart disease, connective tissue disease, and pregnancy. Approximately 25 to 30% of patients with Marfan syndrome develop a dissection. Dissection may also be iatrogenically induced from aortic catherization or cardiac surgery.

Aortic dissections have been classified by two separate systems. The Stanford classification considers any involvement of the ascending aorta a type A dissection and dissections restricted to the descending aorta type B. DeBakey classified type I dissections as those that involve the ascending aorta, the arch, and the descending aorta. Type II involves only the ascending aorta and type III only the descending aorta.

Pseudoaneurysms

Pseudoaneurysms (or "false aneurysms) may occur when there is a violation of the intima, which creates an ulcer into the aortic media. This type of lesion may slowly dilate or cause a deepening of the ulcer and form a pseudoaneurysm; it occurs most commonly in the descending thoracic aorta. Pseudoaneurysms do not commonly evolve into dissections and rarely rupture.[5]

Other Aneurysms

Patients may have aneurysms at anastomoses from prior vascular reconstruction. The aneurysm occurs at the site where the graft is sewn to the artery. Anastomotic aneurysms may occur in the aortic, ileac, or femoral arteries. These aneurysms commonly rupture and cause catastrophic bleeding; however, they may also present with smaller sentinel hemorrhages. Anastomotic aneurysms may erode into the adjacent intestine and form an aortoenteric fistula.

CLINICAL FEATURES

Abdominal Aortic Aneurysms

Symptomatic abdominal aortic aneurysms may present as syncope, back or belly pain, shock, or sudden death. Sudden death most commonly occurs from intraperitoneal rupture of the aneurysm. These ruptures lead to massive, rapid blood loss and it will not be possible to resuscitate the patient. History that is often cited as classic for acute rupture of the abdominal aneurysm is syncope with no warning symptoms followed by severe abdominal or back pain. Syncope is caused by rapid blood loss and a lack of cerebral perfusion. Patients often regain consciousness after their own compensatory mechanisms have been invoked, but they will most often slip again into shock without prompt medical intervention.

Patients will most often present with variations on the classic history.[2] Pain may occur before syncope, and the pain may not be severe in some cases. The pain also may be unilateral and may be located in a flank, costovertebral angle of the groin, or in a single quadrant of the abdomen. Hip pain, tenesmus, and urinary bladder symptoms have been described. Constitutional symptoms such as nausea and vomiting are commonly present.

Physical examination of a patient with acute rupture of an aortic aneurysm may detect the aneurysm. Tenderness to palpation of an aneurysm is commonly interpreted as a sign of rupture. However, a lack of tenderness cannot imply an intact aorta. Patients with an obese abdomen are difficult to exam for the presence of an aortic aneurysm. Very thin patients may have an aorta that is easily palpable, and the diameter of the aorta should be measurable.

Evidence of retroperitoneal hematoma may be seen as periumbilical ecchymosis (Cullen's sign) or flank ecchymosis (Grey-Turner's sign). Retroperitoneal blood may also dissect into the perineum or groin. Scrotal hematomas or inguinal masses may be seen on exam. Retroperitoneal blood may also irritate the psoas muscle and produce an iliopsoas sign. Blood may compress the femoral nerve and present as a neuropathy. The presence or rupture of an AAA does not typically alter femoral arterial pulsations.[6]

Aortoenteric fistulas must be considered in all patients with unexplained gastrointestinal bleeding. A history of aortic graft placement should increase the clinical suspicion of fistula.[7] The duodenum is most frequently involved; and therefore bleeding may manifest as hematemesis, melenemesis, melena, or (if there is rapid transport) hematochezia. These fistulas commonly present as massive, life-threatening bleeding. However, mild "sentinel" bleeding may precede a full-blown rupture. Aortic aneurysms may also erode into the venous vasculature and form aortovenous fistulas, which may present as high-output cardiac failure, decreased arterial blood flow distal to the fistula, and increased central venous volume.

Abdominal aortic aneurysms may uncommonly present as chronic contained ruptures.[8] A retroperitoneal rupture may cause enough fibrosis to limit blood loss. The inflammatory response commonly causes pain, which may continue for a significant length of time. Despite the seriousness of this pathology, the patient may appear remarkably well.

An asymptomatic aneurysm may be found on physical examination or radiologic evaluation. Any aneurysm that is found should be referred for follow-up. Aneurysms greater than 5 cm in diameter are at an increased risk of rupture. Aneurysms of less than 5 cm are unlikely to rupture, however, patients with such asymptomatic aneurysms must be closely followed by their primary care physicians or surgeons. The management of patients with small, asymptomatic aneurysms (including the timing of surgery) is a controversial topic.[2,9] Symptomatic aneurysms of any size should be considered emergent.

Thoracic Aortic Aneurysm

Thoracic aortic aneurysms may become symptomatic by compressing or eroding into adjacent structures. Presenting symptoms can include esophageal, tracheal, bronchial, or even neurologic disorders. A thoracic aneurysm that erodes to an adjacent structure is generally immediately fatal. Rare patients may survive with the assistance of hemodynamic resuscitation.

Dissecting Aortic Aneurysms

Aortic dissections will commonly present (>90 percent) with an abrupt and severe pain in the chest or between the scapulae. Patients often describe the pain as tearing or ripping. Pain in anterior chest is often associated with involvement of the ascending aorta. Back pain may indicate involvement of the descending aorta. Dissection often presents with dynamic pathology; therefore, pain patterns often change as the anatomic injury migrates.[10]

The aortic dissection will cause a spectrum of symptoms based on the anatomic course of the lesion. Dissection into a carotid artery may lead to a classic stroke presentation. Some 40 percent of patients with dissection will have neurologic sequelae. Paraplegia may occur if the arterial blood supply to the spinal cord is interrupted. Abdominal or flank pain may be caused by dissection into the abdominal aorta, renal arteries, or ileac arteries. Dissection may lead to pericardial effusion and tamponade.

Systemic constitutional symptoms may occur with the dissection. Nausea, vomiting, and diaphoresis are common. Patients are frequently apprehensive and express their feelings of impending doom.

Physical examination may help to eliminate some differential diagnoses but will most likely reveal a normal heart and lung. The diastolic murmur of aortic insufficiency may be heard. Decreased pulsation in the radial, femoral, or carotid arteries should significantly raise the suspicion of an aortic lesion and is present in 50 percent of patients.[10] Specific threshold values of blood pressure changes between extremities have not been defined. Hypertension and tachycardia are commonly present, but the dissection may also cause hypotension. Hypotension may accompany pericardial tamponade or coronary artery interruption. Tamponade may result in muffled heart tones, elevated jugular venous pressure, and pulsus paradoxus. Compression of the recurrent laryngeal nerve or the superior cervical sympathetic ganglion may cause either hoarseness of voice or Horner syndrome, respectively.

DIAGNOSIS

Abdominal Aortic Aneurysms

The differential diagnoses for abdominal aneurysms include the causes of syncope, abdominal pain, back pain, and shock. The presentation of syncope with back pain or shock should strongly suggest aortic disease. However, the diagnosis will be difficult to make in shock or syncope without a significant complaint of pain. Other cardiac, abdominal, and retroperitoneal diseases need to be considered, including renal disorders, hepatobiliary disorders, and pancreatic disease. Unfortunately, some patients may appear well enough to receive benign diagnoses such as musculoskeletal back pain or enteritis and be discharged from the emergency department (ED).

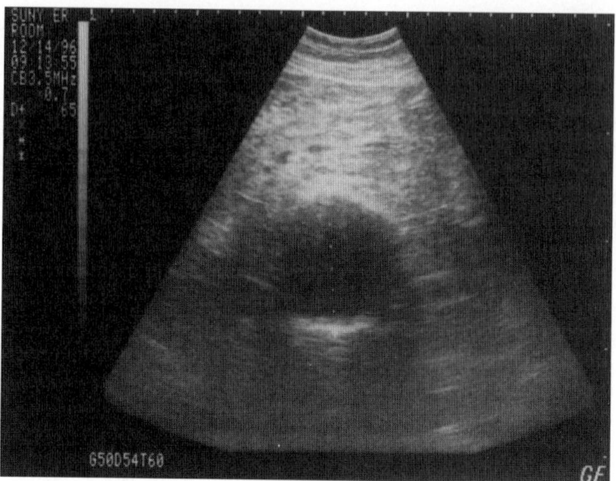

FIG. 54-1. Bedside ultrasound image of an abdominal aortic aneurysm. This aneurysm measures 6.5 cm.

The diagnosis may be further confused by coexisting pathology. Coronary artery disease and chronic lung disease are often present, and these features may distract the physician from the diagnosis of aneurysmal disease. This is especially true in patients without significant pain.

Aneurysms of large arteries other than the aorta may expand or rupture. Ileac aneurysms are notoriously difficult to diagnose because they may be confused with urologic, bowel, or groin disorders. Splenic artery aneurysms may present as undifferentiated shock or intraabdominal catastrophe. A rupture of the splenic artery has a poor prognosis owing to its intraperitoneal location.

Radiologic studies may be very helpful in confirming a ruptured AAA, but since radiographs often unnecessarily delay operative repair, the decision to obtain confirmatory studies must be made carefully.

Radiologic evaluation may include plain radiography, ultrasound (Fig. 54-1), or computed tomographic (CT). Plain abdominal films may show a calcified, bulging aortic contour implying the presence of an aneurysm. Approximately 65 percent of patients with symptomatic aortic aneurysmal disease will have a calcified aorta. Some propose that a cross-table lateral film of the abdominal aorta will have a higher yield for calcifications.[1] The lateral view will allow the aorta to be visualized without overlying the vertebral column. An AP projection may show an arch of calcification, most commonly on the patient's left. Rarely, a chronic aneurysm may erode into a vertebral body. Plain film cannot exclude the presence of AAA.

Rapid bedside ultrasonography is ideal for unstable patients who cannot undergo CT scanning. A technically adequate ultrasound study has virtually 100 percent sensitivity for demonstrating the presence of an aneurysm and measuring its diameter.[11] Obesity or bowel gas may make the study difficult to perform. Rupture cannot be reliably seen.

CT with intravenous contrast is useful to demonstrate the anatomic details of the aneurysm and associated retroperitoneal hemorrhage. CT should be obtained on stable patients. Should unusual circumstances occur (such as the presence of other prominent acute abdominal conditions) and a CT become necessary, the patient should be accompanied by the surgeon, who could expedite an emergent operation if necessary.

Dissecting Aneurysms

The ischemic end-organ manifestations associated with many dissections may confuse the differential diagnosis, which includes myocar-

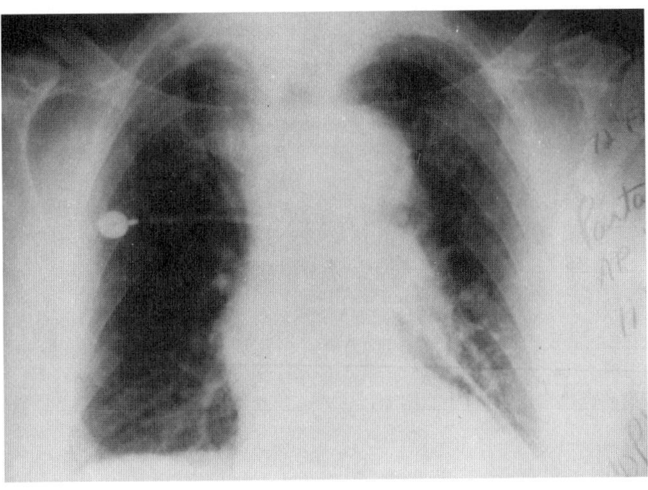

FIG. 54-2. Chest x-ray of a descending saccular thoracic aneurysm.

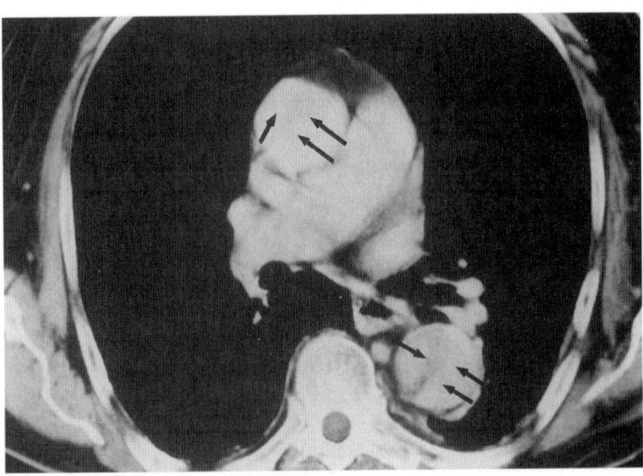

FIG. 54-4. Computed tomographic scan of same patient revealing false (double arrows) and true aortic lumens in both ascending and descending aorta.

dial infarction, pericardial disease, pulmonary disorders, stroke, musculoskeletal disease of the extremities, spinal cord injuries, and intraabdominal disorders. Ischemic manifestations may change with time (as the dissection progresses) distracting the physician from making the correct diagnosis. Rupture of the dissection into the true lumen may cause a cessation of symptoms, and the correct diagnosis may then be inappropriately dismissed.

Thoracic dissecting aneurysms will most commonly (90 percent) have an abnormal aortic contour on chest x-ray. Widening of the mediastinum and deviation of the trachea, mainstem bronchi, or esophagus may also be seen (Figs. 54-2 and 54-3). Intimal calcium may be visible and distant from the edge of the aortic contour (calcium sign).

CT scanning may reliably make the diagnosis of aortic dissection (Fig. 54-4).[12,13] Sensitivity for dissection ranges from 83 to 100 percent and specificity ranges from 87 to 100 percent.[12] Spiral CT with rapid intravenous boluses of contrast may be more sensitive.[13] However, CT scan cannot reliably give anatomic details of other arterial branches off the aorta and cannot address aortic valve competence.

Angiography can be considered the ''gold standard'' for diagnosis and will provide more anatomic detail than a CT scan.[12,13] Aortography also will reliably show complications of dissection, including involvement of branch vessels, aortic valve incompetence, and coronary artery involvement. However, the angiogram is not a perfect study. Erbel[14] found aortography to have a specificity of 94 percent and a sensitivity of 88 percent. Risks of the procedure include the use of intravenous contrast agents and the delay in assembling an angiography team.

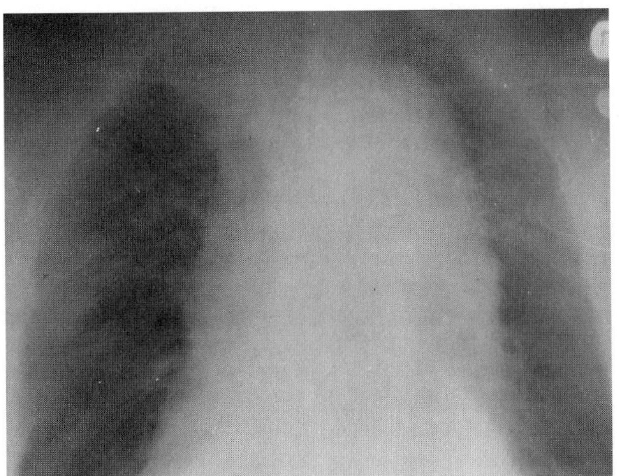

FIG. 54-3. Chest x-ray of a dissecting thoracic aneurysm.

In experienced hands, a transesophageal echocardiogram (TEE) may be as sensitive and specific as angiography.[15–17] Sensitivity for dissection ranges from 97 to 100 percent, specificity 97 to 99 percent.[12] Some 3 percent of patients cannot tolerate the procedure, which should be performed under sedation or general anesthesia. Known esophageal disease is a relative contraindication. Disruption of sound transmission by air in the trachea or left bronchi may cause difficulty in evaluating the ascending aorta. Among the imaging techniques mentioned above, TEE has the highest diagnostic variability between operators or observers. Therefore, the imaging procedure of choice may vary between institutions.[12] In contrast with AAAs, suspected dissections must be confirmed radiologically prior to operative repair.

Thoracic aortic saccular aneurysms are generally uniformly identified on chest x-ray. Rarely, the presence of thoracic, pleural, or parenchymal densities may make the diagnosis more difficult. CT scan will delineate these aneurysms reliably.

EMERGENCY DEPARTMENT TREATMENT

Abdominal Aortic Aneurysm

The emergency physician's role in the care of a patient with an acute rupture of an AAA lies largely in making the diagnosis and assisting with rapid transfer to the operating room.

Any suspected ruptured aneurysm requires immediate operative repair. One-half of patients with a ruptured aneurysm who reach the operating room die.[9] Imaging modalities should be restricted to patients who are considered unlikely to have a ruptured aorta. Standard resuscitative maneuvers (two large-bore intravenous catheters, a cardiac monitor, and supplemental oxygen) are required. The patient suspected of having an AAA may require resuscitation for blood loss. However, overly vigorous fluid resuscitation may be harmful (see Chap. 27), and the appropriate amount of intravenous fluids to be given is controversial.

Aortic Dissection

Patients with suspected aortic dissection will commonly require antihypertensive treatment, which must be provided without increasing the shear force on the intimal flap of the aorta. Therefore, medications with negative inotropic effects must be given initially. β blockers (esmolol, metoprolol, or propranolol) are commonly used for this purpose. The optimal blood pressure is undefined and must be tailored to each patient. However, systolic pressure of 120 to 130 mmHg may be a convenient starting point.

Esmolol may be given as an infusion of 500 μg/kg over 1 min followed by an infusion of 50 to 150 μg/kg per minute. Metoprolol may be given intravenously in three 5-mg doses every 2 min followed by 2 to 5 mg/h. Labetolol, 20 mg (or 0.25 mg/kg) IV over 2 min, repeated q10 min to desired effect or a total dose of 300 mg; or labetolol 2 mg/min to desired effect or total dose 300 mg, can also be given. Calcium channel blockers may be used if a contraindication to β blockers is present.

Vasodilators (such as nitroprusside) may be added for further antihypertensive treatment after the successful administration of a negative inotrope. Nitroprusside may be infused intravenously at 0.3 to 10 μg/kg per minute. Administration should be provided by a pump to ensure precise measurement of drug. Patients should clearly have evidence of adequate β-receptor or calcium channel blockade prior to starting a vasodilator. Close monitoring of the pulse rate is required, as this is a convenient indicator of blockade in most patients. Aortic dissections may cause hypotension, which requires fluid or blood product resuscitation.

Rapid referral to a surgeon is mandatory. Dissections with involvement of the ascending aorta require prompt surgical repair. Patients with dissecting aneurysms of only the descending aorta are worse surgical risks, and indications for repair are controversial.[18]

Asymptomatic abdominal and thoracic aortic aneurysms require prompt outpatient referral. Other interventions are generally not needed.

REFERENCES

1. Crawford ED, Hess KR: Abdominal aortic aneurysm. *N Engl J Med* 321:1040, 1989.
2. Henney AM, Adiseshiah M, et al: Abdominal aortic aneurysm: Report of a meeting of physicians and scientists, University College London Medical School. *Lancet* 341:215, 1993.
3. Berridge DC, Chamberlain J, Guy A, et al: Prospective audit of abdominal aortic aneurysm surgery in the northern region from 1988 to 1992. *Br J Surg* 82(7):906–910, 1995.
4. Faggioli GL, Stella A, Gargiulo M, et al: Morphology of small aneurysms: Definition and impact on risk of rupture. *Am J Surg* 168:131, 1994.
5. Harris JA, Kostaki G, Glover J, et al: Penetrating atherosclerotic ulcers of the aorta. *J Vasc Surg* 19:90, 1994.
6. Satta J, Laara E, Immonen K, et al: The rupture type determines the outcome for ruptured abdominal aortic aneurysm patients. *Ann Chirurg Gynaecol* 86:24, 1997.
7. Batounis E, Georgopoulos S: The validity of current vascular imaging methods in the evaluation of aortic anastomotic aneurysms developing after abdominal aortic aneurysm repair. *Ann Vasc Surg* 10:537, 1996.
8. Jones CS, Reilly MK, Dalsing MC, Glover JL: Chronic contained rupture of abdominal aortic aneurysms. *Arch Surg* 121:542, 1986.
9. Nevitt MP, Ballard DJ, Hallett JW Jr: Prognosis of abdominal aortic aneurysms: A population-based study. *N Engl J Med* 321:1009, 1989.
10. Larson EW, Edwards WD: Risk factors for aortic dissection: A necropsy study of 161 cases. *Am J Cardiol* 53:849, 1984.
11. Graham M, Chan A: Ultrasound screening for clinically occult abdominal aortic aneurysm. *Can Med Assoc* 138:627, 1988.
12. Cigarroa JE, Isselbacher EM, DeSanctis RW, et al: Medical progress: Diagnostic imaging in the evaluation of suspected aortic dissection—old standards and new directions. *N Engl J Med* 328:35, 1993.
13. Naidich JB, Crystal KS: Diagnosis of dissecting hematoma of the aorta: A choice between good and better (editorial; comment). *Radiology* 190:16, 1994.
14. Erbel R, Engberding R, Daniel W, et al: Echocardiography in diagnosis of aortic dissection, *Lancet* 1:457, 1989.
15. Erbel R, Oelert H, Meyer J, et al: Effect of medical and surgical therapy on aortic dissection evaluated by transesophageal echocardiography: Implications for prognosis and therapy. *Circulation* 87:1604, 1993.
16. Blanchard DG, Kimura BJ, Dittrich HC, et al: Transesophageal echocardiography of the aorta. *JAMA* 272:546, 1994.
17. Hartnell G, Costello P, Goldstein S, et al: The Diagnosis of Thoracic Aortic Dissection by Noninvasive Imaging Procedures. *N Engl J Med* 328:1637, 1993.
18. Miller DC: The continuing dilemma concerning medical versus surgical management of patients with acute type B dissections. (Review) (60 refs). Seminars in Thoracic & Cardiovascular Surgery, 5(1):33–46, Jan. 1993.

55 NONTRAUMATIC PERIPHERAL VASCULAR DISORDERS

Anil Chopra

THROMBOPHLEBITIS

Deep venous thrombosis (DVT) is a common, potentially life-threatening condition with an estimated annual incidence of 5 to 20 million cases in the United States. The admission rate for DVT, however, is declining greatly owing to the widespread use of newer outpatient treatments. The most common life-threatening consequence of DVT is pulmonary embolism (PE), which is responsible for approximately 200,000 deaths in the United States every year.[1] The recognition and early treatment of a presumed or known DVT is paramount to reducing the morbidity and mortality from its local and thromboembolic sequelae.

Pathophysiology

The formation of venous clots is related to at least one of Virchow's triad of factors: venous stasis, injury to vessel wall, and hypercoagulable state. Table 55-1 outlines the clinical risk factors predisposing to DVT, which can be remembered by the mnemonic *thrombosis*; Table 55-2 provides a detailed list of associated conditions. Trauma includes multitrauma patients, lower extremity fractures, and burns. Hypercoagulable states include those associated with malignancy; lupus anticoagulant; deficiency of or resistance to protein C, protein S, or antithrombin III; and abnormal plasminogen or plasminogen activators, all of which can lead to clotting. Obstetric risk occurs not only during pregnancy but also in the postpartum period. Medications that predispose to thrombosis include birth control pills and replacement hormones. Major orthopedic, thoracic, abdominal, or gynecologic surgery is a significant risk factor for developing DVT, though the risk is diminished with prophylactic subcutaneous heparin postoperatively. Illness includes cardiovascular diseases—myocardial infarction (MI), congestive heart failure (CHF), and cerebrovascular accident (CVA)—

TABLE 55-1 Clinical Risk Factors for Deep Venous Thrombosis

T	Trauma
H	Hypercoagulable, hormone replacement
R	Recreational drugs (iv drugs)
O	Old (age >40)
M	Malignancy
B	Birth control pill, blood group A
O	Obesity/obstetrics
S	Surgery, smoking
I	Immobilization
S	Sickness

TABLE 55-2 Conditions Associated with Deep Venous Thrombosis

Hereditary		
Antiphospholipid antibody syndrome		
Resistance to activated protein C (factor V Leiden)		
Deficiencies:	Antithrombin III	
	Protein C or S	
	Heparin cofactor II	
	Factor XII	
	Plasminogen activator	
Dysfibrinogenemia		
Dysplasminogenemia		
Polycythemia vera		
Primary thrombocytosis		
General		
Age >40		
Blood group A		
Obesity		
Pregnancy and the postpartum period		
Previous thromboembolism		
Smoking		
Acquired		
Heparin-induced thrombocytopenia		
Hormones:	Birth control pills	
	Replacement therapy	
Immobilization:	Casts	
	Illness	
	Long travel	
Malignancy		
Medical illness:	Congestive heart failure	
	Inflammatory disease (bowel disease, vasculitis)	
	Myocardial infarction	
	Nephrotic syndrome	
	Sepsis	
	Stroke	
Surgery:	Abdominal	
	Orthopedic	
	Pelvic	
	Thoracic	
Trauma:	Brain or spinal cord	
	Burns	
	Lower limb	
	Multisystem	
Vascular injury:	Central lines	
	Intravenous drugs	

nephrotic syndrome, inflammatory bowel disease, and vasculitis (lupus, Behçet syndrome).

Thrombi most commonly form at the venous cusps of deep veins in the lower extremities, where altered or static blood flow initiates clot formation. Blood clots are primarily composed of red cells, fibrin, and platelets. An immature thrombus may propagate, dissolve, or embolize, depending on various local and systemic factors related to thrombogenesis (especially venous stasis and activation of the coagulation pathway) and the body's defenses responsible for clot lysis (antithrombin III, protein C, plasmin, and other factors). The signs and symptoms of DVT are typically due to a partially or totally occluded vein, leading to venous outflow obstruction and/or the variable inflammatory response to a clot adhering to endothelium. PE may sometimes be the first and only clinical indication of an existing DVT in 10 percent of patients.

A postphlebitic syndrome (PPS) may develop following the resolution of a DVT and is related to valvular incompetence and persistent venous outflow obstruction. The true incidence of PPS is unknown, but studies have revealed a range of 20 to 60 percent depending on the criteria used for diagnosis.[2]

Superficial Thrombophlebitis

Thrombosis can occur in any superficial vein, especially in varicosities at the saphenous vein or its tributaries. It is a common, benign, self-limiting process but can cause significant incapacitation. Local pain, redness, and tenderness of a cord along the course of the involved vein are typical findings. Bruising or bleeding may also be noted at the involved site. Doppler ultrasound may be used to confirm the diagnosis if there is any ambiguity or if an alternative diagnosis such as a DVT, cellulitis, or lymphangiitis is possible. Demonstration of flow within the involved vein reliably excludes superficial venous thrombosis.

Mild cases can be treated with warm compresses, analgesia, and elastic supports for the involved extremity with the patient continuing daily activities as tolerated. Severe thrombophlebitis where the patient is functionally debilitated by symptoms should be managed with periods of bed rest, elevation of the extremity, support stockings, and analgesia. Anti-inflammatory medications are commonly used to treat superficial thrombophlebitis. Antibiotics and anticoagulants are of no proven benefit. The incidence of DVT and subsequent PE due to a superficial thrombus is extremely low. Improvement with aggressive therapy can be painfully slow, and symptoms may persist for weeks. Definitive treatment for refractory or recurrent disease is excision of the involved vein. Patients with recurrent or migratory thrombophlebitis should be investigated to exclude a malignancy or other hypercoagulable state.

Deep Venous Thrombosis

CLINICAL FEATURES The clinical examination is unreliable for the detection or exclusion of DVT. Assessment of risk factors (Tables 55-1 and 55-2) may be a stronger predictor whenever the diagnosis is entertained. One study showed that a single risk factor is associated with DVT in 24 percent of patients, while those with four or more risk factors are virtually certain to have the diagnosis established.[3] The constellation of pain, redness, swelling, warmth, and tenderness is present in less than half of patients with confirmed DVT. Swelling and tenderness in the involved extremity are the most common findings, occurring in 80 and 75 percent, respectively, of patients with DVT. Though some patients with DVT may have a low-grade fever, one should be careful to exclude an infectious process such as cellulitis. Differences in calf measurements made 10 cm below the tibial tuberosity of greater than 2 cm have been historically suggested as a screening tool for a DVT, but there is no published scientific evidence to validate this practice. Suspicion of DVT by symptoms alone is sufficient to initiate objective investigations even with a negative physical exam. Pain in the calf with forced dorsiflexion of the ankle and the leg straight (Homans' sign) is not reliable for DVT. The physical findings with DVT depend on its location and the degree of venous obstruction, inflammation, and collateral blood flow. For example, significant iliofemoral vein occlusion can present with minimal to absent clinical findings but can result in a catastrophic PE.

Symptomatic DVT will be in the popliteal or more proximal veins in more than 80 percent of cases. An isolated calf DVT will extend proximally only 20 percent of the time, usually within a week of presentation.[4] Unlike proximal DVT, nonextending calf DVT will rarely cause a PE.

Uncommon presentations of DVT include phlegmasia cerulea dolens (painful blue inflammation) and phlegmasia alba dolens ("milk leg"). In the former, the patient presents with an extensively swollen, cyanotic leg from venous engorgement due to massive iliofemoral thrombosis. This high-grade obstruction can compromise perfusion to the foot from high compartment pressures and lead to venous gangrene. Petechiae and bullae may be present on the skin. Phlegmasia alba dolens is also due to massive iliofemoral thrombosis, but the patient's leg is pale or white secondary to associated arterial spasm. Dorsalis pedis and posterior tibial pulses may be diminished or absent, which can lead to a false diagnosis of arterial occlusion. The arterial spasm with milk leg is transient and often followed by venous engorgement, suggesting the correct diagnosis.

The PPS is manifest by signs and symptoms that can be difficult to differentiate from acute DVT. Pain, swelling, and occasionally ulceration of the skin can occur months to years after the resolution of DVT. Long-term follow-up of patients reveals that the syndrome (PPS) can occur in up to 60 percent of patients who have had a previous proximal DVT and one-third of patients with calf DVT.[2]

Diagnosis

Owing to the poor accuracy of clinical methods in identifying DVT, all patients with any signs or symptoms suggesting DVT must undergo an objective diagnostic evaluation. Less than one-third of patients with clinically suspected DVT are found to have the disease following objective investigation.[4] Several investigative techniques are available to search for a deep thrombus, including plasma D-dimer level, impedance plethysmography (IPG), Doppler ultrasound (duplex), contrast venography, radionuclide scintigraphy, and magnetic resonance imaging (MRI).

Venography has represented the historical ''gold standard'' for the detection of DVT. It can be useful for patients with a high clinical probability of DVT when noninvasive tests are negative. However, it is an invasive, often painful, and expensive test that may cause contrast-related reactions or iatrogenic venous thrombus in about 1 to 2 percent of patients. It is difficult to perform and requires considerable expertise. When contrast is seen throughout the deep venous system (not possible in 5 to 10 percent of tests), a venogram reliably excludes DVT. Inadequate visualization of the deep venous system can occur due to difficulties with venous access (e.g., obesity, severe edema, cellulitis), dilution of contrast in the proximal lower limb, or a previous thrombus.

The commonest test used to identify a DVT in North America is ultrasonography. B-mode ultrasound gives two-dimensional images of a vein and its surrounding structures and can directly visualize a clot, while Doppler flow capacity when combined with color images provides a visual and audible evaluation of blood flow for venous obstruction. B-mode ultrasonography combined with Doppler flow is termed a *duplex*. A duplex scan with or without color flow is highly sensitive and specific for a proximal DVT (clot proximal to the popliteal veins). The positive predictive value of ultrasound is higher than IPG for DVTs (94 versus 83 percent, respectively). Both of these tests are portable, noninvasive, safe, quick, readily accessible, accurate for proximal DVTs, and provide immediate information. Ultrasound testing requires more expertise (due to subjective interpretation). It is also more expensive than an IPG but is the test of choice when available owing to its higher accuracy. Both tests are insensitive for calf DVTs and serial testing is required to exclude the extension of clot to proximal veins. Some centers will not routinely scan the leg for a calf DVTs, choosing instead to do a more time-limited study looking only for the more significant proximal clots.

All plethysmographs measure a change in volume. An IPG that can be done at the bedside measures changes in electrical resistance in response to changes in calf volume secondary to venous obstruction. The procedure involves a supine patient with a leg externally rotated and knee partially flexed, having an 8-in. pneumatic cuff placed around the thigh and inflated to 37 to 51 mmHg to preferentially obstruct venous return, causing calf enlargement. Measurements are made with two electrodes on the calf after cuff inflation and then rapid deflation within 3 s of cuff release. Measurements are plotted on a graph and, if they lie above an experimentally determined baseline, the test is negative for a DVT. If the measurements lie below this line, the test is repeated, with increasing periods of cuff inflation (45 to 120 s). If several of these repeat measurements lie below the baseline, the test is considered positive for DVT. Several studies have shown that sensitivity and specificity for proximal DVT are about 95 percent.[5] False positives can occur with PPS, abdominal or pelvic neoplasms, CHF, and pregnancy. Plethysmography is insufficiently accurate to be useful for isolated calf DVT.

Several radioisotope techniques are available for investigating for DVT, including ^{111}In- or ^{99m}Tc-labeled antifibrin monoclonal antibodies, ^{125}I-labeled fibrinogen, and ^{99m}Tc-labeled red blood cells or macroaggregated albumin. These radioisotopes may be incorporated into actively forming thrombus and can be detected by scanning the extremity hours or days after injection. There are several disadvantages to radionuclide venography which make it a suboptimal test for detecting a DVT. While sensitivity for detecting calf DVT is about 90 percent, sensitivity for thigh DVT is as low as 60 percent and even lower for pelvic veins.[5] Still, this test has been used to complement a negative or equivocal ultrasound exam in high risk patients such as those who have undergone surgery or have an indeterminate lung scan for PE. Radionuclide venography is expensive, time-consuming and not as accurate as IPG or a duplex for proximal DVTs.

Some authorities advocate MRI as the ''gold standard'' for imaging the venous system. It is at least as accurate as any other investigational modality and can detect a filling defect in the entire extremity (including calf veins) and pelvic veins, which are sometimes not well visualized by ultrasonography or venography. An MRI visualizes both extremities simultaneously and can identify alternative causes of extremity swelling such as cysts, aneurysms, hematomas, tumors, and other masses. Some of the limitations of MRI include its cost, lack of ready availability, lack of portability, and inability to be used in patients harboring ferromagnetic objects (prostheses, pacemakers).

D-dimer fragments can be measured as an indicator of the presence or absence of DVT or PE. A quantitative enzyme-linked immunosorbent assay (ELISA) D-dimer level less than 250 ng/mL is helpful to exclude a venous thrombosis, but the test takes several hours to perform (latex and immunofiltration techniques are quicker but less sensitive). It is a fairly nonspecific test, as many other conditions such as infections, surgery, trauma, cardiovascular disease, and cancer can elevate a D-dimer level. It follows, then, that despite a sensitivity of over 80 to 90 percent, a D-dimer level is useful only when it is low.[5] The combination of a normal IPG or ultrasound and a low D-dimer level has a negative predictive value of about 99 percent for proximal DVT.[4]

Clinical Approach to Establishing the Diagnosis

Since the diagnosis of DVT is difficult to establish based solely on history or physical exam, some type of imaging modality is necessary. An appropriate initial imaging study would be either duplex scanning or IPG. The choice is more dependent on local availability and expertise, as both are reasonably accurate, noninvasive, and inexpensive. In patients with risk factors in whom either of these tests are positive, anticoagulation therapy may be initiated if there are no contraindications. If the diagnosis is equivocal or there is potential for false-positive results, either contrast venography or MRI can be performed. A poor IPG study or suspicion of false negative results can be verified by a duplex scan. A good quality duplex scan with adequate compressibility of proximal veins excludes the diagnosis of proximal DVT, but can be repeated in a few days if high clinical suspicion of DVT remains. (There is no evidence that an IPG adds further conformation to a negative duplex scan with good compressibility of the femoral & popliteal vein.) The approach at any given institution is dependent on availability, equipment, and local expertise.

Treatment

Traditional therapeutic measures—including bed rest, continuous leg elevation, and elastic stockings—are of unproven benefit when used with anticoagulation in the management of a DVT. Aggressive anticoagulation will prevent extension of clot and allow for its lysis by the usual fibrinolytic pathways. Early ambulation with appropriate analgesia as needed after adequate anticoagulation with heparin is a practical and safe approach. PPS can be treated with periodic leg elevation, compression stockings, and pain medications as required.

Prevention of PE is the primary objective in treating DVT. Given the potential to propagate, a calf DVT should be followed closely with repeat duplex or IPG in 5 to 7 days after initial examination. (Some authorities suggest two repeat examinations at 2 and 7 days after first test.[7]) The potential morbidity and cost of several months of anticoagulation is not justified for an isolated, nonextending calf DVT except in high-risk groups such as patients with a history of a previous proximal DVT or PE, significant cardiovascular comorbidity, a persistent hypercoagulable state, or poor ambulation.

Several recent studies have documented the accuracy of serial duplex examinations and the safety of withholding anticoagulation in patients clinically suspected of having DVT but with a normal initial ultrasound.[4,7]. A repeat duplex should be done in these patients at 5 to 7 days after initial exam or earlier if there is progression of symptoms or signs. The risk of a PE within 7 days of a normal duplex scan in patients with symptoms of DVT of the lower extremity is near zero. The probability of detecting DVT on a second ultrasound when there is a completely normal color-flow duplex scan from a few days earlier is approximately 2 percent.[2,7] Subsequent thromboembolism (typically nonfatal) within 3 months of two normal serial duplex studies occurs in about 0.6 percent of patients, which is comparable to the outcome in patients with normal venograms.[7] It follows that withholding anticoagulation in patients with negative serial ultrasounds is safe, accurate, and cost-effective.

Proven proximal DVT requires immediate anticoagulation to reduce local morbidity and prevent thromboembolism. The initial choice of treatment is becoming a low-molecular-weight heparin (LMWHs), such as dalteparin, enoxaparin, or tinzaparin. These are *weight-adjusted* and given once or twice daily subcutaneously until oral anticoagulation reaches the therapeutic range (100 U/kg q12h or 200 U/kg q24h for dalteparin; 100/mg/kg q12h for enoxaparin; 175 U/kg q24h for tinzaparin based on actual body weight). The available LMWH agents are *not* interchangeable. These drugs have several advantages over unfractionated heparin, including a more predictable anticoagulant effect, ease of administration, longer half-life, lack of a need to monitor the anticoagulation effect, resistance to inhibition by activated platelets, and a lower incidence of major bleeding and heparin-induced thrombocytopenia.[2,8,9] LMWH has a preferential inhibitory effect on factor Xa rather than factor IIa (thrombin) and is at least as effective and safe as unfractionated heparin in the treatment of DVT or PE.[8,9,10] INR or PTT cannot be used to monitor the effect of LMWH and measuring factor Xa levels is expensive, not readily available, and unnecessary given the very predictable effect of these heparins. The ability to discharge most patients home after treatment with LMWH with next-day follow-up makes this the most cost-effective option. The treatment plan must be discussed with the continuing care physician, including follow-up in 24 h and institution of warfarin.

Despite the increasing use of LMWH, some patients will have indications for admission. These include the patient who is unable to ambulate, has poor social supports or unreliable follow-up, has difficulty with education for drug administration, needs lytic or invasive therapy, or needs to have an alternative serious diagnosis investigated or treated (e.g., arterial ischemia, cellulitis, or pelvic mass). The consequences of a suspected or known PE such as hemodynamic instability or significant comorbidity will also require in-hospital treatment. Obviously, there must be a mechanism for providing the patient with the medication before discharge from the ED.

If LMWH is not immediately available, a continuous infusion of unfractionated heparin can be started until LMWH is initiated or oral anticoagulation is therapeutic. Weight-adjusted dosing of 80 U/kg bolus followed by an infusion of 18 U/kg per hour will rapidly achieve a therapeutic activated partial thromboplastin time (aPTT). Traditional dosing of a 5000-U bolus followed by an infusion of 1000 U/h will result in subtherapeutic aPTT at 6 h in two-thirds of treated patients. If weight-adjusted dosing is not used, a higher bolus of 7500 to 10,000 U followed by an infusion of 1250 U/h or greater is recommended. The infusion is altered to keep the aPTT between 55 and 85 s (1.8 to 2.8 times normal). Close monitoring of patients is required to detect bleeding and heparin-induced thrombocytopenia and thrombosis. Serious bleeding due to LMWH is very unusual, but if it occurs, the anti-Xa effect cannot be reversed. Protamine can counteract the minor antithrombin effect of LMWH, but is not useful given its inability to effect factor Xa and its own inherent potential to cause bleeding.

Oral anticoagulation with the vitamin K antagonist warfarin should be started on the same day as heparin for the treatment of a DVT. However, before its delayed effect of reducing prothrombin concentrations occurs, warfarin increases coagulability and thrombogenesis in the first 24 to 48 h owing to its early effect on reducing protein C levels.[2] This has prompted some authors to suggest that warfarin should be started well after initiation of heparin when the aPTT is adequately prolonged, though it is common practice to start both drugs simultaneously. It is clear, however, that if heparin is discontinued early, when the International Normalized Ratio (INR) first becomes therapeutic, the patient is at risk of clot extension, since warfarin has induced a transient hypercoagulable state. The usual recommended loading dose of warfarin is 7.5 to 10 mg, which is twice the expected maintenance dose. Then the daily warfarin dose is adjusted to keep the INR between 2 and 3. Heparin can be discontinued when the INR is in the therapeutic range for at least two consecutive days.

Warfarin is associated with some serious adverse effects and should not be used in certain circumstances. The commonest risk of warfarin is bleeding. This is usually related to the degree of anticoagulation and typically responds to dose reduction. Skin necrosis secondary to warfarin occurs primarily in patients with a deficiency of protein C or protein S.[2] The necrosis is due to thrombotic occlusion of small vessels, usually three to eight days after initiation of this drug. Warfarin is contraindicated in patients who are pregnant, have a serious or active bleeding diathesis, or have had very recent major surgery (thoracoabdominal, nervous system, spine, or eye). It causes fetal bleeding and is teratogenic, but neither unfractionated heparin nor LMWH crosses the placenta and both are safe for the fetus. LMWH is the preferred drug for the treatment of a DVT in pregnancy and warfarin can be safely started in the postpartum period even in breast-feeding women.[2]

The duration of warfarin treatment has to be individualized and is dependent on a previous history of DVT or PE, reversibility of previous thromboembolic risk factors, the effectiveness of warfarin to resolve thrombosis, and on the risk of bleeding. Oral anticoagulation for 3 to 6 months is associated with fewer recurrent thromboembolic events than shorter treatment regimens. There is no evidence that a longer course of warfarin is needed for patients with a PE. Despite adequate treatment of a DVT, there is a 6 percent risk of a recurrent DVT or PE during the first year and 13 percent over 5 years. Patients who present with a new or progressive clot despite adequate anticoagulation with warfarin need to be started on LMWH and investigated for a hypercoagulable state on an urgent outpatient basis. Warfarin resistance is not infrequently encountered in patients with metastatic disease.

The issue of initiating anticoagulation and interference with workup of possible hypercoagulability occasionally arises. Since LMWH does not alter the ability to investigate hypercoagulable states, there is no need to procure additional blood samples beyond routine coagulation studies in patients with a straightforward DVT. Further, acute-phase reactants themselves can alter blood results with an acute DVT/PE. Initiation of unfractionated heparin therapy is likely to interfere with the workup of hypercoagulability. However, such investigations for the underlying etiology of a DVT typically do not alter management. Thus, these patients can be investigated in 3 to 6 months, when anticoagulation is stopped. When a patient presents with a refractory or progressive clot despite warfarin and is treated with LMWH, further hematologic studies can still be carried out and extra blood from the ED can be held for further testing (factor V Leiden, antithrombin III, protein C and S levels, and antiphospholipid anticoagulants). If, for some reason, unfractionated heparin is used to treat a patient with DVT, then at least two extra blood tubes should obtained prior to initiation of treatment and held for further testing by the hematologist.

Thrombolytic and Mechanical Therapy

Currently, no controlled clinical trials have shown a survival benefit of thrombolytics over heparin and warfarin. Some randomized trials suggest reduced morbidity from PPS if complete clot lysis is achieved with thrombolytics.[2] However, as the short-term benefits of lytic agents are generally small and the long-term benefits remain to be proved, the use of these drugs has very limited indications. In practice, they are rarely used to treat a DVT. Thrombolytics have a significantly greater bleeding risk, including fatal intracerebral hemorrhage, than heparin or warfarin. Currently, lytic drugs such as streptokinase, urokinase, and tissue plasminogen activator (tPA) should be restricted to extensive iliofemoral thrombosis such as phlegmasia cerulea dolens in patients with a low risk of bleeding. Systemic thrombolysis may fail to lyse iliofemoral clots due to local stagnant blood flow; in such cases, intravascular catheter-directed thrombolysis is recommended.

An inferior vena cava filter can be placed to prevent a PE when oral anticoagulation is contraindicated, a DVT persists or propagates despite adequate medical treatment, embolization occurs after 1 to 2 weeks of therapeutic anticoagulation, or there is significant bleeding with the use of anticoagulants. Given the greater than 95 percent patency rate of a Greenfield filter at 1 year after placement, its indications can be expanded. A free-floating, nonadherent iliofemoral thrombus greater than 5 cm has an up to 60 percent chance of forming a PE; in such cases, filter placement should be considered.

Surgical thrombectomy was enthusiastically received in previous decades, but owing to high rates of rethrombosis and failure to prevent postphlebitic sequelae due to valve incompetency, it is rarely considered today. When conventional therapy for DVT is contraindicated or ineffective, thrombectomy followed by heparin can achieve long-term patency. Surgical treatment of a DVT is typically reserved for patients when limb viability is jeopardized by a massive venous clot, such as a persistently ischemic leg secondary to phlegmasia cerulea dolens.

The ED management of patients who are adequately anticoagulated but present with propagation or a new clot is fairly straightforward. Since LMWH is significantly more effective for treating DVT, these patients should all be started on LMWH with urgent follow-up by hematology (or, if otherwise indicated, admission). If they fail LMWH or have large free-floating thrombi, a Greenfield filter should be emergently placed by radiology. The investigation of these patients for a hypercoagulable state or malignancy need not be initiated in the ED. There is no evidence in the literature that increasing anticoagulation beyond an INR of 3 is at all effective in treating refractory DVT.

Axillary and Subclavian Vein Thrombosis

Though up to 90 percent of all DVTs occur in the lower extremities, a clot can develop in the axillary or subclavian vein. The risk factors for developing a venous thrombus in the upper extremity are like those outlined in Tables 55-1 and 55-2, a higher incidence being associated with venous catheterization, intravenous drugs, excessive or unusual exercise (effort thrombosis), malignancy, and other hypercoagulable states. A predisposing venous stricture or chronic compression (cervical rib, hypertrophied scalene muscle, congenital web, etc.) is not uncommonly detected as a causal factor. The patient with DVT of an upper extremity can present with an abrupt or gradual onset of swelling in the arm, associated with dilated veins in the hand and forearm. The arm may feel heavy, with pain on physical activity which is relieved with rest. Sudden onset of severe pain and swelling with a change in the color of the arm is a rare presentation. The two primary methods of investigating a suspected venous thrombosis of an upper limb is by duplex ultrasound or venography. Computed tomography (CT) and MRI are occasionally useful in difficult cases.

It is estimated that a PE occurs in 10 to 30 percent of cases involving axillary or subclavian DVT; aggressive therapy is warranted in such instances. Current treatment options include anticoagulation alone or preceded by catheter-directed thrombolysis. The choice of therapy should be discussed with the consulting vascular surgeon and invasive radiologist but should be individualized in every case. The underlying cause, duration of symptoms, comorbidity and contraindications to lytic agents or anticoagulants can help guide the choice of the most appropriate therapy. Resolution of symptoms and signs is dependent not only on therapy but also on the development of collateral flow. Following initial therapy, an underlying compressive abnormality or venous stenosis, if present, must be corrected (e.g., rib resection, balloon angioplasty).

OCCLUSIVE ARTERIAL DISEASE

Acute limb ischemia secondary to thrombosis or embolism is a true emergency requiring immediate therapy to salvage the limb. The ED physician must urgently initiate treatment and investigation of a threatened limb in collaboration with the radiologist and vascular surgeon. A good understanding of the pathophysiology, etiology, and clinical presentation of peripheral vascular disease will help guide management in the effort to restore blood flow to the affected limb.

Epidemiology

Intermittent claudication has a prevalence of between 1 and 7 percent for men above age 50, with symptomless disease existing in up to 25 percent of men scanned with noninvasive testing in this age group.[11] Symptoms of peripheral arterial disease increase with age and are two to four times more common in men than in women. The vast majority of these patients have a history of prolonged smoking. There has been an increase in the incidence of both chronic limb ischemia and arterial embolic disease in the last decade. Given that atherosclerosis is the usual pathology in ischemic limb pain, it is not surprising that at lest half of these patients have coronary or cerebrovascular disease.[11] Embolic occlusion of an artery also occurs primarily in elderly men and postmenopausal women, given the higher prevalence in this group of heart disease, which is the major source of thromboemboli.

Pathophysiology

Acute limb ischemia results from a blood supply that is inadequate to meet tissue oxygen and nutrient requirements. If allowed to persist, it will lead to cell death and irreversible tissue damage. Even after perfusion is partially or completely restored, reperfusion injury can occur as oxygen radicals form and cause further cell injury. Perfusion may not be fully attainable with prolonged arterial obstruction due to distal edema and thrombi forming in the microcirculation. The extent of injury depends on the duration and location of the arterial blockage, the amount of collateral flow, and the previous health of the involved limb. Also, some tissues are more susceptible to anoxia than others, presumably on the basis of differences in cellular respiration and oxygen requirements. Peripheral nerves and skeletal muscle are very sensitive to ischemia; in them, irreversible changes occur within 4 h of anoxia at room temperature.

Nonembolic limb ischemia is secondary to atherosclerosis in the vast majority of patients.[12] Plaque formation within the intima of an artery results from lipid accumulation, proliferation of smooth muscle cells, and fibrogenesis. Narrowing of the vascular lumen occurs with progression of the atheromatous plaque. Complete or high-grade obstruction can occur at this site of stenosis secondary to plaque rupture, hemorrhage, or thrombus formation. An atherosclerotic vessel can give rise to an aneurysm because of its weakened walls. A true aneurysm, involving dilatation of its entire wall, can present clinically with thrombosis, rupture, and hemorrhaging or by its mass effect on adjacent structures.

Etiology

An embolus is the commonest cause of an acute arterial occlusion in the limb and originates from the heart in 80 to 90 percent of cases of embolism. Atrial fibrillation and recent myocardial infarction are the two primary causes of mural thrombus within the heart. Both conditions result in poor wall motion and stagnant blood flow, predisposing to clot formation. The natural history of an embolus is to either fragment and embolize distally or to propagate locally into a larger clot, though associated venous thrombosis can occur possibly secondary to local ischemia, decreased venous flow, and inflammation. Emboli usually lodge where vessels branch or taper, most frequently in the lower extremities. The commonest location for an embolus in the leg is the bifurcation of the common femoral artery and in the brachial artery of the upper limb. Rare cardiac sources of emboli include tumor emboli from atrial myxomas, vegetations from valve leaflets, and parts of prosthetic devices such as mechanical valves.

Noncardiac sources of arterial emboli include thrombi from aneurysms and atheromatous plaques. Mural thrombus in aneurysms of aortoiliac, femoral, popliteal, and subclavian arteries are the most notable sources. Atheroemboli result from plaque fragmentation and cause obstruction of the microcirculation, giving symptoms in the feet (''blue toe syndrome''), hands, or cerebral circulation (transient ischemic attack). These emboli consist of cholesterol-laden debris and platelet aggregates and can be showered to multiple parts of the body.

Thrombosis unrelated to atherosclerotic disease can occur at an area of vessel injury, as with invasive catheters, balloons, sites of bypass grafting or intraarterial drug injection, and with hypercoagulable states. All of these are potential sources of embolization. Femoral artery catheterization for coronary angiography or angioplasty and vascular access can result in ischemia of an extremity secondary to thrombosis or expanding hematoma; symptoms may be altered by preexisting aortoiliac or femoropopliteal plaques. Radial artery injury during blood-gas analysis or the placement of arterial lines rarely leads to tissue ischemia, given the excellent collateral supply from the ulnar artery. Intentional or accidental intraarterial drug injections by medical personnel or for illicit drugs can result in local vasospasm, infectious arteritis, thrombosis, pseudoaneurysms, and mycotic aneurysms. Inert particles or drug crystals can embolize to obstruct end arteries, leading to gangrene of digits, especially as drug addicts tend to delay seeking medical attention.

Peripheral arterial supply can also be obstructed by vasospastic or inflammatory conditions. Raynaud disease involves vasospasm in small arteries and arterioles in response to a stressor such as cold temperature or emotional stress. Symptoms of local pain, pallor followed by cyanosis, numbness, and parasthesias usually involve the fingers and hands and generally resolve within 30 to 60 min, especially with rewarming. Inflammation of arteries in the limb can occur with collagen vascular diseases such as rheumatoid arthritis, lupus, and polyarteritis nodosa. When clinically active, these vasculitides are often associated with systemic symptoms and multiorgan involvement. Necrosis of blood vessels and loss of limb tissue is always a possibility. Thromboangiitis obliterans (Buerger disease) is an idiopathic occlusive disease resulting from segmental inflammation of arteries in all extremities. It occurs almost exclusively in young smokers (age 20 to 40), predominantly males, and is characterized by painful, tender nodules in the limbs with decreased distal flow.

Limb ischemia may occur with nonembolic central causes. A thoracic aortic dissection can propagate into the carotid, subclavian, and iliofemoral system and present with neurologic and extremity findings. The false lumen created by the dissection occludes flow in the involved artery. Takayasu arteritis, which primarily occurs in Asian females, involves the aortic arch and its branches and has a ''pulseless phase'' where peripheral ischemia and necrosis can develop.

More commonly, low cardiac output states with cardiogenic or hypovolemic shock may present with extremity ischemia. Severe left ventricular dysfunction—which can occur with ischemic cardiomyopathy, valvular heart disease, and cardiac tamponade—acutely threatens limb blood flow, particularly in elderly patients with preexisting atherosclerosis. Acute hemorrhage similarly reduces perfusion to the limbs, but, with acute intervention, may be reversible.

Clinical Features

Patients with acute limb ischemia will exhibit one or more of the ''six P's'': pain, pallor, polar (for cold), pulselessness, parasthesias, and paralysis. However, a lack of one or more of these findings does not exclude ischemia. Pain alone may be the earliest symptom. High clinical suspicion is paramount to early intervention to save a limb. Complete arterial obstruction results in visible skin changes, with initial pallor that may be followed by blotchy, mottled areas of cyanosis and associated petechiae and blisters. Severe, steady pain in the involved extremity associated with decreased skin temperature is expected. Hypoesthesia or hyperesthesia due to ischemic neuropathy is typically an early finding, as is muscle weakness. An absent pulse distal is only so helpful. It may be an abrupt new sign of an occlusive clot or a long-standing finding of chronic vascular disease. As ischemic injury progresses, anesthesia and paralysis become evident and foreshadow impending gangrene. Preservation of light touch on skin testing is a good guide to tissue viability. Necrosis of skin and fat is a late finding.

Despite the generally held belief that limb salvage is possible with reperfusion within 4 to 6 h, tissue loss can occur with significantly shorter occlusion times. As important, mild to severe limb dysfunction is possible even with an injury involving only brief anoxia, with potential for lasting disability. The poor predictability of functional outcome after ischemic injury underscores the need to attain rapid reperfusion and not rely on a probable safe time interval until resolution of occlusion. Disability and tissue loss are inevitable after 6 h of occlusive anoxic injury.

Microemboli present clinically with pain and cyanosis in the involved digit, petechiae, and local muscle pain and tenderness at the site of infarction. Several different small areas can be affected with a shower of microemboli originating from a large or unstable source. Though mottling and decreased function may occur, pulses are preserved.

Chronic peripheral arterial insufficiency is characterized by intermittent claudication, which may progress to intermittent ischemic pain at rest. Femoral and popliteal disease often causes reproducible calf pain with activity that is relieved with rest. Pain at rest typically localizes to the foot and is aggravated with leg elevation, improves with standing, and is poorly controlled with analgesics.[11] Shiny, hyperpigmented skin with hair loss and ulceration, thickened nails, muscle atrophy, vascular bruits, and poor pulses is a hallmark of chronic vascular disease. Complete arterial occlusion from thrombosis of a limb in these patients may present subacutely owing to a well-developed collateral circulation.

Diagnosis

A thorough clinical evaluation is the most useful diagnostic tool for the assessment of occlusive arterial disease. A history of an abruptly ischemic limb in a patient with atrial fibrillation or recent myocardial infarction is highly suggestive of an embolus. Acute ischemia in the limb of a patient known to have advanced peripheral vascular disease is more likely due to thrombosis or a low cardiac output state.

At the bedside, blanching the involved extremity with finger pressure and noting a delay in the return of blood as compared with the uninvolved extremity indicates decreased perfusion. However, several factors can influence capillary refill; thus one cannot rely on the presence or absence of this finding alone.

A hand-held Doppler can document the amplitude of flow or its absence when held over the dorsalis pedis, posterior tibial, popliteal, or femoral arteries in the lower limb and over the radial, ulnar, brachial, or axillary arteries in the arm. If time permits or the diagnosis of arterial occlusion is in question, duplex ultrasonography can be undertaken to detect an obstruction to flow. Cardiac monitoring and an electrocardiogram will detect an dysrhythmia and an echocardiogram can be done to look for an intracardiac thrombus if such is clinically suspected.

In consultation with a vascular surgeon and during the period of preoperative and/or medical management, an arteriogram can be done to confirm the diagnosis, define the vascular anatomy and perfusion, and guide aggressive management. A particular advantage of arteriography is the ability to perform this test on the operating room table before and during surgery. Scanning a limb with a spiral CT or MRI, though accurate and noninvasive, is not usually practical, given the time constraints, in the face of an acutely ischemic limb. However, when an aortic dissection or sources of microemboli such as aortoiliac or femoral aneurysms are suspected, an aorotogram, CT, or MRI can be useful. Transesophageal echocardiography is gaining acceptance as the choice modality for detecting cardiac or aortic root pathology.

Management

When the diagnosis of acute limb ischemia is known or suspected, immediate intravenous heparinization should be started if no contraindications exist. This may help prevent clot extension, recurrent emboli, venous thrombosis, and the appearance of microthrombi distal to the obstruction.[12] Fluid resuscitation and treatment of heart failure and dysrhythmias is necessary to improve limb perfusion.

Definitive treatment of an obstructing clot should be done in conjunction with a vascular surgeon. Prompt surgical embolectomy is the optimal therapy for an acute arterial embolism causing limb-threatening ischemia. Catheter embolectomy has been the choice technique for removal of clot ever since the development of the Fogarty balloon catheter in 1963.[12] It has reduced mortality from arterial emboli by 50 percent and need for amputation by 35 percent. Overall mortality from an arterial embolus is about 15 percent and is usually due to the underlying cardiovascular disease. The limb salvage rate ranges from 62 to 96 percent.[12]

Intraarterial thrombolysis with streptokinase, urokinase, or tPA infused near or into the clot for a few hours to days is an alternative to surgery, with a rate of successful reperfusion of 50 to 85 percent.[12] It should be considered for distal thromboembolic occlusions in surgically inaccessible small arteries, acute thrombosis in a limb with chronic arterial insufficiency and adequate collateral flow, or in poor surgical candidates. Follow-up balloon angioplasty or surgical grafts may be needed to prevent rethrombosis in patients with atherosclerotic plaques. Systemic thrombolysis has been compared with intraarterial lytic agents in randomized trials and has been shown to produce inferior results.[12]

Since thrombotic occlusion usually occurs in arteries with advanced atherosclerosis and a developed collateral supply, it is often not a dramatic event and is occasionally silent.[12] Management of these occlusions therefore is conservative, with heparin alone. An angiogram is helpful to direct therapy and exclude embolic occlusion (radiologically seen as an abrupt cutoff of blood flow) when limb viability is acutely threatened. It is still unclear whether heparin improves outcome in the clinical circumstances of thrombosis in a plaque-laden artery.

Aneurysms of the Extremity

Over 80 percent of all peripheral arterial aneurysms arise in the popliteal artery and the vast majority are due to atherosclerosis. More than 95 percent of patients with popliteal aneurysms are elderly males.[13] Acute symptoms develop with thrombosis or distal embolization and rupture is rare.

False aneurysms of the femoral artery, consisting of encapsulated hematomas adjoining the vessel lumen, arise from iatrogenic injury and occur more frequently than true femoral aneurysms. Duplex ultrasonography, CT scan, or an MRI can confirm the clinical diagnosis and detect mural thrombus. The risk of ischemic complications from an asymptomatic popliteal aneurysm ranges from 8 to 100 percent (mean 36 percent). Thus, elective surgery following arteriography is recommended for all cases.[13] As 37 percent of patients with a single popliteal aneurysm have an aortic aneurysm and half have a contralateral popliteal aneurysm, a thorough search is indicated after detection of a single aneurysm.

Subclavian artery aneurysms occur from atherosclerosis, trauma, or thoracic outlet obstruction. Rupture of a proximal subclavian aneurysm can cause death from exsanguination. Thromboembolism gives rise to typical signs and symptoms of distal ischemia, but it may also produce central neurologic deficits from retrograde propagation of clot into the vertebral and carotid circulation. Because of their severe potential morbidity, these aneurysms should be surgically removed promptly after diagnosis.

REFERENCES

1. Barloon TJ, Bergus GR, Seabold JE: Diagnostic imaging of lower limb deep venous thrombosis. *Am Fam Phys* 56:791, 1997.
2. Ginsberg JS: Management of venous thromboembolism. *N Engl J Med* 335:1816, 1996.
3. Venta ZA, Venta ER, Mumford LM: Value of diagnostic tests for deep venous thrombosis: A decision analysis model. *Radiology* 174:433, 1990.
4. Kearon C, Julian JA, Math M, et al: Noninvasive diagnosis of deep venous thrombosis. *Ann Intern Med* 128:663, 1998.
5. Hirsch J, Hull RD, Roskob GE: Clinical features and diagnosis of venous thrombosis. *J Am Coll Cardiol* 8:114B, 1986.
6. Becker DM, Philbrick JT, Bachhuber TL, et al: D-dimer testing and acute venous thromboembolism. *Arch Intern Med* 156:939, 1996.
7. Birdwell BG, Raskob GE, Whitsett TL, et al: The clinical validity of normal compression ultrasonography in outpatients suspected of having deep venous thrombosis. *Ann Intern Med* 128:1, 1998.
8. Harrison L, McGinnis J, Crowther M, et al: Assessment of outpatient treatment of deep-vein thrombosis with low-molecular-weight heparin. *Arch Intern Med* 158:2001, 1998.
9. Simonneau G, Sors H, Charbonnier B, et al: A comparison of low-molecular-weight heparin with unfractionated heparin for acute pulmonary embolism. *N Engl J Med* 337:663, 1997.
10. Buller HR, Gent M, Gallus AS, et al: Low-molecular-weight heparin in the treatment of patients with venous thromboembolism. *N Engl J Med* 337:657, 1997.
11. Golledge J: Lower-limb arterial disease. *Lancet* 350:1459, 1997.
12. Clagett GP, Krupski WC: Antithrombotic therapy in peripheral arterial occlusive disease. *Chest* 108:431s, 1995.
13. Dawson I, Sie RB, vanBockel JH: Atherosclerotic popliteal aneurysm. *Br J Surg* 84:293, 1997.

CARDIAC TRANSPLANTATION

Michael R. Mill
Michelle S. Grady

The first clinically successful cardiac transplant was performed in December 1967. Since then, advances in the immunosuppression and postoperative care of these patients have resulted in dramatically im-

TABLE 56-1 Etiology of Heart Failure in Transplant Recipients

Adult	Occurrence	Pediatric	Occurrence
Coronary artery disease	44.8%	Congenital heart disease	46.4%
Dilated cardiomyopathies	46.2%	Dilated cardiomyopathies	44.3%
Valvular	3.5%	Retransplantation	2.9%
Retransplantation	2.1%	Miscellaneous	6.4%
Congenital	1.8%		
Miscellaneous	1.6%		

proved patient survival. This has been accompanied by a tremendous growth in the number of procedures performed. Data from the registry of the International Society of Heart and Lung Transplantation (ISHLT) and the United Network for Organ Sharing (UNOS) reveals that 45,993 heart transplants were performed at 301 centers throughout the world between January 1, 1983, and March 1, 1998.[1] This total includes more than 2000 heart transplants per year in the United States since 1990. The actuarial survival after transplantation reported by UNOS is 85 percent at 1 year, with 3-year and 5-year actuarial survivals of 76 percent and 69 percent, respectively.[2] Given the increased number of patients undergoing transplantation and their excellent long-term survival, these patients will come to the attention of physicians in the emergency department (ED) with increasing frequency.

TRANSPLANT RECIPIENTS

Cardiac transplantation has been applied successfully to patients of all ages, from newborns through persons in their late sixties. Heart transplantation is indicated for patients with end-stage heart failure not remediable by standard medical or surgical therapy. The etiology of heart failure in transplant recipients as reported by the ISHLT/UNOS registry is listed in Table 56-1.[1] The majority of adult patients have either idiopathic dilated cardiomyopathies or end-stage coronary artery disease. Many in the latter group will have undergone previous coronary artery bypass surgery. The predominant diagnoses in children undergoing transplantation are dilated cardiomyopathies and congenital heart disease. Many of the children with congenital heart disease will have undergone previous palliative or corrective operations. Patients are carefully evaluated to rule out other irreversible end-organ dysfunction and other systemic illnesses that would separately limit survival.

CARDIAC PHYSIOLOGY AFTER TRANSPLANTATION

The physiologic basis upon which cardiac transplantation is grounded is the ability of the denervated heart to support normal circulation. The lack of sympathetic and parasympathetic innervation does, however, induce an altered physiologic state. The denervated heart has a normal sinus rhythm with a heart rate between 90 and 100 beats per minute. Denervation results in the absence of the initial centrally mediated tachycardia in response to stress or exercise. The heart remains responsive to circulating catecholamines of either endogenous or exogenous origin. The cardiac response to stress or exertion is therefore blunted. With the onset of exercise, the heart rate initially remains unchanged, then gradually increases to a level of approximately 80 percent of predicted over 10 to 15 min. After termination of exercise, this exercise-induced tachycardia will persist for approximately 20 to 30 min before slowly returning to the patient's baseline rate. Patients may complain of fatigue or shortness of breath with the onset of exercise that resolves with continued exertion as an appropriate tachycardia develops. In order to accommodate this response, patients are trained to perform warmup exercises prior to vigorous exertion to initiate an increase in their heart rate. They are also cautioned to allow appropriate time for recovery at the end of exertion.

Cardiac hemodynamics after transplantation as measured by cardiac catheterization reveal a normal to mildly depressed cardiac output at rest. With exercise, cardiac output increases in response to increased venous return (preload) and circulating catecholamines. Maximal cardiac outputs of 80 to 100 percent of normal have been measured. Patients are able to resume normal activity levels, including vigorous exercise, following transplantation. A number of posttransplant patients have completed marathons and participated in other rigorous physical activities, and at least one such individual has competed as a professional athlete.

Cardiac denervation results in an altered response to some medications used in emergency resuscitation.[3] In patients with supraventricular tachycardias, the lack of sympathetic innervation obviates the utility of carotid sinus massage. Atropine, which acts by abolishing reflex vagal slowing, will have no effect on heart rate in patients with symptomatic bradyarrhythmias. Conversely, denervated hearts are quite sensitive to the chronotropic effects of β-adrenergic agents such as isoproterenol, dopamine, and dobutamine. Because these are normal hearts, they are resistant to the proarrhythmic effects of these drugs. Isoproterenol is used preferentially to increase donor heart rates because it has the greatest chronotropic effects and can easily be titrated to achieve the desired heart rate. The typical dose range is 1 to 4 μg/min administered by continuous intravenous infusion.

CARDIAC EVALUATION OF THE POSTTRANSPLANT PATIENT

Electrocardiograms (ECGs) obtained on transplant recipients should demonstrate normal sinus rhythm. The donor heart is implanted with its sinus node intact to preserve normal atrioventricular conduction. The technique of cardiac transplantation also results in the preservation of the recipient's sinus node at the superior cavoatrial junction. The atrial suture line renders the two sinus nodes electrically isolated from each other. Thus, ECGs will frequently have two distinct P waves (Fig. 56-1). The sinus node of the donor heart is easily identified by its constant 1:1 relationship to the QRS complex, while the native P wave marches through the donor heart rhythm independently. The presence of the two separate P waves may lead to confusion about the patient's rhythm. The ECGs may be interpreted erroneously as showing atrial fibrillation, atrial flutter, or frequent premature atrial complexes. The use of calipers aids in the definition of the two distinct P waves. Sinus node dysfunction in the posttransplant heart occurs in approximately 4 to 5 percent of patients and is manifest by either sinus brachycardia with heart rates of equal to or less than 50 beats per minute or sinus standstill with a junctional escape rhythm with heart rates of 60 to 70 beats per minute. This dysfunction occurs in the early postoperative period and resolves spontaneously in most patients. For patients in whom sinus node dysfunction persists, treatment consists of either theophylline, which accelerates the sinus bradycardia in some patients, or implantation of a permanent transvenous pacemaker. The type of pacemaker implanted varies depending on institutional preference but generally is either an atrial pacemaker programmed in the AAIR mode or a ventricular pacemaker programmed in the VVIR mode. Use of an atrial rate-responsive pacemaker preserves atrioventricular conduction in addition to providing physiologic rate responsiveness.

Posttransplant chest radiographs show evidence of a prior sternotomy but otherwise are generally normal. Some patients may have

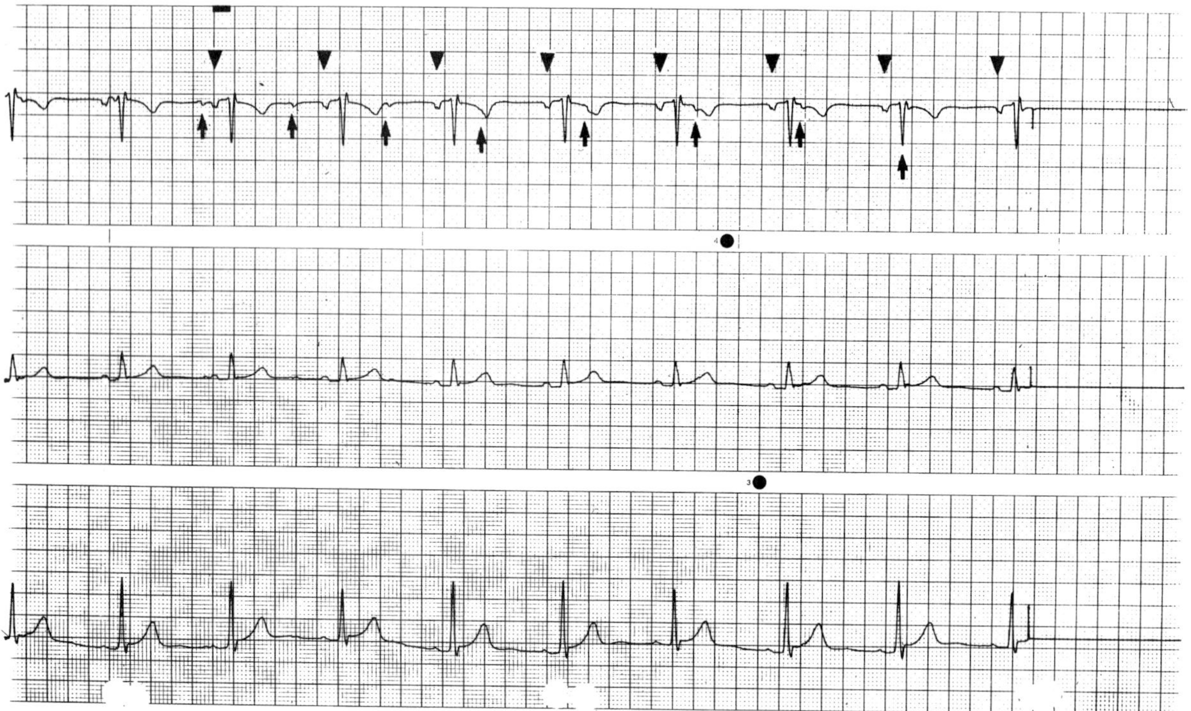

FIG. 56-1. Electrocardiogram demonstrating donor and recipient P waves. ∇ donor P wave; ↑ recipient P wave.

evidence of "cardiomegaly" related to the transplantation of a heart from a donor who was larger than the recipient (Fig. 56-2).

Echocardiography is a useful tool for evaluating cardiac function post-transplantation. Interpretation of the echocardiogram is routine with the exception of the evaluation of the atrial size. Because the atrial anastomoses incorporate the posterior walls of the recipient's native atria, echocardiography will show atrial enlargement, but this has no significant effect on cardiac function. Early rejection results in diastolic dysfunction, although the echocardiographic indices may be subtle and difficult to detect. Severe rejection will be accompanied by signs of biventricular enlargement with global hypocontractility and significant atrioventricular valve regurgitation.

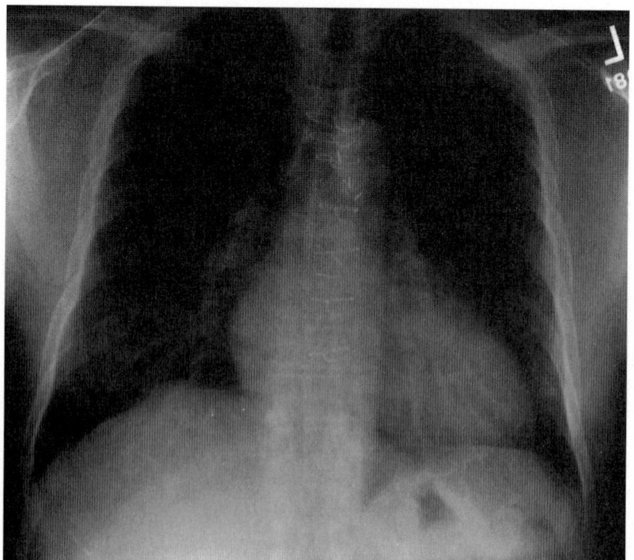

FIG. 56-2. Chest radiograph of healthy posttransplant patient with typical postoperative changes.

IMMUNOSUPPRESSION FOR CARDIAC TRANSPLANTATION

As with all types of solid organ transplantation, lifelong immunosuppression is required to prevent acute graft rejection. One of the most significant challenges of clinical transplantation is to maintain an adequate level of immunosuppression to prevent rejection while preserving adequate immunocompetence to avoid serious infectious complications. Since the mid 1980s, standard immunosuppression has employed a triple drug regimen consisting of cyclosporine (Sandimmune, Sang-Cya), prednisone, and azathioprine (Imuran). The combination of these agents has resulted in superior graft and patient survival rates, has decreased the mortality from infectious complications, and has minimized the side effects of the individual agents. Recently, the newer immunosuppressive agents tacrolimus (Prograf) and mycophenolate mofetil (Cellcept) have been used in place of cyclosporine and azathioprine, respectively. In addition, some programs use induction therapy in the early postoperative period, employing cytotoxic antibody preparations targeted against the T lymphocytes. The most commonly used agents include OKT3, a murine monoclonal antibody, and polyclonal preparations such as antilymphocyte serum (ALS) and antilymphocyte globulin (ALG).

Cyclosporine remains one of the mainstays of immunosuppressive regimens. This fungal metabolite is a potent inhibitor of T-lymphocyte activity and interferes with the generation of interleukin 2 (IL-2). It is a lipophilic substance that is metabolized in the liver by the cytochrome P-450 system. Cyclosporine is usually taken twice daily, and doses are adjusted based on serial blood levels. Target trough levels vary depending on the specific laboratory assay used. Levels are maintained in the range of 300 to 400 ng/dL early after transplantation and then lowered to levels of approximately 150 ng/dL long term. The list of drugs that interact with cyclosporine (Table 56-2) continues to grow yearly, and careful consideration is required before adding or withdrawing medications for an individual patient. Such changes

TABLE 56-2 Cyclosporine Drug Interactions

Drugs increasing cyclosporine blood levels
Clarithromycin
Diltiazem
Erythromycin
Fluconazole
Itraconazole
Josamycin
Ketoconazole
Methylprednisolone
Metoclopramide
Nicardipine
Verapamil
Drugs decreasing cyclosporine blood levels
Carbamazepine
Phenobarbital
Phenytoin
Rifampin
Ticlopidine
Drugs causing enhanced/additive nephrotoxicity
Acyclovir
Amphotericin B
Ganciclovir
Gentamicin
Nonsteroidal anti-inflammatory drugs
Trimethoprim/sulfamethoxazole
Tobramycin

should always be made with the knowledge and input of the patient's transplant physician. Acute increases in cyclosporine levels may be associated with severe renal dysfunction, and acute decreases may result in the development of acute rejection.

Commonly encountered side effects of cyclosporine are listed in Table 56-3. Hypertension occurs in the majority of patients and frequently requires combination therapy to achieve adequate control. Renal insufficiency is also quite common and is mediated at least in part by the vasoconstrictive effects of cyclosporine on the proximal renal tubule. Management of cyclosporine-induced renal insufficiency requires careful monitoring, because worsening renal insufficiency results in elevated cyclosporine levels, leading to more renal dysfunction, thus creating a vicious cycle. Although early renal insufficiency is frequently reversible, some patients have developed end-stage renal disease requiring dialysis or renal transplantation.

Formally known as FK-506, tacrolimus is a macrolide antibiotic with an immunosuppressive mechanism similar to that of cyclosporine.

TABLE 56-3 Common Cyclosporine Side Effects

Hypertension
Renal insufficiency
Hirsutism
Tremor
Gingival hyperplasia
Hyperkalemia
Hypomagnesemia
Hyperuricemia
Glucose intolerance
Seizures

Tacrolimus prevents rejection of the transplanted organ by inhibiting the expression of IL-2 in T cells and inhibiting T-cell growth and proliferation. Studies show that replacing cyclosporine with tacrolimus as a primary or rescue immunosuppressant may result in fewer episodes of rejection, less clinically relevant hypertension, and lower doses of maintenance corticosteroids.[4] Initial studies with tacrolimus after cardiac transplantation suggest that tacrolimus is a safe and effective immunosuppressant alternative to cyclosporine. Oral doses of tacrolimus are typically 0.15 mg/kg twice daily. Doses are adjusted to achieve a goal trough blood level of 10 to 15 ng/dL for the first several months posttransplant and then 5 to 10 ng/dL long term. The most common side effects of tacrolimus are similar to those of cyclosporine, as shown in Table 56-3, with the exception of hirsutism and gingival hyperplasia, which have not been reported. Based on the mechanism by which tacrolimus is metabolized, drugs known to interact with cyclosporine and erythromycin should be considered potential interactants for tacrolimus until proven otherwise.

Azathioprine is a 6-mercaptopurine derivative that acts as a false metabolite in the proliferation of bone marrow stem cells. The typical dose is 1 to 2 mg/kg per day, adjusted to maintain a white blood cell count greater than 5000/mm^3. The most common side effect is bone marrow suppression manifest as neutropenia. In some patients, anemia and thrombocytopenia may be present. The most common drug interaction is with allopurinol, which may be prescribed to treat acute gouty arthritis, itself a side effect of cyclosporine therapy. If allopurinol is to be prescribed, the dose of azathioprine should be decreased by half and frequent follow-up white blood cell counts should be obtained to avoid profound bone marrow suppression.

Mycophenolate mofetil (MMF), another new immunosuppressant, is a potent inhibitor of de novo purine synthesis inhibiting T- and B-lymphocyte proliferation.[5] MMF has been approved by the Food and Drug Administration (FDA) for the prophylaxis of organ rejection in renal transplantation when used concomitantly with cyclosporine and prednisone. MMF is being promoted as an improvement over azathioprine, replacing it in the standard triple-drug immunosuppressive regimen. Clinical studies of MMF after cardiac transplantation suggest that it is a safe and effective alternative to azathioprine in maintenance immunotherapy and possibly more effective in the treatment of refractory and persistent rejection.[6] Dosing of MMF is typically 1.0 to 1.5 g twice daily. The most common side effects include diarrhea, vomiting, leukopenia, and an increase in opportunistic infections, especially involving cytomegalovirus (CMV), both tissue-invasive disease and viremia. Should neutropenia develop, the MMF dosage should be adjusted or the therapy discontinued. Drugs that interact with MMF include antacids and cholestyramine, which decrease absorption of MMF and therefore should not be taken at the same time.

Steroids remain an integral part of posttransplant immunosuppression. Prednisone is begun initially at high doses (1.0 to 1.5 mg/kg per day) posttransplant and weaned over 6 to 8 weeks to a maintenance dose of 0.2 mg/kg per day (about 15 mg/day in the average adult recipient). Many programs now attempt to wean patients off steroids in an effort to avoid the well-known deleterious effects of chronic steroid therapy. Steroid withdrawal is successful in approximately 50 percent of cases.

REJECTION

Rejection after cardiac transplantation is a lifelong risk, although the incidence of rejection decreases with time. Rejection can be divided into three types, based on mechanism of rejection and time after transplantation. *Hyperacute rejection* is mediated by preformed anti-HLA antibodies directed against the donor tissue. Hyperacute rejection results in immediate and irreversible donor heart failure and is a fatal complication unless the patient can be maintained with a mechanical assist device until a new donor heart is located. With the use of ABO blood group–compatible donors and screening of transplant candidates

TABLE 56-4 Standardized Cardiac Biopsy Grading System

Grade	Histologic Description
0	No rejection
1	A = focal (perivascular or interstitial) infiltrate without necrosis B = diffuse but sparse infiltrate without necrosis
2	One focus only with aggressive infiltration and/or focal myocyte damage
3	A = multifocal aggressive infiltrates and/or myocyte damage B = diffuse inflammatory process with necrosis
4	Diffuse aggressive polymorphous infiltrate ± edema, ± hemorrhage, ± vasculitis, with necrosis

for elevated levels of preformed anti-HLA antibodies, hyperacute rejection is very rare in cardiac transplantation.

Acute rejection, the most common type of rejection encountered, occurs in approximately 75 percent of all patients at some time after transplantation. The incidence of acute rejection is greatest within the first 6 weeks posttransplantation as immunosuppressive medications are weaned to chronic maintenance levels. Rejection can occur at any time after transplantation. Late episodes can usually be correlated with some change in the patient's immunosuppressive status, such as an acute illness or noncompliance with medications. Acute rejection is a cellular phenomenon resulting in the infiltration of lymphocytes into the myocardium, with subsequent destruction of individual myocytes. Because most episodes of rejection do not cause clinically detectable graft dysfunction, surveillance endomyocardial biopsies are performed on a routine basis after transplantation. Biopsy specimens are examined histologically and graded according to a grading system (Table 56-4) developed by a working group of the ISHLT.[7] Mild to moderate episodes of rejection (grades 0 to 2) are generally not accompanied by clinical symptoms or hemodynamic changes. Severe rejection (grade 4) can result in profound myocardial dysfunction and death. Patients with grade 2 or higher rejection are treated with augmented steroids or cytotoxic therapy, as outlined below.

Chronic rejection is believed to be manifested in the heart by the development of graft atherosclerosis. This antibody-mediated phenomenon is thought to result in injury to the endothelial lining of the coronary arteries, with the subsequent development of intimal hypertrophy. The lesions may be focal but are more often diffuse and concentric, involving the entire length of the epicardial and intramyocardial vessels. Because the heart is denervated, myocardial ischemia does not present with angina. Instead, recipients present with heart failure secondary to silent myocardial infarctions or with sudden death. Transplant recipients who present with new-onset shortness of breath, chest fullness, or symptoms of congestive heart failure should be evaluated for the presence of myocardial ischemia or infarction. This is done in routine fashion with ECG and serial cardiac enzymes. Echocardiography can be used to look for segmental wall motion abnormalities. If evidence for myocardial ischemia or infarction is found, cardiac catheterization with ventriculography and coronary angiography is indicated. The rate of development of graft coronary disease is quite variable, occurring months to years after transplantation; consequently, cardiac transplant programs employ annual follow-up coronary angiograms to detect its presence. The diffuse nature of graft coronary artery disease generally precludes standard methods of myocardial revascularization such as percutaneous transluminal coronary angioplasty, stent implantation, or coronary artery bypass surgery. Retransplantation is the most effective treatment.

Although most episodes of acute rejection are asymptomatic, symptoms can occur. The most common presenting symptoms are dysrhythmias and generalized fatigue. The development of either atrial or ventricular dysrhythmias in a cardiac transplant recipient must be assumed to be due to acute rejection until proven otherwise. Arrangements should be made for prompt performance of an endomyocardial biopsy. If patients are hemodynamically compromised by their dysrhythmias, empiric therapy for rejection with methylprednisolone (Solu-Medrol), 1 g IV, may be given. If the diagnosis of rejection is confirmed, standard antirejection therapy should be completed. Atrial dysrhythmias may respond to treatment with digoxin or calcium channel blockers. Ventricular dysrhythmias may respond to lidocaine or other class I-C agents. Frequently the dysrhythmias will be controlled only with antirejection therapy.

Untreated acute cardiac rejection results in progressive myocardial dysfunction. Diastolic dysfunction occurs first, followed by systolic dysfunction as the degree of myocardial damage increases. Diastolic dysfunction causes symptoms of congestive heart failure with shortness of breath, fatigue, and malaise. Progressive myocardial dysfunction results in low-output syndrome, with symptoms including nausea, vomiting, and/or diarrhea. Severe rejection leads to hypotension and circulatory collapse. Symptoms of rejection may be mistakenly attributed to a viral syndrome or gastroenteritis. Physical examination reveals signs of heart failure, including distended neck veins, an S_3 gallop on cardiac auscultation, rales on pulmonary auscultation, and occasionally the presence of ascites or peripheral edema. Chest x-rays show enlargement of the cardiac silhouette and pulmonary vascular congestion. ECGs may demonstrate—in addition to dysrhythmias—a decrease in amplitude and widening of the QRS complex.

Patients with signs or symptoms suggestive of acute rejection should be admitted to the hospital with continuous ECG monitoring. Arrangements should be made for performance of an endomyocardial biopsy at the earliest possible time. If facilities for obtaining and interpreting biopsy specimens are not available, transfer to the nearest transplant center should be arranged. Low-output syndrome and/or hypotension should be treated with inotropic agents such as dopamine or dobutamine while specific treatment for rejection is instituted. Treatment for rejection without biopsy confirmation is contraindicated except when the patient is hemodynamically unstable. This is especially true in patients whose symptoms are due to an occult infection because of the potential adverse consequences of high-dose steroid therapy. Empiric treatment for rejection should be employed only after consultation with the patient's transplant center.

Standard therapy for acute rejection includes intravenous methylprednisolone 1 g/day for 3 days. In patients with refractory rejection, treatment with specific T-cell cytotoxic agents such as OKT3, ALS, or ALG is required. Occasionally, patients have been successfully supported with mechanical assist devices for profound circulatory collapse while undergoing therapy for rejection, with resultant complete recovery of normal ventricular function.

INFECTIOUS COMPLICATIONS AFTER CARDIAC TRANSPLANTATION

Infectious complications are fairly common after transplantation, particularly in the early posttransplant period, when the highest doses of immunosuppressive medications are employed. The infectious complications after cardiac transplantation are similar to those following all types of solid-organ transplantation and those in other immunocompromised hosts.[8] The infections most commonly encountered are listed in Table 56-5. Prophylactic regimens are employed by most transplant centers. Pretransplantation, patients are vaccinated with pneumococcal, *Haemophilus influenzae,* and hepatitis B vaccines. Peri-operatively, routine antistaphylococcal antibiotics are used. Postoperatively, mycostatin mouthwash is used to prevent oral and esophageal candidiasis while the patients are on high-dose steroids and is reinstituted when augmented steroid therapy is required to treat rejection. *Toxoplasma gondii* can infect the transplanted heart; it may result from reactivation of a latent recipient infection or be transmitted with the

TABLE 56-5 Common Infections after Cardiac Transplantation

Early posttransplant infections (first month)
Pneumonia
Gram-negative bacilli
Mediastinitis
Staphylococcus epidermidis
Staphylococcus aureus
Gram-negative bacilli
Intravenous lines
Staphylococcus epidermidis
S. aureus
Gram-negative bacilli
Candida albicans
Urinary tract infections
Gram-negative bacilli
Enterococcus
C. albicans
Skin
Herpes simplex virus
Late posttransplant infections (after first month) and for duration of immunosuppression
Viral
Cytomegalovirus (CMV)
Herpes simplex
Varicella zoster
Non-A, non-B hepatitis
Bacteria
Listeria
Nocardia
Legionella
Mycobacterium
Fungi
Aspergillus
Cryptococcus
Candida
Mucor (Phycomyces)
Protozoa
Pneumocystis carinii
Toxoplasma gondii

Source: Horn JE, Barlett JG: Infectious complications following heart transplantation, in Baumgartner WA, Reitz BA, Achuff SC, (eds): *Heart and Heart-Lung Transplantation.* Philadelphia: Saunders, 1990, p 223.

donor organ. *Toxoplasma* titers are measured in all recipients and donors, and pyrimethamine is administered prophylactically for 6 weeks posttransplantation if titers are elevated. Beginning approximately 2 months posttransplantation, trimethoprim/sulfamethoxazole (Septra, Bactrim) is used as prophylaxis against *Pneumocystis carinii* pneumonia (PCP). Antibiotic prophylaxis for any invasive procedure (e.g., dental work, endoscopy, or surgical procedures) is recommended for the lifetime of the patient. Annual flu shots are recommended. Live attenuated virus vaccines such as those for measles, mumps, and rubella are contraindicated in transplant recipients.

Any patient with a history of solid-organ transplantation who presents with symptoms of an infection must be evaluated in an aggressive and thorough manner. Appropriate stains and cultures should be obtained to allow identification of bacterial, fungal, and viral pathogens. There should be a low threshold for instituting antimicrobial therapy while awaiting culture results and for admitting patients to the hospital for further evaluation and intravenous antibiotics. Patients with evidence of pulmonary infiltrates but without productive sputum require bronchoscopy with bronchoalveolar lavage and transbronchial biopsy for definitive diagnosis. Pulmonary infections that are frequently encountered include *P. carinii, Nocardia, Legionella pneumophilia,* and *Aspergillus;* these require special stains and studies for accurate diagnosis. Patients with gastroenteritis and nausea, vomiting, and/or diarrhea require special attention. Inability to ingest or adequately absorb immunosuppressive medications may result in the development of an episode of rejection. If there is any question about a recipient's ability to maintain adequate oral intake, the patient should be hospitalized and immunosuppressive medications be administered intravenously.

Antibiotic therapy for documented infections should be guided by appropriate culture and sensitivities and must take into account underlying renal insufficiency and potential interactions with cyclosporine or tacrolimus.

Of special note is the risk of CMV infection after cardiac transplantation. CMV is a common virus to which the majority of adults have been exposed, as demonstrated by the presence of anti-CMV IgG antibodies in the serum. Posttransplantation, CMV infections can occur due either to the reactivation of latent virus in a previously infected recipient or the development of a new infection with a different viral strain transmitted with the donor organ. The latter situation is much more serious and potentially life-threatening, particularly in recipients who were CMV-negative prior to transplantation. Routine posttransplant surveillance for CMV infection is performed utilizing serial IgG and IgM antibody testing and throat, urine, and serum buffy coat cultures. The recent development of CMV antigenemia assays has enhanced the early detection of CMV infection. CMV disease can occur in either a mild or severe form. Mild disease is manifested by a flulike illness with low-grade fever, fatigue, malaise, and nausea. Severe disease may include profound leukopenia; pneumonitis; gastroenteritis including epigastric pain, vomiting, and diarrhea; and hepatitis with elevated transaminases. CMV pneumonitis carries a mortality of greater than 50 percent. CMV infection typically occurs 4 to 12 weeks posttransplantation. The diagnosis is made by the demonstration of cytoplasmic inclusion bodies in biopsy specimens of affected organs. Treatment includes the use of intravenous ganciclovir and, in severe cases, intravenous immunoglobulin infusions. Of particular concern is the documented increased incidence of acute rejection complicating acute CMV infections. Therefore, patients with active CMV disease must be monitored carefully for signs and symptoms of rejection. An endomyocardial biopsy should be performed if there is any suspicion of rejection.

NONINFECTIOUS COMPLICATIONS OF CARDIAC TRANSPLANTATION

In addition to common forms of cancer, those malignancies associated with chronic immunosuppression also occur in cardiac transplant recipients. These include posttransplant lymphoproliferative disorders (PTLDs), which are usually B-cell lymphomas and have been related to the Epstein-Barr virus. PTLDs may occur as early as 1 month posttransplantation and may present with a variety of nonspecific symptoms. If diagnosed in their early stages, they may respond to decreased levels of immunosuppression, chemotherapy, and/or radiation therapy, with long-term survival reported.

Aseptic necrosis of the femoral heads and thoracic and lumbar spine compression fractures are not uncommon manifestations of long-term steroid therapy. The development of hip pain referred to the medial thigh or knee is often indicative of early aseptic necrosis. Magnetic resonance imaging (MRI) is the most sensitive means of detection, and patients should be referred for orthopedic evaluation if this diagnosis is suspected.

PEDIATRIC CARDIAC TRANSPLANTATION

The care and evaluation of pediatric heart transplant recipients is similar to that of adults, with a few special considerations. Rejection surveillance in infants and small children is done primarily with serial echocardiograms. Difficulties with vascular access and the need for anesthesia make serial endomyocardial biopsy procedures impractical.

Acute rejection is more frequently heralded by symptoms in children than in adults. Children will present with a low-grade fever, fussiness, and poor feeding. Echocardiography will demonstrate decreased ventricular contractility, thickening of the posterior wall of the left ventricle, cardiac enlargement, and mitral and tricuspid valve insufficiency. Because the signs of rejection may be subtle and difficult to quantify, serial echocardiographic studies are required throughout the postoperative period in order to establish each patient's baseline echocardiographic characteristics.

Immunosuppression for children is based on standard triple therapy. Because of the more rapid metabolism of cyclosporine and tacrolimus, higher doses and more frequent (thrice daily) dosing is often needed in children. Steroids are withdrawn whenever possible to avoid their deleterious effects on somatic growth.

Childhood infections are frequently encountered and should be treated according to routine practice. Vaccinations with live attenuated virus are avoided. Exposure to chickenpox (varicella) is avoided if possible. If exposure does occur in a recipient without a history of previous infection, treatment with varicellazoster immune globulin (VZIG) is indicated. Recipients who develop chickenpox are treated with intravenous acyclovir (Zovirax).

EMERGENCY DEPARTMENT EVALUATION AND TREATMENT OF THE POSTTRANSPLANT PATIENT

Cardiac transplant recipients are susceptible to all of the acute illnesses that affect the general population. These patients should be treated in the same way as any other acutely ill or traumatized patient. In the assessment of such patients, however, the possibility that symptoms may be due to rejection, infection, or side effects of their immunosuppressive medications must always be considered. Patients on chronic steroids will have adrenal suppression and may need stress coverage if they are severely ill or in need of surgical intervention. Uninterrupted administration of immunosuppressive medications must be assured to avoid the development of acute rejection. Nonsteroidal anti-inflammatory drugs (NSAIDs) should be used with extreme caution because of the potential exacerbation of underlying renal insufficiency secondary to cyclosporine or tacrolimus use.

The evaluation of patients presenting with signs and symptoms of congestive heart failure must include the consideration of rejection, myocardial ischemia, and fluid overload due to renal insufficiency. Echocardiography provides important information regarding cardiac performance and may demonstrate findings suggestive of rejection (global dysfunction) or ischemic dysfunction (segmental wall motion abnormality). Results of routine annual cardiac evaluations are useful in assessing whether echocardiographic abnormalities represent acute changes or chronic conditions. Similarly, the availability of old laboratory test results will aid in assessing the importance and acuity of renal impairment.

Any transplant patient presenting with an acute febrile illness warrants aggressive and complete evaluation. If a specific diagnosis cannot be established by history, physical examination, and readily available laboratory and radiographic tests in the ED, consultation with the infectious disease service is indicated. The patient should be admitted to the hospital for further invasive tests and broad-spectrum intravenous antibiotics until culture results are available and a specific diagnosis is made.

In the event that a transplant recipient presents to the ED in extremis, standard cardiopulmonary resuscitation should be performed. Etiologies for hemodynamic collapse related to the posttransplant state include severe acute rejection and myocardial ischemia due to advanced graft coronary disease. Sudden death due to an dysrhythmia may also result from rejection or ischemia. Because of sympathetic denervation, vagally induced bradycardias do not occur; therefore atropine has no role in the resuscitation of these patients. The empiric administration of high-dose steroids (methylprednisolone 1 g intravenously) may be beneficial if rejection is present. Finally, hyperkalemia due to chronic renal insufficiency may result in acute dysrhythmias and should be corrected with standard pharmacologic intervention.

REFERENCES

1. Hosenpud JD, Bennett LE, Keck BM, et al: The Registry of the International Society for Heart and Lung Transplantation: Fifteenth Official Report—1998. *J Heart Lung Transplant* 17:656, 1998.
2. UNOS: *United Network for Organ Sharing (UNOS) Update,* special edition. Richmond, VA: UNOS, Spring 1998, p 28.
3. Farrell TG, Camm AJ: Action of drugs in the denervated heart. *Semin Thorac Cardiovasc Surg* 2:279, 1990.
4. Kelly PA, Burckart GJ, Venkatarmanan R: Tacrolimus: A new immunosuppressive agent. *Am J Health Syst Pharm* 52:1521, 1995.
5. Hood KA, Zarembski DG: Mycophenolate mofetil: A unique immunosuppressive agent. *Am J Health Syst Pharm* 54:285, 1997.
6. Kirklin JK, Bourge RC, Naftel DC, et al: Treatment of recurrent heart rejection with mycophenolate mofetil (RS-61443): Initial clinical experience. *J Heart Lung Transplant* 13:444, 1994.
7. Billingham ME, Cary NRB, Hammond ME, et al: A working formulation for the standardization of nomenclature in the diagnosis of heart and lung rejection: Heart Rejection Study Group. *J Heart Transplant* 9:587, 1990.
8. Baumgartner WA, Reitz BA, Achuff SC (eds): *Heart and Heart-Lung Transplantation.* Philadelphia: Saunders, 1990.

57 NONINVASIVE MYOCARDIAL IMAGING

David A. Bluemke
Bennett Chin
João A. C. Lima

Diagnostic imaging tests for imaging myocardial disease have grown substantially in sophistication. Recent developments include new scintigraphic diagnostic contrast agents in nuclear medicine, Doppler methods in echocardiography, and rapid magnetic resonance imaging (MRI) of the heart. Since the cost of these diagnostic tests is relatively high, it is essential that the ''correct'' test be selected. Such a test will lead to the most accurate diagnosis in a short period, with few false positives or negatives. This chapter reviews diagnostic modalities for myocardial imaging, with specific emphasis on basic principles of the techniques. Following this discussion, the use of imaging modalities in an array of cardiovascular disorders is presented.

CHEST X-RAY

The chest x-ray is often the first imaging test obtained for patients with suspected cardiovascular disease. Ideally, lateral and posteroanterior (PA) views of the chest are obtained, with film exposure at a distance of 6 ft (1.8 m). Patients should be upright and have a moderately deep inspiration. For patients who are too ill to stand, semierect x-rays are obtained with an anteroposterior (AP) film exposure. The AP film has two disadvantages: the heart demonstrates magnification, and the pulmonary vessels, which show information regarding the extent of congestive failure, are somewhat blurred because of longer exposure times.

Cardiac size can be measured from the chest x-ray with an error of $\pm$ 10 percent. Unfortunately, borderline cases require accurate measurements, and factors such as depth of inspiration, conformation of the chest wall, and pulmonary diseases all may affect the apparent heart size on a chest x-ray. The cardiothoracic ratio is the ratio between the transverse diameter of the heart on a PA chest x-ray and the greatest internal diameter of the thorax. Although there are other formulas for measuring cardiac size, this method is the quickest and easiest. The normal adult heart measures 50 percent or less of the transverse diameter of the chest. Cardiothoracic ratios greater than 50 percent are considered to be cardiomegaly. In children, the normal cardiothoracic ratio is 65 percent in the first year, decreasing to 50 percent by age 5.

On the chest x-ray, the heart and major vessels are visualized in the middle mediastinum and are readily recognized. The heart as well as the great vessels all appear to have the same density, relative to the radiolucent lungs. On the left side, there is usually air around the cardiac border, but, on the right side, the heart blends in with the density of the liver. In normal individuals, two-thirds of the heart lies to the left of the midline.

Chest X-ray Interpretation

On the PA view of the chest, there are three visible cardiac segments (Fig. 57-1a). The lowermost segment, adjacent to the diaphragm, is the lateral and apical walls of the left ventricle. A small rounded density may be lateral to the cardiac apex; this represents the epicardial fat pad. Superior to the left ventricle is a rounded short segment that varies considerably in size. This is the pulmonary artery and its left main branch. Prominence of the pulmonary artery is normal in young women. Just below this level, the left atrial appendage forms a short portion of the lateral portion of the left heart border. Conditions that result in left atrial enlargement will cause a convex bulge in this portion of the cardiac silhouette. The third and most superior portion of the left edge of the cardiac silhouette is formed by the transverse aortic arch. On a properly exposed chest film, the descending aorta can be seen descending behind the heart shadow. Regarding the right side of the cardiovascular silhouette, the lower rounded portion is due to the lateral border of the right atrium. The upper segment is formed by the superior vena cava. In older adults in whom the ascending aorta becomes more rounded and dilated, the upper segment of the right heart border may become convex, representing the lateral border of the ascending aorta.

On the lateral view of the chest, the anterior and superiormost shadow of the cardiac silhouette is formed first by the ascending aorta, and then the pulmonary artery and the pulmonary artery outflow tract, and then the anterior border of the right ventricle (Fig. 57-1b). Posteriorly, the superior shadow is due to the left atrium, with the left ventricle forming the cardiac silhouette inferiorly.

Early left ventricular failure is reflected on the chest x-ray by a ''redistribution'' pattern of blood flow. Normally, the most prominent pulmonary veins are at the lung bases. With the redistribution phase, the vascularity in the upper lung fields is increased, relative to that of the lower lung fields.

As pulmonary capillary wedge pressure elevates to 20 to 25 mmHg (Fig. 57-2), fluid moves from the vascular bed into the interstitial spaces of the lung. The chest x-ray appears hazy at this stage, with short lines appearing perpendicular to the pleura (Kerley B lines). Finally, as pulmonary capillary wedge pressure further increases to 30 to 35 mmHg, frank alveolar edema ensues due to massive fluid movement from the vasculature to the alveolar spaces.

CARDIAC CHAMBER ENLARGEMENT **Left Ventricle** Increased workload by the left ventricle initially results in dilatation of the ventricle, but if it is sustained, hypertrophy of the left ventricular wall occurs. Hypertrophy is a normal response to increased workload. Chest x-ray findings at this time are usually normal. As the ventricle begins to fail, dilatation results, and the cardiothoracic ratio increases. The apex of the heart also becomes more rounded in appearance. The most marked increases in size of the left ventricle result from hypertension, aortic insufficiency, and cardiomyopathy. Pericardial effusion results in generalized cardiac enlargement (Fig. 57-3).

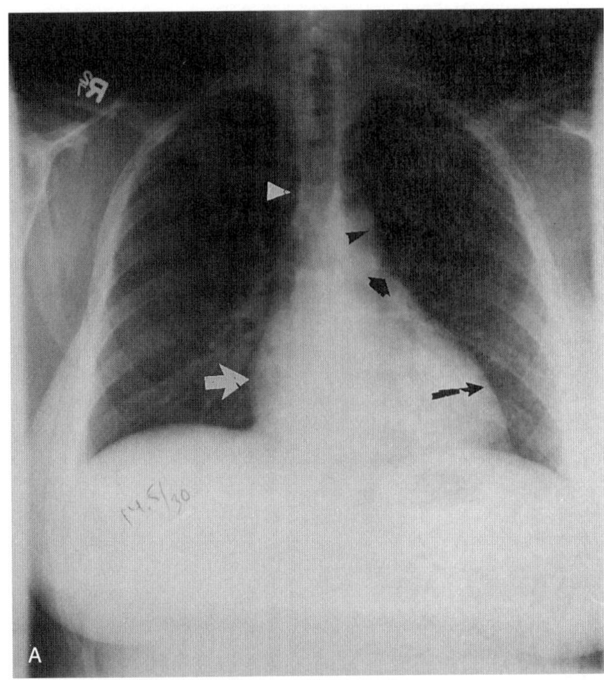

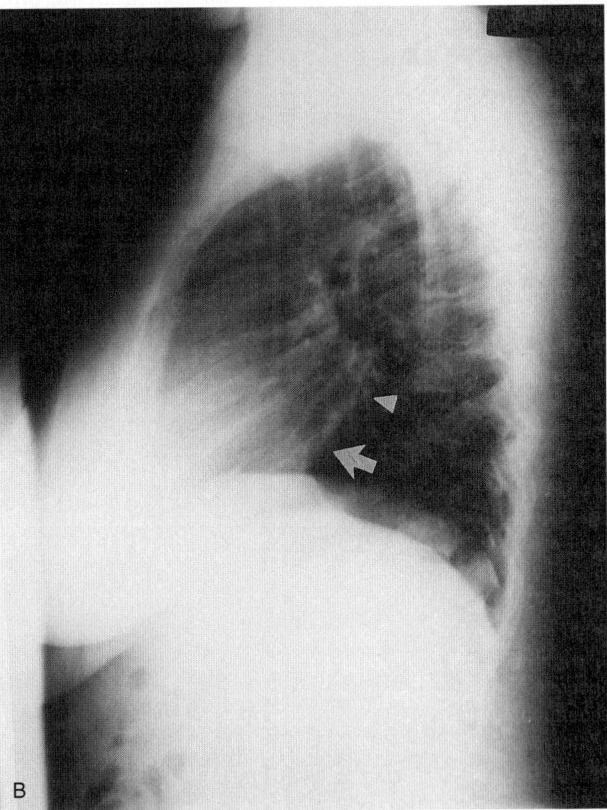

FIG. 57-1. Normal cardiac size and lung fields. **A.** Frontal view. The lateral wall of the left ventricle (*large black arrow*), the pulmonary artery (*small black arrow*), and the aortic arch (*black arrowhead*) form three visible cardiac segments on the left side. On the right side, the right atrium (*white arrow*) and superior vena cava (*white arrowhead*) form lower and upper borders, respectively. **B.** Lateral view. The left ventricle (*arrow*) forms the lower posterior cardiac border, and the left atrium is superior to this (*arrowhead*).

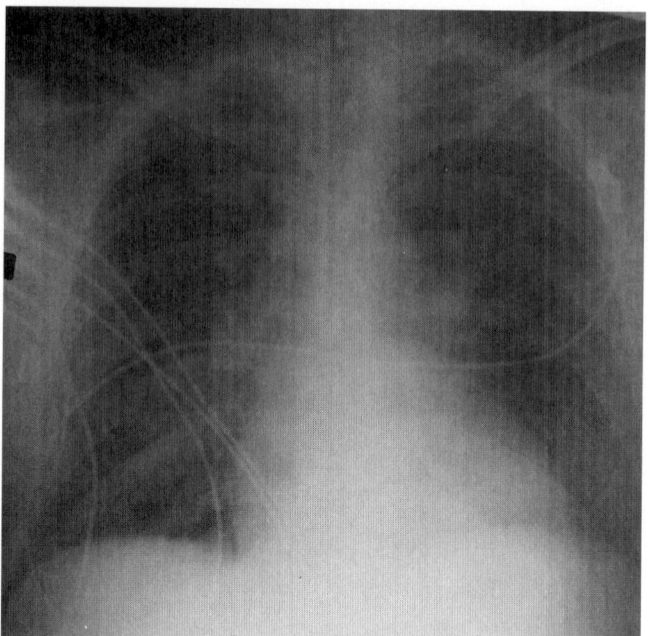

FIG. 57-2. Pulmonary vascular congestion. Bilateral increased lung markings are present, particularly in the lower lung fields, with prominent interstitial lung markings. The pulmonary hila are also enlarged.

Right Ventricle The right ventricle enlarges from processes that increase the work of this chamber, such as pulmonary diseases or pulmonary artery hypertension. Mitral valve disease will also eventually result in right ventricle enlargement. The outflow tract of the right ventricle enlarges first; chest x-ray findings are subtle but include straightening or convexity of the pulmonary artery segment below the aortic knob in the frontal view. Multichamber enlargement is frequent, so that the relative involvement of each cardiac chamber is not easily distinguished on chest x-ray.

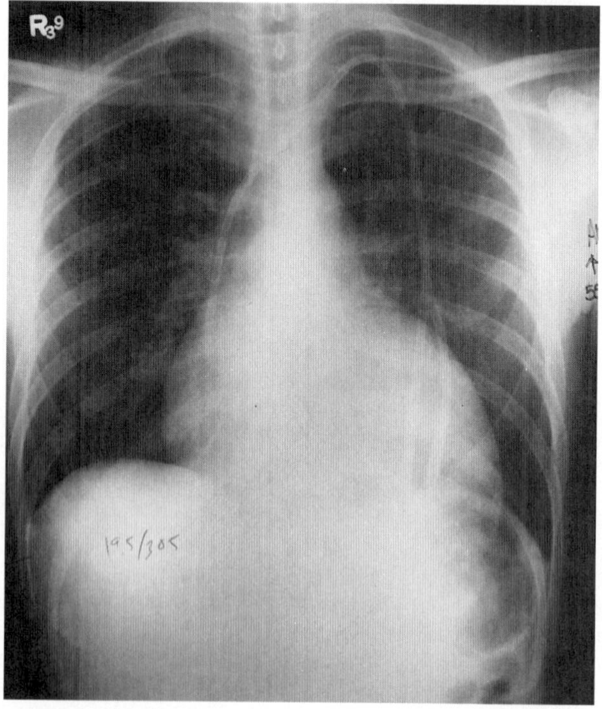

FIG. 57-3. Pericardial effusion. Generalized dilatation of the heart is present, with the cardiothoracic ratio measuring more than 50 percent. Although a similar cardiac silhouette would be present in patients with dilated cardiomyopathy, this patient had documented pericardial effusion.

Left Atrium Common cases of left atrial enlargement include mitral valve disease from rheumatic fever, or congenital defects resulting in left-to-right shunts. The normal left atrium is posterior and does not form any portion of the cardiac silhouette in a normal patient. Moderate enlargement causes the left atrial appendage to become larger and causes a bulge or straightening of the left cardiac border below the pulmonary artery segment. Further enlargement may cause the right-sided border of the left atrium to extend beyond the normal upper aspect of the right atrium and superior vena cava. A double cardiac border is seen on the frontal view on the right side. If the left atrial enlargement is less extreme, a double border may still be seen because of the increased radiodensity of the left atrium. On the lateral view, the upper posterior border of the cardiac silhouette projects more posteriorly than normal.

Right Atrium Enlargement of the right atrium causes enlargement of the lower right cardiac contour with increased convexity. Diseases resulting in right atrial enlargement include atrial septal defect, tricuspid stenosis and insufficiency, and right ventricular failure. In multichamber disease, right atrial enlargement is not separately identified.

COMPUTED TOMOGRAPHY

In evaluation of the heart, the primary role of conventional computed tomography (CT) has been to exclude other abnormalities, such as aortic dissection, that may secondarily affect cardiac function. Because of excellent anatomic resolution, CT is also useful in depicting paracardiac disease processes that involve the myocardium.

Advantages of CT examination of myocardial structures include good resolution of 0.1 to 0.5 mm^2 and rapid imaging times of 5 min or less for the chest. The low-density epicardial fat usually provides excellent contrast to the higher density of the cardiac structures. Calcifications, present at the site of ventricular aneurysms, of the coronary arteries or of atherosclerotic change, are easily depicted. With the advent of helical CT scanners, a full three-dimensional (3D) set of images is obtained, allowing multiplanar reconstruction and 3D viewing. Although conventional CT scanners provide only one image slice each 2 to 5 s, helical CT is increasingly available to emergency departments (EDs). Helical CT and spiral CT are synonyms for the same rapid mode of CT scanning, and are described in more detail below.

Helical Computed Tomography

In conventional (nonhelical) CT scanning, the image acquisition is as follows: scan a slice, move the patient, scan a slice, etc. Thus, there are two distinct parts to the process: turn on the x-ray beam, usually for only about 1 to 2 s, and then move the patient to the next table position. Patient motion to the next position may take an additional 2 to 4 s. Therefore, each slice can take approximately 5 s (1-s scan and 4 s of motion), of which only 20 percent (1 s/5 s) is actually imaging time.

In its most basic form, helical CT consists of scanning a patient *continuously* while the patient is being continuously moved through the CT gantry. In this mode, the x-ray beam is on for perhaps 20 s or more, and the patient is moved for this same duration. The efficiency of scanning is 100 percent. During the scanning process, the x-ray beam source is continuously rotating around the patient, tracing a helical, or a helix, along the patient's body. Implementing this is actually quite demanding of the CT scanner, its computer, and the electronic components. For this reason, helical CT remains a relatively new and developing technology.

Helical CT data sets are truly 3D. Instead of scanning a series of *slices,* a *volume* data set is acquired. This results in

- Vastly improved multiplanar and 3D reconstructions. Since data sets are acquired in a breath hold, respiratory misregistration is eliminated. Data appear "smoother" with fewer "stair-step" artifacts in sagittal and coronal reconstructions.
- Reconstruction of slices at arbitrary intervals. Because of the 3D nature of helical scanning, images can be reconstructed at small intervals, e.g., 2 to 3 mm. This reduces stair-step artifacts in 3D reconstructions.
- Rapid acquisition. Complete helical data sets of a patient's examination are typically acquired within 20 to 30 s, and the patient is then done with the examination.

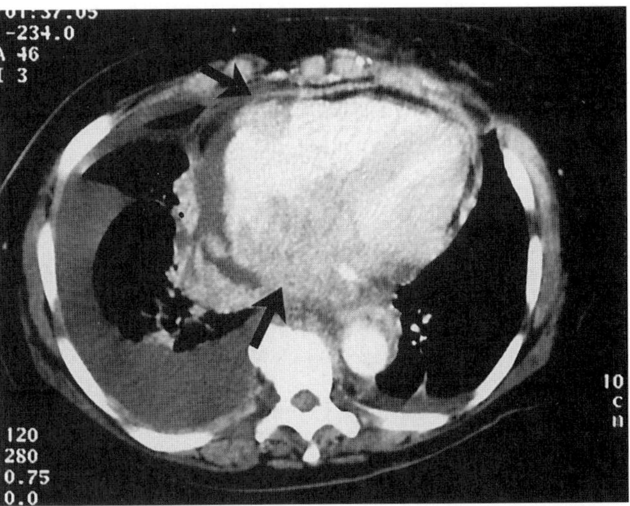

FIG. 57-4. High-grade malignant neoplasm. Helical computed tomographic scan demonstrates right pleural effusion, pericardial effusion, and thickening of the septum and left atrium (*arrows*). (Reprinted from Bluemke and Boxerman,[19] with permission.)

Electron-Beam Computed Tomography

Electron-beam CT technology (Imatron, South San Francisco, CA) operates by a different technology from helical and conventional CT. With those methods, a large detector array and x-ray unit rotate around the patient. The sheer mass of the x-ray apparatus limits the rate of rotation to about once every 0.75 to 1.0 s. With electron-beam CT, electrons are generated and deflected electromagnetically onto tungsten target rings located in the gantry below the patient. X-rays are generated by the electron bombardment of the target rings. The x-rays are then tightly collimated and directed to pass through the patient onto a double ring of detectors in the gantry above the patient. Since mechanical motion is not involved, imaging times are very rapid: images can be acquired every 58 ms (17 images per second). Similar to helical CT, image resolution is excellent: 0.1 to 0.5 mm^2. At this time rate of image formation, very little blurring of cardiac structures takes place. Calcifications involving the coronary arteries are easily detected, and cine images of the myocardium are available.

Electron-beam CT and helical CT require injection of an iodinated contrast medium to enhance blood in the vessels and myocardial cavities relative to the myocardium itself. With helical CT, approximately 120 mL of iodinated contrast is delivered intravenously at a rate of 3 mL/s. Using electron-beam CT, 40 to 80 mL of contrast is given at 2 to 10 mL/s. In both cases, a power injector is used, necessitating large-bore intravenous access.

Radiation exposure is a consideration with all CT scanning methods. With conventional or helical CT, radiation levels are 2 to 4 cGy (2 to 4 rad) per CT slice. If multiple slices are taken at the same level of the heart, then the radiation increases directly in proportion to the number of slices. Electron-beam CT has less exposure to radiation for the patient: each slice has an exposure of 0.54 cGy (540 mrad). However, more imaging slices are acquired with electron-beam CT in obtaining a cine sequence of the heart, so that 10 cine frames would result in an exposure of 5.4 rad. For comparison purposes, a single x-ray of the lumbar spine is approximately equivalent to 1 cGy (1 rad), whereas radiation exposure from a chest x-ray is 0.06 cGy (60 mrad).

Applications

Electron-beam CT is available at only a very few centers across the United States. A major nonemergent application is the detection of coronary artery calcification. The degree of coronary artery calcification bears a strong relationship to the presence of significant coronary artery stenosis. Cardiac anatomy, the relationship between chambers of the heart and great vessels, is readily determined using this modality. Since electron-beam CT can obtain cine images of the heart, cardiac function and focal wall motion abnormalities can be determined. Due to the limited availability of this modality, however, the remaining discussion will focus on non-electron-beam methods.

Although helical CT offers very rapid scanning, it is unable to assess cardiac function, since cine loops of the heart are not obtained. Cardiac anatomy, however, is well assessed. Focal abnormalities of the myocardial wall are indicative of cardiac tumor or thrombus (Fig. 57-4). Differentiation of these possibilities usually requires cine imaging, so that patients with such masses are referred for echocardiography or MRI.

CT offers a good depiction of pericardial disease (Fig. 57-5). Simple pericardial effusions show low density relative to the myocardium, and the extent of effusion can be readily quantified, if necessary. The presence of calcifications of the pericardium is an important factor in the diagnosis of constrictive pericarditis and, with the correct symptoms, improves the specificity of this diagnosis. High-density pericardial fluid collections are likely to represent localized hematomas, either from trauma or surgery.

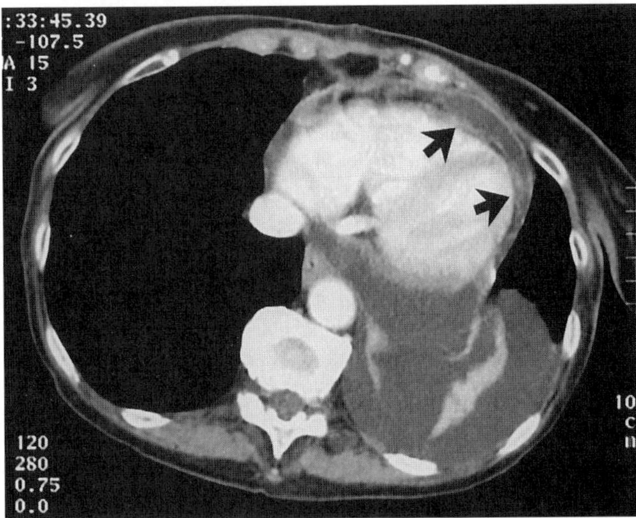

FIG. 57-5. Computed tomographic scan after intravenous contrast administration shows pericardial effusion and enhancement (*arrows*) due to pericarditis, with left pleural effusion and left lower lobe atelectasis. (Reprinted from Bluemke and Boxerman,[19] with permission.)

Helical CT following intravenous administration of contrast is an excellent modality for assessing diseases of the pulmonary arteries. Pulmonary artery emboli appear as low-attenuation defects in the opacified pulmonary arteries. Helical CT can demonstrate emboli not only in the main pulmonary arteries but also in the third- and fourth-order branches, because of high spatial resolution and cross-sectional imaging of these vessels.

NUCLEAR MEDICINE

Nuclear medicine examinations of the heart represent the study of cardiac function and physiology, rather than anatomy. Because of higher spatial resolution, MRI and CT are better suited to anatomic evaluation of the heart. Nevertheless, nuclear medicine examinations of the heart still remain a primary means for assessing cardiovascular function and, in particular, gated radionuclide angiography of the heart is a mainstay of cardiovascular imaging.

Radiopharmaceuticals and Imaging Techniques

ASSESSMENT OF CARDIAC PERFUSION **Thallium-201** Thallium is a potassium analogue that is transported by the Na^+,K^+-ATPase system in cells, in direct proportion to regional blood flow. Approximately 85 percent of each ''pass'' of the contrast agent is extracted from the blood across the capillary bed. Thallium is initially extracted by myocardial cells but then redistributes to maintain an equilibrium with the blood at a rate that is proportional to regional blood flow. Thus, the early images from a thallium scan reflect blood flow, and the later images (redistribution phase) reflect the intracellular K^+ blood pool. The intracellular K^+ blood pool in turn is reflective of cellular viability. The redistribution phase is usually imaged at from 4 to 24 h after the initial injection of thallium.

In combination with exercise or pharmacologically induced coronary hyperemia (from dipyridamole or adenosine), thallium imaging is able to distinguish normal blood flow, ischemia, infarction, and hibernating myocardium. Myocardial tissues distal to a physiologic coronary artery stenosis are unable to increase their blood supply during stress conditions or hyperemia and thus have low radiotracer activity. On 4-h-delayed images, however, the thallium redistributes to these arrows and the radiotracer activity of the myocardium becomes more uniform. With infarction, delayed images show no evidence of radiotracer redistribution, reflecting the lack of intracellular K^+ blood in the area of infarction. With hibernating myocardium, redistribution occurs by 24 h.

Technetium Technetium radionuclides offer greater ease of use and availability for nuclear medicine departments. Whereas thallium requires a cyclotron to produce, technetium agents are widely available and produced by a generator in each nuclear medicine laboratory. The most commonly used technetium agent is technetium-99m sestamibi (^{99m}Tc-sestamibi). This agent is taken up by the myocardium in direct proportion to myocardial blood flow. At this point, the sestamibi molecule becomes trapped within the myocardium and does not redistribute (contrary to the behavior of thallium). Thus, the initial uptake by the myocardium reflects blood flow at the time of injection. Typically, ^{99m}Tc-sestamibi is initially injected at peak exercise, or during the period of maximum coronary vasodilatation (induced by dipyridamole or adenosine).

Since ^{99m}Tc-sestamibi does not redistribute on delayed images, myocardial infarction and decreased flow from physiologically significant coronary stenosis both appear as myocardial defects on images. To differentiate these two possibilities, a second dose of ^{99m}Tc-sestamibi is given while the patient is at rest. If the rest images show uniform radiotracer distribution, then the defect seen on stress images is due to ischemia. Persistent areas of absent radiotracer on rest images indicate areas of myocardial infarction.

GATED RADIONUCLIDE ANGIOGRAPHY Gated radionuclide angiography (RNA) has remained a clinical gold standard for overall assessment of left ventricular function. This test has the advantage of being applicable to nearly all patients, regardless of body habitus or underlying illness. In addition, unlike echocardiography, RNA is relatively operator independent. Radiation exposure is present but insufficient to prevent serial examination of cardiac function in the same patient.

In RNA, a blood sample is labeled with a technetium-based radionuclide, and a series of images of the heart is acquired. These images are gated to the R wave of the electrocardiogram. Function, and measurement of ejection fraction, involve measuring radioactivity counts at multiple time points throughout the cardiac cycle. The number of radioactive counts is directly proportional to the blood volume in the cardiac chamber. Thus, the method is insensitive to the precise geometry of the left ventricle, since only the overall count rates, and thus volumes, are measured. Other than segmentation of the left ventricle from other cardiac cavities, no geometric assumptions regarding left ventricular anatomy are necessary with the technique. Using gated techniques, with display of images as a cine loop, it is possible to assess segmental function of the heart. However, the resolution of the images is limited, and the strength of the examination relies primarily in accurate quantitation of the global left ventricular function.

Ventricular function is assessed by qualitative evaluation of cardiac wall motion, and quantitative assessment of radionuclide counts as a function of time. Computer-generated curves are verified by an experienced observer's interpretation of regional wall motion determined by gated RNA studies. RNA allows particularly good views of the lateral wall of the left ventricle, where there is no overlap from other cardiac segments. Although systolic function is easily assessed, diastolic function of the left ventricle is more commonly performed by echocardiography.

FIRST-PASS CARDIAC STUDIES If the radionuclide is rapidly injected, and the acquisition speed of the nuclear images is rapid, the ''first pass'' of the radionuclide can be tracked, as it passes through the heart. This method relies on tracking of the radionuclide bolus as it passes through the ventricular cavities immediately following contrast injection. In this technique, the acquisition time is very rapid (30 s), although very few heartbeats are evaluated, thus limiting spatial resolution.

Left ventricular ejection fraction measurement is determined by following the passage of the radiotracer between the left and right ventricles. The injection of the radiotracer must be rapid, or poor separation of radiotracer between the two sides of the heart occurs. Patients with dysrhythmias, atrial septal defect, or significant regurgitation across the mitral or tricuspid valves will have poor ejection fraction estimates using this method. First-pass studies using ^{99m}Tc-sestamibi enable cardiac function as well as perfusion to be assessed in the same study.

GATED PERFUSION IMAGING Following injection of ^{99m}Tc-sestamibi, images can be collected such that multiple time points, or cine frames, during the cardiac cycle can be independently collected by gating data acquisition to the cardiac cycle. In this manner, a cine loop, or movie of the cardiac cycle, can be generated. The function of the heart can be qualitatively reviewed to assess for wall thickening or segmental dysfunction. Thus, the perfusion of the heart can be assessed in the same setting as cardiac function. Functional imaging aids in discriminating between true mild perfusion defects and imaging artifact, such as due to attenuation from overlying breast tissue or the diaphragm. When severe perfusion defects are present, due to infarct or significant coronary artery narrowing, accurate estimation of ejection fraction is difficult to measure.

Applications

Myocardial perfusion scintigraphy is a noninvasive modality with high sensitivity for the diagnosis and evaluation of coronary artery disease. Physiologically significant coronary stenoses may be evaluated in populations with known or suspected coronary disease, after therapeutic interventions, preoperatively for risk assessment, and for prognostication after acute ischemia or infarction.

A more recent application of this technique has been made to the patients presenting to the ED with chest pain. In a subset of patients with an intermediate or low probability of coronary artery disease and chest pain (unstable angina), the missed diagnosis of coronary artery disease has been reported as high as 5 to 8 percent.[1-3] As many as a third of patients with acute myocardial infarction do not have electrocardiographic (ECG) changes suggestive or diagnostic of ischemia, many of which have baseline ECG abnormalities.

Several centers around the country have used myocardial perfusion scintigraphy to further classify this subset into high-risk and low-risk categories to reduce the incidence of missed acute ischemic coronary syndromes and the number of unnecessary hospital admissions for noncardiac chest pain. In a large study at the Medical College of Virginia involving 1187 patients, ^{99m}Tc-sestamibi perfusion imaging was used in defining the critical pathways in this population.[4] Used with established clinical criteria, the cardiac event rate at 1-year follow-up for patients with abnormal scan findings was 42 percent versus 3 percent (revascularization) for those with a normal scan findings. In those with abnormal scan findings, 11 percent experienced myocardial infarction and 8 percent suffered cardiac death; in those with normal scan findings, none had myocardial infarction or death. Other centers around the country are reporting similarly favorable results.[5,6]

The nuclear perfusion imaging protocol performed in the ED is very similar to conventional myocardial perfusion stress protocols with the exception that the injections are performed at rest during chest pain. Preliminary reports indicate that timing of injection during chest pain may improve diagnostic sensitivity; however, other centers have reported good results with injections performed up to within 12 h of the chest pain.[7] ^{99m}Tc-sestamibi or tetrofosmin are used because of their favorable imaging properties of minimal redistribution and lower radiation dosimetry compared with ^{201}Tl chloride. After intravenous injection, these ^{99m}Tc tracers are highly extracted and retained for several hours within the myocardium in a distribution proportional to coronary blood flow. This permits imaging several hours later after additional ED evaluation or intervention. Because of the more favorable dosimetry of ^{99m}Tc tracers, a higher dosage approaching 7 to 10 times the injected dose of ^{201}Tl is typically used. This permits high-quality tomographic imaging (single-photon emission computed tomograpy or SPECT) and ECG gating, which provides additional information, including assessment of wall motion, wall thickening, and left ventricular ejection fraction. In patients with a normal findings on resting perfusion study, further evaluation with a stress myocardial perfusion study may be performed with them as outpatients. Preliminary studies have shown the cost effectiveness of this risk stratification, and further studies are currently in progress. Figures 57-6, 57-7 (Plate 7), and 57-8 (Plate 8) illustrate the utility of myocardial perfusion scintigraphy in a patient with acute chest pain.

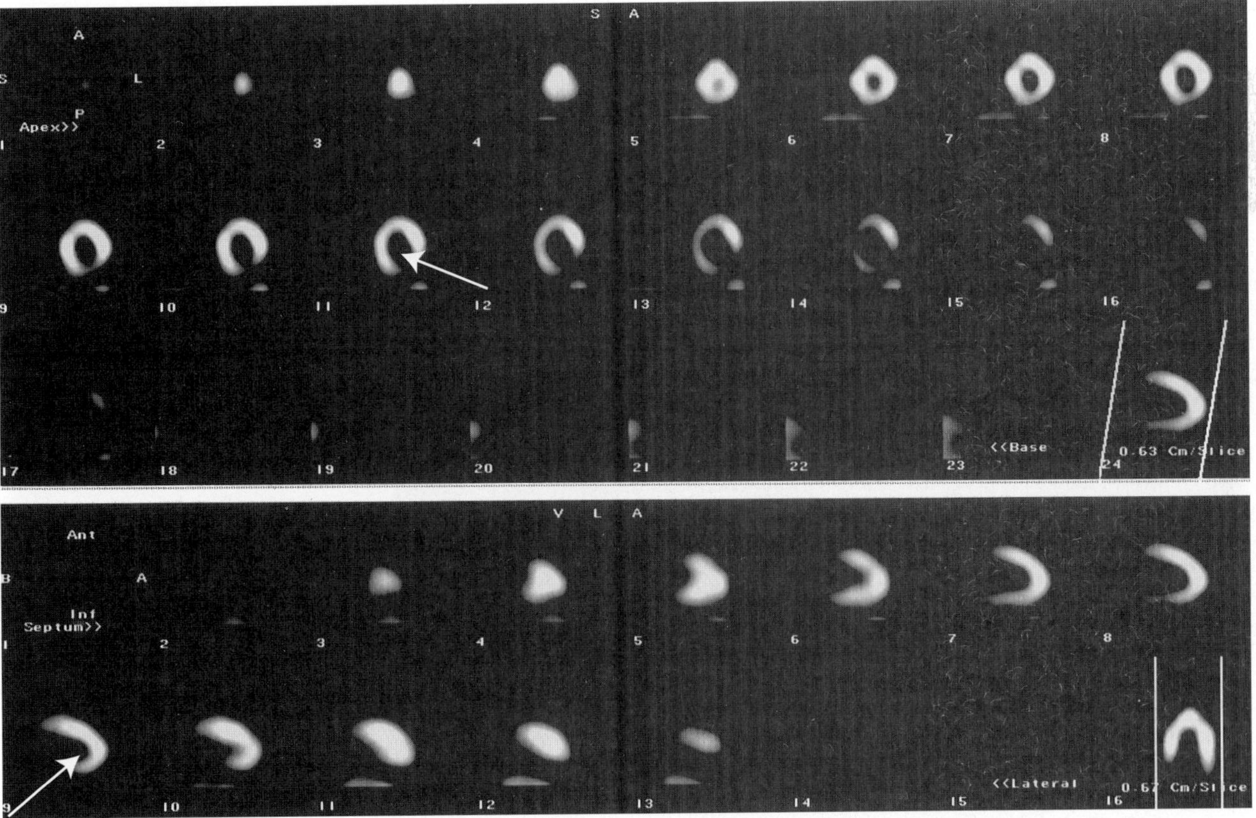

FIG. 57-6. A 59-year-old white hypertensive man who arrived at the emergency department with 6 h of intermittent chest pain. Findings on physical examination and electrocardiography were unremarkable. Initial cardiac enzyme levels (CK-MB, myoglobin, and troponin T) were normal. ^{99m}Tc-sestamibi SPECT perfusion images show a moderate area of hypoperfusion in the middle and proximal inferolateral wall. The patient went directly to catheterization, which showed a 95 percent circumflex marginal stenosis that was successfully treated by angioplasty. (Courtesy of Ethan Spiegler, MD.)

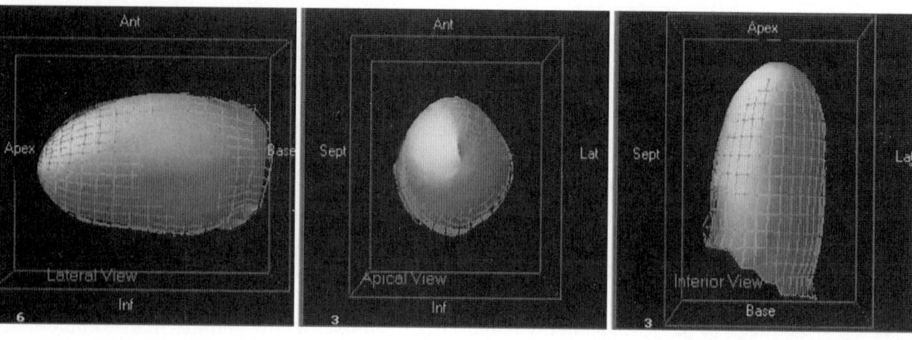

FIG. 57-7 (Plate 7). Three-dimensional representation of gated SPECT data at end diastole.

ECHOCARDIOGRAPHY

Echocardiography is the use of ultrasound to image the heart and great vessels. This general term includes the techniques of M-mode, two-dimensional (2D) imaging, pulsed wave, and color Doppler studies. Frequently, an examination of the heart will apply a combination of these ultrasound methods to the clinical problem at hand.

Echocardiography, after the chest x-ray, represents one of the most commonly applied methods for cardiac diagnosis. Applications of this method include assessment of cardiac chamber size and function, patterns of flow within the ventricles, pericardial assessment, and identification of cardiac masses, including tumors, valve vegetations or calcification, and thrombi (Fig. 57-9). Advantages for this technique include its relatively low cost, portability of the ultrasound equipment, good patient comfort, and safety.

Although the use of echocardiography is extremely widespread, there are limitations to the technique. The method is highly operator dependent. Patient positioning relative to the ultrasound probe is crucial, and specific machine adjustments must be made to optimize the examination to a particular patient. These adjustments may substantially alter the diagnostic ability of the examination. Certain patients have poor ''acoustic windows,'' through which the ultrasound beam ''looks'' to see the cardiac structures. This limits examination quality in patients with chronic obstructive lung disease, obesity, and some

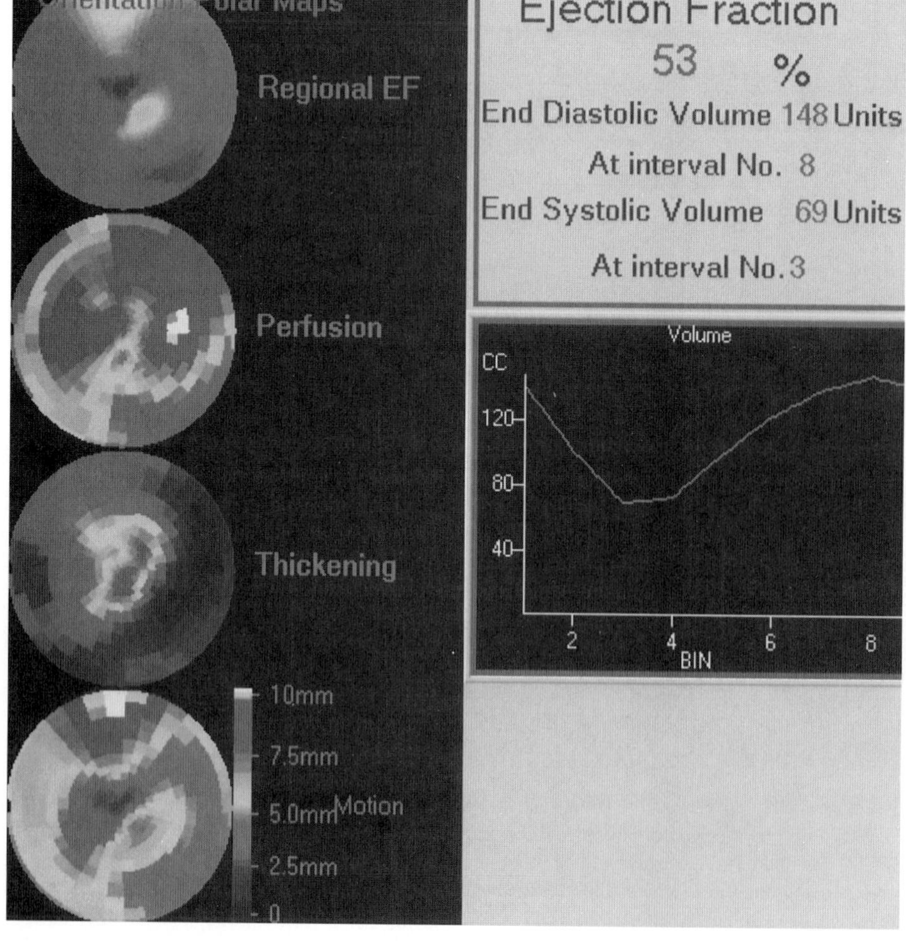

FIG. 57-8 (Plate 8). Bull's-eye representation of gated SPECT data. Hypoperfusion of the proximal inferolateral wall as well as mild hypokinesis and diminished wall thickening. There is preserved global left ventricular function.

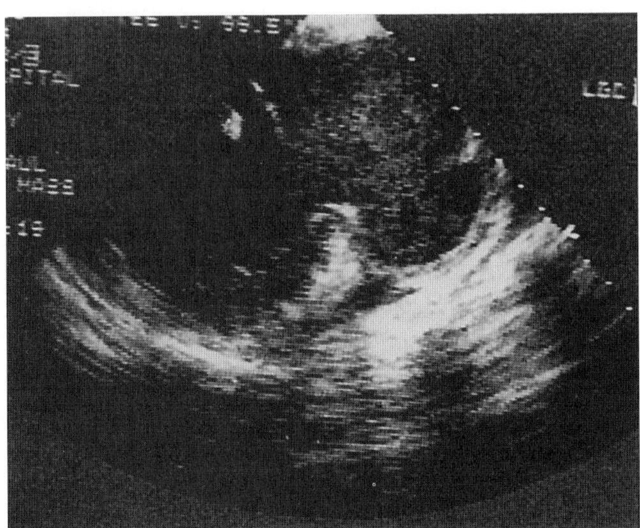

FIG. 57-9. Echocardiography of inferior wall pseudoaneurysm, due to prior rupture of the left ventricular wall. (Reprinted from Burton and Lima,[20] with permission.)

musculoskeletal deformities. The use of transesophageal echocardiography, in part, alleviates the limitations of the technique for these patient populations.

Background

Echocardiography is based on the transmission and disruption of sound waves into the body. These sounds waves are much higher than the normal range of human hearing (20 kHz), and range from 1 to 10 MHz. The relationship between the frequency of the sound wave (f), the velocity of wave (ν), and the wave length (λ) is given by

$$\nu = f\lambda$$

The velocity of sound in the tissues is assumed to be constant, and equal to 1540 cm/s. For typical clinical frequencies of 2 to 5 MHz, the wavelengths are on the order of 0.3 to 0.8 mm. Given the velocity of the wave, pulsed ultrasound methods calculate the distance traveled by the sound wave by measuring the time from the start of the pulse wave to the time taken to reflect from an object and return to the transducer.

ACOUSTIC IMPEDANCE The signal returning to the ultrasound transducer depends on the reflected ultrasound wave. The reflected ultrasound wave is generated at the acoustic interfaces between tissues of different density or through which sounds travel at different velocities. At these tissue interfaces, sound waves are either reflected back to the transducer (specular interface) or scattered into many different directions. The endocardial border represents a specular interface; sound waves are maximally reflected back from this interface when they are incident upon the interface at a 90° angle. As the sound waves become more parallel to the endocardium, the reflected waves are weakest.

Incident ultrasound waves that are scattered as they reflect from red blood cells may be used to assess the Doppler phenomenon, thus measuring the velocity of the red blood cells. The Doppler phenomenon refers to increased frequency of the ultrasound wave when the motion of the red blood cells is toward the transducer, and decreased frequency when the motion is away from the transducer. The Doppler shift, Δf, is related to the velocity of the red blood cells, ν, by the equation

$$\Delta f = (2f_0/C)\nu \cos(\vartheta)$$

where f_0 is the frequency of the incident ultrasound beam, C is the velocity of sound in the tissue, and ϑ is the incident angle of the ultrasound beam relative to the blood vessel of ventricle. In Doppler display mode, blood flowing toward the transducer is coded red; blood flow away from the transducer is shown as blue. Further, the intensity of the red or blue is displayed as proportional to the velocity. According to the foregoing equation, velocities are most accurate when the angle between the ultrasound beam and blood flow is close to 0, since the cosine of 0 is equal to 1. Pulsed wave ultrasound techniques may be used to assess blood velocity: a series of rapid pulses is sent into the tissue, followed by a short segment of time for receiving the reflected waves.

M-MODE DISPLAY M-mode display is unique in medical imaging to echocardiography. The primary advantage of this display mode is that high time resolution, to approximately one-thousandth of a second, can be displayed on the time axis. Compared with this, traditional 2D displays are updated only approximately 30 times per second. Thus, M-mode display has excellent time resolution and can be used to display the periodic motion of, for example, cardiac valves or vegetations. In this display mode, a 2D display is typically first selected. A single line, or slice, of the 2D display is then selected, often across a valve plane. M-mode displays then show the reflected ultrasound signal along this single line, with continual updating every millisecond.

Applications

MYOCARDIAL INFARCTION Echocardiography is more sensitive and specific than history and ECG findings in diagnosing myocardial infarction in patients presenting with chest pain. In several clinical series, left ventricular wall motion abnormalities were observed in 89 to 100 percent of patients with transmural infarction.[8,9] The sensitivity of echocardiography in detecting a nontransmural infarction is somewhat less and depends on the transmural thickness of the infarcted myocardial segment. In addition, patients who had no echocardiographically detected wall motion abnormalities had smaller infarctions and fewer complications.[8,9]

Echocardiography is also useful in the diagnosis and management of chest pain due to causes other than myocardial infarction. Patients with chest pain due to myocardial ischemia usually have echocardiographically detectable wall motion abnormalities with pain, even in the absence of infarction. Other causes of chest pain, including aortic dissection, hypertrophic cardiomyopathy, valvular heart disease, pericarditis, and pulmonary embolism, can frequently be identified or suspected based on transthoracic echocardiography.

In addition to facilitating diagnosis, echocardiography early in the course of acute myocardial infarction provides information important in guiding early management and determining short-term prognosis. The location and size of wall motion abnormalities correlate well with the coronary artery involved in an infarction. Infarction resulting from obstruction of the left anterior descending coronary artery usually causes abnormal function in the anterior, septal, and apical segments of the left ventricle. Akinesis of the basal anterior segment predicts occlusion of the left anterior descending coronary artery, proximal to the first septal perforator, a finding of prognostic significance. There is overlap in the areas of abnormal wall motion in myocardial infarcts involving the left circumflex and right coronary arteries. Occlusion of either vessel can cause abnormal motion in the middle and basilar segments of the posterior and inferior walls. Wall motion abnormalities confined to the posterior and lateral walls are usually caused by obstruction of the circumflex, whereas abnormalities confined to the inferior basal segment are characteristic of obstruction of the right coronary artery.

A number of factors, including the presence of ischemia, stunning, or overload, confound the relationship between the size of regional wall motion abnormalities and the amount of infarcted myocardium. When compared with pathologic examination, echocardiography tends to overestimate the amount of necrosed myocardium early in the course of myocardial infarction. Despite this limitation, echocardiographic estimation of the extent of myocardial infarction correlates well with infarct size as determined by peak creatine kinase, radionuclide imaging, and contrast ventriculography. Echocardiographic evaluation of left ventricular function early in the course of myocardial infarction has been found to be a better predictor of in-hospital mortality than the prognostically strongest clinical parameters. An echocardiographically determined ejection fraction of greater than 40 percent has correlated with a low short-term mortality and could potentially be used to select low-risk patients for early discharge.[10] By contrast, a tall peaked E wave on Doppler evaluation of left ventricular filling has been correlated with elevated left ventricular end-diastolic pressure and worse prognosis.

Echocardiography has been used to assess the efficacy of thrombolytic therapy. The time required for improvement of left ventricular function after reperfusion is related to the duration of ischemia and size of the ischemic zone. In patients with successful reperfusion induced by thrombolytic agents or direct angioplasty, echocardiographically detectable improvement in contractility can occur in the first 24 h. The delay in recovery of function, even after successful reperfusion, limits the utility of echocardiography in acutely assessing the success of thrombolytic therapy.

The widespread use of echocardiography early in the course of myocardial infarction reflects the clinical utility, availability, and safety of this technique. Echocardiography does have a number of potential shortcomings in the early diagnosis and management of acute myocardial infarction. The quality of echocardiographic images depends on the skill of the operator and the habitus of the patient. Images adequate for evaluation of wall motion can not be obtained in 5 to 15 percent of patients in clinical studies of myocardial infarction.[8,9] Abnormal wall motion can be present in patients with Wolfe-Parkinson-White syndrome, bundle branch block, right ventricular overload, and after cardiac surgery. However, in contrast to patients with myocardial infarction, in these patients, wall thickening is usually preserved. On the other hand, myocarditis may cause regional loss of wall thickening and be indistinguishable from infarction by echocardiography. In addition, it is sometimes difficult to differentiate new wall motion abnormalities from preexisting ones by echocardiography.

ACUTE MITRAL REGURGITATION This requires emergent surgery, and has a higher mortality rate than that of chronic mitral valve disease. Etiologies include endocarditis, acute ischemia or myocardial infarction, prosthetic valve failure, and chordal rupture due to myxomatous mitral disease or trauma.

Echocardiographic signs in acute mitral regurgitation include the ''snake'' sign, corresponding to high-frequency fluttering of a ruptured chord in the left atrium. Rupture of the papillary muscle may cause disconnection of the involved tip from the body of the muscle. The direction of the mitral regurgitant distinguishes anterior from posterior flail leaflet: anterior leaflet failure is associated with posteriorly directed jet, and posterior leaflet failure shows anteriorly directed jet. Transesophageal echocardiography appears to be superior to transthoracic imaging for determining the size and etiology of the valvular disorder.

ACUTE AORTIC REGURGITATION Acute aortic regurgitation results from trauma, endocarditis, or aortic dissection. This condition is rapidly fatal and requires immediate surgical repair. Transesophageal echocardiography may be necessary to delineate disruption of valvular or annular architecture in this condition.

For chronic aortic regurgitation, color Doppler demonstrates a regurgitant jet in the left ventricle. In the acute case, however, rapid equilibration of pressures in the aorta and the normal-sized left ventricle causes a small, or no, Doppler jet. The spectral pattern of the continuous wave Doppler will have a low peak velocity and an extremely rapid deceleration slope. These findings correspond to the inaudibility of the murmur of acute regurgitation. In the most severe case, there is little diastolic flow into the ventricle, since the aorta and left ventricle become a continuous chamber. Early closure of the mitral valve or diastolic mitral regurgitation on M-mode or 2D echocardiography are ominous prognostic signs. Early mitral valve closure indicates severe and acute decompensated aortic insufficiency.

MAGNETIC RESONANCE IMAGING

MRI is rapidly becoming the noninvasive gold standard for the assessment of cardiac structure and function. The high contrast between moving blood and the myocardium by MRI, as well as high spatial resolution (Fig. 57-10) and lack of ionizing radiation, results in a superb technique for myocardial assessment. Although availability remains a concern, it is anticipated that major medical centers will increasing have MRI services available for emergency applications in myocardial imaging. Previously, MR machines had been designed to image static areas of the body, specifically, the brain and spine. Currently, all major equipment manufacturers have devoted substantial resources to developing MR equipment specifically for the diagnosis of cardiovascular disorders. This section reviews principles of MRI to provide a basis for emergency medicine professionals in evaluating MR studies. Additionally, the range of emergency medicine applications for cardiac imaging is presented.

Principles of Magnetic Resonance Imaging

The basic process of MRI involves excitation of hydrogen nuclei (i.e., protons) with radio frequency energy. After sending electromagnetic energy into the patient, protons are excited to a higher-energy state. The radio frequency wave is then turned off, and protons ''relax'' to their baseline state. As the protons relax, they emit a radio frequency signal that can be picked up by an antenna, amplified, and used to form an image.

Although hydrogen nuclei are typically used in MRI, other atoms, such as phosphorus (particularly important for cardiac energetics and infarction) can also be used for MRI. Hydrogen is particularly useful for biologic tissues: it is extremely abundant (for example, in water and fat) and is extremely sensitive to the MRI process. In addition, with pathologic processes, the water content of tissues often changes. For example, myocardial infarctions have a higher water content than normal tissues. Therefore, pathologic processes can be readily detected by imaging changes in water content of tissues.

To summarize, the basic MR process involves the following:

- The patient is placed in very high field strength magnet
- The magnetic field causes alignment of protons in the patient
- A radio wave is sent into the patient, disturbing the alignment
- The radio wave is turned off
- The patient emits a radio frequency signal
- The signal is picked up by an antenna and used to form an image

The MR signal is a function of multiple tissue parameters, including T1, T2, proton density, and the rate and type (oxygenated or deoxygenated) of flowing blood. *T1* and *T2* parameters are numbers that characterize the response of biologic tissue to an applied magnetic field. *T1-weighted images* are generally those that help define the *anatomy* that is being viewed (Fig. 57-11). *T2 images* are those that better define the *pathology* of the tissue. *Proton-density images* may also be generated, in which the image intensity is proportional to the number of protons present. Finally, images can be generated that are

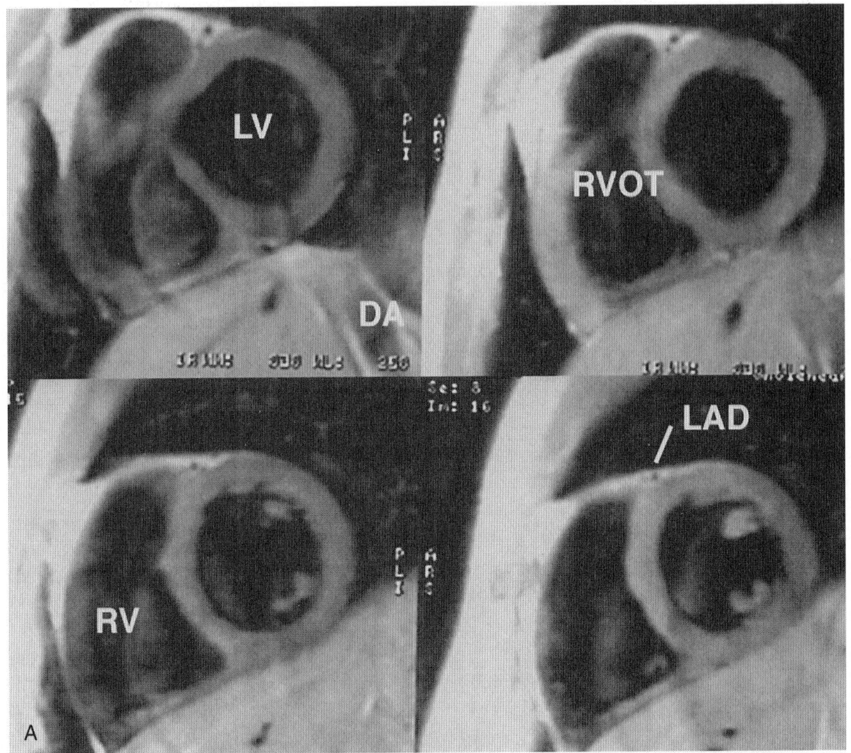

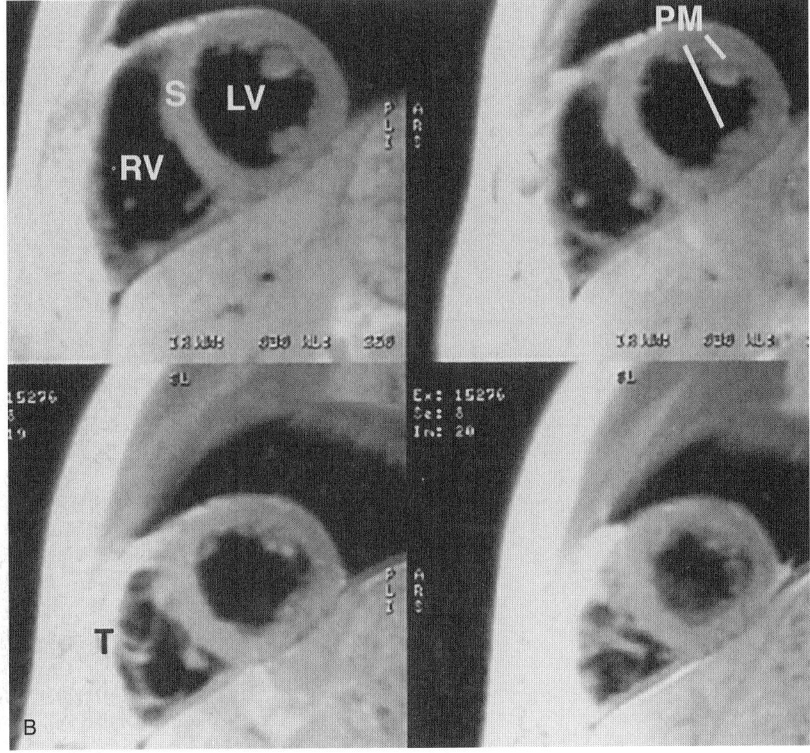

FIG. 57-10. MRI of normal short-axis cardiac anatomy. Short-axis images from the base of the heart **(A)** through the cardiac apex **(B)**. Successive images are displayed left to right, top to bottom. *Abbreviations:* LAD, left anterior descending coronary artery; LV, left ventricle; PM, papillary muscles; RVOT, right ventricular outflow tract; RV, right ventricle; S, septum; T, trabeculations in right ventricle. (Reprinted from Bluemke and Boxerman,[19] with permission.)

sensitive to flowing blood (*bright blood images* or MR angiograms). It is the unique property and strength of MR imaging that four different physical factors (T1, T2, proton density, and blood flow) may be used to derive a variety of imaging results; this is very different from CT scanning or echocardiography, in which only one factor (x-ray attenuation and acoustic attenuation, respectively) is used to generate contrast in images. Although these multiple factors add to the complexity of understanding MR, it also enhances the power of the technique for detecting subtle changes in pathologic tissues relative to normal tissues.

Two parameters are particularly helpful in determining MR image contrast: time to repetition (TR) describes the time between radio frequency pulses, and time to echo (TE) describes the time after each radio frequency pulse when the MR scanner ''listens'' for signal from the patient. By changing the TR and TE values, different types of image contrast are obtained (Table 57-1). For more detailed information

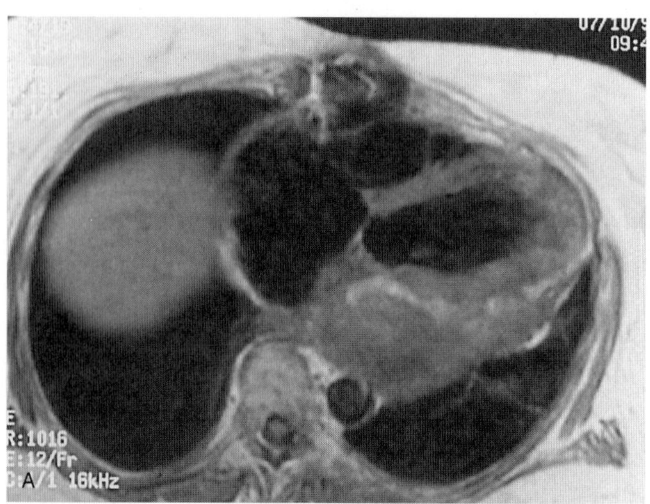

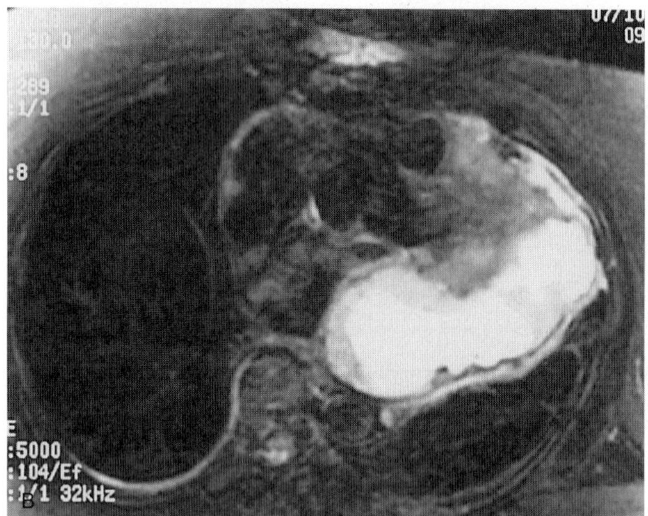

FIG. 57-11. Paracardiac mass demonstrated by MRI. Axial images of the chest demonstrating a mass posterior to the left ventricle. **A.** T1-weighted image, showing thickening of the posterior wall of the left ventricle. **B.** T2-weighted image, showing bright increase signal in the mass. Biopsy revealed hemangiopericytoma. (Reprinted from Bluemke and Boxerman,[19] with permission.)

TABLE 57-1 Appearance of Magnetic Resonance

Image Type	TR (ms)	TE (ms)	Fat Appearance	Water Appearance
T1 weighted	300–600	20–30	Bright	Dark
Proton density	2000–6000	20–30	Intermediate	Intermediate
T2 weighted	2000–6000	80–100	Intermediate*	Bright

*Fat on T2-weighted images are darker than proton-density images. Also, "fat suppression" may often be used with T2 images, resulting in very dark fat signal.

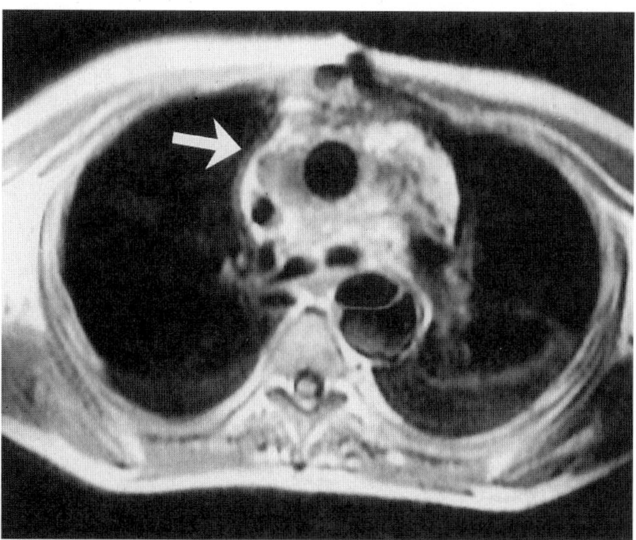

FIG. 57-12. Magnetic resonance imaging of aortic dissection. Axial T1-weighted image shows the site of prior repair of the ascending aorta, following dissection. There is residual soft tissue thickening around the ascending aorta. A residual dissection remains in the descending aorta. The patient had a history of Marfan disease.

regarding MR physics, the reader is referred to standard textbooks on the subject, such as that by Berning and Steensgaard-Hansen.[11]

Magnetic Resonance Pulse Sequences

CONVENTIONAL SPIN ECHO IMAGING The most common pulse sequence traditionally used for cardiac imaging is a conventional spin echo sequence, gated to the cardiac cycle. In this technique, the TR is equal to the duration of the RR interval, and the minimum TE time is used (10 to 20 ms). Since the T1 time of the myocardium is on the order of 800 ms, only moderate T1 weighting is achieved using this method. These images are commonly referred to as *black blood* images, since radio frequency saturation bands are placed above and below the imaging planes, causing blood to lose MR signal and become dark (Fig. 57-12). Since the TR depends on the RR interval, imaging times are typically long (e.g., 6 to 8 min). Image quality is only moderate, and highly dependent on consistent ECG gating and lack of patient motion during the relatively long acquisition times. However, the contrast difference between the heart, the epicardial fat, and the ventricular cavities is relatively good.

T2 weighting for spin echo images is achieved by gating at several multiples of the RR interval, together with a TE time of 80 to 100 ms. Imaging times are quite long if conventional spin echo techniques are used. The image quality of T2-weighted images is lower than that of T1 images, because of lower signal-to-noise ratios typically associated with T2 images. Also, artifacts due to respiratory and cardiac motion may be pronounced because of long imaging times. T2-weighted images are usually not necessary for *anatomic* evaluation of the heart but are more helpful for characterization of cardiac or paracardiac masses (Fig. 57-11b). In these cases, the mass frequently has somewhat restricted motion relative to the myocardium, so that image quality is often adequate. *Fast spin echo* or *turbo spin echo* T2-weighted pulse sequences are available on most new MR sequences. These methods reduce imaging time for T2-weighted images by a factor of 8 to 16. Because of the high signal intensity of fat on fast spin echo images, an additional radio frequency pulse is often added to cause fat to be very dark. This in turn helps to highlight nonfatty structures.

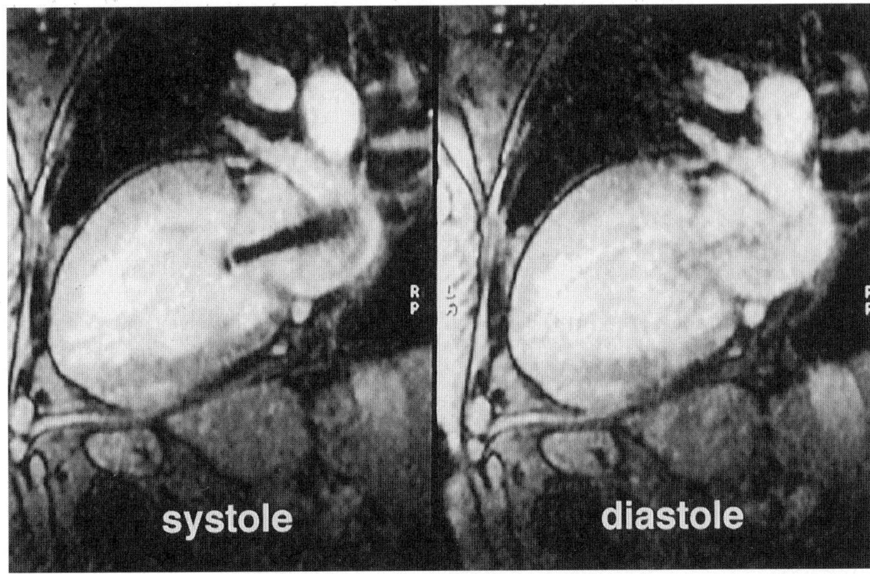

FIG. 57-13. Magnetic resonance imaging of mitral valve dysfunction. Images during systole and diastole show a dark regurgitant jet extending from the valve plane to the left atrium during systole, compatible with mitral valve regurgitation. (Reprinted from Bluemke and Boxerman,[19] with permission.)

CINE IMAGING Cine imaging for cardiac MRI consists of a motion picture loop of various phases of the cardiac cycle (Fig. 57-13). To generate cine images, images must be gated to the cardiac cycle. In cine acquisitions, the imaging pulse is triggered, or gated, to begin based on the R wave of the electrocardiogram. *Segmented k-space* pulse sequences are very rapid, cardiac gated pulse sequences in which a complete cine sequence of the heart is acquired within a breath hold of 12 to 18 heartbeats. This consists of a fast gradient echo acquisition with relatively short TR (e.g., 5 to 10 ms) combined with very short TE (approximately 2 ms), and a flip angle of 10° to 15°. The TR and TE are usually the minimum values achievable by the MR gradient system, so that the system software may automatically set these parameters. The above acquisition parameters result in saturation of background, stationary tissues, while flowing blood has a higher and brighter signal. Breath-hold cine imaging of the heart can be performed in any anatomic plane, e.g., parallel to the long axis and short axis of the heart.

The Magnetic Resonance Environment and Safety Considerations

The MR environment for high-field-strength MR scanners is potentially hostile for ED personnel and their patients. Standard support devices necessary for patient monitoring, such as pulse and blood oxygenation monitoring, blood pressure measurement, and electrocardiogram evaluation, are incompatible with operation inside the MR suites. Cardiac disease patients are typically transported with oxygen cylinders: steel oxygen cylinders will act as high-speed projectiles inside the MR suite if allowed near the MR scanner. Finally, electromechanical infusion pumps for delivery of medication are not certified to operate properly near strong magnetic fields. Because of these considerations, the preparation of patients for MR imaging involves the teamwork of both the ED staff and the MR technologists who can advise on device compatibility and provide MR compatible equipment (Table 57-2).

ED personnel as well as their patients must be "cleared" for MR compatibility prior to entering the MR suite. A number of implanted medical devices are not MR compatible. The most common of these are certain brain aneurysm clips, cardiac pacemakers, cochlear implants, and internally placed pumps or electrical stimulators. Regarding brain aneurysm clips, the specific manufacturer of the clip and the model number should be provided to MR department personnel, who can advise on MR compatibility. Patients are also questioned to determine whether they have had injuries or a typical work history that would place them at risk for having metal fragments in or near the orbit or brain. Because of space limitations, all such devices cannot be reviewed in this chapter, and readers are advised to consult with MR personnel for any implanted device or device transported with the patient. Finally, although there is no known biohazard to humans or fetuses at approved energy levels specified by the Food and Drug Administration, pregnant hospital personnel are advised to stay out of the MR suite. Patients who are pregnant are requested to sign a consent form prior to MR imaging. These consent forms state that the potential benefit of the MR test for that patient greatly outweighs the potential risk to the fetus and mother, which appears to be extremely

TABLE 57-2 Emergency Department Patients in the Magnetic Resonance (MR) Environment

Device/Equipment	Action/Substitute
Pulse monitoring	MR-compatible pulse monitor*
Blood oxygenation	MR-compatible blood oxygen monitor*
Blood pressure	MR-compatible blood pressure device*
Oxygen therapy	Wall O_2 in the MR suite, or aluminum MR oxygen cylinders
Medication infusion pumps	Multiple high-pressure extension tubings, to place the infusion pump outside of the high-gauss magnetic field
Anesthesia pump	MR-compatible anesthesia pump*
Swan-Ganz catheters	Not MR compatible
External fixation devices, halo devices	Some compatible; consult with MR personnel and provide type/manufacturer
Electrocardiogram monitoring	Diagnostic waveforms are not available in the MR environment; low-level capability for identifying prominent arthymias is available

*Available from MR department personnel.

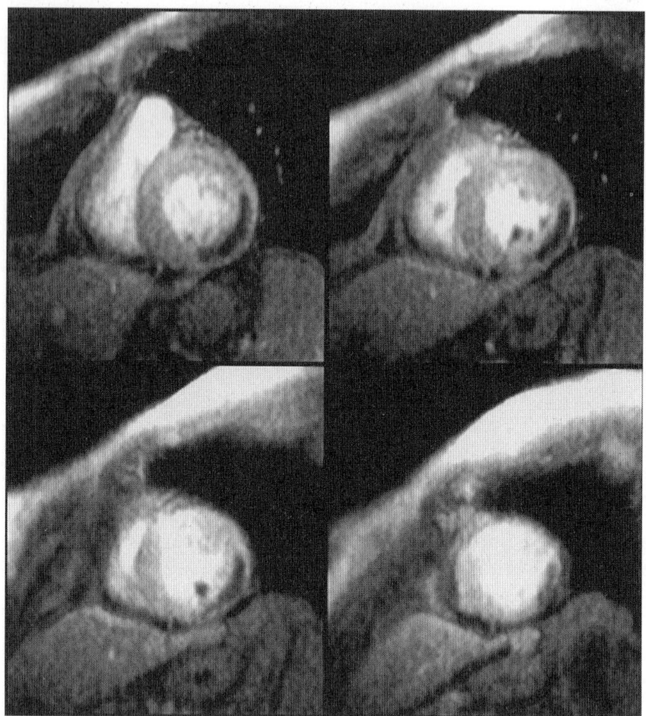

FIG. 57-14. Magnetic resonance imaging of myocardial infarction. Short-axis images of the heart show a focal area of decreased signal in the circumflex artery territory of the left ventricle. Images were acquired in a breath hold, after injection of a gadolinium contrast agent.

low or negligible (particularly, for example, compared with known risks of ionizing radiation with nuclear imaging studies or computed tomography). Contrast agents used for MRI are contraindicated during pregnancy.

Specific Applications of Magnetic Resonance Imaging

ACUTE MYOCARDIAL INFARCTION Infarction can be visualized following intravenous administration of a contrast agent: gadolinium-DTPA. Within the infarct, there is a central ''core'' of tissue within which there is microvascular obstruction, despite patency of the epicardial vessel (Fig. 57-14). Surrounding this is nonviable tissue, with yet a still larger area of myocardium that remains ''stunned.'' Signal intensity of myocardial territory corresponding to microvascular occlusion is reduced (*hypoenhanced*) compared with normal myocardium immediately after contrast administration. In reperfused infarcts, myocardial image intensity is increased (*hyperenhanced*).[12,13] The ability to discern these changes with fidelity may play a role in the detection of myocardial infarcts and the determination of their size. Large human infarcts, associated with prolonged obstruction of the infarct-related artery, frequently have central areas of hypoenhancement during the first several minutes after myocardial infarction. Smaller, reperfused infarcts tend to demonstrate more uniform signal hyperenhancement.[13]

First-pass MRI myocardial perfusion methods may be applied to the assessment of coronary flow reserve. *Coronary flow reserve* is defined as the ratio of blood flow at maximal vasodilatation, divided by flow at rest. Maximal flow is measured under conditions of vasodilatation, as achieved with dipyridamole or adenosine. Typically, coronary flow reserve ranges from 3 to 5 in normal individuals. In the presence of fixed coronary stenoses, coronary flow reserve is markedly reduced.[14] Coronary flow reserve may be measured with an intracoronary Doppler flow ultrasound probe, but first-pass contrast MR has also been found to be useful for flow reserve assessment. In both animal and patient studies, a linear relationship between coronary flow reserve and first-pass MR imaging has been found This indicates that patients with microvascular dysfunction, either from epicardial vascular disease or diseases altering the microvasculature, such as hypertension or diabetes, may be assessed by using these methods.[15]

CHRONIC MYOCARDIAL INFARCTION This results in thinning of the left ventricular wall (remodeling) that is distinct from the normal myocardial wall thickness. These changes are better seen during systole, because of increased thickness of normal myocardium relative to the region of infarction. This finding is specific for chronic myocardial infarction on MRI.[16,17]

Left ventricular aneurysms may occur following myocardial infarction and are depicted as areas of focally protruding myocardium (Fig. 57-15), with transmural thinning and associated with mural thrombus. Although distinguishing between a true aneurysm and false aneurysm (ruptured myocardium contained by pericardium) is usually straightforward by echocardiography, MR is useful in cases in which an adequate acoustic window is not obtained. Pseudoaneurysms are characterized by a relatively small neck communicating with the left ventricular cavity, whereas true aneurysms have a relatively wide neck.[18]

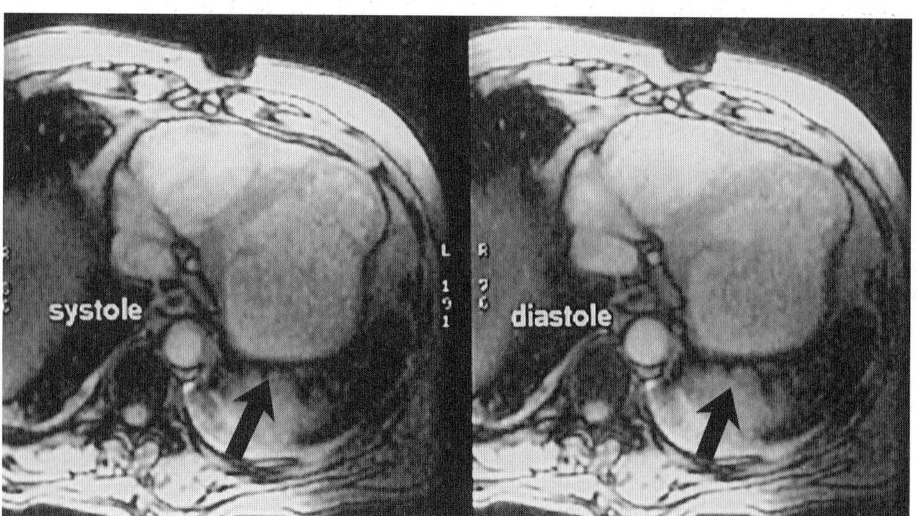

FIG. 57-15. Magnetic resonance imaging of left ventricular aneurysm. A focal outpouching of the left ventricle is present (*arrow*) during both systole and diastole. The patient had a prior myocardial infarction, with resulting thinning of the ventricular wall and aneurysm formation. (Reprinted from Bluemke and Boxerman,[19] with permission.)

REFERENCES

1. Lee TH, Cook EF, Weisberg MC, et al: Acute chest pain in the emergency room: Identification and examination of low-risk patients. *Arch Intern Med* 145:65, 1985.
2. Lee TH, Rouan GW, Weisberg MC, et al: Clinical characteristics and natural history of patients with acute myocardial infarction sent home from the emergency room. *Am J Cardiol* 60:219, 1987.
3. McCarthy BD, Bechansky JR, Agonstino RB, et al: Missed diagnosis of acute myocardial infarction in the emergency department: Results from a multicenter study. *Ann Emerg Med* 22:579, 1993.
4. Tatum JL, Jesse RL, Kontos MC, et al: Comprehensive strategy for the evaluation and triage of the chest pain patient. *Ann Emerg Med* 29:116, 1997.
5. Spiegler EJ, Civelek AC, Bahr R, et al: The use of technetium-99m sestamibi in the emergency room: Can it assist in the triage of patients with chest pain? *Clin Nucl Med* 18:807, 1993.
6. Hilton TC, Thompson RC, Williams HJ, et al: Technitium-99m sestamibi myocardial perfusion imaging in the emergency room evaluation of chest pain. *J Am Coll Cardiol* 23:1016, 1994.
7. Varetto T, Cantalupi D, Altieri A, et al: Emergency room technetium sestamibi imaging to rule out acute myocardial ischemic events in patients with nondiagnostic electrocardiograms. *J Am Coll Cardiol* 22:1804, 1993.
8. Peels CH, Visser CA, Kupper AJ, et al: Usefulness of two-dimensional echocardiography for immediate detection of myocardial ischemia in the emergency room. *Am J Cardiol* 65:687, 1990.
9. Sabia P, Afrookteh A, Touchstone DA, et al: Value of regional wall motion abnormality in the emergency room diagnosis of acute myocardial infarction: A prospective study using two-dimensional echocardiography. *Circulation* (abstract). 84:I85, 1991.
10. Berning J, Steensgaard-Hansen F: Early estimation of risk by echocardiographic determination of wall motion index in an unselected population with acute myocardial infarction. *Am J Cardiol* 65:567, 1990.
11. Stark DD, Bradley WG Jr (eds): *Magnetic Resonance Imaging*. Philadelphia, CV Mosby, 1998.
12. Saeed M, Wendland M, Masui T, Higgins C: Reperfused myocardial infarctions on T1- and susceptibility-enhanced MRI: Evidence for loss of compartmentalization of contrast media. *Magn Reson Med* 31:31, 1994.
13. Lima JA, Judd RM, Bazille A, et al: Regional heterogeneity of human myocardial infarcts demonstrated by contrast-enhanced MRI: Potential mechanisms. *Circulation* 92:1117, 1995.
14. Wilke N, Simm C, Zhang J, et al: Contrast-enhanced first pass myocardial perfusion imaging: Correlation between myocardial blood flow in dogs at rest and during hyperemia. *Magn Reson Med* 29:485, 1993.
15. Wilke N, Jerosch-Herold M, Wang Y, et al: Myocardial perfusion reserve: Assessment with multisection, quantitative, first-pass MR imaging. *Radiology* 204:373, 1997.
16. McNamara MT, Higgins CB: Magnetic resonance imaging of chronic myocardial infarcts in man. *AJR* 146:315, 1986.
17. Higgins CB: MRI in ischemic heart disease: Acute infarction, chronic infarction and contrast media in ischemic myocardial disease. *Radiol Med* 79:680, 1990.
18. Gomes AS, Lois JF, Child JS, et al: Cardiac tumors and thrombus: Evaluation with MR imaging. *AJR* 149:895, 1987.
19. Bluemke DA, Boxerman JL: MRI of acquired cardiac disease, in Stark DD, Bradley WGJ (eds): *Magnetic Resonance Imaging,* 3d ed. Philadelphia, CV Mosby, 1998 pp 409–438.
20. Burton AA, Lima JAC: Echocardiography in patients with acute myocardial infarction, in Lima JAC (ed): *Diagnostic Imaging in Clinical Cardiology.* London, Martin Dunitz, 1998, p 53.

PULMONARY EMERGENCIES

58 RESPIRATORY DISTRESS

J. Stephan Stapczynski

Common respiratory symptoms that bring patients to the emergency department include dyspnea (with the associated findings of hypoxia and hypercapnia), wheezing, and cough. Hiccups are an infrequent presenting symptom but, when persistent, very distressing to the patient. Cyanosis can be associated with pulmonary and vascular, as well as hematologic, pathologic conditions. This chapter discusses these symptoms and signs as they relate to evaluation of emergency patients. It is worth noting that, despite the increasing availability of and reliance on ancillary tests, the assessment of patients still begins with an accurate history and a careful physical examination in order to make the wisest use of ancillary tests.[1]

DYSPNEA

Dyspnea is a subjective feeling of difficult, labored, or uncomfortable breathing. This common emergency department complaint is often described as "shortness of breath," "breathlessness," "not getting enough air," and a variety of other phrases. Dyspnea does not result from a single pathophysiologic mechanism and may result from many disorders. Approximately two-thirds of patients presenting to the emergency department with dyspnea have either a cardiac or a pulmonary disorder. An emergency physician can usually distinguish these on the basis of history, physical examination, and, occasionally, ancillary tests.

Dyspnea must be distinguished from a number of other signs and symptoms. Tachypnea is rapid breathing; it may or may not be associated with dyspnea, and dyspnea is not always accompanied by tachypnea. Orthopnea is dyspnea in the recumbent position. It is most often the result of left ventricular failure and may be associated with diaphragmatic paralysis or chronic obstructive pulmonary disease (COPD). Paroxysmal nocturnal dyspnea is orthopnea that awakens the patient from sleep. Trepopnea is dyspnea associated with only one of several recumbent positions. Trepopnea can occur with unilateral diaphragmatic paralysis, with ball-valve airway obstruction, or after surgical pneumonectomy. Platypnea is the opposite of orthopnea: dyspnea in the upright position. Platypnea results from the loss of abdominal wall muscular tone and, in rare cases, from right-to-left intracardiac shunting, as occurs from a patent foramen ovale. Hyperpnea is essentially hyperventilation and is defined as minute ventilation in excess of metabolic demand. Hyperpnea may not be associated with dyspnea, and dyspnea is not always associated with increased minute ventilation.

Pathophysiology

Dyspnea is a complex sensation that involves both objective and subjective elements. Unlike other noxious sensations, dyspnea does not have a defined neural pathway, and the perceived difficulty probably arises from several pathophysiologic mechanisms.[2] The following processes are involved in the sensation of dyspnea:

1. A sense of voluntary skeletal muscular effort occurs with increased work of breathing. Muscle spindle receptors found in the muscles of respiration, as well as the associated Golgi tendon organ receptors, contribute to the sense of dyspnea when stimulated.
2. Hypercapnic chemoreceptors in the central medulla are stimulated.
3. Hypoxic chemoreceptors, primarily in the carotid body in concert with those in the aortic arch, are stimulated. However, there is a poor correlation between hypoxia and dyspnea, and dyspneic patients with hypoxia often have little improvement after correction of hypoxia.
4. Upper-airway mechanical and thermal receptors are stimulated.
5. A variety of lung receptors respond to various stimuli. They include intraparenchymal pulmonary stretch receptors, airway irritant receptors, and unmyelinated receptors that respond to interstitial edema or a change in compliance. Afferent signals from these receptors reach the brainstem by way of the vagus nerve and supply the majority of neurologic input that results in dyspnea.
6. Peripheral vascular receptors, including the right atrial and left atrial mechanoreceptor and the pulmonary artery baroreceptor, contribute to dyspnea in a poorly defined way.

Input from any or all of these receptors is integrated in a complex manner in the central nervous system (CNS) at both the subcortical and cortical level. Many authors believe that dyspnea results from afferent mismatch, when feedback from these peripheral receptors indicates that the work of breathing is greater than would be expected by the patient's level of activity.[3]

Clinical Features

Dyspnea has many causes but can be divided into general categories (Table 58-1). Because of its mainly subjective component, the presence or degree of dyspnea is difficult to measure, although categorical scales (e.g., the Borg scale) and visual analogue scales can be used in individual patients to gauge changes in the degree of distress in response to therapy. The initial assessment of any patient with dyspnea should be directed toward identifying imminent respiratory failure. The physician should specifically evaluate for tachypnea, tachycardia, stridor, and use of the accessory respiratory muscles, including the sternocleidomastoid, sternoclavicular, and intercostals. Other signs and symptoms of imminent respiratory failure are inability to speak due to the breathlessness, agitation or lethargy due to hypoxia, and paradoxical abdominal wall movement (abdominal wall retracts inward) with inspiration, indicating diaphragmatic fatigue. In patients with any of these signs or symptoms, oxygen should be administered and the need for airway control and mechanical ventilation must be anticipated. Lesser degrees of dyspnea allow for a more detailed medical history, physical examination, and indicated ancillary tests.

Diagnosis

A detailed medical history often identifies the primary process resulting in dyspnea.[3–6] Patients often have underlying chronic disorders and can frequently specifically and accurately self-diagnose their exacerbations. The medical history should include recent infectious and environmental exposures that may impair respiratory function. Patients who require daily medications for symptom control should be questioned carefully about compliance and possible drug interactions.

A number of ancillary tests aid in determining the severity and specific cause of dyspnea. Pulse oximetry is a rapid but insensitive screening test for disorders of gas exchange, and results may be normal in acute dyspnea. Arterial blood gas (ABG) analysis is more sensitive for detecting impaired gas exchange, but results may also be normal in acute dyspnea, and ABG analysis cannot evaluate the work of breathing. Rarely, patients who appear dyspneic or tachypneic but

TABLE 58-1 Common Causes of Dyspnea

Airway	Cardiac	Lung Parenchymal	Pleural and Chest Wall	Vascular	Neuromuscular	Miscellaneous
Airway mass	Left ventricular failure	Asthma	Pneumothorax	Pulmonary embolism	Cerebrovascular accident	Anemia
Foreign body	Myocardial ischemia	COPD	Pleural effusion	Air embolism	Phrenic nerve paralysis	Metabolic acidosis
Angioedema	Pericarditis	Pneumonia	Pleural adhesions	Fat embolism	Guillain-Barré syndrome	Shock
Airway stenosis	Pericardial tamponade	Pulmonary edema	Chest wall injury	Amniotic embolism	Tick paralysis	Low cardiac output states
Bronchiectasis	Arrhythmia	Pulmonary contusion	Abdominal distention	Pulmonary hypertension	Botulism	Hypoxia
Tracheomalacia	Myocarditis	Atelectasis	Kyphoscoliosis	Veno-occlusive disease	Neuropathy	Carbon monoxide poisoning
	Cardiomyopathy	Alveolitis	Pectus excavatum	Sickle cell disease	Myopathy	Methemoglobinemia
	Intracardiac shunt	Pulmonary fibrosis	Pregnancy	Vasculitis		Deconditioning
	Left ventricular outflow obstruction	Adult respiratory distress syndrome		Arteriovenous fistula		Fever
	Valvular disorder	Sarcoidosis				Hyperthyroidism
	Hypertensive crisis					Hypothyroidism
						GE reflux
						Psychogenic hyperventilation

who exhibit no evidence of hypoxia or pulmonary disease are shown to be hyperventilating from metabolic acidosis on ABG testing. A chest radiograph may indicate the general category of primary disease (infiltrate, effusion, and pneumothorax) but also may be normal. Bedside spirometric analysis (peak expiratory flow, or PEF) before and after bronchodilator therapy can be used to diagnose and treat dyspnea resulting from asthma or COPD, although it requires voluntary effort that might be difficult for dyspneic patients. Other potentially useful tests include an electrocardiogram and determination of hemoglobin level. Uncommonly, the specific process resulting in dyspnea cannot be identified by the history, the physical examination, and these simple ancillary tests, and specialized testing, including cardiac stress testing, echocardiography, formal pulmonary function testing, computed tomography scanning of the chest, or combined cardiopulmonary exercise testing, is indicated.

Treatment

Just as there is no single cause of dyspnea, there is no single treatment. In severe dyspnea, the primary treatment goal is maintenance of the airway and oxygenation with a Pao_2 greater than 60 mmHg (arterial oxygen saturation, or Sao_2, approximately 90% or greater). After this is ensured, or for patients with lesser degrees of dyspnea, disorder-specific treatment along with supplemental oxygen can be provided in the emergency department. Patients with unrelieved dyspnea at rest, particularly those with terminal malignancies, may benefit from benzodiazepines and/or opiates.[7]

HYPOXEMIA

Hypoxia is insufficient delivery of oxygen to the tissues. The amount of oxygen available to the tissues is a function of the arterial oxygen content (Cao_2) and blood flow to the tissues.

$$Cao_2 = 0.0031 \times Pao_2 + 1.38 \times Hb \times Sao_2$$

Tissue hypoxia occurs in states of low cardiac output, low hemoglobin concentration, or low Sao_2. The percent oxygen saturation of arterial hemoglobin is, in turn, dependent on the Pao_2, as described by the oxygen-hemoglobin dissociation curve. Hypoxemia is an abnormally low arterial oxygen tension. Under most situations, cardiac output is within a normal range, and hypoxemia is the most common cause of hypoxia. Although the terms *hypoxia* and *hypoxemia* are generally used interchangeably, one can occur without the other. For example, in states of low Pao_2 (hypoxemia) with concomitant polycythemia, the patient may have no tissue hypoxia. Alternatively, very anemic patients may suffer tissue hypoxia despite a normal Pao_2. Hypoxemia is arbitrarily defined as a Pao_2 less than 60 mmHg. As noted above, patients with hypoxemia may not necessarily have dyspnea, and patients with dyspnea may not have hypoxemia.

Relative hypoxemia is the term used when the arterial oxygen tension is lower than expected for a given level of inhaled oxygen. The degree of relative hypoxemia can be assessed by calculating the alveolar-arterial (A-a) oxygen partial pressure difference. This A-a gradient measures how well alveolar oxygen is transferred from the lungs to the circulation. Alveolar oxygen partial pressure is determined by the inhaled oxygen concentration (21% for room air), atmospheric pressure (760 mmHg at sea level), and displacement by water vapor (47 mmHg for full saturation) and carbon dioxide. Gas in the alveolus is fully saturated with water vapor, and the amount of alveolar oxygen is further reduced by carbon dioxide that freely diffuses from the pulmonary capillaries in an amount determined by the ratio between oxygen consumption and carbon dioxide production, or the respiratory quotient (R). On a typical diet, the respiratory quotient is 0.8. Thus, alveolar oxygen from breathing room air at sea level has a $PA_{O_2} = 0.21 \times (760 - 47) - PA_{CO_2}/0.8$. The A-a gradient at sea level for room air is $P(A\text{-}a)_{O_2} = 149 - Pa_{CO_2}/0.8 - Pa_{O_2}$. A simplified formula is often used (Ch. 22): $PA_{O_2} = 145 - Pa_{CO_2}$. A normal $P(A\text{-}a)_{O_2}$ is under 10 in young healthy patients and increases with age. The predicted A-a gradient is approximately $P(A\text{-}a)_{O_2} = 2.5 + 0.21$ (age) mmHg, with age in years and a standard deviation of 11 mmHg. This value for the normal A-a gradient is for healthy, asymptomatic individuals measured in an upright or sitting position. The supine position alone, as well as many chronic cardiac or pulmonary diseases, may raise the A-a gradient. Thus, many patients seen in the emergency department already have an elevated A-a gradient due to position or underlying chronic diseases, making it difficult to evaluate increases in the gradient that may be due to an acute pathologic condition.

Pathophysiology

Hypoxemia results from any combination of five distinct mechanisms.

1. *Hypoventilation.* Hypoventilation from a variety of disorders may result in hypoxemia. Regardless of its specific etiology, hypoxemia resulting from hypoventilation without any other cause for hypoxemia is always associated with an increased P_{CO_2}, and the $P(A\text{-}a)_{O_2}$ is normal. In the case of pure hypoventilation, the additional CO_2 displaces the inhaled oxygen and lowers the amount in the alveolus. This lowered amount, however, diffuses normally and mixes normally into the arterial blood.
2. *Right-to-left shunt.* Right-to-left shunting occurs when blood enters the systemic arteries without traversing ventilated lung. There is always a small degree of right-to-left shunting because of the direct left ventricular return of deoxygenated blood from both the coronary veins and the bronchial arteries. Increased right-to-left shunting occurs in a variety of conditions, including pulmonary consolidation, pulmonary atelectasis, and vascular malformations. Regardless of the specific cause of the right-to-left shunt, there is always an increase in the $P(A\text{-}a)_{O_2}$. In addition, right-to-left shunting does not increase Pa_{CO_2}. In fact, patients with a right-to-left shunt may have an abnormally low Pa_{CO_2}. A hallmark of significant right-to-left shunting is the failure of arterial oxygen levels to increase in response to supplemental oxygen. Although a small improvement is observed with supplemental oxygen, hypoxemia is never fully eliminated because of the continuing mixture of nonoxygenated blood into the systemic circulation.
3. *Ventilation-perfusion mismatch.* Ideal pulmonary gas exchange depends on a balance of ventilation and perfusion. Any abnormality resulting in a regional alteration of either ventilation or perfusion can adversely affect pulmonary gas exchange, resulting in hypoxemia. A wide variety of etiologies may result in these regional impairments, including pulmonary emboli, pneumonia, asthma, COPD, and even extrinsic vascular compression. Regardless of its specific etiology, hypoxemia from ventilation-perfusion mismatch is associated with an increased $P(A\text{-}a)_{O_2}$ gradient and improves with supplemental oxygen.
4. *Diffusion impairment.* Pulmonary gas exchange also depends on diffusion across the alveolar-blood barrier. Any condition that influences this diffusion (e.g., adult respiratory distress syndrome, pneumonia, or pulmonary edema) may result in hypoxemia. Regardless of the specific cause of the diffusion impairment, the $P(A\text{-}a)_{O_2}$ is increased, and hypoxemia improves with supplemental oxygen.
5. *Low inspired oxygen.* Decreased ambient oxygen pressure results in hypoxemia. This is most commonly seen at high altitude or in nonobstructive asphyxia. The $P(A\text{-}a)_{O_2}$ is normal, and hypoxemia improves with supplemental oxygen. For example, Denver, at 5400 ft above sea level, has an atmospheric pressure of 620 mmHg and an inhaled oxygen partial pressure of only $0.21 \times 620 = 130$ mmHg, as opposed to 160 mmHg at sea level.

There are three distinct acute compensatory mechanisms for hypoxemia. Initially, minute ventilation increases. Next, pulmonary arterial vasoconstriction decreases perfusion to hypoxic alveoli. While vasoconstriction balances ventilation and perfusion in order to restore arterial oxygenation, it may also cause acute right heart failure and is ineffective with diffuse lung disease. Finally, sympathetic tone increases and improves oxygen delivery by increasing cardiac output, usually with an increased heart rate. Chronic compensatory mechanisms include an increased red blood cell mass and decreased tissue oxygen demands. These compensatory mechanisms appear to be activated at different levels of hypoxemia for different individuals. However, the acute compensatory mechanisms are always activated when Pa_{O_2} reaches 60 mmHg, and compensatory mechanisms fail when Pa_{O_2} falls below 20 mmHg.

Clinical Features

The signs and symptoms of hypoxemia are nonspecific. CNS manifestations include agitation, headache, somnolence, coma, and seizures. While tachypnea and hyperventilation are often present, at a Pa_{O_2} less than 20 mmHg, there is a central depression of respiratory drive. Cyanosis is not a sensitive or specific indicator of hypoxemia. Patients with chronic compensatory mechanisms may display polycythemia or alterations in body habitus (e.g., pulmonary cachexia).

Diagnosis

The diagnosis of arterial hypoxemia requires objective measurement. Because hypoxemia is defined as a Pa_{O_2} of less than 60 mmHg, formal diagnosis requires ABG analysis. Pulse oximetry is useful in screening for gross alterations in Pa_{O_2}. Although decreased oxygen saturation readings accurately predict significant hypoxemia, normal oxygen saturation readings do not exclude hypoxemia.

Treatment

Regardless of the specific cause of hypoxemia, the initial approach remains the same: ensuring a patent airway and providing supplemental oxygenation with a goal of maintaining a Pa_{O_2} of greater than 60 mmHg. Except in patients with right-to-left shunts, arterial oxygenation responds to supplemental oxygen.

HYPERCAPNIA

Hypercapnia is exclusively due to alveolar hypoventilation and is arbitrarily defined as a Pa_{CO_2} greater than 45 mmHg. Alveolar hypoventilation can be due to a variety of disorders, including rapid shallow breathing, small tidal volumes, underventilation of the lung, or reduced respiratory drive; it is never due to increased CO_2 production (Table 58-2).

Pathophysiology

A portion of each tidal volume remains in the non-gas-exchange area of the respiratory system—termed the "dead space"—and is usually fixed by the anatomic size of the conducting airways (trachea and bronchi). The portion of the tidal volume that reaches the alveoli is that which remains after the dead space volume is subtracted: Ta =

TABLE 58-2 Causes of Hypercapnia

Depressed central respiratory drive
Structural CNS disease
Sedating drugs
Exogenous toxins
Endogenous toxins
Thoracic cage disorders
Kyphoscoliosis
Extreme obesity
Neuromuscular diseases
Intrinsic lung disease associated with increased dead space
COPD

TV − Td. Alveolar ventilation per minute is the volume multiplied by the rate: A = Ta × R = (TV − Td) × R. Alveolar hypoventilation can result from a decrease in respiratory rate, a decrease in tidal volume, or an increase in dead space.

Since the medullary chemoreceptors stimulate both respiratory rate and tidal volume in response to increased CO_2, alveolar ventilation is finely controlled to maintain $Pa{CO_2}$ within a narrow range under most circumstances. In essence, alveolar ventilation is balanced relative to the production of CO_2 to maintain the $Pa{CO_2}$ within a narrow range. Decreased respiratory drive is associated with CNS lesions and toxic depression (Table 58-2). Thoracic cage and neuromuscular disorders produce hypoventilation by allowing a slower respiratory rate and/or a decreased tidal volume relative to the production of CO_2. Intrinsic lung diseases, such as COPD, produce alveolar hypoventilation due to an increase in dead space.

Clinical Features

The signs and symptoms of hypercapnia depend on the absolute value of $Pa{CO_2}$ and its rate of change. Acute elevations result in increased intracranial pressure, and patients may complain of headache, confusion, or lethargy. With severe hypercapnia, seizures and coma can result. Extreme hypercapnia can result in cardiovascular collapse, but this is usually seen only with acute elevations of $Pa{CO_2}$ to over 100 mmHg. As opposed to acute hypercapnia, chronic hypercapnia, even over 80 mmHg, may be well tolerated.

Diagnosis

Diagnosis of hypercapnia requires ABG analysis. The results of pulse oximetry analysis can be normal, depending on other factors. With acute hypercapnia, the serum bicarbonate level increases slightly due to mass action through the CO_2-bicarbonate equilibrium: bicarbonate increases about 1 meq/L for each increase of 10 mmHg in the $Pa{CO_2}$. Patients with chronic hypercapnia have an elevated serum bicarbonate concentration due to the renal response to increased $Pa{CO_2}$: the serum bicarbonate concentration increases about 3.5 meq/L for each increase of 10 mmHg in the $Pa{CO_2}$.

Treatment

Treatment of hypercapnia requires maneuvers to increase minute ventilation, both the rate and the tidal volume. This involves ensuring a patent airway and may require mechanical ventilation. The disposition of hypercapnic patients depends primarily on the underlying cause and severity. In general, patients with hypercapnia that causes CNS symptoms should be hospitalized. Also, patients with neuromuscular disease—either congenital or acquired—who present with acute hypercapnia should be hospitalized. Some COPD patients have chronic hypercapnia and do not require admission provided they are stable. Conversely, patients with COPD who display worsening hypercapnia despite maximal therapy require hospital admission.

WHEEZING

Wheezes are adventitious lung sounds that can be best described as ''musical,'' produced by airflow through the central and lower airways.[8] Wheezes have sinusoidal acoustics, over a wide frequency range, typically 100 to 1000 Hz. The duration is prolonged, typically longer than 80 ms. Wheezes differ from the other two main adventitial lung sounds: rhonchi and crackles (rales). Rhonchi are a series of damped sinusoidal sounds, of lower frequency (<300 Hz) and prolonged duration (>100 ms). Crackles are a series of intermittent individual sounds, typically of less than 20 ms duration.

Pathophysiology

The current theory is that wheezes are produced by airway flutter and vortex shedding from the central and distal airways, although movement of airway secretions may play a small role.[9] While flutter and vortex shedding are possible in normal airways, these processes are more pronounced in obstructed airways. Airway obstruction is associated with the processes of bronchial smooth muscle contraction (bronchospasm), smooth muscle hypertrophy, increased mucus secretion, and peribronchial inflammation.

Clinical Features

Wheezing is not synonymous with airflow obstruction, and it must be remembered that

1. Wheezing can occur in normal adults and children without evidence of airflow limitation during quiet inspiration.
2. Forced expiration can produce wheezing in normal individuals, rendering its presence diagnostically useless.
3. Patients with obstruction may not have wheezing; the sensitivity of wheezing in detecting bronchial hyperreactivity with airflow limitation of greater than 20 percent is at best 75 percent, and patients with profound obstruction (<20 percent of normal) may have not enough gas movement to generate a sound.

These facts notwithstanding, wheezing is usually associated with asthma and other obstructive pulmonary diseases characterized by bronchial obstruction due to muscular spasm and inflammation (Table 58-3).

TABLE 58-3 Causes of Wheezing

Upper airway (more likely to be stridor, may have element of wheezing)
Angioedema: allergic, ACE inhibitor, idiopathic
Foreign body
Infection: croup, epiglottis, tracheitis
Lower airway
Asthma
Transient airway hyperreactivity (usually due to infection or irritation)
Bronchiolitis
COPD
Foreign body
Cardiovascular
Cardiogenic pulmonary edema (''cardiac asthma'')
Noncardiogenic pulmonary edema (adult respiratory distress syndrome, or ARDS)
Pulmonary embolus (rare)
Psychogenic

The duration of wheezing, or, more precisely, that portion of the expiratory phase occupied by wheezing, has been used to quantify the severity of airflow obstruction in moderate-to-severe acute asthma. As noted above, patients with the most profound obstruction may not wheeze, but their condition can be detected by noting markedly decreased lung sounds.

Most patients with bronchospastic disease (either asthma or COPD) relate a history of previous attacks and response to bronchodilators. The finding of wheezing in a symptomatic patient without such a history is a clue that another process may be present.[10]

Diagnosis

Airflow obstruction can be assessed by bedside spirometric analysis using portable machines; either PEF or forced expiratory volume at 1 s (FEV_1) is measured. Accurate measurement requires a cooperative patient and several (usually three) maximal-effort expirations. Severely dyspneic patients are often not able to perform the maneuver. Likewise, children may not understand the directions well enough to give a maximal effort. Since this test is effort dependent, only the maximal value should be reported. The obtained value should be compared to predicted normal values. The predicted value for spirometric measurements is dependent primarily on age, gender, and height, with only a small and clinically inconsequential adjustment for weight and ethnic background. For practical purposes, PEF or FEV_1 values greater than 80 percent of the predicted value are within the normal range. Values between 50 and 80 percent of the predicted value constitute minor airflow obstruction, values between 25 and 50 percent constitute moderate airflow obstruction, and values less than 25 percent constitute severe airflow obstruction. However, the severity of clinical symptoms is dependent as much on the rapidity of the development of obstruction as on its absolute value. Conversely, relief of symptoms is correlated more closely with the relative degree of airflow improvement than with the absolute value.

Spirometric analysis can also be used to monitor response to treatment. Because of variations in effort and measurement, a change in spirometric value of up to 6 percent can be within the error range of the test. Thus, an improvement or decline in PEF or FEV_1 of more than 8 to 10 percent from one measurement to another is significant.

A chest radiograph may be useful in assessing wheezing, particularly for patients without a history of asthma.[10] As noted elsewhere, patients with uncomplicated acute asthma do not require routine chest radiographs during their emergency department assessment and treatment. Conversely, patients with COPD and congestive heart failure who present with dyspnea and wheezing should have chest radiographs to evaluate for severity and complications.

ABG analysis is useful if clinical examination suggests hypoxemia, hypercapnia, or metabolic acidosis. The ABG analysis may also provide baseline values for further testing and treatment. However, most patients with mild-to-moderate asthma and wheezing can be assessed by spirometric analysis and do not require routine ABG analysis.

Treatment

Treatment of wheezing is directed by the underlying disorder and often involves aerosols of β_2 agonists (e.g., albuterol) and/or anticholinergics (e.g., ipratropium bromide). Patients with peribronchial inflammation are often treated with systemic (oral or intravenous) or inhaled steroids.

COUGH

Cough is a common and nonspecific symptom that may bring patients to the emergency department, particularly if the cough interferes with activity or sleep.

Pathophysiology

Cough is a protective reflex that acts to clear secretions and foreign debris from the tracheobronchial tree.[11] Coughing is initiated by stimulation of irritant receptors located largely in the larynx, trachea, and major bronchi. These receptors are stimulated by inhaled irritants (e.g., dust), allergens (e.g., ragweed pollen), toxic substances (e.g., gastric acid), hypo- or hyperosmotic liquids, inflammation (e.g., asthma), cold air, instrumentation, and excess pulmonary secretions.[12] Minor cough receptors located in the upper respiratory tract (sinuses and pharynx) and chest (pleura, pericardium, and diaphragm) may stimulate coughing. Signals from these receptors travel via the vagus, phrenic, and other nerves to the cough center in the medulla.

Once stimulated, the cough center initiates the stereotypical cough pattern: a deep inspiration followed by attempted expiration against a closed glottis that suddenly opens, providing for a forceful exhalation of gas, secretions, and foreign debris from the tracheobronchial tree. Extremely high peak airway velocities have been measured with coughing. The coughing sound is generated at the larynx and resonates in the nasal cavity and the lungs.[11]

Coughing patterns vary widely according to the underlying pathologic condition of the lung, the presence or absence of secretions, and whether the cough is voluntary or involuntary. Thus, it is not surprising that the frequency, duration, and quality of coughing vary among patients.

Clinical Features

For the purposes of differential diagnosis, cough has been subdivided into acute and chronic, although this distinction is primarily used to separate the self-limited syndromes of acute bronchitis and upper respiratory infection (URI) from other causes. For the purposes of discussion, chronic cough is defined as a cough that is present for more than 3 weeks without any periods of resolution. Cough has also been divided into nonproductive and productive with excess sputum production. That distinction may be artificial because, at least for cases of chronic cough, the same disorders produce both nonproductive and productive coughing; the distinction is without diagnostic utility.[13]

Excluding environmental exposures, acute cough is most often due to URI, lower respiratory tract infection, and allergic reactions. Common URIs are associated with a combination of rhinorrhea, sinusitis, pharyngitis, and laryngitis, with the cough due to drainage from the nasopharynx onto cough receptors in the pharynx and larynx. A productive cough is the hallmark of acute bronchitis. While pneumonia generally produces a cough, pulmonary secretions may be scant; thus, the cough is not productive and the presentation may be dominated by other symptoms (e.g., altered mental status, fever, and dyspnea). Mycobacterial and fungal pulmonary infections may produce cough, but the presentation is usually more subacute or chronic. Acute asthma is often associated with cough, but symptoms of wheezing and dyspnea usually dominate. Occasionally, a patient with asthma may present with coughing, as opposed to wheezing, as a manifestation of airflow obstruction.

Chronic cough is due to a wide variety of disorders, but studies have found that most patients have chronic cough due to (1) smoking, often with chronic bronchitis, (2) postnasal discharge, (3) asthma, (4) gastroesophageal (GE) reflux, and (5) angiotensin-converting enzyme (ACE) inhibitor therapy (Table 58-4).[14–16] The association of smoking, chronic bronchitis, and persistent cough is so obvious as to merit little discussion, other than to firmly point it out to patients. Smoking-induced coughing is usually worse in the morning and, with chronic bronchitis, usually productive. Rhinitis with postnasal discharge is associated with mucus drainage from the nose, a history of "allergies or sinus problems," and frequent clearing of the throat or swallowing of mucus. Chronic cough associated with asthma is usually worse at night, exacerbated by irritants, and associated with episodic wheezing

TABLE 58-4 Causes of Cough

Acute	Chronic: common	Chronic: less common
Upper respiratory infection: rhinitis, sinusitis, pharyngitis, laryngitis	Smoking and/or chronic bronchitis	Heart failure
Lower respiratory infection: bronchitis, pneumonia	Postnasal discharge	Bronchiectasis
Allergic reaction	Asthma: reactive airway disease	Lung cancer, other intrathoracic mass lesions
Asthma	GE reflux	Emphysema
Environmental irritants	ACE inhibitor	Pertussis (perhaps more common)
Transient airway hyperresponsiveness		Mycobacterial and fungal infection
		Recurrent aspiration
		Foreign body
		Occupational and environmental irritants
		Interstitial lung disease
		Cystic fibrosis

and dyspnea. Asthma can be exacerbated by β-blocker therapy and present with nocturnal coughing. Cough associated with GE reflux often has a history of heartburn, is worse when lying down, and improves with antiacid therapy (antacids or H_2 blockers). The incidence of ACE inhibitor cough is approximately 10 to 12 percent, although higher values have been published.[17] All ACE inhibitors have been reported to induce cough; it is not clear whether certain agents have a higher likelihood of inducing cough than others. ACE inhibitor cough is thought to result when the blockade of ACE leads to accumulation of bradykinin and substance P, which stimulate the pulmonary cough receptors and enhance the formation of irritating prostaglandin metabolites. Extreme variability characterizes ACE inhibitor cough: early (1 week) or later (1 year) onset after starting treatment, only slightly bothersome to debilitating symptoms, and variation during the day. The association of pertussis in adults with persistent cough (>2 weeks) was documented from a convenience sample from one emergency department.[18] The therapeutic implication of this finding is unclear; antibiotic treatment of adults with pertussis is controversial, and late treatment has no proven benefit. Table 58-4 lists the major causes of cough.

Diagnosis

Most causes of acute cough do not warrant routine ancillary tests. A chest radiograph may be used in patients with purulent sputum and/or fever, and spirometric analysis may be used to document the presence of airflow obstruction in patients with asthma,

Patients with chronic cough are usually treated based on clinical assessment first, and ancillary tests are performed only if symptoms persist.[14,15] Nasolaryngoscopy can be used to document the presence of mucosal inflammation and excessive mucus drainage. Sinus radiographs or computed tomography scanning can document the presence of sinusitis. A chest radiograph can detect focal or diffuse lung disease. Spirometric analysis can identify airflow obstruction, although, in cases of asthma-associated cough, the spirometric values are normal between attacks. GE reflux can be documented by a number of methods; esophageal pH monitoring is probably the most useful.

Treatment

In addition to disease-specific therapy, patients with acute cough may occasionally benefit from antitussives, which block the cough reflex at various locations. Mild cough suppressants, such as the antihistamine diphenhydramine, should be tried first. However, the most effective cough suppressants are the opiates: dextromethorphan, codeine, and oxycodone.[7,19] While cough suppressants are usually restricted to patients with a dry cough and avoided in patients with significant sputum production, there is only tradition to support this practice. Demulcents, part of most proprietary cough preparations, soothe the pharynx and somewhat suppress the cough reflex. Inhaled local anesthetics are effective cough suppressants but also suppress protective lung reflexes and may induce bronchospasm; they should be used only with great caution and under careful supervision.[20]

Because chronic cough is most often due to a few common disorders, an algorithmic approach to treatment using sequential steps appears to be effective:[21]

1. Reduce exposure to lung irritants (e.g., smoking) and discontinue ACE inhibitors and β blockers.
2. Treat for postnasal discharge with an oral antihistamine-decongestant and/or an inhaled nasal steroid. If the cough improves, continue treatment and evaluate for sinus disease with imaging studies.
3. Evaluate and treat for asthma.
4. Obtain chest and sinus radiographs if not already done.
5. Evaluate and treat for GE reflux.
6. Refer the patient for bronchoscopy.

Using a sequential approach, tailoring treatment to the clinical symptoms and the patient's responses, over 95 percent of patients achieve resolution of their cough.[16,21]

HICCUPS

Hiccup, or singultus, is an involuntary respiratory reflex with spastic contraction of the inspiratory muscles against a closed glottis, producing the characteristic sound. As opposed to coughing, where the reflex serves the useful purpose of expelling secretions and debris from the pulmonary tree, a specific protective purpose has not be elucidated for hiccups.[22]

Pathophysiology

The afferent arm of the hiccup reflex consists of the phrenic and vagus nerves as well as the thoracic sympathetic chain. There is no well-defined central hiccup center; instead, there is an intensive interconnection among the hypothalamus, medullary reticular formation, respiratory center, and cranial nerve nuclei. The efferent limb of the reflux uses the phrenic nerve, the recurrent laryngeal branch of the vagus nerve, and the motor nerves to the anterior scalene and intercostal muscles.

As noted above, hiccups are produced by spasmodic contraction of the inspiratory muscles (diaphragm and intercostals) against a closed glottis, a breakdown in the normal relationship between inspiration and glottic closure. Inspiration normally inhibits glottic closure and maintains an open airway. During swallowing, the stimulation of glottic closure inhibits inspiration, preventing aspiration. In some manner, the hiccup reflex disrupts the connection between these two processes so that 30 to 40 ms after the onset of inspiration, glottic closure is stimulated.[23] In most cases where a specific cause can be assigned, hiccups appear to result from stimulation, inflammation, or injury to one of the nerves of the reflex arc.

Clinical Features

For diagnostic classification, hiccups are divided into benign self-limited and persistent, or intractable (Table 58-5).[22,24]

Benign hiccups are generally initiated by gastric distention from food, drinking (especially carbonated beverages), or air. Alcohol ingestion appears to precipitate hiccups by relaxing the relationship between inspiration and glottic closure, making it easier for other stimuli to trigger the reflex. Excessive smoking, a sudden change in environmental temperature, and psychogenic events (excitement or stress) are sometimes associated with hiccups.

TABLE 58-5 Causes of Hiccups

Acute: benign, self-limited	Chronic: persistent, intractable
Gastric distention	Central nervous system
Alcohol ingestion	Structural lesions
Excessive smoking	Trauma
Abrupt change in environmental temperature	Vagal nerve branches
Psychogenic	Inflammation
	Mass lesion
	Phrenic nerve
	Inflammation
	Mass lesion
	Metabolic
	Uremia
	Diabetes
	Gout
	Fever
	Alcohol
	Electrolyte abnormalities
	General anesthesia
	Surgical procedures
	Thoracic
	Abdominal
	Prostate and urinary tract
	Craniotomy

Persistent hiccups are usually due to damage or irritation to a branch of the vagus or phrenic nerve. A wide variety of events have been implicated in producing persistent hiccups. One rare but readily treatable stimulus is a foreign body (often a hair) in the external auditory canal that is pressing against the tympanic membrane and stimulating the auricular branch of the vagus nerve. Several drugs—most often steroids and benzodiazepines—have been implicated in inducing hiccups, but a recent review found evidence of etiologic association unconvincing.[25]

Diagnosis

Most patients with benign hiccups resolve spontaneously or with simple maneuvers, do not seek medical attention, and do not require specific diagnosis. Patients with persistent hiccups often seek medical attention, occasionally in the emergency department.[26]

The evaluation of persistent hiccups should start with a history to determine whether a specific event was associated with the onset. Are the hiccups persistent during sleep? Persistence during sleep suggests an organic cause, and resolution during sleep suggests a psychogenic cause, although this distinction is not absolute.[24] Inquiries should be made concerning general anesthesia, surgical procedures, and several metabolic diseases that are associated with persistent hiccups. As noted above, the external auditory canal should be carefully examined. A chest radiograph should be done to evaluate for possible intrathoracic pathology. Fluoroscopy can be useful to evaluate to unilateral versus bilateral diaphragmatic movement during hiccups.

Treatment

A wide variety of physical maneuvers have been used to terminate an acute episode of hiccups. Many of these measures are based on the concept that stimulating the pharynx will block the vagal portion of the reflex arc and abolish the hiccups.[27] No one method appears to be more effective than another. Swallowing a teaspoon of granulated sugar dry is about as effective as others and does not involve the infliction of noxious or painful stimulation.

Drug treatment also works by inhibiting the reflex arc.[27] A large number of agents have been described as effective, but mostly only as case reports. Of the recommended drugs, only chlorpromazine has been tried enough to have achieved US Food and Drug Administration approval for treatment of intractable hiccups. The recommended dose is 25 to 50 mg intravenously, with a repeated dose in 2 to 4 h if needed. If improvement is noted, oral therapy with 25 to 50 mg tid or qid should be given. Metoclopramide 10 mg intravenously or intramuscularly and, if effective, followed by 10 to 20 mg qid for 10 days appears to be effective. The advantage of both these drugs is that effectiveness is usually evident in 30 min, unlike with other agents. The major disadvantages are extrapyramidal symptoms with both drugs and hypotension with chlorpromazine.

For more gradual control and with perhaps less risk of adverse reactions, oral treatment can be initiated with nifedipine (10 to 20 mg tid or qid), valproic acid (15 mg/kg per day taken tid), or baclofen (10 mg tid). Initiation and maintenance of these agents is best done in concert with a primary care physician who will follow up with the patient.

CYANOSIS

Cyanosis is a bluish color of the skin and mucous membranes that results from an increased amount of reduced hemoglobin (deoxyhemoglobin) or hemoglobin derivatives. The detection of cyanosis can be highly subjective and is not considered a sensitive indicator of the state of arterial oxygenation. In fact, cyanosis is determined by the absolute amount of reduced hemoglobin in the blood; the amount of oxygenated hemoglobin is of little influence.

Pathophysiology

Standard teaching has been that cyanosis is usually present when there is 5 g or more of reduced hemoglobin in 100 mL of capillary blood. However, this figure has been questioned recently when it was demonstrated that central cyanosis can be detected when the deoxyhemoglobin concentration is as low as 1.5 g/100 mL.[28] The increase in the amount of reduced hemoglobin in the cutaneous vessels can result from an increase in the quantity of venous blood in the skin, dilatation of the venules, or a decrease in the oxygen saturation in the capillary blood. In some instances, cyanosis can be detected when the arterial saturation has fallen to 85 percent; in others, it may not be detected until saturation is 75 percent. The absolute, rather than the relative, amount of reduced hemoglobin produces cyanosis.[29]

Various physiologic, anatomic, and physical factors other than the amount of reduced hemoglobin may influence the appearance of cyanosis, making an accurate clinical detection of the degree or even the presence of cyanosis difficult. Physiologic factors include the oxygen content of the blood, level of tissue oxygenation, degree of oxygen extraction, and oxyhemoglobin dissociation curve. Anatomic factors include the status of the cutaneous microcirculation, pigmentation, and thickness of the skin. Physical factors include the lighting under which the patient is examined and the skill of the physician. The tongue is considered one of the most sensitive sites for observing central cyanosis, and the earlobes, conjunctivae, and nail beds are considered much less reliable.

Clinical Features

Clinically, the presence of cyanosis suggests the possibility of tissue hypoxia, and possible causes for hypoxia should be considered. Unexplained cyanosis, particularly in association with normal arterial oxygen tension ($Pa{O_2}$), suggests the possibility of abnormal hemoglobin, such as methemoglobin. However, the absence of cyanosis does indicate adequate tissue oxygenation; severe states of tissue hypoxia are possible without the presence of cyanosis

Cyanosis is traditionally divided into two categories: central and peripheral. The central type is seen under conditions with unsaturated arterial blood or abnormal hemoglobin. The mucous membranes and skin are both affected. In contrast, peripheral cyanosis is due to the slowing of blood flow to an area and an abnormally great extraction of oxygen from normally saturated arterial blood. Congestive failure, peripheral vascular disease, shock states, and cold exposure all create states of vasoconstriction and decreased peripheral blood flow. The differentiation between central and peripheral cyanosis may not be possible in conditions where there may be an admixture of mechanisms (Table 58-6).

Diagnosis

The presence of cyanosis suggests the possibility of hypoxemia, and pulse oximetry analysis is readily available to assist the physician in the early diagnosis of hypoxemia and provide continuous oxygen saturation measurements. However, an exception occurs when the hemoglobin is in a state in which it is unable to bind to oxygen (i.e., methemoglobin or carboxyhemoglobin). In such situations, pulse oximetry analysis not only overestimates the oxygen saturation but also reflects a diminished response to any supplemental oxygen. ABG analysis with co-oximetry is still the gold standard in the assessment of any patient with suspected cyanosis. In central cyanosis, the oxygen saturation of the ABGs is decreased due to the underlying hypoxia. In peripheral cyanosis, assuming normal cardiopulmonary and hemoglobin status, the oxygen saturation should be normal. If methemoglobinemia or carboxyhemoglobinemia is suspected, the ABG analysis will show a normal $Pa{O_2}$ (reflecting a normal amount of dissolved oxygen in the plasma), a normal calculated oxygen saturation (from the normal $Pa{O_2}$), and a decrease in measured oxygen saturation (due to decreased number of oxygen binding sites).

Few tests are as vulnerable to errors introduced by improper sampling, handling, and storage as are ABG analyses. The technical difficulties with obtaining an arterial sample via percutaneous puncture accounts for much of the high preanalytic error rate for isolated ABG samples obtained in the emergency department, compared to a low error rate for samples obtained from an indwelling arterial catheter.

Special attention should be given to the following sources of preanalytic error with ABG samples:

1. Heparin is the anticoagulant of choice, and one make sure that the syringe is flushed with heparin and then emptied thoroughly. This will allow adequate anticoagulation of a 2- to 4-mL blood sample with assurance that the results will not be altered by the anticoagulant. Excessive heparin affects the pH, $P{CO_2}$, and $P{O_2}$ as well as the hemoglobin determination.
2. Air bubbles that mix with the blood sample will result in gas equilibration, significantly lowering the $P{CO_2}$ values with an increase in pH and $P{O_2}$. Any sample obtained with more than minor air bubbles should be discarded.
3. Reducing the temperature of the blood by placing the sample immediately in an ice slush will significantly deter changes in the $P{CO_2}$ and pH for a period of several hours. If the sample is not iced immediately, changes can be significant. As a general rule, arterial blood samples should be analyzed within 10 min or cooled immediately. Failure to properly cool the sample is a common source of preanalytic error.

Hypoxemia, anemia, and polycythemia can be diagnosed by means of hemoglobin and ABG determination. The red cyanosis of polycythemia vera occurs because the increase in the number of red blood cells and the hemoglobin concentration results in sludging of blood flow in cutaneous capillaries and venules. Similarly, cyanosis is enhanced in chronic hypoxemia accompanied by polycythemia.

If the $Pa{O_2}$ and the hemoglobin concentration are normal, the cyanosis may be due to abnormal skin pigmentation or abnormal hemoglobin. The term pseudocyanosis is used to describe a blue, gray, or purple cutaneous discoloration that may mimic cyanosis. Pseudocyanosis can be caused by heavy metals [e.g., iron (hemochromatosis), gold, silver, lead, or arsenic] or drugs (e.g., phenothiazines, minocycline, amiodarone, or chloroquine). Chrysiasis is a specific type of pseudocyanosis that is characterized by a gray, blue, or purple pigmentation of areas exposed to light. It is a rare dose-dependent complication of gold treatment that tends to cause permanent discoloration of the skin. Another example of pseudocyanosis is argyria, which is a slate blue-to-gray coloration of the skin resulting from either chronic ingestion or chronic local application of silver salts or colloidal silver. In pseudocyanosis the skin does not blanch with pressure, in contrast to true cyanotic skin, which does blanch. Carboxyhemoglobinemia does not cause cyanosis. Occasionally, however, carboxyhemoglobinemia does produce a cherry-red flush of the skin, retina, or mucous membranes.

Cyanosis can be caused by methemoglobinemia and sulfhemoglobinemia. Most cases are due to chemicals or medications. Although a wide range of drugs can produce methemoglobinemia, benzocaine, nitrates, and nitrites are the most common agents implicated in drug-induced methemoglobinemia. Sulfhemoglobinemia most commonly results from either phenacetin or acetanilid (Bromo Seltzer). Industrial aniline compounds may produce either sulfhemoglobinemia or methemoglobinemia.

The incidence of acquired methemoglobinemia secondary to industrial exposure to aniline dyes and aromatic amino and nitro compounds has decreased with improvement in occupational health standards. Hereditary methemoglobinemia is a rare genetic disorder affecting

TABLE 58-6 Causes of Cyanosis

Central Cyanosis	Peripheral Cyanosis
Decreased arterial oxygen saturation	Reduced cardiac output
Decreased atmospheric pressure: high altitude	Cold exposure
Impaired pulmonary function	Redistribution of blood flow from extremities
Alveolar hypoventilation	Arterial obstruction
Uneven relationships between pulmonary ventilation and perfusion	Venous obstruction
Impaired oxygen diffusion	
Anatomic shunts	
Certain types of congenital heart disease	
Pulmonary arteriovenous fistulas	
Multiple small intrapulmonary shunts	
Hemoglobin with low affinity for oxygen	
Hemoglobin abnormalities	
Methemoglobinemia: hereditary, acquired	
Sulfhemoglobinemia: acquired	
Carboxyhemoglobinemia (not true cyanosis)	

Source: From Braunwald E, in Wilson J, Braunwald E, Isselbacher KJ, et al (eds): *Harrison's Principles of Internal Medicine,* 12th ed. New York, McGraw-Hill, 1991. Used by permission.

the enzyme NADH-methemoglobin reductase, resulting in structural alterations of the hemoglobin molecule. This enzyme is the major pathway responsible for converting methemoglobin to its reduced state. This pathway plays a clinically significant role in the treatment of methemoglobinemia because it is the pathway by which the antidote, methylene blue, is able to enhance the reduction of methemoglobin. Patients with NADH-methemoglobin reductase deficiency appear cyanotic but are usually compensated and asymptomatic.

Methemoglobinemia produces visible cyanosis with as little as 1.5 g of methemoglobin per 100 mL of blood. Since methemoglobin is incapable of binding with oxygen, the symptoms of methemoglobinemia are secondary to hypoxia, and the severity is related to the quantity of methemoglobin present, the rapidity of onset, and the patient's cardiopulmonary system. Cyanotic patients without cardiovascular or pulmonary disease should be suspected of having methemoglobinemia, especially if cyanosis is not relieved by oxygen administration. An additional clue is that venous blood will appear chocolate brown. Spectrophotometric analysis is required for identification of the pigment and its quantity.

Sulfhemoglobin is inert as an oxygen carrier and can produce deep cyanosis at a level of less than 0.5 g of sulfhemoglobin per 100 mL of blood. Unlike methemoglobinemia, sulfhemoglobinemia is irreversible. Treatment is directed toward symptomatic and supportive care as well as the identification and removal of suspected agents.

Treatment

Patients with central cyanosis should be started on supplemental oxygen. Failure to improve suggests either impaired circulation (shock), abnormal hemoglobin, or pseudocyanosis.

In acquired methemoglobinemia, no treatment is necessary unless signs of hypoxia (i.e., angina, arrhythmias, hypotension, stupor, or coma) are present. Methylene blue in a dose of 1 to 2 mg/kg of body weight given intravenously over 5 min as a 1% solution (0.1 to 0.2 ml/kg) is the antidote for acquired methemoglobinemia. Caution should be taken whenever methylene blue is used; by itself, at high doses, it can cause hemolysis or even precipitate methemoglobinemia and possibly worsen the patient's condition.

REFERENCES

1. Sharma OP: Symptoms and signs in pulmonary medicine: Old observations and new interpretations. *Dis Mon* 41:577, 1995.
2. Manning HL, Schwartzstein RM: Pathophysiology of dyspnea. *N Engl J Med* 333:1547, 1995.
3. American Thoracic Society: Dyspnea. Mechanism, assessment, and management: A consensus statement. *Am J Respir Care Med* 159:321, 1999.
4. Mulrow CD, Lucey CR, Farnett LE: Discriminating causes of dyspnea through clinical examination. *J Gen Intern Med* 8:383, 1993.
5. Joffe D, Berend N: Assessment and management of dyspnoea. *Respirology* 2:33, 1997.
6. Morgan WC, Hodge HL: Diagnostic evaluation of dyspnea. *Am Fam Physician* 15:711, 1998.
7. Davis CL: ABC of palliative care: Breathlessness, cough, and other respiratory problems. *BMJ* 315:931, 1997.
8. Pasterknap H, Kraman SS, Wodicka GR: Respiratory sounds: Advances beyond the stethoscope. *Am J Respir Crit Care Med* 156:974, 1997.
9. Meslier N, Charbonneau G, Racineux JL: Wheezes. *Eur Respir J* 8:1942, 1995.
10. Holden DA, Mehta AC: Evaluation of wheezing in the nonasthmatic patient. *Cleve Clin J Med* 57:345, 1990.
11. Piirila P, Sovijarvi ARA: Objective assessment of cough. *Eur Respir J* 8:1949, 1995.
12. Lalloo UG, Barnes PJ, Chung KF: Pathophysiology and clinical presentations of cough. *J Allergy Clin Immunol* 98:S91, 1996.
13. Smyrnios NA, Irwin RS, Curley RS: Chronic cough with history of excessive sputum production: The spectrum and frequency of causes. Key components of the diagnostic evaluation and outcome of specific therapy. *Chest* 108:991, 1995.
14. Tan RA, Spector SL: Chronic cough. *Compr Ther* 23:467, 1997.
15. Philip EB: Chronic cough. *Am Fam Physician* 56:1395, 1997.

16. Smyrnios NA, Irwin RS, Curley FJ, French CL: From a prospective study of chronic cough: Diagnostic and therapeutic aspects in older adults. *Arch Intern Med* 158:1222, 1998.
17. Pylypchuk GB: ACE inhibitor versus angiotensin II Blocker-induced cough and angioedema. *Ann Pharmacother* 32:1060, 1998
18. Wright SW, Edwards KM, Decker MD, Zeldin MH: Pertussis infection in adults with persistent cough. *JAMA* 273:1044, 1995.
19. Chung KF: Methods of assessing cough and antitussives in man. *Pulm Pharmacol* 9:373, 1996.
20. Fuller RW, Jackson DM: Physiology and treatment of cough. *Thorax* 45:425, 1990.
21. Pratter MR, Bartter T, Akers S, DuBois J: An algorithmic approach to chronic cough. *Ann Intern Med* 119:977, 1993.
22. Launois S, Bizec JL, Whitelaw WA, et al: Hiccup in adults: An overview. *Eur Respir J* 6:563, 1993.
23. Askenasy JJ: About the mechanism of hiccup. *Eur Neurol* 32:159, 1992.
24. Rousseau P: Hiccups. *South Med J* 88:175, 1995.
25. Thompson DF, Landry JP: Drug-induced hiccups. *Ann Pharmacother* 31:367, 1997.
26. Kolodzik PW, Eilers MA: Hiccups (singultus): Review and approach to management. *Ann Emerg Med* 20:565, 1991.
27. Friedman NL: Hiccups: A treatment review. *Pharmacotherapy* 16:986, 1996.
28. Gross GA, Hayes JA, Burden JGW: Deoxyhaemoglobin concentrations in the detection of central cyanosis. *Thorax* 43:212, 1988.
29. Martin L, Khalil H: How much reduced hemoglobin is necessary to generate central cyanosis? *Chest* 97:1, 1990.

59 BRONCHITIS AND PNEUMONIA

Donald A. Moffa, Jr.
Charles L. Emerman

ACUTE BRONCHITIS

Epidemiology

Acute bronchitis may occur in outbreaks as a respiratory virus spreads through a population, or it may be sporadic. It accounts for more than seven million outpatient physician visits among patients older than age 18. Antibiotics are prescribed more than half of the time to treat this condition even though most cases are self-limited and antibiotic therapy has not been shown conclusively to alter outcomes.

Pathophysiology

Acute bronchitis, an infection of the conducting airways of the lung, produces inflammation, exudate, and sometimes bronchospasm of the involved airways. The majority of acute bronchitis is caused by viruses, including influenza A and B, adenovirus, parainfluenza virus, rhinovirus, respiratory syncytial virus (RSV), coxsackievirus A21 and, less commonly, measles, rubella, herpesviruses, or coronaviruses.[1] Enteroviruses such as coxsackievirus and echovirus may cause acute bronchitis, primarily in the summer, whereas rhinovirus may be suspect year round. Most other viruses cause bronchitis from early fall to spring. Influenza is more prevalent during the winter. Adults who have contact with children may develop acute bronchitis and pneumonia from RSV.[2] Measles and herpes simplex viruses may cause severe cases. Bacteria known to contribute to acute bronchitis include *Bordatella pertussis, Mycoplasma pneumoniae, Chlamydia pneumoniae,* and possibly *Streptococcus pneumoniae.*[3]

Clinical Features

The hallmark of acute bronchitis is cough, usually productive, in patients without evidence of pneumonia, sinusitis, or chronic pulmonary disease. Patients may have rhinitis (nasal congestion and discharge), myalgias, and fever.[1] Sputum may be clear or colored, and the presence of colored sputum does not necessarily indicate a bacterial infection. Patients may complain of dyspnea or wheezing; usually due to bronchospasm.

Acute bronchitis caused by influenza A and B usually includes the abrupt onset of fever, chills, headaches, and myalgias that subside over 3 to 4 days, followed by 1 to 2 weeks of nonproductive cough and malaise. Less commonly, patients present with pharyngitis or tracheobronchitis. One-quarter may have rales or wheezes. Outbreaks occur from October to April.

Bordatella pertussis as a cause of acute bronchitis in adults has been increasing since 1981 and has been implicated as a causative agent in adults with chronic cough.[3] Protection owing to childhood immunization diminishes within 4 to 12 years. Cough is usually preceded by low-grade fever, rhinorrhea, and conjunctivitis, but adults usually lack the characteristic "whoop" heard in children. Commonly, available culture and direct fluorescence antibody test of nasopharyngeal swabs are uniformly negative.[3]

Mycoplasma pneumoniae affects mainly older children and young adults and may occur throughout the year, with epidemics occurring every 4 to 7 years. The incubation period is 16 to 30 days. Given the usual brevity of symptoms and relatively quick resolution of illness, diagnostic tests are usually not warranted unless pneumonia is suspected.

Chlamydia pneumoniae, which may cause wheezing associated with acute bronchitis and chronic asthma, has a 30-day incubation period and is found mainly in the elderly. Patients may be afebrile and produce minimal sputum, and laryngitis may be more common than with mycoplasmal or viral infections. Symptoms may persist even after adequate antibiotic therapy.

Diagnosis

Clinical diagnosis is appropriately made when these findings are present: (1) an acute cough (for less than 1 week), (2) no prior lung disease, (3) normal arterial oxygenation, and (4) no auscultatory abnormalities. As noted previously, wheezing in patients without prior history of asthma indicates bronchospasm stimulated by the bronchitic inflammation.

A chest radiograph is not required for straightforward cases of acute bronchitis. As noted below, the absence of fever, tachycardia, tachypnea, or auscultatory abnormalities reduces the likelihood of a radiographic infiltrate to less than 1 percent. Pulse oximetry is indicated if a patient complains of dyspnea or is noted to be cyanotic or short of breath. Bedside spirometry [peak expiratory flow (PEF) or forced expiratory volume in 1 s (FEV_1)] should be done if a patient complains of dyspnea or wheezing or if wheezing is heard on examination. Blood tests are not indicated in routine cases. Sputum cultures are not indicated in immunocompetent patients.

Treatment

Nine randomized, double-blind, placebo-controlled trials were undertaken between 1966 and 1995 to determine antibiotic effectiveness in treating acute bronchitis.[4,5] Whereas two studies reported improvement in symptoms, and a trend toward resolution of cough and clinical improvement at follow-up were noted, systematic review did not find statistical benefit for antibiotic treatment. Most cases of acute bronchitis are self-limited, and patients recover at the same rate regardless of antibiotic treatment. Even if there is evidence of bacterial infection with *B. pertussis, M. pneumoniae, C. pneumoniae,* or *S. pneumoniae,* there is no evidence that antibiotic treatment hastens improvement. There is some evidence that older adults and patients with underlying chronic obstructive pulmonary disease (COPD) benefit from antibiotic treatment for acute bronchitis.[5,6] However, until controlled trials are performed, routine antibiotic use even in these patients cannot be recommended.

There is evidence that bronchodilators are useful in treating acute bronchitis, compared with either placebo or erythromycin. Patients' report decreased cough and faster return to work when treated with oral or inhaled albuterol.[7,8] A significant bronchodilator response, as measured by an improvement in PEF or FEV_1 of greater than 10 to 12 percent, may be useful in determining whether outpatient treatment is useful. The administration of inhaled (metered dose inhaler, 2 puffs q 4 to 6 h) or oral (2 mg tid to qid) albuterol should be considered in acute bronchitis, especially if reversible bronchospasm is present.

Amantadine has been shown to shorten the duration and severity of influenza A in up to half of patients who receive it within 48 h of symptom onset (see Chap. 150, "Common Viral Infections"). Amantadine or rimantadine may be effective in treating acute bronchitis caused by this agent. Aerosolized ribavirin may also be helpful in patients with acute bronchitis due to RSV.

Disposition

Patients with acute bronchitis should be discharged with appropriate instructions for rest, for hydration, and to watch carefully for symptoms of worsening: dyspnea, fever, and lethargy. It usually takes 3 to 4 weeks for cough to resolve completely and for general well-being to return.

TABLE 59-1 Risk Factors for Pneumonia

Aspiration risk
Swallowing and esophageal motility disorders
Stroke
Nasogastric tube
Intubation
Seizure and syncope
Bacteremia risk
Indwelling vascular devices
Intrathoracic devices (e.g., chest tube)
Debilitation
Alcoholism
Extremes of age
Neoplasia
Immunosuppression
Chronic diseases
Diabetes
Renal failure
Liver failure
Valvular heart disease
Congestive heart failure
Pulmonary disorders
Chronic obstructive pulmonary disease
Chest wall disorders
Skeletal muscle disorders
Bronchial obstruction
Bronchoscopy
Viral lung infections

PNEUMONIA

Epidemiology

Community-acquired pneumonia (CAP) is a common medical problem accounting for about 4 million visits to physicians and 600,000 adult hospitalizations per year.[9] Pneumonia is the sixth leading cause of death and is particularly lethal among very young children and older adults, in whom the disease is more common. Whereas older studies of pneumonia pointed to pneumococcus as the most common cause of pneumonia, there is an increasing frequency of atypical or opportunistic infections.[10,11] Unfortunately, although the classic presentation of pneumococcal pneumonia is generally apparent, atypical infections, infections in compromised hosts, and infections in extremes of age may present with more subtle findings.[12] Older patients often present with a change in mental status and often do not manifest respiratory symptoms. Pneumonia may occur through a variety of routes of infection. Pathogenic organisms may be inhaled or aspirated directly into the lungs. Alternatively, some bacteria, such as *Staphylococcus aureus* or pneumococcus, may develop as a result of hematogenous seeding. With this in mind, patients most at risk for pneumonia are those with a predisposition to aspiration, impaired mucociliary clearance, or risk of bacteremia (Table 59-1).

Pathophysiology

Pneumonia is an infection of the alveolar or gas-exchange portions of the lung. Some types of pneumonia produce an intense inflammatory response within the alveoli that leads to filling of the airspace with organisms, exudate, and white blood cells. Pneumonia can spread throughout the lung by the bronchial tree or through the pores of Kohn. Bacterial pneumonia, with an intense inflammatory response, tends to cause a productive cough, whereas other atypical organisms do not lead to such an intense inflammatory response and may only be associated with mild nonproductive cough.

Most of our knowledge about the etiology of pneumonia has been derived from studies of hospitalized patients where pneumococcus was the overwhelming cause. Prospective studies of both inpatients and outpatients with CAP often (up to 40 to 60 percent of the time) fail to identify a specific pathogen.[10,11] When an etiology is found, pneumococcus is still the most common single agent, followed by viruses and the atypical agents such as *Mycoplasma, Chlamydia,* and *Legionella.* In up to 5 percent, multiple agents are identified. Special populations, including nursing-home residents, chronic alcoholics, and HIV-infected patients, may have a somewhat different spectrum of disease.

Clinical Features

Pneumonia can present with a variety of clinical features, many of which overlap with other entities. There is wide variability in the presence of individual symptoms and physical findings.[13] The typical presentation of pneumococcal pneumonia is a sudden onset of illness with fever, rigors, dyspnea, bloody sputum production, chest pain, tachycardia, tachypnea, and abnormal findings by lung examination. Many other types of pneumonia do not have such a sudden and characteristic presentation. Especially in the elderly, the immunocompromised, and children, dramatic presentations are unusual. Sputum production is not necessarily present, particularly with mycoplasmal or viral agents. Pneumonia may be preceded by symptoms of a viral upper respiratory infection with coryza, low-grade temperature, rhinorrhea, or nonproductive cough. Weight loss, malaise, dizziness, and weakness may be associated with pneumonia. Some of the atypical agents are associated with dramatic presentations of headache or gastrointestinal (GI) illness. Occasionally, pneumonia is associated with extrapulmonary symptoms, including joint pain, hematuria, or skin rashes.

The physical examination may show evidence of alveolar fluid (inspiratory rales), consolidation (bronchial breath sounds), pleural effusion (dullness and decreased breath sounds), or bronchial congestion (rhonchi and wheezing). Tachypnea, tachycardia, fever, and hypotension are associated with severe illness and may not be present in all cases.

PNEUMOCOCCAL PNEUMONIA The pneumococcus, although it affects all age groups, is particularly prevalent with the extremes of age.[14] Classically, patients present with sudden onset of disease with rigors, bloody sputum, high fever, and chest pain. This presentation commonly occurs in young adults, particularly in those in crowded living situations such as may occur in a military camp. In this setting, patients will frequently have lobar pneumonia, with parapneumonic pleural effusions occurring in about 25 percent of patients. Patients with functional or anatomic asplenism or patients being treated with immunosuppressive drugs, such as transplant patients, may have a very rapid progression of disease, with acute prostration and septic shock progressing to multisystem organ failure. Patients with chronic lung disease, nursing-home patients, or otherwise healthy elderly patients may have a slower progression of the disease. They may present with malaise and dehydration associated with minimal cough or sputum production. Along with the frequent finding of leukocytosis, elevation of the serum bilirubin or other liver enzymes may be seen. In addition, hyponatremia may be a finding in many causes of pneumonia, including pneumococcal pneumonia.

Pneumococcal pneumonia will respond to a variety of antibiotics, although there is an increased incidence of penicillin-resistant pneumococci. The risk factors for penicillin resistance include patients at the extremes of age, day-care attendance, immunosuppression from alcoholism or cancer, or travel to areas where penicillin resistance is common, including the Mediterranean. In addition to penicillin resistance, there is increasing resistance to other common antibiotics, including tetracycline, azithromycin, and trimethoprim-sulfamethoxazole (TMP-SMX). Patients with intermediate penicillin-resistant pneumococci may still be effectively treated with routine antibiotics so long as an adequate dose is administered. Patients with highly penicillin-resistant pneumococci require treatment with either vancomycin, imipenem, or levofloxacin.

STAPHYLOCOCCAL PNEUMONIA *Staphylococcus aureus* is a consideration in patients with chronic lung disease, patients with laryngeal cancer, immunosuppressed patients, nursing-home patients, or others at risk for aspiration pneumonia. *Staphylococcus aureus* may occur in otherwise healthy patients following viral illness, such as during an influenza epidemic. But even there, pneumococcus is still more common. Patients with staphylococcal pneumonia typically have an insidious onset of disease with low-grade fever, sputum production, and dyspnea. The chest radiograph usually demonstrates extensive disease with empyema, pleural effusions, and multiple areas of infiltrate.

OTHER BACTERIAL PNEUMONIA *Klebsiella* pneumonia usually occurs in compromised patients: patients at risk of aspiration, alcoholics, the elderly, and other patients with chronic lung disease. In contrast to *S. aureus,* patients with *Klebsiella* have acute onset of severe disease with fever, rigors, and chest pain. Herpes labialis is occasionally associated with *Klebsiella* pneumonia. Patients with *Klebsiella* may develop abscesses, although more commonly they have a lobar infiltrate.

Pseudomonas causes a severe pneumonia with cyanosis, confusion, and other signs of systemic illness. The chest radiograph usually shows bilateral lower lobe infiltrates, occasionally associated with empyema. *Pseudomonas* is not a typical cause of CAP, but may be seen in patients who have had prolonged hospitalization or are nursing-home residents.

Haemophilus influenzae pneumonia may be seen both in pediatric patients and in the elderly and should be considered in patients with chronic lung disease, sickle cell disease, or immunocompromised disorders and in alcoholics and diabetics. Patients may either have a gradual progression of disease with low-grade fever and sputum production or occasionally have the sudden onset of chest pain, dyspnea, and sputum production. Bacteremia may be seen in older adults. Pleural effusions and multilobar infiltrates are common findings in *H. influenza* pneumonia.

Moraxella catarrhalis pneumonia has clinical features similar in spectrum to those of *H. influenzae.*[15] Typically, patients with *M. catarrhalis* present with an indolent course of cough and sputum production. Generally, pneumonia with this organism occurs during the winter. Fever and pleuritic chest pain are common clinical symptoms. The chest radiograph usually shows diffuse infiltrates.

ATYPICAL PNEUMONIA Atypical agents are being recognized more frequently as a cause of pneumonia in older children, in young adults, and in the elderly. Because these agents lack a cell wall, they do not respond to β-lactam antibiotics, and current recommendations for empiric antibiotic treatment of CAP take this into account, using either a macrolide or newer-generation fluoroquinolone.

Legionella can cause a range of illness from benign self-limited disease to multisystem organ failure with acute respiratory distress syndrome. Patients at particular risk include cigarette smokers, patients with chronic lung disease, transplant patients, and immunosuppressed patients. There is no seasonality to *Legionella* pneumonia, making it a more common cause of pneumonia in the summer. *Legionella* pneumonia is commonly complicated by GI symptoms, including abdominal pain, vomiting, and diarrhea. In addition, *Legionella* can affect other organ systems, causing sinusitis, pancreatitis, myocarditis, and pyelonephritis. The chest radiograph frequently shows a patchy infiltrate, with the occasional appearance of hilar adenopathy and pleural effusions.

Chlamydia pneumonia is a common cause of respiratory infection, with about half of the population demonstrating antibodies by the age of 15. Infection with *Chlamydia* usually causes a mild subacute illness with sore throat, mild fever, and nonproductive cough, although occasionally patients have a more severe course. Patients with *Chlamydia* pneumonia frequently have abnormal physical examination findings, with rales or rhonchi. The chest radiograph usually shows a patchy subsegmental infiltrate. Chlamydial infection has been associated with the development of adult-onset asthma.

Mycoplasma pneumonia also occurs year round, although it tends to cluster in epidemics every 4 to 8 years.[16] As is the case with *Chlamydia,* it may cause a subacute respiratory illness with cough, sore throat, and headache. *Mycoplasma* pneumonia is frequently associated with retrosternal chest pain. Unlike *Legionella, Mycoplasma* usually is not associated with GI symptoms. The chest radiograph shows patchy infiltrates, with the common occurrence of hilar adenopathy and pleural effusions. *Mycoplasma* occasionally causes extrapulmonary symptoms, including bullous myringitis, rash, neurologic symptoms, arthritis and arthralgia, hematologic abnormalities and, rarely, renal failure.

Diagnosis

Pneumonia is suspected based on a constellation of symptoms and signs, but individual symptoms and clinical findings lack accuracy for precise diagnosis.[13] Attempts have been made to combine some of the symptoms and signs into a scoring system that predicts the probability of pneumonia, and four different decision rules were compared in a study of adult outpatients (Table 59-2). The results of these attempts indicate that clinical criteria are most useful for "ruling out" pneumonia; that is, if a patient has none of the positive predictors, the probability of pneumonia is very low, from 1 to 4 percent. However, clinical criteria are inaccurate for "ruling in" pneumonia; even if a patient has all of the positive clinical predictors, these scoring systems predict pneumonia with a maximal probability of 40 to 50 percent.[13] Thus, for accurate diagnosis, a chest radiograph is required.

Patients with complaints of dyspnea or physical signs of respiratory distress (tachypnea, use of accessory muscles, wheezing, etc.) should have oxygen saturation measured by pulse oximetry. In young, other-

TABLE 59-2 Prediction Rules for Pneumonia in Adult Patients with Cough

Author and Rule	Threshold Score	Sensitivity, %	Specificity, %	Positive Predictive Value, % (Prevalence = 7%)
Diehr et al[32] Points: −2 for rhinorrhea −1 for sore throat 1 for night sweats 1 for myalgia 1 for sputum all day 2 for respiratory rate > 25 2 for temperature > 38°C (100°F) Total score, −3 to 7	0	67	67	14
Singal et al,[33] Probability = $1/(1 + e^{-y})$, where $y = -3.095 + 1.214$ (cough) + 1.007 (fever) + 0.823 (rales) Each variable = 1 if present and 0 if absent	All three, cough and fever, or cough and rales	76	55	12
Gennis et al[34] Positive, if any: T > 37.8°C (100.04F) Heart rate > 100 Respiratory rate > 20	Any abnormality	62	76	17
Heckerling et al[35] Points (one each for): Absence of asthma Temperature > 37.8°C (100.4°F) Heart rate > 100 Decreased breath sounds Rales Total score, 0 to 5	+2	71	67	15

Source: From Emerman et al,[31] with permission.

wise healthy, mildly ill, ambulatory patients, no further ancillary testing may be necessary. If a patient requires admission, additional tests recommended include complete blood count and determination of serum electrolyte, blood urea nitrogen, creatinine, and glucose levels.[9] Evaluation of arterial blood gas is indicated if patients are hypoxic or have moderate to severe respiratory distress. No single set of recommendations for diagnostic testing can encompass all patients, and additional ancillary studies should be obtained according to appropriate indications.

In patients with fever, cough, and radiographic abnormalities, the etiology of the infection is confirmed by identification of a pathogenic organism from the blood, sputum, or pleural fluid. Atypical agents may be demonstrated by a variety of sophisticated laboratory techniques, including evaluation of titers from acute and convalescence sera or by direct fluorescent antibody testing. In hospitalized patients with CAP, about 10 percent will have a positive blood culture, most of which are pneumococcal.[10] The incidence of positive blood cultures in nonhospitalized patients with CAP is lower, pathogen identification does not alter treatment, and the overwhelming majority of patients respond to empiric antibiotic treatment.[11] Thus, blood cultures are recommended only for patients who require hospitalization.

The value of sputum examination in CAP has been debated.[9] The yield of a sputum Gram stain is reduced in the 10 to 30 percent of patients unable to produce sputum, in the 15 to 30 percent of patients who have already received antibiotic therapy, and in the 30 to 65 percent of patients who have a negative Gram stain despite a positive culture. Taken together, the sputum Gram stain is positive in only 10 to 40 percent of cases with CAP. The test is noninvasive and inexpensive, however, so it is often advocated.[9–11] Pneumococcal pneumonia may be suspected in patients with more than 10 gram-positive, lancet-shaped diplococci from an adequate sputum sample. *Haemophilus influenzae* may also be occasionally demonstrated on Gram stain. There are few indications for performing transtracheal aspiration or bronchial washings in the emergency department.

The differential diagnosis of patients with cough and radiographic abnormality includes a number of disorders, such as lung cancer, tuberculosis, pulmonary embolism, chemical or hypersensitivity pneumonitis, connective tissue disorders, granulomatous disease, and fungal infections.

A chest radiograph may provide clues to the underlying organism.[17] Pneumococcal pneumonia typically presents with lobar segmental pneumonia. Occasionally, patients may present with the so-called round infiltrate of pneumococcal pneumonia. In general, patients with bacterial pneumonia are more likely to have unilobar or focal infiltrates than patients with viral or atypical pneumonia. Hilar adenopathy is more common in patients with atypical pneumonia. Pleural effusions occur more commonly in patients with bacterial pneumonia, although occasionally patients with viral pneumonia or atypical agents may have small effusions. Cavitary lesions occur in patients with bacterial or tuberculous lesions. Lung abscesses are rare complications of pneumonia in the antibiotic era, but they occur due to *S. aureus* or *Klebsiella.* Pneumonia may mimic the appearance of lung masses particularly when the pneumonia is pneumococcal and staphylococcal. Other atypical pneumonia such as Q fever and tularemia may present with discrete masses.

Specific Issues

PNEUMONIA IN COPD PATIENTS Patients with COPD have a higher incidence of pneumonia than other outpatient populations who have no identifiable predisposition to pneumonia.[18] Frequent antibiotic use has been blamed for colonization of the respiratory tract by more pathogenic organisms. As a result, there has been more frequent identification of aerobic gram-negative rods and a decline in pneumococcal disease.

Inflammation of large and small airways, bronchial wall distortion, and bullae formation are pulmonary changes affecting patients who have COPD. The lower respiratory tract, which is ordinarily sterile in healthy nonsmokers, in COPD becomes colonized with potentially pathogenic bacteria, and it is assumed that these organisms may cause pneumonia. The risk factors for gram-negative colonization in COPD include advanced age, serious underlying illness, cigarette smoking, recent antibiotic use, endotracheal intubation, malnutrition, viral tracheobronchitis, corticosteroid use, prolonged hospitalization, and advanced pulmonary disease. Patients with stable chronic bronchitis are predominantly colonized with *S. pneumoniae* and nontypeable *H. influenzae.* Although pneumococcal pneumonia occurs more commonly in COPD than in other outpatient groups, its relative frequency appears to be declining. The incidence of pseudomonal pneumonia is low, but certain therapies such as frequent use of broad-spectrum antibiotics and corticosteroids, endotracheal intubation, and instrumentation of the lower respiratory tract may introduce *Pseudomonas aeruginosa* and other bacteria into the lower respiratory tract.

Clinical manifestations of pneumonia in COPD patients may include dyspnea, cough with sputum production, bronchial hyperactivity, or severe fixed airflow obstruction, pleuritic chest pain, and altered mentation. Fever, leukocytosis, and respiratory symptoms are unreliable indicators of pneumonia and may be absent in as many as half of the patients. Physical examination may show signs of lung consolidation. These signs and symptoms are nonspecific in the setting of preexisting lung disease. The classic presentation of pneumococcal pneumonia of acute fever, chills, and pleuritic chest pain may not occur in COPD patients. Instead, symptoms may be more insidious and appear to represent an exacerbation of the underlying disease. The chest radiograph may show a bilateral patchy bronchopneumonia more frequently than lobar pneumonia.

COPD patients with *H. influenzae* pneumonia typically present with gradually increasing cough, sputum production, and shortness of breath. Fever is mild, and arthralgias and myalgias are common. The chest radiograph may initially be considered unchanged, but a patchy bronchopneumonia pattern is common.

COPD patients treated with frequent courses of corticosteroids may develop nonbacterial infections that mimic bacterial pneumonia, including those caused by *Aspergillus fumigatus, Strongyloides stercoralis,* and *Mycobacterium tuberculosis. Aspergillus* causes both a rapidly progressive, necrotizing pneumonia or an indolent form with a less fulminant course. *Strongyloides* can cause bronchospasm, pneumonia, pulmonary infarction, or respiratory failure. The chest radiograph may show alveolar infiltrates, nodular infiltrates, cavitary lesions, or lung abscess.

PNEUMONIA IN DIABETICS Diabetes is associated with an increased risk of recurrent bacterial pneumonia, more serious infection, and higher hospitalization rates.[19] Diabetic patients with pneumococcal disease are more likely than nondiabetics to develop bacteremia, and bacteremia doubles the mortality rate. Diabetics have a higher risk of developing complications from gram-negative pneumonia, such as empyema, lung necrosis, metastatic infections, and bacteremia.

There are two patterns of susceptibility to lower respiratory tract infections in diabetic hosts. First, pulmonary infections that occur with *increased frequency* include those caused by *S. aureus,* gram-negative bacteria, *M. tuberculosis,* and mucormycosis. These infections may occur from aspiration of bacteria from a colonized pharynx, hematogenous spread from an extrapulmonary infection, or contaminated equipment such as nebulizers. Second, pulmonary infections associated with *increased morbidity and mortality* include those caused by *S. pneumoniae, Legionella,* and influenza. Vascular insufficiency, cardiovascular disease, chronic renal insufficiency, or malnutrition may contribute to increased morbidity and mortality.

As with other populations, diabetic patients with pneumonia are often treated empirically, though treatment should be guided by pathogen isolation whenever possible. An alternative to aminoglycosides should be used whenever possible in diabetics who may already have neuropathy or nephropathy from diabetes.

PNEUMONIA IN PREGNANCY Pneumonia in the peripartum period poses threats to the developing fetus as well as the expectant mother and is the most common nonobstetric infection to cause maternal mortality during that period.[20] Antepartum respiratory infection is associated with preterm delivery and fetal loss. Studies have shown a decline in antepartum pneumonia from one case per 367 deliveries during the early 1970s to one case per 2288 deliveries in the late 1980s. Preterm labor is more likely when pneumonia occurs between weeks 20 and 36 of gestation.

Physiologic changes during pregnancy and various therapeutic interventions, such as tocolytics that increase lung water, may predispose pregnant patients to pneumonia. Pneumonia in the postpartum period is commonly attributed to aspiration during labor and delivery. Unusual pathogens that may cause pneumonia in pregnancy include mumps virus, Epstein-Barr virus, swine influenza, influenza A, varicella, *Coccidioides immitis,* and other fungi.

Varicella infection in pregnancy is infrequent (0.7 cases per 1000 pregnancies), but as many as 9 percent of primary varicella infections during pregnancy develop varicella pneumonia. Patients with varicella pneumonia may have cough, dyspnea, pleuritic chest pain, and hemoptysis a few days after the onset of fever, rash, and malaise. The chest radiograph typically shows diffuse miliary or nodular infiltrates that resolve within 2 weeks but may show fulminant pneumonitis or acute respiratory distress syndrome. The mortality rate from varicella pneumonia in nonpregnant patients is 11 to 17 percent, but the rate may be higher in pregnancy.

Penicillins, cephalosporins, and erythromycin, excluding the estolate form, are safe in pregnancy. Clindamycin is likely safe. Tetracycline given in the third trimester may cause fulminant hepatitis in the mother or cause bony and dental abnormalities in the developing fetus if given anytime during pregnancy. Sulfonamides may cause fetal kernicteris if given shortly before delivery. Chloramphenicol can cause fetal bone marrow suppression and gray baby syndrome. Aminoglycosides and vancomycin should be used only when absolutely necessary to avoid fetal renal toxicity and ototoxicity.

Bacterial pneumonia complicating influenza or other viral infections should be treated with antibiotics directed at the likely superinfecting organism. Oral amantadine or inhaled ribavirin may be used if viral pneumonia complicates an influenza infection and for prophylaxis in pregnant women at high risk for influenza infection. Ribavirin is active against influenza A and B, whereas amantadine is active only against influenza A. Varicella pneumonia must be treated early and aggressively with hospitalization and intravenous acyclovir 10 mg/kg every 8 h for 5 days. Varicella immune globulin may help prevent pneumonia in pregnant women infected with varicella but who have no prior immunity, but will not prevent prenatal fetal infection or congenital varicella syndrome.

PNEUMONIA IN THE ELDERLY Pneumonia is the most common infection and represents the fifth leading cause of death among the elderly.[21] The incidence of lower respiratory tract infection in the elderly range from 25 to 44 cases per 1000 in the general population, with the mortality rate approaching 40 percent. COPD, congestive heart failure (CHF), cardiovascular and cerebrovascular disease, lung cancer, dementia, diminished gag reflex, and other disorders that may predispose the elderly to aspiration may make them more susceptible to infection.

The elderly are three times more likely to have pneumococcal bacteremia than younger patients. The mortality from pneumococcal pneumonia is three to five times greater in the elderly (up to 40 percent) than in those younger than age 65. Although becoming more frequent in the elderly, atypical pathogens such as *Mycoplasma* are still more common in younger populations. *Legionella* is the most common atypical agent in the elderly and responsible for up to 10 percent of CAP. Influenza is the most common serious viral infection in the elderly. Postinfluenza bacterial pneumonia is most commonly caused by *S. pneumoniae, S. aureus,* and *H. influenza.*

Instead of respiratory symptoms, elderly patients with pneumonia may complain about falling, weakness, tremulousness, functional decline, or GI symptoms and may exhibit delirium or confusion. Elderly patients are more likely to be afebrile on presentation but are more likely than younger adults to have a serious bacterial infection when temperature is higher than 38.3°C (100.9°F). Tachypnea may predate the diagnosis of pneumonia by 3 to 4 days.

In bacterial pneumonia, the chest radiograph may show a bronchial pattern rather than a classic lobar consolidation. Multiple lung segments are often involved, and patients over age 65 are more likely to show radiographic progression of disease (48 percent) compared with younger patients (11 percent). Early consolidation is more likely to indicate a bacterial etiology than atypical or viral infection. Coexisting conditions such as CHF, lung cancer, or pulmonary embolism may mask pneumonia.

Up to one-third of elderly patients with CAP will not manifest leukocytosis. Poor prognostic indicators include hypothermia or a temperature greater than 38.3°C (100.9°F), a low white blood cell count, immunosuppression, gram-negative or staphylococcal infection, cardiac disease, bilateral infiltrates, and extrapulmonary disease. Elderly patients with pneumonia frequently require hospitalization and about 10 percent may require intensive care.

PNEUMONIA IN NURSING-HOME PATIENTS Nursing-home-acquired pneumonia may be considered a distinct clinical entity, intermediate in severity between CAP and nosocomial pneumonia.[22] Pneumonia in nursing-home patients is a leading cause of hospitalization and along with bronchitis accounts for 30 percent of all nursing-home infections. The mortality rate of nursing-home-acquired pneumonia approaches 50 percent.

The major pathogenic mechanism is aspiration of colonizing oropharyngeal organisms with the resultant pneumonia depending on the organism's virulence, inoculum size, and health of the host's defense system. Nursing-home residents have an increased frequency of colonization by gram-negative bacteria. Altered sensorium, swallowing and esophageal disorders, tracheostomy tubes, nasogastric feeding tubes, and sedative medications may promote aspiration in these patients.

Streptococcus pneumoniae is the most common pathogen (20 percent), but gram-negative organisms as a group are more common (30 percent).[10] Outbreaks of *H. influenzae,* influenza A, influenza B, *Chlamydia,* and RSV have been reported. Staphylococcal pneumonia is seen more frequently in the nursing-home setting (7 to 12 percent) than in the general population (1 percent). Pseudomonal, *Legionella,* and *Mycoplasma* pneumonia are rare in the nursing-home environment.

In nursing-home patients, signs and symptoms of pneumonia are frequently atypical, with altered mental status as the presenting complaint more than one-fifth of the time. Other subtle symptoms may include difficulties with gait, bowel or bladder incontinence, decreased appetite, or a new requirement for feeding. Most patients will have a slightly elevated temperature, respiratory rate, and cough. Pulmonary consolidation is often absent, especially if a patient is dehydrated, and the initial chest radiograph will often fail to show the pneumonia, which may be masked by CHF, COPD, malignancy, or prior lung disease.

Frequently, empiric broad-spectrum antibiotic therapy must be started with consideration of sputum Gram stain results, likely pathogen, host comorbid disease, and recent antibiotic use. Antibiotics should cover pneumococcal, staphylococcal, and gram-negative bacillary infection. Depending on the capability of the nursing home, it may be appropriate to manage patients there, where overall function may be better preserved than in the hospital. The most important indicators for hospitalization are tachypnea with a respiratory rate of more than 30 bpm, temperature greater than 38.3°C (100.9°F), and altered mental status. Patients should certainly be admitted if hemodynamically unstable or if hydration, oxygen, nutritional, or respiratory therapy requirements cannot be met at the nursing home. Patients with diabetes or underlying cardiopulmonary disease frequently require admission.

PNEUMONIA IN HIV PATIENTS Recurrent bacterial pneumonia, pulmonary tuberculosis, and opportunistic pneumonia are AIDS-defining criteria for patients with HIV infection. Although *Pneumocystis carinii* pneumonia (PCP) is the most common AIDS-defining infection, bacterial pneumonia is more common.[23] CAP is 10 times more frequent in HIV-positive patients compared with those who are HIV seronegative, but the overall mortality from bacterial pneumonia is no different between HIV-positive and HIV-negative patients.

The incidence of pneumococcal pneumonia ranges from 20 to 95 per 1000 in HIV-positive patients compared with 3 to 4 per 1000 in HIV-negative patients. *Haemophilus influenzae* type B and nontypeable strains also cause pneumonia in HIV patients. Viral pneumonitis may occur independently or more commonly in association with another pathogenic agent.

Opportunistic infections are uncommon when the CD4 count is above 800 cells/μL and bacterial infections are the likely cause of pneumonia. The likelihood of both bacterial and opportunistic pneumonia increases as the CD4 count falls. Between 250 and 500 cells/μL, there is a greater risk of infection from *M. tuberculosis, Cryptococcus neoformans,* and *Histoplasma capsulatum.* Below 200 cells/μL, there is an increased risk of PCP.

HIV patients with bacterial pneumonia typically present with symptoms and findings similar to those in HIV-seronegative patients. PCP usually presents with rapid exacerbation of symptoms, often after weeks of increasing cough and dyspnea. The chest radiograph in PCP usually reveals bilateral alveolar and interstitial infiltrates, but unusual findings, such as nodular densities, cystic lesion, lobar infiltrate, or pneumothorax, may be seen. Extrapulmonary dissemination and atypical radiographic features (upper lobe involvement) have been associated with patients taking aerosolized pentamidine. Knowledge of a patient's CD4 count may help the clinician formulate a differential diagnosis and diagnostic approach. PCP is unusual with CD4 counts greater than 200 cells/μL, but at less than 100 cells/μL increases greatly. For mild cases of PCP (those patients able to take oral medications and with $Pa_{O_2} > 70$ mmHg) oral treatment with TMP-SMX, trimethoprim-dapsone, clindamycin-primaquine, or atovaquone for 21 days may be used. For moderate to seriously ill patients with PCP, treatment regiments include TMP-SMX orally or intravenously (IV); clindamycin IV plus primaquine orally; or pentamidine isethionate IV for 21 days. Adjunct corticosteroid treatment will most likely benefit patients with a $Pa_{O_2} < 70$ mmHg and reduces the likelihood of respiratory failure, increased oxygen requirement, and death among patients with moderate to severe PCP. Oral prednisone may be used in the following regimen: 40 mg bid for the first 5 days, 40 mg/day for the next 5 days, then 20 mg/day for the next 11 days.

Cryptococcus neoformans is found throughout the world and is the most common fungus causing life-threatening infection in AIDS. Typically causing meningitis, *C. neoformans* may also cause pneumonia presenting with fever, cough, and dyspnea. The chest radiograph may show diffuse or localized infiltrates, cavitation, nodules, miliary disease, lymphadenopathy, or pleural effusions.

TABLE 59-3 Antibiotics Used in Adults with Community-Acquired Pneumonia

Drug	Class	Oral	Intravenous
Doxycycline	Tetracycline	100 mg bid	100 mg bid
Erythromycin	Macrolide	500 mg qid	1.0 g qid
Clarithromycin	Macrolide	500 mg bid	
Azithromycin	Macrolide	500 mg on day 1 and 250 mg on day 2–5	500 mg/day
Trimethoprim-sulfamethoxazole (TMP-SMX)	Sulfonamide	DS tablet = 160/800 mg 1 DS tablet bid	TMP component 8–10 (mg/kg)/day divided bid to qid
Ampicillin-clavulanate	Penicillin + β-lactamase inhibitor	875/125 mg bid	
Ampicillin-sulbactam	Penicillin + β-lactamase inhibitor		1.5–3.0 g qid
Sparfloxacin	Fluoroquinolone	400 mg on day 1 and 200 mg/day thereafter	
Levofloxacin	Fluoroquinolone	500 mg/day	500 mg/day
Trovafloxacin	Fluoroquinolone		200 mg/day
Cefprozil	Second cephalosporin	500 mg bid	
Cefuroxime	Second cephalosporin	500 mg bid	
Cefpodoxime	Third cephalosporin	200 mg bid	
Cefoperazone	Third cephalosporin		4–8 g/day divided qid
Cefotaxime	Third cephalosporin		4–8 g/day divided tid or qid
Ceftazidime	Third cephalosporin		3–6 g/day divided bid or tid
Ceftriaxone	Third cephalosporin		2–4 g/day divided bid
Cefepime	Fourth cephalosporin		2–4 g/day divided bid
Imipenem/clastatin	Carbapenem		500 mg qid
Meropenem	Carbapenem		1.0 g tid
Vancomycin	Miscellaneous		1.0 g bid

Histoplasma capsulatum infection is usually subacute, and chest radiograph may show a diffuse, miliary pattern or a localized infiltrate. HIV patients from endemic areas (the Ohio and Mississippi River valleys, the Caribbean islands, and Central and South America) may present with disseminated disease. *Histoplasma* antigen may be found in urine or blood, and *Histoplasma* may be cultured from respiratory specimens, bone marrow, liver, or blood.

Life-threatening pulmonary aspergillosis may develop in patients with advanced immunosuppression, generally in those patients with absolute neutropenia, CD4 count below 30 cells/μL, or prior corticosteroid use. Disseminated disease is common.

Patients with AIDS from endemic areas may develop disseminated coccidioidomycosis and blastomycosis. Pulmonary disease may present with cough, fever, and dyspnea. Chest radiograph may show nodular, cavitary, or diffuse disease, and antibodies to *Coccidioides immitis* found in the blood may assist diagnosis. Cytomegalovirus (CMV) often can be isolated from lungs of HIV patients but rarely causes clinically significant disease. Patients with CMV pneumonitis may present with dyspnea, nonproductive cough, and fever. The chest radiograph may look similar to that with PCP with diffuse pulmonary infiltrates. Coinfection with CMV does not appear to alter the course of therapy when patients are treated for other pathogens.

PNEUMONIA IN TRANSPLANT PATIENTS Posttransplantation pulmonary infections may occur with both solid organ and bone marrow transplant patients. Factors such as type of transplant, time after transplant, invasive procedures during hospitalization, and prior travel to endemic areas determine the infection that may occur. Pneumonia may result from a newly acquired pathogen or reactivation of a dormant infection such as *M. tuberculosis, Toxoplasma gondii, H. capsulatum, C. immitis, S. stercoralis,* herpes simplex virus, CMV, and varicella-zoster virus.[24]

Immunosuppression of cellular and humoral immunity, airway colonization, hematogenous spread from distant infection, and liberal use of broad-spectrum antibiotics have been blamed for the development of pneumonia in transplant patients. Other risk factors include intubation, pulmonary edema, blood or blood product transfusion, central venous catheter infections, the use of polyurethane film dressings, intensive care unit admission, and use of agents that increase gastric pH.

Certain infections tend to occur during three time periods after transplantation and are related to a patient's degree of immunosuppression during each. These time periods are the first month, 30 to 120 days, and more than 120 days after transplantation.

Pneumonia that occurs during the first 30 days after transplant is usually bacterial and typically of nosocomial origin similar to that in

TABLE 59-4 Assignment to Risk Class I

Age ≤ 50 years
No comorbid conditions
Neoplastic disease
Congestive heart failure
Renal disease
Liver disease
No physical examination abnormalities
Altered mental status
Pulse > 125
Systolic blood pressure < 90 mmHg
Temperature < 35°C (95°F) or > 40°C (104°F)

Source: Adapted from Fine et al,[30] with permission.

any immunocompetent host. Gram-positive and gram-negative pathogens (including *S. aureus* and *Legionella* pneumophila) are encountered, and hematogenous spread from central venous catheters or aspiration of oropharyngeal contents during prolonged intubation may be the cause. Opportunistic infections are rare during this time.

Patients are most severely immunocompromised from 30 to 120 days after transplant. Because of marked depression of cell-mediated immunity, patients are susceptible to infection by viruses (CMV, herpes simplex virus, and adenovirus), fungi (*Candida albicans, A. fumigatus,* and mucormycosis), and protozoa (*P. carinii* and *Toxoplasma gondii*). CMV is the most common infection after kidney, liver, and bone marrow transplantation, usually occurring 4 to 6 weeks after transplantation. CMV pneumonitis in lung transplant patients may present like an acute rejection. Pulmonary infections caused by *P. carinii, A. fumigatus,* mycobacteria, and *Nocardia* are more likely during this period.

More than 120 days after kidney transplantation, immune function improves as a result of withdrawing immunosuppressive therapy, and organisms more typical of CAP are seen. Most patients maintain some degree of immune suppression. Therefore, *C. neoformans, P. carinii,* and other opportunistic organisms may be encountered.

Treatment

Emergency physicians will most often initiate empiric treatment for patients who have CAP. Four different specialty societies have developed guidelines for the treatment of adults with CAP: the American Thoracic Society (ATS), the British Thoracic Society, the Canadian Infectious Disease Society, and the Infectious Disease Society of America.[25–28] Slight differences exist between the guidelines, particularly regarding etiologic diagnosis and antimicrobial therapy. For emergency physicians, the ATS guidelines are most germane because they take into account the low risk of mortality in otherwise healthy patients under the age of 60, emphasize empiric antibiotic selection, and discourage ancillary testing which has little influence on patient management. All four guidelines recognize that although pneumococcal pneumonia is still the single most common cause of CAP, atypical agents are increasingly more common and empiric therapy should include antibiotics that are active against organisms that lack a cell wall (Table 59-3). Recommended agents include doxycycline, a macrolide, or one of the newer fluoroquinolones orally for 7 to 10 days for treatment of bacterial infection, although there is evidence that treatment for up to 21 days is helpful for atypical infections. Doxycycline is an excellent antibiotic because of its tolerance, bioavailability, low price, and easy compliance with twice-a-day dosing. Erythromycin is a very cost-effective agent for CAP, but is associated with GI side affects in about 25 percent of adult patients. Clarithromycin has fewer GI side effects and the advantage of twice-a-day dosing. Azithromycin has the advantage of once-a-day dosing for only 5 days. Both clarithromycin and azithromycin are many times more expensive than erythromycin or doxycycline. The newer fluoroquinolone agents, including sparfloxacin, levofloxacin, and trofloxacin, have extended coverage that includes both common bacterial agents and atypical agents and the advantage of once-a-day dosing. Because of increasing *S. pneumoniae* resistance to doxycycline and the macrolides (approaching 30 percent in some areas), some societies are revising their recommendations to use a fluoroquinolone, such as levofloxacin, as the initial agent for empiric treratment of CAP.

The ATS guidelines recommend that patients over age 60 or those with concomitant disease should be treated with extended-spectrum antibiotics, such as a second-generation cephalosporin, a combination of penicillin plus β-lactamase inhibitor, or TMP-SMX. Although such agents are considered to have an "extended spectrum," they do not cover atypical agents. Clinical trials indicate that, even in older patients, the inclusion of an antibiotic that is active against atypical agents leads to lower mortality and morbidity rates. This suggests that emergency physicians should use a newer fluoroquinolone alone or a macrolide agent plus an "extended spectrum" cephalosporin or penicillin in older or compromised patients with CAP.

Emergency physicians play a prominent role in the initiation of treatment for patients being hospitalized with CAP. Recent evidence indicates that early administration of antibiotics, within the first 8 h of presentation, leads to a lower mortality rate and a shorter hospital stay. Although the yield is low, admitting physicians may benefit from the results of the sputum Gram stain, sputum culture, or blood culture obtained in the emergency department. For patients hospitalized with CAP, therapy should be initiated with a second- or third-generation cephalosporin or penicillin plus β-lactamase inhibitor, usually with a macrolide to provide coverage against *Legionella* or other atypical agents. Coverage can also be provided by a fluoroquinolone alone with the advantage that the newer quinolones such as levofloxacin

TABLE 59-5 Assignment to Risk Classes II to V

Criteria	Points
Demographics	
Female gender	−10
Nursing-home resident	10
Coexistent illness	
Neoplastic disease	30
Congestive heart failure	20
Cerebrovascular accident	10
Renal disease	10
Liver disease	10
Physical examination	
Abnormal mental status	20
Pulse ≥ 125	20
RR ≥ 30	20
Blood pressure ≤ 90 mmHg	15
Temperature < 35° (95°F) or > 40°C (104°F)	10
Ancillary studies	
pH < 7.35	30
Blood urea nitrogen ≥ 30 mg/dL	20
Na ≤ 130 meq/L	20
Glucose ≥ 250 mg/dL	10
Hematocrit < 30%	10
Pao_2 < 60 mmHg	10
Pleural effusion	10

Source: Adapted from Fine et al,[30] with permission.

TABLE 59-6 Prediction of Mortality from Pneumonia

Class	Points	Mortality, %	Treatment Recommendation
I	No predictors	0.1	Outpatient
II	<70	0.6	Outpatient
III	71–90	2.8	Inpatient (briefly)
IV	91–130	8.2	Inpatient
V	>130	29.2	Inpatient

Source: Adapted from Fine et al,[30] with permission.

achieve very high serum levels after oral administration, matching those achieved with intravenous administration. Patients with severe CAP should receive a macrolide plus an extended-spectrum antibiotic with antipseudomonal coverage (ceftazidime, cefoperazone, cefepime, imipenem, meropenem, levofloxacin, or trovafloxacin).

Disposition

An estimated 75 percent of patients with CAP do not require hospitalization. In young adults, the pathogenic organism is frequently viral or atypical and associated with low morbidity and mortality rates. Many factors influence the prognosis and outcome of CAP.[29] In general, physicians tend to overestimate the risk of pneumonia mortality. Fine and coworkers have developed a decision tree that can be used to estimate the risk of death from pneumonia and predict the need for hospitalization[30] (Tables 59-4 to 59-6). With this decision rule, patients are assigned to one of five risk categories, with the lowest category having a mortality rate of around 0.1 percent. Although not a prominent part of this decision rule, patients who are immunocompromised as a result of AIDS or chronic alcohol use may require hospitalization. In addition, a chest radiograph that demonstrates bilateral effusions, bilateral infiltrates, moderately large pleural effusions, or extensive pulmonary involvement is associated with a higher risk of mortality. Patients should be considered for admission to an intensive care unit if they are markedly tachypneic or have high oxygen requirements, evidence of shock, or very extensive pulmonary involvement (more than 50 percent of the lung). For patients in risk category II, admission may be chosen based on the presence of relative hypoxemia, social factors, and the inability to complete a course of oral antibiotics.

Emergency physicians play a role in educating patients about their disease. Most patients will achieve some measure of resolution within 3 to 5 days after the initiation of antibiotics. Large population studies have demonstrated, however, that many patients are still symptomatic at 30 days, with a significant minority of patients experiencing chest pain, malaise, or mild dyspnea even 2 to 3 months after treatment. Patients should be educated about the importance of smoking cessation and moderation of alcohol use. Patients should receive instructions about rest, nutrition, hydration, and follow-up. Patients at risk should be educated about the importance of vaccination against pneumococcus and influenza.

REFERENCES

1. Wilson R, Rayner CF: Bronchitis. *Curr Opin Pulm Med* 1:177, 1995.
2. Dowell SF, Anderson LJ, Gary HE, et al: Respiratory syncytial virus is an important cause of community-acquired lower respiratory infection among hospitalized adults. *J Infect Dis* 174:456, 1996.
3. Wright SW, Edwards KM, Decker MD, Zeldin MH: Pertussis infections in adults with persistent cough. *JAMA* 273:1044, 1995.
4. MacKay DN: Treatment of acute bronchitis in adults without underlying lung disease. *J Gen Intern Med* 11:557, 1996.
5. Fahey T, Stocks N, Thomas T: Quantitative systematic review of randomized controlled trails comparing antibiotic with placebo for acute cough in adults. *BMJ* 316:906, 1998.
6. Grossman RF: Guidelines for the treatment of acute exacerbations of chronic bronchitis. *Chest* 112(suppl):310S, 1997.
7. Hueston WJ: A comparison of albuterol and erythromycin for the treatment of acute bronchitis. *J Fam Pract* 33:476, 1991.
8. Hueston WJ: Albuterol delivered by metered-dose inhaler to treat acute bronchitis. *J Fam Pract* 39:437, 1994.
9. Bartlett JG, Mundy LM, Orloff J: Community-acquired pneumonia. *N Engl J Med* 333:1618, 1995
10. Fang GD, Fine M, Orloff J, et al: New and emerging etiologies for community-acquired pneumonia with implications for therapy. *Medicine (Baltimore)* 69:307, 1990.
11. Marrie TJ, Fine MJ, Coley CM: Ambulatory patients with community-acquired pneumonia: The frequency of atypical agents and clinical course. *Am J Med* 101:508, 1996.
12. Metlay JP, Schulz R, Li YH, et al: Influence of age on symptoms at presentation in patients with community-acquired pneumonia. *Arch Intern Med* 157:1453, 1997.
13. Metlay JP, Kapoor WN, Fine MJ: Does this patient have community-acquired pneumonia? Diagnosing pneumonia by history and physical examination. *JAMA* 278:1440, 1997.
14. Marfin AA, Sporrer J, Moore PS, Siefkin AD: Risk factors for adverse outcome in persons with pneumococcal pneumonia. *Chest* 107:457, 1995.
15. Barreiro B, Esteban L, Prats E, et al: *Branhamella catarrhalis* respiratory infections. *Eur Respir J* 5:675, 1995.
16. Atmar RL, Greenberg SG: Pneumonia caused by *Mycoplasma pneumoniae* and the TWAR agent. *Semin Respir Infect* 4:19, 1995.
17. Macfarlane JT, Miller AC, Smith WHR, et al: Comparative radiographic features of community acquired legionnaires' disease, pneumococcal pneumonia, mycoplasma pneumonia, and psittacosis. *Thorax* 39:28, 1984
18. Griffith D, Mazurek G: Pneumonia in chronic obstructive lung disease. *Infect Dis Clin North Am* 5:467, 1991.
19. Koziel H, Koziel MJ: Pulmonary complications of diabetes mellitus: Pneumonia. *Infect Dis Clin North Am* 9:65, 1995.
20. Rodrigues J, Niederman MS: Pneumonia complicating pregnancy. *Clin Chest Med* 13:679, 1992.
21. Sims RV: Bacterial pneumonia in the elderly. *Emerg Med Clin North Am* 8:207, 1990.
22. Stein D: Managing pneumonia acquired in nursing homes: Special concerns. *Geriatrics* 45:39, 1990.
23. Rosen MJ: Pneumonia in patients with HIV infection. *Med Clin North Am* 78:1067, 1994.
24. Conces DJ: Opportunistic pneumonia. *Curr Probl Diagn Radiol* 22:3, 1993.
25. Niederman MS, Bass JB, Campbell GD, et al: Guidelines for the initial empiric therapy of community-acquired pneumonia: Proceedings of an American Thoracic Society Consensus Conference. *Am Rev Respir Dis* 148:1418, 1993.
26. The British Thoracic Society: Guidelines for the management of community-acquired pneumonia in adults admitted to the hospital. *Br J Hosp Med* 49:346, 1993.
27. Mandell LA, Niederman M: The Canadian Community-Acquired Pneumonia Consensus Conference Group: Antimicrobial treatment of community-acquired pneumonia in adults—A conference report. *Can J Infect Dis* 4:25, 1993.

28. Bartlett JG, Breiman RF, Mandell LA, File TM: Guidelines from the Infectious Diseases Society of America: Community-acquired pneumonia in adults—Guidelines for management. *Clin Infect Dis* 26:811, 1998.
29. Fine MJ, Smith MA, Carson CA, et al: Prognosis and outcomes of patients with community-acquired pneumonia: A meta-analysis. *JAMA* 274:134, 1996.
30. Fine MJ, Auble TE, Yealy DM, et al: A prediction rule to identify low-risk patients with community-acquired pneumonia. *N Engl J Med* 336:243, 1997.
31. Emerman CL, Dawson N, Speroff T, et al: Comparison of physician judgment and decision aids for ordering chest radiographs for pneumonia in outpatients. *Ann Emerg Med* 20:1215, 1991.
32. Diehr P, Wood RW, Bushyhead J, et al: Prediction of pneumonia in outpatients with acute cough—A statistical approach. *J Chronic Dis* 37:215, 1984.
33. Singal BM, Hedges JR, Radack KL: Decision rules and clinical prediction of pneumonia: Evaluation of low-yield criteria. *Ann Emerg Med* 18:13, 1989.
34. Gennis P, Gallagher J, Falvo C, et al: Clinical criteria for the detection of pneumonia in adults: Guidelines for ordering chest roentgenograms in the emergency department. *J Emerg Med* 7:263, 1989.
35. Heckerling PS, Tape TG, Wigton RS, et al: Clinical prediction rule for pulmonary infiltrates. *Ann Intern Med* 113:664, 1990.

ASPIRATION PNEUMONIA, LUNG ABSCESS, AND PLEURAL EMPYEMA

Eric Anderson
Maxime Alix Gilles

ASPIRATION PNEUMONIA

Epidemiology

Aspiration pneumonia is an infectious inflammatory condition that results from the inhalation of oral contents into the lungs. The oral contents can be food, vomitus, inedible objects (e.g., toys, screws, etc.), or oral secretions. One of the earliest recorded aspiration deaths was in 475 B.C. when the Greek poet Anacreon died as a result of aspirating a grape seed.[1] Mendelson in 1946, described 66 obstetrical patients who developed respiratory failure as a result of aspiration of stomach contents during obstetric anesthesia.[2] The pulmonary effects of aspiration are due to the presence of foreign bodies, chemical irritants, and bacterial pathogens in the material aspirated.[3]

The true incidence of pathologic aspiration into the lungs is difficult to determine. Small volumes of aspiration that do not lead to infection or pulmonary disease have been documented in approximately 50 percent of normal subjects during sleep.[4]

Such chronic debilitating conditions as stroke, dysphagia, tube feeding, and altered mental status with decreased level of consciousness place patients at increased risk for aspiration (Table 60-1). Of patients studied within 5 days after an acute stroke, 38 percent demonstrated evidence of aspiration.[5] One-third of those who aspirated had silent aspiration without evidence of cough or gag. Risk factors and predictors for silent aspiration included dysphagia, dysarthria, voice change after swallow, and abnormal gag reflex (Table 60-2).

Patients discharged back to long-term care facilities are at persistent risk for aspiration. Patients who aspirate are at three times the risk of dying compared with patients who did not aspirate.[6]

Pathophysiology

Risk factors for aspiration among emergency patients includes transient or permanent altered mental states with depressed glottic reflexes, anomalies of the esophagus, alcohol or illicit drug intoxication, seizure, tube feedings, anesthesia, advanced age, and supine position. It is not uncommon to see more than one of these risk factors in a single patient. For example, an elderly nursing home patient in a persistent vegetative state with a gastrostomy tube arrives for evaluation of fever. Caretakers may not appreciate aspiration, since the event may be occult secondary to the lack of gag or cough reflex at the time of aspiration.

The severity of the symptoms is related to the volume of material aspirated, the amount of bacterial contamination, and the pH of

TABLE 60-1 Risk Factors for Aspiration Pneumonia and Lung Abscess

NEUROLOGIC
Alcohol intoxication
Intoxication from illicit drug use
Therapeutic drug overdose
Seizure
Chronic decreased level of consciousness
Stroke Poststroke dysphagia Dysarthria
GASTROINTESTINAL
Gastroesophageal reflux disease
Esophageal dysmotility syndrome
Esophageal stricture or obstruction
Zenker diverticulum
Dysphagia
Tube feeding Nasogastric tubes G tubes J tubes
Tracheoesophageal fistula
OTHER
Elderly
Debilitated, chronically in supine position
Cystic fibrosis
General anesthesia
Periodontal disease

TABLE 60-2 Physical Findings in Patients at Risk for Aspiration

Findings
Dysarthria
Cough after swallow
Dysphonia
Voice change after swallowing
Abnormal or absent gag reflex
Neck contracture with neck extended

the material aspirated. Liquids with a pH lower than 2.0 are associated with a much higher mortality rate than are liquids with a higher pH. Aspirated bacteria usually come from oropharyngeal contents, with anaerobic bacteria predominating. Patients in hospitals or long-term care facilities may become colonized by gram-negative bacilli, and these bacteria may make their way into the aspirated inoculum.

Normal mechanisms that protect the airway include the sneeze, gag, and cough reflexes. Particles deposited in the distal nasal epithelium are removed by a sneeze. Lower airways are protected by mucus produced by cells that line the airways. This mucus traps airborne particles of 10-μm diameter. Once trapped by the mucous coating, these larger particles are swept proximally by the mucocillary escalator to the oropharynx, where they are expectorated or swallowed. Alveolar macrophages, polymorphonuclear leukocytes, or lymphocytes destroy infectious particles that are small enough to reach the alveoli.

Many of the symptoms of aspiration pneumonia are elicited by the body's inflammatory response to the infectious or irritative material. Proinflammatory cytokines, which increase capillary permeability and are cytotactic, cause migration of fluids and inflammatory cells into the area of irritation.[7] The inflammatory response is responsible for the symptoms of fever, productive cough, and radiographic findings. These findings may not be present when aspiration occurs in an immunocompromised patient who may not be able to mount the inflammatory responses.

Solid material, such as sand, dirt, toys, and other small objects, can cause rapid asphyxiation secondary to mechanical blockage of the trachea. Patients with total or near-total obstruction of the glottis or trachea will be unable to cough or call for help because of the lack of air movement.

Clinical Features

The typical patient has had problems with oral secretions or coughing with meals, suggesting gastroesophageal reflux.[8] Patients who require tube feedings are at risk for aspiration.[8] In the elderly, localizing symptoms may be minimal, and the complaint may be a change in baseline mental status. There may be a specific witnessed episode of aspiration.

Physical findings include those common to pneumonia: fever; cough; localized rales, wheezes, or rhonchi; tachycardia; and tachypnea. Cyanosis can develop quickly in patients with underlying lung disease or in patients with overwhelming pulmonary bacterial contamination. Aspiration of large volumes of fluid can also precipitate the rapid development of cyanosis.

Chest radiographs may show an interstitial or alveolar pattern. The right lower lobe is the most common area for the development of aspiration pneumonia when aspiration occurs in an upright sitting posture because the right main stem bronchus has a more direct course from the trachea than does the left main stem bronchus (Fig. 60-1). Aspiration in a supine position may produce infection in any lobe, although the posterior pulmonary segments are more susceptible.

Laboratory tests may demonstrate an elevated white blood cell count. In elderly patients the typical leukocytosis may be blunted. In these situations it is helpful to assess the differential and look for a left shift with an increased percentage of immature forms. An elevated C-reactive protein level is a nonspecific indicator of an inflammatory process and may be the only indication of an aerobic infectious pulmonary process resulting from an aspiration.[9] Arterial blood gas measurements may reveal hypoxia if the aspiration or inflammatory process is large enough to significantly interfere with alveolar gas exchange. Oxygen content may be normal early in the course of the illness, but evidence of pulmonary injury can be found by detecting hyperventilation (decreased Pa_{CO_2}) and ventilation-perfusion mismatching (elevated A-a gradient).

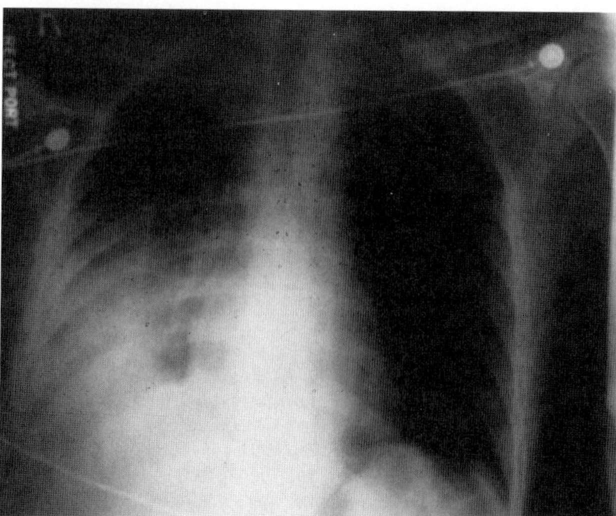

FIG. 60-1. Aspiration pneumonia of the right lower lobe.

Treatment

Prevention of aspiration is particularly important for those patients at risk. Treatment of illicit drug use and alcohol addiction will significantly decrease the individual patient's chance of intoxication and subsequent aspiration. Feeding in an upright position will decrease the risk of aspiration in patients with dysphagia, on tube feedings through nasogastric or orogastric tubes, or with gastrostomy or jejunostomy tubes. Increasing the gastric pH by the use of antacids (four times a day) or proton pump inhibitors (omeprazole 20 mg/d orally) will decrease the pulmonary damage from silent serial aspirators.[10]

Prokinetic agents that increase lower esophageal sphincter tone and stimulate gastric emptying are useful in treating gastroesophageal reflux disease and would be useful in preventing aspiration in patients at risk. These agents include bethanecol 25 mg qid, metoclopramide 10 mg before meals and at bedtime, and cisapride 10 mg before meals and at bedtime. These agents are useful in gastroesophageal reflux disease, but they have some troublesome side effects. The side effects of bethanecol are related to its cholinergic effects: abdominal cramps, salivation, urination, and blurred vision. Cisapride has been reported to cause Q-T interval prolongation and ventricular dysrhythmias, including torsade de pointes, in patients receiving other medication (e.g., ketoconazole and other antifungals). In addition to the desirable antiemetic central nervous system effects of metoclopramide, there are also undesirable effects: mild anxiety, nervousness, insomnia, depression, confusion, disorientation, and hallucinations. Other troublesome side effects of metoclopramide include the extrapyramidal effects of tremor; akathisia; tardive dyskinesia, a Parkinson-like syndrome; gynecomastia; and reversible amenorrhea.[8]

For patients who have experienced an acute, symptomatic aspiration, immediate removal of any airway obstruction and rapid assessment of ventilation is needed. Hypoxia should be corrected by oxygenation, ventilation, and intubation if necessary. Aerosolized bronchodilators are useful for aspiration-induced bronchospasm. For patients in shock, aggressive intravenous (IV) fluid administration and, if appropriate, vasopressors are used.

Healthy patients who aspirate but who are not hypoxic and have no infiltrate on x-ray may be observed for development of signs of infection and may not require antibiotic treatment. Elderly or chronically ill patients who present with signs and symptoms of infection should have antibiotic therapy instituted. In general, appropriate cultures of blood, urine, and sputum (if available) should be obtained in the emergency department, and antibiotic therapy should be initiated. Anaerobes predominate in aspiration pneumonia, and antibiotics that are proven effective include clindamycin 450 to 900 mg IV every 8 h, cefoxitin 2.0g IV every 8 h, ticarcillin-clavulanate 3.1 g IV every 6 h, or piperacillin-tazobactam 3.375 g IV every 6 h.

Bronchoscopy may be indicated for patients who aspirate large objects that move into the distal airways. Patients with viscous materials or tenacious secretions may require direct bronchoalveolar lavage for removal. Patients who develop copious hemoptysis may require bronchoscopy for both diagnosis and treatment.

Disposition

Patients who have had a witnessed episode of aspiration and who are otherwise healthy and exhibit no signs of infection or respiratory compromise may be discharged home with instructions to follow up with their primary care physician in 1 to 2 days. They should be instructed to watch for shortness of breath, fever, chest pain, unusual fatigue, or the development of a cough and to return to the emergency department or see their primary care physician promptly if any of these symptoms develop.

Patients who appear stable but have risk factors for worse or very aggressive disease (diabetes, old age, dialysis, recent stroke, chronic pulmonary disease, active cancer, HIV, etc.) should be admitted to either a hospital or an observation unit. Oxygen, fluids, and possibly antibiotics should be started and the patient followed carefully for 12 to 24 h. If stable after 12 to 24 h of treatment and observation, such patients can be sent home and instructed to follow up as described above and to return if any sign of deterioration develops. Patients with definite evidence of infection should be admitted and antibiotic treatment started. Patients who exhibit hemodynamic or respiratory instability require admission to an intensive care unit.

LUNG ABSCESS

Epidemiology

A pulmonary abscess is a localized area of suppuration and necrosis involving one or more areas of the lung parenchyma and leading to cavity formation and the characteristic radiographic finding of an air-fluid level.[11]

The most common risk factors for lung abscess in adults are a history of alcohol abuse, a history of aspiration pneumonia, dental caries, and poor dental hygiene (Table 60-1). About 90 percent of patients with lung abscess have obvious periodontal disease or some predisposition to aspiration.[11,12]

Limited data exist on lung abscesses in children, especially with regard to bacteriology, diagnosis, and management. In normal children with no known underlying disease, the most common organisms are *Streptococcus pneumoniae,* anaerobic bacteria, nontypable *Haemophilus influenzae,* and *Staphylococcus aureus*.[13] Anaerobic bacteria are the predominant organisms isolated from children with underlying neurologic disorders.[11]

Patients with HIV infection are at risk for lung abscesses, especially those with advanced disease and a low CD4 count (less than 50).[14] The microbiologic etiology of lung abscess in patients with advanced HIV infection differs from that in HIV-negative patients. *Pseudomonas aeruginosa* is one of the most commonly isolated pathogens from patients with advanced HIV infection or AIDS-defining illnesses. Lung abscesses in patients with advanced HIV infection respond poorly to antibiotic therapy.

Pathophysiology

Primary lung abscess usually results from aspiration of anaerobic oropharyngeal bacteria into the dependent portions of the lung. Any breakdown of the normal protective mechanisms predisposes patients to aspiration, which is also the predominant cause of a lung abscess in infants and children.[13] Aspiration of the bacteria leads to pneumonitis, which impairs drainage of fluids and/or aspirated material and results in inflammatory vascular obstruction, leading to tissue necrosis, abscess formation, or empyema. Lung abscesses resulting from bacteremia are usually due to *S. aureus* that enters the blood via skin lacerations, soft tissue infection, and injected drug use.

Clinical Features

Patients typically have an intermittent febrile course, chest pain, cough, tachypnea, dyspnea, weight loss, malaise, and night sweats.[11] Oral examination may reveal gingivitis and poor oral hygiene. Approximately 1 to 2 weeks after the initial aspiration, the lung abscess cavitates, resulting in putrid expectoration in 40 to 75 percent of patients, a finding highly suggestive of an underlying lung abscess.[11]

Diagnosis

The diagnosis and management of lung abscess continues to challenge physicians as more patients present with complex coexisting diseases, often including profound immunosuppression. The diagnosis of a lung abscess is most commonly established by chest radiograph, including both upright and lateral views (Fig. 60-2). These views typically show

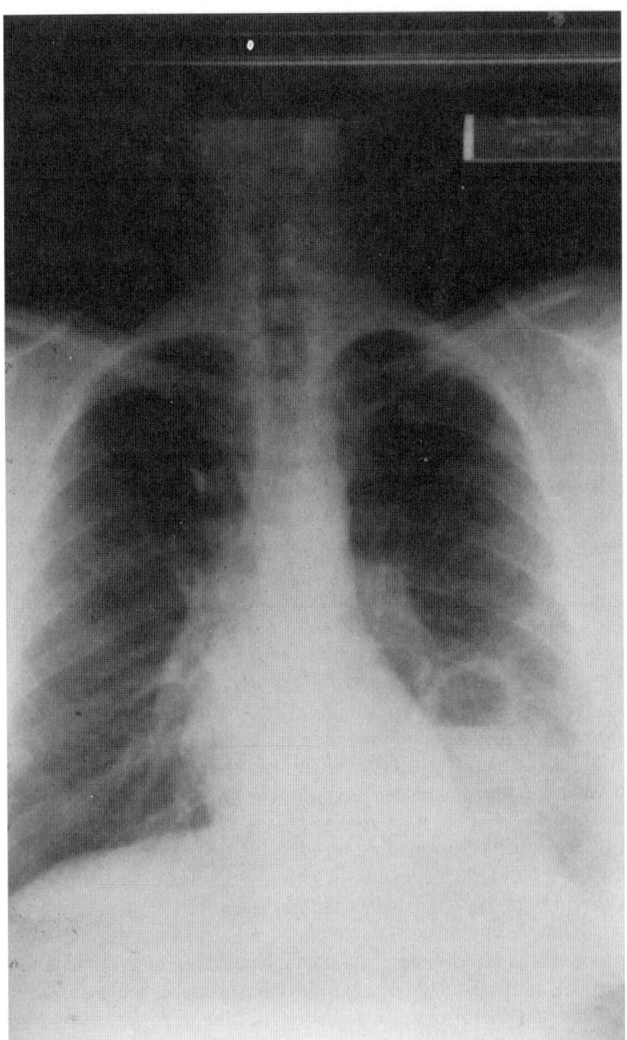

FIG. 60-2. Lung abscess of the left lower lobe.

TABLE 60-3 Noninfectious and Infectious Causes of Lung Abscess

Noninfectious	Infectious
Neoplastic	Anaerobic bacteria
Pulmonary infarction	Gram-negative aerobic bacteria *Klebsiella* *Pseudomonas*
Vasculitis Wegener granulomatosis Rheumatoid nodules	Gram-positive aerobic bacteria *Staphylococcus aureus* *Legionella* *Pseudomonas pseudomallei*
Congenital Bullae, cysts, blebs Sequestration	Fungal
	Amoebic
	Mycobacteria (tuberculosis)
	Actinomycosis/nocardiosis
	Echinococcosis (hydatid cyst)
	Infected bulla
	Right-sided endocarditis

an inflammatory infiltrate of the pulmonary parenchyma with one or more cavities containing an air-fluid level.

Analysis of expectorated sputum is an important first step in the evaluation of patients with a lung abscess.[11] Sputum should be cultured for aerobic and acid-fast organisms, and fungi. While sputum analysis is not reliable in determining the anaerobic bacteria causing a lung abscess, it is useful in detecting or excluding alternative diagnoses.

Anaerobic bacteria remain the most frequent cause of lung abscess, followed by polymicrobial infections (63 percent with anaerobes as coisolates) and *S. aureus*. In addition to bacteria, there are several other infectious and noninfectious causes of lung abscess (Table 60-3).

Fiberoptic bronchoscopy and/or bronchial alveolar lavage are useful diagnostic adjuncts.

Treatment

The treatment of choice for lung abscesses is conservative medical management, with the length of therapy dictated by the patient's clinical course and documented radiographic improvement. Radiographic resolution of an abscess cavity may take up to 2 months. Current first-line therapy for lung abscess is antibiotic therapy directed at anaerobes or mixed aerobic and anaerobic bacteria. This is effective in 80 to 90 percent of patients.[15]

In earlier studies, most patients with lung abscess responded to oral or parenteral doses of penicillin or tetracycline.[11] However, over the past two decades several strains of anaerobic bacteria have evolved resistance to penicillin and tetracycline. Although penicillin has long been the antibiotic of choice, recent trials show clindamycin to be superior.[11] Clindamycin should now be considered the first-choice therapy for anaerobic lung abscess unless otherwise specified by culture results. The adult dosage for clindamycin is 600 mg IV every 6 to 8 h until a clinical response is achieved. Oral clindamycin 300 mg tid or qid can be started once an initial clinical response is noted. Depending on the microbiologic characteristics of the specimens obtained, other antibiotics, such as aminoglycosides, imipenem, chloramphenicol, antipseudomonal penicillins, and cefoxitin, may be effective.

Patients who display no radiographic improvement, show signs of persistent sepsis, or develop complications, such as hemoptysis, bronchopleural fistula, and empyema, require external drainage or resection.[15] The incidence of operative management of lung abscesses has decreased dramatically over the last 40 years and is now less than 10 percent.[11]

Most lung abscesses communicate with the tracheobronchial tree fairly early in the course of the infection and drain spontaneously. Unfavorable conditions, such as a large cavity (greater than 6 cm), necrotizing pneumonia with multiple small abscesses, an elderly or immunocompromised patient, an associated bronchial obstruction, or aerobic bacterial pneumonia may require surgical management despite adequate medical therapy.[11] External drainage or resection of a lung abscess is indicated if fever and toxicity persist despite adequate antibiotic therapy and internal drainage. External drainage is the preferred method of treatment for pleural-based abscesses, particularly in patients with a high risk of surgical mortality.[15]

Overall, surgical and image-guided percutaneous drainage has been successfully used for treatment of lung abscesses. The patient must be placed in a gravity-dependent position whenever possible in order to avoid soiling the normal lung. Placement of a relatively large-bore catheter (12-French or greater outer diameter) is essential in establishing adequate external drainage and maintaining catheter patency. The catheter is positioned in the abscess cavity, aspirated manually, and subsequently irrigated with saline solution.[15] The drainage catheter is irrigated daily in order to maintain patency and placed at −20 cm of water suction.

Disposition

The treatment of choice for lung abscesses is conservative medical management, with the length of therapy dictated by the patient's clinical course and documented radiographic improvement. Most uncomplicated cases require admission to a hospital and a 2- to 3-week course of parenteral antimicrobial therapy.

Most patients with a lung abscess who respond to conservative medical management usually recover with no adverse sequelae. Patients typically become afebrile in 7 to 10 days with appropriate antimicrobial treatment. If patients respond to therapy, they can complete oral antibiotic therapy over a period of 4 to 8 weeks. If a patient is seriously ill or fails to improve after a course of appropriate antibiotic therapy, other interventions may be required to facilitate drainage. Such interventions, previously discussed, may include thoracentesis and percutaneous drainage of the abscess with computed tomography (CT) or fluoroscopic guidance.

PLEURAL EMPYEMA

Epidemiology

Pleural empyema is gross pus in the pleural space or a parapneumonic effusion, documented by Gram stain or culture to be infected, that requires drainage for definitive treatment.[11] Pleural empyema can be found in all age groups.

Empyema of the chest is associated with considerable morbidity and mortality rates despite treatment.[16] Infected pleural fluid collections develop as a complication of pulmonary abscess, chest trauma, or surgical procedures. Other causes include secondary infection from a preexisting hydrothorax, hemothorax, esophageal perforation, or mediastinitis; or direct extension from vertebral osteomyelitis or subdiaphragmatic abscess.[11] These complications preceding an empyema are usually a result of direct hematogenous or lymphatic spread from the primary source.

Pathophysiology

Most empyemas develop from an underlying pulmonary infection and are thought to be secondary to subclinical aspiration of organisms in the dependent portions of the affected lung.[15] Alcohol abuse is a recognized risk factor for pleural empyema, primarily because of the increased incidence of aspiration pneumonia.[17] *Klebsiella pneumoniae* empyema may occur in alcoholic males with multiple host defense defects that impair containment of or perception of disease until it is well advanced.[18] Immunocompromised patients are prone to pleural involvement with fungal or aerobic gram-negative bacillary infection. In patients with a malignancy, fungal or tuberculous foci may be reactivated, and empyema develops. Fungal or mycobacterial empyema may also develop in transplant recipients and patients with AIDS. The most common organisms in healthy adults, children, or patients who have had chest trauma or surgery include *Streptococcus pneumoniae* and *Streptococcus pyogenes.*[17,18] Other bacterial isolates include gram-negative aerobic bacilli in hospitalized patients and anaerobes such as fusiform bacilli, *Bacteroides*, anaerobic *Streptococcus*, and *Clostridium* species.

Pleural empyema represents a continuum of disease ranging from thin pleural fluid microscopically contaminated by organisms to gross pus in the pleural space. Approximately 20 to 30 percent of patients with bacterial pneumonia develop a radiographically apparent pleural effusion.[11] The stages of a parapneumonic empyema are exudative, fibrinopurulent, and organizing. In the early phase, the effusion is thin, watery, and easily drained by thoracostomy. In the exudative and intermediate fibrinopurulent stages, the lung retains its compliance and capacity to fully expand. As infection progresses, the initially serous fluid becomes thick and purulent with organisms, fibrin, and white blood cells. In the fibrinopurulent stage, the deposition of fibrin on the parietal pleura retards the resorption of blood, preventing access to lymphatics and retarding fluid resorption.[19] Fibrin deposition in the presence of bacteria provides an ideal environment for the development of pleural empyema. Over a period of 4 to 6 weeks after the start of an empyema, the fibrin layer becomes organized and forms a thick peel (the thickened pleura that develops around a pleural empyema) in the chronic organizing phase.[16] Early management of empyema may prevent the progression of this process to the more advanced stages, where multiple loculations and scarring complicate drainage.

Clinical Features

The clinical presentation of empyema generally blends with that of an underlying pneumonia. Community-acquired *S. aureus* pneumonia is usually preceded by a viral upper respiratory infection or right-sided endocarditis in intravenous drug users. Patients with empyema are initially seen by a variety of physicians due to the indolent course of the disease. Typical symptoms include pyrexia, pleuritic chest pain, cough, dyspnea, and general malaise. Atypical presentations may include weight loss and anemia. Patients may have decreased breath sounds and dullness to percussion on examination of the chest. Symptoms are often masked by protracted treatment with antibiotic therapy for upper respiratory tract infections, which may result in the delayed diagnosis.

Diagnosis

The diagnosis of a parapneumonic effusion is usually suggested by typical findings on conventional posteroanterior and lateral chest radiographs. Lateral decubitus radiographic views are extremely valuable in the detection of subpulmonic effusions and can distinguish free from loculated pleural effusions.[11] Other radiographic findings suggestive of a pleural effusion or empyema include lower lung zone opacification, blunting of the costophrenic angle, and elevated hemidiaphragm with subpulmonic effusions. Extension of the air-fluid level to the chest wall, a tapering border of the air-fluid collection, thickened pleura, and the presence of edema in the extrapleural tissues suggest the presence of an empyema rather than a lung abscess. Virtually all patients with a parapneumonic effusion should undergo a diagnostic thoracentesis. Microbiologic analysis of the pleural fluid provides important information and helps determine whether drainage is necessary. Infected parapneumonic effusions typically have a pH less than 7.20, a lactate dehydrogenase level greater than 1000 IU/L, and a glucose level lower than 40 mg/dL. [17] Neutropenia, neutrophilia, hypoxia, azotemia, anemia, acidosis, thrombocytopenia, disseminated intravascular coagulopathy, or evidence of multiorgan failure are findings associated with severe infection.

Treatment

The presence of infection, as documented by Gram stain or culture, is an indication for admission and drainage. Image-guided drainage is selected by the availability and convenience of the various techniques and by the size and location of the fluid collection. Ultrasonography, CT, and fluoroscopy can all accurately guide drainage catheter placement. Ultrasonography is the technique of choice to guide thoracentesis and pleural drainage. Thoracic ultrasound is rapid and safe, and can differentiate solid from liquid components and detect subpulmonic or subphrenic pathologic conditions. CT is useful for specific characterization of complex intrathoracic processes, including loculated pleural collections associated with underlying parenchymal consolidation. CT can also be used to guide safe catheter placement into the collection. If fluoroscopy is readily available, it can be used to assess free-flowing loculated collections in supine patients. Radiographically guided pleural drainage procedures have shown success rates ranging from 72 to 80 percent.[15]

The optimal method of establishing external drainage remains controversial.[15] Catheters ranging from 8 to 30 French in outer diameter may be placed under imaging guidance. For serous collections, a 10- or 12-French catheter provides adequate drainage. Thicker collections of purulent or bloody material may require catheters 24 to 48 French in diameter. Most empyema drainage tubes have large round or oval side holes to promote drainage of particulate matter.

Therapy for thoracic empyema requires appropriate antibiotics, prompt drainage of the infected pleural space and lung reexpansion.[17] Empirical antimicrobial therapy is initiated on the basis of its anticipated bactericidal activity against the suspected microbial pathogens. Broad-spectrum antibiotic therapy with clindamycin 450 mg to 900 mg every 8 h IV and a third-generation cephalosporin (e.g., ceftriaxone) can be started with the diagnosis of an empyema and modified according to Gram stain and culture results. In general, antibiotics are given in high doses for 2 to 4 weeks, but more prolonged therapy may be necessary if drainage is not optimal.[18]

Successful treatment of empyema is determined by the stage of the disease process. Tube thoracostomy remains the first treatment option despite variable success rates in the treatment of chronic organizing empyema. Tube thoracostomy, image-directed catheterization, intrapleural thrombolytics, thorascopic drainage, decortication, and chronic open drainage have all been used with success rates ranging from 10 to 90 percent.[17] Generally, the initial exudative stage is amenable to antibiotics and thoracentesis or tube thoracostomy. In the fibrinopurulent stage, antibiotics with drainage by a properly positioned chest tube may resolve the empyema. Most patients with chronic empyema are not cured by medical therapy alone and require surgical intervention. A diffuse organized thick fibrous intrathoracic empyema may require thoracotomy, debridement, irrigation, pleurectomy, decortication, and prolonged open drainage.

The use of intrapleural thrombolytics as an adjunct to the evacuation of loculated pleural effusions has a success rate ranging from 50 to 100 percent,[20] and is associated with low morbidity and mortality rates. Fibrinolysis is likely to be more successful in patients with multiloculated empyemas.[21] Both streptokinase and urokinase are commonly used to convert plasminogen to plasmin. Plasmin dissolves fibrin and produces the dissolution of loculations and early peels, allowing complete evacuation of purulent pleural contents.[21] Urokinase is the agent of choice due to the lower risk of anaphylaxis and to the complications typically associated with streptokinase. The optimal doses of streptokinase and urokinase are unknown; however, mean doses of 275,000 IU and 121,000 IU, respectively, have been used. These agents are injected through drainage tubes, which remain clamped for 6 to 8 h, prior to suction drainage.[11]

Recently, thoracoscopy has been used for the evacuation of hemothorax and the drainage of thoracic empyema with a success rate of approximately 60 percent.[17] Video-assisted thoracic surgery can effectively treat pleural empyema by lysing adhesions, draining the abscess cavity, and decorticating the pleural peel.[19]

Disposition

Admission for early and complete drainage is the fundamental step in the management of an empyema. If primary tube thoracostomy fails, thoracotomy with early decortication has gained favor as therapy for empyema because of the realization that surgery can be safely performed at any stage with low morbidity and mortality rates.[17] After the initiation of antibiotic therapy, the clinical and radiographic response is gradual.

REFERENCES

1. Gleeson K, Reynolds HY: Life-threatening pneumonia. *Clin Chest Med* 15:581, 1994.
2. Mendelson CL: The aspiration of stomach contents into the lungs during obstetric anesthesia. *Am J Obstet Gynecol* 52:191, 1946.
3. Lomotan JR, George SS, Brandstetter RD: Aspiration pneumonia. *Postgrad Med* 102:225, 1997.
4. Gleeson K, Eggli DF, Maxwell SL: Quantitative aspiration during sleep in normal subjects. *Chest* 111:1266, 1997.
5. Daniels SK, Brailey K, Priestly DH, et al: Aspiration in patients with acute stroke. *Arch Phys Med Rehabil* 79:14, 1998.
6. Pick N, McDonald A, Bennett N, et al: Pulmonary aspiration in a long-term care setting: Clinical and laboratory observations and an analysis of risk factors. *J Am Geriatr Soc* 44:763, 1996.
7. Nagase T, Ohga E, Sudo E, et al: Intracellular adhesion molecule-1 mediates acid aspiration-induced lung injury. *Am J Respir Crit Care Med* 154:504, 1996.
8. Kazi N, Meborhan S: Enteral feeding associated gastroesophageal reflux and aspiration pneumonia: A review. *Nutr Rev* 54:324, 1996.
9. Adnet F, Borron SW, Vicaut E, et al: Value of C-reactive protein in the detection of bacterial contamination at the time of presentation in drug induced aspiration pneumonia. *Chest* 112:466, 1997.
10. Matthay MA, Rosen GD: Acid aspiration induced lung injury: New insights and therapeutic options. *Am J Respir Crit Care Med* 154:504, 1996.
11. Wiedemann HP, Rice T: Lung abscess and empyema. *Sem Thorac Cardiovasc Surg* 7:119, 1995.
12. Hammon JMJ, Potgieter PD, Hanslo D, et al: The etiology and antimicrobial susceptibility patterns of microorganisms in acute community-acquired lung abscess. *Chest* 108:937, 1995.
13. Tan TQ, Seilheimer DK, Kaplan SL: Pediatric lung abscess: Clinical management and outcome. *Pediatr Infect Dis J* 14:51, 1995.
14. Furman AC, Jacobs J, Sepkowitz KA: Lung abscess in patients with AIDS. *Clin Infect Dis* 22:81, 1996.
15. Klein JS, Schultz S, Heffner JE: Interventional radiology of the chest: Image-guided percutaneous drainage of pleural effusions, lung abscess, and pneumothorax. *Am J Radiol* 164:581, 1995.
16. Lawrence DR, Ohri SK, Moxon RE, et al: Thoracoscopic debridement of empyema thoracis. *Ann Thorac Surg* 64:1448, 1997.
17. Lemense GP, Strange C, Sahn SA: Empyema thoracis: Therapeutic management and outcome. *Chest* 107:1532, 1995.
18. Bryant RE, Salmon CJ: Pleural empyema. *Clin Infect Dis* 22:747, 1996.
19. Mandal AK, Thadepalli H, Mandal AK, Chettipalli U: Posttraumatic empyema thoracis: A 24-year experience at a major trauma center. *J Trauma* 43:764, 1997.
20. Chin NK, Lim TK: Controlled trial of intrapleural streptokinase in the treatment of pleural empyema and complicated parapneumonic effusions. *Chest* 111:275, 1997.
21. Temes RT, Follis F, Kessler RM, et al: Intrapleural fibrinolytics in management of empyema thoracis. *Chest* 110:102, 1996.

TUBERCULOSIS

Janet M. Poponick
Joel Moll

EPIDEMIOLOGY

Tuberculosis remains an important infectious disease in the world today. It is the leading infectious cause of death in people older than 5 years and is estimated to cause 6 percent of deaths worldwide.[1] In the United States, new cases of tuberculosis steadily declined from the late 1800s until 1984. From 1984 to 1992, tuberculosis cases increased at alarming rates. Factors believed to be responsible for this resurgence of tuberculosis include an increase in the number of homeless persons, the human immunodeficiency virus (HIV) epidemic, drug abuse, increased immigration, the inability of local and state governments to maintain tuberculosis control programs, and the increase of multidrug-resistant tuberculosis.[2]

From 1993 to 1997, tuberculosis was once again on the decline, primarily due to stronger tuberculosis control programs, which targeted high-risk individuals. During 1997, there was a 7 percent decrease in reported cases compared with 1996, and a 26 percent decrease from 1992, when tuberculosis cases peaked.[3] Tuberculosis remains more common in urban areas. The case rate for foreign-born persons remains four to five times higher than that for US-born persons.[3]

Continued improvement in tuberculosis control and prevention requires recognition and treatment of high-risk populations (Table 61-1), continued funding of programs for surveillance and treatment of noncompliant patients, continued basic research into the pathogenesis and immunologic response, and continued development of new pharmacologic agents.[2,3]

PATHOPHYSIOLOGY

Mycobacterium tuberculosis is a slow-growing aerobic rod that has a unique, multilayered cell wall that contains a variety of lipids that account for its acid-fast property. Transmission occurs through inhalation of droplet nuclei into the lungs. Persons with active tuberculosis who excrete stainable mycobacteria in saliva or sputum are the most infectious.[4]

Once the organisms reach the lungs, host defenses are activated.[5] In immunocompetent persons, such defenses may kill off the inhaled mycobacteria and prevent infection. Some organisms may survive, however, and be transported to the regional lymph nodes, where the host's cell-mediated immunity is further activated to contain the infection. Granulomas, known as tubercles, may form as a result of this process, which involves activated macrophages. Tubercles are a sign

TABLE 61-1 Patients with a High Prevalence of Tuberculosis

1. Elderly and nursing-home patients
2. Immigrants from high-prevalence countries
3. HIV-infected patients
4. Alcoholics and illicit drug users
5. Residents and staff of prisons or shelters for the homeless

of primary infection and may progress to caseation necrosis and calcification leading to the Ghon complex.[4] In most cases, the bacteria are contained in the tubercles, but some organisms enter the thoracic duct and spread throughout the body, where they may remain dormant for many years. This is referred to as latent infection and is manifested by a positive tuberculin skin test.[5] In most cases of dissemination in immunocompetent hosts, the organisms do not find a suitable area to proliferate. Survival is favored in areas of high oxygen content or blood flow, such as the apical and posterior segments of the upper lobe and the superior segment of the lower lobe of the lung, the renal cortex, the meninges, the epiphyses of long bones, and the vertebrae.[4] In immunocompromised hosts, hematogenous spread occurs early, as normal host defenses are unable to contain the organisms, and disseminated disease occurs.[4]

The latent infection may reactivate when a host's immune system is no longer capable of containing the foci of previous hematogenous spread. The young, the elderly, or patients with other chronic debilitating diseases are at higher risk for such reactivation disease. For immunocompetent hosts with latent infection, there is a 5 to 10 percent chance of developing reactivation tuberculosis over a lifetime.[5] The population at risk for HIV infection is also at risk for tuberculosis. As the host defense system weakens, latent infection may progress to reactivation tuberculosis. The incidence of reactivation tuberculosis in HIV patients is reported at 7 percent per year.[5]

Current research centers around the basic science involved in the host response to mycobacteria. The key cells are the alveolar macrophages and T lymphocytes, especially the T-helper cells, and the various cytokines and interleukins that are released into circulation. One of the key cytokines released by macrophages is interferon 8 (IFN-8) which seems to correlate with clinical findings.[6] For patients with active tuberculosis, but whose sputum smear is negative and whose chest radiograph is without cavitation, IFN-8 levels are high and there is a lymphocytic cell predominance in the bronchoalveolar lavage fluid. IFN-8 increases in patients who are improving with treatment for tuberculosis. As information on the role of cytokines is revealed by research, more specific new therapies may be developed to enhance or block important mediators.

CLINICAL FEATURES

Primary Tuberculosis

The initial infection is usually asymptomatic and only identified by a positive reaction to purified protein derivative (PPD) .[4] A pneumonitis may result that is similar to a viral or bacterial infection. Hilar adenopathy is present, but rarely massive. In some cases, especially in immunocompromised patients, the primary infection may be rapidly progressive and fatal.

Reactivation Tuberculosis

The majority of cases of tuberculosis are reactivation of latent infection. Symptoms can be divided into systemic and pulmonary. The most common symptom is fever, followed by night sweats, malaise, fatigue, and weight loss. Productive cough, hemoptysis, and pleuritic chest pain develop as the infection grows in the lungs. When the infection is extensive, shortness of breath may develop. The results of a physical examination are generally not helpful, but rales may be noted over areas of pulmonary infection.[4]

While the majority of cases of tuberculosis are pulmonary, up to 15 percent of cases will have extrapulmonary manifestations.[4] Common sites include the adrenal glands, bones and joints, gastrointestinal tract, genitourinary tract, lymph nodes, meninges, pericardium, peritoneum, and pleura.

Miliary tuberculosis is the result of wide hematogenous spread during the primary infection, or secondary seeding of the other organs in an immunocompromised host. Fever, cough, weight loss, hepatomegaly, splenomegaly, lymphadenopathy, and signs of multisystem illness should cause one to suspect miliary disease. Laboratory abnormalities include hyponatremia, anemia, thrombocytopenia, and leukopenia. The chest radiograph shows diffuse nodular infiltrates.[4]

The most common extrapulmonary site of tuberculosis is the lymphatic system and may involve any of the lymph nodes. Tuberculous adenitis causes symptoms at the site of lymph node enlargement. Fever is usually absent, and the lymphadenopathy is painless. The nodes may develop draining sinuses. Diagnosis is made by lymph node biopsy.[4]

A tuberculous pleural effusion usually occurs after primary infection, when a subpleural node ruptures into the pleura.[4] Some cases occur during hematogenous spread. Symptoms are usually fever, shortness of breath, and pleuritic chest pain. The fluid is exudative in nature, and analysis may not reveal the organisms on acid-fast staining. A pleural biopsy reveals granulomas.

Pericarditis and peritonitis as a result of tuberculosis are difficult to diagnose and often require biopsy. Complications of tuberculous pericarditis include tamponade and constrictive pericarditis.[4]

The central nervous system may become seeded during primary infection, leading to several tuberculous (Rich) foci in the meninges, spinal cord, or the brain parenchyma. Rupture of a Rich focus into the subarachnoid space may result in meningitis. In children, the disease is acute, whereas a more indolent course is noted in adults. Fever, signs of meningeal irritation, and cranial nerve deficits are seen. Typical cerebrospinal fluid analysis reveals mononuclear cells and a low glucose level, but early samples may have a predominance of neutrophils.[4]

Pediatric Tuberculosis

Tuberculosis in the pediatric population occurs in the same risk groups as in the adult population (Table 61-1). Primary tuberculosis is usually an asymptomatic disease and generally found during school screening or household screening programs.[4] The classic symptoms of fever, night sweats, and weight loss may be seen in older children, but, in those younger than age 5, presentation may be that of miliary tuberculosis, meningitis, or a pneumonia that does not respond to therapy.[4] The most common radiographic findings include hilar adenopathy, mediastinal lymphadenopathy, or consolidated pneumonia. The most common extrapulmonary presentation is cervical lymphadenitis, but meningitis and bone and joint involvement may also occur.

Tuberculosis and HIV

Tuberculosis (pulmonary and extrapulmonary) often can be the initial clinical manifestation of immunodeficiency and is considered an AIDS-defining illness. HIV infection increases the risk of reactivation disease and the likelihood that initial infection will result in active disease.[7] The incidence of tuberculosis in HIV-infected patients varies according to community prevalence, but is much higher than in the general population. Physicians considering a diagnosis of tuberculosis should offer patients HIV testing, which may provide early diagnosis and therapy.

Pulmonary involvement may be difficult to distinguish from other HIV-associated lung disorders. Tuberculosis must be in the differential of any HIV-associated respiratory disorder and can present atypically on chest radiographs. The incidence of extrapulmonary tuberculosis is higher in patients diagnosed with AIDS (greater than 70 percent) and in those with less advanced HIV infection (24 to 45 percent) than in individuals not infected with HIV.[7] The most common forms of extrapulmonary disease are lymphadenitis and miliary disease.[7]

Treatment of tuberculosis in coinfected individuals is generally effective, but some reports have indicated higher mortality rates in coinfected patients.[7] The incidence of adverse drug reactions to antituberculosis chemotherapy is higher in HIV-infected than in HIV-negative patients.[8] Due to the number of medications taken by patients with HIV, potential drug interactions must also be of concern.

Multidrug-Resistant Tuberculosis

The incidence of multidrug-resistant tuberculosis (MDR TB) peaked during the resurgence of tuberculosis. The majority of cases involved those coinfected with HIV and was associated with a high mortality rate. With the increased surveillance of high-risk groups, the incidence of drug resistance has stabilized.[3] MDR TB continues to be a concern, however, especially to health care workers assigned to patients with resistant strains. *Mycobacterium tuberculosis* becomes resistant by spontaneous genetic mutation, often as a result of inadequate drug therapy or noncompliance with initial treatment.[2,9] The most powerful predictor of drug resistance remains a history of previous tuberculosis.[9]

The vast majority of MDR TB outbreaks have been in the HIV population. Clinically, the most common pattern is resistance to isoniazid and rifampin.[4] Available data suggest no difference in isoniazid resistance among those patients with or without HIV. Rifampin monoresistant tuberculosis has become a problem, especially in those with AIDS.[10] Cases with rifampin monoresistance were more commonly seen in patients who had previously had tuberculosis, a history of diarrhea, rifabutin use, or antifungal therapy.[10]

For those HIV-negative patients who acquire MDR TB strains, or who are noncompliant with therapy, the course is less well defined. A study prior to the HIV epidemic reported a long-term response rate of 56 percent and a mortality rate of 22 percent.[11] The patient population in this study had tuberculosis for a long period and were heavily pretreated for the disease by the community physician prior to referral. A more recent study from New York demonstrated a more promising course.[12] MDR TB was diagnosed more quickly (mean, 44 days) and, therefore, appropriate treatment started earlier. There were 25 HIV-negative patients in this group: eight were health care workers, and eight had a previous tuberculosis history. Overall, 96 percent had a good clinical response, with 64 percent completing a full course of therapy without relapse.[12]

Treatment of MDR TB remains challenging and depends on the sensitivity patterns from culture. The majority of regimens include four to six drugs with treatment as long as 18 to 24 months after sputum conversion. The flurorquinolones have been used successfully in treatment of MDR TB.[9,12] Side effects of multiple-drug regimens are a common problem. When drug therapy fails, resectional surgery is considered to eradicate the disease.

DIAGNOSIS

The diagnosis of tuberculosis can present a challenge to emergency physicians. In the past, physicians mainly considered the diagnosis when presented with a young or older patient with reactivation disease. With the increased incidence of tuberculosis and the appearance of multidrug-resistant strains, one must consider the diagnosis in anyone with respiratory complaints or any extrapulmonary symptoms. The variable clinical presentation along with the time required to culture the organism makes emergent diagnosis difficult. A heightened awareness of the disease along with potential new rapid diagnostic tests can ensure that these patients are not returned to the community without proper therapy.

All prehospital and emergency department personnel must be trained to suspect tuberculosis, institute appropriate precautions, and notify health care providers of their suspicions. Triage workers should ask appropriate questions to detect potential cases. Patients with suspected tuberculosis should be placed in separate waiting areas, wear surgical masks, and be instructed to cover the mouth and nose when coughing. Any immunocompromised patient with respiratory symptoms should be isolated until tuberculosis can be excluded. Prompt evaluation will ensure a minimal amount of time spent in the ambulatory care setting and a minimal risk of exposure to health care providers and other patients.[13,14]

TABLE 61-2 Interpretation of Purified Protein Derivative Skin Test

1. ≥5 mm in duration is positive in
   a. Patients with HIV infection
   b. Patients with close contact with a tuberculosis-infected individual
   c. Patients with abnormal chest radiograph suggestive of healed tuberculosis
2. ≥10 mm in duration is positive in patients not meeting the above criteria, but who have other risks
   a. Intravenous drug users
   b. High-prevalence groups (immigrants, long-term-care facility residents, persons in local high-risk areas)
   c. Patients with conditions that increase the risk of progression to active disease
3. ≥15 mm in duration is positive in all others
4. Detection of newly infected persons in a screening program
   a. ≥10-mm in duration increase within any 2-year period is positive if younger than age 35
   b. ≥15-mm in duration increase within any 2-year period is positive if age 35 or older
5. If the patient is anergic, other epidemiologic factors must be considered

Note: A positive reaction does not necessarily indicate disease.

Skin Test

The most common method to detect exposure to *M. tuberculosis* is a skin test. The Mantoux test, which involves the intracutaneous injection of 0.1 mL of PPD in the forearm, relies on a delayed-type hypersensitivity reaction that is triggered if past exposure to tuberculosis has occurred. The test is read between 48 and 72 h after administration by measuring the extent of skin induration at the test site. Erythema or other skin changes are not assessed. Table 61-2 summarizes the American Thoracic Society's standards for interpretation of test results.[15] All persons with a positive PPD reaction or recent conversion should be referred for possible preventive therapy.

In a few situations, however, the PPD test may be nondiagnostic. Individuals who have received bacille Calmette-Guérin (BCG) immunization for tuberculosis prevention would be expected to have a positive response. Some individuals with remote BCG immunization lose PPD reactivity over time, but if a second PPD is placed within a few weeks of the first, a falsely positive booster effect may be seen.[13] Exposure to nontuberculosis mycobacteria can also result in a false-positive PPD reaction.

A competent immune system is required to yield a positive response to the PPD if there has been exposure to *M. tuberculosis*. Therefore, individuals with abnormal immune systems, such as in HIV, may lose their ability to mount a delayed-type hypersensitivity reaction required to produce a positive PPD reaction. Although the Centers for Disease Control (CDC) no longer recommend routine anergy testing among HIV-positive individuals,[16] some clinicians utilize control agents such as mumps or candida to assess at-risk patients for anergy. Controls are placed on the opposite forearm, and failure to respond with induration may indicate anergy and thus an unreliable PPD. False negatives have also been demonstrated with improper PPD administration. Nonreactivity to a PPD has been occasionally reported in patients with active culture-positive tuberculosis; therefore, a PPD test may occasionally be unreliable in acute stages of the disease.

Chest Radiograph

The chest radiograph is utilized to screen for disease in individuals with positive PPD skin test and for those with signs and symptoms of active infection. In the past, the classic findings of tuberculosis were those associated with reactivation disease. Cavitary or noncavitary lesions in the upper lobe or superior segment of the lower lobe of the lungs are classic findings. Cavitation can be associated with increased infectivity.[4] Calcification of the lesions may be a later finding.

With the resurgence of tuberculosis, radiographic findings of primary disease are becoming more common. In primary infection, parenchymal infiltrates in any area of the lung may be found.[4] Isolated ipsilateral hilar or mediastinal adenopathy is sometimes the only finding. Miliary tuberculosis as either primary or reactivation disease frequently shows small (1 to 3 mm) nodules throughout the lung fields. Pleural effusions, which are usually unilateral, can occur alone or in association with parenchymal disease. Atelectasis, fibrotic scarring, tracheal deviation, and signs of prior thoracic surgery are other findings. Because tuberculosis has a wide variety of appearances on chest radiographs, comparison to previous films is extremely helpful in determining the significance of an abnormal or unusual finding.

Immunocompromised patients, such as those with advanced HIV, are more likely to have radiographs typical of primary infection or with atypical findings. Normal radiographs in the presence of active disease are seen more frequently in HIV-infected patients.[4,7]

Microbiology

Culture for tuberculosis is the ''gold standard'' for diagnosis.[4] Sputum is commonly collected to detect the presence of *M. tuberculosis* by both culture and smear. In the absence of a satisfactory sputum sample, gastric aspirates, pleural and other body fluids, and tissue samples may be employed for culture and other diagnostic tests. Bronchoscopy may also be used to obtain more direct respiratory samples for both smear and culture. Staining of the specimen for acid fastness (i.e., Ziehl-Neelsen stain) or a fluorochrome procedure is the quickest and least expensive method to provide a presumptive diagnosis of tuberculosis. Approximately 60 percent of culture-positive cases of tuberculosis will have smears where acid-fast bacilli are detected, although this may be lower in individuals with HIV.[13]

Newer methods are under development to aid in the speed and sensitivity of diagnosing tuberculosis. Although not widely available, techniques that employ radiometric technology, DNA probes, polymerase chain reaction, reverse transcription, or other technologies may someday provide definitive results in a matter of hours.[4]

TREATMENT

Because of the possibility of resistance, the treatment of active tuberculosis involves the use of a combination of antimycobacterial medications. The emergence of MDR TB prompted the CDC recommendation of treating patients with at least four drugs (and in some cases, six drugs) until susceptibility tests are available.[17] Beginning therapy usually includes isoniazid (INH), rifampin, pyrazinamide, and either streptomycin or ethambutol for 2 months. CDC recommended options for treatment include

1. Daily four-drug therapy for 8 weeks and then 16 weeks of daily or two or three times per week. In this case, treatment is continued for at least 6 months and 3 months after culture conversion.
2. Daily four-drug therapy for 2 weeks followed by two times per week for 6 weeks with subsequent INH and rifampin two times per week for the remaining 16 weeks.
3. Four-drug therapy three times per week for 6 months.

More prolonged therapy is recommended for immunocompromised patients, such as those with HIV or those with extrapulmonary disease. Initial therapy may be modified once drug susceptibilities are available. The importance of directly observed therapy (DOT), where patients are observed taking their antituberculosis medications to ensure compliance, cannot be overstated.[18] The CDC recommends that all two or three times per week regimens should be by DOT.[17]

Although the standard medications used to treat tuberculosis are generally efficacious and safe, occasionally side effects or drug interactions may be significant. INH, the most frequently used antituberculosis agent, has hepatitis as its major toxicity. Although advancing age is thought to be a significant risk factor for the development of hepatitis,[4] the association with age has not always been clear.[8] Preexisting liver disease, pregnancy, ethanol use, HIV, and hepatitis C infection have been associated with an increased risk for hepatotoxicity from INH.[8,15] In addition, those with preexisting medical conditions requiring multiple medications may be at higher risk for drug interactions with antimycobacterial chemotherapy agents. Table 61-3 summarizes commonly used drug dosages and side effects.

With the emergence of multidrug resistance, other treatment modalities have been employed to treat infection that does not respond to antimycobacterial chemotherapy. Among them, surgical resection for multidrug-resistant tuberculosis is a treatment modality that has been shown to have good results, with cure rate of up to 90 percent.[9]

Preventive therapy with INH should be considered for patients with recent conversion to PPD-positive status, for persons who have been in close contact with an individual with active tuberculosis, for anergic individuals with known tuberculosis contact, or if the prevalence of tuberculosis is 10 percent or higher in the community.[16] The decision to institute therapy should be based on the likelihood that the positive PPD reaction represents true exposure to *M. tuberculosis,* the risk of progression to active disease, and the likelihood of INH-induced hepatitis. Therapy should continue for a minimum of 6 months for adults, 9 months for children, and 1 year for those with immunosuppression or HIV.[15] Those at risk for INH hepatotoxicity should be closely monitored for its development if treatment is elected. For those exposed to INH-resistant strains, or those who are intolerant to its use, rifampin and other antimycobacterial agents have been used, but experience is limited.

DISPOSITION

Admission

All hospitalized patients with suspected tuberculosis must be placed in respiratory isolation until the diagnosis is certain.[13] Admission is important in cases where the social situation makes it difficult to obtain a proper diagnosis and for therapy to be instituted. When a patient is proven to have active MDR TB, hospital admission is also indicated to institute therapy and observe for drug toxicity. Other indications for admission include uncertain diagnosis or patient noncompliance. Physicians need to be aware of their own state laws regarding involuntary hospitalization and treatment.[19]

Outpatient Treatment

The vast majority of patients with tuberculosis are treated initially as outpatients. Emergency physicians should contact physicians or public health services providing long-term care prior to discharge. Discharge instructions include home isolation procedures and sites of medication (if DOT is used) and ongoing care. Antituberculosis medications should be instituted by health care professionals who will coordinate the treatment and monitor adverse effects of the medication. Such medications should not be routinely instituted in the emergency department without these measures.

TABLE 61-3 Dosages and Common Side Effects of Some Drugs Used in Tuberculosis (Adults)

Drug	Daily (maxium)	Three times weekly DOT (maximum)	Two times weekly DOT (maximum)	Potential side effects
Isoniazid (INH)	5 mg/kg PO (300 mg)	15 mg/kg PO (900 mg)	15 mg/kg PO (900 mg)	Hepatitis, peripheral neuropathy, drug interactions
Rifampin	10 mg/kg PO (600 mg)	10 mg/kg PO (600 mg)	10 mg/kg PO (600 mg)	Hepatitis, fevers and chills, thrombocytopenia, GI disturbances, drug interactions
Pyrazinamide	15–30 mg/kg PO (2 g)	50–70 mg/kg PO (3 g)	50–70 mg/kg PO (4 g)	Arthralgia, hyperuricemia, hepatitis
Ethambutol	15–25 mg/kg PO	25–30 mg/kg PO	50 mg/kg PO	Optic neuritis, peripheral neuropathy and headache
Streptomycin	15 mg/kg IM (1 g)	25–30 mg/kg IM (1.5 g)	25–30 mg/kg IM (1.5 g)	Eighth cranial nerve damage, rashes, renal failure
Amikacin	7.5–10 mg/kg IM			Eighth cranial nerve damage, renal failure
Ciprofloxacin	750 mg PO bid			GI disturbances, CNS disturbances, arthropathies
Ofloxacin	400 mg PO bid			GI disturbances, CNS disturbances, arthropathies
Sparfloxacin	200 mg PO			Not FDA approved, phototoxicity, nausea and diarrhea
Capreomycin	15 mg/kg IM (1 g)			Nephrotoxicity and ototoxicity
Cycloserine	15 mg/kg PO bid to qid			CNS disturbances with possible seizures, peripheral neuropathy
Ethionamide	10–15 mg/kg PO qd to tid			Nausea, vomiting, diarrhea, abdominal cramps
Para-aminosalicylic acid (PAS)	200 mg/kg PO bid or tid			GI disturbances, hypersensitivity reactions, hematologic disturbances, goiter

Abbreviations: CNS, central nervous system; DOT, directly observed therapy; FDA, Food and Drug Administration; GI, gastrointestinal.

PREVENTION

Prevention of tuberculosis transmission in health care facilities is of extreme importance. Guidelines for prevention of transmission have been published and are available through the CDC. These recommendations include early detection and treatment of active cases, education and screening of health care workers, and engineering controls.[13] Ambulatory care facilities that frequently see tuberculosis patients will need isolation rooms available. Personnel who work in emergency or ambulatory settings where patients with tuberculosis are treated should have routine PPD testing to detect occupational exposure and be offered preventative therapy if appropriate.[13,14] Table 61-4 lists some controls that prevent transmission of disease.

TABLE 61-4 Engineering Controls to Reduce the Transmission of Tuberculosis

1. High air flow (at least six room exchanges per hour) with external exhaust
2. High-efficient particulate filters (HEPAs)
3. Ultraviolet germicidal irradiation
4. Negative-pressure isolation rooms
5. Respiratory protection: HEPA filter masks or respirators

REFERENCES

1. Raviglione MC, Snider DE, Kochi A: Global epidemiology of tuberculosis: Morbidity and mortality of a worldwide epidemic. *JAMA* 273:220, 1995.
2. Brudney K, Dobkin J: Resurgent tuberculosis in New York City. *Am Rev Respir Dis* 144:745, 1991.
3. CDC: Tuberculosis morbidity: United States, 1997. *MMWR* 47:253, 1998.
4. Rossman MD, MacGregor RR: *Tuberculosis.* New York, McGraw-Hill, 1995.
5. Schluger NW, Rom WN: The host immune response to tuberculosis. *Am J Respir Crit Care Med* 157:679, 1998.
6. Condos R, Rom WN, Liu YK, Schluger NW: Local immune responses correlate with presentation and outcome in tuberculosis. *Am J Respir Crit Care Med* 157:729, 1998.
7. Barnes PF, Bloch AB, Davidson PT, Snider DE Jr: Tuberculosis in patients with human immunodeficiency virus infection. *N Engl J Med* 324:1644, 1991.
8. Ungo JR, Jones D, Ashkin D, et al: Antituberculosis drug-induced hepatotoxicity. *Am J Respir Crit Care Med* 157:1871, 1998.
9. Iseman MD: Treatment of multidrug-resistant tuberculosis. *N Engl J Med* 329:784, 1993.
10. Ridzon R, Whitney CG, McKenna MT, et al: Risk factors for rifampin monoresistant tuberculosis. *Am J Respir Crit Care Med* 157:1881, 1998.
11. Goble M, Iseman MD, Madsen LA, et al: Treatment of 171 patients with pulmonary tuberculosis resistant to isoniazid and rifampin. *N Engl J Med* 328:527, 1993.
12. Telzak EE, Sepkowitz, K, Alpert P, et al: Multidrug-resistant tuberculosis in patients without HIV infection. *N Engl J Med* 333:907, 1995.
13. CDC: Guidelines for preventing the transmission of *Mycobacterium tuberculosis* in health-care facilities, 1994. *MMWR* 43(RR-13):1994.

14. Behrman AJ, Shofer FS: Tuberculosis exposure and control in an urban emergency department. *Ann Emerg Med* 31:370, 1998.
15. American Thoracic Society: Diagnostic standards and classification of tuberculosis. *Am Rev Respir Dis* 142:725, 1990
16. CDC: Anergy skin testing and preventive therapy for HIV-infected persons: Revised recommendations. *MMWR* 46(RR-15):1997.
17. CDC: Initial therapy for tuberculosis in the era of multidrug resistance: Recommendations of the Advisory Council for the Elimination of Tuberculosis. *MMWR* 42(RR-7): 1993.
18. Chaulk CP, Kazandjian VA: Directly observed therapy for treatment completion of pulmonary tuberculosis: Consensus statement of the Public Health Tuberculosis Guidelines Panel. *JAMA* 279:943, 1996.
19. Gostin LO: Controlling the resurgent tuberculosis epidemic: A 50-state survey of TB statues and proposals for reform. *JAMA* 269:255, 1993.

SPONTANEOUS AND IATROGENIC PNEUMOTHORAX

William Franklin Young, Jr.
Roger Loyd Humphries

Pneumothorax occurs when air enters the potential space between the visceral and parietal pleura. The cause may be blunt trauma, penetrating trauma, or spontaneous. Iatrogenic pneumothorax occurs secondary to a diagnostic or therapeutic procedure and is really a subset of penetrating traumatic pneumothorax. Primary spontaneous pneumothorax (PSP) occurs in individuals without known lung disease and accounts for two-thirds of spontaneous pneumothoraces. Secondary spontaneous pneumothorax (SSP) occurs in patients with underlying lung disease, especially chronic obstructive pulmonary disease. Emergency department evaluation and management of pneumothorax center on immediate management of complications such as tension pneumothorax or ventilatory failure, eliminating the intrapleural air, optimizing pleural healing, and preventing recurrences.

SPONTANEOUS PNEUMOTHORAX

Epidemiology

An estimated 20,000 new spontaneous pneumothoraces occur each year in the United States, and there is evidence that the rate is increasing.[1,2] However, the true incidence of spontaneous pneumothorax is unknown, with estimates that up to 20 percent of such patients do not seek medical help.[3] Spontaneous pneumothorax is primarily a disease of male smokers who have larger height-to-weight ratios.[4] Male sex carries a 6 : 1 relative risk compared with the risk for females, although more recent studies show a trend to increased cases among women, perhaps due to smoking trends.[2] Smoking is an important risk factor with an overall greater than 20 : 1 relative risk compared with nonsmokers.[5] Spontaneous pneumothorax occurs among all age groups, with three peaks: among neonates (due to hyaline membrane disease or aspiration), among 20- to 40-year-olds (such cases tend to be primary), and among those older than age 40 (typically secondary cases). A genetic component is evidenced in the 11 percent of patients who have family members with spontaneous pneumothorax.[6] Contrary to common belief, only 10 to 20 percent of cases occur with exertion.[4] Spontaneous pneumothorax may rarely be associated with menses (catamenial).[4]

Pathophysiology

The pleurae are serous membranes that surround each lung: the parietal pleura lines the thoracic wall continuous with visceral pleura closely applied to the lung surface. At the hilum of each lung, the parietal and visceral pleurae are contiguous. The intrapleural space has subatmospheric pressure due to the inherent tendency of the chest wall to expand and the lung to collapse from elastic recoil.

Primary spontaneous pneumothorax seems to result from rupture of a subpleural bleb, usually in an upper lobe.[7] These blebs are multiple and have increased wall tension allowing distention and eventual rupture. The mechanism of bleb formation remains unknown, but higher upper lobe transpulmonary pressure, local ischemia from decreased upper lobe blood flow, and subclinical emphysema-like changes have been postulated.[3,7]

Chronic obstructive pulmonary disease (COPD) accounts for most cases of secondary spontaneous pneumothorax.[4] Other causes include cystic fibrosis, pulmonary infections, interstitial lung disease, AIDS, neoplasms, and drug use. Pneumothorax occurs in 5 percent of AIDS patients, is associated with subpleural necrosis from *Pneumocystis* infection, and carries a high mortality.[8] Because of necrosis of lung tissue and continued air leak, simple aspiration and nondrainage techniques fail in this group of patients.[8]

Once there is a break in the pleura, air travels down a pressure gradient into the intrapleural space until pressure equilibrium occurs with partial or total lung collapse.[9] Altered ventilation perfusion relationships and decreased vital capacity then contribute to dyspnea and hypoxemia.

Clinical Features

Symptoms are related to the size of the pneumothorax and rate of development. Patients with mild symptoms may not come for evaluation, whereas those with underlying lung disease may arrive in extremis. Patients with secondary spontaneous pneumothoraces present more dramatically than those with primary pneumothoraces. Tension pneumothorax is rare in PSP/SSP but requires immediate treatment by needle decompression and expeditious chest tube thoracostomy based on clinical signs. Pneumothorax is an important differential diagnosis in patients with chest pain, since it can mimic ischemia causing ST changes and T-wave inversion on the ECG.[3]

Acute pleuritic chest pain occurs in 95 percent of patients and localizes to the side of the pneumothorax in > 90 percent of cases.[6] Dyspnea occurs in 80 percent and predicts a larger pneumothorax.[6] Patients with COPD may acutely decompensate, with 1 to 17 percent mortality. Decreased breath sounds occur over the affected lung 85 percent of the time, but only 5 percent have tachypnea of more than 24 breaths per minute or tachycardia of more than 120 beats per minute.[6] Hyperresonance occurs in fewer than one-third. Tracheal deviation and hemodynamic compromise are the hallmarks of tension pneumothorax that demands immediate treatment.

Diagnosis

Tension pneumothorax diagnosed on clinical grounds requires immediate treatment by needle decompression and expeditious chest tube thoracostomy before radiographic evaluation. The traditional "gold standard" for diagnosis of pneumothorax continues to be the 6-foot upright posteroanterior chest radiograph, although the sensitivity of this examination is 83 percent.[10] A radiolucent line is seen to separate the parietal and visceral pleurae. Pseudo-pneumothorax due to a skinfold, scapular border, or tubing is differentiated from true pneumothorax by looking for vascular markings outside the confines of the radiolucent line and the blending of these lines into the chest wall rather than following the borders of a collapsed lung. Large bullae have been mistaken for pneumothoraces, but bullae and cysts have concave inner margins and rounded edges. Pneumothorax is much more difficult to detect on a supine anteroposterior radiograph. On the anteroposterior view, a deep sulcus sign, representing a deep lateral costophrenic angle, sometimes is a clue to a pneumothorax.[10] Expiratory radiographs by themselves are no more sensitive than inspiratory

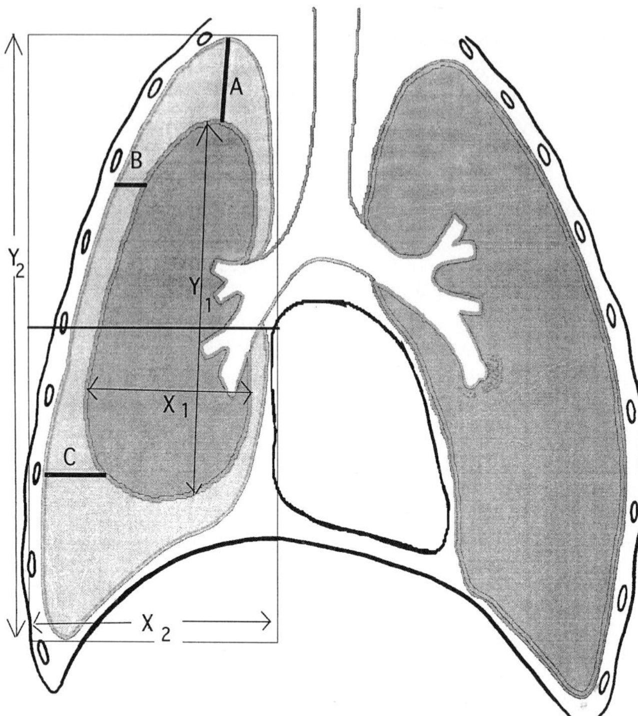

FIG. 62-1. Measurements used in pneumothorax size evaluations.

films and provide inferior evaluation of lung parenchyma.[10] However, comparison of paired inspiratory and expiratory films may be more sensitive than either view alone.[11] Chest computed tomography (CT) may be more sensitive than plain radiographs in detection of pneumothorax, but most studies compare supine chest x-ray film (CXR) with chest CT in the setting of trauma. This is useful if the plain film is equivocal. Ultrasound, although portable and easy to perform, is not useful for the diagnosis of pneumothorax, because ultrasound sensitivity is 73 to 95 percent and its specificity is 68 to 91 percent.[12]

Spontaneous pneumothorax should be included in the differential diagnosis of acute chest pain or acute deterioration in a patient with COPD. ST-segment and T-wave changes may be mistaken for ischemia. Occasionally, severe bullous COPD may mimic pneumothorax, and careful review of the CXR is needed with confirmatory CT if the patient is stable. A thoracostomy with the chest tube inserted into a bulla mistaken for a pneumothorax results in a large pneumothorax, associated bronchopulmonary fistula, and its complications.[3]

The size of the pneumothorax may be calculated, and some physicians use size as a guide to therapy. Radiologist "best guess" estimates show substantial interobserver disagreement and lack of reproducibility.[13] Using the lung area ($x_1 \times y_1$) to hemithorax area ($x_2 \times y_2$) ratio to estimate the size of the pneumothorax has a poor correlation ($r = 0.7$) with actual size[14] (Fig. 62-1). Estimating the amount of collapse by using the ratio of the cube of the pneumothorax diameter (x_1) to the cube of the hemithorax diameter (x_2) also shows poor correlation ($r = 0.7$).[14] Rhea and colleagues[13] describe a nomogram by using the average intrapleural distance, and Collins and coworkers[15] describe a formula using three intrapleural distances measured in centimeters:

$$\%\ \text{pneumothorax} = 4.2 + 4.7\ (\text{A} + \text{B} + \text{C})\ (\text{Fig. 62-1})$$

Whatever method is chosen, the same formula should be used so that sequential calculations are consistent. Chest CT volume measurements represent the current "gold standard," but the patient's clinical status and not the pneumothorax size should determine treatment options.[1]

Treatment

Treatment goals are the elimination of intrapleural air, optimization of pleural healing, and prevention of recurrences. However, there is marked practice variation, and no consensus exists, although attempts have been made.[1,16] Observation, oxygen, catheter aspiration (either single or sequential), tube thoracostomy (either minicatheter or standard chest tube), pleurodesis, video-assisted thoracoscopy (VAT), and thoracotomy are all options, but only the latter three procedures reduce the risk of future pneumothorax recurrence.

Since 1.25 percent of intrapleural air is reabsorbed each day, stable patients with an asymptomatic primary small spontaneous pneumothorax who have ready access to health care may be observed as outpatients after a 6-h period of observation and a repeat chest radiograph showing no increase in pneumothorax size. Extended outpatient observation is needed because a 25 percent pneumothorax would take about 20 days to resolve. Critics of this treatment plan point to the 23 to 40 percent of patients treated by observation who eventually require tube thoracostomy.[1]

Observation may be a reasonable approach for those patients with a contraindication to invasive therapy, such as coagulopathy. Concomitant oxygen administration at 3 to 4 L/min increases pleural air resorption three- to fourfold and should always be used in the emergency department.[1]

Catheter aspiration is underutilized for treatment of spontaneous pneumothorax. Multiple techniques, equipment, and protocols are described, making a consensus statement difficult. Success rates from 37 to 75 percent are described with the greater success seen in PSP.[1] Techniques include simple one-time aspiration with small plastic 16- to 18-gauge intravenous catheters, repeated aspirations through the same catheter, and small-caliber chest tube with aspiration. Minicatheter tube placement uses a specially designed catheter with multiple side ports eliminating the problem of single-lumen obstruction seen with intravenous catheters. The technique involves placing a small catheter either into the second anterior intercostal space in the midclavicular line or laterally at the fourth or fifth intercostal space in the anterior axillary line after local anesthesia and sterile preparation. A three-way stopcock is applied, and a 60 mL syringe is used to aspirate the pleural space until resistance is met and the patient coughs. The stopcock is closed, the tube is secured, and a chest radiograph is obtained to assure reexpansion. Aspiration of more than 4 L suggests continued air leak and failure of simple aspiration. Failure to fully expand warrants another aspiration attempt. If the procedure is successful, patients should be observed for 6 h and, if no recurrence is seen, discharged to close follow-up within 24 h. If the procedure is not successful, a Heimlich valve is attached, with an improved success rate for failed simple aspiration.[17]

Patients who fail to reexpand even with the Heimlich valve can be placed on low suction or undergo formal large-bore chest tube thoracostomy. These patients require admission, although outpatient chest tube management has been described. Standard chest tube thoracostomy with underwater seal drainage is the most commonly used therapy and remains the standard in many hospitals. Proponents point to a low complication rate and a high success rate of 95 percent.[17] Patients with secondary spontaneous pneumothorax, those with recurrent pneumothorax, and those who fail simple catheter aspiration with Heimlich valve require formal large-bore, >28 French chest tube thoracostomy.[17] A proposed treatment algorithm is presented in Fig. 62-2.

Short-term complications of spontaneous pneumothorax include tension pneumothorax, failure to reexpand, persistent air leak, and complications related to the removal of intrapleural air, such as infection, technical errors, and reexpansion pulmonary edema. Reexpansion pulmonary edema is multifactorial, poorly studied, and reports are largely anecdotal.[1] Younger patients with larger pneumothoraces rapidly expanded with suction are at most risk. Pulmonary edema generally occurs on the side of the reexpanded lung. Treatment is supportive.

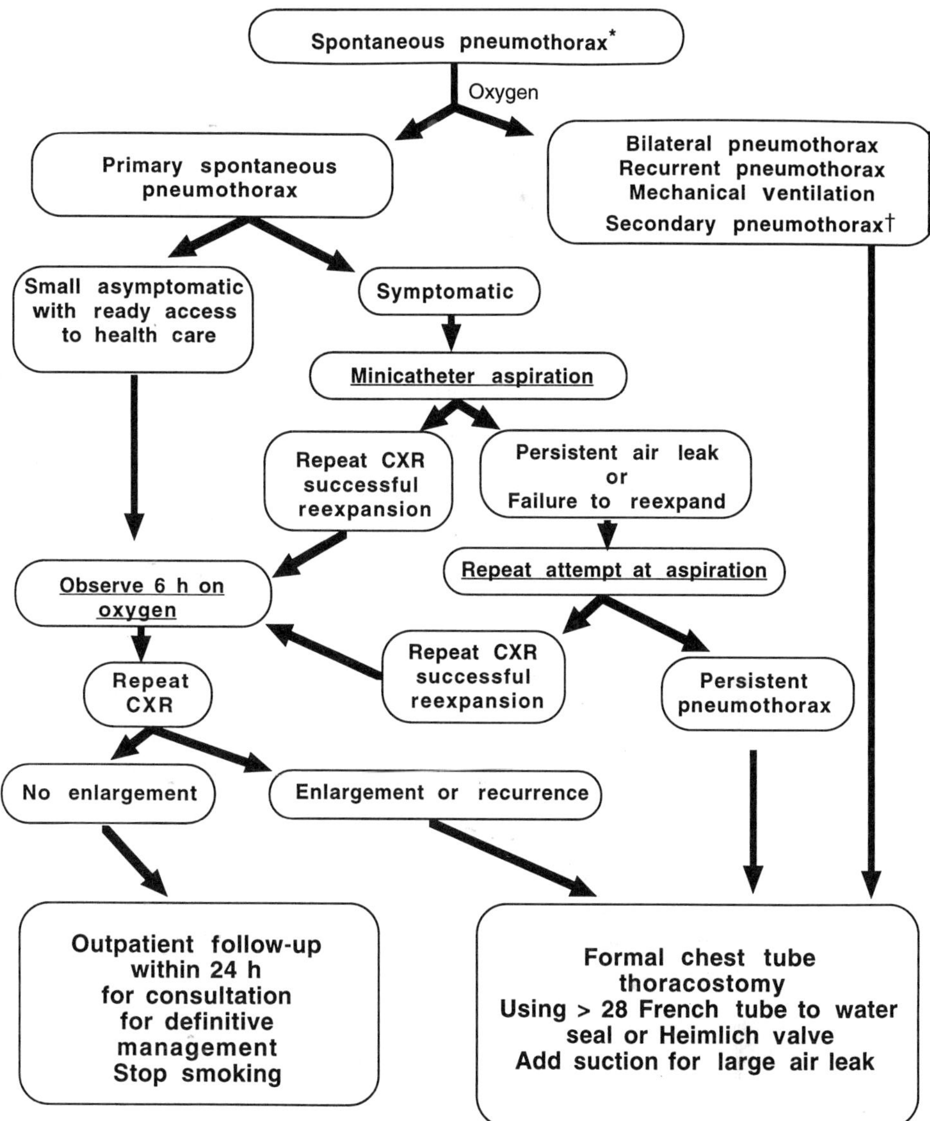

FIG. 62-2. Treatment summary (see the text).
*Symptoms of tension pneumothorax demand immediate decompression.
†Secondary: chronic obstructive pulmonary disease (COPD), AIDS, cystic fibrosis, asthma, or other known prior lung disease.

Disposition

After successful emergency treatment of a spontaneous pneumothorax, referral or consultation regarding definitive management with pleurodesis with or without VAT or thoracotomy should be done. Some authors recommend VAT for the first spontaneous pneumothorax due to the relative high rate of pneumothorax recurrence, lower overall cost, and success rate of the procedure, but this seems overly aggressive.[17] Recurrence after VAT requires open thoracotomy with pleurectomy or pleural scarification.[8]

Recurrence of the pneumothorax is the major long-term complication and the reason that all patients with spontaneous pneumothorax require referral for potential definitive therapy. Primary spontaneous pneumothorax recurs in about 30 to 40 percent and is independent of the method chosen to remove the intrapleural air.[6] Two-thirds of such cases occur within the first year.[6] Smoking cessation reduces this risk by half.[2] Secondary spontaneous pneumothorax recurs in 40 to 50 percent of patients.

IATROGENIC PNEUMOTHORAX

Iatrogenic pneumothorax occurs more than spontaneous pneumothorax and is a subset of traumatic penetrating pneumothorax. Transthoracic needle procedures (transthoracic needle biopsy and thoracentesis) account for more than 50 percent of cases, and subclavian vein catheterization accounts for 22 percent.[18] Given that one central venous line is placed every minute in the United States, and pneumothorax occurs after 1 to 12 percent of subclavian line attempts, iatrogenic pneumothorax must be common.[18–20] Some of the factors increasing the frequency of iatrogenic pneumothorax include the patient population, underlying disease, body habitus, and experience of the operator.[18] Ultrasound guidance for thoracentesis has been shown to reduce the pneumothorax complication rate from 18 to 3 percent[21] and appears promising to reduce the incidence of pneumothorax with central venous line placement.[22]

Chest radiograph is standard after central line placement or transthoracic needle procedures, but may miss an iatrogenic pneumothorax because of the use of a supine technique or inadequate time for the pneumothorax to develop. Delayed pneumothoraces are common after subclavian line placement; up to 4 percent are delayed for up to 96 h.[23] Emergency department experience with other penetrating chest trauma recognizes the risk of delayed pneumothorax of up to 6 h.[24]

Treatment for iatrogenic pneumothorax parallels that for spontaneous pneumothorax, with some important caveats. Patients on mechanical ventilation require large-bore chest tube thoracostomy.[20] Conversely, patients sustaining a small pneumothorax after a needle puncture and not receiving positive pressure ventilation can be initially treated with simple catheter aspiration, which will be adequate in up to 60 percent of patients. These patients need to be admitted to the hospital, with the catheter in place for observation, because prolonged air leak may occur in some patients.[25] Recurrence is not an issue in these patients, but deaths have occurred from iatrogenic pneumothorax.[20]

REFERENCES

1. Baumann MH, Strange C: Treatment of spontaneous pneumothorax: A more aggressive approach? *Chest* 112:789, 1997.
2. Sadikot RT, Greene T, Meadows K, Arnold AG: Recurrence of spontaneous pneumothorax. *Thorax* 52:805, 1997.
3. Kirby TJ, Ginsberg RJ: Management of the pneumothorax and barotrauma. *Clin Chest Med* 13:97, 1992.
4. Jantz MA, Pierson DJ: Pneumothorax and barotrauma. *Respir Emerg* 15:75, 1994.
5. Schramel FM, Postmus PE, Vanerschueren RG: Current aspects of spontaneous pneumothorax. *Eur Respir J* 10:1372, 1997.
6. Abolnik IZ, Lossos IS, Gillis D, Breuer R: Primary spontaneous pneumothorax in men. *Am J Med Sci* 305:297, 1993.
7. Baumann MH, Strange C: The clinician's perspective on pneumothorax management. *Chest* 112:822, 1997.
8. Light RW, Hamm H: Pleural disease and acquired immune deficiency syndrome. *Eur Respir J* 10:2638, 1997.
9. Paape K, Fry WA: Spontaneous pneumothorax. *Chest* 4:517, 1994.
10. Seow A, Kazerooni EA, Pernicano PG, Neary M: Comparison of upright inspiratory and expiratory chest radiographs for detecting pneumothoraces. *Am J Roentgenol* 166:313, 1996.
11. Aitchison F, Bleetman A, Munro P, et al: Detection of pneumothorax by accident and emergency officers and radiologists on single chest film. *Arch Emerg Med* 10:343, 1993.
12. Sistrom CL, Reiheld CT, Gay SB, Wallace KK: Detection and estimation of the volume of pneumothorax using real-time sonography: Efficacy determined by receiver operating characteristics analysis. *Am J Roentgenol* 166:317, 1996.
13. Rhea JT, DeLuca SA, Greene RE: Determining the size of pneumothorax in the upright patient. *Diagn Radiol* 144:733, 1982.
14. Engdahl O, Toft T, Boe J: Chest radiograph: A poor method of determining the size of a pneumothorax. *Chest* 103:26, 1993.
15. Collins CD, Lopez A, Mathie A, et al: Quantification of pneumothorax size on chest radiographs using interpleural distances: Regression analysis based on volume measurements from helical CT. *Am J Roentgenol* 165:1127, 1995.
16. Miller AC, Harvey JE: Guidelines for the management of spontaneous pneumothorax. *BMJ* 307:114, 1993.
17. Light RW: Management of spontaneous pneumothorax. *Am Rev Respir Dis* 148:245, 1993.
18. Sassoon CS, Light RW, O'Hara VS, Moritz TE: Iatrogenic pneumothorax: etiology and morbidity. *Respiration* 59:215, 1992.
19. Damascelli B, Patelli G, Frigerio LF, et al: Placement of long-term central venous catheters in outpatients: Study of 134 patients over 24,596 catheter days. *Am J Roentgenol* 168:1235, 1997.
20. Despars JA, Sassoon CS, Light RW: Significance of iatrogenic pneumothoraces. *Chest* 105:1147, 1994.
21. Raptopoulos V, Davis LM, Lee G, et al: Factors affecting the development of pneumothorax associated with thoracentesis. *Am J Roentgenol* 156:917, 1991.
22. Nash A, Burrell CJ, Ring NJ, Marshall AJ: Evaluation of an ultrasonically guided venepuncture technique for the placement of permanent pacing electrodes. *Pacing Clin Electrophysiol* 21:452, 1998.
23. Plaus WJ: Delayed pneumothorax after subclavian vein catheterization. *J Parenter Enter Nutr* 14:414, 1990.
24. Kiev J, Kersstein MD: Role of three hour roentgenogram of the chest in penetrating and nonpenetrating injuries of the chest. *Surg Gynecol Obstet* 175:249, 1992.
25. Schoenenberger RA, Haefeli WE, Weiss P, Ritz R: Evaluation of conventional chest tube therapy for iatrogenic pneumothorax. *Chest* 104:1770, 1993.

63 HEMOPTYSIS

William Franklin Young, Jr.
Michael W. Stava

Hemoptysis is expectoration of blood from the respiratory tract below the level of the larynx. Hemoptysis presents a diagnostic dilemma due to its multiple causes, ranging from minor to life threatening. Up to 25 percent of cases remain undiagnosed even after extensive evaluation. Priorities in the evaluation of hemoptysis are (1) ensuring adequate oxygenation and ventilation, (2) confirming a pulmonary source of bleeding, (3) looking for neoplasia and systemic disease (e.g., pulmonary embolism or Wegener granulomatosis), (4) appropriate radiographic imaging, and (5) appropriate disposition.

EPIDEMIOLOGY

Hemoptysis may be defined as mild, moderate or massive. The precise degree of hemoptysis required for each categorization is arbitrary and not standardized. Despite lack of clinical utility, mild hemoptysis is usually defined as less than 5 mL of blood in 24 h, moderate hemoptysis is defined as 5 to 600 mL in 24 h, and massive hemoptysis is greater than 600 mL in 24 h.[1] Often patients are unable to accurately estimate the degree of bleeding, and the emergency department time frame requires a more appropriate time categorization. A reasonable amount of hemoptysis considered massive in volume would be greater than 50 mL in a single expectoration.

In a retrospective meta-analysis of six prior studies of hemoptysis, Marshall found an infectious nontubercular cause in approximately 25 percent of cases, tuberculosis in 5 percent, neoplasia in 28 percent, miscellaneous and multiple causes in 13 percent; and an undetermined cause in 28 percent.[2] In another study, cardiovascular causes account for 3 percent of total hemoptysis cases, most due to congestive heart failure, and trauma accounts for less than 3 percent.[3] In summary, out of every four cases of hemoptysis, one neoplasm, one nontubercular infectious case, one miscellaneous case, and one idiopathic case may be expected.

Hemoptysis is described in both sexes, with a 60 : 40 male predominance, and in all age groups.[4] It is rare in children and increases in frequency with age. The true incidence is unknown, since many cases are unreported. Lifestyle activities, such as smoking, predispose patients to lung disease and an increased risk of hemoptysis. Male gender, age over 40, and history of smoking are risk factors for a neoplastic cause of hemoptysis.[2]

PATHOPHYSIOLOGY

The lung has a dual blood supply: (1) bronchial vessels under systemic circulatory pressure supply the supporting structures of the lung, and (2) pulmonary vessels under low pressure perform the specialized oxygen-carbon dioxide exchange in the alveoli.[5] Bleeding may be from either source by three mechanisms: (1) increased intravascular pressure, (2) erosion by an inflammatory process into a pulmonary or bronchial blood vessel, and (3) a complication of a bleeding diathesis.

Hemoptysis due to increases in pulmonary vascular pressure most often arise from primary cardiac abnormalities, such left-sided congestive heart failure (constituting 75 percent of cases) or mitral stenosis. Hemoptysis is usually well tolerated and scant in rheumatic heart disease.

Inflammatory causes of hemoptysis include bronchitis, bronchiectasis, mycetoma, foreign-body aspiration, pulmonary embolism, pneumonia, and malignancy. Fifty percent of malignant lesions are metastatic; the other half are primary lung neoplasms.[4] Erosion into the bronchial vessels under systemic circulatory pressures, with resultant severe hemoptysis, appears to be more common in tuberculosis, bronchiectasis, and mycetomas from fungal infection.[6] Although classically associated with pulmonary embolism, hemoptysis is seen in only 3 to 20 percent of cases and has a sensitivity of only 14 percent for a positive finding on radionuclide scanning.[7] Hemoptysis from vasculitis is usually alveolar in location and part of a larger systemic vasculopathy, such as systemic lupus erythematosus, Wegener granulomatosis, polyarteritis, or Goodpasture syndrome. Extrapulmonary symptoms, especially hematuria, are often seen.

Hemophilia, thrombocytopenia, anticoagulants, and thrombolytics may cause hemoptysis. Thrombolytic-induced hemoptysis occurs in less than 1 percent of patients receiving thrombolysis and is usually self-limited.[8] However, its occurrence should prompt investigation for an underlying cause.

Hemoptysis without a discovered cause tends to resolve spontaneously within 6 months in 90 percent of cases.[2]

CLINICAL FEATURES AND DIAGNOSIS

A history of underlying lung disease provides important clues to the underlying cause of hemoptysis. An abrupt onset of cough with bloody purulent sputum, with or without fever, may indicate acute pneumonia or bronchitis. A chronic productive cough may reflect chronic bronchitis or bronchiectasis. Although typically seen with tuberculosis, fevers, night sweats, and weight loss may represent other infections. Anorexia, weight loss, and change in cough may reflect bronchogenic carcinoma. While some tumors present with new-onset cough and hemoptysis, 80 percent of neoplastically caused hemoptysis had duration of greater than 1 week. Smoking, male gender, and age over 40 are the predominant risk factors for neoplasm. Alveolar hemorrhage syndromes from vasculitis present with dyspnea and mild hemoptysis associated with renal disease and hematuria. As noted earlier, hemoptysis is an insensitive marker for pulmonary embolism and the symptom of hemoptysis is usually overshadowed by anxiety, dyspnea, and chest pain.

The physical examination is useful in determining the severity of hemoptysis, but is unreliable in localizing the site of bleeding. Fever usually suggests an infectious cause. Tachypnea may reflect respiratory compromise with hypoxemia due to the interference of intrapulmonary blood with gas exchange or from underlying lung disease with altered ventilation-perfusion relationships. Blood pressure is usually not changed, except in massive hemoptysis. The nasal cavity and oropharynx should be carefully examined for extrapulmonary causes of hemoptysis (termed pseudohemoptysis) as well as signs of extrapulmonary vasculitis. The cardiac examination may reveal the diastolic murmur of mitral stenosis. The pulmonary examination may reveal fine inspiratory rales associated with alveolar blood or inspiratory and expiratory rhonchi associated with airway secretions and blood. There may be wheezing from bronchial narrowing. Digital clubbing suggests chronic lung disease. Supraclavicular adenopathy and muscle wasting suggest neoplasia.

Upon initial contact, the patient's ventilatory stability should be assessed to the ensure adequate oxygenation and ventilation. The airway may be inadequate and require intubation. Pulse oximetry is necessary to assess oxygenation. Ventilation is assessed by the clinical appearance of tidal volume and mental status. For patients with ongoing massive hemoptysis, immediate intervention with supplemental oxygen, intravenous access, and typing and cross-matching of blood, and urgent consultation with a pulmonologist or thoracic surgeon for emergency bronchoscopy are indicated. Patients who are stable (no respiratory distress and lesser degrees of hemoptysis) should have their sputum evaluated to differentiate true hemoptysis from pseudohemoptysis due to an ear, nose, throat, or gastrointestinal source. A bright red color, frothy appearance, alkaline pH, and presence of macrophages indicating a pulmonary source suggest true hemoptysis. Gastrointestinal blood typically is acidic and dark red, although swallowed epistaxis may be mistaken for gastrointestinal bleeding. Ten percent of pseudohemoptysis is due to lesions of the upper aerodigestive tract.[3]

The laboratory evaluation should be guided by clinical indications. For example, a healthy young person who presents with an acute cough and streaky hemoptysis does not require routine laboratory testing. A complete blood count should be obtained and serum electrolytes, blood urea nitrogen, creatinine, and glucose measured in patients with massive hemoptysis and in the setting of chronic illnesses. Coagulation studies are indicated in patients with liver disease or using anticoagulants. Arterial blood gas analysis should be performed on patients with respiratory distress or altered mental status. Bacterial sputum cultures are indicated with clinical or radiographic evidence of pneumonia. Mycobacterial sputum cultures are indicated with fever, weight loss, night sweating, and cavitary lung masses.

It is generally agreed that all patients with true hemoptysis require radiographic imaging, starting with a chest x-ray, for evaluation.[2,9] Up to 90 percent of individuals with neoplasm as a cause of hemoptysis have abnormal chest x-rays. However, 20 to 30 percent of patients presenting with hemoptysis have a normal chest radiograph, and details of further workup of these patients remains controversial.[2] No definitive diagnosis is reached in up to 90 percent of patients who have normal chest x-rays. Conversely, hemoptysis with a normal chest radiograph carries a small (less than 5 percent) risk of neoplasm.

Chest computed tomography (CT) is felt to have a greater sensitivity than plain radiography in detecting carcinoma or bronchiectasis.[2] Bronchoscopy or laparoscopic biopsy may also be needed. Fiberoptic bronchoscopy and chest CT have complementary roles. Close consultation with the follow-up physician is important to coordinate the timing of these evaluations.

Bronchoscopic evaluation continues to have a pivotal role in the evaluation of ongoing hemoptysis. Patients who are unstable with airway problems or have massive hemoptysis generally require rigid bronchoscopy to evacuate clots and determine the source of bleeding (Fig. 63-1).

TREATMENT

Treatment in the emergency department depends on the severity of the hemoptysis and the likelihood of a malignant cause. All patients with massive hemoptysis, and some patients with minor hemoptysis due to tuberculosis, mycetoma, or bronchiectasis, who are at significant risk of developing massive hemoptysis in the near future, require urgent management and hospitalization. All such patients require intravenous access, supplemental oxygen to ensure adequate arterial saturation, and typing and cross-matching of blood.

Patients with ongoing massive hemoptysis from one lung should be positioned with the bleeding lung dependent to minimize soiling of the contralateral lung. Tracheal intubation with a large-diameter endotracheal tube (8 French or larger to allow for bronchoscopy) is indicated if there is respiratory failure or if the patient is unable to clear the blood from the airways. Double-lumen endotracheal tubes have smaller lumina, which limit suctioning and ventilation.[2] If bleeding persists despite initial measures, the endotracheal tube may be advanced to the main-stem bronchus of the nonbleeding lung to minimize further aspiration of blood. The right main-stem bronchus is easily entered by advancing a standard orotracheal tube. This procedure will occlude the right upper lobe tertiary bronchus and ventilate the right middle and right lower lobes only.[2] The left main-stem bronchus is more sharply angled from the trachea, and selective intubation usually requires special equipment and technique. Mechanical ventilation should be instituted as necessary to support ventilation.

Fresh-frozen plasma should be administered to correct coagulopathy, and platelet transfusions are indicated for thrombocytopenia. Cough suppression with codeine or opioids might be helpful to prevent dislodging of hemostatic clots but carries the risk of suppressing ventilation and increases the risk of aspiration.

Emergency consultation is indicated with a pulmonologist or thoracic surgeon who may arrange for bronchoscopy, high-resolution

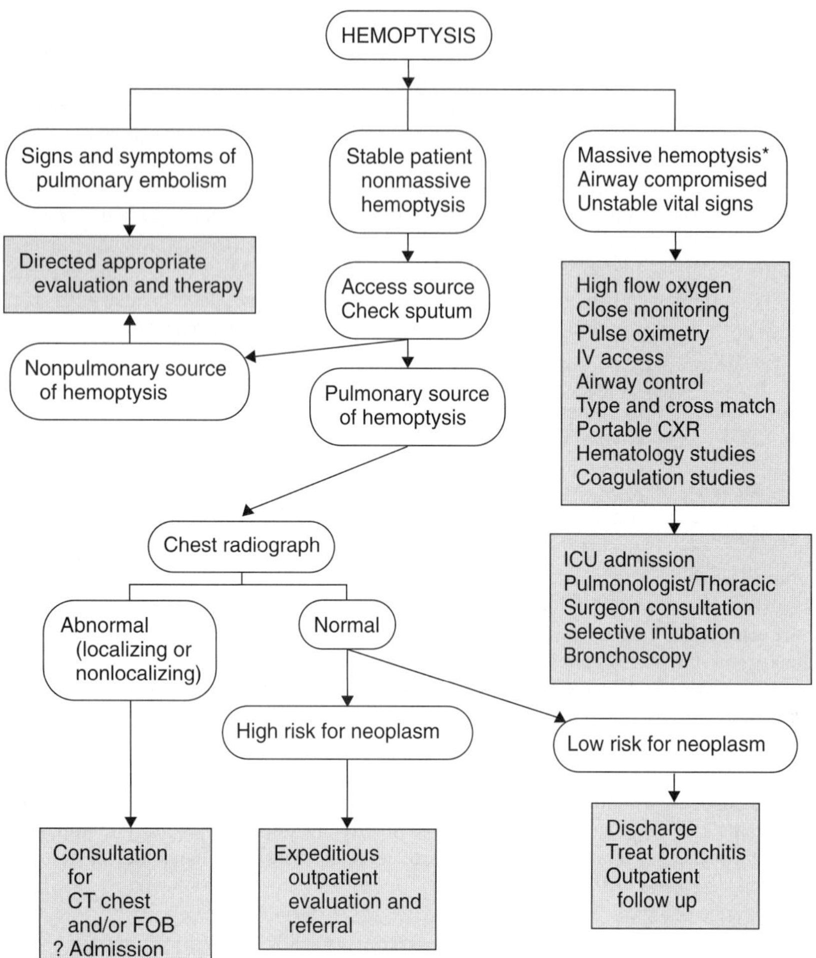

FIG. 63-1. Evaluation of hemoptysis.
* Massive, >50 mL per single expectoration.
† Age >40, smoker, male gender, and weight loss (two or more risk factors).
FOB = fiberoptic bronchoscopy.

chest CT scan, or bronchial artery angiography to localize the specific bleeding site.[10] Patients with massive hemoptysis that has subsided are at high risk of recurrence and require similar intensive management and hospital admission, usually to an intensive care unit. Massive hemoptysis is less common in children, but similar evaluation and management are appropriate.

Patients with minor hemoptysis due to bronchitis should be treated for the underlying disease as appropriate. Smoking cessation, oral antibiotics, and inhaled β-agonist bronchodilators have a role in the treatment in acute bronchitis. Patients at high risk for neoplasm should have a follow-up consultation with their primary care physician or a pulmonary subspecialist.

REFERENCES

1. Nelson JE, Forman M: Hemoptysis in HIV-infected patients. *Chest* 110:737, 1996.
2. Marshall TJ, Flower CDR, Jackson JE: Review: The role of radiology in the investigation and management of patients with haemoptysis. *Clin Radiol* 51:391, 1996.
3. DiLeo MD, Amedee RG, Butcher RB: Hemoptysis and pseudohemoptysis: The patient expectorating blood. *Ear Nose Throat J* 74:822, 1995.
4. Hirshberg B, Biran I, Glazer M, Kramer MR: Hemoptysis: Etiology, evaluation, and outcome in a tertiary referral hospital. *Chest* 112:440, 1997.
5. Cahill BC, Ingbar DH: Massive hemoptysis: Assessment and management. *Chest* 15:147, 1994.
6. Thompson AB, Teschler H, Rennard SI: Pathogenesis, evaluation, and therapy for massive hemoptysis. *Chest* 13:69, 1992.
7. Kemp PM, Tarver DS, Batty V, Lewington V: Pulmonary embolism: Is the clinical history a useful adjunct to aid the interpretation of the equivocal lung scan? *Clin Nucl Med* 21:203, 1996.
8. Chang YC, Patz EF, Goodman PC, Grange CB: Significance of hemoptysis following thrombolytic therapy for acute myocardial infarction. *Chest* 109:727, 1996.
9. Haponik EF, Chin R: Hemoptysis: Clinicians' perspectives. *Chest* 97:469, 1990.
10. Patel U, Pattison CW, Raphael M: Management of massive haemoptysis. *Br J Hosp Med* 52:2, 1994.

ACUTE ASTHMA IN ADULTS

Rita K. Cydulka
Sorabh Khandelwal

Asthma is a chronic inflammatory disorder characterized by increased responsiveness of the airways to multiple stimuli. Many cells and cellular elements, such as mast cells, eosinophils, T lymphocytes, macrophages, neutrophils, and epithelial cells, play a role in the development of the inflammatory response. In susceptible individuals, the inflammation causes recurrent episodes of wheezing, breathlessness, chest tightness, and coughing, particularly at night or in the early morning. These episodes are usually associated with widespread, but variable, airflow obstruction, that is often reversible either spontaneously or with treatment.

Most acute attacks are reversible and improve spontaneously or within minutes to hours with treatment. Although patients appear to recover completely clinically, evidence suggests that asthmatic patients develop chronic airflow limitation.[1] The recognition that asthma is a chronic inflammatory disorder of the airways has significant implications for the diagnosis, management, and potential prevention of its acute exacerbation.

EPIDEMIOLOGY

Asthma affects approximately 4 to 5 percent of the population in the United States.[2] It is the most common chronic disease of childhood, with a prevalence of 5 to 10 percent.[3] On the other end of the spectrum, asthma affects 7 to 10 percent of the elderly, accounting for 68,000 admissions to hospitals in 1991.[4] About one-half of cases of asthma develop before the age of 10 and another one-third before the age of 40. The 2:1 male to female preponderance of asthma in childhood equalizes by age 30. Self-reported prevalence rates for asthma in the United States increased by 75 percent from 1980 to 1994, with the most substantial increase occurring among children aged 0 to 14 years.[2] Similar prevalence rates are reported in developed nations throughout the world.[5] During the same period, the estimated annual number of office visits for asthma in the United States more than doubled from 4.6 million to 10.4 million, hospitalization rates increased from 386,000 to 466,000, and mortality rates associated with asthma, which had been decreasing from 1960 through 1962 and again from 1975 through 1977, increased in all race, gender, and age strata.[2] Death rates were consistently higher among blacks and among the elderly. The economic implications of asthma are substantial despite advances in treatment. In the United States alone, the estimated direct and indirect cost of asthma in all age groups was 6.2 billion dollars in 1990.[6]

PATHOPHYSIOLOGY

The pathophysiologic hallmark of asthma is a reduction in airway diameter caused by smooth muscle contraction, vascular congestion, bronchial wall edema, and thick secretions. These changes are reflected in pulmonary function changes, increased work of breathing, and abnormal distribution of pulmonary blood flow (Table 64-1). Both large and small airways often contain plugs composed of mucus, serum proteins, inflammatory cells, and cellular debris. On a microscopic level, airways are infiltrated with eosinophils and mononuclear cells. Evidence of microvascular leakage, epithelial disruption, and vasodilation is frequently noted. The airway smooth muscle is hypertrophied and characterized by new vessel formation, an increased number of epithelial goblets cells, and deposition of interstitial collagen beneath the epithelium.[7] Subepithelial fibrosis, an increase in the thickness of the reticular layer of the basement membrane, is characteristically increased in both the large and small airways.[7] Recent data collected from transbronchial biopsy, alveolar lavage, and specialized airway imaging techniques suggest that inflammation affects all bronchial pulmonary structures.[8]

TABLE 64-1 Physiologic Consequences of Airflow Obstruction

Increased airway resistance
Decreased maximum expiratory flow rates
Air trapping

Increased airway pressure
  Barotrauma
  Adverse hemodynamic effects

Ventilation-perfusion imbalance
  Hypoxemia
  Hypercarbia

Increased work of breathing
  Pulsus paradoxus
  Respiratory muscle fatigue with ventilatory failure

Current hypothesis states that airway inflammation may be acute, subacute, or chronic. The acute response is determined by early recruitment of cells to the airway. Antigens come in contact with mast cells in the submucosa and cause elaboration of mediators, such as histamine, leukotrienes (including leukotriene B_4), chemokines, tryptase, interleukin 5 (IL-5), IL-8, proinflammatory cytokines, and IL-4, which produce an intense inflammatory reaction, with bronchoconstriction, vascular congestion, edema formation, increased mucus production, and impaired mucociliary transport. Eosinophils, platelets, and polymorphonuclear leukocytes are recruited to the site, activated, and contribute further to the inflammatory cycle that has already been initiated. The immunoglobulin E (IgE) response is controlled by T and B lymphocytes and activated by the interaction of antigen with the mast cell-bound Ig-E molecules.[9] In the subacute or late phase, recruited and resident cells are activated, causing a more persistent pattern of inflammation.

Chronic inflammation is characterized by a persistent cell damage and an ongoing repair process, contributing to some of the microscopic changes seen in the airway. Mediators target ciliated airway epithelium to cause injury or disruption. As a consequence, epithelial cells and myofibroblasts, present beneath the epithelial layer, proliferate and begin to deposit interstitial collagen in the lamina reticularis of the basement membrane. Fibroblasts contribute to the process by releasing cytokines and chemokines, which may be important in both initiating and maintaining the level of airway inflammation and may explain the apparent basement membrane thickening and irreversible airway changes seen in some asthmatics.[10] Clearly, the inflammatory process is multicellular, redundant, and self-amplifying.

Allergic asthma is frequently associated with a personal or family history of allergic diseases such as rhinitis, urticaria, and eczema. Idiosyncratic, or nonallergic, asthma is associated with no family history or personal history of allergy and normal serum levels of IgE. Many stimuli have been noted to provoke an increase in airway responsiveness. Viral respiratory infections are the most common of the stimuli that invoke acute asthma exacerbation.[11] Increased airway responsiveness secondary to infection may last anywhere from 2 to 8 weeks.[11] Exercise is another common precipitant of acute asthma. Unlike other precipitants of acute exacerbation, long-term sequelae and airway reactivity are not noted as a result of exercise. Environmental conditions, such as atmospheric pollutants and antigens noted in heavy industrial or densely populated urban areas, are associated with higher incidence and severity of asthma. In addition, indoor antigens such as mold, house dust mites, cockroaches, and animal dander, are also associated with acute asthma. Occupational exposures, such as metal salt, wood and vegetable dust, pharmaceutical, industrial chemical and plastic, biological enzyme, vapors, gases, and aerosol, may also stimulate an asthma attack. Multiple pharmaceutical agents, such as aspirin, β blockers (including topical β blockers), nonsteroidal anti-inflammatory agents, sulfating agents, tartrazine dyes, and food additives and preservatives have been implicated in acute asthma. As in exercise-induced asthma, exposure to cold air alone can induce acute bronchospasm. Recent evidence indicates that endocrine factors, such as changing levels of estradiols and progesterone during the normal menstrual cycle and pregnancy, may contribute to the level of airway reactivity.[12,13] Finally, emotional stress can produce an asthma attack.

CLINICAL FEATURES

The symptoms of asthma consist of a triad of dyspnea, wheezing, and cough. Many patients will relay the history of asthma upon presentation, but some will not. Early in the attack, patients will complain of a sensation of chest constriction and cough. As the exacerbation progresses, wheezing becomes apparent, expiration becomes prolonged, and accessory muscle use may become evident. Key historical

TABLE 64-2 Key Historical Elements When Obtaining a History from Patients with Acute Asthma Exacerbation

Symptoms
- Cough
- Wheezing
- Shortness of breath
- Chest tightness
- Sputum production
- Fever

Pattern of symptoms
- Perennial
- Seasonal
- Perennial and seasonal
- Continual
- Episodic
- Onset
- Duration
- Frequency

Aggravating factors

History of disease
- Age of onset and method of diagnosis
- Course of disease
- Present management and medications
- History of oral corticosteroid use
- Intensive care unit admissions
- History of intubation for asthma exacerbation
- Other medical diseases

Family history

Social history
- Condition of home
- Exposure to allergens
- Smoking
- Identification of participating causes

Exacerbation profile
- Usual pattern of exacerbation and outcome

Best spirometry measures

Risk factors for death from asthma
- Past history of sudden severe exacerbations
- Prior intubation for asthma
- Prior admission for asthma to an intensive care unit
- Two or more hospitalizations for asthma in the past year
- Three or more emergency care visits for asthma in the past year
- Hospitalization or emergency care visit for asthma within the past month
- Use of more than two canisters per month on inhaled short-acting β_2-agonist
- Current use of systemic corticosteroids or recent withdrawal from systemic corticosteroids
- Difficulty perceiving airflow obstruction or its severity
- Comorbidity, as from cardiovascular diseases or chronic obstructive pulmonary disease
- Serious psychiatric illness or psychosocial problems
- Low socioeconomic status in urban residents
- Illicit drug use
- Sensitivity to *Alternaria*

Note: Expert Panel Report 2.
Source: Adapted from National Asthma Education and Prevention Program Expert Panel,[17] with permission.

points should be obtained on asthmatics presenting with exacerbation to emergency departments (EDs) (Table 64-2). Acute asthma exacerbation can be categorized based on clinical features (Table 64-3).

Physical examination findings are variable. Patients presenting with a severe asthma attack may be in obvious respiratory distress, with rapid breathing and loud wheezing, whereas patients with mild exacerbation may present with cough and end-expiratory wheezing. At times, wheezing may be audible without a stethoscope. Other conditions may present with wheezing and mimic asthma (Table 64-4). The use of accessory muscles of inspiration indicates diaphragmatic fatigue, while the appearance of paradoxical respirations reflects impending ventilatory failure. Alteration in the mental status—e.g., lethargy, exhaustion, agitation, or confusion—also heralds respiratory arrest.

Directed physical examination reveals hyperresonance to percussion, decreased intensity of breath sounds, and prolongation of the expiratory phase, usually with wheezing. Although wheezing results from the movement of air through narrowed airways, the intensity of the wheeze may not correlate with the severity of airflow obstruction. The ''silent chest'' reflects very severe airflow obstruction, with air movement insufficient to promote a wheeze. A pulsus paradoxus above 20 mmHg is also indicative of severe asthma. Although tachycardia and tachypnea are usually seen with acute asthma, vital signs normalize very quickly as airflow obstruction is relieved. Therefore, a normal heart rate, respiratory rate, and the absence of a pulsus paradoxus do not indicate complete relief of airway obstruction.

DIAGNOSIS

Bedside spirometry provides a rapid, objective assessment of patients and serves as a guide to the effectiveness of therapy. The forced expiratory volume in 1 s (FEV_1) and the peak expiratory flow rate (PEFR) directly measure the degree of large airway obstruction.[14] Patient cooperation is essential in order for these tests to be reliable. Sequential measurements help emergency physicians determine response to therapy. Signs on physical examination and a patient's report of symptoms of asthma do not necessarily correlate well with the severity of airflow obstruction. When possible, management decisions should be based on a patient's personal best PEFR or FEV_1 or, if unknown, percent of predicted. Initial spirometry and response to initial treatment can be used to predict the need for hospitalization with 86 percent sensitivity and 96 percent specificity.[15]

Pulse oximetry is a useful and convenient method for accessing oxygenation and monitoring oxygen saturation during treatment but does not aid in predicting clinical outcomes.[16]

Determination of arterial blood gas (ABG) is not indicated in the majority of patients with mild to moderate asthma exacerbation. The main reason to determine ABG during an asthma attack is to assess for hypoventilation with carbon dioxide retention and respiratory acidosis. Such patients almost always have clinical evidence of severe attacks or spirometry demonstrating a PEFR or FEV_1 of less than 25 percent predicted. With acute attacks, ventilation is stimulated, resulting in a decrease in partial pressure of carbon dioxide (P_{CO_2}). Therefore, a normal or slightly elevated P_{CO_2} (e.g., 42 mmHg or more) indicates extreme airway obstruction and fatigue and may herald the onset of acute ventilatory failure.

A chest radiograph is indicated in patients with asthma exacerbation if there is clinical indication of a complication such as pneumothorax, pneumomediastinum, pneumonia, or other medical concern. Routine radiography is unnecessary, but up to one-third of patients requiring admission will demonstrate an abnormality on chest radiograph.

A routine complete blood cell count is rarely indicated and will likely show modest leukocytosis secondary to administration of β-agonist therapy or corticosteroid treatment. In patients taking theophylline prior to ED presentation, a serum theophylline level should be determined. Routine electrocardiogram is also unnecessary but may reveal right ventricular strain, abnormal P waves, or nonspecific ST-T-wave abnormalities, which resolve with treatment. Older patients, especially those with coexisting heart disease, should have cardiac monitoring during treatment. Asthma index scores have failed to predict outcome better than clinical judgment.

TABLE 64-3 Classifying Severity of Asthma Exacerbations

	Mild	Moderate	Severe	Respiratory Arrest Imminent
Symptoms				
Breathlessness	While walking	While talking	While at rest	
Position	Can lie down	Prefers sitting	Sits upright	
Talks in	Sentences	Phrases	Words	
Alertness	May be agitated	Usually agitated	Usually agitated	Drowsy or confused
Signs				
Respiratory rate	Increased	Increased	Often >30/min	
Use of accessory muscles; suprasternal retractions	Usually not	Commonly	Usually	Paradoxical thoracoabdominal movement
Wheeze	Moderate, often only end expiratory	Loud; throughout exhalation	Usually loud; throughout inhalation and exhalation	Absent
Pulse/minute	<100	100–120	>120	Bradycardia
Pulsus paradoxus	Absent <10 mmHg	May be present 10–25 mmHg	Often present >25 mmHg (adult) 20–40 minHg (child)	Absence suggests respiratory muscle fatigue
Functional Assessment				
Peak expiratory flow % predicted or % personal best	80%	~50%–80%	<50% predicted or personal best or response lasts <2 h	
Pa_{O_2}(on air)	Normal (test not usually necessary)	>60 mmHg (test not usually necessary)	<60 mmHg: possible cyanosis	
Pa_{CO_2}	<42 mmHg (test not usually necessary)	<42 mmHg (test not usually necessary)	≥42 mmHg: possible respiratory failure (see text)	
SaO_2% (on air) at sea level	>95% (test not usually necessary)	91%–95%	<91%	

Note: The presence of several parameters, but not necessarily all, indicates the general classification of the exacerbation. Many of these parameters have not been systemically studied, so they serve only as general guides. Hypercapnia (hypoventilation) develops more readily in young children than in adults and adolescents.

Source: Adapted from National Asthma Education and Prevention Program Expert panel,[17] with permission.

TREATMENT

The goal of treatment of acute asthma in the ED is to reverse airflow obstruction rapidly by repetitive or continuous administration of inhaled β_2 agonists, ensure adequate oxygenation, and relieve inflammation. The National Asthma Education and Prevention Program (NAEPP) Expert Panel has developed guidelines for emergency treatment of asthma (Fig. 64-1).[17] The Canadian Association of Emergency Physicians and the British Thoracic Society have developed similar treatment guidelines.[18,19] The following categories of medications are used in the treatment of acute asthma: β-adrenergic agonists, anticholinergics, and glucocorticoids. Magnesium, heliox (helium-oxygen mixture), and ketamine may be considered when the aforementioned medications fail to relieve bronchospasm. Mast cell-stabilizing agents, methylxanthines, and leukotriene modifiers are currently reserved for maintenance therapy only.

TABLE 64-4 Asthma Mimickers

Congestive heart failure (''cardiac asthma'')
Upper airway obstruction
Aspiration of foreign body or gastric acid
Bronchogenic carcinoma with endobronchial obstruction
Metastatic carcinoma with lymphangitic metastasis
Sarcoidosis with endobronchial obstruction
Vocal-cord dysfunction
Multiple pulmonary emboli (rare)

Adrenergic Agents

β-adrenergic agonists are the preferred initial rescue medication for acute bronchospasm. β-adrenergic receptors are divided into two types: β_1 and β_2. Stimulation of β_1 receptors increases rate and force of cardiac contraction and decreases small intestine motility and tone. β_2-adrenergic stimulation promotes bronchodilation, vasodilation, uterine relaxation, and skeletal muscle tremor.

The mechanism of bronchodilator action of β-adrenergic drugs involves stimulation of the enzyme adenyl cyclase, which converts intracellular adenosine triphosphate (ATP) to cyclic adenosine monophosphate (cAMP). This action enhances the binding of intracellular calcium to cell membranes, reducing the myoplasmic calcium concentration, and results in relaxation of bronchial smooth muscle. In addition to bronchodilation, β-adrenergic drugs inhibit mediator release and promote mucociliary clearance.

The most common side effect of β-adrenergic drugs is skeletal muscle tremor. Patients may also experience nervousness, anxiety, insomnia, headache, hyperglycemia, palpitations, tachycardia, and hypertension. Despite earlier concerns over potential cardiotoxicity, especially when these drugs were used in combination with theophylline, clinical experience has not revealed significant problems. Arrhythmias and evidence of myocardial ischemia are rare, especially in patients without prior history of coronary artery disease.

The β-adrenergic agonists used today are analogues of naturally occurring sympathomimetics (Table 64-5). The ideal bronchodilator in this class of drugs would possess pure β_2-receptor activity—bronchodilation without cardiac effects. The older catecholamine bron-

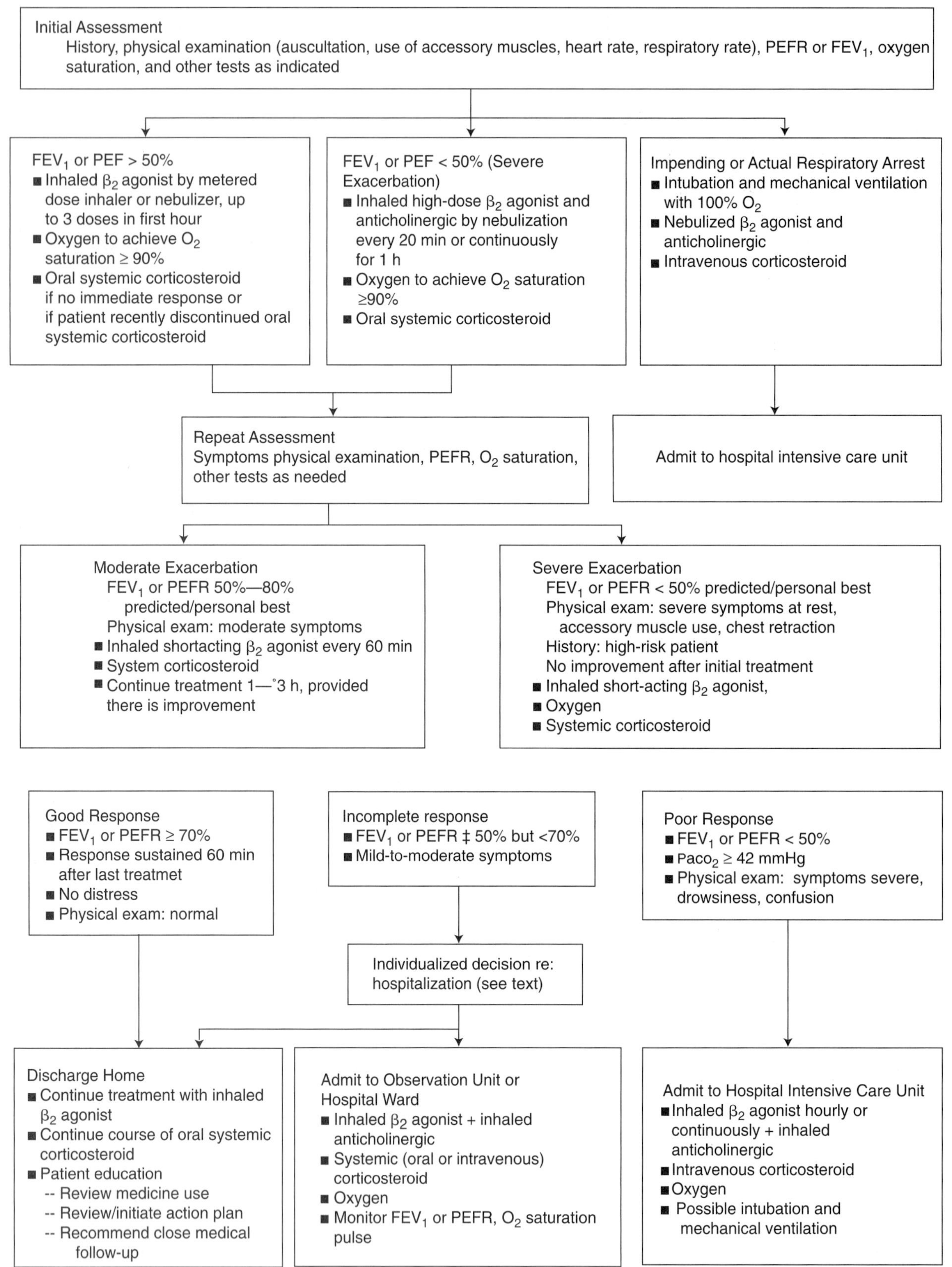

FIG. 64-1. Management of Asthma Exacerbations: Emergency Department and Hospital-Based Care. *Abbreviations:* FEV_1, forced expiratory volume in 1 s; PEFR, peak expiratory flow rate.[17] (Adapted from National Asthma Education and Prevention Program Expert Panel, with permission.)

TABLE 64-5 Dosages of Drugs for Asthma Exacerbations in Emergency Medical Care or Hospital

Medications	DOSAGES Adult Dose	Comments
Inhaled short-acting β_2 agonists		
Albuterol		
Nebulizer solution (5 mg/mL)	2.5–5.0 mg every 20 min for 3 doses, then 2.5–10 mg every 1–4 h as needed, or 10–15 mg/h continuously	Only selective β_2 agonists are recommended. For optimal delivery, dilute aerosols to minimum of 4 mL at gas flow of 6–8 L/min.
MDI (90 μg/puff)	4–8 puffs every 20 min up to 4 h, then every 1–4 h as needed	As effective as nebulized therapy if patient is able to coordinate inhalation maneuver. Use spacer/holding chamber.
Bitolterol		
Nebulizer solution (2 mg/mL)	See albuterol dose	Has not been studied in severe asthma exacerbations. Do not mix with other drugs.
MDI (370 μg/puff)	See albuterol dose	Has not been studied in severe asthma exacerbations.
Pirbuterol		
MDI (200 μg/puff)	See albuterol dose	Has not been studied in severe asthma exacerbations.
Systemic (injected), β_2 agonists		
Epinephrine (1:1000 or 1 mg/mL)	0.3–0.5 mg Sq every 20 min for 3 doses	No proven advantage of systemic therapy over aerosol.
Terbutaline (1 mg/mL)	0.25 mg Sq every 20 min for 3 doses	No proven advantage of systemic therapy over aerosol.
Anticholinergics		
Ipratropium bromide		
Nebulizer solution (0.2 mg/mL)	0.5 mg every 30 min for 3 doses, then every 2–4 h as needed	Should not be used as first-line therapy; should be added to β_2 agonist therapy. May mix in same nebulizer with albuterol.
MDI (18 μg/puff)	4–8 puffs every 6–8 h	Dose delivered from MDI is low and has not been studied in asthma exacerbations.
Corticosteroids		
Prednisone Methylprednisolone Prednisolone	120–180 mg/day in 3 or 4 divided doses for 48 h, then 60–80 mg/day until FEV_1 or PEFR reaches 70% of predicted or personal best	For outpatient "burst," use 40–60 mg per day, for 3–10 days in adults.

Source: Adapted from National Asthma Education and Prevention Program Expert Panel,[17] with permission.
Abbreviation: MDI, metered dose inhaler.

chodilators—isoproterenol and epinephrine—are not β_2 specific and have a short duration of action. Isoetharine is more β_2 selective but still has a short duration of action. These drugs have nearly been replaced by newer agents produced by chemical modification of the parent compound. The resorcinol bronchodilators (metaproterenol, terbutaline, and fenoterol) and saligenin bronchodilators (albuterol and carbuterol) share greater β_2 specificity, as well as longer duration of action and effectiveness through the oral route due to resistance to intestinal sulfatases.

Aerosol therapy with β_2-adrenergic drugs produces excellent bronchodilation and is favored over both the oral and parenteral routes. The aerosol route achieves topical administration of a relatively small dose of drug, producing local effects with minimum systemic absorption and fewer side effects. Aerosol delivery may be achieved with a metered dose inhaler (MDI) with spacing device or a compressor-driven nebulizer. A spacing device attached to the inhaler can improve drug deposition when patient technique is inadequate. Even with optimum technique, however, a maximum of 15 percent of the drug dose is retained in the lungs, regardless of the aerosol method used. Dry-powder delivery devices and MDIs using hydrofluoralkane as propellant have recently replaced chlorinated fluorocarbon (CFC)-driven devices.

Aerosol treatments may be administered every 15 to 20 min or on a continuous basis. Epinephrine or terbutaline may be administered subcutaneously to patients unable to coordinate aerosolized or MDI treatments but their use should generally be avoided in patients with a history of cardiovascular disease. Intravenous β-agonist infusions offer no advantage over aerosolized or MDI-delivered agents and carry potential risk.[20]

Salmeterol xinafoate is a β_2-adrenoreceptor agonist that binds with greater affinity to the β-receptor site than does albuterol. *It is indicated for twice-daily maintenance therapy, should never be used more frequently, and is to be avoided for treatment of acute exacerbation.* Its bronchodilator effect lasts at least 12 h, and tachyphylaxis has not been reported with long-term use. It is an effective treatment for long-term control of asthma, especially nocturnal asthma. Short-acting β_2-adrenoreceptor agonists are generally added for symptoms that occur despite the use of salmeterol.

Corticosteroids

Corticosteroids are highly effective drugs in asthma exacerbation and form one of the cornerstones of treatment. Although the mechanism of action is unknown, many believe that steroids produce beneficial effects by restoring β-adrenergic responsiveness and reducing inflammation. The onset of anti-inflammatory effect is delayed at least 4 to 8 h following intravenous or oral administration.

Corticosteroids should be administered to asthmatics in whom airway obstruction is not immediately relieved after the first nebulized bronchodilator treatment. Although there is considerable disagreement over what constitutes the optimal dose in acute asthma, an initial oral dose of 40 to 60 mg prednisone or an intravenous bolus of 60 to 125 mg methylprednisolone, in patients unable to tolerate oral medications, is sufficient.[21] High-dose corticosteroid therapy offers no advantage.[22] Additional doses should be given every 4 to 6 h until significant subjective and objective improvement is achieved. Patients may be discharged on a 3- to 10-day nontapering burst of oral steroids, 40 to 60 mg prednisone per day, or its equivalent.[23]

Although the role of both oral and inhaled steroids in the long-term prevention of relapse is yet to be identified, all patients with an FEV_1 or PEFR of less than 70 percent predicted after aggressive ED treatment should be prescribed oral steroids.[17]

Anticholinergics

Plants containing anticholinergic alkaloids have been smoked for hundreds, if not thousands, of years to treat respiratory disorders. In recent years, anticholinergics have been rediscovered as potent bronchodilators in patients with asthma and other forms of obstructive lung disease. Although comparisons of bronchodilator response between anticholinergics and β-adrenergic agonists have produced conflicting results, the effects of the drugs used in combination may be additive.[24] This is plausible, because anticholinergics affect large, central airways while β-adrenergic drugs dilate smaller airways.

Anticholinergic drugs competitively antagonize acetylcholine at the postganglionic, parasympathetic effector-cell junction. This process blocks the bronchoconstriction induced by vagal cholinergic-mediated innervation to the larger central airways. In addition, concentrations of cyclic GMP in airway smooth muscle are reduced, further promoting bronchodilation.

Because of significant systemic side effects, atropine sulfate, once the major nebulized anticholinergic used in the United States, has been virtually replaced by the synthetic quaternary derivative: ipratropium bromide (Atrovent, Boehringer Ingélheim). This drug causes far fewer systemic side effects and is very well tolerated. Ipratropium is currently available as both a nebulized solution and an MDI (18 mg/puff) (Table 64-5).

Aerosolized ipratropium bromide, 0.5 mg, should be administered to patients with severe exacerbation.[17] Potential side effects with nebulized anticholinergics include dry mouth, thirst, and difficulty swallowing. Less commonly, tachycardia, restlessness, irritability, confusion, difficulty in micturition, ileus, blurring of vision, or an increase in intraocular pressure are noted.

Theophylline

Theophylline is no longer considered a first-line treatment for acute asthma.[17] Studies have shown that theophylline, in combination with inhaled β_2-adrenergic drugs, appears to increase the toxicity, but not the efficacy, of treatment.[25] Theoretically, theophylline may be a useful adjunct by providing a more sustained bronchodilator effect, contributing to small airway bronchodilation, improving respiratory muscle endurance, and improving resistance to fatigue. Recent data suggest an anti-inflammatory mechanism of action.[26]

The mechanism of action of theophylline remains unknown; 90 percent of theophylline metabolism is hepatic and the remainder is excreted unchanged through the kidneys. A serum theophylline level should be determined for patients who regularly use theophylline. The most common side effects of theophylline are nervousness, nausea, vomiting, anorexia, and headache. At plasma levels greater than 30 μg/mL, there is a risk of seizures and cardiac arrhythmias.

Magnesium

Intravenous magnesium sulfate is being used with increasing frequency in the management of acute, very severe asthma, i.e., FEV_1 of less than 25 percent predicted.[27,28] Its usefulness in mild and moderate exacerbation has not been established. Although the bronchodilating properties of magnesium sulfate can be helpful, it should not be substituted for standard therapy regimens. The dose is 1 to 2 g intravenously over 30 min.

Heliox, Ketamine, and Halothane

Several studies have demonstrated that an 80:20 percent mixture of helium and oxygen (heliox) can lower airway resistance and act as an adjunct in the treatment of very severe asthma exacerbation.[29] At present, heliox is not indicated for use in mild or moderate bronchospasm. Several investigators have reported success with ketamine and halothane in cases where all other treatment modalities have failed. Controlled trials substantiating these claims are lacking.

Mast Cell Modifiers

Both cromolyn and nedocromil exert their anti-inflammatory action by blockage of chlorine channels, thus modulating mast cell mediator release and eosinophil recruitment. These agents also inhibit early and late responses to allergen challenge and exercise. Neither is indicated for treatment of acute bronchospasm.

Leukotriene Modifiers

Leukotrienes are potent proinflammatory mediators that contract airway smooth muscle, increase microvascular permeability, stimulate mucus secretion, decrease mucociliary clearance, and recruit eosinophils into the airway.[1] Two leukotriene modifiers—zafirlukast and zileuton—are currently available as oral tablets for the treatment of asthma. Leukotriene modifiers improve lung function, diminish symptoms, and diminish the need for short-acting β_2 agonists. They are being investigated as an alternative to low-dose inhaled corticosteroid therapy and as steroid-sparing agents. There is currently no indication for the use of leukotriene modifiers in the treatment of acute bronchospasm.

Mechanical Ventilation

When in spite of the emergency physician's best effort to treat an acute asthma exacerbation, when the patient begins to exhibit signs of acute ventilatory failure, noninvasive positive-pressure ventilation may be attempted.[30] However, if the patient manifests progressive hypercarbia and acidosis or becomes exhausted or confused, intubation and mechanical ventilation are necessary to prevent respiratory arrest. Mechanical ventilation does not relieve the airflow obstruction; it merely eliminates the work of breathing and enables the patient to rest while the airflow obstruction is resolved. Fortunately, fewer than 1 percent of asthmatics ever require mechanical ventilation. Direct oral intubation is preferred over the nasotracheal route.

The potential complications of mechanical ventilation in asthmatic patients are numerous. Increased airway resistance may lead to extremely high peak airway pressures, barotrauma, and hemodynamic impairment. Mucous plugging is frequent, often leading to increased airway resistance, atelectasis, and pulmonary infection. Due to the severity of airflow obstruction during the early phases of treatment, the tidal volume may be larger than the returned volume, leading to air trapping and increased residual volume [intrinsic positive end-expiratory pressure (intrinsic PEEP)]. These effects may be partially avoided by utilizing rapid inspiratory flow rates at a reduced respiratory frequency (12 to 14/min), and allowing adequate time for the expiratory phase. One can achieve the goal of ventilatory support—maintenance of an adequate arterial oxygen saturation (90 percent or more)—without concern for ''normalizing'' the hypercarbic acidosis.[31] This approach is called *controlled mechanical hypoventilation* or *permissive hypoventilation*. All patients requiring mechanical ventilation must be admitted to an intensive care unit.

SPECIFIC ISSUES THAT IMPACT DIAGNOSIS, EVALUATION, AND TREATMENT

Age

Diagnosis, evaluation, and treatment of children with asthma are discussed in Chapter 120, ''Asthma and Bronchitis.'' Although newly diagnosed asthma in older populations is not uncommon, differentiation of the etiology of wheezing in older asthmatics may present a challenge. Historical data may help differentiate between congestive heart failure, pulmonary malignancy, and obstructive airway disease, but distinguishing between chronic obstructive pulmonary disease and acute asthma is often difficult.[4]

Treatment of older asthmatics should proceed in the same manner as treatment of younger asthmatics. Age-related changes in pulmonary function must be considered when determining response to treatment in older asthmatics, and care should be taken to avoid medication interactions.

Gender

Recent evidence suggests that men and women interpret changes in pulmonary function differently. Women express a sensation of dyspnea at higher percent predicted PEFR than do men.[32] In addition, cyclic hormonal changes may influence pulmonary function in women.[33]

Pregnancy

Asthma complicates approximately 4 percent of pregnancies. Studies indicate that as many as 42 percent of pregnant asthmatics require hospitalization and that an additional 11 to 18 percent have one or more visits to the ED for exacerbation.[34] In 1993, the NAEPP Expert Panel developed guidelines for the treatment of asthma exacerbation during pregnancy.[34] The principles of managing acute asthma exacerbation are similar to those of managing exacerbation in a nonpregnant state. They consist of repetitive lung function measurements, maintenance of oxygen saturation at greater than 95 percent, administration of repetitive inhaled β_2-agonist and early administration of systemic corticosteroids, along with fetal monitoring. Early intervention during acute exacerbation is key to the prevention of impaired maternal and fetal oxygenation. Uncontrolled asthma is associated with a variety of maternal and fetal complications, including hyperemesis, hypertension, toxemia, vaginal hemorrhage, complicated labor, intrauterine growth retardation, preterm birth, increased perinatal mortality, and neonatal hypoxemia. Although no asthma medication labeled to date qualifies for an FDA use-in-pregnancy category A rating (adequate well-controlled studies in pregnant women have failed to demonstrate risk to the fetus), problems as a result of routine treatment of asthma in the ED have not been reported.

Hyperventilation of pregnancy leads to a higher Pa_{O_2} and a diminished Pa_{CO_2}. Thus, a Pa_{O_2} of less than 70 mmHg in a pregnant women with acute asthma represents fairly severe hypoxemia, and a Pa_{CO_2} of greater than 35 mmHg represents respiratory failure.[35] During asthma exacerbation, the normal alkalosis of pregnancy is aggravated, leading to a decrease in placental blood flow. Hypoxemia is usually more severe in the fetus than in the mother.

β_2 agonists and inhaled corticosteroids are considered safe during pregnancy and are recommended as a routine part of asthma management. As in nonpregnant patients, a short burst of oral steroid (40 to 60 mg prednisone per day) or its equivalent, should be considered for pregnant asthmatics discharged from the ED after treatment for an exacerbation.

DISPOSITION

Disposition decisions should take into account a combination of subjective parameters, such as resolution of wheezing and improvement in air exchange, as assessed by auscultation and patient opinion, and objective measures, such as normalization of FEV_1 or PEFR. The ideal combination of elements needed for successful discharge without risk of early relapse has not yet been determined.[36] Some degree of residual airflow obstruction, airway lability, and inflammation persists after treatment and discharge from the ED.

No single treatment program can be recommended for all patients discharged home from the ED following treatment of exacerbation.

TABLE 64-6 Hospital Discharge Checklist for Patients with Asthma Exacerbations

Intervention	Dose/Timing	Education/Advise	MD/RN Initials
Inhaled medications (metered dose inhaler + spacer/holding chamber) β_2 agonist Corticosteroids	Select agent, dose, and frequency (e.g., albuterol) 2–6 puffs q 4 h 2 puffs QID	Teach purpose Teach technique Emphasize need for spacer/holding chamber Check patient technique	
Oral medications	Select agent, dose, and frequency (e.g., prednisone 20 mg bid for 3–10 days)	Teach purpose Teach side effects	
Peak flow meter	Measure a.m. and p.m. PEFR and record best of three tries each time	Teach purpose Teach technique Distribute peak flow diary	
Follow-up visit	Make appointment for follow-up care with primary clinician or asthma specialist	Advise patient (or caregiver) of date, time, and location of appointment within 7 days of hospital discharge	
Action plan	Before or at discharge	Instruct patient (or caregiver) on simple plan for actions to be taken when symptoms, signs, and peak expiratory flow values suggest recurrent airflow obstruction	

Source: Adapted from National Asthma Education and Prevention Program Expert Panel,[17] with permission.

Although several studies have demonstrated that a short course of oral steroids and β_2-agonist bronchodilators reduce relapse rates among discharged patients,[37] other studies have reported high relapse rates regardless of ED management and use of steroids.[36] Patients with a history of previous ED visits and hospitalization are at highest risk of relapse, regardless of management.[36]

Current guidelines help to determine hospitalization and discharge criteria based on response to aggressive treatment. A good response to treatment is demonstrated by complete resolution of symptoms and a PEFR or FEV_1 of greater than 70 percent predicted. Such individuals can be safely discharged home. Patients with a poor response to treatment are defined as those with persistent symptoms and FEV_1 or PEFR of less than 50 percent predicted. Such patients are likely to have persistent wheezing and dyspnea at rest despite intensive treatment in the ED and should be admitted. An incomplete response to treatment—the midground—is defined as some persistence of symptoms and a PEFR or FEV_1 between 50 to 70 percent predicted. Most asthmatics treated in the ED fall into this category. They may be discharged home safely, provided they have no risk factors for death from asthma (Table 64-2).[17] Patients who fail to improve adequately over a several-hour period because they are in the late phase of their exacerbation and those with significant risk factors for death from asthma should be admitted to either an observation unit or the hospital.[15,17]

The role of observation units in the care of acute asthma exacerbation is currently being determined. Although early studies indicated no reduction in hospitalization rates after treatment in ED observation units, more recent studies indicate that 59 percent of asthmatics admitted to observation units where strict care protocols are followed are successfully treated and discharged.[38,39]

Follow-up care must be arranged following an acute exacerbation to ensure resolution and to review the long-term medication plan for the chronic management of asthma. High relapse rates, despite the routine use of steroids, strongly suggest the need for follow-up within days of the ED visit.[36] Patients with asthma must have an appropriate written plan of action that addresses both routine care and care of worsening symptoms.

Education of patients must become an integral part of ED care. ED personnel should provide basic education on asthma and help link patients with a primary care providers or asthma specialists while providing discharge instructions. Review of patient's discharge medication, use of inhaler technique, and the use of peak flow monitoring are just some of the issues ED physicians can teach and emphasize (Table 64-6).

REFERENCES

1. Busse WW: Leukotrienes and inflammation. *Am J Respir Crit Care Med* 157(suppl):S210, 1998.
2. Mannino DM, Homa DM, Pertowski CA, et al: Surveillance for asthma: United States, 1960–1995. *MMWR* 47:1, 1998.
3. Centers for Disease Control and Prevention: Asthma mortality and hospitalization among children and young adults: United States, 1980–1993. *MMWR* 45:350, 1966.
4. Cydulka RK, McFadden ER, Emerman CL, et al: Patterns of hospitalization in elderly patients with asthma and chronic obstructive pulmonary disease. *Am J Respir Crit Care Med* 156:1807, 1997.
5. International Study of Asthma and Allergies in Childhood (ISAAC) Steering Committee: Worldwide variation in prevalence of symptoms of asthma, allergic rhinoconjunctivitis, and atopic eczema. *Lancet* 351:1225, 1998.
6. Weiss KB, Green PJ, Hodgson TA: An economic evaluation of asthma in the United States. *N Engl J Med* 326:862, 1992.
7. Fabbri LM, Caramori G, Beghe B, et al: Physiologic consequences of long-term inflammation. *Am J Respir Crit Care Med* 157(suppl):S195, 1998.
8. Kraft MR, Djukanovic S, Wilson ST, et al: Alveolar tissue inflammation in asthma. *Am J Respir Crit Care Med* 154(suppl):1505, 1996.
9. Barnes PJ, Pedersen S, Busse WW: Efficacy and safety of inhaled corticosteroids. *Am J Respir Crit Care Med* 157:S1, 1998.
10. Roche WR: Fibroblasts and asthma. *Clin Exp Allergy* 21:545, 1991.
11. Busse WW, Gern JE: Viruses in asthma. *J Allergy Clin Immunol* 100:147, 1997.
12. Agarwal AK, Shah A: Menstrual-linked asthma. *J Asthma* 34:539, 1997.
13. Schatz M, Zeiger RS: Asthma and allergy in pregnancy. *Clin Perinatol* 24:407, 1997.
14. McFadden ER Jr: Clinical physiologic correlates in asthma. *J Allergy Clin Immunol* 77(1 Pt. 1):1–5, 1986.
15. Rodrigo G, Rodrigo C: A new index for early prediction of hospitalization in patients with acute asthma. *Am J Emerg Med* 15:8, 1997.
16. Harden R: Oxygen saturation in adults with acute asthma. *J Accid Emerg Med* 13:28, 1996.
17. National Asthma Education and Prevention Program Expert Panel: *Report 2: Guidelines for the Diagnosis and Management of Asthma.* Bethesda, MD, National Institutes of Health (NIH), 1997; NIH publication 97-4051.
18. Beveridge RC, Grunfeld AF, Hodder RV, Verbeek PR: Guidelines for the emergency management of asthma in adults: CAEP/CTS Asthma Advisory Committee, Canadian Association of Emergency Physicians and the Canadian Thoracic Society. *Can Med Assoc J* 155:25, 1996.
19. British Thoracic Society and others: Guidelines for the management of asthma: A summary. *BMJ* 306:776, 1993.
20. Salmeron S, Brochard L, Mal H, et al: Nebulized versus intravenous albuterol in hypercapnic acute asthma: A multicenter, double-blind, randomized study. *Am J Crit Care Med* 149:1466, 1994.
21. Scarfone RJ, Fuchs SM, Nager AL, Shane SA: Controlled trial of oral prednisone in the emergency department treatment of children with acute asthma. *Pediatrics* 2:513, 1993.
22. Emerman CL, Cydulka RK: A randomized comparison of high vs. moderate dose methylprednisolone in the treatment of acute asthma. *Chest* 107:1559, 1995.
23. Cydulka RK, Emerman CL: A pilot study of steroid therapy in the prevention of early relapse after emergency department treatment of acute asthma: Is a taper needed? *J Emerg Med* 16:15, 1998.
24. Cydulka RK, Emerman CL: Combined treatment with glycopyrrolate and albuterol in acute asthma. *Ann Emerg Med* 23:270, 1994.
25. Rodrigo C, Rodrigo G: Treatment of acute asthma: Lack of therapeutic benefit and increase of the toxicity from aminophylline given in addition to high doses of salbutamol delivered by metered-dose inhaler with a spacer. *Chest* 106:1071, 1994.
26. Evans DJ, Taylor DA, Zetterstrom O, et al: A comparison of low-dose inhaled budesonide plus theophylline and high-dose inhaled budesonide for moderate asthma. *N Engl J Med* 337:1412, 1997.
27. Bloch H, Silverman R, Mancherje N, et al: Intravenous magnesium sulfate as an adjunct in the treatment of acute asthma. *Chest* 107:1576, 1995.
28. Skobeloff EM, Spivey WH, McNamara RM, Greenspon L: Intravenous magnesium sulfate for the treatment of acute asthma in the emergency department. *JAMA* 262:1210, 1989.
29. Manthous CA, Hall JB, Caputo MA, et al: Heliox improves pulsus paradoxus and peak expiratory flow in nonintubated patients with severe asthma. *Am J Respir Crit Care Med* 151(2 part 1):310, 1995.
30. Antonelli M, Conti G, Rocco M, et al: A comparison of noninvasive positive-pressure ventilation and conventional mechanical ventilation in patients with acute respiratory failure. *N Engl J Med* 339:429, 1998.
31. Tuxen DV: Permissive hypercapnic ventilation. *Am J Respir Crit Care Med* 150:870, 1994.
32. Osborne ML, Vollmer WM, Linton KL, Buist AS: Characteristics of patients with asthma within a large HMO: A comparison by age and gender. *Am J Respir Crit Care Med* 157:123, 1998.
33. Skobeloff ME, Spivey WH, St Clair S, Schoffstall JM: The influence of age and sex on asthma admissions. *JAMA* 268:3437, 1992.
34. National Asthma Education and Prevention Program Expert Panel: Report 2: Report of the Working Group on Asthma and Pregnancy—Management of Asthma During Pregnancy. Bethesda, MD, National Institutes of Health (NIH), 1993; NIH publication 93-3279.
35. Schatz M: Pregnancy and asthma. *J Asthma* 34:263, 1997.
36. Emerman CL, Cydulka RK: Factors associated with relapse following emergency department treatment for acute asthma. *Ann Emerg Med* 26:6, 1995.
37. Chapman KR, Verbeek PR, White JG, Rebuck AS: Effect of a short course of prednisone in the prevention of early relapse after the emergency room treatment of acute asthma. *N Engl J Med* 324:788, 1991.

38. Brillman JC, Tandberg D: Observation unit impact on ED admission for asthma. *Am J Emerg Med* 12:11, 1994.

39. Rydman RJ, Isola ML, Roberts RR, et al: Emergency department observation unit versus hospital inpatient care for a chronic asthmatic population: A randomized trial of health status outcome and cost. *Med Care* 36:599, 1998.

CHRONIC OBSTRUCTIVE PULMONARY DISEASE

Rita K. Cydulka
Sorabh Khandelwal

Individuals with chronic obstructive pulmonary disease (COPD) frequently develop severe respiratory distress and are among the most frustrating, frightening, and challenging patients to manage. In a fearful state of mixed anxiety, intense physical effort, and disoriented fatigue, such people face a constant battle against asphyxiation. At other times, presentation is prompted by otherwise uncomplicated medical or surgical disease, which becomes more serious or catastrophic as the impact of chronic respiratory disease is unmasked.

The American Thoracic Society (ATS) defines COPD as a disease state characterized by the presence of airflow obstruction due to chronic bronchitis or emphysema. The airflow obstruction is generally progressive, may be accompanied by airway hyperactivity, and may be partially reversible. Chronic bronchitis is defined as the presence of chronic productive cough for 3 months in each of 2 successive years in a patient in whom other causes of chronic cough have been excluded. Emphysema is defined as abnormal permanent enlargement of the airspaces distal to the terminal bronchioles, accompanied by destruction of their walls and without obvious fibrosis. Note that chronic bronchitis is defined in clinical terms and emphysema in terms of anatomic pathology.[1]

EPIDEMIOLOGY

COPD is a major worldwide respiratory health problem. In North America, COPD is rare in persons younger than age 40, but very common among older individuals, with a prevalence of approximately 10 percent in those aged 55 to 85 years. The disease is more common in men than in women, but is predicted to decrease in incidence in men but not in women, a reflection of gender-based differences in smoking behavior. The World Health Organization estimates that COPD was the sixth leading cause of death in the world in 1990.[2] In the United States, COPD is the fourth most common cause of death, the third most common cause of hospitalization, and the only leading cause of death that is increasing in prevalence.[3]

The mortality of patients hospitalized for a COPD exacerbation is approximately 5 to 14 percent.[4,5] Mortality of COPD patients admitted to an intensive care unit for exacerbation is 24 percent.[6] For patients aged 65 years or older discharged from the intensive care unit after treatment of a COPD exacerbation, the 1-year mortality is 59 percent, nearly double the expected 30 percent.[6]

COPD is an expensive public health problem in terms of direct economic costs (such as hospital admissions and outpatient treatments), indirect economic costs (such as lost years of life, disability, and loss of working capacity), and reduction in quality of life.[1,5–10] The utilization of health care resources by elderly patients with COPD is immense, both during hospitalization and after discharge.[4]

PATHOPHYSIOLOGY

Cigarette smoking accounts for an estimated 80 to 90 percent of the risk of developing COPD. Age of starting, total pack-years, and current smoking status are predictive of COPD mortality.[1] Of note, only 15 percent of smokers develop clinically significant COPD. A variety of other environmental risk factors, such as respiratory infections, occupational exposures, ambient air pollution, passive smoke exposure, and diet, have been suggested, but supporting data is lacking. The only proven genetic risk factor is α_1-antitrypsin deficiency. Airway hyperresponsiveness, which may relate to environmental factors, genetic factors, or both, is a potential risk factor that has received significant attention. However, although airway hyperresponsiveness predisposes individuals to decline in pulmonary function and is a defining component in asthma, the relationship of asthma to COPD is unclear.

The earliest objective changes in the evolution of COPD are clinically imperceptible and are measured as small increases in peripheral airway resistance or lung compliance. The slow, insidious appearance of dyspnea and hypersecretion often requires several decades of disease. The sedentary life habits of many cigarette smokers result in failure to unmask exertional dyspnea, and denial results in suppression of symptoms or attribution of such symptoms to aging, poor conditioning, obesity, or allergies. Further, the respiratory consequences of cigarette smoking are a continuum of slowly evolving and latent effects, unique to each individual, in a complex dose-response relationship. Early in disease evolution, abstinence from smoking may eliminate symptoms and result in physiologic improvement. Once well established, however, abnormalities persist and may still progress despite abstinence.

Pathologic specimens from the patients with early disease demonstrate minor metaplasia of bronchial epithelium and an increase in bronchial gland number and size.[11] As disease evolves, such findings are exaggerated, acute and chronic inflammatory changes in the epithelium are more notable, and acinar expansion, destruction, and coalescence are seen. Elements of emphysematous disease are invariably present in concert with those of bronchitic disease, though one often predominates.

Despite recognition of causative factors, what determines the clinical onset and rate of progression of chronic airflow obstruction, and the direction toward either emphysematous or bronchitic patterns, is uncertain. Clearly, there is a great deal of variability in disease pattern and severity among individuals with seemingly similar predisposition to disease.

The central element in the pathophysiology of chronic airflow obstruction is impedance to airflow, especially expiratory airflow, due to increased resistance or decreased caliber throughout the small bronchi and bronchioles. Airflow obstruction results from a combination of airway secretions, mucosal edema, bronchospasm, and bronchoconstriction from impaired elastance. Impedance to airflow alone accounts substantially for the abnormal physiology of the disease. Exaggerated airway resistance either reduces total minute ventilation or increases respiratory work. To the degree that alveolar hypoventilation occurs, hypoxemia and hypercarbia result. Even without hypoventilation, hypoxemia occurs due to ventilation-perfusion mismatching.

In addition to obstruction of peripheral airways, all forms of advanced chronic airflow obstruction involve other pathophysiologic elements to complete the overall picture. Particularly in dominantly emphysematous disease, destruction and coalescence of alveolar architecture results in reduction of total "matched" alveolar-capillary surface area for diffusion of gas, while vascular destruction results in "unmatched" regions where ventilation is wasted.

Neurochemical and proprioceptive ventilatory responses in chronic airflow obstruction may be aberrant. For example, ventilatory response to hypercarbia may be blunted during sleep, and ventilatory drive and dyspnea may be exaggerated in spite of normal pulmonary inflation. The composition of muscle fiber types, breathing patterns, and resistance to fatigue of respiratory muscles are also altered in advanced chronic airflow obstruction. Finally, pulmonary arterial hypertension supervenes as chronic airflow obstruction progresses. The right ventricle transiently hypertrophies, and then dilates with the evolution of overt cor pulmonale. A low-output state in the pulmonary circulation translates into low left ventricular output. Arterial hypoxemia increases as the effects of right-to-left shunt on poorly oxygenated mixed venous blood are exaggerated. Right ventricular pressure overload is clinically poorly tolerated and associated with atrial and ventricular arrhythmias.

Even though COPD is becoming increasingly recognized as a chronic inflammatory disease of the lower airways, the role of inflammation in its pathogenesis remains a matter of debate. In current COPD guidelines, there is no mention of lower airway inflammation in the definition of COPD.[1,6–10]

CLINICAL FEATURES

Chronic, Compensated COPD

Despite the pathophysiologic segregation of chronic airflow obstruction into categories of pulmonary emphysema, chronic bronchitis, and bronchiectasis, none of these exist as a pure entity in clinical medicine. Most patients demonstrate a mixture of symptoms and signs. The hallmark symptom is exertional dyspnea. Chronic, productive cough is common, and minor hemoptysis is frequent, especially in chronic bronchitis and bronchiectasis.

Physical findings include tachypnea, accessory respiratory muscle use, and pursed-lip exhalation. Airflow obstruction causes wheezing during exhalation, especially during maximum forced exhalation, and prolongation of the expiratory time. In dominantly bronchitic disease, coarse crackles are heard as uncleared secretions move about the central airways. In dominantly emphysematous disease, there is expansion of the thorax, impeded diaphragmatic motion, and global diminution of breath sounds. Weight loss is frequent due to poor dietary intake and excessive caloric expenditure for the work of breathing. Plethora due to secondary polycythemia, and cyanosis; tremor, somnolence, and confusion due to hypercarbia may be seen in advanced disease. Findings of secondary pulmonary hypertension with or without cor pulmonale may be present. The physical signs of left ventricular dysfunction are often disguised or underestimated by the seemingly more overwhelming signs of respiratory disease, or because pulmonary hyperinflation prohibits adequate auscultation.

Acute Exacerbations of COPD

Decompensation is usually due to worsening of airflow obstruction resulting from increased bronchospasm, superimposed respiratory infection or other respiratory pathology, interference with respiratory drive, cardiovascular deterioration, smoking, noncompliance with medications, noxious environmental exposures, use of medications that prevent bronchorrhea, and adverse responses to medication (e.g., anaphylactoid responses or β-adrenergic blockade). Disordered ventilatory drive most commonly arises from misuse of oxygen therapy, hypnotics, or tranquilizers. Metabolic disturbances, as well as inadequate oxygen delivery independent of respiratory function, may cause decompensated COPD.

Exacerbations of COPD usually involve progressive hypoxemia due to bronchospastic worsening of ventilation-perfusion matching. Signs of hypoxemia include tachypnea, cyanosis, agitation and apprehension, tachycardia, and systemic hypertension. The most life-threatening feature of decompensation is hypoxemia where arterial saturation falls below 90 percent. With increased work of breathing, muscle production of carbon dioxide increases and alveolar ventilation is often unable to increase to prevent carbon dioxide retention and respiratory acidosis. Signs of hypercapnia include confusion, tremor, stupor and, finally, hypopnea and apnea.

Patients usually complain of dyspnea and orthopnea. The intensified effort to ventilate is further dramatized by sitting-up-and-forward position, pursed-lip exhalation, accessory muscle use, and diaphoresis. Pulsus paradoxus may be noted during blood pressure recording. Complications such as pneumonia, pneumothorax, or an acute abdomen may be neglected or minimized by the patient's generalized respiratory distress, tachypnea, or global diminution of breath sounds.

DIAGNOSIS

Chronic, Compensated COPD

The most valuable tool in characterizing disease severity is pulmonary function testing, including examination of lung mechanics, analysis of arterial blood gases, description of ventilatory response patterns, tests of respiratory muscle performance, metabolic assessment, and noninvasive survey of hemodynamic reserve. The ratio of forced expiratory volume in 1 s (FEV_1) to forced vital capacity (FVC) should be used to diagnose mild COPD. However, once the disease progresses, the percentage of predicted FEV_1 is a better measure of disease severity.[1,7–10] Various guidelines characterize COPD severity as mild, moderate, or severe, although agreement on precise FEV_1 standards remains arbitrary.[1,8,9]

In the early stages of COPD, arterial blood gas measurements reveal mild-to-moderate hypoxemia without any evidence of hypercapnea. As the disease progresses in severity (especially when the FEV_1 falls below 1 L), hypoxemia becomes more severe and the development of hypercapnia becomes more evident. Not only do arterial blood gas measurements worsen during acute exacerbations, they also may worsen during exercise and sleep.[1]

Radiographic examination is often misleading; mild chronic airflow obstruction is not likely to be radiographically apparent. Dominantly bronchitic disease may be associated with subtle or absent x-ray findings. On the other hand, dominantly emphysematous disease may be associated with remarkable signs of hyperaeration, such as increased anteroposterior diameter, flattened diaphragms, increased parenchymal lucency, and attenuation of pulmonary arterial vascular shadows, despite only mild-to-moderate physiologic alterations. Right or left ventricular enlargement may not produce relative enlargement of the cardiac silhouette. Certainly, radiography is of unquestionable value in diagnosing complications such as pneumothorax, pneumonia, pleural effusion, and pulmonary neoplasia.

Diagnosing heart failure and assessing ventricular function in patients with COPD is difficult. Echocardiography or gated nuclear scans to estimate ejection fractions may prove invaluable. ECGs are useful to identify arrhythmias or ischemic injury but do not accurately assess the severity of pulmonary hypertension or right ventricular dysfunction.

Acute Exacerbations of COPD

Bedside pulmonary function tests provide a rapid, objective assessment of patients and serve as a guide to the effectiveness of therapy. The FEV_1 and the peak expiratory flow rate (PEFR) directly measure the degree of large-airway obstruction. Patient cooperation is essential in order for these tests to be reliable. Sequential measurements help the emergency physician determine response to therapy. Signs on physical examination and physician estimates of pulmonary function are highly inaccurate.[12] Measurement of FEV_1 is preferred over PEFR, because FEV_1 allows comparison with baseline studies and published guidelines.[13]

Although pulse oximetry may identify hypoxemia, it cannot identify hypercapnia or acid-base disturbances. Spirometric criteria that have been used to eliminate the need for arterial blood gases in asthmatic patients cannot be safely applied to patients with COPD. The finding of an arterial pH below that consistent with renal compensation for chronic respiratory acidosis implies either acute exaggeration of hypercapnia or acute metabolic acidosis.

Radiographic abnormalities are common in COPD exacerbation; therefore, radiographs should be strongly considered.[14] ECGs may reveal concurrent disease processes such as ischemia/acute myocardial infarction and signs of cor pulmonale, as well as arrhythmias such as multifocal atrial tachycardia. The theophylline level should be determined in patients whose regimen includes this mediation. Finally, other tests may be indicated to determine the etiology of the exacerbation.

TREATMENT

Chronic, Compensated COPD

The appropriate and optimal management of decompensated chronic airflow obstruction in an emergency department setting requires an appreciation of chronic day-to-day therapy. Specific management limits further insults to the respiratory system, treats reversible bronchospasm, and prevents or treats complications.

HEALTHY LIFESTYLE Elements include regular exercise, weight control, and smoking cessation. Smoking cessation is the only therapeutic intervention that can reduce the accelerated decline in lung function.[15] Smoking cessation (along with long-term oxygen therapy) has been shown to reduce COPD mortality.[1,7–10] Pulmonary rehabilitation can improve exercise capacity and quality of life and is recommended in those patients with moderate to severe COPD.[16] All COPD guidelines recommend yearly influenza vaccination.[1,7–10] Although there is some controversy regarding the pneumococcal vaccine in COPD patients, it is currently recommended by the ATS.[1,7–10,17]

OXYGEN Both the British Medical Research Council (MRC) study and the National Heart, Lung, and Blood Institute's Nocturnal Oxygen Study have demonstrated that long-term oxygen therapy reduces COPD mortality. Oxygen must be started after arterial blood gases document a Pao_2 of 55 mmHg or less, or a Pao_2 between 56 and 59 mmHg when signs of cor pulmonale are present.[1]

PHARMACOTHERAPY There is no evidence that pharmacotherapy can alter the progression of COPD. Inhaled β_2-adrenergic agents used on an as-needed basis may be prescribed for mild to moderately obstructed patients with intermittent symptoms. In those patients with persistent symptoms or in those patients refractory to β_2-adrenergic agents or bothered by side effects, ipratropium bromide is the drug of choice. With increasing symptoms, even after optimization of the above two classes of bronchodilators, theophylline may be helpful. Only about 20 to 30 percent of patients with COPD improve when given chronic oral steroids.[18] Initiating corticosteroid therapy requires careful analysis so as not to subject a nonresponder to the side effects unnecessarily. The European Respiratory Society Study on COPD showed no benefit of inhaled steroids—budesonide 400 μg twice daily—on the annual rate of decline of lung function.[19] Although some subgroups of patients with milder disease may benefit from inhaled steroids, even high doses were of no physiologic or functional benefit in patients with advanced COPD who were nonresponders to oral steroids.[20] Results from other studies using inhaled steroids in COPD are pending. Although some studies support the use of theophylline in stable COPD patients, most current COPD guidelines consider it only an adjunct therapy.[1,7–10]

MOBILIZATION OF SECRETIONS Assurance of generous oral fluid intake and atmospheric humidification, avoidance of antihistamine/decongestant agents, and limitation of antitussive use help mobilize respiratory secretions. The efficacy of specific expectorant products is dubious.

Acute Exacerbations of COPD

The primary goal of emergency therapy in decompensated chronic airflow obstruction is to correct tissue oxygenation. This requires the restoration of the lungs as gas-exchange organs, assurance of hemodynamic efficiency, repletion of red blood cell mass where deficient, and limitation of excessive oxygen demands and carbon dioxide production. Factors that influence drug therapy in the emergency department include (1) the degree of reversible bronchospasm, (2) prior therapy of the patient, (3) recent drug usage and evidence of potential toxicity, (4) the ability of the patient to cooperate in taking inhaled medications, (5) the presence of contraindications to any drug or class of drugs, and (6) specific causes or complications related to the exacerbation.

OXYGEN The first goal in the treatment of COPD is to correct or prevent life-threatening hypoxemia. The goal of oxygen therapy is correction of hypoxemia to an arterial oxygen pressure (Pao_2) of greater than 60 mmHg or an arterial oxygen saturation (Sao_2) of more than 90 percent. This can be accomplished in the emergency department through several devices, including the standard dual-prong nasal cannula, simple face mask, a Venturi mask, and finally a non-rebreathing mask with reservoir and one-way valve. The need to increase Pao_2 must be balanced against the possibility of producing hypercapnia either by one of two suggested mechanisms: respiratory center depression or, more likely, ventilation-perfusion mismatching.[21] Hypercapnia in the face of insignificant acidosis can be tolerated. Improvement after administration of supplemental oxygen may take 20 to 30 min to achieve a steady state after a change in percent of oxygen administered (Fio_2) in patients with COPD. If adequate oxygenation is unachievable without progressive respiratory acidosis, then assisted ventilation may be required.

β_2-ADRENERGIC AGONISTS β_2-Adrenergic agonists remain the first-line therapy in the management of acute, severe COPD. Aerosolized forms are preferred because they minimize systemic toxicity. Limited data exist regarding the optimal dose and frequency of administration. According to ATS guidelines, β_2-adrenergic agents may be administered every 30 to 60 min, if tolerated.[1] Nebulized aerosols administered every 20 min may result in more rapid improvement of FEV_1, but the incidence of side effects is greater.[22] The use of subcutaneous epinephrine or terbutaline in patients with COPD should proceed with great caution because many COPD patients suffer from concurrent coronary artery disease.

Side effects of β_2-adrenergic agonists include tremor, anxiety, and palpitations, so such agonists should be used with care in elderly patients known to have coexisting heart disease. Pao_2 may fall slightly after use of these agents, due to pulmonary vasodilation and resultant ventilation-perfusion mismatch.

ANTICHOLINERGICS Anticholinergics have not yet been adequately assessed as first-step therapy in COPD. However, they are often favored when the history indicates poor responsiveness to β_2 agonists. Ipratropium bromide given by metered dose inhaler with a spacer or as an inhalant solution by nebulization (0.5 mg or 2.5 mL of the 0.02% inhalant solution) is the agent of choice.[18] Evidence suggests that the combination of a β_2-adrenergic agent and an anticholinergic agent may be more effective than albuterol alone in relieving bronchospasm during COPD exacerbation.[23] Repeat doses need not usually be given more often than every 4 to 8 h. Side effects are minimal and appear to be limited to dry mouth and an occasional metallic taste.

CORTICOSTEROIDS There is no firm consensus for the use of systemic steroids in the treatment of COPD exacerbation.[1,7–10] The use of a short course (7 to 14 days) of systemic steroids appears effective in severe exacerbations of COPD with respiratory failure, but their role in mild-to-moderate exacerbations needs to be further delineated.[24] ATS guidelines acknowledge the lack of supporting evidence for the use of steroids in COPD exacerbation, but state that steroids can be useful when an asthmatic component is present.[1] A poor bronchodilator response does not preclude a good response to steroid therapy. Current theory holds that steroid responsiveness is on a continuum rather than an all-or-nothing phenomenon. If used, the optimal effective dose ranges between one and three times the maximal physiologic adrenal secretion rate (i.e., the equivalent of 60 to 180 mg prednisone).

ANTIBIOTICS All current guidelines recommend antibiotics for the treatment of COPD exacerbation, especially if there is evidence of infection (e.g., fever, leukocytosis, change in the chest radiograph, abnormal mucus production).[1,7–10] Recent meta-analysis demonstrates a small, but statistically significant, benefit for antibiotics.[25] Proponents of antibiotic use believe antibiotics have both short-term benefits (i.e., rapid resolution of the symptoms of exacerbation, a rapid return of peak flow rates, avoidance of hospitalization, an early return to work, and prevention of progression of severe airway infection into pneumonia) and long-term benefits (i.e., breaking the vicious cycle of airway infection, inflammation, and loss of lung function; prolonging the time between exacerbations; and preventing secondary infection by resistant organisms). They argue further that differentiating infected from noninfected patients is difficult. Antibiotic choices include macrolides, cephalosporins, trimethoprim-sulfamethoxazole, and the latest-generation fluoroquinolones.

METHYLXANTHINES The role of aminophylline in the treatment of COPD exacerbation remains controversial. ATS guidelines suggest adding theophylline if aerosol therapy cannot be given or proves inadequate.[1] The bronchodilation effect of aminophylline is limited, and its therapeutic range is narrow. A review of the literature reveals a significant effect on spirometry, respiratory muscle strength, resting blood gases, improvement in the sensation of dyspnea, quality of life, cardiac output, and pulmonary vascular resistance, as well as an anti-inflammatory effect.[26] Other study data suggest that aminophylline increases the toxicity but not the efficacy when treating patients with β_2-adrenergic agonists.[27]

In most patients, a serum level of 8 to 12 μg/mL is appropriate. The intravenous loading dose usually required to obtain an initial serum concentration of 10 μg/mL (10 mg/L) is 5 to 6 mg/kg ideal body weight in patients not currently receiving the drug. In patients regularly taking theophylline, a miniloading dose may be alternatively selected: (target concentration − currently assayed concentration) × volume of distribution (i.e., 0.5 times ideal body weight in liters). With the miniload method, the target concentration should be between 10 to 15 μg/mL. The intravenous maintenance infusion rate is 0.2 to 0.8 mg/kg ideal body weight per hour. Lower maintenance rates are given to patients with congestive heart failure or hepatic insufficiency with low clearance rates, whereas higher rates are given to smokers with rapid clearance.

Maintenance theophylline infusion in patients on chronic oral therapy is complex (whether or not a miniloading dose has been given), particularly in attempting to account for enteric drug yet to be absorbed. Both loading and maintenance doses may need to be reduced to minimize the risk of "summation toxicity" due to continued enteric absorption. Standard-release preparations may continue to be absorbed for up to 6 h, and sustained-release preparations may require up to 12 h. Therefore, maintenance infusion rates should be reduced for 6 h after ingestion of a standard-release formulation and 12 h after ingestion of a sustained-release preparation (including 24-h-release forms). Theophylline and aminophylline should not be given orally in an emergency setting unless decompensation is not severe, alimentary motility is assured, and forthcoming ambulatory care is imminent.

ASSISTED VENTILATION Mechanical ventilation is indicated in patients with COPD exacerbation if there is evidence of respiratory muscle fatigue, worsening respiratory acidosis, deteriorating mental status, and in those with clinically significant hypoxemia refractory to supplemental oxygen by usual techniques. The main goals of assisted positive-pressure ventilation in acute respiratory failure complicating COPD are the resting of ventilatory muscles and the restoration of gas exchange to a stable baseline.[1]

Mechanical ventilation is uncomfortable and is associated with a variety of complications including nosocomial pneumonia, sinusitis, pneumothorax, and injury to the trachea and larynx. There are three specific pitfalls in ventilating patients with COPD: (1) overventilation resulting in acute respiratory alkalosis, (2) initiation of complex pulmonary and cardiovascular interactions that may result in systemic hypotension, and (3) creation of intrinsic positive end-expiratory pressure (PEEP), especially if expiratory time is inadequate or if dynamic airflow obstruction exists.[1] The three ventilatory modes most widely used for managing patients with COPD are assist-control ventilation (ACV), intermittent mandatory ventilation (IMV), and pressure support ventilation (PSV). There are some clinical reports that PSV provides increased patient comfort, promotes patient synchrony with the ventilator, and may accelerate weaning, but there is no direct evidence that patient outcome is improved with pressure support modes compared with volume-cycled modes of mechanical ventilation.[1]

Noninvasive positive-pressure ventilation (NPPV) is a term used to describe delivery of gas under positive pressure to the airways and lungs without insertion of an endotracheal tube. It can be delivered via a nasal mask, full face mask, or mouthpiece. NPPV can provide positive pressure to the airways only during inspiration (inspiratory positive airway or IPAP), or the airway pressure can be maintained continuously at the same level (continuous positive airway pressure or CPAP), or NPPV can be delivered so that the airway pressure is higher during inspiration than during expiration, with end-expiratory pressure maintained above atmospheric (bilevel ventilation or BiPAP).[28] NPPV can be delivered using assist-control volume-cycled ventilation, assist-control pressure ventilation, and pressure support ventilation, with or without end-expiratory positive pressure. No particular mode of ventilation or ventilatory device has been shown to be clearly superior.[29] Disadvantages of NPPV include slower correction of gas-exchange abnormalities, risk of aspiration, inability to control airway secretions directly, and possible complications of gastric distension and skin necrosis.[29] Contraindications to the use of NPPV include an uncooperative or obtunded patient, inability of the patient to clear airway secretions, hemodynamic instability, and major gastrointestinal bleeding.[28] Studies suggest a pooled success rate of 76 percent in patients with acute respiratory failure complicating COPD, but the studies consist of small numbers, and failure rates of up to 40 percent have been reported in some studies.[1]

OTHER Tissue oxygen delivery must be maximized by correcting left ventricular failure or arrhythmia to improve cardiac output, replacing red blood cell mass and intravascular fluid to increase arterial oxygen content, and suppressing fever to decrease oxygen consumption.

Future Considerations/New Therapies

Bronchodilators play an important role in the long-term management of patients with COPD, but they do not alter the progression of COPD. Major advances include the development of long-acting β_2-adrenergic agents, such as salmeterol and formoterol, and anticholinergic agents, such as tiotropium bromide. Tiotropium bromide has the benefit of once-daily dosing. Inflammation is being investigated more closely in the pathogenesis of COPD, especially the role of neutrophils.[30] Corticosteroids, chemokine (interleukin 8) inhibitors, leukotriene B_4 inhibitors, adhesion molecule inhibitors, and phosphodiesterase inhibitors are being studied with the goal of inhibiting neutrophil activity. Surfactant replacement is also under investigation. Evidence suggests that the imbalance between proteases in COPD patients may be restored either by inhibiting proteolytic enzymes, such as neutrophil elastase

TABLE 65-1 Indications for Hospitalization for COPD Exacerbation

Admission to Hospital	Admission to Intensive Care Unit
1. Patient has acute exacerbation characterized by increased dyspnea, cough, or sputum production, plus one or more of the following: • Inadequate response of symptoms to outpatient management • Inability to walk between rooms (patient previously mobile) • Inability to eat or sleep due to dyspnea • Conclusion by family and/or physician that patient cannot manage at home, with supplementary home care resources not immediately available. • High-risk comorbid condition, pulmonary or nonpulmonary • Prolonged, progressive symptoms before emergency visit • Altered mentation • Worsening hypoxemia • New or worsening hypercapnia	1. Severe dyspnea that responds inadequately to initial emergency therapy 2. Confusion, lethargy, or respiratory muscle fatigue (the last characterized by paradoxical diaphragmatic motion) 3. Persistent or worsening hypoxemia despite supplemental oxygen or severe/worsening respiratory acidosis (pH < 7.30) 4. Assisted mechanical ventilation is required
2. Patient has new or worsening cor pulmonale unresponsive to outpatient management	
3. Planned invasive surgical or diagnostic procedure requiring analgesics or sedatives that may worsen pulmonary function	
4. Comorbid condition, e.g., severe steroid myopathy or acute vertebral compression fractures, has worsened pulmonary function	

Source: Adapted from American Thoracic Society.[1]

inhibitors, cathepsin inhibitors, matrix metalloproteinase inhibitors, and secretory leukoprotease inhibitors, or by increasing antiproteases, such as α_1-antitrypsin. Evidence also exists that oxidative stress is increased in patients with COPD, and that reactive oxygen species are involved in the pathogenesis of COPD. Therefore, antioxidants such as *N*-acetyl cysteine and spin-trap antioxidants such as α-phenyl-*N*-tertbutyl nitrone may be useful. Pulmonary vasodilators, such as prostacyclin analogues, nitric oxide donors, endothelial antagonists, and angiotensin antagonists, are being studied in the hope of preventing the progression of pulmonary hypertension and cor pulmonale. Mucoregulators, such as tachykinin antagonists, sensory neuropeptide-release inhibitors, mediator and enzyme inhibitors, MUC gene suppressors, and mucolytic agents, may inhibit the hypersecretion of mucus, without affecting normal mucus secretion and normal mucociliary clearance.

DISPOSITION

Admission Criteria

Patients with acute exacerbation of COPD require admission to the hospital if they fail to improve adequately or deteriorate in spite of medical therapy, if they have significant comorbid illnesses, or they are without an intact social support system at home. The primary goals of hospitalization are to manage the acute exacerbation, prevent further deterioration, and educate patients on the nature the disease, current use of medications, and how to deal with the limitations presented by the disease and future exacerbations.

Objective criteria regarding hospital admission, observation unit stay, and emergency department discharge are lacking. Patients with an FEV_1 of 40 percent or more predicted or no clinical evidence of respiratory distress after treatment have a low rate of relapse and may be safely discharged home.[31] The ATS has developed consensus indications for hospitalization of patients with COPD (Table 65-1).

Discharge

Patients with acute exacerbation of COPD have less pulmonary reserve, are more likely to have comorbid diseases, and respond less readily to treatment than patients with acute exacerbations of asthma. Thus, more patients with COPD will likely require admission and, if discharged, more likely relapse. Thus, efforts should be made to ensure success with individuals being discharged with outpatient treatment: (1) adequate supply of home oxygen, (2) adequate and appropriate bronchodilator treatment, and (3) arranged follow-up with their physician.

REFERENCES

1. American Thoracic Society: Standards for the diagnosis and care of patients with chronic obstructive pulmonary disease. *Am J Respir Crit Care Med* 152:S78, 1995.
2. *Lancet*: From what will we die in 2020 [editorial comment]? *Lancet* 349:1263, 1997.
3. Fiel SB: Chronic obstructive pulmonary disease mortality and mortality reduction. *Drugs* 52(suppl 2):55, 1996.
4. Fuso L, Incalzi RA, Pistilli R, et al: Predicting mortality of patients hospitalized for acutely exacerbated chronic obstructive pulmonary disease. *Am J Med* 98:272, 1995.
5. Cydulka RK, McFadden ER Jr, Emerman CL, et al: Patterns of hospitalization in elderly patients with asthma and chronic obstructive pulmonary disease. *Am J Respir Crit Care Med* 156:1807, 1997.
6. Seneff MG, Douglas P, Wagner P, et al: Hospital and 1-year survival of patients admitted to intensive care units with acute exacerbation of chronic obstructive pulmonary disease. *JAMA* 274:1852, 1995.
7. Canadian Thoracic Society Workshop Group: Guidelines for the assessment and management of chronic obstructive pulmonary disease. *Can Med Assoc J* 147:420, 1992.
8. Siafakas NM, Vermeire P, Pride NB, et al, on behalf of the Task Force: Optimal assessment and management of chronic obstructive pulmonary disease (COPD). *Eur Respir J* 8:1398, 1995.
9. Jenkins C, Mitchell C, Irving L, et al, for the Thoracic Society of Australia and New Zealand: Guidelines for the management of chronic obstructive pulmonary disease. *Mod Med Aust* 38:132, 1995.
10. COPD Guidelines Group of the Standards of Care Committee of the British Thoracic Society: BTS guidelines for the management of chronic obstructive pulmonary disease. *Thorax* 52(suppl):1, 1995.
11. Jeffrey PK: Pathology of asthma and COPD: A synopsis. *Eur Respir Rev* 7:111, 1997.
12. Emerman CL, Lukens TW, Effron D: Physician estimation of FEV_1 in acute exacerbation of COPD. *Chest* 105:1709, 1994.
13. Emerman CL, Cydulka RK: Use of peak expiratory flow rate in emergency department evaluation of acute exacerbation of chronic obstructive pulmonary disease. *Ann Emerg Med* 27:159, 1996.
14. Emerman CL, Cydulka RK: Evaluation of high-yield criteria for chest radiography in acute exacerbation of chronic obstructive pulmonary disease. *Ann Emerg Med* 22:680, 1993.
15. Kanner RE: Early intervention in chronic obstructive pulmonary disease: A review of the Lung Health Study results. *Med Clin North Am* 80:523, 1996.
16. Donner CF, Muir JF: Rehabilitation and Chronic Care Scientific Group of the European Respiratory Society.

17. Fine MJ, Smith MA, Carson CA, et al: Efficacy of pneumococcal vaccination in adults: A meta-analysis of randomized controlled trials. *Arch Intern Med* 154:2666, 1994.
18. Celli BR: ATS standards for the optimal management of chronic obstructive pulmonary disease. *Respirology* 2(suppl 1):S1, 1997.
19. Pauwels RA, Lofdahl C, Pride NB, et al: European Respiratory Society study on chronic obstructive pulmonary disease (EUROSCOP): Hypothesis and design. *Respir Eur J* 5:616, 1992.
20. Bourbeau J, Rouleau MY, Boucher S: Randomized controlled trial of inhaled corticosteroids in patients with chronic obstructive pulmonary disease. *Thorax* 53:477, 1998.
21. Dunn WF, Nelson SB, Hubmayr RD: Oxygen induced hypercarbia in obstructive pulmonary disease. *Am Rev Respir Dis* 144:526, 1991.
22. Emerman CL, Cydulka RK: Effect of different albuterol dosing regimens in the treatment of acute exacerbation of chronic obstructive pulmonary disease. *Ann Emerg Med* 29:474, 1997.
23. Cydulka RK, Emerman CL: Effects of combined treatment with glycopyrrolate and albuterol in acute exacerbation of chronic obstructive pulmonary disease. *Ann Emerg Med* 25:470, 1995.
24. Thompson WH, Nielson CP, Carvalho P, et al: Controlled trial of oral prednisone in outpatients with acute COPD exacerbation. *Am J Respir Crit Care Med* 154:407, 1996.
25. Saint S, Bent S, Vittinghoff E, Grady D: Antibiotics in chronic obstructive pulmonary disease exacerbations: A meta-analysis. *JAMA* 273:957, 1995.
26. McKay SE, Howie CA, Thompson AH, et al: Value of theophylline in the treatment of patients handicapped by chronic obstructive lung disease. *Thorax* 48:227, 1993.
27. Rice KL, Leatherman JW, Duane PG, et al: Aminophylline for acute exacerbations of chronic obstructive pulmonary disease. *Ann Intern Med* 107:305, 1987.
28. Nicholson D, Tiep B, Jones R, et al: Noninvasive positive-pressure ventilation in chronic obstructive pulmonary disease. *Curr Opin Pulm Med* 4:66, 1998.
29. Meduri GU: Noninvasive positive-pressure ventilation in patients with acute respiratory failure. *Clin Chest Med* 17:513, 1996.
30. Barnes PJ: New therapies for chronic obstructive pulmonary disease. *Thorax* 53:137, 1998.
31. Emerman CL, Effron D, Lukens TW: Spirometric criteria for hospital admission of patients with acute exacerbation of COPD. *Chest* 99:595, 1991.

THE LUNG TRANSPLANT PATIENT

Thomas P. Noeller

Since the first successful single-lung transplant in 1983 followed by the first successful double-lung transplant in 1986, lung transplantation has become a viable therapeutic modality for end-stage pulmonary disease. Currently 89 centers perform lung transplants in the United States, and in 1997, a total of 942 patients underwent lung transplant nationally.[1] On December 31, 1997, the United Network for Organ Sharing listed 2664 patients on a waiting list for lung transplantation and noted that 409 patients had been removed from a waiting list owing to death during that year. For the most recent year that full data are available, the median waiting time for lung transplantation during 1996 was 566 days after being placed on a waiting list.[2] Overall, survival rates as of September 1997 were 91 percent at 1 month and 77, 58, and 43 percent at 1, 3, and 5 years, respectively.[2] The long-term survival rates were slightly higher at centers performing more than 30 lung transplants per year. Single and double lung transplants as well as heart-lung transplants are most commonly performed for cystic fibrosis, idiopathic pulmonary fibrosis, and emphysema, including alpha$_1$-antitrypsin deficiency. Congenital heart disease and Eisenmenger complex may also be indications for heart-lung transplantation.

MANAGEMENT OF PRETRANSPLANT PATIENTS

Pretransplant patients are likely to present with exacerbations of their underlying disease; assessment and management should be targeted to these processes. The transplant coordinator should always be contacted early in the course of evaluation and treatment to aid in timely disposition (Table 66-1).

TABLE 66-1 Indications for Hospital Admission

Pretransplant patients
Respiratory failure
Infiltrate
Systemic infection
Congestive heart failure or pulmonary edema
Pneumothorax
Posttransplant patients
Respiratory failure
Acute rejection
Rapidly progressive airflow limitation (FEV$_1$ fall of >10% over 48 h)
Infiltrate
Systemic infection
Febrile neutropenia
Pneumothorax

The patient's vital signs, particularly the respiratory rate, should be assessed immediately, along with pulse oximetry and physical examination for the presence of cyanosis, diaphoresis, use of accessory muscles, signs of congestive heart failure, and adequacy of peripheral perfusion. Supplemental oxygen should be applied, intravenous access obtained, and the patient placed on a cardiac monitor. A chest radiograph should be obtained to identify infiltrates or pneumothorax and arterial blood gases may also have to be tested. β_2 Agonists, anticholinergics, and antibiotics should be given as indicated.

Although the perioperative use of corticosteroids was formerly considered to be a contraindication to transplantation, this is changing somewhat. A maintenance dose of 0.2 to 0.3 mg/kg/day of prednisone is acceptable to most centers. If it is felt that a patient requires a corticosteroid burst or an increase in the maintenance dose to treat an acute exacerbation, the transplant coordinator should be contacted. A dose of prednisone greater than 20 mg/day may result in the patient being suspended from the transplant list until such time that the dose can safely be tapered down to 20 mg/day or less. In primary pulmonary hypertension (PPH) and Eisenmenger complex, consideration should be given to therapies that may help to decrease pulmonary vascular resistance, such as morphine sulfate, nitrates, and furosemide. For patients with respiratory failure, noninvasive ventilation or endotracheal intubation with mechanical ventilation may be required, increasing the risk of barotrauma. Ventilator dependence has generally been regarded as a relative contraindication to lung transplantation. Successes have been reported, but ventilator-dependent patients have a much higher mortality after transplantation.

Idiopathic pulmonary fibrosis (IPF) is a common indication for lung transplantation and carries with it the most dismal prognosis. Patients presenting with exacerbations of their disease in the pretransplant phase generally have a worse prognosis. Treatment with high-dose steroids is rarely successful at achieving a remission, and supportive therapy is the mainstay of acute management. The transplant team may recommend cytotoxic drugs such as cyclophosphamide and azathioprine for their steroid-sparing effect.

Chronic infection, especially common in patients with cystic fibrosis (CF), is a major issue with regard to eligibility for transplantation. CF patients tend to be infected with multiple organisms by the time transplantation is considered. The most common organisms include *Pseudomonas* sp., *Burkholderia cepacia, Aspergillus,* and nontuberculous mycobacteria. *Aspergillus* and mycobacterial infections have not been associated with worse outcomes in posttransplant patients. However, infection with *B. cepacia* and panresistant *Pseudomonas* sp. has been associated with poor outcomes and is considered a contraindication to transplantation in some centers. Therefore, emergency physicians need to pay particular attention to infection-control measures and antibiotic selection in pretransplant CF patients. Generally, those patients requiring antibiotics for acute infections require admission for broad spectrum, multiple-drug regimens to prevent the development of panresistant strains.

In patients with PPH, survival correlates with New York Heart Association (NYHA) classification. Recently, prostacyclin was approved for treatment of NYHA class III or IV patients, in whom it has been shown to improve hemodynamics, exercise tolerance and survival. Calcium-channel blockers have been the mainstay of treatment for NYHA class I and II patients for some time. Those patients who fail medical therapy are subsequently listed for transplant. In the acute setting, treatment with agents that may reduce pulmonary vascular resistance—including morphine, nitrates, and furosemide—may help provide stabilization in addition to other supportive measures and identification of precipitating factors.

MANAGEMENT OF POTENTIAL DONORS

Identification and early management of potential donors has become part of the practice of emergency medicine. The establishment of brain death is generally not done in the emergency department (ED); however several steps need to be taken to maximize organ retrieval in appropriate patients. Most organ procurement organizations (OPOs) work closely with their local EDs, providing education in the various facets of organ procurement. Early communication with the OPO is encouraged, as it can help to identify factors that may qualify or disqualify a potential donor, provide assistance in speaking with families about organ donation, and guide the clinicians through the entire complicated process.

Initial management is centered around maintaining the integrity of potential donor lungs by optimizing hemodynamics and preventing aspiration. Accepting centers generally require a clear chest radiograph, Pa_{O_2}>450 mmHg on 100% Fi_{O_2}, and no obvious infection on bronchoscopic evaluation. Mechanical ventilation should maintain arterial P_{O_2}>80 mmHg, P_{CO_2} between 35 and 45 mmHg, and a pH between 7.30 and 7.45. Hemodynamics should be monitored, with a desirable central venous pressure >10 mmHg. If systemic blood pressure cannot be maintained with fluid resuscitation alone without causing pulmonary edema, then dopamine may be used. Transfusions may be used to maintain a hematocrit >30% to optimize tissue oxygenation. However, it is crucial to specify the use of blood that is cytomegalovirus (CMV)-negative blood so as not to infect a CMV-negative recipient.

MANAGEMENT OF POSTTRANSPLANT PATIENTS

Transplant patients are managed by a multidisciplinary team comprising transplant surgeons, pulmonologists, nurse coordinators, pharmacists, physical therapists, dietitians, psychologists, and social workers. At each transplant center, a nurse coordinator is on call to address concerns regarding the care of posttransplant patients in the ED. Patients tend to be well educated and well informed about their disease, but the nurse coordinator may be able to provide additional information regarding recent infection history, medication doses, rejection history, and potential complications in a specific patient. Coordinators should always be called early in the course of patient assessment and management.

Posttransplant patients are at risk for several complications related to their underlying disease, medication side effects, and immunocompromised state. Most centers use cyclosporine, azathioprine, and prednisone for maintenance immunosuppression. In addition, prophylaxis against *Pneumocystis carinii* pneumonia is undertaken with trimethoprim-sulfamethoxazole (TMP-SMX). Prophylaxis against herpes simplex virus (HSV) and CMV is indicated based on the specific immunologic status of the donor and recipient. Patients learn to measure their pulmonary function (FEV_1 and FVC), systemic blood pressure, and temperature daily. They carry a diary with daily vital signs, present medications and doses, names of hospital contacts, and guidelines for contacting the nurse coordinator. Bronchoscopy is necessary to diagnose subclinical rejection and infection. Each transplant center has a protocol concerning bronchoscopy indications. Common warning signs of a fever (>37°C), cough, sputum, or FEV_1 decline >10 percent for over 48 h would prompt a call or visit to the transplant center. Since most patients return to their home communities 2 to 3 months following surgery, they may initially be treated and stabilized in their hometown ED prior to transfer back to the transplant center.

The most frequent complications in the lung transplant patient presenting to the ED are infection and rejection, and they are difficult to differentiate clinically. The patient should be placed in respiratory isolation. Initial assessment is similar to that in the pretransplant patient with regard to stabilization and supportive care. In addition to the standard evaluation of airway, respiratory, and circulatory status, initial assessment should include a chest radiograph, arterial blood gas, complete blood count with differential, serum electrolytes, magnesium, creatinine, and cyclosporine level.

Early Complications

REJECTION Acute rejection is common and may occur three to six times in the first postoperative year. After the first year, the frequency of acute rejection is decreased, but rejection can still be seen several years after transplant. Early after transplant, the diagnosis of rejection is based on clinical parameters. Signs of rejection include cough, chest tightness, fever (>0.5°C above baseline), hypoxemia, decline in FEV_1 (>10%), and the development of infiltrate on the chest radiograph. Radiographic abnormalities are less common more than 6 weeks posttransplant, and an acute rejection episode may actually be "radiographically silent" after this time period. Clinically, acute rejection may be difficult to distinguish from infection. Therefore, bronchoscopy with transbronchial biopsy is frequently necessary to make the definitive diagnosis. During episodes of acute rejection in patients with single-lung transplants, there is a proportional decrease in blood flow to the transplanted lung, which can be monitored with radionucleotide perfusion scans.

Acute rejection is treated with large doses of intravenous methylprednisolone, 500 to 1000 mg on day 1, followed by 500 mg IV qd for 2 days. Clinical response is gauged by improvements in oxygenation, spirometry and radiographic appearance and can be expected to occur within 24 to 48 h after treatment is initiated. Failure to do so should suggest infection as an alternative diagnosis. Following clinical improvement, the maintenance dose of prednisone is increased, with a slow taper back to baseline.

INFECTION Infectious complications are the most common cause of morbidity and mortality in lung transplant patients. Infections may be due to bacteria, fungi, or viruses and most commonly affect the allograft. Bacterial pneumonia is the most common complication in the first 3 months after transplant due to decreased mucociliary clearance, diminished cough reflex, disrupted lymphatics, reperfusion injury, and immunosuppression. Late or recurrent infections are associated with an increased risk of developing obliterative bronchiolitis. Besides airborne transmission, a common route of transmission is from the donor lung. The vast majority of washings from a donor before retrieval will grow at least one organism. Perioperative antibiotics based on culture and sensitivity results have decreased the rate of invasive infection significantly. Infection with panresistant *Pseudomonas* sp. or *B. cepacia* is associated with increased morbidity and mortality and is generally associated with a higher risk of obliterative bronchiolitis. *P. carinii* pneumonia is now rare due to common prophylaxis with TMP-SMX.

Other commonly encountered infectious agents include gram-negative and gram-positive bacteria, *Mycobacterium* sp., *Aspergillus*, CMV, HSV, and Epstein-Barr virus (EBV).

CMV is the most commonly encountered viral agent implicated in posttransplant pulmonary infection. Its clinical spectrum is broad, ranging from asymptomatic shedding to CMV pneumonitis. The risk of infection is directly related to the donor's and recipient's pretransplant immune status. Donor-positive, recipient-negative status is universally associated with the development of CMV infection in the recipient unless aggressive prophylaxis is undertaken with ganciclovir, acyclovir, and intravenous immunoglobulin. If the recipient is CMV-positive, a regimen of ganciclovir followed by acyclovir is used. If the donor and recipient are CMV-negative and either the donor or recipient is HSV-positive, acyclovir only is used. CMV matching has not altered long-term outcome in lung transplant patients, so most centers will transplant regardless of CMV status.

CMV infections occur most commonly between 14 to 100 days posttransplant and manifest as anything from a flulike syndrome to severe multisystem disease including pneumonitis, hepatitis, bone marrow suppression, gastritis, and colitis. Key laboratory features include neutropenia with or without thrombocytopenia, conversion of anti-CMV IgM to positive, and positive CMV cultures from urine, buffy coat, or bronchoalveolar lavage. Definitive diagnosis of CMV pneumonitis requires histopathologic confirmation of tissue obtained by transbronchial biopsy. After confirmation of diagnosis, treatment with ganciclovir or foscarnet is indicated. CMV pneumonitis may be complicated by acute rejection or by bacterial or fungal pneumonia.

Other viral agents, particularly HSV and EBV, have been implicated in posttransplant infections. HSV has a similar presentation to CMV, with diagnosis based on viral culture and differential staining of biopsy specimens. Treatment is with acyclovir. EBV may present as a mononucleosis-type syndrome but is also associated with the development of posttransplant lymphomas.

Fungal infections are less common, but carry a relatively high risk of associated morbidity and mortality. *Candida albicans* is a common airway colonizer but a much less common pathogen. Systemic candidiasis is usually associated with prolonged courses of broad-spectrum antibiotics. The treatment for *C. albicans* is fluconazole, but other *Candida* species may require treatment with amphotericin *B. Aspergillus* sp. may also colonize the airways; this does not require treatment unless associated with invasive disease, evidenced by ulcerations, or histologic evidence of invasion. Itraconazole with amphotericin B is frequently successful in treating early infections, but disseminated disease is usually fatal.

Lung transplant patients are subject to bacterial endocarditis because during the transplant operation the donor pulmonary veins are attached to the atrium by the establishment of a cuff. Therefore, antimicrobial prophylaxis is necessary before dental and other invasive procedures.

OTHER PULMONARY COMPLICATIONS Airway dehiscence and stenosis are now uncommon postoperative complications. Airway dehiscensce, if it occurs at all, is likely to appear within 3 weeks of transplantation, while the patient is still in the hospital. It can be managed expectantly if an omental wrap was used and the omentum is intact. Bronchial stenosis can occur, limiting clearance of secretions and leading to pneumonia. Treatment is with stenting or laser therapy. Spontaneous pneumothorax necessitates the placement of a thoracostomy tube and evaluation of the airways by bronchoscopy.

MEDICATION EFFECTS Various induction agents are used in the perioperative and immediate postoperative period. These include high-dose corticosteroids and T-cell lytic therapy with equine-derived antithymocyte globulin (ATGAM), a polyclonal thymocyte preparation, or OKT-3, a murine monoclonal antibody. The most common posttransplant immunosuppressives include cyclosporine, azathioprine, and prednisone. Major side effects of these medications are summarized in Table 66-2.

TABLE 66-2 Medication Side Effects*

Cyclosporine
Nephrotoxicity
Neurotoxicity
Hyperkalemia
Hyperuricemia
Hypertension
Anorexia
Hyperbilirubinemia
Cholestasis
Gastric dysmotility
Hirsutism
Hypercholesterolemia
Prednisone
Cushing syndrome
Osteoporosis
Adrenal suppression
Hypertension
Hyperglycemia
Peptic ulcer disease
Myopathy
Cataracts
Poor wound healing
Azathioprine
Leukopenia
Thrombocytopenia
Cholestatic jaundice
Alopecia

*Avoid NSAIDs and drugs metabolized by the P-450 system.

Both glucocorticoids and cyclosporine can exacerbate glucose intolerance, worsen osteoporosis, and cause myopathy and systemic hypertension. Commonly, chronic cyclosporine use at the levels employed in lung transplant immunosuppression results in renal insufficiency by decreasing renal blood flow and by a direct effect on the renal tubules, causing in hyperkalemia and hypomagnesemia. Nonsteroidal anti-inflammatory drugs (NSAIDs) should be avoided, since these will act synergistically with cyclosporine to further reduce glomerular filtration. The major side effect of azathioprine is bone marrow suppression. Neutropenia may often result from either azathioprine or CMV infection.

Drugs that are metabolized by the P-450 system will interact with cyclosporine metabolism. Drugs that induce these enzymes (e.g., phenytoin, rifampin, and phenobarbital) may lower cyclosporine levels acutely, possibly precipitating rejection. Drugs that inhibit cyclosporine metabolism (e.g., erythromycin, ketoconazole, cimetidine, and the calcium-channel blockers) may lead to elevation of cyclosporine levels into the toxic range and should be avoided unless appropriate changes in cyclosporine dosing are made to compensate.

Late Complications

OBLITERATIVE BRONCHIOLITIS The most frequent cause of death after the second posttransplant year is obliterative bronchiolitis (OB), characterized by chronic allograft dysfunction and airflow limitation. Current evidence suggests that chronic rejection plays the most important role in the development of OB, but other factors such as CMV infection, toxic fume inhalation, and chronic foreign-body exposure caused by abnormal mucociliary clearance may contribute as well. Diagnostically, the yield from bronchoscopy and biopsy is low. Therefore, diagnosis rests on clinical criteria (i.e., > 20 percent fall in FEV_1 without any other identifiable cause). Since the large airways become bronchiectatic as the small airways are obliterated, episodes of bacterial bronchitis are common. Typically the chest radiograph is clear of infiltrates. Current treatment is augmentation of immunosuppression and high-dose steroids. The prevalence of OB syndrome in long-term survivors is 20 to 50 percent. The course of the disease is highly variable, with some patients stabilizing at a lower level of pulmonary function and others progressing to respiratory failure and death.

Posttransplant Lymphoproliferative Disease (PTLD)

PTLD can be a consequence of T-cell suppression with long-term cyclosporine use. The overall incidence in lung transplant patients is approximately 8 percent. The disease tends to occur with primary EBV infection following lung transplant. Because younger patients are more likely to be EBV-negative at the time of transplantation, they tend to develop EBV infection and PTLD at a higher rate. Presenting features include isolated lymphadenopathy, painful otitis media (secondary to tonsillar involvement), or a viral-like syndrome. PTLD within 1 year of transplantation is usually localized and can be successfully treated with reduced immunosuppression and high-dose acyclovir, with a relatively good prognosis. In contrast, PTLD after 1 year tends to be disseminated, unresponsive to treatment, and usually fatal.

ACKNOWLEDGMENT

Kristine A. Nelson, RN, MN: Executive Director, LifeBanc, Cleveland, OH.

REFERENCES

1. United Network for Organ Sharing web page (www.unos.org): Oct 15, 1998.
2. United Network for Organ Sharing: Data Highlights from the 1997 Annual Report. Transplant Data 1988–1996. Richmond Virginia, 1998.
3. Davis RD, Pasque MK: Pulmonary transplantation. *Ann Surg* 221:14, 1995.
4. Edelman JD, Kotloff RM: Lung transplantation. *Adv Lung Dis* 18:627, 1997.
5. Trulock EP: Lung transplantation. *Am J Respir Crit Care Med* 155:789, 1997.

67 PULMONARY IMAGING

Janet M. Poponick

Imaging of the chest is common practice in the emergent evaluation of patients with dyspnea, chest pain, or trauma. This chapter reviews the indications and limitations of various techniques useful in emergency medicine, including the plain chest radiograph, ventilation-perfusion scans, computed tomography, and echocardiography. The value of a study depends on the technical quality of the procedure and the ability of the physician to interpret the image. Although many studies and findings may have excellent interobserver reliability, others do not. Thus, clinical decisions should be based on knowledge of the value and limitations of image interpretation.

PLAIN RADIOGRAPHY

Chest radiography, which is the most commonly ordered radiologic examination, evaluates the lung parenchyma, cardiac and mediastinal size, and the bony structures of the chest wall. The examination is preferably done in the radiology department with the patient in the standing position. This is the standard posterior-anterior (PA) view (the beam of the x-ray passes posterior to anterior). The patient must be able to take a deep breath and hold while the picture is taken. A "good inspiration" is defined as visualizing the ninth rib above the diaphragm. Adding the lateral film visualizes the posterior lung bases and the retrosternal area, and also helps to localize infiltrates and masses anatomically.

For unstable patients, portable chest radiography is performed at the bedside, with patients sitting upright. Portable chest radiography is limited by the low power of the equipment and variations in radiographic technique. The bedside study is obtained as an anterior-posterior (AP) view (the x-ray beam passes anterior to posterior) and thus magnifies the mediastinal structures. For a trauma victim on a backboard, the portable film may be more difficult to interpret. Skinfolds and clothing under a patient may mimic a pneumothorax. Supine chest radiographs will detect only 40 percent of pneumothoraces,[1] because air rises anteriorly, making the diagnosis of a small pneumothorax very difficult. Likewise, fluid collections layer posteriorly in supine patients, causing a diffuse haziness in the lung fields, which can be confused with infiltrate or contusion. Therefore, chest radiographs are limited by a patient's overall condition, the patient's ability to cooperate with directions, and the technique chosen. The PA and lateral chest radiographs remain the best views.

The chest radiograph should be systematically analyzed so as not to miss key information. To ensure that the radiograph is of the correct patient, always identify the study by patient name. Assess the technique and the quality of the study. In a good-quality study, the trachea is visible in the midline, the medial borders of the clavicle are centrally located over the superior mediastinum, and the thoracic spine is visible through the mediastinal structures. Note the positioning of all lines, the endotracheal tube, and the nasogastric tube. The trachea should be followed to the left and right main-stem bronchi and to the mediastinal structures. Look at the mediastinum for evidence of free air, for density behind the heart, and for cardiac size (which should be less than 50 percent of the thoracic size). Assess position of the diaphragms, looking at position, contour, and subdiaphragmatic free air: the right hemidiaphragm should be slightly elevated compared with the left (0.5 to 2.5 cm is normal). Assess the lung fields and pleura, looking for masses, infiltrates, free air, or effusions. Finally, assess the soft tissue and bones, looking for subcutaneous air or fractures.

Other views may be obtained. The most useful is the *expiratory* film, which may accentuate a free air-lung interface, enabling a small pneumothorax to be diagnosed. Up to 10 percent of small pneumothoraces may be missed in inspiratory film alone.[2] In foreign-body aspiration, the expiratory film shows hyperinflation on the affected side as air is trapped behind the foreign body. The *lateral decubitus* film may be useful to assess a pleural effusion, because free fluid will layer along the dependent portion of the chest.

Specific abnormalities to note on the chest radiograph are pulmonary edema, infiltrates, lung nodules and masses, hilar size and contour, cardiac size and configuration, pleural effusions, and pneumothorax.

VENTILATION-PERFUSION SCANS

The ventilation-perfusion ($\dot{V}/\dot{Q}$) scan is performed on patients with suspected pulmonary embolism (PE). The study has a low incidence of adverse reactions, is noninvasive, and requires no advance preparation.[3] However, it is performed outside of the ED, limiting its use in unstable patients.

The $\dot{V}/\dot{Q}$ scan is a two-step process. First, the ventilation portion of the examination is performed with the patient breathing an aerosolized solution of technetium 99m (^{99m}Tc) diethylenetriaminepentaacetic acid (DTPA). The aerosol is deposited deep into the lungs in proportion to alveolar ventilation. Images are obtained from different projections. The second step is the perfusion study in which ^{99m}Tc-macroaggregated albumin is injected intravenously and becomes trapped within the pulmonary circulation. Again, images are obtained with the patient in multiple positions. Usually, the procedure is quite simple and the test can be finished in 1 h. Procedural problems arise when a patient is

TABLE 67-1 Modified Criteria of the Prospective Investigation of Pulmonary Embolism Diagnosis (PIOPED)

High probability	Two or more large segmental mismatches One large plus two or more moderate mismatches Four or more moderate mismatches
Intermediate probability	One moderate segmental mismatch plus one large mismatch Up to three moderate mismatches One moderate mismatch Unable to categorize as low or high probability
Low probability	Multiple matched defects with some areas of normal perfusion Nonsegmental perfusion defect Chest radiograph abnormality larger than the perfusion defect Normal chest radiograph with small perfusion defects
Normal	No perfusion defects Perfusion outlines the shape of the lungs seen on chest radiograph

Source: From Gottschalk et al,[4] with permission.

unable to lie still. The ventilation study may be limited if a patient cannot take a deep breath or follow instructions or is on a ventilator.

Diagnosis of PE on $\dot{V}/\dot{Q}$ scan is based on documenting perfusion defects in an area of normal ventilation, a *mismatched defect*. Perfusion defects in areas of associated ventilation abnormalities are probably due to vasoconstriction secondary to hypoxia. Such *matched defects* may be due to pneumonia, asthma, or chronic obstructive pulmonary disease. Underlying pulmonary pathology causes abnormalities in both ventilation and perfusion, making interpretation difficult.

The $\dot{V}/\dot{Q}$ scan is reported in terms of probability, correlating the findings of the $\dot{V}/\dot{Q}$ scan with the chest radiograph. Clinicians should understand the definitions for high, intermediate, and low probability used by radiologists when reporting the results of a $\dot{V}/\dot{Q}$ scan (Table 67-1).[4,5] The PIOPED study found that the clinical utility of a $\dot{V}/\dot{Q}$ scan was enhanced when used in conjunction with clinical suspicion of embolism (Table 67-2).[6] For example, if the clinical suspicion for PE is high but the $\dot{V}/\dot{Q}$ scan interpretation is low probability, the probability that a patient may still have PE is 40 percent. Many emergency department patients fall into the intermediate category for clinical suspicion, where a low probability scan does not exclude PE. In this category, 16 percent of the PIOPED study patients had angiographically proven embolism.[6]

The $\dot{V}/\dot{Q}$ scan is most useful when it is either normal or high probability. A normal lung scan has a 4 percent overall probability of a PE; 96 percent of the PIOPED study patients did not have the condition.[6] Unfortunately, normal findings on a $\dot{V}/\dot{Q}$ scan are unusual; only 14 percent of patients in the PIOPED study had normal scan findings. A high-probability scan had an 87 percent overall probability of a PE; the 13 percent of high-probability scans that were later found to have normal pulmonary angiograms were false positive, possibly due to vasculitis or neoplasm.[3,6] Again, a high-probability $\dot{V}/\dot{Q}$ scan is uncommon; only 13 percent of the PIOPED patients had a high-probability scan.[6] The majority of patients undergoing $\dot{V}/\dot{Q}$ scanning will have intermediate- and low-probability scans. The major difficulty in interpreting a $\dot{V}/\dot{Q}$ scan occurs in those with underlying pulmonary disease, such as asthma and emphysema, which alters both ventilation and perfusion. Pretest chest radiographs aid radiologists in such cases. For example, patients with matched defects on $\dot{V}/\dot{Q}$ scan and a corresponding infiltrate on plain chest film may have pneumonia or pulmonary infarct. There is some literature comparing the size of matched defects with the size of the infiltrate on chest radiograph to classify the likelihood of embolism.[7]

Although $\dot{V}/\dot{Q}$ scans remain a common initial test for PE, many patients require further testing, especially those with intermediate or high clinical suspicion and intermediate- or low-probability $\dot{V}/\dot{Q}$ scans.

PULMONARY ANGIOGRAPHY

Pulmonary angiography remains the gold standard for accurately diagnosing PE. The disadvantages include patient discomfort, cost, and complications. Pulmonary angiography has excellent interobserver reliability: the PIOPED study found that review of study angiograms by another radiologist reached the same diagnosis in 96 percent of cases.[8] Complications of pulmonary angiography include (1) fatalities in 0.5 percent, (2) major nonfatal complications such as renal failure, significant hematoma, or respiratory distress in 17 percent, and (3) minor complications such as angina, urticaria, or bronchospasm in 5 percent.[8]

A pulmonary angiogram is performed by a flexible catheter advanced from a peripheral large vein (typically the femoral vein) through the right atrium and ventricle, and into the pulmonary artery. Selective injections of contrast media are made into the lobar pulmonary arteries by using the results of the $\dot{V}/\dot{Q}$ scan to guide which lobar arteries should be inspected first.

A PE is identified by either an abrupt cutoff of dye with a meniscus or contrast media traveling around an intraluminal thrombus. Narrowing or luminal irregularities can be caused by other processes and are not considered diagnostic for PE. Pulmonary angiography can identify emboli out to the subsegmental divisions, beyond the reliability of either $\dot{V}/\dot{Q}$ scanning or dynamic computed tomography (CT).

COMPUTED TOMOGRAPHY

CT provides sharp cross-sectional anatomic displays, which enable identification of fluid collections and distinction between soft tissue

TABLE 67-2 Prevalence of Pulmonary Embolism as Compared with Angiographic Results or Outcome in the Prospective Investigation of Pulmonary Embolism Diagnosis (PIOPED) Trial (Percent)

	CLINICAL PROBABILITY (%)				
$\dot{V}/\dot{Q}$ Interpretation	High (80%–100%)	Intermediate (20%–79%)	Low (0%–19%)	Overall	No. Patients
High probability	96	88	56	87	118
Intermediate probability	66	28	16	30	345
Low probability	40	16	4	14	296
Normal	0	6	2	4	128

Source: Adapted from Kramer and Divgi[3] and the PIOPED Study,[6] with permission.

structures. It eliminates overlap of tissues and thus delineates mediastinal structures very well. A recent upgrade in technology has allowed the scans to be completed more quickly and has the added advantage of being able to evaluate the vasculature by using dynamic and helical techniques.

In the ED, CT scans are useful in assessing the mediastinum to exclude a mediastinal hematoma or aortic injury after blunt trauma, in assessing acute chest pain to exclude the diagnosis of aortic dissection, or in investigating larger pulmonary emboli in unstable patients.

The disadvantages of chest CT include cost, radiation exposure, and adverse reactions to intravascular contrast media. Transporting unstable patients is never easy, but can usually be done safely with monitoring and appropriate personnel accompanying the patient.

Blunt trauma to the chest and abdomen often requires further evaluation by CT. With chest radiographs of supine patients, pneumothorax may be difficult to visualize and be seen only on the upper cuts of the abdominal CT scan.[1] The abdominal CT is done with windows through the lower chest and delineates the air-lung interface very well, identifying even a small pneumothorax.

Aortic injury in the setting of decelerating trauma is suspected by findings on the initial AP chest radiograph of supine patients. Criteria found suggestive of aortic injury include mediastinal widening (greater than 8 cm at the T_4 level), deviation of the nasogastric tube or endotracheal tube to the right, loss of the aortic knob contour, apical capping, or fractures of any of the first three ribs.[9,10] However, the most sensitive finding for aortic injury was the subjective impression of mediastinal widening by the physician viewing the radiograph.[9] When these findings are noted on the chest radiograph, emergent aortography has been used to accurately visualize the aorta and define any injury. However, using sensitive criteria to avoid missing this catastrophic injury means that about 90 percent of aortograms performed to evaluate patients for potential aortic injury are normal. To reduce the incidence of normal studies, some clinicians will attempt to sit the patient up and perform an upright AP or PA chest radiograph before deciding whether there are findings of mediastinal injury.[11] Not all patients can be sat upright, however, and a decision has to be made regarding another imaging study. Two studies have come into clinical practice: transesophageal echocardiography (TEE) and dynamic CT scan.

Dynamic CT scanning with intravenous contrast can be useful, especially in stable patients with possible aortic injury.[12–14] The major advantages of CT are that it is less invasive than aortography and, while on the CT table, the patient can have multiple parts of the body imaged. The major disadvantage is the logistical difficulty in transporting patients who are unstable or on a ventilator to the CT suite. Intravascular contrast media is used with dynamic CT, so a history of a serious reaction remains a contraindication. With appropriate equipment and physicians who can perform and properly interpret the studies, aortography, TEE, or dynamic CT scan are acceptable tests to evaluate aortic injury after blunt trauma.

Dynamic CT scan of the chest may also be helpful in patients with signs and symptoms of aortic dissection: an accurate diagnosis of dissection will be obtained in more than 90 to 94 percent of such patients.[15,16] Dynamic CT scan can accurately identify dissection by visualizing an intimal flap with opacification of the true and false lumens. In patients with type B (descending aorta) dissection, no other study will be necessary. A disadvantage of dynamic CT scan is that, in type A (ascending aorta) dissection, aortography will still be required to assess the aortic valve and major arterial vessels prior to surgery.

Dynamic CT scan has recently been used to diagnose PE. Currently, the $\dot{V}/\dot{Q}$ scan remains the initial imaging modality used, but, with added experience, the dynamic CT scan may replace it. Recent articles report 86 to 91 percent sensitivity and 78 to 95 percent specificity for contrast-enhanced spiral CT in detecting PE out to the segmental divisions of the pulmonary arteries.[17–19] Although dynamic CT can occasionally visualize subsegmental arteries, reliability and interpretation are problematic. Patients must be able to hold their breath, typically for 20 to 24 s, as the CT scan table is moved through the gantry, although scans can be done in 10 to 12 s with thicker image slices. Breath holding may be difficult for dyspneic patients.[19] Another variation is contrast-enhanced electron-beam CT, which has the advantage of a 100-ms scanning time, no need for a breath-holding maneuver, and minimal respiratory or cardiac motion artifact.[20] As radiologists become more familiar with these tests and gain more expertise, the CT scan may become the important noninvasive test for the diagnosis of PE.

TRANSTHORACIC ECHOCARDIOGRAPHY

Echocardiography brought to the bedside of an ED patient is noninvasive, portable, and provides immediate bedside images. Although the techniques of echocardiography are beyond the scope of this chapter, the viewing windows are easy to identify and to access.[21] The subcostal view, at the left intercostal margin at its junction with the xiphoid process, yields information regarding presence of fluid, wall motion, and chamber size. The parasternal view, at the left upper intercostal spaces, gives images of the aorta, cardiac chambers, and heart valves.[22]

Emergency bedside echocardiography is usually performed to detect two conditions: pericardial fluid (in the setting of possible pericardial tamponade) and cardiac wall motion (in the setting of cardiac arrest with maintained electrical activity—pulseless electrical activity or PEA). In both of these settings, the interpretation provided by emergency physician bedside echocardiography has been accurate for clinical decision making.[23,24] Both conditions can be evaluated by performing a limited examination using the subcostal view. A pericardial effusion is identified as fluid following the contour of the heart with the surrounding hyperechoic image of the pericardium. The findings of fluid, hyperdynamic heart, and diastolic collapse of the right atrium and ventricle suggest tamponade.[22] In a pulseless patient with electrical activity on the monitor, echocardiography may accurately identify treatable causes.[24]

Other indications for emergency bedside echocardiography include hypotension of unknown cause, suspected cardiac trauma (blunt or penetrating), and suspected ischemic heart disease. Hyperdynamic wall motion without pericardial fluid suggests hypovolemia. Pericardial fluid suggests cardiac injury. Tension pneumothorax can be suggested by difficulty in visualizing the heart due to an air interface.

Evaluation of patients with possible ischemic chest pain requires a more thorough echocardiographic examination than is usually possible using the equipment and training available to most emergency physicians. Additional training and specific equipment are required to accurately assess cardiac wall motion, cardiac chamber size, and valve function. If the appropriate equipment and physician (usually a cardiologist) are available, though, echocardiography can be very useful in evaluating patients with chest pain.[25] Early echocardiography in the emergency department is more sensitive than an electrocardiogram (ECG) (91 percent versus 40 percent) in predicting acute infarction or revascularization.[25] Echocardiography can identify and assess complications of ischemia: pump failure, mitral valve insufficiency, and pericardial effusion. Along with the medical history, ECG, and serologic markers, echocardiography may aid in the triage process of patients with chest pain.[25]

Other diagnoses that can be made with echocardiography include acute PE, aortic dissection, and cardiac contusion; however, advanced training is necessary to diagnose these conditions accurately.[22]

CHEST ULTRASONOGRAPHY

Ultrasound is not routinely performed to image the thoracic cavity, and does not substitute for the chest radiograph in trauma assessment. However, bedside ultrasound performed by trained emergency physicians was a sensitive as the initial chest radiograph (96 percent) in detecting traumatic hemothorax.[26] The viewing areas used were the right and left intercostal oblique views. Fluid in the pleural space was identified as an anechoic space distal to the hyperechoic line representing the diaphragm.

TRANSESOPHAGEAL ECHOCARDIOGRAM

TEE is useful to image the heart and aorta,[27] and is most commonly used in an emergency department when aortic trauma or dissection is suspected. In both of these conditions, TEE performed by trained physicians has a sensitivity of over 95 percent and specificity over 95 percent.[16,28–33] TEE will also evaluate cardiac function and may disclose unexpected injury.[28] TEE requires extensive training and is usually performed by a cardiologist.

REFERENCES

1. Dee PM: The radiology of chest trauma. *Radiol Clin North Am* 30:291, 1992.
2. Aitchison F, Bleetman A, Munro P, et al: Detection of pneumothorax by accident and emergency officers and radiologists on single chest film. *Arch Emerg Med* 10:343, 1993.
3. Kramer EL, Divgi CR: Pulmonary applications of nuclear medicine. *Clin Chest Med* 12:55, 1991.
4. Gottschalk A, Sostman HD, Coleman RE, et al: Ventilation-perfusion scintigraphy in the PIOPED study: II. Evaluation of the scintigraphic criteria and interpretations. *J Nucl Med* 34:1119, 1993.
5. Ralph DD: Pulmonary embolism: The implications of prospective investigation of pulmonary embolism diagnosis. *Radiol Clin North Am* 32:679, 1994.
6. PIOPED Investigators: Value of ventilation/perfusion scan in acute pulmonary embolism: Results of the Prospective Investigation of Pulmonary Embolism Diagnosis (PIOPED). *JAMA* 263:2753, 1990.
7. Stein PD, Henry JW, Gottschalk A: The addition of clinical assessment to stratification according to prior cardiopulmonary disease further optimizes the interpretation of ventilation/perfusion lung scans in pulmonary embolism. *Chest* 104:1472, 1993.
8. Stein PD, Athanasoulis C, Alavi A, et al: Complications and validity of pulmonary angiography in acute pulmonary embolism. *Circulation* 85:462, 1992.
9. Woodring JH, Dillon ML: Radiographic manifestations of mediastinal hemorrhage from blunt chest trauma [collective review]. *Ann Thorac Surg* 37:171, 1984.
10. Burney RE, Gundry SR, Mackenzie JR, et al: Comparison of mediastinal width, mediastinal-thoracic and cardiac ratios, and ''mediastinal widening'' in detection of traumatic aortic rupture. *Ann Emerg Med* 12:668, 1983.
11. Schwab CW, Lawson RB, Lind JF, Garland LW: Aortic injury: Comparison of supine and upright portable chest films to evaluate the widened mediastinum. *Ann Emerg Med* 13:896, 1984.
12. Madayag MA, Kirshenbaum KJ, Nadimpalli SR, et al: Thoracic aortic trauma: Role of dynamic CT. *Radiology* 179:853, 1991.
13. Richardson P, Mirvis S, Scorpio R, Dunham CM: Value of CT in determining the need for angiography when findings of mediastinal hemorrhage on chest radiographs are equivocal. *AJR* 156:273, 1991.
14. Agee CK, Metzler MH, Churchill RJ, Mitchell FL: Computed tomographic evaluation to exclude traumatic aortic disruption. *J Trauma* 33:876, 1992.
15. Petasnick JP: Radiologic evaluation of aortic dissection. *Radiology* 180:297, 1991.
16. Neinaber CA, von Kodolitsch Y, Nicolas V, et al: The diagnosis of thoracic aortic dissection by noninvasive imaging procedures. *N Engl J Med* 328:1, 1993.
17. Goodman LR, Curtin JJ, Mewissen MW, et al: Detection of pulmonary embolism in patients with unresolved clinical and scintigraphic diagnosis: Helical CT versus angiography. *AJR* 164:1369, 1995.
18. Remy-Jardin M, Remy J, Deschildre F, et al: Diagnosis of pulmonary embolism with spiral CT: Comparison with pulmonary angiography and scintigraphy. *Radiology* 200:699, 1996.
19. Mayo JR, Remy-Jardin M, Muller NL, et al: Pulmonary embolism: Prospective comparison of spiral CT with ventilation-perfusion scintigraphy. *Radiology* 205:447, 1997.
20. Teigen CL, Maus TP, Sheedy PF, et al: Pulmonary embolism: Diagnosis with contrast-enhanced electron-beam CT and comparison with pulmonary angiography. *Radiology* 194:313, 1995.
21. Plummer D: Principles of emergency ultrasound and echocardiography. *Ann Emerg Med* 18:1291, 1989.
22. Hauser AM: The emerging role of echocardiography in the emergency department. *Ann Emerg Med* 18:1298, 1989.
23. Hoffner RJ, Mandavia D, Kelsey J, Henderson SO: The accuracy of bedside echocardiography performed by emergency physicians. *Acad Emerg Med* 5:408, 1998.
24. Corbett SW, O'Callaghan T: Detection of traumatic complications of cardiopulmonary resuscitation by ultrasound. *Ann Emerg Med* 29:317, 1997.
25. Kontos MC, Arrowood JA, Paulsen WH, Nixon JV: Early echocardiography can predict cardiac events in emergency department patients with chest pain. *Ann Emerg Med* 31:550, 1998.
26. Ma OJ, Mateer JR: Trauma ultrasound examination versus chest radiography in the detection of hemothorax. *Ann Emerg Med* 29:312, 1997.
27. Shenoy MM, Dhala A, Khanna A: Transesophageal echocardiography in emergency medicine and critical care. *Am J Emerg Med* 9:580, 1991.
28. Shapiro MJ, Yanofsky SD, Trapp J, et al: Cardiovascular evaluation in blunt thoracic trauma using transesophageal echocardiography (TEE). *J Trauma* 31:835, 1991.
29. Brooks SW, Young JC, Cmolik B, et al: The use of transesophageal echocardiography in the evaluation of chest trauma. *J Trauma* 32:761, 1992.
30. Kearney PA, Smith W, Johnson SB, et al: Use of transesophageal echocardiography in the evaluation of traumatic aortic injury. *J Trauma* 34:696, 1993.
31. Buckmaster MJ, Kearney PA, Johnson SB, et al: Further experience with transesophageal echocardiography in the evaluation of thoracic aortic injury. *J Trauma* 37:989, 1994.
32. Smith MD, Cassidy JM, Souther S, et al: Transesophageal echocardiography in the diagnosis of traumatic rupture of the aorta. *N Engl J Med* 332:356, 1995.
33. Keren A, Kim CB, Hu BS, et al: Accuracy of biplane and multiplane transesophageal echocardiography in diagnosis of typical acute aortic dissection and intramural hematoma. *J Am Coll Cardiol* 28:627, 1996.

GASTROINTESTINAL EMERGENCIES

ACUTE ABDOMINAL PAIN

E. John Gallagher

Most investigators in this field have arbitrarily defined ''acute'' abdominal pain as pain of less than 1 week's duration.[1,2] In keeping with this convention and the American College of Emergency Physicians' Clinical Policies Committee guidelines, this chapter restricts the discussion to postpubescent patients only, excluding individuals with *known* antecedent trauma and women beyond the twentieth week of pregnancy.[2]

EPIDEMIOLOGY

One large cross-sectional study of adults living in the community found that about one individual out of every three reported at least one episode of ''abdominal pain or discomfort'' during the preceding 3 months.[3] The population-based annual incidence of adults presenting to the emergency department (ED) for acute abdominal conditions is approximately 44/1000.

Data from the U.S. National Center for Health Statistics indicate that abdominal pain was the single ''most frequently mentioned'' reason offered by patients for visiting the ED in 1996 (annual incidence approximately 57/1000 adult ED visits.[4] Admission rates for abdominal pain vary markedly, ranging from 18 to 42 percent, with rates as high as 63 percent reported in patients over 65 years of age.[5]

PATHOPHYSIOLOGY

Abdominal pain is traditionally divided into three categories: visceral, parietal, and referred. In general, the visceral (autonomic) and parietal (somatic) types are considered the two basic ''causes'' of abdominal pain. Referred pain can be considered separately as a cortical misperception of either visceral or parietal afferent stimuli. Although each type of pain is thought to have a different neuropathophysiology, the categories are not entirely discrete. For example, visceral pain often blends with parietal pain as a pathologic process evolves. Their shortcomings notwithstanding, these distinctions are clinically useful ways of thinking about abdominal pain.

Visceral Pain

Visceral abdominal pain is usually caused by stretching of fibers innervating the walls or capsules of hollow or solid organs, respectively. Less commonly, it is caused by early ischemia or inflammation. Severity ranges from a steady ache or vague discomfort to excruciating or colicky pain. Because the visceral afferents follow a segmental distribution, visceral pain can be localized by the sensory cortex to an approximate spinal cord level determined by the embryologic origin of the organ involved. For example, foregut organs (stomach, duodenum, and biliary tract) produce pain in the epigastric region; midgut organs (most of the small bowel, appendix, and cecum) cause periumbilical pain; and hindgut organs (most of colon, including the sigmoid) as well as the intraperitoneal portions of the genitourinary system tend to cause pain initially in the suprapubic or hypogastric area.

Because intraperitoneal organs are bilaterally innervated, stimuli are sent to both sides of the spinal cord, causing intraperitoneal visceral pain to be felt in the midline, independent of the right- or left-sided anatomic location of the involved organ. For example, stimuli from visceral fibers in the wall of the appendix enter the spinal cord at about T10. When obstruction causes appendiceal distention in early appendicitis, pain is initially perceived in the midline periumbilical area, corresponding roughly to the location of the T10 cutaneous dermatome.

Parietal Pain

Parietal or somatic abdominal pain is caused by irritation of fibers that innervate the parietal peritoneum, usually the portion covering the anterior abdominal wall. Because parietal afferent signals are sent from a specific area of peritoneum, parietal pain—in contrast to visceral pain—can be localized to the dermatome directly above the site of the painful stimulus. As the underlying disease process evolves, the symptoms of visceral pain give way to the signs of parietal pain, with tenderness and guarding. As localized peritonitis develops further, rigidity and ''rebound'' appear.

Referred Pain

Referred pain is felt at a location distant from the diseased organ. Like visceral pain and in contrast to parietal pain, referred pain produces symptoms, not signs. Unlike visceral pain, referred pain is usually ipsilateral to the involved organ and is felt in the midline only if the pathologic process is also located in the midline. This is because referred pain, in contrast to visceral pain, is not mediated by fibers providing bilateral innervation to the cord. Like those of visceral pain, patterns of referred pain are based upon developmental embryology. For example, the ureter and the testes share the same segmental innervation because these structures were once anatomically contiguous. Both therefore supply afferent fibers to the same lower thoracic and upper lumbar segments of the spinal cord. Thus, acute ureteral obstruction is often associated with ipsilateral testicular pain. Other sites of referred pain reflect similar dermatomal sharing, providing explanations for otherwise puzzling associations between supra- or subdiaphragmatic irritation and ipsilateral supraclavicular/shoulder pain; gynecologic pathology and back/proximal lower extremity pain; biliary tract disease and right infrascapular pain; and myocardial ischemia and midepigastric/neck/jaw/upper extremity pain.

CLINICAL FEATURES

Conceptual Framework

CLASSIFICATION A conceptual framework encompassing undifferentiated acute abdominal pain is summarized in Table 68-1. The classification scheme divides abdominal pain into two main categories: Intraabdominal, i.e., arising from within the abdominal cavity or retroperitoneum, and extraabdominal. Intraabdominal causes are then divided by organ system into the ''3G's'': GI (gastrointestinal), GU (genitourinary), and GYN (gynecologic), plus a fourth, less common but often catastrophic group of *vascular* emergencies. Each of these four organ systems is further subdivided into specific diagnoses within that organ system. Pain of extraabdominal origin, which is substantially less common, is similarly divided into four broad etiologic categories of cardiopulmonary, abdominal wall, toxic-metabolic, and neurogenic.

Broadening the scope of abdominal pain beyond the intraabdominal reminds us that the clinical focus of the ED physician is quite different from that of his or her surgical colleagues. Surgeons, quite appropri-

TABLE 68-1 Conceptual Framework: Undifferentiated Acute Abdominal Pain

Intraabdominal
Gastrointestinal
Appendicitis
Biliary tract disease
Small bowel obstruction
Pancreatitis
Diverticulitis
Genitourinary
Renal colic
Acute urinary retention
Acute scrotum
Gynecologic
Pelvic inflammatory disease
Ectopic pregnancy
Vascular
Abdominal aortic aneurysm
Mesenteric ischemia
Ischemic colitis
Extraabdominal
Cardiopulmonary
Abdominal wall
Hernias
Other abdominal wall syndromes
Toxic-metabolic
Toxic
Infectious
Poisonings
Metabolic
Neurogenic
Nonspecific abdominal pain

ately, approach abdominal pain seeking a binary answer to the question "Does this patient need an operation?" ED physicians, in contrast, must first identify sick or possibly sick patients as early as possible in the course of their illness. Once this determination is made clinically, the ED physician must rapidly decide which additional diagnostic tests, if any, are needed. Although ED physicians may quickly arrive at the same dichotomous question as their surgical counterparts, because they encounter undifferentiated abdominal pain, they must first cast a much broader net that considers causes located both within and outside of the abdominal cavity.

Finally, nonspecific abdominal pain (NSAP), which is the most common "cause" of undifferentiated abdominal pain among ED patients, is listed as a third category. NSAP stands alone since it is unknown to what extent it may represent an underlying intra- versus extraabdominal problem.

ABDOMINAL TOPOGRAPHY By combining the four-quadrant approach traditionally used by U.S. physicians with selected aspects of a strategy widely employed throughout Europe and Asia,[1] a simple model of abdominal topography can be developed. In addition to the standard four quadrants—right upper quadrant (RUQ), right lower quadrant (RLQ), left upper quadrant (LUQ), and left lower quadrant (LLQ)—this model includes four areas of the abdomen that are not discrete but rather constitute combinations of all or part of two or more quadrants: (1) upper half of abdomen (UHA), which includes an area of pain as small as the midepigastrium or as large as the RUQ plus LUQ combined; (2) lower half of abdomen (LHA), which similarly includes an area of pain as small as the midhypogastrium or as large as the RLQ and LLQ combined; (3) central (CTL), which includes an area of pain comprising the centermost "quarters" of all four discrete quadrants, such that carving out these areas from each quadrant defines a periumbilical or "central" quadrant and (4) generalized (GEN), which includes poorly localized pain encompassing much or perhaps most of the abdomen, including at least some portion of all four discrete quadrants.

This topographic configuration is particularly relevant to the broad spectrum of undifferentiated abdominal pain seen in emergency practice. It incorporates both the early (visceral, poorly localized) and late (parietal, better localized) pain of an evolving intraabdominal pathologic process, as well as the more generalized pain associated with toxic-metabolic derangements.

Of greater importance, however, is the inherent limitation in any approach to abdominal pain that relies principally on abdominal topography. Following the first critical examination of the association between the location of overlying pain/tenderness and underlying surgical disease, Staniland and colleagues concluded that "the most striking feature" of their findings was the observation that "the 'stereotype' site of pain is seen to be little more than an *approximate guide to the diagnosis of the disease concerned* [italics added]."[6] Their seminal observation that about one-third or more of cases of abdominal pain that come to operation present in a fashion that clinicians mistakenly regard as "atypical" may represent the largest single reason that the error rate in the clinical diagnosis of abdominal pain is so high. A corollary to this is that one cannot exclude a particular diagnosis based solely on the location of abdominal pain or tenderness.

Historical Features

What follows assumes that the patient is sufficiently stable to allow for a detailed history and goal-directed examination.

Historical data can be conveniently divided into attributes of pain, associated symptoms, and past history.

PAIN ATTRIBUTES The principal characteristics of abdominal pain include location, quality, severity, onset, duration, aggravating and alleviating factors, and change in any of these variables over time.

ASSOCIATED SYMPTOMS These can be subdivided into one of the four main organ systems that are involved in intraabdominal pain, as shown in Table 68-1.

Gastrointestinal Symptoms Anorexia, nausea, and vomiting (unless bloody) are among the least helpful symptoms for specific diagnosis. For example, vomiting has been reported in over 40 percent of patients with salpingitis, and in over 60 percent of patients with renal colic. Lower gastrointestinal (GI) symptoms such as nonbloody diarrhea or constipation are similarly too insensitive and nonspecific to significantly alter the probability of a GI cause of abdominal pain.

Genitourinary Symptoms The hallmark of abdominal pain of genitourinary (GU) origin is the concomitant development of some, often subtle, alteration in micturition—e.g., dysuria, frequency, urgency, hematuria, incomplete emptying, or incontinence (usually overflow). On occasion, non-GU pathology develops in organs contiguous to the GU system, giving the appearance of an intrinsic GU problem. For example, an inflamed appendix lying across the bladder might cause urinary frequency.

Gynecologic Symptoms Distinguishing GI from gynecologic (GYN) causes of acute abdominal pain is one of the most challenging clinical dilemmas in emergency practice. A thorough gynecologic history is indicated, including menses, mode of contraception, fertility, sexual activity, sexually transmitted diseases, vaginal discharge, recent dyspareunia, and a past gynecologic history, including pregnancies, deliveries, abortions, ectopic pregnancies, cysts, fibroids, pelvic inflammatory disease, and laparoscopy.

Vascular Symptoms History of myocardial infarction (MI), other ischemic heart disease or cardiomyopathy, atrial fibrillation, anticoagulation, congestive heart failure, peripheral vascular disease, or a family history of aortic aneurysm are all pertinent historical features in older patients.

PAST MEDICAL HISTORY This includes a history of recent/current medications (including nonsteroidal anti-inflammatory drugs and antibiotics), past hospitalizations, in- or outpatient surgeries, diabetes, other chronic diseases [including human immunodeficiency virus (HIV) status and risk factors], central nervous system (CNS) disease (such as multiple sclerosis), and any history of recent trauma. A social history that includes habits (tobacco, alcohol, and other drug usage), occupation, possible toxic exposures, and living circumstances (e.g., homeless, residing in an unheated dwelling, with no access to running water, living alone, other family members ill with similar symptoms) provides important background and a context within which to place the presenting complaint of acute abdominal pain.

Physical Examination

GENERAL The patient's general appearance—including facial expression, diaphoresis, pallor, and degree of agitation—provides information about the severity of pain. Although this is helpful in determining the immediacy of need for analgesia, severity of abdominal pain bears no necessary relationship to illness severity. For example, the pain of early mesenteric ischemia may be a vague discomfort, in contrast to the sudden onset of the excruciating pain of ureteral colic. Nevertheless, kidney stones have virtually no acute mortality associated with them, while the majority of patients with ischemic small bowel go on to die.

Patients with colicky pain, which is characteristically visceral due to distention of a hollow organ, are often unable to lie still, while those with peritonitis prefer to remain immobile.

VITAL SIGNS A reliable means of obtaining a core temperature is important, although absence of fever, especially in the elderly, has virtually no predictive value. Careful counting of rate and observation of depth of respirations for 15 s is often overlooked. However, it can provide crucial information about tachypnea or hyperpnea, which may be subtle. Pulse and blood pressure should include orthostatic changes if, after obtaining the history, there is any reason to suspect intravascular volume contraction. A pulse change of 30 points lying to standing at 1 min (or the development of presyncope) has been shown to be highly specific for the loss of 1 L of blood or its roughly 3-L equivalent of isotonic solute. Changes in blood pressure have not been shown to be discriminatory, probably because they are late findings that represent failure of the tachycardic response to maintain cardiac output. This threshold does not apply to patients on medications that block a tachycardic response or to the elderly, owing to the effects of aging on the cardiac conducting system.

ABDOMEN **Inspection** The abdomen should be inspected for distention (with air or fluid), scars, and masses.

Auscultation Contrary to conventional teaching, absent or diminished bowel sounds provide little clinically useful information. This is supported by the observation that, in a series of 100 patients with operative confirmation of peritonitis due to perforation of peptic ulcer, about half were noted to have normal or increased bowel sounds.[6] Hyperactive/obstructive bowel sounds, although of limited value, are somewhat more helpful, as reflected by their presence in about half of 100 patients with small bowel obstruction (SBO), in contrast to only 5 to 10 percent of patients with 500 other surgical diagnoses. However, fully 25 percent of those with SBO had absent or diminished bowel sounds.[6] It appears, therefore, that only hyperactive/obstructive bowel sounds have some clinical utility, increasing the likelihood of SBO by about fivefold; however, normal or absent bowel sounds appear very nearly valueless, as evidenced by their occurrence with roughly the same frequency in both SBO and perforated peptic ulcer.

Palpation The vast majority of clinical information obtained from examination of the abdomen is acquired through gentle palpation, using two or three fingers, beginning at a distance from the area of maximum pain. Voluntary guarding (contraction of the abdominal musculature in anticipation of or in response to palpation) can be relieved somewhat by asking patients to flex their knees. Those who remain guarded following this maneuver will often relax if the clinician's hand is placed over the patient's and the patient is then asked to use his or her own hand in palpating the abdomen. In contrast to the symptom of pain, tenderness is a *sign* in which pain is produced by palpation. If tenderness can be confined to a single quadrant, this is preferable. However, this is often not possible, in which case one may have to settle for tenderness encompassing one of the four combined areas noted above. Rigidity (involuntary guarding or reflex spasm of abdominal muscles) is suggestive of underlying peritoneal inflammation, as is pain referred to the point of maximum tenderness when palpating an adjacent quadrant.

''Rebound'' tenderness, often regarded as the clinical criterion standard of peritonitis, has several important limitations. In patients with peritonitis, the combination of rigidity, referred tenderness, and especially, ''cough pain''[7] usually provides sufficient diagnostic confirmation that little is gained by eliciting the unnecessary pain of rebound.[8] False positive rebound tenderness occurs in about one patient in four without peritonitis,[8] perhaps because of a nonspecific startle response. Indeed, more recent work has led some authors to conclude that rebound tenderness, in contrast to cough pain, is of ''no predictive value.''[9]

Enlargement of the liver or spleen and other masses, including a distended bladder, should be sought. The examiner should also examine for hernias, particularly those that are tender, suggesting incarceration or strangulation. Men with abdominal pain should have a GU exam, and it is wise to maintain a low threshold for performing a pelvic examination in the evaluation of abdominal pain, particularly in women of reproductive age, regardless of where in the abdomen the pain is localized.

Although the rectal examination is widely regarded as an essential component of the evaluation of abdominal pain, particularly in suspected appendicitis, there is little evidence that rectal tenderness in patients with RLQ pain provides any useful incremental information beyond what has already been obtained by other, less uncomfortable components of the physical examination.[10] The appearance of the stool—if grossly melanotic, maroon, or frankly bloody—is of value. The test for occult blood, although routinely done, loses sensitivity if not performed serially over several days; similarly, repeated rectal examination by several examiners over a period of hours tends to reduce specificity, presumably due to local trauma. In one series of patients with NSAP, 10 percent were found to have a stool positive for occult blood.[11]

COMPLETE BLOOD COUNT The limited clinical utility of the complete blood count (CBC) can be demonstrated most readily by examining its performance characteristics in the three most common causes of abdominal pain: Appendicitis, biliary tract disease (principally cholecystitis), and NSAP (Tables 68-2 and 68-3). Based upon three studies containing a total of over 1800 patients, a white blood cell (WBC) exceeding the threshold value of 10,000 to11,000/mm^3 only doubled the odds of appendicitis, while a WBC below this cut the odds in half. As noted below in the discussion of likelihood ratios (LRs), an LR(+) less than 2 and an LR(−) greater than 0.4 are of very little clinical value. For acute cholecystitis, the LRs of the WBC count are virtually identical to those seen in appendicitis and are of equally limited clinical value.

TABLE 68-2 Most Common Causes of Acute Abdominal Pain[1,16,34]

Final Diagnosis	Proportion of >10,000 Patients		
Nonspecific abdominal pain	34%		
Appendicitis	28%		
Biliary tract disease	10%		
Bowel obstruction	4%		
Acute gynecologic disease	4%		
		Salpingitis	68%
		Ovarian cyst	21%
		Ectopic	6%
		Incomplete abortion	5%
		Subtotal, gynecoligic	100%
Pancreatitis	3%		
Renal colic	3%		
Perforated peptic ulcer	3%		
Cancer	2%		
Diverticular disease	2%		
Other (≤1% each)	6%		

In one large, well-conducted series of NSAP, 28 percent [95% CI 22 to 34%] of patients were reported to have WBC counts >10,500/mm^3.[11] In an effort to develop a decision rule for the identification of NSAP, it was found that the CBC, or indeed any laboratory test, was not of value in distinguishing patients with NSAP from other, more serious diagnoses. Because of the design of studies on NSAP, it is not possible to calculate a specificity or likelihood ratio for the performance of the WBC count in this setting. However, using 28 percent as the sensitivity of the test, it is possible to estimate that, in order for leukocytosis to be of any value in NSAP (defined as producing LRs that deviate significantly from 1), the WBC count would have to demonstrate substantially better specificity than was seen in either appendicitis or cholecystitis.

TABLE 68-3 Causes of Acute Abdominal Pain Stratified by Age[1,16,34]

Final Diagnosis	≥50 Years Old (N = 2406)	<50 Years Old (N = 6317)
Biliary tract disease	21%	6%
Nonspecific abdominal pain	16%	40%
Appendicitis	15%	32%
Bowel obstruction	12%	2%
Pancreatitis	7%	2%
Diverticular disease	6%	<0.1%
Cancer	4%	<0.1%
Hernia	3%	<0.1%
Vascular	2%	<0.1%
Acute gynecologic disease	<0.1%	4%
Other	13%	13%

All of the above refers only to individual WBC counts. There is some evidence that serial counts may assist in the identification of appendicitis.[12] However, in this setting, it would seem wiser to obtain a more definitive test, such as a CT (see Table 68-4) rather than risk a perforation or other complication while obtaining serial WBCs and waiting for development of a leukocytosis.

As suggested above, perhaps the only way to obtain some utility from the CBC is to use it only for its LR(+), i.e., to pay some attention to it only if elevated, and to recognize that the elevation must be substantial before it is likely to have much meaning. The term *substantial* is purposely left undefined in order to avoid what has been aptly referred to as the "single-cutoff trap," i.e., the binary thinking that is engendered when continuous data, such as the WBC count, are converted into dichotomous categories of normal and abnormal. Entirely consistent with their test performance characteristics, "normal" WBC counts should be regarded as not helpful.

PLAIN ABDOMINAL FILM The plain abdominal radiograph (PAR) is often ordered as an "abdominal series," the meaning of which is not clearly defined. In some institutions, this includes an upright abdomen, in others an upright chest; in still others, only a single supine film is obtained. In a prospective study of 102 consecutive patients admitted with acute abdominal pain, the utility of the erect abdominal film when added to the combination of the supine abdominal and erect chest film was examined. The low yield, misleading findings, and lack of impact on management lead to the conclusion that routine use of the erect abdominal film in the acute abdomen was unnecessary. A similar prospective study of over 250 consecutive patients came to the same conclusion.

In one review of over 1500 abdominal films in patients presenting with suspected appendicitis, NSAP, or urinary tract infection, the authors concluded that "any positive information from these radiographs was less likely to be helpful than incidental or inconsistent (and hence potentially misleading)."

Perhaps the limited utility of the PAR is in part related to the difficulty in interpretation, even among experienced radiologists. One study found that about 40 percent of commonly used radiographic signs and diagnoses showed poor agreement among four qualified diagnostic radiologists when the same 140 films were viewed independently by each.

Recent work has concluded that plain films continue to be markedly overutilized. One study concluded that restriction of the PAR to patients with suspected obstruction, perforation, ischemia, peritonitis, or renal colic would have had no impact on management, and the use of PARs would have been reduced by 80 percent.[13] The authors go on to suggest that more liberal use of ultrasound would decrease unnecessary utilization of plain films. There is evidence that ultrasound is superior to plain chest/abdominal films in the detection of free air,[14] which may be one of the principal uses for the PAR and upright chest film. Still other authors note the superior performance of computed tomography (CT) in identifying virtually any abnormality that can be seen on plain films, particularly SBO and renal colic, in addition to many other findings that can only be seen when the technology of computerized, collimated-beam, tomographic imaging is utilized. Although ultrasound can be extremely helpful, particularly as a screening measure that can be implemented quickly at the bedside, it is highly operator-dependent and limited by overlying gas and obesity. The CT, on the other hand, has none of these technical limitations and would seem to be the key to obviating the need for continued use of the PAR in the future—with or without the aid of sonography.

Just as skull films were once obtained "routinely" in head trauma, were almost always nondiagnostic, and told us virtually nothing about what was going on within the intracranial cavity, the PAR is almost always normal or nonspecific in abdominal pain and similarly tells us

TABLE 68-4 Diagnostic Tests for Appendicitis

Test	Sensitivity[a]	Specificity[b]	LR(+)[c]	LR(−)[d]
Plain abdominal radiograph[1–3]	75% (73%, 77%)[e]	58% (52%, 64%)[e]	2	0.4
Abdominopelvic ultrasound (real-time, graded compression, gray scale)[4–6]	82% (75%, 89%)[e]	93% (88%, 96%)[e]	12	0.2
Abdominopelvic ultrasound (color Doppler added to gray scale)[7]	87% (73%, 96%)[e]	97% (89%, 100%)[e]	26	0.1
Abdominopelvic CT (unenhanced, i.e., no PO, IV, or colonic contrast)[8,9]	88% (82%, 94%)[e]	97% (94%, 99%)[e]	30	0.1
Abdominopelvic CT (PO + IV contrast, no colonic)[4,10]	98% (93%, 100%)[e]	87% (77%, 93%)[e]	7	0.03
Appendiceal CT (limited PO + colonic contrast, no IV)[11]	100% (94%, 100%)[e]	95% (84%, 99%)[e]	21[f]	0.03[f]
Appendiceal CT (colonic gastrograffin contrast only)[12]	98% (90%, 100%)[e]	98% (89%, 100%)[e]	49	0.02
MRI (gadolinium-enhanced)[5]	97% (85%, 100%)[e]	92% (75%, 99%)[e]	12	0.03

[1]Izbicki JR, Knoefel WT, Wilker DK, et al: Accurate diagnosis of acute appendicitis: A retrospective and prospective analysis of 686 patients. *Eur J Surg* 158:227, 1992.
[2]Mittelpunkt A, Nora PF: Current features in the treatment of acute appendicitis: An analysis of 1,000 consecutive cases. *Surgery* 60:971, 1966.
[3]Ramirez JM, Deus J: Practical score to aid decision making in doubtful cases of appendicitis. *Br J Surg* 81:680, 1994.
[4]Balthazar EJ, Birnbaum BA, Yee J, et al: Acute appendicitis: CT and US correlation in 100 patients. *Radiology* 190:31, 1994.
[5]Incesu L, Coskun A, Selcuk MB, et al: Acute appendicitis: MR imaging and sonographic correlation. *AJR* 168:669, 1997.
[6]Rioux M: Sonographic detection of the normal and abnormal appendix. *AJR* 158:773, 1992.
[7]Quillin SP, Siegel MJ: Appendicitis: Efficacy of color Doppler sonography. *Radiology* 191:557, 1994.
[8]Malone AJ Jr, Wolf CR, Malmed AS, Melliere BF: Diagnosis of acute appendicitis: Value of unenchanced CT. *AJR* 160:763, 1993.
[9]Lane MJ, Katz DS, Ross BA, et al: Unenhanced helical CT for suspected acute appendicitis. *AJR* 168:405, 1997.
[10]Balthazar EJ, Megibow AJ, Siegel SE, Birnbaum BA: Appendicitis: Prospective evaluation with high-resolution CT. *Radiology* 180:21, 1991.
[11]Rao RM, Rhea JT, Novelline RA, et al: Helical CT technique for diagnosis of appendicitis: Prospective evaluation of a focused appendix CT examination. *Radiology* 202:139, 1997.
[12]Rao PM, Rhea JT, Novelline RA, et al: Helical CT combined with contrast material administered only through the colon for imaging of suspected appendicitis. *AJR* 169:1275, 1997.
[a]Sensitivity = [TP/(TP + FN)].
[b]Specificity = [TN/(TN + FP)].
[c]LR(+) = positive likelihood ratio = [sensitivity/(1 − specificity)].
[d]LR(−) = negative likelihood ratio = [(1 − sensitivity)/specificity].
[e]A 95% confidence interval was used when data were derived from a single study or when aggregating homogeneous data from different studies.
[f]LR calculations for sensitivity or specificity of 100% are estimated conservatively by using the midpoint of the 95% CI if not doing so would result in an LR(+) = ∞ or an LR(−) = 0.

very little about what is going on within the abdominal cavity and retroperitoneum. Over time, it seems reasonable to speculate that some extension of the helical abdominal CT, or its magnetic resonance imaging (MRI) analog, may replace the abdominal plain film in the very same way—and for the very same reasons—that the head CT/MRI replaced skull films.

DIAGNOSIS

Diagnosis versus Disposition

It is axiomatic in emergency medicine that appropriate disposition and management of acute illness takes precedence over diagnostic accuracy. However, extraordinary technological advances have made rapid, noninvasive diagnosis of many causes of abdominal pain widely available. This has occurred in parallel with the development of an equally sophisticated array of therapeutic options. The net effect of this phenomenon has been to tie diagnosis more closely to disposition and treatment than was the case when the only interventions in abdominal pain were laparotomy vs. observation with medical management.

Diagnostic Error

As accurate diagnosis—as opposed to a discharge or admission decision—becomes more pertinent to emergency medicine, a striking feature of abdominal pain becomes apparent: It is extremely difficult to make the correct diagnosis using only clinical findings and basic laboratory tests. When initial and final diagnoses are compared, diagnostic accuracy is reported as falling somewhere between 50 and 65 percent overall.[15] It is clear that diagnostic error in adults with abdominal pain increases in proportion to age, ranging from a low of 20 percent if only young adults are considered,[15] to a high of 70 percent in the very elderly.[16]

In spite of a high diagnostic error rate, the discharge error rate (proportion of patients mistakenly sent home from the ED) is substantially lower, reported to be 1 percent or less in two series, increasing to 4 percent in patients >65 years old.[5]

Performance Characteristics of Diagnostic Tests

Tables 68-4 through 68-14 provide a summary of the properties of diagnostic tests used for common or serious causes of abdominal pain encountered in the ED. These test properties are displayed as the traditional sensitivity and specificity, accompanied either by confidence intervals or a range of values if the studies from which the data were drawn were too heterogeneous to be combined.

DEFINITION OF LIKELIHOOD RATIOS (LRs)[17] In the far right-hand columns of Tables 68-4 through 68-14, test performance is expressed using positive and negative likelihood ratios (LRs). LRs are defined as the likelihood that a particular test result would be found in a patient *with* the target disorder, relative to the likelihood of that same test result occurring in a patient *without* the target disorder.

Likelihood ratios (LRs) are often divided into positive and negative LRs, expressed as follows: LR of a (+) test = (TPR/FPR) = [(true-positive rate)/(false-positive rate)] = [sensitivity/(1-specificity)]. LR of a (−) test = (FNR/TNR) = [(false-negative rate)/(true-negative rate)] = [(1-sensitivity)/specificity].

The formal definition of an LR(+) is simply a special case of the general definition of LRs: An LR(+) is the likelihood that a *positive* test result would be found in a patient *with* the target disorder, compared with the likelihood of a *positive* test result occurring in a patient *without* the target disorder. The definition of an LR(−) is the likelihood that a *negative* test result would be found in a patient *with* the target disorder, compared with the likelihood of a *negative* test result occurring in a patient *without* the target disorder.

INTERPRETATION OF LRs[17] In general, an LR(+) of 1 to 2, or an LR(−) of 0.5 to 1, alters disease probability by a small and clinically insignificant degree. In contrast, LR(+)s >10, or LR(−)s <0.1 may have a very substantial impact on clinical decision making through meaningful revision of disease probability. LR(+)s of 2 to 10, or LR(−)s of 0.5 to 0.1 may still make some small contribution to management, depending upon their magnitude and the clinical context in which they are applied. Because LRs are odds, a diagnostic test with an LR(−) = 0.1 is as powerful as a diagnostic test with an LR(+) = 10.

CLINICAL APPLICATION OF LRs[17] Likelihood ratios (LRs) combine the stability of sensitivity and specificity with the utility of predictive values, resulting in an index of test performance that can be applied directly to a particular patient at the bedside. This is done by multiplying an LR(+) or LR(−) times the pretest odds of disease, resulting, respectively, in an increased or decreased posttest odds of disease. The larger the LR(+) or the smaller the LR(−), the more powerful the test is.

The performance characteristics of the various tests shown in Tables 68-4 through 68-14 are incorporated into the discussion of specific diagnoses below.

Specific Diagnoses

Table 68-2 is drawn from a combined series of over 10,000 cases of acute (<1 week duration) abdominal pain presenting to over 200 EDs in 17 countries during a 10-year period. The data were collected on a highly standardized instrument.

In virtually all large series of acute abdominal pain, the substantial majority of final diagnoses include nonspecific abdominal pain (NSAP), appendicitis, and biliary tract disease (usually cholecystitis), in that order, accounting for nearly 75 percent of all acute abdominal pain. However, as shown in Table 68-3, as patients age, the triad remains but the order changes to biliary tract disease (again, usually cholecystitis), followed by NSAP and appendicitis.

INTRAABDOMINAL DIAGNOSES (BY ORGAN SYSTEM) **Gastrointestinal** APPENDICITIS In spite of a large number of algorithms and decision rules incorporating many different clinical and laboratory features, an accurate preoperative diagnosis of appendicitis has remained elusive for more than a century. In at least 20 percent of patients with appendicitis, the diagnosis is missed; conversely, normal appendices are found in 15 to 40 percent of all operations performed for suspected appendicitis. Thus, the diagnosis of appendicitis turns out to either be a false positive or false negative just about as often as it turns out to be correct.[18]

Among patients presenting to an ED with acute abdominal pain, the pretest probability, or prevalence, of appendicitis is roughly 10 to 25 percent.[19] Converting this to odds to facilitate multiplication by LRs, the pretest odds of appendicitis in acute abdominal pain is roughly between 0.1 and 0.3. Five clinical features appear to have sufficiently powerful LR(+) values that the presence of *any one* should drive up the clinical odds to the point that an imaging procedure is indicated. Of those radiographic procedures available, appendiceal CT appears to be the best,[20] although there are many imaging alternatives, as listed in Table 68-4. Those clinical features with some predictive value include pain location in the RLQ [LR(+)=8]; pain migration from the periumbilical area to the RLQ [LR(+)=3]; rigidity [LR(+)=4]; pain before vomiting [LR(+)=2 to 3]; and a positive psoas sign [LR(+)=2]. [19] The widely held belief that anorexia is an essential prerequisite of appendicitis is unsupported by evidence. In fact, about one patient in three with surgically documented appendicitis is *not* anorectic preoperatively.[19]

In excluding the diagnosis of appendicitis, the absence of several of the following features is moderately helpful: The absence of RLQ pain [LR(−)=0.2], presence of similar previous pain [LR(−)=0.3], and absence of typical pain migration to the RLQ [LR(−)=0.5].[19] Therefore, clinical exclusion of the diagnosis of appendicitis depends upon a persuasive aggregate of absent features or a strong competing alternative diagnosis. Lacking either of these two conditions, a CT should be seriously considered in the interest of avoiding missed appendicitis. In support of this strategy, a recent report of the impact of targeted appendiceal CT on treatment in suspected appendicitis showed that CT altered management in the majority (59 percent) of cases and represented a substantial cost savings.[20,21]

BILIARY TRACT DISEASE This is the most common diagnosis in ED patients above age 50.[1] Among patients found to have pathologically confirmed acute cholecystitis, the majority lack fever and a significant minority lack a leukocytosis (about 40 percent).[22–24] Pertinent diagnostic tests are shown in Table 68-5.

Recognition that the diagnoses of cholecystitis, "biliary colic," and symptomatic common duct obstruction may represent pathologically distinct entities that cannot be reliably distinguished from one another clinically has led some authors to redefine the *clinical* target disorder as simply "biliary tract disease." Although there is an association between symptomatic biliary tract disease and steady, postprandial upper abdominal pain radiating to the upper back, the likelihood ratios of individual signs, symptoms, and combinations of signs and symptoms are "relatively weak discriminators."[25] Just over one-third of patients have pain isolated to the RUQ, although about two-thirds have tenderness in that location. Most of the remainder complain of diffuse pain in the upper half of the abdomen; among those with pain in the lower abdomen, it is almost invariably in the RLQ. Among the one-third who do not have RUQ tenderness, the distribution is about equally divided between the upper half, the right side, and generalized tenderness throughout the abdomen.[6]

Looking specifically at the common bile duct (CBD), overall clinical accuracy for the identification of obstruction is about 60 percent [95% CI 49 to 70%]. Accuracy is defined here as the proportion of all clinical diagnoses that were correctly identified as obstructed or nonobstructed CBDs.

SMALL BOWEL OBSTRUCTION The central issues in small bowel obstruction (SBO) are diagnosis of the primary disorder and early detection of secondary strangulation or ischemia when present. Only two historical and two physical findings appear to have predictive value: previous abdominal surgery and intermittent/colicky pain plus abdominal distention and abnormal bowel sounds. Although about two-thirds of patients with SBO present with generalized or central abdominal pain and about half have generalized tenderness, the LRs of these findings alone or in combination are such that SBO is another diagnosis that requires imaging confirmation. The general limitations of bowel sounds has been noted previously. As shown in Table 68-6, and also discussed above, the abdominal flat plate is hampered by the large number of indeterminate readings, leaving it with LRs that are of limited usefulness. The CT, however, has an excellent LR(−),

TABLE 68-5 Diagnostic Tests for Biliary Tract Disease

Target Diagnosis	Test	Sensitivity[a]	Specificity[b]	LR(+)[c]	LR(−)[d]
Stones	Plain abdominal radiograph[1–3]	64% (59%, 68%)[i]	68% (52%, 81%)[i]	2	0.5
Stones	Ultrasound metanalysis[4]	84%, 97%[e,f,g] (91%)[h]	95%, 99%[e,f,g] (97%)[h]	30	0.09
Stones	CT[4]	(79%)[h]	(99%)[h]	79	0.3
Acute cholecystitis	Ultrasound meta-analysis[4]	88%, 94%[e,g] (91%)[h]	78%, 80%[e,g] (79%)[h]	4	0.1
Acute cholecystitis	Gray-scale B-mode real-time ultrasound[5]	86% (65%, 97%)[i]	99% (95%, 100%)[i]	86	0.1
Acute cholecystitis	Color velocity imaging and power Doppler ultrasound[5]	96% (77%, 100%)[i]	100% (97%, 100%)[i]	64[j]	0.04[j]
Acute cholecystitis	Radionuclide scanning metanalysis[4]	97% (96%, 98%)[i]	90% (86%, 95%)[i]	10	0.03
Common duct obstruction	Ultrasound[6]	95% (84%, 99%)[i]	93% (81%, 98%)[i]	14	0.05
Common duct obstruction	CT[6]	98% (88%, 100%)[i]	98% (87%, 100%)[i]	41	0.02
Common duct stones	Ultrasound[7]	63% (48%, 76%)[i]	94% (88%, 98%)[i]	11	0.4
Common duct stones	CT[7]	71% (56%, 82%)[i]	97% (91%, 99%)[i]	21	0.3
Common duct stones	HASTE[k] MRI cholangiography[8]	93% (68%, 100%)[i]	100% (63%, 100%)[i]	5[j]	0.07[j]

[1]Gruber PJ, Silverman RA, Gottesfeld S, Flaster E: Presence of fever and leukocytosis in acute cholecystitis. *Ann Emerg Med* 28:273, 1996.
[2]Singer AJ, McCracken G, Henry MC, et al: Correlation among clinical, laboratory, and hepatobiliary scanning findings in patients with suspected acute cholecystitis. *Ann Emerg Med* 28:267, 1996.
[3]Parker LJ, Vukov LF, Wollan PC: Emergency department evaluation of geriatric patients with acute cholecystitis. *Acad Emerg Med* 4:51, 1997.
[4]Shea JA, Berlin JA, Escarce JJ, et al: Revised estimates of diagnostic test sensitivity and specificity in suspected biliary tract disease. *Arch Intern Med* 154:2573, 1994.
[5]Soyer P, Brouland JP, Boudiaf M, et al: Color velocity imaging and power Doppler sonography of the gallbladder wall: A new look at sonographic diagnosis of acute cholecystitis. *AJR* 171:183, 1998.
[6]Baron RL, Stanley RJ, Lee JKT, et al: A prospective comparison of the evaluation of biliary obstruction using computed tomography and ultrasonography. *Radiology* 145:91, 1982.
[7]Sugiyama M, Atomi Y: Endoscopic ultrasonography for diagnosing choledocholithiasis: A prospective comparative study with ultrasonography and computed tomography. *Gastrointest Endosc* 45:143, 1997.
[8]Regan F, Fradin J, Khazan R, et al: Choledocholithiasis: evaluation with MR cholangiography. *AJR* 167:1441, 1996.
[a]Sensitivity = [TP/(TP + FN)].
[b]Specificity = [TN/(TN + FP)].
[c]LR(+) = positive likelihood ratio = [sensitivity/(1 − specificity)].
[d]LR(−) = negative likelihood ratio = [(1 − sensitivity)/specificity].
[e]Limits of range depend upon whether or not meta-analysis is adjusted for verification bias (multivariate adjustment tends to decrease sensitivity and LR(−), and to increase specificity and LR(+).
[f]Because of adjustment, the test properties of ultrasound for detection of gallstones varies from the more commonly published values of about 95% for both sensitivity and specificity.
[g]Range used when aggregating heterogeneous data from different studies.
[h](Best estimate) in parentheses.
[i]A 95% confidence interval was used when data were derived from a single study or when aggregating homogeneous data from different studies.
[j]LR calculations for sensitivity or specificity of 100% are estimated conservatively by using the midpoint of the 95% CI if not doing so would result in an LR(+) = ∞ or an LR(−) = 0.
[k]HASTE MRI = half-Fourier acquisition single-shot turbo spin-echo.

indicating that a negative result makes SBO highly unlikely. The LR(+) of CT is not as powerful as the LR(−), but probable SBO on CT increases pretest odds of this diagnosis by about sixfold (which is slightly better than the abdominal plain film).

Those patients with ischemic bowel secondary to strangulation are extremely difficult to detect clinically or by using plain radiographs. Here again the CT may be of substantial assistance in exclusion of the diagnosis of SBO with ischemia. Unfortunately, there is as yet no radiographic means to confirm the *early* diagnosis of ischemia due to SBO.[26]

ACUTE PANCREATITIS About 80 percent of acute pancreatitis in the United States is caused by alcohol or gallstones, with one etiology predominating over the other depending upon the population studied.[27] The pain and tenderness of acute pancreatitis are limited to the anatomic area of the pancreas in the upper half of the abdomen in only a minority of instances.[6] Most patients' pain and tenderness includes this area; in about half, however, it extends well beyond the upper abdomen to cause generalized tenderness. This may be related to the absence of a capsule that might otherwise contain the inflammation and to the difficulty of localizing pathology that—much like the pathology of an abdominal aortic aneurysm—resides deep in the belly and includes the retroperitoneum. Other features of the history and physical examination—such as the quality of the pain, which is steady and graded as severe in the majority of patients, or vomiting—have not been shown to have sufficient discriminatory power to make them clinically useful. Thus, most patients with upper, central, or generalized abdominal pain and tenderness who lack an alternative explanation for their presentation will require further testing.

TABLE 68-6 Diagnostic Tests for Small Bowel Obstruction

Target Diagnosis	Test	Sensitivity[a]	Specificity[b]	LR(+)[c]	LR(−)[d]
Small bowel obstruction	Supine and erect plain films[1]	41% (29%, 54%) to 86% (76%, 94%)[e,f]	25% (10%, 47%) to 88% (68%, 97%)[e,f]	1 to 3	0.7 to 0.5
Small bowel obstruction	CT with PO and IV contrast[1]	100% (95%, 100%)[f]	83% (63%, 95%)[f]	6[g]	0.03[g]
Small bowel obstruction with ischemia	CT with PO and IV contrast[2]	100% (88%, 100%)[f]	61% (42%, 78%)[f]	3[g]	0.1[g]

[1]Frager D, Medwid SW, Baer JW, et al: CT of small bowel obstruction: Value in establishing the diagnosis and determining the degree and cause. *AJR* 162:37, 1994.
[2]Frager D, Baer JW, Medwid SW, et al: Detection of intestinal ischemia in patients with acute small bowel obstruction due to adhesions or hernia: Efficacy of CT. *AJR* 166:67, 1996.
[a]Sensitivity = [TP/(TP + FN)].
[b]Specificity = [TN/(TN + FP)].
[c]LR(+) = positive likelihood ratio = [sensitivity/(1 − specificity)].
[d]LR(−) = negative likelihood ratio = [(1 − sensitivity)/specificity].
[e]Wide range of sensitivity, specificity, and LR's is due to large numbers of indeterminate readings and whether they are classified as positive or negative. Additional advantage of CT is absence of indeterminate readings.
[f]A 95% confidence interval was used when data were derived from a single study or when aggregating homogeneous data from different studies.
[g]LR calculations for sensitivity or specificity of 100% are estimated conservatively by using the midpoint of the 95% CI if not doing so would result in an LR(+) = ∞ or an LR(−) = 0.

As lipase assays have improved in accuracy and speed over the last several years, serum lipase has largely replaced amylase as the best "everyday" screening test for suspected acute pancreatitis. By setting the threshold for a positive test at twice the upper limit of normal serum lipase, the likelihood ratios for lipase are better than twice as powerful as those of serum amylase in making or excluding the diagnosis of acute pancreatitis.[28] As shown in Table 68-7, there are other biochemical markers for acute pancreatitis that have superior test properties, but these are not yet widely available. Early evidence that ratios of urine to serum amylase or of lipase to amylase improve diagnostic accuracy has not been validated.

Depending upon institutional custom, a diagnosis of acute pancreatitis may be sufficient to determine the appropriate admitting service. However, in settings where not all pancreatitis is admitted to the department of surgery or where it is expected that the ED will make a decision regarding admission to a monitored versus an unmonitored floor bed, it may be necessary for the ED to assess the patient for biliary pancreatitis and, perhaps, for the likelihood of complications. While ultrasound is nearly as good as CT for assessment of common bile duct obstruction (see Table 68-7), CT with contrast enhancement by intravenous bolus is far superior for identifying peripancreatic fluid collections and the extent of glandular necrosis. Both of these findings are associated with increased need for surgery and increased mortality (Table 68-7).

DIVERTICULITIS In one large study, the clinical accuracy of a diagnosis of colonic diverticulitis among patients with abdominal complaints was only 34 percent [95%CI 26 to 42%]. When the "possible/equivocal" clinical diagnoses were removed from analysis and only those patients with a pretest diagnosis of either "highly suspected" or "very unlikely" were included as clinical positives and negatives, respectively, the LR(+) was 2 to 3, and the LR(−) was 0.4, neither of which offers much help in the revision of disease probability. Of those patients with diverticular abscesses, diagnostic performance was somewhat better, with 70 percent categorized as "highly suspected" and the remainder as "possible/equivocal." No documented abscesses were categorized clinically as "very unlikely."[29]

Pain in diverticulitis was confined to the LLQ in less than one-quarter of the documented cases and to the lower half of the abdomen in only an additional one-third of patients. With respect to tenderness, it was as likely to be generalized as it was to be limited to the lower half of the abdomen or to the LLQ. About 10 percent of patients with operatively confirmed diverticulitis did not complain of abdominal pain and 20 percent had no abdominal tenderness whatsoever.[6] Elderly patients are at risk for a severe and often fatal complication of diverticulitis that is only rarely seen in younger age groups: perforation of the colon.[16] Diagnostic imaging tests for acute diverticulitis are shown in Table 68-8.

Genitourinary RENAL COLIC As in appendicitis, a number of clinical decision rules have been developed in an effort to identify patients with the preimaging diagnosis of ureterolithiasis. Most algorithms include features of the pain—e.g., location (unilateral flank), onset (abrupt), quality (colicky), radiation (groin/testicle/labia). Hematuria appears as the only laboratory test in most algorithms. The utility of plain abdominal radiographs, as in other causes of abdominal pain, is highly questionable, as shown in Table 68-9.

A critical examination of ureteral stones documented on intravenous pyelography (IVP) reveals that, in one series, just over half reported colicky pain and groin radiation, with microscopic hematuria seen in about two-thirds.[30] An examination of Table 68-9 shows that the IVP has a specificity comparable to that of helical noncontrast CT; however, because of the IVP's poor sensitivity, CT shows far better LRs, thus making noncontrast helical CT the current criterion standard in the diagnosis of ureteral stones. In older patients, any presentation that resembles renal colic, with or without hematuria, mandates the exclusion of an abdominal aortic aneurysm (AAA) [reported in 18 percent (95% CI 11 to 24%) of suspected AAAs in one series]. This is yet another reason to obtain a noncontrast helical CT, since it performs extremely well in the detection of both ureteral stones and AAAs.

Because the GU tract is mostly retroperitoneal, it uncommonly causes significant anterior abdominal tenderness. One notable exception to this is an impacted stone at the ureterovesical (UV) junction, where the ureter enters the bladder, producing ipsilateral lower-quadrant pain and tenderness. Because stones at the UV junction [like those at the ureteropelvic (UP) junction] are less likely to produce the typical pain of renal colic than are stones located between the top and bottom of the ureter, impaction of a stone at the UV junction on the right may easily mimic appendicitis and will require a noncontrast CT to identify stone disease (Table 68-9). If this shows neither a stone nor evidence of other intraabdominal pathology, an appendiceal CT should be considered to confirm or exclude the diagnosis of appendicitis.[20]

TABLE 68-7 Diagnostic Tests for Acute Pancreatitis

Target Diagnosis	Test	Sensitivity[a]	Specificity[b]	LR(+)[c]	LR(−)[d]
Inflammation	Serum amylase[1]	85%[e] (72%, 93%)[f]	91%[e] (88%, 94%)[f]	9	0.2
Inflammation	Serum lipase (>2× normal)[2]	94% (79%, 99%)[f]	95% (91%, 98%)[f]	19	0.06
Inflammation	Serum isoamylase[3]	90% (74%, 98%)[f]	92% (90%, 94%)[f]	11	0.1
Inflammation	Urinary trypsinogen-2[1]	94% (84%, 99%)[f]	95% (93%, 97%)[f]	19	0.06
Inflammation	Serum trypsin-2 and alpha$_1$ antitrypsin[4]	100% (97%, 100%)[f]	95% (87%, 99%)[f]	20[g]	0.02[g]
Pancreatic necrosis	CT with PO and bolus IV contrast[5,6]	100% (75%, 100%)[f]	100% (92%, 100%)[f]	25[g]	0.1[g]
Drainable collections	Transabdominal ultrasound[7]	54% (23%, 83%)[f]	88% (47%, 100%)[f]	4	0.5
Drainable collections	CT with PO and bolus IV contrast[7]	100% (72%, 100%)[f]	25% (3%, 65%)[f]	1[g]	0.6[g]
Drainable collections	MRI (unenchanced)[7]	100% (72%, 100%)[f]	100% (63%, 100%)[f]	5[g]	0.1[g]
Acute hemorrhagic pancreatitis	Unenhanced CT (criterion standard)	—	—	—	—
Prognosis (morbidity)[h]	CT, bolus IV contrast[8]	91% (71%, 99%)[f]	74% (62%, 84%)[f]	3	0.1
Prognosis (mortality)[i]	CT, bolus IV contrast[8]	100% (48%, 100%)[f]	61% (50%, 72%)[f]	3[g]	0.4[g]

[1]Kemppainen EA, Hedstrom JI, Puolakkainen PA, et al: Rapid measurement of urinary trypsinogen-2 as a screening test for acute pancreatitis. *N Engl J Med* 336:1788, 1997.
[2]Keim V, Teich N, Fiedler F, et al: A comparison of lipase and amylase in the diagnosis of acute pancreatitis in patients with abdominal pain. *Pancreas* 16:45, 1998.
[3]Sternby B, O'Brien JF, Zinsmeister AR, DiMagno EP: What is the best biochemical test to diagnose acute pancreatitis? A prospective clinical study. *Mayo Clin Proc* 71:1138, 1996.
[4]Hedstrom J, Sainio V, Kemppainen E, et al: Serum complex of trypsin 2 and alpha 1 antitrypsin as diagnostic and prognostic markers of acute pancreatitis: Clinical study in consecutive patients. *Br Med J* 313:333, 1996.
[5]Bradley EL III, Murphy F, Ferguson C: Prediction of pancreatic necrosis by dynamic pancreatography. *Ann Surg* 210:495, 1989.
[6]Johnson CD, Stephens DH, Sarr MG: CT of acute pancreatitis: Correlation between lack of contrast enhancement and pancreatic necrosis. *AJR* 156:93, 1991.
[7]Morgan DE, Baron TH, Smith JK, et al: Pancreatic fluid collections prior to intervention: Evaluation with MR imaging compared with CT and US. *Radiology* 203:773, 1997.
[8]Balthazar EJ, Robinson DL, Megibow AJ, Ranson JHC: Acute pancreatitis: Value of CT in establishing prognosis. *Radiology* 174:331, 1990.
[a]Sensitivity = [TP/(TP + FN)].
[b]Specificity = [TN/(TN + FP)].
[c]LR(+) = positive likelihood ratio = [sensitivity/(1 − specificity)].
[d]LR(−) = negative likelihood ratio = [(1 − sensitivity)/specificity].
[e]Accuracy of serum amylase in the diagnosis of acute pancreatitis is inversely related to time elapsed between symptom onset and presentation. Calculation of urine/serum amylase ratios do not appear to improve diagnostic accuracy.
[f]A 95% confidence interval was used when data were derived from a single study or when aggregating homogeneous data from different studies.
[g]LR calculations for sensitivity or specificity of 100% are estimated conservatively by using the midpoint of the 95% CI if not doing so would result in an LR(+) = ∞ or an LR(−) = 0.
[h]Defined as patients requiring drainage or resection of pancreatic abscess or pseudocyst (includes all patients who died).
[i]The initial CT is probably much better in predicting outcome of acute (nontraumatic) pancreatitis than an LR(−) = 0.4 suggests. Half of the 37 patients with mixed-attenuation fluid collections on initial CT (also known as peripancreatic inflammation or phlegmons by various investigators) required surgery, and all deaths occurred in this group.

ACUTE URINARY RETENTION Another situation in which GU disease may cause abdominal tenderness is in the setting of acute urethral obstruction, producing a distended bladder. When the obstruction is truly acute, the bladder often feels like a solid mass rather than a fluid-filled hollow viscus. However, if one always considers this common entity when confronted with a midline mass of variable tenderness arising from the lower half of the abdomen, insertion of a urethral catheter easily makes the diagnosis and treats the acute problem.

ACUTE SCROTUM Testicular torsion is the only cause of acute scrotal pain that must either be confidently excluded from the differential or treated within hours of onset. Consequently, the single target of all diagnostic strategies developed to determine the cause of acute scrotal pain is aimed at identification or exclusion of testicular ischemia. Although the etiology of acute scrotal pain in adults is usually either torsion or epididymitis, there are other causes—including inguinal hernia, acute hydrocele, and torsion of the appendiceal epididymis—none of which threatens testicular survival. Although the pain may radiate upward into the ipsilateral groin and lower quadrant, physical examination in adults leaves little doubt that the primary problem resides in the scrotum and not in the abdominal cavity itself (with the notable exception of torsion in an undescended testis).

Some of the features that favor epididymitis over torsion include the presence of fever, chills, dysuria, pyuria, and, most important, localization of the painful area to a swollen, tender epididymis, located posterior to and palpably separate from the testicle itself. The time course over which the pain began—its onset is characteristically more gradual in epididymitis than in torsion—may be helpful. However, it can also be misleading in patients who torse, detorse, and retorse.

The two diagnostic tests for torsion in common use are radionuclide scrotal scanning (RSI) and color Doppler imaging (CDI) (see Table 68-10). Although CDI appears slightly superior to RSI, particularly in younger patients, these findings are not consistent across studies. Both tests have incorrectly identified normal blood flow to testes later found to be ischemic or necrotic at operation. It is difficult to determine to what extent these errors reflect technologic limitations versus opera-

TABLE 68-8 Diagnostic Tests for Acute Diverticulitis

Target Diagnosis	Test	Sensitivity[a]	Specificity[b]	LR(+)[c]	LR(−)[d]
Abscess	Ultrasonography (high-resolution, graded compression)[1]	98% (90%, 100%)[e]	97% (91%, 100%)[e]	33	0.02
Inflammation or abscess	Helical CT with colinic contrast only (no IV or PO contrast)[2]	97% (89%, 100%)[e]	100% (96%, 100%)[e]	48[f]	0.03[f]

[1]Schwerk WB, Schwartz S, Rothmund M: Sonography in acute colonic diverticulitis. *Dis Colon Rectum* 35:1077, 1993.
[2]Rao PM, Rhea JT, Novelline RA, et al: Helical CT with only colonic contrast material for diagnosing diverticulitis: Prospective evaluation of 150 patients. *AJR* 170,1445, 1998.
[a]Sensitivity = [TP/(TP + FN)].
[b]Specificity = [TN/(TN + FP)].
[c]LR(+) = positive likelihood ratio = [sensitivity/(1 − specificity)].
[d]LR(−) = negative likelihood ratio = [(1 − sensitivity)/specificity].
[e]A 95% confidence interval was used when data were derived from a single study or when aggregating homogeneous data from different studies.
[f]LR calculations for sensitivity or specificity of 100% are estimated conservatively by using the midpoint of the 95% CI if not doing so would result in an LR(+) = ∞ or an LR(−) = 0.

tor skill and experience with CDI. With RSI, the problem appears to be one of image resolution in children whose prepubescent testicles represent smaller targets. Because of these limiting features, most authors suggest that imaging be used adjunctively and not as the criterion standard for deciding which patients require exploration. The most conservative indication for surgery, which is likely to result in the fewest missed torsions and the largest number of negative explorations, is inability to distinguish a normal testis and normal epididymis on physical examination. In many institutions, the time required to obtain a nuclear scan is prohibitive, and unless the urology consultant is rapidly available and proficient at Doppler imaging, torsion will, for the present, remain among the steadily dwindling causes of "abdominal" pain in which the diagnosis is made at surgery.

Gynecologic Pain ACUTE PELVIC INFLAMMATORY DISEASE Absence of a criterion standard has further confounded the already clinically difficult diagnosis of acute pelvic inflammatory disease (PID). Laparoscopic and histopathologic findings, both of which have been proposed as the criterion diagnostic standard, are discordant. Because gross laparoscopic findings have historically been used as the standard in most well-designed studies,[31] the LRs of clinical features, laboratory results, and sonographic findings that follow, unless otherwise noted, have been measured against direct macroscopic inspection of the adnexa.

Symptoms such as lower abdominal pain, which would be expected to have a high LR(−) for PID, have not been studied because they typically represent inclusion criteria for study enrollment. To date, there have been no historical features associated with laparoscopic PID that demonstrate clinically useful LRs in more than one study population.[31] Signs—such as adnexal tenderness (unilateral on laparoscopy in only 5 to 10 percent of cases) and cervical motion tenderness—like lower abdominal pain, have not been well studied because they have been used as inclusion criteria in most investigations. The only physical finding associated with laparoscopic PID across more than

TABLE 68-9 Diagnostic Tests for Renal Colic

Target Diagnosis	Test	Sensitivity[a]	Specificity[b]	LR(+)[c]	LR(−)[d]
Stones	Plain abdominal film[1,2,e]	62% (55%, 68%)[f]	84% (78%, 91%)[f]	4	0.5
Stones	IVP[3]	52% (39%, 64%)[f]	94% (80%, 99%)[f]	9	0.5
Stones	Ultrasound[3]	19% (10%, 30%)[f]	97% (84%, 100%)[f]	6	0.8
Stones	Unenhanced helical CT[3,4]	96% (91%, 98%)[f]	96% (92%, 99%)[f]	24	0.04
Need for intervention (stone removal/nephrostomy/lithotripsy)[g]	Unenhanced helical CT[5]	97% (86%, 100%)[f]	99% (98%, 100%)[f]	97	0.03

[1]Mutgi A, Williams JW, Nettleman M: Renal colic. Utility of the plain abdominal roentgenogram. *Arch Intern Med* 151:1589, 1991.
[2]Elton TJ, Roth CS, Berquist TH, Silverstein MD: A clinical prediction rule for the diagnosis of ureteral calculi in emergency departments. *J Gen Intern Med* 8:57, 1993.
[3]Yilmaz S, Sindel T, Arslan G, et al: Renal colic: Comparison of spiral CT, US and IVU in the detection of ureteral calculi. *Eur Radiol* 8:212, 1998.
[4]Smith RC, Verga M, McCarthy S, Rosenfield AT: Diagnosis of acute flank pain: value of unenhanced helical CT. *AJR* 166:97, 1996.
[5]Dalrymple NC, Verga M, Anderson KR, et al: The value of unenhanced helical computerized tomography in the management of acute flank pain. *J Urol* 159:735, 1998.
[a]Sensitivity = [TP/(TP + FN)].
[b]Specificity = [TN/(TN + FP)].
[c]LR(+) = positive likelihood ratio = [sensitivity/(1 − specificity)].
[d]LR(−) = negative likelihood ratio = [(1 − sensitivity)/specificity].
[e]Combined data from two comparable studies; one concluded that the abdominal flat-plat was of value and the other concluded it was not.
[f]A 95% confidence interval was used when data were derived from a single study or when aggregating homogeneous data from different studies.
[g]Need for intervention includes obstructed patients likely to require treatment, based upon stone size, character, and location.

TABLE 68-10 Diagnostic Tests for Acute Scrotal Pain

Target Diagnosis	Test	Sensitivity[a]	Specificity[b]	LR(+)[c]	LR(−)[d]
Testicular torsion	Testicular radionuclide technetium scan (RSI)[1]	97% (83%, 100%)[e]	100% (94%, 100%)[e]	32[f]	0.03[f]
Testicular torsion	Testicular radionuclide technetium scan (RSI)[2,g]	100% (72%, 100%)[e]	97% (83%, 100%)[e]	33[f]	0.1[f]
Testicular torsion	Color Doppler imaging (CDI)[2,g]	100% (72%, 100%)[e]	77% (58%, 90%)[e]	4[f]	0.2[f]
Testicular torsion	Color Doppler imaging (CDI)[3]	100% (82%, 100%)[e]	100% (96%, 100%)[e]	50[f]	0.1[f]
Testicular torsion	Hand-held Doppler flowmeter with cord compression test[4]	100% (74%, 100%)[e]	97% (85%, 100%)[e]	33[f]	0.1[f]

[1]Melloul M, Paz A, Lask D, Manes A, Mukamel E: The value of radionuclide scrotal imaging in the diagnosis of acute testicular torsion. *Br J Urol* 76:628, 1995.
[2]Paltiel HJ, Connolly LP, Atala A, et al: Acute scrotal symptoms in boys with an indeterminate clinical presentation: comparison of color Doppler sonography and scintigraphy. *Radiology* 207:223, 1998.
[3]Suzer O, Ozcan H, Kupeli S, Gheiler EL: Color Doppler imaging in the diagnosis of the acute scrotum. *Eur Urol* 32:457, 1997.
[4]al Mufti RA, Ogedegbe AK, Lafferty K: The use of Doppler ultrasound in the clinical management of acute testicular pain. *Br J Urol* 76:625, 1995.
[a]Sensitivity = [TP/(TP + FN)].
[b]Specificity = [TN/(TN + FP)].
[c]LR(+) = positive likelihood ratio = [sensitivity/(1 − specificity)].
[d]LR(−) = negative likelihood ratio = [(1 − sensitivity)/specificity.
[e]A 95% confidence interval was used when data were derived from a single study or when aggregating homogeneous data from different studies.
[f]LR calculations for sensitivity or specificity of 100% are estimated conservatively by using the midpoint of the 95% CI if not doing so would result in an LR(+) = ∞ or an LR(−) = 0.
[g]Eight and two indeterminate Doppler and radionuclide studies, respectively, treated as (+) for purpose of conservative calculation of test properties.

one study population is an abnormal vaginal discharge.[31] In spite of this statistical association, the LRs of vaginal discharge range from 0.5 to 2.5, representing very limited power to alter disease probability. Elevated temperature and a palpable mass have been inconsistently associated with PID. The WBC count has not been found to be helpful in any of the studies that examined it. For the performance characteristics of other laboratory tests that have been associated with PID—e.g., the erythrocyte sedimentation rate (ESR) and C-reactive protein (CRP), see Table 68-11. As in the evaluation of ectopic pregnancy (see below), the role of culdocentesis in the diagnosis of PID is *not* supported by evidence.

ECTOPIC PREGNANCY In ruptured ectopic pregnancy, abdominal pain is almost universally present. However, as emphasis in ectopic pregnancy has shifted to identification of patients prior to rupture—with the goal of preserving fertility—pain may be absent at this earlier stage, with vaginal bleeding as the only sentinel complaint. Therefore, any woman of childbearing age who presents to the ED with abdominal pain *or* abnormal vaginal bleeding generally receives a qualitative pregnancy test as a screening measure.

The poor predictive performance of historical features, such as "risk factors," and of the physical examination [sensitivity 19 percent, LR(−)=0.8 among women with a positive hCG], argue strongly that ectopic pregnancy is not a diagnosis that can easily be excluded on clinical grounds.

For this reason, the results of the pregnancy test, independent of most other data, will determine if further testing is indicated to exclude an ectopic pregnancy. If the qualitative hCG is positive, the preferred test is a bedside transvaginal sonogram (TVS). See Table 68-12.

Vascular ABDOMINAL AORTIC ANEURYSM Although abdominal aortic aneurysms (AAAs) have little in common with aortic dissections, these two major forms of catastrophic disease of the aorta are often lumped together. Dissections are uncommon causes of abdominal pain and, because they almost invariably originate in the thoracic aorta, usually produce chest or upper back pain before migrating into the abdomen as the dissection moves distally.

AAAs, on the other hand, tend to enlarge, become aneurysmal over years, and—rather than dissect—leak and rupture. Fewer than half of AAAs present with the triad of hypotension, abdominal/back pain, and a pulsatile abdominal mass. Over three-quarters appear normotensive. Spontaneous containment of bleeding is the principal determinant of prehospital survival. Extent of containment further determines the degree of hypotension, if any, on presentation. The absence of abdominal pain or tenderness is entirely compatible with a contained leak extending into the retroperitoneum. Because the aorta is deep in the abdomen, it is extremely difficult to confirm by palpation that it is too small to represent an AAA, even in thin patients. Neither absence of femoral pulses nor an abdominal bruit have LRs that deviate very far from 1 and therefore lack the power to alter disease probability. Thus, a patient in the retirement-age group presenting with recent onset of abdominal, flank, or low back pain is likely to require either a normal aortic sonogram (performed by an experienced operator) or, preferably, a noncontrast helical CT (criterion standard test) before a AAA can be removed from the working differential diagnosis. Because the direction and extent of leakage or rupture—which can occur anywhere in the abdomen or retroperitoneum—determines the location of pain and tenderness, knowledge of aortic anatomy is not of much help in the diagnosis of AAA. The technology of magnetic resonance angiography (MRA) has not yet reached the stage where MRA can serve as an emergency procedure and conventional angiography has been supplanted by the superior, faster, noninvasive images of the helical CT. As noted earlier, the appearance of renal colic in this age group should be regarded as representing an AAA until the helical CT proves otherwise. See Table 68-13.

MESENTERIC ISCHEMIA Mesenteric ischemia can be divided into arterial and venous disease [mesenteric venous thrombosis (MVT)]. Arterial disease can be subdivided into occlusive and non-occlusive (NOMI or low-flow state). Finally, occlusive arterial disease (generally understood to mean superior mesenteric artery occlusion) may be further categorized into thrombotic or embolic. Several features combine to produce a very high mortality associated with mesenteric ischemia:

TABLE 68-11 Diagnostic Tests for Acute Pelvic Inflammatory Disease

Target Diagnosis	Test	Sensitivity[a]	Specificity[b]	LR(+)[c]	LR(−)[d]
Salpingitis (macroscopic laparoscopy)	Erythrocyte sedimentation rate >15 mm/h[1-3]	75%, 81%[e]	25%, 57%[e]	1 to 2	0.3 to 1
Salpingitis (macroscopic laparoscopy)	C-reactive protein[3,4]	74%, 93%[e]	50%, 90%[e]	2 to 9	0.08 to 0.4
Salpingitis (macroscopic laparoscopy)	Endometrial biopsy[5,6]	70%, 89%[e]	67%, 89%[e]	3 to 6	0.2 to 0.3
Salpingitis (macroscopic laparoscopy)	*Gonococcus* or *Chlamydia* cultured from upper genital tract[6]	65% (41%, 85%)[f]	100% (75%, 100%)[f]	5[g]	0.4[g]
Endometritis (endometrial biopsy)	Transvaginal sonography[7] [(+) = thickened, fluid-filled tube]	85% (54%, 98%)[f]	100% (91%, 100%)[f]	19[g]	0.2[g]
Salpingitis (fimbrial minibiopsy)	Laparoscopy (macroscopic)[8]	50% (29%, 71%)[f]	80% (66%, 90%)[f]	2	0.6
Endometritis (endometrial biopsy)	Laparoscopy (macroscopic)[6]	93% (68%, 100%)[f]	67% (41%, 87%)[f]	3	0.1
Salpingitis/Endometritis (fimbrial minibiopsy or endometrial biopsy)	Laparoscopy (macroscopic)[8]	48% (30%, 67%)[f]	79% (66%, 88%)[f]	2	0.7
Chlamydia cultured from upper genital tract	Laparoscopy (macroscopic)[9]	53% (28%, 77%)[f]	67% (22%, 96%)[f]	2	0.7

[1]Jacobson L, Westrom L: Objectivized diagnosis of acute pelvic inflammatory disease: Diagnostic and prognostic value of routine laparoscopy. *Am J Obstet Gynecol* 105:1088, 1969.
[2]Westrom L: Clinical manifestations and diagnosis of pelvic inflammatory disease. *J Reprod Med* 28(suppl):703, 1983.
[3]Lehtinen M, Laine S, Heinonen PK, et al: Serum C-reactive protein determination in acute pelvic inflammatory disease. *Am J Obstet Gynecol* 154:158, 1986.
[4]Jacobson L, Laurell C-B, Gennser G, Harholev K: Plasma protein changes induced by acute inflammation of the fallopian tubes. *Int J Gynaecol Obstet* 13:249, 1975.
[5]Paavonen J, Aine R, Teisala K, et al: Comparison of endometrial biopsy and peritoneal fluid cytologic testing with laparoscopy in the diagnosis of acute pelvic inflammatory disease. *Am J Obstet Gynecol* 151:645, 1985.
[6]Wasserheit JN, Bell TA, Kiviat NB, et al: Microbial causes of proven pelvic inflammatory disease and efficacy of clindamycin and tobramycin. *Ann Intern Med* 104:187, 1986.
[7]Cacciatore B, Leminen A, Ingman-Friberg S, et al: Transvaginal sonographic findings in ambulatory patients with suspected pelvic inflammatory disease. *Obstet Gynecol* 80:912, 1992.
[8]Sellors J, Mahony J, Goldsmith C, et al: The accuracy of clinical findings and laparoscopy in pelvic inflammatory disease. *Am J Obstet Gynecol* 164:113, 1991.
[9]Stacey C, Munday P, Thomas B, et al: *Chlamydia trachomatis* in the fallopian tubes of women without laparoscopic evidence of salpingitis. *Lancet* 336:960, 1990.
[a]Sensitivity = [TP/(TP + FN)].
[b]Specificity = [TN/(TN + FP)].
[c]LR(+) = positive likelihood ratio = [sensitivity/(1 − specificity)].
[d]LR(−) = negative likelihood ratio = [(1 − sensitivity)/specificity].
[e]Range used when aggregating heterogenous data from different studies.
[f]95% confidence interval was used when data were derived from a single study or when aggregating homogeneous data from different studies.
[g]LR calculations for sensitivity or specificity of 100% are estimated conservatively by using the midpoint of the 95% CI if not doing so would result in an LR(+) = ∞ or an LR(−) = 0.

1. Unless relatively young patients have an arrhythmia (usually atrial fibrillation causing embolization) or a hypercoagulable state (causing MVT), patients with mesenteric ischemia tend to have a substantial degree of age-related comorbidity.
2. The small bowel, which is supplied by the superior mesenteric artery, has a warm ischemia time of only 2 to 3 h.
3. The clinical picture is characterized initially by poorly localized visceral abdominal pain, without tenderness.
4. Patients may become transiently better after a few hours of ischemia, at the time of onset of mucosal infarction, only to later develop peritoneal findings as full-thickness necrosis of the bowel wall becomes apparent.
5. Timely diagnosis requires that an angiogram be obtained very early in the evolution of the pathologic process—so early, in fact, that it may seem clinically premature to order such an invasive test on an elderly patient who may not appear ill.

Elevation of serum phosphate was initially thought to be a sensitive marker for mesenteric ischemia, but this was not confirmed by later work showing a preoperative sensitivity for the diagnosis of acute mesenteric ischemia in the range of only 25 to 33 percent. In contrast, as shown in Table 68-14, serial serum lactates that remain *persistently* normal reduce the clinician's pretest likelihood of diagnosing mesenteric ischemia by more than tenfold. Unfortunately, lactate is elevated in many abdominal and extraabdominal conditions and therefore lacks specificity in the diagnosis of mesenteric ischemia.

There are some distinctions that can be made among the four major forms of mesenteric ischemia: (1) embolic disease is the most abrupt in onset, MVT the most indolent, with the temporal profile of arterial thrombosis somewhere in between; (2) NOMI is usually accompanied by clinical evidence of a low-flow state, typically due to cardiac disease and responding to improvement in cardiac output;[32] (3) MVT may be more amenable to noninvasive diagnosis with CT,[33] occurs in younger patients, has a lower mortality, and can be treated with immediate anticoagulation; (4) following diagnosis, arteriography with papaverine infusion may be an important component of treatment in patients with splanchnic vasoconstriction.

TABLE 68-12 Diagnostic Tests for Ectopic Pregnancy

Target Diagnosis	Test	Sensitivity[a]	Specificity[b]	LR(+)[c]	LR(−)[d]
Pregnancy	Serum hCG (>25 mIU/mL = (+))[1–4]	98%[e,f,g]	99%[e,f,g]	98	0.02
Pregnancy	Serum hCG (>10 mIU/mL = (+))[1–4]	99%[e,f,g]	99%[e,f,g]	99	0.01
Pregnancy	Urine hCG (>50 mIU/mL = (+))[1–4]	(95%)[e,f,g]	99%[e,f,g]	95	0.05
Pregnancy	Urine hCG (>20 mIU/mL = (+))[1–4]	98%[e,f,g]	99%[e,f,g]	98	0.02
IUP[h,i]	TVS[j] on *all* patients (DZ[k] > 1500 mIU/mL hCG)[5]	49% (42%, 57%)[l]	100% (99%, 100%)[l]	98[m]	0.5[m]
IUP[h,i]	TVS[j] *only* on patients with hCG > DZ[k] (DZ > 1500 mIU/mL hCG)[5]	82% (72%, 89%)[l]	100% (99%, 100%)[l]	164[m]	0.2[m]
IUP[h,i]	TVS[j] on *all* patients (DZ[k] > 1500 mIU/mL hCG) + follow-up with serial hCG[5,n]	100% (98%, 100%)[l]	99% (99%, 100%)[l]	200[m]	0.01[m]
Unruptured ectopic[h,o]	TVS[j] on *all* patients (No IUP[i] with DZ[k] > 1000 mIU/mL HCG)[5]	100% (95%, 100%)[l]	89% (83%, 94%)[l]	9[m]	0.03[m]
Ectopic[p]	Culdocentesis[6–8,q,r]	86% (82%, 91%)[l]	37% (20%, 56%)[l]	1.4	0.4
Ruptured ectopic[p]	Culdocentesis[6–8,q,r]	88% (82%, 94%)[l]	16% (9%, 23%)[l]	1	0.8
Unruptured ectopic[p]	Culdocentesis[6–8,q,r]	84% (77%, 91%)[l]	12% (6%, 18%)[l]	1	1.3

[1]O'Connor RE, Bibro CM, Pegg PG, Bouzakis JK: The comparative sensitivity and specificity of serum and urine HCG determinations in the ED. *Am J Emerg Med* 11:434, 1993.
[2]Emancipator K, Cado FF, Burke EM: Analytic versus clinical sensitivity and specificity in pregnancy testing. *Am J Obstet Gynecol* 158:613, 1988.
[3]Alfthan H, Bjorses UAA, Tittinen A, Sternman VH: Specificity and detection limit of ten pregnancy tests. *Scan J Clin Lab Invest* 216:105, 1993.
[4]Brennan DF: Ectopic pregnancy—Part I. Clinical and laboratory diagnosis. *Acad Emerg Med* 2:1081, 1995.
[5]Barnhart K, Mennuti MT, Benjamin I, et al: Prompt diagnosis of ectopic pregnancy in an emergency department setting. *Obstet Gynecol* 84:1010, 1994.
[6]Vermesh M, Graczykowski JW, Sauer MV: Reevaluation of the role of culdocentesis in the management of ectopic pregnancy. *Am J Obstet Gynecol* 162:411, 1990.
[7]Glezerman M, Press F, Carpman M: Culdocentesis is an obsolete diagnostic tool in suspected ectopic pregnancy. *Arch Gynecol Obstet* 252:5, 1992.
[8]Chen PC, Sickler GK, Dubinsky TJ, et al: Sonographic detection of echogenic fluid and correlation with culdocentesis in the evaluation of ectopic pregnancy. *AJR* 170:1299, 1998.
[a]Sensitivity = [TP/(TP + FN)].
[b]Specificity = [TN/(TN + FP)].
[c]LR(+) = positive likelihood ratio = [sensitivity/(1 − specificity)].
[d]LR(−) = negative likelihood ratio = [(1 − sensitivity)/specificity].
[e]hCG measurements expressed in the units of the First International Reference Preparation, the equivalent of the Third International Standard.
[f]Variation in clinically important test performance characteristics have been associated with different manufacturers (Christenson H, Thyssen HH, Schebye O, Berget A: Three highly sensitive "bedside" serum and urine tests for pregnancy compared. *Clin Chem* 36:1686, 1990.
[g]Best estimate.
[h]Includes only patients with (+)hCG and pain or bleeding.
[i]IUP = Intrauterine pregnancy
[j]TVS = transvaginal sonography, performed by experienced operator.
[k]DZ = discriminatory zone, defined as the level of hCG above which transvaginal sonography should detect an intrauterine pregnancy if one is present.
[l]A 95% confidence interval was used when data were derived from a single study or when aggregating homogeneous data from different studies.
[m]LR calculations for sensitivity or specificity of 100% are estimated conservatively by using the midpoint of the 95% CI if not doing so would result in an LR(+) = ∞ or an LR(−) = 0.
[n]Increase of hCG < 66% over 48 h considered abnormal.
[o]About 20% of patients diagnosed as unruptured ectopic had unexpected rupture at surgery.
[p]Among pregnant patients with clinically suspected ectopic.
[q](+) culdocentesis defined as nonclotting blood, hematocrit of aspirate at least 15%; (−) culdocentesis defined as clotting blood or hematocrit of aspirate <15%; dry tap = nondiagnostic culdocentesis.
[r]Conservative analysis excludes patients with nondiagnostic culdocenteses; if included as intermediate results (neither positive nor negative), this would decrease test performance further, thus driving LR's closer to the null point of 1, representing a valueless test.

ISCHEMIC COLITIS Ischemic disease of the large intestine has as little in common with mesenteric ischemia as aortic dissection does with AAA. As is the case with all vascular diseases, ischemic colitis is predominantly a disease of older patients. About 80 percent of individuals have diffuse or lower abdominal visceral pain, accompanied by diarrhea in about 60 percent, often mixed with blood. In contrast to mesenteric ischemia, ischemic colitis is not generally due to large-vessel occlusive disease, angiography is not usually indicated, and, if performed, is typically normal. Not surprisingly, the severity of the presentation appears to be related to the extent of ischemia. In the majority of cases, only segmental portions of the mucosa and submucosa slough. These then go on to heal uneventfully with conservative management. At the opposite end of the spectrum is full-thickness infarction of the colon, occurring in about 10 percent of cases. Bowel necrosis, whether segmental or pancolitic, causes peritonitis, requiring partial or complete colectomy. The mortality in this latter group approaches that of mesenteric ischemia.

TABLE 68-13 Diagnostic Tests for Abdominal Aortic Aneurysm

Target Diagnosis	Test	Sensitivity[a]	Specificity[b]	LR(+)[c]	LR(−)[d]
Uncomplicated abdominal aortic aneurysm (AAA)	Sonography[1,e]	97% (84%, 100%)[f]	100% (88%, 100%)[f]	16[g]	0.03[g]
Leaking/ruptured AAA (intra- or retroperitoneal)	Sonography[1,e]	4% (0%, 21%)[f]	100% (40%, 100%)[f]	0.1[g]	1.0[g]
Uncomplicated or leaking/ruptured AAA (intra- or retroperitoneal)	CT[2-4,h]	97% (85%, 100%)[f]	94% (86%, 98%)[f]	16	0.03
Detailed preoperative anatomy	Conventional angiography[5,j]	No longer a preferred emergency procedure			
Detailed preoperative anatomy	MRI/MRA[5,i,j]	Not a preferred emergency procedure at this time			

[1]Shuman WP, Hastrup W Jr, Kohler TR, et al: Suspected leaking abdominal aortic aneurysm: Use of sonography in the emergency room. *Radiology* 168:117, 1988.
[2]Zarnke MD, Gould HR, Goldman MH: Computed tomography in the evaluation of the patient with symptomatic abdominal aortic aneurysm. *Surgery* 103:638, 1988.
[3]Johnson WC, Gale ME, Gerzof SG, et al: The role of computed tomography in symptomatic aortic aneurysms. *Surg Gynecol Obstet* 162:49, 1986.
[4]Holland BR, Neumann S, Klempa I, Freyschmidt J: Spiral computerized tomography of acute abdominal aortic aneurysm with optimal 3-D image reconstruction. *Chirurgie* 67:44, 1996.
[5]Kaufman JA, Geller SC, Petersen MJ, et al: MR imaging (including MR angiography) of abdominal aortic aneurysms: Comparison with conventional angiography. *AJR* 163:203, 1994.
[a]Sensitivity = [TP/(TP + FN)].
[b]Specificity = [TN/(TN + FP)].
[c]LR(+) = positive likelihood ratio = [sensitivity/(1 − specificity)].
[d]LR(−) = negative likelihood ratio = [(1 − sensitivity)/specificity].
[e]Highly operator-dependent, especially in patients with obesity or bowel gas.
[f]A 95% confidence interval was used when data were derived from a single study or when aggregating homogeneous data from different studies.
[g]LR calculations for sensitivity or specificity of 100% are estimated conservatively by using the midpoint of the 95% CI if not doing so would result in an LR(+) = ∞ or an LR(−) = 0.
[h]Helical noncontrast CT performs at least as good as, and usually better than contrast nonhelical CT in identifying leaking AAAs. Those with no evidence of leak, but with impending rupture, may be particularly difficult to identify. CT performs better than conventional angiography for identification of AAAs in need of urgent intervention.
[i]For identification of detailed preoperative anatomy, MRA is at least as good, and in most institutions, better than conventional angiography.
[j]MRI = magnetic resonance imaging; MRA = magnetic resonance angiography.

In between mucosal/submucosal involvement and full-thickness infarction is an intermediate form of ischemic colitis involving portions of the muscular layer of the large bowel. These areas of deep but incomplete ischemia may later heal with stricture formation, placing the patient at risk for subsequent obstruction of the large bowel. In many instances, the attack of ischemic colitis that lead to the stricture may have been so mild that medical care was not sought at the time and the episode forgotten entirely by the patient. See Table 68-14.

EXTRAABDOMINAL **Cardiopulmonary** If the patient is complaining of pain in the upper half of the abdomen, particularly if the pain is confined to the RUQ or LUQ (with or without tenderness), the chest should be examined for basilar involvement of lung parenchyma or pleura. Because the stethoscope is neither sensitive nor specific for the diagnosis of pneumonia, pulmonary infarction, small pleural effusions, or small pneumothoraces, a chest film should be obtained. Whether a decubitus or expiratory film is requested depends upon clinical suspicion of effusion or pneumothorax, respectively. A negative film, especially if the pain is pleuritic in quality, introduces the differential diagnosis of pulmonary embolism.

If the pain is epigastric and the patient is in an age/gender group where coronary artery disease is prevalent, a further cardiac history and electrocardiogram (ECG) should be obtained. Ischemic cardiac pain referring to the epigastrium is not associated with significant tenderness, although cutaneous dysesthesia may be present, like that found in the upper extremity in other patterns of ischemic cardiac pain.

Abdominal Wall Pain originating from the abdominal wall may be confused with visceral pain because superficial innervation from the lower thoracic roots enters the spinal cord via the same dorsal horn as the deeper visceral afferents. A useful and underutilized test is the sit-up test, also known as Carnett's sign. Following identification of the site of maximum abdominal tenderness, the patient is asked to fold his or her arms across the chest and sit up halfway. The examiner maintains a finger on the tender area, and if palpation in the semi-sitting position produces the same or increased tenderness, the test is said to be positive for an abdominal wall syndrome. The logic of this is that tensing of the abdominal muscles would be likely to protect the underlying organs, thus reducing tenderness if the cause of pain were deep. In patients unable to perform the maneuver, just raising the head and shoulders off the bed may be sufficient.

Abdominal wall syndromes overlap with hernias, neuropathic causes of abdominal pain, and NSAP.

HERNIAS Hernias represent a special type of abdominal wall syndrome characterized by a defect through which intraabdominal contents protrude, often only intermittently during transient increases in intraabdominal pressure. Hernias are ordinarily asymptomatic or, at worst, moderately uncomfortable, but they do not generally cause significant pain unless they have become incarcerated or strangulated. Although the vast majority of hernias are inguinal, there are many other types that must be considered, including incisional, periumbilical, and—especially in women—femoral hernias. In a series of 120 cases,

TABLE 68-14 Diagnostic Tests for Ischemia of the Small and Large Bowel

Target Diagnosis	Test	Sensitivity[a]	Specificity[b]	LR(+)[c]	LR(−)[d]
Mesenteric ischemia	Angiography[1,e]	88% (62%, 98%)[f]	Criterion standard	~90[g]	~0.1[g]
Mesenteric ischemia	Contrast enhanced CT[1,2,h]	71% (57%, 82%)[f]	92% (81%, 100%)[f]	9	0.3
Mesenteric ischemia	Gadolinium-enhanced MRA[3,4,i,j]	100% (78%, 100%)[f]	91% (71%, 99%)[f]	11[g]	0.1[g]
Mesenteric ischemia/infarction	Serum lactate[5–9,k]	96% (80%, 100%)[f]	60% (49%, 70%)[f]	2	0.07
Ischemic colitis[l]	Endoscopy[10,11,m] (Recto-sigmoidoscopy or colonoscopy)	100% (87%, 100%)[f]	100% (96%, 100%)[f]	50[g]	0.06[g]

[1]Klein HM, Lensing R, Klosterhalfen B, Tons C, et al: Diagnostic imaging of mesenteric infarction. *Radiology* 197:79, 1995.
[2]Taourel PG, Deneuville M, Pradel JA, et al: Acute mesenteric ischemia: Diagnosis with contrast-enhanced CT. *Radiology* 199:632, 1996.
[3]Meaney JF, Prince MR, Nostrant TT, Stanley JC: Gadolinium-enhanced MR angiography of visceral arteries in patients with suspected chronic mesenteric ischemia. *J Magn Reson Imaging* 7:171, 1997.
[4]Shirkhoda A, Konez O, Shetty AN, et al: Contrast-enhanced MR angiography of the mesenteric circulation: A pictorial essay. *Radiographics* 18:851, 1998.
[5]Meyer T, Klein P, Schweiger H, Lang W: How can the prognosis of acute mesenteric artery ischemia be improved? Results of a retrospective analysis. *Zentralbl Chir* 123:230, 1998.
[6]Lange H, Toivola A: Warning signals in acute abdominal disorders: Lactate is the best marker of mesenteric ischemia. *Lakartidningen* 94:1893, 1997.
[7]Lange H, Jackel R: Usefulness of plasma lactate concentration in the diagnosis of acute abdominal disease. *Eur J Surg* 160:381, 1994.
[8]Jonas J, Bottger T: Diagnosis and prognosis of mesenterial infarct. *Med Klin* 89:68, 1994.
[9]Bottger T, Jonas J, Weber W, Junginger T: Sensitivity of preoperative diagnosis in mesenteric vascular occlusion. *Bildgebung* 58:192, 1991.
[10]Fanti L, Masci E, Mariani A, et al: Is endoscopy useful for early diagnosis of ischaemic colitis after aortic surgery? Results of a prospective trial. *Ital J Gastroenterol Hepatol* 29:357, 1997.
[11]Brandt CP, Piotrowski JJ, Alexander JJ: Flexible sigmoidoscopy: A reliable determinant of colonic ischemia following ruptured abdominal aortic aneurysm. *Surg Endosc* 11:113, 1997.
[a]Sensitivity = [TP/(TP + FN)].
[b]Specificity = [TN/(TN + FP)].
[c]LR(+) = positive likelihood ratio = [sensitivity/(1 − specificity)].
[d]LR(−) = negative likelihood ratio = [(1 − sensitivity)/specificity).
[e]Conventional arteriography remains the procedure of choice at the present time, often because it is a component of preoperative and nonoperative treatment in nonocclusive arterial ischemia and mesenteric vein thrombosis.
[f]A 95% confidence interval was used when data were derived from a single study or when aggregating homogeneous data from different studies.
[g]LR calculations for sensitivity or specificity of 100% are estimated conservatively by using the midpoint of the 95% CI if not doing so would result in an LR(+) = ∞ or an LR(−) = 0.
[h]There is some evidence in small studies to suggest that IV contrast-enhanced CT may be superior to arteriography in the diagnosis of mesenteric vein thrombosis.
[i]MRA = magnetic resonance angiography.
[j]In the future, conventional angiography may be replaced by rapid MRA.
[k]Metanalysis suggests that a persistently normal lactate over time supports an alternative diagnosis. In contrast, elevated lactate was highly nonspecific, with many false positives and a poor LR(+).
[l]In contrast to mesenteric ischemia, which involves the vascular supply of the small bowel and varying portions of the proximal large bowel, ischemic colitis is confined to the large bowel.
[m]Unlike other vascular causes of abdominal pain, imaging plays a minor role in the diagnosis of ischemic colitis.

sonography of the abdominal wall was shown to be very helpful in identifying hernias and other causes of abdominal wall pain.

OTHER ABDOMINAL WALL SYNDROMES Other causes of abdominal wall pain include rectus sheath hematomas and trauma to other portions of the abdominal wall. In older patients or in those on anticoagulants, the trauma may be very minor and forgotten. In circumstances where the injury is due to stretching causing tearing of muscle fibers, the overlying skin will not show any evidence of bruising that might provide a clue to the presence of bleeding into the abdominal wall.

Toxic-Metabolic TOXIC INFECTIOUS A large number of infectious agents irritate the GI tract, producing pain that is usually crampy. Concomitant vomiting or diarrhea suggests a gastroenteritis or enterocolitis, respectively. Many agents cause both upper and lower tract symptoms; in adults, however, one symptom complex usually predominates over the other. The hallmark of these infections, because most are confined to the lumen (mucosa) of the GI tract, is an absence of significant tenderness. This is because the parietal peritoneum is not irritated by luminal disease. If infarction, penetration, or perforation of the bowel wall occurs, as may happen with some of the invasive dysenteries—e.g., salmonellosis—peritoneal tenderness follows. This is why abdominal tenderness of any significance should never be attributed to uncomplicated "gastroenteritis." Furthermore, because the overall incidence of symptomatic GI infections declines markedly with age, the prior probability of "gastroenteritis" as the basis for abdominal complaints, particularly pain, in the elderly is very low indeed.

Other infections are associated with abdominal pain, although the pathophysiology is less clear. These include group A beta-hemolytic streptococcal pharyngitis (with or without associated scarlet fever), Rocky Mountain spotted fever, and early toxic shock syndrome.

POISONINGS The toxicologic causes of abdominal pain are also legion; they tend to be nonspecific and nondiagnostic in most instances. Some exceptions to this include envenomation by the female black widow spider, which is said to mimic peritonitis. This might represent a diagnostic dilemma if no history was taken and only the abdomen was examined. However, because the rigid abdomen following envenomation is due to muscular spasm, which begins at the site of the bite and gradually spreads to involve other large muscle groups of the back and proximal extremities, the prominence of extraabdominal signs and symptoms, as well as their historical evolution, should point the clinician away from a primary intraabdominal process. Isopropanol-induced hemorrhagic gastritis may be associated with cramping pain from this ingestion. Cocaine-induced intestinal ischemia, progressing to infarction and perforation, has been reported. The first stage of iron poisoning produces abdominal pain and may cause hematemesis due to the direct corrosive effects of iron on the GI tract. Large amounts of iron left in the stomach may also cause perforation. Mercury salts cause severe corrosion of the GI tract, associated with shock. *Acute* inorganic lead toxicity is typically associated with severe, crampy abdominal pain. This is in contrast to *chronic* lead toxicity, in which abdominal pain is minimal or absent. The development of abdominal pain following electrical injury suggests a potentially serious complication and the need for admission. Opiate withdrawal produces abdominal pain, usually crampy in character, associated with diaphoresis and piloerection. In some individuals, the abdominal skin appears dysesthetic to light touch, but significant tenderness should not be present. Mushroom toxicity, though rarely fatal, is commonly accompanied by a chemical gastroenteritis and severe abdominal pain out of proportion to tenderness.

METABOLIC **ACIDOSIS** These causes of abdominal pain include acute anion-gap metabolic acidoses, commonly seen in diabetic ketoacidosis (DKA) and alcoholic ketoacidosis (AKA) and less frequently in lactic acidosis. Although the pain associated with DKA and AKA has been attributed to gastric distention and paralytic ileus, this has not been clearly substantiated. In DKA or AKA, it is critical to consider the possibility that an underlying abdominal problem may have triggered the DKA or AKA, rather than the reverse. This is a particularly challenging clinical problem when amylase or lipase levels are elevated, since both AKA and DKA can be a consequence or a cause of acute pancreatitis. If the acidosis is difficult to ''break'' or the pain persists after normalization of the pH, intraabdominal disease should be sought.

ENDOCRINOLOGIC Of the endocrinopathies associated with abdominal pain, adrenal crisis is the most striking. Patients are often shocky and may exhibit peritoneal signs. The syndrome appears to be principally related to hypocortisolism rather than hypoaldosteronism. Without a history of similar prior episodes following reduced intake or absorption of adrenal steroids, these patients may be indistinguishable from those with an intraabdominal catastrophe in need of urgent exploration. Other endocrinopathies and electrolyte abnormalities associated with abdominal pain include thyroid storm, hypo- and hypercalcemia. This pain is generally crampy, and tenderness is absent unless the hyperthyroid state has caused acute hepatomegaly and distention of the liver capsule. Hypoglycemia has been reportedly associated with abdominal pain, but the evidence supporting this is unconvincing.

SICKLE CELL CRISIS A painful sickle cell crisis is a common cause of abdominal pain, second only to musculoskeletal pain as the most common manifestation of a vasoocclusive crisis in homozygous (SS) sickle cell disease. Occasionally, patients with sickle cell disease and other symptomatic heterozygous forms may present with abdominal pain due to splenomegaly or splenic infarct. Those with heterozygous sickle trait (SA) are almost invariably asymptomatic. The most reliable means of determining whether the abdominal pain is part of a crisis or secondary to an underlying intraabdominal problem is to ask the patient whether or not this is the pain of a ''typical crisis'' or whether it represents a pattern break. If the latter, the problem is usually localized to the RUQ, either secondary to biliary tract disease (about 75 percent of those with SS have bilirubin stones due to chronic hemolysis) or hepatomegaly due to sinusoidal sludging of sickled cells. Additional considerations for SS patients include pancreatitis, salmonellosis, and mesenteric venous thrombosis.

Less common ''metabolic'' entities associated with abdominal pain include virtually all forms of vasculitis, especially systemic lupus and Henoch-Schönlein purpura, porphyria, and familial Mediterranean fever. Each of these may produce peritonitis.

Neurogenic The hallmark of neurogenic abdominal pain is a dysesthetic sensation, particularly in response to light touch in the area of discomfort. This has been characterized by one author as the ''hover'' sign, in which the patient shows signs of discomfort when the examining hand is passed very lightly across the area of dysesthesia. A positive hover sign may be mistakenly interpreted as indicating a generally hyperreactive patient rather than a normal physiologic response to a dysesthetic stimulus.

Because deep and superficial nerve fibers from the same area of the abdomen may enter the cord together, dysesthesias have also been reported with other, more serious intraabdominal disease, such as appendicitis. In the latter, however, the problem is usually more acute, and either upon presentation or subsequently is accompanied by tenderness (in contrast to dysesthesia alone, defined here as an abnormal sensation in response to light touch). This category includes nerve entrapment syndromes, such as rectus nerve entrapment, and iliohypogastric entrapment following a Pfannenstiel incision. A number of other incisional entrapment syndromes have been described. Many of these patients will have a positive Carnett test, but the hover sign is probably more indicative of neurogenic abdominal pain.

Radicular problems causing abdominal pain include diabetic or zosteriform radiculopathy, the latter being characterized by dysesthesias outlining a dermatome, usually with some ''spillover'' into contiguous dermatomes on either side of the involved root. The dysesthesias may present as lancinating, ticlike bouts of shooting pain or continuous burning. Accompanying vesicles confirm the diagnosis, although the pain may precede the cutaneous eruption by several days. Diabetic neuropathic involvement of a root, plexus, or nerve can be confirmed by electromyography.

There is some evidence that greater attention to the examination of the abdominal wall might reduce the frequency with which the diagnosis of nonspecific abdominal pain (NSAP) is made. In one report, about 25 percent of patients with the diagnosis of NSAP were found to have significant tenderness confined to the abdominal wall.

NONSPECIFIC ABDOMINAL PAIN Despite a thorough evaluation, the largest single group of patients seen in the ED will have no definite diagnosis and will receive the designation of NSAP. As Lukens et al point out, the term *undifferentiated abdominal pain* (UAP) would be preferable to *nonspecific,* since the cause of the patient's pain may turn out to be very specific.[11] Unfortunately, the term *NSAP* is relatively entrenched in the English literature. It is essential that diagnostic terms with specific meanings, such as *gastroenteritis* or *gastritis*, not be used as catch-all phrases to describe patients with NSAP.

Although NSAP is a diagnosis of exclusion, there are some clinical features characteristically associated with it. Nausea, present in nearly half the patients, is the most common symptom after abdominal pain. Pain location is often midepigastric or in the lower half of the abdomen. Tenderness is not usually severe, is absent in about one-third of the patients, and localized to the RLQ or midepigastrium in another third. Laboratory tests are usually normal, although a mild leukocytosis is entirely compatible with NSAP. Abdominal radiographs are virtually always normal or nonspecific.[11]

The key to confirming NSAP is reexamination within 24 h (see below).

Special Considerations

THE ELDERLY ABDOMEN In a large combined series of >40,000 patients presenting with acute abdominal pain (<1 week duration), about one patient in four was >50 years old. Diagnostic accuracy in this group fell below 50 percent, reaching a low of about 30 percent in octogenarians, whose corresponding mortality was about 70 times that of patients <30 years old.[16]

Reasons for Increased Diagnostic Error in the Evaluation of the Elderly Abdomen DIFFERENT PREVALENCE OF DISEASE The causes of abdominal pain in elderly patients occur with a substantially different frequency than in younger persons, requiring that the emergency physician approach older patients with a different weighting of prior probabilities than those in younger adults. For example, as shown in Table 68-2, the most common cause of abdominal pain in virtually all consecutive series of adults presenting to the ED is NSAP.[16] When ED patients are dichotomized by age at 50 years, NSAP remains at the top of the list of diagnoses among the younger cohort; however, among the older patients, prevalence is markedly diminished to <20 percent, as shown in Table 68-3.[34]

DIFFERENT KINDS OF DISEASE Another explanation for the increased error and mortality in elderly abdominal pain is that, in addition to an age-related shift in the frequency of certain diseases, there are a number of serious causes of abdominal pain that only rarely arise among younger patients. Specifically, older patients are at risk for vascular causes of abdominal pain—e.g., mesenteric ischemia, AAA, and myocardial infarction.[16,34]

DIFFERENT EVOLUTION OF DISEASE Among common causes of abdominal pain in both young and old, the nature of the presentation and evolution of the same illness is often very different. Using appendicitis as the most common example, those >50 years of age are much more likely to have generalized pain and tenderness (about 14 percent) than are younger patients (about 2 percent).[12] This failure to localize to an area of maximum pain/tenderness may help to account for the nearly 10-fold difference in perforation rate (4 versus 37 percent) in those >60 years of age as compared with their younger counterparts. Later presentation in the course of illness may also contribute to the increased perforation rate (75 percent of the elderly with appendicitis have >24 h of symptoms before seeking care), as may the higher frequency of distention in older patients, making the physical examination more difficult.

DIFFERENT THRESHOLD FOR INTERVENTION An additional contributor to the high incidence of perforation in all causes of elderly abdominal pain is the understandable reluctance to operate upon frail elderly patients without clear-cut signs of peritoneal irritation. This is reflected in the well-established inverse association between negative laparotomies and perforated appendices. At about the age of 45 years, the negative laparotomy rate begins to decrease in parallel with the increase in perforations until each plateaus at about 80 years.[16] Thus, the negative laparotomy rate for appendicitis is lowest in the oldest, who are the group most likely to perforate and therefore most in need of early, expedient surgery.

General Strategies for Evaluation of the Elderly Abdomen ANTICIPATE THE NEED FOR SURGICAL INTERVENTION Assume that the elderly patient with abdominal pain has surgical disease. About 40 percent of all patients >65 years of age presenting to the ED with this complaint ultimately require surgery.

ABDOMINAL AORTIC ANEURYSM Apparent renal colic is an abdominal aortic aneurysm (AAA) until proven otherwise. Do not be misled by the presence of hematuria.

MESENTERIC ISCHEMIA Consider the diagnosis of mesenteric ischemia in all elderly patients with abdominal pain, especially if the pain appears out of proportion to tenderness. The presence of atrial fibrillation, cardiovascular or peripheral vascular disease, especially recent MI, increases the likelihood of mesenteric ischemia. Bloody diarrhea will not be seen until mucosa begins to slough and is far more common in ischemic colitis, which is a relatively benign disease in comparison with mesenteric ischemia.

IMAGING Be liberal with imaging in the elderly who have abdominal pain of unclear etiology. If there is a serious question about important underlying abdominal disease in the setting of a relatively "well-looking" elderly patient, one should have a low threshold for performing an abdominal CT.

GASTROENTERITIS Attributing vomiting or diarrhea in the elderly to gastroenteritis is inadvisable, particularly in association with abdominal pain.

CONSTIPATION Because the prevalence of constipation is so high in the elderly, it is a risky explanation for abdominal pain of sufficient severity to bring an older person to an ED. As a corollary to this, apparent resolution of abdominal pain in the elderly with an enema (which is itself a questionable intervention) should not be taken as evidence of a causal relationship between constipation and abdominal pain.

HIV/AIDS There are several features of patients with HIV and/or acquired immunodeficiency syndrome (AIDS) presenting to the ED with abdominal pain that merit special attention.[35] Abdominal pain is rarely the index event that identifies a patient with HIV disease. Rather, most patients presenting with HIV-associated acute abdominal pain will have previously met criteria for AIDS.

Enterocolitis is the most common cause of abdominal pain in AIDS patients. It is typically accompanied by profuse diarrhea and dehydration. If associated with fecal leukocytes, it is more often accompanied by bacteremia than in immunocompetent patients. Perforation, when it occurs, tends to be large bowel perforation, often caused by *Cytomegalovirus* (CMV).[35] Obstruction presents typically but may be due to an atypical cause such as Kaposi's sarcoma, lymphoma, or atypical mycobacteria.

Biliary tract disease is very common in AIDS patients, presenting in one of two unique forms: (1) AIDS-related cholangiopathy, caused principally by CMV or *Cryptosporidium* sp., which can be treated with sphincterotomy, and (2) AIDS-associated cholecystitis, which is usually acalculous and has a propensity for early perforation.

TREATMENT

General Strategies

HYPOTENSION Clinically important decreases in cardiac output are commonly underdiagnosed in the elderly. This is because many older patients have chronic systolic hypertension, making the traditional threshold value of 100 mmHg systolic an insensitive marker for declaring hypotension or shock in the elderly. Thus, in the setting of abdominal pain, the blood pressure must be interpreted in a clinical context if it is to provide meaningful information.

In abdominal pain with relative hypotension, management depends upon the presumed etiology. In the absence of heavy GI bleeding, which is not typically accompanied by abdominal pain, younger patients are most likely to be volume-contracted from vomiting, diarrhea, decreased intake by mouth, or third-spacing into the GI tract. Treatment is isotonic crystalloid.

In a smaller number of young patients, hypotension may be the result of abdominal sepsis. In this setting, in addition to appropriate antibiotics (see below) and isotonic crystalloid, pressors may be necessary to sustain blood pressure until more definitive intervention can be undertaken. Vasoconstrictors are indicated in septic (vasodilatory) shock, with levophed or high-dose dopamine as the usual choice of agent.

In older patients, in addition to volume contraction and a higher incidence of abdominal sepsis, associated cardiovascular disease represents a third possible cause of decreased cardiac output. Indeed, in the setting of nonocclusive mesenteric ischemia, the diminished cardiac output may be a cause rather than a consequence of the presenting abdominal pain. In this circumstance, if the problem is acute myocardial ischemia, an aortic balloon pump may be used to buy time until the underlying problem can be corrected with angioplasty. Or, if the decreased cardiac output is secondary to congestive heart failure (CHF), appropriate treatment for CHF is indicated.

ANALGESICS In the United States, analgesia is usually withheld from patients with acute abdominal pain until a firm treatment plan is formulated. There is no evidence to support this long-standing practice, which has been attributed to Sir Zachary Cope. More than 75 years ago, Dr. Cope wrote that provision of analgesia to patients with abdominal pain might obscure the diagnosis. However, much has changed since that time in both the diagnosis and treatment of abdominal pain: (1) there have been major advances in diagnostic technology, which is largely independent of the patient's degree of evolving pain and tenderness, and (2) there have been parallel advances in therapeutic technology, including the universal availability of antibiotics and sophisticated intra- and perioperative monitoring.

The most recent edition of Cope's text on the acute abdomen by Silen has softened this recommendation somewhat, but it notes that "it will take many generations to eliminate it [withholding analgesia in abdominal pain] because the rule has become so firmly ingrained in the minds of physicians."[36]

There are four published randomized clinical trials in the English literature, each compatible with the hypothesis that administration of opioids to patients with abdominal pain is at least safe.[37–40] Although none of these trials answers the question definitively, at least one of them suggests that diagnosis and management of abdominal pain may, if anything, be facilitated by opioids. The plausibility of this is supported by an improved ability to obtain a history from a patient relieved of severe pain and the enhanced localization of tenderness through reduction of guarding. These data on opioids cannot be extrapolated to nonsteroidal anti-inflammatory drugs (NSAIDs), such as parenteral ketorolac, because NSAIDs are not pure analgesics and have the potential to mask evidence of early peritoneal inflammation.[41] Pending the definitive study, at the present time available evidence favors judicious use of opioid analgesia in the ED management of acute abdominal pain.

ANTIEMETICS Although metoclopramide (Reglan) appears to be a more effective antiemetic, prochlorperazine (Compazine) is theoretically preferred for control of vomiting in acute abdominal pain because it is less likely to increase motility. Most patients will respond within 10 min to 2.5 mg IV of prochlorperazine, given over 1 min, to be repeated once. Although higher doses have not been tested in the ED setting, 10 to 40 mg prochlorperazine by slow intravenous infusion has been administered to patients receiving chemotherapy, demonstrating a therapeutic dose-response in emesis control with minimal toxicity. Antiemetics may obviate the need for insertion of a nasogastric tube, whose therapeutic value in abdominal pain has never been convincingly demonstrated.

ANTIBIOTICS Antibiotics are indicated in suspected abdominal sepsis and in most patients with localized and all patients with diffuse peritonitis. Endogenous gut flora cause abdominal infections in the GI or GU tract. Primary gynecologic infections, of which PID is the prototype, behave differently and are discussed separately under the treatment of suspected PID (see Chap. 105). In all intraabdominal (nongynecologic) infections, coverage should be targeted at anaerobes and facultative aerobic gram-negative organisms. An exception to this generalization is the need to provide additional coverage for gram-positive aerobes, e.g., *Pneumococcus*, in spontaneous bacterial peritonitis (SBP). SBP, also known as primary peritonitis, occurs in patients with cirrhosis and ascites, probably owing to spontaneous bacteremic seeding of ascitic fluid. The modifier *primary* is used to distinguish SBP from the more common secondary peritonitis of intraabdominal organ inflammation, ischemia, leakage, or perforation.

Historically, a two-drug regimen, attacking gram-negative aerobes with an aminoglycoside (gentamicin or tobramycin, 1.5 mg/kg IV q8h, or amikacin 5 mg/kg IV q8h) and anaerobes with metronidazole (1 g IV loading dose, followed by 500 mg IV q6h, given slowly) or clindamycin (900 mg IV q8h) was used to obtain the requisite coverage for intraabdominal infections. While dual therapy may still be necessary for sicker, older, immunocompromised, or hypotensive patients, monotherapy with a second- eneration cephalosporin, such as cefoxitin (2 g IV q6h) or cefotetan (2 g IV q6h), should be adequate for those who are less ill. Alternative "combined" monotherapy includes ampicillin-sulbactam (3.0 g IV q6h) or ticarcillin-clavulanate (3.1 g IV q6h). For patients requiring a more potent regimen but in whom one is reluctant to use an aminoglycoside, the combination of piperacillin-tazobactam (3.3 g IV q6h) appears to be at least as effective as imipenem-cilastatin (1 g IV q6h, maximum dose), particularly in the treatment of suspected biliary sepsis, and is less likely to cause seizures.

For patients with a history of severe allergy to penicillins/cephalosporins, aztreonam (2 g IV q6h, maximum dose) and clindamycin/metronidazole is a safe alternative. In SBP, monotherapy with a third-generation cephalosporin, such as ceftriaxone (2 g IV q12h, maximum) or cefotaxime (2 g IV q4h, maximum), broadens the spectrum sufficiently to cover for *Pneumococcus* in addition to the gram-negative enteric bacteria, such as *E. coli*.

Perhaps the most persuasive reason to forgo use of an aminoglycoside is not the renal or vestibular toxicity but rather the frequent underdosing of patients because of the fear of toxicity, causing emergence of antimicrobial resistance, particularly of *Enterococcus* species.[42]

DISPOSITION

General Indications for Admission

In addition to those with a specific diagnosis requiring admission, the following patients should be seriously considered as candidates for hospitalization: Those who appear ill; any elderly or immunocompromised (including HIV-positive) patient (with or without comorbidity) in whom the diagnosis is unclear; younger, healthy patients in whom the diagnosis is unclear and any potentially serious cause of abdominal pain has not been comfortably excluded; intractable pain or vomiting; acute or chronic altered mental status; inability to follow discharge or follow-up instructions; undomiciled, living in shelter, or otherwise lacking social supports; excessive alcohol or other drug use.

NONSPECIFIC ABDOMINAL PAIN A substantial number of patients who are discharged with the diagnosis of NSAP are initially admitted as suspected appendicitis. This may be the reason that there appears to be an unexplained predominance of RLQ pain among patients discharged with the diagnosis of NSAP.

Although this entity is poorly understood pathophysiologically, follow-up among patients discharged from the ED with this diagnosis has found that nearly 90 percent are better or asymptomatic at 2 to 3 weeks.[11] Similarly, follow-up of patients discharged from inpatient services with the diagnosis of NSAP has shown that about 80 percent have no further problems and are asymptomatic at 5 years. Of the remainder, about one-third are rehospitalized, of whom one-third have appendicitis. Some of these individuals probably had early appendicitis on their prior admission, with spontaneous resolution due to disimpaction of the appendiceal lumen.[43] Among this group, it is plausible that some later developed recurrent appendicitis that did not resolve and went on to appendectomy. The remaining two-thirds of patients who were neither rehospitalized nor asymptomatic turned out to have "benign" gynecologic and colonic problems, most commonly irritable bowel.[44,45]

The key to confirming NSAP as a working diagnosis is reexamination in 24 h, repeated as necessary if patients remain symptomatic. Whether this occurs on the inpatient service, in the ED observation unit, or at home depends upon the culture of the institution, the clinician's degree of uncertainty about the diagnosis, and the presence of facilities for reliable outpatient follow-up.

REFERENCES

1. de Dombal FT: The OMGE acute abdominal pain survey progress report, 1986. *Scand J Gastroenterol* 23(suppl 144):35, 1988.
2. American College of Emergency Physicians' Clinical Policies Committee: Clinical policy for the initial approach to patients presenting with a chief complaint of nontraumatic acute abdominal pain. *Ann Emerg Med* 23:906, 1994.
3. Agreus L, Svardsudd K, Nyren O, Tibblin G: The epidemiology of abdominal symptoms: Prevalence and demographic characteristics in a Swedish adult population. A report from The Abdominal Symptom Study. *Scan J Gastroenterol* 29:102, 1994.
4. McCaig LF, Stussman BJ: National Hospital Ambulatory Medical Care Survey: 1996 Emergency Department Summary. Advance data from vital and health statistics; no. 293, p 8. Hyattsville, MD: National Center for Health Statistics, 1997.
5. Bugliosi TF, Meloy TD, Vukov LF: Acute abdominal pain in the elderly. *Ann Emerg Med* 19:1383, 1990.
6. Staniland JR, Ditchburn J, de Dombal FT: Clinical presentation of the acute abdomen: Study of 600 patients. *Br Med J* 3:393, 1972.
7. Jeddy TA, Vowles RH, Southam JA: Cough sign: A reliable test in the diagnosis of intra-abdominal inflammation. *Br J Surg* 81:279, 1994.
8. Bennett DH, Tambeur Luc J, Campbell WB: Use of coughing test to diagnose peritonitis. *Br Med J* 308:1336, 1994.
9. Liddington MI, Thomson WH: Rebound tenderness test. *Br J Surg* 78:795, 1991.
10. Dixon JM, Elton RA, Rainey JB, MacLeod DA: Rectal examination in patients with pain in the right lower quadrant of the abdomen. *Br Med J* 302:386, 1991.
11. Lukens TW, Emerman C, Effron D: The natural history and clinical findings of undifferentiated abdominal pain. *Ann Emerg Med* 22:690, 1993.
12. Thompson MM, Underwood MJ, Dookeran KA, et al: Role of sequential leucocyte counts and C-reactive protein measurements in acute appendicitis. *Br J Surg* 79:822, 1992.
13. Anyanwu AC, Moalypour SM: Are abdominal radiographs still overutilized in the assessment of acute abdominal pain? A district general hospital audit. *J R Coll Surg Edinb* 43:267, 1998.
14. Chang-Chien CS, Lin HH, Yen CL, et al: Sonographic demonstration of free air in perforated peptic ulcers: Comparison of sonography with radiography. *J Clin Ultrasound* 17:95, 1989.
15. Simmen HP, Decurtins M, Rotzer A, et al: Emergency room patients with abdominal pain unrelated to trauma: Analysis in a surgical university hospital. *Hepatogastroenterology* 38:279, 1991.
16. de Dombal FT: Acute abdominal pain in the elderly. *J Clin Gastroenterol* 19:331, 1994.
17. Gallagher EJ: Clinical utility of likelihood ratios. *Ann Emerg Med* 31:391, 1998.
18. McColl I: More precision in diagnosing appendicitis. *N Engl J Med* 338:190, 1998.
19. Wagner JM, McKinney P, Carpenter JL: Does this patient have appendicitis? *JAMA* 276:1589, 1996.
20. Rao PM, Rhea JT, Novelline RA, et al: Helical CT combined with contrast material administered only through the colon for imaging of suspected appendicitis. *AJR* 169:1275, 1997.
21. Rao PM, Rhea JT, Novelline RA, et al: Effect of computed tomography of the appendix on treatment of patients and use of hospital resources. *N Engl J Med* 338:141, 1998.
22. Parker LJ, Vukov LF, Wollan PC: Emergency department evaluation of geriatric patients with acute cholecystitis. *Acad Emerg Med* 4:51, 1997.
23. Singer AJ, McCracken G, Henry MC, et al: Correlation among clinical, laboratory, and hepatobiliary scanning findings in patients with suspected acute cholecystitis. *Ann Emerg Med* 28:267, 1996.
24. Gruber PJ, Silverman RA, Gottesfeld S, Flaster E: Presence of fever and leukocytosis in acute cholecystitis. *Ann Emerg Med* 28:273, 1996.
25. Diehl AK, Sugarek NJ, Todd KM: Clinical evaluation for gallstone disease: Usefulness of symptoms and signs in diagnosis. *Am J Med* 89:29, 1990.
26. Frager D, Baer JW, Medwid SW, et al: Detection of intestinal ischemia in patients with acute small bowel obstruction due to adhesions or hernia: Efficacy of CT. *AJR* 166:67, 1996.
27. Steinberg W, Tenner S: Medical progress: Acute pancreatitis. *N Engl J Med* 330:1198, 1994.
28. Keim V, Teich N, Fiedler F, et al: A comparison of lipase and amylase in the diagnosis of acute pancreatitis in patients with abdominal pain. *Pancreas* 16:45, 1998.
29. Schwerk WB, Schwarz S, Rothmund M: Sonography in acute colonic diverticulitis: A prospective study. *Dis Colon Rectum* 35:1077, 1992.
30. Elton TJ, Roth CS, Berquist TH, Silverstein MD: A clinical prediction rule for the diagnosis of ureteral calculi in emergency departments. *J Gen Intern Med* 8:57, 1993.
31. Kahn JG, Walker CK, Washington E, et al: Diagnosing pelvic inflammatory disease. *JAMA* 266:2594, 1991.
32. Lock G, Scholmerich J: Non-occlusive mesenteric ischemia. *Hepatogastroenterology* 42:234, 1995.
33. Rhee RY, Gloviczki P: Mesenteric venous thrombosis. *Surg Clin North Am* 77:327, 1997.
34. Telfer S, Fenyo G, Holt PR, de Dombal FT: Acute abdominal pain in patients over 50 years of age. *Scand J Gastroenterol (Suppl)* 144:47, 1988.
35. Katz MH, French DM: AIDS and the acute abdomen. *Emerg Med Clin North Am* 7:575, 1989.
36. Silen W: *Cope's Early Diagnosis of the Acute Abdomen,* 19th ed. New York: Oxford University Press, 1996, p. 6.
37. Zoltie N, Cust MP: Analgesia in the acute abdomen. *Ann R Coll Surg* 68:209, 1986.
38. Attard AR, Corlett MJ, Kidner NJ, et al: Safety of early pain relief for acute abdominal pain. *Br Med J* 305:554, 1992.
39. Pace S, Burke TF: Intravenous morphine for early pain relief in patients with acute abdominal pain. *Acad Emerg Med* 3:1086, 1996.
40. LoVecchio F, Oster N, Sturmann K, et al: The use of analgesics in patients with acute abdominal pain. *J Emerg Med* 15:775, 1997.
41. Pierik EG, Bruining HA: Non-steroidal anti-inflammatory drugs can disguise an acute abdomen. *Eur J Surg* 160:61, 1994.
42. Farber MS, Abrams JH: Antibiotics for the acute abdomen. *Surg Clin North Am* 77:1395, 1997.
43. Migraine S, Atri M, Bret PM, et al: Spontaneously resolving acute appendicitis: Clinical and sonographic documentation. *Radiology* 205:55, 1997.
44. Jess P, Bjerregaard B, Brynitz S, et al: Prognosis of acute nonspecific abdominal pain. A prospective study. *Am J Surg* 144:338, 1982.
45. Doshi M, Heaton KW: Irritable bowel syndrome in patients discharged from surgical wards with non-specific abdominal pain. *Br J Surg* 81:1216, 1994.

ABDOMINAL PAIN IN THE ELDERLY

Robert McNamara

EPIDEMIOLOGY

There are limited data on the number of emergency department (ED) visits for abdominal pain in the elderly. Patients aged 65 or older accounted for 9 percent of ED visits for abdominal pain in an adult ED population (age > 15).[1] A recent study from a rural ED reported that abdominal pain in those age 65 and greater represented 0.23 percent of all ED visits.[2] In the United States, abdominal pain is the most frequent reason for an ED visit, accounting for 5.1 million of the 96 million ED encounters in 1996.[3] The preceding figures would create estimates ranging from 230,000 to 450,000 elderly patients presenting to U.S. EDs per year with abdominal pain.

Regardless of the current frequency of ED visits for abdominal pain in the elderly, one can count on a steadily rising volume of such cases. The U.S. population is rapidly aging. Current projections predict that those aged 65 and older will rise from 13 percent of the population

TABLE 69-1 Influence of Aging on Abdominal Pain

Increased Risk in the Elderly	Resultant Disease
ASCVD	AAA, mesenteric ischemia, ischemic colitis
Cholelithiasis	Cholecystitis, pancreatitis
Carcinoma	Large bowel obstruction, intussusception
Immobility	Colonic volvulus, Ogilvie syndrome
Medications	Peptic ulcer disease, pancreatitis
Prior surgery	Small bowel obstruction

Key: ASCVD, atherosclerotic cardiovascular disease; AAA, abdominal aortic aneurysm.

in the year 2000 to approximately 20 percent by the year 2030.[4] Since the elderly use the ED more frequently than their proportionate numbers in the general community would indicate, this trend will affect emergency care significantly.[5] Practicing emergency physicians rate abdominal pain as the most challenging clinical situation in this population.[4] Over half of the patients aged 65 or greater who present to the ED with abdominal pain require admission, and one-third or more will require surgical intervention at some point during their hospital stay.[1,3] The mortality rate across all causes of abdominal pain in the elderly is 11 to 14 percent, justifying its anxiety-provoking reputation.[6] The role of the emergency service in the care of these patients is critical, as the mortality rate doubles if the diagnosis rendered in the ED is incorrect.[6,7]

PATHOPHYSIOLOGY

The approach to acute abdominal pain in all age groups requires an understanding of the visceral and somatic pathways of pain perception. Neural pathways are not rerouted as we age; however, it is an accepted axiom that the perception of abdominal pain or at least the reporting of it is altered in the elderly.[7] There is limited proof of this axiom for abdominal pain; however, it is fairly clear that ischemic heart disease is associated with altered pain perception or reporting in the elderly. Other factors such as fear, stoicism, and communication problems may affect the reporting of abdominal pain in older persons.[7,8]

Aging is associated with several factors that influence the prevalence and spectrum of abdominal conditions encountered in this population (Table 69-1). For example, older patients have a statistically increased frequency of abdominal aortic aneurysms that could potentially rupture and present to the ED. The presence of comorbid diseases and their associated therapy certainly contributes to the complexity of care in older patients with abdominal pain. Other important pathophysiologic features to keep in mind regarding this age group include decreased cardiopulmonary reserve, lowered tolerance for hypovolemic shock, and the treatment issues of altered pharmacodynamics and pharmacokinetics.

CLINICAL FEATURES

The History

History taking in older patients with abdominal pain should follow the same general sequence and rules as in younger patients. Unfortunately, an accurate history may be difficult to obtain in this age group. Serious abdominal disease may cause an acute mental status change or distract the patient's attention. Memory deficits or underlying dementia can obscure important aspects, such as the time and nature of the onset of pain.[8] The noise and pace of the ED are often inconsistent with the needs of the older patient who is attempting to relay historical information about his or her abdominal pain. The following historical aspects should be covered:

- *Time of Onset:* Pain awakening the patient from sleep should always be considered significant.
- *Mode of Onset:* A sudden, severe pain should alert the physician to the possibility of serious disease, including a ruptured abdominal aortic aneurysm, aortic dissection, superior mesenteric artery embolus, perforation of a peptic ulcer, or volvulus. It is equally important to remember that these entities may present without a sudden onset. For example, in one prospective series of patients over the age of 70 with perforated ulcers, only 47 percent reported a sudden onset of pain.[6]
- *Progression since Onset:* Steady improvement is reassuring, worsening is not.
- *Location of the Pain:* In general, this seems to be reliable in the elderly. For example, appendicitis in this age group, although diagnostically difficult, generally presents with right-lower-quadrant pain.[9]
- *Character of the Pain:* Severe pain should be taken as an indicator of serious disease. Think of mesenteric ischemia, perforation of a gastric ulcer, vascular accidents, and volvulus.
- *Referral or Radiation of the Pain:* As with location, this aspect of abdominal pain should not change with aging. For example, the referral pattern is helpful in diagnosing older patients with biliary tract disease.[8]
- *Precipitating and Relieving Factors:* Pain with movement suggests irritation of the parietal peritoneum. The results of any self-treatment should be determined.
- *Prior Episodes:* This generally suggests a medical cause with the notable exceptions of mesenteric ischemia (intestinal angina) and cholecystitis.[10]
- *Associated Symptoms:* Anorexia, vomiting, bowel habits, and urinary symptoms are key areas to cover. In general, pain almost always precedes vomiting in surgical causes of abdominal pain, while the converse is true in 75 percent of patients with gastroenteritis or a nonspecific cause of abdominal pain.[1]
- *Further History:* A detailed review of systems is desirable to seek other causes of abdominal pain, especially those of a cardiopulmonary nature. Do not neglect a careful review of medications including over-the-counter nonsteroidal anti-inflammatory agents. Underlying alcohol abuse must also be a consideration in this age group.

The Physical Examination

As with the history, the abdominal examination in the older patient proceeds in the same manner as for younger patients. Complicating factors may include the patient's stoicism or inability to report pain and the less pronounced muscular response to inflammation.[7,8] The following should be addressed:

- *General Appearance:* An ill-appearing older patient with abdominal pain should cause immediate concern, given the high mortality rate in general case series of elderly patients with abdominal pain.[1,6] On the other hand, the clinician can be misled by a deceptively ''well'' appearance in the face of serious underlying disease.[8]
- *Vital Signs:* Reflexively think of a ruptured abdominal aortic aneurysm in the hypotensive older patient with abdominal pain.[11] Determination of a core temperature is advisable; however, lack of fever commonly occurs with serious infectious causes of abdominal pain. Tachypnea and tachycardia are nonspecific findings but should raise the possibility of a cardiopulmonary disorder.
- *Inspection and Auscultation:* Distention is common in large bowel obstruction, including sigmoid and cecal volvulus.[12] High-pitched ''rushes'' suggest small bowel obstruction.

- *Abdominal Palpation:* In general, the location of tenderness is generally reliable in the older patient. Appendicitis usually manifests right-lower-quadrant tenderness,[6,9,13] while cholecystitis and pancreatitis generally cause tenderness in the expected location.[8] Unfortunately, abdominal guarding or muscular rigidity may be lacking despite the presence of chemical or infectious peritoneal irritation. This is partially attributed to the relatively thin abdominal musculature of older patients.[7,8] Disturbingly, of patients over the age of 70 with a perforated ulcer, only 21 percent had epigastric rigidity.[6]
- *Rectal Examination:* This should be performed routinely, and the detection of occult blood should receive follow-up evaluation. In one series of patients over the age of 50, some 10 percent of those discharged from the ED with a diagnosis of nonspecific abdominal pain were diagnosed with cancer, principally of the large bowel, within a year.[14]
- *Further Examination:* There should be careful inspection for hernias, particularly of the femoral canal in the older female patient. Aortic dissection may manifest with unequal femoral pulses. The back should be inspected for herpes zoster. Genital and pelvic examinations may reveal the cause of pain. Assessment of the heart and lungs may yield clues to a nonabdominal cause of the pain.

SPECIFIC DIAGNOSES AND ISSUES

This section reviews the major diagnostic causes of abdominal pain in the older patient and points out specific diagnostic issues to consider in this population. The frequency of each particular disease varies in the reported case series of elderly patients presenting to the ED with abdominal pain. Cholecystitis (12 to 41 percent) is generally the most frequently encountered disease of a surgical nature, followed by bowel obstruction (7 to 14 percent). Nonspecific abdominal pain is also a frequent diagnosis (10 to 23 percent). Perforated viscus, appendicitis, diverticulitis, and pancreatitis each generally represent around 4 to 7 percent, depending on the case series. Aortic aneurysms and mesenteric ischemia are less common.[3,6,8] General coverage of the following conditions can also be found in other chapters.

Appendicitis

Diagnostic problems surrounding appendicitis in the elderly are well known in emergency medicine (see Chap. 74) In one series, only 51 percent of patients over the age of 60 with proven appendicitis had that diagnosis made during the ED phase of their care.[13] Delayed presentation is common and contributes to the higher perforation and complication rate. One must be careful to not exclude appendicitis because of prolonged symptoms, as a small but significant percentage of the elderly will wait more than a week to seek care for this condition.

The abdominal pain is generally reported to be in the right lower quadrant; however, the description may be vague or the pain poorly localized.[9,13] In one study, migration was recorded in only 35 percent of elderly patients with appendicitis.[8] Anorexia, an expected finding in younger patients, may be lacking, while nausea and vomiting are reported in roughly half of elderly patients with appendicitis.[8,9,13] Diarrhea and urinary tract symptoms do not exclude the disease.

Fever may be absent in one-third or more. Tenderness in the right lower quadrant is a frequent finding occurring in 80 to 90 percent of these patients. The presence of peritoneal signs such as rigidity and rebound tenderness have been reported to range from 20 percent to more than 80 percent.[8] Laboratory assessment is potentially misleading, as 20 percent will have a white blood cell count below 10,000.[9,13] Abdominal radiographs rarely add to the diagnostic process and can lead one astray by suggesting small bowel obstruction.[8,9]

It is prudent to include appendicitis in the differential diagnosis of any elderly patient with abdominal pain who has not undergone an appendectomy. The clinician must not expect a neat diagnostic package. In one series, only 20 percent of older patients with appendicitis had all of fever, nausea or vomiting, tenderness in the right lower quadrant, and an elevated white blood count.[13]

Acute Cholecystitis

Acute cholecystitis (see Chap. 81) is the most common surgical emergency in older patients with abdominal pain. Fortunately, physicians have a record of high diagnostic accuracy for this condition in the elderly.[6] The presenting features of acute cholecystitis in the older population are similar to those in younger patients. Right-upper-quadrant or epigastric pain is present in most patients, while radiation to the back or shoulder area occurs in about one-third. Roughly half will report nausea or vomiting, and jaundice will occur in 10 to 30 percent. Fever may be absent in over half of these patients. Laboratory testing may be misleading, as 30 to 40 percent can have a normal white blood cell count. Plain radiographs are of little value; the diagnostic study of choice is ultrasonography. Computed tomography is generally of limited usefulness.[8,10,15]

Conservative management is generally unsuccessful and operative delay increases the complication rate. The older patient can appear deceptively well with acute cholecystitis; however, the overall mortality rate approximates 10 percent.[16] Additionally, a clinical picture of fever, jaundice, and altered mental status without significant abdominal findings has been described in a subset of elderly patients with acute cholecystitis.

Small Bowel Obstruction

The diagnosis of small bowel obstruction is usually straightforward in the older patient (see Chap. 75). Colicky pain, distention, and vomiting that progresses from gastric contents to bile-stained to feculent are the cardinal features. Prior surgery is still the principal risk factor in this age group, and the physician should conduct a careful search for hernias. A missed hernia can lead to a fatal outcome. The mortality rate for small bowel obstruction in the elderly ranges from 14 to 45 percent. Errors in management most frequently relate to misinterpretation of radiographic studies and excessive delays in operative management.[7]

Perforated Peptic Ulcer

Although peptic ulcer disease most frequently presents as gastrointestinal bleeding, perforation is an important cause of abdominal pain in the older patient (see Chap. 73). The expected description of a sudden, acute onset of epigastric pain is reported in only one-half of patients over age 70 with a perforated ulcer.[6] The pain has usually been present only for a matter of hours and is generally severe, constant, and present to some degree in the epigastrium. Free intraperitoneal perforation can cause generalized pain or lower-quadrant symptoms.[8] Vomiting is infrequent. The physical examination is expected to reveal epigastric tenderness, although muscular guarding is variable. In one study, only 21 percent of the elderly with a perforated ulcer had epigastric rigidity.[6] Fever is generally not present early on.

The key diagnostic mistake is excluding this diagnosis because of a lack of "free air" on plain radiographs. Roughly 40 percent of patients with perforated ulcers will not have this finding on their initial radiographs. The left lateral decubitus view or the lateral view of the upright chest radiograph may help to detect the presence of free air. Repeat radiographs after installation of 500 mL of air by a nasogastric tube increases the diagnostic yield of plain radiographs. Computed tomography is capable of detecting small amounts of air in the peritoneal cavity. In one series, missed perforated ulcer was the leading cause of death in elderly patients with abdominal pain, and in each case the plain radiographs did not reveal free air.[7]

Large Bowel Obstruction

A carcinoma is the leading cause of large bowel obstruction, while volvulus and diverticulitis account for most of the remaining cases. All of these precipitating conditions are more common in the elderly. The overall mortality rate approximates 40 percent. Distention is common, vomiting and constipation are reported in about half the patients. Importantly, a significant percentage (up to 20 percent) will report diarrhea. A history of rectal bleeding, altered bowel habits, or weight loss may be present with underlying carcinoma.[12] The pain is usually gradual in onset; however, cecal volvulus can present with the acute onset of severe, colicky pain.[17] Sigmoid volvulus is two to three times more frequent than cecal volvulus and more commonly presents with a gradual onset of pain.[18] Fever or the presence of peritoneal irritation suggests a perforation or gangrenous bowel.

The principal diagnostic study is plain abdominal radiography; however, cecal volvulus may appear as small bowel obstruction and require a barium enema to make the diagnosis.[17] In one large series, a cecal diameter of 10 cm was not useful in predicting perforation. In fact, cecal diameters of up to 20 cm responded to routine decompression methods.[12] Colonic pseudoobstruction, also known as Ogilvie's syndrome, can present in a manner similar to that of large bowel obstruction. This is massive gaseous distention of the colon, generally occurring in chronically ill, immobilized older patients. The abdomen is distended and tympanitic but usually nontender. A cavernous rectal vault is an important clue on physical examination. Old medical records frequently reveal several such presentations. It is important to avoid surgery in these patients as there is no underlying mechanical blockage.[19]

Diverticulitis

The presence of diverticulae increases with age and acute inflammation, diverticulitis, is a common cause of abdominal pain in the older patient (see Chap. 77). This is covered in a separate chapter, however, there are a few important points worth emphasizing. First, computed tomography is the diagnostic study of choice, as a barium enema or colonoscopy can precipitate perforation. Second, diverticulitis can be mistaken for a pelvic mass of gynecologic origin in the older female.

Acute Mesenteric Infarction

The management of mesenteric ischemia is complicated by diagnostic delays that are often associated with a fatal outcome. An aggressive approach is necessary, as early diagnosis markedly improves the chances of survival.[20] The key to making the correct diagnosis is to consider this possibility in the elderly patient with abdominal pain and risk factors for the disease. Superior mesenteric artery occlusion accounts for roughly half of the cases, with embolus and thrombus nearly equal as the source. Nonocclusive infarction accounts for another quarter of the cases, with inferior mesenteric artery occlusion, venous thrombosis, arteritis, and dissection making up the remainder.[21]

The specific risk factors to be aware of are listed in Table 69-2. The principal manifestation of mesenteric infarction is severe abdominal pain, often refractory to narcotic analgesics. Such severe pain combined with a relatively normal abdominal examination is considered the sine qua non of early mesenteric infarction. Despite its vascular nature, the overall spectrum of mesenteric ischemia involves a gradual onset of abdominal pain. If an embolus is the cause, sudden, severe pain may be reported.[20] Prior episodes can be reported, particularly if mesenteric arterial thrombosis is the cause. Associated gastrointestinal symptoms are very common and should not lead the physician astray. Nausea, anorexia, and vomiting are common, and up to half of these patients will report diarrhea. Objective findings on physical examination are inevitable and should be considered an indication of intestinal necrosis and possible perforation. Theoretically, the stool should be guaiac-negative early on. Approximately 60 percent will present with guaiac-positive stools.[21] Laboratory abnormalities such as metabolic acidosis and extreme leukocytosis are likewise indicators of advanced, perhaps irreversible disease.

TABLE 69-2 Risk Factors for Mesenteric Ischemia

Mesenteric Condition	Risk Factors
SMA embolus	Atrial fibrillation, recent MI
SMA thrombosis	Atherosclerosis, low-CO states
Nonocclusive infarction	Low-CO states (esp. CHF), digoxin therapy
Venous thrombosis	Hypercoagulability, prior DVT, liver disease

Key: SMA, superior mesenteric artery; MI, myocardial infarction; CO, cardiac output; CHF, congestive heart failure; DVT, deep venous thrombosis.

The critical aspect of care is to pursue mesenteric angiography based on the history and physical examination without waiting for "hard" evidence on the exam or diagnostic studies. One series reported a 90 percent survival rate when angiography was performed prior to the onset of peritonitis.[20] The usual survival rate is 30 percent or less.

Abdominal Aortic Aneurysm

Rupture of an abdominal aortic aneurysm is a lethal condition that will be more frequently encountered as the population ages (see Chap. 54). The incidence of abdominal aortic aneurysm in men increases rapidly after age 55 and peaks at the age of 80 at 5.9 percent. In women, the incidence rises quickly after age 70, peaking at 4.5 percent at age 90.[22] Early detection and elective repair are associated with a mortality rate of about 4.0 percent. The mortality rate among those who reach the hospital is generally on the order of 50 percent or higher. A favorable outcome depends on a rapid diagnosis and early operative intervention. Unfortunately, initial misdiagnosis is common, occurring in 30 percent of patients in one series.[11]

The most common symptom is abdominal pain, occurring in 70 to 80 percent, and not back pain, which is noted by just over half. The typical pain is sudden and significant. Atypical locations include the hips, inguinal area, and external genitalia. Syncope may be part of the presenting picture with or without significant blood loss from the aneurysm. Because of the lethal nature of this condition, the diagnosis should be considered in any older patient, especially male, with back, flank, or abdominal pain. Hypotension occurs at some point in the majority of these patients. Palpation of a tender, enlarged (>5 cm) aorta is the key physical finding. Unfortunately, the size of the aorta is often difficult to determine on examination.

Management of the unstable patient with a clinically suspected ruptured abdominal aortic aneurysm involves immediate operative intervention without confirmatory testing. A supine plain radiograph of the abdomen will often reveal a clue to the diagnosis, such as a calcified aortic outline or loss of the renal or psoas outline. In the stable patient, ultrasonography can delineate the size of the aorta, while computed tomography gives more information regarding actual rupture.[22] Any such testing should be expeditious and must include careful monitoring of the patient's condition, with appropriate alerting of the operating theater and surgical team.

The most common diagnostic mistake is to diagnose renal colic in these patients. This is understandable given the severe pain and the location of the pain. Furthermore, abdominal aortic aneurysm may present with hematuria. It should be axiomatic that aortic aneurysm be strongly considered in any patient over the age of 50 suspected of having renal colic. An episode of hypotension is often wrongly ascribed to developing sepsis or a ''vagal'' reaction in patients initially misdiagnosed as having renal colic.[11]

Other Conditions and Causes

The list presented above is certainly not comprehensive for abdominal pain in the elderly. Aortic dissection is common in this age group and may cause abdominal pain directly or by causing ischemia of intraabdominal organs, including the bowel. The diagnosis of pancreatitis in this age group is generally straightforward. Tumors can serve as lead points for intussusception in elderly patients. Acute gastric volvulus should be considered in the older patient with sudden epigastric pain, repetitive nonproductive retching, and inability to pass a nasogastric tube. Older patients with underlying vascular disease may develop ischemic colitis, which can be difficult to distinguish from other forms of colitis.

The list of other conditions that can cause abdominal pain in the older patient is extensive, highlighting the need for the comprehensive evaluation of such patients. The most important disease to suspect is acute myocardial ischemia. Some 1 to 2 percent of elderly patients with abdominal pain will be having a myocardial infarction.[10] Virtually all other ''chest'' diseases can cause abdominal pain, including pneumonia, pulmonary embolism, empyema, tuberculosis, congestive heart failure, esophageal rupture, and endocarditis. Genitourinary disease including renal colic, pyelonephritis, epididymitis, and testicular torsion is a possible cause of abdominal pain in the elderly. Diabetic ketoacidosis, herpes zoster, hypercalcemia, addisonian crisis, hemochromatosis, and retroperitoneal or rectus sheath hematomas secondary to anticoagulant therapy are examples of ''medical'' causes of abdominal pain in the elderly.

DIAGNOSTIC CONSIDERATIONS

A comprehensive review of diagnostic testing is available in the individual chapters covering the above conditions, however, certain general and specific points regarding the elderly patient are useful. The most critical axiom is to not let the results of diagnostic testing change your diagnostic thinking in the face of strong clinical evidence of a disease. Laboratory testing can be problematic in this age group. A normal white blood cell count cannot be used to exclude serious intraabdominal diseases, including those with an infectious component. For example, a normal total white blood cell count is found in 20 percent of elderly patients with appendicitis and 30 percent or more of those with cholecystitis. Serum amylase levels are frequently normal in the setting of pancreatitis. Serum lipase is more helpful but still not completely accurate. For the patient's sake, one should hope to see little or no evidence of lactic acidosis in mesenteric ischemia. An elevated bilirubin suggests hepatobiliary disease; however, in the ill older patient, this can be a nonspecific elevation. For example, up to 17 percent of elderly patients with appendicitis can have hyperbilirubinemia.[13] Since undiagnosed cancer is a frequent cause of ''nonspecific'' abdominal pain in older patients, the clinician must be careful not to ignore a low hemoglobin or microcytic indices on the blood count.

Radiographic studies can be equally problematic. Plain radiographs in the setting of perforated ulcer do not show free air in up to 40 percent of the patients. In appendicitis, the abdominal series is often interpreted as supporting the diagnosis of small bowel obstruction. Ogilvie's syndrome will commonly include a radiographic picture consistent with true large bowel obstruction.

Bedside ultrasound in capable hands can assist in rapidly securing the diagnosis of abdominal aortic aneurysm. It can also help clarify the clinical picture in acute cholecystitis and renal colic. Computed tomography is an important diagnostic modality in the older population with abdominal pain. The physician must remember that the unstable patient with a suspected abdominal aortic aneurysm belongs in the operating room and not in the computed tomography suite.

Treatment of the specific entities is covered more thoroughly elsewhere. General measures for the elderly patient with an acute abdominal condition overlap those of younger age groups. Specific useful measures include nasogastric decompression, fluid and blood component resuscitation as indicated, judicious use of narcotic analgesia, and tailored antibiotic coverage.

A period of observation with serial examinations should be considered in the elderly patient with undifferentiated abdominal pain. Depending on the circumstances, this could occur either in the ED, an observation unit, or in an inpatient unit. Patients with severe pain or worsening pain while in the ED should generally not be sent home. Resolved pain is generally reassurring, and such patients who are discharged should receive routine follow-up with their primary care providers. Biliary tract disease and underlying cancer are possibilities in this circumstance.[14]

If an older patient is to be discharged with abdominal pain, the patient should be instructed to return if the symptoms worsen or do not resolve in a brief period of time (6 to 8 h). Similarly, a time limit should be placed on vomiting, as this will quickly resolve in most benign causes. New vomiting after discharge should prompt reevaluation.

REFERENCES

1. Brewer RJ, Golden GT, Hitch DC, et al: Abdominal pain: An analysis of 1,000 consecutive cases in a university hospital emergency room. *Am J Surg* 131:219, 1976.
2. Bugliosi TF, Meloy TD, Vukov LF: Acute abdominal pain in the elderly. *Ann Emerg Med* 19:1383, 1990.
3. McCaig LF: *National Hospital Ambulatory Medical Care Survey: 1996 Emergency Department Summary.* Advance data from vital and health statistics, no. 293. Hyattsville, MD: National Center for Health Statistics, 1997.
4. McNamara RM, Rousseau E, Sanders AB: Geriatric emergency medicine: A survey of practicing emergency physicians. *Ann Emerg Med* 21:796, 1992.
5. Baum SA, Rubenstein LZ: Old people in the emergency room: Age related differences in emergency department use and care. *J Am Geriatr Soc* 35:398, 1987.
6. Fenyo G: Acute abdominal disease in the elderly: Experience from two series in Stockholm. *Am J Surg* 143:751, 1982.
7. Bender JS: Approach to the acute abdomen. *Med Clin North Am* 73:1413, 1989.
8. Fenyo G: Diagnostic problems of acute abdominal pain in the aged. *Acta Chir Scand* 140:396, 1974.
9. Owens BJ, Hamit HF: Appendicitis in the elderly. *Ann Surg* 172:306, 1970.
10. Ponka JL, Welborn JK, Brush BE: Acute abdominal pain in aged patients: An analysis of 200 cases. *J Am Geriatr Soc* 11:993, 1963.
11. Marston WA, Ahlquist R, Johnson G, et al: Misdiagnosis of ruptured abdominal aortic aneurysms. *J Vasc Surg* 16:17, 1992.
12. Greenlee HB, Pienkos EJ, Vanderbilt PC, et al: Acute large bowel obstruction. *Arch Surg* 108:470, 1974.
13. Horattas MC, Guyton DP, Wu D: A reappraisal of appendicitis in the elderly. *Am J Surg* 160:291, 1990.
14. DeDombal FT, Matharu SS, Staniland JR, et al: Presentation of cancer to hospital as ''acute abdominal pain.'' *Br J Surg* 67:413, 1980.
15. Parker LJ, Vukov LF, Wollan PC: Emergency department evaluation of geriatric patients with acute cholecystitis. *Acad Emerg Med* 4:51, 1997.
16. Glenn F: Surgical management of acute cholecystitis in patients 65 years of age and older. *Ann Surg* 193:56, 1981.
17. Andersson A, Bergdahl L, Van Der Linden W: Volvulus of the cecum. *Ann Surg* 181:876, 1976.
18. Anderson JR, Lee D: The management of sigmoid volvulus. *Br J Surg* 68:117, 1981.
19. Hyatt R: Colonic pseudo-obstruction: An important complication in hospitalized elderly patients. *Age Ageing* 16:145, 1987.
20. Boley SJ, Sprayregan S, Siegelman SS, et al: Initial results from an aggressive roentgenological and surgical approach to acute mesenteric ischemia. *Surgery* 82:848, 1977.
21. Ottinger LW: Mesenteric ischemia. *N Engl J Med* 307:535, 1982.
22. Ernst CB: Abdominal aortic aneurysm. *N Engl J Med* 328:1167, 193.

GASTROINTESTINAL BLEEDING

David T. Overton

Gastrointestinal (GI) bleeding is a common problem in emergency medical practice and should be considered potentially life-threatening until proven otherwise.

Acute upper GI bleeding in adults has an overall annual incidence of approximately 100 per 100,000. It is more common among males and markedly more common among the elderly. Its associated mortality rises with age.[1,2] Lower GI bleeding is somewhat less common, with an annual incidence of approximately 20 per 100,000. It, too, is more common among males and among the elderly.[3]

As with all true emergencies, the traditional triad of medical history, physical examination, and diagnosis often must be accomplished simultaneously with resuscitation and stabilization. Factors associated with a high morbidity rate are hemodynamic instability, repeated hematemesis or hematochezia, failure to clear with gastric lavage, age over 60, and coexistent organ system disease.

PATHOPHYSIOLOGY

Causes of Upper Gastrointestinal Bleeding

Upper GI bleeding is defined as that originating proximal to the ligament of Treitz, whereas lower GI bleeding originates more distally.

PEPTIC ULCER DISEASE Peptic ulcer disease, including gastric, duodenal, and stomal ulcers, remains the most common etiology for upper GI hemorrhage, encompassing approximately 60 percent of all cases.[2] Duodenal ulcers, approximately 29 percent of the total, will rebleed in approximately 10 percent of cases, usually within 24 to 48 h. Gastric ulcers, approximately 16 percent of all cases, are more likely to rebleed. Stomal ulcers are uncommon (less than 5 percent of all upper GI bleeds) and are present in only one-third of bleeding patients with a history of prior peptic ulcer surgery.

EROSIVE GASTRITIS AND ESOPHAGITIS Erosive gastritis, esophagitis, and duodenitis together are responsible for approximately 15 percent of all cases of upper GI hemorrhage. Irritative factors, such as alcohol, salicylates, and nonsteroidal anti-inflammatory agents, are predisposing factors.

ESOPHAGEAL AND GASTRIC VARICES Esophageal and gastric varices result from portal hypertension and, in the United States, are most often a result of alcoholic liver disease. Although varices account for only about 6 percent of all cases of upper GI hemorrhage, they are highly likely to rebleed and carry a high mortality rate. Despite this, many patients with end-stage cirrhosis never develop varices, many patients with documented varices never bleed, and many patients with a documented history of varices presenting with upper GI bleeding will be bleeding from nonvariceal sites.

MALLORY-WEISS SYNDROME The Mallory-Weiss syndrome is upper GI bleeding secondary to a longitudinal mucosal tear in the cardioesophageal region. The classic history is repeated retching followed by bright red hematemesis, but coughing and seizures have also been reported as etiologic factors.

OTHER ETIOLOGIES Stress ulcer, arteriovenous malformation, and malignancy are other etiologies of upper GI hemorrhage. ENT (ear, nose, and throat) sources of bleeding can also masquerade as GI hemorrhage. An aortoenteric fistula secondary to an aortic graft is an unusual but important cause of bleeding to keep in mind. Classically, this will present as a self-limited ''herald'' bleed preceding a subsequent massive hemorrhage.

Causes of Lower Gastrointestinal Bleeding

The most common cause of what initially appears to be lower GI bleeding is actually upper GI bleeding. Thus, proximal etiologies should be sought.

Among patients with an established lower GI source of their bleeding, the most common etiology is hemorrhoids. Among nonhemorrhoidal bleeding, angiodysplasia and diverticular disease are most common, followed by adenomatous polyps and malignancies.[4]

DIVERTICULOSIS Diverticular bleeding is usually painless and is thought to result from erosion into the penetrating artery of the diverticulum. Diverticular bleeding may be massive. Patients are often elderly with underlying medical illnesses that contribute to both the morbidity and the mortality rates.

ANGIODYSPLASIA Arteriovenous malformations (angiodysplasia), usually of the right colon, are a common etiology of obscure lower GI bleeding, particularly in the elderly population. They are thought to be more common in patients with hypertension and aortic stenosis.

OTHER ETIOLOGIES Numerous other lesions may result in lower GI hemorrhage. Although carcinoma and hemorrhoids are relatively common causes of bleeding, massive hemorrhage is unusual. Similarly, inflammatory bowel disease, polyps, and infectious gastroenteritis rarely cause severe bleeding. Finally, Meckel diverticulum is an unusual but important etiology to keep in mind.

DIAGNOSIS

Medical History

Although the medical history may suggest the source of bleeding, it is often misleading. Thus, clinicians should strive to maintain a broad differential and clinical approach. Although most patients will volunteer complaints of hematemesis, hematochezia, or melena, GI bleeding may have more subtle presentations. Patients who present with hypotension, tachycardia, angina, syncope, weakness, confusion, or even cardiac arrest may harbor occult, underlying GI hemorrhage.

Historical features such as hematemesis, coffee-ground emesis, melena, or hematochezia should be sought. Classically, hematemesis or coffee-round emesis suggests a source proximal to the right colon, and hematochezia indicates a more distal colorectal lesion. However, exceptions to these rules occur. Weight loss and changes in bowel habits are classic symptoms of malignancy. Vomiting and retching, followed by hematemesis, is suggestive of a Mallory-Weiss tear. A history of an aortic graft should suggest the possibility of an aortoenteric fistula. A history of medication use should be determined, particularly salicylates, glucocorticoids, nonsteroidal anti-inflammatory agents, and anticoagulants. Alcohol abuse is strongly associated with a number of causes of GI bleeding, including peptic ulcer disease, erosive gastritis, and esophageal varices. Ingestion of iron or bismuth can simulate melena, and certain foods, such as beets, can simulate hematochezia. In such instances, stool guaiac testing will be negative. Finally, a prior history of GI bleeding should be sought, although recurrent bleeding episodes often originate from different sources.

Physical Examination

The vital signs may reveal obvious hypotension and tachycardia, or more subtle manifestations such as a decreased pulse pressure or tachypnea. Clinicians should remember that some patients can tolerate substantial volume losses with minimal or no changes in vital signs. Similarly, paradoxical bradycardia can occur in the face of profound hypovolemia.

Skin findings should be noted. Cool, clammy skin is an obvious sign of shock. Spider angiomata, palmar erythema, jaundice, and gynecomastia suggest underlying liver disease. Petechiae and purpura suggest an underlying coagulopathy. Skin findings may be suggestive of the Peutz-Jeghers, Rendu-Osler-Weber, or Gardner syndromes. A careful ENT examination may occasionally reveal an occult bleeding source that has resulted in swallowed blood and subsequent coffee-ground emesis or melena. The abdominal examination may disclose tenderness, masses, ascites, or organomegaly. A rectal examination is indicated to detect the presence of blood, its appearance (bright red, maroon, or melanotic), and the presence of masses.

Laboratory Data

In patients with significant GI bleeding, the most important laboratory test is to type and crossmatch blood. Another important laboratory test is the complete blood count. Additionally, blood urea nitrogen (BUN), creatinine, electrolyte, glucose, and coagulation studies, as well as liver function studies, should be considered. The initial hematocrit level often will not reflect the actual amount of blood loss. Upper tract hemorrhage may elevate the BUN through digestion and absorption of hemoglobin. Coagulation studies, including prothrombin time, partial thromboplastin time, and platelet count, are of obvious benefit in patients taking anticoagulants or those with underlying hepatic disease. An electrocardiogram should be considered in patients in the coronary artery disease age group. Silent ischemia can occur secondary to the decreased oxygen delivery accompanying significant GI bleeding and, thus, supplemental oxygen is advised for such patients.

Diagnostic Studies

Routine abdominal radiographs are often obtained in patients with GI bleeding. In the absence of specific indications, they are of limited value. Similarly, routine admission chest x-rays for patients with acute GI hemorrhage, even those admitted to the intensive care unit, have been shown to be of limited utility in the absence of known pulmonary disease or abnormal findings on lung exam.[5] Barium contrast studies are similarly of limited diagnostic value in an emergency setting. Furthermore, barium limits the use of subsequent endoscopy or angiography.

Angiography can sometimes detect the site of bleeding, particularly in cases of obscure lower tract hemorrhage. Moreover, angiography permits therapeutic options such as transcatheter arterial embolization or the infusion of vasoconstrictive agents. However, to be diagnostic, angiography requires a relatively brisk bleeding rate (0.5 to 2.0 mL/min).

Technetium-labeled red cell scans have also been used to localize the site of bleeding in obscure hemorrhage. Such localization can be used to map the therapeutic approach, whether via angiography or operatively. Scintigraphy appears more sensitive than angiography and can localize the site of bleeding at a rate of 0.1 mL/min.

Another approach is colonoscopy, which may be not only diagnostic, but through the use of endoscopic hemostasis, also therapeutic. In most circumstances, endoscopy is more accurate than arteriography or scintigraphy.

Controversy in the literature remains as to whether scintigraphy, angiography, or colonoscopy, and in which order, should be the initial diagnostic procedure of choice in the evaluation of lower GI bleeding.[6–9] Thus, these decisions are often based on local availability and consultant preference.

TREATMENT

Primary

Immediate resuscitative measures take priority. Patients with profuse upper GI hemorrhage may require definitive airway management to prevent aspiration of blood. Oxygen should be administered, and cardiac monitoring is indicated. Volume replacement should be initiated with crystalloids via large-bore intravenous lines. The decision to administer blood should be based on the clinical findings of volume depletion or continued bleeding, rather that on initial hematocrit values. General guidelines for initiation of blood transfusion are continued active bleeding and failure to improve perfusion and vital signs after the infusion of 2 L of crystalloid. The threshold for blood transfusion should be lower in the elderly. Coagulation factors should be replaced as needed. A urinary catheter is indicated in patients with hypotension.

A nasogastric (NG) tube should be placed in all patients with significant GI bleeding, regardless of the presumed source. Concerns that NG tube passage may provoke bleeding in patients with varices are unwarranted. Bright red or maroon blood per rectum unexpectedly originates from upper GI sources approximately 14 percent of the time.[10] A negative gastric aspirate does not conclusively exclude an upper GI etiology and may result from intermittent bleeding or from pyloric spasm or edema preventing reflux of duodenal blood. If bright red blood or clots are found on NG aspiration, gentle gastric lavage should be performed. To be effective, a large-bore tube, usually oral, must be used. Room temperature water is the preferred irrigant, as iced solutions have no proven benefit and have theoretical disadvantages.[11] The addition of levarterenol to the lavage solution is similarly of unproven benefit. Overvigorous suction should be avoided, because it may produce gastric erosions that can confuse findings on subsequent endoscopy.

Secondary

ENDOSCOPY Upper GI endoscopy is the most accurate technique for the identification of upper tract bleeding sites. It predicts morbidity, and, with the advent of therapeutic endoscopy, is associated with improved outcomes. Early therapeutic endoscopy, where available, should be considered the treatment of choice for significant upper GI bleeding. Thus, early consultation for potential endoscopy should be considered in patients with significant hemorrhage.

Esophageal varices can be endoscopically treated by either band ligation or injection sclerotherapy. Sclerotherapy, which controls acute hemorrhage in up to 90 percent of patients, may decrease the duration of hospitalization and amount of blood transfused when compared with portal-caval shunting. However, complications of sclerotherapy include perforation, sepsis, stricture formation, and portal and mesenteric venous thrombosis. Endoscopic band ligation appears to be as effective as sclerotherapy, but with a decreased incidence of complications, particularly rebleeding and esophageal stricture formation.[12] In addition, band ligation appears superior to sclerotherapy in the long-term management of varices.[13]

Endoscopic hemostasis (with injection sclerotherapy, electrocoagulation, heater probes, and lasers) has been used successfully in a variety of nonvariceal etiologies of upper GI bleeding, as well.

In lower GI bleeding, proctoscopy is often diagnostic in patients with anorectal sources of bleeding, such as hemorrhoids. If an anorectal source is suspected, the patient should be carefully evaluated for significant volume loss or more dangerous proximal sources of bleeding mimicking anorectal bleeding. Colonoscopy can be diagnostic in other forms of lower tract hemorrhage, such as diverticulosis or angiodysplasia, and may also allow ablation of bleeding sites by using the aforementioned technologies.

DRUG THERAPY Infusions of somatostatin and its synthetic, longer-acting derivative, octreotide, have been shown to be effective in reducing bleeding from both varices and peptic ulcer disease. Octreotide has been shown to be as effective as sclerotherapy in acute variceal bleeding.[14] Both agents, when used in addition to sclerotherapy, are more effective than sclerotherapy alone.[15,16] These agents possess the advantages of vasopressin, with considerably fewer side effects. They should be considered useful adjuncts, either before endoscopy or when endoscopy is unsuccessful, contraindicated, or unavailable.[17]

Vasopressin has been used in the past to control GI bleeding, most commonly from varices. However, adverse reactions are common, including hypertension, dysrrhythmias, myocardial and splanchnic ischemia, decreased cardiac output, and gangrene from local infiltration. Although the concomitant use of nitroglycerin has been shown to reduce the incidence of these side effects, the use of vasopressin has been largely supplanted by the use of somatostatin, octreotide, and therapeutic endoscopy.

Studies have also suggested that the proton-pump inhibitor omeprazole may be useful to reduce rebleeding, transfusion requirements, and the need for surgery in the treatment of bleeding peptic ulcers.[18,19]

Other drugs may be of benefit in patients with GI hemorrhage, but are of less concern in the initial emergency department management. For instance, β-blocker therapy has been shown to be beneficial in patients with varices, in preventing both initial variceal bleeds and rebleeding.[20,21] Additionally, the treatment of *Helicobacter pylori* infection with antibiotics reduces the recurrence of peptic ulcer and rebleeding.[22] However, the use of H_2 antagonists in acute upper GI hemorrhage remains of unproven benefit,[23] with no conclusive evidence for reduction in the rates of rebleeding, surgery, or death.

BALLOON TAMPONADE Balloon tamponade with the Sengstaken-Blakemore tube or its variants can provide therapeutic benefit and presumptive diagnostic information. It can control documented variceal hemorrhage in 40 to 80 percent of patients. The device consists of gastric and esophageal balloons and, depending on the variation, may include gastric and/or esophageal aspiration ports. The gastric balloon should be inflated first. If bleeding does not cease, the esophageal balloon should then be inflated, using a manometer to ensure that the pressure does not exceed 40 to 50 mmHg. Radiologic confirmation of proper balloon placement is suggested. The device should be kept in place 24 h after bleeding has ceased. Some authors recommend deflating the esophageal balloon for 30 to 60 min every 8 h to prevent mucosal ulceration.

Like vasopressin therapy, balloon tamponade is frequently associated with adverse reactions, often severe. Mucosal ulceration, esophageal or gastric rupture, asphyxiation from dislodged balloons, tracheal compression secondary to balloon inflation, and aspiration pneumonia have all been reported. Many authors recommend routine prophylactic endotracheal intubation to prevent pulmonary complications. Because of the incidence of adverse reactions, the use of balloon tamponade has decreased considerably and should be considered an adjunctive or temporizing measure supplementing the more definitive modalities of band ligation or sclerotherapy.

SURGERY With patients who do not respond to medical therapy, and in whom endoscopic hemostasis, if available, fails, emergency surgical intervention is indicated. Surgical consultation on any patient admitted to the hospital for GI bleeding is prudent, in case uncontrollable rebleeding occurs.

DISPOSITION

Patients with GI hemorrhage will require hospital admission, and early referral to an endoscopist is advisable. Corley and colleagues[24] found five variables to be independent predictors of adverse outcomes in upper GI bleeding: initial hematocrit less than 30 percent, initial systolic blood pressure lower than 100 mm Hg, red blood in the NG lavage, history of cirrhosis or ascites on exam, and a history of vomiting red blood. Such patients are more likely to require a higher intensity of inpatient care.

On the other hand, other authors have attempted to identify a low-risk subset of patients who might be managed as outpatients. Rockall and coworkers[25] developed a risk score for upper GI bleeding, based on age, presence of shock, comorbidity, diagnosis, and endoscopic findings, to identify a low-risk population. Longstreth and Feitelberg[26] developed similar guidelines. Of note, both of these recommendations are based on the performance of endoscopy prior to discharge to classify patients accurately.

REFERENCES

1. Rockall TA, Logan RF, Devlin HB, et al: Incidence of and mortality from acute upper gastrointestinal hemorrhage in the United Kingdom: Steering Committee and members of the National Audit of Acute Upper Gastrointestinal Haemorrhage. *BMJ* 311:222, 1995.
2. Longstreth GF: Epidemiology and outcome of patients hospitalized with acute lower gastrointestinal hemorrhage: A population-based study. *Am J Gastroenterol* 92:419, 1997.
3. Longstreth GF: Epidemiology of hospitalization for acute upper gastrointestinal hemorrhage: A population-based study. *Am J Gastroenterol* 90:206, 1995.
4. Machicado GA, Jensen DM: Acute and chronic management of lower gastrointestinal bleeding: Cost-effective approaches. *Gastroenterologist* 5:189, 1997.
5. Tobin K, Klein J, Barbieri C, et al: Utility of routine admission chest radiographs in patients with acute gastrointestinal hemorrhage admitted to an intensive care unit. *Am J Med* 101:349, 1996.
6. Suzman MS, Talmor M, Jennis R, et al: Accurate localization and surgical management of active lower gastrointestinal hemorrhage with technetium-labeled erythrocyte scintigraphy. *Ann Surg* 224:29, 1996.
7. Vernava AM, Moore BA, Longo WE, et al: Lower gastrointestinal bleeding. *Dis Colon Rectum* 40:846, 1997.
8. Richter JM, Christensen MR, Kaplan LM, et al: Effective of current technology in the diagnosis and management of lower gastrointestinal hemorrhage. *Gastrointest Endosc* 41:93, 1995.
9. Ng DA, Opekla FG, Beck DE, et al: Predictive value of technetium Tc 99m-labelled red blood cell scintigraphy for positive angiogram in massive lower gastrointestinal hemorrhage. *Dis Colon Rectum* 40:471, 1997.
10. Wilcox CM, Alexander LN, Cotsonis G: A prospective characterization of upper gastrointestinal hemorrhage presenting with hematochezia. *Am J Gastroenterol* 92:231, 1997.
11. Leather RA, et al: Iced gastric lavage: A tradition without foundation. *Can Med Assoc J* 136:1245, 1987.
12. Cello JP: Endoscopy management of esophageal variceal hemorrhage: Injection, banding, glue, octreotide or a combination? *Semin Gastrointest Dis* 8:179, 1997.
13. Avgerinos A, Armonis A, Manokakopoulos S, et al: Endoscopic sclerotherapy versus variceal ligation in the long-term management of patients with cirrhosis after variceal bleeding: A prospective randomized study. *J Hepatol* 26:1034, 1997.
14. Jenkins SA, Shields R, Davies M, et al: A multicenter randomized trial comparing octreotide and injection sclerotherapy in the management and outcome of acute variceal hemorrhage. *Gut* 41:526, 1997.
15. Avgerinos A, Nevens F, Raptis S, et al: Early administration of somatostatin and efficacy of sclerotherapy in acute oesophageal variceal bleeds: The European Acute Bleeding Oesophageal Variceal Episodes (ABOVE) randomized trial. *Lancet* 350:1495, 1997.
16. Beeson I, Ingrand P, Person B, et al: Sclerotherapy with or without octreotide for acute variceal bleeding. *N Engl J Med* 333:555, 1995.
17. Imperiale TF, Birgisson S: Somatostatin or octreotide compared with H_2 antagonists and placebo in the management of acute nonvariceal upper gastrointestinal hemorrhage: A meta-analysis. *Ann Intern Med* 127:1062, 1997.
18. Khuroo MS, Yattoo GN, Javid G, et al: A comparison of omeprazole and placebo for bleeding peptic ulcer. *N Engl J Med* 336:1054, 1997.
19. Schaffalitzky de Muckadell OB, Havelund T, Harding H, et al: Effect of omeprazole on the outcome of endoscopically treated bleeding peptic ulcers:

Randomized double-blind placebo-controlled multicentre study. *Scand J Gastroenterol* 32:320, 1997.

20. Grace ND: Diagnosis and treatment of gastrointestinal bleeding secondary to portal hypertension: American College of Gastroenterology Practice Parameters Committee. *Am J Gastroenterol* 92:1081, 1997.
21. Avgerinos A, Rekoumis G, Klonis C, et al: Propranolol in the prevention of recurrent upper gastrointestinal bleeding in patients with cirrhosis undergoing endoscopic sclerotherapy: A randomized controlled trial. *J Hepatol* 19:301, 1993.
22. Santander C, Gravalos RG, Gomez-Cedenilla A, et al: Antimicrobial therapy for *Helicobacter pylori* infection versus long-term maintenance antisecretion treatment in the prevention of recurrent hemorrhage from peptic ulcer: Prospective nonrandomized trial on 125 patients. *Am J Gastroenterol* 91:1549, 1996.
23. Collins R, Langman M: Treatment with histamine H_2 antagonists in acute upper gastrointestinal hemorrhage: Implications of randomized trials. *N Engl J Med* 313:660, 1985.
24. Corley DA, Stefan AM, Wolf M, et al: Early indicators of prognosis in upper gastrointestinal hemorrhage. *Am J Gastroenterol* 93:336, 1998.
25. Rockall TA, Logan RF, Devlin HB, et al: Selection of patients for early discharge or outpatient care after acute upper gastrointestinal haemorrhage: National Audit of Acute Upper Gastrointestinal Haemorrhage. *Lancet* 347:1138, 1996.
26. Longstreth GF, Feitelberg SP: Outpatient care of selected patients with acute non-variceal upper gastrointestinal haemorrhage. *Lancet* 345:108, 1995.

ESOPHAGEAL EMERGENCIES

Moss H. Mendelson

Patients develop a wide variety of problems related to the esophagus. The complaints of dysphagia, odynophagia, or ingested foreign body immediately point to the esophagus as a source of disease. But the esophagus can be the site of pathology in patients presenting with chest pain, upper gastrointestinal bleeding, malignancy, and mediastinitis. Many esophageal processes can be evaluated over time in an outpatient setting, but several, such as variceal bleeding and esophageal perforation, can be fulminant and rapidly fatal, requiring a unique knowledge base for emergent intervention.

ANATOMY AND PHYSIOLOGY

The esophagus is a muscular tube approximately 20 to 25 cm long. The majority of the esophagus is located in mediastinum, posterior and slightly lateral to the trachea, with smaller cervical and abdominal components as well, as shown in Fig. 71-1. There is an outer longitudinal muscle layer and an inner circular muscle layer. The upper third of the esophagus is made up of striated muscle. Distal to the upper third, smooth muscle appears as well, and the esophagus is all smooth muscle from the lower half down [including the lower esophageal sphincter (LES)]. The cells lining the esophagus are stratified squamous epithelial cells that have no secretory function.

Two sphincters on either end regulate the passage of materials into and out of the esophagus. The upper esophageal sphincter (UES) prevents air from entering the esophagus and food from refluxing out of the esophagus into the pharynx. The LES regulates passage of food into the stomach and prevents stomach contents from refluxing into the esophagus. The UES is composed primarily of the cricopharyngeus muscle. Additional tone is variably provided by the inferior pharyngeal constrictor and the cervical esophagus.[1] The UES has a resting pressure of around 100 mmHg. The LES is not discretely identifiable anatomically. The smooth muscle of the lower 1 to 2 cm of the esophagus, in combination with the skeletal muscle of the diaphragmatic hiatus, functions as the sphincter, with a resting pressure of 25 mmHg.[2] The pressure within the resting esophagus itself closely approximates intrathoracic pressure.[3] Dysfunction of the LES is a major source of esophageal symptoms and is discussed below.

Three major anatomic constrictions exist within the esophagus and are important when considering esophageal foreign bodies and food bolus impaction, discussed below. They are located at the cricopharyngeus muscle, at the level of the aortic arch/left main-stem bronchus, and at the gastroesophageal junction. An empty, collapsed esophagus has no apparent constrictions: only with esophageal filling do the narrowings become apparent.

Innervation of the esophagus is mediated by both the sympathetic and parasympathetic systems and local nerve networks. Both Auerbach's and Meissner's plexuses are present in the esophagus, in the same distribution noted throughout the gastrointestinal tract. Reflex activity and homeostasis are also mediated by parasympathetic afferents and efferents, carried by the vagus nerve. Pain sensation from heat, spasm, distension, or chemical irritation of the esophagus travels exclusively through sympathetic nerve fibers. The heart has a pattern of innervation mirroring that of the esophagus, and there is a convergence of visceral and somatic stimuli within the sympathetic system. This is the anatomic basis that makes esophageal and cardiac chest pain notoriously similar, as discussed below.[4]

The esophageal blood supply is derived from several arterial sources. The inferior thyroid artery, small branches of the thoracic aorta, and ascending branches form the left gastric and inferior phrenic arteries supply the esophagus throughout its length. The esophageal venous circulation includes a submucosal plexus of veins that drains into another plexus of veins surrounding the outside of the esophagus. Blood flows from this plexus into the inferior thyroid, azygos, coronary, and gastric venous systems. The last is one link between the portal and systemic venous systems. Variceal dilatation of the submucosal system can be responsible for massive upper gastrointestinal (GI) bleeding, reviewed below.

Swallowing is initiated voluntarily, then becomes reflex controlled. Control of the swallowing mechanism is provided by both central nervous system (CNS) input and local reflex feedback. As food is moved to the posterior pharynx during the pharyngeal stage of swallowing, the UES relaxes and the bolus passes into the esophagus. Generally this occurs within the first 2 s of swallowing. The food bolus in the upper esophagus subsequently reinitiates constriction of the UES. Peristalsis moves the food bolus down the esophagus (5 to 6 s) to the LES. The LES relaxes (but remains closed) with the onset of swallowing, remains relaxed for the 5 to 10 s it takes for the food bolus to make the trip down, and then recontracts with the peristaltic wave.[5] Simultaneous reflexes outside of the esophagus help to protect the pharynx and larynx from inadvertent reception of food. Impairment of the swallowing mechanism is reviewed below.

DYSPHAGIA

Dysphagia is defined as difficulty with swallowing. The vast majority of patients experiencing dysphagia will have an identifiable, organic process causing their symptoms.

The literature suggests an approach to patients with dysphagia that recognizes two broad pathophysiologic groups, patients with transfer dysphagia and patients with transport dysphagia.[6] Transfer dysphagia occurs very early in the swallowing process as the food bolus moves from the oropharynx through the UES and is often reported as difficulty in initiating a swallow. In transport dysphagia, there is impaired movement of the bolus down the esophagus and through the LES. Transport dysphagia is perceived later in the swallowing process, usually 2 to 4 s or more after swallowing is initiated, and most commonly results in the feeling of food "getting stuck." This initial differentiation between transfer and transport dysphagia provides valuable information regarding the likely underlying esophageal pathology, as noted in Table 71-1. Another useful classification scheme divides dysphagia into obstructive disease versus motor dysfunction. Functional or motil-

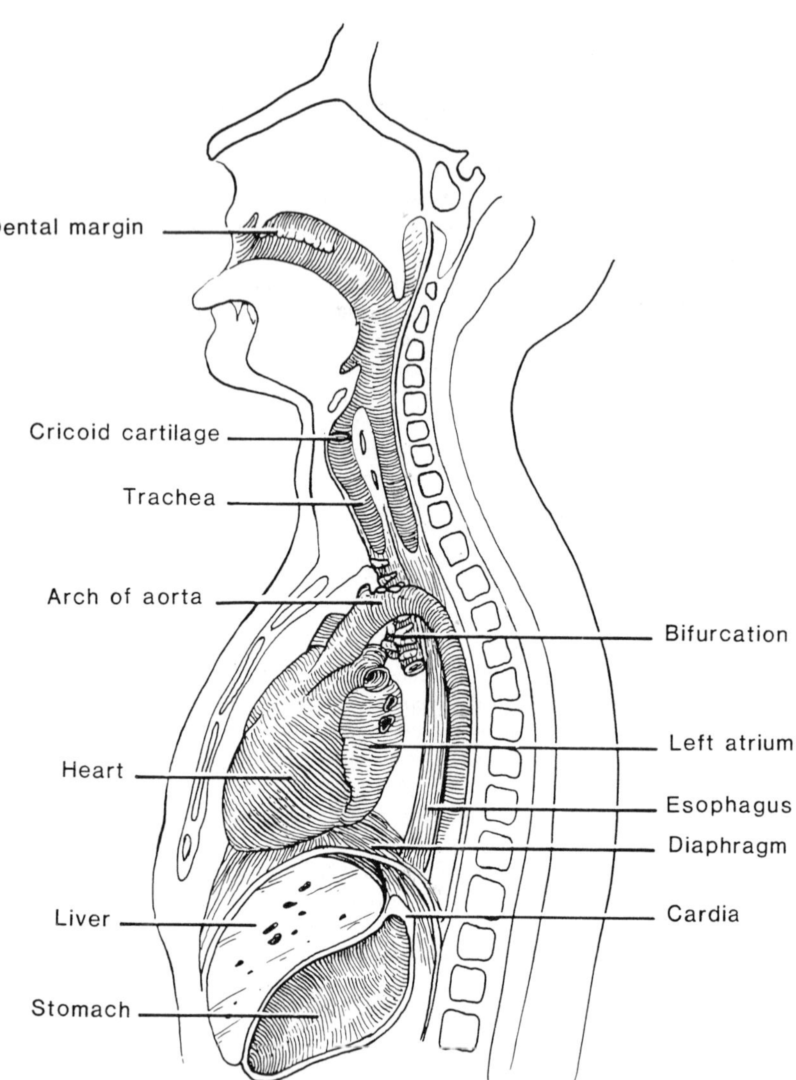

FIG. 71-1. Anatomic relations of the esophagus (seen from the left side). The esophagus is about 25 cm (10 in.) long. The distance from the upper incisor teeth to the beginning of the esophagus (cricoid cartilage) is about 15 cm (6 in.); from the upper incisors to the level of the bronchi, 22 to 23 cm (9 in.); to the cardia, 40 cm (16 in.). Structures contiguous to the esophagus that affect esophageal function are demonstrated.

TABLE 71-1 Dysphagia

Transfer Dysphagia (Oropharyngeal)	Transport Dysphagia (Esophageal)
Discoordination in transferring bolus from pharynx to esophagus	Improper transfer of the bolus from the upper esophagus into the stomach
Swallowing symptoms—gagging, coughing, nasal regurgitation, inability to initiate swallow, need for repeated swallows	Swallowing symptoms—food "sticking," retrosternal fullness with solids (and eventually liquids), possibly odynophagia
Risk of aspiration present	Risk of aspiration present, generally less pronounced than in transfer dysphagia
Long term—weight loss, malnutrition, chronic bronchitis, asthma, multiple episodes of pneumonia	Long term—malnutrition, dehydration, weight loss, systemic effects of cancer
Neuromuscular disease (80%)—cerebrovascular accident; polymyositis and dermatomyositis, scleroderma, myasthenia gravis, tetanus; Parkinson's disease, botulism, lead poisoning, thyroid disease	Obstructive disease (85%)—foreign body; carcinoma, webs, strictures, thyroid enlargement, diverticulum, congenital or acquired large vessel abnormalities
Localized disease—pharyngitis; aphthous ulcers; candidal infection; peritonsillar and retropharyngeal abscesses; carcinoma of tongue, pharynx, larynx; Zenker diverticulum; cricopharyngeal bar; cervical osteophytes	Motor disorder—achalasia, peristaltic dysfunction (nutcracker esophagus), diffuse esophageal spasm, scleroderma
Inadequate lubrication—scleroderma	Inflammatory disease

ity disorders usually cause dysphagia that is intermittent and variable. Mechanical or obstructive disease is usually progressive (solids, then liquids).

Clinical Features

As noted above, historical information is key to the diagnosis of dysphagia. Table 71-1 summarizes some of the clinical features of transfer versus transport dysphagia. Though often occurring as an independent symptom, dysphagia can be associated with odynophagia, which is painful swallowing (suggesting an inflammatory process), or with chest pain that is esophageal in nature and suggests gastroesophageal reflux disease (GERD) or a motility disorder. Additional pertinent historical features to elicit in a patient complaining of dysphagia include the following: Has this been an acute, subacute, or chronic course? Is the dysphagia present for solids, liquids, or both? Is it intermittent or progressive? Is there a sensation of the food being stuck in the esophagus, and where? Is there any past history of esophageal disease? Transport dysphagia that is present for solids only generally suggests a mechanical/obstructive process. Motility disorders typically cause transport dysphagia for solids and liquids.

A poorly chewed meat bolus that impacts in the esophagus is a well-recognized complication of esophageal disease. A preceding history of dysphagia may or may not be obtained. This can be the presenting complaint of a patient with a variety of esophageal pathologies. The bolus may be well localized by the patient; in general, patients able to identify a level of dysphagia below the neck are usually anatomically accurate, whereas those complaining of dysphagia in the neck may be reporting sensations referred from elsewhere in the esophagus.[7] Esophageal filling proximal to the impacted bolus may make the patient unable to swallow secretions and may present an airway/aspiration risk.

Physical examination of patients with dysphagia should focus on the head and neck and the neurologic exam. Signs of previous cerebrovascular accident, muscle disease, or Parkinson's disease can be present. Cachexia and cervical or supraclavicular nodes can be observed in patients with cancer of the esophagus. Watching the patient as he or she takes a small sip of water can also provide very valuable information. Unfortunately, the physical examination is often normal in patients with dysphagia, despite the high yield nature of this complaint.

Diagnosis

The diagnosis of the underlying pathology of dysphagia is most often made outside of the emergency department (ED). The workup is dependent on whether transfer or transport dysphagia is thought to be present, as noted above. Initial evaluation of dysphagia in the ED can include anteroposterior (AP) and lateral neck radiographs, which can be helpful in transfer dysphagia and cases where the transport dysfunction seems proximal. Chest radiography should be obtained in most patients thought to have transport dysphagia. Direct laryngoscopy can be used to identify structural lesions.

Ultimately, oropharyngeal dysphagia is best worked up with videoesophagography, a specialized form of a barium swallow study in which videotaped images are reviewed at low-speed playback to allow detailed analysis. Traditional barium swallow is usually the first test for patients with transport dysphagia. Manometry and esophagoscopy are also employed, depending on the clinical picture. If a foreign body is suspected, the diagnostic workup takes yet another path (see Chap. 72, "Swallowed Foreign Bodies").

Selected Structural/Obstructive Causes

Neoplasms are a common cause of transfer and transport dysphagia. The esophagus or surrounding structures may be the primary site. Esophageal cancer is diagnosed in about 10,000 people a year in the United States. About the same number die from the disease each year as well. Ninety-five percent of esophageal neoplasms are squamous cell; the remaining 5 percent are adenocarcinomas. Men are affected three times as often as women. Risk factors for squamous cell disease includes alcohol, smoking, achalasia, and previous caustic ingestion with lye. Barrett's esophagus predisposes to adenocarcinoma, which has shown an increase in incidence in recent years.[8] There is usually a fairly rapid progression of dysphagia from solids to liquids (6 months). In addition to dysphagia, patients with neoplasm may present with bleeding. Early diagnosis impacts outcome, and for this reason the emergency physician should assume a neoplastic cause in patients over age 40 who present with new-onset dysphagia. These patients need an expedient workup to rule out malignancy. Definitive diagnosis is made by endoscopy with biopsy. Survival is dismal: the median is less than 1 year.

Esophageal stricture occurs as a result of scarring from GERD or other chronic inflammation. Generally they occur in the distal esophagus, proximal to the gastroesophageal (GE) junction. Strictures may interfere with LES function. Symptoms may build over years and are often noted solely with solids. Stricture can serve as a barrier to reflux, so heartburn may decrease as dysphagia increases. Workup involves ruling out malignancy and treatment is dilatation.[9]

Schatzki's ring is the most common cause of intermittent dysphagia with solids. This fibrous, diaphragm-like stricture near the GE junction is present in up to 15 percent of the population, the majority of whom are asymptomatic. The etiology of these rings is debated: they may form over time in response to GERD.[10] Steakhouse syndrome, food impaction in the esophagus due to poorly chewed meat, is a frequent presentation for patients with this obstructive phenomenon. Treatment of Schatzki's ring is dilatation.

Esophageal webs are thin structures of mucosa and submucosa found most often in the mid- or proximal esophagus. They can be congenital or acquired. Esophageal webs are a component of Plummer-Vinson syndrome (along with iron-deficiency anemia), and can be seen in patients with pemphigoid and epidermolysis bullosa. Treatment, again, is dilatation.

Diverticula may be found throughout the esophagus. Pharyngoesophageal, or Zenker's, diverticulum is a progressive outpouching of pharyngeal mucosa, just above the UES, caused by increased pressures during the hypopharyngeal phase of swallowing.[7] Presentation is usually after age 50, as this is an acquired disease. Patients complain of typical transfer dysfunction; additionally, they may have halitosis and the feeling of a neck mass. Diverticula can also be seen in the body of the esophagus, usually in association with a motility disorder.

Selected Motor Lesions Causing Dysphagia

Neuromuscular disorders typically result in misdirection of the bolus, with repeated swallowing attempts. Liquids, especially at the extremes of temperature, are generally more difficult to handle than solids. Symptoms are often intermittent in nature. Cerebrovascular accident (CVA) is the most common cause in this category. Oropharyngeal muscle weakness is often the mechanism, though there can be poor function of the UES as well. Polymyositis and dermatomyositis are the second most common causes of transfer dysphagia in this category.

Achalasia is a dysmotility disorder of unknown cause and the most common motility disorder producing dysphagia. Impaired swallowing-induced relaxation of the LES is noted, along with the absence of esophageal peristalsis. Most patients present between 20 and 40 years of age. Achalasia may be associated with esophageal spasm and chest pain and with odynophagia. Associated symptoms can include regurgitation and weight loss. Dilatation of the esophagus can be massive enough to impinge on the trachea and cause airway symptoms.[11] Therapy involves decreasing the LES pressure by oral medications, the endoscopic injection of botulinum toxin into the muscle of the sphincter, dilatations, or surgical myotomy.

"*Nutcracker esophagus*" is a motility disorder in which there are high-amplitude, long-duration peristaltic contractions in the distal esophagus. Manometric criteria require readings of >180 mmHg. The cause of nutcracker esophagus is unknown and the prevalence of this disease is debated in the literature.[12] Patients with this disorder frequently have associated psychiatric disorders and about one-third have GERD.

CHEST PAIN OF ESOPHAGEAL ORIGIN

Most esophageal causes of chest pain are not immediate threats to life; however, differentiating esophageal pain from ischemic chest pain can be impossible in the ED. Patients with esophageal pain can report spontaneous onset of pain or pain at night, regurgitation, odynophagia, dysphagia or meal-induced heartburn; however, these symptoms are also found in patients with coronary artery disease (CAD), and there is no historical feature that is sensitive or specific enough to routinely make a differentiation between the two.

To minimize missing active ischemic heart disease, clinicians often appropriately set into motion a patient evaluation that proceeds beyond what a traditional ED visit can accomplish, including a provocative test to rule out CAD. The high rate of admission for chest pain of noncardiac etiology is well publicized: ultimately, esophageal disease is frequently determined to be the responsible pathology. The incidence of esophageal disease as the cause of chest pain in patients with normal coronary arteries has been reported as ranging from 20 to 60 percent.[7] The use of ED observation units can help to sort through this process by providing time for a protocol-driven, rapid rule-out of acute myocardial infarction, followed by risk stratification for underlying CAD through the use of some form of stress or radionuclide testing. (See Chap. 45 for further discussion.) At a minimum, an electrocardiogram (ECG) and chest radiographs should be obtained in all patients with ambiguous presentations.

If chest pain is determined to be noncardiac in nature, treatment aimed at esophageal disease is often initiated empirically, without further diagnostic workup. There are no good data on which to base a therapeutic plan for these patients.[13] Outpatient workup options in addition to 6 to 8 weeks of empiric treatment for GERD include an acid infusion test, esophagoscopy, and/or manometry to help clarify pain of esophageal origin.

Gastroesophageal Reflux Disease (GERD)

Reflux of gastric contents into the esophagus causes a wide array of symptoms and long-term effects. It affects up to 25 percent of the adult population, possibly with even higher rates in elderly populations.[14] Classically, a weak LES has been the mechanism held responsible for reflux, and this is seen in some patients. However, it is now accepted that transient relaxation of the LES complex (with normal tone in between periods of relaxation) is a primary mechanism causing reflux. Patients with moderate to severe reflux also often have concomitant hiatal hernia.[2,15] Prolonged gastric emptying, agents that decrease LES, pressure, and impaired esophageal motility predispose to reflux. Table 71-2 highlights some common contributors.

TABLE 71-2 Causes of Gastroesophageal Reflux Disease

Decreased Pressure of Lower Esophageal Sphincter	Decreased Esophageal Motility	Prolonged Gastric Emptying
High-fat food	Achalsia	Medicines (anticholinergics)
Nicotine	Scleroderma	Outlet obstruction
Ethanol	Presbyesophagus	Diabetic gastroparesis
Caffeine	Diabetes mellitus	High-fat food
Medicines (nitrates, calcium channel blockers, anticholinergics, progesterone, estrogen)		
Pregnancy		

As noted, differentiating esophageal symptoms from acute ischemic coronary symptoms is often not possible in the ED. Heartburn is the classic symptom of GERD, and chest discomfort may be the sole manifestation of the disease. The burning nature of the discomfort is probably due to localized lower esophageal mucosal inflammation. Many GERD patients will report other associated gastrointestinal symptoms, such as odynophagia, dysphagia, acid regurgitation, and hypersalivation. The association of pain with meals can be helpful in identifying pain that is due to GERD. Postural changes in pain can also be useful: increasing intraabdominal pressure or negating the esophagus's gravity advantage can exacerbate reflux symptoms dramatically. Antacid-induced relief of symptoms is often noted in reflux disease, though the pain can return after the transient antacid effect wears off, and a certain number of patients with ischemic disease also report improvement. Unfortunately, like cardiac pain, GERD pain may be squeezing, pressure-like, and include a history of onset with exertion and offset with rest. Both types of pain may be accompanied by diaphoresis, pallor, and nausea and vomiting. Radiation of esophageal pain may be felt in either arm, the neck, the shoulders, or the back. Given the serious outcome of unrecognized ischemic disease compared with the relatively benign nature of esophageal pain, a cautious posture on the part of the clinician seems warranted.

Over time complications of GERD can develop that produce dysphagia, such as strictures, as discussed above, or inflammatory esophagitis, discussed below. A severe consequence of GERD, Barrett's esophagus, is present in up to 10 percent of patients with GERD.[16] This condition is identified by biopsy: simple columnar epithelium replaces the normal stratified squamous epithelium in the distal esophagus. Metaplasia and ulceration can be present. This is considered a premalignant condition, with a well-reported association between the development of metaplasia and the onset of adenocarcinoma.[17]

Less obvious presentations of GERD are also well recognized. Pulmonary symptoms, especially asthma exacerbations, and multiple ear/nose/throat symptoms are well described. GERD is present in many asthmatics, and in some can contribute to exacerbation by aspiration of minute amounts of gastric contents, with subsequent inflammation and bronchospasm, and by esophageal activation of reflex vagal tone, with consequent bronchospasm. Unfortunately, a reliable means for identifying asthmatic patients with GERD who will show an improvement in pulmonary symptoms with anti-reflux therapy has not been demonstrated in the literature.[17,18] GERD has been implicated in the etiology of dental erosion, vocal cord ulcers and granulomas, laryngitis with hoarseness, chronic sinusitis, and chronic cough.[19,20]

Comprehensive treatment of reflux disease involves decreasing acid production in the stomach, enhancing upper tract motility, and eliminating risk factors for the disease. As noted above, mild disease is often treated empirically. H_2 blockers or proton-pump inhibitors are mainstays of therapy. Dosage is titrated for each patient. A prokinetic drug may also greatly decrease symptoms. Simple discharge instructions should be given to all patients thought to be experiencing reflux-related symptoms: Avoid agents that exacerbate GERD (ethanol, caffeine, nicotine, chocolate, fatty foods), sleep with the head of the bed elevated (30°), and avoid eating within 3 h of going to bed at night. Management of Barrett's esophagus includes intensive treatment of the underlying GERD with proton-pump inhibition. Often, laser or photodynamic ablation therapy and surgical treatment are employed as well. Close monitoring for dysplastic changes is essential.

Esophagitis

Esophagitis can cause prolonged periods of chest pain and almost always causes odynophagia as well. Diagnosis of advanced esophagitis is by endoscopy. Low-grade disease can be seen by histopathologic examination.

INFLAMMATORY ESOPHAGITIS GERD may induce an inflammatory response in the lower esophageal mucosa. Over time, this can progress to esophageal ulcerations, scarring, and stricture formation. The presence of esophagitis due to reflux warrants aggressive pharmacologic therapy with acid-suppressive medications. If this treatment regimen is not sufficient, surgical options are considered.[17] Barrett's esophagus, mentioned above, can develop as well.

Ingested medications can also be a source for inflammatory esophagitis, usually from prolonged contact of the medication with the esophageal mucosa. Ulceration can be associated with this process. Multiple medications have been implicated: nonsteroidal anti-inflammatory drugs (NSAIDs), potassium chloride, and antibiotics, especially doxycycline, cause a large proportion of medication-related esophageal inflammation.[21] Risk factors for pill-induced esophageal injury include swallowing position, fluid intake, capsule size, and age, with swallowing position being the most important. Withdrawal of the offending agent is generally curative.

INFECTIOUS Patients with immunosuppression [acquired immunodeficiency syndrome (AIDS), iatrogenic causes, cancer] may develop an infectious esophagitis. AIDS especially has made esophageal infection more routine in the ED. The diagnosis of esophageal infection in an otherwise seemingly healthy host should prompt a search for underlying immunocompromise. Candidal species are the most common pathogens, often associated with dysphagia as a primary symptom. Herpes simplex, cytomegalovirus, and aphthous ulceration are also seen and may be more frequently associated with odynophagia. Other agents are rare and include other fungal infections, mycobacteria, and other viral pathogens such as varicella zoster and Epstein-Barr virus. Endoscopy with biopsy and cultures is used to establish this diagnosis.[22]

Esophageal Motility Disorders

Esophageal dysmotility is the excessive, uncoordinated contraction of esophageal smooth muscle. Debate exists over the correlation between symptoms (pain) and observed motor events.[12] Dysmotility disorders can be divided into distinct entities based on manometric criteria. Achalasia and nutcracker esophagus were discussed above. The other motility disorders commonly recognized include diffuse esophageal spasm, hypertensive LES, and nonspecific motor disorder.

Clinically, chest pain is the presenting symptom in the majority of patients with these disorders. The onset is usually in the fifth decade. The pain often occurs at rest and is dull or colicky in nature. Stress or ingestion of liquids at the extremes of temperature may serve as a trigger. An acute episode of pain may be followed by hours of dull, achy, residual discomfort. Thirty to sixty percent of these patients will also experience dysphagia, which is usually intermittent. Pain from spasm may respond to nitroglycerin. Calcium channel blockers and anticholinergic agents can also be employed.

ESOPHAGEAL PERFORATION

Perforation of the esophagus can occur secondary to a number of disparate processes[23] as noted in Table 71-3. Iatrogenic injury is the most frequent cause of esophageal injury, accounting for up to 75 percent of all perforations. Endoscopy, a prime offender, has a lesser rate of perforation when performed on an esophagus free of disease than does endoscopy of a diseased esophagus. Dilation of strictures increases the risk of perforation greatly. Other intraluminal procedures,

TABLE 71-3 Causes of Esophageal Perforation

Causes of Perforation	Comments
Iatrogenic	Intraluminal procedures Endoscopy Dilatation Variceal therapy Gastric intubation Intraoperative injury
Boerhaave's syndrome	"Spontaneous;" usually associated with transient increase in intraesophageal pressure
Trauma	Penetrating Blunt (rare) Caustic ingestion
Foreign body	Includes pill-related injury
Infection	Rare
Tumor	May be intrinsic or extrinsic cancer
Aortic pathology	Aneurysm Aberrant right subclavian artery
Miscellaneous	Barrett's esophagus Zollinger-Ellison syndrome

such as variceal therapy or Sengstaken-Blakemore tubes and palliative laser treatment for cancer, are also associated with perforation. A well-recognized clinical scenario of postemetic perforation, Boerhaave syndrome, is responsible for roughly 10 to 15 percent of esophageal perforations and is discussed below.

Perforation causes a dramatic presentation if esophageal contents leak into the mediastinum. A fulminant, necrotizing mediastinitis with polymicrobic infection that rapidly leads to shock and death can ensue. Perforation into the pleural or peritoneal spaces can occur as well, and contamination of these large potential spaces also tends to result in rapidly progressive infection and shock. If the perforation is small and leakage is contained by contiguous structures, the course may be significantly more indolent. Most spontaneous perforations occur through the left posterolateral wall of the distal esophagus.[24] Proximal perforation, seen mostly with instrumentation, tends to be less severe than distal and can be contained locally as a periesophageal abscess with minimal systemic toxicity.

Pain is classically described as acute, severe, unrelenting and diffuse; reported in the chest, neck and abdomen; and with radiation to the back and shoulders. Back pain may be the predominant symptom. Pain is often exacerbated by swallowing. Dysphagia, dyspnea, hematemesis, and cyanosis can be present as well. Less acute and atypical presentations are also described. Esophageal perforation is often ascribed to acute myocardial infarction (MI), pulmonary embolus, peptic ulcer disease, aortic catastrophe, or acute abdomen, resulting in critical delays in diagnosis, the most important factor in determining morbidity and mortality outcome.

Physical examination varies with the severity of the rupture and the elapsed time between the rupture and presentation. Abdominal rigidity with hypotension and fever often occur early. Tachycardia and tachypnea are common. Cervical subcutaneous emphysema is common in cervical esophageal perforations. Mediastinal emphysema takes time to develop. It is less commonly detected by examination or radiography in lower esophageal perforation, and its absence does not rule out perforation.[25] Hammon's crunch, caused by air in the mediastinum being moved by the beating heart, can sometimes be auscultated. Pleural effusion develops in half of patients with intrathoracic perforations and is uncommon in those with cervical perforations. Pleural fluid can be due to either direct contamination of the pleural space or a sympathetic serous effusion from mediastinitis.

Making the correct diagnosis in a timely manner in an ill patients with esophageal perforation requires suspicion on the clinician's part. Chest radiography and contrast esophagography with water-soluble contrast most often make the diagnosis. Endoscopy, computed tomography (CT) of the chest, and thoracentesis can be useful adjuncts if esophagography (10 to 25 percent false-negative rate) is unrevealing in the face of high clinical suspicion. Endoscopy especially is often done after negative esophagography in penetrating trauma with suspicion of esophageal perforation.

Perforation of the esophagus is associated with a high mortality rate regardless of the underlying cause. The elapsed time between perforation and the initiation of therapy, the location of the perforation, and the etiology all affect outcome. Rapid, aggressive management is key to minimizing the morbidity and mortality associated with esophageal perforation. In the ED, resuscitation of shock, broad spectrum parenteral antibiotics, and emergent surgical consultation should be obtained as soon as the diagnosis is seriously entertained. Patients with systemic symptoms and signs after perforation need operative management. Criteria are developing for the nonoperative management of perforation in select patients.[23]

Instrumentation, especially endoscopic dilatation, has a relatively high rate of perforation; therefore, it is patients with strictures who sustain these injuries, usually perforating distally around the level of the obstruction. A patient with a relatively healthy esophagus undergoing instrumentation will more commonly perforate proximally. Perforation from other instrumentation, including nasogastric tube placement, has been reported.[26]

Boerhaave's syndrome refers to full-thickness perforation of the esophagus following a sudden rise in intraesophageal pressure. The mechanism is sudden, forceful emesis in about three-fourths of the cases; coughing, straining, seizures, and childbirth have been reported as causing perforations as well. Alcohol is frequently an antecedent to this syndrome, which is seen more commonly in males. The perforation is usually in the distal esophagus on the left side.

Trauma to the esophagus accounts for roughly 10 percent of all esophageal perforations. Rupture from blunt injury is rare. Penetrating wounds to the esophagus from neck trauma occur but are often masked by more rapidly fatal injuries to the surrounding critical structures, such as the airway and major vessels. A combination of esophagography and esophagoscopy is used to assess patients for potential esophageal injury.

Foreign-body ingestion may result in perforation of the esophagus as well. The perforation is almost always at one of the sites of anatomic narrowing, where foreign bodies become wedged. The injury can be due to pressure necrosis from the object (coin), penetration from the object (pin, bones), or chemical irritation from the object (battery, pill).

ESOPHAGEAL BLEEDING

The general approach to upper gastrointestinal bleeding (UGIB) from an esophageal source does not differ from the approach for bleeding from other sources and is addressed in more depth in Chap. 70, ''Gastrointestinal Bleeding.'' Resuscitation proceeds concurrently with the diagnostic effort of history, physical examination, and laboratory evaluation. Gastric lavage through a nasogastric tube or larger-bore gastric tube is generally accepted, and early airway management should be considered. Prompt mobilization of resources—including blood products, gastroenterology consult for endoscopy, and an appropriate inpatient level of care—is important.

About 60 percent of variceal bleeding will resolve with supportive care alone.[27] The rate of spontaneous cessation is higher for nonvariceal sources of UGIB. Patients who continue to bleed need specific intervention. Early endoscopy is generally accepted in patients with UGIB for its diagnostic and therapeutic applications. Pharmacologic treatment with an intravenous vasopressin/nitroglycerin combination, somatostatin, or octreotide can be used as well. Balloon tamponade is generally considered a last-resort therapy when pharmacologic management has failed and endoscopy is either not feasible secondary to massive bleeding or is ineffective. Surgical treatment also remains an option.

Varices develop in patients with chronic liver disease in response to portal hypertension. Around 60 percent of patients with chronic liver disease will develop varices. Of patients who develop varices, 25 to 30 percent experience hemorrhage.[28] Patients who develop varices from alcohol abuse have a higher risk of bleeding, especially if there is ongoing alcohol consumption. About two-thirds of patients who have an index bleed experience recurrent hemorrhage, 50 percent occurring within 6 weeks of the initial episode.

With variceal bleeding, endoscopic therapy is often successful in controlling the hemorrhage. Sclerotherapy and ligation are the main alternatives, though in Europe the use of injected Histoacryl (a tissue adhesive) to obstruct the variceal lumen has gained popularity. Shunting procedures performed transvenously or by surgical approach should also be considered.[29] Mortality is significant in esophageal variceal bleeding, quoted at 40 percent.[28] Concurrent hepatic failure is a risk factor for poor outcome.

Mallory-Weiss syndrome is arterial bleeding from longitudinal mucosal lacerations of the distal esophagus/proximal stomach. The majority of these lacerations are located at the GE junction, with only 10 percent found in the lower esophagus proper. Mallory-Weiss tears are responsible for between 5 to 15 percent of upper GI hemorrhage. They can occur at any age but are most common in the fourth through sixth decades. The pathophysiology of Mallory-Weiss syndrome is thought to be a transient, large pressure gradient between thorax and stomach, experienced maximally at GE junction.

Acute onset of upper GI bleeding is the usual presentation, though some patients can present with melana or hematochezia. Rarely the presentation will be one of isolated abdominal pain or syncope. Less than half of patients with Mallory-Weiss tears will report a history of vomiting prior to hematemesis. The spectrum of severity of bleeding is broad, but overall a low relative incidence of surgical intervention or adverse outcome is seen. Initial treatment is supportive as the vast majority of Mallory-Weiss tears stop bleeding spontaneously. Ongoing hemorrhage can require treatment with electrocoagulation, sclerotherapy, and laser photocoagulation. Angiographic embolization or surgical intervention remain options as well.

Esophageal cancer often results in heme-positive stools but is an uncommon cause of significant upper or lower GI bleeding.

REFERENCES

1. Lang IM, Shaker R: Anatomy and physiology of the upper esophageal sphincter. *Am J Med* 103:50S, 1997.
2. Mittal RK, Balaban DH: The esophagogastric junction. *N Engl J Med* 336:924, 1997.
3. Berne RM, Levy MN: *Physiology.* St. Louis, Mosby, 1983.
4. Moore KL: *Clinically Oriented Anatomy.* Baltimore, Williams & Wilkins, 1985.
5. Pope CEN: The esophagus for the nonesophagologist. *Am J Med* 103: 19S-, 1997.
6. Trate DM, Parkman HP, Fisher RS: Dysphagia: Evaluation, diagnosis, and treatment. *Primary Care* 1996; 23:417, 1996.
7. Falk GW, Richter JE: Approach to the patient with acute dysphagia, odynophagia and noncardiac chest pain, in Taylor MB (ed): *Gastrointestinal Emergencies.* Baltimore, Williams & Wilkins, 1997.
8. Pera M, Cameron AJ, Trastek VF, et al: Increasing incidence of adenocarcinoma of the esophagus and esophagogastric junction. *Gastroenterology* 104:510, 1993.
9. Swann LA, Munter DW: Esophageal emergencies. *Emerg Med Clin North Am* 14:557, 1996.

10. Marshall JB, Kretschmar JM, Diaz-Arias AA: Gastroesophageal reflux as a pathogenic factor in the development of symptomatic lower esophageal rings. *Arch Intern Med* 150:1669, 1990.
11. Turkot S, Golzman B, Kogan J, et al: Acute upper-airway obstruction in a patient with achalasia. *Ann Emerg Med* 29:687, 1997.
12. Ouyang A, Cohen S: Motility Disorders of the esophagus, in Haubrich WS, Schaffner F, Berk JE (eds): *Bockus Gastroenterology.* Philadelphia, Saunders, 1995, pp 418–436.
13. Ho K: Noncardiac chest pain and abdominal pain. *Ann Emerg Med* 27:457, 1996.
14. Richter JE: Typical and atypical presentations of gastroesophageal reflux disease: The role of esophageal testing in diagnosis and management. *Gastroenterol Clin North Am* 25:75, 1996.
15. Dent J: Patterns of lower esophageal sphincter function associated with gastroesophageal reflux. *Am J Med* 103 (5A):29S, 1997.
16. Barbezat GO: Recent advances: Gastroenterology. *BMJ* 316:125, 1998.
17. Kahrilas PJ: Gastroesophageal reflux disease. *JAMA* 276:983, 1996.
18. Sontag SJ: Gastroesophageal reflux and asthma. *Am J Med* 103:84S, 1997.
19. Hogan WJ: Spectrum of supraesophageal complications of gastroesophageal reflux disease. *Am J Med* 103:77S, 1997.
20. de Caestecker J: Medical therapy for supraesophageal complications of gastroesophageal reflux. *Am J Med* 103 (5A):138S, 1997.
21. Kikendall JW, Friedman AC, Oyewole MA, et al: Pill-induced esophageal injury: Case reports and review of the medical literature. *Dig Dis Sci* 28:174, 1983.
22. Varghese GK, Crane LR: Evaluation and treatment of HIV-related illnesses in the emergency department. *Ann Emerg Med* 24:503, 1994.
23. Williamson WA, Ellis FHJ: Esophageal perforation, in Taylor MB (ed): *Gastrointestinal Emergencies.* Baltimore, Williams & Wilkins, 1997.
24. Levy F, Mysko WK, Kelen GD: Spontaneous esophageal perforation presenting with right-sided pleural effusion. *J Emerg Med* 13:321, 1995.
25. Janjua KJ: Boerhaave's syndrome. *Postgrad Med J* 73:265, 1997.
26. Ahmed A, Aggarwal M, Watson E: Esophageal perforation: A complication of nasogastric tube placement. *Am J Emerg Med* 16:64, 1998.
27. Terblanche J, Burroughs AK, Hobbs KEF: Controversies in the management of esophageal varices. *N Engl J Med* 320:1393, 1989.
28. Polio J, Groszmann RJ, Taylor MB: Acute management of portal hypertensive hemorrhage from the upper gastrointestinal tract, in Taylor MB (ed): *Gastrointestinal Emergencies.* Baltimore, Williams & Wilkins, 1997.
29. Rossle M, Siegerstetter V, Huber M, Ochs A: The first decade of the transjugular intrahepatic portosystemic shunt (TIPS): State of the art. *Liver* 18:73, 1998.

SWALLOWED FOREIGN BODIES

Wade R. Gaasch
Robert A. Barish

Swallowed foreign bodies, a common presentation in emergency departments, can be innocuous or life-threatening. In the United States, approximately 1500 people die yearly as a result of ingesting foreign bodies. Often thought to be confined to the pediatric population, foreign body ingestion occurs in all age groups. The pediatric age group accounts for approximately 80 percent of all cases, followed by edentulous adults, prisoners, and psychiatric patients. The presence of dentures eliminates the tactile sensitivity of the palatal surface vital to the identification of small items. A correlation exists between age groups and specific types of ingested material. Children most often ingest coins, toys, crayons, and ballpoint pen caps; adults tend to have problems with meat and bones.[1] In addition, psychiatric patients and prison inmates may ingest such unlikely objects as spoons and razor blades.

PATHOPHYSIOLOGY

Although most objects pass spontaneously, 10 to 20 percent require some intervention, and only 1 percent demand surgical treatment.[2] Ingested foreign bodies may be found anywhere throughout the digestive tract, but there are several physiologic ''narrow spaces'' where the majority of articles tend to lodge. The pediatric esophagus has five areas of constriction where coins and other objects may become trapped: cricopharyngeal narrowing (C6), the most common site; thoracid inlet (T1); aortic arch (T4); tracheal bifurcation (T6); and hiatal narrowing (T10–11). Most pediatric obstructions occur in the proximal esophagus; the vast majority of adult impactions arise from esophageal disease in the distal esophagus. Because 97 percent of adults presenting with meat impaction harbor pathologic esophageal conditions, barium swallow must be performed to confirm foreign body clearance and evaluate possible underlying disease.

Once an object has traversed the pylorus, it usually continues to the rectum and is passed in the stool. If, however, the object has irregular or sharp edges, it may become lodged anywhere in the gastrointestinal tract. Objects that lodge in the esophagus (not necessarily limited to sharp or irregular contour) can result in airway obstruction, stricture, or perforation with resulting mediastinitis, cardiac tamponade, paraesophageal abscess, or aortotracheoesophageal fistula. Perforation may be the result of direct mechanical erosion, as with bones, or chemical corrosion, as with button batteries.

CLINICAL PRESENTATION

Objects lodged in the esophagus generally produce anxiety and discomfort. Adult patients often complain of retrosternal pain. Patients are likely to retch or vomit and experience dysphagia, resulting in choking, coughing, or aspiration if they attempt to wash down the object. Eventually, patients may be unable to swallow their own secretions. In the adult, the history often provides all the pertinent information necessary for diagnosis and treatment. However, this is often not true in the pediatric population. In the 16-and-under age group, symptoms include refusal to eat, vomiting (with or without hematemesis), gagging, choking, stridor (''pseudoasthma''), neck or throat pain, inability to swallow, increased salivation, and foreign body sensation in the chest.

Physical examination must include careful evaluation of the nasopharynx, oropharynx, neck, and subcutaneous tissues for air resulting from perforation of a hollow viscus. Laryngoscopy, either direct or indirect, should be done, especially when the patient complains of a sticking sensation or has ingested a bone. Although physical signs are not always present, findings consistent with foreign body ingestion in the 16-and-under age group consist of red throat, dysphagia, palatal abrasion, temperature elevation, anxiety and distress, and peritoneal signs.

EMERGENCY DEPARTMENT MANAGEMENT

General Care

Because the great majority of ingested foreign bodies traverse the entire gastrointestinal tract without any problems, treatment can be expectant once the object has passed through the pylorus.[3] If, however, a foreign body obstructs the esophagus, prevention of aspiration is paramount. This can be accomplished by inserting a tube above the obstructing body to remove unswallowed fluids above the impaction. Conditions warranting consultation with an endoscopist and possible hospital admission are listed in Table 72-1.

The offending object can be located in several ways. A radiopaque object will be demonstrated on standard x-ray films of the neck or abdomen. The procedure of choice for finding and then extracting a foreign body in the esophagus is endoscopy.[4] This procedure has a high success rate and thus avoids progression to surgery.[5] It is also time-efficient.[6] Although many other diagnostic methods are available, they are not as reliable and thorough as endoscopy, so the time spent in arranging for and conducting such tests may not be time well spent for a frightened, uncomfortable patient.

TABLE 72-1 Presentations of Esophageal Foreign Bodies Warranting Endoscopy Consultation and Possible Hospital Admission

Sharp or elongated objects
Multiple foreign bodies
Button batteries
Evidence of perforation
Child with a nickel or quarter at the level of the cricopharyngeus muscle
Airway compromise
Presence of foreign body for more than 24 hours

Source: Adapted from Munter DW: Disorders of the esophagus, in Howell JM, et al (eds): *Emergency Medicine.* Philadelphia: Saunders, 1998, p 318.

If endoscopic equipment and expertise are not available, an esophagogram can be performed. Consultation with an endoscopist is strongly recommended before initiation of any contrast study, because direct visualization of the foreign body after contrast administration may not be possible because of interference from swallowed contrast medium.

The type of contrast agent must be chosen based on the anticipated clinical findings and course.[7] If perforation is suspected, a water-soluble contrast agent (Gastrograffin) should be used. However, since water-soluble agents are pulmonary irritants, barium should be used if aspiration is possible. The least amount of barium possible should be instilled, because barium will block the endoscopic field. If both perforation and aspiration are possible, a nonionic contrast agent is indicated.

Progress of the object through the gastrointestinal tract must be monitored with repeat abdominal x-ray films, usually 2 to 4 h apart. The use of metal detectors, if available, has been advocated as a means of localizing and tracking the progression of metal objects, thereby avoiding repeated radiation exposure. Abdominal examinations should be done frequently to detect early signs of developing peritonitis should perforation occur. Virtually all symptomatic patients will require observation and esophagoscopy. If a nonfood object becomes lodged in the esophagus or is unable to pass through the pylorus, it must be removed as soon as possible, using esophagogastroscopy. Fatal lead encephalopathy has been reported in a child who ingested a lead curtain weight, which supposedly had been in the stomach for an extended time.[8]

Food Impaction

Meat impaction may be treated expectantly, providing the patient can manage his or her own secretions. Time and sedation often will allow the meat to pass into the stomach, but the bolus should not be allowed to remain impacted longer than 12 h. Endoscopy is the preferred method for removal. Alternatives have been suggested if endoscopy is not available.

The use of proteolytic enzymes, such as an aqueous solution of papain (e.g., Adolph's meat tenderizer), to dissolve a meat bolus is *not* recommended, however, because of the number of reported complications and because of increasing availability of and expertise in endoscopy. Several reports in the literature have described esophageal perforation secondary to the enzymatic action of the solution. Mucosal ischemia resulting from distention of the esophageal wall renders the esophagus more susceptible to enzymatic degradation. Hemorrhagic pulmonary edema also has been reported following aspiration of Adolph's meat tenderizer.

Intravenous administration of glucagon to relax esophageal smooth muscle also has been suggested as a method of treating food impaction. A test dose should be given to ensure that hypersensitivity does not exist; then the recommended dose is 1 mg. If the food bolus is not passed in 20 min, an additional 2 mg is given intravenously. An esophagogram must be performed following treatment to ensure passage. This strategy was questioned by Tibbling and associates,[9] who found no statistical difference in disimpaction rates between patients given spasmolytic drugs and those given placebo. For patients with esophageal obstruction caused by food, more efficient approaches to treatment are endoscopy and esophagoscopy.

Bell[10] reports the successful use of nifedipine, which reduces lower esophageal sphincter pressure and the amplitude of the sphincter contractions without changing the amplitude of contractions in the body of the esophagus. By this mechanism, a bolus of food lodged in the vicinity of the gastroesophageal junction may pass. The recommended dose is 10 mg administered sublingually. Sublingual nitroglycerin has also been used successfully, but could cause hypotension.

Coin Ingestion

Because as many as 35 percent of children with a coin lodged in their esophagus will be asymptomatic, some authors recommend that radiographs be performed on *all* children suspected of swallowing coins to determine the presence and location of the object. However, Caravati and colleagues[11] noted no difference in 5-day morbidity rates between children who underwent radiographic evaluation and those who did not after coin ingestion. Coins in the esophagus lie in the frontal plane with the flat side visible on an anteroposterior radiograph; coins in the trachea lie in the sagittal plane.

The use of a Foley catheter, initially reported in the late 1960s, has been promoted as a safe and effective technique for removal when the coin has been impacted for less than 24 h. Before attempting extraction, the airway must be secured with endotracheal intubation. The catheter is passed down the esophagus beyond the object and the balloon inflated. As the catheter is slowly withdrawn, the object is withdrawn along with it. Retrieval of a coin by this technique is less effective after 24 h. Most clinicians prefer using the Foley catheter under fluoroscopy. Foley catheter retrieval of foreign bodies may be complicated by aspiration, and personnel and equipment for airway control must be immediately available. If endoscopic expertise is readily available, Foley catheterization retrieval should be a secondary option.

Button Battery Ingestion

A button battery lodged in the esophagus is a true emergency because of the extremely rapid action of the alkaline substance on the mucosa. Burns to the esophagus have been reported to occur in as little as 4 h, with perforation as soon as 6 h after ingestion. Button batteries in the esophagus require emergency removal if significant morbidity is to be averted. Outcome does not appear to be affected by battery discharge state but is affected by chemical composition.[12] Lithium cells are associated disproportionately with adverse outcome. Mercuric oxide cells tend to fragment more frequently than other cells; however, the threat of heavy metal poisoning has not been supported by the literature or clinical experience. This fact notwithstanding, blood and urine mercury levels should be measured whenever a mercury-containing cell is observed to have split while in the gastrointestinal tract.

Button ingestion can be managed along two main pathways (Fig. 72-1). If the button battery is lodged in the esophagus, its location should be documented by radiograph; then emergent endoscopic removal is mandatory. Given the widespread expertise with endoscopy, we cannot recommend alternative techniques, many of which are associated with significant complications. Ipecac has no place in the management of button battery ingestion.[12] Button batteries that have passed the esophagus need not be retrieved in the asymptomatic patient unless the cell is not passing through the pylorus after 48 h of observation. This is rarely the case unless the battery is of large diameter and the patient is under 6 years of age. In this case, endoscopic retrieval is again the preferred option. Most batteries pass completely through the body within 48 to 72 h, although passage has been reported to take as long as 14 days. All patients with signs and symptoms of gastrointestinal tract injury require immediate surgical consultation.

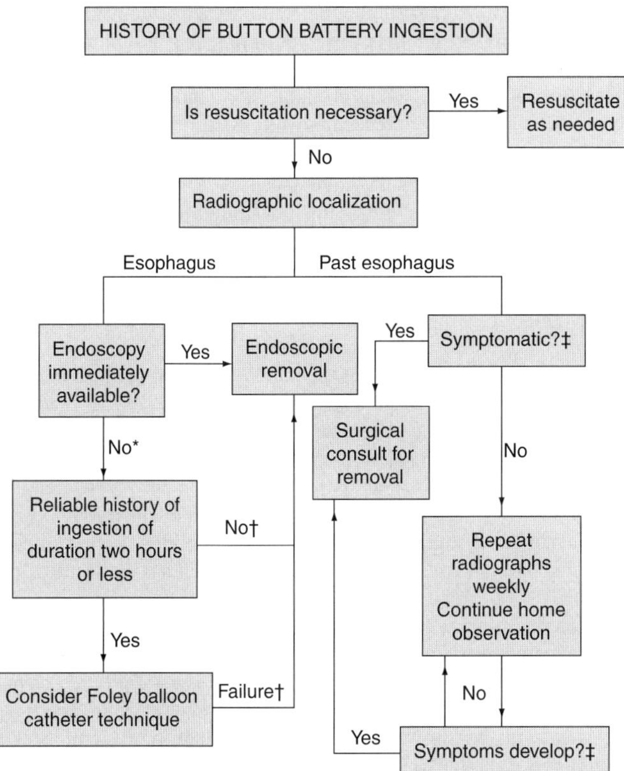

FIG. 72-1. Algorithm for management of button battery ingestion. (Adapted from Kuhns DW, Dire DJ: Button battery ingestions. *Ann Emerg Med* 18:293, 1989.)
*Button batteries in the esophagus must be removed. Endoscopy should be used if available. The balloon catheter technique can be used if the ingestion is less than 2 h old, but should not be used after this because it may increase the amount of damage to the weakened esophagus.
†When the Foley technique fails or is contraindicated due to a greater than 2 h elapsed time period, the button battery should be removed endoscopically. This may require transfer of the patient.
‡Acute abdomen, tarry or bloody stools, fever, persistent vomiting.

Assistance with cell identification may be obtained by calling the National Button Battery Ingestion Hotline (National Capital Poison Center, Washington D.C.) at 202-625-3333.

Ingestion of Sharp Objects

Management of ingested sharp and pointed foreign bodies is controversial. Objects longer than 5 cm and wider than 2 cm rarely will pass the stomach. Objects of that size and those with extremely pointed edges, such as open safety pins or razor blades, must be removed before they pass from the stomach because 15 to 35 percent will cause intestinal perforation, usually in the ileocecal valve.

Paul and Jaffe[13] recommend the following management for children who have swallowed sharp objects. All patients should have an initial radiograph and physical examination. If the patient is symptomatic or has ingested a sewing needle, surgical consultation for possible endoscopy and laparotomy is indicated. Children who have swallowed a sharp object (other than sewing needles) yet are asymptomatic can be managed on an expectant basis. Progression of the sharp object should be documented with serial radiographs. If progression past the stomach is not seen, a water-soluble contrast film may document gastrointestinal perforation. At the first sign of perforation, the object should be removed even if the patient remains asymptomatic. If the object does not progress through the gastrointestinal tract, surgical retrieval is indicated.

Cocaine Ingestion

Cocaine ingestion is an increasingly widespread problem. Carriers will ingest multiple small packets of cocaine in attempts to conceal the drug. A favored packet is the condom, which may hold up to 5 g cocaine. Rupture of even one such packet may be fatal. Webb recommends surgery as the safest method of recovery to avoid the likelihood of packet rupture during endoscopic retrieval. If the packet appears to be passing intact through the intestinal tract, the clinician may choose to observe the patient and wait for the packet to be delivered spontaneously through the rectum.

REFERENCES

1. Webb WA: Management of foreign bodies of the upper gastrointestinal tract: Update. *Gastrointest Endosc* 41:39, 1995.
2. Guideline for the management of ingested foreign bodies. *Gastrointest Endosc* 41:622, 1995.
3. Binder L, Anderson WA: Pediatric gastrointestinal foreign body ingestions. *Ann Emerg Med* 13:112, 1984.
4. Ginsberg GG: Management of ingested foreign objects and food bolus impactions. *Gastrointest Endosc* 41:33, 1995.
5. Blair SR, Graeber GM, Cruzzavala JL, et al: Current management of esophageal impactions. *Chest* 104:1205, 1993.
6. Stack LB, Munter DW: Foreign bodies in the gastrointestinal tract. *Emerg Med Clin North Am* 14:493, 1996.
7. Barsan WG, Lowell JM, Wolf LR: Disorders of the upper gastrointestinal tract, in Rosen P, Barkin R, Danzl DF, et al (eds): *Emergency Medicine: Concepts and Clinical Practice.* St. Louis: Mosby–Year Book 1998, pp 1958–1980.
8. Hugelmeyer CD, Moorhead JC, Horenblas L, Bayer MJ: Fatal lead encephalopathy following foreign body ingestion: Case report. *J Emerg Med* 6:397, 1988.
9. Tibbling L, Bjorkhoel A, Jansson E, Stenkvist M: Effect of spasmolytic drugs on esophageal foreign bodies. *Dysphagia* 10:126, 1995.
10. Bell AF, Eibling DE: Nifedipine in the treatment of distal esophageal food impaction. *Arch Otolaryngol Head Neck Surg* 114:682, 1988.
11. Caravati EM, Bennett DL, McElwee NE: Pediatric coin ingestion: A prospective study on the utility of routine roentgenograms. *Am J Dis Child* 143:549, 1989.
12. Litovitz T, Schmitz BF: Ingestion of cylindrical and button batteries: An analysis of 2382 cases. *Pediatrics* 89:727, 1992.
13. Paul RI, Jaffe DM: Sharp object ingestions in children: Illustrative case and literature review. *Pediatr Emerg Care* 4:245, 1988.

PEPTIC ULCER DISEASE AND GASTRITIS

Matthew C. Gratton

Peptic ulcer disease is a chronic illness manifested by recurrent ulcerations in the stomach and proximal duodenum. Acid and pepsin are thought to be crucial to ulcer development, but it is now recognized that the great majority of peptic ulcers are directly related to infection with *Helicobacter pylori* or nonsteroidal anti-inflammatory drug (NSAID) use.[1,2] Gastritis is acute or chronic inflammation of the gastric mucosa and has various etiologies. Dyspepsia is continuous or recurrent upper abdominal pain or discomfort with or without associated symptoms (nausea, bloating, regurgitation, etc.).[3,4] Dyspepsia may be caused by a number of diseases or may be functional.

EPIDEMIOLOGY

Approximately 10 percent of the US population over 17 years of age have peptic ulcer disease at some time. One-third of them report an active ulcer within the last year.[5,6] Peptic ulcer disease has a high rate of morbidity, with 8 million physicians' visits and 275,000 hospitalizations per year and a high cost to society of $5.65 billion per year in lost wages and medical care.[5] The prevalence of *H. pylori* infection in white Americans below age 35 is about 10 percent, rising to almost 80 percent by age 75. Forty-five percent of black Americans below age 25 are infected.[8] The prevalence of dyspepsia is 25 to 30 percent in the United States.[4,7]

PATHOPHYSIOLOGY

Hydrochloric acid and pepsin destroy gastric and duodenal mucosa. Mucous and bicarbonate ion secretions protect mucosa. Prostaglandins protect mucosa by enhancing mucous and bicarbonate production and by enhancing mucosal blood flow, thereby supporting metabolism. The balance between these protective and destructive forces determines whether peptic ulcer disease will occur. *Helicobacter pylori* infection or NSAIDs are thought to be the causal agents of peptic ulcer disease in almost all cases.[1,2] *Helicobacter pylori* infection is present in 95 percent of duodenal ulcers and 80 percent of gastric ulcers.[9] Although traditional treatment of peptic ulcers by various modalities heals most ulcers, eradication of *H. pylori* reduces recurrence rates from 80 to 15 percent for duodenal and from 50 to 10 percent for gastric ulcers.[9] *Helicobacter pylori* is a spiral, urease-producing, flagellated bacterium that is found living between the mucous gel and the mucosa primarily in the gastric antrum.[6,8] The production of urease, cytotoxins, proteases, and other compounds is thought to disturb the mucous gel and cause tissue injury.[2,8] In the presence of acid and pepsin, ulceration may occur. Chronic active (usually asymptomatic) gastritis is an almost universal finding with *H. pylori* infection, but only 10 to 20 percent of infected people develop peptic ulcer disease.[8,10] It is unclear why most infected persons do not develop symptomatic peptic ulcer disease, but it most likely reflects an interaction of factors, including both host and pathogen (different virulence of strains of bacteria).[10]

Helicobacter pylori has been linked to mucosa-associated lymphoid tissue (MALT) lymphoma, and regression has been documented with eradication of infection. In addition, *H. pylori* infection is considered a definite risk factor for adenocarcinoma of the stomach. However, since the prevalence of gastric cancer in the United States is very low and the *H. pylori* infection rate very high, other factors undoubtedly are involved.[8,9]

NSAIDs inhibit prostaglandin synthesis, thereby decreasing mucous and bicarbonate production and mucosal blood flow, allowing ulcer formation.[2] Gastrin-secreting tumors produce ulceration due to high levels of acid and pepsin production, but acid alone rarely causes ulceration.[10,11] However, inhibition of acid secretion may allow ulcers to heal and is the basis for traditional ulcer treatments.

Hereditary factors cause a predisposition to peptic ulcer disease. There is an association between chronic renal failure, renal transplantation, cirrhosis, and chronic obstructive pulmonary disease and peptic ulceration, but the precise mechanism is unclear. Cigarette smoking is a predisposing factor for peptic ulcer disease, perhaps due to an inhibition of bicarbonate ion production or to increased gastric emptying (but not to increased acid production). Emotional stress may predispose to peptic ulcer disease, but diet and alcohol use do not.

Acute gastritis may be related to ischemia from severe illness (shock, trauma, severe burns, organ failure, etc.) or the direct toxic effects of agents (NSAIDs, alcohol, bile acids, etc.). *Helicobacter pylori* infection causes both acute and chronic gastritis (both usually asymptomatic). Chronic gastritis may also be caused by autoimmune factors that destroy gastric parietal cells, resulting in the loss of acid production and the loss of intrinsic factor production, which in turn cause malabsorption of vitamin B_{12} and therefore pernicious anemia.

CLINICAL FEATURES

Burning epigastric pain is the most classic symptom of peptic ulcer disease. The pain may also be described as sharp, dull, an ache, or an ''empty'' or ''hungry'' feeling. Pain may be relieved by milk, food, or antacids, presumably due to buffering and/or dilution of acid. Pain recurs as the gastric contents empty, and the recurrent pain may classically awaken the patient at night. Pain tends to occur daily for weeks, resolve, and then reoccur in weeks to months. Although no symptoms allow complete discrimination, in a study by Talley et al, peptic ulceration was more likely than nonulcer dyspepsia or cholelithiasis in the presence of night pain; pain relieved by food, milk, or antacids; and a shorter duration of pain.[7] Postprandial pain, food intolerance, nausea, retrosternal pain, and belching are not related to peptic ulcer disease.''[12] Atypical presentations are common in those over age 65, including no pain, epigastric pain not relieved by eating, nausea, vomiting, anorexia, weight loss, and bleeding.[13]

A change in the character of the patient's typical pain may herald a complication. Abrupt onset of severe or generalized pain may indicate perforation with spillage of gastric or duodenal contents and resulting peritonitis. Rapid onset of mid-back pain may be due to posterior penetration into the pancreas, with the development of pancreatitis. Nausea and vomiting may indicate gastric outlet obstruction from scarring or edema. Vomiting bright red blood or coffee-ground emesis, or passing tarry or melanotic stool or hematochezia indicates ulcer bleeding.

On physical examination, the only positive finding in patients with uncomplicated peptic ulcer disease may be epigastric tenderness. This finding is neither sensitive nor specific for the diagnosis.[7] Other physical findings may be indicative of complications: a rigid abdomen consistent with peritonitis in perforation; abdominal distention or a succussion splash due to obstruction; occult or gross blood per rectum or nasogastric tube with ulcer bleeding.

Epigastric pain, nausea, and vomiting may be present with acute gastritis, but the most common presentation is gastrointestinal bleeding, ranging from occult blood loss in the stool to massive upper gastrointestinal hemorrhage. Physical findings may be normal, may reflect only the gastrointestinal bleeding, or may reflect a severe underlying associated illness (as listed above).

DIAGNOSIS

A definitive diagnosis of peptic ulcer disease cannot be made on clinical grounds alone.[12] Uncomplicated peptic ulcer disease can be strongly suspected in the presence of a ''classic'' history including epigastric burning pain; relief of pain with milk, food, or antacids; and night pain accompanied by ''benign'' physical examination findings, including normal vital signs and with or without mild epigastric tenderness. The differential diagnosis of epigastric pain is extensive and in addition to peptic ulcer disease includes gastritis, gastroesophageal reflux disease (GERD), cholelithiasis, pancreatitis, hepatitis, abdominal aortic aneurysm (AAA), gastroparesis, and ''functional'' dyspepsia. A careful history may elicit features that point away from peptic ulcer disease: burning pain radiating into the chest, water brash, and belching may suggest GERD; more severe pain radiating to the right upper quadrant and around the right or left side suggests cholelithiasis; radiation through to the back indicates pancreatitis or AAA; chronic pain, anorexia, or weight loss may indicate gastric cancer. Myocardial ischemic pain may also present as epigastric pain and should be strongly considered in the appropriate clinical setting.

Physical examination findings may also suggest other diagnoses: right upper quadrant tenderness points to cholelithiasis or hepatitis, epigastric mass to pancreatitis (pseudocyst), pulsatile mass to AAA, jaundice to hepatitis, and peritoneal findings to an acute abdomen.

In a patient presenting with epigastric pain, a number of ancillary tests may be helpful to exclude peptic ulcer disease complications and to narrow the differential diagnosis. A normal complete blood count will rule out anemia from chronic gastrointestinal bleeding due to peptic ulcer disease, gastritis, or cancer (but does not rule out acute blood loss). Elevated liver function test results may indicate hepatitis, and elevated lipase levels may indicate pancreatitis. An acute abdominal series may show free air associated with perforation. A ''limited'' emergency department ultrasound examination may show gallstones or an AAA. An electrocardiogram and cardiac enzyme determination are indicated if there is a suspicion of myocardial ischemic pain.

The definitive diagnosis of peptic ulcer disease is made by visualization of the ulcer via upper gastrointestinal barium-contrast radiography or via upper gastrointestinal endoscopy. Endoscopy has a higher yield rate for ulcer and other mucosal pathologic conditions, which may affect clinical care.[1] However, endoscopy also has a higher cost and complication rate.[1]

Since most peptic ulcers are caused by *H. pylori* infection and since eradication of *H. pylori* dramatically decreases ulcer recurrence rate, it is important to note how to diagnose infection. *Helicobacter pylori* can be diagnosed by endoscopic tests, including the *Campylobacter*-like organism (CLO) test; histologic study or culture; and noninvasive tests, including serologic tests and breath tests.[1,10,14] The CLO test detects the presence of urease in a biopsy specimen (presumptive evidence of *H. pylori* infection) with about a 90 percent sensitivity and 100 percent specificity and a cost of about $10. Histologic study using special stains has a sensitivity and specificity above 90 percent and costs about $150. Culture is difficult and has a sensitivity no better than histologic studies (although it has 100 percent specificity if results are positive). The aforementioned costs do not include the cost of endoscopy. Serologic studies detect IgG antibodies to *H. pylori* with very high sensitivity and specificity at a cost of about $50 to $75. It is not useful as a test of cure, since antibodies remain for several years after eradication. The breath test also relies on the presence of urease produced by *H. pylori*. Urea, labeled with carbon 13 or 14, is ingested and in the presence of bacterial urease is broken down into labeled carbon dioxide and ammonia. The labeled carbon dioxide is detected in the breath 30 min later. Sensitivity and specificity are greater than 90 percent, and the cost is $200 to $300. This test is ideal for confirming cure of infection.

TREATMENT

After peptic ulcer disease is diagnosed, the goal of treatment is to heal the ulcer while relieving pain and preventing complications and recurrence. Traditional ulcer therapy heals, relieves pain, and prevents complications but does not prevent recurrence. Treatment of *H. pylori* infection, when present, dramatically decreases the recurrence rate.[9] If NSAID-associated ulcers are present, the offending agent must be stopped to reduce the recurrence rate.

Traditional therapy includes histamine (H_2) receptor antagonists (H_2RAs), proton pump inhibitors (PPIs), sucralfate, and antacids[1,15] (Table 73-1). H_2RAs decrease acid production by blocking the actions of histamine on the parietal cell H_2 receptor. All four drugs heal ulcers approximately equally and are available in over-the-counter preparations.[1,15] Side effects are uncommon, but cimetidine has more significant drug interactions than do the other three due to inhibition of cytochrome P-450 activity.[15] PPIs decrease acid production by blocking hydrogen ion secretion by the parietal cell. PPIs generally heal ulcers faster than do H_2RAs and also have some in vitro inhibitory effect against *H. pylori.*[1,15] Side effects are also rare, but omeprazole has some activity against cytochrome P-450, and both PPIs inhibit absorption of drugs that rely on gastric acidity.[15] Sucralfate appears to protect the ulcer from acid exposure and heals about as well as do H_2RAs.[1,15] Sucralfate has few side effects but does inhibit absorption of a number of medications.[15] Antacids heal ulcers by buffering gastric acid and are as effective as H_2RAs.[1] Due to the simplicity of H_2RAs,

TABLE 73-1 Traditional Drugs for Peptic Ulcers

Drug	Dosage (PO)
H_2 RECEPTOR ANTAGONISTS	
Cimetidine	400 mg bid
Famotidine	20 mg bid
Nizatidine	150 mg bid
Ranitidine	150 mg bid
PROTON-PUMP INHIBITORS	
Lansoprazole	15 mg qd
Omeprazole	20 mg qd
OTHER DRUGS	
Sucralfate	1 g qid
Misoprostol*	200 μg qid
ANTACIDS	
Magnesium hydroxide-aluminum hydroxide-simethicone	
Maalox Extra Strength Antacid (Ciba)	15 mL qid
Mylanta Double Strength (J & J Merck)	2 tablets qid

*FDA-approved only for prevention of NSAID-associated gastric ulcers.
Source: Drugs for treatment of peptic ulcers,[15] with permission.

PPI, and sucralfate dosing requirements, antacids now are used mainly on an as-needed basis for ulcer pain until healing occurs.

Although NSAIDs should be stopped in patients with peptic ulcer disease whenever possible, misoprostol may prevent ulcer formation in those on concurrant NSAID therapy. Misoprostol is a prostaglandin analogue that may act by increasing mucous and bicarbonate production and by increasing mucosal blood flow.

If *H. pylori* infection is diagnosed in the presence of peptic ulcer disease, eradication is clearly indicated.[18,15] Multiple regimens have been proposed and studied mainly using combinations of bismuth subsalicylate, amoxicillin, tetracycline, metronidazole, clarithromycin, an H_2RA (mainly ranitidine), and a PPI (mainly omeprazole). Usual treatment lasts 2 weeks, costs from $30 to $360 and is effective in from 60 to greater than 90 percent of cases.[1,8,10,15]

Patients generally do not present to the emergency department with a definitive diagnosis of peptic ulcer disease but, rather, with a symptom, such as epigastric pain. If appropriate history, physical examination, and laboratory evaluation result in a physician's impression of ''possible peptic ulcer disease'' or ''dyspepsia,'' the physician is left with three main options: empiric treatment with conventional antiulcer medication, immediate referral for definite diagnosis (endoscopic or radiologic study), or noninvasive testing for *H. pylori* followed by antibiotic therapy for patients with positive test results.[1,10]

Traditional emergency department treatment would entail initiating a trial of antacids and/or H_2RAs and early referral to a primary care provider to direct evaluation and subsequent treatment. This still is a reasonable option. Immediate referral for definite diagnosis is mandated if certain ''alarm'' features are present: advanced age, weight loss, long history, anemia, persistent anorexia, early satiety, persistent vomiting, or gastrointestinal bleeding.[1,10,16] Cost-effectiveness analysis supports treatment of *H. pylori*–positive dyspeptic patients with antimicrobial and antisecretory therapy followed by endoscopic study only in those with persistent symptoms.[3,17,18] It would also be reasonable for the emergency department physician to begin symptomatic therapy, order serologic testing for *H. Pylori,* and refer for early follow-up with a primary care provider for initiation of antibacterial therapy if the test results are positive.

COMPLICATIONS

Hemorrhage

In the United States, about 150,000 patients per year are admitted to the hospital with gastrointestinal bleeding due to peptic ulcer disease.[19] Factors predicting death include large initial bleed, continued or recurrent bleeding, older age, and comorbid illness.[19] The mortality rate is 2 to 3 percent for the 80 to 85 percent of patients who do not rebleed, compared to 20 percent or greater for those who do bleed while hospitalized.[19] Shock, low initial hematocrit, red blood in the emesis or stool, and failure of blood to clear with lavage all predict further bleeding.[19]

Treatment for ulcer bleeding should focus on restoring hemodynamic stability by intravenous administration of isotonic saline solution and packed red blood cells. Appropriate blood work should be performed, including a complete blood count and type and crossmatching for several units of packed red cells. Two large-bore intravenous lines should be started and the patient placed on oxygen and a cardiac monitor. A nasogastric tube should be inserted and lavaged with water until clear. This does not slow bleeding but allows monitoring of ongoing bleeding and clears the stomach for endoscopy. An H_2RA or PPI can be started, but there is no proof that either reduce rebleeding rates.

Most patients should undergo upper gastrointestinal endoscopy for diagnostic, prognostic, and treatment purposes. An actively bleeding vessel seen on endoscopy heralds a 35 percent chance of emergency surgery and an 11 percent mortality rate, with decreasing morbidity and mortality rates with findings of a nonbleeding visible vessel; an adherent clot; a flat, pigmented spot; and a low of 0.5 percent emergency surgery and a 2 percent mortality rate if a clear base is found.[19] Treatment through endoscopy includes injection therapy with epinephrine, alcohol, or combinations; heat probe or bipolar electrical coagulation; or laser therapy. All of these treatments stop bleeding, prevent recurrences, and decrease transfusion rates and length of hospital stay. The technique chosen depends on the equipment available and the experience of the endoscopist.[19,20]

The rebleeding rate after endoscopic therapy is about 20 percent and can be treated by repeat endoscopy or emergency surgery. Surgery is also indicated if bleeding cannot be controlled by initial endoscopy. Angiography with arterial vasopressin or embolization can be considered if endoscopy has failed and surgery is thought to be very high risk.[19]

Hospitalization in an intensive care setting is indicated for all patients with significant upper gastrointestinal bleeding due to peptic ulcers. If clinical and endoscopic features suggest a low risk of rebleeding, a ward bed may be acceptable.

Perforation

Perforation is heralded by the abrupt onset of severe epigastric pain as gastric or duodural contents spill into the peritoneal cavity, followed by the development of chemical and then bacterial peritonitis. Patients may not have a prior history of peptic ulcer disease and may in fact have no antecedent history of ulcer-like symptoms. Elderly patients may not have dramatic pain or impressive peritoneal findings.

When the diagnosis is suspected, appropriate laboratory tests, including a complete blood count, type and crossmatch, and a lipase level determination, should be performed; two large-bore intravenous lines started; oxygen and a monitor placed; a nasogastric tube inserted and placed on suction; and an acute abdominal series obtained. Free air is not always present. Some authorities suggest instillation of air into the stomach through the nasogastric tube in order to detect perforation. This procedure may open a sealed perforation, causing more spillage, and if free air is still not visualized, it does not rule out a perforation; thus, it is not recommended. Broad-spectrum antibiotics should be given and a surgical consult promptly obtained. In some cases, nonsurgical therapy has been successful, but operative intervention is the standard in the United States.

Obstruction

Obstruction occurs because of scarring of the gastric outlet due to chronic peptic ulcer disease, edema due to an active ulcer, or some combination of both. Resulting symptoms include abdominal fullness, nausea, and vomiting, and signs may include abdominal distention and a succussion splash. Dehydration and electrolyte imbalances may occur. Treatment includes rehydration with intravenous fluids, correction of electrolyte abnormalities, and relief of distention with nasogastric suction. Hospitalization is almost always indicated. The outlet may open as edema subsides, but surgical correction is often necessary.

DISPOSITION

Patients with complications always require consultation, and most require admission to an appropriate inpatient unit based on the diagnosis and hemodynamic stability. Most patients with epigastric pain or dyspepsia do not leave the emergency department with a definitive diagnosis, but if critical diagnoses (e.g., AAA or myocardial ischemia) are still in the differential, consultation for admission and appropriate workup is indicated. When uncomplicated peptic ulcer disease, gastritis, or dyspepsia is strongly suspected, the great majority of patients can be discharged with antacids and an H_2RA, with or without a seralogic test for *H. pylori,* and close follow-up with their primary care provider. If "alarm" features (indicating possible cancer or bleeding) are present, consultation for early endoscopy is indicated.

Discharge instructions should include an explanation of the diagnosis and home treatment, specific follow-up instructions, and warning symptoms that should prompt immediate reevaluation. The explanation of the diagnosis should specify that peptic ulcer disease is a presumptive diagnosis and that more definitive diagnostic testing may be necessary. Home treatment should include a reminder to take medications as directed; a warning against use of alcohol, tobacco products, and aspirin or other NSAIDs; and a recommendation to avoid foods that appear to upset the individual's "stomach." Specific follow-up should include a name and phone number of the appropriate provider whenever possible as well as a time frame for reevaluation, generally 24 to 48 h if not improving or 1 to 2 weeks if improving. Warning symptoms that merit immediate reevaluation include those that may be attributed to ulcer complications or confounding illness: worsening pain, increased vomiting, hematemesis or melena, weakness or syncope, fever, chest pain, radiation of pain to the neck or back, and shortness of breath.

REFERENCES

1. Soll AH: Medical treatment of peptic ulcer disease: Practice guidelines. *JAMA* 275:622, 1996.
2. Sontag SJ: Guilty as charged: Bugs and drugs in gastric ulcer. *Am J Gastroenterol* 92:1255, 1997.
3. Rabeneck L, Graham DY: *H. pylori:* When to test, when to treat. *Ann Intern Med* 126:315, 1997.
4. Talley NJ, Weaver AL, Tesmer DL, Zinsmeister AR: Lack of discriminant value of dyspepsia subgroups in patients referred for upper endoscopy. *Gastroenterology* 105:1378, 1993.
5. Sonnenberg A, Everhart JE: Health impact of peptic ulcer in the United States. *Am J Gastroenterol* 92:614, 1997.
6. NIH Consensus Development Panel</NM>: *Helicobacter pylori* in peptic ulcer disease. *JAMA* 272:65, 1994.

7. Talley NJ, McNeil D, Piper DW: Discriminant value of dyspeptic symptoms: A study of the clinical presentation of 221 patients with dyspepsia of unknown cause, peptic ulceration, and cholelithiasis. *Gut* 28:40, 1987.
8. Damianos AJ, McGarrity TJ: Treatment strategies for *Helicobacter pylori* infection. *Am Fam Physician* 55:2765, 1997.
9. Forbes GM: Review: *Helicobacter pylori:* Current issues and new directions. *J Gastroenterol Hepatol* 12:419, 1997.
10. Falk GW: *H. pylori* 1997: Testing and treatment options. *Cleveland Clin J Med* 64:187, 1997.
11. Hirschowitz BI: Zollinger-Ellison syndrome: Pathogenesis, diagnosis, and management. *Am J Gastroenterol* 92(suppl):44S, 1997.
12. Werdmuller BFM, Van der Putten ABMM, Loffeld RJLF: Review: The clinical presentation of peptic ulcer disease. *Neth J Med* 50:115,1997.
13. Kemppainen H, Raiha I, Sourander L: Clinical presentation of peptic ulcer in the elderly. *Gerontology* 43:283, 1997.
14. De Boer WA: Diagnosis of *Helicobacter pylori* infection. *Scand J Gastroenterol* 223:35, 1997.
15. Drugs for treatment of peptic ulcers. *Med Lett* 39:1, 1997.
16. Graham DY, Rabeneck L: Patients, payers, and paradigm shifts: What to do about *helicobacter pylori. Am J Gastroenterol* 91:188, 1996.
17. Ofman JJ, Etchason J, Fullerton S, et al: Management strategies for *Helicobacter pylori* seropositive patients with dyspepsia: Clinical and economic consequences. *Ann Intern Med* 126:280, 1997.
18. Fendrick AM, Chernew ME, Hirth RA, Bloom BS: Alternative management strategies for patients with suspected peptic ulcer disease. *Ann Intern Med* 123:260, 1995.
19. Jiranek GC, Kozarek RA: A cost-effective approach to the patient with peptic ulcer bleeding. *Surg Clin North Am* 76:83, 1996.
20. Lee JG, Leung JW: Therapeutic modalities for treatment of peptic ulcer bleeding. *Gastroenterologist* 5:26, 1997.

APPENDICITIS

Denis J. FitzGerald
Arthur M. Pancioli

EPIDEMIOLOGY

Appendicitis has an overall incidence of approximately 1 case per 1000 population per year, with 6 percent of the population experiencing appendicitis at some point in their lifetime. The overall impact is significant, since acute appendicitis results in an estimated 1 million hospital days annually in the United States.[1] Unfortunately, acute appendicitis can be extremely difficult to diagnose, and misdiagnosis remains an important cause of successful malpractice claims against emergency physicians.[2]

PATHOPHYSIOLOGY

Acute appendicitis probably begins with an obstruction of the lumen. The obstruction can result from food matter, adhesions, or lymphoid hyperplasia. Despite the obstruction, mucosal secretion continues, leading to an increase in intraluminal pressure. This pressure will eventually exceed capillary perfusion pressure and will obstruct venous and lymphatic drainage. With such vascular compromise, the epithelial mucosa begins to break down, allowing bacterial invasion by bowel flora. The subsequent inflammatory response and edema further exacerbate the increased intraluminal pressure. Eventually, this increased pressure leads to arterial stasis and tissue infarction. The end result is perforation and spillage of the infected appendiceal contents into the peritoneum.

In order to understand the clinical presentation and the clinical progression of acute appendicitis, it is important to consider the innervation and anatomic variability of the appendix. Presumably, the initial lumenal distention triggers the visceral afferent pain fibers from the appendix, which enter the spinal cord at the tenth thoracic vertebra. As is characteristic of visceral afferent innervation, this pain is generally vague and poorly localized. Based on the anatomic level of these afferent fibers at the tenth thoracic level, the pain is generally perceived by the patient at the periumbilical or epigastric region. Eventually, as the inflammatory process continues, the appendiceal serosa and adjacent structures become inflamed. This inflammation triggers the somatic pain fibers, which innervate the peritoneal structures, typically localizing the pain in the right lower quadrant. This explains the migration of pain from the periumbilical area to the right lower quadrant, classically associated with acute appendicitis.

The clinician must be aware, however, that there are many exceptions to this classic presentation of the pain of acute appendicitis. These exceptions are often due to the variability of the anatomic location of the appendix. In a study of 71,000 human appendix specimens removed over a 40-year period, 26 percent were retrocecal, and 4 percent were located in the right upper quadrant.[3] With the retrocecal appendix, the pain of acute appendicitis may localize to the flank rather than the right lower quadrant. Similarly, in pregnant patients, the gravid uterus may displace the appendix, leading to a presentation of right upper quadrant or flank pain. In male patients, a retroileal appendicitis may irritate the ureter, causing pain in the testicle. A pelvic appendix may irritate the bladder or rectum and cause suprapubic pain, pain with urination, or the feeling of a need to defecate. These anatomically based variations in presentation help to explain the difficulty in making the diagnosis of acute appendicitis.

CLINICAL PRESENTATION

History

The primary symptom in acute appendicitis is abdominal pain. In approximately one-half to two-thirds of patients with appendicitis, the pain evolves in a classic pattern. Beginning in the epigastrium or periumbilical region early in the illness, the pain is initially vague and difficult to localize. Patients may describe their discomfort as indigestion or as a feeling of the need to defecate or pass flatus. As the illness progresses, the pain becomes more localized, typically in the right lower quadrant. As described above, however, the location of the patient's pain varies with the anatomic location of the appendix. One meta-analysis, in which approximately half of the studies focused on patients suspected of having acute appendicitis and half were series of patients examined for abdominal pain, provides characteristics of some common clinical findings in acute appendicitis.[4] In this analysis, right lower quadrant pain was 81 percent sensitive and 53 percent specific for the diagnosis of acute appendicitis. Similarly, migration of the pain from initial periumbilical pain to the right lower quadrant was 64 percent sensitive and 82 percent specific for the diagnosis of acute appendicitis.[4]

In addition to abdominal pain, the classic triad of symptoms in appendicitis includes anorexia, nausea, and vomiting. In acute appendicitis, these symptoms typically appear after the onset of vague abdominal pain. Anorexia is the most common of these symptoms, with 68 percent sensitivity and 36 percent specificity.[4] Vomiting is more variable in acute appendicitis, occurring in about half of patients with acute appendicitis.[4] The significance of the temporal relationship between abdominal pain and onset of vomiting as a predictor of acute appendicitis has not yet been established. Table 74-1 provides a summary of the sensitivity and specificity of many symptoms associated with appendicitis.

Physical Examination

Like the history, the findings upon physical examination of a patient with acute appendicitis depend on the duration of the illness prior to

TABLE 74-1 Summary of Clinical Examination Operating Characteristics for Appendicitis*

Procedure	Sensitivity	Specificity	LR+ (95% CI)	LR − (95% CI)
Right lower quadrant pain	0.81	0.53	7.31–8.46†	0–0.28†
Rigidity	0.27	0.83	3.76 (2.96–4.78)	0.82 (0.79–0.85)
Migration	0.64	0.82	3.18 (2.41–4.21)	0.50 (0.42–0.59)
Pain before vomiting‡	1.00	0.64	2.76 (1.94–3.94)	NA
Psoas sign	0.16	0.95	2.38 (1.21–4.67)	0.90 (0.83–0.98)
Fever	0.67	0.79	1.94 (1.63–2.32)	0.58 (0.51–0.67)
Rebound tenderness test	0.63	0.69	1.10–6.30†	0–0.86†
Guarding	0.74	0.57	1.65–1.78†	0–0.54†
No similar pain previously	0.81	0.41	1.50 (1.36–1.66)	0.323 (0.246–0.424)
Rectal tenderness	0.41	0.77	0.83–5.34†	0.36–1.15†
Anorexia	0.68	0.36	1.27 (1.16–1.38)	0.64 (0.54–0.75)
Nausea	0.58	0.37	0.69–1.20†	0.70–0.84†
Vomiting	0.51	0.45	0.92 (0.82–1.04)	1.12 (0.95–1.33)

*LR+ indicates the positive likelihood ratio with its 95% CI and LR−, the negative likelihood ratio with its 95% CI.
†In heterogeneous studies, the LRs are reported as ranges.
‡Only one study on this is included in the meta-analysis.
Source: From Wagner J, McKinney WP, Carpenter JL: Does this patient have appendicitis? *JAMA* 276:1589, 1996, with permission.

the examination. Early in the course of acute appendicitis, the patient may not have localized tenderness. As the illness progresses, the patient typically develops tenderness, especially to deep palpation, over McBurney's point. This is a point just below the middle of a line connecting the umbilicus and the anterosuperior iliac spine. Pain in the right lower quadrant with palpation of the left lower quadrant (Rosving sign) may also be elicited. As with the subjective pain, the localization of tenderness varies with the anatomic position of the appendix. If the patient has a pelvic appendix, the patient's tenderness may be most pronounced on rectal examination. With a retrocecal appendix, tenderness to palpation may be attenuated by the overlying cecum or may be most pronounced in the right flank. Additional components of the physical examination that may help in the diagnosis of pain resulting from acute appendicitis include rebound tenderness, voluntary guarding, local muscular rigidity over the inflamed area (involuntary guarding), and tenderness on rectal examination. The sensitivity and specificity of these findings are seen in Table 74-1.

Special maneuvers that can aid in the diagnosis of acute appendicitis include the psoas sign and the obturator sign. The examiner checks for a psoas sign by placing the patient in the left lateral decubitus position and extending the right leg at the hip. If an inflamed appendix is overlying the psoas muscle, this maneuver will cause an increase in the patient's pain, thereby eliciting a positive psoas sign. The obturator sign is evaluated by passively flexing the right hip and knee and internally rotating the hip. This action will stretch the obturator muscle. An inflamed appendix may irritate the obturator muscle, and this maneuver will increase pain, indicating a positive obturator sign.

Fever is another relatively late physical finding in acute appendicitis. At the onset of pain, the patient's temperature will probably be normal. If the temperature is taken frequently during the progression of the illness, it will usually rise 1 to 2°C. Temperatures above 39°C (102.2°F) are uncommon in the first 24 h of the illness but not uncommon after rupture of an appendix.

Classic Presentation

The classic clinical presentation of acute appendicitis consists of vague, poorly localized, periumbilical pain followed by anorexia, nausea, and possibly vomiting. Over a period of 4 to 48 h the pain will migrate to the right lower quadrant.[4] Low-grade fever is also a later finding in acute appendicitis. The clinician must be aware, however, that many diagnostic errors occur because the physician fails to consider the variability in the presentation associated with acute appendicitis.

DIAGNOSIS

The diagnosis of acute appendicitis is made primarily with the clinical history and physical examination. Patients with a high clinical probability of acute appendicitis should be surgically explored without the delay of any ancillary testing. Additional studies are largely confirmatory or are used to rule out other pathologic conditions when the diagnosis is less clear. These additional studies include a complete blood count (CBC), urinalysis (UA), pregnancy test for females, and various imaging studies. Clinical observation is another common diagnostic modality.

Complete Blood Count

The CBC has long been used to aid in the diagnosis of acute appendicitis, although its utility is contested.[5–7] The sensitivity of an elevated white blood count (WBC) above 10,000/μL in acute appendicitis is 70 to 90 percent, but the specificity is very low.[7] More important, the positive and negative predictive values of an elevated WBC in acute appendicitis are 92 and 50 percent, respectively.[8] In general, the WBC has limited value in the diagnosis of acute appendicitis. Clearly, overreliance on an elevated WBC will lead the clinician astray and potentially delay necessary surgery. The diagnostic value of C-reactive protein and erythrocyte sedimentation rate have been studied in acute appendicitis with mixed results.[9–11]

Urinalysis and Urine Pregnancy Tests

UA is frequently performed in the workup of possible acute appendicitis. Abnormal UA results, excluding proteinuria, are found in 19 to 40 percent of patients with acute appendicitis.[12,13] Abnormalities include pyuria, hematuria, and bacteriuria, possibly related to the extension of appendiceal inflammation to the ureter. The presence of greater than 20 WBC/hpf (without epithelial cells) in the urine should elevate consideration of urinary tract pathology in the differential diagnosis.[12]

A pregnancy test is an essential component of the workup of abdominal pain in females of childbearing age. It must be clearly stated that pregnant patients and nonpregnant patients have an equal likelihood of getting appendicitis.[14]

Imaging Studies

Imaging studies performed in the workup of possible acute appendicitis include plain radiographs, ultrasound studies, and computed tomography (CT) scans. The utility and role of these studies is controversial.

Plain radiographs of the abdomen are abnormal in 24 to 95 percent of patients with acute appendicitis.[7] Radiographic indicators of possible acute appendicitis include appendiceal fecolith, appendiceal gas, localized paralytic ileus, blurred right psoas muscle, and free air. Since many of these signs are seen in multiple other processes, abdominal radiographs have limited diagnostic value in acute appendicitis.

Graded compression ultrasonography has been widely utilized in the diagnosis of acute appendicitis. This study is safe, noninvasive, and reported to have a sensitivity of approximately 80 to 89 percent.[15] The use of this technique is based on the fact that normal bowel loops and a normal appendix can be compressed with moderate pressure while an inflamed appendix cannot be compressed. The diagnostic criteria for acute appendicitis include the visualization of a noncompressible appendix that has a diameter of 6 mm or greater, demonstration of an appendicolith, or demonstration of a periappendiceal abscess. This technique has limitations with a retrocecal appendix, in that the overlying bowel may limit visualization and compression testing. In addition, an early perforation may be missed, since the diameter of the appendix may be normal after perforation.[16] In addition, color Doppler ultrasound studies may be helpful when the appendix is well visualized but equivocal in size. With this technique, hyperemia in the wall of the appendix has been found to be a sensitive indicator of inflammation.[17]

CT is another adjunctive study used in the diagnosis of acute appendicitis. In one study which directly compared CT to ultrasound in 100 patients, the CT had greater sensitivity (96 versus 76 percent), greater accuracy (94 versus 83 percent), and a greater negative predictive value (95 versus 76 percent). In this study, there was no significant difference when CT was compared to ultrasound with regard to specificity or positive predicitive value.[18] CT findings suggesting acute appendicitis include pericecal inflammation, abscess, periappendiceal phlegmon, or fluid collections. Given its wide availability and usefulness in establishing alternative diagnoses, CT is probably the best choice as initial imaging study, although its radiation exposure limits its application in pregnant patients and children.

Clinical Observation

For patients presenting atypically with suspicion for appendicitis, clinical observation in the emergency department with serial abdominal examinations has proven to be a valuable diagnostic adjunct in clarifying evolving cases of appendicitis.[19,20] Emergency physicians and surgical consultants can both use this option to select the best course of care; emergency physicians can avert inappropriate discharge of a patient and subsequent return with a worsening course, while surgeons can avoid performing unnecessary appendectomies.

SPECIFIC ISSUES THAT AFFECT DIAGNOSIS, EVALUATION, AND TREATMENT

Special Populations

Certain groups are at high risk for appendicitis. Collectively, these patients present atypically and more often have delayed diagnoses as a result, with a concomitant increase in complications, such as appendiceal perforation. Emergency physicians must adopt an aggressive approach to evaluating these patients to reduce morbidity and mortality rates associated with unrecognized appendicitis.

Very young patients present insiduously and have a higher perforation rate. The rate of misdiagnosis is as high as 57 percent in children under age 6 years, with perforation rates approaching 90 percent in some studies.[21,22] Diagnosis in the pediatric population can be confounded by difficulty with communication and atypical symptoms, including concurrent respiratory symptoms. It is important to stress that peritonitis in children can present with such varied signs as lethargy, inactivity, and hypothermia. Appendicitis is a common condition requiring emergency operation in children, and early surgical consultation is recommended in suspicious cases.

The very old may have subtle signs and symptoms even late in the course of appendicitis. Members of this population tend to present late to physicians, often after a period of self-medication. Misdiagnosis rates can surpass 50 percent, with a high incidence of perforation, ranging from 40 to 70 percent.[23–25] Mortality rates for patients over 70 with acute appendicitis approach 30 percent.[26] In addition to late presentation with an advanced course, anatomic changes in the appendix involving the vascular bed and reduced mural thickness are thought to contribute to the fulminant course of appendicitis seen in the elderly.[27] One study found that the most significant predictors of acute appendicitis in the aged were tenderness, rigidity, pain at diagnosis, fever, and previous abdominal surgery.[28] Since extensive laboratory studies may obscure the diagnosis in patients with other concurrent medical problems, a high index of clinical suspicion is needed in the management of these patients.[29]

Pregnant patients can be difficult to diagnose with appendicitis because of variation in presentation resulting from appendix displacement by the gravid uterus as well as the fact that physiologically typical symptoms of appendicitis, such as nausea and vomiting, can be mistakenly attributed to pregnancy. Nonetheless, appendicitis remains the most common extrauterine surgical emergency in pregnancy, and fetal mortality rates can be four times higher if the appendicitis is complicated by perforation and peritonitis.[30] Consequently, the diagnosis of appendicitis must be entertained in any gravid patient presenting with abdominal pain and gastrointestinal symptoms. As an adjunct, ultrasound can be used to aid in diagnosis, particularly in differentiating obstetric causes from appendicitis.

Patients with AIDS are particularly susceptible to complications from appendicitis. Although symptoms are no different for appendicitis in this population,[31] diagnosis can be delayed because of patients' high tolerance for discomfort, the baseline frequency of gastrointestinal symptoms unrelated to appendicitis, and the occurrence of nonsurgical opportunistic pathologic conditions with similar presentations. One study noted a higher incidence of perforation in this population, possibly related to the delay in presentation or to the immunocompromised state.[31] One clear difference in management relates to the WBC, which is generally not elevated even in acute appendicitis. CT remains a good choice for differentiating surgical from nonsurgical pathologic conditions in unclear cases, but the overall management still focuses on basic assessment with aggressive surgical intervention.

Specific Medicolegal Issues

Appendicitis is a leading cause of litigation against emergency physicians. Appendicitis carries a high medicolegal risk because it is difficult to diagnose and there are no definitive diagnostic studies. Several features common to these malpractice cases have been identified.[32] Misdiagnosis of appendicitis more often occurred in patients who presented atypically and who did not receive comprehensive assessments, including rectal examinations. These patients were often given intramuscular narcotics for analgesia, given a diagnosis of gastroenteritis (without manifesting many of the typical symptoms), and discharged without appropriate follow-up care. Based on these considerations, the prudent emergency physician should maintain a high index of suspicion for appendicitis, perform complete examinations, avoid narcotics for unclear diagnoses, use the term *nonspecific abdominal pain* as a diagnosis rather than inappropriate labels for unclear causes, and arrange close follow-up for patients without a clear diagnosis. It is also imperative that all such observations, interventions, and thought processes be clearly documented in the record both to facilitate further care of the patient and to protect against potential litigation.

Transfer Issues

Given the current focus on insurance reimbursement, some authors have noted with concern a trend to transfer uninsured patients with appendicitis to county hospitals for subsequent appendectomy.[33] In a disease process where delayed care has implications for increased morbidity, such a transfer has ramifications for patients' health. Although the Consolidated Omnibus Reconciliation Act (COBRA) restricts transfer of unstable patients, decisions regarding patients' care are increasingly made on the basis of financial concerns. Although no study has yet documented a negative outcome for patients transferred under these conditions, uninsured patients with appendicitis generally have been found to be at increased risk for complications,[34] and the future impact of this practice is not clear.

TREATMENT

Antibiotics

Broad-spectrum antibiotics play an important role in the management of acute appendicitis. Although antibiotics have been found effective alone in treating acute appendicitis,[35] appendectomy remains the standard of care. As a rule, antibiotics should not be given to a patient with undiagnosed abdominal pain, to prevent inadvertent suppression of an evolving clinical presentation. In patients with uncomplicated appendicitis, antibiotics have been found to decrease the incidence of postoperative wound infections. In patients with perforation, early antibiotics have been shown to decrease postoperative abscess formation.[36,37] Antibiotics are most effective when given prior to surgery and should cover anaerobic flora, enterococci, and gram-negative intestinal flora. A common triple-coverage antibiotic combination is metronidazole, ampicillin, and gentamicin. Single coverage with cefoxitin or cefotetan is also an option.[36,38]

Surgery

Appendectomy is the standard of care for acute appendicitis. To prevent complications arising from undiagnosed appendicitis, surgeons accept a 15 to 20 percent negative appendectomy rate. There is some debate regarding an open technique versus a laparoscopic approach in current surgical thought. The postoperative course, morbidity rates, and decreased cost favor the open approach in most cases, with laparoscopic surgery reserved for selected populations.[39] In the emergency department, patients who are being taken to appendectomy should at a minimum be given nothing by mouth, have a peripheral saline IV placed, and be given preoperative antibiotics. Analgesia need not be withheld once the decision for surgery is made. Postoperative care for uncomplicated appendicitis is minimal, with most patients going home 3 days after surgery. In cases of ruptured appendicitis, postoperative care can be complex, requiring multiple interventions to resolve sepsis, paralytic ileus, and abscess formation.

DISPOSITION

The approach to a patient with potential appendicitis varies with the nature of the initial presentation, and it is a paradox in time management. Given the spectrum of appendicitis presentations, the overall goal is to eliminate delay to definitive care in clear cases of appendicitis but to allow time for other potential subtle presentations to evolve into more diagnostic certainty. In general, patients with abdominal pain can be stratified into four groups with respect to their potential for appendicitis. The first group is composed of patients who demonstrate the classic presentation for acute appendicitis. The management of these patients is straightforward, involving prompt surgical consultation and subsequent appendectomy. The emergency department course is focused on preoperative preparation, as outlined previously.

The second group includes those patients with signs and symptoms that are suspicious but not diagnostic for appendicitis. These patients are the most difficult to manage. This group of patients would most likely benefit from imaging studies, either CT or ultrasound, to elucidate the diagnosis. Observation for a 4- to 6-h period with serial examinations may clarify the evolution of the underlying pathologic condition. Surgical consultation is clearly indicated in cases where the examination becomes progressively more characteristic of appendicitis or if a surgical finding is identified on an imaging study.

The third group involves those patients with presentations minimally evoking appendicitis as a diagnostic possibility or for whom appendicitis is not a consideration in the cause of their abdominal complaint. These patients represent the highest medicolegal risk for the emergency practitioner. These patients should be observed in the emergency department for a period, with serial examinations. If the course remains benign and no other contraindications to discharge exist, they should be sent home with no diagnostic label (e.g., nonspecific abdominal pain). Clear follow-up instructions are critical to ensuring optimal outcomes for patients.

For patients with abdominal pain cleared for discharge, follow-up instructions are paramount. Patients should be told that no clear cause for their symptoms was found but that over time their symptoms will either abate or coalesce into a recognizable pattern. Follow-up instructions should include a description of worrisome symptoms that suggest progressive disease and warrant return to the emergency department. Patients should be reevaluated in 12 to 24 h by their primary physician or by the emergency department to ensure resolution of symptoms. Patients should be cautioned to avoid strong analgesics that might mask evolving pathologic processes; instead, they should be instructed to return if their pain increases. In this fashion, the emergency physician establishes a clear continuity of care for the patient with guidelines that minimize the likelihood of an adverse outcome.

The last group is composed of all high-risk special populations presenting with abdominal pain. This group includes elderly, pediatric, pregnant, and immunocompromised patients. As emphasized earlier, these patients require a high index of clinical suspicion and a low threshold for surgical consultation to avoid morbidity and mortality from undetected appendicitis.

REFERENCES

1. Addiss DG, Shaffer N, Fowler BS, et al: The epidemiology of appendicitis and appendectomy in the United States. *Am J Epidemiol* 132:910, 1990.
2. Trautlein IL, Lambert RL, Miller J: Malpractice in the emergency department: Review of 200 cases. *Ann Emerg Med* 13:709, 1984.
3. Collins DC: 71,000 human appendix specimens: A final report, summarizing forty years' study. *Am J Proctol* 14:365, 1963.
4. Wagner J, McKinney WP, Carpenter JL: Does this patient have appendicitis? *JAMA* 276:1589, 1996.
5. Vermeulen B, Morabia A, Unger PF: Influence of white cell count on surgical decision making in patients with abdominal pain in the right lower quadrant. *Eur J Surg* 161:483, 1995.
6. Lyons D, Waldron R, Ryan T, et al: An evaluation of the clinical value of the leucocyte count and sequential counts in suspected acute appendicitis. *Br J Clin Pract* 41:794, 1987.
7. Hoffmann J, Rausmussen O: Aids in the diagnosis of acute appendicitis. *Br J Surg* 76:774, 1989.
8. Marchand A, Van Lente F, Galen RS: The assessment of laboratory tests in the diagnosis of acute appendicitis. *Am J Clin Pathol* 80:369, 1983.
9. Chung J, Kong M, Lin S, et al: Diagnostic value of c-reactive protein in children with perforated appendicitis. *Eur J Pediatr* 155:529, 1996.
10. Peltola H, Ahlqvist J, Rapola J, et al: C-reactive protein compared with white blood cell count and erythrocyte sedimentation rate in the diagnosis of acute appendicitis in children. *Acta Chir Scand* 152:55, 1986.
11. Jaye DL, Waites KB: Clinical applications of c-reactive protein in pediatrics. *Pediatr Infect Dis J* 16:735, 1997.
12. Kretchmar LH, McDonald DF: The urine sediment in acute appendicitis. *Arch Surg* 87:209, 1963.
13. Puskar D, Bedalov G, Fridrih S, et al: Urinalysis, ultrasound analysis, and renal dynamic scintigraphy in acute appendicitis. *Urology* 45:108, 1995.
14. Moawad AH: Acute appendicitis during pregnancy, in Cibels LA (ed): *Surgical Diseases in Pregnancy*. New York, Springer-Verlag, 1990, pp 105–114.
15. Zeiden BS, Wasser T, Nicholas GG: Ultrasonography in the diagnosis of acute appendicitis. *J R Coll Surg Edinburgh* 42:24, 1997.
16. Jeffrey RB, Jain KA, Ngheim HV: Sonographic diagnosis of acute appendicitis: Interpretive pitfalls. *Am J Roentgenol* 162:55, 1994.
17. Lim HK, Lee WJ, Kim TH: Appendicitis: Usefulness of color doppler US. *Radiology* 201:221, 1996.
18. Balthazar EJ, Birnbaum BA, Yee J: Acute appendicitis: CT and US correlation in 100 patients. *Radiology* 190:31, 1994.
19. Graff L, Radford MJ, Werne C: Probability of appendicitis before and after observation. *Ann Emerg Med* 20:503, 1991.
20. Nauta RJ, Magnant C: Observation versus operation for abdominal pain in the right lower quadrant: Roles of the clinical examination and the leukocyte count. *Am J Surg* 151:746, 1986.
21. Golladay S, Sarret JR: Delayed diagnosis in pediatric appendicitis. *South Med J* 81:38, 1988.
22. Rappaport WD, Peterson M, Stanton C: Factors responsible for the high perforation rate seen in early childhood appendicitis. *Am J Surg* 55:602, 1989.
23. Hall A, Wright TM: Acute appendicitis in the geriatric patient. *Am Surg* 44:147, 1978.
24. Klein SR, Layden L, Wright JF, et al: Appendicitis in the elderly. *Postgrad Med* 83:247, 1988.
25. Thorbjarnarson B, Loehr WJ: Acute appendicitis in patients over the age of sixty. *Surg Gynecol Obstet* 125:1277, 1967.
26. Franz M, Norman J, Fabri PJ: Increased mortality of appendicitis with advancing age. *Am Surg* 61:40, 1995.
27. Freund HR, Rubinstein E: Appendicitis in the aged: Is it really different? *Am Surg* 50:573, 1984.
28. Eskelinen M, Ikonen J, Lipponen P: The value of history-taking, physical examination, and computer assistance in the diagnosis of acute appendicitis in patients more than 50 years old. *Scand J Gastroenterol* 30:349, 1995.
29. Horattas MC, Guyton DP, Wu D: A reappraisal of appendicitis in the elderly. *Am J Surg* 160:291, 1990.
30. Mahmoodian S: Appendicitis complicating pregnancy. *South Med J* 85:19, 1992.
31. Flum DR, Steinberg SD, Sarkis AY, et al: Appendicitis in patients with acquired immunodeficiency syndrome. *J Am Coll Surg* 184:481, 1997.
32. Rusnak RA, Borer JM, Fastow JS: Misdiagnosis of acute appendicitis: Common features discovered in cases after litigation. *Am J Emerg Med* 12:397, 1994.
33. Norton VC, Schriger DL: Effect of transfer on outcome in patients with appendicitis. *Ann Emerg Med* 29:467, 1997.
34. Braveman P, Schaaf VM, Egerter S, et al: Insurance-related differences in the risk of ruptured appendix. *N Engl J Med* 331:444, 1994.
35. Eriksson S, Granstrom L: Randomized controlled trial of appendicectomy versus antibiotic therapy for acute appendicitis. *Br J Surg* 82:166, 1995.
36. Bauer T, Vennits B, Holm B, et al: Antibiotic prophylaxis in acute nonperforated appendicitis. The Danish Multicenter Study Group III. *Ann Surg* 209:307, 1989.
37. Antimicrobial prophylaxis in surgery. *Med Lett* 35:91, 1993.
38. Meller JL, Reyes HM, Loeff DS, et al: One-drug versus two-drug antibiotic therapy in pediatric perforated appendicitis: A prospective randomized study. *Surgery* 110:764, 1991.
39. Wilcox RT, Traverso LW: Have the evaluation and treatment of acute appendicitis changed with new technology? *Surg Clin North Am* 77:1355, 1997.

INTESTINAL OBSTRUCTION

Salvator J. Vicario
Timothy G. Price

Intestinal obstruction is an important consideration in patients who present with abdominal complaints to the emergency department. It can be defined as an inability of the intestinal tract to allow for regular passage of food and bowel contents. In turn, this can be secondary to mechanical obstruction or adynamic ileus. Adynamic ileus (paralytic ileus) is the more common entity, but is usually self-limiting and does not require surgical intervention. Mechanical obstruction can be caused by either intrinsic or extrinsic factors and generally requires definitive intervention in a relatively short period of time to determine the cause and minimize subsequent morbidity and mortality.

ETIOLOGY

Small bowel obstruction (SBO) accounts for 20 percent of all acute surgical admissions and results in approximately 9000 deaths per year in the United States. Less commonly, the intestine is obstructed at the large bowel.

Both large and small intestines may be obstructed by various pathologic processes (Table 75-1). Extrinsic, intrinsic, or intraluminal processes precipitate mechanical obstruction. Differentiating SBO from large bowel obstruction (LBO) is important because the incidence, clinical presentation, and modes of therapy vary depending on the anatomic site of the obstruction. The small intestine is characterized by transverse linear densities that extend completely across the bowel lumen (plicae circulares). The colon is situated peripherally in the

TABLE 75-1 Common Causes of Intestinal Obstruction

Duodenum	Small Bowel	Colon
Stenosis	Adhesions	Carcinoma
Foreign body (Bezoars)	Hernia	Fecal impaction
Stricture	Intussusception	Ulcerative colitis
Superior mesenteric artery syndrome	Lymphoma	Volvulus
	Stricture	Diverticulitis (stricture, abscess)
		Intussusception
		Pseudo-obstruction

abdomen, is larger in diameter, and contains short, blunt, and thick projections (haustrae) that arise from the bowel wall and extend only partially into the lumen. Haustrae are less numerous and situated farther apart than plicae circulares.

The most common cause of SBO is adhesions following abdominal surgery.[1-3] Although in most cases several months to years have passed from the time of the previous surgery, SBO may occur within the first few weeks following surgery.[3] The second most common cause of small intestinal obstruction is incarceration of a groin hernia[1,2] (see Chap. 76). This can occur in infants as well as adults and should be suspected anytime there is a complaint of a "knot" or growth in the inguinal region that fails to reduce with manipulation. Other sites that are occasionally responsible for SBO secondary to hernia include the umbilicus, femoral canal, and, rarely, the obturator foramen. Umbilical hernias are more readily apparent and occur in any age group. Obturator or femoral hernias are much less common and may present with femoral or medial thigh pain. Elderly females are particularly susceptible to these defects, and one needs to consider them as a possible cause of SBO in these patients. Finally, a defect in the mesentery itself may cause intestinal obstruction.

Other causes of SBO are much less common and are generally due to intraluminal or intramural processes. Primary small bowel lesions include polyps, lymphoma, or adenocarcinoma. An unusual cause of intraluminal obstruction is gallstone ileus. In this situation, a gallstone has eroded from the gallbladder through the bowel wall and can cause obstruction at the ileocecal valve. Besides the findings of bowel obstruction, one may note air in the biliary tree on abdominal radiographs. Lymphomas may be the leading point of intussusception and present as SBO.

Bezoars are most commonly composed of vegetable matter or pulp from persimmons. Patients who have undergone gastrointestinal pyloroplasty or pyloric resection are most susceptible to intraluminal obstruction by bezoars.

Inflammatory bowel disease may also affect the small bowel at various sites. Likewise, infectious processes including abscesses may obstruct the bowel. Radiation enteritis is also a possible cause of SBO in patients who have undergone radiation therapy.

Colonic obstruction is almost never caused by hernia or surgical adhesions. Neoplasms are by far the most common cause of large bowel obstruction.[4,5] Therefore, anyone who has symptoms of colonic obstruction should be evaluated for a neoplasm. Diverticulitis may create significant secondary obstruction and mesenteric edema. Stricture formation may occur with chronic inflammation and scarring. Fecal impaction is a common problem in elderly, debilitated patients and may present with symptoms of colonic obstruction.

The next most frequent cause of large bowel obstruction after cancer and diverticulitis is sigmoid volvulus. Elderly, bedridden, or psychiatric patients who are taking anticholinergic medication are most often subject to this mechanical problem. A history of constipation may precede the volvulus and presenting symptoms. Radiographic appearance is usually classic (Fig. 75-1). Finally, although much less common, cecal volvulus may also cause large bowel obstruction.

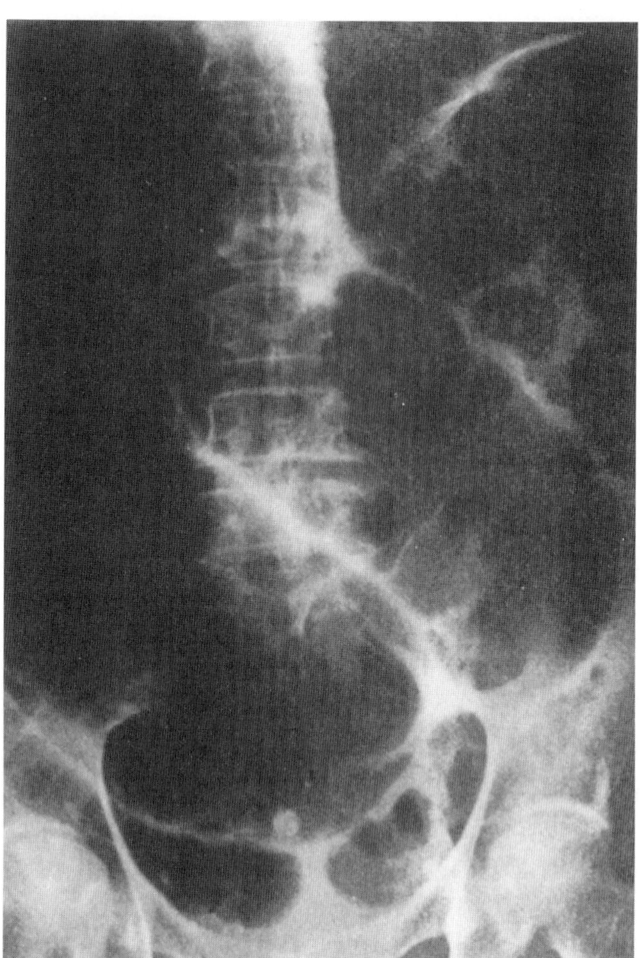

FIG. 75-1. Sigmoid volvulus. Note distension of large bowel and central stripe, giving a "coffee-bean" appearance.

PATHOPHYSIOLOGY

Normal bowel contents contain gas as well as gastric secretions and food. Intraluminal accumulation of gastric, biliary, and pancreatic secretions continues even if there is no oral intake. As obstruction develops, the bowel becomes congested and there is failure of intestinal contents to be absorbed. Vomiting and decreased oral intake follow. The combination of decreased absorption, vomiting, and reduced intake leads to volume depletion with hemoconcentration and electrolyte imbalance, and ultimately can cause renal failure or shock.[5]

Bowel distension often accompanies mechanical obstruction. Distension is due to the accumulation of fluids in the bowel lumen, an increase in intraluminal pressure with enhanced peristaltic contractions, and air swallowing. When intraluminal pressure exceeds capillary and venous pressure in the bowel wall, absorption and lymphatic drainage decrease. At this stage, bacteria may enter the bloodstream, the bowel becomes ischemic, and septicemia and bowel necrosis can develop. Shock rapidly ensues. Mortality approaches 70 percent if bowel obstruction has been allowed to progress this far. With a *closed-loop obstruction* this sequence of events may occur more rapidly. In this instance, there is no proximal escape for bowel contents. Examples of closed-loop obstruction include an incarcerated hernia and complete colon obstruction in the presence of a closed ileocecal valve.

CLINICAL FEATURES

The site and nature of the obstruction and the preexisting condition of the patient will determine the clinical presentation. Almost all patients will have abdominal pain.[4] The pain is generally described as crampy and intermittent. Pain of mechanical SBO is often episodic, usually lasting for a few minutes at a time, and it may be periumbilical or more diffuse. In adynamic ileus, the pain tends to be less intense and more constant. If the obstruction is proximal, vomiting is usually present. The vomitus in proximal obstruction is usually bilious but is feculent in distal ileal obstruction. The pain of large bowel obstruction is usually hypogastric. Large bowel obstructions may be associated with fecal vomiting as well.

Other features that are consistently present with obstruction of small bowel or colon include the inability to have a bowel movement or pass flatus. Care should be taken to avoid the diagnosis of constipation, as this symptom is secondary to partial or complete obstruction. Partial bowel obstruction, however, is often associated with regular passage of stool and flatus.

Physical findings vary, depending on the site, duration, and etiology of the pathologic process. Early symptoms are usually associated with some abdominal distension, often impressive with colonic obstruction yet not readily apparent in cases of incarcerated hernia. Abdominal tenderness may be minimal and diffuse or localized and severe.[3,4] Patients who have developed peritonitis will have severe tenderness. The abdomen may be tympanitic to percussion. Mechanical obstruction will produce active high pitched bowel sounds with occasional ''rushes.'' If obstruction has been present for several hours, peristaltic waves and bowel sounds may be diminished. Patients with an adynamic ileus may have some abdominal distension associated with diminished or absent bowel sounds. Careful search for localized or rebound tenderness is essential to rule out the possibility of gangrenous or perforated bowel, which requires immediate surgical intervention (Fig. 75-2).

Elderly patients have signs and symptoms that are similar to younger patients with intestinal obstruction. Adhesions and hernias are common causes for SBO in this age group, while carcinomas are the most likely etiology of LBO because of the increased likelihood of cancer as people age.[9] Elderly patients who are debilitated or confused, or who are on multiple medications, may be unable to give a detailed history. Careful examination for characteristic bowel sounds, masses or blood in stool, and radiographic investigation will often distinguish bowel obstruction from ileus. There is also evidence that patients over 60 years old are more likely to succumb secondary to complications of bowel obstruction.[3]

All patients with abdominal pain or distension should be examined for signs of organomegaly or masses that may suggest a cause of the obstruction. A rectal examination may identify fecal impaction, rectal carcinoma, occult blood, or stricture. The absence of stool or air in the vault may aid in the diagnosis of bowel obstruction, but its presence does not eliminate a more proximal obstruction, as patients may not be able to evacuate preexisting rectal contents. A pelvic examination should be performed to identify any gynecologic pathology causing obstruction.

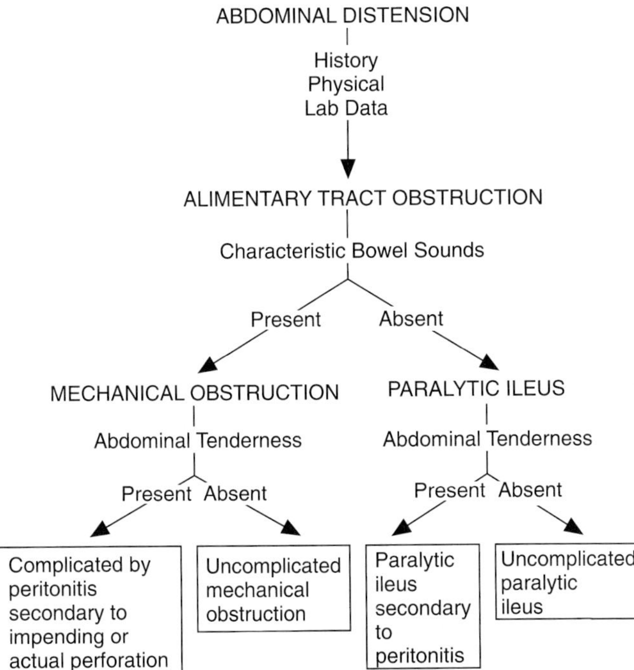

FIG. 75-2. Logic flow diagram emphasizing the clinical importance of abdominal tenderness in alimentary tract obstruction. (From Schwartz GR: *Principles and Practice of Emergency Medicine,* 3d ed, p 1718. Malvern, PA, Lea & Febiger, 1992, with permission.)

LABORATORY AND RADIOGRAPHIC FINDINGS

All patients with suspected obstruction should have a flat and upright abdominal radiograph and upright chest x-ray or a lateral decubitus view if the patient cannot be upright. An abdominal radiograph can confirm the diagnosis, identify free air or masses, and localize the site to large or small bowel (Fig. 75-3*A,B*). Laboratory work usually includes a complete blood count and electrolyte measurements. Depending on the duration of symptoms and site of obstruction or whether there is bowel necrosis, one may find a wide range in white blood cell (WBC) counts and hemoglobin, hematocrit, and electrolyte values. Patients will usually have some elevation in WBC. A white count $>20{,}000/\mu L$ or left shift should make one suspect bowel gangrene, intra-abdominal abscess, or peritonitis.[5] Extreme WBC elevation ($>40{,}000/\mu L$) suggests mesenteric vascular occlusion. The serum anylase and lipase levels may be mildly elevated. Levels of serum electrolytes are usually normal or mildly reduced,[4] depending on whether the obstruction is of short or long duration or whether there is associated emesis. An increase in Hct, BUN, and creatinine are consistent with volume depletion and dehydration. Other indications of the severity of obstruction or secondary complications include increased urine specific gravity, ketonuria, elevated lactate levels, and metabolic acidosis.

Further investigations to determine the site or etiology of obstruction include sigmoidoscopy or barium enema. Upper gastrointestinal studies are rarely indicated. Barium enema can determine the cause and site of large bowel obstruction (Fig. 75-4). Sigmoidoscopy can identify friable mucosa, intraluminal lesions, or the dark-blue gangrenous mucosa associated with dead bowel. If the diagnosis is unclear, repeated examination, preferably by the same examiner, will be necessary. The use of contrast enhanced CT has been advocated to delineate partial from complete bowel obstruction.[7,8]

TREATMENT

If a true mechanical obstruction is diagnosed, then surgical intervention is often required. The frequently quoted adage ''never let the sun rise or set on a mechanical bowel obstruction'' likely refers to the philosophy advocated by surgeons who have noted increased morbidity and mortality when the obstruction has not been treated within 24 h.[6] Prior to surgical intervention, emergency department efforts should be made to decompress the bowel with nasogastric intubation. A nasogastric tube is generally effective in removing excess bowel contents and air. Likewise, because of loss of absorptive capacity, decreased oral intake, and vomiting, most patients will require intravenous fluid replacement. Patients can be monitored prior to surgical intervention by the response of blood pressure and heart rate and measurement of urine output. Surgery should not be delayed unnecessarily by attempting to use long intestinal tubes (Baker, Cantor, or Miller-Abbott) or excessive testing. A volvulus of the sigmoid colon will usually decompress via sigmoidoscopy and insertion of a rectal tube. Should a closed-loop obstruction, bowel necrosis, or cecal volvulus be suspected, then surgical intervention should be performed without delay.[4] All patients with mechanical obstruction require broad-spectrum antibiotic coverage preoperatively, as the risk of infection and septicemia is significant in most conditions.[7,11] If adynamic ileus is the primary problem or the diagnosis is uncertain, conservative measures, including intravenous fluids, naso-

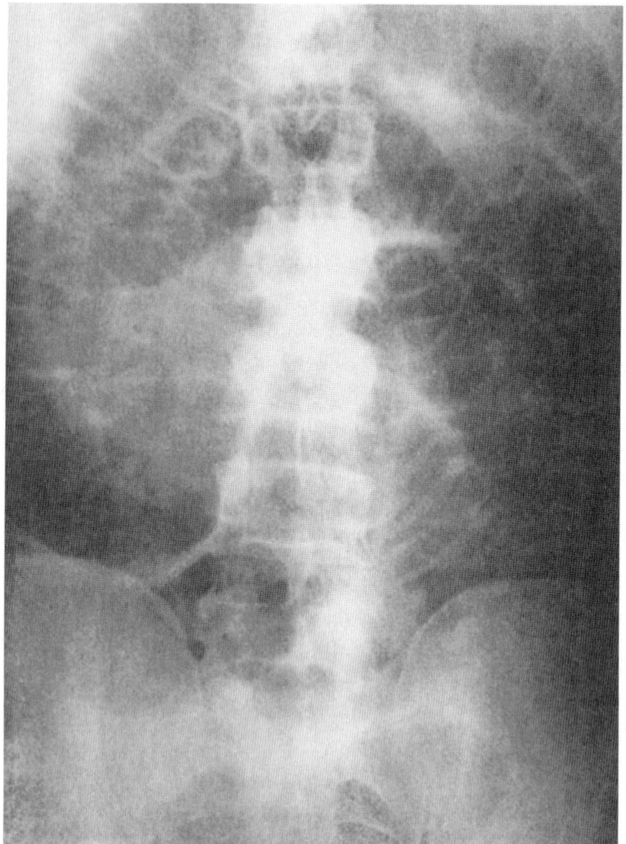

A

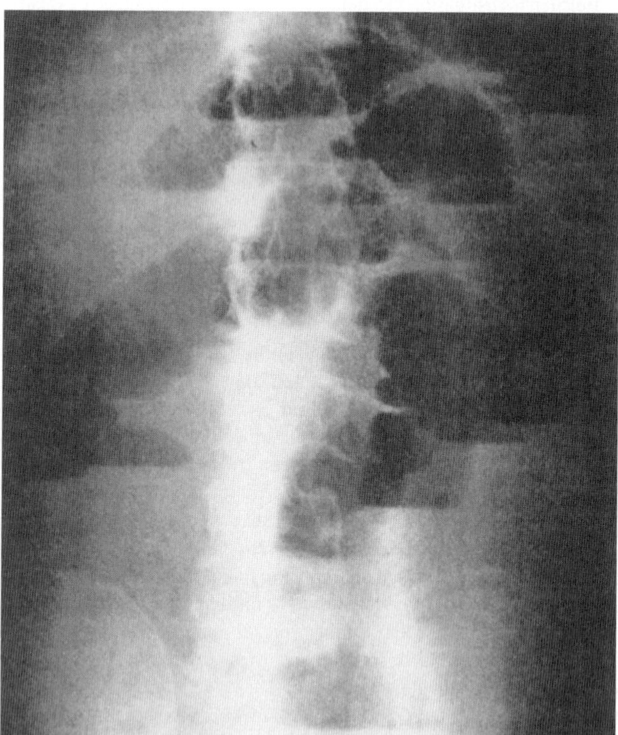

B

FIG. 75-3. A. Flat plate abdominal film illustrates distended loops of small bowel. **B.** Upright film demonstrates multiple air-fluid levels and "step-ladder" appearance. (From Harris JH, Harris WH: *The Radiology of Emergency Medicine,* 3d ed. Baltimore, Williams and Wilkins, 1993, p 843, with permission.)

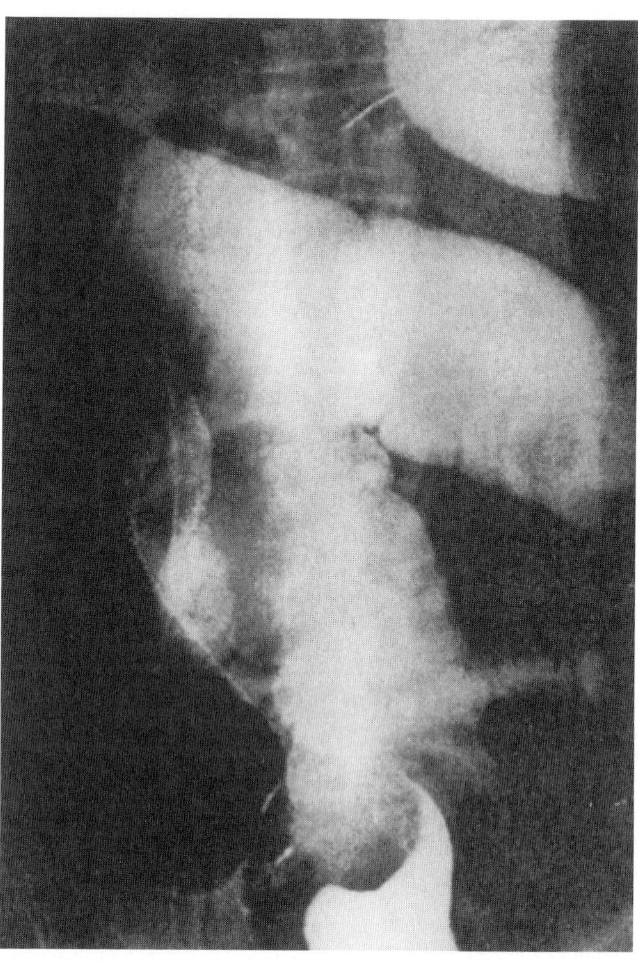

FIG. 75-4. Barium enema examination demonstrating incomplete filling of the sigmoid secondary to volvulus. Note the "parrot-beak" appearance of the point of the volvulus. (From Schwartz GR: *Principles and Practice of Emergency Medicine,* 3d ed. Malvern, PA, Lea & Febiger, 1992, p 1720, with permission.)

gastric decompression, and observation, are generally effective in allowing the bowel to resume normal activity and function. Any medication that inhibits bowel mobility should be discontinued. Radiologic examination to confirm nasogastric tube placement or long-tube location is also advised. Some authors advocate contrast radiography to distinguish partial SBO from ileus or for the differentiation of strangulated from simple SBO.[9,10]

PSEUDO-OBSTRUCTION

Intestinal pseudo-obstruction (Ogilvie's syndrome) may also mimic bowel obstruction. Although any segment of bowel may be affected, low colonic obstruction is the most common clinical presentation. Large amounts of gas will be present in the large intestine. Radiographs reveal a dilated colon with well-defined septae and haustral markings and very little fluid, making air-fluid levels uncommon.[11] Patients may be using anticholinergic or tricyclic antidepressants, which depress motility. One must avoid the use of barium studies as the patient may be unable to evacuate the barium. Preference should be given to colonoscopy after digital rectal examination as an early intervention to rule out true obstruction or significant lesions. Colonoscopy will also treat the pseudo-obstruction by decompression. Surgery is not usually helpful and may be harmful.[11,12]

REFERENCES

1. Leffall LD, Syphax B: Clinical aids in strangulation intestinal obstruction. *Arch Surg* 117:334, 1982.
2. Hofstetter SR: Acute adhesive obstruction of the small intestine. *Surg Gynec Obstet* 52:141, 1981.
3. Becker WF: Intestinal obstruction: An analysis of 1007 cases. *South Med J* 48:41, 1955.
4. Shatila AH, Chamberlain BE, Webb WR: Current status of diagnosis and management of strangulation obstruction of the small bowel. *Am J Surg* 132:299, 1976.
5. Cheadle WC, Garr FE, Richardson JD: The importance of early diagnosis of small bowel obstruction. *Am Surg* 54:565, 1988.
6. Brolin RE, Krasna MJ, Mast BA: Use of tubes and radiographs in bowel obstruction. *Ann Surg* 206:126, 1987.
7. Maglinte DT, Peterson LA, et al: Enterolysis in partial small bowel obstruction. *Am J Surg* 147:325, 1984.
8. Ha HK, Him JS: Differentiation of single and strangulated small bowel obstructions: Usefulness of known CT criteria. *Radiology* 204:507, 1997.
9. Frager D, Baer JW, et al: Detection of intestinal ischemia in patients with acute small bowel obstruction due to adhesions or hernia: Efficacy of CT. *AJR Am J Roentgenol* 166:67-71, 1991.
10. Maglinte DD, Reyes BC et al</AU>. Reliability and role of plain film radiography and CT in the diagnosis of small bowel obstruction. *AJR Am J Roentgenol* 167:1451, 1996.
11. Vanek VW, Al-Salti M: Acute pseudo-obstruction of the colon (Ogilvies syndrome): An analysis of 400 cases. *Dis Colon Rectum* 29:203, 1986.
12. Doudi S, Berry AR, Kettlewell MS: Acute colonic pseudo obstruction. *Br J Surg* 79:99, 1992.

HERNIA IN ADULTS AND CHILDREN

Frank W. Lavoie

A *hernia* is technically defined as an *external* or *internal* protrusion of a body part from its natural cavity. Although internal herniations may be found in cerebral, diaphragmatic, hiatal, or other abdominopelvic locations, the usual use of the term is in reference to the abdominal wall and typically to external presentations. Hernias also may be *interparietal*, within the layers of the abdominal wall. Abdominal wall herniations occur both in adults and children and may be present in groin (inguinal or femoral), umbilical, anterior abdominal, pelvic, or lumbar locations.

PATHOPHYSIOLOGY

General Characteristics

Essential to the understanding of hernias are the anatomic characteristics of the abdominal cavity and, in particular, its fascial and aponeurotic layers. Embryologic development produces localized areas of inherent weakness in the abdominal wall. These include areas where extra peritoneal structures penetrate (as in the inguinal, femoral, and obturator canals, the sciatic foramen, and the umbilical region) and areas devoid of strong multilayer structural support (as in the anterior abdominal wall's linea alba and semilunar line). In addition, surgical incision and trauma may produce areas of abdominal wall weakness.

Herniations may include preperitoneal fat, retroperitoneal organs, and a hernial sac composed of peritoneum containing intraperitoneal structures (e.g., omentum or organs). Clinically significant herniation without a peritoneal sac is uncommon. Hernias may be complicated by inclusion of a viscus forming one wall of the hernial sac. This involves a partially retroperitoneal organ and is called a *sliding hernia*. Sliding inguinal hernias most frequently involve the colon.

The entrapment of the content of a hernia is more likely when the hernia opening is narrow. When the content can be returned to its normal cavity by manipulation, the hernia is *reducible*; when it cannot, it is *irreducible* or *incarcerated*. Incarceration may be *acute* or *chronic*. Incarceration of a single wall of a hollow viscus is known as *Richter hernia*. Incarcerated hernias are subject to inflammatory and edematous changes and are at risk for strangulation. *Strangulation* of a hernia refers to vascular compromise of the incarcerated contents. When strangulation is not relieved in a timely fashion, gangrene develops.

Predisposing Factors

Lack of developmental maturity of anatomic structures is known to predispose to the formation of hernias, as in indirect inguinal and umbilical hernias in premature infants. Family history, undescended testis, and genitourinary abnormalities are additional risks for inguinal hernia. Conditions that increase intraabdominal pressure—such as ascites, peritoneal dialysis, ventriculoperitoneal shunt, cystic fibrosis, chronic obstructive pulmonary disease, and pregnancy—are thought to be associated with hernia.

Specific Hernia Types

INDIRECT INGUINAL HERNIA The inguinal canal is the tract in the abdominal wall through which pass the gubernaculum, testis, and spermatic cord in males or the round ligament in females. The canal is defined by an internal ring defect in the transversalis fascia and transversus abdominis aponeurosis, lateral to the inferior epigastric vessels, and a more medial external ring defect in the external oblique aponeurosis (Figs. 76-1 and 76-2).

Normal passage through the inguinal canal is accompanied by peritoneal evagination known as the *processus vaginalis*. Normal obliteration of the processus occurs in infancy. Passage of contents through a persistent patent processus vaginalis along the inguinal canal leads to an indirect inguinal hernia. Congenital failure of obliteration is the etiology for all indirect inguinal hernias. Acquired myoaponeurotic defects may additionally contribute to indirect inguinal hernia in adults.

Passage of the testis is thought to enlarge the canal and increase the likelihood of inguinal hernia in males. It is more common on the right side due to later passage of the right testis. Indirect inguinal hernias infrequently incarcerate and strangulate, particularly in the first year of life and in females.[1]

DIRECT INGUINAL HERNIA These are protrusions through the transversalis fascia and the external ring, medial to the inferior epigastric vessels. (Figs. 76-1 and 76-3). Direct inguinal hernias are acquired defects that do not involve passage through the inguinal canal and occur predominantly in adults; they rarely incarcerate and strangulate. A hernia with ipsilateral direct and indirect inguinal components may be called a *pantaloon hernia*.

FEMORAL HERNIA A femoral hernia is a protrusion below the inguinal ligament and adjacent to the femoral vessels in the femoral canal (Fig. 76-1). Femoral hernias are more common in women due to the different anatomic structure of the pelvis. Femoral hernias are far less common than inguinal hernias. They do frequently incarcerate and strangulate.[2]

UMBILICAL HERNIA In utero contraction of the umbilical cord insertion forms the fibromuscular umbilical ring. Incomplete development or weakness in the ring allows herniation of abdominal contents (Fig. 76-4).

Congenital umbilical hernias affect 10 to 30 percent of white infants and a higher percentage of children of African descent. They are more common in females. Incarceration and strangulation of childhood umbilical hernias are very rare.[1,3]

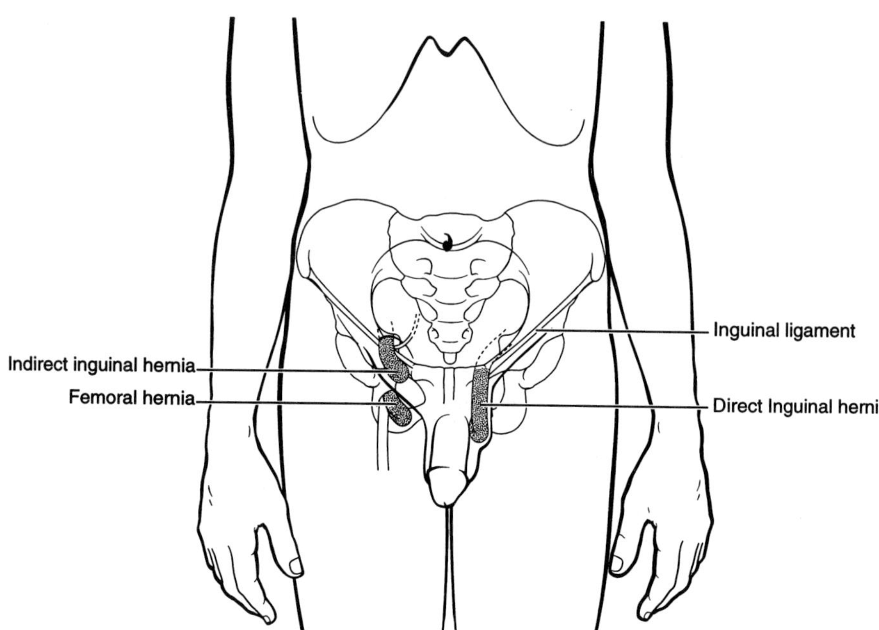

FIG. 76-1. Groin hernias.

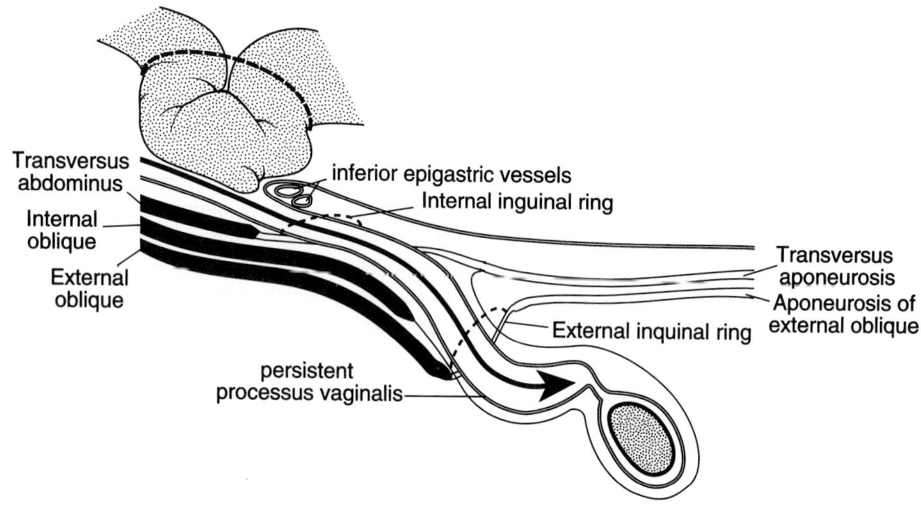

FIG. 76-2. Indirect inguinal hernia.

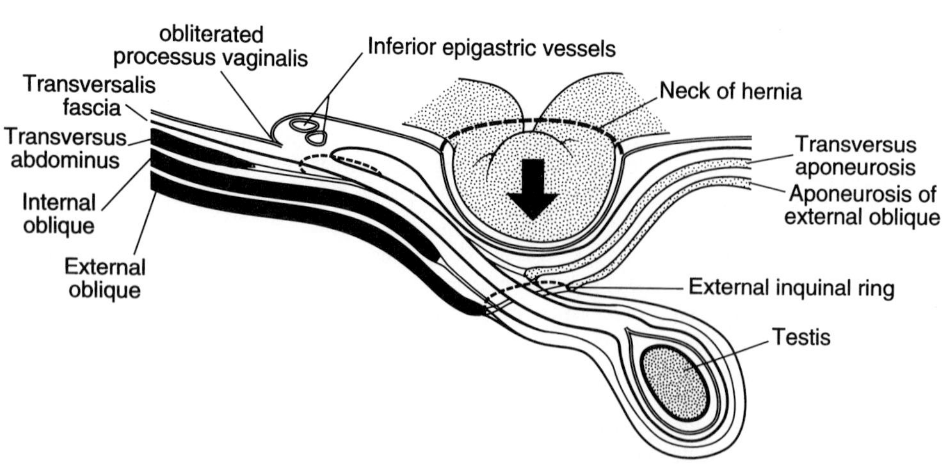

FIG. 76-3. Direct inguinal hernia.

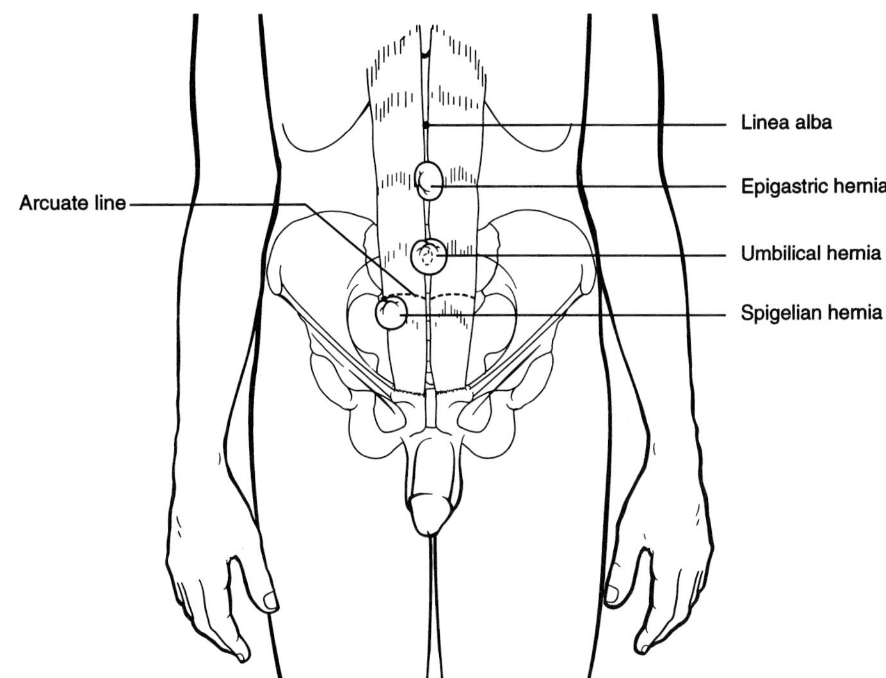

FIG. 76-4. Anterior abdominal wall hernias.

Umbilical hernias may also develop in adults. This acquired defect is more common in women and is associated with obesity, pregnancy, and ascites. Incarceration and strangulation frequently occur.

EPIGASTRIC HERNIA An epigastric hernia involves herniation through the linea alba of the rectus sheath, above the umbilicus (Fig. 76-4).

SPIGELIAN HERNIA Herniation at the site of the semilunar or arcuate line, just lateral to the rectus muscle, through the combined aponeurosis of the transversus abdominis and internal oblique muscles is known as a Spigelian or lateral ventral hernia. This hernia is frequently interparietal, making diagnosis difficult (Fig. 76-4).

PELVIC HERNIA Pelvic hernias are rare. There are *sciatic hernias*, passing through sciatic foramen; *perineal hernias*, passing between perineal muscles; and *obturator hernias*, passing through the obturator canal with the obturator vessels. Obturator hernias frequently incarcerate.[4]

LUMBAR HERNIA Herniation rarely may occur through the inferior or superior lumbar triangles.

INCISIONAL HERNIA Herniation may occur through an incisional area. Infection and obesity contribute to poor wound healing, which increases the likelihood of development of incisional hernia.

TRAUMATIC HERNIA Traumatic herniation involving a variety of organs and locations may be observed. These usually occur without true hernia sacs.[5]

EPIDEMIOLOGY

The incidence of abdominal hernia is estimated to be from 10 to 20 per 1000 births and is greater among premature infants.[6] In the screening of otherwise healthy young adult military recruits, approximately 3 percent are determined to have groin hernias.[7] Currently, approximately 700,000 herniorrhaphies are performed annually in the United States for inguinal hernias alone.[8]

Virtually all groin hernias are more commonly seen in males than in females, whereas hernias of the anterior abdominal wall are of similar incidence (Table 76-1). Consequently, the distribution of hernia types by sex is markedly different (Figs. 76-5 and 76-6).

Indirect inguinal hernias have a bimodal preponderance, with peaks in the first year of life and after the age of 40 years.[9] Direct inguinal hernias are characteristically seen in adults, with a large male preponderance after 40 years of age. Femoral hernias have roughly equal incidence by sex and also tend to occur predominantly after age 40.

Epigastric hernia is of approximately equal incidence by sex. Most occur between the ages of 30 and 70 years. Congenital umbilical hernias are seen in the newborn population and in early childhood.

TABLE 76-1 Hernias in Males and Females, Henry Ford Hospital (1965 and 1967)

	Males		Females	
	Number	%	Number	%
Indirect	887	53.6	107	32.9
Direct	453	27.4	5	1.5
Combination Direct-indirect-femoral	126	7.6	10	3.1
Incisional	57	3.4	57	17.5
Femoral	47	2.8	36	11.1
Umbilical	38	2.3	54	16.6
Hiatal	36	2.2	48	14.8
Epigastric	11	0.7	8	2.46
Total	1655		325	

Source: From Ponka JL: *Hernias of the Abdominal Wall.* Philadelphia, Saunders, 1980, p 82. With permission.

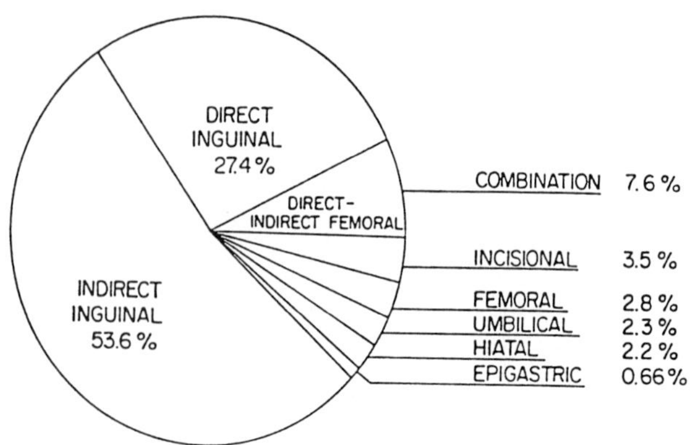

FIG. 76-5. The relative distribution of common hernias seen in 1655 men in 1965 and 1967. The high proportion of indirect and direct inguinal hernias is striking. (From Ponka JL: *Hernias of the Abdominal Wall.* Philadelphia, Saunders, 1980, p 85. With permission.)

Acquired umbilical hernias in adults increase gradually in incidence from age 20 and are rarely seen beyond age 70. They are slightly more common in women and constitute a larger percentage of the hernias in the female population.

There is no difference in the incidence of incisional hernia in males versus females. As in the case of many other hernias, the vast majority of patients diagnosed with incisional hernia are over 40 years of age. The incidence and distribution of other uncommon hernias is less clear.

CLINICAL FEATURES

The majority of hernias are asymptomatic and are detected either on routine physical examination or inadvertently by the patient. Patients with incarceration frequently give a history of hernia; the patient can no longer reduce it and therefore seeks medical attention. If incarceration is acute, pain may develop suddenly. With infants, irritability may be the only presenting complaint. Incarceration may be accompanied by nausea and vomiting if partial or complete bowel obstruction has occurred. Incarcerated hernias are a leading cause of bowel obstruction, second to postoperative adhesions.

When strangulation occurs, the patient may be toxic, along with signs and symptoms of bowel obstruction. In the case of Richter hernia, however, strangulation may occur without intestinal obstruction.[10] Unrelieved strangulation may result in perforation, abscess formation, peritonitis, or septic shock.

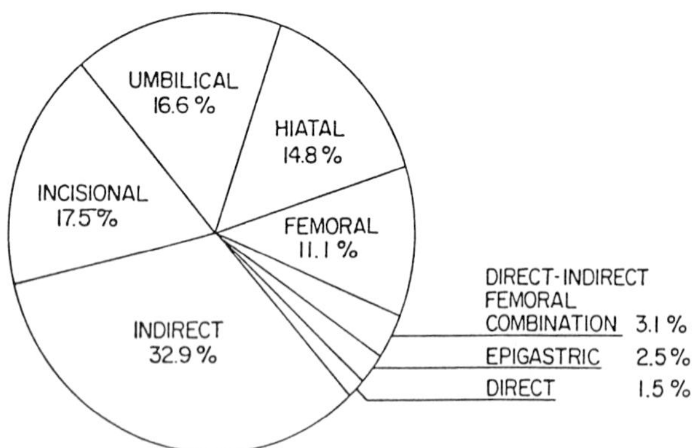

FIG. 76-6. The distribution of common hernias in 325 females in 1965 and 1967. Note the relatively greater frequency of incisional, umbilical, hiatal, and femoral hernias in the female. (From Ponka JL: *Hernias of the Abdominal Wall.* Philadelphia, Saunders, 1980, p 85. With permission.)

TABLE 76-2 Differential Considerations in Groin Hernia

Direct inguinal hernia	Testicular torsion
Indirect inguinal hernia	Retractile or undescended testis
Femoral hernia	Epididymitis
Lymph nodes	Groin cellulitis
Hydrocele	Femoral thrombophlebitis
Spermatic cord tumor	Femoral artery aneurysm
Testicular tumor	

Pain and hypesthesia along the medical aspect of the thigh to the knee are associated with obturator hernias. These patients additionally have intermittent bouts of small bowel obstruction over years. Obturator hernias are more commonly seen in older women.

Physical examination of the patient with a hernia may reveal an abnormal swelling. In inguinal hernias in males, the swelling may extend into the scrotum. The consistency of the mass varies depending upon the content of the hernial sac. If incarceration is present, the swelling is usually tender due to inflammation of the bowel wall or omentum and surrounding tissues. Tachycardia and mild temperature elevation frequently also are present.

DIAGNOSIS

Patients frequently present to the emergency department with a complaint of groin pain. There may or may not be a history of heavy lifting. In males, palpation of the inguinal canal is easily performed by inversion of scrotal skin and passage of a digit through the external ring. Voluntary increase in intraabdominal pressure during this examination reliably detects most inguinal hernias. With the tip of the digit near the internal ring, a tapping sensation is detected at Valsalva or cough. In females, the external ring is generally narrower and the skin of the labium majora is not easily inverted, making introduction of a digit difficult. Therefore, failure to palpate a hernial sac in women is not foolproof.

Groin hernias have a larger number of differential diagnostic possibilities (Table 76-2). They most commonly are confused with tender lymph nodes and hydroceles. Lymph nodes are generally movable, firm, and multiple. Hydroceles may transilluminate and are not tender. Incarcerated hernias will not transilluminate and are tender. If bowel is contained in the hernia sac, bowel sounds may be heard and peristalsis may be seen. In children, retractile or undescended testes may be mistaken for hernias. Testicular torsion or tumor may be confused with incarcerated hernias.

When incarceration is acute, the white blood cell count is slightly elevated with a shift to the left. Electrolyte abnormalities and elevation of the blood urea nitrogen level may occur as a reflection of both the patient's state of hydration and the toxic state. In the elderly and immunocompromised, laboratory studies may not be reliable indicators of the patient's state. Occasionally, as part of a diagnostic evaluation for abdominal pain, a hernia is detected on barium enema.

Upright chest films should be obtained to rule out free air under the diaphragm, which may result from perforation or dead bowel. Flat and upright films of the abdomen, including the groin, should be obtained to assess the possible presence of bowel obstruction. Loops of bowel may be seen entering a hernial sac.

Suspicion of spigelian or pelvic hernias often necessitates use of sonography or CT scanning for diagnosis,[11–13] since detection of herniation is frequently difficult and confusion with other masses is possible.

TREATMENT

If there is a good history that the incarceration is of recent onset, an attempt can be made to reduce the hernia. If there is any question of the duration of the incarceration, no attempt should be made so that no dead bowel is reintroduced into the abdomen. Unfortunately, no specific time line can be delineated.

Before an attempt is made to reduce the hernia, the patient should be placed in the Trendelenburg position and given some mild sedation. A variety of sedating agents can be used, with the benzodiazepines most commonly employed. A warm compress over the area may make the task easier by reducing the swelling and relaxing the abdominal musculature. Only gentle compression of the hernia should be used, and nothing should be forced back. Attempts at reduction should be limited in time and force.

If the incarceration is tender, if it cannot be reduced, or if strangulation is suspected, the patient should not be fed by mouth, and a nasogastric tube should be inserted. Intravenous fluid should be started with the thought of correcting the patient's volume and electrolyte problems.

The treatment of choice for an incarceration which cannot be reduced, or for a strangulation, is surgical. Broad-spectrum antibiotics and vigorous fluid resuscitation may be necessary, but only as a prelude to operation. Mortality is higher in the elderly when emergency surgery is required.

DISPOSITION

Any acutely incarcerated or strangulated hernia, regardless of type or patient age, requires immediate surgical evaluation and repair.

Adult patients with reducible hernias may be discharged and referred for elective surgical repair. They should be advised to avoid conditions that increase intraabdominal pressure, such as lifting activities. Return to the emergency department should be suggested for recurrence that the patient is unable to reduce promptly, emesis, or fever. Following surgical evaluation, patients who are not candidates for operative repair occasionally may be fitted with trusses.

In children, inguinal hernias have a high risk of incarceration, particularly in the first year of life. These hernias should be electively repaired shortly after diagnosis and therefore require timely surgical consultation. Infants with inguinal hernias reduced in the emergency department should generally have repair within a few days.[14]

Umbilical hernias in children very rarely incarcerate. Spontaneous closure of the umbilical ring occurs in 80 percent of these children by age 3 or 4. Discharge and primary care observation is the standard of care for young children with hernias less than 2.0 cm in diameter. Children over age 4 or with larger hernias should be referred for surgical evaluation.

REFERENCES

1. Skinner MA, Grosfeld JL: Inguinal and umbilical hernia repair in infants and children. *Surg Clin North Am* 73:439, 1993.
2. Gallegos NC, Dawson J, Jarvis M, et al: Risk of strangulation in groin hernias. *Br J Surg* 78:1171, 1991.
3. Scherer LR, Grosfeld JL: Inguinal hernia and umbilical anomalies. *Pediatr Clin North Am* 40:1121, 1993.
4. Bergstein JM, Condon RE: Obturator hernia: Current diagnosis and treatment. *Surgery* 119:133, 1996.
5. Sahdev P, Garramone RR, Desani B, et al: Traumatic abdominal hernia. *Am J Emerg Med* 10:237, 1992.
6. Mensching JJ, Musielewicz AJ: Abdominal wall hernias. *Emerg Med Clin North Am* 14:739, 1996.
7. Akin ML, Karakaya M, Batkin A, et al: Prevalence of inguinal hernia in otherwise healthy males of 20 to 22 years of age. *J R Army Med Corps* 143:101, 1997.
8. Millikan KW, Deziel DJ: The management of hernia: Considerations in cost effectiveness. *Surg Clin North Am* 76:105, 1996.
9. Primatesta P, Goldacre MJ: Inguinal hernia repair: Incidence of elective and emergency surgery, readmission and mortality. *Int J Epidemiol* 25:835, 1996.
10. Kadirov S, Sayfan J, Friedman S, et al: Richter's hernia—A surgical pitfall. *J Am Coll Surg* 182:60, 1996.
11. Torzilli G, Carmana G, Lumachi V, et al: The usefulness of ultrasonography in the diagnosis of the spigelian hernia. *Int Surg* 80:280, 1995.
12. Mufid MM, Abu-Yousef MM, Kakish ME, et al: Spigelian hernia: Diagnosis by high resolution real-time sonography. *J Ultrasound Med* 16:183, 1997.
13. Hojer AM, Rygaard H, Jess P: CT in the diagnosis of abdominal wall hernias: A preliminary study. *Eur Radiol* 7:1416, 1997.
14. Gahukamble DE, Khamage AS : Early versus delayed repair of reduced incarcerated inguinal hernias in the pediatric population. *J Pediatr Surg* 31: 1218, 1996.

ILEITIS, COLITIS, AND DIVERTICULITIS

Howard A. Werman
Hagop S. Mekhjian
Douglas A. Rund

CROHN'S DISEASE

Crohn's disease is a chronic inflammatory disease of the gastrointestinal (GI) tract; the exact cause is still unknown. The disease was first described by Crohn, Ginzberg, and Oppenheimer in 1932. In their initial description, the disease was thought to involve only the distal ileum. We now know that Crohn's disease can involve any part of the GI tract from the mouth to the anus. Segmental involvement of the intestinal tract by a nonspecific granulomatous inflammatory process characterizes the disease. The ileum is involved in the majority of cases. In 20 percent, the disease is confined to the colon, making differentiation from ulcerative colitis, at times, a difficult clinical problem. The terms *regional enteritis, terminal ileitis, granulomatous ileocolitis,* and *Crohn's disease* are used to describe the same disease process.

Etiology and Pathogenesis

Environmental, genetic, infectious, and host factors have all been implicated as a cause of both Crohn's disease and ulcerative colitis. Among the environmental factors, smoking has been associated with an increased recurrence rate of Crohn's disease. *Mycobacterium paratuberculosis* and the measles virus have received recent attention and have also been considered as possible etiologies of Crohn's disease. There are few data to support a primary causative role of psychogenic factors. Immunologic factors have received greatest attention. Several mechanisms of injury have been proposed, including autoimmune destruction of the gut mucosal cells as the result of cross-reactivity with antigens from enteric bacteria as well as nonspecific immunologic injury to the gut mucosa as the result of a chronic inflammatory process for both ulcerative colitis and Crohn's disease. Cytokines, including interleukins and tumor necrosis factor, have been invoked in the perpetuation of the inflammatory response. Whether immune factors play a primary or secondary role in the pathogenesis of these diseases is not known. Extraintestinal manifestations suggest a role for immune complexes or an autoantibody response at various involved sites.

Epidemiology

The peak incidence of Crohn's disease occurs in patients between 15 and 22 years of age, with a secondary peak at age 55 to 60 years. The prevalence varies from 10 to 100 cases per 100,000 population and the incidence from 1 to 7 cases per year per 100,000 population in the United States. The incidence of Crohn's disease has been increasing over the past 20 years.[1] There is a 20 to 30 percent increased risk of Crohn's disease among women as compared with men. The disease has a worldwide distribution but is more frequent in people of European extraction. It is four times more common among Jews than non-Jews and is more common in whites than blacks, Asians, or Native Americans. A family history of inflammatory bowel disease is present in 10 to 15 percent of patients. Ulcerative colitis as well as Crohn's disease may be present in other family members, and siblings of patients with Crohn's disease have a higher incidence of the disease.

Pathology

The most important pathologic feature of Crohn's disease is the involvement of all the layers of the bowel and extension into mesenteric lymph nodes. In addition, the disease is discontinuous, with normal areas of bowel (''skip areas'') located between one or more involved areas. On gross inspection, the bowel wall is thickened; subsequent luminal narrowing results in stenosis and obstruction of the intestine. The mesenteric fat often extends over the bowel wall (''creeping'' fat). The appearance of the mucosa varies with the extent and severity of the disease. Longitudinal, deep ulcerations are characteristic. These often penetrate the bowel wall, resulting in fissures, fistulas, and abscesses. Late in the disease, a ''cobblestone'' appearance of the mucosa results from the criss-crossing of these ulcers with intervening normal mucosa.

Microscopically, there is an inflammatory reaction that extends through all layers of the intestine but is most marked in the submucosa. This inflammatory response consists of infiltration by mononuclear cells, lymphocytes, plasma cells, and histiocytes. Fissure ulcers frequently penetrate the muscle layer. Unlike the situation in ulcerative colitis, crypt abscesses are infrequent. Discrete granulomas consisting of epithelioid cells, giant cells, and lymphocytes are seen in 50 to 75 percent of the surgical specimens from Crohn's disease patients. Granulomas are seen uncommonly in mucosal biopsies. Although the finding of granulomas is suggestive, it is not essential for the diagnosis.

Clinical Features

The clinical course of Crohn's disease varies and in the individual patient is unpredictable. Abdominal pain, anorexia, diarrhea, and weight loss are present in 75 to 80 percent of cases. Occasionally, a patient with Crohn's disease may present with acute right-lower-quadrant abdominal pain and fever and, on examination, be found to have a mass in the right lower quadrant. More commonly, the patient experiences an insidious onset of recurrent abdominal pain, fever, and diarrhea that lasts for several years before the definitive diagnosis is established. Approximately one-third of patients develop perianal fissures or fistulas, abscesses, or rectal prolapse, particularly when there is colonic involvement. Finally, patients may also manifest complications of the disease, such as obstruction with vomiting, crampy abdominal pain, and obstipation, or an intraabdominal abscess with fever, abdominal pain, and a palpable mass. In 10 to 20 percent of patients, the extraintestinal manifestations of arthritis, uveitis, or liver disease may be presenting symptoms. Crohn's disease should also be considered in the differential diagnosis of patients with fever of unknown etiology.

The clinical course and manifestations of the disease appear to be related, partly because of its anatomic distribution; in 30 percent, the disease involves only the small bowel; in 20 percent, only the colon is involved; and in 50 percent, both the small bowel and colon are involved. A small percentage of patients present with disease involving the mouth, esophagus, and stomach. Patients with Crohn's disease of the stomach may demonstrate symptoms similar to those associated with peptic ulcer disease (see Chap. 73, ''Peptic Ulcer Disease and Gastritis'').

The recurrence rate for all patients with Crohn's disease is 25 to 50 percent within 1 year for patients whose disease has responded to medical management; the recurrence rate is higher for those patients who require surgery. Patients with ileocolitis have the highest recurrence rate following surgery. The incidence of hematochezia and perianal disease is higher when the colon is involved, as in ileocolitis or Crohn's colitis. A slight increase in the incidence of arthritis may be associated with Crohn's colitis. Except for the additional concern of growth retardation, childhood-onset Crohn's disease seems to have a course similar to that of adult-onset disease.

Extraintestinal manifestations are seen in 25 to 30 percent of patients with Crohn's disease (see Table 77-1), and the incidence of these complications does not differ between patients with Crohn's disease and those with ulcerative colitis. Extraintestinal manifestations are divided among arthritic (19 percent), dermatologic (4 percent), hepatobiliary (4 percent), and vascular (1.3 percent) complications. Peripheral arthropathies are commonly seen in both ulcerative colitis and Crohn's disease and tend to manifest during exacerbations of the underlying disease process. Ankylosing spondylitis can be detected in up to 20 percent of patients with inflammatory bowel disease. Symptoms may occur before, during, and after bouts of Crohn's disease or ulcerative colitis.

Dermatologic complications include erythema nodosum and pyoderma gangrenosum. Ocular manifestations include episcleritis and uveitis.

Hepatobiliary disease is common in patients with inflammatory bowel disease and includes pericholangitis, chronic active hepatitis, primary sclerosing cholangitis, and cholangiocarcinoma. Gallstones are detected in up to 33 percent of patients with Crohn's disease. The incidence of acute and chronic pancreatitis is increased in patients with Crohn's disease and ulcerative colitis.

Vascular manifestations include thromboembolic disease, vasculitis, and arteritis. Patients with thromboembolic complications have a mortality rate of approximately 25 percent. Thromboembolic disease is the result of a hypercoagulable state induced in patients with both Crohn's disease and ulcerative colitis and ranks as the third leading cause of death in patients afflicted with these conditions, behind peritonitis and malignancy. Malnutrition and chronic anemia are seen in many patients with long-standing Crohn's disease. Growth retardation can be seen in children.[2]

Hyperoxaluria is a common and potentially treatable occurrence in patients with ileal disease and steatorrhea. This results from increased colonic absorption of dietary oxalate and accounts for the occurrence of nephrolithiasis in 20 to 25 percent of patients with ileal disease. Finally, myelodysplastic disease, osteomyelitis, and osteonecrosis have been reported as rare complications of ulcerative colitis and, in particular, Crohn's disease.[3,4]

Complications

More than three out of four patients with Crohn's disease will require surgery within the first 20 years of the onset of initial symptoms. Abscess and fissure formation is seen in approximately 30 percent. Abscesses can be characterized as intraperitoneal, retroperitoneal, interloop, or intramesenteric. These patients present with abdominal pain and tenderness typical of their underlying disease but may also have fever spikes and a palpable mass. Patients with retroperitoneal abscesses may present with hip or back pain and difficulty ambulating. Liver abscesses have also been reported in patients with Crohn's disease.

Fistulas are the result of extension of intestinal fissures noted in patients with Crohn's disease into adjacent structures. The most common sites are between the ileum and the sigmoid colon, the cecum, another ileal segment, or the skin. Internal fistulas should be suspected when there are changes in the patient's symptom complex, including

TABLE 77-1 Extraintestinal Manifestations of Inflammatory Bowel Disease

Manifestation	Description
	ARTHRITIC
Peripheral arthritis	Migratory monoarticular or polyarticular pain in peripheral joints (hip, knee, ankle, wrist) with effusion
Ankylosing spondylitis	Pain and stiffness of spine, hips, neck, and rib cage with limitation in truncal motion, loss of lumbar lordosis; decreased chest expansion and forward cervical flexion in advanced disease
Sacroiliitis	Low back pain with morning stiffness, relieved by exercise; progressive joint sclerosis
	OCULAR
Episcleritis	Eye burning or itching without visual changes or pain; scleral and conjunctival hyperemia
Uveitis	Acute blurring of vision, photophobia and pain; perilimbic scleral injection
	DERMATOLOGIC
Erythema nodosum	Painful, red, raised nodules on extensor surfaces of arms or legs
Pyoderma gangrenosum	Ulcerative lesions with a necrotic center and violaceous skin typically found in pretibial region or trunk
	HEPATOBILIARY
Cholelithiasis	Varies from asymptomatic stones to right upper quadrant pain, fever, vomiting
Fatty liver	Mild right-upper-quadrant pain; hepatomegaly
Pericholangitis	Mild elevation in serum alkaline phosphotase, asymptomatic
Chronic active hepatitis	Autoimmune elevation of liver aminotransferase enzymes, may progress to cirrhosis
Primary sclerosing cholangitis	Pruritus progressing to jaundice, fatigue, and lethargy; laboratory findings vary from mild elevations of alkaline phosphatase to cirrhosis, portal hypertension, and liver failure; male predominance
Cholangiocarcinoma	Extrahepatic biliary mass, evidence of biliary obstruction, jaundice, right upper quadrant pain, fever, malaise
Pancreatitis	Varies from painless elevation of serum amylase to clinically apparent central abdominal pain radiating to back; may be associated with drugs such as azathioprine, 6-mercaptopurine, sulfasalazine, mesalamine, olsalazine, metronidazole
	VASCULAR
Thromboembolic disease	Symptoms of deep venous thrombosis and pulmonary emboli; portal vein, mesenteric vein, and hepatic venous thrombosis reported
	OTHER
Malnutrition	Fatigue, malaise, muscular wasting, cachexia
Chronic anemia	Fatigue, malaise, pallor, dyspnea; may be microcytic (blood loss), macrocytic (B_{12} deficiency) or autoimmune hemolytic
Nephrolithiasis	Flank pain, nausea, vomiting, hematuria; stones result from increased dietary oxylate absorption (calcium oxylate stones) and dehydration (urate stones)

bowel movement frequency, amount of pain, or weight loss. Enterovesical fistulas are rare complications of Crohn's disease.

Obstruction is the result of both stricture formation due to the inflammatory process and of edema of the bowel wall. The distal small bowel is the most common site of obstruction. Symptoms include crampy abdominal pain, distention, nausea, and bloating.

Perianal complications are seen in one-third of patients with Crohn's disease and include perianal or ischiorectal abscesses, fissures, fistulas, rectovaginal fistulas, and rectal prolapse. These are more commonly seen in patients with colonic involvement.

While gastrointestinal bleeding is common in patients with Crohn's disease, only 1.3 percent of patients develop life-threatening hemorrhage.[5] In patients with Crohn's disease, bleeding is the result of erosion into a vessel in the bowel wall. Toxic megacolon occurs in 6 percent of all cases of Crohn's disease and is associated with massive gastrointestinal bleeding in over half the cases. Fifty percent of all cases of toxic megacolon occur in patients with Crohn's disease. Free perforation, however, rarely occurs.

When bowel symptoms are present, malnutrition, malabsorption, hypocalcemia, and vitamin deficiency can be severe. In addition to the complications of the disease itself are complications associated with the treatment of the disease with sulfasalazine, steroids, immunosuppressive agents, and antibiotics.

The incidence of malignant neoplasm of the GI tract is three times higher in patients with Crohn's disease than for the general population.

Diagnosis

In the majority of patients, the definitive diagnosis of Crohn's disease is established months or years after the onset of symptoms. Occasionally, the initial presenting complaint is not related to the GI tract but is an extraintestinal manifestation such as arthritis or uveitis. A provisional diagnosis of appendicitis or pelvic inflammatory disease may change to Crohn's disease at the time of surgery. A careful and detailed history for previous bowel symptoms that preceded the onset of acute right-lower-quadrant pain and the absence of true guarding or rebound in patients with Crohn's disease may provide clues to the correct diagnosis before surgery.

A definitive diagnosis of Crohn's disease is confirmed by an upper GI series, an air-contrast barium enema, and colonoscopy. Oral barium studies with fluoroscopy are the most sensitive and specific for detecting ileal involvement. The classic radiographic findings in the small intestine include segmental narrowing, destruction of the normal mucosal pattern, and fistulas. Segmental involvement of the colon with rectal sparing is the most characteristic feature.

Colonoscopy is the most sensitive technique for examining patients with Crohn's colitis. This technique is useful in detecting early mucosal lesions, in defining the extent of colonic involvement, and in surveillance for the occurrence of colon cancer. Air-contrast enemas are also useful in defining mucosal detail. Intraabdominal abscesses, mesenteric inflammation, and fistulas are best diagnosed using either computed tomography (CT) or ultrasound.

Differential Diagnosis

Diseases that should be considered in the differential diagnosis of Crohn's disease (Table 77-2) include lymphoma, ileocecal amebiasis, sarcoidosis, deep chronic mycotic infections involving the GI tract, gastrointestinal tuberculosis, Kaposi's sarcoma, *Campylobacter* enteritis and *Yersinia* ileocolitis. Fortunately, most of these are uncommon conditions and can be differentiated by appropriate laboratory tests. *Yersinia* ileocolitis and *Campylobacter* enteritis may cause chronic abdominal pain and diarrhea similar to Crohn's disease but can be diagnosed by appropriate stool cultures. Acute ileitis should not be confused with Crohn's disease. Young patients with acute ileitis usually recover without sequelae and should not undergo surgery. When Crohn's disease is confined to the colon, ischemic bowel disease (particularly in the elderly) and pseudomembranous enterocolitis as well as ulcerative colitis must be included in the differential diagnosis.

TABLE 77-2 Differential Diagnosis of Ileitis, Colitis, and Diverticulitis

Acute appendicitis
Peptic ulcer disease
Pelvic inflammatory disease
Endometriosis
Ischemic colitis
Leaking aortic aneurysm
Renal calculus
Irritable bowel syndrome
Lactate intolerance
Carcinoma of the colon
Intestinal lymphoma
Kaposi's sarcoma
Gay bowel syndrome
Sarcoidosis
Infectious causes *Campylobacter* enteritis *Shigella* enteritis *Salmonella* enteritis *Yersinia* ileocolitis Hemorrhagic *Escherichia coli* enteritis Intestinal tuberculosis Amebiasis Lymphogranuloma venereum Gonorrheal proctitis Syphilis Actinomycosis *Entamoeba histolytica* Cytomegalovirus Herpes simplex virus
Irradiation colitis
Postirradiation proctosigmoiditis
Fecal impaction
Foreign-body granuloma
Collagen vascular disease

TABLE 77-3 Treatment of Fulminant Colitis

Restore fluid and electrolyte balance
Nothing by mouth
Nasogastric suction for Obstruction Adynamic ileus Suspected toxic megacolon
Parenteral corticosteroids ACTH 120 U/day (if not receiving prior steroids) Hydrocortisone 300 mg/day or methylprednisolone 48 mg/day or prednisolone 60 mg/day
Broad-spectrum antibiotics Ampicillin or cephalosporin Aminoglycoside (gentamicin or tobramycin) Metronidazole or clindamycin
Observe for complications Obstruction Perforation Toxic megacolon Life-threatening hemorrhage Intraabdominal abscess

Treatment

The aim of therapy includes relief of symptoms, suppression of the inflammatory disease, treatment of complications, and maintenance of nutrition. In a disease that is virtually incurable, the emphasis should be on relief of symptoms and avoidance of complications. The pharmacologic agents available for the management of Crohn's disease include symptomatic agents, anti-inflammatory agents, antibiotics, and immunomodulators.

Initial evaluation in the emergency department (ED) should focus on determining the severity of the attack; identifying significant complications such as obstruction, intraabdominal abscess, life-threatening hemorrhage, or toxic megacolon; and eliminating other possible causes of the patient's complaints. Laboratory evaluation should include a CBC, serum electrolytes, BUN, creatinine, and a type and crossmatch where appropriate. Plain radiographs of the abdomen may reveal evidence of obstruction, perforation, or toxic megacolon. Initial treatment (Table 77-3) consists of adequate fluid resuscitation and restoration of electrolyte balance. Nasogastric decompression should be initiated in any patient with evidence of obstruction, peritonitis, or toxic megacolon. Broad-spectrum antibiotics (ampicillin or a cephalosporin, an aminoglycoside, and metronidazole) should be used in patients with fulminant colitis or peritonitis. Patients with severe disease should receive intravenous steroids such as hydrocortisone 300 mg/day or an equivalent dose of methylprednisolone (48 mg/day) or prednisolone (60 mg/day).

Sulfasalazine (Azulfidine), 3 to 4 g/day, has been shown to be effective in treating patients with mild to moderate active Crohn's disease. The mechanism of action is not known but is presumed to be through the topical action of 5-aminosalicylic acid, which is released by the action of colonic bacteria on sulfasalazine. Sulfapyridine is also a by-product of this breakdown. Many of the toxic side effects of sulfasalazine are attributable to sulfapyrizine. These include nausea, vomiting, anorexia, epigastric distress, arthralgias, headache, diarrhea, male infertility, and hypersensitivity reactions (pericarditis, pleuritis, pancreatitis, arthritis, and rash). Because of the toxicity profile associated with sulfasalazine, 5-aminosalicylic derivative agents are now available for either oral or topical use. A slow, timed-release mesalamine (Pentasa) 4 g/day or a pH-dependent release mesalamine (Asacol, Claversal, Salofalk) 2 to 4 g/day have the primary advantage of delivery into the colon. Olsalazine (Dipentum) 1 g/day is a derivative of the sodium salt of 5-aminosalicylic acid, which is converted to two 5-aminosalicylic molecules in the colon and has identical anti-inflammatory properties. Balsalazide (Colazide) 1.5 to 6 g/day has the 5-aminosalicylic acid moiety bound to an inert molecule. Sulfasalazine and all the mesalamine formulations are effective in colonic disease. The topical preparations have limited usefulness and only in the management of Crohn's disease limited to the rectum or the distal 40 cm of rectosigmoid.

Glucocorticoids such as prednisone (40 to 60 mg/day) are reserved for the more severely affected patients and are effective primarily in small intestinal disease as well as in ileocolitis. Immunosuppressive drugs such as 6-mercaptopurine (1 to 1.5 mg/kg/day) or azathioprine (2 mg/kg/day) are useful as steroid-sparing agents, in healing fistulas, and in patients in whom there are serious contraindications for surgery. Recent evidence suggests that they are also effective as maintenance agents. Both agents have been associated with leukopenia, fever, hepatitis, and pancreatitis, necessitating the need for close follow-up, particularly during the initial phase of therapy. The response to immunosuppressives should not be expected before 8 to 12 weeks following the initiation of therapy.

Metronidazole (10 to 20 mg/kg/day) has been shown to be effective in controlled clinical trials and is particularly useful in treatment of patients with perianal complications and fistulous disease. Ciprofloxacin (500 to 750 mg bid) has also been used in this setting as well as in active Crohn's ileitis and ileocolitis. Other agents such as cyclosporine, methotrexate, broad-spectrum antibiotics, monoclonal antibodies against tumor necrosis factor, IL-1 receptor antagonist, interferon alpha, and immunoglobulin therapy must all be considered as experimental forms of therapy at this time because of insufficient experience of therapeutic efficacy in controlled clinical trials.

The role of maintenance therapy in ulcerative colitis is well established. Maintenance therapy and the effectiveness of various therapeutic agents in Crohn's disease is somewhat less certain. Glucocorticoids should not be used for maintaining a remission because of lack of sufficient evidence of their efficacy and the potential for long-term complications. When a patient is responsive to immunosuppressive therapy, it would seem advisable to continue this in a reduced dose for the maintenance of remission. Similarly, a reduced dose of 5-aminosalicyclic acid derivatives is appropriate for the maintenance of remission of colonic disease. The addition of sulfasalazine, azothiaprine, and 6-mercaptopurine to prednisone does not improve the response rate and increases the risk of side effects.

Diarrhea can be controlled by the use of loperamide (Imodium), 4 to 16 mg/day, diphenoxylate (Lomotil), 5 to 20 mg/day, and, in some cases, cholestyramine (Questran), 4 g one to six times daily. The latter is particularly useful as an exchange resin in patients who have limited ileal disease or resection, no bowel obstruction, and mild steatorrhea. The mechanism of action is binding bile acids and eliminating their known cathartic action. The primary aim of dietary therapy is the maintenance of nutrition and the alleviation of diarrhea. Elimination of lactose from the diet is of benefit in patients with lactose intolerance. Reduction in dietary oxalate should be considered in every patient. In addition, supplementation of trace metals, fat-soluble vitamins, and medium-chain triglycerides should be considered in selected patients.

Disposition

Patients who demonstrate signs of fulminant colitis, peritonitis, or complications such of obstruction, significant gastrointestinal hemorrhage, severe dehydration, or fluid/electrolyte imbalance should be hospitalized under the care of a gastroenterologist or surgeon. Hospital admission should be considered in less severe cases that fail outpatient management. Surgical intervention is indicated in those patients with complications of the disease, including intestinal obstruction or hemorrhage, perforation, abscess or fistula formation, toxic megacolon, and perianal disease. In addition, surgery may be indicated in those patients who fail medical therapy. The recurrence rate after surgery approaches 100 percent.

When patients with Crohn's disease are discharged from the ED, alterations in their therapeutic regimen should be discussed with a consulting gastroenterologist. Close follow-up of these patients must be assured prior to discharge.

ULCERATIVE COLITIS

Ulcerative colitis is a chronic inflammatory and ulcerative disease of the colon and rectum characterized most often clinically by bloody diarrhea. The etiology, like that of Crohn's disease, remains unknown, even though extensive investigations into the cause continue.

Epidemiology

Epidemiologic considerations are similar to those of Crohn's disease; the disease is more prevalent in the United States and northern Europe, and peak incidence occurs in the second and the third decades of life. The incidence of ulcerative colitis is about 10 cases per 100,000 and, like the incidence of Crohn's disease, appears to have risen in the last few years.[1] Approximately 250,000 in the United States are afflicted with ulcerative colitis. There is a slight predominance of men among patients with the disease. First-degree relatives of patients with ulcerative colitis have a 15-fold risk of developing ulcerative colitis and a 3.5-fold risk of developing Crohn's disease.

Pathology

Ulcerative colitis involves primarily the mucosa and submucosa. Microscopically, the disease is characterized by mucosal inflammation with the formation of crypt abscesses, epithelial necrosis, and mucosal ulceration. The submucosa, muscular layer, and serosa are often spared. In the usual case, the disease increases in severity more distally, the rectosigmoid being involved in 95 percent of cases. In the early stages of the disease, the mucous membranes appear finely granular and friable. In more severe cases, the mucosa appears as a red, spongy surface dotted with small ulcerations oozing blood and purulent exudate. In very advanced disease, one sees large, oozing ulcerations and pseudopolyps (areas of hyperplastic overgrowth surrounded by inflamed mucosa).

Clinical Features

The clinical features and course of ulcerative colitis vary but are somewhat dependent on the anatomic distribution of the disease in the colon. The disease is classified as mild, moderate, or severe depending on the clinical manifestations.[6] Patients with mild disease have fewer than four bowel movements per day, no systemic symptoms, and few extraintestinal manifestations. Of all patients with ulcerative colitis, 60 percent have mild disease; in 80 percent of cases, the disease is limited to the rectum. Occasionally, constipation and rectal bleeding are the presenting complaints. Progression to pancolitis occurs in 10 to 15 percent of patients with mild disease.

Patients with severe disease constitute 15 percent of those with ulcerative colitis. Severe disease is associated with more than six bowel movements per day, anemia, fever, weight loss, tachycardia, low serum albumin, and more frequent extraintestinal manifestations. Patients with severe disease account for 90 percent of the mortality from ulcerative colitis. Virtually all severely affected patients have pancolitis.

Moderate disease is seen in 25 percent of patients. The clinical manifestations are less severe and patients demonstrate a good response to therapy. These patients usually have colitis extending to the splenic flexure (left-sided colitis) but may develop pancolitis.

Most commonly, ulcerative colitis is characterized by intermittent attacks of acute disease with complete remission between attacks. Such a pattern occurs in the majority of patients. In other patients, the first attack is followed by a prolonged period of inactivity. Infrequently, patients run a chronically active course. The factors associated with an unfavorable prognosis and increased mortality include the severity and extent of disease, a short interval between attacks, and onset of the disease after 60 years of age.

Extraintestinal complications of ulcerative colitis include peripheral arthritis, ankylosing spondylitis, episcleritis, uveitis, pyoderma gangrenosum, and erythema nodosum (see Table 77-1). Clinically apparent liver disease may occur in 5 to 10 percent of patients. The manifestations of liver disease may include any of the following: pericholangitis, chronic active hepatitis, fatty liver or cirrhosis, cholelithiasis, sclerosing cholangitis, and bile duct carcinoma.

Complications

Although blood loss from sustained hemorrhage may be the most common complication of the illness, toxic megacolon is an associated clinical entity that must not be missed.

Toxic megacolon develops in advanced cases of colitis when the disease process begins to extend through all layers of the colon. The result is a loss of muscular tone within the colon, with dilatation and localized peritonitis. If the colon continues to dilate without treatment, signs of toxicity will develop. Plain radiography of the abdomen demonstrates a long, continuous segment of air-filled colon greater than 6 cm in diameter (see Fig. 77-1). Loss of colonic haustra and "thumbprinting," representing bowel wall edema, may also be seen. The distended portion of the atonic colon can perforate, causing peritonitis and septicemia. Mortality from this complication is approximately 50 percent if perforation occurs but less than 10 percent if surgery is undertaken prior to perforation.[7]

A patient with toxic megacolon appears severely ill; the abdomen is distended, tender, and tympanitic. Severe diarrhea (more than 10 bowel movements per day) is often seen. Fever, tachycardia, and signs of hypovolemia are typically part of the clinical picture. Leukocytosis, anemia, electrolyte disturbances, and hypoalbuminemia are the supporting laboratory data.

Some of the more prominent features of toxic megacolon, such as leukocytosis and peritonitis, can be masked in the patient taking corticosteroids. When such therapy is being administered, greater suspicion is required to make the diagnosis. Antidiarrheal agents, hypokalemia, narcotics, cathartics, pregnancy, enemas, and recent colonoscopy have been implicated as precipitating factors in toxic megacolon. Medical therapy with nasogastric suction, intravenous prednisolone 60 mg/day or hydrocortisone 300 mg/day, parenteral antibiotics active against coliforms and anaerobes (ampicillin and clindamycin), and intravenous fluids should be attempted as initial therapy and in preparing the patient for possible surgery. However, prolonged medical treatment of these patients increases mortality; therefore, early surgical consultation must be sought with the aim of performing a colectomy if clinical improvement is not noted in 24 to 48 h with medical treatment.

The fistulas that constitute a hallmark of Crohn's disease occur infrequently in cases of ulcerative colitis. Perirectal fistulas and abscesses are much more common in patients with Crohn's disease but may occur in up to 20 percent of patients with ulcerative colitis.[8] Massive gastrointestinal hemorrhage, obstruction secondary to stricture formation, and acute perforation are other complications of the disease.

There is a 10- to 30-fold increase in the development of carcinoma of the colon in patients with ulcerative colitis. Carcinoma of the colon is the cause of 5 to 15 percent of the deaths attributed to ulcerative colitis. The major risk factors for the development of carcinoma of the colon are extensive involvement and prolonged duration of the disease. The cumulative risk of cancer after 20 and 30 years is 5 to 10 and 12 to 20 percent, respectively. Additional factors that increase the risk of cancer in patients with ulcerative colitis include early onset of the disease and a family history of colon cancer. The availability of fiberoptic colonoscopy allows surveillance of ulcerative colitis patients with periodic colonoscopies and biopsies to detect the high-grade dysplasia thought to predict the development or association of colon cancer. In patients with pancolitis, such surveillance should start 8 to 10 years after the onset of the disease.[9]

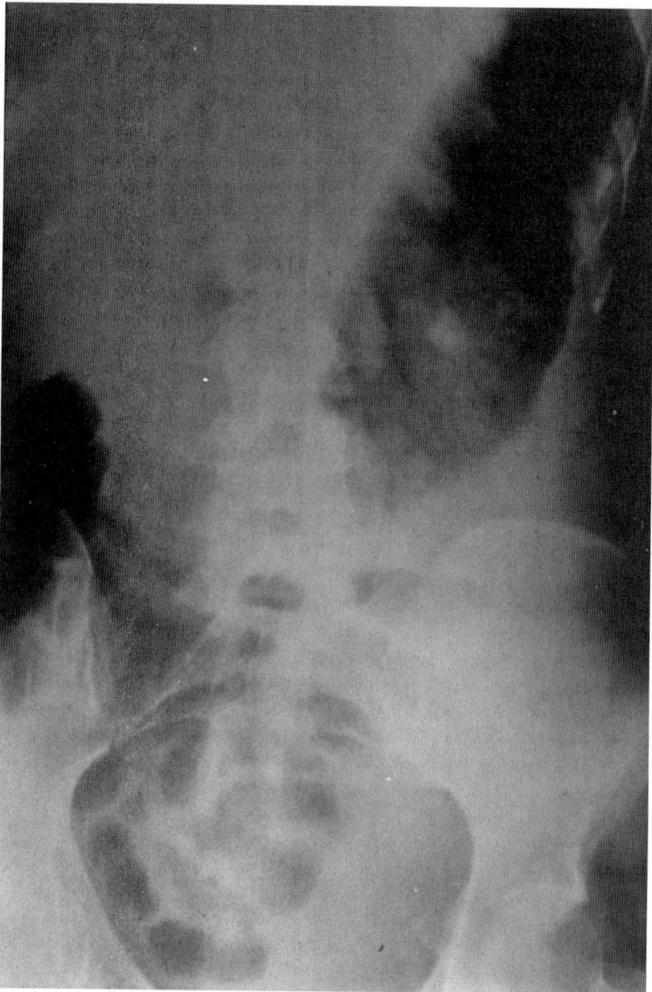

FIG. 77-1. Long, continuous colonic loop in toxic megacolon.

Diagnosis

Laboratory findings in patients with ulcerative colitis are nonspecific; they may include leukocytosis, anemia, thrombocytosis, decreased serum albumin, and abnormal liver function studies. Therefore, the diagnosis of ulcerative colitis rests on the following: a history of abdominal cramps and diarrhea, mucoid stools, stool examination negative for ova and parasites, stool cultures negative for enteric pathogens, and confirmation by sigmoidoscopic or colonoscopic examination. The results of the latter examination are abnormal in 95 percent of the patients with ulcerative colitis. The observed pathologic changes vary depending on the severity and duration of the disease. Granularity, friability, ulceration of the mucosa, and, in more advanced cases, pseudopolyposis are quite characteristic.

Sigmoidoscopy may be done in the office or the ED to confirm the clinical suspicion, but the appearance is not specific. Biopsy may help differentiate acute colitis from chronic colitis and diseases caused by specific etiology, such as amebiasis (see "Pathology," above). Barium enema examination may be useful in differentiating it from Crohn's disease and defining the extent of involvement of the colon. Colonoscopy, however, is the most sensitive method for making the diagnosis and defining the extent and severity of the disease. In addition, colonoscopy is extremely useful in the evaluation of the patient for the development of dysplasia or colon cancer. Barium enema examination should be done with caution or postponed in moderately ill patients. Rigid or fiberoptic proctosigmoidoscopy can be used, however, even in the severely ill patient, provided that it is done gently and without the administration of any enemas or laxatives.

Differential Diagnosis

The major diseases that should be considered in the differential diagnosis of ulcerative colitis include infectious colitis, Crohn's colitis, ischemic colitis, irradiation colitis, and pseudomembranous colitis (see Table 77-2). When the disease is limited to the rectum, particular attention should be paid to sexually acquired diseases, which are frequently seen in the male homosexual population ("gay bowel disease"). Some of the more common diseases in this category include rectal syphilis, gonococcal proctitis, lymphogranuloma venereum, and inflammations caused by herpes simplex virus, *Entamoeba histolytica, shigella,* and *Campylobacter.*

Treatment

Patients with severe ulcerative colitis should be treated with intravenous steroids or adrenocorticotropic hormone (ACTH), replacement of fluids, correction of electrolyte abnormalities, and broad-spectrum antibiotics active against coliforms and anaerobes (ampicillin and clindamycin or metronidazole); hyperalimentation may be considered for the individual patient (Table 77-3). Patients who have not previously been treated with steroids respond best to ACTH, 120 U/day, whereas those on steroids should receive hydrocortisone, 300 mg/day or an equivalent dose of methylprednisolone (48 mg/day) or prednisolone (60 mg/day).[10] Recently, cyclosporine (4 mg/kg/day) has been advocated for cases of fulminant colitis that have failed treatment with intravenous corticosteroids.[11] The use of complete bowel rest and routine administration of parenteral nutrition remains controversial in patients with fulminant disease.[12] When toxic megacolon is suspected, nasogastric suction should be initiated, a surgical consultation obtained, and the patient observed by frequent examinations and flat films of the abdomen. When the diagnosis of toxic megacolon is established and the patient fails to show dramatic clinical improvement within 24 to 48 h, emergency surgery should be considered.

The majority of those with mild and moderate disease can be treated as outpatients. Glucocorticoids are effective in inducing a remission in the majority of cases and constitute the mainstay of therapy in an acute attack. Daily doses of 40 to 60 mg of prednisone are usually sufficient and can be adjusted depending on the severity of the disease. In the treatment of patients with active proctitis, proctosigmoiditis, and left-sided colitis (less than 60 cm of active disease), 5-aminosalicylic acid enemas have been used with great success. Topical steroid preparations (beclomethasone, hydrocortisone, tixocortol, and budesonide) have also been successful. This therapy has also been used to maintain remission in these patients. Once clinical remission is achieved, steroids should be slowly tapered and discontinued. There is no evidence that maintenance dosages of steroids reduce the incidence of relapses.

Sulfasalazine has been used in the treatment of acute attacks but is probably inferior to steroids, especially in the more severe cases. Its primary usefulness is in the form of adjunctive therapy and in the maintenance of a remission. Maintenance doses of 1.5 to 2 g/day significantly reduce the recurrence rate of the disease.

In addition to sulfasalazine, the newer 5-aminosalicylic derivatives are quite effective in inducing remission of ulcerative colitis as well as maintaining it. The main advantage of the newer agents is reduced side effects from the sufapyridine moiety of sulfasalazine. The choice of agents available for the treatment of ulcerative colitis is very similar to that in Crohn's disease [mesalamine (Pentasa, Asacol) and olsalazine (Dipentum)]. Topical glucocorticoid enemas or 5-aminosalicylic enemas (Rowasa, 2 to 4 g/60 mL/day for 3 weeks) or suppositories (500 mg bid) are quite effective in distal protosigmoiditis and have lower systemic side-effect profiles. In refractory cases, a combination of glucocorticoids and immunomodulators such as 6-mercaptopurine (1 to 1.5 mg/kg/day) or azathioprine (2 mg/kg/day) should be considered. The beneficial effects of this combination therapy will not be seen before 8 to 12 weeks, somewhat limiting its usefulness in very sick patients. For these reasons, surgical intervention with elective proctocolectomy may be necessary. Newer agents under investigation for the treatment of ulcerative colitis include nicotine and preparations of short-chain fatty acids.

Supportive measures in the treatment of mild to moderately sick patients include the replenishment of iron stores, a nutritious diet with the elimination of lactose, and adequate physical and psychological rest. Hydrophilic bulk agents such as psyllium (Metamucil) can be used in some patients to improve stool consistency. Antidiarrheal agents should be avoided because they may precipitate toxic megacolon and because they are generally ineffective.

Disposition

Patients with fulminant attacks of ulcerative colitis should be hospitalized for aggressive fluid and electrolyte resuscitation and careful observation for the development of complications. Patients with complications such as significant gastrointestinal hemorrhage, toxic megacolon, and bowel perforation should also be admitted with consultation to both a gastroenterologist and a surgeon.[13] In addition to toxic megacolon, the indications for surgery include colonic perforation, massive lower-GI bleeding, suspicion of colon cancer, and disease that is refractory to medical therapy (large doses of steroids required to control the disease). The surgical treatment options include proctocolectomy with ileostomy, ileostomy with a Koch pouch, proctocolectomy with an ileoanal pouch, or colectomy with ileorectal anastomosis. Age and patient acceptance often influence the choice of surgical procedure, with the increased performance of continent procedures. Unlike the effects of surgery in Crohn's disease, surgical intervention is curative in ulcerative colitis.

Patients with mild to moderate disease can be discharged from the ED. Close follow-up should be arranged with the patient's medical physician or gastroenterologist, and any adjustment in medical therapy discussed. In addition, the patient should be instructed to eat a low-residue diet. Patients should be instructed to return if symptoms do not improve or worsen. Particular attention should focus on the quantity of diarrhea, toleration of oral intake, and associated symptoms such as fever, rectal bleeding, or abdominal pain.

PSEUDOMEMBRANOUS ENTEROCOLITIS

Psuedomembranous enterocolitis is an inflammatory bowel disorder in which membrane-like yellowish plaques of exudate overlie and replace necrotic intestinal mucosa.

Epidemiology

Clostridium difficile is a spore-forming obligate anaerobic bacillus that causes pseudomembranous colitis. *C. difficile* was originally identified as an enteric human pathogen in 1978. The incidence of this disease has been increasing in recent years, coincident with the increased spectrum of antibiotics in use throughout the United States.

Three different syndromes have been described: neonatal pseudomembranous enterocolitis, postoperative pseudomembranous enterocolitis, and antibiotic-associated pseudomembranous colitis. Recent antibiotic use, gastrointestinal surgery or manipulation, severe underlying medical illness, and advancing age have all been identified as risk factors for developing pseudomembranous colitis. Transmission of the organism has been implicated from direct human contact as well as contact with inanimate objects (commodes, telephones, rectal thermometers). *C. difficile* is the most common enteric pathogen associated with nosocomial diarrhea.[14]

Pathophysiology

Hospitalized patients are colonized with *C. difficile* in 10 to 25 percent of cases. Broad-spectrum antibiotics—most notably clindamycin, cephalosporins, and ampicillin/amoxicillin—alter the gut flora in such a way that toxin-producing *C. difficile* can flourish within the colon, producing clinical manifestations of pseudomembranous colitis. It should be remembered, however, that almost any antibiotic (including metronidazole and vancomycin) can lead to pseudomembranous colitis. It should also be noted that chemotherapeutic agents[15] and antiviral agents[16] have been implicated as well. Most strains of *C. difficile* produce two toxins, toxin A, an enterotoxin, and toxin B, a cytotoxin, that interact in a complex and not completely understood manner to produce pseudomembranous colitis and its associated symptoms.

Clinical Features

Pseudomembranous colitis results in a spectrum of clinical manifestations that vary from frequent, mucoid, watery stools to a toxic picture that includes profuse diarrhea (20 to 30 stools per day), crampy abdominal pain, fever, leukocytosis, dehydration, and hypovolemia. Examination of the stool may reveal the presence of fecal leukocytes. These are not generally found in more benign forms of antibiotic-induced diarrhea. Complications of the disease include severe electrolyte imbalance, hypotension, and anasarca from decreased serum albumin. Rarely, toxic megacolon or colonic perforation may occur in patients with pseudomembranous colitis. The disease typically begins 7 to 10 days after the institution of antibiotic therapy, although in some cases symptoms may be noted within a few days or up to 8 weeks after the antibiotic is discontinued. *C. difficile* colitis has now been established as a nosocomial infection in hospitals.

Diagnosis

The diagnosis is suggested by a history of diarrhea that develops during administration of antibiotics or within 2 weeks of their discontinuation. The diagnosis may be confirmed by endoscopy, which reveals characteristic yellowish plaques within the intestinal lumen. Lesions may be seen throughout the entire alimentary tract, although they are typically limited to the right colon. For this reason, colonoscopy may be required in some cases to establish the diagnosis, which may be missed by sigmoidoscopy alone. It should be noted, however, endoscopy is not routinely needed to establish a diagnosis of pseudomembranous colitis.

The diagnosis is confirmed by the demonstration of *C. difficile* in the stool and by the detection of toxin in stool filtrates. The organism is best identified by stool culture using a selective growth medium.[17] This technique has a sensitivity approaching 100 percent but lacks specificity. In addition, culture results take between 28 and 72 h, thus limiting their utilization in establishing the diagnosis in patients with suspected pseudomembranous colitis. Instead, *C. difficile* toxin is detected directly using a number of techniques including tissue-culture assay, enzyme-linked immunosorbent assays (ELISA), latex agglutination, dot-immunobinding assays, and polymerase chain reaction (PCR). Tests vary in their sensitivity, specificity, and time to completion. While tissue-culture assays are considered the "gold standard," most laboratories utilize the ELISA technique to detect the clostridial toxins; it has a sensitivity of 63 to 94 percent and a specificity of 75 to 100 percent.[18]

Treatment

The treatment of pseudomembranous colitis includes discontinuing antibiotic therapy and instituting supportive measures such as the administration of fluids and the correction of electrolyte abnormalities. Twenty-five percent of patients will respond to these measures alone. For those patients with mild to moderate disease who do not respond to supportive measures, metronidazole 250 mg four times daily is the therapy of choice.[19] Vancomycin 125 to 250 mg four times daily is an alternative regimen, although this is considerably more expensive than metronidazole. It should be reserved for cases where the patient has not responded to or is intolerant of metronidazole, where the organism is resistant to metronidazole, or where the patient is pregnant.

Severely ill persons must be hospitalized. Oral vancomycin, 125 to 250 mg four times a day for 10 days, is effective in the majority of severely ill patients.[20] The symptoms usually resolve within a few days. Rarely, emergency colectomy may be required for patients with toxic dilatation of the colon or colonic perforation.

Relapses occur in 10 to 20 percent of patients. The use of antidiarrheal agents may prolong or worsen symptoms in patients with pseudomembranous colitis and should be avoided. Steroids and surgical intervention are rarely needed.

Disposition

Patients with severe diarrhea, symptoms that persist despite appropriate outpatient management, or those with a systemic response (fever, leukocytosis, severe abdominal pain) should be hospitalized. Patients with pseudomembranous colitis who are suspected of having a toxic megacolon or perforation should have an immediate surgical consultation. For those patients who are discharged, discontinuation of any antibiotics and good oral intake must be encouraged. The decision to institute therapy using metronidazole or vancomycin should be made in conjunction with the patient's primary physician.

DIVERTICULITIS

Diverticulitis is an acute inflammatory process caused by bacterial proliferation within an existing colonic diverticulum.

Epidemiology

Acquired diverticular disease of the colon has become an increasingly common disorder of industrialized nations. Diverticulosis coli was first described in the early 1700s by Littre but was not identified as a pathologic entity until the mid-nineteenth century by Cruveilhier. Radiologic studies have suggested that one-third of the population will have acquired the disease by age 50 and two-thirds by age 85.[21] Diverticula are rare in individuals under age 20.

Diverticulitis is estimated to occur in 10 to 25 percent of patients with known diverticulosis. The incidence of diverticulitis increases with age. Only 2 to 4 percent of patients with diverticulitis are under the age of 40. Diverticulitis in the younger age group tends to be a more virulent form of the disease, with frequent complications requiring earlier surgical intervention.[22] Although the frequency of the disease is higher in men, there is an increasing incidence of diverticulitis in women.

Pathophysiology

Colonic diverticula are false diverticula because they do not include all layers of the bowel wall. They consist of mucosa and submucosa with a peritoneal covering that has herniated through a defect in the circular muscle layer of the wall. The sites of herniation are located between the mesenteric and antimesenteric taenia, where intramural blood vessels penetrate the muscularis.

A pathophysiologic mechanism to explain the development of diverticular disease is not apparent. It is still unresolved whether diverticular disease is a disorder of colonic motility, a colonic muscle abnormality, a connective tissue disorder, or a normal concomitant of aging. Low-residue diets have been implicated as a major factor in the pathogenesis of diverticular disease. The most common hypothesis is that acquired diverticula arise because of high intraluminal pressures in areas of relative weakness of the colonic wall. This is based upon observations that the majority of patients have diverticula located within the sigmoid colon. Laplace's law states that the tension on the wall of a hollow cylinder is inversely proportional to the radius of the cylinder multiplied by the pressure within the cylinder. This suggests that the intraluminal pressure in the colon is greatest where the lumen is narrowest. The diameter of the colon is smallest in the sigmoid region, and thus this region of the colon is the most likely location for the development of diverticula.

The complications of diverticular disease that bring the patient to the ED can be divided into two broad categories: (1) inflammation and its associated complications and (2) bleeding (see Chap. 70, "Gastrointestinal Bleeding").

Inflammation, or diverticulitis, is the most common complication of diverticular disease. It results when fecal material becomes inspissated in the neck of an acquired diverticulum, resulting in obstruction of the neck of the diverticulum and subsequent proliferation of colonic bacteria, mucous secretion, and distention of the diverticulum. Clinical diverticulitis always represents microperforation and inflammation of pericolonic tissue. Fortunately, fecal contamination of the peritoneum is usually limited because perforation of a diverticulum occurs into the leaves of the mesentery or because the contamination is walled off by the mobile loops of the sigmoid colon or small bowel and adjacent pelvic structures. Free perforation may occur with generalized peritonitis, but it is uncommon.

Clinical Features

The most common symptom of diverticulitis is pain. This is commonly described as a steady, deep discomfort in the left lower quadrant. Patients will frequently complain of a change in the bowel habits, either in the form of diarrhea or increasing constipation. Tenesmus is another common symptom. The involved diverticulum may irritate the bladder or ureter, causing the patient to have urinary frequency, dysuria, or pyuria. If a fistula develops between the colon and the bladder, the patient may present with recurrent urinary tract infections or pneumaturia. Paralytic ileus with abdominal distention, nausea, and vomiting may develop secondary to intraabdominal irritation and peritonitis. Small bowel obstruction may also occur as adjacent loop of small bowel becomes kinked or narrowed in the inflammatory mass.

Rarely, the clinical presentation may be indistinguishable from acute appendicitis. This may occur when the patient has a redundant sigmoid colon lying on the right side of the abdomen or a right-sided diverticulum that becomes inflamed. The possibility of diverticulitis should always be considered in the patient 50 years of age or older with right lower abdominal pain. Cases of diverticulitis in the cecum or ascending colon have also been reported.

The patient with free perforation will often present with a history of sudden onset of abdominal pain, usually beginning in the lower abdomen and then progressing to generalized abdominal involvement. The patient will appear quite toxic, with signs of diffuse peritonitis. Prior steroid use predisposes the patient to perforation and may mask some of the typical signs and symptoms.

Physical examination frequently demonstrates a low-grade fever, around 38°C (100.4°F). The temperature may, however, be more elevated in patients with generalized peritonitis or in those who have formed an abscess. The abdominal examination reveals localized tenderness, often with voluntary guarding and rebound tenderness. With careful palpation, one may be able to appreciate a fullness or mass over the involved segment of the colon. Rectal examination will often reveal tenderness on the left side. Twenty-five percent of patients may demonstrate occult blood. When free perforation does occur, diffuse abdominal tenderness, rigidity, guarding, and rebound tenderness may be noted. In the female patient, a pelvic examination should always be carried out to eliminate a gynecologic source of symptoms.

Diagnosis

The diagnosis is usually suspected by the clinical history and the findings on physical examination. The presence of peritoneal signs or generalized peritonitis should suggest free perforation or rupture of a peridiverticular abscess. The presence of an abdominal mass associated with occult blood in the stool could indicate colon cancer. Colonic or small bowel obstruction, though uncommon, may necessitate surgical intervention.

Barium contrast studies can easily demonstrate diverticulae but are insensitive in detecting the presence of diverticulitis. In addition, barium introduced under high pressure carries the risk of precipitating a colonic perforation. Abdominal CT is the diagnostic procedure of choice.[23] It can demonstrate inflammation of percolic fat, presence of diverticulae, thickening of the bowel wall, or peridiverticular abscess.[24] Colon cancer is best ruled out by sigmoidoscopy or colonoscopy.

The acute abdominal series may be normal or may demonstrate associated ileus, partial small bowel obstruction, free air indicating bowel perforation, or extraluminal collections of air that might indicate a walled-off abscess. Abdominal ultrasonography is an inexpensive noninvasive method but is operator-dependent and lacks specificity.

Laboratory studies should include routine screening blood tests, urinalysis, and an acute abdominal series. Unfortunately, in many cases laboratory studies are not helpful in the diagnosis. Leukocytosis was seen in only 36 percent of patients with acute diverticulitis.[25] Controversy exists regarding the use of sigmoidoscopy or contrast radiographic studies in the acute inflammatory state. The general opinion in the literature is that these studies should be performed after conservative medical management has been instituted and the acute inflammatory process has subsided.

Differential Diagnosis

In patients over the age of 40 presenting with complaints of abdominal pain, a change in bowel habits, and urinary symptoms, a diagnosis of colonic diverticulitis should be entertained. These symptoms, however, are nonspecific, and a number of pathologic entities may present with similar signs and symptoms (Table 77-2). Some of the most important are discussed below.

Symptoms of irritable bowel syndrome include diffuse crampy or colicky abdominal pain, brought on by meals or emotional upset. The patients may also describe a bloated or distended sensation in the abdomen. The symptoms are usually intermittent and chronic. The passage of flatus or a bowel movement may bring relief. The disease is characterized by alternating bouts of constipation and diarrhea. On physical examination, the patient is afebrile and a cordlike mass may be appreciated in the left lower quadrant corresponding to the sigmoid colon. Signs of localized or generalized peritonitis are not seen. Laboratory studies are normal.

Patients who have colon carcinoma may present with a change in bowel habits, either diarrhea or constipation, and/or abdominal pain that can mimic symptoms of diverticular disease. There may be blood mixed with the patient's stools, and weight loss. Physical examination may reveal a palpable mass, usually nontender. Fever and chills are less common, and laboratory studies may demonstrate anemia without

TABLE 77-4 Treatment of Acute Diverticulitis

Restore fluid and electrolyte balance
Nothing by mouth
Nasogastric suction for Obstruction Adynamic ileus
Broad-spectrum antibiotics Aminoglycoside (gentamicin or tobramycin) Metronidazole or clindamycin Ticarcillin-clavulanic acid or imipenem (alternative therapy)
Observe for complications Obstruction Perforation Intraabdominal abscess

evidence of leukocytosis. An acute abdominal series may demonstrate findings of colonic obstruction. This can be produced by an inflamed diverticula or a carcinoma in an area of the bowel with underlying diverticulosis. Fiberoptic colonoscopy can be useful in differentiating diverticular disease from carcinoma.

Pelvic inflammatory disease may present with abdominal pain, fever, and leukocytosis. The disease is usually found in young women. A careful pelvic examination should be carried out in all female patients with lower abdominal pain. A history of irregular menses and the finding of vaginal discharge should aid in the diagnosis.

Ischemic colitis can present with a broad range of clinical manifestations. Mild transient ischemia may result in mucosal sloughing and painless rectal bleeding. If the disease progresses to gangrene, the patient develops severe abdominal pain and peritonitis. Pain may be out of proportion to physical findings. A plain film of the abdomen may reveal thumbprinting in the region of the involved colonic segment. In more advanced cases, there may be gas within the bowel wall, or, if perforation has occurred, free air in the abdomen. Cautious endoscopic evaluation and contrast x-ray studies are helpful in distinguishing ischemic colitis from diverticulitis.

Treatment

Initial resuscitation of patients with acute diverticulitis should focus on determining the severity of the illness, eliminating other causes of symptoms, and appropriate fluid and electrolyte resuscitation (Table 77-4). In patients who demonstrate signs of toxicity such as fever, tachycardia, leukocytosis and severe abdominal pain, intravenous antibiotics are administered. These should include an aminoglycoside (gentamicin or tobramycin 1.5 mg/kg) and either clindamycin 300 to 600 mg or metronidazole 500 mg. Ticarcillin-clavulanic acid or imipenem have been used as alternative agents. The patient is placed on bowel rest, but in this case, nothing by mouth is given and intravenous fluids are administered. Nasogastric suction is necessary only if the patient manifests signs of bowel obstruction or an adynamic ileus.

Outpatient treatment consists of bowel rest and broad-spectrum oral antibiotic therapy. Patients are instructed to limit activity and to maintain a liquid diet for 48 h. If symptoms improve, low-residue foods are added to the diet. Broad-spectrum antibiotics covering both aerobic and anaerobic bacteria are given. Predominant colonic aerobes include *Escherichia coli, Klebsiella* and *Enterobacter,* while *Bacteriodes fragilis, Peptostreptococcus,* and *Clostridium* are the predominant colonic anaerobes. Common oral antibiotic agents effective against aerobic organisms include ampicillin (500 mg q 6 h), trimethoprim-sulfamethoxasole (2 tablets q 12 h), ciprofloxacin (500 mg q 12 h), or a cephalosporin, such as cefalexin (500 mg q 6 h). One of these agents is taken in combination with metronidazole (Flagyl 500 mg q 8 h), or clindamycin (Cleocin 300 mg q 6 h), which are utilized to treat the anaerobic organisms. Patients are instructed to contact their physician if increasing abdominal pain, fever, or malaise occur. Once the patient has improved, elective evaluation with contrast barium is performed.

Disposition

Patients who have localized pain without signs and symptoms of local peritonitis and without evidence of systemic infection may be treated on an outpatient basis. Careful follow-up should be arranged with the patient's primary physician. The patient should be begun on a clear liquid diet and advance to low-residue foods as symptoms improve. Patients should be instructed to return if fever develops, if they are unable to tolerate oral intake, or if there is worsening abdominal pain.

If a patient has systemic signs and symptoms of infection, has failed outpatient management, or demonstrates signs of localized peritonitis, hospitalization is necessary. Surgical consultation should be obtained at the time of hospitalization. Urgent surgical consultation is indicated if free perforation is found.

REFERENCES

1. Russel M, Stockbrugger RW: Epidemiology of inflammatory bowel disease: An update. *Scand J Gastroenterol* 31:417, 1996.
2. Walker-Smith JA, Savage MO: Effects of inflammatory bowel disease on growth: Growth matters. *Kabi Pharmacia* 12:10, 1993.
3. Hebbar M, Wattel E, Mastrini S, et al: Association between myelodysplastic syndromes and inflammatory bowel diseases: Report of seven new cases and review of the literature. *Leukemia* 11:2188, 1997.
4. Freeman HJ: Osteomyelitis and osteonecrosis in inflammatory bowel disease. *Can J Gastroenterol* 11:601, 1997.
5. Robert JR, Sachar DB, Greenstein AJ: Severe gastrointestinal hemorrhage in Crohn's disease. *Ann Surg* 213:207, 1991.
6. Truelove SC, Witts LJ: Cortisone in ulcerative colitis: Final report on a therapeutic trial. *Br Med J* 2:1041, 1955.
7. Straus RJ, Flint GW, Platt N, et al: The surgical management of toxic dilatation of the colon: A report of 28 cases and review of the literature. *Ann Surg* 184:682, 1976.
8. Farraye FA, Peppercorn MA: Inflammatory bowel disease: Advances in the management of ulcerative colitis and Crohn's disease. *Consultant* 28:39, 46-7, 1988.
9. Kornbluth A, Sachar DB: Ulcerative colitis practice guidelines in adults. *Am J Gastroenterol* 92:204, 1997.
10. Meyers S, Sachar DB, Goldberg JD, et al: Corticotropin versus hydrocortisone in the intravenous treatment of ulcerative colitis. *Gastroenterology* 85:351, 1983.
11. Lichtiger S, Present DH, Kornbluth A, et al: Cyclosporine in sever ulcerative colitis refractory to steroid therapy. *N Engl J Med* 330:1841, 1994.
12. Gonzales-Huix F, Fernandez-Banares F, Esteve-Comas M, et al: Enteral versus parenteral nutrition as adjunct therapy in acute ulcerative colitis. *Am J Gastroenterol* 88:227, 1993.
13. Jewell DP, Caprilli R, Moetenson N, et al: Indication and timing of surgery for severe ulcerative colitis. *Gastroenterol Int* 4:161, 1991.
14. Viscidi R, Willey S, Bartlett JG: Isolation rates and toxigenic potential for *Clostridium difficile* isolates from various patient populations. *Gastroenterology* 81:5, 1981.
15. Silva J, Fekety R, Werk C, et al: Inciting and etiologic agents of colitis. *Rev Infect Dis* 6(suppl 1):S214, 1984.
16. Colarian J: *Clostridium difficile* colitis following antiviral therapy in the acquired immunodeficiency syndrome. *Am J Med* 84:1081, 1988.
17. Demaio J, Bartlett JG: Update on diagnosis of *Clostridium difficile*—associated diarrhea. *Curr Clin Top Infect Dis* 15:97, 1995.
18. Gerding DN, Johnson S, Peterson LR, et al: *Clostridium difficile*—associated diarrhea and colitis. *Infect Control Hosp Epidemiol* 16:459, 1995.
19. Teasley DG, Gerding DN, Olson MM, et al: Prospective randomized trial of metronidazole versus vancomycin for *Clostridium difficile*—associated diarrhea and colitis. *Lancet* 2:1043, 1983.

20. Fekety R, Silva J, Kauffman C, Buggy B, Deery G: Treatment of antibiotic associated *Clostridium difficile* colitis with oral vancomycin: Comparison of two dosage regimens. *Am J Med* 86:15, 1989.
21. Parks TC: Natural history of diverticular disease of the colon. *Clin Gastroenterol* 4:53, 1975.
22. Freischlag J, Bennion RS, Thompson JE: Complications of diverticular disease of the colon in young people. *Dis Colon Rectum* 29:639, 1986.
23. Ferzoco LB, Raptopoulos V, Sileu W: Acute diverticulitis. *N Engl J Med* 338:1521, 1998.
24. Johnson CD, Baker ME, Rice RP: Diagnosis of acute colonic diverticulitis: Comparison of barium enema and CT. *Am J Radiol* 148:541, 1987.
25. Hackford AW, Schoetz DJ, Coller JA, et al: Surgical management of complicated diverticulitis. *Dis Colon Rectum* 28:317, 1985.

78 ANORECTAL DISORDERS

James K. Bouzoukis

Anorectal disorders are varied and multiple and may also be complex, manifesting signs and symptoms of underlying serious local or systemic disorders that could be life-threatening.

ANATOMY

The anorectum is an anatomic structure in which the entodermal intestine unites with and opens into an orifice of ectodermal origin: the anal canal. The junction of these two embryonic structures (the anorectal line) is the dentate line, which marks the anatomic beginning of the anal canal (1 to 2 cm long) and is in continuity with the perianal skin at its distal anal verge. The mucosa of the anal canal consists of stratified squamous epithelium but contains no hair follicles or sweat glands. At the anal verge (perianal region), the anoderm thickens and includes in its structure hair follicles and other cutaneous appendages. Proximal to the dentate line, the rectal ampulla narrows to conform to the opening of the anal canal; in doing so its mucosa takes on a pleated appearance, forming 8 to 14 convoluted longitudinal folds: the columns of Morgagni. Each adjacent column is connected at the dentate line by a flap of mucosa that forms a small anal crypt, normally 1 to 3 mm in longitudinal depth. Infection and inflammation of these crypts and glands become the source of anal sepsis, as characterized by the development of cryptitis, fissures, abscesses, and fistulas.

The anal wall, from its mucosal lining to the intersphincteric plane, which separates the internal from the external sphincters, is a continuation of the usual layers of the wall of the colon and rectum. The innermost lining the mucosa, continues to the anal verge, undergoing a transition just proximal to the dentate line from rectal columnar to cuboidal to squamous epithelium. The submucosa, which normally contains the bulk of the bowel's blood vessels (and autonomic nerves), thickens considerably proximal to the dentate line; its dilated veins in this area are referred to as the internal hemorrhoidal plexus. Likewise, the inner circular muscle layer of the rectum thickens considerably as it terminates distally in the anorectum to form the internal sphincter muscles, while the more attenuated longitudinal muscles of the rectum extend caudally, blending with fibers of voluntary skeletal muscles from the levator ani and external sphincter groups to form the intersphincteric plane (Fig. 78-1).

Additional sphincteric support is provided by an outer layer of voluntary skeletal muscles, the external sphincters, which are divided into three parts: deep, superficial, and subcutaneous. The external sphincters are actually a caudal extension of the puborectalis muscle, which interacts with the levator ani muscle forming the pelvic floor. The puborectalis, the proximal external sphincters, and the internal sphincters form the ring of muscles that one palpates when performing a digital examination of the anorectum.

Lateral to the external sphincters is the ischiorectal space, and superior to the levator ani is the pelvirectal space, where deep, life-threatening infections can occur.

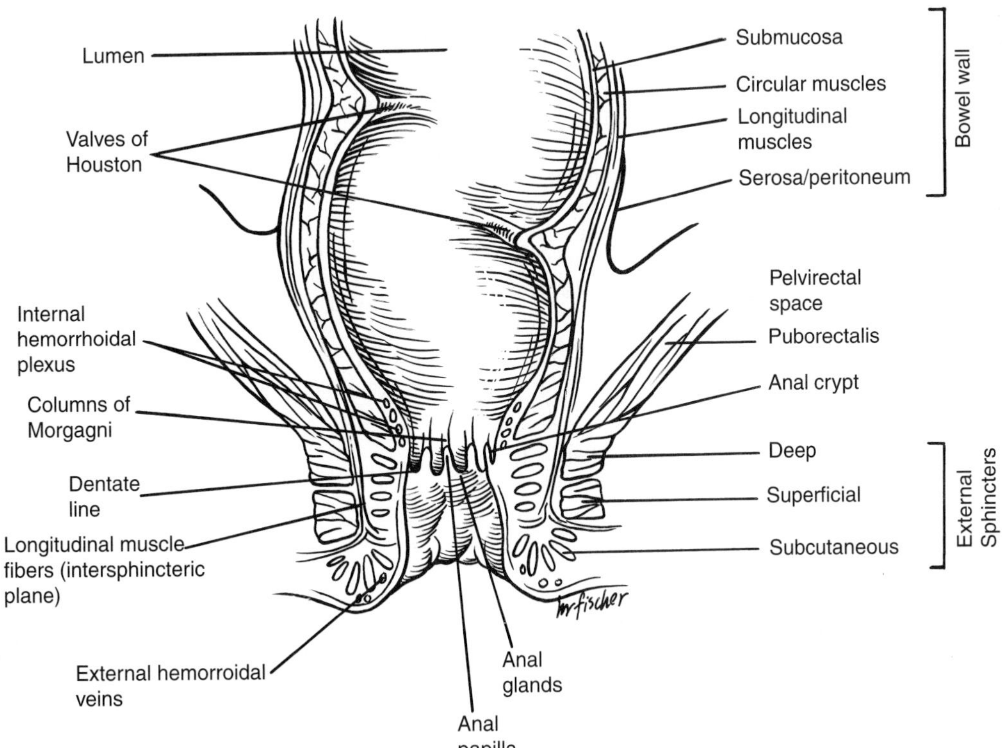

FIG. 78-1. Coronal section of the anorectum.

EXAMINATION OF THE PATIENT

No matter how much historical information is obtained, no definitive diagnosis can be made without a careful examination of the anus and rectum, including anoscopy and, if necessary, proctoscopy.

The lateral, or Sims, position, performed with the patient lying on his or her left side with the left leg extended and the right knee and hip flexed, is probably the most commonly used approach for performing a routine digital rectal examination and is the preferred position for elderly or pregnant patients. From the Sims position, one should elevate the upper right buttock to provide better exposure of the perianal area; if needed, endoscopic examination of the anus and distal rectum can be performed with the patient in this position. In debilitated patients, one may have to perform the examination with the patient in a supine, lithotomy position.

Examining a patient placed in the knee-chest position requires a cooperative patient who is not too ill or in too much distress. This provides for a thorough inspection of the perianal area and is convenient for anoscopy and proctoscopy. Thighs should be at right angles to the table with the feet extended over the end of the table.

A digital examination should always be performed before doing any endoscopic procedure. No bowel preparation is needed to perform an anoscopic examination. After performing a digital examination and determining that the patient will tolerate passage of an anoscope, introduce a well-lubricated, lighted anoscope, remove the obturator, and gently rotate it 360° to view the anorectum circumferentially.

It is usually difficult to perform a proper sigmoidoscopic examination in an emergency department (ED) setting. Ordinarily, the lower bowel must be prepped; a natural bowel movement, spontaneous or induced 1 to 2 h before examination, is usually sufficient preparation. In some acute situations, such as trying to determine the source of lower GI bleeding or obtaining cultures in a case of suppurative proctitis, emergency proctoscopy may be performed. A rigid sigmoidoscope should be utilized, with the patient placed in a Sims position. An inexperienced endoscopist should not attempt to pass the sigmoidoscope beyond the rectosigmoid junction, where the lumen is greatly angulated, because of the risk of perforation.

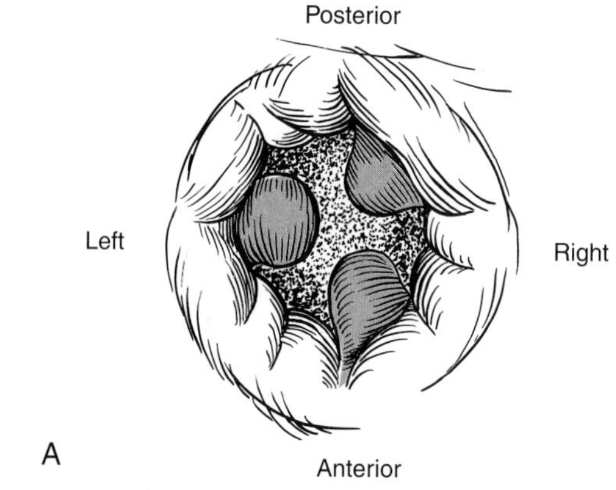

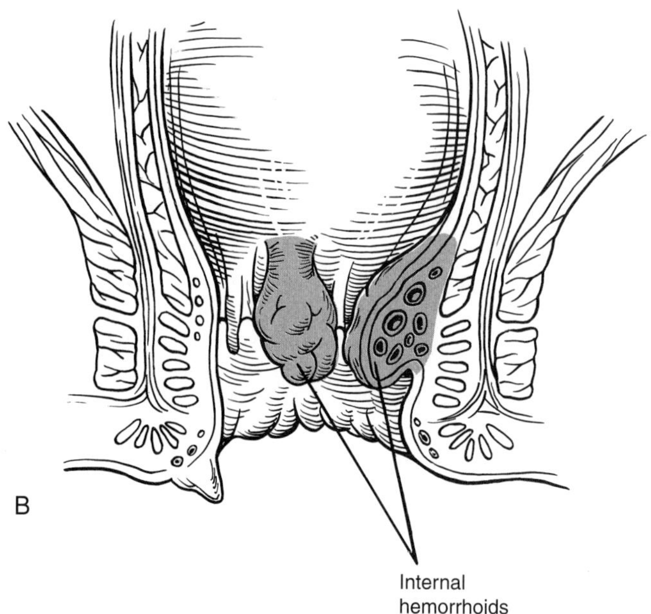

FIG. 78-2. Common sites of hemorrhoids. **A.** Internal hemorrhoids at 2, 5, and 9 o'clock. **B.** Protrusion of anal cushions.

HEMORRHOIDS

The anorectal area is drained by the internal and external hemorrhoidal venous systems. The internal hemorrhoidal veins, which in essence are submucosal vascular cushions that may contribute to anal continence, are located proximal to the dentate line and drain into the portal system through the superior rectal veins and the inferior mesenteric vein. They also communicate freely with the external hemorrhoidal veins, which are subcutaneous to the anoderm and drain primarily through the pudendal and iliac venous systems. When these hemorrhoidal plexuses become excessively engorged, prolapsed, or thrombosed, they are referred to as hemorrhoids—one of the most common problems afflicting human beings.

Internal hemorrhoids, which course along the terminal branches of the superior rectal artery, are constant in their location, coursing longitudinally at the right posterolateral, right anterolateral, and left lateral positions (at the 2-, 5- and 9-o'clock positions when the patient is viewed prone) (Fig. 78-2). Internal hemorrhoids are not readily palpable and can best be visualized through an anoscope. External hemorrhoids are dilatation of veins at the anal verge and can be seen at external inspection.

Although the cause of enlarged hemorrhoids is not always known, there is an association with constipation and straining at stool. They are prevalent during pregnancy and may be the result of sustained increased pressure on the venous drainage of the rectum. One of the physiologic shunts of the portal system involves the hemorrhoidal veins. Consequently, increased portal pressure, occurring as a result of chronic liver disease, may produce marked dilatation and varix formation of the hemorrhoids. The bleeding that can result is extremely difficult to control.

Tumors of the rectum and sigmoid colon, often associated with constipation, tenesmus, and incomplete evacuation, may cause hemorrhoids and must be ruled out in all cases of rectal bleeding in patients over the age of 40.

Clinical Features

Uncomplicated internal hemorrhoids are painless, and the chief complaint is painless, bright-red rectal bleeding with defecation. Bleeding is usually limited, with the blood being found on the surface of the stool, on the toilet tissue, or dripping into the toilet bowl. Although the most common cause of rectal bleeding is hemorrhoids, other, more serious causes should be sought in all patients who present with bleeding as the chief complaint. Clinical signs cannot reliably differentiate colonic lesions from hemorrhoids.[1] Chronic, slow blood loss may go unnoticed but can result in a significant anemia. Pain, when present, is most severe at the time of defecation and subsides with time. Pain is usually associated with thrombosed external hemorrhoids.

As they increase in size, hemorrhoids may prolapse, requiring periodic reduction by the patient (Table 78-1). When prolapse occurs, the patient may develop a mucous discharge and pruritus ani.

If the prolapse cannot be reduced, strangulation can result. Other complications include severe bleeding and thrombosis. Both strangulation and thrombosis are extremely painful and are accompanied by significant edema that must be treated before surgical intervention. Ulceration of the overlying mucosa may also occur.

Treatment

Most treatment is local and nonsurgical unless a complication is present. Hot sitz baths for at least 15 min three times a day and after each bowel movement are the most effective way to relieve pain. Following the bath, the anus must be dried gently but thoroughly to avoid maceration of the perianal skin. Topical analgesics and steroid-containing ointments may provide relief. The patient should not sit for a prolonged period on the commode. Bulk laxatives, such as psyllium seed compounds, or stool softeners should be used after the acute phase is treated. Laxatives causing liquid stool must be avoided; this can result in cryptitis and anal sepsis. The addition of bran or other forms of roughage to the patient's diet should help to prevent future problems.

As a rule, internal hemorrhoids bleed and, if not prolapsed, are not palpable. External hemorrhoids thrombose. Selection of therapy for thrombosed external hemorrhoids depends on the severity of symptoms: if the thrombosis has been present less than 48 h, the swelling is not tense, and the pain is tolerable, the patient may be treated with sitz baths and bulk laxatives. Suppositories, which are placed proximal to the anorectal ring, are of no help. If, on the other hand, thrombosis is acute and recent in origin, significant relief can be provided by excising the clots. With the patient in prone position, the area of the overlying skin to be incised is infiltrated with a local anesthetic using a 30-gauge needle. While applying gentle traction to the skin adjacent to the thrombosed hemorrhoid, an elliptical incision is made in the overlying skin, exposing the thrombosed vein, which is locally excised with the elliptical flap of skin (Fig. 78-3). Because of the multiloculated clots that are invariably present, the technique of unroofing a thrombosed hemorrhoid with an elliptical incision gives far better results than the simple incision and evacuation of a clot. Bleeding is controlled by tucking the corner of a small piece of gauze into the wound and leaving it in place for a few hours. A small pressure dressing may be applied external to the gauze and removed when the patient takes the first sitz bath 6 to 12 h after the drainage procedure. Narcotics may be prescribed, but only judiciously, since they cause constipation and may produce more problems.

Surgical referral and intervention for hemorrhoids is indicated for continued bleeding; incarceration and/or strangulation; severe, unrelenting pruritus; and intractable pain. Surgical treatment can consist of sclerosing injections, the use of rubber-band ligation,[2] or excision. Up to 5 percent of patients undergoing rubber-band ligation may develop acute thrombosis of external hemorrhoids, and immunocompromised patients so treated may develop pelvic sepsis.

TABLE 78-1 Classification of Internal Hemorrhoids

Degree	Symptoms
First	Bleeding; local, compressible swelling
Second	Protrude with defecation, reduce spontaneously, ± bleeding
Third	Protrude with defecation, must be reduced manually, ± bleeding
Fourth	Incarcerated

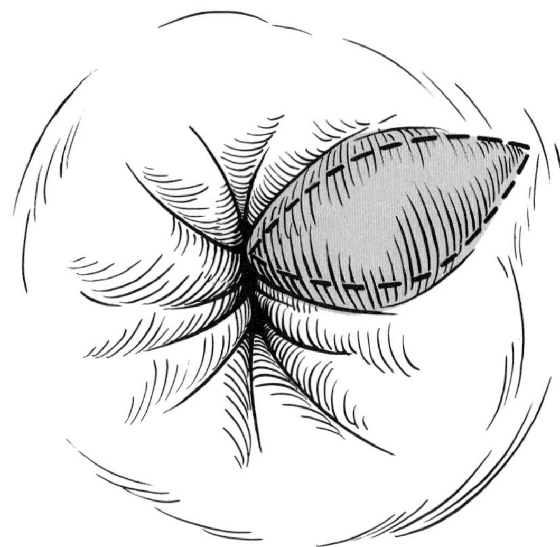

FIG. 78-3. Elliptical excision of thrombosed external hemorrhoid.

CRYPTITIS

Anal crypts are the superficial mucosal pockets that lie between the columns of Morgagni. They are formed by the puckering action of the sphincter muscles and normally flatten out during the passage of a stool. Sphincter spasm and superficial trauma caused by repeated bouts of diarrhea, or trauma produced by evacuation of large, hard stools associated with constipation cause breakdown in the mucosal lining of the crypts. This permits infecting organisms to enter pockets and inflammation to extend into the lymphoid tissue of both the crypts and anal glands. Cryptitis could well be the common denominator for the development of such anal infections as fissure in ano, perirectal abscesses, and fistula in ano.

Associated with cryptitis is the development of hypertrophied anal papillae, which lie between adjacent crypts. When hypertrophy occurs, the papillae may be palpated as small, hard nodules along the wall of the anal canal. Rarely, papillae may hypertrophy and present as a prolapsing polypoid tumor. The crypts most commonly involved are in the posterior half of the anal ring and, in most cases, in the posterior midline, the same location where anal fissures occur.

Clinical Features

Initially, the locally inflamed crypts produce no symptoms, but as the trauma from recurrent diarrhea or passage of large, hard stools continues, the inflammation of the crypts extends to the adjacent papillae, producing an edematous swelling of the sensitive anoderm that lines this part of the canal. At this stage, the patient will experience pain with bowel movements, and if there is an associated papillitis or fissure in ano, there will also be a small amount of bleeding. Anal pain, spasm, and itching with or without bleeding are the cardinal signs and symptoms of cryptitis.

Treatment

Treatment of anal cryptitis, which should be conservative, is based on establishing a definitive diagnosis and ruling out the possibility of more serious anorectal problems. The diagnosis can be suspected clinically from the history and the palpation of the tender, swollen crypt and its associated hypertrophied papillae. Definitive diagnosis of cryptitis is made by anoscopic examination. Gentle insertion of a hooked probe into the crypts brought into view through the anoscope will reveal the involved crypt(s) to be deeper than normal and definitely more tender.

The goal of treatment is to control the trauma of abnormal bowel movements and thus enable the inflammation to subside. Bulk laxatives and additional roughage to the diet to produce formed, soft stools; combined with hot sitz baths they enhance healing by keeping the anus clean and the crypts empty.

Surgical intervention is indicated when the infection has progressed and there is a deep, redundant crypt that will not drain adequately on its own. In these cases, the roof (mucosal surface), as outlined by the passage of a hooked probe, should be infiltrated with local anesthetic and excised. Thus, what had been a deep pocket is converted into an open wound that should heal with proper control of bowel movements and frequent sitz baths.

FISSURE IN ANO (ANAL FISSURE)

This disorder is the result of a linear tear of the anal canal beginning at or just below the dentate line and extending distally along the anal canal. The epithelium in this area consists of anoderm, which has a rich supply of somatic sensory nerve fibers. Consequently, anal fissures are the most common cause of painful rectal bleeding.

Anal fissures are often associated with swelling of the surrounding tissues, producing hypertrophic papillae proximally and the characteristic sentinel pile distally. The latter is frequently misdiagnosed as an external hemorrhoid when in actuality it is the result of edema and fibrosis secondary to the ulcerating fissure. In more than 90 percent of cases, anal fissures occur in the midline posteriorly. In 10 percent of women but in only 1 percent of men, it may be in the midline anteriorly. This almost constant location of anal fissures may be because of the posterior angulation of the rectum on the anus where the posterior midline of the anorectal canal becomes the ''lesser curvature'' for the passage of stool. A fissure not located in the midline should arouse suspicion that another, potentially life-threatening cause may be involved. Such diagnostic possibilities include Crohn's disease, chronic ulcerative colitis, squamous cell carcinoma of the anus, adenocarcinoma of the rectum invading the anal canal, localized anal cancers such as Bowen's disease and extramammary Paget's disease, leukemia, lymphoma, syphilitc fissures, and tuberculous ulcer. Such patients must be referred for a diagnostic biopsy of the ulcer edge, culture of the anal canal, and a systemic evaluation.

Most often, the traditional midline anal fissure is caused by the trauma produced by the passage of a particularly hard and large fecal mass, but it is also seen after acute episodes of diarrhea. Fissures persist because of the severe, chronic internal sphincter spasm that occurs along with the secondary infection of its base.

Clinical Features

Pain of the sharp, cutting variety is the most common symptom. Typically, the pain is most severe during and immediately after a bowel movement. The pain may persist for a few hours after each bowel movement, but invariably it subsides between movements, which is a distinguishing feature of fissures from other forms of painful anorectal disease. The bleeding is bright and small in quantity, usually being noticed only on the toilet paper. In infants, the presence of small amounts of bright blood on the stool or toilet paper is usually the presenting complaint for an anal fissure. Sphincter spasm and pain may be severe enough to make the patient retain stool and avoid defecation.

Diagnosis of anal fissure is usually suggested by the history; however, the anal area must be examined in all cases. With proper exposure, the sentinel pile, if present, and frequently the distal end of the fissure itself, may be seen. The mere retraction of the buttocks and the anal skin may cause considerable discomfort; sphincter spasm may be so severe that the patient will not permit digital examination. Application of a topical anesthetic may provide some relief. If the fissure can be visualized and is present in the posterior midline, rectal examination can be deferred until the patient is having less spasm and pain.

Treatment

Treatment is aimed at providing symptomatic relief, relieving the anal sphincter spasm, and preventing stricture formation. Hot sitz baths for at least 15 min three to four times a day and after each bowel movement will relax the sphincter and provide symptomatic relief. The addition of bran to the diet will serve to prevent stricture formation by providing a bulky stool. Local analgesic ointments provide symptomatic relief. The use of hydrocortisone-containing ointments does provide relief and helps with healing. In a study that compared the effectiveness of these three modalities, most rapid healing of fissures occured with sitz baths and a diet rich in bran, though healing was aided by both an analgesic ointment or a hydrocortisone-containing ointment. Meticulous anal hygiene is imperative; following defecation, the anus must be cleaned thoroughly. Healing is by the development of granulation tissue and the reepithelialization of the ulcerated area. If healing does not occur in a reasonable amount of time, operative treatment consisting of partial sphincterotomy and excision of the fissure may be required.

ANORECTAL ABSCESSES

Abscesses are common in the perianal and perirectal regions, as are fistulas, which are common sequelae. Almost all begin with involvement of an anal crypt and its gland. From there, the infection can progress to involve any of the potential spaces that are normally filled with fatty areolar tissue and have little inherent resistance to the progression of infection. These spaces, which can become infected alone or in combination with each other, are as follows: the perianal space, the intersphincteric space, the ischiorectal space, the deep postanal space (connecting the ischiorectal space on each side posteriorly), and the supralevator or pelvirectal space (Figs. 78-4 and 78-5).

The perianal abscess is the most common anorectal abscess and occurs when pus spreads caudally between the internal and external sphincters. It presents close to the anal verge, post midline, as a superficial tender mass, which may or may not be fluctuant. In contradistinction, ischiorectal abscesses tend to be larger, indurated, and to present more laterally, on the medial aspect of the buttocks. Deeper perirectal abscesses may not manifest cutaneous signs, but rectal pain and tenderness are invariably present. The isolated perianal abscess not associated with deeper, perirectal abscess(es) is the only type of anorectal abscess that can be adequately treated under local anesthesia in an ED setting.

Ischiorectal and other deep abscesses pose a different problem. The ischiorectal fossa forms a large potential space on either side of the rectum, communicating behind it through the deep postanal space, and, in males, has extensions anteriorly above the perineal membrane to the prostate. Infections in this area are insidious and extensive and can point in an area some distance from the anal verge. These abscesses can be large, and yet only a diffuse, nonfluctuant, tender ''mass'' is palpable either through the rectal wall or the overlying skin. If only induration is present, endorectal ultrasonography[3] and/or needle localization under anesthesia may be needed to confirm the diagnosis.

Most abscesses in the anorectal area are the result of obstruction of an anal gland that opens in the base of an anal crypt and normally drains into the anal canal. When obstruction occurs, the gland orifice is blocked, resulting in infection and abscess formation. An element of cryptitis can frequently be identified by anoscopic examination. A variety of diseases are associated with the development of fistulous abscesses, including Crohn's disease, carcinoma of adjacent organs, Hodgkin disease, tuberculosis, and gonococcal proctitis.

Clinical Features

Initially, the patient notices a dull, aching, or throbbing pain that becomes worse immediately before defecation, is lessened after defecation, but persists between bowel movements. The pain is increased by the increased pressure in the rectum that occurs just before defecation.

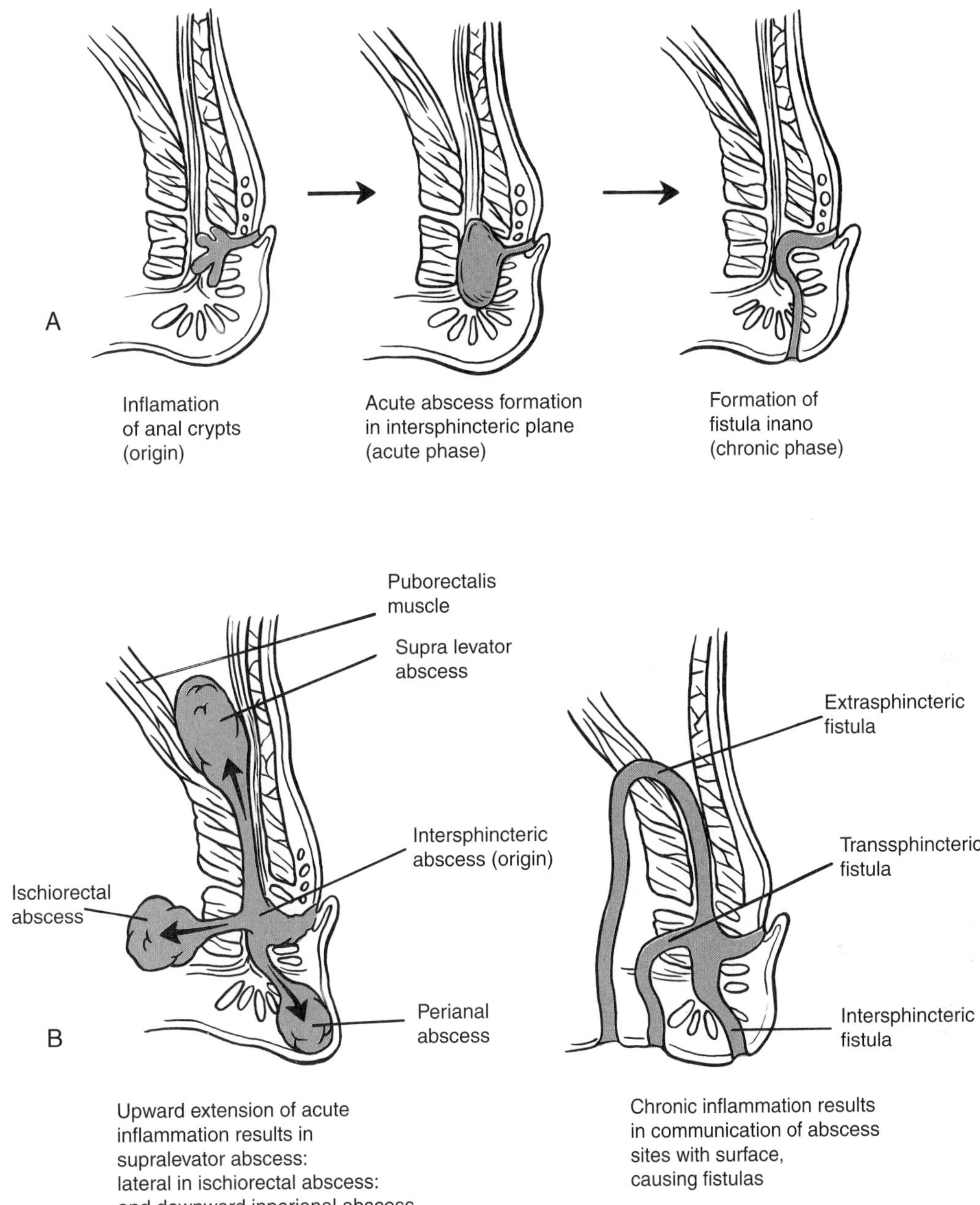

FIG. 78-4. Illustration of mechanism for anorectal abscess and fistula formation.

As the abscess spreads, increases in size, and comes nearer the surface, the associated pain becomes more intense. Pain will be aggravated by straining, coughing, or sneezing. As the abscess progresses, pain and tenderness interfere with walking or sitting.

The patient appears markedly uncomfortable and may be febrile. A tender mass may be present, or there may be a tender, erythematous area with or without fluctuance. On rectal examination, a tender mass or induration is detected. Leukocytosis may be present.

Although clinical evaluation of abscesses is usually sufficient, if pain is out of proportion to physical findings or if the extent of the abscess is uncertain, ultrasonography can be helpful.[3]

Treatment

Treatment is surgical and should be performed as soon as the diagnosis is made, before the abscesses become fluctuant. Drainage should be both early and extensive. All perirectal abscesses should be drained in the operating room. A recent publication revealed that 32 percent of patients who had undergone a simple incision and drainage under local anesthesia were required to have a second operation because of inadequate drainage and recurrence of disease.

Isolated, simple, fluctuant perianal abscesses that are not associated with the presence of any deeper abscesses may be drained using local anesthetics in an ED setting. The local anesthetic should be administered with the finest-gauge needle available (30-gauge) and should be complemented with the administration of systemic analgesia or conscious sedation. To ensure adequate drainage, a cruciate incision should be made over the fluctuant part of the abscess, and the ''dog ears'' resulting from the cruciate incision should be excised so as to prevent premature closure of the cutaneous wall of the abscess (Fig. 78-6). No packing is required, but the wound should be covered with a bulk dressing; sitz baths should be started the next day. If a simple, linear drainage incision is made, the abscess is more likely to recur because of premature closure of skin edges. Whenever this technique

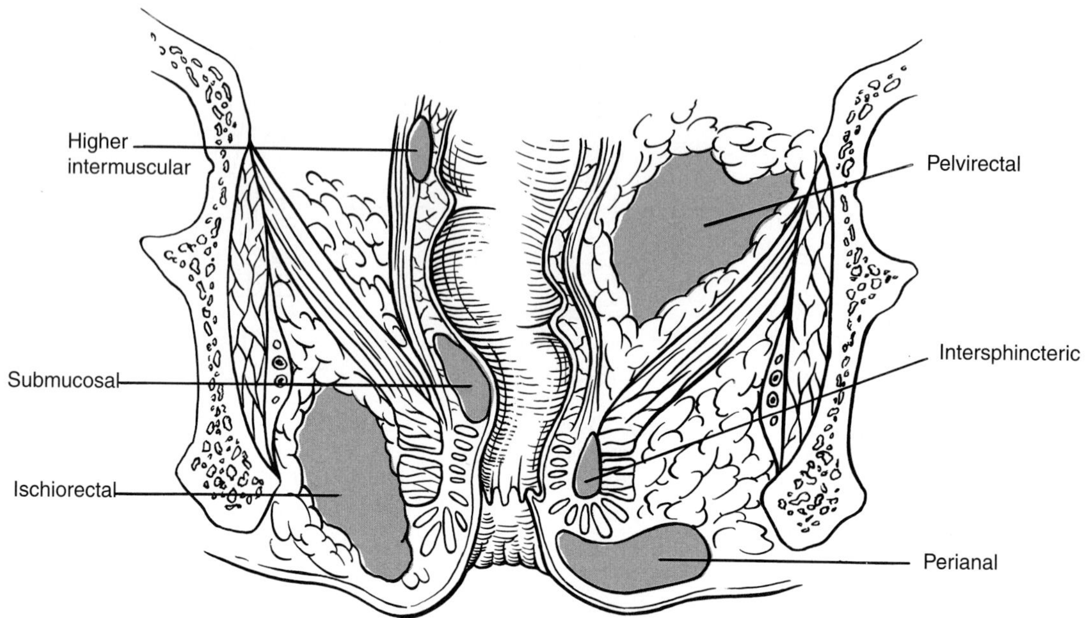

FIG. 78-5. Anatomical classification of common anorectal abscesses.

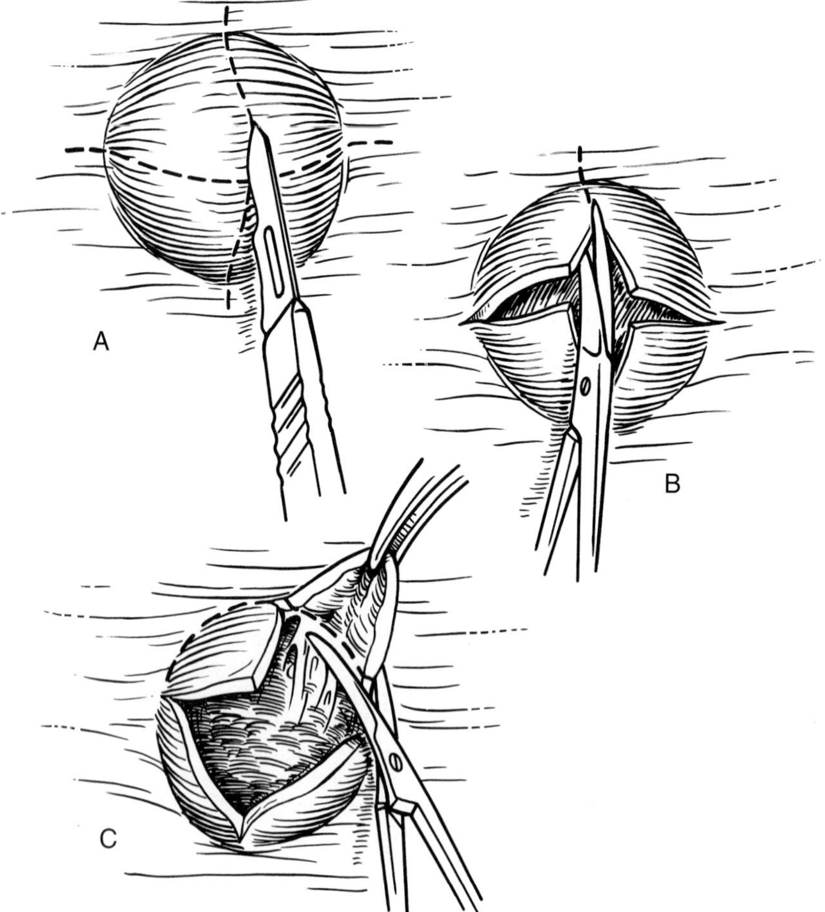

FIG. 78-6. Technique of drainage of perianal abscess.

is used the abscess cavity must be packed initially with strips of gauze for at least 24 h. These patients will require closer follow-up care.

As a rule, antibiotics are not necessary after an abscess has been adequately drained. On the other hand, patients whose immune system may be compromised by diabetes mellitus, AIDS, malignancies, and chemotherapy and/or those patients who have extensive cellulitis should be given broad-spectrum antibiotics.

FISTULA IN ANO

An anal fistula is an abnormal tract that connects the anal canal with the skin and is lined with epithelium and granulation tissue. A fistula in ano most commonly results from a perianal or ischiorectal abscess (Fig. 78-4). It may, however, be associated with ulcerative colitis, Crohn's disease, or tuberculosis. Although anterior-opening fistulas tend to follow a simple, direct course to the anal canal (Goodsall rule), posterior-opening fistulas may follow a devious, curving path, including some that are horseshoe-shaped.

Clinical Features

As long as the tract remains open, there is a persistent, blood-stained, malodorous discharge. More commonly, the tract becomes blocked periodically, producing bouts of inflammation and even local, recurrent abscess formation that is relieved by spontaneous rupture. An abscess may be the only sign of fistula in ano.

Treatment

The only definitive treatment is surgical excision. Improperly excised fistulas may result in permanent fecal incontinence.

VENEREAL PROCTITIS

Sexually transmitted diseases (STDs) of the anorectum are not uncommon among patients who practice anal sex. The infecting organisms, for the most part, are the same ones that are transmitted with vaginal coitus; infection is transmitted and perpetuated almost entirely by men who fail to use condoms (Table 78-2). Exceptions to this occur with women whose lymphogranuloma venereum (LGV) variety of chlamydia infection extends directly to the rectum from the vagina and on occasions when there is a contamination of the anus with gonococcal-laden discharge emanating from the urethra or cervix.

As a rule, if the patient has an anorectal infection caused by one of the STDs, the assumption must be made that another STD may be present; appropriate blood tests must be obtained, and patients should be anoscoped or proctoscoped in order to obtain specimens for Gram stain as well as for viral and bacterial cultures.

Clinical Features

Most venereal diseases involving the anorectal area manifest themselves initially with itching, seepage, and mild pain or irritation. Some infections may persist with mild to minimal symptoms, rendering the patient a carrier of the disease. Most venereal infections, however, will produce significant symptoms of pain, bleeding, and discharge in addition to a bothersome pruritus.

TABLE 78-2 Anorectal Sexually Transmitted Diseases

Bacteria
Neisseria gonorrheae
Chlamydia trachomatis
Treponema pallidum
Virus
Herpes simplex type 2
Human immunodeficiency virus
Papillomavirus

CONDYLOMATA ACUMINATA Condylomata acuminata, commonly known as anal warts, are caused by a papillomavirus and are probably sexually transmitted in more than 90 percent of cases. They begin as discreet, soft, fleshy growths on the skin of the perianal area as well as on the squamous epithelium of the anal canal. Occasionally, the mucosa of the lower rectum becomes involved. Patients usually first notice the presence of a growth in the perianal areas as well as associated pruritus and varying degrees of anal pain. With time, bleeding and anal discharge become part of the symptom complex. Evaluation of a patient with condyloma acuminata must include ruling out the presence of other STDs. These patients should be referred to an appropriate specialist for definitive treatment. Because cases of squamous cell carcinoma arising in association with condyloma acuminata have been reported, multiple biopsies must be taken.

GONORRHEA Symptoms of gonococcal proctitis vary, ranging from none to severe rectal pain with profuse yellow discharge. Patients in the acute phase generally have mild and burning and/or pruritus with some purulent seepage. Proctoscopic examination during this phase of the disease reveals marked hyperemia and edema of the rectal mucosa and diffuse inflammation with purulent discharge from the anal crypts. Unlike nonvenereal cryptitis, infection is not confined to the posterior crypt. Diagnosis is made by Gram's stain and cultures.

CHLAMYDIAL INFECTIONS *Chlamydia trachomatis* is an obligate human intracellular parasite that causes, among other conditions, both urogenital and anorectal infections. The lymphogranulomatous (LGV) variety occurs mainly in tropical and subtropical climates. Infection can involve the rectum by perirectal lymphatic invasion from vaginal seeding or from direct anorectal mucosal infections. The non-LGV chlamydial organisms may infect the rectal mucosa, although they do not cause the extensive rectal scarring and stricturing that its lymph gland–invading cousin from the tropics does. A patient with chlamydial proctitis may be asymptomatic or may present with nonspecific symptoms, including anal pruritus, pain, and purulent discharge. Bleeding may also be present.

The more severe form of proctitis occurring with this infection is usually due to the LGV type of chlamydia. In addition to rectal scarring, which is a late sequel, infection of the perirectal tissue results in perirectal abscesses and chronic fistulas.

Chlamydia may be identified by culture. The LGV forms may be distinguished from the non-LGV variety by the Frei intradermal test or the LGV complement fixation test. Treatment for LGV chlamydial infections should be maintained for at least 21 days.

SYPHILLIS Chancres, the characteristic lesion of primary syphilis, usually manifest themselves at the anal verge or in the anal canal. Rarely will a chancre involve the rectal mucosa, although proctitis due to syphilis can occur in the absence of a chancre. Anal chancres may be very painful. If they are not identified and treated, they will resolve and the patient will proceed to develop secondary and tertiary syphilis. Condylomata lata, which are flatter and firmer than condylomata acuminata, appear in the perianal region as a manifestation of the secondary stage of syphilis.

HERPES Anorectal herpes is almost always caused by the type II herpes simplex virus (HSV-2). Symptoms are itching and soreness in the perianal area progressing to severe anorectal pain. Initially, the virus manifests itself as small, discreet groups of vesicles superimposed on an erythematous base. These vesicles enlarge, coalesce, and rupture, forming exquisitely tender aphthous ulcers that appear on the perianal

TABLE 78-3 Anorectal AIDS-Related Infections

Herpes simplex type 1
Mycobactrium avium-intracellulare
Cytomegalovirus
Salmonella enterocolitis
Shigella
Campylobacter
Entamoeba
Giardia

skin, the anoderm, and even the rectal mucosa. The pain and tenesmus from these lesions may be so intense that the patient is reluctant to have a bowel movement, resulting in constipation and possibly fecal impaction.

AIDS-RELATED INFECTIONS Ironically, infection of the rectum by the human immunodeficiency virus (HIV) per se does not cause any local reaction or symptoms, but its effect on the patient inoculated with this virus can be devastating. Patients who have been rendered immunodeficient by the HIV virus are subject to a variety of opportunistic infections that affect the intestinal, anorectal, and other body systems. Chronic perianal infections with herpes simplex type I as well as type II are commonly seen in AIDS patients. Table 78-3 lists other, more common enteric organisms that infect AIDS patients. Severe rectal pain, diarrhea, and hematochezia are common presenting symptoms.

Treatment

Success in the management of patients with acute venereal proctitis depends on suspecting the diagnosis, obtaining specimens to confirm the diagnosis, and initiating therapy as expeditiously as possible. Patients presenting with symptoms of anorectal pain, rectal discharge, and/or tenesmus should be considered to have proctitis until proven otherwise. Anoscopy or proctoscopy, and a Gram stain should be performed to document the presence of acute proctitis. In addition to the appropriate culture specimens, blood should be drawn to check for syphilis.

Antibiotic therapy should not be delayed, pending the results of cultures. Empirical therapy aimed at eradicating gonorrhea, non-LGV chlamydia, and incubating syphilis should be initiated for any patient presenting with symptoms and physical signs suggestive of acute proctitis. This therapy should be administered to all patients with acute proctitis even if there are concomitant lesions suggestive of herpetic or papilloma virus infections. Uncomplicated cases of venereal proctitis respond to the same antiobiotic regimens used for venereal urethritis or cervicitis. (see Chap. 137). As is the case for STDs in general, these patients must be referred for appropriate follow-up to ensure completion of therapy and eradication of disease.

RECTAL PROLAPSE

Rectal prolapse, known as procidentia, is the circumferential protrusion of part or all layers of the rectum through the anal canal. There are three classes of rectal prolapse: (1) prolapse involving the rectal mucosa only, (2) prolapse involving all layers of the rectum, and (3) intussusception of the upper rectum into and through the lower rectum so that the apex of the intussusception protrudes through the anus.

In the first group, seen primarily in children under the age of 2, the prolapse occurs because of the loose attachment of the mucosa to the submucosal layers, and there is an associated weakness of the anal sphincter. In the second and third groups, prolapse occurs because of the laxity of the pelvic fascia and muscles in addition to a generalized weakening of the anal sphincters. In all cases, the rectum does not conform with, but lies anterior to the sacral concavity, thus obliterating the angulation that normally occurs between rectum and anus. The prolapsing mucosa of a partial prolapse rarely protrudes more than 4 cm beyond the anal verge; the mucosal folds emanate in a radial fashion from the central lumen of the prolapsed mucosa. Mucosal prolapse is frequently associated with third- and fourth-degree hemorrhoids (see Table 78-1).

Complete rectal prolapse (procidentia) occurs at the extremes of life, most commonly in elderly women. Multiparity is not a contributing factor to rectal prolapse; there appears to be a higher incidence of prolapse in women who have had a hysterectomy.

Clinical Features

Most patients are able to detect the presence of a mass, especially following defecation or strenuous activity. In more advanced cases, this may be present when they stand or walk. Irritation to the rectal mucosa caused by recurrent prolapse results in a mucous discharge with some associated bleeding. Some patients may present because of blood-stained mucus on their undergarments, others because of fecal incontinence caused by associated anal sphincter weakness. In pediatric patients, parents often mistakenly believe that the prolapsed mucosa is hemorrhoids.

Treatment

In young children, after appropriate analgesia and sedation, prolapse can be reduced manually by replacing the protruding mucosa proximal to the anorectal ring of sphincter muscles. Every effort should be made to prevent the child from becoming constipated, and the child should be referred for further evaluation.

Surgical intervention is generally indicated in all other age groups unless the prolapse is minimal. A variety of effective surgical procedures is available and may be used depending on the degree of prolapse and the general health of the patient. All adults should be referred to have a proctosigmoidoscopic examination to rule out tumor. In addition, one should check for the possibility of an anterior rectal wall ulcer that may occur in patients with recurrent prolapse.

If vascular compromise appears to have occurred, reduction may be necessary on an emergency basis. Because of the risk of having reduced ischemic bowel that could perforate, these patients must be hospitalized.

ANORECTAL TUMORS

Carcinoma of the anal area represents less than 5 percent of all large bowel malignancy. At the level of the dentate line and extending approximately 1 cm proximal is a transitional zone of epithelium connecting the squamous cell epithelium of the anoderm with the columnar epithelium of the rectum. This transition zone includes columnar, cuboidal, transitional, and squamous epithelial cells that represent the source for a variety of malignancies that arise in the anal canal (Table 78-4). For the purpose of grading malignancies, the United Nations World Health Organization has divided the anal canal into two regions: (1) malignancies of the portion proximal to the dentate line and including the transitional zone are referred to as anal canal neoplasms and (2) tumors arising in the anoderm distal to the dentate line are referred to as anal margin neoplasms.

Anal margin neoplasms have a low-grade malignant potential and are slow to metastasize. Anal canal neoplasms, on the other hand,

TABLE 78-4 Neoplasms of the Anal Region

Anal canal neoplasms (proximal to dentate line)
- Adenocarcinoma of the rectum
- Adenocarcinoma of anal glands and ducts
- Mucoepidermoid carcinoma
- Transitional cloacogenic (basaloid) carcinoma
- Squamous cell carcinoma of the anal canal
- Malignant melanoma
- Kaposi's sarcoma
- Villous adenoma of the rectum

Anal margin neoplasms (distal to dentate line)
- Bowen's disease
- Squamous cell carcinoma of anal margin
- Extramammary Paget's disease
- Basal cell carcinoma
- Giant solitary trichoepithelioma

are far more virulent, metastasize early, and have a poor prognosis. Squamous cell carcinoma of the anal canal has a much poorer prognosis than its anal margin counterpart. Anal canal malignancies metastasize not only to mesenteric lymph nodes and the portal circulation but also to the regional inguinal nodes and via the systemic circulation.

Included among the anal canal neoplasms is Kaposi's sarcoma, the most common AIDS-related malignancy. The anal canal is the third most common site for malignant melanoma (after the skin and the eye), which, when it occurs there, may not be pigmented and is frequently overlooked.

Clinical Features

Early anal canal malignancies usually cause nonspecific symptoms such as pruritus, pain, and bleeding admixed with stool. The sensation and presence of a lump in the anal canal may be erroneously diagnosed as a hemorrhoid. As the neoplasm progresses, the patient experiences anorexia, weight loss, constipation, narrowing of the caliber of the stool, and eventually tenesmus with or without bowel movement. Complete obstruction may also occur.

Anal canal tumors may produce partial rectal prolapse; hemorrhoidal dilatation and prolapse may also occur. More advanced malignancies may present as perirectal abscesses or fistulas.

Villous adenomas, which arise from the rectal columnar epithelium, frequently produce diarrhea and a profuse rectal discharge, with secondary excoriation of skin and pruritus. Patients may suffer a significant loss of electrolytes, resulting in a clinically significant hypokalemia and/or hyponatremia.

Treatment

The anal margin neoplasms may present as persistent ulcers or as chronic dermatologic conditions such as eczema or mycotic infections. Any ulcer that fails to heal within 30 days or any discrete skin lesion that fails to improve with appropriate therapy must be biopsied to rule out the presence of malignancy.

Virtually all anorectal tumors can be detected by careful visual examination of the perianal area, digital palpation of the distal rectum and anal canal, and procto- or sigmoidoscopic examination. In one review of anal malignancies, 80 percent were in the canal and 20 percent at the anal margin. Failure to look, feel, and think would be the only reason not to suspect the presence of these curable but life-threatening lesions.

RECTAL FOREIGN BODIES

The medical literature is replete with the variety of foreign bodies that have been reported to have been inserted into the rectum. Most foreign bodies are in the rectal ampulla and therefore palpable through digital examination and detectable on proctoscopic examination. Any patient presenting with an intrarectal foreign body must have x-rays of the abdomen taken to demonstrate not only the position, shapes, and number of foreign bodies but also the possible presence of free air. Perforation of the rectum or colon is the most frequent and most serious complication. Perforation may be either extraperitoneal or intraperitoneal; both can result in life-threatening sepsis.

Treatment

Although some foreign bodies can be removed in the ED, many require surgical intervention, particularly if they are made of glass or have sharp edges. If the foreign body is removed in the emergency department and is of a size or shape that could cause perforation, a follow-up proctoscopic examination and x-ray studies must be performed. In questionable cases, observations for at least 12 h should be done to ensure that perforation has not occurred. Rectal and anal lacerations may be present and require repair.

Sphincter relaxation is mandatory for removal of large foreign bodies. If the patient's sphincters are taut or otherwise not sufficiently relaxed, local infiltrative anesthesia must be administered to achieve proper relaxation. After the patient has been sedated and placed in the lithotomy position, local anesthetic is injected through a fine, 30-gauge needle to raise an intradermal wheal at the 6- and 12-o'clock positions. The index finger of the physician's nondominant hand is then inserted into the anal canal to act as a guide for a $1\frac{1}{2}$-in., larger-gauge needle through which anesthetic is injected circumferentially along the internal sphincter muscles as they course along the anal canal. Five milliliters of anesthetic should suffice for each quadrant of infiltration. Large bulbar objects create a vacuumlike effect in the rectal ampulla, making it difficult to retrieve the object by simple traction. The vacuum can be overcome by passing a catheter beyond the object and injecting air. A modification of this technique is to insert Foley catheters around the foreign body and, after the vacuum is relieved by injecting air, inflate the balloons of the Foley catheters and use the catheters as traction devices to deliver the foreign body or manipulate it into a more accessible position.

If there is a risk of perforation or if excess manipulation (potential for bacteremia) will be needed to remove the foreign body, the patient should be prepared for emergency surgery, which includes obtaining appropriate laboratory studies, initiating intravenous therapy with crystalloid solution, and administering a loading dose of broad-spectrum (second-generation cephalosporin) antibiotics.

PRURITUS ANI

Pruritus ani is a symptom complex that occurs secondary to a variety of anal and systemic problems. It is not in itself a specific disease process. It effects men far more often than women, and it occurs most commonly during the fifth and sixth decades of life.

There is an entity of primary or idiopathic pruritus ani, the etiology of which is unknown. To make such a diagnosis, one has to rule out the many specific, known causes of secondary pruritus ani. Even so, idiopathic pruritus ani may occur in association with or be precipitated by secondary pruritus ani. Table 78-5 lists the major categories of the various likely causes of secondary pruritus ani.

In Table 78-5 "anorectal disease" includes the various categories that have been discussed in this chapter. The pruritus that accompanies such conditions as fissures, fistulas, hemorrhoids, and prolapses occurs as a result of the perianal skin's being exposed to and macerated by constant mucous and purulent discharge. It is probably the increased perianal moisture caused by these conditions that results in itching. The itching triggers a vicious cycle of scratching, excoriation, and more itching.

TABLE 78-5 Pruritus Ani

Anorectal disease
Dietary factors
Local infection
Local irritants
Dermatologic conditions
Systemic illness
Psychogenic factors

Numerous dietary factors have been implicated and are associated with secondary pruritus ani, although proof of cause is lacking for most of them. Those dietary factors most commonly listed include excessive consumption of caffeine-containing liquids, such as coffee, tea, or colas, and beer, although one recent study failed to demonstrate any correlation between pruritus ani and alcohol consumption. Milk, chocolate, tomatoes, and citrus fruits are other food products that allegedly contribute to pruritus ani. Likewise, certain drugs, such as colchicine and mineral oil, have been associated with pruritus ani. Ingestion of these products can result in increased liquidity and seepage of fecal material, which in itself is a probable cause of pruritus ani.

Infectious agents that have to be considered as causes of pruritus ani include bacteria, viruses, fungi, spirochetes, and parasites. More common bacterial infections, such as staphylococci and streptococci, in addition to all sexually transmitted organisms, will cause pruritus, if not actual pain. Pinworms (*enterobius/vermicularis*) are the most common cause of anal pruritus in children. *Candida/albicans* is commonly found on the perianal skin but is not usually associated with pruritus; the *Trichophyton* species, on the other hand, are always associated with pruritus.

Local irritants, if not the initial cause, commonly contribute to the incidence of pruritus. Fecal contamination, resulting from poor anal hygiene, is by far the most common irritant to the perianal skin. Lysozyme from intestinal mucous secretions, acting together with bacterial exotoxins to raise the stool and skin pH, will cause pruritus. Ironically, patients who compulsively clean their anus, particularly if they use perfumed toilet tissue, soaps, or detergents or hygiene sprays, cause pruritic reactions. Also, wearing of synthetic, tight-fitting underwear retains moisture that normally occurs in the perianal area, another leading cause of pruritus.

Dermatologic conditions contributing to this symptom complex include atopic dermatitis, lichen planus, psoriasis, and seborrheic dermatitis. Any of the anal margin neoplasms, particularly Bowen's disease and extramammary Paget's disease, may initially manifest itself as pruritus.

Finally, certain systemic conditions, such as diabetes mellitus, lymphoma, and certain vitamin deficiencies (vitamins A and D and niacin), because of their secondary effect on the perianal skin, will cause pruritus.

Clinical Features

Appearance of the perianal skin will depend on the severity and chronicity of the underlying conditions that are causing the pruritus. The skin will appear normal with early, mild cases. With acute, more severe exacerbations, the perianal skin will appear reddened, edematous, and moist; frequently, there are excoriations caused by scratching. In chronic cases, the perianal skin takes on a thickened, almost leathery, depigmented appearance. The normal radiating folds of skin thicken into rugae and may include superficial fissures factitiously induced.

Treatment

Pruritus, like any other symptoms, suggests the presence of an underlying cause that should be diagnosed and treated appropriately. Thus, excision of malignancies or surgical correction of fistulas, prolapses, or hemorrhoids would be the definitive treatment for patients with those conditions.

In most cases, specific anorectal lesions are not apparent, and the patient must be referred to a proctologist or dermatologist for probable long-term management.

In the meantime, the patient should be advised to make certain dietary changes, if appropriate, and should be instructed about proper anal hygiene. Scratching of the area must be avoided; if necessary, the patient should be advised to wear gloves at bedtime, when most of the scratching is likely to occur. Patients with maceration of perianal skin should use moist cotton rather than toilet paper. Soaps should be avoided, and the patient should take sitz baths for at least 15 min two to three times a day. The skin should then be thoroughly dried by gently blotting with a soft cloth. Zinc oxide ointment can provide a protective covering for the perianal skin and may enhance the healing. Fungicidal creams should be prescribed for patients with secondary fungal infections. One percent hydrocortisone cream is effective for the allergic component of the inflammation. Finally, as an adjunct to providing symptomatic relief, consider prescribing hydroxyzine hydrochloride (Atarax) as an effective bedtime sedative.

PILONIDAL SINUS

Pilonidal sinus has nothing to do with the anorectum, anatomically or embryologically. Pilonidal sinuses or cysts occur in the midline in the upper part of the natal cleft overlying the lower sacrum and coccyx. Because of their proximity to the anus, infected pilonidal cysts (abscesses) are sometimes mistakenly diagnosed as perirectal abscesses. An abscessed pilonidal sinus is always located in the midline (although there may be secondary fistulous openings on either side of the midline) and does not communicate with the anorectum. On the other hand, long, horseshoe-type fistulas emanating from a perirectal abscess may drain close to the location of a pilonidal sinus but not in the midline.

Although once thought to be congenital in nature, pilonidal sinus is now considered an acquired problem. The sinus is formed by the penetration of the skin by ingrowing hair, which causes a foreign body granuloma reaction. The sinus is perpetuated by the presence of the hair and repeated bouts of infection. Although pilonidal sinuses or infected pilonidal cysts occur most commonly before the fourth decade of life, a small portion of patients may develop this problem in their fourth decade. Pilonidal sinus and abscess formation should be considered a chronic and recurring disease.

Carcinoma is a rare complication of chronic, recurring pilonidal sinus disease. It is more frequent in men and is usually a well-differentiated dermal-type squamous cell carcinoma.

Clinical Features

Depending on whether the disease presents as a cyst or a sinus, the patient generally complains of swelling, pain, or a persistent discharge. When abscess formation occurs, the patient complains of a tender mass. Although there may be more than one sinus with several tiny openings in the midline of the intergluateal cleft, the most common finding is that of a single opening from which hair is protruding. Patients usually present to the ED when an abscess has formed that can no longer drain.

Treatment

Surgery is the treatment of choice. Ideally, a patient should undergo elective excision of the entire pilonidal sinus system and primary closure of skin when there is no infection present in any of the sinuses. Minimal excision, and packing using a local anesthetic in the ED results in reoccurrence. Patients presenting with acute inflammation should have their abscess drained in the ED. Their wounds should be allowed to heal, and then, at least 6 weeks later, if there is no evidence of active infection, they should be referred for definitive surgical excision.

The technique for incising and draining a pilonidal abscess is as follows: Place the patient prone on the proctoscopic table with the buttocks retracted laterally. The patient should receive conscious sedation. Tuck an ABD pad between the lower gluteal cleft to prevent the prep solution from pooling at the anus or genitals. After having prepped the skin, infiltrate the area to be incised with an intradermal injection of anesthetic solution, using a fine-gauge needle. A suction apparatus should be available to aspirate the unusually foul-smelling pus that has accumulated within the abscess. Following drainage, gently break down any loculations that may be present and loosely pack the wound with iodoform gauze. A bulky dressing should then be applied and secured with tape. The patient should be given a prescription for a strong oral analgesic and advised to begin hot sitz baths the following day. Before the sitz bath, the patient should remove the outer dressing but should not attempt to remove the packing until after having soaked in hot water for a few minutes. Ideally, one should allow the warm water current to flush the packing out of the wound. The patient should be seen in 48 to 72 h for evaluation and further advice concerning wound management.

Unless the patient is immunocompromised or there is cellulitis, there is no need to obtain cultures or prescribe antibiotics for an abscess that has been adequately drained.

BIBLIOGRAPHY

Condon ER (Ed): Colon, in Zuideme GD (ed): *Shackelford's Surgery of the Alimentary Tract*, 4th ed. Philadelphia, Saunders, 1996, pp 275–465.

REFERENCES

1. Segal WN, Greenberg PD, Rochay DC, et al: The outpatient evaluation of hematochezia. *Am J Gastroenterol* 93:179, 1998.
2. Bayer I, Nysloraty B, Picovsky BM: Rubber band ligation of hemorrhoids. *J Clin Gastroenterol* 23:50, 1996.
3. Cataldo PA, Scenagore AJ, Luchtfeld MA: Intrarectal ultrasound in the evaluation of perirectal abscesses. *Dis Colon Rectum* 36:554, 1993.

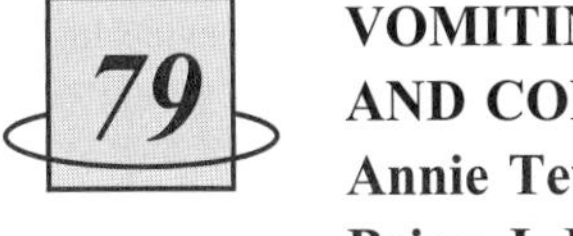

VOMITING, DIARRHEA, AND CONSTIPATION

Annie Tewel Sadosty
Brian J. Browne

Vomiting, diarrhea, and constipation are among the most common complaints of patients presenting to emergency departments. Gastrointestinal dysfunction is the final common pathway for a variety of diseases. Therefore, many patients complaining of vomiting, diarrhea, or constipation have a cause for their symptoms remote from the gastrointestinal system. Emergency physicians must consider not only the gastrointestinal emergencies manifested as vomiting, diarrhea, or constipation but also the nongastrointestinal emergencies manifested as gastrointestinal dysfunction.

An important and often difficult step in the evaluation of patients with vomiting, diarrhea, or constipation is having the patient define the illness. The layperson's definitions of *vomiting, diarrhea,* and *constipation* often differ tremendously from the medical definitions. For example, patients often say "vomiting" when they really mean "coughing up sputum." Some patients complain of "constipation" and mean that they are straining to defecate. Defining the complaint allows the physician to treat patients correctly and in turn increases patients' satisfaction. A complete history of the current illness is the first step toward the correct diagnosis.

After defining the illness, the emergency physician's next step is to determine whether the illness represents an emergency. At the end of the emergency department evaluation, the cause of the patient's symptoms may not be clear. Nevertheless, the physician must decide, based on limited information, whether a patient may be discharged safely and what the initial treatment plan will be.

VOMITING

Pathophysiology

Vomiting is a complex, highly coordinated activity involving the gastrointestinal tract, the central nervous system (CNS), and the vestibular system. In 1952, Wang and Borison identified a medullary vomiting center.[1] The proximity of the medullary vomiting center to other CNS nuclei allows for the coordinated activity of vomiting.[1] Three stages of vomiting have been described: nausea, retching, and emesis.[2] With nausea come hypersalivation and tachycardia. Retching occurs when the pylorus contracts and the fundus relaxes, thereby moving food to the gastric cardia. Finally, emesis occurs when the powerful abdominal muscles contract simultaneously and thus eject food or gastric secretions from the stomach.

Clinical Features

HISTORY There are hundreds of causes of vomiting (Table 79-1). Fortunately, the patient's history often leads the physician to the correct diagnosis. Asking the right questions will help to uncover the etiology.

First, define the vomitus. Is it bloody, bilious or nonbilious, feculent or posttussive? Hematemesis is seen with gastritis, peptic ulcer disease, gastric and esophageal tumors, and Mallory-Weiss tears. Nonbilious emesis occurs with gastric outlet obstruction, as in patients with pyloric strictures secondary to ulcer disease or infants with pyloric stenosis.

Second, determine what symptoms accompany the vomiting. Is the patient febrile? Fever could point toward an infectious or inflammatory source, or it could represent a toxicologic cause, such as salicylate intoxication. Is there associated abdominal pain, back pain, headache, or chest pain that may point to a specific cause? Pancreatitis, cholecystitis, peptic ulcer disease, appendicitis, and pelvic inflammatory disease typically cause abdominal pain. Back pain usually accompanies aortic dissections, rupturing aortic aneurysms, pyelonephritis, and renal colic. Vomiting is one of the signs of increased intracranial or intraocular pressure and may be a foreboding sign in patients complaining of headache. Finally, the complaint of vomiting associated with chest or epigastric pain might suggest a diagnosis of myocardial ischemia. In female patients, obstetric and gynecologic causes of vomiting should always be considered. In a pregnant woman, epigastric pain and vomiting accompanying hypertension may indicate preeclampsia.

Learning more about the patient is as important as defining the illness. What complicating medical conditions does the patient have? Is the patient diabetic? If so, could the vomiting be a manifestation of diabetic ketoacidosis? In a patient with a history of peripheral vascular disease, vomiting may be a sign of mesenteric ischemia. Patients with a history of multiple abdominal surgeries are at risk for intestinal obstruction due to adhesions. Knowledge of the medications to which the patient has access is also critical, since intentional and unintentional poisonings often present first with emesis. Physicians should be suspicious of drug-induced toxicity in patients taking medicines known to have gastrointestinal toxicity (e.g., lithium, digoxin, or theophylline). The social history provides clues, too. Vomiting in

TABLE 79-1 Vomiting and Diarrhea: The GASTROENTERITIS Mnemonic

	Vomiting	Diarrhea
GI	Obstruction: tumor, stricture, hernia, volvulus, intussusception, foreign body, bezoar, extrinsic compression (i.e., SMA syndrome), fecal impaction, etc. Dysmotility: achalasia, scleroderma, gastroparesis, GERD, Ogilvie syndrome, postvagotomy, diabetes, etc. Inflammation: esophagitis, gastritis, PUD, biliary colic, cholecystitis, pancreatitis, hepatitis, inflammatory bowel disease, diverticulitis, etc.	Obstruction: fecal impaction with overflow Dysmotility: irritable bowel syndrome, postvagotomy, short bowel syndrome, etc. Inflammation: inflammatory bowel disease, diverticulitis, sprue, radiation enteritis, etc. Malabsorption (e.g., pancreatic exocrine dysfunction) Lactose intolerance GI bleeding
Appendicitis or **a**orta	Appendicitis/aortic aneurysm or dissection	Appendicitis
Specific diseases	Glaucoma Torsion of testis or ovary	
Trauma	Obstruction (i.e., duodenal hematoma) Dysmotility (i.e., ileus secondary to lumbar compression fractures) Inflammation (i.e., pancreatitis)	
Rx	Medication side effect (e.g., Narcan, opioid analgesics, erythromycin, chemotherapy, ipecac)	Medication side effect (e.g., antibiotics, chemotherapy, laxatives, antacids, sorbitol, colchicine)
Ob-Gyn	Pregnancy (ectopic, uterine, molar) Preeclampsia Hyperemesis gravidarum	
Endocrine or metabolic	Adrenal insufficiency Thyrotoxicosis Diabetic ketoacidosis Alcoholic ketoacidosis Reye syndrome Uremia	Adrenal insufficiency Thyrotoxicosis Uremia
Neurologic	Autonomic neuropathy (e.g., diabetes) Vestibular disorders (cranial nerve VIII) Migraine headache Hypertensive encephalopathy Hydrocephalus Increased ICP (e.g., intracranial neoplasms, subdural or epidural hematoma, subarachnoid hemorrhage, cerebral edema)	Autonomic neuropathy (e.g., diabetes)

(*continued on next page*)

a person who enjoys mushroom hunting may well represent *Amanita* poisoning.

PHYSICAL EXAMINATION Clinical clues may also assist in making the diagnosis. In addition to evaluating the ABCs, much of the physician's initial attention should be directed toward the assessment of hydration status. Severely volume-depleted patients require immediate intervention, lest circulatory collapse be imminent. The abdominal, genitourinary, and pelvic examinations are often revealing. Physicians should search carefully for tenderness, peritoneal signs, hernias, masses, and evidence of obstruction or torsion. The findings of a careful physical examination may point toward unsuspected causes of vomiting, such as bulimia (scars on the dorsum of hands), pneumonia (consolidative findings on lung examination), or Addison's disease (hyperpigmentation). The rectal examination is important. An anal fistula may be the only clue to Crohn's disease in an otherwise healthy teenager with vomiting, or may demonstrate fecal impaction.

Acquire data selectively and smartly. Order diagnostic tests according to the differential diagnosis. In the vomiting, premenopausal woman, consider pregnancy high on the differential diagnosis, and rule it in or out with a pregnancy test. Other laboratory tests that may be of assistance are determination of blood urea nitrogen, creatinine, and amylase levels; liver function tests; determination of blood alcohol and drug levels; and urinalysis. Addisonian crisis can present with vomiting, and the laboratory results may show hyperkalemia and hyponatremia. An electrocardiogram can help if the physician is considering the diagnosis of myocardial ischemia. Chest and abdominal radiography can assist in the determination of the presence or absence of pneumoperitoneum, pneumonia, or intestinal obstruction.

Treatment

Initial management of the acutely ill, vomiting patient is the same, regardless of cause. The ABCs always take precedence. For patients with circulatory collapse secondary to severe dehydration, aggressive volume repletion must begin immediately upon arrival. Two large-bore intravenous catheters should be placed, and crystalloid should be administered aggressively in order to restore circulation quickly.

For patients with less acute conditions, treatment hinges on making the correct diagnosis. A vomiting patient with diabetic ketoacidosis will not respond to symptomatic therapy with antiemetics: vomiting continues until the underlying illness is treated. It is important, therefore, to recognize the illnesses that are not self-limited and to treat them appropriately. However, not all patients with the chief complaint of vomiting are discharged from the emergency department with a clear diagnosis. These patients should be treated symptomatically,

TABLE 79-1 Vomiting and Diarrhea: The GASTROENTERITIS Mnemonic (*Continued*)

	Vomiting	Diarrhea
Toxicology	Acetaminophen Heavy metals (arsenic, mercury, iron, lithium) Alcohol Mushrooms Nicotine Chlorinated hydrocarbon insecticides Organophosphate or carbamates Digoxin Salicylate Isoniazid Theophylline or caffeine	Heavy metals (arsenic, mercury, iron, lithium) Ergot alkaloids Theophylline or caffeine Mushrooms Nicotine Chlorinated hydrocarbon insecticides Thyroid replacement hormone overdose Organophosphate or carbamates
Environmental	Food poisoning Envenomation (e.g., black widow, *Hymenoptera,* scorpion) High-altitude illness Acute radiation syndrome	Food poisoning Envenomation (e.g., black widow, snake, *Hymenoptera*) Acute radiation syndrome
Renal	Obstructive uropathy Renal colic	
Infection	Infectious gastroenteritis (viral, bacterial, parasitic) Pyelonephritis Pneumonia (i.e., pertussis) Pelvic inflammatory disease Meningitis Hepatitis	Infectious gastroenteritis (viral, bacterial, parasitic) Pseudomembranous colitis Pneumonia (e.g., *Legionella*) HIV
Tumors	Gastrinoma	Medullary carcinoma of the thyroid Villous adenoma APUD tumors (e.g., glucagonoma, gastrinoma, carcinoid, VIPoma)
Ischemia	Myocardial infarction Mesenteric ischemia	Mesenteric ischemia Ischemic colitis
Supratentorial	Bulimia	Psychosocial stress

Abbreviations: APUD, amine precursor uptake and decarboxylation; GERD, gastrointestinal reflux disease; GI, gastrointestinal; ICP, intracranial pressure; Ob-Gyn, obstetric and gynecologic; PUD, peptic ulcer disease; Rx, prescription; SMA, superior mesenteric artery; VIPoma, vasoactive intestinal peptide tumor.

and follow-up should be ensured. For patients with mild-to-moderate dehydration who are actively vomiting, we recommend intravenous rehydration and antiemetic therapy in the form of prochlorperazine [Compazine 10 mg IV or IM q8h or 25 mg rectally q12h] or promethazine (Phenergan 25 mg IM, IV, or rectally q6h). Physicians may prescribe the suppository form of these for the patient to use should vomiting continue at home.

Disposition

Patients with life-threatening causes of vomiting should be admitted to the hospital, as should severely dehydrated patients with presumably self-limited causes of emesis. The patient in whom the diagnosis is unclear, but who the physician feels confident does not have a life-threatening cause of emesis, may be discharged safely, provided the patient tolerates fluids in the emergency department and that follow-up the next day, if vomiting continues, is ensured. A dehydrated patient who cannot tolerate oral intake should not be discharged.

DIARRHEA

Epidemiology

At the turn of the twentieth century, diarrhea was one of the leading causes of death in the United States. In the 1990s, however, diarrhea accounted for less than 0.5 percent of all deaths in the United States.[3] Most diarrheal deaths occur in the elderly and the young.[3,4] Worldwide, however, diarrhea remains one of the leading causes of death. In fact, in 1990, diarrhea was listed as the fourth leading cause of death globally and was responsible for a total of 2.9 million deaths.[5] Despite the low US mortality rate, diarrhea causes significant morbidity. It is the second most common reason for work absenteeism and is estimated to cost $608 million in lost productivity per year.[6,7]

Pathophysiology

There are four basic mechanisms of diarrhea: increased intestinal secretion, decreased intestinal absorption, increased osmotic load, and abnormal intestinal motility. Knowledge of normal intestinal function assists in understanding these various mechanisms. Normally, the jejunum receives between 6 and 8 L/day of fluid in the form of oral intake and gastric, pancreatic, and biliary secretions. Dietary intake actually constitutes a small portion of the jejunal load (1.5 L). A healthy small intestine absorbs nearly 75 percent of the fluid to which it is exposed. The 2 L of fluid not absorbed by the small intestine then enter the colon, where fluid is absorbed at an even higher rate. The absorptive power of the colon approaches 90 percent efficiency and far exceeds that of the small intestine. In fact, the colon can make up for a decrease in small-intestinal absorption. Under normal conditions, very little fluid (<100 mL) is lost in the stool each day.[8]

In diarrheal states, normal intestinal physiology is disrupted. At a cellular level, intestinal absorption occurs through the villi, while secretion occurs through the crypts. Often, in diarrheal states, enterotoxins, inflammation, or ischemia damage the intestinal villi preferentially. As a result, diarrhea occurs because of diminished intestinal villi absorption *and* unopposed crypt secretion (the crypts are more resilient after injury).[9] Diarrhea also accompanies the delivery of an osmotic load to the intestine. For example, administration of a laxative results in the collection of an osmotically active, nondigestible agent within the intestinal lumen. Osmosis occurs, drawing fluid into the intestinal lumen, and results in diarrhea. Finally, increased intestinal motility causes diarrhea, as in patients with irritable bowel syndrome, neuropathies, or a shortened intestine secondary to surgery.

Clinical Features

HISTORY The definition of diarrhea varies within the medical literature, so it is not surprising that patients' definitions vary too. Many patients come to the emergency department complaining of "diarrhea" when what they really have is soft stools or two stools per day compared with their usual one. Strictly speaking, diarrhea is present when the daily stool weight exceeds 200 g.[10] Practically speaking, however, diarrhea is present when the patient is making more stools of lesser consistency, more frequently.

Once a true diarrheal illness is confirmed, the physician's focus should change toward attempting to ascertain the cause of the diarrhea. As already mentioned, there are many causes of diarrhea (Table 79-1). Fortunately, the history usually leads the physician to the etiology. The first step is to determine whether the diarrhea is acute (<3 weeks) or chronic (>3 weeks). The acute diarrheas are of greatest concern to the emergency physician, for they are more apt to be a manifestation of an immediately life-threatening illness (infection, ischemia, intoxication, or inflammation).[10] The next step is to define the diarrhea. Is it bloody or melanotic? Is it associated with the ingestion of certain foods, such as milk or sorbitol? What symptoms accompany the diarrhea? Is there fever or abdominal pain, which may suggest diverticulitis or infectious gastroenteritis? Seizures accompanying diarrhea often point toward shigellosis but could also indicate theophylline toxicity. Does the patient have heat intolerance and anxiety, suggesting thyrotoxicosis, or paresthesias and reverse temperature sensation, suggesting ciguatera?

Finally, define the host. A patient's medical and surgical history often assists in narrowing the differential diagnosis. For example, diarrhea resulting from malabsorption secondary to pancreatic exocrine insufficiency need not be considered in an otherwise healthy host. Conversely, the differential diagnosis for diarrhea is broadened for a patient with acquired immunodeficiency syndrome (AIDS). Medications commonly have diarrhea as a side effect or sequel. Is the patient taking medication that may have contributed to the diarrhea (e.g., antibiotics, lithium, chemotherapy, colchicine, and laxatives)? Has the patient traveled outside the United States or to the countryside recently? Rural hiking places the patient at risk for *Giardia*, particularly if water purification procedures were not strictly followed, and travel to Third World countries increases the chances of parasitic infection. Sexual and occupational histories are also important. A patient's sexual preference or occupation may be the physician's only clue to a diagnosis of gay bowel disease or organophosphate poisoning.

PHYSICAL EXAMINATION As with a vomiting patient, the examination begins with the ABCs. Thus, assessment of hydration status occurs shortly after the physician arrives at the bedside. Like the history, a careful physical examination can help narrow the differential diagnosis. Only by doing a thyroid examination can the physician discover a thyroid mass that may be contributing to diarrhea. Abdominal and rectal examinations are critical. Especially in the elderly, fecal impaction may result in diarrhea as liquid stool passes around the impaction. Special attention should be given to the presence or absence of surgical scars, tenderness, masses, or peritoneal signs. Checking the stool for the presence or absence of blood is also important, since bloody diarrhea can be caused by inflammation, infection, or ischemia. An elderly patient with bloody diarrhea and abdominal pain out of proportion to the physical examination may have mesenteric ischemia—a true emergency.

DIAGNOSTIC STOOL EVALUATION Tests specific to the emergency department evaluation of a patient with diarrhea include Wright's stain for fecal leukocytes; stool culture for bacteria, ova, and parasites; and stool analysis for *Clostridium difficile* toxin. Diagnostic testing, while rarely helpful to the emergency physician, occasionally is helpful to the primary care physician. Who should be tested? Stool cultures for bacteria should be obtained in children, toxic patients, patients with a protracted diarrheal illness lasting longer than 3 days, and immunocompromised patients in whom infectious diarrhea is suspected. A request for an ova and parasite evaluation can be made for patients at risk for parasitic disease. In adddition, patients at risk for *C. difficile* colitis should have a stool sample sent for *C. difficile* toxin assay.

Wright's Stain When applied to a stool sample, Wright's stain allows detection of fecal leukocytes. A positive Wright's stain has a sensitivity of 82 percent and a specificity of 83 percent for the presence of bacterial pathogen.[11] Historically, Wright's stain for fecal leukocytes has been used to differentiate invasive and noninvasive infectious diarrheas. In the past, this was an important distinction because physicians were reluctant to prescribe antibiotics for patients with infectious diarrhea because of the fear of prolonging the *Salmonella* carrier state. They therefore reserved antimicrobial treatment for the toxic patients who they felt *truly* had invasive diarrhea. Recently, this dictum has been questioned, and many physicians now treat patients with diarrheal illness with antibiotics regardless of whether or not the diarrhea is invasive or bacterial in origin.[15] Therefore, ascertaining the presence or absence of fecal leukocytes is superfluous if it does not change management.

Bacterial Stool Culture Bacterial stool culture is an expensive and labor-intensive diagnostic test that plays a minor role in the emergency department evaluation of a patient with diarrhea. Most laboratories culture for only three common bacterial pathogens: *Salmonella*, *Shigella*, and *Campylobacter*. Because of a low sensitivity for detecting pathogens, each positive routine stool culture costs the laboratory approximately $950 to $1200, depending on the number of samples tested and the number of tests run on each sample.[9] To limit cost and increase yield, diagnostic testing should be limited to patients with high pretest probabilities of bacterial disease: severely dehydrated or toxic patients, children, immunocompromised patients, and patients with diarrhea lasting longer than 3 days.[9] In addition, if other enteric pathogens are suspected, the laboratory should be notified so that appropriate testing may be performed.

Ova and Parasitic Evaluation Patients in whom a parasitic cause of diarrhea is suspected should have stool sent for evaluation for ova and parasites. These tests lack sensitivity, since many parasites are fastidious. Recently, direct immunoflouresence staining has been shown to improve the sensitivity for detecting *Giardia* and *Cryptosporidium*.[12]

***Clostridium Difficile* Toxin Assay** Diarrhea in a patient with an antecedent history of antibiotic use may be caused by pseudomembranous colitis from *C. difficile* infection. This is diagnosed with the *C. difficile* toxin assay. Unfortunately, this assay has a 10 percent false-negative rate and is rarely available to the emergency physician, since the turnaround time on the test approaches 24 h.[13]

Other Diagnostic Tests If diarrhea is not felt to be infectious in origin, data acquisition should be dictated by the differential diagnosis. Rarely are serum chemistry results or complete blood count results diagnostic or necessary. Electrolyte measurements are warranted in severely dehydrated patients, regardless of the cause of dehydration. They can also be helpful in patients experiencing an addisonian crisis. Serum drug levels can assist the physician in making the diagnosis of theophylline, lithium, or heavy metal intoxication. In patients with a history of abdominal surgery, abdominal films may help rule out partial obstruction as a cause of diarrhea. Finally, a chest radiograph may help diagnose an occult pneumonia (i.e., *Legionella*) in a patient with diarrhea and a cough. For patients in whom mesenteric ischemia is suspected, mesenteric angiography is the test of choice.

Treatment

Initial treatment of any patient begins with the ABCs. Patients with diarrhea are no different. Diarrhea of any type can cause circulatory collapse. Rehydration of severely dehydrated patients should begin immediately after large-bore intravenous access is achieved. Thereafter, treatment is dictated by the differential diagnosis. The emergency medicine approach to a patient with diarrhea, therefore, hinges on treating or excluding the life-threatening causes of diarrhea. Because infectious diarrhea is the most common cause of acute diarrhea, after the differential diagnosis is considered, physicians most commonly are left considering that diagnosis.

NONINFECTIOUS DIARRHEA Almost all true diarrheal emergencies (e.g., gastrointestinal bleed, adrenal insufficiency, thyroid storm, toxicologic exposures, acute radiation syndrome, and mesenteric ischemia, all discussed elsewhere in this textbook) are of noninfectious origin. The emergency physician must be ever mindful of them because patients with those conditions require intensive treatment and hospitalization. The less emergent, noninfectious causes of diarrhea are listed in Table 79-1. They, too, are covered elsewhere in this textbook.

INFECTIOUS DIARRHEA Viruses cause the vast majority of infectious diarrheas, followed by bacterial and parasitic organisms. Treatment of infectious diarrhea involves antibiotic therapy, antimotility agents, restoration of fluid balance, and avoidance of agents that worsen diarrhea. For the past 30 years, two pervasive myths involving the use of antibiotics and antimotility agents in the treatment of infectious diarrhea have dictated the management of large numbers of patients with diarrhea. These myths are discussed in detail below, and a discussion of the modern medical approach to infectious diarrhea follows.

Antibiotics MYTH For years, physicians avoided antibiotic use in the treatment of infectious diarrhea because of a fear of prolonging the *Salmonella* carrier state. This fear arose from an article published in 1969 in which the duration of *Salmonella* excretion following a salmonellosis epidemic was studied.[14] The study compared the length of excretion in patients who received antibiotics (ampicillin or chloramphenicol) with that of patients who were not treated and found that *Salmonella* excretion was longer in the cohort that received antibiotics. The authors concluded that, because of a prolonged carrier state, antibiotics should not be given to patients suspected of having a diarrheal illness due to *Salmonella*.

MODERN MEDICINE For adults with domestically acquired diarrhea in whom the origin is felt to be infectious, antibiotics [ciprofloxacin 500 mg by mouth (PO) bid for 5 days] shorten the duration of illness by approximately 24 h. Regardless of the causative agent, all patients—even those who had a negative Wright's stain, negative stool culture, and a low diarrheal illness score, suggesting less clinically significant disease and/or a viral cause—improved on ciprofloxacin.[15] Even though most infectious diarrheas are self-limited, because of the inconveniencing and occasionally life-threatening nature of the disease, we recommend ciprofloxacin treatment for all patients believed to have an infectious diarrhea who do not have a contraindication to antimicrobial treatment (e.g., pediatric age group, allergy, pregnancy, or drug interaction). Single-dose and 3-day ciprofloxacin regimens have been proposed but deserve further investigation. Trimethoprim-sulfamethoxazole (Bactrim DS on tablet PO bid for 5 days) also shortens the duration of infectious diarrhea in adults but was proven to be inferior to a 5-day course of ciprofloxacin in the above-mentioned study.

Antimotility Agents MYTH Since the early 1960s, the use of antimotility agents in the treatment of diarrhea has been denounced by most of the medical community. This dictum emerged out of a 1963 study published by Formal and colleagues.[16] In this study, guinea pigs were starved and poisoned to make them susceptible to *Shigella* infection (an organism to which guinea pigs are not usually susceptible). They were then innoculated with *Shigella,* and a subset of the study was then given opium. The authors discovered an association between opium administration and fatal *Shigella* infection. From these data, the authors concluded that a major defense mechanism of the guinea pig is its peristaltic activity and that antimotility agents (opium) might increase susceptibility to enteric infection.

A study in 1973 on human volunteers perpetuated the myth. In this study, DuPont and Hornick examined, among other things, the effect of diphenoxylate and atropine (Lomotil) on shigellosis.[17] The authors found that Lomotil seemed to diminish the number of unformed stools but in so doing may have increased patients' susceptibility to invasive infection, since fever was prolonged only in the patients receiving Lomotil. However, the sample size in this study was 25, and there were four treatment arms, making the number of patients in each treatment arm approximately six. The authors admitted that the study was inconclusive due to its small sample size and suggested that further investigation occur before conclusions could be made regarding the use of Lomotil in infectious diarrhea. Nevertheless, the two studies led to a nearly universal avoidance of the use of antimotility agents in patients with infectious diarrhea.

MODERN MEDICINE In 1990, Ericsson, DuPont, Mathewson, and colleagues[18] published a paper that addressed the use of loperamide (Imodium) in the treatment of traveler's diarrhea. In a study of 227 adults with acute diarrhea, combination treatment with Bactrim and loperamide was proven to be both safe and effective in treating traveler's diarrhea. In 1993, a randomized, placebo-controlled, double-blind study was performed in Thailand comparing the use of ciprofloxacin and loperamide with ciprofloxacin and placebo in the treatment of adults with bacillary dysentery.[19] The study showed that loperamide combined with ciprofloxacin decreased the number of diarrheal stools and shortened the duration of illness in adult patients with dysentery due to *Shigella* or enteroinvasive *Escherichia coli.* No complications were seen in the group treated with loperamide. Although the study size was small ($n = 88$), it was much larger than DuPont's 1973 study,[17] and it was the first of its kind to suggest the safety of antimotility agents in the treatment of adult invasive diarrheas. We therefore recommend the prescription of loperamide 4 mg PO initially, then 2 mg PO after each diarrheal stool to a maximum of 16 mg/d, since it has clearly been proven to shorten duration of symptoms when combined with an antibiotic regimen. Diphenoxylate and atropine (Lomotil) is a more potent antidiarrheal whose modern-day safety is less well studied. For patients with severely inconveniencing diarrhea refractory to loperamide, diphenoxylate and atropine (Lomotil two tablets PO qid) may be helpful. It should be used with caution, however, in patients with a history of constipation or cardiac disease.

TABLE 79-2 World Health Organization Recipe for Oral Rehydration Therapy

1 L sterile water (boiled or bottled)
1 cup orange juice
4 tsp sugar
1 tsp baking powder
$\frac{3}{4}$ tsp salt

Source: From Park and Giannella,[9] with permission.

Rehydration For patients presenting to the emergency department with significant dehydration, intravenous fluid therapy is indicated. For a mildly dehydrated patient who is not vomiting, oral rehydration therapy is recommended. Glucose-containing, caffeine-free beverages are the fluids of choice. For patients who can afford to buy it, Gatorade is a good rehydration choice. Otherwise, the World Health Organization recipe for oral rehydration solution can be followed easily and inexpensively (Table 79-2). Mildly dehydrated patients should aim to drink 30 to 50 mL/kg over the next 4 h. For moderate dehydration, patients should drink 100 mL/kg over the next 4 h.[10]

Dietary Restrictions Patients should be counseled to avoid caffeine, sorbitol-containing chewing gum, lactose, and raw fruits until after the diarrhea subsides.

Disposition

Patients with the noninfectious emergencies outlined above warrant hospitalization. Most other patients can be discharged home safely. When deciding whether to admit a patient with diarrhea, conservatism should be the rule with the young and the elderly. They do have higher morbidity and mortality rates and should be evaluated with a careful eye. Regardless of age, any toxic patient should be admitted, as should any patient who cannot convincingly comply with oral rehydration guidelines. Upon discharge, patients with infectious diarrhea should be counseled on limiting the spread of disease through the use of judicious hand washing. Work excuses should be given liberally to patients employed in the food, day care, and health care industries.

CONSTIPATION

Epidemiology

Constipation is the most common digestive complaint in the United States and accounts for more than 2.5 million physician visits per year.[20,21] There is an age-related increase in the incidence of constipation, with 30 to 40 percent of adults over age 65 citing constipation as a problem.[21,22]

Pathophysiology

The cause of constipation is usually multifactorial. Dietary intake affects bowel motility. Diminishing intake of fiber associated with decreased fluid intake can result in constipation. In addition, exercise, medical conditions, and medications affect gut motility. Sedentary patients often become constipated. Medical conditions such as hypothyroidism, hyperparathyroidism, lead poisoning, and chronic neurologic disorders are well-known causes. Some anal pathologic conditions cause painful defecation and in turn can result in constipation due to consequent fear, particularly in children. Patients confined to a hospital bed after an orthopedic injury, for example, may become constipated due to their inability to use a bedpan successfully. Certain medications, such as calcium-channel blockers, iron, narcotic analgesics, and antipsychotics, are also common causes of constipation. Indeed, constipation is a complicated condition with multiple causes (Table 79-3).

Clinical Features

HISTORY As with diarrhea, part of the challenge of treating patients with the complaint of constipation is determining whether they actually are constipated. The easiest, most practical definition of *constipation* is the following: the presence of hard stools that are difficult to pass. Some patients become bowel fixated and feel they are constipated if they do not have a daily bowel movement. They are not.

Once a physician determines that a patient truly is constipated, the physician must attempt to determine the cause. The differential diagnosis is broad (Table 79-3). Determining the onset of the constipation helps narrow the differential diagnosis. Acute constipation represents intestinal obstruction until proven otherwise. Tumors, strictures, and volvuli can all present as acute constipation. Physicians often mistake subacute for chronic constipation. The important distinction here is to determine exactly when bowel habits changed. Generally, acute and subacute conditions have the same differential diagnosis. Chronic constipation, that is, a lifelong or persistent habit, is usually less ominous and, if uncomplicated, can often be managed on an outpatient basis. The presence or absence of associated symptoms may help guide decision making. Vomiting rarely accompanies benign constipation. Inability to pass flatus also raises concern about obstruction. A history of gradually diminishing stool caliber may suggest colon cancer, especially if accompanied by weight loss. The physician should ask the patient about recent changes in dietary fiber or fluid intake. What other medical problems does the patient have? Is there a history of hypothyroidism or diabetes? An antecedent history of diverticulitis may point toward inflammatory stricture. A history of nephrolithiasis could suggest hyperparathyroidism as a cause for constipation. A quick review of the patient's medication list may also point to the culprit.

PHYSICAL EXAMINATION The physical examination should concentrate on ruling out organic causes of constipation. First and fore-

TABLE 79-3 Differential Diagnosis of Constipation

ACUTE OR SUBACUTE
Gastrointestinal: obstructing cancer, volvulus, stricture, hernia, adhesion, pelvic or abdominal masses
Medicinal: addition of new medicine (e.g., antipsychotic, anticholinergic, narcotic analgesic, antacids)
Environmental: change in defecation regimen (e.g., forced to use bedpan)
Exercise and diet: decrease in level of exercise, fiber intake, fluid intake
CHRONIC
Gastrointestinal: slowly growing tumor, colonic dysmotility, anal pathology
Medicinal: chronic laxative abuse, antipsychotics, anticholinergics, narcotic analgesics
Neurologic: neuropathy, Parkinson's disease, paraplegia, cerebral palsy
Endocrine: diabetes, hypothyroidism, hyperparathyroidism
Rheumatologic: scleroderma
Toxicologic: lead poisoning

most, intestinal obstruction must be ruled out. The patient should be examined carefully for the presence or absence of hernias and abdominal or pelvic masses. Rectal and pelvic examinations are necessary. In addition to detecting the presence or absence of an obstructing rectal mass, rectal examination also enables the physician to ascertain whether there is fecal impaction. Anal fissures are also detected during the rectal examination. In addition, rectal examination allows the physician to determine whether the stools are bloody. Guaiac-positive stools can be seen in both functional constipation and constipation resulting from colon cancer. With constipation resulting in fecal impaction, rectal mucosa often ulcerates, forming stercoral ulcers on the rectal walls, which yield guaiac-positive stools. With constipation caused by tumor, stools are also often guaiac positive. Constipation and new ascites in postmenopausal women should prompt evaluation for ovarian or uterine carcinoma. Signs of hypothyroidism may also be evident during the physical examination.

The evaluation of a constipated patient depends on the clinician's level of concern for organic causes of constipation. Patients with a long-standing history of constipation often require little, if any, data acquisition, provided the history and physical examination do not point toward an organic process. An upright chest film and abdominal flat and erect films should be obtained in patients who are at risk for intestinal obstruction: patients with prior abdominal surgery, associated vomiting, significant abdominal distention, abdominal pain, and an acute or subacute history of constipation. In addition to assessing the presence or absence of intestinal obstruction, abdominal films allow the physician to assess stool burden. In patients in whom an organic cause for constipation is suspected, a complete blood count should be obtained to screen for anemia. In addition, thyroid function tests may be helpful with patients in whom the physician suspects hypothyroidism. Electrolyte abnormalities, specifically hypokalemia and hypercalcemia, can be associated with constipation and are worth checking with patients suspected of having an organic cause.

Treatment

FUNCTIONAL CONSTIPATION The treatment of functional (chronic) constipation involves a multidisciplinary approach. Many patients come to the emergency department looking for medication. Medications often employed in the treatment of constipation are listed in Table 79-4. However, the most important part of treatment is dietary and behavior modification. The most important prescription a patient with constipation receives is for a strict dietary and exercise regimen, for without adequate fluid (1.5 L/day), fiber (10 g/day), and exercise, medicinal methods usually fail.[21] In addition, patients should be urged to take advantage of the gastrocolic reflex by attempting to defecate daily after a certain meal.

In its extreme form, functional constipation can result in a variety of potentially life-threatening complications. Fecal impaction and in-

TABLE 79-4 Medicinal Adjuncts Used in the Treatment of Constipation

Type	Generic Name	Trade Name	Prn Doses	Side Effects	Mechanism
Fiber	Bran	NA	1 cup/day	Bloating, flatulence	Increase stool bulk or transit time, increase gut motility.
	Psyllium	Metamucil	1 tsp tid	Bloating, flatulence	
Hyperosmolar agents	Lactulose	Chronulac	15–30 mL qd to bid	Cramps, flatulence	Osmotically active nonabsorbable sugars pull fluid into gut.
	Sorbitol	NA	15–30 mL qd to bid		
	Polyethylene glycol	Golytely	1 gal/4 h	Incontinence	
Suppository	Glycerin suppository	NA	1 PR qd	Rectal irritation	Local rectal stimulation prompts defecation.
Stimulants	Bisacodyl	Dulcolax	10 mg PR tid	Incontinence, rectal burning	Stimulate myenteric plexus, thereby increasing intestinal motility.
	Anthraquinones	Peri-Colace	1–2 tablets PO qhs	Melanosis coli, degeneration of myenteric plexus	
Saline laxative	Magnesium	Milk of Magnesia	15–30 mL qd to bid	Magnesium toxicity	Colonic transit time is shortened.
Enemas	Tap water	NA	500 mL PR	Local trauma	Colonic distention encourages evacuation.
	Soapsuds	NA	1500 mL PR	Local trauma	
	Phosphate	Fleets	1 U PR	Local trauma, hyperphosphatemia (especially in patients with renal failure)	

Abbreviation: NA, not applicable.
Source: Modified from Romero et al,[21] with permission.

testinal pseudo-obstruction are two sequelae of which the emergency physician should be acutely aware.

Fecal Impaction Patients with fecal impaction must be disimpacted manually prior to leaving the emergency department. Manual disimpaction is not a glamorous procedure, and, as a result, many physicians avoid doing it. This is unfortunate, since enemas—the alternative therapy—rarely work for fecal impaction. It must be remembered that manual disimpaction can be a painful procedure for which patients at times require sedation. After disimpaction, a host of medicines may be used to assist the patient in achieving normal fecal flow (Table 79-4). The agents listed in the table start with the least potent and end with the most potent.

Intestinal Pseudo-Obstruction Intestinal pseudo-obstruction is a condition seen in patients with a long-standing history of colonic dysmotility. Patients present in a manner that mimics intestinal obstruction: abdominal distention, crampy abdominal pain, and obstipation. Abdominal x-ray films may reveal a severely dilated colon. Treatment is varied and is best determined in consultation with a surgeon. Sometimes the symptoms resolve with conservative management. Other times, however, patients require operative or colonoscopic decompression of the very dilated intestine.

ORGANIC CONSTIPATION The treatment of organic constipation is dictated by the cause of the constipation. In the emergency department, the precise cause of the constipation is not always known. Emergency physicians often suspect organic causes, such as hypothyroidism and hyperparathyroidism, but seldom actually confirm these diagnoses in the emergency department. Patients in whom an organic cause of constipation is suspected and who are without evidence of obstruction may start a bowel-cleansing regimen in accordance with Table 79-4. Fecal impaction occurs with organic constipation (i.e., hypothyroidism or hyperparathyroidism) also and must be managed aggressively, as outlined above.

Constipation caused by intestinal obstruction is an emergency. Definitive treatment is dictated by the cause of the obstruction. For example, sigmoid volvulus can often be reduced by means of rigid sigmoidoscopy. Large-bowel obstruction resulting from colon cancer requires operative management. Regardless of the cause, intestinal obstruction warrants surgical consultation to assist with management decisions.

Disposition

Patients with functional constipation with or without fecal impaction can be managed safely as outpatients provided patients with fecal impaction are disimpacted manually prior to discharge. Patients with organic constipation of a nonobstructive cause can also be managed safely as outpatients. The primary care provider should be contacted to ensure follow-up and to communicate concern for an organic process. If thyroid function tests were performed, the primary care doctor should be informed so that they may be followed up.

Referral to a gastroenterologist is warranted for patients with constipation of recent onset; chronic constipation associated with weight loss, anemia, or change in stool caliber; refractory constipation; and constipation requiring chronic laxative use.[21]

Finally, patients with organic constipation of obstructive origin require hospitalization and surgical evaluation. The type of bed to which the patient is admitted is dictated by the patient's clinical picture.

REFERENCES

1. Wang SC, Borison HL: A new concept of organization of the central emetic mechanism: Recent studies on the sites of action of apomorphine, copper sulfate and cardiac glycosides. *Gastroenterology* 22:1, 1952.
2. Lumsden K, Holden WS: The act of vomiting in man. *Gut* 10:173, 1969.
3. Lew JF, Glass RI, Gangarosa RE, et al: Diarrheal deaths in the United States, 1979 through 1987. *JAMA* 265:3280, 1991.
4. Bennett RG, Greenough WB: Approach to acute diarrhea in the elderly. *Gastroenterol Clin North Am* 22:517, 1993.
5. Murray CJL, Lopez AD: Mortality by cause for eight regions of the world: Global Burden of Disease Study. *Lancet* 349:1269, 1997.
6. Siegel D, Cohen PT, Neighbor M, et al: Predictive value of stool examination in acute diarrhea. *Arch Pathol Lab Med* 111:715, 1987.
7. Brownlee HJ: Introduction: Management of acute nonspecific diarrhea. *Am J Med* 88(suppl 6A):1S, 1990.
8. Binder HJ: Pathophysiology of acute diarrhea. *Am J Med* 88(suppl 6A):2S, 1990.
9. Park SI, Giannella RA: Approach to the adult patient with acute diarrhea. *Gastroenterol Clin North Am* 22:483, 1993.
10. Kroser JA, Metz DC: Evaluation of the adult patient with diarrhea. *Primary Care* 23: 629, 1996.
11. DuBois D, Binder L, Nelson B: Usefulness of the stool Wright's stain in the emergency department. *J Emerg Med* 6:483, 1988.
12. Hines J, Nachamkin I: Effective use of the clinical microbiology laboratory for diagnosing diarrheal diseases. *Clin Infect Dis* 23:1292, 1996.
13. Bartlett JG: Antibiotic-associated diarrhea. *Clin Infect Dis* 15:573, 1992.
14. Aserkoff B, Bennett JV: Effect of antibiotic therapy in acute salmonellosis on the fecal excretion of *Salmonellae*. *N Engl J Med* 281:636, 1969.
15. Goodman LJ, Trenholme GM, Kaplan RL, et al: Empiric antimicrobial therapy of domestically acquired acute diarrhea in urban adults. *Arch Intern Med* 150:541, 1990.
16. Formal SB, Abrams GD, Schneider H, et al: Experimental *Shigella* infections:. Role of the small intestine in an experimental infection in guinea pigs. *J Bacteriol* 85:119, 1963.
17. DuPont HL, Hornick RB: Adverse effect of Lomotil therapy in shigellosis. *JAMA* 226:1525, 1973.
18. Ericsson CD, DuPont HL, Mathewson JJ, et al: Treatment of traveler's diarrhea with sulfamethoxazole and trimethoprim and loperamide. *JAMA* 263:257, 1990.
19. Murphy GS, Bodhidatta L, Echeverria P, et al: Ciprofloxacin and loperamide in the treatment of bacillary dysentery. *Ann Intern Med* 118:582, 1993.
20. Sonnenberg A, Koch TR: Physician visits in the United States for constipation: 1958 to 1986. *Dig Dis Sci* 34:606, 1989.
21. Romero Y, Evans JM, Fleming KC, et al: Constipation and fecal incontinence in the elderly population. *Mayo Clin Proc* 71:81, 1996.
22. Abyad A, Mourad F: Constipation: Common-sense care of the older patient. Geriatrics 51:28, 1996.

80 JAUNDICE

Richard O. Shields, Jr.

Jaundice is a physical finding that emergency physicians see both as a presenting complaint and as an abnormal finding during the evaluation of other complaints and symptoms. Except in neonates, jaundice itself causes no adverse effects; it serves as a clinical marker of a defect in the metabolism and excretion of bilirubin. The emergency physician must identify those jaundiced patients who require inpatient treatment of the underlying problem and initiate the laboratory or imaging studies on those who will be worked up as outpatients and arrange for their follow-up care.

PATHOPHYSIOLOGY

Jaundice (also called icterus) is the yellowish discoloration of the sclera, skin, and mucous membranes caused by the deposition of bile pigments associated with elevated levels of bilirubin in the blood (hyperbilirubinemia). Jaundice can usually be clinically detected when serum bilirubin levels reach 2.0 to 2.5 mg/dL or above, about twice the upper level of normal. It is usually first noticed in the sclera because scleral tissue contains a large amount of elastin, which has a high affinity for bilirubin. Jaundice is easier to detect in people with light complexions and in the presence of significant anemia. The brownish discoloration of the sclerae in many people with darker complexions may be confused with scleral icterus and makes it more difficult to detect. A greenish tint to the skin indicates long-standing jaundice during which some of the bilirubin deposited in the skin has been metabolized to biliverdin. A yellow-orange discoloration of the skin can be caused by the presence of high levels of carotene in the blood (resulting from the dietary intake of large amounts of beta-carotene) or by longstanding hemochromatosis. Neither of these will discolor the sclera, however.

Bilirubin, a breakdown product of hemoglobin from injured or senescent red blood cells and other heme-containing proteins, is produced in the reticuloendothelial system and then released into the plasma, where it is bound to albumin. Hepatocytes take up the bilirubin, conjugate it (mostly as the mono- and diglucuronide) and excrete it through the bile channels into the small intestine. In the gut, bacterial enzymes release some of the bilirubin and reduce it to urobilinogen and the other pigments that give fecal material its typical color. Some urobilinogen is reabsorbed into the portal circulation, where most is taken up by the liver and reexcreted into the bile. A small amount reaches the kidneys and is excreted unchanged into the urine. Hyperbilirubinemia and jaundice, therefore, can be produced by an overproduction of bilirubin in the reticuloendothelial system, a failure of hepatocyte uptake of bilirubin, a failure of the hepatocyte to conjugate or excrete bilirubin, or an obstruction of biliary excretion into the intestine (Table 80-1).[1]

Depending on whether the defect occurs before or after the conjugation phase in the hepatocyte, two types of hyperbilirubinemia can be produced: unconjugated and conjugated. If increased production of bilirubin exceeds the ability of the liver to process it or if there is a defect in bilirubin uptake or conjugation, then levels of the unconjugated form will rise, producing unconjugated hyperbilirubinemia. Causes include hemolysis from hemoglobinopathies, hemolytic anemias, or transfusion reactions, and in-born errors of bilirubin metabolism.

If the liver can produce but not normally excrete conjugated bilirubin because of a metabolic defect or intra- or extrahepatic obstruction, conjugated hyperbilirubinemia and cholestasis results. Intrahepatic cholestasis is caused by decreased excretion of conjugated bilirubin, hepatocellular damage, or damage to the biliary endothelium. Obstruction of biliary outflow by a congenital defect, inflammation, a mass lesion, or gallstones produces extrahepatic cholestasis.

Jaundice can also be classified as hemolytic (or prehepatic), hepatocellular (or hepatic), and obstructive (or posthepatic), depending on the location of the pathologic mechanism.[1] More than one type can be present in a given patient.

TABLE 80-1 Causes of Jaundice

UNCONJUGATED HYPERBILIRUBINEMIA
Hemolytic anemia
Hemoglobinopathy
Transfusion reaction
Gilbert syndrome
Crigler-Najar syndrome
Prematurity in neonates
Congestive cardiac failure
Sepsis
CONJUGATED HYPERBILIRUBINEMIA
Intrahepatic
Infection
Viral hepatitis
Leptospirosis
Infectious mononucleosis
Toxic
Drugs (ethanol, acetaminophen, etc.)
Chemical (carbon tetrachloride, etc.)
Familial
Rotor syndrome
Dubin-Johnson syndrome
Other
Sarcoidosis
Lymphoma
Liver metastases
Amyloidosis
Cirrhosis
Biliary cirrhosis
Cholestatic jaundice of pregnancy
Extrahepatic
Gallstones
Pancreatic tumors or cysts
Cholangiocarcinoma
Bile duct stricture
Sclerosing cholangitis
Ampullary carcinoma

CLINICAL FEATURES

A careful history and physical examination coupled with judicious use of the clinical laboratory enables the emergency physician to determine whether jaundice is produced by a hemolytic process, hepatocellular disease, or a potentially surgically correctable obstructive process. Often, more extensive diagnostic procedures are needed before the precise etiology of jaundice can be determined.

The sudden appearance of jaundice in a previously healthy young person, especially if preceded by a brief prodrome of fever, malaise, and myalgias, is likely to be caused by a viral hepatitis. Inquire about body fluid exposure over the previous few months, including transfusion of blood products, intimate contact with someone with hepatitis or jaundice, promiscuous sexual activity, intravenous drug use, accidental needle-stick injuries or mucosal contact with body fluids, travel to countries where hepatitis is prevalent, raw shellfish ingestion, and recent tattoos or body piercing. Many times, however, no history of exposure can be elicited. Right upper quadrant pain and tenderness and hepatomegaly may be present, but pruritis is usually absent. Examine for needle tracks, since patients may not volunteer a history of drug use.

Jaundice that develops gradually and is accompanied by weakness, peripheral muscle wasting, ascites, spider angiomata, pruritus, and symptoms of portal hypertension is frequently caused by alcoholic liver disease and cirrhosis. A history of sustained, significant alcohol intake should be elicited from the patient or from family and friends. A history of any previous episodes of jaundice, pancreatitis, or hematemesis should be obtained. Fever, vomiting, and right upper quadrant tenderness accompany episodes of alcoholic hepatitis. The presence of asterixis, fetor hepaticus, or encephalopathy indicates advanced disease.

Toxic hepatitis should be suspected if a history of ingestion or exposure to a known hepatotoxin is obtained. Signs of hepatocellular damage may be present with toxicity from agents such as acetaminophen, halothane, methyldopa, isoniazid, or phenytoin. Cholestatic changes predominate in toxicity from anabolic steroids, oral contraceptives, and chlorpromazine. Mushroom poisoning, carbon tetrachloride, and phosphorus can produce massive hepatic necrosis.

A family history of jaundice or a history of recurrent mild jaundice that resolves spontaneously is most consistent with a familial cause, such as Gilbert's syndrome. Most patients with sickle cell disease develop chronic jaundice, but in the presence of abdominal pain, vomiting, and fever, acute cholecystitis or biliary obstruction must be strongly suspected. The patient should also be asked about other hemoglobinopathies or prior episodes of hemolysis.

Jaundice that develops acutely with abdominal pain, vomiting, fever, and right upper quadrant tenderness is strongly suggestive of acute biliary obstruction from choledocholithiasis. A history of fatty food intolerance and typical biliary colic is supportive. Cholecystitis alone does not produce jaundice. Painless jaundice in an older patient, especially if accompanied by an epigastric mass and weight loss, strongly suggests biliary obstruction from a malignancy. A history of known gastrointestinal malignancy accompanied by a hard, nodular liver indicates metastatic disease as the cause of jaundice. A history of prior biliary tract surgery, pancreatitis, cholangitis, or inflammatory bowel disease should be elicited, since they may be associated with the development of biliary obstruction.

Hepatomegaly with pedal edema, jugular venous distention, and a gallop rhythm makes congestive cardiac failure the likely cause of jaundice.

Laboratory Evaluation

The initial laboratory evaluation of the jaundiced patient should include determinations of the serum bilirubin level (both total and the direct-reacting fraction), the serum liver aminotransferase levels, and the serum alkaline phosphatase level; urinalysis for bilirubin and urobilinogen; a complete blood count; and any other pertinent tests suggested by the physical examination and history (e.g., determinations of serum amylase or lipase levels, and prothrombin time). The serum bilirubin level is measured by the van den Bergh reaction using two techniques to measure both total bilirubin and conjugated bilirubin (the direct fraction). The indirect fraction can then be calculated by subtracting the direct fraction from the total.

If the patient has unconjugated hyperbilirubinemia, the bilirubin is usually only mildly elevated and consists predominately (more than 85 percent) of the indirect fraction. Since unconjugated bilirubin is tightly bound to albumin, it does not appear in the urine. Liver aminotransferase levels will be normal, and the blood count and smear may show evidence of anemia or hemolysis. A Coombs test and hemoglobin electrophoresis may be helpful if no history of hemolytic anemia or hemoglobinopathy is known. Gilbert's syndrome is the most common cause of mild unconjugated hyperbilirubinemia. This is an inherited deficiency in bilirubin conjugation that produces no symptoms other than variable elevations of bilirubin and no adverse effects. Factors that can cause bilirubin to rise include fever, heavy physical exertion, fasting, surgery, and heavy alcohol consumption.

A direct-reacting fraction of at least 30 percent (and usually much higher) is present with conjugated hyperbilirubinemia. Conjugated bilirubin is water soluble and appears in the urine at very low serum concentrations. Urobilinogen will be absent from the urine if significant cholestasis is present. If liver enzyme levels are normal, the jaundice is caused by sepsis or recent systemic infection, in-born errors of bilirubin metabolism (such as Rotor syndrome or Dubin-Johnson syndrome), or pregnancy rather than by primary hepatic disease. If liver enzyme levels are abnormal, which is much more common, the pattern of abnormality suggests the cause. Predominance of aminotransferase elevation is more suggestive of hepatocellular disease, such as viral or toxic hepatitis or cirrhosis, while marked elevations of alkaline phosphatase (two to three times normal) and γ-glutamyl transpeptidase suggest intra- or extrahepatic obstruction, such as malignancy or gallstones.

Further laboratory testing and imaging studies should be undertaken next, directed by which type of jaundice is present. If the initial laboratory studies suggest hepatocellular disease and the clinical examination suggests viral hepatitis, then serologic studies for viral hepatitis should be done. If the clinical picture points to alcoholic liver disease or other toxins, then prothrombin time, platelet count, and serum albumin levels should be determined to help estimate the degree of liver injury. If results of the serologic studies are negative, there is no improvement with withdrawal of the suspected toxic agent, or there is no other obvious etiology, liver biopsy should be considered.[2]

If the clinical examination and initial laboratory findings suggest intrahepatic cholestasis or extrahepatic biliary obstruction, ultrasound studies should be performed to look for gallstones, dilated extrahepatic biliary ducts, or masses in the liver, pancreas, or portal area. Computed tomography can also be used but is usually more costly, involves radiation exposure, and is less sensitive than is ultrasound at detecting stones in the gallbladder.

DISPOSITION

Jaundice alone is not an indication for admission. A hemodynamically stable patient with new-onset jaundice without evidence of liver failure or acute biliary obstruction can be discharged from the emergency department if the appropriate laboratory studies have been ordered and follow-up has been arranged. Surgical consultation should be obtained if extrahepatic biliary obstruction is suspected. For other admission indicators, refer to the appropriate chapters in this text (Chaps. 81 and 82).

REFERENCES

1. Sherlock S, Dooley J: *Diseases of the Liver and Biliary System*, 10th ed. London, Blackwell Science Ltd., 1997, p. 201.
2. Frank BB: Clinical evaluation of jaundice. *JAMA* 262:3031, 1989.

CHOLECYSTITIS AND BILIARY COLIC

Tom P. Aufderheide
William J. Brady
Judith E. Tintinalli

Biliary tract emergencies result primarily from obstruction by biliary calculi in the gallbladder and bile ducts. The four major biliary tract emergencies related to gallstones include biliary colic, cholecystitis, gallstone pancreatitis, and ascending cholangitis. While gallstones are common, most are asymptomatic. The incidence of new-onset biliary pain among patients with previously asymptomatic gallstones is about 2 percent per year for the first 5 years and 15 percent at 10 years.[1] Although the classic patient with symptomatic biliary tract disease is an obese female aged 20 to 40 years, the disease occurs in all age groups and must be especially considered in diabetics and the elderly.[2] In both men and women, age over 60, right upper quadrant (RUQ) pain has the highest positive predictive value (11 to 16 percent) for gallstones.[3]

A number of risk factors are associated with cholecystitis and calculi, including increased age, female sex, parity, obesity, diabetes, profound weight loss, prolonged fasting, cystic fibrosis, intestinal malabsorption syndromes, various medications (particularly oral contraceptive agents and clofibrate), and a familial tendency. Clinical characteristics associated with an increased risk of the development of pigment stones are Asian descent, chronic biliary tract infection, parasitic infection (e.g., *Ascaris lumbricoides*), chronic liver disease (particularly related to alcohol), and chronic intravascular hemolysis (sickle cell anemia and hereditary spherocytosis). Hepatitis A, B, C, and E; HIV; and the herpesviruses are associated with viral cholangitis and hepatitis.[4]

PATHOPHYSIOLOGY

Bile is manufactured in and secreted from hepatocytes and transported to the gallbladder for storage via the canaliculi, ductiles, and bile ducts. The bile ducts become progressively larger and eventually coalesce to form the right and left hepatic ducts, which unite to form the common hepatic duct. The common hepatic duct joins with the cystic duct from the gallbladder to form the common bile duct, which empties into the duodenum through the ampulla of Vater. The pancreatic duct often merges with the common bile duct immediately prior to entering the duodenum. The wall of the gallbladder is innervated with sympathetic and parasympathetic nerves from the celiac plexus.[5]

Bile is composed primarily of water (80 percent), bile acids (10 percent), lecithin and other phospholipids (4 to 5 percent), cholesterol (1 percent), conjugated bilirubin, electrolytes, mucus, and various proteins. The major stimulus for release of bile is the gastrointestinal hormone cholecystokinin, which is secreted from the small intestinal mucosal cells when fats and amino acids enter the duodenum. Cholecystokinin causes forceful contraction of the gallbladder, relaxation of the sphincter of Oddi, increased hepatic bile production, and ultimately release of bile into the duodenum for digestion of a meal. Approximately 95 percent of bile is conserved via enterohepatic circulation.

Gallstones, crystalline structures formed from both normal and abnormal bile components, are divided into three major types: cholesterol (70 percent), pigment (20 percent), and mixed (10 percent). Cholesterol stones, the most commonly encountered gallstones, contain more than 70 percent cholesterol monohydrate. The formation of such stones is complex, involving cholesterol supersaturation of the bile; the formation of monohydrate crystals, with aggregation into successively larger structures; and delayed gallbladder emptying, with bile stasis. Pigment stones are subdivided into black and brown varieties. Black stones are noted in patients with advanced liver disease and hemolytic disorders, while brown stones are found commonly in patients of Asian descent, usually resulting from bacterial or parasitic infection. Both subtypes of pigment stones result from abnormal solubilization of unconjugated bilirubin coupled with the precipitation of calcium salts. The calcium content of cholesterol stones is much lower than that of pigment stones, making cholesterol stones most frequently radiolucent and pigment stones radiopaque. Anatomically, cholesterol gallstones are found in the gallbladder, cystic duct, intrahepatic ducts, and common bile duct. Brown pigment stones have a distribution similar to that of cholesterol gallstones, while black stones occur exclusively in the gallbladder.

The pathogenesis of symptomatic cholelithiasis involves stone migration from the gallbladder into the biliary tract and eventual obstruction. The stone, once lodged in either the cystic or common bile duct, produces increased intraluminal pressure and distention of the hollow viscus, resulting in pain, nausea, and vomiting. Forceful, repetitive contractions of the entire biliary system may relieve the obstruction. If obstruction persists, particularly in either the cystic duct or the infundibulum of the gallbladder, acute cholecystitis may develop. The inflammatory response in acute cholecystitis results from a combination of three factors: mechanical, chemical, and infectious. The mechanical factor produces the rise in intraluminal pressure and distention of the viscus, which culminates in visceral ischemia. Chemical inflammation occurs with the release of various mediators (lysolecithin, phospholipase A, and prostaglandins), resulting in direct mucosal injury. The contribution to the inflammatory response by bacterial agents is variable, occurring in 50 to 80 percent of patients with acute cholecystitis. Bacterial pathogens include enterobacteriaceae (70 percent, particularly *Escherichia coli* and *Klebsiella* species), enterococci (15 percent), bacteroides (10 percent), *Clostridium* species (10 percent), group D *Streptococcus*, and *Staphylococcus* species. The inflammatory process may progress to gangrene of the gallbladder wall with or without perforation.

Gallstone pancreatitis is similarly multifactorial, since it is experimentally produced by injecting bile, bacteria, and trypsin under pressure.[6]

CLINICAL FEATURES

Patients with acute biliary colic display a wide range of symptoms. Location, radiation, and duration of pain are all poor discriminators of gallbladder disease. There is overlap of signs and symptoms with peptic ulcer disease, gastritis, esophageal reflux, and nonspecific dyspepsia. In addition, it has been difficult to determine which symptoms are attributable to biliary tract disease.[7,8] RUQ pain is a common symptom in patients with and without gallstones.[3,9] Up to 25 percent of postcholecystectomy patients may experience RUQ pain of unknown cause.

Biliary tract disease is an important consideration in the evaluation of dyspepsia.[10] Biliary dyskinesia or increased resting pressure of the sphincter of Oddi, or incoordination between gallbladder contraction and relaxation of the sphincter of Oddi, has been proposed as a cause of biliary tract induced dyspepsia.[10]

One study has reported that epigastric pain was the predominant symptom of biliary tract disease in over 60 percent of patients studied,[9] thus accounting for the difficulty in using clinical signs and symptoms to make or exclude the diagnosis. The same study found that radiation of pain to the left upper back appears to be more commonly associated with biliary tract disease than with other upper gastrointestinal disorders, with a likelihood ratio of 4.0 for gallbladder pathology.[9]

The duration and character of the pain are also nonspecific, but the pain of biliary colic is reported to persist for 2- to 6 h. Pain quality is generally persistent, not colicky, and pain episodes are infrequent, occurring at intervals greater than a week.[9] Gallstone pain is not related to meals in at least one-third of patients,[9,11] and clinical studies have not been able to identify an association with fatty food intolerance that is different from its association with a number of other upper gastrointestinal disorders.[3,9,11] Investigators have noted a circadian rhythm to biliary colic,[11] with a peak of symptoms occurring around midnight to 1 A.M., and a time distribution from 9 P.M. to 4 A.M. Attacks tend to reoccur at the same time. This circadian rhythm has obvious diagnostic implications for patients who present with upper abdominal pain during the midnight shift.

Acute cholecystitis usually begins with pain similar to that of biliary colic but that persists beyond the typical 6 h. Associated nausea, vomiting, and anorexia are noted; a history of fever and/or chills is not uncommon. Patients may have either a history of similar attacks or documented gallstones. As the inflammatory process progresses, the patient's pain changes in character and location from visceral (dull and poorly localized mid-upper abdominal) to parietal (sharp and localized RUQ). The examination reveals a patient in moderate-to-severe distress with signs of systemic toxicity, including tachycardia and fever. The abdomen is tender in the RUQ, at times with evidence of localized peritoneal irritation, distention, and hypoactive bowel sounds. Generalized peritonitis with rigidity is rare and, if found, suggests perforation. The Murphy sign—worsened pain or inspiratory arrest resulting from deep, subcostal palpation on inspiration—has been estimated to be 97 percent sensitive for acute cholecystitis.[3] Volume depletion is frequently found. Jaundice, usually not present, may be found in patients with prolonged biliary obstruction with late onset of inflammation or in cases of chronic intravascular hemolysis.

Acalculous cholecystitis, which occurs in 5 to 10 percent of patients with acute cholecystitis, tends to have a more rapid, malignant course. Patients frequently are elderly and have a history of diabetes mellitus. Other risk factors include multiple trauma, extensive burn injury, prolonged labor, major surgery, gallbladder torsion, systemic vasculitic states, and bacterial or parasitic infections of the biliary tract. Patients with acalculous cholecystitis are indistinguishable from those with calculous cholecystitis with two major exceptions: acalculous cholecystitis frequently occurs as a complication of another process (e.g., multiple trauma or extensive burns), and patients frequently are gravely ill on initial presentation.

DIFFERENTIAL DIAGNOSIS

The differential diagnosis of biliary colic includes other conditions associated with upper abdominal pain, including gastritis, gastroesophageal reflux, pancreatitis, hepatitis, and peptic ulcer disease. Atypical myocardial infarction should be considered in older patients. Acute renal colic can be associated with upper abdominal and upper back pain. Both conditions can also be associated with flank tenderness, nausea, and vomiting. Renal colic does not have a circadian rhythm, and the pain is colicky, not continuous, as in biliary colic. Nonetheless, it can be difficult to distinguish biliary from renal colic, and definitive imaging studies may be needed to make the correct diagnosis. Acute pyelonephritis, like cholecystitis, can be associated with flank and upper quadrant pain, but pyuria confirms the former diagnosis. Appendicitis can sometimes be associated with RUQ pain, especially in pregnancy or in patients with a retrocecal or redundant appendix. In women of childbearing age, the differential diagnosis is expanded to include a wide variety of gynecologic disorders, including pelvic inflammatory disease, perihepatitis (Fitzhugh-Curtis syndrome), and ectopic pregnancy. Pregnancy testing, gynecologic history, and pelvic examination should focus on the correct diagnosis. Finally, pneumonia or pleural effusion can be associated with RUQ pain. Diagnosis is confirmed by chest x-ray. However, pancreatitis can also be associated with pleural effusions, usually on the right.

DIAGNOSTIC STUDIES

Results of laboratory studies in patients with biliary colic are frequently normal. The hemogram may reveal chronic anemia with or without evidence of hemolysis in patients with pigment stones. The white blood cell count, serum bilirubin level, alkaline phosphatase level, and aminotransferase levels are often normal. The serum lipase level should be obtained to rule out pancreatitis. The urine must be examined to exclude other causes of abdominal pain. In females, serum or urine pregnancy testing should be performed to rule out obstetric causes of abdominal pain. A negative pregnancy test result also enables one to proceed safely with radiologic studies, if indicated.

The presence of leukocytosis or abnormal liver function study results or lipase levels are often used as indicators for the diagnosis of acute cholecystitis. However, no single test or combination of laboratory tests has a sufficiently high sensitivity to detect acute cholecystitis.[12] A retrospective review of emergency department patients with acute cholecystitis found that 32 percent lacked a white blood cell count greater than 11,000 cells/mL.[13] Typical signs, symptoms, and laboratory findings may not be present in patients over age 60. The sensitivity of Murphy's sign is only 48 percent in the elderly.[14] In a cohort of geriatric emergency department patients with abdominal pain who were determined at surgery to have acute cholecystitis, 56 percent were afebrile, 41 percent had no leukocytosis, and 13 percent were both afebrile and had normal values on routine laboratory tests.[15]

Additional studies in patients with biliary colic may be performed to support the diagnosis and rule out other causes of upper abdominal pain with nausea. Plain film radiographs of the abdomen demonstrate gallstones in only 10 to 20 percent of cases. The majority of stones are cholesterol and therefore radiolucent. Pigment and mixed stones containing at least 4 percent calcium by weight are radiopaque. Abdominal films are more useful in excluding other causes of pain. A chest radiograph should be obtained to identify right lower lobe pneumonia or pleural effusions. A 12-lead electrocardiogram should be obtained in all older patients to exclude myocardial ischemia or infarction.

Ultrasonography is now the initial diagnostic modality of choice. It may show the presence of stones as small as 2 mm, gallbladder distention, wall thickening, and pericholecystic fluid, and during the procedure a sonographic Murphy sign may be elicited. Ultrasonography has a sensitivity of 94 percent and a specificity of 78 percent for the diagnosis of acute cholecystitis.[16]

Computed tomography (CT) scanning can be most useful in the diagnosis of acute cholecystitis when other intraabdominal disorders are considerations in the differential diagnosis. Wall thickening, pericholecystic fluid, and subserosal edema can be identified. However, the sensitivity of CT scanning is insufficient (as low as 50 percent) for it to replace ultrasonography as the diagnostic procedure of choice.[17]

Radioisotope cholescintigraphy using technetium-iminoacetic acid analogues (HIDA), has a sensitivity and specificity of 97 percent and 90 percent, respectively.[16] The study is performed by injecting radioisotopes intravenously. The material is absorbed by the hepatocytes and secreted into the biliary tract. A normal patient will have a clearly outlined gallbladder and cystic duct within 1 h. Failure to demonstrate the gallbladder within this time frame is consistent with cystic duct obstruction. The HIDA scan can only be used in patients with a serum bilirubin level of less than 5 mg/dL. With serum bilirubin above this level, an alternative radioisotope study, the DISIDA scan, is preferred.

COMPLICATIONS

Fluid and electrolyte deficits due to protracted vomiting and anorexia, and upper gastrointestinal hemorrhage from emesis-related Mallory-Weiss tears can coexist with biliary tract emergencies. Complications associated with cholelithiasis include gallstone pancreatitis, ascending cholangitis, and cholecystitis. Patients with cholecystitis may further develop a number of serious complications, including gallbladder empyema and emphysematous (gangrenous) cholecystitis.

Approximately 70 percent of cases of acute pancreatitis are due to either gallstones or alcohol. Depending on the population studied, gallstones are involved in 30 to 70 percent of patients with acute pancreatitis. Of all patients with gallstones, 15 to 20 percent will develop pancreatitis as a result of biliary calculi. Patients with pancreatitis due to gallstones will present similarly to patients with pancreatic inflammation caused by ethanol, with epigastric or diffuse abdominal pain radiating to the back, associated with nausea and vomiting. Patients may manifest symptoms of both acute cholecystitis and acute pancreatitis. Management includes intravenous fluids, nasogastric decompression, analgesics, and parenteral antibiotics with subsequent surgery. In patients who present in extremis or in those who demonstrate clinical deterioration, urgent biliary decompression (surgical or endoscopic) is mandatory.

Ascending cholangitis is a life-threatening emergency with a mortality rate approaching 100 percent in untreated or improperly treated patients. The process results from complete biliary obstruction in the presence of bacteria (gram-negative organisms as well as enterococcal and various anaerobic species). As the obstruction persists, intraluminal pressure increases, resulting in reflux of bacteria into the lymphatic vessels and hepatic veins, with eventual entrance into the systemic circulation. The obstruction most often is due to choledocholithiasis (gallstone obstruction of the common bile duct) and less often to biliary tract strictures, surgical anastomotic strictures, various postprocedural complications, and extrinsic compression from malignancy. Patients present with jaundice, fever, RUQ pain, mental confusion, and shock. The classic Charcot triad of fever, jaundice, and RUQ pain is noted in only 25 percent of patients. Management includes initial volume resuscitation with vasopressor support in cases unresponsive to crystalloid infusion alone, broad-spectrum parenteral antibiotics, and rapid decompression (surgical or endoscopic) of the biliary tree.

Gallbladder empyema, a life-threatening complication of cholecystitis, results from complete obstruction of the cystic duct with bacterial infection of the stagnant bile and abscess formation within the gallbladder wall. Risk factors include age, diabetes mellitus, trauma, burns, vasculitis, and bacterial or parasitic infections of the biliary tract. The presentation is similar to cholangitis, with fever, RUQ pain, altered mentation, and hypotension. Patients frequently develop gram-negative sepsis and require immediate broad-spectrum antibiotic coverage, fluid resuscitation, and urgent surgical consultation for cholecystectomy. The outcome is poor without prompt definitive care.

Gangrene of the gallbladder wall may be focal or diffuse. Focal gangrene results from segmental ischemia of the gallbladder wall caused by severe distention, acute inflammation, empyema, torsion with arterial compromise, or coexisting vasculitis. Patients with diabetes mellitus are at risk for this complication. Perforation of the wall may occur in a contained fashion (into the omentum) or free (into the peritoneal cavity).

Gangrene of the entire gallbladder, also known as emphysematous cholecystitis, is an uncommon complication, occurring in approximately 1 percent of patients with cholecystitis. Emphysematous cholecystitis is acalculous in 30 percent of patients. The gallbladder wall becomes ischemic, with eventual bacterial infection and gangrene. Patients present in extremis with fever, RUQ pain, and septic shock. Plain-film radiographs may demonstrate air in the gallbladder itself, the gallbladder wall, or the biliary tree because of the frequent presence of gas-forming organisms. An abdominal CT scan is the suggested imaging study. The bacteriology of either focal or diffuse gallbladder gangrene includes gram-negative, gram-positive, and anaerobic organisms. Polymicrobial infection is common. Management is similar to that of gallbladder empyema. Mortality rates for gangrenous cholecystitis are very high because of associated sepsis and attendant comorbidity in the typical elderly diabetic patient.

TREATMENT

Patients with accurately diagnosed uncomplicated symptomatic cholelithiasis do not necessarily require immediate surgical intervention. Patients presenting with biliary colic and emesis are best treated with antispasmodic agents (glycopyrrolate), opiate analgesics (meperidine), and antiemetics (promethazine). Meperidine is the analgesic of choice because it produces significantly less spasm of the sphincter of Oddi than do other narcotic agents, such as morphine. Gastric decompression with nasogastric suction may be warranted for protracted vomiting. Volume deficits and electrolyte imbalance can be corrected with isotonic intravenous fluids. With an accurate diagnosis, resolution of symptoms, correction of intravascular volume deficits, and a demonstrated ability to maintain hydration orally, the patient may be discharged from the emergency department. Prior to discharge, the case should be discussed with a surgical consultant or the patient's primary care physician to arrange for timely outpatient follow-up. Patients may be given oral narcotic-acetaminophen pain medication for the common residual abdominal aching. If the symptoms do not resolve within a 4- to 6-h period in the emergency department, the diagnosis of biliary colic must be questioned. Such prolonged pain may represent early, acute cholecystitis.

Ketorolac tromethamine, an injectable nonsteroidal anti-inflammatory drug, has been shown effective in relieving the pain of gallbladder distention. This distention causes the release of prostaglandins, which are associated with the production of pain. Ketorolac inhibits the production of prostaglandins, which may explain why it is effective in this situation. It is not as effective in relieving pain in the presence of infection. When ketorolac does not relieve pain in the clinical setting of symptomatic cholelithiasis, the clinician should reconsider the diagnosis.

Patients with uncomplicated symptomatic cholelithiasis have several options for definitive treatment, including open or laparoscopic cholecystectomy, medical dissolution therapy, and gallstone lithotripsy. Open cholecystectomy with intraoperative cholangiogram provides definitive cure for patients with biliary colic. The laparoscopic technique is rapidly replacing the traditional open cholecystectomy as the procedure of choice. Patients with frequent or severe attacks of biliary colic, a history of associated complications of gallstones, large biliary calculi (>2 cm in diameter), a congenitally abnormal hepatobiliary system, diabetes mellitus, or a desire for rapid cure are best managed with open or laparoscopic cholecystectomy or endoscopic retrograde cholangiopancreatography with possible endoscopic sphincterotomy (ES). Approximately 5 percent of patients have complications from cholecystectomy. The majority of these adverse outcomes are wound infections. Abscess, hemorrhage, bile leakage, and fistula formation are infrequent.[18] Approximately 8 percent of patients develop complications from ES. Pancreatitis and hemorrhage are the most common complications within 30 days of the procedure. Complications, occurring months to years later, such as recurrent stones and cholangitis, are seen in about 10 percent of patients.[19] Medical dissolution therapy with oral bile acid treatment is an option for those with small radiolucent stones (about 10 percent of patients).

Treatment of calculous and acalculous acute cholecystitis is surgical. Basic supportive medical therapy occurs in the emergency department prior to hospital admission and/or surgery. As with biliary colic, patients with acute cholecystitis require volume resuscitation with intravenous isotonic fluid, pain control with opiate analgesics, and bowel rest with nasogastric suction and antiemetic agents. Antibiotic treatment is recommended despite the questionable role of acute infection in all cases of early acute cholecystitis. In patients presenting without sepsis, single-agent therapy with a third-generation cephalosporin is adequate. Patients with obvious infection should receive broadened coverage with ampicillin, gentamicin, and clindamycin, or the equivalent. A minority of patients (usually those with either acalculous or emphysematous cholecystitis or a complication of cholecystitis) present in septic shock and require aggressive resuscitation. All patients with acute cholecystitis must be admitted to the hospital for continued intravenous fluid therapy and antibiotics. Approximately 75 percent of patients treated medically have a complete remission of symptoms within 2 to 7 days of hospitalization; the remainder of patients experience either a progression of the inflammatory process or a complication of acute cholecystitis within this time frame. Most often, surgery is performed 24 to 72 h after admission, once symptoms have resolved. Surgical options include open or laparoscopic cholecystectomy. Patients with a toxic presentation or clinical deterioration require immediate surgery.

REFERENCES

1. Gracie WA, Ransohoff DF: The natural history of silent gallstones: The innocent gallstone is not a myth. *N Engl J Med* 307:798, 1982.
2. Ikard RW: Gallstones, cholecystitis, and diabetes. *Surg Gynecol Obstet* 171:528, 1990.
3. Jorgenson T: Abdominal symptoms and gallstone disease: An epidemiological investigation. *Hepatology* 9:856, 1989.
4. Burgart LJ: Cholangitis in viral disease. *Mayo Clin Proc* 73:479, 1998.
5. Snell RS, Smith MS: *Clinical Anatomy for Emergency Medicine*. St. Louis, Mosby, 1994, pp 431–432.
6. Mergener K, Baillie J: Fortnightly review: Acute pancreatitis. *BMJ* 316:44, 1998.
7. Sondenaa K, Nesvik I, Solhaug O, et al: Randomization to surgery or observation in patients with symptomatic gallbladder stone disease: The problem of evidence-based medicine in clinical practice. *Scand J Gastroenterol* 32:611, 1997.
8. Fenstr LF, Lonborg R, Thirlby R, et al: What symptoms does cholecystectomy cure? *Am J Surg* 169:533, 1995.
9. Diehl AK, Sugarek NJ, Todd K: Clinical evaluation for gallstone disease: Usefulness of symptoms and signs in diagnosis. *Am J Med* 89:29, 1990.
10. Fisher RS, Parkman HP: Management of nonulcer dyspepsia. *N Engl J Med* 339:1376, 1998.
11. Rigas B, Torosis J, McDougall C, et al: The circadian rhythm of biliary colic. *J Clin Gastroenterol* 12:409, 1990.

12. Singer AJ, McCracken G, Henry MC: Correlation among clinical, laboratory, and hepatobiliary scanning findings in patients with suspected acute cholecystitis. *Ann Emerg Med* 28:267, 1996.
13. Gruber PJ, Silverman RA, Gottesfield S, et al: Presence of fever and leukocytosis in acute cholecystitis. *Ann Emerg Med* 28:273, 1996.
14. Adedji OA, McAdam A: Murphy's sign, acute cholecystitis, and elderly people. *J R Coll Surg Edinburgh* 41:88, 1996.
15. Parker LJ, Vukov LF, Woolan PC: Emergency department evaluation of geriatric patients with acute cholecystitis. *Acad Emerg Med* 4:51, 1997.
16. Shea JA, Berlin JA, Escarce JJ, et al: Revised estimates of diagnostic test sensitivity and specificity in suspected biliary tract disease. *Arch Intern Med* 154, 1994.
17. Fidler J, Paulson EK, Layfield L: CT evaluation of acute cholecystitis: Findings and usefulness in diagnosis. *AJR* 166:1085, 1996.
18. Meyers WC: A prospective analysis of 1518 laparoscopic cholecystectomies. *N Engl J Med* 324:1073, 1991.
19. Sugiyama M, Atami Y: Follow-up of more than 10 years after endoscopic sphincterotomy for choledocolithiasis in young patients. *Br J Surg* 85:917, 1998.

82 HEPATIC DISORDERS AND HEPATIC FAILURE

Rawden W. Evans

This chapter will briefly highlight important issues regarding the epidemiology, pathophysiology, and clinical features of acute and chronic liver disease. A rational approach to the interpretation of liver function serologies will be outlined. Specific presentations of hepatobiliary disease will be reviewed, including jaundice, cirrhosis, and complications of end-stage liver disease (ESLD), gallbladder and biliary tract disease, and vascular liver disease. Content will be limited primarily to immediate diagnostic and therapeutic concerns, avoiding discussion of the science of hepatopathology so as to focus on issues most pertinent to the practice of emergency medicine.

ACUTE AND CHRONIC LIVER DISEASE

Epidemiology

The prevalence of chronic liver disease, cirrhosis, and ESLD is steadily increasing. Chronic liver disease is currently the tenth leading cause of death among adults in the United States and accounts for 25,000 deaths yearly, or 1 percent of all deaths. The majority of ESLD (approximately 50 percent) is related to alcohol abuse. However, in recent decades, an increasing number of cases can be attributed to chronic viral hepatitis.[1–3]

Currently, hepatitis C virus (HCV) infection is the most common of all bloodborne infections in the United States, with approximately 28,000 to 180,000 new cases yearly. An estimated 3.9 million (1.8 percent) Americans have been infected. Chronic HCV infection occurs in 85 percent of patients, and chronic liver disease follows in as many as 70 percent of patients. It is further estimated that 40 percent of chronic liver disease is now related to HCV infection and results in 8000 to 10,000 deaths yearly. For perspective, HIV-related deaths number approximately 14,000 yearly. The majority of HCV-infected individuals are in the age group 30 to 49 years, and infection is often subclinical, with symptoms of chronic liver disease and cirrhosis delayed 1 to 2 decades. Therefore, it is anticipated that the number of cases of chronic liver disease related to HCV will increase sharply in the next 10 to 20 years.[4,5]

Effective vaccination against hepatitis B virus (HBV) has lead to a decline in the prevalence of related disease in the general population. Still, there are an estimated 140,000 to 320,000 cases of HBV infection yearly, with 140 to 320 deaths due to acute infections. Chronic HBV infection occurs in 6 to 10 percent of patients, with 5000 to 6000 related deaths yearly. There are currently 1 to 1.25 million Americans with chronic HBV infection.[6]

The hepatitis D virus (HDV) is uncommon and described as a defective agent because infection depends on concomitant or preexisting chronic infection by HBV. In individuals with chronic HBV infection, superinfection with HDV often results in a rapidly progressive or fulminant form of liver disease carrying a high short-term mortality rate. This variety of infection is most commonly associated with intravenous drug use.[2,3]

Hepatitis A virus (HAV) is commonly encountered by Americans, with 33 percent of the population having acquired immunity secondary to exposure. There are approximately 125,000 to 200,000 cases of HAV infection reported yearly, with an estimated 100 related deaths. Fulminant liver failure is a rare complication of HAV infection, and chronic infection does not occur.[2,7]

Acute illness with liver function test abnormalities also occurs with infection by other hepatotropic viruses such as cytomegalovirus (CMV), herpes simplex virus, Coxsackie virus, and Epstein-Barr virus (EBV), although these agents are unlikely to cause clinically evident hepatitis and jaundice in otherwise healthy individuals.

Alcoholic liver disease and viral hepatitis comprise the vast majority of cases of acute and chronic liver disease. Other causes include a variety of toxins, idiosyncratic drug reactions, and autoimmune and metabolic hepatobiliary diseases (Tables 82-1 and 82-2). The epidemiology and clinical features of these disorders are not discussed but are referenced.[1,7–9]

Pathophysiology

Hepatobiliary diseases are classified according to the main pathologic processes involved and include hepatocellular, cholestatic, immunologic, and infiltrative disorders. Considerable overlap occurs among these different processes, with a common result being progressive hepatic dysfunction along with attendant complications. The liver is the largest organ and serves as the command and control center for all major metabolic functions. The liver is central to glucose homeostasis, plasma protein and coagulation factor synthesis, lipid and lipoprotein

TABLE 82-1 Causes of Acute and Chronic Hepatitis

Condition	Cause	Examples
Acute hepatitis	Viral	Hepatitis A, B, C, D EBV CMV
	Toxins	Alcohol Carbon tetrachloride Mushroom poisoning (*Ammanita phalloides*)
	Drugs	Acetominophen Isoniazid Halothane anesthesia Chlorpromazine Erythromycin
Chronic hepatitis (>6 months)	Viral	Hepatitis B, C, D
	Drugs	Methyldopa Amiodarone Isoniazid
	Idiopathic	Autoimmune features (lupoid hepatitis) No autoimmune features
	Metabolic liver disease	Wilson disease α_1-Antitrypsin deficiency

TABLE 82-2 Causes of Chronic Liver Disease and Cirrhosis

Alcohol		
Hepatitis B and C		
Drugs	Methyldopa Methotrexate Amiodarone	
Autoimmune chronic active hepatitis		
Biliary cirrhosis	Primary	
	Secondary	Bile duct strictures Sclerosing cholangitis Biliary atresia Bile duct tumors Cystic fibrosis
Chronic hepatic congestion	Budd-Chiari syndrome Chronic right-sided heart failure Constrictive pericarditis	
Genetic metabolic diseases	Hemochromatosis Wilson's disease α_1-Antitrypsin deficiency Galactosemia	
Cryptogenic		

synthesis, bile acid synthesis and secretion, vitamin storage (B_{12}, A, D, E, and K), and the biotransformation, detoxification, and excretion of an array of both endogenous and exogenous substances.

Common to essentially all causes of chronic liver disease is ongoing hepatocellular injury and death with the progressive disruption of the functional microanatomy of the liver. Deposition of collagen in tracts of scar tissue accompanies this process and characterizes cirrhosis. Eventually, the metabolic function of the liver becomes both compromised and isolated, resulting in nutritional deficiencies, bleeding diatheses, and the accumulation of toxic metabolic wastes. The cirrhotic liver becomes increasingly resistant to blood flow from the splanchnic circulation, contributing to development of portal hypertension and portosystemic shunting of splanchnic blood through collateral veins into the general circulation. Portal hypertension results in splenomegaly and the development of gastroesophageal varices. These varices are thin-walled submucosal vessels prone to ulceration and hemorrhage. Splenomegaly contributes to anemia and thrombocytopenia. Ascites develops secondary to portal hypertension and abnormalities in renal sodium and water excretion caused by diminished glomerular filtration rate (GFR) and elevations in both aldosterone and antidiuretic hormone. Ascites is often massive, worsens chronic fatigue, and compromises respiratory function. Furthermore, ascites sets the stage for recurrent episodes of spontaneous bacterial peritonitis. Add to this the particularly debilitating occurrence of encephalopathy related to the accumulation of a variety of neurotoxic substances in the circulation. Each of these complications will be further addressed below.[1,10]

Clinical Features

Clinical presentation of acute liver disease is variable. Symptoms of hepatocellular necrosis accompanying viral hepatitis include anorexia, nausea, vomiting, and low-grade fever. Cholestatic disease is accompanied by jaundice of varying degree, pruritus, clay-colored stools, and dark urine. Biliary colic implies acute obstructive cholestasis of extrahepatic or mechanical etiology, as in common duct gallstones or rapidly growing tumors. Cholestasis resulting from intrahepatic processes and infiltrative disease presents more insidiously with the slow development of jaundice and few other constitutional complaints.

Chronic liver disease often presents with complications of advancing cirrhosis and portal hypertension that include abdominal pain, ascites, gastrointestinal bleeding, fever, and altered mental status. However, progressive generalized fatigue is not uncommonly the only symptom of chronic liver disease in the absence of supervening complications.

Features of history are sometimes useful: sexual behaviors, travel, volume and duration of alcohol use, illicit drug use, consumption of nutritional supplements (vitamin A), history of blood transfusions, needle-stick blood exposures, herbal remedies, mushroom ingestion, or raw oyster consumption. Family history may be revealing. Gilbert's syndrome is a relatively common and benign familial condition revealed by periodic modest elevations in unconjugated bilirubin, particularly in response to the stress of an acute illness. Family history of jaundice (elevated conjugated bilirubin) may indicate the presence of Dubin-Johnson or Rotor syndrome. The differential diagnosis of familial severe premature liver disease includes Wilson's disease, hemochromatosis, or α_1-antitrypsin deficiency. These uncommon disorders are mentioned because the emergency physician routinely sees and hence screens a large number of patients and is therefore more likely to encounter such diseases.

Physical findings of acute hepatitis are often limited to moderate enlargement of the liver and tenderness. Chronic liver disease is accompanied by a host of physical findings, including sallow complexion, appendicular wasting, palmar erythema, distinctive cutaneous spider nevi, parotid gland enlargement, and testicular atrophy and gynecomastia in males. The liver may be uniformly enlarged and firm or, in advanced cirrhosis, shrunken and grossly nodular. Splenomegaly and ascites accompany portal hypertension.

Liver Function Tests

Liver function tests might better be termed simply *liver tests,* since routine test panels do not assess function as much as serving as general markers of hepatobiliary disease. Liver tests are obtained frequently in emergency medicine practice, and abnormalities of an incidental nature are common. Abnormal liver tests results are found in as many as one-third of those screened, with the incidence of clinically significant liver disease in this fraction only about 1 percent. Questions often arise regarding what to make of the isolated abnormality and, further, how to interpret a pattern of abnormalities to aid in making a specific diagnosis. Each test will be discussed briefly, with an emphasis placed on results that provide specific diagnostic utility.[12,13]

Bilirubin Bilirubin is a breakdown product of hemoglobin and the other heme-containing proteins myogobin and the cytochromes. Unconjugated bilirubin is a poorly soluble anion that travels in the circulation bound tightly to albumin. Unconjugated bilirubin is efficiently taken up by the liver, where it undergoes conjugation and secretion into the bile. The majority of bilirubin is excreted in stool, and a fraction is reabsorbed through the enterohepatic circulation. Test panels usually report total bilirubin and the ''indirect'' fraction representing unconjugated bilirubin. The conjugated fraction is derived simply as the difference between total and indirect. (Note: *Direct* and *indirect* fractions refer to reagent reactivity in the bilirubin assay and have no pathophysiologic meaning.) Total serum bilirubin is normally less than 1.1 mg/dL, and the indirect fraction (unconjugated) is 70 percent. Any disease state increasing bilirubin production or interfering with hepatic bilirubin metabolism and secretion can result in elevations in total bilirubin and variable elevations in the conjugated and unconjugated fractions. The differential diagnosis of these conditions is discussed below.

Transaminases Serum transaminases aspartate aminotransferase (AST) and alanine aminotransferase (ALT) are markers of both hepatocellular disease and hepatobiliary dysfunction. Serum AST derives primarily from the liver but is also released by the heart, smooth muscle, kidney, and brain and is thus relatively nonspecific. A number of medications cause increased AST, including acetaminophen; nonsteroidal anti-inflammatory drugs (NSAIDs); ACE inhibitors; nicotinic acid; the antibiotics isoniazid, sulfonamides, and erythromycin; and the antifungals griseofulvin and fluconazole. ALT is a more specific marker of hepatocellular disease. Mild elevations of the transaminases in the hundreds of units per liter indicate ongoing inflammatory hepatocellular damage as in viral hepatitis and subclinical exposure to hepatotoxic drugs and chemicals. Values in the thousands suggest acute hepatocellular necrosis and signify extensive liver injury as characterizes more fulminant disease or ischemia (so-called shock liver). The value in measuring both enzymes is in consideration of AST : ALT ratios. Ratios greater than 2 are common in alcoholic hepatitis because AST production is stimulated by alcohol. In acute and chronic viral hepatitis, the ratio is generally less than 1. In the absence of ongoing alcohol use, mild elevations of AST and ALT with a ratio greater than 1 suggests the presence of underlying cirrhosis.

Alkaline Phosphatase Elevated alkaline phosphatase (AP) is associated with biliary obstruction and cholestasis. However, mild to moderate elevations accompany virtually all hepatobiliary disease. As a rule of thumb, AP elevations greater than four times normal indicate cholestasis as opposed to primary hepatocellular processes such as hepatitis. Elevations also may be a nonspecific finding because AP is derived from bone, placenta, intestine, kidneys, and leukocytes. Specificity can be increased by comeasurement of the enzyme gamma-glutamyl transpeptidase (GGTP), which when elevated supports the diagnosis of a cholestasis. However, like AST, GGTP production is stimulated by alcohol consumption and is also elevated by drugs inducing hepatic microsomal enzyme activity such as phenobarbital and warfarin. GGTP elevations are also seen in acute and chronic pancreatitis, acute myocardial infarction, uremia, chronic obstructive pulmonary disease, rheumatoid arthritis, and diabetes mellitus. Isolated significant elevations of AP in the absence of marked hyperbilirubinemia (AP : bilirubin of 1000 : 1) is characteristic of infiltrative and granulomatous liver disease such as lymphoma, fungal infections, sarcoidosis, and tuberculosis. The uncommon conditions primary biliary cirrhosis and primary sclerosing cholangitis also produce AP elevations disproportional to bilirubin levels. AP levels in healthy children are often two- to threefold higher than the upper limit of normal for adults. Likewise, doubling of AP levels is common and normal in pregnancy. Incidental findings of three- to fivefold elevations in transaminase levels and doubling of AP in otherwise healthy diabetics and the obese suggest the presence of nonalcoholic steatohepatitis (NASH). Other conditions associated with NASH include jejunoileal bypass, total parenteral nutrition, hyper- and hypothyroidism, and the antiarrhythmic drug amiodarone.[14]

Lactate Dehydrogenase Lactate dehydrogenase (LDH) is often included in liver test panels, although its lack of specificity is limiting. Moderate elevations are seen in all hepatocellular disorders and cirrhosis, but less so in purely cholestatic conditions. LDH may become significantly elevated as a result of hemolysis and accompany a related increase in unconjugated bilirubin. The isoenzyme LDH-5 is specific to the liver and sometimes useful, though not widely available.

Ammonia Metabolism of nitrogen-containing compounds results in the generation of ammonia, which is further metabolized to urea via the Krebs cycle in the liver. Elevated serum ammonia may occur in acute and chronic liver disease as a manifestation of hepatic metabolic failure. Very high ammonia levels are seen in fulminant liver failure, contributing to overall toxicity and signifying poor prognosis. In cirrhosis with worsening portal hypertension and isolation of remaining functional hepatic tissue, ammonia formed by colonic bacteria is carried into the general circulation. This process is worsened by large intestinal protein loads as occurs with gastrointestinal bleeding. However, elevated serum ammonia levels do not reliably correlate with acute worsening of hepatic function in the cirrhotic and serve more as a marker of generalized decline than as a useful diagnostic tool or therapeutic end point.

Prothrombin Time Prolongation of prothromin time (PT) in liver disease reflects the decreased synthesis of the vitamin K–dependent coagulation factors II, VII, IX, and X and as such serves as a real measure of liver function. Prolonged PT is seen typically as a complication of advancing cirrhosis, although it also may be seen in acute hepatitis and exacerbations of chronic, but otherwise compensated, liver disease. When present in acute viral hepatitis, prolonged PT often indicates more severe disease reflecting widespread hepatocellular necrosis. There is a degree of correlation between the extent of PT prolongation and clinical outcome in fulminant liver disease. Abnormalities in PT are also seen in conditions affecting lipid assimilation by the gut because vitamin K is fat soluble. Cholestatic syndromes interfere with fat absorption and thereby promote vitamin K deficiency. Distinguishing vitamin K deficiency from liver synthetic dysfunction can be accomplished by administering parenteral vitamin K (phytonadione 10 mg IM), which should result in a 30 percent reduction in PT within 24 h.

Albumin Like PT, albumin level is a reflection of liver synthetic function. It may be decreased in advancing cirrhosis or severe cases of acute hepatitis, serving as a marker of poor short-term prognosis. Albumin level is not as useful in evaluating fulminant liver disease because its serum half-life is approximately 3 weeks, whereas PT becomes prolonged in a matter of days. Serum albumin is also a reflection of overall nutritional status, and a low value may be nonspecific in a chronically ill individual.

Viral Hepatitis Serology Serum testing for viral hepatitis is often offered as screening panels by hospital laboratories. In hepatitis A, the IgM anti-HAV is detectable at the onset of clinical illness. Hepatitis B serology is somewhat more complicated. Hepatitis B surface antigen (HBsAg) is measurable before clinical illness and elevations in tranaminases are seen, and remains elevated for 1 to 2 months. Antibodies to the hepatitis B core antigen (anti-HBc) appear 2 weeks after HBsAg, and their presence is useful in defining the so-called window period before antibody to the surface antigen (anti-HBsAg) appears. Thus anti-HBc may be the only reliably positive test in the window period and also provides a rough estimate of the time of exposure for epidemiologic purposes. Antibody testing for hepatitis C has become standardized in recent years and is now part of all viral hepatitis screening panels. The alphabetized nomenclature is expanding as more infectious agents responsible for acute and chronic liver disease are recognized. However, hepatitis A, B, and C remain the principal varieties of concern to practitioners in North America.[2,3]

Nonhepatic Causes of Abnormal Liver Tests Hypoalbuminemia accompanies protein wasting enteropathies, malnutrition, and nephrotic syndrome. Alkaline phosphatase elevations occur with a variety of bone diseases, pregnancy, and malignancies. AST elevations accompany acute myocardial infarction and rhabdomyolysis. Bilirubin elevations occur in severe hemolysis, sepsis, and syndromes involving abnormal erythropoesis. PT elevations occur in vitamin K deficiency, chronic antibiotic use, warfarin therapy, and long-standing steatorrhea.

SPECIFIC CLINICAL SYNDROMES

Jaundice

Defined, *jaundice* is simply the yellow pigmentation imparted to the skin, sclera, and mucous membranes by bilirubin when elevated in a host of diseases. Jaundice develops when there is an overproduction of bilirubin and/or a defect in hepatic bilirubin uptake, conjugative metabolism, or biliary excretion. Clinical jaundice reflects hyperbilirubinemia. The clinical syndromes of jaundice are broadly divided into those characterized by predominate elevations in unconjugated or conjugated bilirubin. Unconjugated hyperbilirubinemias are less common and reflect overproduction, decreased hepatic uptake, and decreased conjugation. Conjugated hyperbilirubinemias result from a variety of processes that cause cholestasis, broadly divided as intrahepatic and extrahepatic. Table 82-3 outlines the distinguishing clinical features of these general classifications, and Table 82-4 provides a differential diagnosis useful once a categorical diagnosis is made.

Generalizations may benefit the emergency practitioner. A degree of unconjugated hyperbilirubinemia accompanies all hepatocellular diseases, but primary elevations in unconjugated bilirubin are rare and mostly limited to the infant pediatric population, as in neonatal jaundice and Crigler-Najjar syndrome. In the absence of severe underlying or concomitant liver disease, hemolysis does not result in jaundice. Jaundice presenting in the acutely ill and febrile patient will reflect either viral hepatitis or bacterial cholangitis; a distinction may be made by noting that cholangitis is usually accompanied by much greater elevations in alkaline phosphatase. The subacute presentation of jaundice in the patient without a history of chronic liver disease is most likely the result of infiltrative disease or slowly obstructing extrahepatic tumor, as in the head of the pancreas.[15,16]

A patient with fulminant liver failure (acute hepatic necrosis) presents as acutely ill with jaundice and often complications related to impaired hepatic function, including encephalopathy, coagulopathy, and water, electrolyte, and acid-base metabolic disorders (Table 82-5). Progression of disease to complete liver failure often occurs in 8 weeks or less. The appropriate emergency response to such patients involves recognizing the severity of the illness, instituting appropriate resuscitation, assembling an appropriate database including liver serologies and toxicology screens, and arranging for appropriate inpatient care as indicated by the acuity of the presentation. Appropriate guidelines for inpatient management should be based on age, underlying medical conditions, hemodynamic stability on presentation, and response to initial resuscitation measures. General hospital admission is indicated for management of refractory nausea, vomiting, and dehydration; intensive care unit admission is reserved for patients with encephalopathy, hemorrhage, or hemodynamic instability, especially when a question of sepsis is entertained; and transfer of the patient with fulminant liver failure to a tertiary facility with transplant capabilities would be appropriate.[17,18]

Cirrhosis and Complications of End-Stage Liver Disease

Hepatic cirrhosis results from fibrous scarring mixed with hepatocellular regeneration in response to sustained inflammatory, toxic, metabolic, and congestive insults. Over time, the functional anatomy of the liver is replaced by scar tissue isolating nodules formed by foci of regenerating hepatocytes. Normal function of the liver is dependent not only on preservation of hepatocyte number but also on the elaborate microscopic architecture of the functional hepatic units. In addition to progressive loss of synthetic and metabolic function, scarring and degeneration of the liver contribute to increased resistance to blood flow from the splanchnic circulation, contributing to portal-systemic shunting and portal hypertension. Shunting isolates the remaining functional tissue of the liver, further contributing to the metabolic derangements that characterize progressive and end-stage liver disease. Emergent complications of cirrhosis and end-stage liver disease include gastroesophageal variceal hemorrhage, refractory ascites and spontaneous bacterial peritonitis, hepatorenal syndrome, and hepatic encephalopathy.[1,19]

Gastroesophageal Varices and Hemorrhage Cirrhosis results in a progressive increase in resistance to portal blood flow through the liver and shunting of blood through venous collaterals into the systemic circulation. Increased blood flow and pressure in these collateral veins contribute to the formation of submucosal varices in the gastric fundus

TABLE 82-3 Classification of Jaundice and Clinical Findings

	Types of Jaundice			
Diagnostic Factors	Hemolytic	Hepatocellular	Intrahepatic Cholestatic	Extrahepatic Cholestatic
Symptoms	None, or back ache and joint pain	Nausea, vomiting, fever, anorexia	Deep jaundice, dark urine, light stools, pruritus	Deep jaundice, dark urine, light stools, pruritus, cholangitis, biliary colic
Physical findings	Splenomegaly	Tender hepatomegaly ± splenomegaly	Tender hepatomegaly	Hepatomegaly ± palpable gallbladder
LFTs				
Bilirubin				
Total	<6 mg/dL	Variable	Variable (may be >30 mg/dL)	<30 mg/dL
Direct	<20%	>50%	>50%	>50%
ALT	Normal	>5 × normal	2–5 × normal	<2–3 × normal; >3–5 × normal in presence of cholangitis
Alkaline phosphatase	Normal	<2–3 × normal	>3–5 × normal	>3–5 × normal
PT	Normal	Prolonged*	Prolonged†	Prolonged†
Ultrasound: Biliary dilation?	No	No	No	Yes

*When condition is severe and/or sustained and advanced, implies hepatocellular synthetic failure.

TABLE 82-4 Differential Diagnosis of Hyperbilirubinemias

Classification	Pathophysiology	Specific Conditions
Unconjugated hyperbilirubinemia (bilirubin >80% indirect)	Overproduction	Hemolysis Spherocytosis Autoimmune disorders Erythropoetic disorders
	Decreased hepatic uptake	Gilbert's syndrome Drug related Rifampin Contrast agents Neonatal jaundice
	Decreased conjugation	Gilbert's syndrome Crigler-Najjar syndrome Neonatal jaundice Hepatocellular disease Drug inhibition—chloramphenicol
Conjugated hyperbilirubinemia (bilirubin >50% direct)	Intrahepatic cholestasis (impaired hepatic secretion)	Familial disorders (Rotor syndrome, Dubin-Johnson, benign recurrent cholestasis, cholestasis of pregnancy) Hepatocellular disease Drug-induced cholestasis (phenothiazines, OCP, erythromycin, methyltestosterone) Primary biliary cirrhosis Gram-negative sepsis Postoperative
	Extrahepatic cholestasis (mechanical obstruction to bile flow)	Common duct gallstones Bacterial cholangitis Tumors Pancreatic head Bile duct Ampulla of Vater Strictures Postoperative Primary sclerosing cholangitis Congenital

and esophagus. These superficial and thin-walled varices are prone to ulceration and hemorrhage. Gastroesophageal variceal hemorrhage is a common and dangerous complication of hepatic cirrhosis and portal hypertension. The prevalence among cirrhotics is approximately 25 to 70 percent. Acute hemorrhage carries a 30 to 60 percent mortality rate.

Hemorrhage is heralded by hematemesis, hematochezia, and/or melena, plus varying degrees of hemodynamic instability. Complicating factors include preexisting anemia, thrombocytopenia, and coagulopathy. The differential diagnosis of acute gastrointestinal hemorrhage in the cirrhotic is less important than identification of a condition that requires aggressive managment and appropriate consultation. Basic priorities in management include airway protection and appropriate intravenous access for the infusion of fluids and blood products. Significant coagulopathy should be assumed, and placement of central venous catheters should be performed with extreme caution. Gastric lavage is indicated when active bleeding is suspected to evacuate the stomach and help alleviate repeated vomiting, which can exacerbate hemorrhage. Gastric lavage provides some indication of the location of hemorrhage and a gross assessment of ongoing blood loss. The presence of known gastroesophageal varices is not a contraindication

TABLE 82-5 Fulminant Liver Failure

Presentation	Causes/Associations	Complications	Treatment Priorities
Acute hepatocellular necrosis with rapid development of encephalopathy and liver failure developing in <8 weeks	Hepatitis B, C, D Hepatitis A (rare) Hepatotoxins Acetominophen Isoniazid Halothane Valproic acid Mushrooms Carbon tetrachloride (Reye's syndrome and acute fatty liver of pregnancy resemble fulminant liver failure, but microvesicular fatty infiltation occurs without hepatocellular necrosis)	Encephalopathy Hypoglycemia Hyponatremia Hypokalemia GI hemorrhage Renal failure Cerebral edema	Supportive Correction of electrolyte abnormalities Blood products to correct losses and coagulopathy Dialysis Hyperalimentation Care at appropriate tertiary facility anticipating transplantation

TABLE 82-6 Pharmacologic Adjuncts to Management of Acute Gastroesophageal Variceal Hemorrhage

Agent	Dosing	Cautions
Vasopressin (pitressin, ADH)	Bolus therapy 20 units in 100 cc D_5W IV over 20 min, repeating at 2–4 h intervals. or Continuous infusion 100 units in 250 cc D_5W (0.4 units/cc) IV at 6–24 units/h (16–60 cc/h)	Arterial vasospasm* Myocardial ischemia/infarction Arrhythmias CVA Mesenteric ischemia Limb ischemia
Terlipressin	1–2 mg q4–6h IV	Similar to vasopressin*
Somatostatin	Bolus 250 μg IV, then 250–500 μg/h continuous IV infusion	Minimal adverse side effects
Octreotide (Sandostatin)	Bolus 50 μg IV, then 50 μg/h continuous IV infusion	Minimal adverse side effects

*Adverse side effects may be attenuated by coadministration of nitroglycerin by IV drip, titrating upward for a systolic blood pressure >100 mmHg.

to the careful placement of a nasogastric or orogastric tube. Consultation for emergent endoscopy should be arranged as soon as possible. Endoscopy provides a definitive diagnosis and often a direct means for hemorrhage control by sclerotherapy. Unavailability of such consultation should prompt consideration of early transfer.[20]

In addition to the replacement of blood loss with fluids and blood products, the pharmacologic agents vasopressin and somatostatin have been shown to be useful short-term measures to stem variceal hemorrhage (see Table 82-6). Both agents produce a reduction in portal venous blood pressure, although by importantly different mechanisms. Vasopressin causes splanchnic arteriolar constriction, reducing portal venous inflow and pressure. Somatostatin decreases splanchnic blood flow by causing a direct and selective relaxation of mesenteric vascular smooth muscle. Vasopressin action is nonspecific and has potential for undesireable cardiac and hemodynamic side effects, particularly in older individuals. Coronary vasospasm can cause cardiac ischemia, infarction, and arrhythmias. There is also potential for stroke and mesenteric and limb ischemia. To attenuate these complications, some authorities recommend the coadministration of nitroglycerin by continuous intravenous infusion starting at 40 μg/min and titrating upward for a systolic blood pressure of more than 100 mmHg. Terlipressin is a synthetic derivative of vasopressin that is slowly converted to vasopressin in vivo. Terlipressin has a much longer half-life than vassopressin and has been shown to be superior in a comparison study. This drug is not widely available, but the studied treatment protocol used 1 to 2 mg IV every 4 to 6 h and was compatible with the coadministration of intravenous nitroglycerin.[20–22]

Somatostatin has been demonstrated to be effective in reducing variceal bleeding without significant adverse side effects. The short half-life of somatostatin (1–2 min) has limited its usefulness. Octreotide (Sandostatin), an analogue of somatostatin, has been demonstrated to be as effective as injection sclerotherapy in the management of acute variceal hemorrhage and is considered by many to be a useful primary therapy and adjunct to sclerotherapy. Octreotide may be particularly beneficial in the management of hemodynamically unstable patients undergoing resuscitation but unable to tolerate emergent endoscopy. Octreotide has minimal hemodynamic side effects, giving it a distinct advantage over vasopressin[20–23] (Table 82-6).

Balloon tamponade with inflated gastroesophageal obturators such as the Sengstaken-Blakemore tube is used infrequently because of the high rate of complications and the increasing effectiveness and availability of endoscopic sclerotherapy. Principal complications of these devices include bronchopulmonary aspiration and esophageal rupture. β Blockers and portosystemic shunt surgery or transjugular intrahepatic portosystemic shunts (TIPS) are effective prophylactic measures in some patients with gastroesophageal varices but have no proven role in the management of acute gastroesophageal hemorrhage.

Ascites and Spontaneous Bacterial Peritonitis Ascites and anasarca occur in hepatic cirrhosis as a result of portal hypertension, impaired renal sodium and water excretion, and hypoalbuminemia. When extreme, ascites may cause immobility, abdominal pain, and respiratory compromise. Umbilical hernia is common in this setting, and hernia ulceration with rupture, although rare, is a life-threatening complication.[24] Primary or spontaneous bacterial peritonitis (SBP) is the most frequently encountered complication of cirrhotic ascites, with a yearly risk of approximately 29 percent. The presentation of SBP usually includes fever, abdominal pain, and diffuse abdominal tenderness, but it may be relatively silent and present only with subacute functional decline or worsening in baseline encephalopathy[26,27] (Table 82-7).

SBP is diagnosed by sampling the ascitic fluid by paracentesis. Ideally, ascitic fluid is localized and marked for paracentesis by ultrasound to ensure fluid recovery and avoid encountering intestine during the procedure. In the absence of ultrasound, ascitic fluid can be localized with relative safety by percussion of dullness in the lateral aspects of the lower quadrants with the patient semirecumbant. Alternately, the patient is positioned supine, resting partially on the side where the paracentesis is to be performed. In choosing the site for puncture, avoid areas proximate to remote surgery. The site is prepared and

TABLE 82-7 Diagnosis and Treatment of Spontaneous Bacterial Peritonitis

Setting	Cirrhosis with ascites
Presentation	Fever, abdominal pain and tenderness ± worsening encephalopathy
Diagnosis	Ascitic fluid WBC > 1000/mm³ PMN > 250/mm³
Treatment	Cefotaxime 2 g IV, or Standard dosages of TC/CL,* PIP/TZ,* or AMP/SB* Alternate: ceftriaxone 2 g IV, or ofloxacin 400 mg PO bid†
Disposition	Hospitalize, unless clinically well, compliant, with access to timely follow-up†

*TC/CL = ticarcillin-clavulanate (Timentin), PIP/TZ = piperacillin-tazobactam (Zosyn), AMP/SB = ampicillin-sulbactam (Unasyn).
†Oral therapy with ofloxacin reserved for clinically well and compliant patients with ready access to timely follow-up.

draped in a sterile fashion, and lidocaine is infiltrated locally for anesthesia. An 18- or 20-gauge angiocatheter on a 20-cc syringe is adequate for fluid sampling. Postprocedural leaking of ascitic fluid can be lessened by advancing the catheter in a Z fashion through the skin, subcutaneous fat, and abdominal wall or by placing traction on the overlying skin prior to puncture so that on removing the catheter there is a lateral distance between the skin puncture and the peritoneum. Ascitic fluid is a transudate with protein content generally less than 3 g/dL. Culture results are frequently negative; however, yield can be improved by drawing 10 cc of fluid and processing it as a blood culture. Cell count with white blood cell (WBC) differential is ordered. A total WBC count in excess of $1000/mm^3$ and/or neutrophil count (PMNs) greater than $250/mm^3$ is considered diagnostic for SBP. The Enterobacteriaceae account for 63 percent of infections, *Streptococcus pneumoniae* 15 percent, enteroccoci 6 to 10 percent, and anaerobes less than 1 percent. Appropriate antibiotic regimens are outlined in Table 82-7.[35]

Occasionally patients present with refractory and incapacitating ascites as a primary complaint. Associated symptoms include extreme fatigue, increased respiratory effort, and orthopnea. These individuals often have failed maximal diuretic therapy and have undergone high-volume paracentesis in the past. Before performing this procedure, it is useful to consult with the patient's primary care provider or hepatologist to review a protocol. As much as 6 to 8 L of ascitic fluid can be drained over a 60- to 90-min interval with the concomitant peripheral infusion of albumin (6–8 g/L of ascites collected). Many practitioners believe the albumin infusion is unnecessary when peripheral edema is present because mobilization of edema fluid attenuates intravascular volume loss. Complications of the procedure are not infrequent and include hemorrhage, infection, acute renal failure, and hemodynamic compromise. Such patients may be ideal candidates for an observation unit or short-stay admission.[28]

Hepatorenal Syndrome Hepatorenal syndrome is characterized by acute renal failure in the cirrhotic patient in the presence of histologically normal kidneys. The exact pathophysiology is elusive but is tied in with the metabolic derangments of end-stage liver failure, decreased effective circulating blood volume, and elevated aldosterone and antidiuretic hormone secretion. GFR drops, as does urine sodium secretion, and azotemia worsens with blood urea nitrogen–creatinine ratios usually greater than 20. This characteristic and refractory form of renal failure complicates cirrhosis with ascites and can be precipitated by any acute illness resulting in dehydration and/or sepsis or as a complication of overzealous diuresis or high-volume paracentesis. The ill cirrhotic patient with evidence of acute or worsening renal insufficiency should be hospitalized for appropriate consultation and carefully monitored intravenous fluid administration and diuretic therapy adjustment.[29]

Hepatic Encephalopathy Hepatic encephalopathy is a complex syndrome that often accompanies acute or fulminant liver failure and frequently complicates the course and management of cirrhotics. In acute or fulminant liver failure, encephalopathy occurs in response to the metabolic insults of the disease and also cerebral edema. In chronic liver disease, fluctuating encephalopathy occurs in response to the accumulation of a variety of nitrogenous metabolic wastes normally cleared by the liver and also the prolonged effects of incompletely metabolized substances ingested such as prescription drugs and other more overt hepatotoxins such as acetominophen, NSAIDs, and alcohol.[30]

To appreciate the presence or worsening of baseline encephalopathy, one must determine the patient's underlying functional status. Questions related to changes in personality, worsening dementia, alterations in level of consciousness, and neuromuscular function should be pursued. The staging of hepatic encephalopathy is outlined in Table 82-8. Asterixis characterizes stage II and is a manifestation of neuromuscular weakness made evident when the patient tries to maintain a certain posture. Typically, the hands begin to "flap" when the patient is asked to hold the hands up and extended at the wrist ("stop traffic"). Alternately, the tongue moves back and forth like a snake when the patient is asked to keep his or her tongue extended. Serum ammonia level is often measured in this setting and is frequently significantly elevated. However, this is a nonspecific finding, and ammonia levels are notoriously inaccurate. Thus ammonia may serve as a marker but not as an index of encephalopathy. The list of potential causes of encephalopathy in the cirrhotic patient is long and includes gastrointestinal bleeding, increased dietary protein intake, constipation, infection/sepsis, drugs (frequently benzodiazepines, opiates, or commonly prescribed "muscle relaxers"), acute worsening of hepatic function, or electrolyte and acid-base disturbances. Falls are not uncommon in this population and, along with coagulopathy, place them at increased risk of head injury and intracranial bleeding. Therefore, computed tomographic (CT) imaging of the head is appropriate in the evaluation. The majority of cirrhotics presenting with acute or worsening encephalopathy are best served by hospitalization. There is the occasional patient presenting with a baseline of variable encephalopathy who appears otherwise well (stage I or II) and has an unrevealing workup for serious causes of mental deterioration who may be managed successfully as an outpatient. The cathartic lactulose is prescribed at a dose of 30 cc three times daily until one or two soft stools are produced daily. Lactulose traps ammonia within the lumen of the gut by decreasing intestinal pH and stimulates bacterial uptake of ammonia into fixed bacterial proteins. The antibiotic neomycin is an alternative therapy that decreases intestinal bacterial number, thus reducing toxic substances generated by bacterial protein degradation. Neomycin can be prescribed as 1 g four times daily; infrequent side effects include oto- and nephrotoxicity.

TABLE 82-8 Staging of Hepatic Encephalopathy

Stages	Features
I	General apathy
II	Lethargy, drowsiness, variable orientation, asterixis
III	Stupor with hyperreflexia, extensor plantar reflexes
IV	Coma

Gallbladder and Biliary Tract Disease

Gallstones are the most common cause of biliary tract disease in the United States. Gallstones occur in 20 to 35 percent of the population by age 75 years but in the majority are asymptomatic. Acute colicky pain localizing to the right upper quadrant accompanied by nausea and vomiting, sometimes with a finding of a palpable and tender gallbladder, characterizes gallstone obstruction of the cholecystic duct. The acutely ill patient frequently will give a history of past episodes of postprandial pain, although less severe or prolonged. Typically, pain is of rapid onset and slow resolution with a pattern of radiation to the right lower scapula or right shoulder. Fever and toxicity suggest infection and cholecystitis. Gallstone obstruction of the common bile duct produces pain, frequently mild jaundice, and serologies suggesting biliary obstruction, hepatocellular injury, and pancreatitis. Fever and toxicity suggest infection and cholangitis. The diagnosis usually can be made by clinical presentation, serologies, and ultrasonography. There is an approximate 5 percent incidence of "acalculus cholecystitis" that is usually a late complication of concurrent severe illness or injury, prolonged fasting, or surgery or is related to hyperalimentation.

Gallbladder disease is common in the elderly, who often present late in the course of their illness with a higher rate of infectious complications, perforation, and subsequent mortality. Symptoms in the elderly are often nonspecific and nonlocalizing, requiring greater vigilance on the part of the emergency practitioner. When infection is an apparent complication, initial antibiotic therapy should cover Enterobacteriaceae, enterococci, *Bacteroides,* and *Clostridium* species. See Table 82-9 for specific antibiotic recommendations.[31,35]

Vascular Disease of the Liver

Vascular diseases of the liver are relatively uncommon when compared with the aforementioned conditions, and their diagnoses are unlikely to be made during an evaluation in the emergency department. However, these conditions warrant brief inclusion because their consideration in the evaluation of the acutely ill patient is key to timely diagnosis, treatment, and ultimately improved outcome. These conditions include portal vein thrombosis, hepatic vein thrombosis (Budd-Chiari syndrome), and nonthrombotic venoocclusive disease.

Portal vein thrombosis can result as a late complication of abdominal trauma, sepsis, pancreatitis, and hypercoagulable states and in neonates with umbilical vein infection. Portal hypertension and related complications develop in a subacute manner. Splenomegaly may occur in the absence of hepatomegaly, and liver histology is normal. The diagnosis is made by angiography, and therapy is surgical.[32]

Hepatic vein thrombosis, or Budd-Chiari syndrome, has both acute and chronic presentations that include abdominal pain, hepatomegaly, ascites, and usually mild alterations in liver serologies. Causes and associations include a history of abdominal trauma, oral contraceptive use, polycythemia vera, paroxysmal nocturnal hemoglobinuria, hypercoagulable states, and congenital webs of the vena cava. Diagnosis can be made by Doppler ultrasound of the hepatic veins, and therapy includes anticoagulation.[33]

Nonthrombotic occlusion of hepatic venules creating a small-vessel variant of Budd-Chiari syndrome is associated with the ingestion of certain medicinal teas containing pyrrolozidine alkaloids. These alkaloids are found in *Senecio* and *Crotalia* genera of plants.[34] Venoocclusive hepatic disease also occurs rarely as a complication of chemotherapy and bone marrow transplantation.

TABLE 82-9 Antibiotic Treatment of Cholecystitis and Cholangitis

Regimens	Antibiotics
Primary	Ticarcillin or piperacillin 4.0 g IV plus Metronidazole 1.0 g IV or Ampicillin 2.0 g IV plus Gentamicin 2 mg/kg IV plus Metronidazole 1.0 g IV or Single agents: Imipenem Meropenem TC/CL* PIP/TZ* AMP/SB*
Alternative	Third-generation cephalosporin plus metronidazole or clindamycin or Aztreonam plus clindamycin

*TC/CL = ticarcillin-clavulanate (Timentin), PIP/TZ = piperacillin-tazobactam (Zosyn), AMP/SB = ampicillin-sulbactam (Unasyn).

REFERENCES

1. Williams EJ, Iredale JP: Liver cirrhosis. *Postgrad Med J* 74(870):193, 1998.
2. Centers for Disease Control and Prevention: Hepatitis home page: *www.cdc.gov/ncidod/diseases/hepatitis/index.htm.*
3. Bondesson JD, Saperston AR: Hepatitis. *Emerg Med Clin North Am* 14(4):695, 1996.
4. Alter MJ, Margolis HS: Recommendations for prevention and control of hepatitis C virus (HCV) infection and HCV-related chronic disease. *MMWR* 47(RR-19):1, 1998.
5. Gross JB Jr: Clinician's guide to hepatitis C. *Mayo Clin Proc* 73(4):355, 1998.
6. Lee WM: Medical progress: Hepatitis B virus infection. *N Engl J Med* 337(24):1733, 1997.
7. Koff R: Hepatitis A. *Lancet* 351(9116):1643, 1998.
8. Lee WM: Medical progress: Drug-induced hepatotoxicity. *N Engl J Med* 333(17):1118, 1995.
9. Krawitt EL: Medical progress: Autoimmune hepatitis. *N Engl J Med* 334(14):897, 1996.
10. Kaplan MM: Medical progress: Primary biliary cirrhosis. *N Engl J Med* 335(21):1570, 1996.
11. Friedman S: Seminars in medicine of the Beth Israel Hospital, Boston: The cellular basis of hepatic fibrosis. Mechanisms and treatment strategies. *N Engl J Med* 328(25):1828, 1993.
12. Kamath PS: Clinical approach to the patient with abnormal liver test results. *Mayo Clin Proc* 71(11):1089, 1996.
13. Aranda-Michel J, Sherman KE: Tests of the liver: Use and misuse. *Gastroenterologist* 6(1):34, 1998.
14. O'Connor BJ, Kathamna B, Tavill AS: Nonalcoholic fatty liver (NASH syndrome). *Gastroenterologist* 5(4):316, 1997.
15. Gordon SC: Jaundice and cholestasis: Some common and uncommon causes. *Postgrad Med* 90(4):65, 1991.
16. Frank BB: Clinical evaluation of jaundice: A guideline of the Patient Care Committee of the American Gastroenterological Association. *JAMA* 262(21):3031, 1989.
17. Lee WM: Medical progress: Acute liver failure. *N Engl J Med* 329(25):1862, 1993.
18. Caraceni P, Van Thiel DH: Acute liver failure. *Lancet* 345(8943):163, 1995.
19. McGuire BM, Bloomer JR: Complications of cirrhosis: Why they occur and what to do about them. *Postgrad Med* 103(2):209, 1998.
20. Roberts LR, Kamath PS: Pathophysiology and treatment of variceal hemorrhage. *Mayo Clin Proc*71(10):973, 1996.
21. Burroughs AK: Pharmacologic treatment of acute variceal bleeding. *Digestion* 59(suppl 2):28, 1998.
22. Conn HO, Lebrec D, Terblanche J: The treatment of oesophageal varices: A debate and a discussion. *J Intern Med* 241(2):103, 1997.
23. Lamberts SWJ, van der Lely A, de Herder WW, Hofland LJ: Drug therapy: Octreotide. *N Engl J Med* 334(4):246, 1996.
24. Belghiti J, Durand F: Abdominal wall hernias in the setting of cirrhosis. *Semin Liver Dis* 17(3):219, 1997.
25. King PD, Rumbaut R, Sanchez C: Pulmonary manifestations of chronic liver disease. *Dig Dis* 14(2):73–82, 1996.
26. Runyon BA: Current concepts: Care of patients with ascites. *N Engl J Med* 330(5):337, 1994.
27. Guarner C, Soriano G: Spontaneous bacterial peritonitis. *Semin Liver Dis* 17(3):203, 1997.
28. Forouzandeh B, Konicek F, Sheagren JN: Large-volume paracentesis in the treatment of cirrhotic patients with refractory ascites: The role of post-paracentesis plasma volume expansion. *J Clin Gastroenterol* 22(3):207, 1996.
29. Roberts R, Kamath PS: Ascites and hepatorenal syndrome: Pathophysiology and management. *Mayo Clin Proc* 71(9):874, 1996.
30. Riordan SM, Williams R: Current concepts: Treatment of hepatic encephalopathy. *N Engl J Med* 337(7):473, 1997.
31. Johnston DE, Kaplan MM: Medical progress: Pathogenesis and treatment of gallstones. *N Engl J Med* 328(6):412, 1993.
32. Cohen J, Edelman RR, Chopra S: Portal vein thrombosis: A review. *Am J Med* 92(2):173, 1992.
33. Shill M, Henderson JM, Tavil AS: The Budd-Chiari syndrome revisited. *Gastroenterologist* 2(1):27, 1994.
34. Ernst E: Harmless herbs? A review of the recent literature. *Am J Med* 104(2):170, 1998.
35. Gilbert DN, Moellering R Jr, Sande MA, eds: *The Sanford Guide to Antimicrobial Therapy,* 29th ed. Vienna: Antimicrobial Therapy, 1999.

ACUTE AND CHRONIC PANCREATITIS

Robert J. Vissers
Riyad B. Abu-Laban

ACUTE PANCREATITIS

Pancreatitis is a common cause of abdominal pain, and the lack of a pathognomonic clinical presentation and the absence of a diagnostic gold standard make this disease a diagnostic challenge. Its clinical presentation can vary from mild abdominal pain to refractory shock, and many of its signs and symptoms are shared by other intraabdominal conditions.

Epidemiology

Acute pancreatitis is secondary to cholelithiasis or alcohol abuse in up to 90 percent of cases in the United States, but the etiology varies in different countries.[1] The overall prevalence is estimated to be 0.5 percent, but this also depends on the setting and patient population. Patients with biliary pancreatitis are more commonly female, over 50 years of age, and represent the most common form of pancreatitis in a community hospital setting. Alcoholic pancreatitis presents more frequently to urban emergency departments and is seen most commonly in men between the ages of 35 and 45.[2]

The list of other factors associated with the development of acute pancreatitis is extensive, including drugs, infection, inflammation, trauma, and metabolic disturbances (Table 83-1). Drugs account for up to half of the remaining cases after alcohol and biliary diseases have been excluded (Table 83-2).

Pathophysiology

Although there are many distinct etiologies for acute pancreatitis, the specific mechanism that leads to the disease state remains unclear. The central pathophysiologic cause is believed to be the intracellular activation of digestive enzymes and subsequent autodigestion of the pancreas.[1,3] A number of factors (e.g., endotoxins, toxins, ischemia, infections, and anoxia) are believed to trigger the activation of proenzymes. Activated proteolytic enzymes, such as trypsin, then digest cellular membranes within the pancreas and cause edema, interstitial hemorrhage, vascular damage, coagulation, and cellular necrosis.[1] This noninfectious destruction of the pancreatic parenchyma rapidly causes a local inflammatory reaction that further contributes to the vascular dilatation, permeability, and edema.

The autodigestion theory replaces a previously held belief that the cause was primarily due to an anatomic ''common channel'' between the common bile duct and the pancreatic duct, in actuality a rare occurrence. Alternatively, it was proposed that obstruction at the ampulla of Vater was the primary initiating event in acute pancreatitis, but this does not produce pancreatitis in the experimental setting. Only by injecting bile, bacteria, and trypsin under pressure can pancreatitis be experimentally induced.[2]

Adult pancreatitis is distinguished from most other intraabdominal diseases by its propensity to cause remote systemic effects. It is believed that this represents an extension of the localized process into a generalized systemic inflammatory response.[4] This may lead to shock, adult respiratory distress syndrome (ARDS) and, eventually, multisystem organ failure. Recently, pancreatitis research has focused on the identification of systemic inflammatory mediators. A number of compounds has been implicated, including bradykinin, compliment, platelet-activating factor, nitrous oxide and, most recently, inflammatory cytokines.[4] Inflammatory mediators presently hold the most promise for the identification of better prognostic markers and potential therapies for acute pancreatitis.[5]

TABLE 83-1 Etiologic or Contributing Factors in Acute Pancreatitis

Drugs and toxins
Biliary tract disease
Trauma, penetrating or blunt
Penetrating peptic ulcer
Postoperative
Following ERCP
Obstruction secondary to neoplasms, diverticula, roundworms, benign polyps
Perisphincteric fibrosis
Cystic fibrosis
Metabolic disturbances Hyperlipidemia (Frederickson types I, IV, and V) Hypercalcemia Diabetes mellitus, diabetes ketoacidosis Uremia Hemochromatosis Hereditary pancreatitis
Viral infections Mumps Hepatitis A, B, C Infectious mononucleosis Coxsackie group B Rubella Cytomegalovirus Epstein-Barr virus HIV *Varicella* Echovirus Adenovirus
Pregnancy—any trimester, postpartum
Collagen vascular disease Systemic lupus erythematosus Polyarteritis nodosa
Infection Typhoid fever *Salmonella typhimurium* infection Scarlet fever Streptococcal food poisoning Dysentery Ascariasis Clonorchiasis *Mycobacterium tuberculosis* *Mycoplasma* *Mycobacterium avium, intracellulare* *Legionella* Leptospirosis *Campylobacter*

Clinical Features

The major symptom of acute pancreatitis is mid-epigastric or left upper quadrant pain. It is most commonly described as a constant, boring pain that often radiates to the back as well as the flanks, chest, or lower abdomen. Although usually described as severe, the intensity can be extremely variable and does not correlate with the severity of the disease.[1] The pain is exacerbated in the supine position and can be relieved when sitting with the trunk and knees flexed. Colicky discomfort is atypical and suggests another etiology. Nausea and vomiting are common, and abdominal bloating from gastric and intestinal hypomotility is a frequent complaint.

Physical examination usually reveals a patient in moderate distress. Low-grade fevers and tachycardia are frequently present, and hypotension is not unusual.[1] About 10 percent of patients have respiratory symptoms secondary to atelectasis, pleural effusion (usually left sided) and, rarely, ARDS. Abdominal examination is notable for epigastric tenderness. Peritonitis is a late finding, presumably due to the retroperitoneal location of the organ. Bowel sounds may be diminished from an associated ileus. Cullen sign, a bluish discoloration around the umbilicus, and Grey Turner sign, a bluish discoloration of the flanks are characteristic but rare signs of hemorrhagic pancreatitis.

Patients with pancreatitis may present in hypovolemic shock and multisystem organ failure. Hypotension can result from fluid third-spacing, hemorrhage, increased vascular permeability, vasodilatation, cardiac depression, and vomiting.[2]

Diagnosis

The absence of a pathognomonic clinical syndrome often precludes a diagnosis based solely on presentation. Unfortunately, the only diagnostic gold standard is pathologic examination of the pancreas. Laboratory and radiographic investigations can be helpful in the diagnosis of acute pancreatitis, but both suffer from limited diagnostic accuracy.

LABORATORY TESTS Serum amylase and lipase are the most widely used laboratory tests used in the evaluation of acute pancreatitis (Table 83-3). Both enzyme markers, released during pancreatic inflammation, lack the sensitivity and specificity to be the sole indicators of disease and must be interpreted in the context of the clinical setting.[6,7]

TABLE 83-2 Drugs Associated with the Occurrence of Acute Pancreatitis

Oral contraceptives
Estrogens
Phenformin
Azathioprine
Glucocorticoids
Rifampin
Tetracyclines
Isoniazid
Thiazides
Furosemide
Donidine
Salicylates
Indomethacin
Dextropropoxyphene
Calcium
Warfarin
L-Asparaginase
Paracetamol
Ethacrynic acid

TABLE 83-3 Laboratory Utilization in Suspected Acute Pancreatitis

Test Characteristic	Amylase	Lipase
Sensitivity	80%–90%	90%
Specificity	75%	90%
Suggested best cutoff	3× upper limit of normal	2× upper limit of normal
Prognostic value	Poor	Poor
Rate of rise	Rapid	Rapid
Return to baseline	3–4 days	7–14 days
Other	No additional benefit to ordering both amylase and lipase.	

Amylase This digestive enzyme, used to cleave starch into smaller carbohydrates, is primarily found in the pancreas and salivary glands. Low levels of amylase can also be found in numerous other tissues, including the fallopian tubes, ovaries, testes, adipose tissue, small bowel, lung, thyroid, skeletal muscle, and certain neoplasms. As a result, serum amylase can be elevated in many conditions, making this test relatively nonspecific.

Amylase levels are expressed in either Somogyi units (SU) or international units, with the normal ranges generally reported as 60 to 160 SU/100 mL or 110 to 300 IU/L, respectively.[8] Amylase has a half-life of about 2 h and, although the elimination is incompletely understood, it is at least partially cleared by the kidneys, leading to elevated levels in renal failure.

Not only are there many extrapancreatic causes of an elevated amylase, but serum amylase levels may be normal in proven cases of acute pancreatitis.[9] The lack of a diagnostic gold standard has made estimates of the sensitivity of this test difficult, but most studies suggest a sensitivity of 80 to 90 percent if blood is sampled within 36 h of symptom onset.[10] Amylase rises quickly but, because of its short half-life, returns to normal in 3 to 4 days (even in the presence of ongoing inflammation), making it less sensitive after the first 36 h.

The main difficulty in using serum amylase for the diagnosis of acute pancreatitis is its poor specificity. Depending on the cutoff used, the specificity of amylase ranges from 40 percent when the normal range is used to greater than 90 percent at a cutoff of five times the upper limit of normal. The best accuracy appears to occur at a cutoff of three times the upper limit of normal, which improves the specificity to 75 percent without greatly compromising the sensitivity.[7,8]

Lipase This enzyme, which catalyzes the breakdown of triglycerides into free fatty acids, is predominantly found in the pancreas, but lipase activity is present in the gastric and intestinal mucosa and in the liver. An elevated serum lipase level has been noted in a number of nonpancreatic diseases, most of which are intestinal or hepatobiliary disorders.[7,11] Heparin may cause a release of endothelial membrane-bound lipase into the serum, resulting in a measurable increase in lipase activity within minutes of heparin administration. Lipase is cleared by the kidneys and can be elevated to three times the upper limit of normal in renal failure. The half-life is approximately 7 h, and serum lipase will remain elevated for several days after amylase has returned to baseline. Lipase activity is expressed in units per liter, and the normal range varies greatly, depending on the assay that is used.

Many of the reservations regarding the utility of lipase in pancreatitis were based on the use of older, less specific assays of lipase activity. The recent addition of colipase to these assays has improved the specificity to greater than 90 percent (specificity ranges from 80 to 99 percent, depending on the cutoff used). In addition, the sensitivity of lipase is at least as good as amylase (greater than 90 percent). The most appropriate cutoff in the emergency department appears to be two times the upper limit of normal.[7,8]

Lipase is clearly a more accurate test than amylase in the diagnosis of acute pancreatitis. Although lipase suffers from imperfect sensitivity, a recent study of over 5000 patients in whom both amylase and lipase tests were ordered found that the addition of amylase was not warranted.[12] It is also not cost-effective to order amylase or lipase indiscriminately in all cases of undifferentiated abdominal pain.[6]

Other enzymatic markers have been investigated, including isoenzymes of amylase, but variables such as time, cost, and test accuracy have prevented their use in clinical practice. Lipase-amylase ratios and amylase-creatinine clearance ratios add little to the diagnosis of acute pancreatitis beyond lipase alone.[2,3]

RADIOLOGY Plain radiographs of the chest and abdomen are most useful in excluding other diseases that may be confused with pancreatitis. Calcification of the gland is suggestive of chronic pancreatitis. A sentinel loop secondary to small bowel ileus, or a colon-cutoff sign suggesting local colonic ileus, may be present but neither is diagnostic. Chest radiographs may reveal an elevated hemidiaphragm or a pleural or pericardial effusion.

Ultrasonography is most helpful in the identification of gallstones or dilatation of the biliary tree, which has both diagnostic and therapeutic implications in pancreatic disease. Although pancreatic edema and associated pseudocysts may be visualized on ultrasound, it is generally an insensitive test for the diagnosis of acute pancreatitis, particularly in nonbiliary etiologies. Overlying bowel gas or adipose tissue and the retroperitoneal location of the pancreas frequently impair adequate imaging.[2]

Computed tomography (CT) cannot be used to rule out pancreatitis, as it is insensitive in early or mild disease. Because of better anatomic definition, CT scanning may facilitate grading the severity of the disease and enable better prognostication.[13]

Endoscopic retrograde cholangiopancreatography (ERCP) is rarely employed in the emergency department evaluation but can be very useful for patients in whom the etiology of the pancreatitis remains unclear after initial assessment. Magnetic resonance imaging is being investigated in this role.

Prognostic Markers

For most patients, acute pancreatitis is a self-limited disease, but 5 to 10 percent suffer from significant associated morbidity and mortality.[2,14] It can be difficult to identify patients at risk, although signs of a systemic response suggest a more complicated course. Ranson has identified multiple diagnostic criteria used to predict patient outcome (Table 83-4).[15] The number of factors present is then used to predict mortality. Patients with fewer than three criteria have a 1 percent mortality, those with three to four criteria have a 16 percent mortality, those with five to six criteria have a 40 percent mortality, and those with more than six criteria have 100 percent mortality. Although the presence of several risk factors in the emergency department portends a worse prognosis, the Ranson criteria require an assessment of clinical values within the first 48 h of hospitalization and therefore have limited utility in the initial evaluation. Other scoring systems have been used to predict severity in pancreatitis, such as the acute physiology and chronic health evaluation (APACHE II) score, but complexity and poor sensitivity on initial presentation limit their role in the emergency department.[1] In general, the presence of extraabdominal complications or comorbid conditions indicates an increased mortality risk. Hypotension, tachycardia of more than 130 bpm, a Po_2 of less than 60 mmHg, oliguria, increasing blood urea nitrogen or creatinine, and hypocalcemia are key indicators of a potentially complicated course.[1,3,15]

TABLE 83-4 Ranson Criteria for Predicting Mortality Risk from Acute Pancreatitis

On Admission	48 Hours Later
Age over 55	Change in HCT (falling) decreased more than 10 percent
Blood sugar > 200 mg/dL	Rise in BUN over 5 mg/dL
WCB > 16,000/μL	↓ CA^{2+} below 8 mg/dL
SGOT > 250 Sigma-Fankel units/L	↓ Arterial Po_2 below 60 mmHg Rapid fluid sequestration over 6 L
LDH > 700 IU/L	Base deficit over 4 meq/L

There is no specific serum marker predictive of outcome in acute pancreatitis, although cytokines show great promise.[4] The absolute level of serum amylase or lipase does not correlate with severity.[3,7]

A CT scan, particularly if contrast enhanced, may provide valuable estimates of the severity and prognosis in cases of moderate to severe acute pancreatitis.[13] A CT severity index score has been described. It is suggested that CT scan be performed on patients with three or more Ranson's criteria, significantly ill patients, and patients with clinical deterioration.[16]

Complications include phlegmons, abscesses, or pseudocysts,[16] usually in the first 2 to 3 weeks after the onset of pancreatitis. Systemic complications include pulmonary, cardiovascular, renal, hematologic, central nervous system, and metabolic abnormalities (Table 83-5).[14]

Treatment

Of patients with acute pancreatitis, 90 percent recover without complications and require supportive measures only.[1] The general principle is to ''rest the pancreas.'' Although the use of a nasogastric tube is

TABLE 83-5 Complications of Acute Pancreatitis

Pulmonary
- Pleural effusions, usually left sided
- Atelectasis
- Hypoxemia
- Adult respiratory distress syndrome (>50% mortality)

Cardiovascular
- Myocardial depression
- Hemorrhage, hypovolemia, and myocardial depressant factor

Metabolic
- Hypocalcemia
- Hyperglycemia
- Hyperlipidemia
- Coagulopathy, disseminated intravascular coagulopathy

Other
- Hemorrhage
- Colonic perforation
- Renal failure
- Erythema-nodosum dermatitis
- Arthritis
- Pseudocyst
- Abscess

widely advocated, no studies have demonstrated that its presence alters the course of the illness. It is traditionally recommended to withhold all oral intake, but clear liquids do not appear to be harmful in mild to moderate disease.

The mainstay of treatment for acute pancreatitis is fluid resuscitation. A balanced electrolyte solution, such as normal saline, should be administered for rehydration. Amounts should be given to ensure renal perfusion and good urine output of about 100 mL/h. In unstable patients, hemodynamic monitoring may be required, and pressors are indicated for persistent hypotension despite adequate fluid resuscitation.

Other aspects of supportive care include parenteral narcotics and antiemetics.

In biliary pancreatitis, urgent decompression is indicated if there is persistent biliary obstruction, ideally by endoscopic sphincterotomy of the ampulla of Vater.[1,2] If the obstruction is transient, most patients can be managed with supportive care, and elective cholecystectomy may be performed once inflammation subsides.

Empiric antibiotics are not indicated in mild to moderate pancreatitis but should be given if secondary infection is suspected. Although many other drugs have been used as a potential therapeutic agent in acute pancreatitis, such as H_2 blockers, steroids, nonsteroidal anti-inflammatory drugs, and glucagon, none has demonstrated benefit in controlled, prospective trials.[2]

Peritoneal lavage may provide short-term clinical improvement but does not appear to alter clinical outcome. Acute fluid collections are rarely symptomatic and frequently resolve spontaneously.[16] Laparotomy is indicated for hemorrhage control and abscess drainage. Abscesses and pseudocysts may also be drained radiologically or endoscopically, if indicated.

Disposition

Patients with mild pancreatitis, no evidence of systemic complications, and a low likelihood of biliary tract disease may be managed as outpatients if they are able to tolerate oral fluids and their pain is well controlled. A clear-liquid diet is recommended, oral analgesics should be prescribed, and follow-up in 24 to 48 h is needed. All other patients with acute pancreatitis should be admitted to the hospital. Patients with significant systemic complications, shock, or extensive pancreatic necrosis will need an intensive care setting. Evidence of a pancreatic abscess requires surgical consultation.

CHRONIC PANCREATITIS

Chronic pancreatitis is a chronic inflammatory condition that causes irreversible damage to pancreatic structure and function.

Epidemiology

Table 83-6 lists the causes of chronic pancreatitis. Of these, alcohol abuse is the most important, accounting for 70 to 80 percent of cases.[17] Most of the remaining cases are idiopathic. The mean ages of onset and death in chronic pancreatitis are 42 and 52 years, respectively.[18] Because the disease can be undiagnosed, the true prevalence is unknown, with estimates ranging from 0.04 to 5 percent.[19] As with alcohol abuse, chronic pancreatitis is most common in men. Gallstones are not a cause of chronic pancreatitis, despite their role in the acute form of the disease.[20,21] It is believed that acute pancreatitis does not progress to chronic disease unless complications such as pseudocysts or ductal strictures are present.[19]

Pathophysiology

The pathophysiology of chronic pancreatitis remains poorly understood.[19] In contrast to acute pancreatitis, the pancreas is pathologically abnormal in chronic pancreatitis, both before and after exacerbation. In alcohol-induced disease, it is thought that either alcohol is directly toxic to acinar cells or induces pathologic changes in secretory function.[20] The risk of alcohol-induced chronic pancreatitis is clearly related to the amount and duration of alcohol consumption.[17] Once established, the disease may progress despite abstinence, although the mortality rate is reduced.[18,20] Chronic pancreatitis, regardless of the etiology, results in interstitial inflammation with duct obstruction and dilatation leading to parenchymal loss and fibrosis. This causes pain and eventual impairment of both exocrine and endocrine pancreatic functions, with endocrine impairment occurring later in the disease process.[19] Clinically significant malabsorption does not occur until more than 90 percent of glandular function is lost.[17] The etiology of pain is likely multifactorial and may include parenchymal inflammation, pressure on acinar tissue or small ducts, perineural inflammation, and duodenal or common bile duct stenosis.[20] It is controversial whether pain "burns out" as chronic pancreatitis progresses.[19]

TABLE 83-6 Causes of Chronic Pancreatitis

Alcohol abuse
Malnutrition ("tropical pancreatitis")
Hyperparathyroidism
Pancreas divisum
Ampullary stenosis
Cystic fibrosis
Hereditary
Trauma
Idiopathic

Clinical Features

The hallmark of chronic pancreatitis is abdominal pain, but in about 10 percent of cases the disease may be painless.[21] As in acute pancreatitis, pain is usually mid-epigastric and may radiate to the back, although abdominal tenderness is often less prominent.[2] Nausea and vomiting may be present. In the early stages of chronic pancreatitis, discrete attacks of pain (formerly called "relapsing pancreatitis") occur, lasting days to weeks.[17] Pain is frequently worse after alcohol ingestion or a fatty meal. As the disease progresses, pain-free periods become less frequent and often disappear completely.[2] In distinction to acute pancreatitis, patients with chronic pancreatitis appear chronically ill and may have signs and symptoms of pancreatic insufficiency, including weight loss, steatorrhea, clubbing, and polyuria. Stigmata of chronic liver disease may be present if the etiology is alcohol abuse.

Diagnosis

Differentiating acute and chronic pancreatitis may be difficult during an exacerbation, since the primary distinction is based on disease reversibility.[2] Laboratory investigations are nonspecific in chronic pancreatitis. Amylase and lipase levels may be elevated but have no prognostic significance and are usually normal, particularly when fibrosis is advanced. Glucose tolerance is often impaired, occasionally with an elevated fasting blood sugar level. In 5 to 10 percent of patients with chronic pancreatitis, compression of the intrahepatic portion of the bile duct leads to elevations of bilirubin and alkaline phosphatase levels.[19] Pancreatic calcification on abdominal radiographs is considered pathognomonic for chronic pancreatitis and is present in some 30 percent of patients, particularly those with alcohol-induced disease.[17,22]

Lists of diagnostic criteria for chronic pancreatitis have been developed since no single gold standard exists.[23] Either CT or ultrasound may be indicated to identify local complications of chronic pancreatitis, such as abscess or pseudocyst. The differentiation between chronic pancreatitis and pancreatic cancer can be challenging and is an essential component of imaging interpretation.

Treatment

The management of chronic pancreatitis in the emergency department involves ruling out other diagnoses or complications and includes supportive care. Intravenous narcotic analgesics and antiemetics are usually required. Fluid and electrolyte abnormalities should be corrected. The long-term goals of treatment are pain control, relief of mechanical obstruction or complications, correction of malabsorption, and alteration of the disease course. Pancreatic extracts are frequently administered to improve absorption and reduce pain. Cessation of alcohol ingestion is essential because the 5-year mortality rate of chronic pancreatitis in patients who continue to abuse alcohol is 50 percent.[17] If pain is increasing or intractable, imaging should be performed to assess for complications such as pseudocyst or mechanical obstruction. Surgery, either open or endoscopic, can be helpful in such cases. Other complications include mechanical obstruction of the duodenum or common bile duct, fistulae, ascites or pleural effusions, splenic vein thrombosis, and pseudoaneurysm. Celiac plexus nerve block is frequently performed for long-term pain control.

Disposition

Many patients with chronic pancreatitis can be safely discharged from the emergency department once complications have been ruled out or addressed. Appropriate follow-up is particularly important if pain management is poor or significant weight loss or symptom changes have occurred. Hospital admission may be required during severe pain exacerbation.

REFERENCES

1. Mergener K, Baillic J: Fortnightly review: acute pancreatitis. *BMJ* 316:44, 1998.
2. Moscati RM: Pancreatitis. *Emerg Med Clin North Am* 14:719, 1996.
3. Steinberg W, Tenner S: Acute pancreatitis. *N Engl J Med* 330:1198, 1994.
4. Norman J: The role of cytokines in the pathogenesis of acute pancreatitis. *Am J Surg* 175:76, 1998.
5. Inagaki T, Hoshino M, Hayakawa T, et al: Interleukin-6 is a useful marker for early prediction of the severity of acute pancreatitis. *Pancreas* 14:1, 1997.
6. Hoffman JR, Jaber AJ, Schriger DL: Serum amylase determination in the emergency department evaluation of abdominal pain. *J Clin Gastroenterol* 13:401, 1991.
7. Tietz NW: Support of the diagnosis of pancreatitis by enzymatic tests: Old problems, new techniques. *Clin Chem* 257:85, 1997.
8. Wong ECC, Butch AW, Rosenblum JL, et al: The clinical chemistry laboratory and acute pancreatitis. *Clin Chem* 39:234, 1993.
9. Orebaugh S: Normal amylase levels in the presence of acute pancreatitis. *Am J Emerg Med* 12:21, 1994.
10. Clavien P, Robert J, Meyer P: Acute pancreatitis and normalamylasemia. *Ann Surg* 210:614, 1989.
11. Rosenblum J: Serum lipase is increased in disease states other than acute pancreatitis: amylase revisited. *Clin Chem* 37:315, 1991.
12. Vissers RJ, Dagnone J, Abu-Laban R, Walls RM: Serum amylase offers no additional benefit to serum lipase in the ED diagnosis of acute pancreatitis. *Acad Emerg Med* 4:396, 1998.
13. Balthazar EM: CT diagnosis and staging of acute pancreatitis. *Radiol Clin North Am* 27:19, 1989.
14. Pitchumoni S, Agarwal N, Jain NK: Systemic complications of acute pancreatitis. *Am J Gastroenterol* 83:597, 1988.
15. Ranson JHC: Etiologic and prognostic factors in human pancreatitis: A review. *Am J Gastroenterol.* 77:663, 1982.
16. Bacon TH, Morgan DE: The diagnosis and management of fluid collections associated with pancreatitis. *Am J Med* 102:555, 1997.
17. Mergener K, Baillie J: Chronic pancreatitis. *Lancet* 350:1379, 1997.
18. Levy P: Mortality factors associated with chronic pancreatitis. *Gastroenterology* 96:1165, 1989.
19. Steer ML, Waxman I, Freedman S: Medical progress: Chronic pancreatitis. *N Engl J Med* 332:1482, 1995.
20. Holt S: Chronic pancreatitis. *Southern Med J* 86:201, 1993.
21. Naruse S, Kitagawa M, Ishiguro H, et al: Chronic pancreatitis: Overview of medical aspects. *Pancreas* 16:323, 1998.
22. Ammann RW: Evolution and regression of pancreatic calcification in chronic pancreatitis: A prospective long term study of 107 patients. *Gastroenterology* 95:1018, 1988.
23. Homma T: Criteria for pancreatic disease diagnosis in Japan: Diagnostic criteria for chronic pancreatitis. *Pancreas* 16:250, 1998.

COMPLICATIONS OF GENERAL SURGICAL PROCEDURES

Edmond A. Hooker

Outpatient surgical procedures are commonplace, and, with increasing pressure for cost containment, admitted patients are being discharged earlier in their postoperative course. As a result, more patients are presenting to the emergency department with postoperative fever, respiratory complications, genitourinary complaints, wound infections, vascular problems, and complications of drug therapy (Table 84-1). This chapter reviews the complications common to all surgical procedures as well as procedure-specific complications.

The operating surgeon should be called when one of his or her patients appears in the emergency department with a surgical complication. This is not just courtesy but provides continuity of care important for the patient's well-being.

FEVER

Fever is a common presenting complaint (Table 84-2). A mnemonic for the common causes of postoperative fever is the "five W's": wind (atelectasis or pneumonia), water (urinary tract infection), wound, walking (deep vein thrombosis), and wonder drugs (drug fever or pseudomembranous colitis.[1] Fever during the initial 24 h is usually caused by atelectasis; however, necrotizing streptococcal and clostridial infections also occur in surgical wounds early in the postoperative course. Respiratory complications, such as pneumonia and atelectasis, and intravenous catheter-related problems, such as thrombophlebitis, are the predominant causes of fever in the 24- to 72-h time period.

Urinary tract infections become evident 3 to 5 days postoperatively. Seven to ten days postoperatively, clinical manifestations of wound infections develop. Deep venous thrombosis can result in fever any time but usually not until the fifth postoperative day. Antibiotic-induced pseudomembrane colitis occurs up to 6 weeks postoperatively. An approach for evaluating and managing fever in postoperative patients is presented in Table 84-3.

RESPIRATORY COMPLICATIONS

Respiratory complications occur in many surgical patients and range from atelectasis and pneumonia to pneumothorax or pulmonary embolism.

Atelectasis

Atelectasis, the collapse of pulmonary alveoli, is very common. Contributing factors include inadequate clearance of secretions following

TABLE 84-1 Complications of General Surgical Procedures

Complication	Important Points
Fever	Wind, water, wound, walking, wonder drugs
Pulmonary complications	
Atelectasis	<24 h, treat with pulmonary toilet, discharge unless ill or hypoxemic
Pneumonia	24–96 h, polymicrobial, most require admission
Pneumothorax	Multiple causes, consider expiratory views, consider needle aspiration
Pulmonary embolism	Dyspnea is main symptom, high index of suspicion
Gastrointestinal complications	
Intestinal obstruction	Obtain radiographs, search for causes
Intraabdominal abscess	CT diagnosis, early broad-spectrum antibiotics
Pancreatitis	Always consider in postoperative patients with abdominal pain
Cholecystitis	Usually in older patients, can be acalculous
Fistulas	Can be high output, admit if concerns over output
Genitourinary complications	
Urinary tract infection	3–5 days, oral antibiotics, most discharged
Urinary retention	Rapid catheter drainage, most discharged
Acute renal failure	Prerenal, renal, and postrenal causes, most admitted
Wound complications	
Hematoma	Caused by poor hemostasis, can drain most, but be careful with neck hematomas and hematomas after vascular surgery
Seroma	Painless swelling, clear fluid, drain and discharge
Infection	Open, drain, and culture; be careful with wounds associated with respiratory, gastrointestinal tract, genitourinary tract, or secondary to trauma
Necrotizing fasciitis	Pain out of proportion to physical findings
Dehiscence	Careful with abdominal incisions (evisceration)
Vascular complications	
Superficial thrombophlebitis	Usually aseptic, local therapy and discharge
Deep venous thrombosis	Upper and lower extremity, Doppler studies
Complications of drug therapy	
Diarrhea	Consider pseudomembranous colitis
Drug fever	Many drugs implicated, requires admission
Tetanus	Can occur after gastrointestinal surgery
Procedure-specific complications	See text

general anesthesia, decreased intraalveolar pressure, and postoperative pain, which results in hypoventilation. While atelectasis can occur following any procedure, it frequently occurs following upper abdominal and thoracic surgery. The presentation varies from an isolated fever to tachypnea, dyspnea, and tachycardia.

TABLE 84-2 Causes of Postoperative Fevers in General Surgical Patients

Atelectasis	Pseudomembranous colitis
Pneumonia	Hepatitis
Urinary tract infections	Peritonitis
Skin and soft tissue injury	Pulmonary embolism
Thrombophlebitis (septic and sterile)	Transfusion reaction
Deep vein thrombosis	Thyrotoxicosis
Intraabdominal abscesses	Pheochromocytoma
Unrelated bacterial infection	Adrenal insufficiency

Evaluation includes a chest radiograph, pulse oximetry, and a complete blood count (CBC). Chest radiographs may be normal or show platelike linear densities, triangular-shaped densities, or lobar consolidation. Mild hypoxemia from ventilation-perfusion mismatch is common, but hypercarbia is uncommon. Patients with mid atelectasis and

TABLE 84-3 Evaluation and Management of Postoperative Fever

HISTORY
Presenting signs and symptoms
Onset of symptoms, time since procedure
Procedures performed and complications
Medications
History of blood transfusion
PHYSICAL EXAMINATION
Particular attention to Operative sites and contiguous areas Sites of catheters and invasive monitors Signs of deep venous thrombosis and pulmonary embolism Decubiti Lungs
ANCILLARY STUDIES
Complete blood count with differential
Chest radiograph
Gram stain and culture of wound exudate
Urinalysis (culture if infected)
Sputum Gram stain and culture
Blood cultures
If diarrhea present, consider immunoassay of specimen for *Clostridium difficile* toxin
Further tests as indicated (e.g., computed tomography, radionuclide studies, venography, arteriograms)
TREATMENT
If source identified, start antibiotics; admission based on condition of patient
If no source identified, consider admission, change and culture all catheters, stop all medication that might cause fever

no evidence of hypoxemia may be managed as outpatients with pain control and increased deep breathing. Admission is indicated for aggressive pulmonary toilet and supplement oxygenation in debilitated patients, patients with underlying lung disease, patients with hypoxemia, or those in whom the diagnosis is in question.

Pneumonia

Pneumonia usually presents between 24 and 96 h postoperatively. Predisposing factors include prolonged ventilatory support and atelectasis. Presenting symptoms can include dyspnea, chest pain, productive cough, fever, and tachypnea. Postoperative pneumonia is likely to be polymicrobial. After cultures of sputum and blood are obtained, parenteral antimicrobial therapy with an aminoglycoside and an antipseudomonal penicillin should be administered. Admission to the hospital is generally indicated.

Pneumothorax

Pneumothorax can occur as a complication of thoracic wall surgery, breast biopsy, laparoscopic abdominal surgery, abdominal paracentesis, nasogastric and feeding tube insertion, thoracic surgery, central venous catheter insertion, endoscopic procedures, shoulder arthroscopy, and tracheostomy. The pathophysiology varies with these different procedures, but clinical features are similar. Patients complain of chest pain, shoulder pain, and/or dyspnea. Physical findings can include tachypnea, hyperresonance to percussion, and decreased breath sounds on the affected side. Diagnosis is confirmed by chest x-ray with expiratory views.

Pulmonary Embolus

Pulmonary embolism may present any time during the postoperative period. A lower-extremity or pelvic thrombus dislodges and migrates to the pulmonary vasculature. The presenting signs and symptoms vary, depending on the size of embolus and the underlying cardiopulmonary status of the patient. Patients have varying degrees of dyspnea, chest pain, cough, and anxiety. Hemoptysis is usually seen only late in a patient's course and with massive pulmonary embolism. The patient may have essentially normal vital signs or be tachypneic and tachycardiac.

Diagnosis of pulmonary embolism is difficult because of the poor sensitivity of noninvasive tests. While hypoxemia and a widened alveolar-arterial (A-a) oxygen gradient are frequently found with larger emboli, patients may have normal oxygen content and a normal A-a gradient. Diagnosis requires venous Doppler ultrasonography, ventilation-perfusion scan, pulmonary computed tomography (CT) scan, or pulmonary angiography. Patients with low clinical suspicion, normal vital signs, good oxygenation, and a low probability scan can be discharged, provided other causes of their symptoms have been addressed.

GENITOURINARY COMPLICATIONS

The most common postoperative genitourinary complication is urinary tract infection. However, patients may present with acute urinary retention and acute renal failure (ARF).

Urinary Tract Infection

Urinary tract infections can occur after any surgical procedure. However, there is an increased incidence in patients who have had instrumentation of the genitourinary tract or bladder catheterization. The cause is direct contamination of the urinary bladder, most commonly with *Escherichia coli.* Other organisms isolated include *Staphylococcus aureus, Staphylococcus epidermidis, Proteus mirabilis, Klebsiella, Pseudomonas,* and enterococci. Oral antibiotics are appropriate for most infections; however, elderly or debilitated patients and patients with evidence of sepsis require admission for parenteral antibiotics.

Urinary Retention

Acute urinary retention occurs in about 4 percent of all surgical patients.[2] It is postulated that urinary retention occurs as the result of catecholamine stimulation of α-adrenergic receptors in the bladder neck and urethral smooth muscle. Increased incidence of urinary retention is likely to occur in elderly males, with excessive fluid administration during surgery, and with the use of spinal or epidural anesthesia.

Patients with urinary retention present with lower abdominal discomfort, urinary urgency, and inability to void. The diagnosis is confirmed by placement of a Foley catheter. The bladder can be safely drained quickly without clamping, since there appears to be no foundation for the fears of hematuria, postobstructive diuresis, and hypotension.[3] For patients with normal renal function and no anatomic obstruction, continued catheter drainage is not necessary. For patients with retention after genitourinary procedures, the urologist must be consulted before disposition. Prophylactic antibiotics can be given if the genitourinary tract has been instrumented, if retention is prolonged, or if the patient is at risk for infection.

Acute Renal Failure

ARF is classified according to the primary cause: prerenal, intrinsic, and postrenal. Volume depletion is the most common prerenal cause. Intrinsic causes include acute tubular necrosis and drug nephrotoxicity. Obstructive uropathy is the cause of postrenal ARF. Patients with ARF have either oliguria or anuria, and, depending on the degree of ARF, may have signs of uremia and electrolyte abnormalities.

Patients should be examined for signs of hypovolemia and have a urinary catheter placed. Indwelling urinary catheters must be irrigated or replaced. If the patient is hypotensive, a fluid bolus is given to determine whether the cause is prerenal. In patients with urinary outlet obstruction, the urinary catheter is both diagnostic and therapeutic. If there is doubt about the cause of the renal failure, central venous pressure and pulmonary capillary wedge pressure measurements can be helpful. The presence of postobstructive uropathy above the urinary bladder can be confirmed using abdominal ultrasound. When no prerenal or postrenal cause can be identified, there is likely to be an intrinsic cause of ARF.

WOUND COMPLICATIONS

Wound complications are frequent and include hematomas, seromas, infections, necrotizing fasciitis, and dehiscence. The patient's surgeon should be notified of all wound complications.

Hematomas

Wound hematomas result from unrecognized inadequate hemostasis. Patients have pain, pressure, and swelling within the wound. Patients with wound hematomas may be febrile and have sanguineous or serous wound drainage. Differentiating between hematoma and wound infection can be difficult. A few sutures are removed to allow the hematoma to drain, and cultures are obtained. If there is no evidence of infection and hemostasis can be maintained, the patient can be discharged. In patients with a hematoma of the neck or who have undergone vascular surgery, extreme caution and consultation are appropriate.

Seromas

A seroma, a collection of serous fluid, is usually the result of inadequate control of lymphatics during dissection but can also occur under split-thickness skin grafts and areas with large dead spaces (e.g., axilla, groin, neck, or pelvis). Patients have painless swelling below the wound or graft, and needle aspiration yields a serous fluid. Aspiration confirms the diagnosis and alleviates the problem, although it may have to be repeated later.

Infection

Systemic factors (e.g., extremes of age, poor nutrition, or diabetes) contribute to wound infections; however, local factors (e.g., necrotic tissue, poor perfusion, foreign bodies, and hematomas) are of greatest significance. In nontraumatic, uninfected operative wounds in which the respiratory, alimentary, and genitourinary tract were not entered, infection rates are low. In these cases, the infecting organism is usually from the skin but can originate from remote infected sources (e.g., urinary tract infection). If there is a remote infected source, the organism is probably the same in both infections. Wounds associated with entering the respiratory, alimentary, or genitourinary tract or secondary to trauma have a higher risk of infection.

Presenting signs and symptoms of wound infections include increasing pain, erythema, swelling, drainage, and tenderness at the incision site. Wounds not inolving the perineum and not associated with entry into the gastrointestinal or biliary tract are most often infected with *S. aureus* or streptococci. Such wounds can be safely managed with drainage, culture of the wound, irrigation, loose packing with gauze, and outpatient antibiotics. Wounds involving the perineum or associated with the gastrointestinal or biliary tract are often infected with multiple organisms, including gram-negative bacteria and anaerobes. Parenteral broad-spectrum antibiotics are administered, and admission is necessary.

Necrotizing Fasciitis

Necrotizing fasciitis is a feared complication. The usual cause is direct contamination of the wound with group A streptococcus or *S. aureus;* however, mixed aerobic and anaerobic infections have been reported. Risk factors include diabetes mellitus, alcoholism, immunosuppression, and peripheral vascular disease, but necrotizing fasciitis also occurs in young, otherwise healthy individuals. Early clinical differentiation from cellulitis can be difficult. CT may show asymmetric fascial thickening, gas tracking along fascial planes, or focal fluid collections; however, the actual sensitivity and specificity of CT in the diagnosis of necrotizing fasciitis has not been defined.[4] Magnetic resonance imaging has been shown to be highly sensitive but not totally specific for necrotizing fasciitis and can be a useful adjunct.[5] The presence of marked systemic toxicity and pain out of proportion to local findings indicates fasciitis. In more advanced cases, there may be deep pain with patchy areas of surface hypesthesia, crepitance, or bullae. Treatment should include antibiotics and immediate surgical debridement. Antibiotic choice is controversial but should probably include a penicillin or cephalosporin, an aminoglycoside, and clindamycin.[6]

Wound Dehiscence

Wound dehiscence can be superficial or can extend into the deeper fascial planes. Dehiscence is caused by either inadequate closure or intrinsic host factors, such as malnutrition, glucocorticoid use, or diabetes. The patient may have serosanguineous fluid leaking from the wound. Dehiscence of abdominal incisions has the potential for evisceration. If evisceration is not present, conservative management using abdominal binders is appropriate. However, if there is any uncertainty, operative exploration is indicated.

VASCULAR COMPLICATIONS

Postoperative vascular complications include thrombophlebitis and deep venous thrombosis. Superficial thrombophlebitis usually occurs in the upper extremities, secondary to prolonged cannulation of the vein or infusion of irritating fluids. Deep venous thrombosis is secondary to stasis, endothelial damage, or hypercoagulopathy.

Superficial Thrombophlebitis

Superficial thrombophlebitis of the lower extremities is most frequently secondary to stasis in varicose veins. It is usually aseptic. The patient complains of redness and warmth of the affected vein. If there is no evidence of surrounding cellulitis or lymphangitis, the patient is treated with local heat and elevation. Suppurative superficial thrombophlebitis is characterized by erythema, palpable tender cord, lymphangitis, and pain. Suppurative thrombophlebitis requires excision of the affected vein.

Deep Venous Thrombosis

When lower-extremity superficial thrombophlebitis is seen, the possibility of concurrent deep venous thrombosis must be considered. Swelling of the extremity is the most specific physical sign, and its presence requires diagnostic evaluation. Doppler ultrasonography is generally the preferred diagnostic test. Patients with normal color-flow study results should be treated with elevation and bed rest. Repeat color-flow Doppler ultrasound studies should be performed in 3 days if symptoms persist but sooner if symptoms worsen.

COMPLICATIONS OF DRUG THERAPY

Many medicines have been reported to cause drug fever (Table 84-4).[7] The mechanisms proposed are hypersensitivity reactions, pyogenic effect, and disturbed thermoregulation. In patients in whom no source for the fever can be found, it is appropriate to consider stopping medications known to cause drug fever.

Many antibiotics can cause diarrhea; however, the greatest concern in postoperative patients is pseudomembranous colitis (PMC). PMC is due to the toxin produced by the bacterium *Colstridium difficile.* PMC is related to antibiotic use, which destroys the normal enteric bacterial flora, allowing an overgrowth of the *C. difficile.* Even short courses of antibiotics have been associated with PMC. Patients have watery, and sometimes bloody, diarrhea, elevated temperature, and crampy abdominal pain. Although tissue culture for *C. difficile* is the diagnostic gold standard, the diagnosis is usually made by detecting *C. difficile* cytotoxin in the stool.[1] This immunoassay is slightly less sensitive than is the tissue culture, but it is technically easier to do and provides an answer within 2 to 3 h. If results on the first specimen are negative and the diagnosis is still suspected, a second sample should be sent for immunoassay. When severe illness is present, consider empiric therapy with metronidazole while awaiting diagnostic studies.

COMPLICATIONS OF BREAST SURGERY

Breast biopsy is a common procedure. While complications are infrequent, patients can develop minor wound infections and hematomas. Rarely, pneumothorax has been reported. Wound hematomas frequently require operative control for proper evacuation and hemostasis.

Early complications seen with mastectomies include wound infection, necrosis of skin flaps, and the accumulation of seromas. The most common late complication is lymphedema of the arm. The incidence of postmastectomy lymphedema ranges from a low of 5.5 percent to a high of 80 percent. Most patients can be managed using a combination of fitted compression garments, nighttime elevation, and minor activity restrictions.[8]

TABLE 84-4 Medications Associated with Drug Fever

Allopurinol	Methyldopa
Amphetamine	Metoclopramide
Amphotericin B	Nifedipine
Antihistamines	Nitrofurantoin sodium
Asparaginase	Nomifensine
Azathioprine	Oxprenelol
Barbiturates	Para-aminosalicylic acid
Benztropine	Penicillins
Bleomycin sulfate	Phenytoin sodium
Carbamazepine	Procainamide
Cephalosporins	Propylthiouracil
Chlorpromazine	Prostaglandin E_2
Cimetidine	Quinidine sulfate
Clofibrate	Rifampin
Cocaine derivatives	Ritodrine
Folate	Salicylates
Haloperidol	Streptokinase
Hydralazine hydrochloride	Streptomycin sulfate
Ibuprofen	Sulfonamides
Interferon	Tetracycline
Iodides	Thioridazine
Isoniazid	Tolmetin
Levamisole	Triamterene
Lincomycin	Trifluoperazine
Lysergic acid	Vancomycin hydrochloride
Mebendazole	

COMPLICATIONS OF GASTROINTESTINAL SURGERY

Patients who have undergone any gastrointestinal surgery may have intestinal obstruction, intraabdominal abscess, pancreatitis, cholecystitis, fistulas, and tetanus. Certain procedures, such as anastomoses, gastric surgery, placement of gastrostomy tubes, biliary tract surgery, other laparoscopic surgery, stomas, colonoscopy, and rectal surgery have specific complications.

General Considerations

INTESTINAL OBSTRUCTION Ileus, a functional obstruction of the bowel, is postulated to be the result of stimulation of the splanchnic nerves, leading to neuronal inhibition of coordinated intrinsic bowel wall motor activity. It is expected after any operation in which the peritoneal cavity is violated. Following gastrointestinal surgery, small bowel tone usually returns to normal within 24 h, and colonic function within 3 to 5 days.[9] While ileus can also occur following nongastrointestinal procedures, it is usually secondary to anesthetic agents, and function returns to normal after 24 h.[9] Prolonged ileus can be caused by peritonitis, intraabdominal abscess, hemoperitoneum, pneumonia, electrolyte imbalance, sepsis, and medications.

Presenting symptoms of ileus include nausea, vomiting, obstipation, constipation, abdominal distention, and abdominal pain. When these symptoms are present in the first few days after surgery, they are most often due to adynamic ileus. The symptoms of adynamic ileus are most often mild and respond to nasogastric suction, bowel rest, and intravenous hydration. However, in cases of prolonged ileus, the physician must always look for an underlying cause. Evaluation of patients with suspected ileus includes abdominal radiographs to identify air-fluid levels, chest x-ray, CBC, electrolytes, and urinalysis for secondary causes of ileus.

Mechanical ileus of the bowel is most often secondary to adhesions. Small bowel obstruction above the ligament of Treitz is associated with frequent bouts of bilious emesis. In cases of more distal obstruction, pain and distention become more severe, the frequency and volume of vomiting decrease, and emesis becomes more feculent. Abdominal radiographs demonstrate multiple air-fluid levels and a paucity of gas in the colon; however, with high obstruction, above the ligament of Treitz, there may be no air-fluid levels. In the emergency department, differentiating between functional ileus and mechanical bowel obstruction can be difficult. Both disorders result in varying degrees of abdominal pain, distention, nausea, vomiting, and constipation. Once the diagnosis of mechanical obstruction is confirmed or suspected, surgical consultation is indicated.

INTRAABDOMINAL ABSCESS Intraabdominal abscess is caused most frequently by preoperative contamination, spillage of bowel contents during surgery, contamination of a hematoma, or postoperative anastomotic leaks. Patients may have abdominal pain, nausea, vomiting, ileus, abdominal distention, fever, chills, anorexia, and abdominal tenderness. If the diagnosis is suspected, CT or ultrasound studies of the abdomen are required. The patient should receive broad-spectrum antibiotics. Although some abscesses are amenable to percutaneous drainage, many patients require surgical exploration.

PANCREATITIS Pancreatitis following abdominal surgery is secondary to direct manipulation or retraction of the pancreatic duct. It most commonly occurs following gastric resection, biliary tract surgery, and endoscopic retrograde cholangiopancreatography (ERCP). Clinical presentation varies from mild nausea, vomiting, and abdominal discomfort to intractable vomiting, leukocytosis, and left pleural effusion. Severe hemorrhagic presentation can cause lumbar pain accompanied by blue-gray discoloration of the skin in the flank area (Turner sign) or similar changes around the umbilicus (Cullen sign). While the serum amylase level rises in acute pancreatitis, it is also elevated in patients with severe cholecystitis, renal insufficiency, intestinal obstruction, perforated ulcer, or ischemic bowel. A serum lipase measurement may help to identify those with true pancreatitis, although it may be elevated in a patient with a perforated viscus. Abdominal radiographs may show localized ileus in the region of the pancreas (sentinel loop). CT is useful in defining pancreatic fluid collections or abscesses. Generally, the treatment of postoperative pancreatitis is similar to the treatment of nonoperative pancreatitis: bowel rest, antiemetics, and nasogastric suction.

CHOLECYSTITIS Patients may present during the postoperative period with biliary colic, acute calculous cholecystitis, or acute acalculous cholecystitis. The etiology of these disorders in the postoperative period is not clear. Ultrasound studies of the gallbladder and pancreas should be performed to aid in the diagnosis.

Acalculous cholecystitis is of particular concern in the postoperative period. While it may occur in any age group, it seems to be more common in elderly males. Signs and symptoms are similar to those for calculous cholecystitis, but ultrasound studies fail to reveal gallstones.

Liver function studies and the neutrophil count may be normal. Important findings on ultrasonography include gallbladder enlargement, wall thickening, and pericholecystic fluid collection. Hepatobiliary scintigraphy may be helpful. Early diagnosis is critical because early operative intervention can reduce morbidity and mortality rates.

FISTULAS Enterocutaneous fistulas can occur almost anywhere in the gastrointestinal tract and are usually the result of technical complications or direct bowel injury. High-output fistulas can result in electrolyte abnormalities and volume depletion. Fistulas involving the proximal gastrointestinal tract are frequently high output and are of the greatest concern. Sepsis is the other major complication. Most patients require admission, although many fistulas ultimately close spontaneously.

TETANUS While most cases of tetanus in the United States occur after minor trauma, there have been numerous reports of tetanus following general surgical procedures. *Clostridium tetani* is found in the gastrointestinal tract of 1 percent of the population.[10] During gastrointestinal surgery, there is spillage of *C. tetani.* Proliferation of the organism is facilitated by the presence of devitalized tissue, blood clots, and surgical suture. Incubation can take from 1 to 54 days, at which time the toxin leads to clinical tetanus.[11] The classic symptoms of tetanus, trismus and opisthotonos, may not be manifested at initial presentation. Patients may present with nonspecific symptoms of abdominal discomfort, fever, and abdominal wall rigidity. Diagnosis is based on physical examination and a history of inadequate immunization.

Specific Considerations

ANASTOMOSIS Anastomotic leaks occur most frequently after esophageal and colonic surgery and least frequently after gastric and small intestinal anastomoses. The cause of anastomotic leakage is mainly related to surgical technique.

Intrathoracic esophageal anastomotic leaks usually manifest within 10 days of surgery. The presentation is dramatic, with fever, chest pain, tachypnea, tachycardia, and possibly shock. Chest x-ray may reveal a pneumothorax with pleural effusion. Disruption can be confirmed by contrast esophagography using a water-soluble contrast agent. Even with immediate reoperation, morbidity and mortality rates are high.

The signs and symptoms of gastric anastomotic leaks include abdominal pain, fever, leukocytosis, gastric outlet obstruction, hyperamylasemia, hyperbilirubinemia, peritonitis, and shock. Plain radiographs may reveal pneumoperitoneum or air-fluid levels. The patient should have immediate volume resuscitation, parenteral broad-spectrum antibiotics, and nasogastric tube drainage. Immediate surgery is required.

Small-intestinal anastomoses infrequently leak because of the excellent blood supply and rapid healing of the area. However, if a leak occurs, the patient usually presents with local abscess formation or peritonitis. Treatment is immediate reoperation.

Colorectal anastomoses are prone to disruption because of the large number of pathogenic bacteria, propensity for colonic distention, and single thin layer of circular muscle to support sutures. The patients usually present 7 to 14 days postoperatively with evidence of intraabdominal or pelvic abscess. CT studies can be helpful in diagnosis. Patients should receive broad-spectrum parenteral antibiotics, nasogastric tube drainage, and adequate fluid resuscitation in preparation for surgery.

GASTRIC SURGERY Patients who have undergone partial or complete gastrectomy can present with a few distinct syndromes: dumping syndrome, alkaline reflux gastritis, afferent loop syndrome, and postvagotomy diarrhea. While these complications are rare, the symptoms can be disabling.

Dumping syndrome can occur either early or late after a meal. While the precise etiology of dumping symptoms is unclear, it occurs when the pylorus is either bypassed or removed. The hyperosmolar chyme contents of the stomach are dumped into the jejunum, resulting in rapid influx of extracellular fluid and an autonomic response.

Patients experience nausea, epigastric discomfort, palpitations, abdominal colic, diaphoresis, and, in some cases, dizziness and syncope. Patients with early dumping symptoms experience diarrhea, while those with late dumping symptoms, 2 to 4 h postprandial, usually do not. The late dumping syndrome is felt to be due to a reactive hypoglycemia. The mainstay of treatment is dietary modification; eating small, dry meals; and separating solids from liquids. In refractory cases, pyloroplasty can be tried. Most of these patients do not require admission.

Patients with alkaline reflux gastritis present with continual burning epigastric pain that is aggravated by meals and unrelieved by vomiting. The syndrome is caused by reflux of bile into the stomach. Diagnosis is made by endoscopic examination.

Patients with afferent loop syndrome also present with severe epigastric pain 1 to 2 h after eating, which is relieved by vomiting. The vomitus will be bilious, without food. The syndrome occurs in patients who have undergone gastroenterostomy (Billroth II) reconstruction after partial gastrectomy. Diagnosis is made by contrast radiography or endoscopy. Operative reconstruction is required.

Although most patients undergoing truncal vagotomy have increased bowel movements, some will have diarrhea. The precise etiology is not clear. Patients present with diarrhea that is variable in its occurrence and not associated with food intake. It is often unpredictable and explosive, which can lead to weight loss and malnutrition as well as severe social complications. The incidence of the diarrhea decreases with time, and treatment is mostly symptomatic.

GASTROSTOMY TUBES Most gastrostomy tubes are now placed by either an endoscopist via percutaneous endoscopy or by a radiologist via percutaneous fluoroscopy. If the patient has undergone a laparotomy, the general surgeon may place a gastrostomy tube at the time of surgery. If the tube was placed by the surgeon and has not been replaced, it will have a bumper holding the tube in place. The tube has to be cut and the bumper allowed to pass, or the bumper has to be removed by endoscopic technique. For further discussion, see Chap. 85, ''Complications of GI Devices.''

BILIARY TRACT SURGERY More than half of all cholecystectomies are now performed laparoscopically. There are complications seen after both open and laparoscopic cholecystectomy (Table 84-5) and

TABLE 84-5 Complications of Cholecystectomy

Bile leak
Bile duct stricture
Bleeding
Bowel injury
Intraabdominal abscess
Myocardial infarction
Pancreatitis
Pulmonary complications
Retained common duct stones or stones spilled into peritoneum
Umbilical hernia
Wound infection

TABLE 84-6 Complications of Laparoscopy

RELATED TO PNEUMOPERITONEUM
Cardiac arrhythmias during the procedure
Subcutaneous emphysema
Pneumothorax
Pneumomediastinum
CO_2 embolization
RELATED TO INSERTION OF NEEDLE AND TROCAR
Bleeding from trocar site
Gastrointestinal tract injuries Laceration Intestinal burns
Genitourinary tract injuries
Major vessel injuries
Hernia from trocar site
Wound infection
MISCELLANEOUS
Retained intraabdominal gallstones Biliary cutaneous fistula Chronic pain Infertility Cholelithiasis
Metastases to the trocar site

complications related to the laparoscopic technique (Table 84-6).[12,13] Patients are likely to present to the emergency department with nonspecific abdominal symptoms.

The evaluation of abdominal pain after cholecystectomy depends on the clinical condition of the patient. If there are signs of peritoneal irritation or fever, an injury to the biliary system is likely. The patient should have a CT scan of the abdomen in addition to a CBC, electrolyte measurements, liver function tests, and a serum lipase test. ERCP will be required to identify the site of the injury; however, a collection of bile can be seen in a CT scan. Depending on the ERCP results, reoperation may be necessary. Small collections of bile may require only observation or percutaneous drainage.

Patients presenting soon after cholecystectomy with pain, pancreatitis, and/or jaundice may have retained common duct stones. If the CT scan does not reveal an intraabdominal collection of fluid, an ERCP should be performed. Endoscopic sphincterotomy is usually an effective means of dealing with retained stones. Patients presenting late after cholecystectomy with fever, pain, and jaundice may have bile duct stricture. Diagnosis requires ERCP. While stents are usually tried at first, surgical repair may be necessary. A more recent concern has been the spillage of gallstones into the peritoneal cavity at the time of surgery. Initially, such stones were thought to be innocuous. However, they have been linked to abdominal pain, pelvic pain, dysmenorrhea, intraabdominal abscess, colocutaneous fistula, and implantation into the ovary with subsequent infertility.[14]

OTHER LAPAROSCOPIC SURGERIES Laparoscopic techniques are now being used for an increasing number of procedures. In addition to cholecystectomy, they have been used for appendectomy, colon resection, antireflux surgery, herniorrhaphy, fundoplication, and most gynecologic surgical procedures, including hysterectomy. The complications associated with these procedures have not been completely identified; however, they are likely to be similar to those seen with cholecystectomy.

STOMAS The two most common stomas placed are the ileostomy and the colostomy. Problems with these stomas can be quite debilitating. Most complications are related to technical errors as to where the stomas are placed; however, there can be problems of new disease within the stoma (e.g., Crohn's disease or cancer). Possible complications include ischemia and stomal necrosis, peristomal skin irritation, peristomal hernia, and stomal prolapse.

Ischemia and stomal necrosis are manifested very early in the postoperative course. The cause is inadequate blood supply to the stoma. Normally, the stoma is pink, without any evidence of cyanosis. Any evidence of compromised blood flow requires surgical evaluation.

Peristomal maceration and skin destruction are most likely secondary to a poor seal of the stomal appliance. Consultation with an enterostomal therapist for a properly fitting appliance is indicated.

Prolapse can occur with both ileostomies and colostomies. The cause is usually inadequate fixation of the intraabdominal portion or too large an abdominal wall opening. Patients present with the stoma protrusion, with or without pain. The stoma must be examined to determine viability. The stoma should be pink and painless. Reduction should be attempted if the tissue is viable, followed by consultation with a surgeon. Definitive therapy requires surgical revision.

Parastomal hernias are secondary to too large an abdominal wall opening. As with any hernia, the physician should determine whether the hernia is incarcerated, attempt reduction, and consult a surgeon. Definitive therapy requires local reconstruction of the orifice.

COLONOSCOPY Potential complications of colonoscopy include hemorrhage, perforation, retroperitoneal abscess, pneumoscrotum, pneumothorax, volvulus, postcolonoscopy distention, bacteremia, and infection.

Hemorrhage is the most common complication and can be secondary to the polypectomy procedures, biopsies, laceration of the mucosa by the instrument, or tearing of the mesentery or spleen. If the bleeding is intraluminal, the patient will present with rectal bleeding. Patients with mesenteric or splenic injury will present with signs of intraabdominal bleeding. Treatment of intraluminal bleeding depends on the magnitude of hemorrhage. Signs of intraabdominal bleeding require emergency laparotomy.

Perforation of the colon with pneumoperitoneum usually is evident immediately but can also take several hours to manifest. Perforation is usually secondary to intrinsic disease of the colon (e.g., diverticulitis) or to vigorous manipulation during the procedure. Most patients will require immediately laparotomy; however, in some patients presenting late (1 to 2 days later) without signs of peritonitis, expectant management may be appropriate.

RECTAL SURGERY Patients who have undergone hemorrhoidectomy frequently have problems with postoperative urinary retention, the management of which has been previously discussed. Three other problems that can occur are constipation, rectal hemorrhage, and rectal prolapse.

The management of constipation in a patient who has undergone rectal surgery is no different from that of any other patient with constipation. Gentle rectal examination is indicated, and enemas can still be used. Posthemorrhoidectomy rectal hemorrhage can occur immediately postoperatively but may also be delayed (4 ± 2 days).[15] Proposed causes of delayed bleeding include sepsis of the pedicle, disruption of a clot, and sloughing of tissue.[16] The patient may present with minimal bleeding or massive hemorrhage. While ligation of the affected vessel is needed, a temporary tamponade with a Foley catheter may be helpful.

Patients may present with mucosal prolapse or complete rectal prolapse. Mucosal prolapse occurs when the surgeon has not removed all redundant mucosa during hemorrhoidectomy and is much more common than rectal prolapse. Local treatment by a surgeon is usually corrective. Rectal prolapse can occur after any anorectal surgical procedure and probably is related to injury of the puborectalis muscle. The patient will present with the sensation of protrusion and may complain of pain. The treatment is reduction and surgical consultation.

Infection following anorectal surgery is surprisingly uncommon. The patient usually complains of increasing pain and fever. Examination of the area is necessary to detect an abscess or cellulitis. Fournier's gangrene may follow anorectal surgery. If this is suspected, broad-spectrum parenteral antibiotics are given immediately. The patient requires immediate surgical debridement.

REFERENCES

1. O'Grady NP, Barie PS, Bartlett J, et al: Practice parameters for evaluating fever in critically ill adult patients. *Crit Care Med* 26:392, 1998.
2. Tammela T, Kontturi M, Lukkarinen O: Postoperative urinary retention: I. Incidence and predisposing factors. *Scand J Urol Nephrol* 20:197, 1986.
3. Nyman MA, Schwenk NM, Silverstein MD: Management of urinary retention: Rapid versus gradual decompression and risk of complications. *Mayo Clin Proc* 72:951, 1997.
4. Wysoki MG, Santora TA, Shah RM, Friedman AC: Necrotizing fasciitis: CT characteristics. *Radiology* 203:859, 1997.
5. Schmid MR, Kossmann T, Duewell S: Differentiation of necrotizing fasciitis and cellulitis using MR imaging. *AJR* 170:615, 1998.
6. Gilbert DN, Moellering RC, Sande MA: *The Sanford Guide to Antimicrobial Therapy,* 28th ed. Dallas, Antimicrobial Therapy, 1998.
7. Johnaon DH, Cunha BA: Drug fever. *Infect Dis Clin North Am* 10:85, 1996.
8. Brennan MJ, Depompolo RW, Garden FH: Focused review: Postmastectomy lymphedema. *Arch Phys Med Rehabil* 77(suppl 3):S74, 1996.
9. Nachlas MM, Younis MT, Roda CP, Wityk JJ: Gastrointestinal motility studies as a guide to postoperative management. *Ann Surg* 175:510, 1972.
10. Meyer KA, Spector BK: Incidence of tetanus bacilli in stools and on regional skins of one hundred urban herniotomy cases. *Surg Gynecol Obstet* 54:785, 1932.
11. LaForce FM, Young LS, Bennett JV: Tetanus in the United States: 1965–1969. *N Engl J Med* 280:569, 1969.
12. Callery MP, Strasberg SM, Soper NJ: Complications of laparoscopic general surgery. *Gastroint Endosc Clin North Am* 6:423, 1996.
13. Lujan JA, Parrilla P, Rabies R, et al: Laparascopic cholecystectomy vs. open cholecystectomy in the treatment of acute cholecystitis: A prospective study. *Arch Surg* 133:173, 1998.
14. Patterson EJ, Nagy AG: Don't cry over spilled stones? Complications of gallstones spilled during laparoscopic cholecystectomy: Case report and literature review. *Can J Surg* 40:300, 1997.
15. Basso L, Pescatori M: Outcomes of Delayed hemorrhage following surgical hemorrhoidectomy [letter]. *Dis Colon Rectum* 37:288, 1994.
16. Rosen L, Sipe P, Stasik JJ, et al: Outcome of delayed hemorrhage following surgical hemorrhoidectomy. *Dis Colon Rectum* 36:743, 1993.

COMPLICATIONS OF GASTROINTESTINAL DEVICES

Edmond A. Hooker

The gastrointestinal (GI) device that is most commonly used by emergency physicians is the nasogastric (NG) tube. Other GI devices encountered in the emergency department (ED) include large-bore orogastric tubes, small-bore nasointestinal ("feeding") tubes, and transabdominal feeding tubes (gastrostomy, jejunostomy, and gastrojejunostomy tubes). Although complications from the use of these are rare, they must be anticipated and prevented if possible.

NASOGASTRIC TUBES

The NG tube is probably the most common device placed in the GI tract. Tubes range in size from 6 to 18 Fr (1 Fr = 0.333 mm). These devices are relatively easy to place blindly in an alert, cooperative patient. Obtunded patients or those without an active gag reflex may require endotracheal intubation prior to NG insertion. It is important to note that the presence of an endotracheal tube with an inflated balloon does not prevent passage of these tubes into the respiratory tract.

TABLE 85-1 Complications of Placement of Nasogastric and Nasoenteric Tubes

Epistaxis
Intracranial placement
Bronchial placement
Pharyngeal perforation
Esophageal obstruction or rupture
Bronchial or alveolar perforation
Pneumothorax
Charcoal instillation into the lungs and pleural cavity
Gastric or duodenal rupture

Major complications have been reported with the use of NG tubes (Table 85-1). Improper placement is the principal cause of these complications, and different techniques have been proposed to help identify improper placement of nasogastric tubes (Table 85-2).[1] However, according to published research, none of the techniques have proven effective. The technique that is probably most commonly used, insufflation of air into the NG tube while listening over the stomach, has many reported failures.

Placement of the NG tube into the respiratory tract can result in pneumonia or pneumothorax. If charcoal is instilled, the outcome can be fatal. While not the standard of care, chest radiographs may aid in the confirmation of NG placement prior to instilling charcoal or other medications. If the tube is identified in the chest cavity, it must be determined whether it entered through the lungs or through the esophagus. All possible charcoal should be removed by suctioning prior to removing the NG tube or, in the case of charcoal thorax, by chest tube drainage.

There are numerous reports of intracranial placement of NG tubes.[2] Most cases have been reported in trauma patients; however, there is at least one report of intracranial placement in a nontrauma patient.[3] As with any catheter insertion, force should never be used, and nasogastric tubes should be inserted through the mouth in trauma patients who may have facial or basilar skull fractures. Any time a NG tube is placed and cannot be easily removed, an x-ray should be obtained to determine the location of the tube.

TABLE 85-2 Techniques for Identifying Nasogastric and Nasointestinal Feeding Tube Placement

Indicates gastric placement
Epigastric auscultation of air insufflated through the tube
Aspiration of visually recognizable gastrointestinal secretions
pH testing of aspirates (pH ≤ 6 indicates gastric placement)
Indicates tracheobronchial placement
Coughing or choking
Inability to speak
Air bubbles when proximal end of tube is placed in water

OROGASTRIC LAVAGE TUBES

Large-bore tubes (28 to 40 Fr) are used for gastric decontamination and charcoal instillation. The use of these tubes has come into relative disfavor in recent years.[4] This was not because of complications but rather because of a lack of proven efficacy. Complications have only been rarely reported with the use of the tubes but have included esophageal tears and inability to remove the tube secondary to esophageal spasm. If an orogastric lavage tube cannot easily be removed, the patient should undergo fluoroscopic examination with contrast in order to determine its exact location and any kinking. If the tube is simply stuck because of esophageal spasm, glucagon can be given to assist in its removal.[5]

NASOINTESTINAL TUBES

The small-bore nasointestinal tubes (more commonly called feeding tubes) are usually placed to support nutrition. Complications of these tubes include all of those described with NG tubes (Table 85-1), but the former are also more easily dislodged and clogged. With numerous reports of placement of these tubes into the respiratory tract and subsequent intrapulmonary instillation of tube feedings, most institutions require radiographic confirmation of tube placement.[6,7] Since patients can easily dislodge these tubes after initial confirmation of placement, some recommend pH testing prior to each usage.[8]

Replacement of a dislodged tube should be performed using the manufacturer's instructions and radiographic confirmation should be obtained (Table 85-3). When one of these tubes is clogged from buildup of sediment, the physician can attempt to unclog the tube by instilling saline or cola drink into the tube and leaving it for 30 min; however, replacement will frequently be necessary.[9]

TRANSABDOMINAL FEEDING TUBES

While the techniques for the initial placement of transabdominal feeding tubes (gastrostomy, jejunostomy, and gastrojejunostomy) are beyond the scope of emergency physicians, complications related to these tubes need to be recognized (Table 85-4). These tubes can be placed by a surgeon via open technique, by a gastroenterologist via endoscopic technique [percutaneous endoscopic gastrostomy (PEG)], or by a radiologist via percutaneous techniques. The radiographic technique has been associated with fewer complications than either open or endoscopically assisted placement.[10,11]

Frequent minor complications are associated with the use of these tubes, including purulent drainage and leakage around the stomal site, clogging, dislodgement, and vomiting and diarrhea.

Drainage from the stomal site is a common finding and represents a foreign-body reaction due to the catheter. As long as there is no evidence of cellulitis or necrotizing fasciitis, local skin care with hydrogen peroxide and warm water will usually clear up the problem. If there is granuloma formation with localized bleeding from friable skin, local treatment with silver nitrate will usually help.

Leakage of gastric contents can become a problem. This is managed by careful insertion of a larger tube. Care should be used not to force too large a tube into the stoma, as this can cause separation of the stomach wall from the abdominal wall.

Prevention is the best treatment for clogging of gastrostomy (G) and jejunostomy (J) tubes. Frequent flushing with water and careful crushing of pills will usually prevent this problem. Vomiting and diarrhea can be relieved by decreasing the amount of the feedings and/or diluting them.

TABLE 85-3 Method for Inserting a Nasointestinal Feeding Tube*

Step 1:	Prepare nares with topical anesthetic and lubricant. Restrain uncooperative patients. Lubricate and insert the stylet into the feeding tube (ensure that the stylet does not protrude beyond tip of tube).
Step 2:	Place tube through nares into hypopharynx. If patient starts coughing or choking, tube may be in respiratory tract or coiled up in hypopharynx. The cooperative patient may swallow liquids to assist passage.
Step 3:	After successful passage, remove stylet from tube and obtain a chest x-ray that includes the epigastric area. If tube is in proper position, start feedings.

**Warnings:* Never reinsert a stylet into a feeding tube while the tube is still in the patient and never use a feeding tube prior to radiographic confirmation of placement.

TABLE 85-4 Complication Seen with Transabdominal Feeding Tubes

Complication	Initial Considerations
Purulent drainage from stoma	Local care with hydrogen peroxide unless cellulitic
Leakage from stoma	Carefully replace with larger tube
Tube occlusion	Attempt irrigation, most often just replace
Dislodged tubes	Gently replace, confirm placement with x-rays
Pneumothorax	High index of suspicion, consider needle aspiration
Bacteremia	Consider as potential source in septic patient
Bleeding from tract	If recently inserted, consider local injection, consult
Bleeding from granuloma buildup	Local therapy with silver nitrate
Infection of surrounding skin	Consultation, pull tube, IV antibiotics
Necrotizing fasciitis	Consider MRI to help confirm, surgical debridement
Peritonitis	Determine if fistula exists, consultation, IV antibiotics
Pulmonary aspiration of feedings	Reduce flow rate, half-strength feeds, consider J tube
Vomiting or diarrhea	Reduce flow rate, half-strength feeds, stop feeds
Gastroesophageal reflux	Reduce flow rate, half-strength feeds, consider J tube
Intestinal obstruction	Stop feedings, NPO, admit and observe
Gastric outlet obstruction	Reposition tube
Gastric volvulus	Surgical consult
Gastric perforation	Surgical consult
Esophageal perforation	Surgical consult
Colonic perforation	Surgical consult
Colocutaneous fistula	Surgical consult
Electrolyte abnormalities	Change feedings or increase free water
Gastrointestinal bleeding	Endoscopy and therapy directed at cause

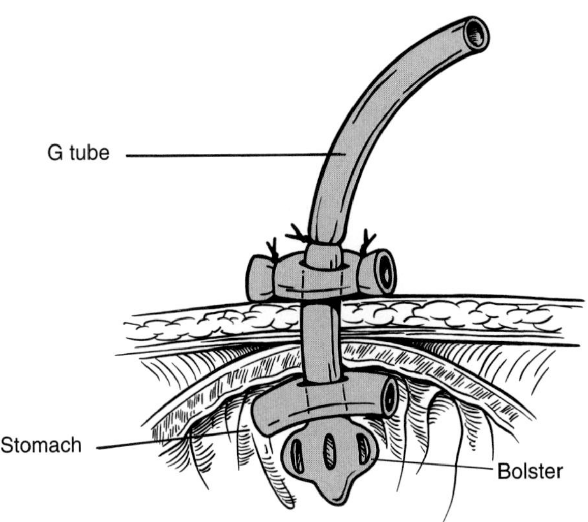

FIG. 85-1. Percutaneous endoscopic gastrostomy tube with a mushroom bolster in place. (Adapted from Gauderer MWL, Ponsky JL: A simplified technique for constructing a tube feeding gastrostomy. *Surg Gynecol Obstet* 152:83, 1981, with permission.)

If the tube cannot be unclogged or if it has fallen out, replacement will be necessary. If the tube was placed by a surgeon or gastroenterologist and has not been replaced, it will probably have a bolster (also called a mushroom) holding the tube in place (Fig. 85-1). This will prevent the tube from being removed. The tube must either have the bolster removed endoscopically or the tube may be cut off and the bolster allowed to pass through the GI tract.[12] The latter technique is generally safe in adults; however, its use in children has been associated with more frequent complications.[13] Endoscopic removal is advisable when there is suspected or potential obstructive disease of the GI tract, such as pyloric stenosis, intestinal pseudoobstruction, and intestinal stricture (e.g., due to radiation, ischemia, or inflammatory bowel disease). If the tube is cut, an abdominal radiograph should be obtained 1 week later to confirm passage of the internal component. Most reported complications from a retained internal bolster have occurred when the bolster did not pass within 1 to 2 weeks.[14]

When the feeding tube has already been replaced or was originally placed via radiographic technique, it should have a balloon holding it in place. The balloon can usually be deflated and the tube easily removed. If there is a problem with removal, the tube can be cut off halfway down; this will usually allow the balloon to deflate. If the catheter still cannot be removed easily, it can be cut off at the skin and the internal component allowed to pass. It should be replaced as quickly as possible to prevent closure of the tract. While there is no published research stating how long it takes for a tract to mature, tracts that are 7 to 10 days old will probably remain open long enough to allow replacement. The physician must first determine, if possible, which type of tube is being used. If the tube is available, replacement with the same size is usually possible. If the tube is not available, it can be difficult to determine whether the tract is for a jejunostomy or gastrostomy tube. Location on the abdominal wall is not helpful. A tract for a G tube is usually larger. Old records may be useful and should be obtained if possible. After determining the type of tract and size of tube used previously, insertion should be performed by the physician using a water-soluble lubricant. If the size of the tube being replaced cannot be ascertained, it is reasonable to start with a 16-Fr replacement gastrostomy tube or Foley catheter. The lubricated tube should pass easily into the stoma without any additional equipment. If resistance is met, the attempt should be abandoned. A smaller tube can be tried to keep the tract open. After replacing the tube, a 20- to 30-mL bolus of a water-soluble contrast material (e.g., Gastrografin) should be instilled through the tube and a supine abdominal x-ray obtained within 1 to 2 min.[15] The x-ray should demonstrate rugae of the stomach for a G tube and flow into a small bowel for a J tube. If there is any question of improper placement, immediate consultation should be obtained.

A special caution regarding jejunostomy tubes should be noted. Jejunostomy tracts are smaller, and smaller-size tubes are used (8 to 14 Fr). These tubes are usually not sutured in place and frequently become dislodged. They can be replaced with catheters made specifically for jejunostomies or with Foley catheters. If a Foley catheter is used to replace a lost jejunostomy catheter, the balloon should never be inflated because it can cause a bowel obstruction or damage the jejunum. The tube is lubricated, inserted into the stoma, and advanced 20 cm. These tubes are easily replaced if the tract is mature: however, if resistance is met, referral to a radiologist for fluoroscopic placement using guidewires is recommended.[16]

REFERENCES

1. Metheny N: Measures to test placement of nasogastric and nasointestinal feeding tubes: A review. *Nurs Res* 37:324, 1988.
2. Marlow TJ, Goltra DD, Schabel SI: Intracranial placement of a nasotracheal tube after facial fracture: A rare complication. *J Emerg Med* 15:187, 1997.
3. Freij RM, Mullett ST: Inadvertent intracranial insertion of a nasogastric tube in a nontrauma patient. *J Accid Emerg Med* 14:45, 1997.
4. Vale JA: Position statement: Gastric lavage. American Academy of Clinical Toxicology; European Association of Poison Centres and Clinical Toxicologists. *J Toxicol Clin Toxicol* 35:711, 1997.
5. Thoma ME, Glauser JM: Use of glucagon for removal of an orogastric lavage tube. *Am J Emerg Med* 13:219, 1995.
6. Bankier AA, Wiesmayr MN, Henk C, et al: Radiographic detection of intrabronchial malposition of nasogastric tubes and subsequent complications in intensive care unit patients. *Intens Care Med* 23:406, 1997.
7. Lipman TO, Kessler T, Arabian A: Nasopulmonary intubation with feeding tubes: Case reports and review of the literature. *J Parenter Enter Nutr* 9:618, 1985.
8. Metheny N, Reed L, Wiersema L, et al: Effectiveness of pH measurement in predicting feeding tube placement: An update. *Nurs Res* 42:324, 1993.
9. Nicholson LJ: Declogging small-bore feeding tubes. *J Parenter Enter Nutr* 11:594, 1987.
10. Wollman B, D'Agostino HB: Percutaneous radiologic and endoscopic gastrostomy: A 3-year institutional analysis of procedure performance. *AJR* 169:1551, 1997.
11. Wollman B, D'Agostino HB, Walus-Wigle JR, et al: Radiologic, endoscopic, and surgical gastrostomy: An institutional evaluation and meta-analysis of the literature. *Radiology* 197:699, 1996.
12. Korula J, Harma C: A simple and inexpensive method of removal or replacement of gastrostomy tubes. *JAMA* 265:1426, 1991.
13. Chait PG, Weinberg J, Connolly BL, et al: Retrograde percutaneous gastrostomy and gastrojejunostomy in 505 children: a 4½ year experience. *Radiology* 201:691, 1996.
14. Yaseen M, Steele MI, Grunow JE: Nonendoscopic removal of percutaneous endoscopic gastrostomy tubes: Morbidity and mortality in children. *Gastrointest Endosc* 44:235, 1996.
15. Wolf EL, Frager D, Beneventano TC: Radiologic demonstration of important gastrostomy tube complications. *Gastrointest Radiol* 11:20, 1986.
16. Boland MP, Patrick J, Stoski DS, Soucy P: Permanent Enteral Feeding in Cystic Fibrosis: Advantages of a Replaceable Jejunostomy Tube. *J Pediatr Surg* 22:843, 1987.

THE LIVER TRANSPLANT PATIENT

Steven Kronick

DEMOGRAPHICS AND SURVIVAL

Worldwide, approximately 7000 liver transplantations are performed yearly. In the United States, more than 4000 liver transplantations are performed at more than 100 centers each year. At present, the number of transplantations performed is limited only by the availability of organ donors. Before the 1980s, 1-year survival after liver transplantation was approximately 30 percent. Improvements in surgical techniques, immunosuppression protocols, and patient selection have increased mean patient survival to 87 percent at 1 year and 77.4 percent at 3 years.[1] Transplantation is the treatment of choice for end-stage liver disease (ESLD) refractory to all other interventions and is considered an effective means to improve quality of life as well as survival.[2] As this population of patients continues to grow, so will the number of patients with liver transplantation who present to the emergency department (ED) with transplant- and non-transplant-related problems. The incidence of transplant-related problems is high (Table 86-1) and evaluation is made difficult by the fact that many of the complications present with similar signs, symptoms, and laboratory abnormalities. Most transplant-related problems will require, at a minimum, direct communication with the transplant center for consultation and follow-up.

TRANSPLANT PROCEDURE

Indications for liver transplantation are listed in Table 86-2. The harvested liver can tolerate ischemia up to 24 h, but it functions best if ischemia time is less than 8 h. The risk of preservation injury increases after this time. Most patients undergo bilateral subcostal incision with upper midline extension to the xiphoid process. After recipient hepatectomy, the donor liver is placed in the recipient typically in the same (orthotopic) location as the liver it is replacing (Fig. 86-1). Venovenous bypass, used in most centers, may predispose the patient to thrombosis and pulmonary embolism. Normal color and consistency return to the organ in approximately 15 min. Early bile production after vascular reanastomosis is most indicative of graft function.[3] The preferred method for biliary tract reconstruction is an end-to-end choledochocholedochostomy. The use of a percutaneous biliary drain varies by center and when used typically stays in place 3 to 6 months. In children and in those whose anatomy will not allow choledochocholedochostomy, Roux-en-Y hepaticojejunostomy is performed. Newer techniques being used increasingly in pediatric patients include reduced-size liver transplant, split liver transplant, and living-related transplantation.[4]

TABLE 86-1 Common Complications Following Liver Transplantation

Complication	% with Complication
Infection	>60
Rejection	>50
Neurologic	≤47
Vascular clot, stenosis	≤30
Renal insufficiency	≤25
Hemorrhage	≤20
Biliary stenosis, leak	≤20
GI	≤15
PTLD	4

Abbreviations: GI, gastrointestinal; PTLD, posttransplant lymphoproliferative disorder.

TABLE 86-2 Indications for Liver Transplantation

Primary biliary cirrhosis
Primary sclerosing cholangitis
Fulminant and subfulminant hepatitis
Cirrhosis due to hepatitis B or C virus
Alcoholic cirrhosis
Children: biliary atresia (accounts for >50%) selected inborn errors of metabolism
Controversial indications
Hepatocellular carcinoma
Contraindications
Extrahepatic malignancy
Liver metastases
Extrahepatic organ failure
Noncompliance
Active substance abuse
AIDS

POSTOPERATIVE COMPLICATIONS

Immediate postoperative complications are not seen in the ED, since patients typically remain hospitalized for approximately 2 weeks. Postoperative problems seen in the ED are most commonly related to bleeding, biliary, vascular, and wound complications.

Bleeding Complications

The vast majority of postoperative bleeding complications in patients will occur in the first week and will not be seen in the ED. More likely is gastrointestinal bleeding, which should be managed in the usual fashion but may signal graft dysfunction and be accompanied by profound hypoglycemia and progressive coagulopathy.[3] Portal hypertension is reversed by liver transplantation and gastrointestinal (GI) bleeding from varices postoperatively may be indicative of portal vein thrombosis. Another contributing factor that may predispose patients to GI bleeding is high-dose steroids. Cytomegalovirus (CMV), herpes simplex virus (HSV), and candidal infection can also lead to significant bleeding.

Biliary Complications

Biliary problems account for a significant proportion of complications, and incidence may be as high as 29 percent.[5] Leaks, strictures (ductal narrowing), and obstruction (ductal blockage) account for 80 percent of these complications. In general, leaks occur early, with 38 percent in the first 30 days and most (80 percent) within the first 6 months.[6] Early leaks tend to be more severe owing to duct disruption and higher immunosuppression and are notoriously difficult to treat. Leaks after the first month are invariably associated with either elective or inadvertent removal of an indwelling biliary catheter.[7] In children, stricture and obstruction are responsible for 90 percent of complications.[6] For patients with Roux-en-Y, the leak tends to occur at the anastomosis, whereas for the majority of patients who have choledochocholedochostomy, the leak is at the anastomosis early or the T-tube site later.[8] The cause of biliary injury is either immunologic or preservation

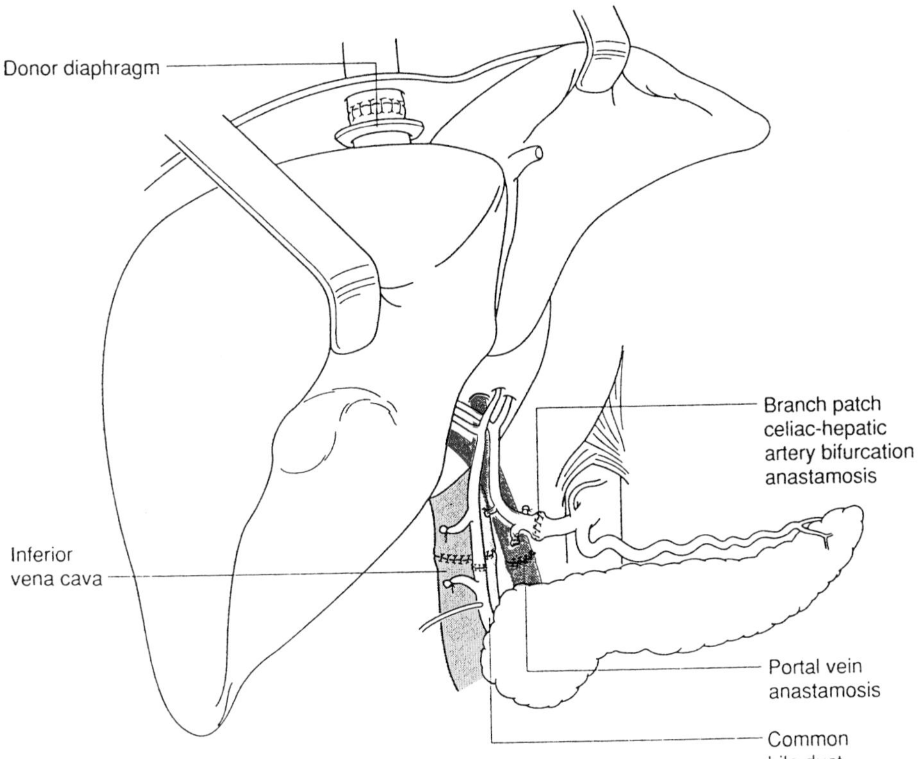

FIG. 86-1. End-to-end choledochocholedochostomy. If the recipient's system permits, this is the preferred method for reconstruction of the biliary system, the last part of the operative phase in liver transplantation.

injury, infection, or ischemia. Biliary leaks present most commonly with peritonitis, fever, abdominal pain, constipation, and abdominal distention, but signs and symptoms may be subtle or masked owing to the use of immunosuppressive agents. Laboratory abnormalities include leukocytosis, hyperbilirubinemia, and increased alkaline phosphatase. If abdominal drains are still in place, you may see bile in the drain, or if a T-tube is present, bile may appear at the tube site.[5] Evaluation should include Doppler ultrasound, as there is an association with hepatic artery thrombosis (HAT). Treatment of the leak includes drainage of abscess, if present, and intravenous antibiotics. Broad-spectrum antibiotic coverage should be directed against gram-positive, gram-negative, and anaerobic organisms.[6] Bacterial infections tend to be polymicrobial and include *Enterobacter, Enterococcus, Bacteroides, Clostridium,* species, and *Pseudomonas.*[3] Biliary leakage is associated with high mortality.

After 12 months, stricture and/or obstruction account for the vast majority of biliary complications. Development of a biliary complication is heralded by three typical presentations. Most common is intermittent episodes of fever and fluctuating liver function tests. The second presentation is gradual asymptomatic worsening of liver function tests. Finally, biliary complication may present as acute bacterial cholangitis with fever, chills, abdominal pain, jaundice, and bacteremia. Stricture or narrowing of the bile duct frequently develops insidiously.[7] The presentation of biliary complication can be difficult to distinguish clinically from rejection, HAT, CMV infection, or a recurrence of a preexisting disease (especially hepatitis).

Liver transplant recipients with suspected biliary complications should be referred to a transplant center. All patients should have a complete blood count (CBC) with platelet count and differential; serum chemistries including electrolytes, blood urea nitrogen (BUN), creatinine, liver function tests, amylase, and lipase levels; cultures of blood, urine, bile, and ascites if present; chest x-ray; and abdominal ultrasound with Doppler flow studies. Ultrasound rules out the presence of fluid collections, screens for the presence of thrombosis of the hepatic artery or portal vein, and identifies any dilation of the biliary tree. The intrahepatic ductal system rarely appears dilated appreciably by ultrasound, even in the presence of complete obstruction. Patients often require cholangiography for complete evaluation. Those patients with choledochocholedochostomy are best evaluated by endoscopic retrograde cholangiopancreatography (ERCP) because it permits both a radiographic diagnosis and the potential for nonoperative intervention. Patients who have Roux-en-Y hepaticojejunostomy or those who cannot have ERCP must undergo percutaneous cholangiography. Early broad-spectrum prophylactic antibiotics should be administered prior to any biliary tract manipulation.

Vascular Complications

Vascular complications are less common than biliary complications but are associated with high morbidity, mortality, and graft failure. HAT is the most common vascular complication and tends to occur within the first 3 weeks after transplantation. The incidence reported is between 5 and 40 percent and tends to be higher in children. For this reason, children are frequently treated prophylactically with antiplatelet agents.

The presentation of HAT may be signaled by elevated prothrombin (PT) and transaminase levels, little or no bile production, liver abscess, unexplained sepsis, or as a biliary tract problem (leak, obstruction, abscess, or breakdown of the anastomosis). HAT may present with massive hepatic necrosis, sepsis, fever, and bacteremia after early thrombosis; bile leak, since the hepatic artery is the sole blood supply; relapsing fever with bacteremia secondary to focal abscesses or biloma; or it can be asymptomatic if collaterals have formed.[5] HAT is ominous, and frequently requires retransplantation. Occasionally, if diagnosed early, immediate thrombectomy and revision of the anastomosis may preclude the need for retransplantation. Pediatric patients are more susceptible to HAT and have a much more varied presentation, with an incidence as high as 26 percent in children and 31 percent in neonates.[9] Duplex ultrasonography (Doppler ultrasound with real-time scanning) has a sensitivity of 92 percent.[10] If ultrasound is not diagnostic and suspicion remains, one should proceed to angiography.[11] Hepatic artery rupture is uncommon and generally associated with intraabdominal sepsis and poor prognosis.[5] Portal vein thrombosis is less common and affects 2 to 3 percent of patients. The diagnosis is suggested by variceal hemorrhage, massive ascites, or other signs of portal hypertension. Initially, effort is directed toward reducing the portosystemic pressure gradient, but retransplantation may be necessary.

Wound Complications

Wound problems are probably underreported and include infection, hematomas, and seromas as the most common complications. Presentation may be subtle. Fever, chills, incisional pain, swelling, erythema, or drainage may not always be present due to immunosuppressive diminution of signs of inflammation. Infection can lead to necrotizing fasciitis. An increased degree of suspicion is necessary. Early broad-spectrum antibiotic coverage should be considered.

REJECTION

Acute allograft rejection is most commonly seen at 7 to 14 days. The incidence of acute rejection varies from 40 to 80 percent during the first posttransplant year. After several months, the incidence of acute rejection decreases steadily, but it may be triggered at any time by tapering of immunosuppressive agents.[12] Though frequently subtle in presentation, a syndrome of acute rejection includes fever, liver tenderness, lymphocytosis, eosinophilia, liver enzyme elevation, and a change in bile color or production. In the perioperative period, the differential diagnosis must include infection, acute biliary obstruction, and vascular insufficiency. The diagnosis can be made with certainty only by excluding other causes of graft dysfunction and biopsy, which usually requires referral back to the transplant center for management and follow-up. Acute rejection is typically treated by high-dose glucocorticosteroid bolus followed by a rapid taper over 5 to 7 days. This treatment is effective in 65 to 80 percent of transplant recipients.[3] Secondary therapy includes the infusion of antilymphocyte globulin (e.g., OKT3), which is accompanied by a variety of potential side effects. Both these therapies are best managed at an experienced transplant center.

Chronic allograft rejection occurs in approximately 5 to 10 percent of recipients and is a major cause of late graft failure. The primary manifestation of chronic rejection is a persistently cholestatic liver injury pattern with elevated serum alkaline phosphatase and bilirubin, which can be associated with pruritus. Significant loss of hepatic synthetic function is often not evident until late in the course of chronic rejection. The diagnosis is made by biopsy.

INFECTION

General Considerations

The vast majority of liver transplant recipients have at least one episode of infection at some time after their transplantation and many have more than one episode. Infections or their complications are believed to account for most of the deaths. Vigilance for infection must remain high, since immunosuppression-induced blunting of the inflammatory response may mask the classic signs and symptoms of infection. Timing of infection after transplantation can be organized into three segments: less than 1 month, 1 to 6 months, and greater than 6 months. Infection in the first 30 postoperative days is primarily from bacteria and fungi. The patient is typically at the greatest levels of immunosuppression and the anastomoses are at their most vulnerable during the first month. The vast majority of infectious agents seen in less than 1 month are the same nosocomial agents seen in similar surgical patients. Opportunistic organisms are notably absent in the first month. CMV is discussed below.

During the first postoperative month, intraabdominal infections—including cholangitis, peritonitis, as well as liver and other intraabdominal abscesses—predominate. Presentation is marked by fever, abdominal pain and distension, ascites, and occasionally jaundice. Workup should include CBC with differential, liver function tests, urinalysis, chest x-ray, abdominal ultrasound, and blood and fluid cultures. Evaluation may include ultrasound, CT scan, T-tube cholangiography, ERCP, liver biopsy, and cultures of blood, urine, or aspirated fluid. The organisms responsible tend to be enterococci, gram-negative aerobes, anaerobes, *Staphylococcus,* and *Candida* species. Patients may also present with pneumonia or urinary tract infections related to intubation or indwelling bladder catheterization while hospitalized. Cultures may need to be held in order for fungi, viruses, CMV, *Nocardia* species, and *Mycobacterium tuberculosis* to grow. Shell-vial cultures should be obtained if there is any suspicion of CMV disease.

From 1 to 6 months, most infection is from viruses [reactivation, donor transmission, Epstein-Barr virus (EBV)] or opportunistic organisms. After 6 months, the incidence of serious infection declines, with cholangitis predominating. Risk of infection after 6 months approaches that of the general population, although morbidity and mortality may be higher.[13] A high index of suspicion should be maintained whenever immunosuppression is high.[14] Close monitoring is essential, as rapid deterioration can take place while the patient is still in the ED.

Bacterial Infection

Bacterial infection is most common in the first month, with gram-negative enteric organisms accounting for over 50 percent. Although gram-negative organisms predominate (especially *Pseudomonas aeruginosa*), gram-positive and anaerobic organisms are not uncommon. Broad-spectrum antibiotics should be considered early in the patient's course. Bacterial infection is frequently associated with the vascular or biliary anastomosis, especially hepatic artery thrombosis but also portal vein thrombosis. Ischemia may lead to bile leak and abscess or deep soft tissue infection. After the first month, the incidence of bacterial infections decreases and the incidence of opportunistic infection increases, but vigilance for bacterial illnesses should remain high. Community-acquired pneumonia is most likely due to *Streptococcus pneumoniae* and *Haemophilus influenzae.* Meningitis shows a high preponderance of Listeria monocytogenes as well as *S. pneumoniae, Staphylococcus aureus,* and gram-negative rods. Empiric antibiotic coverage should be aimed at this flora.

Fungal Infection

Although uncommon, fungal disease is seen most within the first 2 months; it can be disseminated and is accompanied by high mortality. Fungal disease can present with multiple organ involvement, peritonitis, fungemia, pneumonitis, or asymptomatic colonization. The incidence of fungal disease is continuing to decrease, but mortality remains high. Mortality is up to 78 percent if disease is systemic. *Candida* species are responsible for up to 75 percent of fungal illnesses. The diagnosis is by culture or biopsy, and the fungus may be difficult to isolate. Disseminated infection is present when infection is found in two or more sites and is associated with even higher morality. Fungal infection becomes more likely with retransplantation, Roux-en-Y, preoperative steroid use, accompanying vascular complications, the use of three or more intravenous antibiotics, and when the transplant is performed emergently.[12] Endemic mycoses (coccidioidomycoses, histoplasmosis, blastomycosis) are always possible in the immunocompromised host but are rarely seen in liver transplant patients.[3]

Viral Infection

Viral illnesses tend to present within the first few months. Viral and bacterial illnesses are often seen concurrently. The most common viral agent, and the most common cause of infection after transplantation, is CMV, a herpesvirus. It is reported to occur in between 23 and 85 percent of all liver transplant patients. Despite its high incidence and morbidity, it is rarely fatal unless disseminated and rarely has a significant effect on graft survival. It generally occurs within the first 3 months, with the peak incidence in the third and fourth weeks. Later occurrence is generally related to the need to increase immunosuppression for treatment of a prolonged episode of rejection. CMV can cause primary infection, or the infection can be a reactivation. Infection has three basic effects. First, it can produce a mononucleosis-like syndrome with spiking fever, arthralgias, malaise, neutropenia, atypical lymphocytes, and thrombocytopenia, with mild or moderate elevation in transaminase levels. Jaundice is rare. Second, CMV is frequently associated with opportunistic infection, which may be due to an additional immunosuppressive effect of its own. Finally, there is an increased propensity for allograft rejection.

The patient may present with a pneumonitis that, when present, is characterized by bilateral interstitial infiltrates that may lead to adult respiratory distress syndrome. Diagnosis may require bronchoalveolar lavage, but the appearance of the chest x-ray and the clinical picture may be suggestive enough for diagnosis. CMV pneumonitis may be seen in conjunction with *Pneumocystis carinii* pneumonia (PCP). CMV hepatitis may present similarly to rejection, with fever, malaise, anorexia, abdominal pain, hepatomegaly, and liver dysfunction. Liver biopsy is frequently needed for diagnosis but still may not be able to distinguish CMV disease from rejection. Disseminated disease is frequently associated with an increase in immunosuppression, especially with treatment with OKT3. CMV chorioretinitis may present with decreased visual acuity, photophobia, scotomata, floaters, eye redness, or pain. Its presence signals a poor prognosis and the presence of profound immunosuppression.[15]

There are three patterns of CMV infection. The patient at greatest risk is the seronegative recipient of a seropositive donor. Disease may also be caused by reactivation of latent virus that replicates after the initiation of immunosuppression—typically in the seropositive recipient of a liver from a seronegative donor. Finally, a seropositive recipient may receive a liver from a seropositive donor, which may produce either reactivation or superinfection, although it is clinically impossible and irrelevant to distinguish between them.

Effective treatment depends on rapid diagnosis. Treatment is with intravenous ganciclovir for 2 to 4 weeks. Diagnosis has been traditionally based on histology and culture. Standard fibroblast tube cell culture, however, can require 10 to 14 days for incubation. Serologic markers are too insensitive in the immunosuppressed patient, and electron microscopy is cumbersome. The shell-vial technique can detect the presence of CMV after 16 h of incubation. It is an indirect immunofluorescence testing method that uses a monoclonal antibody directed at an early antigen of the virus. Early detection and high antigenemia correlate positively with the severity of the infection.

Other viruses may cause illnesses in the posttransplant patient. Up to 34 percent of all transplant patients develop HSV, and half of these present within the first 3 weeks. Mucocutaneous or genital disease is generally due to reactivation of latent infection. It is generally not severe, and diagnosis can be made with Tzanck smear or culture. EBV can cause primary infection in children or the more common reactivated infection in adults. The disease can be self-limited and cause a mononucleosis-like syndrome, with fever, tonsillitis, and lymphadenopathy, or it may progress to a polymorphous, multiorgan B-cell infiltrative process with high mortality. Finally, it may produce a localized solid tumor. EBV plays a role in the development of a posttransplantation lymphoproliferative disorder and has a high incidence (20 to 30 percent) in patients maintained on immunosuppression and higher (80 percent) in patients who have received antithymocyte antibody.[13] Adenovirus and enteroviruses may cause systemic illness but are uncommon.

Parasitic Infection

Parasites are not common. PCP may present concomitantly with CMV or by itself. Diagnosis may require bronchoalveolar or transbronchial biopsy. Prophylaxis with trimethoprim/sulfamethoxazole (Bactrim) for the first 3 months has greatly reduced the incidence of PCP. Toxoplasma gondii is also uncommon but may cause a meningoencephalitis or single or multiple mass lesions. Toxoplasma infection causes fever, mental status changes, focal neurologic signs, seizures, or visual changes.

COMPLICATIONS OF IMMUNOSUPPRESSIVE AGENTS

Therapeutic immunosuppression is accompanied by a number of side effects and complications. Common and most life-threatening are the variety of infections that occur with the suppression of cell-mediated immunity. The agents of immunosuppression also have a number of nonspecific toxicities that complicate their use. Combined toxicities can produce or worsen preexisting renal insufficiency, hypertension, and hyperglycemia. Hypertension is perhaps the best example of combined toxicity.

Azathioprine interferes with both B- and T-cell responses to antigenic stimulation. Generalized myelosuppression is a common side effect resulting in leukopenia and, to varying degrees, thrombocytopenia and anemia (megaloblastic) and is generally seen within the first few weeks. Other observed toxicities include hepatitis, cholestasis, hepatic vein thrombosis, pancreatitis, dermatitis, and alopecia. Prolonged use also predisposes to malignancies such as squamous cell carcinoma of the skin and lip, cervical carcinoma, and lymphoproliferative disorder.

Glucocorticoids act primarily by inhibiting T-cell and macrophage function. In addition to immune suppression, long-term use of glucocorticoids suppresses endogenous adrenal function, which may produce Cushing syndrome and cause hypertension, glucose intolerance, osteoporosis, avascular necrosis of the hip, cataracts, pancreatitis, peptic ulcer disease, delayed wound healing, behavioral disorders, and malignancies.

Cyclosporine and FK506 inhibit T-cell proliferation. Nephrotoxicity is a common and usually reversible side effect manifest by elevated serum creatinine levels, hypertension, hyperkalemia, hyperuricemia, and gout. Patients are sensitive to dehydration.[12] Other side effects include headache, hirsutism, gingival hyperplasia, hyperglycemia, hypomagnesemia, hypercholesterolemia, hypertriglyceridemia, hepatotoxicity, and hemolytic uremic syndrome. Unlike those of other immunosuppressive agents, blood levels of cyclosporine and FK506 can be monitored along with serum creatinine to avoid serious toxicity; however, random levels are rarely helpful and dose is adjusted based on trough levels.[3]

Nonsteroidal anti-inflammatory agents should be avoided since they may increase nephrotoxicity.[16]

There are numerous drug interactions to consider with the immunosupressive agents. Some of these are summarized in Table 86-3.

INCIDENTAL PROBLEMS

Immunization

Immunization is important in the transplant patient because the prevention of even a common illness may be lifesaving. The key to immuniza-

TABLE 86-3 Reported Drug Interactions with Immunosuppressive Agents

Azathioprine
Allopurinol causes severe leukopenia
Pancuronium may require dose increase
Succinylcholine may require dose reduction
Warfarin (Coumadin) may require dose increase
Avoid drugs that may suppress bone marrow activity: sulfonamides, ganciclovir, cyclophosphamide, methotrexate
CSA(cyclosporine)/FK506(tacrolimus)
Drugs that may increase concentration: erythromycin, metoclopramide diltiazem, nicardapine, verapamil, OCP, ketoconazole, fluconazole, itraconazole, josamycin
Drugs that decrease concentration: octreotide, phenytoin, rifampin, nafcillin, phenytoin, phenobarbital, carbamazepine
Drugs that increase the risk of nephrotoxicity: aminoglycosides, amphotericin B, nonsteroidal anti-inflammatory drugs

Abbreviation: OCP, oral contraceptive pills

tion in the immunosuppressed patient is that all live virus vaccines are contraindicated. Vaccines consisting of denatured protein, carbohydrate, or killed virus are safe, so diphtheria/pertussis/tetanus (DPT), inactivated polio. *H. influenzae* Pittman type, and Heptavax are all safe. Live viral or bacterial vaccines are absolutely contraindicated [oral polio, measles, mumps, rubella, yellow fever, BCG, TY21a typhoid, varicella].[17] All of these may produce clinical disease.

Surgery

If surgery for problems other than those related to the graft is necessary, complications secondary to chronic steroids and immunosuppression should be anticipated. Also, caution must be taken in the presence of a coagulopathy. It is recommended that immunosuppression not be stopped unless there is sepsis, in which case the immunosuppression might need to be reduced. Two series looking at cardiac and general surgery showed no documented decline in graft function and no need for stress dosing of steroids.[18,19]

Bone Disease

Skeletal complications are responsible for significant morbidity and, because of increased survival times, are becoming more prevalent. Osteopenia and osteonecrosis can occur due to immobility, poor nutritional status, decreased muscle mass, steroid use, and immunosuppressive drugs. The first 3 to 6 months posttransplant are accompanied by accelerated bone loss (mostly trabecular). Fractures are common in the first year postoperatively, particularly at sites of trabecular bone (vertebrae and ribs), although long bone and pelvic fractures are also seen. The incidence of vertebral compression fracture may be as high as 38 percent. Patients may develop avascular necrosis of the femoral head from steroid use. Fractures should be treated in the standard fashion.

Neurologic Complications

It is reported that between 19 and 47 percent of all adult liver transplant patients have a neurologic complication at some time during their posttransplant course. Neurologic complications in children, however, are much less common (8 percent).[14] Common presenting problems include headache, seizure, and mental status changes. The etiology is more likely to be noninfectious than infectious. Common noninfectious etiologies are hemorrhage, immunosuppressive toxicity, and metabolic derangement. Central nervous system (CNS) infection is most common in the first few months, with viral and fungal etiologies predominating. CNS CMV infection is rare and CNS herpesvirus infection is seen with the same frequency as in the general population. Bacterial etiologies include *Listeria, Klebsiella, S. aureus, Nocardia,* and *Escherichia coli. Aspergillus, Candida,* and *Cryptococcus* sp. are the more common fungal agents involved. Cryptococcal disease is most common between 2 and 7 months.[16] Patients presenting with headache, seizures, or mental status changes need to evaluated for the presence of metabolic derangement as well as hemorrhage or infection. They will often require computed tomography (CT) of the head and lumbar puncture to rule out these etiologies.[12] Neuropathic pain may be seen and is poorly responsive to opioids. It may respond to tricyclic antidepressants.[16]

Malignancy

There is an increased risk of new malignancy including squamous cell carcinoma, lymphomas, posttransplant lymphoproliferative disorder (PTLD). There is no increased risk of lung, colon, breast, or prostate cancer.[3] The most common posttransplant malignancy is squamous cell cancer of the skin, but sarcoma, Kaposi's sarcoma, and hepatobiliary cancer occur.[20]

REFERENCES

1. UNOS: *Annual Report*, 1998.
2. Geevarghese S, Bradley A, Wright K, et al: Outcomes analysis in 100 liver transplant patients. *Am J Surg* 175:348, 1998.
3. Savitsky E, Uner A, Votey S: Evaluation of orthotopic liver transplant recipients presenting to the emergency department. *Ann Emerg Med* 31:507, 1998.
4. Wood R, Ozaki C, Katz S, Monsour H, et al: Liver transplantation: The last ten years. *Surg Clin North Am* 74:1133, 1994.
5. Ozaki C, Katz S, Monsour H, Dyer C, Wood R: Surgical complications of liver transplantation. *Surg Clin North Am* 74:1155, 1994.
6. Greif F, Bronsther O, Van Thiel D, et al: The incidence, timing and management of biliary tract complications after orthotopic liver transplantation. *Ann Surg* 219:40, 1994.
7. Porayko M, Kondo M, Steers J: Liver transplantation: Late complications of the biliary tract and their management. *Semin Liver Dis* 15:139, 1995.
8. Patenaude Y, Dubois J, Sinsky A, et al: Liver transplantation: Review of the literature: Part 1. Anatomic features and current concepts. *Can Assoc Radiol J* 48:171, 1997.
9. Stafford-Johnson D, Hamilton B, Dong Q, et al: Vascular complications of liver transplantation: Evaluation with gadolinium-enhanced MR angiography. *Radiology* 207:153, 1998.
10. Nolten A, Sproat I: Hepatic artery thrombosis after liver transplanation: Temporal accuracy of diagnosis with duplex US and the syndrome of impending thrombosis. *Radiology* 198:553, 1996.
11. Patenaude Y, Dubois J, Sinsky A, et al: Liver transplantation: Review of the literature: Part 2. Vascular and biliary complications. *Can Assoc Radiol J* 48:231, 1997.
12. Zetterman R: Primary care management of the liver transplant patient. *Am J Med* 96:10S, 1994.
13. Fishman J, Rubin R: Infection in organ-transplant recipients. *N Engl J Med* 338:1741, 1998.
14. Bowen A, Hungate R, Kaye R, et al: Imaging in liver transplantation. *Radiol Clin North Am* 34:757, 1996.
15. Dominguez E: Long-term infectious complications of liver transplantation. *Semin Liver Dis* 15:133, 1995.
16. Carson K, Hunt C: Medical problems occurring after orthotopic liver transplantation. *Dig Dis Sci* 42:1666, 1997.
17. Munoz S: Long-term management of the liver transplant recipient. *Med Clin North Am* 80:1103, 1996.
18. Prabhakar G, Testa G, Abbasoglu O, et al: The safety of cardiac operations in the liver transplant recipient. *Ann Thorac Surg* 65:1060, 1998.
19. Testa G, Goldstein R, Toughanipour A, et al: Guidelines for surgical procedures after liver transplantation. *Ann Surg* 227:590, 1998.
20. Tan-Shalaby J, Tempero M: Malignancies after liver transplantation: A comprehensive review. *Semin Liver Dis* 15:156, 1995.

GASTROINTESTINAL IMAGING

Michael J. Bono

BASIC IMAGING TECHNIQUES

Plain Film Radiography

Plain films remain the workhorse imaging study for the emergency department evaluating a patient with abdominal pain. Plain films can be obtained quickly, cause no discomfort to the patient, and are relatively inexpensive compared to other gastrointestinal (GI) imaging modalities. The emergency physician can interpret plain films. Unlike the chest, where the organs have great differences in water and air content and therefore in radiodensity, the abdomen contains structures of similar radiodensities. Only the presence of air and fat in the bowel or other structures allows indentification of organ boundaries, and the air is transient. A plain film of the abdomen represents a ''snapshot'' of a dynamic system and should be examined systematically. A time-honored technique is to first examine the bones (spine, ribs, pelvis, and hips); then the upper quadrants, flanks, and mid-abdomen for organ masses and calcifications; and finally the lower abdomen. The physician should attempt to look at the area of special interest last.

At most centers, an ''acute abdominal series'' includes a supine film centered at the iliac crest, an upright film centered at the crest, and an upright posteroanterior (PA) chest film. The supine film detects fluid or blood in the peritoneum as well as gas in the bowel, and the upright film displays any air-fluid levels. If the patient is too ill to stand, a left lateral decubitus (left side down) view is acceptable, but a right lateral decubitus is not. On a left lateral decubitus view, free air can be detected between the liver and the peritonuem; this is not possible in a right lateral decubitus view (right side down) because air in the bowel loops will contact the peritoneum. The standard upright PA chest view is best for demonstrating free air in the peritoneal cavity as well as other pathologic conditions of the chest that cause abdominal pain, such as pneumonia, pneumothorax, or atelectasis.

Contrast Radiography

Barium sulfate remains the standard substance for contrast GI imaging. Barium is an insoluble material that is suspended in different carriers by different manufacturers. It has high viscosity and is not absorbed by the GI tract. Gastrograffin is a water-soluble substance, has low viscosity, and, like barium, is not absorbed by the GI tract in most normal adult patients. It is absorbed slightly by the gut in children. Gastrograffin draws substantial amounts of fluid into the bowel lumen, and its low viscosity causes rapid transit through the small bowel into the colon. It therefore has a considerable laxative effect. Gastrograffin is not a recommended oral contrast agent in children, particularly neonates and infants, since the fluid shifts and laxative effect may cause significant fluid and electrolyte disturbances.

Computed Tomography Scanning

Computed tomography (CT) provides imaging of solid organs and, very importantly, a view into the retroperitoneum. Unlike plain radiographs, CT scanning is not dependent on the amount of air and gas in the bowel. Oral contrast material must be given to identify bowel, and intravenous contrast material enhances the density of blood vessels. The introduction of the helical CT scan (spiral CT) has made a significant impact on abdominal imaging due to the speed of the procedure. Routine CT scanning of the abdomen usually requires the patient to lie motionless for 15 to 30 min, while the helical CT scan may be finished in a single breath hold. Helical CT was originally developed to compensate for errors produced by variations in respiratory depth of the patient.[1] The radiation dose to the patient is unchanged. Another advantage of helical CT is improved vascular opacification, which allows excellent imaging of the thoracoabdominal aorta and renal arteries. Data obtained from helical CT can be reformatted in several ways, revealing three-dimensional surface anatomy and obviating the need for arteriography.

Radionuclide Scanning

Radionuclide scanning has been virtually replaced by ultrasonography for emergency department patients with right upper quadrant pain. Technectium-99m–labeled iminodiacetic acid (IDA) is injected intravenously, is taken up by hepatocytes, is secreted into the bile canaliculi, and then flows into the small bowel. Normally there is a small amount of reflux into the cystic duct and gallbladder, but in cholecystitis the cystic duct is frequently occluded. The gallbladder, hepatic duct, and common duct should be visualized within 1 h of IDA administration, but total test time may be several hours.

Ultrasonography

Ultrasound has emerged as a valuable tool for the diagnosis of select conditions in the emergency department. It is noninvasive and inexpensive, and should be readily available to the emergency department physician. Improvements in transducer technology have greatly improved ultrasound imaging. Ultrasound is somewhat operator dependent, and the images are difficult to interpret in obese patients or patients with large amounts of intestinal air or gas. Air is a poor conductor of ultrasound because it scatters, refracts, and reflects the sound waves. Fluid-filled structures transmit sound exceedingly well, and since most of the soft tissues are composed of varing amounts of water, ultrasound is feasible throughout the GI tract and pelvis. A full bladder is an acoustic window into the pelvis, and the liver helps transmit ultrasound in the right upper quadrant.

SPECIFIC GASTROINTESTINAL CONDITIONS

Plain Film Radiography

In the past, tradition dictated the routine use of plain films to screen patients with acute abdominal pain.[2,3] Screening acute abdominal pain patients routinely with plain films is not advisable, since the yield of positive findings that would change clinical management is low, in the range of 10 to 40 percent.[4,5] However, in the proper clinical setting, plain abdominal radiographs are entirely appropriate and are still considered the first test of choice. In patients with a suspected perforated ulcer or free air in the abdomen, plain films demonstrate free air, if present, in a high percentage of patients.[6] Plain films may demonstrate as little as 1 to 2 mL of air.[7] In patients with suspected small bowel obstruction, plain films are the initial method of imaging. Plain films have a sensitivity for revealing high-grade small bowel obstruction of 69 to 82 percent, but, when combined with barium contrast studies, the sensitivity rate may approach 100 percent.[8,9] Low-grade small bowel obstruction is difficult to demonstrate on plain films and has much lower diagnostic rates.[10] Other appropriate conditions for the use of plain film radiographs include moderate or severe abdominal tenderness, suspicion of bowel ischemia, ingestion of radiopaque foreign bodies, and penetrating foreign bodies, such as gunshot wounds.

Abdominal Computed Tomography

CT is the diagnostic tool of choice for many acute abdominal conditions. CT is the first imaging study of choice for patients with suspected diverticulitis, pancreatitis, pancreatic pseudocyst, aortic aneurysm, blunt trauma, and appendicitis. The diagnosis of appendicitis can be made on clinical evaluation, but CT has been proven remarkably sensitive and specific in confirming the diagnosis.[11] Whether patients with suspected appendicitis require oral, intravenous, and/or rectal contrast versus ''no-contrast'' thin cuts through the ileocecal area is debated in the radiology literature.[12] CT is a useful adjunct to plain films in suspected cases of intestinal ischemia, where specific findings may include pneumotosis intestinalis, portal venous gas, mesenteric vessel occlusion, and enlargement of a thrombosed vein.[13] While patients with suspected small bowel obstruction should be imaged initially with plain radiographs, CT has similar sensitivity in revealing obstruction, both high and low grade. When CT correctly showed a small bowel obstruction, the cause of the obstruction was demonstrated in 95 percent of cases. CT offers a further advantage to the emergency physician evaluating the patient with multiple potential causes for acute abdominal pain. While never advocated as a ''screening tool,'' CT scanning can pinpoint a diagnosis in 95 percent of cases where clinical judgment and other imaging studies fail to narrow a wide range of potential diagnoses.[14]

Ultrasonography

Ultrasound is the initial imaging study of choice for evaluation of patients with right upper quandrant pain. Using the liver as an acoustic window, ultrasound can detect cholelithiasis, cholecystitis, choledocholithiasis, biliary duct dilation, and pancreatic masses, both solid and cystic. Ultrasound is also the modality of choice for evaluating patients with pelvic pain. Transvaginal scanning has supplemented the transabdominal approach because of better visualization with higher-frequency endovaginal probe transducers (see Chap. 109, ''Pelvic Imaging''). Ultrasonography of the genitourinary system is discussed in Chapter 97, ''Renal Imaging.''

Graded-compression ultrasound imaging for acute appendicitis has been studied extensively. Sensitivities for appendicitis range from 68 to 93 percent and specificities between 73 and 100 percent, with accuracy in the 95 percent range.[15] Negative laparotomy result rates were reduced significantly using graded-compression ultrasonography.[16] The ultrasonographer is searching for a tubular structure off the cecum that is compressible without pain and is no more than 6 mm in diameter. An infected, inflamed appendix is tender, larger than 6 mm in diameter, fluid filled, and noncompressible. The appendix is difficult to visualize, and the examination is best left to experienced ultrasonographers. Negative ultrasound results in the face of a strong clinical suspicion should never delay surgical intervention. The false-negative rate for graded-compression ultrasonography is from 6 to 14 percent. Other disease processes that can confuse the clinical picture are cecal diverticulitis, inflammatory bowel disease involving the terminal ileum, and periappendiceal phlegmon. Graded-compression ultrasonography is most helpful in the evaluation of patients with atypical right lower quadrant pain and a suspicion of appendicitis.

Barium Enema

Children with signs and symptoms suggestive of intussusception, such as colicky abdominal pain, vomiting, and passage of stool mixed with blood, require stabilization and a barium enema. Plain films may demonstrate signs of intestinal obstruction, such as distended loops, air-fluid levels, and a paucity of bowel gas in the right lower quadrant, the so-called Dance's sign. A barium enema is indicated, and a hydrostatic reduction of the intussusceptum is successful in 50 to 90 percent of cases.[17] A barium enema may be useful for the diagnosis of bowel obstruction, volvulus, appendicitis, and diverticulitis, usually in consultation with surgical colleagues.

Angiography

CT has replaced angiography for imaging patients with suspected abdominal aortic aneurysm. Angiograpy may be helpful in evaluating patients with lower GI bleeding, particularly when combined with colonoscopy to pinpoint the bleeding lesion.[18]

Radionuclide Scanning

Radionuclide scanning can be a useful adjunct to ultrasonography for patients with right upper quadrant abdominal pain. When the ultrasound results are negative or inconclusive in a patient with suspected cholecystitis or cystic duct obstruction, radionuclide scanning may be diagnostic in the absence of stones. These studies involve several hours for the radioisotope to localize to the affected area and may be utilized best in an emergency department observation unit or inpatient setting.

Magnetic Resonance Imaging

Magnetic resonance imaging (MRI) currently has no role in imaging the GI tract in the emergency department patient. MRI is outstanding for imaging the central nervous system and musculoskeletal system, but cost, time in the scanner, and poor image quality due to movement of the bowel limit applicability. MRI is being evaluated as a tool for imaging relatively stationary GI structures, such as the appendix and biliary tree, and has shown some promise.[19,20]

REFERENCES

1. Gupta H, Dupuy DE: Advances in imaging of the acute abdomen. *Surg Clin North Am* 77:1245
2. Lee PW: The plain x-ray in the acute abdomen: A surgeon's evaluation. *Br J Surg* 63:763, 1976.
3. Martin RF, Rossi RL: The acute abdomen: An overview and alogorithms. *Surg Clin North Am* 77:1235, 1997.
4. Eisenberg RL, Heineken P, Hedgcock MW, et al: Evaluation of plain abdominal radiographs in the diagnosis of abdominal pain. *Ann Intern Med* 97:257, 1982.
5. Campbell JP, Gunn AA: Abdominal radiographs and acute pain. *Br J Surg* 75:554, 1988.
6. Grassi R, DiMizio R, Pinto A, et al: Sixty-one consecutive patients with gastrointestinal perforation: Comparison of conventional radiology, ultrasonography, and computerized tomography, in terms of timing of the study. *Radiol Med (Torino)* 91:247, 1996.
7. Miller RE, Nelson SW: The roentgenologic demonstration of tiny amounts of free intraperitoneal gas: Experimental and clinical studies. *AJR* 112:574, 1971.
8. Maglinte DD, Reyes BL, Harmon BH, et al: Reliability and role of plain film radiography and CT in the diagnosis of small bowel obstruction. *AJR* 167:1451, 1996.
9. Anderson CA, Humphrey WT: Contrast radiography in small bowel obstruction: A prospective, randomized trial. *Mil Med* 162:749, 1997.
10. Maglinte DD, Balthazar EJ, Kelvin FM, et al: The role of radiography in the diagnosis of small bowel obstruction. *AJR* 168:1171, 1997.
11. Balthazar EJ, Birnbaum BA, Yee J, et al: Acute appendicitis: CT and US correlation in 100 patients. *Radiology* 190:31, 1994.
12. Rao PM, Rhea JT, Novelline RA, et al: Helical CT technique for the diagnosis of appendicitis: Prospective evaluation of a focused appendix CT examination. *Radiology* 202:139, 1997.
13. Castellone JA, Powers RD: Ischemic bowel syndromes: A comprehensive, state-of-the-art approach to emergency diagnosis and management. *Emerg Med Rep* 18:189, 1997.
14. Taourel P, Baron MP, Pradel J, et al: Acute abdomen of unknown origin: Impact of CT on diagnosis and management. *Gastrointest Radiol* 17:287, 1992.
15. Orr RK, Porter D, Hartmann D: Ultrasonography to evaluate adults for

appendicitis: Decision making based on meta-analysis and probabilistic reasoning. *Acad Emerg Med* 2:644, 1995.

16. Schwerk WB, Wichtrup B, Rothmund M, et al: Ultrasonography in the diagnosis of acute appendicitis: A prospective study. *Gastroenterology* 97:630, 1989.

17. Bisset GS, Kirds DR: Intussusception in infants and children: Diagnosis and therapy. *Radiology* 168:141, 1988.

18. Bono MJ: Lower gastrointestinal tract bleeding. *Emerg Clin North Am* 14:547, 1996.

19. Incesu L, Coskun A, Selcuk MB, et al: Acute appendicitis: MR imaging and sonographic correlation. *AJR* 168:669, 1997.

20. Reinhold C, Bret PM: Current status of MR cholangiopancreatography. *AJR* 166:1285, 1996.

RENAL AND GENITOURINARY DISORDERS

ACUTE RENAL FAILURE

Richard Sinert

Acute renal failure (ARF) is defined as a deterioration of renal function over hours or days that results in the accumulation of toxic wastes and the loss of internal homeostasis. Glomerular filtration rate (GFR) is commonly used as an index of renal function, and rapid declines in GFR are viewed synonymously with ARF. Although this concept of ARF is universally accepted, exact definitions of ARF vary in the medical literature. Laboratory scientists, who can directly measure GFR, define ARF as a 50 percent decline in GFR. Clinicians must rely on indirect measures of GFR to define ARF, such as a 50 percent decline in creatinine clearance or a 50 percent increase in serum creatinine from baseline. Finally, some physicians define only those patients requiring dialysis treatment as having ARF. ARF is very common and emergency physicians play a critical role in the early recognition of ARF and prevention of further iatrogenic injury.

ARF is not a disease by itself, but a potential complication of many other disorders (Table 88-1). The incidence ARF varies widely, reflecting the study of different patient subsets. In general, a patient's age, volume status, and previous history of renal insufficiency significantly influence the risk of ARF (Table 88-2).

PATHOPHYSIOLOGY

The driving force for glomerular filtration is the pressure gradient from the glomerulus to Bowman space of the proximal tubule. Glomerular pressure depends on renal blood flow (RBF) and is controlled by the combined resistances of the renal afferent and efferent arterioles.

Regardless of the cause of ARF, reductions in RBF represent a common pathologic pathway for decreasing GFR.[1] This relationship is most clear in prerenal failure, defined by conditions with normal tubular and glomerular function, where GFR is depressed by compromised renal perfusion. Intrinsic renal failure occurs with diseases of the glomerulus, interstitium, or tubule, associated with the release of renal vasoconstrictors.[2] Postobstructive renal failure initially produces an increase in tubular pressure decreasing the filtration driving force. This pressure gradient soon equalizes, and the maintenance of depressed GFR depends on vasoconstrictors.[3]

Depressed RBF and nephrotoxins result in ischemia and renal cell death. This initial injury triggers the production of oxygen free radicals and release of leukotrienes that continue to cause cell injury. Tubular cellular damage results in disruption of tight junctions between cells, allowing backleak of glomerular filtrate, further depressing effective GFR. In addition, dying cells slough off into the tubules, forming obstructing casts further decreasing GFR and leading to oliguria.

During this period of depressed RBF, the kidneys are especially vulnerable to further insults.[4] Exposure to known nephrotoxins such as radiocontrast agents, aminoglycosides, and nonsteroidal anti-inflammatory drugs (NSAIDs) at this time explains the high rate of iatrogenic causes of ARF[5] (Table 88-2).

Recovery from ARF is first dependent on restoration of RBF. In prerenal failure, restoration of circulating blood volume is usually sufficient. Rapid relief of urinary obstruction in postrenal failure results in a prompt decrease of vasoconstrictors. Clearance of tubular toxins and initiation of therapy for glomerular diseases decrease vasoconstriction and restore RBF in patients with intrinsic renal failure.

Once RBF is restored, the remaining functional nephrons will increase their filtration and eventually hypertrophy. Depending on the size of this remnant nephron pool, GFR will proportionately recover. If the number of remaining nephrons is below a critical value, continued hyperfiltration results in progressive glomerular sclerosis eventually leading to nephron loss. A vicious cycle then ensues where continued nephron loss causes more hyperfiltration until complete renal failure occurs. Hyperfiltration of remnant nephrons explains the commonly observed scenario where progressive renal failure is frequently observed after recovery from ARF.[6]

The differential diagnosis of ARF is classified according to the prerenal, intrinsic renal, and postrenal etiologies of ARF.

Prerenal failure is the most common cause of ARF, accounting for 40 to 80 percent of all cases.[7] Prerenal failure is produced by conditions that decrease renal perfusion (Table 88-3). Besides being an independent cause of ARF, prerenal failure is a common precursor to ischemic and nephrotoxic causes of intrinsic renal failure.[8]

The etiologies of intrinsic renal failure are subdivided anatomically into diseases of the tubules, interstitium, glomeruli, and vessels (Table 88-4). Intrinsic renal failure accounts for approximately 11 to 45 percent of all cases, depending on the population studied. For adults in a community hospital, prerenal failure accounted for 70 percent of ARF cases as compared with only 11 percent from intrinsic renal etiologies.[9] ARF has a different spectrum in the pediatric population: a higher incidence of intrinsic renal causes for ARF (45 percent) secondary to diseases such as glomerulonephritis and hemolytic-uremic syndrome.[10]

Acute tubular necrosis (ATN) secondary to renal ischemia accounts for the majority of cases of intrinsic renal failure. Nephrotoxins are the second most common cause of ATN, accounting for approximately 25 percent. When the etiologies of ARF were reviewed in a multivariate analysis, a synergistic effect was noted for the combination of ischemic and nephrotoxic ATN.[11]

Postrenal failure accounts for 2 to 5 percent of all cases of ARF, but has a significantly higher incidence in selected populations (Table 88-5). In large surveys of elderly men for symptoms of urinary obstruction, prevalence between 20 to 35 percent has been estimated.[12] In young males, renal calculi are the most common cause of obstruction. In young females, cervical carcinoma can cause urinary obstruction. In children, postrenal failure is commonly secondary to congenital malformations such as urethral valves in boys and vesicoureteral reflux in girls.

CLINICAL FEATURES

Morbidity/Mortality from Acute Renal Failure

Reported mortality rates for ARF have remained the same from before to after the advent of dialysis: 40 to 90 percent.[13,14] This statistic reflects a changing epidemiology and etiology of ARF. Before the availability of effective dialysis, many young patients died directly of complications specific to ARF. Now that dialysis effectively treats life-threatening complications of ARF, the patient's age and underlying diseases determine mortality from ARF. ARF has become an index of the severity of patients' other disease processes. With the advent of dialysis, the most common causes of death with ARF are sepsis, cardiac, and pulmonary failure.

This is not to imply that ARF is a benign disease: even in those patients not requiring dialysis, mortality was 31 percent in patients

TABLE 88-1 Incidence of Acute Renal Failure (ARF)

Clinical Setting	Incidence of ARF (%)
Community hospital ward	2–5
Intensive care unit	15–25
Acute pancreatitis	4–6
Trauma	3–9
Rhabdomyolysis	25–30
Severe burns	20–60
Radiocontrast agents	2–30
Aminoglycoside therapy	10–30
Cardiac surgery	5–40

with ARF compared with only 8 percent in matched patients without ARF.[15] Even after adjusting for comorbidity, the odds ratio for dying in patients with ARF was 4.9 compared with patients without ARF.

Mortality rates are generally less for nonoliguric ARF (more than 400 mL/day) compared with oliguric ARF (less than 400 mL/day). This difference is because drug-induced nephrotoxicity and interstitial nephritis usually cause nonoliguric ARF.[16]

Approximately 20 to 60 percent of patients experiencing ARF will require dialysis during their hospital stay.[17] The majority of these patients will recover, with only 25 percent requiring long-term dialysis.[18]

History

A focused history should be obtained using the pathophysiology and differential diagnosis of ARF as a guide.

In prerenal failure, patients commonly present with symptoms related to hypovolemia: thirst, decreasing urine output, dizziness, and orthostatic hypotension. Inquire about a history of excessive vomiting, diarrhea, urination, hemorrhage, or sweating. Third spacing of fluids commonly occurs with burns and with liver and pancreatic diseases. Patients with advanced cardiac failure leading to depressed renal perfusion present with orthopnea, paroxysmal nocturnal dyspnea, and dyspnea on exertion. Insensible fluid losses can result in severe hypovolemia in patients with restricted fluid access and should be suspected in elderly, comatose, or sedated patients.

For intrinsic renal failure, patients can be divided into those with glomerular, interstitial, and tubular etiologies. The nephritic syndrome of hematuria, edema, and hypertension is synonymous with a glomerular etiology of ARF. These patients should be queried about prior throat or skin infections. ATN should be suspected in any patient with a period of hypotension secondary to cardiac arrest, hemorrhage, sepsis, drug overdose, or surgery. A careful search for exposure to nephrotoxins should include a detailed list of all current medications and any recent x-ray examinations (radiocontrast agents). Pigment-induced ARF should be suspected in patients with possible rhabdomyolysis (e.g., muscle tenderness, recent coma, seizures, drug abuse, alcohol, excessive exercise, or limb ischemia) and with hemolysis (e.g., recent blood transfusion). Allergic interstitial nephritis should be suspected with recent drug use associated with fevers, rash, and arthralgias.

Postrenal failure most commonly occurs in elderly men with relatively asymptomatic high-grade prostatic obstruction. Because of their chronicity and slow onset, the classic symptoms of prostatism—urgency, frequency, and hesitancy—are often not communicated to

TABLE 88-2 Iatrogenic Acute Renal Failure: Common Preexisting Conditions and Potential Nephrotoxins

Preexisting Conditions	Potential Nephrotoxins
Hypovolemia	Aminoglycosides Amphotericin Heme–pigments Radiocontrast agents
Angiotensin-converting enzyme inhibitors	Diuretics Small and large vessel renal arterial disease
Nonsteroidal anti-inflammatory drugs	Congestive heart failure Hypertension Renal artery stenosis
Preexisting renal disease (elderly, diabetics, jaundice)	Radiocontrast agents Aminoglycosides Atheroembolism Cardiovascular surgery

TABLE 88-3 Differential Diagnosis of Prerenal Failure

Volume loss
- Hemorrhagic shock
- Vomiting
- Diarrhea
- Diuretics
- Primary hypoaldosteronism
- Salt-losing nephropathy
- Acute tumor lysis syndrome
- Postobstructive diuresis

Fluid sequestration
- Cirrhosis
- Malnutrition (kwashiorkor)
- Nephrotic syndrome
- Pancreatitis
- Burns
- Rhabdomyolysis
- Necrotizing fasciitis
- General anesthesia
- Septic shock

Decreased cardiac output
- Myocardial ischemia/infarction
- Valvular heart disease
- Cardiomyopathy
- Pericardial tamponade
- β adrenergic blockers
- High-output failure (thyrotoxicosis, thiamine deficiency, Paget's disease, arteriovenous fistula)

Renal artery large vessel disease
- Stenosis (atherosclerotic, fibromuscular dysplasia)
- Thrombosis
- Septic emboli

Renal artery small vessel disease
- Cyclosporine and tacrolimus
- Embolic disease (septic, cholesterol)
- Malignant hypertension
- Transplant rejection
- Sickle cell disease
- Preeclampsia
- Hypercalcemia
- Hemolytic-uremic syndrome
- Thrombotic thrombocytopenic purpura
- Vasculitis

TABLE 88-4 Differential Diagnosis of Intrinsic Renal Failure

Tubular diseases
Ischemic acute tubular necrosis
Nephrotoxins: aminoglycosides, radiocontrast, cisplatin, myeloma light chains
Heme pigments: rhabdomyolysis, massive hemolysis
Interstitial diseases
Acute interstitial nephritis: drug reactions methicillin
Autoimmune diseases: systemic lupus erythematosus
Infiltrative disease: sarcoidosis, lymphoma
Infectious agents: Legionnaires' disease, Hantavirus
Acute glomerulonephritis
Rapidly progressive glomerulonephritis: Goodpasture's syndrome, Wegener's granulomatosis, Henoch-Shönlein purpura, Systemic lupus erythematosis, Polyarteritis nodosa
Postinfectious
Membranoproliferative
Vascular diseases
Malignant hypertension
Scleroderma
Thrombotic thrombocytopenic purpura
Polyarteritis nodosa
Hemolytic-uremic syndrome
Renal vein thrombosis

TABLE 88-5 Differential Diagnosis of Obstructive Renal Failure

Infants and children	
Urethra and bladder outlet	
Urethral atresia	Anterior and posterior urethral valves (males)
Phimosis	Calculus (Southeast Asia)
Ureterocele	Neurogenic bladder
Meatal stenosis	Blood clot
Ureter	
Vesicoureter reflux (females)	Retrocaval ureter
Ureterovesical junction obstruction	Retroperitoneal tumor
Ureterocele	Blood clot
Megaureter—prune-belly syndrome	
Adults	
Urethra and bladder outlet	
Phimosis	Benign prostate hypertrophy
Stricture (males)—sexually transmitted diseases	Neurogenic bladder: diabetes mellitus, spinal cord disease, multiple sclerosis, Parkinson disease, anticholinergic drugs, α-adrenergic antagonists
Cancer of prostate, bladder	
Carcinoma of cervix, colon	
Trauma	
Blood clot	
Calculi	
Ureter	
Vesicoureter reflux (females)	Trauma
Calculi	Papillary necrosis: sickle cell disease, diabetes mellitus, pyelonephritis
Uric acid crystals	Inflammatory bowel disease
Blood clot	Pregnant uterus
Aortic aneurysm	Carcinoma of ureter, uterus, prostate, bladder, colon, rectum
Retroperitoneal fibrosis: idiopathic, tumors (cervix, uterus, prostate, colon), tuberculosis, sarcoidosis, methylsergide, propanolol	Retroperitoneal lymphoma
Stricture: tuberculosis, radiation, schistosomiasis, nonsteroidal anti-inflammatory drugs	Accidental surgical ligation
Uterine leiomyomata	
Intrarenal	
Crystals: uric acid, sulfonamide, acyclovir	Protein casts: multiple myeloma, amyloidosis

physicians. In females, a history of prior gynecologic surgery or carcinoma can often be helpful in providing clues to the level of obstruction. Flank pain and hematuria indicate the possibility of renal calculi or of papillary necrosis. Recent use of acyclovir, methotrexate, or sulfonamides suggests the possibility of tubular obstruction by crystals of these medications.

Physical Examination

The patient's volume status must be assessed. Hypotension and tachycardia are obvious clues to decreased renal perfusion. Since hypertension is a common premorbid condition for ARF, knowledge of baseline blood pressures may prove helpful in individualizing a definition of hypotension. Further investigations into the possibility of hypovolemia should include tests for orthostatic hypotension or tachycardia, mucosal membrane moisture, and tissue turgor.

Examination of the *skin* may suggest a systemic vasculitis (livedo reticularis, digital ischemia, butterfly rash, and palpable purpura), allergic interstitial nephritis (maculopapular rash), or endocarditis (track marks of intravenous drug use).

Examination of the *eyes* may find evidence of autoimmune vasculitis (keratitis, iritis, uveitis, and dry conjunctiva), liver disease (jaundice), multiple myeloma (band keratopathy from hypercalcemia), diabetes mellitus, hypertension, or atheroemboli (retinopathy).

Examination of the *ears* can indicate Alport's disease or aminoglycoside toxicity (hearing loss) and Wegener's granulomatosis (mucosal or cartilage ulcerations).

The *cardiac* examination may find potential signs of peripheral arterial emboli (atrial fibrillation), endocarditis (murmurs), and heart failure (jugular venous distention, hepatojugular reflux, and S3 cardiac gallop).

The *pulmonary* examination may find evidence of heart failure or of Goodpasture's syndrome or Wegener's disease (rales). The *abdominal* examination may find evidence of aortic aneurysm, nephrolithiasis or papillary necrosis (flank tenderness), or urinary obstruction (pelvic, rectal masses, prostatic hypertrophy, and distended bladder).

Examination of the *extremities* may find clinical evidence of rhabdomyolysis (limb cyanosis, pulselessness, and edema), vasculitis (palpable purpura), or atherosclerotic disease (diminished pulses).

DIAGNOSIS

Ancillary Tests

Microscopic examination of urine is very useful in establishing the differential diagnosis of ARF (Table 88-6). While changes in urine output are poorly correlated with changes in GFR, the categories of anuria, oliguria, and nonoliguria can be useful in the differential diagnosis of ARF (Table 88-7). Approximately 50 to 60 percent of all causes of ARF is nonoliguric.

TABLE 88-6 Differential Diagnosis of Acute Renal Failure (ARF) According to Urinalysis

Urine Sediment	Etiology of ARF
Normal urinary sediment	Prerenal, postrenal failure, hemolytic uremic syndrome/thrombotic thrombocytopenic purpura, preglomerular vasculitis, or atheroembolism
Hemoglobin without red blood cells	Rhabdomyolysis, massive hemolysis
Albumin	Glomerulonephritis, malignant hypertension
Granular casts	Acute tubular necrosis, glomerulonephritis, interstitial nephritis
Red blood cell casts	Glomerulonephritis, malignant hypertension
White blood cell casts	Acute interstitial nephritis, pyelonephritis
Eosinophiluria	Acute allergic interstitial nephritis, atheroembolism
Crystalluria	Renal calculi, acyclovir, sulfonamides, methotrexate, ethylene glycol, radiocontrast agents

To help differentiate prerenal failure from ATN, chemical analysis of the urine may provide important clues[19] (Table 88-8). The fractional excretion of sodium (FeNa) is a test that is commonly used but, unfortunately, fails to distinguish prerenal causes of ARF from other causes of ARF[20] (Table 88-9).

Blood urea nitrogen (BUN) concentration is poorly correlated with GFR. Since urea is highly permeable to renal tubules, urea clearance varies with urine flow rate: at urine flow rates of less than 30 mL/h, urea clearance is as low as 30 percent of GFR and, with urine outputs greater than 100 mL/h, urea clearance can increase to 70 to 100 percent of GFR. This relation is used clinically to help differentiate prerenal failure from other etiologies of ARF. In prerenal conditions, low urine flow rates favor BUN reabsorption, out of proportion to creatinine (Cr). This results in a disproportionate rise of BUN to relative creatinine, creating a serum ratio of BUN/Cr that is greater than 20 in prerenal failure.

BUN concentration depends on both nitrogen balance and renal function. BUN concentration can rise significantly with no decrement in GFR by increases in urea production with protein loading, trauma, or gastrointestinal bleeding. Corticosteroids and tetracycline increase BUN by decreasing tissue anabolic rates. Basal BUN concentration can be severely depressed by malnutrition or advanced liver disease.

TABLE 88-7 Differential Diagnosis of Acute Renal Failure (ARF) According to Urine Volume

Urine Output (24 h)	Differential of ARF
Anuria (<100 mL/day)	Urinary tract obstruction, renal artery obstruction, rapidly progressive glomerulonephritis, bilateral diffuse renal cortical necrosis
Oliguria (<400 mL/day)	Prerenal failure, hepatorenal syndrome
Nonoliguria (>400 mL/day)	Acute interstitial nephritis, acute glomerulonephritis, partial obstructive nephropathy, nephrotoxic and ischemic acute tubular necrosis, radiocontrast-induced ARF, rhabdomyolysis

TABLE 88-8 Urine Chemical Indices in Differentiating Prerenal from Acute Tubular Necrosis (ATN)

Laboratory Test	Favors Prerenal	Favors ATN
Urine specific gavity	>1.018	<1.012
Urine osmolality (mosm/kg H_2O)	>500	<500
Urine sodium (meq/L)	<20	>40
Plasma blood urea nitrogen/creatinine ratio (mg/dL)	>20	<10–15
Urine/plasma creatinine ratio (mg/dL)	>40	<20
Fractional excretion of Na: FeNa = $U_{Na}/P_{Na} \div U_{Cr}/P_{Cr}$	<1%	>1%

Baseline BUN concentration should be estimated when attempting to correlate changes in BUN with GFR. For example, in a cirrhotic patient with a BUN of 12 mg/dL, a normal range GFR might be assumed, but only with the knowledge of a baseline BUN of 4 mg/dL does the real decrease in GFR become apparent.

Serum creatinine provides the most accurate and consistent estimation of GFR, yet the proper use of creatinine in gauging changes in GFR requires knowledge of its production and clearance.

Creatinine is the breakdown product of the skeletal muscle protein, creatine. Creatinine production is linked to muscle mass, which in turn depends on lean body weight, age, and gender. Muscle mass is a greater percentage of body weight in males and decreases with age.

Variations in muscle mass have important implications in using creatinine to estimate GFR. GFR declines by 1 percent a year after the age of 40 years, but serum creatinine remains unchanged because the decline in GFR is balanced by decreasing muscle mass with age. This implies that older patients have lower GFRs than younger patients with the same serum creatinine. The following formula attempts to compensate for these effects of body weight, age, and gender on the correlation between creatinine and GFR:[21]

For males:

Creatine clearance (mL/min)

$$= \frac{[(140 - \text{age(years)}) \times \text{lean body weight (kg)}]}{[\text{serum creatinine (mg/dL)} \times 72]}$$

For females:

Above formula × 0.85

Some diseases and medications can interfere with the correlation of serum creatinine with GFR. Acute glomerulonephritis causes increased

TABLE 88-9 Exceptions: Intrinsic Renal Failure with FeNa <1%

Urinary tract obstruction
Acute glomerulonephritis
Hepatorenal syndrome
Radiocontrast acute renal failure (ARF)
Myoglobinuric and hemoglobinuric acute renal failure
Renal allograft rejection
Drug-related alterations in renal hemodynamics (captopril and nonsteroidal anti-inflammatory drugs)

TABLE 88-10 Estimation of Glomerular Filtration Rate (GFR) by Serum Creatinine

Creatinine (mg/dL)	GFR (mL/min)
1.0	Normal–baseline
2.0	50% reduction
4.0	70–85% reduction
8.0	90–95% reduction

tubular secretion of creatinine; this falsely depresses the rise in serum creatinine. Trimethoprim, cimetidine, and salicylates all cause decreased creatinine secretion, falsely elevating creatinine with no change in GFR.

A possible error may occur according to the laboratory method used to measure creatinine. The most commonly used method uses alkaline picurate. This method is also called the total chromogen method because it measures all serum chromogens: creatinine plus glucose, fructose, uric acid, acetone, acetoacetate, protein, ascorbic acid, pyruvate, and cephalosporins. At normal serum levels, these noncreatinine chromogens constitute only 5 to 20 percent of the total chromogens. In conditions such as diabetic and isopropyl ketosis, elevations of acetone and acetoacetate falsely elevate serum creatinine. High levels of bilirubin with this method falsely indicate a low creatinine level.

The imidohydrolase method is an enzymatic method for measuring creatinine, which resolves the problem of noncreatinine chromogens and bilirubin with the picurate method. However, the imidohydrolase method has been shown to report falsely high creatinine levels in the presence of high glucose and the antifungal agent flucytosine.

The rate of increase in serum creatinine can be used to estimate GFR. In patients with no renal function (GFR = 0), serum creatinine will increase 1 to 3 mg/dL/day. Lessor increases in serum creatinine indicate remaining renal function (GFR) and larger increases indicate excessive muscle breakdown (e.g., rhabdomyolysis). Under stable conditions, serum creatinine correlates with GFR (Table 88-10).

Knowledge of a patient's baseline creatinine becomes very important: small changes from low baseline levels of creatinine are much more clinically important than large changes from high basal creatinine. For emergency physicians, significant decrements in GFR can occur in the normal range of creatinine: a change of creatinine from 0.6 to 1.2 mg/dL represents a 50 percent decrease in GFR although both values are in the normal range for creatinine, yet a change in creatinine from 8 to 12 mg/dL represents only a 25 percent decline in GFR.

To investigate the possibility of myocardial ischemia and hyperkalemia, an electrocardiogram should be performed on all patients presenting with ARF. Serum electrolytes should be measured. A chest radiograph may also help detect infectious causes of ARF and fluid overload.

Renal Biopsy

Renal biopsy should be considered in all causes of intrinsic ARF, especially in the estimated 10 to 25 percent of patients with ARF that cannot be diagnosed clinically.[22] Retrospective studies have shown that the results of the renal biopsy significantly change the diagnosis and management of ARF in 40 percent of cases.[23] The most common complication of renal biopsy is hematuria, which occurs in almost all patients. Serious complications defined as the need for blood transfusion, nephrectomy, puncture of other organs, or perinephric hematoma occur at a rate of 2.1 percent. Overall mortality for renal biopsy is 0.1 percent.

Imaging Studies

Imaging studies in ARF have their greatest utility in diagnosing urinary obstruction. The goal of the imaging study is to identify the site of blockage and to distinguish anatomic etiologies from merely functional forms of collecting system dilation. The patient's condition (e.g., pregnancy and radiation risks, renal failure and radiocontrast risks) must be taken into consideration in choosing the most appropriate study.

Plain radiographs with or without tomograms (the KUB: kidneys, ureter, and bladder) can provide information on the size and contour of the kidneys. A difference in kidney size of greater than 2 cm is suggestive of unilateral obstruction. Plain radiographs can identify renal blockage approximately 85 to 90 percent of the time and locate ureteral calculi approximately 50 percent of the time. Renal tomograms improve the resolution of renal calculi to 2 mm.

Intravenous pyelography (IVP) is considered the gold standard for defining the extent and anatomy of urinary obstruction, but unfortunately several drawbacks limit its utility for all patients. The nephrotoxicity of radiocontrast dye is of particular importance to patients with chronic renal failure and diabetes mellitus.[24] In patients with a low GFR, sufficient dye for adequate visualization may not excreted until 12 to 24 h after injection. Dilation of the urinary tract is not always indicative of obstruction, and the lack of hydronephrosis does not always rule out obstruction. Functional abnormalities of the urinary system, such as vesicoureteral reflux and the chronic massive diuresis (secondary to diabetes insipidus), can have dilated urinary tracts without obstruction. In addition, intermittent or partial obstructions will often not have hydronephrosis.

Invasive pyelography can be used when the risks of IVP are considered too great. Dye can be injected directly into the renal pelvis (antegrade) or cystoscopically into the ureter (retrograde). These techniques provide the same information as an IVP but without being dependent on renal function and without the nephrotoxicity of intravenous dye. Antegrade and retrograde pyelography also have the same drawback as IVP of not being able to distinguish functional from obstructive causes of urinary system dilation. In addition, these invasive techniques have the added risk of infection.

Ultrasonography—which has excellent sensitivity, safety, low cost, and lack of radiation and nephrotoxic dye—has become the procedure of choice to determine the presence of hydronephrosis, particularly in patients with low GFR. Although ultrasonography has a 90 percent sensitivity for detecting hydronephrosis (compared with the IVP), it may have a high false-positive rate of up to 20 percent.[25] Ultrasonography can misidentify a dilated urinary system as being due to obstruction rather than extrarenal pelvis, calyceal diverticula, congenital megacalyces, diuresis, and ileal conduits. In addition, numerous forms of obstructive uropathy may occur without dilation of the urinary collecting system: intrarenal crystals, nephrocalcinosis, staghorn calculi, and retroperitoneal obstruction.

Radionuclide scanning is performed by the intravenous injection of a radionuclide agent, followed by sequential imaging of its urinary excretion by using a gamma scintillation camera. This technique provides a 90 percent sensitivity in diagnosing upper urinary tract obstruction but without the nephrotoxic risk of IVP dye.[26] However, compared with IVP, radionuclide scanning lacks the resolution to define the exact site of anatomic obstruction adequately. Injection of a diuretic agent during the study will help in the differentiation of a functional versus anatomic obstruction in a dilated collecting system. The finding of increased radionuclide excretion after a diuretic points to a functional rather than an obstructive cause of a dilated collecting system. RBF measurement by radionuclide scanning is becoming the technique of choice to assess the potential for renal recovery after relief of obstruction.[27] However, recovery of renal function is possible even after nonvisualization of the kidney on radionuclide scanning.[28]

Computed tomography (CT) is a sensitive technique for diagnosing hydronephrosis and may delineate the anatomy of obstruction when

TABLE 88-11 Diagnostic Sequence for Acute Renal Failure (ARF)

History and physical examination
Investigate postrenal etiologies of ARF
Bladder catheter
Renal ultrasound
Investigate prerenal etiologies of ARF
Hemodynamic assessment
Urine output
Blood and urine chemistries
Urine chemical indices
Investigate intrinsic-renal etiologies of ARF
Urinalysis
Rheumatologic studies
Renal biopsy

ultrasound and IVP fail to identify an etiology. CT is particularly adept at diagnosing obstruction at the ureteric level compared with ultrasound.[29] A further advantage of CT is that a dilated urinary collecting system is well visualized even without the use of intravenous dye. CT may replace invasive pyelography as the secondary procedure to define the anatomy of obstruction after ultrasound and IVP.

Magnetic resonance (MR) imaging has yet to become fully integrated into the workup of urinary obstruction. Recently reviews have demonstrated MRs potential for the morphologic and functional evaluation of the urinary system. MR urography has demonstrated sensitivity up to 100 percent and specificity of 96 percent for urinary obstruction.[30] The advantages of MR include no radiation exposure, and paramagnetic contrast agents enable renal functional assessment without risks of iodinated contrast materials. MR urography can often differentiate acute from chronic obstruction, by demonstrating perinephric fluid accumulation, which is highly correlated with acute obstruction. Disadvantages of MR include the lack of large-scale accessibility and acceptance. MR can only diagnose obstruction with dilation and cannot differentiate functional dilatation from anatomic obstruction.

Diagnostic Sequence

After obtaining the medical history and performing the physical examination, the following general principles are useful in the diagnosis of ARF (Table 88-11).

Although postrenal failure accounts for only a small proportion of ARFs, it should be the first differential of ARF investigated because of its ease of diagnosis and treatment. A properly positioned bladder catheter can be diagnostic as well as therapeutic for obstruction below the level of the bladder. If no urine is obtained, then placement of the catheter should be tested by irrigation. If fluid returns freely, the catheter tip is most probably in the bladder, and obstruction above the bladder should be investigated. If a question remains, ultrasound may also be used to establish catheter placement.

Large postvoid residuals after catheterization suggest obstruction below the bladder, and catheter drainage should be maintained until the obstruction is relieved. To prevent hypotension and hematuria, the traditional recommendation is for intermittent clamping of the catheter during drainage of a distended bladder, but experimental and clinical evidence provides no support for this tradition.[31] Hematuria upon catheter drainage of a distended bladder is related to the degree of bladder wall damage before relief obstruction and not correlated with the rate of emptying. Urine should be completely and rapidly drained from an obstructed bladder, because prolonged urine stasis only predisposes the patient to urinary tract infection, urosepsis, and renal failure.

Once obstruction below the bladder level has been investigated, obstruction in the upper urinary tract should investigated with a renal ultrasound. If the renal ultrasound detects hydronephrosis, a confirmatory study to define the exact location of obstruction is required: either a CT scan or an IVP. If functional obstruction is still a consideration in the presence of a dilated genitourinary tract, a radionuclide scan before and after diuretics should be obtained.

After excluding postrenal etiologies, investigation of prerenal causes for ARF starts with an assessment of circulating volume. Abnormalities in standard vital signs and the orthostatic tilt test are unreliable detectors of acute volume loss; these tests are significant only when the findings are grossly abnormal.[32,33] More sensitive and reliable indicators of acute changes in circulating volume are base deficit, lactate, and central venous oxygen saturation. Invasive hemodynamic monitoring provides the most reliable means of assessing hemodynamic performance.[34]

Urine output is a generally poor method of gauging blood volume.[35] Oliguria requires differentiating prerenal from intrinsic renal etiologies. Low urine output in prerenal syndromes is the result of normal renal concentrating mechanisms reacting appropriately to hypovolemia, resulting in urine with high specific gravity and high osmolality. To maintain circulating volume, functioning kidneys in a hypovolemic state preferentially reabsorb both urea and sodium, resulting in an increased BUN/Cr ratio and a low FeNa level (Table 88-8). Exceptions to this rule include the etiologies of intrinsic renal failure where the renal concentrating mechanism is preserved or is even stimulated (e.g., glomerulonephritis) (Table 88-9).

Low urine output with intrinsic renal failure is the not result of increased sodium and water reabsorption but, rather, of a decline in GFR. In tubular and interstitial diseases, normal concentrating mechanisms are often lost and decreased GFR is a defense to prevent hypovolemia from excessive renal fluid losses. This results in low urine output, but with isotonic urine that is high in sodium. With intrinsic ARF, the reabsorption of urea and sodium is not augmented as it is in prerenal causes. Intrinsic ARF typically has a parallel rise in both BUN and creatinine that preserves the BUN/Cr ratio and an elevated FeNa level greater than 1 percent.

The classic nephritic triad of hypertension, edema, and red blood cell casts is diagnostic of glomerular forms of intrinsic ARF. These patients require a more detailed evaluation and testing for autoimmune diseases such as poststreptococcal glomerulonephritis and SLE. A renal biopsy should usually be done to define the exact nature of their disease and individualize treatment protocols

TREATMENT

Patients with ARF present challenging fluid-management problems. Hypovolemia potentiates and exacerbates all forms of ARF. The reversal of hypovolemia by rapid fluid infusion is often sufficient to treat and/or ameliorate many forms of ARF,[36] yet rapid fluid infusion can result in life-threatening fluid overload in patients with ARF. Accurate determination of these patients' volume status is essential, often requiring invasive hemodynamic monitoring. The most important treatment for ARF in emergency departments is prompt and appropriate fluid resuscitation.

Patients with nonoliguric compared with oliguric ARF have improved mortality and renal function recovery rates. This has prompted many authors to recommend diuretics in treating oliguric ARF. Unfortunately, randomized double-blind controlled trials have failed to show a benefit in administering diuretics to patients with ARF.[37] These studies concluded that diuretics were only useful in the management of volume-overloaded patients. Care should be taken in prescribing high-dose furosemide because of the association with long-term hearing deficits.

Renal vascular vasodilators in ARF have theoretical and experimental support. Low (''renal'')-dose dopamine [1 to 5 μg/kg/min] has been widely used to treat ARF. Dopamine in these dosages is a potent vasodilator, which increases RBF in the experimental setting of ARF.

Most clinical studies have failed to show that dopamine improves the recovery or mortality rates in patients with ARF.[38] In the majority of ARF studies, dopamine was only associated with an increase in urine output. Current recommendations for dopamine favor its use in ARF patients only with congestive heart failure. Dopamine is proarrhythmic, and controlled studies using dopamine for ARF found an increased mortality associated with its use.[39]

In animal models, calcium channel blockers are protective against ARF if given before the renal insult.[40] In humans, their major benefit has been in preventing ARF in renal transplant patients taking cyclosporine.

If given within 6 h of rhabdomyolysis, infusion of bicarbonate and mannitol has been reported to be protective against myoglobinuric ARF.[41] In addition, mannitol infusion may decrease the rate of ARF if given before radiocontrast agents.[42] There are no controlled studies showing any benefit to mannitol infusion for patients with established ARF. In fact, mannitol given in high doses has been associated as a cause of ARF.[43] There are also significant risks of fluid overload and hyperkalemia in administering large doses of mannitol to ARF patients.

The advent of hemodialysis had a significant impact on the treatment of the life-threatening fluid and electrolyte complications of ARF. However, dialysis may adversely affect remaining renal function. Hemodialysis may decrease RBF or produce hypotension if circulating volume is reduced below normal. Dialysis also causes oliguria that could lead to increased cast formation and further tubular obstruction. Studies comparing intensive dialysis with traditional regimens have failed to show any improvement in outcome of patients with ARF.[44] Hemodialysis should be reserved for complications of ARF unresponsive to medical management. The complications amenable to hemodialysis include acidosis, electrolyte imbalance (e.g., hyperkalemia), fluid overload, uremia (e.g., encephalopathy, pericarditis, and bleeding diathesis), and drug intoxication (e.g., digoxin, aminophylline, aspirin, and lithium).

DISPOSITION

Patients with ARF require admission to the hospital, usually to an intensive care setting where their fluid and medical management can be monitored on an hour-to-hour basis. An appropriate specialist (nephrologist, intensive care specialist, or internist) should be consulted early.

REFERENCES

1. Brezis M, Rosen S: Hypoxia of the renal medulla: Its implications for disease. *N Engl J Med* 332:647, 1995.
2. Thurau K, Boylan JW: Acute renal success: The unexpected logic of oliguria in acute renal failure. *Am J Med* 61:308, 1976.
3. Vaughan ED Jr, Sorenson EJ, Gillenwater JY: The renal hemodynamic response to chronic unilateral complete ureteral occlusion. *Invest Urol* 8:78, 1970.
4. Davidman M, Olson P, Kohen J, et al: Iatrogenic renal disease. *Arch Intern Med* 151:1809, 1991.
5. Conger J: Hemodynamic factors in acute renal failure. *Adv Ren Replace Ther* 4(2 suppl 1):25, 1997.
6. Neuringer JR, Brenner BM: Hemodynamic theory of progressive renal disease: A 10-year update in brief review. *Am J Kidney Dis* 22:98, 1993.
7. Hou SH, et al: Hospital-acquired renal insufficiency: A prospective study. *Am J Med* 74:243, 1983.
8. Shusterman N, Strom BL, Murray TG, et al: Risk factors and outcome of hospital-acquired acute renal failure: Clinical epidemiologic study. *Am J Med* 83:65, 1987.
9. Kaufman J, Dhakal M, Patel B, et al: Community-acquired acute renal failure. *Am J Kidney Dis* 17:191, 1991.
10. Moghal NE, Brocklebank JT, Meadow SR: A review of acute renal failure in children: Incidence, etiology and outcome. *Clin Nephrol* 49:91, 1998.
11. Rasmussen HH, Ibels LS: Acute renal failure: Multivariate analysis of causes and risk factors. *Am J Med* 73:211, 1982.
12. Diokno AC, Brown MB, Goldstein N, et al: Epidemiology of bladder emptying symptoms in elderly men. *J Urol* 148:1817, 1992.
13. Alkhunaizi AM, Schrier RW: Management of acute renal failure: New perspectives. *Am J Kidney Dis* 28:315, 1996.
14. Druml W: Prognosis of acute renal failure 1975–1995 [editorial]. *Nephron* 73:8, 1996.
15. Levy EM, Viscoli CM, Horwitz RI: The effect of acute renal failure on mortality: A cohort analysis [see comments]. *JAMA* 275:1489, 1996.
16. Corwin HL, Teplick RS, Schreiber MJ, et al: Prediction of outcome in acute renal failure. *Am J Nephrol* 7: 8, 1987.
17. Liano F, Junco E, Pascual J, et al: The spectrum of acute renal failure in the intensive care unit compared with that seen in other settings: The Madrid Acute Renal Failure Study Group. *Kidney Int* 66(suppl):S16, 1998.
18. Spurney RF, Fulkerson JW, Schwab SJ: Acute renal failure in critically ill patients: Prognosis for recovery of kidney function after prolonged dialysis support [see comments]. *Crit Care Med* 19:8, 1991.
19. Miller TR, Anderson RJ, Linas SL, et al: Urinary diagnostic indices in acute renal failure: A prospective study. *Ann Intern Med* 89:47,1978.
20. Corwin HL, Schreiber MJ, Fang LS: Low fractional excretion of sodium: Occurrence with hemoglobinuric- and myoglobinuric-induced acute renal failure. *Arch Intern Med* 144:981, 1984.
21. Cockcroft DW, Gault MH: Prediction of creatinine clearance from serum creatinine. *Nephron* 16:31, 1976.
22. Wilson DM, Turner DR, Cameron JS, et al: Value of renal biopsy in acute intrinsic renal failure. *BMJ* 2:459, 1976.
23. Mustonen J, Pasternack A, Helin H, et al: Renal biopsy in acute renal failure. *Am J Nephrol* 4:27, 1984.
24. Parfrey PS, Griffiths SM, Barrett BJ, et al: Contrast material-induced renal failure in patients with diabetes mellitus, renal insufficiency, or both: A prospective controlled study [see comments]. *N Engl J Med* 320:143, 1989.
25. Rao KG, Hacker BH, Woodlief RM, et al: Real-time renal sonography in spinal cord injury patients: Prospective comparison with excretory urography. *J Urol* 135:72, 1986.
26. Powers TA, Grove RB, Bauriedel JK, et al: Detection of obstructive uropathy using ^{99m}technetium diethylenetriaminepentaacetic acid. *J Urol* 124:588, 1980.
27. Kalika V, Bard RH, Iloreta A, et al: Prediction of renal functional recovery after relief of upper urinary tract obstruction. *J Urol* 126:301, 1981.
28. Sherman RA, Blaufox MD: Obstructive uropathy in patients with nonvisualization on renal scan. *Nephron* 25:82, 1980.
29. Katz DS, Lane MJ, Sommer FG: Unenhanced helical CT of ureteral stones: Incidence of associated urinary tract findings. *AJR* 166:1319, 1996.
30. Hussain S, O'Malley M, Jara H, et al: MR urography. *Magn Reson Imaging Clin North Am* 5:95, 1997.
31. Christensen J, Ostri P, Frimodt-Moller C, et al: Intravesical pressure changes during bladder drainage in patients with acute urinary retention. *Urol Int* 42:181, 1987.
32. Abou-Khalil B, Scalea TM, Trooskin SZ, et al: Hemodynamic responses to shock in young trauma patients: Need for invasive monitoring [see comments]. *Crit Care Med* 22:633, 1994.
33. Witting MD, Wears RL, Li S: Defining the positive tilt test: A study of healthy adults with moderate acute blood loss [published errata appear in *Ann Emerg Med* 24:223, 1994, and 25:857, 1995]. *Ann Emerg Med* 23:1320, 1994.
34. Scalea TM, Simon HM, Duncan AO, et al: Geriatric blunt multiple trauma: Improved survival with early invasive monitoring. *J Trauma* 30:129, 1990.
35. Jeng JC, Lee K, Jablonski K, et al: Serum lactate and base deficit suggest inadequate resuscitation of patients with burn injuries: Application of a point-of-care laboratory instrument. *J Burn Care Rehabil* 18:402, 1997.
36. Conger JD: Interventions in clinical acute renal failure: What are the data? *Am J Kidney Dis* 26:565, 1995.
37. Shilliday IR, Quinn KJ, Allison ME: Loop diuretics in the management of acute renal failure: A prospective, double-blind, placebo-controlled, randomized study. *Nephrol Dial Transplant* 12:2592, 1997.
38. Denton M, Chertow GM, Brady HR: ''Renal-dose'' dopamine for the treatment of acute renal failure: Scientific rationale, experimental studies and clinical trials. *Kidney Int* 50:4, 1996.
39. Chertow GM, Sayegh MH, Allgren RI, et al: Is the administration of dopamine associated with adverse or favorable outcomes in acute renal failure? Auriculin Anaritide Acute Renal Failure Study Group [see comments]. *Am J Med* 101:49, 1996.
40. Epstein M: Calcium antagonists and renal protection: Current status and future perspectives. *Arch Intern Med* 152:1573, 1992.

41. Better OS, Rubinstein I: Management of shock and acute renal failure in casualties suffering from the crush syndrome. *Ren Fail* 19:647, 1997.
42. Louis BM, Hoch BS, Hernandez C, et al: Protection from the nephrotoxicity of contrast dye. *Ren Fail* 18:639, 1996.
43. Dorman HR, Sondheimer JH, Cadnapaphornchai P: Mannitol-induced acute renal failure. *Medicine (Baltimore)* 69:153, 1990.
44. Gillum DM, Dixon BS, Yanover MJ, et al: The role of intensive dialysis in acute renal failure. *Clin Nephrol* 25:249, 1986.

EMERGENCIES IN RENAL FAILURE AND DIALYSIS PATIENTS

Richard Sinert

End-stage renal disease (ESRD) is the irreversible loss of renal function, resulting in the accumulation of toxins and the loss of internal homeostasis. Uremia, the clinical syndrome resulting from ESRD, is universally fatal without some form of renal replacement therapy (RRT). At present, RRT consists of two basic modalities: renal transplant and dialysis therapy. This chapter discusses the pathophysiology and clinical features of uremia and the specific techniques and complications related to hemodialysis (HD) and peritoneal dialysis (PD).

EPIDEMIOLOGY

The 1996 annual data report of the United States Renal Data System (USRDS) noted there were 73,091 new cases of ESRD (incidence, 2.7 per 10,000), with 283,932 patients being treated for ESRD (prevalence, 10.4 per 10,000) during that year.[1] The most common age group with ESRD is the 45-to-64 age group, representing 38.7 percent of patients. African Americans make up a disproportionate number of ESRD patients, accounting for 32.3 percent, while making up just 12.2 percent of the US population.

USRDS projects that the incidence of ESRD is growing by 6 to 7 percent per year. An expanding incidence and life span will result in an expected increasing prevalence of ESRD of 8 to 9 percent per year. USRDS projects similar growth rates of ESRD for African Americans and Caucasians but predicts a two times greater growth rate for Native Americans and Asians and Pacific Islanders. The highest growth rate by age occurs in the over-75 age group.

Diabetes mellitus is the most common disease causing ESRD, accounting for 32.5 percent of patients, followed by hypertension (24.5 percent), glomerulonephritis (17.7 percent), and cystic kidney disease (4.7 percent).

The utilization of RRT for ESRD is divided into 62 percent on dialysis therapy and 38 percent with renal transplants.[2] Of the patients on dialysis, 83 percent are on HD and 17 percent on PD. African Americans have significantly lower rates of renal transplantation and PD than do Caucasians and Asians and Pacific Islanders. Pediatric patients ages 0 to 19 have significantly higher rates of renal transplantation and PD than do other age groups.

Overall, ESRD patients have a life expectancy of between 19 and 47 percent of the expected remaining years of life for age-, sex-, and race-matched control subjects without ESRD.[3] One-, two-, and five-year survival rates for ESRD are 78.2, 62.7, and 29.3 percent, respectively. Cardiac causes account for approximately 50 percent of all cases of ESRD death.[4] Infectious causes of death occur in 25 percent of patients in the 20- to 44-year-old age group. Cerebrovascular events make up 6 percent of ESRD deaths, with malignancy accounting for another 1 to 4 percent. Approximately 20 percent of dialysis patients withdraw from therapy before death. Patients over 65 years of age have the highest withdrawal rate, 25 percent. The increasing incidence of withdrawal with age is linked to an increasing severity of comorbid conditions affecting patients' quality of life on RRT.

PATHOPHYSIOLOGY

Piorry, in 1840, was the first to use the term *uremia*, contamination of the blood with urine, to describe the clinical syndrome from ESRD. The concept that uremia is from an excretory failure resulting in toxin accumulation is reinforced by the continued use of the term *azotemia*, the buildup of blood nitrogen.

Excretory Failure

Levels of over 70 chemicals are elevated in uremic plasma, leading to the hypothesis that these toxins, individually or in combination, cause uremic organ dysfunction and produce the symptoms. For over 100 years it has been observed that limiting protein intake markedly improves the symptoms of uremia. Urea, the major breakdown product of proteins, reproduces a few of the neurobehavioral uremic symptoms, but only at very high concentrations. Other potential uremic toxins include cyanate, guanidines, polyamines, and β_2-microglobulin. Ammonia is not a toxin candidate, since ammonia levels are not elevated in ESRD patients.

In conclusion, while toxins from ESRD excretory failure are definitely a factor in uremia, they cannot explain all its clinical features. In addition, if uremia was simply a toxidrome, then dialysis should reverse all its untoward effects. Yet, many uremic organ dysfunctions persist after dialysis, and other processes are clearly important.

Biosynthetic Failure

Biosynthetic failure refers to the aspects of uremia from loss of the renal hormones 1,25 $(OH)_3$ vitamin D_3 and erythropoietin. The kidneys are primarily responsible for the secretion of erythropoietin and 1-α-hydroxylase, which is necessary to produce the active form of vitamin D_3. In ESRD patients, levels of both these hormones are significantly depressed. Since 85 percent of erythropoietin is produced in the kidneys, ESRD patients have depressed levels, contributing to anemia. Vitamin D_3 deficiency results in decreased gastrointestinal (GI) calcium absorption, inducing secondary hyperparathyroidism, responsible for the development of renal bone disease.

Regulatory Failure

Regulatory failure results in an oversecretion of hormones, leading to uremia by disruption of normal feedback mechanisms after renal failure. In response to the accumulation of ions and other waste products with ESRD, the maintenance of internal homeostasis is dependent on a variety of extrarenal processes. These homeostatic responses, while adaptive to one toxin, may have untoward effects outside the system they are attempting to regulate. The "trade-off" hypothesis, first proposed by Bricker, was initially postulated to explain how hyperparathyroidism in ESRD was a trade-off for the beneficial effects of high parathyroid hormone (PTH) levels on controlling phosphate levels. The trade-off for the maintenance of normal calcium and phosphate levels is hyperparathyroidism, causing increased bone turnover and leading to renal bone disease. Bricker has extended this trade-off hypothesis to sodium regulation in ESRD. As the glomerular filtration rate (GFR) decreases in ESRD patients, increasing fractional sodium excretion prevents salt retention. Bricker postulated that the trade-off for this natriuretic factor was a generalized inhibition of sodium transport, which he stated explained many aspects of uremic organ dysfunction.

While Bricker's trade-off hypothesis is still controversial, sodium transport abnormalities have been well documented in uremia. Na^+, K^+-ATPase activity is reduced in the red blood cells, leukocytes, intestinal epithelium, cardiac muscle, and skeletal muscle in uremic patients. Inhibition of Na^+, K^+-ATPase activity results in partial cellular depolarization and increased calcium entry, which are linked to both the high prevalence of hypertension and heart failure in ESRD. Recently an endogenous dialyzable digitalis-like inhibitor of Na^+, K^+-ATPase activity has been isolated in uremic plasma. This defect in Na^+, K^+-ATPase activity is reversed by dialysis.

CLINICAL FEATURES

Uremia should only be viewed as a clinical syndrome; no single symptom, sign, or laboratory test is reliable in diagnosing all aspects of uremia. Although a correlation exists between the symptoms of uremia and a low GFR (8 to 10 mL/min), available laboratory tests [e.g., determinations of blood urea nitrogen (BUN) and creatinine] are inaccurate detecting trends in low GFR. The decision to start chronic dialysis is a clinical decision based on the symptoms of uremia (Table 89-1).[5]

Neurologic Complications

UREMIC ENCEPHALOPATHY Progressive neurologic symptoms of uremia are the most common indications for initiating chronic dialysis. Uremic encephalopathy is a constellation of nonspecific central neurologic symptoms associated with renal failure that respond, in large part, to RRT. Uremic encephalopathy should remain a diagnosis of exclusion after other structural, vascular, infectious, toxic, and metabolic causes of neurologic dysfunction have been investigated. Objective findings of uremic encephalopathy include a significant increase in slow delta waves on the electroencephalogram (EEG) and consistently low scores on psychometric testing. These objective findings of neurologic dysfunction have been linked to inhibition of Na^+, K^+-ATPase activity and increases in brain calcium either from elevated parathyroid hormone levels or abnormal calcium transport in uremic brains. Both symptomatic and objective neurologic findings of uremia improve with dialysis and can be followed to judge the adequacy of RRT.

DIALYSIS DEMENTIA Dialysis dementia (encephalopathy), similar to uremic encephalopathy, consists of a nonspecific set of neuropsychiatric dysfunctions that, unlike uremic encephalopathy, are progressive and eventually fatal. This disorder usually becomes evident after at least 2 years on dialysis and fails to respond to increases in dialysis frequency or renal transplantation. EEG findings can differentiate uremic encephalopathy from dialysis dementia. High brain aluminum levels from oral ingestion of aluminum or high levels of aluminum in dialysate water have been correlated with the development of dialysis dementia. Dialysis dementia has shown some improvement with desferroxamine binding of aluminum.

PERIPHERAL NEUROPATHY Peripheral neuropathy occurs in over 50 percent of HD patients and generally responds poorly to dialysis but can be reversed by renal transplantation. Patients can have both asymmetric (mononeuropathies) and symmetric (polyneuropathies) peripheral deficits. Another common deficit is ''glove-and-stocking'' sensory involvement, presenting with pain or anesthesia affecting the most distal nerves. Electrophysiologic testing of patients with uremia shows depression of motor and sensory nerve conduction. No single pathologic correlate has yet been identified for peripheral uremic neuropathy.

AUTONOMIC DYSFUNCTION Autonomic dysfunction is very common in ESRD patients and presents a significant risk factor for hypotension during dialysis. Resistance to norepinephrine is one postulated mechanism.

SUBDURAL HEMATOMA Subdural hematoma occurs in approximately 3.5 percent of HD patients, presumably related to head trauma, anticoagulants, excessive ultrafiltration, and hypertension. Bilateral subdural hematomas can mimic the symptoms and signs of uremic encephalopathy or dialysis dementia, making the correct diagnosis difficult.

TABLE 89-1 Clinical Features of Uremia

NEUROLOGIC
Uremic encephalopathy
Symptomatic improvement with dialysis
Cognitive defects, memory loss, decreased attentiveness
Slurred speech, reversal of sleep-wake cycle, asterixis
Seizure, coma
Dialysis dementia
Failure to improve with dialysis
Progressive neurologic decline, fatal
Subdural hematoma
Headache, focal neurologic deficits, seizure, coma
Peripheral neuropathy
Singultus (hiccups)
Restless leg syndrome
Sensorimotor neuropathy
Autonomic neuropathy
CARDIOVASCULAR
Hypertension
Heart failure
High-output AV fistula
Uremic cardiomyopathy
Fluid overload
Pericarditis
Uremic
Dialysis-related
Tamponade
HEMATOLOGIC
Anemia, decreased red blood cell survival, decreased erythropoietin levels
Bleeding diathesis
Immunodeficiency (both humoral and cellular)
GASTROINTESTINAL
Anorexia, metallic taste, nausea, vomiting
Peptic ulcer disease, GI bleeding (AV malformations)
Diverticulosis, diverticulitis
Ascites
RENAL BONE DISEASE
Metastatic calcification (calciphylaxis)
Increased bone fractures
Bone cysts
Carpal tunnel syndrome

Cardiovascular Complications

HYPERTENSION Hypertension occurs in 80 to 90 percent of patients starting dialysis. Hypertension represents a significant risk factor for coronary artery disease, cerebrovascular accidents, and heart failure. Hemodynamic profiles of hypertensive ESRD patients show that maintenance of hypertension is dependent on increases in total peripheral resistance. The etiology of the increase in total peripheral resistance appears to be multifactorial. Increases in blood volume, the vasopressor effects of native kidneys, the renin-angiotensin system, and the sympathetic nervous system all have been shown to play a role in ESRD hypertension. Management of hypertension in ESRD patients should begin with the control of blood volume. If that is unsuccessful, most patients' hypertension can be controlled with adrenergic-blocking agents, angiotensin-converting enzyme (ACE) inhibitors, or vasodilating agents, such as hydralazine or minoxidil. Bilateral nephrectomy is rarely necessary for blood pressure control.

HEART FAILURE Congestive heart failure (CHF) occurs for many of the same reasons in ESRD patients as in other patients; hypertension is the most common cause of CHF in ESRD patients, followed by coronary artery disease and valvular defects. Causes of CHF unique to ESRD include arteriovenous (AV) fistula-related high-output failure, uremic cardiomyopathy, and fluid overload. Large AV fistulas can cause high-output CHF, characterized by high cardiac output and low total peripheral vascular resistance. Diagnosis is made by echocardiography, and treatment is by surgical binding of the AV fistula to restrict blood flow.

Uremic cardiomyopathy is a diagnosis of exclusion when all other causes of CHF have been ruled out. In most uremic patients, left ventricular (LV) dysfunction is related to ischemic heart disease, hypertension, and hypoalbuminemia rather than to a uremic toxin. Dialysis rarely improves LV function in uremic patients with CHF.[6] However, parathyroid hormone has been linked to decreased LV function in uremia by studies showing marked improvement of LV function after parathryoidectomy.

Fluid overload in ESRD is a common cause of CHF but not always a requirement for pulmonary edema. Acute myocardial ischemia can cause depressed LV function to the point of causing pulmonary edema even in patients at or below their postdialysis ("dry") weight. In addition, pulmonary edema has been reported in ESRD patients in the absence of high pulmonary artery pressures, seemingly the result of increased pulmonary capillary permeability. Invasive hemodynamic monitoring in ESRD patients with pulmonary edema may be required to guide therapy.

Management of pulmonary edema in ESRD patients is usually similar to treatment in non-ESRD patients. Cornerstones of therapy in both types of patients include oxygen, nitrates, ACE inhibitors, and morphine. Diuretics, such as furosemide, are still effective in treating CHF in ESRD patients even with minimal urine output.[7] In pulmonary edema, intravenous furosemide in doses of 60 to 100 mg provides pulmonary vasodilatation, improving oxygenation. Preload reduction in ESRD patients can also be accomplished by inducing diarrhea with sorbitol and by phlebotomy. Phlebotomy of as little as 150 mL of blood is safe and effective in treating pulmonary edema.[8] For example, phlebotomy of 150 mL in a patient with a hematocrit of 20 percent results in the loss of 120 mL of plasma and 30 mL of packed red blood cells (10 g of hemoglobin). The improved oxygenation by phlebotomy will more than offset the decrease in oxygen-carrying capacity due to the decrease on hemoglobin. Phlebotomized blood should be collected in transfusion bags, enabling plasma to be extracted by the blood bank and transfusion of red blood cells later during dialysis. HD is the ultimate treatment for fluid overload in ESRD patients. PD does not remove volume fast enough to have a significant impact on pulmonary edema.

PERICARDITIS Do not assume that all cases of pericarditis in ESRD patients are due to uremia; patients should be evaluated carefully for other causes. Pericarditis in ESRD can occur both before initiation of dialysis and during dialysis, so-called uremic and dialysis-related pericarditis, respectively. Uremic pericarditis occurs in approximately 16 percent of patients. Uremic pericarditis is most common when the other symptoms of uremia are most severe. The etiology of uremic pericarditis has been linked to fluid overload, abnormal platelet function, and increased fibrinolytic activity. Most cases of uremic pericarditis improve with RRT.

Dialysis-related pericarditis also seems related to the general uremic milieu. This form of pericarditis is most common during periods of increased catabolism (trauma and sepsis) or inadequate dialysis due to missed sessions or vascular access problems. The pathophysiology of dialysis-related pericarditis has been linked to the buildup of middle molecules and hyperparathyroidism.

The clinical features and evaluation of pericarditis in patients with ESRD are similar to those for non-ESRD patients. The classic findings of chest pain, fever, and pericardial friction are more commonly found in dialysis-related than in uremic pericarditis. Mortality rates for ESRD patients with pericarditis are as high as 8 percent.

Management of both uremic and dialysis-related pericarditis in hemodynamically stable patients is by intensive dialysis therapy. HD is preferred over PD because of its higher clearance rates, but the risks of heparin and rapid fluid shifts precipitating tamponade must be taken into account. This therapy is effective in over 55 percent of cases of dialysis-related pericarditis usually after 10 to 14 days. Indomethacin and steroids are of questionable value for ESRD pericarditis. If pericardial effusion persists for more than 10 to 14 days with intensive dialysis, the treatment is considered a failure. Most centers now recommend anterior pericardectomy as the treatment of choice in this condition. Total pericardectomy is reserved for constrictive pericarditis.

Symptoms of pericardial tamponade are often quite subtle in ESRD patients, rarely presenting with the typical Beck's triad. Increased interdialysis weight gain, increased edema, and intradialysis hypotension suggest the early diagnosis of tamponade. Because of the slow accumulation of pericardial fluid, pulsus paradoxus and a pericardial friction rub are absent, and the only clinical suggestions may be weakness, moderate hypotension, and an increasing heart size on x-ray. Ultrasonography is needed to make the diagnosis. Hemodynamically significant pericardial effusions require pericardiocentesis under fluoroscopic or ultrasonographic guidance. Pericardiocentesis, because of its high complication rate, should be used only in hemodynamically unstable patients with pericardial tamponade.

Hematologic Complications

ANEMIA Anemia in ESRD patients is of multifactorial origin, secondary to decreased erythropoietin, blood loss from dialysis, and decreased red blood cell survival times. In addition, wide fluctuations in plasma blood volume seen in dialysis patients often cause factitious anemia. Without treatment, the hematocrit in ESRD patients will usually stabilize at 15 to 20 percent, with normocytic and normochromic red blood cells. Bone marrow will show erythroid hypoplasia with little effect on leukopoiesis or megakaryocytopoiesis. Management of anemia is by the infusion of human recombinant erythropoietin on a regular basis. Erythropoietin replacement therapy has markedly improved the quality of life for ESRD patients by increasing exercise capacity and tolerance. An increase in blood pressure has been reported in approximately 30 to 35 percent of patients receiving erythropoietin.

BLEEDING DYSCRASIA Abnormalities in hemostasis expose ESRD patients to increased risks of GI tract bleeding, subdural hematomas, subcapsular liver hematomas, and intraocular bleeding. The abnormal hemostasis in ESRD is characterized by decreased platelet function and von Willebrand factor defects.[9] Anemia has been determined to be the major etiologic defect causing abnormal hemostasis in ESRD patients. The skin bleeding test is the best predictor of clinically important defects in hemostasis. Improvements in bleeding times can be obtained by infusion of desmopressin, conjugated estrogens, and erythropoietin.

NEUTROPHIL DYSFUNCTION Immunologic deficiency in ESRD patients produces a high mortality rate from infectious diseases. Both leukocyte chemotaxis and phagocytosis are depressed in uremic patients. Abnormal T-cell activation has also been noted in ESRD patients secondary to reduction in interleukin 2 production. Dialysis therapy does not appear to improve the immune function of leukocytes or T cells. In fact, HD may even exacerbate immunodeficiency by complement activation after exposure to the HD filter membrane.

Gastrointestinal Complications

UPPER GASTROINTESTINAL BLEEDING Anorexia, nausea, and vomiting are common symptoms of uremia and are often used as an indication to initiate dialysis and to follow the adequacy of RRT. In the upper GI tract, there is an increased incidence of gastritis and bleeding in ESRD patients, but, it is interesting to note, the incidence of gastric and duodenal ulcers is similar in ESRD patients and the general population. The increased incidence of GI bleeding and rebleeding and the higher mortality rates from GI hemorrhage in ESRD patients are functions more of the bleeding dyscrasia than of a primary GI disease. In addition, ESRD patients are at increased risk from bleeding from angiodysplasias. Successful prevention of recurrent bleeding from GI angiodysplasias has been obtained by use of tranexamic acid and conjugated estrogens, which decrease bleeding time.

DIVERTICULOSIS AND DIVERTICULITIS Chronic constipation is common among ESRD patients secondary to decreased fluid intake and the use of phosphate-bonding gels. ESRD patients have an increased incidence of diverticular disease and colonic perforation, especially patients with polycystic kidney disease.

ASCITES Dialysis-related ascites is an idiopathic form of ascites secondary to fluid overload, portal hypertension from polycystic liver disease, and osmotic disequilibrium. Treatment of refractory ascites is possible with peritoneovenous shunts.

Renal Bone Disease

CALCIPHYLAXIS As the GFR falls, phosphate excretion also falls, resulting in increased serum phosphate levels. When the calcium-phosphate product [Ca (mg/dL) $\times$ PO_4 (mg/dL)] is greater than 70 to 80, metastatic calcification can ensue. Clinically these patients present with complaints of pseudogout secondary to metastatic calcification of synovial joints. Metastatic calcification in small vessels results in skin and finger necrosis. Life-threatening calcifications can occur in the cardiac and pulmonary systems. An increased mortality rate has been observed in ESRD patients with a product greater than 72.[10] Treatment consists of the use of low-calcium dialysate and phosphate-binding gels.

HYPERPARATHRYOIDISM (OSTEITIS FIBROSA CYSTICA) As ESRD progresses, the combination of calciphylaxis and vitamin D_3 deficiency results in depressed ionized calcium levels and stimulation of the parathyroid gland. The increased production of PTH results in high bone turnover. These patients present with weakened bones highly susceptible to fracture. In addition, patients with osteitis fibrosa cystica often complain of bone pain and muscle weakness. High alkaline phosphatase and PTH levels make the diagnosis. Treatment consists of control of serum phosphate with binding gels, vitamin D_3 replacement, and, if necessary, subtotal parathryoidectomy.

VITAMIN D_3 DEFICIENCY AND ALUMINUM INTOXICATION (OSTEOMALACIA) Subsets of ESRD patients present with osteomalacia, a defect in bone calcification. Once vitamin D_3 replacement became universally available, aluminum intoxication became the major cause of osteomalacia in ESRD patients. Sources of aluminum are dialysate diluent and phosphate-binding gels. The signs and symptoms are weakened bones, bone pain, and muscle weakness, similar to those for hyperparathyroidism. Differentiation is made by finding low-to-normal alkaline phosphatase levels and low PTH levels in osteomalacia. Elevated serum aluminum and bone aluminum levels are useful for confirming the diagnosis. Treatment with desferroxamine has been shown to be effective in aluminum bone disease.

β_2-MICROGLOBULIN AMYLOIDOSIS Dialysis-related amyloidosis, or β_2-microglobulin amyloidosis, is seen commonly in dialysis patients over 50 years of age and on dialysis for more than 10 years. Amyloid deposits have been found in the GI tract, bones, and joints. Complications include GI perforations, bone cysts with pathologic fractures, and arthropathies, including carpal tunnel syndrome and rotator cuff tears. Patients with amyloidosis have significantly higher mortality rates than those without this disorder. The etiology of β_2-microglobulin amyloidosis may be related to both decreased clearance and increased synthesis from immunologic reaction to hemodialyzer filters. Switching to more biocompatible filters that have higher clearance of β_2 microglobulin has markedly reduced the incidence of amyloidosis.

TREATMENT

Hemodialysis

HD in humans was first made possible by the invention of the rotating-drum artificial kidney by Kolff et al. in 1943. Access to the patient's bloodstream was not practical until the development of the external AV shunt by Scribner in 1960. Brescia and Cimino in 1966 developed the subcutaneous AV fistula, which made HD safer and more acceptable. RRT became universally available after Congress passed the Medicare entitlement for the treatment of ESRD in 1973.

TECHNICAL ASPECTS The nephron removes toxins and maintains internal homeostasis through an elegant combination of glomerular filtration followed by selective reabsorption and secretion of water and solutes. HD uses the brute force techniques of ultrafiltration and clearance to replace the functions of the nephron. HD substitutes a hemodialyzer filter for the glomerulus to produce a ultrafiltrate of plasma. Adjustment of the pressure gradient across the hemodialyzer filter during HD controls the amount of fluid removal (ultrafiltration). Solute removal (clearance) during HD is dependent on the filter pore size, the amount of ultrafiltration (solute drag), and the concentration gradient across the filter (diffusion). Solute diffusion down chemical gradients from the blood to the dialysis fluid (dialysate) determines their final blood concentration. Since hemodialyzer pore size prevents the filtration of proteins, dialysate consists only of electrolytes (Na^+, K^+, Cl^-, HCO_3^-, Ca^{++}, and Mg^{++}) and glucose, whose concentrations are varied to control their clearance.[11] During HD, blood is removed from the vascular access site by large-bore needles (typically 15 g), circulated through the dialysis machine at rates of 300 to 500 mL/min, and returned to the patient. The dialysate usually flows at a rate of 500 to 800 mL/min through the dialysis filter in the direction opposite to blood flow. Small amounts of heparin, 1000 to 2000 IU, are typically used to prevent thrombosis at the vascular access site. HD sessions typically take 3 to 4 h.

Ultrafiltration and clearance usually occur simultaneously during dialysis but can be separated by adjusting the HD settings. In fluid-overloaded patients, adding suction to the dialysate side of the hemodialyzer filter augments ultrafiltration. Dialysate flow can be lowered, minimizing clearance to prevent hypotension during dialysis. When fluid loss is not desired during dialysis (for patients below their dry weight) balancing dialysate and blood pressures across the filter limits fluid removal. Decreasing the dialysate concentration of the desired solute can augment clearance of specific electrolytes (e.g., potassium).

Long-term successful hemodialysis is dependent on reliable access to the patient's circulation.[12] The external Scribner AV shunt provided adequate vascular access but only lasted on average 1 year. The Brescia-Cimino AV fistula formed by the anastomosis of a native artery and vein in the forearm has a much greater longevity. In cases where a native artery or vein are not suitable for fistula creation, an interposing vascular graft made of an autologous vein, polytetrafluorethylene, or bovine carotid artery must be used for vascular access. These grafts generally have a higher complication rate and shorter functional life expectancies than do natural AV fistulas.

COMPLICATIONS OF THE VASCULAR ACCESS Vascular access is the Achilles heel of HD, and complications of the vascular access account for more inpatient hospital days than any other complication of HD.

Vascular Access Stenosis and Thrombosis Thrombosis and stenosis of the vascular access are the most common complications. Grafts generally have a higher rate of stenosis, secondary to endothelial hyperplasia, than do fistulas. Stenosis or thrombosis presents with loss of bruit and thrill over the access. Stenosis and even thrombosis are not emergencies and can be treated within 24 h by either angiographic clot removal or angioplasty.

TABLE 89-2 Differential Diagnosis of Intradialysis Hypotension

Excessive ultrafiltration
Clearance simultaneous with ultrafiltration
Predialytic volume loss (GI losses, decreased oral intake)
Intradialytic volume loss (tube and hemodialyzer blood losses)
Postdialytic volume loss (vascular access blood loss)
Autonomic neuropathy
Medication effects (antihypertensives, narcotics)
Decreased vascular tone (sepsis, food, dialysate temperature >37°C or 98.6°F)
Cardiac dysfunction (LV hypertrophy, ischemia, hypoxia, arrhythmia)
Pericardial disease (effusion, tamponade)

Vascular Access Infection The vascular access provides the most common portal of entry for infection in dialysis patients. Vascular grafts have a higher incidence of infection than do AV fistulas. Patients with an infected access often present with only signs of systemic sepsis, such as fever, hypotension, or an elevated white blood cell count. Classic signs of pain, erythema, swelling, and discharge from an infected vascular access are often missing. The most common organism is *Staphylococcus aureus,* followed by gram-negative bacteria.[13] Patients with access infections usually require hospital admission. Vancomycin is the drug of choice (1 g intravenously) because of its effectiveness in methicillin-resistant organisms and long half-life (5 to 7 days) in dialysis patients. An aminoglycoside (gentamicin 100 mg intravenously initially and after each dialysis) is usually added empirically to cover gram-negative organisms.

Vascular Access Hemorrhage Hemorrhage from a vascular access can produce life-threatening blood loss. Hemorrhage can result from aneurysms, anastomosis rupture, or overanticoagulation. Bleeding that requires the patient to come to the emergency department should immediately be controlled with digital pressure at the puncture sites for 5 to 10 min, and the patient should be observed for 1 to 2 h afterward. Continued or life-threatening hemorrhage may require the placement of a tourniquet proximal to the access. A vascular surgeon should be consulted if bleeding cannot quickly be brought under control. If overanticoagulation is a concern, the effects of heparin can be reversed by protamine given at a dose of 0.01 mg/IU heparin dispensed during dialysis. If the dose of heparin is unknown, 10 to 20 mg protamine will be sufficient to reverse 1000 to 2000 IU heparin. If bleeding stops, the patient should be observed for 1 to 2 h for rebleeding or thrombosis. Occasionally a newly inserted vascular access will continue to ooze at the insertion despite pressure. DDAVP can be administered as an adjunct to direct pressure. If the emergency physician is unfamiliar with the use of DDAVP in this situation, the nephrologist should be consulted.

Vascular Access Aneurysm Vascular access aneurysms result from repeated puncturing, leading to bulging of the wall. True aneurysms are very rare, occurring in less than 4 percent of fistulas or grafts. Most aneurysms are asymptomatic, with patients occasionally complaining of pain or an associated peripheral impingement neuropathy. Aneurysms rarely rupture, causing hemorrhage.

Vascular Access Pseudoaneurysm Pseudoaneurysms result from subcutaneous extravasation of blood from puncture sites. Patients commonly present with bleeding and infections at access sites. Bleeding from the puncture site is usually controlled by digital pressure or a subcutaneous suture carefully placed at the puncture site. Vascular surgery may be required for continued bleeding or infection.

Vascular Insufficiency Vascular insufficiency of the extremity distal to the vascular access occurs in approximately 1 percent of all patients. The so-called steal syndrome is the result of preferential shunting of arterial blood away from nutrient arteries to the low-pressure venous side of the access. Patients present with exercise pain, nonhealing ulcers, and cool, pulseless digits. Steal syndrome is diagnosed by Doppler ultrasound or angiography and is repaired surgically.

High-Output Heart Failure High-output heart failure can occur when greater than 20 percent of the cardiac output is diverted through the access. Branham's sign, a drop in heart rate after temporary access occlusion, is useful for detecting this complication. Doppler ultrasound can accurately measure access flow rate and establish the diagnosis. Surgical banding of the access is the treatment of choice to decrease flow and treat heart failure.

COMPLICATIONS DURING HEMODIALYSIS TREATMENT **Intradialysis Hypotension** Hypotension is the most frequent complication of HD, occurring during 10 to 30 percent of treatments (Table 89-2). Excessive ultrafiltration from underestimation of the patient's ideal blood volume (dry weight) is the most common cause of intradialysis hypotension.[14] In fact, dry weight is often clinically defined when hypotension prevents further fluid removal. Dry weight is often underestimated because of changes in the ratio of muscle mass to blood volume over time.

Predialysis volume deficiency is an important contributing factor to intradialysis hypotension. Predialysis losses can be suspected when the patient is below dry weight and are usually due to GI bleeding, vomiting, diarrhea, or decreased intake of salt and water. Intradialysis volume loss can occur from blood tubing or hemodialyzer filter leaks.

Factors other than the patient's predialysis volume may cause intradialysis hypotension. Fluid removal during HD averages 1 to 2 L over a 4-h session but removal of up to 2 L/h hour is possible.

Maintenance of normal blood pressure during ultrafiltration is dependent on fluid movement from the interstitial space replenishing the intravascular volume. These fluid shifts are direct consequences of the decrease in intravascular hydrostatic pressure and the increase in serum osmolality caused by ultrafiltration. Blood pressure stability during ultrafiltration is also dependent on increased systemic vascular resistance, heart rate, and contractility caused by increased autonomic tone.

Defenses against intradialysis hypotension can be defeated by a large number of factors. Hypotension often occurs when ultrafiltration and clearance are carried out simultaneously. During clearance, serum osmolality decreases, limiting interstitial fluid refilling of the intravascular space. Autonomic dysfunction, especially common in diabetic patients, may result in failure to increase cardiac output and peripheral resistance during ultrafiltration. Decreased sympathetic tone also increases nitric oxide production, potentiating hypotension. Hypotension is also caused by increased nitric oxide generated in platelets and endothelial cells by an as yet unidentified uremic toxin. Antihypertensive medications and narcotics can both block sympathetic reflexes, resulting in hypotension. Decreases in vascular tone during hemodialysis occur in patients with sepsis, after eating, and when dialysate temperatures are greater than 37°C. Cardiac dysfunction during hemodialysis secondary to dysrhythmias, LV hypertrophy, hypoxia, and myocardial ischemia can prevent reflex increases in heart rate and contractility. Finally, pericardial effusion and tamponade decrease cardiac preload, thus potentiating intradialysis hypotension.

Often, the timing of hypotension is helpful in the differential diagnosis. Hypotension early in the dialysis session usually occurs with patients who are below dry weight from preexisting hypovolemia. Hypotension near the end of dialysis is usually the result of excessive ultrafiltration, but pericardial or cardiac disease is still a possibility.

Intradialysis hypotension produces nausea, vomiting, and anxiety. Orthostatic hypotension, tachycardia, dizziness, and even syncope may occur.

Treatment of intradialysis hypotension includes placing the patient in the Trendelenburg position and stopping HD. If hypotension persists, the patient is given salt by mouth (broth) or normal saline solution 100 to 200 mL intravenously. If these conservative measures fail, excessive ultrafiltration is very unlikely, and a more extensive evaluation is justified. These patients are commonly transferred to the emergency department for further evaluation.

The emergency physician should conduct a detailed investigation of volume status, cardiac function, pericardial disease, infection, and GI bleeding that may be producing or contributing to hypotension. Remember that estimation of this patient's blood volume by clinical criteria has already failed in the dialysis unit. The decision to undertake further volume expansion or administer vasopressors to support blood pressure may require invasive hemodynamic monitoring in an intensive care setting.

Dialysis Disequilibrium Dialysis disequilibrium is a clinical syndrome occurring at the end of dialysis characterized by nausea, vomiting, and hypertension, which can progress to seizure, coma, and death. This syndrome should be distinguished from other neurologic disorders, such as subdural hematoma, stroke, hypertensive crisis, hypoxia, and seizures. Dialysis disequilibrium is produced when large solute clearances occur during HD, as during the patient's first dialysis session or in hypercatabolic patients. The cause of dialysis disequilibrium is believed to be cerebral edema from an osmolar imbalance between the brain and the blood. During high solute removal, the blood has a transiently lower osmolality than the brain, favoring water movement into the brain and causing cerebral edema. This condition can be prevented by limiting solute clearance when initiating HD. Treatment consists of stopping dialysis and administering mannitol intravenously to increase serum osmolality.

Air Embolism Air embolism is always a risk when blood is pumped through an extracorporeal circuit. The clinical presentation depends on the patient's body habitus at the time of the air embolism. If the patient was sitting, air will pass retrograde through the internal jugular vein to the cerebral circulation, causing symptoms of increased intracranial pressure. In a recumbent position, air will go into the right ventricle and pulmonary circulation, causing pulmonary hypertension and systemic hypotension. The passage of air through a right-to-left (e.g., patent foramen ovale) creates an arterial air embolism, which can lodge in the coronary or cerebral circulation, causing myocardial infarction or stoke.

Patients with an air embolism typically present with symptoms of acute dyspnea, chest tightness, and unconsciousness, sometimes progressing to full cardiac arrest. Physical examination may show cyanosis and a churning sound in the heart from air bubbles in the blood.

Treatment consists of clamping the venous bloodline and placing the patient supine. Traditional recommendations have often included the Trendelenburg position with the left side down, presumably to favor air trapping in the right ventricle. However, experimental and anecdotal clinical evidence does not indicate any special benefit of this position. Other suggested therapies for vascular air embolism include percutaneous aspiration of air from the right ventricle, intravenous steroids, full heparinization, and a hyperbaric chamber to reduce bubble size and promote resorption.

Hemolysis and Electrolyte Shifts In the United States, dialysate is prepared by proportionally mixing a dialysate concentrate with water. Errors in proportional mixing can produce severe electrolyte abnormalities, resulting in rapid osmolar shifts and hemolysis.

Hypercalcemia and Hypermagnesemia In some communities, water contains high concentrations of calcium and magnesium and produces a final dialysate high in these minerals. This dialysate can result in the ''hard water syndrome,'' characterized by clinically significant hypercalcemia and hypermagnesemia in HD patients. These patients present with nausea, vomiting, headaches, burning skin, muscle weakness, lethargy, and hypertension. Treatment consists of properly filtering the dialysis water to lower calcium and magnesium concentrations.

EVALUATION OF HEMODIALYSIS PATIENTS Patients on HD may present to the emergency department for complications related to their ESRD or HD, or these conditions may be incidental to the reason for the visit. The past medical history is very important in HD patients, since many of the same diseases that caused ESRD (e.g., hypertension, diabetes, etc.) persist after the patient's kidneys have failed. Questions should be asked about the patient's ESRD and HD (Table 89-3). Repeated episodes of intradialysis hypotension may provide important early clues to pericardial tamponade or myocardial ischemia. Repeated access infections may represent a worsening immunologic status.

Patients should be asked about their HD schedule. The majority of HD patients in the United States are on an every-other-day schedule (Monday, Wednesday, and Friday or Tuesday, Thursday, and Saturday), each session lasting approximately 4 h. Certain centers have begun using high-flux HD machines with higher blood flows, allowing shorter HD sessions. The physician should document all recent missed sessions and the patient's explanations for missing them. Such history taking may provide important clues concerning worsening medical or social issues that need to be addressed outside of the patient's chief complaint.

Dialysis patients are often quite knowledgeable concerning their dry weights and baseline laboratory test results. If the patient is not forthcoming with this data, the emergency physician can contact the HD center and ask about the dry weight, average interdialysis weight gains, and any recent HD complications. In addition, the dialysis nurses and technicians are very devoted to their patients can provide a great

TABLE 89-3 Key Historical Elements for Hemodialysis Patients

Etiology of ESRD
Recent complications of HD
Dialysis schedule
Any missed dialysis sessions
Dry weight, baseline laboratory values and vital signs
Average interdialysis weight gain
Does patient usually make dry weight by end of HD?
Does patient experience intradialysis hypotension? (Timing of hypotension?)
Which vascular access is currently functioning?
Symptoms of uremia
Retention of native kidneys?

deal of ''soft data'' concerning the patient. Query the patient in detail concerning uremic symptoms as markers of inadequate HD. Finally, ask patients whether they retain their native kidneys, which can be continued sources of hypertension, infection, and nephrolithiasis.

The physical examination of HD patients should always include a careful examination of the vascular access (Table 89-4). Remember, the vascular access is both the patient's lifeline and the Achilles' heel, complications of which are responsible for the majority of ESRD inpatient days. Flow through the access can be established by the presence of a bruit and thrill over the access site. The classic signs of infection—erythema, swelling, tenderness, and purulent discharge—are commonly limited until the infection is far advanced. The bedside Branham's sign may detect patients with CHF due to high-output fistula-related heart failure. The cardiac examination of HD patients deserves some special attention. Signs of CHF, such as peripheral edema, HJR, and JVD, may misleadingly suggest the diagnosis of fluid overload when pericardial tamponade is present. A loud cardiac murmur in HD patients may just represent increased flow secondary to anemia or the AV access. Neurologic dysfunction in HD patients is generally diffuse and nonfocal. Any findings suggestive of a focal neurologic deficit should be investigated for structural, vascular, and infectious causes. Rectal examination to detect GI bleeding is always needed.

TABLE 89-4 Key Elements of Physical Examination of Hemodialysis Patients

Vital signs
Vascular access Bruit Thrill Erythema Increased temperature Swelling Tenderness Discharge Bleeding Branham's sign
Cardiac Signs of heart failure Murmurs Muffled (distant) heart sounds Beck's triad
Neurologic Peripheral neuropathy Asterixis

Peritoneal Dialysis

Ganter accomplished the first PD in 1923. Practical long-term RRT with PD did not become available until 1976, when Popovich and Moncrief worked out the basic concepts of continuous ambulatory peritoneal dialysis (CAPD). Their work was significantly aided by the development of a practical silicon rubber catheter by Tenckhoff in 1968, which is still in use today. Because of its simplicity, PD is the most common form of RRT used outside the United States and Canada.

TECHNICAL ASPECTS PD can be accomplished in either an acute setting or chronically via exchanges of solution throughout the day (CAPD) or through multiple exchanges at night while the patient sleeps [continuous cyclic peritoneal dialysis (CCPD)].[11,15]

Similarly to HD, PD relies on the separate processes of clearance (solute removal) and ultrafiltration (fluid removal) to replace the functions of the nephron. In PD, the peritoneal membrane serves as the blood-dialysate interface. Most solute removal occurs via diffusion down chemical gradients established by altering dialysate electrolyte concentrations. The amount of ultrafiltration is determined by osmotic pressure differences between the blood and dialysate, which are manipulated by varying the dialysate glucose concentration. Dialysate is supplied in either a 1.5 or 4.25% glucose formulation, which can be alternated to increase or decrease ultrafiltration.

Typical CAPD regimens utilize four exchanges daily, with 2 L of dialysate infused and left in place for several hours before draining. During the day, approximately 8 L is infused and about 10 L is drained, for a removal of approximately 2 L/day of fluid. Recent concerns that this type of regimen may be inadequate for patients weighing more than 60 kg has prompted the use of automated PD exchanges during the night in addition to one or two daytime exchanges.

COMPLICATIONS **Peritonitis** Peritonitis is the most common complication of PD. The incidence of peritonitis is about one episode every 15 patient-months.[16] Mortality rates with peritonitis have been reported between 2.5 and 12.5 percent, depending on the center studied. Symptoms and signs of peritonitis in PD patients are no different than those for other patients with peritonitis: fever, abdominal pain, and rebound tenderness. Abdominal tenderness and cloudy effluent suggest the diagnosis of peritonitis. Patients will often bring in a sample of the cloudy dialysate fluid, which should be sent for cell count, Gram stain, and culture. The cell count in PD-related peritonitis is usually more than 100 leukocytes, with more than 50 percent neutrophils. Results of the Gram stain are positive in only 10 to 40 percent of cases of culture-proven PD-related peritonitis. Organisms isolated in PD-related peritonitis are *Staphylococcus epidermidis* (about 40 percent), *S. aureus* (10 percent), *Streptococcus* species (15 to 20 percent), gram-negative bacteria (15 to 20 percent), anaerobic bacteria (5 percent), and fungi (5 percent).

Empiric therapy should begin with a few rapid exchanges of fluid lavaged quickly in and out to decrease the number of inflammatory cells in the peritoneum. The addition of heparin (500 to 1000 IU/L dialysate) will decrease fibrin clot formation. Empiric antibiotics are selected to treat the expected gram-positive and gram-negative organisms. PD-related peritonitis can be treated with antibiotics added to the dialysate; parenteral administration is not required. A first-generation cephalosporin (e.g., cephalothin) can be mixed with the dialysate, 500 mg/L with the first exchange and 200 mg/L with subsequent exchanges. In penicillin-allergic patients, vancomycin can be substituted, with an initial dose of 500 mg/L and maintenance doses of 50 mg/

TABLE 89-5 Key Historical Elements for Peritoneal Dialysis Patients

Etiology of ESRD
Type of peritoneal dialysis (CAPD vs CCPD)
Recent complications of PD
Baseline weight, laboratory values, and vital signs
Symptoms of uremia
Retention of native kidneys?

L per exchange. Gentamicin can be added with a loading dose of 100 mg/L and maintenance doses of 4 to 8 mg/L per exchange. Most protocols recommend treating for 7 days after the first negative culture results, usually for a total of 10 days. The decision to admit these patients or treat them as outpatients is a clinical decision based on how ill the patient appears.

Catheter Infections (Exit Site and Tunnel Infections) Infections around a PD catheter are much less well defined than peritonitis. Patients present with pain, erythema, swelling, and discharge around the catheter exit site. The most common bacteria are *S. aureus* and *Pseudomonas aeruginosa*. Empiric therapy consists of a first-generation cephalosporin or ciprofloxacillin, for outpatient therapy.[17] Patients should be referred back to their CAPD centers for follow-up the next day.

Hernias The prevalence of abdominal-wall hernias in PD patients has been estimated to be between 10 and 15 percent. The literature recommends immediate surgical repair of pericatheter hernias, which have the highest risk of developing an incarceration.

EVALUATION OF PERITONEAL DIALYSIS PATIENTS When a PD patient arrives in the emergency department, certain historical elements are important (Table 89-5). As with HD patients, the disease that caused the renal failure frequently persists. The type of PD and the person who performs the daily care may provide information about the risks of infection. Try to obtain the date of the patient's last episode of peritonitis; frequent relapses may signify a fungal etiology or tunnel infection. Ask the patient about baseline weight and laboratory values; PD patients are selected for their knowledge about their condition and their ability to perform the procedure and monitor their care away from professional supervision. Weight gain may signal heart failure from ischemia or pericardial effusion. Weight gain may also be from ultrafiltration failure, a late sign of peritonitis.

The physical examination of PD patients should focus on the abdomen. The physician looks for infections of the peritoneum, tunnel, and exit site (Table 89-6).

TABLE 89-6 Key Elements of Physical Examination of Peritoneal Dialysis Patients

Abdominal examination
  Inspection for hernia
  Auscultation of bowel sounds
  Test for rebound tenderness

Peritoneal catheter
  Examination of surrounding skin
  Palpation of tunnel

REFERENCES

1. United States Renal Data System: Chapter II: Incidence and prevalence of ESRD. *Am J Kidney Dis* 32(suppl 1):S38, 1998.
2. United States Renal Data System: Chapter III: Treatment modalities for ESRD patients. *Am J Kidney Dis* 32(suppl 1):S50, 1998.
3. United States Renal Data System: Chapter V: Patient mortality and survival. *Am J Kidney Dis* 32(suppl 1):S69, 1998.
4. United States Renal Data System: Chapter VI: Causes of death. *Am J Kidney Dis* 32(suppl 1):S81, 1998.
5. Hakim RM, Lazarus JM: Initiation of dialysis. *J Am Soc Nephol* 6:1319, 1995.
6. Parfrey PS, Foley RN, Harnett JD, et al: Outcome and risk factors for left ventricular disorders in chronic uraemia. *Nephrol Dial Transplant* 11:1277, 1996.
7. Russo DB, Memoli B, Andreucci VE: The place of loop diuretics in the treatment of acute and chronic renal failure. *Clin Nephrol* 38(suppl 1):S69, 1992.
8. Eiser AR, Lieber JJ, Neff MS: Phlebotomy for pulmonary edema in dialysis patients. *Clin Nephrol* 47:47, 1997.
9. Gralnick HR, McKeown LP, Williams SB, et al: Plasma and platelet von Willebrand factor defects in uremia [comments]. *Am J Med* 85:806, 1988.
10. Block GA, Hulbert-Shearon TE, Levin NW, et al: Association of serum phosphorus and calcium × phosphate product with mortality risk in chronic hemodialysis patients: A national study. *Am J Kidney Dis* 31:607, 1998.
11. Pastan S, Bailey J: Dialysis therapy. *N Engl J Med* 338:1428, 1998.
12. Ifudu O: Care of patients undergoing hemodialysis. *N Engl J Med* 339:1054, 1998.
13. Goldman M, Vanherweghem JL: Bacterial infections in chronic hemodialysis patients: Epidemiologic and pathophysiologic aspects. *Adv Nephrol Necker Hosp* 19:315, 1990.
14. de Vries JP, Kouw PM, van der Meer, NJ, et al: Non-invasive monitoring of blood volume during hemodialysis: Its relation with post-dialytic dry weight. *Kidney Int* 44:851, 1993.
15. Viglino G, Cancarini G, Catizone L, et al: Ten years of continuous ambulatory peritoneal dialysis: Analysis of patient and technique survival. *Perit Dial Int* 13(suppl 2):S175, 1993.
16. Bailie GR, Rasmussen R, Hollister A, Eisele G: Incidence of CAPD peritonitis in patients using UVXD or O-set systems. *Clin Nephrol* 33:252, 1990.
17. Twardowski ZJ, Prowant BF: Current approach to exit-site infections in patients on peritoneal dialysis. *Nephrol Dial Transplant* 12:1284, 1997.

URINARY TRACT INFECTIONS

David S. Howes
William F. Young

Urinary tract infection (UTI) is defined as significant bacteriuria in the presence of symptoms. It affects an estimated 20 percent of women at some point in their lifetime, and accounts for a significant number of emergency department visits. In the elderly, UTI is a major cause of nosocomial gram-negative sepsis with a significant mortality.

EPIDEMIOLOGY

The epidemiology of UTI varies with age and sex. There are four groups at risk for infection: neonates, girls, young women, and older men (Fig. 90-1). In neonates, a UTI occurs more often in males (1.5:1 M:F ratio) and is often part of the syndrome of gram-negative sepsis. The incidence of UTI in preschool children is approximately 2 percent, with the incidence in girls at least 10 times greater than the incidence in boys. In schoolage children, the incidence rises to 5 percent, almost exclusively girls.

Bacteriuria is rare in males under the age of 50 and symptoms of dysuria or urinary frequency are usually due to a sexually transmitted disease-related infection of the urethra or prostate. However, in men older than 50 years, the incidence of UTI rises dramatically because of prostatic obstruction or subsequent instrumentation.

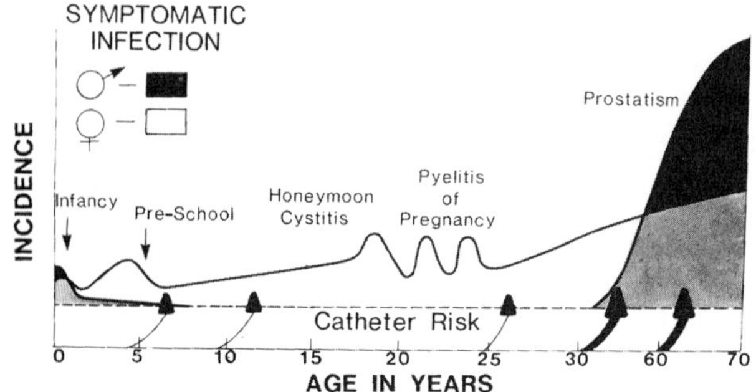

FIG. 90-1. Natural history of urinary tract infections.

Dysuria in females is a common symptom usually due to infection. UTIs are common in otherwise healthy young women, often due to sexual contact. The incidence of infection in postmenopausal women increases with age; the prevalence of bacteriuria among elderly women in nursing homes exceeds 40 percent.

The infecting organisms are generally those found colonizing the perineum, and in women with a traditional "positive" culture of 10^5 colony-forming units (CFU) per mL of urine, *Escherichia coli* is responsible for approximately 80 to 90 percent of infections. However, up to one-half of cases of dysuria in young women are characterized by low bacterial colony count culture results (10^2 to 10^4/mL), which was termed the "acute urethral syndrome." It is now believed that these patients have low-grade or early urinary tract infection due to *E. coli, Staphylococcus saprophyticus,* or *Chlamydia trachomatis.* The definition of UTI based on early studies that reported only upper tract disease established that a colony count of at least 10^5/mL was necessary to indicate the presence of "significant bacteriuria." Recent research suggests that with regard to lower UTI in the presence of symptoms, a colony count of 100/mL or greater may represent significant bacteriuria and merit treatment.[1]

Asymptomatic bacteriuria (ABU) is defined by the presence of more than 10^5/mL of a single bacterial species on two sucessive urine cultures in a patient without symptoms. The requirement for two positive cultures is to eliminate those individuals with transient colonization of the urinary tract. ABU occurs in up to 30 percent of pregnant women and in up to 40 percent of female nursing-home residents. ABU is also common in patients with indwelling urinary catheters and disorders that prevent complete emptying of the bladder.

UTIs in women recur either because of relapse or reinfection. Relapse is caused by the same organism, and symptoms recurring in less than one month represents treatment failure. When symptoms recur in one to six months, it is generally due to reinfection. Reinfection is usually from a different enteric organism or a different serotype of the same organism, and may represent a defect in the defense mechanisms of the host. If a patient has a cluster of infections with more than three recurrences in one year, a more complete workup may be warranted to look for the presence of structural abnormalities, tumor, renal calculi, or associated systemic illness such as diabetes mellitus.

A UTI during pregnancy poses special problems. If untreated, ABU may progress to symptomatic UTI or pyelonephritis, especially in the third trimester, and may lead to preeclampsia, sepsis, or miscarriage. This is the single setting in which treatment of ABU is definitely indicated.

PATHOPHYSIOLOGY

UTI should be thought of as either complicated, that is, occurring in patients with underlying renal or neurologic disease; or uncomplicated, occurring in patients in which no defect can be demonstrated.[2–4] The most common urinary pathogen is *E. coli,* which causes greater than 80 percent of uncomplicated UTIs (Table 90-1). Uropathogenic organisms often have adhesins, fibriae, or pili that allow for bacterial adherence to the uroepithelium. Anaerobic organisms do not grow well in urine and are rarely pathogenic. While complicated UTIs can be caused by *E. coli,* they are more likely to be caused by unusual pathogens, such as *Pseudomonas spp* or enterococcus.

Depending on its pH and chemical constituents, urine is generally a good culture medium. Factors unfavorable to bacterial growth are a low pH (5.5 or less); a high concentration of urea; and the presence of organic acids derived from a diet including fruit juice and methionine, a breakdown product of ingested protein that enhances acidification of the urine. A thin film of urine remains in the bladder after voiding. An intact bladder mucosa removes organisms from the film, probably by the production of organic acids by the mucosal cells and not by antibody formation or phagocytosis. Incomplete bladder emptying renders this mechanism ineffective and is responsible for the increased frequency of infection in patients with a neurogenic bladder, and in postmenopausal women with bladder or uterine prolapse. The latter group also has marked changes in vaginal microflora due to lack of estrogen, with loss of lactobacilli and increased colonization by *E. coli.*

Frequent and complete voiding has been associated with the reduction in recurrence of UTI.[5] Studies have found that the concentration of bacteria in the bladder may increase tenfold after sexual intercourse due to a "milking action" of the female urethra during intercourse. The use of a diaphragm and spermicide is also associated with recurrence in some patients, probably because the spermicide enhances vaginal colonization with *E. coli.*[6] It is recommended, although unproven, that prompt voiding after intercourse may lessen the frequency of UTI. An increased urinary flow also dilutes the bacterial inoculum that occasionally occurs from sexual intercourse.[5,6]

Susceptibility to UTIs may have a genetic basis, that is, women who do not secrete blood group antigens (nonsecretors) have a high incidence of recurrent infection. This appears to be due to the presence of specific uroepithelial cell *E. coli*-binding glycolipids that promote fecal coliform colonization of the vagina.

The majority of uncomplicated UTIs remain in the bladder; the ureteral valves prevent ascent of the bacteria into the kidneys. If these mechanisms fail and ascending infection of the urinary tract occurs, renal defense mechanisms are called into play. Local antibodies are produced in the kidney and kill bacteria in the presence of complement. Local leukocytosis and phagocytosis also help eradicate bacteria.

Urinary infections are categorized into three clinical syndromes. The simplest and most common UTI is acute cystitis, where infection is isolated to the bladder. Subclinical pyelonephritis is characterized by bacterial infection in the upper urinary tract and detected by bladder washout techniques, selective ureteral catheterization, or the presence of antibody-coated bacteria in the urine. However, subclinical pyelone-

TABLE 90-1 Etiologic Agents in Uncomplicated Urinary Tract Infection

Organism	Incidence
Escherichia coli	>80%
Klebsiella sp *Proteus* sp *Enterobacter* sp *Pseudomonas* sp	5–20%
Group D streptococci *Chlamydia trachomatis** *Staphylococcus saprophyticus**	<5%

*Much more common in the "dysuria-pyuria" syndrome where sterile or low colony count culture results are obtained.

phritis is clinically indistinguishable from acute cystitis and it has been estimated about 25 to 30 percent of patients with the acute cystitis syndrome have subclinical pyelonephritis. Several epidemiologic factors correlate with increased risk for subclinical pyelonephritis: lower socioeconomic status; pregnancy; structural urinary tract abnormality; urinary stone; history of relapse after treatment for a UTI; prior history of acute pyelonephritis; frequent UTIs; symptoms for more than seven days; or diabetes or other immunosuppressing conditions.[2] Acute pyelonephritis is characterized by the presence of bacteria in the kidney with localized pain and tenderness and systemic symptoms of infection (fever, chills, nausea, vomiting, and prostration).

The infective process of acute pyelonephritis can progress into three patterns of renal infection not commonly considered part of the UTI spectrum: acute bacterial nephritis, renal abscess, and emphysematous pyelonephritis.[7,8] These tend to be diagnoses made on imaging studies performed on patients who have an inadequate or atypical response to treatment for presumed acute pyelonephritis. On ultrasound or CT imaging studies, acute pyelonephritis is seen as a diffusely enlarged kidney without focal abnormalities. Acute bacterial nephritis produces ill-defined focal areas, sometimes striated or wedge-shaped, of decreased density.[7] Renal abscesses appear as well-defined areas of decreased density.[7] Emphysematous pyelonephritis is a rare gas-forming infection within the kidney, nearly always in diabetics (70 to 90 percent of the time). These patients usually have symptoms and signs of a severe infection, often with dehydration and pyelonephritis.[8]

CLINICAL FEATURES

The clinical symptoms of UTI in an adult are dysuria, frequency, and lower abdominal pain. However, the correlation between symptoms and the presence of infection is inexact as only 50 to 60 percent of women with dysuria have significant bacteriuria.[2,4] Internal dysuria, a burning suprapubic pain during urination associated with bladder tenderness, is more associated with UTIs as compared to external dysuria, the burning sensation as urine passes over inflamed perineal tissue. In females, external dysuria or a history of vaginal discharge is more associated with vaginitis, cervicitis, or pelvic inflammatory disease than with a UTI.

Flank pain, costovertebral angle tenderness, or specific renal tenderness to deep palpation can be associated with cystitis because of referred pain. However, when these are found in association with fever, chills, nausea, vomiting, and prostration, the clinical diagnosis is acute pyelonephritis.

In the male, dysuria with a urethral discharge indicates urethritis.[3] A Gram's stain of the discharge may reveal gram-negative intracellular diplococci, which is virtually diagnostic of gonococcal urethritis. If the Gram's stain is inconclusive, the diagnosis is most likely nonspecific urethritis (NSU), which is mainly chlamydial or another sexually transmitted infection. In either case, laboratory tests for gonorrhea and chlamydia should be obtained, and possibly a serologic test for syphilis. It should be emphasized to the emergency department triage personnel that UTI in young adult males is extremely rare; therefore, a urine specimen should not be obtained until after examination by a physician. Witholding urination may enhance the likelihood of a positive urethral swab in the male patient with minimal discharge. On the other hand, several authors have demonstrated that the presence of urinary leukocytes was more sensitive than urethral Gram's stain in detecting patients who were later found to have chlamydial infection as confirmed by culture. Finally, if bacteriuria is present and is not clinically associated with urethritis or prostatitis, then treatment, followed by urologic referral, is indicated.

DIAGNOSIS

Factors that are independent predictors of a UTI in a patient with dysuria are advanced age, history of a UTI, back pain, pyuria, hematuria, and bacteriuria.[2–4] Among sexually active women, the incidence of symptomatic UTIs is high, and the risk is independently associated with recent sexual intercourse, recent use of a diaphragm with spermicide, and history of a UTI.[5,6]

If UTI is suspected, the first step in establishing the diagnosis is the careful collection of urine for a urinalysis and potentially for culture. The midstream voiding specimen is as accurate as urine obtained by catheterization if the patient is given and follows careful instructions. Instruct the woman to remove her underwear, sit facing the back of the toilet, spread the labia with one hand, cleanse from front to back with povidone-iodine swabs or liquid soap, pass a small amount of urine into the toilet, and then urinate into a sterile cup. Instruct the man to carefully cleanse the urethral meatus, retracting the foreskin if uncircumcised, and obtain a midsteam specimen as described above.

If the sample is properly collected, it should contain no or few epithelial cells. The many sources of contamination include material in the collection bottle, menses, vaginal discharge, urethral or periurethral tissue, and organisms multiplying in the urine after collection. Bacteria in urine double each hour at room temperature; therefore urine should be refrigerated if not sent directly to the laboratory. In addition to special care in cleansing, the use of a tampon also helps women to obtain a clean-catch specimen if menstruation or profuse discharge is present.

Catheterization is indicated if the patient cannot void spontaneously, is too ill or immobilized, or is extremely obese. It may also be performed as part of a urologic evaluation and to relieve obstruction. Many authors promote the ease and accuracy of ''minicath''-obtained urine in women, especially with a vaginal discharge or bleeding. However, unnecessary catheterization should be avoided because 1 to 2 percent of patients develop UTI after a single catheter insertion. This seems to be a problem especially if the catheter insertion is done just prior to delivery.

Although blood or bile may be detected by gross examination of the urine, visual inspection or the smell of the urine is generally not helpful in determining infection. Cloudiness is usually not due to white blood cells (WBC) or bacteria, but to large amounts of protein or amorphous phosphate crystals. Malodorous urine may be caused by diet or medications and is not a reliable sign of infection.

Current emphasis is on the detection of pyuria and bacteriuria in the initial examination of the urine to confirm the diagnosis of a UTI. However, the assessment of pyuria is imperfect. Variables include the specific gravity of the urine, method of centrifuging the specimen, the amount of supernatant in which the sediment is resuspended, and the final volume of urine under the coverslip that is examined. Laboratories that use a WBC counting chamber diminish some of this variability and increase accuracy in assessing both centrifuged and uncentrifuged urine. Using a WBC counting chamber, abnormal pyuria can be defined as the presence of 8 leukocytes or more per mL of uncentrifuged urine. This figure roughly corresponds to 2 to 5 leukocytes per high-power field (hpf or 400×) from a centrifuged specimen.

While some authors feel that low-level pyuria (<10 WBC/hpf) is clinically important, others have suggested that pyuria in women is significant only if there are more than 10 WBC/hpf, and only if bacteria is also present on the microscopic examination. Though the combination of pyuria and bacteruria is likely to be true with typical coliform infection, lower degrees of pyuria with or without bacteriuria may be significant, especially with regard to infection with *Chlamydia*.

As knowledge of UTI in adult women evolves, it is clear that women with symptoms and low-level pyuria (<10 WBC/hpf) do have significant infection that will symptomatically and bacteriologically respond to antimicrobial therapy. In the past, these women were not treated initially and their cultures often did not contain more than 10^5 CFU/mL. Sensitivity to causes of lower UTI other than typical coliforms has brought the designation of the dysuria-pyuria syndrome (also referred to as the acute urethral syndrome), which almost always benefits from treatment.[1] It is in this subgroup of women that the urinalysis may well be more useful than the urine culture. In addition, a positive urinalysis would dictate more immediate management interventions than would awaiting a urine culture.

In men, more than 1 to 2 WBC/hpf can be significant in the presence of bacteria.[3] Again, it must be remembered that urethritis and prostatitis are far more likely causes of pyuria in young males who are sexually active and complain of dysuria, whether or not a urethral discharge is present.

Bacteriuria is also felt to be a sensitive tool for detection of UTI in the symptomatic patient. The presence of any bacteria on a Gram stain of uncentrifuged urine (>1 bacteria per oil-power field or $1000\times$) is significant and highly correlates with culture results of $>10^5$/mL. For Gram-stained centrifuged specimens, more than 15 bacteria per oil-powered field ($1000\times$) is significant. Both of these methods fail to detect low colony count UTI or infection caused by *Chlamydia*. False-positives can occur when vaginal or fecal contamination is present.

Several studies have evaluated urinary dipstick nitrite and leukocyte esterase tests in the diagnosis of UTIs, correlating the results with urinalysis.[9] The urine nitrite reaction has a very high specificity (>90 percent) and a positive result is very useful in confirming the diagnosis of a UTI. However, the urine nitrite sensitivity is low (about 50 percent), rendering it much less useful as a screening examination and a negative result does not exclude the diagnosis of a UTI. The urine leukocyte esterase has been evaluated as an indicator of the presence of pyuria, one marker of UTI. As noted above, there is an inexact correlation between clinical symptoms, results of urine culture, and pyuria as detected by microscopic examination. Initial reports of high sensitivity (near 88 percent) supported use of leukocyte esterase as a screening tool for pyuria. However, these studies were done on symptomatic women with high levels of pyuria. Studies from the emergency department have found a low sensitivity (48 percent) for leukocyte esterase with more common levels of pyuria (6 to 20 WBC/hpf).[9] When the clinical presentation suggests UTI, a positive leukocyte esterase test supports the diagnosis, and treatment should be initiated without the need for microscopic examination. If the leukocyte esterase test is negative, a microscopic examination should be performed to detect lower levels of clinically significant pyuria.

Unfortunately, the clinician is sometimes faced with women who complain of dysuria, have no pyuria or demonstrable pathogen on culture, and who do not respond to antimicrobial treatment. The absence of pyuria in these patients is useful because it indicates that antimicrobial treatment is probably unnecessary. Presuming that vulvovaginitis or cervicitis (gonorrhea, chlamydia, and herpes) has been excluded, causes of dysuria may include inflammation of the urethra from physical trauma or due to the use of chemical agents, such as spermicides, cleansing douches, or other feminine hygiene products.

In a symptomatic patient who has fewer than 2 to 5 WBC/hpf, other causes of false-negative pyuria should be considered. These include ingestion of large amounts of fluids, which wash out the bladder and produce a dilute urine, and, more likely, old or leftover medication, or a drug belonging to another person, being taken by the patient on a self-directed basis, or systemic leukopenia. It should be remembered that, in the case of an infected and obstructed kidney, pyuria may be intermittent or absent.

For the patient with typical symptoms of an uncomplicated UTI and a "positive" urinalysis (pyuria on microscopic examination, positive leukocyte esterase test, bacteriuria on Gram's stain, and/or positive urine nitrite test), urine culture is not required. The vast majority of these patients respond to empiric therapy. Most authors agree that a urine culture should be obtained in these settings: acute pyelonephritis; patients with epidemiologic risk factors for subclinical pyelonephritis; any patient who needs to be hospitalized; those patients who have a chronic indwelling catheter; and all pregnant women, children, and adult males.[2–4] If the patient is symptomatic, a single positive culture is significant. For ABU, two or three positive cultures are necessary before treatment is undertaken, with the exception that treatment for ABU is always indicated in pregnancy.

It is commonly recommended to obtain blood cultures in cases of acute pyelopnephritis, and while they are positive in about 30 percent of patients, the results rarely change management.[10,11] Renal imaging studies are not indicated in otherwise healthy patients with acute pyelonephritis that can be managed as an outpatient. Elderly, diabetic, or severely ill patients with acute pyelonephritis should be considered for imaging, particularly if there is a poor initial response to antibiotic therapy. The kidneys can be imaged with portable ultrasound at the bedside, evaluating for obstruction and focal parenchymal abnormalities.[7] Plain film radiology and ultrasound have poor sensitivity for detection of intrarenal gas formation in emphysematous pyelonephritis; CT is the best imaging modality.[8]

TREATMENT

Acute Cystitis

The selection of antibiotics depends on the suspected bacteriology of the infection, the patient's compliance, potential drug toxicity, and cost.[12] In uncomplicated UTIs, *E. coli* is the offending microorganism in the vast majority of cases, and this and other typical coliform pathogens remain susceptible to a variety of agents: trimethoprim, co-trimoxazole, nitrofurantoin macrocrystals, and the fluoroquinolones (Table 90-2).

Trimethoprim alone or in combination with sulfamethoxazole (co-trimoxazole or TMP/SMX) is generally recommended because these are cheap and effective (Table 90-3). Nitrofurantoin is also effective though compliance with frequent dosing is a problem and nitrofurantoin is not effective against *S. saprophyticus*. Because of increased bacterial resistance, extended-spectrum penicillins (e.g., amoxicillin) and cephalosporins have become less-acceptable alternatives. In cases of treatment failure, or in the host with a structural or immunologic defect, use of amoxicillin with clavulanic acid or one of the fluoroquinolones may be considered. Concern about the emergence of resistant organisms and expense preclude indiscriminate use of the latter agents. In uncomplicated UTIs, the urine should be bacteria-free in 24 to 48 h with substantial relief of symptoms within the same time period. The offer of one to two days of an oral bladder analgesic, such as phenazopyridine, is considerate when urination is painful for the patient.

Until the last decade, the duration of antibiotic treatment for a UTI was 7 to 10 days. Multiple studies of shorter treatment regimens for uncomplicated infections in nonpregnant adult women have been published and three days has become the recommended standard.[2–4,13] Short-course treatment appears to offer a number of advantages: cost and side effects are substantially reduced, compliance improves, and the development of resistant strains of bacteria is less likely. However, 20 to 30 percent of patients given short-course therapy fail treatment and/or quickly relapse. In addition, three-day regimens are not adequate for all patients and a seven-day course is recommended for pregnant women, those with symptoms over a week, patients with diabetes, individuals who had a previous recent UTI, those who are older than 65 years, and women who use a diaphragm.[4]

These recommendations for 3-day treatment courses has also generated concern regarding the entity of subclinical pyelonephritis, which has become increasingly apparent during studies of what was felt to be uncomplicated lower UTI.[2,4] Detection of this entity requires sophisticated differentiation based on analysis of immunofluorescent antibody results or analysis for β-glucuronidase and lactate dehydrogenase isoenzymes, principally research tools not available for routine clinical use. In several series, a number of patients with apparent simple cystitis exhibited tissue invasion as demonstrated by the presence of

TABLE 90-2 Guidelines to Outpatient Management of Uncomplicated UTI

Type of Patient	Presumed Type of Infection	Clinical Characteristics	Antimicrobial Regimens	Comments
Adult female	Lower	Few prior episodes with brief duration of symptoms and no risk factors for subclinical pyelonephritis	1. Co-trimoxazole, 1 double-strength tablet bid × 3 days 2. Nitrofurantoin macrocrystals 100 mg qid × 3 days 3. Amoxicilin/clavulanate 875/125 mg bid × 3 days 4. Trimethoprim 200 mg bid × 3 days 5. Ciprofloxacin 250 mg bid × 3 days 6. Ofloxacin 200 mg bid × 3 days 7. Norfloxacin 400 mg bid × 3 days	Brief-duration regimen Good follow-up available No culture needed
Adult female	Lower/upper	Risk of subclinical pyelonephritis: prolonged symptoms, relapse or recurrent UTI, diabetes mellitus, urinary tract abnormalities, recent pyelonephritis, indigent patients	1. Co-trimoxazole, 1 double-strength tablet bid 2. Amoxicilin/clavulanate 875/125 mg bid 3. Cefpodoxime proxetil 100 mg bid 4. Ciprofloxacin 500 mg bid 5. Ofloxacin 400 mg bid 6. Norfloxacin 400 mg bid	10-day course advised Consider culture Coliforms typical
Adult male	Lower/upper	Suspect underlying anatomic abnormality; R/O urethritis, prostatitis	Same as above	Same as above
Adult female	Lower	Stuttering symptoms, new sexual partner or partner with urethritis, signs and symptoms of cervicitis, pyuria without bacteriuria	1. Doxycycline, 100 mg bid 2. Co-trimoxazole, 1 double-strength tablet bid 3. Sulfamethoxazole, 1 g bid 4. Erythromycin, 500 mg qid (in pregnancy-related cases and will only eradicate *Chlamydia*)	10-day course Culture for gonococcus advisable

antibody-coated bacteria (ACB), that is, unsuspected or subclinical pyelonephritis. This group had a poor response to short-term therapy when compared to patients with ACB who received 10- to 14-day treatment.[4]

On the other hand, it has been suggested that short-course treatment may reliably identify patients with subclinical pyelonephritis as available diagnostic tests. This is because a short-course of antibiotics is less likely to eradicate bacteriuria in the patient with tissue invasion. In practice, women with the diagnosis of uncomplicated acute cystitis would be given a three-day course of co-trimoxazole with the expectation of cure in the vast majority. Those patients with recurrence of symptoms, pyuria, and bacteriuria will be promptly identified as having subclinical renal infection necessitating 14 days of therapy.

In certain emergency department settings, especially those serving indigent populations where there is delay in seeking care, the incidence of subclinical pyelonephritis may approach 70 percent of patients. In this circumstance, short-course therapy is difficult to justify. Before the emergency department physician decides to use a three-day course of treatment, the patient's ability to follow up within one week or return if symptoms persist must be assessed. If follow-up compliance is not expected, or the epidemiologic risk of subclinical pyelonephritis is great, then the patient should be placed on a 10- to 14-day regimen.

One should be suspicious that *Chlamydia* is responsible for symptoms in these settings: a woman with a recent, new sexual partner; a partner with urethritis; examination findings of cervicitis; or when there is low-grade pyuria with no bacteria seen on urinalysis. A seven-

TABLE 90-3 Cost Comparison of Urinary Antimicrobial Agents: 10-Day Course

Generic Name	Cost, $*	Brand Name	Cost, $*
Trimethoprim (TMP)	10.39	Proloprim	30.29
Sulfamethoxazole (SMX)	NA	Gantanol	17.89
Co-trimoxazole (TMP/SMX) DS	11.59	Bactrim DS	34.49
Doxycycline	16.79	Vibramycin	88.79
Nitrofurantoin macrocrystals	23.49	Macrodantin	38.09
Amoxicillin with clavulanate	NA	Augmentin	77.99
Ciprofloxacin	NA	Cipro	82.49
Ofloxacin	NA	Floxin	83.99

*The prices given are retail prices in the Chicago metropolitan area in December 1998 obtained by telephone survey by the author.

day course of doxycycline or a single dose of azthromycin is the preferred treatment.

For recurrent infection, culture and sensitivity tests are essential.[2–4] The infection is often due to a new serotype of *E. coli,* or it may be due to newly resistant organisms that develop as a result of antibiotics excreted into the gastrointestinal tract. Empirical therapy for recurrent infections includes co-trimoxazole, nitrofurantoin macrocrystals, or the fluoroquinolones. However, successful management depends on sensitivity testing. Again, it must be emphasized that these patients need referral when identified as having recurrent infections. In addition to evaluation of the urinary tract, chronic suppressive therapy is usually instituted.

Aggressive therapy is warranted for pregnant women with pyuria or bacteriuria, whether or not associated symptoms are present. Most clinicians prefer a cephalosporin for outpatient treatment. Co-trimoxazole may be considered except within two weeks of the estimated delivery date and in those with glucose-6-phosphate dehydrogenase deficiency. All regimens should be continued for seven days. Inpatient management is stressed for suspected pyelonephritis because the incidence is higher in pregnancy, and maternal and fetal morbidity is substantial.

Adjunctive therapy should include plenty of fluids to enhance diuresis, fruit juices containing vitamin C to acidify the urine, a proper diet, and frequent voiding (at least every two hours) to diminish tissue contact with bacteria.[14] Women should be reminded that postintercourse voiding may be helpful in reducing recurrent infection.

Once the infection is eradicated, management should be directed toward prevention of reinfection; up to 80 percent of women who have had one UTI develop another one at a later time. Because many factors are involved in reinfection and some of these are correctable, appropriate referral is essential.

Acute Pyelonephritis

Classically, acute pyelonephritis is characterized by shaking chills and fever, flank pain, and costovertebral angle tenderness following several days of dysuria and frequency.[2,4] The urine often demonstrates WBC casts and clumps, as well as bacteria. Sometimes the presentation may not be dramatic, and it might be difficult to distinguish lower from upper UTI.

Factors associated with an increased risk for pyelonephritis include pregnancy, prolonged symptoms prior to seeking care, three or more infections in the past year, immunocompromised state, and diabetes mellitus.[2,4] Less often, the patient may have a congenital or acquired anatomic urinary tract abnormality, neurogenic problems that result in incomplete bladder emptying, recent urinary tract instrumentation, renal calculi and nephrocalcinosis, prostatic hypertrophy, or prostatitis as precipitating factors for acute pyelonephritis.

Young, otherwise healthy females with uncomplicated acute pyelonephritis may be candidates for outpatient management.[15] Conversely, oral outpatient treatment cannot be recommended for patients who are immunocompromised, pregnant, diabetic, or chronically ill. Although unproven, a popular regimen at many institutions is to treat the patient with antipyretics, intravenous fluids, and the first dose of antibiotic (either oral or parenteral) while undergoing a brief period of observation in the emergency department to ensure that further oral therapy will be kept down, which is assessed by having the patient drink water.[16] Outpatient therapy for selected patients (young, otherwise healthy, able to keep down fluids and antibiotics) is as safe and effective, and considerably less expensive, than comparable patients treated on an inpatient basis. Acceptable antibiotics include the fluoroquinolones, amoxicillin/clavulanate, or co-trimoxazole, although *E. coli* are demonstrating increasing resistance to co-trimoxazole in some regions.[12] Outpatient treatment should be continued for 10 to 14 days. Patients should be instructed to return if increasing pain, fever, or vomiting. Overall, 80 to 90 percent of selected patients with acute pyelonephritis respond to outpatient oral therapy.[15,16]

The decision to admit a patient with acute pyelonephritis is based on age, host factors, and response to initial emergency department interventions. Fluid replacement and parenteral antibiotics are necessary if the patient is vomiting or dehydrated. Unremitting fever and/or loss of vasomotor tone mandate inpatient therapy. In an otherwise healthy host with no prior or recent history of UTI, the typical offending bacteria would often be *E. coli,* or another coliform bacteria. Acceptable intravenous antibiotic regimens include a fluoroquinolone (ciprofloxacin, levofloxacin, or ofloxacin), ampicillin plus gentamicin, a third-generation cephalosporin (cefotaxime, ceftazidine, or ceftriaxone), or extended spectrum penicillin plus β-lactamase inhibitor (ticarcillin/clavulanate or ampicillin/sulbactam).[12] The selection of which drugs to use depends on cost considerations and on local sensitivity patterns.

Younger patients without complicating factors have the least morbidity or mortality. Overall, about 1 to 3 percent of patients with acute pyelonephritis die from the infection. Factors associated with an unfavorable prognosis are old age and general debility, renal calculi or obstruction, a recent history of hospitalization or instrumentation, diabetes mellitus, evidence of chronic nephropathy, sickle cell anemia, underlying carcinoma, or intercurrent cancer chemotherapy. In patients with these factors, it is imperative that broad-spectrum antibiotic coverage to include *Pseudomonas sp* be provided. A urologic or infectious disease consultation should be considered as part of the initial management of such patients.

Complications of acute pyelonephritis include acute papillary necrosis with possible ureteric obstruction, septic shock, and perinephric abscesses. Imaging studies to detect ureteral obstruction are essential in the management of these complications. Adequate fluid resuscitation must be emphasized.

REFERENCES

1. Kunin CM, Van Arsdale White L, Tong HH: A reassessment of the importance of "low-count" bacteriuria in young women with acute urinary symptoms. *Ann Intern Med* 119:454, 1993.
2. Johnson JR, Stamm WE: Urinary tract infections in women: Diagnosis and treatment. *Ann Intern Med* 111:906, 1989.
3. Lipsky BA: Urinary tract infections in men: Epidemiology, pathophysiology, diagnosis, and treatment. *Ann Intern Med* 110:138, 1989.
4. Stamm WE, Hooton TM: Management of urinary tract infections in adults. *N Engl J Med* 329:1328, 1993.
5. Hooten TM, Scholes D, Hughes JP, et al: A prospective study of risk factors for symptomatic urinary tract infection in young women. *N Engl J Med* 335:468, 1996.
6. Strom BL, Collins M, West SL, et al: Sexual activity, contraceptive use, and other risk factors for symptomatic and asymptomatic bacteriuria: A case control study. *Ann Intern Med* 107:816, 1987.
7. Huang JJ, Sung JM, Chen KW, et al: Acute bacterial nephritis: A clinicoradiologic correlation based on computed tomography. *Am J Med* 93:289, 1992.
8. McHugh TP, Albanna SE, Stewart NJ: Bilateral emphysematous pyelonephritis. *Am J Emerg Med* 16:166, 1998.
9. Propp DA, Weber D, Ciesla M: Reliability of a urine dipstick in emergency department patients. *Ann Emerg Med* 18:560, 1989.
10. Leibovici L, Greenshtain S, Cohen O, et al: Predictors of bacteremia and resistant pathogens in urinary tract infections. *Arch Intern Med* 152:2481, 1992.
11. Thanassi M: Utility of urine and blood cultures in pyelonephritis. *Acad Emerg Med* 4:797, 1997.
12. Abramowicz M: The choice of antibacterial drugs. *Med Lett Drug Ther* 40:33, 1998.
13. Hooten TM, Winter C, Tiu F, Stamm WE: Randomized comparative trial and cost analysis of 3-day antimicrobial regiments for treatment of acute cystitis in women. *JAMA* 273:41, 1995.
14. Avorn J, Monane M, Gurwitz JH, et al: Reduction of bacteriuria and pyuria after ingestion of cranberry juice. *JAMA* 271:751, 1994.

15. Pinson AG, Philbrick JT, Lindbeck GH, Schorling JB: Oral antibiotic therapy for acute pyelonephritis: A methodologic review of the literature. *J Gen Intern Med* 7:544, 1992.
16. Pinson AG, Philbrick JT, Lindbeck GH, et al: Emergency department management of acute pyelonephritis in women: A cohort study. *Am J Emerg Med* 12:271, 1994.

MALE GENITAL PROBLEMS

Robert E. Schneider

One of the most anxiety-provoking problems presenting to an emergency department is the male with acute genital pain. The extensive sensory innervation of this area produces severe symptoms, and the close relationships of the abdominal and genital sensory afferent pathways in the male account for the common association of abdominal pain with some acute genitourinary disorders.

ANATOMY

Penis

The penis is composed of three cylindrical bodies: the two corpora cavernosa, which form the main bulk of the penis, and the corpus spongiosum, which surrounds the urethra (Fig. 91-1). The corpora cavernosa are the major erectile bodies, extending distally from the pubic rami and capped by the glans penis. These two cylindrical structures are encased in a thick tunic of dense connective tissue, the tunica albuginea. All three cylinders are collectively covered by a thinner Buck's fascia, which fuses with Colles's fascia at the level of the urogenital diaphragm.

The blood supply is primarily from the internal pudendal artery, which branches to form the deep and superficial penile arteries. Lymphatic drainage is into the deep and superficial inguinal nodes.

Scrotum

The prepubertal scrotal skin is thin and thickens with subsequent hormonal stimulation. Immediately beneath the skin are the smooth muscle and elastic tissue layers of the Dartos fascia, similar to the superficial fatty layer (Camper's fascia) of the abdominal wall. The deep membranous layer (Scarpa's fascia) of the abdominal wall extends into the perineum, where it is referred to as Colles' fascia and forms part of the scrotal wall (Fig. 91-2). The blood supply is primarily derived from branches of the femoral and internal pudendal arteries. Lymphatics from the scrotum drain into the inguinal and femoral nodes.

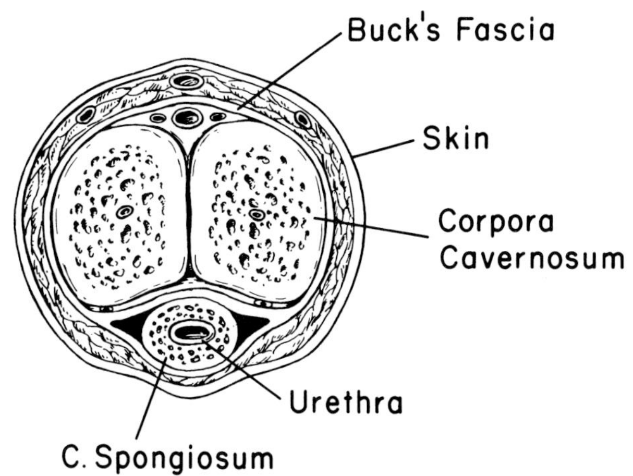

FIG. 91-1. Cross section of the penis.

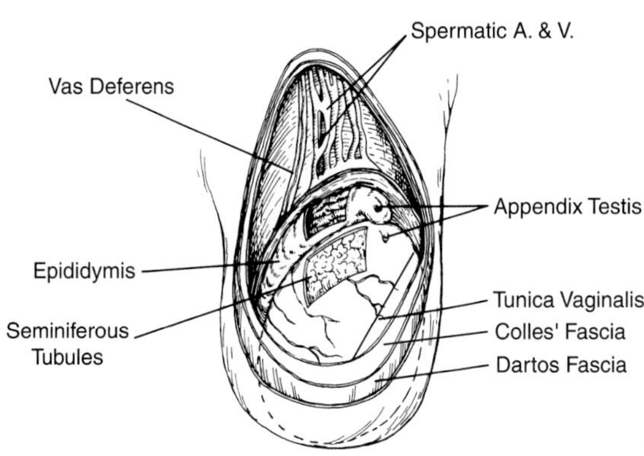

FIG. 91-2. Anatomy of the scrotum and the testis.

Testes

The testes usually lie in an upright position with the superior portion tipped slightly forward and outward. The average size is between 4 and 5 cm in length, and approximately 3 cm in width and depth. The overall volume is about 25 mL. Each testis is encased in a thick fibrous tunica albuginea except posterolaterally, where it is in tight apposition with the epididymis. The enveloping tunica vaginalis anchors each testis and epididymis to the posterior scrotal wall. Inferiorly, the testis is anchored to the scrotum by the scrotal ligament (gubernaculum). A lack of firm posterior fixation leaves both the testes and epididymis at risk for torsion. The posterior (visceral) leaf of tunica vaginalis is contiguous with the tunica albuginea testis. A potential space exists between this visceral leaf and the anterior (parietal) tunica vaginalis. Any traumatic or inflammatory event will impede the normal parietal tunica vaginalis from absorbing viscerally secreted fluid, resulting in a hydrocele (Fig. 91-3).

The blood supply is by the internal spermatic and external spermatic arteries, which travel together in the spermatic cord. Venous return is primarily by the internal spermatic, epigastric, internal circumflex, and scrotal veins. The lymphatics drain toward the external, common iliac, and periaortic nodes.

The epididymis is a single, fine, tubular structure approximately 4 to 5 m long compressed into an area of about 5 cm. The function the epididymis is to promote sperm maturation and motility. Vestigial embryonic structures, the appendix epididymis and the appendix testis, which have no known physiologic function, are often associated with the testes and epididymis. The appendix epididymis, a remnant of the epigenitales, is found attached to the head of the epididymis, or globus major. The appendix testis, a pear-shaped structure of müllerian duct origin, is usually situated on the uppermost portion of the testis at the junction of the testis and the globus major of the epididymis.

The vas deferens, a prominent part of the adnexa of the scrotal contents, is a distinct muscular tube that is easily palpable within the scrotal sac. It extends cephalad in the spermatic cord from the tail of the epididymis (globus minor) traversing the inguinal canal and crossing medially behind the bladder over the ureters to form the ampullae of the vas, where it joins with the seminal vesicles to form the paired ejaculatory ducts in the prostatic urethra.

Prostate

The prostate originates from the urogenital sinus at approximately the third month of embryonic life. It is continually enlarging and

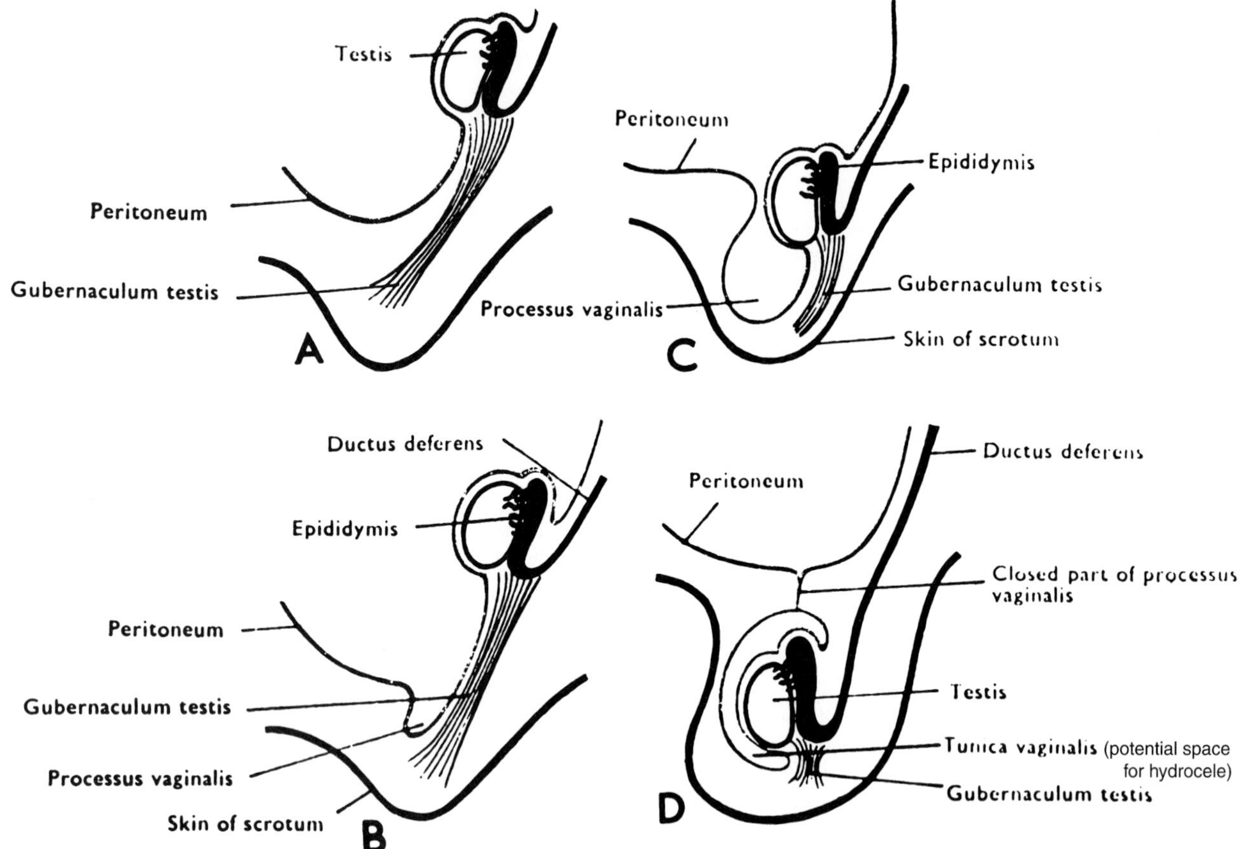

FIG. 91-3. Embryonic retroperitoneal testis descends into the scrotum and invaginates into the tunica vaginalis, which anchors it to the posterior scrotal wall. Note the potential space in the tunica vaginalis for development of a hydrocele.

in the young male is approximately 10 to 15 g, often not definable on rectal examination. As a man matures, the prostate may enlarge dramatically, resulting in significant bladder outlet obstruction. The prostate is divided into five lobes: anterior, median, posterior, and two lateral lobes.

PHYSICAL EXAMINATION

Physical examination should be carried out with the patient in both the supine and upright positions in a well-illuminated, warm room. If the scrotum is contracted despite proper room temperature, a warm towel placed over the genitalia permits the scrotum to relax and the testes to descend and be comfortably examined.

Examination should always begin with visual inspection. In uncircumcised males, the foreskin should be fully retracted to inspect the glans, coronal sulcus, and preputial areas for ulceration or malignant lesions. The location of the urethral meatus and presence of discharge should be noted. The penile shaft should be carefully palpated for plaques, cysts, or early abscesses.

The supine or modified lithotomy (frogleg) position is more comfortable for both the patient and the examiner and allows a more thorough examination of each testis, epididymis, the prostate, seminal vesicles, and rectal ampulla. During the critical evaluation of a scrotal mass, patient relaxation and cooperation in the supine position are paramount. Testicular nodularity or firmness should be considered carcinoma until proven otherwise. The epididymis usually lies on the posterolateral aspect of the testis and, if not inflamed or involved with other pathologic entities, has a soft, fleshy feel similar to that of the earlobe. Many males experience pain and tenderness with palpation of a normal globus major (head), body, and globus minor (tail) of the epididymis. All males experience some discomfort during palpation of a normal prostate. The supine position helps prevent an infrequent vasovagal response to the scrotal or prostate examination. The prostate has a heart-shaped contour with its apex located more distally, abutting the urogenital diaphragm (anatomic soft spot). The consistency of the normal prostate has the same resiliency as the cartilaginous tip of the nose, while suspicious carcinogenic areas feel more like the bony prominence of the chin. The posterior lobe is small and thin, allowing palpation of the median raphe that distinguishes the two lateral lobes. A normal rectal examination does not exclude bladder outlet obstruction secondary to an obstructing median bar or large intravesical prostate. The seminal vesicles, lying just superior to the prostate, cannot normally be distinguished unless there is inflammation, induration, or enlargement.

Examination of the inguinal canals for hernias and the scrotal spermatic cords for varicoceles is best done in the upright position, with the patient straining at the designated time. When the patient is upright, it should be determined whether the testes are aligned along a vertical or horizontal axis. Horizontally aligned testes are at greater risk for torsion.

Some genital disorders may require urine collection and analysis. The uncircumcised male should retract his foreskin and wash the glans penis with cleansing towels before collecting a midstream specimen. Failure to do so will result in preputial contamination. The often-described three-cup specimen used to localize male lower urinary tract infections is time-consuming and requires patient compliance, factors that tend to limit its usefulness in the emergency department.

COMMON GENITOURINARY DISORDERS

Scrotum

Because the scrotal skin is loose and elastic, dramatic enlargement of the scrotum may occur secondary to either scrotal or testicular pathologic conditions.

SCROTAL EDEMA Simple, isolated scrotal edema is uncommon. It usually occurs secondary to insect or human bites, contact dermatitis, or, in young boys, to idiopathic scrotal edema. Contiguous scrotal and penile edema occurs in older men in conjunction with lower extremity edema in fluid overload states (congestive heart failure), hypoalbuminemia, and generalized anasarca.

SCROTAL ABSCESS The important distinction with a scrotal abscess is whether the phlegmon is localized to the scrotal wall, i.e., simple hair follicle abscess, or involves, and even perhaps originates from, infection in one of the primary intrascrotal organs, i.e., testis, epididymis, bulbous urethra. This distinction can be very difficult late in the course of the disease process when a scrotal mass may be the only discernible finding.

A simple hair-follicle scrotal-wall abscess can be managed by incision and drainage. Oftentimes wound care can be simplified by circumferential excision of the entire roof of the abscess. This allows access for wound care and sitz baths and assures healing from the base outward. Antibiotics are rarely needed in an immunocompetent male.

Contiguous involvement of the scrotal skin by an inflammatory mass in the testis or epididymis is best evaluated by ultrasound. A retrograde urethrogram will delineate the integrity of the urethra. Definitive care of any complex abscesses should be directed by a urologist.

FOURNIER'S GANGRENE Fournier's gangrene is a polymicrobial, synergistic infection of the subcutaneous tissues that originates from one of three sites: skin, urethra, or rectum. This infectious process typically begins as a benign infection or simple abscess that quickly becomes virulent, especially in an immunocompromised host, and leads to end-artery thrombosis in the subcutaneous tissue that promotes widespread necrosis of previously healthy tissue (Fig. 91-4).

The diabetic male seems to be most at risk. Prompt recognition of Fournier's gangrene in its early stages should prevent extensive tissue loss that accompanies delayed diagnosis. Aggressive fluid resuscitation; gram-positive, gram-negative, and anaerobic antibiotic coverage; and wide surgical debridement sometimes in conjunction with pre- and postoperative hyperbaric oxygen therapy are the mainstays of treatment. Urologic consultation is often required when periurethral abscess is the inciting event, or when other etiologies have secondarily invaded the urinary tract and supravesical urinary drainage is needed. It is imperative that emergency physicians maintain a very high index of suspicion for this entity in immunocompromised patients who present complaining of scrotal, rectal, or any genitalia pain out of proportion to their physical examination findings. Surgical consultation is strongly recommended in all such patients, rather than deciding on symptomatic treatment and discharge from the emergency department.

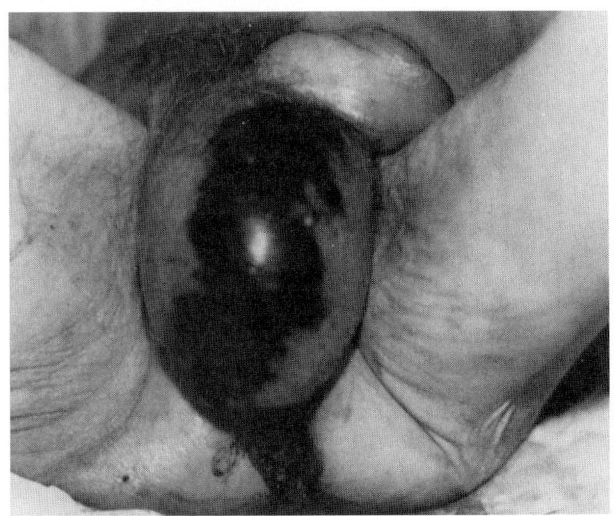

FIG. 91-4. A patient with Fournier's gangrene of the scrotum. Note the sharp demarcation of gangrenous changes and the marked edema of the scrotum and the penis.

Phimosis

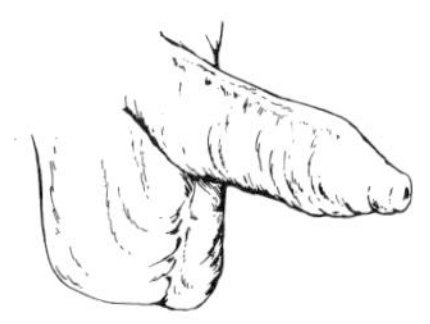

Paraphimosis

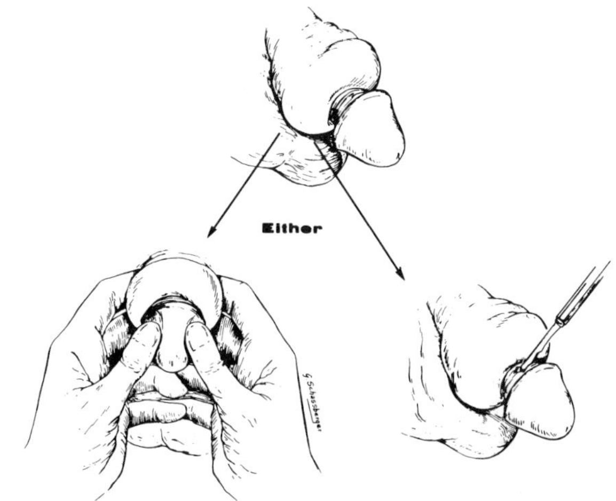

FIG. 91-5. Phimosis and paraphimosis. (The lower figure depicts the method of reduction.)

Penis

BALANOPOSTHITIS Balanitis is inflammation of the glans penis. Posthitis is inflammation of the foreskin. Balanoposthitis is inflammation of both the glans and foreskin. When foreskin retraction is attempted, the glans and apposing prepuce appear purulent, excoriated, malodorous, and tender. When recurrent, it can be the sole presenting sign of diabetes. Treatment consists of cleansing the area with mild soap, assuring adequate dryness, application of antifugal creams (nystatin or clotrimazole), and possibly circumcision. If secondary bacterial infection is present, a broad-spectrum antibiotic, usually a cephalosporin, should be prescribed.

PHIMOSIS Phimosis is the inability to retract the foreskin proximally and posterior to the glans penis (Fig. 91-5). Causes include infection, poor hygiene, or previous preputial injury with scarring. Scarring at the tip of the foreskin can occlude the preputial meatus, infrequently causing urinary retention. Hemostatic dilation of the preputial ostium

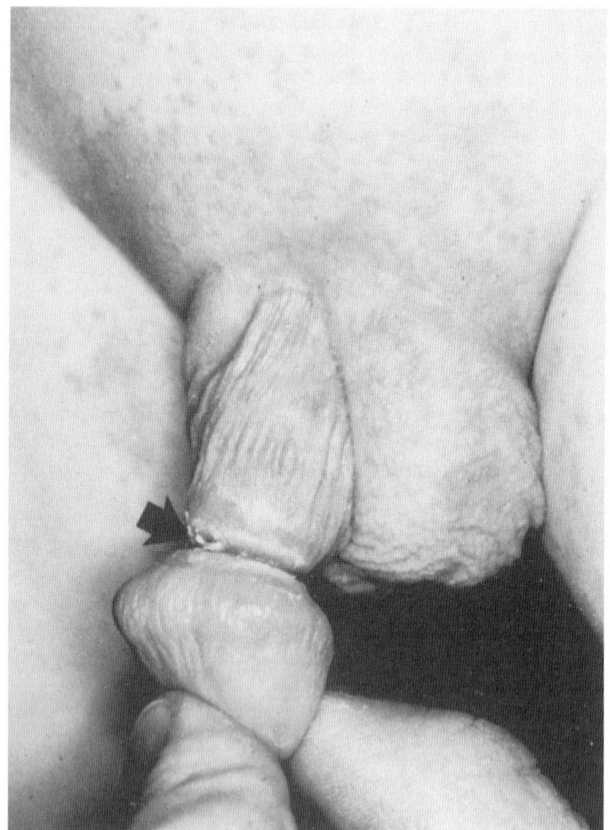

FIG. 91-6. Hair is entrapped behind the coronal sulcus (*arrow*), constricting and progressively amputating the glans.

relieves the urinary retention until definitive dorsal slit or circumcision can be done.

PARAPHIMOSIS Paraphimosis is the inability to reduce the proximal edematous foreskin distally over the glans penis into its naturally occurring position (Fig. 91-5). The resulting glans edema and venous engorgement can progress to arterial compromise and gangrene.

Paraphimosis is a true urologic emergency. Paraphimosis can often be reduced by compression of the glans for several minutes to reduce edema and allow for successful reduction of the foreskin back over the now smaller glans. Tightly wrapping the glans with a ×2-inch elastic bandage for 5 min is one method to reduce edema. Infrequently, several puncture wounds with a small needle (22 to 25 g) can help edema fluid be expressed out the glans. A local anesthetic block of the penis is also helpful if the patient cannot tolerate the pain of compression. If these methods are unsuccessful, local infiltration of the constricting band with 1% plain lidocaine followed by superficial vertical incision of the band will decompress the glans and allow foreskin reduction. This procedure should be done by an emergency physician unless a urologist is immediately available.

ENTRAPMENT INJURIES Various objects can be placed around the penis, initially occluding the venous, and subsequently the arterial, blood supply. String, metal rings, and wire have been wrapped around the penis for sexual, experimental, or accidental reasons. One of the most insidious objects that can become entrapped behind the coronal ridge is human hair, usually found in young circumcised boys aged two to five years (Fig. 91-6). The child presents with swelling of the glans. The offending hair may be invisible within the edematous coronal sulcus. If the hair has been chronically occluding, the urethra and dorsal nerve supply of the penis may be partially or completely involved. Removal of the offending object requires ingenuity and care. Urethral integrity (retrograde urethrogram) and distal penile arterial blood supply (Doppler) must be assured prior to emergency department discharge.

FRACTURE OF THE PENIS An acute tear or rupture of the corpus cavernosa tunica albuginea is rare but easily diagnosed. The penis is acutely swollen, discolored, and tender. The history is of trauma during intercourse or other sexual activity, when a sudden ''snapping sound'' occurs. Even though the urethra is infrequently injured, a retrograde urethrogram may be necessary to assure urethral integrity. Surgical treatment consists of hematoma evacuation and suture apposition of the disrupted tunica albuginea.

PEYRONIE'S DISEASE The patient complains of gradual onset of dorsal penile curvature with erections; it is painful and may preclude successful vaginal penetration during intercourse. Examination of the dorsal penile shaft will disclose a thickened plaque involving the tunica albuginea of the corpora bodies without urethral involvement. Reassurance and urologic referral are warranted. Peyronie's disease of the penis has been noted in association with Dupuytren's contractures of the hand.

PRIAPISM Priapism is a urologic emergency that presents as a painful, hard, pathologic erection in which both corpora cavernosa are engorged with stagnant blood. Even though the glans penis and the corpus spongiosum are characteristically soft and uninvolved, urinary retention may develop. Impotence has been reported to occur in 35 percent of cases who have sustained erections for prolonged periods of time; thus, expedient treatment and early urologic consultation is required. The potential for medical-legal liability mandates meticulous documentation in these cases.

A large number of cases of priapism in adults are pharmacologically related, either to intracavernosal injection for impotence or oral agents for hypertension or mental disorders. Most cases of priapism in children are due to hematologic disorders, usually sickle cell disease. Case reports have attempted to relate a variety of other drugs, metabolic conditions, and trauma to priapism, although the pathophysiologic mechanisms are speculative in most cases.

Priapism is classified into high-flow (nonischemic) priapism and low-flow (ischemic) priapism. The former is rare, most often nonpainful, and usually results from traumatic fistulae between the cavernosal artery and the corpus cavernosum. The latter is more common, is usually quite painful, and is diagnosed by the aspiration of dark acidic intracavernosal blood from the corpus cavernosum.

Low-flow priapism is further categorized as reversible or nonreversible depending upon etiology and the response to medical treatment (Table 91-1). Regardless of specific etiology, initial therapy with terbutaline, 0.25 to 0.5 mg subcutaneously in the deltoid area, repeated in 20 min as needed, is the most effective therapy. Traditional therapies of sedation or ice water enemas are ineffective. Pseudoephedrine 60 to 120 mg orally has been reported effective in some cases that present early (less than 4h). Priapism due to sickle cell disease is most consistently reversed by simple or exchange transfusion. Corporal aspiration followed by irrigation (either with plain saline or with α-adrenergic agonists, i.e., phenylephine (neosynephrine)) is the primary treatment method for persistent priapism. The urologic consultant usually performs this procedure, but if one is not readily available, the emergency physician may need to intervene. Reversible priapism may respond to these treatments, while nonreversible priapism usually does not respond and requires surgery.

CARCINOMA Carcinoma of the penis is a rare disease occurring in about 1 of every 100,000 malignancies reported, usually appearing in the fifth or sixth decade in an uncircumcised male. Carcinoma may appear as a nontender ulcer or warty growth beneath the foreskin in

TABLE 91-1 Causes and Treatment of Low-Flow Ischemic Priapism

Reversible Causes
- A. Sickle cell anemia
  - Treatment: Terbutaline, 0.25–0.5 mg subcutaneously in the deltoid muscle; packed red blood cell transfusion; hydration and alkalization may be beneficial
- B. Iatrogenic injection of PGE1, papaverine, or phentolamine for impotence
  - Treatment: Terbutaline, 0.25–0.5 mg subcutaneously in the deltoid muscle; aspirate 30–70 mL corporal blood, then inject 30–70 mL phenylephrine 20 μg/mL (10 mg in 500 mL normal saline), maximum dose = 1500 μg
- C. Leukemic infiltration
  - Treatment: Terbutaline, 0.25–0.5 mg subcutaneously in the deltoid muscle; specific chemotherapy

Nonreversible Causes
- A. Idiopathic
- B. High spinal cord lesion
- C. Medications (phenothiazines, hydralazine, prazosin)
  - Treatment of all nonreversible causes: Terbutaline, 0.25–0.5 mg subcutaneously in the deltoid muscle; corporal aspiration, phenylephrine instillation; heparin irrigation; shunt surgery

the area of the coronal sulcus or glans penis. It is often hidden by an inflamed phimotic foreskin.

Testes and Epididymis

TESTICULAR TORSION The differential diagnosis of acute scrotal pain includes testicular torsion, torsion of the appendix testis, appendix epididymis, and epididymitis. Testicular torsion must be the primary consideration (Fig. 91-7). While the peak incidence of intravaginal torsion occurs at puberty in conjunction with maximal hormonal stimulation, it may occur at any age.

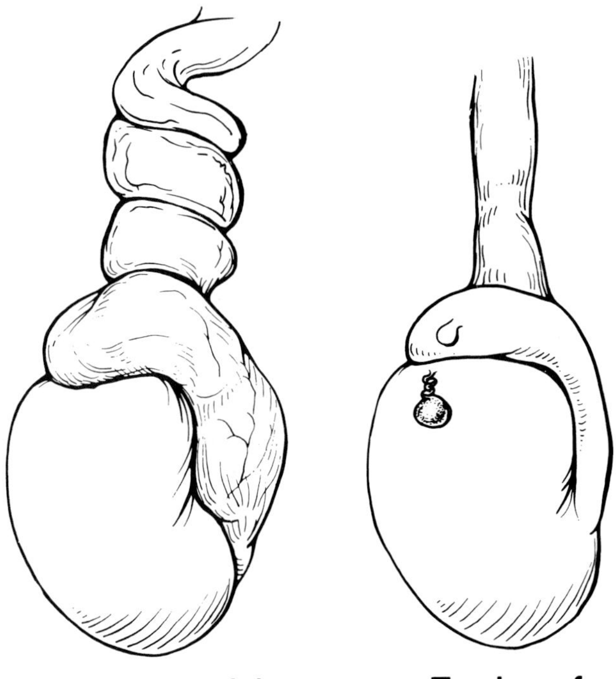

FIG. 91-7. Diagrams of testicular torsion and torsion of the appendix testis.

Torsion of the testis or spermatic cord results from bilateral maldevelopment of fixation between the enveloping tunica vaginalis and the posterior scrotal wall. Characteristically, the at-risk testis is aligned along a horizontal rather than a vertical axis. The axis of alignment can be determined only with the patient in an upright position, and even then the determination may be difficult.

Frequently there is a history of an athletic event, strenuous physical activity, or trauma just prior to the onset of scrotal pain. However, a fair number occur during sleep. Unilateral cremaster muscle contraction results in testicular torsion. The pain usually occurs suddenly, is severe, and is usually felt in either lower abdominal quadrant, the inguinal canal, or the testis. While the pain may be constant or intermittent, it is not positional in nature as testicular torsion is primarily an ischemic event that becomes inflammatory only after the testis has infarcted.

In obvious cases of testicular torsion, emergent urologic consultation and surgical exploration are recommended. The often quoted 4-h warm-ischemia time for testicular salvage comes from controlled animal studies and cannot be extrapolated to clinical medicine. There are no readily available clinical or laboratory parameters to judge either the degree or the duration of testicular ischemia. Therefore, no matter how long the patient has been symptomatic and no matter what the presenting physical examination suggests, if testicular torsion cannot be excluded by history and physical examination, emergency scrotal exploration is the definitive diagnostic test and procedure of choice.

Color-flow duplex Doppler ultrasound and radionuclide scintigraphy are two imaging modalities used to evaluate patients with indeterminate clinical presentations. Both may be useful, but their routine clinical use is limited by timely availability and operator experience in interpreting the images. These studies are considered "positive" for testicular torsion when they demonstrate absent or clearly reduced blood flow to the painful side when compared to the opposite testicle, and "negative" when flow is normal or increased. Both studies have nearly identical reported sensitivity (80 to 90 percent) and specificity (75 to 95 percent) for testicular torsion. Ultrasound has the advantage of demonstrating scrotal anatomy (which may indicate alternate diagnosis) but has the disadvantage of the greater number of indeterminate results when compared to scintigraphy. Within these limitations, both modalities may be useful when promptly available for patients with unclear clinical presentations but should never delay attempted manual detorsion and scrotal exploration.

While awaiting transportation of the patient to the operating room, the emergency physician should attempt manual detorsion of the affected testis. Most testes torse in a lateral to medial fashion. Therefore, detorsion should initially be done in a medial to lateral motion. It must be explained to the patient that detorsion is a painful procedure and while local anesthesia of the affected spermatic cord can initially make the patient more comfortable, it also removes an important endpoint of the detorsion maneuver, i.e., relief of pain. Detorsion is done in a manner similar to opening a book (Fig. 91-8). If one were to stand at the patient's feet, the patient's right testis would be rotated in a counterclockwise fashion (Fig. 91-9); the patient's left testis in a clockwise fashion (Fig. 91-10). Any relief of pain is a positive endpoint. A worsening of the patient's pain would dictate that detorsion be done in the opposite direction. Successful detorsion converts an emergent procedure to an elective one, but one that must be done to correct a potential bilateral anatomic disaster. The timing of the elective surgical correction should depend on the patient's compliance and responsibility.

Young boys may present to the emergency department with nonspecific abdominal pain suggestive of gastroenteritis only to return one to two days later with testicular torsion. Whether these patients had undisclosed testicular torsion at their initial evaluation is not known, but emergency physicians must think about testicular torsion in the

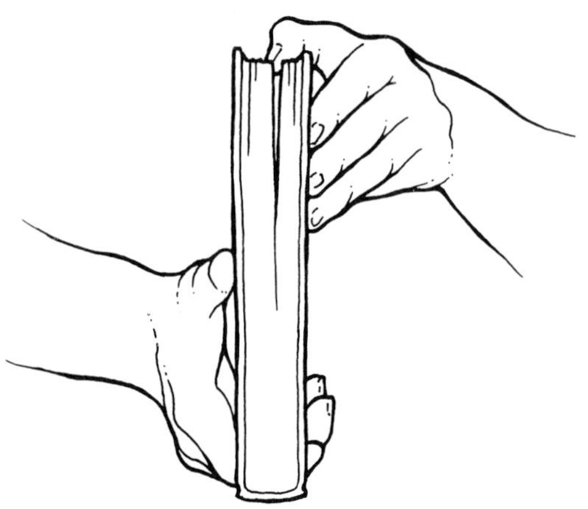

FIGS. 91-8, 91-9, 91-10. Testicular detorsion. This procedure is best done standing at the foot of or on the right side of the patient's bed. The torsed testis is detorsed in a fashion similar to opening a book (Fig. 91-8). That is, the patient's right testis is rotated counterclockwise (Fig. 91-9), the left testis is roated clockwise (Fig. 91-10).

differential diagnosis of any male presenting with a complaint of abdominal pain!

TORSION OF THE APPENDAGES The appendages of the epididymis and testis have no known physiologic function. These pedunculated structures are, however, capable of torsion, and in prepubertal boys probably torse more often than the testes. If the patient is seen early, the pain is more intense near the head of the epididymis or testis, and an isolated tender nodule can often be palpated. When the involved infarcted appendage is brought close to the thin, prepubertal nonhormonally stimulated scrotal skin, a blue reflection may be seen when light shines upon it. This "blue dot sign" is pathognomonic of torsion of the appendix testis or epididymis. If the diagnosis can be absolutely assured and confirmed by color Doppler ultrasound showing normal intratesticular blood flow to the involved testis, immediate surgery is not necessary, because most appendages will calcify or degenerate over 10 to 14 days and cause no harm. If late in the process and testicular swelling is present, or if the color Doppler ultrasound is equivocal, then urologic consultation and surgical exploration may be necessary to exclude testicular torsion.

EPIDIDYMITIS The onset of pain in epididymitis or epididymo-orchitis is usually more gradual than that of testicular torsion because of

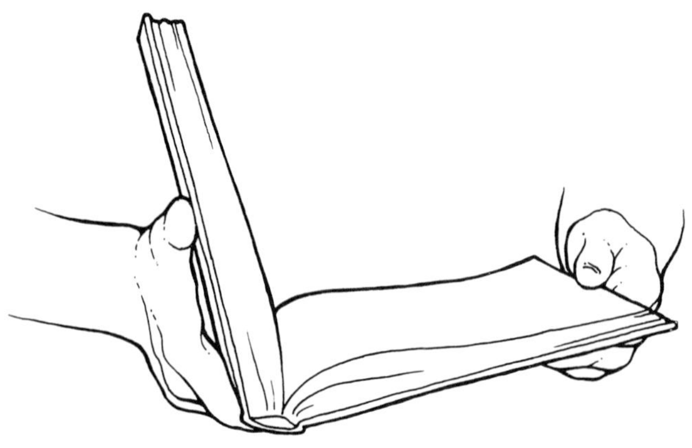

FIG. 91-9. See legend to Fig. 91-8.

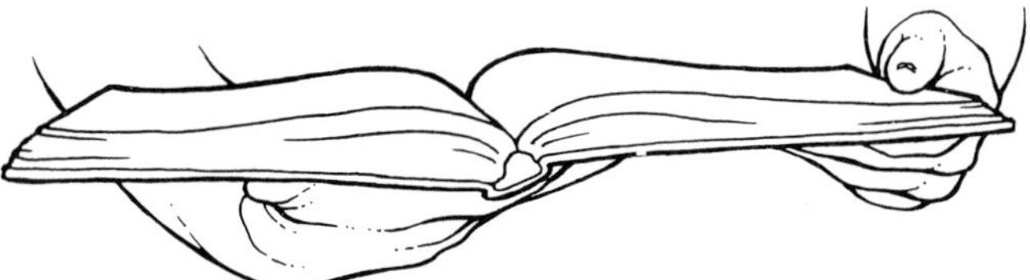

FIG. 91-10. See legend to Fig. 91-8.

its inflammatory etiology. Bacterial infection is the most common cause and tends to be age-dependent. In young boys with documented epididymitis or epididymo-orchitis, congenital anomalies of the lower urinary tract in addition to chemical epididymitis secondary to retrograde reflux of sterile urine into the globus minor (tail of the epididymis) must be considered. In patients less than 40 years of age, epididymitis is primarily due to sexually transmitted diseases (STDs) or their complications, i.e., urethral stricture. In gay men with epididymitis or epididymo-orchitis, fungal infection of the lower urinary tract in addition to the more common STD organisms must be considered. In patients over 40 years of age, epididymitis is caused by common urinary pathogens such as *Escherichia coli* and *Klebsiella.* These patients will most often have pyuria on urinalysis, but the absence of white cells or bacteria does not exclude the diagnosis. Older men with epididymitis due to infected urine must be evaluated for the cause of their lower urinary tract infection, i.e., benign prostatic hypertrophy (BPH) or urethral stricture disease. Oftentimes the answer may be found by passing a 14F or 16F Foley or Coudé catheter into the bladder. Easy passage precludes a stricture. A large residual urine should alert the physician to outlet obstruction as the cause of the patient's infection.

Epididymitis causes lower abdominal, inguinal canal, scrotal, or testicular pain alone or in combination. The retrograde progression of infection from the prostatic urethra to the epididymis explains the location and progression of pain. Patients with epididymitis are more prone to lower urinary tract irritative voiding symptoms and may note transient relief of their pain in the recumbent position with scrotal elevation, due to the inflammatory nature of the disease. Initially, isolated firmness and nodularity of the affected globus minor is noted on examination. As the disease progresses, the sulcus between the epididymis and testis becomes obliterated, and the inflammatory epididymal mass may become contiguous with the testis, producing a large, tender scrotal mass (epididymo-orchitis) that cannot be differentiated from testicular torsion or carcinoma. At this stage the patient may appear toxic and require admission for IV antibiotic therapy (see Table 91-2). Adjunctive diagnostic modalities such as color-flow duplex Doppler sonography or radionuclide scintigraphy will demonstrate increased or preserved blood flow to the testes.

Admission criteria for epididymitis include fever with elevated white blood cell count and subjective toxicity, all of which can be indicative of epididymal or testicular abscess formation. A urologist will dictate inpatient management, which should include: (1) absolute bedrest for the first 24 to 48 h, with scrotal elevation and ice application (10 to 15 min every 4 to 6 h) to the involved testis/epididymis; (2) nonsteroidal anti-inflammatory drugs (NSAIDs); (3) intravenous antibiotics based on etiology (Table 91-2); and (4) narcotics for pain control, with concomitant stool softeners. These measures will prevent further progression of the inflammatory process. Once the bedridden patient is pain-free, he should begin ambulation with a scrotal supporter, being careful not to lift heavy objects or strain when having a bowel movement, both of which will increase intraabdominal pressure and exacerbate the inflammatory cycle. Any significant deviation from this plan will prolong the recovery period. Outpatient management is identical to inpatient management except that oral antibiotics are prescribed initially for 10 to 14 days. A urologist will need to

TABLE 91-2 Etiology and Treatment of Epididymitis and Epididymo-orchitis

Etiology	Treatment		
Chemical	Tetracyclines		
Gonococci	Cephalosporins, fluoroquinolones, macrolides		
Chlamydia	Tetracyclines, macrolides, fluoroquinolones		
Gram-negative bacilli	Fluoroquinolones, TMP/SMX		
Candida	Fluconazole		
Age <35: treat for gonococci (choose one) Ceftriaxone 125 mg IM × 1 dose Cefixime 400 mg po × 1 dose Ofloxacin 400 mg po × 1 dose Ciprofloxacin 500 mg po × 1 dose Spectinomycin 2 g IM × 1 dose	PLUS	Chlamydia (choose one) Doxycycline 100 mg po bid × 10 days Azithromycin 1 g po × 1 dose Tetracycline 500 mg po qid × 10 days	
	OR Azithromycin 2 g po × 1 dose Ofloxacin 300 mg bid × 7–10 days		
Age >35: treat for gram-negative bacilli Ciprofloxacin 500 mg po bid × 10–14 days Ofloxacin 200 mg po bid × 10–14 days TMP/SMX (trimethoprim/sulfamethoxazole) DS 1 tablet bid × 10 days			

reevaluate the patient in five to seven days and then ultimately decide when the patient may return to work based on his job description, i.e., a sedentary worker would be able to return sooner than a laborer.

ORCHITIS Isolated orchitis, or inflammation of the testicle, is quite rare. It usually occurs in conjunction with other systemic diseases, such as mumps, other viral illnesses, or syphilis. Orchitis usually presents as bilateral testicular tenderness and swelling over a few days' duration. Treatment is symptomatic and disease-specific with urologic follow-up.

TESTICULAR MALIGNANCY Any asymptomatic testicular mass, firmness, or induration is the hallmark of testicular carcinoma. Ten percent of tumors will present with pain secondary to acute hemorrhage within the tumor. Metastatic testicular tumors can be insidious and must be suspected in any male with unexplained supraclavicular lymphadenopathy, abdominal mass, or chronic nonproductive cough that appears resistant to antibiotic or other supportive therapy. Testicular examination may be diagnostic. While not a urologic emergency, any unexplained testicular mass must be approached as a tumor, with urgent urologic referral.

Urethra

URETHRAL STRICTURE Urethral strictures are becoming more prevalent secondary to the rising incidence of STDs. Increasingly, in teenagers and young adults, gonococcal and chlamydial infections have resulted in bulbous urethral obstruction (Fig. 91-11), while trauma and urethral instrumentation are less common and tend to be localized to areas where a traumatic event has occurred. In the older population, postendoscopy meatal stenosis or localized urethral strictures are more common.

If a patient requires measurement of his residual urine, has difficulty voiding, or is in urinary retention, and a 14F or 16F Foley or Coudé catheter cannot be easily placed into the bladder, the differential diagnostic possibilities include urethral stricture, voluntary external sphincter spasm, bladder neck contracture, or BPH. If time permits, retrograde urethrography can be done, which will define the location and extent of a urethral stricture. Only endoscopy can confirm a bladder neck contracture or the extent of an obstructing prostate gland. Suspected voluntary external sphincter spasm can be overcome by holding the penis upright and encouraging the patient to relax his perineum and breathe slowly during the procedure (Fig. 91-12).

When a urethral stricture is encountered, copious anesthetic lubrication is placed intraurethrally after the foreskin has been controlled

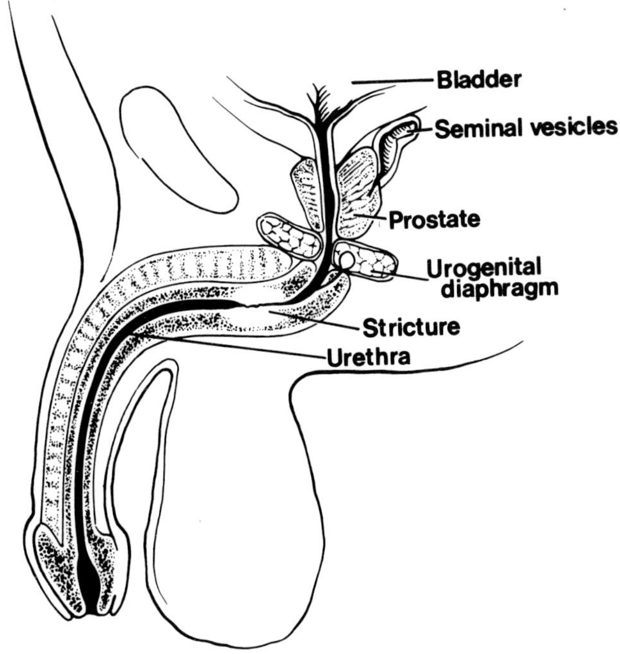

FIG. 91-11. Stricture of the bulbous urethra.

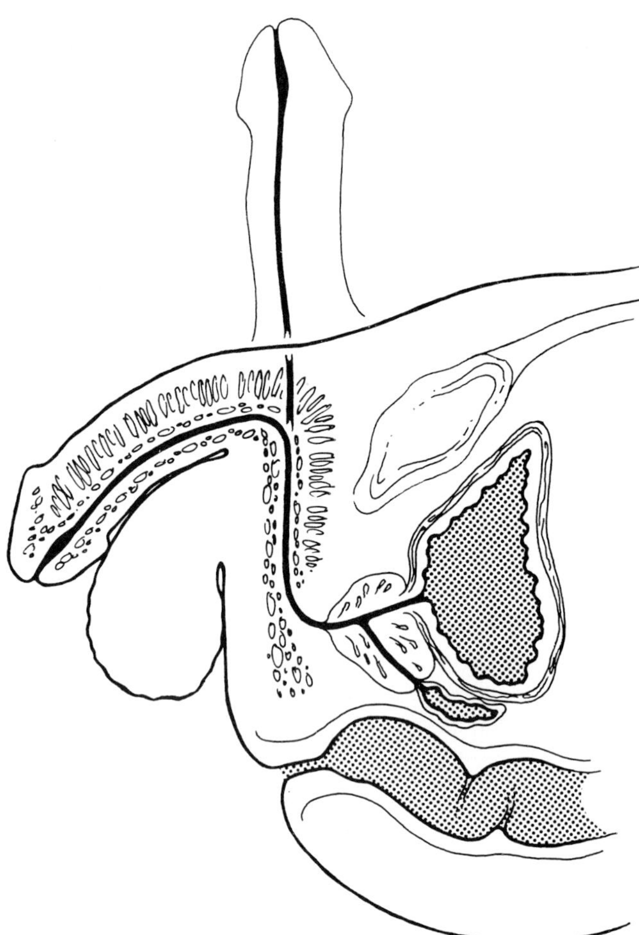

FIG. 91-12. Foley catheter placement. Holding the penis upright will help eliminate urethral folding and reduce external sphincter spasm, both of which can impede catheter placement.

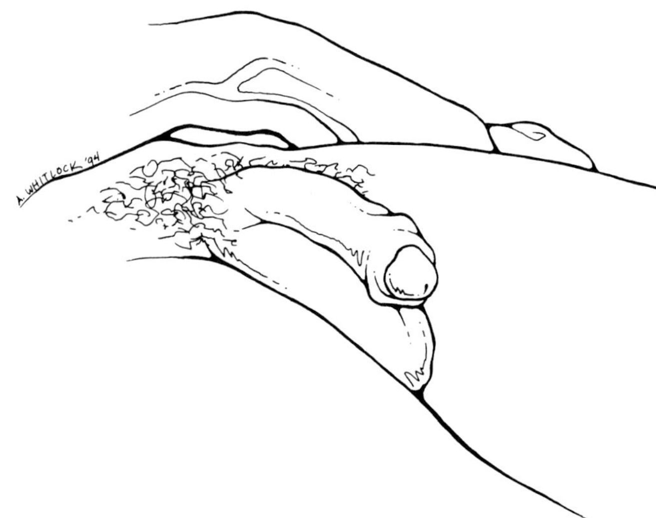

FIG. 91-13. Foley catheter placement. Improper foreskin retraction and immobilization leads to difficulty with catheterization. The uncircumsized patient's foreskin should be fully retracted and immobilized with a folded 4 × 4.

with a folded 4 × 4. This latter maneuver is especially important in uncircumcised patients (Fig. 91-13). A 12F or 14F Coudé catheter may negotiate the strictured area, since this catheter has an angled bend near its tip (Fig. 91-14). If there are previous false passages from attempts at dilation or unsuccessful instrumentation, passage of the Coudé catheter may be difficult. Further urethral manipulation may create new false passages, leading to unnecessary hemorrhage and possible gram-negative bacteremia. If two or three gentle attempts to pass the catheter fail, urologic consultation is indicated. Under no circumstance should a catheter guide or urethral sound be used by anyone other than a urologist (Fig. 91-15).

In an emergency situation, suprapubic cystostomy, utilizing the Seldinger technique, can be performed with the least amount of morbidity. The infraumbilical and suprapubic area is prepped with povidone-iodine solution. A 25- to 27-g spinal needle is used to locate the bladder (Fig. 91-16). This step is especially important in cases of previous lower abdominal surgery where normal anatomic relationships may be distorted. Commercially available introducer cystostomy kits are readily available and utilize the Seldinger technique, which allows easy access to the bladder with a balloon catheter for temporary drainage. After the bladder has been accessed with a syringe and needle, the syringe is removed and a guidewire is passed through the needle into the bladder. The needle is then removed and the fascial dilator with an overlying 14F to 18F peel away sheath is passed over the wire into the bladder. The wire and dilator are then removed leaving the hollow peel-away sheath. An appropriate-sized Foley balloon catheter is passed through the peel-away sheath into the bladder, urine is aspirated from the catheter to assure proper placement, and the balloon is inflated with water. The sheath is then removed from the bladder and peeled away leaving the indwelling catheter, which should be withdrawn until it snugly approximates the cystostomy site. Appropriate urologic follow-up is necessary in two to three days.

URETHRAL FOREIGN BODIES Patients of all ages, but especially young children, may be victims of innocent urethral exploration or attempts to heighten sexual experiences utilizing a variety of foreign bodies such as bobby pins; long, thin paint brushes; or ball point pens. Bloody urine combined with infection and slow, painful urination should suggest a possible foreign body in the lower urinary tract. An x-ray of the bladder and urethral areas may disclose the presence of a foreign body.

Foreign bodies often require endoscopic removal or even open cystotomy. Occasionally a gentle milking action of the proximal end of the urethral foreign body by an experienced examiner will allow its retrieval from the distal urethral meatus. Even then, retrograde urethrography or endoscopic confirmation of an intact, nontraumatized urethra is indicated.

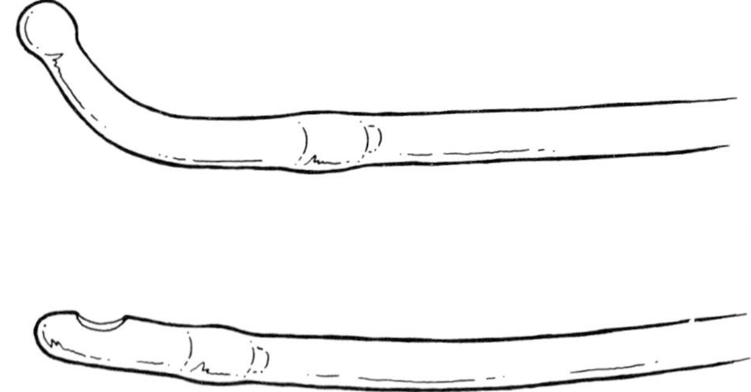

FIG. 91-14. Goudé (top) and straight-tipped (bottom) catheters.

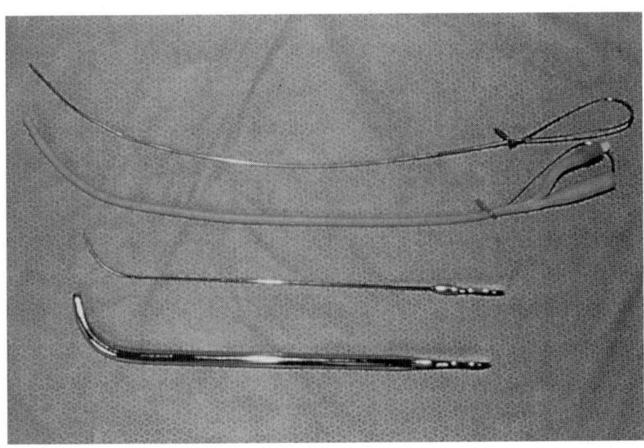

FIG. 91-15. Catheter guides and urethral sounds should be used only by a urologist.

Urinary Retention

Obstructive uropathy causes a wide expanse of signs and symptoms. Overt urinary retention represents one end of the spectrum, while symptoms of insidious overflow incontinence will often fool an unsuspecting examiner. Prior to acquiring a detailed genitourinary history, questions regarding chronic systemic medical illnesses or carcinomas that have as sequelae sensory or motor neurogenic side effects or complications must be addressed. A detailed medication history, including over-the-counter cold and dietary medications, will often reveal the ingestion of a sympathomimetic agonist that has secondarily caused outlet obstruction due to its muscle-constricting effect on the abundant α-agonistic fibers in the bladder neck. Inconvenient, and

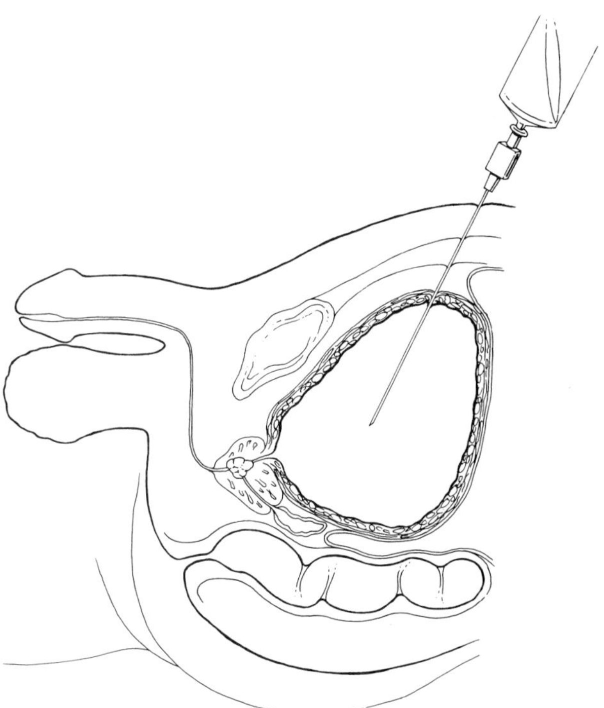

FIG. 91-16. Suprapubic cystostomy. Bladder position is verified with a syringe and needle.

TABLE 91-3 Etiology of Outlet Obstruction

Meatal stenosis
Urethral stricture
Bladder neck contracture
Benign prostatic hyperplasia

therefore infrequent, voiding during a prolonged car trip by a vacationing patient with borderline obstructive symptoms may be just enough to result in urinary retention.

A thorough voiding history begins with questions regarding problems holding or initiating the urinary stream, voiding completely with one continuous stream rather than starting and stopping of the stream, a feeling of complete bladder emptying as opposed to incomplete emptying and postvoid residual, and the relative frequency of nocturia. Ultrasonography is a noninvasive, accurate way to determine the postvoid residual. Most men do not void as well or completely empty their bladders when sitting down to urinate, which happens most often during the night. Infrequent ejaculation may lead to secondary prostatic congestion and subsequent spurious symptoms of irritation and outlet obstruction. Unless specific questions are asked about the latter circumstances, these easily treatable causes of obstructive symptoms can be missed.

The most difficult evaluation involves the patient with silent prostatism. Historically, voiding symptoms have gradually worsened over the years, but at such a pace that the patient often makes adjustments and then perceives each worsening state as ''normal'' for him. The ultimate result is retention, with a large palpable bladder and often 1600 to 2000 mL residual urine. An intact sensory examination, anal sphincter, and bulbocavernosus reflex differentiate chronic outlet obstruction from the sensory or motor neurogenic bladder and spinal cord compression.

Intraurethral causes of urinary retention are the same as those of outlet obstruction (Table 91-3). Appropriate physical examination requires inspection of the meatus for stenosis; palpation of the entire urethral length for masses or fistulas consistent with urethral stricture disease or abscess formation; lower abdominal examination for palpation of a suprapubic mass; and rectal examination to evaluate anal sphincter tone and the size and consistency of the prostate. Outlet obstruction due to a large intravesical prostate can result in a palpably normal prostate on rectal examination. Similarly, rectal examination in a patient in urinary retention may initially reveal a spuriously enlarged, nodular prostate that will shrink considerably once bladder decompression is achieved.

Most patients with bladder outlet obstruction are in distress, and passage of a urethral catheter alleviates both their pain and their urinary retention. Copious intraurethral lubrication must be used, and if attempts at passage of a straight 16F Foley catheter fail, a 16F Coudé catheter should be passed. Be certain to pass either catheter to its fullest extent, obtaining a free flow of urine, and only then inflate the catheter balloon. This will prevent balloon inflation in the prostatic urethra. If the catheter drainage holes become obstructed with lubricating jelly, gentle irrigation with sterile saline or water will quickly establish urinary drainage. Spontaneous, complete drainage of a distended bladder can be accomplished rapidly without the need for repeated clamping of the catheter. Occasionally, when a bladder has been chronically distended, bladder mucosal edema develops. Rapid decompression following catheter placement may result in transient gross hematuria. The transient hematuria is usually self-limited, of little consequence, and responds to orally induced diuresis. Postmicturitional or bladder decompression syncope is rare and should be treated symptomatically.

The catheter should be left indwelling and connected to a portable leg drainage bag. The patient or his family must be instructed in the care and drainage of this simple device. The initiation of antibiotic therapy depends on the presence or absence of infected urine and on the length of time catheter will be left indwelling. The patient or a family member should be instructed on Foley balloon deflation, should it become necessary to remove the catheter because of bladder spasms that are not responsive to oral anticholinergic medication.

If urinary retention has been chronic or insidious, postobstructive diuresis may occur secondary to osmotic diuresis or interstitial tubular dysfunction. Postobstructive diuresis may occur in the presence of normal BUN and creatinine levels and may become an emergency if the patient suddenly becomes hypovolemic or hypotensive without warning. Thus, close monitoring of urine output is essential, with appropriate fluid replacement. For these reasons, all patients with chronic or insidious obstructive voiding symptoms and urinary retention should either be observed for 4 to 6 h or be admitted, with particular attention paid to hourly intake, urinary output, vital signs, and urine and serum electrolytes. Osmotic diuresis will dissipate or the dysfunctional tubules will recover within 24 to 48 h. In all cases of urinary retention, consultation and follow-up with a urologist for a complete genitourinary evaluation are necessary.

BIBLIOGRAPHY

Barone JG, Fleisher MH: Treatment of paraphimosis using the "puncture" technique. *Pediatr Emerg Care* 9:298, 1993.

Cattolica EV: Preoperative manual detorsion of the torsed spermatic cord. *J Urol* 133:803, 1985.

Clayton MD, Fowler JE, Sharifi R, Pearl RK: Causes, presentation and survival of fifty-seven patients with necrotizing fasciitis of the male genitalia. *Surg Gynecol Obstet* 70:49, 1990.

Coldiron BM, Jacobson C: Common penile lesions. *Urol Clin North Am* 15:671, 1988.

Docimo SG, Rukstalis DB, Rukstalis MR, et al: Candida epididymitis: Newly recognized opportunistic epididymal infection. *Urology* 41:280, 1993.

Hendrikx AJ, Dang CL, Vroegindeweij D, Korte JH: B-mode and color-flow duplex ultrasonography: A useful adjunct in diagnosing scrotal diseases? *Br J Urol* 79:58, 1997.

Lewis AG, Bukowski TP, Jarvis PD, et al: Evaluation of acute scrotum in the emergency department. *J Pediatr Surg* 30:277, 1995.

Likitnukul S, McCraken GH, Nelson JD, Votteler TP: Epididymitis in children and adolescents. *Am J Dis Child* 141:41, 1987.

Lindsey D, Stanisic TH: Diagnosis and management of testicular torsion: Pitfalls and perils. *Am J Emerg Med* 6:42, 1988.

Mulhall JP, Honig SC: Priapism: Etiology and management. *Acad Emerg Med* 3:810, 1996.

O'Brien WM: Percutaneous placement of a suprapubic tube with peel away sheath introducer. *J Urol* 145:1015, 1991.

Paltiel HJ, Connolly LP, Atala A, et al: Acute scrotal symptoms in boys with an indeterminate clinical presentation: Comparison of color Doppler sonography and scintigraphy. *Radiology* 207:223, 1998.

Pryor JL, Watson LR, Day DL, et al: Scrotal ultrasound for evaluation of subacute testicular torsion: Sonographic findings and adverse clinical implications. *J Urol* 151:693, 1994.

Shanta TR, Finnerty DP, Rodriguez AP: Treatment of persistent penile erection and priapism using terbutaline. *J Urol* 141:1427, 1989.

Williams JC, Morrison PM, Richardson JR: Paraphimosis in elderly men. *Am J Emerg Med* 13:351, 1995.

UROLOGIC STONE DISEASE

Joel Moll
W. F. Peacock IV

Stones form throughout the urinary tract; however, the most frequent presentation to the emergency department occurs when renal stones migrate down the ureter. This acutely painful condition is called *renal colic.* While bladder stones do occur, they are much less common.

RENAL AND URETERAL STONES

Epidemiology

Urologic stone disease is a common condition with an incidence estimated as high as 12 percent.[1] Stones occur three times more often in males, usually in the third to fifth decades of life.[2] There is a genetic predisposition to stone development, and some hereditary diseases (e.g., renal tubular acidosis, hyperparathyroidism, and cystinuria) increase the frequency of kidney stones.[2]

Lifestyle factors may also augment stone growth. Patients in mountainous, desert, or tropical regions and those in sedentary jobs suffer a higher frequency of stone disease.[2] There is also an increased incidence during the warmest 3 months of the year for any geographic location.[2] In the United States the southeast region has a higher incidence than the remainder of the country.[3] Finally, increased water intake is associated with a decreased incidence of calculi.[4]

Some medications predispose to stone disease. Most recently, the protease inhibitor indinavir sulfate, used to treat HIV infection, has been associated with a 4 percent incidence of symptomatic urolithiasis. Diuretic use has also been shown to increase the prevalence of renal stones.[3]

Children under 16 years of age constitute approximately 7 percent of all cases of renal stones.[2] Unique to this age group is a 1:1 sex distribution.[2,5] The most common causes in this age group involve metabolic abnormalities (50 percent), urologic anomalies (20 percent), infection (15 percent), and immobilization syndrome (5 percent).[2] The remainder are diagnosed as idiopathic.

In patients with a history of a kidney stone, up to a third suffer recurrence within 1 year, with the recurrence rate at 5 years near 50 percent.[2] This is probably because the underlying abnormality that created the first stone is still present.

Pathophysiology

The precise cause of urinary stones is unknown. Theories regarding urinary calculi formation include urinary supersaturation of solute followed by crystal precipitation, or a decrease in the normal urinary proteins that inhibit crystal growth. Urinary stasis from physical anomaly, neurogenic bladder, or catheter placement, and the presence of foreign bodies (e.g., surgical suture) may provide the environment for stone growth.

Approximately 75 percent of calculi are composed of calcium, occurring in conjunction with oxalate, phosphate, or a combination of both.[2] These stones may develop as a result of increased urinary excretion of a given solute. Calcium excretion is elevated in conditions such as high dietary calcium intake, immobilization syndrome, or hyperparathyroidism. Oxalate excretion is enhanced in patients with bowel disease (e.g., Crohn's disease or ulcerative colitis) and as a result of small-bowel bypass surgery. Ten percent of stones are magnesium-ammonium-phosphate (struvite).[2] These stones are often associated with infection by urea-splitting bacteria and are the most common cause of staghorn calculi. Staghorn calculi are large stones that form a cast of the renal pelvis. Antibiotics are ineffective, since there is poor penetration into the calculus. Uric acid causes 10 percent of uroliths.[2] Cystine and other uncommon minerals comprise the remainder.[2]

Passage of stones through the urinary tract may be slowed or halted by areas of anatomic narrowing or bending. Progressing proximally to distally, common areas of impaction include the renal calyx, ureteropelvic junction (where the ureter passes over the pelvic brim and arches over the iliac vessels), and the ureterovesical junction (UVJ). The UVJ has the smallest diameter of the urinary tract and is a common location for impacted stones. The posterior pelvis in women, especially where the ureter is crossed anteriorly by the pelvic blood vessels and broad ligament, may slow the passage of a calculus.

If a stone causes acute ureteral obstruction, after an initial rise of renal blood flow and intraureteral pressure, both parameters decline. Concurrently, there is a proportional increase in renal blood flow to the contralateral kidney. These effects are reversible in acute unilateral obstruction if the obstruction is relieved. However, after prolonged obstruction (several weeks), irreversible renal damage occurs.[2] The contralateral kidney is usually able to maintain excretory requirements throughout the course. Therefore, blood urea nitrogen and creatinine levels do not rise even though there is only one functional kidney.

The probability of spontaneous passage of stones is determined by multiple factors, including size, shape, location, and degree of ureteral obstruction. Stones with diameters less than 4 mm will pass in approximately 90 percent of cases, while 50 percent of stones 4 to 6 mm in diameter pass, and only 10 percent of stones exceeding 6 mm pass spontaneously.[2] Bizarrely shaped or irregular stones with spicules and sharp edges will have a lower passage rate. Rates of passage based on the location of the stone at first diagnosis are approximately 20, 50, and 70 percent for the proximal, middle, and distal ureter, respectively.[6] Finally, with complete obstruction there is a lower rate of spontaneous passage than if the blockage is partial.

Clinical Features

Uroliths may be asymptomatic until there is at least partial obstruction of the urinary tract. The usual episode occurs while the patient is sedentary or at rest. Patients describe the acute onset of severe pain. Although subacute presentations occur, the usual rapidity of symptom onset is in contradistinction to many other diagnoses that may be considered.

Typically the pain originates in either flank, radiates anteroinferiorally around the abdomen, and progresses toward the ipsilateral testicle or labia majora. The discomfort can be extreme in intensity and may be associated with nausea, vomiting, or diaphoresis. Patients may be unable to find a comfortable position to relieve their symptoms. Consequently, they are sometimes anxious, pacing, and reluctant to lie still on the examining table. The ''writhing of renal colic'' is a useful point in the construction of a differential diagnosis.

The characteristic radiating pattern of renal colic pain results from autonomic nerve fibers serving both the kidney and respective gonad. However, atypical presentations with pain referral patterns to the hip, thigh, or knee are rarely reported.[2] As a stone progresses to the midureter, anterior abdominal pain may radiate back toward the flank. With passage near the bladder, the patient may develop urinary frequency and urgency. Symptoms can be remarkably episodic due to intermittent obstruction of the urinary tract. If the stone passes or the obstruction is temporarily relieved, the patient will have immediate relief of symptoms.

Patients are frequently cool and diaphoretic, and a history of fever is unusual. Its presence should prompt a thorough investigation for urinary tract infection or other causes of febrile illness.

In children, symptoms can vary with age. Older children are more likely to present in similar fashion to the adult. Younger children may have a more nonspecific presentation, such as abdominal or pelvic pain. Although renal colic is rare in infants, symptoms may be mistakenly attributed to intestinal colic.[5] Overall, 20 to 30 percent of children may have only painless hematuria.[2]

Patients with known stone disease may present after treatment with extracorporeal shock wave lithotripsy (ESWL). ESWL fractures stones into small particles using focused sound waves. The resulting ''sludge'' is passed in the urine. When there are large fragments, an acute episode of renal colic occurs. The presentation is identical to ''de novo'' episodes of renal colic.

Diagnosis

PHYSICAL EXAMINATION Special attention should be given to the abdominal and cardiovascular portions so that potential catastrophes mimicking acute renal colic are excluded. The vital signs should be carefully noted. There may be elevations of blood pressure and pulse secondary to extreme discomfort. The presence of fever or hypotension should suggest the possibility of concurrent infection or a diagnosis other than renal colic.

The abdominal examination is extremely important. It should specifically include a search for the presence of bruit or a pulsatile mass to ensure that a rupturing or dissecting aortic aneurysm is not missed. Likewise, the pulses in the distal extremities should be carefully examined. If they are diminished, absent, or asymmetric, this suggests a potential vascular catastrophe.

Mild tenderness may be noted over the site of an impacted stone. However, true peritoneal findings (e.g., guarding or rebound) are not a component of acute renal colic. If peritoneal signs are found, the differential diagnosis should be expanded to include those pathologic conditions known to result in discomfort at that anatomic region. Similarly, abdominal distention is not a feature of renal colic. If present, it suggests an alternative explanation of the patient's presentation.

Of equal importance during the physical examination is the genitourinary examination. Costovertebral angle tenderness is not unusual, but, when present with fever or other signs of urinary tract infection, it may suggest pyelonephritis. Pyelonephritis can occur simultaneously with stone disease. In addition, since the radiating pattern of discomfort in renal colic includes the testicle or labia majora, these areas should be evaluated for a potential incarcerated hernia. In a male patient, the testicles should be inspected and palpated to exclude torsion or infection. A pelvic examination should be performed in females when the diagnosis is not clear to assess for ovarian cyst, torsion, infection, or, of importance in pregnant patients, ectopic pregnancy.

Other portions of the physical examination should address the cardiac, respiratory, musculoskeletal, and dermatologic systems. An abnormal cardiopulmonary examination may suggest an alternative diagnosis, such as lobar pneumonia or pulmonary embolus. Musculoskeletal complaints may result in flank pain similar to that caused by renal stones; however, comprehensive extremity and neurologic examinations are usually sufficient to exclude these conditions. Finally, the presence of a vesicular rash overlying a flank dermatome may suggest the onset of herpes zoster.

LABORATORY TESTS All patients with suspected renal colic require a urinalysis. The presence of blood in the urine supports the diagnosis of renal colic. However, there is no correlation between the amount of hematuria and the degree of urinary tract obstruction.[7] Some patients demonstrate gross hematuria, but in up to 15 percent microscopic hematuria is absent.[8] A urine dipstick is an expedient method to aid in the initial diagnosis. The dipstick has excellent sensitivity for detecting red blood cells; however, hemoglobin and myoglobin will also test positively for blood. Therefore, a microscopic analysis should be performed on all dipstick-positive urines. A urinalysis may also help in excluding other alternative or associated conditions, such as infection. Patients with fever, pyuria, or a history of fever and chills should also have a urine culture obtained. Blood cultures, although not routinely required in uncomplicated pyelonephritis,[9,10] should be considered with concurrent obstruction, underlying comorbidity, or systemic toxicity. Urinary crystals, usually oxalate or rarely urate, may indicate the etiology of the present attack and the composition of the stone. However, because such crystals may be seen without association with renal stones, their presence is not diagnostic and should be interpreted cautiously. An elevated urine pH (>7.6) associated with infection may indicate the presence of a urea-splitting organism. An alkaline urine is also seen in renal tubular acidosis or following ingestion of large amounts of alkali. Urine should be collected and strained for the identification of any passed stones. All collected stones should be retained for pathologic analysis.

A pregnancy test specific for the β-HCG subunit should be performed on women of childbearing age. A positive β-HCG test result may indicate an important alternative cause of the patient's complaints, such as ectopic pregnancy. In addition, a positive test result will affect the choice of imaging study to confirm the diagnosis of renal colic.

A complete blood count is indicated if the history or physical examination suggests the possibility of anemia or infection. In straightforward cases of renal colic, a complete blood count is not indicated. If obtained, a complete blood count may demonstrate mild leukocytosis. This indicates white blood cell demargination from stress. A very high white blood cell count may represent infection.

Other laboratory evaluations can be individualized. Serologic testing of renal function (e.g., determination of blood urea nitrogen and creatinine levels) may be required in patients at risk for nephrotoxicity (elderly patients, those with renal insufficiency, diabetic patients, and hypovolemic patients) if a radiocontrast dye study is planned. In addition, diabetic patients should have a glucose level determination to ensure the stress of renal colic has not caused significant hyperglycemia. Diabetics with significant nausea and vomiting may be at risk for hypoglycemia.

DIAGNOSTIC IMAGING The choice of an imaging modality to confirm the diagnosis of urolithiasis should be made with an understanding of the strengths and limitations of each test in conjunction with the characteristics of the patient and the capabilities of the institution. Historically, the standard for diagnosis of renal colic has been the intravenous pyelogram (IVP). With the advent of newer-generation computed tomography (CT) scanners, the use of noncontrast helical CT scanning in the evaluation of flank pain has dramatically increased. In some institutions helical CT has replaced IVP as the initial diagnostic imaging study. Helical CT is generally the emergency department procedure of choice except with pregnant patients, for whom ultrasound is preferred to minimize radiation exposure. Other modalities that may assist in the diagnosis include ultrasound, radionuclide renal scan, and plain abdominal radiographs.

It is controversial whether all patients require emergency department imaging for suspected renal colic. For young, healthy patients in whom the diagnosis is not in question, it may be appropriate to delay the workup, which can be conducted later on an outpatient basis.[11] For older patients, especially those in whom the differential diagnosis includes aortic abdominal aneurysm (AAA), the diagnosis should be confirmed by some imaging modality.

COMPUTED TOMOGRAPHY The noncontrast helical CT scan has been shown to be both sensitive (95 to 97 percent) and specific (96 to 98 percent) in the detection of renal stones.[12,13] Its accuracy is comparable or superior to that of the IVP.[14] Images are obtained from the top of the kidney to the base of the bladder. Refocused images can be obtained in smaller increments through levels of suspicious calcifications and areas of ureteral caliber change. Secondary signs of ureteral obstruction, such as ureteral dilatation, stranding of perinephric fat, dilation of the collecting system, and renal enlargement, can also be helpful in making the diagnosis. In combination, unilateral ureteral dilatation and perinephric stranding have a positive predictive value of 96 percent for stone disease.[13,15] When both are absent, the negative predictive value is 93 to 97 percent.[13,15]

Noncontrast helical CT has several advantages over other imaging modalities, including the avoidance of exposure to radiocontrast agent, greater potential for identifying causes other than stone disease, and superior speed. However, because oral and intravenous radiocontrast agents are not used, the specificity and sensitivity for other diseases, such as AAA or gastrointestinal disorders, are not as great as with imaging protocols employing contrast. Interpretation of a "negative" noncontrast CT scan, when obtained to evaluate the possibility of urologic stone disease, should be done cautiously and with consideration of the limitations of the study. Most newer-generation CT scanners can complete the study within 5 min.[13]

Several disadvantages exist in the use of CT. Helical CT does not evaluate renal function or provide physiologic information about the degree of obstruction. Furthermore, its diagnostic ability relies on a newer-generation CT scanner with a radiologist skilled in using this modality to evaluate stone disease. At some institutions the cost of CT may be greater than that of other imaging modalities.

Abdominal CT scanning is the modality of choice if suspicion of a perinephric abscess exists. However, the use of radiocontrast agents may be required for adequate detection of a potential abscess.

INTRAVENOUS PYELOGRAM The IVP yields information regarding both renal function and anatomic morphology. Its ability to detect renal calculi has been found to be less than that of CT, with a sensitivity of 64 to 90 percent and specificity of 94 to 100 percent.[16,17]

When performing the IVP, intravenous fluid is administered to ensure that the patient is hydrated and will sustain adequate urinary flow throughout the procedure. Maintaining adequate urine output by the administration of intravenous fluids prior to radiocontrast media may decrease the risk of renal injury from radiocontrast dye. After radiocontrast media is administered, an initial scout radiograph is obtained, followed by repeat films at 5, 10, and 20 min. The first and most reliable indication of the presence of obstruction is a delay in the appearance of the nephrogram. Since the ureter is a peristaltic structure, it is usually not completely seen on any one radiograph. Visualization of the entire ureter is suggestive of obstruction.

The location of a radiolucent obstructing stone can often be determined by a ureteral dye-column cutoff. Adjuncts to the diagnosis of renal colic include the presence of a prolonged nephrogram, renal enlargement, dilatation of the collecting system or ureter, and dye extravasation.[18] If extravasation of dye is noted, it should be considered evidence of an obstruction that has decompressed into the perinephric tissue. Extraurinary collections of urine (urinoma) have the potential for infection and abscess formation.

A postvoid film is useful for identifying stones at the UVJ or distal ureter that are otherwise obscured by a full bladder. Multiple delayed films may be required to precisely determine the level of obstruction.

The main advantage of the IVP over other imaging modalities is its ability to give information on both renal function and anatomy. In addition, IVP may be more widely available than CT, depending on the institution. It may also be valuable as an adjunct to CT when functional information and knowledge of the degree of obstruction are required.

The most important potential disadvantage of the IVP is use of radiocontrast dye. Side effects of radiocontrast dye, allergic reaction and nephrotoxicity, must always be considered when ordering an IVP. Prior to obtaining an IVP, the patient should be closely questioned regarding the presence of allergy to radiocontrast media. Appropriate material for managing acute anaphylaxis should be immediately available for unexpected allergic reactions. A history of dye allergy should prompt the selection of an alternative diagnostic modality.

Radiocontrast-agent nephrotoxicity is most likely to occur in patients with preexisting renal insufficiency or diabetes mellitus.[18] These patients have a 9 percent risk of nephrotoxicity attributable to radiocontrast dye.[18] Other predisposing factors include dehydration, hypovolemia, hypotension, advanced age (over 70 years), multiple myeloma, hyperuricemia, hypertension, a history of intravenous radiocontrast media within 72 h, and the use of diuretics to treat cardiovascular disease. In patients at risk for nephrotoxicity when the administration of a radiocontrast agent is not otherwise contraindicated, the dye administration should be deferred until normal blood urea nitrogen and creatinine levels are documented. Although they are also nephrotoxic, nonionic contrast agents may result in a lower frequency of kidney damage. Finally, radiocontrast media should be used with caution in patients taking metformin, which has been associated with severe lactic acidosis and nephropathy in combination with radiocontrast material. Other imaging modalities, such as noncontrast CT or ultrasound, may be preferred for these patients.

Another disadvantage of the IVP is the potential time required to complete the study. If evidence of obstruction exists, serial delayed films are often obtained to delineate the level of obstruction. This may require several hours and multiple repeat radiographs and may delay the final diagnosis. Also affecting the quality of the IVP is the state of the bowel. Since emergency department practice does not allow for a bowel preparation, the IVP can be adversely affected by obstipation or ileus.

A false-negative IVP infrequently occurs when there is a small or radiolucent, partially obstructing stone. The IVP will also be "negative" if the ureteral stone passes into the bladder before radiocontrast dye is excreted by the kidneys. If this happens, the patient usually experiences nearly complete relief of pain. The IVP may also show evidence of ureteral spasm after passage of a stone.

ULTRASOUND With patients who are not candidates for IVP or CT due to concerns of exposure to radiocontrast media (e.g., allergy) or radiation (e.g., with pregnant patients or children), ultrasound may assist in the diagnosis of urolithiasis. It is useful in the detection of larger stones; however, it may miss smaller (less than 5 mm in diameter) ureteral stones.[19] Ultrasound is helpful in diagnosing stones in the proximal and distal ureter. However, it does a poor job of visualizing mid-ureteral stones. Overall it has been shown to be 63 to 85 percent sensitive and 79 to 100 percent specific in diagnosing renal stones.[16,17] Ultrasound is very sensitive (98 percent) in detecting hydronephrosis, which may be a result of a renal calculus; however, the presence of hydronephrosis has a much lower specificity (78 percent).[18] Up to 22 percent of apparent cases of hydronephrosis by ultrasound do not represent obstruction.[18] Causes of false-positive results include normal variations, an extrarenal pelvis, a full bladder, an intravenous fluid bolus, and renal cysts.[18] Ultrasound studies can also obtain information on renal size and, with Doppler scanning, renal blood and urine flow. Limited information may also be obtained regarding other pathologic conditions mimicking urologic stone disease.

Ultrasound has many advantages: it is noninvasive, utilizes no radiocontrast dye or radiation, and has no known side effects.[18] It may also be superior to an IVP in detecting stones at the UVJ.[20] Ultrasound is, however, limited to anatomic findings only. It yields no information on renal function. In addition, the accuracy of ultrasound studies is operator and equipment dependent, body habitus (e.g., obesity) may interfere with obtaining good-quality scans, and ultrasound may miss obstructive signs in the early phase of renal colic. In addition, the rapid bolus infusion of crystalloid can result in a false-positive finding of hydroureter on ultrasound examination.

RENAL SCAN With the increased utilization of CT and ultrasound and the reduced availability of renal scanning, the use of the latter is limited as an initial imaging modality in renal colic.[18]

PLAIN ABDOMINAL RADIOGRAPHS The composition of most urinary calculi makes them sufficiently dense that the majority (90 percent) are radiopaque.[2] Calcium phosphate and calcium oxalate stones have a density similar to that of bone. Magnesium-ammonium-phosphate (struvite) calculi are slightly less radiodense, followed by cystine, which is only partially radiodense. Uric acid and matrix stones are essentially radiolucent. Most stones associated with medications are radiolucent as well, including those associated with the protease inhibitor indinavir.[21] However, because of their small size and the overlapping soft-tissue and bone shadows seen on abdominal radiographs, urinary stones are visible much less frequently on plain films. Plain abdominal radiographs alone have a low sensitivity (29 to 58 percent) and specificity (69 to 74 percent) compared to other imaging modalities.[17,22,23] In addition, a low negative predictive value (23 percent) makes a "negative" radiograph of little value in ruling out stone disease.[22] While a plain abdominal radiograph can assist in localizing some large radiopaque stones, its greatest utility is in the exclusion of other pathologic conditions. However, a plain abdominal radiograph may be helpful in patients with dye allergy, when other imaging modalities are unavailable, or in follow-up of known radiopaque stones. In patients for whom the diagnosis is already established (recent IVP, CT, or ESWL), a plain abdominal radiograph may suffice in localizing a migrating stone.

Differential Diagnosis

A number of diagnoses can be confused with renal colic. The history and physical examination can help to narrow the differential. However, this may be difficult, since the patient's discomfort can interfere with the usual history and physical examination. Crucial to the evaluation of these patients is to ensure that a catastrophe mimicking renal colic is not missed.

The most critical alternative diagnosis to consider is an aortic dissection or ruptured AAA. Renal colic and AAA may have a similar presentation. Focal abdominal tenderness, abdominal distention, pulse disparity, and hemodynamic instability are not found in renal colic. These findings suggest a leaking or ruptured AAA. If a dissection or rupture is suspected, an emergency vascular surgical consultation should be obtained. If an AAA has not been excluded from the differential diagnosis, appropriate monitoring equipment, intravenous access, and professional staff should be sent from the emergency department with the patient for an imaging study.

Pyelonephritis may also cause flank pain; however the prodrome is less acute and the discomfort usually not as severe as renal colic. Fever is not a finding with kidney stones, and the urinalysis of renal colic does not demonstrate bacteriuria or pyuria in the absence of a concurrent infection. If renal obstruction is suspected concurrently with pyelonephritis, obstruction must be excluded by IVP, CT, or ultrasound. Antibiotics have poor penetration into an obstructed kidney. If infection in the presence of obstruction is confirmed, emergency urologic consultation for prompt obstruction relief should be obtained.

Papillary necrosis presents much as renal stones do. It is most frequently seen in patients with sickle cell disease, diabetes, nonsteroidal analgesic abuse, or infection. The urinalysis may appear to represent infection, with hematuria and pyuria. An IVP or CT can demonstrate sloughed renal papillae as a lucency within the renal pelvis. Urologic consultation and hospitalization are usually required.

Renal infarction, resulting from vascular dissection or arterial embolus, may present with acute flank pain. Urinalysis can demonstrate hematuria, and imaging will show decreased or absent function of the affected kidney. Emergency angiography is indicated. In renal vein thrombosis, there may be increased kidney size with decreased function. Urinalysis shows proteinuria and microscopic hematuria. All of these conditions require emergency urologic consultation.

Other pathologic conditions may cause compression or obstruction of the ureter, producing symptoms similar to those of renal colic. Any intrabdominal mass, including neoplasm or vascular structure, can potentially cause external compression of the ureter. A mass located within the urinary system may also cause obstruction and/or pain due to expanding size or in association with hemorrhage or necrosis. Therefore, a neoplasm is always within the differential diagnosis of renal colic.

Patients with severe abdominal pain out of proportion to the findings upon physical examination (especially if elderly or if the pain is in association with atrial fibrillation, congestive heart failure, liver disease, or low-flow vascular states) should raise suspicion of intestinal ischemia.

Gallstone pain can be very similar to that of renal colic and should generally be considered in all patients with any right upper quadrant abdominal tenderness. Unlike the symptoms of renal colic, biliary colic symptoms are often associated with oral intake, last for several hours before remitting, and include vomiting. Pancreatitis is suggested by left upper quadrant or midepigastric pain, especially in the presence of risk factors (e.g., alcohol consumption or cholelithiasis). A perforated peptic ulcer may present with severe pain in the midepigastrum or either upper quadrant. However, these patients have marked tenderness on examination and develop peritoneal signs over time. Appendicitis shares the unilateral presentation with renal colic, but the subacute prodrome usually excludes urolithiasis. Ventral hernias should also be considered in the differential diagnosis and sought on physical examination. Diverticulitis usually causes pain in lower quadrants, more commonly the left, and is associated with abdominal tenderness, fever, diarrhea, possibly hematochezia, but a more insidious prodrome than renal colic.

In women, gynecologic disorders can mimic renal colic. Ruptured ectopic pregnancy can present with acute pelvic and flank pain. A history of amenorrhea, tenderness on pelvic examination, and a positive pregnancy test result suggest this diagnosis rather than renal colic. Hemoperitoneum from a ruptured ectopic pregnancy may cause radiation of pain similar to that of renal colic as blood tracks along the abdominal cavity. Salpingitis usually has a more insidious onset, with cervical motion and uterine tenderness, and purulent discharge on pelvic examination. A tuboovarian abscess usually presents as salpingitis does, along with adenexal tenderness and mass on pelvic examination. An enlarging or ruptured ovarian cyst or ovarian or pelvic mass torsion should also be considered.

In men, other etiologies involving the genitourinary system must also be considered. Although renal colic can often cause pain radiating to the testicle, the findings on physical examination of the affected testicle should be normal. The presence of pain, redness, or swelling on examination should indicate another cause. Testicular torsion can present with the same sudden onset as renal colic; however, physical examination localizes the pathology to the testicle. Other entities, including infections such as epididymitis, prostatitis, and Fournier's gangrene, may have a more insidious onset, and the physical examination will differentiate them from renal colic. Finally, an incarcerated or strangulated hernia should be excluded by examination of the inguinal canals and scrotum.

Drug seekers may present with factitious episodes of renal colic. They can be remarkably inventive in the complexity of their ruse, and there is no specific method of detecting them. A history of multiple medical allergies to nonnarcotic analgesics and radiocontrast media is frequently given. Such patients may report having a known radiolucent stone and may simulate hematuria by placing blood in their urine. The vital signs may suggest this behavior if changes in blood pressure and heart rate do not match the extreme discomfort demonstrated. When the clinician is unsure, it is better to give analgesia than to deprive a patient suffering from true renal colic.

Treatment

The mainstay of emergency department treatment is pain control. Because in most cases the diagnosis is clinical, a rapid urine dipstick test for heme may provide sufficient information, coupled with clinical findings, to initiate analgesic therapy. Pain medication should not be delayed pending test results. Adequate analgesia frequently requires multiple doses of intravenous narcotics, titrated to the patient's level of discomfort. Narcotics may be accompanied by nonsteroidal anti-inflammatory drugs (NSAIDs) but NSAIDs should not be used in place of narcotics. The time of onset of NSAIDs is slower than that of intravenous narcotics. NSAIDs should be used with caution in patients with suspected compromise in overall renal function (elderly patients, diabetics, those with known renal insufficiency, and hypovolemic patients) so as not to precipitate or accelerate a decline in renal function. An antiemetic is an appropriate adjunct when emesis accompanies the symptoms or when nausea accompanies narcotic use. Intravenous fluids, usually normal saline solution, should be administered. For patients with evidence of associated infection, parenteral antibiotics should be administered promptly in the emergency department, and emergency urologic consultation should be obtained.

Disposition

Admission to the hospital is indicated if there is (1) infection with concurrent obstruction, (2) a solitary kidney and complete obstruction, (3) uncontrolled pain, or (4) intractable emesis.[2] Patients with an infection and concurrent obstruction have the potential for severe systemic toxicity and represent a urologic emergency. Patients with renal impairment are candidates for consideration of a drainage procedure, since they have little functional renal reserve. Because of lower rates of spontaneous passage, patients with large (>5 mm), irregular, or proximal stones should be considered for admission. If there is severe concurrent underlying disease (e.g., angina or chronic obstructive pulmonary disease) or in the fragile elderly, when the patient may be unable to tolerate the stress of renal colic, a lower admission threshold is indicated. When the IVP or CT scan demonstrates complete obstruction, or dye extravasation, the admission decision requires individualization and discussion with a urologist. Patients who have previously been diagnosed and managed as outpatients are more likely to require admission if they return with continued pain. A careful history and physical examination are indicated to ensure that the diagnosis is correct, but repeat imaging is probably unnecessary.

In most situations, unilateral renal obstruction has minimal acute or permanent effects. Discharge is appropriate in patients with smaller, rounded stones, in the absence of infection, and when pain is controlled by oral analgesics. Patients should be given a urinary strainer with instructions to save any stones that are passed for pathologic evaluation. Patients should be counseled to return promptly for fever, vomiting, or uncontrolled pain, and they require a prescription for an oral narcotic. Follow-up with a urologist should be arranged within 7 days.[24] Patients whose stone passes in the emergency department require no further treatment. Elective urologic consultation should be arranged so that the etiology of the stone can be determined and a prophylactic strategy arranged. Patients with hematuria, negative imaging study findings, and no other attributable source require urologic follow-up to determine the etiology of their hematuria.

The management of patients with protease-inhibitor-induced urolithiasis is similar to the management of other causes of stone disease; however, adequate hydration is particularly important.[21] In addition, discontinuation of the offending agent for a short period of time may be necessary. Such a decision should be made in consultation with a urologist and an infectious disease specialist. Disposition should be discussed with a urologist if there is (1) renal insufficiency, (2) severe underlying disease, (3) an IVP showing extravasation or complete obstruction, (4) multiple visits, (5) a large stone, or (6) sloughed renal papillae.[2]

BLADDER (VESICAL) STONES

Vesical calculi may occur at any age and are endemic in some developing countries.[25] In endemic areas and historically, the vast majority occur in males and develop in early childhood. In western, industrialized countries, 90 percent occur in males, and 80 percent occur in patients over 50 years of age. Calculi are associated with outflow obstruction or neuropathic bladder disease in 70 percent of cases. Urinary tract infection, vesical diverticuli, and the presence of foreign bodies (e.g., sutures, catheters, or implants) also predispose to bladder calculi. Bladder calculi have been reported in children and adults as a complication of urologic surgery. Calcium oxalate is the most common constituent of bladder stones, but urate and struvite stones also occur. Stones are usually solitary, but multiple stones occur in 25 to 30 percent of cases.[26]

Bladder calculi may be asymptomatic, especially in patients with underlying prostatic obstruction. Typical symptoms are intermittent dysuria and terminal hematuria. The greatest discomfort usually occurs at the end of micturition as the stone impinges upon the bladder neck. In bladder outlet obstruction, there is interruption of the urinary stream, with frequency and urgency commonly reported. There may be associated dull, aching low abdominal pain, unrelated to urination, that is exacerbated by exercise and abrupt movement. Pain is usually referred to the penile tip or scrotum by the second and third sacral nerves. Occasionally pain is referred to the low back or heel. With passage of the calculus, urethral obstruction can occur. Pain is referred to the rectum, the perineal area, or the site of urethral impaction. Patients report interruption of urinary flow followed by pain and urgency.

Physical examination is of little help in diagnosing a bladder calculus. Rarely, exceptionally large stones may be palpated during the rectal, vaginal, or abdominal examination. Urinalysis may demonstrate hematuria, pyuria, or bacteriuria. If there is coexistent infection, a complete blood count may show leukocytosis. Plain radiographs reveal vesical stones in approximately 50 percent of cases. While ultrasound may demonstrate bladder stones, cystoscopic examination is the most accurate method of detection.

Other cystic pathologic conditions can mimic vesical stones, including a foreign body, carcinoma, neurogenic bladder, bladder diverticula, or fistula. Complications include chronic bladder irritation, fistula formation, and urethral obstruction. Pericystitis may develop in chronic cases, and this can result in adherence of the bladder to the adjacent pelvic fat. Bladder perforation is a rare complication.

Bladder calculi require emergency therapy when they result in urinary obstruction or there is associated infection. Acute urethral obstruction requires either the successful removal of the stone or the placement of a catheter. Very distal stones may be able to be gently milked from the penis or removed by forceps. More proximal stones require emergency urologic consultation. If there is coexistent infection, antibiotics should be administered in the emergency department. Most patients with vesical calculi require cystoscopic stone removal. Any patient demonstrating signs of sepsis, urinary infection, or uretheral obstruction requires emergency hospitalization. Patients with symptomatic but nonobstructing bladder stones may be discharged with referral to a urologist.

REFERENCES

1. Seftel A, Resnick MI: Metabolic evaluation of urolithiasis. *Urol Clin North Am* 7:159, 1990.
2. Drach GW: Urinary lithiasis: Etiology, diagnosis, and medical management, in Walsh PC, Retik AB, Stamey TA, Vaughn ED (eds): *Campbell's Urology*, 6th ed, vol 3. Philadelphia, Saunders, 1992.
3. Souchie JM, Coates RJ, McClennan W, et al: Relation between geographic variability in kidney stones prevalence and risk factors for stones. *Am J Epidemiol* 143:487, 1996.
4. Borghi L, Meschi T, Amato F, et al: Urinary volume, water and recurrences in idiopathic calcium nephrolithiasis: A 5-year randomized prospective study. *J Urol* 155:839, 1996.
5. Kroovand LR: Pediatric urolithiasis. *Urol Clin North Am* 24:173, 1997.
6. Morse R, Resnick M: Ureteral calculi: Natural history and treatment in an era of advanced technology. *J Urol* 145:263, 1991.
7. Stewart DP, Kowalski R, Wong P, Krome R: Microscopic hematuria and calculus-related ureteral obstruction. *J Emerg Med* 8:693, 1990.
8. Press SM, Smith AD: Incidence of negative hematuria in patients with acute urinary lithiasis presenting to the emergency room with flank pain. *Urology* 45:753, 1995.
9. McMurray BR, Wrenn KD, Wright DW: Usefulness of blood cultures in pyelonephritis. *Am J Emerg Med* 15:137, 1997.
10. Thanassi M: Utility of urine and blood cultures in pyelonephritis. *Acad Emerg Med* 4:797, 1997.
11. Tasso SR, Shields CP, Rosenberg CR, et al: Effectiveness of selective use of intravenous pyelography in patients presenting to the emergency department with ureteral colic. *Acad Emerg Med* 4:780, 1997.
12. Smith RC, Dalrymple NC, Neitlich J: Noncontrast helical CT in the evaluation of acute flank pain. *Abdom Imaging* 23:10, 1998.
13. Smith RC, Verga M, McCarthy S, Rosenfield AT: Diagnosis of acute flank pain: Value of unenhanced helical CT. *AJR* 166:97, 1996.
14. Smith RC, Rosenfield AT, Choe KA, et al: Acute flank pain: Comparison of non-contrast-enhanced CT and intravenous urography. *Radiology* 194:789, 1995.
15. Smith RC, Verga M, Dalrymple NC, et al: Acute ureteral obstruction: Value of secondary signs on helical unenhanced CT. *AJR* 167:1109, 1996.
16. Sinclair D, Wilson S, Toi A, Greenspan L: The evaluation of suspected renal colic: Ultrasound scan versus excretory urography. *Ann Emerg Med* 18:556, 1989.
17. Svedstrom E, Alanen A, Nurmi M: Radiologic evaluation of renal colic: The role of plain films, excretory urolography, and sonography. *Eur J Radiol* 11:180, 1990.
18. Koelliker SL, Cronan JJ: Acute urinary tract obstruction: Imaging update. *Urol Clin North Am* 24:571, 1997.
19. Juul N, Brons J, Torp-Pederson S, Fredfeldt KE: Ultrasound versus intravenous urography in the initial evaluation of patients with suspected obstructing urinary calculi. *Scand J Urol Nephrol Suppl* 137:45, 1991.
20. Kolbeck SC, Watson LR, Jenkins AD: Sonographic detection of ureteral calculi patients with normal excretory urography. *J Urol* 148:1084, 1992.
21. Gentle DL, Stroller ML, Jarrett TW, et al: Protease inhibitor-induced urolithiaisis. *Urology* 50:508, 1997.
22. Mutgi A, Williams JW, Nettleman M: Renal colic: Utility of plain abdominal roentgenogram. *Arch Intern Med* 151:1589, 1991.
23. Boyd R, Gray AJ: Role of the plain radiograph and urinalysis in acute ureteral colic. *J Accid Emerg Med* 13:390, 1996.
24. Singal RK, Denstedt JD: Contemporary management of ureteral stones. *Urol Clin North Am* 24:59, 1997.
25. Ashworth M: Endemic bladder stones. *BMJ* 301:826, 1990.
26. Schweizer W, Stutz P, Moll W: More than 104 urinary bladder stones. *Trop Doctor* 22:45, 1992.

HEMATURIA AND HEMATOSPERMIA

David S. Howes
Mark P. Bogner

HEMATURIA

Normal urine contains a small number of red blood cells (RBCs), usually too small to be detected by routine chemical dipstick testing or microscopic urinalysis. Hematuria—blood detected by routine methods—may be visible to the eye (gross or frank hematuria) or invisible (microscopic hematuria). The appearance of blood in a patient's urine often motivates the patient to come to the emergency department with a presenting symptom of gross hematuria. Microscopic hematuria is usually detected in the course of evaluating other symptoms. Hematuria may be associated with pain during urination and often accompanies urinary tract infections. Painless hematuria is more often due to neoplastic, hyperplastic, and vascular causes. Gross or microscopic hematuria warrants an attempt at definitive diagnosis, since underlying disease can be found in a substantial percentage of cases. The emergency physician's task is to rule out a life-threatening

TABLE 93-1 Most Common Causes of Hematuria

Etiology	Associated Age
Infections	Women, >15, men >45
Nephrolithiasis	Usually >20
Neoplasms	Typically >40 (except Wilms)
Benign prostatic hypertrophy	Males >40
Glomerulonephritis	Mostly young patients and children
Shistosomiasis	Any, most common cause worldwide

cause, make a diagnosis if possible, initiate treatment, educate the patient, and ensure continued appropriate treatment, disposition, follow-up, and referral.

Epidemiology

Gross hematuria is easy to define: the urine is colored red. However, other pigments, particularly myoglobin, may discolor the urine, or the urine may be contaminated by bleeding from a nonurinary source. It takes approximately 1 mL of whole blood per liter of urine to result in grossly visible hematuria. Gross hematuria may also result in false proteinuria, since 1 mL of whole blood equals about 5 billion RBCs or 50 mg of albumin. This must be taken into account when protein-losing diseases (e.g., nephritic or nephrotic syndromes) are considered in the differential diagnosis. About 3 percent of the general population has had an episode of gross hematuria.[1] The incidence is higher in women (due to urinary tract infections), older adults (due to neoplasia), and older men (due to prostatic hyperplasia).

Microscopic hematuria is more difficult to define. Approximately 1 million RBCs pass into the urine each day. This amount is detected as 1 to 3 RBCs/hpf (400 ×) in centrifuged urine sediment. While various definitions have been proposed, the most common (and arbitrary) definition of microscopic hematuria is more than 5 RBCs/hpf. Population-based studies of healthy young individuals have found at least one episode of transient microscopic hematuria in up to 40 percent of men and 13 percent of women.[2–5] The incidence of microscopic hematuria in children and adolescents is up to 6 percent for one specimen and 1 to 2 percent for two positive specimens.[6,7]

Pathophysiology

Any process that results in infection, inflammation, or injury to the kidneys, ureters, bladder, prostate, male genitalia, or urethra may result in hematuria (Tables 93-1 and 93-2). In false hematuria, the urine appears bloody, but dipstick test results are negative for blood, and there are no RBCs on microscopic evaluation (Table 93-3). Free hemoglobin, myoglobin, or porphyrins in the urine result in a positive urine test strip reaction for blood but no RBCs on microscopic evaluation.

Clinical Features

It is useful to identify when the blood appears during micturition. Initial hematuria is the appearance of blood at the beginning of micturition, with subsequent clearing, and suggests urethral disease. Hematuria occurring between voidings and noticed only as staining of underclothes with blood, while voided urine is clear, indicates lesions at the distal urethra or the meatus. Total hematuria is visible throughout micturition and corresponds to disease of the kidneys, ureters, or bladder. Terminal hematuria, occurring at the end of micturition after initially voiding clear urine, occurs with disease at the bladder neck or prostatic urethra.

Gross hematuria more often indicates a lower-tract cause, while microscopic hematuria tends to occur with kidney disease. Brown or smoky-colored urine along with RBC casts and proteinuria suggests a glomerular source. Red, clotted blood in the urine indicates a source below the kidneys. Hematuria that varies with menstruation and is associated with severe dysmenorrhea may indicate endometriosis involving the urinary tract.

In younger patients, microscopic hematuria is most often caused by nephrolithiasis or urinary tract infection. It is also important to consider such disorders as glomerulonephritis, immune complex disease, Goodpasture's syndrome, Henoch-Schönlein purpura and Wilms' tumor in children, and sickle cell anemia or trait. Poststreptococcal glomerulonephritis is more common in children and typically follows a throat or skin infection. Symptoms appear 7 to 14 days after the primary infection, and the subsequent findings can vary from isolated hematuria to severe nephritis. Unfortunately, treatment of the primary streptococcal infection with antibiotics does not prevent poststreptococcal glomerulonephritis. IgA nephropathy develops several days after a viral respiratory infection and is often accompanied by proteinuria secondary to glomerular damage from immune-complex deposition.

In older patients, infections and nephrolithiasis remain common causes of hematuria, but after age 40 any hematuria, even with a clear diagnosis of urinary tract infection or stone, warrants close follow-up

TABLE 93-2 Differential Diagnosis of Hematuria

UROLOGIC (LOWER TRACT)
Any location
Iatrogenic, postprocedure
Trauma
Infection
Stones, calculi
Erosion, mechanical obstruction by tumor
Ureter(s)
Dilatation, stricture
Bladder
Transitional cell carcinoma
Vascular lesions, malformations
Chemical cystitis
Pancreas transplant drained into bladder
Emphysematous cystitis (associated pneumaturia)
Prostate
Benign prostatic hypertrophy
Prostatitis
Urethra
Stricture
Diverticulor
Foreign body
Endometriosis (cyclic hematuria with menstrual pain)
RENAL (UPPER TRACT)
Glomerular
Poststreptococcal glomerulonephritis
Other glomerulonephritis
IgA nephropathy (Berger's disease)
Thin-membrane nephropathy
Lupus nephritis
Hereditary nephritis (Alport's syndrome)
Fabry's disease (familial glycolipid disease)
Toxemia of pregnancy
Sjögren's syndrome
Serum sickness
Erythema multiforme

TABLE 93-2 Differential Diagnosis of Hematuria (Continued)

RENAL (UPPER TRACT)
Nonglomerular
Interstitial nephritis
Pyelonephritis
Papillary necrosis: sickle cell disease, diabetes, NSAIDs
Vascular: AV malformations or emboli, aortocaval fistula, vasculitis (systemic lupus erythematosus, Goodpasture's syndrome, Henoch-Schönlein purpura)
Malignancy: Wilms' tumor, renal cell carcinoma, other
Cystic disease: polycystic kidney disease, medullary sponge disease
Tuberculosis
Renal trauma
HEMATOLOGIC
Primary coagulopathy (e.g., hemophilia)
Pharmacologic anticoagulation
Sickle cell disease
Sickle thalassemia
MISCELLANEOUS
Eroding AAA
Malignant hypertension
Loin pain–hematuria syndrome
Renal vein thrombosis
Exercise-induced hematuria
Cantharidin (Spanish fly, sexual stimulant) poisoning
Bites or stings of various insects and reptiles with venom with anticoagulant properties (rare in United States)

Abbreviations: AAA, abdominal aortic aneurysm; AV, arteriovenous; NSAIDs, nonsteroidal anti-inflammatory drugs.

and retesting of urine because renal, bladder, and prostate cancer increase in frequency and may coexist with urinary tract infection or kidney stone. Risk factors for uroepithelial cancer in addition to age over 40 include excessive analgesic use, tobacco use, occupational exposures (e.g., to dyes, benzenes, or aromatic amines), pelvic irradiation, and cyclophosphamide use. Similarly, hematuria in a patient on oral anticoagulants should not be attributed to the anticoagulant alone, since the incidence of underlying disease may be as high as 80 percent.[8] Expanding abdominal aortic aneurisms (AAAs) may erode into the urogenital tract or cause inflammation or obstruction from direct pressure. Signs and symptoms include back or flank pain, with or without hematuria.

TABLE 93-3 False Hematuria

Munchausen syndrome, malingering, drug seeking: patients may add blood to voided urine
Medications: NSAIDs, phenytoin, phenothiazines, quinine, rifampin, nitrofurantoin, sulfasalazine
Foods and dyes: beets, berries, rhubarb
Serratia marcescens infection
Amorphous urates
Hemoglobinuria, myoglobinuria, porphyrins

Abbreviation: NSAIDs, nonsteroidal anti-inflammatory drugs.

Malignant hypertension, embolic renal infarction, and renal vein thrombosis (RVT) are other serious diagnoses that can cause hematuria. Pregnancy, dehydration, nephrotic syndrome, lymphoma, and renal cell or other types of carcinoma are all predisposing disorders for RVT. RVTs are commonly asymptomatic, with minimal or no pain. Children with RVT are typically volume depleted and have some other cause of a hypercoagulable state. In adults with RVT there is usually underlying nephropathy and obvious nephrotic syndrome. In pregnancy, hematuria can be associated with urinary tract infection, nephrolithiasis, or preeclampsia.

The reported incidence of hematuria in HIV-infected patients is 18 to 50 percent.[9] Causes include subclinical viral renal infection, early glomerulonephritis, urinary tract infection, chlamydial and gonococcal urethritis, chronic hepatitis B infection, neurogenic bladder, thrombocytopenia, subclinical uroepithelial Kaposi's sarcoma, and urethral trauma. However, up to 80 percent of HIV-positive patients with an episode of asymptomatic hematuria have no specific etiology found after complete urologic evaluation.[9]

Diagnosis

Consider the patient's age, gender, demographic characteristics, habits, potential risk factors, recent genitourinary instrumentation, and comorbidities.[3]

Is the hematuria traumatic or atraumatic, gross or microscopic, initial, terminal, or total? When did it start? Are there associated symptoms, such as menstruation; flank, back, or abdominal pain; dysuria; nausea; or fever? Is the patient pregnant? Are there risk factors for cancer or RVT? Has the patient had a recent respiratory or other infection that might predispose to IgA nephropathy or poststreptococcal glomerulonephritis? Has the patient recently traveled outside the United States, particularly to the Middle East or Africa, raising the risk of schistosomiasis? Was there recent instrumentation of the urinary tract or urinary or renal disease? Are there comorbid conditions, such as diabetes, hypertension, sickle cell disease, HIV, tuberculosis, cancers, lupus, or other diseases associated with vasculitis? A complete medication history is important to identify the use of anticoagulants or nephrotoxic agents. Strenuous exercise is a common cause of benign hematuria in healthy young individuals.[10,11]

The physical examination should note the vital signs and the patient's appearance. A younger and otherwise healthy patient without fever, writhing in pain on the cart, unable to find a comfortable position, exhibiting tachycardia and hypertension, and complaining of severe flank pain radiating to the perineum most likely has nephrolithiasis. Hypertension and edema imply nephrotic syndrome. A new heart murmur (endocarditis) or atrial fibrillation increase the likelihood of embolic disease and renal infarction. Dysuria and suprapubic pain and tenderness with or without fever suggest hemorrhagic cystitis. Perineal pain, dysuria, and a tender, boggy prostate in older men indicate prostatitis. A nodular prostate suggests the possibility of cancer. Flank or back pain with fever and costovertebral angle tenderness suggests pyelonephritis. Flank or back pain without fever suggests nephrolithiasis, asymptomatic AAA, renal infarction, or obstruction secondary to tumor. In an older patient, the examiner should palpate for a pulsatile abdominal mass and listen carefully for bruits. Hematuria with rash, arthritis, and abdominal pain may be the result of Henoch-Schönlein purpura in children. Polycystic kidney disease or renal malignancy may result in a large, palpable kidney.[12] External genitalia in males should be examined for obvious tumor or trauma. A pelvic examination should be performed to rule out a vulvar or vaginal source of hematuria.

A clean-catch midstream urine collection is appropriate for most patients. Catheter-collected specimens are recommended for women with a vaginal discharge, menstrual or vaginal bleeding, or perineal disease. While urethral catheterization may induce hematuria in about 15 percent of patients, the amount rarely exceeds 3 RBCs/hpf.[13]

Convenient, commercially available bedside urine dipstick and pregnancy tests provide useful initial screening examinations. A urine dipstick test for blood can detect as little as 150 μg/L of free hemoglobin, corresponding to 5 to 20 intact RBCs/μL on microscopic analysis. False-negative results may be obtained with urine dipstick tests for blood if the urine has a high concentration of ascorbic acid (more than 5 mg/dL) or a high specific gravity. False-positive results occur when oxidizing agents are present (e.g., household bleach used in cleaning containers) and in the presence of free hemoglobin, myoglobin, or porphyrins. Povidone-iodine may also result in a false-positive urine dipstick test result for blood. The urine dipstick test also provides useful information regarding infection (positive leukocyte esterase or nitrite test results), proteinuria, glycosuria, and ketonuria.

When results of the initial urine dipstick screening examination are positive or unavailable, or the clinical picture is highly suspicious for a urinary tract cause, a formal urinalysis is indicated. Abnormal RBC morphologic characteristics, RBC casts, and proteinuria suggest a glomerular source and the need for further nephrologic or hematologic workup.[14] Such patients typically do not require emergent renal imaging. The finding of normal RBCs on microscopic examination of the urine together with bacteriuria and leukocytes in a young healthy patient supports urinary tract infection as the probable cause of hematuria. If leukocytes are plentiful (more than 20 WBCs/hpf) and clumped, and the patient also has back pain and fever, then pyelonephritis is likely. The presence of normal RBCs without evidence of infection should prompt further urologic evaluation to determine the site of bleeding.

Strenuous exercise is a frequent cause of hematuria and follow-up is recommended even in cases of prompt resolution.[1,10,11,16] Patients taking anticoagulants must have appropriate hematologic studies performed in the ED with imaging studies indicated in follow-up for most older patients in order to exclude malignancy.[8]

A minority of patients (5 to 15 percent) with acute symptomatic urinary lithiasis have no hematuria, as measured by a urine dipstick test or formal urinalysis.[15] Thus, those with a clinical picture indicative of nephrolithiasis still require further evaluation. Further laboratory examination depends on the results of the history, physical examination, and presumptive differential diagnosis.

Renal imaging is done with one of three complementary studies:[16] intravenous pyelography (IVP),[17] helical computed tomography (CT) scanning,[18] or renal ultrasound.[19,20] IVP often clearly delineates renal tumor, obstruction, or stones and their precise location.[17] Renal function studies should be obtained first in older patients, diabetics, and those with preexisting renal disease. The IVP does not directly assess the aorta, retroperitoneum, and pelvis.

Helical (ultrafast) CT scanning without contrast material is highly sensitive and specific in identifying nephrolithiasis.[18] In cases where no stone is identified, intravenous contrast infusion may also be performed and other structures evaluated at the same time.

Renal ultrasound is useful when screening for obstruction, hydronephrosis, or AAA. It is the study of choice in pregnant patients with suspected nephrolithiasis.[19,20] The presence of two kidneys can be confirmed, and they can be measured and screened for tumors or cysts. The pelvis, abdomen, and retroperitoneum can be scanned for free fluid, mass, or aneurysm. However, renal ultrasound rarely identifies or locates stones in the ureters that are not large enough to give findings of obstruction.

Gross hematuria in patients with blunt or penetrating trauma to the abdomen, flank, or back warrants an aggressive approach to identify the source of bleeding and to guide management.[21,22] For detailed discussion, see Chaps. 252, 253, and 254. The incidence of significant urinary injury after blunt trauma is much lower, and imaging may not be required in all patients. Some trauma centers use the degree of hematuria, quantified as the number of red blood cells per high-power field, to decide which patients to image. While such an approach is not universally accepted, the studies indicate that patients with relatively minor blunt trauma to the back or flank (e.g., punched, kicked, fall of less than 10 ft) with low levels of microscopic hematuria (less than 20 RBCs/hpf) rarely have significant urinary injury. If they are stable, such patients can be discharged with careful return instructions and referred for repeat urinalysis.

Treatment and Disposition

Treatment of hematuria is directed at the cause. Urinary tract infections should be treated with appropriate antibiotics. Nephrolithiasis should be treated with hydration and analgesics. Systemic diseases should be appropriately treated. Outpatient management and referral for follow-up are appropriate in hemodynamically stable patients without an apparently life-threatening cause. Patients who are discharged should have no or minimal symptoms; be able to tolerate oral fluids, antibiotics, and analgesics as indicated; and have no significant comorbid conditions. Patients should not have significant anemia or acute renal insufficiency.

Patients under 40 years of age should be referred to a primary care physician for repeat urinalysis 1 to 2 weeks after treatment. Persistent hematuria warrants urologic evaluation. Stable patients over 40 otherwise fitting the low-risk profile outlined above can also be evaluated as outpatients, but in these cases cancer is higher on the differential diagnosis list, and referral to a urologist for more immediate outpatient workup is indicated. Children should have pediatric consultation or referral. HIV-positive patients with asymptomatic microscopic hematuria who have a benign urologic history and normal renal function can be safely referred for outpatient follow-up and repeat urinalysis.

Patients with intractable pain, intolerance of oral fluids and medications, significant comorbid illness, evidence of hemodynamic instability, or possibly life-threatening causes of hematuria should be admitted. Patients with suspected or newly diagnosed glomerulonephritis are at high risk of developing complications, such as pulmonary edema, volume overload, azotemia, or hypertensive emergency, and should be admitted with immediate consultation. In pregnant women, hematuria can accompany preeclampsia, pyelonephritis, or obstructing nephrolithiasis, and consultation and admission are indicated.

HEMATOSPERMIA

Hemospermia, or hematospermia, is a disturbing symptom that produces extreme anxiety in sexually active males. Most seek medical attention after one or two occurrences. Any process that results in trauma or other injury (e.g., tumor with erosion), inflammation, or infection of the male ejaculatory system may result in bloody semen.[23] The most common cause of hematospermia is iatrogenic trauma from instrumentation of the urinary tract or radiation therapy. Patients over 40 in particular may have tumors of the prostate or elsewhere in the ejaculatory system. Benign prostatic hypertrophy can cause hematospermia. In patients under 40, common causes are infections and inflammatory conditions, including prostatitis, seminal vesiculitis, urethritis, sexually transmitted diseases, epididymo-orchitis, calculi with inflammation, and tuberculosis. Testicular tumors occur in the younger population. Vascular abnormalities and cysts causing ductal obstruction are less common causes. As with hematuria, systemic factors may cause hematospermia, including hemophilia, other coagulopathy, oral anticoagulation, severe hypertension, leukemia or other hematologic disease, lymphoma, and scurvy.

A careful history, including sexual history, recent urologic procedures, medications, and HIV and tuberculosis risk factors, should be taken in the emergency department. The patient's general health and condition, vital signs, abdomen, external genitalia, and prostate should be examined. Because hematospermia may be the initial and only presenting complaint in underlying urologic disease, a urinalysis is generally warranted, and treatment and disposition are directed by the urinalysis findings (see ''Diagnosis,'' under ''Hematuria,'' above).

Hematospermia has long been considered a benign condition and is usually diagnosed as idiopathic even after a complete urologic workup. It is not uncommon after vigorous sexual activity. Infection, including sexually transmitted disease, should be considered and treated appropriately in the emergency department. In the absence of other reasons for an expedited workup or admission, patients should be referred to a urologist for follow-up and further outpatient evaluation. Patients under 40 can be reassured that the vast majority of cases of hematospermia in their age group are benign, self-limited, and idiopathic. While all patients with hematospermia should be referred to a urologist, those over 40 are at higher risk for cancer and should be strongly advised to seek further evaluation by a urologist even when there is spontaneous resolution of hematospermia.

REFERENCES

1. Sutton JM: Evaluation of hematuria in adults. *JAMA* 263:2475, 1990.
2. Ahmed Z, Lee J: Asymptomatic urinary abnormalities: Hematuria and proteinuria. *Med Clin North Am* 81:641, 1997.
3. Clarkson AR: Microscopic hematuria: Whom to investigate. *Aust NZ J Med* 26:7, 1996.
4. Fogazzi G, Ponticelli C: Microscopic hematuria: Diagnosis and management. *Nephron* 72:125, 1996.
5. Fracchia JA, Mottoa J, Miller LS, et al.: Evaluation of asymptomatic microhematuria. *Urology* 46:484, 1995.
6. Feld LG, Waz WR, Perez LM, Joseph DB: Hematuria: An integrated medical and surgical approach. *Pediatr Clin North Am* 44:1191, 1997.
7. Mahan JD, Turman MA, Mentser M: Evaluation of hematuria, proteinuria, and hypertension in adolescents. *Pediatr Clin North Am* 44:1573, 1997.
8. Van Savage JG, Fried FA: Anticoagulant associated hematuria: A prospective study. *J Urol* 153:1594, 1995.
9. Cespedes RD, Peretsman SJ, Blatt SP: The significance of hematuria in patients infected with the human immunodeficiency virus. *J Urol* 154:1455, 1995.
10. Gambrell RC, Blount BW: Exercise-induced hematuria. *Am Fam Phys* 53:905, 1996.
11. Jones GR, Newhouse I: Sports related hematuria: A review. *Clin J Sport Med* 7:119, 1997.
12. Beebe DK: Autosomal dominant polycystic kidney disease. *Am Fam Physician* 53:925, 1996.
13. Hockberger RS, Schwartz B, Connor J: Hematuria induced by urethral catheterization. *Ann Emerg Med* 16:550, 1987.
14. Schramek P, Schuster F, Georgopolous M, et al.: Value of urinary morphology in assessment of symptomless microhematuria. *Lancet* 2:1315, 1990.
15. Press SM, Smith AD: Incidence of negative hematuria in patients with acute urinary lithiasis presenting to the emergency room with flank pain. *Urology* 45:753, 1995.
16. McCarthy JJ: Outpatient evaluation of hematuria: Locating the source of bleeding. *Postgrad Med* 101:125, 1997.
17. Chen MYM, Zagoria RJ, Dyer RB: Radiologic findings in acute urinary tract obstruction. *J Emerg Med* 15:339, 1997.
18. Sommer FG, Jeffrey RB, Rubin GD, et al.: Detection of ureteral calculi in patients with suspected renal colic: Value of reformatted noncontrast helical CT. *AJR* 165:509, 1995.
19. Houshiar AM, Ercole CJ: Urinary calculi during pregnancy: When are they cause for concern? *Postgrad Med* 100:131, 1996.
20. Swanson SK, Heilman RL, Eversman WG: Urinary tract stones in pregnancy. *Surg Clin North Am* 75:123, 1995.
21. Miller KS, McAninch JW: Radiographic assessment of renal trauma: Our 15-year experience. *J Urol* 154:352, 1995.
22. Morey AF, Bruce JE, McAninch JW: Efficacy of radiographic imaging in pediatric blunt renal trauma. *J Urol* 156:2014, 1996.
23. Munkelwitz R, Krasnokutsky S, Lie J, et al.: Current perspectives on hematospermia: A review. *J Androl* 18:6, 1997.

COMPLICATIONS OF UROLOGIC PROCEDURES

Elaine B. Josephson
Anthony Gomez

Urologic surgical procedures are being more commonly performed with outpatients or with inpatients who are discharged from the hospital earlier in their postoperative course. Thus, patients often come to the emergency department with complications common to these urologic surgeries: urinary tract infection (UTI), acute renal failure (ARF), wound infection, urinary retention, pain, and fever. Whenever possible, the urologist who performed the original operation should be contacted when one of their patients comes to the emergency department with a complication from the procedure.

Although various problems in the postoperative phase are common to many procedures, the specific complications of surgery involving the prostate, renal/ureteral system, and vasectomies warrant special attention.

PROSTATE SURGICAL PROCEDURES

Prostate surgery is usually performed for either benign prostatic hyperplasia (BPH) or prostate cancer. Common surgical techniques employed include transurethral resection of prostate (TURP), transurethral incision of prostate (TUIP), transurethral laser/vaporization, and transurethral microwave thermotherapy.

Surgical procedures of the prostate typically involve direct manipulation of the urinary outflow tract. Therefore, common complications include hematuria, clots with subsequent urinary retention, urethral strictures, and urinary tract infections. Some patients experience obstructive or irritative voiding symptoms that may include incontinence, hesitancy, dribbling, urgency, and frequency.[1–4]

The overall rate of serious complications is low.[1–4] If bleeding is significant, however, patients should be evaluated for hemodynamic stability, intravenous fluids administered, and appropriate laboratory studies ordered [complete blood cell count (CBC), renal function (BUN/creatinine), and urinalysis (U/A)]. Outflow obstruction should be relieved by placing a triple-lumen urethral catheter and irrigating with saline to remove clots. If infection is present, antibiotics should be administered. An urologist should be consulted.

RENAL/URETERAL SURGICAL PROCEDURES

Lithotripsy (ESWL)

Extracorporeal shock wave lithotripsy (ESWL) involves the use of high-intensity sound waves to break up calculi within the genitourinary system. The main advantage with this technique in dealing with nephrolithiasis is its noninvasive nature. Overall morbidity with ESWL is quite low. Typically, patients with post-ESWL complications may come to the emergency department with the following signs and symptoms: nausea, vomiting (especially 48 h after the procedure), skin ecchymosis, pain, or ureteral colic and fever.[5–8]

Steinstrasse (''street of stone'') refers to the post-ESWL dispersal of calculi usually located within the ureters. It is when an accumulation of these calculi, or a single large fragment becomes lodged that subsequent groin pain, urinary obstruction, and superimposed infection can ensue.[6,7] Steinstrasse is usually visible on a plain abdominal radiograph.

A potentially more serious post-ESWL entity, although rare, is a perirenal hematoma, usually secondary to subcapsular renal hemorrhage. Perirenal hematoma is suspected when there is significant and severe flank pain and evidence of hemorrhage (flank hematoma or fall in hematocrit). The diagnosis is made with computed tomography (CT) or ultrasound. Patients require close monitoring of hemodynamic status and laboratory studies to assess for decreasing hematocrit and renal function.[5,6,8]

In managing postprocedural complications of ESWL patients, supportive therapy is important: intravenous fluid hydration, antiemetics (if needed), and pain management, as well as antibiotic therapy, if indicated. An urologist should be contacted early on for possible surgical intervention if there is a concern regarding complicated Steinstrasse or a perirenal hematoma.

VASECTOMIES

Vasectomies are often done in an outpatient setting. Acute complications that may present to the emergency department include local wound infection (cellulitis or abscess), scrotal hematoma, and epididymitis.[9] Some patients may present months to years later with chronic testicular pain.[10]

Patients should receive appropriate pain management and antibiotics, when indicated, especially in cases of immunosuppression. When there is no evidence of bleeding or wound infection, treatment options for postvasectomy epididymitis include ice packs, scrotal support and analgesia with nonsteroidal anti-inflammatory medications. For patients with suspicion of testicular abscess (diffuse pain and swelling, often with fever), scrotal ultrasound should be used. An urologist should be consulted for testicular abscess, and scrotal hematoma in case surgery is needed to control bleeding.

REFERENCES

1. Soonawalla PF, Pardanani DS: Transurethral incision versus transurethral resection of the prostate: A subjective and objective analysis. *Br J Urol* 70:174, 1992.
2. Cowles RS, Kabalin JN, Childs S, et al: A prospective randomized comparison of transurethral resection to visual laser ablation of the prostate for the treatment of benign prostatic hyperplasia. *Urology* 46:155, 1995.
3. Kaplan SA, Santarosa RP, Te AE: Transurethral electrovaporization of the prostate: One-year experience. *Urology* 48:876, 1996.
4. Blute ML, Tomera KM, et al: Transurethral microwave thermotherapy for management of benign prostatic hyperplasia: Results of the United States prostate cooperative study. *J Urol* 150:1591, 1993.
5. Knapp PM, Kulb TB, et al: Extracorporeal shock wave lithotripsy-induced perirenal hematomas. *J Urol* 139:700, 1988.
6. Ehreth JT, Drach GW, et al: Extracorporeal shock wave lithotripsy: multicenter study of kidney and upper ureter versus middle and lower ureter treatments. *J Urol* 152:1379, 1994.
7. Coptcoat MJ, Webb DR, et al: The complications of extracorporeal shockwave lithotripsy: Management and prevention. *Br J Urol* 58:578, 1986.
8. Swanson SK, Larson TR, et al: Clinical trials of the Northgate SD-3 Dual-Purpose Lithotriptor for renal calculi. *J Urol* 148:1047, 1992.
9. Kendrick JS, Gonzales B, et al: Complications of vasectomies in the United States. *J Fam Pract* 25:245, 1987.
10. McMahon AJ, Buckley J, et al: Chronic testicular pain following vasectomy. *Br J Urol* 69:188, 1992.

COMPLICATIONS OF UROLOGIC DEVICES

C. Richard Ross
Edward Lee

Urologic devices are frequently encountered in the emergency department; these range from a Foley catheter to an artificial urinary sphincter. Complications of these devices are not uncommon and as they can occur in a relatively dramatic manner (e.g., urinary retention) or produce intense pain in a very sensitive region (e.g., unremovable penile ring). Patients typically present in an emergent manner and often are very distraught. Early recognition of the complication, along with timely treatment and consultation, are the goals of emergency physicians.

TABLE 95-1 Common Bacterial Pathogens in Short-Term Catheter-Associated Urinary Tract Infection

Escherichia coli
Enterococci
Pseudomonas aeruginosa
Klebsiella pneumoniae
Proteus mirabilis
Enterobacter sp.
Staphylococcus epidermidis
Staphylococcus aureus

COMPLICATIONS OF URINARY CATHETERS

Infection

Urinary tract infection (UTI) is the most common nosocomial infection, accounting for 40 percent of hospital-acquired infections. As many as 25 percent of patients admitted to academic hospitals have a catheter placed during their stay and, of these, between 10 and 30 percent will develop bacteriuria. Nearly all patients catheterized for longer than 30 days will develop a bacteriuria.[1]

The bacteriuria appears to be as a result of direct inoculation along the inner and outer surfaces of the catheter. Women tend to be infected via the periurethral route, with approximately 70 percent of UTIs being caused by rectal flora, whereas the majority of UTIs in men occur through the intraluminal route. Prevention of bacteriuria in the setting of indwelling catheterization is best accomplished through routine cleaning of the urethral meatus and use of closed drainage systems.

A large number of patients are catheterized while hospitalized, and a portion of those will develop a UTI after discharge and may return to the emergency department with symptoms. The most common pathogens associated with short-term catheter-related UTIs are well known (Table 95-1). Although more than 70 percent of patients will clear a bacteriuria after catheter removal, symptomatic patients should receive antimicrobial treatment.

Most catheter-related UTIs experienced in the emergency department setting are seen in patients with long-term indwelling catheters. It has been estimated that as many as 100,000 patients in nursing homes in the United States are catheterized at any given time. The prevalence of bacteriuria in this population is 100 percent, with as many as 95 percent of patients growing two or more strains of bacteria. Pathogens present in long-term catheterized patients are similar to those present in the short-term catheterization population, with the addition of *Providencia stuartii, Morganella morganii, Pseudomonas* sp., and *Candida* sp.

Most patients requiring long-term catheterization have underlying illnesses and, as such, are subject to increased morbidity and mortality as a result of catheter-related complications. In elderly catheterized patients, as many as two-thirds of febrile illnesses are a result of UTI.[2] Despite this, little has been shown to reduce bacteriuria and its complications significantly in patients with indwelling catheters. Routine antibiotic prophylaxis has been shown to postpone bacteriuria but does not prevent it in long-term catheterized patients and can result in infection with resistant organisms. Similarly, treatment of asymptomatic bacteriuria is not indicated. Chronic intermittent catheterization has a lower rate of bacteriuria and, as such, is an alternative to long-term catheterization in select patients.

Traumatic Complications

Trauma to the urethra can occur during catheterization. A false lumen can be created if excessive force is applied during insertion, especially in patients with underlying urethral stricture or prostatic enlargement. This usually occurs at the level of the proximal bulbous urethra. Signs of false lumen include bleeding, pain, and lack of urine output. This complication can be avoided by using either a large catheter (20 French or larger) or a Coudé-tipped catheter in order to pass an obstruction while using less force. Prolonged suprapubic or transurethral drainage can correct most false lumens, but surgical intervention may be required.

The urethra can also be damaged by inflation of the retention balloon within the urethra. Pain or resistance encountered during balloon inflation may indicate that the balloon is located within the urethra. Forceful removal of the catheter with the balloon fully or partially inflated will also cause urethral damage and edema. Prompt recatheterization is indicated in this situation to avoid subsequent urethral obstruction.

The erosion of the glans penis and necrosis of the urethra that can develop in patients with long-term catheterization can be avoided by properly anchoring the catheter so as to lessen any tension that is exerted on the meatus or urethra. Patients with penile prostheses are at particular risk for urethral necrosis and erosion as a result of urethral compression. Scarring at the site of urethral necrosis can lead to stricture formation. This is much more common in male patients and often presents as difficulty in catheterization. Diagnosis is made by retrograde urethrogram, and treatment frequently requires cystoscopic repair.

Damage to the bladder as a result of catheterization can range from mild bladder wall irritation to bladder perforation. Chronic indwelling catheters produce histologic changes to the bladder wall. Polypoid cystitis, a benign inflammatory reaction, develops after approximately 30 days but is readily reversible upon catheter removal. Squamous cell carcinoma can also develop as a result of long-term catheterization, however, and should be considered in patients who have hematuria with long-term indwelling catheters.

Perforation of the bladder can also result from catheterization. Long-term indwelling catheters can erode through the bladder wall and perforate the bladder. Catheters may also be passed through the bladder wall during catheterization. Although this is uncommon, its risk is increased if the bladder wall is distended or inflamed. Patients with bladder perforations typically have decreased urine output, pyuria, hematuria, and peritoneal signs. Diagnosis is best made by cystogram, and urologic consultation is required for definitive treatment. Many patients respond well to conservative treatment consisting of bladder drainage and decompression, but operative repair is often required.

Nondraining Catheter

Patients with nondraining catheters can present with incontinent leakage around the catheter or with abdominal distention and pain as a result of acute urinary retention. Although acute retention is direct evidence for obstruction, pericatheter leakage as a result of catheter blockage must be differentiated from either decreased urethral tone or spontaneous detrusor contractions. This can be accomplished by flushing the catheter with sterile water. Obstruction is suggested if the catheter does not easily flush or if there is no return of the irrigant.

Obstruction of the catheter by blood clots often creates a situation in which the catheter is easily flushed, but little or no irrigant is returned. If this occurs, the catheter can be replaced with a triple-lumen catheter so that the bladder can be easily irrigated. If, after clearing the bladder of all clots, evidence of continued bleeding is present, urologic consultation is recommended for possible cystoscopy. Some physicians advocate the use of single-lumen catheters to lavage the bladder, as its larger lumen may aid in the evacuation of larger clots.

Obstruction in long-term indwelling catheters can be caused by encrustation of the areas of the catheter exposed to urine. Ammonium magnesium phosphate (struvite), calcium phosphate, Tamm-Horsfall protein, and bacteria can all be components of encrustation.[3] *Proteus mirabilis* and other urea-splitting organisms contribute to obstruction by promoting struvite crystal formation. Routine catheter changes continue to be the mainstay of prevention, although multiple bladder irrigation solutions are currently in use to extend catheter-change intervals.

Non-Deflating Retention Balloon

A number of factors can lead to a frustrating inability to deflate the retention balloon on a Foley catheter. Mechanical obstruction, which is the most common cause of a non-deflating balloon, can occur as a result of clamping or crushing the inflation channel or can be due to a faulty balloon port valve. Also, filling of the balloon with a fluid other than water can lead to crystal formation with resultant blockage of the inflation channel.

Several techniques have been advanced to deflate retained balloons. If the obstruction is distal, the result of a crush or defective valve, the catheter can be cut proximal to the defect. If this does not deflate the balloon, a lubricated guidewire can be introduced into the cut inflation channel in an attempt to clear the obstruction. If this still fails to deflate the balloon, more invasive techniques can be employed. The balloon can be ruptured within the bladder by a number of techniques. The balloon can be overinflated with sterile water, often requiring 10 to 20 times the normal balloon volume. Chemical disruption can be accomplished by injecting ether, acetone, or mineral oil into the balloon port, or the balloon may be ruptured via a percutaneous suprapubic or transvaginal approach using a 25-gauge spinal needle with or without ultrasound guidance. Catheters should be examined closely for missing balloon fragments, which will often need to be removed by cystoscopy. Prior to attempting any of these techniques, the bladder should be filled with 150 to 200 mL normal saline to minimize injury from balloon fragments and chemical irritation.

Other Complications

Other less common complications of long-term catheterization include urethral fistulae, epididymitis, scrotal abscess, prostatitis, and prostatic abscess.

ALTERNATIVES TO LONG-TERM CATHETERIZATION

As has been previously mentioned, one alternative to long-term catheterization is intermittent catheterization. Another option is the placement of a suprapubic catheter. This type of bladder decompression reduces the incidence of certain complications associated with urethral catheterization. Because the suprapubic catheter does not exert pressure on the urethra or external genitalia, erosion and necrosis of these structures are eliminated. Damage to the urethra during insertion is similarly reduced, although injuries from suprapubic catheter insertion can include perforation of intraabdominal structures, as well as urinoma or abscess formation. Rates of bacteriuria from suprapubic catheters are lower as a result of the lower density of organisms at the catheter's abdominal insertion site.[4]

External urinary drainage devices (condom catheters) are also used for the long-term management of incontinence in men. By virtue of the noninvasive nature of these devices, urethral damage is minimized and introduction of external pathogens is greatly reduced. These devices do not, however, decompress the bladder and are therefore most useful in patients with either a hyperreflexic neurogenic bladder or with incontinence not due to neurogenic causes. Use of the condom catheter is also limited by the ability of the catheter to fit securely to the penis. Complications from these devices most commonly result from pressure necrosis at the area of the roller ring of the condom. These complications can range from nonhealing ulcers to distal penile necrosis.

COMPLICATIONS OF URETERAL STENTS

The common use of ureteral stents has greatly increased since the 19th century, when Gustav Simon first placed a tube into the ureteral opening during an open cystostomy. Ureteral stents are primarily used to support internal upper urinary tract drainage, especially in cases where healing is required. Such uses for stents occur in cases of urinary obstruction from nephrolithiasis, as well as obstruction from external malignancies. Stents can also be placed after surgery involving the urinary tract, as adjunctive therapy to extracorporeal shock-wave lithotripsy (ESWL), or in cases involving trauma to the ureter. Ureteral stents have radiopaque markers and are constructed from polymers, such as polyethylene, C-flex and polyurethane, and silicone, which are flexible and resist encrustation with mineral deposits to varying degrees. Stents employ various shapes at one or both ends to help anchor the stent in the renal pelvis and/or bladder, and prevent migration. The shapes most commonly used are "J" curves or pigtail loops.[5]

In patients with nephrolithiasis, stones that do not pass are often treated with ESWL, and adjunctive ureteral stents are often used to assist in urine flow and passage of stone fragments. In response to the presence of the stent, the ureter often dilates, allowing for extraluminal as well as intraluminal flow of urine and stone debris.[6] For larger stones and remaining fragments, stents may remain in for further treatment with ESWL. In nephrolithotomy or other open procedures for the removal of stones, stents are used to decrease the urinary leakage that commonly occurs.

Ureteral stents may relieve obstruction caused by primary or metastatic carcinomas, as well as other pathology (for instance, ureteral fibrosis) that leads to mechanical obstruction. Stents are also used in many surgical and percutaneous procedures involving the upper urinary tract, including nephrolithotomy and percutaneous nephrostomy tube insertion. Easily removable stents assist in maintaining a consistent lumen and outlet for urine, especially in surgical anastomoses of the ureter. Complications from a variety of surgical procedures can result in iatrogenic injury to the ureter, where stents may again be used. In fact, to offset obstruction that may be caused by any resultant ureteral edema, stents are often left indwelling for a period of 24 h after ureteroscopy.[7] Further, any other traumatic injury to the upper urinary tract may call for the use of an ureteral stent to help maintain ureteral patency and/or urinary drainage.

Ureteral stents may remain in place for weeks to months and often function without complication. However, stents can become encrusted with mineral deposits, depending on the length of time a stent has been in place, the characteristics of the stent itself, and the chemical composition of the urine. Encrustation can be minimized by keeping the urine at an acidic pH, uninfected, and dilute, with patients being instructed to maintain fluid intake of at least 2 L/day. Limited encrustation is not in itself an emergency, since dilation of the ureter often allows urine to flow around the stent, thus bypassing an obstructed lumen. Complete obstruction of urine flow is possible, although this tends to occur more often in patients with long-term stents. These patients typically require urologic consultation and in some cases may require stent replacement. In patients who received ureteral stents to treat obstruction from malignancy, 46 to 53 percent fail to drain properly, whereas those stents used as adjunctive therapy for renal stones have a much higher success rate.

Although peristaltic movements of the ureters stop with the placement of the ureteral stent, respiratory movements of the kidneys do not. These movements can result in migration of the stent, either upward toward the kidneys or downward into the bladder. Upward migration can lead to renal injury, obstruction and, in cases of infection, septicemia. Correction may entail pyelotomy, nephrostomy drainage and even, in extreme cases, nephrectomy. Changing abdominal or flank pain, or bladder discomfort, may be indicative of stent migration. X-ray examination is indicated to evaluate stent position, and urologic consultation with further studies may eventually be necessary.

Placement of the ureteral stent itself initiates a foreign-body reaction and can predispose patients to an increased risk of urinary tract infection—up to a 7.5 percent incidence of positive urine cultures in patients with stents. Studies have shown that a higher rate of UTI exists as long as 1 month after the removal of the stent. When a UTI does occur, stent removal is not mandatory, because most infections can be managed with outpatient antibiotics. If pyelonephritis or systemic infection is evident, however, then further evaluation and emergent intervention are indicated. Plain x-ray examination and urologic consultation for evaluation of stent migration/malfunction are indicated. Antibiotic therapy should also be initiated in a timely manner.

Dysuria, urinary urgency, frequency, and abdominal and flank discomfort are common complaints in patients with ureteral stents. The use of analgesics and anticholinergics provides some relief. In some extreme cases, though, a few days of belladonna and opiate suppositories may be effective. The baseline discomfort in a functioning, well-positioned stent can range anywhere from minimal to debilitating. In some cases, the pain may be so great as to necessitate removal of the stent. However, an abrupt change in the character, location, or intensity of the pain requires further evaluation for stent malposition/malfunction. Along with these irritative symptoms, asymptomatic microscopic hematuria is often present, though clinically insignificant. Gross hematuria, with or without clots, may be the result of stent erosion through a segment of the urinary tract, stent migration, or the passage of a renal stone and requires further investigation, including urologic consultation.

COMPLICATIONS OF PERCUTANEOUS NEPHROSTOMY TUBES

While initially developed as emergent procedure for the relief of urinary obstruction, the use of percutaneous nephrostomy (PCN) has expanded beyond urinary diversion to a variety of other diagnostic procedures and therapeutic interventions. Patients with nephrostomy catheters may present to the emergency department days after placement, with complications relating either to the procedure or to the device itself. Other patients may present with complications related to the long-term use of nephrostomy catheters.

The indications for use of percutaneous nephrostomy include supravesicular obstruction or urine leak, adjunctive therapy for ESWL, or percutaneous ultrasonic lithotripsy. PCN is also used in cases of ureteral strictures, or for nephroscopy or antegrade ureteroscopy, often in conjunction with ureteral stents, as well as in cases of patients who have contraindications to surgical interventions. PCN may be indicated in cases where patients have failed ureteral stenting to relieve obstruction, especially in cases involving malignancy, or in cases of pyonephrosis, where the drainage from the kidney may be too viscous to be adequately drained by ureteral stent. Patients with urinary tract fistulas or other injuries may occasionally have PCN for postprocedure urinary diversion while the fistula closes or injury heals.

Complications in patients who have had percutaneous nephrostomy include hemorrhage, hematuria, infection (including septicemia), urinoma, obstruction, or catheter dislodgment. Complications requiring specific treatment or prolonged hospitalization occur in 4 to 8 percent of PCNs. Although patients can have other serious complications from PCN, including pneumothorax, bowel perforation, and liver or splenic injuries, these complications tend to be detected in the postoperative period and are rarely seen by emergency physicians. Hemorrhage tends to be more likely and more severe in patients with a coagulopathy. If a patient has sufficient bleeding to produce clots large enough to obstruct the nephrostomy catheter, then gentle intermittent irrigation with normal saline can be attempted to maintain the catheter's lumen until the bleeding either slows or clears. Hemorrhage—including pelvocalyceal and retroperitoneal hemorrhage—may also occur in the days following PCN. Although the large majority of patients with clinically significant hemorrhage will be recognized in the period during or shortly after PCN, patients with a history of recent percutaneous nephrostomy should trigger a higher level of suspicion. Hematuria, either transient or persistent, occurs commonly (especially after stone extraction) and is not a cause for alarm, provided that the patient is hemodynamically stable, the hematocrit is stable, and that urinary drainage is maintained. If any of the latter criteria are not met, then an arterial injury should be considered. If significant hemorrhage occurs, then aggressive blood transfusion/fluid resuscitation should be followed with urologic consultation, as the patient may require transcatheter embolization or further surgical procedures.

One to 2 percent of patients having PCN to treat pyonephrosis develop septicemia from release of bacteria or endotoxin from the renal parenchyma or collecting system into the blood. These patients can also develop perinephric abscesses. Therefore, patients with indwelling nephrostomy catheters who present to the emergency department with fever, pain, or other signs of systemic illness should have further evaluation, including urologic consultation.

Patients also may present with persistent urine leak from the nephrostomy site: up to 2 percent of patients have more than 1 week of such urinary drainage from the flank. These patients should have urologic consultation and, after treatment by ureteral catheter insertion or continued nephrostomy drainage, usually recover fully. Urinomas are a relatively infrequent complication and may be managed by ensuring that there is adequate drainage from the nephrostomy catheter. Observation and a possible second percutaneous catheter may be inserted by an urologist or a radiologist. In cases of catheter obstruction, the catheter can be intermittently irrigated with normal saline. If this does not resolve the obstruction, then an urologist should see the patient. If the catheter has become dislodged, in most cases a new puncture must be performed. If the catheter has been left indwelling for many weeks, then the renal parenchymal portion of the nephrostomy tract may be negotiated with either a guidewire or a new catheter, with varying rates of success. Any attempt at recannulation should be carried out by an urologist or a radiologist.

COMPLICATIONS OF PENILE PROSTHESES

The use of urologic implantable prostheses has increased since the modern forms became available in the early 1970s. Penile prostheses are generally of two types: semirigid penile prostheses (SRPPs) and inflatable penile prostheses (IPPs).

SRPPs provide rigidity at all times. They are paired cylindrical devices, which are implanted within the corpus cavernosa. The devices are activated by means of a hinged segment or by repositioning a flexible metal core. Two types of SRPP commonly in use are the Finney and the Small-Carrion. These types of prostheses are less expensive and more durable than the IPP type. Disadvantages of the SRPP include reduced ability to conceal the device and need for proper sizing of the device prior to implantation. Incorrect sizing can lead to sagging of the glans if the device is too small or pressure necrosis if the device is too large.

IPPs can inflate and deflate by a hydraulic mechanism. These devices are composed of paired inflatable cylinders within the corpus cavernosa, and a pump and reservoir that are commonly located within either the corpora or the scrotum. Many types of IPPs exist that use different versions of the general concept. As would be expected by the increased complexity of IPP devices, they tend to be more expensive and have a greater rate of mechanical failure. Because of the more natural appearance of this type of device, however, IPPs are still widely used despite their drawbacks.

Erosion, which is a complication of both types of prostheses, occurs through a number of mechanisms, the most prominent being the anatomic relationship of the corpus cavernosa to the urethra. The corpus cavernosa are physically in closest contact with each other in the region of the fossa navicularis. Therefore, the highest degree of pressure exerted by the prostheses to the urethra occurs in this region. Given their constantly rigid state, SRPPs have a higher rate of erosion, which is often worsened by inappropriate sizing of the device. This is particularly the case with either patients who have indwelling catheters or those who perform intermittent catheterizations. Introduction of the catheter into the lumen of the urethra adds to the local pressure and can lead to necrosis.

Because a large percentage of patients requiring penile prostheses have an underlying neurologic deficit, erosions will often present as a prosthetic device protruding from the urethral meatus. Patients with intact sensation frequently complain of pain or discomfort at the site of necrosis. In the case of SRPPs, the protruding device can usually be removed by simple extraction with forceps, followed by careful urethral catheterization and urologic follow-up.

Infection is the most devastating of complications associated with penile prostheses and nearly always results in removal of the prostheses, with long-term antibiotic coverage and wound drainage. Inability to clear the infection fully, as well as scar tissue formation, can limit the possibility of reimplantation of another device.

Penile prostheses incite a foreign body reaction within the host. An inflammatory reaction occurs shortly after implantation and results in the formation of a scar-tissue capsule. Though this capsule helps hold the device in place, it also acts as a potentiator of infection. The surface of the prosthesis provides a site for bacterial adherence, as well as a local environment that is resistant to host defenses. The periprosthetic space created between the prostheses and the capsule acts as an ideal site for the growth of bacteria and the production of an extracellular matrix. This extracellular matrix, along with the relative avascular nature of the capsule, limits the ability of immune cells and antibiotics to penetrate and eradicate infection.

The vast majority of prosthetic infections occur at the time of implantation. This being the case, it makes sense that most infections present within the postoperative period and that the most common infective agents are gram-positive cocci like *Staphylococcus epidermidis.*[8] Reduction of prosthetic infection rates is thus aimed at perioperative precautions, including the use of prophylactic antibiotics. Late infection of established prosthetic devices does occur, however. Hematogenous seeding can occur, so it is currently recommended that patients with penile prostheses be treated in accordance with the American Heart Association's bacterial endocarditis prophylaxis guidelines during procedures likely to induce bacteremia.

COMPLICATIONS OF THE ARTIFICIAL URINARY SPHINCTER

The artificial urinary sphincter (AUS), a device used to treat urinary incontinence, has undergone five revisions since first being described in use in 1972. All types of artificial sphincters perform similar functions: to open partially when bladder pressure exceeds physiologic limits, to equalize pressures of stress, to open fully when operated, to fail in the open position, and to allow catheterization without further operations on the device.[8] The most current model, the AS-800 (American Medical Systems, Minnetonka, MN), introduced in 1982, consists of three parts: an inflatable cuff, a pressure-regulating balloon, and a pump. The cuff is typically placed around the urethra and is filled with fluid, via a pump/reservoir mechanism, providing continence through encircling compression of the urethra. For a patient to urinate, the fluid is pumped from the cuff to the reservoir. The fluid may then be pumped back into the cuff to provide continence or left in the reservoir leaving the cuff in the "open" position. All models enable catheterization without open modification of the device. The AS-800 is equipped with a deactivation button, which allows the device to be left in the "open" state. The device is reactivated by a sharp squeeze on the pump, opening a valve, which enables fluid transfer from the balloon to the cuff.

As subsequent versions of the AUS have been developed, reliability has improved. Mechanical failure rates range between 8 and 20 percent.[9] Examples of mechanical failure include fluid leaks, tube kinking, and pump failure. Fluid leaks present as the sudden onset of incontinence, with the cuff often being the source of the leaking fluid. Tube kinking is often the result of excessive tube length. These patients present in acute urinary retention, as they are unable to deflate the urethral cuff. Pump failure also manifests as a decreased ability or total inability to deflate the urethral cuff. This is usually the result of obstruction of the device's tubing by blood or other debris. Urologic consultation is necessary in these cases to further evaluate the source of the mechanical failure and treat the patient for urinary retention. These patients tend to require only replacement of the defective portion of the apparatus. Another complication, particularly seen in the use of AUS in the pediatric population, is bladder hypertonicity, which occurs after initial placement of the device. Hypertonicity may lead to renal failure, so these cases require close monitoring by nephrology and urology.[10] When the clinical presentation warrants, patients in the emergency department who have a history of AUS implantation should be evaluated for the possibility of renal failure.

Cuff erosion, which is the most common cause of total sphincter failure, tends to occur more commonly in female patients, especially when either the bladder or the vagina has been injured during the implantation procedure. The incidence ranges between 1.3 and 18 percent but has decreased in recent years. After implantation, the device is left in the deactivated state postoperatively for 8 to 12 weeks to allow perivesicular inflammation to decrease as well as to allow the urethra to restore vascularity before regular use of the AUS. Further risk factors for cuff erosion include increased cuff pressure, decreased cuff size, and urethral catheterization, all of which may lead to cuff erosion secondary to pressure necrosis. Patients with cuff erosions tend to present several months postoperatively and may present with any of the following: perineal pain, urethral discharge, gross hematuria, dysuria, urinary urgency or frequency, or recurrent incontinence. Urologic consultation is necessary, with the diagnosis being confirmed by retrograde urethrography and cystourethroscopy. Treatment includes cuff removal with possible reimplantation at a later date, antibiotics, and catheterization.

Infection is infrequent with the AUS, especially in the more recent models. Recent studies report an incidence of infection in the range of 1.2 to 2.7 percent. Like any foreign body, the AUS causes a tissue reaction, which may facilitate infection if bacteria are present. *S. epidermidis* and coliform bacteria tend to be the most common etiology for bacterial infection of the device. A patient's presentation may be subtle in cases of infection and requires a thorough history and physical examination, as well as a heightened degree of suspicion. Patients may be afebrile, lack an elevated white blood cell count, and have sterile blood and urine cultures. Others may have pain, swelling, erythema, or induration around the mechanism. In male patients, there may be thinning of the scrotal skin overlying the pumping mechanism (the most common site of infection), and induration or tenderness along the length of tubing may be palpable in the patient. Treatment of this complication includes urgent removal of the apparatus, with the possibility of reimplantation of a new device after healing.

Patients who present with recurrent urinary incontinence may have difficulties at a variety of sites in the urinary tract. Problems involving the cuff of the AUS include erosion or urethral atrophy and/or rigidity, all of which interfere in the compressibility of the urethra and lead to further incontinence. Treatments involve exchanging various parts of the AUS device itself and may be done electively. Occasionally, detrusor instability leads to increased bladder pressures that overwhelm the urethral cuff. This instability may be treated with medication. Mechanical failure of the urethral cuff may be treated with urologic follow-up and elective replacement of the defective component.

TABLE 95-2 Penile Strangulation Injuries

Grade 1	Edema of distal penis. No evidence of skin ulceration or urethral injury.
Grade 2	Injury to skin and constriction of corpus spongiosum but no evidence of urethral injury. Distal penile edema with decreased sensation.
Grade 3	Injury to skin and urethra but no urethral fistula. Loss of distal penile sensation.
Grade 4	Complete division of corpus spongiosum leading to urethral fistula and constriction of corpus cavernosum with loss of distal penile sensation.
Grade 5	Gangrene, necrosis, or complete amputation of distal penis.

COMPLICATIONS OF PENILE RINGS

Penile strangulation can occur from pressure around the entire penile circumference by rings, hair, or other devices. Since delay in relief of strangulation can lead to vascular compromise and other serious consequences, these devices *must* be removed rapidly. Penile-strangulating objects have been placed for masturbatory purposes, as adjuncts to vacuum erection devices, to prolong erections, enhance sexual performance, and often by children during experimentation. Such devices have also been used to prevent enuresis and nocturnal emissions. In the pediatric population, the possibility of child abuse must also be considered.

Patients often delay seeking medical attention secondary to embarrassment and present to the emergency department with extreme pain. Other presenting symptoms include edema, ulceration, urinary retention, and vascular compromise with and without necrosis. As strangulation occurs, decreased venous and lymphatic drainage leads to edema and swelling of the penis distal to the site of constriction. Further swelling may lead to compromised arterial flow and gangrene of the penile tissue. Necrosis tends to involve mainly the skin and the subcutaneous tissue. However, because each corpus cavernosum has its own artery and these deeper vessels are protected by the Buck's fascia and overlying corporal tissue, gangrene of the corpora cavernosa is rare. Grades of penile strangulation have been described (Table 95-2).

Evaluation of penile strangulation should include assessment of temperature, color, sensation, ability to void, and pulses (preferably by Doppler ultrasound). Some cases of penile strangulation, especially in children, the offending object, such as a hair, may be nearly invisible in the surrounding edema. Penile pain and swelling in children should trigger an increased suspicion of child abuse.

Various devices have been used to remove objects from the penis, including the standard ring cutter, wire cutters, saws, dental drills, hand-held grinding tools, and even orthopedic pneumatic drills. In the use of the latter motorized devices, continuous cool-water irrigation should be used to prevent heat injury to patients. If possible, a makeshift guard should be placed between the ring and the skin, thus isolating the action of the cutting device and preventing secondary injury to the penis. The method chosen for removal depends on the material involved, the size/thickness, and the duration that the item has been in place. Patients with grade 2 or greater injuries should have urologic consultation, and further possible evaluation for urethral injury, including a retrograde urethrogram or a Wood's lamp examination after intravenous administration of fluorescein. In extreme cases, where the constricting object cannot be removed in the emergency department, patients may require admission, with removal of the object in the operating room being followed by possible excision of devitalized tissue and skin grafting.

COMPLICATIONS OF GENITAL PIERCINGS

Body piercing—the use of needles, steel posts, rings, or other adornments—has become increasingly popular in recent years for both sexual and aesthetic reasons. An important element of history to obtain from patients is where the piercing was done (i.e., piercing parlor, doctor's office, store, by a friend, or by one's self), to assess whether aseptic technique was followed and needles were single use and sterilely packaged. If the piercing is performed by a novice, often it is too shallow, increasing injury and the chance that the body will reject the jewelry. Also, emergency physicians should attempt to ascertain the composition of the jewelry material, since contact metal-allergic dermatitis may occur with exposure to nickel or even surgical steel and gold. The resultant inflammation may in cases be so extreme as to envelop the jewelry. Lymphadenopathy and granulomatous tissue formation have occurred as a result of piercing, as has keloid formation over the long term. Genital piercing is also subject to trauma and may rupture the urethra. Trauma to the genitalia secondary to genital piercing may require urologic consultation and further evaluation if anything other than superficial injury is involved.

Infectious complications of genital piercing tend to occur at certain times:

1. When the piercing is performed, possibly with nonsterile technique and/or instruments. The instruments may include improperly sterilized spring-loaded finger-stick devices or piercing guns.
2. In the immediate postpiercing period, if the wound is not kept clean or is handled by the patient.

Embarrassment may cause patients with genital piercing to delay seeking medical attention for potential infection. *Staphylococcus aureus* is the organism most often responsible for piercing infections. However, group A β-hemolytic streptococci (GABHS) and *Pseudomonas aeruginosa* have also been isolated from infected piercing. Body piercing may be responsible for transmission of hepatitis B, hepatitis C, human papillomavirus (leading to recurrent condyloma accuminatum) and, although no cases in the literature currently exist, even HIV. Patients with relatively recent body piercing who present with unexplained hepatitis, endocarditis, or otherwise unexplained evidence of systemic infection should have a closer history of piercing obtained. Tetanus prophylaxis status should be determined for all recently pierced patients. In cases involving bacterial infection, culture specimens should obtained from the piercing site to identify the organism involved and direct appropriate antibiotic therapy. Removal of the jewelry may also be necessary in some cases.[11]

REFERENCES

1. Cancio LC, Sabanegh ES, Thompson IM: Managing the Foley catheter. *Am Fam Physician* 48:829, 1993.
2. Warren JW, Damron D, Tenney JH, et al: Fever, bacteremia, and death as complications of bacteriuria in women with long-term urethral catheters. *J Infect Dis* 155:1151, 1987.
3. Kunin CM: Blockage of urinary catheters: Role of microorganisms and constituents of the urine on formation of encrustations. *J Clin Epidemiol* 42:835, 1989.
4. Carson CC: Infections in genitourinary prostheses. *Urol Clin North Am* 161:139, 1989.
5. Saltzman B: Ureteral stents: Indications, variations, and complications. *Urol Clin North Am* 15:483, 1988.
6. Culkin D, Price VH, Zitman R, et al: Anatomic, functional, and pathologic changes from internal ureteral stent placement. *Urology* 40:386, 1992.
7. Adams J: Renal stents. *Emerg Med Clin North Am* 12:750, 1994.
8. Shandera KC, Thompson IM: Urologic prostheses. *Emerg Med Clin North Am* 12:729, 1994.
9. Montague DK: The artificial urinary sphincter (AS-800): Experience in 166 consecutive patients. *J Urol* 147:380, 1992.
10. Levesque PE, Bauer SB, Atala A, et al: Ten-year experience with the artificial urinary sphincter in children. *J Urol* 156:626, 1996.
11. Samantha S, Tweeten M, Rickman LS: Infectious complications of body piercing. *Clin Infect Dis* 26:738, 1998.

96 THE RENAL TRANSPLANT PATIENT

Richard Sinert

EPIDEMIOLOGY

Renal transplants make up the majority of solid organ transplants in the United States. For 1997, there were 19,971 solid organs transplanted, of which 12,229 were kidneys.[1] However, approximately 30,000 patients were left waiting for a kidney transplant at the end of 1997, and unfortunately, during the year approximately 1800 patients died waiting for a kidney transplant.

The knowledge that there are currently over 57,000 patients waiting for a solid organ transplant is important for emergency medicine. Since emergency physicians routinely care for victims of head trauma and other neurologic injuries, they are often in a position to identify possible donors. The potential for organ donation is often lost to the demands of caring for the severely injured. At such times, it should be remembered that 4000 patients die annually waiting for solid organ transplants.

Graft prognosis is directly related to the source of the donor kidney; recipients of cadaveric kidneys generally have more episodes of rejection and lower graft survival rates. The graft survival rate for kidneys from living donors is about 93 percent at 1 year and 77 percent at 5 years; the graft survival rate kidneys from cadaveric donors is 86 percent at 1 year and 61 percent at 5 years. The major causes of morbidity after renal transplant are hypertension (46 percent of all renal transplants), cataracts (24 percent), avascular necrosis (18 percent), malignant neoplasm (14 percent), urinary tract infection (UTI; 17 percent), chronic hepatitis (6 percent), peptic ulcer disease (4 percent), diverticulitis (3 percent), myocardial infarction (4 percent), and cerebrovascular accident (2 percent).[2]

Generally, recipients from living, related donors have lower mortality rates than recipients from cadaveric donors, probably related to fewer rejection episodes and thus lower immunosuppression requirements. Patients' survival rate after transplantation from a living donor is 98 percent at 1 year and 91 percent at 5 years, compared to survival after cadaveric donation of 94 percent at 1 year and 81 percent at 5 years. The causes of death in renal transplant patients vary among transplant centers.[3] Common causes include coronary artery disease (14 to 50 percent), sepsis (7 to 28 percent), neoplasm (9 to 28 percent), and liver failure (0 to 28 percent). During the first year, most deaths are from infectious causes. Long-term mortality rates are more closely related to the development of coronary artery disease.

This chapter discusses issues related to organ procurement, reviews the pathophysiology of graft rejection, and covers the most common medical complications seen in renal transplant patients, with special emphasis on the evaluation of the renal transplant patient with infections and acute renal failure (ARF).

ORGAN PROCUREMENT

Emergency physicians should be familiar with their departmental policies on brain death and organ procurement. Telephone and beeper numbers for the regional organ procurement organization (OPO) should be readily available.

An increasing demand for donor organs, coupled with improvements in transplant immunology, has greatly expanded the pool of patients eligible for organ donation. The donation of tissue such as skin, bones, and corneas can occur even postmortem. Recently the success of solid organ transplantation using non-heart-beating donors promises to expand the possible donor pool by 20 percent.[4] Absolute contraindications for transplant donors include HIV, sepsis, and malignancy other than primary central nervous system tumors. Advanced age is a relative contraindication; most OPOs do not harvest solid organs from individuals older than 75.

The Uniform Determination of Death Act provides guidelines outlining the neurologic criteria for the diagnosis of brain death: complete and irreversible loss of brain and brainstem function. Cerebral unresponsiveness, brainstem areflexia, and apnea are necessary to diagnose brain death. Reversible causes of brainstem depression, such as hypothermia and drug intoxication, need to be excluded. OPOs should be notified early of potential organ donors, and the OPO coordinator on call should be called even before the formal declaration of brain death.

Discussion of organ donation with the family is best done separately from discussion and acceptance of brain death. Once brain death has been declared, the OPO coordinator, who is highly trained for this delicate discussion, should broach the subject of organ donation. The emergency physician should focus on identifying possible donor candidates and giving the family a realistic prognosis for the patient. Organ donation consent rates vary widely among OPOs and from hospital to hospital. Consent rates are highest when the family initiates the discussion of organ donation. Consent rates are also higher if the discussion about organ donation is decoupled from the explanation of brain death, as described above. For multiple reasons, families may perceive a mixed message if the physicians caring for their seriously ill relative also initiates discussion of organ donation before the patients are "officially dead."

Following brain death, a number of physiologic changes occur that necessitate intervention to preserve donor organ perfusion.[5,6] Increasing cerebral edema after trauma or a cerebrovascular accident results initially in elevated catecholamine release and hypertension. With brainstem necrosis, catecholamine levels drop rapidly to 10 percent of normal values, causing hypotension, which must be corrected with fluids and vasopressors. Pituitary necrosis occurs in approximately 75 percent of organ donors, resulting in diabetes insipidus, which, if untreated, can result in significant hypovolemia. Antidiuretic hormone and free-water deficits should be rapidly replaced in these patients.

Body temperature control is often lost due to ischemia of the hypothalamus, with approximately 86 percent of donors developing hypothermia. Hypothermia has many detrimental effects on potential donor organs, including coagulopathy, shifting of the oxygen-hemoglobin dissociation curve, and hepatic and cardiac dysfunction.

PATHOPHYSIOLOGY OF TRANSPLANT REJECTION

The immune system has evolved to protect us against invasion from foreign pathogens and not renal grafts, and many of the same immune mechanisms that protect us against pathogens are also responsible for graft rejection. Enough divergence does exist between the immune response to transplants and pathogens that complete immunosuppression is not required for graft survival. Transplant research has shown that suppression of cellular, not humoral, immunity is critical for graft survival.

A newly transplanted graft is immediately identified as foreign by circulating T-lymphocytes that recognize class II human leukocyte antigen (HLA) on the surface of the donor organ. Once bound to these antigens, the T-lymphocytes differentiate, proliferate, and produce a wide array of soluble proteins called lymphokines. Lymphokines feed back to increase T-lymphocyte activation and stimulate B-cell antibody production against the graft. Specialized helper T-lymphocytes called cytotoxic T-lymphocytes are stimulated to directly attack the graft by attaching to cell-surface HLA class I antigens.

Identification of the specific components of the immune system responsible for graft rejection allows for a targeted approach to immunosuppression. Pharmacologic protocols have been developed to selectively inhibit those components of the immune system responsible for graft rejection.[7] The doses of these immunosuppressants are then carefully adjusted to balance the risks of graft rejection with the risks of infection.

Azathioprine is a purine analogue. Metabolites of azathioprine are incorporated into DNA and RNA strands, inhibiting their synthesis and function. The immunosuppressant action of azathioprine occurs through blocking gene activation of stimulated T-lymphocytes. Azathioprine is prescribed at a dose of 2 mg/kg/day on a continuous basis as maintenance antirejection therapy. Noncompliance with azathioprine has been associated with a high rejection rate. Deleterious effects of azathioprine include leukopenia, thrombocytopenia, hepatotoxicity, and increased risk of neoplasm.

Corticosteroids have a role both in antirejection maintenance and during acute rejection episodes. Corticosteroids inhibit antigen-stimulated T-lymphocyte proliferation and inhibit lymphokine production. A major drawback of the use of steroids is their nonselectivity of immunosuppression, effecting both the cellular and humoral immunity and resulting in significantly increased risk of infection. Other deleterious effects of steroids include osteoporosis, hyperglycemia, hyperkalemia, and growth suppression in children.

Cyclosporine (CYA) and Tacrolimus (FK506) are both macrolide antibiotics produced by fungi. Although structurally unrelated, both CYA and FK506 agents block the proliferation of helper and cytotoxic T cells and inhibit lymphokine release. Unlike azathioprine and steroids, CYA and FK506 do not interfere with activation and proliferation of suppressor T lymphocytes. In fact, their major immunosuppressant effect may be directly related to their activation of suppressor cells. Both CYA and FK506 have similar toxic profiles, including, nephrotoxicity, hemolytic uremic syndrome, and hypertension. CYA has a vital role in maintenance antirejection therapy: CYA trough whole blood levels between 150 and 300 ng/mL are associated with graft survival.

INFECTIOUS COMPLICATIONS

Infection is the most common cause of early (less than 1 year) mortality and morbidity for transplant patients. Approximately 80 percent of transplant patients experience at least one infection during the first posttransplant year.

Viral Infections

Viral infections produce significant morbidity and mortality in the renal transplant recipient. The most common viral infections come from the herpes group of viruses: cytomegalovirus (CMV), Epstein-Barr virus (EBV), herpes simplex virus (HSV), and varicella-zoster virus (VZV). Transplant patients are also more susceptible to and have a worse outcome from infections with other viruses, such as adenovirus, influenzavirus, and hepatitis virus.

CMV is responsible for more than two-thirds of febrile episodes in the first 6 months posttransplant. Transmission of CMV occurs with an organ transplant from a seropositive donor. With the primary direct CMV infection, patients often present with fever, malaise, hepatitis, pneumonitis, primary chorioretinitis, lymphadenopathy, arthralgias, and myalgias. An important indirect effect of CMV infection is augmented immunosuppression of the host, which increases the incidence of opportunistic infections such as *Pneumocystis carinii*, *Listeria*, and *Aspergillus*. Diagnosis of CMV infection is established by viral culture and antibody titers. Untreated CMV has been associated with 10 to 15 percent mortality rates. Intravenous ganciclovir and foscarnet are both effective in treating CMV.

EBV infection in the renal transplant patient can present in two distinct clinical syndromes, either as the typical uncomplicated mononucleosis syndrome (characterized by fever, mild hepatitis, and leukopenia with atypical lymphocytosis) or as posttransplant lymphoproliferative disease (PTLD).[8] PTLD can range from a mild benign polyclonal disease to a rapidly progressive monoclonal form, which carries a poor prognosis. Other symptoms and signs of EBV are fever of unknown origin, weight loss, hepatotoxicity, pulmonary infiltrates, and gastrointestinal bleeding and perforation. Diagnosis of EBV is established by histologic examination of infected tissue. Primary EBV infection is treated by reducing immunosuppression and administering intravenous acyclovir. Treatment of PTLD is generally ineffective, leading to a substantial mortality rate.

VZV also presents with two distinct clinical syndromes in the renal transplant patient. The majority of transplant patients with VZV present with the typical reactivation-type infection limited to skin eruptions. A primary VZV infection occurs when tissue from a seropositive donor is transplanted to a seronegative host. This primary VZV infection produces a chickenpox syndrome that can be quite virulent, causing hemorrhagic pneumonia, encephalitis, hepatitis, and pancreatitis, with a high mortality rate. Direct immunofluorescence or viral culture is required to make the diagnosis of VZV. Acyclovir, valacyclovir, and famciclovir are all effective for both primary and reactivated VZV.

HSV infection is very common during the first transplant month. The usual presentation of reactivation disease is mucocutaneous ulcerations, which can be complicated by bacterial superinfection. Primary HSV infection can present as a disseminated disease with pneumonitis, esophagitits, or hepatitis. Diagnosis is based on direct immunofluorescence, viral culture, or serologic studies. Treatment with oral or intravenous acyclovir, ganciclovir, and foscarnet is effective.

Hepatitis viruses B and C are responsible for a 10 to 15 percent incidence of chronic liver disease in transplant patients. Disease transmission is from a seropositive donor or by contact with infected individuals. Immunosuppressive therapy directly stimulates viral replication. Both hepatitis B and C can progress to active hepatitis, cirrhosis, and hepatocellular carcinoma. In addition, infection with these viruses can suppress the host's immune defenses. Diagnosis is based on serologic and histologic studies. Therapy with interferon and lamivudine has shown limited success.

Bacterial Infections

UTIs associated with indwelling catheters are the most common bacterial infection in all transplant recipients, occurring in 30 to 40 percent.[9] The organisms responsible for UTIs in transplant patients are similar to those in nontransplant patients: *Escherichia coli*, enterococci, and *Pseudomonas aeruginosa*. UTIs in the first 6 months posttransplant have a high incidence of progressing to urosepsis and usually require longer courses of intravenous agents. UTIs during this period should all be investigated for the possibility of complicating obstruction and stone formation. Infections occurring after this period can be treated for shorter periods with less intensive courses.

The gastrointestinal tract is the next most common source of bacterial infection in the renal transplant patient. Acute bacterial gastroenteritis secondary to *Salmonella*, *Campylobacter*, and *Listeria* is common in these patients. While these bacteria usually have a benign course, occasionally *Salmonella* can spread hematogenously, resulting in endocarditis requiring a prolonged, intensive antibiotic course.

Diverticulitis, often complicated by perforation, is the other common gastrointestinal infection encountered in transplant patients.[10] Patients commonly present with findings of vague abdominal pain as the only symptom of this potentially life-threatening disease. A high index of suspicion should be maintained when evaluating transplant recipients with abdominal pain.

Listeria monocytogenes is a common opportunistic bacterial infection usually acquired by ingesting contaminated foods. Presentation is with diarrhea and abdominal cramps, which can quickly progress to pneumonia, enophthalmitis, and meningitis. Treatment consists of ampicillin and gentamicin, or trimethoprim-sulfamethoxazole (TMP-SMX).

Nocardia asteroides in renal transplant patients typically presents with fever, cough, and pulmonary infiltrates, eventually spreading to skin and central nervous system.[11] *Nocardia* can be effectively treated with TMP-SMX.

Mycobacteria tuberculosis occurs in renal transplant patients both as a primary and as a reactivation disease.[12] Risk factors for mycobacterial infection include malnutrition, history of inadequate treatment, or recent exposure to a contact with tuberculosis. There is no typical presentation for a transplant patient with tuberculosis. Instead, a highly variable presentation has been described, including cavitary pulmonary disease, miliary disease, and multiorgan involvement. Diagnosis is rarely aided by tuberculin skin testing. Definitive diagnosis is by organism identification and culture from sputum, pleural effusions, and bronchoalveolar lavage, lung, or bone marrow biopsy. Therapeutic options are complicated because of the CYA drug interactions with many antituberculosis medications.

Fungal Infections

Candida albicans infection is the result of immunosuppression (especially from steroid use) causing overgrowth of an endogenous gut flora. Mucocutaneous disease affecting the oropharynx, esophagus, and vagina is the most common presentation. Candidal urinary tract infections, usually associated with indwelling catheters, can run a benign course with just cystitis or spread to pyelonephritis. Disseminated candidiasis often results in endocarditis, aortitis, osteomyelitis, meningitis, and brain abscess. Finding the organism in tissues, blood, or urine makes the diagnosis. Treatment of mucocutaneous candidiasis is with nystatin, clotrimazole, or oral fluconazole. Amphotericin is an effective agent for disseminated disease, but intravenous fluconazole may be preferable because of less nephrotoxicity.

Mucormycosis is caused by infections from fungi of *Rhizopus*, *Absidia*, and *Mucor* species. Risk factors include diabetes mellitus, steroid use, and deferroxamine therapy. The most feared complication is invasive rhinocerebral disease. Biopsy and histologic studies confirm the diagnosis. Amphotericin is the only available therapy, but mortality rates remain quite high.

Aspergillus fumigatus and *Aspergillus flavus* cause infections of the lungs, skin, and central nervous system in renal transplant patients.[13] Risk factors for infection include steroids, CMV infection, and neutropenia. Diagnosis is by organism identification from bronchoalveolar lavage and lung biopsy. Treatment is with amphotericin and surgical débridement of isolated lung focus if found.

Cryptococcosis occurs in 2.5 to 3.5 percent of renal transplant patients.[13] *Cryptococcus neoformans* enters through the lung and can spread to the skin and central nervous system, resulting in meningitis. Diagnosis is made by testing for cryptococcal antigen in serum and cerebrospinal fluid. Treatment consists of a combination of amphotericin and fluconazole.

Parasitic Infections

Pneumocystis carinii pneumonia (PCP) occurs in 5 to 10 percent of renal transplant patients not receiving prophylactic therapy. Risk factors include recent increases in the level of immunosuppression and concurrent CMV infections. PCP most often presents during the first 6 months posttransplant with fever, dry cough, dyspnea on exertion, and interstitial pulmonary infiltrates. Diagnosis is based on recovery

TABLE 96-1 Key Historical Elements in Evaluation of Renal Transplant Patients

History of recent temperature elevations
Date of transplantation surgery
Graft source: donor living related versus cadaveric
Rejection history: number of rejection episodes, date of last rejection episode, any recent changes in dosages of antirejection medications
History of chronic infections: CMV, EBV, hepatitis B and C, etc.
Recent exposure to patients with infections: chickenpox, CMV, tuberculosis, etc.
Complete list of immunosuppressant medications, compliance
Complete list of medications, even if unrelated to renal transplant, including over-the-counter medications
Baseline: blood pressure, body weight, serum creatinine level, cyclosporine level

of the organism on bronchoalveolar lavage or lung biopsy. Treatment is with high-dose intravenous TMP-SMX or pentamidine.

Toxoplasma gondii affects cardiac more often than renal transplant patients. Infection results in meningitis, brain abscess, pneumonia, myocarditis, endocarditis, and chorioretinitis. Diagnosis is based on histologic demonstration of trophozoites in a biopsy specimen. Treatment is with pyrimethamine with folinic acid in combination with sulfadiazine or clindamycin.

Strongyloidiasis can result in a hyperinfection syndrome of the gastrointestinal tract from *Strongyloides stercoralis*. Symptoms are usually limited to the gastrointestinal tract, with diarrhea and abdominal pain. With increased immunosuppression, strongyloidiasis can flare, producing hemorrhagic enterocolitis and pneumonia. Diagnosis is often first suspected by eosinophilia and confirmed by finding larvae in stool, body fluids, and tissue specimens. Strongyloidiasis is treated with thiabendazole.

Patient Evaluation

HISTORY The most common reason for a transplant recipient to present to the emergency department is fever.[14] Certain important historical elements should be collected (Table 96-1). While fever is the most common symptom of infection, it may be masked by steroids, uremia, or hyperglycemia, which suppress baseline body temperature. While fever suggests infection, the absence of fever should never be used to rule out possible infection in a transplant patient.

The risk of infection in a transplant patient is related to the state of immunosuppression. In general, renal grafts from living related donors have less risk of rejection, require less immunosuppression, and have less risk of infection. The degree of immunosuppression can be gauged by calculating the length of time from the transplant. Immunosuppression is at its highest level during the first 6 months posttransplant, with the greatest risk of rejection. After this period, rejection is less likely, and dosages of immunosuppressants are usually tapered down. The continued adjustment of immunosuppression over time has allowed a scheme to be developed that predicts the infectious agent by considering the age of the renal graft (Table 96-2).[15]

A history of recent or repeated rejections may also suggest the presence of increased levels of immunosuppression. During a rejection episode, increased immunosuppression is commonly used, which increases the risk of infection.

Infection in a transplant recipient may be either reactivation of a chronic infection or a new infection from exposure to contagious contacts. A complete exposure history of the patient and the patient's recent contacts can provide important clues to possible infections.

PHYSICAL EXAMINATION Renal transplant patients are immunocompromised; a high index of suspicion is required to find infections in unusual sites (Table 96-3). In addition to the common sites of infection (skin, pulmonary tract, and genitourinary tract), the head, neck, rectum, and abdomen should be closely scrutinized for infection. Infections during the first 12 weeks posttransplant are most commonly related to the surgical procedure of engraftment. Special attention should be given to the renal graft, and the examiner should look for signs of wound infection, pyelonephritis, and urine leakage with infection.

ANCILLARY TESTS The workup for renal transplant patients with suspected infection should include routine testing (Table 96-4). Additional tests should be performed based on the patient's presenting complaint, history, and physical examination. Common sites of infection, such as the genitourinary and pulmonary tracts, should be evaluated in all patients with a urinalysis and chest radiograph. A complete blood count; determinations of electrolyte, blood urea nitrogen, and creatinine levels; and liver function tests, while rarely diagnostic, may provide clues to the infectious agent and assess function of the renal graft. A complete blood count may disclose a leukocytosis with a left shift, seen with bacterial infections, unless the immunosuppressive agents have depressed the bone marrow. In addition, leukopenia with an increase in atypical lymphocytes is commonly seen with viral infections, especially CMV. Liver function tests may show mild transaminase elevations with CMV and EBV infections. Much higher elevations of transaminase are associated with hepatitis B. Bacterial cultures of blood and urine should be obtained.

If indicated, blood, urine, other body fluids, and tissue can be obtained for bacterial, mycobacterial, viral, and fungal studies. Serologic studies are especially important for the diagnosis of a wide variety of viral, fungal, and parasitic infections. Renal graft ultrasound

TABLE 96-2 Etiology of Infection by Time from Transplant

FIRST POSTTRANSPLANT MONTH: INFECTIONS RELATED TO SURGERY
UTIs (*Escherichia coli*)
Intravenous lines (*Staphylococcus aureus, Streptococcus viridans*)
Wound infections (*S. aureus, S. viridans*)
Pneumonia (*Streptococcus pneumoniae*)
6 POSTTRANSPLANT MONTHS: HIGHEST INCIDENCE OF OPPORTUNISTIC INFECTIONS
Viremia (CMV, EBV)
PCP
Meningitis (*Listeria monocytogenes*)
Sepsis (*Aspergillus fumigatus*)
AFTER 6 POSTTRANSPLANT MONTHS: THREE SUBGROUPS OF PATIENTS
1. Patients with good graft function on minimal immunosuppressants have the same risk of infection as the general population.
2. Patients chronically infected with latent viruses (e.g., CMV, EBV, hepatitis B and C) often have significant and ongoing end-organ damage (e.g., cirrhosis) secondary to these infections.
3. Patients with poorly functioning grafts who have sustained multiple episodes of rejection, now requiring large dosages of immunosuppressants, commonly have acute and chronic opportunistic infections (e.g., PCP, *Candida*, etc.).

TABLE 96-3 Key Physical Examination Elements for Renal Transplant Patients

VOLUME STATUS
Vital signs, change from baseline body weight, skin turgor, orthostatic pulse and blood pressure changes; invasive hemodynamic monitoring (Swan-Ganz catheterization) may be only reliable means of determining volume status.
HEENT
Periorbital edema (glomerulonephritis), retinal examination (CMV retinitis), sinuses (*S. aureus,* mucormycosis), mouth (*Candida,* or thrush), nuchal rigidity (meningitis due to *Listeria* or gram-negative organisms, retropharyngeal abscess, group A *Streptococcus*), lymphadenopathy (CMV, EBV, and hepatitis)
SKIN
Rashes commonly seen in viral syndromes (e.g., hepatitis B, EBV); look for cellulitis from indwelling catheter sites.
LUNG
Pneumonia is a common source of infection. Pneumococcus and other community-acquired agents are still common sources, but opportunistic infections (e.g., PCP, *Aspergillus,* tuberculosis) should be suspected.
HEART
Pericardial friction rubs can be heard as complications of uremia and a wide range of viral infections.
ABDOMEN
Peritonitis, commonly without a defined source, is one of the most common infections. Right upper quadrant tenderness is associated with hepatitis from hepatitis B or C, CMV, EBV. Peritoneal dialysis catheters, if left in place, can be sources of infection.
RENAL GRAFT
Usually placed in lower quadrant of abdomen; should be inspected, palpated, and auscultated. Inspection: look for signs of wound infection. Palpation: graft tenderness and swelling are often seen in acute rejection, outflow obstruction, and pyelonephritis. Auscultation: bruits suggest renal artery stenosis or arteriovenous malformations.
RECTAL
Perirectal abscess is common yet often overlooked source of infection.
EXTREMITIES
Access sites for hemodialysis can be sources of infection. Peripheral edema can represent recurrent vs de novo glomerulonephritis, graft failure, cirrhosis, nephrotic syndrome (from native kidneys), renal vein thrombosis extending to leg veins, malnutrition, cellulitis, heart failure.

studies should be reserved for patients suspected of having urinary obstruction, pyelonephritis, perinephric abscess, urine leak, or wound infection. A very low index of suspicion should be maintained for lumbar puncture in transplant patients because of the high incidence of *Listeria* meningitis.

ACUTE RENAL FAILURE

Failure of renal allografts is one of the most common causes of end-stage renal disease, accounting for 25 to 30 percent of all patients awaiting renal transplants.[16] Renal transplants can fail for the same reasons that native kidneys fail as well as for some unique causes (Table 96-5).

ARF within the first 1 to 12 weeks posttransplantation is most likely secondary to complications of the transplant surgery itself, usually due to obstruction of a renal artery, vein, or ureter.

Rejection is related to activation of T cells, which in turn stimulate specific antibody production against the graft. Varying clinical syndromes of rejection can be correlated with the length of time after transplantation.

Hyperacute rejection occurs immediately in the operating room, when the graft becomes mottled and cyanotic. Hyperacute rejection is secondary to unrecognized ABO compatibility or a positive T-cell crossmatch.

Acute rejection appears within the first 3 months posttransplant and affects about 30 percent of cadaveric and 27 percent of living-donor transplants.[17] Approximately 15 to 20 percent of transplant patients experience recurrent rejection episodes. Patients present with decreasing urine output, elevated blood pressure, a rising creatinine level, and mild leukocytosis. Fever, graft swelling, pain, and tenderness may be seen with severe rejection episodes. Rejection is secondary to prior sensitization to donor alloantigens (occult T-cell crossmatch) or a positive B-cell crossmatch. Diagnosis depends on graft biopsy.

Late acute rejection commonly occurs 6 months after transplantation and is highly correlated with withdrawal of immunosuppressive therapy.

Chronic rejection occurs 1 year after transplantation secondary to both cellular and humoral immunologic factors. Progressive loss of renal function occurs.

TABLE 96-4 Ancillary Tests for Evaluation of Renal Transplant Patients with Suspected Infection

ROUTINE
Urinalysis
Chest radiograph
Complete blood count
Electrolytes, blood urea nitrogen, creatinine
Liver function tests
Blood culture
Urine culture
INDIVIDUALIZED ANCILLARY TESTS
Mycobacterial, viral, and fungal cultures of blood, urine, and infected tissue
Stool cultures and examination for ova and parasites
Sputum cultures for bacteria and mycobacteria
Serologic studies for CMV, EBV, hepatitis, toxoplasmosis, *Cryptococcus*
Renal ultrasound
Lumbar puncture

TABLE 96-5 Differential Diagnosis of ARF Unique to Renal Transplant Patients

Complications of surgery
  Renal artery stenosis or thrombosis
  Urinary tract obstruction
  Renal vein thrombosis

Rejection syndromes
  Hyperacute rejection
  Acute rejection
  Late acute rejection
  Chronic rejection

Cyclosporine and Tarcolimus nephrotoxicity
Recurrent renal disease

TABLE 96-6 Cyclosporine Drug Interactions

INCREASES LEVELS OF CYA:
Calcium-channel antagonists: diltiazem, verapamil, nicardipine
Antibiotics: erythromycin, clarithromycin, doxycycline, ketoconazole
DECREASES LEVELS OF CYA:
Antibiotics: nafcillin, TMP/SMX (IV), isoniazid, rifampin
Anitconvulsants: phenytoin, phenobarbital, carbamazine
ENHANCES NEPHROTOXICITY WITHOUT ALTERING BLOOD LEVELS OF CYA:
Antibiotics: amphotericin B, acyclovir
Nonsteroidal anti-inflammatory drugs: all formulations

Nephrotoxicity from CYA and Tracolimus (FK506) is related to hemodynamic factors.[18,19] Acute toxicity (CYA levels greater than 300 ng/mL whole blood) causes vasoconstriction and renal ischemia, which can be reversed with decreasing the drug dosage. Chronic toxicity results in fixed vascular lesions and irreversible renal ischemia.

Patient Evaluation

HISTORY A detailed transplant history is important for all patients presenting with ARF. Since many of the clinical rejection syndromes are correlated with the age of the graft, the date of the transplant surgery should always be obtained. The donor source is also an important risk factor for ARF because cadaveric kidneys have higher incidences of ARF and rejection. A history of recent and repeated infections also gives important clues to the patient's level of immunosuppression. In patients with infections, it is common practice to decrease immunosuppressants, which increases the risk of rejection. A complete drug history is very important because many medications affect the levels and toxicity of CYA (Table 96-6).[20]

PHYSICAL EXAMINATION The physical examination in transplant patients with ARF should start with an evaluation of the patient's volume status; the vital signs, the patient's weight, skin turgor, and orthostatic pulse and blood pressure changes may be helpful in identifying hypovolemia. Peripheral edema in these patients is often a misleading sign of fluid overload and can occur in hypovolemic patients due to hypoalbuminemia or venous stasis. Examination of the renal graft can often disclose swelling and tenderness associated with acute rejection, renal vein thrombosis, and obstruction.

ANCILLARY TESTS Renal failure in transplant patients is defined as a 20 percent rise from baseline serum creatinine levels, as opposed to a 50 percent rise in other patients with ARF. As in all cases of ARF, the workup begins with a urinalysis (Table 96-7). Red blood cell casts and proteinuria are commonly seen in recurrent or de novo glomerulonephritis. The presence of white blood cells, bacteria, and nitrites is helpful in diagnosing UTIs. Routine determinations of electrolyte, blood urea nitrogen, and creatinine are rarely diagnostic of the etiology of ARF but may be helpful in determining volume status and identifying hyperkalemia, occasionally seen with CYA toxicity. CYA blood levels should be determined for all patients because of the high incidence of CYA-induced ARF. Renal ultrasound is the best test to rule out urinary obstruction. Renal biopsy is the gold standard for diagnosing rejection.

TABLE 96-7 Evaluation of ARF in Renal Transplant Patients

Urinalysis
Electrolytes
Blood urea nitrogen and creatinine levels
Cyclosporine level
Ultrasound study of renal graft
Renal biopsy

CARDIOVASCULAR DISEASE

Overall, the risk of coronary artery disease posttransplant is three- to fivefold that for age- and sex-matched control subjects. Risk factors for coronary artery disease include (1) pretransplant coronary artery disease, (2) hyperlipidemia secondary to antirejection medications, (3) hypertension, (4) steroids, (5) insulin-dependent diabetes mellitus, (6) erythrocytosis with increased blood viscosity, (7) smoking, and (8) frequent rejection episodes.[21]

Hypertension is found in approximately 50 percent of all transplant patients. Possible causes of hypertension include (1) graft rejection, (2) CYA toxicity, (3) glomerulonephritis (recurrent and de novo), (4) graft renal artery stenosis, (5) essential hypertension from native kidneys, (6) hypercalcemia, and (7) steroids.[22] Calcium channel blockers (CCB) have been shown to be particularly efficacious in treating hypertension in renal transplant patients on CYA, although CCBs interfere with CYA metabolism.

OTHER COMPLICATIONS

Chronic liver disease is an important cause of morbidity and mortality for renal transplant patients.[23] Causes of hepatic dysfunction include (1) viral hepatitis (CMV is leading cause, followed by hepatitis C and B) and (2) antirejection drugs (both azathioprine and CYA cause cholestatic jaundice).

By 15 years after transplantation, there is approximately a 50 percent incidence of malignancy. The most common sites of cancer are the skin (35 to 40 percent) and the viscera (10 to 15 percent). Lymphoproliferative malignancies, such as leukemia and lymphomas, are more prevalent among transplant patients than the general population.[24] Transplant patients are at significantly higher risk for cancers than the general population because of (1) chronic immunosuppression, (2) chronic antigenic stimulation, (3) increased susceptibility to oncogenic viral infections, and (4) direct neoplastic action of immunosuppressants.

DISPOSITION

Transplant patients are chronically immunosuppressed, attempting to balance between underimmunosuppression, with the risk of graft rejection, and overimmunosuppression, with the risk of infection. When these patients present to the emergency department with fever, increasing edema, decreased urine output, graft pain or swelling, or increasing fatigue, they should be evaluated for infection and renal graft function. These patients are complex, and it is often difficult to determine on initial assessment the presence of a serious infection or complication. It is recommended that the patient's physician or transplant coordinator be consulted to help the emergency physician in making the disposition decision.

REFERENCES

1. United Network for Organ Sharing (UNOS) Scientific Registry, July 26, 1998. Internet address: *www.unos.org*
2. Braun WE: Long-term complications of renal transplantation [clinical conference]. *Kidney Int* 37:1363, 1990.

3. Mahony JF: Long term results and complications of transplantation: The kidney. *Transplant Proc* 21(part 2)1433, 1989.
4. D'Alessandro AM, Hoffman RM, Knechtle SJ, et al: Successful extrarenal transplantation from non-heart-beating donors. *Transplantation* 59:977, 1995.
5. Novitzky D: Donor management: State of the art. *Transplant Proc* 29:3773, 1997.
6. Novitzky D: Detrimental effects of brain death on the potential organ donor. *Transplant Proc* 29:3770, 1997.
7. Gerber DA, Bonham CA, Thomson AW: Immunosuppressive agents: Recent developments in molecular action and clinical application. *Transplant Proc* 30:1573, 1998.
8. Preiksaitis JK, Diaz Mitoma F, Mirzayans F, et al: Quantitative oropharyngeal Epstein-Barr virus shedding in renal and cardiac transplant recipients: Relationship to immunosuppressive therapy, serologic responses, and the risk of posttransplant lymphoproliferative disorder. *J Infect Dis* 166:986, 1992.
9. Tolkoff-Rubin NE, Cosimi AB, Russell PS, Rubin RH: A controlled study of trimethoprim-sulfamethoxazole prophylaxis of urinary tract infection in renal transplant recipients. *Rev Infect Dis* 4:614, 1982.
10. Lederman ED, Conti DJ, Lempunt N, et al: Complicated diverticulitis following renal transplantation. *Dis Colon Rectum* 41:613, 1998.
11. Santamaria Saber LT, Figueiredo JF, Santos SB, et al: *Nocardia* infection in renal transplant recipient: Diagnostic and therapeutic considerations. *Rev Inst Med Trop São Paulo* 35:417, 1993.
12. Aguado JM, Herrero JA, Gavalda J, et al: Clinical presentation and outcome of tuberculosis in kidney, liver, and heart transplant recipients in Spain: Spanish Transplantation Infection Study Group, GESITRA. *Transplantation* 63:1278, 1997 [published erratum appears in *Transplantation* 64:942, 1997].
13. Tolkoff-Rubin NE, Rubin RH: Opportunistic fungal and bacterial infection in the renal transplant recipient. *J Am Soc Nephrol* 2(suppl):S264, 1992.
14. Bromberg JS, Grossman RA: Care of the organ transplant recipient. *J Am Board Fam Pract* 6:563, 1993.
15. Rubin RH, Wolfson JS, Cosimi AB, Tolkoff-Rubin NE: Infection in the renal transplant recipient. *Am J Med* 70:405, 1991.
16. Evans RW: The demand for transplantation in the United States, in Terasaki PI (ed): *Clinical Transplantation 1990*. Los Angeles, UCLA Tissue Typing Laboratory, 1991, pp 319–327.
17. Cecka JM, Terasaki PI: Early rejection episodes. *Clin Transplant* 425, 1989.
18. Myers BD, Newton L: Cyclosporine-induced chronic nephropathy: an obliterative microvascular renal injury. *J Am Soc Nephrol* 2(suppl 1):S45, 1991.
19. Shapiro R: Tacrolimus (FK-506) in kidney transplantation. *Transplant Proc* 29:45, 1997.
20. Campana C, Regazzi MB, Buggia I, Molinaro M: Clinically significant drug interactions with cyclosporin: An update [comments]. *Clin Pharmacokinet* 30:141, 1996.
21. Kasiske BL, Guisarro C, Massay ZA, et al: Cardiovascular disease after renal transplantation. *J Am Soc Nephrol* 7:158, 1996.
22. Luke RG: Hypertension in renal transplant recipients [clinical conference]. *Kidney Int* 31:1024, 1987.
23. Rao KV, Anderson WR: Liver disease after renal transplantation. *Am J Kidney Dis* 19:496, 1992.
24. Sheil AG, Disney AP, Mathew TG, et al: Malignancy following renal transplantation. *Transplant Proc* 24:1946, 1992.

97 RENAL IMAGING

Dan E. Wiener
Jennifer Marrast Host

The recent years have seen an explosion in the modalities available to the emergency physician to image the urinary system. This chapter reviews the different methods and discusses their role in the management of patients in the emergency department (ED).

IMAGING MODALITIES

Plain-Film Radiography

The KUB (kidneys, ureters, and bladder) is a plain full-length film of the abdomen. The kidneys can be visualized because the perinephric fat gives them a lucent outline. Renal calculi can usually be visualized, but small ureteral calculi may be hidden by bowel shadows. Calculi in the lower ureters may be confused with phleboliths and can be difficult to differentiate. The KUB by itself rarely adds to patient care in the ED and is most useful in conjunction with ultrasound or intravenous pyelography (IVP) (see below).

Ultrasound

Ultrasound is a rapid, painless method to visualize the urinary tract. The patient requires no preparation and is not exposed to the potentially harmful effects of radiation or contrast material. The limitations of this modality include poor visualization of the ureter and difficulty in imaging obese patients. The quality of the study is both operator- and equipment-dependent. Ultrasound is an anatomic study and provides no data regarding kidney function. Renal ultrasound can document the presence, location, and size of the kidneys and detect focal parenchymal lesions such as cysts and tumors. Hydronephrosis and on occasion dilated ureters and calculi can be demonstrated (Fig. 97-1). Fluid collections surrounding the kidney can also be seen. With Doppler flow capability, vascular problems in the kidney can be identified.

Ultrasound is performed using a 3.5-MHz transducer. With the patient in a supine position, the transducer is placed subcostally from the lateral approach. The operator sweeps the ultrasound plane to locate the kidney. Rotation of the probe permits documentation of the longitudinal and transverse renal axes. The liver is usually used as an acoustic window to visualize the right kidney and the spleen to visualize the left. Images on the right are technically superior to those on the left because the liver provides a better acoustic window than the spleen. An air-filled stomach and dilated loops of bowel can hinder visualization. The kidneys move with respiration, and having patients hold their breath after a maximal inhalation often enhances visualization.

Gerota's fascia, the renal cortex, the collecting system, the renal sinus, as well as proximal and distal calculi can be visualized. Gerota's fascia is associated with perinephric fat and is visualized as a bright area surrounding the kidney. The renal cortex is homogeneous in appearance and more reflective (brighter) than the renal medulla. The renal pelvis is centrally located and appears echogenic. Dilation of

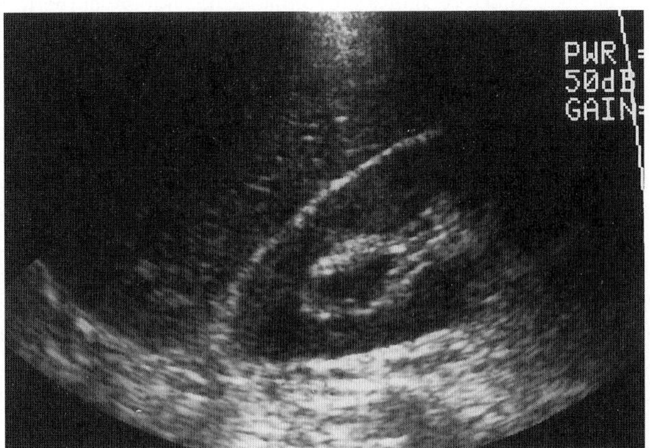

FIG. 97-1. Sonogram, right uterovesicular stone with hydronephrosis. (Photograph courtesy of David Frager, M.D.)

the collecting system by fluid (echo-free) is thus readily apparent. The normal ureter is not visualized, but the dilated ureter can sometimes be seen. In the longitudinal plane, the normal kidney is football-shaped and measures 9 to 12 cm. In the transverse plane, the normal kidney is C-shaped and measures 4 to 5 cm. The kidneys normally measure within 2 cm of each other in the longitudinal axis.

Intravenous Pyelography

The IVP provides both anatomic and functional information about the kidney. It is most commonly utilized in the setting of flank pain and hematuria and has long been considered the ''gold standard'' for visualizing renal calculi. The disadvantages of the study include the necessity of transporting the patient to x-ray, the time demand of the study, and the administration of contrast material. Concern regarding poor images in ED patients because of the lack of bowel preparation is unwarranted.[1]

Before initiation of the IVP, the patient is asked to void and the abdomen is compressed. The standard series of films taken during an IVP include the following:

1. The scout film, a plain radiograph from the level of the kidneys to the bladder prior to the administration of contrast. This allows visualization of stones that may be obscured by contrast material. The compression device is released after the scout film.
2. The nephrogram, a coned view of the kidneys 1 min after injection of contrast. This film is examined for the absence or delay in visualization, homogeneity, and duration of the nephrogram.
3. The pyelogram, two films taken 5 and 10 min after injection. Calyceal dilation or effacement, ureteral dilation, intraluminal filling defects, and the extravasation of contrast material can be seen.
4. The bladder film, taken 20 min after injection.
5. The postvoid film, used to evaluate postvoid residual bladder volume and visualize any retained contract that may have been hidden by the full bladder. Multiple views and tomograms are often used to enhance the quality of the study. When a calculus is suspected, two views are required to distinguish a peristaltic contraction from a tumor or a stricture. Delayed views are necessary in instances of obstruction or nonvisualization.

Computed Tomography

Computed tomography (CT) scanning provides both anatomic and functional information about the kidney. The renal parenchyma, collecting system, extrarenal space, ureters, and bladder can all be visualized. Renal perfusion can be assessed with the administration of contrast material. CT can identify extrarenal pathology or injury not clinically suspected. As the method of choice in assessing stable patients with suspected renal trauma, it determines the extent of the parenchymal injury, demonstrates urine extravasation or perirenal hemorrhage, and evaluates the integrity of renal vascular pedicle and status of adjacent organs. The disadvantage of CT is the time required to perform the study and the need to administer contrast if optimal results are to be obtained.

With CT, images of the kidney and urinary system are reconstructed from information collected by focused x-ray beams arranged on a plane that cuts through the patient's body in a transverse or horizontal direction. The patient lies on a movable table that passes through the CT gantry, which contains the tightly focused x-ray beams. As these beams pass through the patient, they are absorbed by a ring of detectors on the opposite side of the gantry. The intensity of the x-ray beam that reaches the detector is dependent on the absorption characteristics of the intervening tissue. The radiodensity of a small area of tissue can then be calculated from the absorption pattern of multiple beams crossing the area from different directions.

During spiral CT, the x-ray tube is in continuous rotation while the patient is moved smoothly, at a constant speed, through the scanning field. This technique improves the detection of small lesions, as scanning is performed during a single breath-hold, thus reducing the movement of intraabdominal organs and motion artifact, which occurs when imaging is performed during respiration. Data from multiple scanning planes can be used to produce three-dimensional reconstruction of lesions. In trauma, information about the extent of renal disruption, trauma to the renal pedicle, and viability of disrupted fragments can be provided. In addition, shaded surface displays allow volume surface analysis of parenchymal organs and maximal-intensity projections provide analysis of the vasculature. The selected slice thickness of a scan depends on the clinical presentation. Trauma scans are usually 8 to 10 mm thick and are obtained from the diaphragm down to the bottom of the pelvis. CT scans for renal colic utilize 5-mm slices from the top of the kidneys down to the bladder. If there is an area of subtle or equivocal findings, the radiologist may elect to make smaller cuts for clarification.

Intravenous Contrast Enhancement

The IVP and CT use intravenous contrast material containing iodinated compounds that absorb x-rays. These agents allow the vessels and organs to be more easily differentiated from adjacent nonenhancing structures. A typical imaging protocol involves the administration of 150 mL of intravenous contrast by a power injector into an intravenous catheter of adequate size, typically an 18-gauge catheter in the antecubital vein.

Intravenous contrast media are classified according to two characteristics: ionic versus nonionic and high-osmolar versus low-osmolar. Nonionic media are approximately ten times more expensive then ionic media but cause fewer lethal and adverse reactions. The relative risk of adverse reactions with ionic media is about four times greater than that seen with nonionic media.[2] High-osmolar contrast media (HOCM) are all ionic as opposed to low-osmolar contrast media (LOCM), which can be ionic or nonionic.[3] Intravenous contrast media are nephrotoxic; the least nephrotoxic is nonionic LOCM. In patients with normal renal function, there is no measurable impairment of renal function between the use of either HOCM or LOCM.[4] However, in patients with preexisting renal insufficiency and diabetes, nonionic LOCM causes less impairment to renal function than HOCM. Therefore, LOCM should be considered as the first choice of contrast media in patients with the following risk factors: age greater than 50 to 60 years, debilitation, known severe cardiovascular disease, asthma, previous allergy to contrast, renal failure, and/or diabetes.[5] For further discussion, see Chap. 294.

Oral Contrast Enhancement

Oral contrast is used with the abdominal CT scan for a patient suspected of having intraabdominal injuries. This barium- or iodine-based solution markedly increases the density of the gastrointestinal tract, differentiating bowel from other pathology. When there is a suspicion of renal injury, both oral and intravenous contrast is used. Oral contrast is a minimal threat to the kidneys and can be used in patients with depressed renal function.

Dynamic CT Scanning

In dynamic CT scanning, a series of rapid images using helical CT is obtained during peak vessel contrast enhancement. As with IVP, the kidney is visualized in the (1) vascular phase, when major vessels are visualized; (2) nephrogram phase, when contrast reaches the tubules and medullary opacification occurs; and (3) pyelogram phase, when calyceal and pelvic filling is observed. In trauma, dynamic CT is useful in demonstrating compromise of parenchymal perfusion and parenchymal fracture margins. Dynamic CT can also differentiate abscesses and hematomas.

Retrograde Urethrogram

The retrograde urethrogram is the test of choice when there is uncertainty about urethral integrity, usually due to trauma. It is an invasive procedure requiring the use of contrast material.

Using sterile procedure, the foreskin is retracted and the penis is stretched perpendicularly across the patient's thigh to prevent urethral folding. Contrast solution (Renografin 60 or Hypaque 50%, either full or half strength) is injected into the penis using the catheter tip of a 60-mL syringe or through a nonlubricated 16- or 18-Fr Foley catheter inserted just inside the urethral meatus. If a Foley is utilized, the balloon of the catheter is inserted 2 to 3 cm past the meatus and 1 to 2 mL of saline is injected into the balloon to secure the catheter in the fosa navicularis. In the direct syringe technique, slow constant pressure is used to inject 50 to 60 mL of contrast material. With the Foley technique, gravity is used to infuse the contrast medium from the filled syringe with the plunger removed and attached to the catheter, held above the patient's bed. If the medium will not flow, slow, constant pressure can be used, as with the direct syringe approach. The examination is best performed under fluoroscopic visualization. For patients with multiple injuries, fixed or portable radiographic equipment is frequently used. Radiographs are taken during the injection of approximately the last 10 mL of contrast.

In instances when a Foley catheter has already been inserted into the bladder and there is a suspected urethral injury, it is necessary to confirm that the urethra is intact and the catheter is in the bladder. The catheter should not be removed; instead, the urethrogram should be performed around it. Using a lubricated pediatric feeding tube placed alongside the existing Foley catheter, contrast material can slowly be injected to demonstrate the presence or absence of extravasation.

Cystogram

Cystography is the standard examination for bladder trauma. It is an invasive procedure requiring the use of contrast material. An anteroposterior (AP) pelvic or KUB film should be obtained as a scout film before contrast material is introduced.

Using sterile technique, a 16- or 18-Fr Foley catheter is carefully placed into the bladder. A 60-mL pistonless catheter-tip syringe is attached to the Foley and contrast material is poured into the syringe. Contrast is then allowed to enter the bladder via gravity as the syringe is placed above the level of the patient's bladder. The bladder is allowed to fill until extravasation occurs or the bladder is filled (400 mL). If bladder contraction occurs during filling, an additional 50 mL is injected by hand. In children below age 11, estimated bladder capacity is calculated based on the formula (age in years $+2) \times 30$. Incomplete filling of the bladder can limit the quality of the study. To accurately exclude bladder rupture and extravasation, the bladder must be filled with at least 250 mL of contrast material.

Cystograms should be done using fluoroscopy or plain films in the AP oblique, and lateral projections. If there is an associated pelvic fracture, the patient should be kept in the supine position to avoid possible disruption of any retropubic hematomas. To detect posterior perforations, an AP film should always be obtained after bladder drainage.

Angiography

Angiography is the test of choice for defining vascular injuries of the kidney. It is highly invasive, requiring cannulation of the femoral artery and the use of intravascular contrast material. Indications include the absence of a functioning kidney on IVP or CT, findings of a large retroperitoneal hematoma, major renal fractures, or segmental areas of renal nonenhancement. In some instances injuries to the parenchyma and arteries can be treated using interventional angiography to stop hemorrhage.

The femoral artery is accessed by the Seldinger technique (flexible catheter advanced over a guidewire). The tip of the catheter is placed in the aorta and a midstream aortogram obtained to evaluate the number and status of the renal arteries. The catheter tip is then placed at the upper level of the proximal artery and films are obtained to capture the arterial, capillary, and venous phases.

Renal Cortical Scintigraphy (RCS)

RCS, using dimercaptosuccinic acid (DMSA), is a radionuclear study that evaluates kidney function. RCS is most commonly used in the evaluation of children with suspected pyelonephritis and, occasionally, assessment of a renal transplant.

Two hours after administration of Tc^{99m}-DMSA, scanning is performed using a gamma camera. DMSA binds to the renal tubules and accumulates in the functioning renal cortex. Intrarenal blood flow and proximal tubular cell membrane transport determine cortical uptake. Focal or diffuse areas of decreased cortical uptake of tracer without any loss of volume indicate the presence of pyelonephritis. Areas of decreased uptake with volume loss indicate old scars. Images are evaluated for the size of the kidneys, their shape and location, and differential renal function as well as the distribution of cortical uptake.

CONDITIONS

Renal Colic

The ideal imaging study in renal colic would (1) determine the size and location of the stone, (2) define the presence and degree of ureteral obstruction, and (3) identify other causes of flank pain and hematuria when renal calculi have been excluded.

Some 90 percent of renal calculi are radiopaque and theoretically visible on plain radiographs. Studies in the 1930s and more recent textbooks report visualization of stones in 85 to 90 percent of cases. These studies did not specify if the visualized ''stone'' was related to the patient's symptoms or confirmed by other radiographic studies. Recent comparisons between plain-film radiography and IVP (the ''gold standard'') found that plain radiography had a sensitivity of only 58 percent.[6] Compared with helical CT, plain radiography had a sensitivity of 45 percent and specificity of 77 percent.[7] Plain radiography alone has low utility and should not be used in the evaluation of patients with suspected renal colic; it does, however, play a role as an adjunct to IVP and ultrasound.

IVP has long been considered the ''gold standard'' for the evaluation of renal colic. The location of a calculus can be seen by a dye cutoff in the ureter, the size of the calculus can usually be determined, and visualization of the entire ureter secondary to a lack of peristaltic contractions is suggestive of obstruction. Identifying stones at the UV junction or the distal ureter can be difficult but is enhanced by assessment of the postvoid film. Secondary findings of stone disease include delay in the appearance of the nephrogram, distention of the renal pelvis, calyceal distortion, dye extravasation, or hydronephrosis.

Recent studies have compared the efficacy of ultrasound to IVP in the diagnosis of renal stones in ED patients presenting with renal colic[8–11] (Table 97-1). These studies used passage of stones, stone recovery at surgery, or repeat IVP as the gold standard and used the finding of a stone and/or evidence of hydronephrosis as a positive test result for the diagnosis of renal calculi. Both modalities are slightly better at identifying obstruction than localizing a stone. Using either stone identification or detection of obstruction, both modalities have essentially the same range of sensitivity and specificity, although ultrasound has a wider range of sensitivity, reflecting the greater dependence on operator skill and limitations of the modality. Plain-film radiographs can be used as road maps to focus the ultrasound study, with a reported 100 percent sensitivity and 95 percent specificity in

TABLE 97-1 Imaging Modalities in Renal Colic

	IDENTIFICATION OF STONE AND/OR HYDRONEPHROSIS		IDENTIFICATION OF STONE		IDENTIFICATION OF HYDRONEPHROSIS	
	Sensitivity	Specificity	Sensitivity	Specificity	Sensitivity	Specificity
IVP	81–85%*	90–100%*	64%‡	100%‡	90%‡	94%‡
Ultrasound	66–91%*	90–100%*	64%‡	100%‡	85%‡	100%‡
Helical CT	95–98%†	96–100%†			83%†	94%†

*Refs. 11–13.
†Ref. 15.
‡Ref. 14.

identifying ureteral calculi.[12] Theoretically, ultrasound has an advantage in imaging radiolucent stones (about 10 to 20 percent of total), but if there is no dilation of the ureter, it becomes more difficult to place the visualized density correctly. Furthermore, ultrasound has particular difficulty in visualizing dilations of the upper and midureter. The distal ureter is more accessible, since the bladder acts as an acoustic window within the ureter. Ultrasound may also be limited by the delayed appearance of hydronephrosis; in a series of 216 cases of renal calculi causing obstruction, the initial sonogram was negative in 24 percent, but all these patients showed evidence of hydronephrosis when the sonogram was repeated 8 to 12 hours later.[13]

Published studies indicate that emergency physicians can perform bedside ultrasound examinations in patients with renal colic and detect hydronephrosis with 97 percent sensitivity as compared with an IVP.[14] The availability of ultrasound equipment for use in the ED and training of more emergency physicians has the potential to expand the use of this modality and reduce the use of IVP studies for patients with acute renal colic.

Selecting IVP or ultrasound for an individual patient requires some clinical judgment. Certainly patients with contraindications to radiation and the administration of contrast should have an ultrasound. The clinician will have to further weigh the importance of ascertaining functional information about the kidney as well as the increased likelihood of identifying the location of the stone versus the added time and radiation exposure necessary to complete an IVP. One approach would be to obtain ultrasound in all patients presenting with signs and symptoms of renal colic and only proceed to IVP if the patient is deemed to require surgical intervention or if the diagnosis remains unclear.

Helical CT without intravenous contrast has become the imaging modality of choice in many institutions for patients with acute renal colic. The helical CT takes only 5 min to perform and can identify the presence and location of calculi of all compositions, not only providing prompt and accurate diagnosis in most patients with calculi but also identifying extrarenal disorders in patients without calculi. The average dose of radiation at the skin from a helical CT is 3 to 5 cGy, comparable to 1.5 to 3 cGy (0.25 to 0.3 cGy per radiograph) from an IVP. One limitation of the helical CT is that it does not provide functional information about the degree of obstruction.

Studies demonstrate that helical CT has excellent sensitivity and specificity in the diagnosis of renal colic[15] (Table 97-1). One limitation is distinguishing phleboliths from renal calculi, but secondary signs can be used to help make this distinction. For renal colic, these signs include ureteral dilation (sensitivity 90 percent and specificity 93 percent), perinephric stranding (sensitivity 82 percent and specificity 93 percent), collecting system dilation (sensitivity 83 percent and specificity 94 percent), and renal enlargement (sensitivity 71 percent and specificity 89 percent).[16] The presence of ureteral dilation and perinephric stranding had a positive predictive value of 99 percent, and the absence of both had a negative predictive value of 95 percent (both were present or absent in 181/220 patients). Edema of the ureteral wall surrounding the calculus (rim sign) is up to 100 percent sensitive and 94 percent specific in distinguishing renal stones from phleboliths. Helical CT should be considered positive for calculi when any of the following are seen: (1) a stone, (2) both ureteral dilation and perinephric stranding, or (3) a tissue rim sign. Urologists were able to use helical CT without further imaging in 91/105 patients who underwent lithotripsy or endoscopic stone removal.[17] The utilization of this valuable modality will depend on its institutional availability as well as its degree of acceptance among urologists.

Renal Transplant

Renal transplant failure can be secondary to graft rejection or renovascular complications. Modalities available to evaluate the transplanted kidney include angiography, ultrasound with color-flow Doppler and duplex Doppler, and renal scintigraphy. The choice of modality will depend on the clinician's index of suspicion for graft rejection or vascular compromise.

The most common vascular complication of transplant is renal artery stenosis (RAS), with an incidence of 3 to 15 percent in the first 3 years after transplant.[18] Renal artery and vein thromboses are rare, usually occur in the perioperative period, and are generally catastrophic, resulting in loss of the renal graft. In contrast, identification and treatment of RAS can result in graft salvage. Patients with RAS often present with hypertension and worsening renal function. Posttransplant patients are reported to have a 50 to 60 percent incidence of hypertension unrelated to RAS. Therefore, it is the renal transplant patient with hypertension that is progressive or difficult to control with medical therapy who should be considered at risk for RAS. The gold standard for diagnosing RAS is angiography. However, angiography is limited by its invasive nature, the use of nephrotoxic contrast agents, the risk of an adverse reaction to contrast media, and complication rates of 0.5 to 2.3 percent (hemorrhage, intimal flaps, and arteriovenous fistulas).

The conventional sonogram has limited utility but may detect some anatomic abnormalities suggesting a vascular or nonvascular diagnosis. Duplex and color-flow Doppler have been utilized to evaluate the renal artery but are technically difficult and the subject of controversy in the literature about their diagnostic accuracy. Color Doppler has the advantage of sampling long segments of vessels but cannot accurately quantitate flow disturbances. When identified, flow disturbances must be quantified by duplex Doppler. Utilizing peak flow rates, studies have attempted to define a rate of flow that can accurately predict RAS greater than 50 percent. The threshold flow-rate value that provides the best combination of sensitivity and specificity is controversial. Peak systolic velocity of 190 to 250 cm/s has a sensitivity of 90 to 100 percent for RAS greater than 50 percent.[19,20] However, specificity has varied from as low as 55 percent to as high as 95 percent.[21] The overall accuracy can be improved by using peak systolic velocity in conjunction with analysis of the waveform (rounded, smaller-amplitude waveform with stenosis) in detecting significant proximal RAS.

Renal scintigraphy is a test of vascular perfusion, parenchymal extraction, and excretion. Abnormal findings from this study include (1) impaired uptake and visualization, which is consistent with vascular obstruction or hyperacute rejection and is a poor prognostic sign; (2) normal uptake and visualization but with parenchymal retention, which is associated with poor urine flow and the retention of the secreted isotope in the tubules; and (3) decreased uptake with normal parenchymal transit time and absent or minimal cortical retention, which is consistent with chronic rejection or renovascular hypertension. Unfortunately, the effects of renal artery stenosis, graft rejection, and cyclosporine toxicity cannot be distinguished using renal scintigraphy.[22]

Captopril-augmented renal scintigrams have been utilized to distinguish physiologic from nonphysiologic RAS. Patients with normal captopril renal scintigrams are not likely to respond to angioplasty, while patients with abnormal captopril renal scintigrams will likely have a significant improvement following angioplasty. Captopril renal scintigrams can replace renal vein renin sampling in identifying patients with lesions amenable to intervention.[23]

Urinary Tract Infection (UTI)

There is considerable controversy regarding the appropriate imaging of children with UTI to identify predisposing functional and anatomic abnormalities. Sometimes, an emergency evaluation is required because of diagnostic confusion based on atypical presentations, a negative urinalysis, or treatment failure based on persistent fever and toxicity 72 h following the initiation of therapy.

Renal cortical scintigraphy (RCS) using Tc^{99m}-DMSA is the most sensitive imaging modality for establishing the diagnosis of pyelonephritis.[24] In animal models, RCS has a sensitivity of 91 percent and specificity of 99 percent as compared with histopathology.[25] Results in humans with culture-positive UTI have shown a sensitivity of only 50 to 66 percent.[26] While its sensitivity is low, RCS is more sensitive than ultrasound, CT, or IVP.[27] Controversy exists concerning the necessity of documenting renal scarring and pyelonephritis in a child with an apparently simple UTI.[28,29] Some clinicians advocate treating all patients with a 10-day course of antibiotics, as opposed to the usual 5- to 7-day course, to avoid the need to document the presence of pyelonephritis.[30] Also, patients with vesiculoureteral reflux do not always demonstrate scarring on RCS; therefore, a normal RCS does not obviate the need to proceed with voiding cystography. RCS has more accepted utility in following renal scarring in patients with recurrent UTI and pyelonephritis, where progressive renal scarring can result in renal failure or hypertension. An advantage of RCS is that it can be used in children and neonates with poor renal function.

The voiding cystogram is used to demonstrate vesicoureteral reflux, the most common abnormality found in the urinary tract of children, which is seen in approximately 35 percent of children with UTI. Children at risk for vesicoureteral reflux include those with a family history of reflux and Caucasians. Voiding cystography can be done by radiographic or radionuclide technique. The radionuclide voiding cystogram utilizing technetium pertechnetate has the advantage of less radiation exposure but the disadvantage of poor visualization of urethral and bladder abnormalities, which are more commonly seen in boys. The radionuclide voiding cystogram is the imaging modality of choice in girls and is useful for the follow-up of patients and for screening siblings. Boys should undergo radiographic cystography. However, the relationship between vesicoureteral reflux and pyelonephritis remains controversial, with as many as 50 percent of children estimated to have another route of infection. Evaluation of patients with RCS-documented pyelonephritis found only a 37 percent incidence of vesicoureteral reflux on voiding cystograms.[31]

Ultrasound is an insensitive method for diagnosing pyelonephritis or vesicoureteral reflux but can provide anatomic information unavailable in other modalities. It can visualize renal abscesses, hydronephrosis, and obstruction at either the ureterovesical or uteropelvic junction. CT scan can accurately diagnose renal parenchymal lesions but is less sensitive than RCS is detecting pyelonephritis. CT signs of pyelonephritis include renal enlargement, poor corticomedullary definition, and patchy areas of decreased definition. Renal and perinephric abscesses are well visualized on CT. CT is not recommended in children because of the proximity of the gonads and their radiosensitivity before puberty.

Adults with pyelonephritis require only imaging studies if there is a suspicion of complications, including obstruction and perinephric abscess. CT is the imaging modality with the highest yield in demonstrating anatomic and functional renal abnormalities caused by acute pyelonephritis.

Trauma

RENAL INJURIES Blunt trauma is the etiology in 80 to 90 percent of renal injuries. Significant renal injury is usually associated with gross hematuria or signs of shock. Although gross hematuria occurs frequently with major renal injuries, the absence of gross hematuria does not rule out significant injury.[32] The emergency physician should suspect renal injury in patients with flank masses, flank ecchymosis, eleventh- and twelfth-rib fractures, and fractures of the upper lumbar transverse processes. Patients with blunt trauma may have microscopic hematuria without a clinically significant urinary injury; imaging these patients would therefore not be useful. Other approaches have been advocated to reduce the incidence of normal studies in patients with microscopic hematuria after blunt trauma. In adults, imaging can be restricted to those with microscopic hematuria and signs of shock. In children, imaging can be restricted to those with associated major injuries or hematuria of more than 50 red blood cells per high-power field.[33] Penetrating trauma is different; those with stab wounds near the urinary system and gunshot wounds require radiographic evaluation for any degree of hematuria.

Decisions regarding imaging of the kidneys and urinary tract in cases of trauma are usually secondary to the management and stabilization of life-threatening injuries. In the hemodynamically stable patient with suspected intraabdominal injury, the test of choice is a CT scan of the abdomen with administration of IV and oral contrast. The CT scan is more sensitive and specific than IVP and has the advantage of imaging the entire abdomen and retroperitoneum.[34] In hemodynamically unstable patients, an intraoperative IVP is often the only imaging modality available. Ultrasound is neither sensitive nor specific for the detection of renal injuries, although it can be utilized as a screening tool for the detection of intraperitoneal fluid.

The injury pattern to kidneys includes contusions, lacerations, lacerations with extension into the collecting system, and disruptions of the renal vasculature. The renal injury scale developed by the Organ Injury Committee of the American Association for Surgery of Trauma grades these injuries on a scale of 1 to 5[35] (Table 97-2; Fig. 97-2). Radiographic staging is used in conjunction with the clinical situation to differentiate injuries requiring surgical management from those that can be managed nonoperatively. Grade I, II, and III renal injuries will heal spontaneously and are best managed conservatively without surgery, as opposed to grade V lesions, which should be managed surgically. There is no universal agreement on the management of grade IV lesions.

In unstable patients, the ''one-shot'' IVP (a single radiograph of the abdomen taken 5 to 10 min after contrast injection) can identify major renal and urinary injuries. With early repair, this is the most effective way to preserve renal function.[36] The IVP can establish the presence or absence of bilateral kidneys, delineate the renal paren-

TABLE 97-2 Classification of Renal Injuries

Grade I: Contusions that appear as amorphous interstitial extravasation of blood. A hematoma is a well-demarcated, hyperdense collection of blood.
Grade II: Lacerations that are superficial and limited to the renal cortex. These injuries are sometimes accompanied with a subcapsular hemorrhage (a small crescentic formation that flattens the underlying renal contour) or a perirenal hemorrhage, which infiltrates or displaces the perirenal fat.
Grade III: Lacerations greater than 1 cm depth, not involving the collecting system.
Grade IV: Lacerations extending into the medulla and communicating with the collecting system. They are almost always accompanied by a perirenal hemorrhage with extravasation of urine into the perirenal parenchyma or into the perirenal space.
Grade V: The kidneys are shattered and there may be injury to the vasculature of the renal pedicle. A shattered kidney is depicted on CT as multiple fractured planes, with separation of functioning or devitalized tissue. If renal artery occlusion has occurred, the kidney demonstrates no enhancement.

chyma, and define the collecting system and ureter. Findings of contrast extravasation or nonfunction correlate with the presence of major renal injuries.[37] There is currently no role for the standard IVP in renal trauma; a review of the literature from the pre-CT era demonstrated that IVP has a diagnostic accuracy of 50 to 90 percent for renal injuries.[38]

Angiography is used to document and treat renovascular injuries. It is indicated for patients with CT findings of large retroperitoneal hematomas, major renal fractures, and segmental areas of renal nonenhancement. Angiography can also be considered in patients with persistent or recurrent posttraumatic hematuria.[39] If a source of bleeding is identified, the patient can be treated with selective embolization.

Traumatic thrombosis, intrarenal hematomas, and vessel vasospasm are visualized by angiography as sharply demarcated defects, reflecting devitalized tissue. At the margins of the injury, homogeneous staining of the parenchyma indicates an adequate vascular supply, while heterogeneous staining indicates the presence of vessel spasm or traumatic thrombosis. Subcapsular and intrarenal hematomas are visualized as faint staining of the parenchyma and cortex in the nephrographic phase. Infarction of the kidney secondary to vessel thrombosis may be focal or global. It is recognized by the maintenance of a small rim of peripheral perfusion around the subcapsular cortex and the lack of central perfusion. Segment infarcts, depending on the distribution of the occluded vessel, may be either wedge-shaped or hemispheric. Wedge-shaped infarcts are oriented with the base toward the renal capsule and the apex toward the hilum. Arterial injuries are seen as extravasation of contrast material persisting into the venous phase. Arterial injuries should be distinguished from intrarenal urinary extravasation, which has a similar dense pattern. Injuries to the renal artery are characterized by the abrupt termination of the renal artery, just beyond its origin. Traumatic arterial aneurysms (arteriovenous fistulas) are diagnosed by opacification of the anastomosed vein after the administration of contrast into the artery.

Duplex and color Doppler ultrasound studies can detect renal infarcts, vascular pedicle injuries, and arteriovenous fistulas. Segmental or focal infarcts appear as hypoechoic wedge-shaped masses. Arteriovenous fistulas appear as increased flow velocity with arterial pulsations in the draining vein. Color Doppler demonstrates a mass of torturous vessels consisting of multiple colors indicative of the lack of organization and turbulent flow of the vessels. In renal artery occlusion, Doppler will not demonstrate flow to the kidney.

BLADDER INJURIES The bladder is located within and protected by the pelvis. Up to 85 percent of bladder injuries are associated with a pelvic bone fracture, almost always caused by a bony spicule penetrating the bladder. Of patients with bladder rupture, 50 to 85 percent have an extraperitoneal rupture, 15 to 45 percent have an intraperitoneal rupture, and 0 to 12 percent have both. The imaging modality of choice to detect urethral and bladder injuries is a retrograde cystogram. Indications for a retrograde cystogram include (1) inability to void, (2) gross hematuria in the presence of a pelvic bone fracture, and (3) blood at the external urinary meatus. In males, a retrograde urethrogram is usually obtained first to ensure that the urethra is intact before the Foley catheter is advanced into the bladder for the cystogram study. In females, the Foley catheter can usually be placed without a urethral imaging study unless gross blood is visible at the urethral meatus. Bladder injuries are classified as types 1 to 5 (Table 97-3).

URETHRAL INJURIES Injury to the female urethra is rare owing to its short length and mobility. If it is injured, the most common type is avulsion of the proximal urethra, occasionally involving the bladder

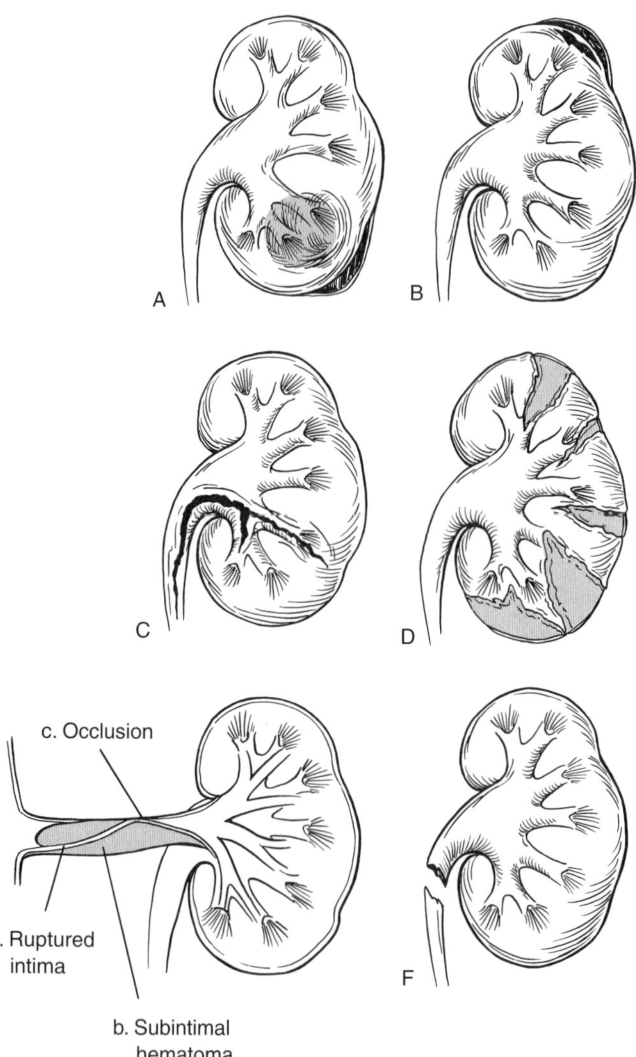

FIG. 97-2. Classification of renal injuries. **A.** Grade I injury. Renal contusion (with subcapsular hematoma). **B.** Grade II injury. Superficial renal laceration (with subcapsular hematoma). **C.** Grade IV injury. Deep laceration extending into the collecting system. **D.** Grade V injury. Shattered kidney. **E.** Thrombotic occlusion of renal artery. There is a rupture of the intima (*a*) complicated by a subintimal hematoma (*b*). This has resulted in complete occlusion of blood flow in the artery (*c*). There is also propagation of blood clot proximally toward the aorta, as well as distally. **F.** Avulsion of UPJ.

TABLE 97-3 Classification of Bladder Injuries

Type 1: Bladder contusion. An incomplete or unperforated tear of the bladder mucosa. This injury is associated with a pelvic hematoma and is the most common type of injury. The radiographic appearance is normal.

Type 2: Intraperitoneal bladder rupture at the junction of the mobile and stationary areas of the bladder and at the peritoneal reflection of the bladder dome. This occurs when the bladder is distended and sustains a blunt abdominal trauma, which leads to an increase in the intravesical pressure. Patients at risk for this injury include those involved in automobile crashes who are wearing lap seatbelts. This injury is characterized radiographically by contrast material running freely, surrounding loops of bowel and intraperitoneal viscera, and filling the paracolic gutters.

Type 3: Interstitial bladder injury. This type of injury is rare. It is an incomplete perforation of the serosa, leaving the mucosa intact. Retrograde cystography reveals an irregularity in the bladder wall without extravesicular leakage of contrast.

Type 4: Extraperitoneal ruptures. These are divided into simple and complex injuries. With simple injuries, extravasation of contrast material is limited to the pelvic extraperitoneal space, while complex injuries are characterized by spread of contrast material beyond the pelvic extraperitoneal space, into the retroperitoneum, scrotum, and the anterior abdominal wall.

Type 5: Combined bladder injury.

neck. Urethral injury should be suspected in females who present with pelvic fractures, blood at the introitus, deep periurethral laceration, difficulty in voiding or inability to void, unsuccessful attempts at catheterization, and the development of vulvar edema after removal of a urinary catheter. One review of 130 cases of pelvic fractures in females found that 4.6 percent had urethral injuries.[40]

The male urethra is divided into the anterior portion, which consists of the penile and bulbous urethra, and the posterior portion, consisting of the membranous and prostatic urethra. The urogenital diaphragm separates these two portions.

Injuries to the anterior urethra are associated with straddle injuries: the bulbous urethra and surrounding corpus spongiosum are crushed against the inferior aspect of the pubis resulting in a contusion and/or partial rupture of the bulbous urethra. Retrograde urethrography is the test of choice to evaluate these injuries. With partial anterior urethral rupture, the retrograde urethrogram demonstrates extravasation of contrast with maintained urethral continuity. Complete anterior disruption is rare and is identified by extravasation of the contrast medium and failure to visualize the anterior urethra completely up to the urogenital diaphragm.

In posterior urethral injuries, the prostatomembranous urethra ruptures above the urogenital diaphragm secondary to shear forces. The classic clinical findings are blood at the urethral meatus, inability to void spontaneously, a palpable bladder, and a superiorly displaced prostate on digital rectal examination. Three patterns of posterior urethral injuries have been described (Table 97-4).

TABLE 97-4 Classification of Posterior Urethral Injuries

Type I: The posterior urethra is stretched but intact. Hematoma collects in the prostatic fossa and the bladder is elevated high in the pelvis.

Type II: The urethra is disrupted at the membranoprostatic junction above the urogenital diaphragm. Contrast material is present in the extraperitoneal space of the pelvis.

Type III: Disruption of the membranous urethra, with extension on the injury into the proximal bulbous urethra and/or diaphragmatic rupture. Depending on the degree of the urogenital diaphragmatic injury, contrast may be visible in the perineum.

URETERAL INJURIES In ureteral injuries, CT scanning with intravenous contrast or IVP usually demonstrates contrast extravasation and hydronephrosis. The most common type of injury is avulsion of the ureter at the uteropelvic junction, often occurring from falls. These injuries will show normal renal parenchyma with failure of the ureter and bladder to opacify and the accumulation of contrast material in the perirenal space.

REFERENCES

1. George CD, Vinnicombe SJ, Balkissoon ARA, et al: Bowel preparation before intravenous urography: Is it necessary? *Br J Radiol* 66:17, 1993.
2. Katayama H, Yamaguchic K, Kozuka T, et al: Adverse reactions to ionic and nonionic contrast media: A report from the Japanese committee on the safety of contrast media. *Radiology* 175:621, 1990.
3. McClennan BL: Preston M. Hickey Memorial Lecture: Ionic and nonionic iodinated contrast media: Evolution and strategies for use. *Am J Roentgenol* 155:225, 1990.
4. Barrett BJ, Carlisle EJ: Metaanalysis of the relative nephrotoxicity of high- and low-osmolality iodinated contrast media. *Radiology* 188:171, 1993.
5. Hartman GW, Hattery RR, Witten DM, et al: Mortality during excretory urography: Mayo clinic experience. *Am J Roentgenol* 139:914, 1982.
6. Mutgi A, Williams JW, Nettleman M: Renal colic: Utility of plain abdominal roentgenogram. *Arch Intern Med* 151:1589, 1991.
7. Levine JA, Neitlich J, Verga M: Ureteral calculi in patients with flank pain: Correlation of plain radiography with unenhanced helical CT. *Radiology* 204:27, 1997.
8. Haddad MC, Sharif HS, Shahed M, et al: Renal colic: Diagnosis and outcome. *Radiology* 184:83, 1992.
9. Hill MC, Rich JI, Mardiat JG, et al: Sonography vs excretory urography in acute flank pain. *Am J Roentgenol* 144:1235, 1985.
10. Middleton WD, Dodds WJ, Lawson TL, Foley WD: Renal calculi: Sensitivity for detection with US. *Radiology* 167:239, 1988.
11. Sinclair D, Wilson S, Toi A, et al: The evaluation of suspected renal colic: Ultrasound scan versus excretory urography. *Ann Emerg Med* 18:556, 1988.
12. Erwin BC, Carroll BA, Sommer GF: Renal colic: The role of ultrasound in initial evaluation. *Radiology* 152:147, 1984.
13. Andressen R, Wegner HEH: Intravenous urography revisited in the age of ultrasound and computerized tomography: Diagnostic yield in cases of renal colic, suspected pelvic and abdominal malignancies, suspected renal mass, and acute pyelonephritis. *Urol Int* 58:221, 1997.
14. Henerson SO, Hoffner RJ, Aragona JL, et al: Bedside emergency department ultrasonography plus radiography of the kidneys, ureters, and bladder versus intravenous pyelography in the evaluation of suspected renal colic. *Acad Emerg Med* 5:666, 1998.
15. Dalrymple NC, Verga M, Anderson KR, et al: The value of unenhanced helical computerized tomography in the management of acute flank pain. *J Urol* 159:735, 1998.
16. Smith RC, Verga M, Dalrymple N, et al: Acute ureteral obstruction: Value of secondary signs on helical unenhanced CT. *Am J Roentgenol* 167:1109, 1996.
17. Preminger GM, Vieweg J, Leder RA, et al: Urolithiasis: Detection and management with unenhanced spiral CT—A urologic perspective. *Radiology* 207:308, 1998.
18. Erley CM, Duda SH, Wakat JP: Noninvasive procedures for the diagnosis of renovascular hypertension in renal transplant recipients—A prospective analysis. *Transplantation* 54:863, 1992.
19. Grenier N, Douws C, Morel D, et al: Detection of vascular complications in renal allografts with color Doppler flow imaging. *Radiology* 178:217, 1991.
20. Baxter G, Ireland H, Moss J, et al: Colour Doppler ultrasound in renal transplant artery stenosis: Which Doppler index? *Clin Radiol* 50:618, 1995.
21. Gottlieb R, Lieberman J, Pabico R, et al: Diagnosis of renal artery stenosis in transplanted kidneys: Value of Doppler waveform analysis of the intrarenal arteries. *Am J Roentgenol* 165:1441, 1995.
22. Dubovsky EV, Russell CD, Erbas B: Radionuclide evaluation of renal transplants. *Semin Nucl Med* 25:49, 1995.
23. Shamlou K, Drane W, Hawkins I, et al: Captopril renography and the hypertensive renal transplantation patient: A predictive test of therapeutic outcome. *Radiology* 190:153, 1994.
24. Jaya G, Bal C, Padhy A, et al: Radionuclide studies in the evaluation of urinary tract infections. *Indian Pediatr* 33:635, 1996.

25. Majd M, Shalaby-Rana E, Rushton H, et al: Diagnosis of experimental acute pyelonephritis in piglets: Comparison of CT and 99m Tc-DMSA scintigraphy. *Radiology* 193:136, 1994.
26. Majd M, Rushton H: Renal cortical scintigraphy in the diagnosis of acute pyelonephritis. *Semin Nucl Med* 22:98, 1992.
27. Bjorgvinsson E, Majd M, Dunne Eggli K: Diagnosis of acute pyelonephritis in children: Comparison of sonography and 99m Tc-DMSA scintigraphy. *Am J Roentgenol* 157:539, 1991.
28. Andrich M, Majd M: Diagnostic imaging in the evaluation of the first urinary tract infection in infants and young children. *Pediatrics* 90:436, 1992.
29. Slovis TL: Is there a single most appropriate imaging workup of a child with an acute febrile urinary tract infection? *Pediatr Radiol* 25:S46, 1995.
30. Schlager T, Lohr J: Urinary tract infection in outpatient febrile infants and children younger than 5 years of age. *Pediatr Ann* 22:505, 1993.
31. Majd M, Rushton H, Jantausch B, et al: Relationship among vesicoureteral reflux, P-fimbriated *Escherichia coli,* and acute pyelonephritis in children with febrile urinary tract infection. *J Pediatr* 119:578, 1991.
32. Mee S, McAninch J, Robinson A, et al: Radiographic assessment of renal trauma: A 10-year prospective study of patient selection. *J Urol* 141:1095, 1989.
33. Morey A, Bruce J, McAninch J: Efficacy of radiographic imaging in pediatric blunt renal trauma. *J Urol* 156:2014, 1996.
34. McAninch J, Federle M: Evaluation of renal injuries with computerized tomography. *J Urol* 128:456, 1982.
35. Pollack AM, Weiss AJ: Imaging of renal trauma. *Radiology* 172:297, 1989.
36. Cass AS, Bubrick M, Luxenberg M, et al: Renal trauma found during laparotomy for intra-abdominal injury. *J Trauma* 25:997, 1985.
37. Cass AS, Luxenberg M: Unilateral nonvisualization on excretory urography after external trauma. *J Urol* 132:225, 1984.
38. Mendez R: Renal trauma. *J Urol* 118:698, 1977.
39. Sciafani SJA, Becker JA, Shaftan GW, et al: Strategies for the radiologic management of genitourinary trauma. *Urol Radiol* 7:231, 1985.
40. Perry MO, Husmann DA: Urethral injuries in female subjects following pelvic fractures. *J Urol* 47:139, 1992.

GYNECOLOGY AND OBSTETRICS

VAGINAL BLEEDING AND PELVIC PAIN IN THE NONPREGNANT PATIENT

Laurie Morrison
Julie Spence

This chapter discusses the emergency department (ED) management of vaginal bleeding and pelvic pain in nonpregnant female patients. A review of the physiology of the normal menstrual cycle, the pathophysiology of abnormal vaginal bleeding, and the physiology of pelvic pain is included. Fluctuation in bleeding and pelvic pain are common in the natural history of the normal menstrual cycle. It is important, therefore, for physicians to differentiate normal variations from pathology.

EPIDEMIOLOGY

ED visits for vaginal bleeding or pelvic pain by women of reproductive-age are common. It is estimated that 5 percent of women aged 30 to 49 years will consult a physician for treatment of menorrhagia.[1] An Australian review of Pap smear requests for women aged 20 to 69 documented that 1 in 20 had abnormal bleeding.[2] Although this data may not be generalizable to the ED, it does emphasize the point that abnormal vaginal bleeding is common. Population-based data are not available for children and adolescents.

In a cross-sectional survey of reproductive-age women who presented to a primary care setting, 90 percent reported some dysmenorrhea, 38 percent experienced dyspareunia sometimes, and 39 percent reported other types of pelvic pain.[3] Overall, pelvic pain is most common in 18- to 30-year-old women. Prevalence does not vary significantly by education, parity, or race.[3] Diagnoses made on the basis of history and physical examination may overestimate the prevalence of pathology. In studies of women with pelvic pain who were referred for laparoscopy, 17 percent of adolescents and 16 percent of reproductive-age women had normal findings on examination.[4,5]

PHYSIOLOGY

Developing Children

In newborn females, the placental transfer of estradiol and gonadotropin is responsible for a mucoid or blood-tinged vaginal discharge, minor breast development, and vaginal flora similar to that in adult women. Uterine bleeding secondary to estrogen withdrawal may occur in the first 6 weeks of life in normal neonates. Bleeding after this time is always abnormal and requires investigation.

By definition, prepubertal children lack secondary sex characteristics. The labia and mons have less fatty tissue than in adults and lack protective hair. The labia minora are thin, and there is less distance between the anus and the vaginal introitus. The thin vaginal epithelium of prepubertal girls is similar to that of postmenopausal women.

Adolescents

Ten years of age tends to be the lower limit for menarche, and the mean age in North America is 12.5 years. Most children develop secondary breast changes 2 years prior to the onset of menarche. At the time of ovarian stimulation, a white or yellow vaginal discharge, which is both nonodorous and nonirritating, may appear. Early cycles are anovulatory and irregular, but unlike adult anovulatory cycles, bleeding is generally not excessive. The hypothalamic pituitary axis takes 1 to 5 years to reach full maturity, and the average time to establish ovulatory cycles is 2 years after menarche.

Normal Menstrual Cycle

The normal menstrual cycle is 28 days and is divided into four phases: follicular, ovulation, luteal or secretory, and menses. The first 14 days are the follicular phase, during which the ovary matures an oocyte for ovulation, and the granulosa cells, lining the follicle, produce estrogen. This stimulates the endometrium to proliferate and thicken (Fig. 98-1). In response to the rising estrogen levels, the pituitary gland secretes follicle-stimulating hormone (FSH) and luteinizing hormone (LH), which stimulate the release of the mature oocyte. The residual follicular capsule forms the corpus luteum. During the luteal phase, the corpus luteum secretes estrogen and progesterone, which maintain the endometrium and make it more receptive to implantation. If fertilization and implantation occur, the developing embryo secretes human chorionic gonadotropin (hCG) into the bloodstream, signaling the corpus luteum to continue the production of progesterone and estrogen necessary to support early pregnancy. In the absence of hCG, the corpus luteum involutes, and estrogen and progesterone levels fall. Hormonal withdrawal causes vasoconstriction in the spiral arterioles of the endometrium. This leads to the final phase, or menses, when the ischemic endometrial lining becomes necrotic and sloughs. The vaginal effluvium contains blood, endometrial tissue, and fluid. The estimated amount of menstrual blood loss ranges from 25 to 60 mL. Judging the amount of bleeding in a menstrual cycle may be difficult. The average tampon or pad absorbs 20 to 30 mL of vaginal effluent, although the number of pads or tampons used is unreliable, as personal habits vary greatly among women. In a normal cycle, fibrinolysis occurs in the uterine cavity and the cervix. In women with heavy bleeding, there may be insufficient time for fibrinolysis, and blood clots may occur. Definitions of commonly used gynecologic terminology have been included in Table 98-1.

Menopause

Menopause results from ovarian ''burnout'' and, on average, occurs at age 51.[6] During the transition phase, or perimenopausal period, there is lengthening or marked variation in the intermenstrual intervals. By age 45, only a few primordial cells remain, and the production of estrogen decreases. As a result, the pituitary continuously produces large quantities of FSH and LH. There is no midcycle rise in estrogen to trigger a further surge of pituitary hormones for ovulation. Estrogens continue to be produced in lower, subcritical levels for a short time after menopause, until the remaining follicles become atretic, and production falls to almost zero.

Pelvic Pain

The distribution of nerves in the pelvis is outlined in Table 98-2. The hypogastric nerve innervates the uterus, adnexae, and bladder dome. The second through fourth sacral nerves provide sensation for the lower segment of the uterus, cervix, bladder trigone, and rectum. Pain of either gynecologic and nongynecologic origin may be referred to the back, buttocks, perineum, or legs.

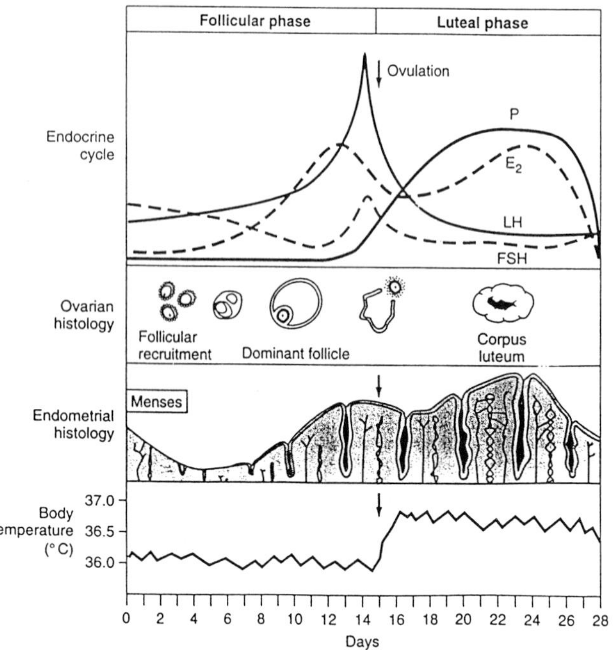

FIG. 98-1. The hormonal, ovarian, endometrial, and basal body temperature changes and relationships throughout the normal menstrual cycle. (From Carr and Wilson,[24] with permission.)

The quality of pain can be characteristic of different etiologies. Visceral or splanchnic pain is colicky and caused by distention of a hollow viscus or stretching of a ligament. Examples include distention of the fallopian tube in ectopic pregnancy, uterine contractions in dysmenorrhea, and stretch of the round ligament with adhesions or in pregnancy. Peritoneal or somatic pain is sharp and localized to the region of inflamed tissue, as in salpingitis, appendicitis, and endometritis. Generalized peritonitis may be seen with larger degrees of inflammation, i.e., with spillage of blood, pus, or gastrointestinal (GI) contents into the peritoneal cavity.

The onset of pain may also provide diagnostic clues. Gradual onset may occur with a slow leak of irritants, as occurs with pelvic inflammatory disease (PID). Sudden onset of pain occurs with ischemia or cyst rupture. Cyclic pain is usually related to the menstrual cycle, and timing is helpful in establishing a diagnosis. Examples include endometriosis and dysmenorrhea (Table 98-3).

TABLE 98-1 Definitions

Vaginal bleeding	Defined temporally as midcycle (ovulatory), premenstrual, menstrual, and postmenstrual.
Abnormal vaginal bleeding	Vaginal bleeding occurring outside the regular cycle
Menorrhagia	Menses >7 days, or menstruation >60 mL, or <21-day recurrence, from any cause
Metrorhagia	Irregular vaginal bleeding outside the normal cycle
Menometrorhagia	Excessive irregular vaginal bleeding
Dysfunctional uterine bleeding	Abnormal vaginal bleeding due to anovulation
Postcoital bleeding	Vaginal bleeding after intercourse, suggesting cervical pathology

TABLE 98-2 Nerves Carrying Painful Impulses from the Pelvic Organs

Organ	Spinal Segments	Nerves
Perineum, vulva, lower vagina	S2–S4	Pudendal, inguinal, genitofemoral, posterofemoral cutaneous
Upper vagina, cervix, lower uterine segment, posterior urethra, bladder trigone, uterosacral and cardinal ligaments, rectosigmoid, lower ureters	S2–S4	Sacral afferents traveling through the pelvic plexus
Uterine fundus, proximal fallopian tubes, broad ligaments, upper bladder, cecum appendix, terminal large bowel	T11–T12, L1	Thoracolumbar splanchnic nerves through uterine and hypogastric plexus
Outer two-thirds of fallopian tubes, upper ureter	T9–T10	Thoracolumbar splanchnic nerves through mesenteric plexus
Ovaries	T9–T10	Thoracolumbar splanchnic nerves traveling with ovarian vessels via renal and aortic plexus and celiac and mesenteric ganglia

Source: From Rapkin,[25] with permission.

PATHOPHYSIOLOGY: THE ANOVULATORY CYCLE

Anovulatory bleeding may be regular but more often is irregular due to fluctuating estrogen levels below the critical level required to maintain endometrial growth. The level of estrogen depends on the age, number, and activity of ovarian follicles. As some follicles degenerate, others resume the production of estrogen and the endometrium continues to proliferate for weeks to months, which may cause glandular hyperplasia (''Swiss cheese'' hyperplasia). This estrogen steady state is insufficient to meet the growing needs of the endometrium and produces a relative estrogen insufficiency, and vaginal bleeding ensues. Alternatively, when follicle degeneration and stimulation are not balanced, absolute estrogen levels fall and withdrawal bleeding occurs. Characteristically, anovulatory cycles present as prolonged amenorrhea with periodic menorrhagia. Due to the lack of progesterone-mediated myometrial contractions and arteriolar vasospasm, anovulatory cycles are rarely associated with cramping.

PREPUBERTAL CHILDREN

History

In children, the history should focus on circumstances of bleeding, times of recurrence, and associated symptoms, including abdominal or pelvic pain. Physicians should also look for signs of precocious puberty. Children who were exposed to diethylstilbestrol (DES) in utero are at risk for adenocarcinoma of the vagina and cervix and

TABLE 98-3 Differential Diagnosis of Acute Pelvic Pain

Gynecologic Disease or Dysfunction

Acute pain
1. Complication of pregnancy
   a. Ruptured ectopic pregnancy
   b. Abortion, threatened or incomplete
   c. Degeneration of a leiomyoma
2. Acute infections
   a. Endometritis
   b. Pelvic inflammatory disease (acute PID)
   c. Tubo-ovarian abscess
3. Adnexal disorders
   a. Hemorrhagic functional ovarian cyst
   b. Torsion of adnexa
   c. Twisted parovarian cyst
   d. Rupture of functional or neoplastic ovarian cyst

Recurrent pelvic pain
1. Mittelschmerz (midcycle pain)
2. Primary dysmenorrhea
3. Secondary dysmenorrhea

Gastrointestinal
1. Gastroenteritis
2. Appendicitis
3. Bowel obstruction
4. Diverticulitis
5. Inflammatory bowel disease
6. Irritable bowel syndrome

Genitourinary
1. Cystitis
2. Pyelonephritis
3. Ureteral lithiasis

Musculoskeletal
1. Abdominal wall hematoma
2. Hernia

Other
1. Acute porphyria
2. Pelvic thrombophlebitis
3. Aneurysm
4. Abdominal angina

Source: From Rapkin,[25] with permission.

require a formal gynecologic consultation. All presentations warrant consideration of sexual abuse.

Physical Examination

As is the case for most pediatric presentations in the ED, children should be completely undressed and thoroughly examined. This enables physicians to look for subtle signs of disease, injury, and abuse. A child's development of secondary sex characteristics should be assessed and compared with the Tanner stages of breast and pubic hair growth. Most premenarchal girls should not undergo a speculum examination or vaginoabdominal palpation except in the event of vaginal bleeding and trauma. The vast majority of examinations and procedures can be done with the parent holding the child.

Young children presenting with vaginal bleeding or trauma can be examined on the parent's lap. Children older than age 3 should be comfortable supine, lying "like a frog," for the examination of the external genitalia (Fig. 98-2*A*). Draping of the legs and perineum is unnecessary and usually cumbersome. Visualization of the vagina is best done by asking the child to "get up on your hands and knees like you are crawling" (Fig. 98-2*B*). She can rest her head on her forearms and look at her parent. The labia and buttocks are gently pressed upward and outward. If the child relaxes the abdominal and back muscles, the resulting lordosis should enable one to see the lower half of the vagina with an otoscope light. Children over age 3 may also be examined while they are supine in the knee-chest position, like a "cannonball."

If cultures are indicated, they should be taken with the child in the supine position with a saline-soaked cotton-tipped swab or a soft medicine dropper. If the findings of the vaginal examination are suboptimal, or if a pelvic mass or foreign body is suspected, a rectoabdominal examination should be performed while the child is in the frog-leg position. The cervix is palpated as a midline button of tissue often described as similar in size and consistency to the eraser on a pencil. The ovaries and uterus should not be palpable. The vagina can be "milked" for blood or discharge.

The use of restraints for pelvic and vulvar examination has no role in modern practice. Conscious sedation or general anesthesia may be required to obtain an adequate examination. A speculum examination should not be performed without appropriate anesthesia.

Differential Diagnosis

The epidemiologic data and the differential diagnosis of vaginal bleeding in the prepubertal child are outlined in Tables 98-4 and 98-5.

Investigations

Most causes of pelvic pain and bleeding in this age group can be diagnosed by taking a complete history and performing a selective physical examination. ED-based investigations are usually unnecessary. Treatment and criteria for consultation are self-evident.

Clinical Conditions in Prepubertal Children

VAGINITIS Vaginitis is the most common cause of pelvic pain and vaginal bleeding in prepubertal children. The immature anatomy and the hypoestrogenic state predispose children to this condition. In this age group, *Staphylococcus epidermidis* and diphtheroids are the predominant vaginal flora. *Lactobacillus,* which metabolizes glycogen to

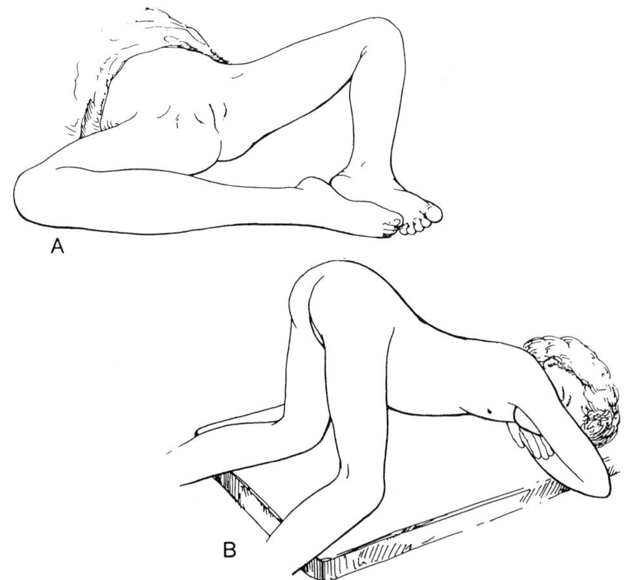

FIG. 98-2. Examination positions for a prepubertal child. (From Paradise,[26] with permission.)

TABLE 98-4 Etiologies for Vaginal Bleeding in Prepubertal Children (Referral Population)

		Incidence
Associated with precocious puberty		21%
True	Idiopathic	
	Cerebral disorders	
	Tuberous sclerosis	
	Congenital adrenal hyperplasia	
	Primary hypothyroidism	
Pseudo	Ovarian tumors	
	Adrenal tumors	
	McCune-Albright syndrome	
	Gonadotropic-producing tumors	
	Iatrogenic	
Not associated with precocious puberty		
Neonatal hormonal withdrawal		
Vaginitis (e.g., shigella, *Streptococcus pyogenes*)		6%
Vulvar lesions (e.g., lichen sclerosus, condyloma)		10%
Trauma		8%
Accidental		
Sexual abuse		
Foreign body		
Tumors		21%
Urethral polyps/prolapse		10%
Precocious menarche		
Unknown		25%

Source: From Hill et al,[27] with permission.

lactic acid in adults, is not found in children. This contributes to the alkaline environment of the prepubertal vagina, and as a consequence, children may develop infections with organisms that are not pathogenic in adults. This topic is covered in greater depth in Chap. 104.

GENITAL TRAUMA Trauma to the genital area must alert physicians to the possibility of sexual assault (see Chap. 289, ''Child Abuse and Neglect''). Perineal trauma represents 0.2 percent of all injuries in children younger than age 15. In an American study of children (mean age, 6.2 years), unintentional injuries to the pelvis were a result of bicycle accidents, straddle injuries, and falls. The labia majora was injured most frequently, and injuries tended to be superficial. Only 3 of 56 children required surgical repair of lacerations.[7] There are case reports of vaginal injuries from water sports, including water skiing, jet-ski accidents, and riding down water chutes. The extent of the injuries range from superficial trauma to deep lacerations with life-threatening retroperitoneal bleeding and abdominal injuries.[8,9] Minor trauma, such as riding a tricycle, may induce ecchymotic bullae that may be misinterpreted as sexual abuse or a straddle injury.

Trauma to the vulva can produce ecchymoses and/or lacerations and may be associated with injury to the vagina and rectum. Straddle injuries may cause severe trauma to the mons, labia majora, buttocks, inner thigh, and periurethral areas. Injuries to the urethra may cause spasm and urinary retention, and it is important to ensure that the child is able to void prior to discharge. The hypoestrogenic skin of the prepubertal vagina tears easily with minor trauma, and there is a risk of wall perforation with a penetrating injury to both the vagina and rectum. All penetrating trauma requires a careful vaginal and rectal examination. It is prudent to refer all children with hymenal injury, or bleeding from the vagina or rectum, for prompt evaluation under anesthesia by a pediatric gynecologist.

Genital trauma management varies with the injury. Hematomas will spread liberally along tissue planes in the perineum, forming large painful masses, and cause pressure necrosis of the overlying skin. Any hematoma should be observed in the ED until it has stopped expanding in size. Small hemostatic lesions heal well with conservative management and wound care. Minor lesions that continue to bleed should respond to pressure dressings or ice packs, and in more severe cases, topical thrombin or Gelfoam (Pharmacia Upjohn, Kalamazoo, MI) absorbable gelatin sponges can be used. Older children may tolerate surgical repair of minor lacerations with local anesthesia. The use of topical anesthetics is contraindicated because of enhanced systemic toxicity. The use of delayed absorbable sutures avoids the discomfort and trauma of subsequent removal. Any crush or penetrating injury secondary to a human bite should be covered with broad-spectrum antibiotics and allowed to heal by secondary intent. There must be a low threshold for admission with subtle injuries, if there is a suspicion of danger at home, or the need for psychological and social support.

TABLE 98-5 Causes of Bleeding and Pelvic Mass by Approximate Frequency and Age Group

BLEEDING

Prepubertal	Adolescent	Reproductive	Perimenopausal	Postmenopausal
Vulvovaginal and external lesions	Anovulation	Pregnancy	Anovulation	Endometrial lesions, including cancer
Foreign body	Pregnancy	Anovulation	Fibroids	Exogenous hormone use
Precocious puberty	Exogenous hormone use	Exogenous hormone use	Cervical and endometrial polyps	Atrophic vaginitis
Tumor	Coagulopathy	Fibroids	Thyroid dysfunction	Other tumor—vulvar, vaginal, cervical
		Cervical and endometrial polyps		
		Thyroid dysfunction		

PELVIC MASS

Infancy	Prepubertal	Adolescent	Reproductive	Perimenopausal	Postmenopausal
Functional ovarian cyst	Germ cell tumor	Functional cyst	Functional cyst	Fibroids	Ovarian tumor (malignant or benign)
Germ cell		Pregnancy	Pregnancy	Ovarian epithelial tumors	Bowel, malignant tumor or inflammatory
		Dermoid/other germ cell tumors	Uterine fibroids	Functional cysts	Metastases
		Obstructing vaginal/uterine anomalies	Ovarian epithelial tumors		
		Epithelial ovarian tumors			

Source: From Hillard,[28] with permission.

VAGINAL FOREIGN BODY Vaginal foreign bodies classically present with intermittent bloody, foul-smelling vaginal discharge. Small wads of toilet paper are most commonly found. Foreign bodies should be suspected when the posterior wall of the lower half of the vagina cannot be visualized when the child is in the "crawling position" (see Fig. 98-2*B*) or knee-chest position (cannonball position). Toilet paper is not palpable on rectal examination, although other foreign bodies such as erasers, beads, and nuts can sometimes be appreciated. Radiographs are usually not helpful. Frequently, the object may be removed by gentle vaginal irrigation with warm water or by "milking" the vagina of any hard objects during rectal exam. Foreign bodies that cannot be removed by simple measures may require examination and removal under anesthesia.

CONGENITAL VAGINAL OBSTRUCTION Vaginal obstruction can be secondary to a transverse vaginal septum or imperforate hymen. Imperforate hymen is found in 1 in 1000 of full-term female neonates, and a transverse vaginal septum is found in 1 in 2000 to 1 in 84,000 females. Diagnosis is made by careful examination of the perineum. Infants may go undiagnosed for weeks until they develop an abdominal mass, difficulty with urination, or a visible bulging membrane at the vagina introitus. In severe forms, children may have constipation, hydronephrosis, respiratory compromise, and edema of the lower extremities. The treatment of hydrocolpos is surgical excision of the obstruction.

PRECOCIOUS PUBERTY AND MENARCHE Children aged 5 to 9 may develop secondary sex characteristics and experience the onset of menarche and accelerated growth indistinguishable from the normal changes of puberty. This is most frequently idiopathic in origin but can be associated with endocrine or neurologic diseases. Referral to a pediatrician is essential.

Premature menarche is cyclic vaginal bleeding in prepubertal children in the absence of pubertal development. It is a diagnosis of exclusion and beyond the purview of emergency physicians. In the ED, it is important to rule out other serious causes of vaginal bleeding prior to referral for further investigations.

URETHRAL PROLAPSE The etiology of urethral prolapse is unknown. It frequently occurs between the ages of 2 and 10 and is more common in black children. It may present as a red or purplish, soft spongy mass approximately 1 to 2 cm in diameter, with a central dimple at the urethral meatus. Urethral prolapse may be discovered surreptitiously during a routine examination of an asymptomatic child. Vaginal bleeding is the presenting complaint in 90 percent of cases. Painless vaginal bleeding may be associated with urinary frequency or dysuria in 25 percent of cases. At times, it is difficult to discern whether the mass is urethral or vaginal in origin. Observing the child urinating on a bedpan may help to determine the etiology and precludes the use of a urinary catheter to confirm the diagnosis. Urethral prolapse is usually treated simply with sitz baths and application of topical estrogen creams. Patients presenting with red or necrotic mucosa may require surgical intervention under anesthesia.

DERMATOLOGIC LESIONS Children with seborrhea and psoriasis may present with bleeding after minor trauma. Lichen sclerosus is seen in hypoestrogenic females. The etiology is unknown. Characteristically, lichen sclerosus appears as an hourglass-shaped depigmented area on the vulva, perianal, and adjacent skin. The skin is thin and atrophic, with tiny ivory papules that coalesce. The patches are usually dry and itchy. Mild forms of lichen sclerosus may be treated with sitz baths and 1% hydrocortisone cream for symptomatic relief. More serious cases should be referred to a dermatologist.

ADOLESCENTS AND ADULTS

History

Adolescent and adult patients presenting to the ED with pelvic pain or bleeding share many common elements of the history and physical examination. Complications related to pregnancy are always possible, and routine inquiries are both appropriate and necessary. Key points that should be routinely addressed when taking the clinical history are age of menarche, menstrual history, date of the last menstrual period (LMP), pattern of abnormal bleeding or discharge, and the presence of dysmenorrhea. Sexually active patients should be asked about contraception, current sexual activity, the use of barrier protection, HIV and hepatitis status, and a history of PID, sexually transmitted diseases (STDs), or ectopic pregnancy. Patients who present with pain should be asked about its quality, timing, location, and radiation, as well as aggravating or alleviating factors. Associated symptoms of the urinary, GI, and musculoskeletal systems, as well as the presence of fever or syncope, should be documented. A history of recent illnesses, psychological stress, weight change, or endocrine problems, including thyroid disease and pituitary tumors, should be obtained. In patients with bleeding, signs and symptoms of a coagulopathy, including nosebleeds, easy bruisability, and menorrhagia, and a family history should be noted in the examination.

Taking the history of adolescent girls is challenging. Honest responses to questioning will require assurances of confidentiality and comfort by the physician. If the patient requests a female physician, honor the request, if at all possible. Always interview the patient without the parent present. Usually this is best done if you ask the parent to leave just prior to the physical examination. Questions regarding STDs and sexual activity can be very disturbing for adolescents. It is important historical information and should be obtained in a nonjudgmental, gentle way that in itself will be educational. It is not realistic to expect an accurate history about the occurrence of periods early in menarche, as the cycle is usually irregular for the first 1 to 2 years and perhaps as long as 5 years.

Physical Examination

Vital signs should be taken in all patients. In cases of heavy bleeding, any postural changes in vital signs should be recorded. A complete examination should include a careful abdominal examination to rule out other nongynecologic causes of pain or bleeding. Femoral and inguinal nodes should be examined for size and tenderness, and the back and hips should be examined to rule out renal, musculoskeletal, or skin pathology. Signs of other illnesses, including hypothyroidism, galactorrhea, and obesity associated with hirsutism, should be documented.

Male physicians should have a chaperone during gynecologic examinations. Female physicians are equally well advised to have a chaperone. At the least, an assistant will be helpful. Prior to beginning the examination, a simple, nonthreatening explanation should be given and verbal consent obtained. Adolescents should be examined without their parents or guardians. The patient should be allowed to empty her bladder and remove any tampons prior to the examination. Positioning and draping should allow the patient to see the physician during the examination. Occasional eye contact is reassuring.

The examination of nonvirginal patients includes a speculum examination, a vaginoabdominal examination (bimanual), and a rectovaginal examination. The vulva and urethral opening should be inspected prior to inserting the warmed and lubricated speculum into the vagina. The site of abnormal bleeding should be determined through careful examination of the perineum, urethra, vulva, and perianal region. The vagina should be inspected for signs of lacerations, fissure, lesions, infection, and foreign bodies. It is imperative that the cervix is well visualized to rule out polyps, inflammation, ulcers, and evidence of cancer and STDs, including condylomata. Cultures are generally taken as part of the routine examination, especially if a mucopurulent discharge is found. The cervical os should be inspected for blood, tissue, an intrauterine device (IUD), pedunculated leiomyomata or polyps, and signs of infection.

On bimanual vaginoabdominal examination, the cervix softness, patency of the os, and pain on movement should be documented. The ovaries and uterus are palpated for size, consistency, pain, and the presence of associated masses. The adnexa and periuterine area should also be carefully examined. The rectovaginal examination is essential and should be done in every patient, especially if the patient cannot tolerate a bimanual examination. The rectovaginal examination enables evaluation of the posterior cul-de-sac for ovarian masses, the posterior wall of the uterus for size and consistency, and the uterosacral ligaments for metastatic nodules or ectopic endometriosis. Stool should be evaluated for the presence of blood.

Virginal patients with menstrual cramps, mittelschmerz, or vaginal discharge do not require a full pelvic examination, because a rectovaginal examination is generally sufficient. In the case of trauma and abnormal vaginal bleeding, a vaginal examination is necessary. It can generally be tolerated by adolescents with intact hymen if a narrow Pederson-type or Huffman speculum is used. Conscious sedation or full anesthesia may be required, depending on psychological response of the patient and the circumstances surrounding the injury or the extent of the injury or disease.

Older patients with a history of pelvic pain and bleeding should undergo a full gynecologic examination. Degenerative changes to the lumbar spine and hips may make the traditional lithotomy position difficult. Alternatively, the patient may be examined supine with knees flexed and legs dropped to the side, or lying on her side with the lower arm behind her back and thighs flexed (the Sims position). A small speculum (e.g., a 1- to 1.5-cm Pederson) should be used if the vulva and vagina appear atrophic. Physicians must remember that the vaginal walls may become adherent in individuals who are not sexually active, and a gentle digital examination may be required to ensure that a speculum examination is possible. Vaginal examination is generally well tolerated in women who are on estrogen replacement. Documentation of the size, shape, and mobility of the uterus is especially important when making a diagnosis in this population. The normal ovary should not be palpable 5 years after menopause, and any enlargement should be considered abnormal.

Differential Diagnosis and Approach to Adolescent, Reproductive-Age, and Postmenopausal Females

Causes of bleeding and pelvic mass by approximate frequency and age group are listed in Table 98-5.

VAGINAL BLEEDING Bleeding in early puberty is usually secondary to anovulatory estrogen withdrawal for the first 2 years after menarche. The amount of blood loss is minimal. Eating disorders, excessive weight loss, stress, and exercise can cause abnormal uterine bleeding. Additionally, medications (e.g., antiseizure medications) that increase the P-450 system of the liver may increase the metabolism of endogenous hormonal glucocorticoids and may cause withdrawal bleeding. Menorrhagia secondary to anovulation is seen in 10 to 15 percent of all gynecologic patients. Nongynecologic causes of vaginal bleeding and pelvic pain must be included in the differential diagnosis, be systematically addressed during the history taking and physical examination, and be pursued with relevant investigations and consultations, if indicated. Primary coagulation disorders account for 19 percent of acute menorrhagia in adolescents. Von Willebrand disease (vWD) is the most common; however, myeloproliferative disorders and immune thrombocytopenia are also possibilities. Otherwise, the differential diagnosis for pelvic pain and/or vaginal bleeding is similar to that in adults.

The causes of vaginal bleeding in nonpregnant, reproductive-age females can be broadly grouped into three categories: nonuterine bleeding, ovulatory abnormal bleeding, and anovulatory abnormal bleeding. Ovulatory bleeding usually results in menorrhagia and intermenstrual bleeding. Nonovulatory cycles may be irregular and heavy (menometrorrhagia) or frequent and light (polymenorrhea) bleeding.

Potential sources of nonuterine bleeding include the cervix, vagina, lower urinary tract, and lower GI tract. Cervical causes include carcinoma, polyps, condylomata, eversion of squamocolumnar junction associated with oral contraceptive pill (OCP) use or pregnancy, trauma, and some infections. Vaginal sources of bleeding include carcinoma, sarcoma, adenosis, lacerations, infections, and retained foreign bodies. Lower urinary tract lesions, such as urethral caruncles and infected urethral diverticula, may mimic vaginal bleeding. Some patients may not be able to determine the source of bleeding, and lower GI causes may need to be investigated.[10]

Ovulatory bleeding is associated with regular menstrual periods that are preceded by breast tenderness, abdominal bloating, and dysmenorrhea. Abnormal bleeding may occur during ovulation, as a result of low estrogen levels. Intermenstrual bleeding may also be caused by structural and inflammatory lesions, including cervical polyps, vaginal lacerations, cervicitis, invasive cervical cancer, endometrial cancer, and fibroids. OCP use remains the most common cause of midcycle bleeding. Premenstrual spotting or delayed menses frequently results from an inadequate luteal phase or persistent corpus luteum. Other causes of abnormal or heavy ovulatory bleeding include pelvic diseases, such as endometriosis, PID, and ovarian neoplasms. Uterine causes include leiomyomas, endometrial polyps, endometrial hyperplasia or malignancy, and adenomyosis. Finally, iatrogenic factors, pregnancy and postpartum complications, and bleeding dyscrasias may result in abnormal bleeding in the woman with ovulatory cycles.[10]

Anovulatory bleeding is irregular shedding of a thickened endometrium. It is a result of chronic stimulation of the endometrium by estrogen and the absence of luteal-phase progesterone. Bleeding is heavy, with long intervals between menstrual periods. Abnormal anovulatory bleeding is seen in perimenarchal and perimenopausal women as well as in patients with endocrine disorders, polycystic ovary syndrome, exogenous hormone use, and liver or renal disease. This pattern of bleeding increases the risk of endometrial hyperplasia and adenocarcinoma.

It is important to distinguish true pathology from dysfunctional bleeding in the perimenopausal and menopausal patients (Table 98-6). Postmenopausal bleeding, i.e., any bleeding that occurs more than 6 months after cessation of menstruation, warrants prompt referral for evaluation. The amount of bleeding does not correlate with the severity of disease. Older patients may not be able to accurately describe the location of pain or bleeding in the proximity of the bladder, uterus, or rectosigmoid. It is imperative that the vagina and cervix be adequately visualized. In perimenopausal or postmenopausal women, malignancy should always be considered, since it is the most important, although not the most common, diagnosis.[11] Bleeding from a vaginal source is uncommon but may be associated with the use of pessaries and douche solutions, which can irritate the mucosa. Cervical polyps may be a source of bleeding. However, an endometrial biopsy is ultimately required to rule out other serious causes of bleeding (Table 98-7).

Hormone replacement therapy is commonly used to relieve symptoms associated with menopause and to reduce the risk of cardiovascular disease. Most therapeutic regimens deliver sequential progestins to induce withdrawal bleeding and protect the endometrium from atypia. Other therapies use continuous administration of estrogen and progesterone to achieve an atrophic endometrium and amenorrhea.[12] In patients treated with sequential hormonal therapy, heavy or prolonged bleeding at the end of the cycle or breakthrough bleeding in two or more cycles should be investigated. Of patients on continuous therapy, 40 percent will have abnormal bleeding in the initial 4 to 6 months.

TABLE 98-6 Factors Frequently Used to Determine the Cause of Abnormal Bleeding in Perimenopausal Women

	CAUSE OF BLEEDING					
Test	Perimenopause	Neoplasia	Fibroid	Adenomyosis	Polyp	Pregnancy Related
History						
Associated hot flashes	Yes	No	No	No	No	No
Increased cramping	No	Sometimes	Sometimes	Yes	No	Sometimes
Bleeding pattern						
Skips and misses	Yes	Possible	No	No	No	—
Amenorrhea	Yes	No	No	No	No	Yes
Regular but shorter interval	Yes	No	No	No	No	No
Regular but heavy	No	No	Yes	Yes	Yes	No
Irregular	Yes	Possible	No	No	Yes	Yes
Physical exam						
Enlarged uterus	No	Sometimes	Yes	Yes	No	Yes
Enlarged and tender uterus	No	No	No	Yes	No	Possible
Ultrasound						
Enlarged uterus	No	No	Yes	Yes	No	Yes
Enlarged uterus with intrauterine mass	No	Yes	Sometimes	No	Yes	Yes
Lab tests						
FSH	Elevated	Normal	Normal	Normal	Normal	Normal
CBC	Usually normal	Normal/low	Normal/low	Normal/low	Normal/low	Normal/low
hCG	Negative	Negative	Negative	Negative	Negative	Positive

Abbreviations: FSH, follicle-stimulating hormone; CBC, complete blood count; hCG, human chorionic gonadotropin.
Source: From Pearlman,[29] with permission.

There is no acceptable criteria for "abnormal bleeding" on these therapies, and investigations are warranted if bleeding continues beyond 6 months or recurs after amenorrhea is established. Although bleeding is frequently caused by an unstable or atrophic endometrium, other causes must be considered. Important conditions in the differential diagnosis include submucosal fibroids, endometrial polyps, endometrial hyperplasia, adenomyosis, and tumors. Most frequently implicated are poor compliance, poor GI absorption, drug interactions, failure to synchronize therapy with endogenous ovarian activity, and coagulation disorders. Emergency therapy should be directed at investigating and treating obvious causes of bleeding. Outpatient ultrasound and endometrial biopsy can then be arranged for stable patients.

PELVIC PAIN The differential diagnosis of pelvic pain is broad and includes pathology of the reproductive, GI, and genitourinary tracts. Gynecologic causes of pain can be subdivided as acute, cyclic, or chronic. Causes of acute pain include inflammation from PID, rupture of ovarian cysts, adnexal torsion, symptomatic fibroid uterus, and degenerative leiomyoma. Cyclic pain may be physiologic or pathologic. Premenstrual syndrome, primary and secondary dysmenorrhea, endometriosis, and adenomyosis are examples of conditions that cause cyclic pain. Pain associated with a fever is frequently from an inflammatory or infectious etiology. Although there are many causes for chronic pelvic pain, it is rarely investigated primarily in the ED, although patients may seek relief from the pain alone. Physicians should be aware, however, that there is an association between chronic pelvic pain and somatization disorders in women with a history of sexual victimization or physical assault.[13]

TABLE 98-7 Etiology of Postmenopausal Bleeding

Factor	Approximate Percentage
Exogenous estrogens	30
Atrophic endometritis/vaginitis	30
Endometrial cancer	15
Endometrial or cervical polyps	10
Endometrial hyperplasia	5
Miscellaneous (e.g., cervical cancer, uterine sarcoma, urethral caruncle, trauma)	10

Source: From Hacker and Moore,[30] with permission.

Investigations

Pregnancy tests should be ordered routinely in women of childbearing age to rule out pregnancy as a cause of pain and bleeding. A complete blood count is essential in most cases of vaginal bleeding and/or pelvic pain. Coagulation studies are ordered only when indicated by the history and physical examination. In individuals with suspected endocrine disorders, determination of thyroid-stimulating hormone and prolactin levels may be helpful, but the levels are rarely available for ED evaluation.

In nonpregnant patients, ultrasound is used to determine total uterine size, presence and location of leiomyoma, and the thickness and characteristics of the endometrium. Ovarian cysts, hydrosalpinx, pelvic adhesions, tubo-ovarian abscesses (TOAs), endometriosis, and ovarian carcinoma may also be seen on pelvic ultrasound. Transvaginal ultrasound may be helpful in further delineating ovarian cysts and fluid in the cul-de-sac. Endovaginal ultrasound is also an inexpensive, noninvasive, and convenient way to visualize the endometrial cavity indirectly and may be performed in perimenopausal women with abnormal bleeding. Depending on the degree of pain and findings on physical examination, ultrasound may be deferred for outpatient evaluation. Computed tomography and magnetic resonance imaging are more expensive and less useful diagnostic modalities and are used primarily for cancer staging.

Referral for follow-up will usually lead to endometrial biopsy in women who are at risk for endometrial cancer and are not pregnant. This procedure is generally indicated for women over the age of 35 with abnormal uterine bleeding or women under the age of 35 with risk factors such as obesity and chronic anovulation.[14] Hysteroscopy is a valuable test that affords a more complete examination of the surface of the endometrium than dilation and curettage (D&C), which may miss 10 to 25 percent of lesions.[15]

Laparoscopy may be used in the evaluation of pelvic pain in nonpregnant women to establish a diagnosis if etiology is uncertain, to visualize an ambiguous adnexal mass, or to confirm the diagnosis of salpingo-oopheritis. It is relatively contraindicated in patients with pelvic masses larger than 12 cm and in patients with peritonitis, ileus, or bowel obstruction.

MANAGEMENT

General Approach

The main approach to nonpregnant patients with pelvic pain or established vaginal bleeding is to determine whether the condition requires general (e.g., resuscitation) or specific ED-based evaluation or intervention. In patients who present primarily with vaginal bleeding, the main issue is to determine whether there has been significant blood loss, and whether a condition exists (such as traumatic injury or bleeding dyscrasia) that places the patient at risk for uncontrolled or significant bleeding. If the bleeding has not led to hemodynamic compromise (and is unlikely to), then, after pregnancy has been ruled out, the only diagnoses that need to be absolutely established in the ED are trauma (including sexual abuse and assault), bleeding dyscrasia, and infection. Foreign bodies may also need to be considered in the prepubescent (particularly young child) and the elderly (e.g., retained pessary). Otherwise, patients can be referred for outpatient investigation, with the timing based on the urgency.

The approach to pelvic pain is similar. Assuming pregnancy has been excluded, acute infectious etiologies, torsion of adnexal anatomy, and nonpelvic surgical etiologies need to be considered for acute ED-based intervention and treatment. Rarely, a ruptured cyst may cause significant internal bleeding, but this is likely evident on evaluation and from the patient's level of pain. If infection is not strongly within the diagnostic possibilities, then the degree of pain may dictate further ED workup. Ultrasound and computed tomography are the most likely useful adjuncts, depending on the diagnoses remaining within consideration. Some patients with significant pain may be observed in an ED that has the capacity and capability for such activities. Reliable patients with moderate pain may be sent home on analgesics with appropriate instructions and a return visit or follow-up arranged within 12 to 24 h. Patients with mild to moderate pain of longer standing (in whom the foregoing considerations have been excluded) may be referred for further outpatient diagnostic evaluation.

The need for inpatient management is self-evident. Significant blood loss or risk thereof, or significant pathology, will usually warrant at least an immediate consultation and likely admission or a further non-ED-based procedure. Patients with intractable pain, or in whom significant pathology cannot be excluded, should be admitted for further evaluation.

Short-Term Management

HEMODYNAMICALLY UNSTABLE Patients who are hemodynamically unstable because of bleeding must be resuscitated according to standard protocols. Attempts should be made to localize the source of bleeding. In women with severe, persistent bleeding, immediate D&C is usually indicated. Uterine packing should be avoided, because it increases the risk of infection and may hide ongoing blood loss.

HEMODYNAMICALLY STABLE Medical management should be considered in hemodynamically stable patients provided the diagnosis is clear. If not, the patient should be referred for further investigation and outpatient management. Short-term hormonal manipulation allows the endometrium to stabilize, which in turn will slow or stop acute bleeding.[10] If the endometrium is thin on ultrasound examination, estrogen may be used to stimulate growth of the denuded, raw surface of the endometrium. With the regimen outlined in Table 98-8, subsequent bleeding may be heavy but should not be prolonged. Oral contraceptives may be used in women who are not pregnant and have no anatomic abnormalities. The progesterone in the OCP decreases the number of available estrogen receptors and, as a result, bleeding may not stop as quickly as when estrogen is used alone. Side effects include nausea and vomiting.[10] Two treatment regimens have been developed using a fixed-dosage pill, with 35 μg ethinyl estradiol and 1 mg norethindrone (Table 98-8). In individuals with persistent light bleeding associated with anovulation, progesterone alone can be used to stabilize an immature endometrium. Bleeding occurs 3 to 10 days after discontinuation and may be heavy due to the large amount of tissue being sloughed.

Long-Term Management

Many therapies are available for the long-term management of vaginal bleeding. Expectant management is appropriate if episodes of heavy or irregular bleeding are infrequent. The OCP is an excellent choice if contraception is required. Ovulatory menorrhagia is decreased by 50 percent, with a similar reduction in the degree of dysmenorrhea. This therapy may be effective in the treatment of patients with fibroids.[14]

Nonsteroidal anti-inflammatory drugs (NSAIDs) are helpful in the treatment of both ovulatory and anovulatory bleeding and dysmenorrhea. All of these medications have the same basic mechanism of action and inhibit cyclooxygenase in the arachidonic acid cascade. The prostaglandin inhibitors alter the ratio of prostaglandin $F_{2\alpha}$, which causes vasoconstriction, and prostaglandin E_2, which causes vasodilation. NSAIDs also increase levels of thromboxane A_2, which causes vasoconstriction and increases platelet aggregation. These medications may reduce blood loss by 20 to 50 percent and reduce dysmenorrhea.

TABLE 98-8 Short-Term Medical Management of Hemodynamically Stable Uterine Bleeding

Estrogen therapy

1. Oral conjugated estrogen (e.g., Premarin) 10 mg/day (2.5 mg qid) or 25 mg IV every 2 to 4 h for 24 h. Note: the efficacy of oral and intravenous estrogens are similar.
2. When bleeding subsides, add medroxyprogesterone acetate (Provera) 10 mg/day.
3. Continue both the conjugated estrogen and the medroxyprogesterone for 7 to 10 days.
4. Stop for a synchronized withdrawal bleed.

Oral contraceptive pill

1. Ethinyl estradiol 35 μg and norethindrone 1 mg—4 tabs for 7 days

or

1. Slow taper (ethinyl estradiol 35 μg and norethindrone 1 mg)
   4 tabs for 2 days
   3 tabs for 2 days
   2 tabs for 2 days
   1 tab for 3 days

Progesterone

Medroxyprogesterone acetate (e.g., Provera) 10 mg/day is used for 10 days.

They have a mild side-effect profile and are inexpensive. Not all women will respond, although 75 percent report a 30 percent decrease in blood loss.[16] NSAIDs are less useful in patients with fibroids.[16] Mefenamic acid (500 mg tid) and naproxen (500 mg bid) are the most well studied, and ibuprofen (400 mg q6h) has been shown to reduce menstrual bleeding in IUD users. NSAIDs should be started on the first day of the period and continued until bleeding stops and pain resolves.

Although virtually never initiated in the ED, clomiphene citrate may be used to decrease bleeding as well as induce ovulation if pregnancy is desired. If there is no risk of pregnancy and no contraindications to estrogen usage, medroxyprogesterone acetate 10 mg daily for 10 days can be used to produce scheduled bleeding. Danazol may be used to decrease bleeding significantly, although it is expensive. Patient acceptance is similar to that of patients on NSAIDs, and reduction of bleeding may be greater.[10] Side effects include musculoskeletal pain, flushing vertigo, backache, breast atrophy, and hirsutism.[16] Patients may still ovulate when using this medication. Gonadotropin-releasing hormone agonists may play a role in the induction of amenorrhea, and women on this therapy become menopausal. Other drawbacks include medication expense and bone loss when used for longer than 6 months.

Hysteroscopy is both diagnostic and therapeutic. It can be used to sample the endometrium, as well as resect polyps and myoma. Endometrial ablation may be performed in patients who do not desire fertility, have no pathologic diagnosis, and for whom medical therapy has failed. This may be performed using laser, electrocautery, or rollerball ablation. Amenorrhea is seen in about 50 percent of women treated, and decreased flow is seen in another 35 percent.[17] Improvement of symptoms of dysmenorrhea is reported in up to 80 percent of patients. Myomectomy may be useful in patients with symptomatic fibroids. Hysterectomy is reserved for selected patient populations.

Clinical Conditions in Adolescents

ABNORMAL UTERINE BLEEDING The most common type of bleeding in adolescents is anovulatory uterine bleeding secondary to the immature hypothalamic-pituitary-ovarian axis. The amount of bleeding is usually minimal and painless. The findings on pelvic and rectovaginal examination are likely to be normal. Investigations are warranted when bleeding persists after 9 days, recurs at intervals of less than 21 days, or produces anemia. Blood loss can be considerable, with monthly losses of 100 to 200 mL resulting in iron deficiency, marrow depletion, and anemia. If bleeding at the onset of menarche is considerable or necessitates blood transfusions, a coagulopathy should be excluded. Acute menorrhagia can generally be controlled with estrogen therapy or the OCP (see Table 98-8). D&C is rarely required.

VAGINAL OBSTRUCTION Adolescents with vaginal obstruction who escape notice as infants usually present after menarche with amenorrhea, cyclic abdominal pain, and on occasion, urinary symptoms. A lower abdominal mass and a bulging bluish membrane at the vaginal introitus are diagnostic of an imperforate vagina. A transverse vaginal septum can be diagnosed with a bimanual vaginal examination. High vaginal obstruction may be more difficult to discern on physical examination and can be confirmed with rectal ultrasound. The treatment for imperforate hymen and vaginal septum is urgent surgical intervention.

DYSMENORRHEA AND MITTELSCHMERZ Primary dysmenorrhea is defined as painful menstruation during ovulatory periods, in the absence of pelvic disease. This significant problem, which may cause 5 to 10 percent of women to miss school or work, occurs shortly after menarche and is most severe in young, nulliparous women. The crampy lower abdominal midline pain of primary dysmenorrhea is secondary to progesterone-mediated myometrial contractions and arteriolar vasospasm. The pain precedes menstrual flow by 12 to 24 h and subsides after menses begins. In severe cases, cramps may be associated with nausea, vomiting, back pain, headache, and irritability. Dysmenorrhea can be relieved with antiprostaglandin therapy (NSAIDs). The OCP should be used as a second-line therapy. Pelvic ultrasound or laparoscopy may be helpful in the assessment of patients with uncertain diagnoses or with pain that does not respond to therapy. Secondary or acquired dysmenorrhea occurs later in life and is associated with recognizable problems with IUDs, infection, leiomyoma, or pelvic adhesions.

Mittelschmerz is defined as transient, midcycle pain at ovulation or after ovulation and is secondary to increasing ovarian capsular pressure before the follicle erupts and chemical spillage into the peritoneum with ovulation. Physical examination may reveal a slightly enlarged ovary on the affected side. The diagnosis of mittelschmerz is clinical, and investigations are unwarranted. It is a difficult diagnosis to establish in an ED setting. However, after significant acute diagnoses have been effectively eliminated, mittelschmerz can be considered among a constellation of other pelvic pain syndromes that do not require urgent ED management. The most important treatment in both mittelschmerz and primary dysmenorrhea is sympathetic reassurance after a complete physical examination to rule out pelvic pathology. Patients should be encouraged to continue all activities, including sports. Adequate pain relief can usually be achieved with NSAID therapy.

GENITAL TRAUMA Vaginal injuries following intercourse is one of the most common injuries. The majority of coital injuries result from vigorous voluntary sexual activity, although violent involuntary sexual activity should be considered. The most common site of injury is the posterior vaginal fornix. Misdiagnosis of coital injuries occurs frequently because either the physician fails to take an adequate history or the patient does not admit to the antecedent activity prior to the injury. Most of the coital injuries are minor, but severe injuries may lead to complications, including hemorrhagic shock.

Clinical Conditions in Reproductive-Age Females

FUNCTIONAL OVARIAN CYSTS Normal ovarian follicles are 2 to 2.5 cm in diameter prior to ovulation, and follicular cysts may reach 8 to 10 cm. In general, these regress spontaneously in 1 to 3 months. Stretching of the capsule is the source of discomfort. Follicular cysts may rupture upon pelvic examination or with intercourse and cause immediate, sharp pain, which resolves rapidly or gradually improves over days. There may be associated peritoneal signs as a result of irritation from cystic fluid or blood.

Corpus luteum cysts are much less common and may grow to 5 to 10 cm in diameter. During the normal development of a corpus luteum, capillaries invade the granulosa cells and spontaneously bleed into the central cavity. If the degree of hemorrhage is large, the capsule is stretched, causing pain. In general, most cysts regress at the end of the menstrual cycle. Symptoms may occur from persistent corpus luteum cysts and include unilateral pelvic pain, amenorrhea, delayed menstruation, or menorrhagia. Cyst rupture is associated with sharp pain, peritoneal irritation, and bleeding. Without an hCG level determination, cyst rupture may be difficult to differentiate from an ectopic pregnancy. Hemorrhage is usually self-limited but rarely can cause marked pain, anemia, hypovolemia, and fluid in the cul-de-sac. Patients must be admitted for careful observation and to have serial hematocrits performed. Surgery is often indicated.

TORSION OF ADNEXA Pain associated with torsion of an ovarian cyst, fallopian tube, or paratubal cyst is acute, severe, and unilateral. It is felt in the lower abdomen and pelvis and may be related to a change in position. On occasion it may be intermittent. Of patients presenting with a torsion, 90 percent will have a mass, which progressively enlarges as arterial flow continues and venous flow is compromised. Nausea and vomiting are common, and patients may have an elevated white blood cell count (WBC) or low-grade temperature. The common differential diagnosis is appendicitis. Ovarian torsion may occur with normal adnexa, but there is an increased risk with ovarian enlargement. Tumors are found in 50 to 60 percent of patients. Benign cystic teratomas (dermoids) are the most common tumors. Torsion from enlargement of other cysts, ovulation induction, or parovarian cysts may also occur. It is rarely associated with malignant tumors, which are usually fixed to the pelvis. Early surgical intervention is required.

ENDOMETRIOSIS After dysmenorrhea, endometriosis is the second most common cause of cyclic pain in reproductive-age females.[18] A prevalence of 5 to 10 percent is widely accepted, although it has been reported in up to 60 percent of patients with infertility. There is a genetic predisposition for endometriosis, and the mean age at diagnosis is 25 to 30 years.[13] In patients with endometriosis, endometrial glands and stroma develop outside the endometrial cavity, initially causing pain with menses. As the disease progresses, pelvic adhesions develop and pain occurs throughout the cycle. If located within the ovarian capsule, endometriomas, or chocolate cysts, may result. The precise pathophysiology of endometriosis is not clear, but it is commonly believed to arise from retrograde menstruation and seeding of menstrual glands. Pain is cyclic or constant and may vary in character and intensity. It is generally worse just prior to or during menses. The number of adhesions and severity of disease correlate poorly with symptoms.[18] The hallmark of the disease is tender nodules felt along thickened uterosacral ligaments, the posterior uterus, and the cul-de-sac. Obliteration of the cul-de-sac with a fixed retroverted uterus is seen in women with extensive disease. Women with endometriomas may present with ovarian enlargement and adnexal tenderness. Alternatively, even a careful physical examination may not find an abnormality. Although the diagnosis may be suggested by history and physical examination, it can only be made upon direct visualization. Laparoscopy is the diagnostic procedure of choice.[18] Ultrasound may reveal endometriomas but is not helpful in defining focal endometriotic lesions. Therapy depends on the severity of symptoms, age, stage of the disease, and desire for future fertility. Hormonal therapy may be instituted to mimic pseudopregnancy, chronic anovulation, or pseudomenopause.[13] Endometriomas may be treated expectantly if they are less than 3 cm in diameter. Pregnancy itself leads to remission and sometimes cure.

ADENOMYOSIS In patients with adenomyosis, dysmenorrhea occurs just prior to or at the time of menstruation. In this condition, endometrial glands grow deeply into the underlying myometrium. Menorrhagia is common and is felt to be a result of aberrant tissue impairing the normal uterine contractility. Symptoms gradually increase in the fourth and fifth decades of life. On pelvic examination, there may be a large fibroid-like mass, or adenomyoma, but more commonly it is a diffuse, infiltrative process. Therapy is symptomatic, and simple analgesics are prescribed. Some cases require surgical management.[18]

LEIOMYOMAS Leiomyomas (fibroids) are benign tumors of muscle cell origin and are the most frequently occurring pelvic tumor. They are found in one of four white women and in one of two black women.[10] Commonly, there is more than one fibroid present. The etiology of leiomyomas is unclear, and theories include the proliferation from a single muscle cell from a small embryonic rest or a defined region of tissue with a higher level of estrogen receptors. They decrease in size during menopause, and enlargement is seen early in pregnancy and, in some cases, OCP use. Up to 30 percent of patients with leiomyomas experience pelvic pain and abnormal bleeding. Acute pain is rare, but severe pain may be experienced with torsion or degeneration. Degeneration is a result of rapid growth and loss of blood supply. This is almost exclusively seen in early pregnancy.

The diagnosis of leiomyoma is made on physical examination. A mass or commonly multiple masses are palpable. In patients with acute degeneration, tenderness, rebound guarding, a fever, and elevated WBC may be seen. Pedunculated subserosal leiomyomas may undergo torsion or cause uterine cramping. Rapid growth at any age or growth after menopause is highly suspicious for malignant transformation. Treatment depends on the size of the fibroid and the severity of symptoms. Generally, fibroids are observed, and pain is managed appropriately. Medical management includes administration of NSAIDs, medroxyprogesterone acetate or depo-medroxyprogesterone acetate, and gonadotropin-releasing hormone agonists. Pedunculated intracavitary leiomyomas may be removed by hysteroscopy. Surgical removal is associated with a 25 to 30 percent rate of recurrence and significant bleeding complications. A percutaneous interventional technique involving uterine artery embolization shows promise in observational trials. Embolization appears to alleviate symptoms and cause fibroid shrinkage.[19]

BLOOD DYSCRASIAS Bleeding disorders may become apparent with an initial presentation of abnormal menstrual bleeding. Uterine hemostasis is not well understood, and any disorder of blood vessels, platelet abnormalities, and coagulation disorders, including vWD, may result in excessive menstrual bleeding. Of historical interest, the first described case of vWD was in a 13-year-old who died as a result of uncontrollable uterine bleeding.[1] The prevalence of objectively confirmed abnormal uterine bleeding is increased in patients with vWD, carriers of hemophilia, and factor XI deficiency, at 73, 57, and 59 percent, respectively, when compared with a 9 to 11 percent rate in a population-based sample. Treatment options include use of antifibrinolytics and the OCP. The latter raises factor VIII and vWF levels and is an effective and popular form of therapy. Antifibrinolytics such as tranexamic acid reduce both plasminogen activator activity and plasmin activity to reduce the amount of bleeding. Desmopressin acetate (DDAVP,® Ferring) stimulates endogenous release of factor VIII and vWF and may be used prophylactically for minor procedures or treatment of bleeding episodes and menorrhagia. DDAVP is given intranasally, parenterally, or by subcutaneous injection. It is important that vWD patients are typed prior to instituting DDAVP, because DDAVP may induce thrombocytopenia in certain subgroups. NSAIDs are ineffective and may increase blood loss.[1]

POLYCYSTIC OVARY SYNDROME Polycystic ovary syndrome, one of the most common endocrine disorders, is the association of hyperandrogenism and anovulation without underlying disease of the adrenal or pituitary glands. A triad of obesity, hirsutism, and oligomenorrhea is classically described, although obesity is not universally seen. When menses occurs, it is heavy and prolonged.[20] The syndrome is further characterized by acne, androgen-dependent alopecia, elevated serum concentrations of androgens, and hypersecretion of LH with a normal or low FSH level. Typical ovarian morphology, which may be seen on ultrasound, is not necessary for the diagnosis and may in fact represent a response of the ovary to chronic anovulation. The differential diagnosis includes hyperprolactinoma, acromegaly, congenital adrenal hyperplasia, and androgen-secreting tumors of the ovary or adrenal gland. Management of menorrhagia in women who do not desire fertility includes low-dose oral contraceptives or cyclic progestin administration.

OTHER CONDITIONS Periods of physical or psychological stress, illness, malnutrition, rapid weight gain or loss, and intense physical

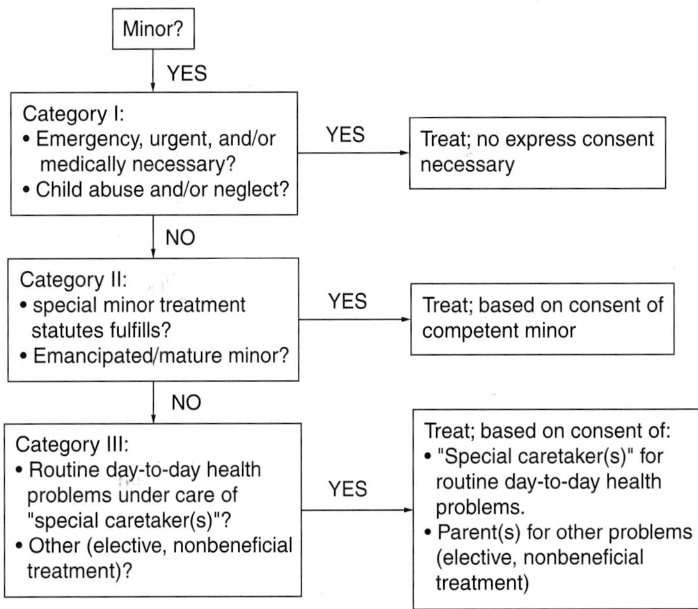

FIG. 98-3. Initial approach to consent for treatment. (From Tsai et al,[31] with permission.)

regimens affect the hypothalamus and disrupt the normal pattern of gonadotropin release. This usually causes amenorrhea but may result in irregular, heavy bleeding. In obese women, menorrhagia may be a result of increased circulating levels of estrogen from peripheral conversion of androstendione to estrone in fatty tissue.[14] Patients with liver and renal disease may also develop irregular bleeding.

Special Considerations

THE LEGALITIES OF TREATING ADOLESCENTS WITHOUT PARENTAL CONSENT Consent is not required to evaluate and initiate treatment in an emergency. State consent statutes and case law vary, so emergency physicians should know and follow their state law and hospital policy with respect to consent. There should be a mechanism in place to obtain consent from the courts when necessary. The American College of Emergency Physicians policy on consent is summarized in Figure 98-3. All states allow minors to consent to diagnosis and treatment of STDs and drug abuse without parental consent. Many states have similar statutes allowing minors independent direct access to prenatal care, termination of pregnancy, and medical care for crime-related injuries. Special considerations are included in some state legislation for emancipated and mature minors. Common sense and appropriate documentation should prevail above all with respect to issues of consent. An a priori awareness of the statutes and policies and established liaisons with local child protection services and the courts should assist emergency physicians in the ongoing provision of timely emergency care.

HIV-INFECTED WOMEN In general, there is no need to change the approach to pelvic pain and bleeding in HIV-positive women. Physicians must look for associated infections and complications of chronic illness. The rate of vaginal and pelvic infections as well as cervical dysplasia is high in this cohort of patients. In a cross-sectional survey of 386 women younger than age 50, with and without HIV, neither infection nor immunosuppression affected menstruation or the rate of abnormal vaginal bleeding.[21] This was also seen in a study of 85 seropositive women, although the power of the study was low.[22]

COMPLICATIONS OF IN VITRO FERTILIZATION Ovarian hyperstimulation syndrome complicates 5 to 10 percent of in vitro fertilization cycles, although only few cases become severe.[23] Particular vigilance is needed with such patients presenting to the ED. The syndrome is characterized by ovarian enlargement and fluid loss from ovarian capillaries into the extravascular compartment. This leads to ascites, abdominal distention, hydrothorax, and localized or generalized tissue edema. Complications include hypovolemia, hemorrhage, and thromboembolism. The cause of the increased capillary permeability, fluid sequestration into the peritoneal cavity, and angiogenesis is not known. Presentation varies with severity. Patients with mild forms present with weight gain, increased thirst, and abdominal discomfort. More severe forms may include hypovolemia, acute respiratory distress due to the ascites and hydrothorax, pericardial effusions, hepatorenal failure, and/or thromboembolic phenomena. Factors associated with increased risk of developing ovarian hyperstimulation include age less than 35, the administration of hCG to trigger the ovulatory response, or endogenous hCG release in early pregnancy.[23]

Elevated WBC level, hemoconcentration, hyponatremia, and hypoalbuminemia may be seen in moderate and severe cases. Ultrasound examination is usually indicated and should be helpful in demonstrating the extent of ovarian enlargement, size and number of corpora luteal cysts, and degree of pelvic and abdominal fluid. Pregnancy may have occurred in patients with ovarian hyperstimulation. Investigations and treatment should be adjusted accordingly. The treatment of mild to moderate cases includes increased fluid intake, close observation, and safe analgesia. Severe cases should be followed closely with serial hematocrits. A coagulation screen, liver function tests, renal function tests, and chest x-ray should also be obtained. Management includes intravenous fluids and, in some cases, the administration of heparin. The use of diuretics should be avoided, and paracentesis, using ultrasound guidance, may be indicated for relief of respiratory distress. Pleural effusions rarely need to be tapped. Pericardial effusion should be imaged and drained under echocardiographic guidance as indicated. Although aggressive resuscitation may be required in severe cases, death remains rare.

REFERENCES

1. Anonymous: A meeting held in London, 12–13 January 1998, to discuss bleeding disorders in women. *Hemophilia* 4:145, 1998.
2. Mitchell H, Medley G: Abnormal vaginal bleeding is common, malignancy is rare. *Med J Aust* 162:164, 1995.

3. Jamieson DJ, Steege JF: The prevalence of dysmenorrhea, dyspareunia, pelvic pain and irritable bowel syndrome in primary care practices. *Obstet Gynecol* 87:55, 1996.
4. Goldstein DP, deCholnoky C, Emans SJ, Leventhal JM: Laparoscopy in the diagnosis and management of pelvic pain in adolescents. *J Reprod Med* 24:251, 1980.
5. Anteby SO, Schenker JG, Polishuk WZ: The value of laparoscopy in acute pelvic pain. *Ann Surg* 181:484, 1975.
6. Jones JS, Montgomery M: Gynecologic disorders in the older patient. *Acad Emerg Med* 1:580, 1994.
7. Bond GR, Dowd MD Landsman I, Rimsza M: Unintentional perineal injury in prepubescent girls: A multicenter, prospective report of 56 girls. *Pediatrics* 96:628, 1994.
8. Mushkat Y, Lessing JB, Jedwab GA, Menachem PD: Vaginal trauma occurring while sliding down a water chute. *Br J Obstet Gynaecol* 102:933, 1995.
9. Perlman SE, Hartwick SP, Wolfe WM: Water-ski douche injury in a premenarcheal female. *Pediatrics* 96:782, 1995.
10. Wells E: Abnormal uterine bleeding, in Pearlman M, Tintinalli JE (eds): *Emergency Care of the Woman.* New York, McGraw-Hill, 1998, pp 481–491.
11. Brenner PF: Differential diagnosis of abnormal uterine bleeding. *Am J Obstet Gynecol* 175:166, 1996.
12. Spencer CP, Cooper AJ, Whitehead MI: Management of abnormal bleeding in women receiving hormone replacement therapy. *BMJ* 315:37, 1997.
13. Lu PY, Ory SJ: Endometriosis: Current management. *Mayo Clin Proc* 70:453, 1995.
14. Wathen PI, Henderson MC, Witz CA: Abnormal uterine bleeding. *Med Clin North Am* 79:329, 1995.
15. Gimpelson R, Rappold H: A comparative study between panoramic hysteroscopy with directed biopsies and dilation and curettage. *Am J Obstet Gynecol* 158:489, 1988.
16. Duncan KM, Hart LL: Nonsteroidal antiinflammatory drugs in menorrhagia. *Ann Pharmacother* 27:1353, 1993.
17. Carlson KJ, Schiff I: Alternatives to hysterectomy for menorrhagia. *N Engl J Med* 335:198, 1996.
18. Muse KN: Cyclic pelvic pain. *Obstet Gynecol Clin North Am* 17:427, 1990.
19. Worthington-Kirsch RL, Popky GL, Hutchins FL: Uterine arterial embolization for the management of leiomyomas: Quality of life assessment and clinical response. *Radiology* 208:625, 1998.
20. Franks S: Medical progress: Polycystic ovary syndrome. *N Engl J Med* 333:853, 1995.
21. Ellerbrock TV, Wright T, Bush T, et al: Characteristics of menstruation in women infected with human immunodeficiency virus. *Obstet Gynecol* 87:1030, 1996.
22. Shah PN, Smith JR, Wells C, et al: Menstrual symptoms in women infected by the human immunodeficiency virus. *Obstet Gynecol* 83:397, 1994.
23. Brinsden P, Wada I, Tan S, et al: Diagnosis, prevention and management of ovarian hyperstimulation syndrome. *Br J Obstet Gynaecol* 102:767, 1995.
24. Carr BR, Wilson JD: Disorders of the ovary and female reproductive tract, in Isselbacher KJ, Braunwald E, Wilson JD, et al (eds): *Harrison's Principles of Internal Medicine,* 13th ed. New York, McGraw-Hill, 1998, p 2101.
25. Rapkin AJ: Pelvic pain and dysmenorrhea, in Berek JS, Adashi EY, Hillard PA (eds): *Novak's Gynecology,* 12th ed. Baltimore, Williams and Wilkins, 1988, pp 400–405.
26. Paradise JE: Paediatric and adolescent gynecology, in Fleisher GR, Ludwig S (eds): *Textbook of Pediatric Emergency Medicine,* 2d ed. Baltimore, Williams and Wilkins, 1988, p 711.
27. Hill NCW, Oppenheimer LW, Morton KE: The aetiology of vaginal bleeding in children: A 20-year review. *Br J Obstet Gynaecol* 96:467, 1989.
28. Hillard PA: Benign diseases of the female reproductive tract: Symptoms and signs, in Berek JS, Adashi EY, Hillard PA (eds): *Novak's Gynecology,* 12th ed. Baltimore, Williams and Wilkins, 1988, p 333.
29. Pearlman MD: Menopause, in Pearlman MD, Tintinalli JE (eds): *Emergency Care of the Woman.* New York, McGraw-Hill, 1998, p 625.
30. Hacker NF, Moore JG: *Essentials of Obstetrics and Gynecology.* Philadelphia, WB Saunders, 1986, p 467.
31. Tsai AK, Schafermeyer RW, Kalifon D, et al: Evaluation and treatment of minors: Reference on consent. *Ann Emerg Med* Volume 22:1212, 1993.

NORMAL PREGNANCY

Christina E. Hantsch
Donna L. Seger

Regardless of the chief complaint, the possibility of pregnancy must be considered in every woman of reproductive age who presents to the emergency department. Pregnancy may be the cause of a patient's symptoms and signs, or pregnancy may alter the diagnosis and management of other conditions. History and physical examination alone are not adequate in excluding pregnancy, and other diagnostic information is frequently required. In one study, over 7 percent of women, who stated that there was no chance they were pregnant and reported an on-time and normal last menstrual period, were pregnant.[1] The use of oral contraceptives or contraceptive implants does not guarantee pregnancy prevention. Although the failure rate is less than 1 per 100 with compliant use of oral contraceptives, nearly 30 percent of women who rely on oral contraceptives alone to prevent pregnancy are not consistently compliant.[2] Among women with levonorgestrel implants, the annual pregnancy rate is 0.8 per 100 during the first 5 years of therapy. The failure rate of implants further increases with time.[3]

TERMINOLOGY

In obstetrics, *gravidity* denotes the total number of pregnancies regardless of duration and outcome. *Parity* denotes the number of pregnancies completed to delivery during the viable period. Parity is not increased for a pregnancy resulting in multiple births or decreased for a stillborn fetus. Notation of obstetric history typically lists the gravidity, abbreviated *G* and followed by the appropriate number, and then the parity, abbreviated *P* and followed by the appropriate number. After the gravidity and parity there may be a listing of the number of term deliveries, preterm deliveries, abortions, and living children. The latter four numbers are separated by hyphens and listed in parentheses. For example, the obstetric history of a woman during her seventh pregnancy who has had 4 term deliveries, 1 preterm delivery, and 1 abortion and has 5 living children is abbreviated G7 P5 (4-1-1-5).

The duration of pregnancy is approximately 40 weeks. By convention, gestational age (or menstrual age) is calculated from the first day of the last normal menstrual period. Pregnancy is typically divided into three trimesters of approximately equal length. The first trimester is from conception to 14 weeks; the second trimester is from 14 to 28 weeks; the third trimester is from 28 to 42 weeks. A term pregnancy requires completion of at least 37 weeks of gestation.

PHYSIOLOGY

Knowledge of the physiologic alterations that occur during pregnancy enables emergency physicians to address pregnancy-related issues as well as to differentiate the normal features of pregnancy from complications and unrelated problems. Physiologic changes depend on the stage of pregnancy.

Cardiovascular System

Maternal cardiovascular changes during pregnancy include a 40 to 45 percent increase in circulating blood volume, a 43 percent increase in cardiac output, and a 17 percent increase in resting heart rate.[4] Systemic vascular resistance is 20 percent lower. Blood pressure decreases to a nadir during the second trimester. The diastolic decrement (10 to 15 mmHg) is greater than the systolic decrement (5 to 10 mmHg). Hemodynamic measurements should be taken with the patient in the left lateral decubitus position, since body position has a significant influence on hemodynamic values. The left lateral position increases venous return by relieving the pressure of the uterus on the inferior vena cava. The increase in cardiac output is detectable from the first trimester until after delivery when readings are taken with the patient in this position.[5]

The heart is displaced up and to the left because of elevation of the diaphragm. This displacement produces a larger cardiac silhouette on chest radiograph and a slight left axis deviation on the electrocardiogram. A small, benign pericardial effusion may also contribute to the enlarged cardiac silhouette.

Respiratory System

Many women experience dyspnea during pregnancy. Although the respiratory rate is unchanged, this symptom may be the result of a hormone-induced 40 percent increase in tidal volume and the related Pco_2 decrease (normal value in pregnancy, 30 mmHg). Functional residual capacity is decreased because of a rise in the level of the diaphragm.[5]

Gastrointestinal System

Pregnancy-induced changes in the gastrointestinal system are due to both progressive displacement of the abdominal viscera and hormone-mediated functional alterations. Gastric reflux commonly occurs as a result of delayed gastric emptying, decreased intestinal motility, and decreased lower esophageal sphincter tone. The size and morphologic characteristics of the liver are not altered by pregnancy, but the presence of placental alkaline phosphatase may produce the increased alkaline phosphatase activity observed on analytical evaluation of maternal liver function. Bilirubin concentration and aspartate aminotransferase and alanine aminotransferase activities are unaltered. Hepatic enzyme systems are induced during pregnancy. Gallbladder emptying is delayed and less efficient, and pregnancy therefore increases the risk of cholesterol gallstones.

Urinary System

Pregnancy-related renal changes include increases in kidney size, renal blood flow, and glomerular filtration rate (GFR). By the second trimester, the GFR may be as much as 50 percent higher than it was preconception. Consequently, blood urea nitrogen and creatinine levels decrease. Dilation of ureteral and renal calyces or pelves due to ureteral compression is also frequently seen on imaging studies. These changes are often less pronounced on the left side, since the sigmoid colon cushions the left ureter from the pressure of the enlarging uterus.

Hematopoietic System

During pregnancy, circulating blood volume expands by an average of 40 to 45 percent due to an increase in both plasma volume and the number of erythrocytes.[6] Hemoglobin concentration decreases due to hypervolemia but should not fall below 11 g/dL. Maternal erythropoiesis combined with fetal erythropoiesis produce the high iron requirements of pregnancy. Reticulocyte count is also slightly increased during the second half of pregnancy, the period of marked erythropoiesis. Leukocyte counts during pregnancy range from 5,000 to 12,000 cells/mL. Dilutional effects on blood volume may also contribute to the variation in leukocyte counts.[7] Beginning in the second trimester, leukocyte function is usually depressed, and increased susceptibility to infection may occur.[8] Patients with chronic autoimmune conditions may improve clinically. Circulating coagulation factor concentrations and erythrocyte sedimentation rate increase during pregnancy. Platelet count may decrease slightly due to increased consumption. However, thrombocytopenia should prompt further evaluation for a pathologic cause.

Endocrine System

Pregnancy-related hormonal changes and feedback mechanism adjustments are incompletely understood. Characteristic changes in carbohydrate metabolism lead to hyperinsulinemia and fasting hypoglycemia. The altered response to glucose ingestion produces postprandial hyperglycemia and ensures a sustained glucose supply to the fetus. Mineral (especially iron), protein, and fat metabolism are also changed. Thyroid alterations include increased vascularity and mild hyperplasia, but clinically detectable goiter is not a normal finding in pregnancy. To assess thyroid function during pregnancy, free thyroxine and thyroid-stimulating-hormone concentrations should be measured, since they are not affected by physiologic changes of normal pregnancy.

Uterus

Uterine weight and intrauterine volume increase during pregnancy from 70 to 1100g and 10 to 5000 mL, respectively. These changes occur through marked stretching and hypertrophy of existing muscle cells rather than formation of new cells. By 12 weeks of gestational age, the uterus exceeds the capacity of the pelvis and expands into the abdominal cavity. There is a progressive increase in uterine blood flow to approximately 450 to 650 mL/min by term.

Breasts

Many women note breast tenderness and tingling from early in the first trimester. The breasts enlarge and become more nodular. Nipple size and pigmentation increase. Striations similar to those often seen on the abdominal wall may develop on the breasts.

HISTORY AND PHYSICAL EXAMINATION

Obstetric and gynecologic history, including menstrual status and contraceptive use, should be obtained on every woman of reproductive age. Cessation of menses, as well as such symptoms as nausea, vomiting, fatigue, and urinary frequency, may be suggestive of pregnancy. The date of the last normal menstrual period aids in determination of gestational age (although it may be misleading if, for example, contraceptive use was recently discontinued). Quickening, the first maternal perception of fetal movement, could also help establish gestational age. Primigravida women note fetal movement between 18 and 20 weeks' gestation. With subsequent pregnancies, quickening typically occurs about 2 weeks earlier (i.e., between 16 and 18 weeks' gestation). The patient's history of prenatal care and the course of current and past pregnancies, as well as the essential components of any medical history (past medical history, medications, allergies, social history, family history, and review of systems), should be obtained.

Physical examination of pregnant women should include routine assessment of maternal well-being as well as an evaluation of fetal status. When a fetal stethoscope is used, fetal heart tones can be heard by 16 to 19 weeks' gestation. The normal fetal heart rate ranges from 120 to 160 beats per minute. Since the fetus easily changes position, the site on the maternal abdomen where the fetal heart tones are best detected varies. Pulsation of the maternal aorta should be distinguished from the fetal heart tones.

A pelvic examination should be performed whenever pregnancy is part of the differential diagnosis. Appearance of the cervix and the presence of discharge or blood in the vaginal vault should be noted. Wet preparation and culture for Neisseria gonorrhoeae and Chlamydia trachomatis may be indicated. Bimanual examination determines size and tenderness of the uterus and adnexa.

By the end of the first trimester, the size of the uterus can also be assessed by abdominal examination. At 12 weeks' gestation, the fundus should be palpable at the level of the symphysis pubis. At 16 weeks, the fundus should be midway between the symphysis and the umbilicus; at

20 weeks, it should be at the umbilicus. From 20 to 32 weeks, the height (in centimeters) of the fundus above the symphysis approximates the gestational age. For an accurate measurement, the pregnant patient should have an empty bladder when fundal height is determined. Later in pregnancy, the presenting part of the fetus should also be determined by palpating the maternal abdomen.

DIAGNOSIS

Accurate diagnosis or exclusion of pregnancy is essential in emergency medicine. Standard analytical techniques screen blood or urine for human chorionic gonadotropin (HCG), a glycoprotein produced by the trophoblast after implantation. Since implantation occurs about 1 week after conception, these screening tests are particularly helpful in establishing or excluding early pregnancy. At 4 to 5 weeks' gestation and beyond, definitive diagnosis can be made by sonographic visualization of the embryo or fetus (see Chap. 109, ''Pelvic Ultrasonagraphy''). Alternatively, in later stages detection (by fetal stethoscope or sonogram) of fetal heart activity distinct from maternal heart activity or detection of palpable fetal movement may confirm pregnancy.

Analytical Techniques

HCG is composed of α and β subunits. The HCG α subunit is indistinct from the α subunit of several other glycoproteins, including luteinizing hormone. The β subunit is unique to HCG. Qualitative enzyme-linked immunosorbent assays (ELISAs) that detect β-HCG in urine can be completed in minutes at the patient's bedside. Available commercial tests can detect β-HCG concentrations as low as 10 to 20 mIU/mL. These tests have a false-negative rate of only 1 percent in detecting pregnancy as early as 1 week after conception. However, to achieve this level of sensitivity, the analysis must be performed on a urine specimen that is not dilute. When urine is dilute, a false-negative result may be obtained for women with early pregnancy (serum HCG < 50 IU/mL).[9] Serum analysis should be performed in clinical situations when pregnancy is a concern but the urine result is questionable. Quantitative serum values are obtained by ELISA technique and can be completed in 1 to 2 h. There are several international standards for serum β-HCG, and the specific reference range should be appropriate for the standard employed.

A positive result on a pregnancy test, whether qualitative or quantitative, does not confirm a normal intrauterine pregnancy. Ectopic pregnancy, recent spontaneous or induced abortion, and HCG-secreting tumors may also produce a positive result. Single quantitative β-HCG determinations in combination with pelvic ultrasonography may differentiate intrauterine pregnancy from these conditions.[10] Serial quantitative serum β-HCG determination may be useful in some outpatient situations, since serum β-HCG levels double every 1.4 to 2.0 days following implantation in early normal pregnancy. Failure of the HCG concentration to double in this time period suggests an ectopic pregnancy or a nonviable pregnancy.

Pelvic Ultrasonography

More detailed discussions of ultrasonography and its application in emergency medicine can be found in Chap. 109. The earliest definitive sonographic finding in pregnancy is a gestational sac. Using transabdominal technique, the gestational sac can be detected at 5.5 to 6 weeks' gestation. With transvaginal technique, the gestational sac can be detected at 4 to 5 weeks' gestation. Other ultrasound markers of pregnancy and the gestational age at which they may be detected by transvaginal ultrasound include the yolk sac at 5 to 5.5 weeks' gestation, fetal pole at 5.5 to 6 weeks, and cardiac activity at 6 weeks. Correlation of these markers with specific, quantitative serum β-HCG values varies with the capabilities of the equipment and the skill of the ultrasonographer.[10]

SPECIFIC ISSUES IN PREGNANCY

Abdominal Discomfort

Many pregnant women experience abdominal discomfort. Round ligament tension and vascular congestion may cause lower abdominal discomfort from early in pregnancy. Braxton-Hicks contractions are irregular, palpable contractions that may occur throughout pregnancy. The differential diagnosis of abdominal pain varies with the stage of gestation and must include all the possibilities in a nonpregnant patient as well as those unique to pregnancy. Understanding of the physiologic changes of pregnancy avoids a delay in definitive diagnosis and management of pregnant patients with abdominal pain.

Medication Use

Therapeutic drug use may be necessary during normal pregnancy. Multiple factors, including gestational age and stage of development, dose and duration of exposure, and individual susceptibility, influence the potential effects of drug exposure during pregnancy. Teratogenesis is defined as the dysgenesis of fetal organs, as evidenced either structurally or functionally. Typical manifestations include restricted growth, fetal death, carcinogenesis, and malformations.[11] The fetus is most vulnerable to teratogenic effects at 4 to 12 weeks' gestation, the period of organogenesis. Exposure early in pregnancy may lead to spontaneous abortion. Exposure later in pregnancy is a less common problem but may also be teratogenic secondary to alterations in placental blood flow as well as direct potential fetal effects. Medication use during pregnancy may also have consequences in the neonate, such as central nervous system (CNS) depression, seizure, respiratory depression, kernicterus, or premature closure of the ductus arteriosus. Manifestations depend on the specific medication. Neonatal withdrawal may occur after maternal use of opiates or benzodiazepines during pregnancy. Finally, the adverse effects of fetal exposure to some medications (e.g., tetracyclines, which produce discoloration of teeth and bone, and diethylstilbestrol, which produces female genital tract abnormalities) may not be evident until later in the life of the child.

Pharmaceutical companies do not test drugs in pregnant women to determine potential fetal effects. Much of the available information on teratogenesis is based on animal studies, inadvertent human exposure during unrecognized pregnancies, and case reports or epidemiologic studies of pregnancy outcome after therapeutic drug administration. Exposure-related risk may be difficult to distinguish from spontaneous occurrence rates. Manufacturer labeling and drug reference books therefore often contain ambiguous statements concerning use of drugs in pregnancy. The US Food and Drug Administration (FDA) currently employs a system that classifies drugs in five risk categories based on available information (Table 99-1). Because of ambiguity and potential inaccuracy within this system, alternative ways of outlining estimated fetal risk for both physicians and the general population are being investigated.[11]

ANTIMICROBIAL AGENTS Antimicrobial medications are frequently used during pregnancy. All of these agents enter the fetal circulation to some extent. The potential teratogenic effects are unknown for some antimicrobials. Information on the safety of newer extended-spectrum or late-generation agents is limited.[12] Table 99-2 lists known pregnancy-related contraindications to some frequently used antibiotics.

Penicillin and cephalosporins are generally regarded as safe for use in any trimester. Neither group has been associated with teratogenesis in either animals or humans. Erythromycin does not cause known

TABLE 99-1 Food and Drug Administration Categorization of Drug Risk in Pregnancy

Drug Category	Risk during Pregnancy
A	Controlled studies have failed to demonstrate a fetal risk in the first trimester (and there is no evidence of risk in later trimesters), and the possibility of fetal harm is remote.
B	*Either* animal studies have not demonstrated a fetal risk but there are no controlled human studies, *or* animal studies have demonstrated an adverse effect that was not confirmed in controlled human studies in women in the first trimester (and there is no evidence of risk in later trimesters).
C	*Either* animal studies have revealed adverse effects on the fetus (teratogenic or embryocidal) and there are no controlled studies in humans, *or* no human or animal studies are available. Drugs should only be used if the potential benefit justifies the potential fetal risk.
D	Evidence of human fetal risk exists, but the benefits of use in pregnant women may be acceptable despite the risk.
X	Studies in animals or humans have demonstrated fetal risk, or there is evidence of fetal risk based on human experience. The risk of use in pregnancy clearly outweighs any possible benefit. Drugs are contraindicated for use in women who are or may become pregnant.

adverse fetal effects, but the estolate formulation is contraindicated in pregnancy, since it may cause maternal cholestatic hepatitis. Sulfonamides (including the sulfamethoxazole component of trimethoprim-sulfamethoxazole) are not known human teratogens. Maternal use close to term, however, may cause complications in the neonate. Sulfonamides compete with bilirubin for albumin binding. The fetus clears free bilirubin via the placenta, but in the neonate free bilirubin accumulates and may cause kernicterus. Trimethoprim, the other component of this combination antibiotic, should be avoided in the first trimester, since it is a folate antagonist and may cause neural tube abnormalities. If trimethoprim-sulfamethoxazole offers a clear advantage over other antibiotics, it is reasonable to use; however, the period of gestation should be considered in making such a decision. Tetracyclines are contraindicated in pregnancy, since they chelate calcium and cause abnormalities in fetal bone development and teeth discoloration.

TABLE 99-2 Pregnancy-Related Contraindications of Some Frequently Used Antibiotics

Antimicrobial Agent	Known Maternal or Fetal Concern
Erythromycin estolate	Maternal hepatotoxicity
Fluoroquinolones	Fetal cartilage abnormalities
Kanamycin	Fetal cranial nerve VIII damage
Metronidazole	Fetal midline facial defects (first trimester)
Streptomycin	Fetal cranial nerve VIII damage
Sulfonamides	Fetal hemolysis, neonatal kernicterus (near term)
Tetracyclines	Fetal bone and teeth abnormalities
Trimethoprim	Folate antagonism (first trimester)

Source: From American College of Obstetricians and Gynecologists.[12]

Maternal hepatic and renal toxicity have also been caused by tetracyclines. Fluoroquinolones have led to fetal cartilage abnormalities in animals and as of this writing remain contraindicated throughout pregnancy.[12]

ANALGESIC AGENTS Acetaminophen is the agent of choice for analgesia or antipyresis in pregnancy. Aspirin should be avoided during pregnancy. Although evidence is conflicting, aspirin use in the first trimester has been associated with congenital defects. Use later in pregnancy may cause coagulation abnormalities with hemorrhagic complications in both the neonate and mother. Premature ductus arteriosus closure and cardiovascular complications in the neonate may also be a result of maternal aspirin use late in pregnancy. Aspirin and other nonsteroidal anti-inflammatory drugs (NSAIDs) may prolong gestation and labor through inhibition of cyclooxygenase. Unfortunately, nonaspirin NSAIDs cannot be employed as tocolytic agents, since they, like aspirin, cause premature ductus closure and subsequent pulmonary hypertension.[11] Use of NSAIDs (especially indomethacin) has also been associated with oligohydramnios, intestinal perforation, hydrops fetalis, and renal failure.

GASTROINTESTINAL AGENTS Many pregnant women, particularly those in the first trimester, suffer nausea and vomiting. Conservative measures, such as reduced meal size and avoidance of specific foods, frequently ease symptoms. Intravenous fluids and electrolyte replacement may alleviate symptoms, but in some cases medications may be necessary. As with most medications, the safety of antiemetics has not been studied in prospective human trials, but the benefit of improved metabolic conditions and maternal well-being should be considered in the management decision.[13] Phenothiazines, such as promethazine and prochlorperazine, may be considered. Several other antiemetics, including metoclopramide and ondansetron, are presumed safe based on data from animal studies.

Physiologic changes in pregnancy often lead to dyspepsia during the third trimester. Most over-the-counter antacid preparations are regarded as acceptable.[11] The histamine antagonists cimetidine and ranitidine have no known teratogenic effect in animals. Although they have not been evaluated in humans, their use in general is considered safe.

ANTIHISTAMINES Sufficient data on fetal outcome after diphenhydramine exposure are lacking. An association with cleft palate has been reported, but in subsequent studies the frequency was not increased above background rates. Use of diphenhydramine is probably safe after the first trimester and until the last 2 weeks of pregnancy. Antihistamines in general should not be used during the last 2 weeks of pregnancy, since fetal exposure during that time has been associated with an increased risk of retrolental fibroplasia. Risks of the newer nonsedating antihistamines are not known.

COLD PREPARATIONS Over-the-counter cold preparations are frequently combination medications containing sympathomimetic agents. All sympathomimetic drugs have vasoconstrictive properties and may lead to vascular-mediated congenital defects. Data on specific agents and their teratogenic potential are inconclusive. Conservative measures for control of symptoms during upper respiratory infections are preferred. When medication is necessary, each component of a combination preparation should be considered before a choice is made. First-trimester exposure to dextromethorphan or guaifenesin has not been associated with adverse fetal effects.

ANESTHETICS Proper use of most agents for local or regional anesthesia, including subcutaneous infiltration of lidocaine, has not been associated with detrimental fetal effects. Combination preparations such as TAC (tetracaine, adrenaline-epinephrine, and cocaine) and

LAT (lidocaine, adrenaline, and tetracaine) should not be used due to the potential risks of absorbed cocaine and adrenaline-epinephrine.

CONTRACEPTIVES Pregnancy may occur in women taking oral contraceptive agents either due to a failure of therapy or to noncompliance. While there is no demonstrated risk of fetal malformation due to contraceptive use in early pregnancy, they should be discontinued as soon as pregnancy is recognized.[3,11]

Radiation Exposure

Teratogenic potential depends on the total radiation dose as well as the gestational age at exposure. The absorbed dose of radiation is measured in grays (Gy), the SI unit, or rads (1 Gy is equivalent to 100 rad). A dose of more than 50 to 100 mGy (5 to 10 rad) and/or exposure at a gestational age of 8 to 15 weeks is of the most concern. Cumulative doses may also be hazardous to the developing embryo or fetus. Table 99-3 lists the radiation doses of some common emergency department radiographic tests.[14] For procedures in which radioactive material is administered, the dose absorbed by the fetus is variable. Fetal exposure may be minimized by adequate hydration to minimize bladder concentrations, maintain brisk urine output, and enhance clearance of the material. Exposure from a lung ventilation-perfusion scan using xenon 133 and technetium 99m is typically less than 5 mGy. Ultrasound and magnetic resonance are the only radiation-free imaging techniques. The short-term electromagnetic field exposure with magnetic resonance imaging has not been shown to have teratogenic effects.[15]

Immunizations

Indications for tetanus toxoid (alone or with diptheria toxoid) are unchanged in pregnant women, since there is no evidence of teratogenicity.[16] Live-virus vaccines, including measles, mumps, rubella, poliomyelitis, and varicella, should be avoided in all trimesters of pregnancy as well as for 3 months preconception.[17] The influenza vaccine is an inactivated (killed-virus) vaccine that can be administered during pregnancy. The Advisory Committee on Immunization Practices, the Center for Disease Control and Prevention, recommends vaccination against influenza for women who will be in the second or third trimester during the influenza season, since women at those stages of pregnancy are at increased risk of influenza-related complications.[18] Immunoglobulins, including tetanus, hepatitis, rabies, and varicella immunoglobulin, can be administered when indicated regardless of the stage of gestation.[16]

TABLE 99-3 Radiation Exposure to the Uterus and Fetus

Procedure	Absorbed Dose, mGy*
Chest radiograph (two views)	<0.01
Pelvic radiograph	1.7
Single abdominal radiograph (KUB)	2.9
Lumbar spine series (three views)	3.5
Intravenous pyelogram	3.6
Chest CT scan	0.06
Pelvic CT scan	26
Abdominal CT scan	8.0

Abbreviations: CT, computed tomography, KUB, kidney, ureter, and bladder.
*1 mGy is equivalent to 0.1 rad.

PREVENTIVE MEDICINE AND COUNSELING

Nutrition and Nutritional Supplementation

Maternal nutrition is important to pregnancy outcome. Total weight gain as well as the pattern of weight gain affect newborn birth weight. Maternal weight gain begins in the first trimester and is most significant during the first half of pregnancy. Average total gain is 12.5 kg (28 lb). A balanced diet with sufficient caloric intake for appropriate weight gain supplies necessary vitamins. Routine supplementation with a multivitamin, therefore, is not necessary.[19] Vitamin supplementation may be necessary for women with special nutritional needs or those who follow a restricted diet (e.g., vegetarian). Since folic acid supplementation prepregnancy and during early pregnancy may prevent neural tube defects, the Centers for Disease Control recommends a regular daily folic acid intake of 400 μg for all fertile women.[20] As soon as pregnancy is established, this supplementation of 1 mg/day should be started. For women with a previous pregnancy affected by neural tube defect, the supplementation should be further increased to 4 mg/day.[20] Appropriate use of vitamin preparations is not harmful (and often folic acid supplementation is provided by a multivitamin preparation) in any trimester of pregnancy, but excess intake of some vitamins (e.g., A, D, C, and B_6) may lead to congenital defects.[19]

With the exception of iron, minerals do not need to be supplemented during normal pregnancy if dietary intake is appropriate. Since most women of childbearing age have poor iron stores and normal dietary intake cannot meet the increased demand during pregnancy, iron supplementation is recommended. Gastrointestinal side effects can be reduced, while still providing iron during the period of greatest demand, by initiation of iron supplementation after the first trimester. Zinc deficiency may be associated with neural tube defects. Daily intake of zinc during pregnancy should be 15 mg.[20,21]

Caffeine

Results of human studies on the effects of caffeine use during pregnancy are conflicting, particularly regarding the potential association between caffeine intake and early fetal loss.

Aspartame

Aspartame (Nutrasweet™) is metabolized to phenylalanine. Phenylalanine crosses into fetal circulation and at very high concentrations can lead to mental retardation. Except in cases of excessive maternal dietary intake or maternal heterozygous carriers of phenylketonuria, fetal toxicity is unlikely.

Substance Abuse

Substance abuse is one of the greatest threats to normal pregnancy.[22] Illicit substances as well as alcohol and tobacco may affect pregnancy outcome through their effects on both the mother and the fetus. Frequently, multiple substances are involved, since substance abusers rarely use a single substance.

ILLICIT SUBSTANCES Use of cocaine, opiates, or amphetamines is associated with multiple complications of pregnancy and congenital abnormalities. Data on other substances, such as hallucinogens and "designer drugs," is inconclusive. Effects of abused substances as well as the general health and well-being of the mother are of concern when treating a pregnant substance abuser.[22] A multidisciplinary approach is important.

NICOTINE Cigarette smoking, a habit to which 25 to 30 percent of reproductive-age women admit, increases the risk of many pregnancy complications. Only 20 percent of smokers quit by the time of the first prenatal evaluation.[23] Although the mechanism by which nicotine produces some of these adverse outcomes is incompletely understood, exposure to nicotine is associated with higher rates of spontaneous abortion, abruption, preterm labor, and low birth weight. Smoking cessation by 16 weeks' gestation may ameliorate adverse effects.[22] Attempts at cessation should first be made without pharmacologic intervention. Recommendations for the use of nicotine gum (pregnancy category C) and nicotine patches (pregnancy category D) should be individualized. Prior cessation attempts and total number of cigarettes per day should be considered in assessing the potential risks and benefits of such interventions.[23]

ALCOHOL Ethanol readily crosses the placenta and enters the CNS of the developing fetus. Fetal exposure to ethanol produces a characteristic clinical condition known as fetal alcohol syndrome, which includes CNS dysfunction, growth retardation, and facial abnormalities. CNS abnormalities including microcephaly, mental retardation, and behavioral disorders are typically the most severe. This syndrome may result from ethanol use during any period of gestation; however, the greatest risk is with first-trimester exposure. Furthermore, although evidence supports a dose-related response to ethanol exposure, there is no established safe quantity of alcohol that may be consumed.[22]

Travel

In general, a normal pregnancy does not prevent women from traveling to reasonable destinations. The possibility of travel-related diseases or the development of complications while in remote areas is an issue that should be addressed before travel is begun. High-altitude stays of a few days' duration have not been associated with risk to the fetus, but exposure for longer duration increases the chance of fetal growth retardation, maternal high blood pressure, and premature delivery. Travel in pressurized aircraft has not been associated with adverse outcome in an otherwise uncomplicated pregnancy. Some commercial airlines, however, enforce restrictions limiting travel during the third trimester. Frequent ambulation is important during travel of long duration regardless of the period of gestation. Protective restraint devices should be used at all times in automobiles and airplanes. Lap belts should have a snug, comfortable fit under the abdomen and across the upper thighs.[24]

Exercise

Although exercise for both fitness and recreation has become a routine activity for many women, the effects of physical exertion on pregnancy outcome are not known, since there has not been a prospective, randomized trial studying this issue. Decreased rate of weight gain and subcutaneous fat deposition in the third trimester has been demonstrated in one (nonrandomized) study, although overall weight gain remained within the normal range.[25] In general, uncomplicated pregnancy should not limit the ability to engage in moderate physical exercise. The American College of Obstetricians and Gynecologists recommends some modifications in exercise routines in view of the physiologic and morphologic changes of gestation.[5] Non-weight-bearing activity and activities that minimize the chance of even mild abdominal trauma are preferable. Exercise in the supine position should be avoided completely after the first trimester due to potential for decreased cardiac output. Although there does not appear to be a need to alter goal intensity as judged by heart rate, exercise should be stopped at the onset of fatigue rather than continuing to exhaustion. Extra attention should be given to augmentation of heat dissipation, hydration, and appropriate clothing during activities. Adequate dietary intake should be ensured. As for all individuals, regular activity is preferable to sporadic exertion. Subjective benefits of exercise both preconception and during early pregnancy have been reported.[26] Specific recommendations for exercise during pregnancy need to be individualized and made with the knowledge that there is no conclusive evidence on which to base recommendations.

TABLE 99-4 Symptoms and Signs in Pregnancy that Mandate Prompt Evaluation

Change in fetal movement pattern
Fever, chills
Refractory emesis
Visual disturbance
Abdominal pain
Significant headache
Anasarca
Dysuria
Vaginal bleeding and fluid loss
Abnormal vaginal discharge

DISPOSITION

Whenever pregnancy is diagnosed in the emergency department, timely access to prenatal care should be arranged. Recommendations for prenatal care for a normal pregnancy include an initial obstetric evaluation no later than 6 to 8 weeks' gestation. Management plans need to be made in view of the condition. Discharge instructions should include recommendations about symptoms and signs for which the patient should be urgently reevaluated (Table 99-4). Recommendations on activities, lifestyle, and appropriate use of prescription and over-the-counter medications should be given.

Obstetric consultation should be obtained whenever there is uncertainty regarding issues, such as specific travel, immunization, medication, or management options. Gestational age, fetal heart tones (if gestational age >16 to 19 weeks), analytical values, parity, and general maternal information should be provided to the consultant.

ACKNOWLEDGMENT

The authors would like to thank Douglas Brown, MD, Assistant Professor of Obstetrics and Gynecology at Vanderbilt University Medical Center, for his review of this manuscript.

REFERENCES

1. Ramoska EA, Sacchetti AD, Nepp M: Reliability of patient history in determining the possibility of pregnancy. *Ann Emerg Med* 18:48, 1989.
2. US Department of Health and Human Services: *Fertility, Family Planning, and Women's Health: New Data from the 1995 National Survey of Family Growth.* DHHS publication PHS 97, 1995.
3. American College of Obstetricians and Gynecologists: Hormonal contraception. Technical bulletin 198. *Int J Gynaecol Obstet* 48:115, 1995.
4. Clark SL, Cotton DB, Lee W, et al: Central hemodynamic assessment of normal term pregnancy. *Am J Obstet Gynecol* 161:1439, 1989.
5. American College of Obstetricians and Gynecologists: Exercise during pregnancy and the postpartum period. Technical bulletin 189, 1994.
6. Whittaker PG, Macphail S, Lind T: Serial hematologic changes and pregnancy outcome. *Obstet Gynecol* 88:33, 1996.
7. Baboonian C, Griffiths P: Is pregnancy immunosupressive? Humoral immunity against viruses. *Br J Obstet Gynaecol* 90:1168, 1983.

8. Krause PJ, Ingirdia CJ, Pontius LT: Host defense during pregnancy: Neutrophil chemotaxis and adherence. *Am J Obstet Gynecol* 157:274, 1987.
9. Gibbon BN, Hemphill RR, Santen SA: Do we still have to worry when the urine is dilute? *Ann Emerg Med* 32:287, 1998.
10. American College of Obstetricians and Gynecologists: Gynecologic ultrasonography. Technical bulletin 215. *Int J Gynaecol Obstet* 52:293, 1996.
11. Koren G, Pastuszak A, Ito S: Drugs in pregnancy. *N Engl J Med* 338:1128, 1998.
12. American College of Obstetricians and Gynecologists: Antimicrobial therapy for obstetric patients. Washington, DC: Educational bulletin 245, 1998.
13. Nelson-Piercy C: Treatment of nausea and vomiting in pregnancy. *Drug Safety* 19:155, 1998.
14. International Commission on Radiological Protection: Summary of the current IRCP principles for protection of the patient in diagnostic radiology. *Ann ICRP* 22:vii, 1991.
15. Elster AD: Does MR imaging have any known effects on the developing fetus? *AJR* 162:1493, 1994.
16. American College of Obstetricians and Gynecologists: Immunization during pregnancy. Washington, DC: Technical bulletin 160, 1991.
17. Advisory Committee on Immunization Practices: Prevention of varicella. *MMWR* 45:1, 1996.
18. Advisory Committee on Immunization Practices: Prevention and control of influenza. *MMWR* 47:1, 1998.
19. American College of Obstetricians and Gynecologists: Nutrition during pregnancy. Washington, DC: Technical bulletin 179, 1993.
20. American College of Obstetricians and Gynecologists: Nutrition and women. Washington, DC: Educational bulletin 229, 1996.
21. Gonzalez MJ, Schmitz KJ, Matos MI, et al: Folate supplementation and neural tube defects: A review of a public health issue. *PRHSJ* 16:387, 1997.
22. American College of Obstetricians and Gynecologists: Substance abuse in pregnancy. Washington, DC: Technical bulletin 195, 1994.
23. American College of Obstetricians and Gynecologists: Smoking and women's health. Educational bulletin 240. *Int J Gynaecol Obstet* 60:71, 1997.
24. Rose SR: Pregnancy and travel. *Emerg Med Clin North Am* 15:93, 1997.
25. Clapp JF, Little KD: Effect of recreational exercise on pregnancy weight gain and subcutaneous fat deposition. *Med Sci Sports Exerc* 27:170, 1995.
26. Wang TW, Apgar BS: Exercise during pregnancy. *Am Fam Physician* 57:1846, 1998.

ECTOPIC PREGNANCY

Richard S. Krause
David M. Janicke

Ectopic pregnancy (EP) occurs when a conceptus is abnormally implanted outside of the uterine cavity. It is a leading cause of pregnancy-related maternal death. Today, earlier diagnosis and hence decreased morbidity and mortality have been made possible by transvaginal sonography and improved sensitivity of serum pregnancy markers. As a result more patients may be eligible for conservative medical and surgical therapies.

PATHOPHYSIOLOGY AND EPIDEMIOLOGY

Fertilization of the oocyte usually occurs in the ampullary segment of the fallopian tube. In normal pregnancy, the zygote passes along the fallopian tube and implants into the endometrium of the uterus, with subsequent development of the placenta. An EP occurs when the zygote is implanted in any location other than the uterus; 95 percent of ectopic pregnancies occur in the fallopian tube. Extratubal sites include the abdominal cavity, cervix, and ovary. Abdominal ectopic pregnancies most commonly derive from early rupture or abortion of a tubal pregnancy, with subsequent reimplantation in the peritoneal cavity.

The fallopian tube is 10 to 12 cm long and is divided into four anatomic segments (proximal to distal): interstitial (cornual), isthmic, ampullary, and fimbrial. The ampullary segment is the longest. The most common site for EP is the ampullary segment, and the second most common site the isthmic segment. Interstitial (cornual) EP is uncommon (>3 percent) and fimbrial EP is rare. Operative description of tubal rupture reveals that it is more common with isthmic than with ampullary implantations. Ectopic pregnancies that have identifiable embryos or fetuses are more frequently associated with rupture. Rupture during the first few weeks of pregnancy is usually located in the isthmic segment of the tube, whereas interstitial rupture is seen later in pregnancy, typically at 9 to 16 weeks of gestation.

Tubal gestations that reach stages of fetal viability are rare (<5 percent of cases), and live-born offspring are extreme rarities. A normal placenta is found in only about 10 percent of ectopic pregnancies, possibly accounting for the much higher incidence of a blighted ovum in extrauterine pregnancies. Tubal abortion occurs when the vascular supply to the placenta is disrupted with bleeding into the fallopian tube and hematoma formation. Intermittent distention of the fallopian tube with blood can occur with leakage of blood from the fimbriated end of the fallopian tube into the peritoneal cavity. The aborting EP and associated hematoma can be completely or partially extruded out of the end of the fallopian tube or through a rupture site in the tubal wall. Tubal rupture is thought to be spontaneous; however, precipitating factors may include trauma associated with coitus or a bimanual examination.

EP represents about 2 percent of pregnancies. The postulated etiology of EP can be divided into two main categories: (1) mechanical or anatomic alterations in the tubal transport mechanism and (2) functional/hormonal factors that alter the fertilized ovum. Possible causes of mechanical or anatomic alterations in tubal transport include pelvic inflammatory disease (PID), previous surgical procedures on the fallopian tube, previous EP, intrauterine contraceptive devices (IUDs), previous induced abortions, peritubal adhesions (secondary to postabortal or puerperal infection, appendicitis, or endometriosis), and diethylstilbestrol (DES) exposure (possibly resulting in tubular diverticula or hypoplasia). PID results in damage to the mucosa of the fallopian tube. The most common cause of PID is infection resulting from sexually transmitted diseases. PID has been reported to increase the risk of EP six- to sevenfold. Each episode of PID increases the probability of EP. PID represents the most common and clear-cut risk factor in the development of EP.[1]

Tubal ligation is also a risk factor for EP. The more tissue-destructive the ligation procedure, the higher the EP rate. Extrauterine pregnancy rates as high as 51 percent of pregnancies have been reported with laparoscopic tubal electrocautery, as compared with rates of 12 percent using nonlaparoscopic methods. Infertility surgery on the fallopian tube has a reported 2 to 7 percent incidence of subsequent EP. Any patient who requires surgery for treatment of an EP is also at a higher risk of developing a subsequent EP. In general, future pregnancies following any prior tubal surgery should be suspected of being ectopic. It is not clear whether this higher incidence of EP is secondary to the underlying disease state or a result of the surgical procedure. IUDs have also been implicated in EP, with 3 to 4 percent of pregnancies occurring with an IUD in place estimated to be ectopic. Increased risk of EP is independent of the type of device. Following discontinuation of the IUD, the risk of EP is no longer significantly increased. Functional and hormonal mechanisms associated with an increased incidence of EP include assisted reproduction with chemical ovulation induction (clomiphene citrate, follicle-stimulating hormone, luteinizing hormone), gamete intrafallopian transfer (GIFT) and in vitro fertilization, altered tubal motility from the effects of estrogen and progesterone, and inherent defects in the fertilized ovum.

The incidence of EP has increased over the last two decades from 4.5 per 1000 reported pregnancies (0.45 percent) in 1970 to 19.7 per 1000 reported pregnancies (nearly 2 percent) in 1992. Reported pregnancies included live births, legally induced abortions, and ectopic pregnancies. An overestimation of the incidence of EP is possible, since the denominator, reported pregnancies, could be biased by lack of reporting of illegally terminated pregnancies or undetected spontaneous abortions. Some possible reasons postulated for the increased incidence of EP include the increased incidence of sexually transmitted tubal infections, unsuccessful tubal sterilizations, assisted reproductive techniques, previous pelvic surgery, and more sensitive and earlier diagnostic techniques. Overall, EP is more common in nonwhite than white women and in women above 35 years of age.[1]

The case-fatality rate per 10,000 ectopic pregnancies decreased from 35.5 in 1970 to 8.8 in 1980 to 3.8 in 1989. This trend was observed in both white and nonwhite women. However, nonwhite women overall had a 3.4 times greater risk of death than white women. Teenagers were the age group with the highest mortality rate. The observed decreased mortality is attributed largely to improved diagnostics and also a heightened awareness among medical personnel. However, EP remains the leading cause of maternal death in the first trimester of pregnancy and is the second leading cause of maternal mortality overall.[1]

CLINICAL FEATURES

The classic triad of symptoms in EP is abdominal pain with vaginal bleeding or spotting in a woman with amenorrhea. While frequently seen in cases of EP, the positive predictive value of this presentation is low, as it is more commonly seen in threatened or spontaneous abortion than in EP and may occur in nonpregnant women due to other causes. Many other presentations occur and range from sudden abdominal pain with life-threatening hypovolemic shock to an absence of symptoms with an EP discovered incidentally on ultrasound exam. To achieve the goal of early diagnosis in as many cases as possible, EP should be considered in all women of childbearing potential who present with abdominal or pelvic complaints or with unexplained signs or symptoms of hypovolemia.

History

Elements of the history that increase the risk for EP are absent in nearly 50 percent of cases and are therefore useful only in increasing clinical suspicion in equivocal cases. The menstrual history is often abnormal, with amenorrhea of between 4 and 12 weeks reported in approximately 70 percent of cases. No missed menses are reported in approximately 15 percent of cases; thus neither a normal menstrual history nor prolonged amenorrhea has a sufficient negative predictive value to rule out an EP.[2]

Abdominal pain is expected in EP with tubal rupture but may be absent without rupture. Overall, up to 10 percent of ED patients with EP may not report pain. The classic pain of rupture is lateralized, sudden, sharp, and severe. However, many atypical pain patterns occur. A ruptured EP may present with shoulder pain from referred diaphragmatic irritation. This was reported in up to 20 percent of patients in one study. Pain may be absent even with rupture, as 4 percent of women in one study with hemoperitoneum from ruptured EP did not report pain. When nonruptured EP is painful, the pain is presumably from tubal distention. With the goal of early diagnosis, the absence of pain is not sufficient to exclude EP from consideration in a patient with other signs or symptoms of the disorder.[2]

Vaginal bleeding is noted in up to 80 percent of cases of EP. Bleeding is usually scanty, but other patterns may occur. Classically, light bleeding occurs at or about the time of expected menses and may be mistaken for a normal period. Bleeding usually precedes pain. The duration of bleeding ranges from 1 day to several months before diagnosis. Heavy bleeding should increase suspicion for threatened abortion or another complication of an intrauterine pregnancy but does not rule out an EP. Typical early pregnancy symptoms may occur and may not differ from symptoms of previous normal intrauterine pregnancies.[2]

Physical Examination

The physical examination in EP is highly variable. In cases of ruptured EP, patients may present in shock, with an adnexal mass and tenderness. Peritoneal signs will usually be present due to peritoneal irritation from blood and is seen in about 90 percent of patients. Relative bradycardia may occur, as in other causes of intraabdominal hemorrhage, as a consequence of vagal stimulation. In cases of rupture without hemodynamically significant bleeding, less prominent peritonitis without significant alteration of vital signs would be expected. Fever is rare, occurring in less than 2 percent of cases. In the more common situation of an unruptured EP, the vital signs are likely to be normal. An adnexal mass or fullness with tenderness is seen in approximately two-thirds of patients. Interestingly, at surgery, the EP may be on the opposite side from the mass. This has been noted in up to 20 percent of patients and is most often secondary to a corpus luteum cyst. Cervical motion tenderness is often seen and blood is often present in the vaginal vault. The cervix may have a blue coloration, as in a normal pregnancy. An enlarged uterus may also be detected, misleading the examiner into believing that the pregnancy is intrauterine. Pelvic examination may be completely normal in cases of ectopic pregnancy. Fetal heart tones are very seldom audible in cases of EP.[2,3]

DIAGNOSIS

The differential diagnosis for women of childbearing potential who present with abdominal or pelvic symptoms or abnormal vaginal bleeding is broad (Table 100-1). In these patients, no combination of signs or symptoms has sufficient negative predictive value to rule our ectopic pregnancy. Pregnancy testing is therefore mandatory. If pregnancy is detected, EP should remain part of the differential diagnosis unless another diagnosis can be made with a high level of certainty. When another diagnosis is not made or when EP is considered along with another diagnosis, EP must be ruled out with a combination of laboratory and imaging studies.

Pregnancy Testing

The diagnosis of pregnancy is central to the diagnostic workup of possible EP. When a patient is not pregnant, there is no ectopic pregnancy. Pregnancy tests currently in use rely on the detection of the β subunit of human chorionic gonadotropin (βhCG) in the urine or serum. Human chorionic gonadotropin (hCG) is a hormone produced by the trophoblast and is normally undetectable in the serum. Intact hCG consists of the α and β subunits. Tests based on detection of the intact molecule or the α subunit cross-react on immunologic assays

TABLE 100-1 Differential Diagnosis of Ectopic Pregnancy

All Patients	Pregnant Patients
Appendicitis	Normal (intrauterine) pregnancy
Inflammatory bowel disease	Threatened abortion
Ovarian pathology Cyst Torsion	Inevitable abortion Molar pregnancy Heterotopic pregnancy
Pelvic inflammatory disease	
Endometriosis	
Sexual assault/trauma	
Urinary tract infection	
Ureteral colic	

with hormones found in the nonpregnant individual and are thus less specific then tests for the βhCG subunit.

Human chorionic gonadotropin preparations are currently standardized in relation to the International Reference Preparation (IRP). Other standard preparations are not equivalent. A preparation often referred to in earlier literature is the Second International Standard (2nd IS). The IRP is roughly equal to 1.7 times the 2nd IS. To avoid confusion when interpreting the literature, attention must be paid to the standard used. In this chapter, hCG and βhCG concentrations are in reference to the IRP unless otherwise noted.[3]

Very early in either an intrauterine pregnancy (IUP) or an EP, detectable amounts of βhCG are released into the serum and filtered into the urine. The concentration of βhCG is fairly closely correlated in the urine and serum, with urinary concentration also depending upon urine specific gravity. Qualitative urine and serum tests for pregnancy usually use the enzyme-linked immunosorbent assay (ELISA) methodology. In the laboratory setting, ELISA tests can detect βhCG at concentrations below 1 mIU/mL. Qualitative tests in clinical use are typically reported as "positive" when the βhCG concentration is ≥20 mIU/mL in urine and ≥10 mIU/mL in serum. A "positive" qualitative test therefore implies that βhCG is present in at least this concentration. At this level of detection, the false-negative rate for detection of pregnancy will not be more than 1 percent for urine and 0.5 percent for serum and may be less. In clinical use, the performance of urine qualitative testing has been found to be from 95 to 100 percent sensitive and specific as compared with serum tests. One study showed that in 100 percent of 95 patients with EP, pregnancy was correctly diagnosed with a sensitive qualitative urine test (Hybritech Tandem ICON II).[4] Urine tests can be performed rapidly at the bedside, and kits from some manufacturers may be used for either urine and serum. A bedside test for urine is therefore the best first test for pregnancy when EP is suspected. Dilute urine may cause a false-negative urine pregnancy test.[5] This is most likely to occur early in pregnancy when βhCG levels are low (<50 mIU/mL). If urine is not available, use of a bedside serum test may be considered. When a bedside urine test is negative and EP is still being considered, a quantitative serum test should be performed. The sensitivity of quantitative serum testing for the diagnosis of pregnancy is virtually 100 percent when an assay capable of detecting ≥5 mIU/mL of βhCG is used.[4,5]

Laboratory Tests and Ectopic Pregnancy

The final diagnosis of EP is made either by ultrasound (US) or direct visualization via the laparoscope or at surgery. Laboratory tests are used as part of an overall diagnostic and management scheme to either raise or lower the level of suspicion for EP. All laboratory tests must be interpreted in light of the clinical picture and findings from US. No single diagnostic test or combination of laboratory tests is currently considered to have sufficient negative predictive value to completely rule out EP or abnormal IUP or positive predictive value to definitively diagnose them.

Much is known about the dynamics of βhCG production in normal and pathologic pregnancy. Early in pregnancy, βhCG levels rise rapidly. βhCG levels decline in nonviable pregnancies and in successfully treated EP. Absolute levels of βhCG tend to be lower in pathologic pregnancies than in IUP, but there is much overlap. Owing to the variability in absolute levels and the overlap between normal and pathologic pregnancies, no single βhCG level can reliably distinguish between a normal and a pathologic pregnancy. *Doubling time* refers to the time needed for βhCG concentration in the serum to double. In normal pregnancy, serum levels of βhCG increase by at least 66 percent every 48 h in 85 percent of patients. Absolute levels of βhCG are lower and doubling times longer in EP and other abnormal pregnancies. This and many other observations has lead to the widely used rule of thumb stating that the serum concentration of βhCG approximately doubles every 2 days early in a normal pregnancy and that longer doubling times indicate pathologic pregnancy. Varying degrees of sensitivity and specificity are obtained using different criteria for evaluating βhCG levels. Sensitivities for the diagnosis of EP between 36 and 75 percent with specificities of 63 to 93 percent have been reported. Even in EP, approximately 13 percent of patients will have an increase in serum βhCG of at least 66 percent in 2 days. A serum βhCG which fails double in 48 h is thus suggestive but not diagnostic of an EP or an abnormal IUP. Serial measurements of βhCG are therefore used to either heighten or lower the suspicion for EP but are not diagnostic.[6]

Progesterone (P) is a steroid hormone secreted by the ovary, adrenal glands, and placenta during pregnancy. During the first 8 to 10 weeks of pregnancy, ovarian production of P predominates and serum levels remain relatively constant. After the tenth week of pregnancy, placental production increases and serum levels rise. Absolute levels of P are lower in pathologic pregnancies and fall when a pregnancy fails. This observation has led multiple authors to propose various P levels as a diagnostic aid in differentiating an early normal from a pathologic pregnancy. As with other diagnostic tests, the sensitivity of P testing increases and the specificity decreases as a lower threshold value is selected. Most pathologic pregnancies have P levels ≤10 ng/mL. For P ≤ 5 ng/mL, nearly 100 percent of pregnancies will be pathologic; there are no normal pregnancies reported with P ≤ 2.5 ng/mL. Progesterone levels >25 ng/mL have a 97 percent sensitivity for viable IUP. An intermediate value of P ≤ 15 ng/mL is 70 percent sensitive and 73 percent specific for EP. A recent metanalysis revealed that 91.7 percent of pregnancies had P ≤ 17.5 ng/mL. For patients with P > 17.5 ng/mL, the authors concluded that clinical follow-up and no further diagnostic workup was needed.[7] As can be appreciated from the above, there is considerable overlap between P levels in normal and pathologic pregnancy. Very low values for serum P thus should increase the clinical suspicion for EP or abnormal IUP, but no value is diagnostic or can completely exclude the diagnosis. Certain authors strongly advocate protocols using serum P levels instead of or as an adjunct to quantitative βhCG levels. However, P levels may not be routinely available on an urgent basis and, as noted, many patients have intermediate values, thus limiting the usefulness of the test. Consequently, the role of serum progesterone assays is currently unclear and it is undergoing further evolution and evaluation.

Numerous other serum markers for the diagnosis of EP have been investigated. These include secretory endometrial protein, estradiol, the pregnancy-associated proteins A to D, and others as well as routine laboratory tests such as amylase, creatine kinase, sedimentation rate, and others. None have been accepted as superior to βhCG measurements at this time.

Sonography and Ectopic Pregnancy

Sonography plays an essential role in the diagnosis of EP. The primary goal of sonography in suspected EP is to determine if an IUP is present. Sonographic findings may also be useful in planning therapy when an EP is discovered. Noninvasive therapies are often reserved for EPs in which no cardiac activity is seen or those in which the mass is less than a specified size, though this area is undergoing rapid change. In addition, sonography provides information regarding fetal age and viability when an IUP is present. It has previously been assumed that if an IUP exists, the diagnosis of EP has been excluded. This assumption is based on the historical incidence of heterotopic pregnancy (combined IUP and EP), reported to occur once per 30,000 pregnancies. This is no longer a completely safe assumption, with heterotopic pregnancy now occurring in up to 1 in 3000 pregnancies in the general population. In vitro fertilization and other efforts to enhance fertility with the use of ovulation-inducing drugs has resulted in a higher incidence of heterotopic pregnancy. Studies have reported up to a

1:95 incidence in the in vitro fertilization population. In this group heterotopic pregnancy should be considered even when sonography demonstrates an IUP. For other patients, demonstrating an IUP still provides a high degree of confidence in ruling out EP. This confidence should be somewhat tempered when a patient has risk factors for EP.[8]

Advances in sonographic imaging include improved portability, decreased cost, and improved image quality of newer machines. Use of transvaginal scanning allows earlier detection of an IUP or an EP. These advances have contributed to increasing use of real-time, bedside sonography in the emergency department (ED) performed by emergency physicians. ED sonography has the further advantage of allowing a potentially unstable patient to remain under continuous observation in the ED. ED sonography in the first trimester of pregnancy has been shown to be accurate and to contribute to earlier diagnosis and treatment of EP. It has been endorsed by the American College of Emergency Physicians (ACEP) and the Society for Academic Emergency Medicine (SAEM). However sonography is a highly operator-dependent procedure. Widespread validation in the community setting of the positive results obtained in academic teaching hospitals does not yet exist. Sonography is a valuable adjunct to the physical examination and laboratory data in the diagnosis of EP when used by emergency physicians, but the limitations of the procedure, equipment, and operator must be kept in mind.[9–11]

Identification of an IUP with sonography is dependent upon operator and technical factors and gestational age as reflected in βhCG levels. Technical factors include the approach [transabdominal (TA) versus transvaginal (TV)], body habitus (possible interference from abdominal wall fat), patient preparation (full bladder needed for TA scanning) and equipment characteristics. Higher-quality equipment produces better images, which are easier to interpret. The quality of the image and the accuracy of the interpretation also depend on the skill of the person who obtains and interprets the images. All of these must be considered when making clinical decisions based upon sonographic results.[11–13]

The sequencing of TA versus TV sonography is situation- and operator-dependent. Usually, TA scanning is performed first. Among other differences, TA scanning is less invasive and offers a wider field of view and easier orientation to the pelvic organs. A full bladder is required for an appropriate acoustic window. TA scanning is often diagnostic. When TA sonography is not diagnostic, TV scanning should be performed. With TV scanning, the shallower depth of field and higher frequencies made possible by the lack of interposed abdominal fat allows better visualization of small structures such as early pregnancies. Orientation to the pelvic organs is more difficult with TV scanning than with TA. A full bladder is not required. There are reports of negative TV but positive TA sonography in cases of EP, so both studies should be performed if the study performed first is not diagnostic.[12,14]

When sonography reveals an unequivocal IUP and no other abnormalities, EP is effectively excluded unless heterotopic pregnancy is a consideration. A living IUP may be definitely diagnosed when cardiac activity is seen within the uterine cavity (cardiac activity usually can be seen by 6 weeks in TV and 7 weeks in TA). It may still be necessary to consider another diagnosis to explain the chief complaint when an IUP is found. If an embryo without cardiac activity is visualized, the diagnosis of fetal demise can be made provided that the crown-rump length is at least 5 mm. Again, there may be other coexisting diagnoses. Diagnosis of an IUP when cardiac activity is not seen is less certain. A gestational sac found early is seen as a small, sonolucent structure surrounded by an echogenic ring (see Fig. 109-8 in Chap. 109). This is normally seen by 5 weeks since the last normal menses. At approximately 6 weeks, the yolk sac becomes visible. The yolk sac is a bright (echogenic) ring within the gestational sac. By 7 weeks, cardiac activity is usually visible within the embryo, with both the embryo and yolk sac visible (see Fig 109-9 in Chap. 109). An intrauterine pregnancy with cardiac activity is referred to as a viable IUP. Generally, the gestational sac, yolk sac, and fetal pole can be visualized by TV at 4.5, 5.5, and 6 weeks respectively. Visualization by TA is approximately one week later.

No further diagnostic testing is needed when sonographic findings confirm or are highly suggestive of EP. An empty uterus with embryonic cardiac activity visualized outside the uterus is diagnostic of EP. This is seen in less than 10 percent of EP using TA scanning but in up to 25 percent of cases when the TV approach is used. When a pelvic mass or free pelvic fluid are seen in conjunction with an empty uterus, EP is considered highly likely. One study suggests that the combination of an echogenic adnexal mass with free fluid in the setting of an empty uterus confers a 100 percent risk of EP, while a large amount of free fluid alone has a 95 percent and a mass alone a 71 percent risk (Table 100-2).[15] A metanalysis of studies published regarding TV sonography for EP suggests that in addition to a living extrauterine pregnancy, an extrauterine gestational sac is highly predictive of EP. The analysis also suggested that any adnexal mass (other than a simple cyst) has a 99 percent specificity and a 96 percent positive predictive value with 84 percent sensitivity for the diagnosis of EP.[16] It has also been suggested that the thickness of the endometrial stripe is predictive of EP when no diagnostic findings are noted on sonography. A large retrospective study found that the average thickness of the endometrial stripe was 6 mm in cases later proved to be EP, while in cases of IUP the stripe measured about 13 mm on average.[17]

If sonography fails to reveal a definite IUP or fails to show findings strongly suggestive or diagnostic of an EP, the test should be considered indeterminate and interpreted in light of quantitative serum βhCG levels. The concept of the "discriminatory zone" was developed by Kadar and colleagues to relate βhCG levels and sonography findings in a clinically useful way.[18] The discriminatory zone is the level of βhCG at which findings of an IUP are expected on sonography. If the βhCG level is higher than the discriminatory zone and the uterus is empty, this is interpreted as suggestive of an EP. An empty uterus with a βhCG level below the discriminatory zone is an indeterminate finding representing an early IUP, an EP or other pathologic pregnancy. The actual level of βhCG representing the discriminatory zone is operator- and technique-dependent. With TV scanning, a conservative discriminatory zone is 1800 to 2000 mIU/mL. For TA scanning, an IUP should be detectable when the βhCG level reaches about 6000 mIU/mL.[14,16] Clinicians should understand this concept and collaborate closely with imaging specialists in equivocal cases to avoid confusion. When EP is suspected, sonography should be performed even in patients with low βhCG levels. Dart and colleagues found that approximately one-third of patients presenting to an ED with the eventual diagnosis of EP and βhCG $>$1000 mIU/mL were identified by TV sonography. They were also able to identify patients with IUP and low βhCG levels.[19]

Diagnostic algorithms using the concept of the discriminatory zone have been proposed and tested. A study of 1263 consecutive ED patients with clinically suspected EP by Barnhart et al. found 205 cases of EP, of whom 81.5 percent were hemodynamically stable.[21] In stable patients, they correctly diagnosed 49.1 percent of EP and 96

TABLE 100-2 Ancillary Ultrasound Findings Suggestive of Ectopic Pregnancy in High-Risk Patients

Ancillary Findings	Risk of Ectopic Pregnancy
Small amount of free pelvic fluid	52%
Echogenic adnexal mass	70%
Moderate/Large amount of free pelvic fluid	86%
Any mass plus echogenic fluid	97%

percent of IUP on the initial visit with a combination of βhCG levels and TV sonography. They used a level of 1500 mIU/mL as their discriminatory zone. If the βhCG level was >1500 mIU/mL and the uterus was empty, dilation and curettage (D&C) or laparoscopy was used to diagnose EP. [A D&C was performed on patients not wishing to continue the pregnancy. If chorionic villi were present, IUP was considered confirmed]. When the βhCG level was <1500 mIU/mL and the uterus empty, they performed serial βhCG measurements every 2 days. If βhCG failed to increase by at least 66 percent in a 2-day period, an operative procedure was used to diagnose possible EP. TV sonography was repeated if the βhCG level was >1500 mIU/mL. With use of this protocol, 100 percent of EP were identified without any complications (sensitivity = 100 percent). The specificity of the protocol was 99.9 percent.[20] In another prospective study, Braffman and colleagues studied 1427 ED patients with suspected EP. Patients with βhCG >1500 mIU/mL had sonography which was diagnostic in 1158 (81 percent).[21] The study was indeterminate in 269 (19 percent). Sixty-five (24 percent) of the patients with indeterminate scans were later found to have an EP.[21] The lack of definitive findings on sonography thus should not be regarded as a benign finding if a patient is suspected of having an EP.

Invasive Diagnostic Techniques

Culdocentesis has been largely supplanted by tests for βhCG in combination with sonography, but it may have use in some circumstances, primarily when sonography is unavailable. Laparoscopy may be both diagnostic and therapeutic. D&C may provide a definitive diagnosis of IUP, thus excluding EP except in cases of heterotopic pregnancy.

Culdocentesis

Culdocentesis is the technique of needle aspiration of the rectovaginal cul-de-sac through the posterior fornix of the vagina. Possible results include a dry aspiration, which has no diagnostic value. If clear, nonbloody peritoneal fluid is aspirated, the tap is considered negative. Aspiration of nonclotting blood constitutes a positive tap, considered indicative of an EP. However, there is no consensus regarding the criteria for a positive test. Volumes between 0.3 mL and 10 mL with hematocrit from 3 to 15 percent have been proposed by various authors. The pathophysiologic basis for culdocentesis is that a ruptured EP will bleed into the pelvic peritoneal cavity. Some 85 to more than 90 percent of patients with a ruptured EP will have a positive culdocentesis. Surprisingly, up to 70 percent of patients with an unruptured EP will also have a positive result. A basic limitation of the technique is thus that it is less sensitive in the diagnosis of nonruptured than ruptured EP. Another cause of a false-negative results is that in cases of rapid bleeding, intraperitoneal blood may clot due to lack of sufficient dwell time to produce defibrination. False-positive results occur because of technical errors (entering a vein or other vascular structure with the needle) or a ruptured corpus luteum cyst. Aspiration of purulent material may indicate another diagnosis, such as PID.

A study by Vermesh and colleagues evaluated 252 consecutive patients, most of whom had culdocentesis followed by surgery for suspected EP.[22] A total of 210 patients (83 percent) had a positive culdocentesis defined by fluid with a hematocrit ≥15 percent. Of these, 191 patients (91 percent) had an EP verified at surgery. Twenty-seven of the patients who were discharged after a negative culdocentesis were later found to have an EP, illustrating the poor sensitivity of this procedure for detection of EP. The authors concluded that culdocentesis has less value than noninvasive tests in the management of suspected EP.[22]

Krol and Abbott have reviewed and discussed culdocentesis in the diagnosis of suspected EP in the ED setting.[23] Their conclusion was that in spite of the limitations of the procedure, it has two remaining indications: in unstable patients suspected of a ruptured EP, culdocentesis may be valuable when bedside sonography is not available, and in stable patients, culdocentesis should be considered when sonography is not available. Their logic is that a positive test would facilitate an appropriate, rapid surgical intervention.[23] These conclusions seem reasonable except that few emergency physicians today have regular experience with culdocentesis. As with any invasive procedure, complications as well as false-negative and false-positive results are expected to increase with operator unfamiliarity.

Laparoscopy

Laparoscopy is primarily useful in patients with suspected EP and a nondiagnostic sonogram. It may provide an earlier diagnosis and a possible route for definitive treatment when compared with serial βhCG measurements and sonography. Laparoscopy has a high sensitivity for the diagnosis of EP with low false-negative rates, reported to occur in 3 to 4 percent of cases. False-negative tests are presumably more common early in the course of EP. False-positive rates are somewhat greater, with rates of 1.6 to 6.2 percent; reported. As with other invasive techniques, results will vary with the skill of the operator and the quality of the available equipment. If a laparoscopist is available who is skilled in the diagnosis and laparoscopic treatment of EP, laparoscopy is a viable alternative, which may be accomplished rapidly and with low morbidity.

Dilatation and Curettage

Uterine curettage provides a method for the definitive diagnosis of an IUP when chorionic villi are obtained from the uterine cavity. EP is thus excluded unless a heterotopic (combined) pregnancy is present. The procedure can be performed in a outpatient setting with intravenous sedation. The procedure terminates an IUP if present and is thus applicable only when termination of pregnancy is desired or when a nonviable pregnancy has been documented. A progesterone level of ≤5 ng/mL or stable or falling βhCG levels provide good though not certain evidence of nonviability. The specimen obtained at D&C is examined for the presence of chorionic villi. This may be done at the bedside by suspending the specimen in saline. Villi are observed to float, and absence of material that floats is presumptive evidence of absent villi and thus suggestive of an EP. One study reported a 6.6 percent; false-negative rate (i.e., villi were reported as present in cases later proved to be EP) with this method and there are false-positive tests as well. The results should thus be interpreted cautiously and formal histologic exam of the specimen is needed in addition to bedside suspension of the specimen.

TREATMENT

The traditional treatment of EP has been laparotomy and salpingectomy. Over the last two decades, more conservative surgical and medical approaches have been developed that allow fallopian tube preservation, outpatient treatment, or shorter hospital admissions, and decreased medical expenditures. The treatment of EP can be divided into surgical or medical approaches. Most authors would agree that if laparoscopy is needed for diagnosis, a surgical approach is most appropriate. For unruptured EP, the most frequently used surgical approach is laparoscopic salpingostomy; the most frequently used medical approach is methotrexate treatment. For ruptured EP, laparotomy is the treatment of choice in hemodynamically unstable patients, although laparoscopic approaches have been utilized when the bleeding can be readily controlled.[24]

Surgical Approach

Overall, laparoscopy as compared with laparotomy has emerged as the preferred surgical approach in the treatment of EP in a hemodynamically stable patient. Laparoscopy has been shown to be associated with less blood loss, reduced postoperative adhesion formation, reduced analgesic requirements, reduced hospital stay and convalescence period, and reduced medical expenditures as compared with laparotomy. In a review of studies examining salpingostomy via a laparoscopic or laparotomy approach, the rates of persistent EP for the laparoscopic approach (3 to 20 percent) versus laparotomy (zero to 11 percent) were reported to be comparable. Reproductive outcomes for patients attempting to conceive after the procedure [intrauterine pregnancy (61 percent) and recurrent EP (15 percent)] also were reported to be similar. Laparotomy is reserved for cases that are too difficult for laparoscopic surgery, for hemodynamically unstable patients, and where the operator is inexperienced with operative laparoscopy. Surgical methods for the treatment of tubal EP include salpingectomy, salpingostomy, salpingotomy, segmental tubal resection and anastomosis, and fimbrial evacuation. Fimbrial evacuation of distal ectopic pregnancies is not recommended because of the higher recurrence rate of EP and high incidence of persistent trophoblastic tissue. Which of the other approaches is used depends on hemodynamic stability, the portion of the fallopian tube involved, and the patient's desire for future pregnancy. Segmental tubal resection and anastomosis is recommended for an unruptured pregnancy in the isthmic portion of the fallopian tube because of associated scarring and narrowing of the tube using other methods (e.g., salpingostomy or salpingotomy).[24]

In cases where future fertility is of no concern or the patient is hemodynamically unstable, salpingectomy is the definitive surgical method. Laparoscopic salpingostomy is recognized as the preferred surgical method for the treatment of unruptured EP in patients where future fertility is desired. This more conservative approach has been reported to result in a higher rate of subsequent intrauterine pregnancies (61 versus 38 percent). However, salpingostomy compared to salpingectomy is associated with an increased risk of persistent EP (3 to 20 percent) and recurrent EP (15 versus 10 percent, respectively). Salpingostomy is performed via laparoscopy by making a linear incision (by electrocautery, scissors, or laser) over the antimesenteric side of the fallopian tube overlying the EP. The products of conception are removed (by forceps or suction) and the incision is left open to heal by secondary intention. The tubal incision can also be sutured (salpingotomy).[24]

Specific indications for laparoscopic salpingostomy include hemodynamic stability, ectopic size ≤5 cm, unruptured or ruptured fallopian tube with minimal tubal destruction, appropriate location of the conceptus (ampullary, infundibular, isthmic), surgical accessibility of the fallopian tube, and the patient's with to preserve reproductive potential. Laparotomy can also be used to perform a linear salpingostomy and should be utilized for patients who are hemodynamically unstable or for whom the laparoscopic approach is difficult (e.g., secondary to adhesions).

To assess for a persistent EP following laparoscopic salpingostomy, a weekly hCG level is obtained. By the second postoperative week, the hCG level should be undetectable or less than 20 mIU/mL. If hCG values are above 20 mIU/mL 2 weeks postoperatively, then a repeat sample shoud be obtained 2 weeks later to establish absence of hCG concentrations. Persistent trophoblastic tissue can be found in the fallopian tube or peritoneum; it is most commonly found in the proximal portion of the fallopian tube. Persistent ectopic pregnancies have been successfully treated by surgical reoperation, methotrexate treatment, or expectant management.[24,25]

Medical Treatment

Methotrexate administration is the most common medical treatment for EP. Other compounds have been used for local injection, including prostaglandins, hyperosmolar glucose, potassium chloride, and mifepristone (RU486). Expectant management with serial hCG levels and ultrasound is also a medical option.

Methotrexate is a potent folate antagonist that inhibits the enzyme dihydrofolate reductase, blocking DNA synthesis prior to cell division. Methotrexate effectively inhibits cell division in rapidly dividing cells such as trophoblastic tissue. Many different methotrexate regimens have been used, including both systemic and direct injection into the ectopic gestational sac under ultrasound guidance or laparoscopy. Somewhat higher success rates have been reported for single-dose intramuscular administration of methotrexate (92 percent) versus local injection under ultrasound (81 percent) or laparoscopy (79 percent). Systemic and local administration of methotrexate produced similar peak plasma concentrations and areas under the curve.[24,25]

Systemic treatment has evolved as the most commonly used methotrexate treatment in selected patients, avoiding possible additional cost and/or morbidity from laparoscopic or US guidance techniques for local injection. Both single-dose (methotrexate 50 mg/m^2) and multiple-dose (1 mg/kg IM every other day for 4 days or 48 h) regimens have been used. Possible side effects associated with methotrexate treatment include bone marrow suppression, acute and chronic hepatotoxicity, stomatitis, pulmonary fibrosis, alopecia, and photosensitivity. Leucovorin has been commonly coadministered to diminish the possible side effects; however, some clinicians report that it is not needed. Precautions are taken following methotrexate treatment to minimize the danger of tubal rupture, including only one pelvic exam by one examiner (similar to placenta previa).[26,27]

Abdominal pain (lasting 4 to 12 h) is common (33 to 59 percent) 3 to 7 days after initiation of methotrexate treatment and is thought to be secondary to methotrexate-induced tubal abortion. This can represent a clinical dilemma in that it is difficult to differentiate expected pain from therapeutic tubal abortion and pain from rupturing persistent EP. Patients presenting with abdominal pain in this time frame following methotrexate administration should have a complete blood count and US to rule out significant free fluid in the cul-de-sac and should be evaluated for other causes of abdominal pain. Such patients may need admission to the hospital for observation. Hemodynamic instability and/or falling hematocrit would require surgical intervention.[26,27]

Single-dose intramuscular administration of methotrexate for the treatment of EP in selected patients represents an outpatient approach that can be initiated in the ED. A treatment protocol should be developed jointly with the emergency and ob/gyn departments. Patients should be instructed that (1) treatment failure occurs in at least 5 to 10 percent of cases, (2) failure is more likely in pregnancies past 6 weeks gestation and tubal mass greater than 3.5 cm in diameter; (3) elective surgery may be necessary if medical therapy fails and emergent surgery may be necessary if tubal rupture occurs (approximately a 5 percent chance); (4) vaginal bleeding, abdominal and/or pleuritic pain, weakness, dizziness, or syncope (possible signs of tubal rupture) should be reported immediately; (5) no sexual intercourse (which can possibly increase the risk of tubal rupture) until hCG concentrations are absent (usually 14 to 21 days following methotrexate); (6) no alcohol or multivitamins with folic acid should be consumed.[26,27]

Stovall et al. reported the largest (120 women) prospective series of patients receiving a single-dose of intramuscular methotrexate.[26] In that favorable series, a nonlaparoscopic diagnostic algorithm was used. Inclusion criteria for single-dose intramuscular methotrexate treatment included hemodynamic stability, TV ultrasound demonstrating an unruptured EP (if identified) ≤3.5 cm in the greatest diameter, hCG titers increasing after curettage (if performed), and patient's desire for

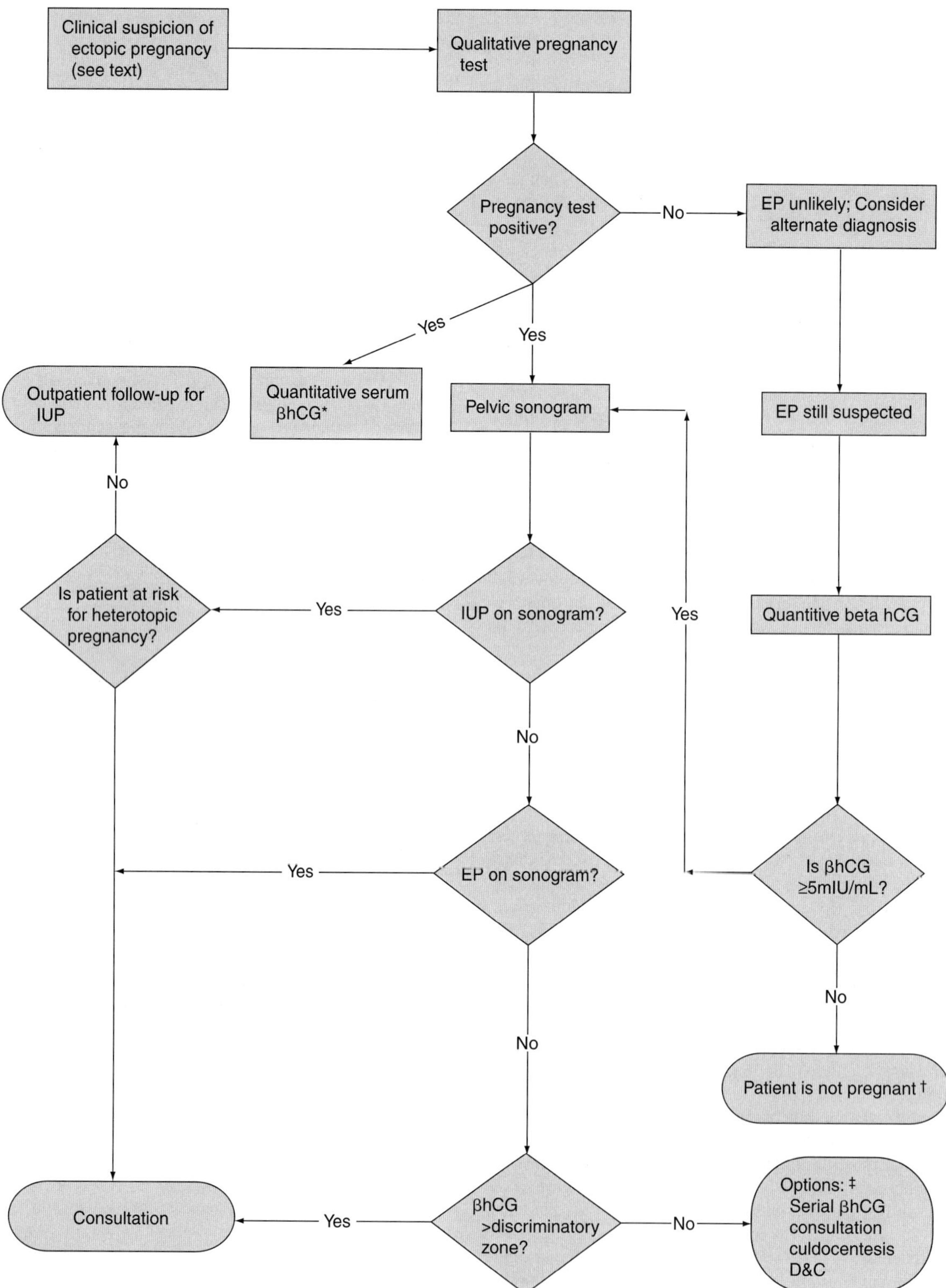

*Quantitative βhCG measurement *prior* to sonography may facilitiate rapid patient disposition by saving time.

†There have been extremely rare reports of pregnancy with βhCG <5 mIU/mL.

‡Serial outpatient βhCG measurements are recommended only for stable patients judged low risk for ruptured EP (see text).

FIG. 100-1. Diagnostic pathway for suspected ectopic pregnancy.

future fertility. The protocol consists of:

Day 0: Lab tests (CBC, quantitative hCG, Rh, serum creatinine), intramuscular methotrexate (50 mg/m^2); if Rh negative, give Rhogam 300 μg.
Day 4: Quantitative hCG.
Day 7: Quantitative hCG, CBC, transaminases; if <15 percent decline or rise in hCG between days 4 to 7, repeat methotrexate (50 mg/m^2).

Weekly hCG titers should be obtained until negative. If hCG titer has diminished less than 50 percent over a 2-week period, then a repeat dose of methotrexate should be given.[26]

In a recent review of the treatment of EP by Yao, more stringent guidelines were recommended, including only treatment in women with hCG <2000 mIU/mL, tubal diameter <2 cm, and absence of fetal cardiac activity.[24] Certain prognostic factors have been identified that are associated with a higher failure rate of methotrexate treatment, including larger tubal diameter, higher hCG concentrations, severe abdominal pain, and presence of fetal cardiac activity. However, no clear consensus has been established for exact tubal diameter or hCG concentration thresholds. Methotrexate is contraindicated in patients with hepatic dysfunction (transaminases greater than twice normal), renal disease, WBC <2000, or platelet count <100,000.[27] Following methotrexate administration, it is not uncommon to observe a transient rise in hCG concentrations between days 1 and 4. Serial ultrasound exams have revealed that the tubal EP may actually increase in size and vascularity before its resolution, and that hCG resolution does not correlate with sonographic resolution.[24]

One randomized trial to date has compared systemic methotrexate (intramuscular; four-dose treatment over 1 week) to laparoscopic salpingostomy in the treatment of tubal pregnancy in 100 patients with laparoscopically confirmed unruptured EP. Primary treatment with either methotrexate or laparoscopic salpingostomy revealed similar success rates (82 versus 72 percent of patients, respectively); homolateral fallopian tube patency rates (3 months after treatment) were also comparable (55 versus 59 percent of patients, respectively). Long-term fertility outcome from this study has not yet been reported.[28]

CLINICAL APPROACH AND DISPOSITION

With the goal of early diagnosis, when a patient with signs or symptoms suggestive of EP is found to be pregnant, further testing to determine if the pregnancy is intrauterine should be undertaken. The nature and timing of additional diagnostic measures depends upon the clinical condition of the patient. Unstable patients suspected of ectopic pregnancy should receive resuscitation, urgent consultation, and operative intervention. Surgery may be both diagnostic and therapeutic if an EP is found or may reveal another cause for the patients condition. When bedside ED sonography is available, it may be valuable even in unstable patients if it does not interfere with resuscitation, consultation, and rapid transfer to the operating room.

Ideally, all pregnant patients with suspected EP should receive immediate sonography. However, issues of availability during off hours may make this impractical. Stable patients who are judged to be at low risk for EP can be considered for discharge and outpatient follow-up. At a minimum, such patients should have a quantitative βhCG level obtained to facilitate subsequent management. Culdocentesis remains an option where sonography is unavailable but at this time is used infrequently.

There are a number of options for stable patients with a βhCG level outside the discriminatory zone and negative sonography. These include consultation or discharge for follow-up in 2 days for reexamination and repeat βhCG levels. Culdocentesis, D&C, and laparoscopy are also options in this circumstance. The flowchart illustrates a suggested diagnostic approach (Fig. 100-1).

REFERENCES

1. Goldner TE, Lawson HW, Xia Z, Atrash HK: Surveillance for ectopic pregnancy—United States, 1970–1989. *MMWR* 42:73, 1993.
2. Stovall TG, Kellerman AL, Ling FW, et al: Emergency department diagnosis of ectopic pregnancy. *Ann Emerg Med* 19:1098, 1990.
3. Kaplan BC, Dart RG, Moskos M, et al: Ectopic pregnancy: prospective study with improved diagnostic accuracy. *Ann Emerg Med* 28:10,1996.
4. Kingdom JC, Kelly T, MacLean AB, et al: Rapid one step urine test for human chorionic gonadotropin in evaluating suspected complications of early pregnancy. *BMJ* 302:1308, 1991.
5. Norman RJ, Buck RH, Rom L, Joubert SM: Blood or urine measurement of human chorionic gonadotropin for detection of ectopic pregnancy? A comparative study of qualitative and quantitative methods in both fluids. *Obstet Gynecol* 153:724, 1988.
6. Kadar N, Romero R</AU>. Further observations on serial human chorionic gonadotropin patterns in ectopic pregnancies and spontaneous abortions. *Fertil Steril* 50:367, 1988.
7. McCord ML, Muram D, Buster, JE, et al: Single serum progesterone as a screen for ectopic pregnancy: Exchanging specificity and sensitivity to obtain optimal test performance. *Fertil Steril* 66:513, 1996.
8. Tal J, Haddad S, Gordon N, Timor Tritsch I: Heterotopic pregnancy after ovulation induction and assisted reproductive technologies: A literature review from 1971 to 1993. *Fertil Steril* 66(1):1, 1996.
9. Jehle D, Davis E, Evans T, et al: Emergency department sonography by emergency physicians. *Am J Emerg Med* 7:605, 1989.
10. Mateer J, Plummer D, Heller M, et al: Model curriculum for physician training in emergency ultrasound. *Ann Emerg Med* 23:95, 1994.
11. Schiager D, Lazzareschi G, Whitten D, Sanders AB: A prospective study of ultrasonography in the ED by emergency physicians. *Am J Emerg Med* 12:185, 1994.
12. Mateer JR, Aiman EJ, Brown MH, Olson DW: Ultrasonographic examination by emergency physicians of patients at risk for ectopic pregnancy. *Acad Emerg Med* 2:867, 1995.
13. Wojack JC, Clayton MJ, Nolan TE: Outcomes of ultrasound diagnosis of ectopic pregnancy—Dependence on observer experience. *Invest Radiol* 302:115, 1995.
14. Zinn HL, Cohen HL, Zinn DL: Ultrasonographic diagnosis of ectopic pregnancy: Importance of transabdominal imaging. *J Ultrasound Med.* 16:603, 1997.
15. Nyberg DA, Mack LA, Laning F, et al: Early pregnancy complications: Endovaginal monographic findings correlated with human chorionic gonadotropin levels. *Radiology* 167:619, 1988.
16. Brown DL, Doubilet PM: Transvaginal sonography for the diagnosis of ectopic pregnancy: Positivity and performance characteristics. *J Ultrasound Med* 13:259, 1994.
17. Spandorfer SD, Barnhart KT: Endometrial stripe thickness as a predictor of ectopic pregnancy. *Fertil Steril* 66:474, 1996.
18. Kadar N, DeVore G, Romero R: Discriminatory hCG zone: Its use in the sonographic evaluation for ectopic pregnancy. *Obstet Gynecol* 58:156, 1981.
19. Dart RG, Kaplan B, Cox C: Transvaginal ultrasound in patients with low beta-human chorionic gonadotropin values: How often is the study diagnostic? *Ann Emerg Med* 30:135, 1997.
20. Barnhart K, Mennuti MT, Benjamin I, et al: Prompt diagnosis of ectopic pregnancy in an emergency department setting. *Obstet Gynecol* 81:1010, 1994.
21. Braffman BH, Coleman BG, Ramchandani P, et al: Emergency department screening for ectopic pregnancy: A prospective US study. *Radiology* 190:797, 1994.
22. Vermesh M, Graczykowski J, Sauer M: Revaluation of the role of culdocentesis in the management of ectopic pregnancy. *Am J Obstet Gynecol* 162:411, 1990.
23. Krol LV, Abbott T: The current role of culdocentesis. *Am J Emerg Med* 10:354, 1992.
24. Yao M, Tuland T: Current status of surgical and nonsurgical management of ectopic pregnancy. *Fertil Steril* 67:421, 1997.
25. Carson SA, Buster JE: Ectopic pregnancy. *N Engl J Med* 329:1174, 1993.
26. Stovall TG, Ling FW: Single-dose methotrexate: An expanded clinical trial. *Am J Obstet Gynecol* 168:1759, 1993.
27. Ander DS, Ward KR: Medical management of ectopic pregnancy—The role of methotrexate. *J Emerg Med* 15:177, 1997.
28. Engelsbel HPJ, Mol S, Van der Veen F, et al: Randomized trial of systemic methotrexate versus laparoscopic salpingostomy in tubal pregnancy. *Lancet* 350:774, 1997.

EMERGENCIES DURING PREGNANCY AND THE POSTPARTUM PERIOD

Gloria J. Kuhn

Pregnant women are susceptible to all of the diseases seen in nonpregnant women as well as diseases present only in the gravid and postpartum periods. In 1994, 8 percent of American women aged 14 to 44 were pregnant and delivered approximately 3.9 million live births. While the majority of pregnancies result in the delivery of a healthy infant from a healthy mother, there are conditions that can complicate the natural course of pregnancy. This chapter discusses diseases that have the potential of complicating pregnancy and increasing morbidity and mortality rates for either the mother or the fetus.

MORTALITY AND MORBIDITY RATES

The lethal triad in pregnancy has been hemorrhage, infection, and preeclampsia. In the United States, maternal mortality and morbidity rates have been significantly reduced, but these three diseases remain the most common complications of pregnancy.

Direct maternal death includes the death of the mother due to obstetrical complications of pregnancy, labor, or the puerperium. Indirect maternal death includes death not directly due to obstetrical causes but resulting from previously existing disease or a disease that developed during the gravid period or was exacerbated by the pregnancy.[1]

The maternal mortality ratio (number of maternal deaths per 100,000 live births) decreased from 582 per 100,000 live births in 1935 to 8.5 per 100,000 live births in 1994 for white women. Unfortunately, the ratio for African-American women is about three times as high. This difference appears to result from socioeconomic factors that result in lack of prenatal care and dietary deficiencies. In 1990, 40 percent of black mothers did not receive prenatal care, compared to 20 percent of white mothers.[2] The black-white mortality rate differential is greatest for diseases seen in the first trimester: ectopic pregnancy, spontaneous abortion, induced abortion, and gestational trophoblastic disease (GTD).

Maternal mortality rates greatly increase with increasing age in all races. The leading causes of maternal death are pulmonary embolus (mostly thromboembolic), ectopic pregnancy, pregnancy-induced hypertension (leading to cerebrovascular accident), hemorrhage (mainly postpartum), and infection.

The disorders most commonly associated with stillbirths are hemorrhage (mainly abruptio placentae), pregnancy-induced hypertension, and pulmonary embolism (primarily amniotic fluid embolism). The gravest threats to the neonate are preterm birth and low birth weight. Low birth weight varies on a racial basis. For white women it is 60 per 1000 live births, while for blacks it is 120 per 1000 births, which accounts for the differences in infant mortality rates between the two groups. Low birth weight also contributes to morbidity rates as a result of respiratory distress, intraventricular hemorrhage, septicemia, necrotizing enterocolitis, bronchopulmonary dysplasia, and retinopathy of prematurity.

Preterm infants who weigh at least 500 g and are born at 24 weeks gestation are considered to be at the lower limit of viability but have much higher rates of mental retardation and severe visual impairment than do full-term, normal-birth-weight infants.

EMERGENCIES DURING THE FIRST HALF OF PREGNANCY

While pregnancy is usually considered in terms of trimesters, when discussing patterns of emergencies, dividing pregnancy into halves is advantageous. Emergencies during the first half include ectopic pregnancy, vaginal bleeding, GTD, urinary tract infection (UTI), and hyperemesis gravadarum.

Vaginal Bleeding

The differential diagnosis of vaginal bleeding during the first trimester should include abortion (most common cause), ectopic pregnancy, and GTD. Other causes include implantation bleeding (physiologic) seen around or just after the time of expected menses due to the burrowing of the embryo into the highly vascular decidual tissue, cervical ectropion, and cervicitis due to infection from gonorrhea, *Chlamydia,* or bacterial vaginosis.

Any woman of childbearing age who presents with a chief complaint of abdominal pain or vaginal bleeding and has not had a hysterectomy should be tested for pregnancy. If a serum or urine pregnancy test result is positive, further evaluation for ectopic pregnancy or spontaneous abortion is indicated. Risk factors for ectopic pregnancy include prior ectopic pregnancy, tubal surgery, history of salpingitis, or assisted fertility. Likewise, women of childbearing age with syncope, hypotension, or mental status changes should have pregnancy testing and evaluation for ectopic pregnancy (see Chap. 100).

SPONTANEOUS ABORTION Estimates of pregnancies that abort spontaneously range from 20 to 40 percent. About 75 percent of spontaneous abortions occur before 8 weeks of gestation. The World Health Organization defines spontaneous abortion as loss of pregnancy before 20 weeks or loss of a fetus weighing less than 500 g. Inevitable abortion will occur in the face of vaginal bleeding and dilatation of the cervix. Incomplete abortion is defined as passage of only parts of the products of conception and is more likely to occur between 6 and 14 weeks of pregnancy. Complete abortion is passage of all fetal tissue, including trophoblast and all products of conception, before 20 weeks of conception. Missed abortion is a fetal death at less than 20 weeks without passage of any fetal tissue for 4 weeks after fetal death. Septic abortion is evidence of infection during any stage of abortion.

The most common cause of fetal wastage is chromosomal abnormalities, accounting for 50 to 60 percent of all losses. Other risk factors include advanced maternal age, prior poor obstetric history, concurrent medical disorders, previous abortion, certain infections, including syphilis and HIV, and some anatomic abnormalities of the upper genital tract. Exposure to some agents, such as certain anesthetic agents, certain heavy metals, and tobacco, is also thought to contribute to the incidence of abortion.

A pelvic examination is mandatory as part of the history and physical examination in order to determine the amount and site of bleeding, whether the cervix has dilated, and whether any tissue has been passed. The amount of bleeding as pads used per hour, last menstrual period, and past medical and obstetric history should be part of the history obtained.

If hemodynamic instability is present, fluid resuscitation should be immediately started. A complete blood count (CBC), blood type, Rh factor and antibody screen, urinalysis (UTI has been associated with increased fetal wastage), and quantitative β serum human chorionic gonadotropin (βhCG) level should be obtained. Vaginal ultrasound studies should be performed to rule out ectopic pregnancy, as a prognostic tool for fetal viability, and to diagnose retained products of conception.

If the patient is bleeding heavily, a Yankower tip is useful to suction blood from the vaginal vault. All material in the vaginal vault should be examined to determine whether it is blood clot or products of conception. Products of conception should be sent for pathologic examination. If tissue is protruding from the cervical os, its careful removal with ring forceps may allow the os to close and decrease bleeding. However, care must be taken to ensure that the tissue is not the rare cervical ectopic pregnancy. If profuse bleeding continues in the face of inevitable abortion, 20 U of oxytocin can be added to a liter of normal saline solution and infused at 150 to 200 mL/h to obtain hemostasis until dilatation and curettage can be performed.

The quantitative βhCG analysis may be very helpful. The β subunit of βhCG is first detectable as early as 9 to 11 days following ovulation (usually 24 days after the last menstrual period) and reaches 200 IU/mL at the expected time of menses.[3] An abnormally high βhCG level suggests advanced pregnancy, multiple gestation, GTD, or, rarely, an ovarian tumor.

Ultrasound studies combined with determinations of βhCG levels can be both diagnostic and prognostic. If the βhCG level is greater than 2000 IU/mL, an intrauterine gestation should be visible. A yolk sac is seen at 36 days, and a heatbeat is noted 41 to 47 days after the last menstrual period. Gestational sacs with a mean diameter greater than 25 mm without an embryo or greater than 20 mm without a yolk sac are definitely abnormal, and loss of pregnancy will result.[3]

Patients with a diagnosis of threatened abortion can be safely discharged if close follow-up is ensured. While low level of activity and even bed rest are sometimes advised, there is no proven effectiveness of this practice. Generally speaking, a miscarriage cannot be avoided. Intercourse and tampons are to be avoided to minimize likelihood of infection. The patient with an incomplete abortion should have the uterus evacuated. The patient with a complete abortion, as shown by ultrasound and/or complete passage of products of conception, can be safely discharged after follow-up is ensured to ascertain that the bleeding has stopped. The patient with a nonviable fetus can either be admitted or discharged to be followed up within a week by her physician, depending on the comfort level of the patient and physician with this decision. Warnings should be given to return immediately if there is heavy bleeding (more than one pad per hour for 6 h), pain, or fever.

All pregnant patients with vaginal bleeding who are Rh negative should be treated with Rh immunoglobulin (Rhogam) if unsensitized. A dose of 300 μg is recommended. Ideally, Rhogam should be administered prior to discharge, but it can also be administered within 72 h by the primary care physician or obstetrician when the woman presents several days or weeks after vaginal bleeding has begun.[4]

GESTATIONAL TROPHOBLASTIC DISEASE GTD is a neoplasm that arises in the trophoblastic cells of the placenta. It complicates 1 in 1700 pregnancies in North America and is more common in Asian women. The noninvasive form of the disease is the hydatidiform mole, which is either complete or partial. Complete moles are more common, and in this form there is no actual fetus, while in the partial mole a deformed, nonviable fetus is present. Both moles and invasive forms of GTD are composed of trophoblasts that produce βhCG.

Symptoms include vaginal bleeding in the first or second trimester (75 to 95 percent of cases) and hyperemesis (26 percent). GTDs, or molar pregnancies, that persist into the second trimester are associated with preeclampsia. When pregnancy-induced hypertension is seen prior to 24 weeks of gestation, the possibility of a molar pregnancy should be considered. The uterus is excessive in size for gestational age and shows a placenta with many lucent areas interspersed with brighter areas on ultrasound study. If GTD is suspected because of abnormally high βhCG levels, a uterine size either larger or smaller than expected, and ultrasound findings suggestive of the diagnosis, obstetric consultation should be obtained. Treatment is by suction curettage in the hospital setting because of risk of hemorrhage. After evacuation, βhCG levels should be monitored, and failure to fall is evidence of persistent or invasive disease necessitating chemotherapy.[5] Metastasis to lung, liver, and brain may occur. Trophoblastic embolization, although extremely rare, may occur, with resulting rapid onset of respiratory distress resembling amniotic fluid embolus.

Urinary Tract Infection

Infections of the urinary tract are the most common bacterial infections during pregnancy. The highest incidence of bacteriuria has been reported in African-American multiparas with sickle-cell trait, while the lowest incidence is seen in affluent white women of low parity.

Pregnant women with UTI are at increased risk for pyelonephritis, and pyelonephritis is a risk factor for preterm labor and low birth weight. The increased risk of pyelonephritis is the result of hydroureter, dilatation of the renal pelvis, and consequent urinary stasis. Pregnant patients with asymptomatic bacteriuria identified on microscopic analysis should have a urine culture performed and be treated if the culture is positive. Untreated, 25 percent will develop symptomatic infection, while treatment will decrease the incidence of symptomatic UTI by 80 to 90 percent.[6]

Symptomatic UTI requires a urine culture and antibiotic therapy. There are various regimens, although only 7-day regimens are recommended during pregnancy. The recurrence rate during pregnancy for all regimens is about 30 percent.

Treatment choices include nitrofurantoin (one tablet bid), ampicillin; or cephalexin. Trimethoprim-sulfamethoxazole is relatively contraindicated in the first trimester because of antifolate properties of trimethoprim, and sulfonamides are contraindicated in the third trimester due to risk of fetal hyperbilirubinemia.

Reliable patients with asymptomatic bacteriuria can be discharged after urine culture, with treatment withheld pending results of culture. If there is any question as to compliance with follow-up, such patients should be treated with the same antibiotic regimen prescribed for pregnant patients with UTI. Patients with pyelonephritis should generally be hospitalized.

Nausea, Vomiting, and Hyperemesis Gravidarum

Nausea and vomiting of pregnancy are generally seen in the first 12 weeks. Both are extremely common, with nausea seen in 70 percent of patients and vomiting in 50 percent, and symptoms are mild in most. Hyperemesis gravidarum is intractable vomiting with weight loss and laboratory values that show hypokalemia or ketonemia. The cause is not known. Women who lose more than 5 percent of prepregnancy body weight have an increased risk of intrauterine growth restriction and low-birth-weight infants. Patients with GTD may also present with intractable vomiting.

The presence of abdominal pain in nausea and vomiting of pregnancy or hyperemesis gravidarum is highly unusual and should suggest another diagnosis. Occasionally, women with ruptured ectopic pregnancies present with nausea and vomiting as well as diarrhea and abdominal pain. After the first trimester, the volume of the gallbladder increases during fasting and postcontraction after a meal. Also, biliary sludge seems to increase in pregnancy in 30 percent, predisposing to stone formation.[7] Cholelithiasis and cholecystitis are more common in pregnant women than in women of comparable age and health status who are not pregnant. Differential diagnosis of vomiting or vomiting with abdominal pain should include cholecystitis, cholelithiasis, gastroenteritis, pancreatitis, hepatitis, peptic ulcer, pyelonephritis, ectopic pregnancy, and fatty liver of pregnancy.

Findings upon physical examination are usually normal except for signs of volume depletion. Rectal examination should be performed to rule out fecal impaction and occult blood. A pelvic examination should be performed if there is pelvic pain, vaginal bleeding, or discharge.

If the examination reveals only loss of volume, laboratory tests to consider include CBC, serum electrolyte determinations, blood urea nitrogen (BUN) and creatinine determinations, and urinalysis. The finding of ketonuria is important, since it is an early sign of starvation. Serial measurement of urinary ketones can be used to determine success of therapy.

TABLE 101-1 Antiemetics

Antiemetic	Brand Name	FDA Category	Oral	Rectal	Intravenous
		ACUTE INTERVENTION FOR BOTH N/V AND HG			
Promethazine	Phenergan	C	25 mg q4h	25 mg q4h	25–50 mg IV push 50 mg in 500 mL 0.9% normal saline over 2 h
Prochlorperazine	Compazine		10 mg q6–8h	25 mg q12h	10 mg over 2 min Maximum of 40 mg q24h
Chlorpromazine	Thorazine	C	10–25 mg q4–6h	100 mg q6–8h	25 mg in 500 mL 0.9% normal saline at 250 mL/h
		MAINTENANCE THERAPY FOR N/V			
Doxylamine with pyridoxine	Unisom Vitamin B_6		25 mg every evening 25 mg q8h		
Diphenhydramine	Benadryl	B	25–50 mg q6h		
Cisapride	Propulsid	C	10 mg q6h		
		MAINTENANCE THERAPY FOR HG			
Metoclopramide	Reglan	B			10 mg over 1–2 min q4–6h or 1 mg/kg in 50 mL D_5 in 0.45% normal saline, over 30 min
Trimethobenzamide	Tigan	C	250 mg q6–8h	200 mg q6–8h	Should not be given IV May be given 200 mg IM q6–8h

Abbreviations: FDA, US Food and Drug Administration; HG, hyperemesis gravidarum; N/V, nausea and vomiting of pregnancy.
Source: From Pearlman M, Tintinalli JE (eds): *Emergency Care of the Woman.* New York, McGraw-Hill, 1998, with permission.

Treatment consists of intravenous fluids containing 5% glucose in either lactated Ringer's or normal saline solution to reverse dehydration and ketonuria. A number of antiemetic drugs can be used (Table 101-1) for patients who remain nauseated or continue to vomit after fluid hydration. Initially, the patient should be given nothing by mouth. Oral fluids should be started after the nausea and vomiting are controlled and prior to discharge.

The patient may be discharged after reversal of ketonuria, correction of electrolyte imbalance, and a successful trial of oral fluids. Discharge with antiemetic medication is usually necessary. Admission guidelines include uncertain diagnosis, intractable vomiting, persistent ketone or electrolyte abnormalities after volume repletion, and weight loss over 10 percent of prepregnancy weight.

EMERGENCIES DURING THE SECOND HALF OF PREGNANCY

Hypertension, Preeclampsia, Eclampsia, and the HELLP Syndrome

Hypertension complicating pregnancy accounts for 18 percent of maternal deaths. It is also implicated in abruptio placentae and in the birth of preterm and low-birth-weight infants. Hypertension is defined as a blood pressure 140/90 mmHg or greater, a 20-mmHg rise in the systolic, or 10-mmHg rise in the diastolic blood pressure. Thus, a normal-appearing blood pressure may in fact be in the preeclampsia range for a given patient. Pregnancy-induced hypertension (PIH) is elevated blood pressure that develops as a result of pregnancy and regresses postpartum. It cannot be distinguished from transient hypertension during pregnancy except retrospectively. Accordingly, the American College of Obstetricians and Gynecologists no longer use the term PIH, preferring the following, more useful classification: (1) chronic hypertension, (2) preeclampsia superimposed on chronic hypertension, (3) transient hypertension, and (4) preeclampsia or eclampsia.[8] Transient hypertension develops after the midtrimester, is mild, does not compromise the pregnancy, and regresses postpartum but may return in subsequent gestations. Preeclampsia is the combination of hypertension, pathologic edema, and proteinuria.[9] The cause of preeclampsia is not known, but recent research suggests that, in women who will develop preeclampsia, there are fewer placental cytotrophoblasts. These do not invade as deeply, remaining in an early stage and failing to take on the characteristics of blood vessel cells.[10]

Eclampsia is the superimposition of seizures on preeclampsia or aggravated hypertension. Seizures are defined as eclamptic if they occur from the twentieth week of gestation to 7 days after delivery but have been reported as late as 26 days after delivery. All chronic hypertensive disorders, regardless of their cause, predispose to development of preeclampsia or eclampsia (Table 101-2). Blood pressure alone is not always a dependable indicator of severity of disease and must be evaluated in the context of other signs and symptoms[11] (Table 101-3).

Presenting complaints of preeclampsia include headache, visual disturbances, edema, or abdominal pain. It always occurs after 20 weeks of gestation unless GTD is present.

TABLE 101-2 Risk Factors for Development of Hypertension during Pregnancy

Nulliparity
Age >40 years
Prepregnancy hypertension
Chronic renal disease
African-American heritage
Diabetes mellitus
Multiple gestation
Gestational trophoblastic disease

TABLE 101-3 Criteria for Hypertension, Preeclampsia, and Eclampsia

Hypertension	BP >140/90 measured twice at least 6 h apart
Transient hypertension	BP >140/90 without other signs of preeclampsia or eclampsia
Preeclampsia	BP >140/90, >20-mmHg rise in systolic, or >10-mmHg rise in diastolic BP Proteinuria (300 mg/24 h or 1 g/mL) Generalized or pedal edema or weight gain of at least 5 lb over 1 week
Eclampsia	Above findings plus generalized seizure

Abbreviation: BP, blood pressure.

The HELLP syndrome (an acronym for *h*emolysis, *e*levated *l*iver enzymes, and *l*ow *p*latelets) is an important clinical variant of preeclampsia that has a predilection for the multigravid patient, in contrast to the primigravida, in whom preeclampsia is more common. In the HELLP syndrome, the blood pressure is variable and may not be elevated initially. This fact, combined with the usual complaint of epigastric or right upper quadrant pain, makes it easy to mistake the HELLP syndrome for other causes of abdominal pain, such as gastroenteritis, hepatitis, pancreatitis, or pyelonephritis. The HELLP syndrome should be considered in any pregnant or postpartum patient who presents to the emergency department with a chief complaint of abdominal pain. The diagnosis can be made based on clinical findings coupled with laboratory results (Table 101-4).

All patients with a sustained blood pressure of 140/90 or greater and any symptoms that may be secondary to hypertension should be hospitalized. Patients with severe hypertension whose blood pressure is greater than 140/90, and who have epigastric or liver tenderness, visual disturbance, or severe headache are managed in the same way as patients with eclampsia, with administration of magnesium sulfate,[12] antihypertensives as needed, and delivery of the fetus. The dose of intravenous magnesium sulfate is 4 to 6 g over 15 min followed by intravenous infusion of 1 to 2 g/h. Reflexes and serum magnesium levels should be followed to avoid neuromuscular depression. Angiotensin-converting enzyme (ACE) inhibitors should never be used because of fetal side effects. Table 101-5 lists pharmacologic agents for the treatment of hypertension in preeclampsia and eclampsia.

Complications of severe preeclampsia, HELLP syndrome, and eclampsia include spontaneous hepatic and splenic hemorrhage, end-organ failure, abruptio placentae, intracranial bleeding, and death of the fetus. Emergency obstetrical consultation should be obtained, or transfer to a tertiary care hospital should be arranged as soon as the patient is stabilized.

TABLE 101-4 Laboratory Evaluation for Suspected Preeclampsia or HELLP Syndrome

Test	Findings in HELLP Syndrome
CBC and peripheral smear	Schistocytes
Platelet count	<100,000 but suspicious if <150,000
Liver function tests (AST, ALT)	Elevated but below levels in viral hepatitis (<500 IU/L)
Renal function tests	Normal or elevated BUN and creatinine levels
Coagulation profile	Abnormal

Abbreviation: AST, serum aspartate aminotransferase; ALT, serum alanine aminotransferase.

Methyldopa is the drug most often used to treat pregnant patients with chronic hypertension as use of this drug does not adversely affect the fetus.[11] Dosage can be started at 250 mg every 6 h and titrated for control of blood pressure. Sedation may occur during initiation of therapy or when dosage is increased but is usually transient. Close follow-up should be assured for patients placed on methyldopa therapy.

Vaginal Bleeding during the Second Half of Pregnancy

The differential diagnosis of vaginal bleeding during the second half of pregnancy includes abruptio placentae, placenta previa, preterm labor, and bleeding from various lesions of the cervix and lower genital tract. One-third of fetuses die when vaginal bleeding occurs after 20 weeks of gestation.[13]

ABRUPTIO PLACENTAE Abruptio placentae, the premature separation of the normally implanted placenta from the uterine wall, accounts for 30 percent of bleeding in the second half of pregnancy. This complication can occur either spontaneously or as the result of trauma to the abdomen. The spontaneous form is far more common, with hypertension the most common risk factor. Other risk factors include hypertension, increased maternal age, multiparity, smoking, cocaine use, and previous abruptions. Abruption can be complete, partial, or concealed. In concealed abruption, there is little or no vaginal bleeding. However, shock may ensue as the actual blood loss is not evident, and establishing the diagnosis may be delayed. The diagnosis of abruption may be difficult, since clinical signs and symptoms depend on the size of the abruption and the amount of blood loss.

Signs and symptoms include vaginal bleeding (unless concealed), abdominal pain, back pain, uterine tenderness, and uterine irritability. Fetal distress, hypotension, and disseminated intravascular coagulation can develop. Abruptio placentae is frequently misdiagnosed as preterm labor. Complications include fetal death, maternal death from hemorrhage or disseminated intravascular coagulation, fetomaternal transfusion, and amniotic fluid embolism. Laboratory tests that should be ordered include CBC, type and crossmatch, coagulation profile, and renal function studies. Crystalloids should be given to maintain maternal volume status. Emergency obstetrical consultation is necessary whenever abruption is suspected. Cardiotocodynamometry and ultrasound studies are used to monitor fetal well-being, and emergency delivery may be necessary. Some centers may elect to treat small abruptions expectantly. Tocolytics should not be given by the emergency physician in the presence of suspected abruption.

PLACENTA PREVIA Placenta previa, the implantation of the placenta over the cervical os, accounts for 20 percent of bleeding episodes in the second half of pregnancy. Incidence is increased with multiparity and prior cesarean section. The patient presents with painless bright-red bleeding. This complication should be distinguished from the ''bloody show,'' which is passage of a very small amount of bright-red blood mixed with mucus at the onset of labor. Since disruption of the placenta by digital or speculum examination can lead to catastrophic bleeding, digital and speculum examination should be avoided.[14] The safest course is to perform emergency ultrasound studies first.

PREMATURE LABOR AND PREMATURE RUPTURE OF MEMBRANES Preterm (premature) labor is defined as labor prior to 37 weeks' gestation,[15] while premature rupture of membranes (PROM) is rupture of membranes prior to onset of labor. Preterm labor, occuring in 10 percent of deliveries, is the leading cause of perinatal death and disease, accounting for approximately 85 percent of neonatal deaths not due to lethal genetic or congenital abnormalities. Three major

TABLE 101-5 Pharmacologic Agents for Antihypertensive Therapy in Preeclampsia and Eclampsia

Generic Name	Trade Name	Mechanism of Action	Dosage	Comment
Magnesium sulfate		Smooth muscle relaxation	4–6 g IV over 15 min, then 1–2 g/h	Neuromuscular depression
Hydralazine hydrochloride	Apresoline	Arterial vasodilator	2.5 mg IV, then 5–10 mg IV for 20 min up to 40 mg total dose; IV infusion 5–10 mg/h titrated	Must wait 20 min for response between IV doses; possible maternal hypotension
Labetalol	Normodyne Trandate	Selective α and nonselective β antagonist	20 mg IV, then 40–80 mg IV for 10 min to 300 mg total dose; IV infusion 1–2 mg/min titrated	Less reflex tachycardia and hypotension than with hydralazine
Nitroglycerin	Nitrostat IV Tridil Nitro-Bid IV	Relaxation of venous (and arterial) vascular smooth muscle	5μg/min infusion, double q5min	Requires arterial line for continuous blood pressure monitoring; potential methemoglobinemia
Sodium nitroprusside	Nipride Nitropress	Vasodilator	0.25 (μg/kg)/min infusion, increase 0.25 (μg/kg)/min q5min	Potential cyanide toxicity

Source: Modified from Dildy GA, Cotton DB: *Acute Care* 26:14–15, 1988–1989, with permission.

factors contribute to spontaneous or induced delivery before 34 weeks: (1) PROM, (2) spontaneous preterm labor without PROM, and (3) complications that jeopardize fetal or maternal health, mandating early delivery.

Many known factors are associated with preterm labor. More common ones include: PROM, abruptio placentae, drug abuse (particularly of cocaine and amphetamines), multiple gestations, polyhydramnios, cervical incompetence, and infection. Sexually transmitted diseases, including syphilis, gonorrhea, *Chlamydia,* and bacterial vaginosis are two to three times more likely to be associated with preterm labor. The presence of low-grade infection is felt to be one of the most important causes of PROM because bacterial colonization can reduce the tensile strength of membranes.[16] Of importance is the association of digital pelvic examinations and increased frequency of PROM. As a result of this finding, cervical examinations should not be performed from 37 weeks gestation unless the results of the examination will clearly influence clinical management. Of course, all digital examinations during pregnancy should be done using sterile gloves.

Labor is defined as regular uterine contractions resulting in progressive cervical effacement and dilatation. When a woman presents to the emergency department with the suspected onset of labor, the date of the last menstrual period should be ascertained and the estimated date of delivery calculated. The gestational age is the number of weeks from the first day of the last menstrual period. If that date is not known, gestational age can be estimated clinically (see Chapter 99). The patient should be asked about the frequency and duration of contractions, about passage of blood-stained mucus (''bloody show''), and whether there has been rupture of membranes, usually signaled by a gush of fluid or constant leakage of fluid.

In addition to the routine physical examination, the fundal height should be measured, fetal heart tones auscultated, and a sterile speculum examination performed. A pooling of fluid in the vaginal vault or leakage of clear fluid from the cervix is evidence of PROM. If there is no fluid, the woman should be asked to press on the fundus or perform a Valsalva maneuver to determine whether there is leakage of fluid. Any fluid should be tested with nitrazine paper (pH > 6.5 indicates amniotic fluid) and swabbed on a glass slide to be examined for ferning, indicating amniotic fluid. The presence of blood or semen may interfere with both of these tests. On visual examination, if the cervix is posterior in the vagina, thick, and closed, it is not yet ripe for labor. If, in contrast, it is midposition to anterior within the vagina, moderately effaced, and approximately 2 cm dilated, the uterus is undergoing changes preparatory to expulsion of the fetus. Tests for *Chlamydia,* gonorrhea, and group B streptococcus should be performed and secretions examined for bacterial vaginosis. If PROM is suspected or confirmed, digital examination should be deferred if possible or, if performed, should be done using sterile gloves.

A number of critical questions must be considered. Has PROM occurred? Is the woman in premature labor? What is the best estimate of gestational age? Is there fetal distress? Is the woman a candidate for tocolytic therapy? All women suspected of premature labor or PROM require obstetric consultation.

Viability of the fetus is possible at 23 weeks of gestation, but mortality and morbidity rates are extremely high. A number of drugs have been used to inhibit labor, but none is completely effective, and there is potential for serious side effects (Table 101-6). Tocolysis was the third most common cause of adult respiratory distress syndrome and death in pregnant women in Jackson, Mississippi, over a 14-year period.[17] Since tocolytic drugs can delay delivery by only a few days, the purpose of tocolytic therapy is to allow time for administration of glucocorticoids to speed fetal lung maturity[18] and transport of the mother to a center equipped to provide intensive care for the fetus. If a patient presents to an emergency department in preterm labor and the fetus is not mature enough to do well (prior to 34 weeks' gestation), the patient should be transported to a tertiary care facility that has a high-risk ICU for mother and child. Tocolytic therapy should be started prior to transport rather than attempting to deliver the infant at the initial emergency room.[19]

Candidates for tocolysis are women in preterm labor between 24 and 34 to 36 weeks of gestation. Prior to 23 weeks, chances of survival of the fetus are remote and the probability of permanent disability high. At about 25 weeks, even a 2-day increase in length of gestation can add 10 percent to the likelihood of neonatal survival. Beyond 34 to 36 weeks, the infant should be mature enough to do well without specific treatment, and the possible side effects of tocolysis are to be avoided.

The decision to institute tocolysis should be made only after consultation with the obstetrician who will be caring for the patient and who can explain the risks and benefits (see Table 101-6). Tocolytics should not be given if abruption is suspected.

Protocols for tocolysis are shown in Table 101-7. β-adrenergic agents have been shown to have serious side effects. However, terbutaline (Brethine), 0.25 mg given subcutaneously and repeated hourly as needed until contractions stop, is commonly used. Common side effects

TABLE 101-6 Potential Complications of Tocolytic Agents

β-ADRENERGIC AGENTS
Hyperglycemia
Hypokalemia
Hypotension
Pulmonary edema
Cardiac insufficiency
Arrhythmias
Myocardial ischemia
Maternal death
MAGNESIUM SULFATE
Pulmonary edema
Respiratory depression*
Cardiac arrest*
Maternal tetany*
Profound muscular paralysis*
Profound hypotension*
INDOMETHACIN
Hepatitis†
Renal failure†
Gastrointestinal bleeding†
NIFEDIPINE
Transient hypotension

*Effect rare, seen with toxic levels.
†Effect rare, associated with chronic use.
Source: From the American College of Obstetricians and Gynecologists: *Preterm Labor.* Technical bulletin 206. Washington, 1995, with permission.

include tachycardia, hypotension, palpitations, headaches, and tremor. Terbutaline should be withheld if the maternal pulse exceeds 140 beats per minute. The combination of magnesium sulfate and nifedipine is potentially dangerous, since nifedipine can enhance the toxicity of magnesium and result in neuromuscular blockade, interfering with both pulmonary and cardiac function. Careful monitoring of the mother and fetus with use of any of these agents, alone or in combination, is mandatory.

The use of prostaglandin synthase inhibitors, particularly indomethacin, has been found to be effective in delaying delivery by 48 h, but there have been increased rates of neonatal morbidity, with complications including closure of the ductus arteriosus, necrotizing enterocolitis, and intracranial hemorrhage. Recommendations for routine use of this agent for tocolysis must await further investigations.

Since preterm infants are at increased risk of developing group B streptococcus infection and there is reason to suspect that the infection may cause preterm labor, 5 million units of penicillin G is given intravenously unless the patient is allergic to it.[16]

EMERGENCIES DURING THE POSTPARTUM PERIOD

Postpartum hemorrhage and infection continue to be the most common emergencies seen during the postpartum period, but amniotic fluid embolism, while rare, is important because of its high morbidity and mortality rates for both mother and fetus. Eclampsia may occasionally present during this period. Peripartum cardiomyopathy (PPC) is seen during the last month of pregnancy or within 5 months of delivery.

Puerperal Hemorrhage

Postpartum hemorrhage is implicated in approximately 28 percent of pregnancy-related deaths. Since most postpartum hemorrhages occur in the first 24 h postdelivery, unless the delivery takes place at home or in a freestanding birthing center, such patients are unlikely to present to the emergency department. However, delayed hemorrhage may be seen days to weeks postpartum.

The differential diagnosis of hemorrhage in the period immediately following delivery includes uterine atony, uterine rupture, laceration of the lower genital tract, retained placental tissue, uterine inversion, and coagulopathy. After 24 h, retained products may cause bleeding. Other causes include uterine polyps or a coagulopathy, most commonly von Willebrand disease.

A history as to length and amount of bleeding should be obtained because physiologic bleeding takes place in the postpartum period and may be of variable duration, not uncommonly extending for periods of up to 5 weeks after delivery. The patient should be questioned about difficulty delivering the placenta. Manual delivery of the placenta increases risk of postpartum hemorrhage.

A careful history and physical examination should elicit the diagnosis in the majority of cases (Table 101-8). The commonest cause of bleeding within the first 24 h is uterine atony. Normally, after delivery the uterus is firm, globular in shape, and palpable at or below the umbilicus. When uterine atony occurs, the uterine fundus is ''doughy'' in consistency and possibly palpable above the umbilicus. The best way to diagnose this is by abdominal palpation and bimanual examination. If the tone of the uterus is good but blood is seen to be coming from the cervical os, the possibility of retained products of conception or uterine rupture must be considered. Uterine rupture is more common after prior cesarean section as a result of separation of the scar. Prior uterine surgery and multiparity can also predispose to this complica-

TABLE 101-7 Tocolytic Therapy Protocols

Agent	Initial Dose	Maintenance	Monitor
Terbutaline (Brethine)	0.25 mg SC	0.25 mg/h SC until contractions stop	Vital signs, FHTs, uterine contractions
Magnesium sulfate	4–6 g IV over 20 min	2–4 g/h titrated to stop contractions	Vital signs, DTR, FHTs, uterine activity; have calcium gluconate for reversal
Nifedipine (Procardia)	10 mg sublingual q20min up to 4 doses or until contractions stop	20 mg PO q6h	Vital signs, FHTs, uterine activity
Glucocorticoids for fetal lung maturity	Betamethasone (Celestone Soluspan) 12 mg IM q24h for 2 doses or dexamethasone (Decadron) 6 mg IM q6h for 4 doses and weekly thereafter		

Abbreviations: FHTs, fetal heart tones; DTR, deep tendon reflexes.

TABLE 101-8 Physical Findings, Cause, and Treatment of Postpartum Hemorrhage

Finding	Cause	Treatment
Enlarged, doughy uterus	Uterine atony	Oxytocin 20–30 U/L at 200 mL/h or methylergonovine maleate 0.2 mg IM and 0.2 mg PO q6h
Globular, firm uterus	Retained products of conception	Dilatation and curettage
Inability to palpate uterus	Uterine inversion	Manual reduction
Blood in vagina but not coming from uterus	Laceration of lower genital tract	Repair in emergency department or operating room
History of cesarean section	Possible uterine rupture	Surgery
Blood does not clot in red-top tube	Coagulopathy	Fresh-frozen plasma

tion. Very rarely, rupture occurs in the face of no prior risk factors. Another cause of bleeding is inversion of the uterus, which occurs most commonly after strong traction is placed on the umbilical cord in an effort to deliver the placenta. Replacement of the fundus is emergent and may require anesthesia. Diagnosis of the cause will allow proper treatment (Fig. 101-1).

The management of postpartum hemorrhage is dependent on stabilization of the patient and diagnosis of the cause of bleeding (see Table 101-8). If bleeding is massive, two large-bore intravenous lines should be started, CBC and clotting studies performed, and the patient typed and crossmatched for blood. A red-top tube should be kept by the bedside, and if a clot has not formed by 7 min, a coagulopathy, either causing the bleeding or resulting from the blood loss, may be present.

Good lighting and suction should be maintained. A speculum examination should be performed to inspect for trauma to the vaginal, vulvar, or cervical tissues. Any lacerations should be repaired after local anesthesia is provided. If a laceration is extensive, the patient should be taken immediately to the operating room.

If a mass is seen in the vaginal vault and the uterus cannot be palpated on the abdominal examination, the possibility of uterine inversion is strong. Emergency obstetric consultation is required.

If blood is seen to be coming from the cervix, the possibility of atony or retained products of conception is high. If atony is present and the uterus is large and doughy, the patient should be treated with oxytocin. It is administered by diluting 20 to 30 U in 1 L of normal saline or lactated Ringer's solution and infusing the fluid at 200 mL/h. Methylergonovine maleate, an alternative agent, can be given at a dose of 0.2 mg intramuscularly, has an onset of action of 7 min, and lasts for 2 h. This agent should not be used if hypertension or preeclampsia is present. Once bleeding is controlled, the patient can be discharged on an oral maintenance dose of 0.2 mg q6h.

If the uterus has good tone, the possibility of retained products of conception is high. An ultrasound study confirms the diagnosis.

Postpartum Infections

Pelvic infection is the most common serious complication of the puerperium. Any persistent fever over 38.0°C (100.4°F) should be considered to be caused by genital tract infection until proven otherwise. Extragenital causes of fever include respiratory tract infection (more common after cesarean section), pyelonephritis, mastitis, and thrombophlebitis.

The route of delivery is the single most significant risk factor for uterine infection, with the vast majority of endometritis occurring secondary to cesarean section. Other risk factors include lower socioeconomic level, multiple gestations, younger maternal age, longer duration of labor and membrane rupture, and internal fetal monitoring. Women with all of these risk factors who were not given antibiotics prophylactically have been found to have a 90 percent rate of pelvic

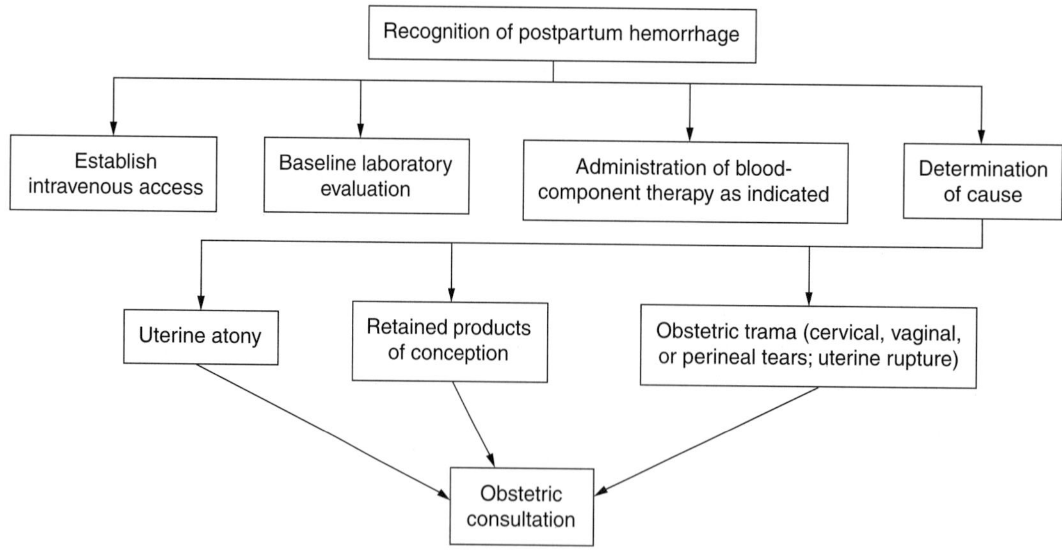

FIG. 101-1. Management plan for postpartum hemorrhage. (From American College of Obstetricians and Gynecologists: *Postpartum Hemorrhage.* Washington, 1998, with permission.)

infection. Digital examination after 37 weeks' gestation is thought to predispose to infection.

The most common pathogens are those that normally reside in the bowel and also colonize the perineum, vagina, and cervix. Both gram-positive and gram-negative aerobes, anerobes, *Mycoplasma hominis,* and *Chlamydia trachomatis* are seen. *Gardnerella vaginalis* is isolated more often in younger women. Many infections are polymicrobial.

Signs and symptoms of postpartum endometritis are foul-smelling, profuse, and bloody discharge and abdominal pain. Only scant discharge may be present, especially in patients with group A β-hemolytic streptococci. Shaking chills suggest bacteremia. Uterine and adnexal tenderness is found upon bimanual examination.

Infection may be localized to the decidua and adjacent myometrium and, if this is the case, responds readily to antibiotic therapy. Complications include parametrial phlegmons; surgical, incisional, and pelvic abscesses; infected hematomas; septic pelvic thrombophlebitis; necrotizing fasciitis; and peritonitis. Necrotizing fasciitis is a feared complication with high mortality and morbidity rates. Risk factors for this complication are obesity, diabetes mellitus, and hypertension.

The mainstay of treatment is antibiotic therapy, drainage of any collections of purulent material, and debridement of necrotic tissue. Routine vaginal cultures are of little clinical utility because of contamination with local flora. Blood culture results are positive in the minority of patients.

Oral antibiotics can be used on an outpatient basis for mild illness when disease is confined to the decidua and myometrium. Any patient who appears toxic or moderately ill, has had a cesarean section, or has underlying comorbid conditions should be hospitalized for parenteral therapy. There are many regimens of therapy. The combination of ampicillin and gentamicin is sufficient for 90 percent of patients. The β-lactam antimicrobials have the advantages of being safe and requiring administration of only one drug, thus being cost-effective. Cephalosporins that can be used include cefoxitin, cefotetan, and cefotaxime. Other regimens include clindamycin and gentamicin or metronidazole plus ampicillin and an aminoglycoside.

AMNIOTIC FLUID EMBOLUS Mortality rates between 60 and 80 percent have been reported for amniotic fluid embolism. Neurologic morbidity rates are even higher, and few patients are without sequelae.[19] In a national registry of patients with amniotic fluid embolus, if the amniotic fluid had meconium staining, no mother survived without neurologic deficit. If the infant is still in utero at the time of the embolus, both mortality and neurologic morbidity rates are high. The factors that cause this catastrophe are not known. The only significant relationship found thus far is fetal male sex.

Onset is sudden, with the mother displaying cardiovascular collapse. Seizure or seizure-like activity at the time of collapse is common. Patients display profound cardiovascular instability, severe hypoxemia, and, if survival is long enough, disseminated intravascular coagulation. Death is rapid, with many patients dying within 1 h of onset of symptoms. It has been suggested that the syndrome resembles that seen with anaphylactic or septic shock. Histologic findings at autopsy usually show material of fetal origin, such as squamous cells, hair, fat droplets, trophoblasts, and other nonspecific cellular debris as well as proteinaceous material, in the maternal circulation. The cause is unknown.

Care is supportive, with use of high concentrations of oxygen and treatment of disseminated intravascular coagulation if the patient survives long enough. Delivery of the infant should be immediate, but infant mortality and morbidity rates remain high even with immediate delivery.[20]

PERIPARTUM CARDIOMYOPATHY PPC is the development of heart failure during or shortly after labor with no apparent cause. Most women have an underlying cause found during workup for PPC.[20] Causes include chronic hypertension, mitral stenosis, obesity, viral myocarditis, and preeclampsia. Terbutaline for tocolysis has been found in many patients who have congestive heart failure but no underlying heart disease. Still, there is a small group of women for whom no cause can be found. PPC appears to be similar to the idiopathic cardiomyopathy seen in young, nonpregnant women. Biopsy shows evidence of myocarditis in up to 30 percent.

Patients present with signs and symptoms of congestive heart failure. Dyspnea, orthopnea, cough, palpitations, and chest and abdominal pain are common complaints. Massive cardiomegaly is seen on chest radiograph and echocardiograph. Treatment is with diuretics and fluid restriction. Digitalis should be used with caution, since 60 percent of patients have complex ventricular dysrhythmias. Afterload reduction has been used, but ACE inhibitors should be avoided if the patient is undelivered. Because of the high association of pulmonary embolus with PPC, anticoagulation with heparin is often recommended. If no underlying cause can be found, the prognosis is very poor, with mortality of almost 50 percent at 1 year. Many survivors demonstrate diminished contractile reserve when studied with dobutamine challenge in periods remote from pregnancy.[21]

REFERENCES

1. Gardner P, Hudson BL: *Advance Report of Final Mortality Statistics: 1993.* National Center for Health Statistics, monthly vital statistics report. Hyattsville, MD, 41(suppl):1–52, 1996.
2. US Department of Health and Human Services: *United States Public Health Service: Promoting Health, Preventing Disease: Year 2000 Objectives for the Nation.* Washington, 1989.
3. Cacciatore B, Tiitenen A, Stenman U, Ylostalo P: Normal early pregnancy: Serum βhCG levels and vaginal ultrasonography findings. *Br J Obstet Gynaecol* 97:899, 1990.
4. Yashar CM: Bleeding in the first 20 weeks of pregnancy, in Pearlman MD, Tintinalli JE (eds): *Emergency Care of the Woman.* New York, McGraw-Hill, 1998.
5. Lurain JR: High-risk metastatic gestational trophoblastic tumors: Current management. *J Reprod Med* 39:217, 1994.
6. Lucas ML, Cunningham FG: Urinary infection in pregnancy. *Clin Obstet Gynecol* 36:855, 1993.
7. Maringhini A, Marceno MP, Lanzarone F, Caltagirone M: Sludge and stones in gallbladder after pregnancy: Prevalence and risk factors. *J Hepatol* 5:218, 1987.
8. National High Blood Pressure Education Program Working Group: Report on high blood pressure in pregnancy. *Am J Obstet Gynecol* 163:1689, 1990.
9. American College of Obstetricians and Gynecologists: *Hypertension in Pregnancy.* Technical bulletin: 219. Washington, 1996.
10. Zhou Y, Damsky C, Fisher SJ: Preeclampsia is associated with failure of human cytotrophoblasts to mimic a vascular adhesion phenotype: One cause of defective endovascular invasion in this syndrome? *J Clin Invest* 99:2152, 1997.
11. Sibai BM: Treatment of hypertension in pregnant women. *N Engl J Med* 335:257, 1996.
12. Eclampsia Trial Collaborative Group: Which anti-convulsant for women with eclampsia? Evidence from the Collaborative Eclampsia Trial. *Lancet* 345:1455, 1995.
13. Ajayi RA, Soothill PW, Campbell S, Nicolaides KH: Antenatal testing to predict outcome in pregnancies with unexplained antepartum haemorrhage. *Br J Obstet Gynaecol* 99:122, 1992.
14. Hertzberg BS, Bowie JD, Carroll BA, et al: Diagnosis of placenta previa during the third trimester: Role of transperineal sonography. *AJR* 159: 83, 1992.
15. American College of Obstetricians and Gynecologists: *Preterm Labor.* Technical bulletin 206. Washington, 1995.
16. Lewis R, Mercer BM: Adjunctive care of preterm labor: The use of antibiotics. *Clin Obstet Gynecol* 38:755, 1995.
17. Perry KG, Martin RW, Blake PC, et al: Maternal outcome associated with adult respiratory distress syndrome. *Am J Obstet Gynecol* 174:391, 1996.
18. National Institutes of Health: NIH consensus development statement: Effect of corticosteroids for fetal maturation on perinatal outcomes. NIH Consensus Development Conference, Bethesda, MD, 1994, pp 4–18.

19. Kierse MJ: New perspectives for the effective treatment of preterm labor. *Am J Obstet Gynecol* 173:621, 1996.
20. Clark SL, Hankins GDV, Dudley DA, et al: Amniotic fluid embolism: Analysis of the national registry. *Am J Obstet Gynecol* 172:1158, 1996.
21. Witlin AG, Mabie WC, Sibai BM: Peripartum cardiomyopathy: An ominous diagnosis. *Am J Obstet Gynecol* 176:182, 1997.

COMORBID DISEASES IN PREGNANCY

Jessica L. Bienstock
Harold E. Fox

This chapter provides an overview of the management of chronic medical conditions in pregnant women, outlining the differences in management strategies that may be considered in view of the physiologic changes of pregnancy and the presence of a second "patient," the fetus.

DIABETES

Diabetes mellitus complicates approximately 2 to 3 percent of all pregnancies. Diabetes in pregnancy is falls into two categories: approximately 90 percent of pregnant diabetic patients have gestational diabetes and 10 percent have diabetes that predates the pregnancy. Those with gestational diabetes are subdivided into classes A_1 and A_2, the former being controlled by diet alone and the latter requiring insulin therapy. Patients with preexisting diabetes, even if they were previously managed with oral hypoglycemic agents, are all treated with insulin therapy during pregnancy. Oral hypoglycemic agents are not used during pregnancy as they do not provide an adequate level of glucose control. In addition, some of these agents have been associated with an increased risk of congenital anomalies, hyperbilirubinemia, and irreversible β-cell hyperplasia in exposed infants. Pregnant diabetic patients are at increased risk for fetal death *in utero,* particularly patients with preexisting vascular disease and preeclampsia as well as those with poor glycemic control.

The goals of glucose control for all patients with gestational diabetes is a fasting plasma glucose level of <90 mg/dL and one hour postprandial blood glucose levels of <140 mg/dL. Those patients with gestational diabetes who are managed by diet alone rarely develop acute glycemic complications because their glucose values rarely reach levels consistent with diabetic ketoacidosis.

Among patients with insulin-dependent diabetes, the need for insulin tends to increase throughout the course of pregnancy. In general, during the first trimester, the initial insulin requirement is 0.7 U/kg per day. By late pregnancy, patients generally require 1 U/kg per day. Generally two-thirds of the total insulin dose is given in the morning and one-third in the evening. Usually, two-thirds of the morning dose consists of NPH and one-third of regular insulin. The evening dose consists of half NPH and half regular insulin. Occasionally, this regimen may result in nocturnal hypoglycemia between 1 and 3 A.M. Administering the predinner NPH at bedtime has been suggested as a way of remedying the problem.

Pregnant diabetics are at increased risk for several pregnancy complications, including hypertensive diseases, preterm labor, spontaneous abortion, and pyelonephritis in addition to hypoglycemia and diabetic ketoacidos (DKA).

About 10 percent of insulin-dependent diabetics will develop ketoacidosis at some point during pregnancy.[1] Ketoacidosis has been reported to occur more rapidly and at lower glucose levels in pregnant patients as compared with nonpregnant patients. While classically the diagnosis of ketoacidosis requires a plasma glucose of >300 mg/dL, DKA may develop in pregnancy at lower glucose value. Beta sympathomimetic agents used for tocolysis, such as ritodrene and terbutaline, have been associated with an increased risk of diabetic ketoacidosis. Pregnant women in DKA are treated with a constant low-dose insulin infusion. General management guidelines are the same as for nonpregnant patients (see Chap. 203).

With contemporary medical management, fetal loss is less frequent, although the literature reports a fetal mortality rate in patients treated for DKA 50 to 90 percent. It is not uncommon to find pathologic patterns of fetal heart rate during DKA; these tend, however, to improve as maternal status improves. Steps should be taken to improve uterine blood flow, such as administration of oxygen, and left lateral uterine displacement.

Up to 45 percent of insulin-dependent diabetics will require evaluation for severe hypoglycemia at some time during the course of their pregnancy.[2] Hypoglycemia generally presents as sweating, tremors, blurred or double vision, weakness, hunger, confusion, paraesthesias, anxiety, palpitations, nausea, headache, or stupor. Hypoglycemic episodes are generally well tolerated by the fetus. Mild hypoglycemia—that is, a glucose <70 mg/dL—in a patient who is able to follow commands can be treated by administration of one cup of low-fat milk together with bread or crackers every 15 min. This regimen is preferred over more highly concentrated glucose solutions because it avoids "overshoot" and subsequent hyperglycemia. In patients who are unable to cooperate with oral therapy owing to severe hypoglycemia, parenteral therapy may be begun using one ampule (50 mL) of a 50 percent dextrose solution given via intravenous push. Alternatively, the patient may be treated using glucagon 1 to 2 mg IM or SC. In addition, intravenous therapy should be instituted with D_5W at a rate of 50 to 100 mL/h. Consideration should be given to the avoidance of subsequent hyperglycemia from glycogen mobilization with acute glucose administration. The goal is normoglycemic control without wide swings.

HYPERTHYROIDISM

Hyperthyroidism in pregnancy is associated with an increased risk of preeclampsia and for neonatal morbidity, including low birth weight and possibly congenital malformations. Symptoms of hyperthyroidism closely mimic symptoms of normal pregnancy and may consist of nervousness, palpations, heat intolerance, and inability to gain weight despite a good appetite. Thyrotoxicosis in pregnancy may also present as hyperemesis gravidarum.

Hyperthyroidism in pregnancy is treated with propylthiouracil (PTU). The time to onset of action of PTU is generally 4 to 6 weeks to achieve maximum effect. PTU is started at a dose of 100 to 150 mg three times a day and increased as needed to a maximum dose of up to 200 mg three times a day. The goal of therapy is to maintain a free T4 level at the upper range of normal. Approximately 2 percent of patients taking PTU will experience a mild purpuric skin rash within the first 4 weeks of therapy. If this occurs, the PTU should be stopped and replaced with methimazole. Agranulocytosis occurs in about 0.3 percent of patients treated with PTU. If agranulocytosis develops, the PTU should be stopped and methimazole should not be started.

THYROID STORM

Patients with thyroid storm present with fever, volume depletion, cardiac decompensation. Thyroid storm has been associated with a mortality rate of up to 25 percent. Patients are treated with intravenous fluids, oxygen, antipyretic agents, as well as PTU 400 mg PO q8 h and sodium iodide 1 gm IV in 500 mL of intravenous fluid each day. Long-term use (>10 days) of sodium iodide results in a high incidence of fetal goiter and hypothyroidism. Propranolol 40 mg PO q6 h is administered unless evidence of cardiac failure is present. Acetaminophen is used for treatment of hyperthermia; a cooling blanket may also be used. Steps should be taken to improve uterine blood flow, such as administration of oxygen as well as maintenance of adequate maternal hydration and left lateral uterine displacement. Radioactive iodine therapy is not used, as the fetus will concentrate iodine 131 after the tenth to twelfth week of gestation, and congenital hypothyroidism results.

HYPERTENSION

Hypertension in pregnancy can be divided into chronic hypertension and preeclampsia. In addition, patients with chronic hypertension not uncommonly develop superimposed preeclampsia. This section discusses only the management of chronic hypertension. Preeclampsia is discussed elsewhere (see Chap. 101).

Chronic hypertension complicates 4 to 5 percent of all pregnancies. It is diagnosed by sustained elevation of arterial blood pressure >140/90 mmHg before the twentieth week of gestation. Pharmacotherapy for pregnant hypertensive patients is generally started when the systolic blood pressure exceeds 160 mmHg or the diastolic blood pressure exceeds 100 mmHg. Commonly used agents for the treatment of chronic hypertension in pregnancy include alpha methyldopa (Aldomet), labetalol, and nifedipine. Antihypertensive agents that are generally not used in pregnancy include diuretics, because of their association with a reduction of uteral placental blood flow, and angiotensin-converting enzyme (ACE) inhibitors, owing to their teratogenic effects as well as fetal/neonatal hypotension and anuria. Maternal mortality associated with chronic hypertension is usually the result of severe hypertension and associated congestive heart failure or cerebrovascular accident. Fetal perinatal outcome is most closely associated with the development of superimposed preeclampsia or placental abruption. However, antihypertensive therapy has not been shown to alter the incidence of fetal complications.

Management of an acute hypertensive crisis in pregnancy is most commonly accomplished with intravenous labetalol (10 mg every 5 to 10 min up to a total dose of 300 mg). Hydralazine (5 to 10 mg every 15 min) given as intravenous bolus injections is an alternative still used by many obstetricians. The aim of antihypertensive therapy in pregnancy is to maintain the blood pressure between 140 and 150 mg systolic and 90 to 100 mg diastolic. Persistent blood pressure levels below this range may jeopardize placental perfusion. Acute intervention for blood pressure control should include fetal monitoring as well as careful assessment of fetal well-being. In all chronic hypertensives, the possibility of superimposed preeclampsia must always be considered (see Chap. 101).

DYSRHYTHMIAS

Significant cardiac dysrhythmias are rare in pregnancy. However, medications such as lidocaine, digoxin, and procainamide may be used for the usual indications and in the usual therapeutic doses and have not been shown to be harmful to the fetus. Use of β blockers for acute tachydysrhythmias has not been associated with adverse neonatal outcomes,[3] but maintenance β blockers are a group C drug and should be prescribed in consultation with a cardiologist and obstetrician. Verapamil has been shown to be effective in the conversion of supraventricular tachycardia to sinus rhythm without adverse fetal effects. Anticoagulation using unfractionated or low-molecular-weight heparin for the treatment of atrial fibrillation in pregnancy appears safe and may be used if the patient meets the criteria for anticoagulin described for nonpregnant patients. Cardioversion also appears safe for the fetus.[4] The presence of an artificial pacemaker has not been shown to affect the course of pregnancy.[5]

THROMBOEMBOLISM

The incidence of deep venous thrombosis in pregnancy ranges between 0.5 and 0.7 percent. Factors associated with an increased risk of venous thromboembolism in pregnancy include advanced maternal age, increasing parity, multiple gestation, operative delivery, bed rest, obesity, history of previous thromboembolism, antithrombin III deficiency, protein S or protein C deficiency, and the lupus anticoagulant syndrome. Postpartum deep venous thrombosis is reported to occur 3 to 5 more times more often than antepartum deep venous thrombosis and 13 to 16 times more frequently after cesarean section as opposed to vaginal delivery.

The clinical diagnosis of deep venous thrombosis (DVT) is similar in pregnant patients to that in nonpregnant patients. Pregnant patients commonly complain of swelling and leg discomfort; duplex Doppler studies should be done to confirm the diagnosis. Impedance plethysmography may also be safely used in pregnancy. Iodine-125 fibrinogen scanning should not be used because unbound iodine crosses the placental barrier and enters the fetal circulation, where it may concentrate in the fetal thyroid. Radionuclide venography using particles of technetium 99m is of no risk to the fetus and can be used to obtain studies of the lower extremity as well as to perform perfusion lung scans.

Diagnosis of pulmonary embolism in pregnancy is similar to that in the nonpregnant patient. Ventilation perfusion ($\dot{V}/\dot{Q}$) scans may safely be performed in pregnancy. No adverse fetal effects of xenon-133 or technetium-99m lung scanning have been reported. Pulmonary arteriography may also be performed in pregnant women if $\dot{V}/\dot{Q}$ scanning is indeterminant. The diagnostic efficiency of spiral CT scanning has not been studied in pregnancy. Treatment for both DVT and pulmonary embolism in pregnancy is with intravenous heparin, with the goal of maintaining the PTT at $1\frac{1}{2}$ to 2 times control. Low-molecular-weight heparin may also be used for both the prophylaxis and treatment of thromboembolic disease at a dose of 1 mg/kg enoxaparin subcutaneously twice a day. Warfarin is not used in pregnancy, as it crosses the placenta and is associated with embryopathy in the first trimester; in the second and third trimester it may lead to a variety of central nervous system and opthamalogic abnormalities. Protamine sulfate may be safely used in pregnancy for patients who require rapid reversal of their heparin anticoagulation. Although there is minimal experience with the use thrombolytic therapy in pregnancy, its use may be entertained in life-threatening situations.

ASTHMA

Asthma complicates between 0.4 and 1.3 percent of all pregnancies. In general, however, there are no differences in the outcome of pregnancies in well-controlled asthmatics versus the general population. Severe asthmatics with poorly controlled disease, however, do have a slight increase in the risk of preterm birth, stillbirth, and low-birthweight babies. Approximately one-third of patients with asthma worsen in pregnancy, approximately one-third remain stable, and one-third improve.[6]

The presentation of asthma in pregnancy is similar to that of the nonpregnant state, with the usual triad of cough, wheezing, and dyspnea. Unfortunately, pulmonary embolism (PE) can also present with similar symptom, and—as noted because of the hypercoagulable state of pregnancy, pregnant women, are at increased risk for PE. Therapeutic agents that are safely used in pregnancy include inhaled glucocorticoids, such as beclomethasone, and cromolyn sodium by inhaler. These agents are used as preventive therapy. For acute therapy of asthma exacerbations β_2 agonists such as salbutamol, metaproterenol, albuterol, and isoproterenol may be given via nebulizer. Intravenous methylprednisolone and oral prednisone can be used in pregnancy, as they do not cross the placenta. Any time glucocorticoids are used, maternal hyperglycemia should be considered in acute management (see discussion of diabetes, above). Epinephrine 0.3 mL (1:1000 dilution) can be given subcutaneously. Oxygen should be administered and titrated to maintain an arterial $P_{O_2} \geq 65$ mmHg. Fetal monitoring should be done after 20 weeks of gestation.

Clinical management of a pregnant asthmatic patient is best guided by the use of the peak expiratory flow rate to assess the severity of the obstruction and monitor the response to therapy. Peak expiratory flow rate is not altered by pregnancy, with mean peak expiratory flow rates in normal pregnant women ranging between 380 and 550 L/min. Peak expiratory flow rates do not change significantly as pregnancy progresses.[7] Peak expiratory flow rates of less than 100 L/min or that demonstrate <10 percent improvement with treatment are a sign of a potentially poor prognosis. Aggressive management is warranted.

The interpretation of arterial blood gases in a pregnant asthmatic must take into account the results in light of the normal values for pregnancy. The normal maternal P_{O_2} ranges between 101 and 108 mmHg early in pregnancy and falls to 90 to 100 mmHg near term. The normal $Paco_2$ in pregnancy ranges from 27 to 32 mmHg and the normal pH ranges from 7.40 to 7.45. The patient should be placed in a near sitting position with a leftward tilt, as up to 25 percent of normal pregnant women in third trimester with develop moderate hypoxia in the supine position. There should be a low threshold for obtaining arterial blood gas assessment as part of the evaluation of pregnant women with asthma, particularly patients who present with obvious hypoventilation and cyanosis whose asthma does not improve after initial therapy or who have peak flow of <200 L/min.[10] Goals of therapy include maintenance of a Po_2 >65 mmHg or an oxygen saturation of >95 percent on an F_io_2 of 35 to 60 percent.

Indications for intubation of the pregnant asthmatic with status asthmaticus include (1) inability to maintain the Pao_2 >65 mmHg (90 percent hemoglobin saturation) despite supplemental oxygen; (2) inability to maintain a $Paco_2$ < 40 mmHg; (3) evidence of maternal exhaustion; (4) significant acidosis (pH < 7.20 to 7.25) refractory to initial management with bronchodilator therapy; and (5) altered mental status.[8] Standard agents for rapid-sequence intubation can be used.

Medications for asthma that may have adverse fetal effects include iodides, which may be associated with neonatal hypothyroidism and goiter, as well as sodium bicarbonate, which, without adequate ventilation, can diminish the transfer of carbon dioxide from the fetus to the mother. Glucocorticoids may also cause alterations in carbohydrate metabolism, although this is a secondary concern in the acute setting. Essentially, acute management should be guided by consideration for the mother. The best outcome for the developing fetus is based on optimal treatment of the mother.

CHRONIC RENAL DISEASE

Maternal risks associated with renal disease are linked to the degree of renal compromise. As renal function diminishes, fertility decreases. Pregnancy rarely occurs in women who have a preconception serum creatine of >3 mg/dL. Preterm delivery and superimposed preeclampsia frequently complicate pregnancies of patients with underlying renal disease. Patients with chronic pyelonephritis may have an increased number of recurrences due to bacteriuria, increased glucosuria, and mechanical compression of the ureter in the third trimester pregnancy. Those with a history of reflux nephropathy are at increased risk of sudden escalating hypertension and worsening renal function. Urolithiasis is associated with more frequent urinary tract infections. Patients with lupus nephropathy are at greatly increased risk for exacerbations of the disease and superimposed preeclampsia, particularly if their disease was not in remission for at least 6 months prior to conception.

CYSTITIS AND PYELONEPHRITIS

The increased urinary stasis associated with pregnancy makes the urinary tract the most common infection during pregnancy. After midpregnancy, mild right-sided hydronephrosis can be found in 75 percent of patients and mild left-sided hydronephrosis is seen in 33 percent of patients. Asymptomatic bacteriuria is present in between 2 to 10 percent of pregnant women. Acute cystitis occurs in about 1 percent of pregnant women, whereas acute pyelonephritis occurs in approximately 2 percent of all pregnancies. The presentation of both cystitis and pyelonephritis is similar in pregnant and nonpregnant women. Causative organisms are similar to those in the general population, with *Escherichia coli* being the etiology in approximately 75 percent. It is not uncommon for acute pyelonephritis to precipitate preterm labor. Therefore prompt therapy is imperative. In addition, pregnant women are at increased risk for the development of bacteremia and septic shock as compared with the nonpregnant population.

Patients with simple cystitis may be treated with a 10-day course of oral nitrofurantoin, ampicillin, or a cephalosporin. Trimethoprin, a folate antagonist, is used by many obstetricians after the first trimester. Single-dose antibiotic therapy is not used for the treatment of cystitis in pregnant patients owing to the high rate of treatment failure. Treatment of pregnant patients with pyelonephritis is much more intense than that of nonpregnant patients. Patients are generally hospitalized, aggressively hydrated, and treated with intravenous antibiotics. The intravenous antibiotics of choice are generally a cephalosporin, such as cefazolin, or ampicillin plus gentamicin. Intravenous antibiotics are continued until the patient is afebrile for at least 48 h and costovertebral angle tenderness has resolved. Patients are then discharged home on oral antibiotics to complete a 10-day course of therapy. Many providers choose to continue women with a history of pyelonephritis during the course of their pregnancy on antibiotic suppression for the remainder of their pregnancy. This is generally accomplished using nitrofurantoin at a dose of 50 to 100 mg/day.

INFLAMMATORY BOWEL DISEASE

Pregnant patients with inflammatory bowel disease are at increased risk for nutritional and metabolic abnormalities that may put the fetus at increased risk for intrauterine growth restriction. Pregnancy itself, however, seems to have little effect on inflammatory bowel disease. When an exacerbation does occur during pregnancy it most frequently happens in either the first trimester or the postpartum period. It is hypothesized that this is due to a correlation with levels of circulating corticosteroids during pregnancy.

In general, the treatment of the pregnant patient with inflammatory bowel disease is the same as that of the nonpregnant patient. Antidiarrheal drugs including codeine, opium, paregoric, and Lomotil may also be used safely in pregnancy. While sulfasalazine and corticosteroids may be safely used in pregnancy, the possibility of the development of gestational diabetes must be considered in all patients on steroid therapy. Sulfa drugs are theoretically contraindicated in the third trimester due to concerns about neonatal hyperbilirubinemia, but they are used fairly commonly by obstetricians without adverse effect. It is important to supplement women who are taking sulfasalazine with folic acid, as sulfasalazine is known to inhibit the absorption and metabolism of folate. The use of suppressive therapy with azathioprine or 6-mercaptopurine has been reported to be safe during pregnancy, but experience with these agents is very limited. Total parental nutrition is a potentially useful adjunct to therapy in some patients who have severe nutritional deficiencies, and it may be safely used in pregnancy. Metronidazole for the treatment of perianal fistulas in patients with Crohn disease is generally not recommended until after completion of the first trimester.

SICKLE CELL DISEASE

Women with sickle cell disease are at increased risk for miscarriage, preterm labor, and other complications due to impaired oxygen supply and sickling infarcts in the placental circulation. Pregnant women are at increased risk for vascular occlusive events, particularly during the third trimester and the postpartum period. Painful crises present similarly in the pregnant and the nonpregnant state. Treatment of painful crises in pregnancy is similar to that for nonpregnant patients.

Cornerstones of management include aggressive hydration and analgesic therapy. Both oral and intravenous narcotics can be used. Caution should be exercised when using nonsteroidal antiinflammatory agents, particularly after 32 weeks of gestation, because of oligohydramnios and a significant risk of premature closure of the fetal ductus arteriosus. Hydroxyurea should not be used in pregnancy because of its teratogenic effects. Sickle cell crisis that does not respond to conservative management is commonly managed using partial exchange transfusion via automated erythrocytapheresis. Simple transfusion alone can be helpful when the hemoglobin level is <6g/dL.[9] The incidence of fetal death in utero can be minimized during sickle cell crisis by using information from continuous electronic fetal monitoring in a woman with a potentially viable fetus. While fetal heart rate patterns are frequently nonreassuring during the acute episode of vasoocclusive crisis, fetal heart rate patterns tend to normalize as the crises improve. In utero resuscitation (oxygen, intravenous hydration, left lateral uterine displacement, fetal scalp manipulation) should be initiated prior to consideration of emergency delivery.

While the majority of sickle cell crises in pregnancy are vasoocclusive crises, aplastic crises present a unique problem as they are usually caused by parvovirus B19 infection, which has been associated with hydrops fetalis. This disease thus presents a risk to both the pregnant woman and her fetus. Careful sonographic fetal assessment should be performed to evaluate the fetus for evidence of parvovirus infection. Once patients with sickle cell disease has been exposed to parvovirus B19, they are unlikely to acquire the infection a second time due to acquired immunity.[10] Then the pregnant patient with a past history of aplastic crisis is unlikely to experience it again.

MIGRAINE

Pregnancy usually improves classic migraines. However, when migraines do occur, they are difficult to treat, because ergot alkaloid should not be used and there has been little experience with the use of sumatriptan in pregnancy. Treatment therefore rests upon the use of analgesics and antiemetic agents. Acetominophen, codeine, and meperidine have all been shown to be safe for use in pregnancy.

Prophylactic therapy using β blockers, such as propanol (40 to 160 mg/day) or atenolol (50 to 100 mg/day), have also been shown to be effective.

SEIZURE DISORDERS

Seizure disorders occur in 0.15 to 1.0 percent of all women of childbearing age. Seizure frequency tends to increase slightly in pregnancy because of the increased volume of distribution, an increase in plasma clearance, and poor medication compliance. Management of a pregnant patient with a known seizure does not differ from that of a nonpregnant woman. Consideration of potential adverse effects of antiseizure medication mandates the use of single-drug therapy when possible. Approximately 45 percent of patients will experience an increase in seizure frequency during pregnancy. Medication doses may need to be increased in pregnancy; however, the serum therapeutic levels do not change. The use of valproic acid is generally avoided in pregnancy because of its association with 1 to 3 percent risk of neural tube defects.

A single maternal grand mal seizure may be followed by fetal bradycardia lasting for up to 20 mins. While transient maternal hypoxia and acidosis are potential threats to the fetus, there is usually no apparent harm caused by isolated seizures. Steps should be taken to optimize the intrauterine environment, including administration of oxygen and left lateral uterine displacement. In contrast, status epilepticus poses a real threat to both mother and fetus with 50 percent of fetuses and 33 percent of mothers not surviving the event. Aggressive management with intubation and ventilation should be considered early in the management of pregnant women with status epilepticus.

HUMAN IMMUNODEFICIENCY VIRUS (HIV)

All pregnant HIV-infected patients beyond 14 weeks gestation should be on zidovudine therapy in an effort to decrease the risk of vertical transmission. Randomized clinical trials of zidovudine have documented a reduction in the vertical transmission rate from 25 to 8 percent.[11] Pregnancy does not appear to alter the natural course of HIV disease, nor do uninfected babies born to HIV-positive women appear to be at increased risk for neonatal complications when compared with appropriate control patients. Patients with CD4+ counts of <200 should be maintained on prophylaxis for *Pneumocystis carinii* pneumonia using trimethoprim/sulfamethoxazole (TMP/SMX; Bactrim DS). Alternatively, aerosolized pentamidine may also be used in pregnant patients. Treatment of overt opportunistic infections in HIV-infected pregnant women should be addressed just as in those who are not pregnant. Patients may present with respiratory insufficiency. The prompt initiation of artificial ventilation in such patients may improve the intrauterine environment and therefore the outcome for the fetus.

SUBSTANCE ABUSE

All pregnant women identified in the ED as substance abusers should be referred to a high-risk obstetrics clinic and be offered substance-abuse counseling. The incidence of a positive urine toxicology test for cocaine ranges from 6 to 27 percent in urban and suburban hospitals. Cocaine use has been associated with an increased risk of placental abruption and fetal death in utero as well as an increased risk of intrauterine growth restriction, preterm labor, premature rupture of membranes, spontaneous abortion, and cerebral infarcts in the fetus. Maternal complications of cocaine use include myocardial infarction, hypertension (which can result in aortic dissection), pulmonary edema, and cardiac dysrhythmias. Subarachnoid hemorrhage, ruptured aneurysms, and strokes have all been reported in cocaine users and are most likely related to transient hypertension. Treatment of acute cocaine intoxication is handled in the usual manner.

Pregnant women in opiate withdrawal are currently treated with methadone or clonidine. There is currently insufficient evidence regarding the use of buprenorphine in pregnancy. Pregnant women should not have methadone discontinued during pregnancy, as it may increase the risk of fetal death in utero and tends to decrease compliance with prenatal care. Patients in withdrawal may be treated with clonidine 0.1 to 0.2 mg sublingually every hour up to 0.8 mg until signs of withdrawal resolve. The maintenance dose is then 0.8 to 1.2 mg/day in divided doses for the first 7 days and tapering for the following 3 days. Treatment for acute opiate overdose is discussed in Chap. 287.

The incidence of alcohol abuse during pregnancy is difficult to determine as most studies have been limited to single hospitals or urban settings, but it probably ranges between 1 and 2 percent. In the largest study, almost 7 percent of women had detectable alcohol in urine samples taken at the time of delivery.[12] It is felt that two or more drinks a day may contribute to increased rates of spontaneous abortion, low-birthweight infants, preterm deliveries, and perinatal mortality. Alcohol use in pregnancy can result in fetal alcohol syndrome, the incidence of which is 0.1 to 0.3 percent of live births. Patients who present in coma due to acute alcohol intoxication or in alcohol withdrawal are managed similarly to nonpregnant patients. Short-acting barbiturates such as pentobarbital can be used for withdrawal, although benzodiazepines should be avoided in early pregnancy if at all possible because of possible teratogenicity. Disulfiram (Antabuse) is a potential teratogen and should be avoided in pregnancy.

Domestic Violence

Between 14 and 17 percent of pregnant women experience domestic violence during the course of their pregnancy.[13] It is a particularly

TABLE 102-1 Therapeutic Agents Commonly Used in Emergency Settings with Known Adverse Effects in Human Pregnancy

Drug	Effect
ACE inhibitors	Renal failure, oligohydramnios
Aminoglycosides	Ototoxicity
Androgenic steroids	Masculinize female fetus
Anticonvulsants	Dysmorphic syndrome, anomalies
Antithyroid agents	Fetal goiter
Aspirin	Bleeding, antepartum and postpartum
Cytotoxic agents, i.e., methotrexate	Multiple anomalies
Isotretinoin	Hydrocephalus, deafness, anomalies
Lithium	Congenital heart disease (Ebstein anomaly)
Methotrexate	Anomalies
Nonsteroidal anti-inflammatory drugs (prolonged use after 32 weeks)	Oligohydramnios, constriction of fetal ductus arteriosus
Tetracycline (after first trimester)	Discoloration of deciduous teeth, inhibits bone growth
Thalidomide	Phocomelia
Warfarin	Embryopathy—nasal hypoplasia, optic atrophy

vulnerable time during which ''intimate violence'' may escalate. Late entry into prenatal care, unintended pregnancy, drug and alcohol use, depression, and housing problems have all been associate with an increased risk of domestic violence. Pregnant women who are the victims of domestic violence are at an increased risk for placental abruption, fetal fractures, uterine rupture, and preterm labor. It is imperative to keep a high index of suspicion and be prepared to initiate appropriate referrals to social service and law enforcement agencies. In addition, for Rh-negative women who have experienced blunt abdominal trauma, consideration should be given to the administration of Rhogam to prevent isoimmunization. (see Chap. 101 for a detailed discussion.)

Effect of Pregnancy and Lactation on Medication Considerations for Concurrent Illness

The classic teratogenic period is from day 31 after the last menstrual period (LMP) in a 28-day cycle to 71 days from the LMP. During this critical time, organs are forming, and teratogens may cause overt malformation. Administration of drugs early in the period of organogenesis will affect the organs developing then, such as the heart or neural tube. Closer to the end of the classic teratogenic period, the ear and palate are forming and may be affected by a teratogen.

Before day 31, exposure to a teratogen produces an all-or-none effect. With exposure around conception, the conceptus usually either does not survive or survives without anomalies. If the organism remains viable, organ-specific anomalies do not develop because repair or replacement permits normal development. A similar insult at a later stage may produce organ-specific defects; after the first trimester, chronic exposure may produce growth restriction.

The Food and Drug Administration (FDA) lists five categories of labeling for drug use in pregnancy:

TABLE 102-2 Drugs Contraindicated during Breast-Feeding

Amphetamines
Aspirin (high doses)
Bromocriptine (Parlodel)
Cytotoxic agents
Ergotamine
Lithium
Radiopharmaceuticals

Source: American Academy of Pediatrics, with permission.

Category A: Controlled studies in women fail to demonstrate a risk to the fetus in the first trimester, and the possibility of fetal harm appears remote.
Category B: Animal studies do not indicate a risk to the fetus, there are no controlled human studies, or animal studies do show an adverse effect on the fetus, but well-controlled studies in pregnant women have failed to demonstrate a risk to the fetus.
Category C: Studies have shown the drug to have animal teratogenic or embryocidal effects, but no controlled studies in women are available or no studies are available in either animals or women.
Category D: Positive evidence of human fetal risk exists, but benefits in certain situations (e.g., life-threatening situations or serious diseases for which safer drugs cannot be used or are ineffective) may make the use of the drug acceptable despite its risks.
Category X: Studies in animals or humans have demonstrated fetal abnormalities, or evidence demonstrates fetal risk based on human experience, or both, and the risk clearly outweighs any possible benefit.

Tables 102-1 to 102-4 list medications to be avoided in pregnancy. Table 102-5 lists categories of drugs generally considered safe during breast-feeding.

Complicating Effects of Radiation

The major factor determining the degree of risk to the fetus in an imaging technique is the amount of ionizing radiation involved in the test. Exposure to ionizing radiation occurs with plain x-ray films, angiography, fluoroscopy, nuclear medicine, and computed tomography (CT). Nonionizing studies include magnetic resonance imaging (MRI) and ultrasound.

The risks of radiation exposure vary with gestational age.

The predominant deterministic effect due to exposure during the first 2 weeks of pregnancy is resorption of the embryo.

The second to eighth week postconception is the period of organogenesis. Significant x-ray exposure during this period may result in

TABLE 102-3 Drugs Whose Effects on Nursing Infants Is Unknown but May Be of Concern

Metronidazole (Flagyl)
Psychotropic drugs
Antianxiety drugs
Antidepressant drugs
Antipsychotic drugs

Source: American Academy of Pediatrics, with permission.

TABLE 102-4 Drugs Potentially Affecting Milk Supply

Decongestants
Diuretics
Combination oral contraceptives

teratogenesis (birth defects). Examples include gross malformation and growth retardation, the latter of which can occur both at term and later at adulthood. Neuropathology and small head size may also occur as a result of significant exposures during weeks 2 to 8.

The embryo has developed into a fetus at about the seventh to eighth week, and neurologic development occurs during the next 7 weeks. Significant x-ray exposure at this time (between weeks 8 and 15) may result in mental retardation, small head size, and decreased IQ. Other possible but less likely effects due to significant exposure during this period include growth retardation as an adult and sterility. Even less likely but still possible are cataracts, neuropathology, and growth retardation at term.

Most of the deterministic effects mentioned above are either not observed or observed much less frequently when the fetus receives significant radiation dose beyond 15 weeks postconception. Mental retardation has been observed as a result of significant exposure during the eighth to twenty-fifth weeks but not beyond. Other effects that have been observed because of exposure after week 15 include sterility and growth retardation as an adult. Less likely effects that have been demonstrated are cataracts, neuropathology, and growth retardation at term.

The most recent evidence suggests that 10 rad is a threshold for human teratogenesis, and the fetus appears to be most vulnerable at 8 to 15 weeks' gestation. The American College of Radiology's position states that there is no single diagnostic test that results in radiation doses that threaten the well-being of the developing embryo or fetus. However, cumulative doses from multiple procedures may enter the harmful range.

The radiation doses involved in commonly used diagnostic tests are given in Table 102-6.

A common nuclear medicine imaging study used by the emergency department physician is the ventilation/perfusion scan. Total fetal exposure to xenon 133 and technetium 99m is about 0.5 rad, and they can be used safely in pregnancy. Fetal exposure from other studies using technetium 99 range from 0.03 to 0.06 rad/mCi and are safe in pregnancy. Because the excretion of these radionuclide particles is often via the maternal bladder, which is close to the fetus, hydration and frequent voiding need to be encouraged.

The two nonionizing imaging studies used frequently are ultrasound and MRI. Ultrasound has been studied extensively over the past 25 years and has no known teratogenic effect. There is much less experience with MRI, but thus far there are no known harmful effects.

TABLE 102-5 Drugs Usually Considered Compatible with Breast-Feeding

Analgesics	Antihypertensives
Antiasthmatics	Antithyroid agents
Antibiotics (most)	Corticosteroids
Anticoagulants	Digoxin
Anticonvulsants	Narcotics
Antiemetics	Oral contraceptives
Antihistamines	Sedatives

Source: American Academy of Pediatrics, with permission.

TABLE 102-6 Radiation Exposure to the Uterus/Fetus

Dosage, rad	Procedure
0.00005	Chest radiography (two views) with shielding of the maternal abdomen.
0.686–1.398	Intravenous pyelogram full series; in the case of a suspected stone a one-shot pyelogram should be used when a renal ultrasound is inconclusive or unavailable
.1	Kidney, ureter, bladder—single abdominal film
0.51–0.126	Lumbar spine series (three films)
0.168–0.359	Lumbosacral spine series (three films)
0.007–0.02	Mammography—diagnostic for suspected breast cancers
0.01	Cerebral angiography
0.056	Upper gastrointestinal series
1.9–3.9	Barium enema
<0.1	Head computed tomography (CT)
<0.2	Chest CT
5.0	Abdominal CT
7.0	Lumbar spine CT
0.50	Pelvimetry CT

REFERENCES

1. Cousins L: Pregnancy complications among diabetic women 1965–1985. *Obstet Gynecol Surv* 42:140, 1987.
2. Coustan DR, Reece RA, Sherwin R, et al: A randomized clinical trial of insulin pump vs intensive conventional therapy in diabetic pregnancies. *JAMA* 255:631, 1986.
3. Frishman WH, Chesner M: Beta-adrenergic blockers in pregnancy. *Am Heart J* 115:147, 1988.
4. Schroeder JS, Harrison DC: Repeated cardioversion during pregnancy. *Am J Cardiol* 27:445, 1971.
5. Jaffe R, Gruber A, Fejgin M, et al: Pregnancy with an artificial pacemaker. *Obstet Gynecol Surv* 42:137, 1987.
6. Clark SL and the National Asthma Education Program Working Group on Asthma in Pregnancy, National Institutes of Health, NHBLI: Asthma in Pregnancy. *Obstet Gynecol* 82:1036, 1993.
7. Brancazio LR, Laifer SA, Schwartz T: Peak expiratory flow rate in normal pregnancy. *Obstet Gynecol* 89:383, 1997.
8. National Asthma Education Working Group: *Management of Asthma during Pregnancy: Report of the Working Group on Asthma and Pregnancy.* NIH pub. no. 93-3279. Bethesda, MD, National Heart Lung and Blood Institute, NIH, USDHHS. 1993.
9. Koshy M, Burd L, Wallace D, et al: Prophylactic red cell transfusion in pregnant patients with sickle cell disease. *N Engl J Med* 319:1447, 1988.
10. Serjeant GR, Serjeant BE, Thomas PW, et al: Human parvovirus in homozygous sickle cell disease. *Lancet* 341:1237, 1993.
11. Recommendations of the USPHS task force on the use of zidovudine to reduce the perinatal transmission of HIV. *MMWR* 43:1, 1994.
12. Vega WA, Kolady B, Hwong J, Noble A.: Prevalence and magnitude of perinatal, substance exposure in California. *N Engl J Med* 329:852, 1993.
13. Mayer L, Liebschutz: Domestic violence in the pregnant patient: Obstetric and behavioral interventions. *Obstet Gynecol Surv* 53:627, 1998.

EMERGENCY DELIVERY

Michael J. VanRooyen
Julia B. VanRooyen

The anxiety experienced by the emergency physician caring for a woman in active labor is not simply due to infrequent experience with normal deliveries in routine practice but also to awareness of the potential for serious and rarely fatal complications of labor. In addition, the initial management of such third-trimester emergencies as preeclampsia, eclampsia, and hemorrhage has major consequences for maternal and child survival. It is therefore important for emergency physicians to be prepared for actively laboring patients or for patients presenting during late pregnancy.

Despite advances in prenatal care and nearly ubiquitous availability of obstetric units in the United States, precipitous deliveries do occur with some frequency in emergency departments (ED). Out-of-hospital delivery may occur because patients are poorly educated, have had no prenatal care, lack transportation, residence in a remote location, or experience premature labor or delivery. A relatively recent and controversial practice is intentional precipitous labor, in which a woman desiring to avoid hospital charges delays care until the final stages of labor.

TABLE 103-1 Equipment and Supplies for Emergency Delivery*

Surgical scissors
Placenta basin
Rubber bulb syringe
Neonatal airways
Towels
Hemostats
Cord clamps
Sterile gloves
Gauze sponge (4 × 4)
Syringes (10-mL)
Needles (23-gauge)

*Excludes standard adult and neonatal resuscitation equipment.

PREHOSPITAL MANAGEMENT

Regardless of the reason for precipitous delivery, this and other third-trimester emergencies require preparedness by both hospital and prehospital providers. Emergency medical system (EMS) personnel must be trained to recognize active labor and manage the precipitous delivery appropriately. Pregnancy-related complications that may occur in the prehospital setting include preeclampsia, eclampsia, maternal hemorrhage, and complications of labor such as cord prolapse and fetal distress. Prehospital personnel need to be aware of available obstetric and neonatal units in the system's catchment area. The development of specialty centers has led to a significant decline in neonatal mortality, particularly among infants weighing less than 1500 g at birth. High-risk maternal units have proliferated as well. As a consequence, transport of pregnant patients for reasons of maternal bleeding, eclampsia or preeclampsia, fetal distress, multiple gestations, fetal anomalies, and other maternal health problems including traumatic injuries has increased markedly. The most common reason for the transport of patients to tertiary care centers is simple premature rupture of membranes.

Prehospital units transporting patient in active labor should be prepared by carrying sterile delivery packs and medical supplies and medications for maternal and neonatal emergencies. The transport team should be trained to assist in the precipitous delivery of an infant and educated in the use of basic obstetric supplies. Prehospital protocols should be reviewed often so that EMS personnel remain prepared for the rare but potentially catastrophic pregnancy-related event.

EMERGENCY DEPARTMENT PREPAREDNESS

Every ED should be prepared for emergency delivery by preparing a basic delivery kit (Table 103-1) and having an infant warmer/isolette and supplies for neonatal resuscitation (see Chap. 9, on neonatal resuscitation). Medications for emergency delivery are listed in Table 103-2. Because of the relative infrequency of ED delivery, extra care must be taken to educate physicians and nursing staff through periodic didactic and equipment orientation sessions.

EVALUATING THE PREGNANT PATIENT

Any pregnant woman beyond 20 weeks gestation who arrives in the ED with signs of active labor should be carefully evaluated to determine the condition of both mother and fetus. An important component of this is the medical and obstetric history of the patient, including parity and estimated date of delivery (EDD). If the last menstrual period (LMP) is known and a pregnancy wheel is not available, the EDD can be calculated by adding 9 months and 7 days to the LMP. Although useful for providing a rough estimate, ultrasound examination late in the third trimester is not an accurate predictor of gestational age, as estimates of EDD can vary up to 3 weeks. Fundal height also provides a rapid estimate of gestational age in the patient who does not recall her LMP or EDD. Fundal height is measured in centimeters (centimeters = weeks of gestation ± 2 weeks) from the pubic symphysis to the top of the fundus as palpated by the examiner. This measurement can lead to overestimation in obese patients. One must obtain pertinent medical information on such matters as allergies, medications, drug and alcohol use, and prenatal care as well as to elicit any past history of complications with prior deliveries or precipitous labor.

Every patient presenting with signs of active labor should receive immediate monitoring of maternal vital signs and fetal heart rate. Maternal blood pressure should be monitored, and Doppler heart tones are helpful to confirm normal fetal heart rate (120 to 160 beats per minute). A persistently slow fetal heart rate (less than 100 beats per minute) is an indicator of fetal distress, and emergent obstetric consultation is necessary.

DISTINGUISHING TRUE FROM FALSE LABOR

The confirmation of true labor as opposed to false labor is an important initial step in the management of the term or near-term pregnant patient. False labor is defined as uterine contractions that do not lead to cervical changes. False labor is characterized by irregular, brief contractions usually confined to the lower abdomen. These contractions, commonly called Braxton-Hicks contractions, are irregular in both intensity and duration. False labor may persist for several days. It is most commonly treated in the outpatient setting by hydration and rest. Uncommonly, admission may be required for supportive care.

True labor is characterized by painful, regular contractions of steadily increasing intensity and duration leading to progressive cervical dilatation. True labor typically begins in the fundal region and upper abdomen and radiates into the pelvis and lower back. True labor also leads to progressive descent of the fetus into the pelvis in preparation for delivery and to cervical dilatation and effacement.

TABLE 103-2 Medications for Emergency Delivery and Indications for Use

Medication	Dose	Indication
Oxytocin 10 μg/mL	Infuse 2 L of 20 U/L 0.9 normal saline solution	Give routinely for uterine contraction and hemostasis immediately postpartum
Methyl ergonovine (methergine)	0.2 mg IM	Control of postpartum hemorrhage
Hydralazine 20 mg/mL	5–10 mg IV push q 20–30 min to treat diastolic BP > 110 mmHg	Control of hypertensive crisis (to diastolic BP 80–90 mmHg)
Labetalol HCL	25–50 mg IV push, followed by 10 mg increments up to a total dose of 1 mg/kg	Alternative to Hydralazine
Magnesium sulfate (50% solution) 5 g/10 mL	bolus 4–6 g IV over 20 minutes	First-line control of eclamptic seizures
Calcium gluconate 10%	1 ampule (10 mL) IV push	Magnesium toxicity (iatrogenic administration)
Phenytoin	10 mg/kg loading, followed by second loading dose of 5 mg/kg 2 h later	Second-line drug for eclamptic seizures
Terbutaline sulfate 1 mg/mL	0.25 mg SC q3 h	Tocolysis
Fentanyl 50 μg/mL	50 μg (1 mL)/h	Short-acting narcotic analgesic
Lidocaine (Xylocaine) 1%	1–10 mL locally	Local anesthetic
Prochlorperazine (Compazine) 10 mg/mL	5–10 mg IV	Nausea and vomiting
Naloxone (Narcan) 0.4 mg/mL	0.8 mg–2 mg IV	Narcotic overdose

PHYSICAL EXAMINATION

Patients without vaginal bleeding should be examined both bimanually and with a sterile speculum. Patients presenting with vaginal bleeding should initially be evaluated with ultrasound prior to any speculum or bimanual examination to rule out placenta previa (see below).[1] If ultrasound is not available for an actively bleeding patient in labor, careful examination with sterile speculum may be performed to estimate the degree of cervical dilatation. However, no digital exam should be performed, and emergent obstetric consultation should be obtained. If spontaneous rupture of membranes (SROM) is suspected, examination with a sterile speculum should be performed and digital exam avoided, as studies have shown an increased risk of infection after a single digital examination.[2] It is particularly important to avoid digital examinations in the preterm patient where prolongation of gestation is desired. Sterile speculum examination allows confirmation of SROM, visualization of the cervix as well as estimation of dilatation and collection of cervical cultures, particularly group B streptococcus, *Neisseria gonorrhoeae* and *Chlamydia*. For pelvic examination, the lithotomy position is typically used. Stirrups are not necessary, although they are helpful. Alternatively, a bedpan may be employed to elevate the patients buttocks enough to allow speculum examination. Lubricant should be avoided unless rupture of membranes has been confirmed, as lubricant may produce a false-positive nitrazine test.

The abdomen should be inspected and palpated to determine fundal height. The cervix is then examined to determine effacement, dilatation, and station. Effacement of the cervix is the process of thinning that occurs during labor. Effacement has conventionally been described in terms of a percentage of normal cervical length. This method is confusing and has poor interrater reliability. More recently, the preferred method is to describe the degree of effacement in terms of actual length of remaining cervix in centimeters. Cervical dilatation describes the diameter of the cervical os and is an indicator of the progression of labor. The index and middle finger of the examining hand are used to determine the diameter, expressed in centimeters (fingertip to 10 cm); 10 cm indicates full dilatation. The station indicates the level that the fetus occupies in the pelvis, with the reference point being the maternal ischial spines, palpable on either side of the vaginal canal at about 4 and 8 o'clock. If the fetus remains above the ischial spines, the station is described as negative. Once the fetal head has reached the level of the ischial spines, the station is zero, with further descent into the pelvis described as +1 or +2. A +3 station corresponds to visible scalp at the introitus, indicating a fetal position consistent with impending delivery.

Both digital exam and Leopold maneuvers provide information about the presentation of the child and can indicate a potential breech presentation or cord prolapse. Leopold maneuvers involve the palpation of the fetus through the maternal abdomen to determine fetal position and presentation. Such maneuvers are relatively unreliable in inexperienced hands. A pregnant woman should not be kept flat on her back for a prolonged period of time, since compression of venous return by the gravid uterus can lead to maternal hypotension and fetal hypoperfusion. After examination, the patient should be placed in the left lateral position.

Rupture of Membranes

Determining whether membranes have ruptured is an important predictor of the likelihood of imminent labor as well as the potential for complications such as infection or cord prolapse.[3] SROM occurs during the course of active labor in most patients, although it may occur prior to the onset of labor in 10 percent of third- trimester patients. SROM typically occurs with a gush of clear or blood-tinged fluid. It can be confirmed by using nitrazine paper to test residual fluid in the fornix or vaginal vault while a sterile speculum examination is performed. Amniotic fluid has a pH of 7.0 to 7.4 and will turn nitrazine paper dark blue. Vaginal fluid typically has a pH of 4.5 to 5.5 and will make the nitrazine strip remain yellow. False-positive tests may occur with blood, lubricant, or other contaminants. Another test used to confirm rupture of membranes (ROM) is ferning, or observing sodium chloride crystals on a slide as amniotic fluid dries.

If membranes are intact, an amniotomy should not be performed in the ED, as this may lead to precipitous labor and increase the potential for cord prolapse. Note whether meconium appears after the ROM, indicated by the presence of thick, greenish-brown fluid. ROM occurring prior to the onset of labor is called premature ROM. Prolonged ROM occurs if delivery does not take place within 18 h of ROM. ROM that occurs before 37 weeks is called preterm ROM.

Third-Trimester Bleeding

Patients who present with third-trimester bleeding require urgent and very careful evaluation. It is important to distinguish serious causes of third-trimester bleeding from the ''bloody show'' that can accompany normal labor, although this can be difficult (Table103-3). The most helpful characteristic is the amount of bleeding. With bloody show, there is typically a small amount of blood on the perineum or undergarments, while previa and abruption can cause active bleeding of significant amounts.

Placenta Previa

Placenta previa occurs when the placenta partially or completely overlies the internal cervical os. Because of the rich vasculature of the placenta, disruption of the placenta by minor manipulation, even a bimanual examination or early cervical dilatation, may induce catastrophic maternal hemorrhage. The presence of placenta previa should be suspected in any third-trimester patient presenting with painless vaginal bleeding, particularly bright red blood per vagina. The primary risk factor for placenta previa is a history of prior cesarean section(s). If previa is suspected, an emergent ultrasound prior to speculum or bimanual examination is required.[4] (Also see Chap. 108, ''Complications of Gynecologic Procedures.'') If previa is present on ultrasound and the patient is actively laboring, no further examination should be performed and arrangements should be made for immediate transport to labor and delivery for cesarean section. Patients who are not in labor and bleeding only minimally can sometimes be managed conservatively by observation.

Placental Abruption

Abruptio placenta (or placental abruption) is the separation of the placenta from its implantation site prior to delivery. This may lead to massive blood loss, although bleeding may be concealed within the uterus up to 20 percent of the time. Placental abruption is classically characterized by the vaginal bleeding, a ''rock-hard'' painful uterus, and fetal distress (decrease in fetal heart rate to <100 beats per minute).[5] Maternal coagulopathy may also be present in abruption (Table 103-3). Risk factors for abruption include maternal hypertension, smoking, cocaine use, and trauma.

Fetal Distress

Fetal distress may occur during active labor, and care must be taken to evaluate the fetal status as often as possible. Indicators of fetal distress include decelerations in fetal heart rate. This is defined as a persistent drop in fetal heart rate during contractions persisting more than 30 s after a contraction. While many EDs do not have fetal monitoring devices, Doppler heart tones should be measured after each contraction to detect the presence of decelerations. Episodic bradycardia persisting for more than 5 min is an indication for immediate cesarean section.

EMERGENCY DELIVERY

The initial step in the management of a woman in active labor is to obtain vital signs and initiate supportive therapy, including obtaining venous access and monitoring the mother and fetus if fetal monitoring is available. A sample for ''type and screen'' should be sent to the blood bank to determine maternal Rh status and ABO blood type. If the pelvic examination reveals no remaining cervix and fetal presentation at the introitus, delivery is imminent. Labor can progress very rapidly in multiparous patients. The stage of labor and the parity of the patient should be taken into account when transport of a laboring patient to another facility is being considered.

As the cervix becomes fully dilated and effacement becomes complete, the fetus continues to descend and the patient experiences the urge to push. Patients delivering in the emergency setting may have difficulty controlling these expulsive efforts, and they are in even greater need of assistance, reassurance, and instruction. Preoccupation with the delivery should not exclude the needs of the mother or minimize the importance of maternal cooperation to accomplish a controlled delivery.

Determination of fetal position is best accomplished in the emergency setting by evaluation of the presenting portion of the infant. Pelvic examination should reveal evidence of the infant's position, including palpable skull sutures and fontanelles (Fig. 103-1) or, in the case of breech delivery, the infant's buttock or extremity. Confirmation may be accomplished by personnel familiar with Leopold maneuvers.

The typical delivery position is the dorsal lithotomy position, which allows maximum visualization and control of the delivery. As time allows, the perineum may then be prepared by washing with mild soap and water and swabbing with povidone-iodine. Drapes should be placed over the patient, and gowns, masks, and sterile gloves donned by medical personnel attending the patient. Pediatric and obstetric services should be notified as appropriate for the institution.

The process of fetal descent during labor and delivery is described by six cardinal movements: (1) engagement, (2) flexion, (3) descent,

TABLE 103-3 Differentiating Etiology of Third-Trimester Vaginal Bleeding in the Actively Laboring Patient

Examination	Placenta Previa	Placental Abruption	Bloody Show
Vaginal discharge	Moderate to large amount of bright red blood	Varying amounts of dark, clotted blood	Small amounts of blood or pink blood-tinged fluid
Abdominal exam	Nontender	Marked tenderness, constant, unremitting uterine pain	Nontender, intermittent pain
Bimanual exam	Contraindicated	Contraindicated	Sterile exam
Laboratory tests	Possible decreased hematocrit	Coagulopathy, disseminated intravascular coagulation possible	Normal
Confirmatory test	Ultrasound	No accurate confirmatory test (ultrasound <10% sensitive)	None
Fetal status	Usually normal	Fetal distress (HR < 100)	Normal

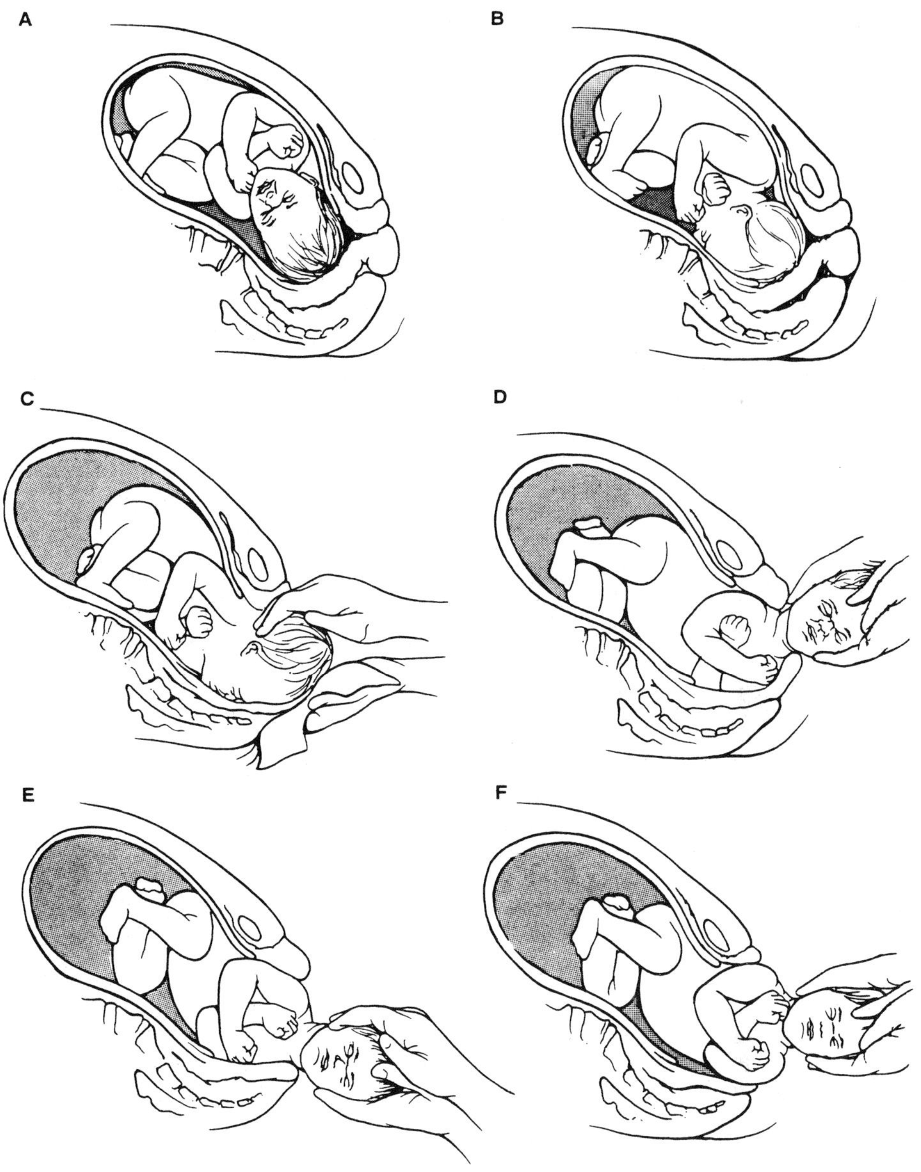

FIG. 103-1. Movements of normal delivery. Mechanism of labor and delivery for vertex presentations. **A.** Engagement, flexion, and descent. **B.** Internal rotation. **C.** Extension and delivery of the head using the modified Ritgen maneuver. After delivery of the head the infant's nose and mouth should be suctioned and the neck checked for encirclement of the umbilical cord. **D.** External rotation bringing the thorax into the anteroposterior diameter of the pelvis. **E.** Delivery of the anterior shoulder. **F.** Delivery of the posterior shoulder. Note that after delivery, the head is supported and used to gently guide delivery of the shoulder. Traction should be minimized.

(4) internal rotation, (5) extension, and (6) external rotation (Fig. 103-1). As the fetus descends through the birth canal and reaches the introitus, the perineum bulges to accommodate the fetal head. Delivery can be aided by gentle digital stretching of the inferior portion of the perineum. The perineum will undergo gradual thinning and stretching to enable the passage of the fetus. The use of routine episiotomy for a normal spontaneous vaginal delivery has been discouraged in recent years and increases the incidence of third- and fourth-degree lacerations at the time of delivery.[6,7]

If an episiotomy is necessary, it may be performed as follows. A solution of 5 to 10 mL of 1% lidocaine is injected with a small-gauge needle into the posterior fourchette and perineum. While protecting the infant's head, a 2- to 3-cm cut is made with scissors to extend the vaginal opening. The incision must be supported with manual pressure from below, taking care not to allow the incision to extend into the rectum.

Control of the delivery of the neonate is the major challenge. As the infant's head emerges from the introitus, the physician should support the perineum with a sterile towel placed along the inferior portion of the perineum with one hand while supporting the fetal head with the other. Mild counterpressure is exerted to prevent the rapid expulsion of the fetal head which may lead to third- or fourth-degree perineal tears.

As the infant's head presents, the left hand may be used to control the fetal chin while the right remains on the crown of the head, supporting the delivery. This controlled extension of the fetal head will aid in the atraumatic delivery. The mother is then asked to breathe through contractions rather than bearing down and attempting to push the baby out rapidly. Immediately following delivery of the infant's head, the infant's nose and mouth should be suctioned. This is particularly important in infants presenting with meconium in order to prevent aspiration. A simple bulb will assist in the routine clearing of the infant's nose and mouth. After suctioning, the neck should be palpated for the presence of a nuchal cord. This is a common condition, found in 25 percent of all cephalad-presenting deliveries. If the cord is loose, it should be reduced over the infant's head; the delivery may then proceed as usual. If the cord is tightly wound, it may have to be clamped in the most accessible area by two clamps in close proximity and cut to allow delivery of the infant.

After the airway is cleared, delivery of the body is allowed to progress. After delivery of the head, the head will restitute, or turn to one side or the other. As the head rotates, the physician's hands are

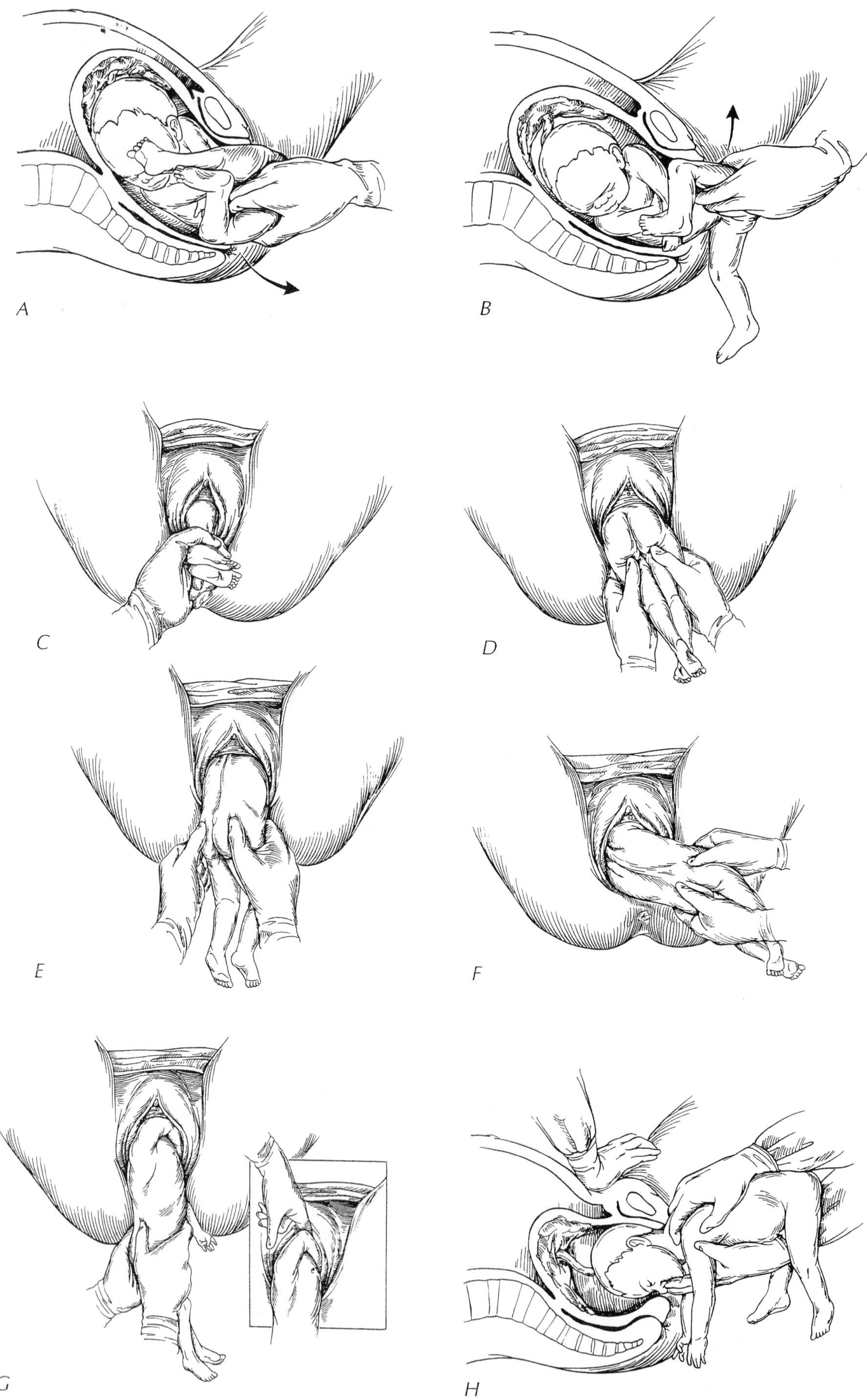
A
B
C
D
E
F
G
H

placed on either side of it, providing gentle downward traction to deliver the anterior shoulder. Care should be taken to provide only gentle traction, as jerky or forceful movements may cause a brachial plexus injury. The physician's hand then gently guides the fetus upward, delivering the posterior shoulder and allowing the remainder of the infant to be delivered. At this point, it is very important to control delivery of the body to prevent perineal lacerations.

A point of practical concern is the need to maintain control of the newly born infant. The combination of amniotic fluid, blood, and white, cheesy desquamation called vernix makes the infant very slippery. It is useful to prepare for the delivery by placing the posterior (left) hand underneath the infant's axilla prior to delivering the rest of the body. The anterior hand may then be used to grasp the infant's ankles and ensure a firm grip. In obstetric training, the student is often instructed to hold the infant close to his or her chest "like a football."

The infant is then loosely wrapped in a towel and stimulated as it is dried. In the setting of an uncomplicated delivery, the mother may immediately hold the child while the cord is being cut provided that the child has responded well to initial stimulation and has a clear airway and good respiratory effort. The umbilical cord is double clamped and cut with sterile scissors; the infant is then further dried and warmed in an incubator, where postnatal care may be provided and Apgar scores calculated at 1 and 5 min after delivery. Scoring includes general color, tone, heart rate, respiratory effort, and reflexes.

In the case of suspected meconium aspiration, the infant is delivered, the cord is double clamped and cut immediately, and the infant is placed in an incubator for airway assessment and possible intubation prior to being stimulated to breathe spontaneously. Intubation allows for the trachea to be suctioned adequately prior to spontaneous breathing, thus reducing the risk of meconium aspiration. If a cyanotic or apneic child is delivered and does not immediately respond to stimulation, neonatal resuscitation is instituted (see Chap. 9, "Neonatal Resuscitation and Emergencies").

COMPLICATIONS OF DELIVERY

Cord Prolapse

In the event that the bimanual examination reveals a palpable, pulsating cord, the examiner's hand should not be removed, but rather should be used to elevate the presenting fetal part to reduce compression of the cord.[8] Immediate obstetric assistance is then necessary, as a cesarean section is indicated. The examiner's hand should remain in the vagina while the patient is transported and prepped for surgery in order to prevent further compression of the cord by the fetal head.[9] No attempt should ever be made to replace a prolapsed cord.

Shoulder Dystocia

Shoulder dystocia is the impaction of fetal shoulders at the pelvic outlet after delivery of the head. Typically, the anterior shoulder is trapped behind the pubic symphysis, leading to delay of delivery of the rest of the infant. It usually occurs in the delivery of larger infants with disproportionately large shoulders compared with the fetal head. Although rare, shoulder dystocia is a serious concern because of the risk of fetal morbidity and mortality if it is not managed promptly and appropriately. Complications of shoulder dystocia include brachial plexus injury from overaggressive traction and fetal hypoxia from impaired respirations and compression of the umbilical cord, leading to compromised fetal circulation.

Shoulder dystocia is first recognized after the delivery of the fetal head, when routine downward traction is insufficient to deliver the anterior shoulder. After delivery of the infant's head, the head retracts tightly against the perineum (the "turtle sign").[10] Upon recognizing shoulder dystocia, the physician should suction the infant's nose and mouth and call for assistance to position the mother in the extreme lithotomy position, with legs sharply flexed up to the abdomen (the McRoberts maneuver) with the legs held by the mother or an assistant. The bladder should be drained if this has not already been done. A generous episiotomy may also facilitate delivery. Next, an assistant should apply suprapubic pressure to disimpact the anterior shoulder from the pubic symphysis. It is important to remember never to apply fundal pressure, as this will further force the shoulder against the pelvic rim.[11]

To deliver the impacted anterior shoulder, a corkscrew maneuver (Wood's maneuver) is the first manipulation attempted. The physician grasps the posterior scapula of the infant with two fingers and rotates the shoulder girdle 180° in the pelvic outlet in an attempt to rotate the posterior shoulder into the anterior position and in the process deliver the shoulder. Gentle traction may then be applied as the patient pushes, and the infant is delivered through an oblique pelvic diameter. If the corkscrew maneuver fails to reduce the dystocia, the physician may then attempt to deliver the posterior shoulder. The physician's hand is passed posteriorly into the vagina until the infant's posterior arm is felt. The elbow is grasped and flexed, and the arm is delivered with the posterior shoulder. The anterior shoulder usually follows.

Breech Presentation

Breech presentations occur in 3 to 4 percent of term pregnancies and are associated with a morbidity rate three to four times greater than that of cephalad presentations. Breech presentations most frequently occur in premature infants, since final rotation in the pelvis may not have occurred. The major concern in breech deliveries is head entrapment. In a normal cephalic delivery, the larger head dilates the cervical canal, thus ensuring that the rest of the infant follows. With breech deliveries, however, the head emerges last and then may become trapped by an incompletely dilated cervix (Fig. 103-2).

Breech presentation is associated with a greater incidence of fetal distress and umbilical cord prolapse. Breech presentations may be classified as frank, complete, incomplete, or footling. The frank breech and the complete breech presentation serve as a dilating wedge nearly as well as the fetal head, and delivery may proceed in an uncomplicated fashion. Footling and incomplete breech positions are not safe for

FIG. 103-2. Management of the vaginal breech delivery. **A.** The Pinard maneuver. The operator's hand is placed behind the fetal thigh, putting gentle pressure at the knee and allowing delivery of the leg. **B.** A similar maneuver of the opposite leg. **C.** The feet are grasped with the thumb and third finger over the lateral malleolus and the second finger is placed between the two ankles. **D.** With maternal expulsive efforts, the breech is delivered to the level of the umbilicus. The sacrum should be kept anterior. **E.** Again, with maternal expulsive efforts, the infant is delivered to the level of the clavicles, keeping the sacrum anterior. Excessive outward traction by the operator will frequently result in the nuchal arms. **F.** The fetus is rotated 90° allowing visualization of the now anterior right arm. **G.** The arm is well visualized and a single digit is used to deliver it. Delivery of the opposite arm is accomplished by rotating the fetus 180° in a clockwise direction and repeating the maneuver. **H.** Delivery of the fetal vertex is accomplished by placing the operator's fingers over the maxillary processes of the fetus, keeping the body parallel to the floor. The body should never be lifted above parallel to prevent hyperextension of the neck. An assistant applies suprapubic pressure, aiding flexion of the fetal head and accomplishing delivery.

vaginal delivery. The main point in a frank or complete breech presentation is to allow the delivery to progress spontaneously. This lets the presenting portion of the fetus dilate the cervix maximally prior to the presentation of the fetal head. It is recommended that the examiner refrain from touching the fetus until the scapulae are visualized. Then the infant may be gently supported by wrapping a towel around its lower half. The infant is then gently rotated until one arm emerges and then rotated the opposite way to allow delivery of the other arm. Do not pull on the fetus, as this may put pressure on the head within the pelvis or entrap the extended fetal arm.

Footling and incomplete breech positions are not considered safe for vaginal delivery because of the possibility of cord prolapse or incomplete dilatation of the cervix. In any breech delivery, immediate obstetric consultation should be requested.

Preterm Delivery

Preterm delivery is a major cause of precipitous childbirth and is often the cause of emergency delivery. Preterm infants also more often present in the breech position, which is associated with a greater incidence of infant morbidity and mortality. Carefully control the delivery to reduce the likelihood of trauma to the fragile preterm infant. Deliver the infant slowly and immediately dry and warm it while performing the initial assessment, as the premature infant is much more likely to require resuscitation. The decision to initiate resuscitative efforts in the ED is often difficult, as patients may deliver extremely premature fetuses of unknown gestational age. One sign of extreme prematurity is eyelids that are still fused. In general, even very premature deliveries (18 to 22 weeks) should receive initial resuscitative efforts until determination of viability is made.

POSTPARTUM CARE

Immediately after the delivery of the infant, the umbilical cord is clamped. The placenta should be allowed to separate spontaneously, assisted with gentle traction. This process can take several minutes, and often the mother and baby have already been moved from the ED to the labor and delivery suite before the placenta delivers. Aggressive traction on the cord risks uterine inversion, tearing of the cord, or disruption of the placenta, which can result in severe vaginal bleeding.[12]

After the removal of the placenta, the uterus should be gently massaged to promote contraction. Oxytocin (20 U in 1 L of 0.9 normal saline) is infused at a moderate rate to maintain uterine contraction (Table 103-2). Uterine atony may follow a precipitous delivery and may lead to excessive vaginal bleeding. Additional oxytocin may be administered, as well as methyl ergonovine (Methergine) 0.2 mg [intramuscularly (IM) only] or prostaglandin F-2 alpha (Hemabate) 0.25 mg IM. With significant postpartum hemorrhage, vigorous bimanual massage should be continued while contractile agents are administered. Episiotomy or laceration repair may be delayed until an experienced obstetrician is able to close the laceration and inspect the patient for fourth-degree (rectovaginal) tears.[13]

REFERENCES

1. Leerentveld RA, Gilberts EC, Arnold MJ, Wladimiroff JW: Accuracy and safety of transvaginal sonographic placental localization. *Obstet Gynecol* 76:759, 1990.
2. Johnston MM, Sanchez-Ramos L, Vaughn AJ, et al: Antibiotic therapy in preterm, premature rupture of membranes: A randomized prospective double blind trial, *Am J Obstet Gynecol* 163:743, 1990.
3. Mercer BM, Lewis R: Preterm labor and premature rupture of membranes: Diagnosis and management. *Infect Dis Clin North Am* 11:177, 1997.
4. Iyasu S, Saftlas AK, Rowley DL, et al: The epidemiology of placenta previa in the United States. *Am J Obstet Gynecol* 168:1424, 1987.
5. Lowe TW, Cunningham FG: *Clin Obstet Gynecol* 33:406, 1990.
6. Borgatta L, Picning SJ, Cohen WR: Association of episotomy and delivery position with deep perineal laceration during spontaneous delivery in nulliparous women. *Am J Obstet Gynecol* 160:294, 1989.
7. Shino P, Klebanoff MA, Corey JC: Midline episiotomics: More harm than good? *Obstet Gynecol* 75:765, 1990.
8. Barnett WM: Umbilical cord prolapse: A true obstetrical emergency. *J Emerg Med* 7:149, 1989.
9. Critchlow CW, Leef TL, Benedetti TJ, et al: Risk factors and infant outcomes associated with umbilical cord prolapse: A population based case-control study among births in Washington state. *Am J Obstet Gynecol* 170:613, 1994.
10. Naef RW, Martin JN: Emergency management of shoulder dystocia. *Obstet Gynecol Clin North Am* 22:247, 1995.
11. Nocon JJ, McKenzie DK, Thomas LJ, et al: Shoulder dystocia: An analysis of risks and obstetric maneuvers. *Am J Obstet Gynecol* 168:1732, 1993.
12. Combs CA, Murphey EL, Laros RK: Factors associated with postpartum hemorrhage with vaginal birth. *Obstet Gynecol* 77:69, 1991.
13. Zahn CM, Yoemans ER: Postpartum hemorrhage, placenta accreta, uterine inversion, and puerperal hematomas. *Clin Obstet Gynecol* 33:422, 1990.

VULVOVAGINITIS

Gloria J. Kuhn

Vulvovaginitis is inflammation of the vulva and vaginal tissues. It is usually characterized by a vaginal discharge and/or vulvar itching and irritation. A vaginal odor may be present. It accounts for 10 million visits to physicians per year in the United States, and is the most common gynecologic complaint in prepubertal girls.[1]

The most common causes of acute vulvovaginitis include (1) infections, (2) irritant or allergic contact vulvovaginitis, (3) local response to a vaginal foreign body, and (4) atrophic vaginitis.

The three most frequent infectious causes are trichomoniasis (caused by *Trichomonas vaginalis*), bacterial vaginosis (BV; caused by replacement of normal flora by overgrowth of anaerobes and *Gardnerella vaginalis*), and candidiasis (usually caused by *Candida albicans*).[2] BV is the most common cause of vaginal discharge or malodor. Polymicrobial infection in women with vaginitis is not uncommon. Vulvovaginal candidiasis, contact vaginitis, and atrophic vaginitis may occur in virgins and after menopause, but other forms of infectious vulvovaginitis are generally found only in sexually active women.[2]

A detailed gynecologic history should be obtained and a pelvic examination performed. Microscopic evaluation of fresh vaginal secretions using both normal saline solution (demonstrating clue cells for BV and motile *T. vaginalis* for trichomoniasis) and 10% potassium hydroxide (KOH) slide preparation (demonstrating yeast or pseudohyphae for candidiasis) and fishy odor in BV (whiff test) will, in most instances, provide a diagnosis (Table 104-1). Culture for *T. vaginalis*

TABLE 104-1 Diagnosis of Vaginitis Based on Vaginal Secretions

Test	Finding	Diagnosis
pH	>4.5	Bacterial vaginosis
pH	>4.5	Trichomoniasis
Normal saline solution	Clue cells	Bacterial vaginosis
Normal saline solution	Motile trichomonads	Trichomoniasis
KOH preparation	Pseudohyphae and/or buds	Candidiasis
KOH preparation	Fishy odor (whiff test)	Bacterial vaginosis

is more sensitive than microscopic examination. One of the most helpful diagnostic tools is measurement of the pH of the vaginal secretions. Secretions should be tested for pH using nitrazine paper. A pH greater than 4.5 is typical of BV or trichomoniasis, while a pH below 4.5 represents physiologic discharge or a fungal infection.[3]

Signs of vulval inflammation and minimal discharge in the absence of vaginal pathogens suggest the possibility of mechanical, chemical, allergic, or other noninfectious causes of vulvovaginitis.

All treatment recommendations are taken from the 1998 guidelines for the treatment of sexually transmitted diseases from the Centers for Disease Control and Prevention (CDC).[3]

NORMAL VULVOVAGINAL ENVIRONMENT

In females of childbearing age, estrogen causes the development of a thick vaginal epithelium with a large number of superficial cells serving a protective function and containing large stores of glycogen. Glycogen is used by the normal flora, consisting of lactobacilli and acidogenic cornynebacteria, to form lactic and acetic acids. The resulting acidic environment favors the normal flora and discourages the growth of pathogenic bacteria. Lack of estrogen or a dominence of progesterone results in an atrophic condition, with loss of the protective superficial cells and their contained glycogen. This is turn results in loss of the acidic environment. Normal vaginal secretions may vary in consistency from a thin, watery material to one that is thick, white, and opaque. The quantity may also vary from scant to a rather copious amount. This material is odorless and produces no symptoms. The normal vaginal pH varies between 3.5 and 4.1. Alkaline secretions from the cervix before and during menstruation and semen, which is alkaline, reduce acidity, predisposing to infection. Before menarche and after menopause, the vaginal pH varies between 6 and 7. Because of scant nerve endings in the vagina, the patient usually does not have symptoms until both the vagina and vulva are involved in an inflammatory or irritant process.

BACTERIAL VAGINOSIS

BV is a clinical syndrome that occurs when the normal H_2O_2-producing *Lactobacillus* species in the vagina are replaced by high concentrations of anaerobic bacteria, *G. vaginalis,* and *Mycoplasma hominis.* BV is the most common cause of a malodorous discharge, but over half of the women who meet the clinical criteria for diagnosis are asymptomatic. The cause of this microbial alteration in the normal vaginal flora is not understood. While BV is rarely seen in women who have never been sexually active, it is not clear whether the disease is the result of a sexually transmitted pathogen.

Bacterial vaginosis can be diagnosed by the use of clinical and microscopic criteria. The CDC states that for the disease to be diagnosed, three of the following signs or symptoms must be present: (1) a homogeneous, white, noninflammatory discharge that smoothly coats the vaginal walls; (2) presence of clue cells on microscopic examination (epithelial cells coated by bacteria); (3) pH greater than 4.5; and (4) a fishy odor to the discharge after addition of KOH (whiff test).[3] Gram staining, which demonstrates a concentration of bacterial morphotypes characteristic of BV, is an acceptable laboratory method of diagnosing BV. Culture of *G. vaginalis* is not recommended.[3]

Research has demonstrated an association between BV and adverse pregnancy outcomes due to preterm labor and premature rupture of membranes (PROM), leading to recommendations that high-risk patients (i.e., those who previously delivered a premature infant) be screened for BV during the second trimester of pregnancy.[4] BV has also been associated with pelvic inflammatory disease, endometritis, and vaginal cuff cellulitis after surgical procedures.

Recommendations for treatment are controversial for asymptomatic patients. Several drug regimens are available (Table 104-2).[3] All symptomatic patients, unless allergic to the drug, should be treated with metronidazole regardless of pregnancy status.[3] Because of the association of BV with postsurgical infection, strong consideration should be given to prophylactic treatment of infected women prior to surgical abortion.

TABLE 104-2 Treatment Regimens for Bacterial Vaginosis

Agent	Dose
RECOMMENDED REGIMENS	
Metronidazole*	500 mg orally bid for 7 d
Clindamycin cream 2%	One full applicator intravaginally qhs for 7 d
Metronidazole gel 0.75%	One full applicator intravaginally bid for 5 d
ALTERNATIVE REGIMENS†	
Metronidazole	2 g PO in a single dose
Clindamycin	300 mg PO bid for 7 d
REGIMENS FOR PREGNANT WOMEN	
High-risk patients	
Metronidazole‡	250 mg PO tid for 7 d
Alternative regimens†	
Metronidazole‡	2 g PO in a single dose
Clindamycin	300 mg PO bid for 7 d
Low-risk symptomatic patients	
Metronidazole‡	250 mg PO tid for 7 d
Alternative regimens†	
Metronidazole‡	2 g PO in a single dose
Metronidazole gel 0.75%	One full applicator intravaginally bid for 5 d
Clindamycin	300 mg PO bid for 7 d
Clindamycin cream 2%	One full applicator intravaginally qhs for 7 d

*Avoid alcohol during and 24 h after treatment.
†Lower efficacy.
‡Contraindicated in first trimester of pregnancy.

Treatment of BV in infected pregnant women who are at high risk for premature labor has decreased the incidence of this complication. Currently, according to the US Food and Drug Administration (FDA), oral metronidazole is contraindicated in the first trimester of pregnancy but can be used in the second trimester. However, intravaginal metronidazole (0.75%) gel is designated a category B drug by the FDA, allowing its use throughout pregnancy.[3–6] However, this and other alternative pharmacotherapies are less effective (Table 104-2). A large randomized clinical trial is currently under way to determine whether all asymptomatic pregnant women should be treated for BV.

Overall cure rates 4 weeks after treatment did not differ significantly between a 7-day regimen of either oral metronidazole, metronidazole vaginal gel, or clindamycin vaginal cream. Metronidazole vaginal gel has the benefit of fewer side effects (i.e., gastrointestinal disturbance and unpleasant taste).[4] All patients on oral metronidazole should avoid alcohol during and for 24 h, and in some cases longer, after treatment because of the disulfiram-like reaction that can occur. Based on frequency of cure rates, alternative treatments are not as efficacious.

CANDIDA VAGINITIS

Candida species are a common cause of vaginitis. While there are no reliable figures as to prevalence of vulvovaginal candidiasis (VVC) because the disease is not reportable, it is estimated that 75 percent of women will experience at least one infection during their childbearing years (with the highest attack rate during the third trimester of pregnancy), making it the second commonest vaginal infection.[2] A small subpopulation of women, less than 5 percent, have repeated episodes of disease with no apparent factors being responsible for recurrent infection.

The organism can be isolated from up to 20 percent of asymptomatic, healthy women of childbearing age, some of whom are celibate. Therefore, this infection is not considered a sexually transmitted disease (STD), although it can be transmitted that way. Factors that favor increased rates of asymptomatic vaginal colonization include pregnancy, oral contraceptives, uncontrolled diabetes mellitus, and frequent visits to STD clinics (perhaps as a result of antimicrobial therapy). It is rare in premenarchial girls[4] and has a decreased incidence after menopause unless replacement estrogen is being used, emphasizing the hormonal dependence of VVC. Immunity to *Candida* infections is primarily cell mediated.

Candida albicans strains account for 85 to 90 percent of those isolated from the vagina, while *Candida glabrata* and *Candida tropicalis* are the commonest non-albicans strains and are often more resistant to conventional therapy. Candidal organisms gain access to the vaginal lumen and secretions predominantly from the adjacent perianal area. Candidal organisms must first adhere to the vaginal epithelial cells for colonization to take place, and *C. albicans* adheres in greater numbers than do other strains.

Factors that enhance the germination of *Candida* (e.g., pregnancy and estrogen therapy) tend to precipitate symptomatic vaginitis, while conditions that inhibit germination (normal flora and local mucosal cell-mediated immunity) prevent acute vaginitis in carriers of yeast. The growth of *Candida* is held in check by the normal vaginal flora, and symptoms of vaginitis usually occur only when the normal balance is upset. Conditions that inhibit growth of normal vaginal flora, particularly *Lactobacillus* species (e.g., systemic antibiotics, especially broad-spectrum agents), diminish the glycogen stores in vaginal epithelial cells (e.g., diabetes mellitus, pregnancy, oral contraceptives, and hormonal replacement therapy), or increase the pH of vaginal secretions (e.g., menstrual blood or semen) may cause increased colonization by *Candida,* which is an opportunistic organism, and subsequent symptomatic infection. Tight-fitting, particularly synthetic, undergarments may also contribute to the problem because of increased temperature, moisture, and local irritation.

TABLE 104-3 Treatment Regimens for Vulvovaginal Candidiasis

Agent	Formulation	Dosage Regimen
	UNCOMPLICATED VVC	
Butoconazole	2% cream	5 g/d for 3 d
Clotrimazole	100-mg vaginal tablet	2 tablets/d for 3 d
Miconazole	200-mg vaginal suppository	1 suppository/d for 3 d
Nystatin	100,000-U vaginal tablet	1 tablet/d for 14 d
Tioconazole	6.5% ointment	5 g intravaginally in a single dose
Fluconazole	150-mg tablet PO	1 tablet as a single dose
	COMPLICATED VVC	
Fluconazole	100-mg tablet PO	1 tablet weekly
Ketoconazole	200-mg tablet PO	1 tab/d for 1–2 weeks
Clotrimazole	500-mg vaginal suppository or tablet	1 suppository or tablet weekly

Note: Not all possible regimens are listed.

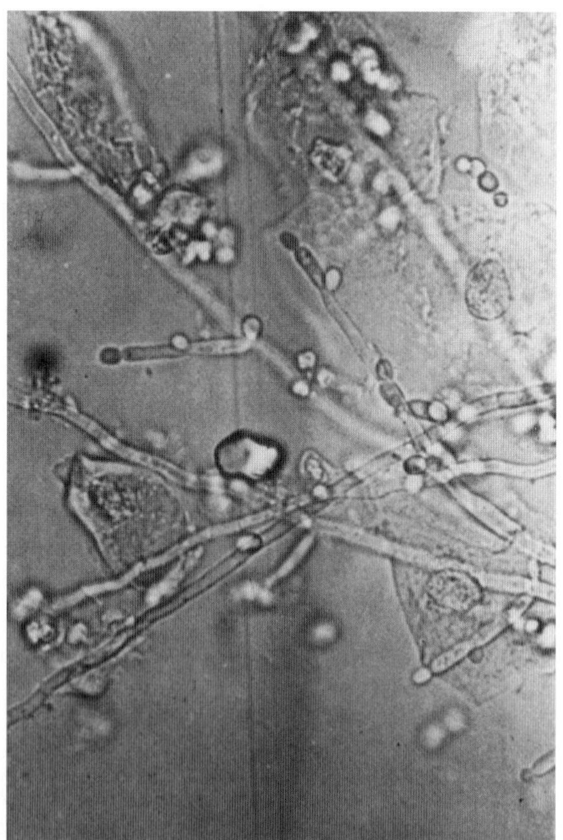

FIG. 104-1. Hyphal elements of *C. albicans* seen on high-power magnification during saline microscopy. The patient had florid candidal vaginitis.

Clinical symptoms include leukorrhea, severe vaginal pruritus (commonest symptom), external dysuria, and dyspareunia. Symptoms vary in severity, but exacerbation is frequently seen in the week prior to menses or with coitus. Odor is unusual.

Gynecologic examination may reveal vulvar erythema and edema, vaginal erythema, and, occasionally, thick ''cottage-cheese'' discharge, seen most often in pregnant patients. The discharge may vary from none to watery to homogeneously thick.

The diagnosis of *Candida* vaginitis is made by microscopically examining a wet mount or normal saline sample of vaginal secretions for yeast buds and pseudohyphae (Fig. 104-1; sensitivity 40 to 60 percent). Two drops of 10% KOH added to the vaginal scretions dissolves the vaginal epithelial cells, leaving yeast buds and pseudohyphae intact, increasing the sensitivity (80 percent) of microscopic examination and yielding almost 100 percent specificity. Culture should only be done in a symptomatic patient with negative findings on microscopic examination.[3]

Most treatment regimens (Table 104-3) are effective in relieving symptoms, but recurrence of infection is common.[3] The topically applied azole drugs are more effective than nystatin, with relief of symptoms in 80 to 90 percent of patients who complete treatment. Creams, lotions, sprays, vaginal tablets, suppositories, and coated tampons are all equally efficacious, and the choice of vehicle should depend on the patient's preference. The azole drugs are all available over the counter (OTC) with durations of 1, 3, or 7 days. One-day treatment with oral fluconazole is as effective as use of topical preparations.[7,8] Partners should not be treated unless the woman has frequent recurrences.

Self-medication should only be advised in women with previously diagnosed VVC and recurrence of similar symptoms. If symptoms persist or recur within 2 months, the patient should be seen so that vaginal and microscopic examinations can be performed. Cultures should be considered for patients with frequent recurrences. All possible precipitating factors, such as high blood glucose levels, should be controlled. However, the majority of women with recurrences do not have obvious precipitating causes.

Uncomplicated VVC (i.e., mild-to-moderate symptoms, sporadic, nonrecurrent disease in a normal host with normally susceptible *C. albicans*) responds to all azoles, including single-dose therapy. Complicated VVC (i.e., severe symptoms, recurrent disease, abnormal host, or resistant organism, such as *C. glabrata*) requires therapy lasting from 10 to 14 days with topical or oral azoles.[3]

Management of women with frequent recurrences is aimed at control, rather than cure, with a long-term suppressive prophylactic regimen. Diagnosis should be certain, oral contraceptives stopped, and blood glucose level checked in diabetics.

Other than initial burning and irritation, side effects of local agents are unusual. Oral agents occasionally cause nausea, abdominal pain, and headaches. Ketoconazole can cause liver toxicity as well as adverse drug interactions with a variety of other medications.

TRICHOMONAS VAGINALIS

Trichomoniasis is caused by the protozoan *T. vaginalis*. Trichomonads are frequently found in the urethra and Skene glands and may be recovered from urine. It is estimated that 2 to 3 million American women contract the disease annually. Trichomonas is almost always a STD, and its prevalence correlates with the overall level of sexual activity of the population studied.[2,9] Recent epidemiologic surveys indicate a possible decline in prevalence. Vaginal trichomoniasis may be associated with adverse pregnancy outcomes, particularly PROM and preterm delivery.[10,11] Trichomoniasis is also reported to facilitate the transmission of HIV.

Seventy percent of men having intercouse with infected women demonstrated the organism within 48 h, while 85 percent of women whose male partners were infected developed trichomonas infection. There is a high prevalence of gonorrhea in women with trichomoniasis. Oral contraceptives, spermicidal agents, and barrier contraceptives are all thought to reduce transmission.

Infection ranges from asymptomatic carrier state to severe, acute inflammatory disease. A vaginal discharge is reported by 50 to 75 percent of patients. It may vary in character from the classic picture of a yellow-green frothy discharge, seen in 20 to 30 percent of patients, to a gray discharge to scant or no discharge. Other symptoms include vulvovaginal soreness and irritation (25 to 50 percent); pruritis, which may be severe (25 to 50 percent); dysuria (25 percent); and malodorous discharge (25 percent). A sense of vulvovaginal fullness may be intense or mild. As many as half of symptomatic women complain of some degree of dyspareunia. Symptoms may be more severe before, during, or after menstruation when the vaginal pH is more alkaline. Lower abdominal pain is rare and should alert the physician to the possibility of other diseases.

Just as symptoms vary in severity, so do the findings on examination. Gynecologic examination reveals the classic "strawberry cervix" secondary to diffuse punctate hemorrhages in only 2 percent of patients. Diffuse erythema is seen in 10 to 33 percent of patients.

The diagnosis of trichomoniasis vaginitis is made through use of the "hanging-drop" slide test, which has a sensitivity of 80 to 90 percent in symptomatic patients. A cotton swab is used to obtain a specimen of secretions from the vaginal vault (not the endocervix) and is placed within a drop of normal saline solution on a glass slide. Microscopic examination reveals many polymorphonuclear leukocytes (PMNs) and motile, pear-shaped, flagellated trichomonads, which are slightly larger than the leukocytes. As a screening test in asymptomatic individuals, the microscopic test may only be 40 percent sensitive, but has virtually 100 percent specificity. Cultures are about 95 percent sensitive and should be considered in symptomatic patients with elevated pH, PMN excess, and absence of motile trichomonads and clue cells.

TABLE 104-4 Treatment Regimens for Trichomoniasis

Agent	Dose
RECOMMENDED REGIMEN	
Metronidazole	2 g PO in a single dose
ALTERNATIVE REGIMEN	
Metronidazole	500 mg PO bid for 7 d

Note: Avoid alcohol during and for at least 24 h after treatment. Metronidazole can be used in pregnant women but not approved by the US Food and Drug Administration until the second trimester.

The causative organism is a flagellated protozoan that may live quiescently in the paraurethral glands and from this nidus of infestation cause overt infection in the susceptible vagina. *Trichomonas vaginalis* may survive up to 24 h in tap water, in hot tubs, in urine, on toilet seats, and in swimming pools, but the usual sequence of events begins with a large deposit of inoculum of organisms contained in the alkaline semen at time of intercourse. Because up to 25 percent of women and 90 percent of men harboring the organisms are asymptomatic, it is difficult to control spread of disease. The cornerstone of therapy remains metronidazole (Table 104-4).[3,12] Recurrence of disease is frequent and may necessitate more than one course of treatment. There is a 90 percent cure rate with either the single- or multiple-dose regimen. The single-dose treatment is preferable because of lower cost, fewer side effects, and greater patient compliance.

GENITAL HERPES

Genital herpes is a sexually transmitted infection caused by a DNA-containing virus specific to human beings. Sexual transmission can occur during asymptomatic periods. Usually, genital herpes is the most frequently encountered of the diseases causing genital ulcers and is thought to be associated with an increased risk for HIV infection.[3] There are two antigenic groups: herpes simplex virus 1 (HSV-1) and herpes simplex virus 2 (HSV-2). Initially, HSV-1 caused oral lesions and HSV-2 genital lesions, but this is no longer the case. Overall, 85 to 90 percent of genital herpes infections are caused by HSV-2, but some studies have found up to 30 percent are caused by HSV-1. Symptomatic genital herpes is the most frequent cause of painful lesions of the lower genital tract in American women. Neonatal infection with high mortality and morbidity rates after passage through an infected birth canal has been seen. Although the actual prevalence is not known, it may be one of the most frequent sexually transmitted diseases. It remains a recurrent disease with no cure at this time.

Initial presentation occurs 1 to 45 days (mean 5.8 days) after exposure. Usually, initial infection is more severe and lasts longer than do subsequent recurrences. There may be both local and systemic manifestations. The lesions begin as painful, fluid-filled vesicles or papules, which progress to well-circumscribed, occasionally coalescent, shallow-based ulcers. They then heal by reepithelialization of mucous membranes or by crusting by the epidermal surface. Symptoms peak in 8 to 10 days and decrease over the next week. Ulcers last 4 to 15 days, with total healing in 21 days. Lymphadenopathy is usually present, and when the deep inguinal nodes are involved, severe pelvic pain may result. Urethritis is usually present, causing severe dysuria, which may cause urethral spasm and urinary retention. Initial disease involves the cervix in over 80 percent of cases. Pharyngitis and secondary spread of lesions to other body sites, usually below the waist, have been reported in up to two-thirds of patients. Systemic symptoms, such as fever, malaise, headache, and myalgias, are common. Hepatitis, aseptic meningitis, and autonomic nervous system dysfunction can occur. Aseptic meningitis has been seen more frequently with HSV-

2 than with HSV-1 infection and has been reported in about 30 percent of patients. Sacral autonomic nervous dysfunction is rare but can result in decreased cutaneous sensation and bladder and bowel dysfunction. After the attack is over, the inactive virus resides in the sacral dorsal root ganglia. Under various stimuli, both exogenous and endogenous, the virus travels down the sensory nerve root to the lower genital area, where it replicates and becomes symptomatic.

Recurrent episodes are usually milder than the initial disease, and the patient usually does not have systemic symptoms. A recurrence may be heralded by genital tingling. Recurrent genital lesions are fewer, smaller, and more often unilateral. Lesions may be ulcerative or resemble a fissure or excoriations. Recurrences tend to occur in the same location and have the same appearance from episode to episode. Symptoms last 4 to 8 days, and the lesions have usually disappeared by 10 days. Frequency of attacks and intervals between attacks are highly variable. The average number of symptomatic recurrences is 5 to 8 per year. Asymptomatic infections, defined as culture-positive viral shedding in the absence of symptoms or lesions, have been documented.

Approximately 25 percent of initial presentations occur in women with preexisting antibody to herpes simplex virus. The initial episodes tend to be less severe and resemble recurrent infections. They may in fact represent recurrent infections in patients who had previous asymptomatic infections. Clinically, it is impossible to distinguish between HSV-1 and HSV-2 infections, but HSV-1 usually causes milder initial disease, results in recurrence less frequently, and results in milder recurrent episodes.

Diagnosis is suspected by clinical presentation and confirmed by either culture or polymerase chain reaction, which is extremely sensitive in detecting low concentrations of viral DNA but not yet widely available. The virus can be isolated from vesicle fluid and the base of a wet ulcer. Intact vesicles, if present, should be unroofed and the fluid cultured directly. Scrapings of an ulcer may be taken for a Pap smear or Tzanck preparation. A Tzanck smear stained with either Wright or Giemsa stain is positive if multinucleated giant cells are present, which may be seen in up to 50 percent of cases. Serologic analysis is useful in classifying the initial herpetic episode as primary or nonprimary but is usually not indicated.

Treatment is not curative. Multiple antiviral agents and regimens are available (Table 104-5). Systemic antiviral agents provide partial control of the signs and symptoms and accelerate healing of the lesions, but do not affect the frequency or severity of recurrences. Topical therapy is not effective.[3] Patients with severe disease may need hospitalization and intravenous therapy. In recurrent episodes, treatment should be started during the prodrome or within 1 day of onset of lesions if treatment is to be beneficial. For patients with frequent recurrences (six or more episodes per year) daily suppressive therapy can be used but should be discontinued after 1 year to allow assessment of the patient's recurrent episodes. Daily suppressive therapy reduces the frequency of recurrences by at least 75 percent. Suppressive therapy does not lessen the rate of viral shedding, and therefore patients should be advised of their continued risk of infecting sexual partners.

TABLE 104-5 Treatment of Genital Herpes

Agent (Oral Tablets or Caplets)	Dose
INITIAL EPISODE	
Acyclovir	400 mg tid for 7–10 d
Famciclovir	250 mg tid for 7–10 d
Valacyclovir	1 g bid for 7–10 d
EPISODIC RECURRENT INFECTION	
Acyclovir	400 mg tid for 5 d
Famciclovir	125 mg bid for 5 d
Valacyclovir	500 mg bid for 5 d
DAILY SUPPRESSIVE THERAPY	
Acyclovir	400 mg bid
Famciclovir	250 mg bid
Valacyclovir	1 g daily
INTRAVENOUS THERAPY FOR SEVERE INITIAL PRESENTATION	
Acyclovir	5–10 mg/kg qid for 5–7 d

Note: All agents categorized class B may be used for pregnant patients.

The safety of acyclovir and valacyclovir during pregnancy has not been established. In pregnant patients with life-threatening disease, such as encephalitis, pneumonitis, or hepatitis, intravenous acyclovir should be used. It should not be used for recurrent episodes or as suppressive therapy. Pregnant women treated with the drug should be reported to the Glaxo-Wellcome registry, which is kept in cooperation with the CDC (1-800-722-9292, extension 38465). Current registry findings do not indicate an increased risk for major birth defects after acyclovir treatment.[2,3,12]

Systemic analgesics may be needed. Some patients have severe dysuria when the urine comes in contact with vaginal and vulvar tissues. Pouring warm water over these tissues during urination may provide symptomatic relief.[12,13]

CONTACT VULVOVAGINITIS

Contact dermatitis results from the exposure of vulvar epithelium and vaginal mucosa to a primary chemical irritant or an allergen. In either case, characteristic local erythema and edema occur. Severe reactions may progress to ulceration and secondary infection. Common irritants and/or allergens include chemically scented douches; soaps; bubble baths; deodorants; perfumes, dyes, and scents in toilet paper, tampons, and pads; feminine hygiene products; topical vaginal antibiotics; and tight slacks, pantyhose, and synthetic underwear.

Clinically, patients report local swelling and itching or a burning sensation. The gynecologic examination reveals an erythematous and edematous vulvovaginal area. Local vesiculation and ulceration are seen more commonly with allergens or when primary irritants are used in strong concentrations. Vaginal pH changes may promote colonization and infection with *C. albicans,* thus obscuring the primary cause.

Diagnosis of contact vulvovaginitis is made by ruling out an infectious cause and by identifying the offending agent. Most cases of mild vulvovaginal contact dermatitis resolve spontaneously when the causative agent is withdrawn. For patients with severe, painful reactions, cool sitz baths and wet compresses of dilute boric acid or Burow's solution may afford relief. Topical corticosteroids, such as hydrocortisone acetate, fluocinolone acetonide, or triamcinolone acetonide relieve symptoms and promote healing. Oral histamines may be helpful if a true allergic reaction is present. If superinfection with *C. albicans* has complicated the case, it needs to be treated.

VAGINAL FOREIGN BODIES

Children and adolescents may insert objects intravaginally during periods of genital exploration or sexual stimulation. In young girls, the most commonly inserted foreign bodies are rolled-up pieces of toilet paper, toys, and small household objects.[1] In adolescents and adult women, it is often a forgotten tampon or sponge contraceptive. Foreign objects left in place for more than 48 h can cause severe localized infections due to *Escherichia coli,* anaerobes, or overgrowth of other vaginal flora. Patients present with a foul-smelling and/or bloody vaginal discharge. The only treatment necessary for vaginitis secondary to the presence of a foreign body is removal of the object.[1] In most cases, the vaginal discharge and odor will disappear without further therapy within several days.

PINWORMS

Pinworms (*Enterobius vermicularis*) may migrate from the anus to the vagina in children and cause intense pruritus that is often most intense during the night, when gravid female worms pass out from the intestinal tract to lay eggs on the perineal skin. Cellophane tape can be used to obtain material for a slide, which can be examined microscopically for the presence of ova, which are large and double walled in appearance. The child and all family members need treatment with an antiparasitic agent, either mebendazole [Vermox (Janssen Pharmaceutica, Inc.)], a single oral dose of 100 mg chewed well, or pyrantel pamoate [Antiminth (Pfizer, Inc.)], a single oral dose of 11 mg/kg (maximum 1 g). Repeat treatment 2 weeks later should be administered, since mature worms seem more vulnerable to treatment than do young worms.[14]

ATROPHIC VAGINITIS

During menarche, pregnancy, and lactation and after menopause, the vaginal epithelium lacks the stimulation of estrogen. The maturation of the vaginal and urethra mucosa depends on the presence of estrogen and can be altered by the absence of estrogen or the presence of antiestrogenic factors, such as hormones, drugs, or diseases. Menopause results in a vaginal mucosa that is attenuated, pale, and almost transparent as a result of decreased vascularity. The vagina loses its normal rugae. The squamous epithelium atrophies, the glycogen content of the cells decreases, and the vaginal pH ranges from 5.5 to 7.0. The mucosa is only three or four cells thick and is less resistant to minor trauma and infection. Marked atrophic changes can cause atrophic vaginitis. It is important to distinguish between symptomatic atrophic vaginitis, which is rare, and an atrophic vagina that is a result of physiologic changes of menopause. When symptomatic vaginitis occurs, the vaginal epithelium is thin, inflamed, and even ulcerated. Symptoms include vaginal soreness, dyspareunia, and occasional spotting or discharge, which may be a thin, scant, yellowish or pink material. The cervix atrophies and retracts and may become flush with the apex of the vault. The upper one-third of the vagina constricts, and the entire vagina becomes shorter in length and loses its elasticity. The increased vaginal pH may permit the growth of nonacidophilic coliform organisms, bacteria not normally found in the vagina, and the disappearance of *Lactobacillus* species. This can lead to the development of a clinical vaginal infection with copious purulent discharge. Unless estrogenic replacement therapy is used, *Candida* and *Trichomonas* infections are rare. The changes seen vary widely from one patient to another. A Pap smear of the cervix and vagina is mandatory in the face of bleeding to rule out carcinoma. A wet preparation will show erythrocytes and increased PMNs associated with small, round epithelial cells, which are immature squamous cells that have not been exposed to sufficient estrogen. The treatment of atrophic vaginitis consists primarily of topical vaginal estrogen. Nightly use of half or all of the contents of an applicator for 1 to 2 weeks should be sufficient to alleviate symptoms.[3] An alternative regimen is use of oral estrogen (0.625 mg conjugated estrogen). Estrogen should not be prescribed for any patient with a past history of cancer of any of the reproductive organs. Atrophic vaginitis is usually not seen in patients who are already on systemic estrogen replacement therapy. Patients should be referred for follow-up to monitor therapy and for the results of the Pap smear.

REFERENCES

1. Farrington PF: Pediatric vulvovaginitis. *Clin Obstet Gynecol* 40:135, 1997.
2. Sobel J: Vaginitis, in Pearlman MD, Tintinalli JE (eds): *Emergency Care of the Woman.* New York, McGraw-Hill, 1998, pp 535–549.
3. Centers for Disease Control and Prevention: 1998 guidelines for treatment of sexually transmitted diseases: Recommendations and reports. *Morb Mortal Wkly Rep* 47:1, 1997.
4. McCoy MC, Katz VL, Kuller JA: Bacterial vaginosis in pregnancy: An approach for the 1990s. *Obstet Gynecol Survey* 50:482, 1995.
5. Schwebke JR: Metronidazole: Utilization in the obstetric and gynecologic patient. *Sexually Transmitted Dis* 22:370, 1995.
6. Seamens CM: Treating sexually transmitted diseases in the emergency department. *Crit Decision Emerg Med* 12:1, 1998.
7. Andersen GM, Barrat J, Bergan T: A comparison of single-dose oral fluconazole with 3-day intravaginal clotrimazole in the treatment of vaginal candidiasis: Report of an international multicentre trial. *Br J Obstet Gynaecol* 96:226, 1989.
8. Droegemueller W, Adamson DG, Brown D, Cibley L: Three-day treatment with butoconazole nitrate for vulvovaginal candidiasis. *Obstet Gynecol* 64:530, 1984.
9. Miller KE: Sexually transmitted diseases. *Primary Care* 24:179, 1997.
10. Fiscella K: Racial disparities in preterm births: The role of urogenital infections. *Public Health Rep* 111:104, 1996.
11. Goldenberg RL, Andrews WW, Yuan AC, MacKay HT: St. Louis ME: Sexually transmitted diseases and adverse outcomes of pregnancy. *Infect Perinatol* 24:23, 1997.
12. Sexually transmitted diseases, in Cunningham FC, Gant NF, MacDonald PC: *William's Obstetrics.* Stamford, Appleton & Lange, 1997, pp 1317–1338.
13. Soper DE: Genitourinary infection and sexually transmitted diseases. In Berek JS, Adashi EY, Hillard PA: *Novak's Gynecology.* Baltimore, Williams & Wilkins, 1996, pp 425–445.
14. Kazura JW: Enterobiasis, in Behrman RE, Kliegman RM, Arvin AM: *Nelson Textbook of Pediatrics.* Philadelphia, Saunders, 1996, p 997.

PELVIC INFLAMMATORY DISEASE

Amy J. Behrman
Suzanne Moore Shepherd

INTRODUCTION

Pelvic inflammatory disease (PID) comprises a spectrum of infections of the female upper reproductive tract. It is a common and serious sexually transmitted disease, generally initiated by ascending infection from the cervix and vagina. The inflammatory processes falling within the rubric of PID may include salpingitis, endometritis, and tubo-ovarian abscess, and extend to produce pelvic peritonitis, and perihepatitis. The annual rate of PID in industrialized countries has been reported to be as high as 10–20 per 1000 women of reproductive age, with over one million cases estimated to occur per year in the United States.[1] These numbers clearly underestimate the true incidence because of both atypical and wide variability of symptoms and the relatively poor reliability of the clinical diagnosis. Long term sequellae, including tubal factor infertility (TFI), ectopic pregnancy, and chronic pain, may occur in as many as 25 percent of patients. The annual direct and indirect costs of the acute disease and its sequella are projected to rise to $10 billion/year by 2000.

Patients with PID frequently present to emergency departments with non-specific complaints and findings. Early diagnosis and aggressive treatment may provide rapid clinical and microbiologic improvement, identify co-existent disease, decrease transmission, and minimize the likelihood of serious sequellae.

ETIOLOGY

Neisseria gonorrhoeae and *Chlamydia trachomatis* can be isolated in many, if not most, cases of PID, and therapy has traditionally been directed primarily against these organisms. However, newer, more sensitive and specific evaluative tools have become available which have significantly improved our understanding of PID. Polymicrobial infection, including anaerobic and aerobic vaginal flora, has clearly been demonstrated in studies relying on cultural material from the upper reproductive tract.[2] Earlier culdocentesis studies suggested that 80 percent of PID was polymicrobial, but there is evidence that this may represent a degree of contamination of the cul-de-sac by the procedure. Laparoscopy cultures more conservatively point to mixed infection in 30 to 40 percent of cases. Pathogenic organisms may include anaerobes, *Gardnerella vaginalis,* enteric gram-negative rods, *Hemophilus influenzae, Streptococcus agalactine, Mycoplasma hominis,* and *Urea urealyticum. N. gonorrheae* and *C. trachomatis* may often be instrumental in the initial infection of the upper genital tract, while anaerobes, facultative anaerobes, and other bacteria are increasingly isolated as inflammation increases and abscesses form. *Gardnerella vaginalis* may also play a role in the initiation of ascending infection.[3] The microbiology of PID also reflects the predominant sexually transmitted diseases present within a given population.

Pathology and Risk Factors

Most cases of PID are presumed to originate with sexually transmitted disease (STD) of the lower genital tract followed by ascending infection of the upper tract. The original STD may not be symptomatic. It is estimated that 10 to 20 percent of untreated gonococcal or chlamydial cervicitis may progress to PID. The precise mechanisms by which infection in the upper genital tract is initiated and propagated remain unclear. The female genital tract is an open system; therefore a vehicle to transport potential pathogens is unnecessary. Although the cervical mucus serves as a functional barrier to ascending infection much of the time, its efficacy may be decreased by hormonal changes during ovulation and by retrograde menstruation. Bacteria may also be carried by or along with sperm into the uterus and tubes. Uterine infection is usually limited to the endometrium but may be more invasive in a gravid or post-partum uterus. Initial gonorrheal adherence is to non-ciliated cells, but it is felt that surface components of the organism affect neighboring ciliated cells. Tubal infection initially affects only the mucosa, but acute, complement-mediated transmural inflammation may develop rapidly. Inflammation may extend to uninfected parametrial structures including the bowel. If purulent material from the tubes spills into the abdomen, frank pelvic peritonitis may result. Infection may extend via direct or lymphatic spread beyond the pelvis to involve the hepatic capsule with acute perihepatitis and focal peritonitis (Fitzhugh-Curtis syndrome).

Risk factors for PID within a sexually active population include multiple sexual partners, history of other STDs, substance abuse, and frequent vaginal douching. Younger age is associated with increased risk, possibly because of a larger zone of cervical ectopy in young women, increased cervical mucosal permeability, lower prevalence of protective chlamydial antibodies, risk-taking behavior, or a combination of these factors.[4] Barrier contraception is associated with lower risk of PID. IUD use is associated with a 2 to 9 fold increased risk for PID, with the highest risk in the first four months after insertion.[5,6] Oral contraceptive pills (OCPs) increase the risk of endocervical infection, probably by increasing the zone of cervical ectopy. However, OCPs decrease the risk of symptomatic PID, possibly by increasing the viscosity of cervical mucus, decreasing menstrual blood flow (and hence decreasing retrograde menstruation), or modifying local immune responses.[7] Bilateral tubal ligation (BTL) does not provide protection from PID, but patients with BTL may have a clinically milder form of the disease.[8] Bacterial vaginosis (BV) is associated with an increased risk of PID, and BV organisms are frequently cultured from upper genital tract specimens in PID. Pregnancy decreases the risk of PID as the cervical os is protected by a mucous ''plug.'' However, PID can occur during the first trimester and may cause fetal loss.

Complications

PID is associated with a number of serious clinical sequelae. Tubo-ovarian abscess is reported in up to one-third of women hospitalized for PID.[9,10] Infection and inflammation can lead to scarring and adhesions within tubal lumens. The rate of potentially fatal ectopic pregnancy is 12 to 15 percent higher in women who have had PID. TFI is increased 12 to 50 percent in women with a past diagnosis of PID, and the incidence of TFI increases with the number and severity of past PID episodes. Asymptomatic or ''silent'' PID appears to be associated with TFI, as well: 50 percent of women with TFI have no history of PID but do have scarring of the fallopian tubes and exhibit antibodies to *N. gonorrhoeae* and/or *C. trachomatis.*[11] Chronic pelvic pain and/or dyspareunia has been reported in 18 percent of women with past histories of PID.[12]

DIAGNOSIS

Clinical Findings

Lower abdominal pain is the most frequent presenting complaint in PID. Other symptoms may include abnormal vaginal discharge, vaginal bleeding, post-coital bleeding, dyspareunia, irritative voiding symptoms, fever, malaise, nausea, and vomiting. PID may be minimally symptomatic or asymptomatic.[9]

The physical examination is usually notable for lower abdominal tenderness, mucopurulent cervicitis, cervical motion tenderness, and bilateral adnexal tenderness. However, women with PID often present with mild pelvic pain, which can be overlooked by the clinician. Disproportionate unilateral adnexal tenderness and/or adnexal mass or fullness may indicate an ovarian abscess. Abdominal guarding and rebound tenderness will develop with peritonitis. Right upper quadrant tenderness, particularly with jaundice, may indicate Fitzhugh-Curtis syndrome. Signs of other STDs should be noted and evaluated.

Laboratory evaluation in the ED should always include a pregnancy test. The possibility of ectopic pregnancy or septic abortion must be considered, and concurrent pregnancy will affect the treatment for PID. Saline-treated and potassium hydroxide-treated wet preparations of vaginal secretions should be examined for leukorrhea (more than 1 pmn/epithelial cell), trichomoniasis, and clue cells. The absence of leukorrhea has been suggested to be a good negative predictor for PID.[13] Endocervical swabs should be sent for culture and can be gram stained for gonococci. DNA probes for gonorrhea and chlamydia are useful, if available. Elevated white blood cell counts, sedimentation rates, and/or C-reactive protein support the diagnosis of PID. The syphilis test for rapid plasma reagin should be performed. Patients should be counseled on testing for hepatitis and HIV. HIV-infected women with PID may present with more severe symptoms and more frequent coinfection with Candida and human papillomavirus.[14]

Due to the need for early treatment to minimize serious sequelae in vulnerable populations, the diagnosis of PID is usually based on clinical criteria with or without laboratory evidence. The wide range of clinical findings may lead to under or over diagnosis. Table 105-1 details the current Centers for Disease Control and Prevention (CDC) diagnostic criteria for PID.[14]

Procedures

If greater accuracy for the diagnosis of PID is desirable, a number of procedures can be performed. These procedures are not necessary, nor are they indicated, in every case of presumptive PID. In fact, transvaginal pelvic ultrasound is the only procedure that may be considered part of routine evaluation whenever PID is considered within the differential diagnosis.

Transvaginal pelvic ultrasound may demonstrate thickened, fluid-filled fallopian tubes or free pelvic fluid in acute, severe PID.[15] These

TABLE 105-1 Diagnostic Criteria for Pelvic Inflammatory Disease

All major criteria below must be present
Lower abdominal pain
Tenderness on lower abdominal examination
Cervical motion tenderness
Adnexal tenderness
In addition, one or more of the following criteria, will enhance the specificity of the diagnosis
Temperature >101°F (38.3°C)
Abnormal cervical or vaginal discharge
Laboratory evidence of *Chlamydia trachomatis* or *Neisseria gonorrhoeae*
Elevated erythrocyte sedimentation rate or C-reactive protein
The following definitive criteria are warranted in selective cases
Positive transvaginal ultrasound, or other imaging technique, showing thickened, fluid filled tubes with or without tuboovarian abscess or free pelvic fluid, *or*
Positive endometrial biopsy, *or*
Positive laparoscopy

Source: Adapted from Centers for Disease Control and Prevention.[14]

findings alone are not specific enough to make a definitive diagnosis. However, pelvic abscesses may be seen as complex adnexal masses with multiple internal echoes. Pelvic ultrasound will also be useful in evaluating the possibility of ectopic pregnancy in those patients where the differential includes both entities.

Endometrial biopsy can also be used for the definitive histopathologic diagnosis of endometritis. Endometritis is uniformly associated with salpingitis. Specimens for culture may also be obtained but will frequently be contaminated with vaginal flora. The procedure is performed with an endometrial suction pipelle curette and is well tolerated. Endometrial biopsy is approximately 90 percent specific with similar sensitivity. Although this procedure is not difficult, few emergency practitioners are currently trained to do it. Thus, it is best deferred to a gynecologist. Further, its diagnostic utility in the ED setting is limited as results are not immediately available.

Culdocentesis can also be performed rapidly in the ED. However, its utility is also limited. The potential positive findings of leukocytes and bacteria are non-specific and may be a product of other inflammatory processes, such as appendicitis or diverticulitis, or due to contamination with vaginal contents.

Laparoscopy is the current gold standard for the diagnosis of PID.[16] It is significantly more sensitive and specific than clinical criteria alone. The minimum criteria to diagnose PID laparoscopically include visible hyperemia of the tubal surface, tubal wall edema, and the presence of exudate on the tubal surface and fimbriae. Pelvic masses consistent with tubo-ovarian abscess or ectopic pregnancy can also be directly visualized. Hepatic capsule exudate and/or adhesions may be demonstrated. Material may be obtained for definitive culture without the risk of vaginal contamination. However, the procedure is invasive and expensive, requiring an operating room and anesthesia. Findings on laparoscopy do not necessarily correlate with the severity of illness, because the laparoscopist can see only the surface of structures. Laparoscopy may fail to define up to 20 percent of cases.

Differential Diagnosis

The differential diagnosis for PID may include any of the following processes, depending on the specific constellation of signs and symptoms present: cervicitis, ectopic pregnancy, endometriosis, ovarian cyst, ovarian torsion, spontaneous abortion, septic abortion, cholecystitis, gastroenteritis, appendicitis, diverticulitis, pyelonephritis, or renal colic.

TABLE 105-2 Outpatient Antibiotic Management of Pelvic Inflammatory Disease

Ceftriaxone 250 mg IM, *or*
Cefoxitin 2 g IM plus probenecid 1 g PO, *or*
Other parenteral third-generation cephalosporin
plus
Doxycycline 100 mg PO bid × 14 days
or alternative regimen:
Ofloxacin 400 mg PO bid × 14 days
plus
Metronidazole 500 mg PO bid × 14 days

Source: Adapted from the Centers for Disease Control and Prevention.[14]

THERAPY

Treatment

Treatment of PID is aimed at relieving acute symptoms, eradicating current infection, and minimizing the risk of long-term sequelae. There is no clear role for anti-inflammatory drugs per se at this time, but effective analgesia should be administered.[10,17] Therapy initiated in the emergency department must include intravenous hydration and empiric, broad-spectrum antibiotics to cover the full range of likely organisms. All regimens should be effective against anaerobes, gram-negative facultative organisms, and streptococci, as well as *N. gonorrheae* and *C. trachomatis*. A variety of inpatient regimes with broad spectrum coverage have been shown to be effective in eliminating acute symptoms and to effect microbiologic cure (84 to 98 percent cure rates). It is less clear that these regimens can reduce long-term sequelae. However, evidence suggests that long-term outcomes are improved if antibiotics are begun within 48 h of symptom onset. Current CDC recommendations are shown in Tables 105-2 and Table 105-3. Few investigators have assessed and compared parenteral and oral antibiotic regimens, or inpatient versus outpatient regimens, with regard to documented elimination of endometrial and tubal infection.[18,19] Several new regimens, including azithromycin, appear promising in terms of adequacy of coverage and potential patient compliance but are not currently recommended by the CDC because of lack of

TABLE 105-3 Inpatient Antibiotic Management of Pelvic Inflammatory Disease

Cefotetan 2 g IV q12h, *or*
Cefoxitin 2 g IV q6h
plus
Doxycycline 100 mg IV/PO q12h
or alternative regimen:
Clindamycin 900 mg IV q8h
plus
Gentamycin loading dose IV/IM (2 mg/kg) and then maintenance 1.5 mg/kg q8h

Source: Adapted from Centers for Disease Control and Prevention.[14]

data. However, many ED practitioners have already included this in their armamentarium.

If an IUD is present, it should be removed after antibiotics have been started. Parenteral antibiotics may be switched to oral antibiotics 24 h after evidence of clinical improvement. All patients should be re-evaluated in 72 hours for evidence of substantial clinical improvement (defervescence, decreased abdominal tenderness, decreased uterine, adnexal, and cervical motion tenderness) and compliance with their regimen.[20–22] Patients who do not improve within this time frame should be re-evaluated for possible laparoscopic or surgical intervention, i.e., drainage of pus loculations or tubo-ovarian abscess, or to reconsider other possible diagnoses.

Surgical Intervention

The majority of tubo-ovarian abscesses (60 to 80 percent) will resolve with antibiotic administration alone. If patients do not respond clinically to antibiotics, laparoscopy may be useful to identify pus loculations requiring drainage or alternative pathologies. An enlarging pelvic mass may indicate bleeding secondary to vessel erosion or a rupturing abscess. Unresolved abscesses may be drained percutaneously, laparoscopically, or surgically.[10,15]

Disposition

As the incidence of PID has risen, the rate of hospitalization has fallen. With the increasing availability of outpatient parenteral therapy, hospitalization rates may fall further. There is little data to demonstrate whether outpatient treatment is as effective as inpatient treatment in optimizing long-term clinical outcomes. Admission decisions in the ED are based on severity of illness, likelihood of compliance with outpatient medications, likelihood of major anaerobic infection (IUD, suspected pelvic or tubo-ovarian abscess, or history of recent uterine instrumentation), certainty of diagnosis, coexistent illness and immunosuppression, pregnancy, patient age, and other major fertility issues. Admission is warranted in a number of circumstances (see Table 105-4).

PREVENTION

Uncomplicated endocervical infections with *N. gonorrheae* and *C. trachomatis* are under-diagnosed and undertreated in emergency departments.[23] Improving education, diagnosis, and empiric treatment rates for these infections, as well as for minimally symptomatic PID, should result in lower incidence and prevalence of PID and should decrease the incidence of major long-term sequelae, such as infertility and ectopic pregnancy.

Patients discharged with PID are frequently noncompliant with medications, frequently do not understand their diagnoses, and frequently do not obtain partner treatment.[24,25] Patients should be educated about these issues, as well as the advisability of testing and treatment for other STDs, including syphilis and HIV. Patients should understand the use of barrier contraceptives and other ''safe sex'' techniques to lessen their risk of re-infection.

Partners of PID patients should be empirically treated for *N. gonorrheae* and *C. trachomatis* if they have had sexual contact with the patient in the 60 days preceding the onset of her symptoms. Sexual contact should be avoided until one full course of treatment is completed.

TABLE 105-4 Admission Criteria for Pelvic Inflammatory Disease

Pregnancy
Surgical emergencies, such as appendicitis, which cannot be ruled out
Immunosuppression (including HIV infection with low CD4)
Pelvic abscess demonstrated or suspected
Intrauterine device in place
High fever, or severe nausea and vomiting
Compliance with an outpatient regimen unlikely
Failed outpatient therapy
Adolescence
Significant fertility issues present

Source: Adapted from Centers for Disease Control and Prevention.[14]

REFERENCES

1. Aral SO, Mosher WD, Cates WI: Morbidity associated with pelvic inflammatory disease. *JAMA* 266:2570, 1991.
2. McNeeley SG, Hendrix SL, Mezzoni MM, et al: Medically sound, cost-effective treatment for pelvic inflammatory disease and tubo-ovarian abscess. *Am J Obstet Gynecol* 178:1272, 1998.
3. Peipert JF, Montagno AB, Cooper AS, Sung CJ: Bacterial vaginosis as a risk factor for upper genital infection. *Am J Obstet Gynecol* 177:1184, 1997.
4. Padian NS, Washington AE: Pelvic inflammatory disease: A brief overview. *Ann Epidemiol* 4:128, 1994.
5. Grimes DA: Intrauterine devices and pelvic inflammatory disease: Recent developments. *Contraception* 36:97, 1987.
6. Washington AE, Cates W, Wasserheit JN: Preventing pelvic inflammatory disease. *JAMA* 266:2574, 1991.
7. Ness RF, Keder LS, Soper DE, et al: Oral contraception and the recognition of endometritis. *Am J Obstet Gynecol* 176:580, 1997.
8. Abbuhl SB, Muskin EB, Shofer FS: Pelvic inflammatory disease in patients with bilateral tubal ligation. *Am J Emerg Med* 15:271, 1997.
9. Hadgu AH, Westrom L, Brooks CA, et al: Predicting acute pelvic inflammatory disease: A multivariate analysis. *Am J Obstet Gynecol* 155:954, 1986.
10. Landers DV, Sung ML, Bottles K, et al: Does addition of anti-inflammatory agents to antimicrobial therapy reduce infertility after murine chlamydial salpingitis? *Sex Trans Dis* 20:121, 1993.
11. Sellors SW, Mahony JB, Chernesky MA, et al: Tubal factor infertility: An association with prior chlamydial infection and asymptomatic salpingitis. *Fertil Steril* 49:451, 1988.
12. Westrom L: Pelvic inflammatory disease: Bacteriology and sequelae. *Contraception* 36:11, 1987.
13. Peipert JF, Boardman L, Hogan JW, et al: Laboratory evaluation of acute upper genital tract infection. *Obstet Gynecol* 87:730, 1996.
14. Centers for Disease Control and Prevention: 1998 Guidelines for treatment of sexually transmitted diseases. *MMWR* 47(RR 1):79, 1998.
15. Bulas DI, Ahlstrom PA, Sivit CJ, et al: Pelvic inflammatory disease in the adolescent: Comparison of transabdominal and transvaginal sonographic evaluation. *Radiology* 183:435, 1992.
16. Morcos R, Frost N, Hnat M, et al: Laparoscopy versus clinical diagnosis of acute pelvic inflammatory disease. *J Reprod Med* 38:53, 1993.
17. Abbuhl S, Shofer F, Reyes I, Chansky M: Pelvic inflammatory disease: Do we treat for pain? *Ann Emerg Med* 21:640, 1992.
18. Hemsell DL, Nobles BJ, Heard MC, Hemsell PG: Upper and lower reproductive tract bacteria in 126 women with acute pelvic inflammatory disease: Microbial susceptibility and clinical response to four therapeutic regimens. *J Reprod Med* 33:799, 1988.
19. Sweet RL, Bartlett JG, Hemsell DL, et al: Evaluation of new anti-infective drugs for the treatment of acute pelvic inflammatory disease.*Clin Infect Dis* 15(suppl 1):S53, 1992.
20. Augenbraun M, Bachmann L, Wallace T, et al: Compliance with doxycycline therapy in sexually transmitted disease clinics. *Sex Trans Dis* 25:1, 1998.
21. Brookoff D: Compliance with doxycycline therapy for outpatient treatment of pelvic inflammatory disease. *South Med J* 87:1088, 1994.

22. Sweet RL, Schachter J, Landers DV, et al: Treatment of hospitalized patients with acute pelvic inflammatory disease: Comparison of cefotetan plus doxycycline and cefoxitin plus doxycycline. *Am J Obstet Gynecol* 156:736, 1988.
23. Yearly DM, Greene TJ, Hobbs GD: Underrecognition of cervical *Neisseria gonorrheae* and *Chlamydia trachomatis* infections in the emergency department. Acad Emerg Med 4:962, 1997. *Acad Emerg Med* 4:962, 1997.
24. Abbuhl S, Sternhagen A, Campbell E: Emergency department patients with PID: Do they understand their diagnosis? *Ann Emerg Med* 18:436, 1989.
25. Spandorfer SD, Sawin SW, Reyes I, et al: Factors associated with compliance with follow-up in patients treated for outpatient pelvic inflammatory disease. *Clin Pract Sex* 55, 1995.

BREAST DISORDERS

Carol A. Terregino
Rachelle A. Greenman

Few if any breast disorders could be considered imminently life-threatening. However, the psychological and personal issues associated with this part of the anatomy classify such disorders as emergent for the patient. This chapter begins with a functional anatomic and physiologic review appropriate to emergency medicine, reviews the physical examination of the breast and common abnormalities detected by inspection and palpation, and then focuses on infectious, inflammatory, and neoplastic entities that emergency physicians may encounter in their practices. Few evidence-based recommendations exist concerning the management of breast disorders beyond the management of breast carcinoma.

ANATOMY

The human breast is formed from the milk stream, an ectodermally derived tissue, which eventually atrophies, leaving behind the nipple bud. The glandular part of the organ develops subcutaneously. Breast ducts extend down from the nipple into the glandular portion of the breast. The mature breast lies between the deep and the superficial layers of the superficial pectoral fascia. Within the axillary space lie multiple groups of nodes, which are of great interest to the surgeon. Knowledge of the lymphatic drainage of the breast allows prediction of sites of metastatic spread.

Three tissue types make up the mature breast: epithelium, fibrous stroma, and fat. The fat composition of the breast increases with age, allowing improved radiographic detection of abnormalities by mammography. Cooper's ligaments are strands of dense connective tissue that extend from the skin through the fat to the underlying deep fascia. Any contraction or impingement on these ligaments, as commonly occurs with cancer, causes a dimpling pattern of the skin. The glandular portion of the breast is composed of ducts that extend downward from the nipple areolar complex and branch radially, terminating in spaces called ductal glandular units, the milk-producing glands of the lactating breast. At the surface of the nipple are 15 to 30 orifices lined with low columnar or cuboidal epithelium that meets with squamous epithelium at the surface.

In prepubescence, the breast tissue is composed of dense fibrous stroma and scattered ducts. Increase in adipose tissue and glandular development are under hormonal influence. The development of breast buds in a prepubescent female unaccompanied by other changes of puberty is called prepubertal gynecomastia, and this entity should not be confused with puberty. During phases of the menstrual cycle, the breast undergoes cyclic changes, including hypertrophy of the stroma and the epithelium and intralobular fluid accumulation corresponding to perimenstrual breast engorgement. During pregnancy there is an increase in lobular units; this is termed adenosis of pregnancy. In lactating females, prolactin stimulates milk production. Milk expulsion is under the control of oxytocin stimulation of myoepithelial cells.

EXAMINATION OF THE BREAST

A systematic approach to the breast examination is essential. The breasts must be inspected for size and symmetry, although some degree of asymmetry is not uncommon and is usually normal. The contour of the breast must be inspected, with special attention to dimpling, masses, or flattening. In order to accentuate potential dimpling, have the patient raise her hands above her head. The color, venous pattern, and any edematous changes should be noted. Nipple inversion of long standing is common and usually normal. Areolar or nipple rashes or ulcerations should be noted. For palpation of the breast, the patient must be in a supine position. Placement of a pillow under the patient's shoulder on the examination side and her arm above her head helps to spread the breast tissue over the chest and make palpation of nodules easier. A patterned approach should be used to ensure that all breast tissue is palpated. The pads of the three middle fingers should be used with a rotatory motion. The consistency of the breast changes with age and the hormonal milieu. Nodules should be described according to their quadrant (upper and lower, outer and inner), shape, size, relationship to surrounding tissue, and tenderness. The nipple should be palpated and compressed for discharge.

ABNORMAL LACTATION

Lactation is the response to normal hormonal stimulation associated with pregnancy and the postpartum period. Prolactin secretion is under a negative control; its levels are determined by neurohormonal transmitters affecting its inhibitory factors, the most important one being dopamine. High levels of estrogen and progesterone during pregnancy inhibit the release of prolactin inhibitory factor. The rising estrogen levels also increase the growth of pituitary lactotrophs. While the prolactin secreted during pregnancy prepares the breast for lactation, lactation does not occur until estrogen levels fall precipitously after delivery. Multiple hormones, including thyroid hormone, insulin, growth hormone, placental lactogen, and cortisol in addition to prolactin, progesterone, and estrogen, prime the breasts to prepare for lactation by stimulating proliferative and secretory activity of the breast alveolar cells. Within 20 to 30 min of nursing, prolactin levels rise to 60 times normal. The discharge is milky, white, and thin and usually involves multiple ducts. Rarely, a bloody lactation, due to the high estrogen levels of pregnancy, may be seen. When weaning, it may take weeks for lactation to cease. However, if the nipples continue to be stimulated manually, the discharge may continue for years.

Galactorrhea is an inappropriate nonlactational milky white nipple discharge. Spontaneous galactorrhea usually indicates hyperprolactinemia, especially when there is concomitant amenorrhea. However, in approximately 30 percent of cases, prolactin levels are normal. Physiologic hormonal alterations that occur at menarche and early menopause can sometimes cause galactorrhea. Hormonal preparations can stimulate the breast tissue directly, elevating prolactin levels and stimulates milk production.

Increased prolactin levels can also be caused by nipple stimulation, chest wall trauma, reduction mammoplasty, breast augmentation, herpes zoster infection of the breast, and postherpetic neuralgia. Rare oncologic causes include ectopic secretion by renal adenocarcinoma, bronchogenic carcinoma, and other prolactin- or estrogen-secreting neoplasms. Increased physical exertion, sexual intercourse, seizures, and hypoglycemia can also stimulate prolactin release.

Pathologic hyperprolactinemia is a frequent cause of the amenorrhea-galactorrhea syndrome. As discussed above, prolactin secretion is predominantly inhibited by dopamine, which is transported along the hypophyseal stalk from the hypothalamus to the pituitary gland, where it directly inhibits synthesis and secretion. Any damage to the hypothalamus or hypophyseal stalk by lesions, such as tumors, radiation scarring, or trauma in addition to congenital, vascular, ischemia, or inflammatory lesions, may result in increased serum prolactin levels.[1]

Drugs that alter dopamine secretion can also cause hyperprolactinemia. The most common causes of hyperprolactinemia include psychotropic agents, such as phenothiazines, haloperidol, tricyclic antidepressants, and fluoxetine. Reserpine and α-methyldopa may cause hyperprolactinemia due to depletion of dopamine reserves. Other drugs shown to increase prolactin levels include calcium channel blockers, angiotensin-converting enzyme inhibitors, cocaine, opiates, marijuana, and H_2 antagonists. Although estrogen therapy can increase prolactin levels, typically oral contraceptives do not increase serum prolactin levels.

Certain medical conditions, such as chronic renal disease and, rarely, liver failure, can cause increased prolactin levels. Hypothyroidism can lead to hyperprolactinemia, galactorrhea, and amenorrhea due to the effects of thyrotropin-releasing factor on the pituitary gland.

Prolactinomas, prolactin-secreting pituitary tumors, are a frequent cause of hyperprolactinemia. Pituitary adenomas secreting other hormones, such as growth hormone and ACTH along with prolactin, may also cause galactorrhea. Therefore, patients with galactorrhea should be evaluated for acromegaly and Cushing disease. Assessment includes visual field and extraocular movement testing. Cranial nerve involvement or diplopia could indicate extension of the tumor into the cavernous sinus. Patients with symptoms or signs of intracranial mass such as headache, nausea, vomiting, or visual abnormality, need immediate neuroimaging studies (computed tomography or magnetic resonance imaging) and neurosurgical consultation.

Routine determination of prolactin levels is not indicated in the emergency department without endocrinologic consultation. Pituitary tumors usually generate prolactin levels greater than 200 μg/L; however, random prolactin levels may not reflect an abnormality. Prolactin levels less than 100 μg/L units are usually not of tumor origin and are probably related to drugs.[1]

Management of galactorrhea in the emergency department should include determination of the urine or serum β-human chorionic gonadotropin level, evaluation for neuroophthalmologic abnormalities and imaging as previously discussed. Further hormonal workup, including serial determination of prolactin, thyroid-stimulating hormone, and growth hormone levels, can be left to the discretion of the primary care provider or specialist. The majority of patients require no intervention other than reassurance and perhaps cessation of drugs. Almost all patients with pituitary-induced hyperprolactinemia can be effectively treated with the dopamine agonist bromocriptine, which normalizes prolactin levels in 80 to 90 percent of patients, restores menses, and halts galactorrhea.[1] Bromocriptine is also useful for treating galactorrhea in patients with normal prolactin levels. Although an understanding of the basis and effects of such treatment is useful, it is not within the purview of emergency medicine.

NIPPLE DISCHARGE

Nipple discharge is a common complaint in benign breast disease. Pathologic processes must be distinguished from the more common physiologic ones. Physiologic discharges usually require manual compression, involve multiple ducts, and are bilateral. The fluid may be clear, white, yellow, or dark green. Discharges of long duration are less likely to be clinically significant.[2]

On the other hand, pathologic nipple discharge is spontaneous, usually unilateral, confined to a single duct, bloody, and associated with a mass. The most common cause of pathologic nipple discharge is intraductal papilloma, followed by duct ectasia (discussed below).[2] While most nipple discharges associated with cancer are bloody, cancer has been shown to be the cause of only 6 percent of cases of bloody discharge.[2]

The precise incidence of breast cancer in women with nipple discharge is unknown.[3] If a palpable mass is associated with a discharge, the likelihood of carcinoma is greatly increased. In a series of women presenting with nipple discharge, over 60 percent of patients with a palpable mass and spontaneous nipple discharge had carcinoma, compared to 6 percent in patients with nipple discharge only.[3]

Workup of spontaneous nipple discharge or a nipple discharge with a mass should include a complete breast examination and referral of all women over age 35 for a mammogram and evaluation by a breast surgeon. Nonspontaneous nipple discharge without a mass can be referred to a primary care provider for arrangement of a mammogram.[3] All postmenopausal discharges are significant. If practical, the discharge should be assessed for the presence of occult blood, which can be done using either a white gauze or reagent stick. Sending the discharge for cytologic analysis may be helpful if the results are positive; the absence of malignant cells does not exclude carcinoma.

SKIN DISORDERS AFFECTING THE NIPPLE AND BREAST

Any disorder of the skin can affect the breast. Some of the more important ones specific to the breast and nipple are discussed below.

Colonization of the nipples or the lactiferous ducts by *Candida albicans* may cause chronically sore nipples during or after lactation. The appearance of the nipple may be normal; however, more commonly, scaling, fissuring, and erythema are present. Predisposing factors for candidal colonization include antibiotic use, vaginal candidiasis, mastitis, and nipple trauma occurring in the early lactation period. Definitive diagnosis may be made by fungal culture, but that should not be necessary. The nipples may be treated with topical antifungal creams.[4] Vaginal candidiasis in the patient, as well as any clinically evident oral candidiasis in the infant, should also be treated.

Atopic dermatitis, which may affect one or both nipples, is manifested by areas of fissuring, weeping skin, or lichenification. This condition occurs in both pregnant and nonpregnant women, most commonly between the ages of 15 and 30. This dermatitis is more common in atopic individuals. Underlying causes of these skin changes include scabies, contact allergy, local medication reaction, and irritation secondary to friction.[5]

Paget's disease is an uncommon neoplastic disorder that usually begins at the nipple and spreads outward, secondarily involving the areola. This is an important distinction, since benign skin conditions begin on the areola. The appearance ranges from that of an eczema-like erosion of the nipple to a red, raw surface, with a copious, clear discharge. Both the areola and nipple have chronic, moist eczematous changes. Paget's disease is estimated to occur in 1 to 2 percent of breast cancers.[4] Most cases are diagnosed in postmenopausal women. Unfortunately, early symptoms, such as an itching or burning sensation of the nipple, may be subtle and may have been present for years before the diagnosis is made. Paget's disease is usually unilateral. Patients may note a small crusted area, with staining of the clothing, or an overt serous or bloody discharge from the nipples. Dermatologic changes of the nipple and areola progress slowly. In later cases, there may be a sharply demarcated area on the nipple areola complex. The nipple may become retracted or deformed.

The histology of Paget's disease is an intraductal carcinoma occurring in the large sinuses beneath the nipple. The carcinomatous cells invade across the nipple epithelium. Paget's disease of the nipple has an associated palpable underlying mass in 50 percent of cases, and 90 percent of these patients have invasive intraductal carcinoma of the breast. Seventy percent of these patients without a palpable mass have in situ intraductal breast carcinoma; the remainder are diagnosed with invasive disease at a later date.[6]

Treatment for intraductal carcinoma associated with Paget's disease is related to the underlying carcinoma. The long-term outcome for treated patients is excellent. Referral to a breast surgeon is mandatory. Topical steroids should never be prescribed because the anti-inflammatory effects may delay the diagnosis.

Mondor's disease of the breast is a superficial phlebitis of the veins in the subcutaneous tissue of the breast. This condition may occur postoperatively or after minor trauma. The patient presents complaining of a painful induration across the costal margin. A cord may be present. The phlebitis may be tender for several weeks. No treatment other than analgesia is required. Follow-up evaluation with a surgeon is indicated.[4]

An ''orange-peel'' appearance of the skin, or *peau d'orange,* is produced by skin edema emphasizing the skin sweat glands. Such a breast appearance indicates underlying breast carcinoma with both stromal infiltration and lymphatic obstruction, causing skin edema. Referral to a breast surgeon for appropriate diagnostic testing and treatment is always indicated.

Erosive adenomatosis of the nipple is an uncommon, benign tumor of the nipple that generally occurs in the fourth decade. It is a proliferation of the lactiferous ducts that usually occurs unilaterally but may occur bilaterally. The onset is insidious and may begin with a serous or bloody nipple discharge that worsens in the premenstrual period. Occasionally, there may be a palpable nodule, but usually the nipple appears eroded or eczematous. There is no accompanying axillary lymphadenopathy. The patient should be referred to a breast surgeon. Complete excision, which may include the entire nipple if it is involved, is curative.

BENIGN BREAST DISEASE

Benign breast disease is traditionally considered to be due to hormonal influence. Prolonged hormonal imbalance leads to proliferation of breast tissue, leading to edema and discomfort. The clinical characteristics of benign breast disease include mastalgia or cyclic breast pain, isolated unilateral or bilateral breast lumps (either cysts or fibroadenomas), bilateral nodularities in the perimenstrual period, fibrocystic disease, and nipple discharge, as discussed above.[7] The patient should be referred to a breast specialist for confirmation of this diagnosis.

NONLACTATIONAL INFLAMMATION (MASTITIS)

Nonlactational mastitis and duct ectasia, or dilated ducts filled with stagnant secretions, make up a clinical complex. A discussion of the confusion in disease classification arising from these independently described conditions is beyond the scope of this chapter. Hughes provides a clear overview of the clinical conditions and their management.[8] Duct ectasia is generally a subclinical condition, with nipple discharge that is either serosanguineous or occultly positive for blood, as the most common clinical manifestation. Patients with mastitis have an average age of 40 years. In some series, up to one-third of patients have type II diabetes mellitus.[9]

Mastitis originates in the subareolar ducts and extends outward in the breast. The cause is generally infectious, and the organisms include gram-negative organisms and anaerobes in addition to *Staphylococcus aureus.* Occasionally, mastitis occurs in areas of cystic breast tissue without an infectious cause. Periductal mastitis may be an evanescent tender breast mass that resolves spontaneously or persistent inflammatory reaction that progresses to abscess formation. Mastitis is manifested by pain, erythema, and warmth of the overlying skin, with exquisite tenderness. Nipple retraction or fistula formation at the edge of the areola occurs frequently with recurrent episodes of periductal mastitis with or without abscess formation.

Management is generally conservative, with heat and antibiotics in an outpatient setting. Referral for mammography is impractical, given the degree of compression necessary to get an adequate image of the inflamed breast. For detection of an abscess cavity, breast ultrasound is more sensitive. Patients should always be referred to a breast specialist for follow-up, since the diagnosis of inflammatory carcinoma must be excluded. All cases should be followed for complete resolution of signs or symptoms.

BREAST ABSCESS

Pathophysiology

Breast abscess may be difficult to distinguish from breast mastitis, a more generalized cellulitis. Due to the compartmentalized structure of the breast, regions of necrosis and avascularity, the abscess may lie deep to the overlying tissues. Typical fluctuance may be difficult to appreciate. The pathophysiology of this entity is not precisely known. However, it has been suggested that it may be due to plugging of the ductal openings by keratin at the junction of squamous cell with cuboid epithelium or due to duct ectasia. Bacterial invasions, more commonly by *staphylococcus,* leads to abscess development. However, as in mastitis, other microorganisms have also been associated with breast abscess. In one case series, monomicrobial aerobic bacteria were most frequently identified with a significant percentage of *proteus mirabilis* isolates. Additionally, polymicrobial anaerobic cultures, most frequently *Peptostreptococcus spp.* and *Bacteroides sp.,* are commonly found in recurrent breast abscesses.[10] The most common site for breast abscesses to occur is in the subareolar tissue. These are difficult to treat and have a high incidence of recurrence.

Diagnosis

The diagnosis of breast abscesses should be considered in all patients who present with painful breast mass, particularly inflammatory conditions. Some recommend ultrasonographic assessment of suspected breast abscess as not all women have an obvious collection of focal pus.[11] Alternatively, as long as carcinoma is not suspected, aspiration for diagnosis can be attempted. A negative aspiration does not exclude the diagnosis of abscess. The technique of aspiration is the same as for suspected abscess at other near-surface body sites.

Treatment

Treatment is determined by the degree of inflamation and the stage of abscesses development.[12] Patients presenting to the ED with small, early subareolar abscess should be treated conservatively with antibiotics alone for a 2-week period. Broad spectrum antibiotics should be prescribed given the high percentage of anaerobes and other aerobes other than *staphylococcus aureus.* Warm compresses and analgesia should be prescribed for pain relief. More severe infections may require hospitalization with intravenous antibiotics, especially in patients with systemic toxicity, diabetes mellitus, or immunocompromise. The patient treated with antibiotics as an outpatient should be referred to a surgeon for follow-up within 24 to 72 h to monitor resolution of signs and symptoms.

The appropriate surgical management of breast abscess is debated.[12] If the patient presents with a fluctuant abscess, one that has drained spontaneously, or if the abscess cannot be treated by antibiotics alone, some recommend a procedure under general anesthesia with wide incision.[12] Commonly, a more conservative incision is recommended. Although some emergency physicians will perform an incision and drainage procedure in the ED, given the potential for multiloculation and the difficulty in achieving adequate analgesia required for appropriate drainage, this procedure is best performed by a breast surgeon under more ideal circumstances. Needle aspiration may be attempted. However, as noted, the abscess is usually multiloculated and the procedure is unlikely to be successful. Some recommend another conservative management approach to breast abscess with ultrasonographic assessment and aspiration.[11]

When evaluating a patient for breast abscess, search for a history of recurrent infection. Case series of women with subareolar abscesses have shown that recurrences occur both in patients treated with antibiotics alone and with incision and drainage in addition to antibiotics.[12]

Recurrent infections may best treated by incision of the ducts, at the discretion of the breast surgeon.

LACTATIONAL MASTITIS

Postpartum mastitis is much more common than nonpuerperal mastitis. The pathophysiology involves obstruction of the duct, inspissation of milk, and secondary bacterial invasion. The patient has localized warmth and tenderness of the affected breast. She may even have systemic symptoms and signs, such as fever, malaise, and leukocytosis. The condition is so painful that it may threaten continuation of breast-feeding. Most authors recommend a conservative approach to mastitis in postpartum patients. Analgesia, warm or cold compresses, and increased pumping of the affected breast have all been recommended. The most commonly identified organism is *S. aureus*. Antibiotics are frequently recommended for lactational mastitis, and the best choice is a penicillinase-resistant penicillin. However, if abscess is present, anaerobes may be involved, and clindamycin is a better choice. Lactating mothers question whether it is safe to continue to nurse with mastitis. Clearly, emptying of the breast, either by a mechanical pump or manually, leads to quicker resolution of the condition. The affected breast milk will not harm the baby, although, with breast abscess, ongoing nursing on the unaffected side with expression of milk on the affected side seems to be the best management approach.[13]

MASTITIS VERSUS INFLAMMATORY CARCINOMA

The differential diagnosis of an inflamed breast in a lactating woman includes acute mastitis, abscess, and, very rarely, cancer. Breast infection in a nonlactating woman, on the other hand, is not as common. The differential diagnosis of inflammation includes duct ectasia, nonpuepural breast abscess, and cancer. Inflammatory breast cancer must be distinguished from mastitis. Whereas the breast tissue changes of mastitis are typically well circumscribed, inflammatory breast cancer generally involves at least one-third of the breast tissue, and edges are not well demarcated.[14] There may or may not be a palpable mass in inflammatory breast carcinoma. However, the breast usually increases in size. Due to the diffuse invasion of lymphatic channels by tumor cells, axillary nodal metastases are almost always present at the time of diagnosis. The classically described *peau d'orange* appearance of the breast is due to edema and thickening of the skin. The breast discoloration may have a uniform appearance or be seen in the dependent part of the breast. Nipple retraction, with dermatologic findings, may occur as the disease progresses. Prolonged use of antibiotics in patients thought to have mastitis may cause significant delays in the diagnosis and treatment of breast cancer. A breast specialist should be consulted for chronic breast infections.[14]

BREAST CANCER

The report by the American Cancer Society that one in eight women will develop breast cancer is actually misleading, in that the risk is cumulative, with half of the risk occurring after the age of 65. The risk for African-American women is only 7 to 8 percent. Such statistics contribute to the anxiety experienced by patients with a breast mass. While the specifics of diagnostics, treatment, and prognosis in breast carcinoma are beyond the scope of this chapter and beyond the purview of emergency medicine, the emergency physician should be familiar with general issues concerning risks, cancer type, and therapy in order to counsel patients in the department.

The etiology of breast cancer is multifactorial. Family history is an important determinant if a mother or a sister develops breast cancer during the premenopausal years or when the disease occurs bilaterally. Genetic mutations have been identified. However, only 5 to 10 percent of all breast cancers are due to such mutations.[2] Specific risks for carrying the BRCA1 and BRCA2 mutations, and the subsequent risks for development of disease have been reviewed by others.[2] Such specifics are best left to genetic counselors or breast specialists, and genetic testing should not be ordered in the emergency department. Less well-defined, and more universally applicable risk factors for breast cancer include nulliparity, late first pregnancy or late menopause, increased fat intake, exogenous estrogen, and ethanol use.

The major subdivisions of breast carcinoma are noninvasive and invasive tumors. Ductal carcinoma in situ (DCIS) is a noninvasive cancer that remains in the ducts without invasion to the surrounding tissue. Presentations of DCIS include a mammographic mass, microcalcifications, nipple discharge, Paget's disease of the breast, or a palpable mass. Treatment options for DCIS include excision, excision and radiation, or mastectomy. The National Surgical Adjuvent Breast Protocol showed decreased recurrence in patients treated with irradiation, as compared to lumpectomy alone, and a recurrence rate equal to that of mastectomy.[15]

Infiltrative ductal carcinoma is the most common type of invasive breast cancer, accounting for 65 to 85 percent of cases. Infiltrative lobular carcinoma accounts for 5 to 10 percent of cases. Its presentation may be a subtle thickening of the breast, rather than a mass. For early-stage carcinomas, the National Cancer Institute Consensus has determined breast conserving therapy to be appropriate.[16] An important meta-analysis of 133 breast cancer trials involving 75,000 women has formed the basis of current recommendations for adjuvant chemotherapy in breast cancer.[17] Risk reduction depends on the patient's absolute risk for recurrence. Axillary node dissection for metastatic spread assessment clarifies the risk; however, 20 to 30 percent of node-negative women die of their disease. Emergency medicine management issues regarding the patient receiving adjuvant chemotherapy for breast cancer are included in Chap. 217, ''Emergency Complications of Malignancy''.

Evaluation of an Isolated Breast Mass

Detection of a palpable breast mass, solid or cystic, is of great concern to patients and may prompt an emergency department visit. The emergency physician should examine the patient systematically, as described above, and determine whether a true mass exists. The normal glandular breast tissue has a nodular consistency. Both the upper outer quadrant of the breast and the inframammary ridge have increased nodularity. When a nodularity is persistent throughout the menstrual cycle, it may well be a true mass and may represent a number of entities, including cyst, fibroadenoma, fibrocystic change, or carcinoma. Usually, a patient with a breast malignancy presents with a solitary mass in the upper outer quadrant. Poorly defined masses or thickenings may also be cancer. The breast may be indurated, with thickened skin and nipple retraction. A serosanguineous nipple discharge may be present.

The patient should always be referred for mammography and evaluation by a specialist, even if a mass cannot be detected on examination.

Aspiration of solid or cystic breast masses is best left to a specialist or a provider of continuity of care. A necrotizing breast carcinoma may present identically to abscess, and some authors recommend biopsy of the abscess wall at the time of abscess drainage,[9] a procedure clearly beyond the scope of emergency medicine practice. Some authors recommend that the same person who performs the fine-needle aspiration procedure be the evaluating cytopathologist,[18] especially since the feel of the lesion (e.g., the rubbery consistency of a fibroadenoma, the gritty consistency of a malignancy, or the resistant nature of a fibrocystic lesion) has diagnostic importance. In addition, nuances in technique are best left to the specialists (e.g., obtaining a dermal specimen when inflammatory disease of the breast is suspected). The consensus statement of a National Cancer Institute conference has identified the specific indications and training and credentialing recommendations for fine-needle aspiration of breast masses.[19]

ACKNOWLEDGMENT

The authors wish to thank Maureen Kling, MD, for her thoughtful review of the manuscript.

REFERENCES

1. Katznelson K, Klibanski A: Prolactinomas, in Arnold A (ed): *Endocrine Neoplasms*. Boston, Kluwer Academic, 1997, pp 41–55.
2. Hansen N, Morrow M: Breast disease. *Med Clin North Am* 82:203, 1998.
3. Gülay H, Bora S, Kiliçturgay S, et al: Management of nipple discharge. *J Am Coll Surg,* 178:471, 1994.
4. Amir LH, Garland SM, Dennerstein L, et al: *Candida albicans:* Is it associated with nipple pain in lactating women? *Gynecol Obstet Invest* 41:30, 1996.
5. Ward KA, Burton JL: Dermatologic diseases of the breast in young women. *Clin Dermatol* 15:45, 1997.
6. Dixon JM, Sainsbury JR, Rodger A: Breast cancer: Treatment of elderly patients and uncommon conditions. *BMJ* 309:1292, 1994.
7. Sitruk-Ware R: Benign breast disease. *Curr Ther Endocrinol Metab* 6:396, 1997.
8. Hughes LE: Non-lactational inflammation and duct ectasia. *Br Med Bull* 47:272, 1991.
9. Leveque J, Lorino CO, Ferrara JJ: Inflammatory disease of the breast. *Recent Results Cancer Res* 119:18, 1990.
10. Meguid MM, Oler A, Numann PJ, et al: Pathogenesis-based treatment of recurring subareolar breast abscesses. *Surgery* 118:775, 1995.
11. Alados JC, Perez M, Fontes J: Bacteriology of non-puerperal breast abscesses. *Int J Gynaecol Obstet* 48:105, 1995.
12. O'Hara RJ, Dexter SP, Fox JN: Conservative management of infective mastitis and breast abscesses after ultrasonographic assessment. *Br J Surg* 83:1413, 1996.
13. Banapurmath CR, Banapurmath SC, Mallikarjuna HB, et al: Successful management of breast abscess with ongoing breast feeding. *Indian Pediatr* 32:488, 1995.
14. Dahlbeck SW, Donnelly JF, Theriault RL: Differentiating inflammatory breast cancer from acute mastitis. *Am Fam Physician* 52:29, 1995.
17. Fisher B, Costantino J, Redmond C, et al: Lumpectomy compared with lumpectomy and radiation therapy for the treatment6 of intraductal breast cancer. *N Engl J Med* 328:1591, 1993.
16. National Institute of Health Consensus Development Panel: Consensus statement: Treatment of early-stage breast cancer. *J Nat Cancer Inst Monogr* 11:11, 1992.
17. Early Breast Cancer Trialists Collaborative Group: Systemic treatment of early breast cancer by hormonal, cytotoxic, hormone therapy: 133 randomized trials involving 31,000 recurrences and 24,000 deaths among 75,000 women. *Lancet* 339:71, 1993.
18. Sanchez MA, Stahl RE: Fine-needle aspiration of the breast. *Pathology* 4:253, 1996.
19. NIH Consensus Development Conference: The uniform approach to breast fine-needle aspiration biopsy. *Am J Surg* 174:371, 1997.

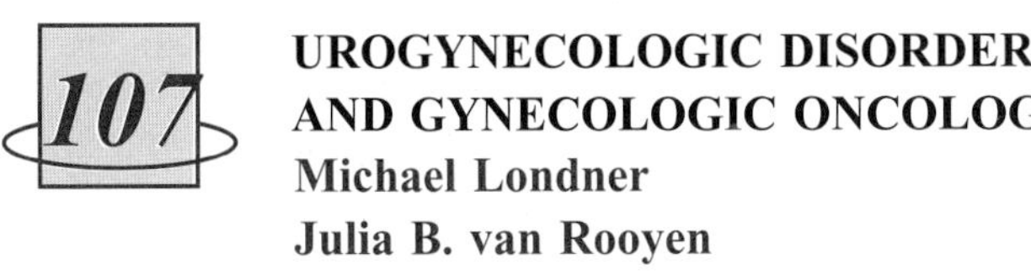

UROGYNECOLOGIC DISORDERS AND GYNECOLOGIC ONCOLOGY

Michael Londner
Julia B. van Rooyen

This chapter discusses the urogynecologic problems of incontinence, prolapse, and urethral syndrome and reviews the more common gynecologic malignancies and their complications.

INCONTINENCE

Although different authors categorize incontinence in various ways, the four most common groupings are

1. Urinary stress incontinence
2. Urge incontinence
3. Total incontinence
4. Overflow incontinence

The six main anatomic structures contributing to continence are

1. The detrusor muscle, a meshwork of fibers surrounding the bladder.
2. The urethra, a 3- to 4-cm tube surrounded mainly by smooth muscle.
3. The urethral sphincter, which provides the secondary defense to urinary incontinence and about 50 percent of total urethral resistance.
4. Two posterior pubourethral ligaments, which suspend the urethra, holding it close to the pubic bone.
5. The autonomic nervous system, the parasympathetic and sympathetic nerves that supply the lower genitourinary tract. Parasympathetic fibers S_2 to S_4 cause detrusor contraction (cholinergic drugs do the same). Sympathetic fibers T_{10} to L_2 have α- and β-adrenergic components. Alpha fibers stimulate the bladder neck and urethral contraction while relaxing the detrusor muscle. Beta fibers relax the urethra and the detrusor muscle.
6. Pudendal innervation provides voluntary urethral contraction.

Continence is maintained because intraurethral pressure exceeds intravesical pressure. The levator ani, surrounding fascia, and ligaments help maintain urethral anatomy in times of abrupt changes associated in intraabdominal pressure.

Stress urinary incontinence occurs when urine is involuntarily lost as a result of increased intraabdominal pressure, i.e., when the intraurethral pressure is less than the intraabdominal pressure. It is caused by multiparity, vaginal delivery, pregnancy, menopause, chronic cough (i.e., chronic obstructive pulmonary disease), or other forms of pelvic relaxation. Symptoms include leaking of urine during cough, straining, laughing, sneezing, running, or other causes of increased intraabdominal pressure. Diagnosis involves ruling out infection, neurologic disease, medications, or other systemic illness as possible causes of stress urinary incontinence. A thorough history and physical examination are required, including full vaginal examination with inspection of all the vaginal walls. Further workup by the consulting gynecologist includes stress testing and, if necessary, urodynamic testing. Treatment options are both nonoperative and operative. Nonoperative options include Kegel exercises, estrogen, α-adrenergic stimulants, intravaginal weights, and *urethral plugs.* Operative management is the approach used most commonly. The purpose of incontinence surgery is to correct the defect and restore the anatomy of the urethra. Surgery may be laparoscopic, vaginal, abdominal, or a combination of these. The list of procedures and variations are very long, but the most common include the Marshall-Marchetti-Kranz, Burch, Pereyra, Stamey, and Raz procedures, collagen injections, and sling suspensions.

Urge incontinence occurs in the setting of detrusor muscle instability. The incidence of this entity is around 15 to 20 percent of all women with incontinence but markedly increases with increasing age. It is often seen in conjunction with stress urinary incontinence also known as *mixed incontinence.* The precise etiology of urge incontinence is unknown, but it is seen in the presence of foreign bodies (suture inadvertently placed in the bladder), intravesical stones, and/or infection. Symptoms include urinary urgency, frequency, nocturia, and incontinence. Observing involuntary detrusor contractions during cystometrics or urodynamic studies is diagnostic. Treatment includes pharmacologic agents (e.g., anticholinergics, β-sympathomimetics, musculotrophics, TCAs, or dopamine agonists), bladder training, biofeedback, and functional electrical stimulation.

Total incontinence is usually the result of a urinary fistula. Fistulas usually occur as a result of pelvic surgery, radiation, and in underdeveloped countries, obstetrical injuries. Greater than 50 percent of fistulas occur after a hysterectomy. Patients present with constant, painless leaking of urine and/or recurrent infections. Placing a tampon into the vagina and instilling methylene blue into the bladder helps to make the diagnosis. In the event that a vesicovaginal fistulae is present, the tampon will stain blue. If there is no staining, then indigo carmine is injected intravenously. If the tampon then stains blue, a ureterovaginal fistula is present. An intravenouspyelogram (IVP) should be obtained in either situation to help define the anatomy and rule out other multiple fistulas. Treatment is initiated with insertion of a diverting Foley catheter and may lead to spontaneous healing if the injury is recent but probably will require operative repair.

Overflow incontinence is a result of urinary retention from a hypotonic detrusor muscle. This is seen in the setting of neuropathy secondary to diabetes, spinal cord injuries, outflow obstruction, postoperatively, or lower motor neuron diseases (i.e., multiple sclerosis). Symptoms include postvoid bladder fullness (the ''feeling'' of never having an empty bladder), small quantities on micturition, and leaking. Diagnosis is made through complete history and physical examination with emphasis on the neurologic examination and determination of postvoid residual volume. Therapy is directed at treating the underlying cause and teaching intermittent self-catheterization.

PROLAPSE

The female pelvic organs, i.e., vagina, uterus, bladder, and rectum, are held in proper alignment by supporting ligaments, fascia, and the pelvic floor muscles. When any or all of these structures fail, the pelvic organs may prolapse within and occasionally protrude through the vagina. This prolapse or displacement may occur singly or more commonly combined. Prolapse can be divided into two broad categories, uterine and vaginal.

Uterine prolapse is graded as first through third degree.

First degree: The cervix remains within the vagina.
Second degree: The cervix protrudes beyond the introitus.
Third degree: This implies descent of the entire uterus outside the vulva, also known as *procidentia.*

This classification system is actually slowly being replaced with staging of all pelvic prolapses through one pelvic organ prolapse quantification (POPQ) profile, now standardized terminology.

A prolapsed, elongated, inflamed, edematous cervix may be mistaken for uterine prolapse if careful evaluation is not undertaken. Procidentia represents complete failure of all supporting structures. The vagina can prolapse without accompanying uterine prolapse, but the uterus cannot prolapse without bringing the upper vagina with it.

Vaginal prolapse is best subdivided into four basic quadrants:

1. Upper anterior vaginal wall: cystocele (represents weakness of the pubocervical fascia)
2. Lower anterior vaginal wall: urethral displacement
3. Upper posterior vaginal wall: enterocele (usually associated with herniation into the pouch of Douglas)
4. Lower posterior vaginal wall: rectocele

In addition, inversion of the vagina is known as *vault prolapse.* Most commonly prolapse results from attenuation of pelvic fascia, ligaments, and muscles following extensive stretching during vaginal delivery. However, prolapse can occur after easy labor or in the nulliparous woman, in which case it is considered a congenital or developmental weakness of pelvic connective tissue. Virtually any cause of repeated increased intraabdominal pressure may lead to prolapse, including chronic cough, ascites, heavy lifting, or habitual straining on defecation. These mechanisms should raise concern to search for occult malignancy, e.g., lung cancer in a person with chronic cough or colonic cancer in someone straining to defecate. Atrophy of the supporting tissue plays a significant role in initiation or worsening of this condition.

The degree of symptomatology is quite variable. The most common complaint is a ''feeling of heaviness or fullness in the pelvis.'' Others may describe ''something falling out.'' More diffuse complaints include backache, pelvic discomfort, and discomfort or straining with defecation or urination. Cystocele may present with frequency, urgency, incontinence, or ultimately, retention (especially if displacement causes kinking of the ureter), whereas rectocele may present with difficulty evacuating the rectal vault.[1] A characteristic not to be overlooked is the worsening of symptoms with prolonged standing followed by alleviation when lying down. Women may become extremely tolerant of prolapse symptoms and present with advanced complications such as infection of the prolapsed segment, decubitus ulceration, bleeding, and carcinoma of the cervix.

Diagnosis revolves around a thorough history and physical examination including vaginal examination. Use of a Sim's speculum or separating the two halves of the standard Grave's speculum and using the posterior blade allows for adequate vaginal inspection. Depress the posterior vaginal wall and ask the patient to bear down. This will demonstrate descent of the anterior vaginal wall in the setting of cystocele and/or urethral displacement. Reversing the speculum to elevate the anterior vaginal wall allows visualization of the intruding posterior wall during straining demonstrative of enterocele or rectocele. A rectal examination often will help to distinguish rectocele from enterocele.

Treatment modalities are grouped into nonoperative and operative.[2] The patient's age, future fertility, degree of sexual activity, and degree of prolapse must be considered in defining a management plan. Nonoperative treatments generally are tried first if future childbearing is desired, the degree of pathology is mild, or the patient is a poor surgical candidate. These options include Kegel (pelvic floor strengthening) exercises, pessaries, estrogen, and electrical muscle stimulation. Operative management options are used in patients failing nonoperative treatments, those with severe prolapse, and those who are symptomatic. The overall goal of surgery is to return the pelvic anatomy to as close to normal as possible. Procedures include anterior/posterior colporrhaphy, enterocele repair, hysterectomy, obliteration of the vaginal vault, urethropexies, urethral sling procedures, and/or suspension of the vaginal vault.

URETHRAL SYNDROME

The term *urethral syndrome* describes a complex of symptoms involving the lower urinary tract including urinary frequency, urgency, dysuria, suprapubic discomfort, postvoid fullness, incontinence, and/or dyspareunia with no objective findings of urologic pathology. Grandmultiparity, delivery without episiotomy, two or more abortuses, and pelvic relaxations appear to predispose.[3] The true incidence of urethral syndrome in the United States among adult women is unknown, as is the cause. The most widely accepted etiology of this enigmatic syndrome is an inflammatory process. Other etiologies include psychogenic factors, *Chlamydia* or *Mycoplasma* infection, atrophic urethritis in the perimenopausal/postmenopausal patient, fastidious organism bacterial infection, urethral stenosis and/or spasm, allergy, neurogenic, and trauma during intercourse. The diagnosis is one of exclusion founded on a thorough history and physical examination, followed by urine microscopic examination and culture. Referral is often obtained then for dynamic cystourethroscopy and urodynamic studies. Treatment encompasses many modalities because the etiology is uncertain.[4] The first approach is often pharmacologic, with antibiotics (doxycycline) or anticholinergics, followed by instillation of dimethyl sulfoxide, periurethral injection of triamcinolone, serial urethral dilation with or without massage, cryosurgery (internal urethrotomy and urethrolysis), bladder neck reconstruction, biofeedback, and psychotherapy. Recent research has led to the use of urethral suppositories with multiple medications including lidocaine, hydrocortisone, and topical estrogens. Lastly, supportive therapy is helpful in all patients.

GYNECOLOGIC MALIGNANCIES

The female reproductive tract cancers account for 13 percent of all cancers in women, following breast, lung, and colon cancer. Symptoms occurring as a result of natural progression of malignancy include bleeding, nausea and vomiting, obstructive uropathy, failure to thrive, and/or paraneoplastic syndromes. Treatment with surgery, chemotherapy, and radiation can themselves cause complications. Surgical complications include bowel and urogenital tract injury, thromboembolism, and bleeding. Chemotherapy-related complications include anemia, febrile neutropenia, thrombocytopenia, neuropathy, uropathy, nausea and vomiting, extravasation injury, and stomatitis. Radiation-related complications focus mainly on injury to the gastrointestinal and genitourinary tracts.

Ovarian Cancer

Cancers of the ovary and fallopian tube are discussed together because of the rarity of fallopian tube cancer and similarity in gross and microscopic appearance, pattern of spread, and disease process. Approximately 26,800 women were diagnosed with ovarian cancer in 1997 in the United States, with about half dying from the disease. A woman has a 1 to 2 percent chance of developing ovarian cancer in her lifetime with no family history. Peak incidence occurs between the ages of 55 and 65 although some types occur earlier. The following risk factors have been identified: infertility, low parity, high-fat diet, lactose intolerance, history of breast or colon cancer, and a family history of site-specific ovarian cancer or its associated syndromes. Oral contraceptives seem to be protective against ovarian cancer. Cancers of the ovary and fallopian tube come in three main histologic types: epithelial (85 percent), germ cell tumors (10 percent), and sex-cord stromal tumors (5 percent). Certain epithelial tumors may involve one ovary, and peak incidence is 10 to 15 years younger. Germ cell tumors include dysgerminomas, endodermal sinus tumors, embryonal carcinomas, immature and mature teratomas, choriocarcinoma, and mixed germ cell tumors. These are usually found in women under the age of 30. Sex-cord stomal tumors are usually divided into female and male types. Granulosa cell tumors secrete estrogen and may result in endometrial hyperplasia and/or cancer with average age of incidence about 50 years. Sertoli-Leydig tumors produce androgens, often resulting in masculinization and often occurring at age 25 years.

Patients often present after the disease has spread beyond the ovary, with symptoms such as abdominal pain, bloating, ascites, early satiety, weight loss, and/or respiratory distress secondary to effusion. It is most important to recognize that a woman presenting to the emergency department with ascites has a gynecologic malignancy until proven otherwise. As a first diagnostic step after pelvic examination, computed tomographic (CT) scanning can be done in the emergency department. Aspiration of ascitic fluid should not be done.

The single most important factor in the large death rate is the advanced stage at diagnosis. Diagnosis and staging of ovarian cancer are based on surgical evaluation. The International Federation of Gynecology and Obstetrics (FIGO) devised an extensive and universal staging classification. In summary (a simplification),

Stage I: Growth limited to one or both ovaries
Stage II: One or both ovaries with pelvic extension
Stage III: One or both ovaries with growth outside the pelvis
Stage IV: One or both ovaries with distant metastasis

Treatment of ovarian cancer may involve surgery, chemotherapy, and/or radiation therapy.

Uterine Cancer

Uterine cancer is the most common gynecologic malignancy. In 1997, 32,800 cases were diagnosed. The average age of incidence is 58 years of age. Endometrial cancer is the most common histologic type, and of these, the most common type is adenocarcinoma of the endometrium. Other histologic types of endometrial cancer that occur less frequently are papillary serous, clear cell, adenosquamous, and adenocanthoma. Sarcomas are malignancies of the uterine muscle. They behave very aggressively and have a worse prognosis than endometrial cancer.

Multiple risk factors have been associated with endometrioid adenocarcinoma of the uterus such as early menses, late menopause, nulliparity, obesity, diabetes, hypertension, and unopposed estrogen use. The use of progestins has drastically reduced the risk of endometrial cancer by 50 percent. Tamoxifen, an antiestrogen that competes with estrogen at its receptor site, has been shown to increase the risk of adenocarcinoma of the uterus.

The most common symptom of endometrial cancer is bleeding. Seventy-five percent of these cancers occur in postmenopausal patients, thus presenting with postmenopausal bleeding. Sarcomas, however, may present with bleeding but also with abdominal pain or prolapse of friable tissue through the cervical os.

The diagnosis of uterine cancer is made by sampling the endometrium. This may be achieved through office endometrial biopsy, a dilatation and curettage specimen, or hysteroscopy. A pathologic specimen must be obtained for proper diagnosis and further treatment planning. A sonogram measuring the endometrial stripe greater than 10 mm, in post-menopausal women, must be evaluated.

Staging for uterine cancer is as follows: (summary of staging)

Stage I: Confined to the uterine corpus
Stage II: Involvement of the cervix
Stage III: Extends to uterine serosa, ovary, vagina, and paraaortic/pelvic lymph nodes
Stage IV: Involvement of the bladder/bowel, inguinal/intraabdominal lymph nodes

Staging is surgical. Treatment involves surgery and also may include radiation and chemotherapy.

The vaginal cuff, vagina, and pelvis are common sites for recurrence. Patients with recurrence often present with vaginal bleeding, vaginal or pelvic masses, or uremia secondary to ureter obstruction. Pulmonary metastases are less common in recurrent uterine cancer but still need to be considered, in a women presenting with respiratory symptoms and a history of uterine cancer.

Cervical Cancer

Currently, 15,800 new cases of cervical cancer are diagnosed per year. The average age at the time of diagnosis is 54. Risk factors include early coitus, multiple sexual partners, high-risk male partners, smoking, human papillomavirus, and HIV infection (or other immunosuppressive states). The diagnosis of cervical cancer in an HIV-positive patient is now considered an AIDS-identifying illness. Smoking increases the risk of cervical cancer in women by 3.5 times, and even passive smoke increases the risk threefold. Approximately 90 percent of cervical cancers are of squamous histologic type, but adenocarcinoma, which comprises 5 to 10 percent of cervical cancers, is increasing and has a worse prognosis.

Cervical cancer, in decreasing order, most often presents with postmenopausal bleeding, abnormal vaginal bleeding, postcoital bleeding, vaginal discharge, pain, or leg swelling. Diagnosis must be made by cervical biopsy. Often, on speculum examination, a mass or ulcerative lesion is seen on the cervix. A Pap smear must never be done if a suspicious lesion is seen! Instead, the gynecologic consultant should be called to perform a biopsy, cone biopsy, or loup electrosurgical excision procedure (LEEP).

Staging of cervical cancer, as opposed to uterine and ovarian cancer, is performed clinically. Once a diagnosis is made by biopsy, a thorough physical examination must be performed, including an examination under anesthesia (cystoscopy and proctoscopy) of the parametrium, pelvic sidewalls, bladder, and rectum, and a chest x-ray. These results are combined to clinically stage the individual. The tumor tends to spread by direct extension causing parametrial thickening and by lymphatic spread to obturator nodes then to pelvic and paraortic nodes.

The staging of cervical cancer is complex, but the following is a brief overview:

Stage I: Confined strictly to the cervix
Stage II: Beyond the cervix but not to the pelvic sidewall
Stage IIA: No parametrial involvement
Stage IIB: Parametrial involvement
Stage III: Extends to pelvic sidewall
Stage IV: Beyond the true pelvis, bladder or rectum involvement

Treatment of cervical cancer requires a team of gynecologic oncologists and radiation oncologists. In stage I to IIA cervical cancer, radical hysterectomy or radiation therapy has demonstrated similar 5-year survival rates (90 percent). Any persons with stage IIB or greater must be treated with radiation.

Recurrent or persistent cancer causes devastating problems for patients, their families, and clinicians. Patients have a 1-year survival rate of 15 percent and a 5-year survival rate of 5 percent when recurrence occurs. Recurrent cervical cancer can be treated palliatively or with some hope of a cure. Curable lesions are those which are easily resected, i.e., single lesions located at the vaginal apex or in the lung or lesions located centrally in the pelvis without lymph node involvement. Curative, exenterative surgery is successful 50 to 60 percent of the time for patients with central recurrences. Pelvic exenterative surgery is very extensive surgery removing the bladder, rectum, uterus (if not already done), and vagina. A colostomy is required, and a neovagina and urinary diversion are created. Recurrent cervical cancers often present to the emergency department with vaginal bleeding, uremia secondary to ureter obstruction or invasion, deep venous thrombosis, leg swelling, or pain.

Vaginal Cancer

Vaginal cancer accounts for only 1 to 2 percent of all gynecologic malignancies. The true definition of primary vaginal cancer is that it must arise from the vagina and not be an extension or metastasis from the cervix or vulva. The main histologic type is squamous cell carcinoma, which comprise 80 percent of all vaginal cancers. Squamous lesions usually occur in postmenopausal woman, whereas other histologic types (rhabdosarcoma, endodermal sinus tumor, adenocarcinoma, and clear cell adenocarcinoma from diethylstilbestrol) usually occur in younger women. The last diethylstilbestrol (DES) administration was around 1971, which would place these women in their forties. The mean age of occurrence for vaginal cancer is 60 to 65 years of age. Epidemiologic factors contributing to the occurrence of vaginal cancer are immunosuppression, chronic irritation (long-term pessary use or prolapse of female organs), decreased socioeconomic status, radiation for cervical cancer, hysterectomy for dysplasia, multiple sexual partners, or DES exposure. The tumor usually presents in the posterior upper third of the vagina. Abnormal vaginal bleeding is the presenting symptom 50 to 75 percent of the time. Some complain of abnormal discharge or postcoital bleeding.

Staging for vaginal cancer is summarized as follows:

Stage I: Vaginal wall involvement
Stage II: Parametrial involvement
Stage III: Pelvic wall involvement
Stage IV: Bladder/rectum or beyond pelvic involvement

Most vaginal cancers are best treated with radiation therapy. The survival rate when radiation is used is 93 percent at 5 years and 87 percent at 10 years. Most recurrences occur within 3 years, but later recurrences are also possible.

Embryonal rhabdomyosarcomas (sarcoma botryoides) occur in children less than 5 years of age and present with vaginal bleeding, discharge, or grapelike masses protruding from the vagina. These cancers respond very well to the chemotherapeutic regimen of vincristine, dactinomycin, and cyclophosphamide, with either surgery or radiation. Complications associated with vaginal cancers are bleeding, infections, fistulas, or complications from chemotherapy, radiation, or surgery.

Vulvar Cancer

Vulvar cancer is responsible for only 1 to 4 percent of all gynecologic malignancies and less than 1 percent of all cancers. Approximately 500 women die from vulvar cancer annually in the United States. Seventy-five percent of women diagnosed with vulvar cancer are greater than 55 years of age, with a third of them greater than 75 years of age. The most common histologic type is squamous cell carcinoma (90 percent), followed by melanoma, basal cell carcinoma, adenocarcinoma, sarcoma, Bartholin gland tumors, and metastasis. Luckily, the prognosis is generally good because recognizable symptoms allow for early diagnosis. The most common presenting symptoms include a mass, pruritus, pain, or ulceration (in decreasing order of frequency). The cause for vulvar cancer is still unknown, but there have been associations of vulvar cancers with other cancers of the anogenital tract. Human papillomavirus (HPV) types 16, 18, 31, 35, and 39 have all been suggested as causative factors.

It seems that the etiology is multifactorial, and HPV alone is not the culprit. Other possibilities include immunodeficiency, vulvar dystrophy, smoking, and exposure to aniline dyes such as benzene. Multicentric lesions are seen more commonly in younger women, whereas unifocal lesions are seen most often in older women. On physical examination, the lesions may appear white, pigmented, raised, thickened, nodular, or ulcerative. A vulvar biopsy should be performed liberally in women with any suspicious lesions. Treatment depends on the stage at the time of diagnosis. More recent years have welcomed the advent of more conservative treatment modalities. The treatment of choice is surgery with adjuvant radiotherapy in more advanced stages.

Staging is summarized as follows:

Stage I: Confined to the vulva or perineum and <2 cm
Stage II: Confined to vulva or perineum and >2 cm
Stage III: Any size lesion spread to lower urethra, vagina, or anus with unilateral positive nodes
Stage IV: Involvement of the upper urethra, bladder, rectum, or pelvic bone with positive bilateral nodes

Radical subtotal vulvectomy is the treatment of choice for patients with lesions less than 2 cm. The use of postoperative radiation may decrease the incidence of recurrence and improve survival in women with lesions larger than 2 cm and positive lymph nodes. The morbidity from surgery is groin wound breakdown and lymphedema from lymph node dissections. Recurrent vulvar cancer may be local, distant, or involve lymph nodes. Patients often present with bleeding, lymphedema, deep venous thrombosis, or metastasis (usually to bone or lung).

Gestational Trophoblastic Disease

Gestational trophoblastic disease (GTD) is a disease of trophoblastic placental tissue. GTD represents a spectrum of diseases ranging from benign to frank malignancy.[5] There are four forms of this process:

1. Hydatidiform mole
2. Invasive mole

3. Choriocarcinoma
4. Placental site tumors

The incidence of molar pregnancy is 1 in 2000 pregnancies; however, the incidence is much higher in Asian women, at 1 in 800. The risk of developing a second molar pregnancy is 1 to 3 percent, sometimes approaching 40 percent. Molar pregnancy is seen with a bimodal distribution. Persons younger than age 20 and older than age 40 are at greatest risk. GTD may be benign or malignant and, when malignant, can be divided into metastatic and nonmetastatic.

The benign form of this disease is hydatidiform mole, either partial or complete. This following summary table includes some of the major differences between partial and complete moles (Table 107-1).

Treatment of hydatidiform mole is suction curettage or hysterectomy. Hyperthyroidism or hypertension must be stabilized prior to surgery. Follow-up is essential because dilation and curettage alone is curative in only 80 percent of patients, leaving 20 percent at risk for persistent trophoblastic disease.

Gestational trophoblastic neoplasm (GTN) includes invasive mole and choriocarcinoma. These tumors can progress to malignancy and ultimately death if left untreated. Luckily, they are highly responsive to chemotherapy, which in turn leads to a cure rate of 90 percent.

Invasive mole is the myometrial invasion of the hydatidiform mole. Common sites for metastasis of this cancer are the lungs and vagina, which occurs in 15 percent of patients. Invasive moles occur in 1 of 15,000 pregnancies, and 15 percent of hydatidiform moles result in invasive moles. Diagnosis is confirmed by consistently elevated or rising beta human chorionic gonadotropin (hCG) levels after a molar evacuation.

Choriocarcinoma is characterized by atypical trophoblastic hyperplasia with direct and vascular invasion into the myometrium and distant sites, most commonly the lungs, brain, liver, pelvis, or vagina. The incidence of choriocarcinoma is approximately 1 per 40,000 pregnancies. Twenty-five percent follow abortion or ectopic pregnancies, 25 percent are seen with term gestations, and the remaining 50 percent result from hydatidiform moles. However, only 2 to 3 percent of hydatidiform moles result in choriocarcinoma.

Symptoms of GTN are continued bleeding after dilation and curettage for hydatidiform mole or bleeding after a pregnancy event (e.g., vaginal delivery, cesarean section, ectopic pregnancy, miscarriage, or abortion). Patients with metastasis may present with dyspnea, cough, chest pain, central nervous system abnormalities, or vaginal mass. The most common site for metastasis is the vagina, followed by the lung.

Treatment depends on the presence of metastasis. Patients with no metastatic disease who wish to preserve their fertility are treated with single-agent chemotherapy, methotrexate, or dactinomycin; otherwise, hysterectomy is the treatment of choice. This initial therapy leads to cure in 85 to 90 percent of patients. When metastatic disease is present, combination chemotherapy is given.

TABLE 107-1 Some Major Differences between Partial and Complete Moles

	Complete Mole	Partial Mole
Symptoms	90% present with vaginal bleeding, 30% with uterine size greater than dates, 15% bilateral theca–lutein cyst enlargement, 10% hyperemesis, 1% preeclampsia (<20 weeks), hyperthyroidism, trophoblastic embolization, nonfetal heart tones auscultated	90% present with incomplete or missed abortion, 70% with vaginal bleeding, all the symptoms of complete abortion may be present but are very rare
Diagnosis	Ultrasonography reveals "snow storm" appearance coupled with a high βhCG level	Usually on histologic examination from tissue obtained from a missed or incomplete abortion

COMPLICATIONS

The complications of gynecologic malignancies are related to the natural progression of disease, surgery, chemotherapy, or radiation. Any combination of these complications can occur depending on the type and stage of neoplasm and treatment modality.

The complications related to the natural progression of disease often represent the symptoms that help to diagnose the disease. These include, but are not limited to, genital tract bleeding, gastrointestinal obstruction, masses or ascites, fistulas (both genitourinary and gastrointestinal), obstructive uropathy, metastasis, lymphedema, and hypercoagulable states leading to deep venous thrombosis or pulmonary embolism.

By far the most common oncologic complication (most frequently seen with cervical or uterine cancer) is bleeding. It may be acute or chronic, massive or minimal, external or internal. Sources include friable tissue, tumor erosion into iliac or femoral vessels, adnexal mass rupture, or coagulopathies that develop secondary to chemotherapy or radiation. Assessment and management begin with the principles of emergency care. Then a thorough history and physical examination including prior diagnoses and treatment should be undertaken to find the likely source and cause of bleeding. Where externally accessible sites of bleeding occur, apply direct pressure. If this fails to control the bleeding, next use topical silver nitrate or Monsel's solution. If bleeding persists, topical absorbable hemostat material can be applied such as Gelfoam, Instal, or Surgicel. Where the vagina is the source of bleeding, vaginal packing may become necessary. Use a long strip of continuous gauze, and place a Foley catheter to prevent retention. Regardless of the causes of bleeding, after stabilization, the gynecology service should be consulted.

Patients occasionally present with abdominal distention and discomfort. This often is concomitant with other complications of cancer and therefore may be accompanied by early satiety, nausea, vomiting, anorexia, weight loss, constipation or diarrhea, urinary frequency, urgency, incontinence, dyspnea, or orthopnea. As always, the first step is complete history and physical examination, including both pelvic and rectal examinations. Diagnostic testing may reveal worsening of known disease, recurrence of cancer, new cancer, torsion of a large ovary, bowel perforation, or intraabdominal hemorrhage. Consultation with a gynecologist, gynecologic oncologist, or surgeon is indicated.

Gastrointestinal complications include obstructions and fistulas. Obstruction is common as a progressive symptom of malignancy, especially with ovarian and uterine tumors that are associated with enlarging masses or ascites. The resulting obstruction may be mechanical or due to tumor ileus from encasement of the nerve plexus leading to dysfunction of a segment of bowel. Patients often present with nausea, vomiting, early satiety, abdominal pain, distention, constipation, and/or obstipation. The normal management scheme for obstruction applies (as discussed in Chap. 75 in more depth). Surgical palliation may give temporary symptomatic relief, but recurrence rates are extremely high. Consultation with a gynecologist, gynecologic oncologist, or surgeon is indicated to discuss and provide permanent proximal decompression and supplemental nutrition.

Fistula formation occurs secondary to bowel encasement or obstruction. Fistula may drain to the abdominal wall, peritoneal cavity, vagina, uterus, or bladder. Instillation of colored medium (e.g., charcoal, food dye in tube feeds), upper gastrointestinal series, barium enema, or a fistulogram often aids diagnosis. Consultation with a gynecologist, gynecologic oncologist, or surgeon is indicated to determine the best treatment.

Urinary tract complications also include obstruction and fistula. Ureteral obstruction classically is seen in cervical cancer but also

TABLE 107-2 Chemotherapeutic Agents and Their Toxicities

Agent	Toxicity	Type of Cancer Treated
	ALKYLATING AGENTS	
Cyclophosphamide	Myelosuppression, cystitis, hepatitis, alopecia	Ovarian, breast, sarcoma
Ifosfamide	Myelosuppression, CNS abnormalities, bladder and renal toxicity	Ovarian, cervical
Chlorambucil	Myelosuppression, dermatitis, hepatitis, gastrointestinal dysfunction	Ovarian
Nitrogen mustard	Nausea, vomiting, myelosuppression	Ovarian, malignant effusions
Cisplatin (alkylating like)	Nephrotoxicity, tinnitis, hearing loss, myelosuppression, peripheral neuropathy, nausea, vomiting	Ovarian, cervical, germ cell
Carboplatin (alkylating like)	Neuropathy, ototoxicity, myelosuppression, nephrotoxicity	Ovarian, germ cell
	ANTIMETABOLITES	
Methotrexate	Myelosuppression, hepatitis, pneumonitis, stomatitis	Breast, ovarian, choriocarcinoma
5-Fluorouracil	Myelosuppression, alopecia, nausea, vomiting	Breast, ovarian
Hydroxyurea	Nausea, vomiting, anorexia, myelosuppression	Cervical
	PLANT ALKALOIDS	
Vinblastine	Myelosuppression, alopecia, nausea, vomiting, neurotoxicity	Germ cell, choriocarcinoma
Vincristine	Myelosuppression, gastrointestinal, alopecia, neurotoxicity	Germ cell, cervical, sarcoma
Paclitaxel (Taxol)	Myelosuppression, alopecia, arrhythmias, hypersensitivity rxn	Ovarian, breast
Etoposide (VP-16)	Myelosuppression, alopecia, hypotension	Germ cell, choriocarcinoma
	ANTITUMOR ANTIBIOTICS	
Bleomycin	Fever, anaphylaxis, pulmonary fibrosis, dermatitis	Cervical, germ cell, malignant effusions
Doxorubicin (Adriamycin)	Myelosuppression, alopecia, cardiotoxicity, nausea, vomiting	Ovarian, breast, uterine
Mitomycin-C	Nephrotoxicity, stomatitis, nausea, vomiting, myelosuppression	Breast, ovarian, cervical
Actinomycin-D (Dactinomycin)	Nausea, vomiting, dermatitis, myelosuppression, stomatitis	Germ cell, choriocarcinoma

occurs with progression or recurrence of other pelvic malignancies. Radiation also may cause permanent scarring of the lumen leading to obstruction. Patients may present with acute renal failure and require percutaneous or cystoscopic emergent decompression. A vesicovaginal or ureterovaginal fistula may develop at the site of untreated cancer or recurrent cancer or after radiation therapy. Fistulas follow radical pelvic surgery about 1 percent of the time and radiation therapy approximately 2.6 percent of the time.

Chronic mild lymphedema of the lower extremities often follows inguinal node resection. Pedal lymphedema is seen after pelvic radiation therapy. Aside from the associated discomfort, the greatest concern is deep veinous thrombosis, especially if lymphedema is unilateral. Duplex ultrasound is necessary. Lymphedema is treated supportively with elevation and support stockings.

Thromboembolic disease has long been associated with gynecologic malignancies and is discussed in Chap. 55.

Most of the side effects of chemotherapeutic agents are predictable and can be lessened with adjuvant medications. Risk factors for poor tolerability of chemotherapy are advanced age, advanced disease, poor nutritional status, or severe systemic involvement. Chemotherapeutic agents may have debilitating effects on many organ systems (Table 107-2).

The complications related to radiation are temporally divided into acute and chronic. The chronic manifestations may be further broken into gastrointestinal, genitourinary, and pulmonary. Acute findings include nausea, vomiting, diarrhea, cystitis, nephritis, pneumonitis, and myelosuppression. Gastrointestinal symptoms are often self-limiting and are controlled with supportive therapy including antiemetics, antidiarrheals, and avoidance of high-fiber diets. Newer studies point to glutamine-rich diets, and the use of sucralfate may further reduce diarrhea. The genitourinary symptoms range from infection to hemorrhagic cystitis with extreme pain. Treatment of these symptoms includes adequate hydration, surveillance for infection, and bladder irrigation with analgesia or steroids. Resolution of myelosuppression is often spontaneous and begins after radiation has been completed.

Chronic findings are divided into gastrointestinal, genitourinary, and pulmonary. The most common complication is radiation enteritis, which presents with chronic diarrhea, malabsorption, or digestive difficulty. Other chronic gastrointestinal complications include strictures, fistulas, perforations, obstructions, and hematochezia. These findings often occur within 2 years of treatment. Management should be a collaborative effort between the oncologist, surgeon, and gastroenterologist. Emergency management includes adequate hydration and symptomatic relief. Genitourinary complications include incontinence, fistula formation, stricture formation, and hemorrhagic cystitis. Incontinence and fistulas were discussed earlier. The most severe complication of stricture formation is obstructive uropathy. This always should be considered as recurrence of disease until proven otherwise and as a result of radiation by diagnosis of exclusion. Both hemorrhagic cystitis and stricture require cystoscopy for evaluation. An oncologist and urologist should institute appropriate treatment.

Lastly, secondary malignancies may arise from radiation therapy. This results from the local nonmalignant tissue being exposed to ionizing radiation. The resulting damage to genetic material leads to mutation that is the presumed mechanism for carcinogenesis. The secondary malignancy is often observed years after the initial radiation therapy, and accuracy in predicting its occurrence is difficult at best.

REFERENCES

1. Romanzi LJ, Chaikin DC, Blaivas JG: The effect of genital prolapse on voiding. *J Urol* 161(2):581, 1999.
2. Cundiff GW, Addison WA: Management of pelvic organ prolapse. *Obstet Gynecol Clin North Am* 25(4):907, 1998.
3. Gurel H, Gurel SA, Atilla MK: Urethral syndrome and associated risk factors related to obstetrics and gynecology. *Eur J Obstet Gynecol Reprod Biol* 83(1):5, 1999.
4. Wesselmann U, Burnett AL, Heinberg LJ: The urogenital and rectal pain syndromes. *Pain* 73(3):269, 1997.
5. Newlands ES, Paradinas FJ, Fisher RA: Recent advances in gestational trophoblastic disease. *Hematol Oncol Clin North Am* 13(1):225, 1999.

COMPLICATIONS OF GYNECOLOGIC PROCEDURES

Michael A. Silverman
Karen J. Morrill Hardart

This chapter provides an overview of the common complications of gynecologic procedures that are likely to lead to an ED visit.

Because of convenience, cost effectiveness, and apparent safety, the number of ambulatory surgeries continues to increase. The indications appropriate for ambulatory surgery also continue to increase. These trends are accompanied by a decrease in the length of hospitalization following major gynecologic surgery. Unanticipated hospital admission after ambulatory surgery occurs in approximately 1 percent of cases and is an important measure of outcome.[1] Gynecologic outpatient surgery has been associated with an unscheduled admission rate of 3.64 percent, with postoperative emesis being the most common reason for admission.[2]

HISTORY AND PHYSICAL EXAMINATION

The most common reasons for emergency department visits during the postoperative period following gynecologic procedures are pain, fever, and vaginal bleeding. A focused but thorough evaluation should be performed. The history should include the surgical procedure performed (abdominal versus vaginal), the reason for it, time of symptom onset and its proximity to the surgery, complications already experienced, patient's postsurgical history, and medications prescribed. The interval between the surgery and the onset of symptoms is very important in determining their cause. For example, most cases of early postoperative fevers are not infectious, and causes may include pulmonary atelectasis, hypersensitivity reactions to antibiotics, pyogenic reactions to tissue trauma, or hematoma formation.

Relevant examination of all appropriate systems should then be performed. It should not be assumed that the etiology of the complaint is gynecologic. Other potential explanations of the symptoms should be investigated. The surgical wound should be examined, and a pelvic examination should be performed, including both a sterile speculum and a bimanual examination. The sterile speculum examination should visualize the cervix or, if it is absent, the vaginal cuff, and any evidence of bleeding, discharge, erythema, or cuff or labial cellulitis should be noted. Cervical cultures should be considered. Bimanual examination after a vaginal or abdominal hysterectomy should evaluate for tenderness, masses, and an intact cuff. Following hysteroscopy or dilation and curretage, cervical motion, uterine, and adnexal tenderness should be evaluated. A rectal examination should always be performed to evaluate tenderness or masses.

Laboratory studies should be directed towards the patient's complaints. A complete blood count with a manual differential count is almost always indicated. A serum β human chorionic gonadotropin level should be obtained for all women of childbearing potential. A catheterized urine specimen, along with urine, blood, wound, and cervical (if present) cultures, should be obtained if the patient is febrile. A chemistry panel may be necessary to evaluate hepatic and renal function.

Imaging procedures are often necessary. A chest radiograph can confirm pneumonia or inappropriate air under the diaphragm. Supine and erect abdominal series help confirm bowel obstruction. Pelvic sonogram remains the gold standard for visualizing the pelvic structures. However, a computed tomography (CT) scan may be necessary, especially if an abscess is suspected.

COMPLICATIONS OF ENDOSCOPIC PROCEDURES

Laparoscopy

Both diagnostic and therapeutic gynecologic laparoscopy accomplished by passing a rigid endoscope through a trocar that is inserted bluntly through a small subumbilical incision into the abdominal cavity after a Veress needle has been used to insufflate the abdomen with carbon dioxide. The pneumoperitoneum must be sufficient to displace the bowel and is maintained throughout the surgery. Additional trocars can be placed so that other accessories can be used during the surgery. Laparoscopy is almost always an ambulatory surgical procedure and is performed under general anesthesia with endotracheal intubation.

There are numerous indications for gynecologic laparoscopy, ranging from diagnosing gynecologic disorders (e.g., endometriosis or ectopic pregnancy) to performing complex gynecologic surgery. The most common surgical procedure in the United States is female sterilization, and more than 60 percent of the procedures are performed laparoscopically. In one study, 82 percent of diagnostic laparoscopies were performed because of infertility.[3] Laparoscopy is also used for lysis of adhesions, CO_2 laser ablation of endometriosis, uterine surgery (including myomectomy), tubal surgeries (including salpingectomy), ovarian surgery (including oophorectomy and oophorocystectomy), paraovarian cyst excision, laparoscopic vaginal hysterectomy, and retropubic urethroplexy.

All of these procedures entail the same potential complications, but more complex surgeries carry considerably more risk. The incidence of major complications in the United States for laparoscopy may be as low as 0.22 percent.[4] In 1993, the American Association of Gynecologic Laparoscopists reported complications for 45,042 procedures as follows: hemorrhage 1 percent, unintended laparotomy 1 percent, blood transfusion for hemorrhage 0.45 percent, and bowel or urinary tract injury 0.41 percent. In 1996, the overall incidence of complications in major operative laparoscopy was reported as 10.4 percent.[5] This rate is still significantly less than the 25 to 50 percent overall complication rate of abdominal surgery, such as hysterectomy or oophorectomy through abdominal incisions, although data related to the two approaches are not directly comparable because of other factors that may mandate a traditional surgical procedure.

The major complications associated with laparoscopy are thermal injury of the bowel, perforation of a viscus, bleeding or other vascular injury, ureteral or bladder injuries, and incisional hernia or wound dehiscence.

Thermal injury is the most serious potential complication. While many significant complications of laparoscopy are recognized in the operating room under direct visualization, patients with thermal injury may not develop symptoms for several days and up to several weeks postoperatively. Various series have reported the incidence of electrothermal injuries to be in the range of 0.5 to 3.2 per 1000 cases. Patient presentations may include bilateral lower quadrant pain and tenderness, fever, elevated white blood cell count, or peritonitis. Plain radiographs may show an ileus or free air under the diaphragm. Air or insufflated CO_2 should be completely absorbed by the third postoperative day. Patients with greater than expected pain after laparoscopy should be considered to have a bowel injury until proven otherwise. Early gynecologic consult is critical if a thermal injury is suspected.

Traumatic injury to the bowel is usually less serious than thermal injury. The very small diameter Veress needle is usually the cause of a bowel perforation, which is recognized on withdrawal of the needle. A sharp trocar may cause more damage. Gastric perforation may result, usually due to stomach distention from aerophagia or a difficult intubation. The large or small bowel may also be perforated. These injuries are usually noted during the operation. On rare occasions, perforation may occur through a single loop of bowel adherent to the anterior abdominal wall. Complications include peritonitis, abscess, enterocutaneous fistula, and septic shock.

Vascular injury occurs between 0.1 and 6.4 per 1000 cases.[6] While such injuries may be immediately life threatening, they are almost universally recognized during the operation. Patients may present with a postoperative hematoma. Local compression, if feasible, is the initial treatment. If the mass enlarges or signs of hypovolemia occur, the wound must be explored by the gynecologist.

Bladder and ureteral injuries may occur from mechanical or thermal trauma. Trocar or dissection injuries to the bladder are typically recognized intraoperatively. Thermal injuries, however, may not be initially apparent and may present with peritonitis or fistula. The diagnosis of a ureteral injury is usually delayed. Thermal injury may present up to 14 days postoperatively with abdominal or flank pain, fever, and peritonitis. There may be an elevated white blood cell count, and an intravenous pyelogram (IVP) shows extravasation of urine or a urinoma. Mechanical obstruction of the ureter from sutures or staples may be recognized intraoperatively by direct visualization but may present up to 1 week postoperatively with fever and flank pain. An IVP helps define the site and degree of obstruction.

Incisional hernias and dehiscence are rare complications after laparoscopy. Incisional hernias are more common when defects larger than 10 mm are made. Intestinal hernia may develop within the first postoperative week. Patients may be asymptomatic or may present with pain, mass, evisceration, or signs and symptoms of a mechanical bowel obstruction. Fever may occur if the bowel is incarcerated, and peritonitis may develop following bowel perforation. Dehiscence usually involves protrusion of the omentum, and, in rare cases, the small bowel passes through the opening. Immediate incisional repair by a gynecologist is usually sufficient; however, a laparotomy may be necessary if the bowel is incarcerated or perforation is a risk.

Wound infection after laparoscopy is uncommon and often not a serious complication. Most are minor skin infections that can be managed expectantly, with oral antibiotics, or with drainage. The risk of infection after laparoscopy is much lower than that after abdominal or vaginal surgery. Excluding minor skin infections, pelvic infection is reported in fewer than 1 in 1000 cases. Pelvic cellulitis and abscess can occur, and severe necrotizing fasciitis, while rare, has been reported. Most infections are probably secondary to a subacute coexisting infection present prior to the procedure or secondary to skin contamination. Broad-spectrum antibiotics typically provide a rapid response.

Hysteroscopy

Hysteroscopy is the direct visualization of the uterine cavity using a rigid or flexible fiberoptic instrument. Hysteroscopy can be done as an office procedure under intravenous sedation or in an operating room under general anesthesia, spinal or epidural anesthesia, or intravenous sedation. Hysteroscopy is done for both diagnostic and therapeutic purposes. The most common indication for hysteroscopy is abnormal vaginal bleeding. Other indications include uterine leiomyomata, intrauterine adhesions, proximal tubal obstruction, removal of intrauterine devices, müllerian anomalies, and infertility evaluation. Therapeutic applications include directed biopsies, removal of small myomata, and endometrial ablation for menorrhagia. Complications of hysteroscopy occur in approximately 2 percent of cases and include fluid overload, uterine perforation with possible damage to intraabdominal organs, infection, toxic shock syndrome, anesthesia reaction, postoperative bleeding, and embolism.[7]

Fluid overload is rare but can occur from absorption of electrolyte and nonelectrolyte solutions during lengthy procedures. The entry of dextran into the circulation can lead to pulmonary edema and disseminated intravascular coagulation. For this reason, no more than 500 mL dextran should be used during a procedure. A lack of recovery of distention medium in excess of 1000 mL also places the patient at risk for fluid overload. If fluid overload is suspected, hyponatremia should be anticipated. A rapid decrease in the serum sodium level can result in generalized cerebral edema, seizures, and death.

Uterine perforation is a relatively common complication. A midline uterine perforation generally does not have significant sequelae. A lateral perforation may lacerate uterine vessels and cause substantial bleeding. Most often, the perforation is noted at the time of surgery, and a laparoscopy is done to investigate for bleeding and/or damage to bowel or bladder. If the complication is not noted at the time of surgery, the patient may present with peritoneal signs if the bowel has been injured or pain and/or bleeding if the vessels were lacerated.

Infection is very rare and most commonly occurs in patients with concurrent genital tract infections. Endometritis or even toxic shock can result.

Postoperative bleeding may be uterine or cervical in origin. Cervical lacerations may be caused by forceful dilation or tears from the tenaculum. Uterine bleeding can result from resection procedures. After hemodynamic stabilization of the patient, the gynecologist can place a Foley or balloon catheter into the uterine cavity and fill it with approximately 10 to 15 mL of water or saline solution. One technique is to remove one-half the fluid from the balloon after 1 h and the other half after 2 h. If bleeding remains stopped, the patient can usually be discharged. If bleeding persists, the patient should be admitted. The catheter is reinflated and left overnight, or occasionally reeploration is required.

Embolism is the most feared complication of using CO_2 gas as a distention medium. The risks of such an occurrence are low when the principles of low flow and low pressure are followed.

COMPLICATIONS RELATED TO MAJOR ABDOMINAL SURGERY

Complications from major abdominal procedures that lead to ED visits usually occur at least 3 days postoperatively. Expected complications include, but are not confined to, wound infection and related morbidity, phlebitis (both superficial and deep), urinary tract infection, bladder and ureteral injury, ileus and bowel obstruction, pneumonia, and atelectasis.

Hysterectomy remains one of the most common major surgical procedures in the United States. It also carries a significant morbidity, with postoperative infection rates reported between 3.9 and 50 percent for abdominal hysterectomies and 1.7 to 64 percent for laparoscopic vaginal hysterectomies. There are numerous risk factors for postoperative infections. Lower socioeconomic status is a risk factor for infection in gynecologic surgery, which may be related to inadequate nutrition or poor hygiene. Obesity also carries an increased risk of infection, possibly due to poor hygiene, altered nutrition, or increased operative time. Additional risk factors include altered immunocompetence, diabetes, lack of prophylactic antibiotics when indicated, premenopausal stage, or excessive amount of operative blood loss.

Wound Infection

CLINICAL FEATURES Wound infections may occur early post-operatively or up to several months after the surgery. Greater than 90 percent occur within the first 2 postoperative weeks. Early infections are characterized by fever, tachycardia, increased wound tenderness, and local cellulitis. As the infection progresses, the wound may be fluctuant or indurated. Wound breakdown and dehiscence can occur if treatment is not initiated rapidly. The infected incision is swollen, erythematous, edematous, and tender. There may be spontaneous purulent drainage from the wound. Initial management consists of opening the incision, probing with a sterile cotton swab to maintain fascia integrity, vigorous cleaning with a fifty-fifty mixture of hydrogen peroxide and saline solution, and packing with saline-soaked wet-to-dry dressings. If staples have been placed, they should be removed. Aerobic and anaerobic cultures could be obtained. The operating gynecologist should always be informed about the patient. Late-onset infections are characterized by persistent low-grade fevers and purulent drainage from the incision. Local wound care, as described above, is appropriate.

DISPOSITION Parenteral therapy with a penicillin-based antibiotic and aggressive local wound care are typically used for early postoperative infections, particularly when there is underlying cellulitis. Most patients are readmitted.

Infected Vaginal Cuff Hematoma, Cellulitis, or Abscess

CLINICAL FEATURES A vaginal cuff is formed during a hysterectomy and is composed of the contiguous retroperitoneal space immediately above the vaginal apex and the surrounding soft tissue. This cuff may become infected, leading to cellulitis, hematoma, or abscess.

Vaginal cuff cellulitis is a common complication following both abdominal and vaginal hysterectomy. Symptoms and signs usually present between postoperative days 3 and 5, and may begin in the hospital, or just after discharge. Patients often complain of lower abdominal pain, pelvic pain, back pain, fever, and abnormal vaginal discharge. Induration, tenderness of the vaginal cuff, and possibly a purulent discharge or labial edema or erythema are prominent during the pelvic examination. The white blood cell count is usually elevated.

A vaginal cuff abscess usually presents early in the postoperative course. Patients complain of fever, chills, pelvic pain, and rectal pressure. On examination, lower abdominal and vaginal cuff tenderness is present. A tender fluctuant mass near the cuff may be palpable, and purulent drainage from the cuff may be seen.

Infected cuff hematomas may present later in the postoperative course and are associated with a decrease in the patient's hemoglobin and hematocrit levels. The hematoma may not be palpable on examination.

DISPOSITION Patients should be readmitted for drainage and intravenous antibiotics. Broad-spectrum antibiotics should be started early, with coverage for gram-negative, gram-positive, and anaerobic organisms. A CT scan may be necessary for diagnosis or to better define an abscess or hematoma.

Postoperative Ovarian Abscess

CLINICAL FEATURES Patients with fever and abdominal and pelvic pain shortly after discharge from the hospital may have a pelvic abscess. Such abscesses are usually ovarian in nature. A sudden increase in pain may be a signal that the abscess has ruptured. This is a surgical emergency and requires a laporatomy. If time permits or the diagnosis is in question, a CT scan can aid in identifying the size and location of the abscess.

DISPOSITION Patients with a pelvic abcess need to be admitted. Some abscesses respond to broad-spectrum antibiotics, and others may require drainage either by an interventional radiologist or by colpotomy.

Dehiscence and Evisceration

CLINICAL FEATURES Wound disruption is a failure of normal healing and includes the breakdown of any layers of a surgical incision. Dehiscence is disruption of all layers, including fascia and peritoneum. Evisceration occurs when there is complete breakdown of the healing processes through all levels of the abdominal wall and the omentum or bowel presents through the incision.

The classic signs of impending dehiscence is the sudden outpouring of serosanguineous blood from the abdominal incision. Most often this occurs between postoperative days 5 and 8. The patient may describe a ''pop'' or tearing sensation. About one-third of the cases of wound dehiscence are associated with evisceration. While gynecologic surgery has a lower wound disruption rate than the 1 to 3 percent reported following major abdominal surgery, the mortality rate is high, with a median of 18.1 percent.[8–10]

DISPOSITION When evisceration has occurred, the abdomen should be covered with moist sterile towels and supported with tape to prevent further extrusion of the gut.

The patient should be taken directly to the operating room for closure. In cases in which there is a sudden appearance of blood but no bowel, it is best to follow the same procedure because evisceration usually is imminent.

Ureteral Injury

CLINICAL FEATURES Operative injury to the ureter results from one of three types of trauma: crushing, transection, or ligation. Each type of injury may be either partial or complete. This complication occurs more often during the performance of abdominal hysterectomy than during any other pelvic surgery. In patients who develop flank pain shortly after surgery, ureteral injury should be suspected. Patients may have fever and costovertebral angle tenderness. A urinalysis should be performed, and if obstruction is suspected, an IVP should be obtained. If obstruction is noted on IVP, it is usually near the ureterovesical junction.

DISPOSITION Patients should be admitted for attempted ureteral catheterization under cystoscopic guidance and possibly exploratomy laporotomy. Percutaneous nephrostomy with delayed repair may also be considered.

OTHER COMPLICATIONS OF GYNECOLOGIC SURGERY

Urinary Retention

Urinary retention in a healthy female after gynecologic surgery is uncommon. However, many women experience either an inability to void or incomplete emptying of the bladder during the postoperative period. Urinary retention is usually a temporary result of pain or bladder atony resulting from anesthesia.

CLINICAL FEATURES Inability to void is more frequent after operations that involve the urethra and bladder neck, i.e., anterior repair or any modification of the retropubic urethropexy. Most problems with voiding following any of these procedures resolve with time and without medication.

DISPOSITION Retention can be initally relieved with insertion of a Foley catheter for 12 to 24 h. Most patients are able to void after this period. An alternative method is intermittent straight catheterization. Patients are instructed to attempt to void on a timed schedule at intervals of less than 3 h. Patients should be taught to perform self-catheterization if they are unable to void. Self-catheterization can be taught in the emergency department, and the patient should be reassured that voiding function will return in time. If a patient still has trouble voiding after temporary placement of a Foley catheter, the problem may be ureteral spasm, which can be treated with phenazopyridine or oxybutynin.

Vesicovaginal Fistula

CLINICAL FEATURES Vesicovaginal fistulas may occur after total abdominal hysterectomy. Patients present 10 to 14 days after surgery with a watery vaginal discharge. The diagnosis can be confirmed by inserting a cotton tampon into the vagina and then instilling methylene blue or indigo carmine dye via a transurethral catheter. If the tampon stains blue, a vesicovaginal fistula is present. If no staining occurs, a ureterovaginal fistula must be ruled out by injecting 5 mL of indigo carmine dye intravenously. If a ureterovaginal fistula is present, the tampon should stain blue within 20 min.

DISPOSITION Gynecologic consultation is necessary. A Foley catheter should be inserted for prolonged drainage if a vesicovaginal fistula is present. With continuous drainage, up to 15 percent close spontaneously within 4 to 6 weeks.

Osteomyelitis Pubis

CLINICAL FEATURES Osteomyelitis pubis is a rare complication of pelvic surgery that presents 6 to 8 weeks after surgery with pain and tenderness along the symphysis pubis, especially with ambulation. Osteomyelitis pubis results from direct or contiguous seeding of the periosteum from pelvic surgery. It has been seen in the past following certain types of bladder neck suspension. Patients have a low-grade fever, elevated sedimentation rate, and leukocytosis. Blood should be drawn for culture, since the results are sometimes positive.

DISPOSITION Patients should be admitted for parenteral antibiotics and possibly surgical debridement.

Wound Hematoma

CLINICAL FEATURES Hematomas are a common complication of wound closure and are more frequent in transverse than in vertical incisions. The wound itself may swell and be painful.

DISPOSITION In general, smaller hematomas can and should be managed expectantly. If there are any signs of infection, the wound should be opened and drained. An ultrasound examination of the incision may be helpful if hematoma is suspected. The patient should be instructed to return if signs of infection develop.

Wound Seroma

CLINICAL FEATURES Wound seromas are relatively uncommon in gynecologic incisions, with the exception of groin dissection. A wound seroma is a collection of serous fluid and may drain spontaneously. In general, it is the presence of drainage, not fever or pain, that prompts patients to seek emergency care.

DISPOSITION If the wound remains intact after gentle probing, the seroma can be watched and usually disappears. If the seroma has reached a large size, drainage can be performed by aspiration and light pressure over the lymphocyst. Wound infection precautions should be given.

Postconization Bleeding

CLINICAL FEATURES High-grade squamous intraepithelial lesions of the cervix may be treated by loop electrocautery or cold-knife cone. The most common complication of these procedures is bleeding. If delayed hemorrhage occurs, it usually occurs 7 days postoperatively. Bleeding following this procedure can be rapid and severe.

DISPOSITION Visualization of the cervix is the key to controlling such bleeding. Application of Monsel solution is a reasonable first step if it is readily available. If this is not successful, a gynecologist should be consulted for suturing of the bleeding arteriole. Often, the patient must be taken to the operating room for repair because adequate visualization is difficult in the emergency department.

Septic Pelvic Thrombophlebitis

CLINICAL FEATURES Septic pelvic thrombophlebitis (SPT) is a diagnosis of exclusion complicating 0.1 to 0.5 percent of gynecologic procedures. The diagnosis is made when a patient with a postoperative fever does not respond to appropriate antibiotics in the absence of an undrained abscess or infected hematoma. Patients with SPT rarely present to the emergency department, since the complication typically presents in the hospital and delays discharge.

There are two forms of SPT. The classic form occurs 2 to 4 days after abdominal surgery and is characterized by fever, tachycardia, gastrointestinal distress, and unilateral abdominal pain. A palpable abdominal cord is seen in 50 to 67 percent of cases. The enigmatic form complicates vaginal delivery and pelvic surgery. Patients have spiking fevers despite clinical improvement on antibiotics. Findings upon pelvic examination may be normal in patients with either form.

DISPOSITION Heparin for 7 to 10 days is the mainstay of treatment. Long-term anticoagulation is not needed unless septic pulmonary emboli have occurred. Antibiotics against heparinase-producing *Bacterioides* species should be given to all patients.

Induced Abortion

There are three major methods for termination of a pregnancy: instrumental evacuation by the vaginal route, stimulation of uterine contraction, and major surgical procedures. Complications occur in between 1 and 5 percent of cases,[11,12] and can be immediate, delayed, or late. Immediate complications, less than 24 h after the abortion, include bleeding and pain. Most immediate complications are arrested at surgery, but many present within 24 h to the emergency department. Retained products of conception, uterine perforation, and cervical lacerations are the most common causes of immediate bleeding and pain. Delayed complications occur between 24 h and 4 weeks postabortion and include excessive bleeding, primarily due to retained products of conception, and post-abortive endometritis. Late complications include post-abortal amenorrhea, psychological problems, including depressions, and Rh isoimmunization.

If a cervical laceration is noted, treatment includes pressure followed by application of Monsel solution or use of silver nitrate sticks. Suturing may be necessary if there is no resolution of bleeding. Uterine perforation occurs in approximately 1 to 3 per 1000 abortion procedures. Most perforations are noted at the time of surgery and are asymptomatic. However, those that go unnoticed can present with pain and/or bleeding and possibly signs of shock. The incidence of retained products of conception is 0.5 to 1.0 percent. On physical examination, the cervical os is generally open. The uterus is usually boggy, enlarged, and tender. A pelvic sonogram should be obtained to evaluate the uterine cavity for retained products. Repeat dilatation and curretage is necessary. If coexistent endometritis is present, treatment with antibiotics is required for 10 to 14 days. Usual therapy includes "triple antibiotics" (ampicillin, gentamycin, and clindamycin) until the patient is afebrile for 24 to 48 h.

Post-abortal endometritis not associated with retained products of conception presents with a firm, yet tender uterus and closed cervical os. Uncomplicated endometritis requires antibiotics, as previously discussed, and possible reaspiration based on sonographic findings. Rh immune globulin should be given to Rh negative women after a spontaneous or induced abortion. If it is not prescribed, the overall risk of sensitization in the second pregnancy is approximately 3 percent.

Brachytherapy

Brachytherapy is the treatment of malignant tumors by radioactive sources that are implanted, typically under general anesthesia, close to (intercavitary) or within (interstitial) the tumor. It may be used as adjuvant therapy following surgery or as primary therapy if the malignancy is advanced. Currently, radiation therapy is geared mainly toward cervical and uterine cancers and remains limited in ovarian cancer.

The normal tissues of the cervix and uterus can tolerate very high doses of radiation. In contrast, the sigmoid, rectosigmoid, and rectum do not and, therefore, are more susceptible to radiation injury. Usually the small bowel is spared because it is in motion. Acute radiation cystitis can occur in the immediate postoperative period. Symptoms of cystitis are present but cultures are negative. Treatment is to increase oral intake and take a urinary analgesic. Chronic radiation cystititis with hematuria requires continuous bladder irrigation.

Radiation induced soft tissue necrosis can also be a significant complication. It is thought to be due to a progressive end arteritis leading to decreased blood flow and eventually hypoxia. Often this leads to inflammation, infection, tissue breakdown, and fistula formation. The use of hyperbaric oxygen has been shown to enhance healing.

Assisted Reproductive Technology

Transvaginal ultrasonographically guided aspiration of oocytes is used universally during in vitro fertilization. Previously, laparoscopic oocyte collection had been used, carrying the occasional complications of laparoscopic surgery, including those related to general anesthesia. Complications related to ultrasound-guided retrieval of oocytes are rare and include ovarian hyperstimulation syndrome, pelvic infections, intraperitoneal bleeding, and adnexal torsions.[13–15] However, the acute abdomen has developed hours to weeks after the procedure and has required prompt surgical intervention.

Ovarian hyperstimulation syndrome can be a life-threatening complication of induction of ovulation. The incidence in the moderate-to-severe form is 1 to 2 percent. Symptoms include abdominal distention, ovarian enlargement, and weight gain in the mildest form. In the most severe form, patients have massive third-spacing of fluids into the abdominal cavity, which can lead to ascites, electrolyte imbalances, pleural effusions, and hypovolemia. Clinically, one sees increased coagulability and decreased renal perfusion. The decreased renal perfusion leads to increased salt and water reabsorption in the proximal tubule, leading to oliguria. Abdominal and pelvic examinations are contraindicated due to extremely fragile ovaries that are at high risk of rupture or hemorrhage. Patients are also at high risk for ovarian torsion because of the size of their ovaries. Electrolyte studies, renal function tests, a complete blood count, coagulation studies, and blood for type and cross match should be obtained. An electrocardiogram to evaluate potential hyperkalemic changes should also be obtained. The gynecologist should be consulted for admission. Treatment is conservative, and diuretics are contraindicated. Volume repletion may be necessary.

REFERENCES

1. Gold BS, Kitz DS, Lecky JH, Neuhaus JM: Unanticipated admission to the hospital following ambulatory surgery. *JAMA* 262:3008, 1989.
2. Meeks GR, Waller GA, Meydrech EF, Flautt FH: Unscheduled hospital admission following ambulatory gynecologic surgery. *Obstet Gynecol* 80:446, 1992.
3. Bateman BG, Kolp LA, Hoeger K: Complications of laparoscopy: Operative and diagnostic. *Fertil Steril* 66:30, 1996.
4. Hulka J, Peterson HB, Phillips JM, Surrey MW: Operative laparoscopy: American Association of Gynecologic Laparoscopists' 1993 membership survey. *J Am Assoc Gynecol Laparosc* 2:133, 1995.
5. Saidi MH, Vancaillie TG, White AJ, et al: Complications of major operative laparoscopy: A review of 452 cases. *J Reprod Med* 41:471, 1996.
6. Chapron CM, Pierre F, Lacroix S, et al: Major vascular injuries during gynecologic laparoscopy. *J Am Coll Surg* 185:461, 1997.
7. Hulka JF, Peterson JB, Phillips JM, Surrey MW: Operative hysteroscopy: American Association of Gynecologic Laparoscopists 1991 membership survey. *J Reprod Med* 38:572, 1993.
8. Richards PL, Balch CM, Aldrete JS: Abdominal wound closure. *Ann Surg* 197:238, 1983.
9. Martyak SN, Curtis LE: Abdominal incision and closure. *Am J Surg* 131:476, 1976.
10. Poole GB: Mechanical factors in abdominal wound closure: The prevention of fascial dehiscence. *Surgery* 97:631, 1985.
11. Hakim-Elahi E, Tovell HMM, Burnhhill MS: Complications of first trimester abortion: A report of 170,000 cases. *Obstet Gynecol* 76:129, 1990.
12. Jacot FRM, Poulin C, Bilodeau AP, et al: A five-year experience with second-trimester induced abortions: No increase in complication rate as compared to the first trimester. *Am J Obstet Gynecol* 168:633, 1993.
13. Dicker D, Ashkenazi J, Feldberg D, et al: Severe abdominal complications after transvaginal ultrasonographically guided retrieval of oocytes for in-vitro fertilization and embryo transfer. *Fertil Steril* 59:1313, 1993.
14. Govaerts I, Devreker F, Delbaere A, et al: Short-term medical complications of 1500 oocyte retrievals for in-vitro fertilization and embryo transfer. *Eur J Obstet Gynecol Reprod Biol* 77:239, 1998.
15. Bergh T, Lundkvist O: Clinical complications during in-vitro fertilization treatment. *Hum Reprod* 7:625, 1992.

PELVIC ULTRASONOGRAPHY

Robert F. Reardon
Dietrich V. K. Jehle

Ultrasonography is a standard diagnostic tool used in the evaluation of pregnancy and female pelvic pathology.[1] Bedside pelvic ultrasound is commonly used in the emergency department (ED) in order to guide the evaluation of women with pelvic pain, pregnancy problems, and maternal trauma. The use of early pelvic ultrasound is essential for the timely diagnosis of ectopic pregnancy and placenta previa. Recent studies have demonstrated that bedside transvaginal ultrasound performed by emergency physicians improves early detection and decreases morbidity of patients with ectopic pregnancy.[2–4] The availability of bedside pelvic sonography decreases the ED length of stay for women with early pregnancy.[5] This chapter describes many other indications for ED bedside pelvic sonography, all of which may be useful to the practicing emergency physician. Since training and experience with pelvic sonography is highly variable among emergency physicians, a cautious approach to ''ruling out'' serious conditions should be employed initially. For example, ordering a ''formal'' ultrasound to be performed in the radiology or ob/gyn department is reasonable when no intrauterine pregnancy is identified in a symptomatic pregnant patient.

IMAGING TECHNIQUES

General discussion of the principles of ultrasonagraphy are found in Chap. 295. Transabdominal and transvaginal imaging are complementary studies in evaluating the female pelvis. Transabdominal sonography gives a good overview of the pelvis but requires a full urinary bladder. When the bladder is full, it acts as an acoustic window to the pelvis for transabdominal scanning. If empty, retrograde filling of the bladder with 300 to 500 mL of saline, with careful avoidance of introducing air, may be necessary to obtain adequate visualization. In contrast, transvaginal sonography is performed with an empty bladder, which is more comfortable for the patient. Transabdominal scanning of the pelvis is usually performed with lower-frequency transducers (3 to 3.5 MHz) that provide a larger field of view and deeper penetration but with lower resolution. Transvaginal images generally provide better resolution with a smaller field of view, since the transducer is placed closer to the area of interest and utilizes a higher-frequency probe (5 to 7.5 MHz). The standard transabdominal views are longitudinal and transverse and the orientation of the pelvic anatomy is relatively simple (Figs. 109-1 and 109-2). Standard transvaginal views are sagittal and coronal; however, orientation of pelvic anatomy is initially more difficult (Fig. 109-3). Identifying the anatomy of the uterus before searching for other pelvic structures may assist in obtaining transvaginal images.

SONOGRAPHIC PELVIC ANATOMY

Transabdominal versus Transvaginal Imaging

Transabdominal midline images of the pelvis in the longitudinal plane will show the long axis of the uterus posterior to the distended bladder.

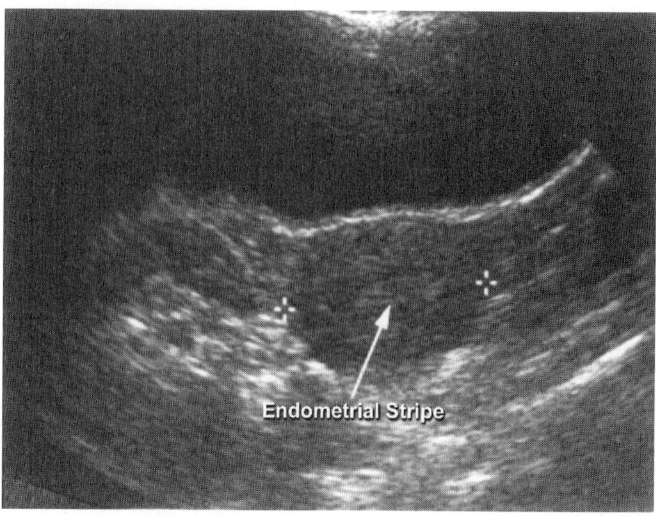

FIG. 109-2. Normal transverse pelvic anatomy. The uterus is seen posterior to the bladder on a transabdominal scan in the transverse plane. The margins of the uterus are marked by plus signs and the arrow points to the endometrial stripe.

The cervix will be visualized immediately posterior to the angle of the bladder. The posterior cul-de-sac (pouch of Douglas) is a potential space where free intraperitoneal fluid may be found, posterior to the uterus (Fig. 109-4). When a normal anteverted uterus is imaged, the uterus meets the vagina at an angle of 90° or greater, dependent on the amount of bladder distention. Retroversion of the uterus is a normal variant and can make transabdominal visualization of the uterine fundus difficult. The position of the uterus is less important when the transvaginal probe is used.

Uterus

Normal uterine size for a nulliparous menstruating female is up to 8 cm in length and 3 to 5 cm in transverse and AP diameter. Maximal uterine size for multiparous women may be 1 to 2 cm greater in each plane. The empty uterus is a thick-walled, muscular organ with moderate echogenicity. It contains a central hyperechoic (endometrial)

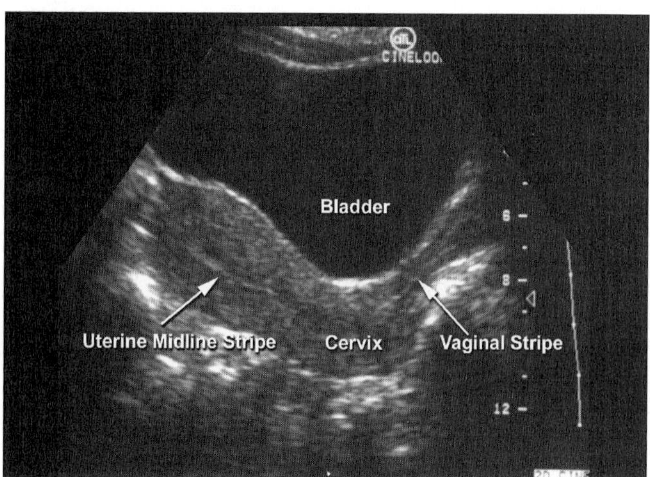

FIG. 109-1. Normal longitudinal pelvic anatomy. The uterus (*left*) and the vagina (*right*) are seen posterior to the anechoic bladder on a transabdominal longitudinal view. The cervix lies immediately posterior to the angle (deepest part) of the bladder.

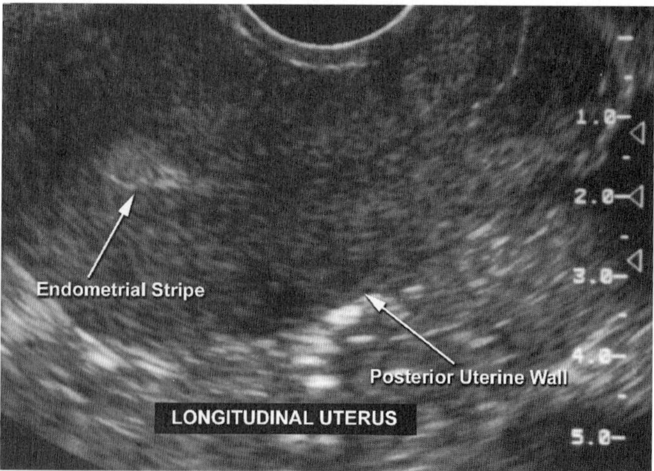

FIG. 109-3. Normal uterus. The midline endometrial stripe is seen at both ends of the uterus on a transvaginal sagittal view. The posterior uterine wall is clearly seen. The tip of the ultrasound probe is very close to the anterior wall of the uterus on this view.

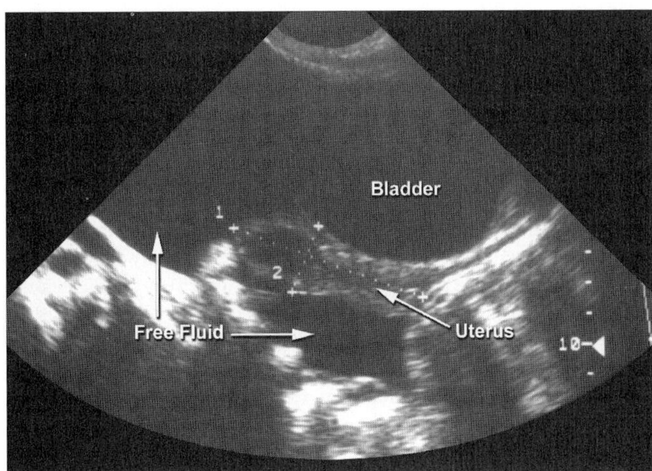

FIG. 109-4. Free fluid. The markers indicate the uterine dimensions on this transabdominal scan in the longitudinal (sagittal) plane. The anechoic bladder is seen anteriorly and anechoic free fluid is seen posteriorly (pouch of Douglas) and on the left side of the image.

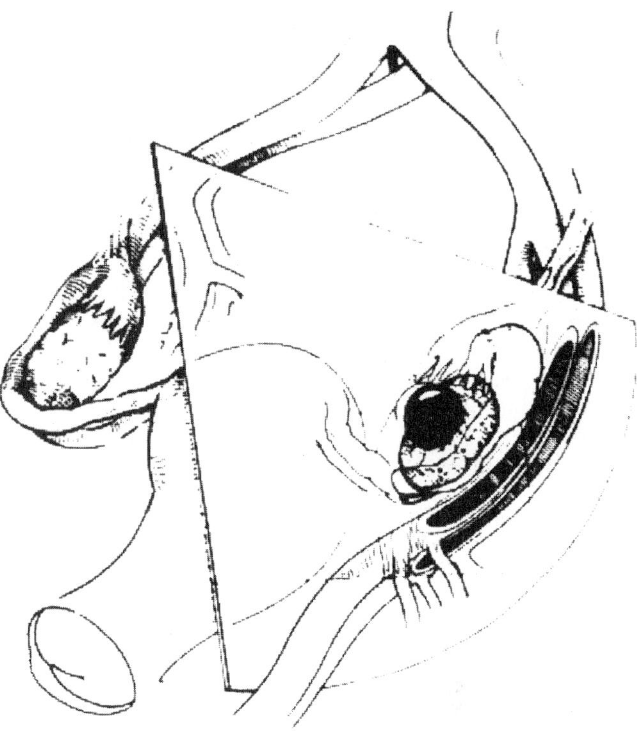

FIG. 109-6. Anatomy of pelvis. This drawing shows the normal anatomic relationship between the ovary and the iliac vessels, with the iliac vessels drawn in longitudinal section. See Fig. 109-7.

stripe that represents the opposed surfaces of the endometrial cavity. In the nonpregnant patient, the appearance of the endometrium is variable depending on the phase of the menstrual cycle. Early in the cycle the proliferative endometrium usually measures 4 to 8 mm in width (Fig. 109-1). Later during the secretory phase, the endometrium generally measures 7 to 14 mm and displays increased echogenicity (Fig. 109-5). The echogenicity and size of the menstrual endometrium are variable and dependent on the amount of blood and clot present within the uterus. The endometrium of the postmenopausal patient without hormonal replacement therapy is generally less than 9 mm in width. The combination of postmenopausal vaginal bleeding and increased endometrial width is suspicious for endometrial carcinoma and requires further evaluation. A markedly thickened postpartum endometrium suggests the presence of retained products of conception.

Ovaries

The ovaries can usually be found lateral to the body of the uterus, anterior to the internal iliac vessels, and anteromedial to the external iliac vessels (Figs. 109-6 and 109-7). There is variability in the position of the ovaries in women who have been pregnant. The distended bladder, which is required for transabdominal imaging of the ovaries, may displace them more cephalad. The size of each ovary is about 2 by 2 by 3 cm, although this may vary widely. Each ovary contains several small hypoechoic cysts, which are the maturing follicles. The sonographic appearance of the ovary changes throughout the menstrual cycle as several follicles are recruited and then a dominant follicle emerges, followed by the development of a corpus luteum.

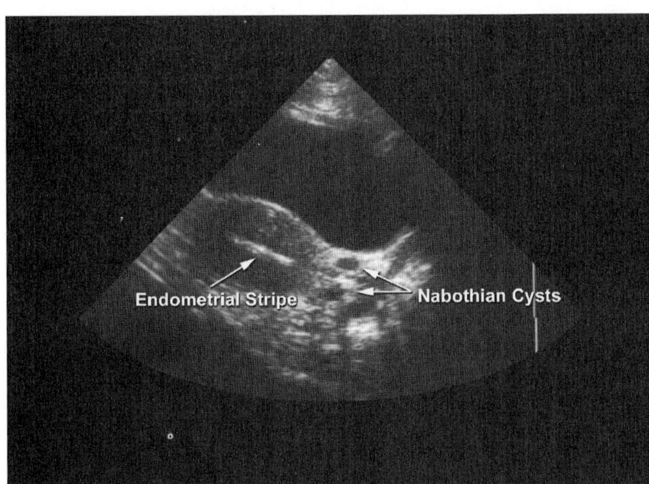

FIG. 109-5. The uterus with a thickened and hyperechoic endometrial stripe (secretory phase) is visualized on this transabdominal image in the longitudinal plane. Two nabothian cysts can be seen at the cervix, immediately posterior to the angle of the bladder.

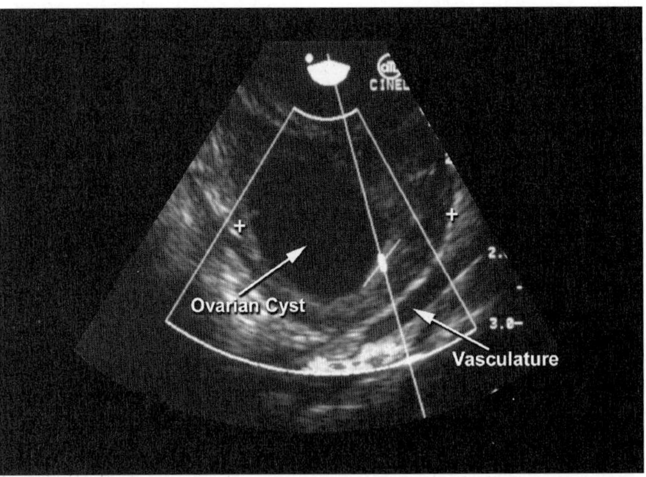

FIG. 109-7. Ovarian cyst. Sonographic image of the structures drawn in Fig. 109-6. A large cyst is visualized in the left ovary (plus signs mark borders). This demonstrates the normal position of the ovary in relation to the iliac vessels.

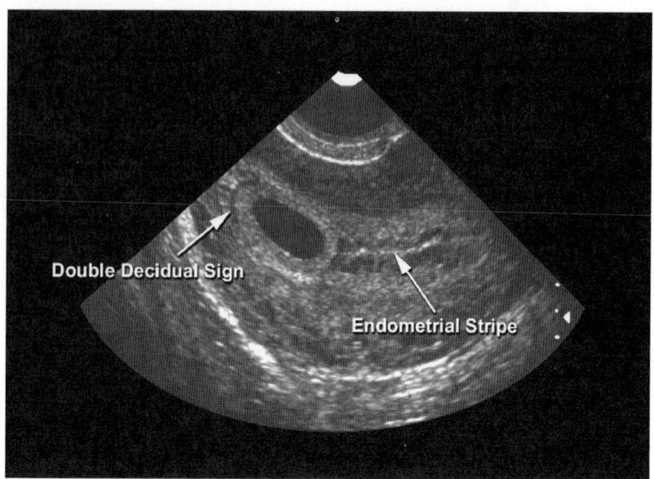

FIG. 109-8. Early intrauterine pregnancy. A gestational sac with a clear double decidual sign (*arrow*) between the two decidual layers on a transvaginal image in the sagittal plane.

NORMAL EARLY PREGNANCY

Ultrasound Findings

The first sonographic finding in early pregnancy is the gestational sac. This is a hypoechoic structure that is slightly eccentric in its location within the uterine cavity. The decidua capsularis and decidua vera are seen as two distinct hypoechoic layers surrounding the early gestational sac; this is known as the double decidual sac sign (Fig. 109-8). The yolk sac is the next embryonic structure to be visualized. It appears as a small ringlike structure within the gestational sac. Finally, the fetal pole can be recognized adjacent to the yolk sac (Fig. 109-9).[6] Cardiac activity can usually be observed if a fetal pole is present. The normal fetal heart rate seen in early pregnancy is 112 to 136 beats per minute, slower than heart rates observed in the second and third trimesters. If the ovaries are imaged early in pregnancy, a corpus luteum cyst may be seen (Fig. 109-9). These cysts usually measure 2 to 4 cm in diameter (can be up to 10 cm) with 3 to 4 mm walls. Corpus luteum cysts are generally anechoic; however, if they are hemorrhagic, they will contain internal echoes.

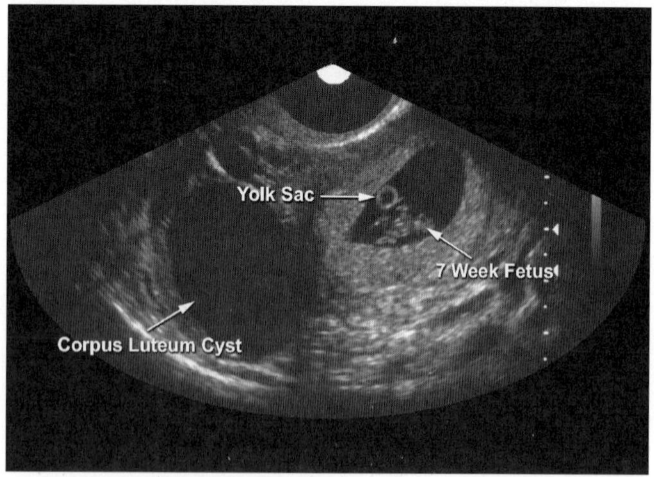

FIG. 109-9. Early intrauterine pregnancy. The ovary with a corpus luteum cyst is seen adjacent to the uterus. A yolk sac and fetal pole are present within the gestational sac.

Pregnancy Testing

The biochemical diagnosis of pregnancy may be made very early with the use of qualitative serum βhCG tests of blood and urine. Modern tests can detect serum βhCG levels of 20 mIU/mL or lower in urine and can diagnose pregnancy within 7 to 10 days after conception, at 3 weeks of gestational age. Gestational age is measured from the first day of the last menstrual period. Quantitative serum βhCG levels correlate with the gestational age of the normal pregnancy. At any given gestational age, serum βhCG titers are markedly higher when twins (or multiple gestations) are present. Table 109-1 indicates the approximate gestational age at which different sonographic and serum markers appear in early pregnancy.[7] The standards shown in the table are those of the International Reference Preparation (IRP). Some institutions may use an older standard called the Second International Standard, with values approximately one-half of the IRP values.

Determining Gestational Age

When sonographic evidence of an early pregnancy is definitive, the gestational age of the pregnancy can be estimated by measurements of the gestational sac, crown-rump length, or biparietal diameter. Mean sac size and crown-rump length provides the best estimates of gestational age during the first trimester. Measurements of sonographic structures very early in pregnancy give better estimates of gestational age than later measurements because the growth of the embryo during the first trimester is consistent between individuals and not dependent on genetic or nutritional factors. Mean sac diameter (MSD) is the average of three gestational sac measurements in millimeters: MSD = (length + width + depth) /3; gestational age (days) = 30 + MSD. In measuring crown-rump length (CRL) it is important to obtain the maximal embryo length, excluding the extremities and yolk sac. Gestational age (weeks) = 6.5 + CRL when CRL is measured in centimeters. Both MSD and CRL give very accurate estimates of gestational age. A significant discrepancy between CRL and MSD suggests a failing pregnancy. After the first trimester, gestational age should be estimated by measuring the (biparietal diameter) BPD of the fetal skull. The BPD is a transverse measurement of diameter at the level of the thalamus. The markers are positioned at the inside of one side of the skull and the outside of the opposite skull surface. Modern ultrasound software is capable of calculating gestational age automatically when the above measurements are marked on the display.

ECTOPIC PREGNANCY

The diagnosis of (ectopic pregnancy) EP is among the most challenging for the emergency physician. Significant morbidity and mortality may result from a missed or delayed diagnosis. (See Chap. 100 for a detailed discussion of ectopic pregnancy.) About half of all ectopic pregnancies

TABLE 109-1 Estimated Sonographic and Serum βhCG Landmarks[7]

Gestational Age	Transabdominal Landmarks	Transvaginal Landmarks	S BhCG Level, IRP*
4–5 weeks	±Gestational sac	Gestational sac	1000 mIU/mL
5 weeks	Gestational sac ± yolk sac	Gestational sac with yolk sac, ±fetal pole	1000–7000 mIU/mL
6 weeks	Yolk sac and fetal pole	Yolk sac and fetal pole with cardiac activity	10,000–23,000 mIU/mL

*IRP = International Reference Preparation.[7]

are missed on first presentation to the ED.[3,8] The use of protocols that rule out ectopic pregnancy incorporating transvaginal pelvic sonography and the βhCG discriminatory zone, can decrease the rate of missed ectopic pregnancies.[2,3,9]

Ectopic Location

EP occurs when the fertilized ovum implants anywhere except in the endometrium of the intrauterine cavity. Approximately 95 percent of EPs occur in the fallopian tube, with the ampulla being the most common location of implantation. Sites of implantation outside of the tube include uterine cornua, abdomen, ovary, and cervix. Cornual and abdominal ectopics may present late with profuse hemorrhage and probably represent the majority of pregnancies in which the patient dies before reaching the hospital. Cornual and cervical ectopics can be easily confused with a normal intrauterine pregnancy on the ultrasound examination. In addition, a cervical pregnancy may be confused with a nabothian cyst.

Initial Evaluation of Patients at Risk for EP

Female patients with complaints of vaginal bleeding, abdominal pain, dizziness, or syncope present very commonly in any ED. A high index of suspicion for EP is required, since about one-third of patients with EP are nontender on exam and about 10 percent have no complaint of abdominal pain.[9] A urine βhCG test should be the first step in the evaluation of such patients. Patients with a positive test require further evaluation. A negative urine test followed by a negative serum βhCG, virtually rules out the possibility of EP.[8] If the qualitative βhCG test is positive, an EP may be present. A protocol to rule out EP that includes bedside transvaginal sonography and a serum βhCG discriminatory zone allows emergency physicians to evaluate high-risk patients more quickly and effectively (see Chap. 100).[3–5]

Ultrasound Evaluation

Transvaginal sonography is more sensitive and specific than transabdominal sonography in evaluating first-trimester pregnancies. Transvaginal sonography can differentiate between intrauterine pregnancy (IUP) and EP in 75 percent of pregnant women who present with pain or bleeding. Transvaginal sonography has 69 percent sensitivity and 99 percent specificity for diagnosing EP.[9] If a definite IUP or EP is seen, the workup is complete. The finding of an IUP rules out the diagnosis of EP as long as there is a single gestation. Patients on fertility drugs may have multiple gestations. The presence of a yolk sac, fetal pole, or cardiac activity within an intrauterine gestational sac confirms the presence of an IUP. Visualization of a gestational sac alone should not be relied upon to make the diagnosis of an early IUP unless a double decidual sign is clearly seen. The presence of an EP is immediately established in about 15 percent, by either visualization of cardiac activity or an obvious gestational sac, yolk sac, and fetal pole outside of the uterus. The finding of a tubal ring in the adnexa is highly suggestive of an EP (Fig. 109-10). An EP is strongly suspected when pelvic free fluid and/or a complex adnexal mass is seen.[10–12] Consider ordering a ''formal'' pelvic ultrasound when no IUP is seen on bedside sonography, since the ancillary findings of EP may be subtle.

Quantitative Serum βhCG and Discriminatory Zone

When no IUP is noted and no sonographic ''ancillary findings'' of EP exist, a quantitative serum βhCG should be obtained if not already done. In using quantitative serum βhCG in a protocol to rule out ectopic pregnancy, the concept of discriminatory zone is important. A discriminatory zone is the serum βhCG level above which an intrauterine pregnancy is expected to be visualized sonographically. A

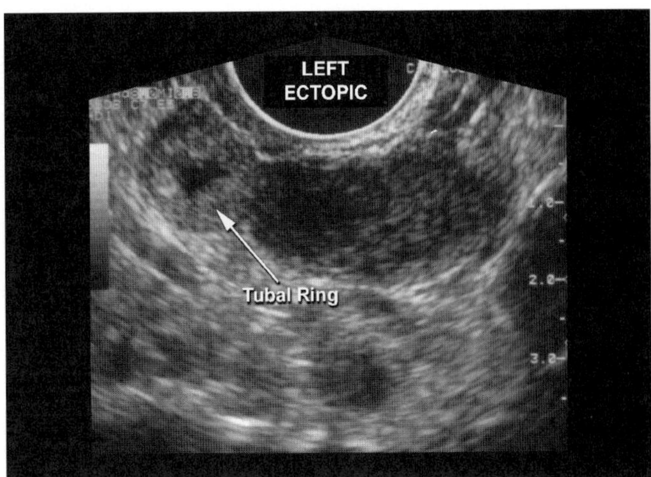

FIG. 109-10. Tubal ring. This represents hypertrophy of the left fallopian tube in a patient with an ectopic pregnancy.

discriminatory zone serum βhCG level of 2000 mIU/mL is commonly used.[2–4] A pregnancy with a serum βhCG level above 2000 mIU/mL without sonographic evidence of an IUP should be considered an ectopic pregnancy until proven otherwise and an ob/gyn consult should be obtained. With a low serum βhCG (<2000) and no IUP or ''ancillary findings,'' most gynecologists recommend a conservative approach with repeat serum βhCG titers and ultrasound studies in 3 to 7 days.[3] The discriminatory zone serum βhCG level may be adjusted depending on institutional variation and preference.

Potential Errors in the Diagnosis of EP

Several common errors should be avoided in evaluating a patient with a potential EP. Not considering the possibility of an EP is the first obstacle to making the diagnosis. A high index of suspicion for this diagnosis must be maintained. Reliance on the protocol to rule out EP, serum βhCG level, and pelvic sonography while ignoring significant physical signs can be a serious mistake. A history of ''passing tissue'' vaginally should not be considered evidence of a spontaneous abortion.[8] Only identification of chorionic villi or obvious fetal parts confirms abortion and rules out EP. Misinterpretation of pelvic sonography can lead to a delayed diagnosis of EP, with disastrous results.[8] An anechoic fluid collection without a clear double decidual reaction (gestational pseudosac) may be misinterpreted as an IUP. A gestational pseudosac is present in about 10 to 20 percent of patients who have an ectopic pregnancy.[8,13] A pseudosac is the result of endometrium that is stimulated by trophoblastic hormones and intrauterine bleeding (Fig. 109-11). The double decidual sac sign can be used to differentiate a true gestational sac from a pseudosac.[14] Finally, misjudging the intrauterine or extrauterine location of a pregnancy is a serious mistake. The location of the uterus should be clearly identified before a gestational sac, yolk sac, and/or fetal pole is called an IUP or EP. A normal pregnancy should be located in the fundus of the uterus. Interstitial and cervical pregnancies can be difficult to differentiate from IUP and should be considered when a patient presents in shock with an apparent IUP by ultrasound. Abdominal and ovarian pregnancies are obviously outside the uterus but may have the appearance of a viable fetus. Not recognizing the ectopic location of an apparently viable pregnancy is likely to have grave consequences, since an advanced EP is likely to cause severe hemorrhage upon rupturing.

Heterotopic Pregnancy

Usually the presence of an intrauterine pregnancy is sufficient evidence that an EP does not exist. However, in the case of patients who are

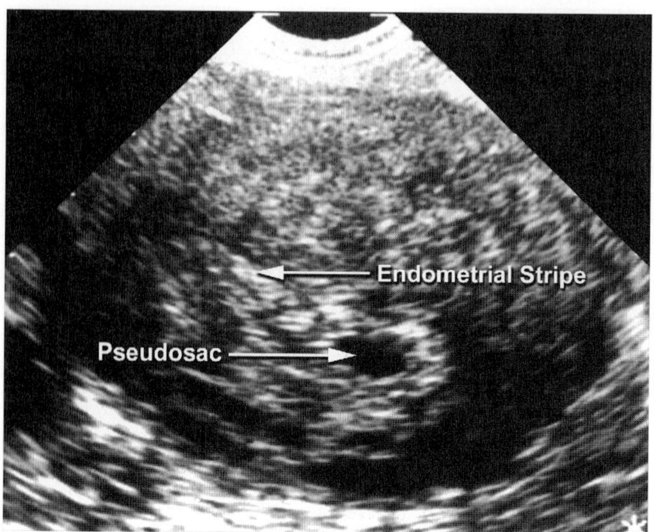

FIG. 109-11. Pseudosac. There is a hypoechoic sac inside the uterus, without a double decidual sign, yolk sac, or fetal pole in a patient with an ectopic pregnancy.

taking progestational/fertility agents, this assumption should not be made. The incidence of simultaneous intrauterine and extrauterine pregnancy (heterotopic pregnancy) in the general population is now thought to be as high as 1 per 4000 pregnancies, although historically this was only reported in 1 per 30,000 pregnancies. Those taking medications to enhance fertility are at much higher risk for heterotopic pregnancy. Patients who have a history of in vitro fertilization may have an incidence as high as 1 per 100 to 200 pregnancies.[15] For this reason sonographic imaging of the entire pelvis should be completed even after identification of an obvious IUP.

Ectopic Pregnancy with Low Serum βhCG

Low-serum βhCG EPs are common, and this is the weakness of the protocol described above. Simply assuming that a patient has a very early IUP because of a low serum βhCG level can be a major mistake. All patients need to have transvaginal sonography, even if they have a very low serum βhCG level. About 50 percent of symptomatic patients with an EP have a quantitative serum βhCG level below the discriminatory zone. In fact EPs with serum βhCG levels < 100 mIU/mL have been reported. EPs with low serum βhCG levels may rupture and cause bleeding just like other EPs.[16] Patients with low serum βhCG and significant risk factors or findings suggestive of EP should be closely observed. (See Chapter 100 for a detailed discussion of risk factors.) Those with low serum βhCG and no risk factors or evidence of EP may be sent home with close follow-up in 24 to 48 h. Pelvic sonography and quantitative serum βhCG are repeated on follow-up. During a normal early pregnancy, the serum βhCG will double about every 2 days. Abnormal pregnancies, ectopic or intrauterine, have a prolonged doubling time.[17]

ABNORMAL FIRST-TRIMESTER INTRAUTERINE PREGNANCY

Spontaneous Abortion

Spontaneous abortion occurs in as many as 40 percent of gestational events and approximately 15 percent of clinically apparent pregnancies. Most pregnancy losses occur early in the first trimester and few are lost after fetal cardiac activity is noted sonographically.[6] A completed abortion occurs when all of the products of conception have left the uterus. After a completed abortion, the cervical os may be opened or closed. If the os is closed and products of conception are not clearly identified, one should be skeptical about the diagnosis. An incomplete abortion occurs when some of the products of conception have been expelled and some still remain within the uterus. After a completed abortion, an empty uterus should be visualized sonographically; thus a postpartum endometrial stripe greater than 10 mm in a symptomatic patient suggests the presence of retained products of conception (Fig. 109-12). An inevitable abortion occurs when the cervical os is open but the products of conception have not yet been expelled.[1] A missed abortion occurs when the fetus is dead and is retained for greater than 4 to 8 weeks.

Threatened Abortion

Threatened abortion is vaginal bleeding in the pregnant patient before 20 weeks gestation. It complicates about 25 percent of all pregnancies. Vaginal bleeding is usually light and is accompanied by crampy pelvic pain. On examination, abdominal, adnexal, and cervical motion tenderness is usually absent and the cervix is closed. The pivotal step in the workup of a patient with first-trimester vaginal bleeding is pelvic sonography. If a live IUP is seen and there is a single gestation, expectant management is the rule. Although limitation of activity is recommended, there is no proven therapy for early threatened abortion.

Viability of an Early IUP

There are several sonographic criteria that can be used to decide whether an early IUP is viable or whether early fetal demise has occurred. Major criteria are those that uniformly predict fetal demise. Inability to visualize a yolk sac or embryo in a large gestational sac is a major criterion for demise; this is referred to as a blighted ovum (Fig. 109-13). Specifically, absence of a yolk sac when MSD is ≥ 10 mm using transvaginal sonography (TVS) or when MSD is ≥ 20 mm using transabdominal sonography (TAS) indicates certain fetal demise.[6] In addition, absence of an embryo when MSD is ≥ 16 mm using TVS or when MSD ≥ 25 mm using TAS predicts fetal demise with confidence.[6] Visualization of a grossly distorted gestational sac

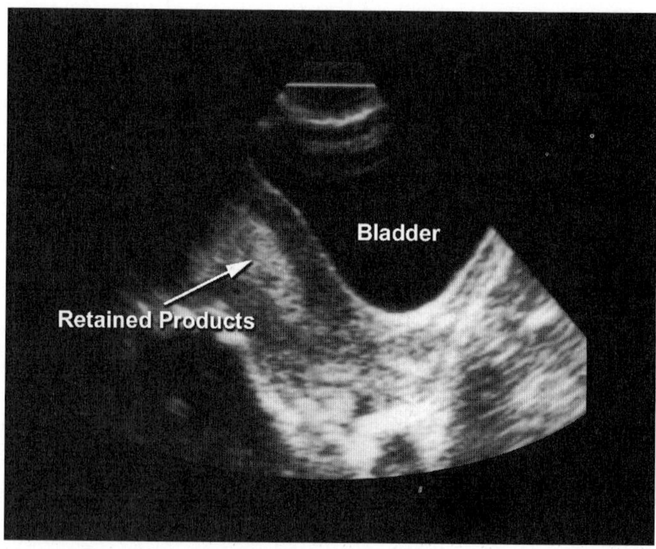

FIG. 109-12. Retained products of conception. There is a very thick (hyperechoic) endometrial echo measuring approximately 3 cm within the uterus on this transabdominal midline longitudinal view. This represents retained products of conception in a patient who had aborted a 10-week IUP. (Courtesy of J. Mateer, M.B. Phelan, and the Department of Emergency Medicine, Medical College of Wisconsin.)

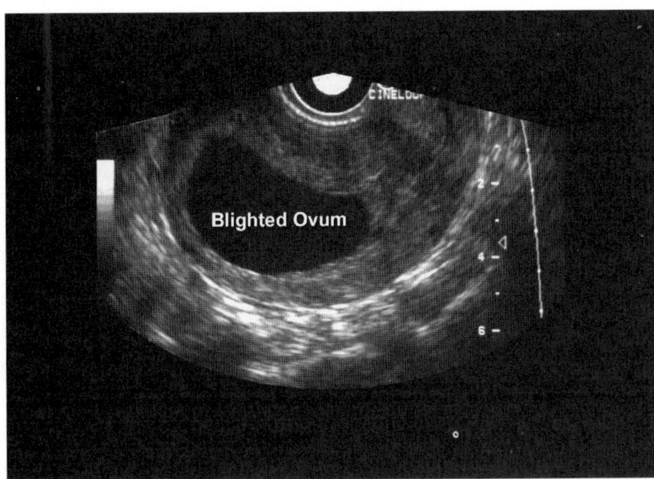

FIG. 109-13. Blighted ovum. There is a large, regularly shaped intrauterine sac without yolk sac or fetal pole.

uniformly predicts fetal demise but is somewhat subjective (Fig. 109-14). A gestational sac located in the lower portion of the uterus adjacent to the cervix is probably in the process of aborting.[6] An irregular, thin, or weakly echogenic choriodecidual reaction surrounding the gestational sac, decreased amniotic fluid volume, or a fetal heartbeat below 90 beats per minute after 6 weeks gestational age are all suggestive but not diagnostic of a failing pregnancy.

Subchorionic Hematoma

An intrauterine hematoma is present in about one-fourth of those with threatened abortion. In the first trimester, blood may accumulate in the endometrial cavity between the chorionic membranes and the uterine wall; this is known as a subchorionic hematoma or implantation bleed (Fig. 109-15 and 109-16). The presence of a subchorionic hematoma may more than double the chances of pregnancy loss in threatened abortion. The size and location are important factors in judging the significance of such bleeding. Small hematomas under the placenta are more important than larger hematomas elsewhere.

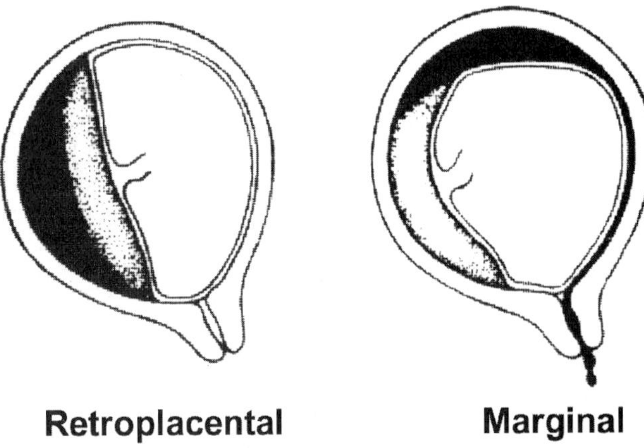

FIG. 109-15. Drawings of retroplacental and marginal hematomas.

Vaginal Bleeding with No IUP

The sonographic finding of an empty uterus in a patient with vaginal bleeding and a positive pregnancy test poses a difficult diagnostic dilemma. Very early IUP and completed spontaneous abortion are possible, but about 25 percent of these patients will have an EP.[13] When echogenic material is seen within the uterus, retained intrauterine products from an incomplete abortion or from partial resorption after fetal demise may be present; this should not be confused with intrauterine blood and clots, which can occur with an ectopic pregnancy. Completed spontaneous abortion is confirmed only by passage of obvious products of conception or identification of chorionic villi pathologically. Serial quantitative serum βhCG levels may be helpful in this setting. After spontaneous abortion, serum βhCG levels fall rapidly during the first 7 days. Close follow-up with serial sonography and serum βhCG levels may be needed before a final diagnosis can be made.

Molar Pregnancy

Gestational trophoblastic neoplasia is a proliferative disease of the trophoblast. The incidence in the United States is about 1 per 1500 live births. Most cases (80 percent) present as a hydatidiform mole

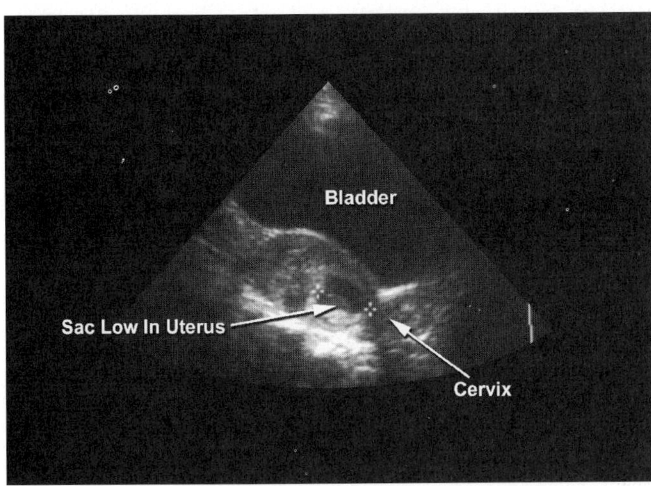

FIG. 109-14. Inevitable abortion. Irregularly shaped intrauterine sac low in the uterus.

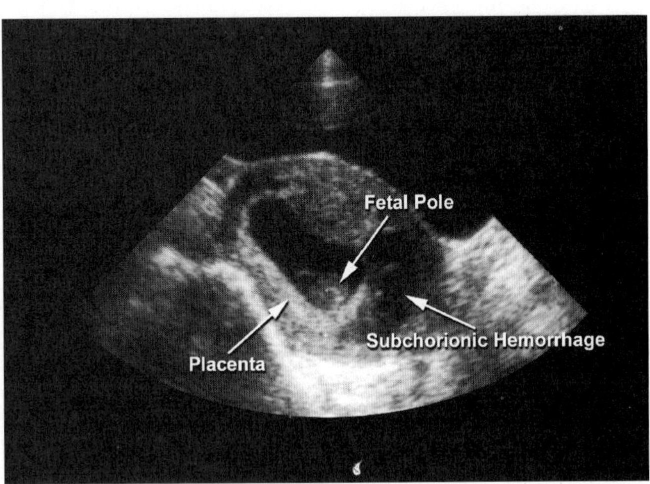

FIG. 109-16. Subchorionic hemorrhage. The anechoic region adjacent to the edge of the placenta represents a subchorionic hemorrhage. The placenta is the hyperechoic structure on the posterior wall of the uterus.

and follow a benign course. More malignant forms of the disease are invasive mole (12 to 15 percent) and choriocarcinoma (5 to 8 percent). Patients with a hydatidiform mole most commonly present with vaginal bleeding but may present with early preeclampsia or hyperemesis gravidarum. A larger-than-expected uterus for gestational age and markedly elevated serum βhCG level (>100,000 mIU/mL) are risk factors for malignant disease and are important clues to making this diagnosis. Most cases of molar pregnancy involve the entire placenta, but molar disease involving only part of the placenta or fetus have also been described. Pelvic ultrasound is the initial study of choice when a molar pregnancy is suspected.[1] Sonographically, a hydatidiform mole is an intrauterine echogenic mass with multiple small hypoechoic vesicles interspersed (Fig. 109-17). It is said to have a characteristic "snowstorm" appearance. However, the appearance of first-trimester moles may be confused with a blighted ovum or threatened abortion. A theca lutein cyst may be seen on examination of the ovaries in as many as half of the cases of gestational trophoblastic disease (GTD). They are large, multiseptated ovarian cysts caused by markedly high levels of serum βhCG. A benign mole usually resolves after evacuation of the uterus. Choriocarcinoma may metastasize to the lung, vagina, brain, or liver and is very sensitive to chemotherapy.

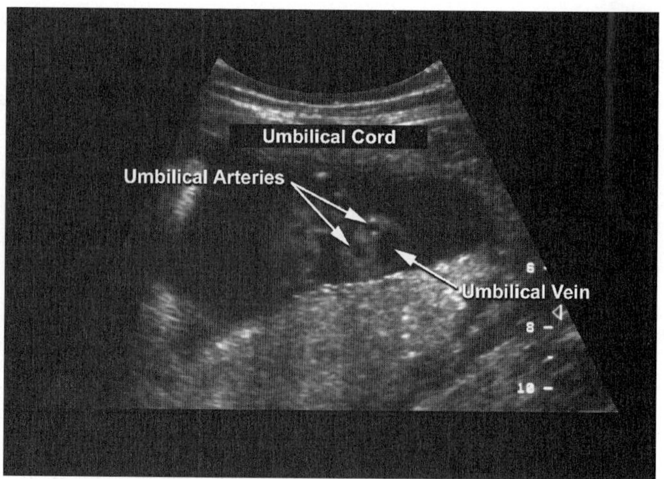

FIG. 109-18. Umbilical cord. Three loops of cord are seen in this image. An umbilical vein and two smaller arteries are seen in each loop of umbilical cord.

Second- and Third-Trimester Pregnancy

Ultrasound evaluations of second- and third-trimester pregnancies are often done in order to evaluate fetal well-being when maternal problems arise. Maternal vaginal bleeding, preeclampsia, diabetes, drug abuse, and trauma may all compromise the fetus. Ultrasound can be used to quickly evaluate several important structures that may have a bearing on the final outcome of the pregnancy. Although emergency physicians are not relied upon to perform routine ultrasound examinations during late pregnancy, many of the structures and abnormalities seen in late pregnancy are easily recognizable, even to those with little ultrasound training.

Immediate Fetal Viability

The visualization of fetal movements and fetal heart rate (normal = 120 to 180 beats per minute) takes priority in the acute setting.[1] The diagnosis of fetal death is established by careful sonographic imaging of the fetal chest for at least 3 min, with lack of cardiac activity. Two experienced sonographers should confirm the diagnosis.

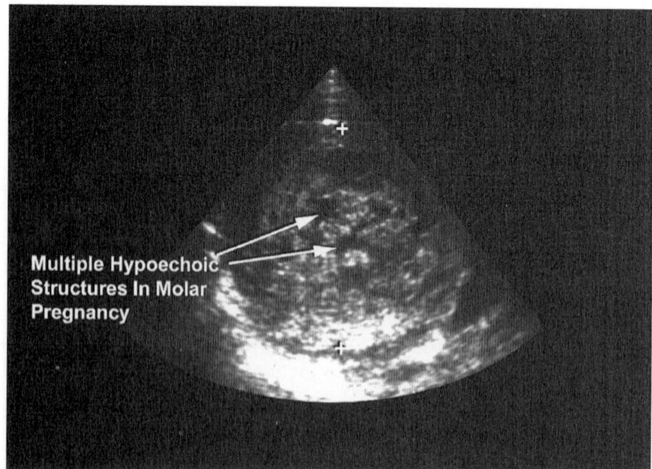

FIG. 109-17. Molar pregnancy. The two plus signs mark the borders of this molar pregnancy, which contains numerous grapelike hypoechoic structures.

Oligohydramnios and Polyhydramnios

The amount of amniotic fluid should be estimated. Subjective estimates of amniotic fluid volumes are best left to experienced sonographers, but extremes of polyhydramnios and oligohydramnios may be obvious to the neophyte. Amniotic fluid volume is large compared with fetal volume in normal early pregnancy; this should not be mistaken for polyhydramnios. A single measurement of the length of the deepest pocket of amniotic fluid gives a gross estimate of the volume and may be the best method of measurement for the inexperienced sonographer. A pocket more than 8 cm deep indicates polyhydramnios and a pocket less than 1 cm deep indicates oligohydramnios. A four-quadrant index can also be used to estimate the volume of amniotic fluid. The uterus is divided into four quadrants and the deepest pocket in each quadrant is measured. If the sum of the four measurements is less than 5 cm, oligohydramnios is present. If the sum is greater than 20 cm, polyhydramnios is present. An obstetrician should be consulted immediately when oligohydramnios is found, since it is associated with fetal renal malformation, severe growth retardation, and fetal death. Polyhydramnios may be associated with fetal anomalies, preterm labor, and premature rupture of membranes, but it is generally considered less serious.

Umbilical Cord

Sonographic examination of the umbilical cord should reveal two arteries and a single larger vein (Fig. 109-18). A cord that contains only one artery is associated with a 25 to 50 percent chance of fetal abnormalities. The cord vessels are best counted at the cord insertion into the fetus, since the two umbilical arteries may normally fuse at the placental end of the cord.

Fetal Gender

Both male and female genitalia are easily recognizable but should be clearly identified before the gender of the fetus is revealed. Lack of visualization of the penis and scrotum without clearly identifying the female labia is not adequate, and in this case no estimate of fetal gender should be made. Errors in sonographic sex determination occur relatively frequently; thus emergency physicians should avoid forecasting gender, as it adds little to emergency care.

Fetal Structures and Abnormalities

Fetal anatomy can be visualized quite easily in the second and third trimesters. Identification of the fetal head, chest, abdomen, and extremities is possible even for those with little ultrasound experience. Most major fetal anomalies can be recognized if ultrasound examination is done during the twentieth week of gestation or beyond. More subtle abnormalities can be recognized when a specific anomaly is suspected and a targeted examination of a single anatomic region is performed. Most routine fetal ultrasound examinations and all targeted examinations are done by physicians who specialize in fetal sonography.

THIRD-TRIMESTER BLEEDING—PLACENTA PREVIA

During the evaluation of third-trimester bleeding, the greatest utility of sonography is to establish the presence or absence of placenta previa. Since the sensitivity of sonography for the diagnosis of placental abruption is very poor, a presumptive diagnosis of placental abruption is often made after placenta previa has been ruled out. Placenta previa occurs when the blastocyte implants on the endometrium close to the cervical os and the placenta covers the os (Fig. 109-19). Painless vaginal bleeding in the third trimester is the classic clinical presentation. Placenta previa is fairly common and complicates about 0.5 percent of pregnancies at the time of delivery. Risk factors include multiparity, prior cesarean section, advanced maternal age, and abnormal fetal presentations. Attempted vaginal delivery in the presence of placenta previa may result in massive hemorrhage and death of the fetus, mother, or both. Cesarean section is required in complete placenta previa. Complete placenta previa is diagnosed when the placenta is implanted on both sides of the cervical os. A partial placenta previa covers part of the cervical os but does not bridge it. A marginal placenta previa abuts the cervical os but does not cover it. Since partial and marginal previas can both cause bleeding and ultrasound cannot distinguish between the two diagnoses, they are commonly grouped together. A low-lying placenta that does not cover or abut the cervical os may still cause bleeding, but not as frequently or severely as placenta previa.

Ultrasound Exam for Suspected Placenta Previa

Ultrasound is highly sensitive in detecting placenta previa, but a significant number of false-positive examinations occur. Since the consequences of placenta previa are so serious, it is important not to underdiagnose the condition. The standard examination for placenta previa uses TAS and a longitudinal projection with a full urinary bladder. In order to rule out placenta previa, the cervical os must be clearly visualized and must be free of overlying placenta. Visualization of the placenta at a site distant from the os makes previa unlikely but does not rule it out, since an accessory placental lobe may also be present. When the relationship between the internal cervical os and the placenta cannot be clearly established using the standard examination, other sonographic approaches may be attempted. Traction on the fetal head with the patient in the Trendelenburg position may allow an improved view of the cervical os in late pregnancy. Completely emptying the urinary bladder may improve transabdominal images of the cervical os in some cases. Transvaginal sonography gives better visualization of the cervix and is preferred in patients who have not had vaginal bleeding. The theoretical risk of dislodging clots and causing significant bleeding by introducing a probe into the vagina has led some clinicians to use transperineal sonography instead. Transperineal sonography is performed by placing the abdominal transducer on the perineum between the urethra and the vagina. This method has been found to be very accurate for diagnosing placenta previa.[18]

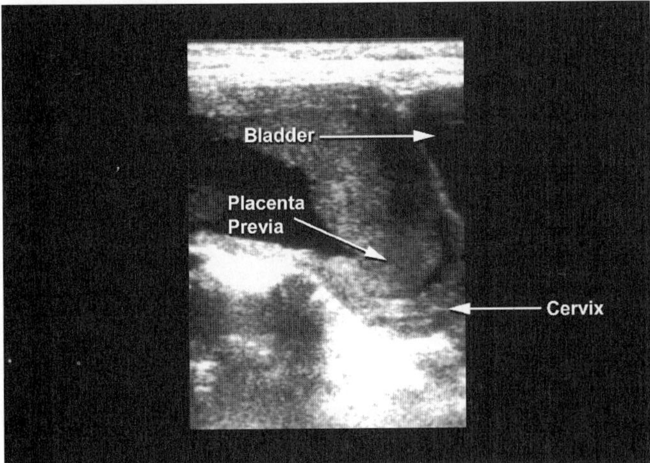

FIG. 109-19. Placenta previa. The cervix is seen on the right side of the image and is covered by the edge of the placenta. The placenta is the homogeneous structure on the anterior wall of the uterus.

False-Positive Diagnosis of Placenta Previa

Sonographic false-positive diagnoses of placenta previa may occur for a number of reasons. An overly distended urinary bladder may cause a low-lying placenta to appear as a previa. A myometrial contraction may mimic the placenta or push the edge of the placenta into the proximity of the cervical os. Diagnosing placenta previa at an early gestational age makes a false-positive diagnosis more likely. Many placentas that appear to cover or abut the cervical os during the second trimester are found to be a safe distance from the os on later exams. This apparent migration of the placenta is probably due to different growth rates of the placenta and the lower uterine segment. Most previas diagnosed before 20 weeks resolve prior to delivery.

THIRD TRIMESTER BLEEDING—PLACENTAL ABRUPTION

Premature separation of the placenta from the wall of the uterus is called *placental abruption.* Abruption can be severe or mild, acute or chronic, and retroplacental or marginal. Abruption causes varying degrees of pain and bleeding. Severe acute abruption classically causes severe, unremitting pain and vaginal bleeding, but bleeding may be mild or absent. Small abruptions may present as vaginal bleeding with little or no pain. Abdominal trauma, maternal hypertension, vascular disease, diabetes, smoking, fibroids, fetal anomalies, and cocaine use are thought to predispose patients to placental abruption. Abruption is found in about 5 percent of all placentas on pathologic examination; however, most small hematomas are asymptomatic and the clinical symptoms of abruption complicate only about 1 percent of all pregnancies. Sonography has very poor sensitivity for diagnosing placental abruption and lack of sonographic evidence certainly does not rule out abruption. However, a clinical presentation suggestive of placental abruption without sonographic evidence of a placenta previa should be assumed to be an abruption until proven otherwise.

Retroplacental Hematoma

Retroplacental hematoma separates the placenta from the uterine wall centrally and is likely the result of bleeding from spiral arteries (Fig. 109-20). Sonographically it appears as a hypoechoic stripe between the placenta and underlying myometrium, but it may have variable echogenicity depending on the age of the bleeding. An acute hematoma may be isoechoic with the placenta, so it may appear as simply a thickened region of the placenta. It will become hypoechoic in 1 to 2 weeks. A retroplacental contraction may mimic a hematoma, and

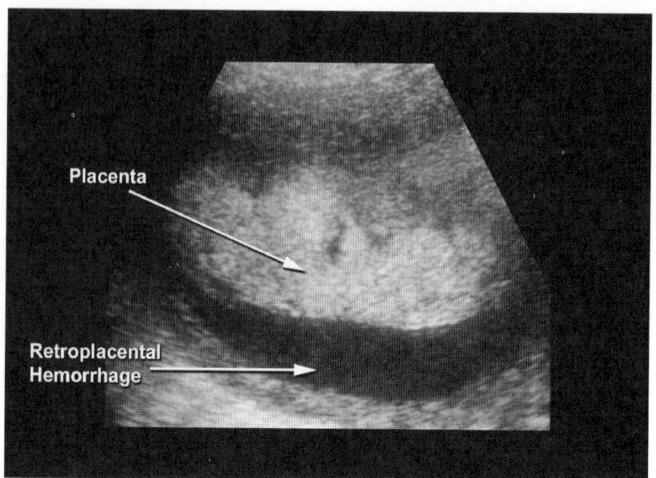

FIG. 109-20. Placental abruption. This retroplacental hemorrhage is visualized in a patient during the third trimester of her pregnancy. Retroplacental abruptions carry a poorer prognosis than marginal abruptions. See Fig. 109-15.

an old heterogeneous hematoma may look like a retroplacental fibroid. Retroplacental hematomas cause placental infarction and may result in fetal growth retardation, fetal death, and massive maternal hemorrhage. When a retroplacental hematoma is apparent sonographically, fetal mortality is directly related to the size of the hematoma.

Marginal Hematoma

Marginal hematomas occur at the edge of the placenta in the subchorionic plane. They are probably the result of bleeding from veins at the margin of the placenta. They are generally associated with less severe complications than retroplacental hematomas, but bleeding may still be severe. Some physicians have claimed that marginal hematomas are of no consequence to the fetus; however, some studies have shown that large hematoma volumes are associated with poor fetal outcomes.

TRAUMA IN PREGNANCY

When trauma occurs during pregnancy, the first priority is the stabilization of the mother. The most common cause of fetal death is maternal death. Ultrasound of the maternal abdomen should be accomplished early after significant blunt trauma.[1] The uterus is well protected within the pelvis during the first trimester of pregnancy; however, during the second and third trimesters, it is at much greater risk of injury due to its intraabdominal position. The sonographic appearance of intraperitoneal blood may be noted in the pelvis before it is detected in the Morison's pouch or elsewhere. Signs of fetal distress may be the first warning sign of occult maternal hemodynamic compromise. After maternal stabilization, the well-being of the fetus should be evaluated. Placental abruption and direct fetal injury must be suspected following significant maternal trauma in the second and third trimesters.

Fetal Sonographic Evaluation

Ultrasound can be used to assist in the initial evaluation of the fetus after maternal trauma.[1] First, ultrasound can aid in making a quick estimate of gestational age. Knowledge of the gestational age is important, since subsequent management decisions will be based on it. Next, a sonographic determination of immediate fetal viability can be made. If the fetus is dead (no cardiac activity and no fetal movement), the management of the mother will become the sole priority. Gross injury to the fetus, placenta, or uterus may be apparent on the initial ultrasound examination. Oligohydramnios following maternal trauma suggests uterine injury or premature rupture of the membranes. Large placental abruptions may be visualized and fetal distress (fetal heartbeat above 180 or below 120) may indicate unrecognized maternal, fetal, or placental injury. Urgent delivery of the significantly compromised fetus is indicated if the gestational age is at least 24 to 26 weeks. Traumatic uterine rupture is usually accompanied by massive bleeding and requires repair or hysterectomy regardless of gestational age. Although sonographic imaging may detect some large abruptions and gross fetal injury, cardiotocographic monitoring is a much more sensitive indicator. Fetal bradycardia, late decelerations, and loss of beat to beat variation are signs of distress. Fetal distress and frequent uterine contractions nearly always appear within 4 h following significant traumatic placental abruption.

PELVIC MASSES

Uterine Masses

A leiomyoma (uterine fibroid) is a benign proliferation of the smooth muscle and connective tissue of the uterus. It is the most common cause of uterine enlargement not related to pregnancy. Fibroids have a variety of sonographic appearances, ranging from hypoechoic masses with irregular uterine contours to echogenic structures with distinct calcified borders (Fig. 109-21). When a fibroid degenerates, multiple small cystic spaces are visualized within the fibroid. Fibroids can be intramural, submucosal, subserosal, or pedunculated. A fibroid may outgrow its blood supply, leading to necrosis and severe pain, especially during pregnancy. Rarely a fibroid degenerates into a uterine sarcoma. In addition, endometrial or ovarian carcinoma may invade the myometrium. Therefore complex or cystic uterine masses require further investigation.

Cervix and Vagina

The vagina and cervix are best visualized with transabdominal sonography. Visualization of the cervix with the transvaginal probe requires that the probe be withdrawn into the distal vagina. Nabothian cysts are benign growths that can commonly be seen in the region of the cervix (Fig. 109-5). Gartner duct cysts are also benign and may be seen at the anterior and lateral walls of the vagina. Imperforate hymen causes primary amenorrhea, lower abdominal pain, and urinary symp-

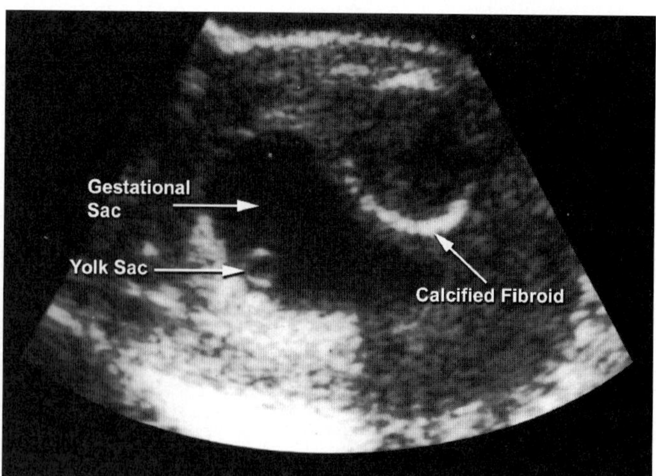

FIG. 109-21. Early intrauterine pregnancy. A yolk sac is seen within gestational sac (*left*). On the right side of the image, there is a calcified fibroid in the anterior wall of the uterus. Acoustic shadowing is seen posterior to the fibroid.

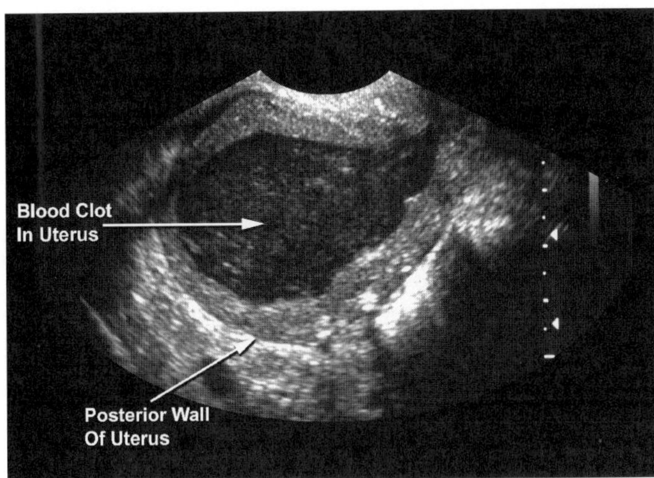

FIG. 109-22. Hematometra. A large amount of hypoechoic blood (clot) is seen within the uterus. This can be seen with an imperforate hymen or as a postoperative complication of gynecologic surgery.

toms during puberty. A tender lower abdominal mass may be palpable on physical examination and pelvic sonography will confirm that the vagina is filled with blood; this is called *hematocolpos.* A distended urinary bladder and a blood-filled distended uterus, or *hematometra,* may also be noted (Fig. 109-22). Perineal examination will reveal a bulging hymen; incision and drainage are required.

Adnexal Masses

Developing ovarian follicles may measure up to 2 cm at midcycle. Functional ovarian cysts measure greater than 2.5 cm and are well defined, thin walled, and anechoic. Most simple ovarian cysts resolve spontaneously, and serial sonographic exams are helpful to follow their progression. In postmenopausal patients, even well-defined anechoic ovarian cysts require further workup, especially if they are greater then 5 cm in diameter. Sonographically, polycystic ovary disease appears as bilaterally enlarged ovaries with multiple small follicles or a small number of very large follicles (Fig. 109-23). In some cases, the follicles are so tiny that they cannot be seen sonographically; thus a normal appearance of the ovaries does not rule out the diagnosis.

Complex Adnexal Masses

Hemorrhagic ovarian cysts have a variable appearance but are often difficult to differentiate sonographically from endometriomas, tubo-ovarian abscesses, benign ovarian tumors, or malignancies (Fig. 109-24). Dermoids appear sonographically as focal bright echoes in a complex adnexal mass. In general, septated, complex, irregular, and hyperechoic adnexal masses are more commonly malignant and require further investigation. The combination of a large, complex adnexal mass and ascites makes the likelihood of ovarian carcinoma very high.

OTHER CONDITIONS

Pelvic Inflammatory Disease and Tuboovarian Abscess

The diagnosis of pelvic inflammatory disease (PID) is usually made clinically, without the aid of ancillary studies. Ultrasound findings are unlikely to be noted early in the course of PID. In cases of severe PID, the ultrasound examination may demonstrate free fluid in the cul-de-sac or pyosalpinx. Pyosalpinx is an enlarged pus filled fallopian tube, which appears sonographically as a distinct circular structure with low-level echoes in the lumen when imaged in cross section. Pyosalpinx may appear to be a multicystic mass if multiple loops of distended tube are lying adjacent to one another. Sonographic evidence of pyosalpinx has been shown to be specific for the diagnosis of PID.[19] Tuboovarian abscess (TOA) is a complication of PID that can be accurately diagnosed using pelvic ultrasound. An abscess will appear sonographically as a complex mass with both cystic and solid components (Fig. 109-24). Percutaneous or transvaginal drainage of a TOA may be facilitated by ultrasound guidance.

Ovarian Torsion

Doppler ultrasound is commonly used for the evaluation of suspected ovarian torsion; however, the diagnostic accuracy of Doppler studies for ovarian torsion is poor. When torsion is present, the lack of internal ovarian blood flow on Doppler examination probably indicates that an ovary is beyond salvage. Also, the absence of blood flow to the ovary can be seen in a variety of cystic ovarian lesions when torsion is not present. Massive ovarian edema is an entity caused by intermittent or partial adnexal torsion. Doppler flow is present and resolution of the edema often occurs after detorsion of the adnexa. Simple gray-

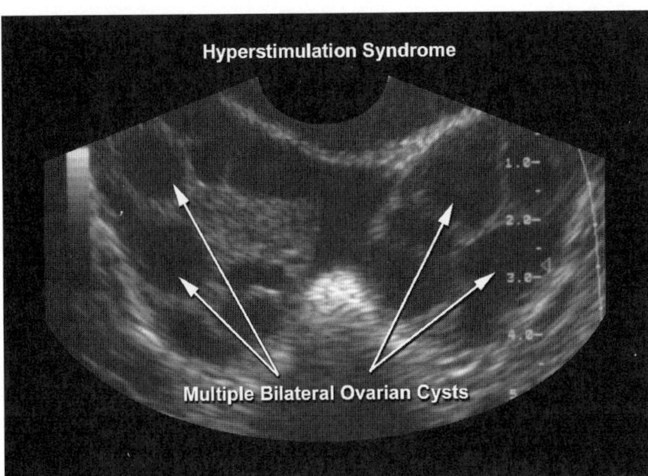

FIG. 109-23. Ovarian hyperstimulation syndrome. Multiple large anechoic cysts are visualized in both ovaries in this image. Ovarian hyperstimulation syndrome or polycystic ovary disease may have this appearance.

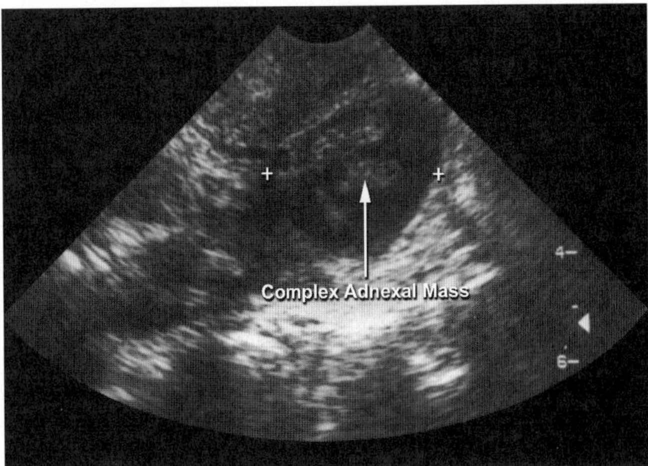

FIG. 109-24. Complex mass. This adnexal mass (plus signs mark borders) has multiple hypoechoic and hyperechoic regions. This could represent a tubo-ovarian abscess, ectopic pregnancy, hemorrhagic ovarian cyst, or ovarian tumor.

scale pelvic sonography is helpful when adnexal torsion is suspected, since most cases of torsion are secondary to large ovarian cysts or masses. The finding of a normal-sized ovary makes adnexal torsion unlikely.

REFERENCES

1. American College of Emergency Physicians: Clinical policy for the initial approach to patients presenting with a chief complaint of vaginal bleeding. *Ann Emerg Med* 29:3, 1997.
2. Mateer JR, Aiman EJ, Brown M, et al: Ultrasonographic examination by emergency physicians of patients at risk for ectopic pregnancy. *Acad Emerg Med* 2:867, 1995.
3. Mateer JR, Valley VT, Aiman EJ, et al: Outcome analysis of a protocol including bedside endovaginal sonography in patients at risk for ectopic pregnancy. *Ann Emerg Med* 27:283, 1996.
4. Durham B, Lane B, Burbridge L, Balasubramaniam S: Pelvic ultrasound performed by emergency physicians for the detection of ectopic pregnancy in complicated first-trimester pregnancies. *Ann Emerg Med* 29:3, 1997.
5. Shih CHY. Effect of emergency physician-performed pelvic sonography on length of stay in the emergency department. *Ann Emerg Med* 29:3, 1997.
6. Dart RG: Role of pelvic ultrasonography in evaluation of symptomatic first-trimester pregnancy. *Ann Emerg Med* 33:3, 1999.
7. Cacciatore B, Tiitinen A, Stenman U, et al: Normal early pregnancy: Serum hCG levels and vaginal ultrasonography findings. *Br J Obstet Gynaecol* 97:899, 1990.
8. Abbott J, Emmans LS, Lowenstein SR: Ectopic pregnancy: Ten common pitfalls in diagnosis. *Am J Emerg Med* 8:515, 1990.
9. Kaplan BC, Dart RG, Moskos M, et al: Ectopic pregnancy: Prospective study with improved diagnostic accuracy. *Ann Emerg Med* 28:1, 1996.
10. Nyberg DA, Hughes MP, Mack LA, et al: Extrauterine findings of ectopic pregnancy at transvaginal US: Importance of echogenic fluid. *Radiology* 178:823, 1991.
11. Brown DL, Doubilet PM: Transvaginal sonography for diagnosing ectopic pregnancy: Positivity criteria and performance characteristics. *J Ultrasound Med* 13:259, 1994.
12. Cacciatore B: Can the status of tubal pregnancy be predicted with transvaginal sonography? A prospective comparison of sonographic, surgical, and serum hCG findings. *Radiology* 177:481, 1990.
13. Dart R, Howard K: Subclassification of interdependent pelvic ultrasonograms: Stratifying the risk of ectopic pregnancy. *Acad Emerg Med* 5:313, 1998.
14. Nyberg DA, Laing, FC, Filly RA, et al: Ultrasonographic differentiation of the gestational sac of early intrauterine pregnancy from the pseudogestational sac of ectopic pregnancy. *Radiology* 146:755, 1983.
15. Dimitry E, Subak-Sharpe R, Mills M: Nine cases of heterotopic pregnancies in four years of in vitro fertilization. *Fertil Steril* 53:107, 1990.
16. Dart RG, Kaplan B, Cox C: Transvaginal ultrasound in patients with low beta-human chorionic gonadotropin values: How often is the study diagnostic? *Ann Emerg Med* 30:2, 1997.
17. Carson SA, Buster JE: Ectopic pregnancy. *N Engl J Med* 329:1174, 1993.
18. Dawson WB, Dumas MD, Romano WM, et al: Translabial ultrasonography and placenta previa: Does measurement of the os-placenta distance predict outcome? *J Ultrasound Med* 15:441, 1996.
19. Cacciatore B, Leminen A, Ingman-Friberg S, et al: Transvaginal sonographic findings in ambulatory patients with suspected pelvic inflammatory disease. *Obstet Gynecol* 80:912, 1992.

FEVER

Carol D. Berkowitz

Fever is the single most common chief complaint of children presenting to the emergency department, accounting for about 30 percent of pediatric outpatient visits. Physicians evaluating febrile children must differentiate mildly ill from seriously ill children, a challenge that may be compounded when no focus of infection is apparent. The extent of the diagnostic workup and the institution of appropriate management, including the use of antibiotics and the need for hospitalization, must be determined. Many factors—such as clinical assessment, physical findings, age of the patient, and height of the fever—influence the evaluation and management decisions.

PATHOPHYSIOLOGY

Fever is defined as a rise in deep body temperature associated with a resetting of the body's thermostat.[1] This thermostat is located in the preoptic region of the anterior hypothalamus near the floor of the third ventricle. Exogenous fever-producing substances (pyrogens)—such as bacteria, bacterial endotoxin, antigen-antibody complexes, yeast, viruses, and etiocholanolone—may stimulate the formation and release of endogenous pyrogens. Endogenous pyrogens are produced by neutrophils, monocytes, hepatic Kupffer cells, splenic sinusoidal cells, alveolar macrophages, and peritoneal lining cells and are believed to induce the synthesis of prostaglandins in the hypothalamus. Endogenous pyrogens include interleukin 1, interleukin 6, and tumor necrosis factor.[2] The body's thermostat is then reset at a higher setting, and the patient, whose own temperature is below that of the body's thermostat, experiences a chill. Peripheral vasoconstriction, shivering, central pooling, and behavioral activity (e.g., putting on a sweater or drinking hot tea) lead to an increase in body temperature.

CLINICAL FEATURES

The possible beneficial effects of fever have been debated for many years.[3] Aside from these considerations, it is important to recognize that fever represents a symptom of some underlying disease, and one must determine what this disease is.

An initial question is "What degree of temperature elevation represents a fever?" One survey conducted among pediatric training programs revealed a wide variability in the temperature considered a "fever" in infants younger than 2 months of age.[4] This figure has ranged from 38° to 39.4°C (100.4° to 103°F). It is important to recognize that oral temperatures are generally 0.6°C (1°F) lower than rectal temperatures and axillary temperatures are 0.6°C (1°F) lower than oral temperatures. Temperatures taken using infrared thermometers that scan the tympanic membrane are of variable reliability and reproducibility.[5] Body temperature normally varies from morning to evening with the body's circadian rhythm. The degree of variation, which is greater in young women and small children, is about 1.1°C (2°F).

Current practice guidelines suggest a temperature of 38°C as a sufficient fever to warrant an evaluation.[6] The relationship between height of fever and incidence of bacteremia is discussed below. In general, higher temperatures are associated with a higher incidence of bacteremia.[7] A retrospective study of hyperpyrexia reported that the incidence of meningitis was twice as high in children with fever above 41.1°C (105.9°F), compared with children with fever between 40.5° and 41.0°C (104.9° and 105.8°F).[8] The incidence of pneumonia and bacteremia was the same in the two groups.

Other studies, many of which have also been retrospective, have had variable results and indicated that children with higher temperatures have more diagnostic studies ordered but the same incidence of different diseases.[9–11]

INFANTS UP TO 3 MONTHS

Diagnosis

The age of the patient influences the extent of the workup. Early studies suggested that infants younger than age 3 months were at high risk for life-threatening infection.[12,13] Recent studies based on outpatients show that the incidence of serious bacterial infection, including bacteremia and meningitis, is about 3 to 4 percent, although serious nonbacterial infections (e.g., aseptic meningitis) are a frequent cause of fever in this age group.[14–16]

Presentation History

The history often provides a clue to the diagnosis. When evaluating infants younger than the age of 1 to 2 months, it is critical to review the birth history because the etiology of the infant's infection may be birth related. The key points to question include the length of the gestation, the use of antibiotics in the mother or infant, and the presence of any neonatal complications, such as fever or tachypnea. Although an organ-specific list of inquiries may be helpful in treating older infants, it is less useful in younger ones because the signs and symptoms of sepsis may be very nonspecific. For instance, vomiting and diarrhea accompany many problems, including gastroenteritis, otitis media, urinary tract infections, and meningitis.[16] Cough or respiratory symptoms would be consistent with a respiratory infection. Frequency of urination is important to assess as a measure of the state of hydration.

Physical Examination

Infants should be undressed completely to enable a full assessment. Vital signs are important to evaluate. For instance, tachypnea may be a clue to lower respiratory tract infection. Crying and the ease of consolability should be evaluated. Inconsolable crying, or increased irritability when handled, is frequently seen in infants with meningitis. Although fullness of the anterior fontanelle may be noted in some of these infants, other signs of meningeal irritation, such as nuchal rigidity, are most often absent. A head-to-toe evaluation should be carried out to determine whether there is a focus of infection, such as an inflamed eardrum or evidence of cellulitis.

Clinical assessment of the severity of illness of young, febrile infants is, however, problematic. Young infants lack social skills, such as the social smile, and their ability to interact with examiners is limited. There is a report in the literature of an infant with group B streptococcal bacteremia who was judged by house staff and faculty to be clinically well.[12] The absence of any diagnostic abnormalities in the medical history or on physical examination suggests the need for extensive laboratory tests to detect occult infection. These tests would include a complete blood count (CBC) and differential, erythrocyte sedimentation rate (ESR), blood culture, lumbar puncture, chest x-ray, urinalysis and culture, and a stool culture if there is a history of diarrhea, particularly if leukocytes are noted on a stool smear. Some authors also recommend a quantitative C-reactive protein as an index of serious bacterial infection.[17,18] Urinary tract infections may not produce symptoms other than fever, and so a urinalysis and culture should be included routinely in the evaluation. Urinary tract infections may be associated with bacteremia in up to 30 percent of infected infants[19,20] and are the single most common bacterial infection in this age group.

The recognition of occult serious infection in well-appearing young, febrile infants is problematic. Most investigators agree that no single variable can correctly identify these infants. Combinations of variables are more helpful in the differentiation process. Criteria have been identified by a number of investigators, but are generally referred to as the Rochester criteria for low risk for serious bacterial infection in infants younger than 3 months of age. These criteria include nontoxic appearance, no soft tissue infection, white blood cells (WBCs) between 5000 and 15,000/mm^3, bands less than 1500/mm^3, normal urinalysis, and stool with less than 5 WBCs/hpf (high power field) in infants with diarrhea.[17,18] The risk of serious bacterial infection in the absence of these variables is about 0.2 percent.

Management

The appropriate management of young febrile infants presents another area of disagreement.[21] There appears to be no ''community standard of practice'' regarding the need for hospitalization; some physicians hospitalize all febrile infants younger than age 3 months, and others hospitalize only those under age 1 month. Because the differentiation between sick and well infants is so difficult, all such febrile infants need extensive septic workups. The decision not to hospitalize a small febrile infant must be made after careful clinical and appropriate laboratory assessment and after ensuring the reliability of follow-up.

Current management strategies include the administration of ceftriaxone at a dose of 50 mg/kg to febrile infants between 1 and 3 months of age who are judged to be at low risk for serious bacterial infection when the above criteria are used.[22] A caretaker with a telephone is an additional criterion for such outpatient management. Similarly, Baskin and colleagues[23] proposed inpatient management of febrile infants who are between 2 and 4 weeks of age and also judged to be at low risk, using parenteral ceftriaxone and only 24 h of observation. Infants could be discharged if cultures were negative after 24 h.

INFANTS OF 3 TO 24 MONTHS

Diagnosis

Many of the considerations noted in the evaluation of infants younger than 3 months of age apply for older infants. Patients between 3 and 36 months have been the focus of considerable research because this group appears to be at higher risk for occult bacteremia. These studies have sought to identify clinical and laboratory characteristics of bacteremic patients.[7,24,25]

Clinical judgment appears to be more reliable in the assessment of older infants. Characteristics that evaluating physicians should note are willingness of patients to make eye contact, playfulness and positive response to interactions, negative response to noxious stimuli, alertness, and consolability. Toxic infants will not respond appropriately.[26]

Presentation History

Again, the medical history and physical examination will frequently reveal the source of infection. Viral illnesses, including respiratory infections and gastroenteritis, account for the majority of febrile illnesses and usually have system-specific symptoms, such as vomiting, diarrhea, rhinorrhea, cough, or rashes. In this age group, such symptoms are more often indicative of an organ-specific infection. Bacterial infections of the respiratory tract include most notably otitis media, pharyngitis, and pneumonia. Otitis media is generally caused by *Streptococcus pneumoniae* or *Haemophilus influenzae*, and antibiotic therapy, such as amoxicillin, should be directed at these organisms.[27] Although pneumonia is commonly of viral etiology, it is appropriate to institute antibiotic therapy with amoxicillin or erythromycin. The physical signs of meningitis, such as nuchal rigidity and Kernig or Brudzinski signs, may be inapparent in children even up to the age of 2 years. A bulging fontanelle, vomiting, irritability that increases when the infant is held, inconsolability, or a febrile seizure may be the only signs suggestive of meningitis. Infants with aseptic meningitis should generally be hospitalized and ensured adequate long-term follow-up because they are at higher risk for subsequent neurologic and learning disabilities. The presence of petechiae on physical examination should alert physicians to the potential presence of a serious underlying infection. Up to 20 percent of children may have bacteremia or meningitis most frequently with *Neisseria meningitidis* or *H. influenzae*.[28,29] Petechiae in association with high fever (≥40°C), ESR at or above 30 mm/h, and WBCs of at least 15,000/mm^3 are most frequently correlated with bacteremia.

Bacteremic infants may or may not have an obvious focus of infection. The height of the fever is a clue to which infants are bacteremic. Although bacteremia may be seen at lower temperatures, a temperature of over 39.5°C (103.1°F) in infants aged 3 to 36 months is associated with a higher incidence of bacteremia. Certain laboratory tests have been recommended to assist in further identifying bacteremic patients. WBCs over 15,000/mm^3, band counts of at least 500/mm^3, total polymorphonuclear counts at or above 10,000/mm^3, and band plus polymorphonuclear counts equal to or greater than 10,500/mm^3 are associated with an increased incidence of bacteremia, although bacteremia also occurs in the absence of these findings.[30] The incidence of bacteremia in children 3 to 24 months of age with a temperature of 39.5°C (103.1°F) or over is about 5 to 6 percent. The incidence increases to 12 to 15 percent in patients with WBCs of 15,000/mm^3 or over. An ESR at or above 30 mm/h has the same significance as WBCs of 15,000/mm^3 or greater.[7,25,26] The organism most commonly causing bacteremia in this age group is *S. pneumoniae. Haemophilus influenzae* has been rarely implicated in cases of occult bacteremia since the availability of *H. influenzae* vaccine.

Is it important to perform a blood culture to detect occult bacteremia?[31] Opinions vary on the answer to this question. It is apparent that bacteremic patients do better if they receive antibiotics early on.[32] Many bacteremic children do have a focus of infection and so are treated anyway. Additionally, in at least 25 percent of bacteremic patients with no focus of infection, the bacteremia is resolved without any antibiotics. Others develop soft tissue infections, which are then appropriately managed. The ability of oral antibiotics to prevent the development of meningitis in bacteremic children is still unclear. The blood culture appears to be useful for following patients who may not be returning for periodic evaluations. Therefore, from a medical and epidemiologic standpoint, blood cultures are indicated in high-risk infants or those in whom the physician suspects an infection.

Management

Is there a role for the use of expectant antibiotics in children suspected of having occult bacteremia? Retrospective studies have all shown that early antibiotics diminished the incidence of persistent bacteremia. In a prospective randomized study comparing oral penicillin to no antibiotics, no improvement was reported in any bacteremic child who did not receive antibiotics.[33] Other investigators report more equivocal results. Outpatient daily injections of ceftriaxone are being used by some physicians for children at increased risk of occult bacteremia. Controlled trials investigating the efficacy of this therapy have demon-

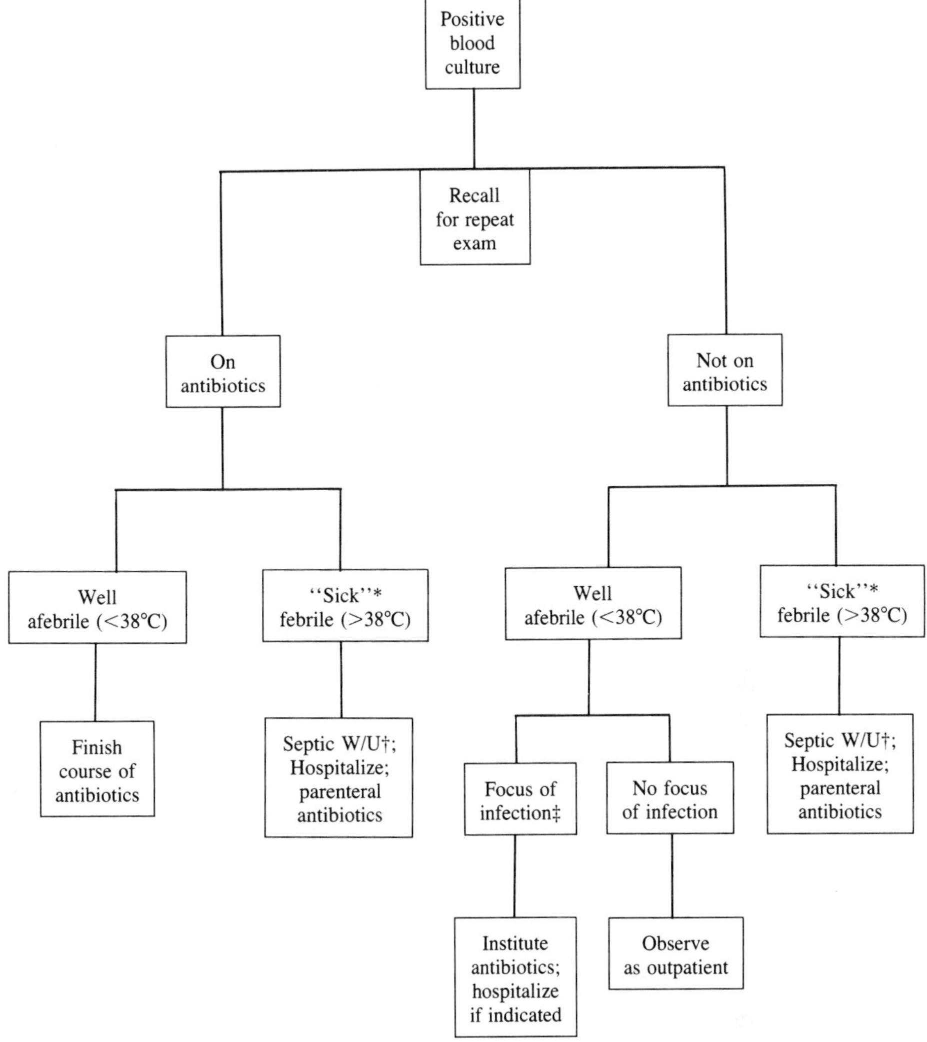

FIG. 110-1. Management of bacteremic children; *"Sick": irritable, lethargic, anorexic, vomiting; †septic W/U (workup): blood culture, lumbar puncture, chest x-ray, complete blood count, differential, urinalysis, urine culture; ‡focus of infection: otitis media, pneumonia, cellulitis.

strated a reduction in the incidence of meningitis in bacteremic children treated with ceftriaxone compared with those treated with oral or no antibiotics. Parenteral ceftriaxone should never be initiated without appropriate antecedent diagnostic studies. Treatment should be discontinued if cultures are negative. The risk from the overuse of ceftriaxone is the emergence of resistant organisms, a phenomenon that has already been observed.[34] Current recommendations suggest that well-appearing infants between 3 and 36 months of age, with no focus of infection, and fever greater than or equal to 39.5°C (103.1°F) and WBCs over 15,000 or a temperature over 40.0°C (104°F), regardless of the white count, may be candidates for expectant antibiotic treatment with ceftriaxone at a dose of 50 mg/kg given twice 24 h apart. If cultures are negative after 48 h, no further treatment is needed. Any child who appears ill or toxic should be admitted to the hospital. Likewise, children who are felt to be at risk for a serious bacterial infection, and do not have reliable follow-up or the ability to return to the hospital, should also be admitted for inpatient management.[35]

An additional dilemma surrounds the management of positive blood culture results. All patients with positive blood cultures should be recalled for repeat evaluation. If they are receiving appropriate antibiotics, are clinically well, and have been afebrile, they should be instructed to complete the course of therapy. If they are afebrile and clinically well but have never been treated with antibiotics, opinions differ regarding the need for additional blood cultures and antibiotic therapy. Generally, neither is necessary unless the child has developed a specific focus of infection. However, any patient who remains febrile or does poorly even if on antibiotics should receive complete septic evaluation (CBC, blood culture, lumbar puncture, chest film, and urine culture), be hospitalized, and receive parenteral antibiotics (Fig. 110-1).

OLDER FEBRILE CHILDREN

Diagnosis

Children over the age of 3 are easier to evaluate. They can specify their complaints and have illnesses similar to younger children, particularly upper respiratory infections and gastroenteritis. The risk of bacteremia appears lower in this age group, but the incidence of streptococcal pharyngitis is higher, especially in children between the ages of 5 and 10 and those with hyperpyrexia.[11] Infectious mononucleosis may present with fever, tonsillar hypertrophy, and exudate, like streptococcal pharyngitis. Marked lymphadenopathy or hepatosplenomegaly would support the diagnosis. Pneumonia in this age group may be caused by *Mycoplasma pneumoniae*. These children present with cough and fever. Rales may not be apparent early in the illness, although the chest film would show evidence of an infiltrate. Bedside cold agglutinins, if positive, provide a clue to the correct diagnosis. Children with pneumonia secondary to mycoplasma should be treated with erythromycin, 30 to 40 mg/kg per day (maximum dose, 1 g).

EMERGENCY DEPARTMENT CARE

Managing the Fever

Once the issue of fever as a symptom has been addressed, it is appropriate to determine the need for fever-reducing measures.

Many parents are concerned about the harmful effects of the fever; many are aware of the risk of febrile seizures. Children who are prone to febrile seizures are not benefited by antipyretics alone because the seizure frequently occurs early in the illness, often before the parents are aware that the child is ill. Aside from febrile seizures, fever is not known to produce any harmful effects in children. Many children, however, feel uncomfortable during the fever, and so it is appropriate to institute measures directed at symptomatically reducing the fever.

The body loses heat in four ways: (1) radiation (60 percent), heat loss from the body to the air in the surrounding environment; (2) evaporation (25 percent), heat loss through the evaporation of perspiration, water, or any liquid applied to the body surface; (3) convection (10 percent), heat loss when air currents blow over the skin; and (4) conduction (approximately 5 percent), heat loss through contact with solid surface. Heat loss through conduction is increased by the use of cooling blankets.

One can facilitate heat loss in children by using any combination of these measures. Unwrapping a bundled child increases heat loss through radiation, and rehydrating a dehydrated child will increase the heat loss through evaporation. Sponging also helps to reduce fever by evaporation. Sponging should be done slowly, using tepid water only. Very rapid cooling by sponging can result in peripheral vascular collapse, and death among small, critically ill infants, has been reported. Sponging with ice water is uncomfortable for children and results in shivering, and sponging with alcohol carries the risk of intoxication, hypoglycemia, and coma. Vigorous rubbing of the skin induces vasodilatation and improves heat loss.[36]

Studies have shown that sponging and antipyretics used together are more effective than either modality used alone. Acetaminophen, ibuprofen, and aspirin are equally effective and appear to work centrally to block prostaglandin synthesis. Heat is lost through peripheral vasodilatation and sweating.

Drug dosage for aspirin or acetaminophen is 10 to 15 mg/kg per dose at 4-h intervals (maximum dose, 600 mg). Increasing the dose does not result in a better or more-sustained effect. Administration of either drug by rectal suppository results in a slight delay in absorption. No studies have evaluated the efficacy of alternating the two drugs at 2-h intervals in an effort to avoid the recrudescence of fever. Administration of the drugs simultaneously at the usual dosage produces a reduction in temperature that is sustained for 6 h rather than 2 to 4 h.[37] The dosage of ibuprofen is 5 mg/kg for fevers less than 39°C (102.2°F) and 10 mg/kg for fevers over 39°C (102.2°F). Ibuprofen may be given every 6 to 8 h, with a maximum daily dose of 40 mg/kg.[38] The key to assuring a good outcome is judicial management, follow-up, and reassessment. It is not appropriate to simply administer ceftriaxone and assume that any infection an infant may have has been appropriately covered. Emergency physicians must be certain that infants can be reevaluated to assure that other problems have not emerged.

The use of aspirin has been curtailed following reports linking aspirin and Reye syndrome. Aspirin should not be used in children with chickenpox or with influenza-like illnesses. The effects of aspirin are cumulative, and more than half of the reported overdoses involve therapeutic misuse. Other side effects of aspirin include gastrointestinal upset and hemorrhage and coagulation disturbances. Acetaminophen is also toxic if taken in inappropriate doses, but there is no cumulative effect, and children are less prone than adults to hepatotoxicity. Side effects of ibuprofen are similar to those of aspirin and include gastrointestinal ulceration, bleeding, and perforation. Platelet disturbances are also reported but are felt to be reversible with cessation of therapy.

REFERENCES

1. Bernheim HA, Block LH, Atkins E: Fever: Pathogenesis, pathophysiology, and purpose. *Ann Intern Med* 91:261, 1979
2. Kluger MJ: Fever revisited. *Pediatrics* 90:846, 1992.
3. Kluger MJ: The evolution and adaptive value of fever. *Am Sci* 66:38, 1978.
4. Berkowitz C, Orr D, Spencer M, et al: Variability in the management of febrile infants. *J Emerg Med* 3:345, 1985.
5. Petersen-Smith A, Barber N, Coody D, et al: Comparison of aural infrared with traditional rectal temperatures in children from birth to age three years. *J Pediatr* 125:83, 1994.
6. Baraff LJ, Bass JW, Fleisher GR, et al: Practice guidelines for the management of infants and children 0 to 36 months of age with fever without source. *Ann Emerg Med* 22:1198, 1993.
7. McCarthy PL, Jekel JF, Dolan TF: Temperature less than or equal to 40°C in children less than 24 months of age: A prospective study. *Pediatrics* 59:663, 1977.
8. McCarthy PL, Dolan TF: Hyperpyrexia in children. *Am J Dis Child* 130:849, 1976.
9. Alpert G, Hibbert E, Fleisher GR: Case-control study of hyperpyrexia in children. *Pediatr Infect Dis J* 9:161, 1990.
10. Bonadio WA, Gronske L, Smith DS: Systemic bacterial infections in children with fever greater than 41°C. *Pediatr Infect Dis J* 8:120, 1989.
11. Marcinak JF: Evaluation of children with fever ≥104°F in an emergency department. *Pediatr Emerg Care* 4:92, 1988.
12. Roberts KB: Fever in the first eight weeks of life. *Johns Hopkins Med J* 141:9, 1977.
13. McCarthy PL, Dolan TF: The serious implications of high fever in infants during their first three months. *Clin Pediatr* 15:794, 1976.
14. Krober MS, Bass JW, Powell JM, et al: Bacterial and viral pathogens causing fever in infants less than 3 months old. *Am J Dis Child* 139:889, 1985.
15. Caspe WB, Chamudes O, Louie B: The evaluation and treatment of the febrile infant. *Pediatr Infect Dis J* 2:131, 1983.
16. Berkowitz CD, Uchiyama N, Tully SB, et al: Fever in infants less than two months of age: Spectrum of disease and predictors of outcome. *Pediatr Emerg Care* 1:128, 1985.
17. Dagan R, Powell KR, Hall CD, et al: Identification of infants unlikely to have serious bacterial infection although hospitalized for suspected sepsis. *J Pediatr* 107:855, 1985.
18. Dagan R, Sofer S, Phillip M, Shachak E: Ambulatory care of febrile infants younger than 2 months of age classified as being at low risk for having bacterial infections. *J Pediatr* 112:355, 1987.
19. Ginsburg CM, McCracken GH: Urinary tract infections in young infants. *Pediatrics* 69:409, 1982.
20. Hoberman A, Wald ER: Urinary tract infections in young febrile children. *Pediatr Infect Dis J* 16:11, 1997.
21. Lieu TA, Baskin MN, Schwartz S, Fleisher GR: Clinical and cost-effectiveness of outpatient strategies for management of febrile infants. *Pediatrics* 89:1135, 1992.
22. Baskin MN, O'Rourke EJ, Fleisher GR: Outpatient treatment of febrile infants 28 to 89 days of age with intramuscular administration of ceftriaxone. *J Pediatr* 120:22, 1992.
23. Baskin MN, O'Rourke EJ, Fleisher GR: Management of febrile infants 15 to 28 days of age with parenteral ceftriaxone and 24 hours of in-patient observation. *Arch Pediatr Adolesc Med* 148:49, 1994.
24. McGowan JE, Bratton L, Klein JO, et al: Bacteremia in febrile children seen in a walk-in pediatric clinic. *N Engl J Med* 288:1309, 1973.
25. Bratton L, Teele DW, Klein JO: Outcome of unsuspected pneumococcemia in children not initially admitted to the hospital. *J Pediatr* 90:703, 1977.
26. McCarthy PL, Sharpe MR, Spiesel SZ, et al: Observation scaled to identify serious illness in febrile children. *Pediatrics* 70:802, 1982.
27. Bluestone CD: Modern management of otitis media. *Pediatr Clin North Am* 36:1371, 1989.
28. Nguyen QV, Nguyen EA, Weiner LB: Incidence of invasive bacterial disease in children with fever and petechiae. *Pediatrics* 74:77, 1984.
29. Mandl KD, Stack AM, Fleisher GR: Incidence of bacteremia in infants and children with fever and petechiae. *J Pediatr* 131:398, 1997.
30. Barron MA, Fink HD: Bacteremia in private practice. *Pediatrics* 66:171, 1980.
31. Dershewitz RA, Wigder HN, Wigder CM, Nadelman DH: A comparative study of the prevalence, outcome, and prediction of bacteremia in children. *J Pediatr* 103:352, 1983.

32. Carroll WL, Farrell MK, Singer JI, et al: Treatment of occult bacteremia: A prospective randomized clinical trial. *Pediatrics* 72:608, 1983.
33. Jaffe DM, Tanz RR, Davis AT, et al: Antibiotic administration to treat possible occult bacteremia in febrile children. *N Engl J Med* 317:1175, 1987.
34. Bradley JS, Scheld WN: The challenges of penicillin-resistant pneumococcal infection. *Clin Infect Dis* 24:S213, 1997.
35. Fleisher GR, Rosenberg N, Vinci R, et al: Intramuscular versus oral antibiotic therapy for the prevention of meningitis and other bacterial sequelae in young febrile children at risk for occult bacteremia. *J Pediatr* 124:504, 1994.
36. Steele RW, Tanaka PT, Lara RP, Bass JW: Evaluation of sponging and of oral antipyretic therapy to reduce fever. *J Pediatr* 77:824, 1970.
37. Steele RW, Young FH, Bass JW, Shirkey HC: Oral antipyretic therapy: Evaluation of aspirin-acetaminophen combination. *Am J Dis Child* 123:204, 1972.
38. Wilson JT, Brown RD, Kearns GL, et al: Single-dose, placebo-controlled comparative study of ibuprofen and acetaminophen antipyresis in children. *J Pediatr* 119:803, 1991.

ASSESSMENT OF THE CHILD IN THE EMERGENCY DEPARTMENT: A PRACTICAL APPLICATION OF NORMAL CHILD DEVELOPMENT

Peter Mellis

Children account for approximately 30 percent of visits in most emergency departments. The majority have minor or self-limited illness, which may optimally be cared for in a nonemergent setting. However, the differentiation of critically ill pediatric patients from the larger number of less ill children with similar complaints represents one of the most important and challenging diagnostic skills for emergency physicians. The key to mastering this process of identifying ill children is a knowledge of child development as applied to the emergency setting.

GENERAL PRINCIPLES OF THE DEVELOPMENTAL APPROACH

Although there are many specific aspects of the developmental approach, a few general principles are applicable to all age groups of children and their families.

Communicate with the Child

Children are best approached in a positive and gentle manner, with an awareness that the first impression sets the tone for the encounter. Review the emergency record for patient name and age so that an introduction and a developmentally structured interaction may be planned. An awareness of the child's age-related communication skills and perspective will result in a more meaningful evaluation. Whenever possible, look at the child from his or her own eye level. Use the child's motor skills, vocabulary, and specific life experiences as reference points. Hunger, discomfort, fear of separation or pain, and feelings of loss of control should be directly addressed. Recognize that the emergency department is a strange and threatening environment and, whenever possible, isolate the child from the sights and sounds of other patient care experiences that may heighten their own anxiety. Most importantly, be honest with children regarding expectations for their experience so that trust can be established.

Communicate with the Family

Assess and treat the child in the context of his or her family, avoiding separation whenever possible. Emergency department policy should encourage parental accompaniment of children to the clinical area. It is optimal to consider that there are two patients, child and parent(s), each with expectations that must be addressed. Caregivers have essential historical information and, in the case of infants and toddlers, are physically necessary to the performance of a meaningful physical assessment. At all ages, children watch their parents for cues with respect to how to respond to the medical staff. Parents who understand and accept the sequence of events involved in emergency care become allies in enlisting their child's cooperation. Whenever possible, parents should be encouraged to remain present during procedures, maintaining visual and physical contact from a sitting position. Appropriate exceptions include parental discomfort and critical illness. Finally, because parents are intimately familiar with their child's range of verbal and nonverbal behavior, the examiner must take the phrase "this is not my child" as parental concern for abnormal level of consciousness. This reliance on parental knowledge is particularly applicable to the assessment of a child with developmental delay.

Assess by Means of Observation

Every effort should be made to gain information regarding a young child prior to interacting with him or her directly. Infants and young children communicate a normal level of consciousness through age-appropriate motor and social responses to their environment. Observe the child's behavior from a distance, preferably without his or her awareness. This can often be accomplished while obtaining the history from the caretakers. Antipyretic therapy and satisfying hunger are often crucial to achieving this period of optimal observation. Often more is learned regarding neurologic status from a brief period of observation than from the traditional physical examination. Nonemergent, uncomfortable examination components and procedures should be performed last.

Obtain Meaningful Vital Signs

Normal ranges for heart rate, respiratory rate, and blood pressure vary significantly with age and must be interpreted in the context of a child's activity at the time (Table 111-1). Anxiety, pain, fever, and crying will increase all values, and these states should be documented if present. Optimal vital signs are obtained without eliciting an adverse reaction to the examiner (e.g., respiratory rate taken by observing abdominal movements, and heart rate auscultated through clothing). If fever is a concern, temperature should be obtained rectally in infants, toddlers, and uncooperative children, because the oral, axillary, and tympanic routes are less reliable. Temperature measured by the oral route is likely to be feasible and accurate in children by 4 to 5 years of age. Blood pressure should be measured on previously well children who are 5 years of age and older (school age), children with chronic disease associated with hypertension (e.g., renal disease), and all children who are critically ill. Weight is a pediatric vital sign because of dosing considerations and the importance of growth as an indicator of chronic disease in children. Appropriate scales and growth charts should be available in emergency departments. For resuscitation purposes, bedside estimates of weight are frequently inaccurate, and length-based resuscitation resources (e.g., Broselow tapes) are recommended.

GROWTH AND DEVELOPMENTAL STAGES

The process of development is not unique to children, but the pace at which change occurs and the implications for patient care are maximal during this period of life. *Developmental stages* are described with associated age ranges, but these are best viewed as a sequence of events with significant individual variation in rate of progression. For purposes of facilitating patient care in the ED, two aspects of each developmental stage must be considered. *Physical aspects* include

TABLE 111-1 Pediatric Vital Signs (Awake and Resting)

Age	Heart Rate/min, Upper Limit	Respiratory Rate/min, Upper Limit	Blood Pressure,* Lower Limit	Weight,† kg
0–1 Month	180	60	60/40	3–4
2–12 Months	160	50	70/45	5–10
12–24 Months	140	40	75/50	10–12
2–6 Years	120	30	80/55	13–25
6–12 Years	110	20	90/60	25–40
>12 Years	100	20	90/60	40–60

*May be estimated by
systolic blood pressure (5th percentile) = 70 + [2 × (age in years)]
†May be estimated by
≤12 months: weight (kg) = 4 + (age in months/2)
1–12 years: weight (kg) = 10 + [2 × (age in years)]

growth and physiologic parameters unique to a given developmental stage, a knowledge of which is essential to provide excellent care. *Neurologic aspects* include motor, language, and social/psychological milestones that impact on both patient assessment and responses during acute illness or injury. These milestones and their related strategies are summarized in Table 111-2. Based on a knowledge of these, the examiner is well equipped to proceed with a developmentally *age-specific approach.*

Early Infancy (0 to 6 Months)

PHYSICAL ASPECTS Rapid growth rate is a characteristic feature of young infants, for whom the major work is eating. After a 5 to 10 percent loss over the first 3 days of life, term infants regain birth weight by 10 days of age. A 20- to 30-g/day weight gain is the best overall sign of health. Normal infants double their birth weight by 5 months. Young infants have a high surface area to body mass ratio with a proportionally large head, resulting in a high rate of heat loss and risk of hypothermia. The normal anterior fontanelle is slightly depressed when a child is upright. Young infants are obligate nose breathers and may experience partial airway obstruction with abnormal positioning or viral upper respiratory tract infections. Normal neonates may exhibit periodic breathing, or 5 to 10 s pauses followed by tachypnea, due to immature central control of respiration. Both cardiac output and minute ventilation are relatively rate dependent in early infancy. A heart rate greater than 180/min and a respiratory rate greater than 60/min should be considered abnormal. Blood pressure is well maintained by compensatory mechanisms at this age, with hypotension a very late finding in shock. The pulmonary vascular bed dilates over the first 6 weeks of life, so that congenital heart lesions resulting in a left-to-right shunt, for example, ventricular septal defect, will present after this age. Finally, the primary series of immunizations, including diphtheria-pertussis-tetanus (DPT), oral poliovirus (OPV), and *Haemophilus influenzae* type b (HIb), are completed by 6 months of age (Table 111-3). The rotavirus vaccine had been added to the primary immunization series, but recent reports of possible association with intussusception have resulted in temporary cessation of use.

TABLE 111-2 Developmental Stages and Emergency Department Assessment Strategy

Stage	Milestone	Strategy
Early infancy (0–6 months)	Motor: lifts head, reaches Verbal: cooing Social: responsive smile	Observation Examine in parent's arms Direct approach
Late infancy (6–18 months)	Motor: reaches/obtains, sits, walks Verbal: jargon, few words Social: stranger anxiety/dependence	Observation Examine in parents arms Indirect approach
Toddler (18–36 months)	Motor: walks well, scribbles Verbal: speaks in phrases Social: stranger anxiety/autonomy	Observation Indirect approach
Preschool (3–5 years)	Motor: runs well, colors Verbal: speaks in sentences Social: magical thinking	Indirect or direct approach Explain briefly just prior to procedures
School age (5–12 years)	Motor: schoolwork, sports Verbal: concrete reasoning Social: task oriented	Direct approach Explain in detail prior to procedures
Adolescence (12–17 years)	Motor: adult Verbal: abstract reasoning Social: autonomy, rebellion	Direct approach Confidentiality Treat as adult

NEUROLOGIC ASPECTS Motor development is the major indicator of neurologic health and proceeds in a cephalocaudal fashion. Neonates demonstrate involuntary "primitive" reflexes, such as the suck, grasp, and Moro (startle) responses, which may be elicited to demonstrate muscle tone and should always be symmetric. By 1 month of age, infants can lift their heads, follow a moving object, and demonstrate a social smile. By 4 months, head control is steady, the child will reach for and grasp objects with the whole hand, a cooing response may be elicited, and rolling over has begun. During this period, normal infants learn trust from their parents and will respond positively to a gentle examiner. This is the period of least parental confidence, and many emergency department visits are made because of lack of knowledge and a need for reassurance.

AGE-SPECIFIC APPROACH Assessment is optimally made by direct interaction using a pleasant, confident tone of voice and smiling face directed toward the infant. Observation of muscle tone, spontaneous activity, eye contact, responsive smile, and recognition of parents is most important. Examination of the infant is best performed in the parent's lap, with use of brightly colored or pleasant-sounding objects

TABLE 111-3 Recommended Schedule of Childhood Immunizations*

Age	DTP	OPV	HIb	MMR	HepB†	VZV	RotaV‡
Birth					HepB		
2 Months	DTP	OPV	HIb		HepB		RotaV‡
4 Months	DTP	OPV	HIb				RotaV‡
6 Months	DTP		HIb		HepB		RotaV‡
12–15 Months			HIb	MMR			
15–18 months	DTP	OPV				VZV	
4–6 Years	DTP	OPV					
11–12 Years				MMR†			
14–16 Years	Td						

**Streptococcus pneumoniae* conjugate vaccine shortly to be recommended at 2, 4, 6, and 15 months.[1]
†Second MMR may be given at 4–6 years or 11–12 years of age. Current recommendations are unclear because mercury in the vaccine could be toxic to neonates and infants. It should not be given in this schedule until a new vaccine is developed.
‡The CDC recommends postponing administration of rotavirus vaccine because there may be an association with intussusception (*MMWR* 48(27), 1999). http://www2.cdc.gov/mmwr
Abbreviations: DTP, diphtheria-tetanus-pertussis; OPV, oral poliovirus (live); HIb, *Haemophilus influenzae* type b conjugate; MMR, measles-mumps-rubella (live); HepB, hepatitis B (live); Td, tetanus toxoid with diphtheria adjuvant (adult); VZV, varicella zoster virus; RotaV, rotavirus (live).

to elicit a motor response. Feeding the infant or eliciting the sucking reflex with a finger will often result in greater cooperation. Optimal examination is done in order of least to most invasive interactions, i.e., observation, auscultation, and palpation, being careful to avoid uncomfortable procedures such as ear and throat examination until the child's level of consciousness is established. Parental confidence should be directly reinforced. Young infants should be carefully monitored during procedures involving conscious sedation or abnormal positioning, because of the risk of airway compromise. Finally, the motor abilities of young infants result in a limited potential for self-inflicted accidental injury. Whenever an injury is developmentally inconsistent with the stated mechanism, the potential for child abuse must be investigated.

Late Infancy (6 to 18 Months)

PHYSICAL ASPECTS Normal infants triple their birth weight by 1 year of age, but the rate of growth slows during this period. The primary teeth begin to erupt by 6 months of age, with an average rate of acquisition of one per month. Head size, center of gravity, and surface area to mass ratio remain large in comparison to adults. The anterior fontanelle is closed by 18 months of age. The measles-mumps-rubella (MMR) vaccination is given at 12 to 15 months of age, and the varicella vaccine is given at 12 to 18 months of age. The DPT and HIb boosters are given during this same period (Table 111-3).

NEUROLOGIC ASPECTS The normal infant sits with minimal support, transfers objects from hand to hand, and babbles by 6 months. By 9 months of age, the infant is crawling, pulling to a standing position, and verbalizing with nonspecific jargon. By 12 months, the infant has a mature pincer-type grasp, begins to walk, and acquires specific words. The developmental combination of mobility and grasp results in increasing risk of toxic and foreign-body ingestion. Between 9 and 12 months, a strong sense of ''stranger anxiety,'' related to fear of separation from parents, is acquired and complicates every aspect of physical assessment. Conversely, the failure of an older infant or toddler to recognize and preferentially respond to parents suggests significant disease.

AGE-SPECIFIC APPROACH Assessment of an older infant and toddler begins with observation, preferably without the child's awareness of the examiner's presence. The child should be undressed to obtain a meaningful respiratory rate and to observe the work of breathing. Spontaneous motor activity, such as sitting and pulling up, and purposeful responses to parental overtures, such as reaching for objects and smiling, are indicators of a normal level of consciousness. The child should see the examiner approach gradually and engage his or her caretakers first. An entire examination requiring any degree of cooperation is best performed while the child is held on the parent's lap or shoulder so that perception of separation is avoided. As for younger infants, the examination proceeds from least to most invasive interactions. Procedures in this age group require adequate physical restraint. Although parental restraint is acceptable for nonpainful examination procedures, parents should not be asked to immobilize their child for invasive procedures. Caretakers should be encouraged to remain present to reassure their child during procedures if it is their desire to do so. The high level of anxiety at this age frequently results in persistently uncooperative behavior despite adequate analgesia. Sedation for procedures may require a significantly higher per-kilogram dose of anxiolytic/analgesic drug to achieve the desired effect.

Toddler (18 to 36 Months)

PHYSICAL ASPECTS Decelerating growth rate and decreased appetite are seen during this period, although the head approaches its adult size. The 20 primary teeth are in place by 36 months, and dental caries are common. High center of gravity, mobility, and curiosity lead to increasing risk for head and orthopedic injuries. A toddler's open growth plates are far more likely to sustain epiphyseal fracture than ligamentous injury. Traction injuries to the arm will frequently result in subluxation of the annular ligament of the radial head (i.e., ''nursemaid's elbow'').

NEUROLOGIC ASPECTS By 18 months of age, most children can walk well, feed themselves, follow simple commands, and use four to six words to indicate their desires. Stranger anxiety peaks at this age but remains important throughout the toddler period. By 24 months, most children can run, climb stairs, and speak with three-word phrases, although only 50 percent of speech is intelligible to nonfamily members. Toddlers understand far more than their spontaneous speech would indicate and learn by imitating the behavior of their family members. When given opportunity to draw, a toddler will scribble with a brief attention span. Parents consistently underestimate the mobility and problem-solving ability of a toddler, resulting in a peak risk for falls and ingestions at this age.

AGE-SPECIFIC APPROACH An examination strategy of indirect observation followed by direct interaction in the safety of the parent's arms should be followed, as described for older infants. The examiner should encourage the parent to have the toddler walk and follow commands as an important component of the assessment for acute systemic or neurologic disease. Allow the child a favorite object, such as a doll or blanket, for comfort during the examination. Talk to the child in simple language about what you will do and offer to let the child touch or hold the examination instruments in order to gain their trust. Older toddlers may indicate the site of pain specifically, but many will be unable to communicate localized pain or tenderness. As described above, perform the physical assessment in order of least to most invasive examination components. As for older infants, restraint is routinely indicated for painful procedures and a higher per-kilogram dose of anxiolytic/analgesic drug may be required. Because of likelihood of epiphyseal fracture, a young child with tenderness over the growth plate following injury should be immobilized with a splint, even if x-ray films are negative.

Preschool Age (3 to 5 Years)

PHYSICAL ASPECTS Growth rate slows significantly during this period, and appetite decreases further. Children develop a more lean body habitus. The incidence of injuries increases with increasing activity. The preschool child is no longer restrained in a car seat and is at risk for defined injury complexes from improperly fitting lap and shoulder belts. A DPT booster is given shortly before beginning school, between the ages of 4 and 6 (see Table 111-3).

NEUROLOGIC ASPECTS Preschool children develop progressive autonomy in terms of mobility and self-care. Attraction to books, drawing, and coloring is common. Expressive language skills expand rapidly, and children this age are often able to identify site(s) of specific complaint. However, a strong sense of fear of pain remains, and the level of anxiety remains high in the emergency setting. Preschool children live in the present and have a limited sense of time and history, so that prior symptoms are frequently forgotten. Self-centered "magical" reasoning is the rule, so that many preschool children believe that emergency department care is punishment for misbehavior. This is occasionally reinforced by parents who state they will "have the doctor give you a shot," which should be discouraged.

AGE-SPECIFIC APPROACH Many preschool children may be directly approached and examined in the traditional systematic fashion. However, some will require the indirect approach described for toddlers, and the nearby presence of a parent is typically essential for cooperation. The examiner should always talk directly with the preschooler to establish rapport and confirm the general complaint. Identification of recent positive experiences such as birthdays or favorite cartoon characters is frequently helpful in gaining cooperation. However, preschool children should be expected to identify only the current complaint, and reliance on parental history should remain. Cooperation during the physical examination is likely, although less comfortable components are still best performed at the end. The performance of painful procedures requires a careful approach. It is always best to be honest regarding discomfort, but information should be given immediately before performing the procedure to minimize the effects of fantasy regarding pain and causality as well as delaying tactics. Comfort and distraction by the parent is frequently effective for minor procedures; however, restraint as for toddlers is typically necessary. Rewards such as verbal praise and a sticker for bravery often significantly enhance the memory of the experience for the child and family.

School Age (5 to 12 Years)

PHYSICAL ASPECTS The school years represent the slowest period of growth in childhood, and the body habitus is typically slender. The primary teeth are loosening and the secondary teeth erupt. The lymphatics reach maximal dimensions relative to body size by 6 years of age. There is increased physical activity, including organized sports, during this period, and injuries become common.

NEUROLOGIC ASPECTS School-age children experience rapid language growth and maturing motor ability. Concrete reasoning ability emerges with an ability to understand cause and effect. The child is increasingly aware of his or her body and develops a sense of modesty. Task-oriented behavior is common, and school and sports activity are typically the central events of the child's life. School-age children are eager to please and often reluctant to express their fears of pain and death.

AGE-SPECIFIC APPROACH The direct examination approach is typically successful for school-age children. Parental accompaniment and respect for modesty should be maintained. Historical information should be elicited from child as well as parent. An effort to inquire about school or extracurricular interests will enhance rapport. Change in school performance is a helpful indicator of chronic disease. Painful procedures are best preceded by explanations to both parent and child, given well in advance with honesty regarding discomfort. The child should be given some degree of choice in the manner in which the procedure is completed, such as a comfortable position, in order to minimize the sense of loss of control.

Adolescence (12 to 17 Years)

PHYSICAL ASPECTS The teen years mark a second period of rapid growth, beginning at age 10 in girls and age 12 in boys. Secondary sexual development begins shortly after beginning the growth spurt, with menarche starting between 10 and 16 years in girls. Sexual activity and drug use are common during adolescence, and many teens are parents themselves, complicating both the differential diagnosis and issues of maturity and reliability in carrying out the follow-up plan.

NEUROLOGIC ASPECTS Abstract reasoning ability progressively develops during adolescence, paired with a self-centered worldview and self-consciousness regarding appearance. Feelings of immortality and denial of the consequences of risky behavior are common. Loss of autonomy is the greatest fear of an adolescent, and mistrust of and rebellion toward authority is normal. Previously well-controlled chronic disease frequently becomes unstable as a result of these developmental issues. Psychiatric disease and suicidal behavior are increasingly recognized in this age group. The parents of teenagers are frequently angered by these changes and may project these feelings on the emergency department staff.

AGE-SPECIFIC APPROACH The traditional history and physical examination with respect for modesty is effective in the assessment of adolescents. The examiner should communicate to the teenager that he or she will be treated "like an adult." Choices must be allowed, such as parental presence during the examination, with proper limit

TABLE 111-4 Consent for Treating Minors

The age of majority varies by state. A minor should not receive care in an emergency department without consent obtained by parent or legal guardian with the following exceptions:

1. Life-threatening emergency
2. State-protected rights to treatment
   - Child abuse
   - Pregnancy
   - Sexually transmitted disease
   - Substance abuse
3. State-defined ''emancipated minor'' status
   - Married
   - Member of armed forces
   - Self-supporting and living on his or her own

setting regarding cooperative behavior. The parent's concerns must be addressed individually and, if necessary, in private. Confidentiality should be stressed, particularly as the law requires with respect to pregnancy and sexually transmitted disease.

MEDICAL CONSENT AND THE TREATMENT OF MINORS

Consent for evaluation and treatment must be obtained for medical care to be delivered in a lawful manner. State laws vary regarding the age of majority at which consent may be given by a patient, varying between 18 and 21 years of age. In the case of minor children, consent must be obtained from the legal guardian (typically a parent, unless custody has been removed) prior to initiation of treatment. This does not apply, however, to triage and examination, and children should be evaluated without delay to determine the nature of the illness or injury. If the child is not accompanied by persons able to provide consent, the parent or guardian should be contacted by phone and witnessed consent obtained. Such attempts should be documented in the medical record. Written documentation from the parent or legal guardian granting consent may suffice in many states, but this should not obviate attempted phone contact for permission to treat. In the absence of consent, the patient should be evaluated sufficiently to determine the presence or absence of an emergent situation. In the setting of an emergency situation in which delay in treatment may threaten the life or health of the child, consent can be assumed and care initiated with ongoing attempts to locate the parent or guardian. If any doubt exists, the emergency physician and patient are best served by providing treatment with documentation of efforts to determine the presence of an emergency and obtain consent for treatment. In the absence of an emergency, further care should not be provided unless specifically permitted under state law (Table 111-4). Most states permit minors to seek treatment for child abuse, substance abuse, sexually transmitted diseases, and pregnancy-related complaints without parental consent. Most states consider a child ''emancipated'' and able to provide consent if a member of the armed forces, married, or self-supporting and living on his or her own. Some states permit older minors to give consent for nonemergent care. Many states have a process for obtaining concurrent judicial review and consent. Emergency physicians are encouraged to become familiar with the specific state laws applicable to consent issues.[2] As a matter of courtesy and necessity, verbal consent should be obtained from older minors as well, typically at age 12 and older.

Parental refusal of consent for care in the setting of possible life-threatening emergency or child abuse presents emergency physicians with a significant challenge. If parental consent cannot be obtained, a court order should be obtained through the appropriate local mechanism to to allow the provision of necessary care for the well-being of the child.

REFERENCES

1. American Academy of Pediatrics, Committee on Practice and Ambulatory Medicine: Recommended childhood immunization schedule: United States, January–December 1998. *Pediatrics* 101:154, 1998.
2. Selbst S: Treating minors without their parents. *Pediatr Emerg Care* 1:168, 1986.

COMMON NEONATAL PROBLEMS

M. Yousuf Hasan
Niranjan Kissoon

The assessment of neonates in the emergency department is more difficult than that of older children and adults. Symptoms are usually vague and nonspecific. Signs are usually subtle and, even when recognized, may not be helpful in pinpointing a diagnosis. For example, respiratory distress may be due to primary respiratory or cardiac disease, generalized sepsis, abdominal pathology, or metabolic derangements. Examination of neonates is time-consuming and requires special skills in the approach to the infant as well as the anxious parent.

The prerequisites for the proper evaluation of neonates are a great deal of patience and an appreciation of the marked variations in normal vegetative functions. Many visits are initiated because of parental concerns related to feeding patterns; weight gain; stool frequency, color, and consistency; and breathing patterns. Physicians involved in the care of neonates in the emergency department should therefore be knowledgeable about patterns of normal vegetative functions in the neonatal population.

NORMAL VEGETATIVE FUNCTIONS

Feeding Patterns

The feeding of infants requires practical interpretation of specific nutritional needs and the widely varying limits of a normal baby's appetite and behavior regarding food. Variation in times between feedings is to be expected in the first few weeks during the establishment of a self-regulation plan. By the end of first month, more than 90 percent of infants establish a suitable and reasonably regular schedule. Most healthy bottle-fed infants want six to nine feedings every 24 h by the end of first week of life; breast-fed infants prefer shorter intervals.[1,2]

Feedings should be considered as having progressed satisfactorily if the infant is no longer losing weight by 5 to 7 days and is gaining weight by 12 to 14 days. Parents usually need reassurance that their infant is obtaining adequate nutrition because of the wide variation in the intakes of normal infants. It is important to appreciate that infants cry for reasons other than hunger and that they need not be fed every time they cry.

Weight Gain

While it is difficult to precisely judge the caloric intake of breast-fed infants and feeding frequency varies widely, intake is adequate if the neonate is gaining weight appropriately and appears content between feedings. Normal newborns may lose 5 to 8 percent of their birth weight during first 3 to 7 days of life. A weight loss of up to 10 percent is acceptable if the infant's examination findings and behavior are normal. On average, infants gain between 20 and 30 g/day in first 3 months of life and 15 to 20 g/day for the next several months. It is important to weigh the infant completely undressed.

An infant's weight between 3 and 12 months of age can be calculated approximately by the following formula:

$$\frac{\text{age (months)} + 9}{2} = \text{expected weight (kg)}.$$ [3]

Stool Patterns

The number, color, and consistency of bowel movements may vary greatly in the same infant and among infants regardless of diet or environment. Breast-fed infants frequently will have 6 or 7 stools per day, while formula-fed infants generally have 1 to 2 stools per day. The first stool, which consists of meconium, is usually passed within first 24 h after birth. Transition stools, which are greenish brown, appear after initiation of milk feeding and are replaced by typical milk stools 3 to 4 days later. Infrequent bowel movements do not necessarily mean constipation, since breast-fed infants may occasionally go 5 to 7 days without a bowel movement. Stool color has no significance unless blood is present. Occasionally, an infant may not have a bowel movement on a given day. The stools of breast-fed infants are softer than those of formula-fed infants. Excessive intake of human milk or maternal use of laxatives further increases the water content of the infant's stool. Overfeeding or use of formula that is too concentrated or too high in sugar content also can produce loose stools.[2,4]

Breathing Patterns

The respiratory rate ranges between 30 and 60 breaths per minute in infants. For premature infants it is higher and fluctuates more widely. Because fluctuations are rapid, the respiratory rate should be counted for a full minute with the infant in full resting state, preferably asleep. A rate consistently over 60 breaths per minute during periods of regular breathing should be evaluated further.

Since the breathing of newborn infants is almost entirely diaphragmatic, the soft front of the thorax usually is drawn inward during inspiration, while the abdomen protrudes. In a quiet infant, this paradoxical pattern has no clinical significance, but when it changes to predominantly thoracic breathing, intraabdominal or intrathoracic pathology should be suspected. On the other hand, an increase in abdominal breathing suggests pulmonary disease.

Newborn infants, especially those born prematurely, may exhibit periodic breathing, characterized by alternating periods of breathing at a normal rate and periods of a markedly slow rate of respiration, which may cease three or more times for 3 s or longer. Such alternating respiratory patterns have been observed in 30 to 95 percent of premature babies during sleep, but less frequently in term infants. Periods of apnea greater than 20 s or accompanied by bradycardia or cyanosis should be evaluated.[5,6]

Sleeping Patterns

Infants are not born with the ability to sleep through the night. Instead, they awaken every 20 min to 6 h, and sleep periods are spread evenly across day and night. By 3 months of age, most of their sleep occurs at night, and by 6 months, most infants are sleeping through the night.

Night waking is defined as waking and crying once or more between midnight and 5 A.M. at least four of seven nights per week for at least four consecutive weeks. This occurs in approximately 25 percent of infants usually under 12 months of age. This prevalence rises to about 50 percent among breast-fed infants. When the child cries during the night, parents can check to ensure that there is no physical reason for the crying. Having determined that there is no physical problem, parents should ignore the crying so that the child learns to fall asleep on his or her own. If parents usually feed the child at that time and the child is older than about 6 months, the volume of the night feedings should be tapered until they are discontinued and all nourishment is given during the daytime.[7,8]

REASONS FOR EMERGENCY DEPARTMENT VISITS

A review of presenting complaints in our pediatric emergency department, a tertiary-care referral center, over a 6-month period indicates the spectrum most likely to be seen by the emergency physician (Table 112-1). Complaints in neonates are usually not single; rather, they are often symptom complexes. Such symptom complexes reflect the nonspecific nature of signs and symptoms in neonates and the similar presentation of many diseases of diverse etiology.

Crying, Irritability, and Lethargy

The symptom complex of crying, irritability, and lethargy is fairly common yet difficult to treat, even in the presence of an identifiable cause. Most neonates exhibit varying degrees and periods of crying during a 24-h period. However, infants who present with an episode of acute, inconsolable crying should be observed closely for an underlying cause (Table 112-2).[2]

Intestinal Colic

Colic is a paroxysm of crying for 3 h/day or more for 3 days/week or more over a 3-week period. The incidence of colic is about 13 percent, with no seasonal variation. Colic is a symptom complex consisting of the sudden onset of paroxysmal crying lasting several hours, a flushed face, circumoral pallor, tense abdomen, drawn up legs, cold feet, and clenched fists. It usually begins soon after birth but seldom lasts beyond 3 months of age. A careful history is important in diagnosis of colic; findings upon physical examination are normal, and laboratory tests are not required. However, when the diagnosis is unclear, a careful history, physical examination, and appropriate laboratory investigations are necessary to rule out conditions listed in Table 112-2. In doubtful situations, admission for observation or return for reassessment is reasonable.

The cause of colic is unknown. Proposed causes include excessive intake of air, insufficient intake of fluid, allergy to protein, and maternal

TABLE 112-1 Common Presenting Complaints

Crying, irritability, lethargy (see Table 112-2)

Gastrointestinal tract symptoms
  Feeding difficulties
  Regurgitation
  Vomiting
  Diarrhea
  Abdominal distention
  Constipation

Cardiorespiratory symptoms
  Rapid breathing
  Cough and nasal congestion
  Noisy breathing and stridor
  Apnea, periodic breathing
  Blue spells, cyanosis

Jaundice
Eye discharge, redness
Diaper rash, oral thrush
Fever and sepsis
Sudden infant death

TABLE 112-2 Conditions Associated with Uncontrollable Crying, Irritability, and/or Lethargy in Neonates

Intestinal colic
Traumatic conditions
Battered child syndrome (e.g., fractures, burns, etc.)
Falls (e.g., skull or extremity fractures)
Open diaper pin
Strangulation of digit or penis
Corneal abrasion or foreign body
Infections
Meningitis
Generalized sepsis
Otitis media
Urinary tract infection
Gastroenteritis
Surgical
Incarcerated hernia (umbilical or inguinal)
Testicular torsion
Anal fissure
Improper feeding practices

stress. Just as the cause remains obscure, no single treatment has been proven effective for all infants who have colic. Changing formula, applying heat to the abdomen, decreasing external stimulation, and rocking the infant all have been advocated as useful interventions by various authorities at various times. Administration of drugs (including sedatives) rarely is beneficial or indicated. Reassuring the parents that colic is a common, self-limited problem in young infants and encouraging them to share care-giving responsibilities during this time can be helpful.

The emergency physician can also be helpful by making the following suggestions:

- Changes in care-taking styles (e.g., increased carrying and rocking, feeding more frequently, and use of a pacifier)
- Changes in environment (e.g., background music or car and stroller rides)
- Changes in feeding for refractory cases (e.g., removal of cow's milk from the diet of an infant who has visible peristalsis, persistent regurgitation, and symptoms after ingesting cow's-milk protein; removal of cow's milk from the diet of a mother of a breast-fed baby; but not switching to formula from breast milk or changing formula).[8–10]

Abuse and Trauma

Distinguishing between accidental and intentional injuries is vital. By making an accurate determination, the practitioner achieves two equally important objectives:

- Protecting victims of abuse from future harm, which is often more severe than the present injuries; and
- Avoiding the damage done by unwarranted suspicion of abuse and the time-consuming investigative process that ensues.

Recognition of abuse and neglect is likely only if the possibility is entertained in the differential diagnosis of the presenting condition. The approach to the family should be supportive, empathic, and nonaccusatory. (See Chap 289 for a detailed discussion.)

Approximately one-third of the cases of child abuse occur in extrafamilial settings, such as with a babysitter or friend. Suspected abuse of a child should trigger immediate concern for the safety of the child's siblings. Spousal abuse often occurs with the abuse of the child. Particular attention should be given to the general appearance of the child and all growth parameters, especially in cases of failure to thrive. Nonorganic failure to thrive and physical or sexual abuse can coexist in the same child.

An inconsistent or implausible history may lead the physician to strongly suspect the diagnosis of child abuse, while the physical examination may reveal unexplained injuries (e.g., bruises of varying ages, skull fractures, extremity fractures, or cigarette burns). If the diagnosis is suspected, the child should be admitted for protection and further investigation.

Intentional trauma to the central nervous system remains the most serious injury, with high rates of morbidity and mortality. Unintentional head injuries in children younger than 2 years of age are common, but motor vehicle accidents and falls from extreme heights typically cause severe brain injury. Scalp hematomas, lacerations, or head bruises should alert the physician to the possibility of inflicted head trauma and brain injury. Vigorous shaking (shaken baby syndrome) may lead to epidural, subdural, and subarachnoid hemorrhages with no external signs of trauma and can be life threatening. The modes of presentation may vary, depending on the severity of central nervous system injury. In acute, severe cases the presenting complaints include choking, apnea, respiratory distress, seizures, altered level of consciousness, or cardiopulmonary arrest. When the injury is milder, presentations may be less acute, with one or more of the following: vomiting, irritability, an inappropriate increase in head circumference with split cranial sutures, failure to thrive, and developmental delay with more social than motor findings.

Physical findings in shaken infants may also include lethargy, poor sucking, irritability, rhythmic eye opening, eye deviation, bicycling movements, decerebrate or decorticate posturing, full fontanel, seizures, and alterations in muscle tone and responsiveness to voice, touch, or pain. An examination of the eye, although difficult, is essential, since presence of retinal hemorrhage, especially in the absence of external signs of trauma, suggests a whiplash injury due to severe shaking. When central nervous system injury is strongly suspected, imaging studies, such as a head computed tomography scan, should be done for confirmation. In addition, a skeletal survey should be done to rule out other injuries. Multiple skeletal fractures at various stages of healing, metaphyseal chip or bucket-handle fractures, and posterior rib fractures in infants are highly suggestive of intentional injuries.

Physical injuries and sexually transmitted disease, if present, should be treated immediately. Children with failure to thrive on the basis of emotional neglect need to be placed in a setting where they can be fed. In every state of the United States, practitioners (and many other professionals who come in contact with children) are "mandated reporters." If abuse or neglect is suspected, a report must be made to a local or state agency designated to investigate such reports. Emergency departments would be well served if protocols for management of such conditions were available.[11–14]

Infections

Neonatal infections are manifested by a variety of symptoms and signs, such as feeding difficulties, fever, jaundice, and respiratory distress. Neck rigidity and Kernig and Brudzinski signs are usually absent in neonates with meningitis. A septic neonate may present with a normal or subnormal temperature. Urinary tract infections are often associated with nonspecific signs, such as irritability, diarrhea, or poor feeding, and diagnosis is established by urine culture rather than urinalysis. There is general consensus that all neonates with possible sepsis should be hospitalized and given broad-spectrum antibiotic therapy pending results of appropriate cultures (e.g., urine, blood, and cerebrospinal fluid). See "Fever and Sepsis" below.

Surgical Lesions

Surgical conditions in neonates can present with wide variety of symptoms, including respiratory distress, fever, lethargy, weight loss, and poor feeding. Progression of symptoms can be helpful in decision making but may not be easily or accurately elicited from an infant or poorly observant parent.

The surgically correctable causes of respiratory distress in newborns are less frequent and include choanal atresia, micrognathia (Pierre Robin syndrome), laryngomalacia, tracheomalacia, tracheoesophageal fistula, and vascular rings. Most of these anomalies are identified in the newborn nursery, but in the emergency department these possibilities should be entertained in any infant with respiratory distress. In the neonate with abdominal symptoms, the most common diagnoses include necrotizing enterocolitis and congenital anomalies such as malrotation with midgut volvulus, duplication, gastroschisis, and omphalocele. Pyloric stenosis typically presents between 2 and 6 months of age. Incarcerated inguinal hernias and intussusception are most common after 2 months of age. Incarcerated hernia and intussusception account for most of abdominal surgical emergencies in the 2-month-old to 1-year-old group; the former decreases in incidence after 1 year of age.

The diagnosis of abdominal emergencies is challenging in the emergency department. A systematic approach helps to minimize missed diagnoses. The most common signs are irritability and crying, followed by poor feeding, vomiting, constipation, and abdominal distention. Prudent and directed use of laboratory and imaging studies will minimize misdiagnosis. The early involvement of a surgeon in the care of pediatric patients who have significant abdominal symptoms is recommended.[15,16]

Improper Feeding Practices

Improper feeding practices may result in an irritable infant with periods of inconsolable crying. These symptoms usually result from overfeeding without adequate burping during feedings. The infant swallows large amounts of air, resulting in bowel distention and occasionally respiratory distress. Instruction in proper feeding practices usually alleviates the problem.[1]

GASTROINTESTINAL TRACT SYMPTOMS

Common presenting gastrointestinal symptoms are listed in Table 112-1.

Feeding Difficulties

Most visits for feeding difficulties are due to parental perception that the infant's food intake is inadequate. The neonate's pattern of intake is not fully established until about 1 month of age. If weight gain is satisfactory and the infant is satisfied after feedings, intake is adequate. Parents can usually provide accurate information of the intake of bottle-fed infants. The weighing of breast-fed infants before and after feedings is not advised, since weights may be inaccurate. In addition, weighing may have adverse psychological effects on a mother whose infant is doing poorly.

Rarely, anatomic abnormalities can cause difficulty in feeding and swallowing. A careful history usually pinpoints such difficulties as having occurred from birth. The infants appear malnourished and dehydrated. The most likely causes are esophageal obstruction (e.g., stenoses, strictures, laryngeal clefts, or cleft palate) and compression of the esophagus or trachea by a double aortic arch. Infants with a recent decrease in intake have an acute disease, usually an infection.[1]

Regurgitation

Regurgitation of small amounts is common in neonates due to reduced lower esophageal sphincter pressure and relatively increased intragastric pressure. Parents may confuse regurgitation with vomiting. Vomiting results from forceful contraction of the diaphragm and abdominal muscles, whereas regurgitation is independent of any effort and probably represents the ultimate degree of gastrointestinal reflux. If the neonate is thriving, parents can be reassured that regurgitation is of no clinical significance and will decrease as the infant grows. Infants who are not thriving or having respiratory symptoms should be investigated for anatomic causes of regurgitation or chronic aspiration.

Regurgitation rarely results from pathologic processes, such as intrinsic compression of the esophagus or occasionally compression of the trachea, in which case it is usually accompanied by stridor and cough. Dysphagia, irritability, anemia due to chronic blood loss, and malnutrition are sequelae of chronic regurgitation with esophagitis, but this condition is rare. Investigations such as scintigraphy, pH monitoring, endoscopy, and biopsy are utilized to confirm the diagnosis of reflux esophagitis. These invasive tests are not justified in patients who are healthy and are not done on an emergency basis. Such infants usually respond well to thickening of feedings. The infant's upper body can be elevated after feedings added if thickening of feedings alone does not resolve the regurgitation.[4,17]

Vomiting

Vomiting results from a variety of causes and is rarely an isolated symptom. ++During the first few weeks of life, vomiting is uncommon and is often confused with regurgitation. Vomiting from birth is most likely due to an anatomic abnormality, such as tracheoesophageal fistula, upper gastrointestinal obstruction, or midgut rotation. More commonly, acute vomiting may be part of the symptom complex of some diseases (Table 112-2), especially increased intracranial pressure, and infections (e.g., sepsis, urinary tract infections, and gastroenteritis).

Projectile vomiting is usually seen in infants with pyloric stenosis and usually assumes its characteristic pattern after the second and third week of life. This condition usually occurs in firstborn males and is characterized by projectile vomiting at the end of feeding or shortly thereafter. The vomitus does not contain bile or blood. Examination of these infants should be done with the infant relaxed and the stomach empty. Prominent gastric waves may be seen going from the left to right. A firm olive mass may be felt by palpating under the liver edge. Malnutrition and dehydration may be evident. Hospitalization is necessary for rehydration and surgical treatment.

In any infant who is vomiting, signs of dehydration and candidiasis of the mouth should be sought. Hepatobiliary (e.g., jaundice), urinary tract, and central nervous system disease can also cause vomiting. Vomiting due to inborn errors of metabolism may present with hypoglycemia and metabolic acidosis. Infants who are vomiting should be admitted for evaluation and therapy.[18,19]

Diarrhea and Dehydration

Diarrhea refers to stools that are abnormally frequent and liquid. The modifier *abnormal* is critical because stools can normally be frequent and liquid in young children. Acute diarrheal illnesses account for more than 3 million ambulatory pediatric visits, 10 million sick days, and 100,000 hospital admissions per year in the United States. In the United States, rotavirus predominantly affects infants between 3 to 15 months. The peak incidence is in the winter months, and rotavirus accounts for as many as 50 percent of the cases of acute diarrhea in winter. Enteric adenoviruses (serotypes 40 and 41) are the second most common viral pathogen in infants. In summer most of the cases of diarrhea are caused by bacteria (including *Escherichia coli, Salmonella,* and *Shigella*). Parasitic causes of diarrhea are rare in neonates. A history of bloody diarrhea strongly suggests a bacterial pathogen, particularly in an older infant or a child. It is important to know that, in infants less than 6 months of age, the most common causes of blood in the stool are cow's milk intolerance and anal fissures.

In diarrheal illness, the history and physical examination serve as an initial screen to narrow the diagnostic possibilities. The choice of

TABLE 112-3 Clinical Assessment of Severity of Dehydration

Signs and Symptoms	Mild Dehydration	Moderate Dehydration	Severe Dehydration
Body weight loss, %	3–5	6–9	10 or more
General appearance and condition; infants and young children	Thirsty, alert, restless	Thirsty; restless or lethargic but irritable to touch or drowsy	Drowsy; limp, cold, sweaty, cyanotic extremities; may be comatose
Radial pulse	Normal rate and strength	Rapid and weak	Rapid, feeble, sometimes impalpable
Respiration	Normal	Deep, may be rapid	Deep and rapid
Anterior fontanel	Normal	Sunken	Very sunken
Systolic blood pressure	Normal	Normal or low	Low, may be unrecordable
Skin elasticity	Pinch retracts immediately	Pinch retracts slowly	Pinch retracts very slowly
Eyes	Normal	Sunken	Grossly sunken
Tears	Present	Absent or reduced	Absent
Mucous membranes	Moist	Dry	Very dry
Urine flow	Normal	Reduced amount and dark	Anuria, severe oliguria
Capillary refill	Normal	±2 s	>3 s
Estimated fluid deficit, mL/kg	30–50	60–90	100 or more

laboratory tests depends on the results of the history and physical examination. The history should assess the infant's state of hydration and possible causative agents. Information regarding oral intake, frequency and volume of stools, general appearance of the infant, mental status, and frequency of urination can help in assessing hydration. The parent should be asked about fever, antibiotic therapy, and exposure to day care or other children and adults with diarrheal illness.

All children with diarrhea should be carefully weighed unclothed for comparison of previous weight and to provide a baseline for monitoring subsequent weights during the course of the disease. In an infant, the normal extracellular fluid volume is 25 percent of body weight; therefore, a loss of 8 percent of body weight as extracellular fluid would result in manifestations of severe dehydration. The actual weight loss is greater than that because of concomitant loss of cellular water.

The physical examination should begin with a global assessment, with particular attention to the state of hydration (Table 112-3). Mucous membranes, more than the lips, should be evaluated for moistness. The appearance of the anterior fontanel and eyes should be assessed. The skin hydration and turgor may give a sense of the degree of dehydration. The finding of doughy and tented skin is associated with hypernatremic dehydration. Finally, the child's mental status with regard to interaction with the examiner and the parent can be used as a measure of seriousness of illness and dehydration.

Temperature, pulse, and blood pressure all provide information concerning the degree of illness. The rest of the physical examination should focus on signs of concurrent viral illness, such as upper respiratory tract infections, that may be associated with gastroenteritis, as well as abdominal findings. A rectal examination is often useful in obtaining a stool sample for detection of occult blood, culture, examination for leukocytes, measurement of pH, and detection of reducing substances. It can also rule out anal fissures as the cause of bloody stools.

Serum electrolyte levels, particularly sodium and bicarbonate levels, should be assessed in any child considered significantly dehydrated. A markedly elevated blood urea nitrogen concentration with a relatively normal creatinine value may indicate recent or rapid dehydration. Serum creatinine values tend to be low in infants and young children, and a creatinine value of 1 mg/dL in this age group may represent a doubling in the normal value. The rest of the diagnostic workup should include a stool sample for the abovementioned tests and a urine sample for culture and analysis.

The decision to rehydrate the child as an inpatient or outpatient or orally or intravenously is dependent upon several factors. Children with greater than 10 percent dehydration, hypernatremic (Na > 150 meq/dL) dehydration, or symptomatic hyponatremia (Na < 130 meq/dL) should be admitted to the hospital. Oral hydration for these children may be attempted in the hospital, depending on the circumstances and cardiovascular stability of the patient. However, if there are any indications of significant peripheral vascular compromise or pending shock, intravenous hydration is mandatory. For a child who is isotonically 5 to 10 percent dehydrated, the choice of inpatient versus outpatient management is dependent on the ability of the person caring for the child to administer oral fluids. Children with this degree of dehydration tend to do well with oral hydration, and this approach may be attempted initially.

Contraindications to oral rehydration are severe vomiting or a required regimen of oral feedings. For the child with less than 5 percent dehydration, oral rehydration should be attempted. If the infant has been breast-fed, feeding should be continued and oral electrolyte-glucose solution given in addition until diarrhea subsides. If the infant has been fed a cow's-milk-based diet, feedings should be resumed slowly after initial feedings with oral rehydration solutions as tolerated, preferably with a lactose-free formula. Increased stool output may occur as feedings are increased, but a gradual increase of caloric intake over 4 or 5 days should avoid exacerbation of diarrhea. The total fluid intake of oral electrolyte solution and regular diet should be approximately 150 mL/kg/day.[20–25]

Abdominal Distention

Abdominal distention is normal in neonates and is usually due to lax abdominal musculature and relatively large intraabdominal organs. It may also be accentuated by excessive gas within the bowel. If the infant is comfortable and feeding well and the abdomen is soft, there is no need for concern. Abdominal distention may also occur in association with bowel obstruction, constipation, or ileus due to sepsis or gastroenteritis. Congenital organomegaly (e.g., hepatomegaly, splenomegaly, or renal enlargement) undetected in the perinatal period may also present as abdominal distention.[4,26]

Constipation

Infrequent bowel movements in neonates do not necessarily mean that the infant is constipated. Breast-fed infants may occasionally go without a bowel movement for 5 to 7 days and then pass a normal stool. However, if the infant has never passed stools, the possibility of intestinal stenosis or atresia, Hirschsprung disease, or meconium ileus or plug should be considered.

Constipation occurring after birth but within the first month of life suggests Hirschsprung disease, hypothyroidism, or anal stenosis. The diagnosis of Hirschsprung disease is supported by absence of feces on rectal examination and abrupt change in bowel luminal size on barium enema and is confirmed by a rectal biopsy demonstrating absence of ganglion cells. Infants with hypothyroidism present with feeding problems; a weak, hoarse cry; hypothermia; hypotonia; and peripheral edema. The child should be admitted for further evaluation and treatment.[27]

CARDIORESPIRATORY SYMPTOMS

Neonates are prone to respiratory problems for a variety of reasons. Anatomic causes are a barrel-shaped chest, a flattened diaphragm, limitation of diaphragmatic movement by abdominal compression, smaller airway diameter, and higher closing volumes. The high compliance of the chest wall, low compliance of the lungs, and less fatigue-resistant fibers in the diaphragm and intercostal muscles are also significant contributory factors. Cardiorespiratory symptoms are also more common in this age group since structural and functional abnormalities of the airway and heart are more likely to present at this time.

Cardiorespiratory symptoms in neonates are nonspecific and may be due to primary organ failure (cardiovascular or respiratory) or secondary to a variety of systemic diseases, such as sepsis, metabolic acidosis, abdominal pathology, and severe meningitis. Regardless of the cause, the assessment and stabilization of the airway, breathing, and circulation are priorities and should be accomplished before or concurrently with establishing a diagnosis.

Rapid Breathing

Rapid breathing can be due to minor problems, such as abdominal distention, or life-threatening illnesses, such as sepsis. Rapid breathing or grunting should always be considered a medical emergency. Admission for investigations, monitoring, and therapy should be considered in all but the mildest cases. When a cause cannot be identified on initial presentation, a full sepsis workup (full blood count, blood culture, urinalysis, chest x-ray, and cerebrospinal fluid examination) should be done and broad-spectrum antibiotics administered (Table 112-4).

TABLE 112-4 Causes of Rapid Breathing in Neonates

Pneumonia
Bacterial
Viral
Chlamydia
Aspiration
Bronchiolitis
Illness in other organ systems
Septicemia
Central nervous system (e.g., meningitis)
Abdomen (e.g., distention, gastroenteritis)
Metabolic acidosis
Congenital diseases
Repiratory disease
Delayed presentation of diaphragmatic hernia
Tracheoesophageal fistula
Lobar emphysema
Tracheal stenosis, webs
Heart disease
Cardiac failure (e.g., hypoplastic left heart, critical coarctation of aorta, aortic stenosis, patent ductus arteriosus)
Cyanotic disease (e.g., transposition of great arteries)
Vascular ring
Neuromuscular disease
Infantile botulism
Muscle weakness

Pneumonia

The lungs are the most common site of infection in neonates. Group B streptococcus is the most common cause of lower respiratory infection in newborns. The infection is most likely acquired in utero from a contaminated amniotic environment. Affected infants frequently develop fulminant illness within hours of birth. Other common bacterial pathogens in newborns and infants include *Streptococcus pneumoniae* and *Haemophilus influenzae* serotype B. Chlamydial pneumonia usually occurs after 3 weeks of age and is accompanied by conjunctivitis in 50 percent of cases. Infants with bacterial as well as viral pneumonia may present with fussiness, stuffy nose, decreased appetite, abrupt onset of high fever (<39°C), nasal flaring, grunting, retraction, tachypnea, and tachycardia.

Patients with chlamydial pneumonia are usually afebrile and tachypenic and have a prominent cough. Respiratory syncytial virus (RSV), adenovirus, and parainfluenzavirus can also cause pneumonia in otherwise well infants. In addition, infections with *Bordetella pertussis* may cause paroxysms of cough in an otherwise well-appearing infant. The cough may not be accompanied by characteristic whoop. Pertussis always must be considered in infants who have severe, paroxysmal cough and posttussive vomiting. Because many adults are susceptible to infection with pertussis, such an infection should be ruled out if the caretaker has a persistent cough.

The approach to febrile infants with suspected bacterial pneumonia should include a full evaluation for potential sepsis (blood and urine cultures, chest radiographs, and complete blood count). The blood culture results are typically negative, but obtaining two culture samples instead of one during the initial evaluation may increase the diagnostic yield fourfold. A lumbar puncture should be done if there are no contraindications.

Infants who have fever and pneumonia should be hospitalized and receive parenteral antibiotics against staphylococci and potential gram-negative pathogens. Infants suspected of having chlamydial or *B. pertussis* pneumonia should receive erythromycin or sulfamethoxazole. Infants who are afebrile with pneumonia may be treated as outpatients when a viral pathogen is suspected. Inability to eat, respiratory distress, and hypoxemia are criteria for hospitalization. Patients observed on an outpatient basis should be seen daily until symptoms are resolving.[28,29]

Bronchiolitis

Bronchiolitis is acute wheezing-associated respiratory illness in early life preceded by signs and symptoms of an upper respiratory infection. Bronchiolitis is a highly seasonal disease, with comparatively few cases seen during summer months and activity peaks during winter months. Serious cases of bronchiolitis occur most commonly in infants younger than 1 year of age, particularly in the first 3 months of life. In the general population of the United States, the incidence of bronchiolitis is 11.4 cases per 100 children-years during the first year of life. Bronchiolitis is more commonly seen in families of low socioeconomic status or infants who have not been breast-fed.

RSV is the most common cause and is probably transmitted by direct contact with nasal secretions of infected individuals much more frequently than by aerosol spread. Shedding of the virus can be documented 1 to 2 days before symptoms occur and for 1 to 2 weeks thereafter. Those exposed are probably not contagious for the entire period of time but should be considered contagious 24 to 48 h before the onset of symptoms and for several days thereafter.

A number of other viral agents also can cause bronchiolitis, although the illness is milder. The parainfluenza viruses are the second most common cause of bronchiolitis and are responsible for autumn and spring epidemics, usually preceding and following RSV outbreaks. Influenza type A virus can also precipitate bronchiolitis, along with adenovirus, rhinovirus, and *Mycoplasma pneumoniae*. The latter two agents are responsible for an increasing number of cases of wheezing-associated respiratory illness with increasing age, but RSV and parainfluenza viruses have been shown to provoke wheezing at all ages.

Acute bronchiolitis presents in infancy with serous nasal discharge accompanied by sneezing. These symptoms are followed by diminished appetite, cough, dyspnea, irritability, and, commonly, periods of apnea. Apnea is more common in neonates and usually presents within the first 3 days of illness. Physical examination reveals a rapid respiratory rate (>60 breaths per minute), cyanosis, air hunger, hyperinflation, intercostal and subcostal retractions, and a palpable liver and/or spleen due to hyperinflation of the lungs. Fever is usually low grade or absent, except in the presence of otitis media, when a temperature as high as 40°C may be present. Chest x-rays usually show hyperinflation with patchy atelectasis.

The diagnosis of bronchiolitis is usually made clinically. A wheezing infant with a history of the aforementioned symptoms for several days, particularly during the peak season for RSV, can be assumed to have bronchiolitis. Previous recommendations of a trial of subcutaneous epinephrine to distinguish bronchiolitis from asthma in wheezing infants is now discouraged because a small number of infants who have true bronchiolitis respond to first-course of β-adrenergic agents, while many patients with status asthmaticus do not. Immunofluorescence or enzyme-linked immunosorbent assays performed on respiratory secretions are very sensitive and specific for detection of RSV. Other diagnostic tests, such as blood gas analysis or cell counts, are directed by clinical assessment but rarely necessary.

Most cases of bronchiolitis are mild and can be managed without hospitalization. Infants recover without β-adrenergic agents or other medications used for relief of wheezing. The decision to hospitalize an infant with bronchiolitis should be based on a number of clinical criteria in addition to other considerations, such as reliability of parents, duration of present illness, and likelihood of obtaining acceptable follow-up. Infants who are born prematurely, have underlying heart or lung disease, are in first 3 months of life, or have low initial oxygen saturation (≤92 percent) are more likely to develop progressive or life-threatening illness. In addition, infants who are not feeding well or who are dehydrated should be considered for hospitalization. If respiratory distress is not severe and the infant is feeding reasonably well, hospitalization is not needed.

Infants for whom hospitalization is being considered should receive at least one course of β-adrenergic agent [albuterol 0.1 to 0.15 mg/kg/dose, up to 5 mg, hourly as required for the first few doses, then every 4 to 6 h]. If the response is good, the drug may be continued. The continued use of such agents in the absence of an initial beneficial response is controversial. It is not possible to predict which individuals with bronchiolitis will respond well to β-adrenergic agents. The hazards of administrating these agents are relatively minor; therefore, it is reasonable to administer β-adrenergic agents by aerosol, at least during first 24 h of hospitalization, and to continue to do so if the response is good.

The use of corticosteroids has never been evaluated adequately. Although a beneficial role for corticosteroids cannot be excluded, most infants with bronchiolitis respond satisfactorily without them. The use of antibiotics generally does not affect the clinical course of bronchiolitis because bacterial infection is almost never simultaneously present. The presence of unexplained high fever in the course of illness may be an indication for temporary antibiotic coverage.[30–32]

ILLNESS INVOLVING OTHER ORGAN SYSTEMS

The search for pathologic conditions in other organ systems is mandatory, since the presence of respiratory symptoms may divert attention from a significant underlying problem. For example, generalized sepsis, meningitis, gastroenteritis, and metabolic acidosis may present with respiratory distress as the predominant symptom.

CONGENITAL DISEASES

Respiratory Disease

Occasionally an H-type tracheoesophageal fistula may present in the first month of life or later with recurrent pneumonia, respiratory distress after feedings, and problems in clearing mucus. Tracheal stenosis may present initially with noisy breathing or a high-pitched cry and tremendous respiratory difficulty even after mild upper respiratory infections. Similarly, neonates with chronic respiratory insufficiency, such as bronchopulmonary dysplasia, may present in respiratory failure even after mild upper respiratory infections.[33,34]

Heart Disease

Rapid breathing due to cardiac disease is usually not associated with significant retractions and use of accessory muscles. As a general rule, a well-developed neonate who presents with unexplained cyanosis and tachypnea should be suspected of having congenital cardiac disease. In neonates with transposition of the great arteries and ventricular septal defect or critical coarctation of the aorta, congestive cardiac failure may be the presenting feature. Signs of heart failure may be very subtle but are life threatening and require emergency referral.[35]

Neuromuscular Disease

Any form of muscle weakness may be associated with shallow breathing and an increase in respiratory rate as a compensatory mechanism.

Cough and Nasal Congestion

Cough may be a prominent feature of most of the primary respiratory conditions listed in Table 112-4. It may also be the initial presentation of a variety of congenital anomalies, including cleft palate, laryngotracheomalacia, laryngotracheal cleft, tracheal webs, tracheoesophageal fistula, tracheal hemangiomas, and vascular rings. Although congenital malformation resulting in cough and nasal congestion is more likely to occur in neonates, in most instances, cough is due to a viral upper respiratory infection and may be associated with sneezing and nasal congestion. It may also be a prominent feature of bronchiolitis and chlamydial and pertussis infections. Treatment of the underlying condition is required. Cough suppressants should be used with extreme caution in neonates. Nasal congestion is best treated with instillation of saline drops when necessary.[32]

Noisy Breathing and Stridor

Noisy breathing is a common presenting complaint in neonates and is usually benign. Stridor is usually due to congenital anomalies (e.g., webs, cysts, stresia, stenosis, clefts, or hemangiomas) extending anywhere from the nose to the trachea and bronchi. Infants who were intubated in the neonatal period are prone to develop subglottic stenosis. Infection (e.g., croup, epiglottis, and abscess) as a cause of stridor in neonates is rare. Stridor worsening with cry suggests laryngomalacia or subglottic hemangioma; stridor and feeding difficulties suggest vascular ring, laryngeal cleft, or tracheoesophageal fistula; stridor with hoarseness suggests vocal cord paralysis. Laryngomalacia is the most common cause of stridor in the neonate. It is characterized by noisy, crowing inspiratory sounds, which usually improve during the first year of life. When the cause is in doubt, the infant should be admitted for evaluation to determine the cause.[36,37]

Apnea and Periodic Breathing

Periodic breathing, which may occur in normal neonates, should be differentiated from apnea. However, periodic breathing may precede apnea, and both may occur in the same patient. Apnea is a cessation of respiration for 10 to 20 s with or without bradycardia and cyanosis. It signifies critical illness and warrants prompt investigation and admission for monitoring and therapy.

Apnea may be precipitated by any of the disease conditions listed in Table 112-4 and usually indicates respiratory muscle fatigue and impending respiratory arrest. Resuscitation, including airway support and ventilation, should be followed by a thorough search for the inciting condition. If no obvious cause is found, the neonate should be assumed to be septic. Cultures should be obtained and broad-spectrum antibiotics started.[38,39]

Cyanosis and Blue Spells

An infant with cyanosis and blue spells usually presents a diagnostic challenge, since such findings may be due to many disorders. If breathing is rapid but not labored, the most likely cause is cyanotic congenital heart disease with right-to-left shunting. Methemoglobinemia, although rare, may have a similar presentation. Irregular or shallow breathing may be associated with sepsis, meningitis, cerebral edema, or intracranial hemorrhage and may also be accompanied by cyanosis. If breathing is labored (e.g., grunting or indrawing), pulmonary disease (e.g., pneumonia or bronchiolitis) is likely. All infants with cyanosis should be admitted for monitoring and further investigation.[40,41]

Jaundice

Jaundice (Table 112-5) may appear at varying times during the neonatal period and requires a complete diagnostic evaluation. Jaundice during the first 24 h rarely presents to the emergency department. The commonest causes of jaundice seen in the emergency department are physiologic jaundice, jaundice due to sepsis, or breast-milk jaundice. Occasionally, infants with hemolysis due to autoimmune congenital causes may present to the emergency department.

Physiologic jaundice is due to the breakdown of fetal red blood cells, and bilirubin rises at a rate of less than 5 mg/dL per 24 h, with a peak of 5 to 6 mg/dL during the second to the fourth day of life, returning to <2 mg/dL by 5 to 7 days. Septic infants with hyperbilirubinemia also have other features of sepsis, such as vomiting, abdominal distention, respiratory distress, and poor feeding. Jaundice associated with breast-feeding is thought to be due to the presence of substances that inhibit glucuronyl transferase in breast milk; it may start as early as the third to fourth day and reaches a peak of 10 to 27 mg/dL by the third week of life. Cessation of breast-feeding causes rapid decline in 2 to 3 days.

TABLE 112-5 Causes of Jaundice in Neonates

<24 h	ABO, Rh incompatibility Sepsis Congenital infections (e.g., rubella, toxoplasmosis, cytomegalovirus infection) Excessive bruising from birth trauma (cephalhematoma or intramuscular hematoma)
2–3 days	Physiologic
3 days to 1 week	Septicemia Syphilis, toxoplasmosis, cytomegalovirus infection
>1 week	Septicemia, congenital atresia of bile ducts, serum hepatitis Congenital hemolytic anemias (sickle cell anemia, spherocytosis) Hemolytic anemia due to drugs (e.g., in glucose-6-phosphate dehydrogenase deficiency) Rubella, herpetic hepatitis Hypothyroidism Breast-milk jaundice

A proper history and physical examination provide clues to the causes of jaundice. A well-looking child who is gaining weight and feeding well is unlikely to be septic. Laboratory evaluation should include a full blood count to test for anemia, a smear for hemolysis, direct and total bilirubin determinations, a reticulocyte count, and a Coombs test. Admission to the hospital, appropriate cultures, and antibiotics are ordered for neonates who are unwell and have any of the signs or symptoms listed in Table 112-5. In all cases, arrangements should be made for monitoring of bilirubin and hemoglobin levels. While most well infants can be monitored out of the hospital, infants who are anemic or have bilirubin levels approaching transfusion levels (approximately 20 mg/dL) should be admitted.[42–44]

Eye Discharge, Redness, and Conjunctivitis

Neonates with red eyes are most likely suffering from conjunctivitis. Neonatal conjunctivitis occurs in 1.6 to 12 percent of newborns during the first month of life. The chemical irritation from antimicrobial prophylaxis against bacterial infection is the most frequent cause, followed by *Chlamydia trachomatis* infection. Other important pathogens in this setting are *H. influenzae* and *Streptococcus pneumoniae. Neisseria gonorrhoeae* is no longer a major cause of neonatal conjunctivitis in the United States because of mandated use of neonatal ocular prophylaxis. The failure rate of antimicrobial prophylaxis is 1 percent. However, because *N. gonorrhoeae* can damage the eye severely, it is important to always test for this pathogen as the possible cause of neonatal conjunctivitis. Viruses rarely cause isolated neonatal conjunctivitis as an isolated problem. They usually cause conjunctivitis as part of a generalized viral syndrome affecting many organs. For example, herpes simplex virus causes neonatal keratoconjunctivitis as part of a generalized viremia with infection at other sites such as skin, mucous membranes, or with disseminated disease. The finding of vesicles anywhere on the body in association with neonatal conjunctivitis suggests the possibility of herpes simplex infection.

An important consideration in the evaluation of neonatal conjunctivitis is the time of onset. Chemical conjunctivitis secondary to ocular prophylaxis usually occurs on the first day of life. Gonococcal conjunctivitis generally has its peak time of onset between 3 and 5 days after birth. By the end of first week of life and throughout the first month of life, *Chlamydia* becomes the most frequent cause of conjunctivitis. It is important to note that these times of onset assume rupture of amniotic membrane at or near the time of delivery.

The conjunctiva can be inoculated before birth by an ascending bacterial infection.

Chlamydial conjunctivitis can vary in severity, ranging from mild-to-severe hyperemia with a thick mucopurulent discharge and psuedomembrane formation. Gonococcal conjunctivitis can present as typical bacterial conjunctivitis. However, in its full-blown form, it presents as hyperacute conjunctivitis with profuse discharge. There often is severe edema of both lids. In marked contrast to other forms of bacterial conjunctivitis, *N. gonorrhoeae* has the capacity to invade superficial layers of the conjunctiva, causing ulceration of the cornea. If it is not treated, it can result in the loss of eye from corneal complications.

A Gram stain and culture should always be obtained in instances of neonatal conjunctivitis to make certain that the conjunctivitis is not due to *N. gonorrhoeae.* Since isolation of *C. trachomatis* requires specialized tissue cultures, proper technique should be employed in collecting those specimens (e.g., Dacron swabs) and specimens for antigen detection.

Gonococcal opthalmia neonatorum is treated best with ceftriaxone (25 to 50 mg/kg per day intravenously or intramuscularly, not to exceed 125 mg) given once or a single dose of cefotaxime (100 mg/kg intravenously or intramuscularly). When disseminated disease is suspected, the duration of treatment is 7 days. Cefotaxime is recommended for hyperbilirubinemic infants. If meningitis is documented, treatment should be continued for 10 to 14 days. Infants with gonococcal opthalmia should have their eyes irrigated with saline solution immediately and at frequent intervals until the discharge is eliminated. Topical antibiotic treatment alone is inadequate and is unnecessary when recommended systemic antibiotic treatment is given.

Chlamydial conjunctivitis and pneumonia in young infants are treated with oral erythromycin (50 mg/kg/day in four divided doses) for 14 days. Oral sulfonamides may be used after the immediate neonatal period for infants who do not tolerate erythromycin. Topical treatment of conjunctivitis is ineffective and unnecessary. Since the efficacy of erythromycin therapy is approximately 80 percent, a second course is sometimes required. A specific diagnosis of *C. trachomatis* infection in an infant should prompt the treatment of the mother and her sexual partners.

The neonate with a red eye and irritability may also be suffering from a corneal irritation or abrasion, usually due to an eyelash. Acute glaucoma, although rare, also presents as a red, teary eye. In these instances, the cornea may be stained or cloudy, the anterior chamber shallow, and the intraoccular pressure increased. Prompt opthalmologic referral of all suspected cases of glaucoma is mandatory. Infectious causes should be treated (Table 112-6) and follow-up care ensured.[45–48]

Diaper Rash and Oral Thrush

Candidal diaper dermatitis is an erythematous plaque with a scalloped border and a sharply demarcated edge that is studded by satellite lesions. It usually occurs in the moist, occluded diaper area and intertriginous zones and usually results from the action of organisms harbored in the gastrointestinal tract. Treatment consists of a topical anticandidal agent with each diaper change or four times daily. Protection of the area with zinc oxide paste overlying the cream will prevent friction, and local treatment with Nystatin cream will prevent spread of the infection. In addition, an oral course of Nystatin is usually warranted to prevent colonization of the gut (Table 112-6).

Oral lesions are white and flaky, covering the tongue, lips, gingiva, and mucous membranes. These lesions are common in debilitated infants and in those on antibiotics. Oral lesions may affect oral intake because of pain and discomfort. Treatment of ill infants consists of treating the underlying pathology, oral antifungal therapy, and an anesthetic gel prior to feeding. Cool liquids may prevent discomfort and pain.[49,50]

TABLE 112-6 Antibiotic Therapy for Infections

Indications	Drugs
Sepsis and meningitis Initial therapy, organism unknown Urinary tract infection	Ampicillin (200 mg/kg/day div q6h IV) *and* gentamicin (2.5 mg/kg/day for 0–7 days of age div q12h IV and for >7 days of age q8h IV) *or* cefotaxime (200 mg/kg/day div q6h)
Pneumonia (bacterial)	Ampicillin (100 mg/kg/day div q6h) *or* cefotaxime (200 mg/kg/day div q6h) *or* ceftriaxone (50–75 mg/kg/day div q12–24 h IM or IV)
Pneumonia (chlamydial)	Erythromycin (40 mg/kg/day div q6h PO)
Pneumonia (pertussis)	Erythromycin (40 mg/kg/day div q6h for 5–10 days PO) *or* ampicillin (200 mg/kg/day div q6h IV if PO medication not retained)
Conjunctivitis (chlamydial)	Erythromycin (50 mg/kg/day div q6h × 14 days)
Conjunctivitis (gonococcal)	Ceftriaxone, 25–50 mg/kg/day IV or IM *or* Cefotaxime, 100 mg/kg/day IV or IM] A single dose of antibiotics may be effective in uncomplicated infection
Necrotizing enterocolitis	Ticarcillin [300 mg/kg/day q6h IV or IM] *and* gentamicin (2.5 mg/kg/day for 0–7 days of age, div q12h IV and for >7 days of age q8h IV)
Oral thrush	Oral nystatin suspension 100,000 U, 1–2 drops to each side of the mouth q4–6h after feedings for 7–14 days
Candidal dermatitis	Nystatin cream 100,000 U/gm or Amphotericin B cream 3%, to affected area q4–6h for 7–14 days

Abbreviations: div, divided; IM, intramuscularly; IV, intravenously; PO, by mouth.

Fever and Sepsis

Fever (Table 112-6) is most commonly due to acute infections. Fever is present when an infant's rectal temperature is 100.4°F or greater, as reportedly measured by a caretaker, or 38°C or more, as measured by a health care professional. The risk of infection rises with the height of fever, especially in infants over 4 weeks of age. The risk is about 3 percent with fever above 39.4°C, 6 percent with fever over 40°C, 13 percent with over 40.5°C, and 26 percent with fever over 41.1°C.

Recognizing neonatal bacterial sepsis early is a difficult task. Neonates have about twice the risk of serious bacterial infection as do infants 4 to 8 weeks of age. Neonatal sepsis tends to appear as either an ''early-onset'' or a ''late-onset'' syndrome, but some cases are difficult to classify. Early-onset disease is seen in first few days of life, tends to be fulminant, and is usually associated with maternal or perinatal risk factors, such as maternal fever, prolonged rupture of membranes, and fetal distress. On the other hand, late-onset disease usually occurs after 1 week of age, tends to develop more gradually, and is less likely to be associated with risk factors. Septic shock and neutropenia are more common with early-onset syndrome, and meningitis is more common in late-onset disease.

Clinical signs of either type of sepsis are not specific (Table 112-7). Septic infants may exhibit any of a variety of symptoms, including

TABLE 112-7 Signs and Symptoms of Neonatal Sepsis

Temperature instability
Central nervous system dysfunction
Respiratory distress
Feeding disturbance
Jaundice
Rashes
Fever, hypothermia
Lethargy, irritability, seizures
Apnea, tachypnea, grunting
Vomiting, poor feeding, gastric distention, diarrhea

lethargy, poor feeding, vomiting, temperature instability (hypothermia more often than hyperthermia), unexplained apnea, respiratory distress, seizures (with or without meningitis), cyanosis, tachycardia, bleeding diathesis, and hypotension.

The bacterial causes of neonatal sepsis tend to reflect the organisms that colonize the female genital tract and nasal mucosae of caregivers. In general, the two groups of pathogens most frequently encountered have been gram-positive cocci, such as β-hemolytic streptococci, and enteric organisms, such as *E. coli* and *Klebsiella* species, and *H. influenzae. Listeria monocytogenes,* a gram-positive rod, is a very common pathogen that causes sepsis and meningitis in neonates. Viral infections are also common and are most likely due to enteroviruses (coxsackievirus and echovirus) acquired at the time of delivery or RSV and influenza A virus acquired postnatally.

When a neonate is thought to be septic, microscopic analysis of cerebrospinal fluid, blood, and urine, and cerebrospinal cultures should be obtained. The infant should be admitted and intravenous antibiotics started. Initial treatment of a neonate with suspected bacterial septicemia or meningitis entails a combination of ampicillin and an aminoglycoside. An alternative regimen of ampicillin and a cephalosporin (e.g., cefotaxime or ceftazidime) is active against most etiologic gram-negative bacilli and can be used in cases when gram-negative meningitis is strongly suspected.

Febrile infants between 4 to 8 weeks of age who satisfy the following criteria are candidates for outpatient management:

- No focus of bacterial infection (middle ear, skin, soft tissue, bone, or joint) on physical examination
- Well appearing (alert, active, and with good muscle tone), well hydrated and tolerating oral fluids adequately, no respiratory distress (respiratory rate <60 breaths per minute, no grunting respiration or retractions)
- Cerebrospinal fluid total white blood cell count less than 10/μL, complete blood count total white blood cell count less than 15,000/μL, urinalysis white blood cell count less than 10 cells/hpf, and negative results for bacteriuria, leukocytes, esterase, and nitrite
- No pulmonary infiltrates on chest radiograph
- Reliable caretaker ensuring close outpatient follow-up.

The decision to administer empiric ceftriaxone pending culture results depends largely on the physician's level of comfort. We prefer to treat, since potentially serious complications, such as focal bacterial infection progressing to bacteremia and septicemia, and seeding of central nervous system can result from misdiagnosed (''occult'') serious bacterial infection that is not treated promptly. Therefore, the therapeutic benefit of administrating ceftriaxone pending culture results outweighs both therapeutic risk and cost considerations. It should be emphasized that thorough and frequent reevaluations of these infants are essential to monitor changes in the clinical course and culture results.[51–56]

Apparent Life-Threatening Events

An apparent life-threatening event (ALTE) (Table 112-8) is an ''episode that is frightening to the observer and is characterized by some combination of apnea (central or occasionally obstructive), color change (usually cyanotic or pallid but occasionally erythematous or plethoric), marked change in muscle tone (usually marked limpness), choking, or gagging. In some cases the observer fears that the infant has died.''

ALTE is not a diagnosis. It is simply a description of a characteristic clinical presentation. The usual age of occurrence is 2 to 3 months, but ALTE can occur at any age. Approximately 1 to 3 percent of infants in the general population are reported to experience ALTEs. The incidence is increased among infants who die of sudden infant death syndrome (SIDS) to about 5 to 6 percent. It can be reassuring to families that only about 1 of 20 SIDS cases occurs in the population who experience ALTE and, except for the most severe ALTE episodes, fewer than 1 to 2 percent of these infants succumb to SIDS. Most infants presenting with the history of ALTE have had relatively mild events and probably are not at increased risk of subsequent infant death compared with general population. Data do indicate a high risk of subsequent infant death following more severe ALTE presentations. The risk of subsequent infant death among all infants who experience an ALTE probably is 1 to 2 percent, but the risk increases to 8 to 10 percent for the relatively rare subgroup of infants who present with ALTE occurring during sleep and who are perceived to require some form of cardiopulmonary resuscitation. Those who experienced more than one such severe episode requiring either cardiopulmonary resuscitation or vigorous stimulation were reported in one study to have a 28 percent subsequent mortality rate despite the prescription of home monitors.

An ALTE may be caused by anything that could give the impression that the infant is extremely ill and in danger of dying. The most common general categories of the causation for ALTEs and their prevalence among ALTE infants are infection (5 to 40 percent, de-

TABLE 112-8 Differential Diagnosis of Acute Life-Threatening Episodes

Infectious	Viral (e.g., RSV, other respiratory viruses) Bacterial (e.g., sepsis, pertussis)
Gastrointestinal	Gastroesophageal reflux with or without obstructive apnea
Respiratory	Airway abnormality (e.g., vascular rings, pulmonary slings, tracheomalacia) Pneumonia
Neurologic	Seizure disorder Central nervous system infection (e.g., meningitis, encephalitis) Vasovagal response Leigh's encephalopathy Brain tumor
Cardiovascular	Congenital malformation Dysrhythmias Cardiomyopathy
Nonaccidental trauma	Battering Drug overdose Munchausen-by-proxy syndrome
No definable cause	Apnea of infancy

pending on the season), gastroesophageal reflux (GER) and other causes of laryngeal chemoreceptor stimulation (20 percent), seizures and other neurologic disorders (15 to 20 percent), and idiopathic (40 to 60 percent). Because most infants who have significant GER do not experience ALTEs, establishing the diagnosis of GER does not prove that it is the cause of ALTE. An unusually strong laryngeal chemoreceptor reflex can significantly increase an infant's susceptibility to ALTE due to GER, even with only minor reflux. This reflex is stimulated by acid or nonisotonic fluids, and the reflex response is apnea, bradycardia, and central pooling of blood.

Another type of ALTE, infantile breath-holding response, is also known as prolonged expiratory apnea or infantile syncope. Normal infants, both premature and full term, often perform a Valsalva maneuver in response to pain or fright, during vigorous activity, and during crying, coughing, and defecation. This maneuver normally decreases minute ventilation but is usually without consequence. However, some infants perform prolonged Valsalva maneuvers that persist until cyanosis, unconsciousness, and even seizures develop. These spells are presumed to be a more severe version of the simple breath-holding spells in which a crying child holds his or her breath until cyanosis develops but resumes breathing. Severe breath-holding spells have been estimated to occur in up to 5 percent of normal children at some time before 6 years of age.

There is no routine evaluation for ALTE. In general, after obtaining vital signs and history and performing a physical examination, further diagnostic testing should be individualized, depending on initial findings and clinical suspicions. If the infant appears to have cardiovascular and respiratory symptoms at the time of presentation, a very careful history should be taken and physical examination performed. If at all possible, a detailed description of the infant at the time of discovery, the specific stimulation and resuscitation measures used, and the infant's response should be obtained directly from those present at the time. Great care must be taken to ensure that the terms used by lay observers to describe the event are interpreted appropriately by the physician. It is useful to determine whether the infant has been chronically ill or essentially well. A report of several days of poor feeding, temperature instability, or respiratory or gastrointestinal symptoms suggests an infectious process.

Reports of "struggling to breathe" or "trying to breathe" imply airway obstruction. Association of the episode with the feeding implies uncoordinated swallowing, GER, or airway obstruction. Episodes that typically follow crying may be related to breath holding. Association of the episode with sleeping may also suggest GER or apnea of infancy. Attempts should be made to determine the duration of episode, but this is often difficult. The physician should also search for past medical problems and any family history of such problems. In addition to a normal, careful physical examination, particular focus should be directed toward the neurologic examination, observation of breathing during sleep and feeding, and evidence on cardiac examination of pulmonary hypertension or structural cardiac abnormalities.

Most infants who present acutely after an ALTE should be hospitalized for monitoring and further evaluation. Some episodes occur in clusters; if they occur in the hospital, observation by medically trained observers may help clarify the severity and cause of the episodes, and availability of trained medical personnel may be necessary for resuscitative efforts. In addition, the family and caretaker may be extremely anxious about the vulnerability of their infant and may benefit from reassurance, assessment, and counseling.[36,57–62]

Sudden Infant Death Syndrome

Neonates may occasionally present in cardiorespiratory arrest. Although SIDS should be considered, catastrophic deterioration is more likely to be due to infectious causes (e.g., septicemia or meningitis), trauma (e.g., intracranial bleeding or child abuse), and inborn errors of metabolism (e.g., medium-chain acyl dehydrogenase deficiency).

In most cases, cardiopulmonary resuscitation is unsuccessful, since the myocardium has suffered severe hypoxic ischemic damage. The physician's role in such cases is to provide supportive care for the family. In most cases, this entails reassurance that all appropriate efforts were made to save their child's life and that the infant has been treated with dignity. Other personnel (e.g., chaplain, social worker, or family physician) may also be required to provide support.

When the cause of death is not known, physicians should obtain appropriate samples (blood, urine, skin biopsy, etc.) and obtain permission for an autopsy. Such postmortem studies are very important because of the genetic implications of metabolic disease. A postmortem protocol for sudden neonatal deaths should be available in all emergency departments.[63,64]

REFERENCES

1. Barnes LA, Curran JS: The feeding of infants and children, in Behrman RE, Kliegman RM, Arvin AM (eds): *WE Nelson Textbook of Pediatrics,* 15th ed. Philadelphia, Saunders, 1996, pp 151–166.
2. Schmitt BD: The first week at home with your new baby. *Contemp Pediatr* 10:77, 1993.
3. Vaughan VC: Assessment of growth and development during infancy and early childhood. *Pediatr Rev* 13:88, 1992.
4. Ulshen M: Normal digestive tract phenomena, in Behrman RE, Kliegman RM, Arvin AM (eds): *WE Nelson Textbook of Pediatrics,* 15th ed. Philadelphia, Saunders, 1996, pp 1031–1032.
5. Hoekelman RA: The physical examination of infants and children, in Bates B (ed): *A Guide to Physical Examination and History Taking,* 4th ed. Philadelphia, Lippincott, 1988.
6. Kleigman RM: Physical examination of the newborn infant, in Behrman RE, Kliegman RM, Arvin AM (eds): *WE Nelson Textbook of Pediatrics,* 15th ed. Philadelphia, Saunders, 1996, pp 434–437.
7. Ferber R: Sleeplessness, night awakening, and night crying in the infant and toddler. *Pediatr Rev* 9:6, 1987.
8. Blum NJ, Carey WB: Sleep problems among infants and young children. *Pediatr Rev* 17:87, 1996.
9. Lehtonen L, Korvenranta H: Infantile colic: Seasonal incidence and crying profiles. *Arch Pediatr Adolesc Med* 149:533, 1995.
10. Adams LM, Davidson M: Present concepts of infant colic. *Pediatr Ann* 16:817, 1987.
11. Davis HW, Zitelli BJ: Childhood injuries: Accidental or inflicted? *Contemp Pediatr* 12:94, 1995.
12. Sirotnak AP, Krugman RD: Physical abuse of children: An update. *Pediatr Rev* 15:394, 1994.
13. Krugman RD: Child abuse and neglect, in Hay WW JR, Groothuis JR, Hayward AR, Levin MJ (eds): *Current Pediatric Diagnosis and Treatment,* 13th ed. Stamford, CT, Appleton & Lange, 1997, pp 210–214.
14. Ibrahim-Gonzalez E: Diagnostic points in child abuse. *Resident Staff Physician* 42:12, 1996.
15. Hechtman DH, Stylianos S: Surgical conditions in the newborn. *Pediatr Ann* 23:231, 1994.
16. Pollock ES: Pediatric abdominal surgical emergencies. *Pediatr Ann* 25:448, 1996.
17. Orenstein SR: Gastroesophageal reflux. *Pediatr Rev* 13:174, 1992.
18. Ramos AG, Tuchman DN: Persistent vomiting. *Pediatr Rev* 15:24, 1994.
19. Garcia VF, Randolph JG: Pyloric stenosis: Diagnosis and management. *Pediatr Rev* 11:292, 1990.
20. DeWitt TG: Acute diarrhea in children. *Pediatr Rev* 11:6, 1989.
21. Harrison HE: Dehydration in infancy: Hospital treatment. *Pediatr Rev* 11:139, 1989.
22. Adelman RD, Solhung MJ: Fluid therapy, in Behrman RE, Kliegman RM, Arvin AM (eds): *WE Nelson Textbook of Pediatrics*, 15th ed. Philadelphia, Saunders, 1996, pp 206–210.
23. Avner ED: Clinical disorders of water metabolism: Hyponatremia and hypernatremia. *Pediatr Ann* 24:23, 1995.
24. Limbos MAP, Lieberman JM: Management of acute diarrhea in children. *Contemp Pediatr* 12:68, 1995.
25. Bernard J: Gastrointestinal disorders due to cow's milk consumption. *Pediatr Ann* 26:244, 1997.
26. Kendig JW: Care of normal newborn. *Pediatr Rev* 13:262, 1992.
27. Fitzgerald JF: Constipation in children. *Pediatr Rev* 8:299, 1987.

28. Schidlow DV, Callahan CW: Pneumonia. *Pediatr Rev* 17:300, 1996.
29. Rosenberg AA, Thilo EH: The newborn infant, in Hay WW JR, Groothuis JR, Hayward AR, Levin MJ (eds): *Current Pediatric Diagnosis and Treatment,* 13th ed. Stamford, CT, Appleton & Lange, 1997, pp 42–46.
30. Welliver JR, Welliver RC: Bronchiolitis. *Pediatr Rev* 14:134, 1993.
31. Hall CB: Respiratory syncytial virus: What we know now. *Contemp Pediatr* 10:92, 1993.
32. Benitz WE, Tatro DS: Pulmonary drugs, in *The Pediatric Drug Handbook.* St. Louis, Mosby, 1995, pp 145.
33. Korones SB, Bada-Ellzey HS (eds): Tachypnea, in *Neonatal Decision Making.* St. Louis, Mosby, 1993, pp 66–67.
34. Taeusch HW: Initial evaluation: History and physical examination of the newborn, in Taeusch HW, Ballard RA, Avery ME (eds): *Shaffer and Avery's Diseases of the Newborn,* 6th ed. Philadelphia, Saunders, 1991, pp 207–224.
35. Rossi AF: Pediatric cardiac intensive care, in Chang AC, Hanley FL, Wernovsky G, Wessel DL (eds): *Cardiac Diagnostic Evaluation.* Baltimore, Williams & Wilkins, 1998, pp 37–43.
36. Korones SB, Bada-Ellzey HS (eds): Stridor, in *Neonatal Decision Making.* St. Louis, Mosby, 1993, pp 68–69.
37. Custer JR: Croup and related disorders. *Pediatr Rev* 14:19, 1993.
38. Carroll JL, Marcus CL, Loughlin GM: Disordered control of breathing in infants and children. *Pediatr Rev* 14:51, 1993.
39. Korones SB, Bada-Ellzey HS (eds): Apnea, in *Neonatal Decision Making.* St. Louis, Mosby, 1993, pp 62–65.
40. Korones SB, Bada-Ellzey HS (eds): Cyanosis, in *Neonatal Decision Making.* St. Louis, Mosby, 1993, pp 58–59.
41. Lees MH, King DH: Cyanosis in the newborn. *Pediatr Rev* 9:36, 1987.
42. Gartner LM: Neonatal jaundice. *Pediatr Rev* 11:422, 1994.
43. Rosenthal P, Sinatra F: Jaundice in infancy. *Pediatr Rev* 11:79, 1989.
44. Korones SB, Bada-Ellzey HS (eds): Jaundice, in *Neonatal Decision Making.* St. Louis, Mosby, 1993, pp 54–57.
45. Gigliotti F: Acute conjunctivitis. *Pediatr Rev* 16:203, 1995.
46. Gonococcal infections, in *Report of the Committee on Infectious Diseases, American Academy of Pediatrics,* 24th ed. 141 Northwest Point Blvd, PO Box 927, Elk Grove Village, IL, 1997, pp 212–219.
47. *Chlamydia trachomatis,* in *Report of the Committee on Infectious Diseases, American Academy of Pediatrics,* 24th ed. 141 Northwest Point Blvd, PO Box 927, Elk Grove Village, IL, 1997, pp 170–174.
48. Wagner RS: Eye infection and abnormalities: Issues for the pediatrician. *Contemp Pediatr* 14:137, 1997.
49. Singalvanija S, Freiden IJ: Diaper dermatitis. *Pediatr Rev* 16:422, 1995.
50. Rasmussen JE: Cutaneous fungus infections in children. *Pediatr Rev* 13:152, 1992.
51. Bonadio WA: Keeping febrile young infants out of the hospital. *Contemp Pediatr* 11:73, 1994.
52. Poland RL, Watterberg KL: Consultation with the specialist: Sepsis in the newborn. *Pediatr Rev* 14:262, 1993.
53. Avner JR: Occult bacteremia: How great the risk? *Contemp Pediatr* 14:53, 1997.
54. Dagan R, Hall CB, Powell KR, Menegus M: Epidemiology and laboratory diagnosis of infection with viral and bacterial pathogens in infants hospitalized for suspected sepsis. *J Pediatr* 115:351, 1989.
55. Nelson JD: *Pocket Book of Pediatric Antimicrobial Therapy,* 13th ed. Baltimore, Williams & Wilkins, 1998.
56. Barone MA: *The Harriet Lane Handbook,* 14th ed. St. Louis, Mosby, 1996.
57. National Institutes of Health Consensus Development Conference on Infantile Apnea and Home Monitoring: Consensus statement. *Pediatrics* 79:292, 1987.
58. Brooks JG: Consultation with the specialist: Apparent life-threatening events. *Pediatr Rev* 17:257, 1996.
59. Carroll JL, Loughlin GM: Sudden infant death syndrome. *Pediatr Rev* 14:83, 1993.
60. Larsen GL, Abman SH, Fan LL, et al: Disorders of the control of breathing: Respiratory tract and mediastinum, in Hay WW JR, Groothuis JR, Hayward AR, Levin MJ (eds): *Current Pediatric Diagnosis and Treatment,* 13th ed. Stamford, CT, Appleton & Lange, 1997, pp 471–472.
61. Willinger M: SIDS prevention. *Pediatr Ann* 24:358, 1995.
62. Evans OB: Breath-holding spells. *Pediatr Ann* 26:410, 1997.
63. Gilbert-Barness E, Barness L: Sudden infant death: A reappraisal. *Contemp Pediatr* 12:88, 1995.
64. Shaefer SJM, McClain ME: Supporting families after sudden infant death. *Pediatr Ann* 24:373, 1995.

113 THE NICU GRADUATE

Daniel G. Batton

Graduates of the neonatal intensive care unit (NICU) may be frequent visitors to the emergency department and often require rehospitalization during the first few months following discharge.[1–3] Most NICU graduates are low-birth weight infants who may have a variety of complications related to prematurity. These infants should be evaluated based upon *postconceptional,* not chronologic, age. For example, a 32-week-gestation premature infant with an 8-week chronologic age since birth is evaluated as a term infant.

Premature infants are usually discharged from the hospital at a postconceptional age of 33 to 38 weeks, although a few infants are well beyond 40 weeks. The normal respiratory rate at this age is 30 to 40 breaths per minute, although an infant with bronchopulmonary dysplasia may breathe 60 to 70 times per minute. The heart rate ranges from 120 to 160 beats per minute but can be considerably lower during quiet sleep. Most laboratory values are similar to adults' values, although the hematocrit can be as low as 20 to 25 percent because of physiologic anemia. Neurodevelopmental milestones most appropriate for a given infant are those corresponding to the postconceptional age. When caring for NICU graduates, attention must be paid not only to the presenting signs and symptoms but also to general problems related to prematurity.

GENERAL CONSIDERATIONS

Cold Stress

Following hospital discharge, premature infants remain susceptible to cold stress when exposed to lower environmental temperatures, primarily because of decreased subcutaneous tissue.[4] Infants who are cold-stressed are not capable of responding by shivering but, rather, attempt to maintain body temperature by increasing their metabolism of brown fat, which results in heat production. However, this increases oxygen consumption and can lead to hypoglycemia. If this compensatory increase in metabolic rate is insufficient to overcome the low environmental temperature, then body temperature will fall. A normal body temperature, however, does not eliminate the possibility of cold stress, since body temperature may be maintained at considerable metabolic expense. The best way to avoid cold stress is to provide an adequate environmental temperature for the infant who is being evaluated in the emergency department. If the room temperature cannot be adjusted appropriately, a heat lamp should be available. Commercial heat lamps are available that have automatic timers and can be adjusted to provide varying amounts of heat. Such lamps should be standard equipment in emergency departments that treat infants and children.

Hypoglycemia

Premature infants are at risk of developing hypoglycemia with an acute illness. This risk may be due in part to increased glucose consumption, cold stress, poor enteral intake during the illness, or suboptimal glycogen stores.[4] Since hypoglycemia can have severe consequences, glucose testing is necessary for all premature infants presenting with an acute illness. If the blood sugar is less than 45 mg percent, intravenous glucose therapy (10% dextrose in water at 100 mL/kg/day) should be initiated.

Hypertension

Longitudinal studies of convalescing premature infants have demonstrated that systemic hypertension may develop in as many as 9 percent.[5] The possible causes include thromboembolic renal artery occlusion following umbilical artery catheterization and bronchopulmonary dysplasia.[6] Although the normal range is age dependent, a systolic blood pressure greater than 120 mmHg or a diastolic pressure greater than 75 mmHg warrants consideration of systemic hypertension.[7]

Fractures

Because of decreased bone mineralization (osteopenia) related to prematurity, fractures of the long bones and ribs are not uncommon in premature infants during their initial hospitalization. Usually by the time of hospital discharge, bone mineralization has improved to such an extent that new fractures are uncommon, but there may be evidence of healing fractures on x-ray examination. This fact should be kept in mind if fractures are incidentally noted on an x-ray, to avoid possible misinterpretation as signs of child abuse. Comparison of current x-rays with previous films may help to clarify the issue.

Failure to Thrive

The establishment of consistent weight gain with oral feedings is a standard criterion for discharge from the hospital for most premature infants. However, this does not ensure that the pattern of weight gain will continue following discharge. Failure to thrive may occur either because of an ongoing chronic disease (e.g., bronchopulmonary dysplasia, malabsorption, or central nervous system disease) or because of dysfunctional parenting. NICU graduates should be consuming at least 150 mL/kg/day of a standard formula if not breast feeding and should be consistently gaining approximately 20 to 30 g/day. A comparison of the current weight with the discharge weight (which parents usually remember) allows for a quick evaluation of this problem, or appropriate growth curves can be utilized.[8,9] Any infant with failure to thrive requires a thorough diagnostic evaluation and often hospitalization for accurate documentation of caloric intake. It should be remembered that prematurity itself is not an adequate explanation for postdischarge failure to thrive.

Immunizations

The recommendation by the American Academy of Pediatrics is to immunize premature infants on the same schedule as normal full-term infants.[10] However, because of prolonged hospitalization and complicated follow-up, it is possible that immunizations might be missed. Inquiry about the immunization status may uncover such a situation. Although it may not be desirable to immunize an infant during an acute illness, appropriate recommendations for follow-up should be made.

ACUTE RESPIRATORY DETERIORATION IN INFANTS WITH BRONCHOPULMONARY DYSPLASIA

Although acute respiratory deterioration can occur in any NICU graduate, this discussion focuses on those infants with ongoing pulmonary disease, such as bronchopulmonary dysplasia (BPD). BPD is usually a sequela of prematurity, hyaline membrane disease, and mechanical ventilation, although it may be associated with other conditions.[11] Features of BPD include tachypnea, hypercarbia, suboptimal oxygenation, and sometimes reactive airway disease. In more severe cases, pulmonary hypertension, pulmonary edema, and cor pulmonale are prominent. The cornerstones of therapy for BPD are oxygen and nutrition. It is essential to take a medication history, since chronic use of diuretics or bronchodilators is seen in selected patients, although their value remains poorly defined. Systemic glucocorticoids are used more commonly as chronic therapy and can lead to adrenal suppression.

TABLE 113-1 Causes of Acute Respiratory Deterioration in Infants with BPD

Respiratory infection

Aspiration
  Gastroesophageal reflux
  Incoordinate sucking or swallowing

Bronchospasm
Pulmonary edema

Dehydration
  Gastroenteritis
  Diuretic therapy

Anemia
Cor pulmonale

Acute deterioration in patients with BPD is usually manifested by an increase in respiratory rate, an increase in respiratory effort, a decrease in oxygenation, and poor feeding. The most common causes of acute respiratory deterioration in infants with BPD are listed in Table 113-1. A careful history can usually delineate the likely cause. For example, a history of an upper respiratory infection or fever suggests an infectious cause, which is the most common reason for an acute respiratory deterioration in a patient with BPD. Although many viruses or bacteria can be responsible for such infections, respiratory syncytial virus (RSV) infection is particularly common in premature infants with BPD.[2,12] It is important to recognize how quickly infants with BPD can deteriorate during an RSV infection due to acute bronchospasm. Such infants usually require rehospitalization for close observation, since many worsen to the point of requiring mechanical ventilation. Although the recent recommendation to use RSV immunoglobulin prophylactically in premature babies with BPD is designed to decrease the frequency of RSV infection,[13,14] it is likely to remain an important cause of acute respiratory deterioration in NICU graduates, particularly those with underlying BPD.

Sudden respiratory deterioration in a patient with BPD is usually due to aspiration, either from gastroesophageal reflux or to a poorly coordinated suck/swallow reflex. Exposure to cigarette smoke or other environmental pollutants may precipitate acute bronchospasm. An increase in pulmonary edema is usually accompanied by the development of peripheral edema and excessive weight gain.

Dehydration is an important cause of acute respiratory deterioration, since many infants possess an altered myocardial compliance (Starling curve shifted to the right), making cardiac output more dependent on end-diastolic filling. Therefore, if an infant becomes dehydrated secondary to vomiting and diarrhea or to aggressive diuretic therapy, cardiac output will decrease and secondary respiratory deterioration will follow. When evaluating and treating an infant with BPD with respiratory distress, there is often a temptation to use diuretics. However, one must be sure that the infant is not already hypovolemic, since in that case diuretics make the infant worse.

Anemia may also exacerbate respiratory distress in an infant with BPD and is suggested by the presence of pallor. Acute cor pulmonale can develop secondary to hypoxemia from any of the above-mentioned causes, and deterioration can be very rapid. The only effective way to treat acute cor pulmonale in infants with BPD is to treat the hypoxemia and its underlying cause.

The usual evaluation of an infant with BPD who has acute respiratory deterioration includes a complete blood count, arterial blood gas determination, appropriate cultures, and a chest x-ray. However, the chest x-ray can be difficult to interpret because of the presence of chronic abnormalities. Therefore, it is essential to compare the current x-ray with previous films to identify acute changes.

Therapy should be directed toward the specific cause of deterioration, but oxygenation is the cornerstone of treatment. Although BPD infants often have chronic CO_2 retention, there is no evidence that respiratory drive is decreased with oxygen administration. Therefore, oxygen should be used liberally while definitive diagnosis and treatment are debated. Specific therapies for BPD have recently been extensively reviewed.[11] Care in an emergency department often centers on the treatment of acute bronchospasm. The most commonly used medications for acute bronchospasm are aerosolized β_2 agonists (e.g., albuterol and terbutaline) with or without glucocorticoids. The majority of infants with BPD who deteriorate sufficiently to need acute bronchodilator therapy require hospitalization and observation.

APNEA AND HOME APNEA MONITORS

Most infants resolve apnea of prematurity before discharge and do not require apnea monitoring at home.[15] However, home monitoring is sometimes utilized for premature infants with severe apnea or if apnea persists beyond 38 weeks' postconceptional age.[16,17] Infants may be brought to an emergency department because of an actual apneic episode or because the parents are not sure of the significance of an alarm. Studies have demonstrated that the majority of alarms at home are not associated with a change in cardiorespiratory status and probably represent monitor dysfunction, such as loose leads.[16] However, caution must be exercised before attributing an alarm to a mechanical problem with the monitor.

All episodes associated with cyanosis or bradycardia, directly observed episodes of apnea, and any episode requiring intervention, such as stimulation or mouth-to-mouth resuscitation, should be thoroughly evaluated and require admission. A recurrence of apnea in a premature infant who was discharged apnea-free warrants admission and a thorough search for the cause. The differential diagnosis (Table 113-2) includes respiratory infection (especially with RSV or pertussis), sepsis, gastroesophageal reflux and aspiration, aspiration with feedings, anemia, and metabolic problems, such as hypoglycemia. Other, more unusual causes include seizures, cardiac dysrhythmias, and posthemorrhagic hydrocephalus. Therapy is directed toward the specific cause.

POSTHEMORRHAGIC HYDROCEPHALUS

Premature infants who have had an intraventricular hemorrhage may develop posthemorrhagic hydrocephalus in the newborn period.[18] Hydrocephalus can progress during the initial hospitalization, in which case the infant is usually discharged with a ventriculoperitoneal shunt in place, or hydrocephalus may develop gradually following discharge.

TABLE 113-2 Most Common Causes of Apnea and Bradycardia at Home in NICU Graduates

Respiratory infection (RSV or pertussis)
Sepsis
Gastroesophageal reflux and aspiration
Aspiration with feedings
Anemia
Hypoglycemia
Seizures
Cardiac arrhythmias
Posthemorrhagic hydrocephalus

Such infants may present to an emergency department because of progressive hydrocephalus if unshunted, or shunt obstruction or infection. Infants with infection usually have nonspecific signs, such as poor feeding, lethargy, irritability, fever, and vomiting, similar to those of any other child with central nervous system infection. Infants with obstructed shunts most often have a tense fontanelle and a history of vomiting, although the infant usually does not appear particularly ill. A comparison of the current head circumference with the head circumference at discharge (if available) is helpful in evaluating for progressive hydrocephalus. A computed tomography scan may be necessary to properly evaluate the size of the ventricles. Empiric antibiotic therapy should be utilized whenever a shunt infection is suspected, pending culture reports. Shunt infections usually require removal of the foreign body, although successful treatment without removal has been reported for *Staphylococcus epidermidis* infections. For both shunt infections and hydrocephalus, neurosurgical consultation is required.

THE EXPECTED HOME DEATH

Some infants are discharged for the NICU with lethal conditions for which further medical intervention is futile, and the parents are expecting the child to die at home. In many cases the parents are instructed to take the infant to the emergency department to be pronounced dead by a physician. The parents should be given a letter at the time of the original hospital discharge by their physicians delineating the infant's problems to provide guidance to the emergency physician facing such a situation.

This is a very traumatic time for the parents, and a futile resuscitation effort is not indicated and can prolong the parents' agony. However, it is very important to request autopsy permission to completely delineate the infant's problems and to provide optimal counseling for future pregnancies.

REFERENCES

1. Mutch L, Newdick M, Lodwick A, Chalmers L: Secular changes in rehospitalization of very low birth weight infants. *Pediatrics* 78:164, 1986.
2. Cunningham CK, McMillian JA, Gross SJ: Rehospitalization for respiratory illness in infants of less than 32 weeks' gestation. *Pediatrics* 88:527, 1991.
3. Yüksel B, Greenough A: Birth weight and hospital readmission of infants born prematurely. *Arch Pediatr Adoles Med* 148:384, 1994.
4. Klaus MH, Martin RJ, Fanaroff AA: The physical environment, in Klaus MH, Fanaroff AA (eds): *Care of the High-Risk Neonate,* 4th ed. Philadelphia, Saunders, 1993.
5. Sheftel DN, Hustead V, Friedman A: Hypertension screening in the follow-up of premature infants. *Pediatrics* 71:763, 1983.
6. Abman SH, Bradley AW, Lum GM: Systemic hypertension in infants with bronchopulmonary dysplasia. *J Pediatr* 104:928, 1984.
7. Tan KL: Clinical and laboratory observations: Blood pressure in very low birth weight infants in the first 70 days life. *J Pediatr* 266, 1998.
8. Ballard RA: *Pediatric Care of the ICN Graduate.* Philadelphia, Saunders, 1988.
9. Bernbaum JC, Hoffman-Williamson M: *Primary Care of the Preterm Infant.* St. Louis, Mosby, 1991.
10. Peter G: Immunization in special clinical circumstances, in Peter G (ed): *1997 Redbook: Report of the Committee on Infectious Diseases,* 24th ed. Elk Grove Village, IL, American Academy of Pediatrics, 1997, p 48.
11. Rush MD, Hazinski TA: Current therapy of bronchopulmonary dysplasia. *Clin Perinatol* 19:563, 1992.
12. Groothuis JR, Gutierrez KM, Lauer BA: Respiratory syncytial virus infection in children with bronchopulmonary dysplasia. *Pediatrics* 82:199, 1988.
13. Groothuis JR, Simoes E, Hemming VG, et al: Respiratory syncytial virus (RSV) infection in preterm infants and the protective effects of RSV immune globulin (RSVIG). *Pediatrics* 95:463, 1995.
14. American Academy of Pediatrics Committee on Infectious Diseases, Committee on Fetus and Newborn: Respiratory syncytial virus immune globulin intravenous: Indications for use: *Pediatrics* 99:645, 1997.
15. Miller MJ, Martin RJ: Apnea of prematurity. *Clin Perinatol* 19:789, 1992.

16. Spitzer AR, Givson E: Home monitoring. *Clin Perinatol* 19:907, 1992.
17. Consensus statement: National Institutes of Health Consensus Development Conference on Infantile Apnea and Home Monitoring, Sept 29 to Oct 1, 1986. *Pediatrics* 79:292, 1987.
18. Volpe JJ: *Neurology of the Newborn,* 3d ed. Philadelphia, Saunders, 1995, pp 431–435.

SUDDEN INFANT DEATH SYNDROME

Carol D. Berkowitz

Sudden death may affect persons of any age, but it is especially devastating when it affects previously healthy individuals. In the past, between 5000 and 10,000 infants (1 to 2 per 1000 live births) succumbed yearly to sudden infant death syndrome (SIDS), also known as "crib death." With recent changes related to infant position during sleep, the number of deaths has decreased to about 3000 and the rate to about 0.8 deaths per 1000 infants.

The term *SIDS* was officially designated in 1963 to describe a syndrome of unexpected death in infants under 1 year of age for which no pathologic cause could be determined by a thorough postmortem examination. The syndrome has been a leading cause of death of infants between 1 month and 1 year of age.[1]

An understanding of SIDS is essential for emergency physicians so that they can recognize the syndrome, initiate resuscitation, manage infants who have experienced an apparent life-threatening event (ALTE, previously termed *"near miss" SIDS*) and counsel the family of the victim.[2]

PATHOPHYSIOLOGY

Over 70 different theories for SIDS has been proposed, including suffocation from sleeping with a parent, milk allergy, and thymic enlargement (status thymicolymphaticus). The main disturbance in some victims appears to be with the infant's ventilatory response, and SIDS and infantile apnea appear related, although the exact nature of this relation is uncertain.[3] Death is due to respiratory rather than cardiac arrest, and some potential SIDS victims may be successfully resuscitated with ventilation alone. Dysrhythmias probably occur only as a terminal event, and syndromes such as prolonged QT interval or Wolff-Parkinson-White syndrome are rare associations.[4] Prospective studies monitoring normal infants showed no antecedent dysrhythmias in infants who eventually succumbed to SIDS. Conversely, approximately 2 percent of premature and low-birth-weight infants experienced bradycardia (fewer than 50 bpm) without apnea 1 week after discharge.[5]

Information implicating ventilation disturbances and hypoxemia has been obtained from two sources: autopsies of infants who succumbed to SIDS, and studies of those who experienced an ALTE but survived. This later group represents infants who were found limp, cyanotic, pale, and lifeless, without any respiratory effort, but who were successfully resuscitated.

Autopsies of some SIDS victims reveal pathologic changes initially felt to be indicative of long-standing hypoxemia. These changes include smooth muscle thickening in small pulmonary arteries, right ventricular hypertrophy, hematopoiesis in the liver, increase in periadrenal brown fat, adrenal medullary hyperplasia, and abnormalities of the carotid body. The only marker now reported with regularity is brainstem gliosis.[6]

Recently, much attention has been given to SIDS and sleeping in the prone position.[7–10] Epidemiologic studies indicate that the incidence of SIDS is lower in countries where infants sleep supine or in the side-down position, and that a reduction in the incidence of SIDS follows a reduction in prone sleeping. Concern about aspiration in infants sleeping in the supine position are unfounded. Two mechanisms linking SIDS to prone sleeping are noted. With prone sleeping, infants will assume a face-down position, particularly in response to a cold stimulus on the face. This may result in upper airway obstruction. However, upper airway obstruction has not been observed in clinical trials; rather, it has been noted that infants rebreathe expired air and experience hypercarbia.[11] Because of these observations related to the prone position, the American Academy of Pediatrics now recommends a supine or side sleeping position for normal infants.

The link between child abuse, SIDS, and ALTE has also received renewed interest.[12–16] Familial cases of SIDS raise the possibility of abuse. Some investigators report that 10 percent of SIDS cases are due to abuse. Some children with ALTE have been purposefully asphyxiated, and in some cases the complaints have simply been fabricated. These problems are referred to as *Munchausen syndrome by proxy*. Child abuse is the diagnosed cause of death in 2000 cases a year. The presence of bruises, long-bone fractures, rib fractures, internal hemorrhages, evidence of physical neglect, or trauma around the nares suggests abuse. Rib fractures in infants are not induced by cardiopulmonary resuscitation. A history inconsistent with the usual events surrounding a SIDS death may also raise the suspicion of abuse. An interesting report on death-scene investigations revealed that in 23 of 26 infants studied, circumstantial evidence of accidental death was present.[17] It is beyond the scope of emergency physicians to conduct such investigations. However, more and more communities are convening Child Death Review Boards to assure the full evaluation of sudden and unexpected death among children. It is important, however, to be aware of the possible role of accidental or intentional trauma in some SIDS victims.

SIDS and Apnea

Four groups of infants who appear at increased risk of SIDS have been identified: (1) term infants who have had a life-threatening episode of apnea, or ALTE; (2) premature infants of low birth weight; (3) siblings of infants who have succumbed to SIDS; and (4) infants of substance-abusing mothers.[18–20]

Studies of infants with ALTE may reveal (1) hypoventilation ($P_{CO_2} > 45$ mmHg) and chronic hypoxemia, (2) a depressed ventilatory response to CO_2 breathing, (3) prolonged sleep apnea (>15 s, associated with cyanosis or pallor), (4) bouts of frequent short apnea, (5) increased periodic breathing (characterized by repeated 3-s pauses in breathing followed by normal breathing for less than 20 s with bradycardia), (6) obstructive apnea, and (7) mixed obstructive and central apnea.[21]

Southall has described three separate components associated with respiratory abnormalities in infants.[22]

First, there is central apnea, in which immaturity, tumor, head injury, infection, or congenital malformation leads to primary failure of respiratory center control. In addition, peripheral chemoreceptors act abnormally, particularly in response to hypercarbia and hypoxia. The dive reflex may contribute to apnea on a central basis. Young monkeys receiving a cold or wet stimulus to the face in the area of the trigeminal nerve stop breathing. This situation may be analogous to a young infant lying in a regurgitated feeding. Alternatively, this stimulus may lead to a face-down sleeping position and airway obstruction.

Airway obstruction is a second component. Obstructive apnea may occur in response to nasal occlusion, as with an upper respiratory infection, and is noted with tonsillar enlargement, hypotonia of the hypopharynx, or glossoptosis. It is a contributing factor in about 5 percent of ALTE episodes. It is detected by the presence of increased chest wall movement, with bradycardia and decreased P_{O_2} (by surface oximeter). It is a contributing component to SIDS in infants with upper respiratory infection.

The third and most significant component is expiratory apnea. Prolonged expiratory apnea is associated with sudden atelectasis. Ventilation perfusion inequalities, hypoxia, and sudden cyanosis occur within 5 to 10 s. There is a rapid loss of consciousness. These episodes may occur even in the face of nasotracheal intubation. In older children, they may occur with crying, as cyanotic breath-holding spells.

Acute hypoxic episodes are felt to occur in 80 percent of SIDS cases.

EPIDEMIOLOGIC FACTORS

The diagnosis of SIDS is confirmed by autopsy, but many clinical and epidemiologic features characterize the syndrome. Although the overall incidence is now about 0.8 per 1000 live births, there is variation among different ethnic groups, with an incidence of 0.51 per 1000 among Asian Americans and 5.93 per 1000 among Native Americans. Victims range in age from 1 month to 1 year, with peaks at $2\frac{1}{2}$ months and at 4 months. The infant frequently has been premature or small for gestational age. Although initial reports suggested a higher incidence of SIDS among premature infants with bronchopulmonary dysplasia, this association has not been confirmed by more recent studies.[23,24]

The syndrome is rare in the first month of life, probably because the neonate has a better anaerobic capacity for survival, and with a gasp may be able to raise his or her arterial P_{O_2} over 20 mmHg and continue breathing. Of the infants who are otherwise healthy, 30 to 50 percent have some acute infection, usually of the upper respiratory tract, at the time of the event. Infection with respiratory syncytial virus has been associated with apnea, particularly in premature infants and those with an antecedent history of apnea.[25,26] Otitis media and gastroenteritis have also been associated with SIDS. Infected infants tend to be older than noninfected infants, and males outnumber females in the infected group by 2:1. The sex ratio is equal in the noninfected group. There is a disproportionate number of babies from the lower socioeconomic group, although this is true for deaths in infancy from all causes. Mothers frequently are younger than 20 years of age and unwed, smoke, use drugs, and have made few prenatal and postpartum visits. Both prenatal and postnatal maternal smoking increase the incidence of SIDS.[27,28] SIDS is more likely to occur during the winter months and when the infant is asleep.

CLINICAL FEATURES

A number of scenarios may confront physicians in the emergency department. These scenarios mirror the range of problems that may be broadly categorized under the heading of SIDS or of ALTE.

Some infants are completely well appearing at the time they are examined, and the parents relate a history of cessation of respiration. The physician must then determine whether the event represented an episode of apnea, was severe enough to be life-threatening, or represents a different disorder.

The sequence of events prior to the episode may be a clue to the cause (see Table 114-1). If the infant stiffened or exhibited clonic movements, the cessation of respiration may have been postictal apnea following a seizure. With a seizure, an infant is frequently awake before becoming apneic. Gastroesophageal reflux may lead to apnea and also may occur in awake infants following a feeding. A history of an upper respiratory infection followed by paroxysmal cough with an apneic episode would be suggestive of pertussis. Hypoglycemia may also be associated with apnea, with or without a seizure. The differential diagnosis also includes infection (sepsis or meningitis) and cardiomyopathy. Infantile botulism may be the cause in 5 to 10 percent of SIDS victims.

The evaluation of healthy-appearing infants with a history of apnea is problematic. Occasionally, parents may have misinterpreted acrocyanosis, postprandial regurgitation, or color changes with stooling as an episode of apnea. The parents should be carefully questioned about what they did to revive the baby, for example, stimulation or mouth-to-mouth resuscitation. No resuscitative efforts suggest a benign event. Conversely, the need for mouth-to-mouth resuscitation bespeaks a more serious event. The finding of irregular respiration or poor muscle tone on physical examination would assist in the diagnosis of an ALTE.

Some infants who have experienced an ALTE have not been fully resuscitated in the field. They should receive the benefit of vigorous cardiopulmonary resuscitation, unless signs of irreversible death (livedo reticularis, blood pH of 6, or boxcar venous pooling in the fundi) are apparent. Frequently the heart will resume beating after prolonged arrest. The infant heart is a remarkably resistant organ and may be revived after irreversible brain damage.

TABLE 114-1 Conditions that May Present as an Apparent Life-Threatening Event

Cardiac arrhythmias/anomalies
Child abuse
Gastroesophageal reflux
Infantile botulism
Inborn errors of metabolism
Intracranial hemorrhage
Pertussis
Respiratory syncytial virus infection
Seizure
Sepsis

DIAGNOSIS

The evaluation of an infant who has experienced an ALTE should include a complete medical history, particularly of the event itself, and take into account the perinatal and epidemiologic factors associated with SIDS and ALTE. A history of other infant deaths in the family should be obtained because of the familial incidence of SIDS. Familial cases of SIDS suggest the possibility of child abuse, as noted above, or of inborn errors of metabolism, such as disorders of fatty acid metabolism.[29,30] Autopsy results in a small subset of infants who have succumbed to SIDS reveals findings such as microvesicular steatosis of the liver, a sign of a disorder of fatty acid metabolism. Sometimes, sudden unexpected death has occurred in other siblings within these affected families. Initial reports suggested that siblings of SIDS victims are at increased risk (about 10-fold) for subsequent SIDS. More recent studies show at most a twofold increase in the incidence of SIDS among SIDS siblings.[31,32]

The physical examination should be complete, with special emphasis on the neurologic evaluation and the presence of any injuries. The initial laboratory assessment should include a complete blood cell count; determination of levels of serum electrolytes, blood sugar, calcium, phosphate, and magnesium; and a 12-lead electrocardiogram. A septic workup including blood culture, cerebrospinal fluid analysis, urine culture, and chest x-ray is indicated in most cases, although studies have shown a negligible yield in the absence of associated findings such as fever. In an infant with an ALTE, the stool should be sent for clostridial culture and botulinum toxin testing, expecially if hypotonia is present. Other studies should be done if suggested by the history and physical examination; these include determination of serum ammonia, urinary organic acids, sleep and awake electroencephalograms, skull x-rays, barium swallow, and computed tomography.

TREATMENT

Initial treatment in the emergency department involves continued resuscitation of the infant, if necessary, and stabilization. In general, all ALTE victims and infants with a history of apnea and/or cyanosis should be admitted to the hospital. The evaluation of these infants is designed to rule out treatable causes of apnea and to determine whether, in the absence of these other causes, the infant is at risk for SIDS, an event reported in from 20 to 100 percent of infants with an ALTE.

Apnea should be monitored in the hospital. Most hospitals are able to obtain pneumograms, which provide evidence of abnormalities related to periodic breathing or episodes of apnea. Polysomnography measures the amount of air flowing in at the mouth and nose and can detect obstructive apnea; the test is complicated and is generally done in a sleep laboratory. Certain tertiary care centers are equipped to evaluate responses to CO_2 breathing and diminished inspiratory oxygen.

HOME MONITORING

Two major treatment modalities are recommended for infants who have experienced an ALTE or are at risk for SIDS. Xanthine derivatives such as caffeine and theophylline are used frequently in treating apnea of prematurity because of their central excitatory effect. Their use is associated with the normalization of the respiratory pattern in over 80 percent of such children. Their efficacy in the prevention of SIDS is unclear. A pragmatic approach to the use of theophylline would be to limit it to infants with abnormal pneumograms. Reversal of these abnormalities with theophylline would be an indication for its use. Theophylline is given at 6 mg/kg per day, and a serum level of 5 to 15 mg/mL should be maintained.

Home apnea monitoring is the second modality that can be offered. Three groups have been defined in a National Institutes of Health Consensus Statement in 1986 as being candidates for home monitoring.[33] Group 1 consists of term infants with unexplained apnea of infancy, usually manifested by a life-threatening episode and/or abnormal pneumogram. The absence of an abnormal pneumogram does not preclude home monitoring. The second group consists of preterm infants who have continued to manifest apnea beyond term (i.e., after 40 weeks postconception). The third group consists of subsequent siblings of two or more SIDS victims, but not of one SIDS victim. Twins of SIDS victims were reported in the past to have a 20-fold increase in their risk for SIDS. More recent studies suggest their chance is the same as for nontwin siblings. Additional candidates for home monitoring include infants with bronchopulmonary dysplasia, especially if oxygen dependent, and infants who require tracheostomy for airway support.

Home-monitoring devices usually measure chest wall movement and heart rate. The detection of bradycardia is particularly important in infants with an obstructive component because chest wall movement is not diminished with obstructive apnea. Parents must be instructed in equipment maintenance, interpretation of the alarm, and cardiopulmonary resuscitation. Home monitoring does not mean simply supplying a family with a mechanical device. It involves the development of a medical team to support the family, interpret any episodes of apnea, and decide when home monitoring can be discontinued. Technicians who are available 24 h a day to maintain the equipment are also required.

Emergency physicians are frequently consulted about monitor alarms. Infants are brought to the emergency department because of alarm triggering. Physicians must be able to differentiate a false alarm from a true episode. The need for vigorous stimulation or mouth-to-mouth resuscitation again suggests a serious episode. If there is concern about equipment malfunction, technical assistance should be obtained from the monitoring company.

The use of home monitors has increased dramatically in recent years. The estimated cost of monitoring (including initial assessment) ranges from $3000 to $5000 per infant, with monthly rental and maintenance costs ranging from $150 to $300. Although parental anxiety is frequently reduced, the reduction in the incidence of subsequent SIDS in monitored infants is questioned. Reports have shown a mortality rate of as high as 50 percent among infants on home monitoring. In many cases, technical errors and parental noncompliance contributed to the infant's demise. Some infants, however, simply failed to respond to aggressive cardiopulmonary resuscitation.

The decision to discontinue monitoring is usually made by an infant's primary physician. In general, most infants remain on a monitor for 6 to 8 months. Criteria for discontinuing the monitor include 2 to 3 months with no episodes requiring stimulation or resuscitation, 3 months without apnea of 20 s or longer, no apnea associated with an upper respiratory infection or immunization, and an improvement in any neurologic problem for which the monitoring was instituted (e.g., apnea associated with seizures).

THE SIDS VICTIM

The management of a nonresuscitatable SIDS infant and his or her family is equally challenging for a physician. The emergency department physician is confronted by the distraught mother who had fed her infant several hours earlier, went to check the sleeping infant, and found the baby cold, blue, and lifeless. Frequently, valiant though unsuccessful efforts are carried out in the emergency department, or the infant is revived briefly, only to succumb after several hours in the intensive care unit.

The major responsibility of the physician is then to notify, counsel, and educate the family. In most jurisdictions, victims of sudden and unexplained deaths must be referred to the coroner's office, where an autopsy is performed at the coroner's discretion.[35] Some jurisdictions have infant death teams that fully evaluate the circumstances surrounding the unexpected death of young infants. If the physician believes the infant is a victim of SIDS, the family should be so advised but told that the final confirmation awaits the autopsy report. The emergency physician should assure the family about their lack of responsibility for the infant's death and assuage their feelings of guilt. He or she should then serve as a facilitator maintaining contact with the family to advise them of the autopsy results. The hospital chaplain or social worker may provide additional support, but the physician's empathy is especially supportive to the family. Most communities have organizations for parents of SIDS victims, and information about these organizations can be obtained from the National Foundation for Sudden Infant Death, 101 Broadway, New York, New York 10036. Parents should be referred to these organizations. Additional information can be obtained from the National Sudden Infant Death Syndrome Resource Center, 8201 Greensboro Drive, Suite 600, McLean, Virginia 22102, telephone (703) 821-8955.

REFERENCES

1. Goyco PG, Beckerman RD: Sudden infant death syndrome. *Curr Probl Pediatr* 20:297, 1990.
2. Merritt TA, Bauer WI, Hasselmeyer EG: Sudden infant death syndrome: The role of the emergency room physician. *Clin Pediatr* 14:1095, 1975.
3. Shannon DC, Kelly DH: SIDS and near-SIDS [second of two parts]. *N Engl J Med* 306:1022, 1982.
4. Scwartz PJ, Strambla-Badiale M, Segantini A, et al: Prolongation of the QT interval and the sudden infant death syndrome. *N Engl J Med* 338:1709, 1998.
5. Guntheroth WG: Sudden infant death syndrome (crib death). *Am Heart J* 93:784, 1977.

6. Shannon DC, Kelly DH: SIDS and near-SIDS [first of two parts]. *N Engl J Med* 306:959, 1982.
7. Kahn A, Groswasser J, Sottiaux M, et al: Prone or supine body position and sleep characteristics in infants. *Pediatrics* 91:1112, 1993.
8. Ponsonby AL, Dwyer T, Gibbons LE, et al: Factors potentiating the risk of sudden infant death syndrome associated with the prone position. *N Engl J Med* 329:377, 1993.
9. American Academy of Pediatrics, Task Force on Infant Sleeping Position and SIDS: Infant sleep position and sudden infant death syndrome (SIDS) in the United States: Joint Commentary from the American Academy of Pediatrics and selected agencies of the federal government. *Pediatrics* 93:820, 1994.
10. Willinger M, Hoffman HJ, Hartford RB: Infant sleep position and risk for sudden infant death syndrome: Report of meeting held January 13 and 14, 1994, National Institutes of Health, Bethesda, MD. *Pediatrics* 93:814, 1994.
11. Chiodini BA, Thach BT: Impaired ventilation in infants sleeping facedown: Potential significance for sudden infant death syndrome. *J Pediatr* 123:686, 1993.
12. Berger D: Child abuse simulating "near-miss" sudden infant death syndrome. *J Pediatr* 95:554, 1979.
13. Rosen CL, Frost JD, Glaze DG: Child abuse and recurrent infant apnea. *J Pediatr* 109:1065, 1986.
14. Meadow R: Suffocation, recurrent apnea, and sudden infant death. *J Pediatr* 117:351, 1990.
15. Emery JL: Child abuse, sudden infant death syndrome, and unexpected infant death. *Am J Dis Child* 147:1097, 1993.
16. Reece RM: Fatal child abuse and sudden infant death syndrome: A critical diagnostic decision. *Pediatrics* 91:423, 1993.
17. Bass M, Kravath RE, Glass L: Death-scene investigation in sudden infant death syndrome. *N Engl J Med* 315:100, 1986.
18. Carroll JL, Loughlin GM: Sudden infant death syndrome. *Pediatr Rev* 14:83, 1993.
19. Malloy MH, Hoffman HJ: Prematurity, sudden infant death syndrome, and age of death. *Pediatrics* 96:464, 1995.
20. Ward SLD, Bautista D, Chan L, et al: Sudden infant death syndrome in infants of substance-abusing mothers. *J Pediatr* 117:876, 1997.
21. Shannon DC, Kelly DH, O'Connell K: Abnormal regulation of ventilation in infants at risk for sudden infant death syndrome. *N Engl J Med* 297:747, 1977.
22. Southall DP: Role of apnea in the sudden infant death syndrome: A personal view. *Pediatrics* 80:73, 1988.
23. Werthammer J, Brown ER, Neff RK, Taeusch HW Jr: Sudden infant death syndrome in infants with bronchopulmonary dysplasia. *Pediatrics* 69:301, 1982.
24. Gray PH, Rogers Y: Are infants with bronchopulmonary dysplasia at risk for sudden infant death syndrome? *Pediatrics* 93:774, 1994.
25. Bruhn FW, Mokrohisky ST, McIntosh K: Apnea associated with respiratory syncytial virus infection in young infants. *J Pediatr* 90:382, 1977.
26. Church NR, Anas NG, Hall CB, Brooks JG: Respiratory syncytial virus-related apnea in infants. *Am J Dis Child* 138:247, 1984.
27. Mitchell EA, Ford RPK, Stewart AW, et al: Smoking and the sudden infant death syndrome. *Pediatrics* 91:893, 1993.
28. Schoendorf KC, Kiely JL: Relationship of sudden infant death syndrome to maternal smoking during and after pregnancy. *Pediatrics* 90:905, 1992.
29. Boles RG, Buck EA, Blitzer MG, et al: Retrospective biochemical screening of fatty acid oxidation disorders in postmortem livers of 418 cases of sudden death in the first year of life. *J Pediatr* 132:924, 1998.
30. Cederbaum SD: SIDS and disorders of fatty acid oxidation: Where do we go from here? *J Pediatr* 132:913, 1998.
31. Brady JP, McCann EM: Control of ventilation in subsequent siblings of victims of sudden infant death syndrome. *J Pediatr* 106:212, 1985.
32. Peterson DR, Sabotta EE, Daling JR: Infant mortality among subsequent siblings of infants who died of sudden infant death syndrome. *J Pediatr* 108:911, 1986.
33. National Institute of Health: Consensus Development Conference on Infantile Apnea and Home Monitoring, Sept 29 to Oct 1, 1986. *Pediatrics* 79:292, 1987.
34. Weese-Mayer DE, Brouillette RT, Morrow AS, et al: Assessing validity of infant monitor alarms with event recording. *J Pediatr* 115:702, 1989.
35. American Academy of Pediatrics–Committee on Child Abuse and Neglect and Committee on Community Health Services: Investigation and review of unexpected infant and child deaths. *Pediatrics* 92:734, 1993.

115 PEDIATRIC HEART DISEASE

C. James Corrall

Pediatric cardiovascular disorders are decidedly uncommon in emergency medicine. The incidence of congenital heart disease is only about eight cases per 1000 live births and contrasts sharply with the increasing prevalence of cardiovascular disease in adult populations.[1] Because of the relative unfamiliarity of such disorders, most emergency medicine physicians have encountered these disorders only in their initial training. The combination of the low incidence and the age-related differences in clinical presentation make timely recognition, stabilization, and appropriate tertiary referral a challenge for primary care physicians. In the emergency department, problems may range from an asymptomatic discovery of a murmur to the life-threatening presentation of a cyanotic infant in cardiogenic shock.

Congenital heart disease is usually classified based on physiology (presence or absence of cyanosis, with or without persistent fetal circulation) or on the nature of the anatomic defect (shunt, obstruction, transposition, or complex). Most pediatric heart disease is congenital, but acquired conditions also occur and include complications secondary to rheumatic fever, Kawasaki disease, and severe chronic anemias, as well as myocarditis, pericarditis, endocarditis, and the tachydysrhythmias.

Pediatric heart disease can also be classified by clinical presentation. The six common clinical presentations to primary care physicians are cyanosis, congestive heart failure, pathologic murmur in asymptomatic patients, abnormal pulses, hypertension, and syncope. Table 115-1 lists the most common lesions in each category. While this is informative in the formation of a broad differential diagnosis in very ill pediatric patients, it is perhaps best to classify heart disease according to the clinical presentation in the emergency department. Most often, this presentation is in children with previously undiagnosed heart disease and to a lesser degree in those with previously diagnosed heart disease or reparative surgery for the same.

Children with previously undiagnosed heart disease can be broadly classified into three categories: unstable, stable but symptomatic, and stable and asymptomatic. Unstable infants usually require immediate and decisive stabilization and aggressive management before diagnostic studies or tertiary referral can be made. Pediatric cardiology consultation should be emergently sought from the regional tertiary care

TABLE 115-1 Clinical Presentation of Pediatric Heart Disease

Cyanosis	TGA, TOF, TA, Tat, TAVR
Congestive heart failure	See Table 115-3
Murmur/symptomatic patient	Shunts: VSD, PDA, ASD Obstructions Valvular incompetence
Abnormal pulses	
Bounding	PDA, AI, AVM
Decreased with prolonged amplitude	Coarctation, HPLV
Hypertension	Coarctation
Syncope	
Cyanotic	TOF
Acyanotic	Critical AS

Note: AI, aortic insufficiency; AS, aortic stenosis; ASD, atrial septal defect; AVM, arteriovenous malformation; HPLV, hypoplastic left ventricle; PDA, patent ductus arteriosus; TA, truncus arteriosus; Tat, tricuspid atresia; TAVR, total anomalous venous return; TGA, transposition of the great arteries; TOF, tetralogy of Fallot; VSD, ventricular septal defect.

center before pharmacologic intervention, if at all possible. Stable and symptomatic infants require less aggressive measures, so there is time to focus on physiologic derangement and correction of abnormalities of oxygenation and metabolism and time for tertiary referral. A baseline electrocardiogram (ECG) and chest radiograph are indicated in such infants particularly when a murmur appears to be pathologic (grade 3 or louder, holosystolic or diastolic in timing, and/or radiating away from the heart). Stable but asymptomatic infants can easily be referred routinely based on findings on general examination. Such infants can be electively evaluated without specific testing in the emergency department. Recent, well-publicized cases of pediatric sudden death from unrecognized pediatric heart disease are rare, but such infants arrive in extremis at the emergency department. This represents a final presentation type of pediatric heart disease that is tragic because such infants cannot often be resuscitated, even by physicians with expertise in pediatric heart disease.

Children with known heart disease arrive at the emergency department for treatment of routine illnesses as well as for problems related to their unique disease. Rarely, they arrive with acute life-threatening cardiovascular complications. Once the knowledge of preexisting heart disease is known, the physician can anticipate complications related to the unique disease, such as hemoconcentration due to polycythemia, bacterial endocarditis, or embolism. Only infrequently do such infants have abnormal immune systems, and most handle routine pediatric illnesses well.

CARDIOVASCULAR PHYSIOLOGY

It is important to understand the interplay between normal cardiovascular dynamics in pediatric patients and the age-related changes that occur during transition to the extrauterine environment. This understanding is necessary in order to recognize the signs and symptoms of pediatric heart disease and to plan therapy appropriate to the physiologic derangement.

Perhaps the most dramatic change that occurs at birth is the transition from fetal to postnatal circulation. Immediately following birth, flow through the umbilical arteries ceases and the venous flow through the cord slows and then stops. These vascular changes are mediated by the rapid increase in arterial oxygen partial pressure (PAO_2) that occurs during lung inflation. Following lung expansion, pulmonary vascular resistance falls and pulmonary blood flow increases. The pulmonary vascular resistance will continue to fall with increases in blood flow over the next 30 to 45 days of extrauterine life. The ductus arteriosus also closes with the rise in arterial PO_2, and blood shunted through a patent foramen ovale ceases. In time, these shunt channels permanently close but, until then, may reopen under conditions of decreased PO_2 or other stresses.[2]

Cardiac output, which is the amount of blood that the heart pumps each minute, is normally the product of the heart rate and the stroke volume of the ventricles. Physiologically, the role of the heart is to facilitate and maintain a cardiac output that is adequate for the metabolic needs of the body by the provision of substrates for adequate cellular function and removal of by-products of metabolism. Since neonates and small children have limited ability to increase stroke volume due to the relatively noncompliant ventricular walls, they rely on changes in heart rate to adjust the cardiac output. Thus, sinus tachycardia is usually the first response to stress in infants and children and is mediated by the intrinsic pacemaker in the sinoatrial node and by various adrenergic, hormonal, and neural mediators.

Several physiologic terms are important to understand, particularly with regard to therapy. *Preload* is normally considered the amount of blood that the heart receives to distribute to the body. Decreasing the amount of blood flowing into the heart lowers the cardiac output. Preload can be reduced due to pharmacologic means such as by the use of intravenous nitrates or by blood loss. Similarly, increasing the amount of blood into the heart will increase the cardiac output in accordance with Starling forces, until the point of maximum compliance of the ventricular wall. At this point, cardiac output decreases dramatically and congestive heart failure occurs. *Afterload* refers to the resistance to blood flow out of the heart. Afterload may be increased anatomically in neonates by an obstructive lesion, such as aortic stenosis or critical coarctation of the aorta. Afterload depends on the size of the ventricle and its compliance or elasticity. The compliance in the neonatal heart is limited, so afterload reaches critical values early. Afterload also depends on the amount of arteriolar resistance in the case of pediatric hypertension unrelated to obstructive lesions in the proximity of the heart and great vessels. Treatment of afterload problems is directed at arterial vasoconstriction or vasodilatation. *Contractility* or *inotropy*, which is the ability of the cardiac muscle to pump blood out of the heart, refers to the force or power of the contraction and determines the amount of work that the heart can perform. Increasing the cardiac contractility increases the stroke volume and hence the cardiac output.

Cardiac contractility is normally regulated by neural or humoral mechanisms. It may be altered pharmacologically by such medications as digoxin or dobutamine. *Cardiac rate* or *chronotropy* is the ability of the heart muscle to pump blood out of the heart per fixed unit of contraction. In the typical circumstance, chronotropy and inotropy can not be differentiated with regard to therapeutic maneuvers. Typically, both the cardiac rate and the relatively fixed contractility of the neonatal heart contribute to the overall cardiac output, with the former contributing more of the output. In pediatric hearts older than 4 to 5 years, there is a more balanced contribution to cardiac output, with the contractility playing a much more prominent role.

THERAPEUTIC IMPLICATIONS

All of the medical management provided to children with heart disease is directed toward increasing cardiac output in low-output states by alteration of the heart rate, preload, afterload, or inherent contractility. As mentioned previously, some of these parameters may be rather fixed due to the inherent limitations of the neonatal ventricular noncompliance.[3]

Heart rate is the most malleable of the cardiac physiologic parameters. Symptomatic bradycardias of all types are treated with oxygenation, atropine and, in severe cases, with epinephrine and/or isoproterenol followed by transthoracic pacemaker and transvenous pacemaker usage. Symptomatic tachycardia must be differentiated into sinus, supraventricular, or ventricular before specific therapy can be initiated.

Preload disorders are common in children and are most frequently due to shock states with resultant hypovolemia that causes the decreased preload. The hypovolemia may be due to increased loss of total body water, such as occurs in excessive diarrhea or vomiting, or it may be a relative loss of volume due to maldistribution. In the latter circumstance, distributive forms of shock such as in sepsis, neurogenic spinal shock, or anaphylaxis produce relative hypovolemia secondary to increased vasodilation and decreased venous return to the heart. In congestive heart failure, preload is markedly increased when the left atrial pressure becomes elevated. The resulting Starling forces produce pulmonary edema and its resultant hypoxemia. The hypoxemia reduces contractility, further increasing the left atrial pressure and accentuating the increased preload state. Treatment of such a state requires diuretics and vasodilation to reduce preload.

Adequate oxygen delivery is necessary for the myocardium during the diastolic filling phase. The oxygen supply depends on the PO_2 of the blood, the hemoglobin concentration, and the coronary perfusion pressure. Hypoxemia results from deoxygenated venous blood entering the systemic circulation by vascular shunts that may be present at any location. Hypoxemia caused by most vascular shunts responds poorly to increasing ambient inspired oxygen. In contrast, most respiratory causes of hypoxemia respond to increasing oxygen.

Anemia profoundly decreases the amount of oxygen available to the tissues by decreasing the amount of oxygen bound to hemoglobin per unit of cardiac output. Transfusions of 10 mL packed red cells per kilogram will raise the hemoglobin approximately 1.5 g/dL and provide improved oxygen-carrying capacity to the tissues. In special circumstances, other competing agents, such as methemoglobinemia and carboxyhemoglobinemia, with increased affinity for oxygen must be excluded.

Myocardial perfusion can only occur during the relaxation phase provided during diastole. The perfusion is markedly impaired under conditions of low cardiac output. Because the coronary perfusion pressure is the difference between the diastolic pressure minus the coronary sinus venous pressure, it follows that any situation that lowers diastolic pressure to 30 to 40 mmHg can lead to poor coronary perfusion, myocardial ischemia, and subsequent ECG changes reflecting injury. Treatment of low diastolic pressure includes infusion with α-adrenergic agents such as phenylephrine, norepinephrine, and epinephrine to raise the diastolic pressure and coronary artery perfusion.

Other factors are also important to augment contractility, but are not as amenable to therapy by emergency physicians. Acidosis adversely affects myocardial contractility and may be persistent after hypovolemia has been corrected. Sodium bicarbonate may rapidly improve contractility in such situations. If acidosis is due to respiratory failure, airway control with endotracheal intubation and mechanical ventilation is useful to correct the hypercapnia and decrease the metabolic demand generated by trying to overcome respiratory failure. Temperature control is also important because elevations can cause an increase in oxygen consumption by 400 percent, causing a marginal cardiovascular system to fail. Ideally, a neutral thermal environment should be maintained to avoid such stress. Hypoglycemia frequently occurs during stressful events, and neonates are less able to respond because of decreased glycogen stores and minimal fat necessary for gluconeogenesis. Low serum glucose of less than 40 mg/dL should be corrected with an infusion of either 25% or 10% dextrose solution. Electrolyte disturbances can interfere with both inotropic and chronotropic responses to decreased cardiac output. Appropriate monitoring of concentrations of potassium, calcium, magnesium, sodium, chloride, phosphate, and bicarbonate is prudent. Finally, attempts must be made to minimize stress in ill neonates. Alleviation of external stressors such as tubing manipulation or skin care should be minimized to increase oxygen availability by decreasing agitation. All attempts to provide for parental care and the minimization of blood drawing are crucial to this goal.

PHARMACOLOGIC ENHANCEMENT OF CARDIAC OUTPUT

In addition to the normalization of preload and metabolic parameters, patients with severe heart failure or cardiogenic shock require aggressive pharmacologic support with vasoactive infusions to enhance contractility and output. From a historical perspective, dopamine hydrochloride has served as the first-line treatment of low cardiac output. In lower dosages of 2 to 5 μg/kg/min, blood flow to the kidney and bowel is increased, and a paradoxical fall in blood pressure is noted. Midrange dosages of 6 to 10 μ/kg/min result in β-adrenergic effect, and heart rate and contractility are improved. In dosages in excess of 10 μ/kg/min, α effects predominate, and vasoconstriction results in correction of hypotension.

Epinephrine has replaced dopamine as the initial infusion of choice in hypotensive states. Predominant β-adrenergic effects are noted at lower dosages of 0.05 to 0.5 μ/kg/min, whereas α-adrenergic effects are noted at higher dosages, which can result in rapid reversal of hypotension. Dobutamine is another useful drug that increases contractility without increasing heart rate or systemic vascular resistance. Its vasodilatory effects and lack of α effect at higher dosage ranges limit its usefulness as a single agent to counteract extremely low cardiac output with normal blood pressure. Nitroprusside can be useful in increasing stroke volume by the mechanism of afterload reduction. It is administered by continuous infusion with arterial and central venous pressure monitoring to detect hypotension and the need for volume expansion. Its use, in doses of 0.5 to 5 μ/kg/min, is always reserved for intensive care situations.

Isoproterenol administration produces a marked decrease in total peripheral vascular resistance predominantly due to vasodilation in skeletal muscle vascular sites. Diastolic and mean blood pressures fall. The effects on the heart are similar to those with epinephrine, but with enhanced heart rate and stroke volume due to the decrease in mean blood pressure and reflexively decreased vagal tone.

Norepinephrine causes marked vasoconstriction of all vascular beds on both the venous side and the arterial side. Consequently, there is a net increase in total peripheral vascular resistance that results in a marked rise in both systolic and diastolic blood pressure. Due to complex actions on the heart, which depend in part on the amount of parasympathetic activity, the overall contribution to chronotropy is negligible and the inotropic response is only minimally increased.

Phenylephrine, which is not a naturally occurring catecholamine, has actions similar to those of norepinephrine, with minimal activity on chronotropic or inotropic function. Like norepinephrine, it causes marked increase in systemic vascular resistance due to direct vasoconstriction of all vascular beds. The difference between this drug and norepinephrine is predominantly in its metabolism. Overall, it has activity that is two to three times the duration of norepinephrine, making it highly effective in situations in which blood pressure elevation is likely to be depressed for long intervals. It is seldom used today, because of its narrow therapeutic window of benefit and its toxicity.

ASSESSMENT OF CHILDREN SUSPECTED OF HAVING HEART DISEASE

The initial evaluation of ill children begins with the process of assessment and triage. Often, children present with symptoms unrelated to the underlying disease, and careful neurologic, pulmonary, and cardiac assessment must be performed to determine the stability of patients and the need for supportive care. From a cardiovascular perspective, this assessment determines whether the cardiac output is low, normal, or hyperdynamic. Concurrent conditions often exist, making definition of physical findings challenging. For instance, the symptoms and signs of increasing pulmonary venous pressure and the signs of a viral upper respiratory tract infection appear similar. What appears to be a feeding disorder with easy fatigue during routine feeds may represent congestive heart failure, particularly if diaphoresis is present with labored breathing.

The physical examination of children with significant congenital heart disease is often not as dramatic as the diagnosis of congestive heart failure in adolescents. In the author's experience, unrecognized congenital heart disease in small infants is often not diagnosed until the second or third visit to the emergency department for the same illness. Most often, that illness is misdiagnosed as a viral upper respiratory illness or a feeding intolerance.

When a child with known cardiac problems presents to the emergency department, the historical information that must be obtained by the emergency physician is problem focused and directed toward known complications of the congenital defect. A detailed history of medications administered and recent changes in dosages and timing of administration are important in such children. New illnesses, particularly of the upper respiratory tract, should be identified. Simple common pediatric illnesses such as croup, pneumonia, or bronchiolitis may cause sudden decompensation in a child with limited cardiac reserves. These illnesses may be difficult or impossible to differentiate clinically from an exacerbation of known cardiac disease. The symptoms and signs of increased right heart failure and critical pulmonary venous pressure states and respiratory illness often overlap and are indistinguishable without echocardiography.

Exertional dyspnea is often present, but overlooked, in older children with cardiac disease. In infants, feeding intolerance is the most reliable marker of exercise tolerance. Historical evidence of slow feeding, increased tachypnea with feeding, persistent staccato cough with feeding, and diaphoresis at midfeeding all suggest borderline cardiac reserves.

In small infants, tachypnea is often the first sign manifested, followed by rales that are more typical of congestive heart failure. Hepatomegaly usually develops late and is always in excess of splenomegaly. In small infants, edema is usually generalized and not associated with jugular venous distention. Accurate blood pressure measurement in infants requires an appropriately sized cuff (approximating two-thirds of the extremity). Ideally, blood pressure should be measured in both upper and lower extremities. Cardiac murmurs should be graded according to location, timing in the cardiac cycle, and loudness. There may be significant cardiac pathology in the absence of murmur and, conversely, a very loud murmur may be innocent and nonpathologic. The pediatric-sized stethoscope bell and diaphragm should be used to discern the exact location of murmurs. Heart sounds should also be assessed particularly for fixed splitting of the second heart sound.

Focused cardiac examination must address the difference between pathologic and innocent cardiac murmurs. Typically, 30 percent of children will have innocent flow murmurs that are incidental findings on routine examination. Usually, innocent flow murmurs are of low intensity and do not radiate. They are brief in the cardiac cycle and usually systolic in timing. They are never holosystolic and are usually accentuated by head position or Valsalva maneuver.[4]

The Still's murmur, which is the most common innocent murmur, is usually early systolic in timing, located at the apex or the lower left sternal border, and is often confused with the murmur of a ventricular septal defect (VSD). It usually does not radiate to the back like the murmur of a VSD. Pulmonary systolic ejection murmur, which is equivalent to the Still's murmur, is extremely harsh and is usually heard loudest in the second and third intercostal spaces on the left. A unique murmur, often heard in neonates, is that of peripheral pulmonic stenosis. This murmur is usually of low intensity, is usually heard in both axillae and the back, and usually vanishes by 3 to 6 months of age. It is often misdiagnosed as a congenital lesion in sick infants and results in inadvertent administration of cardiotonic medication. Significant cardiac murmurs are usually holosystolic, continuous or diastolic in timing and usually associated with radiation.[5]

Laboratory studies are usually not initially helpful in acutely ill, hemodynamically unstable patients, but may be of some benefit in more stable pediatric patients. Such studies are usually confined to chest radiograph, ECG and, in some centers, bedside emergency ultrasound.

Chest radiographic studies are essential in assessing the size and shape of the heart and in evaluating pulmonary blood flow. The chest radiograph also provides some information about the position of the aortic arch, which should be normally left sided. In the normal left-sided aortic arch, there is rightward displacement of the esophagus and trachea to the right. An abnormal right position of the aortic arch may be a clue to the diagnosis of the congenital cardiac lesion. Right-sided aortic arches are seen in truncus arteriosus, transposition of the great vessels, tetralogy of Fallot, tricuspid atresia, and total anomalous pulmonary venous return. The chest radiograph is critical to the assessment of pulmonary vascularity. In small left-to-right shunts, the pulmonary vascularity is normal. Pulmonary vascularity can also be normal in conditions that cause pulmonary stenosis, such as valvular pulmonic stenosis or functional pulmonic stenosis associated with tetralogy of Fallot. Increased pulmonary vascularity may be seen with any cause of left-to-right shunting or in any cause of left-sided failure, such as ischemia or outflow obstruction.

The ECG is useful to evaluate cardiac conduction and, in particular, the rhythm, electrical axis, and chamber size. Such information is clearly age related and will require one to have access to a standard text of normal values of pediatric ECG voltages and criteria for ventricular hypertrophy.[6] The electrical force axis most often defines abnormal chamber diameters and usually does not suggest cardiac ischemia as in the adult population.

Hemodynamically Unstable Patients

Clinical signs of low cardiac output are manifested by signs of dysfunction of one or more organ systems. Shock is diagnosed by determination of skin perfusion and mental status appropriate for age. Additional information may be obtained by assessment of the distal pulse quality, amplitude, and duration. Pallor, cyanosis, and skin mottling are usually present. The infant's hands and feet appear cold, and there is delayed capillary refill that is very distinct from acrocyanosis present in some infants. Mental status changes appear as fluctuating signs of apathy, irritability, or failure to respond to painful stimuli or to parental presence. Body positioning is that of prostration with loss of head control and is preferred to that of upright sitting or standing. Sinus tachycardia is the first response to maintenance of cardiac output, followed by tachypnea in an attempt to correct the acidosis of poor perfusion and oxygen delivery. Hypotension occurs late, is dramatic in its onset, and can occur without warning. Laboratory studies are unhelpful because their results are usually normal.

Noncardiac causes of shock and low cardiac output states must be considered, diagnosed, and treated in tandem with delineation of the possibility of congenital heart disease. Congenital heart lesions that present with low cardiac output are usually classified as shunt dependent and must be treated definitively and quickly. Up to 1 percent of infants are born with one or more congenital heart anomalies. Many of these lesions are of trivial or mild consequence, but a significant number are severe enough to become incompatible with life once the ductus arteriosus begins to close. As this occurs, blood can no longer reach the lungs and distal circulation. These infants present in shock within the first 2 weeks of life. Both cyanotic and acyanotic lesions may present in this fashion. The former include severe coarctation of the aorta, critical aortic stenosis, and hypoplastic left ventricle. Transposition of the great vessels, pulmonary atresia, and hypoplastic right heart syndrome are examples of the latter presentation.

Shunt-dependent lesions mandate immediate surgical referral for repair or palliation of the anatomic condition. It may be necessary to stabilize and restore some function to the shunt-dependent lesion while awaiting transport to a tertiary care facility. One method of providing this care is with the use of prostaglandin infusion to reopen the shunt pharmacologically. Prostaglandin E_1 infusions are successful in reopening the ductus arteriosus in nearly 95 percent of such patients and may allow for less emergent repair of the underlying defect. It is infused at a rate of 0.05 to 0.1 μg/kg/min initially. If there is no improvement within several minutes, it is increased progressively in 0.2 μg/kg/min increments. The minimal effective dosage should be used, because of adverse effects that include fever, skin flushing, diarrhea, and periodic apnea. Intubation and ventilatory support are often necessary as well.

Cardiogenic shock can also occur as a result of dysfunctional myocardium and may mimic the signs and symptoms seen with shunt-dependent anatomic lesions. Such cardiomyopathies are uncommon in pediatric patients, but can be easily confused with anatomic lesions. Cardiomyopathies are usually defined into two groups in children: dilated and hypertrophied. Presentation varies from asymptomatic cardiomegaly discovered on routine chest radiograph to congestive heart failure, cardiogenic shock, or sudden death. Typically, such children self-limit their activities at home and then, during an acute febrile illness, decompensate rapidly and arrive in profound shock. The dilated cardiomyopathies more often cause congestive heart failure, whereas the hypertrophied cardiomyopathies cause sudden death. Emergent medical management includes supportive care as previously outlined in an attempt to enhance contractility. Tragically, little can be done to assist those unfortunate children who suffer sudden death.

TETRALOGY OF FALLOT Although not in itself a cause of hemodynamic instability due to sudden loss of blood flow, tetralogy of Fallot often presents in a dramatic fashion due to hypercyanotic episodes or "tet spells" that mimic other more significant structural lesions. Tetralogy of Fallot is the most common cause of cyanotic congenital heart disease in children older than 4 years of age. Anatomically, it is characterized by obstruction of the right ventricular outflow tract, VSD, dextroposition of the aorta, and right ventricular hypertrophy. Functionally, obstruction of the right ventricular outflow tract and the presence of VSD have the greatest physiologic consequences. Due to the outflow tract obstruction, blood is forced from right to left, resulting in desaturation and compensatory polycythemia and hyperviscosity.

The other cardinal features on physical examination are a holosystolic VSD murmur in the third intercostal space at the left sternal border and a diamond-shaped systolic murmur of pulmonary stenosis in the second intercostal space at the left sternal border. The history may reveal exercise intolerance relieved by squatting. The main radiographic findings are a boot-shaped heart with decreased pulmonary vascular markings. A right-side aortic arch is present in 25 percent of tetralogies. Right ventricular hypertrophy with right axis deviation is the primary ECG abnormality.

The greatest threat to these patients is the hypercyanotic or tet spells. These episodes, dramatic in presentation, are characterized by episodes of paroxysmal dyspnea with labored respiration, increased cyanosis, and syncope. These episodes in concert with polycythemia lead to seizures, cerebrovascular accidents, and death. They occur due to exertion of feeding, crying, or straining at stool and last from a few minutes to hours. The rapid, deep hypernea results from an increase in cardiac output with exertion against fixed right ventricular outflow tract obstruction. The fixed obstruction causes increased shunting across the VSD and increased hypoxia, hypercarbia, and acidosis. The hypoxia and acidosis cause a decrease in systemic vascular resistance that further potentiates the shunt and stimulates the respiratory center to maintain and deepen the hypernea.[7]

Management of hypercyanotic spells consists of positioning and pharmacologic management. Infants should be placed in a knee-chest position. This positioning allows for an increase in venous return to the heart and an increase in systemic vascular resistance. Pharmacologic management includes administration of oxygen to decrease the hypoxemia, and injection of morphine sulfate subcutaneously or intramuscularly at a dosage of 0.2 mg/kg/dose. Many consider the administration of propranolol a contraindication to bypass surgery, so it should not be given without consultation. In extreme cases, phenylephrine infusion 10 μg/kg initial infusion, followed by infusion of 0.5 to 2 μg/kg/min is used to increase the systemic vascular resistance and increase blood pressure.

Lack of recognition of the hypercyanotic episode and timely intervention could result in significant complications, including seizures, cerebral thrombosis, profound lactic acidosis, deterioration in cardiac rhythm, and subsequent death.

TRANSPOSITION OF THE GREAT VESSELS This is the most common cyanotic defect that appears in the first week of life. Infants with this defect who are brought to the emergency department usually have dusky lips noted by parents or have an increased respiratory rate or feeding difficulty. While not as dramatic in presentation as a hypercyanotic spell of tetralogy of Fallot, the defect is easily missed on a single emergency department visit, because of the lack of cardiomegaly or murmur.

Anatomically, in transposition of the great vessels, the aorta originates from the right ventricle, and the pulmonary artery originates from the left ventricle. The systemic veins drain as they usually do into the anatomically correct right atrium, and the pulmonary veins drain into the left atria. Thus, in transposition, the systemic and pulmonary blood flows are not admixed and exist in parallel unless alternative flow is established. To maintain life, mixing of blood occurs either at the level of the atria via an atrial septal defect or at the level of the ventricles by a VSD. If neither of these is present, flow must be maintained by a persistent ductus arteriosus.

Clinically, cyanosis and tachypnea appear within the first several days of life, but may be prolonged when a patent ductus arteriosus fails to close. Ironically, cardiomegaly is often absent and no murmur is noted. The chest radiograph is usually normal, but may show a narrow, small heart due to the overlapping of the abnormally positioned aorta and pulmonary artery. The ECG shows normal right-sided-force dominance. Rarely, depending on the anatomy, frank congestive heart failure will be present.

Treatment of this condition is initially palliative in the cardiac catheterization laboratory and involves the creation of a large artificial atrial septal defect by using a balloon catheter (Rashkind septoplasty). Initially, most emergency physicians who suspect this entity are justified in beginning an infusion of prostaglandin E_1, as previously outlined, while arranging transport to a facility capable of palliation. The definitive surgery that is performed later is the Mustard operation, in which an artificial baffle is created at the atrial level to direct systemic venous return into the left ventricle and the pulmonary return to the right ventricle. The left ventricle then pumps blood to the lungs, and the right ventricle pumps blood to the systemic circulation.[8]

LEFT VENTRICULAR OUTFLOW OBSTRUCTION SYNDROMES No clinical presentation can match the rapidity of onset of cardiogenic shock, hypotension, and acidosis as seen in infants with this group of disorders. In these infants, systemic blood flow depends on a large contribution of shunted blood via a patent ductus arteriosus. When the ductus closes, cardiac output falls, perfusion becomes negligible, and a state of profound cardiogenic shock ensues. Such lesions are often complex, but include hypoplastic left heart syndrome, tricuspid atresia, and critical coarctation of the aorta. Other variants include transposition of the great vessels, as discussed previously, and some tetralogy of Fallot variants.[9]

Such infants present with decreased or absent perfusion, hypotension, and severe acidosis. When these infants present in the first week of life, they must be considered for an infusion of prostaglandin E_1, as outlined earlier. The infusion is begun at 0.1 μg/kg/min preferably by a central line, although any access in such ill infants is acceptable. The dosage may be reduced as perfusion and color return. Side effects of the infusion include hypotension and mandate close observation of blood pressure. Other effects are apnea, focal seizures, and fever that may mimic sepsis. Due to the critical nature of these infants, immediate referral and transfer to a tertiary care facility are necessary.

Hemodynamically Stable, Symptomatic Patients

Some infants arrive at the emergency department with respiratory distress and are found on examination to have findings suggestive of congenital heart disease, usually with evidence of congestive heart failure. These infants have near normal blood pressure and usually display normal skin perfusion, but may have cyanosis. Several congenital cardiac conditions may present in this fashion.

TRUNCUS ARTERIOSUS This congenital anomaly is characterized by a single, large arterial trunk originating from the ventricular portion of the heart. This common vascular trunk supplies blood to both the systemic and the pulmonary circulation. A large VSD is usually present and may account for the murmur that is often heard. Because of the large amount of flow from both ventricles into the single large arterial conduit, flow to the pulmonary tree is greatly enhanced due to decreased flow resistance. This results in little or no cyanosis until pulmonary resistance increases and then cyanosis appears.

Clinically, these infants present with signs of increased pulmonary blood flow, dyspnea, and, occasionally, frank congestive heart failure. Chest x-ray demonstrates cardiomegaly and increased pulmonary vascularity or pulmonary edema. The ECG is initially normal until pulmonary vascular resistance increases and then signs of strain, left ventricular hypertrophy, or biventricular hypertrophy are evident.

VENTRICULAR SEPTAL DEFECT This is the most common cardiac defect, and symptoms displayed depend on the size of the defect. Small defects are often found on routine physical examination. More than 60 percent of these close spontaneously in older childhood.

Moderate-sized VSDs cause elevated right ventricular pressure and subsequent increased pulmonary artery pressure. Infants with this defect present with increased cough with mild upper respiratory tract infections and may have mild increase in pulmonary vascularity and early congestive heart failure. Typically, the chest radiograph is interpreted as mild congestive heart failure, and treatment consists of furosemide and, occasionally, digoxin.

Large VSDs present with congestive heart failure early in infancy, resulting in early and severe pulmonary artery pressure that, if uncorrected, will result in pulmonary hypertension. Such pulmonary hypertension will result in reversal of left-to-right shunt and frank cyanosis in a condition known as the Eisenmenger complex. Originally felt to be surgically irreversible, some centers now are routinely repairing such defects in adolescents who had inadequate management in infancy.[10]

COARCTATION OF THE AORTA This represents localized narrowing of the aortic lumen, most often distal to the origin of the left subclavian artery and in close proximity to the ductus arteriosus or its postnatal remnant, the ligamentum arteriosus.

In infancy, symptomatic infants present with congestive heart failure and feeding difficulty. Decreased pulse amplitude and duration are noted in the lower extremities, and hypertension is noted in the upper extremities. Cardiac examination reveals a systolic ejection murmur at the cardiac base, with interscapular radiation.

Older children present with decreased exercise tolerance and, occasionally, claudication to the lower extremities. In children older than 6 to 7 years of age, a characteristic rib notching of the inferior border of posterior ribs is evident. Such notching is bilateral and usually caused by hypertrophied collateral vessels.[11]

Hemodynamically Stable, Asymptomatic Patients

This class of patients presents to the emergency department for reasons that are not referable to the heart and are discovered to have findings suggestive of cardiac disease. Some of the more common cardiac defects have already been mentioned including mildly affected tetralogy of Fallot, small to moderate-sized VSDs, and coarctation of the aorta. Several common structural defects warrant mention here.

ATRIAL SEPTAL DEFECT Most children remain symptomatic throughout childhood until adolescence, when signs of increased pulmonary hypertension develop. Characteristically, the physical examination of such children reveals a split second heart sound that does not vary with inspiration. Often a soft systolic murmur heard at the upper left sternal border may mimic the pulmonary flow murmur mentioned earlier. Initially, the chest radiograph is normal but, with time, shows an increased size of the right atria and later the right ventricle. The ECG shows a characteristic prolongation of the PR interval and a incomplete or complete right bundle branch block pattern. Cardiomegaly represents a late finding that is usually seen in adults.[12]

CONGENITAL AORTIC STENOSIS This is a less dramatic form of left-sided outlet obstruction than described previously. Children with this defect usually arrive at the emergency department with fatigue, decreasing exercise tolerance, exertional dyspnea, or syncope. The diagnosis is suspected based on the greatly diminished pulse amplitude and duration and the characteristic murmur, which is usually systolic in timing and loud with radiation to the neck. Treatment consists of decreasing activities, particularly sports, and referral for evaluation of surgical intervention. In all circumstances, these children should refrain from any significant physical activity, as sudden death can result.[13]

CONGESTIVE HEART FAILURE

Recognition

The most common cause of congestive heart failure (CHF) in children is congenital heart disease, which often masquerades as other problems, such as pneumonia or sepsis. The distinction between pneumonia and congestive heart failure in infants requires a high index of suspicion. Pneumonia can cause a previously stable cardiac condition to decompensate, so that both problems exist simultaneously. The predominant symptoms include poor feeding, excessive diaphoresis, irritability or lethargy with feeding, weak cry and, in severe cases, grunting and nasal flaring. Pulmonary congestion with rales, ronchi, and wheezing may mimic common lower respiratory viral infections. Gallop rhythms may be difficult to ascertain due to the presence of tachycardia. The common symptoms and signs of an infant with congestive heart failure are outlined in Table 115-2.

Both increased pulmonary blood flow in left-to-right shunts and pulmonary edema decrease lung compliance and thus cause tachypnea in an attempt to maintain minute ventilation. Tachypnea is a cardinal sign of left-sided failure in infants. Unlike tachypnea caused by respiratory viruses, this tachypnea is usually effortless in children with congestive heart failure, due to lack of airway obstruction. Since feeding is the infant's primary form of exertion, dyspnea and sweating during feeding can often be elicited in the history. Peripheral edema, jugular venous distention, and rales are unusual and late signs in infants.

Hepatomegaly appears long before ascites, anasarca, or peripheral edema in right-sided failure in infants, but is usually a late sign. Hepatomegaly exists when the liver is more than 2 cm below the right costal margin in the absence of downward displacement by hyperexpanded lungs. In hepatomegaly, the liver border is rounded rather than sharp.

In congestive heart failure, the details of any murmur detected on physical examination contribute to the diagnosis. The chest radiograph may reveal cardiomegaly, increased or decreased vascular markings, or pulmonary edema. Often, due to the presence of a thymic shadow, the cardiac size is not readily apparent on routine posterior-anterior radiographs of the chest, but can be assessed on the lateral view by obliteration of the retrocardiac window by the enlarged heart. On the posterior-anterior view, the thymic shadow can be distinguished from

TABLE 115-2 Recognition of Congestive Heart Failure in Infants

	Right Sided Failure	Left-Sided Failure	Both
Cardinal Signs	Hepatomegaly	Tachypnea Dyspnea and sweating on feeding Rales	Cardiomegaly Failure to thrive Tachycardia
Unusual Signs	Jugular venous distension Peripheral edema Anasarca		

the cardiac silhouette by the "sail sign," if present, and by the scalloped border that is produced by compression of the thymus against the rib cage. The ECG is often nonspecific, but may reveal only evidence of abnormal electrical axis, rhythm disturbances or, more often, chamber hypertrophy.

Physiologic Correlates of Congestive Heart Failure

Typically, most cases of congestive heart failure in children are caused by afterload increases in the pressure dynamics of one or both chambers of the heart. In these conditions, pressure builds in one chamber of the heart due to an obstructive lesion in the outflow tract of the affected chamber. Several of the more common entities early in the first weeks of life are the left ventricular outflow obstruction syndromes, followed by congenital aortic stenosis and moderate-to-severe coarctation of the aorta. With these lesions, the systemic circulation has inadequate perfusion, and renal flow is diminished. The combination of increased fluid retention and chamber dilatation results in cardiac failure. Treatment of afterload increases is aimed at vasodilatation with either specific load-altering medications, such as nitroprusside or nitroglycerin, or the use of furosemide, which has both a diuretic effect and a vasodilatory effect. Correction of the mechanical obstruction is viewed as the ideal solution.[14]

Less often, congestive heart failure can be related to increases in preload representing an overall volume overload without obstructive pressure consequences. Typical entities include large VSDs, and persistent patent ductus arteriosus in premature infants. Anemias of different etiologies should be considered, especially iron deficiency anemia in small cow-milk-fed infants. Sickle cell anemia and thalassemia variants should also be considered. In the former group of conditions, decreasing the vascular volume with diuretics is beneficial. In addition, the use of digoxin may be beneficial prior to surgical repair. In the latter cases, transfusion is warranted along with judicious use of fluid restriction and diuresis.

Poor contractility is not usually considered a major cause of congestive heart failure in small infants, because the ventricular walls are still relatively noncompliant. In older pediatric patients, though, poor contractility becomes an issue. Kawasaki syndrome, idiopathic endocardial fibroelastosis, pulmonary hypertension associated with Eisenmenger syndrome, and toxic-metabolic causes should be considered in adolescent patients with congestive heart failure. Less frequent inflammatory causes include myocarditis, constrictive pericarditis, and collagen vascular diseases. Treatment is geared toward increasing contractility with dobutamine or digoxin.[15]

Differential Diagnosis

CONGENITAL ANATOMIC HEART DEFECTS Once congestive heart failure is recognized, age-related categories simplify further differential diagnosis as outlined according to time of development in Table 115-3. In the first few minutes of life, congestive heart failure occurs from a variety of noncardiac origins such as asphyxia, acidosis, hypoglycemia, hypocalcemia, anemia, or sepsis. In critically ill premature neonates, a patent ductus arteriosus is the most common cause of congestive heart failure. Among full-term newborns, a hypoplastic left ventricle is the most common cause in the first week of life and coarctation of the aorta is the most common cause in the second week of life. Transposition of the great arteries presents within the first 3 days of life, with either cyanosis or congestive heart failure.[16]

VSDs alone do not cause congestive heart failure in the first weeks of life but, when complicated by transposition of the great arteries, truncus arteriosus, critical aortic stenosis, or coarctation can present with failure at any time during the first few weeks of life. Large, uncomplicated VSDs can present with congestive heart failure after weeks 3 to 4 of life as pulmonary artery pressure continues to fall,

TABLE 115-3 Differential Diagnosis of Congestive Heart Failure Based on Age of Presentation

Age	Spectrum	
1 min 1 hour	Noncardiac origin: anemia, acidosis, hypoxia, hypoglycemia, hypocalcemia, sepsis	Acquired
1 day 1 week 2 weeks 1 month	PDA in premature infants HPLV Coarctation Ventricular septal defect	Congenital
3 months 1 year 10 years	Supraventricular tachycardia Myocarditis Cardiomyopathy Severe anemia Rheumatic fever	Acquired

For meanings of acronyms, refer to Table 115-1.

increasing the left-to-right shunt. Onset of failure is insidious between 1 and 3 months of age, when the left-to-right shunt increases as the pulmonary vascular resistance decreases further from the high fetal values.

Clinical assessment also involves estimation of the degree of severity of the congestive heart failure. For example, depending on the size of the defect, a VSD may present in a variety of ways, ranging from mild tachypnea to chronic compensated congestive heart failure accompanied by growth failure and frank pulmonary hypertension in later years. The finding on clinical examination of a small VSD is often out of proportion to the size of the VSD: a small VSD may have with a loud holosystolic murmur that is hemodynamically insignificant, and a large defect may produce no murmur initially.

In contrast to the gradual onset of heart failure with a VSD, coarctation of the aorta can present with abrupt onset of congestive heart failure precipitated by a delayed closure of the ductus arteriosus during week 2 of life. The severity of the symptoms is directly proportional to the degree of obstruction and can vary from mild tachypnea to cardiogenic shock. Milder degrees of coarctation, on the other hand, present later in life with isolated hypertension and diminished pulses in the lower extremities.

The onset of congestive heart failure after 3 months of age usually signifies acquired heart disease as opposed to congenital heart disease. The exception to this rule occurs when pneumonia, subacute bacterial endocarditis, or other complicating factors cause a previously stable congenital lesion to decompensate. Before 2 years of age, myocarditis, cardiomyopathies, and severe anemia are the most common diseases in the differential diagnosis. Rheumatic fever, once a common cause of congestive heart failure, is seen among children who are 8 to 12 years of age. It is unusual now, except in certain ethnic groups.

MYOCARDITIS AND CARDIOMYOPATHIES Myocarditis affects children of all ages and is the leading cause of end-stage cardiomyopathy requiring transplantation. Viral etiologies include enteroviruses (coxsackie, echovirus, and poliovirus), as well as mumps, influenza virus, and *Varicella zoster*. An emerging cause is HIV-associated myocarditis and chronic Epstein-Barr myocarditis. Many bacterial species have been associated with myopericarditis, but not myocarditis alone. Noninfectious causes include lupus erythematosus, toxins such as tricyclic antidepressants, and cocaine. Myocarditis is often preceded by a viral respiratory illness and needs to be differentiated from pneumonia. As with the latter diagnosis, presenting signs and symptoms are often respiratory distress, fever, tachypnea, and tachycardia. Clues that suggest myocarditis include generalized malaise, fever, and myalgias in age-appropriate children.[17,18]

Cardiomyopathies are uncommon, but significant due to the high mortality and severe disability that they produce. They are usually classified into two groups: either dilated or hypertrophic. The dilated cardiomyopathies display impaired cardiac contractility and ventricular dilation. Most cases are idiopathic or viral in etiology. Most infants who arrive at the emergency department have respiratory symptoms, and a chest radiograph reveals an enlarged heart and vascular congestion. In a small percentage of these infants, acute cardiovascular collapse can result from severe congestive heart failure or dysrhythmia. Infants become acutely symptomatic when their disease is accentuated by intercurrent febrile illness. The hypertrophic cardiomyopathies display thickened myocardium and very plastic immobile contractile state. Often, minor febrile illness may result in sudden unexplained death that could not have been predicted by a previous examination.[19]

Chest radiographs show cloudy lung fields either from inflammation or pulmonary edema. ECG may reveal ST-T-segment changes that are generalized to all leads or rhythm disturbances. Evidence of ectopy signals severe diffuse disease and a high risk of sudden death. Cardiomegaly with poor distal pulses and prolonged capillary refill, however, distinguish it from common pneumonia. Once cardiomegaly is discovered, admission and echocardiogram are warranted. The latter will show a dilated, poorly contracting left ventricle with a low ejection fraction with or without a pericardial effusion. In dilated cardiomyopathies, both ventricles are usually affected and substantial dilatation is apparent at diagnosis.

At this point, the cause of myocarditis must be further delineated in a hospital, and endomyocardial biopsy may be warranted to do so. Parents must be thoroughly versed in cardiopulmonary resuscitation and be aware that a lethal dysrhythmia could cause sudden death. Infants are best kept comfortable in an upright position in an infant seat. Oxygen is administered in a nonthreatening fashion appropriate for age, and a neutral thermal environment is established. If congestive heart failure is apparent, a diuretic is administered. Severe congestive heart failure is initially treated with inotropic infusions (for example, dopamine hydrochloride or dobutamine) along with fluid restriction, diuresis, and supplemental oxygen. Intubation and mechanical ventilation often become necessary during the hospital phase of the illness. Treatment is directed to the underlying cause in addition to the supportive therapy outlined previously.

Such infants require management by pediatric cardiologists in an intensive care setting. Digoxin therapy is often initiated. Intravenous immune serum globulin is used by some experts. Definitive proof of treatment effect is lacking in such therapy in controlled trials. In severe cases, failure of improvement in left ventricular function in weeks 1 to 6 can lead to death unless cardiac transplantation is sought, and remains the only definitive treatment.

PERICARDITIS Usually, this presents as cardiomegaly that is discovered incidentally on chest radiograph. Clinical signs such as chest pain, muffled heart sounds, and a friction rub may be present. In older patients and adolescents, classic pleuritic or positional chest pain, abdominal pain, and tachycardia may be seen. An echocardiogram is performed on an urgent basis to distinguish a pericardial effusion from dilated or hypertrophic myocarditis. The most common etiology is in association with coxsackie viral myocarditis. Bacterial pericarditis from *Haemophilus influenzae* is rare today and was uncommon even before the availability of *H. influenzae* type B conjugated vaccines. Typically, most cases of bacterial pericarditis present with profound toxicity and muffled heart sounds and jugular venous distention. If not appropriately drained in addition to antibiotic treatment, constrictive pericarditis will result in tamponade. Pericarditis that accompanies rheumatic fever, lupus erythematosus, or chronic renal failure is usually secondary and does not produce the main symptomatology. Since diagnostic pericardiocentesis can be complicated by hemorrhage, cardiac tamponade, and arrest, it is usually deferred to a pediatric cardiologist or intensivist for drainage. Pericardiocentesis with an 18-gauge over-the-needle catheter is indicated in the emergency department if an infant with large heart becomes rapidly unstable with loss of pulse. As in adults, the needle is placed in the subxiphoid region and aimed toward the left shoulder. As little as 30 to 50 mL pericardial fluid can cause tamponade, and removal with immediate improvement is diagnostic.[20]

Typically, uncomplicated pericarditis responds to a prolonged course of anti-inflammatory medication and decreased activity or bed rest. Most cases are self-limited and require specialty consultation only for the initial evaluation.

COR PULMONALE If an infant presents in pure right-sided congestive heart failure, the primary problem is most likely to be pulmonary in origin. Hepatomegaly and anasarca may be present, but most often, in early stages, lid edema is the first noticeable sign. Moreover, the lid edema is likely to be appreciated by the parents more than by the physician and must be specifically searched for on examination. Often it will have to be elicited by asking "Do your child's eyes look puffy?" If the underlying problem is bronchopulmonary dysplasia resulting from prematurity and infantile respiratory distress syndrome, the infant may already be on appropriate home oxygenation and diuretic therapy. Upper airway obstruction from hypertrophied adenoidal and tonsillar tissue can produce cor pulmonale, presenting as edema or anasarca. The clinical features of airway obstruction, however, are subtle; a careful history will reveal continuous mouth breathing while awake and sleeping, with or without snoring. Sleep studies and tonsillectomy are indicated. Cor pulmonale from upper airway obstruction in infants usually responds to diuresis and oxygen alone, without the need for digoxin.

Initial Stabilization

The degree and severity of congestive heart failure dictate the types of therapeutic interventions necessary for the initial stabilization phase. Infants who present with mild tachypnea, hepatomegaly, and cardiomegaly simply need to be seated upright in a comfortable position and kept in a neutral thermal environment to minimize preload and to avoid metabolic stress. If the work of breathing is appreciably increased by an increased pulmonary blood flow, 1 to 2 mg/kg furosemide parenterally is indicated. If pulmonary edema is present, then the hypoxemia can usually be corrected by fluid restriction, diuresis, and an increase in ambient oxygen.

Severe degrees of congestive heart failure can present with signs of low cardiac output or cardiogenic shock. Aggressive management is often necessary in secondary derangement, including respiratory insufficiency, acute renal failure, lactic acidosis, disseminated intravascular coagulation, hypoglycemia, and hypocalcemia.

For definitive diagnosis and treatment of congenital lesions presenting in congestive heart failure, cardiac catheterization followed by surgical intervention is often necessary. Stabilization and improvement of left ventricular function can often first be accomplished with inotropic agents. Digoxin is used in milder forms of congestive heart failure. Initial digitalization is performed intravenously, giving one-half the daily dosage followed by one-fourth of the daily dosage intravenously at 6- to 8-h intervals. Maintenance dioxin consists of one-eighth the daily dosage given intravenously or orally at 12-h intervals. For full-term infants up to 2 years of age, the dosage is 0.03 to 0.05 mg/kg/day. Hence, 0.02 mg/kg would be the appropriate first digitalizing dose to be given in the emergency department.

At some point, congestive heart failure progresses to cardiogenic shock, in which distal pulses are absent and end-organ perfusion is threatened. In such situations, continuous infusions of inotropic agents such as dopamine or dobutamine are indicated instead of digoxin. The initial starting range is 5 to 10 μg/kg/min. The "rule of six" simplifies the necessary calculations. A total of 6 mg/kg of body weight of either dopamine or dobutamine is placed in a microdrip chamber and filled to 100 mL with 5% dextrose in water (D_5W) or normal saline; 1 mL/h equals 1 μg/kg/min, so it is administered via a pump initially at 5 mL/h (5 μg/kg/min). Prior to starting a continuous inotropic infusion such as this, the acid-base status should be checked by arterial blood gas analysis. Any abnormality should be corrected with 1 to 2 mEq/kg of sodium bicarbonate as needed and cautious volume expansion with 10 mL/kg of normal saline if necessary.

If inotropic support is inadequate, the use of combination therapy with vasodilatory therapy is warranted. The combination of dopamine and nitroprusside has been used extensively in situations of low cardiac output and low ejection fraction states. Another combination is nitroglycerin, which is readily available to even the smallest emergency departments.

When pharmacologic management is unsuccessful, other measures must be considered. Typically, most emergency physicians will be able to support ventilation with endotracheal intubation and positive end-expiratory pressure. Further care after tertiary referral includes balloon-assist counterpulsation devices or membrane oxygenation until definitive surgical care of the underlying cardiac defect can be undertaken.

DYSRHYTHMIA

This may rarely cause congestive heart failure. Most often, disorders of rate and rhythm are relatively benign except in postoperative cardiac patients. In general, children are able to tolerate higher rates without the usual ischemic phenomenon often present in adults. The treatment in children is usually directed at the underlying structural aspect of the intracardiac conduction system and less at prevention of cardiac ischemia related to rate.

Dysrhythmia appears to be increasing in incidence due to the increase in successful postoperative cardiac repair and survival. The fact that many of these children are now returned to the care of their primary care physicians makes it extremely likely that emergency physicians will encounter them and have the opportunity to deal with the dysrhythmias. Dysrhythmias can occur in the absence of any underlying structural heart disease or metabolic condition. Many conditions that occur in the adult population—such as hypoxia, electrolyte imbalance, collagen vascular diseases, and overzealous use of sympathomimetic agents—rarely occur in children. Because much of the prognosis with regard to the reoccurrence of a dysrhythmia depends on the nature of any underlying structural cardiac defect, noninvasive study is mandated in all first-time occurrences of dysrhythmia.[21]

Recognition of dysrhythmia is age dependent, and dysrhythmia often masquerades as other cardiac entities. In small infants, poor feeding and irritability may be the only signs of illness, with signs of poor cardiac output at higher rates evident later as edema and poor capillary refill. Older children may have more specific symptoms because of their increased ability to verbalize. In such instances, more classic adult symptoms of palpitations may be elicited, as well as syncope due to increased rate.

Typically, dysrhythmias are classified as in adults and are ideally viewed as rates that are either too slow or too fast for adequate cardiac output.

Slow Cardiac Rates

FIRST- AND SECOND-DEGREE ATRIOVENTRICULAR BLOCKS First-degree atrioventricular (AV) block is seen frequently and has no real serious consequence unless it occurs in the presence of another cardiac anomaly such as an atrial septal defect. Second-degree AV block requires a more thorough evaluation. Typically, Mobitz type I second-degree AV block is of no consequence and can be a normal variant. Mobitz type II, however, is always of significance and always requires a minimum noninvasive evaluation and prolonged monitoring.[22]

COMPLETE ATRIOVENTRICULAR BLOCKS Complete AV block can occur and can be either congenital or acquired. Congenital complete AV block is associated with congenital heart disease or may occur independently. In the former, the prognosis is extremely guarded until the underlying defect is corrected. Often the associated congenital defect is so severe (common AV canal) that it is uncorrectable. In the latter condition, AV block occurs during gestation and is usually secondary to maternal connective tissue disease with autoimmune destruction of the AV tracts in infants. The diagnosis is usually suspected prenatally, and treatment is instituted during gestation. Postnatal therapy includes transthoracic pacemaker and transvenous pacemaker use. Acquired AV block can occur without cause in older children, occur as a manifestation of inflammatory diseases of the myocardium, or occur postpartum in adolescent patients. In this category, syncope is usually the initial presenting complaint, and prompt recognition and referral are mandatory. Treatment is with an implantable pacemaker to prevent sudden death.[23]

Fast Cardiac Rates

SINUS TACHYCARDIA Although usually a benign event, the differentiation from the more significant supraventricular tachycardia (SVT) is difficult. Typically, ventricular rates in excess of 230 bpm are highly unusual and should be presumed to be the latter entity. The rate in SVT is usually fixed, with little variability with manipulation of the infant. Vagal maneuvers may be attempted to try to slow the cardiac rate. If slowing can be accomplished, P waves may be visible. The presence of P waves during slowing supports the diagnosis of sinus tachycardia. Other causes of sustained high-rate sinus tachycardia must be sought, including diarrheal dehydration, febrile illness, hyperthyroidism, sepsis, and drug effect from substance abuse or iatrogenic medication administration.

SUPRAVENTRICULAR TACHYCARDIA This is the most common dysrhythmia in the pediatric age range. In infants, SVT presents with a 4- to 24-h history of poor feeding, tachypnea, pallor, and lethargy. In older children, palpitations and chest pain can be prominent in the symptomatology. Physical examination reveals weak pulses and a tachycardia that can be too rapid to be counted accurately. Depending on the time since onset of SVT, other physical signs can vary from congestive heart failure to cardiogenic shock with pending arrest. Low cardiac output is secondary to inadequate ventricular diastolic filling time.

Most children younger than 3 or 4 months of age will have no cause for the tachycardia that can be easily identified. Children over this age often have underlying structural defects or precipitators, such as fever or exposure to sympathomimetic cold remedies. Older children and adolescents are more likely to have accessory pathways. Recurrence rates for accessory pathway disease are as high as 90 percent, and recognition allows for more directed therapy at the AV node.

An ECG rhythm strip shows an unvarying ventricular rate between 220 and 360 bpm, as opposed to a range of 150 to 200 bpm in adults with SVT. The QRS complexes are narrow and regular. P waves are absent or abnormal. Any wide complex rhythm that is seen is considered ventricular in origin, because SVT with aberration is usually extremely rare in children.

SVT must be distinguished from sinus tachycardia, which is the most common tachyarrhythmia in children. In sinus tachycardia, P waves are present. The normal range for heart rate in newborns is 120 to 200 bpm. Under age 5, it is not unusual to find a sinus tachycardia up to a rate of 200 bpm, due to fever, stress, or hypovolemia. The latter requires prompt recognition and adequate volume expansion.[24]

Initial management of *unstable* patients with narrow complex tachycardia consists of immediate synchronized cardioversion at 0.5 J/kg with increases in power output to 2 J/kg as needed. Cardioversion should be undertaken at the lowest possible output in children on digoxin. There is a greater risk of subsequent ventricular fibrillation in such patients, so prophylactic lidocaine hydrochloride should be administered in a dose of 1 mg/kg before cardioversion. If cardioversion is unsuccessful, overdrive pacing is indicated. Once cardioversion is completed, suppressive therapy with digoxin is required.

Intravenous adenosine (0.1 mg/kg followed by 0.3 mg/kg boluses every 1 to 2 min until tachycardia resolves) is now the standard treatment in most pediatric cardiology centers. Because the half-life of adenosine is a matter of seconds, it is administered as a rapid bolus via a peripheral intravenous line. Two syringes can be timed in delivery of the medication: the first syringe contains the adenosine, and the second contains 5 to 10 mL of saline flush. Both syringes can be sequentially emptied in less than 5 s. A brief (3 to 10 s) period of asystole is sometimes seen before return of a normal sinus rhythm. If necessary, the dosage can be doubled, tripled, or quadrupled to convert the rhythm (maximum dosage, 12 mg).[25]

Vagal maneuvers to convert SVT can be attempted, but are usually not successful until after the first dose of digoxin. The diving reflex, which is elicited by submersing the face in ice water, usually produces the greatest vagal tone. An alternative to submersion is to place the ice water in a plastic bag that can be lowered briefly on the infant's face.

Digoxin has been the time-honored standard of medical management of SVT in infants. Since it takes 4 to 6 h before the rhythm converts, however, it is used more for chronic management than for acute conversion. The dosage is the same as that previously listed for congestive heart failure.

Management of a stable SVT in any child over 1 year of age presents a management dilemma, particularly if therapy with adenosine has failed. Verapamil may be used in a dose of 0.1 mg/kg bolus in older children, with preparation for any associated hypotension with calcium chloride at 10 mg/kg ready at the bedside. If verapamil fails, then pharmacologic cardioversion with either propranolol or procainamide should be attempted. Propranolol administration prolongs conduction at the AV node in both antegrade and retrograde fashion and thus is extremely useful in Wolff-Parkinson-White syndrome. It is administered at a dosage of 0.1 mg/kg/dose every 6 h. Procainamide blocks only retrograde conduction and may be beneficial if the rhythm appears to be ventricular in origin. It is administered as a 5- to 15-mg/kg bolus over 20 to 30 min.[26]

ATRIAL FLUTTER This is associated with congenital heart disease approximately 90 percent of the time. The atrial rates generated typically range from 200 to 300 bpm in practice but rates as high as 500 bpm have been reported. With such high rates, the flutter waves are often difficult to visualize unless vagal maneuvers result in slowing long enough to capture the flutter waves. Conduction to the ventricles is variable and can be as high as 1 : 1 to a more usual 3 : 1 or 4 : 1 block.

In the stable patients, control of rate is a first priority and can usually be accomplished by the use of digitalization to slow the ventricular response. The ultimate goal of therapy is to eliminate the flutter waves and to decrease the conducted response of the atria. Evidence suggests that patients with congenital heart disease have a four to five times higher rate of sudden death if flutter persists. In 50 percent of patients, digoxin alone is effective, but other patients require combination therapy with digoxin, usually with procainamide. Combination therapy is usually never appropriate for emergency physicians to undertake, because slowed junctional bradycardia or asystole may occur.[27]

ATRIAL FIBRILLATION This is another supraventricular rhythm that is seen in children. Unlike adult atrial fibrillation, which is usually secondary to ischemic heart disease or pulmonary disease with chamber dilatation, childhood disease is secondary to rheumatic heart disease or dilated cardiomyopathy. Atrial fibrillation in children usually manifests as an irregular rhythm with variable conduction. Rate control is rarely problematic unless rates are in excess of 200 bpm. In unstable patients, immediate cardioversion is usually successful at energy levels of 0.5 J/kg. Overdrive pacing is useful for those that do not convert.

Unlike adult cardioversion, anticoagulation is never necessary prior to the termination of atrial fibrillation. Medical therapy with digoxin is rarely effective, and not enough experience is available with newer agents such as diltiazem or ibutalide. Even in stable patients, cardioversion is usually required. Rarely, electrophysiologic studies are warranted and ablation of the focus is required.[28]

VENTRICULAR TACHYCARDIA This is usually seen in the presence of underlying congenital heart disease. Intentional or inadvertent drug overdose should also be suspected. Occasionally, ventricular tachycardia may be idiopathic and discovered on routine examination in asymptomatic children. In the latter case, complete investigation should include a search for myocarditis, cardiomyopathy, or the prolonged QT syndrome.

Despite the poor prognosis that this rhythm holds in adults, stable asymptomatic children are usually left untreated if the heart is normal. Symptomatic children who present with syncope or chest pain require further study, but treatment should not be instituted by emergency physicians until after these studies are performed.

If patients are unstable in any way, synchronized cardioversion should be performed at an energy of 1 to 2 J/kg. If stability for transfer is uncertain, medical management with lidocaine hydrochloride is warranted. The dosage is usually 1-mg/kg loading followed by a 0.5 mg/kg reload in 20 to 30 min and then a maintenance infusion of 0.01 to 0.04 mg/kg/min infusion. Procainamide can also be used, but must be given over 30 to 60 min at a dose of 15 mg/kg intravenously. Other considerations include phenytoin or propranolol administration.[29]

VENTRICULAR FIBRILLATION As in adult patients, this rhythm is incompatible with life and mandates immediate defibrillation. The initial energy for defibrillation is 2 J/kg and can be doubled, if necessary. Other causes include hypoxia, acidosis, and underlying cardiomyopathy, and their correction may increase the success of defibrillation. A trial of bretylium given as a 5-mg/kg infusion followed by defibrillation may be warranted followed by doubling of the dosage. Failure to respond after two infusions of bretylium followed by three defibrillation attempts usually indicates that the heart is unresuscitatable. Electrophysiology studies are indicated for any children who survive such a rhythm.[30]

CONGENITAL LESIONS THAT PRODUCE SYNCOPE

A child's sudden loss of consciousness is usually due to a previously unrecognized seizure and seldom due to dysrhythmia. When syncope does occur, children are often brought to the emergency department for initial evaluation. An accurate history from a reliable witness is essential to establish cardiac causes as the exact etiology. Typically, the history describes a child who has an initial change in skin color with or without cyanosis, a controlled fall, and then loss of consciousness.

The differential diagnosis includes tetralogy of Fallot, critical aortic stenosis, sick sinus syndrome, hypertrophic cardiomyopathy, and prolonged QT syndrome. Each are discussed in detail next.

Tetralogy of Fallot

This common cyanotic lesion may escape detection in the nursery, so it is important for emergency medicine physicians to recognize this lesion, as well as to recognize and treat hypercyanotic spells as discussed earlier. The degree of cyanosis is directly proportional to the severity of the pulmonary stenosis. In fact, cyanosis may be subtle or absent at rest and clinically obvious only when infants are active or crying.

Dynamic obstruction below the pulmonary valve can lead to an acute increase in the right-to-left shunt, producing a hypercyanotic spell or syncope with cyanosis. Prolonged or recurrent syncope due to tetralogy of Fallot can be a life-threatening emergency, so referral after initial stabilization is indicated for further diagnostic evaluation and possible urgent surgical intervention.

Critical Aortic Stenosis

This noncyanotic lesion can be life threatening and may present at any age. Older children may have a history of exercise intolerance with easy fatigability and chest pain. Prominent physical findings are a systolic ejection click and a diamond-shaped murmur that radiates to the neck and is associated with a suprasternal thrill. Left ventricular hypertrophy with strain can be present on ECG, and the chest x-ray may show poststenotic dilatation of the aorta, although neither of these signs is present consistently.

Syncope without cyanosis caused by critical aortic stenosis can portend a sudden life-threatening dysrhythmia. Patients should be kept strictly at rest and should be sedated, if necessary. Immediate referral for further diagnosis and possible urgent surgical repair is indicated.

Sick Sinus Syndrome

This is a pleomorphic group of dysrhythmias that result from enlargement of the right atrium, which typically is poorly distended due to the low-pressure state of the chamber. Enlargement can occur due to diseases of the lung, in particular, bronchopulmonary dysplasia and cystic fibrosis that result in the adult equivalent of cor pulmonale. Anatomic enlargement can occur in Epstein anomaly, an abnormal atrialization of the right ventricle. Such conditions result in wandering atrial pacemakers and sinus arrest. Occasionally, bursts of atrial flutter result in low-output states that may result in syncope.

Hypertrophic Cardiomyopathy

This can occur in children of any age, but is most often seen in adolescents. Nearly one-half have abnormal ECG findings, usually of a supraventricular origin (atrial flutter or fibrillation are most common). The disease is caused by a primary hypertrophied, undilated left ventricle without structural lesion and is usually inherited, so a family history will be helpful. Typically, most children present with chest pain, exertional dyspnea, and syncope. Occasionally, sudden death is the only clinical finding.

The cause of most cases of sudden death is unknown and may be the consequence of hemodynamic, structural, and electrophysiologic consequences. Although supraventricular rhythms are more common, electrophysiologic studies indicate that ventricular dysrhythmias are the cause of sudden death.

Once recognized, therapy should be instituted with β blockade to ameliorate symptoms. The goal of therapy is to improve left ventricular filling during diastole. β Blockade results in heart rate reduction to allow for more time for diastolic filling. Blockade also decreases myocardial muscle tension and improves compliance and eases filling. Other agents may be useful, but are usually instituted after conduction studies are performed. Surgery may be useful to eliminate some of the symptoms. Neither surgery nor medical management will prevent sudden death. There is not enough evidence to suggest that implantable defibrillation devices will prevent the sudden death of these children.[31]

Prolonged QT Syndrome

This is searched for more than any other etiology as a cause of syncope in young healthy children. In nearly all cases, the syndrome is inherited and is associated with deafness in about 75 percent of cases. Secondary, noncongenital cases result from anorexia, bulimia, or chronic ingestion of antidysrhythmic medications. Undiagnosed, untreated, or undertreated congenital prolonged QT syndrome results in a mortality rate in excess of 90 percent.

The syndrome is characterized by episodes of paroxysmal ventricular tachycardia often with torsades de pointes morphology. The usual precipitators, which include emotional lability or stress, can progress to ventricular fibrillation and sudden death without warning. The syndrome is thought to arise from an imbalance of sympathetic innervation to the heart with left-side predominance. Other considerations include electrolyte channel defects.

Therapy is directed toward prevention, and patients should be treated with β blockade to prevent the asymmetric sympathetic activity. Treatment is continued for life, and compliance must be stressed to adolescents, because lack of compliance can result in sudden death. Other medical management includes phenytoin administration. Implantable pacemakers or internal defibrillators may prove beneficial.

Treatment of the life-threatening ventricular tachycardia includes synchronized cardioversion and magnesium sulfate intravenously for refractory torsades de pointes. Referral for emergency cardiology consultation is mandatory for previously unrecognized cases.[32]

ANTICIPATING PROBLEMS IN CHILDREN WITH CONGENITAL HEART DISEASE

Children with congenital heart disease are brought to the emergency department for routine accident care, as well as for childhood illnesses. Some childhood illnesses may predispose patients to acute cardiovascular complications. A significant number of these children are treated with digoxin, diuretics, and anticoagulants that can make care of acute problems difficult. Special problems must be anticipated and complications of therapy for other conditions avoided.

Hypoxemic Spells

Most emergency department procedures involve fear and apprehension, as well as pain in the preparation of wounds and fracture splint placement or reduction. Infants with uncorrected tetralogy of Fallot can have hypoxemic episodes when total oxygen demand during painful procedures exceeds that which the restricted pulmonary blood flow can support. Strain also increases the right-to-left shunt through a VSD, as well as the reduced pulmonary blood flow. As described previously, loss of consciousness can result. Pediatric consultation should be obtained, if at all possible, before attempting conscious sedation.

Surgical Shunt Dysfunction

Due to palliative shunt procedures performed in the neonatal period prior to definitive operative repair of complex congenital heart disease, shunts can malfunction. Typically, infants in such a situation are in acute distress with increasing cyanosis. Although not as dramatic as with ductus-dependent lesions, symptoms develop when the shunt flow narrows to less than 50 percent of usual. Ordinarily, a continuous murmur is heard over the side of the shunt. Diminution or disappearance of the murmur suggests occlusion of the shunt. Typically, emergency physicians can do nothing for these infants. Palliative therapy with 100 percent oxygen is utilized, and transfer to a tertiary center is expedited. The use of thrombolytic therapy has been tried, but should be used by only pediatric cardiologists by direct shunt instillation or systemically. In all cases, possible replacement of the shunt or definitive surgical repair might be the only option.

Pulmonary Hypertensive Crisis

Many children with congenital heart disease have increased pulmonary artery pressure, particularly those with large VSDs. With painful procedures, these patients can experience pulmonary vasospasm. In such conditions, cyanosis and lethargy can develop and can mimic the hypercyanotic episodes of tetralogy of Fallot. Treatment is directed toward alkalinization with intravenous sodium bicarbonate and 100 percent oxygen to facilitate pulmonary vasodilation. Anxiolysis and analgesia are useful.

Diuretic Complications

Diuretics may be inadequate for the weight of the child because of normal growth and present as congestive heart failure. Conversely, during times of excess extraneous losses such as diarrhea or vomiting, dehydration can occur with subsequent hemoconcentration that could compromise cardiac function or shunt integrity. Careful monitoring of potassium levels is imperative during such losses.

Digoxin Toxicity

Because of the narrow therapeutic window between treatment and toxicity, digoxin toxicity can easily develop. In infants, toxicity is manifested most often by bradycardia and occasionally by other dysrhythmias. The usual adult patterns of atrial and ventricular tachycardia are not seen, except in adolescents. It is always good practice to monitor digoxin concentrations expectantly during any visit where blood will be drawn.

Usually, increased serum concentrations can be managed by withholding dosages of digoxin. Rarely, pharmacologic intervention is required for bradycardias. Ventricular dysrhythmias are managed medically with lidocaine or phenytoin. For severely intoxicated children, the use of digoxin immune globulin is indicated and will reverse toxicity rapidly. Usually, the dosage can be calculated readily based on the amount of digoxin elevation in nanograms above normal (see Chap. 168, "Digitalis Glycosides"). A 1-ng increase in digoxin is assumed to reflect a burden of 1 mg digoxin. Each vial of digoxin-specific antibody binds 0.4 mg digoxin. Therefore, a digoxin level that is 5 ng above expected would require 12.5 vials of digoxin-specific antibody. Care should be taken to avoid volume overload.

Anticoagulation Problems

Some children with congenital heart disease are on anticoagulant therapy to prevent shunt occlusion or thrombosis of surgically implanted valves or grafts. The risk of serious bleeding is small with routine emergency department visits, but must be considered for any elective repair of fractures or lacerations. Prothrombin time and the international normalized ratio (INR) must be monitored. Reversal of anticoagulation with the administration of either vitamin K or fresh-frozen plasma should be undertaken only after consultation with a pediatric cardiologist.

Anemia and Polycythemia with Cyanotic Congenital Heart Disease

Children with this problem require an increase in hemoglobin concentration to compensate for hypoxemia. Children develop tachycardia, feeding difficulty, or congestive heart failure when hemoglobin concentrations fall to normal. Often, anemia will be compensated for by polycythemia, which will cause increased viscosity and the potential for cerebrovascular complications. Iron supplementation is important for prevention of anemia. When polycythemia occurs, therapeutic phlebotomy may be warranted.

Viral Infections with Congenital Heart Disease

Although few normal children have problems with common viral pathogens such as influenza virus, parainfluenza virus, or respiratory syncytial virus, children with congenital heart disease are at unique risk for major sequelae. Distinguishing minor early infections with these agents and differentiating them from the symptoms of congestive heart failure is a challenge, even for seasoned clinicians. Children with lesions that increase pulmonary blood flow are far more at risk because of pooling of alveolar secretions. The pooled secretions allow for stasis and secondary bacterial overgrowth. Dramatic increases in mortality and morbidity are evident among affected infants. No effective therapy is available for parainfluenza and influenza virus, and prophylaxis against influenza B with amantadine analogues is not approved for small children. Hospitalization and specific treatment of infants affected by respiratory syncytial virus has been difficult to justify due to conflicting studies regarding efficacy of the antivirals and ribavirin and the expense of respiratory syncytial virus-specific immune globulin. Most infants will benefit from admission for bronchodilator therapy, but the prophylactic use of antibiotics to prevent secondary bacterial pneumonia is not justified. Admission may help sort out the distinction between congestive heart failure and underlying pulmonary infection.[33]

Subacute Bacterial Endocarditis

Children with congenital heart disease are at great risk of developing endocarditis. Transient bacteremia produced by iatrogenic procedures such as dental work or gastrointestinal or urologic manipulation can lead to localized colonization and infection. Although the thrust of most primary care providers is toward prevention of this disease, cases still occur. Typically, the usual presentation is of unexplained fever in children with known congenital heart disease. Appropriate evaluation includes multiple blood cultures, urine culture and analysis, and complete blood count. Parenteral or oral antibiotics should be administered in consultation with a pediatric cardiologist familiar with the child's history. In cases of known source of infection, such as otitis media or pneumonia, multiple blood cultures should be obtained, and appropriate therapy should be directed at the site of primary infection.

Acutely ill children with high fever mandate hospitalization, multiple blood cultures, and echocardiographic study of the heart. Usually, treatment is instituted following the obtainment of cultures and is directed toward the most common pathogens. Established diagnosis is followed by 4 to 6 weeks of intravenous antibiotic therapy.[34]

ENDOCARDITIS PROPHYLAXIS PRIOR TO PROCEDURES

Prophylactic treatment is recommended for patients with congenital heart malformations and rheumatic fever with valvular disease who are undergoing surgical or dental procedures and instrumentation involving mucosal surfaces. The administration of the medication should be timed such that an effective serum level will be present during the 15 min after the mucosal manipulation, when the transient bacteremia occurs. Amoxicillin 50 mg/kg (maximum, 2 g) is given 1 h before the procedure and 25 mg/kg (maximum, 1.5 g) 6 h later. For patients with valvular disease, 2 mg/kg gentamicin is given intravenously or intramuscularly 30 min before the procedure and 8 h later, in addition to the amoxicillin. Erythromycin 20 mg/kg orally (maximum, 800 mg erythromycin ethylsuccinate or 1 g stearate) can be given 2 h before the procedure, with half the dose given 6 h later.

The indications for prophylaxis and treatment options are well outlined in the American Heart Association guidelines for prophylaxis of endocarditis. Cases of endocarditis can occur despite appropriate prophylaxis. Vigilance in performing appropriate blood cultures is warranted in any children with symptoms suggestive of endocarditis.[35]

EVALUATION OF FEVER IN INFANTS WITH HEART DISEASE

Infants and children with known heart disease are prone to the same illnesses as other children. When they are brought to the emergency department for treatment of febrile illnesses, they are most likely to be hemodynamically stable and capable of handling the illness. Any signs of congestive heart failure are indications for an admission. Otherwise, blood cultures should be obtained, as well as a complete blood count, as would be performed for any infant between the ages of 6 months and 24 months. Although occult bacteremia has the same probability for occurrence in a child with congenital heart disease, concern for bacterial endocarditis must be greater. Oral or parenteral antibiotics should be administered with great care if presumptively treating early bacteremia or subacute bacterial endocarditis. It is more prudent to arrange admission, repeated cultures, and expectant therapy for such infants than to begin antibiotic therapy blindly simply because of the presence of congenital heart disease. A follow-up visit is mandatory in 12 to 24 h for any children who are discharged home without hospital admission.

REFERENCES

1. Grabitz RG, Joffres MR: Congenital heart disease incidence in the first year of life: The Alberta Pediatric Cardiology Program. *Am J Epidemiol* 128:318, 1988.
2. Lister G, Apkon M, Fahey JT: Shock, in Emmanouilides GC, Riemenschneider TA, Allen HD, Gutgesell HP (eds): *Moss & Adam's Heart Disease in Infants, Children and Adolescents: Including the Fetus and Young Adult,* 5th ed. Baltimore, Williams and Wilkins, 1725, 1994.
3. Matthay MA: Invasive hemodynamic monitoring in critically ill patients. *Clin Chest Med* 4:233, 1983.
4. McNamara DG: Value and limitation of auscultation in the management of congenital heart disease. *Pediatr Clin North Am* 37:93, 1990.
5. Rosenthal A: How to distinguish between innocent and pathologic murmurs in childhood. *Pediatr Clin North Am* 31:1229, 1984.
6. Park MK, Gunteroth W: *How to Read Pediatric ECG's.* St. Louis, CV Mosby, 1982.
7. Van Roenkens CN, Zuckerman AL: Emergency management of hypercyanotic crises in tetralogy of Fallot. *Ann Emerg Med* 25:256, 1995.
8. Kirklin JW, Colvin EV, McConnell ME, et al: Complete transposition of the great arteries: Treatment in the current era. *Pediatr Clin North Am* 37:171, 1990.
9. Starnes VA, Griffin ML, Pitlick PT, et al: Current approach to hypoplastic left heart syndrome: Palliation, transplantation or both? *J Thorac Cardiovasc Surg* 104:189, 1992.
10. Weidman WH, Blount SG Jr, DuShane JW, et al: Clinical course in ventricular septal defect. *Circulation* 56:156, 1977.
11. Bernstein D: The cardiovascular system: Chapter 386.17, Acyanotic congenital heart disease: Coarctation of the aorta, in Behrman RE, Kliegman RM, Arvin AM: *Nelson Textbook of Pediatrics,* 15th ed. Philadelphia, WB Saunders, 1996, pp 1301–1304.
12. Makoney L, Truesdell SC, Krzmarzick TR, et al: Atrial septal defects that present in infancy. *Am J Dis Child* 140:1115, 1986.
13. Doyle EF, Arumugham P, Lara E, et al: Sudden death in young patients with congenital aortic stenosis. *Pediatrics* 53:481, 1974.
14. Perkin RM, Levin DL: Shock in the pediatric patient: I. Clinical pathophysiology. *J Pediatr* 101:163, 1982.
15. Perkin RM, Levin DL: Shock in the pediatric patient: II. Therapy. *J Pediatr* 101:319, 1982.
16. Dickerman JD, Lucey JF: *Smith's The Critically Ill Child,* 3d ed. Philadelphia, WB Saunders, 1985.
17. Greenwood RD, Nadas AS, Fyler DC: The clinical course of primary myocardial disease in infants and children. *Am Heart J* 92:549, 1976.
18. Friedman RA, Duff DF: Myocarditis, in Feigin RD, Cherry JD (eds): *Pediatric Infectious Disease,* 4th ed. Philadelphia, PA, WB Saunders, 1997, pp 349–367.
19. Caforia AS, Stewart JT, McKenna WJ: Idiopathic dilated cardiomyopathy: Rational treatment awaits better understanding of pathogenesis. *BMJ* 300:890, 1990.
20. Gersony WM, Hordof AH: Infective endocarditis and diseases of the pericardium. *Pediatr Clin North Am* 25:831, 1978.
21. Dick M, Campbell RM: Advances in the management of cardiac arrhythmias in children. *Pediatr Clin North Am* 31:1175, 1984.
22. Genitz MH, Vetter VL: Cardiac emergencies, in Fleisher GR, Ludwig S (eds): *Pediatric Emergency Medicine,* 3d ed. Baltimore, Williams and Wilkins, 1993, pp 533–573.
23. Michaelsson M, Engle MA: Congenital complete heart block: An international study of the natural history. *Cardiovasc Clin* 4:86, 1972.
24. Binder LS, Boeche R, Atkinson D: Evaluation and management of supraventricular tachycardia in children. *Ann Emerg Med* 20:51, 1991.
25. Overhold ED, Rheubas KS, Gutgesell HP, et al: Usefulness of adenosine for arrhythmias in infants and children. *Am J Cardiol* 61:336, 1988.
26. Gillette PC, Garson PC, Kugler JD: Wolff-Parkinson-White syndrome in children: electrophysiologic and phasmacologic characteristics. *Circulation* 60:1487, 1979.
27. Garson PC, Garson A Jr, Biuk-Boelkens M, Hesslein PS: Atrial flutter in the young: A collaborative study of 380 cases. *J Am Coll Cardiol* 6:871, 1985.
28. Freed MD: Advances in the diagnosis and therapy of syncope and palpitations in children. *Curr Opin Pediatr* 6:368, 1994.
29. Gow R: Ventricular arrhythmias in infants and children. *Curr Opin Pediatr* 2:963, 1990.
30. Perry JC, Garson A Jr: The diagnosis and treatment of arrhythmias. *Adv Pediatr* 36:177, 1989.
31. Maron BJ, Tajik AJ, Ruttenberg HD, et al: Hypertrophic cardiomyopathy in infants: Clinical features and natural history. *Circulation* 65:7, 1982.
32. Towbin JA: New revelations about the long-QT syndrome. *N Engl J Med* 333:384, 1985.
33. Fixler DE: Respiratory syncytial virus infection in children with congenital heart disease: A review. *Pediatr Cardiol* 17:163, 1996.
34. Saiman L, Prince A, Gersony WM: Pediatric infective endocarditis in the modern era. *J Pediatr* 122:847, 1993.
35. Dajani AS, Bisno AL, Chung KJ, et al: Prevention of bacterial endocarditis: Recommendations by the American Heart Association. *JAMA* 277:1794, 1997.

OTITIS AND PHARYNGITIS IN CHILDREN

Kimberly S. Quayle
Susan Fuchs
David M. Jaffe

OTITIS MEDIA AND EXTERNA

Otitis Media

Otitis media, or inflammation of the middle ear, is one of the most common pediatric diagnoses. Each year there are 24.5 million office visits and over 3.7 million emergency department visits, with direct and indirect costs of $5.7 billion a year.[1–3] Acute otitis media (AOM) (acute suppurative, purulent, or bacterial) is associated with signs and symptoms of inflammation of the middle ear, such as otalgia, otorrhea, fever, irritability, anorexia, or vomiting.[4] Otitis media with effusion (OME) (secretory, nonsuppurative, serous, or mucoid) is a relatively asymptomatic collection of fluid in the middle ear. The duration (not the severity) of OME can be divided into acute (<3 weeks), subacute (3 weeks to 3 months), and chronic (>3 months).[5] The most important distinction between OME and AOM is that the signs and symptoms of acute infection (otalgia, otorrhea, and fever) are lacking in OME, but hearing loss may be present in both conditions.[5]

ACUTE OTITIS MEDIA Infants and young children are at greatest risk for the development of otitis media, with the peak incidence occurring between 6 and 18 months.[1] By 3 years, more than two-thirds of children have had at least one episode of AOM, and one-third have had three or more episodes.[6] The incidence is higher in males, Native Americans, Alaskan and Canadian Eskimos, and children who attend day care, are exposed to tobacco smoke, have a cleft palate or other craniofacial anomaly (e.g., Down syndrome), sleep in a prone position, use a pacifier, have older siblings or parents with a history of ear infections, had their first episode of AOM at less than 6 months of age, or have congenital or acquired immunodeficiency.[1] The incidence is lower in breast-fed infants.[1]

Middle ear effusion may persist for weeks to months after an episode of AOM. Antibiotic therapy generally sterilizes the effusion but does not clear it from the middle ear space. After the first episode of AOM, 70 percent of children still have a middle ear effusion at 2 weeks, 40 percent at 1 month, 20 percent at 2 months, and 10 percent at 3 months.[4]

Etiology Bacteria are the most common cause of AOM and can be isolated in a pure culture from the middle ear exudate in 60 to 75 percent of cases. These organisms colonize the nasopharynx and enter the middle ear via the eustachian tube. *Streptococcus pneumoniae* and *Haemophilus influenzae* are the most common pathogens [*Strep. pneumoniae* 30 to 50 percent (most common serotypes, 19, 23, 6, 14, 3, and 18), *H. influenzae*—primarily nontypable strains—15 to 30 percent], and *Moraxella* (formerly *Branhamella*) *catarrhalis* the third most common organism (7 to 20 percent).[6] Of importance is a major change in the increased prevalence of β-lactamase-producing *M. catarrhalis* (70 to 90 percent) and *H. influenzae* (30 to 40 percent), which affects antibiotic therapy decisions.[7] *Strep. pyogenes* (group A) and *Staphylococcus aureus* are each found in 2 percent of cultures.[4] *Chlamydia pneumoniae* may also be a causative organism, especially in those less than 6 months of age.[8] However, in infants 6 weeks or less, gram-negative enteric bacilli and *S. aureus* account for 10 to 20 percent of isolates. Although viruses are rarely recovered from middle ear effusions, recent studies have shown an increased risk of OME following an upper respiratory tract infection due to rhinovirus, respiratory syncytial virus, adenovirus, and influenzavirus A or B.[4,6]

Pathophysiology Abnormal function of the eustachian tube appears to be the dominant factor in the pathogenesis of middle ear disease. Two types of tube dysfunction may result in otitis media: obstruction and abnormal patency. Obstruction can result from persistent collapse of the eustachian tube due to increased tubal compliance, an inadequate active opening mechanism, or both. Infants and younger children are susceptible to eustachian tube obstruction because the cartilage that supports the eustachian tube is less stiff than in adults. In addition, an upper respiratory tract infection or allergies can obstruct the eustachian tube and decrease its function. The obstructed eustachian tube prevents equilibration of air pressure between the middle ear and the atmosphere and creates conditions favorable to the development of purulent or sterile effusions. The other type of dysfunction is abnormal patency, which may allow reflux of nasopharyngeal secretions.[5]

Clinical Features Classic signs and symptoms of AOM include ear pain (otalgia), otorrhea, and fever; however, ear pulling and irritability may be the only clues in an infant. The most important diagnostic tool is the pneumatic otoscopic examination. Before adequate visualization of the external canal and tympanic membrane (TM) can be achieved, cerumen must be removed from the canal by blunt curettage or by irrigation with warm water.[9] The presence or absence of discharge and the position, color, and degree of translucency and mobility of the TM must be assessed. The light reflex is of no diagnostic value. The normal eardrum is translucent and pearly gray but may become reddened with crying. The eardrum should be freely mobile in response to positive and negative pressure by the pneumatoscope; however, retracted TMs have reduced mobility. The TM of AOM is usually opaque, hyperemic, and sometimes bulging, and bony landmarks (long and short process of the malleus) are not easily discernible. However, the most significant sign is the loss of or decrease in mobility of the TM.[5,9]

Tympanometry is a noninvasive diagnostic technique used to determine the compliance of the TM and the middle ear. A fixed tone at a given intensity is delivered through a probe snugly placed in the external ear canal as the air pressure in the canal is varied from positive to negative. The tympanogram is a recording of the acoustic compliance of the middle ear, and patterns obtained are useful in distinguishing a normal ear from one with an effusion.[5,9] Acoustic reflectometry is a technique that in the uncooperative infant or child is easier to perform than tympanometry (since the instrument does not need to seal the auditory canal). When fluid is present in the middle ear, sound reflection is increased.[6]

Aspiration of the middle ear is the most definitive method of verifying the presence and type of middle ear effusion and infecting organism; however, its use for this purpose in the emergency department setting is rarely practical. It may be beneficial in (1) children with overwhelming sepsis, (2) immunologically deficient children, (3) neonates, (4) children with persistent symptoms of AOM after more than 48 to 72 h on antimicrobial therapy, or (5) otitis media with confirmed or potential suppurative complications.[5] Diagnostic tympanocentesis may be performed by inserting an 18-gauge spinal needle or catheter over a needle attached to a syringe through the inferior portion of the TM. The aspirate should be cultured in blood culture broth and on blood and chocolate agar plates. When therapeutic drainage is required, a myringotomy should be performed. The incision should be made in the lower half of the TM and should be large enough to allow adequate drainage and aeration of the middle ear. Myringotomy may relieve unusually severe otalgia, either at initial examination or at any time during the course of the disease. In addition, it should be performed when a suppurative complication (e.g., meningitis, facial paralysis, or mastoiditis) is present.[5,6]

Treatment Selection of the appropriate antibiotic is based on several factors: (1) knowledge of the likely etiologic agent or recovery of a specific pathogen from middle ear fluid, (2) the efficacy of certain antibiotics against the organism responsible for AOM, (3) antibiotic penetration into middle ear fluid, (4) a history of drug allergy, (5) compliance issues, (6) drug side effects, and (7) treatment failure or success of previous drug regimens for that child.[1,4] Despite the approval of 14 antibiotics by the US Food and Drug Administration for the treatment of AOM (see Table 116-1 for doses and frequency) and the changing antibiotic susceptibility patterns that have emerged over the past few years, amoxicillin [40 to 50 (mg/kg)/day divided tid for 10 days] remains the drug of choice. The preference for this drug is based on calculations that show that amoxicillin would result in clinical treatment failure in 8 to 10 percent of cases of AOM (based on data on organism prevalence, spontaneous clearance rates, and antimicrobial resistance).[1]

However, if β-lactamase-producing *H. influenzae* or *M. catarrhalis* is suspected or documented, appropriate antibiotics include trimethoprim-sulfamethoxazole (TMP-SMZ; Bactrim or Septra), erythromycin and sulfasoxazole (Pediazole), cefaclor (Ceclor), amoxicillin-clavulanate (Augmentin), cefuroxime axetil (Ceftin), and cefixime (Suprax). Other oral agents include ceftibuten (Cedax), cefproxil (Cefzil), cefpodoxime (Vantin), loracarbef (Lorabid), azithromycin (Zithromax), and clarithromycin (Biaxin), since all are active against β-lactamase-producing organisms.[1,4,10]

In infants 6 weeks of age or less, several factors should be taken into account. If the infant is younger than 2 weeks (or is older but has remained in a newborn nursery for a prolonged period), group B streptococcus, *Staph. aureus* and gram-negative bacilli are the most likely pathogens. A child of this age warrants a full septic workup (complete blood count, blood culture, urinalysis, urine culture, lumbar puncture with cerebrospinal fluid analysis and culture, and possibly a chest radiograph) and admission for parenteral antibiotics (ampicillin

TABLE 116-1 Treatment Options for Acute Otitis Media

Generic Name (Trade Name)	Dose, (mg/kg)/day	Frequency*
Amoxicillin (Amoxil)	40 mg/kg/d	tid
Trimethoprim-sulfamethoxazole (TMP-SMZ, Bactrim, Septra)	8/40 mg/kg/d	bid
Erythromycin and sulfasoxazole (Pediazole)	50/150 mg/kg/d	qid
Amoxicillin-clavulanate (Augmentin)	45 mg/kg/d	bid
Second-generation cephalosporins		
Cefaclor (Ceclor)	40 mg/kg/d	bid or tid
Cefuroxime axetil (Ceftin)	30 mg/kg/d	bid
Cefprozil (Cefzil)	30 mg/kg/d	bid
Third-generation cephalosporins		
Cefixime (Suprax)	8 mg/kg/d	qd or bid
Ceftibuten (Cedax)	9 mg/kg/d	qd
Cefpodoxime (Vantin)	10 mg/kg/d	qd
Loracarbef (Lorabid)	30 mg/kg/d	bid
Macrolides		
Azithromycin (Zithromax)	5 mg/kg/d, but 10 mg/kg/d on day 1, for a total of 5 days	qd
Clarithromycin (Biaxin)	15 mg/kg/d	bid
Ceftriaxone, intramuscular (Rocephin)	50 mg/kg	One dose

*All for 10 days, except as noted.

plus gentamicin, cefotaxime, or ceftriaxone). For infants between 2 and 6 weeks of age who have been discharged for more than 2 weeks from a nursery, *Strep. pneumoniae* and *H. influenzae* are the most likely organisms.[5] While a full septic workup is warranted, decisions about admission and treatment options are based on the results of these tests, the appearance of the infant, availability of close follow-up, and prevailing policies.

If the child is allergic to penicillin, erythromycin and sulfoxazole in combination, TMP-SMZ, clarithromycin, or azithromycin are recommended. When deciding which antibiotic to use, there are several issues to consider:

1. The efficacy of cefaclor is lower than that of amoxicillin-clavulanate, cefuroxime axetil, or cefixime.[10]
2. The efficacy of cefixime and ceftibuten against *Strep. pneumoniae* is less than that of other cephalosporins, but former are preferred when a β-lactamase-producing organism is suspected.[10]
3. When *Strep. pneumoniae* is suspected, cefproxil, erythromycin, clarithromycin, and azithromycin have superior activity.
4. The recent approval of intramuscular ceftriaxone may be of benefit when a child cannot take oral antibiotics due to emesis, when absorption of an oral antibiotic is in doubt (e.g., with malabsorption or inflammatory bowel disease), or when compliance is questionable.[11–13]

There has been a great increase in the prevalence of *Strep. pneumoniae* resistant to penicillin (and amoxicillin) in Europe as well as the United States in the past few years. Recent data demonstrate resistance levels of 16 to 41 percent in US cities.[8,14,15] Some key pieces of information to consider are the degree of resistance in the community and data on relative-resistance versus high-resistance organisms (since highly resistant *Strep. pneumoniae* are also resistant to TMP-SMZ, erythromycin, most cephalosporins, and ciprofloxacin).[8,14,15] Initially in the United States, the distribution of the two types of organisms was equal, but it has begun to follow the pattern in Europe, where relative resistance is two- to threefold higher than high resistance.[8]

The risk of being colonized or infected with penicillin-resistant *Strep. pneumoniae* is higher in younger children, those who have had several episodes of AOM, and those who have received multiple courses of antibiotics.[8] Some of the recent resistance patterns include the following:

1. Second-generation cephalosporins have good in vitro activity against penicillin-resistant *Strep. pneumoniae* and group A streptococcus.[8]
2. Cefprozil, cefpodoxime, and cefuroxime axetil are the only oral agents with some activity against penicillin-resistant *Strep. pneumoniae,* but the first 2 days are not effective against highly resistant strains.[8]
3. Although there is apparent resistance in vitro against azithromycin and clarithromycin for highly resistant *Strep. pneumoniae,* middle ear fluid concentrations exceed the minimum inhibitory concentrations (MIC) needed to eradicate it.[8]
4. At least 3 days of intramuscular ceftriaxone are needed to successfully treat highly penicillin-resistant *Strep. pneumoniae.*[14]

In areas where drug resistant *Strep. pneumoniae* has become a concern, amoxicillin remains the drug of choice for the treatment of acute otitis media. However, since the standard dose (40 mg/kg/day) may not eradicate penicillin resistant organisms, a higher dose, (80 to 90 mg/kg/day) has been recommended for high-risk patients. These include those less than 2 years of age, those with recent (prior month) antibiotic exposure, and attendance in day care. (Of note, the Food and Drug Administration has not approved amoxicillin at these higher doses.)[16]

Although there is recent literature to support a short-course (5-day) therapy for selected children (those >2 years of age with a mild episode and an otitis-free history), the standard length of treatment remains 10 days, except for azithromycin, which is given for 5 days.[16,17]

In the numerous trials of antibiotics in the treatment of otitis media, adverse reactions requiring the discontinuation of the drug have occurred in fewer than 5 percent of patients. With ampicillin, amoxicillin, and amoxicillin-clavulanate, diarrhea is the most common side effect, followed by rash. TMP-SMZ can also cause diarrhea and skin rash (including Stevens-Johnson syndrome), but the major concern is the development of neutropenia and thrombocytopenia. In addition, a patient with glucose 6-phosphate dehydrogenase deficiency should not receive sulfonamides. Erythromycin often causes gastrointestinal symptoms, including abdominal cramps, nausea, vomiting, and diarrhea. Besides possible cross-sensitivity in patients with penicillin allergy, cefaclor can cause a serum sickness–like reaction consisting of a rash, arthralgia or arthritis, and fever.[1]

Additional therapy, including antipyretics and analgesics, may be helpful in alleviating some of the acute symptoms. A topical analgesic [antipyrine, benzocaine, and glycerin (Auralgan)] instilled into the external ear canal often provides some relief from otalgia, but it should not be used when a TM perforation is present.[18] Decongestants, antihistamines, or glucocorticoids have no demonstrable role in the treatment of AOM.[4] With appropriate antimicrobial therapy, most children with AOM are significantly improved within 48 to 72 h. Persistent or recurrent pain or fever after 48 to 72 h indicates a need for reexamination of the child and the possible selection of another antimicrobial agent. Reasons for response failure include a resistant organism, noncompliance, and host-related structural or immunologic abnormalities.[6,18]

Standard practice has been that children with an uncomplicated course should be reexamined within 10 to 14 days of the completion of antibiotic therapy. Recent studies have demonstrated that this visit may be delayed to 3 to 6 weeks in certain cases.[1,18] However, in view of the fact that an emergency physician is not usually providing long-term follow-up care for such patients, phone contact with the patients' physician to arrange for a follow-up visit is recommended.

Recurrent AOM Many children have repeated episodes of AOM. Recurrent AOM is three or more episodes of AOM in 6 months or four episodes in 12 months, with at least one episode within the past 6 months.[4] Some children develop symptoms and a new ear effusion, often associated with an upper respiratory tract infection, after a previous effusion has resolved, while others develop symptoms of AOM with no documented resolution of a previous effusion. There is a correlation between such "otis-prone" children and the onset of AOM before 1 year of age. Other risk factors include day-care attendance and genetic susceptibility: a sibling or parent with a history of severe or recurrent AOM. Due to the risk of long-term sequelae, such as hearing loss and speech impairment, prevention of further episodes is desirable.[19] A more thorough physical examination and laboratory x-ray studies should be performed to rule out sinusitis, allergies, immune deficiencies (C3 and C5 deficiency), submucous cleft palate, or a tumor of the nasopharynx. If none of these is present, the preferred method of prevention for this particular group of patients is prophylaxis with antibiotics: amoxicillin [20 (mg/kg)/day at bedtime] or sulfasoxazole (75 mg/kg in one or two divided doses) for 3 to 6 months, with rechecks every 1 to 2 months. Prophylaxis is especially important during the fall and winter, when respiratory tract infections tend to occur; for children less than 2 years of age; and for those in day care. Although there is concern that the use of prophylaxis results in increased nasopharyngeal carriage of resistant pneumococci in this population, the benefits must be weighed against the risks and other options.[17] Active immunization is still being studied. Some investigators have had success with the use of the current 23-valent capsular polysaccharide pneumococcal vaccine in children greater than 2 years of age with recurrent AOM. Others have used an influenza A vaccine and shown a decreased incidence of AOM in children in day care.[1,18]

Myringotomy with tympanostomy tube insertion is the next step for children who fail antibiotic prophylaxis, although some physicians would have chosen myringotomy instead of antibiotic prophylaxis. Adenoidectomy is recommended at the time of myringotomy tube placement for children with severe nasal obstruction.[1]

Persistent AOM Persistent AOM is defined as the persistence of AOM within 6 days of initiating therapy or the recurrence of signs and symptoms within a few days of completing a 10-day course of antibiotics. This condition may be caused by the same pathogen (relapse) or a new bacterial species (reinfection).[5] Ideally, tympanocentesis for culture and identification of the organism should be performed, although this is not always feasible. A search for a suppurative complication of otitis media (e.g., mastoiditis) or a concurrent infection (e.g., meningitis) should be done before changing antibiotic therapy. If these conditions are not present, another medication can be prescribed, taking into account the spectrum of the initial choice (specifically, coverage of β-lactamase-producing organisms), as well as the antibiotic resistance patterns in the community. If penicillin resistant *Strep. pneumoniae* is an issue, the best antibiotic choices are: high dose amoxicillin-clavulanate (80 to 90 mg/kg/day of the amoxicillin component; with 6.4 mg/kg/day of clavulanate), cefuroxime axetil (30 mg/kg/day) or intramuscular ceftriaxone.[16] The patient should be followed closely, with a recheck in 2 to 3 days and another after 10 to 14 days.[5,6]

Chronic Suppurative Otitis Media The persistence (greater than 6 weeks) of a chronic purulent ear discharge in the presence of a nonintact TM is known as chronic suppurative otitis media. It is thought to be a sequela of partially treated or untreated AOM or recurrent AOM. *Pseudomonas aeruginosa*, gram-negative bacilli, and *S. aureus* are the most common causative organisms, although anaerobes have also been cultured.[5,19] It is thought that the organisms gain access to the middle ear through the perforated TM and become pathogens in the middle ear. A thorough examination is imperative, since chronic ear drainage can be a manifestation of a cholesteatoma (which requires surgery). In the absence of a cholesteatoma, recent studies suggest that the following steps result in a more rapid improvement in ear drainage and a decreased need for tympanomastoid surgery: (1) parenterally administered broad-spectrum, antipseudomonal antibiotics [ticarcillin, ticarcillin-clavulanate (Timentin), mezlocillin, or ceftazidime (Fortaz, Tazicef, or Tazidime)] either on an inpatient or an outpatient basis; and (2) daily cleansing and aspiration of the external and middle ear followed by instillation of ear drops [Cortisporin suspension (polymyxin B, neomycin, and hydrocortisone) or Coly-Mycin (colistin, neomycin, and hydrocortisone)].[5,7,19]

Complications and Sequelae of Otitis Media The complications and sequelae of otitis media predominantly involve the middle ear and adjacent structures within the temporal bone, but in rare instances intracranial complications may occur. The aural or intratemporal complications and sequelae include hearing loss, perforation or retraction pocket of the TM, tympanosclerosis, adhesive otitis media, ossicular discontinuity and fixation, chronic suppurative otitis media, cholesteatoma, mastoiditis, petrositis, labyrinthitis, and facial paralysis. Suppuration in the middle ear, mastoid, or both may extend into the intracranial cavity, producing the following intracranial complications: meningitis, extradural abscess, subdural empyema, focal encephalitis, brain abscess, and lateral (sigmoid) sinus thrombosis. These complications are uncommon except in neglected cases.[5,19]

OTITIS MEDIA WITH EFFUSION OME is a collection of fluid in the middle ear, without acute clinical signs and symptoms, that often follows an episode of AOM.[3] Hearing loss is by far the most prevalent complication and morbid outcome of OME. The extent of hearing loss is dependent on the volume of the effusion rather than the physical properties of the effusion and OME is associated with a mild-to-moderate conductive hearing loss of 20 dB or more.[18] Auditometry is of limited value as a diagnostic method for the identification of OME, but it can be helpful in the evaluation of the effect of middle ear disease on hearing.[20] The relationship between persistent or episodic conductive hearing loss and impairment in the cognitive linguistic and speech development of children has been reported. However, the degree and duration of the hearing loss required to produce such deficits have not been defined.[3,18]

Other factors that should be considered in addition to hearing loss when deciding whether to treat OME include (1) occurrence in young infants, since they are unable to communicate their symptoms and may have suppurative disease, (2) an associated acute purulent upper respiratory infection, (3) permanent conductive or sensorineural hearing loss, (4) vertigo, (5) alterations in the tympanic membrane (severe atelectasis and/or a deep retraction pocket in the posterosuperior quadrant or the pars flaccida), (6) middle ear changes, such as adhesive otitis or ossicular involvement, (7) persistence of the effusion for more than 3 months (chronic OME), (8) occurrence of the episodes so close together that the child has OME for 6 out of 12 months, (9) the presence of craniofacial abnormalities, and (10) impaired or deficient immunologic status.[1,20] A thorough search for an underlying cause (e.g., sinusitis, allergy, submucous cleft, or tumor) should be attempted before treatment is begun.

There are several management options for children between 1 and 3 years of age with OME that persists for less than 3 months: observation (no treatment) or treatment with an antibiotic for 10 to 14 days.[3] Because most episodes of OME clear spontaneously and because of the concern for antibiotic resistance, the no-treatment option is currently preferred.[16,17] However, if antibiotic therapy is chosen, since bacteria that cause OME are similar to those found in AOM, the antibiotics used are the same. Amoxicillin, amoxicillin-clavulanate, trimethoprim-sulfamethoxazole, cefaclor, erythromycin, and sulfasoxazole.[3]

The Agency for Health Care Policy and Research (AHCPR) recommends that, for children with an effusion for 3 months and a hearing loss of 20 dB or more, referral to an otolaryngologist for myringotomy with tympanostomy tube placement is another option (in addition to the abovementioned options).[3] However, many reserve myringotomy and tube placement for patients who have failed an antibiotic trial first.[1,16,18,20]

The other nonsurgical methods available, including the use of decongestants, antihistamines, and immunotherapy, have not been shown to be effective in clinical trials.[20] The addition of an oral corticosteroid [prednisone 1 (mg/kg)/day in two doses for 7 days] to the use of oral antibiotics for 14 to 21 days remains controversial. Steroids should not be used in a susceptible child who has been exposed to Varicella in the past month, due to a risk of disseminated disease.[18]

Myringotomy with tympanostomy tube placement improves the conductive hearing loss for longer periods of time than myringotomy alone.[4,5] Tympanostomy tubes remain in place for a few weeks to several years, with an average of 6 months. Possible complications of myringotomy tubes are scarring (tympanosclerosis), localized atrophy, persistent perforation, and the rare development of a cholesteatoma.[4] For children 4 years old or more who have recurrent chronic otitis media with effusion and who have had one or more myringotomy and tympanostomy tube operations in the past, adenoidectomy is a reasonable option.[3] The presence of upper airway obstruction, recurrent acute or chronic adenoiditis, or both is another indication to consider adenoidectomy.[1,20]

Otitis Externa

External otitis (OE) is any inflammatory condition of the auricle, external ear canal, or outer surface of the TM. It can be caused by infection, inflammatory dermatoses, trauma, or combinations of the three.

PATHOPHYSIOLOGY The flora of the normal ear canal are the same as those of normal skin. They include *Staphylococcus epidermidis,* diphtheroids, β-hemolytic streptococcus, *Staph. aureus,* anaerobes, and fungi.[21,22] Compromise of any of the protective features of the ear canal (e.g., shape and cerumen) can lead to OE due to colonization and invasion by pathogenic organisms, especially gram-negative enteric bacteria, *Pseudomonas,* and fungi. Causes include (1) high environmental temperature and humidity, (2) hyperhydration and maceration of epithelial tissue in the canal, (3) absorption of moisture by the stratum corneum, (4) lack of cerumen through blocked gland ducts and/or mechanical removal (scratching), (5) obstruction of gland ducts by edema and keratin debris, (6) invasion by exogenous or endogenous organisms through breaks in the damaged epithelial surface, and (7) trauma.[21,22]

CLINICAL FEATURES The mildest form of OE is characterized by itching or a sense of fullness in the ear. As it progresses, increasing pain, itching, redness, swelling, tenderness of the canal, and cheesy or purulent discharge occur. Inward pressure on the tragus or pulling the auricle up and back usually results in discomfort. If the TM can be visualized, it is often red, thick, and covered with the flat vesicles or areas of desquamating epithelium.[21] In the severe stage, pain is intense and can be caused by any movement of the jaw or the ear. There is often disseminated infection, with the presence of enlarged and tender lymph nodes. Further anterior spread of the infection affects the parotid gland and subcutaneous tissue. Posterior spread involves the mastoid, and medial spread involves cranial nerves IX through XII, with possible osteomyelitis of the skull.[21,22]

When there is localized OE (furunculosis), although pain, itching, and signs of infection, such as erythema, are present, a localized abscess is often seen. The organism responsible is usually *Staph. aureus.*[22] When OE is caused by fungi (otomycosis), intense itching is usually present.[21,22]

DIAGNOSIS The hardest part of the diagnosis is to distinguish between OE and otitis media. Ideally, clinical inspection of the TM with a pneumatic otoscope helps establish the diagnosis; however, the TM of a child with OE may be as red and distorted as that of a child with otitis media, although mobility of the TM is normal or slightly decreased in OE. In addition, visualization of the TM may be difficult because of edema of the canal in OE. Tympanometry can be helpful if the canal is clear and a tight seal for the earpiece can be formed without too much discomfort. Parotitis, periauricular adenitis, mastoiditis, dental pain, and temporomandibular joint dysfunction should be considered when the discomfort is poorly localized and the ear canal and TM appear normal. In addition, pain can be referred from pharyngitis or tonsillitis, but such pain is often made worse by swallowing or eating. Foreign bodies in the ear can also cause OE.[21]

TREATMENT A thorough and atraumatic cleansing of the ear canal is the most important part of therapy. For mild infections, dry mopping using a small tuft of cotton attached to a wire applicator is sufficient and may be curative. If the canal is inflamed, edematous, and occluded by debris, cleansing can be done with gentle suctioning: a soft plastic infant feeding tube (with an opening at the tip) attached to a DeLee trap can be used. If there is no perforation of the TM, irrigation with warm hypertonic (3%) saline solution, or 2% acetic acid in Burow's solution (Otic Domeboro) is helpful. Acidified isopropyl alcohol (equal parts vinegar and alcohol) or hydrogen peroxide can also be used, followed by drying with suction, compressed air, or a hair dryer. The use of cotton swabs to clean the ears should be strongly discouraged.[21,22] If the canal cannot be cleaned sufficiently, an otowick can be placed in the canal to act as a passage for the use of drops. It can be left in place for 2 to 3 days, at which point reexamination and removal can be performed.[21,22]

Acetic acid ear drops are the easiest and least expensive way to eliminate the infecting agent. A 2% solution is effective and available commercially in aqueous (Otic Domeboro) or propylene glycol (Vosol or Orlex) solutions. These drops should be used three to four times a day for at least 1 week. However, when OE is accompanied by a TM perforation, burning or stinging will occur with the use of acid- or alcohol-containing medication; thus, an antibiotic preparation containing neomycin, polymyxin B, and hydrocortisone (Cortisporin Otic suspension) is less irritating. Another option is the use of Cortisporin ophthalmic suspension, which is free of both acid and alcohol. Ophthalmic gentamicin or tobramycin are alternative drugs; however, when these agents are administered systemically, they have ototoxic properties, although hearing loss due to their topical use has not been documented.[21] Another option is the use of ophthalmic quinolone drops (ciprofloxacin, ofloxacin, and norfloxacin, all 0.3%).[22] Although quinolones are not approved for children via the oral route, these drops can be used in children over 1 year of age. Otic chloramphenicol should be avoided because of the risk of aplastic anemia. Swimming should be prohibited during the course of treatment. After brief showers (with infrequent hair washing), drops should be instilled into the ear.

The basic treatment of otomycosis is similar to that for acute bacterial OE, with cleansing followed by 2% acetic acid or M-cresyl acetate (25%) preparations. Patients who do not respond can be treated with topical ophthalmic suspensions of miconazole, nystatin, clotrimazole, or amphotericin B. Glucocorticoids are present in many topical otic preparations, but their value is unproven. Topical benzocaine and lidocaine may be useful to reduce the itching, but they are inadequate for the relief of moderate to severe pain, for which oral analgesics may be required.[21,22]

Children who fail to respond within 48 h of treatment should be reexamined. If the ear is not clear and dry, other causes, such as cellulitis, abscess, sensitization to the antibiotic, local dermatoses, or even noncompliance, should be excluded.[21] In some cases, oral antibiotics active against *Staph. aureus* (e.g., dicloxacillin or cephalexin) may be required (ciprofloxacin, the only oral antipseudomonal drug, is not approved for children <18 years of age).[22]

Patients with progressive, unresponsive, or severe infection may require parenteral (intravenous) therapy. Cultures of canal secretions should be taken and a combination of an aminoglycoside (gentamicin or tobramycin) and an antipseudomonal penicillin (ticarcillin or piperacillin) started. If the clinical findings and course of the illness suggest an infection due to *Staph. aureus,* a penicillinase-resistant antibiotic [nafcillin, oxacillin, vancomycin, or ampicillin sulbactam (Unasyn) for those over 12 years of age] should also be given.[21]

PHARYNGITIS

Pharyngitis, infection of the pharynx and the tonsils, is a very common pediatric problem. It is estimated that $300 million are spent annually in its diagnosis and treatment.[23] Despite physicians' long-standing familiarity with pharyngitis, there remains wide variability in approach. Controversies and new developments pertain to (1) selection of patients for throat culture and antibiotic treatment, (2) use of rapid diagnostic tests for group A β-hemolytic streptococcus (GABHS), (3) increased incidence of serious systemic streptococcal disease, and (4) occurrence of bacteriologic and clinical failure with penicillin treatment of GABHS.

Nonstreptococcal Pharyngitis

ETIOLOGY Most cases of acute pharyngitis in children are caused by viral infections. Examples include adenovirus, Epstein-Barr virus (see below), influenza virus, parainfluenza virus, rhinovirus, herpes simplex virus, and enterovirus. Although many of these viruses cause symptoms in addition to sore throat and fever, such as cough, coryza, conjunctivitis, or mucosal ulcerations, some viral infections can be clinically difficult to distinguish from GABHS.

Mycoplasma and *Chlamydia* have been suggested as uncommon causes of pharyngitis in adults and adolescents, however neither organism appears to be an important cause of pharyngitis in children.[24,25] Many organisms—viral, bacterial, fungal, and even protozoal—have been associated with pharyngitis; however, only a relatively few are of practical significance to the emergency evaluation of pharyngitis in the immune competent child. Recent studies have suggested that *Arcanobacterium haemoliticum* (formerly *Corynebacterium haemoliticum*) might be a cause of non-GABHS tonsillopharyngitis with or without a scarlatiniform rash.[26] Erythromycin is the treatment of choice; however, no prospective therapeutic studies are available. Among bacterial pathogens, GABHS is clearly the most important, accounting for 15 to 40 percent of all pharyngeal infections in school-age children. GABHS pharyngitis is unusual in children under 3 years of age, and rheumatic fever is rare in this age group.[25,27]

DIAGNOSIS AND TREATMENT The few non-GABHS organisms that occasionally require specific diagnosis are *Corynebacterium diphtheriae, Neisseria gonorrhoeae,* EBV, and human immunodeficiency virus type 1. Despite the many etiologic possibilities, in school-age children the diagnostic task is most often reduced to distinguishing GABHS, which requires specific antibiotic therapy, from nonstreptococcal pharyngitis.

Diphtheria is a rare but serious cause of pharyngitis in developed countries. Immunization in infancy with an alum-precipitated toxoid combined with pertussis antigen and tetanus antigen (DPT) has been effective in nearly eliminating diphtheria in childhood, but it can occur in crowded conditions where there are socioeconomic barriers to immunization. Morbidity occurs because of both infectious and toxic reactions. Infectious invasion and spread occur with enough tissue necrosis to produce a pseudomembrane that can progress to cause airway obstruction. The *C. diphtheriae* bacteria also produce an exotoxin that can cause widespread organ damage, including myocarditis and cardiac dysrhythmia, neuritis with both bulbar and peripheral paralysis, nephritis, and hepatitis. Diagnosis must be clinical in order to expedite effective therapy; however, the bacteria can be grown on Loeffler media. Treatment is directed at both killing the bacteria and neutralizing the exotoxin. Therefore, both antibiotic (penicillin or erythromycin) and horse-serum antitoxin must be given.

N. gonorrhoeae is an infrequent but important cause of pharyngitis in sexually active adolescents. Gonococcal pharyngitis in younger children strongly suggests child sexual abuse. Gonococcal pharyngitis may either be asymptomatic or cause very mild symptoms with occasional exudative tonsillitis and/or cervical lymphadenopathy. Pharyngeal throat swabs should be plated on Thayer-Martin medium to recover the organism. Rectal and vaginal or urethral cultures as well as serum to test for syphilis and hepatitis B should be obtained whenever gonorrhea is suspected or documented. Gonococcal pharyngitis in children and adolescents should be treated with ceftriaxons (125 mg intramuscularly once). Children who cannot tolerate ceftriaxone may be treated with a 5-day regimen of trimethoprim-sulfamethoxazole. Children 9 years or older should also receive oral doxycycline (100 mg bid for 7 days) for presumptive *Chlamydia* infection. Children 8 years or younger should receive erythromycin [40 mg/kg/day in divided doses]. Azithromycin (20 mg/kg, 1 g maximum) orally in a single dose is an alternative treatment for *Chlamydia* in all age groups.[28]

EBV is a herpesvirus that is a common cause of infection in childhood and adolescence. While EBV has been associated with a variety of clinical syndromes, most children infected with EBV are asymptomatic or have only mild nonspecific symptoms. EBV can cause isolated tonsillopharyngitis and pharyngitis as a manifestation of infectious mononucleosis (IM). Clinically, the classic IM syndrome begins with malaise, fatigue, and sore throat. Fever and adenopathy are the most common signs. Splenomegaly and hepatomegaly are also present in the majority of infected children, while skin rash, enanthem, eyelid edema, and jaundice occur much less commonly. Pharyngitis occurs in nearly all children with IM. The appearance of the throat can resemble that of bacterial GABHS disease. Dual infection with EBV and GABHS has also been documented. Classic IM is much less common in children under the age of 2 years, when EBV tends to cause a nonspecific febrile illness. However, recently IM has been reported to occur in toddlers more commonly than was once thought. These younger children most often have a syndrome characterized by fever, tonsillitis, lymphadenopathy, and hepatosplenomegaly.[29,30]

The laboratory can be helpful in establishing the diagnosis of IM. There is an increase in both the proportion and the absolute number of atypical lymphocytes in the peripheral blood smear (generally ≥ 50 percent lymphocytes and ≥ 10 percent atypical lymphocytes). Liver transaminase levels show moderate elevation [generally aspartate aminotransferase (AST) is <600 U/dL]. The heterophil antibody is present (and can be demonstrated by rapid slide test methods) in over 90 percent of children over the age of 5 with IM, but in only 75 percent between the ages of 2 and 4, and in fewer than 30 percent under the age of 2. EBV-specific serologic testing can provide information as to the likelihood of acute, postacute, old quiescent, and reactivation-type infection. These determinations are made on the basis of the presence of specific patterns of IgM and IgG responses to viral capsid antigen and IgG responses to EBV early antigen and the Epstein-Barr nuclear antigen.[31]

IM is generally a benign, self-limited, but somewhat prolonged illness. In general, treatment involves nonspecific supportive modalities (fluids, acetaminophen, and rest). Fatal complications are rare. Death can be caused by neurologic complications (e.g., meningoencephalitis or Guillain-Barré syndrome), splenic rupture and hemorrhage, and bacterial and fungal sepsis. Immunocompromised children may have unusual susceptibility to fulminant EBV infection. Airway obstruction secondary to tonsillar hypertrophy can also occur. This complication responds rapidly to glucocorticoid administration (dexamethasone 1 mg/kg to 10 mg maximum; then 0.5 mg/kg every 6 h) and rarely requires intubation. Airway obstruction is the only complication for which the use of steroids is widely accepted.

Human immunodeficiency virus type 1 is a recently recognized cause of acute pharyngitis. Primary retroviral infection can produce a mononucleosis-like illness with fever, sore throat, and lymphadenopathy that can last for a few days or a few weeks. Such findings as gastrointestinal symptoms or mucocutaneous lesions occur more commonly with acute HIV infection and are very unusual with mononucleosis caused by EBV. Primary HIV infections should be considered in high-risk populations.[32]

Streptococcal Pharyngitis

GABHS pharyngitis is the most common treatable cause of pharyngitis in children. The peak months of infection are January to May, but, because of the high frequency of occurrence in school-age children, the beginning of school in the fall is also associated with GABHS pharyngitis in many areas. The peak ages are 4 to 11 years, with GABHS infection being uncommon under the age of 3 years.

DIAGNOSIS No set of symptoms or signs is completely specific for GABHS. Nonetheless, there are findings that are typically, but not exclusively, associated with GABHS. Generally, the infected child experiences sudden onset of sore throat and fever. The tonsils and pharynx appear markedly red and have a moderate-to-large amount of exudate. The soft palate and uvula are also red and may have petechiae. The anterior cervical lymph nodes are enlarged and tender. The presence of a scarlatiniform rash and pharyngitis is virtually diagnostic of GABHS. Headache, vomiting, abdominal pain, meningismus, and torticollis can occur as well. These are of little diagnostic importance but must be recognized as possibly attributable to GABHS. The presence of significant coughing, rhinorrhea, or both suggests an alternative diagnosis. Diagnostic accuracy on the basis of clinical findings alone is reported at about 50 to 75 percent for children thought to have GABHS and 75 to 85 percent for children thought not to have GABHS.[33] There is general agreement that clinical diagnosis alone would result in an unacceptably high rate of misdiagnosis.

The mainstay of laboratory diagnosis is still the throat culture, although rapid antigen-detection techniques are gaining popularity in pediatric offices and emergency departments. The tonsil or posterior pharyngeal wall should be swabbed vigorously. In many centers, the swab is sent to the laboratory in appropriate culture medium for further handling. The sample is plated on a blood agar culture medium with neomycin and nalidixic acid added. Colonies that show β hemolysis are identified as group A by bacitracin disk tests, fluorescent antibody staining, or latex agglutination. The rate of false-negative results from single throat culture is about 10 percent. Recovery rates are maximized by good swabbing technique, multiple cultures (rarely actually performed), and incubation in a carbon dioxide-enriched environment. Positive cultures may indicate either an acute GABHS infection or the carrier state. Rates of GABHS carriage vary with the season but have been reported to be as high as 15 percent. There is imperfect correlation between the amount of growth (generally reported on a scale of 1+ to 4+) and the likelihood of true infection. Chronic carriers of GABHS are not at increased risk for developing true GABHS pharyngitis or suppurative and nonsuppurative (e.g., rheumatic fever and nephritis) sequelae, nor do they pose an increased risk for disease transmission.

Incubation of throat cultures takes 24 to 48 h, during which time management must occur with uncertainty as to the diagnosis. Antigen-detection procedures are often available in emergency departments and practitioners' offices. The tests involve extraction of group A carbohydrate antigen from a throat swab and then combining the antigen with a latex agglutination, coagglutination, or enzyme-linked immunosorbent assay. Recently a chemilluminescent DNA probe test and optical immunoassay have become commercially available. The nonculture tests take 10 to 30 min to perform and are generally more expensive per test than direct plate culturing. Sensitivity under controlled laboratory conditions using the culture as the gold standard ranges from 85 to 90 percent, and specificity ranges from 98 to 100 percent. Unfortunately, when measured in the field under less well-controlled circumstances, sensitivity of the latex agglutination test has been as low as 50 percent.[34] In other words, the false-positive rate is low, but the false-negative rate may be unacceptably high. Recent reports have shown that the optical immunoassay tests are nearly as sensitive as blood agar plate culture and more sensitive than other rapid tests for GABHS; this includes one study done in an office-based setting.[35,36] Any emergency department or office planning to use a rapid diagnostic test must assess the performance of the test on site. A safe and commonly used approach is to obtain swabs for both throat culture and rapid test simultaneously. Children with positive rapid test results are treated for GABHS. If the results are negative, the throat culture is processed and the children are managed according to an acceptable strategy while awaiting throat culture results. Some have advocated using optical immunoassay tests alone without culture confirmation of negative antigen test results;[35,37] however, as of this writing, the American Heart Association and the American Academy of Pediatrics have not yet supported that policy.[38]

TREATMENT The objectives of treatment for GABHS are (1) to prevent rheumatic fever, (2) to prevent suppurative complications (e.g., peritonsillar abscess and cellulitis, suppurative cervical lymphadenitis, and retropharyngeal abscess), and (3) to hasten clinical recovery. GABHS is highly sensitive to penicillin, and there has been no evidence of development of resistance in vitro despite decades of use. A single dose of intramuscular penicillin G benzathine—600,000 U if the patient weighs 27 kg (60 lb) or less and 1.2 million U if the patient weighs more than 27 kg—is effective but causes significant local discomfort in over 50 percent of recipients. A preparation containing 900,000 U of penicillin G benzathine and 300,000 U of penicillin G procaine (CR Bicillin 900/300, introduced in 1976) is effective for children who weigh 64 kg (140 lb) or less and significantly reduces the magnitude and frequency of local reactions. Oral penicillin V is a popular alternative. A regimen of 250 mg two to three times daily for 10 days effectively eradicates infection and prevents rheumatic fever.[38,39] Variable levels of compliance have been reported. Improvements in compliance can be achieved with careful parent education at the time of discharge. If compliance or follow-up are problematic, the intramuscular route should be used. Alternatives to penicillin for children with penicillin allergy include erythromycin, cephalosporins, clindamycin, azithromycin, and clarithromycin.

An increased number of apparent treatment failures with penicillin have been reported.[40] GABHS remains susceptible to penicillin in vitro. Alternative explanations for these findings may involve children who are carriers of GABHS and develop a viral pharyngitis, patients who reacquire the organism from a family member or another close contact, or patients who are noncompliant with the prescribed penicillin. Other proposed mechanisms include development of GABHS penicillin tolerance and the production of β lactamases from other normal pharyngeal flora.[41,42] The evidence does not support the diminished efficacy of penicillin therapy for GABHS pharyngitis. Reports of the proposed therapeutic failures have prompted many recent studies comparing the efficacy of penicillin to that of other antibiotics. In general, penicillin remains the recommended antibiotic of choice based on past experience, cost, and historically successful prevention of rheumatic fever.[38,41,43]

The overall incidence of rheumatic fever has been declining in the developed countries and is now less than 1 per 100,000 in the continental United States.[44] A number of scattered outbreaks of acute rheumatic fever were reported in the United States during the latter part of the 1980s.[45,46] There is ample justification for adherence to the American Heart Association recommendations that one of the abovementioned antibiotic regimens for documented GABHS pharyngitis must be provided. Antibiotic treatment begun within 9 days of the onset of infection is effective in preventing rheumatic fever.

Poststreptococcal glomerulonephritis is a nonsuppurative complication of GABHS disease that is not preventable with antibiotic therapy. Its occurrence is related to infection with nephritogenic strains of streptococci.

Research has also clearly demonstrated the beneficial effects of early antibiotic therapy on reduction of signs and symptoms of GABHS pharyngitis.[47] In addition, because it is recommended that children with GABHS receive antibiotics for 24 h prior to returning to school or day care, early treatment benefits both the children and their parents, especially parents who work outside the home. Based on these considerations, many strategies for testing and treatment have been proposed, ranging from treating all children with pharyngitis with antibiotics to withholding antibiotics from all pending culture results. Cost-effectiveness studies employing decision-analysis methods have been performed to compare some of these strategies.[37,48] The best strategy for a given institution depends on the local prevalence of GABHS, the availability and accuracy of rapid antigen testing, and the ability to follow up successfully on untreated children found to have positive culture results. A widely accepted strategy that incorporates the latest technology is to perform rapid antigen testing on all children with pharyngitis and to treat all with positive results. In addition, children with classic clinical findings or a scarlatiniform rash should be treated regardless of the result of rapid testing. Those with a negative rapid test result and equivocal or atypical clinical features for GABHS should have a throat culture performed, but treatment may be withheld pending culture results. Positive culture results indicate the need for treatment. It is not necessary to reculture to test for eradication of GABHS in asymptomatic children. Children with recurrent or persistent symptoms and those with previously documented rheumatic fever do require reculturing. Children with persistent positive culture results in this context can be treated with a different antibiotic such as amoxicillin-clavulanate, a cephalosporin, or clindamycin. The asymptomatic carrier state need not be treated except in certain circumstances. These exceptions include a family history of rheumatic fever, an outbreak of rheumatic fever or glomerulonephritis, or multiple documented symptomatic episodes of streptococcal pharyngitis occurring within a family or closed community. Clindamycin, amoxicillin-clavulanate, or a combination of penicillin and rifampin have been shown to be effective in eradicating GABHS in carriers.[49]

Some authors have suggested that early treatment of GABHS pharyngitis due to the availability of a positive nonculture test may lead to more frequent recurrences, possibly secondary to suppression of the immune response.[50] Other studies have not supported this view.[51] An intentional delay in the initiation of penicillin therapy for GABHS pharyngitis is not recommended at present.

Indications for tonsillectomy remain uncertain and controversial. One study showed that, for children with many recurrent episodes of pharyngitis (seven or more episodes in 1 year, five or more annually for 2 years, or three or more annually for 3 years), tonsillectomy reduces the incidence of pharyngitis for the subsequent 2 years compared with nonsurgical management. However, five of six children in the nonsurgical groups experience significant improvement as well.[52] The decision regarding tonsillectomy for such children should be individualized to account for various considerations of risks, benefits, and quality of life, including the quality of available anesthetic and surgical services, impact of recurrent illness versus surgery on the child and parents, school performance, and comparative costs to the family.

Recent outbreaks of pharyngitis caused by groups G and C streptococci have been reported often associated with contaminated food sources.[53–55]. Although the acute clinical syndromes associated with these organisms are identical to those of GABHS pharyngitis, they are unlikely to cause preventable nonsuppurative sequelae. However cases of acute glomerulonephritis following infection with group G streptococci have been described.[56]

A recent resurgence of invasive GABHS infections has been noted.[44,57,58,59] Serious illnesses include septicemia, toxic shock–like syndrome, pneumonia, cellulitis, lymphangitis, and nerotizing fasciitis. Such systemic infections may produce an extraordinarily virulent syndrome progressing rapidly to shock and death. Data suggest an appearance of new serotypes of GABHS but also an increased strain-associated virulence, rather than virulence related to a given serotype. The pathogenetic mechanism by which these virulent strains produce severe disease is not well understood.

Symptomatic therapy for both GABHS and nonstreptococcal pharyngitis includes acetaminophen for analgesia. A throat spray (e.g., Chloraseptic) can be used before meals and bedtime if further analgesia is required. Lozenges should be avoided in the children under 5 years because of the possibility of aspiration.

REFERENCES

1. Klein JO, Bluestone CD: Management of otitis media in the era of managed care. *Adv Pediatr Infect Dis* 12:351, 1997.
2. Weiss HB, Mathers LJ, Forjuoh SH, et al: *Child and Adolescent Emergency Department Visit Databook.* Pittsburgh, Center for Violence and Injury Prevention, Allegheny University of the Health Sciences, 1997.
3. Stool SE, Berg AO: *Clinical Practice Guideline: Otitis Media with Effusion in Young Children.* Publication 94-0622. Rockville, MD. Agency for Health Care Policy and Research, 1994.
4. Klein JO: Otitis media. *Clin Infect Dis* 19:823, 1994.
5. Bluestone CD, Klein JO: *Otitis Media in Infants and Children,* 2d ed. Philadelphia, Saunders, 1995.
6. Maxson S, Yamauchi T: Acute otitis media. *Pediatr Rev* 17:191, 1996.
7. Steele RW: Management of otitis media. *Infect Med* 15:174, 1998.
8. Block SL: Causative pathogens, antibiotic resistance and therapeutic considerations in acute otitis media. *Pediatr Infect Dis* 16:449, 1997.
9. Paradise JL: Otitis media in infants and children. *Pediatrics* 65:917, 1980.
10. Pichichero ME: Assessing the treatment alternatives for acute otitis media. *Pediatr Infect Dis J* 13:S27, 1994.
11. Barnett ED, Teele DW, Klein JO, et al: Comparison of ceftriaxone and trimethoprim-sulfamethoxazole for acute otitis media. *Pediatrics* 99:23, 1997.
12. Barnett ED, Teele DW, Klein JO, et al: Comparison of ceftriaxone and trimethoprim-sulfamethoxazole for acute otitis media [reply to letter]. *Pediatrics* 100:158, 1997.
13. Varsano I, Volovitz B, Horev Z, et al: Intramuscular ceftriaxone compared with oral amoxicillin-clavulanate for treatment of acute otitis media in children. *Eur J Pediatr* 156:858, 1997.
14. Block SL, Harrison CJ, Hendrick JA, et al: Penicillin-resistant *Streptococcus pneumoniae* in acute otitis media: Risk factors, susceptibility patterns and antimicrobial management. *Pediatr Infect Dis J* 14:751, 1995.
15. Appelbaum PC: Epidemiology and in vitro susceptibility of drug-resistant *Streptococcus pneumoniae. Pediatr Infect Dis J* 15:932, 1996.
16. Dowell SF, Butler JC, Giebink GS, et al: Acute otitis media: Management and surveillance in an era of pneumococcal resistance—A report from the Drug-Resistant *Streptococcus pneumoniae* Therapeutic Working Group. *Pediatr Infect Dis J* 18:1, 1999.
17. Dowell SF, Marcy SM, Phillips WR, et al: Otitis media: Principles of judicious use of antimicrobial agents. *Pediatrics* 101:165, 1998.
18. Berman S: Otitis media in children. *N Engl J Med* 332:1560, 1995.
19. Fliss DM, Leiberman A, Dagan R: Medical sequelae and complications of acute otitis media. *Pediatr Infect Dis J* 13:S34, 1994.
20. Bluestone CD, Klein JO: Clinical practice guidelines on otitis media with effusion in young children: Strengths and weaknesses. *Otolaryngol Head Neck Surg* 112:507, 1995.
21. Marcy SM: Infections of the external ear. *Pediatr Infect Dis* 4:192, 1985.
22. Bojrab DI, Bruderly T, Abdulrazzak: Otitis externa. *Otolaryngol Clin North Am* 29:761, 1996.

23. Tompkins RK, Burnes DC, Cable WE: An analysis of the cost-effectiveness of pharyngitis management and acute rheumatic fever prevention. *Ann Intern Med* 86:481, 1977.
24. Gerber MA, Randolph MF, Chanatry J, et al: Role of *Chlamydia trachomatis* and *Mycoplasma pneumoniae* in acute pharyngitis in children. *Diagn Micro Infect Dis* 6:263, 1987.
25. McMillan JA, Sandstrom C, Weiner LB, et al: Viral and bacterial organisms associated with acute pharyngitis in a school-aged population. *J Pediatr* 109:747, 1986.
26. Karpathios T, Drakonaki S, Zervoudaki A, et al: *Arcanobacterium haemolyticum* in children with presumed streptococcal pharyngotonsilitis or scarlet fever. *J Pediatr* 121:735, 1992.
27. Bisno AL: Acute pharyngitis: Etiology and diagnosis. *Pediatrics* 97(suppl):949, 1996.
28. American Academy of Pediatrics: Gonococcal infections, in Peter G (ed): *1997 Red Book: Report of the Committee on Infectious Diseases,* 24th ed. Elk Grove Village, IL, American Academy of Pediatrics, 1997, pp 212–219.
29. Grose C: The many faces of infectious mononucleosis: The spectrum of Epstein-Barr virus infection in children. *Pediatr Rev* 7:35, 1985.
30. Sumaya CV, Ench Y: Epstein-Barr virus infectious mononucleosis in children: I. Clinical and general laboratory findings. *Pediatrics* 75:1003, 1985.
31. Sumaya CV, Ench Y: Epstein-Barr virus infectious mononucleosis in children: II. Heterophil antibody and viral-specific responses. *Pediatrics* 75:1011, 1985.
32. Vanhems P, Allard R, Cooper DA, et al: Acute human immunodeficiency virus type 1 disease as a mononucleosis-like illness: Is the diagnosis too restrictive? *Clin Infect Dis* 24:965, 1997.
33. Breese BB, Disney FA: The accuracy of diagnosis of beta-hemolytic streptococcal infection on clinical grounds. *J Pediatr* 44:670, 1954.
34. Lieu TA, Fleisher GR, Schwartz JS: Clinical performance and effect on treatment rates of latex agglutination testing for streptococcal pharyngitis in an emergency department. *Pediatr Infect Dis J* 5:655, 1986.
35. Gerber MA, Tanz RR, Kabat W, et al: Optical immunoassay test for group A beta-hemolytic streptococcal pharyngitis: An office-based, multicenter investigation. *JAMA* 277:899, 1997.
36. Kaltwasser G, Diego J, Welby-Sellenriek PL, et al: Polymerase chain reaction for *Streptococcus pyogenes* used to evaluate an optical immunoassay for the detection of group A streptococci in children with pharyngitis. *Pediatr Infect Dis J* 16:748, 1997.
37. Webb KH: Does culture confirmation of high-sensitivity rapid streptococcal tests make sense? A medical decision analysis. *Pediatrics* 101:e2, 1998; http://www.pediatrics.org/cgi/content/full/101/2/e2.
38. Dajani A, Taubert K, Ferrieri P, et al: Treatment of acute streptococcal pharyngitis and prevention of rheumatic fever: A statement for health professionals. *Pediatrics* 96:758, 1995.
39. Bass JW: A review of the rationale and advantages of various mixtures of benzathine penicillin G. *Pediatrics* 97(suppl):960, 1996.
40. Pichichero ME, Margolis PA: A comparison of cephalosporins and penicillins in the treatment of group A beta-hemolytic streptococcal pharyngitis: A meta-analysis supporting the concept of microbial copathogenicity. *Pediatr Infect Dis J* 10:275, 1991.
41. Markowitz M, Gerber MA, Kaplan EL: Treatment of streptococcal pharyngotonsillitis: Reports of penicillin's demise are premature. *J Pediatr* 123:679, 1993.
42. Pichichero ME: Group A streptococcal tonsillopharyngitis: Cost-effective diagnosis and treatment. *Ann Emerg Med* 25:390, 1995.
43. Bisno AL, Gerber MA, Gwaltney JM, et al: Diagnosis and management of group A streptococcal pharyngitis: A practice guideline. *Clin Infect Dis* 25:574, 1997.
44. Kaplan EL: Recent epidemiology of group A streptococcal infections in North America and abroad: An overview. *Pediatrics* 97(suppl):945. 1996.
45. Veasy LG, Weidmeier SE, Orsmond GS: Resurgence of acute rheumatic fever in the intermountain area of the United States. *N Engl J Med* 316:421, 1987.
46. Wald ER, Dashefsky B, Feidt C, et al: Acute rheumatic fever in western Pennsylvania and the tristate area. *Pediatrics* 80:371, 1987.
47. Randolph MF, Gerber MA, DeMeo KK, et al: Effect of antibiotic therapy on the clinical course of streptococcal pharyngitis. *J Pediatr* 106:870, 1985.
48. Lieu TA, Fleisher GR, Schwartz JS: Cost-effectiveness of rapid latex agglutination testing and throat culture for streptococcal pharyngitis. *Pediatrics* 85:246, 1990.
49. American Academy of Pediatrics: Group A streptococcal infections, in Peter G (ed): *1997 Red Book: Report of the Committee on Infectious Diseases,* 24th ed. Elk Grove Village, IL, American Academy of Pediatrics, 1997, pp 483–494.
50. Pichichero ME, Disney FA, Talpey WE: Adverse and beneficial effects of immediate treatment of group A beta-hemolytic streptococcal pharyngitis with penicillin. *Pediatr Infect Dis J* 6:635, 1987.
51. Gerber MA, Randolph MF, DeMeo KK, et al: Lack of impact of early antibiotic treatment for streptococcal pharyngitis on recurrence rates. *J Pediatr* 117:853, 1990.
52. Paradise JL, Bluestone CD, Bachman RZ: Efficacy of tonsillectomy for recurrent throat infection in severely affected children. *N Engl J Med* 310:674, 1984.
53. Gerber MA, Randolph MF, Martin NF, et al: Community wide outbreak of group G streptococcal pharyngitis. *Pediatrics* 87:598, 1991.
54. Turner JC, Fox A, Fox K, et al: Role of group C beta-hemolytic streptococci in pharyngitis: Epidemiologic study of clinical features associated with isolation of group C streptococci. *J Clin Microbiol* 31:808, 1993.
55. Meier FA, Centor RM, Graham L, et al: Clinical and microbiological evidence for endemic pharyngitis among adults due to group C streptococci. *Ann Intern Med* 150:825, 1990.
56. Gnann JW, Gray BM, Griffin FM, et al: Acute glomerulonephritis following group G streptococcal infection. *J Infect Dis* 156:411, 1987.
57. Davies HD, McGeer A, Schwartz B, et al: Invasive group A streptococcal infections in Ontario, Canada. *N Engl J Med* 335:547, 1996.
58. Cockerill FR, MacDonald KL, Thompson RL: An outbreak of invasive group A streptococcal disease associated with high carriage rates of the invasive clone among school-aged children. *JAMA* 277:38, 1997.
59. Stevens DL: Invasive group A streptococcal infections: The past, present, and future. *Pediatr Infect Dis J* 13:561, 1994.

SKIN AND SOFT TISSUE INFECTIONS

Richard Malley

This chapter discusses several of the more common skin and soft tissue infections of childhood, including conjunctivitis, impetigo, sinusitis, and cellulitis. Because of its particular severity, orbital/periorbital cellulitis will be highlighted in a section separate from the general discussion of cellulitis; however, the pathophysiology and clinical manifestations that are shared will not be repeated.

CONJUNCTIVITIS

Definition

Conjunctivitis is an inflammation of the conjunctivae, the membranes that line the surface of the eye. This inflammation may be the result of infection, allergy, or mechanical or chemical irritation. Keratoconjunctivitis involves the cornea as well as the conjunctivae.

Etiology

The etiology of infectious conjunctivitis differs between the newborn and the older child (Table 117-1). In the newborn, pathogens that reside in the birth canal play a major role in ocular infections. *Chlamydia trachomatis* is the most frequent, but *Neisseria gonorrhoeae* poses the greatest threat to the integrity of the eye. Later in childhood, the respiratory tract pathogens predominate, particularly *Hemophilus* species. Trachoma, a recurrent chlamydial conjunctivitis seen in tropical regions, will not be discussed.

Epidemiology

Conjunctivitis is the most common ocular infection of childhood. It may occur at any age. Neonates acquire most infections during passage through colonized birth canals; in older children, respiratory tract

TABLE 117-1 Etiology of Infectious Conjunctivitis

Frequency	Neonate	Child
Very frequent	*Chlamydia trachomatis*	Adenoviruses *Hemophilus* species
Moderately frequent	*Streptococcus pneumoniae* *Streptococcus fecalis* (enterococcus) *Neisseria gonorrhoeae*	*Streptococcus pneumoniae*
Infrequent	*Hemophilus influenzae* Herpes simplex *Staphylococcus aureus*	*Neisseria gonorrhoeae* *Neisseria meningitidis* *Chlamydia trachomatis* Herpes simplex *Staphylococcus aureus* *Corynebacterium diphtheriae*

pathogens spread from person to person. Conjunctivitis is usually a sporadic disease, but epidemics of viral illness may occur.

Pathophysiology

Pathogens introduced into the conjunctival sac may proliferate and produce hyperemia and an inflammatory exudate. This exudate may be purulent, fibrinous, or serosanguineous. With certain organisms, corneal involvement (keratitis) also may occur.

Clinical Features

Older children with conjunctivitis may complain of photophobia, ocular pain or pruritus, a sensation of a foreign body in the eye, crusting of the eyelids, or conjunctival erythema. Infants and young children are usually brought by their parents for ''pink eye'' or crusting. The duration of symptoms with infectious conjunctivitis is most often 2 to 4 days but may be longer in cases which are untreated or resistant to therapy.

As with any ocular complaint, the physician should perform a thorough examination of the structure and function of both eyes, including, when age appropriate, examination of visual acuity, visual fields by confrontation, extraocular muscle function, periorbital area, eyelids (with eversion), conjunctivae, cornea with fluorescein staining, pupillary reflex, anterior chamber, and fundus. Erythema and increased secretions characterize conjunctivitis. Chemosis may be seen. Intense erythema and purulent discharge are more common with an infectious rather than an allergic cause. The cornea does not stain with fluorescein in children with conjunctivitis unless an associated keratitis has developed, as with herpes simplex or adenoviruses. Most importantly, visual acuity is normal.

Fever and/or other systemic symptoms do not occur with isolated conjunctivitis. However, conjunctivitis may be only one manifestation of a viral upper respiratory tract infection, in which case the temperature may be elevated.

Diagnosis

The diagnosis of infectious conjunctivitis rests primarily on the clinical examination. A Gram stain, which should be performed in neonates or in confusing cases, usually shows more than five white blood cells per oil immersion field and, in many cases, bacteria. The finding of gram-negative intracellular diplococci presumptively identifies *N. gonorrhoeae* in the first few weeks of life. Conjunctival scrapings and/or cultures may be performed in selected circumstances to diagnose *C. trachomatis* or specific viral and bacterial pathogens.

Differential Diagnosis

The differential diagnosis of the ''red (or pink) eye'' includes conjunctivitis, orbital/periorbital infection, foreign body, corneal abrasion, uveitis, and glaucoma. Periorbital and orbital infections cause obvious swelling and tenderness around the eye and/or loss of ocular mobility. Foreign bodies should be visible on direct examination, often only following eversion of the upper eyelid. Thus the differential diagnosis usually revolves around four conditions: conjunctivitis, corneal abrasion, uveitis, and glaucoma (Table 117-2). Both uveitis and glaucoma are uncommon. The erythema in these conditions is concentrated around the limbus, and the discharge consists primarily of tears. Additionally, the vision is decreased in glaucoma, and the cornea may be cloudy. A corneal abrasion is easily identified by the uptake of fluorescein.

Finally, conjunctivitis may be only one manifestation of a systemic disorder, such as measles and Kawasaki disease.

Complications

Conjunctivitis is generally self-limited, with the notable exceptions of herpes simplex and *N. gonorrhoeae.* The potential complications are corneal ulceration and scar formation leading to visual impairment.

Treatment

Bacterial and viral conjunctivitides are far and away the most common cause for the complaint of a red eye in childhood. Once the diagnosis of conjunctivitis is established on the basis of diffuse injection, purulent

TABLE 117-2 Differential Diagnosis of the ''Red Eye''

	Conjunctivitis	Corneal Abrasion	Uveitis	Glaucoma
History	URI	Trauma, contact lens	JRA, sarcoid, trauma	Prematurity, Marfan's syndrome, homocystinuria
Visual acuity	Normal	Normal or decreased	Normal or decreased	Decreased
Ocular exam				
External	Watery or purulent discharge	Watery discharge	Watery discharge	Watery discharge
Cornea	Usually normal; staining if keratitis	Staining	Normal or band keratopathy	Cloudy, staining
Anterior chamber	Normal	Normal	Cells, hypopyon, hyphema	Normal or shallow
Pupil	Normal	Normal	Small	Fixed
Intraocular pressure	Normal	Normal	Variable	Increased

Abbreviations: URI, upper respiratory infection; JRA, juvenile rheumatoid arthritis.

TABLE 117-3 Differential Diagnosis of Allergic and Infectious Conjunctivitis

	Allergic	Infectious
History		
Pruritus	Yes	No
Chronic	Yes	No
Recurrent	Yes	No
Seasonal	Yes	No
Sneezing, rhinorrhea	Yes	Variable
Exam		
Discharge	Watery	Watery or purulent
Chemosis	Present	Usually absent
Fluorescein	Negative	Negative, except keratitis
Lab		
Gram stain	Negative	White cells, bacteria

TABLE 117-4 Treatment of Conjunctivitis by Pathogen

Viruses	
Herpes simplex	Trifluridine, vidarabine, or acyclovir, topically (neonates may also have systemic infection)
Other	Supportive
Chlamydia	
Chlamydia trachomatis	Erythromycin, 50 mg/kg per day orally, for 14 days
Bacteria	
Neisseria gonorrhoeae	Child: ceftriaxone 125 mg IM or IV Adult: ceftriaxone 250 mg IM or IV
Neisseria meningitidis	Child: penicillin, 50,000 units/kg/day, IV, for 7 days Adult: penicillin, 10 million units/day, IV, for 5 days
Hemophilus influenzae, Streptococcus pneumoniae, and others	Topical antibiotic ointments: sulfonamide, erythromycin, etc.

discharge, and normal vision, infectious and noninfectious causes are next separated. Allergic conjunctivitis is usually distinguished by chronicity, seasonality, pruritus, and associated symptoms of allergic rhinitis; if the physician is uncertain, a Gram stain should be done (Table 117-3).

In approaching infectious conjunctivitis (Fig. 117-1), the physician must decide whether the ocular disorder is one manifestation of a systemic illness such as measles or is occurring in relative isolation. Isolated conjunctivitis may be due to various viruses and bacteria, of which herpes simplex and *N. gonorrhoeae* are particularly severe, or to *C. trachomatis,* especially in the first 3 months of life.

Fluorescein staining always should be performed in an effort to identify the dendritic corneal ulcerations characteristic of herpetic disease. If they are identified, treatment is with acyclovir or other antiviral agents under the supervision of an ophthalmologist. Because *N. gonorrhoeae* is usually acquired during passage through the birth canal, infants under 1 month of age must always be tested for this pathogen with a Gram stain and culture. If gram-negative intracellular diplococci are seen on smear, a single intramuscular injection of ceftriaxone (125 mg) is indicated.[1]

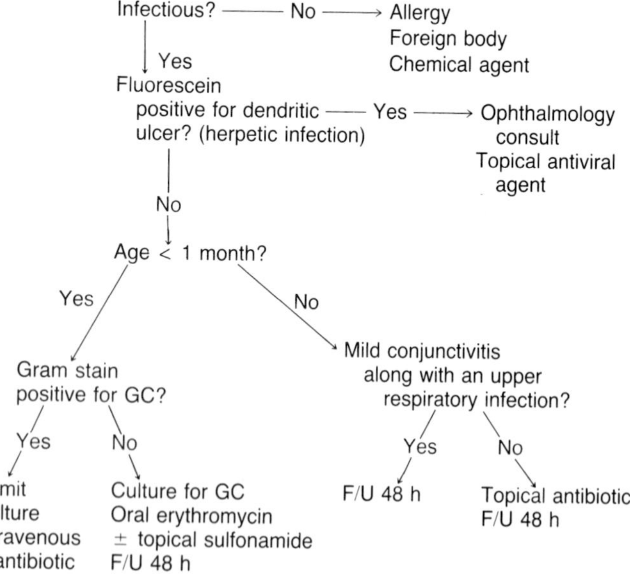

FIG. 117-1. Approach to the child with an isolated, infectious conjunctivitis. *Abbreviations:* F/U, follow-up; GC, gonorrhea culture.

Infants beyond 1 month of age and older children with an obvious clinical diagnosis of conjunctivitis do not routinely require smears or cultures. In patients under 3 months of age, treatment is instituted with erythromycin (50 mg/kg/day) orally for *C. trachomatis* (Table 117-4). Older children require only topical antibiotic instillation into the conjunctival sac. A child who has unusually severe disease or who fails to respond to therapy within 48 h may benefit from a laboratory investigation. Appropriate studies in the infant under 1 month of age would include a Gram stain and bacterial culture and either a scraping or culture for *C. trachomatis.* Older children require only a Gram stain and bacterial culture. Diagnostic tests for herpes simplex are not usually rewarding in the absence of corneal ulceration; culture for adenoviruses may be helpful in persistent or severe hemorrhagic infections to avoid unnecessary additional testing, but there is no specific treatment. All children with conjunctivitis should be reevaluated within 48 h. Failure to improve warrants further investigation and continued, careful follow-up.

IMPETIGO

Definition

Impetigo is a superficial bacterial infection of the skin confined to the epidermis. Deeper spread to the dermis leads to ecthyma. There are two varieties of impetigo: impetigo contagiosa and bullous impetigo.

Etiology

Traditionally, group A β-hemolytic streptococcus (GABHS) was considered the major pathogen in impetigo contagiosa. However, recent studies have suggested that *Staphylococcus aureus* often can be the primary infecting agent and that therapy which does not include coverage for this organism is significantly less effective. In particular, in bullous impetigo, the primary pathogen is *S. aureus.*[2]

Epidemiology

Impetigo is the most common skin infection seen in the emergency department. The prevalence is greatest in young children, particularly those under the age of 6 years. Impetigo may occur sporadically or, occasionally, in epidemics. Conditions favoring epidemic spread include warm weather, overcrowding, and poor hygiene. Bullous impetigo is less common than impetigo contagiosa.

Pathophysiology

The intact epidermis forms a relatively impervious barrier to bacteria. The development of impetigo follows a breach in the integument; this may be an obvious abrasion or an inconspicuous insect bite. Bacteria then invade the skin and elaborate toxins, such as streptolysins, which promote local spread.

Clinical Features

The chief complaint of children with impetigo is most often that of sores on the body. There are no associated systemic manifestations such as fever or malaise. Regional lymph nodes may be minimally enlarged.

The typical lesion of impetigo contagiosa begins as an erythematous papule. Small vesicles may follow transiently, but rapid progression to crusted lesions occurs. These crusts, which are initially honey-colored and fine in consistency, may appear on any area of the body; between the upper lip and the nose is a very characteristic site. The lesions enlarge over days to weeks, and the crusts become thicker. Erythema is mild. No induration is present.

In bullous impetigo, the characteristic skin lesions are superficial bullae filled with purulent material. The bullae range in size from 0.5 to 3 cm and have minimal, if any, surrounding erythema.

Diagnosis

The diagnosis of impetigo rests with the visual appearance of the lesions. Rarely are laboratory tests needed.

In cases where the diagnosis of impetigo is uncertain, Gram stain of the lesions is helpful, showing abundant polymorphonuclear leukocytes and gram-positive bacteria. Local culture may be obtained from patients whose disease does not respond to standard therapy. If performed, the peripheral white blood cell count is normal.

Differential Diagnosis

Several dermatologic disorders may resemble either impetigo contagiosa or bullous impetigo. These include tinea corporis, nummular eczema, small burns or abrasions, allergic contact dermatitis, eczema herpeticum (with underlying atopic dermatitis), and scalded skin syndrome.

Complications

Impetigo may spread locally or, in the case of streptococcal infections, lead to remote, nonsuppurative sequelae. Occasionally, impetigo may progress to cellulitis or lead to lymphadenitis in the regional nodes. The attack rate for acute poststreptococcal glomerulonephritis has been as high as 1 percent in certain epidemics; however, the disease is unusual following sporadic skin infections.

Treatment

The treatment of impetigo is oral antibiotic therapy or an appropriate topical antibiotic for limited eruptions. A first generation oral cephalosporin such as cephalexin (50 mg/kg/day) or erythromycin (50 mg/kg/day) provides effective oral therapy. Mupirocin is the only topical agent with proven efficacy.[3] Combination topical and systemic therapy is unnecessary. Vigorous scrubbing, in addition to topical or systemic antibiotic agents, offers no advantage; routine cleanliness is sufficient.

Antibiotic therapy hastens the resolution of impetigo and limits suppurative complications. Although the incidence of glomerulonephritis may be reduced, it has not been possible to demonstrate this effect with certainty in clinical studies due to the low incidence of this disease.

SINUSITIS

Definition

Sinusitis is an inflammation of the paranasal sinuses: maxillary, ethmoid, frontal, or sphenoid. This inflammation may be on the basis of infection or allergy; it may be acute, subacute, or chronic.

Etiology

The major pathogens in acute bacterial sinusitis in childhood are *Streptococcus pneumoniae, Moraxella catarrhalis,* and nontypable *Hemophilus influenzae.*[4] The incidence of *H. influenzae* sinusitis in children would be expected to decline with Hib vaccination.[5] Other potential etiologic agents found in a minority of infections include group A streptococcus, group C streptococcus, α-hemolytic streptococcus, and *Peptostreptococcus.* Similar clinical investigations in adults have been in general agreement, finding nontypable *H. influenzae* and *S. pneumoniae* in 60 to 70 percent of the cases. Although *S. aureus* and anaerobic organisms are isolated occasionally, they rarely play a role in acute infections in childhood. Severe sinusitis is not a common illness in children, but mild or subacute disease may occur more frequently.

Pathophysiology

The ethmoid and maxillary sinuses are present at birth, but the frontal and sphenoid sinuses do not become aerated until 6 or 7 years of age. The sinuses are lined primarily by ciliated columnar epithelium and connect with the nasopharynx via narrow ostia. Normally, the epithelium is coated by a double layer of mucus: a viscid gel layer superficially and a more fluid layer underneath. Resistance to infection depends on the patency of the ostia, the function of the ciliary mechanism, and the quality of the secretions.

Obstruction of the ostia results either from mucosal swelling or, less commonly, mechanical obstruction. By far the most frequent offenders are viral upper respiratory infection and allergic inflammation. Less common causes include cystic fibrosis, trauma, choanal atresia, deviated septum, polyps, foreign body, and tumor.

Factors that impair normal mucociliary function include viral infections, cold or dry air, certain chemicals or drugs, and, rarely, inborn errors of motility. Alterations of the mucus occur in asthma and cystic fibrosis.

The bacteria that cause sinusitis often colonize the nasopharynx of healthy children. Disruptions in one or more of the barriers described above allow these organisms to ascend through the ostia and multiply within the sinuses.

Clinical Features

The spectrum of sinusitis has not been completely defined as it relates to clinical manifestations. However, there are two major types of infection which can usually be distinguished on clinical grounds: acute, severe sinusitis, and mild, subacute sinusitis (Table 117-5).

Acute, severe infections of the sinuses are infrequent during childhood. Such patients often have a history of headache and an elevated temperature. Findings include fever, localized swelling and/or erythema, and facial tenderness. A mucopurulent discharge usually accompanies severe sinusitis but may also indicate a nasal foreign body when unilateral.

Mild, subacute sinusitis is encountered more commonly than the severe form during childhood. This type of infection usually manifests

TABLE 117-5 Signs and Symptoms in Children with Sinusitis

	Acute, Severe Disease	Mild, Subacute Disease
Headache	+++	++
Fever	+++	+
Facial tenderness	++	—
Facial swelling	++	—
Nasal discharge	+++	++++

TABLE 117-6 Antibiotic Therapy for Sinusitis

	Acute, Severe Sinusitis	Mild, Subacute Sinusitis
Initial	Cefuroxime, 100 mg/kg/day IV *or* Ceftriaxone, 75 mg/kg/day IV *or* Ampicillin-sulbactam, 200 mg/kg of ampicillin/day IV	Amoxicillin, 40 mg/kg/day PO
Persistent	Antibiotics as above plus surgical drainage	Cefprozil, 30 mg/kg/day PO *or* Erythromycin-sulfisoxazole; 40 mg/kg/day of erythromycin PO
Penicillin allergic	Cefuroxime, 100 mg/kg/day IV	As for persistent cases

as a protracted ''cold.'' Rather than improving in 3 to 7 days, these children persist with the symptoms of an upper respiratory infection beyond 2 weeks. They have a nasal discharge, which may be serous or mucopurulent. Fever is infrequent.

Bacterial infection of the sinuses must be contrasted with congestion of brief duration found in association with some viral upper respiratory infections. Such congestion per se does not constitute a purulent infection.

Diagnosis

The diagnosis of sinusitis is usually made on clinical grounds without any laboratory or radiographic studies. In older children and adolescents, transillumination of the maxillary or frontal sinuses may provide assistance.

Standard radiographs, including anteroposterior, lateral, and occipitomental views should be obtained in patients with an uncertain clinical diagnosis and in cases of severe sinusitis. The most diagnostic findings for purulence are an air-fluid level or complete opacification. Mucosal thickening greater than 4 mm is usually indicative of infection but may accompany viral upper respiratory disease, particularly in the first year of life. A normal radiograph suggests, but does not prove, that a sinus is free of disease.

Several studies have shown that ultrasonography may be useful for the diagnosis of sinusitis, but there is not sufficient experience to recommend this modality for routine use. The anatomy of the paranasal sinuses is superbly defined by computed tomography (CT). However, the cost of CT does not justify its substitution for plain radiography, except in cases where complications are suspected.

Ultimate confirmation of infection within the paranasal sinuses rests with demonstration of organisms by Gram stain and quantitative culture of aspirated secretions. Aspiration is not routinely indicated but can be performed in selected cases of maxillary sinusitis in the outpatient setting via the intranasal route. Appropriate circumstances for aspiration include (1) life-threatening complications, (2) immunosuppressive conditions, (3) clinical unresponsiveness, and (4) unusually severe disease. The presence of organisms on Gram stain and a count of at least 10^4 colony-forming units point to bacterial infection.[4]

Differential Diagnosis

Sinusitis may cause local swelling, facial pain, or nasal discharge. Other causes of swelling include superficial infection (cellulitis), trauma, cold injury, and allergic edema. Facial pain may be neurogenic, odontogenic, or related to the temporomandibular joint. Nasal discharge, particularly unilateral, should lead to a suspicion of a foreign body within the nares.

Complications

The proximity of the paranasal sinuses to the brain sets the scene for the occurrence of life-threatening complications from sinusitis; however, the use of antibiotics has reduced the incidence of such complications. Infection may spread from the sinuses to surrounding structures through the diploic veins, which have no valves, or by erosion through bone.

The most commonly encountered complications are periorbital cellulitis and orbital cellulitis/abscess. Periorbital infection causes swelling around the eye, while intraorbital accumulation of pus may be recognized on the basis of proptosis and decreased ocular motion. Infection may also produce osteomyelitis of the surrounding bone; in the frontal region this is referred to as Pott's puffy tumor. Less commonly, complications follow intracranial extension and may include epidural, subdural, or brain abscess; meningitis; and cavernous sinus thrombosis. Meningitis rarely follows sinusitis; it more commonly occurs after bacteremia. Focal intracranial involvement can be demonstrated by CT.

Treatment

In deciding on appropriate therapy, the first step is to differentiate bacterial sinusitis from nasal congestion accompanying viral upper respiratory tract disease. Although the latter resolves spontaneously or may be treated with decongestants, sinusitis requires therapy with antibiotics (Table 117-6). Mild, subacute infections respond well to oral therapy for 10 to 14 days; as for otitis media, amoxicillin (40 mg/kg/day) remains the first-choice antimicrobial (Fig. 117-2). Failure to improve with amoxicillin therapy suggests infection with pathogens

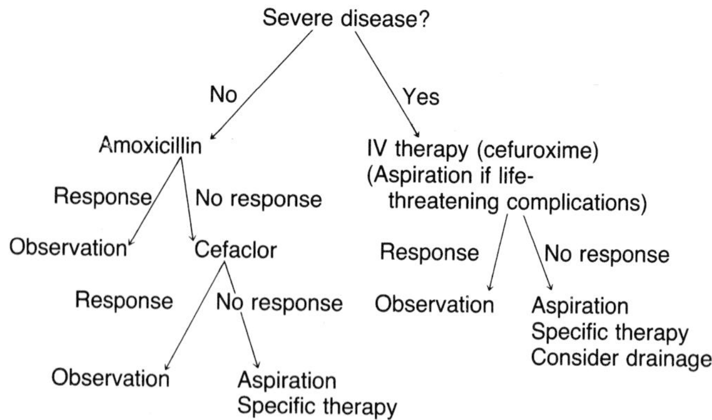

FIG. 117-2. Approach to sinusitis in the immunocompetent child.

TABLE 117-7 Etiology of Cellulitis

	Most Likely	Less Likely
	IMMUNOCOMPETENT HOST	
Trunk/extremity	*S. aureus* *Streptococcus pyogenes*	*H. influenzae*
Face* (periorbital/buccal); unimmunized	*H. influenzae*	*S. aureus* *S. pneumoniae*
Face* (periorbital/buccal); immunized	*S. aureus* *S. pneumoniae*	*H. Influenzae*
Any site/animal bite	*S. aureus*	*Pasteurella multocida*
Any site/human bite	Anaerobic organisms	*S. aureus*
	IMMUNOCOMPROMISED HOST	
Any site	*S. aureus,* gram-negative rods	Anaerobic organisms

* Definitive epidemiology awaits further studies since the advent of the widespread immunization against *H. influenzae* type B.

that are often resistant to this drug, such as *M. catarrhalis* or *H. influenzae,* or perhaps with penicillin-resistant *S. pneumoniae.* A second course of treatment with erythromycin/sulfisoxazole, newer oral second and third generation cephalosporins such as cefprozil or cefpodoxime, or amoxicillin-clavulanic acid should then be instituted; aspiration for culture may be useful for those patients in whom the infection still persists after a second course of therapy.

Acute, severe sinusitis may result in life-threatening complications and requires intravenous antibiotic therapy directed at *S. pneumoniae,* amoxicillin-resistant *H. influenzae,* and less commonly *S. aureus.* Cefuroxime (100 mg/kg/day) and ceftriaxone (75 mg/kg/day) represent single-drug regimens effective for this disease; ampicillin-sulbactam (200 mg/kg/day) is an alternative for the nonallergic patient. Failure of severe disease to respond promptly to antibiotic therapy or the occurrence of complications indicates the need for surgical consultation in regard to drainage procedures.

CELLULITIS

Definition

Cellulitis is an infection of the skin and subcutaneous tissues. It extends below the dermis, differentiating it from impetigo, but does not involve muscle (pyogenic myositis) or bone (osteomyelitis). Any region of the body may be involved, but two divisions are important in regard to predicting the most likely pathogens: (1) the trunk and extremities and (2) the face (buccal and periorbital cellulitis).

Etiology

The organisms that play an important role in the immunocompetent host under normal circumstances include *S. aureus, S. pyogenes* (group A β-hemolytic streptococcus), and *H. influenzae* (Table 117-7). In general, *S. aureus* is the most common and *H. influenzae* the least among the three major pathogens, particularly in children immunized against *H. influenzae* type B.[5] However, in certain anatomic locations, particularly for young or unimmunized children, *H. influenzae* remains an important consideration. Additionally, unusual organisms may cause cellulitis in immunocompromised hosts or following their introduction in special types of wounds (Table 117-7).

Epidemiology

Cellulitis is a frequent infection, particularly in the warm weather. The precise incidence is unknown; however, in a study at an urban children's hospital, this infection accounted for 1 of every 500 visits. Children of any age may develop cellulitis, but, as noted above, disease due to *H. influenzae* has become rare, affecting mainly infants under the age of 6 months.

Pathophysiology

Cellulitis may occur either when a pathogen is directly inoculated into the subcutaneous tissue or following an episode of bacteremia. The majority of infections involve local invasion after a breach in the integument. The organisms responsible are usually *S. aureus* and *S. pyogenes.* In contradistinction, *H. influenzae* disseminates hematogenously.

Clinical Features

The child with cellulitis manifests a local inflammatory response at the site of the infection, including erythema, edema, warmth, and tenderness. There may be a history of a preceding wound or a complaint related to loss of function, such as limp with an infection of a lower extremity. Fever is unusual except in infections due to *H. influenzae* (Table 117-8).

Inspection of the area of cellulitis usually shows intense erythema. A violaceous hue suggests *H. influenzae* but has been reported with other pathogens including *S. pneumoniae.* Red streaks may radiate proximally along the course of the lymphatic drainage, and the regional nodes may enlarge.

Diagnosis

The diagnosis of cellulitis is made by inspection. Laboratory studies including a WBC count, blood culture, and aspirate culture are obtained for specific indications: immunocompromise, fever, severe local infection, facial involvement, and failure to respond to therapy.

The WBC count is normal in most cases of infection due to *S. aureus* or *S. pyogenes,*, which are locally invasive. On the other hand, cellulitis due to *H. influenzae* results from bacteremia and is usually accompanied by a polymorphonuclear leukocytosis. In one study of children with cellulitis, the WBC count was over 15,000/μL in 3 of 4 children infected with *H. influenzae,* and 0 of 19 infected with *S. aureus* or *S. pyogenes.*[6] Among 194 patients with *H. influenzae* cellulitis reported in the literature as reviewed in 1983, the WBC count was greater than 15,000/μL in 84 percent, with a mean of 20,850/μL.[7]

TABLE 117-8 Usual Clinical and Laboratory Features of Children with Cellulitis

Characteristic	*H. influenzae*	*S. aureus*
Age	$<$3 yrs	Any
Fever	Yes	No
Color of lesion	Violaceous	Erythematous
Location	Cheek, periorbital	Trunk, extremity
Preceding wound	No	Yes
WBC count	$>$15,000/μL	$<$15,000/μL
Bacteremia	Yes	No

The blood culture is usually negative in infections due to *S. aureus* and *S. pyogenes*. On the other hand, *H. influenzae* as a rule causes a bacteremic infection.

Aspirate cultures are best obtained close to the center of an infected lesion, as the periphery may consist primarily of edema fluid devoid of organisms. The needle should be sufficiently large to permit the evacuation of purulent material—22 gauge for the face and 19 gauge for the trunk and extremities. Using a 5- or 10-mL syringe prefilled with 1 mL of sterile, nonbacteriostatic saline, the needle is directed into the subcutaneous tissue to a depth of approximately 0.5 to 1.0 cm, and aspiration is attempted. If there is no return, the saline is injected and reaspirated. The material obtained is used for culture and Gram stain.

Differential Diagnosis

Cellulitis must be differentiated from other causes of erythema and edema, including trauma and allergic reaction. Allergic edema is not tender and usually only mildly erythematous. Traumatic lesions may be easily distinguished when there is a history of injury and absence of fever. Cold injury, especially on the cheeks (''popsicle panniculitis''), may be confused with cellulitis.

Complications

Cellulitis due to *S. aureus* and *S. pyogenes* may at times spread locally or involve the regional lymph nodes; distant foci occur only rarely. Bacteremic *H. influenzae* infections are more likely to spread hematogenously, involving the central nervous system, epiglottis, joints, or pericardium.

Treatment

The treatment of cellulitis is the administration of systemic antibiotic therapy. Although most patients respond rapidly to oral antistaphylococcal agents, the clinician must identify those individuals who require broad-spectrum or intravenously administered drugs (Fig. 117-3).

Obviously, signs of sepsis are indicative of hematogenous dissemination and demand treatment as an inpatient. Additionally, children under 6 months of age and those with impaired immunity are unable to contain local bacterial infections and will benefit from intravenous therapy.

Among otherwise healthy children over 6 months of age, only those who are clinically ill-appearing, or in whom bacteremic disease is suspected, need to be admitted to the hospital. Prior to the advent of the *Hemophilus* vaccine, physicians could identify patients at risk for invasive *H. influenzae* disease fairly reliably on the basis of anatomic location, presence of fever, and a WBC count greater than 15,000/μL. Although the incidence of this disease has dropped considerably, it is important to remember that young infants are still at some risk of being infected with this organism.

The usual therapy for patients discharged from the emergency department is an antistaphylococcal antibiotic, such as dicloxacillin or cephalexin. Broad-spectrum therapy is recommended presumptively for patients who are immunocompromised or suspected to have bacteremia, pending a definitive isolate (Table 117-9).

PERIORBITAL/ORBITAL CELLULITIS

Definition

Cellulitis as previously defined may involve the tissues anterior to the orbital septum (periorbital cellulitis) or within the orbit (orbital cellulitis).

Etiology

S. aureus, S. pneumoniae, and *H. influenzae* are the principal etiologic agents. Orbital infections are most often caused by *S. aureus.*

Epidemiology

Children under the age of 3 years are more likely to become bacteremic than those who are older; thus, they experience the highest incidence of periorbital disease. Orbital cellulitis may occur at any age.

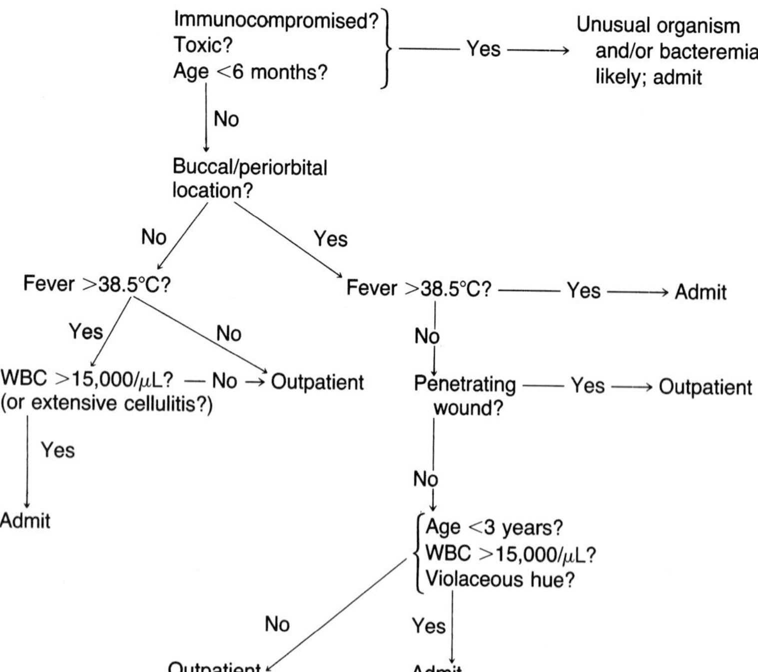

FIG. 117-3. Approach to the child with cellulitis.

TABLE 117-9 Initial Antibiotic Therapy for Cellulitis

	Drug	Dose
Presumptive immunocompetent		
Extremity or buccal/periorbital		
Afebrile	Dicloxacillin	50–100 mg/kg/day PO
	or	
	Cephalexin	50–100 mg/kg/day PO
Febrile/leukocytosis	Ampicillin/sulbactam	200 mg/kg as ampicillin/day IV
	or	
	Cefuroxime	100 mg/kg/day IV
	or	
	Ceftriaxone	75 mg/kg/day IV
Immunocompromised		
Any site	Oxacillin	150 mg/kg/day IV
	or	
	Cefazolin	100 mg/kg/day IV
	and	
	Gentamicin	5–7.5 mg/kg/day IV
	or	
	Tobramycin	5–7.5 mg/kg/day IV
Specific organism		
Streptococcus pyogenes	Penicillin	100,000 units/kg/day PO *or* IV
Staphylococcus aureus	Dicloxacillin	50–100 mg/kg/day PO
	or	
	Oxacillin	150 mg/kg/day IV
Haemophilus influenzae		
Ampicillin-sensitive	Ampicillin	200 mg/kg/day IV
Ampicillin-resistant	Cefuroxime	100 mg/kg/day IV
	or	
	Ceftriaxone	75 mg/kg/day IV

Pathophysiology

Organisms reach the periorbital area either hematogenously or by direct extension from the ethmoid sinus. In the case of orbital disease, contiguous spread is most common.

Clinical Features

Orbital and periorbital cellulitis cause the periorbital area to appear red and swollen. The periorbital edema is usually more prominent with preseptal infections. Proptosis or limitation of extraocular muscle function indicates orbital involvement. Fever is more common with periorbital cellulitis.

Diagnosis

Periorbital and orbital cellulitis are distinguished from noninfectious disorders on the basis of the clinical findings and the WBC count. Leukocytosis occurs frequently with cellulitis, more often with bacteremic preseptal infections. A blood culture is often positive.

CT is performed when orbital involvement is likely. An inflammatory mass is easily demonstrated when present using this modality.

Differential Diagnosis

As for cellulitis in other regions, allergic and traumatic causes for edema must be considered. Additionally, tumors and metabolic disease may cause swelling, discoloration, and/or proptosis. Thyrotoxicosis usually occurs in adolescents. The most likely tumor is metastatic neuroblastoma. Pseudotumor occurs rarely.

Complications

Periorbital cellulitis may serve as a focus for metastatic bacterial disease; of particular concern is the occurrence of meningitis. Orbital cellulitis may evolve into a subperiosteal abscess; this condition threatens the integrity of the eye and should be considered a surgical emergency. Intracranial extension may occur rarely.

Treatment

Admission and treatment with intravenous antibiotics is the rule. Blood cultures should always be done, and an aspirate culture is indicated for any ill child. In a child under 6 months of age, strong consideration of a lumbar puncture is indicated whenever infection with *H. influenzae* is suspected. Beyond 6 months of age, in the immunized child, although the possibility of meningitis remains, a decision regarding a lumbar puncture can be based on the clinical status and examination of the patient. Presumptive therapy of periorbital or orbital cellulitis is directed against *S. aureus* and *H. influenzae* (Table 117-9). Surgical drainage may be necessary with abscess formation or sinusitis.

REFERENCES

1. Laga M, Naamara W, Brunham RC, et al: Single-dose therapy of gonococcal ophthalmia neonatorum with ceftriaxone. *N Engl J Med* 315:1382, 1986.
2. Sadick NS: Current aspects of bacterial infections of the skin. *Derm Clin* 15(2):341–349, 1997.
3. Barton LL, Friedman AD, Sharkey AM, et al: Impetigo contagiosa: III. Comparative efficacy of oral erythromycin and topical mupirocin. *Pediatr Dermatol* 6:134, 1989.
4. Bussey MF, Moon RY: Acute sinusitis. *Pediatr Rev* 20(4):142, 1999.

5. Adams WG, Deaver KA, Cochi SL, et al: Decline of childhood *Hemophilus influenzae* type b (Hib) disease in the Hib vaccine era (see comments). *JAMA* 269:221, 1993.
6. Fleisher G, Ludwig S, Henretig F, et al: Cellulitis: Initial management. *Ann Emerg Med* 10:356, 1981.
7. Fleisher G, Heeger P, Topf P: *Hemophilus influenzae* cellulitis. *Am J Emerg Med* 1:274, 1983.

BACTEREMIA, SEPSIS, AND MENINGITIS IN CHILDREN

Peter Mellis

For emergency physicians who frequently care for young children, the identification and treatment of potentially life-threatening systemic infectious disease represents a continuing challenge. Although most children have either self-limited viral or minor focal bacterial infection, a subset will have serious bacterial disease with potential for morbidity and mortality. This chapter provides an overview of the presentation and management of bacteremia, sepsis, and meningitis in pediatric patients in the ED. Although each is discussed separately, it must be kept in mind that these entities represent different points along a spectrum and may occur concurrently as a result of progression of disease.

BACTEREMIA AND SERIOUS BACTERIAL INFECTION

Pathophysiology

Children between the ages of birth and 3 years old are at relatively increased risk for bloodborne bacterial disease due to immaturity of the reticuloendothelial system. The term *bacteremia* refers to the presence of a positive blood culture without reference to specific clinical symptomatology. Bacteremia may resolve spontaneously, progress to *septicemia,* or be associated with focal *serious bacterial infection* (SBI), most often involving the meninges, lung, kidney, bowel, bone, or joint.

The risk of bacteremia decreases with age, with the highest incidence in the first 3 months of life (Table 118-1). Neonates with fever, defined as a rectal temperature of 38.0°C or higher, have a 5 percent risk for bacteremia and 15 percent incidence of SBI due to pathogens encountered at the time of birth.[1–3] Bacteremia in this age group either results in a fulminant septicemic process within hours to days of birth (*early-onset disease*) or a focal SBI developing weeks to months later (*late-onset disease*). Group B *Streptococcus* is by far the most common bacterial pathogen in this age group, followed by *Escherichia coli, Listeria monocytogenes,* and *Enterococcus* sp. Infants aged 30 to 90 days are at a progressively lesser risk for late-onset infection from these neonatally acquired pathogens but are increasingly susceptible to community-acquired pathogens. This age group thus represents a transition period from neonates and those infants aged 3 months and older.

TABLE 118-1 Age-Related Risk Groups and Causes of Bacteremia in Children

Group	Risk	Pathogens
Neonates	High risk	Group B *Streptococcus* *Escherichia coli* *Listeria monocytogenes* *Enterococcus* sp.
Young infants 30–90 days	Intermediate risk	Neonatal pathogens (above) Community-acquired pathogens (below)
Older infants 3–36 months	Low risk	*Streptococcus pneumoniae* *Neisseria meningitidis* *Haemophilus influenzae* b (unimmunized) Group A *Streptococcus* *Escherichia coli* (pyelonephritis) *Salmonella* sp. (gastroenteritis) *Staphylococcus aureus* (osteomyelitis)

TABLE 118-2 Serious Bacterial Infections Associated with Bacteremia

Meningitis
Pneumonia
Pyelonephritis
Bacterial enteritis
Facial cellulitis
Septic arthritis
Osteomyelitis

Children aged 3 months and older are susceptible to infection from community-acquired pathogens and are at relatively less risk for bacteremia and SBI in comparison to younger infants. Bacteremia in this age group is either a result of SBI or may precede the development of focal serious infection. Focal SBI that may be associated with bacteremia includes meningitis, pneumonia, pyelonephritis, bacterial enteritis, facial cellulitis, septic arthritis, and osteomyelitis (Table 118-2). The reader is referred to subsequent chapters for description of the pathogenesis and microbiology of these infections in children. Pneumonia is most frequently viral in etiology in older infants and children, with less than 3 percent incidence of associated bacteremia, most often due to *Streptococcus pneumoniae*.[4] Urinary tract infection (UTI) is usually caused by *E. coli* ascending infection, with associated bacteremia most commonly noted in infants younger than 6 months of age.[5] Bacterial enteritis caused by *Salmonella* sp. as well as septic arthritis and osteomyelitis caused by *Staphylococcus aureus* and *Streptococcus pneumoniae* carry some risk of bacteremia in infancy. The development of generalized septicemia without a primary focus is quite rare in immunologically competent children, occurring primarily with *Neisseria meningitidis* infection.

Bacteremia may also occur in the 3- to 36-month age group without clinically recognized septicemia or focal SBI. This "occult" bacteremia (OB) has been found to have an incidence of 3 percent of children 3 to 36 months of age with rectal temperatures of 39°C or higher, a well clinical appearance, and no major focal bacterial infection.[6,7] The most common organism responsible is *Streptococcus pneumoniae*, which accounts for 90 percent of OB. *Streptococcus pneumoniae* OB most often resolves spontaneously but carries a 10 percent risk of complicating SBI, including a 3 percent risk of meningitis.[8] *Haemophilus influenzae* type b (HIB) has historically been reported to account for 10 percent of OB, with a 50 percent risk of progression to SBI, including a 25 percent risk of meningitis.[9] However, the impact of the HIB vaccine on the incidence of HIB-related bacteremic disease has been dramatic, virtually eliminating this organism as a potential pathogen in adequately immunized patients.[10] Other organisms, such as *Neisseria meningitidis* and *Salmonella* sp., contribute a minority of cases but with a high rate of subsequent focal SBI. Although uncommon, group A β-hemolytic streptococcus has been reported as a cause of bacteremia, often associated with primary varicella infection.[11] Initial studies reported that untreated OB, without reference to the specific etiology, carries a 10 percent risk of progression to complicating focal meningitis.[12] However, no studies have been performed since the universal introduction of the HIB vaccine, and the actual risk of progression from OB to complicating focal SBI in adequately immunized children is likely much lower.[8] Two developments will profoundly develop the future management of bacteremia and SBI due to *S. pneumoniae*. The widespread emergence of penicillin- and cephalosporin-resistant strains of *S. pneumoniae* has complicated the choice of optimal therapy for bacteremia, SBI and meningitis in particular. Antibiotic treatment within the prior month has been demonstrated to be a risk factor for infection due to a resistant strain.[13] Of potentially greatest importance to the emergency physician caring for a febrile child, a newly developed polyvalent pneumococcal vaccine has recently completed phase III clinical trials and was shown to reduce by 90 percent the incidence of all pneumococcal bacteremia and meningitis in immunized infants.[14]

Clinical Features

Historical risk factors for neonatally acquired bacterial infection in infants less than 3 months of age include premature delivery, ruptured amniotic membranes for more than 24 h prior to delivery, and maternal amnionitis prior to or following delivery. Specific symptoms suggestive of a focus of infection in this age group are rare. High fever is uncommon in this age group, and serious illness may be present in the setting of low-grade fever or normal temperature.[2] Infant temperatures should be obtained via the rectal route in the ED, as the axillary and auditory canal routes are less reliable in the identification of fever.[15] A history of fever measured by the parent via the rectal route carries the same significance as fever detected in the ED, although the perception of tactile fever at home in the setting of a normal temperature in the ED does not.[16] Of greatest utility to emergency physicians, *the symptoms and signs suggestive of bacteremia and SBI most frequently produce an overall ill appearance*. Parents may note poor feeding, decreased responsiveness, or irritability in response to attempts to console. Physical examination findings suggestive of an ill appearance include poor eye contact and muscle tone, including weak suck, poor head control, and indifferent response to stimuli. Signs of respiratory distress and poor perfusion parameters are suggestive of septicemia and should be specifically sought. Although uncommon, findings suggestive of a specific focus of infection, such as otitis media, skin, soft tissue, bone, or joint inflammation, place young infants in a higher-risk group for SBI. However, due to the nonspecific nature of the signs and symptoms of illness at this age, the history and physical examination alone are unreliable screening tools for bacteremia and SBI in neonates, with marginally improved predictive value in infants 30 to 90 days old.[17]

Children 3 months of age and older found to have bacteremia and SBI most often are noted to have fever with rectal temperatures of 39.0°C or higher,[18] although serious infection can uncommonly occur without the finding of fever.[19] As for younger infants, the most important historical and physical findings are related to overall appearance. *Parental report of persistent lethargy or irritability with associated fever raises significant concern for SBI with associated bacteremia.* Symptoms of respiratory, gastrointestinal, soft tissue, bone, or joint inflammation should be elicited. The reader is referred to subsequent chapters for a complete description of the symptoms suggestive of focal SBI in children. Historical risk factors of importance include immunization status, prior infections, and underlying conditions that impair immune response, such as sickle cell anemia and HIV. The physical examination is performed in two phases. The first is a global assessment of the child's appearance performed in order to categorize the child as "ill" versus "well," optimally after antipyretic therapy has been administered. This assessment should specifically include *mental status,* evaluated by observing response to parental physical and social stimulation, and *perfusion and hydration parameters.* A *well appearance* is evidenced by an awake, responsive infant or child with good eye contact, developmentally appropriate social interaction with family members, normal muscle tone, and vigorous cry. An *ill appearance* is evidenced by lethargy or irritability, failure to respond to or be consoled by family members, weak cry, poor muscle tone, or abnormal peripheral perfusion parameters. If the examination findings are equivocal, the child should be reassessed in a short period of time and, if unchanged, considered "ill-appearing." The performance of an overall assessment of appearance has been shown to improve the sensitivity of the history and physical examination in detecting SBI.[20] The second phase of physical examination is devoted to eliciting signs of specific SBI as well as minor focal infection. Signs of meningitis are reviewed later in this chapter. The finding of a minor focus of infection, such as upper respiratory infection, otitis media, pharyngitis, or gastroenteritis, does not exclude the possibility of bacteremia or SBI.

TABLE 118-3 Low-Risk Criteria for Febrile Infants 30–90 Days of Age

History
• Full term
• No underlying medical problems
• No prior antibiotics
Physical examination
• "Well appearance"
• No focus of infection (otitis, skin, soft tissue, bone, or joint)
Laboratory
• WBC 5000–10,000/μL with < 1500 bands/μL
• Urinalysis < 10 WBCs/hpf, negative for leukocyte esterase, nitrite
• Stool smear < 5 WBCs/hpf (if diarrhea present)
• Normal chest x-ray (if clinically indicated)
Follow-up
• Reliable parents
• Home telephone and transportation

Source: Rochester Criteria, from Dagan et al,[22] with permission.

The clinical presentation of the patient at risk for OB includes age 3 to 36 months, rectal temperature of 39°C or higher, a well appearance, and either no other signs of infection or signs of minor focal infection only. However, only 3 percent of patients with these findings will have a positive blood culture. A well-appearing child with a rectal temperature less than 39°C is extremely unlikely to be bacteremic. By definition, it is impossible to distinguish children with OB from those without bacteremia by clinical features alone.[21]

Diagnosis

Because of the relatively greater risk for bacteremic illness and lack of sensitivity of the clinical examination, the febrile or ill-appearing neonate, regardless of temperature, should be comprehensively evaluated for SBI via a *sepsis workup.* This should include complete blood count, urinalysis, cerebrospinal fluid (CSF) cell count, Gram stain, evaluation of protein and glucose levels, and culture and sensitivities of the urine (suprapubic or catheterized), blood, and CSF. Respiratory symptoms or signs are indications for chest x-ray. The differential diagnosis for septic-appearing neonates includes congenital cardiac disease, metabolic disease, nonaccidental trauma, and bowel obstruction.

Infants 30 to 90 days of age are optimally evaluated via a *low-risk* versus *high-risk* stratification that combines both clinical and routine laboratory assessments[22] (Table 118-3). Low-risk infants are those who were born at full term, have no underlying medical problems, and have not previously been treated with antibiotics. On physical examination, these young infants must have a well appearance with no identified focus of possible bacterial infection to specifically include otitis media, skin, soft tissue, joint, or bone infection. To be considered low risk, these young infants must additionally have negative laboratory screening tests. These are defined as white blood count of 5000 to 15,000/μL with less than 1500 bands/μL, urinalysis revealing less than 10 white blood cells per high-power field (WBCs/hpf) and negative for leukocyte esterase and nitrite, and, when diarrhea is present, stool smear with less than 5 WBCs/hpf. Cultures of the blood and urine (suprapubic or catheterized) should be performed. Stool should be cultured if diarrhea is bloody or WBCs are present as above. A chest x-ray is indicated only if there are significant respiratory findings such as severe cough, tachypnea, grunting respirations, or rales.[23] Lumbar puncture should be performed routinely in febrile infants less than 60 days of age and strongly considered for those 60 to 90 days because of limited sensitivity of the clinical assessment at these ages for the detection of meningitis. Febrile infants aged 30 to 90 days who meet low-risk criteria have less than a 1 percent risk of bacteremia and less than a 2 percent risk of SBI. In contrast, young infants categorized as high risk are reported to have a 2 to 10 percent risk of bacteremia and 10 to 15 percent risk of SBI, with ill appearance weighing heavily toward the higher respective risks.[24] Infants 30 to 90 days of age considered high risk by either clinical or laboratory parameters should have a complete evaluation for sepsis as for neonates.

The laboratory assessment of children 3 to 36 months of age and older should be individualized based on the overall appearance of the child, clues from the history and physical examination, and a knowledge of the incidence of bacteremia and SBI in this age group. Most importantly, *an ill-appearing febrile child, regardless of age, should be stabilized and comprehensively evaluated for sepsis* as just described. In contrast, *a well-appearing febrile infant should have laboratory evaluation based on clinically identified risk factors for SBI with bacteremia.* The reader is referred to subsequent chapters for a discussion of the laboratory evaluation for specific focal bacterial infections in children. Blood culture is of limited utility in the outpatient management of radiographically identified pneumonia but should be considered in those patients ill enough to warrant admission.[4] Similarly, blood cultures are indicated in febrile children aged 6 months or less who have UTI or those with clinical features of pyelonephritis indicating admission.[5] Blood cultures are also appropriate for febrile pediatric patients with presumed bacterial enteritis, facial cellulitis, septic arthritis, and osteomyelitis. All febrile patients who are immune-compromised, such as with sickle cell anemia and HIV, should also have blood cultures obtained (Table 118-4). The identification of a clearly recognizable viral syndrome such as bronchiolitis renders the yield of laboratory testing for bacteremic disease negligible.[25]

The complete blood count is a nonspecific test that may assist in the identification of bacteremia and SBI but is not diagnostic and must be interpreted in the clinical context. Although the incidence of bacteremia rises with white blood counts of 10,000/μL or more, there is no threshold value of the white blood count (WBC) that distinguishes between bacteremic and nonbacteremic patients or identifies patients with SBI with adequate sensitivity and specificity. A WBC of 5000/μL or less in ill-appearing infants is suggestive of overwhelming bacterial sepsis but in well-appearing infants suggests benign viral illness with transient bone marrow suppression. The choice of a threshold of WBC of 15,000/μL or more for obtaining a blood culture in the setting of a well-appearing child with temperature of 39°C or higher and no or minor focus of infection will identify only 65 percent of those with OB. Moreover, only 7.5 percent of such children who meet these clinical criteria will prove to be bacteremic. Decreasing the WBC threshold for obtaining a blood culture to improve sensitivity markedly decreases the specificity and predictive value of the test.[26] Other available screening tests, such as absolute band count, erythrocyte sedimentation rate, and C-reactive protein, have failed to provide significantly greater sensitivity or specificity. Although the blood culture is the "gold standard" for the identification of bacteremia, its result cannot be predicted by a screening test with any degree of confidence at the time of initial ED evaluation. *The pursuit of OB should not distract emergency physicians from carefully evaluating febrile infants for focal serious bacterial infections, including UTI, pneumonia, meningitis, and soft tissue, bone, or joint infection.*

TABLE 118-4 Indications for Blood Cultures in Children

• Unexplained ill appearance, regardless of age or fever
• Febrile neonates
• "High-risk" febrile infants aged 30–90 days
• Meningitis
• Pneumonia (requiring admission)
• Pyelonephritis (age ≤ 6 months or febrile requiring admission)
• Bacterial enteritis (age < 2 years)
• Facial cellulitis
• Septic arthritis
• Osteomyelitis
• Underlying immune deficiency with fever

Treatment

EMERGENCY The treatment plan for febrile infants, like the diagnostic evaluation, must be stratified by patient age and directed toward the age-related and organ system–specific probable pathogens (Figs. 118-1 and 118-2 and Table 118-5). Febrile neonates, after being fully

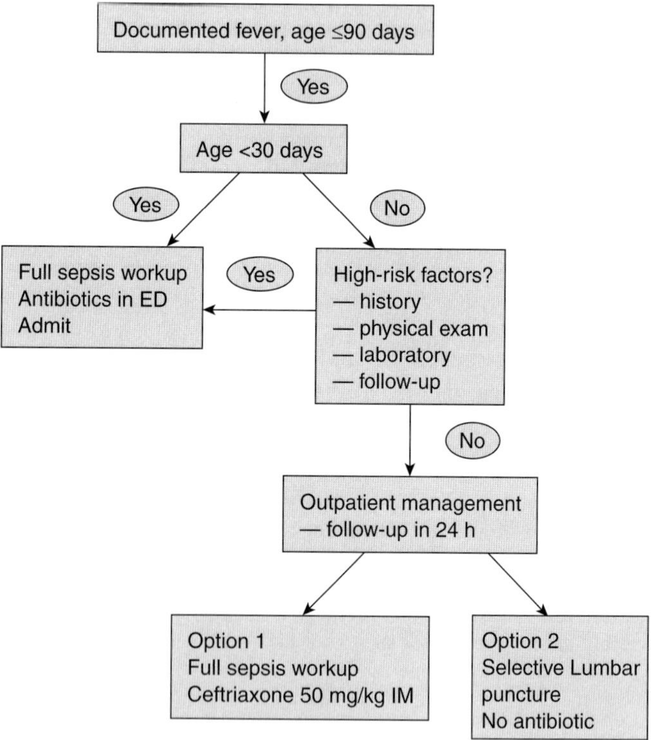

FIG. 118-1. Management scheme for febrile infants aged 0 to 90 days. *Abbreviations:* ED, emergency department.

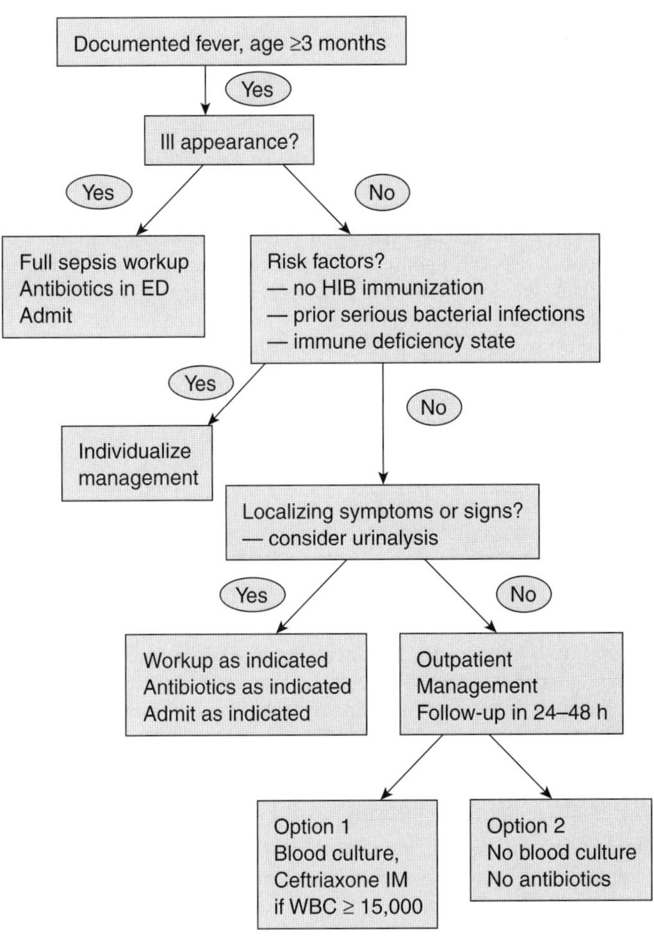

FIG. 118-2. Management scheme for febrile infants aged 3 months or older. *Abbreviations:* ED, emergency department; HIB, *Haemophilus influenzae* type b.

evaluated for sepsis as described above, should be stabilized with supportive care and treated with broad-spectrum intravenous antibiotics to cover group B *streptococcus, E. coli, Listeria monocytogenes,* and *Enterococcus* sp. pending culture results. Optimal therapy includes ampicillin 100 mg/kg and either cefotaxime or ceftriaxone 50 mg/kg IV, with initial doses given in the ED prior to admission. Young infants aged 30 to 90 days considered to be high risk for SBI based on the foregoing clinical or laboratory parameters should be similarly evaluated for sepsis and treated with ampicillin and either cefotaxime or ceftriaxone to cover both neonatal and community-acquired pathogens. Young infants aged 30 to 90 days considered low risk for SBI based on clinical and laboratory parameters may be reasonably managed as outpatients in two ways if follow-up is feasible based on physician judgment of parental reliability and availability of a home telephone and source of transportation. The more traditional and conservative approach is to perform a lumbar puncture on all such young infants to exclude bacterial and aseptic meningitis definitively and treat with ceftriaxone 50 mg/kg IM prior to discharge.[27] Alternatively, it has been shown that well-appearing infants in this age group considered low risk may be safely managed with selective lumbar puncture and without antibiotics, providing strict adherence to clinical, laboratory, and follow-up criteria is maintained.[28]

The treatment of febrile infants 3 to 36 months of age remains a subject of considerable controversy. As for all infants, *an ill-appearing febrile child should be stabilized with supportive care and fully evaluated for sepsis, and broad-spectrum intravenous antibiotics such as cefotaxime or ceftriaxone should be administered in the ED.* Fortunately, most penicillin- and cephalosporin-resistant strains of *S. pneumoniae* demonstrate only intermediate resistance at this time and may be adequately treated with a third-generation cephalosporin. Treatment of focal SBI presumptively identified by diagnostic testing in the ED depends on the likely pathogens and is reviewed in subsequent chapters. Treatment of meningitis is reviewed later in this chapter. The optimal treatment for children at risk for OB has not been established. Published observational retrospective studies,[29,30] prospective randomized trials,[7,31] and meta-analyses of pertinent prior studies[12,33,34] have concluded that expectant antibiotic treatment of patients at risk for OB resulted in a shorter duration of fever and a lower rate of subsequent focal SBI. However, no study has shown that oral antibiotics alter the rate of subsequent development of meningitis.[8,12,30] Initial therapy for pediatric patients at risk for OB with ceftriaxone 50 mg/kg IM has been recommended because of a reported significant reduction in the incidence of subsequent culture-positive meningitis compared with oral antibiotics or observation without therapy.[7,12] However, critical reviews of these studies have revealed significant methodologic flaws that seriously undermine the conclusion that antibiotic therapy prevents subsequent SBI, in particular the failure to include partially treated meningitis as an adverse outcome.[33,34] At the present time, there is no standard of care for the treatment of well-appearing febrile children 3 to 36 months of age who are at risk for OB.[35] Reasonable approaches include (1) blood culture if WBC is 15,000 or greater, followed by ceftriaxone 50 mg/kg IM, and (2) no blood culture and antibiotic therapy only for clinically identified infection, e.g., otitis media, in either case with follow-up within 24 h. If antibiotic treatment for OB is chosen, *emergency physicians should be wary of both the efficacy of antibiotic treatment in preventing focal SBI and the potential for delayed diagnosis for partially treated infection with altered presentation,* e.g., UTI or meningitis.[36]

OUTPATIENT Follow-up within 24 h and clear instructions regarding indications for early return are the cornerstones of management of

TABLE 118-5 Antibiotic Dosages for Bacteremia and Meningitis*

Age Group	Bacteremia/Sepsis	Meningitis
Neonates	Ampicillin 100 mg/kg plus Cefotaxime 50 mg/kg or Ceftriaxone 50 mg/kg	Ampicillin 100 mg/kg plus Cefotaxime 50 mg/kg or Ceftriaxome 50 mg/kg
Young infants 30–90 days	Ampicillin 100 mg/kg plus Cefotaxime 50 mg/kg or Ceftriaxone 50 mg/kg‡	Ampicillin 100 mg/kg plus Cefotaxime 100 mg/kg plus vancomycin 15 mg/kg† or Ceftriaxone 100 mg/kg plus vancomycin 15 mg/kg†
Older children	Cefotaxime 50 mg/kg or Ceftriaxone 50 mg/kg‡ plus *consider* Vancomycin 15 mg/kg†	Cefotaxime 100 mg/kg plus vancomycin 15 mg/kg† or Ceftriaxone 100 mg/kg plus vancomycin 15 mg/kg†

*All doses are IV unless specified otherwise.
†Vancomycin indicated only in suspected *bacterial* meningitis or sepsis with critical illness.
‡Preferred for outpatient treatment of occult bacteremia and serious bacterial disease due to long half-life; may be given IM.

well-appearing febrile infants 3 to 36 months of age. Young infants 30 to 90 days of age may be similarly managed as outpatients if all low-risk criteria have been met. Communication with a patient's primary physician to facilitate such follow-up represents optimal management. In the absence of a primary physician, consideration should be given to performing such follow-up in the ED. The parents should be educated regarding the effective use of antipyretics and instructed to return with the child to the ED immediately for symptoms of ill appearance suggestive of SBI. Patients who return to the ED with the report of a positive blood culture for *S. pneumoniae* who are afebrile and well appearing on follow-up may be managed as outpatients with repeat blood culture, oral antibiotic therapy, and follow-up in 24 h.

ADMISSION All febrile neonates and ill-appearing infants should be admitted for observation and parenteral antibiotic treatment pending culture results. Young infants aged 30 to 90 days who fail to meet low-risk criteria should also be admitted and treated. Infants 3 months of age or older who return to the ED with either (1) a report of any gram-negative organism on blood culture or (2) persistent fever or ill appearance with a report of positive blood culture for *S. pneumoniae* should have a complete evaluation for sepsis, parenteral antibiotic therapy in the ED, and admission for continued treatment.

SEPSIS

Pathophysiology

Sepsis is a clinical syndrome defined by bacteremia with clinical evidence of invasive, systemic infection that can progress with variable rapidity to circulatory failure. Sepsis can occur in isolation or with focal bacterial disease such as meningitis. The pathophysiology of sepsis is related to (1) colonization with a bacterial pathogen, usually nasopharyngeal, (2) invasion of the blood by encapsulated organisms and release of inflammatory mediators, and (3) host defense-response failure. This process results in systemic manifestations that are clinically detectable. Circulatory consequences may include alteration in systemic vascular tone and decreased myocardial contractility. Neurologic effects include decreased cerebral perfusion pressure and abnormal temperature homeostasis. Sepsis may also result in a microvascular angiopathy and disseminated intravascular coagulopathy involving the kidneys, lungs, skin, and central nervous system.

Host defense risk factors for sepsis include impaired splenic function (e.g., congenital absence, surgical removal, or functional impairment in sickle hemoglobinopathy) and congenital metabolic disease (e.g., galactosemia), as well as the more rare primary or acquired humoral and cellular immunodeficiency states. The presence of an indwelling foreign body or obstruction to drainage of a body cavity represents additional risk factors.

The likely pathogens for sepsis demonstrate an age-related distribution. In the first month of life, group B *Streptococcus* and *E. coli* dominate and are capable of causing an explosive sepsis syndrome that may increasingly be recognized in the ED with the trend to early newborn discharge. The risk presented by these organisms falls dramatically by the third month of life. In infancy and early childhood, HIB and *N. meningitidis* predominate as pathogens for sepsis, although the incidence of HIB disease has fallen markedly since the introduction of the HIB vaccine. *Streptococcus pneumoniae* is more likely to cause focal disease but may also result in sepsis syndrome, particularly with sickle cell disease and other causes of asplenia. In school-age children, *N. meningitidis* predominates as the cause of sepsis, but group A β-hemolytic *Streptococcus* has increasingly been implicated. Rocky Mountain spotted fever, caused by *Rickettsia rickettsii* and acquired following tick bite in endemic areas of the United States, must not be overlooked as possible cause of sepsis in the summer and fall seasons.

Clinical Features

The sepsis syndrome may present with either a subtle or obvious, rapidly progressive clinical picture. Neurologic symptoms most frequently include altered mental status with irritability, confusion, or lethargy. Poor feeding, lack of spontaneous motor activity, and hypotonia are common findings. Hyperpyrexia, defined as a rectal temperature higher than 41.1°C, may occur, although this is not specific for sepsis. Hypothermia may occur, particularly in infants under 3 months of age, and is a grave finding. Tachypnea and retractions may reflect hypoxia or the development of metabolic acidosis. Early septic shock is accompanied by subtle findings of resting tachycardia, widened pulse pressure, warm distal extremities, and brisk capillary refill. Subsequently, classic signs of hemodynamic compensation occur, including weak distal pulses, delayed capillary refill, and cool extremities. Ultimately, these are followed by signs of decompensation with decreased sensorium and hypotension. Cutaneous findings may include petechiae, which may progress to coalescent purpura over hours to days.

Diagnosis

Sepsis represents a *clinical* diagnosis of exclusion in the ED, pending the results of cultures and treatment, because of the potential for rapid progression of disease. Obvious septic shock rarely presents a problem of diagnosis but rather of management. In more subtle cases, the combination of altered mental status and abnormal vital signs should suggest to the emergency physician the possibility of sepsis. Because of the characteristically nonspecific presentation, febrile or ill-appearing neonates should be considered septic until proven otherwise. No laboratory test is diagnostic, although a WBC greater than 20,000/μL is supportive of bacterial sepsis. However, the presence of a WBC in the "normal" range in the setting of an ill-appearing child is not reassuring. A WBC less than 5000/μL or platelet count less than 150,000/μL is a grave prognostic sign, particularly for disease due to *N. meningitidis*. Cultures of the blood, urine, CSF, and diarrheal stool, if present, should be obtained to identify a primary focus of infection and guide future therapy. Gram-stained smears made from CSF and petechial scrapings may provide immediate diagnostic information regarding the identity of the organism.

The differential diagnosis for a "septic-appearing" child includes infectious, cardiac, metabolic, and traumatic disease. Major focal bacterial infections, such as meningitis and pericarditis, and systemic viral disease may present with findings of fever, altered mental status, and cardiorespiratory compromise. Young infants with congenital heart disease or viral myocarditis may present in cardiogenic shock with respiratory distress and signs of poor perfusion. Toxic ingestion and congenital metabolic disease may present with altered mental status as the major complaint. Finally, child abuse with head or abdominal injury may present with altered mental status, temperature instability, and signs of poor perfusion without historical or cutaneous evidence of trauma.

Treatment

EMERGENCY Stabilization must take priority over completion of the diagnostic workup. Restoration of oxygenation and perfusion are the first priorities in the initial management of sepsis. An ill-appearing child should be provided high-flow oxygen and monitoring of heart rate, respirations, and blood pressure, and oxygen saturation should be initiated. Attention to airway patency should continue throughout the assessment, with particular emphasis during procedures such as lumbar puncture. Secure vascular access should be obtained early and, in the setting of signs of poor perfusion, fluid resuscitation performed with 20 mL/kg boluses of normal saline with serial reassessments. In such cases, an indwelling Foley catheter should be placed to ensure adequate response to fluid resuscitation by establishment of urine output of 1 to 2 mL/kg/h. In young infants in particular, hypoglycemia should be identified early by bedside testing and corrected with intravenous 25% dextrose (D25 or 25 gm/100 mL) 0.5-g/kg bolus(es). Endotracheal intubation and mechanical ventilation are indicated if a patient is judged to have advanced respiratory or circulatory failure and neurologic compromise with potential for loss of airway control. Intubation should also be considered for septic-appearing patients who require interhospital transport. If serial fluid bolus therapy does not restore evidence of adequate perfusion, inotropic support with dopamine in the setting of normal blood pressure or epinephrine in hypotensive states is indicated.

The diagnostic evaluation of septic-appearing infants in the ED should include cultures of the blood, urine, and CSF. Diarrheal stool should be stained for white blood cells and cultured, if present. A complete blood count, electrolyte panel, and determination of blood glucose level are routinely indicated. A chest x-ray and arterial blood-gas measurement are indicated for signs of respiratory distress or critical illness. Liver functions, coagulation studies, and fibrin split product analysis should be considered for critically ill children.

Antibiotic therapy should initiated in the ED as soon as possible and should not be withheld pending lumbar puncture if the patient is unstable. Antibiotic selection is made according to the likely age-related pathogens (Table 118-5). In the first 2 months of life, ampicillin 100 mg/kg and either cefotaxime or ceftriaxone 50 mg/kg IV are indicated. Adequate initial therapy for children 3 months and older is cefotaxime or ceftriaxone 50 mg/kg IV. Because of the widespread emergence of penicillin- and cephalosporin-resistant strains of *S. pneumoniae*, vancomycin 15 mg/kg IV should be considered as part of initial therapy for critically ill, septic children, particularly in the setting of an underlying immune deficiency state.[37] In endemic areas during the summer and early fall, chloramphenicol 25 mg/kg IV should be considered for children with possible Rocky Mountain spotted fever. Care must be taken to monitor patients following antibiotic administration for abrupt vascular collapse due to acute bacterial lysis with release of endotoxins.

ADMISSION All children with suspicion for bacterial sepsis should be admitted for monitoring and treatment pending culture results. Disposition decision making for a possibly septic child must specifically include choice of the appropriate pediatric inpatient unit. A child with limited suspicion for sepsis who is alert and requires no cardiorespiratory stabilization in the ED may be admitted to a pediatric floor unit for antibiotic therapy pending culture results. A child with evidence of cardiorespiratory or neurologic compromise requiring stabilization in the ED should be admitted to a pediatric intensive care unit (PICU) because of the risk of progression of disease. If interhospital transfer to a PICU is necessary, a pediatric transport team should be utilized.

MENINGITIS

Pathophysiology

In most cases, meningitis occurs as a complication of a primary bacteremia. The inflammatory response to the products of bacterial multiplication may result in alteration of the permeability of the blood-brain barrier with extension of infection and inflammation to the brain itself. The resulting brain edema, increased intracranial pressure, decreased cerebral blood flow, and vascular thrombosis produce neuronal injury. Less commonly, meningitis occurs via the hematogenous route from a distant primary focal infection, direct extension from adjacent infection, or following head injury with cribriform plate fracture. The incidence of meningitis is highest between the ages of birth and 2 years, with age-related peak risks during the neonatal period and between 3 and 8 months. Host defense factors resulting in impaired splenic function or immunodeficiency are associated with increased risk for sepsis and meningitis.

The pathogenic organisms responsible for bacterial meningitis parallel those responsible for sepsis. In the neonatal period, group B *Streptococcus* and *E. coli* predominate. In older infants and children, *S. pneumoniae* and *N. meningitidis* are the likely pathogens. Although penicillin-resistant strains of *S. pneumoniae* are increasing in frequency, there is no evidence that these organisms are more virulent.[38] Infants and children who have not received the HIB vaccine continue to be at risk for HIB meningitis.

Clinical Features

Because the presenting symptoms are subtle and overlap with those of less serious infection, a high index of suspicion for meningitis is crucial. Two modes of presentation are seen. The most frequently encountered pattern is an insidious progression of a febrile illness over several days. Less commonly, a fulminant progression to septic shock and meningitis may occur over hours, most commonly caused by *N. meningitidis*.

Symptoms and signs of bacterial meningitis depend on patient age and duration of illness. No single complaint or physical finding is specific. However, the findings of *fever associated with altered mental status constitutes a reasonable basis for suspicion for meningitis.* Infants typically present with nonspecific symptoms including decreased responsiveness, poor feeding, and vomiting. Although common, fever is not universally present at the time of diagnosis. Signs of ''paradoxical irritability'' despite parental comforting attempts; decreased responsiveness to visual, verbal, and painful stimuli; hypotonia; bulging fontanelle; or respiratory distress may be seen. Older children will usually complain of headache, photophobia, nausea, and vomiting. As for infants, signs of lethargy and confusion are primary indicators for suspicion of meningitis, and fever may not be consistently present. Nuchal rigidity and the classic findings of the Kernig sign (neck pain elicited with passive knee extension) and Brudzinski sign (involuntary lower extremity flexion elicited with passive neck flexion) are helpful only if positive. Seizures occur early in the course of 25 percent of patients with bacterial meningitis and are typically initially generalized but may be focal.[38] Focal neurologic findings, focal or prolonged seizures, and presentation with obtundation or coma suggest an adverse outcome. Pretreatment with oral antibiotics is associated with an altered presentation characterized by less consistent findings of fever or altered level of consciousness and longer duration of symptoms before diagnosis.[36]

Diagnosis

On the basis of reasonable clinical suspicion, a lumbar puncture must be performed to make or exclude the diagnosis of meningitis. The WBC is not an adequate screen for meningitis. In the absence of fever, a computed tomography (CT) scan of the brain may be necessary to exclude intracranial mass lesion prior to lumbar puncture. If meningitis is strongly suspected, the CT scan should not delay antibiotic therapy. CSF should be obtained for culture and sensitivity, protein and glucose levels should be determined, and cell count and Gram stain should be rapidly performed. CSF leukocytosis with a predominance of polymorphonucleocytes, CSF protein level greater than 100 mg/mL, and CSF glucose level less than 50 percent of blood glucose level are considered positive screening test results for bacterial meningitis. The Gram stain has a 70 percent sensitivity for preliminary identification of the offending organism and should be reported to the emergency physician as soon as available. Because of the emergence of penicillin-resistant strains of *S. pneumoniae*, it is prudent to perform CSF latex agglutination for specific bacterial antigens on all patients with abnormal CSF to facilitate early identification of high-risk patients. If prior treatment with antibiotics has occurred, the emergency physician should have a lower threshold for performing a lumbar puncture, and rapid antigen techniques are routinely indicated as these are often essential to diagnosis.[39] A bedside blood glucose level, complete blood count, electrolyte panel, and cultures of blood and urine should be obtained before performing the lumbar puncture. Indications for deferring lumbar puncture in the ED include cardiorespiratory compromise or risk of increased intracranial pressure. In such cases, antibiotic therapy should be given in the ED and lumbar puncture performed as soon as possible in the inpatient setting.

The differential diagnosis for bacterial meningitis includes the same spectrum of systemic disease as described for sepsis. Aseptic meningitis refers to evidence of meningeal inflammation with negative CSF cultures and is far more common than bacterial meningitis. Most frequently, this is due to viral meningeal infection, but other causes such as tuberculosis or syphilis should be considered. Parameningeal infection or brain abscess may rarely mimic the presentation and laboratory features of meningitis. Central nervous system (CNS) mass lesion, nonaccidental head injury, and toxic drug ingestion should also be considered in afebrile patients.

Treatment

EMERGENCY As for clinically septic children, treatment for meningitis begins with stabilization of oxygenation, ventilation, and perfusion parameters. Provision of supplemental oxygen and monitoring of heart rate and oxygen saturation during and following lumbar puncture are appropriate with careful attention to prevention of airway compromise.[40] Children with meningitis are often septic and may require vigorous initial isotonic fluid bolus therapy to restore systemic and CNS perfusion. However, subsequent fluid should be provided at a maintenance rate to minimize brain edema. Neurologic complications are frequent and must be treated aggressively to prevent secondary CNS injury. Seizures are treated with lorazepam 0.1 mg/kg IV and, if necessary, phenytoin 15 mg/kg or phenobarbital 10 mg/kg IV, along with correction of hypoglycemia or other underlying metabolic disorder. Severe respiratory distress and decreasing mental status with risk of loss of control of airway protective reflexes should prompt elective endotracheal intubation. Suspicion for increased intracranial pressure is a sufficient indication for hyperventilation and, if hemodynamic stability permits, mannitol 1 g/kg IV.

Empirical antibiotic therapy for the likely age-related pathogens should be initiated as soon as possible in the ED. Recommended antibiotic dosages are higher with meningitis because of poor drug penetration across the blood-brain barrier and concern for the possibility of antibiotic resistance. In the first 3 months of life, ampicillin 200 mg/kg and cefotaxime or ceftriaxone 100 mg/kg IV are indicated. Children 3 months of age and older should receive cefotaxime or ceftriaxone 100 mg/kg (maximum, 2 g) IV (see Table 118-5). Due to the widespread emergence of penicillin- and cephalosporin-resistant strains of *S. pneumoniae*, vancomycin 15 mg/kg IV should also be routinely administered as initial therapy to children older than 1 month who have presumed bacterial meningitis.[37,41]

Steroid therapy has been shown to decrease the incidence of neurologic complications significantly in bacterial meningitis due to HIB if given before or at the time of initial antibiotic therapy. However, this benefit has not been demonstrated for meningitis due to *S. pneumoniae* or *N. meningitidis,* and steroid therapy may actually worsen neurologic sequalae.[37] Current guidelines are to *consider* steroid therapy in cases of suspected bacterial meningitis, specifically administering dexamethasone 0.15 mg/kg IV either before or immediately after the initial antibiotic dose to children 1 month of age or older.[37]

Prophylaxis of contacts to eliminate carriage of organisms from the upper respiratory tract is indicated following identification of an index case of meningitis caused by organisms capable of causing epidemic disease. For HIB disease, a regimen of rifampin 20 mg/kg (maximum, 600 mg) once per day for 4 days is indicated for (1) household members if there is a home contact aged less than 4 years and (2) day-care center staff and enrollees resembling households, defined as children less than 2 years of age with contact of 25 h per week or more. For *N. meningitidis* disease, a regimen of rifampin 10 mg/kg (maximum, 600 mg) twice per day for 2 days is indicated for all household members, day-care center contacts, and medical personnel who have had direct physical exposure to the index case prior to antibiotic therapy. There is no indication or effective prophylaxis for *S. pneumoniae* disease.

ADMISSION All pediatric patients with identified or presumed meningitis should be admitted for supportive care, monitoring for complications, and antibiotic therapy. As for sepsis, the disposition decision for children with meningitis must also include choice of the appropriate pediatric inpatient unit. Stable patients may be admitted to a monitored isolation bed on a pediatric floor unit for antibiotic therapy pending culture results. Children with evidence of cardiorespiratory or neurologic compromise should be admitted to a PICU because of the risk of progression of disease. If transfer of such a patient is necessary, a pediatric transport team should be utilized for referral to a tertiary care center.

REFERENCES

1. Wasserman GM, White CB: Evaluation of the necessity for hospitalization of the febrile infant less than three months of age. *Pediatr Infect Dis J* 9:163, 1990.
2. Caspe WB, Chamudes O, Louie B: The evaluation and treatment of the febrile infant. *Pediatr Infect Dis J* 2:131, 1983.
3. Bonadio WA, Webster H, Wolfe A, et al: Correlating infectious outcome with clinical parameters of 1130 consecutive febrile infants aged zero to eight weeks. *Pediatr Emerg Care* 9:84, 1993.
4. Hickey RW, Bowman MJ, Smith GA: Utility of blood cultures in pediatric patients found to have pneumonia in the emergency department. *Ann Emerg Med* 27:721, 1996.
5. Bachur R, Caputo GL: Bacteremia and meningitis among infants with urinary tract infections. *Pediatr Emerg Care* 11:280, 1995.
6. Jaffe DM, Tanz RR, Davis AT, et al: Antibiotic administration to treat possible occult bacteremia in febrile children. *N Engl J Med* 317:1175, 1987.
7. Fleisher GR, Rosenberg N, Vinci R, et al: Intramuscular versus oral antibiotic therapy for the prevention of meningitis and other bacterial sequelae in young, febrile children at risk for occult bacteremia. *J Pediatr* 124:504, 1994.
8. Rothrock SG, Harper MB, Green SM, et al: Do oral antibiotics prevent meningitis and serious bacterial infections in children with *Streptococcus pneumoniae* occult bacteremia? A meta-analysis. *Pediatrics* 99:438, 1997.
9. Korones DN, Marshall GS, Shapiro ED: Outcome of children with occult bacteremia caused by *Haemophilus influenzae* type b. *Pediatr Infect Dis J* 11:516, 1992.
10. Adams WG, Deaver KA, Plikaytis BD, et al: Decline of childhood *Haemophilus influenzae* type b (Hib) disease in the Hib vaccine era. *JAMA* 269:221, 1993.
11. Doctor A, Harper MB, Fleisher GR: Group A β-hemolytic streptococcal bacteremia: Historical overview, changing incidence, and recent association with varicella. *Pediatrics* 96:428, 1995.
12. Baraff LJ, Oslund S, Prather M: Effect of antibiotic therapy and etiologic microorganism on the risk of bacterial meningitis in children with occult bacteremia. *Pediatrics* 92:140, 1993.
13. Tan TQ, Mason EO, Kaplan SL: Penicillin-resistant systemic pneumococcal infections in children: A retrospective case-control study. *Pediatrics* 92:761, 1993.

14. Black S, Schinefield H, Ray P, et al: Efficacy of heplavalent conjugate pneumococcal vaccine (Wyeth-Lederle) in 37,000 infants and children: Results of the Northern California Raiser Permanente Efficacy Trial. 38th Interscience Conference on Antimicrobial Agents and Chemotherapy, Sand Diego, Sept. 24–27, 1998 (abstract).

15. Schuman AJ: The accuracy of infrared auditory canal thermometry in infants and children. *Clin Pediatr* 6:347, 1993.

16. Bonadio WA: Incidence of serious infections in afebrile neonates with a history of fever. *Pediatr Infect Dis J* 6:911, 1987.

17. Baker MD, Avner JR, Bell LM: Failure of infant observation scales in detecting serious illness in febrile 4- to 8-week-old infants. *Pediatrics* 85:1040, 1990.

18. Teele DW, Pelton SI, Grant MJ, et al: Bacteremia in febrile children under 2 years of age: Results of cultures of blood of 600 consecutive febrile children seen in a ''walk-in'' clinic. *J Pediatr* 87:227, 1975.

19. Kline MW, Lobin MI: Bacteremia in children afebrile at presentation to an emergency room. *Pediatr Infect Dis J* 6:197, 1987.

20. McCarthy PL, Lembo RM, Fink HD, et al: Observation, history, and physical examination in diagnosis of serious illnesses in febrile children ≤ 24 months. *J Pediatr* 110:26, 1987.

21. Teach SJ, Fleisher GR: Efficacy of an observation scale in detecting bacteremia in febrile children three to thirty-six months of age, treated as outpatients. *J Pediatr* 126:877, 1995.

22. Dagan R, Powell KR, Hall CB, et al: Identification of infants unlikely to have serious bacterial infection although hospitalized for suspected sepsis. *J Pediatr* 107:855, 1985.

23. Bramson RT, Meyer TL, Silbiger ML, et al: The futility of the chest radiograph in the febrile infant without respiratory symptoms. *Pediatrics* 92:524, 1993.

24. Baraff LJ, Oslund S, Schriger DL, et al: Probability of bacterial infections in infants less than three months of age: A meta-analysis. *Pediatr Infect Dis J* 11:257, 1992.

25. Kupperman N, Bank DE, Walton EA, et al: Risks for bacteremia and urinary tract infections in young febrile children with bronchiolitis. *Arch Pediatr Adolesc Med* 151:1207, 1997.

26. Jaffe DM, Fleisher GR: Temperature and total white blood cell count as indicators of bacteremia. *Pediatrics* 87:670, 1991.

27. Baskin MN, O'Rourke EJ, Fleisher GR: Outpatient treatment of febrile infants 28 to 89 days of age with intramuscular administration of ceftriaxone. *J Pediatr* 120:22, 1992.

28. Baker MD, Bell LM, Avner JR: Outpatient management without antibiotics of fever in selected infants. *N Engl J Med* 329:1437, 1993.

29. Woods ER, Merola JL, Bithoney WG, et al: Bacteremia in an ambulatory setting. *Am J Dis Child* 144:1195, 1990.

30. Harper MB, Bachur R, Fleisher GR: Effect of antibiotic therapy on the outcome of outpatients with unsuspected bacteremia. *Pediatr Infect Dis J* 14:760, 1995.

31. Bass JW, Steele RW, Wittler RR, et al: Antimicrobial treatment of occult bacteremia: A multicenter cooperative study. *Pediatr Infect Dis J* 12:466, 1993.

32. Baraff LJ, Bass JW, Fleisher GR, et al: Practice guideline for the management of infants and children 0 to 36 months of age with fever without source. *Pediatrics* 92:1, 1993.

33. Kramer MS, Shapiro ED: Management of the young febrile child: A commentary on recent practice guidelines. *Pediatrics* 100:128, 1997.

34. Long SS: Antibiotic therapy in febrile children: ''Best-laid schemes...'' *J Pediatr* 124:585, 1994.

35. Ros SP, Herman BE, Beissel TJ: Occult bacteremia: Is there a standard of care? *Pediatr Emerg Care* 10:264, 1994.

36. Rothrock SG, Green SM, Wren J, et al: Pediatric bacterial meningitis: Is prior antibiotic therapy associated with an altered clinical presentation? *Ann Emerg Med* 21:146, 1992.

37. American Academy of Pediatrics, Committee on Infectious Diseases: Therapy for children with invasive pneumococcal infections. *Pediatrics* 99:289, 1997.

38. Arditi M, Mason EO, Bradley JS, et al: Three-year multicenter surveillance of pneumococcal meningitis in children: Clinical characteristics and outcome related to penicillin susceptibility and dexamethasone use. *Pediatrics* 102:1087, 1998.

39. Bhisitkul DM, Hogan AE, Tanz RR: The role of bacterial antigen detection tests in the diagnosis of bacterial meningitis. *Pediatr Emerg Care* 10:67, 1994.

40. Fiser DH, Gober GA, Smith CE, et al: Prevention of hypoxemia during lumbar puncture in infancy with preoxygenation. *Pediatr Emerg Care* 9:81, 1993.

41. Ahmed A: A critical evaluation of vancomycin for treatment of bacterial meningitis. *Pediatr Infect Dis J* 16:895, 1997.

VIRAL AND BACTERIAL PNEUMONIA IN CHILDREN

Kathleen Brown
Thomas E. Terndrup

EPIDEMIOLOGY

Pneumonia is defined pathologically as an inflammation of lower tract lung tissue. Clinically, pneumonia is defined by the presence of pulmonary infiltrates on a chest radiograph, usually associated with a combination of clinical signs, such as cough, fever, chest pain, tachy pnea, and a variety of abnormal auscultatory findings. Most commonly, pneumonia is caused by an infectious agent, although aspiration of irritants and interstitial inflammation are also referred to as such.

Pneumonia develops more often in early childhood than at any other age. The incidence of pneumonia in children decreases as a function of age. In North America it has been estimated at 40 per 1000 in preschool children and approximately 9 per 1000 in 10-year-olds.[1,2] Infectious causes often display seasonal variation. Parainfluenza occurs predominantly in the fall, respiratory syncytial virus (RSV) in the winter, and influenza in the spring. Bacterial pneumonia is more common in the winter, when indoor crowding promotes respiratory transmission of microbes. Several risk factors increase the incidence or severity of pneumonia: prematurity, malnutrition, low socioeconomic status, passive exposure to smoke, and attendance at day-care centers. The mortality rate of childhood pneumonia is less than 1 percent in industrialized nations, but pneumonia accounts for up to 5 million deaths annually in children less than 5 years of age in developing countries.[3]

PATHOPHYSIOLOGY

The majority of pneumonias are acquired through aspiration of infective particles into the lower respiratory tract. There are a number of protective mechanisms preventing infection with aerosolized infective particles. Aerosolized particles are filtered in the nasal cavities or entrapped and cleared by the normal mucus and ciliated epithelium of the upper respiratory tract. Aspiration is further prevented by laryngeal reflexes and coughing. In the lower respiratory tract, alveolar macrophages and various immune mechanisms prevent further invasion by infectious agents. These defense mechanisms include the ingestion and killing of bacteria by macrophages, the activation of complement and antibodies that neutralize bacteria, and the transportation of particles from the lung by lymphatic drainage. Abnormalities in any of these protective mechanisms predispose patients to acquired pneumonia. Anatomic abnormalities of the respiratory tract, immune deficiencies, neuromuscular weakness, airway abnormalities that predispose the child to aspiration, and alterations in the quantity or quality of mucus secretion (e.g., cystic fibrosis). Passively acquired maternal antibodies may further prevent respiratory tract infection by pneumococcal and *Haemophilus influenzae* infections.

Suppression of the normal respiratory physiologic and anatomic defenses may occur secondary to a preceding viral infection of the upper respiratory tract. Coexistence of viral and bacterial pathogens in children has been demonstrated in 50 percent or more of cases.[4,5] Bacteria that cause pneumonia include many of the same organisms that colonize the child's upper airway. In addition, organisms that are transmitted person-to-person by airborne droplet spread may cause pneumonia. Less commonly, bacterial and certain viral (e.g., herpes simplex virus, varicella, rubella, rubeola, and Epstein-Barr virus) microbes may cause pneumonia through hematogenous or contiguous spread.

Parenchymal invasion by bacteria results in an acute inflammatory response that includes exudation of fluid; deposition of fibrin; and infiltration of the alveoli with fluids, polymorphonuclear leukocytes, and, soon, macrophages. Accumulation of excess alveolar fluid creates the characteristic consolidation seen on chest radiograms. Viral agents, mycoplasma, and chlamydia typically cause inflammation characterized by a predominately mononuclear infiltrate involving submucosal and interstitial tissues.

Etiology

The specific etiologic agent of pneumonia cannot be identified in up to 40 to 60 percent of patients.[4–10] The predominant pathogens that cause pneumonia in pediatric patients are a function of the patient's age, the presence of underlying disease, the vaccination status, and attendance in day care. Since clustering of cases of pneumonia due to a particular microbe are common, it is helpful to be aware of recent local outbreaks. When an etiologic agent is identified, the best predictor of the agent is age. The most common etiologic agents causing pneumonia according to age groups are illustrated in Table 119-1 and discussed below.

TABLE 119-1 Common Causes of Pneumonia

Age Group	Pathogens (in Order of Decreasing Frequency)
0–1 month	Group B streptococcus *Escherichia coli* *Klebsiella* or Enterobacteriaceae *Listeria*
1–3 months	Pneumonitis syndrome (afebrile pneumonia) *Chlamydia trachomatis* RSV or other respiratory viruses *Bordetella pertussis* *Ureaplasma urealyticum*
1 month to 2 years	RSV or other respiratory viruses *Streptococcus pneumoniae* *Haemophilus influenzae* type B (HIB), Non-type-B *H. influenzae* (NTHI), *C. trachomatis, Mycoplasma pneumoniae*
2–5 years	Respiratory viruses *S. pneumoniae* *Haemophilus influenzae* type B (HIB) or Non-type-B *H. influenzae* (NTHI) *M. pneumoniae* *Chlamydia pneumoniae*
6–18 years	*M. pneumoniae* *S. pneumoniae* *C. pneumoniae* Non-type-B *H. influenzae* (NTHI) Adenovirus or respiratory virus
All ages	Severe pneumonia *S. pneumoniae* *S. aureus* Group A streptococcus *Haemophilus influenzae* type B (HIB) *M. pneumoniae* Adenovirus Immunocompromised (all of the above plus): *P. carinii* Cytomegalovirus Fungi

NEWBORNS: BIRTH TO 1 MONTH The newborn age group is the only developmental period when bacterial infections are more common than viral agents as the leading cause of pneumonia. The majority of infections in this age group are caused by aspiration of the maternal genital organisms present during labor and delivery. The predominant pathogen is group B streptococcus, followed by *Escherichia coli, Klebsiella* species, and other gram-negative enteric bacilli from the Enterobacteriaceae family. Other, less commonly encountered organisms include nontypeable *H. influenzae,* other streptococci (group A and α-hemolytic species), enterococci, *Listeria monocytogenes,* Bordetella pertussis, and anaerobic bacteria.[11]

INFANTS: 1 TO 24 MONTHS During the first 2 years of life, viruses are the most common etiologic agent of pneumonia. RSV, parainfluenzavirus, influenzavirus, and adenovirus account for most lower respiratory tract infections, including pneumonia, in this age group.[1,2,4,7] There are at least 14 other viral agents isolated in children with pneumonia, which include rhinoviruses, enteroviruses, coronavirus, measles, varicella, rubella, herpes simplex virus, and Epstein-Barr virus.[7,8,12] Bacterial pneumonia due to *Streptococcus pneumoniae, Streptococcus pyogenes, Staphylococcus aureus,* and *H. influenzae* should be considered in infants and toddlers who are severely ill, have rapid onset and progression of symptoms, or have lobar or diffuse infiltrates, large effusions, or abscesses on radiograph.[13]

Very young infants (1 to 3 months) may present with what is often referred to as afebrile pneumonitis, or atypical pneumonia. This syndrome is typified by cough, tachypnea, and sometimes progressive respiratory distress in the absence of fever. Apneic episodes can occur with RSV, chlamydia, and pertussis. There is often radiographic evidence of bilateral diffuse pulmonic infiltrates with air trapping. The viruses listed above are the most common etiologic agents.[14] *Chlamydia trachomatis* is also often identified in this scenario.[10,14] *Ureaplasma urealyticum, Mycoplasma hominis, Pneumocystis carinii,* and *B. pertussis* have also been implicated in this syndrome, but the extent of their role is not as well defined.[10,15]

PRESCHOOL: 2 TO 5 YEARS As age increases, the overall incidence of pneumonia decreases, but the relative frequency of bacterial pathogens, particularly *S. pneumoniae,* as etiologic agents increases. Despite this, respiratory viruses, particularly influenzavirus A and B and adenovirus, remain the most common cause of pneumonia in this age group. The most common bacterial pathogen encountered is *S. pneumoniae.* In the recent past, *H. influenzae* type B (HIB) was encountered nearly as frequently; however, since implementation of widespread immunization against this agent, its incidence as an agent of invasive disease is thought to be much less.[16,17] However, non-type-B *H. influenzae* (NTHI), which is not protected against by the vaccine, may be an increasingly common agent of bacterial pneumonia.[18] Other bacteria that are isolated less commonly include of *S. aureus,* group A streptococcus, and *Moraxella catarrhalis.*[1,4,7] *Mycoplasma pneumoniae* has been found more frequently in this age group in recent studies.[19,20]

SCHOOL AGE AND ADOLESCENCE Once children reach school age, *M. pneumoniae* is the most frequent bacterial cause of pneumonia.[1,20,21] The peak incidence is between 10 and 15 years of age.[22] *Streptococcus pneumoniae* also remains a common pathogen in this age group.[1] *Chlamydia pneumoniae* is estimated to be the cause of up to 19 percent of pneumonias in school-aged and adolescent patients.[9,10,19,20] These infections are usually mild or asymptomatic.[20] *Staphylococcus aureus* pneumonia can occur at any age but tends to be most frequent in older children.[23] Respiratory viruses, especially adenovirus, can also cause pneumonia in this age group.

ALL AGES: SPECIAL CONSIDERATIONS The most common etiologic agents causing severe pneumonia (requiring admission to an intensive care unit) in all age groups beyond the neonatal period include *S. pneumoniae, S. aureus,* group A streptococcus, HIB, adenovirus, and *M. pneumoniae. Staphylococcus aureus* is notorious for causing rapidly progressive disease, often with pulmonic abscesses. A resurgence of virulent group A streptococci has been associated with sporadic cases of invasive disease, including necrotizing fasciitis with pneumonia and empyema in children.[24] Increased severity of *M. pneumoniae* infections in children with sickle cell disease has been described.

Gram-negative bacilli, including *Pseudomonas,* should be considered in patients who have recently been hospitalized. Anaerobic infections should be considered in children with neurologic or anatomic defects that predispose them to aspiration. Unusual causes of bacterial pneumonia in children include *Mycobacterium tuberculosis, Legionella pneumophila, Chlamydia psittaci, Francisella tularensis,* and rickettsial infections. Children with progressive or unresponsive pneumonia should be evaluated for evidence of these microorganiams. An immunocompromised host is susceptible to all of the infections listed above as well as to opportunistic infections, such as *P. carinii,* cytomegalovirus, and fungal diseases.

CLINICAL FEATURES

Clinical findings in a child with pneumonia are highly variable and are dependent on the specific respiratory pathogen, age, the severity of the disease, and any underlying illnesses. Tachypnea is the most frequent sign of pneumonia in children and may be an otherwise isolated finding. The best physical examination finding for ruling out pneumonia in an infant or child is the absence of tachypnea.[25] However, tachypnea is a nonspecific symptom and may occur secondary to fever, anxiety, metabolic disease, cardiac disease, or other respiratory problems. Fever can increase an infant's respiratory rate by 10 breaths per minute for each degree centigrade of elevation.[26] Respiratory rates should be counted over 1 min. Several studies have shown that rates counted over less time tend to overestimate the rate. Generally accepted standards for tachypnea in an infant or child are shown in Table 119-2.[27]

Auscultation of the lungs may reveal localized rales, wheezing, and decreased air entry in the affected area. However, auscultatory findings may not be reliable in children. When a group of pediatricians was asked to examine children with lower respiratory tract symptoms, there was only fair agreement about most auscultatory findings.[28] In younger children, decreased breath sounds, rather than rales, are often heard, since the involved areas tend to be ventilated poorly. Observable findings, such as respiratory rate and work of breathing, are more reliable.[25] Signs of increased work of breathing may include retractions, chest indrawing in infants, or paradoxical (seesaw) breathing. Grunting respirations are frequently present, particularly in infants with pneumonia.[29] Abdominal distention and pain may be present secondary to a paralytic ileus or diaphragmatic irritation in lower-lobe pneumonias.[30]

TABLE 119-2 Standards for Tachypnea in Infants and Children

Age, Months	Upper Limit of Normal Respiratory Rate, Breaths per Minute
<2	55
2–12	45
>12	35

The clinical presentation may be suggestive of the etiologic agent. Two classic presentations have been described for pneumonia: typical pneumonia and atypical pneumonia. Typical pneumonia is characterized by abrupt onset of fever, chills, pleuritic chest pain, and productive cough. Associated physical examination findings include high-grade fever, localized findings on chest examination, and a toxic appearance. Atypical pneumonia is characterized by gradual onset (over days) of headache, malaise, nonproductive cough, and low-grade fever. Associated physical examination findings may include wheezing, prolonged expiration, rhinitis, conjunctivitis, pharyngitis, and rash. The typical pattern is generally thought to be associated with a bacterial pathogen, and the atypical pattern is thought to be more characteristic of a viral infection; however, significant overlap exists, and identification of a causal agent based on clinical presentation is not always reliable.[31]

Typical clinical presentations have been described for some specific pathogens. Pneumonia due to *S. aureus* is notorious for being particularly rapid in the progression of clinical findings. Patients with *B. pertussis* pneumonia typically develop prodromal symptoms, including mild cough, conjunctivitis, and coryza, that lasts 1 to 2 weeks. A severe, paroxysmal cough often associated with emesis and dehydration, because coughing prevents eating and drinking, is characteristic of the catarrhal phase of pertussis infections. The inspiratory whoop is generally present only in older children. A history of maternal pelvic or conjunctival chlamydial infection is present in up to 50 percent of cases in which the infant develops *C. trachomatis* pneumonia. An infant with a chlamydial infection is usually afebrile, has a distinct staccato cough (i.e., short, abrupt onset), and diffuse rales on auscultation. Such infants rarely appear systemically ill. Chlamydial pneumonia in adolescents is usually insidious in onset and often includes complaints of sore throat and dysphagia. Mycoplasmal infections generally present with the gradual onset of malaise, fever, and headache. A hacking, nonproductive cough usually begins 3 to 5 days after the onset of illness and is present in up to 98 percent of children. Mycoplasmal infection may produce pharyngitis, and rales are present in approximately 75 percent of patients. A variable rash, which may be papular, vesicular, urticarial, or erythema-multiforme-like, is present in about 10 percent of patients with *M. pneumoniae.*

The age of the patient may also affect the clinical presentation. Pneumonia often occurs in association with a sepsis syndrome in neonates.[11,22] Infants frequently lack the classic symptoms and present with a variety of nonspecific findings. Nonspecific symptoms and signs of pneumonia in infants include fever without a localizing source, apnea, poor feeding, abdominal pain, vomiting or diarrhea, hypothermia, grunting, bradycardia, lethargy, and shock. Sputum production is uncommon in nontracheostomized children less than 8 years of age.

The severity of pneumonia may be judged by clinical features. More severe pneumonia is associated with deterioration of the patient's mental status, the use of accessory muscles, and the presence of retractions, nasal flaring, splinting, and cyanosis. Infants with poor feeding and lethargy may have more severe disease. A patient with a history of immunosuppressive therapy, a history of primary immune deficiencies, or a history suggestive of an immune deficiency may have more severe pneumonia, often caused by unusual pathogens. Children with underlying illnesses, such as congenital heart disease, chronic pulmonary disease, or sickle cell disease, are often more severely compromised by pneumonia.

DIAGNOSIS

Initially it is important to differentiate pneumonia from noninfectious pulmonary conditions, such as congestive heart failure, atelectasis, primary and metastatic tumors, and congenital abnormalities, such as pulmonary hypoplasia or congenital lobar emphysema. The wide variety of conditions that may simulate pneumonia include radiologic imaging problems (e.g., poor inspiration or a prominent thymus), recurrent or acute aspiration, atelectasis, tumors, collagen vascular disorders, allergic alveolitis, chronic pulmonary diseases (e.g., cystic fibrosis or asthma), and congenital abnormalities (e.g., pulmonary sequestration). A thorough history and physical examination usually help to exclude many of these conditions.

Radiographs

The chest radiograph is considered the pragmatic reference standard for making the diagnosis.[25] The finding of consolidation on radiograph is thought to be a reliable sign of pneumonia.[32]

Differentiating the various microbiologic causes of pneumonia is often more difficult. Typical patterns of clinical presentation and epidemiologic data on incidence have been described above but often overlap. Radiographically, viral pneumonias tend to appear as diffuse interstitial infiltrates, frequently with hyperinflation, peribronchial thickening, and areas of atelectasis. Bacterial pneumonias tend to have lobar or segmental consolidation. Pneumatocele formation and a combination of pneumothorax and empyema are highly suggestive of *S. aureus* infection. However, bacterial pneumonias with perihilar interstitial and nodular patterns on radiographs have been reported.[33,34] *Chlamydia trachomatis* infections usually lead to hyperexpansion and diffuse alveolar or perihilar interstitial infiltrates. Radiographic patterns in *M. pneumoniae* infections are variable. Lower-lobe streaky or patchy infiltrates are the most common, but many other patterns are possible, including lobar infiltrates in 10 to 25 percent of cases. Viral pneumonias can also cause lobar or segmental consolidations.[34] Several studies have looked at the accuracy of the chest radiograph in differentiating viral from bacterial disease. A recent review of these studies found sensitivities ranging from 42 to 80 percent and specificities of 42 to100 percent.[25]

Laboratory Studies

The white blood count is usually elevated with a left shift in bacterial pneumonia, especially early in the illness.[35] Typically, viral, chlamydial, and pertussis pneumonias produce lymphocytosis. However, it is not unusual for viral pneumonia to initially provoke a significant polymorphonuclear cell response. In patients with mycoplasmal pneumonia, the total white blood count and differential count are usually normal, but the erythrocyte sedimentation rate may be elevated. Chlamydial infections or parasitic infections often produce eosinophilia.

Blood culture results are rarely (5 to 10 percent) positive in children with pneumonia, even when it is proven to be bacterial.[4,8,22] Blood cultures should be obtained in infants who have high fever, appear ill, or require hospitalization. Sputum cultures may also help in identifying the causative organism but are difficult to obtain from nontracheostomized children, particularly those less than 8 years of age.

Cultures of the nasopharynx and throat for viral pathogens, chlamydia, pertussis, and mycoplasma often reveal the causative agent in patients with pneumonia caused by these organisms. Bacterial cultures of these regions have no diagnostic value.[6] Fluorescent antibody tests for *C. trachomatis* and *B. pertussis* are preferable to culture in some settings. Rapid viral antigen tests exist for a number of organisms, including RSV and influenza. Bacterial antigen testing is available in some centers but has a poor sensitivity and specificity in diagnosing the cause of pneumonia.[4,23] Serologic testing can be done for viruses, mycoplasma, parasites, and fungi in persistent or puzzling cases. Skin testing for tuberculosis should also be considered in patients not responding to traditional therapy or with apical, cavitary pneumonia. More invasive diagnostic procedures, such as obtaining endotracheal cultures, percutaneous lung aspiration, bronchoalveolar lavage, or open-lung biopsy, may be necessary in patients with severe disease that is unresponsive to empiric therapy. Results of tests for cold agglutinins are positive in 72 to 92 percent of patients with *M. pneumoniae* infection. Cold agglutinin test results may also be positive in viral infections and are less consistently positive in young children. To perform the bedside test for cold agglutinins, place several drops of blood in a blue-stopper coagulation profile tube, and place it in icewater for 15 to 30 s. The presence of floccular agglutination is considered a positive result, and agglutination should disappear with rewarming.

TABLE 119-3 Antibiotic Therapy for Children with Pneumonia

Age Group	Inpatient Therapy	Outpatient Therapy
0–1 month	Ampicillin and gentamicin or ampicillin and cefotaxime	N/A
1–3 months	Pneumonitis syndrome: erythromycin or clarithromycin Other: cefuroxime	N/A N/A
3 months to 5 years	Cefuroxime (consider adding erythromycin or clarithromycin)*	Amoxicillin, or erythromycin, or clarithromycin
6–18 years	Erythromycin or clarithromycin (consider adding cefuroxime)*	Erythromycin or clarithromycin, or azithromycin
All ages	Add vancomycin if resistant *S. pneumoniae* is suspected	

*Add additional coverage in severely ill patients.

TREATMENT

All patients with pneumonia should be assessed for hypoxia, and oxygen provided if indicated. Cyanosis is often not present in hypoxic children.[28] Oxygen saturation correlates well with clinical outcome and length of hospital stay.[36] Children with an oxygen saturation of 90 percent or less should receive supplemental oxygen. Additional respiratory support should be provided as dictated by the patient's clinical condition. Hydration status should be assessed and supplemental fluid administered if needed. In patients requiring hospital admission for suspected bacterial pneumonia, intravenous antibiotics should be administered in the emergency department. Empiric coverage should be guided by the age of the patient and the epidemiologic data discussed above. Table 119-3 contains suggested inpatient and outpatient antibiotic therapy. In newborns, ampicillin (150 to 300 mg/kg/day) in combination with either an aminoglycoside (gentamicin 2.5 mg/kg per dose) or a third-generation cephalosporin (cefotaxime 100 to 150 mg/kg/day) is preferred. The ampicillin provides coverage against *Listeria* and enterococcal species. For infants with pneumonitis syndrome or afebrile pneumonia (see above), erythromycin (40 mg/kg/day qid) is the drug of choice. In children 3 months to 5 years of age, ampicillin (150 mg/kg/day qid) or cefuroxime (150 mg/kg/day tid) alone is usually sufficient. In children who are unresponsive to this therapy or who have a suggestive clinical presentation, mycoplasma and chlamydial infections should be considered. Appropriate coverage for these infections include erythromycin (40 mg/kg/day qid) or clarithromycin (15 mg/kg/day bid). In children over 5 years of age, erythromycin or clarithromycin alone is usually sufficient. In severely ill hospitalized children in this age group, the addition of cefuroxime should be considered. In all age groups, if resistant *S. pneumoniae* is suspected, vancomycin should be added.[36]

Children with fulminant viral pneumonia, such as an immunocompromised patient with varicella, may require treatment with acyclovir. In RSV pneumonia, ribavirin therapy should be considered for selected high-risk children, such as those with significant underlying cardiopulmonary or oncologic diseases and those with severe RSV pneumonia. Lymphocytic interstitial pneumonia in HIV-positive children should include a combination of prednisone and zidovudine. Bone marrow and solid organ transplant patients with cytomegalovirus pneumonia may require ganciclovir and gammaglobulin. In a recent study, ceftazidime or ceftriaxone eradicated nosocomial pneumonia in 90 percent of cases, but ceftazidime had improved efficacy against *Pseudomonas aeruginosa.* Children with cystic fibrosis often develop acute infectious exacerbations secondary to *Pseudomonas* and *S. aureus,* often with reduced antimicrobial resistance to standard antibiotics.

Most children with uncomplicated pneumonia can be treated as outpatients. If a bacterial cause is suspected, the patient should be placed on an appropriate antibiotic. The choice of oral antibiotic should be based on the considerations discussed above regarding the most likely etiologic organisms based on the age and clinical presentation of the patient. For outpatient treatment, amoxicillin (40 mg/kg/day tid) is preferred for children between 3 months and 5 years.[36] Alternatively, daily intramuscular ceftriaxone may be used.[36,38] After 5 years of age and in penicillin-allergic children, erythromycin (40 mg/kg/day qid) or tetracycline (in children >9 years of age) are the preferred initial agents. Recent data indicate similar cure rates, fewer side effects, and reduced termination of therapy with clarithromycin compared to erythromycin.[39,40] Azithromycin has also been shown to have a cure rate equal to that of erythromycin in children with community-acquired pneumonia.[41] It should be noted that both of these drugs are significantly more expensive than erythromycin or tetracycline.

If viral pneumonia is suspected, no specific antibiotic therapy is warranted. Symptomatic treatment should include fever control and hydration. Patients with viral pneumonia often have a mixture of airway and air-space disease. If the patient has prominent airway disease (bronchiolitis-like) symptoms, bronchodilator therapy should be considered.

All patients discharged with a diagnosis of pneumonia should have routine follow-up with a primary care provider within 1 to 2 days. The duration of therapy varies with the clinical response, predisposing host factors, and suppurative complications. Ten days of antimicrobial treatment should suffice for most uncomplicated cases.

DISPOSITION

Admission Criteria

Suggested criteria for admission of children with pneumonia include hypoxia (oxygen saturation ≤90 percent), respiratory distress, a history of apneic episodes or cyanosis, toxic appearance, dehydration, age less than 3 months, impaired immune function, and infections unresponsive to oral therapy. The presence of underlying disease and the ability of the care givers should also be considered. The finding of a pleural effusion or pneumatocele or findings suggestive of a bacterial infection in a child less than 1 year of age suggest a pathogen other than *S. pneumoniae* (particularly HIB or *S. aureus*). Since such infections can progress rapidly and are not well tolerated, hospitalization is generally required. Infants with suspected *B. pertussis* or *M. tuberculosis* should be admitted. Children with moderate or severe complications from pneumonia should be hospitalized. Indications for admitting patients with RSV pneumonia are the same as for RSV bronchiolitis.

Complications

Most viral pneumonias will resolve spontaneously without specific therapy. Complications are similar to those for bronchiolitis and include dehydration, bronchiolitis obliterans, and apnea. Apnea is commonly seen in very young infants with RSV, chlamydial, or pertussis infections. Pleural effusions can occur with viral pneumonias but are not common.

Uncomplicated bacterial pneumonia usually responds rapidly to antibiotic therapy. A delay in improvement or a worsening condition after therapy has begun should prompt an evaluation for possible complications. Complications of bacterial pneumonia include pleural effusions, empyemas, pneumothorax, pneumatoceles, dehydration, and development of additional infectious foci. Pneumococcal pneumonias are accompanied by pleural effusions in about 10 percent of cases. Pneumonia due to HIB is complicated by pleural effusions in from 25 to 75 percent of cases. Other foci of infection are frequently seen with HIB and can include meningitis, septic arthritis, epiglottitis, soft tissue infections, and otitis media. Pneumonias secondary to *S. aureus* have a high rate of complications, including empyemas (80 percent) and pneumatoceles (40 percent). Mycoplasmal pneumonia is only rarely complicated by pleural effusions, meningitis, encephalitis, arthritis, and hemolytic anemia. Whenever pneumonia is complicated or prolonged, roentgenographic follow-up is recommended to assure complete resolution, which may take 4 to 6 weeks or longer.

Discharge Instructions

All children released to go home from the emergency department with a diagnosis of pneumonia should receive specific advice on the dosage and scheduling of medications and the signs of worsening respiratory distress. Children who become unable to ingest adequate amounts of fluid or prescribed antibiotics should be instructed to return for further care. All children discharged with the diagnosis of pneumonia should have follow-up scheduled with the primary care provider within 24 to 48 h.

REFERENCES

1. Murphy TF, Henderson FW, Clyde WA Jr, et al: Pneumonia: An eleven-year study in a pediatric practice. *Am J Epidemiol* 113:12, 1981.
2. Wright AL, Taussig LM, Ray CG, et al: The Tucson Children's Respiratory Study: II. Lower respiratory tract illness in the first year of life. *Am J Epidemiol* 129:1232, 1989.
3. Grant JP: The state of the world's children, 1990: UNICEF. Oxford, Oxford University Press, 1990.
4. Turner RB, Lande AE, Chase D, et al: ''Pneumonia in pediatric outpatients: Cause and clinical manifestations.'' *J Pediatr* 111:194, 1987.
5. Hietala J, Uhari M, Tuokko H, Leinonen M: Mixed bacterial and viral infections are common in children. *Pediatr Infect Dis J* 8:683, 1989.
6. Isaacs D: Problems in determining the etiology of community acquired childhood pneumonia. *Pediatr Infect Dis J* 8:143, 1989
7. Paisley JW, Lauer BA, Mcintosh K, et al: Pathogens associated with acute lower respiratory tract infection in young children. *Pediatr Infect Dis J* 3:14, 1984.
8. Nohynek H, Eskola J, Laine E, et al: The causes of hospital-treated acute lower respiratory tract infection in children. *Am J Dis Child* 145:618, 1991.
9. Ruuskamen O, Nohynek H, Zeigler T, et al: Pneumonia in childhood: Etiology and response to antimicrobial therapy. *Eur J Clin Microbiol Infect Dis* 11:217, 1992.
10. Davies HD, Matlow A, Petric M, Glazier Rwang EEL: Prospective comparative study of viral, bacterial and atypical organisms identified in pneumonia and bronchiolitis in hospitalized Canadian infants. *Pediatr Infect Dis J* 15:371, 1996.
11. Bohin S, Field DJ: The epidemiology of neonatal respiratory distress. *Early Hum Dev* 37:73, 1994.
12. Boyer KM, Cherry JD: Nonbacterial pneumonia, in Feigin RD, Cherry JD (eds): *Textbook of Pediatric Infectious Diseases,* 3d ed. Philadelphia, Saunders, 1992.
13. Jadavji T, Law B, Lebel MH, et al: A practical guide for the diagnosis and treatment of pediatric pneumonia. *Can Med Assoc J* (suppl) 156:703S, 1997.
14. DeMuri GP: Afebrile pneumonia in infants: *Prim Care* 23(4):849, 1996.

15. Matlow AG, Richardson SE, Quinn PA, Wang EEL: Isolation of *Ureaplasma urealyticum* from neonatal respiratory tract specimens in a pediatric institution. *Pediatr Infect Dis J* 15:371, 1996.
16. Lee GM, Harper MB: Risk of bacteremia for febrile young children in the post-*Haemophilus influenzae* type B era. *Arch Pediatr Adoles Med* 152:624, 1998.
17. Bower C, Condon R, Payne J, et al: Measuring the impact of conjugate vaccines on invasive *Haemophilus influenzae* type B infection in Western Australia. *Aust N Z J Pub Health* 22:67, 1998.
18. Urwin G, Krohn JA, Deaver-Robinson K, et al: Invasive disease due to *Haemophilus influenzae* serotype F: Clinical and epidemiologic characteristics in the *H. influenzae* serotype B vaccine era. The *Haemophilus influenzae* Study Group. *Clin Infect Dis* 22:1077, 1996.
19. Block S, Hedrick J, Hammerschlag MR, Cassell GH, et al: *Mycoplasma pneumoniae* and *Chlamydia pneumoniae* in pediatric community-acquired pneumonia: Comparative efficacy and safety of clarithromycin vs erythromycin ethylsuccinate. *Pediatr Infect Dis J* 14:189, 1995.
20. Hammerschlag MR: Atypical pneumonias in children. *Adv Pediatr Infect Dis* 10:1, 1995.
21. Broughton RA: Infections due to *Mycoplasma pneumoniae* in childhood. *Pediatr Infect Dis* 5:71, 1986.
22. Schidlow DV, Callahan CW: Pneumonia. *Pediatr Review* 17:300, 1996.
23. Schutze GE, Jacobs RF: Management of community acquired bacterial pneumonia in hospitalized children. *Pediatr Infect Dis J* 11:160, 1992.
24. Novotny W, Faden H, Mosovich L: Emergence of invasive group A streptococcal disease among young children. *Clin Pediatr* 31:696, 1992.
25. Margolis P, Gadomoski A: Does this infant have pneumonia? *J Am Med Assoc* 279:308, 1998.
26. Gadomoski A, Permutt T, Stanton B: Correcting respiratory rate for the presence of fever. *J Clin Epidemiol* 47:1043, 1994.
27. Taylor JA, Del Beccaro M, Done S, et al: Establishing clinically relevant standards for tachypnea in febrile children less than 2 years. *Arch Pediatr Adoles Med* 149:283, 1995.
28. Margolis P, Ferkol T, Marsocci S, et al: Accuracy of the clinical exam in detecting hypoxemia in infants with respiratory illness. *J Pediatr* 124:552, 1994.
29. Poole S, Chetham M, Anderson M: Grunting respirations in infants and children. *Pediatr Emerg Care* 11:158, 1995.
30. Kanegaye JT, Harley JR: Pneumonia in unexpected locations: An occult cause of pediatric abdominal pain. *J Emerg Med* 13:773, 1995.
31. Fang GD, Fine M, Orloff J, et al: New and emerging etiologies for community-acquired pneumonia with implications for therapy. *Medicine* 69:307, 1990.
32. Davies HD, Wang EE, Manson D, et al: Reliability of the chest radiograph in the diagnosis of lower respiratory infections in young children. *Pediatr Infect Dis J* 15:600, 1996.
33. Simpson W, Hacking P, Court S, Gardner P: The radiologic findings in respiratory syncytial virus infections in children: II. *Pediatr Radiol* 2:155, 1974.
34. Wildin S, Chonmaitree T, Swisschuk L: Roentgenographic features of common viral respiratory tract infections. *Am J Dis Child* 142:43, 1988.
35. Triga MG, Syrogiannopoulos GA, Thoma KD, et al: Correlation of leukocyte count and erythrocyte sedimentation rate with the day of illness in presumed bacterial pneumonia. *J Infect* 36:63, 1998.
36. Harris JA: Antimicrobial therapy of pneumonia in infants and children. *Semin Respir Infect* 11:139, 1996.
37. Shann F, Barker J, Poore P: Clinical signs that predict death in children with severe pneumonia. *Pediatr Infect Dis J* 8:852, 1989.
38. Dagan R, Philip M, Watemberg NM, et al: Outpatient treatment of serious community-acquired pediatric infections using once-daily intramuscular ceftriaxone. *Pediatr Infect Dis J* 6:1080, 1987.
39. Block S, Hedrick J, Hammerschlag MR, et al: *Mycoplasma pneumoniae* and *Chlamydia pneumoniae* in pediatric community-acquired pneumonia: Comparative efficacy and safety of clarithromycin vs. erythromycin ethylsuccinate. *Pediatr Infect Dis J* 14:471, 1995.
40. Chein SM, Pichotta P, Siepman N, et al: Treatment of community-acquired pneumonia: A multicenter, double-blind randomized study comparing clarithromycin with erythromycin. *Chest* 103:697, 1993.
41. Roord JJ, Wolf BH, Gossens MM, et al: Prospective, open randomized study comparing efficacies and safeties of a 3-day course of azithromycin and a 10-day course of erythromycin in children with community-acquired acute lower respiratory tract infections. *Antimicrob Agents Chemother* 40(12):2765, 1996.

PEDIATRIC ASTHMA AND BRONCHIOLITIS

Maybelle Kou
Thom Mayer

ASTHMA

Asthma is a chronic disease of the tracheobronchial tree characterized by airway obstruction, inflammation, and hyperresponsiveness. Triggers for cytokine-mediated inflammation and hyperresponsiveness are well known and can be as innocuous as changes in barometric pressure. The cascade of events leading to mucous plugging, airway edema, and obstruction is generally reversible with appropriate, aggressive therapy. Symptoms of asthma can vary from overt wheezing to paroxysmal dyspnea to cough. In the absence of audible wheezing, the child may frequently go undiagnosed, which may lead to high morbidity as the disease goes untreated. The need for parents, caretakers, and physicians to correctly assess the severity of the disease and provide adequate and timely treatment is paramount to the care of children with asthma.

The National Institutes of Health (NIH) 1997 Expert Panel Report 2 (EPR-2), *Guidelines for the Diagnosis and Management of Asthma*,[1] is a publication with which all physicians should be familiar. It provides treatment algorithms for use in the acute-care setting and clear guidelines to outpatient management (Fig. 120-1). However, most institutions will need to tailor these protocols to meet regional, local, and individual hospital needs.

Epidemiology

Asthma affects 14 million Americans, 4.8 million below 18 years of age.[2] The prevalence of asthma has increased in all age groups by 40 percent in the last decade. In 1995, there were more than 1.8 million emergency department (ED) visits for asthma, 570,000 of which were patients from 0 to 14 years of age.[3] The estimated number of admissions in this same age group approached 70 per 10,000. An investigation of over 113,000 pediatric asthma admissions from 1986 to 1993 revealed that although the number of discharges paralleled the general increase in population, the percentage of patients with adverse outcomes [mainly intubation, but also need for cardiopulmonary resuscitation (CPR)] as well as death almost tripled.[4] Between 1993 and 1995 there were 170 deaths due to asthma in the age group from 0 to 14.[5] Some authors interpret these data as a sign that the emphasis upon outpatient management of asthma may be leading to increased morbidity and mortality.

Specific risk factors associated with the development of asthma in children include low birth weight, family history of asthma, urban household, low-income household, and race (children of African-American, Asian, and Hispanic descent).[6,7] These factors also have an influence on when hospitalization might be required during exacerbation. Most children presenting with asthma do so before the age of 8, with male predominance in the prepubertal age group. During adolescence, this ratio equalizes.

Risk factors that contribute to the deaths of children with asthma include socioeconomic background, limited access to health care, improper medication administration, and unrecognized severe disease. Extreme lability of disease, nocturnal asthma, and history of respiratory failure with previous intubation have also contributed to these deaths.[8]

Pathophysiology

Bronchial hyperreactivity appears to have a genetic basis; however, the difficulty in distinguishing atopy from asthma has resulted in limited studies of this area. Nonetheless asthma is classified as extrinsic (IgE-mediated), intrinsic (infection-induced), and mixed (both IgE-

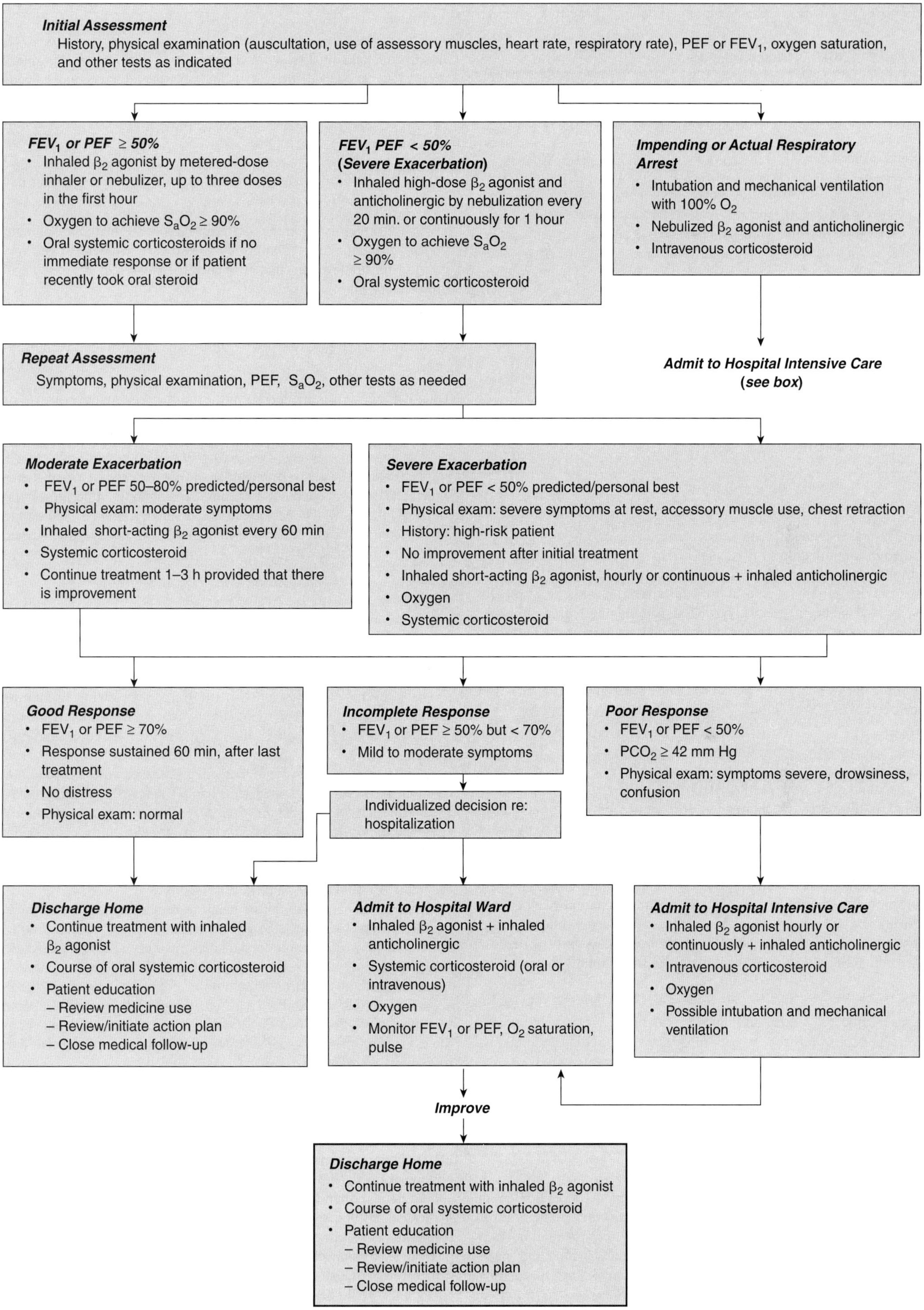

Initial Assessment
History, physical examination (auscultation, use of assessory muscles, heart rate, respiratory rate), PEF or FEV_1, oxygen saturation, and other tests as indicated

FEV_1 or PEF ≥ 50%
- Inhaled β_2 agonist by metered-dose inhaler or nebulizer, up to three doses in the first hour
- Oxygen to achieve $S_aO_2 \geq 90\%$
- Oral systemic corticosteroids if no immediate response or if patient recently took oral steroid

FEV_1 PEF < 50% (Severe Exacerbation)
- Inhaled high-dose β_2 agonist and anticholinergic by nebulization every 20 min. or continuously for 1 hour
- Oxygen to achieve $S_aO_2 \geq 90\%$
- Oral systemic corticosteroid

Impending or Actual Respiratory Arrest
- Intubation and mechanical ventilation with 100% O_2
- Nebulized β_2 agonist and anticholinergic
- Intravenous corticosteroid

Admit to Hospital Intensive Care (see box)

Repeat Assessment
Symptoms, physical examination, PEF, S_aO_2, other tests as needed

Moderate Exacerbation
- FEV_1 or PEF 50–80% predicted/personal best
- Physical exam: moderate symptoms
- Inhaled short-acting β_2 agonist every 60 min
- Systemic corticosteroid
- Continue treatment 1–3 h provided that there is improvement

Severe Exacerbation
- FEV_1 or PEF < 50% predicted/personal best
- Physical exam: severe symptoms at rest, accessory muscle use, chest retraction
- History: high-risk patient
- No improvement after initial treatment
- Inhaled short-acting β_2 agonist, hourly or continuous + inhaled anticholinergic
- Oxygen
- Systemic corticosteroid

Good Response
- FEV_1 or PEF ≥ 70%
- Response sustained 60 min, after last treatment
- No distress
- Physical exam: normal

Incomplete Response
- FEV_1 or PEF ≥ 50% but < 70%
- Mild to moderate symptoms

Individualized decision re: hospitalization

Poor Response
- FEV_1 or PEF < 50%
- $PCO_2 \geq 42$ mm Hg
- Physical exam: symptoms severe, drowsiness, confusion

Discharge Home
- Continue treatment with inhaled β_2 agonist
- Course of oral systemic corticosteroid
- Patient education
  - Review medicine use
  - Review/initiate action plan
  - Close medical follow-up

Admit to Hospital Ward
- Inhaled β_2 agonist + inhaled anticholinergic
- Systemic corticosteroid (oral or intravenous)
- Oxygen
- Monitor FEV_1 or PEF, O_2 saturation, pulse

Admit to Hospital Intensive Care
- Inhaled β_2 agonist hourly or continuously + inhaled anticholinergic
- Intravenous corticosteroid
- Oxygen
- Possible intubation and mechanical ventilation

Improve

Discharge Home
- Continue treatment with inhaled β_2 agonist
- Course of oral systemic corticosteroid
- Patient education
  - Review medicine use
  - Review/initiate action plan
  - Close medical follow-up

FIG. 120-1. Management of asthma exacerbations: emergency department and hospital-based care. (From the National Institutes of Health, National Heart, Lung, and Blood Institute.)

TABLE 120-1 Asthma Triggers

Air pollution
Tobacco smoke
Rhinitis/sinusitis
Gastroesophageal reflux
Viral respiratory infections
Medications
Exercise
Anxiety/stress
High/low environmental temperature
High humidity
Allergens Mold Animal dander/feces Pollen

and infection-induced). Since environmental factors are strongly implicated in the initiation of bronchial hyperreactivity, it should come as no surprise that 66 to 75 percent of asthmatic children are "allergic,"[9] many with serum IgE elevation. Concurrent sinusitis and bronchospasm secondary to chronic postnasal drip may be present. Whereas allergens and irritants are the most common and preventable triggers of asthma in children above 2 years of age, viral respiratory infections are felt to be predisposing in those below age 2. Respiratory syncytial virus is one of many viruses that can cause wheezing; this is discussed below, under "Bronchiolitis" (Table 120-1).

AIRWAY INFLAMMATION Bronchial smooth muscle cells are regulated by the autonomic nervous system. Sympathetic β_2 receptors cause bronchodilation, whereas parasympathetics govern bronchoconstriction. While the exact neurogenic mechanism for hyperreactivity is unknown, IgE-mediated inflammation is well characterized as a contributor in the pathogenesis of an asthma attack. Mast cells release histamine, leading to the formation of arachidonic acid metabolites and the inflammatory cytokine cascade. Asthma is a two-stage process: (1) bronchoconstriction due to histamine and leukotriene release (early stage) and (2) airway mucosal edema with mucous plugging (late phase). Since resolution depends largely on the degree of mucosal inflammation, an asthma attack may persist from days to weeks.

AIR TRAPPING, $\dot{V}/\dot{Q}$ MISMATCH, AND HYPOXEMIA Bronchospasm, mucosal edema, and mucous plugging cause variable and reversible airflow obstruction with subsequent air-trapping and impaired oxygen exchange. While increased lung volumes and pulmonary overdistention may help maintain airway patency, the resultant tidal volume approaches the volume of the pulmonary dead space and results in alveolar hypoventilation. Concurrently, $\dot{V}/\dot{Q}$ mismatch in areas of atelectasis contributes to hypoxia.

CARBON DIOXIDE RETENTION AND RESPIRATORY FAILURE In the early stages of a severe exacerbation, symptoms of CO_2 retention may not be clinically obvious due to effective alveolar capillary diffusion. Indeed, compensatory hyperventilation may cause a fall in Pa_{CO_2} and even a respiratory alkalosis. More severe obstruction and inadequate alveolar ventilation ultimately result in marked CO_2 retention, respiratory acidosis, and respiratory failure.[11] *Pseudonormalization* of Pa_{CO_2} is therefore ominous: the apparently "normal" Pa_{CO_2} of 40 mmHg coupled with altered mental status is a clear sign of respiratory failure. The acidosis that results from hypoxia and hypercapnea leads to pulmonary vasoconstriction, pulmonary hypertension, and right heart strain.

PEDIATRIC ANATOMIC DIFFERENCES The untreated pediatric asthma patient is ultimately at higher risk of respiratory failure due to these anatomic differences:

- Increased compliance of the infant rib cage and immature diaphragm result in paradoxical respiration: inward displacement of the ribs during inspiration contributes to increased work of breathing and respiratory muscle fatigue.
- Young lung tissue lacks elastic recoil and is more prone to atelectasis. This then contributes to $\dot{V}/\dot{Q}$ mismatch.
- Airway walls are thicker and result in greater narrowing with bronchoconstriction.

Thus if expiration is hampered by obstruction, complete collapse of alveoli and lung segments may occur.[12]

Postmortem specimens of pediatric asthma patients show the lungs to be pale and hyperinflated. Microscopy reveals smooth-muscle hyperplasia of bronchial and bronchiolar walls, thickened basement membrane, and mucosal edema. Submucosal eosinophilic infiltration is the hallmark of asthma. The leukocyte-laden mucous plugs occluding the airway contain eosinophils, polymorphonuclear cells, lymphocytes, and shed epithelial cells; there is an absence of mast cells.

Evaluation

To avoid delays in treatment, a brief physical examination should be performed before a detailed history is obtained. Treatment with inhaled β_2 agonists should not be withheld while the initial evaluation is in progress, even if the patient is in the triage area owing to lack of availability of a treatment room. Examination of vital signs should include respiratory rate, pulse, blood pressure, temperature, and pulse oximetry (Sa_{O_2}). Pulse oximetry, "the fifth pediatric vital sign," is an excellent noninvasive device for detecting severe airway obstruction. A room-air oxygen saturation of less than 91 percent in an infant may predict the need for hospitalization. *Oxygen supplementation should never be delayed for any child in apparent respiratory distress for the sake of obtaining a pulseox.* Oximetry may also be inaccurate in states of poor perfusion and fails to reflect a decrease in Pa_{CO_2} until the value of 80 mmHg is reached.

After initial stabilization, the health care provider must perform a complete exam, trying not to upset the child further. Children who are nonverbal and in respiratory distress may cry and be excessively clingy. The patient's chest must be visible for complete examination. Inspection and auscultation should be performed to assess alertness, accessory muscle use, and work of breathing. The severity of disease may be underestimated in the silent or "quiet wheezer," in whom the expiratory phase is usually prolonged and wheezing is absent due to extreme air trapping.

The "tripod position" is a significant indicator of distress: the child sits forward, hands over knees, on the edge of the bed. The nostrils should be inspected for presence or absence of nasal flaring, foreign bodies, and concurrent sinusitis. Hallmark "musical" polyphonic inspiratory and expiratory wheezes may not always be present on lung exam and are not prognostic of severity of disease. Extremities should be inspected to assess cyanosis and clubbing. Insensible fluid losses may result in delayed capillary refill and poor skin turgor. Pulsus paradoxus in severe exacerbation is usually 20 to 40 mmHg and may be reflected by significant jugular venous distention, which is otherwise difficult to appreciate in the pediatric examination.

Parents should be asked specifically if the child has previously had spells of wheezing (asthma attacks) and of what severity (Table

TABLE 120-2 Pertinent Questions to Ask about Asthma History

How long has the child been wheezing? Coughing?
When did the attack begin? Fever? Triggers?
How does this attack compare with previous attacks?
What are the child's current medications? Inhaled or oral bronchodilators? Chronic/acute use? Inhaled or oral steroids? What is the dosing schedule? Has the child been compliant with medication?
What medications have been required when the child was sick in the past? Is peak flow used to assess the child at home? What is normal? What has it been today?
Was the child ever In the ED for asthma? Hospitalized? Intubated? For how long?
Exposure to triggers? Pets?
Are there smokers in the house?
Exercise tolerance? Development?
Questions specific to the neonatal intensive care unit (NICU) What was the child's estimated gestational age? How long did he or she spend in the NICU? Was the child on a ventilator? How long? Was he or she given a diagnosis or bronchopulmonary disease? Was the child on oxygen? At home? Did the child have fluid on the lungs? Do medications include Lasix or Aldactone?

120-2). A history of asthma may be denied because pediatricians who are reluctant to give the diagnosis of asthma use *reactive airway disease* as alternative nomenclature. History of previous hospitalizations, intubation, and tracheostomy should be actively sought, including old records when the parent is unable to give information owing to a language barrier or ignorance of the situation. History of prematurity, bronchopulmonary dysplasia (BPD), and oxygen requirement is especially significant. Specific questions should be asked of information that the parent may not automatically volunteer—for example, regarding a stay in the neonatal intensive care unit (NICU) (see Table 120-2). In the adolescent, specific questions regarding, for example, use of inhalants, tobacco, or drugs (especially amphetamine and cocaine) should be asked, as well as over-the-counter purchases of bronchodilators that their parents may not be aware they have been using. History of aspiration or choking, as well as possible ingestion should be included for all ages. Family history of asthma and allergy can also give a sense of whether or not the parent or caretaker will be able to continue treatment once the ED visit terminates.

CLINICAL SCORING SYSTEMS IN ASTHMA The Wood-Downes-Lecks[13] clinical scoring system had been used in the past but is now replaced by the Expert Panel Report of the NIH (Table 120-3). The authors feel that scoring systems are not helpful in predicting outcome, since asthma is a dynamic and not static illness; they recommend that scoring systems be used only as a guide for progression of treatment.

MEASUREMENT DEVICES FOR PEAK EXPIRATORY FLOW RATE (PEFR) The 1997 EPR-2 advocates use of the PEFR (or peak flow) meters in the ongoing assessment and management of asthma. The newer hand-held spirometers are designed for personal use and portability and are readily available in the ED. Forced expiratory volume in 1 s (FEV_1) is estimated by measuring PEFR and correlates with the degree of airway obstruction; PEFR is already decreased by 25 percent once wheezing is detected by stethoscope (see Table 120-4). PEFR values in liters per minute are based on the child's height. A PEFR of less than 50 percent indicates severe obstruction, less than 25 percent indicates possible hypercarbia. In the ED, PEFR is an excellent tool to evaluate mild asthma or for reevaluating patients after treatment, especially those who know their "personal best" score. Pre- and posttreatment values should be obtained when possible.

Use in children below age 5 is limited by patient cooperation. In older children, the ability to perform deep inspiration and forced expiration may not be feasible during an acute exacerbation (Table 120-5).

Arterial blood gas analysis should be obtained to determine $Paco_2$ in children with impending respiratory failure, if the patient is hypoventilating, if PEFR is less than 30 percent of predicted, or if the patient is not responding as expected to treatment. It may also be helpful in determining which children should potentially be admitted to an intensive care unit versus a regular floor.

Complete blood count and chemistries are usually unnecessary unless there is a concurrent febrile illness or coexisting disease. Chronic steroid use can cause leukocytosis and elevated band count. Chronic use of albuterol can cause significant hypokalemia. If the child is on theophylline, a level should be obtained.

Chest x-ray is not routinely recommended but should be performed in new-onset asthma or to rule out pneumonia, pneumothorax, foreign body, or pneumomediastinum. A chest x-ray should also be obtained when a patient is admitted to the hospital. Findings typical of asthma are hyperinflation, flattened diaphragm, increased AP diameter, peribronchial cuffing, and atelectasis.

Differential Diagnosis

NEW-ONSET ASTHMA In the new-onset "wheezer," upper and lower respiratory and nonrespiratory causes must be differentiated (Table 120-6).

INFECTION Fever and focal wheezing implicate infectious etiologies such as pneumonia or bronchiolitis. Nocturnal wheezing, nocturnal cough, and poor exercise tolerance may be clues of more chronic illness. Sinusitis can exacerbate asthma symptoms; a history of nasal congestion and nocturnal cough or snoring should be treated with at least a 2-week course of antibiotics and nasal steroids. Recurrent attacks, failure to thrive, and a history of sinusitis and chronic ear infections should raise suspicion of cystic fibrosis as an etiology.

CARDIAC LESIONS: CONGENITAL AND ACQUIRED Infants with history of BPD may present with mild illness with rapid deterioration. Prolonged mechanical ventilation in the neonatal period causes smooth muscle hypertrophy and pulmonary hypertension, leading to cardiac disease. It may be necessary to distinguish pulmonary edema as a cause of wheezing; usually a history of diuretic use will aid in diagnosis. Congenital heart lesions causing congestive heart failure will also present with wheezing that may have been mistaken for asthma, exacerbated by concurrent viral infection. Other clues—such as feeding difficulties, failure to thrive, hepatosplenomegaly, genetic syndromes, and radiographs revealing abnormal cardiac silhouettes—point to a cardiac etiology. Workup to exclude viral myocarditis should be considered in the previously well child.

UPPER AIRWAY OBSTRUCTION A monophonic fixed inspiratory wheeze at the level of the vocal cords suggests upper airway obstruction

TABLE 120-3 Classifying Severity of Asthma Exacerbations*

	Mild	Moderate	Severe	Respiratory Arrest Imminent
Symptoms				
Breathless	While walking	While talking (infant—softer, shorter cry; difficulty feeding)	While at rest (infant—stops feeding)	
	Can lie down	Prefers sitting	Sits upright	
Talks in	Sentences	Phrases	Words	
Alertness	May be agitated	Usually agitated	Usually agitated	Drowsy or confused
Signs				
Respiratory rate	Increased	Increased	Often >30/min	
		Guide to rates of breathing in awake children: *Age* / *Normal rate*: <2 months <60/min; 2–12 months <50/min; 1–5 years <40/min; 6–8 years <30/min		
Use of accessory muscles; suprasternal retractions	Usually not	Commonly	Usually	Paradoxical thoraco-abdominal movement
Wheeze	Moderate, often only end expiratory	Loud; throughout exhalation	Usually loud; throughout inhalation and exhalation	Absence of wheeze
Pulse/min	<100	100–120	>120	Bradycardia
		Guide to normal pulse rates in children: *Age* / *Normal rate*: 2–12 months <160/min; 1–2 years <120/min; 2–8 years <110/min		
Pulsus paradoxus	Absent <10 mmHg	May be present 10–25 mmHg	Often present 20–40 mmHg (child)	Absent

Source: Expert Panel Report 2: Guidelines for the Diagnosis and Management of Asthma, 1997. National Institutes of Health Publication no. 98-4051. Bethesda, MD: NIH, 1997.

such as that secondary to croup, which may be more prominent on expiration (the seal-like cough). Careful history can indicate tracheomalacia, either congenital or secondary to prolonged intubation. A toxic child in tripod position with inspiratory stridor, absent cough, and inability to tolerate secretions is more likely to have retropharyngeal abcess or epiglottitis. Lateral and AP neck radiographs will aid in differentiation; if epiglottitis is suspected, the patient should never be left unattended. Vocal cord dysfunction can be voluntary, producing an inspiratory wheeze, shortness of breath, and parental anxiety. The wheeze is usually extinguishable with a β_2 agonist and behavioral modification (removal of stressor).

FOREIGN-BODY ASPIRATION Sudden onset of unilateral wheezing in the previously healthy child suggests foreign-body aspiration, most commonly in the right mainstem bronchus. If chest x-ray fails to reveal a radiopaque density, an expiratory film may show hyperinflation on the side of the obstruction due to air-trapping (ball-valve mechanism). A lateral decubitus film is more helpful in the small child who cannot follow commands. The dependent lung, usually deflated due to external compression from the x-ray table, will appear normal or hyperinflated if a foreign body is present. Infection and abcess must be suspected if fever is present.

GASTROESOPHAGEAL REFLUX DISEASE (GERD) A history of postprandial wheezing or coughing is indicative of GERD with microaspiration of liquid into the tracheobronchial tree. Severe GERD has been implicated in apnea and sudden infant death syndrome. Recurrent microaspiration can result in fever and pneumonia. Most children with reflux can be managed conservatively; however, a history of cyanotic spells after feeding warrants admission for barium swallow and upper gastrointestinal (GI) series. Tracheoesophageal fistula should be suspected in the newborn who experiences choking and cyanosis after feeding, although most cases should be diagnosed in the nursery: these can be missed due to shorter hospitalizations following delivery.

Treatment

β_2-RECEPTOR AGONISTS **Albuterol** (salbutamol) is the treatment of choice. Dosage is as follows: unit dose (0.5 percent solution) by nebulizer, O_2 flow at 6 to 7 L/min up to 2.5 mg/20 min or three unit doses by continuous nebulizer over 1 h. This may be repeated to a total of six unit doses. Continuous cardiac monitoring is required.

β_2 receptors are widely distributed on bronchial smooth muscle and airway epithelial cells. β_2-receptor agonists activate adenylate cyclase, increase cyclic adenosine monophosphate (cAMP) levels, cause bronchial smooth muscle relaxation due to increased binding of intracellular calcium to the endoplasmic reticulum, and decrease myoplasmic calcium. The development of specific β_2-receptor agonists such as albuterol (salbutamol in Canada, not to be confused with the long-acting Salmeterol) has revolutionized treatment of asthma, reducing the β_1 side effects of tachycardia and dysrhythmias seen with isoproterenol, which is now rarely used. Tachycardia and ''jitteriness'' are common side effects (more so with oral medication than inhaled), and, rarely, dysrhythmias have been reported. During an acute attack, use of a β_2-receptor agonist may cause transient drops in PO_2 due to pulmonary vasodilatation and ventilation-perfusion mismatch. Anecdotally, nebulized terbutaline (0.25 mL) has no advantage over albuterol and may be useful in patients who respond. Salmeterol (Serevent), a long-acting β_2 agonist that has been shown to reduce the need for

TABLE 120-4 Classification of Asthma Severity: Clinical Features before Treatment

	Days with Symptoms	Nights with Symptoms	PEFR or FEV_1*	PEFR Variability
Step 4 Severe Persistent	Continual	Frequent	≤60%	>30%
Step 3 Moderate Persistent	Daily	≥5/month	>60%–<80%	>30%
Step 2 Mild Persistent	3–6/week	3–4/month	≥80%	20–30%
Step 1 Mild Intermittent	≤2/week	≤2/month	≥80%	<20%

*Percent predicted values for forced expiratory volume in 1 second (FEV_1) and percent of personal best for peak expiratory flow rate (PEFR) (relevant for children 6 years old or older who can use these devices).
Notes: Patients should be assigned to the most severe step in which *any* feature occurs. Clinical features for individual patients may overlap across steps.

An individual's classification may change over time.

Patients at any level of severity of chronic asthma can have mild, moderate, or severe exacerbations of asthma. Some patients with intermittent asthma experience severe and life-threatening exacerbations separated by long periods of normal lung function and no symptoms.

Patients with two or more asthma exacerbations per week (i.e., progressively worsening symptoms that may last hours or days) tend to have moderate-to-severe persistent asthma.
Source: NIH Guidelines.[1]

TABLE 120-6 Differential Diagnosis of Asthma

Bronchopulmonary dysplasia (BPD)

Cystic fibrosis

Bronchiectasis

Pneumonia
- Bacterial
- Viral

Varicella

Pneumonitis

Gastroesophageal reflux disease
- Aspiration pneumonia

Anatomic defects of the airway
- Tracheoesophageal fistula
- Tracheomalacia
- Bronchial stenosis
- Bronchogenic cyst
- Pulmonary sequestration

Vocal cord dysfunction

Cardiovascular defects
- Congestive heart failure
- Tricuspid atresia and transposition
- Vascular ring

Miscellaneous
- Foreign-body aspiration
- Anaphylaxis
- Hyperventilation syndrome

Salicylate ingestion

β-blocker ingestion

''as needed'' albuterol dosing, is not indicated for use in acute exacerbations.

Tachyphylaxis has been documented with chronic and improper use of β_2 agonists[17] and appears to be related to saturation of β_2 receptors from frequent dosing intervals and/or decreased downregulation of the number of β_2 receptors on leukocytes of asthmatic patients. In this setting, increasing doses of β_2 agonists prove to be ineffective. Efficacy is preserved as long as the medication is used as needed and not on a scheduled basis. Overuse of such medications as aerosolized epinephrine (available over the counter as Primatene Mist) has also been implicated in the deaths of asthmatics due to tachyphylaxis and cardiac dysrhythmias. Furthermore, most physicians do not recommend the use of such products for even mild bronchial asthma. Physicians and pharmacists should educate patients to use medications only under a doctor's supervision.

TABLE 120-5 Predicted Average Peak Expiratory Flow for Normal Children and Adolescents, Male and Female

Height, in.	L/min	Height, in.	L/min
43	147	56	320
44	160	57	334
45	173	58	347
46	187	59	360
47	200	60	373
48	214	61	387
49	227	62	400
50	240	63	413
51	254	64	427
52	267	65	440
53	280	66	454
54	293	67	467
55	307		

Source: From Polger G, Promedhat V: *Pulmonary Function Testing in Children: Techniques and Standards.* Philadelphia: Saunders, 1971, with permission.

METERED-DOSE INHALER (MDI) Continuous aerosolized therapy with albuterol is a safe,[14] fast, and effective way to deliver medication directly to the lung capillary beds and may be associated with a reduction in hospital admission.[15] Although the literature has stated that MDI therapy is just as effective as nebulizer treatment in children above 6 years of age,[16] patient compliance may be the rate-limiting factor in administering MDI in the emergency setting. Failure to improve with home MDI use occurs in children due to tachypnea, inability to take a breath and hold it, and inability to form a seal around the chamber mouthpiece, at which point nebulized medication becomes a necessity.

SUBCUTANEOUS EPINEPHRINE If a patient is unresponsive to the above therapy or respiratory distress increases, subcutaneous epinephrine should be administered while line placement is attempted. Give 0.01 mL/kg aqueous epinephrine 1 : 1000 to a maximum of 0.3 mL. This may be repeated every 20-30 minutes for a total of 3 doses.

TERBUTALINE More β_2-specific than epinephrine, terbutaline can be given subcutaneously in place of epinephrine as 0.01 mL/kg of 1-mg/mL solution up to 0.25 mL.

Terbutaline is the only intravenous β_2 agonist available in the United States (intravenous albuterol is available in Europe and Canada). Its use should be considered in children who have not responded to conventional therapy who are admitted to a monitored unit. Side effects will be seen more frequently with intravenous than aerosolized administration. The use of terbutaline in exacerbations of pediatric asthma is limited in older children, where myocardial ischemia has occurred secondarily to tachyarrhythmias caused by the drug. Intravenously, terbutaline is given as 0.05 to 0.1 μg/kg per minute. Continuous cardiac monitoring is recommended.

CORTICOSTEROIDS Glucocorticoids are well known to inhibit the secretion of inflammatory leukotrienes and prostaglandins and to prevent and reverse the increase in vascular permeability that leads to airway edema. In vitro studies have shown that glucocorticoids cause an increase in density of β_2 receptors on leukocyte cell membranes and reverse tolerance to β_2 agonists.[18,19] Early administration during the course of an acute exacerbation is recommended for all patients unless the PEF is >50 percent and there is an immediate response to the first treatment (Fig. 120-1) and except when exercise-induced attacks occur in a previously well child. If the parent has already administered a dose at home, the dose can be repeated in the ED. Orally, prednisone or prednisolone is administered as 2 mg/kg. Prednisolone formulations are as follows: Pediapred 5 mg/5 mL and Prelone 15 mg/5 mL. Intravenous methylprednisolone is available as Solumedrol, single 2 mg/kg.

The current literature states that there is no advantage in giving intravenous versus oral glucocorticoids in the acute setting.[20] If a child has vomited oral medicines or is already intubated, then intravenous administration is preferred. Intramuscular administration is also an option.

It is well known that outpatient maintenance glucocorticoid therapy reduces the severity of attacks and thus reduces the need for hospitalization. A few controlled studies in pediatric patients have compared early ED administration of steroids versus placebo and have found that hospitalizations were less frequent in the treatment group than in those who did not receive treatment,[21,22] albeit the samples studied were small. Conversely, studies have shown no significant difference in the hospitalization rate when glucocorticoid treatment is begun in the ED.[23–25] While these data may be somewhat conflicting, the authors' position is that steroids treat inflammation, reduce relapse attacks, and therefore should be administered as early as possible in the acute attack to prevent prolonged hospitalization.

Inhaled glucocorticoids are increasingly recognized as the mainstay of asthma prevention in the population with mild to severe asthma, but they play a lesser role in treatment of the acute attack. There is still underuse[26] of inhaled glucocorticoids despite their well-documented efficacy in long-term control, prevention of ''rescue'' utilization of medication, and role in airway remodeling.[27] Side effects are less serious than with chronic oral glucocorticoids, although a few cases of adrenal suppression have been reported in the literature. Oral candidiasis can be prevented by diligent lingual hygiene (tongue brushing) and rinsing of the oral cavity after use. On an anecdotal basis, usage of nebulized dexamethasone is not recommended, as the molecule is too big to be absorbed at the alveolar-capillary level. Initial Canadian studies of nebulized budesonide, however, do suggest a benefit in treatment of asthma.[28,29]

Emergency physicians treating new-onset asthmatics may occasionally encounter parents who are skeptical about the use of glucocorticoids. The parents may often be fearful of the side effects and/or may confuse these with anabolic formulations. The parents should be educated about the reasons that warrant glucocorticoid therapy and reassured that short-term treatment is not usually associated with long-term sequelae.

INTRAVENOUS FLUIDS Most children presenting in status asthmaticus will be dehydrated because of increased insensible losses. It is worthwhile to administer a bolus of fluid (20 mL/kg of normal saline) to aid in thinning secretions and repleting lost volume, especially in those patients for whom admission seems inevitable.

ANTICHOLINERGIC THERAPY Studies in children suggests that use of nebulized ipratropium bromide (Atrovent) potentiates the effects of albuterol[30,31] and has the added advantage of compatibility when mixed with albuterol solution for combined administration via nebulizer. The anticholinergic action of such treatment is thought to prevent bronchoconstriction induced by cyclic guanosine monophosphate. Continued debate has led to many studies in adults that reveal no significant differences in efficacy from the use of ipratropium bromide with albuterol, although anecdotally the response is variable. It is a safe drug with few side effects and may be given to patients of all ages. It is available in liquid and MDI form. An MDI in combination with albuterol (Combivent) is at this time indicated for adult use only. The dosage of ipratroprium bromide is 250 μg in 2 mL of NaCl. It may be mixed with albuterol solution and administered as 250 μg every 6 h, or it may be added to first continuous nebulizer treatment.

MAGNESIUM SULFATE Intravenous magnesium sulfate has been used for the treatment of acute asthma exacerbations for many years; it may be administered to patients who are slow responders to conventional therapy and to intubated asthmatic patients. The exact mechanism of action is unknown but may resemble the tocolytic effects of magnesium sulfate on uterine smooth muscle. Several small studies have shown that patients who receive intravenous magnesium show improvement in short-term pulmonary function without adverse effects, such as low blood pressure.[32,33] Magnesium sulfate may be given as 25 to 50 mg/kg IV over 20 min; this may be repeated once to a serum magnesium level of 4 mg/dL. The maximum dose for children is 2 g.

HELIOX Heliox is generally available as 80 : 20 or 60 : 40 mixtures of helium and oxygen. If available, it may be initiated in the ED. It is recommended for the asthmatic who does not improve with conventional treatment but in whom intubation is not imminent.[34] The lower density and high diffusivity of the gas allows easier passage through turbulent obstructed airways. The peak flow rate increases while airway resistance and work of breathing decrease. It is possible to continue to administer β_2 agonists during Heliox treatment.

OTHER THERAPIES Theophylline is a competitive phosphodiesterase inhibitor that was thought to aid bronchodilation by increasing cAMP. While it is mentioned here for completeness, the authors do not recommend its routine use in the ED. Routine addition of theophylline to conventional therapy shows no benefits in the treatment for acute bronchospasm. It has an extremely narrow therapeutic-to-toxic ratio as well as side effects such as central nervous system (CNS) irritability and tachycardia. Drug interactions with P-450 metabolites also make its use undesirable. It is reserved for patients who clearly respond to it or for those who remain refractory to other modes of treatment. Aminophylline 6 mg/kg (85% theophylline) is given in 25 to 50 mL of NaCl over 20 min IV. If the patient is already on theophylline, a loading dose is given [(mg) = (desired level − measured level)/2 × kg].

Inhaled anesthetics such as halothane have also been used as inpatient treatment. Selected patients have been placed on cyclosporine, gold, hydroxychloroquine, and other immunomodulators. Health care professionals should be aware of the recent popularization of herbal remedies and inquire about their use: as of yet, no clinical studies have been performed on these medicines.

Chest physical therapy is of no proven benefit in the setting of acute asthma. Mucolytics may exacerbate symptoms by causing worsening of airway obstruction by loose particles. Sedation, unless in the setting of intubation, should be avoided to help protect airway reflexes.

Agents for Adjunct Ambulatory Treatment

Cromolyn sodium has long been used to inhibit mast-cell degranulation and histamine release. It is not recommended in the acute attack.

Nedocromil (Tilade) works similarly; however, it may be effective only if strict compliance is maintained. A primary feature is that it reduces the cough component of asthma; it is also considered to be "steroid sparing."

Leukotriene receptor inhibitors (LTRIs) are increasingly popular agents for use in the outpatient prophylactic management of asthma. These medications do not supersede steroid use in the acute attack. They are classified as 5-lipoxygenase inhibitors or 5-lipoxygenase–activating protein inhibitors, of which montelukast is approved for pediatric use; zafirlukast may be used in children of age 12 and above. Currently only limited data are available, but the initial response is encouraging and suggests less need for medication and chronic steroid use. A trial comparison to inhaled steroids will provide more information. Although initial studies have revealed a relatively good safety profile, zafirlukast has been linked to several adult cases of Churg-Strauss syndrome[36] (granulomatous necrotizing vasculitis). Interleukin 4–receptor medications are not currently approved for pediatric use.

Most *hand-held aerochamber devices* have a one-way valve and mouthpiece for children over age 4. A slow 3- to 5-s inhalation is required for each MDI actuation. For children below age 4, a mask attached to the end of the chamber is fitted over the nose and mouth. The appropriate size should be given. The MDI is attached to the other end of the chamber and medication is delivered. The mask is held to the child's face for five inhalations. Teaching should be performed before the child is discharged.

Complications of Moderate and Severe Asthma Exacerbation

Respiratory failure may occur even if treatment is in progress, mainly from muscle fatigue. Atelectasis is common and may be responsible for the overdiagnosis of pneumonia in pediatric asthmatic patients. While pneumomediastinum is rare, children may present with vague chest pains for which a radiograph can reveal the diagnosis. Most can be managed on an outpatient basis provided that there is good follow-up. Generally, mediastinal air will resorb over 2 to 3 days. A large pneumomediastinum and/or pneumothorax requiring chest tube thoracostomy will require admission for close monitoring and observation.

Reassessment and Disposition

Treatment algorithms greatly simplify the decision of whether or not a child should be admitted. Disposition can be made after 2 to 4 h of therapy for patients who remain stable (Table 120-7). A child who does not respond after 2 h of continuous treatment whose Pa_{CO_2} is greater than 40 mmHg should be admitted to an intensive care unit (ICU) for continuous therapy. Children with oxygen requirements, refractory asthma, and/or dyspnea on exertion may be admitted to the floor. If parents of children with newly diagnosed asthma do not feel comfortable taking care of their children even with adequate teaching, admission may be warranted (this also applies to patients with mild attacks requiring nebulization but with limited resources and inability to obtain nebulizers on weekends and at night).

An intubated patient or patient requiring continuous nebulization should be transported to a facility with pediatric intensivist capability by advanced life support providers with pediatric airway experience.

TABLE 120-7 Admission Criteria

Respiratory failure requiring intubation
Status asthmaticus: Persistent retractions, tachypnea O_2 requirement after 2 h of therapy
Return ED visit within 24 h
Limited home resources
Pneumothorax
Complete lobar atelectasis
Large pneumomediastinum
Underlying cardiopulmonary disease

Discharge Instructions and Ambulatory Treatment

Children responding well to conventional therapy may be discharged after 2 to 4 h of treatment. A short ED observation period is recommended for patients with an incomplete response but acceptable PEFR. Detailed discharge instructions should outline medication administration, inhaler use, and follow-up (Table 120-8). No child should be discharged without an MDI and spacer (Fig. 120-2), and prescriptions for oral glucocorticoids are generally recommended unless the attack was extremely mild (resolved with minimal treatment) or exercise-induced. Studies suggest that a tapered dose is not generally needed for "burst dose" (3- to 10-day) therapy,[35] since the side effect of adrenal suppression with prolonged use is unlikely to occur. Of the two most common forms of methylprednisolone, Pediapred is reported to taste better than Prelone; however, its lower concentration requires that three times the volume of Prelone be given for the same dose.

A courtesy call to the private pediatrician of the child who has been treated for asthma in the ED should be made, as it facilitates continuity of care for the child and ensures follow-up. All children should be referred to their pediatrician for follow-up within 24 h.

BRONCHIOLITIS

Bronchiolitis, or inflammation of the bronchioles, is the term applied to the clinical syndrome of wheezing, chest retractions, and tachypnea in children below age 2; it causes more significant illness in infants less than 6 months of age.

Epidemiology

Peak prevalence is from late October to May. Over 90,000 children are hospitalized at an average cost of $70,000 per child, with 4500 deaths annually from RSV infection. The peak age of incidence in urban populations is 2 months and results in hospitalizations lasting 5 to 7 days. Disease in older children is usually milder. Bronchiolitis has also been shown to be a cause of severe pneumonitis in elderly populations.

This highly infectious virus is transmitted by direct contact with large droplets of secretions and self-inoculation by contaminated hands via the eyes and nose (no significant transmission occurs by small-particle aerosol). RSV-infected secretions remain infectious on countertops for more than 6 h. Strict attention to hand washing and use of masks and gloves can prevent transmission. RSV is shed from the respiratory tract of symptomatic and asymptomatic patients for up to 9 days. Immunocompromised patients may continue to shed for up to 6 weeks.

TABLE 120-8 Discharge Treatment Dosage Guidelines

Sympathomimetic agents: adrenergic agonists
Short-acting β_2 agonists
Albuterol (= salbutamol)
Nebulizer solution (5 mg/mL) 0.05 mg/kg (min 1.25, max 2.5 mg) in 2 to 3 mL of normal saline q4–6h
Or premixed 2.5 mg/3 mL of normal saline q4–6h
MDI (*Proventil HFA, Ventolin,* generic) 90 μg per puff 1–2 puffs q3–4
Suspension 2 mg/5 mL, 0.1 mg/kg per dose, q6–8h
Long-acting β_2 agonists
Albuterol extended-release tablets (Repetabs, Volmax) 0.1–0.2 mg/kg q12h
Salmeterol (*Serevent*) 21 μg per puff q12h
Anticholinergic agents
Ipatropium bromide (*Atrovent*)
Nebulizer (0.25 mg/mL) 0.25–0.5 mg q6h
MDI (18 μg per puff) 1–2 puffs q6h
Treatment of inflammation
Glucocorticoids
Prednisone (5-, 10-, and 20-mg tablets) 1–2 mg/kg PO qd
Prednisolone (*Prelone, Pediapred*)
(5 mg/5 mL, 15 mg/5 mL) 1–2 mg/kg PO qd
"Burst dose" max 60 mg/day × 3–10 days
Inhaled steroid preparations
Beclomethasone
Vanceril DS (84 μg per puff) 2 puffs bid
Beclovent (42 μg per puff) 4 puffs bid
Triamcinolone (*Azmacort*) (100 μg/puff) 2 puffs bid
Flunisolide (*Aerobid*) (250 μg per puff) 2 puffs bid
Budesonide (*Pulmicort Turbuhaler*) (100, 200, and 400 μg per puff) 200–400 μg bid
Fluticasone (*Flovent*) (44, 10, and 220 μg per puff) 2 puffs bid
Unclassified anti-inflammatory agents
Cromolyn sodium (*Intal*)
MDI (800 μg per puff) 2–4 puffs qid
Neb (10 mg/mL) 20 mL qid
Nedocromil (*Tilade*)
MDI (1.75 mg per puff) 2 puffs qid
Leukotriene receptor inhibitors
5-Lipoxygenase inhibitors
Zileuton (*Zyflo*) 600 mg qid (not for children age 12 and under)
5-Lipoxygenase-activating protein inhibitors
Zafirlukast (*Accolate*) 20 mg bid (children age 12 and up)
Montelukast (*Singulair*) 5 mg qd (children age 6 and up) 10 mg qd (ages 12 and up)

Pathophysiology

Respiratory syncytial virus (RSV) causes 50 to 70 percent of clinically significant bronchiolitis.[37] First isolated in the 1950s, it is a significant cause of infant morbidity and is one of the major causes of hospital admission in infants below 1 year of age. Symptoms can vary from minimal rhinorrhea to bronchiolitis or pneumonia. Of the two antigenic subtypes of RSV, A and B, the former is generally more severe but less common. Two surface proteins, G (attachment) and F (fusion), are necessary for RSV to cause infection. Research is concentrating on F protein antibodies, which show less antigenic diversity than G proteins and neutralize both RSV subtypes. Immunity to the virus is variable owing to antigenic diversity; therefore reinfection does occur. No vaccine has yet been identified.

Non-RSV bronchiolitis is caused by influenza virus, parinfluenza virus, echovirus, and rhinovirus. *Mycoplasma pneumoniae* and *Chlamydia trachomatis* also produce symptoms. Adenovirus causes a particularly destructive form, bronchiolitis obliterans, observed in Native Canadian Eskimo populations.

Mucous plugging results from necrosis of the respiratory epithelium and destruction of ciliated epithelial cells. This and submucosal edema lead to peripheral airway narrowing and variable obstruction, with areas of patchy atelectasis or overdistention in lung segments. Progressive disease causes severe pneumonia, with extensive destruction of respiratory epithelium, parenchymal necrosis, and formation of hyaline membranes. Bronchiolar regeneration occurs within 3 to 4 days; however, cilia may take as long as 15 days to regenerate.

Increased airway resistance and decreased compliance result in increased work of breathing. Like the infant with lower airway obstruction, the infant with bronchiolitis breathes at higher lung volumes due to uneven resistance within the lung. Alteration of gas exchange results from the patchy atelectasis and airway obstruction. $\dot{V}/\dot{Q}$ mismatch is variable and severe hypoxemia may result.

Clinical Features

Infection begins with nasal discharge, pharyngitis, and cough. Fever accompanies the first few days of illness, with temperatures as high as 40°C (104°F). The parent brings the child to the ED because of increased respiratory symptoms, nasal congestion, and difficulty feeding.

Symptoms reach a peak at 3 to 5 days, generally resolving in 2 weeks with normalization of pulmonary function. It must be noted that resultant wheezing can persist for weeks to months. Respiratory isolation precautions should be entertained owing to the severity of illness that can occur in children with a history of prematurity, cystic fibrosis, congenital heart disease, or immunocompromise. These latter children are more at risk for apnea also.

Physical findings include tachypnea greater than 50 to 60 breaths per minute, tachycardia, mild conjunctivitis, chest retractions, prolonged expiration with hyperresonant chest, wheezes throughout, and hypoxemia. The most reliable clinical finding that correlates with hypoxemia is tachypnea, which signifies serious impairment of gas exchange. The hypoxemic child with bronchiolitis may not show cyanosis. The severity of wheezing or intercostal retractions will also not correlate with the severity of hypoxemia. Respiratory rate must be followed, but this may be difficult, as variation occurs with fever and crying. Pulse oximetry is the single best objective predictor of severe disease, and most children with saturations of less than 91 percent will probably need admission. If respiratory rate cannot be determined in the very small or dehydrated child, an arterial oxygen saturation should be obtained.

YOUNG INFANTS AND APNEA The mechanism inducing RSV-related apnea in young infants is not completely understood but may be related to hypoxemia and upper airway obstruction.[51] Infants at highest risk are less than 6 weeks old, have a history of prematurity, apnea of prematurity, and low O_2 saturation on admission. It is difficult to predict apneic events. The severity of wheezing and retractions does not correlate with frequency of apnea, and most infants less than 1 month of age will have atypical disease, where they may present without wheezing and retractions. Apneic infants generally require intubation during the course of the illness, sometimes requiring mechanical ventilation for up to a week or more. Postextubation, these infants are not at higher risk of apnea and may be discharged without apnea monitors.

Children with underlying diseases such as bronchopulmonary dysplasia, cystic fibrosis, immunodeficiency, or congenital heart defects are at increased risk of severe RSV. Care must be taken in treating infants with a history of BPD, as many will have a tendency toward chronic CO_2 retention. Since hypoxemia remains the major respiratory stimulus in this population, supplemental oxygen may cause further CO_2 retention, therefore saturations of 94 to 95 percent are acceptable.

Numerous retrospective analyses and observations note that children with bronchiolitis as infants frequently develop asthma later on.[52]

Please demonstrate your inhaler technique at every visit.

1. Remove the cap and hold inhaler upright.
2. Shake the inhaler.
3. Tilt your head back slightly and breathe out slowly.
4. Position the inhaler in one of the following ways (A or B is optimal, but C is acceptable for those who have difficulty with A or B. C is required for breath-activated inhalers):

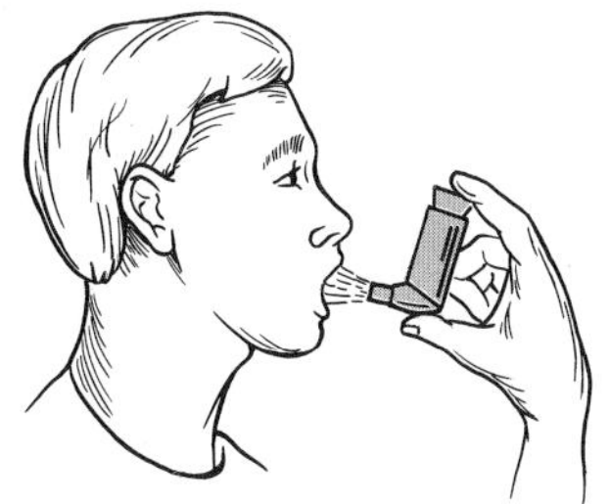

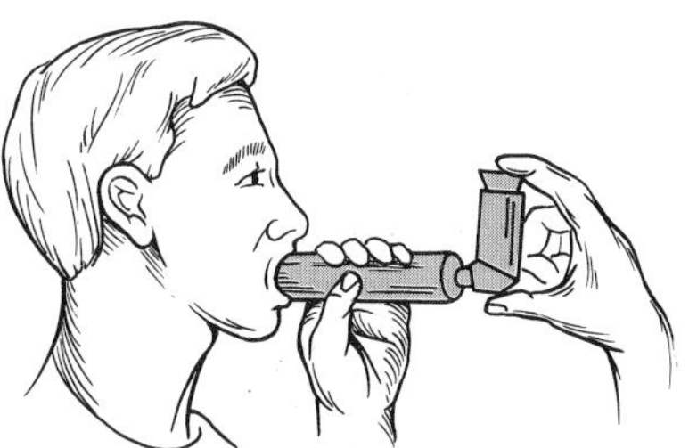

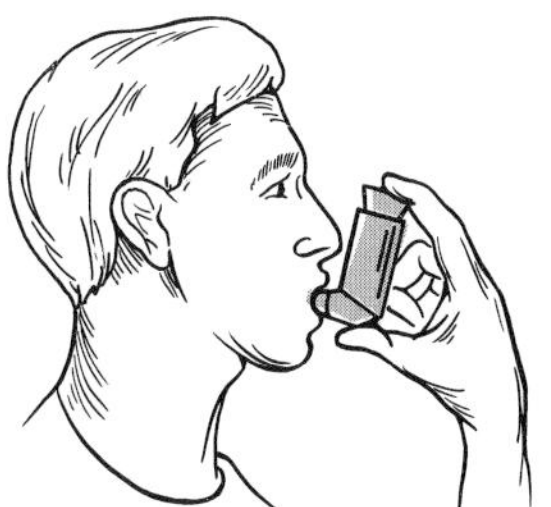

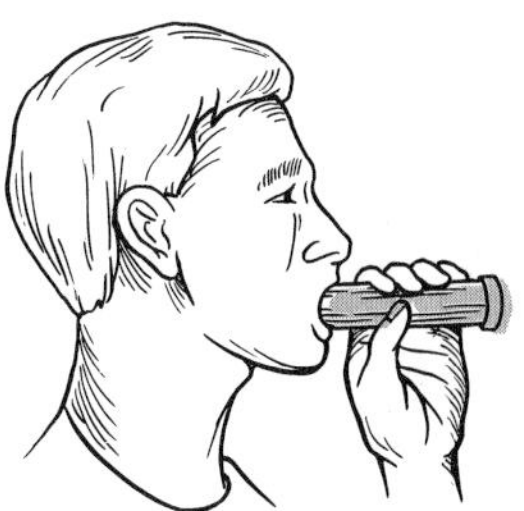

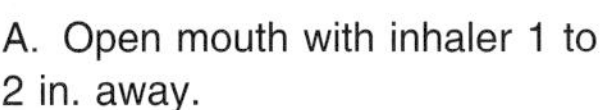

A. Open mouth with inhaler 1 to 2 in. away.

B. Use spacer/holding chamber (that is recommended especially for young children and for people using corticosteroids).

C. In the mouth. Do not use for corticosteroids.

D. NOTE: Inhaled dry powder capsules require a different inhalation technique. To use a dry powder inhaler, it is important to close the mouth tightly around the mouthpiece of the inhaler and to inhale rapidly.

5. Press down on the inhaler to release medication as you start to breathe in slowly.
6. Breathe in slowly (3 to 5 s).
7. Hold your breath for 10 s to allow the medicine to reach deeply into your lungs.
8. Repeat puff as directed. Waiting 1 min between puffs may permit second puff to penetrate your lungs better.
9. Spacers/holding chambers are useful for all patients. They are particularly recommended for young children and older adults and for use with inhaled corticosteroids.

Avoid common inhaler mistakes. Follow these inhaler tips:

- Breathe out *before* pressing your inhaler.
- Inhale *slowly.*
- Breathe in through your mouth, not your nose.
- Press down on your inhaler at the *start* of inhalation (or within the first second of inhalation).
- Keep inhaling as you press down on inhaler.
- Press your inhaler only *once* while you are inhaling (one breath for each puff).
- Make sure you breathe in evenly and deeply.

NOTE: Other inhalers are becoming available in addition to those illustrated above. Different types of inhalers may require different techniques.

(From the *Expert Panel Report 2: Guidelines for the Diagnosis and Management of Asthma.* National Asthma Education and Prevention Program, National Heart, Lung, and Blood Institute, 1997.)

FIG. 120-2. Steps for using your inhaler. (From the Expert Panel Report 2: Guidelines for the Diagnosis and Management of Asthma. National Asthma Education and Prevention Program, National Heart, Lung, and Blood Institute, 1997.)

Diagnosis

The diagnosis of bronchiolitis is suggested by clinical presentation, patient age, and history of RSV exposure or community epidemic. Immunofluorescence assays currently available are extremely sensitive but not necessary for all patients. Since the prevalence of RSV during an epidemic is so high, routine testing is costly and is best reserved for children with predisposing medical conditions or complicated courses of disease.

Complete blood counts (CBCs) and chemistries may not be helpful in diagnosis. The white blood cell count can be normal or elevated with a left shift. An elevated band count may be present. Chemistries should be obtained if there is poor feeding or evidence of dehydration. Salicylate ingestion may present with respiratory distress, and mixed metabolic acidoses and respiratory alkelosis and β-blocker ingestions can exacerbate wheezing, so the history should include questioning about possible injestion. Chest x-ray may reveal patchy atelectasis, segmental atelectasis, hyperinflation, and peribronchial thickening.

Emergency Department Management

Most cases of bronchiolitis are treated on an outpatient basis, for which close follow-up with a private pediatrician is essential. During RSV epidemics, the emergency physician will be exposed to a broad spectrum of patients at varying stages of disease and must be able to identify those who need admission and who are at risk for apnea. Infants in respiratory failure will require emergent intubation and admission to the ICU. Treatment is mainly supportive and consists of oxygen, fluid replacement, fever management, and optimal bronchodilators. The most important therapy is supplemental humidified oxygen. At concentrations of 28 to 40 percent, arterial hypoxemia is improved in most infants.

Increased insensible fluid loss occurs from increased work of breathing and can cause significant dehydration that warrants a 20 mL/kg bolus. Patients with poor fluid intake due to congestion may also require intravenous hydration and admission (especially if parents are unable to feed the child owing to uncontrollable secretions). Beyond initial resuscitation, fluid replacement should not exceed maintenance due to the potential for the development of pulmonary edema in some of these children.

Fever should be controlled with acetaminophen or ibuprofen. Children with concurrent otitis media should receive the appropriate course of oral antibiotics. Those who appear toxic with temperature above 38.5°C should have a CBC drawn to rule out other intercurrent infections. A 9-year prospective study of 565 children with documented RSV showed the risk of secondary bacterial infection was low; subsequent secondary bacterial infections were seen more frequently in the group treated with antibiotics.[38]

BRONCHODILATORS A trial of bronchodilator therapy is optional and reasonable in the treatment of bronchiolitis and can be aborted if the child fails to show a response. Much research points to the fact that unless there is a history of asthma, there is a limited role for bronchodilator therapy in treatment of bronchiolitis. Many studies of oral and nebulized albuterol alone show that it fails to improve oxygen saturation or to reduce the length of hospitalizations,[39–41] leading some authors to question the cost/benefit of such therapy. Ipatropium also does not affect the natural course of the disease,[42] although anecdotes suggest it may have a role in drying up secretions.

Racemic epinephrine has been compared with albuterol and found to reduce hospitalizations in children with bronchiolitis.[43] It can improve symptom scores of respiratory rate, wheezing, and retractions at 15 min compared with nebulized saline.[44] It can be used safely in hospitalized children up to every 2 h. If used in the ED, the authors recommend an observation period of 4 h before a disposition decision is made.

HELIOX Heliox can be considered for children with severe obstructive symptoms and works for the same reasons as in asthma. A recent study[45] showed that its use increased Sa_{O_2} in children when compared with oxygen alone. At this juncture, its use can provide a useful bridge in reducing the need for intubation in certain populations of infected children.

GLUCOCORTICOIDS Controlled studies have failed to demonstrate any proven benefit in the use of glucocorticoids, including studies on oral prednisolone and dexamethasone.[46] The authors recommend the use of glucocorticoids only if there is a history of asthma; these drugs have been helpful in infants with a history of BPD. Initial reports on budesonide, a smaller molecule that has been widely studied in Europe and Australia, suggest a benefit. In a Finnish study[47] of 100 patients, budesonide was seen to reduce the number of hospital admissions and subsequent wheezing episodes as compared with controls. A more recent study on nebulized budesonide[48] stated that its effects in preventing postbronchiolitic wheezing were unremarkable. It is currently being introduced in the United States in a MDI form and more studies need to be performed.

RIBAVIRIN Ribavirin is a guanosine-resembling synthetic nucleoside analogue generally used as inpatient therapy. When delivered as a small-particle aerosol, it has produced improvement in oxygenation. It is thought to work by decreasing viral protein synthesis. Candidates for such treatment are those with immunodeficiency, cystic fibrosis, congenital heart disease, and severe illnesses of infancy. Since the introduction of intravenous immunoglobin, the use of ribavirin appears to be less frequent.

RESPIGAM RSV IMMUNE GLOBULIN INTRAVENOUS (HUMAN) RespiGam has been in use for the past few years as outpatient passive immunization for infants at risk for severe RSV disease. The treatment involves monthly intravenous infusion of immunoglobulin during RSV season. It is recommended for infants with documented BPD and for those with a gestational age of less than 35 weeks (at the discretion of the physician). The PREVENT[49] study demonstrated a reduction of the incidence and duration of RSV hospitalization and severity of illness.

PALIVIZUMAB (SYNAGIS) The FDA approved Synagis in mid-1998 for prevention of RSV in pediatric patients. It is the first monoclonal antibody that can be given by intramuscular injection to provide protection against infection[50] (protein binding neutralizes the virus). Like RespiGam, it is administered monthly to those patients at highest risk and is desirable for those children in whom vascular access is a challenge. The Impact-RSV trial[50] showed a 55 percent reduction in hospitalization in a group of 1500 patients, with few adverse effects. These results and the ease of administration are encouraging in reducing the morbidity of the disease.

OTHER MODALITIES The anecdotal theory that mist helps to dilute secretions has not been proven; in fact, very little water reaches the lower airways to begin with. Infants with high temperatures and documented RSV are unlikely to require workup for occult bacteremia unless they appear septic. Studies have failed to show any utility in obtaining blood cultures in children with fever attributable to RSV. Antibiotics should be reserved for concurrent otitis media or other identifiable bacterial infections.

Disposition

Infants with visible moderate to severe respiratory distress, apneic spells, or dehydration should be admitted to the ICU. Infants without wheezing but sustained tachypnea (RR > 60) should also be admitted, preferably to a step-down unit. Hospitalization should be considered in all infants with a history of BPD, congenital heart disease, and immunocompromise.

Those with mild disease who are taking fluids well and whose parents are capable of taking care of them may be released with good follow-up instructions. Home health visits and nebulizers may be instituted if deemed necessary. Albuterol in syrup form can also be initiated for children who respond. Parents should be instructed on how to perform aggressive nasal suctioning and evaluate respiratory distress. Use of vapor solutions available over the counter should be discouraged, and parents who smoke cigarettes should be cautioned that tobacco smoke can worsen the illness. Decongestants and antihistamines are of questionable benefit; their use in infants less than 6 months of age is not recommended.

REFERENCES

1. Expert Panel Report 2: *Guidelines for the Diagnosis and Management of Asthma.* 1997 National Institutes of Health Publication No. 98-4051. Bethesda, MD: NIH, 1997.
2. Surveillance for Asthma—United States 1960–1995. *MMWR* 47:6, 1998.
3. Surveillance for Asthma-United States 1960–1995. *MMWR* 47:14, 1998.
4. Calmes D, Leake BD, Carlisle DM: Adverse outcomes among children hospitalized with asthma in California. *Pediatrics* 101:845–850, 1998.
5. Surveillance for Asthma—United States 1960–1995. *MMWR* 47:7, 1998.
6. Surveillance for Asthma—United States 1960–1995. *MMWR* 47:16, 1998.
7. Goodman DC, Stukel TA, Chang CH: Trends in Pediatric asthma hospitalization rates: regional and socioeconomic differences. *Pediatrics* 101:208, 1998.

8. Kercsmar C: Asthma in Chernick V, Boat T (eds): *Kendig's Disorders of the Respiratory Tract in Children,* 6th ed. Philadelphia: Saunders, 1998, pp 688–699.
9. Davis WB: Eosinophilic alveolitis in acute respiratory failure: A clinical marker for a non-infectious etiology. *Chest* 90:7, 1986.
10. McFadden ER, Gilbert IA: *N Engl J Med* 327:1928, 1992.
11. Kercsmar C: *Asthma* in Chernick and Boat (eds): *Kendig's Disorders of the Respiratory Tract in Children* 6 ed., Saunders, 1998; p 688.
12. Wohl M: *Developmental physiology of the respiratory system* in Chernick V, Boat T (eds): *Kendig's Disorders of the Respiratory Tract in Children,* 6th ed., Philadelphia: Saunders, 1998, p 19.
13. Wood DW, Downess JJ, Lecks HI: A clinical scoring system for the diagnosis of respiratory failure. *Am J Dis Child* 123:227, 1972.
14. Katz RW, Kelly HW, Crowley MR, Grad R, et al: Safety of continuous nebulized albuterol for bronchospasm in infants and children. *Pediatrics* 92:666, 1993.
15. Buck M: Administration of albuterol by continuous nebulization. *AACN Clin Iss* 6:279, 1995.
16. Williams JR, Bothner JP, Swanton RD: Delivery of albuterol in a pediatric emergency department. *Pediatr Emerg Car* 12:263, 1996.
17. Suissa S, Ernst P, Boivin JF, Horwitz RI, et al: A cohort analysis of excess mortality in asthma and use of inhaled beta-agonists. *Am J Respir Crit Care Med* 149:604, 1994.
18. Davis AO, Lefkowitz RJ: Corticosteroid-induced differential regulation of beta-adrenergic receptors in circulating human polymorphonuclear leukocytes and mononuclear leukocytes. *J Clin Endocrinol Metab* 51:599, 1980.
19. Hui KK, Conolly ME, Tashkin DP: reversal of human lymphocyte B-adrenoceptor desensitization by glucocorticoids. *Clin Pharmacol Ther* 32:566, 1982.
20. Barnett PL, Caputo GL, Baskin M, Kuppermann J: Intravenous versus oral corticosteroids in management of acute asthma in children. *Ann Emerg Med* 29:212, 1997.
21. Tal A, Levy N, Bearman JE: Methylprednisolone therapy for acute asthma in infants and toddlers: A controlled clinical trial. *Pediatrics* 86:350, 1990.
22. Scarfone RJ, Fuchs SM, Nager AL, Shane SA, et al: Controlled clinical trial of oral prednisone in emergency department treatment of children with acute asthma.*Pediatrics* 92:513, 1993.
23. Rodrigo C, Rodrigo O: Early administration of hydrocortisone in emergency room treatment of acute asthma. *Respir Med* 88:755, 1994.
24. Wolfson DH, Nypaver MM, Blaser M, Hogan A, et al: A controlled trial of methyl-prednisolone in early ED treatment of acute asthma in children. *Pediatr Emerg Care* 10:335, 1994.
25. Lin RY, Resola GR, West fal RE, Bakalchuk L, et al: Early parenteral corticosteroids administration in acute asthma. *Am J Emerg Med* 15:621, 1997.
26. Dales RE, Schweitzer I, Kerr P, Crougeon L, et al: Risk factors for recurrent emergency department visits for asthma. *Thorax* 50:520, 1995.
27. Laitinen LA, Laitinen A: Remodeling of asthmatic airways by glucocorticosteroids. *J Allergy Clin Immunol* 97:153, 1996.
28. deBlic J, Delacourt C, Le Bourgeois M, Mahut B, et al: Efficacy of nebulized budesonide in treatment of severe infantile asthma; A double blind study. *J Allergy Clin Immunol* 98:14, 1996.
29. Sung L, Osmond MH, Klassen TP: *Acad Emerg Med* 5:209, 1998.
30. Schuh S, Johnson DW, Callahan S, Canny G, et al: Efficacy of frequent nebulized Ipatropium bromide added to frequent high dose albuterol therapy in severe childhood asthma. *J Pediatr* 126:639, 1995.
31. Qureshi F, Pestian J, Davis P, Zaritsky A: Effective nebulized ipratropium on the hospitalization rates of children with asthma. *N Engl J Med* 8:1030, 1998.
32. Ciarallo L, Sauer AH, Shannon MW: IV Mg therapy for moderate to severe pediatric asthma: Results of a randomized, placebo-controlled trial. *J Pediatr* 129:809, 1996.
33. Devi PR, Kumar L, Singhi SC, Prasad R, et al: IV MgSo4 in acute severe asthma not responding to conventional therapy. *Indian Pediatr* 34:389, 1997.
34. Kudukis TM, Manthous CA, Schmidt GA, Hall JB, et al: Inhaled heliox revisited: Effect of inhaled helium oxygen mixture during treatment of status asthmaticus in children. *J Pediatr* 130:217, 1997.
35. Cydulka RK, Emerman CL: A pilot study of steroid therapy after emergency department treatment of acute asthma: is a taper needed? *J Emerg Med* 16:15, 1998.
36. Holloway J, Ferriss J, Groff J, Craig TJ, et al: Churg-Strauss syndrome associated with zafirlukast. *J Am Osteopath Assoc* 98:275, 1998.
37. Wohl ME: Bronchiolitis, in Chernick V, Boat T (eds): *Kendig's Disorders of the Respiratory Tract in Children,* 6th ed., Philadelphia: Saunders, 1998, p 473.
38. Hall CB, Powell KR, Schnabel KC, Gala CL, et al: Risk of secondary bacterial infection in infants hospitalized with RSV infection. *J Pediatr* 113:266, 1988.
39. Dobson JV, Stephens-Groff SM, McMahon SR, Stemmler MM, et al: The use of albuterol in hospitalized infants with bronchiolitis. *Pediatrics* 101 (3pt 1):361, 1998.
40. Lugo RA, Salyer JW, Dean JM: Albuterol in acute bronchiolitis-continued therapy despite poor response? *Pharmacotherapy* 18:198, 1998.
41. Cengizlier R, Saraclar Y, Adalioglu G, Tuncer A: Effect of oral and inhaled salbutamol in infants with bronchiolitis. *Acta Paediatr Jpn* 39:61, 1997.
42. Chowdury D, al Howasi M, Khalil M, al-Frayh AS, et al: The role of bronchodilators in the management of bronchiolitis: A clinical trial. *Ann Trop Paediatr* 15:77, 1995.
43. Menon K, Sutcliffe T, Klassen TP: A randomized trial comparing the efficacy of epinephrine with salbutamol in the treatment of acute bronchiolitis. *J Pediatr* 126:1004, 1995.
44. Reijnonen T, Korppi M, Pitkakangas S, Tenhola T, et al: The clinical efficacy of nebulized racemic epinephrine and albuterol in acute bronchiolitis. *Arch Pediatr Adolesc Med* 149:686, 1995.
45. Hollman G, Shen G, Zeng L, Yngsdal-Krenz R, et al: Helium-oxygen improves clinical asthma scores in children with acute bronchiolitis. *Crit Care Med* 26:1731, 1998.
46. Klassen TP, Sutcliffe T, Watters LK, et al: Dexamethasone in salbutamol treated inpatients with acute bronchiolitis: A randomized controlled trial. *J Pediatr* 130:191, 1997.
47. Reijnonen T, Korppi M, Kuikka L, Remes K, et al: Anti-inflammatory therapy reduces wheezing after bronchiolitis. *Arch Pediatr Adolesc Med* 150:512, 1996.
48. Richter H, Seddon P, et al: Early nebulized budesonide in treatment of bronchiolitis and prevention of post-bronchiolitis wheezing. *J Pediatr* 132:849, 1998.
49. The PREVENT Study Group: *Pediatrics* 99:93, 1997.
50. Palivizumab: A Humanized RSV monoclaonal antibody reduces hospitalization from RSV infection in high risk infants. The IMpact-RSV Study Group: *Pediatrics* 102:531, 1998.
51. Church NR, Anas NG, Hall CB, Brooks JG: RSV-related apnea in infants: Demographics and outcome. *Am J Dis Child* 138:247, 1984.
52. Korrpi M, Kuikka L, Reijomen T, Remes K, et al: Bronchial asthma and hyperreactivity after early childhood bronchiolitis or pneumonia. An 8-year follow up study. *Arch Pediatr Adolesc Med* 148:1079, 1994.

SEIZURES AND STATUS EPILEPTICUS IN CHILDREN

Michael A. Nigro

Approximately 2 percent of the United States population have some form of epilepsy. Many more experience seizures in association with febrile illnesses or other acute problems. In children aged 0 to 9 years, the prevalence is 4.4 cases per 1000, and in those 10 to 19 years, the prevalence is 6.6 cases per 1000. Simple febrile convulsions constitute a separate category, with an incidence of 3 to 4 percent in children.

These numbers alone do not reveal the most important features of the seizure phenomenon—the increased morbidity and mortality rates that are a direct result of seizures, their cause, or their treatment. Epidemiologic studies indicate an overall mortality rate two to three times higher in epileptic patients than in nonepileptics. The earlier the onset of seizures and the more deprived the social environment, the higher the morbidity and mortality rates.

Typically, a patient with seizures arrives at the emergency department with one of the following:

1. The initial or a recurrent seizure
2. Status epilepticus
3. Complications of medication

TABLE 121-1 International Classification of Epileptic Seizures

Partial seizures (seizures beginning focally)
- Partial seizures with elementary symptomatology (generally without impairment of consciousness)
  - With motor symptoms (includes Jacksonian seizures)
  - With special sensory or somatosensory symptoms
  - With autonomic symptoms
  - Compound forms
- Partial seizures with complex symptomatology (generally with impairment of consciousness)
  - With impairment of consciousness only
  - With cognitive symptomatology
  - With affective symptomatology
  - With "psychosensory" symptomatology
  - With "psychomotor" symptomatology
  - Compound forms
- Partial seizures secondarily generalized

Generalized seizures (bilaterally symmetric without localized onset)
- Absences (petit mal)
- Bilateral massive epileptic myoclonus
- Infantile spasms
- Clonic seizures
- Tonic seizures
- Tonic-clonic seizures (grand mal)
- Atonic seizures
- Akinetic seizures

Unclassified epileptic seizures

Source: From Gastaut,[1] with permission.

4. A history of seizures with an acute, underlying disease—e.g., sickle cell anemia, metabolic disease, or febrile illness—that needs treatment

Emergency care should include (1) safely stopping the seizure, (2) identifying and correcting immediately treatable or reversible causes, and (3) initiating appropriate diagnostic studies and arranging follow-up. If management is difficult, the patient should be admitted. There are significant enough differences in the treatment of children that unless the physician is experienced in pediatric management or able to readily obtain pediatric consultation, the child should be transferred to a pediatric facility. Treatment and diagnostic studies may be complex, and time is important in reducing morbidity.

DEFINITION

A *seizure* is an episodic alteration in motor activity, behavior, sensation, or autonomic function. It represents an abrupt change in brain function. The term *epilepsy* indicates recurring seizures without a simple discernible and reversible cause. Physiologically, a seizure is an abnormal, sudden, and excessive electric discharge of neurons (gray matter) that propagates down the neuronal processes (white matter) to affect end organs in a clinically measurable fashion. The International Classification of Epileptic Seizures is accepted as the contemporary standard (Table 121-1).

EEG

Electroencephalographic (EEG) recording on an emergent basis is becoming more commonplace as the phenomenon of nonconvulsive status epilepticus (NCSE) is appreciated. In this condition, the patient seems to be seizure free but unresponsive and the EEG indicates a condition of subclinical status epilepticus and warrants more aggressive treatment to improve the EEG abnormality, if this is possible. In a child who unexpectedly remains comatose or in a neonate where clinical seizures may be difficult to detect, immediate and continuous EEG monitoring may more reliably direct aggressive antiepileptic drug (AED) treatment.

NEUROIMAGING IN EPILEPSY

The choice of central nervous system (CNS) imaging depends in part on the circumstances and the age of the patient:

1. Cerebral ultrasound is most advantageous in the evaluation of neonates and young infants as a quick and relatively reliable method to identify intraventricular and parenchymal hemorrhage, periventricular leukomalacia, major malformations, cerebral edema, and hydrocephalus. It is not as useful in identifying more discrete cerebral migrational defects.
2. Computed tomography (CT) has its best application in evaluating seizures associated with head trauma.
3. Magnetic resonance imaging (MRI) is the preferred imaging technique in evaluating causes of epilepsy including migrational defects, mesial temporal sclerosis, acute parainfectious disseminated encephalomyelitis, stroke, and neoplasm.
4. Magnetic resonance angiography (MRA) is of value in defining vascular abnormalities of stroke and stroke-like events.
5. Transcranial doppler can be helpful in determining impending cerebrovascular occlusive disease of sickle cell anemia.

NEWER ANTIEPILEPTIC DRUGS (AEDs)

Newer AEDs are indicated in the management of seizures as add-on drugs, although there are currently numerous studies determining their application as initial and monotherapy.

Gabapentin

Gabapentin (Neurontin) was released in 1994 as adjunctive therapy for partial seizures. It is a novel AED with ill-defined mechanism of action, although it was initially designed as a GABAergic agent, i.e., increasing the effect of γ-aminobutyric acid (GABA), the major cerebral inhibitor. It has no drug interactions, is not metabolized, and is not protein bound. Normal renal function is desirable, since it is excreted solely via the renal system. A short half-life of 5 to 6 h, and limited intestinal absorption capability necessitates frequent dosing of 3 to 4 times a day. Dosage is 20 to 60 mg/kg/day, and maximal dosage can be reached in several days. Side effects are mild, self-limiting, and usually consist of vertigo, light-headedness and, infrequently, behavioral changes. Rarely, myoclonic seizures have been provoked soon after initiating the drug. AED levels are not useful in determining therapeutic and toxic effects. It is available in 100-, 300-, and 400-mg capsules.

Lamotrigine

Lamotrigine (Lamictal) probably acts on voltage-sensitive sodium channels and excitatory amino acid neurotransmitters. Two very important features of lamotrigine include its predilection to produce a significant rash, which could progress to Stevens-Johnson syndrome, and the effects of comedication. The half-life of lamotrigine is reduced by 50 percent when administered with enzyme inducers such as phenytoin, carbamazepine, and phenobarbital and doubled when used in conjunction with valproate. The combination with valproate has been associated with most of the adverse reactions. In children, it should be started very slowly and increased very gradually. It is indicated in the treatment of partial and generalized epilepsy, including absence, drop, and myoclonic seizures. When administered with enzyme inducers, the dose begins at 2 mg/kg/day and is increased over 6 to 8 weeks to a maximum of 15 mg/kg/day. When used with valproate

(Depakote), it should be started at 0.2 mg/kg every other day, increased by 0.2 mg/kg/day to 1 mg/kg/day, and then, over the next 6 weeks, increased to a maximum of 5 mg/kg/day. When changes are made in reducing or introducing comedication, the lamotrigine dose will have to be modified in most instances. Given as monotherapy, the half-life is 25 to 30 h. It has minimal protein binding. Blood levels do not reflect toxic or therapeutic effects. There is no reported significant hepatic or hematologic side effect.

Topiramate

Topiramate (Topamax) became available in 1997. Its mechanism of action is uncertain, but it appears to be effective in preventing propagation of the seizure from its focus. The half-life is 19 to 23 h, and 85 percent of the drug is eliminated unchanged through the renal system. The remaining 15 percent is metabolized by P-450 hepatic metabolism. With the relatively long half-life, the drug is given in a twice-daily dosage. It is indicated in the treatment of partial seizures and is being evaluated as monotherapy. In children, the drug is begun slowly at 1 mg/kg/day and over 8 to 12 weeks is gradually increased to a maximum of 10 mg/kg/day or 400 mg/day if necessary. The major side effect limiting dosage and rate of incrementing dosage is the effect on memory and name recall.

Tiagabine

Tiagabine (Gabitril) is a GABA reuptake inhibitor resulting in higher levels of cerebral GABA available for inhibition of the epileptic excitatory activity. With a relatively short half-life of 5 to 8 h ultimate dosage should be administered tid. Absorption is slower and the drug more easily tolerated when given with meals. Metabolism is via the P-450 mechanism and, as a result, the half-life is significantly reduced by coadministration with enzyme inducers such as carbamazepine, phenytoin, and phenobarbital. The maximum effective dose in children at this time is estimated to be 1 mg/kg/day. This dose should be started at 0.1 mg/kg/day and gradually increased over the next 6 to 10 weeks. Because of high protein binding, free levels of coadministered AEDs should be monitored (phenytoin, carbamazepine, and valproate). Most common side effects are sedation and behavioral. Activation of myoclonic seizures can also occur.

Vigabatrin

Vigabatrin (Sabril) is an enzyme-induced irreversible inhibitor of GABA aminotransferase resulting in increased cerebral GABA levels. It is rapidly absorbed, unaffected by food consumption. It is not protein-bound and is excreted unmetabolized by the renal system. It has no significant drug interactions. Blood levels are not useful in determining therapeutic effect or toxicity. Abnormalities of cerebral myelin have not been substantiated in humans; however, recently investigators identified visual changes in adults using vigabatrin. Dosage is initated at 30 mg/kg/day and gradually increased over 4 weeks to a maximum of 100 mg/kg/day (bid dosage) if necessary for improved seizure control. European studies initially found it very effective in the treatment of infantile spasms associated with tuberous sclerosis. More common side effects include dizziness, ataxia, and behavioral changes in children. As with all AEDs, seizure activation has been reported but cannot be predicted with any reliability.

Oxcarbazepine

Oxcarbazepine (Trileptal) is a 10-keto analogue of carbamazepine but is not oxidatively metabolized. As a result, there is little, if any, induction of hepatic enzymes and no autoinduction of metabolism, allowing for a more rapid titration to maximum dosage. Its active metabolite is a monohydroxy derivative (MHD) that has a half-life of 10 h, allowing for a bid dosing. It is begun at 20 mg/kg/day and increased to a maximum of 60 mg/kg/day or to tolerance and seizure control. It will probably be approved for use as adjunctive treatment of partial epilepsies. It can be used in combination with any of the existing AEDs, including carbamazepine. Unlike carbamazepine, it has no epoxide metabolites and is not affected by erythromycin.

Depacon

Depacon is the intravenous preparation of valproate, and recent experience indicates it is well tolerated by children. It is usually administered IV when the oral maintenance dose cannot be tolerated and can also be used at a higher induction dose when rapid levels are desired and the patient is naive to the drug. Dosage is the usual maintenance dose administered IV over 15 min. Loading dose for naive patients is 10 to 30 mg/kg IV over 15 min.

Extended Release Agents

Carbatrol and Tegretol XR are extended-release forms of carbamazepine that permit bid or 12-h dosing.

Fosphenytoin

Fosphenytoin (Cerebyx) is a prodrug of phenytoin that contains a disodium phosphate ester that is cleaved during hydrolysis, yielding a molecule of phenytoin. Phosphatases are ubiquitous and present in newborns, so fosphenytoin can be used at any age. It is water soluble and can be given IV and intramuscularly (IM) without the side effect of infusion-related complications attributed to phenytoin extravasation. A 1 mg phenytoin equivalent (PE) is the therapeutic equivalent of 1 mg of phenytoin. Fosphenytoin can be infused at 3 mg PE/kg/min with therapeutic free phenytoin levels achieved by 7 to 8 min following infusion and 30 min following IM use. Rapid infusion in alert patients may produce perineal pruritis.

ADDITIONAL ADVANCES IN EPILEPSY TREATMENT THAT WARRANT CONSIDERATION

Increasingly, children with intractable epilepsy are undergoing implantation of the Cyberonics vagus nerve stimulator (Neurocybernetic Prosthesis System). This devise is programmed to deliver a stimulus at a specific intensity and frequency for a specific interval (e.g., 15 s every 3 min). Although the mechanism of action is uncertain, electrical stimulus of the left vagus nerve can significantly reduce seizure frequency. Common side effects include hoarseness and difficulty swallowing during stimulation. Problems with instrumentation are unlikely to warrant an emergency department visit. A malfunctioning stimulator can be temporarily turned off by taping a magnet over the subcutaneous pacemaker.

The ketogenic diet has been used with increasing frequency in the management of childhood epilepsy. Ketones are an alternative energy source for cerebral metabolism. By severely restricting glucose and increasing fat intake, ketosis can be maintained and seizure control improved. There are several concerns about an emergency department visit that warrant mention. It is necessary to maintain ketosis and, as a result, glucose infusions should be avoided if possible, and prescriptions given should have no measurable carbohydrate content. This is most easily managed by consultation with the prescribing neurologist, associated dietician, and pharmacist. Hematuria and flank pain may be due to renal calculi. Pancreatitis is an uncommon occurrence in children on the ketogenic diet.

TABLE 121-2 Critical Pathway: New-Onset Seizure with Neurologic Compromise

Clinical Assessment	History and Physical Examination
Tests	Complete blood count Urinalysis Calcium, magnesium Electrolytes Urine drug screen
Procedures	Neuroimaging: computed tomography or magnetic resonance imaging. EEG
Admit	To neurology if no primary care physician. Anticipate 2-day admission.
Nutrition/hydration	Keep vein open as indicated per age.
Meds IV	If rapid AED induction is warranted, use either phenobarbital or fosphenytoin 20 mg PE/kg at 3 mg PE/kg/min.
Meds PO	Less rapid AED induction can be achieved with the same dosage PO in 3 divided doses over 6 h.
Monitoring ancillaries	Vital signs and neurologic checks every hour if loading and then as indicated. Cardiac monitor, pulse oximeter, resuscitative equipment available.
Education	Discuss possible cause of seizure, potential risk for more seizures, and need for AEDs.
Discharge planning	Arrange out patient follow-up.

Abbreviations: AED, antiepileptic drug; PE, phenytoin equivalent.

THE FIRST SEIZURE

The first seizure in a child usually causes some degree of panic in the parents, and an accurate description of the seizure and preseizure events may not be obtainable. If it lasts seconds to minutes, and if others in the family have experienced seizures, an emergency visit may not be made. Unless the child is in status epilepticus, or seizures recur in the emergency department (Table 121-2), the physician can defer immediate anticonvulsant treatment and concentrate on defining the cause and the risk of recurrence (Fig. 121-1).

Hauser and coworkers[2] categorized seizure recurrence for all ages according to the presumed cause. Of their patients, 73 percent were categorized as having idiopathic seizures and 27 percent as having remote symptomatic seizures. Idiopathic seizures recurred in 17 percent of the patients by 20 months after the initial seizure and in 26 percent of the patients by 36 months after the first seizure, but the recurrence rate was greater in patients with generalized spike-wave EEGs and in patients with siblings who had had seizures. In patients with prior neurologic insult (cerebrovascular accident, meningitis, etc.), the recurrence rate was 34 percent by 20 months after the initial seizure.

Immediate diagnostic evaluation (Table 121-3) is initiated in the emergency situation. If the seizure was brief and appears to be idiopathic, the decision to initiate anticonvulsant therapy can be deferred until the appropriate neurologic assessment is completed. The causes of a first seizure vary, but idiopathic seizures account for 26.3 to 47 percent of children seen with seizures, depending on the study cited. Secondary seizures occur for a wide variety of reasons (e.g., inflammatory, structural, metabolic, or secondary to general illness).

In any group of seizure patients, there is a subgroup in which the seizure is a symptom of an underlying disorder and is not due to idiopathic epilepsy. In such cases, correction of the primary problem makes seizure recurrence unlikely. Thus, the primary goal must be to uncover disorders that are readily identifiable and reversible. Symptomatic seizures of hypoglycemia, hypocalcemia, and electrolyte imbalance can be treated immediately. There is little risk of recurrence and no need for anticonvulsant use. Seizures occurring as a result of intracranial infections and craniocerebral trauma may require only immediate or short-term anticonvulsant use. Symptomatic seizures of systemic lupus erythematosus (SLE), sickle cell anemia, leukemia, arteriovenous malformations, and neoplasms may be the heralding symptoms of a complex, yet treatable, underlying disease. Seizures have been reported in children after topical application of *N, N*-diethyl-*m*-toluamide (DEET) and lindane (Kwell). Ingestion of rare and common agents has been associated with new-onset seizures, including camphor, theophylline, isoniazid, tricyclic antidepressants, oral and parenteral meperedine, cyclosporine, stimulants such as methylphenidate, and lead and mercury exposure. These seizures may be brief and self-limiting or may progress to status epilepticus and result in permanent neurologic sequelae and epilepsy. Identification and specific treatment of the underlying problem are most important to achieve full recovery. Aseptic and bacterial meningitis, viral encephalitis, brain abscess, and more uncommon problems such as cat-scratch fever and mycoplasma-related encephalopathy may present with seizures. In a child with a ventriculoperitoneal shunt, seizures are more likely to arise from associated cerebral abnormalities (epilepsy) rather than shunt malfunction.

If the initial seizure is prolonged or emerges into status epilepticus, appropriate therapy and diagnostic workup must be initiated (Tables 121-3 to 121-5). If seizures are acutely repetitive or occur in the presence of associated or preexisting neurologic deficit and the patient is at a higher risk for recurrence of seizures, then anticonvulsant management can be initiated immediately (Table 121-4). For partial seizures, carbamazepine, phenytoin, and phenobarbital are most commonly used and equally efficacious whereas, in primary generalized seizures, valproate is most commonly used. However, the other AEDs are also effective and may need to be used because of intolerance or ineffectiveness. For the most part, these AEDs can be used interchangeably.

Side-effect profile, physician preference, and parental experience and comfort usually dictate which AED will be used initially. Phenytoin and carbamazepine have a similar mechanism of action and effectiveness; therefore, their side-effect profiles will determine which to initiate. Phenobarbital is quite effective and, though a sedative, in some may create more problems of irritability and limit its effectiveness. Nonetheless, it can be well tolerated in the majority of infants and children and has a wide spectrum of effectiveness. See Table 121-2 for the clinical pathway in management of new-onset seizures.

Absence seizures (petit mal) rarely require emergency care, and an EEG should be obtained for confirmation before one starts AEDs, since absence seizures could mimic partial status and an AED such as ethosuximide will be ineffective. Valproate, ethosuximide and, more recently, lamotrigine are the appropriate AEDs for absence epilepsy chronic management, with the benzodiazepines effective in the acute management of status absence epilepticus.

FEBRILE SEIZURE

Febrile seizure is a unique and common form of seizure in childhood. Although various types occur (tonic, tonic-clonic, and clonic), the characteristics of a simple febrile seizure separate it from other symptomatic and idiopathic seizure disorders. The National Institutes of Health (NIH) Consensus Development Conference of Febrile Seizure defined it as an event in infancy or childhood usually occurring between 3 months and 5 years of age, associated with fever but without evidence of intracranial infection or defined cause.[3] Typically, these seizures are generalized and last less than 10 min, and there is no postictal

FIG. 121-1. New onset seizure. General treatment plan.

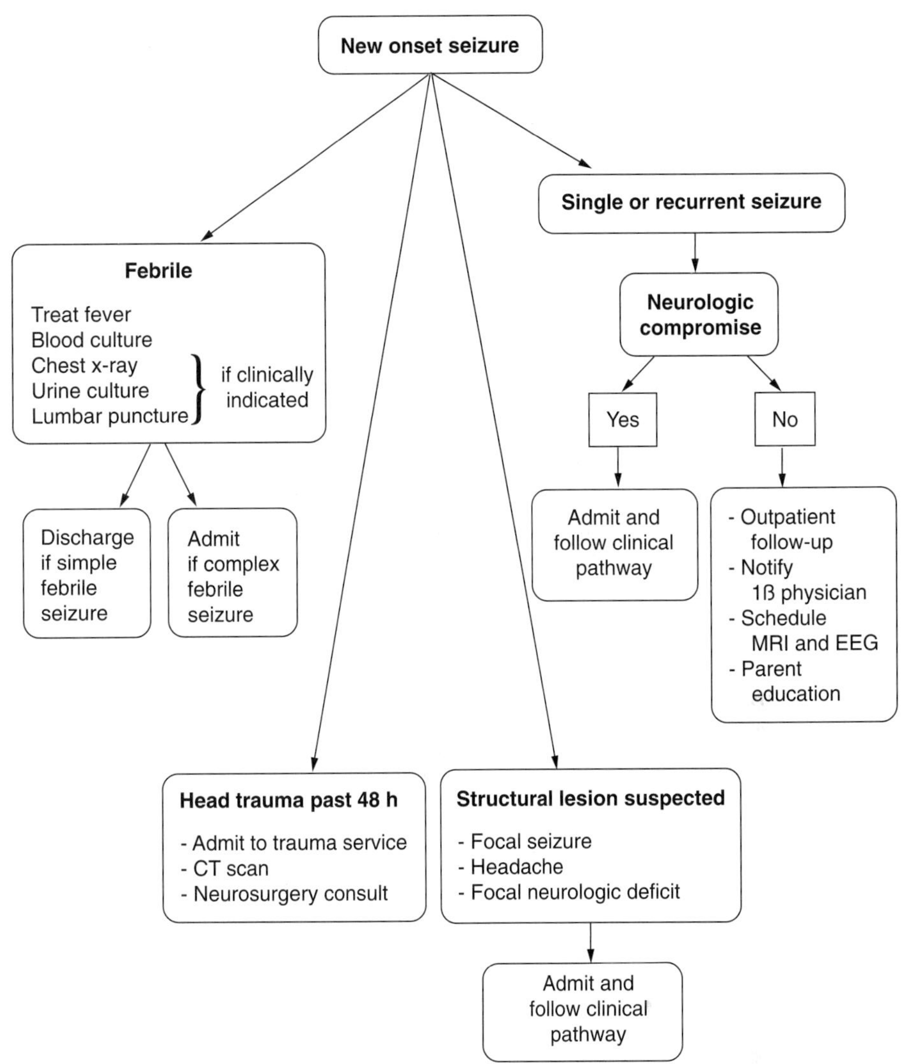

focal neurologic deficit. The EEG usually does not reveal paroxysmal (epileptic) activity, and there often is a family history of similar seizures. Typically, a rapid rise in temperature, usually above 38.8°C (101.8°F), occurs at the onset of the illness and, on occasion, recurs several times in the course of the illness. Three to four percent of young children experience febrile seizures and, of these, 30 to 40 percent have recurrences, especially when the first seizure occurs when a child is younger than 1 year of age. The mortality from simple febrile seizures is extremely low.

Evaluation

The first febrile seizure warrants the most concern, because the benign nature of the illness has not yet been established. More concern regarding intracranial infection is justified with the first febrile seizure before the propensity for recurring simple febrile convulsions has been established. The initial evaluation concentrates on serious causes, such as meningitis, encephalitis, and bacterial sepsis. Lumbar puncture is warranted whenever intracranial infection appears likely. If a cause is not found and the child is ill, admission, workup, and therapy are warranted. Underlying diseases should be diagnosed. Toxic encephalopathy with fever as a symptom should be identified and treated. An EEG can be done electively and, when indicated by family history or atypical presentation, may be helpful in determining whether AED treatment is warranted.

Treatment

Therapy for the cause of the fever is the main goal. A simple febrile seizure does not warrant treatment with AEDs. Information from the NIH collaborative study pointed out the lack of benefit of chronic AED use, the greater likelihood of AED-related side effects, and the good prognosis in untreated patients. If a child exhibits repetitive seizures with this or prior febrile seizures, then phenobarbital can be administered and maintained until the child improves. Chronic AED prophylaxis with phenobarbital or valproate is limited to children with (1) complex febrile seizures (prolonged or focal), (2) a preexisting neurologic deficit, e.g., cerebral palsy, (3) onset under 6 months of age, (4) repeated seizures in the same illness, (5) prior nonfebrile seizures, and (6) more than three febrile seizures in 6 months.

Rectally or orally administered diazepam has been used successfully to prevent seizures when given at the onset of a febrile illness. Usual dosage is 0.2 to 0.5 mg/kg as a single dose.

If acute treatment is warranted, the following protocol is recommended:

1. Interrupt the fever gradually with tepid baths (no alcohol) and acetaminophen or ibuprofen administration.
2. Identify the source of infection and perform a lumbar puncture if meningitis or encephalitis is suspected.
3. If indicated, administer a loading dose of phenobarbital 15 mg/kg IV, followed by 4 to 6 mg/kg/day to attain therapeutic levels of 15 to 40 μg/mL.

TABLE 121-3 Diagnostic Studies in Seizure Patients

Study	Neonatal Seizure	First Seizure in Children	Status Epilepticus	Recurring Breakthrough (Nonstable)
Complete blood count with differential	X	X	X	—
Random blood sugar	X	X	X	X
Electrolytes	X	X	X	X
Creatinine	X	—	X	—
Magnesium	X	X	X	—
Calcium	X	X	X	X
Blood urea nitrogen	X	X	X	—
Blood gases	X	—	X	—
Serum ammonia	X*	—	—	—
Urine and serum amino acid screen	X*	X*	—	—
TORCH titers	X*	—	—	—
Lumbar puncture	X*	X*	X*	—
Anticonvulsant levels	—	—	X	X
EEG	X	X	X*	—
Echoencephalogram (real-time cerebral ultrasound)	X	—	—	—
Computed tomography	X*	X*	X*	X*
Magnetic resonance imaging	X*	X*	X*	X*
Chest x-ray	X*	X*	X*	X*
Skeletal x-ray survey	—	X*	X*	X*
Toxicology screen	X*	X*	X*	X*
Cardiac/pulmonary evaluation	X*	—	X	—
Evaluation for superimposed medical problems, infectious disease	X	X	X*	X

* When history or physical examination warrants it.
Note: X, diagnostic studies to be performed; —, studies need not be performed.

4. Arrange for follow-up studies with the child's family physician.
5. Admit the ill child without an easily treatable problem or one in whom recurrent seizures have occurred within several hours or 1 day.
6. Obtain an EEG when appropriate. An EEG may be helpful (if abnormal) as an indication of a convulsive disorder.

An alternative AED regime has been the administration of oral or rectal diazepam at the onset of a febrile illness prior to the onset of seizures. The Tufts University study by Rosman and colleagues[4] proved diazepam efficacy in seizure prevention when oral diazepam 0.33 mg/kg was administered every 8 h during all febrile illnesses in at-risk children. Importantly, 39 percent experienced side effects such as lethargy, ataxia, and irritability.

NEONATAL SEIZURES

Seizures in neonates are difficult to identify and often require aggressive therapy. All neonates experiencing seizures should be considered to be at serious risk from the underlying disorder and the effect of unremitting seizures and also to be at increased risk for epilepsy. Electroconvulsive activity should be of as much concern as the outward clinical signs of seizure. Prompt, effective anticonvulsant therapy and other specific therapies lessen the impact of short-term detrimental effect on long-term neurologic functioning. In many instances, the seizure itself is less important for its immediate effects than it is as an indicator of significant underlying disease (e.g., infection, metabolic disorder, or CNS malformation) that will ultimately have more effect on the morbidity and mortality rates.

The difference in seizure presentation is due to the lack of arborization of the immature brain, which prevents rapid propagation of electrical epileptic activity, and to the particular illnesses to which newborns are subject (hypoxic ischemic encephalopathy, and metabolic and dysplastic conditions). Multifocal or fragmentary seizures occur more commonly at this age, and clonic or tonic movements independently affect the limbs simultaneously or fleetingly.

Progressive migratory partial seizures (Jacksonian) are rarely seen at this age. Autonomic seizures manifest as variable changes in respira-

TABLE 121-4 Initial and Maintenance Doses in the First Seizure (Nonstatus Partial and Tonic, Clonic, and Tonic-Clonic Seizures of Childhood)

Drug	Route	Initial Dose, mg/kg/day	Maintenance Dose, mg/kg/day	THERAPEUTIC LEVEL Total	Free	Half-life, h
Phenytoin (Dilantin)[1]	PO/PR	8	4–8	10–22	1.0–2.2	24
Fosphenytoin (Cerebyx)	IV/IM	15–20 mg PE	4–8 mg PE	10–22	1.0–2.2	18
Carbamazepine (Tegretol, Carbatrol)	PO/PR	10	10–40	6–12	1.8–2.2	14[2]
Valproate (Depakote, Depakene)	PO/PR	10	20–60	50–130	10–25	10
Valproate (Depacon)	IV	10	20–60	50–130	10–25	10
Primidone (Mysoline)	PO/PR	5	10–20	5–12	NA	12
Ethosuximide (Zarontin)	PO/PR	20	20–30	50–100	NA	30
Gabapentin (Neurontin)	PO	20	20–60	NA	NA	6
Lamotrigine (Lamictal)[3,4]	PO	0.2–5.0	5–15	NA	NA	12–60
Topiramate (Topamax)	PO	1.0	8–10	NA	NA	14–23
Tiagabine (Gabitril)	PO	0.1	1	NA	NA	7
Clonazepam (Klonopin)	PO	.05	0.1–0.3	NA	NA	18–50
Acetazolamide (Diamox)	PO	10	10	NA	NA	24–42
Felbamate (Felbatol)[5]	PO	15	45	NA	NA	19
Oxcarbazepine[6]	PO	10	40–60	NA	NA	10
Vigabatrin[6]	PO	20	40–100	NA	NA	

[1]Higher free phenytoin levels when administered with valproate.
[2]With chronic use.
[3]6–8 weeks to achieve maintenance dose.
[4]Coadministration with valproate requires very low dosage initially, whereas coadministration with an enzyme inducer requires higher initial dosage.
[5]Not recommended for routine use.
[6]Likely to be available in 1999.
Abbreviation: PE, phenytoin equivalent; PR, per rectum.

tion (tachypnea, depression, or apnea), temperature, and color (cyanosis), and also as cardiac dysrhythmias and pupillary changes. Myoclonic seizures usually have hypoxic or metabolic causes and indicate a poor prognosis unless the cause is easily identifiable and readily reversible (e.g., hypocalcemia or hypoglycemia). Myoclonic seizures can, however, be refractory in metabolic disorders such as urea cycle defects and nonketotic hyperglycinemia. Unilateral (partial or focal) seizures may be associated with structural lesions, and permanent neurologic deficit may be associated with them. The causes of neonatal seizures are diverse, but the majority of the seizures are attributable to a few well-defined causes.

Evaluation

Common neurologic nonepileptic problems encountered in newborns are hyperexcitability in tremulous infants, nonepileptic cerebral manifestations of sepsis, cardiac disease, hypoxia, apnea of prematurity, and benign myoclonus. A rare condition seen in neonates is hyperekplexia. It is usually autosomally dominantly inherited and presents with exaggerated startle reactions to tactile stimuli over the face and trunk, resulting in tonic extension of the limbs, flexion of the head, and apnea. It is responsive to clonazepam.

The workup includes early assessment for treatable causes. Sepsis and metabolic derangements are frequent causes of neonatal seizures. The highest incidence of neonatal seizures is in infants with hypoxia/ischemia, sepsis, or hypoglycemia. Hereditary neonatal seizures (''fifth day fits'') are autosomal dominant, variably expressed, and usually require chronic AEDs, often with a good outcome.

Complex hereditary metabolic disorders—e.g., urea cycle defects with hyperammonemia, maple syrup urine disease, and methylmalonic acidemia—usually become evident days or weeks after feedings with protein are initiated. Others may appear symptomatic in utero or soon after delivery—e.g., nonketotic hyperglycinemia, in which the mother reports fetal hiccoughs—and soon after birth the infant is flaccid, exhibiting myoclonic seizures. Seizures in these metabolic disorders are a signal of possibly significant CNS impairment.

Some of these disorders may be completely controlled or the effects may be reversed with appropriate dietary management (galactosemia and urea cycle defects) or coenzyme replacement (pyridoxine dependency, biotinidase deficiency, subtypes of folate, and vitamin B_{12} responsive methylmalonic acidemia).

In evaluating an infant, the cause of the seizures may be readily apparent. Dysmorphic newborns could have a chromosomal defect (trisomy or deletion) or be identifiable only by the combination of unusual features (Cornelia de Lange syndrome). Neurocutaneous diseases infrequently cause seizures in newborns but are readily identifiable by certain signs, e.g., encephalotrigeminal hemangiomatosis in Sturge-Weber syndrome, or achromic patches in tuberous sclerosis.

TABLE 121-5 Doses for Status Epilepticus in Children

Drug	Recommended Loading Dose	Route	Repeat	Rate	Maximum Dose
Diazepam	0.2 mg/kg	IV	3 times	1 mg/min	5 mg 0–2 years 10 mg 2 years and older
Lorazepam	0.1 mg/kg	IV	4 times	Over 2 min	0.4 mg/kg
Midazolam	0.2 mg/kg	IV	1 time	Over 2 min	0.4 mg/kg
Midazolam infusion		IV	Continuous	0.04–0.05 mg/kg/h	Until seizure cessation
Phenobarbital	20.0 mg/kg	IV	0		400 mg
Fosphenytoin	20.0 mg PE/kg	IV	0	3 mg PE/kg/min	Until effective therapeutic level reached.
Paraldehyde	0.3 mL/kg	Rectal	q4h		15 mL
Clonazepam	0.3 mg/kg	NG	1 time		10 mg
Valproic acid	60.0 mg/kg	IV	0	Over 15 min	
Pentobarbital	5 mg/kg	IV	Continuous	0.5–3.0 mg/kg/h	Until 3- to 6-s burst suppression
Lidocaine	2.0 mg/kg	IV		5–10 mg/kg/h	

Abbreviation: PE, phenytoin equivalent.

Cutaneous herpes with seizures is an indication that herpes simplex encephalitis is present. Chorioretinitis is a clear sign of intrauterine infection that could cause seizures (e.g., herpes, toxoplasmosis, cytomegalovirus, or rubella). Cerebral imaging is warranted in neonates to help define cerebral hemorrhage and structural abnormalities. Ultrasound may be sufficient for diagnosis in some cases, but MRI is the best study for migrational defects of the CNS (e.g., lissencephaly, heterotopia, and agenesis of the corpus callosum).

Treatment

Several factors influence treatment in neonates: (1) variations in the metabolic half-lives of drugs, (2) associated etiologic conditions (e.g., hypoxia prolongs the half-life of many drugs and may affect the renal or gastrointestinal clearance rate), and (3) greater difficulty in identifying the end point of seizure control in neonates.

Effective seizure control is obtained by rapidly achieving therapeutic blood levels of the anticonvulsant chosen. Newborns have different rates of metabolism and excretion of anticonvulsants from older infants and children. In infants younger than 7 days of age, the half-life of phenobarbital, the drug of first choice, is 100 h and, after 28 days of continuous therapy, the half-life of the drug is reduced to 60 to 70 h.

In the presence of hypoxia with tissue acidosis and associated renal and hepatic dysfunction, anticonvulsant half-lives may be increased, with therapeutic and toxic levels achieved more readily, and requiring lower dose and less frequent administration of AEDs.

Blood levels of phenobarbital of 16 to 40 μg/mL are necessary to achieve seizure control in the majority of cases. Levels of 40 to 80 μg/mL have been maintained in resistant cases with inconsistent benefit. Dosages of phenobarbital of 3 to 4 mg/kg/day maintain mid to high therapeutic levels and prevent toxicity.

Phenytoin is the second drug of choice in treating neonatal seizures. Fosphenytoin is well tolerated in neonates and can be used for induction and maintenance therapy without the problems associated with phenytoin administration. Loading doses of fosphenytoin are 15 to 20 mg PE/kg at 3 mg PE/kg/min with IV maintenance of 4 to 8 mg PE/kg/day. When converting to oral dosage of phenytoin, 8 to 12 mg/kg/day is typically required. Free phenytoin levels up to 2.2 μg/mL may be necessary for adequate seizure control.

Pyridoxine (vitamin B_6) 100 mg/day is empirically used when no reasonable cause for seizures has been identified and the seizures remain uncontrolled. Seizure reduction rather than EEG improvement is the best indication of B_6 response. Biotin 10 mg/day is the long-term replacement therapy for biotinidase deficiency.

In status epilepticus of neonates, diazepam or lorazepam must be used with caution, since its half-life may be prolonged, and respiratory depression superimposed on an immature and possibly compromised respiratory apparatus should be anticipated. Diazepam may exaggerate hyperbilirubinemia by uncoupling the bilirubin-albumin complex and should be used with caution in jaundiced babies.

Treatment principles in the management of neonatal seizures are as follows:

1. Identify and correct treatable causes (hypocalcemia, hypoglycemia, and electrolyte imbalance).
2. Identify and treat associated problems such as sepsis, hyperbilirubinemia, and acidosis.
3. Initiate anticonvulsant therapy with appropriate loading doses, and carefully observe blood levels to adjust the maintenance dosage (Table 121-6).

INFANTILE SPASMS

Infantile spasms are a unique form of seizures. The onset is typically between 3 and 9 months of age but may begin as late as 18 months. Concurrently, the child exhibits regression in development. The spasms are very brief, lasting a split second, often with flexion or extension of the head and trunk. They occur singly or repeatedly in bursts of 5 to 20 spasms at a time, usually several times per day and more often upon arousal from sleep or with sudden auditory or physical stimulation. The EEG is abnormal in virtually every case (hypsarrhythmic in 50 percent). Mental retardation in patients with this disorder is as high as 85 percent. Parents are often frustrated because medical professionals fail to recognize these spasms as seizures.

There are many causes of infantile spasm (secondary type), including migrational defects, prior CNS trauma, hypoxia, neurocutaneous disorders, and infectious and metabolic disorders. The idiopathic type is the most alarming because it affects children with no prior neurologic

TABLE 121-6 Drug Regimen for Neonatal Seizures

25% glucose, 2 mL/kg IV bolus given to infants with proven hypoglycemia or when highly suspect because of circumstances.
Calcium gluconate (10%) 200–500 mg/kg/d divided in 4 doses (in proven hypocalcemic infants).
Magnesium sulfate 25–50 mg/kg IV or IM. Repeat q 4–6 h for 3–4 doses if necessary to normalize magnesium.
Phenobarbital 20 mg/kg at rate of 1 mg/kg/min, then 3–4 mg/kg/day.
Fosphenytoin 20 mg PE/kg at rate of 3 mg/kg/min, then 4–8 mg PE/kg/day in 2 divided doses IV or PO. Phenytoin maintenance 8–12 mg/kg/day in 2 divided doses to maintain a free level of 1.0–2.2.
Lorazepam 0.10 mg/kg over 2 min. Repeat twice at 10-min intervals if necessary.
Midazolam 0.2 mg/kg over 2 min. Repeat once if necessary. If refractory seizures use midazolam continuous infusion at 0.04–0.5 mg/kg/h.
Pentobarbital as an alternative to continuous midazolam infusion. Initial pentobarbital dose is 5 mg/kg bolus followed by continuous infusion of 0.5–3.0 mg/kg/h to maintain electroencephalographic burst suppression at 3- to 6-s intervals.

Abbreviation: PE, phenytoin equivalent.

disorder and no etiology is identified. Differential diagnosis includes benign myoclonus, dyskinesia due to gastroesophageal reflux, and tics.

Treatment

Early diagnosis and aggressive management may minimize the neurologic deficit associated with infantile spasms. Although adrenocorticotropic hormone (ACTH) remains the treatment of choice because of favorable outcome, the frequency and severity of complications warrant consideration of alternative AEDs. Clonazepam and valproate have been effective in limited cases and warrant consideration in refractory cases or when the potential side-effect risk is too great with ACTH (e.g., active cytomegalovirus infection). Vigabatrin has particular effectiveness in infantile spasms associated with tuberous sclerosis.

Once infantile spasms are recognized, prompt neurologic referral is recommended. It is necessary to initiate a basic assessment including electrolytes, calcium, glucose, complete blood count, creatinine and lumbar puncture (LP). The LP is warranted to identify the rare syndrome of glucose transporter defect, which is a potentially treatable cause of infantile spasms. If the cerebrospinal fluid (CSF) glucose is less than 60 percent of blood glucose, this disorder should be highly suspected. The best course of treatment is the ketogenic diet. More complex metabolic testing is not necessary in the emergency department situation. MRI is the preferred neuroimaging study and can be done electively.

HEAD TRAUMA AND SEIZURES

Head trauma can result in seizures of three types: immediate seizures, early posttraumatic seizures, and late posttraumatic seizures. Immediate seizures result from impact and presumably are due to traumatic depolarization of neurons. The risk of recurring seizures in these patients is minimal unless there are more serious prognostic factors such as prolonged coma and penetrating head injury.[5] Anticonvulsants are sometimes used because of the unknown potential for immediate recurring seizures. In a patient who recovers rapidly, chronic anticonvulsant use is usually not indicated. An exception would be a patient with a prior seizure history or a family history of epilepsy.

Early posttraumatic seizures occur within the first week after trauma, and epilepsy results in 20 to 25 percent of these patients. These early seizures are presumed to result from the focal effects of contusions or lacerations and the associated hypoperfusion, which causes ischemia and related metabolic changes.

Treatment of immediate and early posttraumatic seizures requires the correction of neurologic problems, e.g., depressed fracture or hematoma, the reduction of cerebral edema, proper oxygenation (airway maintenance and correction of shock), and the careful administration of anticonvulsants. With immediate and early posttraumatic seizures when impaired consciousness already prevails, it is helpful to avoid the use of significantly sedative medication (barbiturates or diazepam), if possible. Phenytoin may be used successfully with relative safety (Table 121-4). The dosage is determined by the clinical presentation. Rapid loading is warranted to obtain immediate therapeutic levels in patients in whom repeated seizures are occurring or likely to recur, especially when a seizure may further aggravate associated medical or surgical conditions.

Immediate posttraumatic seizures warrant anticonvulsant therapy for initial control, whereas long-term management of immediate seizures remains controversial.

Late posttraumatic seizures occur after 1 week and may be seen as late as 10 years after the trauma. Structural changes such as atrophy with gliosis and permanent local vascular changes, altered dendrite branching, and presumably modified neurotransmitter function account for the development and permanence of these seizures. Of these seizures, 40 percent are focal or partial seizures and 50 percent are temporal lobe seizures, indicating the predilection for traumatic injury and known epileptogenic properties of this structure. The risk of recurring seizures in this group is reported to be as high as 70 percent.

Early and late posttraumatic seizures warrant long-term anticonvulsant therapy in view of the risk of immediate and later recurrence. Late-onset posttraumatic seizures are most likely to recur, and long-term anticonvulsant therapy is necessary. Patients at greater risk for chronic posttraumatic seizures include those with depressed skull fractures, posttraumatic amnesia more than 24 h after the trauma, dural penetration, acute intracranial hemorrhage, early posttraumatic epilepsy, and a foreign body in a cerebral wound. The more severe the seizure and the later the onset, the less likely remission will occur.

Emergency management of seizures related to trauma should emphasize neurosurgical assessment; the rapid, careful administration of nonsedative anticonvulsants; the interruption of the seizures; and the stabilization of the general medical condition.

BREAKTHROUGH SEIZURES IN KNOWN EPILEPTICS

When seizures recur in known epileptics, something has occurred to alter the balance of the excitation-inhibition complex, causing the seizure threshold to be lowered. Complete seizure control is not always possible. A child with mental retardation, cerebral palsy, and complex partial seizures with or without secondary generalization is most likely to have recurring seizures. Tonic-clonic (grand mal) seizures are the most dramatic and often lead to emergency treatment. The usual causes of seizure breakthrough can be summarized as follows: lowered anticonvulsant blood levels, change in habits, complicating factors of epilepsy management, and progression of the underlying cause. Superimposed head trauma may also precipitate seizures. And, finally, an unprovoked episode of seizures may occur in a well child with adequate levels of anticonvulsants.

Lowered Anticonvulsant Blood Levels

1. Due to noncompliance. This is a common cause, most often in a preteen or teen who has been given the responsibility for self-medication, more often seen with tid and qid dosing.

2. Related to intercurrent infection. Anticonvulsant levels fall during acute infections (viral or bacterial) with or without fever. Quite often, a child's seizure recurrence is an indication of the infection before the acute problem is evident, e.g., varicella or otitis media.
3. The interaction of different drugs. An example is the reduction of the phenytoin level by the induction of parahydroxylation when barbiturates are used concomitantly (see the section on "Problems of Anticonvulsant Use").

Change in Habits

1. Altered sleep patterns because of trips, holidays, or parties.
2. A job, exams, or an emotional stress may lead to seizures in active teens. If a pattern develops, knowledge of the pattern is quite helpful in defining treatment.
3. Alcohol use can lower the seizure threshold and can also increase noncompliance.
4. The use of illicit drugs or prescription drugs that lower the threshold. Examples are neuroleptic agents, lindane (Kwell), theophylline, phencyclidene (PCP), LSD, cyclosporine, isoniazid, meperidine, tricyclic antidepressants, stimulants, and certain anesthetic agents (e.g., ethrane).

Complicating Factors of Epilepsy Management.

1. Toxic levels of drugs. An example is phenytoin intoxication, which can increase seizure frequency. Carbamazepine and other AEDs in therapeutic dosage have been found to infrequently increase seizures. Tiagabine and gabapentin may increase myoclonic seizures.
2. The use of phenytoin in some myoclonic epilepsies.
3. Anticonvulsant-induced osteomalacia with hypocalcemia (rickets). This uncommon problem may increase the seizure frequency and typically occurs after 5 to 7 years' use.
4. Downregulation of benzodiazepine receptor sites with decreasing antiepileptic response (e.g., clonazepam and nitrazepam).
5. Carbamazepine-induced hyponatremia.

Progression of the Underlying Cause

Examples are subacute focal (Rasmussen) encephalitis, neoplasm, arteriovenous malformation, and degenerative disease (ceroid lipofuscinosis—Huttenlocher-Alpers). Blume and coworkers[6] reported that 16 of 38 children undergoing cerebral resection for intractable seizures were found unexpectedly to have a cerebral tumor.

Treatment

When a child known to have epilepsy presents with recurring seizures, several steps may minimize the treatment time and disclose the reason for the breakthrough. The physician should first assess the obvious factors: the airway and the vital signs. Next, if the patient is having seizures at the time, the physician should test for the levels of anticonvulsants, electrolytes, calcium, and glucose and should obtain a complete blood cell count with differential. An IV catheter should be inserted if the child is not alert, so that medication can be administered as necessary. If the patient is febrile, a source of infection should be sought.

Once these procedures have been completed, anticonvulsant management is initiated. Assume the anticonvulsant levels are low and give a partial loading dose. If the patient is compliant, give the daily dose of phenobarbital or phenytoin orally if the patient is able to swallow, or intravenously if not. If the patient is known to be noncompliant or if the levels of the anticonvulsant are found to be significantly below the therapeutic range, give double the daily dose (e.g., in a child on 60 mg of phenobarbital, give 120 mg initially and repeat the dose if the seizures recur despite levels in the low therapeutic range).

If the anticonvulsant levels are within a high therapeutic range and the child is well without an obvious source of infection or other cause of breakthrough, then one can decide whether another anticonvulsant is necessary. One may decide to wait and see whether there is a trend toward increased seizure frequency, warranting additional medication, or whether this is a solitary episode, warranting observation, monitoring of drug levels, and follow-up. If the levels are within the high therapeutic range and seizures recur, additional anticonvulsants are warranted in appropriate loading doses (Table 121-4).

Recurring or frequent tonic, tonic-clonic, or clonic seizures warrant loading doses that produce therapeutic levels safely and rapidly. Phenobarbital or fosphenytoin can be administered IM and IV while Depacon (valproate) can be given IV to achieve this effect. Rectal administration of liquid preparations of valproate, phenobarbital, phenytoin, primidone, and carbamazepine can result in therapeutic levels within 4 h. Using large enough doses of primidone, carbamazepine, topiramate, and tiagabine will most likely result in significant CNS toxicity and a greater likelihood of sedation, ataxia, and confusion. Because of the greater risk of serious rash, lamotrigine should not be given in an emergency situation for immediate seizure control.

Seizures that begin with focal features, partial or complex partial (temporal lobe, psychomotor), may appear less dramatic and typically warrant a slower modification of drug therapy unless the seizures are prolonged or postictal Todd paralysis occurs. If a patient requires additional drugs, phenobarbital, phenytoin, and valproate can be used interchangeably without producing uncomfortable side effects. Patients with petit mal (generalized absence) epilepsy rarely are brought to the emergency department, since the seizures are not alarming to the parents. If some injury occurs because of the absence spells, or if the parent is unusually concerned and brings the child for emergency treatment, determining the blood levels of anticonvulsants is most useful. Addition of another anticonvulsant can be initiated, e.g., lamotrigine (Lamictal), ethosuximide (Zarontin), valproate (Depakote), clonazepam (Klonopin), or acetazolamide (Diamox).

Most often, epileptic patients with breakthrough seizure can be sent home, and modification of the drug regimen can be carried out by the attending physician. Following the initial evaluation, modification of drug therapy, and treatment for any superimposed problems, the emergency physician should (1) arrange for follow-up evaluation by the attending physician, (2) emphasize the need for compliance, and (3) provide continued treatment for infections.

STATUS EPILEPTICUS

Status epilepticus (SE) represents a state of "epileptic seizure that is so frequently repeated or so prolonged as to create a fixed and lasting epileptic condition."[7] This definition applies to continuous seizures lasting at least 30 min. As a practical measure, seizures are usually treated as SE if they persist more than 10 min. Classification of status seizures is listed in (Table 121-7).

About 5 to 10 percent of children with epilepsy and 60,000 to 100,000 total epileptics experience one bout of status grand mal (SGM). This condition is a neurologic emergency that could be fatal. The longer the SGM persists, the greater the morbidity and the mortality rates and the more difficult it is to control the seizures. In patients with no neurologic sequelae, the mean duration of SGM is $1\frac{1}{2}$ h. Neurologic sequelae result when SGM lasts an average of 10 h. The mean duration of SGM in patients who die is 13 h.

Effects of Status Grand Mal

Experimental models in animals provide evidence of the neurologic effects of SGM. Selective permanent cell damage in the hippocampus, amygdala, cerebellum, thalamus, and middle cerebral cortical layers

TABLE 121-7 Classification of Status Seizures

Primary generalized convulsive status grand mal (continuous and noncontinuous)
Tonic-clonic status
Myoclonic status
Clonic-tonic status
Secondary generalized convulsive status (continuous and noncontinuous)
Tonic-clonic status with partial onset
Tonic status
Simple partial status
Partial motor status including epilepsia partialis continua
Partial sensory status
Partial status with vegetative or autonomic symptoms
Partial status with cognitive symptoms
Partial status with affective symptoms
Complex partial status
Absence (petit mal) status

Source: Modified from Delgado-Escueta and Bajorek,[13] with permission.

develops after 60 min of seizure activity. Even with artificial ventilation and correction of existing metabolic derangements, most changes still occur. This cell death results from the increased metabolic demands and the exhaustion of the continuously firing neurons. In addition, there are secondary effects that probably exaggerate the adverse effects of SGM. After unremitting SGM, the cerebral P_{O_2} and amounts of cytochrome A and cytochrome A3 reductase decrease, enhancing the risk of cell damage. Increases in calcium, arachidonic acid, arachidonic diglycerol, prostaglandin, and leukotriene levels in the neurons exaggerate or cause cerebral edema or cell death. Increased levels of cyclic AMP and increased release of prolactin, growth hormone, ACTH, cortisol, insulin, glycogen, epinephrine, and norepinephrine may contribute to the progression of cell damage with the loss of physiologic responsiveness.

Late secondary effects include lactic acidosis, elevated CSF pressure, hyperglycemia followed later by hypoglycemia, dysautonomia with hyperthermia, diaphoresis, dehydration, hypertension followed by hypotension, and eventually shock. In addition, excessive muscle activity leads to myolysis, myoglobinuria, and renal failure. Neuropathologic studies indicate nucleovacuolation and ischemic nerve cell damage leading to neuronal dissolution.

Treatment

Treatment is best initiated when the type of seizure is identified. To obtain the most effective and rapid cessation of SE, the following evaluation and therapeutic goals must be reached:

1. Specific delineation of the type and subtype of SE so that appropriate treatment can be chosen. For example, tonic-clonic generalized SE is very responsive to diazepam or phenytoin; noncontinuous clonic or tonic-clonic seizures may be refractory to diazepam.
2. Identification and treatment of the reversible precipitating cause of SE, e.g., cerebral infection, trauma, electrolyte disturbance, brain abscess, hypoglycemia, or sickle cell crisis.
3. Rapid cessation of SE to prevent secondary effects that both prolong the seizures and cause irreversible neuronal damage.
4. Full support of medical systems to prevent unwarranted complications of the seizures or the treatment, e.g., respiratory depression, dysrhythmia, aspiration pneumonia, shock, and myoglobulinuria.

In treating patients with SE, the end point of therapy is cessation of the clinical seizures, with return of normal function. When a patient fails to arouse, the possibility of nonconvulsive status must be entertained and then the end point is improvement in the EEG abnormality. The amount of benzodiazepines (BZDs) necessary to stop the seizures has been derived from studies that confirm an essential point, i.e., complications of BZDs occur in markedly ill patients with complex disorders or with prior use of high doses of other hypnotic drugs.

Rapid-acting BZDs remain the drug of choice in SGM. BZDs are effective in SE via several mechanisms: (1) agonist binding at the BZD receptor causes an increase in GABA for its receptor and GABA acts as a receptor for a longer period, and (2) BZDs block sustained high-frequency discharges of epileptic neurons. BZDs are effective because they have high lipophilicity, rapid brain penetration, and brain receptor binding. Multiple studies have compared the safety and effectiveness of lorazepam, diazepam and, more recently, midazolam. Each has its own merit in terms of onset and duration of action. Treiman and colleagues[9] recently reported on a comparison of three therapies in the treatment of SE. They found lorazepam superior to phenytoin and equal to phenobarbital alone and phenytoin in combination with diazepam. The ease of IV lorazepam use made it the recommended initial treatment in SE.

Currently, lorazepam is used as the initial treatment because of its pharmacokinetic properties, exhibiting a slightly slower onset of action (latency) but a longer duration, allowing for a more prolonged seizure-free interval following initial infusion. Lorazepam is begun at 0.1 mg/kg given over 2 min and repeated for a maximum of 8 mg. To maintain the seizure-free state, a long-term AED is started simultaneously with phenobarbital 20 mg/kg at 1 mg/kg/min. Alternatively, fosphenytoin 20 mg PE/kg at 3 mg/kg/min can be used.

In an open study by Lacey and coworkers,[10] lorazepam was administered to 31 children with SE. The initial dose was 0.05 mg/kg, with 20 patients requiring two injections and one patient requiring three injections. The median dose was 0.05 mg/kg, with a total median cumulative dose of 2.0 mg. The median latency was 10 min; control lasted at least 3 to 6 h in 83 percent of the patients and 24 h in nearly 50 percent of the patients. In a double-blind randomized trial by Leppik and coworkers,[11] 78 adult patients were treated with either lorazepam (4 mg) or diazepam (10 mg). Latency (2 to 3 min), efficacy (76 to 89 percent), and adverse effects (12 to 13 percent) did not differ significantly in both groups.

Diazepam was the BZD used initially in the modern era of epilepsy management and can be used in addition to or instead of lorazepam. A starting diazepam dose of 0.2 to 0.5 mg/kg, given at a rate of 1 mg/min and repeated as needed to a maximum of 2.6 mg/kg, is recommended to stop continuous tonic-clonic and clonic seizures. This higher dose is rarely used, since most patients stop seizing at lower doses and additional drugs such as phenytoin may be employed.

The safety of diazepam at the maximum dose of 2.6 mg/kg over the course of treatment has been substantiated. Smith and Masotti[12] described an effective dose of diazepam as 0.08 to 2.72 mg/kg in infants and young children, with an average effective dose of 0.68 mg/kg. Many authors recommend initial doses of 1 mg per year of age, with a maximum total dose of 5 mg in infants and 10 mg in children. Eckert[13] reported maximum doses in adolescents as 35 mg in brief periods and 100 mg in 24 h.

Midazolam (MDZ) is a more rapid-acting BZD and has the advantage of relatively rapid IM absorption. It has been used via IV, IM, nasal, and rectal routes in the treatment of SE. We are currently completing a study on its effectiveness and safety in childhood SE in comparison to lorazepam. MDZ is water soluble at physiologic ph (open ring) and becomes lipid soluble (ring closure) after injection. It has a distribution half-life of 1.5 to 3.5 h. The initial dosage is a 0.2-mg/kg bolus, which can be repeated in 15 min. Because of its short half-life, it has been used as a continuous infusion at 0.05 to 0.4 (mg/kg)/h to treat continuous unresponsive seizures, but this has not been extensively tested. When given IM, seizure control occurred within 2 to 3 min of injection. In a study by Chamberlain and colleagues,[14] more rapid cessation of seizures occurred with MDZ (7.8–4.1 vs 11.2–3.6 min) in comparison to IV diazepam. This was attributed to the ease of administration of the IM MDZ as compared with the time needed for IV site acquisition with the diazepam.

The following steps should be followed when treating continuous SGM (tonic-clonic SE) (Table 121-5):

1. Assess basic functions immediately and maintain blood pressure, airway, and pulse.
2. Obtain blood to be tested for levels of anticonvulsants, electrolytes, blood urea nitrogen, calcium, and glucose, and for a complete blood count with differential while inserting an IV catheter for fluid administration.
3. Administer a bolus of 25 percent glucose, 2 mL/kg.
4. Administer IV lorazepam, 0.1 mg/kg, and repeat up to a total dose of 8 mg or early signs of respiratory depression. Alternatively, administer IV diazepam, 0.2 mg/kg over 2 min, repeating in 15 min and 30 min, if necessary, to a total dose of 2.6 mg/kg.
5. Administer IV phenobarbital, 20 mg/kg at 1 mg/kg/min, as BZD is being infused.
6. Administer IV fosphenytoin, 20 mg PE/kg at 3 mg/kg/min, if phenobarbital is ineffective. When a patient reaches this level, transfer to the intensive care unit is warranted.
7. If seizures persist, give additional 10 mg/kg of phenobarbital to reach levels of 60 μg/mL.
8. Administer paraldehyde rectally, 0.3 mL/kg, mixed with an equal amount of mineral oil, if available and the above are ineffective.
9. Under intensive care monitoring, administer pentobarbital, 2 mg/kg bolus, followed by maintenance of 1 to 2 mg/kg/h, to effect 3 to 6 s of EEG burst suppression.
10. In noncontinuous SGM, administer continuous MDZ at a dose of 0.04 to 0.05 mg/kg/h.

Noncontinuous SE can be more difficult to treat since the end point is more elusive. Rapidly acting drugs such as diazepam and lorazepam are less effective, and a more sustained effect is necessary. Often noncontinuous SE is not responsive to appropriate therapeutic levels of phenytoin and phenobarbital. MDZ can be given as a continuous infusion of 0.04 to 0.05 mg/kg/h. Alternatively, large doses (0.2 to 0.6 mg/kg) of clonazepam via nasogastric tube may be used to produce the desired effect of cessation of noncontinuous seizures and the anticonvulsant effect can be maintained by additional drugs (phenytoin or phenobarbital) and clonazepam (0.1 to 0.3 mg/kg/day).

Paraldehyde rectally administered can be very effective in treating SE and acute repetitive seizures. Paraldehyde should be administered only with glass syringes and rubber tubing in view of its degradation to toxic by-products in the presence of certain plastics.

In absence SE, the BZDs are highly effective. The child usually appears dazed and may exhibit repetitive eye blinking.

Epilepsia partialis continua is a serious neurologic condition, although it does not appear life threatening at first. The patient exhibits repeated continuous or minimally interrupted clonic jerking of one side of the body and usually one part of an extremity for days, weeks, or months. It is typically due to encephalitis or cerebrovascular accident or associated with heterotopias and indicates a relatively poor prognosis. Initial management is similar to that of SE.

The use of propofol has been advocated in adults with refractory SE,[15] but its prolonged use in children with refractory SE was associated with progressive severe metabolic acidosis and rhabdomyolysis, which the authors concluded was due to propofol.[16]

DIFFERENTIAL DIAGNOSIS OF SEIZURES

It is necessary to identify nonepileptic paroxysmal disorders to prevent confusion with epilepsy. The differential diagnosis of seizures must take into account many disorders that can produce loss of consciousness, unusual movements, impaired awareness, or bizarre behavior. Many of these disorders are age-specific.

In newborns, the problems partly reflect the intrauterine experience. Jitteriness or hyperexcitability appears as high-amplitude tremulousness easily brought out by passive movement of the extremities or jarring of the crib. Drug-withdrawn infants are irritable and tremulous and may have diaphoresis, vomiting, and diarrhea. In addition, seizures may occur. Sepsis, hypoglycemia, and hypocalcemia may produce nonepileptic paroxysmal activity in addition to seizures. Hyperekplexia, or startle disease, mimics tonic and clonic seizures. Near-miss sudden infant death syndrome (SIDS) remains a multifactorial condition in which seizures are part of the differential diagnosis and might be considered part of the cause.

In older infants, it is more common to see cyanotic and pallid breath-holding spells, which typically occur following an abrupt trauma (a fall or a minor spanking) or a verbal reprimand. The infant gives a sudden cry followed by prolonged inhalation or exhalation, resulting in no air exchange, and a Valsalva maneuver, often with bradycardia. A brief tonic nonepileptic seizure often occurs. Drug intoxication manifested by hyperkinesis, impaired awareness, or altered behavior (hallucinations) is usually accidental at this age. In adolescence, PCP intoxication mimics complex partial seizures and may result in seizures with more severe overdoses.

Congenital heart disease can produce paroxysmal events at all ages. Abrupt mental status changes may occur in patients with pulmonary hypertension, aortic stenosis, tetralogy of Fallot, single ventricle, cardiac rhabdomyomas, etc. Acquired cardiomyopathy may result in decreased cardiac output (Adams-Stokes disease) or cerebrovascular accident. The prolonged QT syndrome and neurocardiogenic syncope may cause nonepileptic seizures or syncopal episodes. They should be evaluated for when epilepsy is unsubstantiated or the more obvious problems of diaphoresis, light-headedness, and skin color/temperature changes precede or accompany unconsciousness. In adolescents, syncope due to stretching and yawning or following hair combing (vasovagal) is more common. Many children experience syncope when standing in church.

Hyperkinetic movement disorders can be difficult to differentiate from complex partial seizures. Sydenham's chorea is infrequently seen today, and drug-induced chorea (ethosuximide, carbamazepine, or diphenhydramine hydrochloride) and lupus-induced chorea are likewise very uncommon. Tourette syndrome is more frequently seen, but rarely does the child appear acutely ill. Kinesogenic chorea is a movement disorder brought on by action and mimics simple motor partial seizures.

Immediate posttraumatic migraine may recur after relatively minor injury and cause confusional states mimicking concussion or complex partial seizures.

Pseudoseizures represent a particular problem for the treating physician because the "seizures" appear to represent a significant threat to the patient's safety, and vigorous anticonvulsant therapy is often initiated. Unfortunately, pseudoseizures often occur in patients with documented epilepsy. Secondary gain should become evident in these cases. The "seizures" are atypical in that the patient may waken fully in the interictal phase and require repeated large doses of anticonvulsants even to the point of protracted drug-induced depression. Another form of pseudoseizures consists of those described by the parent and never observed by other witnesses (Münchausen by proxy).

To distinguish pseudoseizures from the true epileptic spells, a bedside technique may be dramatic and diagnostic, and prevent overtreatment. One method is to insert a nasopharyngeal tube and observe the patient's response. A pseudoseizure patient will become responsive immediately. Experience dictates referral, or even hospitalization, for patients with a diagnosis of pseudoseizure, to prevent recurrences, provide family education, and lessen the likelihood of inappropriate treatment.

Simple sleep myoclonus and night terrors are of concern to parents but are easily distinguished from nocturnal seizures. REM sleep disorder may mimic seizures.

Preventing misdiagnosis and mistreatment is an essential part of the emergency management of seizures and related disorders.

PROBLEMS OF ANTICONVULSANT USE

Unwanted features of anticonvulsants may be seen soon after the drug is initiated or may develop weeks, months, or years later. These problems may turn up during evaluation for other illnesses (e.g., macrocytic anemia) or be the basis for emergency treatment.

Immediate side effects often subside in time. Lethargy is usually dose related and subsides with chronic use and can occur with the oldest AED (phenobarbital) as well as the newest AEDs (topiramate and tiagabine). Irritability and changes in cognition can persist and be significant but are unrelated to drug levels (valproate). Rashes may occur within days or weeks of initiation of therapy but must be differentiated from concurrent viral exanthem. Pruritic and/or morbilliform rashes usually require cessation of medication. Stevens-Johnson syndrome, with bullous skin lesions affecting mucous membranes, is a serious potential reaction. There is a risk of serious sequelae—blindness, esophageal stenosis, or loss of life.

With valproic acid use, hepatic failure may occur within days or up to 2 years after first use. The drug reaction results in behavior alteration, increasing lethargy, and vomiting. Levels of liver enzymes may be minimally to markedly elevated, and hyperammonemia with or without symptoms of hepatic failure may be found. Immediate cessation of valproate, hospitalization, and observation are necessary if symptomatic hepatic reaction is evident. In asymptomatic patients with enzyme level elevations, a reduction of the dosage and careful observation are warranted. Gastrointestinal side effects are common with initial use of valproic acid and may be so severe that more serious hepatic problems are considered. These side effects can be avoided by taking the drug with meals, by avoiding carbonated beverages and citric juices, and by using the enteric-coated form or sprinkles. Pancreatitis secondary to valproate use may occur with initial and chronic use.

Toxicity due to overdosage at any time can produce some readily identifiable symptoms and signs. Phenytoin toxicity occurs when serum levels exceed 25 μg/mL in most patients (above 20 μg/mL in some). Nausea, dysarthria, diplopia, and ataxia are seen early, with progression to impaired levels of consciousness and decerebrate posturing. Virtually all anticonvulsants produce ataxia and lethargy with significant overdosage. Cardiopulmonary monitoring during high-dose drug use in SE should be employed, since cardiac dysrhythmia, hypotension, or respiratory depression can occur. The use of fosphenytoin has eliminated the problem of venous and subcutaneous extravasation-related phenytoin side effects. Chronic phenytoin use can result in folate deficiency with macrocytic anemia, acquired osteomalacia (increased vitamin D turnover), neutropenia (often transient), peripheral neuropathy, lupus-like syndromes, and myasthenic weakness.

Valproate-induced thrombocytopenia is a significant side effect warranting lowering or discontinuation of the drug if platelet levels are significantly lowered or bleeding is evident. Lower carnitine levels due to valproate metabolism may be a contributing factor of valproate hepatotoxicity.

Drug interactions may be quite dramatic. Valproate and aspirin use can result in a bleeding diathesis. Antihistamines used in conjunction with barbiturates can be very sedating, warranting smaller doses of the antihistamine. When erythromycin is used, particular care must be exercised, since the carbamazepine levels may rise to toxic levels rapidly. Toxicity is greater when carbamazepine and lithium are used together, and blood levels may be in the therapeutic range. Total phenytoin levels are typically reduced when valproic acid and tiagabine are also used, but free phenytoin usually remains therapeutic and it is essential to measure free phenytoin. When barbiturates are used concomitantly with phenytoin, increased parahydroxylation can cause enhanced metabolism of phenytoin so that therapeutic levels fall, resulting in seizure breakthrough. Hyperbilirubinemia and hypoalbuminemia can affect anticonvulsant binding and blood levels.

Movement disorder (e.g., chorea) can result after several weeks' or months' use of ethosuximide and carbamazepine. The movements may be profound and usually respond to the reduction or discontinuation of the drug and, if necessary, the use of diphenhydramine (Benadryl), 12.5 to 25 mg IV. Clonazepam and diazepam can cause acute bladder dysfunction with urinary retention.

Many problems of dose-related toxicity can be avoided by maintaing therapeutic blood levels. Blood level determinations should be done randomly to determine compliance at times of increased seizure frequency or when signs of toxicity develop. In some patients, side effects develop at therapeutic levels. Idiosyncratic effects cannot be predicted, but families must be made aware that significant side effects can develop with little warning, and evaluation by a physician is recommended before a drug is dismissed. Obtaining the patient's history, consulting with the primary physician or consultant, and reviewing readily available drug information in the package insert or *Physicians' Desk Reference* make emergency evaluation and treatment of anticonvulsant drug reactions simpler.

ERRORS IN EMERGENCY MANAGEMENT OF SEIZURES

After a patient arrives for treatment, the initial assessment may be incomplete, resulting in inappropriate or inadequte therapy. Not identifying treatable infections, electrolyte imbalance, child abuse, and accidental trauma can lead to rapidly progressive deterioration and demise, or may make seizure control difficult. By not ascertaining anticonvulsant levels in a patient with epilepsy, the physician loses an opportunity to determine whether the anticonvulsant is ineffective or simply at too low a level.

If the emergency physician communicates with the primary physician, unnecessary studies and drugs that either were ineffective or produced some side effects can be avoided. Additionally, it is important to consult with the patient's physician when prescribing nonanticonvulsants that might interfere with anticonvulsants or produce unwanted side effects.

In the aggressive treatment of seizures (SE and recurring breakthrough seizures), inadequate loading doses or improper drug selection may prolong the seizure and worsen the prognosis. Excessive dosage can result in respiratory depression or hypotension and, in rare instances, can exacerbate the seizures. If nonepileptic paroxysmal disorders are not recognized, the patient is put at the additional risk of unnecessary medication and inadequate treatment of the real disorder.

Emergency physicians cannot deal with all the problems facing patients with epilepsy. Follow-up care by the primary physicians or appropriate consultants ensures better compliance and, hopefully, lessens emergency situations in the future.

REFERENCES

1. Gastaut H: Clinical and electroencephalographic classification of epileptic seizure. *Epilepsia* 11:102, 1970.
2. Hauser WA, Anderson VE, Levenson RB, et al: Seizure recurrence after a first uprovoked seizure. *N Engl J Med* 307:522, 1982.
3. Consensus Development Conference on Febrile Seizures. Proceedings. *Epilepsia* 2:377, 1981.
4. Rosman NP, Colton T, Labazzo J, et al: A controlled trial of diazepam administered during febrile illnesses to prevent recurrence of febrile seizures. *N Engl J Med* 329:79, 1993.
5. Rosman NP, Herskowitz J, Carter AP, O'Connor JF: Acute head trauma in infancy and childhood. *Ped Clin N Am* 26:707–736, 1979.
6. Blume BT, Gerven JP, Kaufmann JCE: Childhood brain tumors presenting as chronic uncontrolled focal seizures. *Ann Neurol* 12:538, 1982.
7. Commission on Classification and Terminology of the International League Against Epilepsy: Proposal for revised clinical and electroencephalographic classification of epileptic seizures. *Epilepsia* 22:489, 1981.
8. Delgado-Escueta AV, Bajorek JG: Status epilepticus: Mechanisms of brain damage and rational management. *Epilepsia* 23(suppl 1):S29, 1982.
9. Treiman DM, Meyers PD, Walton NY, et al: A comparison of four treatments for generalized convulsive status epilepticus. *N Engl J Med* 339:792, 1998.

10. Lacey DJ, Singer WD, Horwitz SJ, et al: Lorazepam therapy of status epilepticus in children and adolescents. *J Pediatr* 108:771, 1986.
11. Leppik IE, Derivan AT, Homan RW, et al: A double blind study of lorazepam and diazepam in status epilepticus. *JAMA* 249:1452, 1983.
12. Smith BT, Masotti RE: Intravenous diazepam in the treatment of prolonged seizure activity in neonates and infants. *Dev Med Child Neurol* 13:630, 1971.
13. Eckert C: Neurologic emergencies, in *Emergency Room Care,* 4th ed. Boston, Little, Brown, 1981, pp 409–420.
14. Chamberlain JM, Altieri MA, Futterman C, et al: A prospective, randomized study comparing intramuscular midazolam with intravenous diazepam for the treatment of seizures in children. *Pediatr Emerg Care* 13:92, 1997.
15. Lowenstein DH, Alldredge BK: Status epilepticus. *N Engl J Med* 338:970, 1998.
16. Hanna JP, Ramundo ML: Rhabdomyolysis and hypoxia associated with prolonged propofol infusion in children. *Neurology* 80:301, 1998.

BIBLIOGRAPHY

Berg AT, Shinnar S, Hauser WA, et al: A prospective study of recurrent febrile seizures [see comments]. *N Engl J Med* 327:1161, 1992.

Boeve BF, Wijdicks FM, Benarroch EE, Schmidt KD: Paroxysmal sympathetic storms (''diencephalic seizures'') after severe diffuse axonal head injury. *Mayo Clin Proc* 73:148, 1998.

Delgado-Escueta AV, Treiman DM,</AU> Walsh GO: The treatable epilepsies (first of two parts). *N Engl J Med* 308:1508, 1983.

Delgado-Escueta AV, Treiman DM, Walsh GO: The treatable epilepsies (second of two parts). *N Engl J Med* 308:1576, 1983.

Dieckmann RA: Rectal diazepam for prehospital pediatric status epilepticus. *Ann Emerg Med* 23:216, 1994.

Dreifuss FE, Rosman NP, Cloyd JC, et al: A comparison of rectal diazepam gel and placebo for acute repetitive seizures. *N Engl J Med* 338:1869, 1998.

Farwell JR, Lee YJ, Hertz DG, et al: Phenobarbital for febrile seizures: effects on intelligence and on seizure recurrence. *N Engl J Med* 322:364, 1990.

Gross TV, Shinnar S: Convulsive status epilepticus in children. *Epilepsia* 34(suppl 1):12, 1993.

Maytal J, Novak GP, King KC: Lorazepam in the treatment of refractory neonatal seizures. *J Child Neurol* 6:319, 1991.

Millichap JG, Colliver JA: Management of febrile seizures: Survey of current practice and phenobarbital usage. *Pediatr Neurol* 7:243, 1991.

Nypuaver MM, Reynolds SL, Tanz RR, Davis AT: Emergency department laboratory evaluation of children with seizures: Dogma or dilemma? *Pediatr Emerg Care* 8:13, 1992.

Pellock JH: Management of acute seizure episodes. *Epilepsia* 39:S28, 1998.

Rivera R, Segnini M, Baltodano A, Perez V: Midazolam in the treatment of status epilepticus in children [see comments]. *Crit Care Med* 21:955, 1993.

Seizure temporally associated with use of DEET insect repellent: New York and Connecticut. *MMWR* 38:678, 1989.

Shorvon SD: The use of clonazepam, midazolam and nitrazepam in epilepsy. *Epilepsia* 39:S15, 1998.

Tassinari CA, Daniele O, Michelucci R, et al: Benzodiazepines: Efficacy in status epilepticus. *Adv Neurol* 34:465, 1983.

122 VOMITING AND DIARRHEA IN CHILDREN

Christopher M. Holmes
Ronald D. Holmes

Vomiting is the forceful ejection of stomach contents through the mouth and is always a cause for concern. Associated symptoms, the age of the child, the pattern of vomiting, and the duration of symptoms help to determine the etiology. The causes of acute vomiting are listed in Table 122-1.

Most infants and children who come to the emergency department because of vomiting have a self-limited viral disorder. Only a small percentage of these patients will require assessment beyond obtaining a careful medical history and performing a physical exam, and a smaller number will require specific treatment. For most children, the only treatment will be the recommendation to provide additional fluids and to continue age-appropriate feedings. It is important to remember that vomiting need not resolve before a rehydrated or well-hydrated child may be discharged from the emergency department.

TABLE 122-1 Differential Diagnosis of Vomiting

Infection
Viral
Bacterial
Meningitis
Sepsis
Appendicitis
Otitis media
Urinary tract infection
Other infections
Intestinal obstruction
Pyloric stenosis
Toxic ingestion
Contaminated food
Metabolic disorder
Diabetic ketoacidosis
Hyperammonemia
Head injury/increased intracranial pressure
Hepatitis
Cholecystitis
Pancreatitis
Pregnancy
Abdominal trauma
Munchausen by proxy

Diarrhea is defined as an excessive loss of water in the stool. Most cases of diarrhea result from self-limited enteric infections. Infectious diarrhea may be either inflammatory (dysentery) or noninflammatory. Inflammatory infectious diarrhea is commonly due to bacterial or parasitic infections/infestations. These organisms tend to localize in the colon or distal small bowel and result in dysentery, which is characterized by frequent bowel movements containing blood, mucus, or pus. Noninflammatory infectious diarrhea is caused by viruses and parasites that localize to the proximal small bowel, or by toxin-producing bacteria. In these cases, the diarrhea is profuse, watery, and commonly associated with nausea and vomiting. Fever is less likely. The term *gastroenteritis* is applied to this group of infections, although the stomach is rarely involved.

Other causes of acute diarrhea are uncommon but must be considered. In agricultural areas, poisoning with anticholinesterase insecticides, organophosphates, and carbamates must be considered, especially if diarrhea is accompanied by profuse sweating, lacrimation, hypersalivation, and abdominal cramps. Vomiting and diarrhea may also be a nonspecific presentation for other infectious diseases, such as otitis media, urinary tract infection, or other more serious conditions, including intussusception, malrotation, increased intracranial pressure, and metabolic acidosis.

EPIDEMIOLOGY

In the United States, children younger than 3 years of age have 1.3 to 2.3 episodes of diarrhea each year. The prevalence is higher in children attending day-care centers. Up to one-fifth of all acute-care outpatient visits to hospitals are by families with infants or children affected by acute gastroenteritis, and 9 percent of all hospitalizations of children younger than 5 years of age are for diarrhea.[1] Most enteric infections are self-limited, but excessive loss of water and electrolytes, resulting in clinical dehydration, may occur in 10 percent and is life threatening in 1 percent.[2]

Pathogenic viruses, bacteria, or parasites may be isolated from nearly 50 percent of children with diarrhea. Viral infection is the most common cause of acute diarrhea. Bacterial pathogens may be isolated in 1 to 4 percent of cases. While infants and children who attend day-care centers are most likely to acquire viral gastroenteritis, they are at increased risk of acquiring a variety of enteric infections/infestations by *Shigella*, *Campylobacter*, *Clostridium difficile, Salmonella*, *Cryptosporidium*, and *Giardia lamblia*. The attack rate during outbreaks may range from 30 to 100 percent, and shigellosis is particularly contagious.[3]

Enteric infections causing diarrhea are spread by the fecal-oral route by contaminated food, water, and fomites. Rotaviruses, Norwalk viruses, the enteric adenoviruses, calicivirus, and astroviruses are the most recognized viral pathogens that affect children. Of these, rotavirus is the most common, typically occurring in the cooler months of the year in North America (October to April), and infecting every child in the United States by age 4 years. This virus causes potentially lethal dehydration in 0.75 percent of children younger than 2 years of age.[4] Older children and adults have acquired immunity against the rotaviruses and are less likely to develop the severe dehydrating syndrome. Symptomatic enteric adenovirus (EAd) infection with serotypes 40 and 41 causes diarrhea that is associated with concurrent respiratory symptoms. Infections, with no clear peaks, occur throughout the year and may be responsible for 5 to 20 percent of hospitalizations for childhood diarrhea.[5] Outbreaks of EAd infection occur second only to rotavirus infection in prevalence. Norwalk virus infection is also implicated in causing epidemic gastroenteritis. In addition to developing nausea, vomiting, diarrhea, and abdominal cramps, affected children and adults may have headache, fever, chills, and myalgias. Vomiting is more prevalent in children, whereas diarrhea is more common in adults.

The major bacterial enteropathogens in the United States are *Campylobacter jejuni*, *Shigella* species, *Salmonella* species, *Yersinia enterocolitica, Clostridium difficile*, *Aeromonas hydrophila,* and *Escherichia coli*. *Escherichia coli* is the most common bacterial organism causing diarrhea in children around the world but is less common in the United States. Diarrhea due to *E. coli* may be watery and caused by enterotoxigenic *E. coli* (ETEC) or enteropathogenic *E. coli* (EPEC), or present as a dysentery-like disease due to infection with enterohemorrhagic *E. coli* (EHEC).

Giardia lamblia is a common cause of diarrhea in infants and young children in day-care centers. As many as 50 percent of infected children may be asymptomatic. *Cryptosporidium* infestations occur in a similar epidemiologic pattern. Although *Cryptosporidium* was first recognized as an opportunistic pathogen in immunocompromised children, it is now recognized as a cause of protracted watery diarrhea in otherwise healthy children. *Entamoeba histolytica* causes diarrhea, proctitis, dysentery, or hematochezia. Symptomatic infection in children results from exposure by travel to a geographic locale endemic for the organism or in adolescents through sexual transmissions.

PATHOPHYSIOLOGY

Viral pathogens cause acute gastroenteritis by tissue invasion and a directly cytopathic effect to small intestinal villous cells. As a consequence, there is villous damage and decreased intestinal absorption of nutrients, electrolytes, and water, resulting in watery diarrhea. Villous injury also results in reduced disaccharidase levels and diminished total mucosal glucose-coupled sodium transport. The end result is a decrease in intestinal water absorption. The volume of fluid delivered from the lumen of the damaged small intestine exceeds the colon's limited ability for fluid absorption, and the net result is watery diarrhea.

Bacteria cause diarrhea by a variety of mechanisms, including production of enterotoxins and cytotoxins and invasion of the mucosal absorptive surface. Enteric infections with *E. coli* are prototypic for understanding several of these pathogenic processes. ETEC and EPEC adhere to the mucosa and produce enterotoxins or damage the microvilli, respectively. Certain strains of EHEC invade the colonic mucosa, resulting in inflammation and an illness similar to shigellosis. EHEC serotype O157 : H7 typically produces a hemorrhagic colitis with little inflammation and may produce verotoxins that have been implicated in causing hemolytic-uremic syndrome (HUS).[6] Antibiotic-associated diarrhea and colitis due to cytotoxigenic *Clostridium difficile* may result in a similar pattern of diarrhea.

Bacterial toxins may also be ingested directly in food. The most common are heat-stable toxins produced by *Staphylococcus aureus* present in improperly stored or prepared meats, poultry, and dairy products. *Bacillus cereus* also produces a heat-stable toxin typically ingested with boiled or fried rice. Although *Shigella* is considered a prototype organism causing dysentery, it can also produce a toxin that causes watery diarrhea, encephalopathy, or seizures. Parasitic infestations may cause diarrhea by a variety of mechanisms similar to those discussed for viral gastroenteritis.

CLINICAL FEATURES

Evaluation of a child's state of hydration is most important. If possible, it is best to determine the degree of fluid loss by comparing the child's current weight to a recent previous weight. When objective measurements are not available, the state of hydration can be assessed by physical examination. Combinations of physical signs, including ill general appearance, capillary refill of longer than 3 s, dry mucous membranes, and absent tears, are good predictors. The presence of two or more signs predicts 5 percent or greater dehydration, whereas three or more signs predict 10 percent or greater dehydration.[7] Severe dehydration accompanied by lethargy, hypotension, and delayed capillary refill requires immediate administration of parenteral fluids. Although capillary refill may be affected by conditions other than dehydration, it should be considered a sign of significant dehydration until proven otherwise.[8] Guidelines for assessing dehydration are listed in Table 122-2.

Bacteria that invade the mucosa of the terminal ileum and colon can cause dysentery, which is characterized by frequent bowel movements that contain blood, mucus, or pus. The diarrhea is often accompanied by fever, tenesmus, and painful defecation. Infants and children who have bloody or mucousy diarrhea after having received antibiotics may have antibiotic-associated pseudomembranous colitis due to infection with cytotoxigenic *C. difficile*. Infestations with *Entamoeba histolytica* may also cause dysentery. Table 122-3 lists the enteric infections that cause children to have bloody diarrhea.

DIAGNOSIS

The approach to diagnosis and successful treatment involves obtaining a medical history carefully, and selective laboratory testing. Most hospital laboratories provide various cultures and immunoassays of stool for the presence of the enteric pathogens. Routine stool culture for bacterial pathogens now includes *Campylobacter jejuni*, *Y. enterocolitica*, and *Aeromonas* in addition to *Salmonella* and *Shigella*. Subculturing for *E. coli* serotypes or stool assays for *Clostridium difficile* toxin activity are available. Enzyme immunoassays also are available to test stool for the presence of rotavirus, enteric adenovirus, and astrovirus.

TABLE 122-2 Assessment of Dehydration

Variable	Mild, 3%–5%	Moderate, 6%–9%	Severe, >9%
Blood pressure	Normal	Normal	Normal to reduced
Quality of pulses	Normal	Normal or slightly decreased	Moderately decreased
Heart rate	Normal	Increased	Increased
Skin turgor	Normal	Decreased	Decreased
Fontanelle	Normal	Sunken	Sunken
Mucous membranes	Slightly dry	Dry	Dry
Eyes	Normal	Sunken orbits	Deeply sunken orbits
Extremities	Warm, normal capillary refill	Delayed capillary refill	Cool, mottled
Mental status	Normal	Normal to listless	Normal to lethargic or comatose
Urine output	Slightly decreased	<1 mL/kg/h	≪1 mL/kg/h
Thirst	Slightly increased	Moderately increased	Very thirsty or too lethargic to indicate

Source: From the American Academy of Pediatrics.[14]

Most children have a nonspecific gastroenteritis and not dysentery. Clinicians must assess the likelihood of defining a treatable etiology and, as a consequence, the indication for performing a stool culture. The presence of fecal leukocytes or positive guaiac testing has been used as a screening tool to identify children at increased risk for invasive bacterial enteric infection, but fecal leukocytes have poor sensitivity and guaiac testing has poor specificity.[9] Therefore, it is best to combine these tests with the clinical findings to determine the need for stool cultures. If a child is febrile and has abrupt onset of diarrhea occurring more than four times per day or blood in the stool, the illness is more likely to have been caused by a bacterial pathogen and stool cultures are indicated.[10] The likelihood of identifying bacterial pathogens is increased if the patient's stool or accompanying exudate contains polymorphonuclear leukocytes.[11]

Anaerobic stool cultures and assay of stool for *Clostridium difficile* toxin activity should be obtained for children who have been receiving antibiotics and develop bloody diarrhea. A history of hiking or camping should prompt examination for ova and parasites. In addition, a swab of mucus or bloody exudate from the stool should be placed in transport medium and sent to the laboratory for culture of *Shigella* species. *Shigella* is a fastidious pathogen and is more likely to be recovered from a swab than from a fresh stool specimen. In cases of persistent or recurrent diarrhea, especially with weight loss or day-care center exposure or in immunocompromised children, stool samples should be collected in fixative and examined for *G. lamblia, Entamoeba histolytica,* and *Cryptosporidium*. Depending on geographic location or travel history, serologic testing for confirming *E. histolytica* infection may be indicated.

TABLE 122-3 Enteric Pathogens That Cause Dysentery

Salmonella
Shigella
Campylobacter jejuni
Enterohemorrhagic *Escherichia coli* O157 : H7
Entamoeba histolytica
Yersinia enterocolitica
Trichuris trichiura

Dehydration caused by diarrhea is usually isotonic, and measurement of serum electrolytes is not necessary. It is most important, however, to be aware of the physical findings of hypernatremic dehydration (hyperirritability, sunken eyeballs and fontanel, parched mucous membranes, and thickened, doughy skin) and the special requirements for rehydrating these infants following initial fluid resuscitation. In children receiving intravenous (IV) therapy, electrolytes may be measured initially and during therapy.

Protracted vomiting and/or diarrhea occurring in infants and toddlers, in combination with fasting, may increase the risk of hypoglycemia. Measurement of blood glucose may be helpful in managing these patients.

SPECIFIC ISSUES THAT IMPACT DIAGNOSIS, EVALUATION, AND TREATMENT

Age

Infants under 1 year of age pose a more difficult problem because of the risk of rapid dehydration and hypoglycemia. Signs of sepsis in this age group may be nonspecific, but any infant who fails to make eye contact or to respond to a parent's voice or face may be toxic and will likely be admitted to the hospital. Although bilious vomiting may develop in older infants and children who acquire viral gastroenteritis, bilious vomiting in an infant under 2 years of age is a sign of intestinal obstruction until proven otherwise.

Comorbid Medical Conditions

Infants and children who appear to be malnourished are at significant risk of complications of diarrhea and dehydration and should be admitted to the hospital. In addition, high-risk social situations should be identified and consideration given to admitting such children. These situations include the single, often teenage, parent who is without an intact support system, or parents/caregivers who are homeless or unable to provide appropriate fluids to the child. Special consideration must also be given to chronically ill infants who develop acute diarrhea or severely handicapped, developmentally delayed children in whom it is difficult to provide oral fluids.

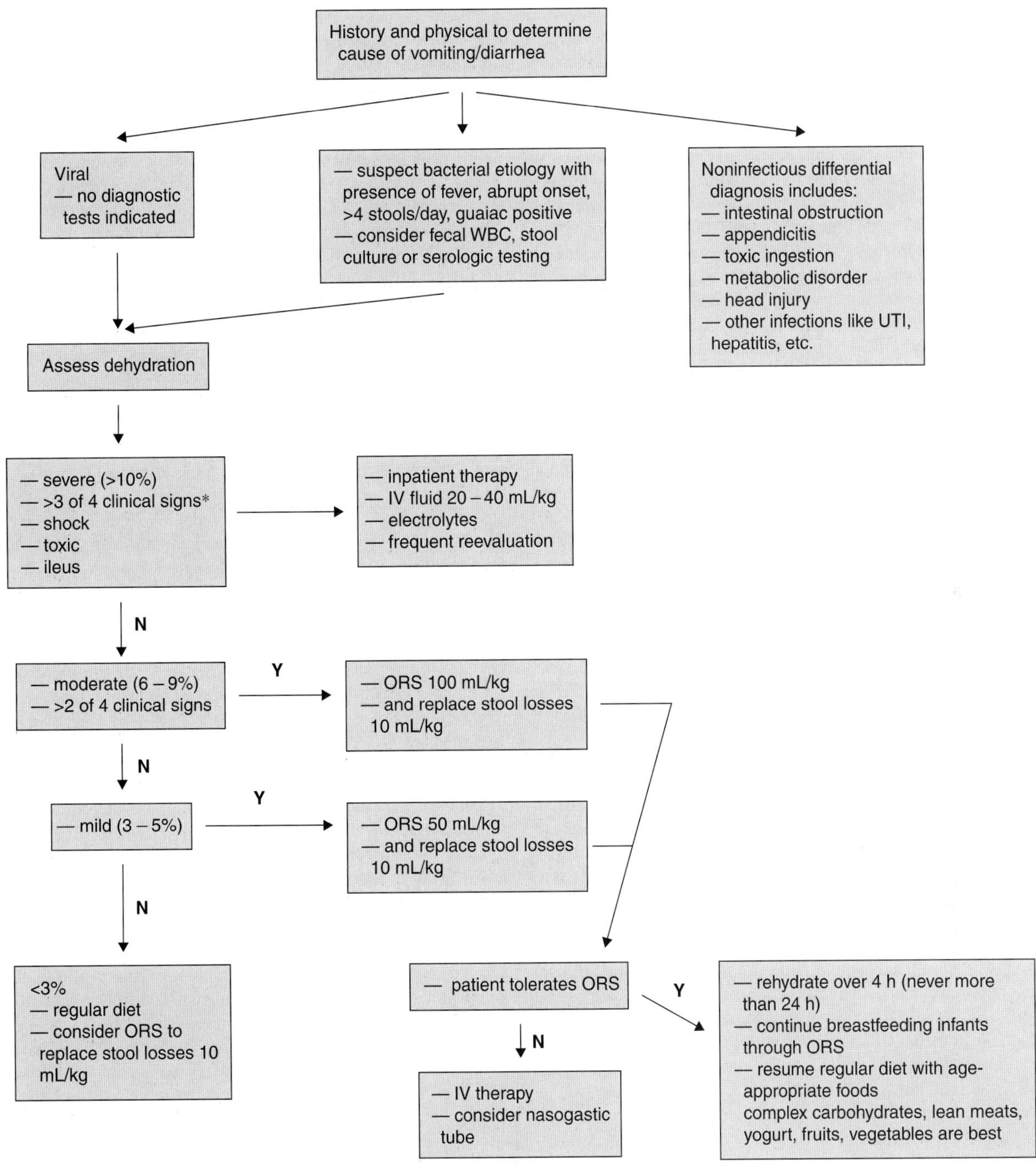

*Four clinical signs include ill general appearance, capillary refill <2 seconds, dry mucous membranes, and absent tears; ORT: oral rehydration therapy like Pedialyte; IV: intravenous; BRAT: bananas, rice, applesauce, toast; UTI: urinary tract infection. Adapted from Practice parameter: The management of acute gastroenteritis in young children. Pediatrics 97: 424, 1996. * Adopted from American Academy of Pediatrics.[14]

FIG. 122-1. Evaluation and treatment of diarrhea in children.

EMERGENCY TREATMENT

Gastroenteritis

Treatment of diarrhea changed in the mid-1960s with the introduction of oral rehydration solution (ORS) as an alternative to administration of IV fluids. Although ORS is still not universally used in the United States, it has been proven to be effective and to result in fewer complications than IV therapy. ORS successfully rehydrates 90 percent of children in whom it is used.[11]

The majority of children with diarrhea and vomiting who become dehydrated may be treated with ORS (Fig. 122-1). This treatment capitalizes on the fact that glucose-coupled sodium and water absorption remains sufficiently intact during most infections. Glucose-electrolyte solutions, like Pedialyte, are commonly available in the United States. The glucose concentration of these solutions does not exceed the sodium concentration in millimolar units by more than 2:1. In addition, the osmolality of commercial hydration solution is relatively low and about 310 mosm/L. In contrast, other clear fluids, such as soft drinks, juices, and Jell-O water, are largely carbohydrate based, are typically deficient in Na^+ and Cl^-, and have osmolalities ranging from 510 to 1225. The routine use of such highly osmolar sugar-based solutions to treat acute diarrhea will predictably amplify net small intestinal fluid secretion and increase diarrhea.

Vomiting is not a contraindication to administering ORS. The key in the treatment of vomiting children is to give small volumes of glucose-electrolyte solution, often starting with 5 mL at a time given every couple of minutes. ORS may also be given in the form of a popsicle. Giving ORS in this manner is labor intensive, though, and, if parents or staff are not available, then IV therapy may be necessary. For IV rehydration, between 20 and 40 mL/kg of Ringer's lactate or normal saline may be given over 1 to 3 h. Following parenteral rehydration, many children may be discharged home for regular feedings and supplemental ORS solution, provided follow-up is available, they do not appear toxic, and the caregiver is reliable. The daily volume of ORS should not exceed 150 mL/kg/day.[12] Breast milk or infant formula should be used if additional fluid is needed to satisfy thirst.

Children who have mild diarrhea and no dehydration may continue age-appropriate feedings and supplemental fluids as needed to replace ongoing stool loss (10 mL/kg/stool). ORS may be used to replace stool loss: although the solution is salty and may be refused, children who are dehydrated rarely refuse ORS. Mild dehydration (3 to 5 percent) may be treated by giving 50 mL/kg ORS plus replacement of ongoing losses over a 4-h period. Moderate dehydration (6 to 9 percent) is treated with 100 mL/kg plus replacement of ongoing losses over 4 h. Age-appropriate feedings should be reintroduced after a child is rehydrated. Severe dehydration (more than 10 percent) is a medical emergency, and the child should be given bolus IV fluids (20 mL/kg) using normal saline. The bolus may be repeated as needed to restore circulating volume and the child admitted to the hospital.

In general, reinstatement of food should begin after the 4-h rehydration phase is completed and never delayed more than 24 h. Recent studies have shown that the introduction of full-strength formula or unrestricted diet immediately following rehydration is associated with decreased duration of diarrhea, positive nitrogen balance, and increased weight gain. Breast-feeding should be routinely continued for infants with acute gastroenteritis. Infants who have been receiving formula feedings and who are not dehydrated may rapidly return to their feeding. There is no need to give dilute formula. Some practitioners have recommended the BRAT diet (bananas, rice, applesauce, and toast), but this diet does not provide adequate energy, fat, or protein. Instead, complex carbohydrates, lean meats, yogurt, fruits, and vegetables should be encouraged. Fatty foods and foods high in simple sugars like juices and soft drinks should be avoided. Some ethnic groups may prefer to use traditional home remedies like herbal teas or rice water. Since the osmolality of these solutions is variable, they may worsen the diarrhea. Finally, there is little evidence to support a lactose-free diet. Over 80 percent of children with acute diarrhea can tolerate full-strength milk safely.[13]

Vomiting

The use of antiemetics is controversial. The consensus opinion of a panel convened by the American Academy of Pediatrics and published in 1996 is that antiemetic drugs are not needed. If vomiting persists despite efforts to give ORS, then IV hydration is indicated. Physicians who prescribe antiemetics should be aware of the potential adverse effects of these drugs.[14]

Dysentery

Antibiotic therapy does not affect the clinical course in most cases of acute diarrhea. Patients with uncomplicated *Salmonella* gastroenteritis should not be given antibiotics unless they appear septic or are bacteremic, have a hemoglobinopathy, or have an underlying chronic gastrointestinal disorder. However, infants younger than 6 months of age are generally treated with antibiotics because of their overall risk of bacteremia or suppurative disease. If a child has had diarrhea lasting longer than 10 to 14 days and has a significant fever, systemic complaints, and inflammatory cells or blood in the stool, then empiric antimicrobial treatment may be indicated after sending a stool sample for bacterial culture. Therapy should provide coverage for the usual dysenteric agents (*Shigella, Salmonella,* and *Campylobacter*), and either ampicillin or trimethoprim-sulfamethoxazole are reasonable choices. Debilitated patients, children with underlying gastrointestinal disorders, immunocompromised children, and children with severe bloody diarrhea should be treated with oral antibiotics[15] (Table 122-4).

Children who have been receiving antibiotics and develop bloody diarrhea may have antibiotic-associated colitis. Most cases of antibiotic-associated colitis caused by *Clostridium difficile* resolve spontaneously when antibiotics are discontinued. Infants and children with protracted diarrhea that has not improved after discontinuing antibiotics may benefit from receiving cholestyramine [2 (g/kg)/day divided into three equal doses]. Cholestyramine is an anion-exchange resin that adsorbs *C. difficile* cytotoxin.

Several antidiarrheal drugs are available to alter intestinal motility, decrease secretions, and adsorb toxins or fluids to reduce diarrhea. Few published data are available, though, to support the use of these agents for treating acute diarrhea in children. Antimotility agents should not be used to treat acute diarrhea in children.[16]

DISPOSITION

Indications for Hospital Admission

All infants who appear toxic should be admitted. Patients with 10 percent dehydration, intractable vomiting, or altered consciousness should be given an infusion of normal saline or Ringer's lactate, regardless of the serum osmolality, and admitted. Infants who are less ill, but whose families may not be able to follow the guidelines for administering ORS, should also be admitted.

Infants who are malnourished and have acute diarrhea require special attention. They more often need to be admitted to the hospital and may require consultation. Malnourished infants are likely to develop metabolic acidosis accompanied by an increase in the anion gap and renal dysfunction. The increased anion gap is due to the accumulation of unmeasured anions, lactate, and phosphate and is accompanied by normochloremia. This is in contrast to most well-nourished infants, who develop hyperchloremic acidosis due to fecal loses of bicarbonate. The latter group of infants can be expected to improve with oral therapy.

Infants and children with bloody diarrhea may have a gastrointestinal infection due to *Escherichia coli* O157:H7 and are at risk of developing HUS. The source most frequently identified in outbreaks has been exposure to undercooked ground meat, undercooked poultry, eggs, or unpasteurized milk. Person-to-person transmission, especially in child day-care centers, is also a well-recognized risk factor for childhood HUS. The risk is highest for children under 5 years of age who are infected with *E. coli* O157:H7 and may approach 13 percent.[6] Any child who presents with acute bloody diarrhea and laboratory evidence of hemolytic anemia, thrombocytopenia, and/or elevated serum creatinine should be admitted.

Most cases of acute gastroenteritis do not require consultation. In cases of suspected intestinal obstruction, appendicitis, or intussusception, surgical consultation is indicated. Many surgeons prefer consultation prior to radiologic confirmation of intussusception. Ingestions of toxins often require consultation with a poison control center or toxicologist. In cases where abuse or neglect is suspected, social service and the primary care physician should be involved. Chronic diarrhea

TABLE 122-4 Clinical Features, Diagnostic Aids, and Treatment of Diarrhea

Agent	Clinical Features/Historical Clues	Diagnostic Aids	Treatment
Viral			**Rehydration**
Rotavirus	Watery diarrhea, winter, most common agent	Enzyme immunoassay available, but of little help in acute management	
Enteric adenovirus	Watery diarrhea, and/or concurrent respiratory symptoms		
Norwalk	Watery diarrhea, epidemic gastroenteritis, with associated fever, headache, myalgias		
Bacterial			**Rehydration *plus***
Campylobacter jejuni	Fever, abdominal pain, watery or bloody diarrhea, may mimic appendicitis, animal reservoir	Fecal WBC, stool culture	Erythromycin ethylsuccinate (EES) 50 mg/kg/day divided qid
Shigella	Fever, abdominal pain, headache, mucoid diarrhea, possible seizure, toxic megacolon, small inoculum and very contagious	Fecal WBC, stool culture, swab culturette	TMP-SMX (Bactrim) 8/40 mg/kg/day divided bid or ampicillin 50–100 mg/kg/day divided qid
Salmonella	Fever, dysentery, animal reservoir, large inoculum	Fecal WBC, stool culture	Antibiotics prolong carrier state and indicated only if complicated (septic, hemoglobinopathy), TMP-SMX (Bactrim) 8/40 mg/kg/day divided bid
Escherichia coli			
Enterotoxigenic ETEC	Watery diarrhea (enterotoxin), cholera-like	Culture, ELISA	TMP-SMX (Bactrim) 8/40 mg/kg/day divided bid
Enteropathogenic EPEC	Water diarrhea (enterotoxin), chronic	Fecal WBC, culture	Neomycin 100 mg/kg/day PO divided qid
Enterohemorrhagic EHEC	Dysentery, serotype O157:H7 associated with HUS	Fecal WBC, culture, PCR, serotype with HUS check, CBC, BUN, creatinine	Supportive care, no antibiotics
Vibrio cholera	Rice-water diarrhea (enterotoxin)		TMP-SMX (Bactrim) 8/40 mg/kg/day divided bid
Yersinia enterocolitica	Fever, vomit, diarrhea, abdominal pain, may mimic appendicitis, animal reservoir	Stool culture, serology	Ceftriaxone (Rocephin) 50 mg/kg/day (controversial)
Clostridium difficile	Recent antibiotic use	Fecal WBC, culture, toxin assay	Metronidazole (Flagyl) 15–40 mg/kg/day divided tid, discontinue other antibiotics
Staphylococcus aureus	Food poisoning (toxin mediated)		No antibiotics
Parasitic			**Rehydration *plus***
Giardia lamblia	Diarrhea, flatulence, mountain streams, day care	Stool ova and parasite	Furazolidone or metronidazole (Flagyl) 15–40 mg/kg/day divided tid
Entamoeba histolytica	Bloody, mucoid stools, hepatic abscess	Serologic test	Metronidazole (Flagyl) 15–40 mg/kg/day divided tid

Abbreviations: BUN, blood urea nitrogen; CBC, complete blood count; EHEC, enterohemorrhagic *E. coli;* ELISA, enzyme-linked immunosorbent assay; EPEC, enteropathogenic *E. coli;* ETEC, enterotoxigenic *E. coli;* HUS, hemolytic-uremic syndrome; PCR, polymerase chain reaction; TMP-SMX, trimethoprim-sulfamethoxazole; WBC, white blood cell count.

or chronic vomiting should be discussed with the child's primary care provider to determine whether consultation is indicated.

DISCHARGE INSTRUCTIONS

Infants and children who are not dehydrated or who have responded well to oral or IV hydration may be discharged with instructions to take ORS solutions and age-appropriate feedings. The family should be instructed to return to the emergency department or to their own physician if the child becomes unable or unwilling to drink the ORS solution, begins to vomit, has increased emesis, develops bilious emesis, or shows signs of dehydration, such as decreasing urine output or decreased tearing, or if there is a decrease in the child's level of activity or state of alertness. Infants and small children should be reevaluated within 24 h especially if they continue to have diarrhea. The family should be instructed to telephone their primary care provider and he or she should decide if a visit is necessary. If the family does not have a primary care physician, then the family should contact the emergency department.

REFERENCES

1. Cicrello HG, Glass RI: *Pediatr Infect Dis* 5:163, 1994.
2. Glass RJ, Lew JF, Gangorosa RE, et al: Estimate of morbidity and mortality rates for diarrheal diseases in American children. *J Pediatr* 118(suppl): 527, 1991.
3. Barlett AV, Moore M, Gary GW, et al: Diarrheal illness among infants and toddlers in day care centers: I. Epidemiology and pathogens. *J Pediatr* 107:495, 1985.

4. Ho MS, Glass RI, Pinsky PF, Anderson LJ: Rotavirus as a cause of diarrheal morbidity and mortality in the United States. *J Infect Dis* 158:1112, 1988.
5. Van R, Wun CC, O'Ryan ML, et al: Outbreaks of human enteric adenovirus types 40 and 41 in Houston day care centers. *J Pediatr* 120:516, 1992.
6. Rowe PC, Orrbine E, Lior H, et al: Risk of hemolytic uremic syndrome after sporadic *Escherichia coli* 0157:H7 infection: Results of a Canadian collaborative study. *J Pediatr* 132:777, 1998.
7. Gorelick MH, Shaw KN, Murphy KO: Validity and reliability of clinical signs in the diagnosis of dehydration in children. *Pediatrics* 99:e6, 1997.
8. Gorelick MH, Shaw KN, Murphy KO, Baker D: Effect of fever on capillary refill time. *Pediatr Emerg Care* 13:305, 1997.
9. Hiricho L, Campos M, Rivera J, Guerrant RL: Fecal screening tests in the approach to acute infectious diarrhea; a scientific overview. *Pediatr Infect Dis J* 15:486, 1996.
10. DeWitt TC, Humphrey KF, McCarthy P: Clinical predictors of acute bacterial diarrhea in young children. *Pediatrics* 76:551, 1985.
11. Santosham M, Daum RS, Dillman L, et al: Oral rehydration therapy of infantile diarrhea: A controlled study of well-nourished children hospitalized in the United States and Panama. *N Engl J Med* 306:1070, 1982.
12. American Academy of Pediatrics Committee on Nutrition: Use of oral fluid therapy and posttreatment feeding following enteritis in children in a developed country. *Pediatrics* 75:358, 1985.
13. Brown KH, Peerson JM, Fontaine O: Use of nonhuman milks in the dietary management of young children with acute diarrhea: A meta-analysis of clinical trials. *Pediatrics* 93:17, 1994.
14. American Academy of Pediatrics, provisional Committee on Quality Improvement, Subcommittee on Acute Gastroenteritis Practice Parameter: The management of acute gastroenteritis in young children. *Pediatrics* 97:424, 1996.
15. Richards L, Claeson M, Pierce N: Management of acute diarrhea in children: Lessons learned. *Pediatr Infect Dis J* 12:5, 1993.
16. World Health Organization. *The Rational Use of Drugs in the Management of Acute Diarrheoea in Children.* Geneva: World Health Organization, 1990.

123 PEDIATRIC ABDOMINAL EMERGENCIES

Robert W. Schafermeyer

Evaluation of abdominal emergencies in childhood presents a diagnostic challenge. Some diseases are common to both adults and children and others are age specific, such as congenital anomalies, volvulus, and Hirschsprung disease. One must understand the differential diagnoses of the presenting symptoms, recognize the clinical manifestations of the more common and life-threatening diseases, and be sensitive in approaching infants and children.

One can classify abdominal disease processes in several ways. Is the child febrile or afebrile? Does the disease appear to be obstructive or nonobstructive, abdominal or extraabdominal in nature? Is it due to a local process, or is it systemic? Does the child appear healthy and happy or sick and septic?

The child's age influences the presenting signs and symptoms significantly. The spectrum of pathologic gastrointestinal (GI) conditions of a 2-day-old infant is vastly different from that of a 2-week-old, and both are quite different from that of a 2-year-old.

HISTORY

An infant or young child cannot give a complete history, but if the child is verbal, one should try to get historical information from him or her and then obtain and listen carefully to what the parent or caregiver says. Find out the accurate chronology of events, whether fever has been a part of the illness, the quality and location of pain, feeding and bowel habits, and the quality and quantity of vomiting and bowel losses. Inquire whether bleeding has been present in vomitus or stools. Ask about weight changes. A history of prematurity, necrotizing enterocolitis, congenital anomalies, inborn errors of metabolism, cystic fibrosis, intussusception, or sickle cell anemia are all associated with abdominal complications.

Unfortunately, because some children either are too young or too frightened to speak for themselves or have not been under continuous observation, trauma as a factor in the development of a GI emergency may be missed in battered or abused children. A parent or caregiver may mislead and confuse a physician by evasion and lies. Trauma must always be considered by physicians evaluating pediatric patients presenting with what appears to be an abdominal emergency.

EVALUATION

Children vary greatly in their ability to cooperate with a physical examination. One should take a few moments to gain the confidence of the child before any painful examination or procedures occur. Allowing the child to rest or be on the caregiver's lap may help. Remove clothing to avoid missing an incarcerated hernia, petechiae, visible masses, or peristalsis. Look first and then feel. Consider some nontouch maneuvers and observations such as the child's responses during coughing, walking, climbing onto the table, or jumping up and down.

The child can be invited to self-palpate or palpate with the physician. Start in the least painful areas. Also evaluate extraabdominal areas such as the pharynx, mucous membranes, neck, lung fields, inguinal regions, femoral triangles, testes, and scrotum. Failure to do so may result in delayed or missed diagnoses. Never omit the rectal examination and guaiac test. The diagnosis of Hirschsprung disease, volvulus, or intussusception will be missed without them.

The most important studies include a urinalysis, a complete blood count and differential, and a test of the stool for occult blood. Other tests, ultrasound, and x-ray evaluation should be guided by history, physical examination, how ill the child appears, and the differential diagnoses. Electrolyte and amylase studies, a pregnancy test, and chest and abdominal x-rays may be useful in certain cases. Computed tomography and ultrasonography are also helpful in the evaluation of stable patients with acute pain.[1]

Once the history, physical examination, and laboratory studies are completed, one should have a list of differential diagnoses. If a child is critically ill, resuscitation and evaluation must be simultaneous. Early consultation must be part of the child's care. If the child is ill but stable and the findings are equivocal, then the patient should be admitted for observation and reassessment.

KEY SYMPTOMS

The important GI signs and symptoms are pain, vomiting, diarrhea, constipation, bleeding, jaundice, and masses.

Pain

Abdominal pain can be a manifestation of a variety of disease states not necessarily related to the intestinal tract.[2,3] The origin of the pain may be extraabdominal, such as one might see in a 3- to 6-year old with tonsillitis or pneumonia. Therefore, a careful general physical examination is necessary. One should distinguish between two types of pain—peritonitic and obstructive:

1. Peritonitic pain tends to be exacerbated by motion and thus keeps patients relatively immobile, as, for example, in appendicitis.
2. Obstructive pain is usually spasmodic and associated with restlessness and motion, as, for example, with intussusception.

In the very young (up to 2 years of age), pain is usually described by the caregiver in general terms, such as fussiness, irritability, and inconsolableness. With severe peritonitic pain, the caregiver may state that the child is very irritable or lethargic or seems to be grunting as

TABLE 123-1 Etiology of Pain

Under 2 Years	6–11 Years
Appendicitis	Appendicitis
Colic (first 4 months)	Diabetic ketoacidosis
Congenital anomalies	Functional
Gastroenteritis	Gastroenteritis
Incarcerated hernia	Henoch-Schönlein purpura
Intussusception	Incarcerated hernia
Malabsorption	Inflammatory bowel disease
Malrotation	Obstruction
Metabolic acidosis	Peptic ulcer disease
Obstruction	Pneumonia
Sickle cell pain crises	Renal stones
Toxins	Sickle cell syndrome
Urinary tract infection	Streptococcal pharyngitis
Volvulus	Torsion of ovary or testicle
	Toxins
	Trauma
	Urinary tract infection

2–5 Years	Over 11 Years
Appendicitis	Appendicitis
Diabetic ketoacidosis	Cholecystitis
Gastroenteritis	Diabetic ketoacidosis
Hemolytic-uremic syndrome	Dysmenorrhea
Henoch-Schönlein purpura	Ectopic pregnancy
Incarcerated hernia	Functional
Intussusception	Gastroenteritis
Malabsorption	Incarcerated hernia
Metabolic acidosis	Inflammatory bowel disease
Obstruction	Obstruction
Pneumonia	Pancreatitis
Sickle cell pain crises	Peptic ulcer disease
Toxins	Pneumonia
Trauma	Pregnancy
Urinary tract infection	Renal stones
Volvulus	Sickle cell syndrome
	Torsion of ovary or testicle
	Toxins
	Trauma
	Urinary tract infection

if in pain. Peritonitis or pain from intussusception may present as lethargy or an altered level of consciousness. Between 2 and 6 years of age, pain of GI origin is usually referred to the periumbilical region, and diagnosis requires correlation of the patient's observations and the physician's visual and tactile evaluation. Youngsters with pain of peritonitic origin walk with obvious discomfort and prefer to lie still. In contrast, youngsters with obstructive pain may be unable to remain immobile on the examining table. The etiologies of pain vary significantly with age (Table 123-1). Every emergency physician must be familiar with and recognize the life-threatening causes of pain (Table 123-2). The clinician must provide appropriate supportive therapy while completing the diagnostic evaluation and/or consultation.

TABLE 123-2 Life-Threatening Causes of Pain

Appendicitis	Metabolic acidosis
Congenital anomalies	Peptic ulcer disease: complications
Diabetic ketoacidosis	Pneumonia
Ectopic pregnancy	Sepsis
Hemolytic-uremic syndrome	Toxins
Incarcerated hernia	Trauma
Intussusception	Volvulus

Vomiting

Vomiting is a common childhood problem and may be a specific or nonspecific manifestation of a benign process or a serious, life-threatening illness or injury. Vomiting or regurgitation may be a manifestation of a relatively minor problem (e.g., a nervous parent, poor feeding habits, or gastroesophageal reflux) or it may be a sign of a more serious illness. Bilious vomiting is always a serious manifestation in an infant or a child. Vomiting may be a sign of obstructive or nonobstructive GI diseases, or of infections or metabolic disorders (Table 123-3).

Vomiting (bilious or not) is a classic symptom of mechanical intestinal obstruction in children. In the early phases of illness, before a child has developed electrolyte abnormalities (e.g., in a child with pyloric stenosis) or before a child has reached the stage of harboring gangrenous bowel (e.g., internal volvulus), the child's general condition may appear to be good. The child may be hungry immediately after vomiting and even eat vigorously. One must not ignore the possibility of a serious underlying intraabdominal pathologic condition merely because a vomiting child appears to be systemically well.

The emergency physician must evaluate the child's circulatory and volume status and administer boluses of normal saline at 20 mL/kg for any child in shock or dehydrated. A one-time dose of an antiemetic can be given safely to children over 6 months of age. Children with shock or severe dehydration will need consultation. For children who appear systemically well after about 2 h, 30 mL of clear liquids or infant rehydration solution can be provided at 15- to 30-min intervals.

Diarrhea

Diarrhea is an increased number of watery stools over a defined period of time. An infant may have a formed or semiformed stool after each

TABLE 123-3 Causes of Vomiting

Newborn (0–3 Months)	Under 2 Years
Congenital adrenal hyperplasia	Appendicitis
Congenital anomalies	Congenital adrenal hyperplasia
Food poisoning	Diabetic ketoacidosis
Gastroenteritis	Foreign body
Gastroesophageal reflux	Gastroenteritis
Hirschsprung disease	Head trauma
Hydrocephalus	Hirschsprung disease
Inborn errors of metabolism	Hydrocephalus
Incarcerated hernia	Incarcerated hernia
Kernicterus (newborn)	Intussusception
Malrotation	Malrotation
Meconium ileus	Meningitis
Meningitis	Metabolic acidosis
Necrotizing enterocolitis	Neurologic diseases
Obstruction: anatomic causes	Obstruction
Obstruction: renal system	Pneumonia
Pneumonia	Pyloric stenosis
Pyloric stenosis	Sepsis
Sepsis	Toxins
Toxins	Urinary tract infection
Urinary tract infection	Volvulus
Volvulus	

Over 2 and Adolescents	
Appendicitis	Neurologic diseases
Diabetic ketoacidosis	Pancreatitis
Foreign body	Peritonitis
Gastroenteritis	Pneumonia
Head trauma	Pregnancy
Hirschsprung disease	Sepsis
Incarcerated hernia	Toxins
Meningitis	Trauma
Metabolic acidosis	Urinary tract infection

TABLE 123-4 Causes of Diarrhea

Anatomic: Hirschsprung disease
Dietary: allergy, malabsorption, overfeeding
Infectious: bacterial, parasitic, toxic, viral
Inflammatory: Crohn's disease, hemolytic-uremic syndrome, ulcerative colitis
Malabsorption: cystic fibrosis, enzyme deficiencies, celiac disease
Systemic: endocrinopathy, immunodeficiencies
Obstructive: fecal impaction

feeding and this could be normal. Several mechanisms can cause diarrhea in the child, including osmotic, secretory, and transit disorders. Viral and bacterial pathogens cause the majority of episodes of diarrhea. Some tumors, such as neuroblastomas, secrete hormones that can increase stool water content.

When the presenting symptom is diarrhea, one must quantitate the number and volume of stools, consistency, and the presence of blood. Ascertain the norm for the child, since there is great individual variability in frequency and type of stools. Associated symptoms or the presence of diarrheal illness in other members of the family helps in establishing the diagnosis. Dehydration and electrolyte imbalance should be assessed and treated. Diarrhea may represent fluid expelled around an anatomic obstructive mass, such as an impaction, or functional obstruction, as in Hirschsprung disease (absence of parasympathetic ganglia cells in the muscle layers of the colon). Bloody diarrhea may be infectious or a manifestation of a systemic disease (e.g., hemolytic-uremic syndrome; Table 123-4).

Treatment of diarrhea will vary depending on cause. A suspicion of Hirschsprung or Crohn's disease warrants surgical consultation. Malabsorption, hemolytic-uremic syndrome, cystic fibrosis, or persistent diarrhea with weight loss and failure to thrive warrants pediatric consultation. Other causes may only require 24 h of rehydration solution and avoiding fatty or high-carbohydrate-containing foods for 2 or 3 days. Stool cultures are warranted in children with bloody diarrhea, diarrhea for more than 5 days, or toxic appearance or to track an epidemic form of illness.

Constipation

Constipation is infrequent, dry, hard stools that may result from defects in filling or emptying the rectum.

Constipation may be a sign of a pathologic or functional process. Eventually, watery stool works its way around the impaction and causes diarrhea. Thus, rectal examination is very important in the evaluation of both constipation and diarrhea.

Causes of constipation are quite different in infants and older children. In infancy, one must consider causes such as maternal drugs, congenital GI anomalies, cystic fibrosis, Hirschsprung disease, poor intake, and anal fissure. One should note abdominal shape and girth, and the presence of bowel sounds and masses, and check the anal area. Check rectal tone and stool for occult blood. If a bowel obstruction is suspected, surgical consultation is necessary. If no systemic cause or serious illness is suspected, dark thick molasses or corn syrup can be added to the diet. Finally, if the child is listless or hypotonic, one should consider infantile botulism (see Table 123-5).

In older children, one should not automatically think that the cause is functional. Constipation is seen in children who are anorexic or who have cerebral palsy, neuromuscular disease, dehydration, hypercalcemia, hypokalemia, hypothyroidism, or depression or who have ingested drugs such as diuretics, antihistamines, anticholinergics, or narcotics. A thorough history and physical examination, including rectal, are necessary. An empty rectal vault does not rule out constipation. If there are signs of bowel obstruction, tumor, or serious illness, one should consult an appropriate specialist.

Acute constipation is treated by increased oral fluids and possibly a stool softener or milk of magnesia. Chronic constipation is treated in three separate steps, and follow-up with a primary care specialist is important. The steps are cleanout, maintenance, and behavior modification.

Bleeding

Bleeding may be a sign of GI inflammation, duplication, foreign-body infection, or systemic illness, or it may be nothing more than an anal fissure or milk allergy. GI bleeding in the newborn, either vomited or per rectum, may be the result of swallowed maternal blood. The laboratory can differentiate between maternal and fetal blood by the Kleihauer-Betke test or hemoglobin electrophoresis. Rarely, hemorrhagic states cause GI bleeding in the newborn. Small amounts of blood in the stool of an infant, if fresh, may be a manifestation of anal fissures, which are easily identified. In children 2 to 10 years of age, painless bleeding of small to moderate amounts of fresh blood usually mixed through the stool might be an indication of benign GI polyps, or bloody diarrhea may indicate a bacterial infection or inflammatory bowel disease.[4]

The presence of small to moderate amounts of blood in the stool of an infant (particularly associated with vomiting) must lead the physician to consider malrotation of the midgut. This is a life-threatening condition that requires immediate investigation and surgical consultation because volvulus of the midgut can lead to midgut gangrene if the problem is not identified and corrected early in its course.

Major painless upper GI bleeding in infants or children is most commonly the result of bleeding varices secondary to portal hypertension. Major painless lower GI bleeding in infants or children is frequently ascribable to a Meckel's diverticulum.

Frequently, the cause of minimal to moderate amounts of blood in the stool of an infant or a child may never be identified. Repeated episodes of bleeding require GI studies, endoscopic evaluation, and Meckel isotope scanning (Table 123-6).

TABLE 123-5 Acute and Chronic Constipation

NONORGANIC	
Miscellaneous	Drugs
Anorexia nervosa	Anticholinergics
Functional	Antihistamines
Limited fluid intake	Diuretics
Minimal bulk diet	Opiates
Prolonged immobilization	Phenothiazine
Psychogenic	Thorazine
	Vincristine
ORGANIC	
Gastrointestinal	Metabolic
Anal fissure	Dehydration
Anal stricture/stenosis	Hypercalcemia
Chagas disease	Hypokalemia
Cystic fibrosis	Hypothyroidism
Hirschprung disease	Renal tubular acidosis
Obstruction	Neuromuscular
Tumor	Amyotonia congenita
Volvulus	Myotonic dystrophy
Infectious	Spina bifida
Infantile botulism	Spinal cord disease or injury
	Tumors

TABLE 123-6 Causes of Gastrointestinal (GI) Bleeding

Under 2 Months	Under 2 Years	Over 2 Years
	UPPER GI BLEEDING	
Bleeding diathesis Swallowed maternal blood Vascular malformation	Bleeding diathesis Foreign body Gastroenteritis Traumatic hemobilia Vascular malformation Mallory-Weiss tear	Esophageal varices Foreign body Gastroenteritis Mallory-Weiss tear Peptic ulcer disease Traumatic hemobilia Vascular malformation
	LOWER GI BLEEDING	
Congenital duplications Intussusception Meckel's diverticulum Necrotizing enterocolitis Swallowed maternal blood Vascular malformation Volvulus	Anal fissure Congenital duplication Gastroenteritis Hemolytic-uremic syndrome Henoch-Schönlein purpura Inflammatory bowel disease Intussusception Meckel's diverticulum Milk allergy Polyps: benign, familial	Allergy Colitis Gastroenteritis Hemolytic-uremic syndrome Henoch-Schönlein purpura Inflammatory bowel disease Meckel's diverticulum Polyps

Jaundice

Jaundice is an ominous sign, since it represents hepatic dysfunction. It might represent sepsis, congenital infection (TORCHS), or postnatal viral hepatitis. It might represent a minor ABO incompatibility or a major ABO or Rh factor incompatibility, with the possibility of kernicterus or death. It may represent the first signs of cystic fibrosis, galactosemia, or other hepatic enzyme deficiencies, or it could be the harbinger of an anatomic problem such as biliary atresia, a choledochal cyst, or even pyloric stenosis. All jaundiced patients must be evaluated promptly and consultation obtained (Table 123-7).

Masses

The presence of a mass could be the first sign of a congenital anomaly or a tumor (e.g., Wilms's tumor or neuroblastoma). It could be a pyloric "olive" or the intussusception mass if associated with vomiting or a guaiac-positive stool. If a child has an acute surgical or obstructive abdomen, resuscitation and prompt surgical consultation are necessary.

TABLE 123-7 Causes of Bilirubin Abnormalities

Unconjugated	Conjugated
ABO or Rh incompatibility Autoimmune hemolytic anemia Hepatic: Crigler-Najjar syndrome, Gilbert's disease Hypothyroidism Sepsis Sickle cell anemia G6PD deficiency	Anatomic defect: biliary, hepatic Hemolytic-uremic syndrome Hepatic abscess Hepatitis: congenital, acquired Hepatitis: TORCHS Inflammatory bowel disease Metabolic: cystic fibrosis, galactosemia, etc. Sepsis Sickle cell anemia Toxins Urinary tract infections Wilson's disease

TABLE 123-8 Causes of Abdominal Masses

Hepatomegaly
Splenomegaly
Gastrointestinal duplication
Neuroblastoma
Sacral teratoma
Wilms's tumor
Pyloric stenosis
Intussusception mass
Constipation (fecal mass)

Otherwise, emergency evaluation should be followed by pediatric consultation and admission (Table 123-8).

DIAGNOSIS AND MANAGEMENT OF SELECTED EMERGENCIES

Gastrointestinal Emergencies in Infants in the First Year of Life

MALROTATION WITH AND WITHOUT VOLVULUS Volvulus is a major life-threatening complication of malrotation.[5] The complications of malrotation occur most commonly in the first year of life, although malrotation can give rise to symptoms at any time in a person's life. It is the most urgent of GI emergencies in infants and children because of consequent gangrene of the total midgut. The time interval from the first symptom to the development of total midgut gangrene may be only a few hours.

Pathophysiology During gestation, at approximately 6 weeks of age, the elongating intestines prolapse into the yolk sac. Upon reentry at 10 weeks, the midgut undergoes a 270° counterclockwise turn around the superior mesenteric artery. Usually, the duodenum and the cecum become fixed by peritoneal bands, and the small intestine has a broad mesenteric attachment along its base. Abnormal rotation and inadequate fixation can occur during gestation. Incomplete rotation or malrotation can leave the cecum high in the abdomen, with its peritoneal attachments crossing the duodenum in an obstructing manner. The mesentery fails to fan out, and the midgut is suspended and its entire vascular supply travels along a narrow pedicle.

Clinical Features The presenting symptoms are usually vomiting (ultimately becoming bilious), with or without abdominal distention, and streaks of blood in the stool. Infants with symptoms of obstruction or bilious vomiting must receive prompt surgical consultation and active resuscitation. The most dramatic presentation in newborns is the sudden onset of an acute abdomen and shock, with a rigid and discolored abdomen associated with bilious or bloody vomiting and bloody stools, indicating the presence of gangrenous bowel. On physical examination, such infants may appear pale and have grunting respirations, and approximately one-third of the infants will appear jaundiced. The vast majority of cases present within the first month of life. In older children, the pain is usually constant, not colicky. This symptom complex usually occurs in previously healthy children. However, there may have been minor episodes in the past of vomiting or abdominal discomfort. A child suspected of harboring a malrotation with possible midgut volvulus should have flat and upright abdominal x-rays. The presence of a loop of bowel overriding the liver is suggestive of the diagnosis. Occasionally, an upper GI examination may reveal an abnormal location of the ligament of Treitz.

Intussusception, duodenal stenosis, or atresia can produce a clinical picture similar to midgut volvulus.

Treatment An infant with systoms of obstruction or bilious vomiting must receive prompt surgical consultation, active resuscitation, and hospital admission. Intravenous fluid should be started immediately, and a nasogastric tube placed. Blood should be typed and cross-matched. A white blood cell count may identify early gut necrosis. Electrolytes and venous blood gases may identify sodium or potassium abnormalities or ongoing acidosis. Any child with vomiting or bloody stools who is identified as having an incompletely rotated bowel requires urgent laparotomy to prevent the development of midgut volvulus and total midgut gangrene.

INCARCERATED HERNIA **Clinical Features** An incarcerated hernia will not be detected unless the infant or child is totally undressed at the time of examination. The symptoms include irritability, poor feeding, vomiting, and an inguinal or scrotal mass. The differential diagnosis of an inguinal or scrotal mass most frequently includes hydrocele of the cord or the scrotum, undescended testicle, torsion of the testicle, torsion of the appendix testis, inguinal lymphadenopathy, inguinal node abscess, orchitis, and inguinal or scrotal trauma. The incidence of incarceration of inguinal hernias is highest in the first year of life. In both boys and girls, the incarcerated sac may contain small or large bowel. In girls, an ovary may be present in the sac.

Treatment In most instances, provided the child is examined gently and his or her confidence obtained, it is possible to achieve manual reduction of the incarcerated hernia (if it has been present for only a short period of time) without the use of sedation. When this maneuver is unsuccessful, most cases can be successfully reduced following the administration of intramuscular meperidine (up to 2 mg/kg of body weight in the first year of life). Quite often, as a result of the relaxation induced by the meperidine, the hernia spontaneously reduces. In the absence of spontaneous reduction, one should attempt to reduce the hernia. The few patients who do not respond to these maneuvers must undergo surgical reduction.

Once the hernia is reduced, the patient should be referred for surgical repair on an elective basis. Provisions are generally made for pediatric surgical consultation the next day. If it was a difficult reduction, the child should be admitted or observed for 6 to 12 h, and the pediatric surgeon consulted.

INTESTINAL OBSTRUCTION **Clinical Features** Intestinal obstruction presents in infants and young children in the classic manner, with symptoms of pain (manifested by irritability); vomiting; abdominal distention; and, later, absence or diminution of bowel movements. The differential diagnosis of intestinal obstruction in newborns and infants includes intestinal atresia or stenosis, meconium ileus (newborns only), incarcerated inguinal hernia, intussusception, malrotation, malrotation with volvulus, volvulus around a congenital intraabdominal band, duplication cysts of the intestinal tract, imperforate anus, and Hirschsprung disease.

Diagnosis and Treatment Flat and upright films of the abdomen show dilated loops of bowel with air-fluid levels (Fig. 123-1). Such an appearance on the plain x-ray film warrants a barium enema examination with a Hirschsprung catheter, which helps to differentiate between Hirschsprung disease, malrotation, and colonic stenosis and also separates lower large bowel obstruction from upper small bowel obstruction.

Once intestinal obstruction has been diagnosed, the patient should be prepared for surgical intervention by having an intravenous line and a nasogastric tube placed and should be admitted.

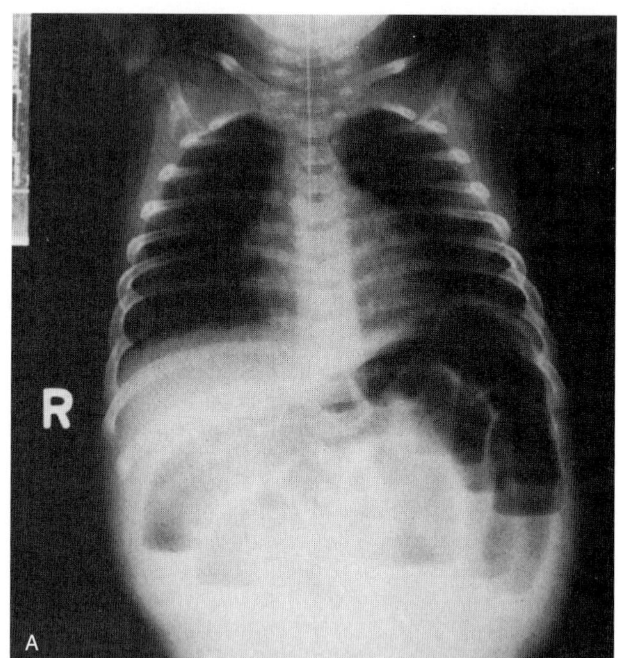

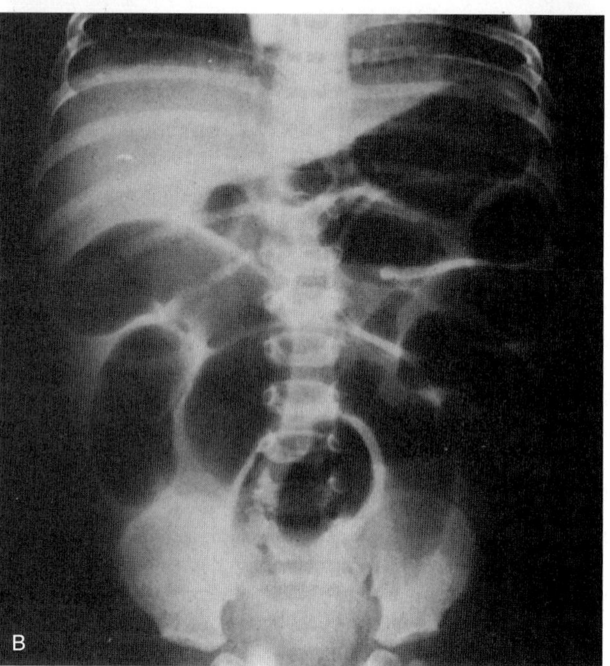

FIG. 123-1. Mechanical intestinal obstruction. *A.* Upright film. *B.* Flat film.

PYLORIC STENOSIS The infant with a history of nonbilious projectile vomiting must be considered to have pyloric stenosis. The disorder affects approximately 1 in 150 male and 1 in 750 female patients. It occurs more frequently in firstborn males, and a familial incidence is noted in approximately 50 percent of patients. It is caused by diffuse hypertrophy and hypoplasia of the smooth muscle that narrows the antrum of the stomach to a small channel that can be easily obstructed.

Clinical Features Onset is rare before the age of 1 week, and the disorder usually begins in the second or third week of life. It seldom develops after the third month of life. Initially, the infant may only regurgitate small amounts of milk, making it difficult to distinguish the cause of vomiting from simple regurgitation, gastric reflux, or milk intolerance. Vomiting usually becomes projectile within a week of onset of symptoms, and the vomitus is never bile stained although it may occasionally have streaks of blood. Vomiting occurs just after or near the end of feeding, and afterward the infant will refeed hungrily unless the child has become malnourished or dehydrated.

Vomiting eventually becomes projectile. Constipation usually is noted because the infant is not retaining enough formula and becomes dehydrated.

Physical examination usually demonstrates a hungry infant who has failed to gain weight over the past several weeks or has lost weight. Jaundice occurs in 1 to 2 percent of cases. If one undresses and then feeds the infant, peristaltic waves can sometimes be seen passing from left to right across the upper abdomen, just prior to an episode of vomiting. Palpation of a pyloric tumor—the "olive"—is pathognomonic. If it is present, one can be sure of the diagnosis. The olive is usually felt near the lateral margin of the right rectus muscle just below the liver edge. Palpation of the olive is very dependent on the amount of hypertrophy of the pylorus and the skill of the clinician.

In advanced cases, the physical examination will reveal dehydration and lethargy. The child may appear moribund, with sunken eyes, decreased elasticity of the skin and loss of subcutaneous tissue.

Diagnosis If the olive is palpated, further studies are not necessary. If no olive is palpated, abdominal ultrasonography is recommended. Accuracy depends on the use of a high-resolution machine and an experienced sonographer. Although false positives are rare, false negatives can occur in up to 20 percent of cases, often due to bowel gas interference. If the diagnosis is highly suspected and the findings on ultrasonography are normal, an upper GI series can be performed. This usually demonstrates delayed gastric emptying and indentation of the antrum by the pyloric olive. The pyloric channel is narrowed and appears like a "string." If pyloric stenosis is not noted, the radiographer can evaluate the infant for gastroesophageal reflux. The major risk from the upper GI series is the potential for aspiration. The barium should be removed after the x-ray to prevent aspiration.

Treatment Once the diagnosis of pyloric stenosis has been confirmed or is highly suspected, surgical consultation should be obtained. Surgery is the treatment of choice, and the procedure is very safe.

Oral intake should be restricted and an intravenous line started. Dehydration and electrolyte abnormalities must be corrected before surgery. Much of the reduced morbidity and mortality from surgery for this disease can be attributed to improved preoperative status. Extensive and protracted vomiting in pyloric stenosis may lead to hypokalemia and hyponatremia. More striking decreases occur in chloride concentration and an increase in pH and carbon dioxide content. This constitutes the characteristic changes of hypochloremic alkalosis. Initial administration of 5% dextrose in normal saline or normal saline to which potassium chloride is added gradually and successfully replaces the calculated deficits of potassium chloride and sodium.

INTUSSUSCEPTION Intussusception occurs when a portion of the alimentary tract is telescoped into another segment. It is the most common cause of intestinal obstruction between 3 months and 6 years of age and is rare under 3 months of age. The male/female ratio is 4:1.

Pathophysiology The causes of most intussusceptions are unknown. There is a seasonal incidence that seems to follow peak viral illness seasons. In some patients, recognizable causes for intussusception are found, such as Meckel's diverticulum, intestinal polyp, duplication, lymphosarcoma, or as a complication of Henoch-Schönlein purpura, but are rarely found in infants under 2 years of age. Rarely, tumors or foreign bodies may cause intussusception. Ileocolic intussusceptions are the most common. The upper portion of the bowel invaginates into the lower portion, bringing the mesentery with it. Constriction of the mesentery obstructs venous return with engorgement of the intussusceptum. With edema and bleeding, there may be bloody stools, with mucus giving rise to the characteristic "currant jelly" stool.

Clinical Features The classic patient is a robust, 6- to 18-month-old infant without prior difficulty. Suddenly, the child appears to be in pain. The youngster may be playing quietly in the playpen and suddenly stop playing, begin to cry, and even roll around in discomfort. Just as suddenly, the pain ceases, and the child appears to be as happy and content as before the onset of pain. Episodes may recur at more frequent intervals, with the duration of the painful attacks increasing. Some children become very still, listless, and pale, and appear to be in a shocklike state due to the visceral pain. Vomiting is rare in the first few hours but usually develops after 6 to 12 h. The classic "currant jelly" stool associated with intussusception is a late manifestation of the disease complex and is present in only 50 percent of cases.[6] Its absence should not delay evaluation for intussusception in the patient. However, a positive stool guaiac test is present in almost every case. Fever can occur and even rise to 41°C (106°F). Respirations may be shallow and grunting in nature.

Apathy or lethargy may be the only presenting sign of intussusception in up to 10 percent of cases. Because of this, some infants will receive a lumbar puncture and other diagnostic studies, thus delaying the diagnosis and management of the child's illness.[7,8]

Examination between attacks may reveal the often-described sausage-shaped tumor mass of intussuscepted bowel in the right side of the abdomen. If this mass is felt in the epigastrium, the long axis is usually horizontal. At least one-third of patients do not have a palpable mass, but the absence of a mass must not delay further investigation. An ileoileal intussusception may have a less typical presentation, with symptoms and signs suggestive of intestinal obstruction.

Diagnosis and Management The presumptive diagnosis of intussusception is made on the basis of the history and may be seriously considered as a result of a telephone description of a child's problem by the caregiver. The apparent well-being of a child in the absence of clinical findings should not mislead the physician. An x-ray examination of the abdomen may show a mass or filling defect in the right upper quadrant of the abdomen (Fig. 123-2*A*). Even in the presence of normal plain x-ray films (which can be 30 percent of cases), the history described demands a barium enema examination, which demonstrates the classic "coiled spring" (Fig. 123-2*B*). The barium enema examination is not only a diagnostic tool in the management of this disease, but is frequently curative.[7] If it is obtained in the first 12 to 24 h of the developing intussusception, up to 80 percent of cases can be corrected by barium enema alone. When barium enema does not resolve the intussusception, surgical intervention is indicated. If the barium enema reduces the intussusception, the parents should be warned of a 5 to 10 percent recurrence rate, usually within the first 24 to 48 h following barium enema reduction.

Recently, air insufflation is being used by radiologists more frequently than barium to diagnose and manage intussusception. This is a safer method particularly if there is a possibility of perforation, since the peritoneum would not be contaminated by barium. It may be as effective as barium and enables better control over colonic pressure used for the reduction.[9] In most hospitals, protocol calls for notification of the pediatric surgeon prior to radiologic reduction of intussusception.

Once reduction occurs, the child should be observed to watch for any recurrence of symptoms or for complications from the reduction. Reliability of the parents or caretaker and other pediatric social concerns may affect length of observation.

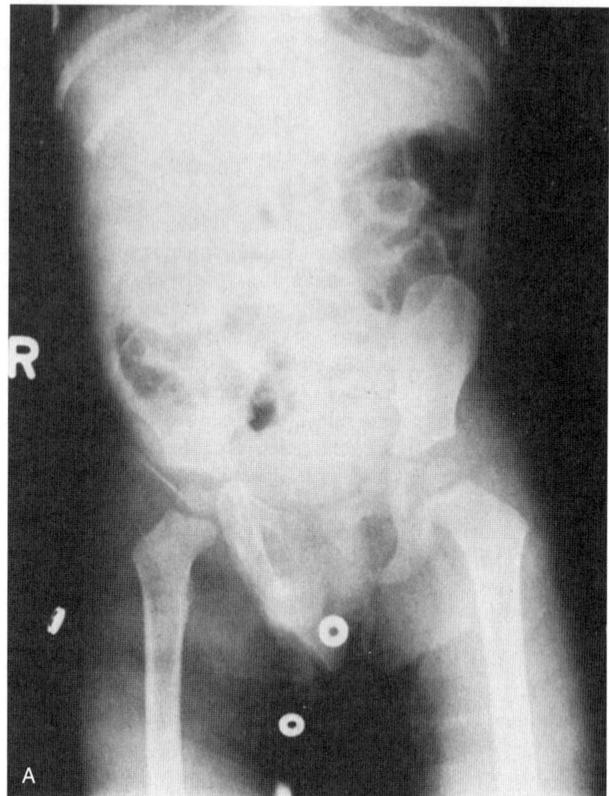

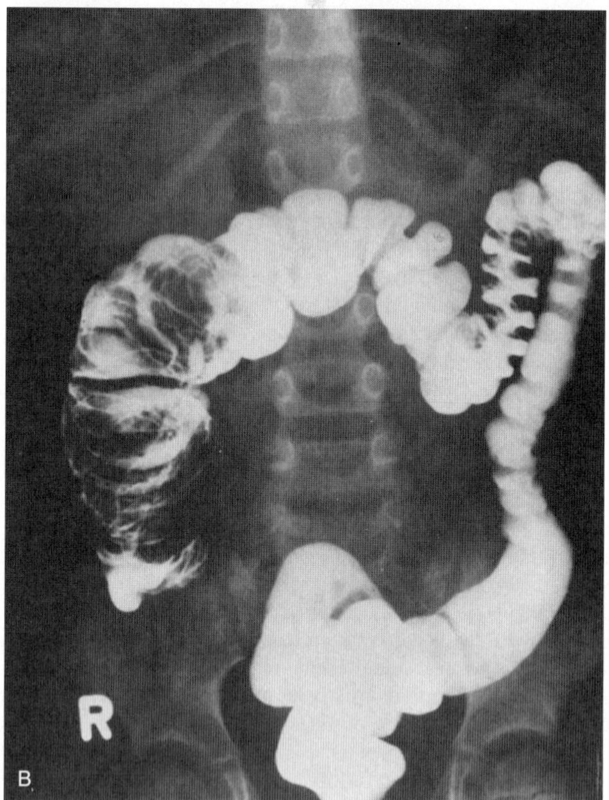

FIG. 123-2. Intussusception. *A*. Plain film with loss of bowel pattern in the right upper quadrant. *B*. With barium enema, showing a "coiled spring" in the ascending colon.

A barium enema reduction is contraindicated if there is free peritoneal air on plain films or if the infant has signs of peritonitis or sepsis. The surgeon and emergency physician should provide intravenous fluid replacement for hypovolemia (due to vomiting, poor intake, and third spacing of fluids) and provision of antibiotics is essential in such a patient.

The recurrence rate after barium enema reduction ranges from 5 to 10 percent and usually occurs within the first 24 to 48 h following reduction. A second attempt at barium reduction can be considered and is usually successful. If another episode of intussusception occurs, then an exploratory laparotomy is necessary.

Gastrointestinal Emergencies in Children 2 Years and Older

APPENDICITIS **Clinical Features** Although appendicitis can occur in children younger than age 2, the presentation is usually one of peritonitis or sepsis because of the delay in diagnosis.[10] Over age 2, appendicitis becomes a more important part of the differential diagnoses of abdominal pain. The classic progression of symptoms associated with appendicitis applies equally to children and adults. The events involve early anorexia followed by the development of mild to moderate periumbilical pain and then vomiting and the movement of the pain to the right lower quadrant of the abdomen. The youngster should be observed walking into the examining room; in most instances, the child appears to be in discomfort as he or she moves along. This discomfort associated with motion can be exacerbated by asking the youngster to jump up and down before he or she lies down on the examining table. On inspection of the patient, the physician may find limited motion of the lower abdomen due to inflammation of the peritoneum and, depending on the duration of the symptoms, there may be abdominal distention. Palpation may reveal the presence of tenderness in the right lower abdominal quadrant. The position of the appendix may vary greatly, and thus tenderness on examination may vary. Guarding and rebound tenderness may or may not be present in this area. The longer the duration of the symptoms, the greater is the possibility of finding a right lower quadrant mass representing localized perforation with the development of an appendiceal abscess. A rectal examination should be performed to detect the presence of a low-lying, intrapelvic, acutely inflamed appendix or to palpate a mass. The child may have a mild fever and an elevated white blood cell count in the range of 11,000 to 20,000. When there is doubt in the overall symptom complex, an x-ray may reveal the presence of an appendicolith (Fig. 123-3).

Diagnosis Symptoms consistent with appendicitis together with the presence of an appendicolith warrant the clinical diagnosis of appendicitis and laparotomy. Intravenous fluids should be given and surgical consultation obtained. The following signs and symptoms make the diagnosis of acute appendicitis difficult:

1. The temperature may be normal.
2. The white blood cell count may be normal.
3. The child may not be anorexic and may actually request food.
4. A heavily built child may manifest minimal right lower quadrant tenderness and minimal tenderness on rectal examination.
5. Gastroenteritis is not infrequently associated with appendicitis. Thus, a child presenting with a several-day history of vomiting and diarrhea, perhaps even with siblings suffering from the same problem, should not have the diagnosis of appendicitis discounted on this basis. Intensification of pain in the presence of a history of gastroenteritis should suggest an acutely inflamed appendix secondary to gastroenteritis.[11]

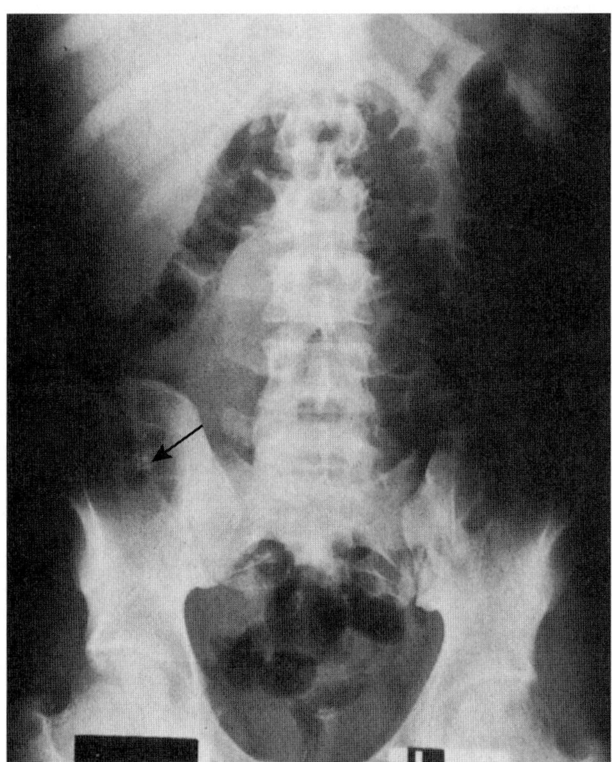

FIG. 123-3. Appendicitis; appendicolith in the right lower quadrant.

6. Appendicitis has been identified in children younger than 1 year of age and is not uncommon in the second year. The incidence of perforation in this age group is much higher because of the difficulty of making the diagnosis and the confusion with gastroenteritis.

Recently, ultrasonography has been a subject of interest in identifying patients with appendicitis. It is, however, operator dependent and has missed not only inflamed appendices but also ruptured appendices. Overall, it has good sensitivity and specificity. It is not yet a gold standard.[12]

Treatment Once the diagnosis of appendicitis is strongly considered or confirmed, surgical consultation should be obtained and the child should be admitted to the hospital. The child should receive any appropriate supportive therapy. If the child is febrile, rectal acetaminophen may be given. The child should not receive any oral fluids or food. Start an intravenous line and administer fluid boluses if the child shows signs of sepsis or shock. Closely monitor the child's vital signs and give pain medication parenterally after consultation with the surgeon.

If the diagnosis is possible but not probable, surgical consultation should be considered and the child reexamined until either resolution of the illness or need for laparotomy is determined.

If a perforated appendix is suspected or the child appears septic, ensure that the patient is adequately oxygenated and ventilated, and hypovolemia is corrected. Ensure adequate circulation and urinary output. Start broad-spectrum antibiotics. Ampicillin, gentamicin, and clindamicin are possible regimens.

MECKEL'S DIVERTICULUM A Meckel's diverticulum can cause a variety of signs and symptoms, such as bleeding, peritonitis, intussusception, and intestinal obstruction. The presence of gastric mucosa in the diverticulum may give rise to an ulcer in the adjacent ileum, which may cause symptoms such as painless rectal bleeding. Bleeding is brisk and usually bright red. The ulcer may perforate and cause peritonitis. Isotope scanning reveals the presence of a Meckel's diverticulum containing gastric mucosa in up to 50 percent of the cases. A scan with normal findings does not eliminate the diagnosis.

Acute inflammation in a Meckel's diverticulum may simulate acute appendicitis or may initiate intussusception. Finally, the vitellointestinal remnant attaching the apex of a Meckel's diverticulum to the intraabdominal umbilical region may be the focus around which volvulus of the small bowel or an internal hernia develops, each of these giving rise to intestinal obstruction. Surgical consultation is necessary.

BLEEDING There are several systemic processes that can result in GI bleeding. Upper GI bleeding is usually the result of peptic ulcer disease, varices, or gastritis. Lower GI bleeding can be due to not only the previously mentioned diseases, but also due to infectious colitis, coagulopathies, ulcerative colitis, and Crohn's disease. Two other illnesses can cause abdominal pain and bleeding: Henoch-Schönlein purpura (HSP) and hemolytic-uremic syndrome (HUS)

In HSP, some children may present with joint pain, abdominal pain, or seizure. Usually, there is a petechial or purpuric rash on the buttocks and lower extremities. Many children have guaiac-positive stools but rarely present with bleeding unless there is associated intussusception. Treatment is usually symptomatic and on an outpatient basis unless the child appears ill or has a complication of the disease.

In HUS, there is usually a history of a gastroenteritis with or without bloody diarrhea up to 2 weeks before onset of illness. Toxigenic strains of *Escherichia coli* have been implicated as a possible link to HUS. Low-grade fever, pallor, hematuria, and hematochezia occur. The central nervous system can be involved. Hypertension occurs in up to 50 percent and seizures in up to 40 percent of cases. Acute bowel perforation, toxic megacolon, intussusception, renal failure, and pancreatitis can occur. These children should be managed by appropriate pediatric specialists or intensivists.

COLON POLYPS Single polyps or multiple or classic familial polyposis may give rise to painless hematochezia. Single polyps are usually benign (juvenile), with no propensity for malignant degeneration. Frequently, the parent describes what is obviously a prolapsed polyp, easily palpated on rectal examination. It is rare for bleeding originating from a polyp to be life threatening. Familial polyposis is rare and is a premalignant syndrome. The child should be referred to a pediatric surgeon.

OTHER CAUSES OF GASTROINTESTINAL BLEEDING Blood represents local irritation or erosion in the majority of children. What appears to be a small amount of blood on the stool or diaper of a healthy child is probably due to an anal fissure or could be related to food substances that have a red or melanotic coloration. A stool test for occult blood and a gentle rectal examination may be all that is needed in a healthy child.

On the other hand, if the child is sick- or ill-appearing or shocklike or has petechiae, one must consider vascular malformation, Meckel's diverticulum, intestinal duplication, or sepsis. In adolescents, one must consider stress ulceration, peptic ulcer disease, and inflammatory bowel disease. Sepsis, severe gastroenteritis, HSP, and HUS should also be part of the differential diagnoses.

In infants, a coagulation survey should be included in the evaluation if the child is ill or shocklike or has a family history of a clotting disorder. Also remember that GI bleeding could be the presentation of intussusception or volvulus. In neonates the differential diagnosis consists of many severe disorders, and consultation may be necessary to exclude them (Table 123-6).

Pancreatitis

Pancreatitis is not common in childhood. The most common cause is abdominal trauma. It can also occur as an idiopathic or postviral process (mumps, influenza, coxsackie, etc.) or be due to drugs or toxins. Systemic diseases such as cystic fibrosis, systemic lupus erythematous and α_1-antitrypsin deficiency can cause pancreatitis.[13]

Clinical findings include central abdominal pain, vomiting and, sometimes, fever. The abdomen may be distended and is tender to palpation. Patients should receive fluids to correct dehydration and any hypovolemia and receive appropriate pain management. Most of the children will need to be admitted for intravenous hydration, pain management, and diagnostic studies.

Intraabdominal Masses

Every child should have a careful abdominal examination because intraabdominal masses grow silently at first until they cause obstruction, bleeding, or hemorrhage into the tumor or until a parent sees a mass protruding in the abdomen. The child should be supine with his or her head turned toward the parent, and one should carefully palpate all quadrants of the abdomen. If a mass is palpated, the child should be referred to a pediatric surgeon and diagnostic imaging studies obtained. A careful rectal examination, especially if the child has constipation or a gait abnormality, must be done to check for a presacral teratoma and for ovarian masses; both of these tumors can show calcifications on plain film x-rays in approximately 50 percent of cases.

Neuroblastomas can arise from adrenal glands or along the sympathetic chain. They often cross to the midline, and the best cure rate is obtained in children under 1 year of age. Computed tomography is the best way to evaluate this tumor. Wilms's tumor is an intrarenal tumor initially and should be considered in children with hematuria. Ultrasound and computed tomography help define this tumor. Bone scan is also needed. Rhabdomyosarcoma occurs in the pelvis or anywhere there is striated muscle, and it is highly malignant.

In girls over the age of menarche, one must consider pregnancy, and if there is lower quadrant pain, one must consider ectopic pregnancy. One should obtain a serum pregnancy test and consider the use of ultrasonography.

Foreign Bodies in the Gastrointestinal Tract

It is safe to generalize that anything that reaches the stomach will eventually traverse the GI tract and be spontaneously evacuated through the rectum. Nails, open safety pins, pieces of glass, and coins are examples of objects that have traveled the intestinal tract completely. It may take weeks for a coin, for example, to complete the trip to the anus. Any foreign body caught in the esophagus must be removed by esophagoscopy (see Chap. 75). Very rarely is surgical removal of a foreign body in the stomach or distal to the stomach warranted. Occasionally, a long, thin foreign body may not traverse the duodenum and may need to be removed surgically. Round objects almost always pass spontaneously.

Portal Hypertension

Portal hypertension is rare in children in the United States, but is one of the common causes of major upper GI hemorrhage. Extrahepatic portal thrombosis, parenchymal liver disease associated with fibrocystic disease, and biliary cirrhosis in youngsters with congenital biliary atresia surviving as a result of portal enterostomy are examples of conditions that can result in portal hypertension and esophagogastric varices. In two-thirds of cases, no specific cause is found.

Massive hematemesis is the usual initial manifestation, along with hematochezia in children, whereas ascites is more common as the presenting sign in infants. Usually, the bleeding is self-limited. A nasogastric tube can be placed to empty the stomach and to monitor for continued bleeding and blood transfusions given as indicated. Correct any coagulation abnormalities. Emergency consultation with a surgeon, pediatric surgeon, or a pediatric gastroenterologist is necessary.

REFERENCES

1. Johnson GT, Johnson P, Fishman EK: CT evaluation of the acute abdomen: Bowel pathology spectrum of disease. *Crit Rev Diagn Imaging* 37:163, 1996.
2. Moir CR: Abdominal pain in infants and children. *Mayo Clin Proc* 71:984, 1996.
3. Mason JD: The evaluation of acute abdominal pain in children. *Emerg Med Clin North Am* 14:629, 1996.
4. Vinton NE: Gastrointestinal bleeding in infancy and childhood. *Gastroenterol Clin North Am* 23:93, 1994.
5. Andrassy RJ, Mahour GH: Malrotation of the midgut in infants and children. *Arch Surg* 116:158, 1981.
6. Yamamoto LG, Morita SY, Boychuk RB, et al: Stool appearance in intussusception: Assessing the value of the term "currant jelly." *Am J Emerg Med* 15:292, 1997.
7. Winslow BT, Westfall JM, Nicholas RA: Intussusception [review]. *Am Fam Physician* 54:213, 220, 1996.
8. Conway EE Jr: Central nervous system findings and intussusception: How are they related? *Pediatr Emerg Care* 9:15, 1993.
9. Kirks DR: Air intussusception reduction: "The winds of change." *Pediatr Radiol* 25:89, 1985.
10. Puri P, O'Donnell B: Appendicitis in infancy. *J Pediatr Surg* 13:173, 1978.
11. Horwitz JR, Gursoy M, Jaksic T, Lally KP: Importance of diarrhea as a presenting symptom of appendicitis in very young children. *Am J Surg* 173:80, 1997.
12. Gupta H, Dupuy DE: Advances in imaging of the acute abdomen [review]. *Surg Clin North Am* 77:1245, 1997.
13. Weizman Z: Acute pancreatitis in childhood: Research of pathogenesis and clinical implications [review]. *Can J Gastroenterol* 11:249, 1997.

THE DIABETIC CHILD AND DIABETIC KETOACIDOSIS

Maribel Rodriguez
Thom A. Mayer

EPIDEMIOLOGY

Diabetes mellitus is classified in two types. Type I, or insulin-dependent diabetes mellitus (IDDM), is seen mostly in children and adolescents. Insulin deficiency characterizes IDDM, and patients need exogenous insulin for survival. Type II, or non-insulin-dependent diabetes mellitus (NIDDM), is the type seen most commonly in older people or those with obesity and is rarely seen in childhood and adolescence. NIDDM is not discussed in this chapter. IDDM is the most common endocrine disorder of childhood and adolescence, affecting at least 1 in 400 children in the United States.[1] Incidence increases with age and peaks in early to mid-puberty. A seasonal distribution of new cases has been reported, with more cases during the cooler months for unknown reasons.[2] Female and male incidence rates are approximately equal.

PATHOPHYSIOLOGY

IDDM is a disease caused by autoimmune destruction of insulin-producing β cells of the pancreatic islets of Langerhans.[3] There is no single diabetes gene, but a genetic predisposition for acquiring IDDM exists. Certain genetic alterations raise or lower the risk of β-cell damage. In white populations, inheritance of the human leukocyte antigen HLA-DR3 or HLA- DR4 is present in 90 percent of type I diabetes, and 1 in 50 persons with both antigens will have the disease.[1] This and other genetic markers help to explain the worldwide differences in prevalence and incidence of type I diabetes.[4]

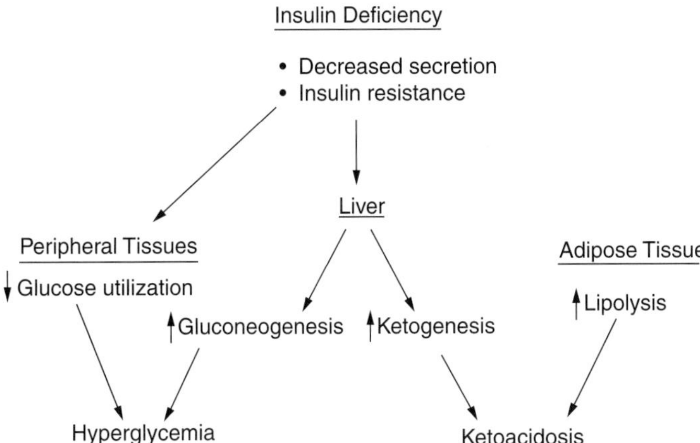

FIG. 124-1. Pathophysiology of diabetic ketoacidosis.

DIAGNOSIS

The diagnosis of IDDM in the pediatric population is usually straightforward. While the triad of polyuria, polydipsia, and polyphagia is the classic presentation, other symptoms include failure to gain weight, weight loss, enuresis, anorexia, and changes in vision, behavior, and school performance. Hyperglycemia in association with glucosuria with or without ketonuria establishes the diagnosis.[5] In rare instances, hyperglycemia in children can be found in association with hyperthyroidism, lead intoxication, Cushing disease, brain tumors, pheochromocytoma, and therapy with corticosteroids.[1]

DIABETIC KETOACIDOSIS

Diabetic ketoacidosis (DKA) is a common complication among children with IDDM, accounting for 14 to 31 percent of all diabetes-related hospital admissions.[6,7] It is the single most common cause of death in diabetic patients under 24 years of age.[7] DKA is considered to be present when there is hyperglycemia (i.e., blood glucose level >250 mg/dL), ketonemia (i.e., ketones >1:2 dilution of serum), and metabolic acidosis (i.e., pH <7.2 and plasma bicarbonate ≤15 meq/L)[5] accompanied by glucosuria and ketonuria. The majority of patients are also moderately to severely dehydrated. Precipitating factors for the initial presentation or for DKA include stress such as trauma, infection, vomiting, and psychological disturbances.[5]

The basic cause of DKA is absolute or relative insulin deficiency (Fig. 124-1). There also are elevated levels of counterregulatory hormones (glucagon, cortisol, growth hormone, epinephrine, and norepinephrine), which antagonize insulin.[2] These hormonal abnormalities result in increased glucose production (promoting glycogenolysis, gluconeogenesis, lipolysis, and ketogenesis) and decreased utilization. With progressive insulin deficiency, glucosuria accompanies the hyperglycemia. The resultant osmotic diuresis produces polyuria, which can result in a profound loss of fluids and electrolytes, dehydration, and compensatory polydipsia. Hyperosmolality is commonly encountered as a result of progressive hyperglycemia, which contributes to the symptoms, especially cerebral obtundation, in DKA. Serum osmolality can be estimated with the following formula:

$$\text{Serum osmolality (mosm/kg)} = (2 \times \text{serum Na}^+ \text{ [meq/L]}) + \frac{\text{glucose (mg/dL)}}{18} + \frac{\text{BUN (mg/dL)}}{2.8}$$

The hormonal interplay of insulin deficiency and glucagon excess shunts free fatty acids into ketone body formation. The rate of formation of these bodies, principally β-hydroxybutyrate and acetoacetate, exceeds the capacity for peripheral utilization and for renal excretion. The combination of ketoacid formation and dehydration results in metabolic acidosis, and, for compensatory alkalosis, rapid deep breathing (Kussmaul respirations) may be manifested at advanced stages. Dehydration with decreased perfusion to the tissues leads to lactic acidosis, which contributes to more profound acidosis. Once patients are sufficiently ketotic and acidotic, they manifest the classic fruity breath odor of ketosis. The state of consciousness may vary from alertness to drowsiness or coma, depending on the severity of DKA. Other findings on physical examination include fever, vomiting, and exquisite abdominal pain with guarding and rigidity, which can mimic an acute abdomen. The clinical findings of acute abdomen usually resolve with the treatment of DKA, but if not, an underlying cause must be sought. DKA should be considered in children who are vomiting and appear dehydrated but continue to urinate excessively.

In known diabetic patients, DKA may be precipitated by acute infections or other stresses but is usually caused by omission of insulin. A thorough search for sources of infection is essential. It is important to note that the degree of hyperglycemia does not correlate with the degree of acidosis, and patients who are only minimally hyperglycemic may be severely acidotic. The early recognition and treatment of DKA should be well known to every emergency physician so that the morbidity and mortality rates associated with this complication of IDDM can be reduced.

TREATMENT OF DIABETIC KETOACIDOSIS

The basic components of DKA treatment are appropriately aggressive fluid and electrolyte replacement (with special attention to potassium) and initiation of insulin therapy, which is essential to arrest further metabolic decompensation (Fig. 124-2). Once the diagnosis is confirmed, determinations of the glucose level, venous pH, and electrolyte levels should be made and checked hourly, with further therapy adjusted accordingly. An electrocardiogram is useful for potential evidence of hyperkalemia. If sepsis is suspected as the precipitating factor, blood and urine cultures, lumbar puncture, and chest x-ray should be performed, and antibiotics should be started if indicated.

Fluid Resuscitation

Appropriate fluid replacement should be instituted promptly. Water and electrolyte losses occur secondary to polyuria caused by the osmotic diuresis produced by glycosuria, hyperventilation, vomiting, and diarrhea. Dry mucous membranes, poor skin turgor, and orthostatic hypotension in the older child are the most accurate clinical indications of dehydration. Virtually all patients with DKA are at least 5 to 10 percent dehydrated and require both maintenance and replacement fluid therapy. However, fluid resuscitation that is too aggressive can result in cerebral edema, the most lethal complication of DKA. For initial rehydration, 10 to 20 mL/kg/h of 0.9% NS solution should be given for the first 1 to 2 h of resuscitation to establish adequate vascular volume and improve tissue perfusion. If signs of shock are present, a 20 mL/kg bolus of 0.9% normal saline solution should be given and may need to be repeated if dehydration and shock are severe. However, for the majority of patients, the initial volume resuscitation of 10 to 20 mL/kg/h for the first 1 to 2 h is adequate to restore perfusion. Once this is accomplished, the remaining fluid deficit can be replaced over the next 24 to 48 h. If possible, the fluid deficit should be calculated by comparing the patient's weight on presentation with a recent, healthy weight. If such an estimate is not possible, it can be assumed that the fluid deficit is 10 percent of the body weight (100 mL/kg) in children in DKA unless the patient is in shock.

Maintenance Fluids

After the initial reexpansion, 0.45% NS is used. In children whose serum osmolality is high, 0.9% NS should be continued until it has

Assessment

Dehydration
- Current/previous weight
- Clinical assessment
- 5–10% minimum

Contributing Stressors
- Infection
- Trauma
- Gastroenteritis
- Drugs/overdose

Baseline Ladoratory
- Glucose (BS)
- pH
- Electrolytes
- Urinalysis
- Serum osmolarity
- Phosphate
- Calcium
- Serum ketones

Therapy of DKA

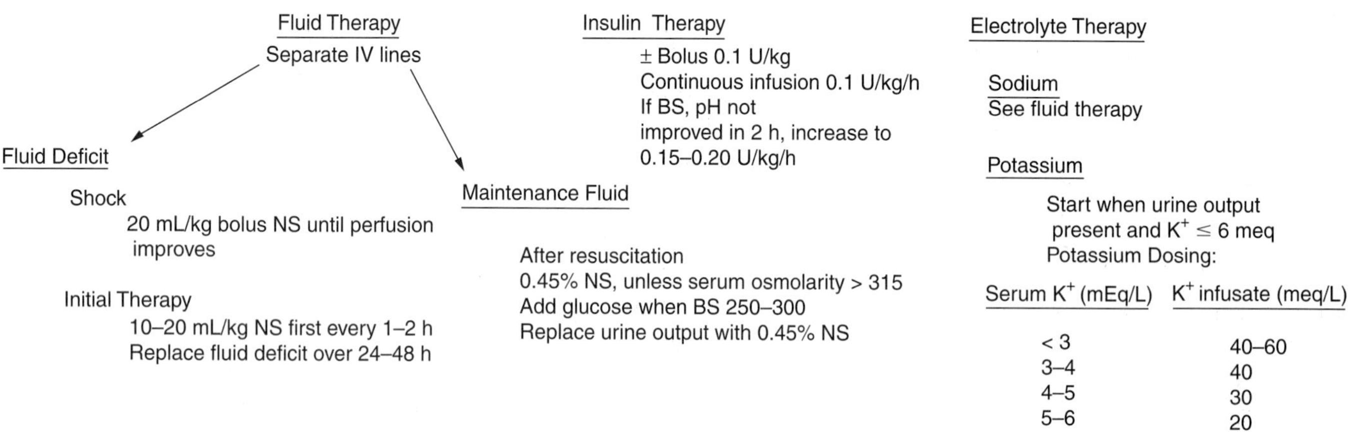

Fluid Therapy
Separate IV lines
Fluid Deficit
Shock
20 mL/kg bolus NS until perfusion improves
Initial Therapy
10–20 mL/kg NS first every 1–2 h
Replace fluid deficit over 24–48 h
Maintenance Fluid
After resuscitation
0.45% NS, unless serum osmolarity > 315
Add glucose when BS 250–300
Replace urine output with 0.45% NS
Insulin Therapy
± Bolus 0.1 U/kg
Continuous infusion 0.1 U/kg/h
If BS, pH not improved in 2 h, increase to 0.15–0.20 U/kg/h
Electrolyte Therapy
Sodium
See fluid therapy
Potassium
Start when urine output present and K+ ≤ 6 meq
Potassium Dosing:
Serum K+ (mEq/L)
K+ infusate (meq/L)
< 3
40–60
3–4
40
4–5
30
5–6
20

FIG. 124-2. Treatment of DKA.

decreased toward normal (<315 mosm/L).[2] After the initial resuscitation is completed, the calculated remaining deficit should be replaced over the next 36 to 48 h depending on the calculated or measured osmolality (>320 mosm/L or >340 mosm/L, respectively).[8] Once the serum glucose level is between 250 and 300 mg/dL,[2,5] intravenous fluids should be changed to 5% dextrose solution (D5) and 0.45% NS. Administration of glucose limits the decline of serum osmolality and reduces the risk of cerebral edema. Insulin should be continued even after dextrose infusion has been started because blood glucose levels are corrected more rapidly than ketoacidosis. As long as acidosis persists, insulin infusion should be maintained at the same rate. Blood glucose levels should be maintained at approximately[5] 250 to 300 mg/dL,[2,5] and urine output should be replaced hourly with 0.45% NS. Oral hydration may be started as soon as nausea and vomiting subside. Fluid resuscitation and correction of metabolic abnormalities should not be undertaken too rapidly in order that such complications as cerebral edema, hypoglycemia, and hypokalemia may be avoided.

Electrolyte Management

Monitoring and correction of electrolyte imbalances are paramount to the treatment of DKA. Despite the common findings of lowered serum sodium and potassium levels on initial presentation, the body stores of these two electrolytes are depleted even more than is obvious, secondary to the osmotic diuresis and renal excretion of anionic ketoacids. In addition, the hyperglycemia and hyperlipidemia of DKA cause spuriously low serum sodium measurements that do not adequately reflect the degree of sodium deficit. While maintenance sodium levels are 3 meq/kg/day, children with DKA have a sodium deficit estimated at 6 meq/kg. Fluid replacement is best accomplished through two intravenous lines: one replacing the fluid deficit as 0.9% NS and a second providing maintenance fluid therapy as 0.45% NS. Decline of the serum sodium level during resuscitation is a potential marker for the development of cerebral edema, and fluid therapy should be adjusted accordingly. Serum sodium levels should be monitored at least every 3 to 4 h during the initial resuscitation phase.

Virtually all patients with DKA also have potassium depletion, regardless of their serum potassium level on presentation. Administration of potassium should be started early, even when serum potassium concentration is normal. If the potassium level is high (>6 meq/L), replacement should be withheld until urine output is established and the serum potassium level begins to fall, in order to avoid iatrogenic hyperkalemia and cardiac dysrhythmias. Although potassium moves from intracellular to extracellular sites during acidosis, the reverse occurs during correction of acidosis. This shift of potassium back to the intracellular compartment may result in life-threatening hypokalemia. Therefore, potassium is added to the fluid resuscitation after boluses of NS once the patient's urine output is adequate. Often, twice-daily maintenance therapy of potassium (3 to 4 meq/kg/d) is needed to replenish potassium stores and achieve acceptable serum levels. An electrocardiogram provides a rapid assessment of serum potassium concentration. T waves are peaked in hyperkalemia and low and associated with U waves in hypokalemia. Because both hypokalemia and hyperkalemia are potential causes of death due to cardiac instability, the serum potassium level should be monitored every 1 to 2 h.[2]

Potassium chloride is the most common form used to replenish potassium deficits, and excess chloride may aggravate acidosis. The extent of acidosis can be reduced by substitution of potassium phosphate, which is also depleted in diabetic ketoacidosis.[5] Potassium replacement may be accomplished with one-half the dose as potassium chloride and phosphate. By contributing to the formation of 2,3-diphosphoglycerate, exogenous phosphate shifts the oxygen dissociation curve to the right, facilitating release of oxygen to tissues and aiding in correction of acidosis. Furthermore, resistance to insulin action is associated with hypophosphatemia.[9] Therefore, the use of phosphate is recommended by most endocrinologists, but its efficacy is debated by others, who recommend phosphate therapy only if the serum level is 2 meq/L or less. Because the excessive use of phosphate may result in hypocalcemia, serum calcium should be monitored periodically.

Insulin Therapy

Continuous low-dose short-acting (regular) insulin by intravenous infusion is the method of choice for treating DKA. Continuous intravenous insulin eliminates the problem of poor absorption from other routes. A priming dose of 0.1 U/kg of regular insulin is followed by a constant infusion of 0.1 U/kg/h. Some authorities debate the necessity or efficacy of the initial intravenous bolus and begin with the infusion. If acidosis has not improved in 2 h, the inravenous insulin rate should be increased to 0.15 to 0.2 U/kg/h.[2] Concern that the insulin may adhere to the glass and tubing has proven to be unfounded, and effective delivery of insulin can be provided without the addition of albumin or gelatin to the infusate.[5] When acidosis is corrected, the continuous infusion may be discontinued.

Ketonemia and ketonuria may persist despite clinical improvement. Nitroprusside, which is routinely used to measure ketones, reacts with acetoacetate and weakly with acetone, but not with β-hydroxybutyrate. With the correction of acidosis, β-hydroxybutyrate dissociates to acetoacetate, which is identified by the nitroprusside reaction. Therefore, the persistence of ketonuria may not reliably reflect the clinical improvement.

Bicarbonate therapy remains highly controversial. With provision of fluids, electrolytes, glucose, and insulin, metabolic acidosis is usually corrected through the interruption of ketogenesis and the generation of bicarbonate by the distal tubule.[5] Concerns that the therapeutic administration of bicarbonate may result in paradoxical central nervous system acidosis and possible cerebral depression, shift of the oxygen dissociation curve to the left (diminishing the release of oxygen to tissues), worsening hypokalemia, and alkalosis underlie the recommendation to avoid bicarbonate therapy unless severe acidosis (pH $<$ 6.9) threatens to cause cardiac dysrhythmias or decreases cardiac contractility.[9] In general, the majority of patients with DKA, even those with severe acidosis, can be adequately resuscitated without bicarbonate therapy, which carries substantial side effects.

Cerebral Edema

Cerebral edema is unpredictable. It usually becomes apparent several hours after the child appears to be improving. A previously alert patient may become lethargic; complain of headache; have abnormal neurologic findings, including papilledema; progress to coma; and have respiratory arrest, with herniation of the brainstem. Recovery may occur with prompt recognition and treatment with intravenous mannitol. Although clinically apparent cerebral edema is often fatal, subclinical cerebral edema is present in many patients during therapy for ketoacidosis.[10] Although the precise pathophysiology of cerebral edema in DKA is unknown, factors associated with increased incidence include excessive fluid administration, precipitous correction of the blood glucose level, failure of the serum sodium level to rise with treatment, and bicarbonate therapy.

Treatment of clinical cerebral edema includes control of intracranial pressure with mannitol therapy, intracranial pressure monitoring, ventriculostomy fluid drainage, fluid restriction, and other therapies to control intracranial pressure, including barbiturate therapy when indicated.

DISPOSITION

The vast majority of patients who present with DKA are sufficiently ill to require admission to the hospital for correction of fluid and electrolyte imbalances over a 24- to 72-h period. A very small and select group of patients can be considered for outpatient management of DKA, provided there is appropriate follow-up and supervision by the patient's parents and the treating physician. Patients with stable vital signs who can easily tolerate oral fluids and have minimal dehydration and electrolyte imbalances can be considered for discharge. Such patients still require 3 to 6 h of emergency department treatment to ensure clear documentation that clinical findings and laboratory values are improving. Most important, discharge instructions and follow-up should be carefully and cautiously coordinated between the caregivers and the patient's primary care physician.

However, the majority of patients with a past history of DKA need to be admitted to the hospital for ongoing therapy, treatment of underlying diseases that may have precipitated the DKA, and normalization of fluid and electrolyte levels. Patients with altered mental status, severe acidosis, or profound fluid and electrolyte deficits should be considered for management in the pediatric intensive care unit. Many hospitals have developed clinical treatment guidelines for patients with DKA, including criteria for admission to the intensive care unit.

REFERENCES

1. Ginsberg-Fellner F: Insulin-dependent diabetes mellitus. *Pediatr Rev* 11:239, 1990.
2. Plotnick L: Insulin-dependent diabetes mellitus. *Pediatr Rev* 15:137, 1994.
3. Atkinson MA: The pathogenesis of insulin-dependent diabetes mellitus. *N Engl J Med* 331:1428, 1994.
4. Sperling MA: Aspects of the etiology, prediction, and prevention of insulin-dependent diabetes mellitus in childhood. *Pediatr Clin North Am* 44:269, 1997.
5. Sperling MA: Diabetes mellitus, in Sperling MA: *Pediatric Endocrinology*. Philadelphia, Saunders, 1996, p 229–242.
6. Kreisberg RA: Diabetic ketoacidosis: An update. *Crit Care Clin* 5:817, 1987.
7. Connell FA: Diabetes mortality in persons under 45 years of age. *Am J Public Health* 73:1174, 1983.
8. Rosenbloom AL: Diabetic ketoacidosis in childhood. *Pediatr Ann* 23:284, 1994.
9. Sperling MA: Diabetic ketoacidosis. *Pediatr Clin North Am* 31:591, 1984.
10. Krane EJ: Subclinical brain swelling in children during treatment of diabetic ketoacidosis. *N Engl J Med* 312:1147, 1985.

HYPOGLYCEMIA

Randolph Cordle

Emergency physicians must be able to recognize the sometimes subtle and other times stunning effects that hypoglycemia may cause, as prompt diagnosis and treatment may spare an otherwise normal child severe brain damage or even death.[1] This is especially true in the first year of life when the diagnosis is difficult to make based on clinical findings alone (Table 125-1).

DEMOGRAPHICS

The definition of hypoglycemia is somewhat controversial. In the past, many believed neonates would tolerate lower levels of glucose than older children. Most agree that, in all pediatric age groups, a blood glucose $<$40 mg/dL should be considered abnormal. Normally the whole blood concentration of glucose is 10 to 15% less than that found in the serum or plasma. This is due to a dilutional effect caused by the red blood cells in whole blood that contain little glucose. Therefore, acceptable serum or plasma glucose levels would be greater than

TABLE 125-1 Cause of Hypoglycemia in Children

Perinatal	
Transient	
Small for gestational age	Congenital heart disease*
Infant of diabetic mother	Hypothermia*†
Erythroblastosis fetalis	Umbilical artery catheter displaced
Polycythemia	Exchange transfusion*†
Infection*†	Cessation of high levels of IV glucose*†
Adrenal hemorrhage or glucocorticoid suppression*†	Hypoglycemia-inducing drug use by the mother
Pre- or postmature infant	Maternal toxemia of pregnancy
Fetal alcohol syndrome	Idiopathic*
Nesidioblastosis	
Fetal distress from any cause	
Infancy	
Those marked * above and	
Substrate-related	Amino acid metabolic abnormality
Starvation	Propionic acidemia
Idiopathic ketotic hypoglycemia	Methylmalonic aciduria
Endocrine	Tyrosinemia
Hypopituitarism†	Others
Glucagon deficiency	Hyperinsulinism
Glucocorticoid deficiency†	Islet cell adenoma†
Hypothyroidism	Functional β-cell secretory defect†
Adrenocorticotropin deficiency†	Factitious insulin use
Growth-hormone deficiency†	Beckwith-Wiedemann syndrome†
Inborn errors of metabolism	Nesidioblastosis†
Types I, III, and VI glycogen storage disease	Islet cell hyperplasia†
Hereditary fructose intolerance†	Factitious sulfonylureas use†
Acyl-CoA dehydrogenase deficiency†	
Carnitine deficiency†	
UMG-CoA lyase deficiency	
Childhood	
Those marked † above and	
Idiopathic ketotic hypoglycemia	Toxin-induced (alcohol, akee fruit)
Drug-induced, especially salicylates	Fulminant hepatic disease
Large nonpancreatic tumors; neuroblastoma	Factitious disorders
	Idiopathic

*Perinatal and infant hypoglucemia.
†Perinatal, infant, and childhood hypoglycemia.

45 mg/dL. Values slightly above this may still be concerning in symptomatic patients.

Pediatric hypoglycemia may be considered a relatively rare disorder if one excludes diabetics and the neonatal population. Hypoglycemia was reported in only 6.54/100,000 children presenting to a pediatric emergency department (ED).[2] Of these, 58 percent had a diagnosis of idiopathic ketotic hypoglycemia. Outside of the neonatal period, idiopathic ketotic hypoglycemia was by far the most common cause of hypoglycemia presenting to the ED. Surprisingly, only 10 percent of the presenting hypoglycemic patients were found to be diabetics having an insulin reaction, possibly because prehospital treatment alone is sufficient for most cases. Outside of the neonatal period, if all children are considered, the highest prevalence of hypoglycemic events is almost certainly in the insulin dependent diabetic population.

PATHOPHYSIOLOGY

Normally a highly sophisticated regulatory system maintains glucose concentrations within a very narrow range. This is truly a steady state system and not an equilibrium. The rate of production does not equal the rate of utilization at any given moment. Both production and utilization change on a minute-to-minute basis. Relative to body weight, glucose production and utilization are much higher in children than in adults. This is due to the higher basal metabolic rate of children, utilization of glucose for growth and development, and greater activity. The quantity of glucose produced and utilized per kilogram of body weight is known as *glucose flux*. This is discussed further below.

All tissues can use glucose for energy metabolism. Tissues such as the heart, other muscles, and the kidneys can use other substrates quite efficiently; however, the brain, red blood cells, lymphocytes, and platelets are nearly totally dependent upon glucose for their metabolism. Pagliara demonstrated that, in the fasted adult model, up to 80 percent of the glucose produced by glycogenolysis and gluconeogenesis is used for brain metabolism.[3] Nearly all the rest is used by the formed elements of blood. An adequate quantity of glucose for the brain's metabolism depends on its degree of utilization and the plasma glucose level.

Relatively speaking, the brain is a much larger organ in children than in adults. Therefore more than 80 percent of the glucose utilization in the fasted child is by this one organ. In fact, studies have demonstrated that glucose utilization correlates better with brain weight than with body weight. In the postabsorptive state, the glucose requirement of small children is up to $2\frac{1}{2}$ times that of the adult, or about 5 to 7 mg/kg per minute. After fasting, this drops to 4 mg/kg per minute, a value still much higher than that in the fasted adult. The majority of brain development has occurred by the end of the second year of life. During the fasting state, nearly all the endogenously produced glucose in children below 2 years of age is required and utilized by the brain. When inadequate quantities of glucose are available, development and growth will stop, so that all sources of endogenous energy can be used strictly for the maintenance of brain metabolism. Therefore normal growth and brain development will not occur if inadequate quantities of glucose are supplied.

During periods of inadequate glucose supply to the brain, alternative sources of energy such as ketones and Krebs cycle intermediates will be utilized. Adult studies have demonstrated that, in the short term, up to two-thirds of the brain's energy requirements can be supplied using these substances. Ketones should not, however, be relied upon to save the brain from injury or death even in the short term. Not surprisingly, many causes of childhood hypoglycemia are associated with the lack of ketone production. Even in normal patients with hypoglycemia, ketone production is a slow process occurring over a period of hours. Ketones are not immediately available when acute changes in blood glucose occur. Neonates and children with free fatty acid utilization abnormalities, carnitine deficiency, and ketone-production-limiting hyperinsulinemias are at particular risk for devastating neuroglycopenia because they lack the ability to effectively produce or utilize ketones as an alternative energy source.

Carrier mediated transport is responsible not only for shuttling glucose through the blood-brain barrier but also moving it from the cerebrospinal fluid (CSF) into the extracellular space, where it can be utilized by the individual cells of the brain. A limiting factor in the movement of glucose from the plasma to the brain is the turnover rate of this carrier system. When the plasma glucose concentration and brain glucose utilization are normal, this carrier-mediated system maintains a three-fold surplus of glucose in the brain. This buffer allows for normal fluctuations of plasma glucose over time. The CSF glucose concentration is maintained at about 65% of that found in the blood while that of the brain's extracellular fluid is maintained at about one-third the CSF glucose concentration. In general, CSF and brain extracellular glucose concentrations remain near constant. When the plasma glucose level drops to about 30 mg/dL, the supply to the brain cells becomes dangerously low. If not rapidly corrected, the extracellular glucose concentration may approach zero and neuronal metabolism will fail. Fortunately, acute changes in the plasma glucose concentration do not immediately affect that of the CSF and brain. Changes here lag behind those in the plasma by a few hours. As the plasma glucose concentration decreases, systemic changes occur, hopefully leading to a resupply of exogenous or endogenously produced glucose. If not, neuroglycopenia will arise. Conversely, when neuroglycopenic patients are given exogenous glucose, it often takes a few hours for their mental status to return to normal even if there are no permanent sequelae. In patients presenting with stroke-like symptoms, it is not uncommon for paresis to last a few hours. Peak CSF glucose levels do not occur until 2 h after intravenous dextrose is given. Equilibrium of glucose between the CSF, brain extracellular space and plasma is typically not achieved for about 4 h. Assuming ongoing carbohydrate provision, plasma equilibrium occurs more quickly.

Although these alternative fuel sources can temporarily maintain cerebral metabolism, rapid return of glucose is necessary for multiple additional reasons. Glucose is utilized exclusively for brain growth and development. It is also required for the development of membrane lipids and structural proteins. Infant brain myelination is dependent on adequate substrate supply, including glucose. Cerebral hypoperfusion has also been linked to episodes of hypoglycemia. Hypoglycemia associated with anoxia or poor cerebral perfusion is more likely to cause permanent brain damage than if associated with normal cerebral perfusion and oxygenation. Prolonged or repetitive episodes of hypoglycemia may cause permanent neurologic sequelae, including mental retardation and death. At the time of presentation, it is not possible to determine clinically which patient's signs and symptoms will be permanent. Some patients develop cerebral edema secondary to prolonged neuroglycopenic seizures. More commonly, cerebral damage from hypoglycemia alone is thought to be due to the release of excitotoxins, which lead to neuronal necrosis. True infarction is relatively rarely seen. This neuronal necrosis selectively affects some parts of the brain while leaving others, such as the brainstem and cerebellum, relatively intact.

With the ingestion of a meal, macromolecules are enzymatically broken down into their component parts. Once absorbed, the elevated glucose concentration causes the release of insulin. Simultaneously, glucagon secretion is suppressed. Depending upon the amount and type of food ingested as well as the degree of glucose utilization, the patient may have ample glucose immediately available for the next few hours. In addition to its effect on glucagon, insulin in concert with an elevated glucose level suppresses glucocorticoid release. The elevated insulin levels also lead to the suppression of ketogenesis, gluconeogenesis, lipolysis, and glycogenolysis. Simultaneously, they induce glycogen production in the liver and muscle from glucose, protein production from amino acids, and fat production from lipids. Fats are also produced from endogenous lipids formed from surplus amino acids and glucose in the liver. Fat is the body's major energy storage form.

In the early fasting state, the remaining free glucose is rapidly utilized for energy. After this, insulin levels drop as glucagon and epinephrine levels increase, inducing glycogenolysis. Assuming that normal glycogen stores are present, children may be able to maintain a normal plasma glucose concentration for 4 to 6 h, only half the time seen in adults. This is primarily due to two factors. Children, as discussed above, have a much higher relative glucose flux than do adults. They also have relatively smaller glycogen stores.

In the late fasting state, children become dependent on gluconeogenesis and, to a lesser extent, alternative fuels. Gluconeogenesis uses amino acids and glycerol as substrates. These substrates are derived primarily from muscle protein and fat. Elevated glucagon, cortisol, and growth hormone in the milieu of a low insulin level stimulate gluconeogenesis. Low levels of insulin and elevated levels of growth hormone, epinephrine, and glucagon stimulate lipolysis to provide glycerol for gluconeogenesis and free fatty acids for ketogenesis. Mitochondrial beta-oxidation of free fatty acids leads to the production of acetyl-CoA and NADH + H^+, substrate inducers of gluconeogenesis. During the late fasted state, free fatty acids are converted to acetyl-CoA faster than the liver can use it to produce ketones. Accumulating acetyl-CoA allosterically stimulates one of the rate-limiting enzymes of gluconeogenesis—namely, pyruvate carboxylase. The NADH + H^+ is then used to reduce newly formed oxaloacetate to malate, which is carried to the cytoplasm, where the rest of gluconeogenesis occurs. Without this reducing substance, oxaloacetate would just build up in the mitochondria and gluconeogenesis would not occur. An additional important precursor for gluconeogenesis is lactate. It is primarily generated from pyruvate. Although almost exclusively occurring in the liver during prolonged fasts, a minor degree of gluconeogenesis may occur in the kidneys as well.

As discussed above, ketogenesis may play a vital role in providing glucose to the brain during the fasted state. Although its direct role is relatively minor, its indirect one may be great. By providing for the energy needs of the heart, kidneys, muscles, and other tissues, it allows a higher percent of endogenously produced glucose to be utilized by the brain. Like gluconeogenesis, the production of ketones is also dependent upon the release of triglycerides from adipose tissue. Once released into the milieu of low insulin and glucose, these triglycerides are degraded to form glycerol and free fatty acids. The glycerol enters the liver and is used for gluconeogenesis and/or glycolysis. The free fatty acids diffuse into hepatocytes, where they are converted to fatty acyl-CoA by thiokinase (fatty acyl-CoA synthetase). Fatty acyl-CoA is then carried through the inner mitochondrial membrane by carnitine. Without this carrier, these polar molecules could not pass through the membrane.

Once in the mitochondria, beta-oxidation occurs. In addition to acetyl-CoA's role in gluconeogenesis, it is also converted in the liver to acetoacetate and beta hydroxybutyrate, the primary ketones utilized for fuel. Therefore, defects in medium or, less commonly, long and short chain acyl-CoA dehydrogenase enzymes may lead to nonketotic hypoglycemia. Nonfunctional lipases, nonfunctional carnitine transferase, and low levels of carnitine may lead to a similar clinical syndrome. Abnormal metabolites of fatty acids may accumulate in the liver. In the past, treatment for these disorders was preventing the occurrence of the late fasting state. This was accomplished with frequent feedings. More recently, carnitine deficiency may be treated with the addition of supranormal levels of carnitine to the diet. Although rare in this country, Jamaican vomiting illness may also present with a nonketotic hypoglycemia. The toxin hypoglycin, found in the unripe akee fruit, prevents proper beta-oxidation of fatty acids. Therefore, acetyl-CoA is not produced, gluconeogenesis is not induced, and ketones are not formed normally.

The complexity of this homeostatic system should be apparent from the above discussion. As the glucose approaches 70 mg/dL, glucagon and epinephrine levels begin to rise. By the time the glucose level reaches 55 mg/dL, an intense counterregulatory chemical response is apparent. In children with insulin-dependent diabetes or chronic hyperinsulinemia, the epinephrine response may be diminished. In these children, activation of this response may not occur until the glucose concentration is about 35 mg/dL. Under conditions of even normal glucose utilization, there may not be time for endogenous mechanisms to prevent severe hypoglycemia. Patients on β blockers are also at particularly high risk. These agents often blunt the counterregulatory catecholamine response leading not only to worsening hypoglycemia but also to a paucity of classic signs often used to make the diagnosis. These patients may present with only neuroglycopenic symptoms and signs, such as seizure, "stroke," or coma. Glucagon's release is normally stimulated by hypoglycemia as well as elevated levels of growth hormone, epinephrine, and cortisol. However, calcium-channel blockers, β agonists, and anticholinergic drugs suppress its release. Therefore, these drugs may predispose individuals to hypoglycemia (Table 125-2). In the fed state, insulin levels may be in the range of 50 to 100

TABLE 125-2 Drugs Related to Hypoglycemia

Ethanol	Sulfonylureas	Salicylates
Insulin	Phenformin/ metformin	Sulfisoxazole
β-blockers	Oxytetracycline	Ethylenediaminetetraacetic acid
Bishydroxycoumarin/ warfarin	Phenylbutazone	Manganese
Propoxyphene	Chlorpromazine	Diphenhydramine
Indomethacin	Para-aminobenzoic acid	Haloperidol

μU/mL. During periods of hypoglycemia, insulin levels are normally suppressed to 5 to 10 μU/mL maximum.

CLINICAL FEATURES

Classically, hypoglycemic patients present with either neuroglycopenic or excessive adrenergic signs and symptoms (Table 125-3). Postprandial hypoglycemia is more likely to present with signs of adrenergic excess whereas fasting hypoglycemia commonly presents with neuroglycopenic symptoms. In general, the more rapid the decrease in glucose concentration, the more adrenergic-type symptoms will be noted. Variability and crossover in symptoms is the rule, however, and not the exception. Neonates and young children may present with poor feeding, jitteriness, emesis, ravenous hunger, lethargy, altered personality, repetitive colic-like symptoms, hypotonia, or hypothermia. In other cases they unfortunately present after an apparent life-threatening event, seizure, or cardiac arrest. As children grow older they begin to present more like adults, with signs of adrenergic excess and then neuroglycopenia. If treatment is not forthcoming, the adrenergic symptoms may abate, leaving only the neuroglycopenic ones. In some cases, as with type I glycogen storage disease, patients may have no obvious symptoms despite an incredibly low blood glucose concentration. Children with unexplained catastrophic presentations such as coma, severe hypothermia, and arrest should have bedside glucose testing performed immediately and, if clinically indicated, a specimen should be sent for formal laboratory evaluation as well. Empirically treating patients after cardiac arrest with glucose may worsen neurologic outcomes, as hyperglycemia is detrimental in cases of cerebral edema and anoxia. Therefore, whenever possible, bedside testing and historical data surrounding the event should guide therapy in this population. Hypoglycemia should be suspected in all moderately to severely injured or ill children. The underlying disease process will often mask the symptoms of hypoglycemia. Children with increased physiologic stress require periodic reevaluation for hypoglycemia, as they are often unable to maintain sufficient glucose influx to meet their increased needs. This is especially true in patients whose illness, injury, or treatment prevents them from being able to express their needs.

TABLE 125-3 Clinical Signs of Hypoglycemia

Adrenergic Excess	Neuroglycopenia
Anxiety	Confusion
Tachycardia	Ataxia
Perspiration	Headache
Nausea	Depressed consciousness
Tremors	Blurred vision
Pallor	Lightheadedness
Chest pain	Focal neurologic deficits
Weakness	Seizures
Abdominal pain	Strabismus
Hunger	Staring
Irritability	Paresthesias

The most common cause of hypoglycemia in non-insulin-dependent children over the age of 1 year is idiopathic ketotic hypoglycemia. It is more a physiologic aberration than a true pathologic syndrome.[2,4] It usually presents in children less than 18 months of age after a period of fasting. Often this is seen on holidays and weekends, when parents sleep late, inadvertently extending the child's usual nighttime fasting period. It is also more common during illnesses preventing normal food intake. These children return to normal after a glucose load and have no suspicious findings in either their history or physical exams.[2,5] Classically, this problem was thought to arise because these children were small for age, but that idea has been called into question by more recent findings.[2,4] Currently, alanine, by far the most important amino acid in gluconeogenesis, is thought to play a major role in this disorder.[3,6] Haymond et al.[5] demonstrated lower serum alanine concentrations in these patients as compared with age-matched control groups during fasting. Giving gluconeogenic precursors to these patients during periods of fasting prevents hypoglycemia, lending further support to the theory outlined above. Children with idiopathic ketotic hypoglycemia present with normal ketonemia and ketonuria. If not tested for early, the ketones may be missed because they dissipate rapidly with treatment of the hypoglycemia. If tested, insulin will be normally suppressed and cortisol as well as growth hormone will be normally elevated during the hypoglycemic period. Treatment is primarily to avoid prolonged fasting. Provision of frequent high-carbohydrate and high-protein meals also helps to prevent recurrence. Some have used feedings of raw cornstarch at bedtime, as described under "Treatment" at the end of this chapter. Monitoring of urine ketones during periods of decreased oral intake, such as illness, is recommended.[4] Should ketones be detected, the patient should be given additional carbohydrate and protein containing foods and/or be brought to medical attention at once.

DIFFERENTIAL DIAGNOSIS

The differential diagnosis of hypoglycemia differs in different age groups. Some disorders are only transiently seen in neonates, while others may start in the neonatal period but extend throughout childhood. Still others are not usually seen until after the neonatal period. For example, some inborn errors of metabolism always present in early infancy while others may not be clinically apparent until the child is a few years old. Table 125-1 lists some causes of hypoglycemia in childhood. A full discussion of each of these is beyond the scope of this chapter. Diagnostic suspicion of many of these should prompt a discussion with and referral to an expert in metabolic diseases.

Many drugs (Table 125-2) may predispose children to hypoglycemia. Some have more supporting evidence and occur more frequently than others. Besides insulin and possibly sulfonylurea type medications, ethanol is by far the most common cause of drug-induced hypoglycemia in children. Ethanol inhibits gluconeogenesis. Hypoglycemia after the ingestion of alcohol may occur in adults but is far more likely in children due to their higher relative glucose utilization and much lower relative quantities of glycogen. As mentioned above, children become more quickly dependent on gluconeogenesis than do adults. This effect on liver metabolism is often seen at alcohol levels too low to cause clinical intoxication. Therefore, any child with a history of alcohol ingestion should be closely monitored for hypoglycemia and given glucose either orally or parenterally. In nonintoxicated patients, this may be accomplished by feeding. Intoxicated-appearing patients should always be evaluated for hypoglycemia at presentation and every few hours thereafter if unable to eat. In young children who will not be able to eat for more than 4 h, maintenance fluids containing dextrose should be given.

Testing for blood glucose has evolved over the recent past. Rapid bedside test strips and colorimetric readers should be available in all EDs. These are most accurate when the glucose concentration is in the normal range. Their specificity decreases at both ends of the concentration spectrum, so they should only be used as a screening tool. All patients with symptoms of hypoglycemia should have a specimen sent to the laboratory for chemical analysis. Bedside test strips occasionally give falsely elevated results. Residual isopropyl alcohol on the skin may lead to false positive low glucose values. The definitive diagnosis and workup should be based on the chemical analysis and not just the screening reagent-strip test. In symptomatic patients, treatment should begin based on the bedside test result. Treatment can be altered, if necessary, upon return of the chemical analysis.

EVALUATION

This is quite complex in some cases and controversial in others. In all cases, a detailed history should be obtained and a meticulous physical exam performed. Inquiry regarding prior episodes of hypoglycemia should occur. Detailed data regarding family, birth, development, and past medical history are needed. History of childhood death from unknown causes in a first- or second-degree relative should be sought. Potential access to insulin, sulfonylureas, β blockers, salicylates, and other toxins should be determined. Physical exam should include a head-to-toe survey for signs of other serious illness as well as findings more specifically related to hypoglycemia. Hypopituitarism may be associated with midline defects such as abnormal incisors, palatal defects, cleft-lip defects, midface abnormalities, or abnormal palpebral fissures. Hyperpigmentation, undescended testes, severe dehydration, and micropenis may be associated with abnormalities arising from the adrenal or pituitary glands. Children with short stature or less than expected recent growth should be evaluated for growth hormone abnormalities.[2,4] Height, weight, and head circumference should be plotted on a standardized growth chart. Tanner stage should be determined. The fundi should be evaluated for signs of optic nerve hypoplasia associated with hypopituitarism. Each patient should have a thorough examination of the abdomen specifically in an attempt to identify large masses such as those from neuroblastoma and, more importantly, hepatomegaly associated with most hypoglycemia causing glycogen storage, fatty acid oxidation, and other metabolic abnormalities.

Emergency physicians should make the diagnosis of hypoglycemia and any other clinically important associated disease processes. They should then institute appropriate therapy. Concurrently, they must differentiate between ketotic and nonketotic hypoglycemia and, based on this information, make decisions regarding the potential need for further studies. In questionable cases, it is practical to collect an extra set of blood tubes and an additional urine specimen for later use if deemed necessary. Many potentially required additional study results are valuable only if they are based on samples obtained when the child is hypoglycemic. This being said, children should not be allowed to remain hypoglycemic for any significant period of time before treatment. Overzealous or time-consuming attempts at laboratory collection should be avoided.

Prehospital protocols for hypoglycemic children should include the collection of appropriate blood specimens prior to treatment whenever possible. Prehospital laboratory specimens should not be discarded except at the discretion of the consultant or admitting physician.

The majority of children who present to the ED, however, probably do not need extensive laboratory evaluation. Infants and especially neonates should be evaluated thoroughly on first presentation unless the cause of hypoglycemia is clear. Developmentally normal children over 1 year of age who have normal head circumference and growth, who make a complete recovery after receiving glucose, have normal electrolytes, and present with findings consistent with idiopathic ketotic hypoglycemia do not usually need a detailed investigation. Patients with hepatomegaly, other signs of illness, significant acidemia, hyperpigmentation, or other clinically significant physical findings require a complete evaluation at presentation. In patients where a full workup is deferred, appropriate tubes of blood and a urine specimen may be collected and held by the lab. Close follow-up should be arranged and the patient's primary care physician made aware of the child's visit and findings. Should hypoglycemia recur or the child's clinical situation change, the held specimens may be extremely valuable. See Fig. 125-1 for a general approach to the laboratory evaluation of these patients. Variance from this is not only acceptable but expected based on the specifics of the individual clinical situation.

SPECIAL ISSUES AFFECTING DIAGNOSIS

1. Mentally challenged children can be especially difficult to evaluate. Often they have dysautonomia as well as feeding difficulties. A low threshold for blood glucose evaluation is appropriate in these patients, especially if the caretakers note a change in baseline behavior or mental status.
2. Most children who present with self-harming thoughts, suicidal threats, or true suicide attempts should have their glucose checked as part of their medical clearance. This is especially true of diabetic children and those with access to a relative's oral hypoglycemic agents. Inpatient monitoring of glucose may be necessary if overdose of an oral hypoglycemic agent is suspected. Most cases, however, will demonstrate hypoglycemia within 6 to 8 h. Management of such overdoses is often complex and is beyond the scope of this chapter.
3. In patients thought to have a factitiously depressed glucose associated with an elevated insulin level, the C-peptide level should be determined.[7,8] Typically the insulin level in these cases will be very high. If exogenous insulin is the cause, the C-peptide level will be inappropriately suppressed.[7] Normally C-peptide is produced in equimolar quantities during the processing of proinsulin to insulin; therefore, its levels should follow those of insulin itself. In cases of insulinoma, for example, both the insulin and C-peptide levels will be high.
4. Patients found to have hypoglycemia and non-glucose-reducing substances in their urine should have galactosemia ruled out. The dipstick urine test will be negative for glucose, but the laboratory evaluation for reducing substances will be positive in this case. This disease usually presents during infancy with failure to thrive, vomiting, hepatomegaly, and jaundice.

TREATMENT

Whenever possible, if the clinical condition allows, children should be treated with oral glucose loading. Clearly this should not occur in children unable to protect their airways. Common methods include orange juice with 2 tsp of sugar added per glass, maple syrup, honey (in older children), and, in mild cases, nondiet soda. Sucrose and fructose should not be given to any child suspected of having hereditary fructose intolerance. Lactose should not be given to children suspected of having galactosemia. Once the glucose concentration is back to the normal range, these children should be given a meal containing complex carbohydrates, proteins, and fats. This is presuming that inborn errors of metabolism have been ruled out.

When oral treatment is not an option, the intravenous route should be used (Table 125-4). Boluses of 0.25 to 0.5 g/kg are most commonly used. This is equivalent to 2.5 to 5 mL/kg 10% D/W, 1 to 2 mL/kg 25% D/W, or 0.5 to 1 mL/kg 50% D/W. If no response is seen within 5 min, this should be repeated and a bedside glucose checked. If the glucose remains <50 mg/dL and three boluses have been given, the clinician should consider using one of the alternative agents listed below. The proper choice should be based upon the clinical and historical findings.

Boluses in neonates should be given with 10% D/W. Infants should receive 10% D/W whenever possible, although 25% D/W is acceptable as well. In older children, 25% D/W may be used. 25% D/W and especially 50% D/W are very hyperosmolar and may cause phlebitis or tissue necrosis, if they extravasate. Even without extravasation, patients commonly complain of pain at the injection site for 1 to 2 weeks. The risk of extravasation is increased when smaller veins, such as those found in infants, are used. In addition to this, hyperosmolar

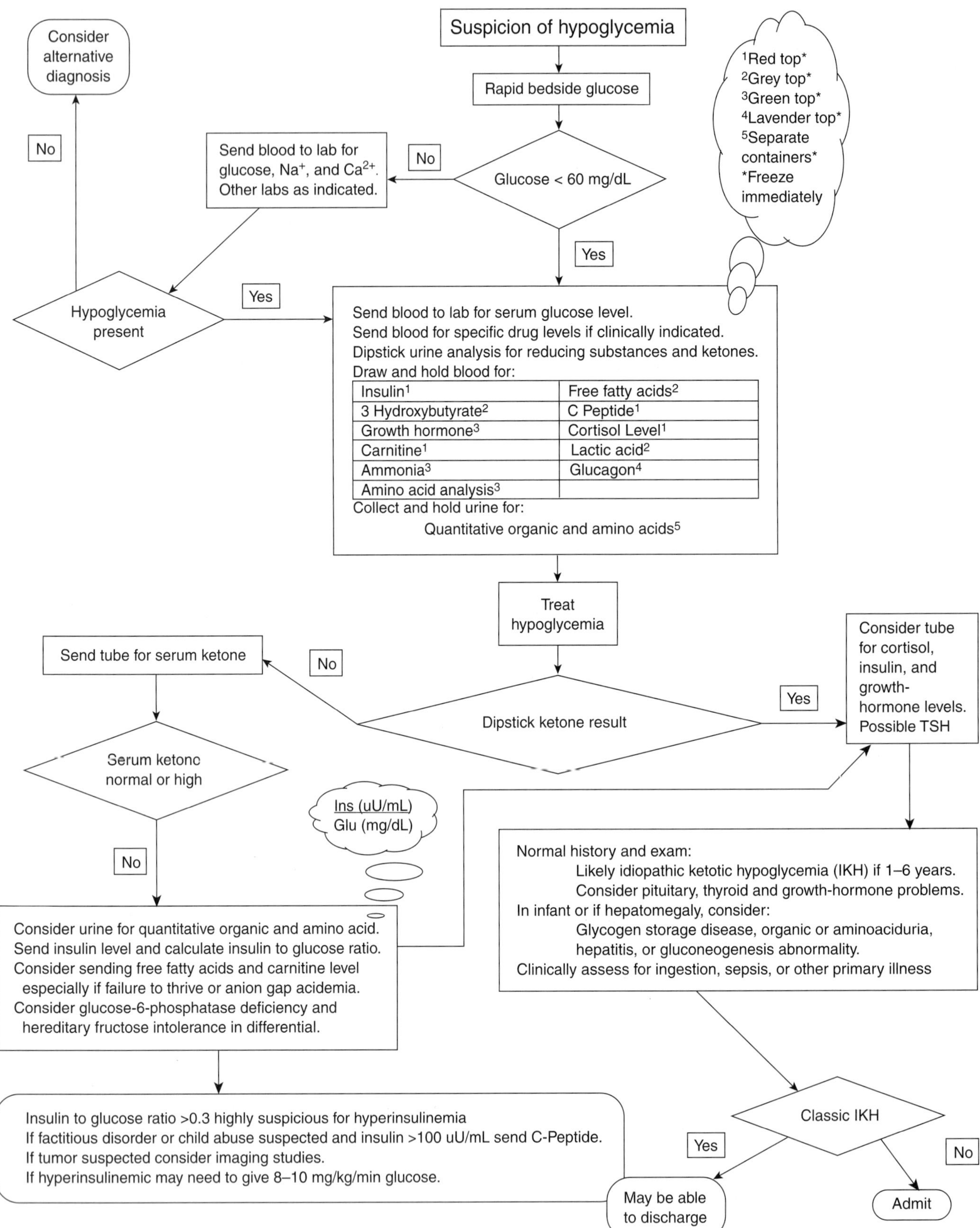

FIG. 125-1. General approach to the lab evaluation of hypoglycemia.

TABLE 125-4 Treatment of Hypoglycemia

Oral (preferred) Consider NG tube if poor IV access in child unable to swallow	
Orange juice with 2 tsp sugar/8 ounces	
2–4 honey packets (not infants)	
Parenteral	
IV Bolus	Maintenance
Infants	
5cc/kg 10% Dextrose* in 0.9% NaCl	4cc/kg/hr 10% Dextrose in 0.9% NaCl
Child	
2cc/kg 25% Dextrose in 0.9% NaCl	3cc/kg/hr 10% Dextrose in 0.9% NaCl
Glucagon (if neither route above available) (Dilute in NS or Sterile Water)† (Max dose 1 mg)	
Infant 50 ug/kg IV, IM, or SQ	
Child 30 ug/kg IV, IM, or SQ	

*10% Dextrose = 100 mg Dextrose/ml NaCl; 25% Dextrose = 250 mg Dextrose/ml NaCl.
†See text.

loading in premature neonates is associated with an increased risk of intracranial germinal matrix hemorrhage and subsequent periventricular leukomalacia. The use of 25% D/W and 50% D/W may also lead to an increased incidence of rebound hypoglycemia due to endogenous insulin release. When time allows, diluting 50% D/W or 25% D/W to 10% D/W with normal saline or half normal saline will decrease the risk of pain, phlebitis, and necrosis at the injection site by decreasing the osmolarity. This practice also prevents the administration of large volumes of free water when multiple boluses are required, as would occur if sterile water were used as the diluent. This volume would be equivalent to a fluid bolus of 2.5 to 15 mL/kg. Since many of these patients are also dehydrated, this amount of electrolyte-containing solution is certainly not excessive and probably somewhat therapeutic.

Once the patient's glucose is brought into the normal range, maintenance fluids should be started. The amount of glucose required for maintenance of euglycemia varies with age, underlying glucose utilization and the patient's insulin level. Neonates commonly require 6 to 8mg/kg per minute or 4 mL/kg/ per hour of a 10% dextrose containing electrolyte solution. In general, children will require 4 to 6 mg/kg per minute or about 3 mL/kg per hour of a 10% dextrose containing electrolyte solution. Plain 10% dextrose should never be used for multiple boluses or maintenance fluids. This practice causes water intoxication, hyponatremia, intractable seizures, and possibly death. Typically, 10% D/0.9% NS or 10% D/0.45% NS (77 mmol/L Na^+ will be appropriate. Alterations may occur once the serum sodium is known. Likewise, potassium may be added once urine output is established and the current serum concentration is known. This is especially important in patients with potential mineralocorticoid deficiency. Patients who are hyperinsulinemic often require maintenance rates of 10 to 12 mg/kg per minute. In some cases, 25 mg/kg per minute will be needed. The clinician will need to use more concentrated glucose-containing electrolyte solutions in these cases. A central line should be considered if a concentration greater than 12.5% dextrose is required.

Glucagon works only if the patient has intact glycogen stores.[4,9] Its use should be considered, especially in the prehospital arena, when an intravenous line cannot be placed. In some children, hypoglycemia is due to depleted, abnormally produced, or unmobilizable glycogen stores.[4] An intraosseous line should be considered in these cases, if an intravenous line is unobtainable so as to allow glucose loading, especially if symptoms of neuroglycopenia are present. Controversy surrounds the use of glucagon in cases of sulfonylurea overdose and hyperinsulinemia. Glucagon stimulates insulin release; therefore, at least theoretically, giving it to these patients could lead to worsening hypoglycemia. The glycemic response to insulin is increased in these patients. At present, there are no prospective controlled studies in this patient group to guide the clinician. Typical dosing is 1 mg glucagon in adults, 30 μg/kg in children, and 50 μg/kg in infants. The maximum single dose is 1 mg for hypoglycemia, although higher doses are used for other indications. It may be given subcutaneously, intramuscularly, or intravenously. Studies have demonstrated effectiveness even when glucagon is given intranasally, although this is not the standard of care at this time.[10–12] If no intravenous line is available, the intramuscular route is probably best. One exception to this is in small neonates who may not have adequate muscle mass. The diluent that is packaged with glucagon contains phenol. When glucagon is given to children, it should be diluted with saline or sterile water. Phenol especially should not be used if glucagon will be given intravenously. If a 50% rise in serum glucose concentration is not seen within 30 min, the clinician should suspect either previous depletion of glycogen stores, an abnormality in fatty acid oxidation, or type I glycogen storage disease. Less commonly, glycogen storage disease types III, VI and IX can present in this fashion as well.

In refractory cases, especially those associated with adrenal insufficiency, steroids may be useful. Hydrocortisone succinate is a good choice owing to its effective glucocorticoid and additional mineralocorticoid effects. The majority of adrenally suppressed patients will have associated mineralocorticoid depression as well. In these cases a steroid such as hydrocortisone must be used instead of one such as dexamethasone, which has almost no mineralocorticoid activity. The dose of hydrocortisone succinate is 1 to 2 mg/kg IV every 6 h. The minimum dose is 25 mg and the maximum dose is 100 mg.

Hyperinsulinemic patients may also be given diazoxide to inhibit insulin release and activity.[6] More recent literature has suggested that octreotide may be a better choice; it is not associated with the rare hypotensive effects of diazoxide. Octreotide dosing for this potential indication is controversial and not yet established. Diazoxide is given intravenously at 3 to 5 mg/kg for neonates and 1 to 3 mg/kg for children every 8 h. Diazoxide should be given over at least 30 min to prevent severe hypotension. In children who are able to eat, feedings every 3 to 4 h will often suffice as well. If given only simple carbohydrates, these children will develop postprandial hyperglycemia with subsequent rebound hypoglycemia secondary to stimulation of insulin secretion. Therefore, their diet should consist of complex carbohydrates, proteins, and fats as well. Feedings of raw cornstarch at night usually maintain safe glucose levels for a number of hours and are not typically associated with the rebound phenomenon discussed above.[13] Starches are absorbed slowly, leading to a lower but more continuous supply of glucose. Children with endogenous hyperinsulinemia due to insulinomas often require near total pancreatectomy.[14]

REFERENCES

1. Burchell A, Lyall H, Busuttil A, et al: Glucose metabolism and hypoglycaemia in SIDS. *J Can Pathol* 45(supplement):39, 1992.
2. Pershad J, Monroe K, Atchison J: Childhood hypoglycemia in an urban emergency department: Epidemiology and a diagnostic approach to the problem. *Pediatr Emerg Care* 14:268, 1998.
3. Pagliara AS, Karl IE, Haymond M, et al: Hypoglycemia in infancy and childhood: Part I. *J Ped* 82:365, 1973.
4. Crigler JF: Intermittent hypoglycemia of children. *Postgrad Med* 51:210,1972.
5. Haymond MW, Pagliara AS: Ketotic hypoglycemia. *Clin Endocrinol Metab* 12:447, 1983.
6. Pagliara AS, Karl IE, Haymond M, et al: Hypoglycemia in infancy and childhood. Part II. *J Ped* 82:558, 1973.
7. Lebowitz MR, Blumenthal SA: The molar ratio of insulin to C-peptide: An aid to the diagnosis of hypoglycemia due to surreptitious (or inadvertent) insulin administration. *Arch Intern Med* 153: 650, 1993.

8. Sheehy TW: Case report: Factitious hypoglycemia in diabetic patients. *Am J Med Sci* 304:298, 1992.
9. Pollack CV: Utility of glucagon in the emergency department. *J Emerg Med* 11:195, 1993.
10. Pontiroli AE, Calderara A, Pajetta E, et al: Intranasal glucagon as a remedy for hypoglycemia: Studies in healthy patients and type I diabetic patients. *Diabetes Care* 12:604, 1989.
11. Slama G, Alamowitch C, Desplanque N, et al: A new non-invasive method for treating insulin-reaction: Intranasal lyophilized glucagon. *Diabetologia* 33:671, 1990.
12. Stenninger E, Aman J: Intranasal glucagon treatment relieves hypoglycemia in children with type I IDDM. *Diabetologia* 36:931, 1993.
13. Chen YT, Cornblath M, Sidbury JB: Cornstarch therapy in type I glycogen storage disease. *N Engl J Med* 310:171, 1984.
14. Synn AY, Mulvihill SJ, Fonkalsrud EW: Surgical disorders of the pancreas in infancy and childhood. *Amer J Surg* 156:201, 1988.

ALTERED MENTAL STATUS IN CHILDREN

Nancy Pook
Natalie Cullen
Jonathan I. Singer

Altered mental status (AMS) in a child is the failure to respond to the external environment in a manner appropriate to the child's developmental level, despite verbal or physical stimulation.[1] Alteration in mental status consists of impairment of awareness and arousal, the two components of consciousness. Patients with AMS require simultaneous stabilization, diagnosis, and treatment. The objectives of treatment are to sustain life and prevent irreversible central nervous system damage. Once the patient is resuscitated, the next objective is to establish the cause of AMS and stop disease progression.

PATHOPHYSIOLOGY

There is a spectrum of alterations of mental status, ranging from confusion or delirium (disorders in perception) to lethargy, stupor, and coma (states of decreased awareness). A lethargic pediatric patient has decreased awareness of self and the environment. In an emergency setting, this translates to decreased eye contact with family members, nursing, and physician personnel.[2] A stuporous pediatric patient has decreased eye contact, decreased motor activity, and unintelligible vocalization. Stuporous patients can be aroused with vigorous noxious stimulation. Comatose patients are unresponsive and cannot be aroused by verbal or physical stimulation, such as phlebotomy, arterial catheterization, or lumbar puncture.[3–5]

Irrespective of the cause, AMS is indicative of either depression of the cerebral cortex or localized abnormalities of the ascending reticular activating system. Both cerebral cortices must be affected in order to cause AMS. Classic causes of bilateral cortical impairment are toxic and metabolic states that deprive the brain of normal substrates. Altered mental status can also be produced through dysfunction of the reticular activating system that is housed in the brainstem and midbrain. This system connects cranial nerve nuclei and extends from the brainstem to the thalamus. It governs respirations, cardiovascular functions, and many aspects of homeostasis, as well as daily wake-sleep cycles. Any abrupt interruption or selective destruction of the reticular activating system may result in AMS.[1,3]

The pathologic conditions that effect awareness and arousal can be described using three broad pathologic categories: supratentorial mass lesion, subtentorial mass lesion, and metabolic encephalopathy.[3,6]

Supratentorial mass lesions cause AMS by compressing the brainstem and/or diencephalon. Signs and symptoms of this type of lesion include focal motor abnormalities that are often present from the onset of the altered level of consciousness. The progression of neurologic dysfunction is from rostral to caudal with sequential failure of midbrain, pontine, and medullary function. Compromise by supratentorial lesions causes slow nystagmus toward and fast nystagmus from a cold stimulus during caloric testing.

Subtentorial mass lesions lead to reticular activating system dysfunction, in which prompt loss of consciousness is generally the rule. There is a discrete level of dysfunction. Cranial nerve abnormalities are frequently found due to the highly packed neurologically eloquent anatomy. Abnormal respiratory patterns such as Cheyne-Stokes respiration, neurogenic hyperventilation, and ataxic breathing are common. With brainstem injury, asymmetric and/or fixed pupils are found. No eye movements occur despite cold stimuli to both auditory canals.

Metabolic encephalopathy usually causes depressed consciousness before depressed motor signs, which, when present, are typically symmetric.[3,7] Respiratory function is involved relatively early, and abnormalities are often secondary to acid-base imbalance. Pupillary reflexes are generally preserved. Pupils may be sluggish, but the movement is intact and symmetric. Exceptions occur with profound anoxia and the influence of cholinergics, anticholinergics, opiates, and barbiturates.

CLINICAL FEATURES

Two individuals are needed to manage a pediatric patient with AMS. One individual should act as historian to perform a methodical and comprehensive interview. The key questions that must be explored concern prodromal events leading to the change in consciousness, recent illnesses, the likelihood of an infectious exposure or exposure to intoxicants, and the likelihood of trauma, including abuse.[1,4] The historian should make inquiries regarding antecedent fever, headache, head tilt, abdominal pain, vomiting, diarrhea, gait disturbance, seizures, drug ingestion, palpitations, weakness, hematuria, weight loss, and rash. For infants and young children with AMS, developmental milestones should be pursued. The past medical history, immunization history, and family history are important in children of all ages. The clinician should be alert for any inappropriate responses or inconsistencies and delays in seeking care that may arouse the suspicion of child abuse. Although it may be possible to obtain a history quickly, in order to be thorough and pay attention to detail, one physician must be dedicated to obtaining the history while the second physician manages the resuscitation.

One should proceed with a general examination only after cardiac and cerebral resuscitation. The objectives of the examination are to identify occult infection, trauma, toxicity, or metabolic disease.[4,6] The neurologic examination should document the child's response to sensory input, motor activity, pupillary reactivity, oculovestibular reflexes, and respiratory pattern. Although several coma scales have been published,[8,9] the most simplified and functional in an emergency setting is the AVPU scale. This is a descriptive tool in which *A* means "alert," *V* means "responsive to verbal stimuli," *P* means "responsive to painful stimuli," and *U* means "unresponsive."

Following a targeted history and a focused examination, the treating physician should anticipate and observe changes in the patient's status that may indicate improvement or deterioration. An additional task of the physician who attends the patient is to make an operational, if not specific, diagnosis of AMS.

DIAGNOSIS

The differential diagnosis for AMS in children is diverse and differs slightly from that for adult patients.[1,4] The familiar mnemonic AEIOU TIPS remains a useful tool for organizing the diagnostic possibilities (Table 126-1).

Alcohol

In younger pediatric patients, alcohol ingestion is typically accidental; intentional ingestion is more likely in adolescents. AMS may occur

TABLE 126-1 AEIOU TIPS: A Mnemonic for Pediatric Altered Mental Status

- **A** Alcohol
  - Acid-base and metabolic disorders
    - Diabetes mellitus
    - Dehydration
    - Hypercapnia
    - Hepatic failure
    - Hypoxia
    - Inborn errors of metabolism
  - Dysrhythmia and cardiogenic causes
    - Ventricular fibrillation
    - Stokes-Adams attack
    - Aortic stenosis
- **E** Encephalopathy
  - Hypertensive
  - Reye syndrome
  - Hemorrhagic shock and encephalopathy syndrome
  - Postimmunization
  - HIV disease
- Endocrinopathy
  - Addison's disease
  - Congenital adrenal hyperplasia
  - Thyrotoxicity
  - Cushing's syndrome
  - Pheochromocytoma
  - Hepatic porphyrias
- Electrolytes
  - Na^+, Ca^{2+}, Mg^{2+}, PO_4^-
- **I** Insulin
  - Hypoglycemia
  - Ketotic hypoglycemia
  - Hyperglycemia
- Intussusception
- **O** Opiates
- **U** Uremia
  - Chronic renal failure
  - Hemolytic uremic syndrome
- **T** Trauma
  - General trauma with hypovolemia
  - Head injury
  - Mass lesion
  - Cerebral edema
  - Cerebrovascular accident
  - Electric shock
  - Decompression sickness
- Thermal
- Tumor
- **I** Infection
  - Meningitis
  - Encephalitis
  - Brain abscess
  - Visceral larva migrans
  - Severe systemic infection
- Intracerebral vascular disorders
  - Subarachnoid hemorrhage
  - Venous thrombosis
  - Arterial thrombosis
  - Intracerebral and intraventricular hemorrhages
  - Cerebral emboli
  - Acute infantile hemiplegia
  - Acute confusional migraine
  - Moyamoya malformation
- **P** Poisoning
- Psychogenic
- **S** Seizure
- Shunt malfunction

with serum levels less than 100 mg/dL. Hypoglycemia may occur concurrently.

Acid Base and Metabolic Disorders

Children with diabetes may present in ketoacidosis. The classic presentation includes weight loss, polyuria, polydypsia, polyphagia, weakness, vomiting, abdominal discomfort, Kussmaul respirations, a fruity acetone breath, and AMS. Patients with diabetic ketoacidosis, as well as many other pediatric disease states associated with a loss of circulating volume, may develop inadequate perfusion. Patients with hypotonic or hypertonic dehydration may develop AMS with and without seizures. Poorly perfused patients or patients with inadequate air exchange have insufficient oxygen delivery to the brain and exhibit insomnia, somnolence, and confusion. Patients who develop hypercapnia as a result of primary lung disease or neurologic dysfunction may also present with AMS. Those with hepatic failure present with nausea, fatigue, and behavioral alterations and may rapidly become obtunded. Patients with inborn errors of metabolism typically present early in life with poor feeding, recurrent vomiting, seizures, metabolic acidosis, lethargy, stupor, and coma.

Dysrhythmia and Other Cardiogenic Causes

Ventricular fibrillation causes unconsciousness by diminished oxygen delivery to the brain. In a Stokes-Adams attack, heart block leads to loss of consciousness. Critical aortic stenosis leads to unconsciousness through decreased cardiac output.

Encephalopathy

Hypertensive encephalopathy may occur in pediatric patients at diastolic pressures of 100 to 110 mmHg. Reye syndrome follows a viral illness, such as influenza or varicella. Patients are afebrile and anicteric, and develop pernicious vomiting. Confusion and delirium may lead to increasing obtundation. Hemorrhagic shock and encephalopathy syndrome is a symptom complex of unknown cause that affects previously healthy infants. The common features include a mild prodromal, nonspecific illness of several days' duration followed by the onset of profuse, watery diarrhea that becomes bloody, and seizures. Patients present poorly perfused, with profound metabolic acidosis and evidence of disseminated intravascular coagulation. Laboratory evidence of hepatic, renal, pancreatic, and myocardial dysfunction is common.

Endocrinopathy

AMS is a rare presentation of these disorders. Patients with Addison disease present with nausea, vomiting, abdominal pain, weakness, malaise, hypotension, and mental status changes, including psychosis. Presumptive evidence is provided by finding hyperpigmentation, depressed sodium and blood sugar levels, an elevated potassium level, and a variably increased calcium level. Infants with congenital adrenal hyperplasia may present in an acute salt-losing, volume-depleted hypotensive crisis or with virilization, characterized by ambiguous genitalia and cortisol insufficiency also manifested as hypoglycemia. Thyrotoxic infants may present with ventricular dysrhythmia. Patients may also exhibit symptoms similar to those of adults, including goiter, irritability, exophthalmos, hyperthermia, high-output congestive heart failure, mania, delirium, psychosis, and, later, apathy and decreasing levels of consciousness. Patients with pheochromocytoma may present with hypertensive encephalopathy.

Electrolytes

Hyponatremic children become symptomatic with plasma levels around 120 meq/L. Manifestations include anorexia, headache, nausea, vomiting, irritability, weakness, cramps, disorientation, seizures, and AMS. Hypernatremic individuals develop muscle weakness, irritability, seizures, and AMS. Disorders of calcium, magnesium, and phosphorus present with neuromuscular signs, including weakness, tetany, seizures, and apathy.

Insulin

Hypoglycemia may be an end product of an endocrinopathy (e.g., adrenal insufficiency, hyperthyroidism, or hypopituitarism) or the result of an exogenous substance, such as ethanol, salicylate, oral hypoglycemics, and insulin. Hypoglycemia may result from a common stress pathway of decreased gluconeogenesis, as seen during sepsis or Reye syndrome. Adrenergic signs of palpitations, hunger, and sweating are seen at levels less than 60 mg/dL. Irritability, confusion, seizures, and coma occur at levels of 40 mg/dL or less. Infants and children are prone to develop ketotic hypoglycemia with fasting, especially with infections in early infancy. AMS from hyperglycemia is rare in children. The most common cause of hyperosmolar central nervous system dysfunction is diabetic ketoacidosis.

Intussusception

Intussusception is readily diagnosed in the small percentage of younger children who present with a classic constellation of abdominal pain, vomiting, abdominal mass, and rectal bleeding. AMS may be the initial symptom and dominant concern of the physician and the parent caring for a child with intussusception. AMS remains until the bowel obstruction is reduced.[10]

Opiates

Children who have ingested opiates may present with miosis, absent bowel sounds, and lethargy. Common opiates that may be present in the household include dextromethorphan, diphenoxylate and atropine (Lomotil), and loperamide (Imodium). Ingestion of clonidine, an α agonist, may also cause signs and symptoms similar to opiate intoxication. Abuse and neglect should always be suspected in children with opiate intoxication.

Uremia

In children with chronic renal failure, neurologic dysfunction may develop secondary to stroke, hypertension, or metabolic derangements. Encephalopathy occurs in over one-third of patients with chronic renal failure and is manifested by headache, irritability, cognitive derangement, and seizures. Hemolytic uremic syndrome is a pediatric disorder characterized by microangiopathic hemolytic anemia and uremia. It follows a prodrome of abdominal pain and diarrhea and is manifested by pallor, thrombocytopenia with purpura, red blood cell fragmentation, and oliguria.

Trauma

Trauma may occur on the cellular or global level. In the context of multisystem trauma, a hypovolemic state may create insufficient cerebral perfusion. Such hypovolemic states may be created by other ''traumatic'' insults, such as primary peritonitis or ruptured appendicitis with hypovolemia. Children may have transient loss of consciousness after closed head injury. Occasionally, a seizure may occur immediately after closed head injury, resulting in AMS from the postictal state. The signs and symptoms of acute epidural hematoma are typically posttraumatic loss of consciousness followed by a lucid interval and then rapid AMS. Acute epidural hematoma can also present with a gradual loss of consciousness associated with ipsilateral pupillary dilatation. As in adults, subdural hematomas may be acute, subacute, or chronic. Most children with subdural hematomas have external signs of trauma. The exceptions are abused infants, typically less than 6 months of age, who may present without external signs of injury. Abused children who are shaken typically present with a history of vomiting, seizures, and changes in respiratory pattern associated with AMS. Retinal hemorrhages or a tense fontanel may suggest the diagnosis. Children with blunt head trauma are more inclined than adults to develop diffuse cerebral swelling, increased intracranial pressure, and AMS without extracerebral or intracerebral collections of blood. While uncommon in childhood, cerebrovascular accidents, including bleeding from arteriovenous malformations, may cause focal neurologic deficits followed by status epilepticus and coma.

Tumor

Primary brain tumor or metastatic or meningeal leukemic infiltration may alter the metabolism of the brain. Intracerebral tumors commonly produce focal neurologic dysfunction, whereas posterior fossa tumors typically block the ventricular system and create signs and symptoms suggestive of hydrocephalus. Both supratentorial and infratentorial tumors may present abruptly with AMS, fever, or meningismus after an intratumor hemorrhage.

Thermal

Extremes of body temperature may also lead to central nervous system dysfunction. Progressive hypothermia leads to insidious AMS. Patients who develop body-core temperatures greater than 41°C (105.8°F) develop headache, weakness, and dizziness followed by confusion, euphoria, combativeness, and AMS. Posturing, seizures, hemiparesis, and pupillary changes may be present.

Infection

Infection is more common as a cause of AMS in children than in adults. The incidence of bacterial meningitis and septicemia is highest in early infancy and considerably higher throughout childhood than in adulthood. Bacterial meningitis should be high on the differential diagnostic list in a pediatric patient with AMS. Unless there are contraindications to lumbar puncture, examination of cerebrospinal fluid (CSF) should be considered in lethargic, febrile pediatric patients (Table 126-2). Similarly, pediatric patients may become encephalopathic due to direct invasion of the brain by multiple pathogens. Patients with encephalitis have fever, headache, and, may have signs of meningeal irritation or neurologic deficits. Herpes viruses, arbovirus, rotavirus, and Epstein-Barr virus are among the most common viral agents associated with encephalitis. Encephalitis may occur in the course of mycoplasmal illness, shigellosis, Lyme disease, or cat-scratch disease. Visceral larva migrans may produce encephalopathy in the young. A brain abscess may create signs and symptoms suggestive of encephalitis. Patients with a brain abscess present with fever and headache that precede changes in presentation and consciousness. Affected patients may also present with generalized or focal seizure activity. Patients at risk for brain abscess include those with sinusitis, cyanotic congenital heart disease, immunodeficiency, and intravenous drug abuse. Any systemic infection associated with vasculitis, or vasodepressant toxins, with shock may lead to AMS secondary to cerebral hypoperfusion.

Intracerebral Vascular Disorders

Subarachnoid hemorrhage may occur following trauma or spontaneous rupture of a berry aneurysm or arteriovenous malformation. Nuchal rigidity is an inconstant finding. Venous thrombosis may follow severe dehydration or a pyogenic infection of the paranasal sinuses, mastoid, or middle ear. Periorbital edema with cranial nerve abnormalities is a clue. Arterial thrombosis is uncommon in children, except in those with homocystinuria. Children with homocystinuria have a marfanoid appearance, dislocated lenses, and mental retardation. Intracerebral and intraventricular hemorrhages may follow birth asphyxia or trauma in neonates, but in older children they may signify a congenital or acquired coagulopathy. Signs of subacute bacterial endocarditis include splinter hemorrhages, splenomegaly, microscopic hematuria, and AMS caused by cerebral emboli. Acute infantile hemiplegia presents with an acute seizure followed by hemiparesis and coma. Acute confusional migraine may be associated with profound alterations in consciousness.

Poisoning

Drugs may be transferred to a fetus transplacentally. Infants and children may receive drugs through neglect, abuse, or accident. Drugs may be utilized as a suicide gesture in adolescents. AMS may be caused by exogenous intoxicants, such as ethanol, ethylene glycol, methyl alcohol, paraldehyde, salicylates, anticholinergics, including antihistamines, cholinergics, opiates, tricyclic antidepressants, carbamazepine, clonidine, sedative-hypnotics, amphetamines, cocaine, cannabis, nicotine, carbon monoxide, hydrocarbons, and phenothiazines. Household and beauty products may also cause AMS.

Psychogenic

Psychogenic unresponsiveness is a rarity in pediatric patients. It is characterized by decreased responsiveness but otherwise normal find-

TABLE 126-2 Procedure: Lumbar Puncture

Relevant anatomy: CSF is produced by the choroid plexus and circulates around the brain and spinal cord within the subarachnoid space. A spinal needle traverses the skin, subcutaneous tissue, supraspinal ligament, interspinal ligament, ligamentum flavum, dura, and arachnoid before entering the subarachnoid space surrounding nerve roots that form the cauda equina in the lumbar region.

Indications: The primary indication for emergent lumbar puncture is the possibility of central nervous system infection. It is also indicated for suspected spontaneous subarachnoid hemorrhage.

Contraindications: Absolute contraindications include the presence of infection in tissues near the puncture site and increased intracranial pressure secondary to a space-occupying lesion. The presence of coagulopathy or lumbosacral deformity is a relative contraindication.

Possible complications: The most serious complication is cardiorespiratory arrest, which may occur if a child's neck is excessively flexed. Concomitant bacteremia during the procedure may lead to seeding of infection in the subarachnoid space. Postspinal headache may rarely be seen in children. Implantation of epidermoid tumors is manifested by pain in the back and lower extremities years after lumbar puncture.

Equipment needed: Necessary equipment consists of a lumbar puncture kit with spinal needle. A 22-gauge $1\frac{1}{2}$-in needle is used for children under the age of 6 years. A 22-gauge $2\frac{1}{2}$-in needle is required for children age 6–12 years, and a 21-gauge $3\frac{1}{2}$-in needle is used over the age of 12. A manometer with a three-way stopcock is used to measure CSF pressure.

Patient positioning: An assistant is generally required to ensure proper positioning of the patient. The classic posture for lumbar puncture is lateral recumbent with spine flexed and knees drawn upward to the chest, with shoulders and back perpendicular to the table. An alternative for a small infant is sitting with the thighs flexed toward the abdomen. It is critical to avoid flexion of the neck.

Steps of procedure

1. The back may be cleansed with providone-iodine surgical scrub, or, alternatively, povidone-iodine solution may be allowed to air-dry on the skin. Sterile draping is optional in infants and best avoided to maximize landmark exposure and proper positioning. Local anesthesia with 1 percent xylocaine should be administered to all children, irrespective of age.
2. The intersection of a line joining the superior portion of the iliac crest and the spine meets at the spinous process of L4. Optimal insertion is at the L3–L4 interspace but may be performed one space above or below.
3. The spinal needle is inserted into the chosen site with the stylet in place through the epidermis and dermis. Then the stylet may optionally be removed for the remainder of the procedure. The clinician may not feel an increasing resistance and ''pop'' into the subarachnoid space in younger children.
4. Manometry may be performed as indicated in cooperative children who have lumbar puncture performed in the lateral decubitus position. Normal relaxed pressure is 5–15 cm H_2O.
5. If the tap is bloody, one may replace the stylet and leave the needle in place. Insert a second spinal needle one interspace cephalad, and collect fluid for analysis. Finally, withdraw both needles. This process minimizes red blood cell contamination in the collected fluid.
6. Place a bandage over the insertion site.

Analysis: Mandatory CSF studies include bacterial culture and Gram stain from tube 1, protein and glucose from tube 2, and cell count and differential from tube 3. Tube 4 may be sent for viral or fungal cultures, or latex agglutination in specific circumstances.

ings on neurologic examination, including normal oculovestibular reflexes. Psychogenic unresponsiveness may occur as a conversion reaction, an adjustment reaction, a panic state, or a manifestation of malingering.

Seizure

Generalized tonic-clonic major motor seizures are associated with prolonged unresponsiveness in pediatric patients. Seizure in a young febrile patient suggests intracranial infection.

DIAGNOSTIC ADJUNCTS

Ancillary procedures for diagnosis of AMS include analysis of blood, gastric fluid, urine, and CSF; electrocardiography; roentgenography; ultrasonography; and computed tomography (CT) scanning.[1,3,5] Diagnostic tests should be guided by the clinical situation. Rapid estimation of the blood glucose level with a glucose oxidase strip is a universally accepted evaluation in pediatric patients with AMS. Confirmation by laboratory analysis of venous blood is recommended. Electrolyte determinations, liver function studies, and renal function studies may provide additional information regarding the state of hydration, suspected endocrine and metabolic derangements, and liver and kidney function. If the history is consistent with a toxic ingestion or a toxidrome is identified, toxicology screening is in order. The white blood cell count and differential blood count as independent evaluations are rarely helpful, except perhaps in management decisions regarding highly febrile children less than 2 years of age. A blood culture should be obtained whenever sepsis is suspected.

An arterial blood gas or capillary blood gas analysis with pulse oximetric analysis may provide useful information in cases of trauma, respiratory distress, or suspected acid-base imbalance.

It is not inappropriate to place an indwelling urinary catheter in an ill pediatric patient. The initial urine specimen can be analyzed and a portion sent for toxicologic screening.

Lumbar puncture with CSF examination should not be delayed if AMS is thought to be secondary to meningitis or encephalitis.[11] The lumbar puncture should not be performed and CT should be performed first if AMS is thought to be secondary to trauma, suspected increased intracranial pressure, subdural or epidural fluid collection, cavernous sinus thrombosis, lateral sinus thrombosis, cerebral hemorrhage, brain tumor, cord tumor, or brain abscess. Shock or hypotension and hypoxia should be corrected before lumbar puncture, and empiric antibiotics should be given if meningitis is suspected.

A 12-lead electrocardiogram should be obtained if there are pathologic auscultatory findings or a rhythm disturbance is evidenced while monitoring the patient. An electrocardiogram may further guide therapy in cases of tricyclic antidepressant overdose.

Radiologic evaluation should be directed by the clinical scenario. Portable cervical spine radiography is mandatory prior to mobilization of the neck in a traumatized patient. A chest x-ray may be used to confirm or clarify examination findings and to document endotracheal tube placement. Abdominal films are indicated for the acute ingestion of radiopaque material if suspected, or if the patient exhibits signs and symptoms of an acute abdomen, including possible intussusception. Abdominal ultrasound studies may useful to screen cases of intussusception with an atypical presentation.[12] Skull films are reserved for traumatized patients in whom a depressed fracture is suspected. A CT scan of the head may be obtained for suspected increased intracranial pressure, vascular disorder, or mass lesion.[13]

Miscellaneous adjuncts that may be of assistance in specific instances are blood ammonia, serum osmolality, blood alcohol level, thyroid function tests, and a blood lead level. Skeletal survey may be of significance in a potentially abused young child. Barium or air enema may be both diagnostic or therapeutic in patients with intussusception and AMS. A portable EEG may prove to be diagnostic in a case of non-motor status epilepticus.

TREATMENT

The first priorities in AMS are stabilization and reversal of acutely life-threatening conditions before specific diagnostic maneuvers, such as lumbar puncture, are undertaken.[1,4,6] Airway, breathing, and circulation must be assured. For suspected cervical injury, spinal immobilization is mandatory, and the airway is opened with the jaw-thrust maneuver.

Hypoxia must be corrected, and continuous pulse oximetric monitoring should be established. There is no contraindication to providing oxygen to pediatric patients. Oxygen is obviously indicated for patients with signs of hypoxemia or hypoperfusion, but hypercapnia must be avoided. Bag-valve-mask ventilation may reverse hypercapnia, but endotracheal intubation is necessary to protect the patient from aspiration.

Fluid resuscitation is necessary in hypotensive comatose patients, since cerebral perfusion is dependent on adequate mean arterial pressure. A fluid bolus of 20 mL/kg of isotonic crystalloid should be given quickly. Poorly perfused patients should be reassessed and boluses repeated up to a total of 60 mL/kg as necessary. Thereafter, pressors should be utilized. In hemodynamically stable patients with suspected head injury, encephalitis, or meningitis, the intravenous fluids should be reduced to an hourly rate that provides two-thirds of the calculated maintenance volume. Empiric therapy may be initiated with 2 mL/kg of a solution of 25% dextrose in water intravenously if hypoglycemia is strongly suspected.[14] Alternatively, the blood glucose level may be rapidly estimated by means of a glucose oxidase stick, and glucose-containing fluids may be indicated by absolute or borderline levels.[15]

If there is clinical suspicion of opiate or clonidine overdose, a narcotic antagonist may be administered. The recommended dose for naloxone is 2 mg/kg as a starting dose.[16] Any dose, if successful, may be repeated as necessary to maintain narcotic reversal. Flumazenil (Mazicon™), a benzodiazepine antagonist, may be used for pure benzodiazepine ingestion in an otherwise healthy child. It is dosed at 0.01 mg/kg intravenously with cardiac monitoring established.[17]

Seizures should be aborted if present. Benzodiazepines are typically first-line drugs. The longer-acting anticonvulsants, such as phenytoin or phenobarbital, may additionally be needed.

The treating physician must restore acid-base balance, primarily by ensuring adequate hydration and compensatory ventilation. Sodium bicarbonate should be utilized sparingly and only in circumstances where the pH is 7.0 or less.

The clinician should control core body temperature. Maintaining euthermia is critical to minimizing metabolic demands. A child's increased body surface area hastens radiant heat loss. Heat loss may be minimized with the use of a heating lamp during resuscitative procedures.

Septic-appearing patients and those suspected of having intracranial infection should receive empiric intravenous antibiotics in a timely fashion.[2,11]

DISPOSITION

All patients with AMS should receive continuing care in an area that can provide physiologic monitoring and repeated physical examinations from caretakers. In general, this requires admission to an intensive care unit or transfer to a tertiary care center with pediatric intensive care capabilities. Only those patients with transient, reversible causes of AMS may be treated, monitored in the emergency department, and discharged following observation. Patients who are discharged (e.g., those with a closed head injury or simple febrile seizure) should receive disease-specific discharge instructions. Patients who are evaluated for AMS and discharged home should have a repeat evaluation within 24 h of discharge.

REFERENCES

1. Rubinstein JS: Initial management of coma and altered consciousness in the pediatric patient. *Pediatr Rev* 15:204, 1994.
2. Singer JI, Vest J, Prints A: Occult bacteremia and septicemia in the febrile child younger than two years. *Emerg Med Clin North Am* 13:381, 1995.
3. Plum F, Posner JB: *The Diagnosis of Stupor and Coma*, 4th ed. Philadelphia, Davis, 1984.
4. Cantor RM: The unconscious child: Emergency evaluation and management. *Int Pediatr* 4:9, 1989.
5. Alguire PC: Rapid evaluation of comatose patients. *Postgrad Med* 87:223, 1990.
6. James HC: Emergency management of acute coma in children. *Am Fam Physician* 48:473, 1993.
7. Roth KS: Inborn errors of metabolism: The essentials of clinical diagnosis. *Clin Pediatr* 30:183, 1991.
8. Yager JY: Coma scales in pediatric practice. *Am J Dis Child* 144:1088, 1990.
9. Tatman A: Development of a modified pediatric coma scale in intensive clinical practice. *Arch Dis Child* 77:519, 1997.
10. Singer JI: Altered consciousness as an early manifestation of intussusception. *Pediatrics* 64:93, 1979.
11. Talan DA: Infectious disease issues in the emergency department. *Clin Infect Dis* 23:1, 1996.
12. Harrington L, Connolly B, Hu X: Ultrasonographic and clinical predictors of intussusception. *J Pediatr* 132:836, 1998.
13. Quayle KS, Jaffe DM, Kuppermann N, et al: Diagnostic testing for acute head injury in children: When are head computed tomography and skull radiography indicated? *Pediatrics* 99:726, 1997.
14. Luber SD: Acute hypoglycemia masquerading as head trauma: A report of four cases. Am *J Emerg Med* 14:543, 1996.
15. Hoffman RS, Goldfrank LR: The poisoned patient with altered consciousness: Controversies in the use of a "coma cocktail." *JAMA* 274:562, 1995.
16. Perry HE: Diagnosis and management of opioid- and benzodiazepine-induced comatose overdose in children. *Curr Opin Pediatr* 8:243, 1996.
17. Sugarman JM, Paul R: Flumazenil: A review. *Pediatr Emerg Care* 10:37, 1994.

SYNCOPE AND SUDDEN DEATH

William E. Hauda II
Thom Mayer

Although syncope is usually benign, it may be a symptom of serious cardiac disease and can predispose individuals to sudden death. The sudden death of a child may be due to cardiac, neurologic, or respiratory illnesses, or trauma. This chapter discusses syncope and sudden death due to cardiovascular causes, although the other causes of sudden death are mentioned briefly.

EPIDEMIOLOGY

Syncope

Syncope is very common in adolescence and less common in younger children. Between 20 and 50 percent of adolescents experience at least one episode of syncope.[1,2] Syncope is a presenting symptom of 0.05 percent of pediatric visits[3] and 6 percent of hospital admissions.[2] Approximately 25 percent of patients referred to a cardiology or neurology specialty clinic for the evaluation of syncope are eventually diagnosed with a serious illness.[4] However, most causes of syncope are benign, the most common cause being neurally mediated syncope.[3] Prior syncopal events are not always associated with an increased risk of future sudden death.[5]

Sudden Death

A distinction must be made between sudden unexpected death and sudden cardiac death, as the first includes many causes, such as a seizure, asthma, or toxic ingestion. Sudden cardiac death includes just those causes that directly relate to cardiovascular dysfunction. The rate of sudden unexpected death in children is 2.3 percent of all deaths or 1.3 cases per 100,000 patient years.[6] Sudden cardiac death encompasses approximately one-third of these deaths, or about 600 deaths per year in the United States. Excluding trauma, sudden cardiac death is the most common cause of sports-related death in young athletes.[7] The sports most frequently associated with sudden death are basketball, football, and track events.[8] The greatest risk for sudden cardiac death is among patients with congenital or acquired structural cardiac disease, including postoperative congenital heart disease. The most frequent causes of sudden cardiac death in children are acute myocarditis, cardiomyopathy, cyanotic and noncyanotic congenital heart disease, valvular heart disease, congenital complete heart block, Wolff-Parkinson-White syndrome (WPW), long QT syndrome (LQTS), Marfan syndrome, coronary artery disease, and anomalous coronary arteries.[9,10] Hypertrophic cardiomyopathy is the most common cause of sudden cardiac death in adolescents without known cardiac disease.[9]

PATHOPHYSIOLOGY

Syncope is the temporary loss of consciousness from reversible disruption of cerebral functioning (Table 127-1) and usually refers to inadequate cardiac output and cerebral hypoperfusion, resulting in a temporary loss of consciousness.

Vascular syncope occurs when a stimulus causes venous pooling in the legs, leading to a decrease in ventricular preload with a compensatory increase in heart rate and myocardial contractility. After fainting, return of consciousness occurs while lying on the floor because gravity no longer contributes to venous pooling of blood. Neurally mediated syncope (NMS) or reflex syncope occurs when receptors in the atria, ventricles, and pulmonary arteries sense a decrease in venous return, and an efferent brainstem response via the vagal nerve causes bradycardia, hypotension, or both. Because the pathophysiology of NMS is related to abnormal circulatory control, this form of syncope is often grouped with other forms of vascular syncope, such as orthostasis and hypovolemia.

Cardiac syncope occurs when there is an interruption of cardiac output from an intrinsic cardiac problem. These causes are divided into tachydysrhythmias, bradydysrhythmias, outflow obstruction, and myocardial dysfunction (Table 127-1).

Any event that causes sufficient cerebral hypoperfusion can lead to sudden death. The most common causes are seizures, cardiac diseases, and metabolic diseases. Little is known regarding the most common dysrhythmias that cause sudden death in children, because such cardiopulmonary arrests are unwitnessed. In children, bradycardic or asystolic arrests are thought to be most common, especially in children younger than 1 year of age, but in older children ventricular fibrillation is also seen.[11] Overall in children, however, the incidence of ventricular fibrillation as the presenting cardiac dysrhythmia is much lower than that in adults.[8,11,12]

CLINICAL FEATURES

Syncope is characterized by a sudden onset of falling with a brief episode of loss of consciousness. Other associated symptoms or signs are usually related to the etiology for the syncopal event. Two-thirds of children experience a prodrome of light-headedness or dizziness prior to the event,[4] but vertigo is much less common. Involuntary motor movements occur with all types of syncopal events but are somewhat more common with seizures.[4] Factors related to more serious causes of syncope are outlined in Table 127-2. Events that may mimic syncope in children are listed in Table 127-3.

Sudden cardiac death is usually an unexpected, unwitnessed, terminal event. In patients who have a witnessed arrest and resuscitation is rapidly started, the likelihood of survival is much greater, approaching 25 percent.[8] Witnesses may be able to describe prodromal symptoms to aid in determining the cause of the event.[13]

DIAGNOSIS

No clinical or historical features reliably distinguish between vasovagal syncope and other causes.[4] However, certain historical features and a careful history and physical exam should increase an emergency physician's suspicion of a potentially serious cause (Table 127-2). Particular attention should be directed to the cardiovascular exam, including palpation of the cardiac impulse, auscultation of the heart, and evaluation of the peripheral pulses. Orthostatic measurements will identify volume depletion or autonomic dysfunction. An electrocardiogram (ECG) should be obtained for nearly all children but will usually be normal.[4] Other laboratory studies are directed by the nature of the history and physical exam.

Many of the diseases that cause syncope also cause sudden death in children. A syncopal event can be the presenting symptom of these more serious illnesses. Up to 25 percent of children who suffer a sudden death have a history of at least one prior syncopal event.[6] Because syncope is a very common event, however, a syncopal event by itself is not associated with an increased risk of sudden death unless certain features are present.[5] The two most common causes of sudden cardiac death among children who do not have known cardiac disease are hypertrophic cardiomyopathy and myocarditis.[6] Primary rhythm disturbances undoubtedly are underrepresented due to the inherent difficulty in identifying these causes after death.

Among athletes who have died suddenly, however, only 10 percent had previously experienced at least one episode of syncope.[13] Even with a standard sports screening evaluation, fewer than 5 percent of athletes who subsequently die are suspected of having cardiac disease.[13] The two most common cardiac lesions associated with sudden death among athletes are hypertrophic cardiomyopathy and aberrant coronary arteries.[13] Other coronary artery abnormalities, Marfan syndrome (ruptured aortic aneurysm), valvular heart disease, myocarditis, and dilated cardiomyopathy are less common.

History

The most crucial step in evaluating a child with a syncopal or near death event is a careful medical history. Interview any family members, friends, or witnesses who were with the child just prior to the event. The events leading up to the incident should be described in detail, as should any apparent change in the child's behavior or symptoms. Pay particular attention to details such as the intake of medications, drugs, fluids, and food. Note the position the child was in when syncope

TABLE 127-1 Causes of Syncope in Children and Adolescents

ABNORMAL CIRCULATORY CONTROL
Neurally mediated syncope
Primary neurally mediated syncope (NMS)
NMS exacerbated by anemia, dehydration, medications
Hypovolemia
Diuretic abuse
Dehydration
Anemia
Orthostatic hypotension
Shy-Drager syndrome (idiopathic autonomic insufficiency)
Postexertional
Riley-Day syndrome (familial dysautonomia)
Medications (diuretic, tricyclic, antihypertensive)
HYPOXIA OF ANY OTHER CAUSE
Pulmonary embolism
Central nervous system depression from overdose
Carbon monoxide poisoning
CARDIAC ABNORMALITIES
Tachydysrhythmias
Long QT syndrome
Romano-Ward syndrome
Jervell-Lange-Nielsen syndrome
Acquired long QT
Medications
Electrolyte abnormalities
Hypokalemia
Hypomagnesemia
Hypocalcemia
Organophosphate exposure
Hypothyroidism
Intracranial bleeding or trauma
Liquid protein diets
Pheochromocytoma
Supraventricular tachycardia
Postoperative atrial surgery
Hyperthyroidism
Ventricular tachycardia
Postoperative ventricular surgery
Cardiomyopathies
Wolff-Parkinson-White syndrome
Supraventricular and ventricular tachycardia
Arrhythmogenic right ventricular dysplasia
Exertional tachycardia
Pacemaker malfunction
Bradydysrhythmias
Atrioventricular block
Congenital atrioventricular block
Postoperative congenital heart disease
Postoperative valve surgery
Idiopathic
Neuromuscular disorders
Lyme disease
Sinus node disease
Pacemaker malfunction
Outflow obstruction
Tetralogy of Fallot
Mitral valve prolapse
Aortic valve stenosis
Pulmonic valve stenosis
Hypertrophic cardiomyopathy
Eisenmenger syndrome
Cardiac tumors
Primary pulmonary hypertension
Pulmonary embolism
Cardiac tamponade
Myocardial dysfunction
Cardiomyopathy
Kawasaki disease
Coronary artery anomalies
ENDOCRINE ABNORMALITIES
Hyperthyroidism
Hypoglycemia
Adrenal insufficiency
NEUROLOGIC DISORDERS
Seizure
Migraine
PSYCHIATRIC DISORDERS
Hysterical faint
Malingering
Hyperventilation
Panic attack
Munchausen syndrome
RESPIRATORY DISORDERS
Breath-holding spell
Apnea
Hypoxemia
GASTROINTESTINAL DISORDERS
Gastroesophageal reflux
MEDICATIONS AND DRUGS
Antihypertensives
Tricyclic antidepressants
Diuretics
Antiarrhythmics
Cocaine

Note: Seizures and all of the cardiac and metabolic diseases are also associated with sudden death.

occurred, because recumbent positioning is less consistent with NMS or other forms of vascular syncope. A history of syncope during exertion or exercise increases the likelihood of the more serious etiologies. The prodromal symptoms will often aide in identifying the cause of the event. The sequence and timing of motor movements, level of consciousness, and postural positioning will help to differentiate primary seizures from NMS or other true causes of syncope. A history of previous syncopal events should be sought. Any known medical problems should be considered, especially known cardiac diseases, diabetes, seizures, medication or drug use, or psychiatric or psychological problems. Ask about a family history of structural cardiac disease, dysrhythmias, sudden death, migraines, or seizures. Statements by the witnesses that the patient appeared dead and required cardiopulmonary resuscitation (CPR) must be evaluated carefully. The duration of pulselessness and the degree of intervention required should be carefully recounted by the witnesses. Anytime that CPR has been performed, even if by an inexperienced layperson, the event should be considered a resuscitated sudden death and evaluated comprehensively.

Physical Examination

Complete cardiovascular, neurologic, and pulmonary examinations are crucial, but the findings are normal in the vast majority of children with syncope, regardless of the seriousness of the etiology. The cardiovascular examination includes assessment of blood pressure, resting heart rate, oxygen saturation, and respiratory rate. Blood pressure and heart rate should also be measured during positional changes (orthostatic vital signs). Auscultation should be performed to identify any murmurs, abnormalities in rhythm, and variations or abnormalities

TABLE 127-2 Risk Factors for a Serious Cause of Syncope

Exertion preceding the event
History of cardiac disease in the patient
Family history of sudden death, deafness, or cardiac disease
Recurrent episodes
Recumbent episode
Prolonged loss of consciousness
Associated chest pain or palpitations
Medications that can alter cardiac conduction

in heart sounds. Any abnormalities in the cardiovascular assessment require an in-depth cardiac evaluation.[14]

Laboratory Assessment

An ECG is recommended for every patient, as it is a relatively inexpensive test that can identify some very serious causes of syncope.[15] Abnormalities found on the ECG may not correlate with the syncopal event, however, and some patients with an arrhythmic cause of syncope will have normal ECGs.[4] Other laboratory tests should be guided by clinical suspicion (for example, a hemoglobin measurement for a patient with possible anemia or a glucose measurement for a patient with diabetes). Routine laboratory studies are not needed in a child with a clear episode of vasovagal syncope. However, patients with an atypical presentation or worrisome associated symptoms should have a serum chemistry panel, hematocrit, thyroid function tests, chest radiograph, and ECG in the emergency department. Hyperthyroidism predisposes patients to supraventricular tachycardias (SVTs), so thyroid function tests must be obtained with any child where an SVT is considered. In adolescents, a serum alcohol level and urine drug screen should be considered due to the possibility of illicit drug use (most commonly cocaine and amphetamines).

An echocardiogram should be obtained for patients with known or suspected cardiac disease. A patient with abnormal heart sounds, cardiac murmurs, evidence of cardiac chamber enlargement or repolarization abnormalities on ECG, or other features that suggest myocardial

TABLE 127-3 Events Easily Mistaken for Syncope

Condition	Distinguishing Characteristics
Basilar migraine	Headache, rare loss of consciousness, other neurologic symptoms
Seizure	Loss of consciousness simultaneous with motor event, prolonged postictal phase
Vertigo	Rotation or spinning sensation, no loss of consciousness
Hyperventilation	Inciting event, paresthesias or carpopedal spasm, tachypnea
Hysteria	No loss of consciousness, indifference to event
Hypoglycemia	Confusion progressing to loss of consciousness, requires glucose administration to terminate.
Breath-holding spell	Crying prior to event, child 6–18 months old

Adapted from Braden and Gaymes,[32] with permission.

Suggested Diagnostic Plan

Classic vasovagal event
- No underlying medical problems
  - Physical exam
  - Orthostatic vital signs
  - Short observation in ED
  - 12-Lead ECG
- Underlying medical problems
  - Physical exam
  - Laboratory assessment determined by underlying problems
  - 12-Lead ECG

Exercise-induced event
- 12-Lead ECG in ED
- CBC, chemistry panel, tox screen in ED
- Chest x-ray in ED
- Consult pediatrician and cardiologist
- Admit to monitored inpatient bed
- Echocardiogram in ED or hospital

Event associated with chest pain, palpitations, cardiac disease, or family history of cardiac disease, recurrent or recumbent episodes
- 12-Lead ECG in ED
- CBC, chemistry panel, tox screen, CPK/MB in ED
- Chest x-ray in ED
- Consult pediatrician and cardiologist
- Admit to monitored inpatient bed
  - Serial CPK/MBs
- Echocardiogram in ED or hospital

Documented dysrhythmia by prehospital or ED personnel
- 12-Lead ECG in ED
- CBC, chemistry panel, tox screen, CPK/MB, thyroid function tests in ED
- Chest x-ray in ED
- Consult pediatrician and cardiologist
- Admit to PICU for dysrhythmias requiring antiarrhythmic therapy or cardioversion
- Admit to monitored inpatient bed for all other dysrhythmias
- Echocardiogram in ED or hospital

Episode of sudden death or a history of cardiopulmonary resuscitation
- 12-Lead ECG in ED
- CBC, chemistry panel, tox screen, CPK/MB, thyroid function tests in ED
- Chest x-ray in ED
- Consult pediatrician and cardiologist
- Admit to PICU
  - Serial CPK/MBs
- Echocardiogram in ED or hospital

All other events
- 12-Lead ECG in ED
- CBC, chemistry panel, tox screen, CPK/MB in ED
- Chest x-ray in ED
- Consult pediatrician and cardiologist
- Discharge if all studies are negative
- Follow-up in a few days with cardiologist for echocardiogram and portable rhythm monitor

Abbreviations: CBC, complete blood count; ECG, electrocardiogram; ED, emergency department; PICU, pediatric intensive care unit.

dysfunction requires a prompt echocardiogram. If an echocardiogram cannot be obtained in the emergency department, then an inpatient evaluation must be performed.

The clinical utility of other tests, such as stress tests, tilt-table tests, electrophysiologic studies, and cardiac catheterization, are usually directed by the pediatric cardiologist and are beyond the scope of this chapter.

Patients resuscitated from sudden death must have a complete evaluation unless a clear cause for the arrest is apparent. The diagnostic possibilities are extensive, so laboratory and radiographic studies should be directed by clinical and historical information. All such patients should have a serum chemistry panel, CPK-MB, complete blood count, serum alcohol level evaluation, urine drug screen, thyroid function tests, chest radiograph, and ECG in the emergency department. Look for complications resulting from the arrest, such as hypothermia, acidosis, rhabdomyolysis, and cerebral edema or hypoxia. The inpatient evaluation can include an echocardiogram, cardiac catheterization, stress test, and electrophysiologic testing.

SPECIFIC CONDITIONS

Neurally Mediated Syncope

This category encompasses the terms vasovagal syncope, vasodepressor syncope, neurocardiogenic syncope, reflex syncope, and simple faint. NMS is the most common cause of syncope in children[3] and usually is preceded by a sensation of warmth, nausea, light-headedness, and a visual grayout or tunneling of vision.[15] This type of syncope frequently lasts less than 1 min.[4] Common precipitating factors include prolonged recumbence just prior to standing or prolonged standing, sight of blood or disfiguring injury (for example, fractures or soft tissue injuries), emotional upset, mild physical trauma or pain, physical exertion, and hot or crowded conditions. Other contributing factors that are less common include hypovolemia, anemia, dehydration, and pregnancy. NMS can also occur with swallowing, urination, defecation, and coughing; breath-holding spells are a variant of this form of syncope. Medications that alter vascular tone or heart rate may contribute to the development of syncope, including β blockers, calcium-channel blockers, and diuretics. Surreptitious use of diuretics is common among athletes, such as wrestlers, who must maintain weight restrictions.

Identifying NMS as the cause of syncope can be difficult in an emergency department. Because NMS is physiologically based on inadequate compensatory mechanisms to maintain blood pressure and cardiac output in a wide range of clinical states, the distinction between syncope from NMS and other causes of orthostatic syncope is often blurred. However, NMS and other orthostatic causes of syncope are generally considered to be benign illnesses.

Three clinical patterns of NMS occur: vasodepressor syncope, cardioinhibitory syncope, and mixed syncope. Any disorder that causes vasodilatation, vagal stimulation, or both can result in syncope.

ORTHOSTATIC SYNCOPE Patients will typically complain of light-headedness and weakness after standing for a period of time ranging from seconds to minutes. Factors that predispose children to orthostatic syncope include anemia, dehydration, and medications, especially calcium-channel blockers and angiotensin-converting enzyme inhibitors.[3] A drop of greater than 20 mmHg in blood pressure with an increase in heart rate of more than 20 beats per minute while checking vital signs with the child in the supine to standing position is often considered diagnostic of orthostatic hypotension.

SITUATIONAL SYNCOPE Urination, defecation, coughing, and swallowing have all been described as causing syncope. The pathophysiology is thought to be related to an exaggerated Valsalva response causing cardioinhibitory syncope. Stretching, neck extension, external neck pressure, and hair grooming have also been described as causing syncope, presumably due to carotid sinus hypersensitivity or abnormal Valsalva responses.[14]

FAMILIAL DYSAUTONOMIA Abnormalities in heart rate and blood pressure control can be inherited as a primary disorder, such as the Riley-Day syndrome. This disorder results from abnormal development of the sensory and autonomic ganglia, perhaps due to a lack of nerve growth factor during embryogenesis. Manifestations include failure to thrive, developmental delay, temperature instability, abnormal sweating, absent lacrimation, breath-holding spells, and seizures.[14]

Cardiac Dysrhythmias

Outpatient continuous portable ECG monitoring (Holter monitoring) only identifies the cause of syncope in 3 percent of pediatric patients.[4] A cardiac dysrhythmia should be suspected if the syncope is associated with an intense sympathetic stimulus such as fright, anger, surprise, or physical exertion.[16] The event will usually start and end abruptly, contrary to nonarrhythmogenic causes such as hypoglycemia or seizures, which are more gradual. Associated symptoms may include palpitations or irregularities of heartbeat.

LONG QT SYNDROME This disorder may be inherited or acquired and is characterized by a prolonged QT interval on the surface ECG. Although the incidence of inherited LQTS is rare (1:5000 births), it is associated with hypertrophic cardiomyopathy and thus accounts for up to half of the cases of sudden cardiac death.[18] Classically, a patient with LQTS should have a corrected QT interval that is longer than 0.44 s on the surface ECG.[16] Other abnormalities on the ECG associated with LQTS include torsade de pointes, T-wave alternans, notched T waves in three leads, and prominent U waves.[14] Patients with a LQTS may have a normal ECG in the emergency department.[4] These patients may be diagnosed by a history of LQTS in a family member (familial LQTS), stress testing (exertional LQTS), or Holter monitoring (intermittent LQTS). The history should also include any recent use of medications that can prolong the QT interval (Table 127-4). The 10-year mortality can be reduced from 70 to 4 percent by appropriate treatment.[17] Genetic studies to date have identified four genetic loci associated with LQTS, all of which encode proteins involved in sodium and potassium transport. Two clinical syndromes not associated with structural heart disease are also recognized: Romano-Ward syndrome is an autosomal dominant condition not associated with deafness, whereas Jervell-Lange-Nielsen syndrome is an autosomal recessive disease associated with deafness.

WOLFF-PARKINSON-WHITE SYNDROME WPW is characterized by antegrade conduction through an accessory pathway causing a reentrant SVT. Symptoms are manifested when conduction down the accessory pathway occurs at very rapid rates leading to a reentrant SVT. An ECG may show the characteristic delta wave, but it can also be normal. Although WPW occurs in only 0.1 percent of the population, it is more common in patients with Ebstein malformation, corrected transposition of the great arteries (levo-TGA), and hypertrophic cardiomyopathy.[14] The risk of sudden death and syncope are highest in patients who have atrial dysrhythmias such as atrial fibrillation and atrial flutter. Patients at greatest risk for death are those who conduct antegrade over the accessory pathway, allowing 1:1 conduction of an atrial dysrhythmia. Atrial fibrillation and atrial flutter are rare prior to adolescence.

ATRIOVENTRICULAR BLOCK This condition is most common in children with congenital heart disease but also occurs as a rare congenital disorder. Atrioventricular (AV) block is most common after heart surgery but also occurs with acquired heart disease, such as hypertro-

TABLE 127-4 Medications That Prolong the QT Interval

Macrolide antibiotics
Erythromycin (many trade names)
Clarithromycin (Biaxin)
Azithromycin (Zithromax)
Tricyclic antidepressants
Imipramine (Tofranil)
Amitriptyline (Elavil)
Amoxapine (Asendin)
Desipramine (Norpramin)
Nortriptyline (Pamelor)
Others
Phenothiazines
Thioridazine (Mellaril)
Pimozide (Orap)
Antifungals
Fluconazole (Diflucan)
Ketoconazole (Nizoral)
Gastrointestinal prokinetics
Cisapride (Propulsid)
Antihistamines
Astemizole (Hismanal)
Terfenadine (Seldane)
Diphenhydramine (Benadryl)
Epinephrine
Local anesthetics used by dentist or physician
Trimethoprim
Trimethoprim-sulfamethoxazole (Bactrim)
Antiarrhythmics
Class IA
Quinidine (many trade names)
Procainamide (Pronestyl)
Disopyramide (Norpace)
Class IC
Ecainide (Enkaid)
Flecainide (Tambocor)

phic cardiomyopathy and myocarditis, and muscular dystrophy.[14] Carditis associated with Lyme disease has an 87 percent incidence of AV block.[18] Congenital AV block was first described by Morquio in 1901, and although the risk of death is highest in infants, asymptomatic children may also die in adolescence.[19] Congenital AV block is also associated with mothers who have connective tissue disease.[14] Syncope from a high-degree AV block not related to positional changes or exertion is called a Stokes-Adams attack. Prophylactic pacemaker insertion is routinely performed in children with either acquired or congenital AV block.

SICK SINUS SYNDROME Sick sinus syndrome is also known as tachycardia-bradycardia syndrome. Isolated sinus node dysfunction rarely causes syncope; a syncopal event is more likely to be due to a reentrant atrial tachycardia.[14] Most commonly, these dysrhythmias are associated with prior heart surgery, especially the Mustard or Senning operation for transposition of the great vessels and the Fontan operation.[14,20] Syncope and sudden death can occur following pacemaker placement, since the pacemaker will prevent bradycardia but not tachycardia.

SUPRAVENTRICULAR TACHYCARDIA Any cause of SVT can lead to syncope while recumbent if the heart rate is high enough to inhibit cardiac filling or if coincident vasomotor abnormalities occur.[21] WPW and atrial fibrillation are the most common causes, but primary SVT can also occur. Episodes of SVT are associated with congenital heart disease, including Ebstein anomaly and l-TGA.

PACEMAKER MALFUNCTION Although pacemakers are not common in childhood, any child with a pacemaker who has syncope or presyncope should be presumed to have a pacemaker malfunction. Syncope can be caused in several ways: lack of pacemaker output (low battery, broken lead, or malfunction), noncapture of myocardium (exit block or lead fracture), retrograde AV conduction (reflex vasodilatation from enhanced jugular venous pulsations with a ventricular pacemaker), and pacemaker-mediated tachycardia (sensed atrial tachycardia or retrograde P waves with atrial sensing pacemaker).

Structural Cardiac Disease

HYPERTROPHIC CARDIOMYOPATHY Also known as idiopathic hypertrophic subaortic stenosis, this disease is both a dynamic and a fixed subvalvular obstruction. Exertional syncope is a common presentation, but infants may present with congestive heart failure and cyanosis. Any child with exertional related syncope must have this diagnosis considered. Onset of symptoms in early childhood is associated with a greater risk of mortality; the 10-year mortality is 50 percent for children diagnosed by 14 years of age.[22] Syncopal events appear to be related to myocardial ischemia and/or ventricular tachycardia, probably as a LQTS. An echocardiogram is necessary to exclude or confirm this diagnosis and should be done in the emergency department or on the inpatient ward. Most authors recommend implantable cardiac defibrillators in children with hypertrophic cardiomyopathy.

DILATED CARDIOMYOPATHY This disorder is unusual in children but can occur by three general mechanisms: idiopathic, with congenital heart disease, or after myocarditis. Syncope and death are thought to be caused by ventricular dysrhythmias or severe myocardial dysfunction.

ARRHYTHMOGENIC RIGHT VENTRICULAR DYSPLASIA This disorder is rare in the United States but is a common cause of adolescent death in Italy. Presentation is more common in older adolescents or adults.[14] Patients usually present with congestive heart failure, cardiomegaly, and syncope or sudden death from an dysrhythmia. ECG abnormalities include left bundle branch block and T-wave inversion, but some patients may have a normal ECG.[14]

CONGENITAL CYANOTIC AND NONCYANOTIC HEART DISEASE Hypercyanotic spells may progress to syncope in tetralogy of Fallot, tricuspid atresia, TGA, and Eisenmenger syndrome. Children with structural heart disease are also prone to ventricular dysrhythmias and AV block.

VALVULAR DISEASES Several valvular lesions are associated with syncope and sudden death. In general, the degree of valve dysfunction correlates with the risk of sudden death. *Aortic stenosis* is usually due to a congenital defect, often associated with a bicuspid valve, although unicommissural or severely dysplastic valves also occur. Other associated cardiac anomalies, particularly coarctation of the aorta, also occur.[23] Most patients are identified by the presence of a murmur. Exertional syncope is due to reduced cerebral blood flow and is commonly associated with chest pain, dyspnea on exertion, and poor exercise tolerance.[23] Mitral valve prolapse (MVP) is probably not by itself associated with an increased risk of sudden death.[24] A child with MVP and syncope requires a more intensive diagnostic workup. Adults with MVP and significant mitral regurgitation have more frequent dysrhythmias, but this has not been shown in children. Ebstein malformation of the tricuspid valve is an uncommon disorder. Sudden death is thought to be due to the development of supraventricular or ventricular dysrhythmias.[25]

PULMONARY HYPERTENSION Primary pulmonary hypertension (without structural heart disease) is uncommon but can present in adolescence. It is often associated with dyspnea on exertion, shortness of breath, exercise intolerance, and syncope. Eisenmenger syndrome is acquired pulmonary hypertension due to a cardiac shunt. High blood flow to the pulmonary circulation from a left-to-right shunt leads to a reactive increase in pulmonary resistance. After months to years, the development of pulmonary hypertension causes the shunt to reverse to a right-to-left shunt and cyanosis becomes apparent. One-half of patients with pulmonary hypertension develop syncope.[14] Physical findings include an increased ventricular impulse, a loud second heart sound, and cyanosis, which is particularly prominent in patients with Eisenmenger syndrome. Syncope and sudden death in these patients are usually related to an dysrhythmia.

CORONARY ARTERY ABNORMALITIES Many of these patients present with sudden death often during exercise or with a prior history of exercise-induced syncope.[26] Abnormalities of coronary artery origin include the left main artery arising from the right sinus of Valsalva or, less frequently, the right artery arising from the left sinus. In both cases, the aberrant artery often passes between the aorta and pulmonary artery, thus placing it at risk for extrinsic compression, especially during physical exertion. Other abnormalities include myocardial overbridging, coronary artery fistulae, coronary artery spasm, and coronary artery aneurysms and stenosis from Kawasaki disease.

Noncardiovascular Causes

SEIZURES Although not truly syncope, a seizure may appear to be a syncopal event even to the medical professional. Seizures often have little or no prodrome and are associated with a loss of consciousness. Seizures usually have a prolonged recovery phase (postictal phase), which most syncopal events lack. Other findings commonly associated with a seizure include onset while supine, convulsions immediately with loss of consciousness, and a warm, flushed, or cyanotic skin color.[14] Many patients who are diagnosed with a syncopal event in the emergency department are later found to have a seizure disorder.[3] Adding to the confusion, up to 71 percent of syncopal events may have associated behavior that could be called a seizure.[27]

BREATH HOLDING Breath-holding spells are thought to be related to NMS. Typically, the children are 6 to 18 months old and have an intense emotional trigger that causes crying and then a breath hold during expiration.[28] The children then become cyanotic or pale and lose consciousness from the progressive cerebral hypoperfusion. Myoclonic activity or seizures may occur. The episode is usually short, requires no specific intervention, and rapidly resolves with gasping respirations and progressive loss of cyanosis or pallor. Up to 20 percent of children with breath-holding spells develop NMS in later life.[28]

ATYPICAL MIGRAINE Basilar artery migraines may be associated with syncope due to poor cerebral circulation during vasospasm. Most patients with this disorder will also have headache, a family history of migraines, symptoms referable to the posterior cerebral circulation (visual changes, dysarthria, tinnitus, vertigo, or ataxia), and a normal heart rate and blood pressure during the event.[29,30]

HYPERVENTILATION Severe hypocapnia can cause syncope by intense cerebral vasospasm that leads to cerebral hypoperfusion. Typically, there is also a history of dyspnea, chest tightness, light-headedness, tunnel vision, carpopedal spasm, or paresthesias.

HYSTERIA Hysterical syncope is an event that occurs without neurologic or cardiovascular changes but otherwise has the visual appearance of syncope. Often these events occur in front of an audience, are independent of posture, and rarely result in injury. The patient may even describe the event, often in an indifferent or unconcerned manner, clearly indicating that consciousness was not lost.

HYPOGLYCEMIA Syncope due to hypoglycemia is more commonly of a gradual onset and is associated with diaphoresis, tachycardia, hunger, and generalized weakness. Unconsciousness resolves with glucose administration but does not usually resolve with the supine position. A history of disorders of glucose production (enzyme or storage deficiencies) or glucose utilization (diabetes) is usually present.

TREATMENT

Syncope

Most children with syncope will be fully recovered by the time they arrive at the emergency department.[3,4] Continued altered level of consciousness should prompt an evaluation for causes other than syncope. Treatment should be tailored to current symptoms. Signs of compromised oxygenation, ventilation, or circulation should be addressed immediately. A cardiac monitor should be applied to the patient while gathering the history and physical findings to document any transient dysrhythmias. Vascular access and blood for laboratory studies should be obtained for all children except those in which a simple vasovagal event explains the symptoms.

Treatment is targeted to specific identified etiologies for the syncopal event. Ongoing cardiac dysrhythmias or seizures should be managed as appropriate. Most patients, however, will have no treatable dysrhythmias in the emergency department.

Sudden Death

A child who survives an out-of-hospital cardiac arrest must be rapidly stabilized, and any identified conditions must be quickly treated. In general the principles of pediatric advanced life support are followed (see Chap. 10, ''Pediatric Cardiopulmonary Resuscitation''). Unstable ventricular or supraventricular rhythms should be immediately cardi overted with direct-current countershocks in either a synchronized or unsynchronized fashion. Wide QRS-complex tachydysrhythmias should not be treated with class 1A agents such as procainamide and quinidine if LQTS is suspected, because these medications act by also prolonging the QT interval. Class IB drugs such as phenytoin or intravenous amiodarone should be used instead.

Treatment in the emergency department is directed at identifying the probable cause for the arrest so that future events can be prevented. The possible etiologies are extensive, so laboratory and radiographic studies are directed by clinical and historical information. All patients should have a serum chemistry panel, complete blood count, serum alcohol level, urine drug screen, thyroid function tests, chest radiograph, and ECG in the emergency department. The inpatient evaluation can include an echocardiogram, cardiac catheterization, stress test, and electrophysiologic testing.

DISPOSITION

Syncope

A child who had a syncopal event can present a challenging disposition decision. When the cause of syncope is not readily apparent from the emergency department evaluation, multiple additional tests are frequently performed but rarely provide further diagnostic information.[31] Unfortunately, few studies have examined the most effective evaluation in the emergency department and the hospital.

Obviously, any child with a dysrhythmia documented by prehospital providers or on the ECG in the emergency department must be admitted. Children who have any of the risk factors in Table 127-2 should also be admitted in consultation with a pediatric cardiologist. Patients with a normal ECG but a history suspicious for an dysrhythmia are candidates for outpatient ambulatory cardiac monitoring.[14] Identified causes of syncope should be treated as appropriate in the emergency department and admission to the hospital should be directed by the need for further evaluation or therapy. All children admitted for a syncope evaluation should be placed on a cardiorespiratory monitor in the hospital.

If, after an appropriately thorough history, physical, and laboratory evaluation, a clear precipitating cause for the syncope cannot be identified in the emergency department, the child may be discharged to home with close follow-up by the child's primary physician or a cardiologist. Because NMS accounts for up to 50 percent of the cases of syncope in children, most pediatric patients without cardiac risk factors or exercise-induced symptoms may be safely evaluated as outpatients.[14,31,32] Many of these children will have addition tests as outpatients, including portable rhythm monitoring, tilt-table testing, and stress testing, although the cost effectiveness of this approach remains in doubt.[31]

Sudden Death

After stabilization, children who have suffered a sudden cardiac arrest should be transferred to a pediatric intensive care unit that is capable of managing cardiac disorders. These children must be transferred with a crew capable of treating cardiac arrest from any dysrhythmia. In general, this should be done with a dedicated pediatric critical care transport team and consultation with the receiving pediatric intensivist.

REFERENCES

1. Kudenchuk PJ, McAnulty JH: Syncope: Evaluation and treatment. *Mod Concepts Cardiovasc Dis* 54:25, 1985.
2. Manolis AS: Evaluation of patients with syncope: Focus of age-related differences. *Am Coll Cardiol Curr J Rev* 3:13, 1994
3. Pratt JL, Fleisher GR: Syncope in children and adolescents. *Pediatr Emerg Care* 5:80, 1989.
4. McHarg ML, Shinnar S, Rascoff H, Walsh CA: Syncope in childhood. *Pediatr Cardiol* 18:367, 1997.
5. Driscoll DJ, Jacobsen SJ, Porter CJ, Wollan PC: Syncope in children and adolescents. *J Am Coll Cardiol* 29:1039, 1997.
6. Driscoll DJ, Edwards WD: Sudden unexpected death in children and adolescents. *J Am Coll Cardiol* 5:118B, 1985.
7. Maron BJ, Epstein SE, Roberts WC: Causes of sudden death in competitive athletes. *J Am Coll Cardiol* 7:204, 1986.
8. Kuisma M, Suominen P, Korpela R: Paediatric out-of-hospital cardiac arrests: Epidemiology and outcome. *Resuscitation* 30:141, 1995.
9. Klitzner TS: Sudden cardiac death in children. *Circulation* 82:629, 1990.
10. McCaffrey FM, Braden DS, Strong WB: Sudden cardiac death in young athletes: A review. *Am J Dis Child* 145:177, 1991.
11. Walsh CK, Krongrad E: Terminal cardiac electrical activity in pediatric patients. *Am J Cardiol* 51:557, 1983.
12. Schoenfeld PS, Baker MD: Management of cardiopulmonary and trauma resuscitation in the pediatric emergency department. *Pediatrics* 91:726, 1993.
13. Maron BJ, Shirani J, Poliac LC, et al: Sudden death in young competitive athletes. *JAMA* 276:199, 1996.
14. Tanel RE, Walsh EP: Syncope in the pediatric patient. *Cardiol Clin* 15:277, 1997.
15. Gutgesell HP, Barst RJ, Humes RA, et al: Common cardiovascular problems in the young: Part I. *Am Fam Physician* 56:1825, 1997.
16. Moss A, Schwartz PJ, Crampton RS, et al: The long QT syndrome: Prospective longitudinal study of 328 families. *Circulation* 84:1136, 1991.
17. Jancin B: Long QT syndrome tracked to a genetic cause. *Pediatr News* 30:8, 1996.
18. McAlister HG, Klementowicz PR, Andrews C, et al: Lyme carditis: An important cause of reversible heart block. *Ann Intern Med* 110:339, 1989.
19. Michaelson M, Jonzon A, Riesenfeld T: Isolated congenital complete atrioventricular block in adult life. *Circulation* 92:442, 1995.
20. Martin TC, Smith L, Hernandez A, Weldon CS: Dysrhythmias following the Senning operation for dextro-transposition of the great arteries. *J Thorac Cardiovasc Surg* 85:928, 1983.
21. Leitch J, Klein G, Yee R, et al: Syncope associated with supraventricular tachycardia. *Circulation* 85:1064, 1992.
22. McKenna WJ, Franklin RCG, Nikoyannopoulos P, et al: Arrhythmia and prognosis in infants, children, and adolescents with hypertrophic cardiomyopathy. *J Am Coll Cardiol* 11:146, 1988.
23. Braunwald E, Goldblatt A, Aygen MM, et al: Congenital aortic stenosis: I. Clinical and hemodynamic findings in 100 patients. *Circulation* 27:426, 1963.
24. Bisset GS, Schwartz DC, Meyer RA, et al: Clinical spectrum and long-term follow-up of isolated mitral valve prolapse in 119 children. *Circulation* 62:423, 1980.
25. Bialostozky D, Horowitz S, Espino-Vela J: Ebstein's malformation of the tricuspid valve: A review of 65 cases. *Am J Cardiol* 29:826, 1972.
26. Liberthson RR, Dinsmore RE, Bharati S, et al: Aberrant coronary artery origin from the aorta: Diagnosis and clinical significance. *Circulation* 50:774, 1974.
27. Lempert T, Bauer M, Schmidt D: The clinical phenomenology of induced syncope. *Neurology* 41:127, 1991.
28. Lombroso CT, Lerman P: Breath holding spells. *Pediatrics* 39:563, 1967.
29. Diamond S: Basilar artery migraine. *Migraine* 81:45, 1987.
30. Moran AM, Arnold LW, Saul JP: Basilar artery migraine: A substrate for non-hypotensive syncope. *Cardiol Young* 6:184, 1996.
31. Gordon TA, Moodie DS, Passalacqua M, et al: A retrospective analysis of the cost-effective workup of syncope in children. *Cleve Clin Q* 54:391, 1987.
32. Braden DS, Gaymes CH: The diagnosis and management of syncope in children and adolescents. *Pediatr Ann* 26:422, 1997.

FLUID AND ELECTROLYTE THERAPY

William Ahrens

INTRODUCTION

Fluid and electrolyte abnormalities are among the most common problems confronting physicians who care for children. This is primarily due to the high incidence of gastroenteritis in the pediatric population, and the vulnerability of children to the loss of water and solutes. In poor countries, diarrheal diseases are common causes of infant death. In the United States, they often result in prolonged emergency department stays and hospitalization. Electrolyte abnormalities are most commonly secondary to fluid imbalances.

FLUID REQUIREMENTS

The key to managing fluids in infants and children is the realization that there are vast differences in the maintenance requirement of water in first 2 years versus the rest of life. There is a direct correlation between caloric requirements and the need for free water, and rapidly growing infants require an enormous amount of calories relative to their body weight. They therefore require a correspondingly enormous amount of water. The daily turnover of free water in infants is up to 3 to 4 times that of adults. This includes increased insensible losses from the skin and respiratory tract, which are usually electrolyte free. Urine accounts for approximately 50 percent of daily fluid requirements and is the predominant cause of sensible losses; because infants have a decreased ability to concentrate urine, they must lose a relatively large amount of free water to excrete waste products. In addition, a relatively large percentage of young infants' total body water is contained in the extravascular space in comparison with older children and adults. This puts them at greater risk for cardiovascular compromise when confronted with sudden fluid losses.

TABLE 128-1 Maintenance Requirements for Fluid and Electrolytes, Based on Body Weight

Body weight	0–10 kg	10 to 20 kg	>20 kg
Total water volume	100 mL/kg	1000 mL + 50 mL/kg for each kg > 10 kg	1500 mL + 20 mL/kg for each kg > 20 kg
Sodium	3 meq/kg	3 meq/kg	3 meq/kg
Potassium	2 meq/kg	2 meq/kg	2 meq/kg
Chloride	5 meq/kg	5 meq/kg	5 meq/kg

Caloric expenditure and therefore fluid requirements can be estimated from body surface area, which is huge in infants when compared with adults. However, weight is a sufficiently accurate and more easily obtained method of calculating fluid requirements. The fundamental formula is

For the first 10 kg: 100 mL/kg/24 h
For the second 10 kg: 50 mL/kg/24 h
For more than 20 kg: 20 mL/kg/24 h

For example,

1. A 10-kg baby requires 100 mL × 10 kg, or a total of 1000 mL/24 h.
2. A 20-kg baby requires 100 mL × 10 kg = 1000 mL + (50 mL × 10 kg) = 500 mL, for a total of 1500 mL/24 h.
3. A 40-kg baby requires 100 mL × 10 kg = 1000 mL + (50 mL × 10 kg) = 500 mL + (20 mL × 20 kg) = 400 mL, for a total of 1900 mL/24 h.

Note that despite a fourfold increase in body weight, the water requirement does not even double; this reflects the relatively small increase in body surface area that accompanies the increase in mass in growing babies. Hypermetabolic states increase the requirement for free water. The most common of these are fever (which increases the free water requirement by approximately 12 percent per degree of elevation in temperature centigrade) and increased sweating.

Electrolyte requirements remain constant throughout childhood and can be estimated by body weight. All infant formulas contain sufficient electrolytes to satisfy these, as do Ricelyte and Pedialyte. The requirement for sodium is 2 to 3 meq/kg/24 h and for potassium is 2 meq/kg/24 h (Table 128-1).[1]

ISOTONIC DEHYDRATION

Isotonic dehydration occurs when there is a proportionately equal loss of sodium and water; the serum sodium thus remains within normal range of 130 to 145 meq/L. It most often results from diarrheal illness and is the most common fluid and electrolyte problem encountered in pediatrics. Fluid is initially lost from the extracellular space. Intracellular fluid then shifts into the vascular tree, which protects circulating blood volume at the expense of intracellular dehydration.

The clinical manifestations of isotonic dehydration depend on the absolute volume deficit, the rate at which fluid is lost, and the age of the patient. When fluid is lost over a relatively long period, a large deficit may be well tolerated and clinical manifestations can be rather subtle, even though up to 40 percent of intracellular fluid may be lost. This most commonly occurs in patients with protracted diarrheal illnesses. In contrast, sudden massive loss of fluid such as occurs in cholera-associated or rotavirus diarrhea can be fatal if not treated aggressively, because most of the volume is lost from the extracellular space and there is insufficient time for intracellular fluid to shift into the vascular tree. This is especially true in young infants, because a relatively large percentage of their total body water is contained in the extracellular space. Rapid fluid loss can result in cardiovascular collapse, whereas older children will remain well compensated.

EVALUATION

The most accurate way to estimate the degree of dehydration is calculating weight loss, which in acute situations amounts to free water deficit. However, this information is rarely available. In practice, estimating the degree of dehydration depends on integrating multiple factors. Patients usually have a history of vomiting and diarrhea. It is useful to quantitate the approximate number of stools and to determine whether the patient is able to tolerate any oral feedings without vomiting. Parents are asked what liquids the child has been given, since excess free water can cause hyponatremia, and "homemade" remedies may contain excess sodium. A history of decreased urine output implies significant fluid loss.

Physical examination has been demonstrated to provide a reliable estimation of the degree of dehydration[2] (Table 128-2). Hypotension indicates hypovolemic shock. The patient's mental status is important: normal mental status usually implies mild dehydration, whereas irritability signifies at least moderate fluid loss. Lethargy implies severe volume loss and/or an electrolyte abnormality, especially hypernatremia. Decreased skin turgor and sunken eyes and fontanelle imply moderate to severe fluid loss and usually occur when intracellular fluid has had time to diffuse into the intravascular space. In these patients, vital signs may be only slightly abnormal and not indicative of the degree of dehydration.

It is important to realize that assessing the degree of dehydration in very young infants is notoriously difficult, and fluid losses are often underestimated.

LABORATORY FINDINGS

In isotonic dehydration, the sodium level is within normal range. The potassium level is usually normal or slightly decreased. The serum bicarbonate level is often decreased: in mild dehydration it is usually in the range of 15 to 20 meq/L, whereas in more severe cases it falls below 10 meq/L. A low serum bicarbonate level reflects stool losses, the presence of ketones from "starvation," and in severe dehydration lactic acidosis. The blood urea nitrogen level usually rises with increasingly severe fluid losses. Urine specific gravity also rises in significant dehydration and may reach 1.030. In young infants, a decreased ability to concentrate urine may result in a falsely low specific gravity. It is not necessary to check the electrolyte level of patients who are mildly dehydrated.[3]

MANAGEMENT

The management of dehydrated children depends on the degree of fluid loss, as well as a patient's ability to tolerate oral liquids. Mildly dehydrated patients (<5 percent) who tolerate Pedialyte can usually be discharged home on clear liquids, with close follow-up. Moderately dehydrated patients generally require intravenous therapy, although oral rehydration (discussed below) is an option.

Severely dehydrated patients require aggressive resuscitation. Boluses of 20 mL/kg of 0.9 normal saline (NS) are given until improved mental status, vital signs, and peripheral perfusion indicate stable intravascular volume.[4] In extreme situations, an intraosseous line may

TABLE 128-2 Estimation of Dehydration

Extent of dehydration	Mild	Moderate	Severe
Weight loss			
Infants	5%	10%	15%
Children	3%–4%	6%–8%	10%
Pulse	Normal	Slightly increased	Very increased
Blood pressure	Normal	Normal to orthostatic, >10 mmHg change	Orthostatic to shock
Behavior	Normal	Irritable, more thirsty	Hyperirritable to lethargic
Thirst	Slight	Moderate	Intense
Mucous membranes*	Normal	Dry	Parched
Tears	Present	Decreased	Absent, sunken eyes
Anterior fontanelle	Normal	Normal to sunken	Sunken
External jugular vein	Visible when supine	Not visible except with supraclavicular pressure	Not visible even with supraclavicular pressure
Skin* (less useful in children >2 years of age)	Capillary refill <2 s	Slowed capillary refill, 2–4 s (decreased turgor)	Very delayed capillary refill (>4 s) and tenting; skin cool, acrocyanotic, or mottled*
Urine specific gravity	>1.020	>1.020; oliguria	Oliguria or anuria

*These signs are less prominent in patients who have hypernatremia.

be necessary. Fluid replacement then consists of replacing 50 percent of the estimated volume deficit in the first 8 h, and the remainder of the deficit in the next 16 h. If diarrhea continues, the ongoing losses must also be replaced. Maintenance fluids are added to the deficit replacement.[5]

For example, a 12-kg infant is estimated to be 10 percent dehydrated. After a 20 mL/kg bolus of 0.9 NS, she is alert and perfusion is adequate. Fluid orders can then consist of

1. Maintenance is 100 mL/kg × 10 kg/24 h = 1000 mL + (50 mL/kg × 2 kg/24 h) = 100 mL, for a total of 1100 mL/24 h or 46 mL/h.
2. Deficit = 10 percent of body weight (1.2 kg) = 1200 mL; replace 600 mL over the first 8 h or 75 mL/h; replace 600 mL over the next 16 h or 38 mL/h.

Thus, for the first 8 h, maintenance + deficit = 121 mL/h; for the next 16 h, maintenance + deficit = 84 mL/h.

Appropriate rehydrating solutions in infants are 5% D/0.2NS or 5% D/0.45NS. In infants, 5% D in 0.2NS is isotonic for maintainance rehydration in isotonic dehydration. In children, 5% D/0.45NS can be used for maintainance rehydration in isotonic dehydration. Glucose is added to the solution to minimize further catabolism. Remember that 0.9NS is used for bolus rehydration. After the patient has urinated, potassium can be added at a maximum concentration of 40 meq/L. Most patients will begin to tolerate oral feeding with clear liquids within 24 h. All severely dehydrated patients are admitted to the hospital.

Patients who are moderately dehydrated can be managed in a number of ways. Oral rehydration is an effective modality, but is labor intensive and time-consuming. Some patients can be aggressively rehydrated with normal saline over a period of 2 to 4 h in the emergency department and safely discharged.[4,6] The success of rapid rehydration may be correlated with an initial serum bicarbonate level of greater than 13 meq/L, but further study is needed to clarify this. Extreme caution should be exercised in using rapid rehydration in neonates and young infants, since the underlying gastroenteritis is likely to continue and these patients are at relatively great risk of cardiovascular compromise. If they are discharged, follow-up must be expedient and absolutely certain. Patients with persistent profuse diarrhea and those with intractable vomiting are candidates for admission. Fluid management is then the same as for severely dehydrated patients, with 50 percent of the deficit replaced in the first 8 h and the remaining 50 percent replaced over the next 16 h.

HYPERNATREMIC DEHYDRATION

Hypernatremic dehydration occurs when there is a relatively greater loss of free water than sodium. It often occurs when patients with gastroenteritis are treated with salt-rich solutions. The predominant clinical problems related to hypernatremic dehydration result from the increase in serum osmolarity. As sodium rises and osmolarity increases, fluid is drawn from the interstitial and intracellular spaces into the vascular tree. This protects circulating blood volume and peripheral perfusion and can result in deceptively normal vital signs, despite severe dehydration. Loss of intracellular fluid causes doughy, tenting skin. Faced with osmotic disequilibrium, brain cells create charged molecules (*idiogenic osmols*) in an effort to preserve intracellular volume and electrical neutrality. Despite this, mental status changes are common, including irritability, lethargy, and seizures.

The most essential aspect of managing hypernatremic dehydration involves replacing lost free water in such a way that the serum sodium falls no more than 10 to 15 meq/L/24 h. A more rapid decrease in serum osmolarity can result in the influx of water into brain cells, resulting in cerebral edema. In patients in whom perfusion is inadequate, a 10- to 20-mL/kg bolus of 0.9 NS is administered. There is no universal agreement on the optimal subsequent hydrating solution to be used, but 5% D/0.45 NS will be adequate in the majority of cases and is probably less risky than the more hypotonic 5% D/0.2 NS. It is most important that rehydration be spread out over 48 to 72 h, rather than the 24 h used for isotonic dehydration. In cases of severe hypernatremia ($Na^+ >$ 165 meq/L), it is reasonable to consult a pediatric intensivist or nephrologist after the patient is stabilized. Even with optimal management, patients with severe hypernatremia are at risk for neurologic sequelae.

DIABETES INSIPIDIS

Diabetes insipidis, which is most commonly caused by a deficiency of the antidiuretic hormone (ADH) arginine vasopressin, usually occurs secondary to damage to the neurohypophyseal unit and commonly occurs after severe head trauma, central nervous system infections, and suprasellar tumors, especially craniopharygiomas. An extremely rare form of diabetes insipidis is characterized by a failure to respond to vasopressin and is referred to as *nephrogenic*.

Clinically, the syndrome is characterized by polyuria, which can be massive. Most patients also manifest polydipsia. The excessive loss of free water can result in hypernatremia. The patient's urine is usually extremely dilute, with a specific gravity of less than 1.005 and an osmolality of 50 to 200 mosm/L. Diagnosis can be made by water deprivation testing or by serum assay of vasopressin.

Diabetes insipidis is treated with desmopressin (DDAVP), an analogue of vasopressin. The dose is individualized, and consultation with a pediatric endocrinologist is advisable.

HYPONATREMIC DEHYDRATION

Hyponatremia is defined as a serum sodium level of less than 130 meq/L. There are many causes of hyponatremia, which are usually categorized on the basis of whether total body water is increased, decreased, or normal. Hyponatremic dehydration most commonly occurs when a parent replaces acute fluid losses from vomiting and diarrhea with free water. Much less common causes of hyponatremic dehydration include adrenal insufficiency states, third-space losses from ascites or pancreatitis, and diuretic use.

In severe cases of hyponatremic dehydration, shock can result. However, the most common clinical manifestations of symptomatic hyponatremia involve the central nervous system. Although a gradual reduction in serum sodium is usually well tolerated, a sudden decrease can result in irritability, lethargy, and seizures. Seizures are most common with a serum sodium level of less than 120 meq/L, but are more dependent on the rate of fall than the absolute value of serum sodium.

The management of hyponatremic dehydration associated with cardiovascular instability consists of the infusion of normal saline in 20 mL/kg boluses until the patient is stable. Many patients with gastroenteritis who suffer hyponatremic-induced convulsions will stop seizing following the administration of a bolus of normal saline alone. Subsequent management is aimed at restoring both the volume and sodium deficits. The standard formula used in correcting serum sodium is

$$(\text{Na desired} - \text{Na measured}) \times 0.6 \times \text{kg body wt}$$

in which 0.6 reflects the fractional distribution of sodium. To prevent overcorrection, the desired sodium is usually 125 meq/L, which corrects osmolarity sufficiently to prevent further seizures. In stable patients, the correction is carried out over several hours, as there is no physiologic advantage to raising the serum sodium rapidly. In patients with profound hyponatremia or persistent seizures, it may be necessary to infuse 3% NS at a dose up to 12 meq/kg; in clinical practice, this is rarely necessary. In patients with profound hyponatremia, rapid correction of serum sodium has resulted in central pontine demyelinolysis.

HYPONATREMIA WITH INCREASED TOTAL BODY WATER

Causes of hyponatremia associated with increased total body water are acute water intoxication, the syndrome of inappropriate antidiuretic hormone (SIADH), edema-forming states including nephrotic syndrome, and cirrhosis.

Acute water intoxication can result in a profound rapid decrease in serum sodium. It is often psychogenic, but can occur in young infants who are accidentally given large amounts of free water. If seizures occur, treatment with 3% saline may be necessary. In most cases, fluid restriction suffices to lower serum sodium.

SIADH occurs in a variety of disease states, including central nervous system infections, and following head trauma. ADH stimulates the resorption of free water, resulting in hyponatremia. The most important laboratory finding in SIADH is a urine osmolarity greater than serum osmolarity. Hypouricemia is also usually present. The fundamental treatment is fluid restriction.

In nephrosis and cirrhosis, hyponatremia is usually mild and chronic. Even though whole body water is increased, intravascular volume may be low due to third spacing. Treatment usually consists of diuresis, with a combination of albumin followed by a diuretic. These patients are best managed in consultation with a pediatric nephrologist.

ORAL REHYDRATION

It has been repeatedly demonstrated that oral rehydration is as effective as intravenous therapy in treating infants with mild to moderate dehydration.[7–10] It has had an enormous impact in developing countries, where prepackaged electrolyte solutions are available in lieu of infinitely more expensive intravenous solutions. Although time constraints may limit oral therapy in emergency departments in the United States, emergency physicians who do work in international medicine must be familiar with its use.

Water and electrolyte solutions created for treating dehydrated patients differ from maintenance solutes primarily in the composition of electrolytes. Rehydration solutions contain 60 to 90 meq/L sodium and 2% to 2.5% glucose, compared with maintenance solutions, which contain approximately 45 to 50 meq/L sodium (Table 128-3). The higher sodium content is thought to facilitate the absorption of water in the small intestine. Some controversy exists regarding the propensity of the World Health Organization's rehydrating formula, containing 90 meq/L sodium, to cause hypernatremia. In dehydrated patients, this appears to be rare, but reformulated oral rehydrating solutions containing 50 to 60 meq/L sodium are in use. Studies continue to investigate the optimum sodium content of oral rehydration solutions, as well as the optimum composition of sugars. Current evidence indicates that reduced osmolarity formulas limit the duration of diarrhea. In practice, maintenance solutions can be effectively used if rehydrating solutions are unavailable.

Fluid replacement is accomplished by administering 50 mL/kg over 4 h to mildly dehydrated patients and 100 mL/kg to patients with moderate dehydration. Vomiting can be reduced by administering the fluid slowly. This can be done be using a teaspoon or eyedropper. Ongoing losses from continuing diarrhea are also replaced. Once adequate hydration is reestablished, supplemental feeding should be encouraged. This is especially important in malnourished infants.

Severe dehydration, persistent vomiting, continuing severe diarrhea, or significant hypernatremia may preclude the use of oral rehydration when intravenous therapy is available. If necessary, however, the vast majority of these patients can be salvaged by persistent administration of small quantities of oral fluids. Fluid can also be administered by nasogastric tube, if necessary.

SPECIFIC SITUATIONS

Pyloric Stenosis

The protracted vomiting that characterizes pyloric stenosis can result in significant losses of hydrogen ion, chloride, potassium and, occasionally, sodium. This leads to the characteristic hypochloremic metabolic alkalosis. Fluid replacement must take into account potentially severe losses of chloride and potassium. Appropriate replacement

TABLE 128-3 Composition of Commercial Oral Hydration Solutions

	Na^+ (meq/L)	K^+ (meq/L)	Cl^- (meq/L)	Base (meq/L)	Carbohydrate (% Weight for Volume)
Maintenance Solutions					
Resol (Wyeth)*	50	20	50	Citrate, 34	2% Glucose
Ricelyte (Mead Johnson)	50	25	45	Citrate, 34	3% Rice syrup solids
Pedialyte (Ross)	45	20	35	Citrate, 30	2.5% Glucose
Rehydrate Solutions					
Rehydralite (Ross)	75	20	65	Citrate, 30	2.5% Glucose
World Health Organization formulation (for use in cholera)	90	20	80	HCO_3^-, 30	2% Glucose

*Includes calcium, 4 meq/L; magnesium, 4 meq/L; phosphate, 5 meq/L.

can be accomplished with 0.9 NS with 40 meq/L potassium. Serum electrolytes should be monitored during therapy.

Adrenogenital Syndrome

The most common cause of adrenogenital syndrome in children is congenital adrenal hyperplasia secondary to deficiency of 21-hydroxylase. Defective steroidogenesis results in a deficiency of cortisol and an overproduction of intermediary metabolites. Affected infant boys appear normal, whereas infant girls have ambiguous genitalia. Adrenal insufficiency can also occur in patients who have been on long-term treatment with steroids.

Patients can present with vomiting, lethargy, and failure to thrive. Profound volume deficit can lead to shock. Glucocorticoid deficiency can result in hypoglycemia, and mineralocorticoid deficiency causes hyponatremia and hyperkalemia. Metabolic acidosis may be present.

Initial resuscitation is with 0.9 NS until adequate perfusion is reestablished. Hypoglycemia is treated with intravenous glucose. In infants, 25% dextrose in a dose of 2 to 4 mL/kg is usually adequate. In older children and adolescents, 50% dextrose in a dose of 1 to 2 mL/kg is appropriate. Neonates are best treated with 10% dextrose at 1 to 2 mL/kg, to avoid rapid shifts in osmolarity. Treatment also consists of initiating glucocorticoid therapy with cortisol at a dose of 50 mg/m^2/dose intravenously every 6 h. Mineralocorticoid therapy is not necessary during the acute adrenal crisis.

Cystic Fibrosis

Patients with cystic fibrosis have an elevated content of sodium and chloride in sweat. During hot weather or strenuous exercise, affected children can suffer severe salt depletion and corresponding electrolyte abnormalities. Intercurrent pulmonary infection may be present. Profound chloride loss is compensated for by a rise in serum bicarbonate, resulting in a metabolic alkalosis. Hyponatremia is present, and serum potassium is decreased. Patients can present with lethargy and signs of hypoperfusion. Treatment is with 0.9 NS, with supplemental potassium. Resuscitation should be aggressive.

Hypokalemia

Potassium is the predominant intracellular cation. Hypokalemia occurs when the serum potassium falls below 3.4 meq/L and most commonly occurs secondary to profuse vomiting with or without diarrhea. Therapy with loop diuretics can also cause hypokalemia. In diabetic ketoacidosis, profound hypokalemia can result from osmotic diuresis, although, in the face of the hydrogen-potassium shift that accompanies acidemia, serum levels may be normal or falsely elevated. Uncommon causes of hypokalemia are renal tubular acidosis and familial hypokalemia-induced paralysis.

Severe potassium depletion can result in skeletal muscle weakness, ileus, and cardiac conduction disturbances. A prominent electrocardiographic (ECG) manifestation is the U wave. Clinical manifestations generally reflect the rate of fall of serum potassium rather than the absolute level.

In most cases, hypokalemia occurs slowly, and it is difficult to predict whole body stores based on the serum level. In general, oral replacement over several days is adequate. Dehydration must be corrected. If intravenous therapy is necessary, 0.2 to 0.3 meq/kg/h is adequate. In extremely urgent situations, such as hypokalemia-induced respiratory insufficiency, 1 meq/kg/h can be administered, with continuous ECG monitoring. This is usually done via a central line. In diabetic ketoacidosis, potassium repletion should begin early in the course of therapy, since diuresis-induced depletion can result in profound hypokalemia as acidosis is corrected and serum potassium shifts into cells.

Hyperkalemia

Hyperkalemia is defined as a serum potassium level greater that 5.5 meq/L. In infants and children, hyperkalemia is most commonly due to hemolysis that occurs during blood drawing and does not reflect serum levels. Causes of true hyperkalemia include renal failure, rhabdomyolysis, the use of potassium-sparing diuretics, and adrenal corticoid insufficiency. Metabolic acidosis can result in hyperkalemia due to the hydrogen-potassium shift.

Cardiac conduction delay is the most common manifestation of hyperkalemia and is potentially life-threatening. Peaked T waves are the first manifestation, followed by prolonged PR interval and then widening of the QRS complex, an ominous finding that can precede ventricular arrhythmias and asystole. All patients with suspected hyperkalemia should receive an ECG evaluation. Any patient with ECG changes requires emergent therapy to reverse cardiac conduction toxicity. Asymptomatic patients with normal ECG usually do well with therapy to enhance potassium excretion. Most commonly, this occurs in patients with renal failure who have sustained a gradual rise in serum potassium.

Treatment of symptomatic hyperkalemia is directed at immediately antagonizing its deleterious effects on cardiac conduction and at enhancing potassium excretion. Calcium gluconate 10% at a dose of 0.5 to 1 mL/kg antagonizes the membrane effects of potassium within minutes, and has a duration of action of approximately 1 h. Sodium bicarbonate at a dose of 1 to 2 meq/kg elevates serum pH and causes an intracellular shift of potassium. It has an onset of action within minutes and a duration of action of up to 2 h. Intravenous insulin and glucose also produce an intracellular shift of potassium, with an onset of action of 30 to 60 min and a duration of action of 4 to 6 h. Glucose is administered at a dose of 0.5 to 1 g/kg, with 1.0 unit of regular insulin for every 3 g of glucose. Patients must then be monitored carefully for the presence of hypoglycemia. Inhaled β-agonist agents in doses used for asthma can also cause an intracellular shift of potassium, with an onset of action within minutes; this may prove an attractive alternative when treating patients with difficult intravenous access.

Sodium polystyrene sulfonate is a resin that exchanges sodium for potassium at a 1:1 ratio and therefore enhances potassium excretion. It can be administered orally or by enema. A dose of 1g/kg will lower serum potassium by up to 1.2 meq/L. When it is administered orally, it is usually given with a cathartic to enhance transit time through the gastrointestinal (GI) tract. Hypernatremia or volume overload are potential complications. In patients with hyperkalemia secondary to renal failure, dialysis is usually necessary. In patients with hyperkalemia secondary to metabolic acidosis, normalization of serum pH usually restores serum potassium to normal levels.

Disorders of Calcium

Normally, 99 percent of total body calcium is contained in bone. Normal serum levels are maintained by a complex interaction between dietary intake, absorption from the GI tract and resorption from bone, and renal excretion. Serum calcium is inversely proportional to serum phosphorus. The active form of vitamin D stimulates absorption of calcium and phosphorus from the GI tract; its formation depends on exposure to sunlight and healthy kidneys. Parathyroid hormone increases calcium resorption from bone in response to hypocalcemia and increases phosphorus excretion. Calcitonin decreases calcium resorption from bone in response to hypercalcemia.

In the serum, 45 to 50 percent of serum calcium exists in the ionized or free form; most of the remainder is bound to albumin. Ph affects the proportion of calcium that is ionized and therefore bioavailable. Acidosis increases and alkalosis decreases the fraction of ionized calcium.

HYPOCALCEMIA This can result from hypoparathyroidism or end-organ resistance to parathyroid hormone. True hypoparathyroidism can be idiopathic, follow thyroid surgery, and can be associated with magnesium deficiency. End-organ resistance to parathyroid hormone is most commonly associated with vitamin D deficiency. The most common causes of this are dietary deficiency and chronic renal failure. Young infants fed cow's milk, which is high in phosphate, can develop significant hypocalcemia. A common cause of hypocalcemia is hyperventilation; the decreased P_{CO_2} results in an acute respiratory alkalosis that rapidly decreases ionized calcium.

Clinical manifestations of hypocalcemia include muscle weakness, vomiting, and irritability. Infants may simply appear "jittery." In severe cases, tetany, larygnospasm, carpopedal spasm, and seizures can occur. Carpopedal spasm is especially common in patients with hyperventilation syndrome. The most characteristic ECG abnormality is a prolonged QT interval.

Laboratory evaluation of hypocalcemia of unknown etiology includes total serum and ionized calcium, phosphate, total protein and albumin, measurement of parathyroid hormone, and blood urea nitrogen and creatinine.

Intravenous calcium is the treatment of choice for symptomatic hypocalcemia. Calcium gluconate 10% is administered in a dose of 0.5 to 1 mL/kg over several minutes, with continuous ECG monitoring. Further management depends on determining the etiology of hypocalcemia.

HYPERCALCEMIA This exists when serum calcium exceeds 11 mg/dL and most often results from increased bone resorption. Probably the most common cause in children is malignancy involving the lymphoreticular system. Less common causes include vitamin D intoxication and hypervitaminosis A.

Clinical manifestations of hypercalcemia include fatigue, irritability, anorexia and vomiting, and constipation. Affected patients may be clinically dehydrated and complain of polyuria. An ECG may reveal bradycardia and a shortened QT interval.

The laboratory evaluation of hypercalcemia includes evaluation of total serum and ionized calcium levels, a complete blood count, and evaluation of total protein and albumin, and alkaline phosphatase. An evaluation of the vitamin D level may also be indicated, depending on the patient's medical history.

The treatment of hypercalcemia depends on the etiology. In the acute scenario, patients with functioning kidneys can be treated by aggressive intravenous hydration followed by furosemide, which will enhance calcium excretion.

Metabolic Acidosis

Metabolic acidosis results from the addition of acids or the removal of alkali. The differential diagnosis in pediatric patients is similar to that in adults, with a few notable exceptions. As in adults, it is useful to distinguish between metabolic acidosis with an elevated anion gap from that in which the anion gap is normal.

In infants and children, the most common cause of metabolic acidosis with a normal anion gap is diarrhea. Diarrheal fluid is rich in bicarbonate and low in chloride, and acidosis occurs when bicarbonate is lost in stool. Laboratory values will reveal a hyperchloremic acidosis. Acidosis resolves with the correction of dehydration.

Renal tubular acidosis (RTA) is the other major cause of non-anion gap acidosis in children. RTA constitutes a group of tubular transport disorders. In type 1, or distal RTA, there is impaired hydrogen secretion in the distal tubule. Inability to secrete hydrogen usually results in a urinary pH greater than 6. In type 2, or proximal RTA, there is inability to resorb bicarbonate at the proximal tubule. Accompanying hypokalemia is common and can be severe. In both types, affected infants commonly present with failure to thrive. They can acutely decompensate during diarrheal illness, when bicarbonate loss in the stool can exacerbate acidosis. Treatment of RTA usually involves the administration of supplemental bicarbonate, which improves acidosis and enables relatively normal growth and development.

The differential diagnosis of metabolic acidosis with an elevated anion gap is substantially the same in children as in adults and implies the presence of an endogenously created or exogenously ingested acid (Table 128-3). The one notable exception is the possibility of an inborn error of metabolism (IEM). Of the IEMs that cause metabolic acidosis, the most common are methylmalonic, propionic, and isovaleric acidemia. The typical emergency department presentation is a neonate with vomiting, lethargy, and failure to thrive. It is extremely difficult to distinguish these infants from those with more common disorders, especially sepsis. Helpful ancillary studies include evaluation of serum lactate, pyruvate, and ammonia levels. Management requires consultation with a pediatric endocrinologist or geneticist.

REFERENCES

1. Nolpe J, Forbes G: Fluids and electrolytes: Clinical aspects. *Pediatr Rev* 17:399, 1996.
2. Gorelick Marc H, Shaw KN, Murphy KO: Validity and reliability of clinical signs in the diagnosis of dehydration in children. *Pediatrics* 99:1, 1997.
3. Teach SJ, Yates EW, Feld LG: Laboratory predictors of fluid deficit in acutely dehydrated children. *Clin Pediatr* 36:395, 1997.
4. Luten RC: Rapid rehydration in pediatric patients. *Ann Emerg Med* 28:353, 1996.
5. Harrison HE: Dehydration in infancy: Hospital treatment. *Pediatr Rev* 11:139, 1989.
6. Reid SR, Bonadio WA: Outpatient rapid intravenous rehydration to correct dehydration and resolve vomiting in children with acute gastroenteritis. *Ann Emerg Med* 28:318, 1996.
7. Santosham M, Faysd I, Abu Zikri M, et al: A double blind clinical trial comparing World Health Organization oral rehydration solution with a

reduced osmolarity solution containing equal amounts of sodium and glucose. *J Pediatr* 128:45, 1996.
8. Mackenzie A, Barnes G: Randomized controlled trial comparing oral and intravenous rehydration therapy in children with diarrhea. *BMJ* 303:393, 1991.
9. el-Mougi M, Henadawi A, Koura H, et al: Efficacy of standard glucose based and reduced osmolarity maltodextrin based oral rehydration solutions: Effect of sugar malabsorption. *Bull WHO* 74:471, 1996.
10. Cohen MB, Mezoff AG, Laney DW Jr, et al: Use of a single solution for oral rehydration and maintenance therapy of infants with diarrhea and mild to moderate dehydration. *Pediatrics* 95:639, 1995.

UPPER RESPIRATORY EMERGENCIES

Randolph Cordle
Nicholas C. Relich

STRIDOR

The physical sign common to all causes of upper respiratory tract (URT) obstruction is stridor.

Stridor is due to Venturi effects created by somewhat linear airflow through a variably collapsible tube, the airway. When one inhales, the relative pressure in the center of the tube becomes greater than that at its edges. This pressure differential leads to collapse of the airway walls. During expiration, the previously collapsed areas are reopened owing to the relative increase in air pressure during expiration. Forced expiration or expiration against a partially closed glottis may cause expiratory stridor even in patients with a normal airway. As one progresses from the supraglottic to the glottic and subglottic and finally the tracheal areas of the airway, there is an increase in physiologic support and therefore a decrease in the amount of collapse that occurs upon inspiration.

Supraglottic obstructions cause inspiratory stridor, with marked inspiratory and expiratory variation; obstructions at the glottic and subglottic areas commonly cause both inspiratory and expiratory stridor of lesser magnitude.[1] Finally, obstructions at the level of the trachea and primary bronchi may be associated with inspiratory or expiratory stridor, although usually of a much lesser degree. Although the posterior walls of the trachea and bronchi are somewhat collapsible, good support is provided by the horseshoe-shaped cartilage within its walls. In premature infants and infants with tracheomalacia, these supports are not well formed and inspiratory and expiratory stridor may be impressive. Expiratory stridor, or wheeze, is common in distal airways, since intrathoracic pressure may become much greater than atmospheric pressure during expiration. The pressure differential creates high relative laminar flow through semicollapsible bronchi, resulting in wheezes. This information can be clinically useful when one is evaluating a wheezing child. Commonly, gentle pressure over the chest wall or midabdomen during expiration will increase the intrathoracic pressure and exacerbate wheezing. This maneuver may also assist in detecting inspiratory stridor because the child will follow this relative forced expiration with a much deeper inspiration than at rest. Patients with marked variation in the pattern of stridor should be considered to have a foreign body in the airway until proven otherwise. The quality of the pitch is not clinically useful for diagnosis. The answers to two questions, the age of the patient and the duration of symptoms, will narrow the differential diagnosis considerably, since stridor in an infant below 6 months of age has different causes that it does in older children (Table 129-1).

Stridor in Children below 6 Months of Age

An infant under 6 months of age with a long duration of symptoms (weeks to months) characteristically has a *congenital* cause of stridor.

TABLE 129-1 Differential Diagnosis of Inspiratory Stridor

Congenital*
Laryngeal or tracheal webs, cysts, tumors
Laryngomalacia*
Vascular ring (double aortic arch, pulmonary sling, aberrant innominate artery)
Ectopic thyroid, thyroglossal duct cyst
Congenital vocal cord paralysis
Tracheomalacia
Tracheal stenosis
Hemangioma
Tracheoesophageal fistulas
Cystic hygroma
CNS malformation
Inflammatory
Viral croup†
Epiglottis†
Retropharyngeal abscess†
Tetanus
Diphtheria
Postextubation edema
Airway thermal injury
Irritant inhalation injury
Subglottic stenosis
Bacterial tracheitis
Peritonsillar abscess
Submental space infection
Noninflammatory
Aspiration or foreign body into airway†
Esophageal foreign body
Gastroesophageal reflux
Tetany, trauma, tumors
CNS insult
Immotile cilia syndrome
Granuloma
Retropharyngeal hematoma
Laryngeal fracture
Allergic reaction
Anaphylaxis
Angioneurotic edema
Teratoma
Papilloma
Laryngeal cyst
Lymphangioma
Neuroblastoma
Rhabdomyosarcoma
Lymphoma

*Common causes under 6 months of age.
†Common causes over 6 months of age.

Laryngomalacia accounts for 60 percent of all neonatal laryngeal problems. It is due to a developmentally weak larynx.[2] Collapse occurs with each inspiration at the epiglottis, aryepiglottic folds, and arytenoids. Generally, the stridor worsens with crying and agitation. It often improves with neck extension and when in the prone position.[2] In over 90 percent of cases, this is a self-limited disorder resolving by 2 years of age. Symptom exacerbations may occur with upper respiratory infections or increased work of breathing due to any cause. It only rarely is associated with respiratory distress, failure to thrive, apnea, or feeding problems. Definitive diagnosis is by fiberoptic laryngeal exam.[2] In rare cases, tracheotomy or epiglottoplasty may be needed.[2]

The next most common cause of neonatal stridor is vocal cord paralysis or paresis. Most infants will have a history of birth trauma, shoulder dystocia, macrosomia, forceps delivery, an abnormal cry, or other intrathoracic anomaly. Diagnosis is typically by flexible fiberoptic laryngoscopy with visualization of the cords during speech or crying. Endotracheal intubation can be quite difficult in a child with bilateral vocal cord paralysis. Placing the bevel of the endotracheal tube parallel to the small remaining glottic opening and rotating the endotracheal tube one-quarter turn while applying gentle pressure may assist in passing the tube. Force should not be used, as this may damage the laryngeal structures. Needle cricothyroidotomy and subsequent tracheotomy may be required to secure the airway. It is unlikely that the laryngeal mask airway (LMA) would be helpful in this case. Use of the LMA is contraindicated in abnormal or obstructed airways because the path of least resistance to flow will likely be around the mask and not into the airway.[3] Retrograde intubation may be difficult as well, owing to the size of the structures and potential difficulty in passing the tube from the trachea into the hypopharynx.

Arnold-Chiari malformation should be considered in children with Down syndrome who present with stridor. Hydrocephalus should also be considered in children with myelomeningocele, sacral epidermal abnormalities, or sacral dimples.

Stridor in Children above 6 Months of Age

The patient above 6 months of age with a relatively short duration of symptoms (hours to days) characteristically has an acquired cause of stridor. Causes are either inflammatory, such as viral croup or epiglottitis, or noninflammatory, such as a foreign-body aspiration. The remainder of the chapter deals with the most common acquired causes of stridor: epiglottitis, peritonsillar abscess, viral croup, foreign-body aspiration, retropharyngeal abscess, and bacterial tracheitis (Table 129-2).

TABLE 129-2 Common Acquired Causes of Stridor

	Viral Croup	Bacterial Tracheitis	Epiglottitis	Peritonsillar Abscess	Retropharyngeal Abscess	Foreign-Body Aspiration
Etiology	Parainfluenza viruses Occasionally RSV Influenza	*Staphylococcus aureus* (most) *Streptococcus pneumoniae* *Haemophilus influenzae*	*Streptococcus pneumoniae* *Haemophilus influenzae*	*Streptococcus pyogenes* *Staphylococcus aureus*	Polymicrobial *Streptococcus pyogenes* *Staph aureus* B-lactamase + GNR* Oral anaerobes	Variable Peanuts Sunflower seeds Balloons/other toys Hot dogs Raisins/Grapes
Age	6 mo–3 yr Peak 1–2 yr	3 mo–13 yr Majority < 3 yr	All ages Classically 1–7 Median now 7	10–18 yr (most) 6 mo–5 yr (rare)	6 mo–4 yr Peak < 1 yr Rare > 4 yr	Any 6 mo–5 yr most common 80% < 3 yr About ⅔ deaths < 1 yr
Onset	1–5 days	2–7 day viral upper respiratory infection Suddenly worse over 8–12 h	Rapid, hours	Antecedent pharyngitis	Insidious over 2–3 days after an upper respiratory infection or local trauma	Immediate or delayed possible
Position effect	None	None	Worse supine Prefer erect	Worse supine	Almost opisthotonic May improve in sniffing position	Usually none Location-dependent
Stridor	Inspiratory and expiratory	Inspiratory and expiratory	Inspiratory	Uncommon	Inspiratory when severe	Location-dependent
Cough	Seal-like bark	Usually Possible thick sputum	No	No	No	Often transient or positional
Voice change	Hoarse Not muffled	Usually normal Possibly raspy	Muffled "Hot potato"	Muffled "Hot potato"	Often muffled "Hot Potato"	Location-dependent Primarily if at or above glottis
Drool	No	Rare	Yes	Often	Yes	Rare—often if esophageal
Dysphagia	No	No	Yes	Yes	Yes	Rare—typically if esophageal
Radiologic appearance	Subglottic narrowing "steeple" Distended hypopharynx	Subglottic narrowing Ragged tracheal air shadow Tracheal foreign bodies	Enlarged epiglottis Vallecular space loss Supraglottic ballooning	May see enlarged tonsillar soft tissue	Thickened bulging pretracheal soft tissue	Often normal Possible radiopaque density Ball-valve effect Segmented atelectasis Air contrast effect may be seen

**Abbreviation:* GNR, gram-negative rods.

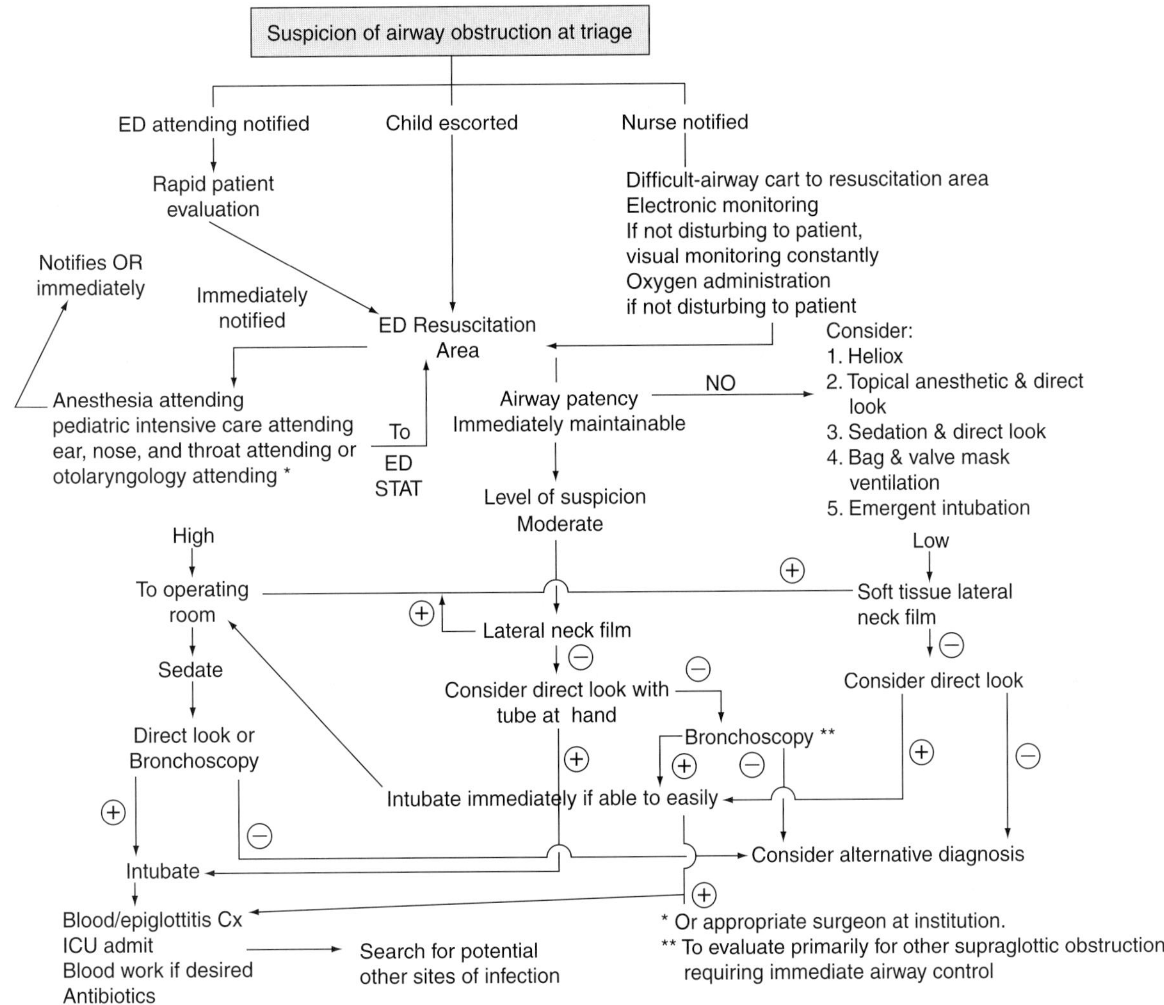

FIG. 129-1. Obstructed airway protocol.

EPIGLOTTIS

Clinical Features

Since the introduction of the *Haemophilus influenzae* vaccine, the incidence and demographics of this disease have changed remarkably. Currently *H. influenzae* is thought to be responsible for less than 25 percent of cases. Now, gram-positive organisms such as *Streptococcus pyogenes*, *Staphylococcus aureus*, and *Streptococcus pneumoniae* are responsible for most cases in immunized children. In immunocompromised children, herpes simplex, *Candida* and varicella must also be considered.

Prior to the introduction of the *Haemophilus* vaccine, the median age of this disease was 3 years, with 25 percent occurring in children under age 2. Although epiglottitis can occur at any age, its median age of presentation is currently 7.[4]

The classic symptoms are an abrupt onset over several hours of high fever, sore throat, stridor, dysphagia, and drooling. Some cases may develop over 1 to 2 days. Physical examination reveals a toxic-appearing, apprehensive child with an ashen-gray color. The child often sits in a tripod position, or the "sniffing" position, with the neck slightly extended and the chin forward. As opposed to the child with croup, there is no cough. The voice may be muffled, but supraglottic foreign bodies, peritonsillar abscess, and retropharyngeal abscess may present similarly. If inflammatory changes extend beyond the epiglottis to include the vocal cords, voice pitch will be altered as well.

Older children and adults may have much more subtle presentations than young children. In fact, some older children will complain of only a severe sore throat. Stridor may or may not be present. The diagnosis is suggested by severe sore throat, the finding of a relatively normal-appearing oropharynx, and striking tenderness with gentle movement of the hyoid. The diagnosis needs to be confirmed by fiberoptic bronchoscopy.

Diagnosis

The ideal approach to the diagnosis of epiglottitis varies depending on the practice environment. Each institution should have a written "Suspected Epiglottitis Management Protocol" (Fig. 129-1). Themes necessary in all protocols include:

1. Immediate recognition and triage to a resuscitation area
2. Continuous monitoring by someone trained in the management of the difficult airway
3. Rapid consultation of appropriate colleagues
4. Consideration and risk-benefit analysis of patient transfer with appropriate personnel present during the transfer
5. Bedside radiology without disturbing patient or, if moved to the x-ray suite, constant monitoring by a physician with appropriate airway equipment

Lateral neck radiographs are usually unnecessary in patients with a classic presentation for epiglottitis. When the diagnosis is uncertain,

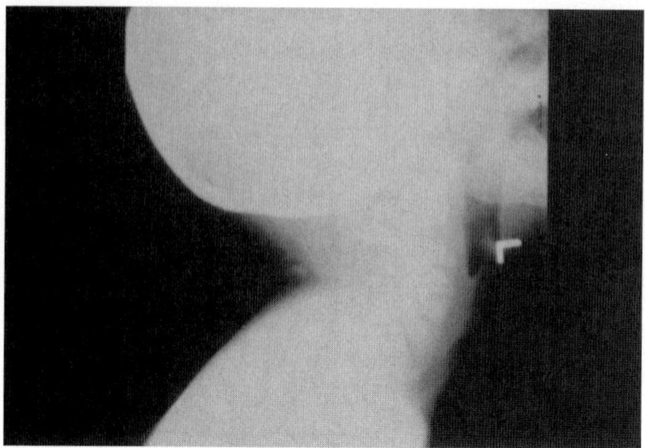

FIG. 129-2. A normal lateral neck x-ray.

radiographs should be taken with the neck extended during inspiration using a high-kilovolt soft tissue technique. The child typically holds its head in the sniffing position and has prolonged inspiration, already making it quite easy to obtain these radiographs. False-positive findings may occur due to normally widened retropharyngeal space structures if the radiograph is taking during expiration or with the head flat. Lateral neck radiographs are not required if the patient is already intubated, and often the typical findings for epiglottitis will not be seen in such cases. False-negative radiographic evaluations do occur. Direct visualization of the epiglottis should occur prior to discharge if suspicion for the diagnosis still exists.

In evaluating lateral neck radiographs, the epiglottis, vallecula, hypopharynx, tracheal air column, arytenoids, and retropharyngeal or prevertebral space should be checked. The epiglottis is normally tall and thin, projecting up into the hypopharynx (Fig. 129-2). Normally there is a poorly delineated space between the epiglottis and the anteriormost aspect of the hypopharynx. In epiglottitis, the epiglottis is swollen and appears squat and flat, like a thumbprint at the base of the hypopharynx (Fig. 129-3). Commonly, the vallecular airspace is obscured. Another common finding is ballooning of the hypopharynx just above the area of the larynx. This is illustrated by the different sizes of the hypopharynx in Figs. 129-2 and 129-3. While not specific for epiglottitis, this distention does indicate significant obstruction of the upper respiratory tract. The retropharyngeal space is normally 3 to 4 mm wide. Commonly it is stated that it should be less than the width of the adjacent vertebral body. The tracheal air column should be of uniform width without densities.

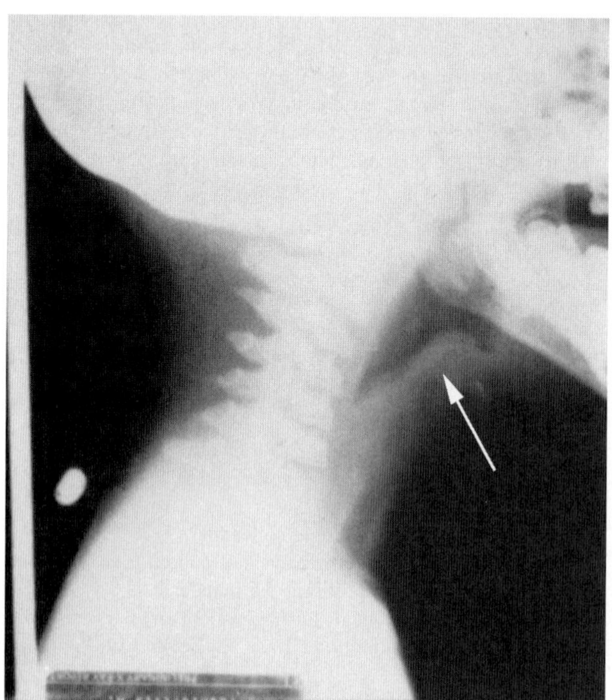

FIG. 129-3. Lateral neck view of a child with epiglottitis.

In some scenarios, gentle direct visualization can be attempted. Most proponents of this practice would agree that it should be performed only at sites where experts in pediatric airway management are present with appropriate equipment to maintain the airway by whatever means necessary. Typically this is done in the following stepwise manner. In his or her position of comfort, the child is asked to open its mouth wide. If the epiglottis is not seen, the child is asked to stick its tongue out, with a tongue blade used to depress the anterior aspect of the tongue in the hope of visualizing the epiglottis. If the epiglottis is still not seen, as is more common, fiberoptic laryngoscopy by an operator skilled in the techique, and with the ability to intubate over the scope, is the safest next step.

Airway Management

Should the child develop ventilatory fatigue or if airway obstruction or apnea occurs before the airway has been secured, bag-valve-mask ventilation can be effective.

Patients with epiglottitis who are initially seen in the office, clinic, or emergency department (ED) without pediatric or ear-nose-throat (ENT) subspecialty support should be transported to a referral center by ground or air, whichever is more appropriate, accompanied by personnel who can manage the airway. Oxygen should be given, and continuous nebulized racemic epinephine can be given to decrease airway edema. The child should be kept seated upright. Heliox can also be a temporizing measure until specialists arrive (see discussion of croup, below). The referral center should be alerted as soon as possible, so that decisions concerning intubation or tracheostomy can be made in advance. Patients usually are intubated by the most skilled individual available as soon as the diagnosis is made. Sedation, paralytics, and vagolytics are used as indicated. To reduce the incidence of postextubation stridor, a tube one size smaller than usual should be used. Tube sizes above and below this size should be immediately available. One can determine that a correct size has been by checking for the pressure at which a leak develops around the tube. The tube should be secured immediately, with as little patient movement as possible afterward so as to minimize the likelihood of tube dislodgement.

Supportive Therapy

A second- or third-generation cephalosporin such as cefuroxime, cefotaxime, or ceftriaxone is generally administered to ensure adequate coverage of *H. influenzae*. With the increasing incidence of *S. pneumoniae* as a cause for epiglottitis and the marked increase in resistance of this organism to cephalosporins, one can empirically give vancomycin also. Some recommend adding nafcillin instead, based on the increasing incidence of gram-positive cocci, including *S. aureus*, as etiologic agents. Blood cultures are positive in 80 to 90 percent of patients. Cultures of the epiglottis itself are much less sensitive. Typically oral antibiotics are continued for 7 to 10 days after the patient is extubated.

VIRAL CROUP

Viral croup (laryngotracheitis or laryngotracheobronchitis) is responsible for more than 90 percent of cases of stridor outside of the neonatal period. About $20 to $76 million per year is spent in the United States alone on health care related to viral croup. Children 6 months to 3 years of age are most commonly affected, with a peak incidence between 1 and 2 years of age.[5] It is uncommon after age 6. This is due to the much greater effect of a small amount of mucosal edema and inflammation in the airway of a small child versus that of an adult. As little as 1 mm of airway edema in an infant may cause a decrease in cross-sectional area of 50 to 60 percent. This leads to increased resistance and work of breathing. In the adult airway, 1 mm of edema is nearly inconsequential. The incidence of true croup is thought to be equal in males and females, but many authors believe that moderate to severe cases are twice as common in males. Most cases occur in the late fall or early winter.

Acute viral croup is thought to be on a continuum with spasmodic croup. It is very difficult or impossible to differentiate them prospectively. Retrospectively, spasmodic croup is seen more commonly in atopic children, has no seasonal variation, usually has almost complete symptom resolution within 6 h, is not characteristically associated with fever, and is often recurrent. Both spasmodic croup and acute viral croup have nocturnal exacerbations.

Etiology

Practically all cases are viral. Parainfluenza virus types I, II, and III are most common by far, but sometimes indistinguishable syndromes can be caused by influenza A or B, respiratory syncytial virus (RSV), rhinoviruses, adenoviruses, and even measles virus. Cases caused by adenovirus may be associated with hemorrhagic cystitis and conjunctivitis. Measles pneumonitis should be considered in atypical cases and, if suspected, treated aggressively. In unimmunized or immunosuppressed adults, measles pneumonitis is not uncommonly fatal. The incubation period for parainfluenza virus is 2 to 6 days. These viruses are usually shed for about 2 weeks. In cases caused by RSV, the shedding may continue for a much longer period and symptoms may take months to clear completely. In children over the age of 5, *Mycoplasma pneumoniae* infection has also been associated with a croup-like syndrome.

Signs and Symptoms

There is typically a 1- to 5-day prodrome consisting of cough, coryza, and occasionally other upper respiratory infection–type symptoms. This is followed by a 3- to 4-day period of barking cough. The cough is typically worse in the late evening and at night and may occur strictly during these times. Children may or may not have a low-grade fever during the illness. The typical duration of symptoms ranges from 3 to 7 days regardless of the treatment. Typically the third and fourth days are the worst, and then the child starts to improve. Children who do not follow this general course should be reevaluated.

Viral croup is classically associated with biphasic stridor, although often the inspiratory component is much greater than the expiratory component. Stridor is unaffected by position but increases with crying or agitation. Intercostal retractions and tachypnea are common signs. The voice is often hoarse but not muffled. If inflammation extends from the trachea to the more distal bronchi, wheezing or crackles will be present.

Diagnosis

Croup is a clinical diagnosis. Generally laboratory tests are unnecessary. The white count is typically normal or with a slight lymphocytosis. Blood cultures or nasopharyngeal washings are not clinically useful, since knowing the exact etiologic agent does not change management.

Radiographs are primarily used to help rule out other causes of stridor in atypical or prolonged cases. A lateral neck film and posteroanterior (PA) chest radiograph should be obtained as appropriate. The aryepiglottic area is normal. The lateral neck radiograph may demonstrate slightly ill-defined tracheal air shadows, narrowing on inspiration greater than that on expiration, and slight distention of the hypopharynx. Typically fixed subglottic obstructions—such as papillomas, foreign bodies, hemangiomas, and subglottic stenosis—cause narrowing of the airway that does not change with the phase of respiration. Many of the latter noncroup causes also cause asymmetry in appearance, whereas croup causes symmetrical changes in the air column. The PA chest x-ray is most useful to rule out radiopaque foreign body. In cases of croup, the normally squared shoulders of the subglottic tracheal air shadow will appear more like a "steeple," "pencil tip," "nail," or "hourglass."

General Treatment

Pulse oximetry should be measured and supplemental humidified oxygen given. Children with croup should not be sedated except in the course of a rapid-sequence intubation. Antibiotics are not indicated for patients with a confident diagnosis of croup. Antipyretics should be given for fever to decrease the required minute ventilation and work of breathing. The least invasive route possible should be used to provide hydration, to replace insensible water losses from respiratory distress and fever. Urine output, or the number of wet diapers, should be monitored and intravenous hydration provided if necessary.

Exposure to humidified air, either cold night air or moist air from a shower, is used to treat this disease, but it is not known why this is effective. Nebulization tents, or "croup tents," are no longer used. A tent isolates the child and enshrouds it in a mist, making the child more anxious and difficult to monitor. Furthermore, it is very difficult to maintain an adequate concentration of oxygen within the tent.

In general, calculating a croup score (Table 129-3) is more useful as a research tool than as an adjunct to clinical practice. Its primary use is to provide a semiobjective scale by which to cohort patients for comparative studies. Its usefulness as a tool for clinical decision making with individual patients is much less clear. The score, if calculated, should only be used as one piece of data in the decision-making process. For example, a child with severe retractions and markedly decreased air entry may have a score of only 5 but would be considered at high risk by most clinicians and treated aggressively. Generally, healthy appearing children with stridor only when agitated do not require treatment with epinephrine. Children with stridor at rest or whom appear in distress should receive epinephrine as discussed below. All children receiving catecholamines should receive steroids as well. The use of steroids, as discussed below, is generally agreed upon in moderate to severe episodes of croup. In mild croup controversy exists regarding the absolute need of steroid treatment but there is some evidence showing benefit in this population as well. The use of steroids in the mildest cases should be decided on an individual case-by-case basis and may vary between reasonable clinicians. Further research, using clinically important endpoints and number-to-treat analysis, should help to clarify their use in this patient population.

Epinephrine

Racemic epinephrine, a nearly equimolar mixture of the two isomers (D and L) of epinephrine, is a mainstay of moderate to severe croup treatment. The majority of its activity is due to the L-isomer. The D-isomer is only about 30 percent as active as the L-isomer. The drug is quite effective when nebulized. Positive effects can be seen in as little as 10 min, with maximal effects seen in about 1 h. In most cases its pharmacologic effects are practically gone by 2 h. Nebulized epinephrine has clearly been shown to decrease airway edema, most likely by vasoconstriction of the boggy mucosal vessels. Its use does not change the natural course of disease, but it does improve ventilation. Use of racemic epinephrine decreases the number of children

TABLE 129-3 Modified Westley Croup Score*

Clinical Indicators	Score
Inspiratory stridor	
None	0
At rest, with stethoscope	1
At rest, no stethoscope required to hear	2
Level of consciousness	
Normal	0
Altered	5
Air entry	
Normal	0
Decreased	1
Severely decreased	2
Cyanosis	
None	0
Agitated	4
Resting	5
Retractions	
None	0
Mild	1
Moderate	2
Severe	3
	Total =

**Note:* Multiple variations of this are used in the literature. When discussing scores, one must know which scale is being used. Score of 8 or greater indicates respiratory failure.
Source: Adapted from Super DM, Cartelli NA, Brooks LJ, et al: A prospective randomized double-blind study to evaluate the effect of dexamethasone in acute laryngotracheitis. *J Pediatr* 115:323, 1989, with permission.

with croup requiring intubation, intensive care unit admission, and general admission to the hospital.

L-epinephrine, a pure isomer, is used as an advanced cardiac life support (ACLS) drug in a 1:1000 concentration. Although only recently subjected to evidence-based scrutiny,[6] this form has been used exclusively in many foreign countries for years. The L-isomer is at least as effective and safe as racemic epinephrine (Table 129-4).[6] Although some forms contain sulfur dioxide, a known respiratory irritant, this has not been reported to cause any significant problems in this patient group.[6] Both racemic and L-epinephrine are relatively contraindicated in patients with severe left ventricular outflow obstruction (idiopathic hypertrophic subaortic stenosis, subvalvular aortic stenosis, etc.) because it may worsen the obstruction.[7] When the drug is used in these patients, very close monitoring is indicated.

Ledwith's group monitored patients for 3 h after epinephrine nebulization and found that 38 percent of the patients who had a recurrence

TABLE 129-5 Discharge Criteria

At least 3 h since last epinephrine
Nontoxic appearance
Able to take fluids well
Not clinically dehydrated (labs not necessary)
Room-air oxygen saturation greater than 90%
Age greater than 6–12 months*
Weather conditions allow rapid return to ED for worsening
Parents have a phone and no social issues of concern
Caretaker seems able to recognize change in child's clinical status
Relatively short transit time from home to hospital

*Controversial.
Source: Adapted from: Kunkel NC, Baker D: Use of racemic epinephrine, dexamethasone, and mist in the outpatient management of croup. *Pediatr Emerg Care* 12:156, 1996.

requiring admission did so between the second and third hour.[8] Prendergast et al. also demonstrated that there was an upward trend in the croup score between the second and third hours only in those patients ultimately requiring admission.[9] The current standard of care for moderate to severe croup is to administer nebulized epinephrine with early steroids (see below) and monitor these patients in the ED for at least 3 h before considering discharge (Table 129-5).

Dexamethasone

The literature clearly demonstrates clinical benefits of steroid use in moderate to severe croup.[10,11] It suggests benefits in mild croup as well. Steroids should be given within 1 h of presentation, and early effects of steroid use may be seen at ½ to 2 h. Most likely this is due to vasocontriction of the edematous mucosa. Their effects on immune modulation and protein synthesis occur later and may be responsible for the longer-term clinical benefits seen with these agents. Certainly any child receiving nebulized epinephrine should also receive steroids.[7]

Dexamethasone, a fluorinated derivative of prednisolone, has anti-inflammatory effects about 25 times greater than those of hydrocortisone at equal doses. It has minimal to no mineralocorticoid effect. Its half-life is about 2 days (range 36 to 72 h).[12] Peak effects are seen in 2 h with persistent effects over the next few weeks. Early studies used 0.6 mg/kg of dexamethasone, so this became the standard to which other doses and interventions were compared. It was then shown that doses greater than 0.3 mg/kg were clearly beneficial, but doses less than this had marginal benefit. More recently, Geelhoed's group demonstrated that 0.15 mg/kg was equivalent to 0.6 mg/kg when given

TABLE 129-4 Epinephrine for Stridor

Drug	Concentration	Accurate Dosing*	Quick Dosing
L-epinephrine	1:1,000 1 mL = 1 mg	0.5 mL/kg (max 5 mL)	2.5 mL < 1 year 5 mL > 1 year
Racemic epinephrine	2.25% = 1.125% L	0.05 mL/kg (max 0.5 mL)	0.25 mL < 6 months 0.5 mL > 6 months

*Diluted if necessary with normal saline to make 3–5 mL total volume.

TABLE 129-6 Steroids for Croup

Steroid	Concentration	Dose	Route	Information
Dexamethasone	0.25, 0.5, 1, 1.5, 2, 4, 6 mg tablets	0.3 mg/kg	PO	Crush in juice, acetaminophen elixir, or applesauce
	4, 10, 20, 24, mg/mL	0.3 mg/kg	IV	Erratic GI absorption
	8, 16 mg/mL	0.3 mg/kg	IM	Minimize volume
	0.5 mg/5 mL elixir	0.3 mg/kg	PO	May contain 5% alcohol Taste varies by brand
	0.1, 1 mg/mL oral solution	0.3 mg/kg	PO	May contain 30% alcohol
Budesonide	2 mg/4 mL	2 mg	Nebulized	Not readily available
Prednisolone	5 mg/5 mL syrup	1 mg/kg	PO	Pediapred 5% alcohol
	15 mg/5 mL syrup	1 mg/kg	PO	Prelone
Prednisone	1, 2.5, 5, 10, 20, 50 mg tablets	1 mg/kg	PO	
	1,5 mg/mL syrup	1 mg/kg	PO	Poor taste

orally.[13] Until further studies confirm these findings, the recommended dose is 0.3 to 0.6 mg/kg.

No direct comparison of oral and parenteral dexamethasone has been made, but there is no reason to suspect that the oral route would be any less efficacious than the intramuscular route. Studies primarily from the adult asthma literature demonstrate near bioequivalence of intravenous and oral steroids. Giving steroids orally has become near standard practice for asthma and is becoming so for croup as well.[14] The greatest problem with giving oral steroids is vomiting and the bitter taste. Various steroid preparations are available (Table 129-6).[11] Using crushed dexamethasone tablets or giving the medication in small aliquots over the first 30 min is said to reduce the number of children who vomit.

More recent studies have investigated the use of nebulized steroids. If steroids could be selectively deposited at the area of inflammation, they could have a greater effect on the disease process with fewer side effects. Johnson's study using dexamethasone resulted in benefits that were not clinically significant and two children in the study developed bacterial tracheitis with associated neutropenia[15]; nebulized parenteral dexamethasone is therefore not recommended. Multiple other studies using budesonide have had more encouraging results[13,14,16–21] In fact, one study of hospitalized children with moderately severe croup was unable to show a difference in efficacy between nebulized budesonide and nebulized epinephrine.[16] A few conclusions can be drawn. Nebulized budesonide is at best equivalent to dexamethasone in the short term but possibly not quite as good if given later in the course of the disease.[13,18,19,22] Klassen's group found an increased number of repeat visits in their budesonide cohorts when compared with their oral dexamethasone cohort.[19] Johnson et al. found an overall decrease in admissions using nebulized budesonide but a further 15 percent reduction was found using intramuscular dexamethasone.[18] Results are mixed regarding an additive effect of nebulized budesonide used with parenteral steroids.[21] Budesonide use is more expensive, requires a nebulizer, increases nursing or respiratory therapy time at the bedside, and may frighten small children. Based on the currently available information, the use of nebulized steroids is not standard care.

A child with resting stridor, increased pCO_2, decreased pO_2, decreased mental status, cyanosis, age less than 1 year (some say 6 months), or a croup score above 8 (Table 129-3) should be considered in early respiratory failure and managed aggressively to prevent progression to pulmocardiac arrest.

Fortunately, if treated aggressively, less than 1 percent of admitted patients will need intubation. Intubation should be performed whenever clinically indicated by the most experienced operator available. A number of findings should prompt the clinician to strongly consider elective intubation. These include:

1. A croup score above 8 without rapid improvement
2. Two catecholamine nebulizations required within 1 h
3. Hourly nebulizations required beyond the second hour
4. Acute mental status changes associated with respiratory distress
5. Worsening respiratory failure despite onging treatment
6. Severe croup in a child with neonatal lung disease
7. Moderately severe to severe croup in a child who needs transfer (especially if by helicopter)

The cricoid cartilage is normally the narrowest part of the young child's airway and will be especially narrow in croup owing to inflammation of the tracheal mucosa. Postintubation subglottic stenosis can be minimized by using a tube that is 0.5 to 1.0 mm smaller than would be expected. Never force a tube through the cricoid ring.

Fiberoptic laryngoscopy should be considered in atypical or recurrent presentations of a crouplike syndrome. It may also be indicated in children who fail to respond to standard therapy and occasionally in the very young to rule out laryngomalacia and other congenital causes of stridor.[7]

Heliox

Helium is much less dense than either oxygen or nitrogen, and replacing the nitrogen in air with helium decreases its resistance to flow. Helium will increase ventilation in patients with nearly all types of upper airway obstruction.[23,24] It may also restore laminar flow, improving ventilation and ventilation/perfusion matching. The work of breathing also decreases. Carbon dioxide diffuses much faster through a helium-oxygen mixture than it does through a nitrogen-oxygen mixture. This may make ventilation more effective. The indications for the use of heliox use are still somewhat controversial.[24] Most would agree that children not requiring high-flow oxygen should be given a trial of heliox for poor ventilation secondary to upper airway partial obstruction. If nothing else, this may serve as a temporizing measure and allow for a more controlled intubation. Following intubation, helium may be given through the ventilator circuit as a mixture with oxygen. Volume and flow readings from the ventilator will be inaccurate if helium is used,[24] since ventilators are calibrated for use with a nitrogen-oxygen mixture.

One easily forgotten point is that oxygen and helium gas cannot occupy the same space. Due to the rule of partial pressures, if the helium concentration is increased, the oxygen concentration must decrease.

Helium's therapeutic effects are found only when its concentration makes up 60 to 80% of the inspired gas. Therefore, an individual who requires greater than 35 to 40% oxygen cannot use this modality. The flow of oxygen and helium must be high enough to exceed the patient's minute ventilation to prevent entrainment of room air and increased dead-space ventilation.

BACTERIAL TRACHEITIS

Bacterial tracheitis, also known as membranous croup or membranous laryngotracheobronchitis, is rare. It is generally caused by bacterial superinfection of an antecedent viral upper respiratory infection. It is most commonly seen in children less than 3 years of age, with a median age of incidence at $4\frac{1}{2}$ years. Nearly all reported cases have arisen in those between 3 months and 13 years of age. Typically, 2 to 7 days of a croup-like syndrome is followed by worsening symptoms and the development of a toxic appearance over a period of several hours. Children appear septic or similar in appearance to those with epiglottitis, with a few important differences.[25] As a rule, children with bacterial tracheitis have severe inspiratory and expiratory stridor, cough with occasional thick sputum production, a raspy or hoarse voice, and no dysphagia. Children with bacterial tracheitis may also complain of a gnawing or burning substernal chest discomfort.

The history, physical, laboratory, and radiologic findings may help diagnose less obvious cases in nontoxic-appearing patients. Most patients will have a markedly elevated white count with an impressive left shift. Blood cultures are typically negative. AP and lateral neck radiographs usually demonstrate subglottic narrowing of the trachea. Irregular densities may be seen within the trachea and its borders may appear ragged and indistinct.

Management is similar to that of epiglottitis. Ideally, these patients should go to the operating room for sedation, intubation, and bronchoscopy. Culture and Gram stain of the mucopurulent secretions should be obtained at this time. Gram-stain findings may help guide antibiotic therapy. In less severe cases without respiratory distress, bronchoscopy may be performed without immediate intubation. This is the exception to the rule, however, as greater than 85 percent of cases will require intubation.

Antibiotics effective against *S. aureus*, *S. pneumoniae*, and beta lactamase–producing gram-negative organisms such as *H. influenzae* and *M. catarrhalis* should be given empirically. Vancomycin and a third-generation cephalosporin, such as cefotaxime or ceftriaxone, are commonly used.

FOREIGN-BODY ASPIRATION

Demographics

The peak incidence of foreign body aspiration is in the 1- to 3-year age group. At least 90 percent of cases are seen in children under age 4, but it has been reported in infants as young as 3 months. In children younger than 6 months, foreign-body aspiration is often secondary to a feeding given by "a helpful sibling."

The most commonly aspirated foreign bodies fall into two groups: foods and toys.[26] The most dangerous objects are those that are cylindrical or small, smooth, and round. Commonly aspirated foods include peanuts, sunflower seeds, raisins, grapes, hot dogs, and smaller sausages.

Because of the large number of deaths due to the aspiration of toys, the federal government instituted the Consumer Product Safety Act of 1979,[27] which has decreased the incidence of toy aspiration. However, watch groups warn that most toys are not properly evaluated for safety prior to marketing. Consumer scrutiny by direct inspection of the toy in addition to reading any warning label and the appropriate age range printed on its carton should be stressed in providing anticipatory guidance to the parents of young children.

Although small, round metal objects typically do not cause tissue reactions, this is not the case with vegetable matter. Aspirated vegetable matter commonly causes an intense pneumonitis and subsequent pneumonia and/or suppurative bronchitis. Aspirated vegetable matter is commonly difficult to remove if not found early, as it swells with the absorption of moisture from the surrounding lung and, if left long enough, may even sprout.

At presentation, many patients with foreign-body aspiration may be completely asymptomatic with a normal physical exam. Some data suggest that the majority will present or have presented previously with symptoms consistent with but not specific for foreign body aspiration. The study of Laks and Barzilay demonstrated fever in 36 percent, wheeze in 35 percent, crackles in 38 percent, and tachypnea in 45 percent of patients at presentation.[29] Although the location of the aspirated foreign body does play a role in determining the symptoms and signs seen on presentation, there is overlap between groups. Classic dogma is that laryngotracheal foreign bodies cause stridor, whereas bronchial foreign bodies cause wheeze. Studies have shown, however, that about 30 percent of laryngotracheal foreign bodies and up to 10 percent of bronchial foreign bodies will demonstrate wheezing and stridor respectively. More importantly, a significant proportion will have no cough, wheeze, or stridor. It is true that the majority of patients presenting with severe immediate onset stridor or cardiac arrest after aspiration will be found to have a laryngotracheal foreign body. Patients with alternating wheezing and stridor may have a mobile foreign body. Other signs and symptoms of foreign-body aspiration may include cough, history of a choking episode, history of persistent or recurrent pneumonia, apnea, pharyngeal pain, or persistent symptoms of croup or asthma remaining after adequate treatment for 5 to 7 days. Foreign-body aspiration should be considered in all children given a diagnosis of "unilateral wheeze." Upper esophageal foreign bodies may impinge upon the posterior aspect of the trachea, leading to signs and symptoms of airway obstruction. Commonly the patient will present with stridor. Contrary to most cases of airway aspiration, patients with an esophageal foreign body typically will have dysphagia.

Diagnosis

Only one-fourth of patients who have aspirated a foreign body present within 24 h of the event. A high index of suspicion is required to diagnose this disorder. Foreign-body aspiration should always at least be considered in a young child with respiratory symptoms. If the clinical scenario clearly indicates the presence of a foreign body or airway obstruction, the hospital's protocol for obstructed airway should be implemented immediately. When a diagnosis is considered in a stable child, plain radiographs may be helpful if positive. Clinicians should never rule out a foreign-body aspiration based only on plain radiographs, as they may be entirely normal in up to one-third of bronchoscopically proven cases of foreign-body aspiration. Friedman's review found that only 7 percent of aspirated foreign bodies were radiopaque.[30]

Nonradiopaque foreign bodies at the laryngeal or tracheal locations may be identified by looking for telltale air contrast of the foreign body in relation to the surrounding normal soft tissues. Computed tomography (CT) may be helpful. In most cases, however, additional radiologic procedures are not ideal, and laryngoscopy and rigid bronchoscopy are indicated.

In cases of complete obstruction, segmental atelectasis may be seen on plain radiographs. In other cases, intermittent or partial obstruction occurs, creating a ball-valve effect (Fig. 129-4). In these cases, additional radiographs or fluoroscopy may be helpful. Partial obstruction, most commonly of the right mainstem bronchus, may cause obstructive emphysema of the involved lung by allowing air past the obstruction on inhalation but preventing its passage on exhalation. In cooperative, stable children, inspiratory and expiratory PA chest radiographs looking for hyperinflation of the involved lung with contralateral mediasti-

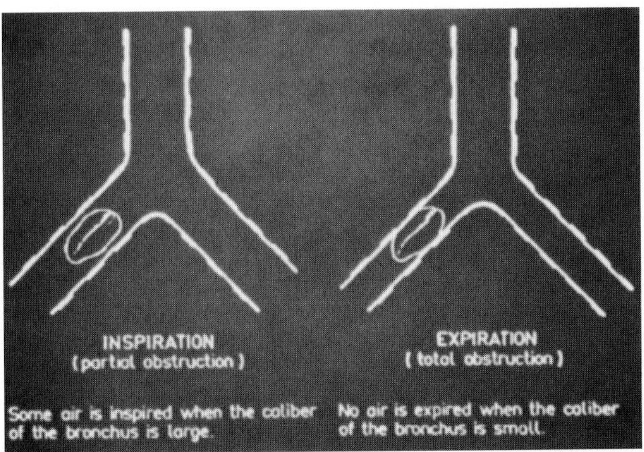

FIG. 129-4. Inspiratory and expiratory films in foreign-body aspiration.

nal shift and decreased excursion of the ipsilateral diaphragm may be indicated. Forced expiration by having a parent gently push on the child's lower abdomen during expiration may increase the sensitivity, but this has not been adequately studied. In young or uncooperative children, the ball-valve phenomenon may best be demonstrated by fluoroscopy. Bilateral decubitus PA chest radiographs may also be used but are less sensitive than fluoroscopy. The obstructed side will remain fully inflated with the ipsilateral diaphragm inferiorly displaced when the involved side is down. When the unobstructed side is down, it will show the normal findings of diaphragmatic elevation, rib splinting, and decreased relative volume compared to the upside (Figs. 129-5 and 129-6). Series have demonstrated that bronchoscopically proven cases of foreign-body aspiration were definitively diagnosed preoperatively in only 60 percent of cases. Clinically suspected foreign-body aspiration should ultimately be ruled out by bronchoscopy.

Although uncommon, esophageal foreign bodies may cause stridor. Esophageal foreign bodies more commonly are radiopaque and are, therefore, more easily seen on plain radiography. In general, narrow, flat foreign bodies such as coins will be oriented in the coronal plane if they are in the esophagus. The tracheal cartilages with the exception of the cricoid ring are incomplete and horseshoe-shaped, with the opening directed posteriorly. These anatomic characteristics cause most narrow, flat radiopaque tracheal foreign bodies to be sagittally oriented on radiography. Certainly exceptions to these generalities do occur. Radiolucent foreign bodies in the esophagus may be suspected in many cases due to an air-fluid level or soft tissue changes in the area just cephalad to the obstruction. Older children may complain of something stuck in the throat. Discussion of esophageal foreign-body management is found in Chap. 72.

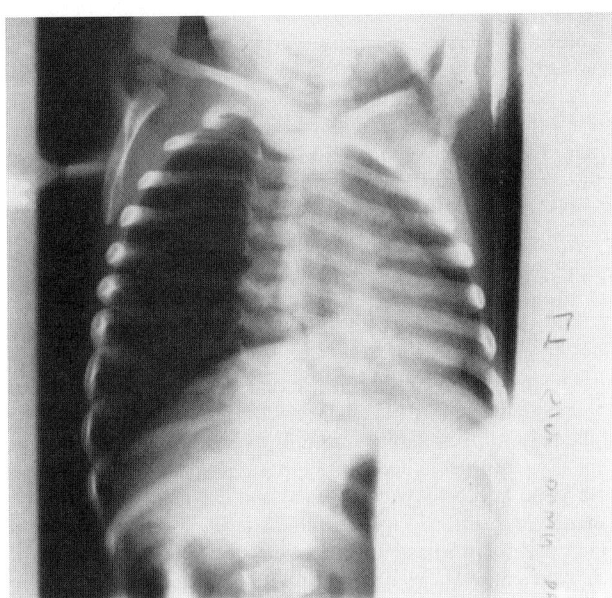

FIG. 129-5. Normal decubitus film with left side down.

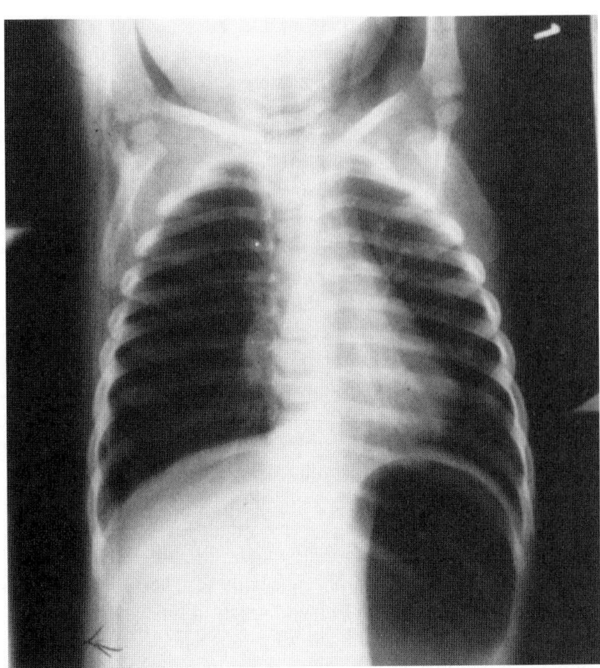

FIG. 129-6. Decubitus film, right side down, with foreign-body aspiration on the right side.

Treatment

If a child who is presumed to have aspirated a foreign body has severe signs and symptoms but is maintaining the airway, alert, and able to speak, the predetermined obstructed airway protocol should be instituted. If local personnel are not able to remove the foreign body, a transport team experienced in the management of the difficult pediatric airway should be summoned to the patient's location. Ideally, the transport team will have a physician member trained and experienced in the removal of foreign bodies and in the management of the difficult pediatric airway. In general, the foreign body should be removed. If not possible, in the case of a supralaryngeal foreign body, the child should be electively intubated prior to transport. Exceptions may occur based on clinical circumstances. Racemic epinephrine or heliox may be an alternative.

The outcome of patients with laryngotracheal foreign-body aspiration and sudden collapse or cardiopulmonary arrest primarily depends upon appropriate bystander basic life support and emergency medical system response. Basic pediatric cardiopulmonary resuscitation (CPR) and foreign-body removal are discussed in Chap. 10. If no spontaneous breathing is detected, two slow breaths should be given. If air does not enter easily, causing a rise of the chest, then the head-tilt chin-lift maneuver should be reapplied and rescue breaths reattempted. If still no air enters the lungs, foreign-body obstruction is likely. The child's mouth should be opened, and if a foreign body is visualized, it should be removed.

Relief of obstruction in the infant is performed by holding the infant in the head-down prone position and giving up to five forceful back blows between the infant's shoulder blades with the heel of one hand. The infant is then turned to the supine position and given five quick chest compressions one finger's breadth below the intermammillary line. Once again, the oropharynx should be opened, and if a foreign body is visualized, it should be removed. If not, the airway should be opened by the jaw-thrust chin-lift maneuver and rescue breathing should be attempted. If air does not enter the lungs, the head should be repositioned and the jaw-thrust chin-lift maneuver reapplied and rescue breathing reattempted. If still no air enters the lungs, back blows and chest thrusts should once again be administered.

In a child over 1 year of age, the same sequence should occur with the exception that no back blows are given and the Heimlich maneuver is used instead of chest thrusts. The Heimlich maneuver should be performed in the standard fashion well below the tip of the xiphoid and slightly above the navel in the midline. Five distinct upward thrusts should be administered followed by reevaluation of the airway and another attempt at rescue breathing. If, after two cycles, the airway in the infant or child is not opened, allowing passage of air during rescue breathing, direct laryngoscopy should be used to locate and remove the foreign body, if possible using McGill forceps.

If, upon laryngoscopy the foreign body is noted to be below the cricoid ring within the trachea, an endotracheal tube should be placed. The child can often be ventilated after this maneuver. One must be absolutely certain that air is actually entering the lungs, however, and not just filling the pharynx and stomach. If, after an endotracheal tube is placed, the child still cannot be ventilated, the endotracheal tube should be gently advanced in hope of pushing the foreign body from the trachea into one of the mainstem bronchi. The endotracheal tube is then withdrawn to its normal position and ventilation is attempted. If the foreign body is visualized at the glottis but cannot be removed, a needle cricothyroidotomy may be lifesaving. Esophageal foreign-body removal is typically a semielective procedure. Those esophageal foreign bodies causing a respiratory embarrassment or serious potential for gastrointestinal injury due to puncture, laceration, or corrosion should be removed by endoscopy. Esophageal foreign bodies not causing respiratory distress and thought to be of low risk to the gastrointestinal system if allowed to pass should be monitored for progression toward the stomach over 8 to 12 h.

PERITONSILLAR ABSCESS

Peritonsillar abscess in children most commonly presents in adolescents with an antecedent sore throat. Often there is a period of improvement prior to the onset of progressive worsening symptoms. Peritonsillar abscess may rarely occur in the younger child. Most commonly, patients appear acutely ill with fevers, chills, dysphagia, trismus, drooling, or a muffled or "hot potato" voice. When present, trismus is thought to be due to secondary inflammation of the neighboring pterygoid muscles. These children may have ipsilateral ear pain and torticollis. Torticollis may represent an attempt to relax the ipsilateral sternocleidomastoid muscle so as to decrease pressure on the peritonsillar space.

The peritonsillar space is not limited to the area surrounding the superior aspect of the tonsil visualized during the oropharyngeal exam. In fact, this potential space extends from the area lateral to the adenoids to the area of the pyriform sinus. Once a tonsillar infection has escaped the boundary of the tonsillar capsule, purulent material may flow relatively freely throughout this area. These anatomic relationships are important to remember, as they help to explain the classic physical findings of this disease process.

Careful visualization of the oral cavity is a must to reliably rule out this infection. The majority of cases will involve the superior aspect of the peritonsillar space, which can lead to discovery with meticulous examination. This may be nearly impossible in the young child with trismus. Diagnosis in this case is much more difficult. In this instance, some have recommended CT scanning of the oropharyngeal and cervical soft tissues, while others believe that this practice may be dangerous as the child could acutely obstruct the airway.[31] One possible alternative is an ultrasound examination at the bedside. Ultrasound has been used for drainage of peritonsillar abscess in difficult or complicated cases for some time with good success.

Typically, however, bilateral tonsillar erythema and exudate will be noted on exam. The uvula and anterior pillar of the tonsil on the affected side may be displaced away from the involved tonsil. The involved tonsil is, as a rule, anteriorly and medially displaced. Cervical adenopathy is often present but does not differentiate this process from the much more common causes of pharyngitis.

When uvular deviation, marked soft palate displacement, severe trismus, airway compromise, or localized areas of fluctuance are noted, the diagnosis of peritonsillar abscess can be made with confidence and no imaging study is required. In less obvious cases with minimal or no trismus, no localized areas of fluctuance, and no displacement of pharyngeal structures, differentiating peritonsillar abscess from peritonsillar cellulitis is difficult. If a child appears toxic, the diagnosis should certainly be considered peritonsillar abscess until proven otherwise. In younger children, imaging may be required to help differentiate these processes (see above). In nontoxic-appearing adolescents with good follow-up, involved parents, and findings most consistent with peritonsillar cellulitis, a trial of antibiotics may be the best choice for initial treatment. Penicillin or clindamycin are most commonly used.

The definitive treatment of peritonsillar abscess has changed significantly over the last decade. Previously, most cases were taken to the operating room for incision and drainage. Today, the majority of cases are treated as outpatients with needle aspiration, antibiotics, and pain control. Clearly, definitive follow-up is a must. The local protocol and individual physician comfort should dictate who performs the peritonsillar abscess aspiration. Very young and uncooperative children may be better served with formal incision and drainage in the operating room. The patient must be under control during needle aspiration to prevent injury the jugular vein and carotid artery.[30] In general, a single episode of peritonsillar abscess is not an indication for tonsillectomy.

RETROPHARYNGEAL ABSCESS

Demographics

Retropharyngeal abscess, although rare, is the second most commonly seen infection of the deep neck space.[33] The usual age range is 6 months to 4 years, with peak incidence in infants. Retropharyngeal abscess is quite rare after age 4 because repeated upper respiratory–type infections have obliterated the retropharyngeal lymph nodes by this age in most children. Most cases of retropharyngeal abscess evolve insidiously over a few days after a relatively minor upper respiratory infection or pharyngitis. Localized trauma to the posterior pharyngeal wall is another cause. This most commonly occurs in children who fall with a stick or similar object in their mouths.

Anatomic Relationships

Two major cervical lymph node chains enter the retropharyngeal space. They drain lymph not only from the nasopharynx but also the adenoids and the posterior paranasal sinuses. The retropharyngeal space is the potential space located between the posterior pharyngeal wall (more properly the buccopharyngeal fascia) and the prevertebral fascia. It extends from the base of the skull to the level of T1 or T2 in the area of the posterior mediastinum. It is the only deep neck space that extends the entire length of the neck. Anatomists believe that it may actually be in continuity with the prevertebral space, which extends to the level of the psoas muscle. For this reason or due to erosion

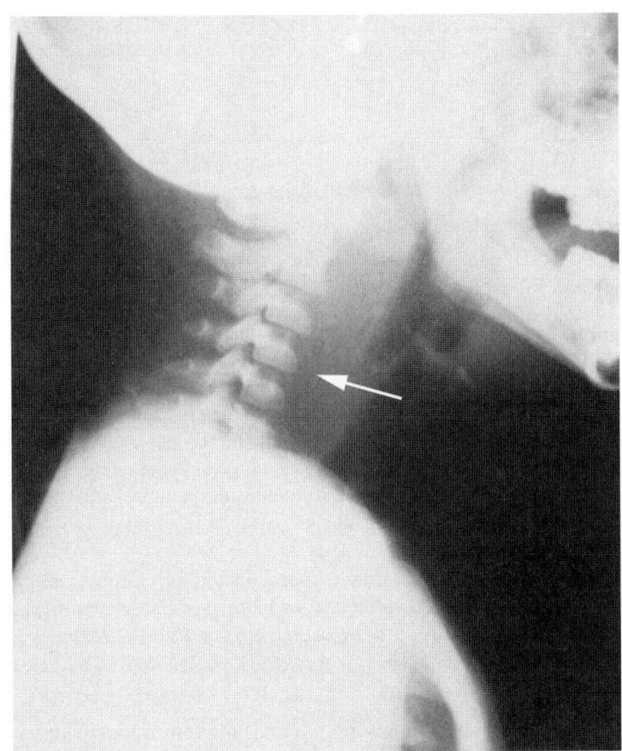

FIG. 129-7. Lateral neck view of a child with retropharyngeal abscess and widened retropharyngeal space.

through the prevertebral fascia, infections in the retropharyngeal space are known to have extended this entire length.

Signs and Symptoms

The symptoms most commonly found in patients with retropharyngeal abscess are, individually, not specific for this disease, but, taken together, they point toward the correct diagnosis. Although the symptoms are not commonly recognized in preverbal children, older children will complain of sore throat and most have a history of high fever. Other symptoms include dysphagia, decreased oral intake, and stiff neck.

In general, children with retropharyngeal abscess appear quite ill. Signs of retropharyngeal abscess include muffled voice, persistently hyperextended neck, inspiratory stridor, meningismus, and, if partial airway obstruction is present, respiratory distress and tachypnea. Ipsilateral cervical adenopathy has also been described but is not specific. Often a unilateral or bilateral retropharyngeal mass can be visualized during examination of the oropharynx. Unilateral masses are typically easier to detect than bilateral ones. Although palpation will commonly demonstrate fluctuance, this practice is dangerous and unnecessary. Laboratory testing is neither sensitive nor specific for retropharyngeal abscess.

Classic teaching is that a lateral neck radiograph should be obtained when one suspects this infection. This radiograph should be taken during inspiration with the neck extended so as to limit false-positive results. Diagnostic criteria for this radiograph are controversial (Fig. 129-7). Most would agree that the normal prevertebral soft tissue should be no wider at the second cervical vertebra than the diameter of the vertebral body at the same level. Radiographs showing slightly wider prevertebral soft tissues at this level without obvious bulging have a low specificity for retropharyngeal abscess. If the criterion for a positive test is considered two times the diameter of the vertebral body at the same level, the sensitivity is about 90 percent, but the specificity still not very good unless air-fluid levels are seen within the retropharyngeal soft tissues.[5] Still others have suggested using values of 7-mm prevertebral soft tissue width at C2 and 14-mm prevertebral soft tissue width at C6 as the criteria for the presence of a retropharyngeal abscess. The sensitivity and specificity of these criteria would seem to be quite dependent on the age and position of the patient. Ravindranath et al. found no correlation between the findings on lateral neck radiographs and CT scans in patients who clinically appeared to have a retropharyngeal abscess.[34] Therefore, definitive diagnosis should be based on CT scan results whenever possible. CT scan differentiates cellulitis from abscess and helps with surgical planning by demonstrating the degree of extension that has occurred.[5] It can also be used to clarify equivocal x-ray findings.[34] CT's sensitivity for retropharyngeal abscess is thought to be near 100 percent.[5] Unstable patients should be intubated before going to the CT scan suite. A physician accustomed to managing the difficult pediatric airway and appropriate equipment should accompany stable patients.

Treatment

After the airway has been stabilized, the patient should receive analgesia and in most cases be prepared for surgery. Retropharyngeal cellulitis and very small localized abscesses may do well with antibiotics alone. All other cases should undergo an incision and drainage procedure. These decisions should be made in consultation with an otolaryngologist.

Most retropharyngeal abscesses are found to contain mixed flora when cultured. Common organisms include *S. aureus*, *S. pyogenes*, *S. viridans*, and beta lactamase–producing gram-negative rods such as *Klebsiella*. Oral anaerobes such as *Peptostreptococcus* species, *Fusobacterium* species, and *Bacteroides* species are also frequently seen. Antibiotic choice is controversial. Single-agent therapy with ampicillin/sulbactam may be best. Others use clindamycin and/or nafcillin with a third-generation cephalosporin. Some believe that high-dose penicillin G is most appropriate. In patients who are not allergic to penicillin, ampicillin/sulbactam provides the broadest coverage of the potential etiologic agents. Penicillin-allergic patients who are not known to be allergic to cephalosporins may achieve the best results with clindamycin and a third-generation cephalosporin.

Most patients do quite well, but complications do occur. Airway obstruction from sudden rupture of the abscess cavity can be rapidly fatal. Aspiration pneumonia, empyema, and frank asphyxia are described. Abscess extension throughout the neck and even to the psoas may occur. With extension, mediastinitis may develop. Erosion into the carotid artery and internal jugular vein thrombosis has been reported.

REFERENCES

1. Rothrock SG, Perkin R: Stridor: A review, update, and current management recommendations. *Pediatr Emerg Med Rep* 1:29, 1996.
2. Mancuso RF: Stridor in neonates. *Pediatr Clin North Am* 43:1339, 1996.
3. Tobias JD: Laryngeal mask airway: A review for the emergency physician. *Pediatr Emerg Care* 12:370, 1996.
4. Gorelick MH, Baker MD: Epiglottitis in children, 1979–1992: Effects of Haemophilus influenzae type B immunization. *Arch Pediatr Adolesc Med* 148:47, 1994.
5. Bank DE, Krug SE: New approaches to upper airway disease. *Emergency Med Clin North Am* 13:473, 1995.
6. Waisman Y, Klein BL, Boenning DA, et al: Prospective randomized double-blind study comparing L-epinephrine and racemic epinephrine aerosols in the treatment of laryngotracheitis (croup). *Pediatrics* 89:302, 1992.
7. Cressman WR, Myer NM III: Diagnosis and management of croup and epiglottitis. *Pediatr Clin North Am* 41:265, 1994.
8. Ledwith CA, Shea LM, Mauro RD: Safety and efficacy of nebulized racemic epinephrine in conjunction with oral dexamethasone and mist in the outpatient treatment of croup. *Ann Emerg Med* 25:331, 1995.
9. Prendergast M, Jones JS, Hartman D: Racemic epinephrine in the treatment of laryngotracheitis: Can we identify children for outpatient therapy? *Am J Emerg Med* 12:613, 1994.

10. Cruz MN, Stewart G, Rosenberg N: Use of dexamethasone in outpatient management of acute laryngotracheitis. *Pediatrics* 96:220, 1995.
11. Tibbals J, Shann FA, Landau LI: Placebo-controlled trial of prednisolone in children intubated for croup. *Lancet* 340:745, 1992.
12. Kunkel NC, Baker D: Use of racemic epinephrine, dexamethasone, and mist in the outpatient management of croup. *Pediatr Emerg Care* 12:156, 1996.
13. Geelhoed GC, Macdonald WPG: Oral and inhaled steroids in croup: A randomized, placebo-controlled trial. *Pediatr Pulmonol* 20:355, 1995.
14. Klassen TP, Rowe PC: Outpatient management of croup. *Curr Opin Pediatr* 8:449, 1996.
15. Johnson DW, Schuh S, Koren G, et al: Outpatient treatment of croup with nebulized dexamethasone. *Arch Pediatr Adolesc Med* 150:349, 1996.
16. Fitzgerald D, Mellis C, Johnson M, et al: Nebulized budesonide is as effective as nebulized adrenalin in moderately severe croup. *Pediatrics* 97:722, 1996.
17. Husby S, Agertoft L, Nortensen S, et al: Treatment of croup with nebulized steroid (budesonide): A double blind, placebo controlled study. *Arch Dis Child* 68:352, 1993.
18. Johnson DW, Jacobsen S, Edney PC, et al: A comparison of nebulized budesonide, intramuscular dexamethasone, and placebo for moderately severe croup. *N Engl J Med* 339:498–503, 1998.
19. Klassen TP, Craig WR, Moher D, et al: Nebulized budesonide and oral dexamethasone for treatment of croup: A randomized controlled trial. *JAMA* 279:1629, 1998.
20. Klassen TP, Feldman NE, Watters LK, et al: Nebulized budesonide for children with mild-to-moderate croup. *N Engl J Med* 331:285, 1994.
21. Klassen TP, Feldman ME, Watters LK, et al: The efficacy of nebulized budesonide in dexamethasone-treated outpatients with croup. *Pediatrics* 97:463, 1996.
22. Collier J: Inhaled budesonide and adrenalin for croup. *Drug Ther Bull* 34:23, 1996.
23. Anderson M, Szartengren M, Bylin G, et al: Deposition in asthmatics of particles inhaled in air or in helium-oxygen. *Am Rev Respir Dis* 147:524, 1993.
24. Tobias JD: Heliox in children with airway obstruction. *Pediatr Emerg Care* 13:29, 1997.
25. Bernstein T, Builli R, Jacobs B, et al: Is bacterial tracheitis changing? A fourteen-month experience in a pediatric intensive care unit. *Clin Infect Dis* 27:458, 1998.
26. Dean KH, Zimmerman PH: Tracheobronchial foreign bodies in children: A study of 94 cases. *Laryngoscope* 100:525, 1990.
27. Reilly JS: Prevention of aspiration in infants and children. Federal regulations. *Ann Otol Rhinol Laryngol* 99:273, 1990.
28. Losek JD: Diagnostic difficulties of foreign body aspiration in children. *Am J Emerg Care* 8:348, 1990.
29. Laks Y, Barzilay Z: Foreign body aspiration in childhood. *Pediatr Emerg Care* 4:102, 1988.
30. Friedman E: Foreign bodies in the pediatric aerodigestive tract. *Pediatr Ann* 17:640, 1988.
31. Friedman NR, et al: Peritonsillar abscess in early childhood. *Arch Otolaryngol Head Neck Surg* 123:630, 1997.
32. Yellon RF, Bluestone CD: Head and neck space infections in children, in Bluestone CD, Stoll SE, Kenna MA (eds): *Pediatric Otolaryngology*, 3d ed. Philadelphia: Saunders, 1996, pp 15–25.
33. Ungkanont K, Yellon RF, Weissman JL, et al: Head and neck space infections in infants and children. *Otolaryngol Head Neck Surg* 112:375, 1995.
34. Ravindranath T, Janakiraman N, Harris V: Computed tomography in diagnosing retropharyngeal abscess in children. *Clin Pediatr* 32:242, 1993.

ACUTE PAIN MANAGEMENT AND SEDATION IN CHILDREN

Erica Liebelt
Nadine Levick

Appropriate and safe treatment of pain and anxiety in children is an integral component of an emergency department's clinical practice. Children are reported to be less adequately treated for pain than their adult ED cohorts.[1]

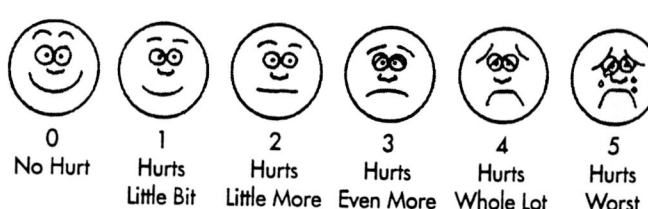

FIG. 130-1. FACES pain scale. (From Wong DL, Hockenberry-Eaton M, Wilson D, et al: *Whaley and Wong's Nursing Care of Infants and Children,* 6th ed. St Louis, Mosby, 1999, p 1153. Copyright © Mosby. Reprinted by permission.)

Pediatric pain experience, perception, and expression is determined by many factors, including the nature of the illness, injury, or procedure, developmental level, emotional and cognitive state, personal concerns, the meaning of pain, family attitudes, culture, and the environment. Basically, anything that is painful for an adult is likely to be painful for a child.

Children experience fear and anxiety in addition to physical pain, and all must be assessed and managed in an age and developmentally appropriate fashion. Parents or caregivers are also distressed about the child's pain. The QUESTT approach is a useful tool in addressing pediatric pain management.[2]

*Q*uestion the child for a description and location of the pain, using age and culturally appropriate and familiar language. Toddlers, and some older children who have difficulty understanding pain scales, can usually locate pain by pointing to the affected part.

*U*se a pain rating scale (Figs. 130-1 and 130-2) to provide a quantitative measure of pain intensity. Scales differ in their developmental appropriateness, i.e., the child's ability to grasp numeracy, abstract thought, pictorial appreciation.

*E*valuate behavior and physiologic responses to pain, such as facial expression. This is particularly useful in nonverbal children.

*S*ecure parents'/caregivers' involvement. They know their child best. Encourage their involvement in pain assessment, and facilitate participation in the management.

*T*ake cause of pain into account. The nature of the pathology or type of procedure permits anticipation of the type, duration, and intensity of pain.

*T*ake action: Ensure that all appropriate modalities are enlisted to treat the specific disorder and the pain, with ongoing assessment and documentation of pain until it is resolved.

A child who presents to the ED without a guardian or adult consent should have life- and limb-threatening conditions and severe pain managed without delay. Each institution should have policies that outline the procedures to follow in such cases.

PAIN ASSESSMENT

Well-validated pain assessment tools are available.[3] Tools specific to an age group or developmental stage should be selected. Children who are developmentally delayed, emotionally disturbed, or non-English speaking require special assessment. Pain severity in infants must be inferred from physiologic and behavioral responses, but for the toddler and older child, subjective measures can be included. Parental involvement in pain assessment can be a valuable adjunct for relieving pain and anxiety.[4] Finally, pain measurement should be repeated and improvement assessed until pain has abated.

Objective (Nonself-Report) Pain Assessment

Physiologic changes from pain include tachycardia, tachypnea, crying, sweating, blood pressure elevation, decreased oxygen saturation, pupil dilation, flushing or pallor, nausea, and muscle tension. These parame-

TABLE 130-1 CRIES—for Neonates and Those 32 to 60 Weeks of Gestation: A Score of 4 or More Requires Intervention

	0	1	2
Cry quality	No	High pitched	Inconsolable
Requires O_2 for sat >95%	No	<30% O_2	>30% O_2
Changes in heart rate (HR) and blood pressure (BP)	= or < Preop	Increase <20% preop	Increase >20% preop
Expression	None	Grimace	Grunt
Sleepless	No	Frequent waking	Constantly awake

Source: Adapted from: Krechel SW, Bildner J. CRIES: a new neonatal postoperative pain measurement score. Initial testing of validity and reliability *Paediatr Anaesth* 5:53, 1995.

ters can be muted in persistent pain and can be confounded by fear, anxiety, or fever. Specific behaviors associated with pain include withdrawal of the painful part, pulling ears, or refusing to use a body part. The characteristic facial features of an infant in pain have been described: brows—lowered, drawn together; forehead—bulge between brows, vertical furrows; eyes—tightly closed; cheeks—raised; nose—broadened, bulging; mouth—open, squarish.

A number of objective numeric scores have been developed and validated for the assessment of pain intensity for infants and nonverbal toddlers. The CRIES scale was developed for the assessment of postoperative pain in neonates, or those 32 to 60 weeks of gestation, with a score of 4 or more requiring intervention (see Table 130-1). The CHEOPS score, a 13-point behavioral score for infants, which ranges from 4 (no pain) to 13 (worst pain) (see Table 130-2), is reliable in children under 5 years of age.

TABLE 130-2 CHEOPS (Children's Hospital of Eastern Ontario's Pain Scale)

Item	Behavior	Score
Cry	No cry Crying/moaning Scream	1 2 for either 3
Facial	Smiling Composed Grimace	0 1 2
Verbal	Positive, without complaints Not talking/nonpain complaints Pain complaints	1 for either 2 0
Torso	Neutral Shifting/tense/upright/shivering Restrained	1 2 for either 2
Touch	Not touching Reaching/touching/grabbing Restrained	1 2 for each 2
Legs	Neutral Squirming/kicking/drawn up/tensed Restrained	1 2 for each 2

13-point behavioral score: score 4 (no pain) to 13 (worst pain).
Source: Adapted from: McGrath PJ, Johnson G, Goodman JJ, et al: CHEOPS: A behavioral scale for rating postoperative pain in children, in Fields HL, Eubner R, Cervero R (eds.): *Advances in Pain Research and Therapy*. New York, Raven Press, 1985, vol 9, pp 395–402.

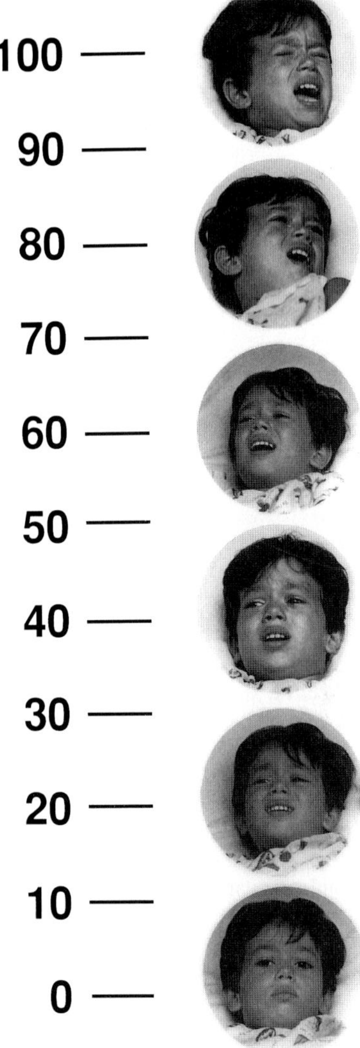

FIG. 130-2. Oucher pain scale. (The Hispanic version of the OUCHER was developed and copyrighted by Antonia M. Villarrael, PhD, RN (University of Pennsylvania) and Mary J. Denyes, PhD, RN (Wayne State University) in 1990. Reprinted with permission.)

Subjective (Self-Report) Pain Assessment

Self-reports can be used reliably for developmentally normal children over the age of four years. The pictorial FACES pain scale, which can be used for children age three years and up, demonstrates six cartoon facial expressions from no distress to extreme distress (Fig. 130-1): Face 0: happy, no hurt; Face 1: hurts a little bit; Face 2: hurts a little more; Face 3: hurts even more; Face 4: hurts whole lot; Face 5: hurts as much as you can imagine. It is useful in the ED setting as the scale is compact, can be purchased in the form of a pin or badge, and can pinned to a coat, making it always available. The Oucher pain scale is a photographic serial representation of children demonstrating the facial appearance of increasing intensity of pain. There are a number of versions of this assessment tool depicting various ethnic/racial groups. There are some limitations to its utility in the ED in that the photographic depiction cards are awkwardly large and are prone to being misplaced or removed. Numeric scales can be used with children age five years and older provided that they can count and have a concept of the relative magnitude of numbers. They also have the advantage of not requiring special photographic images. The Visual Analogue Scale (VAS) is a 0 to 10 numeric scale, which

TABLE 130-3 Nonpharmacological Pain Relief Techniques for Children

Before Procedure	During Procedure	After Procedure
Preparation rehearsal	Parental presence	Medical play
Medical play	Distraction	Positive incentive reward
Breathing/relaxation	Breathing/relaxation	Breathing/relaxation
Guided imagery	Guided imagery	Tactile stimulation
Desensitization	Muscle relaxation	
Thought stopping	Music	
Hypnosis	Hypnosis	
	Positive self-talk	
	Comfort measures	
	Tactile stimulation	

Adapted from: Wyman CI. Conscious sedation: a self study guide. http://gasnet.med.yale.edu/reference/protocols/sedation/index.html

requires a degree of abstract thought, can be used in children age 7 years and older. The VAS and numeric scales are easy to use in the ED, and require no specific equipment.

PAIN TREATMENT

Nonpharmacologic Modalities

Cognitive behavioral and physical techniques are useful nonpharmacological adjuncts to pediatric acute pain management.[5] Several simple, age- and development-specific interventions can significantly decrease a child's anxiety and later pain perception. Cognitive behavioral modalities include reassurance and explanation, relaxation, distraction, music, psychoprophylaxis, biofeedback, and guided imagery. Environmental alterations, such as dimmed lights, a quiet room, or stereo headphones may relieve anxiety. Distraction techniques such as story telling, singing, and games are effective. Guided imagery can be used with children as young as three or four years who have a rich fantasy world and can be encouraged to imagine their favorite place or activity. General strategies for nonpharmacological pain relief techniques are outlined in Table 130-3. Tables 130-4 through 130-8 suggest strategies that are best suited for infants, toddlers, preschoolers, school-age children, and adolescents. Physical techniques include kinesthetic or tactile stimulation, heat and cold applications and massage as well as the more complex modalities of transcutaneous electrical nerve stimulator (TENS), acupuncture, acupressure and electro-acupressure.

TABLE 130-4 Highlights of Child Development and Nonpharmacologic Pain Management Specifics: The Infant (0 to 12 Months)

Cannot verbalize pain

Displays pain by:
- Crying and facial expressions
- Physiologic changes; i.e., heart rate and respirations

Receptive to voice, touch, texture (i.e. warm blanket or heated room)

Benefit from tactile stimulation:
- Rocking, swaddling, patting, stroking and massaging

Comforted by:
- Sucking a pacifier during a procedure
- Sucking on the breast or bottle after a procedure

Can be distracted using bubbles, novel toys

Tables 130-4 through 130-7. All of these tables were constructed based on textual information from the following two sources:
Wyman CI. Conscious sedation: a self study guide. http://gasnet.med.yale.edu/reference/protocols/sedation/index.html
Acute Pain Management Guideline Panel. Acute Pain Management in Infants. Children, and Adolescents: Operative and Medical Procedures. Quick Reference Guide for Clinicians. AHCPR Publication No. 92-0020. February 1993. Rockville, MD: Agency for Health Care Policy and Research, Public Health Service, U.S. Department of Health and Human Services.

TABLE 130-5 Highlights of Child Development and Nonpharmacologic Pain Management Specifics: The Toddler (1 to 3 Years)

Capacity for basic reasoning and some understanding of causality

Age-appropriate language necessary

Benefit from tactile stimulation:
- Holding, patting, stroking, massage of the area

Easily distracted with:
- Books, puppets, music, action rhymes, bubble blowing, or other toys

Parental presence:
- Give parent a task
- Can help to calm a child
- *Not* to hold the child down or to perform any painful procedures

Cognitive/behavioral:
- Guided imagery
- Comfort from a blanket or toy from home
- Medical play with a doll and equipment before procedure
- Toy or small keepsake is a good reward after procedure

Pharmacologic Modalities

The choice of a pharmacologic agent for a pediatric patient's pain management should consider the nature of the procedure, the duration

TABLE 130-6 Highlights of Child Development and Nonpharmacologic Pain Management Specifics: The Preschooler (4 to 5 Years)

Thinks intuitively, believes there is a cause for everything

Does not understand temporal causality

Longer attention span and a higher level of interest than a toddler

Mixes fact with fiction, thinks magically

May still need to be held and stroked

May benefit from a comfort toy/blanket from home

Cognitive/behavioral:
- Some preschoolers like to watch the procedure, can hold pieces of equipment, etc. in preparation
- A doll and medical equipment can be used to explain procedure
- Guided imagery to remember and play out a super hero story or a cartoon character
- Distraction music, story telling, singing a song, remembering a movie, reciting nursery rhymes

A reward of a toy after procedure with discussion of this prior to procedure is effective

TABLE 130-7 Highlights of Child Development and Nonpharmacologic Pain Management Specifics: School Aged Child (6 to 12 Years)

Concrete operation, logical reasoning, can concentrate, delays gratification, knows the function and names of body parts, understands time, and generalizes from experience
May still need and benefit from a hug, a pat or a massage
Procedural rehearsal and preparation is effective
Benefit from: Verbal reward along with a toy or other incentive
Cognitive/Behavioral: Guided imagery used prior to and during the procedure Can be taught breathing and muscle relaxation techniques prior to the procedure Can use thought stopping and positive self-talk during procedure Parental presence is often welcome with this group, but ask the child May like to use a headset and listen to music or watch television or play video game

of the procedure, and the most appropriate route of administration. It should be made in conjunction with nonpharmacological techniques. Pharmacologic analgesic therapy can be systemic (opioids and nonopioids), or nonsystemic (local anesthetic agents with topical, local, or regional administration). There is a continuum between systemic analgesia and sedation. When narcotics are used, closely monitor patients, precalculate the appropriate dose of naloxone, and have resuscitation equipment readily available. Suggested systemic medications, dosages, routes of administration, and comments for non-opioid analgesics are outlined in Table 130-9 and for opioids in Table 130-10. Nonsystemic medications and techniques for administration, such as local anesthetic (LA) topical, local and regional procedures are discussed in detail in Chap. 32.

Avoidance of painful intramuscular and subcutaneous injections is particularly important when treating children. The intravenous route is recommended for titration of narcotic medications. Noninvasive topical or mucosal techniques for the delivery of systemic pharmacologic agents should be used where appropriate.

Systemic Pharmacologic Agents

ACETAMINOPHEN Acetaminophen is a commonly used analgesic and antipyretic that is useful for mild pain and as an adjunct for moderate pain in combination with codeine. Acetaminophen is rapidly absorbed from the gastrointestinal tract and is distributed throughout most body tissues. The plasma half-life is 1.25 to 3 h, but may be increased by liver disease and following overdosage. Elimination of acetaminophen is principally by liver metabolism (conjugation) and subsequent renal excretion of metabolites.

TABLE 130-8 Highlights of Child Development and Nonpharmacologic Pain Management Specifics: Adolescence (>13 Years)

Can deal with reality, uses abstract thinking, can synthesize direct information
Apprehension about self-image
Often does not want a parent in the room for procedures; ask the patient to decide
Any cognitive/behavioral techniques can be used
Discuss openly issues involving pain, and allow the teen to choose useful techniques

ASPIRIN Salicylates such as aspirin exhibit analgesic, anti-inflammatory, and antipyretic activity, and inhibit platelet aggregation. There is a strong association between Reye's syndrome and the use of aspirin in children, but the pathogenesis has not been determined. Aspirin must be used with caution, if at all, in children. Dehydrated patients who are more susceptible to salicylate toxicity even in therapeutic doses. The FDA advises that aspirin not be used in children with varicella or influenza.

NSAIDs Ibuprofen is a racemic mixture of two isomers. It has anti-inflammatory, antipyretic, and analgesic properties. The analgesic effect is related to inhibition of prostaglandin synthesis. It is used for children over six months of age as an alternative to acetaminophen. The most frequent adverse effects involve gastrointestinal (GI) tract irritation and renal dysfunction. Renal failure has been reported. Dehydrated patients are at higher risk for renal failure. There is a rare association with aseptic meningitis and severe hepatic reactions. Safety and efficacy have been established for children over six months of age.

Ketorolac is a pyrrolizine carboxylic acid derivative. It is an anti-inflammatory, antipyretic, and potent analgesic agent with similar actions and side effect profile to other NSAIDs, with slightly less GI irritation when given IV/IM than for oral NSAIDs. Overall, ketorolac has a lower incidence of side effects and longer duration of action than morphine. It acts peripherally, does not affect opiate receptors, and does not cause respiratory depression. Ketorolac is the only IV NSAID approved by the FDA. It may be used in combination with opioids, but has an opioid-sparing effect. Thus, smaller opioid dosages may provide adequate pain relief. It should not be admixed in the same syringe as opiates or hydroxyzine due to incompatibilities. Ketorolac also has good oral bioavailability, but has not been shown to be more efficacious than less expensive NSAID oral preparations. There is limited data on the use in children less than 16 years of age. In addition to GI irritation and platelet effects, ketorolac has been reported to adversely effect renal function, particularly in the dehydrated patient. Additionally, an increased risk of renal failure in patients on diuretics has been reported. Because ketorolac is highly protein-bound, it should be used cautiously in the presence of other protein-bound drugs such as warfarin. Interactions with renal clearance of lithium resulting in increased lithium levels have been reported. There is potential for cumulative adverse effects if ketorolac is combined with aspirin or other NSAIDs. There have been reports of bronchospasm and anaphylactoid reactions in adults. Duration of ketorolac therapy should not exceed five days.

OPIOIDS Narcotic or opioid medications remain the mainstay of analgesic pharmacotherapy for severe pain. Opioids include the phenanthrene derivatives (e.g., morphine, codeine, and hydromorphone), the phenylpiperidine derivatives (e.g., meperidine and fentanyl) and the diphenylheptane derivative (methadone). Close clinical and physiologic monitoring is essential with the use of opioids in the pediatric ED patient, as is an understanding of the relationship between level of pain, narcotic dose, and conscious state. Opioids in general have analgesic effects at lower doses than those required for sedation. A detailed discussion of opioid drugs is outlined in Chap. 34.

Morphine remains the gold standard opioid for the management of moderate to severe acute pain; it is widely used and easily reversed with naloxone. Its oral bioavailability is poor. Infants less than three months old are particularly sensitive to its respiratory depressant effects.

Hydromorphone (Dilaudid) is a hydrogenated ketone of morphine. It is well absorbed following oral, rectal or parenteral administration. It has a more rapid onset and a shorter duration of action than morphine

TABLE 130-9 Non-Opioid Analgesics

Drugs	Dose	Comments/Toxicity/Adverse Reactions
Acetaminophen (Paracetamol)	Oral: 10–15 mg/kg q 4 h Rectal: as above: (25–40 mg/kg 1st dose only)	No antiinflammatory activity Toxic dose: 140 mg/kg in 24 h Max dose: 75 mg/kg/d
Enteral NSAIDS		
Aspirin	Oral: 10–15 mg/kg q 4 h Rectal: as above	Reyes syndrome in children GI irritation, platelet dysfunction Tinnitus Max dose: 4 gm/d
Ibuprofen	Oral: 10 mg/kg q 6–8 h	GI irritation, platelet dysfunction Max dose: 40 mg/kg/day or 2.4 gm/d
Naproxen	Oral: 5–7 mg/kg q 12 h Rectal: as above	GI irritation, platelet dysfunction Max dose: 1.5 gm/d
Parenteral NSAIDs		
Keterolac	IV/IM: 0.5–1.0 mg/kg q 6 h	Platelet dysfunction GI irritation Use cautiously in patients with renal insufficiency or dehydration Do not use >5 d Max single dose: 30 mg IV/60 mg IM Max daily dose (IV)–120 mg/d

when given orally. Side effect profile is similar to morphine but less marked.

Meperidine is a synthetic derivative of morphine and is one-tenth as potent an analgesic per milligram of drug. Onset and duration of action is shorter than morphine and meperidine has slightly better oral bioavailability. Normeperidine (6-*N*-desmethyl-meperidine) is a toxic meperidine metabolite excreted through the kidney. Normeperidine is a cerebral irritant that can cause effects ranging from dysphoria and irritability to convulsions. Because of its unique toxicity, meperidine is contraindicated in patients with impaired renal function and in those receiving antidepressants of the monamine oxidase inhibitor class. These effects have been observed even in young, otherwise healthy patients who were given sufficiently high doses of normeperidine. Therefore, meperidine should be reserved for very brief courses in otherwise healthy patients who have demonstrated an unusual reaction or allergic response during treatment with other opioids, such as morphine or hydromorphone.

TABLE 130-10 Opioid Analgesics

	DOSE			
Drug	Enteral	Parenteral	Duration of Action	Toxicity/Adverse Reactions
Opioids				
Morphine	Oral: 0.3–0.5 mg/kg q 4–6h Onset: 15–30 min	IV: 0.05–0.15 mg/kg Onset: 5–10 min IM/SC: 0.1–0.2 mg/kg Onset: 15–30 min	2–4 h	Respiratory depression, (esp with IV push) Hypotension Nausea, vomiting
Codeine	Oral: 1–2 mg/kg q 4 h Onset: 30–60 min	IM: 0.5–1 mg/kg Onset: 10–30 min	4 h	Nausea Caution in renal failure Not recommended for IV use
Hydromorphone	Oral: 0.03 mg/kg q 4–6h Onset: 15–30 min	IV: 0.015 mg/kg Onset: 15 min	2–4 h	Less pruritus and nausea than morphine
Meperidine	Oral: 1–2 mg/kg q 3–4 h Onset: 15–30 min	IV or IM: 1–2 mg/kg Onset: IV 5–10 min IM 10–15 min	2–3 h	Respiratory depression (esp with IV push) Hypotension Seizures Avoid with MAO inhibitors
Oxycodone	Oral: 0.1 mg/kg q 4 h Onset: 10–15 min	N/A	3 h	Less nauseating than codeine
Fentanyl	Transmucosal: 10–15 μg/kg Onset: 15–20 min	IV: 1–3 μg/kg Onset: 1–2 min	30 min	Respiratory depression (esp with IV push) Chest wall rigidity (See text for treatment) Use $\frac{1}{3}$ dose in children <6 months Emesis with transmucosal prep
Opioid Antagonist				
Naloxone	N/A	IV/IM/IO/ETT: 0.001–0.01 mg/kg	30–40 min	Duration of action is shorter than agonists Potential for hypertension, pulmonary edema, and seizures particularly in opioid-dependent patients

Fentanyl is a short-acting synthetic opioid, 80 to 100 times as potent as morphine. When administered intravenously it has a rapid onset of action of less than 1 min and a short duration of action (15 to 30 min), due to its high lipid solubility and rapid redistribution. The major ED role for fentanyl is as an analgesic component for conscious sedation. In infants, it is less of a cardiovascular and respiratory depressant than morphine, and causes less histamine release, but the respiratory depressant effect may lag behind the analgesic effect. Fentanyl is associated with an idiosyncratic reaction of chest wall rigidity. This is more likely to occur with a high bolus dosing (5 μg/kg), but can occur with lower dosing (1 to 2 μg/kg). Small infants, less than 6 months of age, are at greater risk. The management approach for chest wall rigidity includes: naloxone 0.001 to 0.01 mg/kg or neuromuscular blockade (succinylcholine 2 mg/kg, or rocuronium 0.6 to 1.0 mg/kg, or pancuronium 0.1 mg/kg) and mechanical ventilation with 100 percent oxygen. Given the high concentration of fentanyl, exercise caution to avoid inadvertently flushing a residual bolus of the drug remaining in the IV line.

The new oral transmucosal fentanyl citrate (OTFC) (Oralet) preparation is a raspberry-flavored fentanyl-impregnated lozenge that allows administration of an opioid through oral transmucosal absorption. This nonthreatening ''needleless'' mode of drug delivery has been demonstrated in recent years to be an efficacious and safe method for inducing conscious sedation in children undergoing diagnostic or therapeutic procedures that are painful, such as bone marrow aspiration, laceration repair, gynecologic examination, and fracture reductions.[6] The transdermal fentanyl patch currently has no role in ED acute pain management. Steady-state levels are not reached until 12 to 24 h, and the subdermal depot remains for 24 h after the patch is removed.

Codeine is readily absorbed from the gastrointestinal tract, and a very useful agent in the ED for adjunct oral pain therapy with acetaminophen. Codeine can be given IM, but IV administration is not recommended due to a higher side-effect profile. At therapeutic doses, the analgesic effect reaches a peak within two hours and persists between four and six hours. The plasma concentration does not correlate with brain concentration or relief of pain. Codeine crosses the blood-brain barrier, is found in fetal tissue and breast milk, but is not bound to plasma proteins. The plasma half-life is about 2.9 h. The elimination of codeine is primarily by the kidneys, and about 90 percent of an oral dose is excreted by the kidneys within 24 h of dosing.

ADJUNCTS Benzodiazepines have sedative, anxiolytic, amnestic, and muscle-relaxant properties. They have no analgesic action. They are adjuncts for acute pain management in the child over the age of 10 years where anxiety or muscle spasm is a prominent feature. Benzodiazepines can be given IV, orally, or rectally. Benzodiazepines are discussed in detail in the following sedation section.

Hydroxyzine is an H_1-receptor antagonist that is indicated for anxiety and allergic pruritus; it also has sedative properties. Hydroxyzine has no analgesic action. It is available in oral and IM preparations (dosage 0.5 mg/kg oral or IM); IV administration is not recommended. It should be considered as a second-line drug to benzodiazepines, and IM injections generally should be avoided for pain-control medications. Promethazine (Phenergan) is also an H_1-receptor antagonist, with sedative, anxiolytic, and antiemetic properties, in addition to providing relief of minor allergic conditions. It is not recommended for children less than two years of age. Promethazine can be given orally, rectally, IV (slowly), or IM. The evidence to support a synergistic analgesic effect of H_1-antagonists with opioids is limited, and they may potentiate the sedative effects of opioids.

Nonsystemic Pharmacologic Agents

Nonsystemic topical, local and regional techniques are of great value in the management of painful conditions or procedures for the pediatric ED patient and may minimize the need for use of narcotics and sedatives. The amide and ester local anesthetic medications (lidocaine, bupivacaine, prilocaine, and procaine) and refrigerant agents are the most commonly used nonsystemic agents. Techniques range from topical applications such as tetracaine, adrenaline, and cocaine (TAC); lidocaine, epinephrine, and tetracaine (LET); eutectic mixture of local anesthetic (EMLA); and ethyl chloride, local infiltration of LA, peripheral nerve block, hematoma block, and IV Bier's block. The general discussion of these agents as well as specific comments regarding their use in children is found in Chap. 32.

TABLE 130-11 Universal Practice Guidelines for Sedation in Children

Standardized documentation
History and physical including
ASA physical status class I and II
Mallampati airway evaluation
Informed consent
Record keeping during and after the procedure
Standardized fasting guidelines
Solids/liquids
Personnel
Qualifications, training and responsibilities
Number of personnel required
Monitoring equipment
Pulse oximetry
Continuous electrocardiogram
Blood pressure
Temperature
Emergency drugs and resuscitation equipment
Equipment for venous access
O_2 and O_2 delivery system
Suction
Airway equipment
Resuscitation drugs
Reversal drugs
Recovery facilities and discharge criteria
Personnel
Equipment
Monitoring outcome

Abbreviations: ASA, American Society of Anesthesiologists.
Adapted from: Yaster M, Krane EJ, Kaplan RF, Coté CJ, Lappe DG (eds): Pediatric Pain Management and Sedation Handbook. St. Louis, Mosby, 1997, pp 296–297.

CONSCIOUS SEDATION

Conscious sedation is a medically controlled state of depressed consciousness that allows protective reflexes to be maintained, retains the patient's ability to maintain a patent airway independently and continuously, and permits appropriate response by the patient to physical stimulation or verbal command.

The goals of conscious sedation are to minimize fear and anxiety, maintain patient safety, control behavior, provide amnesia, and return the patient to a state for safe discharge. Factors involved in the selection of the sedation regimen include the specific procedure being performed, duration of procedure, the developmental age and physical condition of the child, and physician experience with the agents. Practice guidelines for the sedation of children are noted in Table 130-11.

In the ED environment, conscious sedation should only be performed by physicians appropriately skilled in airway and resuscitation

TABLE 130-12 ASA Physical Status Classification System

I	Healthy, no underlying organic disease
II	Mild or moderate systemic disease that does not interfere with daily routines
III	Organic disease with definite functional impairment
IV	Severe disease that is life threatening
V	Moribund
E (suffix)	a procedure undertaken as an emergency

Abbreviation: ASA, American Society of Anesthesiologists.

management, and only for patients considered to be class I or class II (Table 130-11). The American Academy of Pediatrics and the American Society of Anesthesiologists (ASA) have published guidelines for monitoring and management of pediatric patients during and after sedation for diagnostic and therapeutic procedures.[7,8] Salient features of these documents are discussed below and should be incorporated into the ED's sedation policy.

Patient Evaluation

The first step is assessment of the patient for sedation in the emergency department. The history should identify any abnormalities of the major organ systems and airway; previous adverse experience with sedation, analgesia, or anesthesia; any neurologic disorder or impairment; medications and allergies; and time and nature of the patient's last oral intake. Focused physical examination should include baseline vital signs and oxygen saturation, evaluation of cardiorespiratory status and the oropharynx and airway.

Appropriate candidates for sedation protocols in the ED are healthy patients or patients with mild systemic disease (Table 130-12). Children with severe systemic disease (ASA III or IV); infants <3 months of age; premature infants <60 weeks postconceptual weeks of age; and children with underlying respiratory/airway disease, neurologic conditions, CNS injury, multiple trauma, or liver/kidney disease are at increased risk for sedation complications and require consultation with an anesthesiologist.

For nonemergent sedation, fasting for two hours from clear liquids and four to eight hours for solids and nonclear liquids, is recommended. Children requiring urgent or emergent sedation despite recent oral intake should not receive deep sedation to avoid depression of protective airway reflexes that may result in aspiration. Procedures should be delayed, if possible, to facilitate gastric emptying that may decrease the risk of regurgitation and aspiration. Ranitidine (1 mg/kg IV) and metoclopramide (0.15 mg/kg IV) given 30 to 60 min prior to sedation may increase gastric pH and reduce gastric volume. Obese patients or patients with a history of gastroesophageal reflux may also benefit from premedication with these drugs.

Informed consent should be obtained from the child's parent or legal guardian with explanations about the procedure, sedation and analgesia plan, and associated risks. All information can be documented on a sedation assessment and monitoring chart.

Equipment and Monitoring

The ED must be appropriately equipped for administering sedation to children of all ages and sizes. An oxygen source capable of delivering >90 percent oxygen and positive pressure ventilation, appropriate size masks, and functioning suction apparatus with Yankauer-tip catheters must be at the child's bedside. Appropriately-sized laryngoscopes, endotracheal tubes, intravenous catheters, and emergency medications must be readily available. Airway management and breathing equipment must be checked before each sedation procedure.

The child should be attached to a cardiac monitor and pulse oximeter. During the procedure, one person whose sole responsibility is monitoring the patient, preferably a registered nurse with basic life support and PALS training, or a physician who is not performing the procedure, must be present. Continuous quantitative monitoring of oxygen saturation (pulse oximetry) and heart rate, and intermittent monitoring of respiratory rate and blood pressure should be recorded at 5- to 10-min intervals. Level of consciousness (response to verbal commands/tactile stimuli) and pulmonary ventilation (observing chest wall excursion and/or auscultation of breath sounds and/or capnography) should also be monitored. All drugs and doses administered must be clearly documented, with special attention to calculation of single and cumulative doses in mg/kg.

After the procedure, the child must be observed and monitored in an area with suitable equipment and vital signs recorded every 15 minutes. Pulse oximetry should be maintained until the patient is fully alert. Observation should be continued until all discharge criteria are met (Table 130-13). Appropriate discharge instructions with follow-up should be conveyed to the child's caretaker.

SEDATION AGENTS AND TECHNIQUES

Indications for sedating infants and children in the emergency department include diagnostic procedures (CT scans) and as an adjunct to analgesia and anesthesia for painful procedures.[9] Table 130-14 lists common pharmacologic options for sedation. Nonpharmacologic techniques should also be considered when preparing to sedate children and should not be forgotten in the midst of a busy emergency department. As previously discussed, parental involvement, verbal preparation, relaxation, tactile stimulation, and distraction techniques are all effective. Manual restraint (sheets or papoose boards) may be required as an adjunct to the nonpharmacologic and pharmacologic approach to procedures for infants and toddlers. Parents should not be requested to provide or be responsible for the restraint of the child, but rather should be encouraged to provide comfort.

An ideal pharmacologic agent for sedation is one that is effective, has rapid onset, is easily titratable with a predictable duration of action, is quickly eliminated or reversible, has no adverse effects, and is easy and painless to administer. Although the ideal agent does not exist, there are several good drugs and regimens that when administered appropriately can provide safe and adequate analgesia and/or anesthesia.

Sedatives can be administered by a variety of routes including IV, IM, oral, rectal, sublingual, transmucosal, and intranasal; each route has advantages and disadvantages. Intravenous administration allows the most precise titration of drug to the desired effect; IM administra-

TABLE 130-13 Recommended Discharge Criteria

Cardiovascular function and airway patency are satisfactory and stable.
The patient is easily arousable, and protective reflexes are intact.
The patient can talk (if age-appropriate).
The patient can sit up unaided (if age-appropriate).
For a very young or handicapped child, incapable of the usually expected responses, the pre-sedation level of responsiveness or a level as close as possible to the normal level for that child should be achieved.
The state of hydration is adequate.

From Committee on Drugs, American Academy of Pediatrics: Guidelines for monitoring and management of pediatric patients during and after sedation for diagnostic and therapeutic procedures. *Pediatrics* 89:1110, 1992. Used with permission of the American Academy of Pediatrics.

TABLE 130-14 Sedative Drugs for the Pediatric Patient

Drug	Route/Dose	Duration of Action	Contraindication
Benzodiazepines			
Midazolam (Versed)	IV: 0.05–0.10 mg/kg (single max dose 2 mg) Subsequent incremental doses at 3 minute intervals to desired effect or up to a total of 0.2 mg/kg IM: 0.3 mg/kg PO: 0.5–0.75 mg/kg (max dose 15 mg) Nasal: 0.3–0.5 mg/kg (max dose 5 mg) PR: 0.5 mg/kg (max dose 15 mg)	30–45 min	Uncontrolled pain CNS depression Shock Hypersensitivity to benzodiazepines
Diazepam (Valium)	IV: 0.1–0.2 mg/kg (max 10 mg) PO: 0.2–0.3 mg/kg PR: 0.5 mg/kg	2–6 h	
Sedative/hypnotic			
Chloral hydrate	PO/PR: 50–75 mg/kg (max 2 g)	2–4 h	Hepatic/renal impairment Hypersensitivity
Barbiturate			
Pentobarbital (Nembutal)	IV/IM: 4–6 mg/kg (max 150 mg) PR: <4 years 3–6 mg/kg >4 years 1.5–3.0 mg/kg	2–4 h	CNS depression Hypersensitivity to barbiturates Hepatic impairment Porphyria
Oral Transmucosal Fentanyl Citrate (Oralet)	10–15 μg/kg (max dose 400 μg)	45–60 min	Children <15 kg Treatment of acute or chronic pain Hypersensitivity to fentanyl Altered mental status/CNS depression MAO inhibitor use
Nitrous oxide	50% N_2O/50% O_2 via inhalation	3–5 min after ceasing inhalation	Previous narcotic sedative within 4 h Impaired mental status Intoxication Nausea/vomiting Pregnancy Pneumothorax Bowel obstruction
Ketamine (Ketalar)	IV: 1.0 mg/kg Administer midazolam (0.05 mg/kg) and atropine (0.01 mg/kg) concurrently IM: 2.0–4.0 mg/kg (combine atropine and midazolam in same syringe) PO: 10 mg/kg (administer with midazolam 0.5 mg/kg and atropine 0.02 mg/kg)	IV: 20–60 min IM: 30–90 min PO/PR: 60–120 min	Age ≤3 months History of airway instability, tracheal stenosis URI/asthma Cardiovascular disease/Hypertension Increased intracranial pressure states (head trauma, hydrocephalus, brain tumor) Poorly controlled seizure disorder Glaucoma or acute globe injury Psychosis, porphyria, thyroid disorder
REVERSAL AGENTS			
Naloxone (Narcan)	IV/IM: 0.01–0.1 mg/kg/dose (max single dose 2 mg) Repeat to desired effect every 2 minutes	20–45 min	Use smaller doses 0.001 mg/kg in children dependent on opioids
Flumazenil (Romazicon)	IV/IM: 0.01 mg/kg/dose (max initial dose 0.2 mg) Repeat at 60-s intervals to desired effect or maximum of 0.05 mg/kg or 1.0 mg	20–45 min	Chronic benzodiazepine therapy for seizures Concomitant use of medications that have the potential to cause seizures (tricyclic antidepressants, theophylline, bupropion, INH) Hypersensitivity to benzodiazepines

tion usually is painful and not titratable. Oral and transmucosal routes are more readily accepted by children than nasal or rectal routes. Despite the options for administration routes, side effects can occur with any route of administration.

Benzodiazepines

Benzodiazepines provide anxiolysis and amnesia but not anesthesia. They can be used alone as a sedative, or in conjunction with a narcotic or local anesthetic for a painful procedure. Midazolam (Versed) is a short-acting benzodiazepine that has an onset of action within 5 min and a duration of action of 30 to 45 min. Midazolam is safe and effective for use in the ED in children undergoing laceration repair, fracture reduction, and other painful procedures.[10] Adverse effects include respiratory depression and paradoxical inconsolability.[11] Anecdotally, this latter effect appears to happen with increased frequency in children with attention deficit hyperactivity disorder, and is reversible with flumazenil.

Diazepam is a longer-acting benzodiazepine that has been used extensively as a sedative for children and has amnestic properties.

Diazepam can be used for extended diagnostic procedures and for muscle relaxation for orthopedic reductions. It has been largely replaced by midazolam.

Sedative/Hypnotics

Chloral hydrate is a pure sedative/hypnotic with no analgesic properties that is used primarily for sedation of infants and young children requiring painless diagnostic procedures.[12] The time to sedation is relatively long (45 to 60 min) and its effects can last several hours because of its active metabolite, making it an impractical agent for use in the ED. Adverse effects include nausea, vomiting, and paradoxical delirium/excitement, which are not reversible. Serious adverse effects including airway obstruction and death have been reported with chloral hydrate use.

The short-acting barbiturates can provide rapid onset of sedation for painless procedures such as computed tomography and magnetic resonance imaging studies in children with no preexisting central nervous system depression.[13] Again, they have no analgesic or amnestic properties. Intravenous pentobarbital has an onset of action within 30 s and children are usually appropriately sedated within 5 min. Its duration of action is 30 to 60 min, making it a better choice for children undergoing emergent procedures. Respiratory and central nervous system depression can occur which can be exacerbated in the presence of other depressants such as opioids and benzodiazepines.

Narcotics

A discussion of individual narcotics is found in the preceding analgesia section. Narcotics can be administered intravenously in conjunction with an anxiolytic such as benzodiazepines for sedation for painful procedures.

The oral transmucosal fentanyl citrate lozenge (Oralet) comes in three dosage strengths (200, 300, and 400 μg) and is administered over 10 to 20 min by asking the patient to suck, not chew, the lozenge. It can be removed by the physician or "self-removed" by the patient when sedation is achieved. Onset of action is within 5 to 15 min with maximum effect occurring in 20 to 30 min. Suitable candidates for OTFC are children at least two years of age, weighing greater than 15 kg. Children receiving MAO inhibitors in the past 14 days should not use this drug. Vomiting is the most frequently reported adverse affect as well as pruritus and hypoventilation.

Nitrous Oxide

Limited studies in children have shown nitrous oxide (N_2O) to be an effective and safe sedative/analgesic either alone or in combination with a local anesthetic for laceration repair, orthopedic procedures, and other minor surgical procedures.[14,15] It offers many advantages over other pharmacologic agents for use in the outpatient setting and emergency department. It provides analgesia, anxiolysis, and sedation without the need for IV line placement, has a low incidence of complications and adverse effects, and can result in shorter ED lengths of stay due to rapid recovery. Nitrous oxide interacts with the endogenous opioid system to confer analgesia and appears to blunt the patient's reaction to pain. It produces a sense of euphoria, relief from anxiety, and an almost "detached" attitude toward pain and the patient's surroundings.

In the outpatient setting, nitrous oxide should be delivered via a fixed-ratio mixture of nitrous oxide to oxygen, usually 50 percent N_2O:50 percent oxygen (oxygen concentration must be a minimum of 30 percent) by a self-administered demand-valve apparatus with a scavenger device. This mode of administration protects against equipment failure and/or human error, which may result in too high concentration of nitrous oxide. The gas is routinely delivered by an inspiratory effort of the patient, minimizing the risk of loss of consciousness and protective reflexes because the mask will fall off when the patient is sedated. The gas/oxygen mixture can be inhaled through a face mask, mouthpiece, or nasal hood in which a flavored Chapstick lining or concentrated "child-friendly" scent can be applied to disguise the odor of the gas. For younger children unable to hold their own mask, the physician or parent can assist in the delivery of the mixture by placing the mask lightly on the child's face.

Nitrous oxide has a rapid onset of action of three to five minutes and a short duration of action on withdrawal of three to five minutes. The gas is not metabolized, and is eliminated by the lungs unchanged. Short-term use has no significant effects on other organs. The most common reported side effects are nausea and vomiting. Diffusional hypoxia is another potential concern since nitrous oxide rapidly diffuses out of the blood and into the alveoli, where it can displace oxygen and cause hypoxia. This theoretical concern has not been supported by clinical evidence. Nevertheless, supplemental oxygen should be administered throughout the recovery phase. Nitrous oxide use in the ED also has the potential for abuse, environmental contamination, and potential teratogenic effects especially with chronic exposure. The use of nitrous oxide is contraindicated in patients with pneumothoraces, bowel obstruction, middle ear effusions, and patients undergoing procedures using balloon-tipped catheters because of its rapid diffusion into gas-collecting areas of the body, which could cause acute expansion, over distension, and perforation. It also should be avoided in patients with head injuries, psychiatric diseases, or drug intoxication. Because of nitrous oxide's opioid agonist properties, it may result in deep sedation or general anesthesia if combined with a sedative or opioid. Thus, extreme caution should be exercised when administering it to a patient with recent administration of either of these medications.[16]

Ketamine

Ketamine is a unique sedative analgesic that has been studied extensively in children undergoing outpatient procedures.[17–19] A derivative of phencyclidine, ketamine produces a dissociative effect resulting in a trance-like cataleptic state, providing a combination of sedation, amnesia, and analgesia. Spontaneous respirations and pharyngeal muscular tone are maintained, as well as protective airway reflexes of coughing and swallowing. Ketamine has very few negative inotropic effects making it a reasonable option for acutely ill patients. Its sympathomimetic actions may produce mild to moderate increases in heart rate, blood pressure, and cardiac output. However, in the catecholamine-depleted child, ketamine may result in hypotension due to unopposed direct vasodilatory effects. It also is a good option for the difficult-to-control child with mental retardation or behavioral disorder where initial IV access can be difficult. Clinical effects from intravenous and intramuscular ketamine occur within several minutes and last about 30 min. It has also been shown to be effective when administered via the transmucosal, oral, and rectal routes.[20]

Because ketamine stimulates salivary and tracheobronchial secretions, it should be administered concurrently with an anticholinergic drug, either atropine or glycopyrrolate. Both agents may be combined in a single IM injection. Hallucinatory emergence reactions have been reported with ketamine although less frequently in children less than 10 years of age. These reactions can be reduced with premedicating the child with a benzodiazepine such as midazolam. However, this combination may prolong the patient's recovery time because benzodiazepines will inhibit ketamine's metabolism. Ketamine can also cause increased intracranial and intraocular pressure because of increased cerebral blood flow.

Other adverse effects are nystagmus, random limb movement, and vomiting. Ketamine has the potential for causing laryngospasm and thus should not be used in patients with upper respiratory or pulmonary infections or who have increased salivary secretions. If laryngospasm occurs, the child should be ventilated with a bag-valve mask. Paralysis and emergent intubation must be performed if this is unsuccessful. Contraindications to ketamine's use are age ≤3 months; history of airway instability or tracheal stenosis; procedures involving stimulation of the posterior pharynx; cardiovascular disease including congestive heart failure and hypertension; head injury associated with loss of consciousness, altered mental status, central nervous system masses, abnormalities, or hydrocephalus; poorly controlled seizure disorder; glaucoma; acute globe injury; or psychosis.

Other Agents

Propofol is an ultrashort-acting intravenous anesthetic marketed in the United States as Diprivan. It has been reported as a safe and effective nonanesthetic sedative for adults undergoing fracture reduction, reduction of joint dislocations, minor surgical procedures (I&D of abscesses), cardioversion, and chest tube placement in the ED.[21] It has been used in children in the ED for difficult fracture reduction, incarcerated inguinal hernia reductions, and cardioversion, although there are no published reports. Propofol's onset of action occurs within seconds and its duration of action is extremely short, requiring continuous infusion for maintenance of clinical effects. After discontinuation of the drug in sedative doses, patients are usually awake and responsive within minutes. It does not possess any analgesic properties in sedative doses and must be used in conjunction with narcotics for painful procedures. Propofol has potent dose-related respiratory depressant effects, may quickly result in deep sedation, and may produce hypotension. More experience is needed before it can be recommended for routine use in children in the ED.

In the past, the "DPT cocktail," consisting of Demerol (meperidine), Phenergan (promethazine), and Thorazine (chlorpromazine), was a popular sedative/analgesic choice for children in the emergency department. Unfortunately, the intramuscular route does not allow for titration of effects and its onset of action is variable. The wide range of doses used and combination of three sedatives adds to confusion and potential for serious respiratory depression. In addition, the efficacy of this "cocktail" can be variable while its duration of action can be several hours, not making it a preferable choice for sedation in the ED.[22]

Reversal Agents

Naloxone is an opioid antagonist and should be readily available for reversal of respiratory depression, apnea, and severe hypotension. It can be administered in incremental doses of 0.01 to 0.1 mg/kg (maximum single dose 2 mg) to the desired reversal of life-threatening effects, because it would not be desirable to reverse all of the analgesia in a patient undergoing a painful procedure. Naloxone's duration of action is short (approximately 45 min); thus, reversal of toxic effects of longer-acting opioids, such as morphine, or large doses of short-acting opioids, such as fentanyl, may require additional doses.

Flumazenil is a benzodiazepine antagonist that reverses the central nervous system depression and, to some degree, respiratory depression secondary to inadvertent excess sedation.[23] Incremental doses of 0.01 to 0.02 mg/kg (maximum single dose 0.2 mg) every 1 to 2 min can be titrated to the desired reversal effect. Respiratory depression and hypoventilation should be managed with standard airway management techniques and assisted ventilation if necessary. Flumazenil has also been shown to reverse the paradoxical delirium secondary to midazolam.[24] In the setting of a polypharmaceutical overdose, flumazenil should not be administered. It should not be used in patients on chronic benzodiazepine therapy or on tricyclic antidepressant medications because of the risk of seizures. Flumazenil's duration of action is about 40 to 60 min. Because the duration and degree of reversal depends on the plasma concentrations of benzodiazepine as well as the amount of flumazenil given, the sedative and respiratory depression effects of the benzodiazepine may last longer than the antagonism produced by flumazenil. Both drugs should be readily available and appropriate doses calculated prior to initiation of the procedure.

REFERENCES

1. Schechter NL: The undertreatment of pain in children: An overview. *Pediatr Clin North Am* 36:781, 1989.
2. Baker CM, Wong DL: Q.U.E.S.T: A process of pain assessment in children. *Orthop Nurs* 6:11, 1987.
3. McGrath P: Pain in the pediatric patient: practical aspects of assessment. *Pediatr Ann* 24:126, 1995.
4. Wolfram RW, Turner ED, Philput C: Effects of parental presence during young children's venipuncture. *Pediatr Emerg Care* 13:325, 1997.
5. Acute Pain Management Guideline Panel. Acute Pain Management in Infants, Children, and Adolescents: Operative and Medical Procedures. Quick Reference Guide for Clinicians. AHCPR Pub. No. 92-0020. February 1993. Rockville, MD: Agency for Health Care Policy and Research, Public Health Service, U.S. Department of Health and Human Services.
6. Schutzman SA, Liebelt E, Wisk M, et al: Comparison of oral transmucosal fentanyl citrate and intramuscular meperidine, promethazine, and chlorpromazine for conscious sedation of children undergoing laceration repair. *Ann Emerg Med* 28:385, 1996.
7. Committee on Drugs, American Academy of Pediatrics. Guidelines for monitoring and management of pediatric patients during and after sedation for diagnostic and therapeutic procedures. *Pediatrics* 89:1110, 1992.
8. American Society of Anesthesiologists. Practice guidelines for sedation and analgesia by non-anesthesiologists. *Anesthesiology* 84:459, 1996.
9. Sacchetti A, Schafermeyer R, Gerardi M, et al: Pediatric analgesia and sedation. *Ann Emerg Med* 23:237, 1994.
10. Connors K, Terndrup TE: Nasal versus oral midazolam for anxious children undergoing laceration repair. *Ann Emerg Med* 24:1074, 1994.
11. Doyle WL, Perrin L: Emergence delirium in a child given midazolam for conscious sedation. *Ann Emerg Med* 24:1173, 1994.
12. Binder LS, Leake LA: Chloral hydrate for emergent pediatric procedural sedation: a new look at an old drug. *Am J Emerg Med* 9:530, 1991.
13. Strain JD, Harvey LA, Foley LC, et al: Intravenously administered pentobarbital sodium for sedation in pediatric CT. *Radiology* 161:105, 1986.
14. Burton JH, Auble TE, Gillman MA: Effectiveness of 50% nitrous oxide/50% oxygen during laceration repair in children. *Acad Emerg Med* 5:112, 1998.
15. Gamis AS, Knapp JF, Mathias S: Nitrous oxide analgesia in a pediatric emergency department. *Ann Emerg Med* 18:177, 1989.
16. Gillman MA: Analgesic (subanesthetic) nitrous oxide interacts with the endogenous opioid system: A review of the evidence. *Life Sci* 39:1209, 1986.
17. Green SM, Rothrock SG, Lynch EEL, et al: Intramuscular ketamine for pediatric sedation in the emergency department: safety profile in 1,022 cases. *Ann Emerg Med* 31:688, 1998.
18. Green SM, Rothrock SG, Harris T, et al: Intravenous ketamine for pediatric sedation in the emergency department: safety profile with 156 cases. *Acad Emerg Med* 5:971, 1998.
19. Green SM, Hummel CB, Wittlake WA, et al: What is the optimal dose of intramuscular ketamine for pediatric sedation? *Acad Emerg Med* 6:21, 1999.
20. Qureshi F, Mellis PT, McFadden MA: Efficacy of oral ketamine for providing sedation and analgesia to children requiring laceration repair. *Pediatr Emerg Care* 11:93, 1995.
21. Swanson ER, Seaberg DC, Mathias S: The Use of propofol for sedation in the emergency department. *Acad Emerg Med* 3:234, 1995.
22. American Academy of Pediatrics Co. Reappraisal of lytic cocktail/demerol, phenergan, and thorazine (DPT) for the sedation of children. *Pediatrics* 95:598, 1995.
23. Sugarman JM, Paul RI: Flumazenil: A review. *Pediatr Emerg Care* 10:37, 1994.
24. Shannon M, Albers G, Burkhart K, et al: Safety and efficacy of flumazenil in the reversal of benzodiazepine-induced conscious sedation. *J Pediatr* 131:582, 1997.

PEDIATRIC EXANTHEMS

Michael S. Weinstock
Michael S. Catapano

Rashes with diverse etiologies can look alike. Assessing the signs and symptoms preceding or presenting with the exanthem and obtaining an accurate history of prior immunizations, potential human or animal contacts, and recent environmental exposure helps to determine the diagnosis. The various etiologic agents and associated exanthems are noted in Table 131-1. Further discussion of cutaneous disorders is found in Section 19, ''Disorders of the Skin.''

BACTERIAL

Bullous Impetigo

Bullous impetigo, or staphylococcal impetigo, is a local skin infection caused by phage group II staphylococci. The staphylococci produce an epidermolytic toxin that acts locally to cause separation of the skin at the granular layer, giving rise to bullae. The infection occurs primarily in newborn infants and young children. The characteristic skin lesions of bullous impetigo are superficial, flaccid, thin-walled bullae that occur most often on the extremities but can occur anywhere. They range in size from 0.5 to 3 cm. They can arise from normal skin or may have a thin, red halo. The bullae are filled with a clear, pale-to-yellow fluid and rupture easily, leaving a moist, denuded base that dries rapidly with a shiny coating. Extensive areas of skin may be involved if untreated.

The clinical appearance of the lesions usually makes diagnosis easy. However, single lesions or extensive involvement may not be as typical. Staphylococci cultured from fluid from aspirated bullae will establish the diagnosis.

Systemic antistaphylococcal antibiotics, usually oral, along with local wound cleansing and topical antibiotics (such as neosporin) are effective in eradicating the infection. Prognosis for complete recovery is good.

Impetigo Contagiosum

Impetigo is a superficial pyoderma caused by infection with staphylococci, although group A β-hemolytic streptococci may also be cultured. It is a common skin infection, primarily affecting young children, especially in warm, humid conditions. Impetigo can arise at the site of insect bites or superficial cutaneous trauma; sometimes there is no apparent predisposing skin lesion. Fever and systemic signs are uncommon.

The skin lesions start as small erythematous macules and papules. These develop into discrete, thin-walled vesicles which become pustular and quickly rupture (see Fig. 131-1). As the vesicles rupture, a yellow fluid forms an exudate, which dries to form a stratified golden, yellow crust that accumulates. The crusts can be readily removed, leaving a smooth, red surface. The crusts can spread the infection to other parts of the body. Initially, the lesions are discrete, but they may enlarge and become confluent. Local adenopathy may be present. The infection occurs most frequently on the face, neck, and extremities.

The diagnosis of impetigo can be readily made on the basis of the typical clinical appearance. Cultures are generally not necessary. Systemic antibiotic therapy must be combined with wound scrubbing and cleansing and application of neosporin or mupirocin ointment for optimal results. Effective antibiotics include oral antibiotics such as erythromycin, clindamycin, cephalosporins, and dicloxacillin.

Erysipelas

Erysipelas, or St. Anthony's fire, is cellulitis and lymphangitis of the skin caused by group A, β-hemolytic streptococci. It is frequently accompanied by fever, chills, malaise, headache, and vomiting.

The rash is characterized by local redness, heat, swelling, and a raised, indurated border. There is marked involvement of the superficial dermal lymphatics. The rash starts as an erythematous plaque that rapidly enlarges by peripheral extension. At first, it is scarlet, hot, brawny, swollen, and tender. The edge is raised and sharply demarcated. The rash can vary in appearance from a transient hyperemia to intense inflammation, vesiculation, and bulla formation. The face is the most frequent site. A skin wound, fissure, or ulcer may act as a portal of entry.

TABLE 131-1 Different Diagnosis of Exanthems

Vesiculopustules	Maculopapules	Urticaria	Petechiae
Drug eruption	Drug eruption	Varicella (urticaria around vesicle)	Drug eruption
Herpes simplex	Secondary lues	Coxsackie A5, A9	Bacterial endocarditis
Variola	Scarlet fever	Infectious hepatitis	Echovirus
Vaccinia	Echovirus 9, 16	Mononucleosis	Coxsackie A5, A9
Varicella	Coxsackie A5, A9, A16, B5	*Mycoplasma pneumoniae*	Mononucleosis
Generalized zoster	Reovirus 2	Hepatitis	Rubella
Rickettsialpox	Erythema infectiosum		Thrombocytopenia with many acute infections
Coxsackie A and B	Gianotti-Crosti syndrome		
Reovirus 2	Rubella		
Mycoplasma pneumoniae	Rubeola		
Echovirus 4	Hepatitis		
Contagious ecthyma (orf)	Infectious mononucleosis		
	Arbovirus (dengue)		
	Rickettsioses		

Source: From Burnett JW, Crutcher WA: Viral and rickettsial infections, in Moschella SL, Hurley, HJ (eds): *Dermatology.* Philadelphia, Saunders, 1985, vol 1, chap 12, pp 673–738, with permission.

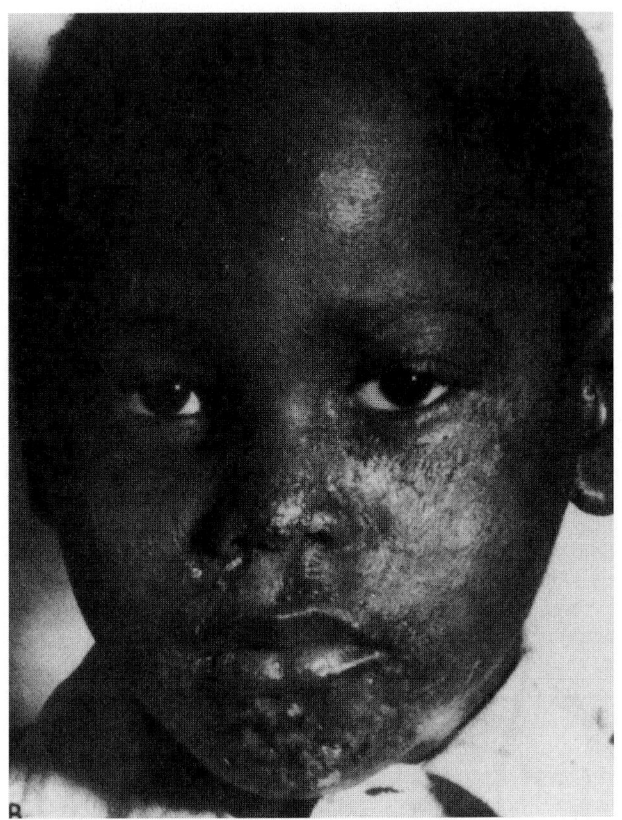

FIG. 131-1. Impetigo contagiosum. [From Marples RR, Leyden JL: Bacterial infections, section I. Fundamental cutaneous microbiology, in Moschella SL, Hurley HJ (eds): *Dermatology*. Philadelphia, Saunders, 1985, vol 1, chap 11, pp 590–642, with permission.]

Diagnosis is made on clinical grounds, although aspiration of the leading edge of the lesion will frequently demonstrate streptococci. A brief course of parenteral penicillin is usually warranted because of the rapid advancement of the infection, the acutely toxic state of the patient, and the possibility of suppurative complications. Rapid clinical response is usually obtained. Erythromycin may be used in patients unable to take penicillin.

Mycoplasma Infections

Mycoplasma pneumoniae infections are a common cause of pneumonia, upper respiratory infections, and bronchitis in children between 5 and 19 years of age. The most frequent presenting clinical findings in children and adults are fever, cough, sore throat, malaise, headache, chills, and rash. An erythematous maculopapular rash, the most frequent presentation, is located on the trunk and may be discrete or confluent. However, the most frequently reported exanthem is consistent with erythema multiforme and Stevens-Johnson syndrome, with lesions occurring primarily on the trunk, legs, and arms. The rash occurs most commonly during the febrile period. An enanthem of generalized ulcerative stomatitis or pharyngitis-tonsillitis associated with the exanthem is common. The diagnosis can be confirmed by the use of either serum cold agglutinins or several specific antibody tests.

Mycoplasma responds to several antimicrobials, including erythromycin, tetracycline, chloramphenicol, and aminoglycosides. Infection with *M. pneumoniae* should be suspected in patients with pneumonia and a rash.

Scarlet Fever

Scarlet fever is an acute febrile illness, primarily affecting young children, caused by group A β-hemolytic streptococci. Recently group C streptococci have been implicated as well. Clinical manifestations include acute onset with fever, sore throat, headache, vomiting, and abdominal pain followed by a distinctive exanthem in 1 to 2 days.

There are both an exanthem and an enanthem associated with scarlet fever. They are caused by an erythrogenic toxin elaborated by the streptococcal organism. The tonsils and pharynx are red and covered with exudate, although occasionally pharyngeal findings are minimal. The tongue has a white coating through which red and hypertrophied papillae project, creating the appearance of a "white strawberry tongue." The white coating disappears by day 4 or 5, and the tongue acquires a bright-red appearance, the "red strawberry tongue." Bright-red or hemorrhagic spots may be seen on the soft palate or anterior pillars of the tonsillar fossae.

The exanthem of scarlet fever begins 1 or 2 days after the onset of the illness. It starts on the neck, axillae, and groin, spreading to the trunk and extremities. The rash is red and finely punctate, consisting of 1- to 2-mm papules giving the rash a characteristic rough, sandpaper feel. It is sometimes easier to identify the rash by palpation. The rash blanches with pressure. Linear petechial eruptions, Pastia's lines, are often present in the antecubital and axillary folds. There is facial flushing with circumoral pallor. A brawny desquamation occurs at 2 weeks, yielding fine flakes of dry skin.

The diagnosis of scarlet fever is readily made on clinical grounds. Throat swabs usually culture group A β-hemolytic streptococci, although group C may be cultured as well. Treatment with antibiotics is necessary to reduce the incidence of rheumatic fever and nephritis and will probably ameliorate the course of the disease. Penicillin is the antibiotic of choice, or erythromycin for those who are penicillin-allergic.

RICKETTSIAL

Rocky Mountain Spotted Fever

Rocky Mountain spotted fever (RMSF) is an infectious disease caused by *Rickettsia rickettsii* which is transmitted by ticks. The prominent clinical manifestations of RMSF can be directly related to the primary pathologic lesion in the endothelial cells lining small blood vessels where the rickettsia multiply. Rash, headache, mental confusion, terminal heart failure, and shock are manifestations of the generalized vasculitis.

The incubation period is from 2 to 12 days with either a sudden or gradual onset of symptoms. Peak severity usually occurs within 1 to 2 weeks. Headache, fever, toxicity, rash, and myalgia are the major clinical features. The rash (Fig. 131-2), a pathognomonic feature of the disease, usually appears on the second or third day. The initial lesions first appear on the wrist and ankles spreading rapidly to the extremities and trunk. These lesions also are found on the palms and soles of the patient. Initially, lesions are small, erythematous macules which blanch on pressure. They rapidly become maculopapular and petechial.

Laboratory diagnostic confirmation is difficult during the early phase of the disease, frequently mandating treatment based on clinical criteria. Serologic tests are used to confirm the diagnosis of RMSF. Some laboratory data may be helpful in establishing the presumptive diagnosis early, such as hyponatremia, leukopenia, and thrombocytopenia.

Specific therapy consists of tetracycline or chloramphenicol. In seriously ill children 100 mg/kg per 24 h of chloramphenicol up to 3 g total dose is advised. As improvement is noted, therapy can be changed to 50 mg/kg per 24 h in four divided doses orally. Treatment can be terminated 2 or 3 days after fever returns to normal for 24 h.

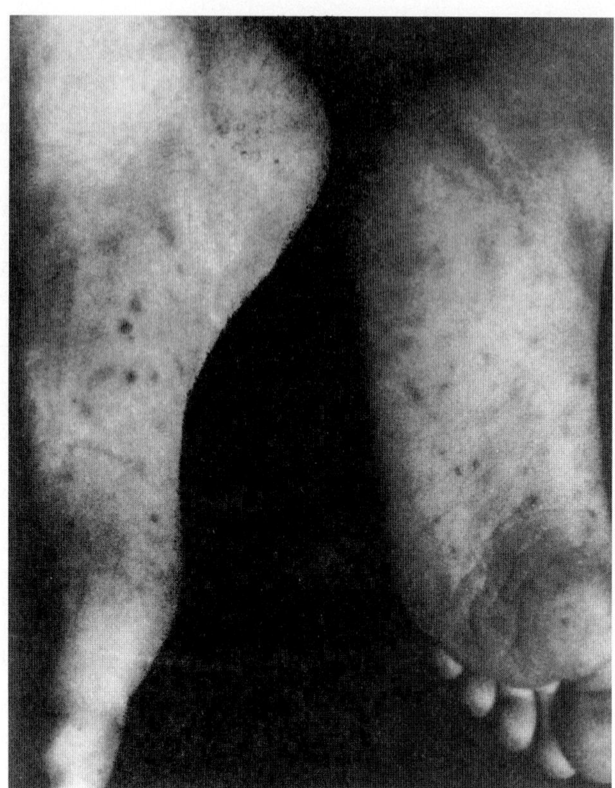

FIG. 131-2. Rocky Mountain spotted fever. [From Burnett JW, Crutcher WA: Viral and rickettsial infections, in Moschella SL, Hurley HJ (eds): *Dermatology*. Philadelphia, Saunders, 1985, vol 1, chap 12, pp 673–738, with permission.]

The mortality of RMSF in the United States has held steady for a decade at 3 to 6 percent of identified cases despite treatment.

VIRUSES

Enteroviruses

Enteroviruses are an exceedingly common cause of illness and exanthem in young children. Enteroviruses are small, single-stranded RNA viruses belonging to the picornavirus group and consist of polioviruses and nonpolioviruses (coxsackievirus and echovirus). There are many types of coxsackieviruses and echoviruses that have been associated with illnesses. They usually occur in epidemics and are most prevalent in the summer and early fall. Transmission usually occurs by fecal-oral route and possibly by the respiratory route.

The clinical manifestations of infection with coxsackieviruses and echoviruses are extensive. The spectrum of disease includes nonspecific febrile illness, upper respiratory infection, parotitis, croup, bronchitis, pneumonia, bronchiolitis, vomiting, diarrhea, abdominal pain, hepatitis, pancreatitis, conjunctivitis, pericarditis, myocarditis, orchitis, nephritis, arthritis, meningitis, and encephalitis.

Similarly, the associated skin manifestations include an array of exanthems. Diffuse macular eruptions, morbilliform erythema, vesicular lesions, petechial and purpural eruptions, rubelliform rash, roseola-like rash, and scarlatiniform eruptions have been reported.

Strict clinical-virologic associations have been difficult to demonstrate. A single clinical syndrome can be associated with many types of coxsackieviruses and echoviruses. On the other hand, some types of coxsackieviruses and echoviruses have been associated with multiple illnesses and exanthems.

Hand, foot, and mouth disease is an acute infectious illness, caused by enteroviruses, that primarily affects children. Initial manifestations include fever, anorexia, malaise, and sore mouth. Oral lesions appear 1 to 2 days later and cutaneous lesions shortly thereafter. The oral lesions begin as vesicles on an erythematous base which ulcerate. The vesicles are usually 4 to 8 mm in size, and are very painful. They are located on the buccal mucosa, tongue, soft palate, and gingiva. The exanthem starts as red papules which change to gray vesicles about 3 to 7 mm in size. They are found on the palms and soles but may occur on the dorsum of the feet and hands and on the buttocks, as well. They may be oval, linear, or crescentic and may run parallel to skin lines. They heal in 7 to 10 days.

Herpangina is a febrile disease of children associated with many types of coxsackieviruses and echoviruses. The onset is acute with fever to 40°C, headache, sore throat, dysphagia, anorexia, and, occasionally, stiff neck. In the pharynx, there are one or more yellowish-white 2-mm vesicles with hyperemic borders. They are located in the posterior pharynx on the tonsils, uvula, soft palate, and anterior faucial pillars. The vesicles will usually ulcerate, leaving a shallow, gray-yellow crater 2 to 4 mm in size. The lesions persist for 5 to 10 days.

Boston exanthem is caused by echovirus 16. It is an acute illness with fever, anorexia, pharyngitis, and lymphadenopathy. An enanthem similar to herpangina may be present. The exanthem begins as small, discrete, pink macules that develop into papules. It appears on the face and chest, spreads centrifugally, and may involve the palms and soles. As in roseola, the rash may appear with defervescence of the fever.

Infection due to echovirus 9 is common and produces a typical enteroviral illness. Clinical manifestations include fever, headache, nausea, vomiting, abdominal pain, cough, coryza, pharyngitis, and nuchal rigidity. The exanthem is rubelliform, a maculopapular rash beginning on the face and neck or extending to the trunk and feet and sometimes the palms and soles. Occasionally, there are lesions on the buccal mucosa and soft palate that resemble Koplik spots. Petechiae may occur. The appearance of this rash and the presence of nuchal rigidity makes this illness occasionally mimic meningococcemia. The exanthem persists for about 5 days.

Infection with coxsackievirus A9 is a common cause of exanthem. It is an acute febrile illness with a discrete erythematous maculopapular rash that begins on the face and neck and extends to the trunk and extremities. Aseptic meningitis may occur. The rash may also be vesicular or urticarial.

The clinical differentiation of enteroviral disease is difficult. Since there is no specific therapy for enteroviral infection, it is more important to consider bacterial diseases in the differential diagnosis in order to exclude treatable causes of sepsis, meningitis, myocarditis, and pneumonia. Symptomatic therapy for enteroviral infections includes adequate hydration, antipyretics, and viscous lidocaine gel for painful oral lesions.

Erythema Infectiosum

Erythema infectiosum (fifth disease) is an acute, febrile illness with a unique exanthem. Outbreaks of erythema infectiosum occur primarily in the spring. During epidemics, the attack rate is highest in children 5 to 15 years of age, but all age groups can be affected. The illness is caused by infection with human parvovirus, a single-stranded DNA virus.

The abrupt appearance of the rash is frequently the first manifestation of erythema infectiosum. It begins with a characteristic fiery red rash on the cheeks. The rash is a diffuse erythema of closely grouped tiny papules on an erythematous base. The edges are slightly raised. The erythema is most intense below the eyes and extends over the cheeks in a pattern reminiscent of butterfly wings; it is sometimes referred to as a *slapped-cheek appearance*. There is circumoral pallor as well as sparing of the eyelids and chin. The facial rash fades after

4 to 5 days. Approximately 1 to 2 days after the appearance of the facial rash, a nonpruritic macular erythema or erythematous maculopapular rash occurs on the trunk and limbs. It is at first localized to the deltoid areas, trunk, and forearms but usually extends to involve a large area. This stage of the exanthem may last 1 week. A distinctive aspect of the rash is that it fades with central clearing, giving a reticulated or lacy appearance. The palms and soles are rarely affected.

The exanthem may recur in the ensuing 3 weeks, sometimes briefly. The intensity of the recurrent exanthem varies and may be related to exposure to environmental factors such as sunlight, hot baths, and, perhaps, physical exertion or emotional upset. Associated symptoms frequently occur and may include fever, malaise, headache, sore throat, cough, coryza, nausea, vomiting, diarrhea, and myalgia. Arthralgias and arthritis can occur, but usually only in adults. These symptoms may occur before or after the onset of the rash.

There is no specific treatment for human parvovirus infection. Symptomatic therapy is all that is required. Recovery is usually complete.

Measles

Prior to a nationwide immunization program in 1965 measles was an expected disease of childhood. It is a highly contagious, endemic myxovirus infection. It is a winter-spring disease in temperate climates, but it occurs throughout the world.

After exposure, the incubation period for the disease is about 10 days. The prodromal period lasts approximately 3 days and is characterized by upper respiratory symptoms. The onset of clinical measles is characterized by general malaise, systemic toxicity, fever, coryza, conjunctivitis, photophobia, and cough.

The exanthem develops about the fourteenth day following exposure. The rash first appears behind the ears and at the hairline of the forehead. It spreads in a centrifugal pattern from the head to the feet. It is initially erythematous and maculopapular but rapidly progresses to confluence, especially on the face. Initially the rash is red and blanches on pressure. As it fades, it takes on a copper-to-brownish hue. With healing there may be some fine desquamation. The rash generally lasts 7 days.

Koplik spots are an associated pathognomonic enanthem. The lesions are white, 1-mm discrete spots which first appear on the buccal mucosa opposite the lower molars and then spread to involve the entire buccal mucosa. The treatment of measles is supportive.

Infectious Mononucleosis

The diagnosis of infectious mononucleosis can be entertained in those children, adolescents and young adults who present with fever, sore throat, malaise, and fatigue accompanied by tonsillopharyngitis and lymphadenopathy.

There is strong evidence for Epstein-Barr virus (EBV) as the etiologic agent of the "mononucleosis syndrome." The age of initial (primary) infection varies and appears to depend upon socioeconomic status. The mononucleosis symptom complex is associated with the primary infection. A 2- to 5-day prodromal period of malaise and fatigue with or without fever may precede the full onset of the syndrome. The adenopathy is usually confined to the anterior and posterior cervical chain but may be generalized. There is a 5-percent incidence of a generalized erythematous maculopapular rash associated with an enanthem consisting of petechiae on the soft palate. The incidence of the rash increases to almost 100 percent in those patients taking ampicillin or its congeners. The treatment for infectious mononucleosis is supportive.

Rubella

Rubella (German measles) was once a common childhood disease that had its highest incidence during the spring. The incubation period is 12 to 25 days following exposure with a 1- to 5-day prodrome of fever, malaise, headache, and sore throat.

The exanthem varies and is sometimes difficult to identify. It may present as a short-lived blush, or it may have the more common 2- to 3-day course. The exanthem begins as irregular pink macules and papules on the face spreading to the neck, trunk, and arms in a centrifugal distribution. It coalesces on the face as the eruption reaches the lower extremities and then clears in the same fashion. As enanthem of pinpoint petechiae involving the soft palate (Forschheimer spots) may accompany the rash but is nonspecific.

Lymphadenopathy is a clinical manifestation of rubella, with the enlargement characteristically in the suboccipital and posterior auricular nodes. The clinical diagnosis of the individual case is often difficult, but the epidemic nature of the illness, along with the seasonal variation and high expression rate of the exanthem, help in establishing the diagnosis. A history of inadequate immunizations may assist in the diagnosis. There is no specific therapy.

Varicella

Varicella, or chickenpox, is a result of infection with varicella-zoster virus, a herpes virus. In normal children it is characterized by a pruritic generalized vesicular exanthem with mild systemic manifestations. Cases generally occur in late winter and early spring. It is highly contagious in the prodromal and vesicular stage. Varicella most frequently occurs in children less than 10 years old, but it may occur at any age.

The exanthem starts on the trunk or scalp and first appears as faint, red macules. Within 24 h, the rash acquires the typical vesicular appearance of varicella. The rash consists of teardrop vesicles on an erythematous base, which then dry and crust over (see Fig. 131-3). Successive fresh crops may appear for a few days. The extent of the rash may be minimal but usually will spread centrifugally and become

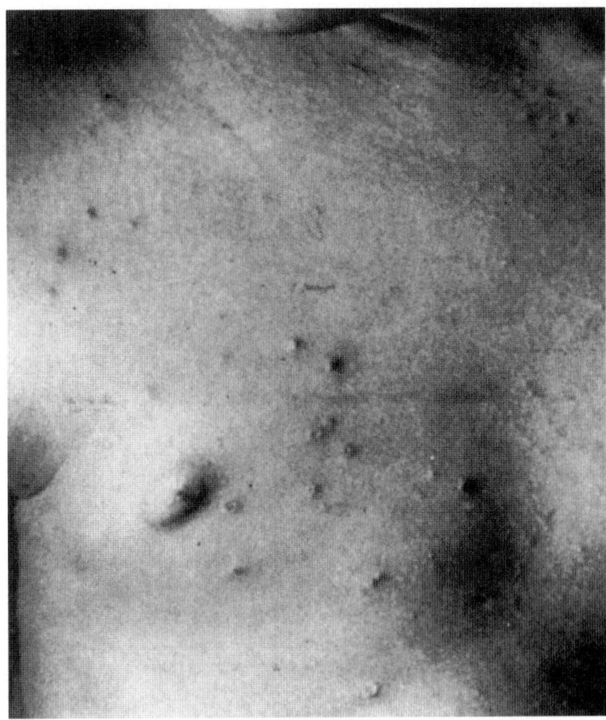

FIG. 131-3. Varicella. [From Burnett JW, Crutcher WA: Viral and rickettsial infections, in Moschella SL, Hurley HJ (eds): *Dermatology*. Philadelphia, Saunders, 1985, vol 1, chap 12, pp 673–738, with permission.]

widespread. Palms and soles are spared. Vesicles may occur on mucous membranes and proceed to rupture and form shallow ulcers. Low-grade fever, malaise, and headache are frequently present but are usually mild. The diagnosis of varicella is usually made clinically on the basis of its distinctive rash. A Tzanck smear of the vesicle contents will demonstrate varicella giant cells with inclusion bodies.

Complications of varicella can occur, including encephalitis, pneumonia, nephritis, and infection of the vesicles with staphylococci or streptococci. Neonates born to mothers with perinatal varicella infection may develop serious illness.

Uncomplicated varicella requires no specific therapy. Acetaminophen may be used as needed, but aspirin should be avoided as it may predispose to the development of Reye syndrome. Oral antihistamines may be useful to reduce itching. Most importantly, lesions should be cleansed regularly to prevent secondary infection. In the absence of central nervous system complications, the prognosis is excellent. Routine use of acyclovir for uncomplicated varicella infections in children is not recommended. While limited data are available on pediatric use, no unusual toxicity or problems have been noted.

Immunocompromised patients with varicella require aggressive treatment with antiviral drugs such as acyclovir. The dose of acyclovir is 80 mg/kg per day in four divided doses up to 800 mg/dose. Administration of varicella zoster immune globulin (VZIG) should be considered for immunocompromised patients exposed to individuals with varicella.

Roseola Infantum

Roseola infantum, or exanthem subitum, is a common acute febrile illness of childhood. There appears to be no seasonal preponderance to its occurrence. The most likely etiologic agent has been identified as the human herpesvirus 6, although other viruses have been associated with a roseola-like illness.

Roseola is characterized by a febrile period of 3 to 5 days, defervescence, and the appearance of a rash for 1 or 2 days. Primarily, young children are affected, with most patients being between 6 months and 3 years. The illness begins abruptly with high fever, sometimes as high as 40.6°C. The child is usually alert and active but may be irritable, especially with very high fever. Associated symptoms are usually mild and may include cough, coryza, anorexia, and abdominal discomfort. Lymphadenopathy may be present. Febrile convulsions may occur. The fever persists for 3 to 5 days, and most often returns to normal by crisis. The child rapidly becomes well.

The exanthem in roseola usually coincides with defervescence of the fever, but it may follow a short afebrile interlude. The rash is an erythematous macular or maculopapular eruption that consists of discrete, rose or pale-pink lesions 2 to 5 mm in size. It is most prominent on the neck, trunk, and buttocks, but the face and proximal extremities may also be involved. The lesions blanch with pressure. There is no mucous membrane involvement. The rash lasts 1 to 2 days but may fade rapidly, usually without desquamation.

There is no specific treatment for roseola. Acetaminophen is useful for fever control and convulsions should be treated vigorously. Recovery is usually complete.

ETIOLOGY UNCLEAR

Erythema Nodosum

Erythema nodosum is an inflammatory exanthem of unknown etiology. It is probably an inflammatory reaction to a stimulus. In the past, erythema nodosum was associated with streptococcal infections, tuberculosis, sarcoid, fungal infections, *Yersinia* infections, vasculitis, inflammatory bowel disease, and leukemia. Now it is more commonly associated with drugs, especially oral contraceptives. Any age can be affected. Constitutional symptoms may be present at the onset, including fever, malaise, myalgias, and arthralgias.

Erythema nodosum presents a distinctive clinical appearance. Bilateral, very tender nodules develop symmetrically. They usually occur on the shins but can occur on the arms, thighs, calves, and buttocks. The nodules are 1 to 5 cm in diameter, and individual lesions may coalesce to form sizable areas of induration. The skin over the nodules is red, smooth, and shiny. No ulceration occurs. After a week or two, the color of the lesions changes from red to blue and may achieve a dull, purple, bruised appearance. The eruption lasts several weeks.

The diagnosis of erythema nodosum is usually readily made on clinical grounds. A thorough history and physical, and perhaps laboratory evaluation, must be performed to exclude an underlying cause. There is no known therapy to alter the course of the disease. Nonsteroidal anti-inflammatory drugs may provide relief from the sometimes significant pain associated with these lesions.

Kawasaki Disease (Mucocutaneous Lymph Node Syndrome)

Kawasaki disease, or mucocutaneous lymph node syndrome (MLNS) is a disease of unclear etiology found predominantly in children under 9 years of age.

The diagnosis of this disorder is based on a constellation of clinical findings. The patient must exhibit a prolonged fever associated with at least four of the following: (1) conjunctivitis, (2) rash, (3) lymphadenopathy, (4) changes in the oropharynx consisting of injection of the pharynx and lips with prominent papillae of the tongue (strawberry tongue), and (5) extremity erythema and edema.

The rash has been described as erythematous, morbilliform, urticarial, scarlatiniform, or erythema multiforme–like. It has a predilection for the perineum. Additional supportive evidence which may help in the presumptive diagnosis are leukocytosis, elevation of acute-phase reactants, elevated liver function tests, arthritis, arthralgia, and irritability.

In the second phase, there is usually a sharp rise in the platelet count, desquamation of the fingers and/or toes, and the most serious complication, the development of coronary artery aneurysm. A small percentage (1 to 2 percent) of patients with coronary artery aneurysm develop sudden cardiac failure, resulting in death from myocardial infarction with coronary artery thrombosis.

The differential diagnosis includes drug allergy, toxic epidermal necrolysis, staphylococcal toxin–mediated syndromes, erythema multiforme, and scarlet fever. The etiologic speculations include a hyperimmune response to a variety of infections, a viral syndrome, allergic or toxic response to pollutants, drugs, toxic agents, and a possibility of a rickettsial disease.

Treatment of Kawasaki disease is controversial and includes various antibiotics, salicylates, and steroids. Intravenous gamma globulin is now routinely recommended. Aspirin may be the most promising therapy. Bed rest, supportive therapy, and frequent monitoring are mainstays of treatment.

Pityriasis Rosea

Pityriasis rosea is a mild inflammatory exanthem of unknown cause. The available evidence suggests a viral etiology. Pityriasis rosea affects all age groups but occurs most commonly in patients 10 to 35 years old. It tends to occur in spring and fall but not in epidemics. Pityriasis rosea is not contagious. A pityriasis rosea–like eruption has been associated with some drugs and viruses. Occasionally there are prodromal symptoms including malaise, headache, sore throat, fatigue, and arthralgia.

The rash of pityriasis rosea evolves over a period of several weeks. It begins with a "herald patch," a solitary, erythematous lesion with a raised edematous border most frequently occurring on the chest or back. It is 2 to 6 cm in diameter. About 1 or 2 weeks later, there is a widespread, symmetrical eruption of pink- or salmon-colored maculopapular lesions. The patches are oval and are covered with dry epidermis which desquamates to form a ring of scale at the periphery. The lesions are 0.5 to 1.5 cm in diameter and are at first discrete, but can become confluent. The long axes of the patches frequently run parallel to lines of skin tension, giving rise to the Christmas tree pattern seen on the back. The eruption is generalized and chiefly affects the trunk, although it can occur anywhere. The lesions can be localized. Mucous membranes can be involved with plaques, hemorrhagic punctate spots, or ulcers. Successive crops of skin lesions can occur, and the entire illness can last 3 to 8 weeks. Healing is complete, without sequelae or evidence of organ involvement.

The diagnosis of pityriasis rosea is made by the clinical appearance. It can be confused with viral exanthem, drug eruptions, syphilis, and seborrheic dermatitis. Potassium hydroxide preparation of skin scrapings will serve to distinguish pityriasis rosea from tinea corporis. A serologic test for syphilis must be done to exclude that diagnosis.

Therapy is directed at alleviating symptoms. No treatment has been shown to shorten the duration of the rash. The rash is sometimes very itchy. Oatmeal baths and oral antihistamines will provide temporary relief. Emollients will help dryness and irritation. Secondary infection must be prevented with thorough cleansing.

BIBLIOGRAPHY

Freedberg IM, Eisen AZ, Wolff K, et al (eds): *Fitzpatrick's Dermatology in General Medicine,* 5th ed. New York, McGraw-Hill, 1999.

MUSCULOSKELETAL DISORDERS IN CHILDREN

Richard A. Christoph

PHYSIOLOGY OF MUSCULOSKELETAL SYSTEM IN CHILDREN

The child's musculoskeletal system differs from the adult's in multiple respects, reflecting the child's active growth and development. These differences relate to the patterns of injury and illness manifested by children presenting to the emergency department. In utero, fetal positioning leads to a flexor pattern in the extremities, with external rotation of the hips and internal rotation of the tibiofibular apparatus. The ankle is in dorsiflexion, and the feet are inverted. Upon the newborn's arrival, motor development progresses predictably in a rostral-to-caudal direction and in a proximal-to-distal direction. Thus, the infant achieves head and trunk control prior to extremity control. Proficiency in movements of the upper extremity precedes lower extremity control.

The joint contractures brought about by fetal positioning and motor development influence the child's gait. The child requires a broad base of support and maintains distinct flexion of hips and knees and dorsiflexion of the ankles, resulting in a high-stepping gait. The arms of the toddler are abducted at the shoulder and flexed at the elbow. The child does not develop reciprocating arm swinging until about 2 years of age.

Simultaneously with development of the central nervous system and the maturation of motor milestones and gait, the child is growing most actively in early childhood. Bone growth occurs through two types of ossification. Growth in circumference occurs at the periosteal surface, as mesenchymal cells differentiate into osteocytes, which lay down new bone in a process known as *intramembranous ossification*. Longitudinal growth is achieved through *endochondral ossification,*, consisting of a proliferation and hypertrophy of cartilage cells at a physis. An organized vascular invasion of this cartilage results in delivery of mesenchymal cells to the area, which then differentiate into osteocytes, completing the transformation of cartilage to bone.

It is helpful to think of long bones as consisting of discrete anatomic areas. Long bones may have physes, or areas of growth cartilage, at both ends (e.g., tibia and femur). Other long bones (e.g., the phalanges) have a physis at only one end. The area of the long bone between a physis and the adjacent joint is the epiphysis, and the area of bone between a physis and a point for muscle or ligamentous attachment is an apophysis. The metaphysis of a long bone represents the area of widening, or flaring, of the long bone between its midshaft (the diaphysis) and the physis.

The long bones of children are generally less dense and more porous than the long bones of adults. The resulting increased compliance contributes to the tendency of children's long bones to respond to mechanical stress by bowing and buckling, rather than fracturing through and through, as in adult fracture patterns. The periosteum of the diaphysis and the metaphysis is thicker in children and is continuous from the metaphysis to the epiphysis, surrounding and protecting the mechanically weaker physis. This physeal weakness is related to the reduced oxygen tension found in the hypertrophic zone of the physis, a location of frequent fractures within the physis. The physis is sensitive to alterations in the blood supply to this hypertrophic zone as well as to nutritional, hormonal, and mechanical influences.

Growth of the musculoskeletal system and its response to illness, injury, and nutrition are also influenced by the growth of muscle and connective tissues. The ligaments of children are stronger and more compliant than those of adults, often tolerating mechanical forces at the expense of apophyseal attachments or epiphyseal integrity. While the absolute number of muscle fibers is fixed at birth, the fibers of tendons can increase in number and in size. The growth of muscle through hypertrophy and the growth of tendons through hypertrophy and proliferation depend on the mechanical forces applied to them.

CHILDHOOD PATTERNS OF INJURY

Physeal Injuries

The weakest zone, or layer, of the physis is its third layer of cells and matrix (hypertrophic cell zone). It is particularly susceptible to shearing, bending, and tension stresses. It represents the layer of the physis that is most consistently fractured. Consequently, the reserve and proliferative cartilage cells in the first two zones of the injured physis usually remain with the epiphysis. This is relevant in that the predominant circulatory support of the cells in these two reproductive zones of the physis arises through the epiphyseal vasculature and thus is more likely to be spared in the event of physeal injury (Fig. 132-1).

It has been demonstrated that compression forces applied to the physis can affect bone growth. This is particularly true when compression forces are applied to the epiphyseal side of the physis. The injury to bone growth caused by compression results from interruption of the epiphyseal circulation to the reproductive cells of the physis.

Although several authors have classified injuries to the physis, the Salter and Harris classification system offers a thorough and practical classification based on the mechanism of injury, the relationship of the fracture line to the germinal (reproductive zone) layer of the physis, and the prognosis for disturbance of bone growth (Fig. 132-2).

TYPE I PHYSEAL FRACTURE In type I physeal fracture (representing 6 percent of physeal injuries), the epiphysis separates from the metaphysis. The cleavage is through the hypertrophic cell zone of the physis. The reproductive cells of the physis remain with the epiphysis. There are no associated fragments of bones, since the thick periosteal attachments surrounding the physis remain intact. However, the epiphysis may be somewhat displaced from the metaphysis. Bone growth is not usually disturbed (Fig. 132-2).

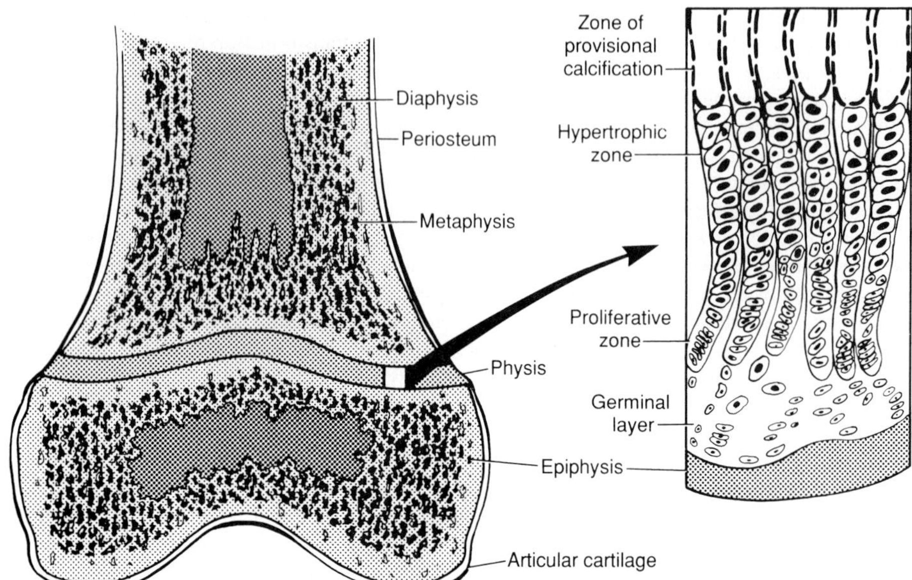

FIG. 132-1. Relationship between anatomic regions of a typical long bone and and the physis. Detail: cellular zones of physis. (Reproduced with permission from Tolo and Wood, 1994.)

Diagnosis is suspected clinically in a child with point tenderness over a physis. Radiographically, the only abnormality may be an associated joint effusion. Any epiphyseal displacement is usually apparent on one or more views. In the absence of epiphyseal displacement, the diagnosis is a clinical one, supported by the appearance of the typical joint effusion.

Treatment consists of immobilization of the suspected fracture using an appropriate splint, the application of cold compresses for 48 h, and elevation. Referral to an orthopedic surgeon is probably warranted in order to render aftercare and to ensure monitoring for bone growth disturbances. Analgesia may be necessary, despite immobilization, for 24 to 72 h, after which time the child usually remains quite comfortable in the immobilization device.

TYPE II PHYSEAL FRACTURE Type II physeal fractures are the most common, representing 75 percent of physeal injuries. The line of fracture extends a variable distance along the hypertrophic cell zone of the physis and then out through a piece of metaphyseal bone. The periosteum on the concave side (overlying the metaphyseal fragment) remains intact, whereas the periosteum on the convex (opposite) side of the fracture is torn away from the diaphysis while remaining adherent to the epiphysis (Fig. 132-2). Growth is preserved, since the reproduction layers of the physis maintain their position with the epiphysis and the epiphyseal circulation. Diagnosis is made radiographically by noting the triangular fragment of metaphysis (Holland sign) unassociated with discernible injury to the epiphysis.

Reduction of the fracture should be gentle and is usually easily achieved. Analgesia with or without sedation should be offered to the child prior to any reduction maneuvers. When using sedation and analgesics, precautions should be taken as to patient selection, premedication assessments, monitoring, and postmedication observation consistent with institutional guidelines. Overreduction of the type II frac-

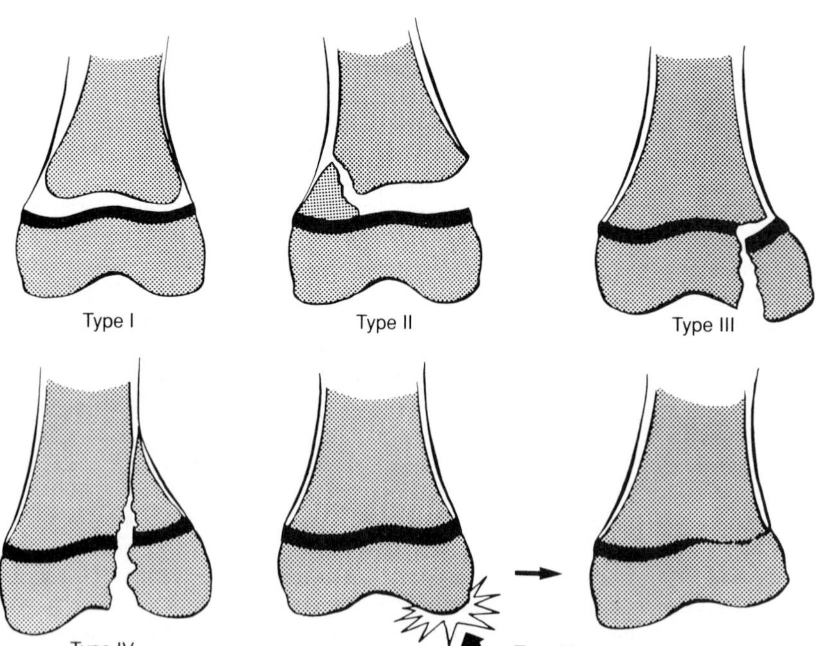

FIG. 132-2. Salter-Harris classification of physeal injuries. (Reproduced with permission from Tolo and Wood, 1994.)

ture is usually prevented by the periosteal hinge remaining on the concave side of the fracture.

Immobilization, cold compresses, and elevation are principles of management, as in the case of type I fractures. Referral to an orthopedic surgeon for aftercare and observation is important, as is the provision of adequate analgesia in the initial days following the fracture.

TYPE III PHYSEAL FRACTURE The hallmark of this injury is an intraarticular fracture of the epiphysis extending to the hypertrophic cell zone of the physis, with the cleavage plane continuing along the physis to the periphery (Fig. 132-2). The injury, usually involving the proximal or distal tibia epiphysis, is caused by severe intraarticular shearing forces. The prognosis for subsequent bone growth is related to the preservation of circulation to the epiphyseal bone fragment and is usually favorable. The type III physeal fracture represents less than 10 percent of physeal injuries.

Diagnosis is a radiographic one based on the appearance of an epiphyseal fragment unassociated with an apparent metaphyseal fracture. There may or may not be an associated periosteal injury.

Reduction of the unstable epiphyseal fragment with careful restoration of the alignment of the articular surface is critically important. Open surgical techniques are frequently necessary in order to ensure the necessary anatomic reduction of the articular surface, especially with severely displaced fractures. This fracture warrants consultation with an orthopedic surgeon in the emergency department.

Decisions regarding admission or operative open reduction are made in consultation with an orthopedic surgeon experienced in the management of physeal injuries. If closed reduction techniques are successfully employed by the orthopedic consultant, aftercare instructions are similar to those offered to patients suffering from type II physeal injuries.

TYPE IV PHYSEAL FRACTURE The fracture line originates at the articular surface and extends through the epiphysis, the entire thickness of the physis, and through the metaphysis (Fig. 132-2). It is an injury pattern most often involving the distal humerus and represents about 10 percent of physeal injuries. Future bone growth is at risk. Perfect anatomic reduction of the articular surface and of the physis is required to minimize the potential for premature bone growth arrest.

The diagnosis is made upon identification of epiphyseal and metaphyseal fragments radiographically. The fragments may or may not be variably displaced. Radiographic interpretation of fractures involving the distal humerus and elbow can be challenging because of the dynamic nature of the ossification centers of the region.

Open surgical reduction should be performed early by an experienced orthopedic surgeon. Internal fixation of the fragments is accomplished using fine, smooth Kirschner wires traversing the physeal growth plate perpendicularly.

TYPE V PHYSEAL FRACTURE This fortunately rare injury pattern (1 percent of physeal injuries) usually involves the knee or ankle. It is the result of severe abduction or adduction to the joint, which transmits profound compressive forces to a local segment of the physis, crushing the reproductive chondrocytes of the reserve zone and proliferative zone. Minimal or no displacement of the epiphysis occurs (Fig. 132-2).

The diagnosis of type V physeal injuries may be very difficult initially. Often, the seriousness of the injury is underappreciated. An initial diagnosis of sprain or possible type I physeal fracture may prove incorrect in view of subsequent development of premature growth arrest. Radiographs may appear normal or may demonstrate focal narrowing of the physeal plate. An associated joint effusion is the norm, although its presence is nonspecific.

Treatment of type V physeal injuries consists of cast support of the knee or ankle, non-weight-bearing for at least 3 weeks and close orthopedic outpatient follow-up in anticipation of the nearly inevitable focal bone growth arrest.

Torus Fractures

The porosity and compliance of the metaphyses of children's long bones, coupled with the relative thickness of the periosteum in this area, confer unique fracture characteristics. Compressive forces often result in a bulging or buckling of the periosteum rather than a more complete fracture line. Cortical, or *torus,* fractures are so named to describe a prominence or bulging of the bony cortex, usually involving the metaphysis.

Diagnosis is based on point tenderness over the site of the torus fracture. While a simple torus fracture does not produce a visible deformity of the extremity, soft tissue swelling routinely overlies the bone injury. In children who are not morbidly obese, the torus fracture is frequently palpable as a ridge over the metaphyseal area of the long bone.

Radiographically, the manifestation of a torus fracture may be somewhat subtle. Interpretation of radiographs is aided by following the contour of the metaphyseal flare, observing any asymmetry, bulging, or deviation of the cortical margin. With magnification, deviations in the trabecular pattern of the cortical markings can be seen to be associated with the bulging prominence of the cortical margin.

Since torus fractures are not typically associated with severe angulation, displacement, or rotational abnormalities, most can be competently managed by the emergency physician. Reduction techniques are rarely, if ever, necessary. The extremity is splinted in a position of function for 3 to 4 weeks. Aftercare can be arranged through the child's primary care physician or an orthopedic consultant, usually in 2 weeks. Analgesia requirements in the immediate days after the injury are usually minimal following the application of the splint.

Greenstick Fractures

Stresses and forces can be applied to the porous, compliant bones of children in such a way as to create an incomplete cortical fracture. A greenstick fracture is characterized by cortical disruption and periosteal tearing on the convex side of the bone, with an intact periosteum on the concave side of the fracture. Greenstick fractures are more stable and somewhat less painful than complete fractures, since the area of intact periosteum protects the child from bony crepitance.

The need for reduction is related to the degree of angulation of the fracture, the age of the child, and the anatomic location of the injury. Orthopedic consultation may be helpful in the decision analysis regarding possible reduction and outpatient management.

Plastic Deformities

Plastic deformities (sometimes known as bowing or bending fractures) are almost exclusively limited to the forearm and lower-leg long bones. Usually this pattern of injury is noted in combination with a completed fracture of the other bone of the forearm or lower leg. The cortex of the diaphysis of the long bone is deformed, with preservation of the periosteum all along the diaphysis. Such injuries result from the compliance and porosity of the child's bones, with the associated tendency to deform (bend) rather than fracture in the traditional sense.

Diagnosis is made radiographically. Proper interpretation of the radiographs requires an awareness of the normal shape of the long bones involved, since fracture lines and disruptions in the periosteum are absent.

Prompt orthopedic consultation is important.

FRACTURES ASSOCIATED WITH CHILD ABUSE

It is important to remember that all of the skeletal injuries associated with accidental trauma can also be inflicted as a result of nonaccidental injury (e.g., child battering, shaken baby syndrome, or child abuse). However, certain injury patterns are encountered consistently as a result of child maltreatment, particularly multiple fractures in various stages of healing. An understanding of the various mechanisms of inflicted injury will facilitate better awareness of the patterns of injury suggesting abuse. Correlation of the child's age, motor capabilities, and the alleged mechanism of injury with the injury pattern being evaluated is fundamental to the evaluation of childhood skeletal injuries, as is the identification of coexisting cutaneous signs suggestive of abuse (e.g., suspicious bruises, burns, etc.).

Direct Blows

Direct blows may result in transverse, oblique, longitudinal, greenstick or torus fractures. All of these fractures are commonly associated with accidental mechanisms and are nonspecific for child abuse. Correlation with the child's age or motor development, however, may arouse suspicions. A transverse or oblique fracture of the humerus of a 2-month-old infant is quite a different situation from an isolated similar fracture in an 8-year-old.

Twisting Injuries

Twisting injuries create spiral fractures in long bones, highly specific for child abuse in children who are not yet ambulatory. Spiral fractures in ambulatory children lose their specificity for child abuse but remain a potential manifestation of abuse and warrant careful consideration. Whereas toddlers (1 to 3 years of age) commonly suffer spiral fractures of the lower one-third of the tibia accidentally as the result of a trivial fall or by twisting themselves on a planted foot (the so-called toddler's fracture), spiral fractures of the tibia may occur with child abuse. Spiral fractures of the femur may be accidental in toddlers but can also be seen in child abuse in this age group. Spiral femur fractures in newborns and preambulatory infants are highly suggestive of nonaccidental trauma. Correlation with the alleged mechanism of injury and a discrete but careful inspection for other evidence of abuse will prove helpful, along with a review of past injuries experienced by the child or the child's siblings.

The injury pattern most closely related to inflicted injury is that of metaphyseal-epiphyseal fractures. More specifically, chip fractures of the metaphyses or epiphyses, particularly in various stages of healing, are seen as the result of twisting or jiggling forces. Callus formation becomes striking during the healing process, along with remarkable new bone deposits along the periosteum. Subperiosteal hemorrhage may create an elevation of the periosteum away from the underlying bony cortex. Fragmentation of the clavicle and acromion and separation of the costochondral junctions of the ribs are especially suggestive of abuse.

Distraction Injuries

Distraction injuries to the long bones create hemorrhagic separation of the distal metaphyses, creating a lucency parallel and proximal to the physis. The result is a bucket-handle fracture.

Shaking Injuries

Shaking injuries create fractures similar to those caused by twisting mechanisms. In addition, retinal hemorrhages, intracranial injuries, and intraabdominal injuries may result. Spinal compression fractures, vertebral subluxations and dislocations, and anterior notching of vertebral bodies can be seen.

Squeezing Injuries

Squeezing injuries create encirclement bruises and rib fractures highly suggestive of abuse. Particular attention should be given to multiple rib fractures and rib fractures in various stages of healing, the presence of which is classically associated with the battered child syndrome. Appreciation of this phenomenon is related to an understanding of normal bone healing and an ability to date the approximate age of any bone injuries identified in the child's workup. By looking for associated soft tissue findings, the appearance of a distinct fracture line, callus formation and calcification, and ossification of newly laid periosteal bone, the physician will be in a better position to detect discrepancies between the alleged history of the injury(ies) and the radiographic evidence of injury.

CLAVICLE FRACTURE

The clavicle, extending from the scapular acromion process to the manubrium sterni, serves as the sole skeletal connection between the upper extremity and the trunk and absorbs all medial forces imposed upon the upper arm. The clavicle consists of a double curve in the horizontal plane. Viewed from the front, the medial two-thirds is convex, while the lateral one-third is concave. The junction between the two curves represents its structurally weakest area and most frequently fractured site. The clavicle is the most commonly fractured bone in children.

Clavicle fractures may occur in the newborn as a result of shoulder compression during a difficult delivery. In the older infant, toddler, or child, the usual mechanism of fracture is a fall onto an outstretched hand or elbow or onto the side of a shoulder. Often, in younger children, the fracture is of the incomplete, or greenstick, type. A direct blow to the clavicle may also cause a fracture.

Diagnosis of clavicular fracture is facilitated by its subcutaneous location and the ease of its palpation on examination. Newborns with clavicle fractures may not be symptomatic. When they are symptomatic, it may come in the form of "pseudoparalysis," or nonuse of the ipsilateral upper extremity. Alternatively, parents or health care providers may notice the bone callus at 2 to 3 weeks of age, indicative of a fracture previously unappreciated.

Older infants and children with clavicular fractures have pain on attempted range-of-motion movement of the neck or upper extremity. Soft tissue swelling, point tenderness, and bone crepitance are indicative of the fracture site. In view of the close proximity of the clavicle to the subclavian vessels and lung, careful assessment of the circulation to the ipsilateral upper extremity and chest auscultation are important. Anteroposterior radiographs of the clavicle and shoulder are principally useful in excluding other associated skeletal injuries, particularly those involving the proximal humerus and scapular prominences. Dislocations of the sternoclavicular joint, particularly posterior dislocations of the proximal clavicle, are optimally visualized by lordotic views.

Care of the child with a clavicle fracture is principally directed toward comfort and analgesia for the child. The child's future bone growth and the modeling potential confer great healing and restorative capability to the fractured clavicle. Even displaced fractures nearly always heal well, whether or not strict anatomic reduction is accomplished in the emergency department.

"Figure-of-eight" shoulder abduction restraints are available in various sizes and can be offered to children outside infancy. Application should ensure a snug, symmetrical fit without excessive tightness or pinching. As is the case with the application of any orthopedic appliance, subsequent assessment of the child's neurovascular status in the upper extremities is mandatory. Some children, however, complain of greater discomfort with the figure-of-eight restraint than without. In such instances, the use of an upper extremity sling-and-swathe or shoulder immobilizer will offer adequate protection from the discomfort associated with shoulder and upper extremity movements.

Children with either type of immobilizing or restraint device are encouraged to wear the restraint day and night for 2 weeks, followed by daytime use for another 2 to 3 weeks. Oral analgesia sufficient to ensure the child's comfort is of paramount importance. Follow-up care can be arranged through the child's primary care physician or an orthopedic surgeon.

SUPRACONDYLAR FRACTURES

The most common elbow fracture in childhood is the supracondylar fracture of the distal humeral metaphysis. It is an important injury pattern not only by virtue of its frequency but also because of its associated potential neurovascular complications. Hyperextension forces during a fall against an outstretched arm displace the distal fragment posteriorly and proximally.

The close proximity of the brachial artery to the supracondylar fracture predisposes the artery to contusion, laceration, or entrapment by fractured fragments. Subsequent arterial spasm or compression by splints, casts, or other dressings may further embarrass the arterial blood supply to the muscles of the forearm and to the hand. A resultant forearm compartment syndrome may ensue, with the development within hours of permanent injury and disability to the function of the involved forearm and hand. This is called *Volkmann's ischemic contracture* and is presaged by (1) pain referred to the proximal forearm upon passive extension of the fingers, (2) "stocking-glove" anesthesia of the ischemic hand, and (3) rock hard forearm swelling. Skin perfusion is usually normal despite the severe ischemic insult to the entire forearm and hand, and pulses may remain palpable at the wrist despite serious vascular compromise. The clinical suspicion of a potential ischemic compartment syndrome involving the forearm necessitates an immediate consultation by an orthopedic surgeon who is prepared to offer a complete and radical forearm decompression if reduction of the fracture does not satisfactorily restore vascular integrity.

The diagnosis of a supracondylar fracture of the distal humerus is suspected when tenderness is elicited upon palpation of the distal humerus and the child complains of pain on passive flexion of the elbow. The child usually prefers to maintain the forearm in pronation. The degree of soft tissue swelling and ecchymosis of the elbow ranges from severe to subtle.

As mentioned above, neurovascular assessment of the hand and forearm is the most critical step in the evaluation of elbow injuries in children. In addition to assessments of vascular integrity, injuries to the ulnar, median, or radial nerves should be noted. Such associated injuries are common, occurring in 5 to 10 percent of children with supracondylar fractures.

Differential diagnostic considerations include fractures to the humeral condyles, intercondylar fractures, fractures of the radial head and the olecranon of the ulna, and subluxation of the radial head ("nursemaid's elbow"). The physical examination of all these conditions may be undistinguishing except for that of nursemaid's elbow.

Definitive diagnosis of supracondylar fractures rests with radiography, which usually delineates the injury. Occasionally the appearance of the fracture line is subtle. Observations of a loss of the usual anterior angulation of the capitellum or of a posterior fat pad sign, indicative of an intraarticular elbow effusion (usually of blood), may confer indirect evidence of a supracondylar fracture if the fracture line itself is inapparent. An anterior humeral line, an imaginary line drawn along the anterior margin of the distal humeral diaphysis, normally bisects the posterior two-thirds of the capitellum in the lateral view of the elbow. In subtle supracondylar fractures with loss of the normal anterior angulation of the capitellum, the anterior humeral line may bisect the anterior portion of the capitellum. In association with a posterior fat pad sign, such a loss of the normal anatomic relationships may well indicate a supracondylar fracture.

Management of a child's supracondylar fracture is begun immediately upon arrival in the department. Splinting of the affected elbow in extension is recommended in order to safeguard against development of secondary injury to the vessels, nerves, and soft tissues surrounding the fracture. Frequent reassessments of neurovascular status of the forearm and hand are important. Consultation with an orthopedic surgeon is necessary in all cases of supracondylar fracture. In cases of neurovascular compromise, immediate fracture reduction is mandatory. Careful monitoring of neurovascular status following fracture reduction and maintenance of the elbow in extension are in order. If an ischemic volar forearm compartment is still suspected over the succeeding 6 h, surgical decompression and/or arterial exploration may be indicated.

In the absence of neurovascular compromise, therapy is influenced largely by the degree of displacement of the distal fragment, associated soft tissue swelling, and the reliability of the follow-up arrangements. Admission is indicated for all children whose supracondylar fracture is displaced, who manifest significant soft tissue swelling, or whose parents cannot ensure reliable outpatient follow-up. Open reduction is indicated if closed reduction techniques are unsuccessful, especially for oblique fractures. Outpatient management is considered for the child whose fracture is nondisplaced and has minimal swelling. The orthopedic surgeon should reexamine such children within 24 h of injury.

Lateral and medial condylar fractures, intercondylar fractures, and transcondylar fractures carry their own associated risks of neurovascular compromise. Children with such fractures typically present with moderate-to-severe soft tissue swelling and tenderness of the elbow, which is maintained in a moderate degree of flexion. Circulatory integrity of the forearm and hand should be assessed immediately. Peripheral nerve function, particularly ulnar nerve function, is at risk.

Immediate orthopedic consultation is indicated, since such fractures often require open reduction and carry risks of long-term sequelae. Neurovascular insults usually resolve nicely with appropriate management of the fracture. Growth arrest is rare.

RADIAL HEAD SUBLUXATION

Radial head subluxation is an extremely common injury (nursemaid's elbow) with a peak incidence between 1 and 4 years of age. It has been recognized for centuries. While a history of linear traction upon a hand or wrist is frequently elicited, it is not uncommon to receive a history of an incidental fall in which the arm, elbow, and forearm were impacted between the ground and the child's trunk. Occasionally there is no history of trauma, and the parents note only nonuse of the affected limb.

The child maintains the arm partially flexed at the elbow and in forearm pronation. Typically, the arm is kept close to the trunk. The child usually is found seated in the parent's lap and appears quite contented and playful but declines to actively move the affected arm.

A slow and pleasant approach to the child's examination demonstrates no tenderness to palpation of the clavicle, shoulder, humerus, elbow, forearm, wrist, or hand. By carefully avoiding movements involving the elbow and forearm, the physician will note painless passive range of motion of the shoulder, hand, and wrist. In contrast, even modest attempts to supinate the forearm or to flex or extend the elbow elicit pain and anguish.

There is seldom clinical doubt if the child's age, mechanism of injury, body positioning, and examination (nonuse as opposed to tenderness to palpation) are consistent with the diagnosis. Radiographs in such a situation are superfluous, since there are no radiographic abnormalities associated with this condition and since the examination effectively excludes other entities. Radiographs should be considered, however, if the child exhibits point tenderness, soft tissue swelling, or ecchymosis of the elbow.

Reduction is usually easily accomplished. The physician's thumb is placed over the child's radial head. The child's hand is grasped by the physician. Beginning with the child's elbow in extension and the forearm in pronation, three simultaneous maneuvers are rapidly accomplished: (1) downward pressure on the child's radial head by the physician's thumb, (2) passive *full* supination of the child's forearm, and (3) passive *full* flexion of the child's elbow. A "click" is often but not always palpated by the physician's thumb as reduction is accomplished. The child cries out for a few seconds but is usually and easily soon distracted. Observation for up to 15 min typically demonstrates a full return to normal function and use, especially if the physician notes the click. If function and use have not normalized within 15 min, a repeated attempt at reduction is recommended. Alternative diagnoses should be considered if the child's arm does not return to normal function and use following a second reduction attempt. Radiographic studies may then be indicated.

For children who recover full, unrestricted use after one or two reduction maneuvers, further therapy is unnecessary. A sling may be offered to the child whose function and use have improved but are not complete. The toddler will often discard the sling within minutes or hours, however. Parents should be gently reminded to avoid lifting the child by the hand, wrist, or forearm and should be informed of the increased risk of recurrence until the child reaches 5 to 6 years of age.

DISORDERS OF THE HIP AND LOWER EXTREMITY

Slipped Capital Femoral Epiphysis

Associated with obesity and puberty, slipped capital femoral epiphysis (SCFE) is of multifactorial etiology, including physeal cartilage fatigue, genetic predisposition, endocrinologic factors, and trauma. There is a male-to-female predominance of 8:3, and it is more common in blacks than in whites. Peak incidence occurs between 12 and 15 years in males and between 10 and 13 years in females. The child with SCFE may present clinically with either a chronic slip or an acute slip.

With a chronic SCFE, the child complains of pain in the groin referred to the anteromedial thigh and knee. The pain is dull, vague, intermittent or continuous, and is exacerbated by physical activity. It may or may not be related to a history of trivial or significant injury. If walking is observed, the lower limb is held in external rotation, and the gait is antalgic. Typically, the examiner notes that attempts at hip flexion are accompanied by lateral rotation of the thigh. Full flexion is restricted, and the child cannot touch his or her thigh to the abdominal wall. Limb shortening of 1 to 2 cm may be noted, as may disuse atrophy of the muscles of the proximal thigh.

Acute SCFE may be the result of an acute traumatic event or may represent an acute-on-chronic slip in which sudden, severe pain and inability to bear weight develop in a patient who has been experiencing weeks to months of pain in the hip-thigh-knee region. Examining a patient with a suggested acute slip elicits great pain. Marked external rotation of the thigh is noted, as well as readily apparent limb shortening. Great gentleness is required of the examining physician, and the hip should not be forced into maximum range of motion, which can aggravate the displacement of the fracture. The child is not asked to walk to observe the gait.

The differential diagnosis includes septic arthritis, toxic tenosynovitis, Legg-Calvé-Perthes disease, and other hip fractures. Differentiating SCFE from septic arthritis is usually not difficult, since the child with SCFE is not febrile or toxically ill appearing and demonstrates no remarkable elevation in peripheral white blood cell (WBC) level or erythrocyte sedimentation rate (ESR). Differentiation from the other entities requires radiographs, including AP films and bilateral "frog-leg" lateral radiographs.

Medial slips of the femoral epiphyses will be noted on the AP views, while the frog-leg lateral films of both hips are used in comparison to detect posterior slips. In the AP view, a line drawn along the lateral (superior) aspect of the femoral neck should transect the lateral quarter of the femoral epiphysis (Fig. 132-3). The slipped epiphysis will not be transected by the line at all or will be transected less than noted on the unaffected hip. Moderate to severe slips will be detected by this method (Fig. 132-4), while mild slips require the interpretation of the frog-leg lateral x-rays of both hips. If the diagnosis of SCFE is suspected, both types of radiographs are necessary.

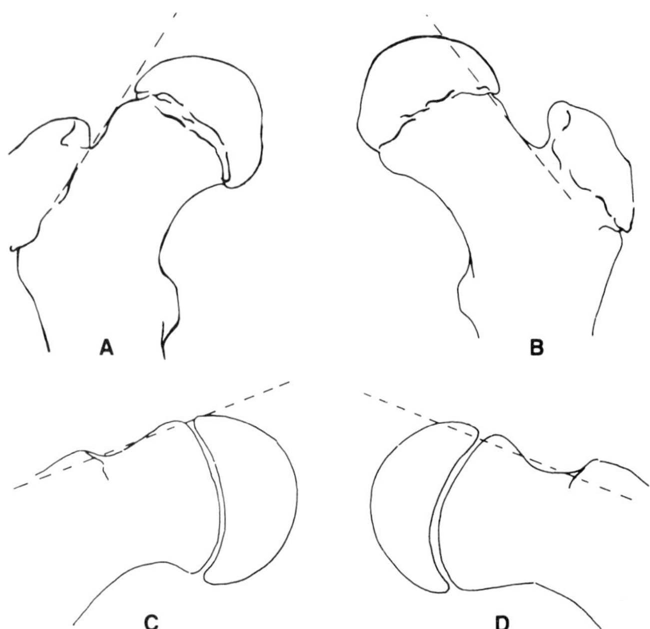

FIG. 132-3. A line drawn along the lateral (superior) aspect of the femoral neck fails to transect the lateral quarter of the femoral head in medial SCFE, seen in **A** and **C**. The normal anatomic relationship is illustrated in **B** and **D**.

Management in the emergency department consists of (1) confirmation of the diagnosis, (2) assurance of absolute non-weight-bearing, (3) orthopedic consultation, and (4) admission to the hospital. No patient with SCFE is treated as an outpatient, even if the intent is to perform surgery the following day. The management of SCFE is operative reduction and fixation, although there exists a certain amount of discussion in the orthopedic literature as to the optimal technical approach. Subsequent immobilization of the hip is maintained for at least 12 weeks, and careful observation for 1 to 2 years thereafter is

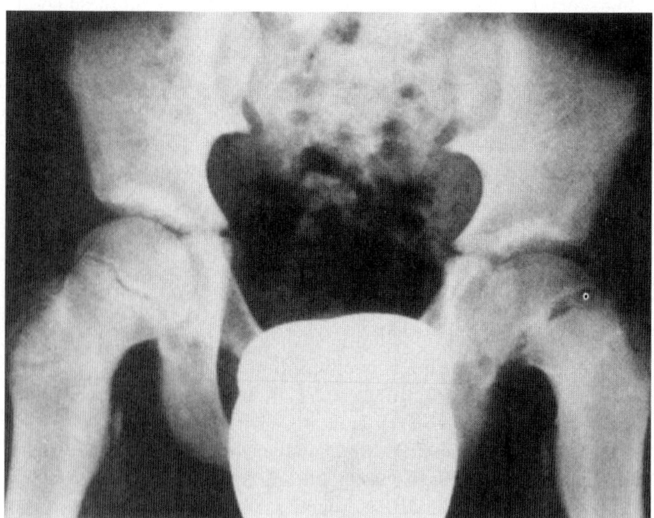

FIG. 132-4. AP radiograph illustrating a medial SCFE involving the left hip.

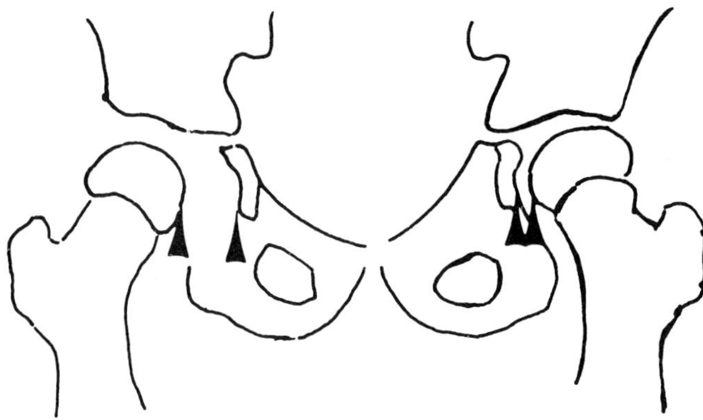

FIG. 132-5. Widening of the joint space, indicating an effusion, is a nonspecific finding seen in children with toxic tenosynovitis, Legg-Calvé-Perthes disease, suppurative arthritis, and hemarthrosis.

necessary in anticipation of the development of this condition's most serious complication, avascular necrosis of the femoral head.

Transient Tenosynovitis of the Hip

Acute transient tenosynovitis of the hip is the most common cause of hip pain in children less than 10 years of age (peak, 3 to 6 years). There is a boy-to-girl predominance that is variously described as 3:2 to 5:1. The right hip is somewhat more commonly affected than the left, and the condition is bilateral in 5 percent of cases. The etiology of the condition is not known, although trauma, viral and bacterial infection, and allergy (hypersensitization) have been proposed by authors to explain the condition.

Symptoms may be acute or gradual in onset. There may be a history of recent upper respiratory symptoms offered by the parent. Considering the age group, such an association is probably best interpreted casually. The child complains of pain in the anteromedial or anterolateral thigh and knee. The gait is antalgic. Tenderness is elicited upon palpation of the anterior hip, and range of motion is limited by the discomfort. The child's systemic temperature is normal or minimally elevated. The child does not appear toxically ill.

The peripheral WBC and ESR are usually normal. If performed, tuberculin skin tests, rheumatoid factor titers, and antistreptococcal antibodies titers are negative. Radiographs of the hip are either normal or demonstrate mild to moderate hip effusion (Fig. 132-5). There are no bone changes associated with the condition.

The differential diagnosis includes SCFE and other hip fractures, Legg-Calvé-Perthes disease, and suppurative arthritis of the hip. Less common differential considerations include rheumatic fever, juvenile rheumatoid arthritis, and, rarely, tuberculosis of the hip.

If the peripheral WBC and ESR are substantially elevated and a hip effusion is noted on the radiograph, a diagnostic arthrocentesis should be performed to exclude suppurative arthritis. Consideration should be given to open irrigation of the hip joint in the operating room by an orthopedic consultant after obtaining samples of synovial fluid for laboratory studies (Gram stain, aerobic and anaerobic cultures, and acid-fast bacilli stain and culture). The synovial fluid in transient tenosynovitis of the hip is clearly transudative, will have negative stains for microorganisms, and will yield sterile cultures.

If further differentiation of transient tenosynovitis of the hip from Legg-Calvé-Perthes disease is necessary, a technetium-99m bone scan or a magnetic resonance imaging (MRI) scan will confirm the absence of avascular necrosis of the femoral head. This aspect of the diagnostic workup can be performed in the ambulatory setting.

Admission to hospital is necessary only for management of SCFE, other hip fractures, and septic arthritis of the hip. Once these diagnostic considerations are effectively eliminated, the child with suspected transient tenosynovitis of the hip can be managed as an outpatient. Weight bearing is eliminated, and anti-inflammatory agents are recommended until the child's hip is painless and range of motion returns to normal (3 to 7 days). Some authors recommend an additional period of rest (7 to 10 days) after symptoms have resolved. Antibiotics are of no value; glucocorticoids are not recommended.

Various authors have noted an association between transient tenosynovitis of the hip and the subsequent development of Legg-Calvé-Perthes disease, ranging from 0.5 to 10 percent. It remains unclear whether the association is one of cause and effect or misdiagnosis of early Legg-Calvé-Perthes disease. Follow-up clinical evaluations of patients with a diagnosis of transient tenosynovitis of the hip should occur at 2 weeks with the child's primary care physician. Subsequent clinical elevations (possibly to include radiographs) are performed by the primary care physician at 2 months and 6 months after the initial episode.

Legg-Calvé-Perthes Disease (Coxa Plana)

The incidence of Legg-Calvé-Perthes disease varies worldwide from 1 in 1200 to 1 in 12,500. The onset of symptoms is between 4 and 9 years of age in 80 percent of patients, with a range of age between 2 and 13 years of age. It is bilateral in 10 percent of cases.

The disease process is characterized as an avascular necrosis of the femoral head complicated by subsequent subchondral stress fracture. Resorption of areas of bone within the femoral head (rarefaction) is followed by the laying down of new bone. Collapse and flattening of the femoral head may ensue, along with the potential for subluxation. The result is a painful hip joint associated with restricted range of motion, muscle spasm, and soft tissue contractures.

Clinically, the child with Legg-Calvé-Perthes disease presents with limp and pain of weeks' to months' duration. Pain is usually mild, chronic, and dull. It is most noticeable in the groin, the anteromedial thigh, and the knee. It is exacerbated by physical activity, relieved by rest, and associated with an antalgic limp. There are no associated systemic symptoms. Hip range of motion is restricted; there may be a flexion-abduction contracture as well. Thigh muscle atrophy, due to disuse, is common.

The radiographic findings associated with Legg-Calvé-Perthes disease depend on the stage of the disease process. During the incipient stage (1 to 3 months), the radiograph of the hip demonstrates only widening of the cartilage space of the affected hip and a smaller size of the ossific nucleus of the femoral head (Fig. 132-6). The second

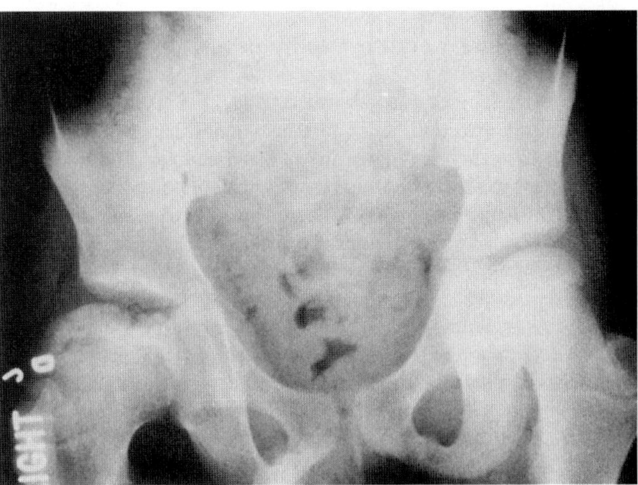

FIG. 132-6. Legg-Calvé-Perthes disease. The right hip illustrates joint-space widening, reduced size of the ossific nucleus of the femoral head, and increased opacification of the femoral head.

radiographic sign is the appearance of the subchondral stress fracture line in the femoral head (Caffey's sign). The third radiologic finding is increased opacification of the femoral head, brought on by deposition of new bone upon avascular trabeculae, calcification of the sclerotic marrow, and collapse and crowding of the avascular trabeculae in the dome of the epiphysis. Ultimately, deformities of the femoral head and neck become apparent, along with subluxation and extrusion of the femoral head from the acetabulum.

The other commonly employed imaging modalities include the technetium-99m bone scan and MRI. The scan demonstrates markedly reduced uptake of nuclide within the affected femoral head. These findings precede apparent plain film radiographic abnormalities. MRI offers superior resolution and sensitivity, with areas of low signal intensity reflecting necrotic regions within the femoral head. Arthrogram-like images of the cartilaginous portions of the femoral head and acetabular rim are produced. Excellent visualization of deformities and flattening of the femoral head is possible as well as subluxation or anterolateral extrusion of the femoral head from the acetabulum.

The differential diagnosis of coxa plana includes toxic tenosynovitis of the hip, which shares many similar features with early Legg-Calvé-Perthes disease. Careful review of the radiographs is necessary to exclude the findings associated with coxa plana, as mentioned previously. If doubt exists, technetium-99m bone scan or MRI imaging studies should be considered.

The differentiation of coxa plana from acute rheumatic fever (ARF) is based on the natural history and responsiveness of ARF to salicylates. Tuberculous arthritis of the hip may mimic coxa plana. Differential screening tests should include a tuberculin skin test and determination of the ESR. Unilateral tumors, such as eosinophilic granuloma, osteoid osteoma, osteoblastoma, and lymphoma, should be considered and excluded by laboratory studies and computed tomography (CT) scan. Bone dysplasias are often confused with Legg-Calvé-Perthes disease. Hypothyroidism, sickle cell disease, and Gaucher disease should also be excluded.

Care in the emergency department involves the consideration or establishment of the accurate diagnosis and orthopedic consultation. Treatment efforts are directed toward restoration of full range of motion of the hip and stabilization of the femoral head within the acetabulum, with resumption of normal activities as rapidly as possible. All except the most mildly affected children are hospitalized initially and treated with traction. The duration of traction and the timing of further therapy directed at containing the femoral head within the acetabulum (orthotics versus surgical containment) depend on the severity of the coxa plana and the responsiveness of the hip irritability to traction therapy.

Other Avascular Necrosis Syndromes

KOHLER DISEASE OF THE TARSAL NAVICULAR This is an uncommon condition affecting boys more commonly than girls (4:1), occurring at about 5 years of age in boys and at about 4 years of age in girls. It appears to result from repetitive compressive forces applied to the tarsal navicular, the last bone of the foot to ossify in normal children. Affected children appear to have a delayed ossification of this bone during a critical phase in its growth, predisposing it to the compressive stresses of preschool ambulation.

The child presents with an antalgic limp, bearing weight on the lateral side of the foot, thus splinting the medial longitudinal arch. The child complains of local pain and tenderness over the navicular bone of the foot and often has induration over the area. There is no fever or other constitutional symptoms. Range of motion of the other joints of the foot is intact.

Radiographically, the picture is classic. The tarsal navicular is narrowed, as seen in the lateral view of the foot and ankle, and flattened, with irregular rarefaction and sclerosis. Comparison of radiographs of the contralateral foot is often helpful.

Treatment is as an outpatient using a short-leg walking cast. The use of crutches to ensure non-weight bearing is recommended for the initial 3 weeks. Orthopedic aftercare should be arranged. The prognosis is very good.

FRIEBERG INFARCTION This condition of adolescents is seen much more commonly in girls (3:1). The usual site of involvement is the head of the second metatarsal, although other metatarsals can be affected, and it is occasionally bilateral. While its etiology is not known with certainty, it is generally presumed to be caused by a vascular insufficiency (aseptic necrosis).

Clinically, the patient complains of pain and tenderness under the affected metatarsal head. This is associated with local soft tissue swelling and restricted range of motion of the metatarsophalangeal joint. Radiographs of the foot demonstrate flattening, sclerosis, and irregularity of the metatarsal head. CT scan or technetium-99m bone scan may serve to clarify the diagnosis in selected patients whose diagnosis remains obscure.

Management is as an outpatient, utilizing a short-leg walking cast for 3 to 4 weeks. Follow-up care is provided by an orthopedist who may recommend a surgical excision of the affected area of metatarsal if conservative therapy is ineffective.

Osgood-Schlatter Disease

This very common syndrome affects preadolescent males three times more often than females. The etiology is a traumatic stress imposed upon the proximal tibial tuberosity by a contracted quadriceps muscle mechanism. The ligamentum patellae detaches cartilaginous fragments from the tibial tuberosity without necrosis. However, an inflammatory process is established by the reparative process, resulting in a patellar tendinitis and a remarkable prominence, induration, and tenderness of the tibial tuberosity. There is no avascular necrosis of the tibial tuberosity.

The patient complains of pain and tenderness over the anterior aspect of the knee and of the tibial tuberosity. It is exacerbated by running, climbing stairs, jumping, and kneeling. Symptoms are relieved with rest. Examination reveals thickening and tenderness of the patellar tendon, with maximum palpation tenderness over the insertion point of the patellar tendon onto the tibial tubercle. The tibial tuberosity is noticeably enlarged and indurated. There is no knee effusion.

Radiographs illustrate patellar tendon thickening and soft tissue swelling over the tibial tuberosity without knee effusion. The irregularity of the ossification of the tibial tubercle is normal for this age group and is *not* a diagnostic feature of Osgood-Schlatter disease. However, prominence of the tibial tuberosity, with or without a small, free bone fragment located anterior and superior to the tibial tubercle, *is* characteristic of the disorder.

The disease is self-limited. Acute symptoms subside following restriction from excessive physical activities for a period of approximately 3 months. Severely painful knees may benefit symptomatically from the use of crutches. Contracted, taut, hypertrophic quadriceps and hamstring muscles require stretching exercises. Rarely, more aggressive strategies to ensure rest of the knee are utilized, such as the use of a knee immobilizer or long leg cylinder cast. Even so, the stretching exercises of the quadriceps and hamstring groups are continued. The use of glucocorticoid injection into the patellar tendon and the parapophyseal soft tissues is controversial and is to be discouraged.

ACUTE SUPPURATIVE ARTHRITIS

Acute suppurative arthritis, an inflammation of a joint caused by pyogenic organisms, occurs in all age groups but is more common in neonates, infants, and children less than 3 years of age. The hip is the most commonly involved joint, followed in frequency by the knee

TABLE 132-1 Causes of Suppurative Arthritis in Children

Newborn (0–2 Months)	% of Cases	Infant (2–36 Months)	% of Cases	Child (>36 Months)	% of Cases
Staphylococcus aureus	35–46	*H. influenza*†	30–35	*Staph. aureus*	30–45
Group B *Steptococcus*	20–25	*Streptococcus* species	12	*Streptococcus* species	18–26
Gram-negative bacilli	10–28	*Staph. aureus*	11	Gram-negative bacilli	10–15
Neisseria gonorrhoeae	5–7	Gram-negative bacilli	10	*Strep. pneumoniae*	7
Haemophilus influenzae	2	Unknown or unidentified	35	*N. gonorrhoeae*	5–10
*Candida albicans**	7–17				

*Hospital acquired.
†Data collected prior to implementation of *H. influenzae* B (Hib) vaccine.

and the elbow. Any joint can be involved. Simultaneous infection of more than a single joint can occur.

Bacteria may access the joint through hematogenous transmission, from direct extension of infection from an adjacent area of infected metaphyseal bone, or via direct inoculation during arthrocentesis, or accidentally during femoral venipuncture. The etiologic organisms encountered in septic arthritis vary with the age of the child (Table 132-1). The relative frequency of *Haemophilus influenzae* is decreasing as a consequence of immunization practices.

The pathophysiology of septic arthritis exemplifies the seriousness of the condition and the risks of long-term sequelae. Synovial edema and hyperemia accompany increased secretion of synovial fluid, which may be serosanguinous early on, cloudy, or suppurative with polymorphonuclear (PMN) leukocyte counts ranging from 5000 to 200,000 and exceeding $50,000/\mu L^3$ after the earliest stages. Synovial fluid glucose concentration is decreased, and the protein content is elevated. The mucin string is poor to very poor. Within days, the synovial fluid becomes frankly purulent, if it was not so initially. The hyaline articular cartilages degenerate initially at points of contact between opposing articular surfaces. The synovium itself is eventually replaced by granulation tissue, and the infection invades surrounding bone, particularly epiphyseal and metaphyseal bone. Adhesions are created within the joint and restrict motion. Subluxation or dislocation may occur in the setting of marked distention of the damaged joint capsule. In the hip joint, avascular necrosis of the femoral head ensues. Eventually, the untreated infection leads to ankylosis or total destruction of the joint.

Although systemic symptoms can be subtle in the newborn, the diagnosis is not usually in doubt in the older infant or toddler. Symptoms are acute in onset and predominantly involve pain in the affected joint. The child with a lower extremity septic arthritis walks with a severely antalgic limp or, more typically, cannot bear weight at all. Profound signs of constitutional and systemic illness are the rule, with high fever [40 to 40.5°C (104 to 105°F)], apprehension, irritability, anorexia, and prostration manifestly apparent. Examination of the affected joint demonstrates warmth, soft tissue swelling, and exquisite palpation tenderness. The child maintains an infected hip in 30° to 60°of flexion, with milder degrees of abduction and external rotation.

Radiographic imaging studies are helpful but nondiagnostic. They are important in order to ensure the absence of changes that would indicate adjacent osteomyelitis, fracture, or other processes. The expected findings are those of joint effusion and distention (Fig. 132-7). Comparison films of the contralateral joint in question are often helpful.

The differential diagnosis includes osteomyelitis, ARF, acute pauciarticular juvenile rheumatoid arthritis (JRA), transient tenosynovitis, cellulitis and suppurative bursitis, hemarthrosis, Legg-Calvé-Perthes disease, and SCFE (when the involved joint is the hip).

Distinguishing suppurative arthritis from osteomyelitis involving an adjacent metaphysis is probably the most difficult problem in the differential diagnosis. Gentle examination may enable the physician to ascertain the area of greatest tenderness. Osteomyelitis is most tender over the metaphysis, while septic arthritis manifests greatest tenderness directly over the joint line. Motion of the joint is much more painful and more restricted in septic arthritis compared to osteomyelitis. Osteomyelitis creates more swelling over the limb as a whole. Arthrocentesis is necessary to establish the diagnosis of suppurative arthritis. Care is necessary during the arthrocentesis to avoid contaminating a noninfected joint by introducing organisms from an infected metaphysis, cellulitis, or bursa. A sympathetic effusion from an area of metaphyseal osteomyelitis usually is serous and contains only a few thousand PMNs.

The other differential diagnostic considerations usually pose fewer problems to the clinician. Transient tenosynovitis does not manifest symptoms and signs of systemic toxicity. The peripheral WBC and ESR are normal or only minimally elevated. Occasionally, arthrocentesis is necessary to adequately exclude the diagnosis of suppurative arthritis, however. JRA of the pauciarticular form may present with an isolated inflamed joint but is usually an illness of gradual onset, and the child does not appear toxically ill. The affected joint is not as tender as in septic arthritis and has better range of motion. Although the WBC is elevated and the mucin string is poor in both conditions, the Gram stain of synovial fluid in JRA is negative and its culture is sterile.

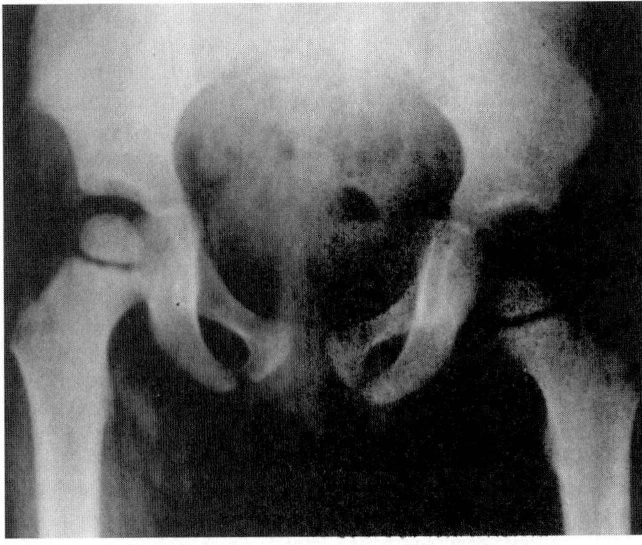

FIG. 132-7. Large left hip effusion in child with suppurative arthritis.

TABLE 132-2 Initial Antibiotic Therapy of Acute Suppurative Arthritis in Children

Age	Suspected Organism	Antibiotics
Newborn (0–2 months)	*Staph. aureus*	Methicillin or nafcillin*
	Group B *Streptococcus*	Ampicillin or penicillin and gentamicin
	Gram-negative bacilli	Cefotaxime/ceftriaxone
	N. gonorrhoeae	Cefotaxime/ceftriaxone
	Unknown	Methicillin or nafcillin* and cefotaxime/ceftriaxone
Infant (2–36 months)	*H. influenzae*	Cefuroxime or cefotaxime/ceftriaxone
	Streptococcus species	Penicillin G
	Staph. aureus	Methicillin or nafcillin*
	Gram-negative bacilli	Cefotaxime/ceftriaxone
	Unknown	Methicillin or nafcillin* and cefotaxime/ceftriaxone
Child (>36 months)	*Staph. aureus*	Methicillin or nafcillin*
	Streptococcus species	Penicillin G, other β-lactams, clindamycin
	Gram-negative bacilli	Cefotaxime/ceftriaxone
	N. gonorrhoeae	Ceftriaxone or penicillin G
	Unknown	Methicillin or nafcillin* and cefotaxime/ceftriaxone

*Vancomycin, if methicillinase-resistant *Staph. aureus* is suspected.

Rheumatic fever is characterized by the fleeting, migratory nature of the arthritis and may be associated with other stigmata, such as carditis, as illustrated by Jones' revised criteria for the diagnosis of ARF (see Table 132-5). There is a remarkable responsiveness of the arthritis of ARF to salicylates. The response of the arthritis to salicylates should be used as a diagnostic tool only after the diagnosis of suppurative arthritis has been excluded by arthrocentesis, with Gram stain and culture of the synovial fluid.

Cellulitis is notable for local skin erythema, induration, and tenderness. The adjacent joint has relatively preserved motion and is less tender. Lymphangitis or regional lymphadenitis is commonly encountered with cellulitis. Often the patient or examiner will note the presence of a minor abrasion, laceration, puncture, or furuncle within the cellulitis, serving as an entrance site for local invasion of bacteria.

Hemarthrosis can rarely pose a problem in the differential diagnosis of septic arthritis. In the absence of a history of trauma, a congenital or acquired coagulopathy is suspected (hemophilia A, factor IX deficiency, Von Willebrand disease, leukemia, etc.). Henoch-Schönlein purpura may present with one or more painful joints prior to manifestation of the other cardinal symptoms of the disease (abdominal pain, nephritis, purpura). The arthralgia with this condition is migratory, however, and represents a periarticulitis rather than an actual arthritis. If the joint of involvement happens to be the hip, a diagnosis of Legg-Calvé-Perthes disease may come to mind. This condition is not, however, associated with high fever, systemic signs of illness, and prostration, and the examination and culture of the synovial fluid will easily distinguish this condition from septic arthritis.

The management of acute suppurative arthritis consists of (1) establishing the diagnosis by obtaining synovial fluid from the infected joint for Gram stain and culture as well as other microscopic and laboratory studies; (2) drainage of the infected joint of bacterial products and infectious debris [suppurative arthritis of the hip requires open surgical drainage (arthrotomy), while more superficial joints can frequently be drained arthroscopically or even through arthrocentesis]; (3) emergent initiation of appropriate initial antibiotic therapy (Table 132-2); and (4) local care of the joint (support by skin traction for larger joints; splinting of the wrist, ankle, and smaller joints).

An analysis of the cerebrospinal fluid (CSF) is indicated in children suspected of suppurative arthritis or osteomyelitis caused by *H. influenzae*. This is necessary, since meningitis is a frequently coexisting illness in children with *H. influenzae* suppurative arthritis and since the antibiotic dosages for meningitis differ from the dosages used in suppurative arthritis. Follow-up considerations (e.g., hearing tests and cognitive tests) will also vary in the setting of coexisting meningitis.

The prognosis of suppurative arthritis is influenced by (1) the length of time between onset of symptoms and initiation of treatment, (2) the joint involved (prognosis is poorer if the hip is involved), (3) the presence of associated osteomyelitis (poorer), and (4) the age of the patient, with neonates and younger infants having a less favorable prognosis than older children due to the typically longer delay in initiation of specific treatment.

STRUCTURAL SCOLIOSIS

Scoliosis is a lateral deviation of a series of vertebral bodies from the normal spinal axis. If scoliosis is progressive, structural deformities occur in the vertebral bodies and the rib cage. Scoliosis is a physical sign and is not itself a diagnosis. Eighty percent of structural scoliosis is idiopathic: it is not related to a paralytic or neurologic etiology, and there are no causative congenital vertebral anomalies.

There are three peak periods of onset of idiopathic structural scoliosis: infantile (0 to 3 years), juvenile (4 years to puberty), and adolescent (onset of puberty to physeal closure). Prevalence data have been obtained in two ways historically: school screening and chest radiographs obtained for screening of tuberculosis. The prevalence of curves of less than 10° is 2 to 3 percent in North America, while the prevalence of more severe curves decreases as the severity of the curve increases. While the prevalence of minor (<10°) curves is equal among boys and girls, there is a distinct female gender predilection for curves exceeding 15° to 20°. This presumably is related to the observation that curve progression is more common in girls.

Large-scale screening programs remain somewhat controversial. Overreferral to orthopedists is common and is to be expected. Use of a scoliometer can dramatically reduce overreferral. The potential for excessive exposure to ionizing radiation is minimized by ensuring that an experienced orthopedic surgeon reexamines all referred patients prior to the ordering of the diagnostic scoliosis radiogram (single, standing AP radiogram of the entire spine with the iliac crests as high as possible). Another difficulty with screening programs is parental noncompliance. Finally, the cost effectiveness of large-scale screening programs is yet to be firmly established.

Despite the difficulties and controversies of large-scale screening programs, primary care physicians and emergency physicians are in a strong position to rapidly and easily identify scoliosis in children presenting to the emergency department for unrelated problems. Children with scoliosis do not usually complain of backache or fatigue. Their complaints, if they have any, relate to concerns of high shoulder; prominent scapula or breast; prominent hip; asymmetry of rib cage, trunk, or flank creases; or poor posture; or they have noticed the curve itself.

When the diagnosis is being considered, the examination of the child and the spine should be orderly. The child is observed standing, first clothed, then unclothed (but with appropriate draping for modesty), for body habitus, posture, and alignment. Lateral deformity of the spine is usually best visualized from behind the standing child. Look for balance of the head, neck, and shoulders over the pelvis. A plumb line held over the spinous process of the seventh cervical vertebra normally should pass right over the intergluteal cleft. Lateral deviation from the midline should be noted and can be measured in centimeters.

The Adams forward bending test optimally demonstrates the degree and direction of any associated rotation of the vertebrae. The patient's knees should be straight and the feet placed together. The child bends forward at the hips with the arms dependent and the palms held in opposition. The child is inspected head on for cervical and thoracic rotation and from the rear for thoracolumbar and lumbar rotation. The right and left posterior rib cage and the paravertebral lumbosacral muscles are inspected and compared for asymmetry. Rotational abnormalities of the vertebral bodies, associated with the lateral curvature of scoliosis, will result in one side (rib cage and paravertebral lumbar muscles) being higher than the other. In structural scoliosis, the vertebral body rotation is toward the convex side of the curve of the scoliosis and toward the elevated side of the rib cage or paravertebral lumbar muscles. This asymmetry can be quantified by use of a scoliometer, a gravity level device that measures in degrees of rotation. Scoliosis manifesting greater than 10° of vertebral rotation warrants referral to an orthopedic surgeon.

Conservative management of scoliosis is employed for structural scoliosis manifesting less than 50° of vertebral rotation or 50° of curve when measured radiographically. Various orthotic braces are utilized with varying success. Nonoperative candidates with more severe curves (35° to 50°) usually obtain better results using orthotic devices worn nearly continuously (23 h daily), compared to nighttime-only braces. All of these devices are fitted to a particular child's torso. They require substantial discipline on the part of the child and the parents, however. Careful follow-up care is provided by the orthopedic surgeon, who must be particularly vigilant for progression of the scoliosis, defined as an increase in the curvature of more than 5° on two or more successive visits. Such curve progression is ominous in that it is associated with the development of more severe curvatures ultimately requiring surgical stabilization.

SELECTED RHEUMATOLOGIC DISORDERS IN CHILDREN

Kawasaki Syndrome

Kawasaki syndrome is a generalized vasculitis involving small and medium size arteries, with characteristic involvement of the coronary arteries. There is growing evidence to suggest that Kawasaki syndrome is caused by superantigen bacterial toxins, which stimulate large populations of T cells expressing particular T-cell receptor β chain variable-gene segments. Superantigen stimulation induces massive proliferation and expansion of the target T cells, with subsequent production of proinflammatory cytokines. Vascular endothelial cells are recruited into this inflammatory process with resulting vascular damage. Toxins elaborated by *Staph. aureus* and *Streptococcus pyogenes* are known to possess superantigen properties. There is increasing evidence to suggest that these organisms elaborate superantigen toxins in children with Kawasaki syndrome.

Epidemiologically, Kawasaki syndrome affects 3000 to 5000 children annually in the United States. There is a male-to-female preponderance of 1.5 to 1. The peak age of onset is 1 to 2 years, with 80 percent of patients being less than 4 years of age.

The diagnosis of Kawasaki syndrome is established by the presence of clinical criteria listed in Table 132-3. The fever is high, spiking, and prolonged, persisting for 1 to 2 weeks in untreated patients. The conjunctivitis is nonpurulent and bilateral and has an onset shortly after the appearance of the fever. The oropharyngeal features are prominent during the acute febrile period. The extremities, particularly the palms and soles, are often quite painful. The polymorphous rash is most commonly a raised, deep-red, plaquelike eruption. Less commonly, it may be scarlatiniform, a morbilliform maculopapular rash, or even a fine pustular eruption. It is most widespread on the trunk and proximal extremities, with particular involvement of the perineum. At least one cervical lymph node measuring 1.5 cm in diameter is necessary to fill the lymphadenopathy criterion. There are a wide variety of associated findings in Kawasaki syndrome, as illustrated in Table 132-4.

TABLE 132-3 Diagnostic Criteria for Kawasaki Syndrome

Fever of at least 5 days' duration (100%)

Presence of at least four of the following five conditions:
1. Bilateral conjunctivitis (85%)
2. Changes of the lips and oral mucosa (90%)
   Dry, red, fissured lips
   Strawberry tongue
   Oropharyngeal edema
3. Changes of the extremities (75%)
   Erythema of palms and soles
   Edema of hands and feet
   Periungual desquamation
4. Polymorphous rash (80%)
5. Cervical lymphadenopathy (70%)

Illness not explained by other known disease process

The acute febrile phase of the disease lasts 7 to 14 days and is marked by the features listed in Table 132-3. The subacute phase, lasting 2 to 4 weeks, is indicated by a gradual resolution of the fever, rash, and lymphadenopathy. The irritability and conjunctival injection may persist. The characteristic desquamation of the fingers and toes occurs during this subacute phase, as does the associated symptom of arthralgia or arthritis. Thrombocytosis approaching $1{,}000{,}000/\mu L^3$ is also noted during this subacute phase, during which time the patient is at greatest risk for the development of coronary artery thrombosis. The convalescent phase begins when all clinical and associated signs and symptoms have disappeared and continues until the ESR and the platelet count return to normal (6 to 10 weeks).

An acute carditis develops in 50 percent of patients, usually manifested by a myocarditis with symptoms of tachycardia and gallop rhythms indicative of mild to severe congestive heart failure. Pericarditis, conduction disturbances, and valvular insufficiencies are less frequent manifestations of carditis.

Most seriously, coronary artery aneurysmal dilatations occur in 20 percent of untreated patients. Coronary artery involvement can be detected as early as the seventh day, with a peak frequency of coronary aneurysm formation occurring 4 weeks after the onset of illness. Untreated, the coronary artery aneurysms are quite prone to thrombosis during the subacute phase because of the hypercoagulable state created by the thrombocytosis. Sudden death can occur in 1 to 2 percent of untreated patients, and the remainder are at risk for long-term consequences such as coronary artery stenosis and subsequent cardiac ischemia.

The laboratory features of Kawasaki syndrome reflect the marked inflammatory and immune activation characteristic of the disease. Such findings, however, are nonspecific. A moderate leukocytosis with a

TABLE 132-4 Associated Features of Kawasaki Syndrome

Cardiovascular system	Genitourinary system
Coronary artery aneurysms	Urethritis with sterile pyuria
Myocarditis-pericarditis	Proteinuria
Mitral or aortic insufficiency	Pulmonary system
Dysrhythmias	Pneumonitis
Peripheral ischemia	Cough, coryza
Central nervous system	Gastrointestinal system
Irritability	Hydrops of the gall bladder
Aseptic meningitis	Hepatitis
Anterior uveitis	Nausea, vomiting, diarrhea
Sensorineural hearing loss	Abdominal pain
Hematologic system	
Thrombocytosis (subacute phase)	
Anemia	

left shift, a remarkable thrombocytosis appearing during the second week of the illness, and other secondary laboratory abnormalities consistent with a diffuse systemic vasculitis may be present.

The care of the child with Kawasaki syndrome in the emergency department consists primarily of establishing the diagnosis. Patients meeting diagnostic criteria with consistent laboratory findings are usually admitted. The use of intravenous immunoglobulin (IVIG) has substantially decreased the morbidity and mortality associated with the disease. Rapid resolution of fever and the other clinical stigmata and reversal of the laboratory abnormalities occur following IVIG infusion. More importantly, the use of IVIG within the first 10 days of the illness reduces the incidence of coronary artery aneurysms to 3 to 4 percent. It also has been demonstrated to be effective in promoting the resolution of established aneurysms. A single infusion of intravenous IVIG in a dose of 2 g/kg infused over a 10-h period has been demonstrated to be the most effective regimen. Aspirin can be used as adjunctive therapy in anti-inflammatory doses of 80 to 100 mg/kg/day until the fourteenth day of the illness. The dose is then reduced to 3 to 5 mg/kg/day for its platelet antiadhesive effect during the period when the child is at risk of clotting coronary artery aneurysms due to the thrombosis. Usually, the low dose aspirin therapy is continued until the platelet count returns to normal. However, patients exhibiting coronary aneurysms despite IVIG therapy should receive low dose aspirin indefinitely or for at least 1 year following the resolution of the aneurysms. Echocardiography, necessary to identify coronary artery aneurysms, provides valuable baseline information for the child who does not initially manifest abnormalities. The echocardiogram is repeated 3 to 6 weeks after IVIG therapy in order to guide further aspirin therapy decisions.

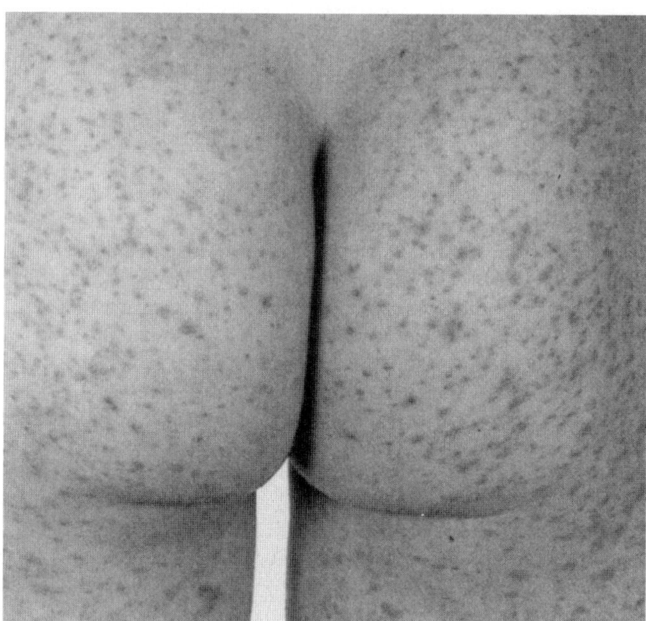

FIG. 132-8. Henoch-Schönlein purpura. Purpuric lesions of dependent body areas, particularly on flanks, buttocks, and lower extremities.

Henoch-Schönlein Purpura

Henoch-Schönlein purpura is a common, self-limited generalized leukocytoclastic vasculitis. Vasculitis involves primarily small vessels and is mediated by immune complexes produced through IgA and the alternate complement pathways. A variety of infectious and noninfectious stimuli appear to precipitate the immunologic mechanisms of the vasculitis.

The disorder is classically characterized by the appearance of a dermovasculitis with a propensity for the lower trunk, buttocks, perineum, and lower extremities, as is characteristic of generalized vasculitides (Fig. 132-8). In addition, the vasculitis includes involvement of the glomeruli, with the subsequent development of hematuria and with the potential for long-term renal sequelae. Involvement of the bowel wall causes recurrent colicky abdominal pain and frequently leads to the development of melena or hematochezia. Eight percent of children with severe abdominal colic caused by Henoch-Schönlein purpura experience massive gastrointestinal hemorrhage or intussusception. Arthritis, or, more specifically, a polymigratory periarticulitis, occurs in most affected children. Rarely, massive pulmonary hemorrhage can occur.

The clinical diagnosis is not usually obscure in those children manifesting all or several characteristics of the disorder. The child with hematuria, abdominal pain, a history of migratory periarthritis, and a palpable, purpuric tender rash on the buttock and lower extremity is not a diagnostic dilemma. Difficulty ensues upon the evaluation of a child manifesting exclusively abdominal colic or apparent arthritis.

Care of the child with suspected Henoch-Schönlein purpura in the emergency department consists of establishing the diagnosis or maintaining a high index of suspicion for the diagnosis. Otherwise, emergency care is entirely supportive. Consideration of specific laboratory or imaging studies is influenced by the specific symptoms manifested by the child. For example, the child presenting exclusively with hematuria and abdominal pain may require a urine analysis and urine culture, a kidney-ureter-bladder abdominal radiograph, assessment of renal function, and a complete blood count. Such circumstances might even serve as an indication for a renal ultrasound or an intravenous pyelogram if the clinician suspects ureterolithiasis as the cause of the child's symptoms. Similarly, a child with migratory polyarthritis might reasonably be expected to undergo an evaluation of arthritis, including plain radiographs of affected joints, complete blood count, rheumatoid factor titer, antinuclear antibody titer (ANA) and complement levels. In summary, the diagnostic evaluation in the emergency department is often influenced by the need to exclude other disease processes that share common features with this generalized vasculitis. When the entire clinical picture presents itself, however, the extent of the diagnostic workup is much reduced.

Children with Henoch-Schönlein purpura are admitted to the hospital when the diagnosis is in doubt, for observation and control of abdominal pain, for monitoring of renal function, and for fluid hydration in the setting of recurrent emesis. Children with extremely mild symptoms can be safely and expectantly observed as outpatients, as long as an experienced primary care provider is available. Arthritis, when present as an isolated symptom, is usually easily controlled with aspirin. Prednisone is not utilized in the management of arthritis when it represents the child's only symptom of active vasculitis. The child's primary care physician maintains contact with the family on a daily basis and evaluates the child in the office at frequent intervals in the initial weeks following the establishment of the diagnosis. Particular attention is directed to the development of symptoms suggestive of abdominal colic, gastrointestinal hemorrhage, intussusception, and the development of chronic renal disease. Chronic renal sequelae are reported in approximately 7 to 9 percent of children with Henoch-Schönlein purpura and do not respond well to glucocorticoid therapy.

Poststreptococcal Reactive Arthritis

As a result of an increase of reported cases of group A β-hemolytic streptococcal infections in recent years, emergency physicians have joined the ranks of clinicians concerned about poststreptococcal nonsuppurative sequelae. In addition to ARF, discussed previously, an understanding has emerged recently that poststreptococcal reactive arthritis represents a distinct clinical entity that may also be seen with increasing frequency.

Reactive arthritis is a sterile inflammatory mono- or oligoarthritis that occurs in association with a primary infection at a distant site. The primary infection associated with reactive arthritis may be caused by a variety of reported organisms. In addition to group A β-hemolytic streptococci, primary infections with *Salmonella, Staphylococcus,* and other groups of *Streptococcus* have been reportedly associated with reactive arthritis. Unlike ARF, reactive arthritis is not associated with carditis.

The differences in pathogenesis between poststreptococcal reactive arthritis (PSRA) and ARF are incompletely understood. Both syndromes occur secondary to group A β-hemolytic streptococcal throat infection. It has been speculated that differences in virulence among streptococcal M serotypes or the presence of coinfecting viruses may explain the development of ARF rather than the more benign reactive arthritis. Human host factors, such age-related and gender-related differences in immune response, may contribute to the different paths of clinical sequelae.

The differentiation between ARF and PSRA rests entirely on clinical grounds. The arthritis of PSRA predominantly affects females, while the arthritis of ARF is more commonly in males. Of poststreptococcal nonsuppurative sequelae, ARF is observed more commonly in younger patients (mean age, 12 +/- 4 years). While the typical patient with reactive arthritis is older, it may occur in children as young as 4 years of age. The arthritis of ARF is classically a migratory polyarthritis, while the arthritis of PSRA is described as a nonmigratory mono- or oligoarthritis. Erythema nodosum and erythema multiforme are frequently associated with PSRA while encountered only sporadically and infrequently in cases of ARF. Both reactive arthritis and ARF have been sporadically reported to be associated with a cholestatic hepatitis with piecemeal necrosis. Finally, patients experiencing the full clinical expression of reactive arthritis suffer a much milder illness than is seen in classic ARF.

Management of PSRA consists of nonsteroidal anti-inflammatory medications, to which the inflammatory arthritis is highly responsive. The issue of penicillin prophylaxis, a mainstay in the long-term management of ARF, is controversial with PSRA, and almost certainly will be resolved only following long-term prospective study.

Acute Rheumatic Fever

An acute inflammatory disease affecting widely disparate organ systems, ARF primarily affects children of school age. The incidence of ARF has steadily fallen in developed countries over the past 50 years. However, a resurgence in cases of group A β-hemolytic streptococcal infections over the past 10 years has increased concerns about ARF and other nonsuppurative sequelae of streptococcal infections. Outbreaks of ARF are regularly reported in North America. It is preceded by infection with certain strains of group A β-hemolytic *Streptococcus* (mucoid types 3, 5, and 18). Different layers of the cell wall of the streptococcal organism appear to stimulate antibody production to variable host tissues. The hallmark histologic feature of rheumatic fever is the Aschoff body, found in the connective tissue and created by edematous, fragmented collagen fibers. The connective tissue of the heart, joints, central nervous system, and subcutaneous tissues and skin are targeted by the immune reaction. The carditis is an endomyocarditis, with valvulitis primarily involving the mitral and aortic valves. The arthritis is characterized by synovial edema and periarticular swelling with joint effusions.

The child develops the disorder 2 to 6 weeks following a streptococcal pharyngitis. While nonspecific symptoms of systemic illness predominate early on, physical examination eventually reveals evidence of arthritis, carditis, choreiform movements, erythema marginatum, or subcutaneous nodules, individually or in combination. Jones' criteria for establishing a diagnosis of acute rheumatic fever are illustrated in Table 132-5. Either two major criteria or one major and two minor criteria plus evidence of an antecedent streptococcal infection are necessary to establish the diagnosis.

TABLE 132-5 Revised Jones' Criteria for the Diagnosis of Acute Rheumatic Fever

Major	Minor
Carditis	Fever
New or changing murmurs	Arthralgia
Cardiomegaly, congestive heart failure	History of previous attack of ARF
Pericarditis	Elevated ESR, C-reactive protein
Migratory polyarthritis	Prolonged PR interval on electrocardiogram
Chorea	Rising titer of antistreptococcal antibodies
Erythema marginatum	
Subcutaneous nodules	

Note: Diagnosis is likely when two major criteria or one major and two minor criteria are met. Group A *Streptococcus* may be documented by a history of scarlet fever, isolation of group A *Streptococcus* from throat culture, or rising titers of antistreptococcal antibodies.

Arthritis (occurring in 60 to 75 percent of initial attacks) is characterized as a migratory, fleeting polyarticular arthritis primarily affecting the large joints. The carditis occurs in a third of new cases and may be mild or severe. Its presence is heralded by any combination of a new cardiac murmur, tachycardia, a gallop rhythm, a pericardial friction rub, congestive heart failure, or a hyperactive precordium. Sydenham's chorea occurs in 10 percent of cases and may have its initial appearance months following a streptococcal infection. Chorea may be the sole manifestation of acute rheumatic fever. The skin rash of acute rheumatic fever (erythema marginatum) is described as serpiginous and persists only for several days. It usually coexists with the presence of carditis in some form. Subcutaneous nodules are more rare and are located on the extensor surfaces of the wrists, elbows, and knees. The greatest morbidity and mortality is associated with the development of carditis.

Diagnostic studies are utilized to clarify the associated antecedent infection by group A streptococcus (a pharyngeal swab for culture, antistreptolysin titers, or streptozyme titers), or are employed to identify and assess the presence and extent of carditis. An electrocardiogram, is obtained to assess for conduction delays or hypertrophy. A chest x-ray serves to identify cardiac dilatation or pulmonary vascular congestion or edema. Echocardiography is utilized to identify evidence of valvulitis or valvular insufficiency and also to exclude other diagnostic considerations.

The differential diagnosis includes JRA, septic arthritis, Kawasaki syndrome, viral or other forms of cardiomyopathy, leukemias, and other forms of vasculitis, including drug reactions. Rarely, tumors of the central nervous system require differentiation from ARF when the child's sole clinical manifestation is chorea.

Treatment of ARF in the emergency department is directed primarily toward the management of complicating features of carditis. In the absence of cardiac or hemodynamic instability (and such is the rule), early consultation with a pediatric cardiologist is recommended, and admission to the hospital is generally advised in the early stages until the diagnosis is confirmed. Arthritis is managed with high-dose aspirin therapy (75 to 100 mg/kg/day) in order to effect a serum salicylate level in the range of 20 to 30 mg/dL. The aspirin dose is reduced after approximately 1 week to 50 mg/kg/day for an additional 4 to 6 weeks. Significant carditis or congestive heart failure is managed with glucocorticoids, usually in the form of prednisone in a dose of 1 to 2 mg/kg/day. This is continued for 2 weeks following the resolution of symptoms and the return of the ESR to normal. The duration of glucocorticoid therapy requires a subsequent taper of the steroids over a 4 to 6 week period. Chorea can be managed with haloperidol, 0.01

to 0.03 mg/kg/day in four divided doses. All children with ARF are treated with penicillin, even if the cultures for group A *Streptococcus* are negative. Benzathine penicillin G can be administered in a single dosage of 1.2 MU. Alternatively, procaine penicillin G 600,000 U can be administered daily for 10 days. Penicillin V 25,000 to 50,000 U/kg/day divided into four doses and administered orally is also effective. Erythromycin may be substituted for the penicillin-allergic patient. All therapy, if pursued, is administered for 10 days. Long-term prophylactic therapy against group A *Streptococcus* is begun upon completion of the acute phase of therapy. Acceptable prophylactic regimens include benzathine penicillin G, 1.2 MU administered intramuscularly every month, penicillin V 200,000 U administered orally twice daily, or sulfadiazine 1 g administered orally each day. The duration of required prophylactic therapy is incompletely understood, but 5 years of prophylactic antibiotics for those children without cardiac involvement represents the minimum. Patients with manifestations of carditis are placed on life-long prophylactic antibiotic regimens.

Juvenile Rheumatoid Arthritis

JRA is not a single entity. Rather, it encompasses a group of disorders characterized by chronic noninfectious synovitis and arthritis and is associated with a wide range of systemic manifestations. The hypothetical etiology of the arthritis is that of an autoimmune response to a number of antigens not yet completely identified.

Pauciarticular disease is the most common form of the disease in children. It usually involves a single large joint, typically the knee. Serologic findings for rheumatoid factor are negative, while ANA titers are positive in 90 percent of patients. Extraarticular manifestations of this form of the disease include the development of iridocyclitis, Reiter's syndrome, and inflammatory bowel disease. Ultimate joint damage occurs only infrequently.

Polyarticular disease occurs in approximately a third of cases. Rheumatoid factor (RF) serology may be positive or negative, while ANA titers are positive in 25 percent of the RF-negative patients and 75 percent of RF-positive patients. There is a female preponderance, and both large and small joints may be affected. Contrary to the case in pauciarticular JRA, long-term morbidity with polyarticular disease is related to progressive joint destruction, particularly of the hips and knees.

Systemic JRA is the least common presentation, occurring in only about 20 percent of children with the disease. This form is associated with the particularly high fevers commonly associated with the disease, which characteristically produces one or two fever spikes per day exceeding 39.5°C, and is often associated with shaking chills. In addition, there are other prominent extraarticular manifestations of the disease including a pale, erythematous coalescing macular rash, primarily on the trunk but also present in other areas including palms and soles. Hepatosplenomegaly, pleuritis, and pericarditis are common. Serology for RF and ANA are negative. The arthritis of systemic JRA may progress substantially, leading to joint destruction in as many as a quarter of patients.

Laboratory evaluations associated with the disease are not highly specific for JRA. Arthrocentesis is often necessary to exclude acute suppurative arthritis, particularly in pauciarticular presentations. Initially, radiographs demonstrate only soft tissue swelling and synovial effusions. The findings associated with bone and joint damage occur later.

Emergency department management focuses primarily upon excluding other diagnostic considerations, especially in children who have not previously received a confirmed diagnosis of JRA. Hospital admission is recommended for those children in whom the diagnosis is in doubt or who are to be treated empirically for suspected acute suppurative arthritis while synovial fluid cultures are pending.

Initial therapy for those with an established diagnosis includes aspirin at a dosage of 80 to 125 mg/kg/day, with careful monitoring of salicylate levels to maintain a therapeutic level between 20 and 30 mg/dL. Other nonsteroidal anti-inflammatory drugs are becoming increasingly popular.

The use of glucocorticoids should be reserved for use exclusively in those patients in whom the diagnosis is categorically certain and whose systemic JRA symptoms have proved unresponsive to aspirin. They are also utilized in the management of decompensated pericarditis or myocarditis and in the management of unresponsive iridocyclitis. Other management strategies, including intraarticular glucocorticoid injections and the use of gold or chloroquine, or cytosine, should be initiated by a pediatric rheumatologist.

BIBLIOGRAPHY

Jansen TL, Janssen M, Van Riel PL: Acute rheumatic fever or post-streptococcal reactive arthritis: A clinical problem revisited. *Br J Rheumatol* 37:335, 1998.

Rowely AH, Gonzalez-Cruzzi F, Shylman ST: Kawasaki syndrome. *Adv Pediatr* 38:51, 74, 1991.

Swischuk LE: Radiographic signs of skeletal trauma, in Ludwig S, Kornberg AE (eds): *Child Abuse*, 2d ed. New York, Churchill Livingstone, 1992, pp 151–174.

Tachdjian MO: *Pediatric Orthopedics*, 2d ed. Philadelphia, Saunders, 1990.

Tolo VT, Wood B: *Pediatric Orthopedics in Primary Care.* Baltimore, Williams & Wilkins, 1994.

Warren RW, Perez MD, Wilking AP, Myones BL: Pediatric rheumatic diseases. *Pediatr Clin North Am* 41:783, 1994.

SICKLE CELL DISEASE

Peter J. Paganussi
Thom Mayer
Maybelle Kou

Sickle cell disease (SCD) is among the most common inherited disorders worldwide. It is the most common pediatric genetic condition encountered in emergency medicine, especially in urban settings. This genetic condition is found primarily in people of African, Mediterranean, Indian, or Middle Eastern heritage.

In the United States about 8 percent of the African-American population carries the hemoglobin (HgbS) gene and about 0.15 percent (approximately 1/500) are homozygous (HgbSS). These individuals have a predominance of "sickled" hemoglobin, thus resulting in symptomatic SCD. Patients with this hemoglobinopathy have both sickle (A_2) and fetal hemoglobin. The most frequently encountered heterozygous sickle genotypes are HgbSA (sickle cell trait), Hgb-beta thalassemia (sickle beta thalassemia), and HgbSC (sickle cell–hemoglobin SCD). These less common variants of the homozygous disorder have similar, but far less severe, clinical manifestations. Patients with sickle cell trait have a normal life expectancy. However, SCD is associated with a significant mortality rate: 20 to 30 percent of all deaths from SCD occur before 5 years, with a mean age at death of 14 years of age. Current survival has been greatly improved as a result of more aggressive infection prophylaxis and advances in therapy. Nonetheless, the highest mortality occurs in children between 1 and 3 years of age, with sepsis being the leading cause of death.

The end-organ pathology created by sickle cell anemia can be found in every organ system. Clinical effects of the disorder can begin in infancy but usually are not seen until 5 to 6 months of age, because high levels of fetal hemoglobin are present following birth, and the beta-Hgb subunit is not predominant until about 3 months of age. SCD is characterized by abnormal sickle-shaped cells that are less deformable than normal red blood cells. Aggregation of these less pliant, abnormally shaped cells leads to obstruction and thrombosis

TABLE 133-1 Types of Sickle Cell Crises

Vasoocclusive crises
Musculoskeletal
Long bones
Lumbosacral
Dactylitis
Abdominal pain
Generalized
Right-upper-quadrant syndrome
Acute chest syndrome
Central nervous system crisis
Renal crises
Priapism
Hematologic crises
Acute splenic sequestration
Aplastic crises
Hemolytic crises
Infectious crises

of small vessels, resulting in ischemia and tissue infarction, leading to end-organ dysfunction.

PATHOPHYSIOLOGY

The genetic abnormality responsible for the sickling process is caused by a single amino acid substitution of valine for glutamic acid in the beta subunit of the hemoglobin molecule. The resultant hemolytic anemia is caused by the abnormal properties of HgbS. Affected red blood cells undergo repeated cycles of sickling and unsickling, with the HgbS strands polymerizing abnormally in response to deoxygenation. Without an attached O_2 molecule, they tend to coalesce and stretch into long monofilaments, thereby resulting in the distorted sickle shape of the red cell membrane. These irreversibly sickled cells diminish blood viscosity, causing hemolysis and obstructing the microcirculation (vasoocclusive phenomenon) of end-organ tissues. Capillary obstruction deprives tissues of oxygen and metabolic nutrition. It has long been presumed that the resultant hypoxia and ischemia cause the pathologic and clinical features of the disease. This entire process is felt to be self-perpetuating and sustains continued sickling. Others have recently proposed that plasma proteins, endothelial cells, and other genetically driven mechanisms play a major role in this complex process. A few investigators have even questioned whether vasoocclusion exists at all, theorizing that tissue ischemia and infarction result from shunting of blood away from end-organ vascular beds rather than occlusion by deformed, sickled cells.

CLINICAL PRESENTATION

Patients with SCD classically present with signs and symptoms classified by the type of crisis they manifest (Table 133-1).

Vasoocclusive crises are the classic ''sickle crises'' characterized by painful events, often involving the back, chest, extremities or abdomen. They are the most common reason for emergency department (ED) visits by children with SCD. These vasoocclusive events account for more of the morbidity and hospitalizations than any other set of complications. The episodes are highly variable from patient to patient, with many patients reporting no crises at all, whereas others experience them on a regular basis, varying in location, duration, and severity. Typical sickle cell patients average about four severe attacks per year; with few patients reporting crises daily.

Some of these vasoocclusive crises seem to have ''triggers.'' Stress (emotional or physical), cold water immersion/exposure (especially as associated with shivering postexposure), dehydration, high altitudes/hypoxia, or infection (bacterial or viral, with the latter being the most common trigger in children under the age of 10).

Most vasoocclusive crises occur without any obvious cause. They result from the classic mechanism of sludging of sickled red blood cells into the microcirculation, resulting in tissue hypoxia and infarction. The associated pain may recur in the same location(s), but it can be anywhere in the body. Young children tend to have pain in the limbs, whereas adolescents more commonly complain of abdominal pain. Overall *musculoskeletal* (first) and *abdominal pain* (second) are the two most common types of vasoocclusive crises.

With *musculoskeletal pain*, the location can be anywhere but mostly involves the long bones—i.e.,the femur, tibia, and humerus. Lumbosacral pain is also commonly reported. Often there are no demonstrative physical findings but point tenderness may be found in the painful locations. Inguinal pain with difficulty in weight bearing and walking should raise the suspicion of avascular necrosis of the femoral head. Radiographs and/or a bone scan will aid in the diagnosis.

Infants may present with *sickle dactylitis*, also known as hand and foot syndrome. This occurs secondary to ischemia and infarction in the bone marrow of the extremities. Nutrient arteries that supply the metacarpals and the metatarsals become occluded and cause avascular necrosis. Clinically one sees swelling and pain of the hands and feet, often with an accompanying low-grade fever (i.e., less than 38.6°C or 101.5°F). One or all four extremities may be involved. Dactylitis is usually seen in children under the age of 2 and is rare after the age of 5.

Abdominal pain is the next most common type of vasoocclusive crisis seen in children with SCD. It is characterized by its abrupt onset, lack of localization, and recurrence. Patients often complain of diffuse, generalized abdominal pain, typically in the absence of significant peritoneal signs. Bowel sounds usually remain present and auscultate normally during these attacks. It can be extremely difficult to differentiate whether the pain is caused by vasoocclusive crisis or by a more common type of surgically correctable condition. While peritoneal signs are often absent in crisis, abdominal guarding and rebound tenderness may be present to cloud the diagnosis. Mesenteric infarction as well as splenic and hepatic infarction are the most likely causes of the pain, but the differential also should include pancreatitis, hepatitis, appendicitis, perforated viscus, and pelvic inflammatory disease/gynecologic pathology. It is important to determine if the abdominal pain in SCD patients has substantially changed in character, quality, duration, severity, and associated symptoms. If such changes are present, infection or other related diagnoses should be explored.

Because of the rapid turnover of red blood cells bilirubin gallstones commonly form. This can result in biliary colic and/or cholecystitis with a secondary gallstone ileus [''right-upper-quadrant (RUQ) syndrome'']. Any sickle cell patient in crisis with RUQ pain should be carefully evaluated for this possibility. Approximately 75 percent of sickle patients have demonstrable bilirubin gallstones; fortunately only about 10 percent become symptomatic.

RUQ syndrome is characterized by the sudden onset of RUQ pain, anorexia, extreme hyperbilirubinemia (greater than 50 mg/dL), and progressive hepatomegaly. RUQ syndrome is usually benign and self-limiting in the pediatric patient population. It is felt to result from intrahepatic cholestasis and seems reversible with intravenous fluids and other supportive measures. However, in a small number of adult patients, this syndrome can progress to liver failure.

With all of the aforementioned conditions, ultrasound examination and/or computed tomography (CT) of the abdomen and pelvis may be useful. Prompt surgical consultation is initiated in patients in whom the diagnosis cannot be clarified.

Infections can cause vasoocclusive crises; therefore, determining the presence of an infectious process is critical. Painful crises are often associated with a low-grade fever and leukocytosis, but any temperature above 101°F/38.4°C (or an absolute band count greater than 300 cells per cubic millimeter) is more likely to represent an infectious etiology than tissue ischemia.

Other Vasoocclusive Types of Crises

ACUTE CHEST SYNDROME/PULMONARY CRISIS Acute chest syndrome is characterized by signs and symptoms of acute lower respiratory tract disease—i.e., cough, chest pain (often pleuritic in nature), leukocytosis, tachypnea, dyspnea, and so on. All are usually accompanied by an infiltrate on chest x-ray (often the infiltrate takes 2 to 3 days to become apparent on a radiograph). The differential diagnosis includes acute chest syndrome/pulmonary infarction, pneumonia (bacterial or viral), and pulmonary thromboembolus. Pulmonary infarcted areas often become secondarily infected, leading to the acute chest syndrome. This is a major cause of mortality in sickle patients of all ages but especially in those above the age of 10. It accounts for about 15 percent of adult deaths and can be seen in about 30 percent of patients with sickle disease.

A standard chest/infiltrative disease workup is indicated with some notable variations. Arterial blood gases, complete blood count (CBC), and sputum analysis are certainly indicated. These patients should all be admitted to the hospital for supplemental oxygen therapy, pulmonary toilet, and empiric parenteral antibiotic therapy. The role and value of noninvasive pulse oximetry has been controversial. Some investigators believe that it accurately reflects arterial oxygen saturation, but others question the accuracy of the readings. It is clear, however, that some totally asymptomatic patients with sickle disease exhibit appreciable oxygen desaturation. This may be due to the abnormal sickle cell morphology of the red blood cell (RBC) and its spectrographic "reflection" on light plethysmography as measured by most standard pulse oximeters. The other issue is pulmonary angiography, which in general is to be avoided, since contrast material seems to cause more pulmonary sickling. A ventilation/perfusion ($\dot{V}/\dot{Q}$) scan may be helpful, especially if a baseline scan is available for comparison. If a significant $\dot{V}/\dot{Q}$ mismatch is discovered, heparinization may be indicated. The major concern is that multiple episodes of chest syndrome can result in pulmonary fibrosis and impair pulmonary function. Patients with multiple episodes often develop pulmonary hypertension and end-stage lung disease as young adults, hence the high morbidity and mortality rates. Any patient with significant cardiopulmonary decompensation should be considered for exchange transfusion therapy.

CEREBROVASCULAR DISEASE/CNS CRISIS Some 5 to 10 percent of children (15 to 25 percent in all age categories) with SCD have a clinically apparent cerebrovascular event, characterized by acute onset of hemiparesis, seizures, headaches, transient ischemic attacks, dizziness/vertigo, sensory hearing loss, cranial nerve palsies, paresthesias, and inexplicable coma. These crises tend to be painless but are abrupt in onset. Cerebral infarction is more common in children, while cerebral hemorrhage is more typical in adults. The overall rate of subarachnoid hemorrhage (SAH) is increased in sickle disease patients. CT scan, lumbar puncture, and magnetic resonance imaging (MRI) are all helpful.

RENAL CRISIS Like cerebrovascular crisis, renal vasoocclusive events are common but generally asymptomatic. Symptoms of renal infarction may include flank pain, renal colic, and costovertebral angle tenderness to percussion/palpation. Gross or microscopic hematuria may be evident, and some patients may actually pass renal tissue in their urine secondary to papillary necrosis. Monitoring of baseline renal function (i.e., BUN/creatinine) is always recommended in sickle patients.

PRIAPISM This painful, sustained erection of the penis in the absence of sexual stimulation is the result of the accumulation of sickled cells in the corpora cavernosa. Severe and prolonged attacks can cause impotence. This occurs in up to 30 percent of males with SCD; surgical decompression is usually required. Newer approaches include oral administration of α-adrenergic agonists (terbutaline and pseudoephedrine) or intrapenile injection (usually with dilute epinephrine) of vasodilators such as hydralazine, and/or needle aspiration of the corpora cavernosa.

TABLE 133-2 Comparison of Findings in Sequestration, Aplastic, and Hemolytic Crises in Sickle Cell Disease

	Sequestration Crises	Aplastic Crises	Hemolytic Crisis
Onset	Sudden	Gradual	Sudden
Pallor	Present	Present	Present
Jaundice	Normal	Normal	Increased
Abdominal pain	Present	Absent	Absent
Hemoglobin level	Very low	Low or very low	Low
Reticulocytes	Unchanged or increased	Decreased	Increased
Marrow erythroid activity	Unchanged or increased	Decreased	Increased

Hematologic Crises

The hallmarks of these crises are an acute drop in serum hemoglobin levels and clinical symptoms of generalized weakness/malaise, fatigue, shortness of breath/exertional dyspnea, progressive congestive heart failure, and/or shock. There are two types of hematologic crisis (Table 133-2).

ACUTE SPLENIC SEQUESTRATION This occurs primarily in infants and young children and is the second most common cause of death in children with SCD under the age of 5. The spleen will enlarge to beyond its baseline size, accompanied by a decline in hemoglobin concentration; hence patients present with splenomegaly and hypovolemic shock. These symptoms may occur suddenly or insidiously, and repeated episodes are common. It is a result of sickled cells blocking splenic outflow and drainage, thus causing pooling of both peripheral blood and sickled cells in the spleen. These crises are often preceded by a viral infection, with parvovirus B19; rhinoviruses and echoviruses have also recently been implicated.

These splenic sequestration crises are often divided into major and minor types. In major sequestration, the spleen enlarges rapidly and the serum hemoglobin levels drop to less than 6 g/dL—or to 3 g/dL from that particular patients' baseline. A minor episode is more insidious and leads to progressive splenomegaly, with hemoglobin levels generally greater than 6 g/dL. Reticulocyte counts tend to be higher than normal, reflecting the compensatory increase in bone marrow activity.

Management includes transfusion of packed RBCs and exchange transfusions. Ultimately splenectomy may become necessary.

APLASTIC CRISIS Among the most life-threatening of all complications related to SCD, this complication occurs when bone marrow erythropoiesis slows or completely ceases, resulting in erythroid aplasia. It is characterized by severe anemia with hematocrit levels of 10 percent or lower, hemoglobin levels of 1 to 3 g/dL or less, and reticulocyte counts of as low as 0.5 percent. White blood cell (WBC) counts and platelet counts tend to remain stable despite the lack of erythropoiesis. It is now known that these crises can be precipitated primarily by viral infections (most notably parvovirus B19), but folic acid deficiency and bone marrow suppressive/toxic drugs such as phenylbutazone have also been implicated. Fortunately these crises tend to occur only once in the lifetime of a patient with SCD and are usually self-limiting. RBC transfusions are usually necessary secondary to the severe anemia. This helps to avoid any secondary cardiopulmonary complications.

Infections/Infectious Crises

Bacterial infection poses a serious threat to the child with sickle cell anemia. In the first 10 years of life the most common infections are bacteremia, pneumonia, osteomyelitis, meningitis, and urinary tract infections. In the group under 5 years of age, it is often fatal; it occurs rapidly and can be overwhelming. The primary pathogens are usually encapsulated organisms: *Streptococcus pneumoniae, Haemophilus influenzae, Escherichia coli,* and *Staphylococcus aureus.* Other common infections include pneumonia caused by *Mycoplasma pneumoniae,* and osteomyelitis due to *Salmonella typhimurium, Staph. aureus,* and *E. coli.*

Repeated splenic infarction resulting in functional asplenia is felt to be the most likely reason for the increased risk of infection. Splenic infarction can occur as early as 5 months and is routine by 5 years of age. The susceptibility to bacterial infections results from deficient antibody formation and impaired phagocytosis. The complement activation system is impaired as well. Serum levels of IgM are also decreased.

During the first 5 years of life, the most common bacterial pathogen appears to be *Strep. pneumoniae*, and sepsis from this organism is the most common cause of death in this age group. The middle ear and the lungs tend to be the typical foci. Beyond 5 years, there tends be an increased frequency of gram-negative infections.

Children with SCD tend to become infected with *H. influenzae* at higher rates than other children. The course of these infections tends to be more insidious than that of those with *Strep. pneumoniae.*

Pneumonia of bacterial etiology is approximately 100 times more common in SCD patients than in the general population. Pneumonia generally causes hypoxia that further exacerbates the sickling. *Strep. pneumoniae* and *H. influenzae* are the two most common etiologic agents, but mycoplasmal infections are also common and should be considered when patients fail empiric (i.e., ''nonmacrolide'') antibiotic therapy. Viral pneumonia is also common, especially under the age of 2.

SCD patients also have an increased incidence of osteomyelitis. Often the etiologic agent is *S. typhirium* (about 50 percent). It can also be caused by *Staph. aureus* and *E. coli.* Also seen in increased frequency from the general population are meningitis and urinary tract infections. Bacterial meningitis and septicemia are approximately 600 times more common in SCD patients than in other children.

DIAGNOSIS

NEWBORN SCREENING In the United States, most states with a sizable African-American population have implemented newborn screening programs to identify affected individuals at birth. Success in preventing early complications and assuring reliable follow-up mechanisms has had a significant effect on reducing overall mortality from the disease. Patients identified through programs such as these are then enrolled for comprehensive treatment. Cord blood can be utilized right in the delivery room.

Hemoglobin electrophoresis is the ''gold standard'' and most accurate diagnostic study to determine and distinguish sickle cell anemia (homozygous Ss), sickle cell trait (HgbSC), and sickle cell thalassemia. In the newborn and infant, this test is always necessary to confirm the diagnosis.

LABORATORY STUDIES As always, prudent laboratory testing is tailored to the clinical signs and symptoms of patients as they present to the ED. The following is a list of some commonly ordered diagnostic studies.

SICKLE PREP If the diagnosis is in question or in previously undiagnosed cases, the emergency physician will need a rapid assay for determining the presence of SCD. The sickle prep is a peripheral blood smear specially prepared so as to induce RBC sickling. These cells are then seen on routine microscopy of the smear. Tests such as the Sickledex and Metabisulfite tests have been used. While these tests can be useful in the ED, they are limited in their ability to diagnose SCD in infants under the age of 4 to 6 months, and they cannot diagnose sickle cell trait.

COMPLETE BLOOD COUNT (CBC) All patients who present to the ED in sickle cell crisis or any other complaint referable to SCD should have a CBC performed; of paramount importance is the serum hemoglobin level. The average hemoglobin in patients with SCD is generally between 6 and 9 g/dL. Obtaining a prior baseline level is critical, because any patient with a drop of 2 to 3 g/dL in hemoglobin or a decline in the serum hematocrit by 4 to 6 percent may reflect severe hematologic crisis or hypovolemia and shock. Platelet counts are usually elevated at baseline. White blood cell (WBC) counts are also often elevated at baseline, ranging from 12,000 to 18,000 μL, usually with a normal differential. Any rise in the total WBCs or leftward shift may indicate the presence of significant underlying pathology. The peripheral smear often shows sickled cells as well as Howell-Jolly bodies, indicative of splenic dysfunction and failure.

RETICULOCYTE COUNT Because of accelerated RBC turnover, reticulocytes appear in greater numbers on the peripheral smear. The mean reticulocyte count is approximately 12 percent (with a range of 5 to 15 percen) in SCD patients. With a reticulocyte count of 3 percent or less, aplastic crisis should be considered. An extremely high count may be indicative of hemolysis. Certainly any decrease of 2 g/dL or greater in serum hemoglobin levels warrants obtaining a reticulocyte count.

BLOOD CULTURES Blood cultures should be obtained in any SCD patient with a temperature higher than 38.4°C (101°F) and in any patient suspected of having bacteremia or sepsis. Any child with radiographic evidence of infiltrative disease should also have blood cultures drawn.

URINALYSIS (UA) Any patient with a fever and/or urinary symptoms (especially dysuria or hematuria) should have a UA (and appropriate culture) obtained. RBCs or tissue in the urine are seen with papillary necrosis/renal crisis. Isosthenuria, the inability to concentrate urine, is typically present, with specific gravities of about 1.010. The specific gravity can be quite low in patients with SCD even when they are dehydrated.

ELECTROLYTES Electrolytes should be obtained in any SCD patient who appears clinically to be dehydrated. Significant imbalances can occur because of isosthenuria.

ARTERIAL BLOOD GAS (ABG) An ABG should be obtained in all SCD patients with chest pain not typical of vasoocclusive crisis or in patients with any respiratory complaints. A large arterioalveolar (A-a) gradient suggests either pulmonary infection, infarction, or potential thromboembolus. It is helpful to have a baseline reference ABG since most adolescents and adults with SCD exhibit a mild to moderate chronic hypoxia. Generally, arterial P_{O_2} levels less than 60 mmHg in adults or 70 mmHg in children are indicative of acute pathology.

LIVER ENZYMES Liver enzymes may be helpful in SCD patients who present with abdominal pain. However, baseline abnormalities are common, especially an elevated indirect bilirubin, which is usually secondary to the chronic hemolytic state of SCD.

CEREBROSPINAL FLUID ANALYSIS A lumbar puncture should be performed when meningitis is a consideration.

Radiologic Studies

CHEST X-RAY Patients with chest pain, suspected pneumonia, or dyspnea/respiratory symptoms should have chest radiographs. It is important to remember that in acute chest syndrome, the x-ray may appear normal for the first 48 h; thus a normal-appearing radiograph does not preclude significant pulmonary pathology.

EXTREMITY X-RAYS Extremity x-rays should be obtained in patients in whom ischemic necrosis of the femoral or humeral head is suspected or in those with localized bony tenderness. Avascular necrosis of the femoral head occurs in up to 12 percent of SCD patients. Small lytic lesions are also seen in patients with sickle dactylitis. Plain radiographs are somewhat limited in diagnosing bony infarction and/or osteomyelitis acutely. It may take 10 to 14 days for the radiographic changes to become evident. A bone scan or MRI can detect changes consistent with osteomyelitis usually within 24 h.

CT/MRI OF THE HEAD CT or MRI of the head should be obtained in SCD patients with any lateralizing neurologic signs or acute/new neurologic deficits.

ABDOMINAL ULTRASOUND OR CT These tests may be helpful in patients with abdominal pain, especially if a surgically correctable cause is suspected. The diagnosis of typical intraabdominal pathology (i.e., appendicitis, cholecystitis, pancreatitis, abscesses, bowel obstruction/infarction) with these imaging modalities is not affected by the presence of vasoocclusive crisis.

TREATMENT

Management of patients with SCD focuses on both acute and chronic illness. It is important to remember that progressive end-organ involvement occurs over time. Of primary importance are ocular, pulmonary, cardiac, hepatic, and renal changes. These—as well as issues of growth, development, and sexual maturation—should be routinely monitored at well-patient visits to the pediatrician/hematologist. In the ED, it is the acute illness that confronts the physician. Complications arising from SCD are managed based upon the nature of the pathology. The ED care of patients with SCD presenting in crisis is generally supportive in nature. The mainstays of therapy have been hydration/fluid replacement, analgesia, supplemental oxygen, and blood transfusion.

FLUID REPLACEMENT All types of sickle cell crisis can be precipitated or exacerbated by dehydration. If the episode is relatively mild, oral fluid replacement may be effective. Patients with severe pain, orthostasis, or change in vital signs will likely require intravenous hydration. The rate of hydration is generally at $1\frac{1}{2}$ times maintenance (about 2250 mL/M^2 per day). Patients need to be carefully monitored to avoid fluid overload and iatrogenic cardiac failure, especially those with cardiopulmonary crisis/acute chest syndrome. Electrolytes should be checked and fluid choice adjusted appropriately.

ANALGESIA Analgesia is of paramount importance and should always be sufficient to control the pain. ''Standard doses'' of narcotic medication may not be enough for the individual patient with SCD. Although narcotic dependence or enhanced narcotic-seeking behavior may be a problem for rare patients, this should never affect the decision to control severe pain. The establishment of treatment guidelines and protocols for the ED management of patients with SCD can help minimize manipulative behavior and change expectations. The approach should be consistent. With the advent of patient-controlled analgesia (PCA) pumps, narcotic usage and dosing can be carefully controlled and reviewed. In the ED, narcotics should be chosen with potential side effects, drug interactions, and serum half-lives in mind.

Oral narcotic preparations such as Tylenol #3, Vicodin, or Percocet are usually adequate for moderate types of pain. Parenteral narcotics are usually required for more severe pain. Demerol (meperidine) in often used, in combination with an antiemetic, as an intramuscular injection. This may be useful, but only in limited doses, since meperidine can lower the seizure threshold. Also, repeated intramuscular injections run the risk of forming sterile abscesses and scarring, which can further exacerbate painful crises; they are therefore to be avoided in treatment of prolonged, painful crises. Intravenous narcotic administration is preferable, and a PCA pump is ideal. Morphine (at 0.15 mg/kg per dose to a maximum of 10 mg) every 2 to 3 h and hydromorphone (Dilaudid, at about 0.02 to 0.05 mg/kg per dose) are good choices. Dilaudid has a slightly more rapid onset and slightly shorter duration of action as compared with morphine. Approximately 1.3 mg of Dilaudid is considered equivalent to about 10 mg of morphine. Both medications should be adjusted to provide about 3 to 4 h of pain relief. The addition of nonsteroidal anti-inflammatory drugs has been shown to be of some benefit; however, these are to be used cautiously or not at all in patients with renal compromise.

OXYGEN Supplemental oxygen has long been considered an important part of treating SCD crises. More recent investigations have shown that it is beneficial only if the patient has demonstrable hypoxia.

CARDIAC MONITORING Cardiac monitoring is necessary if the patient has a history of known cardiac disease, signs and symptoms of acute chest syndrome, or cardiopulmonary compromise. When aggressive fluid replacement is warranted, cardiac monitoring also becomes important.

TRANFUSION THERAPY Blood transfusions are often necessary in children undergoing splenic sequestration crisis and severe aplastic crisis. In addition, transfusions may be needed in the management of cerebrovascular accident (CVA), priapism, or as perioperative management prior to surgery. Naturally, transfusion carries risk: alloimmunization, HIV infection, hepatitis, volume overload, and iron toxicity (secondary to repeated transfusions). Transfusion can also markedly decrease erythropoiesis.

The decision to institute transfusion therapy can be difficult. Clearly, in splenic sequestration crisis with hypotension, blood should be transfused. A hematologist should be consulted emergently to help direct therapy. An initial transfusion of 10 mL/kg of packed RBCs can be started in the ED.

Aplastic crisis may also require a transfusion of packed RBCs. When aplastic, splenic sequestration, or hemolytic crises occur, exchange transfusion is preferable. If the serum hemoglobin is greater than 6 g/dL, transfusion is rarely indicated.

Symptom-Specific Therapy

INFECTIONS Pneumococcal sepsis in children with SCD has a 14 percent mortality rate. Prophylactic oral penicillin, administered daily, has proven to be quite effective in decreasing the incidence of sepsis and death in children under the age of 6. This practice has not been shown to be of value in the adult population with SCD. The polyvalent pneumococcal vaccine is also recommended at 2 years of age. (*Note:*

Some recommend it be given at 6 months, 2 years, and again at 6 years of age.)

Since *Strep. pneumoniae* and *H. influenzae* are the primary bacterial pathogens of SCD, patients should be vaccinated in childhood against them as well as receiving the hepatitis B vaccine. Parenteral antibiotic therapy usually begins with cephalosporins (i.e., cefuroxime or ceftriaxone), which have excellent activity against these two pathogens. Choice of intravenous antibiotic depends upon the given clinical scenario and culture results.

CNS CRISIS Any neurologic signs or symptoms necessitate immediate stabilization and careful monitoring. Admission to an intensive care unit (ICU) setting is most appropriate. A head CT or MRI should be obtained, and—based on those results—lumbar puncture may need to be performed to rule out meningitis or subarachnoid hemorrhage. After an acute central nervous system (CNS) event, exchange transfusion may be indicated, with a goal of lowering the HgbS concentration to less than 30 percent.

PRIAPISM All SCD patients with this condition should have a urologic consultation. Intravenous hydration and analgesic therapy should be instituted immediately. The bladder should be emptied, either by spontaneous void if possible or by catheterization. If the priapism is not relieved after 2 to 3 h, exchange transfusion becomes necessary. If this is not successful, surgical intervention will be required. This is why prompt urologic consultation in the ED for this entity is important.

LOCALIZED BONE PAIN Localized bone pain accompanied by fever and leukocytosis strongly suggests osteomyelitis. Diagnosis can be confirmed by plain film radiographs, bone scan, and/or MRI. The site may be needle-aspirated and cultured. Empiric parenteral antibiotic therapy should begin with coverage provided to treat *Salmonella* species and *Staph. aureus*. Intravenous trimethoprim-sulfamethoxazole (2.5 mg/kg, based on the trimethoprim component, q 6 h) or, as an alternative, ceftriaxone (25 to 50 mg/kg q 12 h), which provides better *Staph.* coverage, can be used.

DISPOSITION

Disposition depends upon ED findings, observation, and response to initial therapy. The following is a list of guidelines to aid ED physicians in determining which children with SCD require hospitalization:

1. Temperature greater than or equal to 103°F/39°C, WBC counts greater than 30,000/mm^3, or left shift and/or other hematologic parameters greatly altered from baseline values.
2. Any signs of respiratory distress, hypoxia, and/or lobar infiltrate on chest x-ray.
3. Any new CNS findings or presence of neurologic crisis.
4. Patients with splenic sequestration or aplastic crisis.
5. An acute abdomen.
6. Prolonged priapism.
7. Any type of vasooclusive crisis that does not respond to intravenous hydration and analgesia (usually after about 4 to 6 h of therapy).
8. Inability to maintain adequate oral hydration.
9. Patients in whom the diagnosis remains uncertain.
10. Follow-up (i.e., telephone contact, return visit, etc.) is uncertain or unlikely because of distance, inconvenience, or poor compliance.

If patients with vasoocclusive crisis are discharged home, they should be advised to maintain adequate oral hydration, take pain medication (a 2- to 3-day supply should be provided), and return immediately if fever over 100.4°F/38°C occurs, the pattern of pain worsens or changes, or vomiting begins. All patients treated and released from the ED should be reevaluated in 24 to 48 h by their private pediatrician/physician or hematologist (generally 24 h for children and 24 to 48 h for adults).

Variants of Sickle Cell Disease

SICKLE CELL TRAIT (SCT) This is the carrier state of SCD and the most frequently encountered sickle cell variant. It is erroneous to consider this a "mild" form of SCD. Hematologically these patients are normal. Their RBCs have a normal lifespan; therefore there is no demonstrable anemia. The peripheral smear should not reveal sickled cells except in the presence of extreme hypoxia.

Clinically these patients have minimal complications, with the kidney being the most commonly affected organ. Hematuria is found in about 1 percent of patients with SCT and is most likely due to papillary necrosis following microinfarcts in the renal medullary tissue. Severe hypoxia and/or exposure to high altitudes can cause splenic infarction and CNS complications; there is also an increased incidence of sudden death in these patients during physical exertion/training. This is thought to be secondary to increased sickling under these extreme conditions. In general, the vast majority of these patients are asymptomatic and lead normal lives with a normal life expectancy.

SICKLE CELL HEMOGLOBIN-SC DISEASE This heterozygous variant results when the gene for HgbS is inherited from one parent and the gene for HgbC is inherited from the other parent. These patients can have a mild to moderate anemia and usually a mild reticulocytosis. Their peripheral smear reveals an abundance of target cells and a few sickle-shaped cells. Additionally HgbC may be seen precipitated as rhomboid crystals in the RBCs. Splenomegaly is the major feature of HgbSC disease and persists into adulthood in about 60 percent of patients.

Patients with HgbSC disease can have painful crises and organ infarcts; they are also at higher-than-normal risk for bacterial infections. Avascular necrosis of the femoral head, ocular complications/visual loss, and renal medullary infarcts have all been reported in these patients. Women with SC disease have an increased incidence of complications during pregnancy. Overall, while some patients have complications as profound as those with SCD, most patients with HgbSC disease have few clinical complications.

SICKLE CELL BETA-THALASSEMIA DISEASE Also a heterozygous sickle cell variant, this occurs when the gene for sickle hemoglobin is inherited from one parent and the gene for beta thalassemia is inherited from the other. The clinical severity of the disease, frequency of complications, and the degree of the resultant anemia depends on the type of beta-thalassemia gene inherited. Approximately 80 to 90 percent of affected individuals have a beta-thalassemia gene that allows for the production of some normal beta chains; thus some normal HgbA is produced. These patients in general do quite well; they have a mild hemolytic anemia (with near normal Hgb levels), suffer few painful crises, and sustain minimal end-organ damage. The remaining 10 to 20 percent of patients inherit a beta-thalassemia gene that produces no beta chains; therefore they have no normal hemoglobin. These individuals have a severe hemolytic anemia and vasoocclusive symptoms similar to those seen with SCD. Splenomegaly is found in 70 percent of patients with this variant.

BIBLIOGRAPHY

American Academy of Pediatrics publishes guidelines on the management of sickle cell disease. *Am Family Physician* 55:1973, 1997.

Ballas SK: Management of sickle pain. *Curr Opin Hematol* 4:104, 1997.

Buchanan GR: Newer concepts in the management of sickle cell disease. *Pediatrics* 1:100, 1995.

Davis H, Schoendorf KC, Gergen PJ, Moore RM Jr: National trends in the mortality of children with sickle cell disease, 1968 through 1992. *Am J Public Health* 87:1317, 1997.

Davis SC: Blood transfusion in sickle cell disease. *Curr Opin Hematol* 3:485, 1996.

Losek JD, Hellmich TR, Hoffman GM: Diagnostic value of anemia, red blood cell morphology, and reticulocyte count for sickle cell disease. *Ann Emerg Med* 21:915, 1992.

Pollack CV Jr: Emergencies in sickle cell disease. *Emerg Med Clin North Am* 11:365, 1993.

Robieux IC, Kellner JD, Coppes MJ, et al: Analgesia in children with sickle cell crisis: Comparison of intermittent opioids vs continuous intravenous infusion of morphine and placebo-controlled oxygen inhalation. *Pediatr Hematol Oncol* 9:317, 1992.

Schiffman MA: Preventable sudden death in children with sickle hemoglobinopathies and fever: The need for a protocolized approach (editorial). *Ann Emerg Med* 20:1043, 1991.

Serjeant GR, Serjeant BE: Management of sickle cell disease: Lessons from the Jamaican Cohort Study. *Blood Rev* 7:137, 1993.

134 EVALUATING THE HANDICAPPED OR DISABLED CHILD

Cheryl H. Hack

There are about 7 million children in the United States who have conditions that impair their ability to function physically or mentally. Some disabilities and handicaps may be medically distinct and self-limited, such as limb deformities, hearing impairments, or spastic diplegia. Others are multidimensional, consisting of multiple medical problems such as meningomyelocele or severe mental impairment with associated severe cerebral palsy. Impaired neurologic functioning, orthopedic deformity, and chronic illness with multiple system involvement result in complex medical problems and greater likelihood that an individual will encounter difficulties and require emergency evaluation and treatment. Caring for handicapped or disabled children in the emergency department (ED) can be a difficult task due to complex ongoing medical problems, limited historical information, altered baseline functioning, and/or the need for the emergency physician to consider the impact of interventions on the course of the underlying disability or impairment.

Evaluating the child with handicapping or disabling conditions in the ED requires more time. Patience in obtaining a good history will assist the physician in decision making. Knowledge of specific medical problems associated with various handicapping or disabling conditions will help to focus the history and examination. Identification of management issues will allow the physician to design interventions that benefit the child and the family in both the long and short term.

Obtaining a medical history in the ED can be difficult, even with a normally healthy child. Obtaining a medical history in a disabled or handicapped child provides even more challenges. A medical condition of importance may not be reported because it is under treatment and is not currently creating any difficulty for the individual (e.g., neurogenic bowel or bladder). Information regarding the use of assistive devices such as braces, hearing aids, glasses, or prosthetics may not be offered because the family does not realize that this may give the physician information needed for making treatment decisions. Directed questioning may be necessary to avoid difficulties.

While obtaining the medical history, attempt to identify all existing medical conditions. Medications currently being used can be helpful in this task. A list of medications commonly used in cerebral palsy is given in Table 134-1. Information regarding the use of assistive devices may be important in management issues. Ask specifically about bracing, hearing aids, glasses, and use of suppositories and enemas. Hearing aids in a child with external otitis media or perforated tympanic membrane must be a consideration. Braces or night splints must be considered when lacerations or skin lesions are present. Children with complex medical problems may receive a variety of medical procedures in the home setting, including suctioning, nebulizer treatments, chest percussion and drainage, clean intermittent catheterization, and fecal disimpactions. Knowledge of these home-based procedures will help in making decisions regarding hospitalization and/or further home treatment. Associated medical conditions may have an impact on development of a differential diagnosis. By using information from the medical conditions associated with individual disorders described below, the physician can better guide questioning regarding associated medical problems.

TABLE 134-1 Medications Commonly Used for Spasticity

Generic Name (Brand Name)	Most Common Side Effects
Baclofen (Lioresal)	Drowsiness, dizziness, weakness, confusion, headache, insomnia, hypotension, nausea, constipation, urinary frequency
Clonidine (Catapres)	Drowsiness, dry mouth, orthostatic hypotension, nausea and vomiting, anxiety, depression, sleep disturbance, nocturia, rash
Dantrolene (Dantrium)	Drowsiness, dizziness, weakness, diarrhea, constipation
Diazepam (Valium)	Drowsiness, ataxia, weakness, confusion, constipation, dysarthria, diplopia, rash, urinary retention

CEREBRAL PALSY

Cerebral palsy is a disorder of movement and posture due to static, nonprogressive injury sustained by the developing brain. The brain damage must occur by 5 years of age. It occurs in 2.5 to 3 per 1000 individuals. Diagnosis before 12 to 18 months of age can be confused with transient tonal problems or progressive degenerative disorders. The movement problems manifest in a variety of forms and can affect the head, trunk, and extremities in a variety of ways. Cerebral palsy is commonly classified by type, distribution, and degree of involvement. Types include spastic, dyskinetic (choreoathetoid), hypotonic, and mixed forms. Distribution relates to the involvement of the extremities. Diplegia, hemiplegia, and quadriplegia are the most common. Rarely one sees a child with monoplegia or triplegia. Severity is rated subjectively as mild, moderate, or severe.

Children with cerebral palsy may have associated medical problems as a direct effect or complication of motor dysfunction or underlying brain damage. Seizures, oral motor dysfunction, gastroesophageal reflux, constipation, urinary tract infections, pneumonia, wheezing, hearing loss, strabismus, visual impairments, scoliosis, contractures, and hip dislocation or subluxation are all seen with increased frequency in children with cerebral palsy. Children with less severe presentations have minimal associated medical problems (i.e., the child with spastic diplegia may have only issues related to spasticity). As the severity of impairment increases to spastic quadriplegia, the incidence and severity of associated problems and need for emergency medical treatment also increase.

In managing the child with severe cerebral palsy in the ED, special attention should be given to seizures, respiratory tract problems, fluid status, nutritional status, bracing, and skin problems.

Seizures

Seizures are present in 50 percent of children with cerebral palsy. With increasing severity of cerebral palsy, there are often more frequent and complex seizures. Multiple seizure types may occur in a single individual. This may cause difficulty in eliciting a complete seizure history if the physician is unaware that different seizure presentations are documented historically. Multiple anticonvulsant medications may be required to adequately control seizures. When multiple anticonvulsants are required, the physician should be alert to the possibility of multiple seizure types, interactions of the various anticonvulsant medications, and the possible fragility of seizure control. Contact with the managing neurologist is strongly advised in such cases. The treatment of medical problems should be evaluated with regard to drug-drug interactions whenever a medication is recommended. Anticonvulsant medications may affect or be affected by many other drugs. Theophylline is known to lower seizure threshold, and erythromycin may elevate drug levels into the toxic range.

Pulmonary Problems

Respiratory tract symptoms are seen commonly in children with severe forms of cerebral palsy. They include chronic congestion, recurrent wheezing pneumonia, microaspiration, and aspiration.[1] The respiratory tract problems are generally related to oral motor dysfunction and gastroesophageal reflux.

Oral motor dyspraxia presents with exaggerated gag and retained bite reflexes, tongue thrust, and oral hypersensitivity, which can lead to choking, gagging, and aspiration.[1,2] Oropharyngeal incoordination manifests early with poor feeding and failure to thrive and contributes to aspiration. Gastroesophageal reflux is associated with aspiration of food and chemical fumes that may be damaging to pulmonary tissues and can be associated with the development of pneumonia. Lack of head control may lead to pooling of secretions in the posterior pharynx with spillage of contents into the vallecula and then into the trachea.

Pneumonia often is due to aspiration. If there is no evidence for secondary bacterial infection, the pneumonia may be chemical in nature and may resolve on its own. Pneumonia often is treated early with antibiotics because of the risk of secondary bacterial infection if the aspiration is of oral contents. With mounting evidence for ongoing microaspiration in many individuals with cerebral palsy that does not result in infection, this concept will need to be reexamined, and treatment may be deferred initially. Secondary bacterial superinfection should be treated promptly. Unilateral pneumonia could involve the possibility of a foreign body retained in the respiratory system, as it would be in the normal child.

Wheezing is a difficult problem in this population. Some children with cerebral palsy have been born prematurely and have a history of respiratory problems stemming from bronchopulmonary dysplasia and reactive airways disease. A small number may have developed tracheomalacia and required tracheostomy. When these children have adventitial respiratory noises, it is important to differentiate clearly what is happening. Wheezing accompanied by impaired air movement should be treated appropriately with bronchodilators. However, the clinician must evaluate the situation carefully for evidence of stridor on inspiration as opposed to wheeze on expiration. Possible reasons for wheezing or stridor include a retained foreign body, tracheal edema, impaired vocal cord function, tracheomalacia, aspiration of gastroesophageal contents, and asthma (Table 134-2). Aspiration should be considered before instituting therapy. Children with spastic quadriplegia in particular are at risk for reactive airways triggered by microaspiration of saliva, food, or gastric fluids. The respiratory tract may be responding to a potential threat, and bronchodilatory treatments may not be effective in resolving the wheezing and would not be a desired treatment. Management of wheezing in the emergent situation should start with an assessment of the contribution of aspiration. A simple initial evaluation should investigate the effect of positioning in severely affected individuals with impaired head control. Placing the head and neck in the "sniffer" position to maximize the airway and minimize the risk of secretions pooling in the posterior pharynx may improve respiratory functioning by decreasing aspiration. Evaluations of air movement, nasal flaring, intercostal retractions, and blood gases to assess respiratory distress are indicated. If significant impairment of air movement is compromising the patient, bronchodilators may be used with caution, remembering that if the wheezing is due to aspiration, there may be little or no improvement. In such cases, reconsideration of treatment options is always warranted. Further evaluation for gastroesophageal reflux leading to aspiration will require multiple radiographic studies and should be done either in the outpatient setting or, if the respiratory distress is severe, on an inpatient basis following resolution of the immediate distress. Medications to reduce reflux or acidity such as metoclopramide, cisapride, and ranitidine may be helpful. Children will need to be hospitalized if secondary pneumonia is suspected or respiratory compromise is evident.

TABLE 134-2 Respiratory Distress in Children

Stridor	Wheezing
Epiglotitis	Asthma
Foreign body aspiration	Tracheomalacia
Spasmodic croup	Gastroesophageal reflux
Allergic reaction	Foreign body aspiration
Laryngomalacia	Tracheal stenosis
Subglottic stenosis	Extrinsic tracheal compression
Vocal cord dysfunction	Microaspiration
Bacterial tracheitis	Bronchiolitis
Trauma	

Drooling

The control of saliva may be impaired in children with severe spastic quadriplegia. Poor head control and oromotor deficits are the cause. With the head held flexed or to the side, there may be pooling of oral secretions in the anterior portion of the oral cavity. If bolus formation is not initiated, these secretions will spill over the lips and onto the face and body. Although primarily thought of as a social or cosmetic issue, drooling may lead to skin problems such as chapping on the face. Families and physicians have used a variety of techniques to stem the drooling when it persists in childhood and is perceived as a problem. As a side effect, some common medications are noted to decrease secretions. These drugs, including scopolamine, atropine, imipramine, trihexyphenidyl hydrochloride (Artane), glycopyrrolate (Robinal), benztropine mesylate (Cogentin), and antihistamines, have been used with limited success.[3] Side effects of these medications, toxicity (if the family should give multiple doses), and possible drug interactions are of concern in the emergency setting. Surgery also has been used for severe drooling. Salivary duct rerouting is the most commonly used procedure at this time.[4] Following surgery, cheek swelling and swallowing dysfunction have been noted. In a small number of patients, ranula formation was noted. In the past, xerostoma has been reported after surgical removal of salivary glands with resulting lesions of the oral mucosa and increased dental caries. None of these issues needs to be handled on an emergent basis and should be referred to the ENT service for long-term management on an outpatient basis.

Growth Failure

Growth failure may be a problem in the child with cerebral palsy. Increased energy requirements and difficulty in handling food in the oral cavity combine to cause growth failure. Energy requirements in the young child with spastic cerebral palsy may be increased to 140 to 160 kcal/kg/day. Chronic failure to thrive decreases energy and strength to accomplish motor tasks and coordinate movement and may impair immunologic function. Children with oromotor dysfunction often have limited skills in handling foods and particularly in handling liquids. These children require high-caloric-density food and may require alternative feedings on a supplemental or primary basis.

Gastrostomy tubes with or without Nissan fundoplications may be in place. Tube feedings may be the primary caloric intake or may be used supplementally (often at night) to improve the nutritional, health, and functional status of the child. Problems with the gastrostomy tube or the skin surrounding it may bring children into the ED. Irritation of the skin site due to movement of the gastrostomy tube may occur with development of granulation tissue and/or leakage of gastric contacts. The stability of the tube needs to be checked, and bumpers holding the tube in place may need to be adjusted. If leakage of acidic contents has caused skin breakdown, the leakage needs to be eliminated, if possible, and a barrier should be used to protect the skin until it heals. Zinc oxide-based creams often are effective, but adherence to the skin can be a problem. An enterstomal therapist may be able to offer assistance in choosing products that offer the best adherence properties. Gastrostomy tubes falling out and being pulled out intentionally or unintentionally also can be an issue. The stoma should be maintained if possible to allow for replacement of an appropriate tube in a controlled manner as soon as possible. Placement of a red rubber feeding tube through the stoma and taping it in place can be effective for up to several days if necessary. If skin irritation or breakdown is a problem, then securing the tube may be a challenge. The physician should attempt to secure the tube without placing tape on macerated skin surfaces.

Dehydration

Marginal or deficient fluid balance may be present in children with severe cerebral palsy and oromotor problems, particularly if gastrostomy tube feedings are not in place. When the child with failure to thrive and a limited fluid status develops a routine gastroenteritis, dehydration and nutritional status become major difficulties. Some children dehydrate with minimal diarrhea or vomiting and have difficulty maintaining hydration until the diarrhea or vomiting resolves. Hypernatremia or hyponatremic dehydration with seizure activity may result if the sodium load is very high or low. Hospitalization decisions should be based on the history of diarrhea, hydration status of the patient in relation to the amount of diarrhea reported, and baseline nutritional status. The further below the 5th percentile for weight a child is, the greater is the concern that the child cannot be orally hydrated if diarrhea or vomiting persists. Obtaining a premorbid weight from the family will assist the physician in estimating fluid loss. Monitoring urine output also will provide information, as will the traditional signs of dry mucous membranes, tachycardia, skin tenting, and sunken eyes. When rapid dehydration occurs in the malnourished child with limited hydration as the baseline, intravenous access may be a problem. If an intravenous line cannot be placed successfully, interosseus line placement should be considered. In addition to treatment with fluid boluses, full feeds should be continued.

Constipation

Constipation occurs secondary to increased tone, impairment of sphincter relaxation, and limited fluid and fiber intake. It may be accompanied by rectal tears, overflow diarrhea, and anorexia. Getting an accurate history is important in the diagnosis of constipation. Families frequently complain of constipation if the child cries, strains, or does not have a bowel movement daily. Constipation is hard balls of stool even if this occurs on a daily basis. There is no constipation if the stools are soft, even if the child cries, appears to strain, or does not have a daily stool. Emergent management of constipation is by suppository if the problem is of brief duration or with an enema if long-standing or if fecal material can be palpated in the abdomen. Saline, Fleets, or oil-based enemas may be used. If constipation is of long duration, a home program will be needed. Contact with the treating physician or a gastroenterologist most likely will be needed.

In children with recurring constipation, avoid the routine use of Fleets enemas so as to prevent electrolyte abnormalities. Avoid chronic use of oral mineral oil in children with oromotor dysfunction because it is associated with a high risk of aspiration and may cause impaired absorption of fat-soluble essential vitamins. If a home program has been developed with frequent use of these products, electrolytes should be monitored and vitamin deficiency syndromes may need to be considered.

Enuresis

Enuresis, or incontinence, may persist due to motor and mental difficulties. In the severely impaired child, as with infants, urinary tract infections should be considered in the uncomfortable, ill-appearing child without clear evidence of other infectious sources. An increased incidence of urinary tract infections has been observed without evidence of urinary tract abnormalities. This has been ascribed to hygiene issues in the past, although a neurogenic bladder with urinary retention should be ruled out. A urinalysis should be done, with care taken to limit external contamination. Contractures of the hips and tight adductors make it difficult at times to clean the vaginal and perineal areas. Referral for radiologic studies to rule out anomalies of the urinary tract is recommended. Most urinary tract infections can be managed on an outpatient basis. If pyelonephritis is suspected, a urology consultation and hospitalization should be considered.

Sensory Problems

Problems with vision and hearing are common and do not generally cause any difficulty on an emergent basis. Hearing loss is present in 5 to 15 percent of children with hemiplegia. In addition, there may be conductive losses in children who are bottle-fed in a supine position. Visual problems include strabismus, hyperopia, cataracts (congenital infections), retinopathy of prematurity, and cortical blindness.

Spasticity Management and Contractures

Spasticity of muscles not only causes functional impairments but also is associated with the development of bony deformity in many children with cerebral palsy. Management occurs in progressive stages depending on the functional impairments. Physiotherapy, orthotics, medications, and then surgeries are used. When left untreated, the child is likely to develop contractures and positional deformities.

Oral medications have been used to treat spasticity in recent years, including benzodiazepines, dantrolene, and baclofen. Their use has been limited by the development of tolerance for dosages, narrow therapeutic ranges, hepatic toxicity, and sedation. Injections of alcohol in the form of nerve-point blocks and botulinium toxin into the muscle also have been used. These treatments are more invasive, can be painful, are of limited duration (3–6 months), and can result in loss of function for a short period of time. They also can be very effective in decreasing spasticity and improving the child's function.

Surgical treatment of spasticity comes from two different directions at this time. Orthopedic surgeons operate to correct skeletal deformities, release contractures, and rebalance muscles to improve function. Tendon lengthening, tendon releases, muscle transfers, and osteotomies are the primary procedures. Neurosurgeons operate to reduce spasticity and prevent bony deformities and functional losses.[5] Neurosurgical procedures include baclofen pumps that can dispense medication directly into the intrathecal sac to eliminate systemic side effects seen in oral medications and selective dorsal rhizotomies that provide a permanent reduction in tone.

The emergency physician may be called on to evaluate pain or loss of function and should be aware of these procedures and medications and their effects. Following injection procedures, there are occasionally muscle imbalances with muscle spasms and pain. Following injection procedures and surgery, there may be loss of function in the affected extremities, and with botulinum toxin, there have been rare cases of systemic effects of short duration (personal observation). The baclofen pump, which has an 18-mL drug reservoir, can be palpated as a circular metal disk in the abdominal wall. In the event of pump failure, there could be a drug overdose. Symptoms of baclofen overdose include drowsiness, light-headedness, dizziness, somnolence, respiratory depression, seizures, rostral progression of hypotonia, and loss of consciousness progressing to coma. See Figs. 134-1 and 134-2 for management of baclofen overdose.

Contractures of the extremities are one of the most commonly perceived difficulties of children with cerebral palsy. When spasticity is not treated, major problems can develop at the hip, ankle, wrist, and hand. In a small number of cases, elbow, shoulder girdle, and knee deformities are of concern. Adductor contractures of the hips may interfere with perineal hygiene and sitting. Hip flexion contractures may interfere with standing and independent transfers. Hip subluxation and dislocation may interfere with ambulation and may result in chronic pain syndromes and arthritis when the child becomes an adult.[6,7] The routine treatment for the pain is the same as for degenerative arthritis. Bracing is used for management of contractures and should be closely evaluated when wounds are sustained in braced areas. Bracing will hold the joint in a different position, and areas of skin tension will change with bracing. Placement of sutures or dressings may be affected by the brace or the altered position of an extremity without a brace. Friction from the brace could impair wound healing, increase the chance of infection, and create new wounds due to the

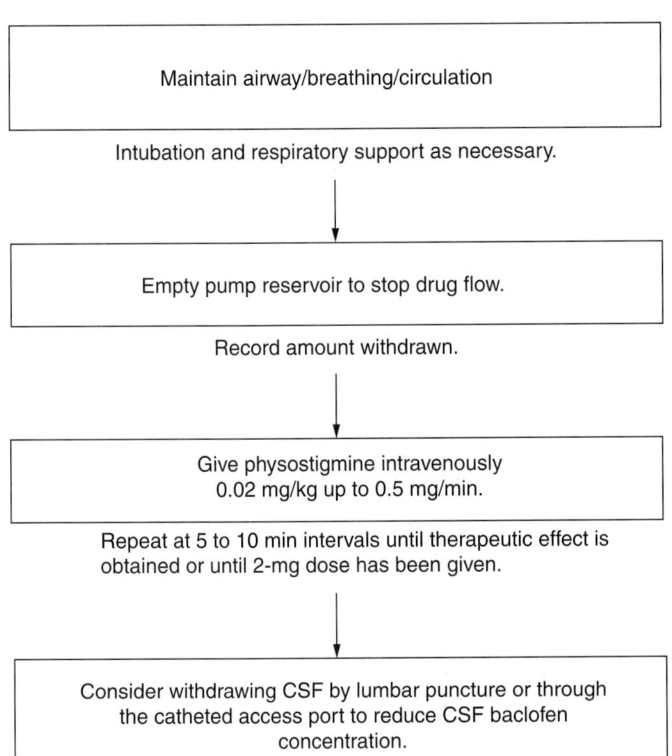

FIG. 134-1. Management of intrathecal baclofen overdose.

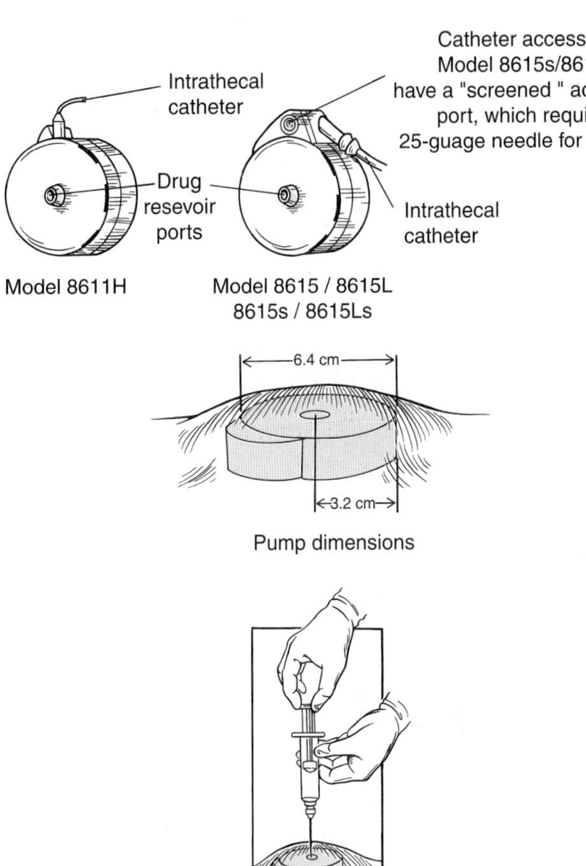

FIG. 134-2. Use of an infusion pump. (With permission of Medtronic Neurological.)

pressure of the brace if proper assessment and attention to the brace is not part of the management. Removal of a brace may be required in early wound management unless a tension problem will complicate management more. Similar problems may occur with serial casting procedures.

Fractures

Osteopenia frequently develops in bones secondary to disuse and nutritional issues.[8] Fractures occur more easily in osteopenic bones. Children with limited movement and osteopenia may sustain fractures without excessive force being used. Lifting or moving an older child may cause fractures when osteopenia is present. Stretching and range-of-motion exercises used to prevent the development of contractures also can result in fractures if the person doing them is unaware of osteopenia and uses an aggressive stance for therapy. Fractures may present with discomfort and swelling of an extremity and should be considered in the irritable, severely impaired child. Fractures may be treated with casting if the child has and uses voluntary movement, but soft wraps may be used in the child with significantly limited voluntary movement. Displaced fractures are uncommon, and, when present, forceful activity is generally involved. Routine handling and therapy generally are not associated with this type of injury. Consultation with an orthopedic surgeon and hospitalization may be required.

Scoliosis

Scoliosis is present in children with quadriplegia and may contribute to respiratory tract problems due to restrictive phenomena. Skin problems also may develop under braces, requiring modification of the brace. Referral for orthopedic management may be required to evaluate the brace, particularly if it is new or very old.

MENINGOMYELOCELE (MYELOMENINGOCELE)

Meningomyelocele is the most common congenital defect of the neural tube. The spinal cord, meninges, and vertebral column are involved due to failure of the neural tube to fuse in early embryogenesis. It causes varying amounts of sensory and motor impairment based on the level of the lesion and accompanying medical problems. Incidence is 0.7 per 1000 live births in the United States. Etiology is considered to be multifactorial, although folic acid deficiency has been associated. Folic acid is currently recommended as a supplement as early as possible during pregnancy. Other neural tube defects are anencephaly, encephalocele, lipomeningocele, spina bifida occulta, sacral agenesis, and meningocele.

Children with meningomyelocele have multiple, complex medical problems due to impairment of nerves at or below the site of the lesion. There is variable impairment of sensory and motor nerves controlling voluntary and autonomic functioning. Associated medical concerns include neurogenic bowel and bladder function, contractures, scoliosis, club feet, hydrocephalus, Chiari II malformation, tethering of the spinal cord, spinal cord syrinx, vesicoureteral reflux, decubitus ulcers, constipation, encopresis, recurrent urinary tract infections, growth failure, latex allergy, gastroesophageal reflux, apnea/stridor syndrome, seizures, partial agenesis of the corpus callosum, strabismus, visual acuity impairment, precocious puberty, and osteoporosis. Individuals also may have cognitive impairments. Mild forms of cognitive impairment may affect visual motor functioning. More severe cognitive impairment has been associated with sparing of verbal skills and a ''cocktail party'' syndrome, in which the children may be able to carry on superficial social conversations with ease but be unable to comprehend and use specific information provided to them or respond to specific questions.

Hydrocephalus

Hydrocephalus is present in 70 to 90 percent of children with thoracic or lumbar level defects and in substantial numbers of those with sacral level defects. It is routinely treated with shunt placement early in life. Concerns regarding shunt function are common in patients presenting to the acute care setting. Signs and symptoms of shunt malfunction are lethargy, irritability, nausea, vomiting, visual problems, cognitive changes, neck pain, headache, swelling along the shunt path, or seizure.[9,10] Not all symptoms need be present to indicate malfunction of the shunt. The symptomatology is nonspecific and can easily be due to a variety of other problems such as sepsis, urinary tract infection, otitis media, gastroenteritis, sinus infection, or viral syndromes. A number of children with massive constipation and a shunt may complain of similar symptomatology, which resolves when the fecal backup is relieved. Evaluation for shunt malfunction should proceed only after infectious and other causes have been eliminated. Preliminary studies for a malfunctioning shunt include a shunt survey (radiographs of the skull, chest, and abdomen) to evaluate connections and the shunt position and head CT to assess ventricular size and position of the proximal end in the ventricle. If questions remain, a shunt tap should be used to evaluate opening pressures and assess for infection. If inconclusive, a shunt clearance study with dye or radioisotope may provide additional information regarding flow through the system. Shunt taps should be done by neurosurgical staff when they are available, unless respiratory or cardiac compromise appears to be life-threatening.

Urinary Tract Problems

Urinary tract problems were at one time a primary cause of morbidity and mortality in children with meningomyelocele. Neurogenic bladder with chronic retention from dyssynergia, overflow incontinence, dribbling incontinence from an open bladder neck, vesicoureteral reflux, renal calculi, and urinary tract infections are common problems in this population. Children may be on prophylactic antibiotics, oxybutynin, or imipramine in an attempt to eliminate infections, minimize upper tract damage, and assist in the development of urinary continence. The side effects of the latter two are given in Table 134-3. Urinary tract colonization has been described in 60 to 70 percent of this population, and in the absence of vesicoureteral reflux, treatment is reserved for those with symptomatic urinary tract infection. Use of nitrofurantoin, trimethoprim-sulfamethoxazole, or amoxicillin is advised until culture results are available to minimize development of resistant strains of bacteria. Prior to treating an infection, it is important to know what antibiotics are currently in use. If broad-spectrum antibiotics have been used recently, there is an increased potential for a monilial infection.

TABLE 134-3 Medications Commonly Used in Meningomyelocele

Generic Name (Brand Name)	Most Common Side Effects
Oxybutynin (Ditropan) Propantheline (Pro-Banthine)	Dry mouth, blurred vision, gastrointestinal intolerance, fever, flushing
Imipramine (Janimine, Tofranil)	Nervousness, sleep disorders, tiredness, mild GI disturbances, constipation, seizures, anxiety, syncope

Clean intermittent catheterization is used to increase continence and manage urinary retention. When used with good technique, it does not increase the incidence of urinary tract infection. On rare occasions, false channels are formed with catheterization. When this occurs, special catheters such as coudé (curved-tip) catheters may be used to facilitate catheterization and minimize the chance of further trauma. It is wise to question the family regarding catheterization, catheter size, and special types of catheters that may be used. Use of indwelling catheters with balloons is not recommended due to problems with latex allergies (see below).

Intractable incontinence may be present due to severe bladder neck or sphincter deficiency and/or a noncompliant, high-pressure, low-capacity bladder. Reconstructive surgery such as bladder augmentation, bladder neck sling, artificial urinary sphincter, or collagen injections to the bladder neck may be required to provide continence and an adequate bladder capacity. Bladder augmentation has been used widely to increase the bladder capacity of some children with small hyperreflexic bladders. Any individual with a bladder augmentation who presents with abdominal pain should be evaluated for rupture of the bladder. Symptoms of bladder rupture include abdominal pain (which may radiate to the shoulder), abdominal distention, and shock. This is a life-threatening event requiring vascular support, antibiotic prophylaxis, and immediate operation. If this is suspected, the urologist should be contacted immediately.

A small number of children may develop renal calculi. If a small stone is being passed, symptomatic treatment for severe pain is required. Larger stones and asymptomatic stones should be noted, and follow-up with the child's urologist is recommended.

Chiari II Malformation

Chiari II malformation is present in the majority of children with meningomyelocele. Chiari II malformation consists of malformation of the cerebellum, hindbrain, and brainstem. Aqueductal stenosis is commonly associated. Symptomatic Chiari malformation is characterized by apnea, vocal cord paralysis, stridor, oral motor dysfunction, visual dysfunction, and upper limb weakness and incoordination in the infant. In older children it presents with visual dysfunction, motor incoordination, headache, and hand weakness.[11] Even mild cervical hyperflexion-extension injuries may result in symptoms. Of greatest concern is the young child or infant who presents to the ED with stridor and meningomyelocele. Suspicion of a Chiari malformation should be present, and evaluation should be ordered on an expedited basis. Stridor may be associated with vocal cord paralysis and may proceed to complete airway obstruction in a small number of patients. Evaluation is by MRI of the craniocervical junction. For children with severe respiratory compromise, immediate hospitalization is required. If respiratory tract function is not severely impaired and the process is static by history, a case-by-case decision should be made regarding hospitalization based on availability of prompt outpatient services from neurosurgery, otorhinolaryngology, and radiology for MRI. When significant respiratory compromise is associated with Chiari II malformation, tracheostomy may be required. Tracheostomy should be reserved for patients in whom intubation is not possible.[12]

Individuals with myelomeningocele and Chiari II malformation may have instability of the craniocervical junction. If the Chiari malformation has been symptomatic, it may have been treated with decompression surgery. The surgery may involve removal of a posterior segment of the cranium at the foramen magnun and/or laminectomy of the cervical vertebrae. Fusion of the cervical vertebrae may be done to improve cervical stability. If the child is in a motor vehicle accident, there should be a high index of suspicion for upper cervical spine injury. Routine precautions should be instituted, and complete evaluation, including flexion and extension films of the neck, should be done if indicated.

Spinal Cord Tethering

Tethering of the spinal cord can occur as the child grows. Tethering may present as ataxia, rapid progression of scoliosis, loss of functional motor level, a change in urinary continence (new-onset incontinence in a child who had previously been dry on a bladder program), or new-onset orthopedic deformities of the lower extremities. For the child who presents with increasing urinary incontinence with no evidence of an acute urinary tract infection, a neurosurgical consult should be considered. This is generally not an emergency, although it should be evaluated promptly in an office setting.

Skin Problems

Burns and pressure sores are seen in insensate areas with increased frequency. Burns occur and can be quite severe due to a lack of protective response triggered by pain. Pressure sores are frequent due to a lack of sensation. Common areas for pressure sores are under braces and in the sacral and ischial regions. Caution should be used in evaluation of pressure sores because healthy-appearing tissue may overlie abscesses or infected tracts extending proximally toward bony structures deep to them. When infections track deep, osteomyelitis may develop, requiring hospitalization, surgical debridement, long-term intravenous antibiotic therapy, and management of the skin surface.

Open areas should be evaluated carefully for evidence of tracts. Other wounds proximate to a pressure ulcer should be documented carefully with a suspicion that they may be connected by tracts. Evaluation should include probing for tracts, looking for undermined areas, obtaining radiographs to assess bony changes of osteomyelitis, and an erythrocyte sedimentation rate (ESR) or C-reactive protein determination. If cellulitis or bone changes are identified, consider admission for institution of intravenous antibiotics and a complete evaluation of bone involvement. Simple pressure ulcers without evidence of infection or extension can be treated successfully with local measures and pressure relief. Superficial wounds can be treated with sulfadiazine or duoderm wafers. Deeper wounds require wet-to-dry or gel dressings. Sulfadiazine, wet-to-dry dressings, and gel dressings are changed two to four times daily. Duoderm wafers are left in place for up to 3 days at a time if they remain dry and intact. Ulcers below braces require discontinuation of the bracing for 3 to 6 weeks to allow healing to occur. Ulcers on the buttocks require staying in a prone or supine position, with all pressure off the wound.

Additionally, the physician should check to ensure that a pressure-relief system is intact and functioning to prevent future skin breakdown. For wheelchair users, cushions to relieve pressure are advised. Air-filled ROHO cushions, gel cushions, and foam cushions are available and used extensively for this purpose. Children are also instructed in wheelchair push-ups to change their position in the chair. Watches with alarms that can be set to go off every 15 to 20 min are advised to remind the individual to do a push-up.

Bowel Problems

Neurogenic bowel is often seen, with resulting fecal incontinence, encopresis, or constipation. Many children are on a routine bowel management program in an attempt to achieve fecal continence. Bowel problems may present in the ED in a number of atypical ways. Children with shunted hydrocephalus often present with complaints of headache or shunt malfunction. This may be due to significant intraabdominal pressure from fecal retention, which may be transmitted via the shunt to the head. Abdominal discomfort also may be a presenting complaint, but frequently the child and family will deny any bowel problems or constipation. Even in children with daily stools, severe fecal stasis may develop due to impaired peristalsis. The child who presents with intermittent diarrhea also may have fecal stasis and buildup with overflow incontinence.

Bowel management techniques in the home include dietary manipulations, Karo syrup in feeds, Senokot, Dulcolax, glycerin suppositories, or a variety of enemas. Due to the chronic nature of this difficulty, mineral oil and Fleets enemas are not used routinely. This is to minimize the chance of families repeatedly using preparations that may cause vitamin deficiency or metabolic disturbances with frequent, ongoing use.

When constipation or fecal stasis is a consideration, a flat plate of the abdomen is helpful in clarifying the problem. Constipation of significant proportion can be handled by a high enema, suppository, or manual disimpaction. High enema is often the most effective. Difficulties may be encountered due to poor rectal tone and the inability of the child to retain an enema or suppository voluntarily. Families who routinely use enemas may have adapters to assist in the retention of an enema. When constipation or fecal stasis is the problem, there is generally no need for hospitalization. Following an initial clean-out procedure in the emergency department, the child can be discharged. Follow-up with the general pediatrician, a comprehensive spina bifida program with specialists knowledgeable about bowel management, or an enterostomal therapist to arrange an ongoing bowel management program is advised.

Sexual Abuse

Sexual abuse questions may come up on occasion in children with meningomyelocele. Care must be taken in the assessment because rectal tone is often impaired, and a patulous anus may result. Rectal tears and prolapse also may be present in the child with constipation.

Latex Allergy

Latex allergy is a concern in children and adults with meningomyelocele. It occurs in 24 to 67 percent of children with meningomyelocele. Increasingly severe allergic-type reactions are being reported related to latex and latex-containing products. Reactions vary from mild local reactions to anaphylaxis. Children may present with local or generalized swelling, hives or edema, itching, or a rash. Runny nose or eyes, coughing, sneezing, wheezing, stridor, and difficulty swallowing or breathing also may be presenting complaints.[13–15] A history of latex allergy or sensitivity should be obtained in all children with meningomyelocele prior to any examination or procedure in which latex gloves or other latex-containing supplies may be used. Many routine medical supplies contain latex, including frequently used supplies on the crash cart. (See Table 134-4 for a list of latex-containing supplies.) Many programs are recommending that identification bands be worn by children with meningomyelocele and latex allergy. If a severe allergic reaction is observed, the child should be discharged with an Epi-Pen, and formal testing for latex sensitivity should be done in the private physician's office. All surgeons providing care and the local anesthesiologist should be notified. This can be done by notifying the local physician or clinic responsible for the child's specialty care.

Fractures

Fractures occur with increased frequency when the child has osteopenia. Children with fractures to the lower extremity should be evaluated for level of sensation. If the child is insensate and paraplegic, casting may not be required. Soft wrapping of the extremity and elevation are the preferred mode of treatment.[16]

Respiratory Tract Problems

Respiratory tract problems generally are not associated with meningomyelocele other than vocal cord paralysis with Chiari II malformations or with the child with severe allergy to latex. Rarely, fibrotic changes in the lung have been associated with oxybutynin use. If chronic respiratory difficulties are present in a child on oxybutynin, discontinuation of the drug should be considered along with acute management.

SPINAL CORD INJURY

Pediatric spinal cord injury is an acute traumatic lesion of the spinal cord and roots resulting in motor and/or sensory deficit occurring between birth and adolescence. About 1100 new pediatric cases occur each year secondary to motor vehicle accidents, sporting accidents, falls, gunshot wounds, and birth trauma.

Spinal cord injury may result in complete or partial loss of neurologic function below the level of the lesion. Pain, heterotopic bone ossification, hypercalcemia, renal calculi, and depression are frequent issues for all children with spinal cord injury.[17] Other associated medical problems are similar to those encountered by children with meningomyelocele. Neurogenic bowel and bladder, decubitus ulcers, spasticity or hypotonicity, gastroesophageal reflux, esophagitis, aspiration, impaired sensation, ureterovesical reflux, scoliosis, contractures, and osteoporosis are common. For children with cervical or thoracic level lesions, respiratory compromise due to impaired phrenic nerves and/or abnormal innervation of abdominal musculature may be present. Autonomic dysreflexia and oral motor dysfunction also may be present. Since many of the issues are well covered in the section on meningomyelocele, this section will cover only the issues specific to spinal cord injuries.

Autonomic Dysreflexia

Autonomic dysreflexia is dramatic paroxysmal hyperactivity of uninhibited sympathetic and parasympathetic nerves in children with spinal cord lesions proximal to thoracic level 6. It is caused by stimulation below the level of the lesion by bladder overdistention, fecal impaction, skin breakdown, or fractures. Presentation is sweating, flushing, pounding headache, hypertension, bradycardia, and piloerection above the level of the lesion. Death or cerebral vascular accident may result.[17]

Dysreflexia is managed by eliminating the stimulus. Moving the child to a sitting position to take advantage of orthostatic hypotension, discontinuation of procedures in progress, emptying the bladder, disimpaction of the bowel, and normalizing body temperature should be used as required. When disimpaction is required, an anesthetic gel or ointment should be used to minimize afferent stimulation. If positional changes and elimination of the stimulus do not suffice, treatment may require sublingual nifedipine or IM or IV hydralazine. Nitropaste in a 1-in patch also may be applied, if available, for emergency reduction of hypertension. It should be removed immediately when blood pressure returns to normal.

Pain

Chronic pain described as dysesthesia or paresthesia is common in adolescents with spinal cord injury but infrequent in younger children. Pain generally is managed with analgesic agents. Long-term use of narcotic analgesics is avoided. Heat, relaxation therapy, and hypnosis also have been useful adjuncts. Care must be taken in the emergency room to avoid prescribing of medications that may be abused.

Heterotopic Bone Formation

Heterotopic bone formation may develop months after spinal cord injuries. It presents with heat, swelling, restricted motion, and pain. Commonly affected joints are the hip, knee, elbow, or shoulder. Ankylosis may develop and make routine activities impossible. This will need to be differentiated from fracture, infection, or other emergent conditions. Management is conservative, with analgesics for pain. Aspirin is sometimes used for prevention of recurrence. When heterotopic bone formation is present, the child and family should be prepared for problems with skin breakdown and secondary infection, which occur rarely.

Respiratory Dysfunction

Respiratory dysfunction is seen in some children with cervical-level lesions. Use of ventilators may be necessary either during the night or full time. Even in those with no need for early ventilator support, respiratory difficulty may develop due to increasing spasticity of abdominal muscles or muscular fatigue. When children present with respiratory difficulty, attention must be paid to pulmonary toilet, use of assistive devices, and the presence of previous respiratory difficulties or progression of respiratory difficulties. Impaired motor control may result in reflux and aspiration, which may contribute to the difficulties being experienced. Pulmonary consultation, if available, may allow the emergency physician to adjust the ventilator and prevent hospitalization. Children with phrenic nerve stimulators may need to be hospitalized for management.

Psychiatric and Psychological Problems

Psychiatric and psychological problems develop related to loss of independence and impairments of body image. Depression, severe uncontrolled anger, panic attacks, and temper tantrums can make care of these children difficult. Most difficulties of this type can be handled on an outpatient basis by a psychologist, social worker, or physician experienced in working with this population. For severe depression, suicidal ideation, or other emotional problems that are out of control, hospitalization and/or psychiatric evaluation may be needed.

DEVELOPMENTAL DISABILITY (MENTAL RETARDATION)

Mental retardation is a substantial limitation in present functioning associated with subaverage intellectual capabilities and limitations in

TABLE 134-4 Latex-Containing Supplies and Alternatives

Latex-Containing Supplies	Latex-Free Alternatives or Adaptations
Airways, masks and straps	Hudson, Vital Signs airways, masks
Ambu bag (black reusable)	Clear bags (Respironics, Laerdal)
Anesthesia bags, tubing	Neoprene bag
Band-aids	Sterile dressing with plastic tape
Blood pressure cuff	Use over clothing or stockinette, Clean Cuff (Vital Signs)
Bulb syringe	
Catheters, condom	Silicone (Mentor, Coloplast)
Catheters, indwelling Foley— even silicone may have a latex balloon	Silicone (Kendall, Argyle, Bard)
Catheter leg bags straps	Velcro, nylon (Mentor, Dale)
Catheters, straight	Mentor, Bard, Coloplast, MMG
Catheters, urodynamics	Bard, Rush, Cook
Catheters, rectal pressure	Cover latex balloons, use vinyl glove
Condoms, diaphragms	Polyurethane, tachylon Natural skin over/under latex condom
Crutches—axillary, hand pads	Cover with stockinette
Disposable diapers	Huggies, Pampers
Dressings—Moleskin (Johnson & Johnson), Coban (3M)	Tegaderm, Duoderm, Steri-strip, Reston foam liner, Comfeel, Xerofoam, PinCare, Bioclusive, Webrill
Elastic bandages, Ace wrap (brown), Esmarch	TEDS, Baxter elastic bandages, white cotton Ace wrap
Electrode pads	Baxter, Conmed EKG, Dantec EMG
Endotracheal tubes	Plastic tubes (Mallinckrodt, Sheridan, Portex)
Feeding nipples	Silicone (Gerber, Evenflo, MAM)
Foam rubber lining of braces	Line with cloth, felt
Gloves, sterile and exam, surgical and medical	Vinyl, neoprene, polymer gloves: Neolon, Senicare, Tru-touch, Tachylon, Tachyl, Dermaprene, Allergard
IV access: injection ports, Y-sites, PRN adapters, needleless systems	Use stopcock to inject medications; cover Y-sites and do not puncture; flush IV tubing before use; Abbott, Baxter, IVAC, Braun tubing; Braun, Clave needleless systems
IV bag ports, buretrols	Do not puncture ports to add medications; B. Braun burette
Jobst spandex products OR garb (masks, hats, shoe covers)	Jobst has a nonlatex material Remove elastic bands
Medication vials	Remove latex stoppers
Pacifiers	Plastic, silicone, and/or vinyl
Penrose drains	Jackson-Pratt, Zimmer Hemovac
Rubber bed pads (washable)	Disposable underpads
Stethoscope tubing	Cover tubing with stockinette
Suction catheters	Mallinckrodt, Yankauer, Davol
Syringes, disposable	Prepare medication in syringe right before use, or use glass syringes; Abboject, Abbott PCA vials
Tape, adhesive	Plastic, silk tape: Microfoam, Micropore, Transpore, Dermaclear, Dermicel, Waterproof
Tourniquet	Place over clothing or stockinette: VelcroPedic, Grafco tourniquets
Theraband strips and tubes (OT)	Cover with cloth
Wheelchair cushions, tires	Neoprene cushions (ROHO), cover seat with fabric, use leather gloves

TABLE 134-5 Medical Conditions Associated with Specific Mental Retardation Syndromes

Down syndrome	Atlantoaxial instability leading to spinal cord compression in the cervical region, congenital heart defects, atrioventricular canal defects, atrial septal defects, ventricular septal defects, tetralogy of Fallot, patent ductus arteriosus, pulmonary hypertension, duodenal atresia, tracheoesophageal fistula, Meckel diverticulum, Hirschsprung disease, imperforate anus, obesity, constipation, hypothyroidism, ureteropelvic junction obstruction, hydronephrosis, undescended testes, hypospadius, leukemia (acute lymphocytic and nonlymphocytic), chronic serous otitis media, chronic sinus infections, tear duct infections, questionable immunologic dysfunction (thyroiditis), alopecia areata, diabetes, rheumatoid-type arthropathy, autoimmune hemolytic anemia, nystagmus, alternating esotropia, congenital cataracts, glaucoma, keratoconus, blepharitis, conductive hearing loss, obstructive sleep apnea, dental malocclusions, short stature, hypotonia resolving with age, Tourette syndrome, Alzheimer disease
Fragile X syndrome	Mitral valve prolapse, seizures, strabismus, frequent ear infections, and self-abusive behaviors
Prader-Willi syndrome	Hyperphagia, obesity, hypoventilation, cor pulmonale, NIDDM, scoliosis, strabismus, inability to vomit, decreased sensitivity to pain, seizure disorder, acanthosis nigricans, hypoxia, right-sided heart failure, pulmonary hypertension, gastric perforation, obstructive sleep apnea
Williams syndrome	Supravalvular aortic stenosis, pulmonic stenosis, coarctation of the aorta, strabismus, joint contractures, hypertension, urethral stenosis, vesicoureteral reflux, constipation, ulcers, and hypercalcemia
Rett syndrome	Hyperventilation, breath-holding, air-swallowing, bruxism, ataxia, muscle wasting, poor circulation, scoliosis, seizures, and intermittent flushing

two or more adaptive skill areas (communication, self-care, home living, social skills, community use, self-direction, health and safety, functional academics, leisure, and work). It is a result of injury, disease, metabolic disorder, or other abnormality of the central nervous system occurring before the age of 18. Mental retardation occurs in 2.5 percent of the population. Etiology is known for certain syndromes associated with mental retardation, but the majority of individuals with mental retardation have no clearly identified etiology. Down syndrome, fetal alcohol syndrome, and fragile X syndrome are the most common known etiologies of mental retardation.

Dealing with the mentally retarded child in the ED is difficult because of the variety of medical problems that may be encountered and because the individual often is not able to clearly communicate the problem to the physician or the care provider. It is important to be aware that a child or care provider who cannot cooperate with questioning or physical examination may be mentally impaired.

Children with mental retardation have a wide variety of associated medical problems. With increasing severity of mental retardation, there is increased incidence of associated problems. Cerebral palsy, visual deficits, seizure disorders, failure to thrive, hypotonia, gastroesophageal reflux, aspiration, and psychiatric disorders have all been seen in the general population with mental retardation. Mental retardation associated with known syndromes may have diagnosis-specific medical problems such as in Down syndrome, the best known of these syndromes. Listings of diagnosis-specific medical problems can be found in Table 134-5.

Pulmonary Problems

Respiratory tract symptoms may be present in severely mentally impaired individuals. Chronic congestion, recurrent pneumonia, and wheezing may occur due to low tone and are similar to the problems seen in the individual with cerebral palsy. Mentally impaired individuals function at an earlier developmental age than the chronologic age. Severely impaired individuals may function at a preschool level and thus are at an increased risk of a foreign body aspiration like an average toddler.

Gastroesophageal Reflux

Gastroesophageal reflux is often present when tone is low. It may contribute to aspiration problems and can be associated with gastritis and esophagitis. Gastroesophageal reflux may present as emesis, nonspecific irritability, discomfort, or a lack of appetite and may contribute to failure to thrive. When the family complains about emesis, the physician needs to clarify their description; they may be seeing clearing of secretions from the upper airways. In the severely impaired child, ''emesis'' may be a stimulated gag and cough to clear secretions from the posterior pharynx. True emesis should contain stomach contents. If the child is tube fed, this will be formula. Often the parent will describe emesis that is composed of mucousy material instead of formula or food.

Evaluation for gastroesophageal reflux generally is not required on an emergent basis, but management information may be useful. Metoclopramide can be used to improve transit time through the stomach when delayed gastric emptying is found on scintigraphic studies of gastric functioning. Ranitidine and other new blocking agents have been used to decrease the acidity of the gastric contents when gastritis or esophagitis is identified. Thickened feedings, positioning, and other techniques have been used with some success but are of questionable assistance in older individuals. In some cases, Nissan fundoplication is required for management of moderate to severe reflux not responsive to medical management.

Children with cognitive impairments may have unusual behaviors such as pica. When indigestible materials are ingested on a routine basis, bezoars may develop consisting of hair, cloth, or other materials. This also may present like reflux due to outlet obstruction. A barium swallow should identify this problem. Surgical removal may be required on an emergent basis. This problem should be evaluated for admission on a case-by-case basis.

Seizures

Seizures are present in 30 percent of children with mental retardation. With increasing severity of mental retardation, there are often increasingly complex seizures. Problems associated with epilepsy are identical to those of children with cerebral palsy described earlier in the chapter. The physician should be alert to the possibility of multiple seizure types, use of multiple anticonvulsants, drug-drug interactions of anticonvulsant medications, and the possible fragility of seizure control. Contact with the managing neurologist is strongly advised in such cases.

Psychiatric and Behavioral Problems

Psychiatric and behavioral problems combined with limited understanding of what is happening to them and an unfamiliar, overstimulating situation often lead to an uncooperative and at times combative child. The prevalence of major psychiatric disorders and attention deficit disorder is two to three times that of the general population. Stereotypy and self-injurious behavior are seen almost exclusively in the mentally retarded population, with increased incidence in children with the most severe cognitive limitations. Treatment of psychiatric and behavioral disorders is similar to treatment of these disorders in the general population.

The most worrisome problem in the ED is self-injurious behaviors. Self-injurious behavior is chronic, repetitive acts that may result in serious medical consequences. Self-injurious behaviors may include head-banging, chewing, hitting, and picking at various body parts. Behavior management, protective strategies, and pharmacologic intervention have all been used with variable success. When dealing with injuries sustained secondary to self-injurious behavior, use protective strategies immediately. Referral to psychiatric, psychological, or developmental services for behavior management and possible pharmacologic intervention is advised. This may be done on an outpatient basis. For children with known problems who are currently being treated for psychiatric disorders or behavioral problems, the side effects of the medications may become an issue. See Table 134-6 for a list of pharmacologic agents and their side effects.

Down Syndrome

Congenital heart defects occur in 40 to 60 percent of children with Down syndrome. Atrioventricular canal defects, ventricular septal defects, atrial septal defects, tetralogy of Fallot, and patent ductus arteriosus are all reported in this population. Pulmonary hypertension may develop in these children, associated with chronic upper airway obstruction and left-to-right shunts. Congestive heart failure has been described even in children without known heart lesions. Mitral valve prolapse and aortic regurgitation are described in adults but not in children.

Gastrointestinal problems are common, including imperforate anus, pyloric stenosis, tracheoesophageal fistula, and Hirschsprung disease. Due to gastrointestinal malformations, hypotonia, and previous surgeries, partial bowel obstruction and constipation may present as problems in the emergency room.

Atlantoaxial instability and dislocation have been identified and are felt to be related to joint laxity. Spinal cord compression may develop, with neck pain, head tilt, torticollis, frequent staggering or falling, increased deep tendon reflexes, clonus, limb weakness, paresthesias, or hemi- or quadriplegia. Symptomatic children require immediate surgical stabilization.

Recurrent upper respiratory infections, chronic sinusitis, and chronic middle ear effusions are seen in many young children with Down syndrome. These can be treated using standard protocols but should be referred to an otorhinolaryngologist or pulmonologist when they occur repeatedly. Sleep apnea and obstructive apnea are described but are not generally problems in the emergency setting.

A variety of other medical problems may be seen on an emergent basis: hypothyroidism, thyroiditis, leukemia, and transient neonatal leukoproliferative disorder. Skin problems are seen including eczema, folliculitis, alopecia areata, and sun hypersensitivity.

TABLE 134-6 Medications Commonly Used in Mental Retardation

Generic Name (Brand Name)	Most Common Side Effects
Diazepam (Valium)	Drowsiness, ataxia, weakness, confusion, constipation, dysarthria, diplopia, rash, urinary retention
Desipramine (Norpramin, Pertofrane)	Drowsiness, incoordination, weight gain, constipation, blurred vision, dry mouth, insomnia, anxiety, confusion, nightmares, delusions, psychosis, blood dyscrasias
Fluphenazine (Permitil, Prolixin), haloperidol (Haldol), Methylphenidate (Ritalin), thioridazine (Mellaril)	Extrapyramidal movement disorders, neuroleptic malignant syndrome, drowsiness, restlessness, nausea, blurred vision, rash, dry mouth, polyuria, altered glucose regulation, weight gain or loss, anorexia, insomnia, rebound, headache, tics, agitation, rash, tachycardia, hypertension, weight loss, decreased growth rate, abdominal pain

Fragile X Syndrome

Fragile X syndrome is an X-linked condition consisting of mental retardation or learning disabilities, connective tissue disorders, and sensory integration dysfunction. It affects 1 in 1000 individuals and affects males more severely than females. There are few associated medical conditions, and generally they do not cause severe problems. Mitral valve prolapse, seizures, strabismus, frequent ear infections, allergies, self-abusive behaviors (particularly biting), and hyperextensible joints are reported in some children. The major difficulties that may be encountered may be related to autistic-like behaviors and self-abusive behaviors.

Prader-Willi Syndrome

Prader-Willi syndrome is a condition characterized by mental retardation, hypotonia, hypogonadism, and obesity. It is a sporadic multisystem disorder with an incidence of 1 in 10,000. It is due to a chromosomal deletion on the 15th chromosome. Presentation in infancy is of poor suck, hypotonia, developmental delay, and early failure to thrive. During childhood, the poor eating habits change to hyperphagia and obesity, which becomes a major problem for health and life. Consequences of obesity include somnolence, hypoventilation, cor pulmonale, and non-insulin-dependent diabetes mellitus. Associated problems are scoliosis, strabismus, and inability to vomit. Occasional problems may include decreased sensitivity to pain, seizure disorder, short stature, skin picking, easy bruisability, fractures from minor trauma, and acanthosis nigricans.

Obesity develops due to hyperphagia, inability to vomit, and decreased caloric requirements. Children become obsessed with food and eating. Abnormal behaviors are manifested with gorging, foraging for food, eating inedibles, and violent temper outbursts when eating is thwarted. Respiratory problems occur secondary to massive obesity. Pickwickian syndrome with hypoventilation, hypercapnia, hypoxia, and right-sided heart failure have been seen in older children. Impaired breathing leads to carbon dioxide retention, acidosis, constriction of the pulmonary arterioles, pulmonary hypertension, and the chance of pulmonary embolus. Non-insulin-dependent diabetes mellitus is seen in some patients related to their obesity. Most people with diabetes can be managed with oral hypoglycemics and/or weight loss. Insulin is rarely required, and response to insulin may be unpredictable. Early atherosclerosis and glomerulosclerosis may occur secondary to the diabetes.

The inability to vomit can be of concern in the ED. Hyperphagia may result in food foraging, consumption of nonfood materials, and toxic ingestions. In this patient population, ipecac should be avoided. Ipecac toxicity can result if the patient is unable to vomit. Gastric aspiration or other techniques should be used.

Respiratory insufficiency with hypoventilation is frequently not responsive to hypercapnia. Medroxyprogesterone acetate may be helpful as a respiratory stimulant in some cases. Gastric perforation as a consequence of overeating is seen in rare cases.

Williams Syndrome

Williams syndrome is a disorder of unknown etiology that presents with elfinlike facies, cardiovascular disease, infantile hypercalcemia, learning disabilities or mild to moderate mental retardation, and an outgoing personality. It appears to develop into a multisystem disease in adulthood.

Cardiovascular difficulties, endocrinologic abnormalities, urinary tract problems, gastrointestinal problems, and arthropathy are observed with increasing incidence over time. Supravalvular aortic stenosis is the most common cardiac problem. Pulmonic stenosis, coarctation of the aorta, strabismus, joint contractures, and hypertension are also reported. Hypercalcemia is seen in infants and recurs in adults. Calcium levels should be monitored. Children who present with polydypsia, polyuria, irritability, and constipation should be evaluated for hypercalcemia. Urethral stenosis, bladder diverticuli, vesicoureteral reflux, renal artery stenosis, constipation, ulcers, diverticulitis, and arthropathy are reported in adults with the syndrome.

Rett Syndrome

Rett syndrome is a form of mental retardation occurring only in females and characterized by normal early development followed by a loss of purposeful hand use, regression in social development, progressive ataxia or spasticity, and development of mental retardation.[18] Hand stereotypies and spontaneous noncommunicative vocalizations or laughter are typical of this syndrome. Incidence is 1 in 10,000 to 15,000 females. Hyperventilation, breathholding, air swallowing, bruxism, ataxia, muscle wasting, poor circulation in the lower extremities, frequent fractures, scoliosis, seizures, and intermittent flushing have been described in association with this syndrome.

These girls may present to the ED with a variety of symptoms, including fainting due to apnea or hyperventilation or with severe abdominal distension due to air swallowing. Apnea has been known to last 30 to 40 s and may involve cyanosis. Screaming attacks may occur in puberty. Children need to be assessed for possible pain due to an acute abdomen, dental pain, kidney stones, or other medical causes. If no source of medical concern is identified, the child may be suffering from a screaming attack.

Seizures are seen often in this population and may be generalized, partial, or mixed. Atypical infantile spasms also have been described. Seizures may be refractory to drug therapy, and individuals are at times prone to adverse reactions to their anticonvulsant medications. Some "seizures" actually may be nonepileptic paroxysmal events unresponsive to antiepileptic medications. Caution is advised in adjusting dosages. Consultation with the treating neurologist or specialist managing the child is strongly advised if seizure is the presenting problem.

REFERENCES

1. Orenstein SR, Orenstein DM: Gastroesophageal reflux and respiratory disease in children. *J Pediatr* 112(6):847, 1988.
2. delRosario JF, Orenstein SR: Evaluation and management of gastroesophageal reflux and pulmonary disease. *Curr Opin Pediatr* 8(3):209, 1996.
3. Blasco PA, Stansbury JC: Glycopyrrolate treatment of chronic drooling. *Arch Pediatr Adolesc Med* 150:932, 1996.
4. Becmeaur F, Horta-Geraud P, Brunot B, et al: Diversion of salivary flow to treat drooling in patients with cerebral palsy. *J Pediatr Surg* 31(12):1629, 1996.
5. Abbott R: The management of cerebral palsy: How can neurosurgery help? *Pediatr Ann* 26(10):591, 1997.
6. Bleck EE: *Orthopaedic Management in Cerebral Palsy.* London: MacKeith Press, 1987.
7. Cornell MS: The hip in cerebral palsy. *Dev Med Child Neurol* 37:3, 1995.
8. Henderson RC, Lin PP, Greene WB: Bone-mineral density in children and adolescents who have spastic cerebral palsy. *J Bone Joint Surg* 77A(11):1671, 1995.
9. Madkikians A, Conway EE Jr: Cerebrospinal fluid shunt problems in pediatric patients. *Pediatr Ann* 26(10):613, 1997.
10. Key CB, Rothrock SG, Falk JL: Cerebrospinal fluid shunt complications: An emergency medicine perspective. *Pediatr Emerg Care* 11(5):265, 1995.
11. Rauzzino M, Oakes WJ: Chiari II malformation and syringomyelia. *Neurosurg Clin North Am* 6(2):293, 1995.
12. Roger G, Dnoyelle F, Garabedian EN: Disorders of laryngeal mobility in children. *Pediatr Pulmonol Suppl* 16:105, 1997.
13. Weido AJ, Wim TC: The burgeoning problem of latex sensitivity. *Postgrad Med* 98(3):173, 1995.
14. Leger RR, Meeropol E: Children at risk: Latex allergy and spina bifida. *J Pediatr Nurs* 7(6):371, 1992.
15. Task Force on Allergic Reaction to Latex: American Academy of Allergy and Immunology: Committee report. *Allergy Clin Immunol* 92(1 pt 1):16, 1993.
16. Karol LA: Orthopedic management in myelomeningocele. *Neurosurg Clin North Am* 6(2):259, 1995.
17. Boyd J, Perrin J: Spinal cord injury, in Molnar G (ed): *Pediatric Rehabilitation,* 2d ed. Baltimore: WIlliams & Wilkins, 1992, pp. 334–362.
18. Hagberg B, Anvret M, Wahlström J (eds): Clinical criteria, stages and natural history, in *Rett Syndrome: Clinical and Biological Aspects.* London: MacKeith Press, 1993, pp 4–20.

135 UROGYNECOLOGIC PROBLEMS IN CHILDREN AND ADOLESCENTS

Richard A. Christoph

UROLOGIC PROBLEMS OF PREADOLESCENT AND ADOLESCENT BOYS

Disorders Involving the Foreskin

Differentiation of the genitalia occurs between the ninth and thirteenth gestational week. The prepuce of the glans penis, which forms the foreskin, is adherent to the underlying glans penis and remains so throughout gestation and during the first several years of postnatal life. The foreskin of the newborn and infant cannot easily be retracted. Doing so shears the attachments between the epithelial layers of the glans penis and the foreskin. This normal adherence of the foreskin of the infant and toddler to the underlying glans penis is referred to as physiologic phimosis and is a part of normal male child physical development and maturation. It can persist in some (3 to 6 percent) boys into the grade-school years, spontaneously resolving during early puberty in the vast majority of boys.

FORESKIN PEARLS Secretions and sloughed epithelial cells (smegma) from the surface of the glans penis accumulate under the foreskin and contribute to the gradual elevation and separation of the foreskin from the surface of the glans penis. The thin foreskin may reveal such accumulations of smegma, referred to as foreskin pearls. They ultimately will decompress at the terminus of the foreskin's attachment to the glans penis. If unassociated with evidence of cellulitis (erythema, warmth, induration, and tenderness), they do not represent an infectious complication and require no treatment beyond an explanation and reassurance for the concerned parent.

PHIMOSIS It is important to differentiate physiologic phimosis, as mentioned above, from pathologic phimosis. Phimosis is pathologic when a previously retractable foreskin is no longer retractable or when foreskin retraction is unachievable beyond puberty. Pathologic phimosis is rare in children. It may complicate circumcision or may result from repeated trauma, infections, or chemical irritation. It may be suspected if, during examination of the comfortably retracted foreskin, the foreskin appears rolled or thickened, rather than thin and effaced as the foreskin is pushed gently toward the base of the penis.

Pathologic phimosis associated with obstruction of urinary stream, recurrent urinary tract infections, or recurrent bouts of balanoposthitis represents an indication for referral to a urologist or pediatric surgeon for elective circumcision. Nonsurgical management of pathologic phimosis has been proposed. Case reports and case series reports of balloon dilatation and topical steroids suggest a limited role for these approaches.

PARAPHIMOSIS Regardless of the reasons for foreskin retraction, timely replacement of the foreskin ring distal to the glans penis is necessary. Failure to do so will result in the formation of painful edema in the foreskin and glans penis secondary to venous congestion caused by the constriction by the preputial ring. Ultimately, vascular insufficiency may threaten the viability of the glans penis and foreskin. This condition, known as paraphimosis, is an emergent urologic condition.

Differential diagnostic considerations include penile infections (balanoposthitis), idiopathic penile edema (insect bites, contact dermatitis, etc.), and, more important, a circumferentially constricting foreign body (hair, clothing, rubber band, etc.). Among the most pressing duties of the examining physician is the identification and removal of any constricting foreign body. The profound edema of the glans penis and the foreskin may make this task exceedingly difficult.

Management rests largely with the control of swelling and of pain, using systemic analgesia, dorsal penile nerve block, or both. Control of edema may be achieved by application of cool, compressive (1-in Surgical Cling) dressings, starting at the distal penis and wrapping proximally. Alternatively, the glans penis may be cooled with ice water-filled latex examination gloves. Reexamination of the penis for the presence of a constricting foreign body should then be performed.

Once the diagnosis of paraphimosis has been confirmed, it is reduced using a variety of techniques. The most commonly successful reduction technique involves the simultaneous distal traction of the foreskin using the index and third fingers of each hand while the thumbs push the swollen glans penis back through the paraphimotic ring of the foreskin. The use of a gauze sponge between the third and index fingers of each hand and the foreskin aids considerably in traction on the foreskin. If this technique is unsuccessful, a surgical release of the edematous foreskin is indicated, ideally in conjunction with urologic consultation. Either a single puncture of the foreskin using a 21-gauge needle or (more definitively) a dorsal slit of the edematous foreskin ring should restore vascular supply to the glans penis.

Discharge from the emergency department is appropriate following demonstration of spontaneous voiding of the bladder. Outpatient consultation with a urologist or a pediatric surgeon is appropriate and should be coordinated through the child's primary care physician.

BALANOPOSTHITIS Balanitis is an inflammation of the glans penis. Balanoposthitis is an inflammatory process that also involves the foreskin. The cause of balanoposthitis in preadolescent boys is usually infection but may occasionally be trauma, including chronic friction, zipper injuries, and contact dermatitis, or a fixed drug eruption (tetracycline or clotrimazole). Even rarer are plasma-cell balanitis and balanitis xerotica obliterans. As many as 3 percent of boys experience balanoposthitis, the vast majority of whom are uncircumcised.

The microbiology of infectious balanoposthitis reveals an abundance of gram-positive and gram-negative organisms. Most infections of the foreskin and glans penis represent invasion by normal flora and are usually polymicrobial. Contributing factors to the development of these infections (e.g., poor hygiene) are unproved and controversial. *Candida albicans* may be the pathogen in prepubertal children, and recurrences of balanoposthitis due to this organism should alert the physician to the possibility of immunocompromise, such as occurs with diabetes mellitus. Group A β-hemolytic streptococcus has been reported as an infectious organism, and its identification (via rapid antigen detection of associated thin, purulent discharge) warrants aggressive and specific antistreptococcal therapy. Sexually transmitted organisms are responsible for many cases of balanoposthitis in older adolescents.

Physical examination of a child with balanoposthitis reveals redness (100 percent), swelling (91 percent), discharge (up to 73 percent in one series but usually far less common), and soreness. Systemic fever and constitutional symptoms are atypical. Any urethral discharge is swabbed for detection of streptococcal antigen, and rapid antigen assays that test negative are cultured. If the rapid streptococcal antigen test result is negative, a smear of the discharge is examined using Gram stain. The presence of polymorphonuclear leukocytes on Gram stain of a urethral smear of a prepubertal boy whose rapid test for *Streptococcus pyogenes* is negative should alert the physician to the possibility of a sexually transmitted infection. The emergency physician should be cognizant of the forensic diagnostic criteria for documentation of infections due to *Neisseria gonorrhoeae* and *Chlamydia trachomatis* in his or her community and should select the appropriate culture methods, DNA probes, or other rapid diagnostic tests accordingly.

Management of the more common nonspecific balanoposthitis involves local hygiene measures, including sitz baths and gentle cleaning of the foreskin sulcus and glans penis. The soothing effect of a warm-water sitz bath also facilitates voiding in many children with voluntary urinary retention due to dysuria from a variety of causes. Some clinicians recommend the application of 0.5% hydrocortisone cream to the affected parts. Antimicrobial topical ointments that do not contain neomycin have been traditionally recommended, but their utility is unproved. Occasionally, 5 to 7 days of amoxicillin or a first-generation cephalosporin may be useful in recalcitrant cases or in cases associated with more advanced cellulitis. Circumcision is considered in cases of recurrent balanoposthitis.

Circumcision Complications

MEATAL STENOSIS Stenosis of the urethral meatus is fairly common. It represents a condition most likely acquired as a result of prolonged exposure of the meatus to moisture from wet diapers. The inflammation from an episode of ammoniacal (diaper) dermatitis causes the tender meatal edges to slough their epithelial surfaces. The urethral meatus becomes adherent to the side-to-side fashion, starting ventrally and progressing dorsally, resulting in a pinpoint meatus at the apex of the glans penis. Meatal stenosis is quite rare in uncircumcised boys.

The clinical presentation of a child with meatal stenosis is typical. It usually comes to the attention of the family of a boy only after the age of toilet training. The family relates that the boy's urine stream is notably difficult to control. There exists a characteristic dorsal deflection of the urinary stream, and the boy may complain of intermittent dysuria, blood spotting on his underwear due to meatal inflammation, and occasionally urinary frequency or a sense of voiding urgency due to residual urethral urine following voiding. Prolonged voiding times are not unusual, and some boys condition themselves to sit while voiding in their efforts to cope with these symptoms.

Management of a symptomatic boy with urethral stenosis usually involves urethral meatotomy, an office procedure in the hands of most pediatric urologists. Subsequently, a regimen designed to maintain separation of the recently divided urethral meatus edges is necessary for up to 6 weeks in order to prevent restenosis.

POSTCIRCUMCISION PHIMOSIS Improper seating of a circumcision bell clamp at the time of foreskin removal may result in excess residual foreskin following the procedure. Since the circumcision site is circumferential in nature, the inevitable contraction of the scar may yield a progressive narrowing of the foreskin orifice. At some point, the narrowed foreskin orifice slides distally over the glans penis, entrapping it. Further contraction of the circumcision scar may result in such a degree of phimosis that urine flow is obstructed. This phenomenon is more common in boys with prominent peripenile fat pads, particularly in boys with a retracted-appearing penis.

Diagnosis rests with the identification of a tight phimotic ring in a boy who has prevously undergone circumcision. Occasionally, early detection of progressive narrowing of the foreskin orifice may afford an opportunity for stretching the foreskin orifice either through aggressive foreskin retraction or the use of a hemostat. More commonly, the child requires a circumcision revision.

SURGICAL PENILE GLANS ADHESIONS Contact of a postcircumcision scar with the recently denuded glans penis may result in a very thick adhesion between the epithelial surface of the glans penis and the circumcision scar. These adhesions cannot be separated by blunt dissection, requiring surgical separation instead. They are prevented by repeated application of antimicrobial ointment to the glans penis for 7 to 10 days following circumcision.

Disorders of the Penile Shaft

HYPOSPADIAS The incidence of hypospadias approximates 1 in 300 live male births in the United States. If the most minor degrees of hypospadias are included in incidence studies, the rate climbs to as high as 1 in 125 live male births. The condition is more common in white boys than in black boys and internationally is most common in Italians and in those of Jewish ancestry. Hypospadias exhibits a polygenic inheritance pattern.

Hypospadias is a congenital defect characterized by an incomplete development of the anterior urethra. The urethral meatus may be located anywhere along the ventral shaft of the penis or may open to the scrotum or perineum. More proximal locations of the urethral meatus are associated with a greater likelihood of ventral shortening and curvature of the penis during erection (i.e., chordee). Hypospadias occurs as a result of varying defects of the urethra, corpus spongiosum, and corpus cavernosa. The ventral skin of the penis is usually thin, and the foreskin is insufficient on its ventral surface.

Several classification systems have been proposed for hypospadias, the most useful of which relate the location of the urethral meatus after any associated ventral curvature has been released. Such a classification system allows boys with hypospadias to be grouped into three categories:

1. *Anterior hypospadias* (50 percent of cases) refers to a urethral meatus position on the inferior surface of the glans penis, on the ventral corona or subcoronal furrow, or somewhere along the distal third of the ventral shaft.
2. *Middle hypospadias* (20 percent of cases) refers to a urethral meatus position along the middle third of the ventral shaft.
3. *Posterior hypospadias* (30 percent of cases) refers to a urethral meatus position along the posterior third of the ventral shaft, at the base of the shaft in front of the scrotum, on the scrotum between the genital swellings, or behind the scrotum or genital swellings.

Hypospadias and chordee are associated with several other anomalies. Undescended testes and inguinal hernia are the most common associated anomalies, ranging from a 9 percent incidence with anterior and middle hypospadias to a 17 percent incidence with posterior hypospadias. A utricle masculinus (a membranous urethral sac) is more frequently associated with more severe and posterior forms of hypospadias. Abnormalities of the higher urinary tract are infrequent in boys with hypospadias, and routine evaluation of the urinary tract is not recommended in boys solely because of the presence of hypospadias.

The treatment of hypospadias and chordee is designed to provide a straight penis with a urethral meatus as close as possible to the glanular tip so as to afford a directionally forward urinary stream and normal coitus. A boy whose urethral meatus is located very anteriorly on the ventral surface of the glans penis and who does not manifest ventral penile curvature probably will be capable of directionally forward urine stream and probably does not require urologic consultation. The identification of any more significant degree of hypospadias suggests an indication for urologic consultation in cooperation with the child's primary care physician. Experienced pediatric urologists can perform a variety of single-staged and multistaged operative procedures to accomplish the goals of treatment outlined above.

PRIAPISM Priapism is a persistent and usually painful engorgement of the paired dorsal corpora cavernosa, resulting in a dorsal penile erection, while the glans penis and the ventral surface remain flaccid. The resultant erection is not necessarily associated with sexual stimulation or desire, and it is not relieved by ejaculation.

In children, the disorder most commonly has a hematologic basis. Sickle cell hemoglobinopathies account for about two-thirds of cases in children. Priapism affects 2 to 6 percent of prepubertal children with sickle cell disease, and the frequency increases upon completion of puberty to as high as 40 percent of adult patients with sickle cell disease. Leukemia is the underlying hematologic disorder in about 11 percent of children with priapism. Other causes include blunt trauma, anticoagulation therapy, diabetes mellitus, and idiopathic causes.

The etiology of the painful engorgement of the corpora cavernosa elements in priapism is thought to center on the autonomic control of blood flow *out of* the emissary venous system of the penis versus the rate of blood flow *into* the arterioles and sinusoids of the corpora cavernosa. The flow of blood into the arterioles and sinusoids of the corporal elements may be characterized as either high flow or low flow, reflected in ^{99m}Tc penile scan flow studies. The mechanism of high-flow priapism was initially described as a consequence of blunt trauma, whereas the priapism associated with sickle cell disease in adults is usually referred to as low-flow, or ischemic, priapism. Some children with sickle cell-mediated priapism have been identified with high-flow ^{99m}Tc penile scans, giving rise to optimism that the penile scans would prove useful in predicting impotence risks. However, the ^{99m}Tc penile scan data on children with sickle cell priapism remain inconclusive in predicting long-term sequelae.

Priapism differs from a normal penile erection in that the glans penis and the ventral surface of the penis remain flaccid. Its onset is most frequently at night or in early morning. While the priapism of sickle cell anemia may represent an isolated finding, associated complications of sickle cell disease, including sequestration, aplastic crisis, infection, and vasoocclusive crisis, should be investigated. The most frequently encountered acute complication is acute urinary retention, which may represent a voluntary effort to avoid pain or may be mechanical in nature. The long-term complication is impotence. Factors contributing to the development of impotence are variable among patients: multiple episodes, prolonged duration, and onset of priapism in older patients have all been associated with development of impotence.

The diagnosis of priapism is strictly clinical. Laboratory data serve to illustrate comorbid conditions or metabolic status. Differential diagnostic considerations include phimosis with erection and paraphimosis, each distinguished from priapism by engorgement of the glans penis. Peyronie's disease results in tissue fibrosis that yields plaques, which may create a painful erection of the penis. A history of anticoagulant use usually indicates anticoagulant-induced priapism. Cervical or thoracic spinal cord lesions may produce an erection due to sympathectomy, but the erection will involve the corpora cavernosa as well as the glans penis and ventral portion of the penis. The use of ^{99m}Tc penile scans is currently limited to research.

Management of priapism centers on pain relief, adequate hydration, and monitoring for urinary retention. All children with priapism are admitted to the hospital. A child whose priapism is associated with an underlying hematologic disorder receives a hematologic-oncologic consultation. The aggressiveness of fluid administration, the indications for and administration of blood transfusions, and the timing of surgical consultation are all matters of debate.

Scrotal Swelling and Scrotal Masses of Childhood

This section reviews diagnostic entities and management specific to prepubertal boys. In particular, painless scrotal masses and swelling are reviewed. The most common causes of painless *cystic* scrotal masses in prepubertal boys are inguinal hernias, hydroceles, varicoceles, and spermatoceles. Less frequently encountered entities include various painless *solid* scrotal masses, such as acute idiopathic scrotal edema, testicular tumors, and soft-tissue tumors of the spermatic cord.

PAINLESS CYSTIC SCROTAL MASSES **Inguinal Hernias and Hydroceles** Inguinal hernias and hydroceles, caused by incomplete or abnormal obliteration of the processus vaginalis, are the most common cause of inguinal and scrotal masses in childhood. The incidence of pediatric inguinal hernias is 10 to 20 per 1000 live births and is much higher in premature and low-birth-weight infants. Inguinal hernias are more common on the right side (60 percent) than on the left (30 percent), and 10 percent are bilateral. They are more common in boys (male-to-female ratio, 4:1). In addition to prematurity and low birth weight, many other conditions are associated with increased incidence of inguinal hernias and hydroceles, including (1) all forms of ascites and increased quantities of peritoneal fluid, (2) a positive family history, (3) hypospadias and epispadias, (4) cryptorchidism, (5) cystic fibrosis, (6) various connective tissue diseases, and (7) the mucopolysaccharidoses.

Hydroceles exist when fluid surrounds the testes, with or without direct communication with the abdominal cavity through the processus vaginalis. Their natural course is distinctly different from that of inguinal hernias. Isolated hydroceles manifest a substantially lower risk of incarceration than inguinal hernias. Most noncommunicating hydroceles are painless, are apparent in the immediate neonatal period, and disappear spontaneously by 1 year of age.

Clinically, a child with an inguinal hernia has a bulge or swelling in the scrotum or groin that is most apparent when the child is crying. At times the parent remarks on symptoms of fussiness, vomiting, or other feeding problems. Examination of the child reveals a smooth mass arising from the external ring, perhaps accompanied by swelling in the ipsilateral hemiscrotum. Unincarcerated hernias are easily reducible. Palpation of the spermatic cord reveals a thickening or the ''silk-sleeve'' sign.

Examination of a child with suspected hydrocele reveals a scrotal fullness that transilluminates. However, the presence of transillumination of the scrotal mass fails to exclude reliably the possibility of coexisting hernia or another pathologic condition. Palpation of the testis confirms descent and is necessary in order to exclude accompanying testicular tumor. If palpation fails to adequately demonstrate a normal-sized and -shaped testis, sonography is indicated to rule out the possibility of an accompanying intratesticular tumor.

A noncompressible, painless cystic mass in a newborn that is unassociated with abnormalities of the testis suggests a diagnosis of noncommunicating hydrocele. Observation of such a child is appropriate, since the majority of cases resolve spontaneously within the first year of life.

Compressibility of the mass suggests a hydrocele communicating with the abdominal cavity through the processus vaginalis. In such a situation and in cases of suspected inguinal hernia, surgical consultation is indicated for the purpose of scheduling surgical repair. Meanwhile, the family is educated about the signs and symptoms of incarceration of an inguinal hernia, including (1) increase in the size of the hernia mass or persistence of a mass, (2) systemic toxicity, (3) abdominal distention, or (4) vomiting, especially bilious vomiting. In cases where a clear clinical diagnosis is not possible, surgical consultation and elective exploration are warranted.

A clinical challenge exists when a child with a hydrocele presents with a coexisting condition that leads to scrotal pain and/or increased scrotal swelling. Inguinal hernia incarceration, testicular torsion, epididymitis, intrascrotal tumors, and acute intraabdominal pathologic conditions may occur in a child with a hydrocele. Careful and gentle examination is usually sufficient to diagnose an incarcerated inguinal hernia or coexistent testicular pathologic condition.

The safest and one of the more effective maneuvers for reducing incarcerated inguinal hernias involves relaxation of the abdominal wall, using sedation if necessary, and subsequent placement of the child in the Trendelenburg position. This results in successful reduction of the incarceration more than 70 percent of the time. Failure of this technique represents an indication for immediate surgical consultation and exploration.

Varicoceles A varicocele is a dilated and elongated network of veins of the pampiniform plexus and apparently is a consequence of spermatic venous valvular incompetence. Found predominantly on the left side (85 to 90 percent), varicoceles are rare in children under 10 years of age, but the incidence increases through early puberty to include 15 percent of adolescents.

Physical examination is best performed in the upright position and reveals a mass posterior, lateral, and superior to the testis extending up the spermatic cord. The mass as been described as feeling like a bag of worms. While usually painless, some boys report a dull ache in their scrotum associated with the varicocele.

The clinical significance of varicocele rests primarily with the association between this condition and adult male infertility. While infrequently an immediate concern of the adolescent, there is ample evidence that the risks of testicular hypotrophy, declining semen parameters, and infertility progress the longer the varicocele remains untreated. Therefore, the identification of a varicocele represents an indication for urologic referral in conjunction with the boy's primary care physician. Urologists recommend surgical repair of varicoceles that are (1) bilateral, (2) painful, or (3) associated with a significant disparity in testicular size of greater than 2 cm^3. Rarely, a varicocele may develop as a consequence of an acute increase in inferior vena caval pressure, in turn the consequence of an intra-abdominal tumor or vena caval thrombosis.

Spermatoceles and Epididymal Cysts Sperm-containing cysts of the rete testis or efferent ducts (spermatoceles), or of the epididymis (epididymal cysts) are the next most common cause of painless scrotal masses in children after hernias, hydroceles, and varicoceles. Located superior and posterior to the testes, they usually transilluminate well. Ultrasound studies confirm the location of the mass, demonstrating a nearly echo-free zone without disorganization of the surrounding parenchyma. Spermatoceles and epididymal cysts are unassociated with infertility and are usually painless. Management consists of confirming the diagnosis with sonographic study if necessary and subsequent parental and patient education. Surgical excision is reserved for enlarging spermatoceles, particularly those associated with discomfort unresponsive to nonsteroidal anti-inflammatory medications.

PAINLESS SOLID SCROTAL MASSES **Idiopathic Scrotal Edema** Idiopathic scrotal edema results in painless scrotal erythema and induration in boys from age 2 to 11 years. Two-thirds of cases are unilateral. The etiology remains obscure. No specific allergen has been identified.

The child has no complaint of pain but may note minimal pruritis and may exhibit a waddling gait. Erythema and swelling may extend to portions of the phallus, abdomen, and groin. Examination reveals a thickened and edematous scrotal skin and underlying tunics, but the boy has little or no tenderness to palpation of the affected areas. There is no fever. The testes, epididymis, and tunica vaginalis are normal, although the degree of swelling of the scrotal skin may preclude adequate examination by palpation. In sonographic studies done in such extreme cases, the underlying scrotal structures and vascular flow appear normal. The urinalysis results and peripheral white blood cell count are normal.

The scrotal edema and erythema resolve in 1 to 4 days, although recurrence rates approach 21 percent. Management involves reassurance of the child and parents. No benefit has been observed from use of steroids, antihistamines, and antibiotics.

Solid Painless Extratesticular Masses Of greatest concern upon identifying a painless solid paratesticular mass in childhood is the diagnosis of paratesticular rhabdomyosarcoma, the most common paratesticular malignancy in childhood. Rhabdomyosarcoma is one of the most common malignant solid tumors of childhood, along with the lymphomas, Wilms tumor, and neuroblastoma. The paratesticular site is the primary location in 10 percent of children with rhabdomyosarcoma. Rhabdomyosarcoma has two peak incidences: one between 2 and 6 years of age, and the other between 14 and 18 years of age.

The clinical presentation is that of a painless, unilateral, solid scrotal mass that initially is distinct from the testis, characteristics that are confirmed by sonographic evaluation. Immediate referral to a pediatric hematologist-oncologist, who will coordinate a multidisciplinary surgical–diagnostic staging and management approach, is mandatory.

There exist a variety of other painless malignant and benign solid tumors of the extratesticular scrotum, but the diagnosis and subsequent management of all of them rest with histologic methods following surgical exploration through an inguinal incision.

Solid Painless Intratesticular Masses Testicular tumors account for less than 1 percent of solid tumors in infants and children. The peak incidence of testicular tumors occurs at 2 years of age. Their significance lies, not in their frequency, but in the relatively frequent development of a secondary hydrocele in 7 to 25 percent of affected patients. This association leads to misdiagnoses and delays initiation of definitive treatment of the underlying tumor. As stated previously, the association of testicular tumors and secondary hydrocele mandates sonographic visualization of the testis if the size or position of the hydrocele precludes an adequate palpation examination of the testis.

Demonstration of a painless intratesticular mass mandates immediate referral to a pediatric hematologist-oncologist, who will coordinate obtaining a surgical diagnosis and determine treatment based on histologic analysis and staging of the tumor.

GYNECOLOGIC PROBLEMS OF PREADOLESCENT GIRLS

Disorders of the Labia

LABIAL AND VULVAR AGGLUTINATION (ADHESIONS) Agglutination (adhesion) of the labia minora or vulva is usually seen in girls 3 months to 6 years of age, although it is occasionally seen in girls who are approaching puberty. This condition is also called vulvar synechiae, gynatresia, vulvar or labial fusion, and labial coalescence. This disorder accounts for about 50 percent of prepubertal gynecologic complaints seen in an outpatient setting.

Prepubertal labia minora, covered by a very thin hypoestrogenized epithelium, are easily inflamed and denuded following infection, local trauma, or irritation. Often, the source of irritation is an environmental source previously tolerated during the diapered neonatal period and during earlier infancy (e.g., bubble bath, baby shampoos, and soaps). In addition, the anterior progression of labial agglutination from its origins at the posterior fourchette may lead to a significant ''pocketing'' of voided urine behind the agglutinated tissues, serving as a nearly constant source of additional irritation.

The girl with labial agglutination is most often asymptomatic, and the diagnosis comes to the physician's attention through parental concern or during routine examination. Some children have symptoms of urethritis; others have difficulties in toilet training due to the tendency for the perineum to remain moist from pocketed urine. Urinary tract infections are common.

The physical examination of a girl with labial agglutination is sufficient to distinguish this condition from its differential diagnostic considerations: ambiguous genitalia and imperforate hymen. The site of midline fusion of the labioscrotal folds seen in ambiguous genitalia, known as the median raphe, is a thick, raised, linear structure. In contrast, the site of midline labial agglutination is very characteristically thin, demonstrating agglutination of medial surfaces of the labia, not fusion of the labioscrotal folds. In addition, the agglutinated labia minora are distinct from and fused in the midline under the clitoral hood, while in ambiguous genitalia the labia minora are incorporated into the clitoral hood. Differentiation of labial agglutination from imperforate hymen is easily accomplished by noting that the hymen is located at the vaginal orifice, which is on the same plane as the urethra, as compared to the more exterior position of and posterior-to-anterior extension of labial agglutination. Occasionally, the presence of labial agglutination may give rise to parental concerns about sexual abuse if the adhesions are forcibly disrupted during straddle activity, resulting in a larger than previously recognized ''opening,'' perhaps with a small amount of oozing blood.

Most girls exhibiting labial agglutination require no treatment, since the adhesions resolve spontaneously during puberty. Girls whose labial agglutination results in recurrent urinary tract infections, toileting difficulties, or difficulties in visualizing the urethra should probably be treated. Almost always, the agglutination responds to removal of the source of the caustic irritation coupled with careful application of topical estrogen cream (0.1% conjugated estrogen vaginal cream) twice daily for 2 to 4 weeks.

LICHEN SCLEROSIS ATROPHICA Although uncommon in prepubertal girls, lichen sclerosis is being increasingly recognized by emergency physicians and pediatricians. This increased recognition is in some measure a reflection of increased concern about and awareness of sexual abuse and the subsequently increased frequency of perineal examination of prepubertal girls. The affected girl complains of itch, irritation, dysuria, perineal and/or perianal pain, and bleeding. There may be a coexistent vaginal discharge. As perianal pain persists, the girl may develop problems with painful defecation, stool retention, constipation, and encopresis.

The characteristic appearance of the vulva is white, atrophic, and finely wrinkled. Ulcerations, blisters, excoriations, and inflammation are seen over the vulva, perineum, and perianal area, often giving rise to the terms *hourglass* or *figure-eight* to describe the pattern of skin involvement. Secondary infection is possible. Progression of the disease leads to distortion, thickening, and scarring of vulvar and perineal architecture. The condition is differentiated from vitiligo by absence of inflammation or atrophy in the latter. The diagnosis of lichen sclerosis atrophica is made on clinical grounds and may be confirmed histologically from biopsy specimen in atypical cases.

The friability of the affected tissues leads to an increased risk of bleeding, even as a consequence of very minor trauma (e.g., the friction associated with bicycling). This has given rise to concerns in some parents about possible sexual abuse. Typically, the child denies such contact. There is no evidence linking lichen sclerosis atrophica to sexual abuse.

Management involves removal of all perineal irritants accompanied by the use of systemic antipruritics and the local application of an emollient ointment, such as A & D ointment. A 2- to 3-month course of treatment with a low-potency topical steroid cream, such as 2.5% hydrocortisone cream, applied two to three times daily, is often useful. Topical antifungal creams and systemic antibiotics are indicated for treatment of yeast and dermatophyte infections, and bacterial superinfections, respectively.

Interlabial Masses

URETHRAL PROLAPSE Urethral prolapse is an uncommon disorder affecting prepubertal girls from the immediate newborn period to 11 years of age in which there is a circular eversion of urethral mucosa through the urethral meatus. It has been estimated to have an incidence of about 1:2880 girls, and almost all (90 to 100 percent) cases occur in black girls.

The etiology of urethral prolapse is not clearly understood. Many hypotheses have been proposed to explain the disorder, most of which center on lax periurethral fascia, vaginal mucosal atrophy, urethral mucosal redundancy or increased urethral width, repeated episodes of increased intraabdominal pressure, and estrogen deficiency of the prepubertal girl. The specific contributions of any of these phenomena to the development of urethral prolapse are conjectural.

Urethral prolapse typically presents with painless "vaginal" bleeding. The diagnosis is made with the observation of a doughnut-shaped mass originating from and encircling the urethral meatus that protrudes through the vulva. The prolapsed tissue is edematous and friable, often ulcerated, and apparently infected. Urethral prolapse is the only diagnosis in which a circular mass surrounds the urethral meatus. It is necessary to identify the urethral meatus with certainty, either by observing the child voiding her bladder or by catheterization if necessary.

While painless vaginal bleeding is the most common complaint at presentation, dysuria, perineal discomfort, and the sensation of a vulvar mass have been reported as isolated symptoms. The often dark, cyanotic, hemorrhagic appearance of the mass and its associated blood clots have been misinterpreted by families and physicians as evidence of sexual abuse. In fact, the correct diagnosis is not commonly made by the physician initially examining the child. The differential diagnostic considerations include prolapsed ectopic ureterocele, prolapsed bladder, prolapsed urethral polyp, ectopic ureter, urethral cysts, hydrocolpos, condyloma acuminatum, periurethral abscess, and sarcoma botryoides. Identifying a round mass encircling the urethral meatus eliminates each of these diagnostic considerations.

A wide range of treatment options have been recommended for urethral prolapse. Conservative therapy appears warranted for a mild degree of prolapse and include sitz baths, application of topical estrogen cream (0.1% conjugated estrogen cream), and serial observations over several months. Surgical treatment options include primary excision of the prolapse (associated with the highest success rate and lowest rates of recurrence), manual reduction under anesthesia, suture ligation of the prolapse over a Foley catheter, and cryosurgery. Failure of conservative therapy serves as an indication for consultation with a urologist, pediatric surgeon, or gynecologist.

HYDROCOLPOS If an imperforate hymen, transverse vaginal septum, or atretic vagina completely prevents the egress of secretions from the uterus and cervical glands, a hydrocolpos results (hydrometrocolpos if the uterus is also distended).

A bulging, shiny, pearly gray "mass" is seen covering the introitus. The mass is actually the remarkably distended hymenal membrane, stretched thin. The urethral meatus is observed to be distinct from the "mass" and is located anterior to it. Examination may reveal an abdominal mass palpable externally as well as a palpable rectal mass. The child may experience urinary retention.

A sonogram reveals a nonmobile, midline, cystic mass behind the bladder. The superior wall of the bladder may exhibit compression by the mass. In the presence of urinary retention or ureteral compression by the mass, the sonogram may reveal hydronephrosis. Treatment consists of aspiration and surgical drainage of the cyst's contents, a grayish-white mucoid material.

PARAURETHRAL CYSTS Paraurethral cysts occur uncommonly in children but are seen occasionally in the neonatal period. Cystic degeneration of the paraurethral glands, Gartner's ducts, müllerian ducts, or Skene's ducts may result in the appearance of a cystic paravaginal or introital mass. Following a careful history and physical examination, the infant with a suspected paraurethral cyst should undergo imaging studies necessary to evaluate the relationship between the cystic mass and the urethra, bladder, ureters, and kidneys. These studies usually begin with a sonogram and may include a voiding cystourethrogram, contrast injection of the cyst itself, and occasionally cystourethroscopy.

SARCOMA BOTRYOIDES Sarcoma botryoides is an embryonal rhabdomyosarcoma arising from a hollow viscous, such as the bladder or the vagina. The name refers to the grapelike configuration of the mass. The peak incidence is at 2 years of age, and over 90 percent of cases occur before 5 years of age.

The tumor arises in the distal vagina in younger girls, whereas in older children it originates more commonly on the anterior wall of the vagina near the cervix. Tumor growth fills the vagina with a mass that assumes the shape of a cluster of grapes, often prolapsing through the urethra or vaginal introitus. All growths with such an appearance should be presumed malignant until proved otherwise. Other symptoms may include vaginal bleeding, abdominal pain, or a palpable abdominal mass.

Early diagnosis is critically important to prognosis. Upon observing a suspicious lesion, immediate referral to a pediatric hematologist-oncologist is indicated.

BIBLIOGRAPHY

Anveden-Hertzberg L, Glauderer MD: Urethral prolapse: An often misdiagnosed cause of urogenital bleeding in girls. *Pediatr Emerg Care* 11:212, 1995.

Brown MR, Cartwright PC, et al: Common office problems in pediatric urology and gynecology. *Pediatr Clin North Am* 44:1091, 1997.

Duckett JW, Snyder H III: The MAGPI hypospadias repair in 1111 patients. *Ann Surg* 213:620, 1991.

Fernandes ET, Dekermacher S, et al: Urethral prolapse in children. *Urology* 41:240, 1993.

Harrison BP: Pediatric penile swelling. *Acad Emerg Med* 3:384, 1996.

Hashmat AI, Raju S, et al: ^{99m}Tc penile scan: An investigative modality in priapism. *Urol Radiol* 11:58, 1989.

Kass EJ, Reitelman C: Adolescent varicocele. *Urol Clin North Am* 22:151, 1995.

Miller ST, Rao SP, et al: Priapism in children with sickle cell disease. *J Urol* 154:844, 1995.

Redmond CA, Cowell CA, et al: Genital lichen sclerosis in prepubertal girls. *Adolesc Pediatr Gynecol* 1:177, 1988.

Schwartz RH, Rushton HG: Acute balanoposthitis in young boys. *Pediatr Infect Dis J* 15:176, 1996.

Skoog SJ: Benign and malignant scrotal masses. *Pediatr Clin North Am* 44:1229, 1997.

Skoog SJ, Conlin MJ, et al: Pediatric hernias and hydroceles. *Urol Clin North Am* 22:119, 1995.

Starr NB: Labial adhesions in childhood. *J Pediatr Health Care* 10:26, 1996.

PEDIATRIC URINARY TRACT INFECTIONS

Michael F. Altieri
Mary Camarca
Thom A. Mayer

EPIDEMIOLOGY

Urinary tract infections (UTIs) are an important cause of febrile illnesses in infants and children in the United States. UTI occurs in 4 to 7 percent of febrile infants.[1] Symptomatic UTIs occur in approximately 2 percent of children from 1 to 5 years of age and in up to 3 to 5 percent of school-aged girls.[2] Since the presenting signs and symptoms are often nonspecific, especially in younger infants, the diagnosis of UTI is often presumptive rather than definitive. The incidence of UTI varies greatly with age, gender, historical factors, such as prematurity, and history of previous UTI. Proper initial evaluation, interpretation of laboratory data, treatment, and follow-up are essential to avoid the long- term complications of renal scarring. The American Academy of Pediatrics has published a practice parameter on this subject, the recommendations from which are reflected in this chapter.[3]

PATHOPHYSIOLOGY

In the neonatal period, UTI originates via hematogenous spread resulting in bacterial seeding of the renal parenchyma. After the neonatal period, bacteria gain access to the urinary tract via perineal and periurethral colonization, with subsequent retrograde contamination of the lower urinary tract structures. Virulence of the pathogen, host immunity, and structural and functional aspects of the urinary tract all play important roles in the development of UTI. Much is known about structural and functional factors contributing to the risk of UTI. Congenital urinary tract anomalies, vesicoureteral reflux, and urolithiasis are associated with a higher incidence of UTI.[3–6] However, it is now clear that pyelonephritis in the absence of vesicoureteral reflux is far more common than previously thought. Behavioral and functional factors, such as poor hygiene, voluntary urinary retention, and constipation, have been associated with increased risk of UTI.[7,8]

CLINICAL FEATURES

Other than fever, few symptoms are consistently found in infants and children diagnosed with UTI. Neonates may present with jaundice, poor feeding, irritability, and lethargy. Older infants and young children commonly present with gastrointestinal complaints, such as abdominal pain, vomiting, and change in appetite. The classic signs of dysuria, urinary frequency, urgency, or hesitancy are more likely to be present in older children and adolescents. The clinical signs and symptoms of UTI also vary with the primary site of infection along the urinary tract. The symptoms of dysuria, frequency, and urgency are more often associated with lower tract (uncomplicated) infections, such as cystitis, and urethritis. More systemic symptoms, such as fever, chills, vomiting, and dehydration, suggest upper tract (complicated) infection. However, recent studies clearly indicate that pyelonephritis often occurs in the absence of such symptoms.[9,10] Unfortunately, the signs and symptoms of infection anywhere along the urinary tract may be nonspecific and overlapping. For these reasons, UTI should be considered in all febrile children, regardless of symptoms or lack thereof. Furthermore, upper tract infection should be considered as well, particularly in febrile children. The utility to distinguish between lower and upper tract disease is relevant when considering treatment options, long-term sequelae, and recommendations for follow-up.

DIAGNOSIS

Gram-negative enteric bacteria are the most commonly isolated organisms in UTI. While P-fimbriated *Escherichia coli* accounts for the vast majority of infections, *Klebsiella, Proteus,* and *Enterobacter* species are also important pathogens. *Enterococcus* species, *Staphylococcus aureus,* and group B streptococci are the most frequently isolated gram-positive organisms and are more likely to be causative organisms in the neonatal period. Coagulase-negative staphylococcal UTI occurs in teens and young adults. Adenovirus may cause acute cystitis, occurs more commonly in young boys, and is clinically indistinguishable in many cases from bacterial disease.

While urine culture is the gold standard in the diagnosis of UTIs in children, culture results are rarely, if ever, available to physicians in the emergency department. Therefore, emergency physicians must rely on clinical data and other laboratory tests while obtaining a urine culture to subsequently confirm the diagnosis.

TABLE 136-1 Interpretation of Positive Urine Culture Results

Method of Collection	Quantitative Culture: UTI Present
Suprapubic aspiration	Growth of urinary pathogens in any number (exception of up to 2–3 $\times$ 10^3 coagulase-negative staphylococci)
Catheterization	Febrile infants or children with $\geq 5 \times 10^4$ CFU/mL of single pathogen*
Midstream clean void	Symptomatic patients with $\geq 10^5$ CFU/mL of a single urinary pathogen
Midstream clean void	Asymptomatic patients with two specimens on different days with $>10^5$ CFU/mL of the same organism

*Infection may be present with counts as low as 10–50 $\times$ 10^3 CFU/mL.
Abbreviation: CFU, cell-forming units.
Source: Adapted from Hellerstein S,[13] with permission.

TABLE 136-2 Management of Urinary Tract Infections

Age, Range and Clinical Status	Management
$<$2–3 months Febrile UTI	Hospitalize; IV antibiotics for 4–5 d with good clinical response, discharge when tolerating oral medication and diet; 10 d of therapeutic doses of medication and then suppressive medication
$>$2–3 months through adolescence Acute pyelonephritis, but not severely ill or dehydrated (uncomplicated UTI)	Hospitalize; IV antibiotics until afebrile 24–36 h and able to take oral medication and fluids; discharge on 10-d course of oral medication If renal scarring on RCS, IV therapy may be extended to 7 d
$>$2–3 months through adolescence Acute pyelonephritis, but not severely ill or dehydrated (uncomplicated UTI)	IM or IV antibiotic; start oral medication at therapeutic doses after 12–18 h; contact physician after 24 h if unable to take oral medication or adequate fluids; contact physician at 48 h for adjustment in medication and to schedule F/U urine and imaging studies If renal scarring on RCS, IV therapy may be extended to 7 d
Infancy to adolescence Acute cystitis	5–7 d of therapeutic doses of oral antibiotic for UTI; urinalysis and culture after 4–5 d Sitz baths and/or analgesia for symptomatic relief
Adolescence Acute cystitis	Single IM or IV dose of ceftriaxone or aminoglycoside; single oral dose of trimethoprim-sulfamethoxazole; 3-d oral regimen with trimethoprim-sulfamethoxazole or nitrofurantoin; follow-up urinalysis and culture after 4–5 d

Abbreviation: F/U, follow-up.
Source: Adapted from Hellerstein,[13] with permission.

TABLE 136-3 Common Antimicrobial Drugs Used in Pediatric Urinary Tract Infections

Drug	Dosage and Interval
PARENTERAL THERAPY	
Ampicillin	100 mg/kg/d 12 h (<1 week) q6–8h (>1 week)
Ceftriaxone*	75 mg/kg/d q12–24h
Cefotaxime	150 mg/kg/d q6–8h
Gentamicin	5 mg/kg/d q12h (<1 week) 7.5 mg/kg/d q8h (>1 week)
ORAL THERAPY	
Amoxicillin†	20–40 mg/kg/d q8h
Augmentin	50 mg/kg/d q8h
Trimethoprim-sulfamethoxazole (TMP-SMX)	6–12 mg/kg/d TMP, 30–60 mg/kg/d SMX q12h
Cephalexin	25–50 mg/kg/d q6h
Cefixime	8 mg/kg/d q12h

*Should not be used in neonates because of potential biliary sludge pseudolithiasis. If cocci are present in urinary sediment, ampicillin should be added until culture and sensitivities are available.

†*E. coli* resistance should be considered.

Source: Adapted from Altieri, MF, Camarca M, Bock G: Pediatric urinary tract infections. *Ped Emerg Med Rep* 2:103, 1977, with permission.

With an incontinent child, a specimen for urinalysis and culture should be obtained through direct bladder sampling (catheterization or suprapubic sampling) or through a cleanly voided specimen in boys and older girls. *Bagged urine specimens are not acceptable because of the high degree of contamination.* Urine specimens from older children with voiding control should be obtained from a cleanly voided midstream clean catch.[5] Parents should be instructed on the proper technique for avoiding contamination of specimens. Periurethral contamination of specimens can be avoided by having girls sit backward (facing the rear of the toilet). This position favors labial retraction and better exposure of the urethral meatus. Because bacterial contaminants grow rapidly at room temperature, a urine specimen that cannot be cultured immediately should be kept on ice or at a temperature of 4°C (39.2°F) until culturing can be accomplished.

While urinalysis is the most common adjunctive diagnostic test for a possible UTI, urine chemical test strips are also a quick means of initial urine screening for the detection of leukocyte esterase and urinary nitrates. Esterases are released into the urine after the breakdown of white blood cells, providing presumptive evidence of infection. Occasionally, false-negative urine test strip results are obtained for very young infants because their leukocyte response may be limited. Nitrates are converted to nitrites by gram-negative urinary pathogens, and urine test strips may also provide indirect evidence of bacteriuria. Hematuria, proteinuria, and pyuria are commonly associated with UTIs but are nonspecific and can occur in the absence of infection. The presence of bacteria in catheterized urinary sediment also lends support to the presence of a UTI. In most studies, the sensitivities of a positive test result for urinary leukocyte esterase or nitrite or a positive urine culture result are less than 50 percent. The combined presence of pyuria (more than five white blood cells per high-power field) and bacteriuria on urine microanalysis improves the sensitivity to approximately 65 percent. The positive predictive value of a urinalysis is 81 percent.

Peripheral white blood cell counts and erythrocyte sedimentation rates are also nonspecific indicators that should only be interpreted in conjunction with the results of the urinalysis and urine culture. A guide to interpreting urine culture results based on the various methods of obtaining urine samples is contained in Table 136-1.

TREATMENT

As mentioned before, early treatment of UTIs, especially in infants and young children, decreases the risk of kidney damage. Table 136-2 summarizes the approach to management of children with UTI. Inpatient management should be instituted for any child less than 3 months of age with a febrile UTI; children who have significant dehydration or appear toxic; those with pyelonephritis, urinary stents or other urinary foreign bodies, or renal insufficiency; or those who are immunocompromised. In addition, if a child's compliance and follow-up is questionable, inpatient or pediatric short-stay unit treatment should be considered.

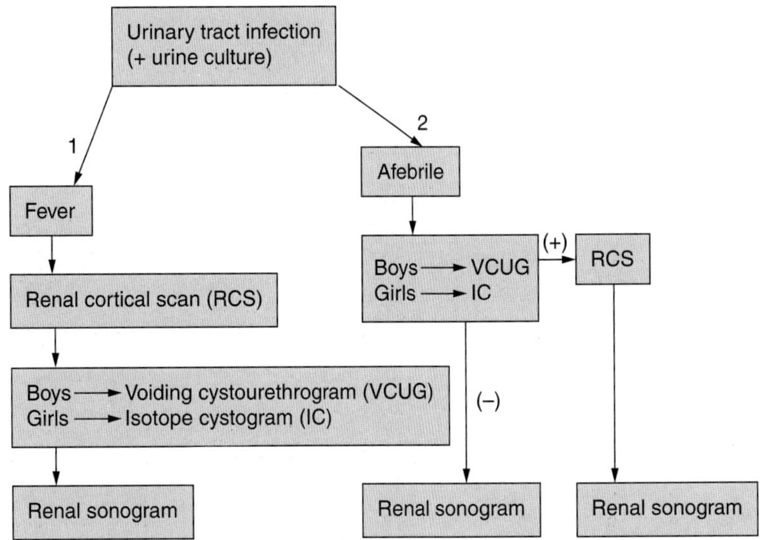

FIG. 136-1. Algorithm for radiographic evaluation of children with their first UTI. (Adapted from Gausche M, in Strange GR, ed: *Pediatric Emergency Medicine: A Comprehensive Study Guide.* New York, McGraw-Hill, with permission.)

Children older than 3 months with febrile UTIs who appear nontoxic and only mildly dehydrated and who do not have persistent vomiting may be rehydrated in the emergency department. These children may initially receive intravenous antibiotic therapy and may then be discharged home on a course of oral antibiotics. Prior to discharge, they should demonstrate adequate oral intake and retention of fluids and have arrangements made for follow-up care within several days either with the primary care physician or the emergency department. Specific antibiotics and their dosing for both inpatient and outpatient therapy are contained in Table 136-3, but therapy should be guided with an understanding of the antibiotic resistance patterns in the hospital and community. Instructions should be given to the caregiver regarding follow-up on culture results.

DISPOSITION

Numerous clinical investigators and clinicians have discussed and debated in recent years the most appropriate radiologic studies for the follow-up of children with UTIs, and various algorithms have been proposed.[9-12] Although imaging studies for UTIs are rarely indicated as part of the diagnostic workup in the emergency department (except in cases where there is a palpable mass), it is important to arrange follow-up for all children with febrile UTIs. A recent evidence-based study of the existing literature suggested that large multicenter studies are needed to more carefully delineate a definitive approach to imaging the genitourinary system in children with UTI.[11] However, until such studies are completed, the following is a reasonable diagnostic approach to imaging. First, the goals of radiologic imaging are to (1) identify existing upper tract disease capable of causing cortical scaring so that appropriate antibiotic therapy can be instituted, (2) identify treatable lesions of the genitourinary system, and (3) guide an approach to prevent further renal scarring and subsequent impairment of renal function.

In the past, indications for imaging of pediatric patients with UTI included neonates, females with recurrent UTI (two or more episodes), and males of any age with UTI. However, more recent studies support the approach outlined in Fig. 136-1, which some institutions utilize even for patients with a first episode of UTI.[12] Acutely febrile and/or toxic children with UTI as the documented or presumed source of fever should have a renal cortical scan (RCS) to assess for renal involvement. If renal scarring and/or active infection is present, the patient should have intravenous antibiotic therapy to reduce scarring and eliminate infection. If the RCS results are negative, males should have a voiding cystourethrogram (VCUG) and females an isotope cystogram (IC) to assess for vesicoureteral reflux. In afebrile children, the VCUG for males and IC for females should initially be assessed, followed by RCS if the results are positive. Renal sonography may be done at the time of RCS, VCUG, or IC to assess for dilatation of the collection system.

While such radiologic imaging is not necessarily coordinated by the emergency department, it is important for emergency physicians to be aware of the necessity of follow-up and the reasons for imaging so that it can be coordinated with the patient's inpatient physician or primary care provider.

REFERENCES

1. Hoberman A, Chao H-P, Keller DM, et al: Prevalence of urinary tract infections in febrile infants. *J Pediatr* 23:17, 1993.
2. Gonzalez R: Urinary tract infections, in Behrman R, Klieman R, Arvin A, et al (eds): *Nelson's Textbook of Pediatrics,* 15th ed. Philadelphia, Saunders, 1996, pp 1528–1532.
3. Committee on Quality Improvements. Subcommittee on Urinary Tract Infection: Practice parameter: The diagnosis, treatment, and evaluation of the initial urinary tract infection in febrile infants and young children. *Pediatrics* 103:843, 1999.
4. Bock GH: Urinary tract infections, in Hockerman R, (ed): *Primary Pediatric Care,* 3d ed. St. Louis, Mosby-Year Book, 1997, pp 1640–1644.
5. Gearhart P, Herzberg G, Jeffs RD, et al: Childhood urolithiasis: Experiences and advances. *Pediatrics* 87:445, 1991.
6. Smellie JM, Normand ICS, Katz G: Children with urinary tract infection: A comparison of those with and those without vesicoureteric reflux. *Kidney Int* 20:717, 1981.
7. Smellie JM, Normand ICS: Urinary tract infections in children. *Postgrad Med* 61:895, 1985.
8. Bethyn AJ, Jenkins HR, et al: Radiologic evidence of constipation in urinary tract infection. *Am J Dis Child* 73:534, 1995.
9. Conway J, Cohn R: Evolving role of nuclear medicine for diagnosis and management of urinary tract infections. *J Pediatr* 124:87, 1994.
10. Goldraich N, Goldraich I: Update on dimercaptosuccinic acid renal scanning in children with urinary tract infection. *Pediatr Nephrol* 9:221, 1995.
11. Dick PT, Feldman W: Routine diagnostic imaging for childhood urinary tract infection: A systematic overview. *J Pediatr* 128:15, 1996.
12. Andrich MP, Majd M: Diagnostic imaging in the evaluation of the first urinary tract infection in infants and young children. *Pediatrics* 90:436, 1992.
13. Hellerstein S: Urinary tract infections: Old and new concepts. *Pediatr Clin North Am* 42:1433, 1995.

SEXUALLY TRANSMITTED DISEASES

Dexter L. Morris

Sexually transmitted diseases (STDs) are commonly encountered in emergency and urgent care settings. It is important to diagnose and treat them to protect the health and future fertility of the patient as well as the health of the patient's sexual contacts. Furthermore, individuals with STDs are more likely to acquire human immunodeficiency virus (HIV) infection than the general population. Thus diagnosis of an STD suggests the need for HIV counseling and testing. This chapter discusses the major STDs with the exception of HIV infection, which is discussed in Chap. 139, and hepatitis B infection, which is discussed in Chap. 82. Vaginosis and pelvic inflammatory disease (PID) are also discussed elsewhere (Chaps. 104 and 105, respectively). In addition to specific antimicrobial treatment for STD patients, the end of this chapter contains important guidelines for follow-up and reporting of STDs. Treatment guidelines for STDs change frequently. *The Morbidity and Mortality Weekly Report* of the Centers for Disease Control and Prevention (CDC) is an excellent source of updates.

DIAGNOSIS

The most important aspect of the diagnosis of STDs is to maintain a high level of awareness. While many patients may present with an obvious STD (lesion on the penis), more commonly the chief complaint may be as vague as dysuria or lower abdominal pain. For example, a study at an inner-city ED suggested that half the patients who were discharged with a diagnosis of urinary tract infection (UTI) had one or more positive STD cultures.

Once a physician suspects an STD, obtaining a history of sexual activity and previous STDs is important. This may clue the physician into examining or culturing oral or anal areas, help differentiate mechanical from infectious lesions, and predict risk for hepatitis and HIV infections. Questions about pregnancy and sexual assault should asked, if appropriate. These questions can be asked in a nonconfrontational manner by explaining to the patient their rationale.

Careful examination of the genital areas (and pelvic examination in women) is important. The foreskin should be retracted, if present, and the physician should be sure to look in skin folds and other areas that may not be readily viewable, particularly in obese persons. Cultures for gonorrhea and chlamydia should be taken if there is a suspicion of STDs to document the infection. Other tests may be appropriate for specific lesions.

STDs without Lesions

CHLAMYDIAL INFECTIONS *Chlamydia trachomatis* is an obligate intracellular bacterium that has a growth cycle that alternates between two morphologic forms. Chlamydial infections present with a wide spectrum of clinical manifestations. In men, infection causes urethritis, epididymitis, and proctitis. In women, urethritis, cervicitis, and PID are common. In both sexes, the prevalence of asymptomatic infection is high, ranging from 3 to 5 percent in the general population to 15 to 20 percent among individuals attending STD clinics. Patients with gonorrhea have an even higher incidence of concomitant chlamydial infection. Untreated chlamydial infections are thought to be an important cause of infertility in women. The incubation period is 1 to 3 weeks, and symptoms, if present, can range from mild vaginal burning or irritation to peritonitis.

Diagnosis Although the organism can be cultured, this has a relatively low yield. Indirect methods using direct immunofluorescence, enzyme-linked immunosorbent assay (ELISA)-type assays, and DNA probes are available.

Treatment Treatment is with azithromycin 1 g PO in a single dose or doxycycline 100 mg PO bid for 7 days. Table 137-1 lists alternative treatment options.

GONOCOCCAL INFECTIONS *Neisseria gonorrhoeae* are gram-negative diplococci that remain sensitive to antibiotics, although recent years have seen the emergence of strains resistant to penicillin (up to 25 percent) and, less commonly, tetracycline. Gonococcal infection presents usually as urethritis in men and cervicitis or PID in women. Epididymitis and prostatitis also can occur in men. Rectal infection occurs in 30 to 50 percent of women with gonococcal cervicitis and can be the only site of infection in homosexual men. *N. gonorrhoeae* also can be isolated from the pharynx, but rarely does it cause a pharyngitis. The incubation period ranges from 3 to 21 days. Disseminated infection also occurs in approximately 2 percent of untreated primary gonorrhea. This manifestation is characterized by skin lesions (tender pustules on an erythematous base, 50 to 70 percent), arthralgias, tenosynovitis, or arthritis (30 to 40 percent), and fever or general malaise (80 percent). Gonococcal infections can decrease fertility in women, presumably by scarring the fallopian tubes. They also increase the chance of ectopic pregnancy by the same mechanism.

Diagnosis Cervical or urethral culture on a selective medium is the standard for diagnosis, having a sensitivity of 80 to 90 percent. A Gram stain of a urethral smear showing intracellular gram-negative diplococci is sensitive and specific in men but much less useful in women. Diagnosis of disseminated gonococcal infection is more difficult with only 20 to 50 percent of blood, lesion, or joint cultures being positive. Obtaining cervical, rectal, and pharyngeal samples may improve the chance of a culture diagnosis.

Treatment Cefixime 400 mg PO, ceftriaxone 125 mg IM or ciprofloxacin 500 mg PO, or ofloxacin 400 mg PO all in single doses are recommended. Patients also should be treated for presumed chlamydial infection. PID or disseminated disease is usually treated with higher doses of ceftriaxone. Decisions to admit patients with symptomatic disease are based on their overall clinical picture as well as their ability to follow up on an outpatient basis.

TRICHOMONAL INFECTIONS *Trichomonas vaginalis* is a flagellated protozoan that causes urogenital infections in men and women. The prevalence is less than 1 percent in women overall but up to 15 percent in those attending STD clinics. Disease is most commonly characterized by vaginosis with discharge. Abdominal pain also can be present. In men, the disease is often asymptomatic, but it can cause urethritis. Incubation ranges from 3 to 28 days.

Diagnosis Microscopic examination of wet preparations of cervical smears or spun urine samples that reveal the classic motile parasites is diagnostic.

Treatment Metronidazole 2 g PO in a single dose is the usual treatment.

TABLE 137-1 Antimicrobial Therapy for STDs

Disease	Recommended Treatment	Alternative(s)
Chlamydial infection	Azithromycin 1 g PO single dose *or* Doxycycline 100 mg PO bid × 7 d	Erythromycin base 500 mg PO qid × 7 d *or* Ofloxacin 300 mg PO bid × 7 d
Gonococcal infections*	Cefixime 400 mg PO single dose *or* Ceftriaxone 125 mg IM single dose *or* Ciprofloxacin 500 mg PO single dose *or* Ofloxacin 400 mg PO single dose	Spectinomyin 2 g IM single dose
Trichomoniasis	Metronidazole 2 g PO single dose	Metronidazole 500 g PO bid × 7 d
Syphilis, primary, secondary, early latent	Benzathine penicillin G 2.4 million units IM single dose	Doxycycline 100 mg PO bid × 14 d
Syphilis, late latent or unknown	Benzathine penicillin G 2.4 million units IM 3 doses 1 week apart	
Herpes simplex infections, first episode	Acyclovir 400 mg PO tid for 7–10 d *or* Famciclovir 250 mg PO tid for 7–10 d *or* Valacyclovir 1 g PO bid for 7–10 d	
Chancroid	Azithromycin 1 g PO single dose *or* Ceftriaxone 250 mg IM single dose *or* Ciprofloxacin 500 mg PO bid × 3 d *or* Erythromycin base 500 mg PO qid × 7 d	
Lymphogranuloma venereum	Doxycycline 100 mg PO bid × 21 d	Erythromycin base 500 mg PO qid × 21 d

*Patients treated for gonococcal infections also should be treated for chlamydial infection.
Abbreviations: bid, twice a day; IM, intramuscularly; IV, intravenously; PO, by mouth; qid, four times a day; tid, three times a day.
Source: Adapted from Centers for Disease Control and Prevention: Guidelines for treatment of sexually transmitted diseases, *MMWR* 47:RR-1, 1998.

STDs with Lesions

The diseases discussed in this section often present with genital lesions that may be difficult to distinguish from one another. Characteristics of the lesions and their accompanying signs and symptoms are provided in Table 137-2. Granuloma inguinale (donovanosis) rarely occurs in the United States, and readers are referred to the Bibliography for more information.

GENITAL WARTS Human papillomaviruses (HPVs) are DNA viruses that cause genital warts by direct transmission. Different geno-

TABLE 137-2 Clinical Features of Genital Ulcers

Disease	Nature of Genital Ulcer	Incubation Period (Range)	Painful	Inguinal Adenopathy
Syphilis	Indurated, relatively clean base; heals spontaneously	2 weeks or longer	No	Firm, rubbery nodes; tender
Herpes simplex infection	Multiple, small, grouped vesicles coalesce and form shallow ulcers; vulvovaginitis	2–7 d	Yes	Tender bilateral adenopathy
Chancroid	Irregular, purulent; undermined edges; not indurated; multiple ulcers	2–12 d	Yes	Present in 50%; usually unilocular; if fluctuant, very painful; may form crater
Lymphogranuloma venereum	Usually not observed; small and shallow; rapid spontaneous healing	5–21 d	No	More common in males; nodes in matted cluster; unilateral or bilateral multi-located

Source: Adapted from Scientific American Medicine: *Sexually Transmitted Diseases.* New York: Scientific American Medicine, December 1997.

types also have been implicated in cervical cancer, but the relationship is far from clear. The warts usually appear after an incubation period of 3 to 4 months and may coalesce to form condylomata acuminata. Although painless, their location or size may cause discomfort.

Diagnosis Diagnosis is clinical, with care to exclude other STDs.

Treatment Treatment decisions are based on the size and number of lesions, the amount of discomfort they are causing, and patient preferences. Recommended treatment is podofilox 0.5% solution or gel applied with a cotton swab or a finger to the visible warts twice a day for 3 days, followed by 4 days of no therapy, with the cycle repeated up to 4 times. Also recommended is imiquimod 5% cream applied at bedtime 3 times a week for up to 16 weeks. The treatment area should be washed 6 to 10 h after treatment with Imiquimod. Cryotherapy in a physician's office is also a common therapy.

SYPHILIS INFECTIONS *Treponema pallidum,* a spirochete, is the causative agent of syphilis as well as yaws and pinta. It enters the body through mucous membranes or nonintact skin. It remains very sensitive to penicillin; thus diagnosis rather than treatment is the main difficulty in controlling this disease. The last 7 years has seen a marked increase in syphilis thought to be secondary to behavior associated with drug use. Syphilis occurs in three stages.

1. *Primary.* The initial stage of infection is characterized by a painless chancre with indurated borders on the penis, vulva, or other areas with sexual contact. The incubation period is about 21 days, with lesions then disappearing after 3 to 6 weeks. There are no constitutional symptoms, and a lesion may even be absent with primary disease.
2. *Secondary.* This stage, which occurs 3 to 6 weeks after the end of the primary stage, includes nonspecific symptoms such as sore throat, malaise, fever, and headaches. Rash and lymphadenopathy are the most common symptoms. The rash often starts on the trunk and flexor surfaces, spreading to the palms and soles. It takes on many forms but is often dull red and papular. This stage also resolves spontaneously.
3. *Tertiary (latent).* Involvement of the nervous and cardiovascular systems is characteristic of this stage, which may occur years after the initial infection. Specific manifestations range from acute meningitis, dementia, and neuropathy (tabes dorsalis) to thoracic aneurysm. Tertiary syphilis is uncommon.

Diagnosis Dark-field microscopy can be used to identify treponemes from primary lesions as well as from secondary lesions. Several serologic tests are available, including nontreponemal tests (rapid plasma reagin, VDRL) and specific treponemal antibody tests (fluorescent treponemal antibody absorption, or FTA-ABS). Nontreponemal tests are positive about 14 days after the appearance of the chancre and false positive in 1 to 2 percent of the population. FTA-ABS tests are slightly more sensitive and specific but more difficult to perform.

Treatment Given the multiple stages and manifestations of syphilis, considering the diagnosis is the most crucial part of treatment. Benzathine penicillin G 2.4 million units IM in a single dose has remained the standard of care. Doxycycline 100 mg PO bid for 2 weeks may be used for allergic individuals. Treatment of latent syphilis is usually three doses of penicillin as above, given 1 week apart.

HERPES SIMPLEX INFECTIONS Herpes simplex virus type 2 (HSV-2) or HSV-1 can cause genital herpes infections by infection of mucosal surfaces or nonintact skin. Primary infections are characterized by painful pustular or ulcerative lesions occurring 8 to 16 days after contact with an infected individual (although infections can be asymptomatic). Systemic symptoms are common and include fever, headache, and myalgias. Dysuria is common, whereas urinary retention secondary to swelling and pain is not uncommon. Approximately 80 percent of patients also have lymphadenopathy, and aseptic meningitis can occur. The untreated illness lasts 2 to 3 weeks to complete healing. Unfortunately, the virus remains latent, and recurrent infections occur in 60 to 90 percent of patients. These are usually milder and of shorter duration.

Diagnosis Clinical diagnosis of the painful vesiculopustular lesions is often possible. A smear may be taken of the lesions and stained to demonstrate large intranuclear inclusions, although this is less sensitive than direct culture. Viral cultures can be done and are positive in 1 to 4 days. New assays using ELISA and polymerase chain reactions are being developed.

Treatment For a first clinical episode, treatment is with acyclovir 400 mg PO tid for 7 to 10 days, acyclovir 200 mg PO 5 times a day for 7 to 10 days, famciclovir 250 mg PO tid for 7 to 10 days, or valacyclovir 1 g PO bid for 7 to 10 days. Treatment duration can be extended if the lesions persist. For treatment of proctitis or oral infections, higher doses are used (acyclovir 400 mg five times a day for 7 to 10 days). Acyclovir at 5 to 10 mg/kg of body weight may be given IV every 8 h for 5 to 7 days to patients requiring hospitalization.

Episodic recurrent infection should be treated for 5 days with acyclovir 400 mg PO tid, acyclovir 800 mg PO bid, famciclovir 125 mg PO bid, or valacyclovir 500 mg PO bid.

CHANCROID *Hemophilus ducreyi* is a pleomorphic gram-negative bacillus that causes genital ulcers and lymphadenitis. It is much more common in developing countries but has seen a resurgence in recent years in the United States. After an incubation period of 3 to 10 days, a tender papule appears at the site of infection, followed by ulceration of the lesion. Multiple lesions may be present in up to 50 percent of patients and may include bubo formation and spontaneous rupture. There are few constitutional symptoms.

Diagnosis Diagnosis can be made on clinical grounds, but other diseases such as syphilis need to be excluded. A swab of a lesion or pus from a bubo can be cultured but only with limited success.

Treatment Azithromycin 1 g PO in a single dose, ceftriaxone 250 mg IM in a single dose, ciprofloxacin 500 mg PO bid for 3 days, and erythromycin base 500 mg PO qid for 7 days are all recommended treatments.

LYMPHOGRANULOMA VENEREUM Specific serotypes of *C. trachomatis* cause this disease, which although endemic in other parts of the world is seen only sporadically in the United States. The primary lesion can take on many forms and be confused with other STDs (see Table 137-2). Ten days to 6 months following the initial lesion, an inguinal bubo forms (unilateral in 60 percent). The buboes continue to grow, either rupturing or forming firm inguinal masses.

Diagnosis Serologic tests and culture are the mainstays of diagnosis.

Treatment Doxycycline 100 mg PO bid for 21 days is the usual regimen. Table 137-1 gives alternative treatments.

TREATMENT DURING PREGNANCY

Pregnant patients with STDs should be referred to the physician providing their prenatal care. In general, penicillin, ceftriaxone, azithromycin, cefixime, metronidazole, and acyclovir are felt to be safe for use during pregnancy. If the safety of treatment is in doubt, an obstetrician should be consulted.

PROPHYLAXIS FOR EXPOSED PATIENTS

Patients who have been sexually exposed to a person known to have an STD should be treated presumptively for gonorrhea and chlamydial infections with one of the regimens described earlier. Cultures are usually taken for documentation purposes. Prophylaxis also should be given for victims of sexual assault. HIV prophylaxis is discussed in Chap. 149, and prophylaxis for herpes simplex infection has not been fully studied.

GENERAL RECOMMENDATIONS FOR TREATMENT AND FOLLOW-UP

When treating patients for STDs in the ED, it is important to remember that many STDs occur together; follow-up and compliance for many ED patients are poor, and lack of treatment can contribute to infertility. For these reasons, a standardized approach is suggested for patients with suspected STDs. This should include

1. Treating even when an STD is only suspected, especially for gonorrhea and chlamydia, with emphasis on single-dose treatments
2. Obtaining a serologic test for syphilis
3. Ascertaining pregnancy status and consulting obstetrics if the patient is pregnant
4. Reporting appropriate diseases to the state health department
5. Counseling patients about prevention of STDs
6. Counseling patients about the advisability of HIV testing
7. Counseling patients about advising partner(s) to seek treatment
8. Arranging for appropriate follow-up
9. Documenting all the preceding on the medical record

BIBLIOGRAPHY

Adimora AA, Hamilton H, Holmes KK, Sparling PF: *Sexually Transmitted Diseases: Companion Handbook.* New York: McGraw-Hill, 1994.

Berg E, Benson D, Haraszkiewicz P, et al: High prevalence of sexually transmitted diseases in women with urinary infections. *Acad Emerg Med* 3(11):1030, 1996.

Centers for Disease Control and Prevention: 1998 Guidelines for treatment of sexually transmitted diseases. *MMWR* 47:RR, 1998.

Scientific American Medicine SAM-CD: *Sexually Transmitted Diseases.* New York: Scientific American, December 1998.

138 TOXIC SHOCK SYNDROME AND STREPTOCOCCAL TOXIC SHOCK SYNDROME

Shawna J. Perry
Ann L. Harwood-Nuss

TOXIC SHOCK SYNDROME

Toxic shock syndrome (TSS) is a severe, life-threatening syndrome characterized by high fever, profound hypotension, diffuse erythroderma, mucous membrane hyperemia, pharyngitis, diarrhea, and constitutional symptoms. It can rapidly progress to multisystem dysfunction with severe electrolyte disturbances, renal failure, and shock. Although first described in 1978 by Todd in seven children with *Staphylococcus aureus* infections, TSS has been associated primarily with tampon use.[1] In 1981, a nationwide epidemic of TSS associated with extended tampon use was widely recognized among otherwise healthy young women.

TABLE 138-1 Case Definition of Toxic Shock Syndrome

An illness with the following clinical manifestations:
- Fever: temperature ⩾102.0°F (⩾38.9°C)
- Rash: diffuse macular erythroderma
- Desquamation: 1–2 weeks after onset of illness, particularly on the palms and soles
- Hypotension: systolic blood pressure ⩽90 mmHg for adults or less than fifth percentile by age for children aged <16 years; orthostatic drop in diastolic blood pressure greater than or equal to 15 mmHg from lying to sitting, orthostatic syncope, or orthostatic dizziness
- Multisystem involvement (three or more of the following)
  - Gastrointestinal: vomiting or diarrhea at onset of illness
  - Muscular: severe myalgia or creatine phosphokinase level at least twice the upper limit of normal
  - Mucous membrane: vaginal, oropharyngeal, or conjunctival hyperemia
  - Renal: blood urea nitrogen or creatinine at least twice the upper limit of normal for laboratory or urinary sediment with pyuria (greater than or equal to 5 leukocytes per high-power field) in the absence of urinary tract infection
  - Hepatic: total bilirubin, alanine aminotransferase enzyme, or asparate aminotransferase enzyme levels at least twice the upper limit of normal for laboratory
  - Hematologic: platelets less than 100,000/mL
  - Central nervous system: disorientation or alterations in consciousness without focal neurologic signs when fever and hypotension are absent

Laboratory criteria: negative results on the following tests, if obtained:
- Blood, throat, or cerebrospinal fluid cultures (blood culture may be positive for *Staphylococcus aureus*)
- Rise in titer to Rocky Mountain spotted fever, leptospirosis, or measles

Case classification
- Probable: a case in which five of the six clinical findings described above are present
- Confirmed: a case in which all six of the clinical findings described above are present, including desquamation, unless the patient dies before desquamation occurs

Source: From Centers for Disease Control,[10] with permission.

The TSS case definition is given in Table 138-1. This definition was formulated in 1980 and revised in 1997, by the Centers for Disease Control and Prevention (CDC) to ensure that cases included in various surveillance studies were the same clinical entity as TSS. In the absence of a definitive laboratory marker, the strict application of the case definition is warranted but undoubtedly excludes the less severe (subclinical) cases.[2]

The incidence of TSS has dropped precipitously over the past 20 years, with the majority of cases unrelated to menses and crossing all segments of society. A similar, but more menacing TSS-like syndrome, streptococcal toxic shock syndrome (STSS), has emerged over the last decade. It is associated with invasive and noninvasive streptococcal infections, has a rapidly progressive course, and a very high case-fatality rate.

Pathophysiology

ETIOLOGY AND PATHOGENESIS Most cases of TSS have been directly associated with colonization or infection with *S. aureus.* An exotoxin, toxic shock syndrome toxin (TSST-1) has been implicated as a significant factor in the production of symptoms associated with TSS, either through direct toxic effects on the host or through stimulation of secondary mediators in response to TSST-1. The biologic properties of TSST-1 include the ability to (1) induce fever directly on the hypothalamus or indirectly via interleukin 1 (IL-1) and tumor necrosis factor (TNF) production, (2) promote T-lymphocyte "super-antigenization" and overstimulation, (3) induce interferon production, (4) enhance delayed hypersensitivity, (5) suppress neutrophil migration and immunoglobulin secretion, and (6) enhance host susceptibility to endotoxins.

Ninety percent of menstrual-related cases of TSS (MRTSS) are caused by *S. aureus* strains that produce TSST-1, which is present in less than half of nonmenstrual-related TSS (NMTSS) cases. Enterotoxins B and C have been identified from isolates of NMTSS and have a biochemical structure almost identical to that of TSST-1. This explains the similarity in clinical manifestations of MRTSS and NMTSS. NMTSS may be mediated by unidentified precursors and toxins or by-products of TSST-1.[3]

The amount of TSST-1 produced by toxigenic strains of *S. aureus* in MRTSS is enhanced by certain vaginal conditions: temperature of 39 to 40°C (102.2 to 104°F), a neutral pH, a Po_2 of greater than 5 percent, and supplemental CO_2. These conditions can be met with the change in vaginal pH from acidic to neutral during menses and an increase in O_2 and CO_2 content of the vagina with the introduction of tampons or intravaginal devices. Other influences include synthetic fibers in tampon composition and a synergistic relationship between *S. aureus* and *Escherichia coli*.[4]

The most impressive aspect of the pathophysiology is the massive vasodilatation and rapid movement of the serum proteins and fluids from the intravascular to the extravascular space. Hypotension is accounted for by (1) decreased vasomotor tone, causing pooling of blood in the periphery and therein decreased central venous pressure and pulmonary capillary wedge pressure; (2) nonhydrostatic leakage of fluid into the interstitium, causing decreased intravascular volume and generalized nonpitting edema, primarily of the head and neck; (3) depressed cardiac function, including decreased wall motion and decreased shortening fraction; and (4) total body-water deficits secondary to vomiting, diarrhea, and fever.

Hypoalbuminemia, hypoferrinemia, and proteolysis caused by IL-1 are consistent with the peripheral edema, anemia, and rhabdomyolysis seen in TSS. TNF induces profound acidosis, shock, and multisystem organ failure in animal models similar to the effects of TSS. The multisystem organ failure may be a reflection of either a direct effect of the toxin on tissues or the rapid onset of hypotension and decreased perfusion.

The immunologic status of an individual plays a role in the pathogenesis of TSS, especially in cases of recurrence. Low convalescent titers to TSST-1 and enterotoxins B and C are found in the majority of patients with TSS for up to 1 year after infection.[3]

EPIDEMIOLOGY CDC surveillance of TSS from 1979 through 1996 reported 5296 definite and probable cases (Fig. 138-1). From 1981 through 1987, there was a dramatic decrease in the number of reported cases. In 1992, only 44 definite cases, 51 probable cases, and 3 deaths occurred from TSS. Of the 44 definite cases, 20 occurred during menstruation. The decrease in cases is presumably due to changes in the composition of tampons, general public awareness of the risks of tampon use, and increased medical awareness and detection. Although the use of contraceptive sponges and diaphragms places the individual at risk, their exact contribution to the development of TSS is unclear.

TSS was initially a disease of young, healthy, menstruating women; 50 percent of cases reported in 1986 and 1987 were found in this group. Tampon use increased the risk of TSS in susceptible females by 33 times. *S. aureus* has been isolated from the vaginas of 98 percent of women with TSS, compared to an 8 to 10 percent carrier rate in control subjects. It is presumed that women who develop menstrual TSS are colonized with *S. aureus* before the onset of menstruation.

The proportion of NMTSS cases has increased since 1980 (59 percent), primarily because of the decrease in the number of menstruation-related cases. The absolute number of cases of NMTSS has remained relatively constant, however. Nearly 25 percent of NMTSS cases are associated with postpartum and *S. aureus* vaginal infections.[5] There is an increasing incidence of NMTSS in males. Men constitute one-third of patients with TSS, with a mortality rate 3.3 times that of MRTSS in women. A 50 percent mortality rate has been reported in non-TSST-1 *S. aureus* infections (i.e., enterotoxin B or C), while a 10 percent rate has been reported in TSST-1–producing *S. aureus* infections.

The means by which *S. aureus* enters the host in TSS are numerous and have been well documented in a wide variety of clinical settings. TSS has also been reported following influenza and influenza-like illnesses and is associated with a significant mortality rate (43 percent). Nasal packing (nasal tampons) is also associated with TSS, with 20 to 40 percent of the adult population carrying *S. aureus* in the nasal vestibule.

Clinical Features

TSS should be considered in any unexplained febrile illness associated with erythroderma, hypotension, and diffuse organ pathology. Diagnostic criteria for TSS are listed in Table 138-1. Patients with MRTSS usually present between the third and fifth day of menses. The median time to onset of illness in postsurgical NMTSS is two postoperative days. There appears to be a spectrum of severity of TSS. Mild cases of TSS may be excluded from the CDC case definition. Mild TSS is generally characterized by fever and chills, myalgias, abdominal pain, sore throat, nausea, vomiting, and diarrhea. Hypotension is usually not present, and the illness is self-limited. Severe TSS is an acute-onset, multisystem disease with symptoms, signs, and laboratory abnormalities reflecting multiple-organ involvement. Headache is the most common complaint. Some patients may experience a prodrome consisting of malaise, myalgias, headache, nausea, vomiting, and diarrhea. Sudden onset of fever and chills occurs approximately 1 to 4 days prior to presentation. Diffuse myalgias, particularly in the proximal aspects of the extremities, abdomen, and back, are reported by virtually all patients; arthralgias are also common. Profuse, watery diarrhea and repeated vomiting are reported by 90 to 98 percent of patients. Orthostatic lightheadedness or syncope may be present. Patients also complain of sore throat, headache, paresthesias, and photophobia. The patient may complain of abdominal pain, cough, or sore throat.

Physical examination reveals hypotension or an orthostatic decrease in systolic pressure of 15 mmHg in all cases. In general, victims of TSS appear acutely ill. The initial state usually lasts about 24 to 48 h; the patient may be obtunded, disoriented, oliguric, and hypotensive. There is an overall body-fluid deficit due to losses from fever, vomiting, diarrhea, and decreased systemic vascular resistance. Depressed cardiac function may also be present. Patients may show nonpitting edema of the face and extremities secondary to nonhydrostatic leakage of intravascular fluid into the interstitium. Other prominent signs may include profound muscle weakness and tenderness or abdominal tenderness. The diarrhea is usually watery and profuse, frequently with associated incontinence. One-half to three-quarters of patients have pharyngitis, with a strawberry-red tongue; conjunctival hyperemia and vaginitis are also seen. Tender, edematous external genitalia, diffuse vaginal hyperemia, "strawberry" cervix, scant purulent cervical discharge, and bilateral adnexal tenderness are seen in 25 to 35 percent of patients with menstruation-related TSS.

The rash of TSS is a diffuse, blanching erythroderma, classically described as painless "sunburn," which fades within 3 days of its appearance and is followed by full-thickness desquamation, especially of the palms and soles, during convalescence. This CDC criterion is most often missed, since it may be subtle or difficult to detect in darkly pigmented patients. Variations include patchy erythroderma and localized maculopustular eruptions. In all cases, a fine, generalized desquamation of the skin, with peeling over the soles, fingers, toes,

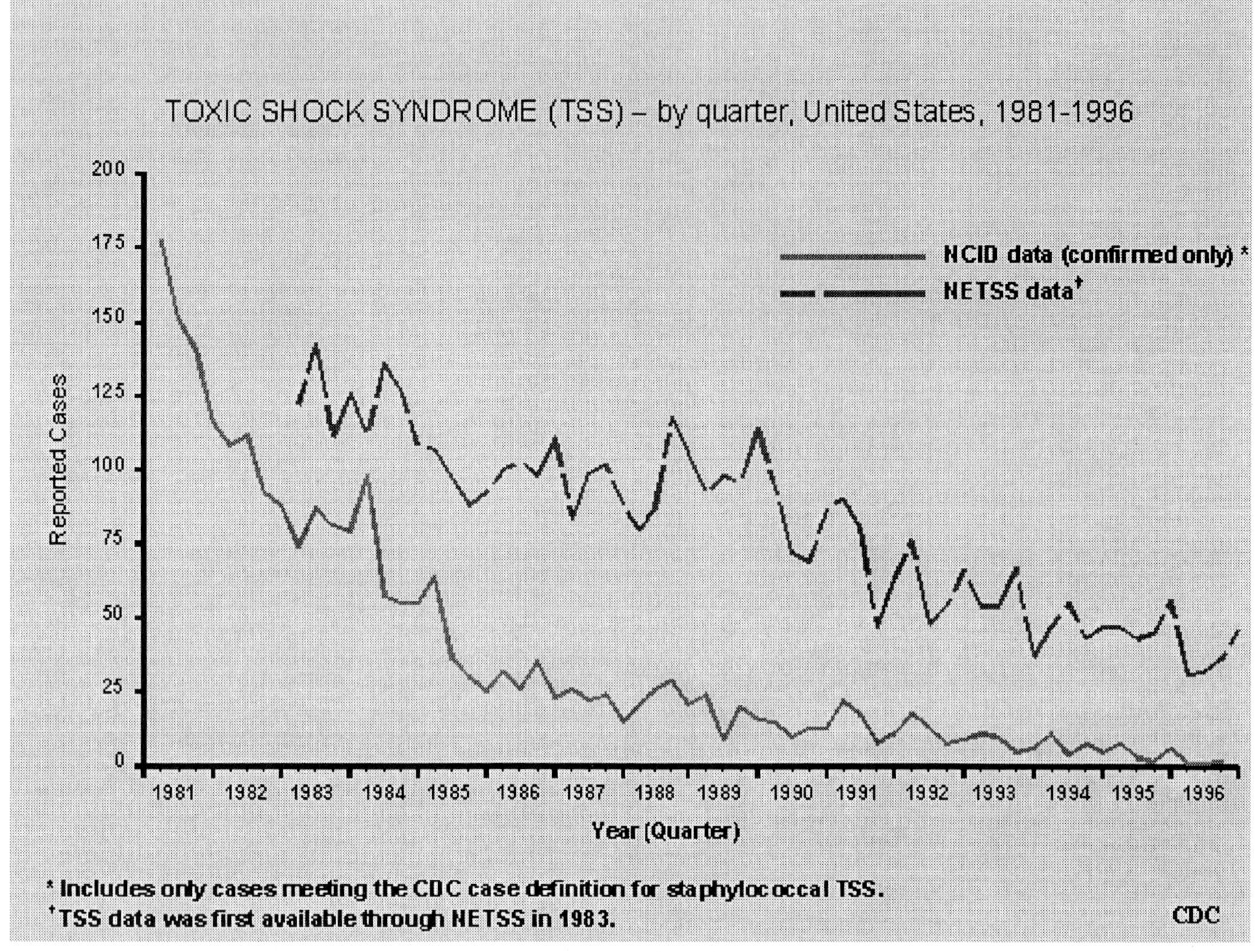

FIG. 138-1. Toxic shock syndrome by quarter in the United States, 1981 to 1996.

and palms, occurs from 6 to 14 days after the onset of illness. Most severely ill patients experience loss of hair and nails 2 to 3 months later.

Specific focal neurologic findings rarely occur. Patients present with varying degrees of altered consciousness. Approximately 75 percent of patients have nonfocal neurologic abnormalities without signs of meningeal irritation. Confusion, disorientation, agitation, hysteria, somnolence, and seizures have been reported, consistent with a toxic encephalopathy from cerebral edema. If the clinical picture is unclear, a computed tomography scan and lumbar puncture should be performed. Figure 138-2 illustrates the temporal relationships of the major manifestations of TSS.

Abnormal laboratory values reflect the multisystem involvement in TSS. Leukocytosis, with an increase in immature forms, is frequently seen; lymphocytopenia has also been reported. A mild anemia with acute hypoferrinemia and abnormal peripheral smears consistent with microangiopathic hemolytic anemia or disseminated intravascular coagulation may be found. Azotemia, myoglobinuria, and abnormal urinary sediment (sterile pyuria and red blood cell casts) are seen as acute renal failure develops. Liver function abnormalities and hyperbilirubinemia are seen in approximately 3 percent of patients with clinical evidence of coagulopathy. Metabolic acidosis secondary to hypotension is also seen. Electrolyte abnormalities, including hypocalcemia, hypophosphatemia, hyponatremia, and hypokalemia, are common. Hypocalcemia is out of proportion to the degree of hypoalbuminemia and may be difficult to correct if there is a concomitant decrease in the serum magnesium level.

Acute renal failure secondary to acute tubular necrosis is a complication of TSS. It appears to be secondary to prerenal deficits, renal ischemia caused by hypotension, rhabdomyolysis, and possibly direct damage from TSST-1 mediators. Ventricular arrhythmias, bundle branch block, first-degree heart block, and T-wave and ST-T-wave changes have been reported. Echocardiography of patients with TSS shows wall motion abnormalities and decreased shortening fraction, suggestive of toxic cardiomyopathy. Adult respiratory distress syndrome (ARDS) with refractory hypotension represents the ultimate end-organ damage secondary to TSS.

Diagnosis

Other systemic illnesses characterized by fever, rash, diarrhea, myalgias, and multisystem involvement resemble TSS (Table 138-2). Kawasaki disease (mucocutaneous lymph node syndrome) is characterized by fever, conjunctival hyperemia, and erythema of the mucous membranes with desquamation. Although the exanthems may be quite similar. Kawasaki disease may present with target lesions resembling erythema multiforme, and the bright-red appearance of the vermillion border is not common in TSS. Furthermore, over 80 percent of those afflicted with Kawasaki disease are under 5 years of age, and Kawasaki disease is not characterized by hypotension, renal failure, or thrombocytopenia.

Staphylococcal scalded skin syndrome (SSSS) is most commonly seen in children less than 5 years of age and is characterized by fever,

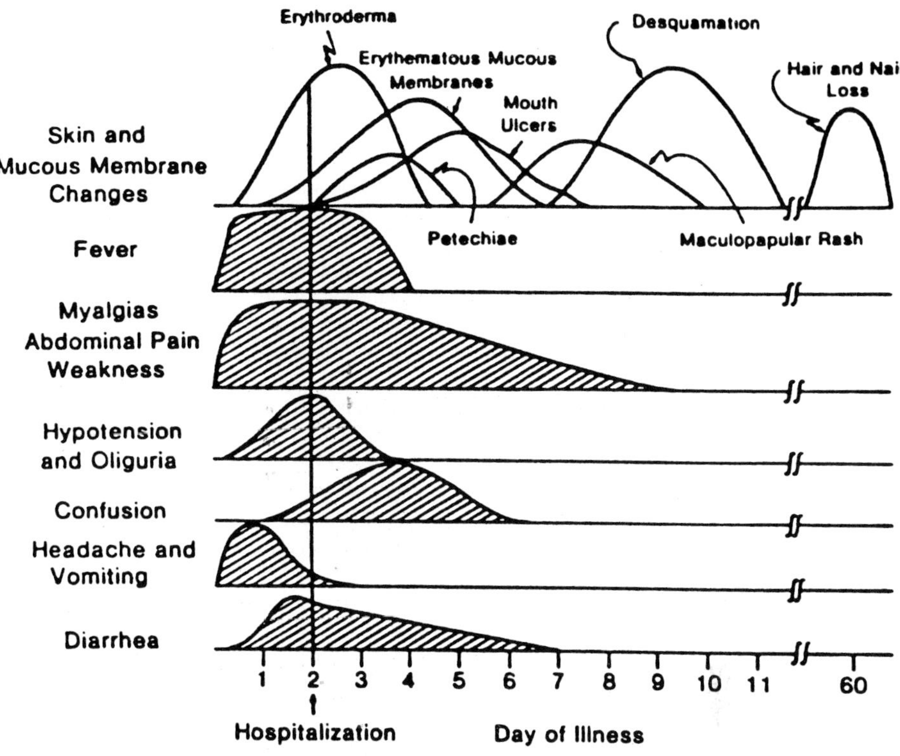

FIG. 138-2. Composite drawing of major systemic, skin, and mucous membrane manifestations of toxic shock syndrome. (From Chesney PJ, David JP, Purdy WK, et al: Clinical manifestations of toxic shock syndrome. *JAMA* 246:741, 1981, with permission.)

generalized painful erythroderma, and conjunctivitis. SSSS may be distinguished from TSS by its lack of multisystem involvement. In contrast, staphylococcal scarlet fever is so similar to TSS, with full-thickness desquamation, that only pathologic specimens or serologic evidence of the exfoliatin toxin will differentiate the two entities. In streptococcal scarlet fever, the "sandpaper" rash is distinct from the macular "sunburn" rash of TSS.

Rocky Mountain spotted fever, a rickettsial infection acquired from tick bites, has a presentation similar to that of TSS, but the rash is usually petechial and delayed in onset. Toxic epidermal necrolysis resembles SSSS and occurs primarily in adults. Non-toxin-mediated, it is related to drug exposure and has a bullous component. Erythema multiforme can be associated with fever, pharyngeal erythema, and toxemia. The rash is multiform, with symmetric involvement of the lower extremities. Immunologically mediated from a drug exposure or infectious agent, it can progress to Stevens-Johnson syndrome.

Septic shock must always be considered in the differential diagnosis of TSS. In general, the appearance of a rash and the laboratory abnormalities associated with TSS will aid in distinguishing these two entities.

TABLE 138-2 Differential Diagnosis of Toxic Shock Syndrome

Acute pyelonephritis	Acute viral syndrome
Septic shock	Leptospirosis
Acute rheumatic fever	Systemic lupus erythematosus
Streptococcal scarlet fever	Rocky Mountain spotted fever
Staphylococcal scarlet fever	Tick typhus
Staphylococcal scalded skin syndrome	Gastroenteritis
Legionnaire disease	Kawasaki disease
Pelvic inflammatory disease	Reye syndrome
Hemolytic uremic syndrome	Toxic epidermal necrolysis
	Erythema multiforme

Treatment

Management of TSS depends on its severity. The most important aspect of initial treatment is the aggressive management of circulatory shock. Continuous monitoring of the heart rate, respiratory rate, blood pressure, oxygen saturation, urinary output, and central venous pressure is essential. Pulmonary capillary wedge pressure monitoring may also be needed in severe cases. During the first 24 h, patients may require 4 to 20 L of crystalloid and fresh-frozen plasma. There have been reports of patients requiring up to 20 L of fluid in the first 24 h of hospitalization. A dopamine infusion beginning at 5 to 20 (μg/kg)/min may be used if volume correction fails to restore normal arterial pressure. Large amounts of intravenous fluid and pressors to treat refractory hypotension can result in the rapid onset of pulmonary edema. ARDS may then complicate TSS and require mechanical ventilation with positive end-expiratory pressure.

Evaluation must include arterial blood gas analysis, complete blood count screen with peripheral smear, serum electrolyte determinations including Mg^{2+} and Ca^{2+}, coagulation studies, urinalysis, and chest radiograph. Patients with abnormal coagulation profiles and evidence of bleeding require colloid replacement, fresh-frozen plasma, or transfusions. Thrombocytopenia may require platelet transfusions. An electrocardiogram and echocardiogram may also be indicated.

A focus of infection should be aggressively sought and promptly treated. Cultures of all potentially infected sites should be obtained, including blood cultures, prior to initiating antibiotic therapy. Women with tampon-related TSS should have the tampon removed. Some authors recommend irrigation of the vagina with saline or povidoneiodine solution. Early consultation with a surgeon or a gynecologist is recommended if drainage or debridement of infectious sites is warranted.

Although antimicrobial agents have not been shown to affect the outcome of the acute illness, they are recommended and have been given to most patients to eradicate the focus of toxin-producing staphylococci as well as to decrease the recurrence rate. Antibiotic selection should include an antistaphylococcal penicillin or cephalosporin with β-lactamase stability. Nafcillin or oxacillin in doses of 1 to 2 g every 4 h provides adequate antimicrobial coverage. Cefazolin, 2 g every 6 h, also provides adequate coverage, but the first-generation cephalosporins are less β-lactamase-stable than the antistaphylococcal penicillins. In penicillin-allergic patients, clindamycin, vancomycin, and first-generation cephalosporins can be used. Vancomycin or trimethoprim-sulfamethoxazole may be used if methicillin-resistant strains are encountered. Although data on the optimum duration of antimicrobial therapy are not available, it seems prudent to administer parenteral antibiotics for at least 3 days or until the patient clinically improves. Oral antistaphylococcal antibiotics (dicloxacillin or clindamycin in penicillin-allergic patients) should then be administered for an additional 10 to 14 days. Methylprednisolone and intravenous immunoglobulin have shown improvement in some cases of TSS.[6]

Most patients become afebrile and normotensive within 48 h of hospitalization. Initial laboratory abnormalities resolve within 1 to 2 weeks, although full anemia correction occurs in 4 to 6 weeks.

Numerous sequelae of TSS have been reported and include late onset of maculopapular rash, decreased renal function, reversible loss of hair and nails, prolonged neuromuscular abnormalities, and cyanotic extremities. Neurologic deficits are common, with 50 percent of patients exhibiting residual memory deficits, decreased ability to concentrate, and diffuse electroencephalographic abnormalities.

The mechanism responsible for these sequelae is not yet clear; it has been suggested that they are due to either the delayed effects of the toxin or circulating immune complexes or are drug-mediated.

Patients not treated with β-lactamase-stable antimicrobial drugs have recurrence of the disease.[7] Most recurrent episodes of MRTSS occur by the second month following the initial episode and happen on the same day of menses as the prior attack, although some have recurred in less than 1 month and some more than 1 year later. In the majority of patients having recurrence, convalescent antibody titers are low and nonprotective. The initial episode is the most severe, although deaths have resulted from recurrences of initially mild cases of TSS.

The risk of MRTSS has decreased as a result of changes in tampon components and public education about correct tampon usage. During the outbreak of the 1980s, some tampons were composed of polyester foam and cross-linked carboxymethcellulose (polyacrylate), which provided increased absorbency and encouraged longer periods of use. Tampons are now composed of cotton and rayon. Since 1990, the US Food and Drug Administration has required a limit on tampon absorbency into one of four ranges (junior, regular, super, and super-plus) corresponding to the level of flow. Tampons should be changed every 4 to 8 h, and patients with a history of MRTSS are discouraged from their use.

STREPTOCOCCAL TOXIC SHOCK SYNDROME

The decline in the incidence of TSS in the late 1980s was closely followed by the emergence of an even more serious illness. Initially classified as streptococcal toxic shock-like syndromes (TSLS) by the CDC, a consensus definition was formulated in 1993. It was identical to the case definition for TSS except that TSLS develops in association with a severe soft-tissue infection and culture results from a normally sterile site must be positive for *Streptococcus pyogenes* [group A streptococcus (GAS)]. In 1995, the CDC published a new case definition for streptococcal toxic shock syndrome (STSS); the current case definition, as published in 1997, is shown in Table 138-3.[8,9]

STSS is defined as any group A streptococcal infection associated with invasive soft tissue infection, the early onset of shock, and organ failure. Similar in presentation to TSS, STSS is associated with a higher mortality rate, may occur in patients of all ages, and may occur in most countries of the world. Labeled the "flesh-eating bacteria," the most serious GAS soft tissue infections associated with STSS are streptococcal necrotizing fasciitis and streptococcal myositis.

TABLE 138-3 Case Definition of Streptococcal Toxic Shock Syndrome

An illness with the following clinical manifestations occurring within the first 48 h of hospitalization or, for a nosocomial case, within the first 48 h of illness:

- Hypotension defined by a systolic blood pressure less than or equal to 90 mmHg for adults or less than the fifth percentile by age for children aged less than 16 years
- Multiorgan involvement characterized by two or more of the following:
  - Renal impairment: creatinine greater than or equal to 2 mg/dL (≥177 μ/L) for adults or greater than or equal to twice the upper limit of normal for age; in patients with preexisting renal disease, a greater than twofold elevation over the baseline level
  - Coagulopathy: platelets less than or equal to 100,000/mL (≤100 × 106/L) or disseminated intravascular coagulation, defined by prolonged clotting times, low fibrinogen level, and the presence of fibrin degradation products
  - Liver involvement: alanine aminotransferase, aspartate aminotransferase, or total bilirubin levels greater than or equal to twice the upper limit of normal for the patient's age; in patients with preexisting liver disease, a greater than twofold increase over the baseline level
  - Acute respiratory distress syndrome: defined by acute onset of diffuse pulmonary infiltrates and hypoxemia in the absence of cardiac failure or by evidence of diffuse capillary leak manifested by acute onset of generalized edema, or pleural or peritoneal effusions with hypoalbuminemia
  - A generalized erythematous macular rash that may desquamate
  - Soft tissue necrosis, including necrotizing fasciitis or myositis, or gangrene

Laboratory criteria for diagnosis
- Isolation of group A streptococcus

Case classification
- Probable: a case that meets the clinical case definition in the absence of another identified etiology for the illness and with isolation of group A streptococcus from a nonsterile site.
- Confirmed: a case that meets the clinical case definition and with isolation of group A streptococcus from a normally sterile site (e.g., blood or cerebrospinal fluid or, less commonly, joint, pleural, or pericardial fluid)

Source: From Centers for Disease Control,[9] with permission.

STSS associated with GAS invasive infections, in contrast to previous reports of GAS bacteremia, most commonly affects individuals between the ages of 20 and 50 *without* predisposing illnesses.[10] There is regional variability in populations at risk for developing STSS and necrotizing fasciitis from GAS infections. Extremes of age, diabetes, alcoholism, drug abuse, and immunodeficiency appear to be risk factors for GAS invasive infections.[11,12]

It is estimated that in the United States each year there are 2000 to 3000 cases of STSS and 500 to 1500 cases of necrotizing fasciitis.[9] The mortality rate is very high for STSS, at 30 to 80 percent.[12] In patients with STSS, 70 percent of the soft tissue infections progress to necrotizing fasciitis or myositis requiring surgical intervention. The morbidity rate of STSS is 65 to 80 percent, associated with surgical intervention to control the infection.[11,12,13] The mortality rate for streptococcal myositis is 85 percent, and that for necrotizing fasciitis is 20 to 50 percent.[12] The rate of recurrence is unknown.

Epidemiology

Although severe invasive infections caused by *S. pyogenes* (GAS) have been reported with increasing frequency during the past decade, it is not entirely clear whether these reports reflect an actual increase in the incidence of disease or increased awareness. The latter is likely, due to the dramatic nature of the infections and the coining of the phrase ''flesh-eating bacteria'' by the tabloid press to describe invasive necrotizing infections caused by GAS. It is believed that there has been a true, recent increase in the GAS virulence properties that may account for the changes in clinical diseases caused by GAS. Few population-based studies exist on its prevalence. Reports on the incidence range from 1.5/100,000 population in Canada to 4.4 /100,000 in the Arizona.[11,13] STSS may be underdiagnosed when associated with GAS invasive infections, since 90 percent of patients are in shock or develop shock within 4 to 6 h of admission. Prospective population-based surveillance studies from Canada from 1991 through 1995 demonstrated an incidence of STSS associated with necrotizing fasciitis to be 13 to 46 percent.[11,13] There have also been recent reports of toxic shock-like syndrome caused by non-group A streptococcal infection, specifically groups B, C, and G. In 1998, a documented group B streptococcal necrotizing fasciitis and STS-like syndrome was reported in three patients with significant underlying disease; the authors postulate that group B streptococcus has acquired an increased ability to cause fasciitis and may be the cause of a new clinical syndrome in adults.[14,15,16]

Pathophysiology

The resurgence of GAS invasive infections appears to be the result of the production of more virulent exotoxins from the M-type isolates of GAS. Streptococcal pyogenic exotoxins (SPEs) are produced by 90 percent of GAS isolates.[16] Three distinct exotoxins (SPEs A, B, C) have been identified. SPE A, also known as the scarlet fever toxin, is the most powerful and most frequently found SPE in STSS. It has a molecular structure similar to that of enterotoxin B of NMTSS. The SPEs A and B display features similar to those of TSS-mediated exotoxins, including pyrogenicity, superactivation of T cells, and synthesis of TNF, IL-1, and IL-6.[16] These powerful cytokines can induce severe acidosis, shock, and multisystem organ failure, as in TSS. The effects of the ''superantigens'' SPE A and SPE B are hypothesized to be similar to yet more profound than those of TSST-1, with greater induction of TNF, IL-1, IL-6, and other cytokines, thereby causing more severe signs and symptoms.[16] The patients suspected of being most at risk for developing STSS are those without immunity to M-type 1 SPE A- or B-producing strains of GAS. The SPE C has been found in fewer GAS isolates, and its role in STSS is not clear.

The portal of entry of streptococci cannot be proven in about 50 percent of cases and can only be presumed in many others.[12] Most commonly, infection begins at a site of minor local trauma, usually without disruption of the skin. Cases have developed from burns, lacerations, abrasions, hematomas, minor nonpenetrating muscle injuries, surgical procedures, and recent infections with varicella or influenza.[12]

Clinical Features

Pain is the most common initial symptom of STSS, usually of abrupt onset, severe, and preceding tenderness or physical findings.[12] Eighty percent of patients have signs of soft tissue infection; this progresses to necrotizing fasciitis or myositis in 70 percent of patients. Although most commonly affecting the extremities, the location of the pain may suggest an intraabdominal process, such as peritonitis or pelvic inflammatory disease, or other conditions, such as pneumonia or pericarditis. Up to 20 percent of patients may experience a prodromal influenza-like episode including fever, chills, myalgias, and diarrhea. Fever is the most common early sign. Confusion is present in 55 percent of patients, and coma or combativeness may also occur. Other early signs and symptoms of STSS may include dizziness, diffuse rash, and abdominal pain. The initial diagnosis of STSS may be difficult, if not impossible, to distinguish from TSS. If necrotizing fasciitis is present, fever, severe pain, swelling, and redness at the site of the wound are seen. Myositis is an uncommon complication of invasive GAS infection, with a very high fatality rate. The most common symptom is severe pain; swelling and erythema may be the only early physical findings. Muscle compartment syndromes may develop rapidly.

On physical examination, fever is the most common presenting sign, followed closely by shock. Shock is apparent at presentation or develops within 4 to 8 h of admission in virtually all patients with STSS. It may be refractory to treatment or require massive volume replacement. The development at the site of the soft tissue infection of vesicles and bullae with progression to violaceous or blue discoloration is considered an ominous sign of necrotizing fasciitis or myositis. ARDS develops in 55 percent of patients, usually following the onset of hypotension; intubation is required in the majority of cases. A diffuse erythematous rash is much less prevalent in STSS (10 percent), but if it does occur, there is desquamation.

Laboratory evaluation shows mild elevation in the white blood cell count (13,000) with a profound bandemia as high as 40 to 50 percent. Liver function test values may be two times normal; decreased platelet levels and disseminated intravascular coagulopathy may be seen. Renal dysfunction persists or progresses in all patients; dialysis is commonly required. Creatinine kinase levels become elevated if the soft tissue infection becomes necrotizing. Blood cultures are positive for GAS in 60 percent of patients, and more than 90 percent of patients with STSS have positive tissue culture results with a known site of infection.[11] One recent report suggests that magnetic resonance imaging may be useful in the early diagnosis of GAS necrotizing fasciitis.[17] Definitive diagnosis of STSS is made by positive GAS culture results from a normally sterile site in addition to the clinical and laboratory parameters defined in the case definition (Table 138-3).

Diagnosis

The differential diagnosis is the same as for TSS (see Table 138-2) with the significant addition of invasive and noninvasive GAS infections, necrotizing fasciitis, myositis, and serious infections caused by *Clostridium perfringens, Clostridium septicum,* and mixed organisms, such as anearobic and aerobic bacteria.

Treatment

The initial treatment of STSS is similar to that of TSS, with aggressive management of shock and early use of vasopressors (see ''Treatment'' under ''Toxic Shock Syndrome''). Antibiotic therapy should be initiated immediately in the emergency department to treat STSS and the associated infection, if present; intravenous penicillin G, 24 million U/day in divided doses, and intravenous clindamycin, 900 mg every 8 h.[12] Erythromycin should be used in penicillin-allergic patients. Intravenous immunoglobulin may be useful in the treatment of invasive GAS infections associated with STSS.[18] Although antibiotics are important, prompt and aggressive exploration and débridement of suspected deep-seated *S. pyogenes* infection are mandatory. If STSS is suspected, immediate surgical consultation is indicated, since 70 percent of patients with STSS require débridement, fasciotomy, or amputation.

Disposition

All patients suspected of having STSS should be admitted to an intensive care unit.

REFERENCES

1. Todd J: Toxic-shock syndrome associated with phage group-1 staphylococci. *Lancet* 2:1116, 1978.
2. Centers for Disease Control: Case definition for toxic shock syndrome. *MMWR* 46:30, 1997.

3. Chance TD: Toxic shock syndrome: Role of the environment, the host and the microorganism. *Br J Biomed Sci* 53:284, 1996.
4. Berkley SF: The relationship of tampon characteristics to menstrual toxic shock syndrome. *JAMA* 258:917, 1987.
5. Kain KC: Clinical spectrum of nonmenstrual toxic shock syndrome (NMTSS): Comparison with menstrual TSS by multivariate discriminant analyses. *Clin Infect Dis* 16:100, 1993.
6. Todd J: Corticosteroid therapy for patients with toxic shock syndrome. *JAMA* 252:3399, 1984.
7. Chesney PJ: Toxic shock syndrome: Management and long-term sequelae. *Ann Intern Med* 96:84, 1982.
8. Centers for Disease Control, National Center for Infectious Diseases, Division of Bacterial and Mycotic Diseases: Group A Streptococcus Fact Sheet. November 20, 1996.
9. Centers for Disease Control: Case definitions for infectious conditions under public surveillance. *MMWR* 46:34, 1997.
10. Stevens DL: Streptococcal toxic-shock syndrome: Spectrum of disease, pathogenesis, and new concepts in treatment. *Emerg Infect Dis* 1(3):1, 1995.
11. Davies HD: Invasive group A streptococcal infections in Ontario, Canada. *N Engl J Med* 335:547, 1996.
12. Kaul R: Population-based surveillance for group A streptococcal necrotizing fasciitis: Clinical features, prognostic indicators, and microbiologic analysis of seventy-seven cases, Ontario Group A Streptococcal Study. *Am J Med* 103:18, 1997.
13. Gardam MA: Group B streptococcal necrotizing fasciitis and streptococcal toxic shock-like syndrome in adults. *Arch Intern Med* 158:1704, 1998.
14. Hirose Y: Toxic shock-like syndrome caused by non-group A beta-hemolytic streptococci. *Arch Intern Med* 157:1891,1997.
15. Stevens DL: Severe streptococcal infections associated with a toxic shock-like syndrome and scarlet fever toxin A. *N Engl J Med* 321:1, 1989.
16. Hackett SP: Superantigens associated with staphylococcal and streptococcal toxic shock syndrome are potent inducers of tumor necrosis factor synthesis. *J Infect Dis* 168:232, 1993.
17. Drake DB, Woods JA, Bill TJ: Magnetic resonance imaging in the early diagnosis of group A beta streptococcal necrotizing fasciitis: A case report. *J Emerg Med* 16:403, 1998.
18. Lamothe F: Clinical usefulness of intravenous human immunoglobulins in invasive group A streptococcal infections: Case report and review. *Clin Infect Dis* 21:1469, 1995.

TABLE 139-1 Indicator Conditions for Case Definitions of AIDS

Esophageal candidiasis
Cryptococcosis
Cryptosporidiosis
CMV retinitis
Herpes simplex virus
Kaposi's sarcoma
Brain lymphoma
Mycobacterium avium complex
PCP
Progressive multifocal leukoencephalopathy
Brain toxoplasmosis
HIV encephalopathy
HIV wasting syndrome
Disseminated histoplasmosis
Isosporiasis
Disseminated MTB disease
Recurrent *Salmonella* septicemia
CD4 cell count <200 cells/μL*
Pulmonary tuberculosis*
Recurrent bacterial pneumonia*
Invasive cervical cancer*

*Added in 1993.

139 HIV INFECTION AND AIDS

Richard E. Rothman
Gabor D. Kelen

HIV causes a wide spectrum of diseases ranging from asymptomatic infection to life-threatening illnesses and may involve virtually any organ system. The signs and symptoms associated with complications are frequently nonspecific, and the social problems faced by this population are unusually complex. While the development of antiretroviral therapies has been found to slow the progression of opportunistic infections, an increasing array of therapeutic complications has emerged.

EPIDEMIOLOGY

The first reported cases of AIDS were described in 1981 when individuals with *Pneumocystis carinii* pneumonia and Kaposi sarcoma were discovered among previously healthy homosexual men. The principal pathologic characteristic of AIDS was subsequently determined to be a defect in cell-mediated immunity. In 1983, isolation of a retrovirus (HIV) established the etiologic basis of AIDS. The development of an antibody assay for HIV in 1985 allowed for serologic diagnosis of infected individuals and led to an appreciation of the major modes and principal risk factors for HIV transmission.

The diagnosis of AIDS is most commonly made with laboratory evidence of HIV infection and the presence of one or more "indicator conditions." The most recent Centers for Disease Control and Prevention (CDC) definition of AIDS for reporting purposes was published in 1993 (Table 139-1).[1] The case definition of AIDS includes either the presence of one or more indicator conditions (now including pulmonary tuberculosis, recurrent bacterial pneumonia, or invasive cervical cancer), or a laboratory measure of severe immunosuppression (CD4 T-lymphocyte count <200 cells/μL).

Worldwide, the number of patients with HIV is continuing to grow dramatically, with current estimates of 30.6 million people living with HIV or AIDS. Since the beginning of the epidemic, 11.7 million people are reported to have died from HIV-related illnesses. If current trends continue, 60 to 70 million people will be infected with HIV by the year 2000. Developing countries, the least equipped to deal with the epidemic, have been hit particularly hard.

In the United States, HIV surveillance has improved as a result of new laws requiring mandatory reporting of HIV seropositivity in over 20 states. As of December 31, 1997, there were an estimated 1.1 million people infected with HIV (approximately 1 in every 250 Americans). Reported cases of AIDS number 641,086, and 390,692 patients with HIV-related deaths have been described.[2] AIDS is now the leading cause of death among American men 25 to 44 years old and the third leading cause of death among women in the same age group. Regional trends have changed markedly over the past decade. While more than 50 percent of AIDS cases occurred in five urban centers through 1987

TABLE 139-2 Distribution of AIDS Cases by Mechanism of Transmission, % Cases

Primary Risk Factor	1981–1987	1988–1992	1993–1995
Male homosexual contact	64.0	54.6	50.8
Injected drug use	17.2	24.2	27.3
Male homosexuality plus injected drug use	8.3	7.0	5.6
Heterosexual contact	2.5	6.1	10.1
Transfusion recipient	2.6	1.9	1.0
Perinatal transmission	1.2	1.5	1.0
Hemophilia	1.0	0.9	0.8
No risk reported	3.2	3.9	9.2

Source: From Centers for Disease Control and Prevention, with permission.[3]

(New York, San Francisco, Los Angeles, Newark, and Miami), the majority of new HIV cases now occur outside these centers, with the most significant increases seen in smaller metropolitan areas.

Risk factors commonly associated with HIV infection include homosexuality or bisexuality, injected drug use, heterosexual exposure, receipt of a blood transfusion prior to 1985, and vertical and horizontal maternal-neonatal transmission. The change in the distribution of AIDS cases by mechanism of transmission since the start of the HIV epidemic is shown in Table 139-2.[3]

Increasing use of emergency department services by HIV-infected persons is due in part to changes in the demographic distribution of HIV cases and AIDS-related illnesses.[4] In homosexual and bisexual men, rates of newly acquired HIV, HIV progression to AIDS, and AIDS-related deaths have all declined (largely due to access to antiretroviral therapy and, in part, to effective prevention strategies). Meanwhile, rates of new HIV infection have continued to rise among young, disadvantaged, minority populations who utilize the emergency department for both primary and emergency care. During the past several years, the highest percentages of increase in reported AIDS cases have occurred among women, minority populations, and children. These changes are principally due to an increase in HIV prevalence among injected drug users and their women partners. Seroprevalence studies in one inner-city emergency department reflect these trends, with rates of HIV infection among unselected adult patients rising from 6 to 11.4 percent over a 4-year period.[4]

PATHOPHYSIOLOGY

HIV is a cytopathic retrovirus that kills infected cells. The viral genes are carried as a single-stranded RNA molecule within the viral particle. Following infection, the virus selectively attacks host cells involved in immune function, primarily CD4 T lymphocytes. Within the host cell, the RNA template is reverse-transcribed into DNA (using the enzyme reverse transcriptase), which then becomes permanently integrated into the host's genome. Once integrated, retroviral DNA may lie dormant or be activity-transcribed and translated to produce virally encoded proteins and new HIV virions. Activation of viral protein precursors into the functional enzymes required for virion infectivity is carried out by HIV protease.

The HIV virion is composed of a central RNA molecule and reverse transcriptase protein surrounded by a core protein encased by a lipid bilayer envelope. Two virally encoded transmembrane proteins, gp41 and gp120, play a critical role in the recognition and attachment of HIV virions to receptors on host CD4 lymphocytes. As a result of infection, immunologic abnormalities eventually occur, including lymphopenia, qualitative CD4 T-lymphocyte function defects, and autoimmune phenomena. Profound defects in cellular immunity ultimately result in a variety of opportunistic infections and neoplasms.

Antiretroviral therapy is directed at reducing levels of HIV RNA by interfering with the activity of the enzyme's reverse transcriptase (nucleoside and nonnucleoside reverse transcriptase inhibitors), and HIV protease (protease inhibitors). Although use of antiretroviral agents has had a significant impact on progression of disease, long-term inhibition of viral replication has remained elusive, due to a combination of factors including drug toxicity and the emergence of mutant, drug resistant strains of HIV.

Transmission of HIV has been shown to occur via semen, vaginal secretions, blood or blood products, breast milk, and transplacental transmission in utero. HIV has also been isolated from saliva, urine, cerebrospinal fluid, brain, tears, alveolar fluid, synovial fluid, and amniotic fluid. Transmission has never been documented to occur by casual contact, although there is one reported case of possible salivary transmission by deep kissing from an HIV-infected male with bleeding gums to a female partner. HIV is a very labile virus and is easily neutralized by heat or common disinfecting agents, such as Lysol, a 1:10 solution of household bleach, 0.3% hydrogen peroxide, 35% isopropyl alcohol, or 50 percent ethanol.

CLINICAL STAGES OF HIV INFECTION

The stages of HIV infection from initial acquisition to end-stage AIDS are described in Table 139-3. Acute HIV infection, essentially indistinguishable from a "flulike" illness, usually goes unrecognized but is reported to occur in 50 to 90 percent of patients.[5] The time from exposure to onset of symptoms is usually 2 to 4 weeks, and the most common symptoms include fever, sore throat, fatigue, myalgias, and weight loss. Many experts now argue that it is beneficial to identify patients at this early stage because it may be the optimal time to begin antiretroviral therapy. The best method of establishing a diagnosis during this window (when HIV antibody serologic test results are usually negative or indeterminant) is by quantitative analysis of plasma HIV RNA. Acute infection is associated with high-level HIV RNA viremia and a precipitous decline in CD4 cell counts, reflecting ongoing destruction of the host immune response. Acute symptoms last an average of 2 weeks, with clinical recovery accompanied by a significant reduction in HIV RNA levels and a moderate increase in CD4 counts.

Seroconversion, reflecting detectable antibody response to HIV, usually occurs 3 to12 weeks after infection, although delays of up to 11 months have been reported. This is followed by a long period of asymptomatic infection during which patients generally have no findings on physical examination except for possible persistent generalized lymphadenopathy, characterized by enlarged lymph nodes involving at least two noncontinuous sites other than inguinal nodes. The mean incubation time from exposure to the development of AIDS is estimated at 8.23 years for adults, and 1.97 years for children under age 5. Virologic studies of patients during this period suggest that a steady state of HIV replication and CD4 cell death and replacement exists until increased levels of HIV replication occur. Variables most predictive of disease stage are viral burden and CD4 counts, with a steeper decline in CD4 count and a higher viral burden associated with rapid progression and poor outcome.[6] Other, indirect risk factors for progression include β_2 microglobulin concentration, low levels of HIV antibody, and low hemoglobin concentration.

Early symptomatic infection is characterized by conditions that are more common and more severe in the presence of HIV infection but, by definition, are not AIDS indicator conditions. Examples include thrush, persistent vulvovaginal candidiasis, peripheral neuropathy, cervical dysplasia, recurrent herpes zoster infection, and idiopathic throm-

TABLE 139-3 Stages of HIV Infection

Stage	CD4 Cell Count, Cells/μL	Clinical Manifestations
Acute infection	Normal	Mononucleosis-like syndrome
Asymptomatic infection	>500	Asymptomatic or persistent generalized lymphadenopathy, aseptic meningitis, myopathy, Guillain-Barré syndrome
Early symptomatic	200–500	Thrush, candidal esophagitis, bacterial pneumonia, herpes zoster, oral hairy leukoplakia, B-cell lymphoma, Hodgkin's disease, idiopathic thrombocytopenic purpura, Kaposi's sarcoma,* TB*
Late symptomatic infection (AIDS)	<200	Opportunistic infections and malignancies (see Table 139-1)
End-stage disease	<50	Disseminated CMV or *M. avium* complex

*Frequently present in patients with CD4 cell counts >200; however, both are classified as AIDS indicator conditions.

bocytopenic purpura. These conditions occur with increased frequency as the CD4 cell count drops below 500 cells/μL.

As the CD4 count drops below 200 cells/μL, the frequency of opportunistic infections dramatically increases. AIDS is defined by the appearance of any indicator condition (Table 139-1) or a CD4 count of less than 200 cells/μL. The average survival time following a diagnosis of AIDS has been estimated to be between 16 to 24 months.[7] Antiretroviral therapy and prophylaxis and treatment of opportunistic infections have been shown to delay the time to onset of complications and death in this group of patients.[8]

Advanced HIV infection exists in patients with a CD4 count of less than 50 cells/μL or clinical evidence of end-stage disease, including disseminated *Mycobacterium avium* complex or disseminated cytomegalovirus (CMV). Patients in this group have a median survival of 12 to 18 months.[7]

DIAGNOSIS

Infection with HIV may be diagnosed by several methods: detection of viral-specific antigen, assays for HIV nucleic acid, isolation of the virus by culture, and detection of antibodies to HIV. The most common assay used to detect viral antibody is an enzyme-linked immunoassay (EIA) and a confirming Western blot test on EIA-positive specimens. EIA is approximately 99 percent specific and 98.5 percent sensitive; the Western blot test is nearly 100 percent sensitive and specific if performed under ideal laboratory circumstances.

Currently, diagnostic HIV testing has no utility in emergency department evaluation or management of patients. A few limited exceptions may exist, such as when health care providers are exposed to patients' blood or in cases of sexual assault.[9,10] Given the narrow window of opportunity for initiating therapy at the earliest stages of infection, the emergency department may yet prove to be an ideal setting for both diagnostic testing and screening.[10,11]

Knowledge of recent CD4 cell counts and HIV viremia load is frequently helpful in placing patients' emergency department presentation in an appropriate context (Table 139-3). When this information is unavailable or the stage of disease is unknown, the total lymphocyte count may be used to approximate the CD4 cell count, since a total lymphocyte count of less than 1000 cells/μL has been shown to be strongly predictive of a CD4 count of less than 200 cells/μL.

CLINICAL FEATURES AND TREATMENT

The spectrum of disease caused by HIV infection varies greatly. Many patients with asymptomatic infection may come to the emergency department for complaints unrelated to HIV disease.[12] Others may have involvement of virtually any organ system, commonly with multiple interrelated problems. Because of the complexity of HIV infection and related opportunistic infections or malignancies, specific diagnoses often cannot be made in the emergency department.

Evaluation of HIV-infected patients should be carried out with the same priority-based logical approach used for all emergency department patients, with attention to concerns particular to this population. Patients with unstable vital signs require attention to the "ABCs" and rapid stabilization. Universal precautions (in some hospitals termed standard precautions) must be used in all cases. The history and physical examination should focus on identifying the clinical stage of disease in order to direct attention to the most likely complications. History gathering must include a thorough review of past and current medications, previous infections, and attention to activities of daily living. Physical findings that might assist with staging (Table 139-3) include the presence of thrush, evidence of temporal wasting, or dementia. Diagnostic and therapeutic maneuvers are directed toward recognition of organ system involvement, assessment of the severity of disease, and institution of symptomatic and specific therapy. Table 139-4 lists some of the common pathogens causing organ system involvement in HIV-infected patients. While it is unlikely in most cases that specific therapy will be initiated by the emergency department physician, familiarity with therapeutic approaches and related complications is important. Table 139-5 contains a summary of common infections and current recommendations for therapy.

Pulmonary Complications

Pulmonary presentations are among the most common reasons for emergency department visits by HIV-infected patients.[10,12] Presenting complaints frequently are nonspecific and include cough, hemoptysis, shortness of breath, and chest pain. Emergency department evaluation should be directed toward determining the likely diagnosis, since early treatment may have a significant impact on morbidity and mortality rates. Appreciation of the epidemiologic characteristics and common findings associated with various pathogens can assist the emergency physician in arriving at an appropriate differential and working diagnosis, leading to sound treatment and disposition decisions.

The most common causes of pulmonary abnormalities in HIV-infected patients include community-acquired bacterial pneumonia, PCP, *Mycobacterium tuberculosis* (MTB), CMV, *Cryptococcus neoformans, Histoplasma capsulatum,* and neoplasms.

In addition to the history and physical examination, evaluation of patients with pulmonary complaints may be assisted by pulse oximetric analysis, arterial blood-gas determination, sputum culture, Gram staining, acid-fast staining, blood culture, and chest x-ray. Pulmonary radiographic findings are helpful in determining likely causes (Table 139-6). Admission should be considered for patients with new-onset

TABLE 139-4 Common Conditions Causing Organ System Involvement in AIDS Patients

Cause	Systemic	Pulmonary	Gastrointestinal	Neurologic
		BACTERIA		
Staphylococcus aureus	X	X		
Streptococcus pneumoniae	X	X		
Clostridium perfringens	X			
Haemophilus influenzae	X	X		
Shigella sp.	X		X	
Salmonella sp.	X		X	
Listeria monocytogenes	X			
Treponema pallidum	X			X
Neisseria gonorrhoeae			X	
Campylobacter jejuni			X	
Nocardia asteroides	X	X		
Chlamydia sp.	X		X	
Legionella sp.	X	X		
Mycobacterium avium complex	X	X		
Mycobacterium tuberculosis	X	X		
Anaerobes	X			
		VIRUSES		
Human immunodeficiency	X		X	X
Hepatitis	X			
Epstein-Barr	X			
Herpes simplex	X	X	X	X
CMV	X	X	X	X
Herpes zoster	X			X
Adenoviruses	X	X	X	
		FUNGI		
Aspergillus sp.	X			
Histoplasma capsulatum	X	X		
Cryptococcus neoformans	X	X		X
Coccidioides sp.	X	X		
Candida sp.	X	X	X	
		PROTOZOA		
Cryptosporidium sp.	X		X	
Toxoplasma gondii	X	X		
Pneumocystis carinii	X	X		
Isospora sp.	X		X	
Entamoeba sp.	X		X	
Giardia lamblia			X	
Strongyloides sp.			X	
		MALIGNANCY		
Kaposi's sarcoma	X	X	X	
Lymphoma	X	X	X	X
Hodgkin's disease	X			

TABLE 139-5 Treatment Recommendations for Common HIV-Related Infections

Organ System	Infection	Therapy
Systemic	*Mycobacterium avium intracellulare*	Clarithromycin 500 mg PO bid + Ethambutol 15 mg/kg/day PO + Rifabutin 300 mg/kg/day PO
	CMV	Gancyclovir 5 mg/kg IV bid or Foscarnet 60 mg/kg IV q8h
Pulmonary	PCP	TMP-SMX 15–20 TMP/kg/day and 75–100 mg SMX/kg/day PO or IV for 3 weeks or Pentamidine 4 mg/kg/day IV or IM for 3 weeks
	MTB	Isoniazid 5 mg/kg/day PO + Rifampin 10 mg/kg/day PO + Pyrazinamide 15–30 mg/kg/day PO + Streptomycin 15 mg/kg/day IM
CNS	Toxoplasmosis	Pyrimethamine 50–100 mg/day PO + Sulfadiazine 4–8 mg/kg/day + Folinic acid 10 mg/day PO
	Cryptococcosis	Amphotericin B 0.7 mg/kg/day IV ± Flucystosine; maintenance therapy required
Ophthalmologic	CMV	Ganciclovir 5 mg/kg bid for 2 weeks; maintenance therapy required
Gastrointestinal	Candidiasis: thrush	Clotrimazole 10 mg 5 times a day, troches OR Nystatin 500 K U 5 times a day, gargle
	Esophagitis	Fluconazole 100 mg/day PO
	Salmonellosis	Ciprofloxacin 500 mg bid PO for 2–4 weeks; maintenance therapy required
	Cryptosporidiosis	No known effective cure
Cutaneous	Herpes simplex	Acyclovir 1000 mg/day PO or Acyclovir 5–10 mg/kg/day IV
	Herpes zoster	Acyclovir 4000 mg/day PO; IV therapy required for ocular involvement or dissemination
	Candida, Tricophyton	Clotrimazole, miconazole, or ketoconazole, topical therapy bid–tid for 3 weeks

Abbreviations: bid, twice a day; CMV, cytomegalovirus; CNS, central nervous system; IM, intramuscularly; IV, intravenously; Mtb, *Mycobacterium tuberculosis;* PCP, *Pneumocystis carinii* pneumonia; PO, by mouth; tid, three times a day; TMP-SMX, trimethoprim-sulfamethoxazole.

pulmonary symptoms, especially those with hypoxia. Decisions regarding patients with known pulmonary involvement are based on comparison to baseline status, the effectiveness of ongoing or previous treatment, and the individual's ability to obtain outpatient follow-up. Specific symptoms are discussed below with selected common causes.

Despite substantial decreases in the incidence of PCP due to effective prophylaxis, it continues to be the most common opportunistic infection among AIDS patients. Approximately 70 percent of HIV-infected patients will acquire PCP at some time during their illness, and PCP is often the initial opportunistic infection that establishes the diagnosis of AIDS. This disease is the most frequent serious complication of HIV infection in the United States and the most common identifiable cause of death in patients with AIDS. The classic presenting symptoms of PCP are fever, cough (typically nonproductive), and shortness of breath (progressing from being present only with exertion to being present at rest).

Symptoms are often insidious and accompanied by fatigue. Chest x-rays most often show diffuse interstitial infiltrates (Table 139-6). Although typical radiographic findings occur in up to 80 percent of cases, negative x-rays are reported in 15 to 20 percent of patients with PCP.[13] In patients with nondiagnostic x-ray findings and signs and symptoms suggestive of PCP, further testing should be pursued. The lactate dehydrogenase (LDH) level is elevated in patients with PCP, but the test for LDH has relatively low sensitivity and specificity, making its use in the emergency department impractical. Arterial blood-gas analysis usually demonstrates hypoxemia and an increase in the alveolar-arterial (A-a) gradient. (Early PCP should be suspected if a patient demonstrates a decrease in pulse oximetric values with exercise.) Presumptive diagnosis of PCP is often assumed in the emergency department if there is hypoxia without any other explanation. Inpatient diagnostic testing may include bronchoscopy with lavage, biopsy, and culture or examination of induced sputum by indirect immunofluorescence using monoclonal antibodies.

Initial therapy for PCP is trimethoprim-sulfamethoxazole (TMP-SMX) TMP 15 mg/kg/day and SMX 75 mg/kg/day) either orally or intravenously for 3 weeks in two or three divided doses [typical oral dosage 2 double strength (DS) tid]. Adverse reactions (most commonly rash, fever, and neutropenia) occur in up to 65 percent of AIDS patients. Pentamidine isothionate 4 mg/kg/day is one of a number of effective alternative agents. Steroid therapy should be instituted for patients with a Pa_{O_2} less than 70 mmHg or an alveolar-arterial gradient greater than 35.[14] The usual regimen is oral prednisone 40 mg bid for 5 days, then 40 mg qd for 5 days, and then 20 mg qd for an additional 11 days. Seventy percent of patients will have reinfection within 18 months. Prophylactic therapy is an important step in preventing reinfection and has also been shown to reduce the risk of developing bacterial pneumonia; oral TMP-SMX 1 DS qd is the preferred agent. Prophylaxis is also recommended in all patients with CD4 counts below 200 cells/μL. Repeat infections may be less responsive to therapy.

The incidence of Mtb is increasing, particularly among the homeless, institutionalized, immigrant, and intravenous-drug-using populations. Reactivation of prior infection is common, and there is a much greater risk of direct progression of disease from recently acquired infection. The incidence of tuberculosis (TB) in the AIDS population is estimated to be 200 to 500 times that in the general population.[15] Prevalence studies demonstrate significant regional variations, attrib-

TABLE 139-6 Chest Radiographic Abnormalities: Differential Diagnosis in AIDS Patients

Finding	Causes
Diffuse interstitial infiltration	PCP CMV Mtb *Mycobacterium avium intracellulare* Histoplasmosis Coccidioidomycosis Lymphoid interstitial
Focal consolidation	Bacterial pneumonia *Mycobacterium pneumoniae* PCP Mtb *Mycobacterium avium intracellulare*
Nodular lesions	Kaposi's sarcoma Mtb *Mycobacterium avium intracellulare* Fungal lesions Toxoplasmosis
Cavitary lesions	PCP Mtb Bacterial infection Fungal infection
Adenopathy	Kaposi's sarcoma Lymphoma Mtb Cryptococcosis

uted to both the demographic characteristics of the populations and the efficacy of local public health control measures.

Clinical manifestations of TB in HIV infection vary significantly according to the severity of immunosuppression. Whereas PCP does not occur until the CD4 count is approximately 200 cells/μL, TB frequently occurs in patients with CD4 counts of 200 to 500 cells/μL. Classic pulmonary manifestations include cough with hemoptysis, night sweats, prolonged fevers, weight loss, and anorexia. With worsening immunosuppression, atypical and extrapulmonary manifestations are more common. Frequent sites of dissemination are peripheral lymph nodes, bone marrow, and the urogenital system. Classic upper lobe involvement and cavitary lesions are less common, particularly among late-stage AIDS patients.[13] Negative purified protein derivative (PPD) TB test results are frequent among AIDS patients due to immunosuppression. Definitive diagnosis may be made by stain and culture of sputum, although in some cases bronchoscopy with biopsy may be required.

In the emergency department, physicians should maintain a high index of suspicion for TB among HIV-infected patients with pulmonary symptoms due to the high rates of person-to-person transmission. Immediate isolation should be instituted until the diagnosis is ruled out. Specific procedures for ruling out TB vary by region and site and have been found to be inadequate in some emergency departments.[16] Any patient identified as high risk based on clinical presentation should be placed in isolation, with the decision for further isolation based on results of chest x-ray and detailed historical and clinical information. Current treatment guidelines recommend a four-drug initial empiric therapy (Table 139-5). Multidrug-resistant TB remains an issue of concern and should increase the awareness of the need for early isolation. All HIV-infected patients with positive PPD test results should receive prophylaxis with isoniazid for 1 year.

Nonopportunistic bacterial pneumonias are the most common pulmonary infections in HIV-infected patients. Common pathogens include *Streptococcus pneumoniae, Haemophilus influenzae,* and *Staphylococcus aureus.* Productive cough, leukocytosis, and the presence of a focal infiltrate suggest bacterial pneumonia, especially in those with earlier-stage disease. The response to empiric therapy tends to be good; a specific diagnosis can be established by Gram staining and culture.

Patients with severe immunosuppression are predisposed to disseminated fungal infections, such as *C. neoformans* and *Aspergillus fumigatus.* Other noninfectious disorders of the lung seen in HIV-infected patients include neoplasms (e.g., Kaposi's sarcoma) and lymphocytic interstitial pneumonitis. CMV or *Mycobacterium avium* complex are unlikely unless the CD4 count drops below 50 cells/μL.

Neurologic Complications

Central nervous system (CNS) disease occurs in 90 percent of patients with AIDS, and 10 to 20 percent of HIV-infected patients initially present with CNS symptoms.[17] Neurologic disease is caused by a variety of opportunistic infections and neoplasms as well as the direct and indirect effects of HIV infection on the CNS. Common presenting symptoms indicative of CNS pathology include seizures, altered mental status, headache, meningismus, and focal neurologic deficits.[17] Emergency department evaluation should include a complete neurologic examination and, when appropriate, computed tomography and lumbar puncture. Specific CSF studies that may be of value include opening and closing pressures, cell count, glucose, protein, Gram stain, India ink stain, bacterial culture, viral culture, fungal culture, toxoplasmosis and cryptococcus antigen, and coccidioidomycosis titer. Even if the emergency department evaluation is unrevealing, all patients with new or changed neurologic signs or symptoms should be admitted to the hospital for further workup. The most common causes of neurologic symptoms include AIDS dementia, *Toxoplasma gondii,* and *C. neoformans.*

AIDS DEMENTIA AIDS dementia complex (also referred to as HIV encephalopathy or subacute encephalitis) is a progressive process commonly heralded by subtle impairment of recent memory and other cognitive deficits caused by direct HIV infection. In the early stages, diagnosis can be confused with depression, anxiety disorders, or substance abuse. Later phases of the illness are characterized by obvious changes in mental status and more severe disturbances, including aphasia and motor abnormalities. When a patient presents to the emergency department with an established diagnosis of AIDS dementia, with progressive signs or symptoms, it is important to rule out other CNS processes. A computed tomography (CT) scan in AIDS dementia typically shows cortical atrophy and ventricular enlargement.

TOXOPLASMOSIS Toxoplasmosis is the most common cause of focal encephalitis in patients with AIDS. Symptoms may include headache, fever, focal neurologic deficits, altered mental status, or seizures. Serologic tests are not useful in making or excluding the diagnosis because antibody to *T. gondii* is prevalent in the general population. The presence of antibody to *T. gondii* in the cerebrospinal fluid is helpful, although there is a high rate of false-negative results. On a noncontrast scan, toxoplasmosis typically appears as multiple subcortical lesions with a predilection for the basal ganglia.

Noncontrast CT scanning is often used as an initial imaging study in the emergency department in HIV-infected patients with neurologic deficits, since the addition of contrast has been shown to be of marginal value in patients with completely normal noncontrast CT scans. In cases in which clinical suspicion for CNS pathology is high but the CT scan is equivocal or negative, contrast enhanced CT scanning should be arranged in the emergency department. With contrast enhancement, toxoplasmosis lesions are ring-enhancing, with surrounding areas of edema. Magnetic resonance imaging is slightly more sensitive than contrast CT in detecting the extent and number of lesions with toxoplasmosis but is usually not indicated in the emergency department.

Other causes in the differential diagnosis of ring-enhancing lesions on contrast CT include lymphoma, fungal infection, and cerebral tuberculosis. In the emergency department, it is often not possible to differentiate these causes based on initial imaging studies, but general patterns in the appearance of lesions, based on underlying pathology, have been described. Toxoplasmosis tends to have a greater number of lesions with a predilection for the basal ganglia and corticomedullary regions, while lymphoma is more often characterized by singular lesions, typically in the periventricular white matter or corpus callosum. TB is distinguished by a characteristic inflammatory appearance on CT, with a thick, isodense exudate filling the basal cisterns.

Patients with suspected toxoplasmosis should be admitted and treated with pyrimethamine (100- to 200-mg load, then 50 to 100 mg/day) and sulfadiazine (4 to 8 g/day), with folinic acid added (10 mg/day) to reduce hematologic toxicity. Steroids are beneficial for significant edema or mass effect. Failure to improve suggests an alternative diagnosis, which may require biopsy. For patients responsive to toxoplamosis therapy, chronic suppressive therapy with pyrimethamine, sulfadiazine, and folinic acid is usually indicated after initial treatment. Oral TMP-SMX (1 DS qd) is recommended for prophylaxis in patients with positive toxoplasmosis serologic test results and CD4 cell counts less than 100 cells/μL.

CRYPTOCOCCOSIS Cryptococcal CNS infection may be seen in up to 10 percent of AIDS patients and may cause either focal cerebral lesions or diffuse meningoencephalitis. The most common presenting signs are fever and headache, followed by nausea, altered mentation, and focal neurologic deficits. Presentation may be subtle. Diagnosis relies on identifying organisms in cerebrospinal fluid by cryptococcal antigen (nearly 100 percent sensitive and specific), culture (95 to 100 percent sensitive), or staining with India ink (60 to 80 percent sensitive); serum cryptococcal antigen is also useful but has slightly lower sensitivity (approximately 95 percent). Patients with CNS cryptococcus shall be admitted for antibiotic therapy; preferred treatment is intravenous amphotericin B 0.7 mg/kg/day for 10 to 14 days. Oral flucytosine 100 mg/kg/day may be added to this therapy. Sixty percent of patients may be expected to respond to therapy, and side effects are frequent, most notably bone marrow suppression. Initial therapy should be followed by 8 to 10 weeks of oral fluconazole. Lifelong maintenance therapy with lower doses of fluconazole is indicated for all patients.

OTHER NEUROLOGIC DISORDERS Other, less common CNS infections that should be considered in the presence of neurologic symptoms include bacterial meningitis, histoplasmosis (usually disseminated), CMV, progressive multifocal leukoencephalopathy, herpes simplex virus, neurosyphilis, and TB. Noninfectious CNS processes include CNS lymphoma (occurring in 5 percent of AIDS patients and typically manifested as a subacute neurologic deterioration over several months), cerebrovascular accidents, and metabolic encephalopathies.

HIV infection is associated with a variety of disorders of the peripheral nervous system. The most common of these is HIV neuropathy characterized by painful sensory symptoms in the feet. Symptomatic relief with pain-modifying agents, such as amitriptyline or phenytoin, should be used judiciously because of their potential for causing delirium in patients with concurrent HIV dementia. Narcotic analgesia may be helpful in severe cases.

Gastrointestinal Complications

Gastrointestinal manifestations of HIV infection are common. Approximately 50 percent of AIDS patients will present with gastrointestinal complaints at some time during their illness. The most frequent presenting symptoms include odonophagia, abdominal pain, bleeding, and diarrhea. Organisms commonly associated with gastrointestinal infection in AIDS patients are shown in Table 139-4. Emergency department evaluation should focus on recognizing the severity of symptoms and obtaining appropriate initial diagnostic studies. Therapy should include volume and electrolyte repletion and initiation of antibiotic therapy when appropriate. Disposition should be based on the duration of symptoms, the clinical appearance of the patient, and the response to emergency department therapy.

Diarrhea is the most frequent gastrointestinal complaint and is estimated to occur in 50 to 90 percent of AIDS patients. It is caused by a wide variety of enteric pathogens that affect the general population as well as other, less virulent organisms that are more common in the immunocompromised population. Emergency department evaluation of patients with diarrhea should include microscopic examination of stool for leukocytes, ova, and parasites; acid-fast staining; and bacterial culture of stool. Common causes include bacterial organisms, such as *Shigella, Salmonella,* enteroadherent *Escherichia coli,* and *Campylobacter;* parasitic organisms, such as *Giardia, Cryptosporidium,* and *Isospora belli;* CMV; *M. avium intracellulare;* and antibiotic therapy.[17]

Clinical clues regarding the cause of diarrheal illnesses may be provided by the patient's history and confirmed by supplementary testing; however, results are usually not available during the emergency department visit. Bacterial pathogens generally follow a more acute and fulminant course, while parasitic infections are more frequently indolent. If bacterial infection is suspected, empiric treatment with ciprofloxacin, which covers the common bacterial pathogens, can be started. *Cryptosporidium* and *Isospora* infection are common parasitic causes and are associated with profuse watery diarrhea. Both can be identified by a modified acid-fast stain. *Isospora belli* is usually responsive to TMP-SMZ, but relapse is common. Cryptosporidiosis tends to be difficult to treat. In patients with end-stage disease, the most common pathogens are CMV and *M. avium intracellulare;* both diagnoses usually require biopsy. Prolonged antimicrobial therapy is indicated for treatment, and resistance and relapse are frequent for both entities. About 15 percent of patients with late-stage AIDS suffer from severe, high-volume, watery diarrhea with no pathogen identified even after thorough investigation. The presumed diagnosis is AIDS-related enteropathy. Patients often require admission for correction of electrolyte abnormalities and rehydration. Octreotide, the somatostatin analogue, may be helpful in some cases.

Emergency department management should be directed toward repletion of fluid and electrolytes. Patients who are nontoxic appearing and can tolerate liquids can be referred for outpatient follow-up of test results. Patients with severe diarrhea who do not require antibiotics may benefit from symptomatic therapy, such as attapulgite (Kaopectate), psyllium (Metamucil) and, if necessary, diphenoxylate hydrochloride with atropine (Lomotil).

Oral lesions are common in HIV-infected patients and frequently contribute to malnutrition. Oral candidiasis or thrush affects more than 80 percent of AIDS patients. The tongue and buccal mucosa are commonly involved, and the plaques characteristically can be easily scraped from an erythematous base. Differentiation from hairy leukoplakia (usually manifested as adherent, white, thickened lesions on the lateral tongue borders) may be challenging for the inexperienced, but microscopic examination on potassium hydroxide smear confirms the diagnosis. The development of oral candidiasis is a poor prognostic sign and is predictive of progression to AIDS. Most oral lesions can be managed symptomatically on an outpatient basis. Clotrimazole or nystatin suspension or troches (five times daily) are the preferred treatment. Refractory or recurrent disease can be managed with oral fluconazole. Amphotericin B is reserved for severe cases.

Other causes of painful oral and perioral lesions include oral hairy leukoplakia, herpes simplex virus, and Kaposi's sarcoma. Herpes simplex can usually be recognized by typical vesicular lesions, with diagnosis confirmed by identifying multinucleated giant cells from scrapings or by culture. Both herpes simplex and hairy leukoplakia are responsive to oral acyclovir. Oral Kaposi's sarcoma appears as a nontender, well-circumscribed, slightly raised violaceous lesion. Diagnosis requires biopsy; topical treatments may be palliative.

Esophageal involvement may occur with *Candida,* herpes simplex, and CMV. Complaints of odonophagia or dysphagia are usually indicative of esophagitis and may be extremely debilitating. Disease typically occurs in patients who have oral thrush and CD4 counts of less than 100 cells/μL. Treatment of esophagitis in the emergency department is usually presumptive. Endoscopy, histologic staining, culture, and biopsy are reserved for patients who fail to respond or have atypical presentations. Presumptive treatment for *Candida,* which accounts for 50 to 70 percent of cases, is with oral fluconazole (200 to 400 mg qd for 2 to 3 weeks) or oral ketoconazole (100 to 200 mg qd for 2 to 3 weeks). Relapses are common, and intravenous amphotericin B may occasionally be required. Treatment failures endoscopically discovered to be caused by CMV and herpes simplex are treated with acyclovir and gancyclovir, respectively.

Hepatomegaly occurs in approximately 50 percent of AIDS patients. Elevation of alkaline phosphatase levels is frequently seen. Jaundice is rare. Coinfection with hepatitis B and hepatitis C is common, especially among injected drug users. Opportunistic infection with CMV, *Cryptosporidium, M. avium intracellulare,* and MTB may also cause signs of hepatitis.

Anorectal disease is common in AIDS patients. Proctitis is characterized by painful defecation, rectal discharge, and tenesmus. Common causative organisms include *Neisseria gonorrhoeae, Chlamydia trachomatis,* syphilis, and herpes simplex. Proctocolitis includes the same symptoms in the presence of diarrhea, and multiple bacterial organisms may be responsible (most commonly *Shigella, Campylobacter,* and *Entamoeba histolytica*). Diagnostic evaluation should include anoscopy, with microscopic examination, Gram stain, and culture of pus and/or stool.

Cutaneous Manifestations

Generalized cutaneous conditions, such as xerosis (dry skin), seborrheic eczema, and pruritus, are common and may be manifested prior to development of opportunistic infections. Treatment is with emollients and, if necessary, mild topical steroids. Pruritus may respond to oatmeal baths and antihistamines. Other infections, including *S. aureus* (manifested as bullous impetigo, ecthyma, or folliculitis), *Pseudomonas aeruginosa* (which may present with chronic ulcerations and macerations), and syphilis are frequently seen and should be treated with standard therapies. Several specific dermatologic conditions are discussed in more detail below.

Kaposi's sarcoma appears more often in homosexual men than in other risk groups. Clinically, it consists of painless, raised brown-black or purple papules and nodules that do not blanch. Common sites are the face, chest, genitals, and oral cavity; however, widespread dissemination involving internal organs may occur. Since cutaneous Kaposi's sarcoma is not generally associated with significant rates of morbidity or mortality, therapy is indicated only for extensive, painful, or cosmetically disfiguring lesions. Cryotherapy or radiation can be used for localized disease; widespread disease may be responsive to chemotherapy with vincristine, vinblastine, or doxyrubicin.

Herpes simplex infections are common and may be localized or systemic. In patients with significant immunosuppression, infection may become progressive, manifested as chronic ulcerative mucocutaneous lesions. Diagnosis and treatment are the same as for other patients with herpes simplex (see Chap. 150, "Common Viral Infections"). Intravenous acyclovir therapy 5 to 10 mg/kg/day is needed for extensive disease.

Reactivation of varicella zoster virus is more common in patients with HIV infection and AIDS than in the general population.[18] The clinical course is prolonged, and complications are more frequent. In HIV-positive patients with oral acyclovir 800 mg five times a day or oral famciclovir 500 mg tid for 7 days is usually sufficient. However, in patients with disseminated disease or ophthalmic zoster, admission is indicated for intravenous acyclovir.

Intertriginous infections with either *Candida* or *Trichophyton* are often seen in patients with HIV and can be diagnosed by microscopic examination of potassium hydroxide preparations of lesion scrapings. Treatment includes topical imidazole creams, such as clotrimazole, miconazole, or ketoconazole. Scabies occurs in about 20 percent of HIV-infected patients, but classic intertriginous lesions are less common. Any patient with a scaly, persistent pruritic eruption should have lesions scraped and examined histologically for scabies mites. Treatment is with permethrin 5% cream or lindane lotion. Human papillomavirus infections occur with increased frequency in immunocompromised patients. Treatment is cosmetic or symptomatic and may include cryotherapy, topical therapy, or laser therapy. Other dermatologic conditions that occur with increased frequency among HIV-infected patients include psoriasis, atopic dermatitis, and alopecia. Referral for dermatologic consultation is appropriate.

Constitutional Symptoms and Febrile Illnesses

OVERVIEW Systemic symptoms, such as fever, weight loss, and malaise, are common in HIV-infected patients and account for the majority of HIV-related emergency department presentations.[12] In the emergency department, systemic infection and malignancy must be excluded. Appropriate laboratory investigation may include electrolyte determinations, complete blood count, blood cultures (aerobic, anaerobic, and fungal), urinalysis and culture, liver function tests, chest radiograph, and serologic testing for syphilis, cryptococcocus, toxoplasmosis, and coccidioidomycosis. Lumbar puncture may also be considered if there are neurologic signs or symptoms or unexplained fever.

When evaluating fever in patients with late-stage HIV and AIDS, it is important to remember that this population may not manifest the typical signs and laboratory findings associated with systemic infection. Clinical impression is therefore critical for determining appropriate disposition; ill-appearing patients should receive fluid resuscitation and empiric antibiotics in the emergency department and then be admitted for further evaluation and management. Outpatient evaluation and treatment may be attempted only when all of the following conditions are met: the source of the fever does not dictate admission, appropriate laboratory studies have been initiated, the patient is able to function adequately at home (e.g., can maintain sufficient oral intake, etc.), and appropriate and timely medical follow-up can be arranged.

COMMON CAUSES OF SYSTEMIC ILLNESS AND FEVER Although fever may indicate any of a variety of infections (including bacterial, fungal, viral, and protozoal pathogens), the most common causes in the HIV-infected population are HIV-related fever, non-Hodgkin lymphoma, and systemic infections, such as *M. avium* complex, CMV, and infective endocarditis. Fever caused by HIV infection alone tends to occur in the afternoon or evening and is generally responsive to antipyretics.

Most non-Hodgkin's lymphomas in the HIV-infected population are high-grade B-cell tumors that present with a rapidly growing mass lesion. New CNS symptoms, particularly a change in mental status in the presence of fever, should be evaluated with neuroimaging. Definitive diagnosis requires biopsy. Radiotherapy and chemotherapy are effective treatment regimens.

Disseminated *M. avium* complex is the most common opportunistic bacterial infection in AIDS patients, causing disseminated disease in up to 50 percent of patients at some time during their illness. Infection occurs predominantly in patients with CD4 counts of 100 cells/μL or less. Persistent fever and night sweats are typical. Associated symptoms include weight loss, diarrhea, malaise, and anorexia. Dissemination to the bone marrow, liver, and spleen result in the common associated laboratory findings of anemia and elevated alkaline phosphatase levels. Diagnosis may be made by acid-fast stain of stool or other body fluids, or by blood culture. *Mycobacterium avium* complex cannot be eradicated, but clarithromycin combined with ethambutol and rifabutin have been shown to significantly reduce bacteremia and improve symptoms.

CMV is the most common cause of serious opportunistic viral disease in HIV-infected patients. Disseminated disease commonly involves the gastrointestinal or pulmonary systems. The most important manifestation is retinitis (see below). Treatment is with foscarnet or ganciclovir; oral ganciclovir can be used for prophylaxis.

Fever in injected drug users should always raise concern for infective endocarditis. Previous studies have failed to identify reliable clinical or laboratory predictors of this disease. The current standard of care, therefore, is to admit all febrile injected drug users and await the results of blood cultures, due to the significant morbidity and mortality rates of missed endocarditis and the difficulties associated with outpatient follow-up in the population.

Psychiatric Disorders

Epidemiologic studies of patients infected with HIV and AIDS show a high lifetime prevalence of psychiatric disorders compared to the general population. Persons at highest risk for HIV infection (i.e., injected drug users and homosexual men) frequently suffer from mood disturbances prior to contracting HIV. Infection with HIV produces brain injury and is associated with a variety of CNS and metabolic disturbances that can produce psychiatric symptoms. HIV infection is also a significant psychosocial stressor, leading to social isolation, poverty, and hopelessness.

Evaluation of psychiatric symptoms in the emergency department should focus on an aggressive search for underlying organic causes of the acute presentation.[19] Delirium suggests the presence of a primary physiologic disease; the workup should include laboratory studies, neuroimaging, and lumbar puncture. The differential diagnosis includes CNS and toxic-metabolic derangements. Frequently, a period of observation may be required if a patient is found to be intoxicated or experiencing withdrawal symptoms.

AIDS psychosis is poorly understood. Patients may present with psychiatric symptoms, such as hallucinations, delusions, or other abnormal behavioral changes. The cause is unclear, and treatment has been identical to that for other psychoses. Acute episodes require admission.

Depression occurs in 20 percent of patients, most commonly in those with lower CD4 counts.[20] Depressive illnesses are often responsive to hospitalization and psychosocial intervention. Antidepressant therapy may be considered if symptoms of depression continue longer than 2 weeks. However, due to the increased propensity to develop medication side effects, close patient monitoring is required. Patients with suicidal ideation usually require inpatient psychiatric management.

An increased incidence of mania is observed in both the early and late stages of HIV. Late-stage mania is closely associated with dementia and carries a poor prognosis.

Management of HIV-positive patients with psychiatric complaints must include attention to violent behavior and suicidality. Assessment and stabilization may require physical restraints and acute pharmacologic intervention. Neuroleptics and benzodiazepines may be used in combination. Haloperidol and diazepam are often used; alternatives include droperidol (which has a rapid onset and short half-life) and lorazepam (which offers improved intramuscular absorption).[21]

Ophthalmologic Manifestations

Seventy-five percent of patients with AIDS develop ocular complications. Although a wide range of ophthalmic diseases occur, recognition of a few is most critical.[22]

The most common ophthalmic finding in patients with AIDS is retinal microvasculopathy, which is characterized by retinal cotton-wool spots identical in appearance to those of diabetes or hypertension. Retinal microaneurysms are also seen, primarily in the periphery. These lesions are believed to be incidental and do not cause visual disturbances. The diagnostic dilemma is to distinguish these findings from early CMV infection, and ophthalmologic consultation is recommended.

CMV retinitis is the most frequent and serious ocular opportunistic infection and the leading cause of blindness in AIDS patients. The prevalence is estimated to be up to 40 percent. Visual loss and blindness occur in all cases without early detection and prompt treatment.[23] The presentation of CMV retinitis is variable. It may be asymptomatic early on but later causes changes in visual acuity, visual field cuts, photophobia, scotoma, or eye redness or pain. Findings on indirect ophthalmoscopy are characteristic, with fluffy white perivascular lesions and areas of hemorrhage within them. First-line treatment (5 mg/kg q8h for 14 to 21 days and then 6 mg/kg/day either oral or intravenous). Even with treatment, there are frequent relapse and progression of disease, with 10 percent of affected patients ultimately going blind.[22]

Herpes zoster ophthalmicus usually presents with paresthesia and discomfort in the distribution of cranial nerve V_1, followed by the appearance of the typical zoster skin rash. Ocular complications include conjunctivitis, episcleritis, iritis, keratitis, secondary glaucoma, and, rarely, retinitis. Early recognition and treatment is essential to prevent ocular damage. In immunocompetent patients, oral acyclovir may be used in consultation with an ophthalmologist. Immunocompromised patients should receive intravenous therapy. Close follow-up with reexamination should be arranged for all outpatients.

A variety of lesions can affect the areas around the eye in HIV patients, most notably Kaposi's sarcoma and molluscum contagiosum. Patients with such lesions may be referred to an ophthalmologist for local excision or cryotherapy.

Cardiovascular Manifestations

Clinically significant cardiac disease among AIDS patients is uncommon. Findings such as pericardial effusion, cardiomyopathy, and congestive heart failure are frequently reported at autopsy but are often clinically silent.

Renal Manifestations

Renal insufficiency among AIDS patients may be secondary to prerenal azotemia, drug nephrotoxicity, or HIV-associated nephropathy, which may cause chronic renal insufficiency due to focal and segmental glomerulosclerosis. Renal tubular acidosis is common and may explain a finding of hyperchloremic metabolic acidosis. Management decisions should be made in conjunction.

Sexually Transmitted Diseases

Sexually transmitted diseases are epidemiologically associated with HIV infection. Diseases that cause genital ulcers, such as herpes, chancroid, and syphilis, are believed to provide vascular portals of entry for HIV. Prevalence studies demonstrate a three- to fivefold increased odds ratio of HIV seropositivity in patients with genital ulcers.[24] A similarly increased risk of HIV infection has recently been found among patients with gonorrhea and chlamydial infections. These studies, along with recent emergency-department-based prevalence surveys, have led to a recommendation for increased surveillance of sexually transmitted diseases as a means of controlling HIV transmission.[25,26] All patients with symptoms suggestive of sexually transmitted disease should be tested for gonorrhea, chlamydia, and syphilis. Primary (chancre) and secondary (rash, mucocutaneous lesions, and adenopathy) syphilis should be treated with a single intramuscular dose of benzathine penicillin, 2.4 million units. For latent syphilis or unknown duration of secondary syphilis, three weekly injections are recommended. Any patient with known or suspected syphilis should be evaluated for the possibility of neurosyphilis, which is known to have an increased incidence in the HIV-infected population. Therapy for other sexually transmitted diseases is based on current CDC guidelines (see Chap. 137, ''Sexually Transmitted Diseases'').

Drug Reactions

A recent series found that 3 to 5 percent of emergency department visits by symptomatic HIV-positive patients were related to complications of pharmacologic therapy.[12] That incidence is likely to increase as the number of new antiretroviral drugs and various combination therapies being prescribed continues to increase.

Table 139-7 illustrates common side effects of medications frequently prescribed for HIV-infected patients. Review of current reference sources and consultation with a hospital pharmacologist and an infectious disease specialist are indicated when drug reactions are suspected.

Immunizations of HIV-Infected Patients

According to the US Public Health Service Immunizations Practices Advisory Committee, HIV-infected persons should not receive live virus or live bacteria vaccines. Killed vaccines pose no danger to immunosuppressed patients.[27] Since symptomatic HIV-infected persons have a suboptimal response to vaccines, all single-dose vaccines are advised to be given as early as possible in the course of HIV infection.[27]

Table 139-8 summarizes the CDC recommendations for common immunizations. Pneumococcal vaccine is recommended for all patients over 2 years of age. Tetanus-diphtheria vaccine is recommended as a booster every 10 years for those who have completed primary series. The measles-mumps-rubella vaccine is contraindicated because measles is a live vaccine with reported serious reactions in HIV-infected patients. Hepatitis B vaccine is recommended for all high-risk individuals, including injected drug users, sexually active homosexual men, and sexually active men and women with sexually transmitted diseases or more than one sexual partner in the past 6 months. Patients should be referred to a primary care provider for routine immunization.

Antiretroviral Therapy

Treatment of patients with HIV has changed substantially in the past several years due to the introduction of potent antiretroviral agents. In 1996, a decline in the number of new AIDS cases and AIDS-related deaths was seen for the first time since the beginning of the epidemic, attributed in large part to the use of these new medications.[2] Extended survival has been linked to dramatic decreases in the incidence of new opportunistic events.

The first antiretroviral agent discovered to have clinical efficacy was zidovudine (AZT) (Retrovir). AZT is a thymidine analog that inhibits HIV replication by interfering with the action of viral RNA-dependent DNA polymerase (reverse transcriptase). This agent is effective in delaying progression to AIDS and decreasing mortality rates for patients with AIDS. These trends are associated with changes in the host immune response demonstrated by increased CD4 cell counts and reduced risks of opportunistic infections. Combination therapy with two nucleoside reverse transcriptase inhibitors and a protease inhibitor results in maximal response of the immune system.[28] Eleven antiretroviral agents are currently licensed for use in HIV infection, and this number is likely to increase in the near future.

The goal of antiretroviral therapy is to reduce HIV viremia as much as possible for as long as possible. The best time to start therapy and the best drugs to use are not known with certainty, and treatment strategies will continue to evolve. General guidelines include initiation of antiretroviral therapy in persons with CD4 cell counts of less than 500 cells/μL. However, therapy must be tailored to individual patients with attention to suppression of viral replication, preservation of immune function, drug side effects, drug interactions, and the patient's preference. Education and counseling also constitute an integral part of antiretroviral therapy. For these reasons, decisions regarding initiation of and changes in antiretroviral therapy should always be made in consultation with the primary care physician and an infectious disease consultant.

ETHICAL CONSIDERATIONS

Many ethical considerations are involved in testing and treatment of HIV-infected patients. While emotionally driven sentiment has advocated on-site emergency department HIV testing, there is no rationale at this time for widespread emergency-department-based testing. Many departments have adopted strict policies against such testing due to the difficulties of ensuring adequate confidentiality, follow-up, and counseling. However, emergency-department-based voluntary HIV screening and counseling programs may play an important role in the national strategies of early HIV detection in the future, due to limitations of health care access for many at risk.[29] At present, recommendations for testing and referral to designated test sites should be made when indicated.

Confidentiality regarding HIV-related diagnoses is paramount in providing appropriate care. Treatment without discrimination, as with all disease states, should be initiated in all patients unless they specifically request otherwise.

Resuscitation of patients with advanced AIDS is a controversial subject, but in reality, decision making is no different than for other debilitating conditions. Since emergency department physicians often have limited information about individual patients, their wishes, and the state of their disease, it is recommended that appropriate therapy and resuscitative measures be undertaken unless advance directives are available. There is, however, a growing consensus not to undertake ''futile'' resuscitation. Care should be taken that the label *HIV* or *AIDS* does not bias the judgment that resuscitation is futile. Contact with a patient's primary care physician and family early during the emergency department stay helps in decision making about care.

Management of patients with possible sexual, injected drug use, or other nonoccupational exposure to HIV has become relevant since the US Public Health Service issued a recommendation for the use of antiretroviral drugs to reduce the risk of acquisition of HIV following occupational exposure (see below).[30] The CDC has withheld making definitive statements regarding postexposure prophylaxis (PEP) for nonoccupational exposures because of the lack of data available regarding the use of antiretroviral agents in this setting. PEP must therefore be considered on a case-by-case basis and should generally be restricted to situations in which the risk of infection is high, the intervention can be initiated promptly (<36 h), adherence to the regimen is likely, and the individual is most likely to maintain risk-reduction behavior over time.[31] Advantages of therapy must also be carefully balanced with the risk of medication side effects. In the emergency department, when the physician is faced with a case in which PEP is being considered, the assistance of experts should be sought. Risks and benefits of therapy should be considered in consultation with an infectious disease specialist and the patient's primary care provider. The CDC has a 24-h telephone hotline for physicians designed to assist with appropriate initiation of PEP (PEP Hotline 1-888-448-4911).

PRECAUTIONS FOR HEALTH CARE WORKERS

Health care workers are often exposed to the blood and body fluids of HIV-infected patients or patients at high risk of harboring the HIV

TABLE 139-7 Common Drug Reactions Seen in HIV-Infected Patients

Drug	Fever	Rash	N/V	Diarr	H/A	ΔMS	Neuropathy	↑Lft	↑Glu	↓Glu	↓Mg	↓K	↓WBC	↓Hct	↓Plt	Other
ANTIRIETROVIRAL																
Zidovudine (AZT)	X	X	X	X	X	X							X	X		
Didanosine		X	X	X	X	X	X									Pancreatitis
Zalcitabine	X	X	X	X	X		X									
Saquinivir		X	X	X												
Ritonavir			X	X	X											Paresthesias
Indinavir		X	X		X											Nephrolithiasis
Lamivudine	X		X	X	X		X									Cough
ANTIBIOTICS																
TMP-SMX	X	X	X					X					X		X	Hepatotoxicity
Pentamidine		X							X	X			X	X		Metallic taste
Clindamycin		X														
Isoniazid	X	X	X				X	X					X	X	X	Hepatitis
Rifabutin		X	X					X					X		X	Skin
Atovaquone	X	X	X	X	X								X	X		
Dapsone	X	X	X		X								X	X		Hepatitis
Azithromycin		X	X	X	X											
Clarithromycin			X	X	X											
ANTIFUNGALS																
Amphotericin	X		X		X						X	X	X	X	X	Nephrotoxicity
Ganciclovir			X	X									X			
Clotrimazole			X	X												
Ketoconazole			X	X				X								
Fluconazole		X	X	X	X			X								
Itraconazole		X	X	X	X			X								
Pyrimethamine													X	X		
ANTIVIRAL																
Ganciclovir	X		X	X									X	X		
Foscarnet	X		X	X							X	X		X		Nephrotoxicity, seizures
ANALGESICS																
Ibuprofen		X	X	X				X					X	X		
Narcotics			X			X										

Note: This table shows only a representative sample of drug reactions that may occur in HIV-infected persons. Note in particular the frequency of gastrointestinal effects of many medications. Additional references should be consulted for complete information.
Abbreviations: diarr, diarrhea; glu, glucose; H/A, headache; hct, hematocrit; Lft, liver function tests; ΔMS, change in mental status; N/V, nausea and vomiting; plt, platelets; WBC, white blood cells.

TABLE 139-8 Immunization Recommendations for HIV-Infected Patients

Vaccine	Asymptomatic	Symptomatic
Diphtheria-pertussis-tetanus (to age 7)	Yes	Yes
Tetanus-diphtheria	Yes	Yes
Oral poliovirus	No	No
Inactivated polio vaccine	Yes	Yes
Measles-mumps-rubella	No	No
Haemophilus influenzae B conjugate	No (but not contra-indicated)	No (but not contra-indicated)
Pneumococcal	Yes	Yes
Influenza (inactivated)	No (but not contra-indicated)	No (but not contra-indicated)

Source: From Bartlett JG: *Medical Management of HIV Infection,* Baltimore, Johns Hopkins University, Department of Infectious Diseases, 1998; and Centers for Disease Control: *MMWR* 38:205, 1989, with permission.

virus. Emergency-department-based studies have demonstrated that substantial numbers of patients continue to have unsuspected HIV infection and that HIV seropositivity cannot be accurately predicted, even with the aid of risk factors assessment.[9] Universal precautions should be practiced, and all contacts with blood or body fluids should be considered potentially infectious. Universal precautions include gloves, gown, mask, and eye protection for any situation with the potential for exposure by splash, spray, touch, puncture, or immersion. These measures are also indicated for all emergency department procedures, including examination of bleeding patients, chest tube placement, central line placement, suturing, wound care, and lumbar puncture.[32]

The risk of acquiring HIV through occupational exposure is low. The likelihood of contracting AIDS after a parenteral exposure has been estimated at 0.32 percent; for mucocutaneous exposure, risk is considered to be at least one-tenth of that. Approximately 80 percent of documented occupational exposure cases have resulted from hollow-bore needle-stick injuries. As of December 1997, the CDC had documented 54 cases of HIV seroconversion following occupational exposure.

Guidelines for PEP of health care workers following an occupational exposure are based on a recent case-control study of needle-stick injuries from an HIV-infected source (which included 33 cases who seroconverted and 739 control subjects). This study reported that AZT prophylaxis was associated with a 79 percent reduction in disease transmission.[33] PEP recommendations for health workers are based on exposure category, and PEP should be administered in consultation with an infectious disease specialist. The highest-risk injuries are deep punctures and injuries caused by large-bore hollow needles. PEP should be initiated as quickly as possible, preferably within 1 to 2 h. The interval after which there is no benefit for starting PEP is not known, although animal studies suggest little benefit if started 24–36 hours after exposure. Antiretroviral therapy can be given for patients presenting more than 36 h after exposure, depending on the risk of transmission. Treatment regimens vary by type of exposure. All include AZT and lamivudine (3TC); indinavir (Crixivan) or nelfinavir (Viracept) is added for high-risk exposures. PEP should probably be given for 4 weeks. However, GI and constitutional side effects can be considerable.

DISPOSITION

Consultation with an infectious disease specialist and sometimes others with expertise in HIV is often necessary to provide proper therapy and disposition. Disposition decisions, as for all patients, are based on the need for definite inpatient evaluation or management and determination of the patient's ability to function as an outpatient (with special consideration regarding oral intake, ambulation, and availability of appropriate medical follow-up). General considerations for admission and discharge are given in Table 139-9.

TABLE 139-9 Considerations for Disposition Decisions for HIV-Infected Patients

Conditions Suggesting Admission	Conditions Suggesting Discharge
New presentation of fever of unknown origin	Normal or baseline vital signs
Hypoxemia (worse than baseline; $Pa_{O_2} < 60$)	Stable medical condition
Suspected PCP	Able to take PO/not orthostatic
Suspected tuberculosis	Follow-up and referral arranged
New CNS symptoms	Patient or care giver understands instructions
Intractable diarrhea	Patient, home care giver, or hospice able to care for patient
Suicidal ideation	
Suspected CMV retinitis	
Herpes zoster ophthalmicus	
Cachexia, weakness	
Unable to care for self or receive adequate care	
Unable to assure appropriate follow-up	

REFERENCES

1. Centers for Disease Control and Prevention: 1993 revised classification system for HIV infection and expanded surveillance case definition for AIDS among adolescents and adults. *MMWR* 41:1, 1993.
2. Centers for Disease Control and Prevention: U.S. HIV and AIDS cases reported through 1997. *HIV/AIDS Surveill Rep* 9:1, 1997.
3. Centers for Disease Control and Prevention: Human immunodeficiency virus in the United States: 1995 update. *MMWR* 4:849, 1995.
4. Kelen GD, Hexter DA, Hansen KN, et al: Trends in human immunodeficiency virus (HIV) infection among a patient population of an inner-city emergency department: Implications for emergency department based screening programs for HIV infection. *Clin Infect Dis* 21:867, 1995.
5. Schacker T, Collier AC, Hughes J, et al: Clinical and epidemiologic features of primary HIV infection. *Ann Intern Med* 125:257, 1996.
6. O'Brien WA, Hartigan PM, Martin D, et al: Changes in plasma HIV-1 RNA and CD4-lymphocyte counts and the risk of progression to AIDS. *N Engl J Med* 334:42, 1996.
7. Vellq W, Chiesi A, Volpi A, et al: Differential survival of patients with AIDS according to the 1987 and 1993 CDC case definitions. *JAMA* 271:1083, 1994.
8. Yarchoan R, Venzon DJ, Pluda JM, et al: CD4 count and the risk for death in patients infected with HIV receiving antiretroviral therapy. *Ann Intern Med* 115:184, 1991.
9. Kelen GD, Fritz S, Quaish B, et al: Unrecognized human immunodeficiency virus (HIV) infection in general emergency patients. *N Engl J Med* 318:1645, 1988.
10. Kelen GD, Digiovanna T, Bisson L, et al: Human immunodeficiency virus infection in emergency department patients: Epidemiology, clinical presentations and risk to health care workers: The Johns Hopkins experience. *JAMA* 262:516, 1989.
11. Kelen GD, Shahan SB, Quinn TL: HIV screening and counseling: Experience with rapid and standard serologic testing. *Ann Emerg Med* 33(2):147, 1999.
12. Kelen GD, Johnson G, Digiovanna TA, et al: Profile of patients with human immunodeficiency virus infection presenting to an inner-city emergency department: Preliminary report. *Ann Emerg Med* 19(9):963, 1990.
13. Huang L, Stanell JD: AIDS and the lung. *Med Clin North Am* 80:4, 1996.
14. NIH-UC Expert Panel for Corticosteroids as Adjunctive Therapy for *Pneumocystis* Pneumonia: Consensus statement for use of corticosteroids as adjunctive therapy for *Pneumocystis* pneumonia in AIDS. *N Engl J Med* 323:1500, 1990.
15. Markowitz N, Hansen NI, Hopewell PC, et al: Incidence of tuberculosis in the United States among HIV-infected persons. *Ann Intern Med* 126:123, 1997.
16. Moran GJ, McCabe F, Morgan TM, et al: Delayed recognition and infection control for tuberculosis in the emergency department. *Ann Emerg Med* 26:290, 1995.
17. Neild PJ, Nelson MR: Management of HIV-related diarrhoea. *Int J STD AIDS* 8:286, 1997.
18. Buchbinder SP, Katz MH, Hessal NA, et al: Herpes zoster and human immunodeficiency virus infection. *J Infect Dis* 166:1153, 1992.
19. Lyketsos CG, Fishman M, Treisman G: Psychiatric issues and emergencies in HIV infection. *Emerg Med Clin North Am* 13:163, 1995.
20. Lyketsos CG, Hoover DR, Guccione M, et al: Depressive symptoms as predictors of medical outcomes in HIV infection. *JAMA* 270:2563, 1993.
21. Pilowsky LS, Ring H, Shine PJ, et al: Rapid tranquilization: A survey of emergency prescribing in a general psychiatric hospital. *Br J Psychiatry* 160:831, 1992.
22. Greenwood J, Graham EM: The ocular complications of HIV and AIDS. *Int J STD AIDS* 8:358, 1997.
23. Baven ER, Wison P, Atkins M, et al: Natural history of untreated CMV retinitis. *Lancet* 346:1671, 1995.
24. Dickerson MC, Johnston J, Delea TE, et al: The causal role for genital ulcer disease as a risk factor for transmission of human immunodeficiency virus. *Sex Transm Dis* 23:429, 1996.
25. Ernst AA, Farley TA, Martin DH: Screening and empiric treatment for syphilis in an inner-city emergency department. *Acad Emerg Med* 2:765, 1995.
26. Yearly DM, Greene TJ, Hobbs GD: Underrecognition of cervical *Neiserria gonorrhoeae* and *Chlamydia trachomatis* infections in the emergency department. *Acad Emerg Med* 4: 962, 1997.
27. Centers for Disease Control and Prevention: Standard for pediatric immunization practices: Recommended by the National Vaccine Advisory Committee. *MMWR* 42:1, 1993.
28. Spooner KM, Lance C, Masur H: Antiretroviral therapy: Reference guide to major clinical trails in patients infected with human immunodeficiency virus. *Clin Infect Dis* 20:1145, 1995.
29. Kelen GD, Hexter DA, Hansen KN, et al:: Feasibility of an emergency department-based risk-targeted voluntary HIV screening program. *Ann Emerg Med* 27:687, 1996.
30. Centers for Disease Control and Prevention: Update: Provisional Public Health Service recommendations for chemoprophylaxis after occupational exposure to HIV. *MMWR* 45:468, 1996.
31. Katz MH, Gerberding JL: Postexposure treatment of people exposed to the human immunodeficiency virus through sexual contact or injection-drug use. *N Engl J Med* 336:1097, 1997.
32. Kelen GD, Hansen KN, Green GB, et al: Determinants of emergency department procedure- and condition-specific universal (barrier) precaution requirements for optimal provider protection. *Ann Emerg Med* 25:743, 1995.
33. Cardo DM, Culver DH, Ciesielski CA, et al: A case-control study of HIV seroconversion in health care workers after percutaneous exposure: Centers for Disease Control and Prevention Needlestick Surveillance Group. *N Engl J Med* 337:1485, 1997.

140 TETANUS

Donna L. Carden

EPIDEMIOLOGY

Tetanus is an uncommon disease in the United States but remains a major health problem worldwide and an important cause of infant mortality in developing countries.[1] The institution of effective and widespread immunization programs for children and routine boosters in adults has resulted in a decline in the average annual incidence of tetanus in the United States from 0.39 per 100,000 persons in 1947 to the current annual incidence of 0.02 per 100,000.[2] Although tetanus is probably underreported in the United States,[3] the incidence of the disease in this country remains considerably less than the global incidence of 18 per 100,000.[1] In the United States, the majority of tetanus occurs in temperate areas, with the states of Texas, California, and Florida responsible for the greatest number of reported cases (34, 20, and 13, respectively).[4] The overall case-fatality rate for tetanus in the United States is about 11 percent where the outcome is known, 2.3 percent among those aged 20 to 39 years; 16 percent among those aged 40 to 59, and 18 percent among those aged 60 years or older.[4] From 1995 to 1997, among the 124 cases reported in the United States, only 13 percent of patients had received a primary series of tetanus toxoid, and only half of those who sought medical care were given toxoid.[4] Intravenous drug users, especially Hispanics in California, are at disproportionate risk of contracting the disease.[4]

PATHOPHYSIOLOGY

Tetanus is an acute, often fatal disease caused by wound contamination with *Clostridium tetani,* a motile, nonencapsulated anaerobic gram-positive rod. *Clostridium tetani* exists in either a vegetative or a spore-forming state. The spores of this organism are ubiquitous and extremely resistant to destruction, surviving in soil or on environmental surfaces for years. *Clostridium tetani* is usually introduced into a wound in the spore-forming, noninvasive state but can germinate into a toxin-producing, vegetative form if tissue is compromised and tissue oxygen tension is reduced. Any factor that lowers the local oxidation-reduction potential, such as the presence of crushed, devitalized tissue, a foreign body, or the development of suppuration, favors the development of the vegetative, toxin-producing form of *C. tetani.*[5]

Once converted into the vegetative form, *C. tetani* produces two exotoxins: tetanolysin, which appears to be clinically insignificant; and tetanospasmin, a potent neurotoxin that is responsible for all the clinical manifestations of tetanus. Although the infection caused by *C. tetani* remains localized at the site of injury, tetanospasmin reaches the nervous system by hematogenous spread of the exotoxin to peripheral nerves and by retrograde intraneuronal transport. Bloodborne tetanospasmin does not cross the blood-brain barrier, but retrograde intraneuronal transport of the exotoxin enables tetanospasmin to gain access to the central nervous system.[1]

Tetanospasmin acts on the motor end plates of skeletal muscle, in the spinal cord, in the brain, and in the sympathetic nervous system. This extremely potent exotoxin prevents the release of the inhibitory neurotransmitters glycine and γ-aminobutyric acid (GABA) from presynaptic nerve terminals, releasing the nervous system from its normal inhibitory control.[6]

CLINICAL FEATURES

With the advent of routine immunization of children in the United States, tetanus has become a disease of the elderly, who are particularly susceptible to tetanus due to failure to receive primary immunization or the recommended decennial immunizations. In fact, the majority of Americans over age 70 lack adequate immunity to tetanus.[7,8]

The exotoxin tetanospasmin is responsible for the clinical manifestations of tetanus, which consist of generalized muscular rigidity, violent muscular contractions, and instability of the autonomic nervous system. Wounds that become infected with toxin-producing *C. tetani* are most often puncture wounds[2] but vary in severity from deep lacerations to minor abrasions.[2,5] Tetanus can also develop after surgical procedures, otitis media, and abortion and can develop in neonates through infection of the umbilical cord and in intravenous drug users.

The incubation period of tetanus, that is, the period from initial inoculation to the onset of symptoms, can range from less than 24 h to longer that 1 month. The shorter the incubation period, the more severe is the disease and the worse is the prognosis for recovery.[1]

Clinical tetanus can be categorized into four forms: local, generalized, cephalic, and neonatal. The different categories of clinical tetanus depend on what population of neurons are involved.

Local tetanus is manifested by persistent rigidity of the muscles in close proximity to the site of injury and usually resolves after weeks to months without sequelae. Local tetanus may progress to the generalized form of the disease.

Generalized tetanus is the most common form of the disease and frequently follows a puncture wound to the foot from a nail.[2] Of those patients who seek medical care for their initial injury, the majority (more than 90 percent) do not receive appropriate tetanus prophylaxis.[2]

The most frequent presenting complaints of patients with generalized tetanus are pain and stiffness in the masseter muscles (lockjaw).[9] Nerves with short axons are affected initially; therefore, symptoms appear first in the facial muscles, with progression to the neck, trunk, and extremities.[9] The transition from muscle stiffness to rigidity leads to the development of trismus and the resultant characteristic facial expression: *risus sardonicus* (sardonic smile) (Fig. 140-1). Reflex convulsive spasms and tonic contractions of muscle groups are responsible for the development of dysphasia, opisthotonos (Fig. 140-2), flexing of the arms, clenching of the fists, and extension of the lower extremities. Patients are completely conscious and alert unless laryngospasm and tonic contraction of the respiratory muscles result in respiratory compromise.

Disturbances of the autonomic nervous system, generally a hypersympathetic state, occur during the second week of clinical tetanus and present as tachycardia, labile hypertension, profuse sweating, hyperpyrexia, and increased urinary excretion of catecholamines.[10] The autonomic complications of generalized tetanus are particularly difficult to manage and contribute significantly to the morbidity and mortality of the disease.

Cephalic tetanus follows injuries to the head or occasionally otitis media and results in dysfunction of the cranial nerves, most commonly the seventh. This form of tetanus has a particularly poor prognosis.

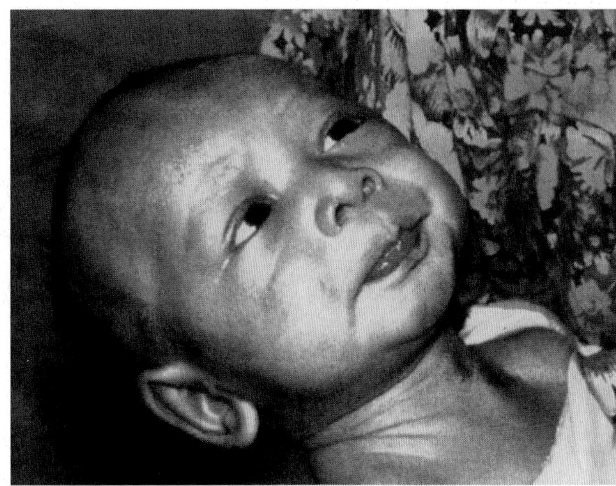

FIG. 140-1. *Risus sardonicus* (sardonic smile) of tetanus. (From photograph reproduced with permission from the Immunization Action Coalition.)

Neonatal tetanus is an important cause of infant mortality in developing countries and carries an extremely high mortality rate (greater than 90 percent).[9] Because passive immunity from maternal antibodies protects an infant from tetanus, neonatal tetanus occurs only if the mother is inadequately immunized. Most cases of neonatal tetanus arise from unsterile handling of the umbilical stump.

Infants with neonatal tetanus present with weakness, irritability, and an inability to suck in week 2 of life.[1] Tetanic spasms, rigidity, opisthotonic posturing, and a hypersympathetic state develop later.[1]

DIAGNOSIS

Tetanus is diagnosed solely on the basis of clinical evidence. Most patients who develop the disease either have an unknown or inadequate immunization history.[2] Tetanus should be immediately suspected in older patients with a puncture wound who present with pain or stiffness in the masseter muscles.

There are no laboratory tests to diagnose tetanus, although serum antitoxin titers of $\geq$0.01 IU/mL are usually protective and may be helpful retrospectively. Wound culture is of limited value, since *C. tetani* may be present in the absence of clinical signs or symptoms of tetanus and cultures are positive in fewer than 50 percent of patients with documented disease.[5,11]

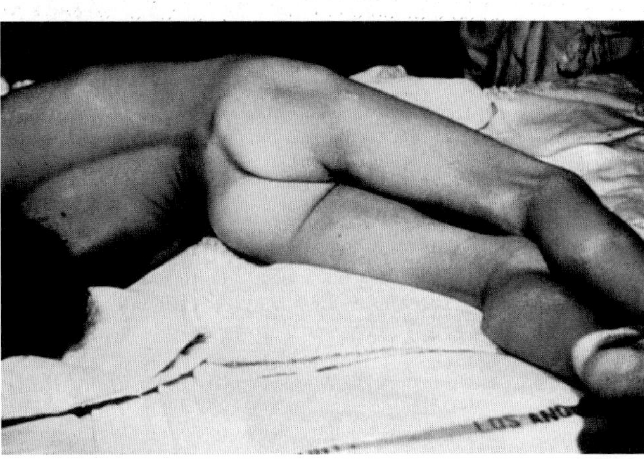

FIG. 140-2. *Opisthotonos* of tetanus. (From photograph reproduced with permission from the Immunization Action Coalition.)

TABLE 140-1 Differential Diagnosis of Tetanus

Strychnine poisoning
Dystonic reaction (phenothiazines, metoclopramide)
Hypocalcemic tetany
Peritonsillar abscess
Peritonitis
Meningeal irritation (bacterial meningitis, subarachnoid hemorrhage)
Rabies
Temporomandibular joint disease

The differential diagnosis of tetanus is presented in Table 140-1. Strychnine poisoning most closely mimics the clinical picture of generalized tetanus.

TREATMENT

Patients with tetanus should be managed in an intensive care unit. Respiratory compromise may require immediate neuromuscular blockade and orotracheal intubation, but tracheostomy provides the best method of prolonged ventilatory control. Environmental stimuli must be minimized to prevent the precipitation of reflex convulsive spasms.

Identification and debridement of the wound through which the clostridial spores were introduced are necessary to minimize further toxin production and to improve the oxidation-reduction potential of the infected tissue. A wound may not be identified in up to 10 percent of patients with tetanus.

Tetanus Immune Globulin

Human tetanus immune globulin (TIG) neutralizes circulating tetanospasmin and toxin in the wound but not toxin that is already fixed in the nervous system. Even though TIG does not ameliorate the clinical symptoms of tetanus, there is evidence that its administration significantly reduces mortality.[12] In a study of 545 cases of tetanus, Blake and colleagues reported that 500 IU was as effective as larger doses of TIG in reducing tetanus-induced mortality.[12] TIG should be administered intramuscularly opposite the site of tetanus toxoid administration. It should be given before wound debridement, since exotoxin may be released during wound manipulation.[11] Repeated doses of TIG are unnecessary, since the half-life of the antitoxin is 28 days.[9]

Antibiotics

Antibiotics, although of questionable utility in the treatment of tetanus, have traditionally been administered. *Clostridium tetani* is sensitive to a number of antibiotics (e.g., penicillins, cephalosporins, tetracycline, and erythromycin), but parenterally administered metronidazole should be considered the antibiotic of choice.[13] Penicillin, a centrally acting $GABA_A$ antagonist may potentiate the effects of tetanospasmin, and therefore its use should be avoided.[1]

Muscle Relaxants

As already noted, tetanospasmin prevents neurotransmitter release at inhibitory interneurons, and therapy of tetanus is aimed at restoring normal inhibition. The benzodiazepines are centrally acting inhibitory agents that have been used for this purpose. Diazepam has been extensively utilized and results in a desirable degree of sedation as well as amnesia. However, the large intravenous doses of benzodiazepines required in tetanus may result in metabolic acidosis secondary to the propylene glycol vehicle. Thus, the water-soluble agent, midazolam, is currently the preferred agent for producing muscle relaxation in patients with tetanus.[9] Other drugs have been used less frequently but are effective muscle relaxants in the treatment of tetanus. Baclofen is a specific $GABA_B$ agonist that restores central inhibition and muscle relaxation when administered intrathecally in patients with tetanus.[14] Dantrolene blocks the release of calcium from sarcoplasmic reticulum and has been used to treat tetanus-induced muscle spasms.[15] However, prolonged use (i.e., use for longer than 60 days) is associated with hepatoxicity.

Neuromuscular Blockade

To control ventilation and muscular spasms as well as to prevent fractures and rhabdomyolysis, prolonged neuromuscular blockade may be required in the treatment of tetanus. Succinylcholine is recommended for emergency airway control, while vecuronium is the neuromuscular blocking agent of choice for prolonged blockade because of its minimal cardiovascular side effects.[16] Concomitant sedation with barbiturates or benzodiazepines is mandatory.

TABLE 140-2 Summary Guide to Tetanus Prophylaxis in Wound Management

	CLEAN, MINOR WOUNDS		ALL OTHER WOUNDS[a]	
History of Adsorbed Tetanus Toxoid (Doses)	Td[b] 0.5 mL IM	TIG, 250 U IM	Td[b] 0.5 mL IM	TIG, 250 U IM
Unknown or less than three	Yes[c]	No	Yes	Yes
Three or more[d]	No[e]	No	Yes[f]	No

[a]For example, wounds >6 h old, contaminated with soil, saliva, feces, or dirt; puncture or crush wounds; avulsions; wounds from missiles, burns, or frostbite.
[b]DPT for children <7 years of age (DT if pertussis vaccine is contraindicated); Td for persons >7 years of age.
[c]The primary immunization series should be completed. Three doses total are required, with the second dose given at least 4 weeks after the first and the third dose 6 months later.
[d]If only three doses of fluid toxoid have been received, then a fourth dose of *absorbed* toxoid should be given.
[e]Yes, if routine immunization schedule has lapsed in a child <7 years of age of if >10 years since last dose.
[f]Yes, if routine immunization schedule has lapsed in a child <7 years of age or if >5 years since last dose. Boosters more frequent than every 5 years may predispose to side effects.
Abbreviations: DPT, diphtheria-pertussis-tetanus; DT, Diphtheria-tetanus toxoids; IM, intramuscular; Td, tetanus-diphtheria; TIG, tetanus immune globulin.
Source: Adapted from the American College of Emergency Physicians,[23,24,25] with permission.

TABLE 140-3 Treatment of Tetanus

Respiratory management	Succinylcholine for emergency intubation; vecuronium for prolonged neuromuscular blockade
Immunotherapy	TIG ≥ 500 U IM as a single dose *and* Tetanus toxoid (DPT or Td depending on age), 0.5 mL IM at presentation, and 6 weeks and 6 months after presentation
Antibiotic therapy	Metronidazole, 500 mg IV every 6 h
Muscle relaxation	Midazolam, 5–15 mg/h continuous IV infusion *or* Lorazepam, 2 mg IV to effect *or* Diazepam, 5 mg IV every 1–3 h to effect
Neuromuscular blockade	Vecuronium, 6–8 mg/h IV
Management of autonomic dysfunction	Labetalol, 0.25–1.0 mg/min continuous IV infusion *or* Magnesium sulfate, 70 mg/kg IV loading, then 1–4 g/h continuous infusion to maintain blood level of 2.5–4 mmol/L Morphine sulfate, 0.5–1.0 mg/kg/h Clonidine, 300 μg every 8 h per nasogastric tube

Treatment of Autonomic Dysfunction

The combined α- and β-adrenergic blocking agent labetalol has been successfully used to treat the manifestations of sympathetic hyperactivity in tetanus. However, several investigators have reported fatal cardiovascular complications in patients treated with β-adrenergic blocking agents alone.[17,18] Adrenergic blocking drugs, although effective in the treatment of the autonomic dysfunction of tetanus, may precipitate dangerous myocardial depression if sympathetic activity transiently diminishes.

Magnesium sulfate inhibits the release of epinephrine and norepinephrine from the adrenal glands and adrenergic nerve terminals, eliminating the source of catecholamine excess in tetanus[19] and providing a rationale for its clinical use.[10] Morphine sulfate has also been demonstrated to be effective in treating the autonomic dysfunction in tetanus[10] by reducing sympathetic α-adrenergic tone and central sympathetic efferent discharge, and by producing peripheral arteriolar and venous dilatation.[9]

Continuous epidural block with bupivacaine provides sympathetic nervous system blockade, muscular relaxation, and analgesia in generalized tetanus.[20] The central α-receptor agonist, clonidine, decreases central sympathetic and peripheral arteriolar tone[21] and has also been used to manage tetanus-induced cardiovascular instability. Finally, it has been suggested that overactivity of the parasympathetic nervous system may contribute to the autonomic instability in patients with tetanus, since many of the clinical manifestations of the disease mimic cholinergic crisis. Evidence supporting this concept is provided by a report that atropine provides cardiac stabilization in patients with severe tetanus.[22]

Active Immunization

Patients who have recovered from tetanus must undergo active immunization, since the disease does not confer immunity. Adsorbed tetanus toxoid (0.5 mL) should be administered intramuscularly at the time of presentation and at 6 weeks and 6 months after injury. Tetanus-diphtheria (Td) should be administered to patients older than 7 years of age,[23] and diphtheria-pertussis-tetanus (DPT) to patients younger than 7 years of age.[24] A summary of the guidelines for active tetanus immunization is presented in Table 140-2. A summary of the management of tetanus is presented in Table 140-3.

REFERENCES

1. Bleck TP: Tetanus: Pharmacology, management, and prophylaxis. *Dis Mon* 37:551, 1991.
2. Izurieta HS, Sutter RW, Strebel PM, et al: Tetanus surveillance: United States, 1991–1994. *MMWR* 46(SS-2):15, 1997.
3. Sutter RW, Cochi SL, Brink EW, et al: Assessment of vital statistics and surveillance data for monitoring tetanus mortality, United States 1979–1984. *Am J Epidemiol* 131:132, 1990.
4. Bardenheier B, Prevots DR, Khetsurian N, et al: Tetanus: Surveillance—United States, 1995–1997. *MMWR* 47(SS-2):1, 1998.
5. Kefer MP: Tetanus. *Am J Emerg Med* 10:445, 1992.
6. Mellanby J, Green J: How does tetanus toxin act? *Neuroscience* 6:281, 1981.
7. Gergen PJ, McQuillan GM, Kiely M, et al: A population-based serologic survey of immunity to tetanus in the United States. *N Engl J Med* 332:761, 1995.
8. Richardson JP, Knight AL: Prevention of tetanus in the elderly. *Arch Intern Med* 151:1712, 1991.
9. Ernst ME, Klepser ME, Fouts M, et al: Tetanus: Pathophysiology and management. *Ann Pharmacother* 31:1507, 1997.
10. Wright DK, Lalloo UG, Nayiager S, et al: Autonomic nervous system dysfunction in severe tetanus: Current perspectives. *Crit Care Med* 17:371, 1989.
11. Alfrey DD, Rauscher LA: Tetanus: A review. *Crit Care Med* 7:176, 1979.
12. Blake PA, Feldman TM, Buchanan TM, et al: Serologic therapy of tetanus in the United States, 1965–1971. *JAMA* 235:42, 1976.
13. Ahmadsyah I, Salim A: Treatment of tetanus: An open study to compare the efficacy of procaine penicillin and metronidazole. *BMJ* 291:648, 1985.
14. Muller H, Borner U, Zierski J, et al: Intrathecal baclofen for treatment of tetanus-induced spasticity. *Anesthesiology* 66:76, 1987.
15. Farquhar I, Hutchinson A, Curan J: Dantrolene in severe tetanus. *Intensive Care Med* 14:249, 1988.
16. Powles AB, Ganta R: Use of vecuronium in the management of tetanus. *Anaesthesia* 40:879, 1985.
17. Buchanan N, Smit L, Cane RD, De Andrade M: Sympathetic overactivity in tetanus: Fatality associated with propranolol. *BMJ* 2:254, 1978.
18. Edmundson RS, Flowers MS: Intensive care in tetanus: Management, complications, and mortality in 100 cases. *BMJ* 1:401, 1979.
19. James MFM, Manson EDM: The use of magnesium sulfate infusions in the management of very severe tetanus. *Intensive Care Med* 11:5, 1985.
20. Southorn PA, Blaise GA: Treatment of tetanus-induced autonomic nervous system dysfunction with continuous epidural blockade. *Crit Care Med* 14:251, 1986.

21. Sutton DN, Tremlett MR, Woodcock TE, et al: Management of autonomic dysfunction in severe tetanus: The use of magnesium sulfate and clonidine. *Intensive Care Med* 16:75, 1990.
22. Dolar D: The use of continuous atropine infusion in the management of severe tetanus. *Intensive Care Med* 18:26, 1992.
23. American College of Emergency Physicians, Scientific Review Committee: Tetanus immunization recommendations for persons seven years of age and older. *Ann Emerg Med* 15:1111, 1986.
24. American College of Emergency Physicians, Scientific Review Committee: Tetanus immunization recommendations for persons less than seven years old. *Ann Emerg Med* 16:1181, 1987.
25. Recommendations of the Immunization Practices Advisory Committee (ACIP): Diphtheria, tetanus, and pertussis: Recommendations for vaccine use and other preventive measures. *MMWR* 40, RR-10, 1–28, 1991.

RABIES

David J. Weber
David A. Wohl
William A. Rutala

Currently, rabies causes an estimated 40,000 to 100,000 deaths each year worldwide.[1] In addition, millions of persons, primarily in developing countries, undergo costly postexposure treatment. In the United States, rabies continues to be endemic in many wild animals. Although human rabies is rare in the United States, postexposure rabies prophylaxis is likely provided to more than 35,000 persons per year.[2] Prevention efforts in the United States are estimated to cost between $230 million and $1 billion dollars.[1]

This chapter briefly reviews the microbiology, epidemiology, clinical presentation, and treatment of rabies. Because animal bites and scratches are commonly seen by primary care and emergency medical physicians, the postexposure management of persons potentially exposed to a rabid animal is reviewed in detail. Comprehensive reviews of rabies have been published in the medical literature[3–7] and in standard infectious disease or microbiology textbooks.[8–13] Current information is available on the "rabies homepage" produced by the Centers for Disease Control and Prevention.[14]

MICROBIOLOGY

Rabies virus is the prototype member of the genus *Lyssavirus,* of the family *Rhabdoviridae,* order *Mononegavirales.*[6] Members of this order have a nonsegmented, negative-stranded RNA genome that is tightly encapsulated into ribonucleocapsid structures. Members of the family *Rhabdoviridae* are grouped on the basis of their conical or bullet shape as visualized by electron microscopy. Their host range includes vertebrates (primarily mammals and fish), invertebrates (primarily arthropods), and plants. The *Rhabdoviridae* that infect animals and humans are divided into two genera, the *Lyssavirus* (Greek *Lyssa,* frenzy) and *Vesiculovirus* (Latin *vesicula,* little bladder).[3] Vesiculoviruses (e.g., vesicular stomatitis virus) cause disease in cattle, swine, horses, and a variety of other vertebrates.[3] Humans occasionally develop infection, which is most commonly characterized by a nonfatal, nonspecific influenza-like viral syndrome.

The rabies group of *Lyssavirus* is comprised of six serotypes, or genotypes, and includes classic rabies virus, Lagos bat virus, Mokola virus, Duvenhage virus, European bat lyssavirus 1, and European bat lyssavirus 2.[6] Rarely have lyssaviruses other than rabies caused human disease (<10 total cases described worldwide).

PATHOPHYSIOLOGY

Once introduced, the initial infection and multiplication occur with local monocytes for the first 48 to 96 h. Subsequently, the virus spreads across the motor end-plate, and ascends and replicates along peripheral nervous axoplasm to the dorsal root ganglia, the spinal cord, and the central nervous system (CNS). Following CNS replication in the gray matter, the virus spreads outward by peripheral nerves to virtually all tissues and organ systems. Viral infection of the salivary glands engenders infectivity of saliva; the infectivity of other body fluids is less well established.

Histologically, rabies is similar to other forms of encephalitis: diffuse and extensive monocellular infiltration with focal hemorrhage and demyelination, predominantly in perivascular areas in the gray matter of the CNS, basal ganglia, and the spinal cord. Negri bodies are the characteristic histologic finding for rabies, which is the site of CNS viral replication. They are eosinophilic intracellular lesions found within cerebral neurons and are highly specific for rabies. Negri bodies are encountered in about 75 percent of proven animal rabies; thus, although their presence is pathognomonic for rabies, their absence does not exclude rabies as a diagnostic possibility.

EPIDEMIOLOGY

Rabies is primarily a disease of animals.[5] The epidemiology of human rabies is a reflection of both the distribution of the disease in animals and the degree of human contact with these animals.[5] In those parts of the world where canine rabies has been controlled (i.e., the United States, Canada, and Europe), dogs account for less than 5 percent of the cases in animals. Where canine rabies has not been controlled (i.e., most developing countries of Asia, Africa, Latin America, and South America), dogs account for 90 percent or more of reported cases in animals. The major wildlife vectors of rabies are: dogs (major vector of rabies throughout the world, particularly Asia, Latin America, and Africa); foxes (Europe, Arctic, and North America); raccoons (eastern United States); skunks (midwestern United States, western Canada); coyotes (Asia, Africa, and North America); mongooses (yellow mongoose in Asia and Africa; Indian mongoose in the Caribbean Islands); and bats (vampire bats from Northern Mexico to Argentina, insectivorous bats in North America and Europe). In 1996, 49 states, the District of Columbia, and Puerto Rico reported 7124 cases of rabies in animals.[15] Wild animals accounted for almost 92 percent of the reported cases: raccoons (50.4 percent); skunks (23.2 percent); bats (10.4 percent); foxes (5.8 percent); and other wild animals including rodents and lagomorphs (2.1 percent). Rabid domestic animals included cats (3.7 percent); cattle (1.8 percent); dogs (1.6 percent); horses and mules (0.65 percent); sheep and goats (0.22 percent); and other animals such as ferrets (0.06 percent).

Animal reservoirs for rabies are found worldwide with the exception of some islands (e.g., Hawaii, Great Britain), Australia, and Antarctica. Rabies infections of mammalian species occur in geographically discrete outbreaks. Disease transmission within an outbreak is primarily intraspecific and involves a single, distinctive rabies variant. The geographic boundaries of current North America reservoirs for rabies are:[6]

1. An expanding reservoir for raccoon rabies that now encompasses the southeastern, mid-Atlantic, and northeastern United States (>3000 cases in 1996).
2. A long-standing reservoir in red and arctic foxes in Alaska, that has spread to include foxes across Canada as far east as Ontario, Quebec, and the upper parts of the northern New England states (usually <100 cases reported each year).
3. Three separate variants that infect striped skunks in long-standing reservoirs in California, the north central states, and the south central states (several thousand cases per year).
4. Two different variants in gray foxes in small but long-standing reservoirs in Arizona and Texas (~10 to 20 cases per year).
5. A recently recognized outbreak of rabies in coyotes in south Texas as a result of spillover infection from domestic dogs in a long-standing reservoir at the Texas-Mexico border.

Transmission of rabies virus usually begins when the contaminated saliva of an infected host is passed to a susceptible host. The most common mode of rabies viral transmission is through the bite of a rabid animal. Other routes of documented transmission have included contamination of mucous membranes (i.e., eyes, nose, mouth), aerosol transmission during spelunking in bat-infested caves or while working in the laboratory with rabies virus, corneal transplants, and iatrogenic infection through improperly inactivated vaccine.[14] Fomites have not been implicated in transmission. The risk of developing rabies following an animal bite or scratch by a rabid animal depends on whether a bite or scratch occurred, the number of bites, the depth of the bites, and the location of the wounds. In the absence of postexposure prophylaxis, the risk ranges from 80 to 100 percent (multiple severe bites around the face), to 15 to 40 percent (single bites), to 5 to 10 percent (superficial bites on the extremities). Contamination of open wounds with saliva carries a risk of approximately 0.1 percent.

The epidemiology of human rabies in the United States between 1946 and 1996 has been well described in a series of reports from the CDC.[15–18] In the United States, deaths in humans caused by rabies totaled 99 in the 1950s, 15 in the 1960s, 23 in the 1970s, 10 in the 1980s, and 22 from 1990 through 1996.[18] The median age of these patients was 27 (range: 4 to 82 years of age) and 20 (63 percent) were male. Cases were reported from 20 states; 7 cases (22 percent) were reported from California and 6 from Texas. Eleven patients were exposed to rabies in eight foreign countries. The onset of illness occurred in all months and with no apparent seasonal pattern.

Of the 32 patients that died of rabies between 1980 and 1996, a definite history of animal exposure was identified in only 7 (22 percent); 6 resulted from a dog bite received in a foreign country and 1 was from a bat bite received in the United States. Contact with an animal was identified in 12 persons; 8 with a bat, 2 with a dog, 1 with a cow, and 1 with a cat. For the remaining 13 patients, a potential source of animal exposure was not identified.

Current epidemiologic patterns of rabies in the United States have been summarized as follows:[18] The annual reports of rabies in wildlife far exceed those of rabies in domestic animals; rabies variants in bats are associated with a disproportionate number of infections in humans (53 percent), although bats constitute only about 10 percent of all reported rabies cases in animals annually; most other cases of human rabies diagnosed in the United States are attributable to infections acquired in areas of enzootic canine rabies in outside of the United States; most persons with a case of rabies that originated in the United States have no history of an animal bite; and rabies is diagnosed after death in more than one-third of the latter group.

Bites of squirrels, hamsters, guinea pigs, gerbils, chipmunks, rats, mice, rabbits, hares, and other small rodents almost never require antirabies postexposure prophylaxis. This author is at variance with Table 141-2 in that he would treat unprovoked attacks by woodchucks, beavers, and other large rodents.

PREEXPOSURE PROPHYLAXIS

Preexposure prophylaxis with rabies vaccine is highly recommended for persons whose recreational or occupational activities place them at risk for acquiring rabies (Table 141-1). Such persons include rabies research laboratory workers, rabies biologics production workers, rabies diagnostic laboratory workers, spelunkers, veterinarians and staff, animal-control and wildlife workers, travelers visiting foreign areas of enzootic rabies for more than 30 days, and veterinary students. Although the initial rabies preexposure vaccine regimen is similar, the need for booster doses, the timing of booster doses, and the need and timing of serologic tests to confirm immunity differ based on the degree of individual risk for exposure to rabies.[19] Emergency medicine health care providers should refer persons at risk for rabies who have not received preexposure prophylaxis to their local physician or health department for appropriate immunization.

Preexposure vaccination does not eliminate the need for additional therapy after a rabies exposure, but simplifies postexposure prophylaxis by eliminating the need for human rabies immune globulin (HRIG) and by decreasing the number of doses of vaccine required (see below).

POSTEXPOSURE PROPHYLAXIS

Postexposure prophylaxis is indicated for persons possibly exposed to a rabid animal. Administration of rabies postexposure prophylaxis

TABLE 141-1 Rabies Vaccine: Criteria for Preexposure Immunizations[19]

Risk Category	Nature of Risk	Typical Populations	Preexposure Regimen
Continuous	Virus present continuously, often in high concentrations. Aerosol, mucous membrane, bite or nonbite exposure possible. Specific exposures likely to go unrecognized.	Rabies research lab workers*; rabies biologics production workers.	Primary preexposure immunization course. Serology every 6 months. Booster vaccination when antibody titer falls below acceptable levels.†
Frequent	Exposures usually episodic with source recognized, but exposure may also be unrecognized. Aerosol, mucous membrane, bite, or nonbite exposure.	Rabies diagnostic lab workers,* spelunkers, veterinarians and staff, and animal control and wildlife workers in rabies enzootic areas. Certain travelers to foreign rabies enzootic areas.	Primary preexposure immunization course. Serologic testing every 2 years, booster for low titers.†
Infrequent (greater than population at large)	Exposure nearly always episodic with source recognized. Bite, or nonbite exposure.	Veterinarians and animal control and wildlife workers in areas of low rabies endemicity. Veterinary students.Travelers to areas where rabies is enzootic and medical care is limited.	Primary preexposure immunization course. No routine booster immunization or serology.
Rare (population at large)	Exposure always episodic, mucous membrane, or bite with source recognized.	U.S. population-at-large, including individuals in rabies-enzootic areas.	No preexposure immunization.

*Judgment of relative risk and extra monitoring of immunization status of laboratory workers is the responsibility of the laboratory supervisor.
†Acceptable antibody level is 1:5 titer (complete inhibition in RFFIT at 1:5 dilution). Boost if titer falls below 1:5.
Abbreviation: RFFIT, rapid fluorescent focus inhibition test.

TABLE 141-2 Rabies Postexposure Prophylaxis Guide[19]

ANIMAL TYPE	EVALUATION AND DISPOSITION OF ANIMAL	POSTEXPOSURE PROPHYLAXIS RECOMMENDATION
Dogs, cats, and ferrets	Healthy and available for 10 days observation	Should not begin prophylaxis unless animal develops clinical signs of rabies*
	Rabid or suspected rabid	Immediate therapy (see Table 141-3)
	Unknown (escaped)	Consult public health officials
Skunks, raccoons, bats, foxes, and most other carnivores	Regard as rabid unless geographic area is known to be free of rabies or until animal is proven negative by laboratory tests†	Immediate therapy (see Table 141-3)
Livestock, small rodents, lagomorphs (rabbits and hares), large rodents (woodchucks and beavers), and other mammals	Consider individually	Consult public health officials.‡ Bites of squirrels, hamsters, guinea pigs, gerbils, chipmunks, rats, mice, other small rodents, rabbits, and hares almost never require antirabies postexposure prophylaxis.

*During the 10-day holding period, begin therapy with human rabies immune globulin (HRIG) and rabies vaccine at first sign of rabies in a dog, cat, or ferret that has bitten someone. The symptomatic animal should be killed immediately and tested.

†The animal should be killed and tested as soon as possible. Holding for observation is not recommended. Discontinue vaccine if immunofluorescence test results of the animal are negative.

‡Bites of squirrels, hamsters, guinea pigs, gerbils, chipmunks, rats, mice, other rodents, rabbits, and hares almost never require antirabies treatment.

is a matter of medical urgency, not a medical emergency.[14] All persons presenting with an animal bite or scratch should be evaluated for the presence of a life-threatening condition, such as arterial laceration, pneumothorax, or respiratory compromise. Appropriate emergency care for animal bites should be provided.[20] Key aspects include tetanus prophylaxis, wound cleansing, measures to prevent bacterial infection, and evaluation for rabies prophylaxis. Cleansing of the wound with a 20% solution of soap and water is an essential first step in rabies prevention. In experimental animals, simple wound-cleansing has been shown to markedly reduce the likelihood of rabies.

All persons bitten or scratched by an animal, whether domestic or wild, should be evaluated for the need to initiate rabies postexposure prophylaxis. The decision to initiate rabies postexposure prophylaxis should be based on the following:[14] geographical location of the incident; the type of animal that was involved; and how the exposure occurred (i.e., provoked or unprovoked), the vaccination status of the animal, and whether the animal can be safely captured and tested for rabies (Table 141-2; Fig. 141-1). Excellent guidelines are often available from the local health department. For the purpose of rabies postexposure prophylaxis, a bite exposure is defined as any penetration of the skin by the teeth of an animal. Bites to the face and hands carry the highest risk, but the site of the bite should not influence the decision to begin therapy.[19] Scratches, abrasions, open wounds, or mucous membranes contaminated with saliva or other potentially infectious material (such as brain tissue) from a rabid animal constitute nonbite exposures. If the material containing the virus is dry, the virus can be considered noninfectious. A fully vaccinated dog or cat is unlikely to become infected with rabies, although rare cases have been reported among animals that had received only a single dose of vaccine. No documented vaccine failures have occurred among dogs or cats that had received two vaccinations.

Other contact by itself, such as petting a rabid animal and contact with blood, urine, or feces (e.g., guano) of a rabid animal, does not constitute an exposure and is not an indication for prophylaxis.[19] Local health departments may vary in their recommendations for salivary exposure, however. Apart from corneal transplantation, bite and nonbite exposures inflicted by infected humans could theoretically transmit rabies, but no such cases have been documented. Persons with suspected rabies may be managed using "standard precautions."[21]

Bats are increasingly implicated as an important wildlife reservoir for variants of rabies virus transmitted to humans. Minor bites by bats and awakening in a room with a bat have been associated with the development of rabies. For this reason, the CDC recommends rabies postexposure prophylaxis for all persons who have sustained a bite, scratch, or mucous membrane exposure to a bat unless the bat is available for testing and is negative for evidence of rabies.[22] Postexposure prophylaxis is also appropriate, even in the absence of a demonstrable bite, scratch, or mucous membrane exposure, in situations in which there is reasonable probability that such contact occurred (e.g., a sleeping person awakens to find a bat in the room or an adult witnesses a bat in a room with a previously unattended child or a mentally disabled or intoxicated person).[22]

The CDC recommends that a healthy dog, cat, or ferret that bites a person should be confined and observed for 10 days.[23] Such animals should be evaluated by a veterinarian at the first sign of illness during confinement. Any illness in the animal should be immediately reported to the local health department. If signs suggestive of rabies develop, the animal should be euthanized, its head removed, and the head shipped under refrigeration (not frozen) for examination of the brain by a qualified laboratory designated by the local or state health department. Any stray or unwanted dog, cat, or ferret that bites a person may be euthanized immediately and the head submitted for rabies examination. Animals other than dogs, cats, or ferrets that might have exposed a person to rabies should be immediately reported to the local health department. Prior vaccination of an animal does not preclude the necessity of euthanasia and testing if the period of virus shedding is unknown for that species.

In the United States, postexposure prophylaxis consists of a regimen of 1 dose of human rabies immune globulin (HRIG) and 5 doses of rabies vaccine over a 28-day period (Table 141-3). Rabies immune globulin and the first dose of rabies vaccine should be given as soon as possible after exposure, preferably within 24 hours. Rabies vaccines available in the United States include human diploid cell vaccine (HDCV) (produced in human diploid cells; Imovax, Pasteur Merieux Connaught), rabies vaccine absorbed (RVA) (produced in fetal rhesus diploid lung cells; Rabies Vaccine Absorbed, SmithKline Beecham), and purified chick embryo cell culture vaccine (PCEC) (produced in chick embryo cells; RabAvert, Chiron).[24] All currently used vaccines are produced in cell culture and are significantly less toxic than older vaccines that were produced in neural tissue. Side effects, including mild erythema, swelling, and pain at the injection site, have been reported among 30 to 74 percent of vaccine recipients. Systemic reactions, such as headache, nausea, abdominal pain, muscle aches, and dizziness, have been reported among 5 to 40 percent of recipients. Serum-sickness-like reactions (type III hypersensitivity) have been noted among approximately 6 percent of persons receiving booster

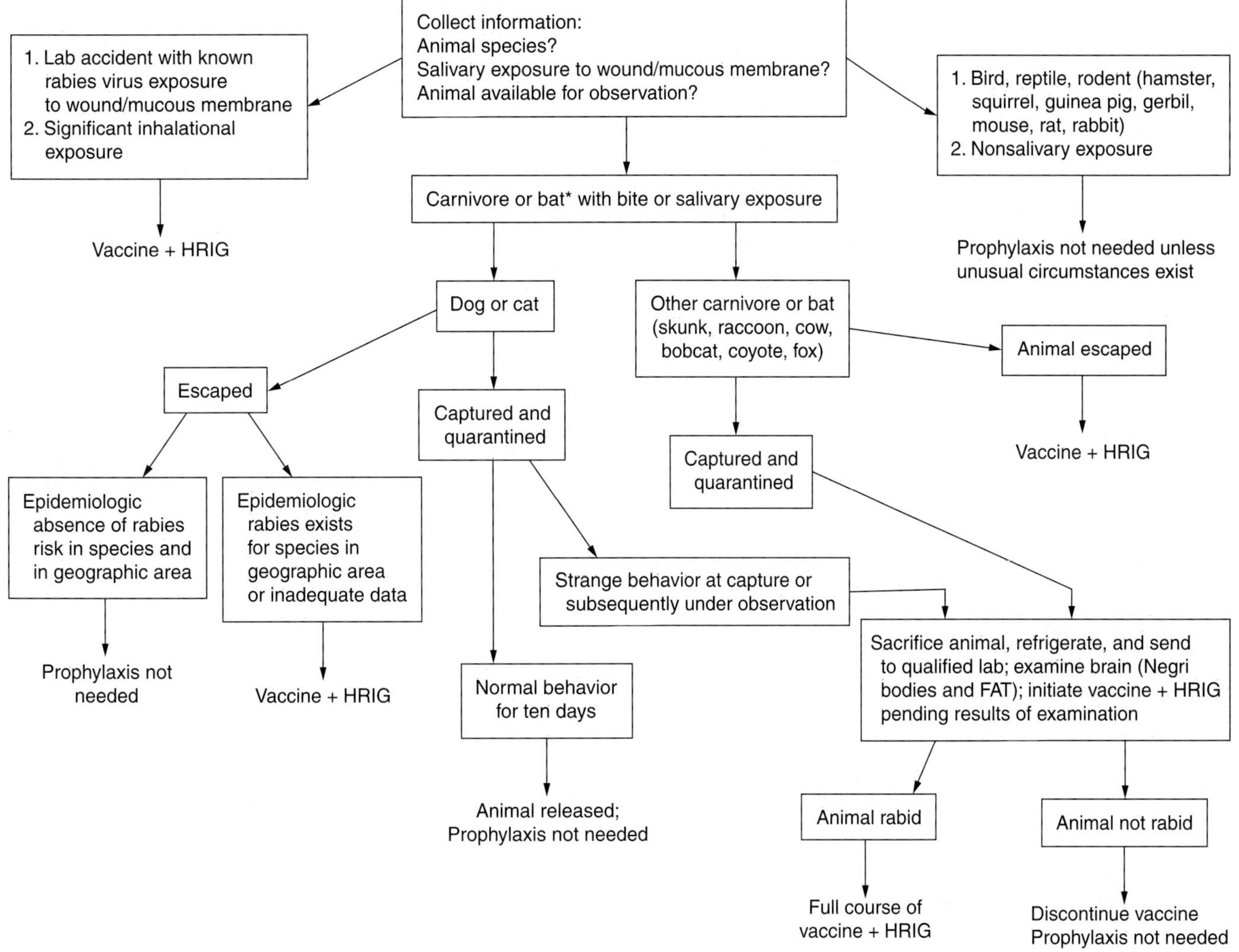

FIG. 141-1. Clinical guidelines for administration of rabies postexposure prophylaxis. FAT, fluorescent antibody test; HRIG, human rabies immune globulin. (Adapted from Mann JR: Rabies risk: Systemic evaluation and management of animal bites. *Compr Ther* 7:53, 1981. Used with permission.)

doses of HDCV, 2 to 21 days after administration of the booster dose. Such reactions have not been life threatening and have not been reported with the RVA or PCEC vaccines. Anaphylaxis and neurologic symptoms have only rarely been associated with the current rabies vaccines. Severe egg allergy is a contraindication to the use of the PCEC vaccine. Once initiated, rabies prophylaxis should not be interrupted or discontinued because of local or mild systemic adverse reactions to rabies vaccine.[19] Usually such reactions can be successfully managed with anti-inflammatory and antipyretic agents. When a person with a history of serious hypersensitivity to rabies vaccine must be revaccinated, antihistamines may be given. Epinephrine should be readily available to counteract anaphylactic reactions, and the person should be observed carefully immediately after vaccination.

HRIG is administered only once (i.e., at the beginning of antirabies prophylaxis) to provide immediate antibodies until the patient responds to rabies vaccine by producing antibodies. Failure to use HRIG has led to rabies, despite appropriate postexposure prophylaxis with human diploid cell vaccine. If HRIG was not given when vaccination was begun, it can be given through the seventh day after administration of the vaccine.[19] Beyond the seventh day, HRIG is not indicated because an antibody response is presumed to have occurred. The CDC recommends that as much as possible of the full dose be infiltrated around the wound.[22] HRIG should never be administered in the same syringe or into the same anatomic site as the vaccine. Even if the wound has to be sutured, it should be infiltrated locally with HRIG. This practice is safe and does not create an additional risk of infection.[25] However, caution is needed when injecting into a tissue compartment, such as the finger pulp, because excessive HRIG can increase compartment pressure and lead to necrosis.[26]

The CDC recommendations for postexposure prophylaxis should be followed EXACTLY. Although no postexposure prophylaxis vaccine failures have been reported in the United States since HDCV's licensing in 1980, 13 persons outside the United States have contracted rabies after postexposure prophylaxis with tissue culture-derived vaccine.[5] Each of these cases involved deviation from the recommended protocol; wounds not cleansed, passive immunization with HRIG not provided, or rabies vaccine injected into the gluteal rather than the deltoid area.

POSTEXPOSURE PROPHYLAXIS IN SPECIAL CIRCUMSTANCES

Prior Rabies Immunization

If exposed to rabies, persons previously vaccinated should receive two intramuscular doses (1 mL each) of vaccine, one immediately and one three days later.[19] Previously vaccinated refers to persons who have

TABLE 141-3 Type of Treatment and Regimen for Rabies Postexposure Prophylaxis by Vaccination Status[19]

VACCINATION STATUS	TREATMENT	REGIMEN*
Not previously immunized	Wound cleansing	All postexposure treatment should begin with immediate thorough cleansing of all wounds with soap and water. If available, a viricidal agent such as povidone-iodine solution should be used to irrigate the wounds.
	Human rabies immune globulin (HRIG)	Administer 20 IU per kg body weight. As much as possible of the full dose should be infiltrated into and around the wound(s), and the remainder should be administered intramuscularly at an anatomic site distant from the vaccine administration. HRIG should not be administered in the same syringe as vaccine. Because HRIG may partially suppress production of antibody, no more than the recommended dose should be given.
	Vaccine	1 mL of human diploid cell vaccine (HDCV), rabies vaccine absorbed (RVA), or purified chick embryo cell culture (PCEC) vaccine administered intramuscularly (deltoid area)† on days 0, 3, 7, 14, and 28 (day 0 indicates the first day of treatment).
Previously vaccinated‡	Wound cleansing	All postexposure treatment should begin with immediate thorough cleansing of all wounds with soap and water. If available, a viricidal agent such as povidone-iodine solution should be used to irrigate the wounds. Human rabies immune globulin (HRIG) should not be given.
	Vaccine	1 mL of HDCV, RVA, or PCEC administered intramuscularly (deltoid area)† on days 0 and 3.

*These regimens are applicable for all age groups, including children.

†The deltoid area is the only acceptable site of vaccination for adults and older children. For younger children, the outer aspect of the thigh may be used. Vaccine should never be administered in the gluteal area.

‡Any person with a history of preexposure vaccination with HDCV, RVA, or PCEC; previous postexposure prophylaxis with HDCV, RVA, or PCEC; or previous vaccination with any other type of rabies vaccine and a documented history of antibody response to the previous vaccination.

received one of the recommended preexposure or postexposure prophylaxis regimens of HDCV, RVA, or PCEC, or those who have received another vaccine and had a documented rabies antibody titer. HRIG is unnecessary and should not be given in these cases because an anamnestic antibody response will follow the administration of a booster regardless of the prebooster antibody titer.[27]

Immunocompromised Persons

Immunization of immunocompromised persons presents special challenges. First, vaccines may represent a danger to the immunocompromised person. Second, the immune response of immunocompromised persons to vaccination may not be as good as that of immunocompetent persons; higher doses or additional immunizations may be required, although even with these modifications, the immune response may be suboptimal. The Advisory Committee on Immunization Practices (ACIP) considers these persons severely immunocompromised: congenital immunodeficiency; human immunodeficiency virus (HIV) infection; leukemia lymphoma; aplastic anemia; generalized malignancy; or therapy with alkylating agents, antimetabolites, radiation, or large amounts of corticosteroids.[28]

Because rabies vaccine is formulated with inactivated virus, it does not represent a danger to immunocompromised persons and may be administered to such persons using the standard recommended doses and schedule (Table 141-3).[28] Further, the recommendations for the use of HRIG are the same in immunocompromised and immunocompetent persons.[28] However, corticosteroids, other immunosuppressive agents, and immunosuppressive illnesses can interfere with the development of active immunity and predispose the patient to developing rabies if exposed. Immunosuppressive agents should not be administered during postexposure prophylaxis, unless essential for the treatment of other conditions. When rabies postexposure prophylaxis is administered to persons receiving steroids or other immunosuppressive therapy, it is especially important that serum be tested for rabies antibody to ensure that an adequate response has developed.[28] To test the adequacy of the immune response, serum collected 2 to 4 weeks after the postexposure prophylaxis should completely neutralize challenge virus at a 1:25 serum dilution by rapid fluorescent focus inhibition test (RFFIT).[19]

Travelers

Preexposure prophylaxis is recommended for international travelers based upon the local incidence of rabies in the countries to be visited, the availability of appropriate antirabies biologics, and the intended activity.[29] Such persons include veterinarians, animal handlers, field biologists, spelunkers, and certain laboratory workers. Chloroquine phosphate (and possibly other structurally related antimalarials such as mefloquine, which is administered for malaria chemoprophylaxis) may interfere with the antibody response to rabies vaccine. Always immunize persons receiving antimalarial chemoprophylaxis by the intramuscular route.

Between 1980 and 1996, six persons died in the United States from rabies after having been bitten by a dog while visiting a foreign country. In that same period, three U.S. citizens died in foreign countries from exposure that occurred in the foreign country. For this reason, all persons who have returned from abroad should be questioned regarding whether they received an animal bite or scratch in an area with endemic rabies. Persons bitten or scratched by an animal in an area with endemic rabies should receive appropriate postexposure prophylaxis if the injury has occurred within the known incubation period (which may extend up to five years).

U.S. citizens and residents who are exposed to rabies while traveling in countries where rabies is endemic may sometimes receive postexposure prophylaxis with regimens or biologics that are not used in the United States. If postexposure prophylaxis is begun outside the United States using a non-FDA-approved regimen or biologic of nerve tissue origin, it may be necessary to provide additional treatment when the patient reaches the United States.[19] State and local health departments should be contacted for specific advice in such cases. The major modification used abroad, usually in an attempt to reduce cost, is the substitution of various schedules for intradermal injection or the use of non-FDA-approved vaccines.

TABLE 141-4 Natural History of Clinical Rabies in Humans

CLINICAL STAGE	DEFINING EVENT	USUAL DURATION	COMMON SYMPTOMS AND SIGNS*
Incubation period	Exposure	20 to 90 days	None
Prodrome	First symptom	2 to 10 days	Pain or paresthesia at site of bite Malaise, lethargy Headache Fever Nausea, vomiting, anorexia Anxiety, agitation, depression
Acute neurological phase	First neurologic sign	2 to 7 days	Anxiety, agitation, depression Hyperventilation, hypoxia Aphasia, incoordination Paresis, paralysis Hydrophobia, pharyngeal spasms Confusion, delirium, hallucinations Marked hyperactivity
Coma	Onset coma	0 to 14 days	Coma Hypotension, hypoventilation, apnea Pituitary dysfunction Cardiac arrhythmia, cardiac arrest
Recovery	Death or initiation of recovery	Months	Pneumothorax Intravascular thrombosis Secondary infections

*Not every symptom or sign may be present in each case.

Pregnancy

Adverse pregnancy outcomes or fetal abnormalities have not been associated with rabies vaccination.[30,31] Because of the potential consequences of inadequately treated rabies exposure, and because adverse events have not been associated with rabies postexposure prophylaxis during pregnancy, pregnancy is not considered a contraindication to rabies postexposure prophylaxis or HRIG.[19] If there is substantial risk of exposure to rabies, preexposure prophylaxis may also be indicated during pregnancy.

Children

The risk of rabies and the management of postexposure prophylaxis in children have been reviewed.[26,32] In infants and children, the dose of rabies vaccine for preexposure and postexposure prophylaxis is the same as that recommended for adults (Table 141-3). The dose of HRIG for postexposure prophylaxis is based on body weight. For small children with multiple bites, the calculated dosage of HRIG may be insufficient to infiltrate all wounds. However, sterile saline can be used to dilute the volume twofold or threefold to permit thorough infiltration.[26]

CLINICAL DISEASE

Rabies virus causes acute encephalitis in all warm-blooded hosts, including humans, and the outcome is almost always fatal. While patients with rabies may manifest a variety of clinical symptoms and signs, the disease tends to follow a characteristic course (Table 141-4).

Rabies infection is most commonly initiated by the bite of a rabid animal. Most commonly, the incubation period ranges from 20 to 90 days.[9] However, incubation periods have been reported as short as 4 days and as long as 19 years. Incubation periods exceeding one year have been well documented in the literature.[33] For patients who died from rabies in the United Sates between 1980 and 1996 and for whom a definite animal bite occurred, the median incubation period was 85 days (range: 53 to 150 days).[18] The incubation period has been reported to be shorter when the site of bite is on the head than when it is on an extremity.[9]

During the prodromal period, the symptoms and signs of rabies are often nonspecific. They include fever, sore throat, chills, malaise, anorexia, headache, nausea, vomiting, dyspnea, cough, and weakness. Early in the course some patients may report symptoms suggestive of rabies such as limb pain, limb weakness, and paresthesias at or near the presumed exposure site. Nonspecific neurologic symptoms may be reported including apprehension, anxiety, agitation, irritability, depression, and psychiatric disturbances.

The prodrome merges into the acute neurologic phase, which begins when the patient develops objective signs of central nervous system disease. Two major forms of acute neurologic disorder have been described: furious and paralytic. Furious rabies is noted in about 80 percent of patients and is characterized by hyperactivity, disorientation, hallucinations, and bizarre behavior. Periods of hyperactivity may alternate with periods of calm. Signs of autonomic dysfunction are frequently present and include hyperthermia, tachycardia, hypertension, and excessive salivation. About 50 percent of patients have classic hydrophobia in which attempts at drinking fluids result in severe spasms of the pharynx, larynx, and diaphragm. Paralytic rabies is noted in about 20 percent of patients and is characterized by paralysis, which may be maximal in the extremity that was bitten, diffuse, and symmetrical, or it may ascend in a pattern similar to Guillain-Barré syndrome. Accompanying signs may include fever and nuchal rigidity.

Coma almost always occurs within 10 days of the onset of symptoms. In the series reported by Noah and colleagues, the median duration of illness was 19 days (range: 7 to 28 days).[18] All patients in the series died. Death occurs from a variety of complications including pituitary dysfunction, seizures, respiratory dysfunction with progressive hypoxia, cardiac dysfunction with dysrhythmias and arrest, autonomic dysfunction, renal failure, and secondary bacterial infections.

Rarely have patients recovered from rabies, but in all such cases the patient had received either postexposure or preexposure prophylaxis with duck embryo vaccine or suckling mouse brain vaccine before the onset of symptoms. Despite intensive therapy, no persons without postexposure prophylaxis have survived in the United States since 1980.

DIAGNOSIS AND TREATMENT

The diagnosis of rabies is frequently made postmortem. This occurs because of the rarity of the disease, the increasing numbers of persons without an obvious exposure, and clinical confusion with other disorders. Important clues to diagnosis include a history of an animal bite and the development of the pathognomonic signs of hydrophobia and aerophobia. Tetanus should not be confused with rabies, because in tetanus the mental status is usually normal and the cerebrospinal fluid is normal. Other diseases that may be confused with rabies include poliomyelitis, Guillain-Barré syndrome, transverse myelitis, postvaccinial encephalomyelitis, intracranial mass lesions, cerebrovascular accidents, and poisoning with atropine-like compounds.

During the incubation period of rabies, no diagnostic test is available for either animals or persons that will indicate infection. Routine laboratory tests are of limited value for the diagnosis of rabies. Specific tests are required to diagnose rabies. Because no single test is uniformly informative, a battery of tests is commonly recommended. Early in the course of illness, the most reliable diagnostic test is a nuchal skin biopsy with immunofluorescent rabies antibody staining. Once clinical symptoms develop, a brain biopsy is universally positive when properly stained, but the invasive nature of this test precludes routine use. RFFIT may be performed on serum to detect rabies antibodies. However, while serum antibody may be present as early as day 5 of clinical illness, it may be absent after 10 to 14 days or more. Rabies virus has been isolated antemortem from human saliva, brain tissue, cerebrospinal fluid, urine, and tracheal secretions. Recently, nested PCR of RNA extracted from saliva has been shown to be a sensitive test. However, further study is required before this test can replace virus isolation as a standard antemortem diagnostic test.

No specific therapy exists to treat rabies. Treatment is directed at the clinical complications of the disease.[9]

REFERENCES

1. Rupprecht CE, Smith JE, Fekadu M, et al: The ascension of wildlife rabies: A cause for health concern or intervention? *Emerg Infect Dis* 1:107, 1995.
2. Krebs JW, Long-Marin SC, Childs JE: Causes, costs, and estimates of rabies postexposure prophylaxis treatments in the United States. *J Public Health Manage Pract* 4:56, 1998.
3. Fishbein DB: Rabies. *Infect Dis Clin North Am* 5:53, 1991.
4. Frenia ML, Lafin SM, Barone JA: Features and treatment of rabies. *Clin Pharm* 11:37, 1992.
5. Fishbein DB, Robinson LE: Current concepts: Rabies. *N Engl J Med* 329:1632, 1993.
6. Smith JS: New aspects of rabies with emphasis on epidemiology, diagnosis, and prevention of the disease in the United States. *Clin Microbiol Rev* 9:166, 1996.
7. Haburchak DR: Rabies reconsidered: Is the increasing zoonotic reservoir a new public threat? *Infect Med* 14:943, 1997.
8. Baer GM, Bellini WJ, Fishbein DB: Rhabdoviruses, in Fields BN, Knipe DM (eds): *Virology.* New York, Raven Press, 1990, p 883.
9. Fishbein DB, Bernard KW: Rabies virus, in Mandell GL, Bennett JE, Dolin R (eds): *Principles and Practices of Infectious Diseases,* 4th ed. New York, Churchill Livingstone, 1995, p 1527.
10. Dietzschold B, Rupprecht CE, Fu ZF, et al: Rhabdoviruses, in Fields BN, Knipe DM, Howley PM (eds): *Virology,* 3rd ed. Philadelphia, Lippincott-Raven, 1996, p 1137.
11. Rupprecht CE, Hanlon CA: Rabies, in Evans AS, Kaslow RA (eds): *Viral Infections of Humans,* 4th ed. New York, Plenum Medical Book Company, 1997, p 665.
12. Bleck TP, Rupprecht CE: Rhabdoviruses, in Richman DD, Whitley RJ, Hayden FG (eds): *Clinical Virology.* New York, Churchill Livingstone, 1997, p 879.
13. Hanlon CA, Rupprecht CE: The reemergence of rabies, in Scheld WM, Armstrong D, Hughes JM (eds): *Emerging Infections I.* Washington, DC, ASM Press, 1998, p 59.
14. http://www.cdc.gov/ncid/dvrd/rabies/
15. Krebs JW, Smith JS, Rupprecht CE, et al: Rabies surveillance in the United States during 1996. *JAMA* 2111:1525, 1997.
16. Held JR, Tierkel ES, Steele JH: Rabies in man and animals in the United States, 1946–1965. *Pub Health Rep* 82:1009, 1967.
17. Anderson LJ, Nicholson KG, Tauxe RV, et al: Human rabies in the United States, 1960 to 1979: Epidemiology, diagnosis, and prevention. *Ann Intern Med* 100:728, 1984.
18. Noah DL, Drenzek CL, Smith JS, et al: Epidemiology of human rabies in the United States, 1980 to 1996. *Ann Intern Med* 128:922, 1998.
19. Centers for Disease Control and Prevention: Human rabies prevention—United States, 1999. Recommendations of the Immunization Practices Advisory Committee (ACIP). *MMWR* 48(RR-1):1, 1999.
20. Weber DJ, Hansen AR: Infections resulting from animal bites. *Infect Dis Clin North Am* 5:663, 1991.
21. Garner JS: Guideline for isolation precautions in hospitals. *Infect Control Hosp Epidemiol* 17:53, 1996.
22. Centers for Disease Control and Prevention: Human rabies—Texas and New Jersey, 1997. *MMWR* 47:1, 1998.
23. Centers for Disease Control and Prevention: Compendium of animal rabies control, *MMWR* 48(RR-3):1, 1999.
24. Anonymous. A new rabies vaccine. *Med Lett Drugs Ther* 40:64, 1998.
25. Wilde H, Bhanganada K, Chutivongse S, et al: Is injection of contaminated animal bite wounds with rabies immune globulin a safe practice? *Trans R Soc Trop Med Hyg* 86:86, 1992.
26. Lang J, Plotkin SA: Rabies risk and immunoprophylaxis in children. *Adv Pediatr Infect Dis* 13:219, 1998.
27. Fishbein DB, Bernard KW, Miller KD, et al: The early kinetics of the neutralizing antibody response after booster immunizations with human diploid cell rabies vaccine. *Am J Trop Med Hyg* 35:663, 1986.
28. Centers for Disease Control and Prevention: Recommendations of the Advisory Committee on Immunization Practices (ACIP): Use of vaccines and immune globulins in persons with altered immunocompetence. *MMWR* 42(RR-4):1, 1993.
29. Centers for Disease Control and Prevention: *Health information for internation travel, 1996–1997.* Atlanta, Department of Health and Human Services, 1997.
30. Chabala S, Williams M, Amenta R, et al: Confirmed rabies exposure during pregnancy: Treatment with human rabies immune globulin and human diploid cell vaccine. *Am J Med* 91:423, 1991.
31. Chutivongse S, Wilde H, Benjavongkulchai M, et al: Postexposure rabies vaccination during pregnancy: Effect on 202 women and their infants. *Clin Infect Dis* 20:818, 1995.
32. Ledwith M, Baltimore RS: Management of rabies exposures in pediatric practice. *Curr Opin Pediatr* 9:478, 1997.
33. Smith JS, Fishbein DB, Rupprecht CE, et al: Unexplained rabies in three immigrants in the United States. *N Engl J Med* 324:205, 1991.

MALARIA

Jeffrey D. Band

With the increase in international travel and the continued shift of travel to tropical locales, it is not surprising that physicians are seeing more patients with infectious diseases acquired in the tropics. Malaria, a protozoan disease transmitted by the bite of the *Anopheles* mosquito, remains one of the most significant of these. Four species of the genus *Plasmodium* infect humans: *P. vivax, P. ovale, P. malariae,* and *P. falciparum.* Annually, over 250 million persons develop malaria, and more than 2.5 million persons die.[1] The incidence of malaria has been increasing in recent years despite worldwide aggressive attempts at control. Not only is the mosquito vector becoming less susceptible to a variety of insecticides, but *Plasmodium falciparum*—the parasite responsible for the most deadly form of malaria—is becoming increasingly resistant to antimalarial medications.

Malaria, especially disease due to *P. falciparum,* represents a medical emergency in any nonimmune host. Its early manifestations are largely nonspecific and can mimic other infectious diseases. Failure to diagnose infection rapidly can be disastrous. Likewise, failure to use specific antimalarial agents to which the individual strain is susceptible can result in early death. A diagnosis of malaria must be considered in any person returning from the tropics with an unexplained febrile illness. Questions regarding recent travel should become routine in emergency departments.

EPIDEMIOLOGY

Malaria transmission occurs in large areas of Central and South America, the Caribbean, sub-Saharan Africa, the Indian subcontinent, Southeast Asia, the Middle East, and Oceania. Certain species may predominate in a given geographic area.[2] For example, *P. vivax* is more common in the Indian subcontinent and in Central America, whereas *P. falciparum* is the most prevalent form in Africa, Haiti, and New Guinea.

The risk of contracting malaria, which varies considerably between regions, is largely dependent on the intensity of transmission in both urban and rural areas, and, for travelers, on the itinerary and time and type of travel. From 1990 to 1994, the Centers for Disease Control and Prevention reported 2580 cases of malaria among US civilians.[3] Of the more than 500 cases in 1994, a total of 303 (58 percent) were acquired in sub-Saharan Africa, 102 (20 percent) in Asia, 74 (14 percent) in the Caribbean and Central America, 24 (5 percent) in Oceania, and only 9 (2 percent) in South America. *Plasmodium vivax* accounted for 46 percent of all cases, and *P. falciparum* for another 46 percent. Mixed infections were uncommon, representing less than 1 percent of all cases. Thus, more than half of all cases of malaria, including the majority of cases due to *P. falciparum,* were acquired from travels in sub-Saharan Africa. Yet, for every traveler to sub-Saharan Africa, at least 10 travelers visit potential malarious areas of Asia and South America each year. Clearly, the intensity of exposure appears to be much higher in sub-Saharan Africa.

Resistance of *P. falciparum* to chloroquine continues to spread (Table 142-1).[4] In addition, strains of *P. falciparum* are resistant to other chemotherapeutic agents, including pyrimethamine-sulfadoxine, quinine, mefloquine, doxycycline, and new agents, including halofantrine and artesunate (the latter two agents are not available in the United States). Recently, strains of *P. vivax* have been isolated from patients who have failed chloroquine therapy.[5] Prior to 1990, no strains of *P. vivax, P. ovale,* or *P. malariae* were resistant to chloroquine.

PATHOPHYSIOLOGY

The organism is transmitted primarily by the bite of an infected female anopheline mosquito. This vector is most frequently found in tropical and subtropical regions below 8200 ft (2500 m) above sea level. Plasmodial sporozoites are injected into the host's bloodstream during the mosquito's blood meal and are carried directly to the liver. The hepatic parenchymal cells are invaded, and asexual reproduction of the parasite begins (preerythrocytic schizogony or exoerythrocytic stage). As thousands of daughter merozoites are formed, the parenchymal liver cell ruptures, releasing daughter merozoites back into the circulation, where they rapidly invade erythrocytes (erythrocytic stage). In *P. vivax* and *P. ovale* infection, a portion of the intrahepatic forms are not released, remain dormant for months, and can later activate and cause clinical relapses.

The clinical manifestations of malaria first appear during the erythrocytic stage. Once merozoites enter this stage, they never reinvade the liver. Merozoites mature within the erythrocyte and take on various morphologic forms, including the early ring forms, trophozoites, and schizonts (which represent a mass of new merozoites). Eventually, the target erythrocyte lyses, and new merozoites invade uninfected

TABLE 142-1 Geographic Distribution of Malaria, Including Resistant Strains

Geographic Region	Areas with Malaria	Countries with Chloroquine-Resistant *Plasmodium falciparum* (CRPF)	Countries with Fansidar-Resistant *P. falciparum*
Central America	All countries	None	None
Caribbean	Dominican Republic and Haiti	None	None
South America			
Temperate	Argentina	None	None
Tropical	All countries	All countries except Paraguay	Interior Amazon Basin
East Asia	China	China	South China
Eastern South Asia	All countries except Brunei and Singapore	All infected areas	Infected areas except Philippines
Middle South Asia	All countries	All countries	Afghanistan and Bhutan
Western South Asia and Middle East	Iraq, Oman, Saudi Arabia, Syria, Turkey, and United Arab Emirates	Oman and Saudi Arabia	None
Northern Africa	All countries except Tunisia	Algeria	None
Sub-Saharan Africa	All countries except Cape Verde, Reunion, Sao Tome/Principe, and Seychelles	Widespread	Widespread
Southern Africa	All countries except Lesotho and St. Helena	Widespread	Occasional
Oceania	Limited to Papua New Guinea, Solomon Islands, and Vanuatu (small foci elsewhere)	Widespread	Widespread

TABLE 142-2 Characteristics of Malaria-Causing *Plasmodium* Species

	P. falciparum	*P. vivax*	*P. ovale*	*P. malariae*
Incubation period (mean)	8–25 days (12)	8–27 days (14)	9–17 days (15)	15–30 days
Asexual erythrocytic cycle	48 h	48 h	48 h	72 h
Relapse	No	Yes	Yes	No
Red blood cell (RBC) preference	Reticulocytes (but can infect RBCs of all ages)	Reticulocytes	Reticulocytes	Older cells
Morphologic characteristics				
Degree of parasitemia	High (multiple rings per RBC)	Low	Low	Low
Ring forms and early trophozoites	Ring forms predominate; threadlike cytoplasm with double-chromatic dots	Amoeboid cytoplasm	Compact cytoplasm	Compact cytoplasm
Mature trophozoites	Rarely seen	Observed	Observed	Observed
Schizonts	Rarely seen	Observed	Observed	Observed
Gametocytes	Banana shaped	Round	Round	Round

red blood cells, continuing the infection and causing clinical manifestations. Lysogeny may become regular, occurring at 2- to 3-day intervals in established and untreated infections, producing the classic periodicity of symptoms.

After several cycles, a proportion of the merozoites develop into sexual forms (gametocytes). Upon ingestion by another feeding anopheline mosquito, male and female gametocytes undergo sexual reproduction and become infective sporozoites ready for their next host.

Each species of *Plasmodium* has specific characteristics, including typical morphologic forms and selective red blood cell tropism (Table 142-2). Many of these characteristics are responsible for important pathophysiologic consequences.

Malaria may also be transmitted by direct transfusion of infected blood or passed transplacentally from mother to fetus. In these cases, an exoerythrocytic phase is absent.

Disease ensues after an incubation period ranging from 8 days in the nonimmune and unprotected host to several weeks or more. Both incomplete suppression by partially active chemoprophylaxis and incomplete immunity can markedly prolong the incubation period to months or even years. Only the asexual intraerythrocytic parasite is responsible for the symptoms and pathophysiologic consequences. The hallmark of malaria is the recurring febrile paroxysm that corresponds to hemolysis of infected erythrocytes and release of antigenic products with activation of macrophages and production of cytokines.

Hemolysis can be high with *P. falciparum* infection, since parasitemia can be overwhelming and erythrocytes of all ages are susceptible. Parasitized erythrocytes lose flexibility and are removed in the microcirculation, with resultant obstruction and tissue anoxia of the lungs, kidneys, brain, and other vital organs. Noncardiac pulmonary edema, renal failure, and cerebral malaria may result. Sequestration accounts for the paucity of observed mature parasites in the peripheral smear of patients infected with *P. falciparum.*

In addition to prolonged high fever, hemolysis, and, in the case of infection with *P. falciparum,* obstruction to capillary flow, immunologic sequelae may also occur, resulting in glomerulonephritis, nephrotic syndrome, thrombocytopenia, and polyclonal antibody stimulation. Lastly, hypersplenism with resultant pancytopenia may occur, especially in cases of prolonged, untreated malaria.

CLINICAL FEATURES

Typically, patients develop a prodrome of malaise, myalgia, headache, and low-grade fevers, often accompanied by chills.[6] In some patients, headache, chest pains, cough, abdominal pain, arthralgias, or diarrhea may be prominent. The early manifestations are quite nonspecific and can easily become confused with a viral syndrome, influenza, hepatitis, and other less severe self-limited clinical entities. Illness usually progresses to severe chills followed by high-grade fevers accompanied by tachycardia, nausea, orthostatic dizziness, and extreme weakness. After several hours, the fever abates and the patient becomes diaphoretic and exhausted. Over time, the paroxysms of malaria—chills and fever followed by diaphoresis—may occur at nearly regular intervals that correspond to the length of the asexual erythrocytic cycles (Table 142-2). The classic paroxysms of malaria are often lacking in malaria due to *P. falciparum* or in persons who received some form of chemoprophylaxis.

The findings on physical examination are also not specific for malaria. Most patients appear acutely ill with high fevers, tachycardia, and tachypnea. Splenomegaly and tender abdomen are commonly present in advanced infection. The liver may or may not be enlarged. Features quite atypical for malaria include lymphadenopathy and a maculopapular skin rash.

Laboratory features include normochromic normocytic anemia with findings suggestive of hemolysis, a normal or mildly depressed total leukocyte count, thrombocytopenia, an elevated erythrocyte sedimentation rate, elevated lactose dehydrogenase, and mild abnormalities in liver and renal functions. Other laboratory abnormalities include hyponatremia, hypoglycemia, and a biologic false-positive VDRL.

Complications of malaria can occur rapidly in untreated infection, especially when the agent is *P. falciparum.*[7] Infections caused by any

TABLE 142-3 Guidelines for Preparing Malaria Smears

1. Use scrupulously clean slides; manufacturers' precleaned slides may have residual debris.
2. Obtain a large drop of blood from the patient's finger by using a blood lancet.
3. Place the cleaned surface of the slide against the drop of blood; with a quick circular motion, make a film the size of a dime. Do not mix excessively or distortion will result. The thick smear should be of such depth that newsprint would be barely legible. (Let the smear air dry for 30 to 60 min.)
4. Obtain a small drop of blood from the patient's finger and, with a second clean slide, spread the blood gently over the slide. Air dry the thin film, fix it with methyl alcohol, and stain it with Giemsa stain.
5. If the thin smear is negative, examine the thick smear. Once air dried, the thick film should not be fixed prior to staining with Giemsa.

TABLE 142-4 Treatment Regimens for Malaria

Clinical Setting	Drug	DOSAGE GUIDELINES Adults	Children
Uncomplicated infection with *Plasmodium vivax, P. ovale, P. malariae,* and chloroquine-sensitive *P. falciparum*	Chloroquine phosphate *plus*	1-g load (600-mg base), then 500 mg (300-mg base) in 6 h, then 500 mg (300-mg base) per day for 2 days (total dose, 2.5 g)	10-mg/kg base to maximum of 600 mg load, then 5-mg/kg base in 6 h and 5-mg/kg base per day for 2 days
	Primaquine phosphate*	26.3-mg load (15-mg base) per day for 14 days upon completion of chloroquine therapy	0.3-mg/kg base for 14 days upon completion of chloroquine therapy
Uncomplicated infection with chloroquine-resistant *P. falciparum*	(a) Quinine sulfate *plus*	600–650 mg PO tid for 5–7 days	8.3 mg/kg PO tid for 5–7 days†
	doxycycline *plus/minus*	100 mg PO bid for 7 days	Contraindicated in children <8 years of age
	pyrimethamine-sulfadoxine (Fansidar)‡	3 tablets (75 mg/1500 mg) PO × 1 dose	Over 2 months old: >50 kg 3 tab; 30–50 kg 2 tab; 15–29 kg 1 tab; 10–14 kg 1/2 tab; 4–9 kg 1/4 tab
	OR (b) Mefloquine *plus*	1250 mg PO × 1	1 tablet/10 kg PO × 1§
	doxycycline‖ *OR*	See above	See above
	(c) Halofantrine#	500 mg 6 h apart for 3 doses (repeat again in 1 week)	8 mg/kg salt orally, given q6h for 3 doses (repeat again in 1 week)
Complicated infection with chloroquine-resistant *P. falciparum*	Quinidine gluconate *plus*	10-mg/kg load over 2 h, then 0.02 mg/kg/min continuous infusion until patient is stabilized and able to tolerate PO therapy (see above)	Same as adults**
	doxycycline	100 mg IV q12h until tolerating PO therapy (see above)	Contraindicated in children <8 years of age

*Terminal treatment for *P. vivax* and *P. ovale* only.
†If unable to administer with doxycycline due to patient's age, extend treatment to full 10 days.
‡Optional; of unlikely value if acquisition in area with Fansidar resistance.
§Not formally approved yet by Food and Drug Administration in this setting.
‖Optional; many experts feel comfortable with mefloquine alone.
#Halofantrine is not commercially available in the United States (contact Smith-Kline Beecham at 1-800-366-8900). Becoming drug of choice for self-treatment of presumptive malaria in Thai-Cambodian and Myanmar borders *if* access to medical care is not available. In these areas, may need to extend treatment to 3 days instead of 1 day.
**Consult an expert in pediatric infectious disease immediately for guidance.

species of *Plasmodium* can result in hemolysis, splenic enlargement and, occasionally, splenic rupture. An immune-mediated glomerulonephritis is also common to all forms but tends to occur most often in *P. malariae* infection. With the ability to cause high parasitemia levels and sequestration with capillary sludging, *P. falciparum* infection can be fatal. Cerebral malaria—characterized by somnolence, coma, delirium, and seizures—is associated with mortality rates in excess of 20 percent. Reversible causes of encephalopathy must be excluded. The cerebrospinal fluid is usually normal, except for a slightly elevated opening pressure and protein concentration. A mild pleocytosis might also be present. Other life-threatening complications associated with *P. falciparum* infection include respiratory failure due to noncardiogenic acute pulmonary edema (similar to adult respiratory distress syndrome), renal failure (acute tubular necrosis), and severe metabolic abnormalities, including lactic acidosis and profound hypoglycemia. Any target organ is susceptible to the effects of severe tissue hypoxia from the cytoadherence between the parasitized erythrocyte and the vascular endothelium of the host.

The very young, the elderly, and pregnant women are at greatest risk for complications due to *P. falciparum.*

DIAGNOSIS

The definitive diagnosis is established by the visualization of parasites on Giemsa-stained thick and thin blood smears. In early infection, especially infection due to *P. falciparum,* in which parasitized erythrocytes are sequestered from the bloodstream, parasitemia may be undetectable. Also, parasitemia fluctuates over time: it generally is highest during chills and as the fever is on the rise. High fevers are schizonticidal. In highly suspicious cases, failure to detect parasitemia is not an indication to withhold therapy. Delay in the diagnosis and treatment of malaria can have disastrous results. If parasitemia is not seen in the stained thin smear, a thick smear that concentrates blood cells may provide the diagnosis[3] (Table 142-3). Extreme care in the preparation of slides is important, since debris may result in false-positive smears. If parasites are not visualized, repeated smears should be obtained at least twice daily for 2 to 3 days to exclude malaria completely. Newer molecular probes for rapid diagnosis and speciation of the invading pathogen are in development.[8,9] The two major questions to be answered by the blood smear are the degree of parasitemia present (correlates with prognosis) and whether *P. falciparum* is responsible

TABLE 142-5 Adverse Effects, Precautions, and Contraindications of Antimalarial Drugs

Drug	Minor Toxicity	Major Toxicity	Precautions/Contraindications
Chloroquine	Nausea/vomiting, diarrhea, pruritus, postural hypotension, rash, fever, headache, dizziness	Rare; hypotension and shock after parenteral therapy; retinopathy after prolonged use	Avoid with patients with severe psoriasis and some types of porphyria
Mefloquine	Nausea/vomiting, cramps, diarrhea, anorexia; dizziness, headaches, bradycardia	Rare unless underlying heart disease with bradycardia or the patient is on selected cardiotoxic medications (dysrhythmias, arrest); acute toxic confusional states may occur, as can seizures	Precaution during pregnancy and in children weighing <10 kg.; avoid if the patient is receiving quinine or quinidine; avoid if the patient has heart conduction disturbance or if underlying seizure disorder
Fansidar (pyrimethamine-sulfadoxine)	GI disturbances, photo toxocity, headaches, dizziness, skin rash	Fatal cutaneous eruptions reported, agranulocytosis	Contraindicated during pregnancy and in infants or if the patient is allergic to sulfonamides or pyrimethamine
Doxycycline	GI disturbances, photo toxicity, vaginal candidiasis	Rare	Contraindicated during pregnancy, in children <8 years of age; may depress prothrombin time in patients receiving anticoagulants
Proguanil*	Generally well tolerated; may develop mouth ulcers, dizziness, or alopecia	Rare, anemia after prolonged use	Contraindicated if the patient is allergic to proguanil; best to avoid use during pregnancy and in young infants
Quinine or quinidine	Cinchonism (nausea and vomiting, headache, tinnitus, dizziness, visual disturbance)	Hypotension, cardiac dysrhythmias, hypoglycemia, Coombs-positive hemolysis, abortions, neuromuscular paralysis (myasthenia)	Contraindicated in cardiac disease; cautiously in pregnancy, myasthenia gravis
Primaquine†	Nausea, vomiting, diarrhea, cramps, methemoglobulinemia	Massive hemolysis in patients with G6PD deficiency, exacerbation of systemic lupus erythematosus or rheumatoid arthritis	Contraindicated in G6PD deficiency, pregnancy
Halofantrine	GI disturbances, headaches, dizziness, pruritus	Similar to mefloquine	Similar to mefloquine but more cardiotoxic

*Not used for acute therapy.
†Terminal treatment for *Plasmodium vivax* and *P. ovale* infections only.
Abbreviations: G6PD, glucose-6-phosphate dehydrogenase; GI, gastrointestinal.

for infection. Most patients with *P. falciparum* infection should be managed in the hospital setting, as should any patient with more than 3 percent parasitemia. Clues to the diagnosis of *P. falciparum* infection include the presence of small ring forms with double-chromatin knobs within the erythrocyte, multiply infected rings in individual red blood cells, a paucity of trophozoites and schizonts on smear, the pathognomonic crescent-shaped (banana-shaped) gametocyte, and parasitemia exceeding 4 percent. Repeated smears should be obtained daily to assess the efficacy of drug treatment.

TREATMENT

Therapeutic decisions are based on the severity of the illness, the agent, and whether the patient may be infected with chloroquine-resistant *P. falciparum*.[2,10] If *P. falciparum* infection can be excluded, most persons can be managed in the ambulatory setting. Close follow-up, including repeated smears, is necessary. Patients with significant hemolysis or who have underlying severe chronic medical problems that can be aggravated by high fevers or hemolysis are best hospitalized. Infected infants and pregnant women are also best managed in the hospital.

Chloroquine is the drug of choice for treatment of infection due to *P. vivax, P. ovale,* and *P. malariae.* Table 142-4 summarizes the treatment regimens for malaria. With treatment, the parasite load should decrease significantly within the first 24 to 48 h. No asexual forms of the parasite should be detectable 3 to 4 days after treatment is completed. Gametocytes, the sexual forms, which do not cause disease in the human host, may persist for several weeks after treatment and are not an indicator of treatment failure. Chloroquine has no effect on the exoerythrocytic parasites, which may be dormant in the liver with infection due to *P. vivax* and *P. ovale.* Unless terminal treatment is administered with primaquine, clinical relapses commonly occur. Primaquine should not be used in patients with glucose-6-phosphate dehydrogenase deficiency, because primaquine may induce massive hemolysis of erythrocytes. Table 142-5 summarizes the commonly described adverse effects and precautions or contraindications of the antimalarial medications. Despite treatment with both chloroquine and primaquine, infection or relapse may persist.

Treatment of *P. falciparum* infection is generally best managed in a hospital setting, particularly if the level of parasitemia exceeds 3 percent. Unless one is certain that the patient could not have chloroquine-resistant *falciparum* infection (based on geographic exposure,

TABLE 142-6 Recommended Chemoprophylactic Regimens for Prevention of Malaria*

Drug	Adult Dose	Pediatric Dose
	TRAVEL TO AREA WHERE CRPF HAS NOT BEEN REPORTED	
Primary drug		
Chloroquine phosphate	300-mg base (500 mg salt) PO, 1/week	5-mg/kg base (8.3 mg/kg salt) PO, 1 week, up to adult dose
Second-line drug		
Doxycycline	100 mg PO qd	>8 years of age: 2 mg/kg PO qd up to adult dose
	TRAVEL TO AREAS WHERE CRPF HAS BEEN REPORTED	
Primary drug		
Mefloquine	228-mg base (250 mg salt) PO, 1 week	>45 kg 1 tab/week 31–45 kg 3/4 tab/week 20–30 kg 1/2 tab/week 12–19 kg 1/4 tab/week 5–11 kg 5 mg/kg base/week
Second-line drugs		
Doxycycline†	See above	See above
Chloroquine	See above	See above
plus		
Fansidar‡ (pyrimethadine sulfadoxine)	See Table 142–5	See Table 142–5
Proguanil§	200 mg PO qd	>10 years adult dose 7–10 years 150 mg/day 2–6 years 100 mg/day <2 years 50 mg/day
	TRAVEL TO AREAS WHERE MULTIPLE-DRUG RPF HAS BEEN REPORTED	
Primary drug		
Doxycycline	See above	See above
Second-line drug		
Halofantrine (self-treatment)	See Table 142–4	See Table 142–4
Artemisinin derivatives‖	Investigational	Investigational

*For prolonged exposure in areas with *Plasmodium vivax* or *P. ovale,* primaquine (Table 142–5) should be added at completion of prophylaxis.
†Doxycycline is the preferred second-line agent for travels except for travels to rural Thailand (border areas along Cambodia and Burma), where it should be considered first-line due to prevalence of mefloquine resistance.
‡Fansidar may be used for unexplained febrile illnesses if medical assistance is not readily available (see a physician as soon as possible) and resistance is not widespread (Table 142–2).
§Some experts add proguanil to chloroquine prophylaxis for alternative prophylaxis in selected sub-Saharan countries (Angola, Burundi, Kenya, Malawi, Mozambique, Rwanda, Tanzania, Uganda, Zaire, and Zambia).
‖Not available in the United States and usually used in combination with other antimalarial agents such as mefloquine or doxycycline.
Abbreviations: CRPF, chloroquine-resistant *Plasmodium falciparum;* RPF, resistant *P. falciparum.*

Table 142-1), it is best to assume the infecting strain is resistant to chloroquine and to initiate treatment with a combination of quinine and doxycycline with or without pyrimethamine-sulfadoxine. Quinine may at times be in short supply, since only firms that specialize in generic drugs currently manufacture the product. Mefloquine is also an effective therapy for chloroquine-resistant *P. falciparum* (and the asexual erythrocyte stages of the other *Plasmodium* species). Halofantrine, a recently introduced antimalarial compound, may have a limited role for self-treatment of presumptive malaria acquired in Southeast Asia or if multiple drug-resistant malaria is suspected.

Persons presenting with complications caused by *P. falciparum* or with high parasitemia but unable to tolerate oral medications due to vomiting should receive intravenous medications. Supportive care is critical for these patients and includes close hemodynamic monitoring, use of judicious fluid replacement, correction of significant metabolic abnormalities, and additional support as needed (dialysis, mechanical ventilation, and so on). Exchange transfusions have been lifesaving in some patients with parasitemia in excess of 10 percent. Glucocorticoids have not been shown to be of benefit in the treatment of cerebral malaria and should not be used.[11] Quinidine is the intravenous drug of choice due not only to its widespread availability but also to its enhanced activity against *P. falciparum.* Parenteral quinine is available only from the Centers for Disease Control and Prevention.

Quinine and quinidine are potent inducers of insulin release and may cause severe hypoglycemia. Sudden changes in orientation, sweating, tremor, tachycardia, or anxiety should prompt measurement of plasma glucose concentration. Cinchona alkaloids are myocardial depressants, so cardiac monitoring is needed during administration. Terminal treatment with primaquine is not needed in patients with *P. falciparum* malaria, due to the absence of dormant asexual forms in the liver.

PREVENTION

Malaria is largely preventable through use of personal protective measures and appropriate chemoprophylaxis. A recent study confirmed that travelers to malarious areas frequently do not use antimosquito measures or take antimalarial drugs.[12] Between dusk and dawn, travelers should remain in well-screened areas, use mosquito nets if needed, and wear long-sleeved clothing. A pyrethrum-containing insect spray should be used during evening hours and before retiring to bed. Permethrin can be sprayed on clothing for additional protection, and an insect repellent containing *N,N*-diethyl-*m*-toluamide (DEET) applied to exposed skin.

Appropriate chemoprophylaxis depends on where one will be traveling. If potential exposure to infected mosquitoes is likely, prophylaxis is warranted even if such exposure will be brief. Table 142-6 summarizes the chemotherapeutic agents of choice.[2,4,13] The Centers for Disease Control and Prevention maintains a 24-h malaria hotline (888–232-3228), which provides up-to-date information on resistance patterns in countries. Chemoprophylaxis should generally be taken for 4 weeks following the last exposure. Studies exploring other chemoprophylactic options, such as proguanil combined with atovaquone or dapsone[10,14] and monotherapy with daily azithromycin,[15] appear promising.

Lastly, even with the religious use of antimosquito measures and chemoprophylaxis, malaria can be contracted or can recur. For reasons discussed earlier, malaria must be considered whenever fever occurs in someone who has traveled to a malarious area or who has received "successful" therapy in the past. Vaccines directed against various antigens of the malaria parasite are currently in trials, but the findings thus far have not been overwhelmingly encouraging.

REFERENCES

1. World Health Organization: World malaria situation in 1994. *Weekly Epidemiol Rec* 72:269, 1997.
2. Centers for Disease Control and Prevention: *Health Information for International Travel 1996–1997.* Atlanta, US Department of Health and Human Services, 1997.
3. Centers for Disease Control and Prevention: CDC surveillance summaries: Malaria surveillance—United States, 1994. *MMWR* 46:1, 1997.
4. World Health Organization (WHO): *International Travel and Health—Vaccination Requirements and Health Advice, 1998.* Geneva, WHO, 1998.
5. Than M, Kyaw MP, Soe AY, et al: Development of resistance to chloroquine by *Plasmodium vivax* in Myanmar. *Trans R Soc Trop Med Hyg* 89:307, 1995.
6. Svenson JE, MacLean JD, Gyorkos TW, Keystone J: Imported malaria: Clinical presentation and examination of symptomatic travelers. *Arch Intern Med* 155:861, 1995.
7. Warrell DA, Molyneaux ME, Beales PF: Severe and complicated malaria. *Trans R Soc Trop Med Hyg* 84(suppl):1, 1990.
8. Beadle C, Long GW, Weiss WR, et al: Diagnosis of malaria by detection of *Plasmodium falciparum* HRP-2 antigen with a rapid dipstick antigen-capture assay. *Lancet* 343:564, 1994.
9. Humar A, Ohrt C, Harrington MA, et al: Para Sight F test compared with the polymerase chain reaction and microscopy for the diagnosis of *Plasmodium falciparum* malaria in travelers. *Am J Trop Med Hyg* 56:44, 1997.
10. White NJ: The treatment of malaria. *N Engl J Med* 335:800, 1996.
11. Hoffman SL, Rustama D, Punjabi NH, et al: High-dose dexamethasone in quinine-treated patients with cerebral malaria: A double-blind placebo-controlled trial. *J Infect Dis* 158:325, 1988.
12. Kain HC, Harrington MA, Tennyson S, Keystone JS: Imported malaria: Prospective analysis of problems in diagnosis and management. *Clin Infect Dis* 27:142, 1998.
13. Lobel HO, Kozarsky PE: Update on prevention of malaria for travelers. *JAMA* 278:1767, 1997.
14. Lell B, Luckner D, Ndjave M, et al: Randomized placebo-controlled study of atovaquone plus proguanil for malaria prophylaxis in children. *Lancet* 351:709, 1998.
15. Anderson SL, Oloo AJ, Gordon DM, et al: Successful double-blinded, randomized, placebo-controlled field trial of azithromycin and doxycycline as prophylaxis for malaria in Western Kenya. *Clin Infect Dis* 26:146, 1998.

COMMON PARASITIC INFECTIONS

Harold H. Osborn

Despite significant advances in medical knowledge and technology over the last half century, parasitic disease remains prevalent worldwide. It is estimated by the World Health Organization that 200 million people, living mostly in the rural tropics, suffer from schistosomiasis and that hookworm infects approximately a quarter of the world's population.[1] Such parasites as *Ascaris* and *Enterobius* each infect 1 billion people. *Ascaris* is said to infect 3 million people in North America; *Enterobius* infection rates among children in the United States vary from 10 to 45 percent.

Worldwide, malaria is the most prevalent infectious disease among humans, affecting over 500 million and killing over 2 million people each year.[2] In the United States, parasitic disease is becoming increasingly recognized. In addition to the persistence of endemic parasites in this country, three factors account for this trend: (1) immigration to the United States of infected individuals from the countries of Asia, Africa, and Latin America; (2) increased travel by Americans, particularly to the underdeveloped parts of the world; and (3) the rise of parasitic infections among immunosuppressed patients, especially those afflicted with HIV.[3]

Serologic surveys in the United States have demonstrated that 20 to 70 percent of the population have antibodies to *Toxoplasma* and over 90 percent have antibodies to *Pneumocystis carinii.* These two parasites can cause significant morbidity and mortality when they reactivate in immunosuppressed individuals and create opportunistic infections.

Finally, *Cryptosporidium* and *Giardia* are now recognized as causes of traveler's diarrhea and have become major causes of diarrhea in immunocompetent individuals in the United States. Person-to-person spread of these parasites has led to diarrheal illness in day care centers and other institutions, and contamination of municipal water supplies has led to major outbreaks. In 1993, 400,000 people in Milwaukee became ill after *Cryptosporidium* contaminated the drinking water, and 54 people died as a result.[4] It is estimated that 10 to 15 percent of the chronic diarrhea and wasting in AIDS patients is due to infection with *Cryptosporidium parvum.* Recently, surveys of water throughout the United States indicate that 50 percent of rivers and lakes may be contaminated with *Cryptosporidium.*[5] This parasite cannot be contained by chlorination, iodination, or ozonation of the water; it must be eliminated by filtration.

Outbreaks of diarrhea in the summer of 1996 due to the consumption of strawberries contaminated with *Cyclospora,* a coccidian, highlights the challenge of emerging parasitic diseases. Another problem in the 1990s was the increasing emergence of drug-resistant strains of various parasites. Malaria provides a notable example of drug resistance and two species (*Plasmodium falciparum* and *Plasmodium vivax*) now demonstrate resistance.[2] In addition, strains of leishmania are resistant to antimonial drugs in many areas, and reports of metronidazole-resistant trichomoniasis and giardiasis are increasingly common.[6]

The agents that cause parasitic diseases belong to three major groups: helminths (worms), protozoa, and arthropods. The multicellular helminths include nematodes (round worms), cestodes (flat worms), and trematodes (flukes). The protozoa are single-celled organisms that cause a variety of diseases ranging from malaria to amebiasis. Arthropods are classified as ectoparasites and are medically important as obligatory intermediate hosts and as mechanical vectors in many diseases. This chapter reviews diseases caused by helminths and protozoa. Malaria is discussed in Chap. 142, "Malaria."

HISTORY

The recognition of parasitic disease begins with the elicitation of a careful history. Specifically, the clinician should inquire about travel to or immigration from high-risk areas. Parasites flourish in warm, moist climates where sanitation is poor and where many of the people share a low socioeconomic status and have inadequate nutrition. Children are infected with parasites more frequently than adults because of their oral behavior, poor hygiene, and limited ability to ward off arthropod vectors.

Parasitic disease should be considered in any patient with unexplained fever, abdominal pain, diarrhea, skin ulcers, rash, or eosino-

TABLE 143-1 Risk Factors for Parasitic Disease

Risk Factor	Parasite
Blood transfusion	*Plasmodium* species, *Trypanosoma, Babesia, Toxoplasma*
Intravenous drug use	*Plasmodium* species
Homosexuality	*Entamoeba* (also seen after colonic irrigation therapy), *Giardia, Cryptosporidium*
Immunocompromised host	*Toxoplasma, Pneumocystis, Strongyloides, Cryptosporidium, Microsporidium, Isospora,* and *Cyclospora*
Hypogammaglobulinemia	*Giardia, Cryptosporidium*
Institutionalization	*Hymenolepsis nana, Entamoeba histolytica, Giardia*
Day-care centers	*Giardia, Cryptosporidium*
Livestock workers	*Cryptosporidium*
Pica	*Toxocara* (visceral larva migrans), hookworm (*Necator americanus*)
Consumption of raw food	
Sushi, sashimi, gefilte fish	*Diphyllobothrium, Anisakis*
Pork	*Taenia solium, Trichinella, Sarcocystis*
Beef	*Taenia saginata, Toxoplasma, Sarcocystis*

philia. The history should include dates of travel or immigration, destination or country of origin, living conditions, and activities. Certain specific areas of the world may implicate particular parasitic agents. Hmong tribesmen, who came to this country from Indochina in large numbers in 1979 and 1980, often harbor *Paragonimus westermani* (lung fluke), whereas visitors to Russia or the Rockies may return with *Giardia.* The history should also include questions about sexual orientation and contacts, drug use, and past illnesses as well as a complete review of systems. The use of pretravel medications, including antimalarial and antidiarrheal agents, should be elicited.

The presence of risk factors can provide a clue to specific parasitic diseases (Table 143-1). Cases of acute Chagas disease (trypanosomiasis) and babesiosis following blood transfusions have been described in the United States and Canada. Institutionalized patients may suffer from amebiasis and can become infected with *Hymenolepsis nana* (the most common tapeworm in the United States) or *Giardia.* Immunocompromised hosts (including those on steroids or antineoplastic agents) are susceptible to infection by *Strongyloides, Toxoplasma, Cryptosporidium,* and *P. carinii* and can develop a life-threatening hyper-infection syndrome with *Strongyloides stercoralis.* It is interesting to note that patients with AIDS, while susceptible to *Toxoplasma, Cryptosporidium, Pneumocystis, Isospora, Microsporidium,* and *Cyclospora,* are not any more susceptible to *Amoeba* and *Strongyloides* than immunocompetent individuals. Finally, the consumption of raw food has been associated with a variety of parasitic diseases, including fish, pork, and beef tapeworm.

PATHOPHYSIOLOGY

Parasites differ in their pathogenicity and in their capacity to produce invasive or systemic disease. The subclass coccidia, for example, includes both *Toxoplasma* and *Isospora.* However, *Isospora* is unable to invade the intestinal mucosa and thus produces only enterocolitis, whereas *Toxoplasma* crosses the intestine and produces severe systemic illness.

Sometimes various forms of the parasite differ in their ability to cause illness. The adult form of *Trichinella spiralis* remains in the intestine, while the larval form crosses and migrates to striated and cardiac muscle. Amebiasis can result in both intestinal and visceral infections. Pathogenicity may vary among strains within a genus. Infection with *Entamoeba* can result in an asymptomatic cyst carrier state or hepatic abscesses, depending on the strain involved.

Finally, organisms differ in their virulence. The infectious dose of *Giardia* and *Cryptosporidium* is on the order of 10^1 to 10^3 organisms. By contrast, the infectious dose of *Vibrio cholerae* and *Salmonella* is 10^5 to 10^8 organisms. This may be an important factor in the genesis of outbreaks in institutions and day-care centers.

CLINICAL FEATURES

Unfortunately, symptoms may be nonspecific, and the latency period between exposure and symptom appearance may be years. Symptoms can be acute or chronic, specific or vague. Parasitic disease can present with relatively common complaints, such as headache, fever, cough, and malaise, or with acute, life-threatening complications, such as seizures, hemoptysis, melena, and intestinal obstruction. A differential diagnosis can be attempted on the basis of history and knowledge of typical symptoms associated with various parasitic agents (Table 143-2).

DIAGNOSIS

Diarrhea is a common complaint that can be a manifestation of an inconsequential and self-limited problem or the hallmark of a serious chronic illness or infection, occasionally with life-threatening potential. Although a variety of systemic illnesses, toxins, drugs, and malabsorption syndromes can cause diarrhea, the infectious causes are of most immediate concern. Although viruses and bacteria are generally the most common causes of infectious diarrhea, parasites constitute a significant cause as well.

The majority of diarrhea-inducing infections are noninflammatory, usually arising in the upper small bowel from the action of an enterotoxin (e.g., *V. cholerae* or enterotoxigenic *Escherichia coli*) or other processes that alter the absorptive function of the villous tip (e.g., *Cryptosporidium, Giardia,* rotavirus, and Norwalk-like virus). In contrast, inflammatory diarrhea, which often presents as dysentery (bloody stools), arises in the colon from an invasive process, sometimes mediated by a cytotoxin (e.g., *Salmonella, Shigella, Campylobacter, Clostridium difficile,* and *Amoeba*).

If diarrhea has persisted for more than a few days, is bloody in nature, or is accompanied by substantial fever, dehydration, or weight loss, the patient should be evaluated more closely. Diarrheal illness lasting 10 days or longer and diarrhea in those with risk factors (see Table 143-1) should prompt a vigorous search for parasites.

Examination of a stool sample for fecal leukocytes has been advocated in these cases, but this procedure is controversial. The presence of fecal leukocytes has been considered a sign of inflammatory diarrhea and has been used to exclude toxigenic bacteria, viruses, and most parasites. However, when studied, the presence of fecal leukocytes has been shown to be neither sensitive nor specific for inflammatory causes.[7]

Examination of a stool specimen for ova and parasites is the best method of detecting intestinal parasites, including the cysts and trophozoites of protozoa and the larvae, eggs, and adults of helminths. Three specimens collected on different days should be examined, and the stool must be free of substances such as bismuth, barium, nonabsorbable antidiarrheal agents, and mineral oil.[8] Antimicrobial agents should be stopped at least 1 week prior to the stool collection. Fresh specimens are best, and specimens over an hour old should be preserved with formalin or polyvinyl alcohol. Multiple stool examinations are particularly important when dealing with formed stool, which usually contains

TABLE 143-2 Symptoms of Parasitic Disease

Symptom	Possible Cause
Abdominal pain	*Ascaris, Clonorchis, Diphyllobothrium, Entamoeba, Fasciola, Giardia,* hookworm, *Hymenolepsis, Schistosoma, Taenia, Trichuris*
Anemia	*Babesia, Diphyllobothrium,* hookworm, *Leishmania donovani, Plasmodium* species, *Trichuris*
Asthma	*Ascaris, Strongyloides, Toxocara*
Conjunctivitis and keratitis	Filariae (*Onchocerca volvulus*), Taenia, *trichinella, Trypanosoma*
Diarrhea	*Dientamoeba, Entamoeba, Fasciola, Fasciolopsis, Giardia,* hookworm, *Hymenolepsis, L. donovani, Palantidium, Schistosoma, Strongyloides, Taenia, Trichinella, Trichuris*
Edema	*Fasciolopsis,* filariae (*Wuchereria bancrofti*), *Trichinella, Trypanosoma*
Eosinophilia	*Ascaris, Dracunculus, Fasciola,* filariae (*W. bancrofti, Brugia malayi*) fluke (*Paragonimus westermani, Chlonorchis sinensis, Fasciolopsis leuski*), *Hymnenolepsis,* hookworm, *Schistosoma, Strongyloides, Taenia, Toxocara, Trichinella, Trichuris*
Fever	*Ascaris, Babesia, Entamoeba, Fasciola,* filariae (*W. bancrofti*), fluke (*C. sinensis*), *Giardia, L. donovani, Plasmodium* species, *Toxocara, Trichi, Trichuris, Trypanosoma*
Hemoptysis	*Ascaris, Echinococcus, Paragonimus*
Hepatomegaly	Fluke, (*C. sinensis, Opisthorchis viverrini, Fasciola*), *L. donovani, Plasmodium* species, tapeworm (*Echinococcus*), *Schistosoma, Toxocara, Trypanosoma*
Intestinal obstruction	*Arcaris, Diphyllobothrium,* fluke (*Fasciolopsis buski*), *Strongyloides, Taenia*
Jaundice	Fluke (*C. sinensis, O. viverrini*), *Plasmodium* species
Meningitis	*Acanthamoeba,* malaria (*Plasmodium falciparum*), *Naegleria,* primary amebic meningoencephalitis, *Toxocara, Trichinella, Trypanosoma*
Myocardial disease	*Taenia, Trichinella, Trypanosoma* (*T. cruzi*)
Nausea and vomiting	*Ascaris, Entamoeba, Giardia, Leishmania, Taenia, Trichinella, Trichuris*
Pneumonia	*Ascaris,* filariae (*W. bancrofti, B. malayi*), fluke (*P. westermani*), *Strongyloides, Trichinella*
Pruritus	*Dientamoeba, Enterobius,* filariae (*O. volvulus*), *Trichuris*
Seizures	*Hymenolepsis, Trichinella, Paragonimus,* tapeworm (*Echinococcus, Cysticercus*)
Skin ulcers	*Dracunculus,* hookworm, *L. donovani, Trypanosoma*
Splenomegaly	*Babesia, Toxoplasma, Plasmodium*
Urticaria	*Ascaris, Dracunculus, Fasciola, Strongyloides, Trichinella*

fewer parasites than do diarrheal specimens. In patients with suspected giardiasis, 7 or 8 specimens may be necessary.

Occasionally *Giardia, Cryptosporidium,* and the larvae of *Strongyloides* may be detected by examining a duodenal aspirate or by having the patient swallow a string with a gelatin capsule (Entero-test). Recent studies suggest that detection of *Giardia* by examination of seven stool specimens is just as effective as examination of duodenal contents.

Special procedures for removing parasites include the following: warm water concentration through a filter for *Strongyloides* (Baermann test), sticky tape swab of the perianal area for *Enterobius* (Swube test), passage of urine through a nucleopore filter for *Schistosoma hematobium,* and use of an acid-fast stain to detect *Cryptosporidium, Isospora,* and *Cyclospora.*

The enzyme-linked immunosorbent assay (ELISA) technique can be used to make a serologic diagnosis of a variety of parasitic infections. In addition, the ELISA technique has been used to detect antigens of *Giardia* and *Cryptosporidia* in stool. Malaria-causing plasmodia, *Babesia,* microfilaria of *Wuchereria* and *Brugia,* and the trypanosomes that cause Chagas disease can be detected by Giemsa-stained thick and thin films of peripheral blood.

Finally, organisms that affect the central nervous system (CNS; e.g., *P. falciparum* which causes cerebral malaria, and *Acanthamoeba* or *Naegleria,* which cause amoebic meningoencephalitis) can be detected by culture or microscopic examination of centrifuged cerebrospinal fluid. *Pneumocystis* is detected by characteristic findings on chest x-ray, elevated lactate dehydrogenase (LDH) levels, and evidence of hypoxemia, and is confirmed by lung biopsy with special stains, while *Toxoplasma* is detected by characteristic findings on computed tomography (CT) scan in association with elevated serum antibody levels and is rarely confirmed by brain biopsy.

HELMINTHS

Nematodes (Roundworms)

Nematodes are cylindrical, unsegmented, elongated white worms. Their mode of entry into the human host varies from ingestion of eggs (*Ascaris* and *Enterobius*) to penetration of the skin (*Necator, Ancylostoma,* and *Strongyloides*) to inoculation by insect bite (*Wuchereria*).

ASCARIS *Ascaris lumbricoides* has a worldwide distribution, and its life span if left treated is 2 to 7 years. Larval invasion follows the ingestion of *Ascaris* eggs, and during this stage the parasite migrates through the lungs. Clinical disease is due to pulmonary hypersensitivity or intestinal complications. Patients may have fever, cough, dyspnea, hemoptysis, and eosinophilia. Obstruction of the common bile duct and the intestine have been described.[9] The chest x-ray may reveal eosinophilic pneumonitis (Loeffler syndrome). The diagnosis is made by finding eggs or, occasionally, an adult worm in the stool. Serologic tests, including bentonite flocculation, ELISA, and indirect hemagglutination, may be helpful. Treatment is with mebendazole, albendazole, or pyrantel pamoate. Intestinal obstruction may necessitate surgery, especially in children.

ENTEROBIUS (PINWORM) Adult *Enterobius* (pinworm) resides in the cecum, appendix, ileum, and ascending colon after its eggs are ingested. The gravid female migrates to the anus, especially at night, where it causes intense pruritus. Autoinfection with hand-to-mouth transmission is possible after scratching. A host of problems from vaginitis to enuresis have been attributed to *Enterobius* infection without good evidence. It is most prevalent in temperate climates during the winter and fall. The diagnosis is confirmed with a cellophane tape swab of the anus. All family members should be examined. Treatment is with pyrantel pamoate, albendazole, or mebendazole and should be repeated after 2 weeks.

NECATOR (HOOKWORM) *Necator americanus* prevails in the southern United States and is often seen in immigrants from warmer climates. Infection is associated with the use of human fertilizer and the lack of shoes and latrines. Because each worm can withdraw 0.03 to 0.2 mL of blood a day, infection often leads to chronic anemia. Pica and geophagy are often seen in infected children. Patients may have cough, low-grade fever, abdominal pain, diarrhea, weakness, weight loss, heme-positive stools, and eosinophilia. The diagnosis is made by finding ova in the stool. In mild infections, multiple stool specimens or concentration techniques may be necessary. The parasite burden may be estimated using the Beaver stool or Kato slide smear method. Infections with less than 2100 eggs per gram of feces (<50 adult worms) are usually not hematologically important, whereas infections with over 11,000 eggs per gram result in significant anemia. Hookworm is best treated with mebendazole, albendazole, or pyrantel pamoate.

STRONGYLOIDES (THREADWORMS) Adult threadworms reside in the mucosa of the small intestine. Because entry of the parasite is through the skin, penetration can lead to allergic manifestations, pruritus, and an erythematous rash. Migration throughout the lungs can produce cough, dyspnea, and pneumonia. The intestinal phase is manifested by abdominal pain, diarrhea with mucus and blood, and eosinophilia. Autoinfection can occur due to internal production of infective larvae. Larval migration in the skin produces larva currens. Fatalities may occur due to hyperinfection in elderly and immunocompromised patients (e.g., patients with leprosy, nephrotic syndrome, hepatic disease, or lymphoproliferative disorders and those on steroids). The diagnosis is confirmed by finding larvae in the stool. Occasionally, use of a formalin ether concentration method or duodenal aspiration may be necessary. Various stages of the parasite may be found in the sputum. An ELISA test is also available. An upper gastrointestinal series may reveal a deformed duodenal bulb, and *Strongyloides* may be confused with ulcer disease. Treatment is with thiabendazole or ivermectin.

TRICHURIS TRICHIURA (WHIPWORM) Like *Ascaris, Trichuris trichiura* is found in rural communities in the southern United States. The infection is most often acquired in childhood because the ova are deposited in the soil where children play and defecate freely. The adult worm resides in the cecum. Patients complain of anorexia, insomnia, abdominal pain (including pain in the right upper quadrant), fever, flatulence, bloody diarrhea, weight loss, and pruritus and may have eosinophilia and microcytic hypochromic anemia. *Trichuris* can result in colitis or rectal prolapse in children. The diagnosis is made with the finding of ova in the stool. Mebendazole or albendazole is the treatment of choice.

TRICHINELLA SPIRALIS Trichinosis is common in Mexico and the United States and results from the consumption of infected pork and, less commonly, bear and walrus meat. In the early stages of infection with *Trichinella spiralis,* the patient may present with acute myocarditis, nonsuppurative meningitis, bronchopneumonia, or catarrhal enteritis. The primary lesions are in striated muscle. Clinical symptoms depend on the site of invasion. Patients may present with nausea and vomiting, diarrhea, fever, urticaria, periorbital edema, (pathognomonic) splinter hemorrhages, myalgia, muscle spasm, stiff neck, headache, and psychiatric disturbances. Laboratory manifestations of trichinosis include leukocytosis, eosinophilia, elevated creatine phosphokinase and electrocardiographic changes. The diagnosis can be confirmed with latex agglutination, skin test, and a bentonite flocculation test. Biopsy of tender muscle may be helpful after the fourth week. Since *T. spiralis* encysts in striated muscle, stool examination is not helpful after the initial gastrointestinal phase in making the diagnosis. The differential diagnosis includes staphylococcal and salmonella food poisoning, shigellosis, and amebiasis. Mebendazole is indicated for treatment of the intestinal phase but may be ineffective after encystment. Steroids are indicated for severe infections, such as CNS disease and myocarditis, but are not advocated routinely because their use can increase the number of circulating larvae. Most cases are mild and never come to medical attention.

Trematodes (Flukes)

Trematodes are leaflike, symmetrical flatworms lacking a body cavity but possessing a ventral sucker to hold their position. They live in intermediate hosts such as snails, crabs, and fish and shed their eggs from the human host in the feces (*Schistosoma, Clonorchis,* and *Fasciola*), urine (*Schistosoma haematobium*), or sputum (*Paragonimus*).

SCHISTOSOMA Schistosomes penetrate the skin, creating a papular pruritic rash. The adult form resides in the venous system. Symptoms of acute disease—fever, lymphadenopathy, and hepatosplenomegaly (so-called Katayama fever)—are rarely seen. More typically, patients present in the chronic stage with granulomas in the liver (portal hypertension) and bladder (obstructive hydroureter). Patients may present with diarrhea, abdominal pain, melena, hepatosplenomegaly, hematemesis, and, in the late stages, ascites and liver failure. With *S. haematobium,* dysuria and hematuria may be found. The diagnosis is suggested by a positive immunofluorescent antibody test result and confirmed by finding eggs in the feces or on rectal biopsy. Treatment is with praziquantel.

Cestodes (Flatworms)

The cestodes are flatworms commonly referred to as tapeworms. They have a scolex, or head, equipped with suckers, or hooks. Cestodes grow by segmentation, extending proglottides from the neck.

TAENIA *Taenia solium* (pork tapeworm) is occasionally encountered in the United States in immigrants or visitors from Central America and the Middle East. *Taenia saginata* (beef tapeworm) is seen more often, especially in those who consume raw beef (e.g., steak tartare). Adult worms live in the small intestine. Infected patients can be asymptomatic or present with nausea and vomiting, headache, abdominal pain, pruritus, constipation, diarrhea, and intestinal obstruction. The larval stage of *T. solium* can cause clinical disease (cysticercosis), which can be serious and sometimes fatal. *Taenia* cysts may be found in subcutaneous tissue, the eye, the brain, and the heart and cause seizures and hydrocephalus. Radiographs of the soft tissues may reveal curvilinear calcifications indicative of cysts, and cysts can be seen in the meninges and brain parenchyma on CT scanning. The diagnosis is made by finding gravid proglottids in the stool. An ELISA or hemagglutination reaction may be helpful, but results of both can be falsely negative if the cysts are calcified. Treatment of the adult (intestinal) stage is with praziquantel. The larval (tissue) stage is treated with albendazole.

DIPHYLLOBOTHRIUM *Diphyllobothrium* (fish tapeworm) has been reported in the Pacific northwest, Minnesota, Michigan, and other areas where raw fish (e.g., sushi and sashimi) and gefilte fish are consumed. *Diphyllobothrium* can compete with the host for vitamin B_{12}, and thus patients can present with pernicious anemia. Treatment is the same as for *Taenia.*

PROTOZOA

Amebas

Amebiasis, which is caused by *Entamoeba histolytica,* occurs worldwide and is associated with poor sanitation. Outbreaks have been reported in institutions for the mentally retarded and in the homosexual

TABLE 143-3 Commonly Used Antiparasitic Drugs

Drug	First-Line Agent	Alternative Agent	Side Effects
Albendazole (Zental)	Tapeworm (*Echinococcus granulosus, Cysticercus*), *Ascaria,* cutaneous larva migrans, *Enterobius, Gnathostoma, Truchuris,* hookworm (*Ascaris duodenale, Necator Americanus*), *Microsporidium*	*Capillaria, Trichostrongylus,* visceral larva migrans	Diarrhea, abdominal pain
Amphotericin B (Fungizone)	Amebic meningoencephalitis (*Naegleria*)	*Leishmania* (*L. braziliensis, L. mexicana*)	Fever, headache, anorexia, nausea, diarrhea, muscle and joint pain, azotemia, anemia, renal tubular acidosis (RTA), leukopenia
Bithionol (Bithin)	Fluke (*Fasciola hepatica*)		Photosensitivity, nausea and vomiting, urticaria
Chloroquine	*Plasmodium* species (except resistant *P. falciparum*)		Pruritus, vomiting, headache, confusion, skin eruptions, myalgias, extraocular movement (EOM) palsies
Clindamycin (Cleocin)	*Babesia,* chloroquine-resistant *P. falciparum*		
Diethylcarbamazine (Hetrazan)	Filariae (*Wuchereira bancrofti, Loa loa,* tropical pulmonary eosinophilia), visceral larva migrans		Allergic reactions, GI symptoms
Iodoquinol (Yodoxin)	*Entamoeba* (*Entamoeba histolytica*), *Dientamoeba*	*Balantidium*	Rash, acne, enlarged thyroid, nausea, diarrhea, anal pruritus; rarely: optic atrophy, peripheral neuropathy
Ivermectin (Mectizan)	Filariae (*Onchocerca volvulus*), *Strongyloides,* cutaneous larva migrans		Fever, pruritus, tender nodes, bone and joint pain, headache
Lindane (Kwell)		Lice, scabies	Eczema, conjunctivitis, aplastic anemia
Mebendazole (Vermox)	*Angiostrongylus, Ascaria, Capillaria, Enterobius,* filariae (*Mansonella perstans*) *Trichuris,* hookworm, *Trichinella*	*Leishmania,* visceral larva migrans	Diarrhea, abdominal pain, agranulocytosis
Mefloquine (Lariam)		Chloroquine-resistant *P. falciparum*	Vertigo, nausea, nightmares, headache
Meglumine (Glucantime)	*Leishmania*		Joint and muscle pain, nausea
Metronidazole (Flagyl)	*Entamoeba* (*E. histolytica, E. polecki*), *Dracunculus, Trichomonas, Blastocystis, Giardia*	*Balantidium*	Nausea, headache, dry mouth, reaction with alcohol; rarely: seizures, ataxia, leukopenia, pancreatitis
Niclosamide (Niclocide)	Fluke (*Fasciolopsis buski*), tapeworm (*Diphyllobothrium, Taenia, Dipylidium*)	Tapeworm (*Hymenolepsis*)	Nausea, abdominal pain
Nifurtimox (Lampit)	*Trypanosoma* (*T. cruzi*)		Anorexia, vomiting, sleep disorder, tremors
Paromomycin (Humatin)	*Dientamoeba, Cryptosporidium*	*E. histolytica, Giardia*	GI disturbance; rarely: eighth nerve and renal damage

community. Amebae inhabit the cecum and large intestine, where they cause ulcers and diffuse inflammation, which can mimic ulcerative colitis. Rarely, an ameboma develops in the liver and presents as a liver abscess. Approximately half of all infected patients are asymptomatic. Symptoms include nausea and vomiting, anorexia, diarrhea, fever, abdominal pain, and leukocytosis. Protozoan infections, including amebiasis, do not produce eosinophilia. The diagnosis is established with stool testing, including testing of postcathartic stools and concentration and staining techniques. Stool specimens should be fixed in polyvinyl alcohol formalin, or merthiolate-iodine-formalin. Serologic tests (ELISA and indirect hemagglutination reaction) can be helpful in the presence of extraintestinal disease. Treatment is with metronidazole or tinidazole.

Giardia

Giardia is probably the most common intestinal parasite in the United States. It inhabits the duodenum and upper jejunum, where the alkaline pH creates a favorable milieu. Cysts are ingested in fecally contaminated water or food or are passed by hand-to-mouth transmission. Waterborne outbreaks have become more common in the United States because the cysts are resistant to chlorination. Day-care centers have been increasingly implicated in promoting giardiasis.

Symptoms depend on the duration of infection at the time of presentation. Patients may complain of explosive, watery, or foul-smelling diarrhea, flatus, abdominal distention, fatigue, and fever or chronic diarrhea with weight loss or general debilitation. Stools should be examined for cysts and trophozoites with routine and concentration techniques. *Giardia* antigen can be detected in the stool with immunofluorescence or ELISA technique. Occasionally, duodenal aspiration, the string test (Entero-test), or small-bowel biopsy is necessary to make the diagnosis. The drug of choice for treatment is metronidazole.

Trypanosoma

American *Trypanosoma* (*T. cruzi*) causes Chagas' disease. Three strains of African *Trypanosoma* cause sleeping sickness. Chagas' disease is usually transmitted by the reduviid (kissing) bug, but infection

TABLE 143-3 *(continued)*

Drug	First-Line Agent	Alternative Agent	Side Effects
Pentamidine isethionate (Pentam)	*P. carinii*	*Trypanosama* (*T. bruceli*), *Leishmania*	Hypotension, hypoglycemia, vomiting, blood dyscrasia, renal damage, GI disturbance
Praziquantel (Biltricide)	Fluke, *Schistosoma,* tapeworm (*Hymenolepsis, Cysticercus*); tapeworm (*Diphyllobothrium latum, Taenia, Dipylidium, Hymenolepsis nana, Cysticercus cellulosae*)		Malaise, headache, dizziness, abdominal upset, fever, eosinophilia
Primaquine phosphate	*P. vivax, P. orale* (prevention of relapse only)		G6PD hemolysis, neutropenia, GI disturbances
Pyrantel pamoate (Antiminth)	*Ascaria, Enterobius,* hookworm, *Trichostrongylus, Moniliformis*		GI disturbances, headache, dizziness, rash, fever
Pyrimethamine (Daraprim)	Chloroquine-resistant *P. falciparum, Toxoplasma*		Blood dyscrasias, folate deficiency; rarely: rash, vomiting, seizures, shock
Quinacrine (Atabrine)		*Giardia*	Dizziness, headache, vomiting, diarrhea, yellow skin, toxic psychosis, insomnia, rash, blood dyscrasias
Quinine sulfate (Quinamm)	*Babesia,* chloroquine-resistant *P. falciparum*		Cinchonism, hemolytic anemia, blood dyscrasias, photosensitivity, hypoglycemia, arrhythmias, hypotension
Sodium stibogluconate (Pentostam)	*Leishmania*		Muscle pain, joint stiffness, nausea, diarrhea, rash, pruritus, liver and heart damage, bradycardia; rarely: hemolytic anenmia, sudden death
Spiramycin (Rovamycin)		*Toxoplasma*	GI symptoms
Suramin sodium (Germanin)	*Trypanosoma* (African)		Vomiting, pruritus, urticaria, paresthesias, neuropathy
Tetracycline (achromycin)	*Dientamoeba*		Nausea, vomiting, metallic taste, discolored teeth in children
Thiabendazole (Mintezol)	*Angiostrongylus, Strongyloides,* visceral larva migrans, cutaneous larva migrans	*Capillaria, Dracunculus, Trichostrongylus*	Nausea, vertigo, rash, leukopenia, hallucinations, erythema multiforme, Stevens-Johnson syndrome, rarely: shock, seizures
Tinidazole (Fasigyn)	*Amoeba* (*E. histolytica*), *Trichomonas*	*Giardia*	Allergic reactions
Trimethoprim-sulfamethoxazole (Septra, Bactrim)	*Isospora, Pneumocystis carinii, Cyclospora*		

Source: Adapted from Drugs for parasitic infections, *Med Lett* 40: 1, 1998, with permission.

can also follow breast-feeding and blood transfusion, as has occurred in the United States. A nodular swelling, or chagoma, develops at the site of inoculation following a bite. The acute phase of the disease can last 2 to 3 months, and patients present with fever, headache, anorexia, conjunctivitis, and myocarditis. Infants can develop meningocephalitis, and heart involvement can lead to congestive heart failure and ventricular aneurysms. The organism can attack the myenteric plexus of the gastrointestinal tract, resulting in megacolon. Chronic infection can result in a cardiomyopathy. Laboratory abnormalities include anemia, leukocytosis, an elevated sedimentation rate, and electrocardiographic changes. During the acute phase, trypomastigotes can be seen on a peripheral smear or cultured from the blood. In the chronic phase, the diagnosis is made with a complement fixation test, ELISA, or biopsy of the liver, spleen, or bone marrow. Treatment of acute Chagas' disease is with nifurtimox or benzindazole. Treatment of sleeping sickness is with suramin sodium.

Babesia

Babesia is a protozoan that, like *Plasmodium* species, possesses an erythrocytic phase. It is transmitted by *Ixodes* ticks and occasionally by blood transfusion. Babesiosis has been reported in the northeastern United States (especially Nantucket, MA, and Long Island, NY). Babesiosis in the northeast is caused by the murine species, *Babesia microtti,* and is transmitted by the deer tick, *Ixodes,* which also serves as a vector for Lyme disease. Patients may have intermittent fever, splenomegaly, hemolysis, and jaundice. Infection can be fatal in splenectomized patients, but its incidence is apparently not increased in immunocompromised patients. Diagnosis can be made on a Giemsa-stained peripheral smear. Occasionally, *Babesia* on smear can be confused with the ring forms of *P. falciparum* malaria. Babesiosis can simulate rickettsial diseases, such as Rocky Mountain spotted fever and Lyme disease. Treatment is with clindamycin and quinine.

Cryptosporidium

Cryptosporidium is a protozoan parasite of the subclass Coccidia, which also includes *Toxoplasma, Isospora, Cyclospora, Eimeria,* and *Sarcocystis. Cryptosporidium parvum* is the species that most commonly causes disease in human beings. Previously regarded only as a disease of immunodepressed individuals (especially those with AIDS),

Cryptosporidium is now recognized as an important and increasingly common cause of diarrhea, including traveler's diarrhea, worldwide.

Like *Giardia, Cryptosporidium* is waterborne, as has been well documented in England and the United States, most recently in Milwaukee. Like *Giardia, Cryptosporidium* causes diarrhea by altering the microvillous tips of the cells lining the small intestine. It can infect other mammals, including cows, and waste water (raw sewage) and runoff from dairies and pastures may be the source of oocysts that contaminate reservoirs and pools.

The diarrhea of cryptosporidiosis, in both immunocompetent and immunocompromised patients, is profuse and watery (cholera-like), usually without blood, fecal leukocytes, and mucus. It is occasionally associated with crampy abdominal pain, nausea and vomiting, low-grade fever, and weight loss. Although the illness is self-limited in most immunocompetent individuals (lasting several days to 2 weeks), it can be relentless and debilitating in the immunocompromised, often resulting in severe dehydration, malabsorption, weight loss, and death. Rarely, *Cryptosporidium* can also cause respiratory and biliary tract disease.

The diagnosis is made by finding oocytes in the stool. Concentration of the stool specimen using formalin ether gives a higher yield. A modified Ziehl-Neelsen acid-fast stain is used to visualize the oocysts. A serum ELISA for antibodies to *Cryptosporidium* is available.

Treatment is mainly supportive (oral or intravenous hydration and antidiarrheal agents). Treatment of immunocompromised patients is difficult, and at present there is no accepted regimen. Paromomycin, a somatostatin-like agent, octreotide, and azithromycin have all been used with some success.

PROTOZOAN INFECTIONS IN IMMUNOCOMPROMISED HOSTS

Respiratory Tract

Pneumonia occurs commonly in immunocompromised patients and is often due to *P. carinii.* Because most normal children have antibodies to *P. carinii, P. carinii* pneumonia probably represents a reactivation of a latent infection. The natural habitat and mode of transmission of *P. carinii* are poorly understood. Patients present acutely with fever, dyspnea, a nonproductive cough, and scant rales. Arterial blood gas analysis may reveal hypoxia or an increased alveolar-arterial (A-a) gradient. The serum LDH level may be elevated. Early, the chest x-ray may be normal. Later, the classical appearance is of symmetrical interstitial infiltrates in the mid and lower lung zones. *Pneumocystis carinii* occurs in premature and debilitated infants, AIDS patients, those receiving organ transplants, and those with inherited immunodeficiencies. Diagnosis is usually made by lung biopsy. The specimen should be stained with methenamine-silver nitrate or toluidine blue. Serologic tests are of limited value because many normal individuals have antibodies. Treatment is with trimethoprim-sulfamethoxazole or pentamidine isethionate. In patients with respiratory compromise (P_{O_2} <70 mmHg or A-a gradient >35 mmHg on room air) the addition of steroids has been shown to be beneficial.

Gastrointestinal Tract

Most patients with AIDS (50 to 98 percent) either present with or later develop diarrhea that is often life-threatening. Gastrointestinal disease in immunocompromised patients is often due to *Cryptosporidium, Isospora, Microsporidium,* and *Cyclospora.*

The diagnosis of *Cryptosporidium* is made with a modified Ziehl-Neelsen acid-fast stain or Kinyoun stain of the stool. Many antimicrobial and antidiarrheal agents have been tried without much success in the treatment of cryptosporidiosis. The high rate of recurrence and relapse of this disease is probably related to the underlying immunodeficiency. *Isospora belli* is another protozoan that can cause significant gastrointestinal disease. As with *Cryptosporidium,* infection with *Isospora* occurs after ingestion of oocysts in contaminated food or water and following sexual contact. Symptoms may vary from acute gastroenteritis in immunocompetent individuals to severe, protracted diarrhea in the immunocompromised. Characteristic oocysts can be detected in the stool with acid-fast stains. Treatment is with trimethoprim-sulfamethoxazole.

Microsporidium is an obligate intracellular protozoan that is becoming more commonly recognized as a pathogen in patients with AIDS and the immunocompetent. Most patients present with diarrhea and a wasting syndrome, but hepatitis, peritonitis, and keratitis have been described. Diagnosis by stool examination is difficult due to the small spore size. Immunologic detection of spores with polyclonal serum has been attempted. Definitive diagnosis usually requires intestinal biopsy and detection with transmission electron microscopy. Treatment is difficult. Patients who do not respond to standard antidiarrheal therapy can be tried on octreotide, albendazole, or metronidazole.

Central Nervous System

Toxoplasma, an intracellular parasite carried by cats and other intermediate hosts, can cause significant disease in immunocompromised patients. Infection can come from the ingestion of oocysts or undercooked meat, by placental transfer, following organ transplant, or during a blood transfusion. Acquired toxoplasmosis is usually asymptomatic. During acute infection, transient lymphadenopathy and splenomegaly may be present. Reactivation can result in encephalitis, chorioretinitis, myocarditis, and pneumonia. Symptoms of cerebral toxoplasmosis can include severe headache, seizures, confusion, and lethargy. Focal deficits may appear, and cerebellar, brainstem, and cranial nerve lesions may be seen. Making the diagnosis may be difficult. Ventricular fluid, brain tissue, or the buffy coat from a blood sample may be inoculated into test animals. The Sabin-Feldman dye test is fairly specific. An ELISA test for IgG and IgM antibodies to *Toxoplasma* is available. CT scanning may reveal characteristic intracerebral lesions with ring enhancement following the use of contrast. Magnetic resonance imaging is also used. Treatment is with pyrimethamine plus sulfadiazine or spiramycin.

TREATMENT

Patients with potentially life-threatening infections (e.g., cerebral malaria, pneumocystic pneumonia, amebic meningoencephalitis, or CNS toxoplasmosis) should be started on antiparasitic treatment immediately in the emergency department (Table 143-3). Patients who are dehydrated from gastrointestinal losses or fever should receive intravenous hydration. Those who can take fluids orally can be rehydrated by mouth.

DISPOSITION

Patients with diarrhea who appear severely ill, toxic, or dehydrated; those who cannot tolerate anything by mouth; and those with organ system involvement (e.g., lung, blood, or CNS) should be admitted for intravenous hydration, further diagnostic evaluation, and antiparasitic drug treatment as indicated. Patients who do not require hospitalization can be treated with antiparasitic agents if a specific diagnosis has been made and should be referred for follow-up. Those who can tolerate oral fluids can be reliably rehydrated with the World Health Organization oral rehydration solution. Such a solution can be prepared by adding 3.5 g sodium chloride (or $\frac{3}{4}$ teaspoon of table salt), 2.5 g sodium bicarbonate (or 2.9 g sodium citrate or 1 teaspoon of baking soda, 1.5 g potassium chloride (or 1 cup of orange juice or two bananas), and 20 g glucose (or 40 g sucrose or 4 tablespoons of sugar) to a liter (1.05 quart) of clean water. This makes a solution of approximately 90 mmol sodium, 20 mmol potassium, 80 mmol chloride, 30 mmol bicarbonate, and 111 mmol glucose per liter.

REFERENCES

1. World Health Organization: *The World Health Report 1996: Fighting Disease, Fostering Development.* Geneva, World Health Organization, 1996.
2. Campbell CC: Malaria: An emerging and reemerging global plaque. *FEMS Immunol Med Microbiol* 18:32, 1997.
3. James SL: Emerging parasitic infections. *FEMS Immunol Med Microbiol* 18:313, 1997.
4. Mackenzie MD: A massive outbreak in Milwaukee of *Cryptosporidium* infection transmitted through the public water supply. *N Engl J Med* 331:161, 1994.
5. Widmer G, Carraway M, Tzipori S: Waterborne *Cryptosporidium:* A perspective from the USA. *Parisitol Today* 12:286, 1996.
6. Upcroft JA, Upcroft P: Drug resistance and *Giardia. Parasitol Today* 9:187, 1993.
7. Huicho L, Sanchez D, Contraras M, et al: Occult blood and fecal leukocytes as screening tests in childhood infectious diarrhea: An old problem revisited. *Pediatr Infect Dis J* 12:474, 1993.
8. Rosenblatt JE: Laboratory diagnosis of parasitic infections. *Mayo Clin Proc* 69:779, 1994.
9. Wittner M, Tanowitz HB: Intestinal parasites in returned travelers. *Med Clin North Am* 76:1433, 1992.

FOODBORNE AND WATERBORNE DISEASES

William T. Anderson

Foodborne and waterborne disease is the most widespread public health challenge facing contemporary medicine. The spectrum of illness is changing with the emergence of new pathogens and reemergence of old ones. Individual outbreaks of foodborne or waterborne illnesses have caused sickness in hundreds of thousands of people. The number of identified outbreaks has increased over the past 20 years.[1] The globalization of the food economy and explosion in international travel have facilitated the transmission of disease between continents.[1] Patients can present with uncommon pathogens and develop life-threatening complications or chronic illnesses. Emergency physicians need to understand the scope and magnitude of foodborne and waterborne illnesses. They should be able to recognize risk factors in the vast population of patients who present with diarrheal illness that compels a more aggressive investigation. Physicians should be cognizant of which pathogens can and cannot be tested for in their laboratory. Finally, emergency physicians should instruct patients on how to reduce their risk in the future. Specific etiologic agents and the general management of infectious diarrhea are covered elsewhere in this text.

Foodborne and waterborne illnesses encompass a variety of clinical and etiologic conditions. Waterborne illness is defined by the Centers for Disease Control and Prevention (CDC) as an illness that occurs after consumption or use of water intended for drinking or as illness associated with recreational water such as swimming pools, whirlpools, hot tubs, spas, water parks, and naturally occurring fresh and marine surface waters.[2] A foodborne-illness outbreak is the occurrence of two or more cases of a similar illness resulting from the ingestion of a common food.[3] Food or water may act as a vehicle for transmission of actively growing organisms or as a transfer medium for nonreplicating viruses, toxins, protozoa, bacteria, or chemical agents.

EPIDEMIOLOGY: FOODBORNE DISEASE

From 1988 to 1992, a total of 2423 outbreaks of foodborne diseases in the United States were reported to the CDC: 77,373 persons developed predominantly diarrheal illness.[3] This number represents only a small fraction of foodborne outbreaks. Most infections are undiagnosed or unreported. It has been estimated that foodborne illness affects 6 to 80 million people in the United States and causes 9000 deaths each year.[4] On a global scale, the prevalence of all diarrheal illnesses has been estimated to be 3 to 5 billion cases per year and is associated with 5 to 10 million deaths per year or approximately 27,000 deaths per day.[5]

The epidemiology of foodborne illnesses has evolved quickly over the past few decades in response to several influences. New pathogens such as *Escherichia coli* O157:H7,[6] enteroinvasive *Klebsiella pneumoniae,*[6] and *Cyclospora cayetanensis*[7] have been recognized as recent causes of foodborne illness. The expanding role of pathogens such as *Campylobacter jejuni, Listeria monocytogenes,* and *Yersinia enterocolitica,* previously unrecognized causes of foodborne illness, has brought them to the forefront.[7] A growing list of foods, previously thought to be safe, have been identified as new vehicles for transmission.

The evolution of foodborne epidemiology over the past few decades has been a reflection of changes in the food supply and population demographics. International trade has allowed people to come in contact with previously unfamiliar pathogens that are native to remote parts of the world.[4] Bacteria, viruses, parasites, and chemical contamination at the site of processing can be disseminated to a multitude of locations thousands of miles away. Low-dose contamination at a central processing site can cause widespread outbreaks that often are undetected.[4,8] Consolidation of the food industry has led to a larger market share and greater geographic distribution of products from a single supplier or distributor.[4] This increases the risk of larger outbreaks of disease. In 1994, a nationwide outbreak of over 224,000 illnesses of *Salmonella* serotype Enteritidis from one distributor occurred when ice cream premix was transported in tanker trucks that had not been completely sanitized after transporting nonpasteurized liquid eggs. No source for contamination was found in the manufacturing plant.[9]

The eating habits of the US population have changed, with a greater emphasis on incorporating fruits and vegetables in the diet.[1] To meet this increased demand, the volume of imported fresh fruits and vegetables has escalated. Imports can account for more than 75 percent of grocery-store fruit and vegetable stock.[1] Outbreaks of foodborne illness have occurred recently in produce such as fresh squeezed orange juice, raspberries, frozen strawberries, sliced tomatoes, and lettuce.[4]

Population dietary patterns have changed as a larger percentage of meals are consumed outside the home.[4] Nearly 80 percent of foodborne outbreaks in the United States from 1988 to 1992 occurred in cafeterias, restaurants, or delicatessens.[3] The number and array of food-service establishments that mass produce food has expanded. Many restaurants rely on transient personnel who have inadequate knowledge of food-handling techniques.[10] In the home, there has been a decline in basic food preparation skills. Many adults who prepare meals do not routinely wash their hands after handling raw meat or poultry.[10]

The number and the percentage of people with increased vulnerability to illness have changed. The United States will continue to experience a demographic shift to an older population base: 20 percent of the population will be over age 65 by the year 2040.[11] Patients with compromised immunity secondary to AIDS, immunosuppressants, chemotherapy, or chronic illnesses also represent an expanding segment of the population with heightened susceptibility to foodborne illness.[4,11]

Travelers are at an increased risk of foodborne illnesses secondary to exposure to new, previously unseen pathogens, increased exposure through meals at hotels and restaurants, and unpredictable standards for public health cleanliness and water-supply systems.[12] The relative risk of foodborne infection with viruses, bacteria, or parasites varies by country, but ranges from 20 to 50 percent for all travelers.[1] Enterotoxigenic *E. coli* is recognized as the major cause of travelers' diarrhea,[5] but other strains of *E. coli* are associated with travel, including enterohemorrhagic and enteroinvasive *E. coli*.[12] The prevalence of *Salmonella typhi* necessitates typhoid immunization for travelers to many countries.[12] *Salmonella* serotype Enteritidis outbreaks have occurred on airlines and railways from contaminated meals.[12] Other pathogens associated with international travel include *Brucella,* hepatitis A,[12] *Vibrio, Shigella, Campylobacter, Giardia lamblia,* and *Cryptosporidium.*[5]

Food-industry influences have contributed to the emergence of new pathogens in foodborne disease. The common use of antibiotics in animal food reservoirs and humans have facilitated an increase of antibiotic resistant strains of *Salmonella* and *Campylobacter jejuni.*[4] The disposal of the more than 1 billion tons of manure and associated pathogens that are an annual by-product of the farm industry is a growing dilemma and can contribute to the contamination of fruits and vegetables at harvest.[4]

National and international surveillance of foodborne illness is subject to constraints that limit reliable information and lead to inaccurate estimates of the magnitude of the problem. Globally, it is estimated that only 1 to 10 percent of the true incidents of foodborne illnesses are reported.[13] Some countries have estimated that foodborne illnesses may be 300 to 350 times more frequent than reported.[13]

There are a variety of reasons for this worldwide underestimation of illness. Many countries have failed to implement even a basic foodborne-disease surveillance system. Cholera is the only foodborne disease that must be reported internationally.[13] It is difficult to compare data from different countries because of the lack of uniform data collection. As well, many governments are reluctant to provide information on foodborne diseases, particularly if a country's economy is based on tourism or food exports.[13] In the majority of countries, foodborne-illness surveillance infrastructures or laboratories are nonexistent or function with inadequate resources making these countries vulnerable to outbreaks or epidemics of foodborne disease.[13]

EPIDEMIOLOGY: WATERBORNE DISEASE

There are 215,000 water systems in the United States classified as public systems that are regulated under the Safe Water Drinking Act and the Surface Water Treatment Rule.[2] These regulations require water utilities to disinfect surface water and groundwater by using parameters such as turbidity, coliform counts, and the presence of human enteric viruses and *Giardia lamblia* cysts as target organisms to assess efficacy of treatment.[2] The surveillance system for waterborne-disease outbreaks is similar to that for foodborne illnesses. Criteria for a waterborne outbreak is the presence of a similar illness in two or more people after the ingestion of drinking water or after exposure to water used for recreational purposes. Epidemiologic evidence must implicate water as the probable source of infection.[2]

The CDC identified 30 outbreaks of waterborne disease in the United States associated with drinking water causing illness in 405,366 people from 1993 to 1994.[2] A single outbreak of cryptosporidiosis, the largest waterborne-disease outbreak ever reported in the United States, accounted for 403,000 cases from which 4400 people were hospitalized. The outbreak was traced to a community water system. Surface water from Lake Michigan had been filtered and chlorinated, but a deterioration in the water quality and the decreased effectiveness of the coagulation-filtration process led to an inadequate removal of *Cryptosporidium parvum* oocysts. The treated water had met all state and federal quality standards that were then in effect. The outbreak was recognized by widespread absenteeism among employees of hospitals and among students and school teachers, a shortage of antidiarrheal drugs citywide, and a marked increase in the number of emergency department visits.[2] A single waterborne outbreak associated with *Salmonella*, infecting 625 people, occurred when municipal water-storage towers were inadequately protected from wild-bird droppings.[2]

PATHOPHYSIOLOGY

Normal physiologic defense mechanisms that exist to prevent disease from foodborne and waterborne pathogens include gastric acid, the normal flora of the gastrointestinal tract, intestinal motility, and mucous glycoproteins of the intestinal mucus. The effectiveness of each of these barriers can be altered by age, concomitant infections, chronic illnesses, medications, and the pathogen itself.

A gastric pH of 3 or less is generally found in most healthy adults and can effectively kill most foodborne pathogens.[14] A reduction in acidity can occur secondary to antacids, medications such as H_2 blockers, and proton-pump inhibitors. Chronic underlying medical conditions such as diabetes mellitus, pernicious anemia, and gastric surgery also reduce gastric pH. Hypochlorhydria has also been demonstrated in *Helicobacter pylori* infections.[14]

Nonpathogenic, indigenous intestinal bacteria inhibit colonization of pathogens by direct competition for nutrients and by the production of fatty acids or chemicals that are bactericidal. Alterations of intestinal flora occur commonly after antibiotic use, as well as secondary to radiation therapy, chemotherapy, and abdominal surgery.[14] Recent antibiotic use lowers resistance to *Salmonella* infections and has been implicated as a risk factor for infection with *E. coli* O157:H7.[14]

The normal motility of the intestinal tract provides an important defense mechanism by minimizing the contact between the mucosal surface and the pathogen. Bowel stasis permits multiplication and overgrowth of foodborne or waterborne pathogens and contributes to retrograde migration from the colon to the small intestine. Antiperistaltic agents, narcotics, and previous radiation therapy theoretically can prolong gut transit time and increase pathogen infectivity.[14]

Bacteria, such as enterotoxigenic *E. coli,* can increase their pathogenicity by adhering to the mucosal surface via surface pili or fimbria that bind to receptors on intestinal epithelial cells.[5] Direct invasion of the mucosal epithelial cells occurs with many foodborne pathogens such as *Shigella, Salmonella,* enteroinvasive *E. coli, Campylobacter,* and *Vibrio parahaemolyticus.*[5] Intracellular multiplication of these organisms is followed by epithelial cell death. Cytotoxins, such as the Shiga toxin of *Shigella dysentariae* or Shiga-like toxins produced by enterohemorrhagic *E. coli* O157:H7, enteropathogenic *E. coli*, and *V. parahaemolyticus* also cause cellular membrane disruption and cell lysis.[5] *Vibrio cholera* and enterotoxic *E. coli* produce protein toxins that alter fluid and electrolyte transfer across epithelial cell membranes and produce large volumes of fluid that exceed the absorptive capacity of the colon. The resultant, excessive diarrhea can lead to rapid dehydration.[5]

The most common pathogens causing foodborne illnesses are *Salmonella, Campylobacter, E. coli* O157, and the Norwalk viruses.[15] Viral gastroenteritis, caused by Norwalk viruses, rotaviruses, enteric adenoviruses, astroviruses, and calciviruses, accounts for the majority of cases of infectious diarrhea seen in the emergency department.[16] Usually transmitted person to person, food and water transmission is not uncommon and should be considered.[17] Viral infections of the gastrointestinal tract cause an enormous amount of diarrhea-related mortality and morbidity and is one of the leading causes of infant death worldwide.[18] Simultaneous infection with more than one viral pathogen is common.

Foodborne viruses are usually transmitted person to person by the fecal-oral route and are infectious in very low doses. Lack of confirmation of a viral etiology leads to an underreporting of viral foodborne outbreaks.[16] Viruses do not multiply or produce toxins, and food items simply act as transfer mediums.[17] Foods may be contaminated either at the source or at the time and place of preparation. Bivalve mollusks (oysters, clams, mussels, and cockles) have been implicated in the transmission of viruses. Their contamination usually occurs at the source in polluted shallow coastal waters.[17,19] Viral contaminants remain active when they are inadequately cooked or consumed raw, particularly in oysters.[17] The application of raw sewage or sludge to fruit and vegetable crops is another source of primary viral contamination.[17]

Viral contamination from infected food handlers occurs after harvesting as food items pass through several hands before reaching consumers. It is largely associated with cold food items that require much handling during preparation (salads and sandwiches) or ice.[17] Surfaces used in food preparation may become contaminated, as well. Food handlers may be asymptomatically shedding virus particles prior to the onset of illness or continue to shed virus particles up to 48 h after recovery.[17] Although unusual, airborne transmission of virus particles has been demonstrated in outbreaks of foodborne illness on cruise ships and in schools.[16] As in bacterial infections, waterborne transmission of virus is an effective mechanism of infectivity. Outbreaks have been associated with contamination of private wells, small water systems, and community water systems.[2,16] Seasonal outbreaks of Norwalk gastroenteritis have been associated with swimming in lakes and pools.[16]

Hepatitis A was the fourth leading cause of foodborne disease among outbreak-associated illness compiled by the CDC for 1988 to 1992.[3] It is the only reportable foodborne viral disease, and the true incidence of illness is underreported.[19] When food samples have become unavailable for testing, hepatitis A outbreaks are likely to be recognized weeks after contaminated food has been consumed. Most infections are the result of consumption of infected bivalves, but outbreaks associated with infected strawberries and raspberries have occurred.[16,17] Diarrhea is not commonly associated with hepatitis A.

Viruses can be eliminated at any step along the food-handling process. Heating is an effective means of inactivating hepatitis A virus particles in mollusks, and their exposure to temperatures of 85° to 90°C for at least 90 s is recommended.[17,19] Viruses are a small target for ionizing radiation. Enteric viruses are often acid resistant, and hepatitis A virus is quite resistant to drying. Viruses in water or on surfaces can be inactivated by chlorine, ozone, or ultraviolet light.[19]

DIAGNOSIS

Recognizing foodborne or waterborne illness can be extremely challenging for emergency physicians. Symptoms associated with foodborne illness are very common and nonspecific except for syndromes associated with chemical agents. Physical examination should be directed at identifying toxic or dehydrated patients, identifying the presence of blood in the stool, and excluding other diarrheal illnesses. A variety of diagnostic tests are available for confirmation of pathogens in suspected outbreaks, but routine testing of patients with infectious diarrhea for ova and parasites and stool cultures is not cost effective.[20] The majority of patients will have a self-limited illness that resolves by the time culture results are available. Diagnostic studies and cultures should be directed toward patients with blood or mucus in the stool, fever or other signs of toxicity, or significant historical risk factors for foodborne illness. When fecal leukocytes are present, the culture yield is higher for bacterial pathogens, but the absence of fecal leukocytes does not exclude a bacterial etiology and limits its diagnostic efficacy.[20]

Obtaining a complete history of an acute diarrheal illness is important. In a presumed foodborne illness, determining the exact time of exposure can help direct the evaluation to particular causative agents, although significant overlap exists between syndromes of foodborne illness (Table 144-1).[3] Extending a history beyond 3 or 4 days will provide only limited benefit in identifying pathogens—such as hepatitis A, *Cryptosporidium*, and *Salmonella*—with prolonged incubation periods.

A history of two or more people within a household becoming ill simultaneously may indicate a foodborne etiology. If additional cases occur within 24 to 36 h, nonfoodborne sources, such as viruses, are more likely. Patients should be questioned about inadequate food-handling practices at home, such as preparation of food several hours prior to consumption, insufficient cooking or reheating of food, cross contamination between raw and cooked foods on common preparation surfaces, or people with poor personal hygiene handling the food.[21]

Patients should be questioned about other activities associated with an increased risk of foodborne disease, such as frequent restaurant meals, exposure to day-care centers, consumption of street-vended food or raw seafood, overseas travel, and camping with the ingestion of lake or steam water.

Host factors that reduce resistance and immunocompetence should be identified. The recent use of antibiotics and medications that reduce gastric acidity, such as H_2 blockers, proton-pump inhibitors, and antacids, should be identified. Identify patients with AIDS or other immunocompromised conditions.

The very young and the elderly have a higher incidence of infection and greater risk of complications from foodborne illnesses. Children

TABLE 144-1 Etiologic Agents for Foodborne Diseases and Usual Incubation Periods

Incubation period / Agent
1–6 h
Norwalk viruses
Astrovirus, calcivirus
Staphylococcus aureus
Bacillus cerus vomiting toxin
Ciguatoxin
Scombroid toxins
Paralytic or neurotoxic shellfish poisoning
Puffer fish, tetrodotoxin
Heavy metals
Monosodium glutamates
Short-acting mushroom toxins
6–24 h
Bacillus cereus diarrheal toxin
Clostridium perfringens
Vibrio parahaemolyticus
Long-acting mushroom toxins
24–48 h
Nontyphoidal *Salmonella*
Enterotoxigenic (ETEC)
Clostridium botulinum
Trichinella spp. intestinal phase
2–6 days
Shigella
Campylobacter
Escherichia coli O157 : H7
Vibrio cholerae
Streptococcus group A
Yersinia enterocolitica
6–14 days
Cryptosporidium parvum
Salmonella typhi
Cyclospora
Giardia lamblia
>14 days
Hepatitis A
Brucella
Listeria monocytogenes invasive disease
Trichinella spp. systemic phase

Source: From CDC,[3] with permission.

younger than age 5 and adults older than age 65 have the highest attack rate for infection with *E. coli* and are at the greatest risk for hemolytic-uremic syndrome.[14] Isolation rates for *Salmonella* reported to the CDC and the risk for bacteremia were highest among children under age 9 and adults over age 80.[14] Residents of chronic care facilities are at increased risk for illness and death because of their close proximity, increased frequency of fecal incontinence, and a general debilitated state with multiple concurrent illnesses.[14]

A recent history of swimming in pools, water parks, lakes, and other recreational water facilities is important and should raise suspicion for cryptosporidiosis, although other pathogens such as enterohemorrhagic *E. coli* have been linked to water-park outbreaks.[2]

Stool cultures should minimally include the most frequent causes of foodborne illnesses: *Campylobacter, Salmonella,* and *Shigella.*[20] The frequency of *E. coli* O157:H7 foodborne illness has increased, and many laboratories routinely culture for it, as well. The Gram stain can identify *Campylobacter,* one of the most common causes of gastroenteritis, with a sensitivity of 66 to 99 percent and still has a role in the diagnosis of diarrheal disease.[20] Cultures for other organisms should be based on prevalence rates in the community or an increased index of suspicion based on history and physical examination. Emergency physicians should be cognizant of which pathogens are and, equally as important, are not routinely cultured for in their laboratories. Optimal sensitivity of the test requires more than a single specimen, preferably obtained in the emergency department, especially for ova and parasites.[20] Rectal swabs are not adequate for specimen collection.

Public health authorities usually become aware of and initiate investigations of potential foodborne or waterborne outbreaks when there is an increase in the frequency of pathogens reported to them by hospitals or a cluster of suspicious cases. Variations of this reporting structure do occur. Emergency physicians concerned about possible outbreaks should communicate with the infection control departments and microbiology laboratories in their hospitals.

CHRONIC SEQUELAE

Chronic secondary complications of foodborne illness occur in about 2 to 3 percent of patients.[22] The true incidence is probably higher because chronic sequelae may be difficult to link to the acute illness and may occur despite successful elimination of the primary organism. Frequently, the host and pathogen have common surface antigens. Host recognition of the foreign antigen initiates an autoimmune response. A low but consistent incidence (0.2 to 2.4 percent) of seronegative reactive arthritis has been noted following outbreaks of *Salmonella typhimurium, Shigella flexneri,* and *Campylobacter jejuni.*[22,23] Superantigens—protein virulence factors that can elicit extreme immune responses in the host—have been isolated from several foodborne bacteria and are thought to be associated with several autoimmune disorders, such as rheumatoid arthritis, multiple sclerosis, Graves disease, and psoriasis.[22] A link between *Campylobacter* and Guillain-Barré syndrome has been suspected for over a decade. It is estimated that possibly 40 percent of Guillain-Barré cases are secondary to primary infection, with *Campylobacter* usually developing 7 to 21 days after resolution of gastrointestinal symptoms.[22,23] Hemolytic-uremic syndrome (HUS), characterized by acute renal failure, thrombocytopenia, and microangiopathic hemolytic anemia, develops in some patients, particularly children, following acute colitis with *E. coli* O157:H7. HUS is caused by toxin-mediated damage to the glomerular epithelial cells and possibly the tubular epithelial cells and is the leading cause of acute renal failure in children.[22,23] Other organisms that have been linked to HUS include other strains of *E. coli, Citrobacter, Campylobacter, Shigella, Salmonella,* and *Yersinia.*[23] Many of the acute symptoms of ciguatera poisoning can persist as a waxing and waning chronic symptom complex that is often misdiagnosed as chronic fatigue syndrome, brain tumor, or multiple sclerosis.[23]

PREVENTION AND SURVEILLANCE

Traditional Surveillance

Effective foodborne-disease surveillance is critical to determine the frequency of cases, identify newly emerging pathogens, and isolate factors that contribute to the disease transmission.[11] Traditional surveillance systems for foodborne illnesses rely on clinical microbiology laboratories reporting identified pathogens or suspected outbreaks to state health departments, which then report them to the CDC.[24] This type of passive surveillance requires a person with a diarrheal illness to seek care from a physician who then in turn obtains a stool culture. The current underreporting of foodborne illnesses is a direct consequence of this interdependent chain of events where an elimination of even one step results in a case not being identified.[24] It is estimated that only 1 in 20 to 100 cases of *Salmonella* are reported to the CDC.[11]

FoodNet

FoodNet is a collaborative project of participating data collection sites in the CDC, US Department of Agriculture, and the US Food and Drug Administration (FDA) that became operational in 1995. It employs an active surveillance strategy for diarrheal illnesses and foodborne illnesses in sentinel populations monitored at over 300 clinical laboratories throughout the United States.[24] FoodNet investigators actively contact these laboratories for confirmed cases of *Salmonella, Shigella, Campylobacter, E. coli* O157:H7, *Listeria, Yersinia, Vibrio, Cyclospora,* and *Cryptosporidium.* They have built a comprehensive database of foodborne illness in these regions.[24] Physician practice patterns for ordering stool specimens have also been monitored. Population surveys create an approximation of the number of patients with diarrheal illness who seek medical care.[24] This information is centrally based at the CDC and facilitates timely recognition and response to foodborne outbreaks.

PulseNet

PulseNet, completed in May 1998, is a national computer network of public heath laboratories that perform DNA fingerprinting on two bacteria: *E. coli* O157:H7 and *Salmonella typhimurium.* Using a standardized methodology for pulsed-field gel electrophoresis (PFGE), designated network laboratories in the United States can rapidly determine whether foodborne illnesses in multiple locations are linked to a common pathogen and food source. Bacterial PFGE patterns are entered into a centralized national electronic database by the state or local health department. Matching patterns from different locations during a defined time period will trigger an alert to a possible multilocation foodborne-illness outbreak.[8]

Prevention

The current system for ensuring food safety is complex, with authority divided between federal, state, and local governments. Currently in the United States, the FDA inspects food-processing plants and, along with the US Department of Agriculture, regulates the interstate commerce of these foods. Final delivery destinations, such as restaurants, supermarkets, and cafeterias, are regulated by local health departments. The movement of food from the farm or water sources follows a predictable process-specific pathway. Contamination can occur at one or more points in the process. Hazard Analysis and Critical Control Points (HACCP) is an applied methodology that identifies and controls the key steps in the process that are vulnerable to contamination. It requires cooperation between government regulatory agencies and the food industry and replaces the simple inspection of a final product. Industry-wide solutions can be implemented once contamination points are identified.[1,7,10,11]

Emergency physicians should advise infected patients of the potential risks they pose to family members or others, particularly if they are food handlers or health care workers.[19] A small number of factors in food handling are responsible for a large percentage of foodborne disease.[21] The most important steps that can be taken in the home to prevent foodborne disease is thorough cooking and eating cooked food promptly. Educate patients that food from animal sources such as meat, dairy, and eggs should be either pasteurized or completely cooked and not eaten undercooked or raw. Cross contamination from the juices or drippings from raw meat, poultry eggs, or shellfish with other foods must be avoided by washing hands or common preparation surfaces with soap and water. Prepared food should not be left for extended periods of time at temperatures that will promote bacteria growth.[4,21] The World Health Organization has established rules for the preparation of safe food in the home that can be accessed via the Internet at http://www.who.int/fsf/gldnrls.htm.

REFERENCES

1. Kaferstein Y, Motarjemi Y, Bettcher D: Foodborne disease control: A transnational challenge. *Emerg Infect Dis* 3:503, 1997.
2. Centers for Disease Control and Prevention (CDC): Surveillance summaries: Surveillance for waterborne disease outbreaks: United States, 1993–1994. *MMWR* 45:SS-1:2, 1996.
3. Centers for Disease Control and Prevention (CDC): Surveillance summaries: Surveillance for foodborne-disease outbreaks: United States, 1988–1992. *MMWR* 45:SS-5:1, 1996.
4. Altekruse S, Cohen M, Swerdlow D: Perspective: Emerging foodborne diseases. *Emerg Infect Dis* 3:285, 1997.
5. Cheny C, Wong R: Acute infectious diarrhea. *Med Clin North Am* 77:1169, 1993.
6. Sabota J, Hoppes W, Ziegler J, et al: A new variant of food poisoning: Enteroinvasive *Klebsiella pneumoniae* and *Escherichia coli* sepsis from a contaminated hamburger. *Am J Gastroenterol* 93:118, 1998.
7. Tauxe R: Emerging foodborne diseases: An evolving public health challenge. *Emerg Infect Dis* 3:425, 1997.
8. Slutsker L, Altekruse S, Swerdlow D: Foodborne diseases, emerging pathogens and trends. *Infect Dis Clin North Am* 12:199, 1998.
9. Hennessy T, Hedberg C, Slutsker L, et al: A national outbreak of *Salmonella enteritidis* infections from ice cream. *N Engl J Med* 334:1281, 1996.
10. Collins J: Impact of changing consumer lifestyles on the emergence/reemergence of foodborne pathogens. *Emerg Infect Dis* 3:471, 1997.
11. Altekruse S, Swerdlow D: The changing epidemiology of foodborne diseases. *Am J Med Sci* 311:23, 1996.
12. Cartwright R, Chahed M: Foodborne disease in travelers. *World Health Stat Q* 50:102, 1997.
13. Motarjemi Y, Kaferstein F: Global estimation of foodborne illness. *World Health Stat Q* 50:5, 1997.
14. Klontz K, Adler W, Potter M: Age-dependant resistance factors in the pathogenesis of foodborne infectious disease. *Aging Clin Exp Res* 9:320, 1997.
15. Centers for Disease Control and Prevention (CDC) Information Service: *Foodborne Bacterial Diseases*. Document 310100. CDC: 24 April 1997.
16. Hedberg C, Osterholm M: Outbreaks of foodborne and waterborne viral gastroenteritis. *Clin Microbiol* 6:199, 1993.
17. Appleton H: Foodborne viruses. *Lancet* 336:1362, 1990.
18. Taterka J, Cuff C, Rubin D: Viral gastrointestinal infections. *Gastroenterol Clin North Am* 21:303, 1992.
19. Cliver D: Virus transmission via food. *World Health Stat Q* 50:90, 1997.
20. Hines J, Nachamkin I: Effective use of the clinical microbiology laboratory for diagnosing diarrheal diseases. *Clin Infect Dis* 23:1292, 1996.
21. World Health Organization (WHO): *The WHO Golden Rules for Safe Food Preparation*. Geneva: WHO. Http://www.who.ch/programmes/fsf/gldnrls.htm.
22. Bunning K, Lindsay J, Archer D: Chronic health effects of microbial foodborne disease. *World Health Stat Q* 50:51, 1997.
23. Lindsay J: Chronic sequelae of foodborne diseases. *Emerg Infect Dis* 3:443, 1997.
24. FoodNet Working Group: Foodborne Diseases Active Surveillance Network (FoodNet). *Emerg Infect Dis* 3:581, 1997.

INFECTIONS FROM ANIMALS

John T. Meredith

The World Health Organization classifies zoonotic infections as those diseases and infections that are naturally transmitted between vertebrate animals and humans.[1] This broad class of diseases includes more than 200 specific diseases and syndromes covering an extremely variable range of clinical syndromes and medical therapy.[2] Zoonotic infections can be transmitted to humans by direct contact with an infected animal or infected animal product, by ingestion of contaminated water or food products, by inhalation, and through arthropod vectors. In North America and Western Europe, many of the serious zoonotic infections either have been eradicated or are beginning to come under control. Rabies, brucellosis, and echinococcosis will probably be eliminated from developed countries within the next 20 years.[3] Nevertheless, zoonotic infections with a relatively low incidence in North America often incur high morbidity and mortality. Pets are the principal reservoirs of zoonoses in North America. Zoonotic infections still represent a significant public health issue in most of the underdeveloped regions of the world, especially those undeveloped regions and countries dependent economically on agricultural animals. As such, the incidence of zoonotic infections is significant, with accompanying high morbidity and mortality. Another concern is the ever-increasing growth and mobility of the world's population. This increase in human mobility has resulted in the appearance of new zoonotic infections and the reemergence of previously eliminated zoonoses. Of significance is that more than 50 percent of the newly identified infectious agents since 1976 are associated with animals.[4] This trend of newly emerging zoonoses is likely to continue. Thus, diversity of presentation, human mobility, and zoonotic reemergence make the diagnosis and management of zoonotic infections a daunting task for emergency physicians.

RISK ASSESSMENT

Zoonotic infections are common in North America, with an estimated 4 million people infected annually.[5] These diseases are underdiagnosed, and the possibility of a zoonotic infection should be an integral part of the differential diagnosis of any patient who presents with an infectious syndrome. Specific occupations and avocations result in an increased risk of zoonotic acquisition by increased exposure to both domestic and nondomestic animals. Farmers, migrant workers, slaughterhouse workers, veterinarians, cattle ranchers, animal researchers and handlers, forestry workers, hunters, pet owners, and outdoor enthusiasts all have an inherent risk of acquiring a zoonotic infection.[6] The type of animal exposure is another important factor. Dressing, skinning, or handling an animal's skin; a history of animal bite or scratch; and ingestion of animal or dairy products all carry an associated risk of zoonotic infection. Recent travel and history of habitation, particularly in an underdeveloped country or rural area, represent particular risk factors for zoonotic infection. Other factors are a patient's immunologic status and the presence of comorbid or debilitating diseases. Patients with acquired immune-deficiency syndrome, diabetes, alcoholism, intravenous drug abuse, asplenism, cancer, and a history of chemotherapy all have an increased risk of acquiring a zoonotic infection. When assessing a patient who might have a zoonotic disease, information regarding occupation, avocation, place of residence, exposure to pets and to domesticated and wild animals, immunologic status, history of debilitating illness or drug and alcohol abuse, travel history, and arthropod exposure is very important to elicit (Table 145-1).[7]

SYSTEMIC ZOONOSES INFECTIONS

Zoonotic infections are caused by an extremely diverse group of microorganisms. A myriad of classification approaches focus on the patho-

TABLE 145-1 Risk Factors for Zoonotic Infection

Risk Category	Examples
Agricultural workers	Farmers, cattle ranchers, sheep ranchers, and migrant workers
Animal-processing workers	Slaughterhouse workers, animal-hide processors, and workers in any manufacturing plant that deals with animal products or by-products
Outdoor enthusiasts	Forestry workers, lumbermen, surveyors, park rangers, hunters, spelunkers, fishermen, and those who regularly engage in outdoor recreational activities
Pet owners	Those with a dog, cat, bird, rodent, rabbit, reptile, or fish
Professionals	Veterinarians, animal researchers, and animal handlers
Immunocompromised patients	Those with congenital immunodeficiencies, diabetes mellitus, alcoholism, renal failure, liver failure, cancer splenectomy or HIV

gen, animal vector, mode of transmission, geographic range, and clinical syndrome. For emergency physicians, the best approach is one of clinical syndrome presentation, but systemic zoonoses are most difficult to diagnose. Often, they present as an undifferentiated febrile illness with pyrexia, cephalgia, myalgia, malaise, and weakness. This presentation is very common in patients in an emergency department and can indicate pathology other than that of a zoonotic infection. The concern is how to differentiate a zoonotic infection from a benign febrile illness. In this regard, risk factors for acquiring a zoonotic infection are very important, as is recognizing the seasonal variation of most zoonotic infections. In the United States, most zoonoses show an increased incidence in the spring and summer.[8] However, systemic zoonotic infections should be included in the differential diagnosis of any seriously ill patient who presents with an undifferentiated fever. Specific zoonoses that can present as an undifferentiated febrile illness or septic presentation include *Aeromonas* spp, *Brucella canis, Capnocytophaga, Chlamydia psittaci, Leptospira* sp., *Francisella* sp., *Salmonella enteritidis, Streptococcus pyogenes, Yersinia pestis, Coxiella burnetii, Ehrlichia* sp., and *Rickettsia rickettsii* (Table 145-2).

TICKBORNE ZOONOTIC INFECTIONS

Tickborne zoonoses deserve special consideration. More zoonotic diseases are transmitted by ticks then by any other vector.[9] Tickborne infections include bacterial, rickettsial, viral, and protozoan infections. As a subset of zoonotic infection, these diseases often go unrecognized in the initial evaluation of febrile patients. Because a high proportion of physicians in the United States know little about tickborne disease, they do not consider this diagnosis in febrile patients.[8] Additionally, not all patients who acquire a tickborne zoonotic infection recall a history of a tick bite.[10] Nevertheless, tickborne zoonoses represent a significant source of mortality and morbidity in the United States—approximately 13,000 cases each year.[11] An understanding of the geographic distribution of tickborne zoonoses is important in diagnosing this zoonotic subset (Table 145-3). The seasonal variation in tickborne zoonoses follows that of other zoonotic infections in North America, the highest incidence being incurred during spring and summer. Rocky Mountain spotted fever (RMSF), Lyme disease, relapsing fever, Colorado tick fever, tularemia, babesiosis, and ehrlichiosis often present with an undifferentiated febrile illness most characteristic of a viral infection, though often accompanied with a rash (Table 145-4).

RMSF is the one of the most frequently reported rickettsial infections in the United States.[12] The causative organism is *Rickettsia rickettsii,* a pleomorphic, obligate intracellular parasite, and the vector is the *Dermacentor* sp. tick. Deer, rodents, horses, cattle, cats, and dogs can serve as zoonotic hosts. RMSF is classically described as a triad of fever, rash, and tick exposure in a majority of infected patients; but a history of tick exposure can only be recalled in approximately 50 percent of these patients. Additionally, RMSF is often misdiagnosed.[13] Other presenting signs and symptoms include malaise, myalgias, lymphadenopathy, abdominal pain, nausea, vomiting, diarrhea, hepatosplenomegaly, cephalgia, conjunctivitis, confusion, meningismus, renal failure, respiratory failure, and myocarditis. The rash of RMSF occurs on days 1 to 15 of the illness but is absent in up to 17 percent of patients.[14] Characteristically, this rash appears maculopapular, occurring on the extremities and around the wrist and ankles. The rash spreads centripetally up the trunk, involves the palms and soles, and can become petechial and, rarely, necrotic. The characteristic presentation of this rash may aid in the diagnosis of RMSF. Laboratory abnormalities are nonspecific and consist of a normal or decreased leukocyte count, thrombocytopenia, elevated liver function studies, and hyponatremia. Laboratory diagnosis is unreliable in the early course of RMSF. Diagnosis can be confirmed with a rise in antibody titer between acute and convalescent serum. Skin biopsy with immunofluorescent testing can also confirm diagnosis, but a negative skin test does not exclude infection.[15] Additionally, a culture of *R. rickettsii* may confirm diagnosis. Treatment is with a tetracycline or chloramphenicol (doxycycline 100 mg PO bid for 14 days or chloramphenicol 500 mg qid for 10 days).

Lyme disease is the leading vector-borne zoonotic infection in the United States.[16] Though most prevalent in the Northeast, all continental 48 states have reported Lyme disease. The responsible organism is *Borrelia burgdorferi,* a spirochete, and the vector is the *Ixodes* spp. tick. Small mammals and deer serve as the principal zoonotic hosts. Typically described in three distinct stages, the initial stage of illness often presents with a macular dermatitis: erythema migrans. This rash associated with early Lyme disease occurs 2 to 20 days at the site of the tick bite and is a result of a vasculitis. Erythema migrans, which is an erythematous plaque with central clearing, may persist for up to 1 month and recur in the secondary stage of Lyme disease.[17] Erythema migrans, though, occurs in only 60 to 80 percent of cases.[18] Untreated erythema migrans resolves spontaneously in 3 to 4 weeks. Nevertheless, erythema migrans may aid in the diagnosis of Lyme disease.[10,18] With the dissemination of the *Borrelia* spirochete, the secondary stage of illness—fever, adenopathy, and flulike symptoms—along with multiple annular dermatologic lesions may occur. The most common neurologic symptom is the development of cranial neuritis, and often facial nerve palsy that can be unilateral or bilateral. This palsy can occur concomitantly with the initial rash of erythema migrans. Other peripheral neuropathies can occur in addition to an asymmetric oligoarticular arthritis of the large joints, with a particular predilection to the knees. Chronic manifestations, the tertiary stage of illness, occur years after the initial infection and consist of chronic arthritis, myocarditis, subacute encephalopathy, axonal polyneuropathy, and leukoencephalopathy. These manifestations account for the tertiary stage of illness.[19] Diagnosis is principally a clinical one, though a two-step serologic test—enzyme immunoassay and Western immunoblot—may help to confirm it. *Borrelia burgdorferi* has been cultured, but that is extremely difficult. Treatment is with doxycycline (100 mg PO bid for 10 to 21 days) in the initial stage of illness.[9] Alternative antibiotic therapy includes amoxicillin, (500 mg PO tid for 10 to 21 days), cefuroxime (500 mg PO bid for 21 days), and clarithromycin (500 mg PO bid for 21 days).[16] Prophylactic treatment is not recommended, since fewer than 10 percent of the bites transmit the disease, and because prophylactic antibiotic administration may depress the immune response to the disease. A vaccine against Lyme disease is now available for high-risk individuals. This vaccine is made from the outer surface protein of *B. burgdorferi* using recombinant technology.

TABLE 145-2 Systemic Zoonotic Infections

Agent	Animal Reservoir	Physical Findings	Diagnostic Tests	Antibiotic Treatment*
Aeromonas sp.	Fish and reptiles	Nonspecific fever, severe crepitant cellulitis with systemic toxicity		Fluoroquinolones or TMP-SMX
Brucella canis	Dogs	Nonspecific fever	Serologic testing and blood culture	Doxycycline *plus* gentamicin, streptomycin, OR rifampin
Capnocytophaga	Dogs and cats	Fever, sepsis, and endocarditis from infected bite	Culture of bite wound	Amoxacillin/clavulanate; OR clindamycin *plus* either a fluoroquinolone, or TMP-SMX
Chlamydia psittaci	Birds	Fever, pneumonia, endocarditis, sepsis	Serologic testing and sputum culture	Tetracycline or erythromycin
Coxiella burnetii (Q fever)	Cats, livestock, and ticks	Fever, pneumonia, hepatitis, meningitis, endocarditis	Serologic testing	Doxycycline or a fluoroquinolone for meningitis
Ehrlichia sp.	Ticks	Nonspecific fever, sepsis, meningitis, hepatitis	Serologic testing, peripheral blood smear, immunocytologic testing, and polymerase chain reaction testing	Doxycycline
Leptospira sp.	Birds, dogs, and rodents	Fever, pneumonia, conjunctivitis, lymphadenopathy	Dark-field microscopic examination of body fluids; serologic testing	Penicillin G intravenously or doxycycline
Francisella sp. (tularemia)	Rabbits, cats, and wild animals	Fever, sepsis, meningitis, pneumonia, hepatitis, rash	Serologic testing	Streptomycin or gentamicin, *plus* chloramphenicol for meningitis
Rickettsia rickettsii	Ticks	Fever, diarrhea	Stool culture	Doxycycline or chloramphenicol
Salmonella enteria	Dogs, cats (rarely), and reptiles (turtles)	Fever, sepsis, cellulitis, meningitis, endocarditis, septic arthritis	Blood culture	Ciprofloxacin or ceftriaxone
Streptococcus	Livestock	Fever, pneumonia, meningitis, lymphadenopathy	Blood culture	Erythromycin, vancomycin, or TMP-SMX
Yersinia pestis	Dogs, cats, and rodents		Blood culture and culture of suspected sites	Gentamicin, streptomycin, doxycycline, or chloramphenicol

Abbreviation: TMP-SMX, trimethoprim-sulfamethoxazole.
* Specific doses are listed within text.

As the tick feeds on an immunized host, antibodies are ingested destroying spirochetes in the gut of the engorging tick prior to the transmission to the host. A course of three injections of vaccine are required for maximal effectiveness in preventing asymptomatic infections.

Relapsing fever is frequently misdiagnosed and underreported.[20] The responsible organisms are *Borrelia* spirochetes, which can alter their surface antigens. The vectors are *Ornithodoros* ticks, and the principle zoonotic reservoirs are wild rodents. Often the initial presentation is that of a rash or pruritic eschar at the site of a tick bite. An average incubation period of 7 days precedes the onset of fever, chills, cephalgia, myalgia, arthralgia, abdominal pain, and general malaise. Characteristically, the febrile episodes are interspersed with afebrile periods. Leukocytosis, thrombocytopenia, and an elevated erythrocyte sedimentation rate are the typical laboratory findings. Diagnosis is confirmed with the appearance of spirochetes on Wrights- or Giemsa-stained peripheral blood smears. Treatment is with doxycycline or erythromycin (doxycycline 100 mg PO bid for 14 days or erythromycin 500 mg qid for 10 to 14 days).[21,22]

Colorado tick fever has an RNA virus as etiology. Endemic to the western mountainous regions of the United States, approximately 300 cases are reported annually. The principal vector is the tick of the *Dermacentor* sp., and the zoonotic reservoirs are deer, marmots, and porcupines. With an incubation period of 3 to 7 days, the onset of illness is characterized by fever, chills, cephalgia, myalgia, and photophobia. Often following the initial presentation is a macular or petechial rash. Rarely, complications occur. Diagnosis is most often clinical, with associated epidemiologic factors, but the virus can be isolated from blood or cerebrospinal fluid (CSF) by inoculating suckling mice.[23] Treatment is supportive care, with infrequently, a long convalescence.

Tularemia, which has been characterized as ''a plague-like disease of rodents,''[24] is caused by a gram-negative, nonmotile coccobacillus: *Francisella tularensis*. The zoonotic vectors are ticks of the *Dermacentor* sp. and the *Amblyomma* sp., and the principal zoonotic reservoirs are rabbits, hares, and deer.[11] However, tularemia can be contracted through open wounds while dressing an infected zoonotic host. The clinical presentation depends on the method of inoculation, with the ulceroglandular form being the most common. This particular form

TABLE 145-3 Tickborne Zoonotic Infections: Geographic Distribution

Disease	Geographic Distribution
Lyme disease	Atlantic central and northcentral USA
Rocky Mountain spotted fever	Most of the continental USA although more prevalent in the southeast and southcentral USA
Ehrlichiosis	Japan, Malaysia, and the USA
Human granulocytic	Eastern, northeastern, and northcentral USA
Human monocytic	Mostly southern USA
Q fever	Worldwide
Relapsing fever	Worldwide
Tularemia	USA (except Hawaii) and Canada
Babesiosis	Coastal areas of MA, RI, and NY; also in MD, VA, MN, WI, GA, WA, and Mexico
Colorado tick fever	Western and northwestern USA and southwestern Canada

is often an ulcer at the site of the tick bite, with painful regional adenopathy. Other forms are a glandular form without ulcerations, and a typhoidal form consisting of fever, chills, cephalgia, and abdominal pain. The oropharyngeal form and pneumonic form are the result of deposition into the eyes or inhalation of *F. tularensis* bacterium. Laboratory findings are nonspecific, and the diagnosis can be determined by culture and enzyme-linked immunosorbent assay (ELISA). Treatment is with streptomycin [15 mg/kg intramuscularly (IM) daily for 10 to 14 days] or gentamicin (3 mg/kg/day in three divided doses daily for 10 to 14 days). A live attenuated vaccine is available for research workers and laboratory personnel.[25]

Babesiosis is a malaria-like disease with the etiologic agents being protozoan parasites: *Babesia microti* and *Babesia equi*.[26] The major zoonotic reservoirs are domesticated mammals, rodents, and deer. *Ixodes* ticks functions as the principal vector. Blood transfusions have been implicated in the transmission of babesiosis.[26] Clinically, the presentation is of generalized malaise, anorexia, fever, and chills often progressing to intermittent sweats, myalgia, and cephalgia. Splenectomy and immunologic impairment are thought to be risk factors for this zoonosis. Additionally, babesiosis can progress, resulting in hemolytic anemia. Laboratory tests often show evidence of hemolysis, liver dysfunction, anemia, thrombocytopenia, and renal failure. Interestingly, approximately 20 percent of the patients with babesiosis have a concurrent infection with Lyme disease. Diagnosis is made by finding intraerythrocytic ring forms on a Giemsa-stained peripheral blood smear, though false-negative results can occur when the level of parasitism is low. Treatment is with oral quinine (650 mg tid for 7 days) plus intravenous or oral clindamycin (600 mg tid for 7 days).[26]

Ehrlichiosis is a zoonotic disease with two principal presentations of *human granulocytic ehrlichiosis* and *human monocytic ehrlichiosis*. The etiologic agent responsible for the granulocytic form is thought be be similar to *Ehrlichia phagocytophila* and *Ehrlichia equi*.[27,28] The predominant form in the United States is the monocytic form caused by *Erlichia chaffeensis*. The ehrlichia bacteria are gram-negative pleomorphic coccobacilli that infect circulating leukocytes.[28] The zoonotic reservoirs are thought to be deer, dogs, and other mammals, with the vectors being *Ixodes* sp. and *Amblyomma* sp. ticks. Characteristic clinical presentation is that of fever, cephalgia, malaise, nausea, vomiting, abdominal pain, anorexia, and myalgia. In a minority of cases, a maculopapular or petechial rash is present involving the soles and palms. Renal failure, respiratory failure, and encephalitis can develop. Diagnosis is with serologic testing. Laboratory studies can demonstrate leukocytopenia, thrombocytopenia, and liver dysfunction. Treatment is with doxycycline, 100 mg PO bid for 7 to 14 days.[28]

Tick removal can present a vexing challenge to the emergency physician. The use of a burning match or any action resulting in crushing the tick should be avoided. These attempts at removal result in the tick regurgitating into the wound site. Additionally, they have the potential for incomplete removal of the tick. The most effective way to remove an imbedded tick is a two-step approach. First, viscous lidocaine is applied to kill the tick and anesthetize the bite site. Second, careful and gentle traction is applied to the tick's head with fine forceps. It is imperative that all parts of the tick be removed. Residual tick body parts can stimulate a granulomatous reaction and persistent infection.

ZOONOTIC ENCEPHALITIS AND MENINGITIS

Zoonotic encephalitis is most often transmitted hematologically as an arboviral infection with an arthropod vector and animal host. Often the vector is a mosquito or tick and the animal host is a small animal or bird. The one exception is rabies, which follows peripheral nerve tracts after inoculation from an infected animal's bite. Additionally, encephalitis may be seen in the nonviral zoonotic infections of *Bartonella henselae, Brucella canis,* borreliosis, *Coxiella burnetii, Ehrlichia* sp., listeriosis, leptospirosis, Lyme disease, RMSF, psittacosis, and toxoplasmosis.[11,29,30] The presentation is one of a prodromal illness with malaise, myalgia, fever and, occasionally, parotiditis. This prodromal phase advances to a sudden decline in mental status associated with headache and fever. Prompt recognition and therapy of encephalitis is important, given the high morbidity and mortality rates. However, it is significant to recognize that there are no pathognomonic signs and symptoms that distinguish the exact etiology of encephalitis. The CSF is often abnormal, showing a slightly elevated opening pressure, normal to slightly elevated protein concentration, normal glucose levels, and predominance of lymphocytes. The patient has an abnormal electroencephalogram with diffuse bilateral slowing interrupted by occasional spike activity. CSF viral cultures are frequently sterile, and the infectious agent is rarely isolated from the CSF.[31–33] ELISA of serum can be used to detect most arboviral infections causing encephalitis. Treatment is supportive and directed toward decreasing the intracranial pressure.

Zoonotic meningitis has an equally varied range of pathogens. Brucellosis, listeriosis, plague, salmonellosis, tularemia, leptospirosis, Lyme disease, ehrlichiosis, Q fever, RMSF, and psittacosis can all be etiologic agents. CSF is almost always abnormal as in zoonotic encephalitis but with a greater concentration of lymphocytes. Treatment is directed toward the specific organism cultured from the CSF. However, empiric antibiotic coverage should be administered immediately in any presumptive case of meningitis in an effort to reduce mortality and morbidity.

RESPIRATORY ZOONOTIC INFECTIONS

Respiratory zoonotic infections can be divided into two distinct syndromes of upper respiratory infections (pharyngitis) and lower respiratory infections (pneumonia). Recurrent culture-proven streptococcal pharyngitis in a household member can have a zoonotic source—often the household pet.[34] For complete eradication of this form of streptococcal pharyngitis from a family, the family pet, in addition to family members, may require a course of antistreptococcal antimicrobial therapy. Prolonged exudative pharyngitis raises the suspicion of a zoonotic origin or atypical pharyngitis, particularly if the exudative pharyngitis includes systemic symptoms and leukocytosis, and is refractory to standard antistreptococcal therapy. In this case, it is pertinent to inquire about animal exposure. Dogs and domesticated farm animals can be the source of *Streptococcus* sp., *Corynebacterium ulcerans, Yersinia*

TABLE 145-4 Tickborne Zoonotic Infections

Disease	Vector	Animal Reservoir	Clinical Features	Antibiotic Treatment
Babesiosis	*Ixodes dammini, I. scapularis,* and *I. pacificus*	Cattle, horses, dogs, cats, rodents, deer	Fatigue, malaise, anorexia, nausea, headache, sweats, rigors, abdominal pain, emotional lability, depression, dark urine, hepatomegaly, fever, petechia, ecchymosis, occasional rash and, occasionally, pulmonary edema	For the seriously ill, quinine + clindamycin
Colorado tick fever	*Dermacentor andersoni*	Deer, marmots, porcupines	Fever, chills, headache, myalgias, nausea, vomiting, photophobia, abdominal pain, and occasional sore throat; also may have conjunctivitis, lymphadenopathy, hepatosplenomegaly, stiff neck, retroorbital pain, weakness, and lethargy	Supportive care
Human granulocytic ehrlichiosis	*Ixodes scapularis*	Dogs, deer, other mammals	Fevers, chills, malaise, headache, nausea, muscle aches, cough, sore throat, and pulmonary infiltrates (especially in children)	Doxycycline or chloramphenicol
Human monocytic ehrlichiosis	*Amblyomma americanum* (lone star tick) and *D. variabilis*	Dogs, deer, other mammals	Fevers, chills, malaise, headache, nausea, muscle aches, cough, sore throat, and pulmonary infiltrates (especially in children)	Doxycycline or chloramphenicol
Lyme disease (*Borrelia burgdorferi*)	*Ixodes dammini*	Deer, sheep, deer mice	Erythema migrans, meningitis, encephalitis, neuropathy, and joint and heart symptoms	Doxycycline, amoxicillin, cefuroxime, azithromycin, clarithromycin, ceftriaxone, or cefotaxime
Rocky Mountain spotted fever (*Rickettsia rickettsii*)	*Dermacentor andersoni* (wood tick) and *D. variabilis* (dog tick)	North American mammals	Petechia, purpura, pulmonary infiltrates, jaundice, myocarditis, hepatosplenomegaly, meningitis, encephalitis, and lymphadenopathy	Doxycycline or chloramphenicol
Relapsing fever (*Borrelia burgdorferi*)	*Ornithodoros* sp.	Human body lice, wild rodents, humans	Fever, chills, headache, myalgias, and arthralgias; pain, nausea, vomiting, and hypotension	Erythromycin or doxycycline
Tularemia (*Fancisella tularensis*)	*Dermacentor* sp., and *Amblyomma* sp.	Rabbits, deer, dogs	Pneumonia, regional lymphadenopathy and headache, cough, myalgias, arthralgias, nausea, vomiting, ulceration at inoculation site, and ocular findings	Streptomycin or gentamycin

sp., and viral vesicular stomatitis. All of these zoonoses can present as an exudative pharyngitis.[5] Nondomesticated animals can be a source of exudative pharyngitis as a result of *Bordetella* sp., *Francisella tularensis, Streptobacillus moniformis,* and *Yersinia pestis*.[5] Both pet birds and wild birds carry *Chlamydia psittaci,* which can cause an atypical exudative pharyngitis in humans.

Zoonotic pneumonia presents as an atypical pneumonia with systemic symptoms. Most often the presentation consists of productive or nonproductive cough, fever, chills, headache, myalgias, and a nonspecific rash. These pneumonias are community acquired. Of concern to emergency physicians is that zoonotic pneumonia can often be rapidly lethal, as is the case in pneumonic plague. Zoonotic pneumonia should be considered in any case of gram-negative community-acquired pneumonia and in any case of atypical pneumonia with systemic symptomatology (Table 145-5).[35] A detailed history provides the data necessary for the consideration of zoonotic pneumonia. Inquiries about animal exposure, occupation, and recent travel are warranted for patients with an atypical pneumonia. Particular attention should be paid to slaughterhouse workers and those individuals exposed to ticks, birds, and other fowl. Additionally, a history of outdoor activity, recreational history, and food-contact history should be obtained.

Anthrax (*Bacillus anthracis*) is extremely rare in North America. The pulmonary form—inhalation anthrax—is acquired most often from handling unsterilized, imported animal hides or imported raw wool. Inhalation anthrax is universally fatal. Not a true pneumonia, inhalation anthrax is a mediastinitis without alveolar involvement. Initial symptoms are flulike in character and progress to respiratory failure in 3 to 4 days, with a marked mediastinal and hilar edema. One of the serious concerns to emergency physicians is the potential use of *B. anthracis* as a biologic warfare agent. Though *B. anthracis* can be readily cultured, the delivery system that can generate 5 μ particles and disperse large volumes of culture material is not easily deployable in a large population center. Currently, active-duty US military personnel are being immunized against anthrax. Treatment is with either ciprofloxacin (750 mg PO bid for 7 to 10 days) or doxycycline (100 mg PO bid for 10 to 14 days). Penicillin or erythromycin can be used as alternative antibiotics.[36]

Brucellosis (*Brucella* sp.) occurs most often in slaughterhouse workers exposed to the aerosol of *Brucella* bacteria. The consumption of unpasteurized dairy products is another way of acquiring brucellosis. Pneumonia with frank pulmonary infiltrates as a result of brucellosis is uncommon. Often the presentation is one of an upper respiratory

TABLE 145-5 Zoonotic Pneumonias

Disease	Organism	Reservoirs	Treatment
Inhalation anthrax	*Bacillus anthracis*	Imported animal hides, raw wool, and sick domestic animals	Vancomycin or penicillin
Brucellosis	*Brucella* sp.	Food animals and product handling, ingestion, and inhalation	Doxycycline *plus* rifampin or gentamicin; TMP-SMX *plus* gentamicin
Psittacosis and ornithosis	*Chlamydia psittaci*	Bird exposure—pet and pet shop, veterinarians, and turkey farms	Doxycycline or erythromycin
Q fever	*Coxiella burnetii*	Inhaled endospores from animal-contaminated soil; cat afterbirth and ticks	Doxycycline
Tularemia	*Francisella tularensis*	Aerosol from dead birds and dead animals; bacteremic spread from bubo; ticks and biting flies	Gentamicin or streptomycin
Leptospirosis	*Leptospira interrogans*	Domestic and wild animals, contaminated water, veterinarians, and farmers	Doxycycline, ampicillin, or amoxicillin intravenously; penicillin for severe cases
Pasteurellosis	*Pasteurella multocida*	Underlying respiratory disease; contact with cats or dogs in the home	Doxycycline, penicillin, or third-generation cephalosporin
Melioidosis	*Pseudomonas pseudomallei*	Penetrating injury in endemic area in rodent-contaminated soil or water	Cefrazidime *plus* TMP-SMX; chloramphenicol or doxycycline
Rocky Mountain spotted fever	*Rickettsia rickettsii*	Tick-associated, typical rash	Doxycycline or chloramphenicol
Toxoplasmosis	*Toxoplasma gondii*	Contact with domestic food animals and pets, ingestion of cysts, and pneumonia in immunocompromised persons	Pyrimethamine, sulfadiazine *plus* folinic acid, or clindamycin
Plague	*Yersinia pestis*	Contact with mammals and fleas; veterinarians; and outdoor activities in endemic area; cats	Aminoglycoside *plus* a tetracycline or chloramphenicol
Viral pneumonias			
Hantavirus pulmonary syndrome	Bunyaviridae	Rodent feces, urine, and saliva	Ventilator oxygenation or ribavirin
Influenza pneumonia	Influenza A	Aquatic fowl, pigs, horses, and marine mammals	Supportive care, amantadine, or rimantadine

Abbreviation: TMP-SMX, trimethoprim-sulfamethoxazole.

infection with a cough, hoarseness of voice, and wheezing. Typically, peritracheal and hilar lymph node involvement is seen. With long-standing resolution, calcified granulomas and lymph nodes are characteristic findings.[37] Doxycycline (100 mg PO bid for up to 6 weeks) combined with rifampin (10 mg/kg/day up to 600 mg per day) is effective therapy.[38]

Chlamydia psittaci is common to most birds and fowl. Psittacosis is also known as parrot fever, parrot disease, or ornithosis. Human acquisition is from the inhalation of dust from dried bird feces, feather dust, or aerosolized avian respiratory secretions. Psittacosis is characterized by an incubation period of 5 to 14 days followed by abrupt onset of fever chills, cephalgia, myalgia, and generalized malaise. Pneumonia is atypical, with a nonproductive cough and lobar or interstitial infiltrates on chest radiograph. Extrapulmonary manifestations involving the heart, central nervous system, liver, and kidney are common. Tetracyclines (doxycycline 100 mg PO bid for 10 to 14 days) are the drugs of choice for treatment, with erythromycin (250 mg PO qid for 10 to 14 days) for patients intolerant to tetracycline.[39,40]

Q fever (*Coxiella burnetii*) is unique because it is the only rickettsial infection acquired by aerosol inhalation rather than by an arthropod vector. Q fever is common among domesticated farm animals in the United States and is shed in urine, afterbirth products, and feces. Feed lots are often contaminated with *C. burnetii,* which is highly resistant to environmental degradation. The disease is often self-limiting, with variable pulmonary manifestations and extrapulmonary findings. In addition to pulmonary infiltrates, pericarditis, myocarditis, endocarditis, and granulomatous hepatitis can occur. Treatment is with doxycycline (100 mg PO bid for 10 to 14 days), with erythromycin (250 mg PO qid for 10 to 14 days) as an alternative antibiotic.[41]

Pasteurellosis (*Pasteurella multocida*) is endemic to the normal oral flora of cats and most dogs. Often associated with necrotizing cellulitis from bite wounds, bronchitis, bronchopneumonia, and suppurative pleural effusion can occur as a result of pulmonary infection. Treatment is with amoxicillin with clavulanate (500 mg/125 mg PO tid for 10 to 14 days), tetracycline (doxycycline 100 mg PO bid for 10 to 14 days), penicillin (penicillin V 500 mg PO qid for 10 days), or a third-generation cephalosporin.[42]

Rocky Mountain spotted fever (*Rickettsia ricketsii*), an arthropod-vectored rickettsial infection, can result in a pulmonary capillary vasculitis with associated bronchiolitis.[11] Often a nonproductive cough is present. The chest radiographic findings vary from a normal radiograph to one that shows diffuse interstitial infiltrates and pleural effusions. A secondary bacterial pneumonia is commonly associated with this rickettsial pneumonia. Treatment is with tetracycline or chloramphenicol.[43]

Plague (*Yersinia pestis*) is endemic to the United States and is most often found in rock squirrels and ground rodents of the Southwest. Cats can also be carriers of plague. The principal vector is the rodent flea. Humans and household pets can become infected when bitten by an infected flea. Often an eschar is found at the site of the flea bite, followed by the development of a bubo, an enlarged proximal lymph node. Sepsis and pneumonia from hematologic spread then follow the bubo formation. The pneumonic form is highly contagious and rapidly fatal if not aggressively treated. Additionally, the pulmonary plague can be disseminated from one person to another through aerosolization of respiratory secretions. Treatment is with gentamicin [2.0 mg/kg intravenous (IV) loading dose followed by 1.7 mg/kg IV tid for 10 to 14 days], streptomycin (1 gram IM bid for 10 to 14 days), or a combination of tetracycline and an aminoglycoside.[44]

Influenza accounts for the major viral zoonotic pneumonia. Influenza viruses of the Orthomyxoviridae family are classed as types A, B, and C, and ''Thogoto-like'' virus. Influenza types A, B, and C infect humans, but zoonotic infections are limited to influenza type A.[45] Migrating aquatic fowl are thought to be the natural animal reservoir for influenza type A. Horses and marine mammals can also serve as reservoirs for this zoonotic virus. Additionally, there is very strong epidemiologic and biologic evidence for transmission of influenza between specific species, such as between pigs and humans.[46] Antigenic drift of the viral surface proteins hemagglutinin and neuraminidase in conjunction with a zoonotic reservoir accounts for the frequent human pandemics of influenza. The most noted of these pandemics have been the Spanish influenza of 1918, the Asian influenza of 1957, and the Hong Kong influenza of 1968. It is estimated that 20 to 40 million deaths worldwide were attributed to the Spanish influenza pandemic.[46] Influenza pneumonia carries a high morbidity for all age groups. The mortality rate is greatest in those older than age 70. This age group accounts for 90 percent of the deaths from influenza.[47] Treatment of influenza pneumonia is supportive care. Though amantadine and rimantadine have shown to be effective against influenza A, these two antivirals are not effective against types B and C. Antibiotic therapy for superimposed bacterial pneumonia can contribute to the reduction of mortality and morbidity from influenza. Prevention is by annual vaccination and by preventing influenza introduction into domestic poultry and pigs.

Hantavirus, identified in 1977, is a viral zoonosis. The recognized etiologic agent in North America is the Sin Nombre virus, which belongs to the Bunyaviridae family of viruses. To date, at least 10 distinctive serotypes have been identified, each with a specific rodent vector, geographic distribution, and clinical manifestation.[47] The deer mouse (*Peromyscus maniculatus*) is the primary vector in the United States.[48] Infected rodents excrete Hantavirus in feces, urine, and saliva. Human infection occurs with the inhalation of dried, particulate feces contact with urine, or by a rodent bite. The majority of Hantavirus serotypes have a predilection for the kidney, and the most common worldwide presentation is that of acute renal failure with concurrent thrombocytopenia, ocular abnormalities, and flulike symptoms. In the United States, the presentation of this zoonosis is that of Hantavirus pulmonary syndrome,[47–49] which consists of an initial flulike prodromal illness of 3 to 4 days' duration, rapidly followed by pulmonary edema, hypoxia, hypotension, tachycardia, and metabolic acidosis. Dizziness, nausea, vomiting, absence of cough, and thrombocytopenia are common and may help to differentiate Hantavirus pulmonary syndrome from adult respiratory disease syndrome, bacterial pneumonia, and influenza pneumonia.[2] Hantavirus pulmonary syndrome carries a very high mortality rate of 50 to 70 percent. Diagnosis is with an immunofluorescent or immunoblot assay. Treatment consists of supportive care with attention to adequate oxygenation and possibly the use of an inhalation solution of ribavirin.[47–49]

GASTROINTESTINAL ZOONOTIC INFECTIONS

With a multitude of etiologies, gastroenteritis is one of the most common illnesses treated by emergency physicians. Many of the parasitic, bacterial, and viral organisms responsible for gastroenteritis share a zoonotic source in addition to a human source. In the evaluation of patients with suspected gastroenteritis, information regarding travel history and animal exposure is extremely important. Occupational exposure to cattle, horses, poultry, sheep, swine, or reptiles and even exposure to a household pet can be significant in determining a zoonotic origin. Dogs in particular are well known to have a 40 percent carriage rate for *Giardia lamblia* and a 30 percent carriage rate for the bacterial enteropathogens *Salmonella* sp. and *Yersinia* sp.[50]

Zoonotic gastroenteritis often presents with fever, headache, and abdominal pain often localizing to the right lower quadrant. Patients may have diarrhea or constipation. Laboratory findings may consist of electrolyte and acid-base abnormalities if diarrhea is severe. Leukocytosis may be seen if an interstitial invasion has occurred, and eosinophilia is often a finding with intestinal parasitic infestation. Most cases of zoonotic gastroenteritis are self-limiting and require only fluid hydration. However, specific pathogens may require specific therapy (Table 145-6).

DERMATOLOGIC ZOONOTIC INFECTIONS

Dermatologic findings are common in zoonotic infections, as the dermis is often the site of inoculation and may display focal findings. The common dermatologic infections of impetigo, ecthyma, and cellulitis can be transmitted zoonotically, as can human infestations with mites and lice. The dermatophytoses *Tinea verrucosum* and *Microsporum canis* account for the majority of zoonotic dermatophyte

TABLE 145-6 Gastrointestinal Zoonotic Infections

Zoonoses	Animal Reservoir	Antibiotic Treatment
Brucellosis	Dogs and farm animals	Doxycycline or TMP-SMX
Campylobacter sp.	Dogs, cats, farm animals, poultry, and unpasteurized milk	Erythromycin or doxycycline
Giardia lamblia	Beavers, dogs, cats, and farm animals	Metronidazole, tinidazole, or quinacrine
Salmonella sp.	Reptiles (turtles), aquatic animals, dogs, cats, and humans (*S. typhi*)	TMP-SMX or ciprofloxacin
Tularemia	Rabbits, cats, and wild animals	Streptomycin, gentamicin, or doxycycline
Yersinia sp.	Dogs and cats	Gentamicin, chloramphenicol, TMP-SMX, doxycycline, or ciprofloxacin
Vibrio cholerae	Shellfish	Doxycycline, ciprofloxacin, or TMP-SMX (strain 0139 resistant to TMP-SMX)

Abbreviation: TMP-SMX, trimethoprim-sulfamethoxazole.

TABLE 145-7 Specific Zoonotic Dermatologic Findings

Zoonoses	Characteristic Rash
Aeromonas sp.	Crepitant cellulitis with systemic toxicity
Lyme disease	Erythema migrans at the focus of the tick bite
Rocky Mountain spotted fever	Maculopapular rash on soles and palms, centripetal spread, and advance characteristic of petechial hemorrhage and necrosis
Viral hemorrhagic fever	Petechial and purpuric rash

infections, with *M. canis* accounting for 15 percent of all human dermatophytoses.[51] Chancriform lesions (ulcerations at the site of inoculation) can result from zoonotic infection of bacterial, mycobacterial, fungal, or viral etiology. The most significant bacterial chancriform zoonotic lesions are *Bacillus anthracis* (anthrax), *Bartonella henselae* (cat-scratch disease), *Erysipelothrix rhusiopathiae* (erysipeloid), *Francisella tularensis* (tularemia), *Listeria monocytogenes* (listeriosis), *Mycobacterium marinum,* and *Pseudomonas mallei* (glanders).[5,30,52] The vast majority of these chancriform zoonotic infections occur in livestock workers, cattle ranchers, veterinarians, stable workers, horse trainers, slaughterhouse workers, poultry workers, and farmers. Significant zoonotic fungal chancriform infection is principally from *Blastomyces dermatitidis* (cutaneous blastomycosis) and *Sporothrix schenckii* (sporotrichosis). Dog and cat owners, along with veterinarians, are most at risk of contracting these two fungal zoonoses.[51] All of the chancriform zoonotic infections most commonly appear at the site of inoculation, often the hands or forearms.

Zoonotic dermatoses of viral etiology include *Vaccinia* sp. (cowpox), *Paravaccinia* sp. (pseudo-cowpox), and bovine papular stomatitis. These cutaneous viral zoonoses often occur on the hands and forearms of patients who work closely with cattle, sheep, goats, or horses.

Systemic zoonoses are also accompanied by dermatologic findings, usually a generalized maculopapular rash, which is common in bartonellosis, lymphocytic choriomeningitis, Colorado tick fever, leptospirosis, psittacosis, and rickettsial infections. However, the maculopapular rash associated with most zoonotic infections is nonspecific and does not facilitate the diagnosis. Those zoonotic infections with specific dermatologic findings aiding in the diagnosis are infections from *Aeromonas* sp., Lyme disease, RMSF *Vibrio* sp., and viral hemorrhagic fevers (Table 145-7).[5,11]

ZOONOSES ACQUIRED FROM HOUSEHOLD PETS

It is estimated that there are more than 110 million dogs and cats, with 70 percent of all households in the United States having these pets. Additionally, up to 20 percent of all households have a pet bird, and more than 20 million homes have an aquarium.[53] There are more than 30 significant human diseases acquired from household pets.[30] Dogs and cats are the two most common household pets in North America and account for the majority of these zoonotic infections. Small rodents, pet birds, reptiles, and aquarium fish account for only a fraction of the zoonotic infections in the United States (Table 145-8).[53] Interestingly, though pet owners often have close contact with their pets, pet-acquired zoonoses are infrequent and not often recognized. Yet these infections have a very diverse etiology and encompass parasitic, bacterial, rickettsial, and fungal infections.

Parasitic infections are very common among household pets, predominantly dogs and cats. Up to 50 percent of dogs are infected with at least one intestinal parasite, and 15 percent of adult dogs actively excrete *Toxocara canis,* the source of toxocariasis, visceral larva migrans.[52] Despite its prevalence in dogs, human toxocariasis is infrequently diagnosed probably because infection is often subclinical. Typically, the only indication of infection is eosinophilia. Children may display fever, cough, and nonspecific rash, as well as an inability to gain weight. Rarely, pulmonary infiltrates, hepatosplenomegaly, and seizures may occur. Diagnosis is by either biopsy of infected tissue or by ELISA. Treatment in the symptomatic patient consists of oral diethylcarbamazine (2 mg/kg tid for 10 days) or albedazole (400 mg bid for 5 days). Corticosteroids can be used to control the allergic component.

Other intestinal parasites that may be transmitted to humans from household pets include *Ancylostoma caninum* (cutaneous larva migrans), *Echinococcus granulosus* (echinococcosis), and *Dipylidium caninum* (dipylidiasis or dog and cat tapeworm).[52] Cutaneous larva migrans is often a self-limiting, pruritic, erythematous serpiginous rash caused as the larva migrates through the skin and is often acquired from fecal-contaminated soil. Topical thiabendazole is effective therapy in shortening the disease course.[34,52] Though dogs and other carnivores are the definitive hosts for *E. granulosus,* echinococcosis is most common in areas of cattle and sheep ranching. This zoonosis involves multiple organ systems: liver, lung, muscle, bone, kidney, and brain. Typically, there is a unilocular cyst containing multiple larvae that enlarge over time. Diagnosis and treatment usually occur at the time of surgical resection. Aspiration of the cyst is contraindicated, because leakage of the cystic fluid can spread the infection and cause an anaphylactic reaction.[52] Dipylidiasis, a tapeworm common to both dogs and cats, is found worldwide. Human infection is rare; when infection does occur, however, it is often in children and presents with the nonspecific symptoms of diarrhea and pruritus ani. Occasionally, the cucumber-shaped proglottides are seen moving in the child's stool. Treatment is with oral niclosamide. Infection with *Dirofilaria immitis* (dog heartworm) is extremely rare in humans.[52]

Cats are the host of the intracellular protozoan *Toxoplasma gondii,* which causes toxoplasmosis. Human toxoplasmosis can occur in three ways: by ingestion of uncooked or raw meat, especially pork or mutton containing the *Toxoplasma* cysts; by ingestion of the oocysts from cat and wild-animal feces; and transplacentally.[30,34,52] Transplacental transmission can result in congenital abnormalities of retinochoroiditis, hydrocephalus, hepatosplenomegaly, and thrombocytopenia in 10 percent of the children infected. The majority of children transplacentally infected with toxoplasmosis display no significant abnormalities. Nevertheless, pregnant women should limit their contact to only indoor cats and avoid contact with cat feces. The encysted trophozoite can become reactivated in a previously infected host if the host becomes immunocompromised.[54]

Bacterial zoonoses from household pets include, but are not limited to, brucellosis, leptospirosis, salmonellosis, and campylobacteriosis. Brucellosis (*Brucella canis*) is an uncommon infection in humans and is most often acquired from dogs. Pigs, cattle, and goats are less frequent transmitters. The typical human course for brucellosis is self-limited, with fever, headache, myalgias, and nonspecific laboratory findings. Tetracycline is the standard therapy in treating human brucellosis, with streptomycin added to tetracycline in the treatment of severe cases.[30,34] Leptospirosis (*Leptospira canicola*) infects almost all mammals, but dogs are the principal vector for humans. Humans become infected through exposure to body fluids, particularly urine, of an infected animal. The acute phase of leptospirosis is characterized by headache, malaise, myalgias, and fever. Nonspecific rash, meningitis, uveitis, myositis, and leptospiruria follow the acute phase. Doxycycline (100 mg PO bid for 10 to 14 days) and high dose penicillin (penicillin G 20 to 24 million units IV qd for 10 to 14 days) are the mainstays of treatment for leptospirosis.[34,52]

Campylobacteriosis (*Campylobacter jejuni*) is a major cause of infectious diarrhea in humans. This zoonotic infection also occurs in dogs, cats, pigs, poultry, cattle, and horses. Human infection from a pet is uncommon, but the presence of a puppy or kitten with a diarrheal

TABLE 145-8 Pet-Associated Zoonotic Infections

Dogs	Cats	Birds	Rodents	Fish and Reptiles
Anthrax	Anthrax	*Cryptococcus*	Leptospirosis	Erysipeloid
Brucellosis	Campylobacteriosis	Erysipeloid	Listeriosis	*Mycobacterium marinum*
Campylobacteriosis	Crytosporidiosis	Listeriosis	Lymphocytic choriomeningitis	Salmonellosis
Crytosporidiosis	Histoplasmosis	*Mycobacterium*	Murine typhus	Vibriosis
Dirofilariasis	Pasteurellosis	Ornithosis (*Chlamydia psittaci*)	Plague	
Echinococcosis	Plague	Salmonellosis	Rat-bite fever (*Streptobacillus moniliformis*)	
Histoplasmosis	Q fever	Tularemia	Salmonellosis	
Leptospirosis	Rabies	Viral encephalitis	Tularemia	
Pasteurellosis	Salmonellosis		Yersiniosis	
Rabies	Toxocariasis			
Rocky Mountain spotted fever	Tularemia			
Salmonellosis				
Toxocariasis				
Tularemia				
Yersiniosis				

illness in the house and human contacts experiencing diarrhea should raise the suspicion of pet-acquired campylobacteriosis. Though the disease is often self-limiting, treatment with erythromycin can facilitate resolution in protracted cases. Nontyphoidal salmonellosis is typically a self-limiting gastrointestinal illness prevalent among dogs. Human transmission is rare. Diarrhea in any pet should alert the pet owner to use increased personal hygiene and to dispose of the pet's feces properly.[30,34]

The ticks and fleas inhabiting dogs and cats can transmit the zoonotic infections of tularemia, plague, and Rocky Mountain spotted fever. Tularemia (*Francisella tularensis*) is a zoonotic infection occurring in humans exposed to infected animals or the vectors of ticks or deer flies. Endemic in the wild-animal population of the southeastern and north-central United States, cats are the primary reservoir of tularemia in human infections. Transmission is often by cat bite, tick bite, or scratch. Dogs do not directly transmit tularemia but do serve as carriers of the ticks that can transmit this zoonosis. Tularemia presents in four different forms, depending on the site of infection. The ulceroglandular form is the most common, followed by oculoglandular tularemia, oropharyngeal tularemia, and pneumonic tularemia. The infrequent but most serious pneumonic form is most common among laboratory workers and animal handlers. This form has the highest mortality. Treatment is with either streptomycin or tetracycline.[30,34,52]

Plague (*Yersinia pestis*) is endemic in the rodent population of the southwestern United States. Dogs and cats can also be sources of this zoonosis. Transmission occurs when bitten by fleas inhabiting an infected rodent, dog, or cat or by eating infected rodents. Plague has three forms: bubonic or suppurative lymphadenopathy (the most common), the pneumonic form, and the septicemic form. Because of the aggressive nature of *Y. pestis,* treatment should not be delayed. Aggressive treatment with gentamicin or streptomycin should be initiated at the first indication of infection. Doxycycline or chloramphenicol are effective alternative antibiotics.[30,43,52]

Rocky Mountain spotted fever (*Rickettsia rickettsii*) is a tick-transmitted, systemic zoonosis, with the tick *Dermacentor* sp. as principal vector and reservoir. Animal reservoirs consist of rodents, rabbits and, infrequently, dogs. Children incur two-thirds of the documented infections of RMSF. With a characteristic rash, this systemic zoonosis often presents with fever and headache. Treatment is with tetracycline or chloramphenicol in young children and pregnant women.[26,32,54]

Zoonotic fungal infections are occasionally acquired by humans. The most common of these infections is a dermatophytosis from *Microsporum canis*. It is estimated that up to 30 percent of human dermatophytoses have a zoonotic origin.[52] Treatment is often with topical antifungals or griseofulvin.

ZOONOSES TRANSMITTED FROM ANIMAL BITES

Well recognized is that up to 1 percent of all emergency department visits are a result of an animal bite.[55] The vast majority of these bites (70 to 93 percent) are from dogs. Conversely, cats account for 3 to 15 percent of all animal bites but carry the highest risk of infection.[55,56] Infection acquired from either a dog bite or a cat bite is typically mixed flora. *Staphylococcus* and *Streptococcus* species predominate, followed by *Corynebacterium* species and *Pasteurella multocida*.[56] Cat bites are notorious for *P. multocida* infection, with 50 to 70 percent of healthy cats having *Pasteurella* isolates.[30,56] Anaerobes account for infection in 41 percent of all animal bites. Appropriate wound care with meticulous irrigation and wound exploration for joint, tendon, vascular, and nerve involvement is a prerequisite. Antibiotic coverage is warranted for wounds at high risk of infection and can typically consist of one of the following antibiotics: amoxicillin with clavulanate (500 mg/125 mg PO tid for 10 to 14 days), ampicillin with sulbactam (1.5 to 3.0 g/0.5 to 1.0 g IV or IM qid for 7 to 10 days), ticarcillin disodium (3 g IV every 3 to 6 h for 7 to 10 days), or piperacillin and tazobactam (3.375 g IV qid for 7 to 10 days). In addition to antibiotic

TABLE 145-9 Zoonotic Infections Among HIV-Positive Patients

Infection	Source	Clinic Findings	Antibiotic Treatment
Cat-scratch disease (*Bartonella henselae*)	Cats	Pyogenic granulomas, regional lymphadenopathy, and fever	Erythromycin or doxycycline
Bordetella (*Bordetella bronchiseptica*)	Dogs	Fever, pharyngitis, and cough	Erythromycin
Campylobacter (*Camplobacter* sp.)	Dogs and cats	Gastroenteritis and diarrhea	Erythromycin, ciprofloxacin, or azithromycin
Cryptococcus (*Cryptococcus neoformans*)	Bird droppings, and cats	Flulike symptoms early, photophobia, headache, cranial nerve symptoms, and meningeal irritation later	Amphotericin B, fluconazole
Cryptosporidium	Dogs	Diarrhea and self-limiting	No effective antimicrobial
Giardia (*Giardia lamblia*)	Dogs and cats	Gastroenteritis and diarrhea	Metronidazole, tinidazole, or quinacrine
Listeria (*Listeria monocytogenes*)	Livestock, and dairy products	Sepsis and meningitis	Ampicillin; penicillin *plus* gentamicin; or TMP-SMX, or vancomycin
Mycobacterium			
M. avium	Pet birds	Pneumonia and gastroenteritis	Azithromycin or clarithromycin
M. marinum	Fish	Cutaneous granulomas and skin ulcerations at distal extremities	Rifampin and ethambutol (some strains susceptible to TMP-SMX and doxycycline)
Rhodococcus (*Rhodococcus equi*)	Farm animals	Pneumonia and cavitating lung lesions	Vancomycin, erythromycin, or imipenem *plus* rifampin
Salmonella (*Salmonella* sp.)	Dogs, cats, reptiles, and farm animals	Gastroenteritis, diarrhea, and sepsis	Ciprofloxacin or norfloxacin
Toxoplasmosis (*Toxoplasma gondii*)	Cats	Pneumonia, brain abscesses, encephalitis, and ocular disease	Pyrimethamine *plus* sulfadiazine

Abbreviation: TMP-SMX, trimethoprim-sulfamethoxazole.

coverage, the current tetanus status should be addressed for every animal bite victim.[30,56]

Rabies deserves special consideration in reference to animal bites. Though rabies is relatively rare among pet dogs and cats, it is increasing in incidence among wild animals. In the United States, seven species account for 97 percent of laboratory-confirmed rabies. In decreasing frequency, these species are skunks (62 percent), bats (12 percent), raccoons (7 percent), cattle (6 percent), cats (4 percent), dogs (3 percent), and foxes (3 percent).[56] Any unprovoked bite, regardless if the animal is a stray or pet, or a bite sustained from a dog or cat without documented rabies immunization, is cause for alarm. Until there is documented proof that the animal is free of rabies, the animal in question is assumed to have rabies.

Of special note is that a history of animal vaccination does not exclude the possibility that rabies has been acquired by the biting animal.[52] The rabies status of an animal can be determined either by quarantining the animal for 10 days and observing it for behavioral changes or by postmortem examination of brain tissue. If it cannot be determined that the animal is free of rabies, then the bite victim should undergo rabies prophylaxis, which consists of human diploid cell vaccine and rabies immune globulin.[52]

ZOONOTIC INFECTIONS AND IMMUNOCOMPROMISED PATIENTS

Immunocompromised patients deserve special consideration and encompass a very large group: patients with congenital immunodeficiencies, diabetes mellitus, chronic renal failure, or liver failure; splenectomized patients; chronic alcoholics; cancer patients; and HIV-positive patients. Of all of these patients, those undergoing chemotherapy and those with AIDS have the greatest risk of acquiring a zoonotic infection.[7] It is estimated that 30 to 40 percent of immunocompromised patients may own pets.[57] *Salmonella* and *Campylobacter* are the two most common infections acquired by immunocompromised patients from their pets,[7] but the overall risk of transmission of *Salmonella* and *Campylobacter* from contact with pets is low. Additionally, *Mycobacterium marinum,* from aquatic pets, and *Bartonella,* from cats, are also commonly acquired by immunocompromised patients. Other acquired zoonotic infections that immunocompromised patients are susceptible to include *Toxoplasma gondii, Cryptosporidium, Giardia, Rhodococcus equi, Bartonella, Mycobacterium marinum,* and *Bordetella bronchiseptica* (Table 145-9). With the exception of *Bartonella* (cat-scratch disease), most of these zoonotic infections are acquired by immunocompromised patients from sources other than exposure to animals.[54] These sources are principally from contaminated food or water. Nevertheless, it is important for emergency physicians to inquire about animal exposure and zoonotic risk factors when evaluating immunocompromised patients. Consultation with an infectious disease specialist and a veterinarian may be warranted in evaluating immunocompromised patients in the emergency department.

ACKNOWLEDGMENT

The author wishes to acknowledge Robert B. Grose and his contribution to the multiple tables in this chapter.

REFERENCES

1. World Health Organization (WHO): *Zoonoses Technical Report Series, 1959.* Geneva, WHO, 1959.
2. Hart CA, Trees AJ, Duerden BI: Zoonoses: Proceedings of the third Liverpool Tropical School Bayer symposium on microbial diseases held on 3 February 1996 [Review Article]. *J Med Microbiol* 46:4, 1997.
3. Veterinary Public Health Unit, Division of Communicable Diseases, World Health Organization: Zoonoses in the world: Current and future trends. *Schweiz Med Wochenschr* 125:875, 1995.
4. Institute of Medicine: *Emerging Infections: Microbial Threats to Health in the United States.* Washington, DC, National Academy Press, 1992.
5. Simpson GL: Vector borne and animal associated infections, in Brillman CJ, Quenzer RW (eds): *Infectious Diseases in Emergency Medicine,* 2d ed. Philadelphia, Lippincott-Raven, 1998:209–229.
6. Weinberg AN, Weber DJ: Animal associated human infections. *Infect Dis Clin North Am* 5:xi, 1991.
7. Angulo FJ, Glaser CA, Juranek DD, et al: Caring for pets of immunocompromised persons. *J Am Vet Med Assoc* 205:1711, 1994.
8. Walker DH, Barbour AG, Oliver JH, et al: Emerging bacterial zoonotic and vector-borne diseases: Ecological and epidemiological factors. *JAMA* 275:463, 1996.
9. Centers for Disease Control: Lyme disease: United States, 1987 and 1988. *MMWR* 38:668, 1989.
10. Doan-Wiggins L: Tick-borne diseases. *Emerg Med Clin North Am* 9:303, 1991.
11. Spach DH, Liles WC, Campbell GL, et al: Tick-borne diseases in the United States. *N Engl J Med* 329:936, 1993.
12. Centers for Disease Control: Rocky Mountain spotted fever: United States, 1990. *MMWR* 40:451, 1991.
13. Kirkland KK, Sexton DJ: Therapeutic delay in Rocky Mountain spotted fever. *Clin Infect Dis* 12:1118, 1995.
14. Woodward TE: Rocky Mountain spotted fever: Epidemiological and early clinical signs are keys to treatment and reduced mortality. *J Infect Dis* 150:465, 1984.
15. Walker DH: Rocky Mountain spotted fever: A seasonal alert. *Clin Infect Dis* 12:1111, 1995.
16. Steere AC et al: Vaccination against Lyme disease with recombinant *Borrelia burgdorferi* outer-surface lipoprotein A with adjuvant. *N Engl J Med* 339:209, 1998.
17. Wright SW, Trott AT: North America tick-borne diseases. *Ann Emerg Med* 17:964, 1988.
18. Steere AC: Lyme disease. *N Engl J Med* 321:586, 1989.
19. Shadick NA, Phillips CB, Logigian EL, et al: The long term clinical outcomes of Lyme disease: A population-based retrospective cohort study. *Ann Intern Med* 121:560, 1994.
20. Fihn S, Larson EB: Tick-borne relapsing fever in the Pacific Northwest: An underdiagnosed illness? *West J Med* 133:203, 1980.
21. Horton JM, Blaser MJ: The spectrum of relapsing fever in the Rocky Mountains. *Arch Intern Med* 145:871, 1985.
22. Butler TC: Relapsing fever, in Gorbach SL, Bartlett JG, Blacklow NR (eds): *Infectious Diseases.* Philadelphia, WB Saunders, 1992, pp 1302–1304.
23. Emmons RW: An overview of Colorado tick fever. *Prog Clin Biol Res* 178:47, 1985.
24. McCoy GW, Chapin CW: Further observation of a plague-like disease of rodents with a preliminary note on the causative bacteria. *J Infect Dis* 10:61, 1912.
25. Evans ME, Gregory DW, Schaffner W, McGee ZA: Tularemia: A 30-year experience with 88 cases. *Medicine (Baltimore)* 64:251, 1985.
26. Boustani MR, Gelfand JA: Babeiosis. *Clin Infect Dis* 22:611, 1996.
27. Bakken JS, Krueth J, Wilson-Nordskog C, et al: Human granulocytic ehrlichiosis (HGE): Clinical and laboratory characteristics of 41 patients from Minnesota and Wisconsin. *JAMA* 275:199, 1995.
28. Dawson JE: Human ehrlichiosis in the United States, in Reminton JS, Swartz MN (eds): *Current Clinical Topics in Infectious Diseases.* Cambridge, MA, Blackwell Science, 1996, pp 164–171.
29. Whitley RJ, Cobbs CG, Alford CA, et al: Diseases that mimic herpes simplex encephalitis: Diagnosis, presentation, and outcome. *JAMA* 262:234, 1989.
30. Tan JS: Human zoonotic infections transmitted by dogs and cats. *Arch Intern Med* 157:1933, 1997.
31. Johnson RT, Mims CA: Pathogenesis of viral infections of the nervous system. *N Engl J Med* 278:23, 1968.
32. Kennard C, Swash M: Acute viral encephalitis: Its diagnosis and outcome. *Brain* 104:129, 1981.
33. Rennels MB: Arthropod-borne virus infections of the central nervous system. *Neurol Clin* 2:241, 1984.
34. Goldstein EJC: Household pets and human infections. *Infect Dis Clin North Am* 5:1177, 1991.
35. Weinberg AN: Respiratory infections transmitted from animals. *Infect Dis Clin North Am* 5:649, 1991.
36. Brachman PS: Inhalation anthrax. *Ann NY Acad Sci* 353:83, 1980.
37. Greer AE: Pulmonary brucellosis. *Dis Chest* 29:508, 1956.
38. Fox MD, Kaufman AF: Centers for Disease Control: Brucellosis in the United States, 1965–1974. *J Infect Dis* 136:312, 1977.
39. Centers for Disease Control: Compendium of measures to control *Chlamydia psittaci* infection among humans (psittacosis) and pet birds (avian chlamydiosis), 1998. *MMWR* 47:1, 1998.
40. Grayston JT, Thom DH: The chlamydial pneumonias. *Curr Clin Top Infect Dis* 11:1, 1991.
41. Sawyer LA, Fishbein DB, McDade JE: Q fever: Current concepts. *Rev Infect Dis* 9:935, 1987.
42. Weber DT, Wolfson JS, Swartz MN, et al: *Pasteurella multocida* infections: Report of 34 cases and review of the literature. *Medicine (Baltimore)* 63:133, 1984.
43. Byrd RP, Vasquez J, Roy TM: Respiratory manifestations of tick-borne diseases in the southeastern United States. *South Med J* 90:1, 1997.
44. Perry RD, Fetherston JD: *Yersinia pestis:* Etiologic agent of plague. *Clin Microbiol Rev* 10:35, 1997.
45. Webster RG, Sharp GB, Claas EC: Interspecies transmission of influenza viruses. *Am J Respir Crit Care Med* 152:525, 1995.
46. Brown IH, Alexander DJ: Influenza, in Palmer SR, Soulsby L, Simpson DIH (eds): *Zoonosis: Biology, Clinical Practice and Public Health Control.* Oxford, Oxford University Press, 1998, pp 365–386.
47. Clement J, McKenna P, van der Groen G, et al: Hantavirus, in Palmer SR, Soulsby L, Simpson DIH (eds): *Zoonosis: Biology, Clinical Practice and Public Health Control.* Oxford, Oxford University Press, 1998, pp 331–352.
48. Centers for Disease Control: Hantavirus pulmonary syndrome: Colorado and New Mexico, 1998. *MMWR* 47:249, 1998.
49. Duchin JS, Koster FT, Peters CJ, et al: Hantavirus pulmonary syndrome: Clinical description of seventeen patients with a newly recognized disease. *N Engl J Med* 330:949, 1994.
50. Bauer D: The capacity of dogs to serve as reservoirs for gastrointestinal disease in children. *Ir Med J* 87:184, 1994.
51. Scott DW, Horn RT Jr: Zoonotic dermatoses of dogs and cats. *Vet Clin North Am* 17:117, 1987.
52. Elliot DL, Tolle SW, Goldberg L, Miller JB: Pet-associated illness. *N Engl J Med* 16:985, 1985.
53. Chomel BB: Zoonoses of house pets other than dogs, cats, and birds. *Pediatr Infect Dis J* 11:479, 1992.
54. Glaser CA, Angulo J, Rooney JA: Animal-associated opportunistic infections among persons infected with the human immunodeficiency virus. *Clin Infect Dis* 18:14, 1994.
55. Douglas LG: Bite wounds. *Am Fam Physician* 11:93, 1975.
56. Weber DJ, Hansen AR: Infections resulting from animal bites. *Infect Dis Clin North Am* 5:663, 1991.
57. Wise JK, Yang JJ: Veterinary services market for companion animals, 1992: 1. Companion animal ownership and demographics. *J Am Vet Med Assoc* 201:990, 1992.

SOFT TISSUE INFECTIONS

Steven G. Folstad

GAS GANGRENE

Gas gangrene or clostridial myonecrosis is a rapidly progressive and serious life- and limb-threatening soft tissue infection caused by one of the spore-forming clostridial species of organism. Severe myonecrosis with gas production and sepsis are the hallmarks of this disease, and early diagnosis and aggressive management are needed to prevent the high risk of mortality associated with this infection.

Epidemiology

Clostridium species are ubiquitous organisms found throughout our environment. It is estimated that a full 30 percent of traumatic injuries are contaminated with one or more of the *Clostridium* species. There is approximately 1000 cases of gas gangrene reported to the Centers for Disease Control and Prevention (CDC) each year in the United States.[1] The incidence of disease secondary to these organisms is decreasing, presumably due to better wound management and more effective antibiotic therapy. For example, the incidence of gas gangrene in battle-related injuries was 5 percent during World War I; this dropped to 0.2 percent during the Korean war and to 0.01 percent during the war in Vietnam.

Pathophysiology

There have been seven *Clostridium* species identified as causing gas gangrene. *Clostridium perfringens* is attributed to 80 to 95 percent of cases, with *C. septicum* being the second most common etiology.[2] The clostridial organisms are large, gram-positive, spore-forming anaerobic bacilli normally found in the soil, gastrointestinal tract, and female genitourinary tract. They produce several exotoxins that are responsible for the cellular destruction as well as the rapid progression and systemic toxicity of the disease. Bacteremia is rare. Secondary toxic effects may be caused by the release of myoglobin, creatine phosphokinase (CPK), and potassium from tissue breakdown.

There are two potential mechanisms for infection with clostridial organisms. The first and most common is through direct inoculation from an open wound. Similar to tetanus, clostridial species thrive best in contaminated wounds with crushed or ischemic edges that tend to offer a favorable anaerobic environment. The second mechanism for infection is via hematogenous spread. Nearly all these patients are relatively immunocompromised from some form of underlying disease such as diabetes mellitus, peripheral vascular disease, alcoholism, drug abuse, or hematologic or gastrointestinal malignancies. Almost a third of these cases of "spontaneous gas gangrene" are caused by *C. septicum*, with an even higher incidence in cases related to malignancies.

Clinical Features

The incubation period is short, usually less than 3 days. The most common presenting complaints in early gas gangrene are pain out of proportion to physical findings, as well as a sensation of "heaviness" of the affected part. On examination, the area may demonstrate a brawny edema with crepitance. The skin will develop a bronze or brownish discoloration with a malodorous serosanguineous discharge, and bullae may be present. Systemic manifestations include a low-grade fever with tachycardia out of proportion to the fever. The patient may be confused or irritable and have a rapid deterioration of the sensorium. Laboratory evaluation may reveal any or all of the following: metabolic acidosis, leukocytosis, anemia, thrombocytopenia, coagulopathy, myoglobinemia and myoglobinuria, and liver or kidney disfunction. Gram stain of the bullae often shows pleomorphic gram-positive bacilli with or without spores, red blood cells, but very few white blood cells. Radiologic studies may demonstrate gas within soft tissue fascial planes and possibly gas within the peritoneal or retroperitoneal space.

Diagnosis

Early diagnosis and treatment are essential in this life-threatening disorder. Familiarity with the disease and its clinical features is important to avoid overlooking the subtle early signs of its presentation. Any patient presenting with pain out of proportion to physical findings, with or without low-grade fever, and significant tachycardia, with or without a cutaneous injury, should be carefully evaluated for possible clostridial infection. Crepitus detectable on physical examination may be a later finding, and its absence does not rule out the diagnosis. Plain radiographs of the affected area may reveal gas within the involved muscle and surrounding soft tissue. A Gram stain of exudate or tissue showing gram-positive rods with a relative lack of leukocytes is considered diagnostic. Surgical exploration is also helpful in the diagnosis. In the early stages, the muscles are edematous and pale but still bleed when cut; in later stages, the muscles lose contractility and on dissection appear beefy red without bleeding and gas bubbles may be evident between the tissues.

The differential diagnosis of clostridial myonecrosis must encompass other gas-forming infections, including necrotizing fasciitis, streptococcal myositis, acute streptococcal hemolytic gangrene, crepitant cellulitis, and synergistic necrotizing cellulitis. The crepitance should be differentiated from other causes of subcutaneous emphysema such as pneumothorax, pneumomediastinum, and fractured larynx or trachea. The edema and pallor, with loss of distal pulses, seen in an affected extremity should be differentiated from vascular thrombosis conditions such as phlegmasia cerulea dolens.

Treatment

Treatment consists of four main phases:

1. *Resuscitation* should begin in the emergency department (ED) immediately on making a presumptive diagnosis. Aggressive fluid resuscitation using crystalloid, plasma, and packed cells is usually needed to replace red blood cells lost due to hemolysis and to correct hypotension due to shock. Volume status should be closely monitored using urine output and central venous pressure readings. Avoid the use of vasoconstrictors when possible due to the possibility of decreasing perfusion to already ischemic muscle.
2. *Antibiotic therapy* using penicillin G 10 to 40 million units per day in divided doses is recommended. Clindamycin, metronidazole, and chloramphenicol are alternative choices for the penicillin-allergic patient. Sodium penicillin is recommended over potassium penicillin to reduce the risk of worsening hyperkalemia in patients with hemolysis and tissue necrosis. Mixed infections with other anaerobes, gram-negative rods, and staphylococci are common. Therefore, multiple-antibiotic therapy using aminoglycosides, penicillinase-resistant penicillins, or vancomycin is recommended. Tetanus prophylaxis should be given as indicated.
3. *Surgical debridement* is a mainstay of therapy and may include fasciotomy, debridement, or amputation. The borders for debridement are guided by the appearance of the muscle.
4. *Hyperbaric oxygen (HBO) therapy* has been a widely used therapeutic modality since the early 1960s. Although there are no prospective human studies, retospective data suggest a twofold reduction in mortality in patients receiving concomitant HBO therapy.[3] The timing of its use in relation to surgical debridement remains somewhat controversial. Standard therapy consists of surgical debridement prior to HBO therapy, partly for confirmation of the diagnosis based on muscle appearance. Some argue that since elevated partial pressures of oxygen are bactericidal in tissues, as well as inhibitory to toxin production, preoperative HBO therapy may allow for sharper demarcation of necrotic tissue at debridement and less loss of tissue to amputation and decreased systemic toxicity. Typical HBO therapy at this time consists of 100% oxygen at 3 atm of pressure for 90 min immediately following surgery, with three dives in the first 24 h followed by two dives a day for 4 or 5 days.

Wound care at the time of initial evaluation and treatment is the most important factor in preventing clostridial infections. Debridement of crushed or dead tissue and copious irrigation prior to wound closure will help prevent the development of an environment favorable to clostridial growth. Prophylactic penicillin administration may be beneficial in preventing subsequent infection.

CELLULITIS

Cellulitis is a local soft tissue inflammatory reaction secondary to bacterial invasion of the skin. The classic symptoms of cellulitis have been attributed previously to bacterial invasion and subsequent proliferation within the local tissues; however, new evidence suggests that the majority of symptoms may instead be secondary to a complex set of immune and inflammatory reactions triggered by cells within the skin itself.[4]

Epidemiology

The term *cellulitis* represents a broad spectrum of disease in both location and severity. Unfortunatelly, general data on prevalence and incidence of disease are difficult to obtain and interpret. Cellulitis is a common disease in all EDs, affecting the elderly, the immunocompromised, and those with peripheral vascular disease at a much higher rate and severity.

Pathophysiology

Cellulitis is a local inflammation of the skin characterized by pain, induration, warmth, and erythema. It is caused by invasion of the tissues with bacteria, most commonly staphylococci or streptococci in adults and *Hemophilus influenzae* in children. In diabetic patients, additional consideration needs to be given to Enterobacteriaceae and rarely clostridia. Lymphangitis and lymphadenopathy are seen occasionally in previously healthy patients, but purely local inflammation is much more common. Systemic involvement with fever, leukocytosis, and bacteremia is seen most typically in patients with underlying immunosuppressive diseases. Traditional thought has been that the symptoms of cellulitis are related to the effects of the bacteria and their proliferation on local tissues. This has been poorly substantiated in that efforts at isolating these organisms from infected tissue have had a very poor yield. Needle aspiration of the leading edge of an area of cellulitis produces organisms in less that 10 percent of cultures, and even punch biopsy from the same area yields organisms in only around 20 percent of cultures. Only areas with suppuration or abscess formation have significantly higher yield. Recent studies now suggest that although bacterial invasion is what triggers the inflammation, the organisms are largely cleared from the site within the first 12 h, and the infiltration of lymphoid and reticular cells and their products is what produces the majority of symptoms.[4] Cells such as Langerhans cells and keratinocytes release the cytokines interleukin-1 and tumor necrosis factor that enhance infiltration of the skin by circulating lymphocytes and macrophages. The net effect of this is much more rapid clearing of bacteria but at the price of a significantly larger inflammatory response. Theoretically, the addition of anti-inflammatory agents to the treatment regime of cellulitis would be beneficial. Further study needs to be done to identify what specific role, if any, such agents should play.

Clinical Features

Patients with cellulitis typically present with localized tenderness, warmth, induration, and erythema. Specific note should be made on physical examination of evidence of lymphangitis or lymphadenitis because this may suggest more serious infection. The presence of high fever and chills suggests bacteremia, especially in patients with underlying medical disorders.

Diagnosis

In otherwise heathy patients, the clinical presentation is sufficient for diagnosing cellulitis. The high likelihood of typical organisms and the low yield of isolation techniques make further efforts unwarranted. In patients with underlying disease or signs of bacteremia, blood cultures and leukocyte counts are indicated. Local means of isolating the organism are controversial, but in the case of a toxic-appearing patient, they may be worthwhile. Differentiating deep venous thrombosis from cellulitis in the lower extremities is often difficult and may require Doppler studies or venogram.

Treatment

Simple cellulitis in otherwise healthy adult patients can be treated as on an outpatient basis with dicloxacillin (500 mg PO q6h), a macrolide (EES 500 mg PO q6h, azithromycin 500 mg PO initial dose then 250 mg PO qd × 4 d, clarithromycin 500 mg PO q12h), or amoxicillin-clavulanate (875/125 mg PO q12h), with all treatments lasting for 10 days except for azithromycin. The exception to this is cellulitis involving the head or neck, for which most patients should be admitted for intravenous antibiotics. Appropriate intravenous antibiotics include parenteral first-generation cephalosporins (cefazolin 1 g IV q6h) and penicillinase-resistant penicillins (nafcillin or oxacillin 2 g IV q4h). In diabetics, a perenteral second- or third-generation cephalosporin (ceftriaxone 1-2 g IV qd) should be used or imipenem (500 mg IV q6h) in severe cases.[5]

Disposition

Patients with evidence of bacteremia and those with underlying diseases such as diabetes mellitus, alcoholism, or other immunosuppressive disorders should be admitted for intravenous antibiotics. Empirical therapy may be started with the antibiotics listed earlier and changed as indicated by culture results.

All patients discharged on oral antibiotics should have close follow-up arranged with their local medical doctor to evaluate the success of treatment. Anti-inflammatory agents for the treatment of cellulitis are experimental at this time, and until further research identifies a specific role, they should be used with caution.

ERYSIPELAS

Epidemiology

There has been a dramatic increase in the incidence in erysipelas over the past 20 years, as well as a change in the locations that are infected most commonly. Previously, erysipelas involved the face more frequently, but now it is primarily an infection of the lower extremities.[6]

Pathophysiology

Erysipelas is a superficial cellulitis with lymphatic involvement that is caused primarily by group A *Streptococcus*. Atypical infections most commonly seen with other groups of streptococci are also noted. Infection is typically achieved through a portal of entry in the skin, with traumatic wounds, ulcers, and infected dermatoses of the lower extremities being the most common sites. Peripheral vascular disease, especially venous insufficiency, is a local risk factor for infection. Most often erysipelas occurs proximal to the portal of entry into the skin.

Clinical Features

The onset of symptoms is usually abrupt, with a sudden onset of high fever, chills, malaise, and nausea. Over the next 1 to 2 days a small area of erythema with a burning sensation develops. As the infection continues, a red, shiny, hot plaque forms. The plaque has a tense, painful induration that is sharply demarcated from the surrounding normal tissue. Lymphangitis and local lymphadenopathy are common.

Purpura, bullae, and small areas of necrosis also are seen. Systemic symptoms continue until antibiotic therapy is initiated. On resolution of the infection, desquamation of the site typically occurs.

Diagnosis

The diagnosis is based primarily on physical findings. Leukocytosis with an increase in the neutrophil count is common. Performing a needle aspiration of the infection site is rarely successful at isolating an organism, but swabbing the portal of entry, when identifiable, may have a higher success rate. Blood cultures are positive in only around 5 percent of patients.[7] Serologic testing to determine ASO and anti-DNAase B titers may be more specific but is of little use acutely in the ED.

The differential diagnosis includes other forms of local cellulitis. Some believe that necrotizing fasciitis is a complication of erysipelas infections and should be considered in all cases.

Treatment

Penicillin G (1–2 million units IV q6h) may be used in nondiabetic patients for initial treatment due to the high incidence of streptococcal infection. Penicillinase-resistant penicillins (nafcillin or oxacillin 2 g IV q4h), parenteral second- or third-generation cephalosporins (ceftriaxone 1–2 g IV qd), or amoxicillin-clavulanate (875/125 mg PO q12h) should be used in diabetic patients and those with facial disease. Imipenem (500 mg IV q6h) is recommended in severe cases. Erythromycin, cephalosporins, or a macrolide should be used in patients with penicillin allergy. Essentially all patients with erysipelas should be admitted to the hospital for intravenous antibiotics.

CUTANEOUS ABSCESSES

The development of cutaneous abscesses most often is caused by a breakdown in the skin's normal protective barrier followed by contamination with local resident bacterial flora. In most cases involving otherwise immunocompetent patients, appropriate surgical incision and drainage are the only treatment required.

Epidemiology

Cutaneous abscesses are a common ED presentation, representing 1 to 2 percent of presenting complaints. There has been little recent investigation into the bacteriology or recommended treatment of simple cutaneous abscesses. This is probably secondary to the excellent outcome with simple incision and drainage regardless of the location or etiology.

Pathophysiology

Intact, healthy skin usually acts as an excellent barrier to bacterial invasion. Cutaneous factors such as constant desquamation of the epidermis continually shedding bacteria and the lower pH of 3 to 5 of the skin also contribute to the skin's protective function. Host cellular and humeral defenses further protect invading bacteria from developing subsequent infection. When favorable host factors are lacking, or in cases of overwhelming bacterial contamination, a break in the skin's integrity either superficially (abrasion, laceration, or thermal injury) or from deep inoculation (laceration, puncture, or bite) may lead to colonization and subsequent infection. Infection typically starts as a local superficial cellulitis. Many organisms that colonize normal skin can cause necrosis and liquefaction with subsequent accumulation of leukocytes and cellular debris. Loculation and subsequent walling off of these products of infection lead to abscess formation. As the infection progresses and the area of liquefaction increases, the abscess wall thins and ruptures spontaneously, draining either cutaneously or into an adjoining tissue compartment.

The bacterial etiology of soft tissue absceses often can be predicted by knowledge of the normal flora colonizing specific areas of the body. Environmental factors such as temperature, humidity, and the general hygiene of a patient play a role in the likelihood of infection, but only by increasing the number of bacteria colonizing the skin. In abscesses involving the scalp, trunk, and extremities, staphylococcal species are the most common infecting organism. *Staphylococcus aureus,* the least common of the staphylococcal species isolated on normal skin, is the most common species causing infection. *S. epidermis* and *S. hominis* are also seen frequently. Streptococci commonly colonize the oral and nasal mucosa and can be seen in abscesses involving the adjoining soft tissues. The intertriginous and perineal areas often are colonized by the gram-negative aerobes *Escherichia coli, Proteus mirabilis,* and *Klebsiella* species. Abscesses involving the axilla are most often infected with *P. mirabilis* for reasons that are not clear. Abscesses in the perirectal and genital areas are most commonly mixed anaerobic and aerobic in nature, with *Bacteroides* species being the most common anaerobe.

In abscesses secondary to foreign bodies, *S. aureus* is the most commonly isolated species. Bite injuries, especially by cats, are at risk for infection with *Pasteurella* multocida but also can involve *S. aureus*, as well as *Streptococcus viridans* and *Eikenella corrodens.* Human bites are less likely to involve *P. multocida* but have a high incidence of involvement with the anaerobe *Bacteroides fragilis* and the gram-positive *Corynebacterium jeikeium,* as well as the usual staphylococcal and streptococcal organisms. In infections associated with intravenous drug abuse, ''mixed'' infections prevail, with anaerobic bacteria predominating.[8] The most common anaerobic organism is the *Peptostreptococcus* species, with *Staphylococcus* and *Streptococcus* species being the predominating aerobic organisms. Interestingly, a significantly higher percentage of anaerobic infections have been noted in patients injecting cocaine. This has been attributed to the relative anaerobic enviroment created by the vasoconstrictive effect of the cocaine.

Clinical Features

Patients present with an area of swelling, tenderness, and erythema. Inspection of the area may reveal fluctuance, induration, or active drainage. Lymphadenitis, localized lymphadenopathy, or fever may indicate systemic involvement of the infection, but in otherwise healthy patients, cutaneous abscesses tend to remain localized. A careful history should be obtained, with special attention given to underlying immunocompromising illnesses, steroid or other immunosuppressive drug use, and alcoholism. Close inspection of the area for evidence of predisposing injury or foreign body is important. Radiography may be indicated to evaluate for certain radiopaque foreign bodies, and ultrasound may be useful in identifying nonradiopaque objects. Ultrasound can accurately identify many small foreign objects or at least a small fluid collection representing surrounding abscess. The limiting factor in the use of ultrasound is that because of the superficial location of most of these objects, a very high frequency ultrasound transducer is required (7.5–10 MHz). Specific abscesses that may be encountered in the ED are discussed below.

BARTHOLIN GLAND ABSCESSES Bartholin gland abcesses are seen primarily in sexually active women. Another diagnosis should be considered in postmenopausal women. The Bartholin or vestibular glands are located at the 5 and 7 o'clock positions of the vaginal vestibule. The glands are secretory in nature, and obstruction of the ducts can cause retention of secretions leading to cyst and eventually abscess formation. The patient presents with a unilateral painful swelling of the labia and with a fluctuant 1- to 2-cm. mass at the location of Bartholin's gland. *Neisseria gonorrhoea* and *Chlamydia trachomatis* are often isolated in these abscesses, and cervical cultures are recommended in all patients with Bartholin's gland abscesses. Treatment is not recommended routinely, except in patients with a high clinical suspicion for sexually transmitted disease. Anaerobes, especially Bacteroides species, are also common, as are the gram-negative organisms typically colonizing the perineal region. Treatment involves incision and drainage along the vaginal mucosal surface. There is a very high incidence of reinfection if more definitive steps are not taken to form a permanent fistulous tract. This can be done by using a Word catheter, a small catheter with a balloon on the distal end used to hold the abscess cavity open during healing, or by marsupializing the abscess walls.

PARONYCHIA AND FELONS Paronychia and felons are discussed in Chap. 277, "Hand Infections."

HIDRADENITIS SUPPURATIVA Hidradenitis suppurativa is a recurrent, chronic infection involving the apocrine sweat glands. Blockage of these glands by keratinous material leads to inflammation, local cellulitis, and subsequent abscess formation. Multiple areas of infection develop in different apocrine glands and coalesce to form chronic draining fistulous tracts. These tracts tend to occur in the axilla and groin, where the apocrine sweat glands predominate. Hidradenitis suppurative is more common in women and blacks, and there appears to be a genetic factor involved in its development. Obesity, shaving, and poor hygiene also contribute. The causative organism is usually *Staphylococcus,* but *Streptococcus* also can be involved. In the groin, gram-negative organisms and anaerobes also may be seen. Patients often will present with multiple lesions in different stages of development and healing but with an acute exacerbation in one or a few areas. ED treatment is directed primarily at incision and drainage of the acute infection with referral to a surgeon for further definitive treatment. This often requires wide excision of the affected area. Oral antibiotics should be used in patients with significant areas of cellulitis.

INFECTED SEBACEOUS CYSTS Sebaceous glands occur diffusely throughout the body. Blockage of the duct of a sebaceous gland may lead to development of a glandular cyst that may exist for a long period of time without becoming infected. Once bacterial invasion occurs, abscess formation is common. These patients typically present with an erythematous, tender cutaneous nodule that is commonly fluctuant. Simple incision and drainage are the appropriate ED treatment. The cyst always contains a capsule that must be removed to prevent further infection. This is usually best done at a later follow-up visit when the initial inflamation has improved or resolved. Occasionally, the wall of the sac can be grasped with a forceps and removed at the time of drainage.

PERIRECTAL ABSCESSES Most, if not all, perirectal infections are felt to arise from mucinous glands located within the anal crypts. Blockage of the ducts to these glands leads to bacterial invasion, infection, and commonly, abscess formation. The location of the subsequent abscess depends on the direction in which the infection spreads. The most common area of infection is the perianal abscess that is located superficially below the anal ring. Ischiorectal abscesses, supralevator abscesses, and intersphincteric abscesses all are caused by spread of infection into deeper perirectal tissues. Perirectal abscesses are more common in middle-aged males with other risk factors, including inflamatory bowel disease, diabetes, and other immunocompromising illnesses. The bacterial etiology of these infections is primarily the normal fecal flora. Mixed anaerobic and aerobic infections predominate, with *B. fragilis* being the primary anaerobe. Perirectal abscesses can represent serious, life-threatening infections, and only the most superficial should be treated with local anesthesia and incision and drainage in the ED.

PILONIDAL ABSCESSES Pilonidal abscesses are located along the superior gluteal fold. It is thought that a pilonidal sinus forms along the gluteal fold possibly at the time of embryogenesis, although others believe it to be secondary to local soft tissue trauma. These sinuses are lined with squamous epithelium and hair. It is blockage of the sinus tract with hair and other keratinous material that leads to bacterial invasion and infection. The causative organisms typically are normal skin flora, with *Staphylococcus* species being the most common. Contamination with peritoneal and fecal organisms is also possible. Patients tend to develop symptoms in their late teens and early twenties, and without definitive surgical treatment, they tend to have recurrent infections, sometimes developing a chronic draining fistulous tract. Patients typically present to the ED with a tender, swollen, and fluctuant nodule located along the superior gluteal fold. Systemic symptoms are rare. The appropriate initial treatment includes incision and drainage using care to remove all excess hair and debris from the abscess cavity. The cavity should be packed with iodoform gauze, and the patient should return in 2 to 3 days for advancement of the packing. Antibiotics generally are not needed. Surgical referral is recommended for more definitive treatment.

STAPHYLOCOCCAL SOFT TISSUE ABSCESSES *Staphylococcus* species are ubiquitous throughout the skin and have a particular affinity for hair follicles, where infection is common. Inflammation of a hair follicle caused by bacterial invasion is known as *folliculitis* and is best treated noninvasively with warm soaks. A deeper invasion into the soft tissue surrounding a hair follicle can lead to a localized abscess formation called a *furuncle* (boil). These are most commonly found on the face, neck, back, axilla, and inner thigh. Unless severe, warm compresses usually are adequate to promote spontaneous drainage. In the thick skin on the back of the neck, several furuncles may coalesce to form a large area of infection containing many interconnected sinus tracts and abscesses. This is known as a *carbuncle* and often requires surgical wide excision for complete resolution. Carbuncles are seen much more commonly in diabetics and may demonstrate signs of systemic involvement.

Diagnosis Most simple cutaneous abscesses in otherwise healthy patients are local infections without need for further evaluation. Clinical presentation of a tender, swollen, often erythematous nodule strongly suggests infection. A palpable area of fluctuance is typically enough for the diagnosis of abscess. Notice should be made of the admitting vital signs, with particular attention to temperature and heart rate. Fever or tachycardia suggests systemic involvement of the infection and may indicate the need for further laboratory testing. In patients with diabetes, alcoholism, and other immunocompromising conditions, the threshold for further diagnostic studies should be lower. A complete blood count and in certain situations (such as possible osteomyelitis) an erythrocyte sedimentation rate usually are all that are needed to evaluate for possible systemic involvement. Diabetic patients routinely should have blood glucose checked.

In simple abscesses involving otherwise healthy patients, a routine culture and sensitivity is not needed. If it is felt that antibiotic treatment is indicated, the causative organisms usually can be predicted by the general location of the abscess. If further certainty is required, a Gram stain of the abscess aspirate most often will lend the required information, and results can be obtained while the patient is still in the ED. Gram-positive cocci in clusters suggest infection with *S. aureus*, whereas many different organisms suggest a mixed anaerobic and aerobic infection. In patients in whom possible deep or chronic infection may complicate the course, early wound cultures with sensitivities may prove useful. Immunocompromised patients demonstrating systemic signs of infection also should have blood cultures drawn. In patients in whom foreign body involvement is a potential issue, plain radiographs or possibly ultrasound should be used to assist in identification.

Treatment Incision and drainage are the only treatment necessary in most cases of superficial and localized abscesses. Often it is difficult to determine clinically if an area of fluctuance is present within an area of induration and swelling. Needle aspiration of the most likely area of induration often can help in the diagnosis. When pus is encountered with aspiration, incision and drainage should be performed. When no pus is located, a trial of antibiotic therapy and warm compresses is appropriate initially. These patients should have a follow-up evaluation scheduled because many will need incision and drainage in the future.

Consideration must be given to the best location for abscess drainage. Abscesses well suited to ED treatment are those which are superficial, well localized, and not in close proximity to nerves or vascular structures. Fluctuant masses should be examined for pulsations or bruits if near vascular structures. Patient comfort is also an important consideration. Infiltration of a local anesthetic most often gives poor pain relief. The lower pH of infected tissue typically greatly reduces the effectiveness of a local anesthetic. Injecting additional fluid into an already swollen and tender area also increases pain. Regional or field blocks can be used effectively at times, and digital blocks to assist in the drainage of a large paronychia or felon are usually all that are needed. Patients with evidence of deeper tissue infection, as in many cases of perirectal abscess, and those in whom adequate analgesia cannot be obtained in the ED should be taken to the operating room for appropriate surgical drainage.

Nitrous oxide has been used with good success in many EDs for years. The parenteral use of rapid and ultra-short-acting sedatives and analgesics for conscious sedation in the ED has been shown to be both safe and effective when they are used appropriately. They are best suited for procedures that are very painful and short in duration. Incision and drainage seem ideal in this regard. Many agents have been used effectively, with the combination of fentanyl and midazolam being one of the more common and effective. Both these agents have a short time to peak effect (3-5 min for midazolam and <1 min for fentanyl) and a short duration of action (each 1 to $1\frac{1}{2}$ h), which allows the patient to be discharged at his or her presedation mental status baseline without a prolonged recovery period. Furthermore, the patient benefits from the analgesic effect of the fentanyl as well as the sedative, anxiolytic, and amnestic effects of the midazolam. Fentanyl, with less than 1 min to peak effect, is very well suited to titration for desired effect during the procedure. For further discussion, see Chap. 33.

Prior to any sedation or analgesia, the procedure should be explained to the patient, including any possible complications. With most superficial abscesses, the risks involved are relatively few. The possibility of severing a cutaneous nerve with residual local numbness, as well as the risk of injury to deeper nerves and blood vessels, should be discussed. The possibility of poor or delayed wound healing should be discussed in patients with diabetes or peripheral vascular disease. Some estimate should be made of the residual scarring that may be anticipated, especially in areas of cosmetic significance. As with all elective and invasive procedures, informed consent should be obtained in all patients. Although the risk of complications is low, informed consent prior to the procedure ensures that the patient has been appropriately educated concerning the risks and benefits, as well as optimizing medicolegal coverage for the clinician. Informed consent in patients receiving conscious sedation is also important and should cover the risk of respiratory depression requiring endotracheal intubation.

The patient should be positioned to ensure appropriate access to the abscess and in the most comfortable position possible. The area should be prepared with Betadine and draped in a sterile fashion. After appropriate anesthesia, the abscess should be opened widely over the area of greatest fluctuance, using a No. 11 or 15 scalpel blade to ensure adequate drainage. As much pus as possible should be expressed by gentle compression. Hemostats are then used to break up any loculated areas within the abscess cavity. The cavity is irrigated with saline and packed loosely with gauze tape to hold it open to promote drainage while the infection resolves. The packing should be left in place long enough for the cavity to heal from the inside out, preventing recollection of the abscess. Patients are discharged with instructions for warm compresses or soaks three to four times a day. A follow-up visit should be scheduled in 2 to 3 days for recheck and advancement or replacement of the packing. Wounds that continue to actively drain at the time of follow-up should have the packing replaced. Replacing the packing performs some degree of debridement of the abscess cavity, as well as providing fresh packing for absorption of pus and debris. Wounds that are not actively draining can have the packing advanced as needed to allow for internal healing while keeping the incision open to promote drainage.

The use of antibiotics in patients with cutaneous abscesses is somewhat controversial. The risk of systemic infection following local incision and drainage appears to be low. A recent ED study demonstrated that in 50 afebrile patients in whom blood cultures were drawn 2 and 10 min after incision and drainage of cutaneous abscesses, none of the cultures was found to be positive.[9] There are no good data suggesting that antibiotic treatment following incision and drainage speeds infection resolution in otherwise healthy patients. Generally, it is felt that in patients without underlying immunocompromising conditions or signs of systemic infection, antibiotics are not indicated following incision and drainage of superficial cutaneous abscesses. With a lack of hard scientific data pointing to clear-cut guidelines for antibiotic therapy, clinical judgment needs to be exercised. In patients with diabetes, alcoholism, or other underlying immunocompromising illnesses, or in those on immunosuppressant medications such as steroids or chemotherapeutics, the threshold for antibiotic use should be much lower. Furthermore, patients who present with signs of systemic disease such as fever and chills and those with cellulitis extending beyond the abscess borders also should be considered for antibiotic therapy. Abscesses involving the hands or face should be treated more aggressively with antibiotics because of the higher morbidity associated with prolonged infection or complications. The specific antibiotic used should be chosen according to the most likely pathogen involved. This can be somewhat predicted by the location of the infection. Duration of therapy should be directed to some degree by the severity of infection but typically should continue for 5 to 7 days.

Of separate concern are patients with underlying structural heart disease at risk for bacterial endocarditis. Certain structural cardiac conditions lead to a higher incidence of bacterial endocarditis. Futhermore, the severity of disease and morbidity are increased in patients with certain underlying cardiac diseases who develop bacterial endocarditis. The American Heart Association recently has updated its guidelines for patients at increased risk for developing bacterial endocarditis.[10] Table 146-1 outlines the cardiac conditions considered to be at high and moderate risk based on predicted outcomes if endocarditis does occur. Note that several types of patients frequently encountered in the ED, namely, patients after coronary artery bypass grafting, those with pacemakers, and those with mitral valve prolapse without valvular regurgitation, are not recommended for endocarditis prophylaxis. Despite the apparent low risk of transient bacteremia following incision and drainage of a simple cutaneous abscess, the American Heart Association recommends prophylactic antibiotics for those patients in the high- and moderate-risk catagories prior to the procedure. No mention is made of postprocedure treatment. The antibiotic selected should be directed at the most likely organism causing the abscess. Table 146-2 outlines suggested antibiotic treatment by organism for soft tissue infections and should be used for preprocedure prophylaxis for endocarditis. An intravenous or intramuscular antistaphylococcal penicillin, clindamycin, or first-generation cephalosporin is appropriate for patients not able to take oral medications. In patients with known methicillin-resistant *S. aureus* infection, vancomycin is recommended for prophylaxis.

Disposition Most patients can be discharged following incision and drainage of a cutaneous abscess. Again, clinical judgment plays an important part in this decision. Patients with severe underlying disease

TABLE 146-1 Cardiac Conditions at Risk for Endocarditis

Endocarditis prophylaxis recommended:
High-risk category:
Prosthetic cardiac valves
Previous bacterial endocarditis
Complex cyanotic heart disease (e.g., single ventricle, transposition of the great vessels, tetralogy of Fallot)
Surgically constructed systemic pulmonary stunts or conduits
Moderate-risk category:
Most other congenital cardiac malformations
Acquired valvular dysfunction (e.g., rheumatic heart disease)
Hypertrophic cardiomyopathy
Mitral valve prolapse with valvular regurgitation and/or thickened leaflets
Endocarditis prophylaxis not recommended:
Negligible-risk category (no greater risk than general population):
Isolated secundum atrial septal defect
Surgical repair of ASD, VSD, or PDA
Previous coronary artery bypass grafting
Mitral valve prolapse without valvular regurgitation
Physiologic, functional, or innocent heart murmur
Cardiac pacemakers

Abbreviations: ASD, atrial septal defect; VSD, ventricular septal defect; PDA, patent ductus arteriosus.

or those with immunocompromising conditions may benefit from admission and intravenous antibiotics. Furthermore, patients with signs of systemic infection or deeper infection such as osteomyelitis should be considered for admission. Appropriate follow-up within 2 to 3 days for those discharged is important.

SPOROTRICHOSIS

Sporotrichosis is a mycotic infection caused by the fungus *Sporothrix schenckii* commonly found on plants and vegetation and in soil. Infection is caused by traumatic inoculation and usually remains within the local soft tissues and lymphatics. Disseminated forms, although more rare, do occur.

Epidemiology

The organism responsible for sporotrichosis occurs worldwide and is found most commonly in soil, sphagnum moss, and decaying vegetable matter. Inoculation into the host most commonly occurs from a spine or barb on a plant puncturing the skin during handling. It is a common disease among florists, gardeners, and agricultural workers. Transmission from infected animals, especially cats, has been documented, and veterinarians and animal handlers are also at increased risk. The largest outbreak of sporotrichosis in the United States involved 15 states and 84 persons, all of whom handled conifer seedlings shipped in sphagnum moss contaminated with *S. schenckii.*[11]

Pathophysiology

S. schenckii is a thermally dimorphic fungus that changes from its mycelial form to its yeast form on entering a body-temperature environment. Local infection occurs in most cases, with disease limited to cutaneous or lymphocutaneous areas.[12] Osteoarticular involvement including osteomyelitis, septic arthritis, bursitis, and tenosynovitis occurs and may be related to a local cutaneous infection or secondary to hematogenous spread. Systemic forms, including pulmonary, meningeal, and disseminated forms, are much more rare.

Clinical Features

The incubation period averages 3 weeks from the time of initial inoculation but varies from a few days to several weeks. After the fungus enters the body through a break in the skin, three types of localized infections may occur. The fixed cutaneous type is characterized by lesions restricted to the site of inoculation and may appear as a crusted ulcer or verrucous plaque. Local cutaneous-type infections also remain local but present as a subcutaneous nodule or pustule. The surrounding skin becomes erythematous and may ulcerate, resulting in a chancre. Local lymphadenitis is common. The lymphocutaneous type is the third and most common type. It is characterized by an initial painless nodule or papule at the site of inoculation that later develops subcutaneous nodules with clear skip areas along local lymphatic channels. The local reactions in all three types of infections tend to be relatively painless but show no signs of improvement without treatment.

Diagnosis

History and physical findings are the key to diagnosis. Histopathologic stains are of little help because the organisms are scarce in tissues. Fungal cultures are the best way to isolate the fungus, and tissue biopsy cultures often are diagnostic. Routine laboratory tests are nonspecific, but an increased white blood cell count, eosinophil count, and erythrocyte sedimentation rate may be noted. The differential diagnosis includes tuberculosis, tularemia, cat-scratch disease, leishmaniasis, staphylococcal lymphangitis, and nocardiosis.

Treatment

The treatment of choice for cutaneous sporotrichosis until recently was potassium iodide (SSKI) 3 to 4 g three times a day to be continued for at least 1 month beyond resolution of clinical symptoms. This was

TABLE 146-2 Antibiotic Recommendations for Soft Tissue Infections (Oral)

Staphylococcus aureus
Dicloxacillin 250–500 mg q6h
Amoxicillin-clavulanate 500/125 mg q8h or 875/125 mg q12h
Cephalexin 250–500 mg q6h
Clarithromycin 500 mg q12h
Azithromycin 500 mg first day, then 250 mg qd × 4 d
Streptococcus species
Penicillin V 250–500 mg q6h
Amoxicillin-clavulanate 500/125 mg q8h or 875/125 mg q12h
Cephalexin 250–500 mg q6h
Clindamycin 150–450 mg q6h
Erythromycin 250–500 mg q6h
Clarithromycin 500 mg q12h
Azithromycin 500 mg first day, then 250 mg qd × 4 d
Amoxicillin-clavulanate 500/125 mg q8h or 875/125 mg q12h
Ciprofloxacin 500–750 mg q12h
Ofloxacin 200–400 mg q12h
Cephalexin 250–500 mg q6h
Bacteroides fragilis
Amoxicillin-clavulanate 500/125 mg q8h or 875/125 mg q12h
Clindamycin 150–450 mg q6h
Metronidazole 500 mg q6h
Pasturella multocida (animal bites, esp. cats)
Penicillin V 250–500 mg q6h
Amoxicillin-clavulanate 500/125 mg q8h or 875/125 mg q12h
Ciprofloxacin 500–750 mg q12h
Ofloxacin 200–400 mg q12h

a cumbersome treatment and was associated with a high incidence of side effects such as metallic taste, anorexia, and swelling of the salivary glands. Recently, itraconazole (100–200 mg qd for 3–6 months) has been shown to be a highly effective and much better tolerated treatment for localized as well as many systemic forms of sporotrichosis.[13] Fluconazole has been shown to be less effective than itraconazole and should be reserved for those few patients not tolerating itraconazole. Ketoconazole has shown even poorer results than fluconazole. Intravenous amphotericin B is effective, but adverse reactions usually limit its use to disseminated forms.

Disposition

Essentially all patients with a cutaneous form of sporotrichosis can be treated on an outpatient basis. Discharge instructions should include basic wound care for open lesions, and close follow-up with a local medical doctor should be arranged. Patients who are acutely ill or have evidence of systemic disease should be admitted to the hospital initially for possible treatment with intravenous amphotericin B.

REFERENCES

1. Riseman J, Zamboni W, Curtis A, et al: Hyperbaric oxygen therapy for necrotizing fasciitis reduces mortality and the need for debridements. *Surgery* 108(5):847, 1990.
2. Corey E: Nontraumatic gas gangrene: Case report and review of emergency therapeutics. *J Emerg Med* 9:431, 1991.
3. Stephens M: Gas gangrene: Potential for hyperbaric oxygen therapy. *Postgrad Med* 99(4):217, 1996.
4. Sachs M: Cutaneous cellulitis. Arch Dermatol 127:493, 1991.
5. Sanford J, Gilbert D, Moellering R, Sande M: *The Sanford Guide to Antimicrobial Therapy,* 29th ed. Dallas: Antimicrobial Therapy, Inc., 1999.
6. Chartier C, Grosshans E: Erysipelas. *Int J Dermatol* 29:459, 1990.
7. Ochs M, Dolwick F: Facial erysipelas: Report of a case and review of the literature. *J Oral Maxillofac Surg* 49:1116, 1991.
8. Bergsein J, Baker E, Aprahamian C, et al: Soft tissue abscesses associated with parenteral drug abuse: Presentation, microbiology, and treatment. *Am Surg* 61(12):1105, 1995.
9. Bobrow B, Pollack C, Gamble S, Seligston R: Incision and drainage of cutaneous abscesses is not associated with bacteremia in afebrile adults. *Ann Emerg Med* 29(3):404, 1997.
10. Danjani A, Taubet K, Wilson W, et al: Prevention of bacterial endocarditis: Recommendations by the American Heart Association. *JAMA* 277(2): 1794, 1997.
11. Dixon D, Salkin I, Duncan R, et al: Isolation and characterization of *Sporothrix schenckii* from clinical and environmental sources associated with the largest U.S. epidemic of sporotrichosis. *J Clin Microbiol* 29:1106, 1991.
12. Rafal E, Rasmussen J: An unusual presentation of fixed cutaneous sporotrichosis: A case report and review of the literature. *J Am Acad Dermatol* 25:928, 1991.
13. Kauffman C: Old and new therapies for sporotrichosis. *Clin Infect Dis* 21(4):981, 1995.

147 REPORTABLE COMMUNICABLE DISEASES

Jane H. Brice

The Centers for Disease Control and Prevention (CDC) in Atlanta publishes a list of reportable communicable diseases that is updated and revised routinely. The most recent update as of this writing (1997) includes 52 nationally reportable diseases and is summarized in Table 147-1.[1] The requirement to report these diseases is mandated by state or territory laws and regulations, and therefore, the list differs for each state or territory.

TABLE 147-1 Nationally Reportable Communicable Diseases

Acquired immunodeficiency syndrome (AIDS)	Lyme disease
Anthrax	Malaria
Botulism	Measles
Brucellosis	Meningococcal disease
Chancroid	Mumps
Chlamydia trachomatis genital infections	Pertussis
Cholera	Plague
Coccidioidomycosis	Poliomyelitis, paralytic
Cryptosporidiosis	Psittacosis
Diphtheria	Rabies, animal
Encephalitis, California serogroup	Rabies, human
Encephalitis, eastern equine	Rocky Mountain spotted fever
Encephalitis, St. Louis	Rubella
Encephalitis, western equine	Rubella, congenital syndrome
Escherichia coli O157 : H7	Salmonellosis
Gonorrhea	Shigellosis
Haemophilus influenzae invasive disease	Streptococcal disease, invasive, group A
Hansen's disease (leprosy)	*Streptococcus pneumoniae,* drug-resistant invasive disease
Hantavirus pulmonary syndrome	Streptococcal toxic shock syndrome
Hemolytic-uremic syndrome, post-diarrheal	Syphilis
Hepatitis A	Syphilis, congenital
Hepatitis B	Tetanus
Hepatitis C/non-A, non-B	Toxic shock syndrome
HIV infection, pediatric	Trichinosis
Legionellosis	Tuberculosis
	Typhoid fever
	Yellow fever

Source: Centers for Disease Control and Prevention: Case definitions for infectious conditions under public health surveillance. *MMWR* 46(RR-10):1, 1997.

The reliability of the national reporting system rests on health care providers, laboratories, and other public health personnel. Without consistent and timely reporting, it becomes very difficult to monitor trends in disease patterns, to detect unusual occurrences or pockets of disease, and to assess the effectiveness of public health interventions to eradicate or contain disease. Data reported by the 50 states, the District of Columbia, and the U.S. territories are summarized in the *Morbidity and Mortality Weekly Report,* which can be accessed online at *www.cdc.gov/epo/mmwr/mmwr.html.*

"The usefulness of public health surveillance data depends on its uniformity, simplicity, and timeliness."[1] What follows here is a summary of the case definitions for each of the specified nationally reportable diseases from the *Morbidity and Mortality Weekly (MMWR)* update on reportable diseases.[1] These case definitions establish uniform reporting criteria and are subject to revision. For the most up-to-date information, go to *www.cdc.gov/epo/mmwr/other/case_def/about.html.*

ACQUIRED IMMUNODEFICIENCY SYNDROME (AIDS)

AIDS is a chronic illness with varying manifestations. The CDC defines this syndrome[2,3] as all human immunodeficiency virus (HIV)-infected adolescents (≥13 years) and adults with (1) a CD4 T-lymphocyte count of less than 200, (2) a CD4 T-lymphocyte percent of total lymphocyte of less than 14 percent, or (3) any of the following: pulmonary tuberculosis, recurrent pneumonia, invasive cervical cancer, or 23 other clinical conditions discussed elsewhere in this text and available on the MMWR Web site.[4]

ANTHRAX

Anthrax is an acute illness with one of several distinct clinical presentations. The cutaneous form is characterized by a skin lesion evolving over 2 to 6 days from a papule to a vesicle to a depressed black eschar. The inhalation form presents with a brief upper respiratory infection followed by hypoxia and dyspnea. On chest radiography, there will be evidence of mediastinal widening from adenopathy. The intestinal form is distinguished by severe abdominal pain and cramping followed by fever and sepsis. Finally, in the oropharyngeal form, a mucosal lesion in the oral cavity develops along with cervical adenopathy, edema, and fever.

The laboratory diagnosis is made by (1) isolation of *Bacillus anthracis* from a clinical specimen, (2) anthrax electrophoretic immunotransblot (EITB) reaction to the protective antigen and/or lethal factor bands in at least one serum specimen obtained after onset of symptoms, or (3) demonstration of *B. anthracis* through immunofluorescence.

BOTULISM

Foodborne An acute illness of varying severity, foodborne botulism is manifested by diplopia, blurred vision, bulbar weakness, or symmetric paralysis that may be of rapid onset. Laboratory confirmation of this illness consists of demonstration of botulinum toxin in serum or stool or in food the subject recently consumed. A positive *Clostridium botulinum* culture from stool also serves as confirmation of the diagnosis.

Infant A constellation of symptoms in an infant under 1 year of age including constipation, poor feeding, and failure to thrive followed by progressive weakness, impaired respiration, and death should suggest infant botulism. Laboratory confirmation of the diagnosis is made in the same manner as described for foodborne botulism.

Wound The symptoms for wound botulism mirror those found in the foodborne form. The laboratory diagnosis is made by finding botulinum toxin in serum or obtaining a positive culture from the wound.

BRUCELLOSIS

Infection with *Brucella* may be either of acute or insidious onset. Brucellosis is characterized by fever, night sweats, undue fatigue, anorexia, weight loss, headache, and arthralgias. The laboratory diagnosis may be made in several ways: (1) culture positive from a clinical specimen, (2) at least a fourfold increase in *Brucella* agglutination titers between the acute and convalescent phases in serum taken at least 2 weeks apart and studied in the same laboratory, or (3) positive immunofluorescence of *Brucella* in a clinical specimen.

CHANCROID

Chancroid is a sexually transmitted disease caused by the organism *Haemophilus ducreyi.* It is manifested by a painful genital ulcer with inflammed inguinal lymph nodes. Isolation of the organism from a clinical specimen confirms the diagnosis.

CHLAMYDIA TRACHOMATIS GENITAL INFECTIONS

Genital infection with *Chlamydia trachomatis* is sexually transmitted and may present in several different manners. There may be evidence of urethritis, epididymitis, cervicitis, or acute salpingitis, or the infection may be completely asymptomatic. It is therefore essential to test for *Chlamydia* whenever there is a suspicion of infection or when there is evidence of other sexually transmitted infection. *Chlamydia* also may cause conjunctivitis or pneumonia in newborns through perinatal transmission. Finally, *Chlamydia* causes lymphogranuloma venerum, which is discussed below. The diagnosis of *Chlamydia* is confirmed through either a positive culture or detection of the antigen or nucleic acid on immunofluorescence.

CHOLERA

Cholera infection is manifested by a diarrheal illness of varying severity. The presence of vomiting does not exclude the diagnosis. Isolation of the toxigenic *Vibrio cholerae* O1 or O139 from stool or emesis confirms the diagnosis. Serologic evidence of recent infection also may confirm a recent illness caused by cholera.

COCCIDIOIDOMYCOSIS

Infection with the fungus *Coccidioides immitis* may manifest in an acute or chronic illness and may, in some persons, be maintained in an asymptomatic state. This fungus is endemic in the southwestern United States. Those demonstrating symptoms usually complain of an influenza-like febrile respiratory illness. The disease may disseminate in approximately 0.5 percent.

Coccidioidomycosis should be considered in those with one or more of the following: (1) influenza-like signs and symptoms (fever, cough, chest pain, myalgia, arthralgia, and headache), (2) pneumonia or other pulmonary lesion on chest radiograph, (3) erythema nodosum or erythema multiforme rash, (4) involvement of bones, joints, or skin by dissemination, (5) meningitis, and (6) involvement of viscera or lymph nodes.

Laboratory confirmation is made through (1) culture, histopathology, or molecular evidence of *C. immitis,* (2) serologic tests including detection of IgM by immunodiffusion, enzyme immunoassay, latex agglutination, or tube precipitation or detection of rising titer of IgG by immunodiffusion, enzyme immunoassay, or complement fixation, or (3) coccidioidal skin-test conversion after onset of symptoms.

CRYPTOSPORIDIOSIS

Diarrhea, abdominal cramps, loss of appetite, low-grade fever, and nausea and vomiting are the cluster of signs and symptoms associated with cryptosporidiosis. The infection may be asymptomatic in some persons. The illness also can be prolonged and life threatening in immunocompromised patients. It is caused by the protozoa *Cryptosporidium parvum.*

In the laboratory, the diagnosis is confirmed by detecting oocysts in stool or demonstrating *Cryptosporidium* in intestinal fluid or small bowel biopsy specimens. Additionally, identifying *Cryptosporidium* antigen in stool by specific immunodiagnostic testing will confirm the diagnosis of cryptosporidiosis.

DIPHTHERIA

Diphtheria is characterized by upper respiratory symptoms including sore throat, low-grade fever, and an adherent membrane to tonsils, pharynx, and/or the nose. There is a cutaneous form of diphtheria that does not need to be reported to the CDC. Isolation of *Corynebacterium diphtheriae* from clinical specimens or a histopathologic diagnosis of diphtheria confirms the illness.

ENCEPHALITIS, ARBOVIRAL

Arboviral encephalitis is characterized by a febrile illness associated with any of the following neurologic signs and symptoms: headache, confusion, altered sensorium, nausea and vomiting, meningismus, cranial nerve palsy, paresis or paralysis, sensory deficit, altered reflexes, seizures, abnormal movements, or coma. The illness may be of varying severity and cannot be distinguished clinically from other central nervous system infections.

The diagnosis is made based on laboratory detection of (1) a fourfold or greater rise in serum antibody titer, (2) isolation of virus or finding viral antigen or genomic sequences in tissue, blood, cerebral spinal fluid, or other bodily fluids, or (3) IgM anitbody detected on enzyme immunoassay from serum or cerebral spinal fluid.

Eastern equine encephalitis, western equine encephalitis, California serogroup encephalitis, or St. Louis encephalitis are reportable to the CDC.

ESCHERICHIA COLI O157:H7

A diarrheal disease of variable severity, *E. coli* O157:H7 has gained national prominence through several food-borne outbreaks. The diarrhea of this disease is often bloody and associated with abdominal cramping. It may be complicated by hemolytic-uremic syndrome or thrombotic thrombocytopenic purpura. It also may be asymptomatic.

In the laboratory, isolation of the bacteria in a clinical specimen, or isolation of Shiga toxin–producing *E. coli* O157:NM from a clinical specimen (strains of O157:H7 that have lost the flagellar H antigen become nonmotile and are called *NM*) is diagnostic.

GONORRHEA

This sexually transmitted disease is characterized by varying manifestations including urethritis, cervicitis, or salpingitis. It may be asymptomatic in some persons or may become disseminated. Laboratory detection of *Neisseria gonorrhoeae* in clinical specimens confirms the diagnosis. Other methods of laboratory confirmation include detection of antigen or nucleic acid in specimens or observation of gram-negative intracellular diplococci in a urethral smear obtained from a male patient.

HAEMOPHILUS INFLUENZAE INVASIVE DISEASE

Invasive disease caused by *H. influenzae* include meningitis, bacteremia, epiglottitis, or pneumonia. Laboratory isolation of *H. influenzae* from a normally sterile site such as blood, cerebral spinal fluid, or joint fluid is necessary to confirm the diagnosis.

HANSEN'S DISEASE (LEPROSY)

Hansen's disease is a chronic infection with *Mycobacterium leprae* involving the skin predominantly but which can include peripheral nerves and the mucosa of the upper airway as well. There are four clinical forms of Hansen's disease. Tuberculoid leprosy is characterized by one or a few well-demarcated, hypopigmented, and anesthetic skin lesions. Often these lesions have active, spreading edges and a clearing center. Peripheral nerve swelling or thickening also may be present. In the lepromatous form, a number of erythematous papules and nodules may be present or an infiltration of face, hands, and feet with lesions in a bilateral and symmetric pattern that progresses to thickening of the skin. The borderline or dimorphous form presents with skin lesions characteristic of both the tuberculoid and lepromatous forms. Finally, in the indeterminate form, early lesions, usually hypopigmented macules, are present that do not develop the more characteristic features of the tuberculoid or lepromatous forms.

Demonstration of acid-fast bacilli in skin or dermal nerves makes the diagnosis. Specimens should be obtained from a full-thickness skin biopsy of a lepromatous lesion, if possible.

HANTAVIRUS PULMONARY SYNDROME

Hantavirus pulmonary syndrome is a febrile illness characterized by bilateral interstitial pulmonary infiltrates and respiratory compromise resembling adult respiratory distress syndrome. There is typically a prodrome of fever, chills, myalgias, headache, and gastrointestinal distress. Common laboratory findings include one or more of the following: hemoconcentration, left shift in white blood cell count, neutrophilic leukocytosis, thrombocytopenia, or circulating immunoblasts.

Hantavirus should be considered in the setting of one or more of the following: (1) febrile illness [temperature greater than 38.3°C (101°F)] in a previously healthy individual with bilateral interstitial edema that may radiographically resemble adult respiratory distress syndrome and respiratory compromise requiring oxygen support developing within 72 h of hospitalization, or (2) unexplained respiratory illness resulting in death and autopsy examination demonstrating noncardiogenic pulmonary edema without identifiable cause.

Detection of hantavirus-specific IgM or rising titers of IgG, detection of hantavirus-specific ribonucleic acid sequences by polymerase chain reaction techniques in clinical specimens, and detection of hantavirus antigen by immunohistochemistry are all acceptable laboratory methods for confirming the diagnosis.

HEMOLYTIC-UREMIC SYNDROME, POSTDIARRHEAL

Hemolytic-uremic syndrome presents as acute onset of microangiopathic hemolytic anemia, renal injury, and low platelet count. Most cases occur within 3 weeks of an acute diarrheal illness. A low platelet count is typical early in the illness (within the first 7 days) but may have normalized by the time the patient seeks care. If the platelet count is not less than 150,000/μL within 7 days of the onset of the gastrointestinal illness, consider another diagnosis. Thrombotic thrombocytopenic purpura has similar features and is distinguished from hemolytic-uremic syndrome by the presence of fever and CNS involvement. Additionally, it may have a more gradual onset. Few cases of thrombotic thrombocytopenic purpura are associated with a diarrheal illness.

In the laboratory, both of the following findings will be present: (1) anemia of acute onset with microangiopathic changes (schistocytes, burr cells, or helmet cells on smear) and (2) acute renal failure with hematuria, proteinuria, or increased creatinine levels (50 percent over the patient's baseline values, or greater than 1.0 mg/dL for a child under 13 years of age, or greater than 1.5 mg/dL for persons over 13 years of age with previously normal renal function).

HEPATITIS

Hepatitis is characterized by acute and discrete onset of symptoms and jaundice or elevated serum aminotransferase levels. At present, hepatitis A, B, C, non-A and non-B, and delta are reportable. The laboratory diagnosis of each of the hepatitis viruses is listed below.

Hepatitis A. Detection of IgM to the hepatitis A virus (anti-HAV).

Hepatitis B. (1) Detection of IgM to hepatitis B core antigen (anti-HBc) or hepatitis B surface antigen (HBsAg) and (2) anti-HAV negative, if done.

Hepatitis C. Detection of antibody against hepatitis C antigen (anti-HCV), (2) serum aminotransferase levels greater than 2.5 times the upper limit of normal, (3) anti-HAV negative, if done, and (4) anti-HBc or HBsAg negative, if done.

Non-A, non-B hepatitis. (1) Serum aminotransferase levels greater than 2.5 times the upper limit of normal, (2) anti-HAV negative, and (3) anti-HBc and HBsAg negative.

Delta hepatitis. (1) HBsAg or anti-HBc positive and (2) detection of antibodies to hepatitis delta virus (not a reportable disease).

Persons with chronic hepatitis, those who are hepatitis B surface antigen positive, or those who are anti-hepatitis C virus positive should not be reported unless they have acute illness compatible with viral hepatitis at the time of the laboratory finding.

PERINATAL HEPATITIS B

In infants aged 1 to 24 months, infection with hepatitis B may range from an asymptomatic state to fulminant hepatitis. On laboratory investigation, the infant will be HBsAg-positive.

HIV INFECTION, PEDIATRIC

Pediatric (13 years of age) infection with human immunodeficiency virus (HIV) runs the gamut from asymptomatic to severely immunocompromised. Case definitions are broken into two age categories:[3]

1. Any child under 18 months of age born to an HIV-positive mother who has positive results on two separate tests (excluding cord blood) from one or more of the following: HIV culture, HIV polymerase chain reaction, or HIV p24 antigen, or who meets criteria for an acquired immunodeficiency deficiency syndrome (AIDS) diagnosis based on the 1987 AIDS surveillance case definition.
2. Any child 18 months of age or older born to an HIV-positive mother or any child infected by blood, blood products, or other known means of transmission who is HIV-positive by repeatedly positive enzyme immunoassay and confirmatory test or meets criteria set forth for children under 18 months of age.

LEGIONELLOSIS

Infection with *Legionella* causes two distinct illnesses: (1) legionnaires' disease, manifested by fever, myalgia, cough, and pneumonia, and (2) Pontiac fever, which is a milder illness without pneumonia. Laboratory confirmation of *Legionella* infection can be made by any of the following methods: (1) isolation of *Legionella* from respiratory secretions, lung tissue, pleural fluid, or other normally sterile site, (2) demonstration of fourfold or greater rise in reciprocal immunofluorescence antibody titer to greater than or equal to 128 against *Legionella pneumophila* serogroup 1 between paired acute and convalescent serum specimens, (3) detection of *L. pneumophila* serogroup 1 in respiratory secretions, lung tissue, or pleural fluid by direct fluorescent antibody testing, or (4) detection of *L. pneumophila* serogroup 1 antigen in urine by radioimmunoassay or enzyme-linked immunosorbent assay.

LYME DISEASE

This tick-borne illness presents with systemic manifestations including those of the dermatologic, rheumatologic, neurologic, and cardiac systems. The best clinical marker is erythema migrans, the initial skin lesion that occurs in 60 to 80 percent of patients. Other acute symptoms include fatigue, fever, headache, mildly stiff neck, arthralgias, and myalgias. Late manifestations are variable and are best discussed by system:

1. *Musculoskeletal.* Recurrent brief and intermittent episodes (over weeks or months) of objective joint swelling in one or several joints, sometimes followed by chronic arthiritis.
2. *Central nervous system.* Any of the following (alone or in combination): lymphocytic meningitis, cranial neuritis (particularly Bell's palsy which is occasionally bilateral), radiculopathy, or rarely encephalomyelitis.
3. *Cardiovascular.* Acute onset of high-grade (second- or third-degree) AV block that resolves in days to weeks and is sometimes associated with myocarditis (note that palpitations, bradycardia, bundle-branch blocks, or myocarditis alone is not enough).

Isolation of the organism *Borrelia burgdorferi* from a clinical specimen or demonstration of antibody (IgM or IgG) against *B. burgdorferi* in serum or cerebral spinal fluid confirms the diagnosis. A two-test approach (enzyme-linked immunosorbent assay followed by Western blot) is recommended.

MALARIA

Malaria is caused by infection with one of the *Plasmodium* species. Most patients have fever. Other complaints include headache, chills, sweats, myalgias, nausea, vomiting, diarrhea, or cough. Untreated infection by *Plasmodium falciparum* can lead to coma, renal failure, pulmonary edema, and death. In the laboratory, malaria parasites can be seen on blood smear.

MEASLES (RUBEOLA)

Measles is an illness characterized by all the following (1) generalized rash lasting more than 3 days, (2) temperature greater than or equal to 38.3°C (101°F), and (3) cough, coryza, or conjunctivitis. The laboratory diagnosis can be made by any of the following: (1) positive serologic tests for measles IgM, (2) significant rise in measles antibody levels by any standard serologic assay, or (3) isolation of measles virus from clinical specimens.

MENINGOCOCCAL DISEASE

Meningococcal disease is most commonly evident as meningitis and/or meningococcemia. It may progress rapidly to purpura fulminans, shock, and death. Isolation of *Neisseria meningitidis* from a normally sterile site such as blood or cerebral spinal fluid confirms the diagnosis.

MUMPS

An illness with acute onset, mumps is characterized by unilateral or bilateral tender, self-limited swelling of parotid or other salivary gland for 2 or more days without other cause. The laboratory diagnosis is evident by (1) isolating mumps virus from a clinical specimen, (2) a significant rise between acute and convalescent titers in serum mumps IgG, or (3) finding mumps IgM in serum.

PERTUSSIS

Pertussis is an illness with cough lasting for 2 weeks or longer without other cause and with one of the following: (1) paroxysms of cough, (2) inspiratory whoop, or (3) posttussive vomiting. The laboratory confirmation is found in isolation of *Bordetella pertussis* from clinical specimens or a positive polymerase chain reaction for *B. pertussis.*

PLAGUE

An illness characterized by fever, chills, headache, malaise, prostration, and leukocytosis, plague manifests predominantly in one of the following clinical forms: (1) bubonic plague, manifested by regional lymphadenitis, (2) septicemic plague, in which there is septicemia without evident bubo, (3) pneumonic plague, where pneumonia results from either inhalation of infectious droplets (primary pneumonic plague) or hematologic spread from bubonic or septicemic cases (secondary pneumonic plague), or (4) pharyngeal plague, in which there is pharyngitis and cervical lymphadenitis resulting from exposure to larger infectious droplets or ingestion of infected tissues.

Presumptive laboratory diagnosis is made by (1) an increase in serum antibody titers to *Yersinia pestis* fraction 1 antigen without plague vaccination or (2) detection of fraction 1 antigen by fluorescent assay. Confirmatory laboratory diagnosis is produced by (1) isolation of *Y. pestis* in clinical specimens or (2) a fourfold or greater rise in serum antibody titer to *Y. pestis* fraction 1 antigen.

POLIOMYELITIS, PARALYTIC

Paralytic poliomyelitis is an illness of acute onset and apparent in the flaccid paralysis of one or more limbs with absent or diminished tendon reflexes in the affected limbs without other cause and without sensory or cognitive losses. Laboratory testing only serves to classify the case into categories set up by the CDC. The clinical case definition is sufficient for reporting.

PSITTACOSIS

Psittacosis is a disease found among bird handlers that presents with fever, chills, headache, photophobia, cough, and myalgia. In the laboratory, any of the following methods will confirm the diagnosis: (1) isolation of *Chlamydia psittaci* from respiratory secretions, (2) a fourfold or greater increase in antibodies against *C. psittaci* by complement fixation or microimmunofluorescence (MIF) to a reciprocal titer of at least 32 between paired acute and convalescent serum samples, or (3) detection of serum IgM to *C. psittaci* by MIF to a reciprocal titer of at least 16.

RABIES, ANIMAL

The laboratory diagnosis of animal rabies is the only necessary item for reporting. The diagnosis is usually made by a positive direct fluorescent antibody test (preferably performed on CNS tissue) or by isolation of rabies virus in cell culture or in a laboratory animal.

RABIES, HUMAN

In humans, rabies is an acute encephalomyelitis that almost always progresses to coma and death within 10 days of the first symptom. Laboratory confirmation of the illness can be made in any of the following manners (although the CDC strongly recommends confirming the diagnosis by *all* the suggested methods): (1) direct fluorescent antibody of viral antigen in clinical specimen (preferably the brain or the nerves surrounding hair follicles in the nape of the neck), (2) isolation in cell culture or in a laboratory animal of rabies virus from saliva, cerebrospinal fluid, or CNS tissue, or (3) identification of a rabies neutralizing antibody titer of greater than 5 in the serum or cerebrospinal fluid of an unvaccinated person.

ROCKY MOUNTAIN SPOTTED FEVER

This is a tick-borne illness of acute onset and characterized by headache, myalgia, fever, and petechial rash that appears on the palms and soles in two-thirds of patients. Laboratory diagnosis may be made by one of several methods: (1) a fourfold or greater rise in antibody titer to *Rickettsia rickettsii* antigen by immunofluorescence antibody, complement fixation, latex agglutination, microagglutination, or indirect hemagglutination antibody test in acute and convalescent specimens taken 4 weeks apart, (2) positive polymerase chain reaction to *R. rickettsii,* (3) positive immunofluorescence of skin lesion (biopsy) or organ tissue (autopsy), or (4) isolation of *R. rickettsii* from a clinical specimen.

RUBELLA

Rubella is characterized by all the following: (1) acute onset of generalized maculopapular rash, (2) temperature greater than 37.2°C (99°F), if measures, and (3) arthralgia/arthritis, lymphadenopathy, or conjunctivitis. Laboratory confirmation is obtained by (1) isolation of rubella virus, (2) significant rise in serum rubella IgG titers between the acute and convalescent phases by any standard serologic assay, or (3) positive serologic test for rubella IgM. It should be noted that rubella IgM tests are occasionally falsely positive in persons with other viral illnesses such as Epstein-Barr virus, cytomegalovirus, or parvovirus infection or in the presence of rheumatoid factor.

RUBELLA, CONGENITAL SYNDROME

The congenital syndrome of rubella is an illness of infancy resulting from rubella virus infection in utero. Infants present with signs and symptoms from the following categories: (1) cataracts/congenital glaucoma, congenital heart disease, hearing loss, and pigmentary retinopathy or (2) purpura, splenomegaly, jaundice, microcephaly, mental retardation, meningoencephalitis, and radiolucent bone disease. Laboratory detection is undertaken by any of the following methods: (1) isolation of rubella virus, (2) demonstration of rubella-specific IgM, or (3) infant rubella antibody levels persistently high for longer than expected from passive maternal antibody transfer. Infant antibodies should decrease by a twofold dilution each month of life.

SALMONELLOSIS

Infection with *Salmonella* causes diarrhea, abdominal pain, and occasionally nausea and vomiting of variable severity. Infections may be asymptomatic or may cause extraintestinal disease. Isolation of *Salmonella* from a clinical specimen confirms the diagnosis.

SHIGELLOSIS

Shigellosis presents with diarrhea, nausea, abdominal cramping, and tenesmus of varying severity or may be asymptomatic. Isolation of *Shigella* from a clinical specimen confirms the diagnosis.

STREPTOCOCCAL DISEASE, INVASIVE, GROUP A

Invasive group A streptococcal disease is associated with any of several clinical syndromes, including (1) pneumonia, (2) bacteremia associated with cutaneous infection (cellulitis, erysipelas, or infection of a surgical or nonsurgical wound), (3) deep soft tissue infection (myositis or necrotizing fasciitis), (4) meningitis, (5) peritonitis, (6) osteomyelitis, (7) septic arthritis, (8) postpartum sepsis (puerperal fever), (9) neonatal sepsis, or (10) nonfocal bacteremia. Laboratory isolation of group A streptococci (*Streptococcus pyogenes*) by culture from a normally sterile site makes the diagnosis.

STREPTOCOCCUS PNEUMONIAE DRUG-RESISTANT INVASIVE DISEASE

Drug-resistant, invasive *S. pneumoniae* is associated with many clinical syndromes depending on the site of infection. Isolation of the organism from a normally sterile site and finding a "nonsusceptible" isolate form the crux of the diagnosis.

STREPTOCOCCAL TOXIC SHOCK SYNDROME

Streptococcal toxic shock syndrome (STSS) is a severe, rapidly progressive illness associated with either invasive or noninvasive group A streptococcal infection. This syndrome may occur with infection at any site but is most often associated with a cutaneous lesion. To be considered as STSS, all the following manifestations must be present within 48 h of hospitalization:

1. Hypotension: systolic blood pressure less than 90 mmHg for adults or less than the fifth percentile by age for children under 16 years of age.
2. Multiorgan involvement with two or more of the following:
   a. Renal: Creatinine greater than 2 mg/dL for adults, or twice the upper limit of normal for age, or twice the baseline value for persons with underlying renal dysfunction.

b. Coagulopathy: Platelets less than 100,000/μL or disseminated intravascular coagulopathy.
c. Hepatic: Total bilirubin, alanine aminotransferase, or aspartate aminotransferase twice the upper limit of normal for age or twice normal baseline values for those persons with underlying liver disease.
d. Respiratory: Adult respiratory distress syndrome.
e. Dermatologic: Generalized erythematous macular rash that may desquamate.
f. Musculoskeletal: Soft tissue necrosis including necrotizing fasciitis, myositis, or gangrene.

The laboratory diagnosis is made by isolating group A *Streptococcus* in a normally sterile site.

SYPHILIS

The manifestations of syphilitic illness vary with the time period between infection and detection. Primary syphilis is recognized by the one or more chancres, usually on the genitalia. Secondary syphilis is identified by the presence of localized or diffuse mucocutaneous lesions. The primary chancre may still be present. Laboratory diagnosis for primary or secondary syphilis rests on demonstrating *Treponema pallidum* by dark-field microscopy, direct fluorescent antibody (DFA-TP), or equivalent method.

Latent syphilis has no clinical symptoms. The early latent period occurs in those infected within the previous 12 months, and the late latent period refers to those infected for greater than 1 year. Persons in whom the period of infection cannot be documented and in whom there are no clinical symptoms are referred to as being latent of unknown duration. Laboratory diagnosis of latent syphilis can be made in one of the following ways: (1) no past diagnosis of syphilis and a reactive nontreponemal test (VDRL or RPR) and a reactive treponemal test (FTA-ABS or MHA-TP) or (2) history of syphilis therapy and current test titer with fourfold increase from last nontreponemal test titer.

Neurosyphilis is evident by the presence of CNS findings in the setting of a reactive serologic test for syphilis and a reactive VDRL in cerebrospinal fluid. Late syphilis with clinical manifestations other than neurosyphilis is manifested by inflammatory lesions of the cardiovascular system, bone, and skin. Rarely, lesions of the upper or lower respiratory tracts, mouth, eye, abdominal organs, reproductive organs, lymph nodes, or skeletal muscles occur. Evidence of late syphilis is seen after more than 15 years of untreated infection.

Syphilitic stillbirth is fetal death after at least a 20-week gestation or in a fetus weighing greater than 500 g in which the mother had untreated or inadequately treated syphilis at delivery. This should be reported as congenital syphilis.

SYPHILIS, CONGENITAL

Infection in utero with *T. pallidum* causes an illness of varying severity in children. Those under 2 years of age may present with hepatosplenomegaly, rash, condyloma lata, snuffles, jaundice (nonviral hepatitis), pseudoparalysis, anemia, or edema from nephrotic syndrome and/or malnutrition. Older children may have the stigmata of syphilis: interstitial keratitis, nerve deafness, anterior bowing of the shins, frontal bossing, mulberry molars, Hutchinson teeth, saddle nose, rhagades, or Clutton joints.

Identification of *T. pallidum* by dark-field microscopy, fluorescent antibody, or other specific stains in specimens from lesions, placenta, cord blood, or autopsy material confirms the diagnosis.

TETANUS

Tetanus has an acute onset and is characterized by hypertonia and/or painful muscular contractions typically of the muscles of the neck and jaw without other cause. Since there are no serologic tests available to confirm the suspicion of tetanus, a clinically compatible case is sufficient for diagnosis.

TOXIC SHOCK SYNDROME

Toxic shock syndrome is an illness manifested by

1. Temperature greater than or equal to 38.8°C (102°F)
2. Diffuse macular erythroderma
3. Desquamation, particularly affecting the palms and soles, 1 to 2 weeks following onset of illness
4. Hypotension, as defined by
   a. Systolic blood pressure less than or equal to 90 mmHg for adults or less than the fifth percentile by age for those persons under 16 years of age
   b. Orthostatic decrease in diastolic blood pressure greater than or equal to 15 mmHg from lying to sitting
   c. Orthostatic syncope or dizziness
5. Multisystem involvement (three or more):
   a. Gastrointestinal: vomiting or diarrhea at outset
   b. Muscular: Severe myalgia or creatinine phosphokinase twice the upper limit of normal
   c. Mucous membranes: Vaginal, oropharyngeal, or conjunctival hyperemia
   d. Renal: Blood urea nitrogen or creatinine twice the upper limit of normal or urinary sediment with pyuria in the absence of urinary tract infection
   e. Hepatic: Total bilirubin, alanine transferase, or aspartate transferase twice the upper limit of normal
   f. Hematologic: Platelets less than 100,000/μL
   g. Central nervous system: Disorientation or alteration in consciousness without focal neurologic signs when fever and hypotension are absent

Although the diagnosis is primarily a clinical one, laboratory evaluation should include no rise in Rocky Mountain spotted fever, leptospirosis, or measles titers, if obtained, and negative blood, throat, and cerebrospinal fluid cultures. Blood cultures positive for *Staphylococcus aureus* is not inconsistent with the diagnosis of toxic shock syndrome.

TRICHINOSIS

Trichinosis presents with variable manifestations. Most commonly a person will complain of fever, myalgia, and periorbital edema. Eosinophilia may be present on white blood cell differential. Trichinosis is caused by ingestion of *Trichinella* larvae in meat most commonly. On laboratory evaluation, *Trichinella* larvae may be found in tissue obtained by muscle biopsy, or the serologic test for *Trichinella* will be positive.

TUBERCULOSIS

Tuberculosis is a chronic infection characterized pathologically by formation of granulomas. Caused by *Mycobacterium tuberculosis,* the most common site of infection is the lungs, although other organs may be involved. The following criteria must be met for a reportable case of tuberculosis: (1) a positive tuberculin skin test, (2) other signs and symptoms compatible with tuberculosis (abnormal chest radiograph or clinical evidence of current disease), (3) treatment with two or more antituberculosis medications, and (4) completed diagnostic evaluation. Laboratory confirmation can be made by any of the following methods: (1) isolation of *M. tuberculosis* from a clinical specimen, (2) detection of *M. tuberculosis* from a clinical specimen by nucleic acid amplification test, or (3) acid-fast bacilli in a clinical specimen when culture has not or cannot be obtained.

TYPHOID FEVER

The insidious onset of fever, headache, malaise, anorexia, relative bradycardia, constipation or diarrhea, and cough are characteristic of typhoid fever. Caused by the bacteria *Salmonella typhi,* typhoid fever may be relatively mild or even asymptomatic. Isolation of *S. typhi* in blood, stool, or other clinical specimen seals the diagnosis.

YELLOW FEVER

This mosquito-borne viral illness presents with acute onset of fever, headache, myalgias, and conjunctival injection. This is followed by brief remission and recurrence of the preceding symptoms along with hepatitis, albuminuria, jaundice, and in some cases renal failure, shock, and generalized hemorrhages. Laboratory diagnosis of yellow fever is made on finding (1) a fourfold or greater rise in yellow fever titer in patients with no recent history of yellow fever vaccination and in whom cross-reaction to other flaviviruses has been excluded or (2) yellow fever virus antigen or genome in tissue, blood, or other body fluids.

REFERENCES

1. Centers for Disease Control and Prevention: Case definitions for infectious conditions under public health surveillance. *MMWR* 46(RR-10):1, 1997.
2. Centers for Disease Control and Prevention: 1993 Revised classification system for HIV infection and expanded surveillance case definition for AIDS among adolescents and adults. *MMWR* 41(RR-17):1, 1992.
3. Centers for Disease Control and Prevention: 1994 Revised classification system for human immunodeficiency virus infection in children less than 13 years of age. *MMWR* 43(RR-12):1, 1994.
4. www.cdc.gov/epo/mmwr/other/case_def/about.html.

148 OCCUPATIONAL EXPOSURES, INFECTION CONTROL, AND STANDARD PRECAUTIONS

Kathy J. Rinnert

The estimated 9.7 million people who receive care in emergency departments (EDs) each year in the United States represent a range of humanity that includes all age, racial, ethnic, and socioeconomic groups.[1] The diverse patient population and unpredictable ED work environment combine to create special hazards for health care personnel and increase their risk of occupational exposure to infectious agents.

This chapter examines standard precautions, infection control practices, and occupational exposures for health care providers in the prehospital setting and the ED. Routes of infectious disease exposure, infectious disease precautions, and use of personal protective equipment (PPE) are also discussed. Finally, occupational exposures commonly encountered in the ED are reviewed.

OCCUPATIONAL RISKS AND EXPOSURES

The Occupational Safety and Health Administration (OSHA) estimates that approximately 5.6 million workers are at risk for contact with blood and other body fluids during the performance of their work duties.[2] Of these, 4.4 million health care workers are at risk of exposure to potentially infectious materials. OSHA defines health care workers to include nurses, physicians, dentists and dental workers, laboratory and blood bank technologists, medical examiners, phlebotomists, ED personnel, intensive care and operating room technicians, orderlies, housekeeping personnel, and laundry workers. OSHA defines an additional 1.2 million non–health care workers also at risk for infectious exposure to include those in law enforcement; fire, rescue, and emergency medical services; correctional facilities; research laboratories; and the funeral industry.

OSHA defines *occupational exposure* as a "reasonably anticipated skin, eye, mucous membrane, or parenteral contact with blood or other potentially infectious materials that may result from the performance of the employee's duties."[2] OSHA defines *blood* as "human blood, blood products, or blood components." *Other potentially infectious materials* are defined as "human body fluids, such as saliva, semen, and vaginal secretions; cerebrospinal, synovial, pleural, pericardial, peritoneal, and amniotic fluids; any body fluids visibly contaminated with blood; unfixed human tissue or organs; HIV- or HBV [hepatitis B virus] containing cell or tissue cultures, culture mediums, or other solutions; and all body fluids where it is difficult or impossible to differentiate between body fluids." Health care workers should treat all bodily secretions, fluids, and tissues as potentially infectious substances.

Sources of exposure for blood-borne, airborne or droplet, and contact-related pathogens are multiple and varied. Low compliance with barrier precautions for blood-borne diseases has been demonstrated in hospital workers, emergency medical personnel, and air medical crews.[3–7] Activities that expose medical personnel to blood-borne diseases include placement of venous access, phlebotomy, needle recapping, specimen handling, administration of injected medications, lumbar puncture, chest tube insertion, airway suctioning, placement of nasogastric and orogastric tubes, intubation, placement of urinary catheters, and hemorrhage control. Health care activities that bring workers into close physical proximity to patients or their environment expose workers to airborne or droplet-dispersed organisms. Dressing changes, wound debridement, and wound irrigation may expose health care workers to contaminated materials or infectious agents. Workplace activities that may expose health care personnel to contact-dispersed organisms or parasites include cleaning patient care areas or equipment, changing linens, caring for incontinent and diapered patients, and physical examination. A seemingly innocuous physical examination (including integument, scalp, eyes, oropharynx, respiratory tract, and wounds) is not an activity without risk depending on the nature of the infectious agent or exposure source.

Many infectious diseases can be transmitted via blood or body fluid contamination, including HIV; hepatitis A virus (HAV), HBV, hepatitis C virus (HCV), and hepatitis D virus (HDV); cytomegalovirus; tetanus; tuberculosis (TB); herpes virus; malaria; Rocky Mountain spotted fever; and Creutzfeldt-Jakob disease. Some of these diseases are fatal (e.g., HIV), some are seriously debilitating and chronic (e.g., hepatitis), and some require protracted multidrug regimens due to drug resistance (e.g., TB).

Disease transmission may also occur by exposure to airborne nuclei, particle droplets, or contact (direct or indirect). Diseases spread by airborne droplet nuclei include measles, varicella and tuberculosis. Diseases transmitted by large particle droplets include *Haemophilus influenzae* type B, *Neisseria meningitidis*, pertussis, adenovirus, influenza, mumps, and rubella. Diseases spread by patient contact (direct contact) or by contact with items within the patient's environment (indirect contact) include *Clostridium difficile,* pediculosis, and scabies. Contact isolation may also apply to those patients with gastrointestinal, respiratory, skin, or wound colonization or infection with multidrug-resistant bacteria determined to be of special clinical and epidemiologic significance. Examples include methicillin-resistant *Staphylococcus aureus* and vancomycin-resistant enterococcus. The Hospital Infection Control Practices Advisory Committee of the Centers for Disease Control and Prevention (CDC) has developed a listing of selected infections and conditions that may be encountered in the ED, along with recommended occupational exposure precautions.[8,9]

While the geographic distribution and population incidence of most infectious diseases are well known, this does not imply that infectivity is limited to specific ethnic groups, races, or subsets of the population.[10–15] As the world population becomes increasingly mobile, patients with geographically isolated diseases may migrate to regions where the disease incidence may be low or nonexistent. In addition, many infectious diseases display heterogeneous and varying symptom complexes, including prolonged latent or asymptomatic stages.[16] Therefore, providing health care to an apparently healthy, asymptomatic patient does not preclude the possibility of disease infectivity and exposure. Since health care workers cannot readily identify those who are infected or risky, it is prudent to employ infection control practices and utilize PPE during all patient care activities. It is on this premise that the concept of standard precautions is based.

Portals for infectious disease entry are percutaneous, mucous membrane (oral, ocular, nasal, or rectal), respiratory, and dermal.

Percutaneous exposures are the most commonly reported and pose the highest risk for the contraction of blood-borne disease. It is estimated that only 10 percent of such injuries are reported.[17] Needle sticks or cuts by sharp objects account for the majority. Needle sticks by hollow needles have a higher rate of infection with HBV and HIV than do those by solid needles. It is postulated that this is due to the larger inoculum transferred to the worker within the bore of a hollow needle. Workplace activities that put personnel at risk for percutaneous injuries include phlebotomy, initiation of intravenous access, manipulation of access devices, suturing, and medication injection. Since the majority of these activities are nursing functions, it is not surprising that many studies document nurses as the most likely recipients of needle-stick injury.[17,18]

Mucous membrane exposures are the second most commonly reported occupational exposure and result from splatters, splashes, and sprays of blood and body fluids. Risk is entailed by such health care tasks as wound management (hemorrhage control, exploration, cleansing, irrigation, and debridement), airway suctioning, nasogastric or orogastric tube placement, intubation, and handling specimen containers of blood or body fluids.

Respiratory exposures result from the inhalation of airborne or droplet particulate materials. Health care workers risk respiratory exposure when they are confined with an expectorating, coughing, or sneezing patient for prolonged periods or in a poorly ventilated environment.

Dermal exposure involves skin contact with patients (direct contact) or environmental surfaces or objects that are contaminated with infectious materials (indirect contact). Risk of infection is increased if the place of worker contact is a large surface area or if the dermis is not intact (abraded, chapped, or excoriated). The emergence of drug-resistant organisms, such as methicillin-resistant *S. aureus* and vancomycin-resistant enterococci, pose additional exposure risk. Transmission of these diseases may be related to contact with infected patients, medical equipment used on them, or both. Workplace activities that place the health care worker at risk include patient examination, turning or moving patients, and changing linens or wound dressings. Parasites of the integument (e.g., scabies, lice, etc.) are also agents of dermal exposure. Other dermal exposures include hypersensitivity reactions of health care workers that may occur with prolonged or repeated exposure to specific inert substances (e.g., latex).

The risk of infection in an exposed health care provider depends on the route (portal) of exposure, the concentration (number of organisms) of pathogen in the infectious material, the infectious characteristics (virility) of the pathogen, the volume (dose) of infectious material, and the immunocompetence (susceptibility) of the exposed individual. Infectious characteristics may vary as the pathogen mutates, becoming resistant to treatment agents (e.g., antibiotics, antivirals, antifungals, etc.) or the host's immune defenses. The potential for infection may be incrementally higher as the route of exposure changes; that is, percutaneous exposures have greater potential for infection than do mucous membrane exposures, respiratory exposures, or dermal exposures.

As the number of organisms of the infectious agent increases, the rate of infectivity increases. For example, a percutaneous exposure to HBV carries a higher risk of infection than does a similar exposure to HIV. This higher rate of disease transmission is probably due to the higher concentration of virus in the blood of infected persons. It is reported that the concentration of virus in a HBV-infected individual is 100,000,000 free virus particles per cubic centimeter of blood, imparting a 6- to 30- percent risk of infection after a single percutaneous exposure. In contrast, there are 1000 free virus particles per cubic centimeter of blood in an HIV-infected patient, which imparts a 0.5 percent risk of infection following a percutaneous exposure. As the infectious disease state progresses, the concentration of microorganisms varies, depending on the immunocompetence or treatment status of the host. The CDC considers blood or blood-containing body fluids to be the "single most important source of HIV and HBV in the workplace setting." The strength (virility) of the infectious agent and the length (time) of exposure may also contribute to the transmission of blood-borne diseases, but the effect of these factors on infectivity is unclear.

INFECTION CONTROL

Infection control practices are designed to prevent transmission of microbial agents and to provide a wide margin of safety for health care workers. These practices were developed for hospital employees and other workers in health care facilities as a result of epidemiologic knowledge of blood-borne exposures and transmission rates.[3–6] Emergency personnel should utilize these practices to minimize infection due to contact with contaminated body secretions, devices, objects, or surfaces. Infection control practices include hand washing; use of personal protective equipment (PPE); cleaning, disinfecting, and sterilizing patient care equipment and environmental surfaces; decontamination and laundering of soiled uniforms, clothing, and patients' linens; disposal of needles, sharps, and infectious waste; and patient placement. Infection control measures that are simple, part of the routine work environment, and uniform across all situations have the greatest likelihood of compliance.

Basic infection control principles serve as a starting point for the prevention of infectious disease transmission. These principles are implemented in concert with other practices to prevent or mitigate exposure to transmissible infectious diseases. A complete infection control program includes administrative controls, equipment engineering, work practice controls, education of the work force, and medical management.

Administrative controls are designed to organize, define, and direct infection control activities. The most important of these activities is the development of a written infection control (exposure) plan. This plan defines all policies, procedures, and activities related to the education, prevention, and management of infectious diseases in the work force. Jobs and specific work tasks are identified and evaluated for potential exposure to infectious diseases. Initial and recurrent training in infectious disease hazards and risk activities must be provided to all health care workers. Risk reduction training and activities must be documented and monitored for adequate compliance. Other administrative controls include written policies and procedures for all infection control activities. Infection control monitoring, compliance, evaluation, modification, and quality improvement are to be clearly defined in policy and procedure documents.

Equipment engineering serves to reduce employee exposure by removing the hazard or isolating the health care provider from exposure. Examples of such equipment include self-sheathing needles, needleless drug administration devices, sharps containers, pocket masks, disposable airway equipment, syringe splash guards, and PPE. PPE is "specialized clothing or equipment which does not permit blood or potentially infectious substances to pass through or reach worker clothing, skin, eyes, mouth, or other mucous membranes under normal conditions of use."[2]

PPE includes such items as examination gloves, face masks, eye protection, face shields, and impervious gowns and aprons. The American Society for Testing and Materials has published specifications for examination gloves and protective clothing materials (gowns and shoe, sleeve, and leg covers).[19–25] In addition, the National Fire Protection Association (NFPA) specifies the minimum documentation, design and performance criteria, and test methods for emergency medical clothing.[26,27] Package labeling for PPE must describe components of the medical garment and indicate compliance with NFPA standards. Several sources make recommendations on the types of PPE to be worn during specific patient care activities.[7,28,29]

The most common barrier devices for infection control and prevention of blood exposures in the ED include examination gloves, eye and face protection, and disposable resuscitation equipment. Disposable, single-use examination gloves are standard in all health care settings. They are utilized when patient care activities involve potential exposure to blood, blood-containing body fluids, or other potentially infectious materials or contact with mucous membranes, tissues, or nonintact skin. Adequate supplies of gloves should be available to allow glove changes if significant contamination or loss of integrity (tears or punctures) occurs. Health care providers should avoid handling personal or common-use items (e.g., telephone, door handles, drinking cups, and combs) while wearing gloves to prevent environmental contamination. Gloves should fit tightly and extend above the wrist to provide maximal barrier protection for the wrist and lower forearm. Choice of glove ultimately depends upon individual preference and task performance needs. The potential for hypersensitivity reactions to glove component materials (latex, powder, etc.) must be taken into account when furnishing PPE for health care workers.

Emergency medical personnel who operate in the out-of-hospital environment (emergency medical services, air medical services, and interfacility transport services) may be exposed to situations where broken glass or sharp metal is exposed. In such cases, gloves with additional protective characteristics are needed. Structural firefighters' gloves are optimal and can be used during rescue and extrication activities. Firefighters' gloves can be replaced by examination gloves when patient care activities commence.

Face masks, eye protection, face shields, and gowns should be present in all EDs and emergency response vehicles. These barrier devices are used when anticipated exposure includes the possibility of splashes, sprays, arterial bleeding, or exsanguinating hemorrhage or when airway management techniques are undertaken. Face masks and eye protection should be worn simultaneously or a face shield employed to protect the ocular, oral, and nasal mucous membranes. Impervious aprons or gowns are appropriate if massive exposures are anticipated. Appropriately sized and adequate numbers of barrier devices should be available if gross contamination or loss of barrier integrity occurs. Additional uniform or work clothing and shower facilities should be available if contamination of clothing or dermal surfaces occurs.

Disposable resuscitation equipment should be readily available for all patient encounters requiring rescue breathing. Most bag-valve-masks, oxygen reservoirs, and tubing are meant to be discarded after each use. Reusable equipment must be cleaned and disinfected after each use. Disinfecting procedures for all reusable equipment (laryngoscope blade and handle, pocket mask, gurney, and patient care area) should be documented in policy and performed after each use.

Pocket masks are designed to isolate the health care provider from contact with blood, saliva, respiratory secretions, and vomitus. These masks vary in type and can be cleaned and disinfected for reuse or discarded after a single use. All personnel who may be called upon to render resuscitative efforts should have ready access to pocket masks.

Work practice controls modify the performance of a task to minimize exposure to blood and blood-containing body fluids and infectious materials. Work practice controls necessitate delineated policies concerning proper disposal of needles and sharps containers (i.e., avoid shearing, bending, recapping, or breaking); proper disposal of contaminated linens, clothing, and infectious waste; appropriate disinfection techniques for reusable equipment; and restriction of employee activities (e.g., avoidance of eating, drinking, smoking, and application of cosmetics) while in work areas that entail a reasonable likelihood of exposure to blood and body fluids.

Education of the work force on topics of infectious disease transmission, epidemiology, disease symptoms, portals of exposure, control methods, administrative compliance mechanisms, appropriate use and cleaning of medical equipment, use of PPE (barrier precautions), and medical management of infectious disease is necessary. In addition, there must be an awareness of the types of PPE to utilize and methods of risk reduction. Health care providers must also be aware that utilization of these devices does not totally eliminate infection risk.[30,31] Members of the work force are more likely to comply with infection control guidelines when they understand the purpose and reasoning that underlie recommendations for the use of PPE and specific risk reduction practices. Mandatory compliance with the utilization of PPE must be established in departmental or hospital policy and enforced in daily practice.

Medical directors and administrators of EDs should classify their work force (e.g., clerical personnel, coders, billers, supervisors, nurses, doctors, physicians' assistants, nurse practitioners, emergency medical technicians, paramedics, electrocardiogram technicians, radiography technicians, etc.), identify risky activities (e.g., hemorrhage control, intravenous access, phlebotomy, suctioning, intubation, etc.), and devise infection control plans. EDs should ensure initial and repeated infection control training programs; establish engineering and workplace controls; and administer postexposure medical evaluation, counseling, prophylaxis, and referral for health care workers with infectious disease exposures.

Medical management practices include preventive vaccinations, acute postexposure medical evaluation, infectious disease counseling, disease prophylaxis, and medical follow-up. Vaccines should be readily available to all health care personnel who may be exposed to infectious disease. OSHA mandates vaccines at initial employee training and within 10 days of employment for all personnel at risk of exposure.[2] In addition, mechanisms for postexposure medical management should be well defined and readily available to health care providers 24 h/day. Once a blood exposure has occurred, policies and procedures for exposure management must be understood and followed by all employees. An exposure incident is a "specific eye, mouth, or other mucous membrane, nonintact skin, or parenteral contact with blood or other potentially infectious materials."[2] An established reporting policy for exposed personnel should include medical assessment, prophylaxis, and follow-up appropriate to the type and source of the exposure.[28,32] As with any medical evaluation, the confidentiality of the source patient and employee must be strictly maintained.[33]

LEGISLATIVE REGULATIONS

OSHA has drafted federal regulations that prescribe safeguards to protect workers and reduce risk of exposure to blood-borne diseases.[34] These standards were first published in Title 29, Code of Federal Regulations, part 1910.1030, in December 1991.[35] Title 29 (the blood-borne standard) requires employers of one or more individuals "who can reasonably be expected to come into contact with blood or specified body fluids during the performance of their duties" to develop programs involving five major initiatives for the mitigation of blood-borne disease transmission: (1) development of a written exposure control plan, (2) utilization of engineering controls to reduce risk by removing the hazard or isolating the worker from exposure, (3) utilization of work practice controls to standardize and maximize the safety with which work tasks are performed, (4) identification of mechanisms for compliance with Title 29 standards, and (5) communication of workplace hazards to those with potential for blood-borne disease exposures. Workplace education should include information about the agents of infectious disease, epidemiology, methods of disease transmission, disease signs and symptoms, risky work tasks, risk reduction strategies, and postexposure management. Such education must occur at initial employment, with repeated training provided at specified intervals.

INFECTION PRECAUTIONS

In 1987, the CDC recommended the use of blood and body substance precautions for all patients through a system called universal precautions. The initial precautions applied to all body substances. These recommendations were revised in 1988 to include only those body fluids associated epidemiologically with transmission of blood-borne pathogens.[36] Exposures related to oropharyngeal or respiratory secretions (airborne or droplet), parasitic infectious exposures, and contact exposures were not considered in the revised precautions. Confusion resulted, with hospitals adopting some but not all aspects of universal precautions or body substance isolation. Such confusion has led to lack of uniformity in infectious disease precautions from facility to facility. The focus of universal precautions and body substance isolation is on blood and blood-containing fluids, and the recommendations inadequately address infections transmitted by air or droplet. Confusion, lack of uniform application of infection control precautions, and the emergence of antibiotic-resistant organisms have promoted the development of a new system that is simple, is easy to apply, and pertains to all methods of infectious disease transmission.

In 1996, the Hospital Infection Control Practices Advisory Committee of the CDC devised a new system of isolation precautions to address all methods of disease transmission and to bring uniformity to hospital infection control practices. The new guidelines contain two tiers of precautions: standard and transmission-based. Standard precautions combine the major features of body substance isolation and universal precautions. Transmission-based precautions are designed for patients with documented or suspected transmissible pathogens for which additional protection beyond standard precautions is required. Transmission-based precautions are of three types: airborne, droplet, and contact. They are to be utilized in addition to, not in place of, standard precautions.[37] Unlike universal precautions, which list specific body fluids that may transmit blood-borne pathogens, or body substance isolation, which considers all body fluids to pose risk for transmission of blood-borne pathogens, standard precautions assume a broader approach to health care and patient protection, by including agents transmitted by routes other than blood.

Standard Precautions

Standard precautions should be exercised when caring for *all* patients and include hand washing, gloves, mask and eye protection or face shield, gowns, handling of patient care equipment and linens, environmental controls, workplace controls, and patient placement.

Hand washing is to be performed after touching blood, body fluids, secretions, excretions, and contaminated items *whether or not* gloves are worn. Hands should be washed immediately after gloves are removed, between patient contacts, and when otherwise indicated to avoid the transfer of organisms to other patients or environments. It may be necessary to wash hands between procedures on the same patient to prevent cross-contamination of various body sites. Plain soap and water are recommended for routine use. Washing with an antimicrobial agent or waterless antiseptic may be utilized for control of outbreaks or hyperendemic infections.

Clean, nonsterile gloves are to be used when touching blood, body fluids, secretions, excretions, and contaminated items. Clean gloves should be used before touching nonintact skin and mucous membranes. Gloves should be changed between tasks and procedures following contact with material that may contain a high concentration of microorganisms. Gloves should be removed and hands washed before touching noncontaminated items, environmental surfaces, or other patients.

TABLE 148-1 Airborne-Spread Infectious Diseases

Rubeola (measles)
Varicella (including disseminated zoster)
Tuberculosis

Source: Modified from Centers for Disease Control and Prevention.[8]

Face masks, eye protection, and face shields should be fluid resistant and are worn to protect mucous membranes of the eyes, nose, and mouth during patient care activities and the performance of procedures likely to generate splashes or sprays of blood, body fluids, secretions, excretions, and infectious materials. Masks that become significantly soiled, moistened by the user's exhaled vapor, or contaminated by fluids should be immediately replaced, since loss of protective function occurs if the barrier device is completely saturated.

Clean, nonsterile gowns should be fluid resistant and used to protect the worker's skin and clothing during patient care activities and the performance of activities likely to generate splashes or sprays of blood, body fluids, secretions, and excretions. The gown selected should be appropriate for the type and volume of fluid likely to be encountered. Soiled gowns should be replaced as soon as possible, since barrier protection is lost if the garment is saturated with contamination. Sleeve protectors, booties, and leggings should be used if a large volume of contamination or infectious material difficult to contain is anticipated.

Patient care equipment and linens soiled with blood, body fluids, secretions, and excretions should be handled to prevent skin and mucous membrane exposure, contamination of clothing, and transfer of microorganisms to other patients and environments. Reusable items should be cleaned and reprocessed to eliminate infectivity. Single-use items should be discarded properly.

Environmental controls relate to hospital procedures for the decontamination of objects in patient care areas. Environmental surfaces, beds, bed rails, bedside equipment, and frequently touched surfaces should be cleaned and disinfected between patient use.

Workplace controls (work practice controls) include proper disposal techniques for needles, scalpels, and other sharp instruments. Proper handling of these devices should stress the avoidance of recapping, excessive handling, and manipulation. Proper disposal should emphasize the use of self-sheathing devices, use of puncture-resistant containers, and routine replacement of sharps containers prior to overflowing. Patients who contaminate the environment or those who cannot assist in their own hygiene should be placed in a private room if available.

Airborne Precautions

In addition to standard precautions, airborne precautions are utilized for patients known to be or suspected of being infected with microorganisms transmitted by airborne droplet nuclei. Airborne precautions also apply to small particle residue (5 μm or smaller) of evaporated droplets containing microorganisms that remain suspended in the air and can be dispersed widely by air currents over a long distance. Examples of infectious agents spread by this method are found in Table 148-1.

As with standard precautions, utilization of previously described techniques for hand washing, gloves, face mask and eye protection or face shield, gowns, equipment and linen, environmental controls, and workplace controls applies. The placement of patients in the ED requires a room with (1) monitored negative air pressure in relation to surrounding areas, (2) 6 to 12 air changes per hour, and (3) discharge of the room air to the outdoors or high-efficiency filtration of the air before it is circulated to other areas in the hospital. The door to the patient's room must be kept closed, and the patient must remain in the room. Movement and transportation of the patient should be limited. If movement is unavoidable, the patient should wear respiratory protection to avoid contamination of other areas within the hospital. Health care providers entering the room must wear respiratory protection, such as a personalized, fitted mask with efficient filters (approved particulate respirator).

Droplet Precautions

In addition to standard precautions, droplet precautions are employed for patients known to have or suspected of having serious illnesses transmitted by large particle droplets (>5 μm in size) that can be generated by the patient during talking, sneezing, or coughing or during the performance of procedures. Examples of infectious agents spread by this method are listed in Table 148-2.

As with standard precautions, utilization of previously described techniques for hand washing, glove, face mask and eye protection or face shield, gown, equipment and linen, environmental controls, and workplace controls applies. Patients should be placed in a private room. Special air handling and ventilation are not required, and the door may remain open. If a private room is not available, the patient may be placed in a room with other patients who have active infections with the same microorganism (i.e., cohorting). When this is not achievable, maintain spatial separation of at least 3 ft between the infected patient and other patients and visitors. Patient transportation should be limited to essential procedures only. Patients who must be moved to other areas of the hospital for testing and procedures should don face masks to minimize the dispersal of droplets. Health care personnel should observe standard precautions and wear face masks when working within 3 ft of the patient.

Contact Precautions

In addition to standard precautions, contact precautions should be utilized with patients known to have or suspected of having serious illnesses easily transmitted by direct patient contact or by contact with items in the patient's environment. Examples of such infectious diseases are seen in Table 148-3.

As with standard precautions, utilization of previously described techniques for hand washing, glove, face mask and eye protection or face shield, gown, equipment and linen, environmental controls, and workplace controls applies. If the examination and care of a patient result in contact with infective materials and a high concentration of microorganisms (wound drainage or fecal material), changing of gloves is required. Hand washing with an antimicrobial agent or waterless antiseptic is required after removal of gloves. After glove removal and hand washing, workers should avoid contact with potentially contaminated environmental surfaces or items in the patient's room.

In addition to wearing a gown as described in the standard precautions, one should wear a clean, nonsterile gown upon entering a patient's room if one anticipates substantial contact with the patient or if the patient is incontinent or has diarrhea, a colostomy, an ileostomy, or wound drainage not contained by dressings. The gown should be removed prior to leaving the patient's room, and care should be taken to avoid contact with potentially contaminated environmental surfaces.

Transportation and movement should be limited to essential purposes only. If the patient must be moved to another treatment area, one should ensure that contamination spread is minimized by large, bulky dressings.

Medical equipment (e.g., blood pressure cuffs, stethoscopes, bedside commodes, etc.) should be dedicated to a single patient (or cohort of similarly infected patients) to avoid sharing between noninfected patients. Health care personnel who use personal medical equipment (e.g., stethoscopes) should thoroughly clean these items between using them on different patients if the possibility of contamination exists.

Specific workplace activities and medical devices may significantly mitigate the occupational exposures experienced by health care personnel. These task-related and device-related recommendations are found in Tables 148-4 and 148-5, respectively.

TABLE 148-2 Droplet-Spread Infectious Diseases

Invasive *Haemophilus influenzae* type B (including meningitis, pneumonia, epiglottis, sepsis)
Invasive *Neisseria meningitidis* (including meningitis, pneumonia, sepsis)
Serious bacterial respiratory infections: Diphtheria (pharyngeal) *Mycoplasma* pneumonia Pertussis Pneumonic plague Streptococcal pharyngitis, pneumonia, scarlet fever
Serious viral infections: Adenovirus Influenza Mumps Parvovirus B19 Rubella

Source: Modified from Centers for Disease Control and Prevention.[8]

TABLE 148-3 Contact Spread Infectious Diseases

Multidrug-resistant infections or colonization (gastrointestinal, respiratory, skin, wound sites)
Enteric infections with low infective dose or prolonged environmental survival: *Clostridium difficile* Enterohemorrhagic *Escherichia coli* 0157:H7 *Shigella* Hepatitis A Rotavirus
Respiratory syncytial virus
Parainfluenza virus
Enteroviral infections
Skin infections that are highly contagious or that may occur on dry skin: Diphtheria (cutaneous) Herpes simplex virus (neonatal or mucocutaneous) Impetigo Major, noncontained abscesses, cellulitis, decubiti Pediculosis Scabies Staphylococcal furunculosis Herpes zoster (disseminated or in an immunocompromised host)
Viral hemorrhagic conjunctivitis
Viral hemorrhagic infections (Ebola, Lassa, Marburg)

Source: Modified from Centers for Disease Control and Prevention.[8]

COMMON OCCUPATIONAL EXPOSURES

Hepatitis

Hepatitis is most commonly caused by a virus. More than 90 percent of cases of viral hepatitis in humans are caused by five viruses: HAV,

TABLE 148-4 Task-Specific Recommendations for Use of PPE

Patient Care Activity	Disposable Gloves	Mask and Protective Eyewear	Impervious Gown
Measuring blood pressure	No*	No	No
Measuring pulse	No*	No	No
Measuring temperature	No*	No	No
Examination of bleeding patient	Yes	No†	No†
Wound management, dressing	Yes	No†	No†
Minor hemorrhage control	Yes	No†	No†
Profuse hemorrhage control	Yes	Yes	Yes
Cardiopulmonary resuscitation	Yes	No†	No†
Venipuncture	Yes	No	No
Intravenous line placement	Yes	No	No
IM, SQ, IV medication administration	Yes	No	No
Cricothyrotomy, needle decompression	Yes	Yes	No
Intubation, airway adjunct placement, suctioning	Yes	Yes	No
Childbirth	Yes	Yes	Yes
Nasogastric or orogastric tube placement	Yes	Yes	No†
Specimen handling	Yes	No	No

*Utilize gloves if task performance includes possible contact with patient's blood, secretions, or body fluids.
†Utilize mask, protective eyewear, and impervious gown if possibility of splashing or spray exists.
Source: Adapted from Kelen et al.[7]

TABLE 148-5 Task-Specific Recommendations for Use of Medical Safety Devices

Patient Care Activity	Self-Sheathing Needles	Needleless Administration Devices	Splash Guards	Sharps Containers
Wound care, lavage	No	No	Yes	No
Venipuncture	Yes	No	No	Yes
Intravenous line placement	Yes	No	No	Yes
IM, SQ, IV medication administration	Yes	Yes	No	Yes
Cricothyrotomy, needle decompression	Yes	No	No	Yes
Intubation, airway adjunct placement, suctioning	No	No	No	No†
Nasogastric or orogastric tube placement	No	No	No	No†
Specimen handling	No*	No	No	No†
Childbirth	No	No	No	No†
Resuscitation activities	Yes	Yes	No	Yes

*Utilize self-sheathing device if specimen has needle permanently attached.
†Utilize sharps container or noncrush container for contaminated hardware, devices, equipment, or specimens.
Source: Adapted from Kelen et al,[7] with permission.

HBV, HCV (or classic non-A, non-B hepatitis virus), HDV (or delta agent), and hepatitis E virus [(HEV) or epidemic non-A, non-B hepatitis virus].

These five viruses are each very different and share only a common tropism for the liver, with the hepatocyte representing the dominant site for viral replication and acute or chronic hepatitis as the major clinical manifestation of infection. The viruses can be divided into two distinct groups based upon the existence of a lipid-containing outer envelope.[38] HBV, HCV, and HDV all possess a lipid-containing outer viral envelope. HAV and HEV, lacking a lipid envelope, are stable when secreted from infected hepatocytes into bile and thus gain entry into the gastrointestinal tract. These viruses are spread by the fecal-oral route and can cause extensive single-source outbreaks of disease. HAV and HEV do not cause persistent infection, nor have they been identified as the causative agents of chronic viral hepatitis. In contrast, HBV, HCV, and HDV, because of their lipid envelope, are probably inactivated by bile. Therefore, these viruses are not shed into the gastrointestinal tract in biologically significant amounts. These viruses are transmitted by several routes, including virus shed from mucous membranes or by percutaneous exposure. HBV, HCV, and HDV may each cause persistent infection, and all three have been identified as etiologic agents in chronic viral hepatitis and cirrhosis. Persistent infections caused by HBV and HCV may ultimately result in the development of primary hepatocellular carcinoma.

HAV is a single-stranded RNA virus within the genus *Hepatovirus* of the family Picornaviridae. HAV is worldwide in its distribution, with the highest prevalence of infection in geographical regions with substandard water and sanitation. It is estimated that there are between 125,000 and 200,000 infections per year in the United States, where risk factors associated with disease acquisition include living in the same household with a hepatitis patient (≈25 percent of patients), close contact with young children attending day-care centers (≈18 percent), sexual activity with oral-anal contact (≈11 percent), and foreign travel to areas where hepatitis A is endemic (≈4 percent).[39] It is noteworthy that approximately 40 percent of patients report no apparent risk factor. While most cases of hepatitis A can be explained by fecal-oral transmission, association with injected drug use has been reported by 2 percent of patients.[38] While this association may reflect the general living conditions and poor sanitation that may be associated with injected drug users, acute infection with HAV is associated with a substantial viremia that may persist for several weeks. Percutaneous transmission of the virus may be possible if individuals share nonsterile needles during the prodromal phase.

Recently developed formalin-killed whole virus vaccines are highly effective in the prevention of hepatitis A. Two such vaccines are being used in the United States: Havrix (Smith-Kline Beecham) and Vaqta (Merck and Company.)[40] These vaccines are given as a single primary immunization with a booster dose at 6 to 12 months. Immunizations should target individuals with increased risk of acquiring hepatitis A or those who are at increased risk of fatal, fulminant disease, including children in communities where hepatitis A is endemic, travelers to developing nations, male homosexuals, and injected drug users. People with underlying liver disease, particularly those over 50, are at increased risk of fulminant hepatitis A and should be immunized. Preventive measures for health care providers include the use of standard precautions with the addition of contact precautions when caring for patients who are incontinent or diapered.

HBV is a partially double-stranded, circular DNA virus of the family Hepadnaviridae. HBV is worldwide in its distribution and is an important cause of acute and chronic hepatitis. Approximately 300,000 new cases of HBV B are reported in the United States each year. It is estimated that 300 million people worldwide are chronic carriers, with approximately 1 million of them in the United States.[41] Ninety-five percent of adult cases resolve spontaneously, while 5 percent of patients develop chronic hepatitis B. In contrast, neonates develop the chronic form in 90 percent of cases.[42] Percutaneous exposure to blood, sexual transmission, and perinatal transmission account for most HBV infections in humans. In 1972, mandatory screening for HBV began on donor blood; as a result, the risk of posttransfusion transmission of HBV is extremely low.

Active prophylaxis against HBV infection has been available since 1982. These highly effective, recombinant vaccines are available in two commercial products: Recombivax HB (Merck and Company) and Engerix-B (Smith Kline Beecham). These vaccines are given as a series of three intramuscular injections at 0, 1, and 6 months. As of this writing, neonatal and infant HBV vaccination has been suspended until a mercury-free vehicle is developed. While the need for booster vaccination is unclear, it has been suggested that revaccination occur after an interval of 10 years. Current recommendations are to vaccinate all newborn infants and all adolescents and adults in high-risk groups. Passive immunity is available using hepatitis B immunoglobulin (HBIG), which is prepared from the pooled serum of patients with spontaneous recovery from acute HBV. HBIG is given simultaneously with HBV vaccine to adults not immune to HBV who have experienced percutaneous or sexual exposures and newborns whose mothers are hepatitis B surface antigen (HBsAg) positive. Highest efficacy is found when HBIG is administered within 12 h of exposure to HBV. Completion of the HBV vaccine series at 1 and 6 months must be performed to ensure long-term (>10 years) immunity. The CDC currently recommends a postvaccination titer be obtained within 1 to 6 months of completing the vaccine series.

Health care workers who are exposed to blood or body fluids in their daily work are at increased risk for acquiring HBV. In the CDC study of HBV infections in sentinel counties, health care providers accounted for only 1 percent of cases, compared to heterosexual contact with multiple partners (27 percent), injected drug use (14 percent), and homosexual contacts (11 percent). The risk of acquiring HBV after an accidental needle stick from a patient with HBV varies from 20 percent if the patient is HBsAg positive to 66 percent if the patient is both HBsAg and hepatitis B e antigen positive.[42] Preventive measures for health care providers include the use of standard precautions and HBV vaccination. Postexposure medical examination, counseling, treatment (HBIG and HBV vaccine), and follow-up are required.

HCV is an enveloped, single-stranded RNA virus of the flavivirus family. It was discovered in 1988 and identified as the agent responsible for most cases of non-A, non-B hepatitis. HCV is the most common chronic blood-borne infection in the United States and a major cause of chronic liver disease worldwide. Throughout the 1980s, an average of 230,000 new infections occurred each year in the United States.[43] Between 1989 and 1996, the annual number of infections declined by more than 80 percent, to 36,000.[43] The Third National Health and Nutrition Examination Survey, conducted between 1988 and 1994, estimates that 3.9 million Americans (1.8 percent) have been infected with HCV.[44] While most acute infections are asymptomatic, serious sequelae result from this infection. Persistent infection develops in most HCV-infected patients (>85 percent). Chronic hepatitis develops in approximately 60 to 70 percent of HCV-infected patients and may progress to cirrhosis (10 to 20 percent) and hepatocellular carcinoma (1 to 5 percent).[45,46] Factors that may influence the severity and progression of disease in patients with chronic HCV infection include alcohol-induced liver disease, older age at the time of infection, male gender, and immunodeficiency.

The most common and the efficient route of transmission of HCV is parenteral. Before the first immunoassays for detecting antibodies to HCV were introduced in 1990, transfusion of blood and blood products accounted for approximately 90 percent of infections. Measures such as deferral of high-risk donors and widespread use of hepatitis antibody testing have decreased the risk of contracting HCV to 1 in 100,000 U transfused. In contrast, injected drug usage has consistently accounted for a substantial portion of HCV infections and currently accounts for 60 percent of HCV transmissions in the United States.[47]

The prevalence of HCV infection among health care workers is no greater than in the general population, averaging 1 to 2 percent, which is 10 times lower than the prevalence of HBV.[48–52] The average incidence of anti-HCV seroconversion after unintentional needle sticks or sharps exposure from an HCV-positive source is 1.8 percent (range, 0 to 7 percent).[53] Since no vaccine currently exists, preventive measures must focus on counseling, screening high-risk populations (injected drug users, recipients of blood clotting factor concentrates before 1987, recipients of blood and solid organ transplants before 1992, and chronic hemodialysis patients), and use of infection control practices. Preventive measures for health care providers include the use of standard precautions.

HDV is a single-stranded, circular RNA virus. The genome of HDV is contained within an envelope provided by HBV. Although HBV surface proteins are required for HDV viral assembly, they are not needed for viral replication. HDV infection can occur simultaneously with HBV infection (coinfection) or as a superinfection of patients with chronic HBV infection. While coinfection increases the initial severity of the acute HBV infection, the progression to an HBV carrier state occurs less frequently. HDV superinfection tends to increase the frequency and severity of clinical sequelae of chronic HBV infection. Currently, no evidence links HDV with progression to hepatocellular carcinoma.

The prevalence of HDV is unclear; serologic markers of HDV in an HBV coinfection become unmeasurable within 1 to 5 years. There is similar difficulty in testing for HDV superinfection. HDV infections are rare in the United States. In countries with increased HBV endemicity, such as Greece, Italy, Jordan, and Egypt, as many as 50 percent of chronic HBV-infected patients may exhibit superinfection with HDV.[54]

HDV is transmitted primarily by parenteral contact with blood. Sexual and vertical transmission of HDV is reported, but it is less efficient than with HBV. Prevention of HDV depends on prevention of HBV infection (immunization) and reducing exposure to blood (reduction of high-risk behaviors). No vaccine for HDV currently exists. Preventive measures for health care providers include the use of standard precautions.

HEV is a nonenveloped, single-stranded RNA virus provisionally classified in the Caliciviridae family. HEV is the major etiologic agent of enterically transmitted non-A, non-B hepatitis worldwide. The virus is endemic and epidemic in developing countries that lack the infrastructure to ensure adequate sanitation and water purification. HEV is spread primarily by the fecal-oral route. The clinical infection mimics HAV, and infections usually resolve without sequelae. The case fatality rate is low except in pregnant women, in whom it may approach 20 percent.[55] No vaccine for HEV currently exists. Preventive measures for health care providers include the use of standard precautions with the addition of contact precautions when caring for patients who are incontinent or diapered.

Hepatitis G virus (HGV), characterized in 1996, is a flavivirus. It is estimated that there are 900 to 2000 infections each year in the United States, the majority being asymptomatic or minimally symptomatic. Transmission has been documented through blood transfusions and vertical transmission from mother to infant in the perinatal period.[56] Coinfection with HBV and HCV is common, probably reflecting similar modes of transmission. HGV is the only identifiable agent in 0.3 percent of community-acquired acute hepatitis.[57] No vaccine for HGV currently exists. Preventive measures for health care providers include the use of standard precautions.

Human Immunodeficiency Virus

HIV is an enveloped genome of two identical, single-stranded RNA molecules. HIV, classified as a retrovirus in the subfamily lentivirus, replicates in activated CD4 T lymphocytes. There are two types of human lentiviruses: HIV-1, the predominant HIV type in most parts of the world, and HIV-2, primarily found in West Africa.[58] As of December 1996, the Joint United Nations Programme on HIV/AIDS estimated that there were a total of 27 million adults and 2.6 million children with HIV infection. Of these cases, 62 percent occurred in sub-Saharan Africa and 23 percent in South and Southeast Asia.[59] As of 1996, there were at least five African nations with adult prevalence of HIV greater than 10 percent. In 1996, there were over 32,000 deaths in the United States due to HIV and/or AIDS, ranking it the eighth leading cause of death in the nation.[60] The capacity of HIV to recombine and generate mosaic genotypes confounds treatment efforts and vaccine development. The virus mutates at varying rates over time in various individuals, and data suggest that the host's ongoing immune response is a driving force for genetic variation.

More than 70 percent of HIV infections are due to unprotected heterosexual intercourse. Other important modes of transmission include unprotected homosexual intercourse, injected drug use, mother-infant vertical transmission, and blood transfusions. Blood screening, use of a voluntary donor pool, and more rational use of blood products has greatly reduced transfusions as a means of infection.

Percutaneous injury with exposure to HIV-infected blood in health care workers accounts for 80 percent of occupational exposures.[17] The average risk of HIV infection from all types of percutaneous exposures to HIV-infected blood is 0.3 percent.[61] Risk of infection is increased for deep injury, injury by a device previously placed in the source patient's artery or vein, visible blood on the device causing the injury, and death of the source patient as a result of AIDS within 60 days postexposure. The risks of acquiring HIV after mucous membrane and skin exposure to HIV-infected blood are approximately 0.1 percent and less than 0.1 percent respectively.[17] As previously mentioned, large-volume exposures, increased viral titer in the source patient, large surface area of contact, and loss of integrity in mucous membranes or skin may increase the risks of acquiring HIV. Chemoprophylaxis should be recommended to exposed workers after occupational exposures associated with highest risk for HIV transmission. The US Public Health Service has published guidelines for the management of health care workers exposed to HIV with recommendations for postexposure prophylaxis (Tables 148-6, 148-7, and 148-8).[62] Chemoprophylaxis should begin as soon as possible after the exposure, ideally within 1 to 2 h. Animal studies show that antiretrovirals are not effective if started later than 24 to 36 h after the exposure event. No vaccine for HIV currently exists. Preventive measures for health care providers include the use of standard precautions. Postexposure medical examination, counseling, treatment (antivirals based on risk evaluation), and follow-up should be readily available to health care personnel.

Tuberculosis

TB is a global epidemic that is expected to result in an estimated 90 million new cases and 30 million deaths during the current decade.[63] Four subspecies of mycobacteria exist, each of which can cause tubercular disease: *Mycobacterium africanum, Mycobacterium bovis, Mycobacterium microti,* and *Mycobacterium tuberculosis.* Mycobacteria are slow-growing, aerobic rods with lipid-laden cell walls, which account for its acid-fast-staining characteristics. *Mycobacterium tuberculosis* is the primary cause of TB in humans.[64] According to the World Health Organization Global Tuberculosis Programme, *M. tuberculosis* kills more adults in the world each year then any other single pathogen.[65] During 1997, approximately 19,900 (7.4 cases per 100,000) cases of TB were reported in the United States.[66] This represents a 7 percent decrease from 1996 and a 26 percent decrease from 1992.[66] In 1997, six states (California, Florida, Illinois, New Jersey, New York, and Texas) reported 57 percent of all TB cases in the United States.[67] From 1992 to 1997, a substantial decline in the number of TB cases has been noted among US-born persons in all age groups. During this same time, the number of cases among foreign-born persons has increased by approximately 6 percent. Approximately 7.6 percent of isolates in 1997 were resistant to at least one antibacterial, isoniazid, and 1.3

TABLE 148-6 Determine Exposure Code (EC)

Exposure* Type	No PEP	EC 1	EC 2	EC 3
Intact skin only†	X			
Mucous membrane or skin integrity, compromised‡ with small volume exposure (e.g., few drops, short duration)		X		
Mucous membrane or skin integrity, compromised‡ with large volume exposure [e.g., several drops, major splash and/or long duration (i.e., several minutes or more)]			X	
Percutaneous exposure, less severe (e.g., solid needle, superficial scratch)			X	
Percutaneous exposure, more severe (e.g., large-bore hollow needle, deep puncture, visible blood on device, needle used in source patient's artery or vein)§				X

*Exposure refers to the source material blood, bloody fluid, or an instrument contaminated with these substances. In cases of exposure to OPIM (other potentially infectious material, e.g., semen or vaginal secretions; cerebrospinal, synovial, pleural, peritoneal, pericardial, or amniotic fluids; or tissue), or an instrument contaminated with one or more of these substances, determination of the need for PEP must be made on a case-by-case basis. OPIM are considered a low risk for transmission in health care settings. Any unprotected contact to concentrated HIV in a research laboratory or production facility is considered an occupational exposure that requires clinical evaluation to determine the need for PEP.
†Contact with intact skin not normally considered a risk for HIV transmission. However, if the exposure was to blood and the circumstances suggest a higher volume exposure (e.g., an extensive area of skin was exposed or there was prolonged contact with blood), the risk of HIV transmission should be considered.
‡Skin integrity is considered compromised if there is evidence of chapped skin, dermatitis, abrasion, or open wound.
§The combination of these severity factors (e.g., large-bore hollow needle *and* deep puncture) contribute to an elevated risk for transmission if the source person is HIV-positive.
Source: From Centers for Disease Control and Prevention,[62] with permission.

percent were resistant to two agents, isoniazid and rifampin (multidrug-resistant TB).[66] Outbreaks of multidrug-resistant TB, particularly among HIV-infected persons, contributed to the resurgence of TB in the late 1980s and early 1990s.

Transmission of TB occurs through inhalation of aerosolized bacilli. Fewer than 1 to 10 bacilli can cause infection, but only about 20 percent of exposed individuals become infected.[68] Infectious individuals expel large droplets by coughing or sneezing. Large droplets are usually trapped in the upper airways of exposed individuals, where mechanical barriers prevent access to the alveoli. Some droplets partially evaporate into smaller droplet nuclei (1 to 5 μm), which remain suspended in the environment for extended periods and are easily carried by air currents. Small droplet nuclei, containing 1 to 3 tubercle bacilli, have an approximately 50 percent chance of reaching the alveoli after inhalation.[68]

Control measures for TB have included the widespread use of bacille Calmette-Guérin (BCG) vaccine and the provision of unsupervised pharmacologic therapy. While the BCG vaccine has the highest coverage of any vaccine in the World Health Organization Expanded Programme on Immunization, randomized and placebo-controlled trials have shown efficacy ranges from 0 to 80 percent.[65] Since evidence exists that the vaccine confers protection against serious forms of childhood TB (disseminated and meningeal TB), which have high rates of morbidity and mortality, the vaccine will continue to be a component of childhood immunization strategies in developing countries. BCG has never been recommended in the United States because of its low efficacy and due to the dermal hypersensitivity it induces with purified protein derivative. Preventive measures advocated by the CDC include environmental controls (negative-pressure ventilation and ultraviolet radiation) in health care settings, application of directly observed therapy, and vaccine development. Occupational exposures for health care providers can be mitigated through use of standard and airborne precautions.

Mumps

Mumps is a systemic disease caused by the mumps virus, which belongs to the paromyxovirus family. Humans are the only known host. Although infection and swelling of the parotid gland (parotitis) is a hallmark of the disease, involvement of the central nervous system and testes occur frequently. Incidence of mumps has decreased steadily since the introduction of live mumps vaccine in 1967, with routine use of the preparation beginning in 1977. In 1995, 906 cases were reported, representing a 99 percent decrease from the 185,691 cases reported in 1968.[69]

Mumps is transmitted by infectious droplets rather than by true airborne spread. While isolation of patients is the mainstay of outbreak control, this mechanism is not effective in preventing subsequent cases. Primary prevention by immunization is preferred. A monovalent mumps vaccine (Mumpsvax, Merck and Company) available in the United States is a live virus-vaccine (Jeryl-Lynn strain) that is prepared in egg culture. This vaccine is 97 percent effective in producing measurable antibody in susceptible individuals to whom the vaccine is administered. Various tri- and bivalent preparations are available as combination vaccines for mumps, measles, and rubella. Current recommendations for infectious disease (including mumps, measles, and rubella) vaccinations are published in the Red Book by the Com-

TABLE 148-7 Determine HIV Status Code (HIV SC)

HIV Status of Exposure Source	No PEP	HIV SC 1	HIV SC 2	Unknown
HIV negative*	X			
HIV positive,† lower titer (asymptomatic and high CD4 count)‡		X		
HIV positive *f*, higher titer (advanced AIDS, primary HIV infection, high or increasing viral load or low CD4 count)‡			X	
HIV status unknown or source unknown				X

*A source is considered negative for HIV infection if there is laboratory documentation of a negative HIV antibody, HIV polymerase chain reaction (PCR), HIV p24 antigen test result from a specimen collected at or near the time of exposure and there is no clinical evidence of recent retroviral-like illness.
†A source is considered infected with HIV (HIV positive) if there has been a positive laboratory result for HIV antibody, HIV PCR, or HIV p24 antigen or physician-diagnosed AIDS.
‡Examples are used as surrogates to estimate the HIV titer in an exposure source for purposes of considering PEP regimens and do not reflect all clinical situations that may be observed. Although a high HIV titer (HIV SC2) in an exposure source has been associated with an increased risk for transmission, the possibility of transmission from a source with a low HIV titer also must be considered.
Source: From Centers for Disease Control and Prevention,[62] with permission.

TABLE 148-8 Determine PEP Recommendation

EC	HIV SC	PEP Recommendation
1	1	PEP may not be warranted. Exposure type does not pose known risk for HIV transmission. Exposed health care worker and treating clinician should decide if the risk of drug toxicity outweighs the benefit of PEP.
1	2	Consider basic drug regimen.* Exposure type poses negligible risk for HIV transmission. A high HIV titer in the source may justify consideration of PEP. Exposed health care worker and treating clinician should decide if the risk of drug toxicity outweighs the benefit of PEP.
2	1	Recommend basic regimen. Most HIV exposures are in this category; no increased risk for HIV transmission has been observed, but use of PEP is appropriate.
2	2	Recommend expanded regimen.‡ Exposure type represents an increased HIV transmission risk.
3	1 or 2	Recommend expanded regimen. Exposure type represents an increased HIV transmission risk.
unknown	unknown	If the source, or in the case of an unknown source, the setting where the exposure occurred suggests a possible risk for HIV exposure and the EC is 2 or 3, consider PEP basic regimen.

*Basic regimen is 4 weeks of zidovudine, 600 mg per day in two or three divided doses, *and* lamivudine, 150 mg twice daily.
†Expanded regimen is the basic regimen plus *either* idinavir, 800 mg every 8 h, *or* nelfinavir, 750 mg three times a day.
Source: From Centers for Disease Control and Prevention,[62] with permission.

mittee on Infectious Diseases of the American Academy of Pediatrics.[70] Adults who may be at increased risk for exposure to and transmission of mumps should be considered for vaccination. These persons include international travelers, persons attending colleges or post-high school educational institutions, and persons who work in health care facilities. Preventive measures for health care providers include use of standard and droplet precautions as well as vaccination if immunization status is unclear.

Measles

Rubeola, or measles, is caused by the measles virus, a paromyxovirus. Worldwide, measles is the most common cause of death among children that is preventable by use of a vaccine.[71] Incidence of measles has decreased steadily since the introduction of measles vaccine in 1963. In the United States, measles incidence is at the lowest level ever measured, with 488 and 135 cases reported in 1996 and 1997, respectively.[72] International importations and cases directly linked to international importations accounted for more than half of the cases reported during these years. This indicates that further reduction of measles incidence in the United States requires international cooperation and improved global control of measles. Obstacles to measles eradication in the United States include increasing numbers of susceptible children and infants who are not immunized and circulation of measles virus from other geographic regions of the world. Measles vaccination levels among the school-aged population in the United States, currently at 98 percent, must be maintained.

Transmission of the measles virus occurs by aerosolization of respiratory secretions. While isolation of patients is the mainstay of outbreak control, this mechanism is not effective in preventing subsequent cases. Primary prevention by immunization is preferred. A monovalent measles vaccine (Attenuvax, Merck and Company) available in the United States is a live virus vaccine that is prepared in egg culture. Various tri- and bivalent preparations are available as combination vaccines for mumps, measles, and rubella. Adults who may be at increased risk for exposure to and transmission of measles should be considered for vaccination. For persons born during or after 1957 who work in health care facilities, adequate vaccination consists of two doses of measles-mumps-rubella vaccine (M-M-RII, Merck and Company) or other live measles-containing vaccine separated by at least 28 days. Preventive measures for health care providers include use of standard and airborne precautions as well as vaccination if immunization status is unclear.

Rubella

Rubella, or German measles, is an exanthematous illness caused by a togavirus. Some of the most important consequences of rubella are miscarriages, stillbirths, fetal anomalies, and therapeutic abortions that result when rubella infection occurs during early pregnancy. When maternal infection occurs during the first 12 weeks of pregnancy, the probability of fetal infection with serious residual defects is 80 percent. When maternal infection occurs at 13 to 14 weeks' gestation, the probability of defects is 67 percent. The probability of fetal anomalies decreases to 25 percent by 26 weeks' gestation.[73] Before rubella vaccine was licensed in 1969, there were over 50,000 cases per year in the United States. In 1988, 225 cases were reported, the lowest since reporting began.[69] Outbreaks in unvaccinated adult populations (e.g., in prisons, colleges, and workplaces) led to more than 1000 cases being reported in 1990 and 1991.

Transmission of rubella is by respiratory droplets. While isolation of patients is the mainstay of outbreak control, this mechanism is not effective in preventing subsequent cases. Primary prevention by immunization is preferred. A monovalent rubella vaccine (Meruvax, Merck and Company) available in the United States is a live-virus vaccine that is prepared in human diploid cells. Various tri- and bivalent preparations are available as combination vaccines for mumps, measles, and rubella. Persons generally can be presumed to possess immunity to rubella if they have received one dose of measles-mumps-rubella or other live rubella vaccine on or after their first birthday, possess laboratory evidence of rubella immunity, or were born before 1957. Adults with unclear serologic evidence of immunity should receive one dose of rubella-containing vaccine. Preventive measures for health care providers include use of standard and droplet precautions as well as vaccination if immunization status is unclear.

Varicella and Herpes Zoster

Varicella zoster virus (VZV) is a double-stranded DNA virus of the Herpesviridae family. Varicella (chickenpox) is the primary manifestation of VZV infection. Once VZV infection has occurred, the virus is permanently established in the dorsal root and trigeminal ganglia, persists in latent form, and recurs when reactivated as herpes zoster (shingles). More than 90 percent of humans become infected with VZV.[74] In the United States, there are over 3.5 million cases of chickenpox and 300,000 cases of herpes zoster per year.[75,76] Chickenpox is highly contagious and poses a serious nosocomial and occupational infection risk.

Varicella (chickenpox) transmission occurs by contact, droplet, airborne, and transplacental routes.[74] Transmission associated with herpes zoster (shingles) occurs with direct contact with vesicular lesions. Airborne transmission of herpes zoster may also occur, especially if the source patient is immunosuppressed.[77,78] VZV infections may be prevented or modified via passive immunoprophylaxis with varicella zoster immunoglobulin (VZIG).[79] Types of exposures to varicella or zoster for which VZIG is indicated (i.e., susceptible people exposed to infected persons) includes residents in the same household, playmates with face-to-face indoor contact, hospitalized patients whose beds are adjacent to or in large wards (varicella), hospitalized patients with face-to-face contact (varicella), hospitalized patients visited by persons deemed to be contagious (varicella), physical contact with persons deemed to be contagious (zoster), and newborn infants with onset of varicella in the mother 5 days antepartum or 48 h postpartum.[80] VZIG is given as an intramuscular injection and should be administered within 48 h of exposure and not more than 96 h after exposure. In 1995, a live attenuated varicella vaccine (Oka, Merck and Company) was approved. The vaccine is recommended by the American Academy of Pediatrics for all susceptible children by their thirteenth birthday. The vaccine is also approved for healthy persons 13 years of age or older who have no previous infection or immunization history. These patients require two doses of varicella vaccine administered 4 to 8 weeks apart.[81] Preventive measures for health care providers include use of standard, airborne, and contact precautions. Health care providers who are susceptible to varicella should not enter the room if other immune care givers are available.

Influenza

Influenza viruses are divided into three types: A, B, and C. Influenza types A and B are responsible for epidemics of respiratory illness that occur every winter. Type A viruses are divided into subtypes based on two surface antigens: hemagglutinin (H) and neuraminidase (N). Three subtypes of H (H1, H2, and H3) and two subtypes of N (N1 and N2) are found among influenza A viruses. Currently circulating subtypes of influenza A are A(H1N1) and A(H3N2).

Two features of influenza virus replication and evolution account for its prominent place among emerging and reemerging diseases. First is the rapid and unpredictable antigenic change (antigenic drift) in the surface proteins, H and N. Antigenic drift occurs as a virus becomes established within the human population, rendering individuals susceptible to new viral strains that are resistant to antibodies formed to previously circulating viruses. Annual epidemics occur because sufficient numbers of individuals in the population are susceptible to the antigenically drifted virus. The second reason for the prominence of the influenza virus is the emergence of novel influenza viruses in humans (antigenic shift). Antigenic shift occurs when animal influenza viruses normally infecting only avian or swine reservoirs are transmitted to humans. This may occur either by direct transmission of an animal strain to humans or by genetic reassortment between influenza viruses of human and animal etiology. Antigenic shift is the appearance of a new influenza virus with novel H and N proteins that are immunologically distinct from those of the influenza viruses previously circulating in the human population. A pandemic occurs when human-to-human transmission of these novel viruses occurs and leads to disease in a large, immunologically susceptible human population.[82] During the twentieth century, three well-known pandemics resulted in high rates of morbidity and mortality in the United States and worldwide: the "Spanish" influenza (1918), killing 20 million worldwide and approximately 500,000 in the United States; the "Asian" influenza (1957), killing 70,000 in the United States; and the "Hong Kong" influenza (1968), killing 34,000 in the United States.[83] Influenza A and B viruses continually undergo antigenic drift. Only influenza A viruses exhibit antigenic shift, accounting for occasional pandemics.

Influenza virus is spread primarily by small particle aerosols of virus-laden respiratory secretions expelled into the air by coughing, sneezing, and talking. Direct contact with secretions also enables transmission of the virus. Two measures are available to reduce the impact of influenza: immunoprophylaxis with inactivated (killed virus) vaccine and chemoprophylaxis with an influenza-specific antiviral agent. Annual vaccination prior to the influenza season is the most effective means of reducing morbidity and mortality rates. Immunization programs focus on individuals at high risk for complications of influenza infection and individuals who may transmit the virus to high-risk populations. High-risk individuals include persons age 65 years and older; residents of chronic care and nursing home facilities; adults and children of any age with chronic disorders of the pulmonary or cardiovascular systems (including asthma); adults and children with chronic metabolic diseases (including diabetes mellitus), renal dysfunction, hemoglobinopathies, or immunosuppression; children and teenagers receiving long-term aspirin therapy (at risk for developing Reye's syndrome after influenza); and women who will be in the second or third trimester of pregnancy during influenza season.[82] Individuals who should receive vaccinations to reduce transmission to high-risk groups include prehospital personnel, nurses, physicians, hospital and clinic personnel who have contact with patients, staff of nursing home and chronic care facilities, home health care providers, and household contacts of those in high-risk populations. A trivalent vaccine is prepared on an annual basis to protect for two strains of influenza A and one strain of influenza B. Typically, one intramuscular injection is sufficient to ensure immunity. Two doses administered 1 month apart may be needed for previously unvaccinated children under age 9 years.[84]

Prophylactic use of the antiviral agents amantadine-hydrochloride and rimantadine-hydrochloride are 70 to 90 percent effective in preventing infection by influenza A virus when administered during the influenza season. Antivirals are useful in individuals who have not been vaccinated or have contraindications to vaccination. Vaccinations or chemoprophylaxis should be obtained for ED personnel on an annual basis. Additional preventive measures include use of standard, airborne, and contact precautions.

Scabies

Scabies is a highly contagious, pruritic skin disorder caused by an arachnid, *Sarcoptes scabiei* var. *hominis.* The human scabies mite is endemic in many developing countries, where the prevalence ranges from 20 to 100 percent. In some areas of Central and South America, the scabies infestation rate among young children is close to 100 percent.[85] Human scabies is transmitted primarily by direct personal or sexual contact with infected individuals. Although less common, transmission may occur by contact with contaminated bedding and clothing. The mite has been found to survive for 2 to 3 days on inanimate objects. The scabies mite is motionless at room temperature and lacks the ability to jump or fly from person to person.[86]

The average person infected with scabies harbors 10 to 15 live adult female mites at any given time.[87] In patients with Norwegian scabies, an atypical, crusted form of scabies, mite populations are in the thousands to millions.[88] This form is often seen in physically or mentally handicapped, immunocompromised, or institutionalized persons. Some sources advise testing patients who exhibit Norwegian scabies for HIV.[89] Preventive measures for health care providers include use of standard and contact precautions in patients with pruritic eruptions.

Pediculosis

Pediculosis is a dermal infestation caused by a parasitic insect (lice). Lice are sucking insects belonging to the family Pediculidae. Infestations in various body regions (e.g., head, thorax, and groin) are caused by the head louse (*Pediculus humanus capitis*), the body louse (*Pediculus humanus corporis*), and the crab louse (*Phthirus pubis*). There are three stages in the life cycle of the louse: the nit, the nymph, and the adult. Nits are louse eggs found firmly attached to hair shafts and take about 1 week to hatch. Nymphs mature to adults in 7 days and survive by feeding on human blood. Adult lice are about the size of a sesame seed and can live up to 30 days on an infested individual. Adult forms also feed on blood and may survive up to 2 days on inanimate objects.

Lice are transmitted by direct contact with infected individuals or common use of infected bedding, clothing, or combs, brushes, or headgear. Worldwide, as many as 6 to 12 million people are infected each year. Preschool- and elementary school-age children and their household contacts are infested most often. Prevention of occupational exposures in health care providers includes use of standard and contact precautions.

Latex Allergy

Latex is a milky cytosol secreted by lactifer cells from the rubber tree, *Hevea brasiliensis.*[90] Trees harvested in Malaysia account for the majority of latex used in the manufacture of medical products. The cytosol contains *cis*-1,4 polyisoprene, which is immunologically inert. A manufacturing process called sulfur heat vulcanization results in the cross-linking of chains of polyisoprene, yielding a polymer that exhibits excellent tensile strength, elasticity, and barrier capacity.[90] Such desirable characteristics have lead to the use of rubber latex in the manufacture of many medical products, including gloves (for surgery, examination, and housekeeping and cleaning), intravascular devices (balloon catheters, intravenous tubing, and ports), airway devices (nasopharyngeal airways, endotracheal tubes, and oxygen masks), tourniquets, blood pressure cuffs, electrocardiogram leads, tape, and dressings.

Immune reactions to latex products may take three forms: irritant, contact dermatitis (type IV), and IgE (type I). Irritant reactions are nonimmune in nature and result in dry dermal erythema limited to the site of contact. Contact dermatitis occurs as a result of dermal exposure to chemicals used in the manufacturing of latex products. Thiurams and thiazoles are the most common chemicals to induce this type IV response.[91] This reaction, which may extend beyond the site of contact, results in a dry dermal erythema, pruritus, weeping, and vesiculation. Such loss of skin integrity permits the access of latex proteins to the immune system and may result in an IgE-mediated response. IgE (type I) response is an immunologic reaction to protein allergens contained in latex. Clinical manifestations of such reactions include urticaria, asthma, rhinitis, angioedema, laryngeal edema, and anaphylaxis. IgE reactions may occur as a result of mucosal, dermal, contact, or inhalational exposure. Cornstarch powder, which serves as a lubricant to ease the donning of latex gloves, binds and aerosolizes protein allergens, leading to inhalation exposure.

At highest risk of developing IgE-mediated latex allergy are individuals with high exposure to latex and those who are atopic. Workers in industries that make rubber products (e.g., tire manufacturers and doll makers) and those who use rubber products (e.g., housekeepers, hairdressers, and health care workers) are at high risk of developing this allergy.[90] While anyone can develop latex allergy, specific patient populations are at higher risk. Individuals likely to develop latex allergy include those with a history of multiple allergies (including dermal, respiratory, oral, or facial reactions to latex or rubber products); asthma (reactive airways disease), eczema, multiple food allergies (especially to bananas, avocados, and other tropical fruit), frequent surgical or dental procedures, multiple urogenital procedures (e.g., bladder, vaginal, and rectal), spina bifida and related conditions of spinal dysraphism, congenital urinary anomalies, or sensitivity to ethylene oxide (a sterilization agent).

Since September 1998, the US Food and Drug Administration has promulgated uniform labeling for all medical products.[90] Many latex-free medical products exist on the market and may be substituted for currently used products. Prevention of disease in health care workers is critical and requires the use of synthetic or low-allergen powder-free gloves.[90] The National Institute for Occupational Safety and Health and the CDC have published several documents that describe the hazards of latex allergy and suggest steps health care providers may take to protect themselves.[92,93] Health care institutions recognize latex allergy as a threat to the work force. As a result of the growing number of reports of anaphylaxis and other allergic reactions to latex, many institutions have drafted policies to increase awareness of latex allergies, identify individuals (patients and staff) who may be at risk, and outline steps to reduce latex exposures.[94,95] Emergency personnel may take the following steps to protect themselves from latex exposure and allergy in the workplace: use nonlatex gloves for workplace activities that do not involve contact with infectious materials; use synthetic or low-allergen powder-free gloves when handling infectious materials; avoid oil-based hand lotions or creams when wearing latex gloves (to prevent glove deterioration); wash hands with mild soap and dry thoroughly upon removal of latex gloves; frequently clean work areas and equipment contaminated with latex-containing dust; obtain education and training regarding latex allergy; and recognize the symptoms of latex allergy. Health care providers should be aware that hypoallergenic latex gloves do not reduce the risk of latex allergy but do reduce reactions to chemical additives in latex.

REFERENCES

1. Centers for Disease Control and Prevention, National Center for Health Statistics: *FASTATS 1995 US Emergency Department Visits.* Advance data 285. Atlanta, 1998.
2. US Department of Labor: *Occupational Exposure to Blood-borne Pathogens: Precautions for Emergency Responders.* OSHA 3130. Washington, DC, 1992.
3. Nelsing S, Nielsen TL, Nielsen JO: Occupational blood exposure among health care workers: I. Frequency and reporting. *Scand J Infect Dis* 25:193, 1993.
4. Nelsing S, Nielsen TL, Nielsen JO: Occupational blood exposure among health care workers: II. Exposure mechanisms and universal precautions. *Scand J Infect Dis* 25:199, 1993.
5. Centers for Disease Control and Prevention: Case-control study of HIV seroconversion in health-care workers after percutaneous exposure to HIV-infected blood: France, United Kingdom, and United States, January 1988–August 1994. *MMWR* 44:929, 1995.
6. Eustis TC, Wright SW, Wrenn KD et al: Compliance and recommendations for universal precautions among prehospital providers. *Ann Emerg Med* 25:512, 1995.
7. Kelen GD, Hansen KN, Green GB et al: Determinants of emergency department procedure- and condition-specific universal (barrier) precaution requirements for optimal provider protection. *Ann Emerg Med* 25:743, 1995.
8. Centers for Disease Control and Prevention, Hospital Infection Control Practices Advisory Committee: Guideline for isolation precautions in hospitals: II. Recommendations for isolation precautions in hospitals. *Am J Infect Control* 24:32, 1996.
9. Centers for Disease Control and Prevention, Hospital Infection Control Practices Advisory Committee: Guideline for isolation precautions in hospitals: I. Evolution of isolation practices. *Am J Infect Control* 24:24, 1996.
10. Centers for Disease Control and Prevention. *HIV/AIDS Surveillance Rep* 7:5, 1995.
11. Centers for Disease Control and Prevention: First 500,000 AIDS cases: United States, 1995. *MMWR* 44:849, 1995.
12. Centers for Disease Control and Prevention: Update: Trends in AIDS diagnosis and reporting under the expanded surveillance definition for adolescence and adults: United States, 1993. *MMWR* 43:826, 1994.
13. Centers for Disease Control and Prevention: Update: HIV-2 infection among blood and plasma donors: United States, June 1992–June 1995. *MMWR* 44:603, 1995.
14. Centers for Disease Control and Prevention: Heterosexually acquired AIDS: United States, 1993. *MMWR* 43:155, 1994.
15. Centers for Disease Control and Prevention: Human immunodeficiency virus transmission in household settings: United States. *MMWR* 43:347, 1994.
16. Molinari JA: Practical infection control for the 1990s: Applying science to government regulations. *J Am Dent Assoc* 125:1189, 1994.
17. Marcus R: CDC Cooperative Needlestick Study Group: Surveillance of health care workers exposed to blood from patients infected with human immunodeficiency virus. *N Engl J Med* 319:1118, 1988.

18. Henderson DK, Fahey BJ, Willy M, et al: Risk of transmission of human immunodeficiency virus type 1 (HIV-1) associated with clinical exposures. *Ann Intern Med* 113:740, 1990.
19. American Society for Testing and Materials: *Standards on Emergency Medical Services.* 03-630094-53. Philadelphia, 1994.
20. American Society for Testing and Materials: *Standard Specification for Rubber Examination Gloves.* ASTM D 3578-91. Philadelphia, 1991.
21. American Society for Testing and Materials: *Test Method for Detection of Holes in Medical Gloves.* ASTM D 5151-92. Philadelphia, 1992.
22. American Society for Testing and Materials: *Test Method for Resistance of Protective Clothing Materials to Synthetic Blood.* ASTM ES 21-92. Philadelphia, 1992.
23. American Society for Testing and Materials: *Test Method for Resistance of Protective Clothing Materials to Penetration by Blood-Borne Pathogens Using Viral Penetration as a Test System.* ASTM ES 22-92. Philadelphia, 1992.
24. American Society for Testing and Materials: *Test Method for Resistance of Protective Clothing Materials to Permeation by Liquids or Gases.* ASTM F 739. Philadelphia, 1986.
25. American Society for Testing and Materials: *Standard Test Method for Resistance of Protective Clothing Materials to Penetration by Liquids.* ASTM F 903. Philadelphia, 1990.
26. National Fire Protection Association: *Standard on Protective Clothing for Emergency Medical Operations.* NFPA 1999. Quincy, MA, 1992.
27. National Fire Protection Association: *Standard on Fire Department Occupational Safety and Health Program.* NFPA 1500. Quincy, MA, 1992.
28. Centers for Disease Control and Prevention: Guidelines for prevention of transmission of human immunodeficiency virus and hepatitis B virus to health-care and public-safety workers. *MMWR* 38(suppl 6):3, 1989.
29. Rinnert KJ: Risk reduction for exposure to blood-borne pathogens in EMS: Position paper of the National Association of EMS Physicians. *Prehosp Emerg Care* 2:62, 1998.
30. US Department of Labor: *Personal Protective Equipment.* OSHA 3077. Washington, DC, 1995.
31. Collins CL, Mullan RJ, Moseley RR: HIV safety guidelines and laboratory training. *Public Health Rep* 106:727, 1991.
32. Centers for Disease Control and Prevention: Update: Provisional public health services recommendations for chemoprophylaxis after occupational exposure to HIV. *MMWR* 45:468, 1996.
33. Steele LJ: When universal precautions fail: Communicable disease notification laws for emergency responders. *J Legal Med* 11:451, 1990.
34. *Occupational Safety and Health Act of 1970.* 91st Cong, Pub L 91-596, section 2193, December 1970, amended by Pub L 101–553, section 3101, Washington, DC, November 1990.
35. US Department of Labor: *Bloodborne Pathogens Standard.* Title 29 CFR, part 1910.130. Washington, DC, July 1, 1992.
36. Centers for Disease Control and Prevention: Update: Universal precautions for prevention of transmission of HIV, HBV, and other bloodborne pathogens in health-care settings. *MMWR* 37:378, 1988.
37. Centers for Disease Control and Prevention: Draft guidelines for isolation precautions for hospitals: I. Evolution of isolation practices, and II. Recommendations for isolation precautions in hospitals: Notice of comment period. *Fed Reg* 59:55552, 1995.
38. Lemon SM: Type A viral hepatitis: Epidemiology, diagnosis, and prevention. *Clin Chem* 43:1494, 1997.
39. Francis DP, Hadler SC, Pendergast TJ, et al: Occurrence of hepatitis A, B and non-A/non-B in the United States: CDC Sentinel County hepatitis study I. *Am J Med* 76:69, 1984.
40. Lemon SM, Thomas DL: Vaccines to prevent viral hepatitis. *N Engl J Med* 336:196, 1997.
41. Alter MJ, Mast EE: The epidemiology of viral hepatitis in the United States. *Gastroenterol Clin North Am* 23:437, 1994.
42. Gitlin N: Hepatitis B: Diagnosis, prevention, and treatment. *Clin Chem* 43:1500, 1997.
43. Centers for Disease Control and Prevention: Recommendations for prevention and control of hepatitis C virus (HCV) infection and HCV-related chronic infection. *MMWR* 47:1, 1998.
44. McQuillan GM, Alter MJ, Moyer LA, et al: A population-based serologic study of hepatitis C virus infection in the United States, in Rizzetto M, Purcell RH, Gerin JL, Verme G (eds): *Viral Hepatitis and Liver Disease.* Turin, Edizioni Minerva Medica, 1997, pp 267–270.
45. Alter MJ, Mast EE, Moyer LA, et al: Hepatitis C. *Infect Dis Clin North Am* 12:13, 1998.
46. Centers for Disease Control and Prevention: Recommendations for prevention and control of hepatitis C virus (HCV) infection and HCV-related chronic disease. *MMWR* 47:1, 1998.
47. Alter MJ: Epidemiology of hepatitis C. *Hepatology* 26:62, 1997.
48. Thomas DL, Factor SH, Kelen GD, et al: Viral hepatitis in health care personnel at the Johns Hopkins Hospital. *Arch Intern Med* 153:1705, 1993.
49. Cooper VW, Krusell A, Tilton RC, et al: Seroprevalence of antibodies to hepatitis C virus in high-risk hospital personnel. *Infect Control Hosp Epidemiol* 13:82, 1992.
50. Panlilio AL, Shapiro CN, Schable CA, et al: Serosurvey of human immunodeficiency virus, hepatitis B virus, and hepatitis C virus infection among hospital-based surgeons. *J Am Coll Surg* 180:16, 1995.
51. Shapiro CN, Tokars JI, Chamberland ME: American Academy of Orthopedic Surgeons Serosurvey Study Committee: Use of hepatitis B vaccine and infection with hepatitis B and C among orthopaedic surgeons. *J Bone Joint Surg* 78A:1791, 1996.
52. Thomas DL, Gruninger SE, Siew C, et al: Occupational risk of hepatitis C infections among general dentists and oral surgeons in North America. *Am J Med* 100:41, 1996.
53. Alter MJ: The epidemiology of acute and chronic hepatitis C. *Clin Liver Dis* 1:559, 1997.
54. London WT, Evans AA: The epidemiology of hepatitis viruses B, C, and D. *Clin Lab Med* 16:251, 1996.
55. Tepper ML, Gully PR: Viral hepatitis: Know your D, E, F, Gs. *Can Med Assoc J* 156:1735, 1997.
56. Feucht HH, Zollner B, Polywka S, et al: Vertical transmission of hepatitis G. *Lancet* 347:615, 1996.
57. Alter MJ, Gallagher M, Morris TT, et al: Acute non-A-E hepatitis in the United States and the role of hepatitis G virus infection. *N Engl J Med* 336:741, 1997.
58. DeCock KM, Adjorlolo G, Ekpini E, et al: Epidemiology and transmission of HIV-2: Why there is no HIV-2 pandemic. *JAMA* 270:2083, 1993.
59. Workshop Report from the European Commission (DG XII, INCO-DC) and the Joint United Nations Programme on HIV/AIDS: HIV-1 subtypes: Implications for epidemiology, pathogenicity, vaccines, and diagnostics. *AIDS* 15:17, 1997.
60. Centers for Disease Control and Prevention, National Center for Health Statistics: *FASTATS AIDS/HIV. Monthly vital statistics report* 46:1 suppl. Atlanta, May 22, 1998.
61. Tokars JI, Marcus R, Culver DH, et al: Surveillance of HIV infection and zidovudine use among health care workers after occupational exposure to HIV-infected blood. *Ann Intern Med* 118:913, 1993.
62. Centers for Disease Control and Prevention: Public Health Service guidelines for the management of health care worker exposures to HIV and recommendations for postexposure prophylaxis. *MMWR* 47:1, 1998.
63. Bradford WZ, Daley CL: Multiple drug-resistant tuberculosis. *Infect Dis Clin North Am* 12:157, 1998.
64. Abernathy RS: Tuberculosis: An update. *Pediatr Rev* 18:50, 1997.
65. Centers for Disease Control and Prevention: Development of new vaccines for tuberculosis: Recommendations of the Advisory Council for the Elimination of Tuberculosis (ACET). *MMWR* 47:1, 1998.
66. Centers for Disease Control and Prevention: Tuberculosis morbidity: United States, 1996. *MMWR* 46:695, 1997.
67. Centers for Disease Control and Prevention: Tuberculosis morbidity: United States, 1997. *MMWR* 47:253, 1998.
68. Demangone D, Karras D: The clinical challenge of tuberculosis: A state-of-the-art review of diagnostic strategies, atypical presentations, and treatment guidelines for the emergency physician. *Emerg Med Rep* 18:235, 1997.
69. Centers for Disease Control and Prevention: Measles, mumps, and rubella: Vaccine use and strategies for elimination of measles, rubella, and congenital rubella syndrome and control of mumps: Recommendations of the Advisory Committee on Immunization Practices (ACIP). *MMWR* 47:1, 1998.
70. Peter G (ed): *1997 Red Book: Report of the Committee on Infectious Diseases.* 24th ed. Elk Grove Village, Il, American Academy of Pediatrics, 1997.
71. Markowitz L, Orenstein W: Measles vaccine. *Pediatr Clin North Am* 37:603, 1990.
72. Centers for Disease Control and Prevention: Advances in global measles control and elimination: Summary of the 1997 international meeting. *MMWR* 47:1, 1998.
73. Gold E: Almost extinct diseases: Measles, mumps, rubella, and pertussis. *Pediatr Rev* 17:120, 1996.

74. Centers for Disease Control and Prevention: Prevention of varicella: Recommendations of the Advisory Committee on Immunization Practices (ACIP). *MMWR* 45:1, 1996.
75. Guess HA, Broughton DD, Melton LJ III, et al: Population-based studies of varicella complications. *Pediatrics* 78(part 2):723, 1986.
76. Preblud SR: Varicella: Complications and costs. *Pediatrics* 78:728, 1986.
77. Garner JS: Guideline for isolation precautions in hospitals. *Infect Control Hosp Epidemiol* 17:53, 1996.
78. Josephson A, Gombert ME: Airborne transmission of nosocomial varicella from isolated zoster. *J Infect Dis* 158:238, 1988.
79. Straus SE, Ostrove JM, Inchauspe G, et al: Varicella zoster virus infections: Proceedings of the National Institutes of Health Conference, 1987 Feb 18, Bethesda, Md. *Ann Intern Med* 108:221, 1988.
80. Peter G (ed): *1997 Red Book: Report of the Committee on Infectious Diseases,* 24th ed. Elk Grove Village, IL, American Academy of Pediatrics, 1997, pp 573–585.
81. Stover BH, Bratcher DF: Varicella zoster virus: Infection control and prevention. *Am J Infect Control* 26:369, 1998.
82. Cox NJ, Fukuda K: Influenza. *Infect Dis Clin North Am* 12:27, 1998.
83. Centers for Disease Control and Prevention, National Center for Health Statistics: *FASTATS Influenza: General Information: National Center for Infectious Disease.* Atlanta, June 4, 1998.
84. Centers for Disease Control and Prevention: Prevention and control of influenza: Recommendations of the Advisory Committee on Immunization Practices (APIC). *MMWR* 47:1, 1998.
85. Rasmussen JE: Scabies. *Pediatr Rev* 15:110, 1994.
86. Molinaro MJ, Schwartz RA, Janniger CK: Scabies. *Cutis* 56:317, 1995.
87. Sterling GB, Janniger CK, Kihiczak G, et al: Scabies. *Am Fam Physician* 46:1237, 1992.
88. Sirera G, Ruis F, Romeru J, et al: Hospital outbreak of scabies stemming from two AIDS patients with Norwegian scabies. *Lancet* 335:1227, 1990.
89. Schlesinger I, Oelrich DM, Tyring SK: Crusted (Norwegian) scabies in patients with AIDS: The range of clinical presentations. *South Med J* 87:352, 1994.
90. Kelly KJ, Walsh-Kelly CM: Latex allergy: A patient and health care system emergency. *Ann Emerg Med* 32:723, 1998.
91. Fisher A: Allergic contact reactions in health personnel. *J Allergy Clin Immunol* 90:729, 1992.
92. Centers for Disease Control and Prevention: *Latex Allergy: A Prevention Guide.* Publication 98-113. Department of Health and Human Services, National Institute for Occupational Safety and Health. Atlanta, 1998.
93. Centers for Disease Control and Prevention: *Preventing Allergic Reactions to Natural Rubber Latex in the Workplace.* Publication 97-135. Department of Health and Human Services, National Institute for Occupational Safety and Health. Atlanta, 1997.
94. Dallas County Hospital District: Latex allergy, in *Parkland Health and Hospital System Safety Manual.* 1998, draft policy, section S, pp 1–5.
95. University of North Carolina Hospitals: Latex allergy, in *UNC Hospital's Latex Allergy Policy.* 1995, pp 1–2.

ANTIBIOTICS IN THE EMERGENCY DEPARTMENT

James H. Bryan
Kenneth C. Dirk
Jonathan Jui

INTRODUCTION

When prescribing antibiotics and using this chapter:

1. Ask the patient about any allergies to medications.
2. Use your judgment about these recommendations especially with regard to drug interactions and side effects.
3. Unless otherwise indicated, the dosages listed here are for adults with normal renal and hepatic function.
4. Hospital admission and parenteral therapy should be considered for any patient who is severely ill, immunocompromised or who may not be compliant with oral medications/follow-up.
5. When needed, multiple drug therapy is noted and indicated by the words **PLUS** or **PLUS/MINUS**.
6. The first-line therapies listed in this chapter are based upon efficacy and cost. If a first-line medication fails, consider switching to a broader-spectrum (and often more expensive) therapy.
7. When using IV vancomycin or an antipseudomonal aminoglycoside, serum levels should be monitored.
8. Frequently used abbreviations: bid, twice a day; DRSP, drug-resistant *Streptococcus pneumoniae;* IM, intramuscularly; IV, intravenously; MRSA, methicillin-resistant *Staphylococcus aureus;* PO, orally; qid, four times a day; qd, every day; tid, three times a day.

PREGNANCY RISK CATEGORIES

Pregnancy risks for all medications listed in the chapter are denoted after each drug dosage. The risk category is contained in brackets, e.g., [B].

Category A: Controlled studies have failed to demonstrate fetal risk during the first trimester.
Category B: Animal studies have not demonstrated a risk, but there are no controlled studies in women; or, animal studies have shown an adverse effect that was not confirmed in controlled studies in women in the first trimester, and there is no risk in later trimesters.
Category C: Animal studies have shown adverse effects and there are no studies in women; or, no animal or human studies are available. Use only if the potential benefit outweighs the risk to the fetus.
Category D: There is positive evidence of human fetal risk. Use only in life threatening situations or for serious illnesses where no alternative medications are effective.
Category X: Contraindicated. Fetal risk outweighs potential benefit.

Medications that Should Be Used with Caution or Are Contraindicated in Pregnancy

- acyclovir (Zovirax): **Category C**— may cause chromosomal breaks at very high concentrations. No data available on risk in breast feeding.
- erythromycin estolate (Ilosone): **Category B** relative to fetus but contraindicated due to maternal risk of cholestatic hepatitis. No risk in breast feeding. All other erythromycin preparations are considered safe in pregnancy and breast feeding.
- lindane (Kwell): **Category C**— less toxic alternatives exist. Considered safe in breast feeding
- metronidazole (Flagyl): **Category B**— contraindicated in first trimester; use in later trimesters if benefits outweigh the risk. Discontinue breast feeding during use—recommend single dose therapy with resumption of breast feeding 12–24 hours after use.
- nitrofurantoin (Macrodantin, Macrobid): **Category B**— contraindicated in third trimester because of possibility of hemolytic anemia. Avoid during breast feeding if infant at risk for G6PD deficiency; otherwise considered safe.
- Quinolones: ciprofloxacin (Cipro), norfloxacin (Noroxin), ofloxacin (Floxin), levofloxacin (Levaquin): **Category C**— may cause arthropathy in fetuses, although recent review does not substantiate this risk.
- sulfonamides: **Category B** in first and second trimesters; **Category D** in third trimester due to possible kernicterus. Avoid during breast feeding in premature infants and infants with hyperbilirubinemia or G6PD deficiency. Considered safe in full term infants without medical problems.
- tetracyclines/doxycycline (Vibramycin): **Category D**— may stain teeth and bone.

- trimethoprim/sulfamethoxazole (Bactrim, Septra): **Category C** in first and second trimesters; **Category D** in third trimester. See sulfonamides, above. Trimethoprim interferes with folic acid metabolism and should be used in the first and second trimesters only if the potential benefits outweigh the risks.

Considered Relatively Safe in Pregnancy

- cephalosporins: **Category B**
- penicillins: **Category B**
- erythromycins (except estolate preparations): **Category B**
- clotrimazole (topical): **Category B**

EAR/NOSE/THROAT

Acute Necrotizing Ulcerative Gingivitis (ANUG)

1. Penicillin V potassium (Pen-VEE K) 500 mg PO qid [B]
2. Tetracycline (Achromycin) 500 mg PO qid [D]
3. Doxycycline (Vibramycin) 100 mg PO bid [D]

Course: 7–10 days
Organisms: spirochetes, fusobacterium

Dental Infections/Periapical and Periodontal Abscesses

1. Clindamycin (Cleocin) 300 mg PO qid [B]
2. Erythromycin 500 mg PO qid [B, except estolate contraindicated]
3. Amoxicillin/clavulanic acid (Augmentin) 875/125 mg PO bid **OR** 500/125 mg PO tid [B]

Course: 7–10 days
Organisms: oral flora

Epiglottitis

A. CHILDREN

1. Cefuroxime (Ceftin) 50 mg/kg IV q8h [B]
2. Cefotaxime (Claforan) 50 mg/kg IV q8h [B]
3. Ceftriaxone (Rocephin) 50 mg/kg IV qd [B]

Organisms: *H. influenzae, S. pyogenes, S. pneumoniae, S. aureus*

B. ADULTS

1. Cefuroxime (Ceftin) 1 g IV q8h [B]
2. Cefotaxime (Claforan) 2 g IV q8h [B]
3. Ceftriaxone (Rocephin) 2 g IV qd [B]

Organisms: group A *Strep, H. influenzae*

Ludwig's Angina

Note: *Requires admission to the hospital, usually to the ICU, for airway monitoring and management.*

Regimen A (*Note **two** drug therapy*)
Penicillin G 4 million units IV q4h [B]
(Administer over 1 h. Rapid infusion may cause seizures.)
PLUS
Metronidazole (Flagyl) 15 mg/kg IV loading dose, maximal dose 1000 mg, then 7.5 mg/kg IV q6h (max 500 mg/dose) [B, contraindicated in 1st trimester]

Regimen B
Cefoxitin (Mefoxin) 2 g IV q8h [B]
Clindamycin (Cleocin) 600 mg IV q8h (if penicillin allergic) [B]
Ticarcillin/clavulanic acid (Timentin) 3.1 g IV q6h [B]
Piperacillin/tazobactam (Zosyn) 3.375 g IV q6h [B]
Ampicillin/sulbactam (Unasyn) 3 g IV q6h [B]

Organisms: *Streptococcus* sp., *Bacteroides* sp., *Eikenella corrodens*, polymicrobic

Otitis Externa

1. Neomycin, polymyxin B, and 1% hydrocortisone otic solution (Cortisporin otic) 4 drops in affected ear tid–qid [C]; dispense 10 mL
   OR (for severe infection)
2. Ofloxacin 0.3% otic solution (Floxin) 10 drops in affected ear bid (use 5 drops bid if child <12 years old) [C]; dispense 10 mL

If refractory:

1. Ciprofloxacin 0.2% and hydrocortisone 1% otic suspension (Cipro HC otic) 3 drops in affected ear bid × 7 days [C]; dispense 10 mL
   OR
2. Dicloxacillin 500 mg PO qid for *S. aureus* [B]

Course: 10 days (except 7 days for Cipro or Dicloxacillin as noted)
Organisms: *Pseudomonas*, Enterobacteriaceae, *S. aureus, Proteus* sp.

Notes:

1. Use Cortisporin otic suspension (not solution) if TM perforated.
2. Cotton wicks placed in the canals aid absorption especially if the canal closes completely due to edema.
3. Consider malignant otitis externa, especially in immunocompromised patients or diabetics. Patients usually appear ill and require admission.

Otitis Media

A. CHILDREN AGE 10 OR UNDER

1. Amoxicillin (Amoxil) 80–90 mg/kg/day PO divided bid or tid [B]
   Easy dose: 40 mg/kg/dose PO bid OR **30 mg/kg/dose PO tid**
   Maximum dose 750 mg/dose bid **OR** 500 mg/dose tid
   Available in suspensions of 125 mg and 250 mg/5 mL
2. TMP/SMX (Bactrim, Septra) 6–12 mg/kg/day TMP and 30–60 mg/kg/day SMX PO divided bid [C; D in 3rd trimester]
   Easy dose: 1 mL/kg/day PO divided bid = 8 mg/kg/day TMP and **40 mg/kg/day SMX**
   Maximum: 20 mL/dose
   Suspension of TMP 40 mg and SMX 200 mg/5 mL
3. Azithromycin (Zithromax) 10 mg/kg PO initial dose, then 5 mg/kg/day for 4 days [B]
   Maximum: 500 mg on day 1 and 250 mg on days 2–5
   Available in suspensions of 100 mg and 200 mg/5 mL
4. Erythromycin/sulfisoxazole (Pediazole) 50 mg/kg/day erythromycin and 150 mg/kg/day sulfa PO divided tid or qid [C; D in 3rd trimester]
   Easy dose: 1.25 mL/kg/day PO divided tid OR **qid**
   Maximum: 10 mL/dose
   Suspension of erythromycin 200 mg and sulfisoxazole 600 mg/5 mL
5. Ceftriaxone (Rocephin) 50 mg/kg IM single dose [B]
   Maximum: 1 g/dose

If severe or refractory:

1. Amoxicillin/clavulanate (Augmentin) 80–90 mg/kg/day as amoxicillin, PO divided bid or tid [B]
   Easy dose: 40 mg/kg/dose as amoxicillin PO bid OR **30 mg/kg/dose as amoxicillin PO tid**
   Maximum: 750 mg/dose as amoxicillin bid **OR** 500 mg/dose as amoxicillin tid
   Available in suspensions of 125 mg and 250 mg amoxicillin/5 mL

2. Cefuroxime axetil (Ceftin) 20–30 mg/kg/day PO divided bid [B]
   Easy dose: 20 mg/kg/day = 10 mg/kg/dose PO bid
   Maximum: 250 mg/dose
   Available in suspension of 125 mg/5 mL
3. Cefpodoxime (Vantin) 10 mg/kg/day PO in 1 dose [B] (probably effective but data limited)
   Maximum: 400 mg/dose
   Available in suspensions of 50 mg and 100 mg/5 mL
4. Cefprozil (Cefzil) 15 mg/kg/dose PO bid [B] (probably effective but data limited)
   Maximum: 250 mg/dose
   Available in suspensions of 125 mg or 250 mg/5 mL
5. Ceftriaxone, 50 mg/kg IV or IM QD for 3 days

B. ADULTS AND CHILDREN OVER AGE 10

1. Amoxicillin (Amoxil) 500 mg PO tid [B]
2. TMP/SMX DS (Bactrim DS, Septra DS) 1 tablet PO bid [C; D in 3rd trimester]
3. Azithromycin (Zithromax) 500 mg PO initial dose, then 250 mg PO for 4 days [B]
4. Amoxicillin/clavulanate (Augmentin) 500 mg PO tid or 875 mg PO bid [B]
5. Cefuroxime axetil (Ceftin) 250–500 mg PO bid [B]
6. Ceftriaxone (Rocephin) 1 g IM/IV single dose [B]

Course: 10 days (except azithromycin and ceftriaxone as noted)
Organisms: *S. pneumoniae* (30–35%), non-typeable *Haemophilus influenzae* (20–25%), *Moraxella (Branhamella) catarrhalis* (10–15%), group A *Strep*, *Staphylococcus aureus* (1–2%) and viral (35%)

Parotitis/Sialoadenitis

1. Dicloxacillin 500 mg PO qid [B]
2. Cephradine (Velosef) 500 mg PO qid [B]
3. Cephalexin (Keflex) 500 mg PO qid [B]
4. Amoxicillin/clavulanic acid (Augmentin) 875/125 mg PO bid **OR** 500/125 mg PO tid [B]
5. Clindamycin (Cleocin) 150–450 mg PO qid [B]
6. Vancomycin (Vancocin) 15 mg/kg IV q12h (for severe penicillin allergy; max 1 g/dose; monitor serum levels) [C]

Course: 7–10 days
Organisms: *Staphylococcus aureus*, anaerobes

Periorbital and Orbital Cellulitis

See Skin and Soft Tissue Infections.

Sinusitis, Acute

A. CHILDREN

Uncomplicated

1. Amoxicillin (Amoxil) 80–90 mg/kg/day PO divided bid or tid [B]
   Easy dose: 40 mg/kg/dose PO bid OR **30 mg/kg/dose PO tid**
   Maximum: 750 mg/dose bid **OR** 500 mg/dose tid
   Available in suspensions of 125 mg and 250 mg/5 mL
2. TMP/SMX (Bactrim, Septra) 6–12 mg/kg/day TMP and 30–60 mg/kg/day SMX PO divided bid [C; D in 3rd trimester]
   Easy dose: 1 mL/kg/day PO divided bid = 8 mg/kg/day TMP and 40 mg/kg/day SMX
   Maximum: 20 mL/dose
   Suspension of TMP 40 mg and SMX 200 mg/5 mL
3. Erythromycin/sulfisoxazole (Pediazole) 50 mg/kg/day erythromycin and 150 mg/kg/day sulfa PO divided tid or qid [C; D in 3rd trimester]
   Easy dose: 1.25 mL/kg/day PO divided tid or qid
   Maximum: 10 mL/dose
   Suspension of erythromycin 200 mg and sulfisoxazole 600 mg/5 mL

If severe or refractory:

1. Amoxicillin/clavulanate (Augmentin) 80–90 mg/kg/day as amoxicillin, PO, divided bid or tid [B]
   Easy dose: 40 mg/kg/dose as amoxicillin, PO bid OR **30 mg/kg/dose as amoxicillin, PO tid**
   Maximum dose: 750 mg/dose as amoxicillin, PO bid **OR** 500 mg/dose as amoxicillin, PO tid
   Available in suspensions of 125 mg and 250 mg amoxicillin/5 mL
2. Cefuroxime axetil (Ceftin) 20–30 mg/kg/day PO divided bid [B]
   Easy dose: 20 mg/kg/day = 10 mg/kg/dose PO bid
   Maximum: 250 mg/dose
   Available in suspension of 125 mg/5 mL
3. Cefpodoxime (Vantin) 10 mg/kg/day PO in 1 dose [B]
   Maximum: 400 mg/dose
   Available in suspensions of 50 mg and 100 mg/5 mL
4. Cefprozil (Cefzil) 15 mg/kg/dose PO bid [B]
   Maximum: 250 mg/dose
   Available in suspensions of 125 mg or 250 mg/5 mL
5. Clarithromycin (Biaxin) 7.5 mg/kg/dose PO bid (for severe penicillin allergy) [C]
   Maximum: 500 mg/dose
   Available in suspensions of 125 mg or 250 mg/5 mL

B. ADULTS, SINUSITIS

Notes:

1. Many ENT consultants consider decongestants an equally important component of therapy, but this is not supported by the literature.

Sprays:
   a. 0.25% phenylephrine (Neo-Synephrine) nasal spray tid to qid for 3 days only [C]
   b. Oxymetazoline 0.05% (Afrin) nasal spray bid for 3 days only [C]

Oral:
   Pseudoephedrine (Sudafed) 30–60 mg PO qid [C]

2. Consider adding antihistamines if an allergic component is suspected.
   a. Diphenhydramine (Benadryl) 25–50 mg PO qid [B, contraindicated in 1st trimester]
   b. Cetirizine (Zyrtec) 10 mg PO qd [B]
   c. Fexofenadine (Allegra) 60 mg PO bid [C]

Uncomplicated

1. TMP/SMX DS (Bactrim DS, Septra DS) 1 tablet PO bid [C; D in 3rd trimester]
2. Azithromycin (Zithromax) 500 mg PO initial dose, then 250 mg PO qd for 4 days [B]
3. Clarithromycin (Biaxin) 250–500 mg PO bid [C]

If severe or refractory:

1. Amoxicillin/clavulanate (Augmentin) 500 mg PO tid or 875 mg PO bid [B]
2. Cefuroxime axetil (Ceftin) 500 mg PO bid [B]
3. Cefpodoxime (Vantin) 200 mg PO bid [B]
4. Cefprozil (Cefzil) 250 mg PO bid [B] **OR** (if severe penicillin allergy or suspect DRSP)

5. Levofloxacin (Levaquin) 500 mg PO qd (if severe penicillin allergy or suspect DRSP; [C])

Course: 7 to 21 days (except azithromycin as noted)
Organisms: *S. pneumoniae, H. influenzae*, group A *Streptococcus, M. catarrhalis*, anaerobes

Tonsillitis/Pharyngitis

A. CHILDREN AGE 10 AND UNDER

Note: If patient exhibits signs or symptoms of severe swelling/edema (e.g., voice change, unable to swallow saliva), consider adding prednisone (1–2 mg/kg PO × 5 days) to the antibiotic regimen.

1. Penicillin V potassium (Pen VEE-K) 25–50 mg/kg/day PO divided tid–qid [B]
   Easy dose: 45 mg/kg/day = 15 mg/kg/dose PO tid
   Maximum: 500 mg/dose
   Available in suspensions of 125 mg and 250 mg/5 mL
2. Amoxicillin (Amoxil) 20–50 mg/kg/day PO divided tid [B]
   Easy dose: 30 mg/kg/day = 10 mg/kg/dose PO tid
   Maximum: 250 mg/dose
   Available in suspensions of 125 mg and 250 mg/5 mL
3. Erythromycin ethyl succinate (EES) 30–50 mg/kg/day PO divided qid [B]
   Easy dose: 40 mg/kg/day = 10 mg/kg/dose PO qid
   Maximum: 500 mg/dose
   Available in suspensions of 200 mg and 400 mg/5 mL
4. Azithromycin (Zithromax) 10 mg/kg PO initial dose, then 5 mg/kg/day for 4 days [B]
   Maximum: 500 mg day 1 and 250 mg days 2–5
   Available in suspensions of 100 mg and 200 mg/5 mL
5. Benzathine penicillin G (Bicillin L-A)—single dose therapy [B]
   In children less than 60 lb: 600,000 units IM
   In children greater than 60 lb: 1.2 million units IM

If severe or refractory:

1. Clindamycin 8–20 mg/kg/day PO divided qid (for penicillin allergic) [B]
   Easy dose: 5 mg/kg/dose PO qid
   Maximum: 300 mg/dose
   Available in suspension of 75 mg/5 mL
2. Cefuroxime axetil (Ceftin) 20–30 mg/kg/day PO divided bid [B]
   Easy dose: 20 mg/kg/day = 10 mg/kg/dose PO bid
   Maximum: 250 mg/dose
   Available in suspension of 125 mg/5 mL
3. Cefpodoxime (Vantin) 5 mg/kg/dose PO bid [B]
   Maximum: 200 mg/dose
   Available in suspensions of 50 mg and 100 mg/5 mL
4. Amoxicillin/clavulanate (Augmentin) 20–40 mg/kg/day (as amoxicillin) PO divided tid [B]
   Easy dose: 30 mg/kg/day = 10 mg/kg/dose PO tid
   Maximum: 500 mg per dose
   Available in suspensions of 125 mg and 250 mg amoxicillin/5 mL

B. ADULTS AND CHILDREN OVER AGE 10

Notes:

1. Sexual history essential to help rule out gonococcus (see Genital Tract Infections—Gonorrhea). Lab tests include latex agglutination (rapid strep test), Gram stain and/or culture.
   If prepubertal, treat for group A *Streptococcus* only.
2. If patient exhibits signs or symptoms of severe swelling/edema (e.g., voice change, unable to swallow saliva), consider adding prednisone (40 mg PO qd × 5 days) to the antibiotic regimen.

1. Penicillin V potassium (Pen-VEE K) 250–500 mg PO tid–qid [B]
2. Erythromycin 250 mg PO qid **OR** 500 mg bid [B, except estolate contraindicated]
3. Erythromycin ethyl succinate (EES) 400 mg PO qid **OR** 30–50 mg/kg/day PO divided qid [B]
4. Azithromycin (Zithromax) 500 mg PO initial dose, then 250 mg PO qd for 4 days [B]
5. Clarithromycin (Biaxin) 250–500 mg PO bid [C]

In refractory cases:

1. Clindamycin (Cleocin) 300 mg PO qid [B]
2. Cefuroxime axetil (Ceftin) 250 mg PO bid [B]
3. Cefpodoxime (Vantin) 200 mg PO bid [B]
4. Amoxicillin/clavulanate (Augmentin) 500 mg PO tid or 875 mg PO bid [B]

Course: 10 days (except azithromycin as noted).
Organisms: *Streptococcus* sp., *Mycoplasma pneumoniae, Chlamydia pneumoniae*, rhinovirus and Epstein-Barr virus

EYE

Blepharitis

Erythromycin ophthalmic ointment (Ilotycin)—apply to lid margins bid–tid [B]; dispense 3.5 g tube
Course: 14 days
Organisms: *S. aureus, S. epidermidis*

Conjunctivitis: Adult and Children

Notes:

1. Sulfacetamide may sting or burn when applied. This often decreases compliance.
2. Ophthalmic ointment is thick and impairs vision when first applied. Although drops require more frequent dosing, patients usually tolerate drops better while awake. Ointment is best used at bedtime.
3. If conjunctivitis is secondary to an imbedded organic material (mascara brush, tree branch), or in contact lens wearers, consider antipseudomonal coverage.
4. Slit lamp exam important to rule out herpes as organism. If herpes or gonococcus suspected, immediate ophthalmologic consultation is indicated.

1. Erythromycin ophthalmic ointment (Ilotycin)—apply to lid of affected eye bid–tid [B]; dispense 3.5 g tube
2. Sulfacetamide (10%) ophthalmic solution or ointment (Bleph-10, Sodium Sulamyd) [C]
   Solution: apply 1–2 drops to affected eye q2h; dispense 5 mL
   Ointment: apply to lid of affected eye qid; dispense 3.5 g
3. Tobramycin (0.3%) ophthalmic solution or ointment (Tobrex) [B]

Solution: apply 1–2 drops to affected eye q 2–4 h; dispense 5 mL
Ointment: apply to lid of affected eye q4h; dispense 3.5 g

For *Pseudomonas* coverage (see Note 3, below)

1. Ciprofloxacin (0.3%) ophthalmic solution (Cipro): 2 drops to affected eye q2h while awake for 2 days, then q4h for 5 days [C]

Course: 7 days
Organisms: *S. aureus, S. pneumoniae, E. coli, Proteus* sp., *Pseudomonas*

Conjunctivitis: Neonatal

(Gram stain and culture necessary)

1. Chlamydia trachomatis (occurs days 3–10)
   Erythromycin 50 mg/kg/day divided qid PO for 14 days
2. Neisseria gonorrhea (occurs days 2–4)
   Ceftriaxone 50 mg/kg IV or IM

Corneal Abrasion

1. Treat same as conjunctivitis, above, except consider antipseudomonal coverage (ciprofloxacin or tobramycin) for abrasions due to organic foreign bodies and contact lenses.
2. Patching of the eye is no longer considered necessary and should be based on patient comfort issues (i.e., discomfort of foreign body sensation versus discomfort of eye patch).
3. If eye is to be patched, use ointment instead of solution.
4. Consider short-acting cycloplegics (e.g., cyclopentolate 1–2 drops to affected eye [C]) if eye is to be patched.
5. A short course of acetaminophen with codeine or hydrocodone is appropriate for pain control.
6. Up to date tetanus prophylaxis is recommended for patients with corneal abrasions.

Course: 3 days

GASTROINTESTINAL

Ascariasis, Giardiasis. See Parasites.

Clostridium difficile/Pseudomembranous Colitis

Regimen A
Metronidazole (Flagyl) 500 mg PO tid [B; contraindicated 1st trimester]
PLUS (to bind toxin)
Cholestyramine (Questran) 4 gm PO tid

Regimen B
Vancomycin (Vancocin) 125–250 mg PO tid [C] (cholestyramine binds vancomycin; do not use)
Course: 10–14 days

Diverticulitis

Note: Treatments listed are for outpatient therapy in patients that appear nontoxic and are without evidence of bowel perforation. If patients appear toxic, are unable to tolerate PO, or perforation is suspected, admission is required.

Regimen A (*Note **two** drug therapy*)
TMP/SMX DS (Bactrim DS, Septra DS) 1 tablet PO bid [C; D in 3rd trimester] **OR**
Ciprofloxacin (Cipro) 500–750 mg PO bid [C]
PLUS
Metronidazole (Flagyl) 500 mg PO qid [B, contraindicated 1st trimester]

Regimen B
Amoxicillin/clavulanic acid (Augmentin) 500/125 mg PO tid **OR** 875/125 mg PO bid [B]
Course: 10–14 days
Organisms: *Enterobacter, Bacteroides,* enterococci

Gastroenteritis

Base treatment on the presence of fecal leukocytes or clinical picture:

1. Ciprofloxacin (Cipro) 500 mg PO bid [C]
2. TMP/SMX DS (Bactrim DS, Septra DS) 1 tablet PO bid [C; D in 3rd trimester]
   PLUS (to cover *Campylobacter*)
   Erythromycin 500 mg PO qid [B, except estolate contraindicated]
3. Amoxicillin/clavulanate (Augmentin) 500 mg PO tid
   PLUS (to cover *Campylobacter*)
   Erythromycin 500 mg PO qid [B, except estolate contraindicated]

Course: 3–5 days
Organisms: *Shigella, Salmonella, Campylobacter,* enteroinvasive *E. coli, Yersinia*

Helicobacter pylori (associated with non-NSAID induced duodenal or gastric ulcers)

Regimen A (*Note **four** drug therapy*)
Bismuth subsalicylate (Pepto-Bismol) 2 tabs PO qid with meals and at bedtime [D]
PLUS
Metronidazole (Flagyl) 500 mg PO bid **OR** 250 mg PO qid with meals and at bedtime [B, contraindicated 1st trimester]
PLUS
Tetracycline (Achromycin) 500 mg PO qid before meals and at bedtime [D] (doxycycline has lower efficacy; do not substitute)
PLUS
Omeprazole (Prilosec) 20 mg PO bid before meals [C]

Regimen B (*Note **three** drug therapy*)
Metronidazole (Flagyl) 500 mg PO bid **OR** 250 mg PO qid with meals and at bedtime [B, contraindicated 1st trimester] **OR**
Amoxicillin (Amoxil) 1 g PO bid **OR** 500 mg PO qid [B]
PLUS
Omeprazole (Prilosec) 20 mg PO bid before meals [C]
PLUS
Clarithromycin (Biaxin) 500 mg PO bid with meals [C]
Course: 7–14 days (90% eradication with 7 days of therapy)
Organism: *Helicobacter pylori*
Note: Usual definition of cure: negative serology urea breath test 1–3 months or longer after treatment.

Spontaneous Bacterial Peritonitis (SBP)

1. Cefotaxime 2 g IV q8h (q4h if life-threatening) [B]
2. Ticarcillin/clavulanic acid (Timentin) 3.1 g IV q6h [B]
3. Piperacillin/tazobactam (Zosyn) 3.375 g IV q6h [B]

4. Ampicillin/sulbactam (Unasyn) 3 g IV q6h [B]
Organisms: Enterobacteriaceae, *S. pneumoniae,* enterococci, anaerobes

GENITOURINARY TRACT INFECTIONS (EXCLUDING SEXUALLY TRANSMITTED DISEASES)

Cystitis

A. CHILDREN AGE 10 AND UNDER

1. TMP/SMX (Bactrim, Septra) 6–12 mg/kg/day TMP and 30–60 mg/kg/day SMX PO divided bid [C; D in 3rd trimester]
   Easy dose: 1 mL/kg/day PO divided bid = 8 mg/kg/day TMP and 40 mg/kg/day SMX
   Maximum: 20 mL/dose
   Suspension of TMP 40 mg and SMX 200 mg/5 mL
2. Amoxicillin (Amoxil) 20–40 mg/kg/day PO divided t.i.d. [B]
   Easy dose: 30 mg/kg/day = 10 mg/kg/dose PO tid
   Maximum: 250 mg/dose
   Available in suspensions of 125 mg and 250 mg/5 mL
3. Amoxicillin/clavulanate (Augmentin) 20–40 mg/kg/day (as amoxicillin) PO divided tid [B]
   Easy dose: 30 mg/kg/day = 10 mg/kg/dose PO tid
   Maximum: 500 mg/dose
   Available in suspensions of 125 mg and 250 mg amoxicillin/5 mL
4. Cefuroxime axetil (Ceftin) 20–30 mg/kg/day PO divided bid [B]
   Easy dose: 20 mg/kg/day = 10 mg/kg/dose PO bid
   Maximum: 250 mg/dose
   Available in suspension of 125 mg/5 mL
5. Cefixime (Suprax) 8 mg/kg/day PO in 1 dose [B]
   Maximum: 400 mg/day
   Suspension 100 mg/5 mL

B. ADULTS AND CHILDREN OLDER THAN 10
Notes:

1. If patient has significant bladder pain, add phenazopyridine (Pyridium) 200 mg PO tid after meals for 2 days [B] (will turn the urine red/orange color)
2. **For uncomplicated cystitis in adult females** (non-pregnant, non-diabetic) with symptoms of short duration, consider short course therapy:
   a. TMP/SMX DS (Bactrim DS, Septra DS) 1 tablet PO bid for 3 days [C; D in 3rd trimester]
   b. Ciprofloxacin (Cipro) 500 mg PO bid for 3 days [C]
   c. Ofloxacin (Floxin) 200 mg PO bid for 3 days [C]
   d. Norfloxacin (Noroxin) 400 mg PO bid for 3 days [C]
   e. Fosfomycin (Monurol) 3 g PO single dose [B]

1. TMP/SMX DS (Bactrim DS, Septra DS) 1 tablet PO bid [C; D in 3rd trimester]
2. Ciprofloxacin (Cipro) 500 mg PO bid [C]
3. Ofloxacin (Floxin) 200 mg PO bid [C]
4. Norfloxacin (Noroxin) 400 mg PO bid [C]
5. Levofloxacin (Levaquin) 500 mg PO qd [C]
6. Amoxicillin/clavulanic acid (Augmentin) 250 mg PO tid [B]
7. Cefuroxime axetil (Ceftin) 250 mg PO bid [B]
8. Ceftibuten (Cedax) 400 mg PO qd [B]

Course: 7 to 10 days (See Notes below)
Organisms: *E. coli,* enterococci, *Staph* sp.

Endometritis

A. EARLY POSTPARTUM [1ST 48 H]
(*Note **three** drug therapy*)

1. Cefoxitin (Mefoxin) 2 g IV q 6–8 h [B]
2. Ticarcillin/clavulanic acid (Timentin) 3.1 g IV q6h [B]
3. Imipenem (Primaxin) 500–1000 mg IV q6h [C]
4. Ampicillin/sulbactam (Unasyn) 3.0 g IV q6h [B]
5. Piperacillin/tazobactam (Zosyn) 3.375 g IV q6h [B]

PLUS

1. Doxycycline (Vibramycin) 100 mg IV or PO q12h [D]
2. Clindamycin (Cleocin) 450–900 mg IV q8h [B]

PLUS

1. Gentamicin (Garamycin) 2 mg/kg IV loading dose, then 1.7 mg/kg IV q8h (monitor serum levels) [D]
2. Ceftriaxone (Rocephin) 2 g IV qd [B]
3. Cefotaxime (Claforan) 2 g IV q8h [B]

Organisms: *Prevotella bivia* and other Bacteroides sp., group B streptococci, *Enterococci, E. coli, Chlamydia trachomatis, Gardnerella vaginalis*

B. LATE POSTPARTUM (48 H TO 6 WEEKS)
Doxycycline (Vibramycin) 100 mg PO or IV bid (discontinue nursing) [D]
Course: 14 days
Organisms: *C. trachomatis, M. hominis*

Epididymitis and Orchitis

A. YOUNGER PATIENTS (LESS THAN 35 YEARS OF AGE)
Treat for gonorrhea and chlamydia—*See Sexually Transmitted Diseases.*

B. OLDER PATIENTS (GREATER THAN 35 YEARS OF AGE)

1. Ciprofloxacin (Cipro) 500 mg PO bid [C]
2. TMP/SMX DS (Bactrim DS, Septra DS) 1 tablet PO bid [C; D in 3rd trimester]
3. Ofloxacin (Floxin) 200 mg PO bid [C]

Course: 10–14 days
Organisms: *E. coli, Proteus* sp.

Prostatitis—Acute

A. YOUNGER PATIENTS (LESS THAN 35 YEARS OF AGE)
Treat for gonorrhea and chlamydia—*See Sexually Transmitted Diseases.*

B. OLDER PATIENTS (GREATER THAN 35 YEARS OF AGE OR HISTORY OF INSERTIVE ANAL INTERCOURSE)

1. Ciprofloxacin (Cipro) 500 mg PO bid [C]
2. TMP/SMX DS (Bactrim DS, Septra DS) one tablet PO bid [C; D in 3rd trimester]
3. Ofloxacin (Floxin) 200 mg PO bid [C]

Course: 14–28 days
Organisms: *E. coli, Enterobacter, Klebsiella, Proteus*

Prostatitis—Chronic

Chronic prostatitis involves similar organisms as acute prostatitis. If patient has already had treatment, a longer course of a different antibiotic is warranted. Referral to urologist recommended as chronic therapy may be needed. **Course:** 1–3 months.

Pyelonephritis

A. UNCOMPLICATED

Young, otherwise healthy patients with pyelonephritis may be treated as outpatients. Use the same medications as listed in Cystitis, except exclude TMP/SMX from treatment regimen (due to resistance). Consider initiating therapy with a single dose of parenteral medication as listed below for complicated pyelonephritis. **Course:** 14 days.

B. COMPLICATED

Admission is recommended for patients with pyelonephritis complicated by elderly, pregnant, renal insufficiency, or structural abnormality (including a single kidney), immunocompromised (e.g., diabetics, HIV, transplant, chemotherapy), intractable nausea/vomiting, sickle cell anemia, renal calculi, toxic appearance, unremitting fever.

1. Ceftriaxone (Rocephin) 2 g IV qd [B]
2. Cefotaxime (Claforan) 1 g IV q12h [B]
3. Ciprofloxacin 400 mg IV q12h [C]
4. Levofloxacin (Levaquin) 500 mg IV qd [C]
5. Ampicillin 2 g IV q4h [B] **PLUS** gentamicin (Garamycin) 2 mg/kg IV loading dose, then 1.7 mg/kg IV q8h **OR** 5.1 mg/kg IV QD (monitor serum levels) [D]
6. Ampicillin/sulbactam (Unasyn) 3.0 g IV q6h [B]
7. Ticarcillin/clavulanic acid (Timentin) 3.1 g IV q6h [B]
8. Piperacillin/tazobactam (Zosyn) 3.375 g IV q6h [B]
9. Imipenem (Primaxin) 500–1000 mg IV q6h [C]

Organisms: *E. coli, Enterococcus,* Enterobacteriaceae

Sterile Pyuria

(Pyuria without bacteria or with negative culture. Consider evaluation for tuberculosis as possible etiology.)

1. Doxycycline 100 mg PO bid [D]
2. Tetracycline 500 mg PO qid [D]
3. Erythromycin 500 mg PO qid [B, except estolate contraindicated]
4. Ofloxacin (Floxin) 200 mg PO bid [C]
5. Levofloxacin (Levaquin) 250 mg PO qd [C]
6. Azithromycin (Zithromax) 500 mg PO initial dose, then 250 mg PO qd for 4 days [B]

Course: 7 days (except azithromycin as noted)
Organisms: *C. trachomatis, Ureaplasma urealyticum,* tuberculosis

HEART

Endocarditis (Culture Results Unavailable)

Note: If patient condition permits, cultures should be obtained before initiating antimicrobial therapy

Infective endocarditis—native valve
Regimen A (*Note **three** drug therapy*)
Penicillin G 3.5 million units IV q4h [B] **OR**
Ampicillin 2 g IV q4h [B]
PLUS
Nafcillin 2 g IV q4h [B]
PLUS
Gentamicin (Garamycin) 2 mg/kg IV loading dose, then 1.7 mg/kg IV q8h (monitor serum levels) [D]

Regimen B (*Note **two** drug therapy*)
Vancomycin (Vancocin) 15 mg/kg IV q12h (max 1 g/dose; monitor serum levels) [C]
PLUS
Gentamicin (Garamycin) 2 mg/kg IV loading dose, then 1.7 mg/kg IV q8h (monitor serum levels) [D]
Organisms: *Strep viridans, Strep* sp., enterococci, *Staph sp.*

Infective endocarditis—prosthetic valve (*Note **three** drug therapy*)
Vancomycin (Vancocin) 15 mg/kg IV q12h (max 1 g/dose; monitor serum levels) [C]
PLUS
Gentamicin (Garamycin) 2 mg/kg IV loading dose, then 1.7 mg/kg IV q8h (monitor serum levels) [D]
PLUS
Rifampin (Rimactane) 600 mg PO qd [C]
Organisms: *Staph epidermidis, Staph aureus, Strep viridans,* enterococci

1. **Infective endocarditis—intravenous drug abusers** (*Note **two** drug therapy*)
   Nafcillin 2 gram IV q4h [B] (preferred)
   OR if penicillin allergic or suspect MRSA
   Vancomycin (Vancocin) 15 mg/kg IV q12h (max 1 g/dose; monitor serum levels) [C]
   PLUS
   Gentamicin (Garamycin) 2 mg/kg IV loading dose, then 1.7 mg/kg IV q8h (monitor serum levels) [D]

Organisms: *S. aureus,* gram-negative bacilli

Endocarditis Prophylaxis

Prophylaxis is **recommended** for patients with

1. **High risk conditions:** prosthetic valves, previous history of endocarditis, congenital heart disease (e.g., transposition or tetralogy), pulmonic shunts/conduits
   OR
2. **Moderate risk conditions:** cardiomyopathy, mitral prolapse with regurgitation

AND undergoing the following procedures: Dental procedures (excluding filling cavities, suture removal, orthodontic removal or adjustment, or dental x-rays), rigid bronchoscopy, sclerotherapy of esophageal varices, dilation of esophageal strictures, biliary tract or intestinal surgery, prostatic surgery, cystoscopy, and urethral dilatation.

In general, prophylaxis is **not recommended** for

1. **Low risk conditions:** ASD or repaired ASD/VSD, PDA beyond 6 months old, mitral valve prolapse without regurgitation/insufficiency, history of CABG, history of rheumatic fever without valve dysfunction, cardiac pacemakers or AICDs.
   OR
2. **Patients undergoing the following procedures:** Intubation, TEE*, flexible bronchoscopy*, EGD without biopsy*, uninfected D&C/TAB, uninfected IUD insertion/removal, uninfected Foley cath placement, cardiac catheterization, angioplasty, coronary stent placement, or skin biopsy. (**Consider prophylaxis in high-risk patients.*)

A. ADULTS AND CHILDREN OVER AGE 10

1. Amoxicillin (Amoxil) 2 g PO 1 h before procedure [B]
2. Clindamycin (Cleocin) 600 mg PO 1 h before procedure [B]
3. Cephalexin (Keflex) 2 g PO 1 h before procedure [B]
4. Azithromycin (Zithromax) 500 mg PO 1 h before procedure [B]

If unable to take PO

1. Ampicillin 2 g IV/IM 30 min before procedure [B]
2. Clindamycin (Cleocin) 600 mg IV 30 min before procedure [B]
3. Cefazolin (Ancef) 1 g IV/IM 30 min before procedure [B]

B. CHILDREN AGE 10 AND UNDER

Note: Do not exceed adult dose

1. Amoxicillin (Amoxil) 50 mg/kg PO 1 h before procedure [B]
2. Clindamycin (Cleocin) 20 mg/kg PO 1 h before procedure [B]
3. Cephalexin (Keflex) 50 mg/kg PO 1 h before procedure [B]
4. Azithromycin (Zithromax) 15 mg/kg PO 1 h before procedure [B]

If unable to take PO

1. Ampicillin 50 mg/kg IV/IM 30 min before procedure [B]
2. Clindamycin (Cleocin) 20 mg/kg IV 30 min before procedure [B]
3. Cefazolin (Ancef) 25 mg/kg IV/IM 30 min before procedure [B]

MENINGITIS/ENCEPHALITIS

Encephalitis

Herpes simplex virus (HSV) encephalitis
Requires admission to hospital
Acyclovir (Zovirax) 10 mg/kg IV q8h (infused over 1 h) [C]

Meningitis

Notes:

1. If meningitis is suspected, do not delay antibiotics while obtaining lumbar puncture or cultures.
2. Some regions have a high incidence of **drug-resistant *Streptococcus pneumoniae* (DRSP)** [susceptible MIC ≤0.1 μg/mL; intermediate >0.1 to ≤1.0; resistant ≥2.0]. If prevalence of DRSP is high (i.e., >2% isolates intermediate or resistant MIC), add vancomycin to regimen.
3. Some authorities recommend dexamethasone in children or adults with positive Gram stain or coma. **Dexamethasone dose: 0.4 mg/kg IV q12h for 4 doses** [C] with first dose given prior to antibiotics (if patient's condition permits, efficacy is improved if given 15–20 min before antibiotics).

A. NEONATAL AND INFANTS (UP TO 8 WEEKS OF AGE)

(*Note **two or three** drug therapy*)

Note: Ceftriaxone is no longer recommended in neonates because of the potential for biliary sludge pseudolithiasis.

Cefotaxime (Claforan) 75 mg/kg IV or IM q6h [B]
PLUS (to cover group B *Strep* and *Listeria*)
Ampicillin 50 mg/kg IV or IM q6h [B]
PLUS/MINUS (to cover DRSP—see notes, above)
Vancomycin (Vancocin) 15 mg/kg IV q6h (monitor serum levels) [C]

Organisms: group B *Strep, E. coli, Listeria, Klebsiella, Enterobacter, S. aureus, H. influenzae*

B. INFANT/CHILD

1. Cefotaxime (Claforan) 75 mg/kg IV or IM q6h [B] **OR**
2. Ceftriaxone (Rocephin) 50 mg/kg IV or IM q12h (max 2 g/dose) [B]
   PLUS/MINUS (to cover DRSP—see notes, above)
1. Vancomycin (Vancocin) 15 mg/kg IV q6h (max 1 g/dose; monitor serum levels) [C]

Organisms: *H. influenzae, S. pneumoniae, N. meningitidis*

C. PEDIATRIC PATIENTS WITH A SEVERE PENICILLIN ALLERGY

Regimen A (*Note **two** drug therapy*)
Vancomycin (Vancocin) 15 mg/kg IV q6h (max 1 g/dose; monitor serum levels) [C]
PLUS
TMP/SMX (Bactrim, Septra) 5 mg/kg IV q12h based on TMP [C; D in 3rd trimester]

Regimen B (*Note **three** drug therapy*)
Vancomycin (Vancocin) 15 mg/kg IV q6h (max 1 g/dose; monitor serum levels) [C]
PLUS
Gentamicin (Garamycin) 2 mg/kg IV loading dose, then 1.7 mg/kg IV q8h (monitor serum levels) [D]
PLUS
Rifampin (Rimactane) 10–20 mg/kg IV qd (max 600 mg/dose) [C]

D. ADULT (18–50 YEARS OF AGE)

1. Ceftriaxone (Rocephin) 2 g IV q12h [B] **OR**
2. Cefotaxime (Claforan) 2 g IV q8h [B]
   PLUS/MINUS (to cover DRSP—see notes, above)
   Vancomycin (Vancocin) 15 mg/kg IV q6h (max 1 g/dose; monitor serum levels) [C]

Organisms: *S. pneumoniae, N. meningitidis*

E. ADULT (>50 YEARS OF AGE, OR IMMUNOCOMPROMISED)

(*Note **two or three** drug therapy*)

1. Ceftriaxone (Rocephin) 2 g IV q12h [B] **OR**
2. Cefotaxime (Claforan) 2 gm IV q8h [B]
   PLUS
   Ampicillin 2 g IV q4h [B]
   PLUS/MINUS (to cover DRSP—see notes, above)
   Vancomycin (Vancocin) 15 mg/kg IV q6h (max 1 g/dose; monitor serum levels) [C]

Organisms: *S. pneumoniae, N. meningitidis, Listeria,* aerobic gram-negative bacilli

F. ADULT PATIENTS WITH A SEVERE PENICILLIN ALLERGY

Regimen A (*Note **two** drug therapy*)
Vancomycin (Vancocin) 15 mg/kg IV q6h (max 1 g/dose; monitor serum levels) [C]
PLUS
TMP/SMX (Bactrim, Septra) 5 mg/kg IV q12h based on TMP [C; D in 3rd trimester]

Regimen B (*Note **three** drug therapy*)
Vancomycin (Vancocin) 15 mg/kg IV q6h (max 1 g/dose; monitor serum levels) [C]
PLUS
Gentamicin (Garamycin) 2 mg/kg IV loading dose, then 1.7 mg/kg IV q8h (monitor serum levels) [D]
PLUS
Rifampin (Rimactane) 10–20 mg/kg IV qd (max 600 mg/dose) [C]

G. MENINGOCOCCAL PROPHYLAXIS (CLOSE CONTACTS)

1. Ciprofloxacin (Cipro) 500 mg PO single dose (must be >18 years) [C]
2. Rifampin 600 mg q12h for 4 doses (pediatric dose: 10 mg/kg PO q12h for 4 doses) [C]
3. Ceftriaxone (Rocephin) 250 mg IM single dose (pediatric dose <15 years: 125 mg IM single dose) [B]

OCCUPATIONAL HIV EXPOSURE

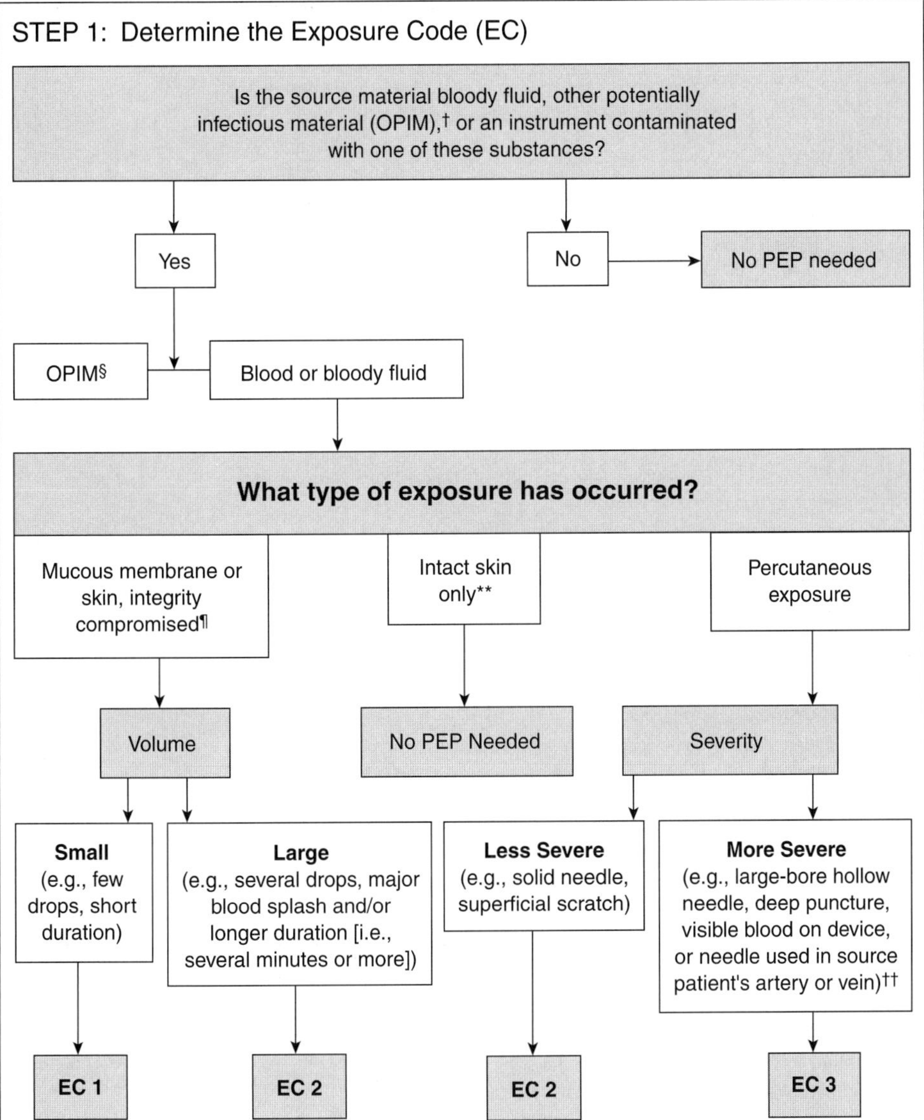

*This algorithm is intended to guide initial decisions about PEP and should be used in conjuntion with other guidance provided in this report.

†Semen or vaginal secretions; cerebrospinal, synovial, pleural, peritoneal, pericardial, or amniotic fluids; or tissue.

§Exposures to OPIM must be evaluated on a case-by-case basis. In general, these body substances are considered a low risk for transmission in health-care settings. Any unprotected contact to concentrated HIV in a research laboratory or production facility is considered an occupational exposure that requires clinical evaluation to determine the need for PEP.

¶Skin integrity is considered compromised if there is evidence of chapped skin, dermatitis, abrasion, or open wound.

**Contact with intact skin is not normally considered a risk for HIV transmission. However, if the exposure was to blood, and the circumstance suggests a higher volume exposure (e.g., an extensive area of skin was exposed or there was prolonged contact with blood), the risk for HIV transmission should be considered.

††The combination of these severity factors (e.g., large-bore hollow needle and deep puncture) contribute to an elevated risk for transmission if the source person is HIV-positive.

FIG. 149-1. Determining the need for HIV post-exposure prophylaxis (PEP) after an occupational exposure.*

STEP 2: Determine the HIV Status Code (HIV SC)

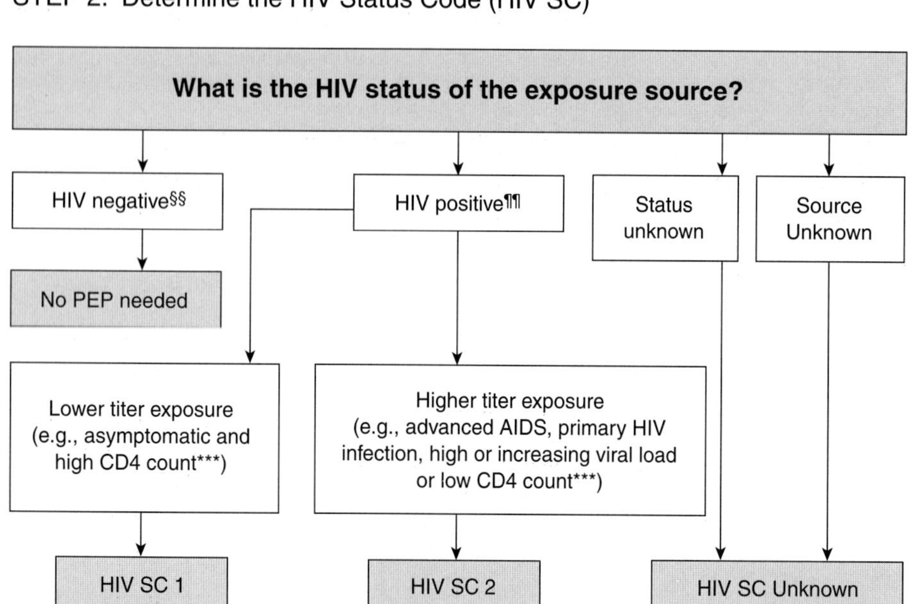

§§ A source is considered negative for HIV infection if there is laboratory documentation of a negative HIV antibody, HIV polymerase chain reation (PCR), or HIV p24 antigen test result from a specimen collected at or near the time of exposure and there is no clinical evidence of recent retroviral-like illness.

¶¶ A source is considered infected with HIV (HIV positive) if there has been a positive laboratory result for HIV antibody, HIV PCR, or HIV p24 antigen or physician-diagnosed AIDS.

*** Examples are used as surrogates to estimate the HIV titer in an exposure source for purposes of considering PEP regimens and do not reflect all clinical situations that may be observed. Although a high HIV titer (HIV SC 2) in an exposure source has been associated with an increased risk for transmission, the possibility of transmission from a source with a low HIV titer also must be considered.

STEP 3: Determine the PEP Recommendation

EC	HIV SC	PEP recommendation
1	1	**PEP may not be warranted.** Exposure type does not pose a known risk for HIV transmission. Whether the risk for drug toxicity outweighs the benefit of PEP should be decided by the exposed HCW and treating clinician.
1	2	**Consider basic regimen.†††** Exposure type poses a negligible risk for HIV transmission. A high HIV titer in the source may justify consideration of PEP. Whether the risk for drug toxicity outweighs the benefit of PEP should be decided by the exposed HCW and treating clinician.
2	1	**Recommend basic regimen.** Most HIV exposures are in this category; no increased risk for HIV transmission has been observed but use of PEP is appropriate.
2	2	**Recommend expanded regimen.§§§** Exposure type represents an increased HIV transmission risk.
3	1 or 2	**Recommend expanded regimen.** Exposure type represents an increased HIV transmission risk.
Unknown		If the source or, in the case of an unknown source, the setting where the exposure occurred suggests a possible risk for HIV exposure and the EC is 2 or 3, consider PEP basic regimen.

††† Basic regimen is four weeks of zidovudine, 600 mg per day in two or three divided doses, and lamivudine, 150 mg twice daily.

§§§ Expanded regimen is the basic regimen plus either indinavir, 800 mg every 8 hours, or nelfinavir, 750 mg three times a day.

CDC, PHS Guidelines for the Management of Health-Care Worker Exposures to HIV and Recommendations for Post-Exposure Prophylaxis. *MMWR* 47 (No. RR-7):14–15, 1998.

FIG. 149-1 (*Continued*). Determining the need for HIV postexposure prophylaxis (PEP) after an occupational exposure.*

PARASITES

Ascariasis

1. Albendazole (Albenza) 400 mg PO single dose [C]
2. Mebendazole (Vermox) 100 mg PO bid for 3 days [C]
3. Pyrantel pamoate (Antiminth) 11 mg/kg PO single dose (max 1 g) [not recommended in pregnancy]

Organism: *Ascariasis lumbricoides*

Giardiasis

1. Metronidazole (Flagyl) 250 mg PO tid for 5 days [B, contraindicated 1st trimester]
2. Furazolidone (Furoxone) 1.5 mg/kg PO qid for 10 days (consider in children; max 100 mg/dose) [C]
3. Paromomycin (Humatin) 10 mg/kg PO tid for 7 days (max 500 mg/dose) [not absorbed from GI tract so may be useful in pregnancy; not FDA approved for this use]

Course: 5 days
Organism: *Giardia lamblia*

Lice, Body

No pharmacologic treatment is required. Body lice live in clothing and only leave for a blood meal. If possible discard clothing, otherwise treat clothing with 1% malathion powder or 10% DDT powder. Untreated nits viable for 1 month. Clothing of sexual partners and other close contacts should also be discarded or treated. **Organism:** *Pediculosis humanus corporis.*

Lice, Head and Pubic (Crabs)

Notes:

1. Lindane (Kwell) is cheaper but less effective and potentially toxic (seizures, aplastic anemia).
2. Lindane is not recommended in patients with extensive dermatitis, children under 2 years old or in pregnant/lactating women; it should **not** be applied following a bath.
3. Bedding and clothing should be washed and dried using heat cycle or removed from body contact for at least 72 h.
4. Sexual partners and other close contacts should also be treated.

1. Permethrin cream 5% (Elimite) [B]
   Wash hair, apply as a liquid and leave on for 10 min, wash off, and comb. Re-treat in 1 week. Also available OTC as Permethrin 1% creme rinse (Nix).
   Dispense 60 mL
2. Pyrethrins with piperonyl butoxide (RID) [C]
   Apply as for permethrin cream, above
   Dispense 60 mL
3. Lindane 1% shampoo (Kwell) [B]
   Apply to hair for 4 min, wash off (see notes, below)
   Dispense 1–2 ounces
4. Ivermectin (Stromectol) 200 μg/kg PO single dose (adults or pediatrics) [C]

Organism: *Pediculosis humanus capitus, Phthirus pubis*

Pinworms

1. Mebendazole (Vermox) 100 mg PO single dose; repeat dose in 2 weeks [C]
2. Pyrantel pamoate (Antiminth, Pin-X) 11 mg/kg PO single dose (max 1 g); repeat every 2 weeks × 2 [not recommended in pregnancy]
3. Albendazole (Albenza) 400 mg PO single dose; repeat dose in 2 weeks [C]

Organism: *Enterobius vermicularis*

Scabies

Notes:

1. Bedding and clothing should be washed and dried using heat cycle or removed from body contact for at least 72 h.
2. Sexual partners and other close contacts should also be treated.

1. Permethrin cream 5% (Elimite)
   Apply to skin from neck down, leave on 8–14 h, wash off; re-treat in 1 week [B]
   Dispense 60 g
2. Crotamiton 10% (Eurax)
   Apply to skin from neck down for 2 nights and wash off 24 h after second application [C]
   Dispense 60 mL
3. Ivermectin (Stromectol) 200 μg/kg PO single dose (adults or pediatrics) [C]

Organism: *Sarcoptes scabiei* (skin mite)

PRESURGICAL ANTIBIOTICS

Note: Must be given within 2 h of surgery to be effective.

Appendicitis (Not Perforated)

1. Cefoxitin (Mefoxin) 2 g IV [B] **OR**
2. Cefotetan (Cefotan) 2 g IV [B]

Organisms: enteric gram negative bacilli, anaerobes

Bowel Perforation/Peritonitis

*(Note **two** drug therapy, **except** Regimen D)*

Regimen A
Cefoxitin (Mefoxin) 2 g IV [B] **OR**
Cefotetan (Cefotan) 2 g IV [B]
PLUS/MINUS
Gentamicin (Garamycin) 2 mg/kg IV [D]

Regimen B
Clindamycin (Cleocin) 600 mg IV [B]
PLUS
Gentamicin (Garamycin) 2 mg/kg IV [D] **OR**
Aztreonam (Azactam) 2 g IV [B]

Regimen C
Cefotaxime (Claforan) 2 g IV [B]
Ceftriaxone (Rocephin) 1–2 g IV [B]
Ceftizoxime (Cefizox) 2 g IV [B]
Cefoperazone (Cefobid) 2 g IV [B]
Ceftazidime (Fortaz) 2 g IV [B]
PLUS
Metronidazole (Flagyl) 1 g IV [B, contraindicated 1st trimester]
OR
Clindamycin (Cleocin) 600 mg IV [B]

Regimen D
Imipenem (Primaxin) 500 mg IV [C]

Organisms: enteric gram negative bacilli, anaerobes, enterococci

Cholecystitis/cholangitis

Regimen A

Ticarcillin/clavulanic acid (Timentin) 3.1 g IV [B]
Ampicillin/sulbactam (Unasyn) 3 g IV [B]
Piperacillin/tazobactam (Zosyn) 3.375 g IV [B]
Imipenem (Primaxin) 500–1000 mg IV [C]
Meropenem (Merrem) 1 g IV [B]

Regimen B (*Note **two** drug therapy*)

Cefotaxime (Claforan) 2 g IV [B]
Ceftriaxone (Rocephin) 1–2 g IV [B]
Ceftizoxime (Cefizox) 2 g IV [B]
Cefoperazone (Cefobid) 2 g IV [B]
Ceftazidime (Fortaz) 2 g IV [B]
PLUS
Metronidazole (Flagyl) 1 g IV [B, contraindicated 1st trimester]
OR
Clindamycin (Cleocin) 600 mg IV [B]

Regimen C (*Note **one or two** drug therapy*)

Ticarcillin (Ticar) 3–4 g IV [B] **OR**
Piperacillin (Pipracil) 3–4 g IV [B]
PLUS/MINUS
Metronidazole (Flagyl) 1 g IV [B, contraindicated 1st trimester]

Regimen D (*Note **two** drug therapy*)
Aztreonam (Azactam) 2 g IV [B]
PLUS
Clindamycin (Cleocin) 600 mg IV [B]
Organisms: Enterobacteriaceae, enterococci, *Bacteroides, Clostridium*

Open Fractures

(*Note **two** drug therapy for **severe** fractures*)

1. Cefazolin (Ancef) 1–2 g IV [B]
2. Vancomycin 15 mg/kg IV (max 1 g) [C]
3. Clindamycin (Cleocin) 600 mg IV [B]

PLUS (*for severe fractures—grade II and above*)

1. Gentamicin (Garamycin) 2 mg/kg IV [D]

Organisms: *S. aureus, S. epidermidis,* gram negative rods

Penetrating Abdominal Wounds

See Presurgical Antibiotics, Bowel Perforation/Peritonitis.

RESPIRATORY TRACT INFECTIONS

Bronchitis

A. ADULTS (NON-SMOKERS, NO UNDERLYING DISEASE OR HISTORY OF RESPIRATORY PROBLEMS)

Notes: Antibiotics are rarely necessary. Treat with inhaled beta-agonist therapy (e.g., albuterol, metaproterenol). If no improvement after 1 week, consider treatment

1. Erythromycin 500 mg PO qid [B, except estolate contraindicated]
2. Erythromycin ethyl succinate (EES) 400 mg PO qid [B]
3. Azithromycin (Zithromax) 500 mg PO initial dose, then 250 mg PO qd for 4 days [B]
4. Clarithromycin (Biaxin) 250–500 mg PO bid [C]
5. Doxycycline (Vibramycin) 100 mg PO bid [D]

(Chlamydia pneumonia (TWAR) has resistance to erythromycin. Consider azithromycin or clarithromycin.)

Course: 7–10 days (except azithromycin as noted)
Organisms: usually viral, *Mycoplasma pneumoniae, S. pneumoniae, Chlamydia pneumoniae* (TWAR)

B. ADULTS (SMOKER OR CHRONIC ILLNESS)

Note: In addition to antibiotics, treat with an inhaled β-agonist (e.g., albuterol, metaproterenol)

1. TMP/SMX DS (Bactrim DS, Septra DS) 1 tablet PO bid [B; D in 3rd trimester]
2. Doxycycline (Vibramycin) 100 mg PO bid [D]
3. Azithromycin (Zithromax) 500 mg PO initial dose, then 250 mg PO qd for 4 days [B]
4. Clarithromycin (Biaxin) 250–500 mg PO bid [C]
5. Amoxicillin/clavulanate (Augmentin) 250–500 mg PO tid [B]
6. Levofloxacin (Levaquin) 250–500 mg PO qd [C]
7. Sparfloxacin (Zagam) 400 mg PO initial dose, then 200 mg PO qd [C]
8. Cefuroxime axetil (Ceftin) 250–500 mg PO bid [B]
9. Cefpodoxime proxetil (Vantin) 200 mg PO bid [B]

Course: 10 days (except azithromycin as noted)
Organisms: *H. influenzae, M. catarrhalis, S. pneumonia, Klebsiella* sp., anaerobes, *E. coli*

Pertussis

Notes:

1. Consider diagnosis in afebrile patients, including adults, with persistent cough.
2. Treatment of household contacts recommended.
3. Differential diagnoses include gastroesophageal reflux, asthma, and postnasal drip.

A. PEDIATRIC

1. Erythromycin estolate (Ilosone) 40 mg/kg/day PO divided bid–tid for 7 days [contraindicated in pregnancy]
   Easy dose: 20 mg/kg/dose PO bid for 7 days
   Maximum: 250–500 mg per dose
   Liquids: 125 mg and 250 mg/5 cc
2. Erythromycin ethyl succinate (EES) 30–50 mg/kg/day PO divided qid for 14 days [B]
   Easy dose: 10 mg/kg/dose PO qid for 14 days
   Maximum: 250–500 mg per dose
   Liquids: 200 mg and 400 mg/5 cc
3. TMP/SMX (Bactrim, Septra) 10 mg/kg/day TMP & 50 mg/kg/day SMX PO divided bid for 14 days [C; D in 3rd trimester]
   Easy dose: 1.25 cc/kg/day PO divided bid for 14 days
   Maximum: 20 cc per dose
   Suspension of TMP 40 mg and SMX 200 mg/5 cc

B. ADULTS

1. Erythromycin estolate (Ilosone) 500 mg PO qid for 7 days [contradicted in pregnancy]
2. TMP/SMX DS (Bactrim DS, Septra DS) 1 tablet PO bid for 14 days [B; D in 3rd trimester]

Organisms: *Bordetellal pertussis, Bordetella parapertussis*

Pneumonia

A. NEONATES (<1 MONTH)

(*Note **two** drug therapy*) Ceftriaxone is no longer recommended in neonates because of the potential for biliary sludge pseudolithiasis.

1. Ampicillin 50 mg/kg IV q6h [B] **OR**
2. Nafcillin 50 mg/kg IV q6h [B]

OR (if suspect **MRSA**)

3. Vancomycin (Vancocin) 10 mg/kg IV q6h (max 1 g; monitor serum levels) [C]
   PLUS

1. Gentamicin (Garamycin) 2 mg/kg IV loading dose, then 1.7 mg/kg IV q8h (monitor serum levels) [D] **OR**
2. Cefotaxime (Claforan) 50 mg/kg IV q6h [B]

Organisms: group B *Strep, Listeria,* coliforms, *Staph. aureus, Pseudomonas, Chlamydia*

B. PEDIATRIC (1 MONTH–18 YEARS)

INPATIENT THERAPY

(*Note **two** drug therapy*)

Erythromycin 10 mg/kg IV q6h (max 1 g/dose) [B, except estolate contraindicated]

PLUS

Cefuroxime 50 mg/kg IV q8h (max 1 g/dose) [B]

OUTPATIENT THERAPY

Note: Consider initiating outpatient therapy with a single dose of the parenteral antibiotics listed above for inpatient therapy.

1. Erythromycin 30–50 mg/kg/day PO divided qid
   Easy dose: 10 mg/kg/dose PO qid
   Maximum: 250–500 mg/dose
   Liquids:
   Erythromycin ethyl succinate (EES) 200 mg and 400 mg/5 mL [B]
   Erythromycin estolate (Ilosone) 125 mg and 250 mg/5 mL (contraindicated in pregnancy)
2. Clarithromycin (Biaxin) 7.5 mg/kg/dose PO bid [C]
   Maximum: 250–500 mg/dose
   Suspensions: 125 mg and 250 mg/5 mL
3. Erythromycin/sulfisoxazole (Pediazole) 50 mg/kg/day erythro and 150 mg/kg/day sulfa PO divided tid **OR** qid [C; D in 3rd trimester]
   Easy dose: 1.25 mL/kg/day PO divided qid
   Maximum: 10 mL/dose
   Suspension of erythromycin 200 mg and sulfisoxazole 600 mg/5 mL

Course: 10–14 days

Organisms: *S. pneumoniae, H. influenzae* (1–24 months), *Chlamydia pneumoniae, Mycoplasma pneumoniae,* RSV (1–24 months), viral

C. ADULTS (60 YEARS OLD OR LESS, COMMUNITY ACQUIRED, NO COMORBIDITY)

INPATIENT THERAPY

Regimen A

(*Note **two or three** drug therapy*)

Cefotaxime (Claforan) 2 g IV q8h [B] **OR**

Ceftriaxone (Rocephin) 2 g IV qd [B]

PLUS

Erythromycin 5 mg/kg/dose IV qid (max 1 g/dose) [B, except estolate contraindicated] **OR**

Azithromycin (Zithromax) 500 mg IV qd [B]

PLUS/MINUS (if suspect drug-resistant *Strep. pneumoniae*)

Vancomycin (Vancocin) 15 mg/kg IV q6h (max 1 g/dose; monitor serum levels) [C]

Regimen B (*Note **one or two** drug therapy*)

Levofloxacin (Levaquin) 500 mg IV qd [C]

PLUS/MINUS (if aspiration suspected)

Clindamycin 600 mg IV q8h [B]

OUTPATIENT THERAPY

Notes:

1. Initial antibiotic selection may differ in areas with community-wide erythromycin (macrolide) resistant *S. pneumoniae.*
2. Erythromycin variably effective against *H. influenzae.*
3. Consider initiating outpatient therapy with a single dose of the parenteral antibiotics listed above for inpatient therapy.

1. Azithromycin (Zithromax) 500 mg PO initial dose, then 250 mg PO qd for 4 days [B]
2. Clarithromycin (Biaxin) 250–500 mg PO bid [C]
3. Erythromycin 500 mg PO qid **OR** erythromycin ethyl succinate (EES) 400 mg PO bid [B, except estolate contraindicated]
4. Levofloxacin (Levaquin) 500 mg PO qd [C]
5. Doxycycline (Vibramycin) 100 mg PO bid [D]

Course: 10–14 days (except azithromycin as noted) (levofloxacin preferred in areas with *S. pneumoniae* macrolide resistance)

Organisms: *S. pneumoniae, Mycoplasma pneumoniae, Chlamydia pneumoniae* (TWAR), *Legionella* sp., *H. influenzae*

D. ADULTS (OLDER THAN 60 YEARS OF AGE, SMOKER, CHRONIC ILLNESS, ALCOHOLIC)

INPATIENT THERAPY

Note: Treat as for adults (60 years old, community acquired, no comorbidity), above.

OUTPATIENT THERAPY

Note: Consider initiating outpatient therapy with a single dose of the parenteral antibiotics listed above for inpatient therapy.

Regimen A

Azithromycin (Zithromax) 500 mg PO initial dose then 250 mg PO qd for 4 days [B]

Clarithromycin (Biaxin) 250–500 mg PO bid [C]

Regimen B (if suspect Drug Resistant *S. pneumoniae*)

Levofloxacin (Levaquin) 500 mg PO qd [C]

Sparfloxacin (Zagam) 400 mg PO initial dose, then 200 mg PO qd [C]

Grepafloxacin (Raxar) 600 mg PO qd [C]

Regimen C (if suspect aspiration)

Amoxicillin/clavulanate (Augmentin) 500 mg PO tid [B]

Course: 10–14 days (except azithromycin as noted)

Organisms: *S. pneumoniae, H. influenzae, M. catarrhalis, Legionella* sp., *Chlamydia pneumoniae,* coliforms

Pulmonary Tuberculosis

(*Chest x-ray positive, active disease*) Many regional variations and conflicting recommendations exist. Unless local/regional sensitivities are well established, consider initiating treatment with **four drug therapy.**

A. CHILDREN

Notes:

1. Patients with positive chest x-rays (active disease) **must be isolated.**
2. All cases **must be reported** to the local health department.
3. Antituberculosis medications have inherent toxicities and side effects: INH (hepatitis, peripheral neuropathy), rifampin (hepatotoxicity, flu-like syndrome, discoloration of body fluids/staining of contact lenses), PZA (arthralgias, hyperuricemia, hepatitis), ethambutol (optic neuritis), and streptomycin (ototoxicity). Close monitoring is essential.
4. Consider adding pyridoxine (vitamin B_6) 25–50 mg PO qd [A] to decrease NIH-induced neuropathy.

Isoniazid (INH) 10–20 mg/kg/day PO (max 300 mg/day) [C]

PLUS

Rifampin (Rimactane) 10–20 mg/kg/day PO (max 600 mg/day) [C]

PLUS

Pyrazinamide (PZA) 15–30 mg/kg/day PO (max 2 g/day) [C]

PLUS

Ethambutol (Myambutol) 15–25 mg/kg/day PO (max 2.5 g/day) [B]

OR

Streptomycin 20–40 mg/kg/day (max 1 g/day) [D]

B. ADULTS

Isoniazid (INH) 5 mg/kg/day PO (max 300 mg/day) [C]
PLUS
Rifampin (Rimactane) 10 mg/kg/day PO (max 600 mg/day) [C]
PLUS
Pyrazinamide (PZA) 15–30 mg/kg/day PO (max 2 g/day) [C]
PLUS
Ethambutol (Myambutol) 15–25 mg/kg/day PO (max 2.5 g/day) [B]
OR
Streptomycin 15 mg/kg/day (max 1 g/day) [D]

Course: Treatment regimens vary. Initiate therapy with all drugs simultaneously, and arrange appropriate follow-up.

SEPSIS

Note: If patient condition permits, cultures should be obtained prior to antibiotic administration.

A. NEONATAL (UP TO 8 WEEKS OF AGE, NORMAL HOST)

(*Note **two** drug therapy*)

Note: Ceftriaxone is no longer recommended in neonates due to the potential for biliary sludge pseudolithiasis.

Cefotaxime (Claforan) 50 mg/kg IV/IM q8h (q12h if < 1 week old) [B]
PLUS (to cover group B *Strep* and *Listeria*)
Ampicillin 25 mg/kg IV/IM q6h (q8h if < 1 week old) [B]

Organisms: group B *Strep, E. coli, Listeria, Klebsiella, Enterobacter, S. aureus, H. influenzae*

B. INFANT/CHILD (NORMAL HOST)

1. Cefotaxime (Claforan) 50 mg/kg IV/IM q8h [B] **OR**
2. Ceftriaxone (Rocephin) 100 mg/kg IV or IM q24h [B]

Organisms: *H. influenzae, S. pneumoniae, N. meningitidis, S. aureus*

C. PEDIATRIC (IMMUNOCOMPROMISED)

Regimen A
(*Note **two or three** drug therapy*)
Ceftazidime (Fortaz) 50 mg/kg IV q8h [B]
Mezlocillin (Mezlin) 50–75 mg/kg IV q 4–6 h [B]
Ticarcillin (Ticar) 50 mg/kg IV q 4–6 h [B]
Piperacillin (Pipracil) 50 mg/kg IV q 4–6 h [B]
Ticarcillin/clavulanic acid (Timentin) 50 mg/kg IV q6h [B]
Piperacillin/tazobactam (Zosyn) 100 mg/kg IV q8h [B]
PLUS
Gentamicin (Garamycin) 2 mg/kg IV loading dose, then 1.7 mg/kg IV q8h (monitor serum levels) [D] **OR**
Tobramycin (Nebcin) 2 mg/kg IV loading dose, then 1.7 mg/kg IV q8h (monitor serum levels) [D] **OR**
Amikacin (Amikin) 5 mg/kg IV q8h (monitor serum levels) [D]
PLUS/MINUS (if indwelling intravascular device present)
Vancomycin (Vancocin) 10 mg/kg IV q6h (max 1 g/dose; monitor serum levels) [C]

Regimen B
(*Note **one or two** drug therapy*)
Imipenem (Primaxin) 30 mg/kg IV q8h [C] **OR**
Meropenem 40 mg/kg IV q8h [B]
PLUS/MINUS (if indwelling intravascular device present)
Vancomycin (Vancocin) 10 mg/kg IV q6h (max 1 g/dose; monitor serum levels) [C]

Organisms: Enterobacteriaceae, *Pseudomonas* sp., *S. aureus, S. epidermidis, S. viridans, Corynebacterium* sp.

D. PEDIATRIC PATIENTS WITH A SEVERE PENICILLIN ALLERGY

(*Note **two** drug therapy*)

Vancomycin (Vancocin) 10 mg/kg IV q6h (max 1 g/dose; monitor serum levels) [C]
PLUS

1. Gentamicin (Garamycin) 2 mg/kg IV loading dose, then 1.7 mg/kg IV q8h (monitor serum levels) [D] **OR**
2. Aztreonam (Azactam) 30 mg/kg IV q8h [B]

E. ADULT (NORMAL HOST)

Regimen A
Ticarcillin/clavulanic acid (Timentin) 3.1 g IV q6h [B]
Piperacillin/tazobactam (Zosyn) 3.375 g IV q6h [B]
Imipenem (Primaxin) 500–1000 mg IV q8h [C]
Meropenem 1 g IV q8h [B]

Regimen B
(*Note **two** drug therapy*)
Cefotaxime (Claforan) 2 g IV q8h [B] **OR**
Ceftriaxone (Rocephin) 2 g IV q12h [B]
PLUS
Metronidazole (Flagyl) 15 mg/kg IV loading dose, max dose 1000 mg then 7.5 mg/kg IV q6h (max 500 mg/dose) [B; contraindicated 1st trimester] **OR**
Clindamycin (Cleocin) 900 mg IV q8h [B]

Regimen C
(*Note **two** drug therapy*)
Ciprofloxacin (Cipro) 400 mg IV q12h [C]
Ofloxacin (Floxin) 400 mg IV q12h [C]
Levofloxacin (Levaquin) 500 mg IV qd [C]
PLUS
Clindamycin (Cleocin) 900 mg IV q8h [B]

Organisms: gram positive cocci, gram negative cocci, anaerobes

F. ADULT (IMMUNOCOMPROMISED)

Regimen A
(*Note **two or three** drug therapy*)
Ceftazidime (Fortaz) 2 g IV q8h [B]
Mezlocillin (Mezlin) 3 g IV q6h [B]
Ticarcillin (Ticar) 3–4 g IV q4h [B]
Piperacillin (Pipracil) 3–4 g IV q4h [B]
Ticarcillin/clavulanic acid (Timentin) 3.1 g IV q6h [B]
Piperacillin/tazobactam (Zosyn) 3.375 g IV q6h [B]
PLUS
Gentamicin (Garamycin) 2 mg/kg IV loading dose, then 1.7 mg/kg IV q8h (monitor serum levels) [D] **OR**
Tobramycin (Nebcin) 2 mg/kg IV loading dose, then 1.7 mg/kg IV q8h (monitor serum levels) [D] **OR**
Amikacin (Amikin) 7.5 mg/kg IV q12h (monitor serum levels) [D] **OR**
Aztreonam (Azactam) 1–2 g IV q8h [B]
PLUS/MINUS (if indwelling intravascular device present)
Vancomycin (Vancocin) 15 mg/kg IV q12h (max 1 g/dose; monitor serum levels) [C]

Regimen B
(*Note **one or two** drug therapy*)
Imipenem (Primaxin) 500–1000 mg IV q8h [C] **OR**
Meropenem 1 g IV q8h [B]
PLUS/MINUS (if indwelling intravascular device present)
Vancomycin (Vancocin) 15 mg/kg IV q12h (max 1 g/dose; monitor serum levels) [C]

Organisms: Enterobacteriaceae, *Pseudomonas, S. aureus, S. epidermidis, S. viridans, Corynebacterium* sp.

G. ADULT PATIENTS WITH A SEVERE PENICILLIN ALLERGY

(*Note* ***two*** *drug therapy*)

1. Vancomycin (Vancocin) 15 mg/kg IV q12h (max 1 g/dose; monitor serum levels) [C]
   PLUS
1. Gentamicin (Garamycin) 2 mg/kg IV loading dose, then 1.7 mg/kg IV q8h (monitor serum levels) [D] **OR**
2. Aztreonam (Azactam) 1–2 g IV q8h [B]

H. INTRAVENOUS DRUG ABUSERS

(*Note* ***two*** *drug therapy*)

1. Nafcillin 2 g IV q4h [B]
   OR (especially if catheter-induced sepsis)
2. Vancomycin (Vancocin) 15 mg/kg IV q12h (max 1 g/dose; monitor serum levels) [C]
   PLUS
1. Gentamicin (Garamycin) 2 mg/kg IV loading dose, then 1.7 mg/kg IV q8h (monitor serum levels) [D]

Organisms: *S. aureus, Pseudomonas,* enterococci

SEXUAL ASSAULT PROPHYLAXIS

Sexually Transmitted Disease Prophylaxis

(*Note* ***two*** *drug therapy to treat* ***gonorrhea and chlamydia***)

Gonorrhea treatment

Notes:

1. Azithromycin (Zithromax) 2 g PO single dose is considered effective for *N. gonorrhoeae* and *Chlamydia*, but GI discomfort is common.
2. May consider prophylaxis for *T. vaginalis* with metronidazole (Flagyl) 2 g PO single dose [B, contraindicated 1st trimester]
3. Recommend initial testing for GC, *Chlamydia*, HIV, syphilis, and pregnancy.
4. Ofloxacin (Floxin) and ciprofloxacin (Cipro) do not have activity against incubating syphilis.

1. Ceftriaxone (Rocephin) 125 mg IM single dose [B]
2. Cefotaxime (Claforan) 500 mg IM single dose [B]
3. Cefixime (Suprax) 400 mg PO single dose [B] (not for pharyngeal infection)
4. Ciprofloxacin (Cipro) 500 mg PO single dose [C]
5. Ofloxacin (Floxin) 400 mg PO single dose [C]
6. Spectinomycin (Trobicin) 2 g IM single dose [B]
   PLUS (for *Chlamydia* coverage)
1. Azithromycin (Zithromax) 1 g PO single dose [B] **OR**
2. Doxycycline (Vibramycin) 100 mg PO bid for 7 days [D]

Pregnancy Prophylaxis

Notes:

1. Consider only if patient is not already pregnant.
2. Must be taken within 72 h of unprotected sex to be effective.
3. May cause severe nausea.

1. Ovral (50 μg ethinyl estradiol + 0.5 mg norgestrel) 2 tablets PO initially, then 2 tablets PO 12 h later [X] **OR**
2. Lo/Ovral (30 μg ethinyl estradiol + 0.3 mg norgestrel) 4 tablets PO initially, then 4 tablets PO 12 h later [X]
3. Levonogestrel (Plan B) 0.75 mg 1 tablet PO initially then 1 tablet PO 12 h later
4. Leven, Nordette (30 μg ethinyl estradiol + 0.15 mg levonorgestrel) 4 tablets PO initially, then 4 tablets PO 12 h later.

SEXUALLY TRANSMITTED DISEASES

Female Genital Infections

Note: Pregnancy test advised prior to initiation of therapy in many cases.

CERVICITIS

A. Chlamydia, Gonorrhea, Herpes Simplex, Syphilis *See General Genital Infections.*

PELVIC INFLAMMATORY DISEASE (PID)

A. Outpatient Management

Regimen A

(*Note* ***two*** *drug therapy*)

Ofloxacin (Floxin) 400 mg PO bid [C]

PLUS

Metronidazole (Flagyl) 500 mg PO bid [B, contraindicated 1st trimester] **OR**

Clindamycin (Cleocin) 450 mg PO qid [B]

Regimen B

(*Note* ***two or three*** *drug therapy*)

Ceftiaxone (Rocephin) 250 mg IM once [B] **OR**

Cefoxitin (Mefoxin) 2 g IM [B], plus probenecid 1 g PO single dose [B]

PLUS

Doxycycline (Vibramycin) 100 mg PO bid for 14 days [D]

PLUS/MINUS (if resistant to therapy)

Metronidazole (Flagyl) 500 mg PO bid [B, contraindicated 1st trimester] **OR**

Clindamycin (Cleocin) 450 mg PO qid [B]

Course: 14 days

B. Inpatient Management

Notes: Hospital admission often advisable for parenteral antibiotics especially in cases with pregnancy, peritonitis, suspected abscess, clarification of diagnosis, immunodeficiency, and failure of outpatient therapy.

Regimen A

(*Note* ***two*** *drug therapy*)

Cefoxitin (Mefoxin) 2 g IV q6h [B] **OR**

Cefotetan (Cefotan) 2 g IV q12h [B]

PLUS

Doxycycline (Vibramycin) 100 mg PO bid for 14 days [D]

OR (if pregnant)

Azithromycin (Zithromax) 500 mg IV qd for 2 days, then 250 mg IV qd for 7 more days [B]

Regimen B

(*Note* ***two*** *drug therapy*)

Clindamycin (Cleocin) 900 mg IV q8h [B]

PLUS

Gentamicin (Garamycin) 2 mg/kg IV or IM loading dose, then 1.7 mg/kg IV/IM q8h (monitor serum levels) [D]

Course: After afebrile for 24 h on IV antibiotics, switch to doxycycline 100 mg PO bid for 14 days [D]. Also, if treating tubo-ovarian abscess, add metronidazole (Flagyl) 500 mg PO bid [B, contraindicated 1st trimester] **OR** clindamycin (Cleocin) 450 mg PO qid for 14 days [B].

Organisms: *N. gonorrhoeae, Chlamydia trachomatis, Mycoplasma hominis,* Enterobacteriaceae, anaerobes

VAGINITIS

Note: 1998 CDC Sexually Transmitted Diseases Treatment Guidelines report that treating partners is unnecessary.

A. Bacterial Vaginosis

Nonpregnant

1. Metronidazole (Flagyl) 500 mg PO bid for 7 days [B, contraindicated 1st trimester]
2. Clindamycin cream (2%) [Cleocin] one applicator (5 g) intravaginally qhs for 7 days [B]
3. Metronidazole gel (0.75%) [Metrogel Vaginal] one applicator (5 g) intravaginally bid for 5 days [B, contraindicated 1st trimester]
4. Clindamycin (Cleocin) 300 mg PO bid for 7 days [B]

Pregnant

Note: Metronidazole contraindicated 1st trimester. Begin treatment in 2nd trimester with

1. Metronidazole (Flagyl) 250 mg PO tid for 7 days [B, contraindicated 1st trimester] **OR**
2. Clindamycin (Cleocin) 300 mg PO bid for 7 days [B]

Organisms: polymicrobic: *Gardnerella vaginalis, Bacteroides, Mycoplasma hominis, Mobiluncus, Peptococcus*

B. Herpes Simplex

See General Genital Infections.

C. Trichomonas

Note: Partners must be treated and should be advised to avoid sex until full course of therapy is completed and both partners are asymptomatic.

Nonpregnant

1. Metronidazole (Flagyl) 2 g PO single dose [B, contraindicated 1st trimester] **OR**
2. Metronidazole 500 mg PO bid for 7 days [B, contraindicated 1st trimester]

Pregnant

Clotrimazole (Gyne-Lotrimin, Mycelex-7) 100 mg intravaginally qhs for 14 days (decreases symptoms, but cure rate only 20%) [B]

D. Vaginal Candidiasis/Yeast

Note:

1. All available over the counter (OTC) except fluconazole.
2. For relapses or treatment failures not resolved in one week, consider fluconazole (Diflucan) 150 mg PO on days 1, 5, 9, and 13. [C]
3. Creams and suppositories are oil-based and may weaken condoms or diaphragms.

1. Fluconazole (Diflucan) 150 mg PO single dose [C, not recommended in pregnancy]
2. Miconazole vaginal suppositories (Monistat 3) 200 mg intravaginally qhs for 3 days [generally accepted in pregnancy]
3. Miconazole 2% vaginal cream (Monistat 7): one applicator (5 g) per vagina qhs for 7 days [generally accepted as safe in pregnancy]
4. Clotrimazole vaginal suppositories (Gyne-Lotrimin, Mycelex-7) 100 mg tablet intravaginally qhs for 7 days **OR** two 100 mg tabs intravaginally for 3 days [B]
5. Clotrimazole 1% vaginal cream (Gyne-Lotrimin, Mycelex-7): one applicator (5 g) per vagina qhs for 7 days [B]
6. Butoconazole (Femstat) 2% cream one applicator (5 g per vagina qhs for 3 days [C]

Course: As listed, however 7 days of treatment are recommended for those medications used during pregnancy.

Male Genital Infections

EPIDIDYMITIS/PROSTATITIS

A. Younger Patients (less than 35 years of age)

Treat for gonorrhea and chlamydia—See General Genital Infections.

B. Older Patients (greater than 35 years of age):

See Genitourinary Tract Infections.

HERPES SIMPLEX

See General Genital Infections.

SYPHILIS

See General Genital Infections.

URETHRAL DISCHARGE/URETHRITIS

Note: Urethral swab Gram stains (which are notoriously inaccurate) may help determine the diagnosis although most centers treat empirically and may or may not send GC and *Chlamydia* culture/antigen tests for confirmation.

A. Gonorrhea and Chlamydia

See General Genital Infections.

B. Trichomonas

Note: Partners must be treated and should be advised to avoid sex until full course of therapy is completed and both partners are asymptomatic.

Metronidazole (Flagyl) 2 g PO single dose [B, contraindicated 1st trimester]

Organisms: *N. gonorrhoeae, C. trachomatis, Ureaplasma urealyticum, T. vaginalis, Mycoplasma hominis*

General Genital Infections (Male and Female)

GENITAL WARTS

1. Liquid nitrogen application to warts.
2. Referral to dermatology or primary care physician for other forms of therapy.
3. Obtain VDRL/RPR.

Organism: human papillomavirus

GONORRHEA/CHLAMYDIA

Notes:

1. Up to 50% of GC positive patients have *Chlamydia trachomatis* as well.
2. Patients may need a repeat culture 4–7 days after treatment if they remain symptomatic.
3. With the emergence of penicillinase-producing *N. gonorrhoeae* (PPNG), there will be regional differences in selecting the *primary* antibiotic.
4. All patients with gonorrhea should have a serologic test for syphilis (VDRL/RPR). Consider testing for HIV.
5. Single dose ofloxacin (400 mg) [C] or azithromycin (2 g) [B] cover both chlamydia and gonorrhea.

A. Uncomplicated Urethral, Endocervical or Rectal

(*Note* ***two*** *drug therapy to treat* ***gonorrhea and chlamydia***)

Gonorrhea treatment

1. Cefixime (Suprax) 400 mg PO single dose [B]
2. Ceftriaxone (Rocephin) 125 mg IM single dose [B]
3. Ciprofloxacin (Cipro) 500 mg PO single dose [C]

4. Ofloxacin (Floxin) 400 mg PO single dose [C]
5. Spectinomycin (Trobicin) 2 g IM single dose (if allergic to cephalosporins and quinolones) [B]

PLUS (for chlamydia treatment)

Non-pregnant (chlamydia treatment)

1. Azithromycin (Zithromax) 1 g PO single dose [B]
2. Doxycycline (Vibramycin) 100 mg PO bid for 7 days [D]
3. Erythromycin 500 mg PO qid for 7 days [B, except estolate contraindicated]
4. Ofloxacin (Floxin) 300 mg PO bid for 7 days [C]

Pregnant (chlamydia treatment)

1. Erythromycin 500 mg PO qid for 7 days OR 250 mg PO qid for 14 days [B, except estolate contraindicated]
2. Amoxicillin (Amoxil) 500 mg PO tid for 7 days [B]
3. Azithromycin (Zithromax) 1 g PO single dose [B, preliminary data indicate probably safe and effective, but data insufficient to recommend routine use]

B. Pharyngeal

Note: Chlamydia coinfection of pharynx is unusual, but coinfection of genitals may occur; therefore it is recommended to treat both GC and chlamydia.

1. Ceftriaxone (Rocephin) 125 mg IM single dose [B]
2. Ciprofloxacin (Cipro) 500 mg PO single dose [C]
3. Ofloxacin (Floxin) 400 mg PO single dose [C]

PLUS (for chlamydia treatment)

1. Azithromycin (Zithromax) 1 g PO single dose [B] **OR**
2. Doxycycline (Vibramycin) 100 mg PO bid for 7 days [D]

HERPES SIMPLEX—GENITAL

A. Primary Episode

1. Acyclovir (Zovirax) 400 mg PO tid **OR** 200 mg PO 5 times a day [C]
2. Famciclovir (Famvir) 250 mg PO tid [B]
3. Valacyclovir (Valtrex) 1000 mg PO bid [B]

Course: 7–10 days.

B. Recurrent Episodes

Treatment beneficial only if instituted within 2 days of onset of lesions.

1. Acyclovir (Zovirax) 800 mg PO bid **OR** 400 mg PO tid **OR** 200 mg PO 5 times/day [C]
2. Famciclovir (Famvir) 125 mg PO bid [B]
3. Valacyclovir (Valtrex) 500 mg PO bid [B]

Course: 5 days

C. Chronic Suppression

1. Acyclovir (Zovirax) 400 mg PO bid [C]
2. Famciclovir (Famvir) 250 mg PO bid [B]
3. Valacyclovir (Valtrex) 500 PO qd **OR** 250 mg PO bid [B]

PUBIC LICE (CRABS) AND SCABIES

See Parasites.

SYPHILIS (PRIMARY, SECONDARY, LATENT <1 YEAR)

Notes:

1. Consider HIV testing.
2. Treatment failures may occur with any regimen. Patients should be reexamined in 3 and 6 months.
3. Three weekly injections of benzathine penicillin are recommended for treatment failures, latent infections >1 year, and for HIV-infected patients.

1. Benzathine penicillin G (Bicillin L-A) strongly preferred, use alternatives only if penicillin allergy (consider desensitization in patients with a penicillin allergy) [B]
   a. a. Children: 50,000 units/kg IM single dose (max 2.4 million units)
   b. b. Adults: 2.4 million units IM single dose

If penicillin allergic:

1. Doxycycline (Vibramycin) 100 mg PO bid for 14 days [D] **OR**
2. Tetracycline 500 mg PO qid for 14 days [D]

Organism: *Treponema pallidum*

SKIN AND SOFT TISSUE INFECTIONS

Note: Consider tetanus status in all patients.

Bites

Note: Consider initiating outpatient therapy with a single dose of IV medication listed under inpatient therapy.

A. CAT (OUTPATIENT THERAPY)

Notes:

1. Cat bites have a high infection rate (30–50%) and frequently require IV antibiotic therapy. Close follow-up is mandatory.
2. Consider x-ray to rule out broken cat tooth.

1. Amoxicillin/clavulanate (Augmentin) 500/125 mg PO tid **OR** 875/125 mg PO bid [B] **OR**
2. Cefuroxime axetil (Ceftin) 500 mg PO bid [B]

If penicillin allergic

(*Note* ***two*** *drug therapy*)

1. Clindamycin 300–450 mg PO qid [B]

PLUS (for *Eikenella* coverage)

1. Ciprofloxacin (Cipro) 500 mg PO bid [C] **OR**
2. TMP/SMX DS (Septra DS, Bactrim DS) 1 tablet PO bid [C; D in 3rd trimester] **OR**
3. Doxycycline (Vibramycin) 100 mg PO bid [D]

Course: 7–10 days

Organisms: *Pasteurella* sp., streptococci, staphylococci, *moraxella, neisseria, fusobacterium, bacteroides, porphyromonas, prevotella, erysiphelothrix.*

B. DOG (OUTPATIENT THERAPY)

Note: Consider need for rabies therapy.

1. Amoxicillin/clavulanate (Augmentin) 500/125 mg PO tid **OR** 875/125 mg PO bid [B]

If penicillin allergic (*Note* **two** *drug therapy*)

1. Clindamycin 300–450 mg PO qid [B]

PLUS (*for capnocytophaga (DF2) coverage*)

1. Ciprofloxacin (Cipro) 500 mg PO bid [C] **OR**
2. TMP/SMX DS (Septra DS, Bactrim DS) 1 tablet PO bid [C; D in 3rd trimester] **OR**
3. Doxycycline (Vibramycin) 100 mg PO bid [D]

Course: 7–10 days

Organisms: *Pasteurella multocida,* staphylococcus, streptococcus, *fusobacterium* sp, *bacteroides* sp, EF4, *Capnocytophaga cynodegmi* (formerly DF2), EF4

C. HUMAN (OUTPATIENT THERAPY)

1. Amoxicillin/clavulanate (Augmentin) 500/125 mg PO tid **OR** 875/125 mg PO bid [B]
2. Cephradine (Velosef) [B] **OR** Cephalexin (Keflex) [B] 500 mg PO qid **PLUS** penicillin 500 mg PO qid [B]

3. Penicillin 500 mg PO qid [B] **PLUS** dicloxacillin 500 mg PO qid [B]

If penicillin allergic
(*Note* ***two*** *drug therapy*)
1. Clindamycin 300–450 mg PO qid [B]
PLUS (for *Eikenella* coverage)
1. Ciprofloxacin (Cipro) 500 mg PO bid [C]
2. TMP/SMX DS (Septra DS, Bactrim DS) 1 tablet PO bid [C; D in 3rd trimester]

Course: 7–10 days
Organisms: *S. viridans, Eikenella corrodens, Staph* sp., *Corynebacterium,* anaerobes (*Peptostreptococcus, Bacteroides*)

D. BITES (HUMAN, DOG, AND CAT)—INPATIENT THERAPY

1. Ampicillin/sulbactam (Unasyn) 1.5 g IV q6h [B]
2. Cefoxitin (Mefoxin) 2 g IV q8h [B]
3. Ticarcillin/clavulanate (Timentin) 3.1 g IV q6h [B]
4. Piperacillin/tazobactam (Zosyn) 3.375 g IV q6h [B]

If penicillin allergic
(*Note* ***two*** *drug therapy*)
1. Clindamycin (Cleocin) 900 mg IV q8h [B]
PLUS
1. Ciprofloxacin (Cipro) 400 mg IV q12h [C]
2. TMP/SMX (Bactrim, Septra) 5 mg/kg IV q12h based on TMP [C; D in 3rd trimester]

Breast Infections

A. Mastitis
Note: Continue nursing to decrease duration of symptoms.

1. Cephradine (Velosef) 500 mg PO qid [B]
2. Cephalexin (Keflex) 500 mg PO qid [B]
3. Dicloxacillin 500 mg PO qid [B]
4. Clindamycin (Cleocin) 300 mg PO qid [B]

Course: 10–14 days
Organism: *Staphylococcus aureus*

B. Breast Abscess
Notes:

1. Incision and drainage usually required.
2. Discontinue nursing.
3. Treat mild cases with oral regimen as listed for Mastitis, above.

1. Cefazolin (Ancef) 1 gram IV q 8 hours [B]
2. Nafcillin 2 grams IV q 4 hours [B]
3. Vancomycin (Vancocin) 15 mg/kg IV q 12 hours (max 1 gram/dose; monitor serum levels) [C]

Organism: *Staphylococcus aureus*

Cellulitis

A. UNCOMPLICATED

Note: Consider initiating outpatient therapy with cefazolin (Ancef) 1–2 g IV/IM. [B]; if cellulitis is severe, schedule wound check in 24 h.

1. Cephradine (Velosef) 500 mg PO qid [B]
2. Cephalexin (Keflex) 500 mg PO qid [B]
3. Dicloxacillin 500 mg PO qid [B]
4. Cefadroxil (Duricef) 500 mg PO bid [B]
5. Clindamycin (Cleocin) 300 mg PO qid [B]

Course: 10–14 days
Organisms: *Staph.* and *Strep.* sp.

Infected Lacerations

A. Non-Contaminated Most infected lacerations are due to Staphylococcal and Streptococcal species and should be treated the same as Cellulitis. Lacerations contaminated by fresh or brackish water have a high incidence of infections by *Aeromonas* and should be treated as outlined below.

B. Contaminated (fresh or brackish water)

1. TMP/SMX DS (Bactrim DS, Septra DS) 1 tablet PO bid]C; D in 3rd trimester]
2. Ciprofloxacin (Cipro) 500 mg PO bid [C]
3. Ofloxacin (Floxin) 200 mg PO bid [C]
4. Norfloxacin (Noroxin) 400 mg PO bid [C]
5. Levofloxacin (Levaquin) 500 mg PO QD [C]

Course: 10–14 days
Organism: *Aeromonas hydrophilia*

B. COMPLICATED: CHRONIC, PERINEAL, OR INFECTIONS IN DIABETICS

Notes:

1. Consider initiating therapy with a long acting cephalosporin, e.g., cefonicid (Monocid) or ceftriaxone (Rocephin) 1–2 g IM/IV.
2. If cellulitis is moderate or severe, schedule a wound check in 24 h to assess need for admission.

1. Ciprofloxacin (Cipro) 500 mg PO bid [C] **PLUS** clindamycin (Cleocin) 300 mg PO qid [B]
2. Amoxicillin/clavulanate (Augmentin) 500 mg PO tid [B]

Course: 10–14 days
Organisms: gram negative rods, anaerobes, *S. aureus, Strep* sp.

Necrotizing Fasciitis

Regimen A (for ''flesh-eating bacteria, gas gangrene, non-groin infections)
Clindamycin (Cleocin) 900 mg IV q 8 hours [B]
PLUS
Penicillin G 4 million Units IV q 4 hours [B]
OR (if penicillin allergic)
Vancomycin (Vancocin) 15 mg/kg IV q 12 hours (max 1 gram/dose; monitor serum levels) [C]
Organisms: Group A, C, G streptococci, *Clostridium* sp., polymicrobic anaerobes and aerobes

Regimen B (for Fournier's gangrene)
Metronidazole (Flagyl) 15 mg/kg IV loading dose (maximum 1 gram) then 7.5 mg/kg IV q 6 hours (max 500 mg/dose) [B; contraindicated 1st trimester]
PLUS
Ticarcillin/clavulanic acid (Timentin) 3.1 gm IV q 6 hours [B] **OR**
Ampicillin/sulbactam (Unasyn) 3 mGM IV q 6 hours [B] **OR**
Piperacillin/tazobactam (Zosyn) 3.375 gm IV q 6 hours [B]
Organisms: *E. coli, Klebsiella,* enterococci, *Bacteroides, Fusobacterium, Clostridium,* polymicrobic anaerobes and aerobes

Fungal Infections

Note: Many antifungal agents are contraindicated in patients taking terfenadine (Seldane) or Cisapride (Propulsid), as this combination may produce life-threatening dysrhythmias. Specific agents implicated at this time include ketoconazole, itraconazole, and fluconazole (at doses of 400 mg/day), but the provider is urged to consult the PDR prior to prescribing these agents.

A. CANDIDA (CUTANEOUS)

1. Clotrimazole 1% cream (Lotrimin, Mycelex)—apply to rash tid–qid [B]
2. Miconazole 2% cream (Monistat-Derm)—apply to rash tid–qid [generally accepted as safe in pregnancy]
3. Nystatin cream (Mycostatin)—apply to rash tid–qid [A]
4. Amphotericin B 3% cream (Fungizone)—apply to rash tid–qid [B]

Course: 14 days

B. CANDIDA (ORAL THRUSH) (NOT AIDS PATIENTS)

1. Fluconazole (Diflucan) 200 mg PO single dose or 100 mg/day for 5 days [C]
2. Itraconazole (Sporanox) oral solution 200 mg (20 mL) PO qd without food for 7 days [C]
3. Nystatin (Mycostatin) 500,000 U swish and swallow qid **OR** two 500,000 U tabs PO tid [B]
   Infant dose: 1 mL each buccal mucosa qid [B]
4. Clotrimazole (Mycelex) 10 mg troche–dissolve in mouth 5 times/day [B]

Course: 14 days (except fluconazole and itraconazole as listed)

C. TINEA CAPITIS

1. Terbinafine (Lamisil) 250 mg PO qd for 2–3 weeks [B]
2. Itraconazole (Sporanox) 3–5 mg/kg per dose PO qd for 30 days [C]
3. Ketoconazole (Nizoral) 200 mg PO qd for 30 days [C]
   Children: 3.3–6.6 mg/kg PO qd for 30 days [C] (monitor for hepatotoxicity)

D. TINEA CRURIS (JOCK ITCH), PEDIS (ATHLETES FOOT), OR CORPORIS

1. Clotrimazole 1% cream (Lotrimin, Mycelex)—apply to rash bid [B]
2. Miconazole 2% cream (Monistat-Derm)—apply to rash bid [generally accepted as safe in pregnancy]
3. Ketoconazole 2% cream (Nizoral)—apply to rash qd [C]

Course: 2–3 weeks or 1 week after itching gone

For severe or refractory infections

1. Ketoconazole (Nizoral) 200 mg PO qd for 4 weeks minimum [C] (monitor for hepatotoxicity) **OR**
2. Fluconazole (Diflucan) 150 mg PO once per week for 1–4 weeks (not FDA approved for this indication) [C]

E. TINEA UNGUIUM (ONYCHOMYCOSIS)

Fingernails

1. Terbinafine (Lamisil) 250 mg PO qd for 6 weeks [B]
2. Itraconazole (Sporanox) 200 mg PO bid for 1 week/month for 2 months [C]

Toenails

1. Terbinafine (Lamisil) 250 mg PO qd for 12 weeks [B]
2. Itraconazole (Sporanox) 200 mg PO qd for 3 months [C]

F. TINEA VERSICOLOR

1. Fluconazole (Diflucan) 400 mg PO single dose [C]
2. Ketoconazole (Nizoral) 400 mg PO single dose **OR** 200 mg PO QD for 7 days (monitor for hepatotoxicity; not FDA approved for this use) [C]
3. Ketoconazole 2% cream (Nizoral) apply to rash qd for 2 weeks [C]
4. Itraconazole (Sporanox) 400 mg PO qd for 3–7 days [C]
5. Selenium sulfide (Selsun) 2.5% lotion—apply as lather, leave for 10 minutes, then wash off. Apply qd for 7 days [C]

Herpes Simplex

A. BELL'S PALSY

(*Treatment considered optional by some authorities*)

Acyclovir (Zovirax) 400 mg PO 5 times a day for 10 days [C]

PLUS/MINUS

Prednisone 30 mg PO bid for 5 days [C]

B. GENITAL

See Sexually Transmitted Diseases, General Genital Infections.

Herpes Zoster (Shingles)

Notes:

1. Above recommendations most effective if started within 3 days of onset of rash.
2. Patients with lesions in multiple dermatomes may require admission and IV therapy (see dose under *Immunocompromised host*, below).

A. NORMAL HOST

1. Acyclovir (Zovirax) 800 mg PO 5 times a day for 7–10 days [C]
2. Famciclovir (Famvir) 500 mg PO tid for 7 days [B]
3. Valacyclovir (Valtrex) 1000 mg PO tid for 7 days [B], plus/minus prednisone 30 mg PO bid for 5–7 days.

B. IMMUNOCOMPROMISED HOST

Acyclovir (Zovirax) 10–12 mg/kg IV q8h; decrease to 7.5 mg/kg in elderly patients (each dose infused over 1 h) [C]

Impetigo

1. Dicloxacillin 12–25 mg/kg/day PO divided qid [B]
   Easy dose: 20 mg/kg/day = 5 mg/kg/dose PO qid
   Maximum: 500 mg/dose
   Available in suspension of 62.5 mg/5 mL
2. Cephalexin (Keflex) 25–50 mg/kg/day PO divided qid [B]
   Easy dose: 40 mg/kg/day = 10 mg/kg/dose PO qid
   Maximum: 500 mg/dose
   Available in suspensions of 125 mg and 250 mg/5 mL
3. Cephradine (Velosef) 25–100 mg/kg/day PO divided qid [B]
   Easy dose: 40–80 mg/kg/day = 10–20 mg/kg/dose PO qid
   Maximum: 500 mg/dose
   Available in suspensions of 125 mg and 250 mg/5 mL
4. Mupirocin 2% ointment (Bactroban)—apply to lesion tid for 3–5 days [B]
5. Erythromycin ethyl succinate (EES) 30–50 mg/kg/day PO divided qid [B]
   Easy dose: 40 mg/kg/day = 10 mg/kg/dose PO qid
   Maximum: 500 mg/dose
   Available in suspensions of 200 mg and 400 mg/5 mL
6. Azithromycin (Zithromax) 10 mg/kg PO initial dose, then 5 mg/kg/day for 4 days [B]
   Maximum: 500 mg on day 1 and 250 mg on days 2–5
   Available in suspensions of 100 mg and 200 mg/5 mL
7. Clarithromycin (Biaxin) 7.5 mg/kg/dose PO bid [C]
   Maximum: 500 mg
   Available in suspensions of 125 mg and 250 mg/5 mL

Course: 10 days (except mupirocin and azithromycin as noted)
Organisms: group A *Strep* (honey-crusted lesions); *S. aureus* (bullous lesions)

Orbital (Postseptal) and Periorbital (Preseptal) Cellulitis

Notes:

1. Periorbital cellulitis is confined to the space anterior to the septum (i.e., eyelids).
2. The infection in orbital cellulitis is posterior to the septum and is characterized by proptosis, ophthalmoplegia, and visual loss.
3. All cases of orbital cellulitis and all but the mildest cases of periorbital cellulitis should be admitted.
4. In the absence of trauma, most cases of orbital and periorbital cellulitis are due to extension of sinus infections.

INPATIENT THERAPY: ORBITAL AND PERIORBITAL CELLULITIS

A. Pediatrics

Regimen A

(*Note* ***two*** *drug therapy*)

Ceftriaxone (Rocephin) 100 mg/kg IV qd [B]
Cefotaxime (Claforan) 40 mg/kg IV q6h [B]
Cefuroxime (Zinacef, Ceftin) 30 mg/kg IV q8h [B]
PLUS
Clindamycin (Cleocin) 10 mg/kg IV q6h [B]

Regimen B (if severe penicillin allergy): (*Note* ***three*** *drug therapy*)
Vancomycin (Vancocin) 10 mg/kg IV q6h (max 1 g/dose; monitor serum levels) [C]
PLUS
Aztreonam (Azactam) 30 mg/kg IV q8h [B]
PLUS
Clindamycin (Cleocin) 10 mg/kg IV q6h [B]

Regimen C

(*Note* ***single*** *drug therapy*)

Ampicillin/sulbactam (Unasyn) 50 mg/kg IV q6h [B]
Ticarcillin/clavulanic acid (Timentin) 50 mg/kg IV q6h [B]
Piperacillin/tazobactam (Zosyn) 100 mg/kg IV q8h [B]

B. Adults Regimen A

Ampicillin/sulbactam (Unasyn) 3 g IV q6h [B]
Ticarcillin/clavulanic acid (Timentin) 3.1 g IV q6h [B]
Piperacillin/tazobactam (Zosyn) 3.375 g IV q6h [B]

Regimen B (if severe penicillin allergy): (*Note* ***two*** *drug therapy*)
Vancomycin (Vancocin) 15 mg/kg IV q12h (max 1 g/dose; monitor serum levels) [C]
PLUS
Clindamycin (Cleocin) 450–900 mg IV q8h [B]

OUTPATIENT THERAPY: PERIORBITAL CELLULITIS ONLY

Note: Only mild cases of periorbital cellulitis should be treated on an outpatient basis, and these require follow-up within 24 h. Initiate therapy with a dose of IV antibiotic listed above for inpatient treatment.

A. Children Less Than 5 Years Old

1. Amoxicillin/clavulanate (Augmentin) 80–90 mg/kg/day (as amoxicillin) PO divided bid or tid [B]
   Easy dose: 40 mg/kg/dose PO bid OR **30 mg/kg/dose PO tid**
   Maximum: 750 mg/dose bid or 500 mg/dose tid
   Available in suspensions of 125 mg and 250 mg amoxicillin/5 mL
2. Cefuroxime axetil (Ceftin) 20–30 mg/kg/day PO divided bid. [B]
   Easy dose: 20 mg/kg/day = 10 mg/kg/dose PO bid
   Maximum: 250 mg/dose
   Available in suspension of 125 mg/5 mL
   OR (if severe penicillin allergy)
3. Clarithromycin (Biaxin) 7.5 mg/kg/dose PO bid [C]
   Maximum: 500 mg
   Available in suspensions of 125 mg and 250 mg/5 mL

OUTPATIENT THERAPY: PERIORBITAL CELLULITIS ONLY

B. Adults and Children Age 5 Years and Older

1. Cephradine (Velosef) 500 mg PO qid
2. Cephalexin (Keflex) 500 mg PO qid
3. Dicloxacillin 500 mg PO qid
4. Cefadroxil (Duricef) 500 mg PO bid
5. Clindamycin (Cleocin) 300 mg PO qid
6. Amoxicillin/clavulanate (Augmentin) 500/125 mg PO tid OR 875/125 mg PO bid [B]

Course: 10–14 days

Organisms: *H. influenzae* (pediatrics), *Staphylococcus aureus, S. epidermidis, Streptococcus pneumoniae, Streptococcus* sp., *M. catarrhalis*, anaerobes

Varicella Zoster (Chickenpox)

Note: Start therapy within 24 h after onset of rash.

A. NORMAL HOST

Notes:

1. Children 2–12 years old are not routinely treated.
2. Acyclovir (Zovirax) 800 mg PO qid or 20 mg/kg/dose, for adults and children >12 years old for 5 days [C]
3. If pregnancy in 3rd trimester or evidence of pneumonia, consider admission and IV therapy (see dose under *Immunocompromised host*, below).

B. IMMUNOCOMPROMISED HOST

Acyclovir (Zovirax) 10–12 mg/kg IV q8h; decrease to 7.5 mg/kg in elderly patients (each dose infused over 1 h) [C]

TICK-BORNE DISEASES

Lyme Disease

A. STAGE I (EARLY)—ERYTHEMA CHRONICUM MIGRANS

1. Doxycycline (Vibramycin) 100 mg PO bid [D]

If pregnant

1. Amoxicillin (Amoxil) 500 mg PO tid [B]
2. Cefuroxime axetil (Ceftin) 500 mg PO bid [B]
3. Clarithromycin (Biaxin) 500 mg PO bid [C]

In children <8 years old

1. Amoxicillin (Amoxil) 20–50 mg/kg/day PO divided tid [B]
   Easy dose: 30 mg/kg/day = 10 mg/kg/dose PO tid
   Maximum: 250 mg/dose
   Available in suspensions of 125 mg and 250 mg/5 mL
2. Cefuroxime axetil (Ceftin) 20–30 mg/kg/day PO divided bid [B]
   Easy dose: 20 mg/kg/day = 10 mg/kg/dose PO bid
   Maximum: 250 mg/dose
   Available in suspension of 125 mg/5 mL
3. Clarithromycin (Biaxin) 7.5 mg/kg/dose PO bid (*for severe penicillin allergy*) [C]
   Maximum: 500 mg/dose
   Available in suspensions of 125 mg or 250 mg/5 mL

Course: 21 days

B. STAGE II OR III—ARTHRITIC, NEUROLOGIC, CARDIAC SYMPTOMS

1. Ceftriaxone (Rocephin) 2 g IV qd for 21 days [B]
2. Consider doxycycline (Vibramycin) 100 mg PO bid [D] **OR** amoxicillin (Amoxil) 500 mg PO tid [B] in very mild cases

Course: 30 days.

Organism: *Borrelia burgdorferi* transmitted via ixodid ticks

Rocky Mountain Spotted Fever

1. Doxycycline (Vibramycin) 100 mg PO bid [D]
2. Chloramphenicol (Chloromycetin) 500 mg PO qid [C]

In children <8 years old and pregnant women
1. Chloramphenicol (Chloromycetin) 50 mg/kg/day PO divided qid [C]

Course: 7 days minimum or until 2 days after fever resolution
Organism: *Rickettsia rickettsii* transmitted via ixodid ticks

ADVERSE EFFECTS AND PRESCRIBING HINTS

Cephalosporins

- **Cephalexin/Cephradine:** Take with meals. May cause nausea and diarrhea.

Erythromycins

- May cause stomatitis, nausea, diarrhea, transient hearing loss with large doses.
- Erythromycin estolate may cause cholestatic hepatitis in adults; this risk increases in pregnancy.
- May interfere with hepatic metabolism of other medications, especially warfarin, phenytoin, valproate, carbamazepine, theophylline, and digoxin.
- Do not prescribe concurrently with terfenadine (Seldane).
- **Erythromycin base:** Take on empty stomach.
- **Non-base erythromycin (e.g., EES):** Take with meals.

Metronidazole

- May cause nausea, vomiting, headache, metallic taste, disulfiram (Antabuse)-like reaction with alcohol.
- Do not use in first trimester of pregnancy.
- It can alter metabolism of warfarin, phenytoin, and phenobarbital.

Penicillins

- May cause nausea and diarrhea (about 10%) and candidal vaginitis in women (about 40%).
- Skin rashes may appear with all penicillins especially in patient with mononucleosis (>50%).
- **Amoxicillin:** Take with meals.
- **Ampicillin:** Take on empty stomach.
- **Dicloxacillin:** Take on empty stomach.
- **Penicillin:** Take on an empty stomach. IV Penicillin is most often supplied as the potassium salt. Monitor for hyperkalemia when giving high doses of penicillin G.
- **Amoxicillin/clavulanate:** Take with meals to reduce GI side effects.

Quinolones

- Contraindicated in patients under 18 years of age or pregnant/nursing mothers (see Table 149-1).
- Avoid antacids.
- May cause increase in theophylline levels, increases warfarin levels; alters phenytoin levels (↑ or ↓).

Tetracyclines

- Avoid dairy products and antacids.
- Do not use in children less than 8 years old or pregnant/nursing mothers.
- May lead to photosensitivity, nausea, cramps or diarrhea.
- **Tetracycline:** Take on empty stomach.

Trimethoprim/Sulfamethoxazole (TMP/SMX)

- May take on empty stomach or with meals.
- May cause rash, nausea, or vomiting.
- May cause acute hemolytic anemia in patients with G6PD deficiency.
- Blood dyscrasias (e.g., thrombocytopenia, megaloblastic anemia, neutropenia) are dose-related.
- TMP/SMX is pregnancy category C in trimesters 1 and 2, and category D in 3rd trimester. Trimethoprim interferes with folic acid metabolism and therefore should be used in the 1st and 2nd trimesters only if the potential benefit outweighs the potential risk. TMP/SMX is contraindicated in the 3rd trimester because it can cause kernicterus.
- Increases phenytoin levels.

TABLE 149-1 Functional Classification of Quinolones

Generation	Prototype	Aerobic Gram Positive	Aerobic Gram Negative	Anaerobic	Mycoplasma, Chlamydia	Phototoxicity	QT Prolongation
First	Naldixic acid	None	Enterobacteria	None	None	No	No
Second	Ciprofloxacin	Some	Yes Enhanced Pseudomonas	None	None	No	No
	Ofloxacin	Some	Yes Enhanced	None	Yes	No	No
	Levofloxacin	Yes, including *S. pneumoniae*	Yes Enhanced	None	Yes	No	No
	Lomefloxacin	None	Yes Enhanced	None	None	Yes	No
	Sparfloxacin*	Yes, including *S. pneumoniae*	Yes Enhanced	None	Yes	Yes	Yes*
Third	Grepafloxacin	Yes, including *S. pneumoniae*	Yes Enhanced	None	Yes	No	Yes*
	Trovofloxacin†	Yes, including *S. pneumoniae*	Yes Enhanced	Yes	Yes	No	No

* Contraindicated in QT prolongation, torades de pointe has been reported.
† Trovofloxacin: Rare hepatic failure.

DRUG INTERACTIONS

In this section, we have attempted to identify some of the most common or potentially dangerous drug interactions. This list is in no way all-inclusive, and the prescriber is reminded to utilize the PDR and other sources for more complete listings.

Ciprofloxacin–Norfloxacin

- Theophylline—increased theophylline levels due to decreased metabolism.
- Warfarin (Coumadin)—although many consider this interaction weak, warfarin levels may increase due to decreased metabolism.
- Alters phenytoin levels (↑ or ↓)

Erythromycin

- Terfenadine (Seldane)—concomitant use may produce cardiac dysrhythmias/sudden death.
- Theophylline—increased theophylline levels due to decreased metabolism.
- Warfarin (Coumadin)—increased warfarin levels due to decreased metabolism.
- Increases phenytoin and valproate levels.

Ketoconazole–Fluconazole–Itraconazole

- Terfenadine (Seldane)—concomitant use may produce cardiac dysrhythmias/sudden death.
- Warfarin (Coumadin)—increased warfarin levels due to decreased metabolism.
- Cisapride (Propulsid)—concomitant use may produce cardiac dysrhythmias/sudden death.

Rifampin

- Theophylline—decreased theophylline levels due to increased metabolism.
- Warfarin (Coumadin)—decreased warfarin levels due to increased metabolism.

Warfarin (Coumadin)

Many antibiotics interfere with Warfarin (Coumadin) metabolism and should be used, if at all, with extreme caution in patients on anticoagulation therapy. These antibiotics include

- ciprofloxacin (many consider this interaction negligible)—potentiates warfarin activity
- dicloxacillin and nafcillin—inhibit warfarin activity
- erythromycin—potentiates warfarin activity
- fluconazole—potentiates warfarin activity
- ketoconazole—potentiates warfarin activity
- metronidazole—potentiates warfarin activity
- miconazole—potentiates warfarin activity
- rifampin—inhibits warfarin activity
- tetracycline/doxycycline—potentiates warfarin activity
- trimethoprim/sulfamethoxazole (Bactrim, Septra)—potentiates warfarin activity

Antiobiotics compatible with warfarin include most oral cephalosporins, penicillins (except dicloxacillin and nafcillin), and clindamycin. Consider ciprofloxacin with monitoring of PT/INR.

Immunosuppressants

Multiple drugs interact with immunosuppressant medications, especially with cyclosporin. Review interactions or contact the transplant physician prior to prescribing new antibiotics to patients on immunosuppressive therapy.

Anticonvulsants

Multiple antibiotics interfere with metabolism of anticonvulsants, especially with phenytoin. Review potential drug interactions before prescribing new antibiotics to patients on anticonvulsant therapy.

CEPH DU JOUR

(A cross reference to cephalosporins)

First Generation

generic (Brand name)	***Brand Name (generic)***
cefadroxil (Duricef, Ultracef)—PO	Ancef (cefazolin)
cefazolin (Ancef)—IM, IV	Cefadyl (cephapirin)
cephalexin (Keflex)—PO	Duricef (cefadroxil)
cephalothin (Keflin)—IM, IV	Keflex (cephalexin)
cephapirin (Cefadyl)—IM, IV	Keflin (cephalothin)
cephradine (Velosef)—PO	Ultracef (cefadroxil)
	Velosef (cephradine)

Second Generation

generic (Brand name)	***Brand Name (generic)***
cefaclor (Ceclor)—PO	Ceclor (cefaclor)
cefamandole (Mandol)—IM, IV	Cefotan (cefotetan)
cefmetazole (Zefazone)—IV	Ceftin (cefuroxime axetil)
cefonicid (Monocid)—IM, IV	Cefzil (cefprozil)
cefotetan (Cefotan)—IM, IV	Kefurox (cefuroxime sodium)
cefoxitin (Mefoxin)—IV	Lorabid (loracarbef)
cefprozil (Cefzil)—PO	Mandol (cefamandole)
cefuroxime axetil (Ceftin)—PO	Mefoxin (cefoxitin)
cefuroxime sodium (Kefurox, Zinacef) IM, IV	Monocid (cefonicid)
loracarbef (Lorabid)—PO	Zefazone (cefmetazole)
	Zinacef (cefuroxime sodium)

Third Generation

generic (Brand name)	***Brand Name (generic)***
cefixime (Suprax)—PO	Cedax (ceftibuten)
cefoperazone (Cefobid)—IM, IV	Cefizox (ceftizoxime)
cefotaxime (Claforan)—IM, IV	Cefobid (cefoperazone)
cefpodoxime (Vantin)—PO	Claforan (cefotaxime)
ceftazidime (Fortaz, Tazidime)—IM, IV	Fortaz (ceftazidime)
ceftibuten (Cedax)—PO	Rocephin (ceftriaxone)
ceftizoxime (Cefizox)—IM, IV	Suprax (cefixime)
ceftriaxone (Rocephin)—IM, IV	Tazidime (ceftazidime)
	Vantin (cefpodoxime)

Fourth Generation

cefepime (Maxipime)—IM, IV	Maxipime (cefepime)

Sources include:
Public Health Service Guidelines for Management of Health-Care Worker Exposures to HIV and *Recommendations for Postexposure Prophylaxis*, Centers for Disease Control and Prevention; *The Sanford Guide to Antimicrobial Therapy 1999*, Antimicrobial Therapy Inc.; *Emergency Medicine Reports*, American Health Consultants; and *Emergency Medicine and Acute Care Essays*, Emergency Medicine Abstracts.

EMRA would like to thank the many residents who sent letters or called with comments, criticisms, and suggestions for this chapter.

COMMON VIRAL INFECTIONS: INFLUENZAVIRUSES AND HERPESVIRUSES

Robert A. Brownstein

Viral illnesses are among the most common reasons that people come to an emergency department. Although some may be trivial, such as the common cold, others are life threatening, such as viral encephalitis, hemorrhagic fever viruses, and HIV, and still others are capable of causing chronic diseases and may contribute to the development of certain malignancies. Effective therapies for some viruses are now available, with more drugs and vaccines undergoing clinical trials. Influenzaviruses and the herpesvirus family are discussed in this chapter.

INFLUENZA A AND B

Influenza viruses are single-stranded RNA viruses of the orthomyxovirus family. There are three types—A B, and C—as determined by their genetic material. Type C does not cause significant human disease and does not warrant further discussion. The virions have surface glycoproteins that contain either hemagglutinin or neuraminidase activity. Different subtypes of influenza (i.e., influenza A-H1N1 versus influenza A-H2N2) have large differences between the hemagglutinin (H) or neuraminidase (N) molecules, whereas different strains of the same subtype have minor differences in the H or N molecules.

Antigenic drift is minor mutations in the RNA genome of either the H or N molecule causing a change in antigenicity. Influenza A has much more frequent drift than B, and H more than N, so that influenza A and H molecules show virtually annual changes accounting for decreased antigenicity and facilitating annual epidemics.

Antigenic shift occurs by genetic reassortment within a host infected by two different influenzaviruses, producing a new virus with little or no antigenic similarity to the old viruses. The population lacks immunity against the new virus, but has high levels of immunity against the old virus, giving the new virus a competitive advantage. This type of shift has occurred three times with hemagglutinin and twice with neuraminidase in this century (thus, we have H1, 2, and 3, and N1 and 2). Antigenic shifts are responsible for the flu pandemics, such as in 1918.

Epidemiology

Flu occurs worldwide, in the winter months in the northern and southern hemispheres, and sporadically year round in the tropics. In the United States, flu generally occurs from November to April. Influenza is spread by droplets generated by coughing. During epidemics, attack rates are in the 20 to 30 percent range, and may be as high as 50 percent during pandemics.[1] The Centers for Disease Control and Prevention and local health departments track influenza activity monthly. Influenza A attack rates are higher for children than for adults or the elderly, but the disease carries a higher mortality rate for young adults and especially for the elderly. Influenza B produces a similar illness with high attack rates for children and lower attack rates for adults, probably because of preexisting immunity due to a lower rate of antigenic drift.

After exposure, the incubation period is usually about 2 days. Viral shedding (contagiousness) starts approximately 24 h before the onset of symptoms, rises to peak levels within 48 h, and then declines over the next 3 to 7 days. In young children. viral shedding is prolonged.

Pathophysiology

Following exposure, the virus enters the columnar cells of the respiratory tract epithelium. Host defenses at this point include mucociliary clearance, nonspecific proteins and, if present, specific immunoglobulin A (IgA) molecules. The invaded epithelial cells release large numbers of virions before cell death; thus, large numbers of virions are available for spread with respiratory secretions. Influenza viral particles are rarely found outside the respiratory tract.

Clinical Features

Classic flu symptoms include fever of 38.6° to 39.8°C (101° to 103°F), with chills or rigor, headache, myalgia, and generalized malaise. Respiratory symptoms include dry cough, rhinorrhea, and sore throat, frequently with bilateral tender, enlarged cervical lymph nodes. The onset of symptoms is typically rapid and dramatic; many patients recall the exact time of onset. Ocular symptoms include eye pain, light sensitivity, tearing, and pain with lateral gaze. Myalgias and arthralgias, but not arthritis, are extremely common. The myalgias often affect back muscles in adults and calf muscles in children. Almost half of affected children have gastrointestinal symptoms, but these are unusual in adults. The elderly do not usually have classic symptoms and may have with only fever, malaise, confusion, and nasal congestion.

The fever generally lasts 2 to 4 days, followed by rapid recovery from most of the systemic symptoms. Cough, fatigue, and occasionally depression may last for several weeks following recovery.

Diagnosis

Traditionally, diagnosis has been through the use of viral cultures or serologic tests, which do not yield results for several days. These tests are not useful in individual patients except to confirm diagnosis after recovery from acute illness, but they do provide useful epidemiologic data. Some studies have shown that a clinical diagnosis of flu during a known outbreak has an accuracy of approximately 85 percent,[2,3] but bacteremia should also be considered in patients with rigor and myalgias. Newer rapid antigen tests are becoming available that may change the approach to flulike illnesses. These tests will enable rapid diagnosis and institution of antiviral agents, and may decrease the empiric use of antibiotics. One commercially available test requires a little more than 1 h to perform and lists a sensitivity of 50 to 70 percent, with a specificity of 93 to 100 percent.[4]

Complications

The complications of acute influenza infection include primary influenza pneumonitis, secondary bacterial pneumonia, croup, exacerbation of chronic obstructive pulmonary disease, and Reye's syndrome. Other rare complications include Guillain-Barré syndrome, myocarditis, and pericarditis.

Primary influenza pneumonitis occurs most commonly in those with preexisting cardiac or pulmonary disease, but in most large outbreaks it has been seen in previously healthy young adults. The initial symptoms are typical flulike symptoms with progression to cough and dyspnea. There is significant hypoxia. Radiologic findings are bilateral infiltrates similar to Adult Respiratory Distress Syndrome (ARDS). Bacterial cultures and Gram stains are negative, and antibiotics do not help. Treatment is primarily supportive. Most clinicians would support the use of anti-influenza agents, but there are no good studies demonstrating efficacy. The mortality rate of influenza pneumonitis remains high.

Secondary pneumonia is clinically similar to pneumonia occurring without antecedent flu. This complication presents 1 to 2 weeks after the flu, with a brief well period in between. Secondary pneumonia is most common in the elderly and in those with diabetes mellitus or preexisting cardiopulmonary disease. Treatment is initially with broad-spectrum antibiotics and pulmonary support, with narrowing of antibiotic coverage when culture results become available.

Reye's syndrome has been associated with influenza B and varicella zoster infections and with the use of aspirin.[5] It occurs primarily in children between the ages of 2 and 16 years and begins with vomiting and progresses to altered mental status or coma. There is hepatomegaly due to fatty infiltration of the liver. There are elevated levels of liver enzymes (alanine aminotransferase and aspartate aminotransferase), elevated ammonia levels, and an elevated prothrombin time. Hypoglycemia is common. The case fatality rate is from 10 to 40 percent. The American Academy of Pediatrics has recommended that aspirin not be used for fevers caused by influenza or varicella.[6,7]

Treatment

Two antiviral drugs—amantadine and rimantadine—are currently approved for the treatment of influenza A. Neither has activity against influenza B. For maximal effectiveness, both need to be started within 48 h of onset of symptoms and can reduce the duration of systemic symptoms by 1 to 2 days. The dose is 100 mg bid for 5 days for both drugs. Amantadine is cleared renally, and the dose needs to be adjusted in the elderly and in renal insufficiency. The recommended dose for persons older than age 65 is 100 mg qd. Amantadine causes an increase in seizure activity in patients with a preexisting seizure disorder. Rimantadine is cleared hepatically, and a 50 percent dose reduction is recommended in severe liver dysfunction. Rimantadine has a significantly lower incidence of central nervous system (CNS) side effects than does amantadine. Neither drug should be used during pregnancy. Both amantadine and rimantadine can be used in children older than the age of 1 year, although only rimantadine is officially approved for prophylaxis in children. Amantadine costs approximately $20 for a course of therapy versus about $140 for a course of rimantadine in adults. A new medication—zanamavir—appears promising in clinical trials and has activity against both influenza A and B.[8]

Prophylaxis

The flu vaccine is formulated annually and contains two strains of influenza A and one of influenza B. It is 70 to 90 percent effective in preventing illness in those under age 65. For patients over age 65 and not in chronic care facilities, it is 30 to 70 percent effective in preventing hospitalizations due to flu and pneumonia. For those in chronic care facilities, it is 50 to 60 percent effective in preventing hospitalizations due to flu and pneumonia, and approximately 80 percent effective in preventing excessive numbers of deaths due to flu and pneumonia.[9] The vaccine is recommended for all persons over age 65; for residents of chronic care facilities; for adults and children with chronic cardiopulmonary disease; for persons with diabetes mellitus and other chronic metabolic diseases, renal disease, or hemoglobinopathies; and for the immunosuppressed and health care workers. Children and teenagers who require aspirin therapy should be immunized because of the risk of Reye syndrome. Women who will be pregnant during flu season should be immunized. The vaccine is safe for pregnant and lactating women. A whole virus vaccine is used in adults, whereas a split virus vaccine is used in children younger than age 12. The only contraindication to immunization is known allergy to egg protein or other vaccine components.

Amantadine and rimantadine are as effective as the vaccine in preventing flu, when used at the same doses as just described but for a prolonged duration. Consideration should be given to instituting chemoprophylaxis in a chronic care facility where flu has been definitively diagnosed, regardless of vaccination status of patients. The medicines should be given for at least 14 days, and then until the outbreak has subsided for a full week. For those at high risk who can not be vaccinated, a 6- to 8-week course of chemoprophylaxis during peak flu season is indicated. Postexposure prophylaxis consists of immunization followed by 14 days of chemoprophylaxis.[8]

HERPESVIRUSES

The herpesviruses are a ubiquitous class of enveloped DNA viruses that cause an expanding list of human illness. The herpesviruses all have the ability to dwell in the host as a lifelong latent infection and may cause clinical disease or recurrent disease at a time distant from the primary infection. Some have been shown to be carcinogenic. Each herpesvirus has distinguishing clinical characteristics and will be discussed individually. Human herpesviruses 6 and 7, both which cause roseola, and human herpesvirus 8, implicated in Kaposi sarcoma, are not discussed in this chapter. As a class, the herpesviruses are transmitted by close contact, since they are unable to survive in the environment and are unable to penetrate intact skin. The varicella zoster virus (VZV) can be spread via aerosolized particles as well as by close contact. Most transmission of the herpes simplex virus (HSV) and of Epstein-Barr virus (EBV) occurs during asymptomatic shedding. Viruses discussed below are HSV, VZV, EBV, and cytomegalovirus (CMV).

HERPES SIMPLEX VIRUSES 1 AND 2

Epidemiology

HSV has been found in all populations throughout the world. Transmission is via contact of infected secretions (saliva or genital) with mucous membranes or with open skin. There is serologic evidence of exposure to HSV-1 in most persons by the time of puberty, and the rates are higher among lower socioeconomic classes. HSV-2 is spread primarily sexually, and its rates are variable among different adult populations, depending on sexual behavior.

Pathophysiology

After exposure, the virus replicates locally in the epithelial cells, causing lysis of the infected cells and producing an inflammatory response. This response results in the characteristic rash of HSV, which is indistinguishable from the rash of VZV. The rash consists of small thin-walled vesicles on an erythematous base. Continued replication may result in viremia in immunocompromised hosts and rarely in normal hosts. Following primary infection, the virus becomes latent in a sensory nerve ganglion.

Clinical Features

ORAL HSV HSV-1 primarily causes oral lesions, but may cause genital infection. HSV-2 causes identical lesions, but primarily genital, and may cause oral lesions. The primary oral infection of HSV-1 is often mild or asymptomatic. In children under age 5, it may present as a pharyngitis or gingivostomatitis associated with fever and cervical lymphadenopathy. The lesions are distributed throughout the mouth, unlike the limited posterior involvement of herpangina. Admission of the young may be necessary due to poor oral intake and dehydration. In teenagers and young adults, there may simply be a posterior pharyngitis or tonsillitis. The primary lesions generally last 1 to 2 weeks. The diagnosis is largely clinical. Viral cultures take days to weeks to be performed and thus are of little use in an emergency department setting. The use of intravenous (IV) acyclovir at a dose of 5 mg/kg has been recommended for severe gingivostomatitis that requires admission and IV hydration.[10] Oral acyclovir has been shown to shorten the duration of symptoms in children if begun within the first 72 h of symptoms. No treatment other than oral hygiene is required for mild or moderate disease.

Recurrent oral lesions occur in 60 to 90 percent of infected individuals and are usually milder and generally occur on the lower lip at the outer vermilion border, but considerable variation exists, with individuals usually having recurrences at the same site as prior recurrences. The recurrences are often triggered by local trauma, sunburn, or stress. The outbreaks are frequently preceded by prodromal symptoms of local adenopathy and pain or tingling. The lesions usually follow the prodrome within the first 48 h and may last for up to 10 days, but are usually crusted over by 48 h. Treatment of recurrent oral herpes labialis with oral acyclovir 400 mg five times per day in adults shortens duration of symptoms. Topical acyclovir is ineffective. Topical pencyclovir applied every 2 h for 4 days shortens duration of symptoms[11] and has recently been approved for this indication. In patients with severe or frequent recurrences, prophylaxis with oral acyclovir can reduce outbreaks by 50 to 75 percent.[10]

GENITAL HSV HSV-1 and 2 cause identical genital infections, with HSV-2 causing the majority. These are covered in detail in the section on sexually transmitted diseases. A few items of importance are presented here. Recurrent genital lesions carry a small threat of intrauterine infection in pregnant patients, as does primary genital HSV (1 or 2),[12] and initiation of oral acyclovir and consultation with an obstetrician or perinatologist and follow-up within 72 h are recommended. Cesarean section is recommended for all women with active lesions present when labor commences, whether primary or recurrent.[13] Primary lesions carry a higher risk of transmission to the neonate.[14]

OCULAR HSV HSV infections of the eye can lead to corneal blindness and are usually caused by HSV. An ulcerative keratitis is the most common manifestation. Herpetic vesicles can be seen on the conjunctiva or on the lid margin as a blepharitis. There is a regional adenopathy. Fluorescein staining may show a diagnostic dendritic ulceration of the cornea. Due to the threat of permanent vision loss, consultation with an ophthalmologist is mandatory and antiviral therapy should be begun immediately. Superficial keratitis usually heals completely in several weeks. Recurrent ocular infections may involve the deeper structures, with a high risk of visual loss, and, if deeper structures are involved, immediate consultation with an ophthalmologist and the administration of IV acyclovir is appropriate. Following the acute treatment, long-term treatment with acyclovir can reduce recurrences of ocular HSV.[15]

ENCEPHALITIS Herpes simplex encephalitis, which is usually caused by HSV-1, is rare, but is one of the most common types of viral encephalitis in the United States. The mechanism of entry into the CNS is not definitely known, but is believed to be along neural routes. The temporal lobes are the major targets, and temporal abnormalities seen by computed tomography (CT), magnetic resonance imaging (MRI), or electroencephalography, though not always present, increase the likelihood of HSV encephalitis.

Clinically, there may be a preceding viral-like illness or the onset may be sudden. There may be no cutaneous manifestation of an HSV infection. There may be headache, fever, and altered mental status, indicated by speech disturbances or focal seizures. Temporal lobe seizures may present as olfactory hallucinations. The cerebrospinal fluid (CSF) findings are nonspecific showing an elevated white blood cell count, with mononuclear predominance. Cultures are usually negative for HSV. Conclusive diagnosis is made by biopsy, with either culture or direct antibody testing. HSV DNA identified in the CSF by polymerase chain reaction has been used, but the sensitivity and specificity have not been well defined and a negative result does not rule out HSV encephalitis. For untreated persons, the mortality rate is close to 70 percent. Treatment should be initiated in the emergency department if the diagnosis is suspected. Treatment is with IV acyclovir at 10 mg/kg/q8.

BELL'S PALSY HSV may affect the peripheral branches of the cranial nerves. HSV-1 is a frequent cause of Bell's palsy, which has classically been described as an idiopathic palsy of the peripheral branch of cranial nerve VII (CN VII). It occurs equally among men and women and occurs most frequently in the middle aged and has been reported in children. CN VII controls motor function of the facial muscles and the stapedius muscle, taste sensation of the anterior two-thirds of the tongue, and lacrimal gland secretory function. Clinical features include facial hemiplegia or hemiparesis, taste disturbance in greater than 50 percent of the cases, decreased blinking, variably dry eyes, or increased tearing, jaw or face pain, as well as numbness of the face and or neck in 60 percent of patients.[16] The diagnosis is made by definite findings of peripheral nerve VII involvement and exclusion of other treatable causes. The motor control of the muscles of the forehead are from bilateral motor cortices to the CN VII motor nuclei, so central CN VII lesions spare the forehead, but cause unilateral weakness of the lower face. A peripheral lesion results in paralysis of the forehead, along with the face. Attempting to close the eye on the affected side results in an upward gaze (Bell's phenomenon). Paralysis of the stapedius muscle results in hyperaccusis on the affected side.

Ruling out of other conditions is important in making the diagnosis. The results of a detailed examination of the cranial nerves should be normal except for the aforementioned findings associated with CN VII. The findings on examination of the ear, tympanic membrane, mastoid, and parotid gland should be normal in order to make a diagnosis of Bell's palsy. A CN VII palsy in association with otitis media, mastoiditis, or parotitis is a potential ear, nose, and throat (ENT) emergency and should prompt immediate consultation. The presence of vesicles on the tympanic membrane or in the ear canal is diagnostic of the Ramsay Hunt syndrome and is discussed in the section on VZV. A history of chronic ear infections, prior ear surgery, or tumor or recent head trauma excludes a diagnosis of Bell's palsy. If the presentation and examination are consistent with Bell's palsy, imaging of the CNS (CT or MRI) is not indicated, but if there are atypical features, recent trauma, or doubt, then imaging is recommended along with ENT consultation. The differential diagnosis includes stroke, tumor, atypical Guillain-Barré syndrome, and Lyme disease, especially if in endemic areas and if bilateral.

Treatment consists of prednisone for anti-inflammatory effect at 60 mg PO qd or 1 mg/kg/day for 5 days and then tapered over the next 5 days, along with acyclovir 400 mg five times per day for 10 days and follow-up with either ENT or neurologic consultation.[17] The prognosis is generally good for total recovery, but patients with total paralysis are at increased risk of long-term or permanent paralysis and should be seen in follow-up within 2 to 3 days, and patients with incomplete paralysis instructed to return if the weakness becomes total paralysis. Among patients with incomplete paralysis, 6 percent will have residual weakness at 1 year. Among the patients with complete paralysis at 1 year, 84 percent had total or good recovery, with 16 percent having poor to fair recovery.[18]

Eye care is important in preventing damage due to impaired blinking and decreased tearing. Artificial tears should be used frequently during the day at any sign of dryness or every 2 h. At night, a lubricating ointment with or without an eye patch should be used. Care of the eye is the most important therapeutic intervention that can be made by emergency physicians.

HERPETIC WHITLOW Herpetic whitlow is a primary or recurrent HSV infection of the finger. HSV-1 is seen in children who autoinnoculate their fingers by putting them in their mouths during an episode of oral herpes. HSV-1 is also seen in health care workers who are exposed to infected oral secretions. HSV-2 is more common among adults due to digital/genital contact in the community. The disease is usually limited to a single digit. Herpetic whitlow is frequently painful and accompanied by axillary adenopathy. Vesicles, which may be recognizable early in the course of the disease, coalesce and may appear to contain pus, but actually contain necrotic epithelial cells causing the purulent appearance. Healing occurs spontaneously over 2 to 3 weeks if local wound care and pain control are used. Whitlow

TABLE 150-1 Oral Dosing Regimens and Comparative Retail Prices for Antiviral Drugs

	ANTIVIRAL DRUGS		
Disease	Acyclovir (oral)	Valacyclovir	Famciclovir
Primary genital herpes	200 mg 5×/day for 10 days	1 g bid for 10 days	Not indicated
Price*	$38.00	$88.00	—
Recurrent genital herpes	200 mg 5×/day for 5 days	500 mg bid for 5 days	125 mg bid for 5 days
Price*	$19.00	$35.00	$33.00
Chickenpox	800 mg qid for 5 days	Not indicated	Not indicated
Price*	$64.00	—	—
Herpes zoster	800 mg 5×/day for 10 days	1 g tid for 7 days	500 mg tid for 7 days
Price*	$129.00	$69.00	$154.00

*Prices based on retail price to consumer at a single national chain in July 1998; current local prices may vary considerably.

may be misdiagnosed as a paronychia and incised, which may delay healing or allow a secondary infection to occur. When incised, no purulent material will be expressed. For patients with frequent painful recurrences suppressive therapy with acyclovir may be effective.[10]

IMMUNOCOMPROMISE Immunocompromised patients (those with organ transplants, HIV, etc.) are at increased risk of disseminated or severe typical and atypical HSV disease, usually resulting from reactivation of latent virus. HSV infection in immunocompromised patients may cause esophagitis, proctitis, colitis, and pneumonitis, as well as encephalitis. Definitive diagnosis is difficult without a biopsy of the affected tissue, because these patients generally all have latent HSV and are frequently shedding HSV in their secretions. Any evidence of disseminated or CNS disease mandates admission and IV acyclovir. The decision to admit or treat the immunocompromised on an outpatient basis with mucocutaneous HSV is based on severity of disease, reliability of the patient, and ability of the patient to stay hydrated; is made on a case-by-case basis; and should be made in conjunction with the patient's primary care provider. Additionally, patients with large areas of skin involvement by burns or eczema are at risk of severe or fatal infection although, most commonly, resolution will occur without treatment. Consultation and consideration for admission for these patients are recommended.

ANTIVIRAL DRUGS There are three agents widely available for HSV: acyclovir (Zovirax and generic), famciclovir (Famvir), and valacyclovir (Valtrex). Only acyclovir is available in oral and IV forms, whereas the others are available only in an oral form. Famciclovir and valacyclovir are more active in vitro, but all have similar clinical efficacy.[7] Oral dosing regimens and comparative retail prices are listed in Table 150-1 (listed are retail prices for consumers from a single national chain in July 1998; current prices may vary considerably). Valacyclovir and famciclovir are pregnancy category B, used only if benefits to the patient outweigh the risk to the fetus. Acyclovir is pregnancy category C, but is generally considered safe in pregnancy. All three medications are indicated for recurrent genital HSV and shingles. Only acyclovir and valacyclovir are indicated for primary genital HSV. Acyclovir is also indicated in primary varicella (chicken pox). IV acyclovir is indicated for CNS or disseminated disease. Other uses of these drugs, such as in treating whitlow or severe oral disease, are off label and not well studied.

HERPES ZOSTER: CHICKENPOX

Epidemiology

Herpes zoster virus (VZV and human herpesvirus 3) is the cause of chickenpox as a primary infection, which may reactivate later in life as zoster (shingles). Prior to the use of the varicella vaccine, 90 percent of primary infection occurred among children at age 10 years or younger, with the majority of these in children younger than age 3. Only approximately 10 percent of individuals over age 15 remain susceptible to VZV. Chickenpox is endemic, occurring year round, but there are annual epidemics in late winter and early spring. After exposure, attack rates are close to 80 percent among susceptible household contacts. The route of spread is presumed to be respiratory. Patients are infectious for approximately 48 h before the appearance of the rash until the vesicles are crusted over, and for about 4 to 5 days after the appearance of the rash.

Pathophysiology

After exposure, viral replication occurs at an unknown site, followed by a viremia. Viral replication in the skin results in degenerative changes in epithelial cells, leading to multinucleated giant cells in vesicles. The rash usually appears 14 to 15 days after exposure. The rash then fades, and the virus becomes latent in a dorsal root ganglion.

Clinical Features

In children, there is typically a prodrome of 1 to 2 days of low-grade fever and malaise, followed by the appearance of lesions on the face and trunk. The lesions initially are maculopapular and then vesicles with clear fluid on an erythematous base. The fluid quickly becomes turbid due to the accumulation of cellular debris. As the lesions continue to age, they scab over. The rash spreads centripetally to involve the extremities. Over the next several days, new lesions appear in crops. A hallmark of chickenpox is the presence of lesions in various stages. Accompanying the rash is fever up to 39.8°C (103°F), malaise, pruritus, and anorexia. The mortality rate among children is less than 2/100,000 cases and death is generally due to encephalitis. Varicella encephalitis is characterized by chickenpox accompanied by an altered level of consciousness, fever, vomiting, headaches, and seizures. Cerebellar ataxia is a more benign CNS complication characterized by ataxia, vomiting, tremor, and altered speech, with complete resolution within a month. Another serious potential complication is Reye syndrome, so parents should be instructed to avoid aspirin and aspirin-containing products.

In adults, the mortality rate of primary varicella infection approaches 30/100,000 cases, and the disease process is more severe and prolonged. Encephalitis may occur, but a more common life-threatening complication is VZV pneumonitis,[19] which presents with cough, tachypnea, and dyspnea approximately 4 days after the onset of illness. Chest x-rays reveal a diffuse pneumonitis. Women in the second or third trimesters of pregnancy are at higher risk of severe pneumonitis. Women in the immediate perinatal period are at increased risk of severe disease, as are neonates. Chickenpox during pregnancy can cause fetal anomalies.[7]

Treatment

Acyclovir is the only medication approved for active chickenpox. For previously healthy children, its benefit is small and, generally, care is supportive, with attention to skin care, including bathing and the use of antipruritic drugs. The American Academy of Pediatrics does not recommend the use of acyclovir in uncomplicated chickenpox in previously healthy children who are younger than age 12. Oral acyclovir is recommended for patients older than age 12 and those with chronic illnesses or on chronic salicylate therapy. For children, the dosage is 20 mg/kg PO qid for 5 days (maximal single dose, 800 mg); adults are given 800 mg PO qid for 5 days. For maximal benefit, acyclovir should be started within 24 h of development of the rash. All patients with varicella encephalitis or pneumonitis should be admitted for IV acyclovir. Treatment of pregnant or peripartum women who develop chickenpox should be discussed with an obstetrician or perinatologist, as some physicians will elect to admit for IV acyclovir. Neonates who develop chickenpox or whose mothers develop postpartum chickenpox should be admitted for IV acyclovir. Immunocompromised patients tend to have more severe disease and should be admitted for IV acyclovir.

Varicella zoster immune globulin (VZIG) is available to confer passive immunity to exposed susceptible adults or immunocompromised children and pregnant women. VZIG should also be given to any neonate with chickenpox or whose mother developed chickenpox within 5 days before delivery or 48 h after delivery.[7]

Varicella vaccine is now recommended for children who are age 1 year or older. It is also recommended for adults with either a reliable history of never having chickenpox or with serologic evidence of susceptibility. The vaccine is a live attenuated cell-free vaccine. Because it is a live vaccine, it is contraindicated in immunocompromised patients, household contacts of immunocompromised patients, and pregnant or lactating women.

HERPES ZOSTER: SHINGLES

Herpes zoster (shingles) is the reactivation of latent VZV infection. There is a lifetime incidence of almost 20 percent, with the majority of cases being among the elderly. It occurs only in people who have had chicken pox. After a single occurrence in an immunocompetent host, there is a 4 percent likelihood of a second occurrence.

The lesions of shingles are identical to those of chickenpox, but are limited to a single dermatome in distribution. Thoracic and lumbar dermatomes are most common. The cranial nerves may be affected as well, with the potential complications of herpes zoster ophthalmicus (HZO) and Ramsay Hunt syndrome. What triggers the reactivation is unknown. The disease begins with a prodrome of pain in the affected area for 1 to 3 days, followed by the outbreak of a maculopapular rash that quickly progresses to a vesicular rash. The course of the disease is usually around 2 weeks, but may persist for a full month.

HZO is due to involvement of the ophthalmic branch of CN V and is a vision-threatening condition. The Hutchinson sign (lesions on the tip of the nose) may be seen before ocular involvement is recognized, but its absence does not rule out HZO.[20] Ocular involvement can be seen in the presence of only a slight rash on the forehead. HZO induces a keratitis and may be followed by involvement of deeper structures. There is usually facial pain, regional adenopathy, and occasionally a red eye preceding the appearance of the rash. A dendriform corneal ulcer can often be identified with fluorescein staining. The presence of a skin rash helps differentiate HZO from ocular HSV. HZO or suspected HZO mandates an ophthalmologic consultation due to the threat to vision.

CN VII can also be affected. Involvement of the maxillary or mandibular branches can result in intraoral lesions. Involvement of the geniculate ganglion of CN VII results in Ramsay Hunt syndrome, which clinically presents as a facial palsy resembling Bell palsy with a unilateral motor weakness, loss of taste on the anterior two-thirds of the tongue, and vesicles in the ear canal or on the tympanic membrane (the only sites of CN VII cutaneous innervation). Ramsay Hunt syndrome has also been described as an infrequent cause of altered mental status in the elderly.[21] This is treated in the same fashion as Bell palsy. Immunocompromised patients should be admitted for IV acyclovir.

The most common complication of shingles is postherpetic neuralgia (PHN). This is uncommon in younger patients, but increases in frequency with age. The pain at times may be so severe as to be debilitating. Occasionally, the anterior horn cells become involved, causing a transient local weakness or paralysis, with these patients being particularly prone to severe pain. PHN occurs in 10 to 20 percent of all patients after an episode of acute zoster, but in up to 70 percent of patients aged 70 years or older. It generally resolves in 1 to 2 months, but may last greater than a year in some patients.

The treatment of zoster in the normal host is aimed at decreasing the risk of PHN, as the antivirals have a clinically small, but statistically significant, effect on the duration of the acute disease. Treatment should begin as soon as possible, and within 72 h of onset of disease for maximal benefit. The present literature shows that all three currently available antiherpes agents are more effective than placebo at reducing the duration of PHN, but not at reducing its incidence.[22–24] There is a suggestion that both famciclovir and valacyclovir may be more effective than acyclovir, but this has not been shown to be clinically significant.[25] Corticosteroids have not been shown to be effective, but have been shown to improve quality-of-life indices in affected elderly, and a 21-day taper beginning at 60 mg PO qd should be considered in patients older than age 50 if no contraindications exist.[26,27]

Initial treatment of patients with PHN is typically systemic analgesia, often narcotics. Patients should be referred back to their primary care provider, because first-line agents often fail, and a trial of amitriptyline or carbamazepine may be tried as second-line therapy.

Immunocompromised patients have an increased risk of disseminated disease. This can be recognized clinically by evidence of the rash involving more than a single dermatome or crossing the midline. Disseminated disease may occur in patients with skin lesions limited to a single dermatome. Patients with disseminated disease may develop pneumonitis, hepatitis, meningoencephalitis, or other organ system involvement and should be admitted for IV acyclovir. Immunocompromised patients with shingles without evidence of dissemination can be treated as outpatients with oral acyclovir at the standard dosing, with instructions to return if the rash spreads or if they develop respiratory symptoms, headaches, or other signs of organ system disease. Close follow-up with their primary care provider is recommended.

EPSTEIN-BARR VIRUS: INFECTIOUS MONONUCLEOSIS

Human herpesvirus 4, known as Epstein-Barr virus (EBV), is the primary cause of the infectious mononucleosis syndrome. EBV is found in humans throughout the world. Serologic testing reveals that 90 to 95 percent of the adult population has developed antibodies to EBV.[28] Approximately half of the population will seroconvert as young children, with a second peak incidence during the teen and young adult years.

EBV is spread by close contact between individuals shedding the virus and a susceptible individual. EBV is not able to survive outside the human host for any significant amount of time, and spread via fomites has not been demonstrated. Transmission among teenagers is often via the exchange of saliva during kissing. Adults may asymptomatically shed EBV for up to 18 months after clinical recovery, and

EBV may be demonstrated in the throats of up to 20 percent of all adults. In immunocompromised persons, up to 50 percent may demonstrate EBV.

After infection, there is a 1- to 2-month incubation period during which viral replication occurs in B lymphocytes in the reticuloendothelial system. The presence of EBV induces the production of specific anti-EBV antibodies, as well as the production of the heterophil antibodies. Heterophil antibodies react with antigens on the red cells of sheep, horses, and cows. Heterophil antibodies are not specific for EBV and can be produced by infection with CMV or toxoplasmosis, as well as other infections. Heterophil antibodies are rarely produced in infants.

Following the asymptomatic incubation, EBV can produce a wide array of illnesses. Classic infectious mononucleosis is manifested by fever, exudative pharyngitis, lymphadenopathy, splenomegaly, and an atypical lymphocytosis. Infants and young children frequently have asymptomatic infections. A prodrome of malaise, fatigue, and fever may be present for several days before the onset of the symptoms in classic mononucleosis. An elevated liver transaminase level is uniformly found in mononucleosis. Hepatomegaly and jaundice are unusual in children and young adults, but common in older adults. A severe sore throat is a common presenting complaint, and the appearance may be of a severe bilateral exudative tonsillitis/pharyngitis. Bilateral tender cervical adenopathy is virtually universal. At some point in the illness, approximately half of the patients will have palpable splenomegaly. Splenomegaly is most prominent during week 2 of illness and then resolves over the next 1 to 2 weeks. The majority of patients have an uncomplicated course and recover fully. Chronic fatigue syndrome is not caused by EBV infection.

Generally, the treatment is supportive in the absence of complications. If ampicillin is given to a patient with EBV to treat a possible strep throat infection, there is an approximately 95 percent incidence of rash due to transient production of EBV-induced antibodies against ampicillin. Acyclovir has in vitro effects on EBV replication, but in vivo clinical studies have failed to show any clinically significant effect.[29]

Complications of EBV infections are uncommon and usually do not result in long-term morbidity. The upper airway in approximately 3 percent of children may be obstructed by severe tonsillitis/pharyngitis.[30] Management includes ENT consultation for airway control, if required. Prednisone, 1 to 2 mg/kg/day, should be given to patients with airway compromise. Humidified oxygen and a nasopharyngeal airway are also helpful. Tonsillectomy is usually not necessary and should be reserved for patients who fail to respond to conservative measures. If endotracheal intubation is required, a prolonged period of intubation should be anticipated due to the extent of edema.

The spleen may rupture spontaneously or secondary to minor trauma. The incidence of splenic rupture is believed to be 0.1 to 0.5 percent of patients with EBV. It most commonly occurs during week 2 or 3 of illness. Presenting complaints may be abdominal pain, left scapular pain, or hypotension. Abdominal pain is unusual in infectious mononucleosis and should prompt consideration of splenic rupture. Patients with EBV should be instructed to avoid contact sports and strenuous activity for 4 weeks following the onset of clinical disease. Patients with splenic rupture should be admitted to a general surgical service.

Hematologic complications include autoimmune hemolytic anemia and thrombocytopenia. Corticosteroids will benefit some patients with hematologic complications and should be initiated in the emergency department for those admitted with severe anemia or severe thrombocytopenia. Refractory severe thrombocytopenia may be treated with splenectomy.

Neurologic complications of EBV are quite rare, but may include encephalitis, meningitis, cranial nerve palsies, and the Guillain-Barré syndrome. The CSF usually contains atypical lymphocytes. Recovery is usually complete.

In immunocompromised patients, EBV may be a cause of B-cell lymphomas and other lymphoproliferative syndromes. EBV has been implicated as a causal agent in African Burkitt lymphoma and in nasopharyngeal carcinomas. Death may be caused by overwhelming EBV infection in patients with Duncan disease (an X-linked recessive disorder), which is clinically silent until EBV infection. Patients with HIV may develop hairy leukoplakia that will respond to acyclovir therapy.

The diagnosis of EBV is based on clinical findings and on nonspecific laboratory tests. Confirmatory EBV-specific antibody testing is available, but same-day results are generally not available, so these tests have little value in the setting of the emergency department. The complete blood count is usually moderately elevated, with elevated percentages of lymphocytes and monocytes. Atypical lymphocytes are usually found and may be up to 30 percent of the white blood cells.

The heterophil antibodies are produced in 80 to 90 percent of patients older than age 4. More than 50 percent of children younger than age 4 will not have detectable heterophil antibodies.[31] Commercially available tests for heterophil antibodies (Monospot, Mono-plus, Monolatex, and Mono-lex) have a sensitivity of 78 to 83 percent, with a specificity of 98 to 100 percent.[32] False negatives may occur more frequently during the first week of illness. Patients with classic symptoms of infectious mononucleosis, atypical lymphocytes, and a positive heterophil antibody test generally require no further testing to confirm the diagnosis. Patients with classic symptoms who have a negative heterophil antibody test should have repeat heterophil testing performed in a week, and if still negative, specific EBV antibody testing may be indicated. Viral capsid antigen (VCA) antibodies of the IgG and IgM classes are present in high titers during acute disease, with IgG persisting for life and IgM persisting for 4 to 8 weeks. The presence of IgM antibodies to VCA is a sensitive and specific indicator of acute EBV infection. Antibodies to Epstein-Barr nuclear antigen develop 4 to 6 weeks after the onset of clinical illness and persist for life, their presence is evidence against acute EBV infection. Other illnesses which may present with a similar clinical picture, but with negative EBV tests include CMV mononucleosis, acute toxoplasmosis, primary HIV infection and strep throat.

CYTOMEGALOVIRUS

Cytomegalovirus (CMV, or human herpesvirus 5) is another ubiquitous virus with worldwide distribution. It is, like the other members of the herpesvirus family, capable of causing a primary illness and then existing in a latent state in the human host indefinitely with the ability to reactivate at a later time. It is present in approximately 1 percent of newborns and in 40 to 100 percent of adults, depending on geographic location, socioeconomic status, attendance at day care, and sexual behavior. There are two peaks of seroconversion, the first in the perinatal period and the second during young adulthood, presumably related to sexually activity. CMV is not easily spread by casual contact, but requires repeated or prolonged intimate contact for transmission. It is found in milk, saliva, urine, semen, and cervical secretions. CMV is also transmitted via blood transfusions containing viable leukocytes or via solid organs or bone marrow during transplantation.

CMV is one of the TORCH agents [*t*oxoplasmosis, *o*ther (viruses), *r*ubella, *C*MV, and *h*erpes (simplex viruses)] and is capable of causing intrauterine infection. Fewer than 25 percent of neonates with intrauterine CMV will display symptoms. Those at highest risk are those whose mother acquires primary disease during the first half of the pregnancy. A seropositive mother's antibodies to CMV appear to provide the fetus some protection. Classic intrauterine CMV (congenital cytomegalic inclusion disease) involves multiple organs, including jaundice, hepatosplenomegaly, microcephaly, petechiae, and inner ear problems, as well as CNS defects. Children who are asymptomatic at birth may still have hearing loss that results in lower IQ scores and learning disabilities later in life.

In contrast to intrauterine infection, perinatal infection (presumably acquired from the cervix of the mother during birth or from breast milk) is usually asymptomatic and has no long-term consequences.

In healthy immunocompetent children and adults, CMV infection is also usually asymptomatic. When CMV does cause disease in this setting, it is typically an illness resembling EBV infectious mononucleosis. Typical presenting complaints include fever, chills, myalgia, and headache. Clinical features include a prolonged fever (1 to 5 weeks), an atypical lymphocytosis, lymphadenopathy, splenomegaly, and mild elevations of the liver transaminase levels. Pharyngitis and tonsillitis are not usually present. There are rarely complications or long-term health consequences. The diagnosis of CMV mononucleosis should be considered in individuals who have a mononucleosis-type illness but are heterophil-antibody negative. The complications of CMV in immunocompetent patients include the Guillain-Barré syndrome, viral pneumonitis, hepatitis, hemolytic anemia, and thrombocytopenia.

In patients with HIV, CMV can cause illness with significant morbidity. Symptomatic infections generally do not occur in patients who are simply HIV positive, but in those with more advanced disease, such as ARC (AIDS-related complex) or AIDS. The most common illness is CMV retinitis, which occurs in more than 10 percent of AIDS patients. Typical complaints are of floaters or of decreased vision. Careful funduscopic examination may reveal characteristic retinal hemorrhages and exudates. Progression to blindness will occur without chronic suppressive therapy with IV ganciclovir or foscarnet. CMV may cause gastrointestinal disease as either an esophagitis or as a colitis. Additionally, CMV can cause an adrenalitis resulting in adrenal insufficiency.

CMV causes significant morbidity and mortality in transplant patients. It can infect numerous different organs, causing colitis, hepatitis, pneumonia, and CNS disease. The most serious infection is CMV pneumonia, which is most common in recipients of bone marrow transplants. The CMV seen in transplant patients may represent primary infection after exposure from the transplanted tissue itself or in transfused blood products, or reactivation of latent infection. The primary infections tend to be more severe. CMV infections occur 4 to 8 weeks after transplant typically, and CMV should be included in the differential diagnosis for patients presenting with a febrile illness within the first 3 months after transplant. CMV may also contribute to rejection of the transplanted organ.

The diagnosis of CMV is difficult because most people are seropositive. The presence of IgM antibodies is helpful, but not very sensitive or specific because of false negatives during some acute infections and their persistence beyond the acute infection in others. To make a definitive diagnosis based on serologies, a conversion from seronegative to seropositive or an acute rise in antibody titer should be seen, and this will require samples from before the illness and during the illness. Another method of diagnosis is by viral culture, which, using the "shell" method, takes only 48 h. Children can shed virus in their urine and respiratory secretions for extended periods following infection, but, in healthy adults, virus is not usually shed in the urine or respiratory tract except during acute illness. Healthy adults may shed virus in semen and cervical secretions. In immunocompromised individuals, a biopsy of the organ suspected to be infected with CMV is the preferred method of diagnosis, because of the prevalence of false-positive cultures in immunocompromised patients. Biopsy specimens of infected organs will show characteristic CMV inclusion bodies. In the emergency department, definitive diagnosis is not available, and suspicion of CMV should be based on clinical grounds such as presentation and time from transplant. A review of transplant records may yield clues, such as the recipient's and donor's CMV status prior to transplantation. The disposition of the patient depends on the clinical setting, not on the diagnosis of CMV, and should be discussed with the patient's primary care provider.

CMV is treated with either ganciclovir or foscarnet. Ganciclovir is approved for therapy of CMV retinitis in AIDS patients and for prevention of CMV in transplant patients. It is also used for treating CMV infections in other organ systems. In AIDS-associated CMV retinitis, ganciclovir is given initially at higher doses for 2 to 3 weeks, followed by lifetime suppressive therapy. For other CMV infections, ganciclovir is given for a period of 2 to 3 weeks and then stopped. Foscarnet is used for resistant CMV infections or for patients unable to take ganciclovir. Neither medication cures patients of CMV, but instead they suppress the acute disease process.

REFERENCES

1. Monto AS, Kioumehr F: The Tecumseh Study of Respiratory Illness: IX. Occurrence of influenza in the community. *Am J Epidemiol* 102:553, 1975.
2. Knight V, Fedson D, Baldini J, et al: Amantadine therapy of epidemic influenza. *Infect Immun* 1:200, 1970.
3. VanVoris LP, Betts RF, Roth FK, et al: Successful treatment of naturally occurring influenza A/USSR/77 H1N1. *JAMA* 245:1128, 1981.
4. ZymeTx: ZstatFlu product package insert. Oklahoma City, ZymeTx, 1988.
5. Waldman RJ, Hall WN, McGee H, VanAmberg G: Aspirin as a risk factor in Reye's syndrome. *JAMA* 247:3089, 1982.
6. Fulginiti VA, and the Committee in Infectious Diseases: Aspirin and Reye's syndrome [special report]. *Pediatrics* 69:810, 1982.
7. American Academy of Pediatrics Committee on Infectious Diseases: *The Red Book: Report of the Committee on Infectious Diseases,* 24th ed. Elk Grove Village, IL, American Academy of Pediatrics, 1997.
8. Hayden FG, Osterhaus AD, Treanor JJ, et al, for the GG167 Influenza Study Group: Efficacy and safety of the neuraminadase inhibitor zanamavir in the treatment of influenza virus infections. *N Engl J Med* 337:874, 1997.
9. Advisory Committee on Immunization Practices: Recommendations of the Advisory Committee on Immunization Practices: Prevention and control of influenza. *MMWR* 46, 1997.
10. Kesson AM: Position paper of the Pediatric Special Interest Group of the Australian Society for Infectious Diseases: Use of acyclovir in herpes simplex virus infections. *J Paediatr Child Health* 34:9, 1998.
11. Spruance SL, Rea TL, Thomig C, et al: Penciclovir cream for the treatment of herpes simplex labialis: A randomized, multicenter, double-blind, placebo-controlled trial. *JAMA* 277:1374, 1997.
12. Hutto C, Arvin A, Jacobs R, et al: Intrauterine herpes simplex virus infections. *J Pediatr* 110:97, 1987.
13. Gibbs RS, Amstey MS, Sweet RL, et al: Management of genital herpes infection in pregnancy. *Obstet Gynecol* 71:779, 1988.
14. Brown ZA, Bendetti J, Ashley R: Neonatal herpes simplex virus infection in relation to asymptomatic shedding at the time of labor. *N Engl J Med* 324:1227, 1991.
15. Herpetic Eye Disease Study Group: Acyclovir for the prevention of recurrent herpes simplex virus eye disease. *N Engl J Med* 339:300, 1998.
16. Adour KK, Byl FM, Hilsinger RL Jr, et al: The true nature of Bell's palsy: Analysis of 1000 consecutive patients. *Laryngoscope* 88:787, 1978.
17. Adour KK, Ruboyianes JM, VanDoersten PG, et al: Bell's palsy treatment with acyclovir and prednisone compared with prednisone alone: A double blind, randomized, controlled trial. *Ann Otol Rhinol Laryngol* 105:371, 1996.
18. Peitersen E: The natural history of Bell's palsy. *Am J Otolaryngol* 4:107, 1982.
19. Fleisher G, Henry W, McSorley M, et al: Life threatening complications of varicella. *Am J Dis Child* 138:896, 1981.
20. Marsh RJ: Herpes zoster ophthalmicus. *J R Soc Med* 90:670, 1997.
21. Rahimi AR: Ramsay Hunt syndrome. *Geriatrics* 53:93, 1998.
22. Jackson JL, Gibbons R, Meyer G, Inouye L: The effect of treating herpes zoster with oral acyclovir in preventing postherpetic neuralgia. *Arch Intern Med* 157:909, 1997.
23. Tyring S, Barbarash RA, Nahlik JE, et al: and the Collaborative Famciclovir Herpes Zoster Study Group: Famciclovir for the treatment of acute herpes zoster: Effects on acute disease and postherpetic neuralgia. *Ann Intern Med* 123:89, 1995.
24. Beutner KR, Friedman DJ, Forszpaniak C, et al: Valaciclovir compared with acyclovir for improved therapy for herpes zoster in immunocompetent adults. *Antimicrob Agents Chemother* 39:1546, 1995.
25. Kost RG, Straus SE: Postherpetic neuralgia: Pathogenesis, treatment, and prevention. *N Engl J Med* 335:32, 1996.
26. Esmann V, Geil JP, Kroon S, et al: Prednisolone does not prevent postherpetic neuralgia. *Lancet* 2:126, 1987.

27. Whitley RJ, Weiss H, Gnann JW Jr, et al, and the NIAID Collaborative Antiviral Study Group: Acyclovir with and without prednisone for the treatment of herpes zoster. *Ann Intern Med* 125:376, 1996.
28. Pereira MS, Blake JM, Macrae AD: Epstein-Barr virus antibodies at different ages. *BMJ* 4:526, 1969.
29. Van der Horst C, Joncal J, Ahronheim G, et al: Lack of effect of peroral acyclovir for the treatment of acute infectious mononucleosis. *J Infect Dis* 164:788, 1991.
30. Sumaya CV, Ench Y, Shapiro ED, et al: Epstein-Barr virus infectious mononucleosis in children: I. Clinical and general laboratory tests. *Pediatrics* 75:1003, 1985.
31. Sumaya CV, Ench Y: Epstein-Barr virus infectious mononucleosis in children: II. Heterophile antibody and viral specific responses. *Pediatrics* 75:1011, 1985.
32. Gerber MA, et al: Evaluations of enzyme-linked immunosorbent assay procedure for determining specific Epstein-Barr virus serology and of rapid test kits for diagnosis of infectious mononucleosis. *J Clin Microbiol* 34:3240, 1996.

GENERAL MANAGEMENT OF POISONED PATIENTS

Jason B. Hack

Robert S. Hoffman

The perception that most people have of a poisonous substance is consistent with common definitions. Mofenson and colleagues established guidelines that must be fulfilled for a substance, and its subsequent exposure, to be categorized as nontoxic (Table 151-1).[1,2] A *poisoning* is an event where a living organism is exposed to a chemical that adversely affects the functioning of that organism. The exposure to the toxin may be occupational, environmental, recreational, or medicinal. A poisoning may result from varied portals of entry, including inhalation, insufflation, ingestion, cutaneous and mucous membrane exposure, and injection. Toxic exposures commonly occur, for example, when substances are tasted or swallowed. Toxins may be in the form of gas or vapors or in a suspension such as dust. Caustics, vesicants, or irritants may affect the skin. A toxin may enter the body transdermally and affect internal structures. Parenteral exposure is also common through intravenous or subcutaneous injection of medications or drugs of abuse.

A poison may affect the body in many ways. It may inhibit or alter normal cellular function, change normal organ function, or may change the normal uptake or transport of substances into or within the organism. The toxin may also exclude essential substrates in the environment from being efficiently utilized by the organism. This chapter discusses the general management of poisoned patients. The following chapters discuss specific approaches to patients exposed to individual classes of drugs.

In 1996, there were 2,155,952 toxic exposures reported to poison centers in the United States: 1,137,295 (52.6 percent) involved children younger than 18 years of age. Some authors currently list poisoning as the third leading cause of death in the United States and, between 1985 and 1995, the incidence of toxin-related deaths is said to have increased approximately 300 percent. Although many of these exposures were referred to as "accidents," most were preventable or avoidable by modalities such as increased awareness and education, increased parental control over children, instituted checks and balances in hospitals and pharmacies, computer networking and recognition of potential drug interactions, better hospital protocols to ensure patient identification, detailed procedures to check proper dosing, better warning labels and packaging on products with potential toxicity, and better access to mental health care by the underinsured. The public must be made aware of the potential tragedy when nonfood (potentially harmful) items are stored in food areas behind insufficiently secured barricades accessible to children, as well as the potential health threat when toxins are stored in empty food containers.

Poison centers should be an integral part of the management of exposed patients. These centers are typically staffed with specialists who are trained in the management of poisoned patients, have extensive reference material at their disposal, and have rapid access to medical toxicologists if more extensive evaluation is required. Routine consultation in cases where toxic exposure is suspected can help focus diagnosis and treatment and reduce cost and unnecessary hospitalizations.

EMERGENCY DEPARTMENT MANAGEMENT OF POISONED PATIENTS

ABCs

The first priorities are always the ABCs. Once the airway and respiratory status is secured, abnormalities of blood pressure, pulse, rectal temperature, and oxygen saturation must be corrected. Although the proper use of antidotes is essential in the treatment of poisoned patients, only in very rare incidences (such as cyanide poisoning) would the administration of an antidote take precedence over completing the primary evaluation and normal attempts to stabilize the ABCs.

Medical History

As much detailed information as possible must be obtained about the medical history. Answers to questions pertaining to the number of exposed persons and the type, amount, and route of exposure are essential. In addition, the patient's intent must be extensively appraised. Clinicians must be aware of the inherent inaccuracies in these types of histories. The patient's motivation, potential for secondary gain, and perceived risk of arrest all may affect the history. Corroborating information should be obtained from the patient's private physician, witnesses, or emergency medical technicians who were on scene. Histories of where in the environment the patient was found, empty pill bottles or containers nearby, smells or unusual materials in the home, the occupation of the person, or the presence of a suicide note all may provide important clues to identifying the exposure.

Toxicologic Physical Examination

The comprehensive physical examination must be performed on a fully undressed patient. This affords the physician every opportunity to check the patient's clothing for substances still retained in the pockets or substances hidden on the patient's body (waistbands, groin, or between skinfolds). In addition, physicians must pay special attention to certain aspects of the physical examination. Care must be taken when searching belongings, particularly pockets, because health care providers have been stuck by uncapped needles.

The skin must be examined for cyanosis or flushing, excessive diaphoresis or dryness, signs of injury or injection, ulcers, or bullae. Bruising may be a clue as to duration of unconsciousness, as well as coagulopathy. Examine the eyes for pupil size, reactivity, nystagmus, dysconjugate gaze, or excessive lacrimation. Hypersalivation or excessive dryness should be noted in the oropharynx. The chest examination should include careful evaluation of the lungs to assess for bronchorrhea, or wheezing, and the heart must be assessed for its rhythm, rate, and regularity. Bowel sounds, urinary retention, and abdominal tenderness or rigidity must also be noted. The extremities must be evaluated for tremor or fasciculation. Cranial nerves, reflexes, resting muscle tone, coordination, cognition, and the ability to ambulate all must be assessed.

Toxidromes

The term *toxidrome* refers to the collection of signs and symptoms that are observed after an exposure to a substance (a toxic "fingerprint"). Toxidromes include grouped, physiologically based abnormalities of

TABLE 151-1 Nontoxic Ingestions

Only one substance is involved in the exposure.
The substance must be absolutely identified.
The substance's product label must not contain any consumer product safety commission signal words indicating a potential hazard of toxicity.
The exposure must have been unintentional.
The route of exposure must be known.
An approximate amount of the substance involved in the exposure must be known.
The exposed individual must be free of symptoms for the extent of the observation period.
Follow-up consultation must be easily available or a responsible parent or guardian must be present.

Note: All of the listed criteria must be fulfilled in order for an ingestion to be classified as nontoxic.
Source: Adapted from Mofenson et al[1] and Mofenson and Grensher.[2]

vital signs, general appearance, skin, eyes, mucous membranes, lungs, heart, abdomen, and neurologic examination that are known for many substances and typically he!pful in establishing a diagnosis when the exposure is not well defined (Table 151-2). Similarly, certain clinical findings may narrow the etiologic possibilities (Table 151-3).

DECONTAMINATION

The general approach to most toxic exposures involves the removal of the patient from the substance or of the substance from the patient. Toxins outside the body must be washed away. Toxins inside the body must be either bound within the gut lumen to make it unavailable for absorption or have its elimination enhanced from the gut, the blood, or the tissues.

Gross Decontamination

Patients may still have the toxin on their skin or clothing. Decontamination is generally achieved by undressing patients completely and washing them thoroughly with copious amounts of water. Patients requiring assistance should be attended to by properly gowned staff in an isolated area. Patients should be scrubbed with soft brushes so as not to injure their skin (thereby allowing the toxin to enter through an injured barrier). The towels used to dry patients, and their clothing, shoes, socks, watches, and jewelry, should all be handled as potentially hazardous waste. This gross decontamination will decrease the likelihood of spreading illness among staff members and other patients.

Eyes

Following ocular exposures, the eyes must be immediately flushed with copious amounts of irrigation solution, after topical analgesia. This irrigation should continue until a copious amount (usually several liters) of irrigant is used and, if appropriate, the pH of the eyes returns to a physiologic range.

Gastrointestinal Decontamination

Each of the methods used to decontaminate the gastrointestinal (GI) tract have potential benefits and risks that must be considered prior to their use. The three general methods of decontamination involve removal of the toxin from the stomach, binding it inside the gut lumen, or mechanically flushing it through the GI tract. The choice of method(s) used is determined by the toxin ingested, the time course, the patient's clinical status, and the skills of the physician available. GI decontamination must never be initiated as a punitive action.

GASTRIC EMPTYING

Emesis

Emesis is achieved by administration of syrup of ipecac. Syrup of ipecac is a plant-derived compound composed of two alkaloidal substances—emetine and cephaeline—which work both peripherally on the stomach and centrally on the chemotactic trigger zone to induce vomiting. Dosing of syrup of ipecac is 15 mL for children 1 to 12 years of age, and 30 mL for adults, usually followed by sips of water. The dose may repeated once if vomiting does not occur after 30 min. Approximately 90 percent of patients vomit within 20 min after the first dose, and up to 97 percent vomit if a second dose is given. A typical patient vomits less than 3 to 5 times, and symptoms usually resolve within 2 h.

The ingested toxin should be suspected as the cause if protracted vomiting occurs. Contraindications to the administration of syrup of ipecac include ingestions with potential to alter mental status; active or prior vomiting; caustic ingestion; a toxin with more pulmonary than GI toxicity (e.g., hydrocarbons); and potential for seizures. Rare but potential complications of syrup of ipecac–induced emesis include aspiration, Boerhaave syndrome, Mallory-Weiss tear, and intractable vomiting.

The clinical situations where syrup of ipecac would be used in the hospital setting are limited. Most patients reach the hospital beyond the time frame when the use of syrup of ipecac would be beneficial, because the toxin has been absorbed or has passed through the pylorus. Also, even when syrup of ipecac is given with activated charcoal in less than 60 min after ingestion, it does not alter outcome when compared to treatment with activated charcoal and a cathartic. Ipecac's administration also prolongs the time to administration of oral antidotes by 1 to 6.5 h.[3]

Syrup of ipecac may still be indicated, especially when it can be given in the home immediately after an ingestion of a known toxin that is still expected to be in the stomach and that does not have the previously listed contraindications. Possible rare hospital indications for its use include very recent ingestions of substances not expected to compromise the airway or lead to altered mental status or hemodynamic derangement or seizure, a recent ingestion of a pill that is known not to be able to fit into the holes of the appropriately sized orogastric tube, or a substance known not to adsorb to activated charcoal (see the following sections).

Orogastric Lavage

The principal method of gastric emptying is orogastric lavage, which is performed with the patient lying in the left lateral decubitus position. A 36 to 40 French tube is used for adults (22 to 24 French tube for children), which is inserted after careful measurement of the depth (from the chin to the xiphoid process). Correct positioning must be assessed by insufflation of air to ensure accurate placement in the stomach. Lavage with room-temperature water is commonly continued until the effluent is clear. Before the tube is removed, activated charcoal should be instilled in a dose of 1 g/kg, if indicated. The contraindications to this procedure include pills that are known not to fit into the holes of the orogastric lavage hose, nontoxic ingestions, non-life-threatening ingestions, caustic ingestions, any patient whose airway integrity is not assured, or toxic ingestions that are more damaging to the lungs than to the GI tract. Complications of this procedure include insertion of the tube into the trachea, aspiration, esophageal or gastric perforation, decreased oxygenation during the procedure,[4] and inability to withdraw the tube once inserted (knot formation).

TABLE 151-2 Toxidromes

Toxidrome	Representative Agent(s)	Most Common Findings	Additional Signs and Symptoms	Potential Interventions
Opioid	Heroin Morphine	CNS depression, miosis, respiratory depression	Hypothermia, bradycardia. Death may result from respiratory arrest, pulmonary edema	Ventilation or naloxone
Sympathomimetic	Cocaine Amphetamine	Psychomotor agitation, mydriasis, diaphoresis, tachycardia, hypertension, hyperthermia	Seizures, rhabdomyolysis, myocardial infarction Death may result from seizures, cardiac arrest, hyperthermia	Cooling, sedation with benzodiazepines, hydration
Cholinergic	Organophosphate insecticides Carbamate insecticides	Salivation, lacrimation, diaphoresis, nausea, vomiting, urination, defecation, muscle fasciculations, weakness, bronchorrhea	Bradycardia, miosis/mydriasis, seizures, respiratory failure, paralysis Death may result from respiratory arrest 2° to paralysis and/or bronchorrhea, seizures	Airway protection and ventilation, atropine, pralidoxime
Anticholinergic	Scopolamine Atropine	Altered mental status, mydriasis, dry/flushed skin, urinary retention, decreased bowel sounds, hyperthermia, dry mucous membranes	Seizures, dysrhythmias, rhabdomyolysis Death may result from hyperthermia and dysrhythmias	Physostigmine (if appropriate), sedation with benzodiazepines, cooling, supportive management
Salicylates	Aspirin Oil of wintergreen	Altered mental status, respiratory alkalosis, metabolic acidosis, tinnitus hyperpnea, tachycardia, diaphoresis, nausea, vomiting	Low-grade fever, ketonuria Death may result from pulmonary edema, cardiorespiratory arrest	MDAC, alkalinization of the urine with potassium repletion, hemodialysis, hydration
Hypoglycemia	Sulfonylureas Insulin	Altered mental status, diaphoresis, tachycardia, hypertension	Paralysis, slurring of speech, bizarre behavior, seizures Death may result from seizures, altered behavior	Glucose containing solution intravenously, and oral feedings if able, frequent capillary blood for glucose measurement
Serotonin syndrome	Meperidine/dextromethorphan + MAOI, SSRI + TCA, SSRI/TCA/MAOI + amphetamine, SSRI overdose	Altered mental status, increased muscle tone, hyperreflexia, hyperthermia	''Wet dog shakes'' (intermittent whole body tremor) Death may result from hyperthermia	Cooling, sedation with benzodiazepines, supportive management, theoretical benefit—cyproheptadine

Abbreviations: CNS, central nervous system; MDAC, multidose activated charcoal; MAOI, monoamine oxidase inhibitor; SSRI, selective serotonin reuptake inhibitor; TCA, tricyclic antidepressant.

Although the perceived benefits of orogastric lavage are the immediate return of small pills or pill fragments, and a reduction in the amount of substance available for further intoxication, studies typically demonstrate drug removal ranging from only 35 to 56 percent. Of three large studies that evaluated the clinical efficacy of orogastric lavage,[3,5,6] only one showed any benefit from the procedure, and only if it was initiated in obtunded patients within 1 h of the ingestion.[3] Indications for this procedure are generally limited to ingestion of a life-threatening toxin that requires ventilatory support, depresses mental status, or may cause seizures.

ADSORPTION OF THE TOXIN IN THE GUT LUMEN

Activated Charcoal

The most appropriate agent to decontaminate the GI tract is activated charcoal, which is produced by pyrolysis of carbonaceous materials and activated by steam cleaning to increase its surface area. Activated charcoal is beneficial because it adsorbs the toxin within the gut lumen, making the toxin less available for absorption into the tissues, and because it enhances elimination. It establishes a free-drug concentration gradient favoring movement back into the GI lumen to enhance elimination (''GI dialysis''),[7] and it can also bind the drug in the bile, interrupting the enterohepatic circulation. The benefits of this technique include its capability to decontaminate the gut without requiring invasive procedures, its rapid administration, and its proven safety in both adults and children.

Activated charcoal is typically given in a slurry of water or juice by mouth or through a nasogastric tube, in an activated charcoal-drug dose of 10:1 (thought to be the smallest dose of activated charcoal that can be given with out reducing its efficacy[8]) or in 1 g/kg, whichever is larger. The first dose of activated charcoal is often given with a cathartic to reduce GI transit time. Sorbitol, and magnesium citrate solution, are the most commonly used cathartics (see the cathartic section).

TABLE 151-3 Agents that May Alter Presenting Signs or Symptoms*

Drugs	Seizures	Change in Blood Pressure	Change in Ventilation	Change in Heart Rate	Temperature Change
Alcohol withdrawal	✓	↑	↑	↑	↑
Amphetamines	✓	↑	↑	↑	↑
Anticholinergic	✓	↑	↑	↑	↑
Baclofen	✓	↓	↓	↑	↓
Caffeine	✓	↑	↑	↑	
Camphor	✓				
Cocaine	✓	↑	↑	↑	↑
Gyrometria esculenta (mushroom)	✓				
Isoniazid	✓				
Lithium	✓				
Methaqualone	✓	↑	↓	↑	
Serotonin syndrome	✓	↑	↑	↑	↑
Theophylline	✓	↑	↑	↑	
Tricyclic antidepressants	✓	↑	↓	↑	
β-adrenergic antagonists	✓	↓		↓	
Calcium-channel blockers		↓		↓	
Clonidine		↓	↓	↓	↓
Ethanol		↓	↓	↑	↓
Phenothiazines		↓	↓	↑	
Opioids		↓	↓	↓	↓
Organophosphates	✓	↓	↓	↓	
Meprobamate		↓	↓		
Monoamine oxidase inhibitor overdose	✓	↑	↑	↑	↓
Phencyclidine		↑	↓	↑	↑
Sedative hypnotic withdrawal	✓	↑	↑		↑
Phenylpropanolamine		↑	↑	↑	
Barbiturates		↓	↓	↓	↓
Ethchlorvynol		↓	↓	↓	
Glutethamide		↓	↓		
Salicylates		↓	↑	↑	↑
Nicotine	✓	↑	↑	↑	
Hydrocarbons		↓	↑	↑†	
Toxic alcohols	✓	↓	↑	↑	
Iron	✓	↓	↑	↑	

*Listed are the most common or most classically seen with the agent.

Contraindications to activated charcoal include isolated ingestion of a substance known not to adsorb to activated charcoal (such as iron, lithium, or lead), or if the patient is to undergo endoscopic evaluation such as would be required following a caustic ingestion. The risks, which are exceedingly rare, include aspiration and intraluminal impaction in patients with abnormal gut motility. Clear indications for administration of activated charcoal are ingestion of any drug known to adsorb to it or after unknown ingestion by patients with protected airways.

Multiple-Dose Activated Charcoal

One dose of activated charcoal is usually sufficient to achieve a therapeutic effect. Multiple-dose activated charcoal, however, should be administered in specific instances, such as after ingestion of very large doses, substances that form bezoars in the GI tract, potentially injurious toxins that slow gut function, or toxins that are released slowly into the gut lumen. Multiple-dose activated charcoal is usually given as follows: the first dose is up to 1 g/kg body weight, which is then followed by subsequent doses of 0.25 to 0.50 g/kg. Repeated doses of activated charcoal should be given in an interval ranging from 1 to 4 h. To prevent excessive fluid loss and electrolyte imbalance, only the first dose of activated charcoal should be given with a cathartic.

Multiple-dose activated charcoal is contraindicated in patients who have decreased gut motility, because the risks of the procedure include aspiration from gastric distention, and impaction of charcoal within the gut. The benefits of multiple-dose activated charcoal include achievement of a 10:1 activated charcoal to drug ratio in patients with very large ingestions and the binding of drugs within the gut lumen after ingestion of substances that have a large enterohepatic or enteroenteric circulation. Patients having ingested life-threatening toxins who have decreased gut motility can receive multiple doses, but the stomach must be suctioned just prior to the administration of the next dose of activated charcoal to minimize distention.

Cathartics

Typically, activated charcoal is administered with an osmotic cathartic, such as a 70% sorbitol solution (1 g/kg), or a 10% solution of magnesium citrate (in a dose of 250 mL for adults and 4 mL/kg for children). Cathartics have been repeatedly shown to decrease the transit time for the passage of the activated charcoal (and presumably the adsorbed toxin) through the GI tract.[9,10] Although most studies fail to show a benefit of administering a cathartic alone,[11,12] several studies suggest that there is a decrease in peak serum plasma concentrations, and area under the curve when the cathartic is administered with activated charcoal.[13,14] No definitive clinical human data, however, suggest that the addition of a cathartic to a dose of activated charcoal either limits the toxin's bioavailability or changes the patient's clinical outcome.

Indications for use of cathartics generally mirror those for the administration of activated charcoal. When multiple-dose activated charcoal is used, only the first dose is accompanied by a cathartic, to limit complications. Complications of cathartic administration include nausea and abdominal pain, severe volume depletion, electrolyte imbalances and fluid shifts, and hypermagnesemia in patients with renal compromise.

Contraindications for cathartic use are, after an ingestion of a substance that will result in diarrhea, children younger than age 5, patients with renal failure (only magnesium-containing cathartics are contraindicated), intestinal obstruction, or an ingestion of any caustic material.

IRRIGATION OF THE BOWEL LUMEN

Whole Bowel Irrigation

Another technique for clearing the gut is whole bowel irrigation, which involves the installation of large volumes of polyethylene glycol in an electrolyte and osmotically balanced solution that neither causes fluid nor electrolyte shifts. This technique is accomplished in adults by the installation of 2 L/h polyethylene glycol solution either by mouth or through an nasogastric tube or, in children, by the installation of 50 to 250 mL/kg/h or as much of polyethylene glycol solution as tolerated. The end point is clear rectal effluent. When done properly, this technique produces a rapid catharsis by mechanically forcing ingested substances through the bowel at a rapid rate.

Contraindications include patients with preceding diarrhea, ingestions that are expected to result in significant diarrhea (except for heavy metals, as these substances do not adsorb well to activated charcoal) and patients with absent bowel sounds or with obstruction. The complications included bloating, cramping, and rectal irritation from frequent bowel movements. Close nursing care is needed to maintain patient cleanliness.

Controlled studies clearly demonstrating improvement in clinical outcome after this procedure are lacking, but many authors describe limited symptomatology following potentially toxic doses of substances known not to adsorb to activated charcoal.[15] Common indications for whole bowel irrigation include ingestion of sustained-release preparations, and ingestions that are known not to adsorb to activated charcoal; substances that form bezoars; in clinical situations where nonobstructive, nonsharp foreign bodies are present in the bowel (such as drug vials); and, in cases of illicit drug body packing.

ENHANCED ELIMINATION

Alkalinization

Urinary alkalinization is beneficial in the treatment of certain ingestions. The urinary pH is manipulated to exploit physiologic properties of specific toxins. Only nonionized substances are free to move passively across membranes. Ionized particles must remain in the fluid-filled compartments in which they were formed. Weak acids are mostly uncharged at physiologic pH, but become charged in alkaline environments. By significantly raising the urinary pH with intravenous sodium bicarbonate, toxins that are weak acids are converted from their nonionized form to their ionized form and are therefore held within the urinary collection system. This "ion trapping" keeps the toxin within the renal tubules, thereby enhancing its excretion. This creates an imbalance in the concentration gradient of the toxin between the blood and the urinary collection system, drawing more toxin into the renal lumen. The ideal toxin that can be eliminated by this technique is one with substantial urinary excretion and with a pK_a less than the serum pH (Table 151-4).

Administer an intravenous bolus of 1 to 2 meq/kg sodium bicarbonate, followed by either intermittent boluses of sodium bicarbonate or a continuous intravenous infusion to achieve a urinary pH of 7.5 to 8.0. Serum pH should not be allowed to rise above 7.5 to 7.55. Pronounced hypokalemia may result from this technique and must be corrected aggressively. Hypokalemia induces the kidneys to reabsorb potassium preferentially. To remain electronegatively neutral, hydrogen ions are excreted, inhibiting the production of an alkaline urine. This may result in a paradoxically acidic urine.

The benefit of urinary alkalinization is a decrease in toxin serum half-life from increased urinary excretion. The risks include congestive heart failure, pulmonary edema, pH shifts, and profound hypokalemia. Therefore, contraindications to this procedure include patients who cannot tolerate the volume or sodium load, hypokalemia, renal insufficiency, and ingestion of a toxin that does not respond to alkalinization.

Hemodialysis

Hemodialysis is generally reserved for specific toxins that must be both potentially life threatening and amenable to removal by this

TABLE 151-4 Agents That Other Modalities May Increase Their Excretion

Drugs	Agents Where Urinary Alkalization Is Commonly Considered	Agents Where Hemodialysis Is Commonly Considered
2-4-D (herbicide)	✓	
Phenobarbital	✓	
Chlorpropamide	✓	
Salicylates	✓	✓
Methanol	✓	✓
Ethylene glycol		✓
Lithium		✓
Theophylline*		✓

*Indicates also removed by hemoperfusion.

method (see Table 151-4). A semipermiable membrane is used to create a concentration gradient to filter out toxins. The benefits include the ability to remove toxins that are already absorbed from the gut lumen, removal of substances that do not adhere to activated charcoal, and the ability to remove both the parent compound and the active toxic metabolites. Hemodialysis is much less effective where the toxin ingested has a large volume of distribution (>1 L/kg), has a large molecular weight (more than 500 Da), or is highly protein bound.

Hemodialysis is rarely absolutely contraindicated, but relative contraindications include hemodynamic instability, very small children, patients with poor vascular access or profound bleeding diatheses. Risks of hemodialysis are typically minimal in experienced centers, but they include large fluid shifts, electrolyte imbalances, infection and bleeding at the catheter site, and intracranial hemorrhage.

Hemoperfusion, which is also used for decontamination of a patient's systemic circulation, involves placing a filter filled with activated charcoal into the circuit of the hemodialysis machine. This filtration alleviates the constraints of protein binding and molecular size, both of which limit the utility of hemodialysis. Toxins that can be removed by this method must adsorb well to activated charcoal and have a small volume of distribution. In practice, it is only commonly recommended for theophylline overdoses.

INITIAL INTERVENTIONS

Patients may be unresponsive or have an altered mental status for many reasons. Four possible diagnoses (hypoxia, opioid intoxication, hypoglycemia, and Wernicke encephalopathy) may be easily overlooked, but are readily treated by the administration of specific antidotes. Within the first few minutes after the patient's arrival, the administration of empiric antidotes [supplemental oxygen, 1.0 to 2.0 mg intravenous naloxone in adults and 0.01 mg/kg in children, 50 mL 50% dextrose in water (50% D/W) for adults and 1 gm/kg glucose as 10% or 25% D/W for children, and 100 mg thiamine in adults] should be considered after taking into account the medical history, vital signs, and laboratory data immediately available. These treatments are simple, inexpensive, and generally without undue risk of an adverse reaction when used appropriately. Thamine is generally not administered for unexplained unresponsiveness in children. However, 1 g/kg of glucose is often administered when serum glucose cannot be rapidly ascertained or hypoglycemia excluded. Naloxone (0.01 mg/kg titrated to effect), may be given, particularly in older children where accidental or intentional opioid exposure cannot be excluded. Intentional poisoning of children as a form of child abuse does occur.

The suggestion that the administration of thiamine should precede the administration of 50% D/W to prevent the precipitation of acute Wernicke encephalopathy is unfounded.[16] The most important management issue with both 50% D/W and thiamine is that both should be given in a timely manner in the emergency department so that these often occult diagnoses are added to the differential diagnosis and are treated promptly.

Although opioid intoxication often presents with the classic triad of central nervous system (CNS) depression, miosis, and respiratory depression, only respiratory status is useful as an indicator of a patient response to naloxone.[17] Many toxins, though, produce miosis or CNS depression, and some opioids classically leave pupil size unaltered, making these findings less useful in isolation.

Naloxone, which is a competitive opioid antagonist that can be administered intravenously or intramuscularly, is appropriate to use for a hypoventilating but nonintubated, opioid intoxicated patient. Extremity restraints for the patient should be considered before administering the drug. Naloxone may completely reverse the symptoms observed, restoring effective ventilations and mental status for 20 to 60 min, so patients should be observed for 2 to 3 h afterward. The risks include the precipitation of an acute withdrawal syndrome. Although acute withdrawal is never life threatening, vomiting from withdrawal can result in aspiration. Thus, the reflexive administration of large doses of naloxone should be discouraged. Patients who become resedated may require additional naloxone doses administered either in intermittent boluses or via a continuous infusion. The latter is achieved by the administration of two-thirds the dose of the naloxone that fully aroused the patient in the initial bolus, but infused over an hour with the dose adjusted to the patient's ventilatory status.

REFERENCES

1. Mofenson HC, Grensher J, Caraccio TR: Ingestions considered nontoxic. *Emerg Med Clin North Am* 2:159, 1984.
2. Mofenson HC, Grensher J: The nontoxic ingestion. *Pediatr Clin North Am* 17:583, 1970.
3. Kulig KW, Bar-Or D, Cantrill SV, et al: Management of acutely poisoned patients without gastric emptying. *Ann Emerg Med* 14:562, 1985.
4. Thompson AM, Robins JB, Prescott LF: Changes in cardiorespiratory function during gastric lavage for drug overdose. *Hum Toxicol* 6:215, 1987.
5. Merigian KS, Woodward M, Hedges JR, et al: Prospective evaluation of gastric emptying in the self-poisoned patient. *Am J Emerg Med* 8:479, 1990.
6. Pond SM, Lewis-Driver DJ, Williams GM, et al: Gastric emptying in acute overdose: A prospective randomized controlled trial. *Med J Aust* 163:345, 1995.
7. Levy G: Gastrointestinal clearance of drugs with activated charcoal. *N Engl J Med* 307:676, 1982.
8. Olkkola K: Effect of charcoal-drug ratio on antidotal efficacy of oral activated charcoal in man. *Br J Clin Pharmacol* 19:767, 1985.
9. Krenzelok EP, Keller R, Stewart RD: Gastrointestinal transit times of cathartics combined with charcoal. *Ann Emerg Med* 14:1152, 1985.
10. Harchelroad F, Cottington E, Krenzelok EP: Gastrointestinal transit times of a charcoal/sorbitol slurry in overdose patients. *J Toxicol Clin Toxicol* 27:91, 1989.
11. Minton NA, Henry JA: Prevention of drug absorption in simulated theophylline overdose. *J Toxicol Clin Toxicol* 33:43, 1995.
12. Al-Shareef AH, Buss DC, Allen EM, Routledge PA: The effects of charcoal and sorbitol (alone and in combination) on plasma theophylline concentrations after a sustained-release formulation. *Hum Exp Toxicol* 9:179, 1990.
13. Picchioni AL, Chin L, Gillespie T: Evaluation of activated charcoal-sorbitol suspension as an antidote. *J Toxicol Clin Toxicol* 19:433, 1982.
14. Goldberg MJ, Spector R, Park GD, et al: The effect of sorbitol and activated charcoal on serum theophylline concentrations after slow-release theophylline. *Clin Pharmacol Ther* 41:108, 1987.
15. Roberge RJ, Martin TG: Whole bowel irrigation in an acute oral lead intoxication. *Am J Emerg Med* 10:577, 1992.

16. Hack JB, Hoffman RS: Thiamine before glucose to prevent Wernicke encephalopathy: Examining the conventional wisdom. *JAMA* 279:583, 1998.

17. Hoffman JR, Schringer DL Votey SR, Luo JS: The empiric use of naloxone in patients with altered mental status: A reappraisal. *Ann Emerg Med* 20:246, 1991.

TRICYCLIC ANTIDEPRESSANTS

Kirk C. Mills

EPIDEMIOLOGY

Tricyclic antidepressants (TCAs) are associated with more drug-related deaths than any other class of prescription medication. Their complex pharmacologic activity, low therapeutic index, and general availability predispose to the development of clinical toxicity. The 1997 Annual Report of the American Association of Poison Control Centers Toxic Exposure Surveillance System indicated that 1 of every 27 adult exposures to a pharmaceutical medication involved a TCA.[1] Over the past 5 years, there have been an average of 19,000 exposures and 120 associated deaths related to TCAs. However, these numbers undoubtedly underestimate the true magnitude of TCA-related drug toxicity. Most reported TCA exposures occur in young adults, with approximately 60 percent of all exposures believed to be intentional.

TCAs are used primarily for the treatment of major depression. In addition, they are prescribed frequently for other psychiatric and medical conditions such as obsessive-compulsive disorder, attention-deficit disorder, panic and phobia disorders, anxiety disorders, eating disorders, chronic pain syndromes, peripheral neuropathies, nocturnal enuresis, migraine headache prophylaxis, and selected drug withdrawal therapy. There are currently eight different TCAs available in the United States (Table 152-1), but many more varieties are available in other countries. The five most commonly reported TCAs involved in drug exposures include amitriptyline (40 percent), imipramine (17 percent), doxepin (14 percent), nortriptyline (12 percent), and desipramine (6 percent). Two related antidepressants, maprotiline and amoxapine, have minor structural differences when compared with traditional TCAs but have similar toxicity in overdose and thus will be included in this chapter. Cyclobenzaprine (Flexeril) is a muscle relaxant that is almost structurally identical to amitriptyline but lacks antidepressant activity. It tends to have less cardiotoxicity than amitriptyline but can still produce significant central nervous system (CNS) sedation and antimuscarinic toxicity in overdose.[2] The average therapeutic dose for TCAs is highly variable. Initially, lower doses are used, followed by gradual increases until the desired therapeutic response is achieved. In addition, this process allows most patients to become acclimated to the typical TCA-induced adverse effects such as CNS sedation and dry mucous membranes.

TCA-related drug toxicity is not just limited to cases of drug overdose. There are at least eight different possible mechanisms for developing TCA-related drug toxicity while taking therapeutic doses. First, mild to moderate toxicity commonly will develop if unacclimated individuals are started on higher therapeutic doses. Second, toxicity can result when TCAs are combined with other medications having similar pharmacologic actions (e.g., antihistamines, antipsychotics). Third, a subset of the population consists of slow metabolizers of TCAs, and as such, these people will develop higher plasma TCA levels for any given dose. Fourth, many drugs have the potential to inhibit the metabolism of TCAs, resulting in elevated TCA plasma levels. Fifth, some TCAs are available as mixed-drug formulations combined with either benzodiazepines or antipsychotic agents, having the potential for additional drug toxicity. Sixth, patients with certain medical conditions such as underlying heart problems or seizure disorders are more susceptible to TCA toxicity at therapeutic doses. Seventh, TCAs have the potential to produce serotonin syndrome, especially in combination with other serotonergic medications (see Chap. 153, ''Newer Antidepressants and Serotonin Syndrome''). Finally, rare cases of neuroleptic malignant syndrome have been reported in association with therapeutic use of TCAs.

TABLE 152-1 Tricyclic Antidepressants

Generic Name	Trade Name(s)	Formulations (mg)	Adult Daily Dose (mg)	Active Metabolites
Amitriptyline	Elavil	10, 25, 50, 75, 100, 150	75–300	Nortriptyline
Amoxapine*	Asendin	25, 50, 100, 150	50–300	7-Hydroxyamoxapine 8-Hydroxyamoxapine
Clomipramine	Anafranil	25, 50, 75	50–200	Desmethylclomipramine
Cyclobenzaprine*	Flexeril	10-mg tablet	20–40	None
Desipramine	Norpramin Pertofrane	10, 25, 50, 75, 100, 150	75–200	None
Doxepin	Adapin, Sinequan	10, 25, 50, 75, 100, 150 Oral solution 10 mg/mL	75–300	Desmethyldoxepin
Imipramine	Tofranil	10, 25, 50	75–200	Desipramine
Maprotiline*	Ludiomil	25, 50, 75	75–150	Desmethylmaprotiline
Nortriptyline	Pamelor, Aventyl	10, 25, 50, 75 Oral solution 2 mg/mL	75–150	None
Protriptyline	Vivactil	5, 10	15–40	None
Trimipramine	Surmontil	25, 50, 100	75–200	Desmethyltrimipramine

*See text for clarification.

TABLE 152-2 Pharmacologic Profile of Tricyclic Antidepressants

Pharmacologic Activity	Potency	Clinical Presentation	Treatment
Antagonism of postsynaptic histamine receptors	++++ to ++	Sedation	Supportive care alone
Antagonism of postsynaptic muscarinic receptors	++++ to ++	Sedation, coma, agitation, confusion hallucinations, seizures, mydriasis, dry mucous membranes, dry skin, tachycardia, mild hypertension, hyperthermia, ileus, urinary retention, tremor	Supportive care alone (physostigmine contraindicated)
Antagonism of postsynaptic α-adrenergic receptors	++++ to ++	Sedation, miosis, orthostatic hypotension, reflex tachycardia	Intravenous fluids Norepinephrine
Inhibition of norepinephrine reuptake	++++ to +	Agitation, mydriasis, diaphoresis, tachycardia, early hypertension	Supportive care alone
Inhibition of serotonin reuptake	++++ to +	Sedation, mydriasis, myoclonus, hyperreflexia (see serotonin syndrome)	Supportive care alone Consider cyproheptadine for treatment of serotonin syndrome
Inhibition of voltage-gated sodium channels	++++ to +	Impaired conduction, wide QRS, other conduction abnormalities; impaired cardiac contractility; wide complex sinus tachycardia, ventricular ectopy	Sodium bicarbonate Hyperventilation Hypertonic saline
		Hypotension	Intravenous fluids Sodium bicarbonate Hypertonic saline
Inhibition of voltage-gated potassium channels	+++ to +	Prolongation of QT interval, ventricular ectopy, torsades de pointes	Magnesium sulfate Cardiac overdrive pacing
Antagonism of postsynaptic serotonin (5-HT) receptors	++ to +	None, possible therapeutic benefit	None
Antagonism of postsynaptic GABA-A receptors	++ to +	Seizures	Benzodiazepines Phenobarbital or Propofol
Antagonism of postsynaptic dopamine receptors	++ to +	Extrapyramidal symptoms ranging from dystonic reactions to neuroleptic malignant syndrome	Supportive care

PATHOPHYSIOLOGY

TCAs have a distinct chemical structure comprised of three aromatic rings: a central seven-member ring, two outer benzene rings, and an aminopropyl side chain connected to the central ring. There are only minor structural differences among the TCAs, usually on the central aromatic ring or aminopropyl side chain. Amoxapine is unique in that it has an aromatic side chain. Maprotiline has an ethylene bridge across a six-member center ring, giving it a tetracyclic chemical structure. It is not surprising that other chemicals that share the same basic tricyclic chemical structure as the TCAs, such as carbamazepine and phenothizaines, would manifest similar toxicity in overdose.

TCAs are nonselective agents that exhibit a multitude of pharmacologic effects (Table 152-2) and have considerable variation in potency. There are subtle and potentially clinically significant pharmacologic differences among the TCAs at therapeutic plasma levels. However, these differences become less important at the higher plasma levels typically seen in overdose. Only a few of their pharmacologic actions are believed to have a direct therapeutic effect, such as inhibition of amine reuptake (norepinephrine, serotonin) and antagonism of postsynaptic serotonin receptors (5-HT2). Thus, the remaining pharmacologic actions are essentially without therapeutic benefit but significantly contribute to TCA-related adverse effects and overdose toxicity. Most clinical findings seen in TCA overdose can be explained by the following seven pharmacologic actions, listed in descending order of general potency.

Antihistaminic Effects

TCAs are potent inhibitors of peripheral and central postsynaptic histamine receptors. Doxepin is a particularly potent antihistamine, but its nonspecific pharmacologic activity makes it impractical as a therapy for seasonal allergies or other allergic conditions. Antagonism of central histamine receptors primarily leads to CNS sedation and may contribute significantly to the development of coma frequently seen in TCA overdose.

Antimuscarinic Effects

TCAs frequently produce antimuscarinic symptoms. They are competitive inhibitors of acetylcholine at central and peripheral muscarinic receptors. This action is commonly referred to as being *anticholinergic,* but the term *antimuscarinic* is more precise because TCAs do not antagonize acetylcholine at nicotinic receptors. Central antimuscarinic symptoms vary from agitation to delirium, confusion, amnesia, hallucinations, slurred speech, ataxia, sedation, and coma. Peripheral antimuscarinic symptoms include dilated pupils, blurred vision, tachycardia, hyperthermia, hypertension, decreased oral and bronchial secretions, dry skin, ileus, urinary retention, increased muscle tone, and tremor. Antimuscarinic symptoms are especially common when TCAs are combined with other medications that also have antimuscarinic activity. Examples include antihistamines, antipsychotics, antiparkinsonian drugs, antispasmodics, and some muscle relaxants.

Physostigmine is an inhibitor of acetylcholinesterase activity and potentially can reverse antimuscarinic symptoms. Historically, it was used to reverse TCA-induced antimuscarinic symptoms, but its use is often associated with life-threatening complications. Although antimuscarinic symptoms are a common finding in TCA overdose, they are not directly responsible for TCA-related deaths. Therefore, antimuscarinic symptoms are an important clinical marker of TCA toxicity, but they do not require specific therapy other than supportive care alone. Physostigmine has no role in the current management of TCA overdose emergency department (ED) patients.

Inhibition of α-Adrenergic Receptors

Inhibition of postsynaptic central and peripheral α-adrenergic receptors is a characteristic action of most TCAs. They do not inhibit β-adrenergic receptors. TCAs have a much greater affinity for α_1- than α_2-adrenergic receptors. Inhibition of α_1 receptors produces CNS sedation, orthostatic hypotension, and pupillary constriction. This action frequently offsets antimuscarinic-induced pupillary dilation. Thus, patients with TCA toxicity can present with constricted, dilated, or midpoint-sized pupils. Orthostatic hypotension is often associated with reflex tachycardia. The antihypertensive effect of clonidine can be negated by TCAs because of their ability to block the binding of clonidine to α_2 receptors.

Inhibition of Amine Uptake

Inhibition of amine reuptake is believed to be the most important mechanism by which TCAs are efficacious in treating depression. TCAs are potent inhibitors of norepinephrine (NE) and serotonin (5-HT) reuptake but have little affinity for inhibition of dopamine (DA) reuptake.[3] Inhibition of neurotransmitter reuptake leads to increased synaptic levels and subsequent augmentation of the neurotransmitter response. Inhibition of NE reuptake is thought to produce the early sympathomimetic effects occasionally seen in some TCA overdoses and may contribute to the development of cardiac dysrhythmias. Serotonin syndrome results from increased 5-HT brainstem activity and has been produced by TCAs that are particularly potent 5-HT uptake inhibitors such as clomipramine and amitriptyline. In general, TCAs must be used in combination with other serotonergic agents to produce serotonin syndrome. Myoclonus and hyperreflexia often are attributed to increased serotonin activity.

Sodium Channel Blockade

TCA-induced cardiotoxicity is the single most important factor contributing to patient mortality. Life-threatening cardiotoxicity results from TCA-induced inhibition of sodium influx through voltage-dependent sodium channels. Inhibition of fast sodium channels in His-Purkinje cells leads to delayed depolarization and conduction abnormalities.[4] Impaired sodium entry into myocardial tissue leads to decreased contractility. Sodium channel blockade is often referred to synonymously as *membrane stabilizing, quinidine-like,* or *local anesthetic effect.* Sodium channel blockade results in a prolongation of phase 0 of the action potential, which becomes more pronounced with rapid heart rates, hyponatremia, and acidosis. This effect expresses itself on the electrocardiograph (ECG) as prolongation of PR and QRS intervals and right-axis deviation (RAD) of the terminal 40 ms. The RAD is most pronounced in the terminal 40 ms of limb leads, as demonstrated on ECG by a terminal R wave in lead aVR and an S wave in lead I. Rapid influx of sodium is necessary for the release of intracellular calcium stores and subsequent myocardial contractility. Some of the negative chronotropic effect of sodium channel blockade can be attenuated by the sinus tachycardia secondary to antimuscarinic activity. Bradycardia is particularly worrisome when accompanied by QRS complex widening because it indicates profound sodium channel blockade. Local changes in electrical conduction can predispose to ventricular dysrhythmias by establishing reentry loops. In summary, severe sodium channel blockade culminates in depressed myocardial contractility, various types of heart blocks, RAD, hypotension, wide QRS, and cardiac ectopy.

Sodium channel blockade can be overcome in part by serum alkalinization (pH 7.50–7.55) and increasing the serum sodium concentration. In humans, intravenous sodium bicarbonate (NaHCO3) is thought to be more effective than either hyperventilation (alkalinizes blood) or sodium chloride (increases Na^+) in treating TCA cardiotoxicity. One explanation for the greater effectiveness of $NaHCO_3$ is that it produces both blood alkalinization and increased serum sodium concentration. The mechanism by which blood alkalinization partially reverses sodium channel blockade remains unknown, but it does not appear to be related to enhancement of plasma TCA serum protein binding. It may decrease the overall inhibition to sodium ion influx. Recent animal data suggest that hypertonic saline (7.5% NaCl) may be more efficacious than sodium bicarbonate or hyperventilation in reversing TCA cardiotoxicity.[5] Whether this finding also will be applicable to humans is currently unknown. Hypertonic saline is believed to act primarily by increasing the extracellular sodium concentration gradient, thus favoring the inward movement of sodium ions.

Potassium Channel Antagonist

TCAs block myocardial potassium channels and inhibit the efflux of potassium ions during repolarization. This effect is seen on ECG as QT interval prolongation, which is more pronounced at slower heart rates. Many TCA overdose patients develop sinus tachycardia, which is partially protective against severe QTc interval prolongation. Torsades de pointes is a life-threatening complication of severe QT interval prolongation, but it is rarely seen in TCA overdoses.[6]

GABA-A Receptor Antagonist

Generalized seizures commonly occur in the setting of TCA overdoses. Possible mechanisms for these seizures include TCA-induced γ-aminobutyric acid receptor A (GABA-A) antagonism, neuronal sodium channel blockade, central anticholinergic activity, and effects on biogenic amines. The exact etiology of these seizures remains speculative, but TCA-induced antagonism of the GABA-A may represent the most important mechanism. All drugs that inhibit GABA-A neurotransmission are associated with seizures. Benzodiazepines and barbiturates are potent GABA-A agonists and are considered the anticonvulsants of choice in treating TCA-induced seizures. Propofol (Diprivan) is a short-acting intravenous anesthetic with anticonvulsant activity. It should be considered for patients with resistive seizures, especially in the setting of hypotension.

PHARMACOKINETICS

All TCAs share similar pharmacokinetic properties. They are highly lipophilic and readily cross the blood-brain barrier, and peak plasma levels occur between 2 and 6 h after ingestion at therapeutic doses. Gastrointestinal absorption can be prolonged because of their antimuscarinic effect on gut motility. Bioavailability is only 30 to 70 percent because of extensive "first pass" hepatic metabolism. They are highly protein bound to α_1 acid glycoproteins. Their apparent volume of distribution is extremely large and ranges from 10 to 50 L/kg. Tissue TCA levels are commonly 10 to 100 times greater than plasma levels. Only 1 to 2 percent of the total body burden of TCAs is found in the blood. These pharmacokinetic properties explain why attempts at removing TCAs by hemodialysis, hemoperfusion, peritoneal dialysis, or forced diuresis are generally unproductive.

TCAs are eliminated almost entirely by hepatic oxidation, which consists of *N*-demethylation of the amine side-chain groups and hydroxylation of ring structures. The removal of a methyl group from the tertiary amine side chain usually produces an active metabolite designated by the desmethyl prefix (see Table 152-1). These active metabolites often will have different pharmacologic activities when compared with the parent compounds. Amoxapine and maprotiline both have active metabolites. Although secondary amines such as desipramine, nortriptyline, and protriptyline are effective antidepressants, their metabolites are generally considered inactive. Clinical toxicity from tertiary TCAs usually lasts longer than that from secondary TCAs alone because of the production of active metabolites. Some TCAs undergo enterohepatic circulation prior to their eventual oxidation, conjugation, and renal elimination, but this does not significantly contribute to their toxicity.

The average elimination half-life of TCAs is approximately 24 h (range 6-36 h) at therapeutic doses, but this can increase to 72 h after overdose. Inhibition of TCA metabolism by other drugs that use the same hepatic enzymes can prolong the half-life of TCAs. This carries the risk of elevating TCA plasma levels and producing clinical TCA toxicity at therapeutic doses. Approximately 7 percent of the U.S. population are genetically slow metabolizers of TCAs. This predisposes them to develop higher plasma levels at any given daily TCA dose.

TOXICITY

Therapeutic doses for TCAs are highly variable and are determined by many factors but range from 1 to 5 mg/kg per day (see Table 152-1). Any dose greater than this has the potential to produce TCA toxicity. Life-threatening symptoms usually occur with ingestions of greater than 10 mg/kg in adults. Pediatric patients are particularly susceptible to the antimuscarinic activity of TCAs. Other patients at higher risk for TCA toxicity include patients who have coingested cardiotoxic or CNS-depressive medications, geriatric patients, and patients with heart disease. Desipramine is the most potent sodium channel blocker among the TCAs.[3] It has twice the fatality rate of other TCAs. Some TCAs, especially desipramine, are able to precipitate severe cardiotoxicity (e.g., wide QRS complex, hypotension) without producing significant antimuscarinic symptoms. TCA-related fatalities are commonly associated with ingestions of greater than 1 g. Most TCA overdose fatalities occur within the initial hours after ingestion, often before the patient reaches the hospital. Fatalities more than 24 h after ingestion are unusual with appropriate medical therapy.

Quantitative plasma TCA levels are very helpful in monitoring chronic drug therapy (e.g., compliance, metabolism) and are frequently used by psychiatrists for this purpose. However, quantitative plasma TCA levels have limited application to ED patients. The results of quantitative levels are rarely available to emergency physicians during the time of patient evaluation and therefore have negligible impact on patient care. Some studies have shown that patients with a combined plasma level of parent TCA and metabolite of greater than 1000 ng/mL are at greater risk for developing seizures and cardiotoxicity. However, the severity of clinical toxicity does not always correlate with the extent of plasma TCA elevation. Patients can develop severe toxicity at plasma levels less than 1000 ng/mL.[8,9] Conversely, patients with plasma TCA levels much greater than 1000 ng/mL may not develop seizures or ventricular dysrhythmias. Serious toxicity rarely develops at therapeutic levels alone (<300 ng/mL). When this occurs, other causes should be entertained to explain the patient's condition. As always, the most important thing is to treat the patient and not the drug level.

An interesting but confounding characteristic of TCAs is their ability to undergo significant postmortem drug redistribution.[10] Plasma levels can increase by as much as 10- to 50-fold after death as tissue binding sites release TCAs back to the blood. This is a time-dependent process. The diagnostic accuracy of postmortem TCA levels is inversely proportional to the time they were obtained after death. The relevance of TCA postmortem drug redistribution to emergency physicians relates to ED deaths of patients taking TCAs therapeutically. The medical examiner may inappropriately assign the cause of death to unrecognized TCA overdose if elevated levels are detected and no other cause of death is uncovered. This, in turn, may raise false concerns about the care provided to the patient during his or her ED resuscitation.

CLINICAL FEATURES

The clinical presentation of TCA toxicity varies tremendously from mild antimuscarinic symptoms to severe cardiotoxicity secondary to sodium channel blockade. In up to 70 percent of TCA poisonings, coingested drugs also are involved, and the additional toxicity from these coingestants should be considered when evaluating these patients. Antimuscarinic symptoms commonly serve as markers for TCA toxicity (e.g., dry mouth and axillae, sinus tachycardia), but they alone are rarely responsible for patient fatalities. Moreover, antimuscarinic symptoms are not uniformly present in TCA toxicity. As an example, sinus tachycardia is the most frequent dysrhythmia noted in TCA toxicity, but it is only present in approximately 70 percent of symptomatic patients. Altered mental status is the most common symptom reported following TCA exposure.

Mild to moderate TCA toxicity may present as drowsiness, confusion, slurred speech, ataxia, dry mucous membranes and axilla, sinus tachycardia, urinary retention, myoclonus, and hyperreflexia. Antimuscarinic syndrome is classically associated with decreased bowel tones and ileus. However, bowel function is fairly resistant to inhibition and active bowel sounds can be present even in seriously ill patients. Therefore, the presence of active bowel tones does not rule out the possibility of antimuscarinic syndrome. Mild hypertension is observed occasionally and rarely requires treatment. Nontolerant individuals occasionally develop coma and respiratory depression after relatively small overdoses without obvious peripheral antimuscarinic effects and without QRS widening. Overflow urinary incontinence may be mistaken for normal micturition in pediatric (diaper-dependent) patients.

Serious toxicity is almost always seen within 6 h of major TCA ingestion and consists of the following symptoms: coma, cardiac conduction delays, supraventricular tachycardia, hypotension, respiratory depression, premature ventricular beats, ventricular tachycardia, and seizures.[8] Secondary complications from serious toxicity include aspiration pneumonia, anoxic encephalopathy, hyperthermia, and rhabdomyolysis. Pulmonary edema is a well-recognized complication of TCA overdose. Seizures are usually generalized and brief in duration. The exception to this rule is seen in amoxapine and maprotiline overdoses. These agents can cause status epilepticus. Amoxapine seizures commonly occur without corresponding QRS widening.

DIAGNOSIS

TCA toxicity should be suspected in all patients with a positive serum TCA drug screen in conjunction with corresponding clinical toxicity and/or characteristic ECG abnormalities. Most cases of TCA toxicity will be associated with elevated quantitative TCA plasma levels. However, these are routinely not available to the emergency physicians, nor do they have an impact on ED care. Conversely, qualitative TCA drug tests are available in most hospitals and have a rapid turnaround time. They can be used to confirm the presence of TCAs but cannot differentiate between therapeutic and toxic levels. False-positive qualitative serum TCA drug screen results can occur with diphenhydramine, carbamazepine, cyclobenzaprine, cyproheptadine, and phenothiazines. Some of these medications also can produce typical TCA electrocardiographic abnormalities and similar clinical toxicity. False-negative serum TCA drug tests are extremely unusual. They should be repeated with a new specimen if there is a high clinical suspicion for TCA exposure. Urine drug testing may be helpful in identifying other toxico-

TABLE 152-3 Differential Diagnosis of Tricyclic Antidepressant Toxicity

Drug	False-Positive Serum Drug Screen	Wide QRS/Right Axis Deviation	Antimuscarinic Activity	Point of Differentiation
Carbamazepine	Possible	At levels greater than 20 μg/mL	Yes	History of seizure disorder Elevated serum carbamazepine level
Cyclobenzaprine	Possible	Very unlikely but theoretically possible	Yes	History of Flexeril use for muscle pain or back problems
Diphenhydramine	Possible	At moderate to high doses	Yes	History of over-the-counter-drug use, allergies, or insomnia
Phenothiazines	Possible	Mesoridazine Thioridazine	Yes	History of psychotic disorder with antipsychotic use
Class IA antiarrhythmics	No	Yes	Yes	History of heart problems History of leg cramps (quinine)
Class IC antiarrhythmics	No	Yes	No	History of heart problems
Propranolol	No	Seen at moderate to high doses	No	Bradycardia almost always seen Positive response to glucagon
Propoxyphene	No	Often seen in overdose	No	Opiate toxidrome Reversal with naloxone
Cocaine	No	At high doses	No	Sympathomimetic presentation Positive urine cocaine drug screen
Lithium	No	At elevated serum levels	No	History of bipolar disorder Elevated serum lithium level
Hyperkalemia	No	At increased serum levels	No	Elevated serum potassium level

logic causes for the patient's condition. The differential diagnosis of TCA toxicity encompasses those drugs which can mimic any one of the three criteria used in making the diagnosis (Table 152-3). However, the quintessential point for emergency physicians is that the initial treatment for all these medications is identical and should not be delayed until definitive drug test results become available.

ECG abnormalities are seen commonly with TCA toxicity and generally are useful in identifying patients at increased risk for seizures and ventricular dysrhythmias. The "classic" TCA electrocardiogram is shown in Fig. 152-1, consisting of sinus tachycardia, right-axis deviation (RAD), and prolongation of the PR, QRS, and QT intervals. This "classic" ECG pattern is seen frequently in moderate to severe TCA toxicity, but its absence does not eliminate the possibility of TCA toxicity during the first 6 h after ingestion. Figure 152-2 is an ECG 4 days later with near-complete resolution of all abnormalities. Moderate prolongation of the QT interval is noted frequently, even at therapeutic TCA doses. Nonspecific ST-segment and T-wave abnormalities are commonly observed in TCA overdose. Less common ECG abnormalities include right bundle branch block and high-degree atrioventricular blocks.

Life-threatening complications can occur in the absence of significant ECG abnormalities.[9] However, these complications are more likely in the presence of a widened QRS greater than 100 ms and/or RAD of the terminal 40 ms of greater than 120°. The risk of seizures increases as the QRS complex exceeds 100 ms, and ventricular dysrhythmias are more likely if QRS prolongation exceeds 160 ms. RAD is commonly demonstrated as a positive terminal R wave in lead aVR and a negative S wave in lead I (Fig. 152-3). Both abnormalities are equally helpful in identifying patients at risk for serious toxicity.[11] They usually occur together but can occur in exclusion of each other. The development of RAD of the terminal 40 ms and/or QRS widening appears to be less predictable of TCA-induced cardiotoxicity in young children.[12] Pediatric ECGs tend to have a wider range of acceptable variant features, and this complicates the ECG identification of TCA toxicity.

ECG abnormalities universally develop within 6 h of ingestion and usually resolve over 36 to 48 h.[13] The identification of either QRS widening greater than 100 ms or terminal RAD greater than 120° warrants sodium bicarbonate therapy and admission to a monitored hospital bed. Unfortunately, up to 10 percent of the population will have a prolonged QRS of more than 100 ms or terminal RAD without exposure to sodium channel blocking drugs. Therefore, these ECG abnormalities in isolation are not 100 percent specific for TCA toxicity. Most patients on TCA therapy do not have prior ECGs available for comparison. Thus, any observed ECG abnormalities must be assumed attributable to TCA exposure until proven otherwise.

TREATMENT

All patients should be evaluated immediately for alterations of consciousness, hemodynamic instability, and respiratory impairment. Every patient requires an intravenous line, continuous ED cardiac monitoring, and an ECG. Serial ECGs will be required in most patients. Suggested laboratory studies include determinations of serum electrolyte, creatinine, and glucose levels. A quantitative serum acetaminophen level is recommended in all overdose patients. Most symptomatic patients will require arterial blood gas measurement. Patients with antimuscarinic symptoms may require a urinary catheter to prevent urinary retention and a nasogastric tube if bowel sounds are absent. Patients who are initially asymptomatic may deteriorate rapidly and therefore should be monitored closely for several hours. Emergency physicians should report all TCA exposures to a regional poison control center.

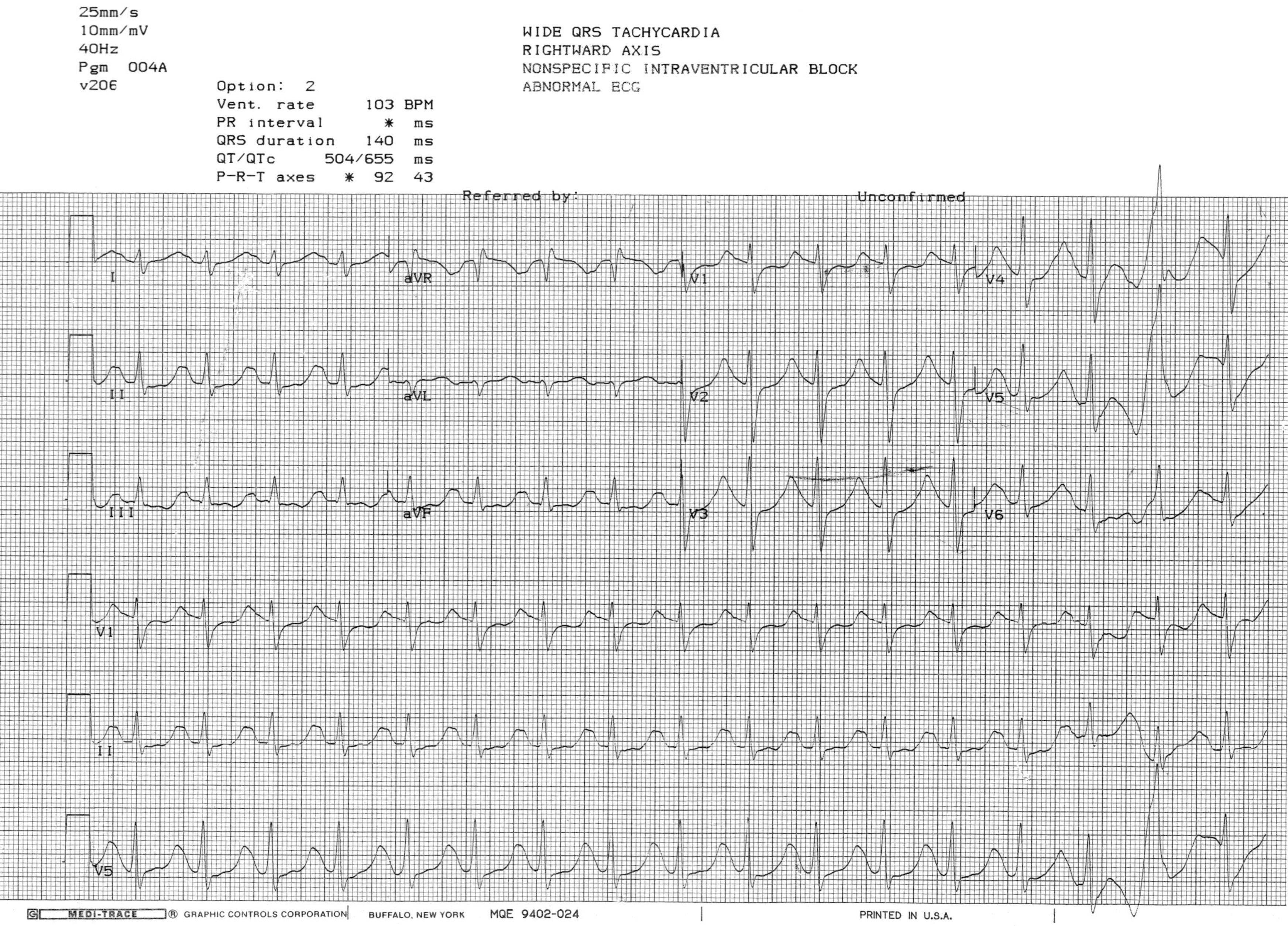

FIG. 152-1. ''Ciassic'' TCA electrocardiographic abnormalities. Sinus tachycardia and prolonged PR, QRS, and QT intervals. Also, right axis deviation (RAD) of terminal 40 ms.

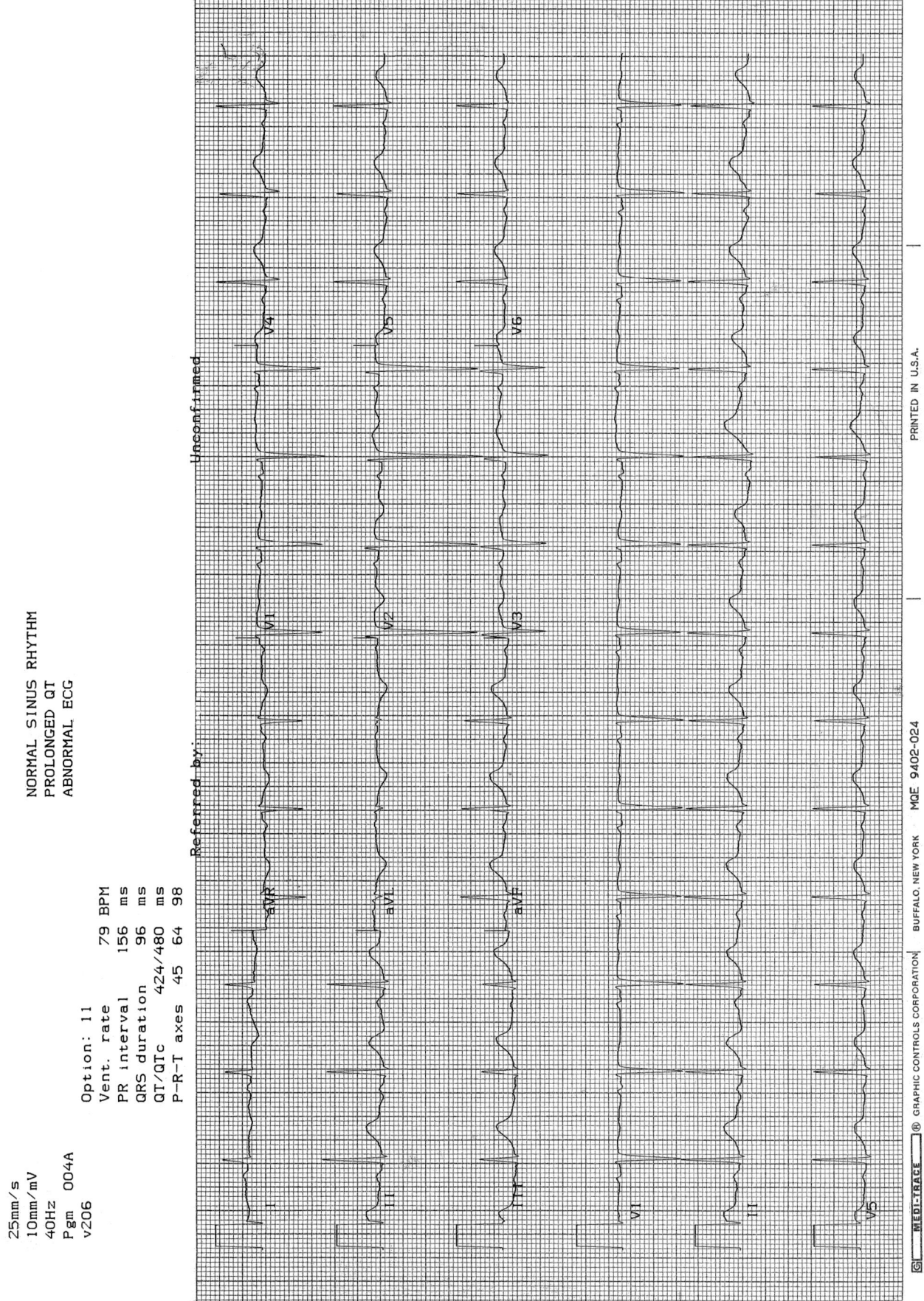

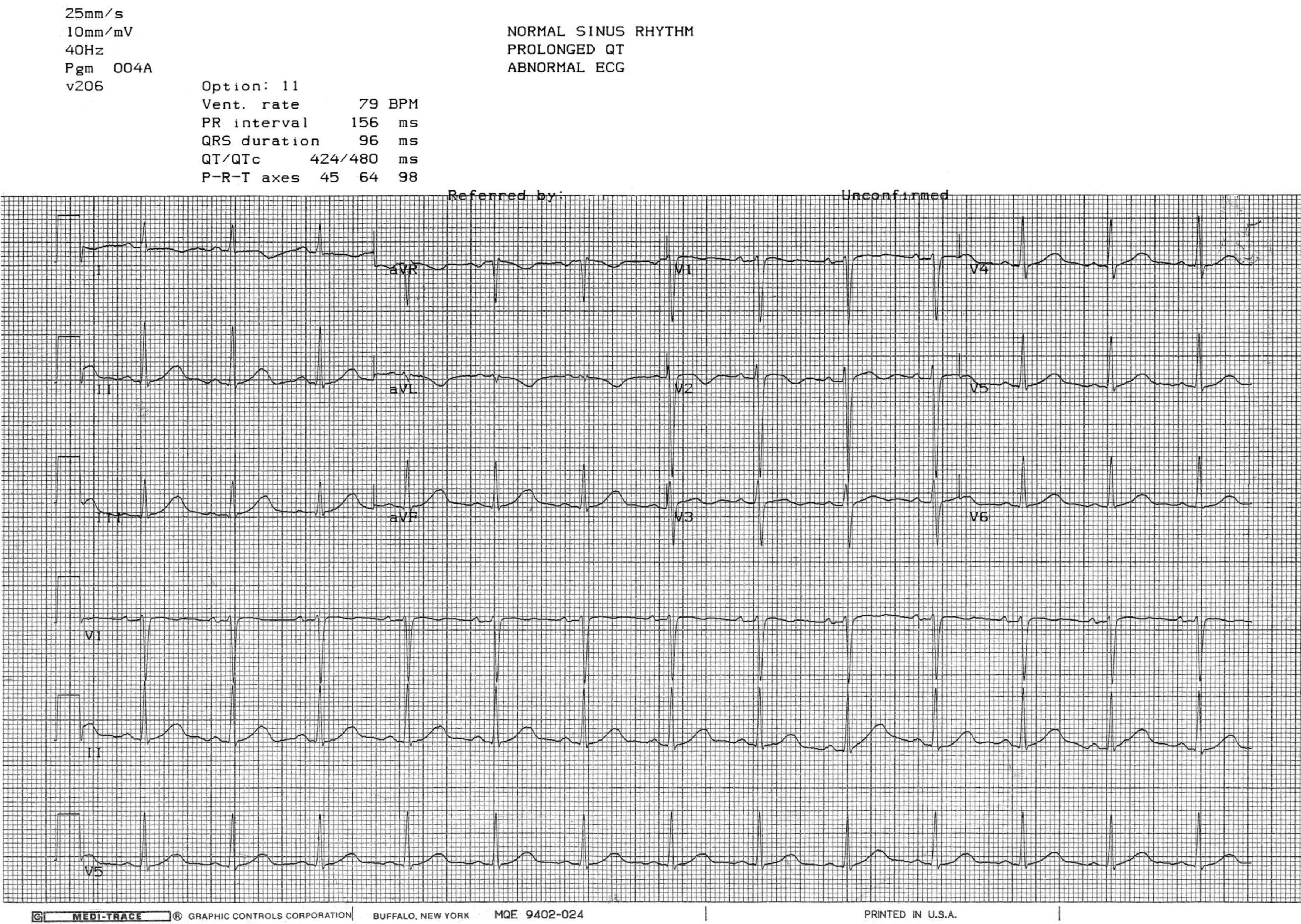

FIG. 152-2. Repeat ECG 4 days later in the same patient as in Fig. 152-1. Only mild QTc prolongation persists.

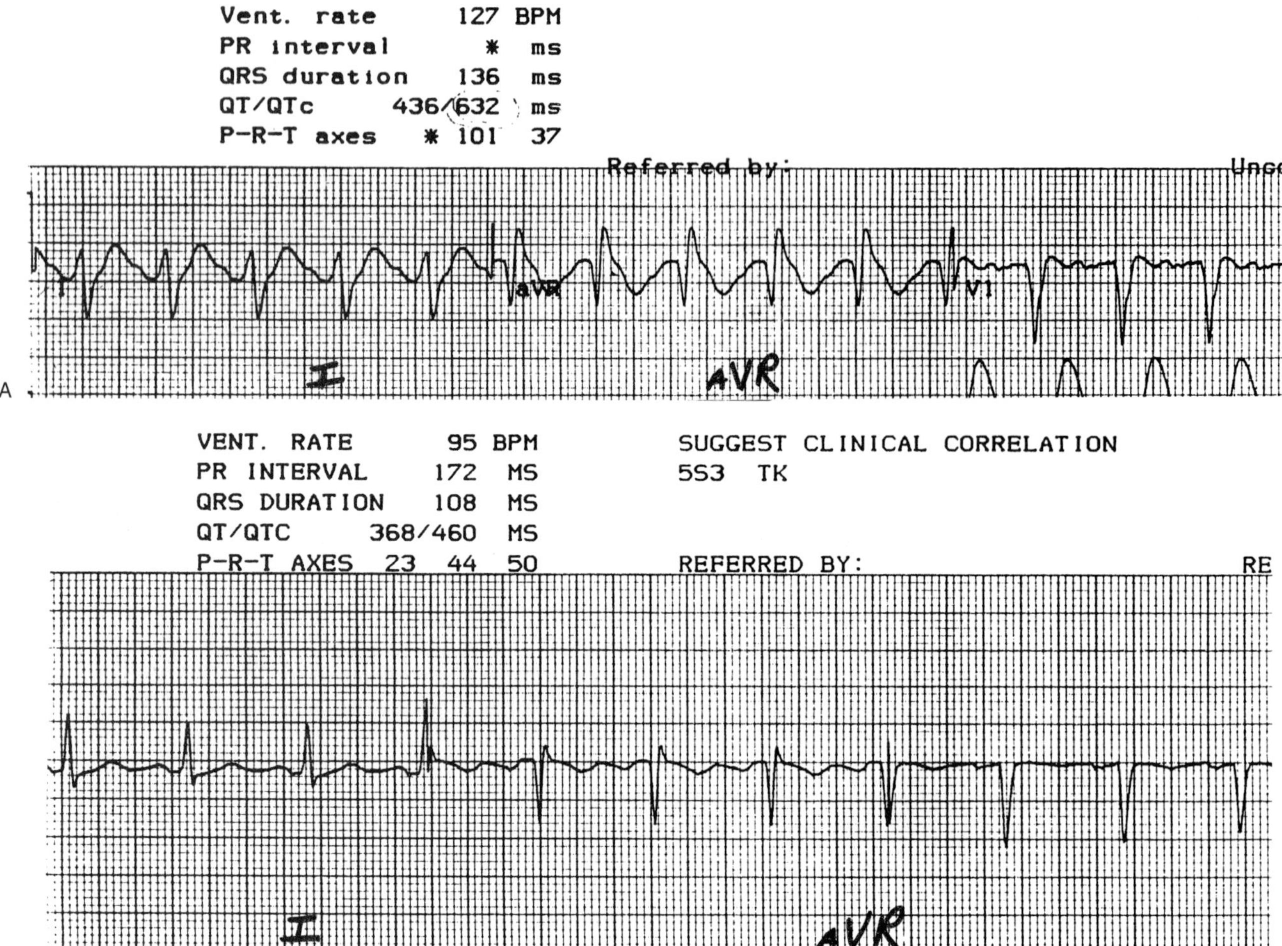

FIG. 152-3. A. An example of terminal 40 ms RAD during TCA toxicity. Note the large R wave in aVR and S wave in lead I. **B.** The same patient after complete resolution of TCA toxicity. Note the decrease in the R wave height in aVR and S wave in lead I.

Gastrointestinal Decontamination

Although the best method of gastrointestinal decontamination in TCA ingestions remains undefined, a few generalizations are still possible.[14] The risks associated with using syrup of ipecac outweigh any beneficial effects, and its use cannot be recommended. Activated charcoal (AC) has been shown to effectively bind TCAs and decrease their absorption. Therefore, all patients should receive 1 g/kg of AC. Whether gastric lavage and AC is better than AC alone remains unproven. Studies have shown that the gastric lavage is most effective when it is performed within the first few hours after ingestion. Most emergency physicians opt to perform gastric lavage and give AC to patients who present relatively early after TCA ingestion. The proper method of performing gastric lavage in alert patients is to place the patient in the left lateral decubitus position to prevent pulmonary aspiration. Obtunded patients require endotracheal intubation prior to performing gastric lavage. Asymptomatic patients with reliable histories of minimal TCA ingestions can be treated with AC alone and observed for toxicity. Some authors have recommended giving repeat doses of AC to enhance TCA elimination, but these recommendations should be viewed cautiously in the setting of decreased intestinal motility.

Sodium Bicarbonate Therapy

Indications for sodium bicarbonate therapy include QRS complex widening greater than 100 ms, hypotension refractory to fluid hydration, and ventricular dysrhythmias. Sodium bicarbonate has been shown to improve conduction, increase contractility, and suppress ventricular ectopy. It is given as an initial bolus of 1 to 2 meq/kg, which can be repeated until patient improvement is noted or until blood pH equals 7.50 to 7.55 (Fig. 152-4). Alkalinization beyond this point can be deleterious and therefore is discouraged. Continuous infusions of sodium bicarbonate are usually administered as 3 ampules (50 meq/50 mL) placed in 1 L of 5% D/W or 2 ampules added to 5% D/0.45 NS (slightly hypertonic with $NaHCO_3$ added) solution and run at a rate of 2 to 3 cc/kg/h. Adjustments in the intravenous rate are made based on blood pH measurements, serum sodium level, and clinical response to therapy. Hypokalemia is an expected complication of $NaHCO_3$ therapy. Intravenous potassium supplementation is usually required, and serum potassium levels should be measured frequently.

Altered Level of Consciousness

Patients with altered level of consciousness require a trial of intravenous dextrose, thiamine, naloxone, and oxygen to rule out reversible causes of CNS depression. Antagonism of postsynaptic muscarinic, histamine, and α-adrenergic receptors contributes to the development of altered mentation in TCA overdoses. Coma from TCA toxicity is typically rapid in onset. Unresponsive patients may have unrecognized head or neck trauma. Flumazenil should not be given to patients suspected of having mixed-drug overdoses involving TCAs and benzodiazepines because this may precipitate generalized seizures. There is a very high incidence of pulmonary aspiration among TCA overdose patients who present comatose to the ED. Agitation is commonly observed prior to the onset of coma, as well as in previously comatose patients as they awaken. Agitation is best controlled with reassurance, decreased environmental stimulation, and benzodiazepines. As mentioned previously, physostigmine should not be administered to patients taking TCAs.

Seizures

Most seizures occur within the first 3 h following ingestion. Typically, these seizures are generalized and brief in duration. Multiple seizures are reported in approximately 10 to 30 percent of TCA overdoses. Focal seizures are atypical and require further neurologic evaluation. Seizures are especially common with maprotiline and amoxapine ingestions and require aggressive management because status epilepticus is frequently associated with these two particular antidepressants. Benzodiazepines (e.g., diazepam, lorazepam) are the anticonvulsants of choice to stop existing seizure activity. Barbiturates (e.g., phenobarbital) are indicated to treat seizures resistant to benzodiazepines. The initial intravenous dose of phenobarbital is 15 mg/kg, but this can be increased in patients with continued seizure activity and adequate blood pressure. Hypotension is a major side effect. Endotracheal intubation and respiratory support will be required when benzodiazepines are combined with barbiturates or propofol. Phenytoin is an ineffective anticonvulsant for stopping TCA-induced seizures. Physostigmine and $NaHCO_3$ do not stop TCA-induced seizures. If seizures continue despite adequate dosing with benzodiazepines and phenobarbital, consideration should be given to paralyzing the patient with a neuromuscular blocking agent. This will stop the physical manifestations of the seizure and its secondary effects, which include metabolic acidosis, hyperthermia, rhabdomyolysis, and renal failure. It does not stop brain seizure activity. Therefore, following the induction of muscle paralysis, these patients require electroencephalographic (EEG) monitoring and continued anticonvulsant therapy.

Hypotension

Hypotension should be treated initially with isotonic crystalloid fluids in increments of 10 mL/kg. In the setting of impaired cardiac contractility, pulmonary edema can develop if excessive fluids are administered. Hypotension that does improve with appropriate fluid challenges should be treated with $NaHCO_3$ (regardless of QRS width). Vasopressors should be used when hypotension is unresponsive to fluids and sodium bicarbonate therapy. The most effective vasopressor is norepinephrine, because it directly competes with TCAs at α-adrenergic receptors. Dopamine is less effective than norepinephrine in reversing TCA-induced hypotension.[15] In many cases, dopamine administration actually will cause a lowering in systolic blood pressure due to its β-adrenergic and dopaminergic actions that promote vasodilation. If used, it should be adjusted at the upper range of the dose (12 to 20 μg/kg/min). A pulmonary artery catheter should be placed in patients whose hypotension is refractory to fluid, $NaHCO_3$, and vasopressor therapy. Mechanical irritation of the heart during pulmonary artery catheter placement may precipitate life-threatening conduction abnormalities and ventricular dysrhythmias. Hypotension induced by TCAs represents a potentially reversible cause of cardiovascular collapse. Mechanical support of the circulation with cardiopulmonary bypass, overdrive pacing, or aortic balloon pump assistance may be warranted in patients with refractory hypotension, although no studies document their effectiveness.

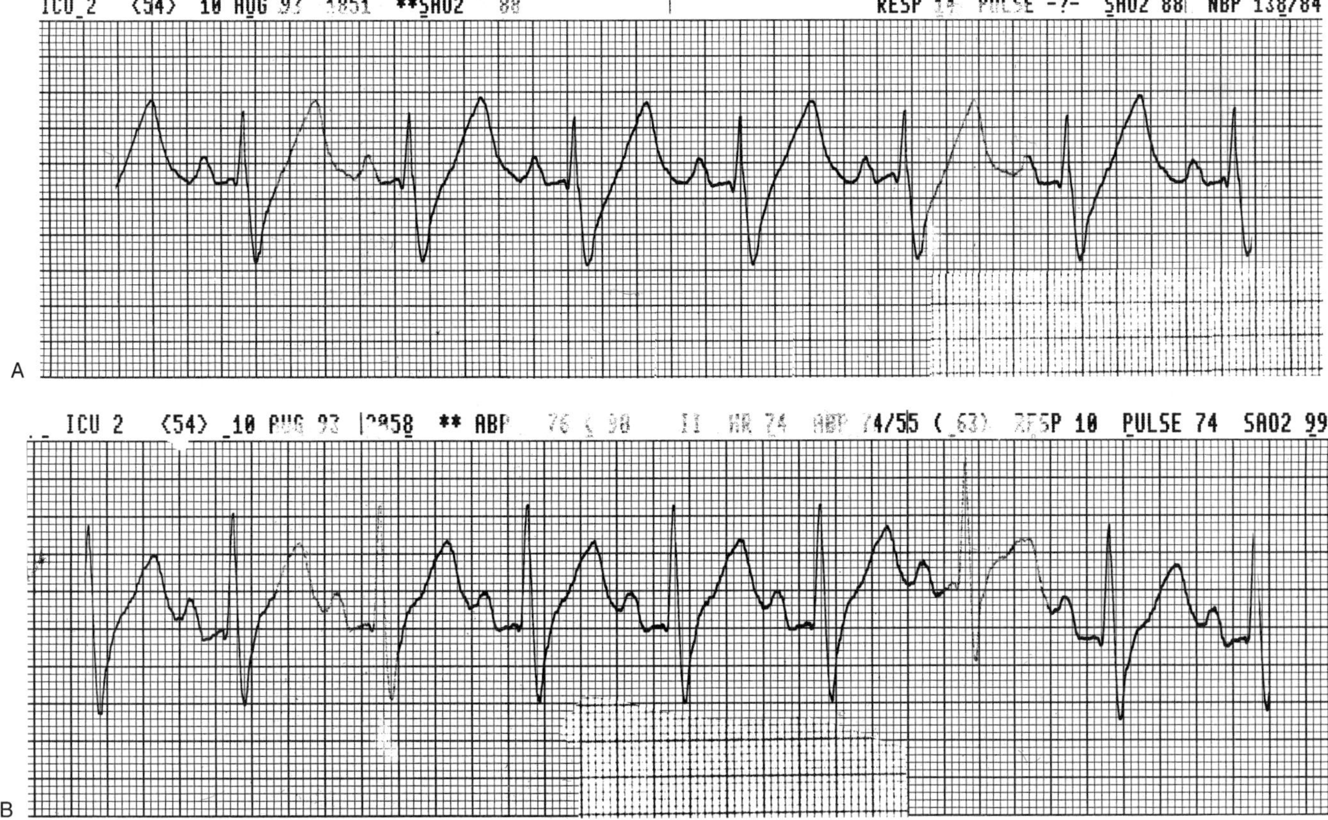

FIG. 152-4. A. Cardiac rhythm strip of a patient with a wide QRS, recorded 3 h after ingesting amitriptyline. **B.** Narrowing of the QRS complex in same patient after receiving an intravenous bolus of sodium bicarbonate.

Dysrhythmias

TCAs frequently alter cardiac rate, conduction, and contractility. Asymptomatic patients with sinus tachycardia, isolated PR and QT prolongation, or first-degree atrioventricular (AV) block do not require specific pharmacologic therapy. Conduction blocks greater than first-degree AV block are worrisome because they can rapidly progress to complete heart block secondary to impaired infranodal conduction. Most patients with QRS prolongation greater than 100 ms should be treated with $NaHCO_3$ therapy, although this is somewhat controversial. This recommendation is made despite the absence of randomized, controlled human trials demonstrating $NaHCO_3$ therapy benefits in otherwise asymptomatic patients with QRS prolongation.[16] Nonetheless, the early use of sodium bicarbonate in the setting of sodium channel blockade has become a common practice for treating QRS widening. Hyperventilation represents a reasonable alternative to sodium bicarbonate therapy in the setting of renal failure, pulmonary edema, or cerebral edema.

Ventricular dysrhythmias should be treated immediately with sodium bicarbonate administration. Lidocaine is the second agent of choice in treating ventricular dysrhythmias. Excessive lidocaine administration is capable of producing seizures. Bretylium is generally considered a third-line drug for ventricular dysrhythmias. Synchronized cardioversion is appropriate in patients with unstable dysrhythmias. Torsade de pointes should be treated initially with 2 g of intravenous magnesium sulfate. Efforts should be made to rule out other causes of torsades de pointes. Overdrive pacing is frequently required to prevent a recurrence of this dysrhythmia. Intravenous isoproterenol may be of some benefit in treating recurrent torsade de pointes when overdrive pacing is not available. The following medications are contraindicated in the treatment of TCA-induced dysrhythmias: all class IA and IC antiarrhythmic agents, beta blockers, calcium channel blockers, and all class III antiarrhythmic agents.

DISPOSITION

Patients who remain asymptomatic 6 h after ingestion do not require hospital admission for toxicologic reasons. They may still require hospital admission because of other coexisting medical or psychiatric conditions. Psychiatric evaluation is warranted for intentional drug ingestions. All symptomatic patients require hospital admission to a monitored bed. Patients demonstrating signs of moderate to severe toxicity should be admitted to an intensive care unit. Hospitalized patients can be cleared medically after 12 h of being asymptomatic: including a normal or baseline ECG, normal mental status, and resolution of all antimuscarinic symptoms.

REFERENCES

1. Litovitz TI, Klein-Schwartz W, Dyer KS, et al: 1997 Annual report of the American Association of Poison Control Centers Toxic Exposure Surveillance System. *Am J Emerg Med* 16:443, 1998.
2. Spiller HA, Winter ML, Mann KV, et al: Five-year multicenter retrospective review of cyclobenzaprine toxicity. *J Emerg Med* 13:781, 1995.
3. Buckley NA, McManus PR: Can the fatal toxicity of antidepressant drugs be predicted with pharmacological and toxicological data? *Drug Safety* 18:369, 1998.
4. Kolecki PF, Curry SC: Poisoning by sodium channel blocking agents. *Crit Care Clin* 13:829, 1997.
5. McCabe JL, Cobaugh DJ, Menegazzi JJ, et al: Experimental tricyclic antidepressant toxicity: A randomized, controlled comparison of hypertonic saline solution, sodium bicarbonate, and hyperventilation. *Ann Emerg Med* 32:329, 1998.
6. Phillips S, Brent J, Kulig K, et al: Fluoxetine versus tricyclic antidepressants: A prospective multicenter study of antidepressant drug overdoses. The Antidepressant Study Group. *J Emerg Med* 15:439, 1997.
7. Preskorn SH: Pharmacokinetics of antidepressants: Why and how they are relevant to treatment. *J Clin Psychiatry* 54(suppl 9):14, 1993.
8. Hulten B-A, Adams R, Askenasi R: Predicting severity of tricyclic antidepressant overdose. *Clin Toxicol* 30:161, 1992.
9. Caravati EM, Bossart PJ: Demographic and electrocardiographic factors associated with severe tricyclic antidepressant toxicity. *Clin Toxicol* 29:31, 1991.
10. Hilberg T, Bugge A, Beylich K-M: An animal model of postmortem amitriptyline redistribution. *J Forensic Sci* 38:81, 1993.
11. Liebelt EL, Francis PD, Woolf AD: ECG lead aV_R versus QRS interval in predicting seizures and arrhythmias in acute tricyclic antidepressant toxicity. *Ann Emerg Med* 26:195, 1995.
12. Berkovitch M, Matsui D, Folgelman R, et al: Assessment of the terminal 40-millisecond QRS vector in children with a history of tricyclic antidepressant ingestion. *Pediatr Emerg Care* 11:75, 1995.
13. Liebelt EL, Ulrich A, Francis PD, et al: Serial electrocardiogram changes in acute tricyclic antidepressant overdoses. *Crit Care Med* 25:1721, 1997.
14. Bosse GM, Barefoot JA, Pfeifer MP, et al: Comparison of three methods of gut decontamination in tricyclic antidepressant overdose. *J Emerg Med* 13:203, 1995.
15. Tran PT, Panacek EA, Rhee KJ, et al: Response to dopamine vs norepinephrine in tricyclic antidepressant-induced hypotension. *Acad Emerg Med* 4:864, 1997.
16. Hoffman JR, Votey SR, Bayer M, et al: Effect of hypertonic sodium bicarbonate in the treatment of moderate-to-severe cyclic antidepressant overdose. *Am J Emerg Med* 11:336, 1993.

NEWER ANTIDEPRESSANTS AND SEROTONIN SYNDROME

Kirk C. Mills

The newer antidepressants are commonly referred to as atypical, heterocyclic, or second-generation antidepressants to distinguish them from monoamine oxidase inhibitors (MAOIs) and tricyclic antidepressants (TCAs). This distinction is important because newer antidepressants are more selective in their pharmacologic activity and have drastically different toxicologic behavior than MAOIs and TCAs. As a group, the newer antidepressants are the most popular form of psychopharmacologic therapy for the treatment of major depression. In addition, they are also commonly prescribed in the treatment of many other psychiatric disorders such obsessive-compulsive disorder, panic disorders, and eating disorders. Although none of the newer antidepressants have been labeled by the Food and Drug Administration for use in children, their use in adolescents and older children is not uncommon.

Emergency physicians are increasingly challenged to evaluate patients who have taken these newer antidepressants. Questions commonly arise as to the extent of management needed to treat these patients appropriately. Therefore, the newer antidepressants are discussed individually in this chapter, highlighting specific treatment recommendations. Importantly, all antidepressants, especially the MAOIs and selective serotonin reuptake inhibitors (SSRIs), have the potential to produce the serotonin syndrome, a recently recognized drug-induced disorder, which is discussed at the end of this chapter. The newer antidepressants that are discussed in this chapter include trazodone (Desyrel), nefazodone (Serzone), bupropion (Wellbutrin), mirtazapine (Remeron), venlafaxine (Effexor), and the SSRIs: fluoxetine (Prozac), sertraline (Zoloft), paroxetine (Paxil), fluvoxamine (Luvox), and citalopram (Celexa).

GENERAL PRINCIPLES OF NEWER ANTIDEPRESSANTS

The newer antidepressants are a heterogeneous group of drugs that differ significantly in chemical structure, mechanism of action, pharmacokinetic characteristics, and adverse effect profile. Nonetheless, they also share many important similarities that are summarized in the following seven points. For brevity within this chapter, most of these points are not repeated for each individual drug:

1. These agents do not significantly inhibit cardiac sodium, calcium, or potassium ion channels. Therefore, they do not demonstrate the same cardiotoxicity or electrocardiographic conduction abnormalities typically seen with TCAs.

2. These agents do not inhibit monoamine oxidase activity and are not associated with tyramine-like reactions. The use of indirect sympathomimetics is not contraindicated.

3. They have negligible affinity for acetylcholine, dopamine, γ-aminobutyric acid (GABA), glutamate, or β-adrenergic receptors. Although their exact mechanism of action remains poorly understood, it is traditionally attributed to inhibition of neurotransmitter reuptake (except mirtazapine).

4. Newer antidepressants (except bupropion) appear to have a much higher safety margin than the MAOIs and TCAs. Nonetheless, they can still cause fatalities, especially at very high doses or when combined with other drugs. Importantly, there is extremely limited human data on the ''typical'' presentation or optimal management of patients having overdosed on newer antidepressants. Therefore, current management recommendations may require modification as more information becomes available. Emergency physicians should routinely contact a regional poison control center (PCC) to report exposures to newer antidepressants. Also, consultation with a medical toxicologist is available through most regional PCCs.

5. Attempts at enhancing the elimination of newer antidepressants via hemodialysis, hemoperfusion, forced diuresis, or multiple-dose activated charcoal are unlikely to be successful and therefore not recommended. Whole bowel irrigation does not offer any advantage over single-dose activated charcoal in providing gastrointestinal decontamination to patients exposed to newer antidepressants.

6. The newer antidepressants are not detected by routine hospital serum and urine drug screens. Certain specialty laboratories do have the capability to measure parent drug and metabolite plasma levels, but this information is only useful for the confirmation of suspected drug overdose. Specific levels are not immediately available to emergency physicians nor do they affect the management of these patients. Postmortem drug redistribution is likely to occur with the newer antidepressants and, thus, postmortem drug level interpretation must take this factor into consideration.

7. Since all of the newer antidepressants are metabolized primarily by the liver, hepatic dysfunction can lead to elevated drug levels and subsequent drug toxicity. Also, drug interactions are possible when the newer antidepressants are combined with other drugs dependent on hepatic metabolism.

TRAZODONE

Trazodone hydrochloride (Desyrel) was released in the United States in 1982 for the treatment of endogenous depression. In 1997, the American Association of Poison Control Centers Toxic Exposure Surveillance System (AAPCC-TESS) recorded 10,460 exposures to trazodone.[1] During the past 5 years, the frequency of reported trazodone exposures has increased by almost 300 percent. Thus, trazodone exposures represent an increasingly common poisoning concern for emergency physicians. Trazodone is relatively safe in overdose when compared with MAOIs and TCAs. The calculated fatality rate for trazodone is 1 in 1200 exposures. This is approximately seven to ten times less than the fatality rate for MAOI or TCA exposures. The average daily therapeutic dose for trazodone is between 150 to 400 mg, with a maximum dose of up to 600 mg restricted to psychiatric inpatients. Trazodone is available as 50-mg, 100-mg, 150-mg, and 300-mg tablets. There is a low potential for trazodone abuse, and a distinct withdrawal syndrome has not been observed with its abrupt discontinuation. Trazodone is a category C risk in pregnancy.

Trazodone is a triazolopyridine derivative that is structurally unrelated to other antidepressants. Its antidepressant action is believed to be due to a combination of serotonin (5-hydroxytryptamine or 5-HT) reuptake inhibition and antagonism of postsynaptic 5-HT_2 receptors.[2] Trazodone is a moderately potent nonselective α-adrenergic receptor blocker with at least five times greater affinity for α_1- than α_2-adrenergic receptors. Consequently, trazodone is frequently associated with orthostatic hypotension, which is maximal within the first 6 h of use and can be minimized by taking the medication at bedtime. Sedation, which is a common side effect of trazodone therapy, is believed to be secondary to inhibition of central α-adrenergic and histamine receptors.

Trazodone is rapidly and completely absorbed, with peak plasma levels occurring between 1 and 2 h following oral administration. It is highly protein bound and has a moderate volume of distribution (1.2 L/kg). The majority of trazodone undergoes hepatic oxidation by the cytochrome P-450 isoenzyme system. It has one active metabolite, *m*-chlorophenylpiperazine (*m*-CPP), which has a complex pharmacologic profile, such as inhibition of 5-HT uptake, stimulation and inhibition of multiple postsynaptic serotonin receptors, and interactions with other neurotransmitter systems. The overall contribution of *m*-CPP to the therapeutic and toxic effects of trazodone is currently under investigation. The half-life of trazodone ranges from 5 to 9 h at therapeutic doses but can increase up to 13 h in overdose.

The adverse effect profile for trazodone is very favorable when compared with other antidepressants except for its association with priapism. Trazodone is the most common cause of drug-induced priapism. The estimated incidence of priapism while on therapeutic doses ranges from 1 in 1000 to 1 in 10,000 patients. Any patient with a history of increased frequency, duration, or inappropriate penile or clitoral engorgement should immediately discontinue trazodone therapy. Human volunteer and laboratory animal studies have proven that trazodone is far less cardiotoxic than TCAs. Therapeutic use of trazodone has been occasionally reported to be arrhythmogenic, especially in patients with underlying cardiac risk factors such as conduction abnormalities or ischemic heart disease. Examples of cardiac rhythm abnormalities reported in association with trazodone therapy include sinus arrest, sinus bradycardia, various atrioventricular blocks, complete heart block, atrial fibrillation, and ventricular dysrhythmias (premature ventricular beats or torsade de pointes). The most frequently reported dose-related adverse effects are drowsiness, dizziness, dry mouth, nausea and vomiting, and orthostatic hypotension. There have been rare case reports of patients experiencing reversible liver enzyme elevation, jaundice, and abnormal liver histology in association with trazodone therapy.

Pharmacokinetic drug interactions are relatively uncommon with trazodone. Trazodone levels may be increased by concurrent fluoxetine administration. Increased serum digoxin and phenytoin levels have been reported in patients receiving trazodone. Elderly patients have a predisposition for developing elevated plasma trazodone levels at any given therapeutic dose. Pharmacodynamic interactions are most common with coingestants such as ethanol, central nervous system (CNS) depressants, or α-adrenergic blockers.

Acute Overdose Toxicity

There is no established toxic dose for trazodone. As a general guideline, serious toxicity in an average adult is unexpected with ingestions of less than 2 g. This safety margin is significantly reduced when other medications are coingested with trazodone. The most common symptom of acute trazodone poisoning is CNS depression. Other CNS-related symptoms include ataxia, dizziness, coma, and seizures. Trazodone rarely produces coma or seizures when it is the only drug ingested. Pupils are usually normal size and remain reactive to light. Infrequently, patients may complain of muscle weakness. Trazodone-induced CNS symptoms show marked improvement within 6 to 12 h after ingestion and are almost always resolved by 24 h. Orthostatic hypotension is the most frequently reported cardiovascular abnormality noted in trazodone overdose and usually responds to fluid administration. Mild abnormalities of sinus rhythm, such as sinus bradycardia and tachycardia, are frequently encountered. The most common electrocardiographic abnormality is moderate prolongation of the QTc interval. Polymorphic ventricular tachycardia (torsade de pointes) has been reported in rare cases. Commonly reported gastrointestinal complaints include nausea, vomiting, and nonspecific abdominal pain. Respiratory depression is infrequently observed with pure trazodone overdoses. Priapism has been reported following an acute overdose of 3.5 g.

Treatment

An intravenous line should be started and cardiac monitoring initiated on all patients. In pure trazodone ingestions, significant neurologic and cardiac toxicity is not expected and supportive care is usually the only treatment required. Specific antidotal therapy is not available. Gastrointestinal decontamination can be applied selectively in cases where the dose ingested can be accurately calculated. Ingestion of 1500 mg or less of trazodone in an adult carries a low risk of toxicity, as long as trazodone is ingested as a single agent and the patient does not have any underlying cardiac or neurologic risk factors. These patients should receive 1 g/kg of activated charcoal, and gastric lavage is probably unnecessary. Ingestions of more than 2000 mg of trazodone poses the greatest risk for associated toxicity and complications. Also, patients having coingested other drugs and/or ethanol have a higher incidence of coma, seizures, and respiratory arrest. Gastric decontamination in these patients is best achieved by early gastric lavage followed by administration of activated charcoal. Hypotension should be initially treated with isotonic intravenous fluid administration. If the use of a vasopressor becomes necessary, direct-acting vasopressors (e.g., norepinephrine) are recommended. Drugs with β-adrenergic receptor activity (e.g., dopamine) can theoretically potentiate the hypotension in the presence of trazodone-induced α-adrenergic receptor antagonism. Patients who have remained asymptomatic for at least 6 h can be safely discharged from the emergency department. This assumes that any necessary psychiatric evaluation has been completed or arranged. All intentional trazodone ingestions should be properly evaluated for the presence of other drugs (e.g., acetaminophen). Patients with neurologic and/or cardiac symptoms persisting longer than 6 h after ingestion will require hospital admission to a monitored bed. In addition, patients with coingestants associated with delayed toxicity will require prolonged observation or formal hospital admission.

NEFAZODONE

Nefazodone (Serzone), was approved in 1995 for the treatment of depression. It is both structurally and functionally related to trazodone. Nefazodone inhibits serotonin reuptake and also antagonizes postsynaptic 5-HT_2 receptors.[3] It has little affinity for other receptors except slight antagonism of postsynaptic α_1 receptors. Nefazodone is available in 100-mg, 150-mg, 200-mg, and 250-mg tablets. The recommended effective dose for nefazodone is between 300 and 600 mg/day. Although nefazodone is rapidly absorbed, it has a bioavailability of only 20 percent due to extensive first-pass hepatic metabolism. Peak levels occur within 1 h, and its elimination half-life ranges from 2 to 6 h. It is 99 percent protein bound, with a relatively small volume of distribution. It has three active metabolites: hydroxynefazodone, desethylhydroxynefazodone, and *m*-CPP. The hydroxynefazodone metabolite is pharmacologically equivalent to the parent compound. The *m*-CPP metabolite is noteworthy only because it is also produced by trazodone. Nefazodone can inhibit the metabolism of terfenadine, astemizole, and cisapride, which in turn can lead to life-threatening prolongation of the QT interval (torsade de pointes). Certain benzodiazepines such as alprazolam and triazolam have marked increased CNS effects in the presence of nefazodone. Overall, nefazodone has a favorable adverse effect profile. Compared with placebo, however, nefazodone has a higher incidence of headache, dizziness, drowsiness, asthenia, tremor, dry mouth, nausea, constipation, and blurred vision. It also predisposes patients to postural hypotension and priapism but not to the same degree as trazodone. Nefazodone has a category C rating in pregnancy.

Treatment

Experience with nefazodone in overdose is extremely limited. Unpublished premarketing data suggest that nefazodone is relatively safe in overdose. The most common symptoms reported include nausea, vomiting, and somnolence. There were no fatalities with pure nefazodone ingestions ranging from 1000 to 11,200 mg. Based on its pharmacokinetic profile, the onset of nefazodone toxicity would be expected to occur within the first 6 h following an overdose. At present, management of nefazodone overdoses should follow the aforementioned guidelines for trazodone.

BUPROPION

Bupropion (Wellbutrin) has been available in the United States since 1989 for the treatment of major depression. The actual incidence and severity of bupropion exposures are unknown because the AAPCC-TESS data do not include a separate category for bupropion exposures. However, since bupropion has recently been approved for the treatment of smoking cessation (Zyban), the potential for bupropion poisoning is considerable. Both Wellbutrin and Zyban tablets are manufactured by the same company and are available in similar 150-mg sustained-release formulations. For smoking cessation, Zyban (150 mg) is administered either once or twice daily for no more than 12 consecutive weeks. Wellbutrin comes in a variety of doses and formulations, including sustained-release tablets (100 and 150 mg) and regular-release tablets (100 and 75 mg). The recommended starting dose of Wellbutrin is 100 mg given twice daily, gradually increasing up to 300 mg/day. The incidence of seizures drastically increases at doses greater than 450 mg/day, and higher doses are therefore prohibited. The combination of the two bupropion preparations, Wellbutrin and Zyban, is contraindicated due to obvious concern for bupropion toxicity. Other contraindications include patients with bulimia, anorexia nervosa, epilepsy, or taking MAOIs. Bupropion is a category B drug in pregnancy. The information in this section is derived from studies utilizing only the Wellbutrin form of bupropion. It is assumed that this information is equally applicable to Zyban exposures, and therefore no further distinction in this chapter is made between these two bupropion products.

Bupropion has a monocyclic phenylaminoketone chemical structure that resembles those of the phenylethylamines (e.g., amphetamine).[4] However, bupropion does not produce stimulant effects or drug-addictive behavior at therapeutic doses. The therapeutic mechanism of action for bupropion is poorly understood but currently believed to be related to its ability to inhibit dopamine neuronal reuptake. It does not directly stimulate postsynaptic dopamine receptors. In vitro studies show bupropion to be a weak inhibitor of norepinephrine and serotonin neuronal reuptake. Bupropion is rapidly absorbed after oral administration and undergoes extensive first-pass hepatic metabolism. It is highly protein bound, has an extremely large volume of distribution, and readily crosses the blood-brain barrier. Peak plasma levels occur within 2 h for regular-release tablets and 3 h for sustained-release preparations. Its elimination half-life ranges between 14 to 20 h. Bupropion has one important metabolite—hydroxybupropion—which is less potent than bupropion, preferentially inhibits norepinephrine reuptake, and may contribute to seizure development.

Bupropion antidepressant therapy is well tolerated. It does not produce CNS depression, orthostatic hypotension, or cardiovascular changes, or impair sexual function at therapeutic doses. The most commonly reported adverse effects are of mild severity and include dry mouth, dizziness, agitation, nausea, headache, constipation, tremor, anxiety, confusion, blurred vision, and increased motor activity. Bupropion has been reported to infrequently produce catatonia, hallucinations, psychosis, and paranoia that are probably related to its dopaminergic activity.

Abrupt discontinuation of bupropion has not been associated with any withdrawal symptoms but may pose a slight theoretic risk of precipitating neuroleptic malignant syndrome, since bupropion is considered a dopamine agonist. Bupropion is relatively free of significant drug interactions. In general, bupropion should not be combined with selective serotonin reuptake inhibitors, lithium, MAOIs, TCAs, dopaminergic drugs (e.g., levodopa), or drugs that are known to lower patient seizure threshold (e.g., phenothiazines).

Acute Overdose Toxicity

Bupropion differs from other new antidepressants in that it has a low toxic to therapeutic ratio. Toxicity can occur at doses equal to or just slightly greater than the maximum therapeutic dose of 450 mg/day. As a general rule, significant toxicity is not expected in pure bupropion overdose with adult ingestions of less than 450 mg. The largest case series of bupropion overdoses reported that symptomatic patients ingested a mean of 2310 mg and the lowest symptomatic dose was 200 mg.[5] Patients who remained asymptomatic ingested a mean of 1325 mg and the largest asymptomatic dose was 4000 mg. The most commonly reported symptoms in pure bupropion overdose include sinus tachycardia (43 percent), lethargy (41 percent), tremor (24 percent), generalized seizures (21 percent), confusion (14 percent), and vomiting (14 percent). Mild hyperthermia is occasionally reported. Sinus tachycardia is the most common electrocardiographic abnormality. An isolated case of moderate QT interval prolongation has been reported in conjunction with a massive bupropion overdose. Otherwise, bupropion does not produce myocardial conduction abnormalities. Hypotension is unexpected in pure bupropion overdoses but has been reported in mixed-drug overdoses. Hypertension is usually of only mild to moderate severity. Coma and cardiac arrest have been reported in severe bupropion overdoses. The hallmark of bupropion toxicity is generalized seizures. The actual incidence of seizures is unknown but is probably greater than the estimated 21 percent obtained by retrospective studies. There is no correlation between the development of seizures and the presence of other symptoms such as sinus tachycardia. Therefore, seizures can develop in otherwise asymptomatic patients. Seizures usually occur within the first 1 to 4 h after ingestion of regular-release bupropion. The average time of seizure onset is 3.7 h, but they may be delayed for up to 8 h. Recent case reports suggest that sustained-release preparations may predispose patients to seizures up to 14 h after exposure. Laboratory study findings are usually normal except for rare cases of mild hypokalemia.

Treatment

Emergency physicians should anticipate the possible early onset of generalized seizures in all cases of bupropion ingestion. A peripheral intravenous line should be established and cardiac monitoring initiated in all patients. Rapid gastrointestinal decontamination is recommended using gastric lavage and administering 1 g/kg of activated charcoal. Syrup of ipecac is contraindicated due to risk of seizures. Significant cardiotoxicity is not expected except in mixed-drug overdoses. Sinus tachycardia is rarely of hemodynamic significance. Seizures that last longer than 5 min, are focal in nature, or repetitive should be aggressively treated with benzodiazepines. Diphenylhydantoin (phenytoin) is generally less effective than benzodiazepines or phenobarbital in stopping drug-induced seizures but was reportedly effective in stopping seizure activity in one case of bupropion-induced status epilepticus. Hospital admission is recommended for all patients with seizures, sinus tachycardia, or lethargy. Asymptomatic patients having ingested only regular-release bupropion can be medically cleared after 8 h of observation. In many cases, a psychiatric evaluation may also be necessary. Similar guidelines for sustained-release bupropion preparations have not been established. Therefore, patients ingesting more than 450 mg of sustained-release bupropion probably require longer periods of monitoring before medical clearance.

MIRTAZAPINE

Mirtazapine (Remeron), a tetracyclic compound structurally unrelated to other currently available antidepressants, has been available in the United States since 1996.[6] In contrast to all other atypical antidepressants, mirtazapine does not inhibit neuronal amine uptake. Instead, it blocks central presynaptic α_2-adrenergic receptors and postsynaptic serotonin receptors, subtypes 5-HT_2 and 5-HT_3. This has the net therapeutic effect of increasing central norepinephrine and serotonin (5-HT_1) neurotransmission. Mirtazapine has a high affinity to block histamine (H_1) receptors and a low affinity for all other postsynaptic receptors. Mirtazapine is commonly associated with somnolence (antihistamine effect) and less often associated with weight gain and increased appetite. It is supplied as 15-mg and 30-mg tablets, with an average daily dose range of between 15 to 45 mg. It is has a category C rating in pregnancy. Because it might cause serotonin syndrome, its use is discouraged in combination with MAOIs. Although not specifically contraindicated, the use of other serotonergic agents (e.g., meperidine, dextromethorphan, and tramadol) should also be avoided in patients taking mirtazapine.

Mirtazapine has a similar pharmacokinetic profile as other atypical antidepressants. It is rapidly and completely absorbed following oral administration. Bioavailability is approximately 50 percent due to significant first-pass hepatic metabolism. Peak levels occur within 2 h after ingestion. Mirtazapine is metabolized by the hepatic oxidase enzyme system (P-450), with only minor active metabolites. Theoretically, since mirtazapine is metabolized by the P-450 enzyme system, drug interactions with other P-450-dependent medications is possible. Presently, no such interactions have been reported, although experience with mirtazapine is very limited. The elimination half-life for mirtazapine averages 26 h for males and 37 h for females. The difference in mirtazapine half-life between men and women is attributed to decreased P-450 metabolism in females. Mirtazapine is highly protein bound (85 percent) and has a large volume of distribution (5 L/kg). Plasma levels are unlikely to be affected by attempts at extracorporeal removal.

Acute Overdose Toxicity

Mirtazapine appears to be associated with limited toxicity in overdose. Presently, only 11 cases of mirtazapine overdose have been reported in the medical literature. The most common presentation includes sedation, confusion, sinus tachycardia, and mild hypertension.[7] Doses up to 1350 mg have been tolerated without significant sequelae. The risk of coma and respiratory depression is greatest at larger doses or when combined with other CNS-depressant drugs. Vital sign abnormalities are rarely of clinical significance and have not required specific treatment.

Treatment

Treatment guidelines have not been established for mirtazapine overdoses. Based on the currently available data, the following recommendations seem logical but may require modification as experience with mirtazapine increases. For this reason, PCC consultation is strongly encouraged for most cases involving the use of mirtazapine. Fortunately, mirtazapine toxicity usually resolves over 24 h with supportive care alone. Single-dose activated charcoal is the gastrointestinal decontamination method of choice. Gastric lavage may be warranted in selected patients presenting early after large overdoses or with significant coingestants. Syrup of ipecac is contraindicated, and whole bowel lavage is unnecessary. Symptomatic patients should be admitted to a monitored bed, but significant cardiac toxicity is unlikely. Electrocardiographic abnormalities other than sinus tachycardia have not been reported. Asymptomatic patients can be medically cleared after 8 h of observation.

SELECTIVE SEROTONIN REUPTAKE INHIBITORS

SSRIs represent a structurally heterogeneous group of drugs that share a selective affinity to inhibit presynaptic serotonin reuptake without significantly affecting norepinephrine or dopamine reuptake. The increase in synaptic serotonin levels may not entirely explain their therapeutic effects.[8] As with most antidepressant agents, acute alterations in biogenic amine levels do not correlate with immediate clinical response to drug therapy. Secondary receptor and cellular compensatory mechanisms are currently believed to play an important role in their mechanism of action. SSRIs are essentially devoid of direct presynaptic or postsynaptic receptor interactions. Thus, they are associated with very few unwanted pharmacologic actions, in contrast to TCAs.

SSRIs represent the most common form of pharmacotherapy for depression in the United States. In 1997, the AAPCC-TESS recorded 27,941 exposures to SSRIs, with 21 associated deaths. This was the first year that the AAPCC-TESS specifically tracked SSRI exposures. It is expected that exposures to SSRI will continue to be a common problem faced by emergency physicians. There are currently five SSRIs available in the United States: fluoxetine (Prozac, released in 1988), sertraline (Zoloft, released in 1991), paroxetine (Paxil, released in 1993), fluvoxamine (Luvox, released in 1994), and citalopram (Celexa, released in 1998). There are slight potency differences between SSRIs, but their clinical efficacy appears to be comparable. The daily equivalent doses of the SSRIs are as follows: fluoxetine, 20 mg; paroxetine, 20 mg; citalopram, 40 mg; sertraline, 50 mg; and fluvoxamine, 150 mg. In pregnancy, some SSRIs (fluoxetine and sertraline) have a category B rating, whereas others (paroxetine and fluvoxamine) have a category C rating.

The SSRIs have similar pharmacokinetic profiles, including rapid and complete oral absorption, peak plasma levels occurring 4 to 8 h after ingestion (citalopram, 2 to 4 h), significant first-pass hepatic metabolism, high degree of protein binding (except citalopram), and large volume of distribution. Fluoxetine is the only SSRI with a clinically significant active metabolite, norfluoxetine, which is equally as potent as fluoxetine. The half-lives of fluoxetine and norfluoxetine are 2 to 4 days and 7 to 14 days, respectively. The effects of fluoxetine may last for up to 5 weeks because of the prolonged period necessary to allow for norfluoxetine metabolism. Sertraline and paroxetine have similar half-lives of approximately 24 h. The half-life of citalopram is estimated at 33 h, whereas fluvoxamine has the shortest half-life at 15 h. The SSRIs are metabolized almost entirely by the hepatic cytochrome P-450 isoenzyme system. It is becoming increasingly recognized that the SSRIs can inhibit the metabolism of other drugs dependent on the cytochrome P-450 isoenzyme system.[9] Clinically significant drug interactions are most likely to occur with drugs that have a low therapeutic index, for example, TCAs, antipsychotics, anticonvulsants, benzodiazepines, opiates, theophylline, warfarin, terfenadine, astemizole, and cisapride. SSRIs are contraindicated in combination with MAOIs. This includes a 2-week abstinence (''washout'') period for most SSRIs and a 5-week abstinence period for fluoxetine. The administration of other serotonergic agents in combination with SSRIs should also be avoided whenever possible.

The most serious drug-related adverse effect of SSRI psychopharmacotherapy is the potential to produce serotonin syndrome (see discussion below). Other CNS-related adverse effects include headache, sedation, insomnia, dizziness, weakness or fatigue, tremor, and nervousness. Seizures are very uncommon but have been reported with all SSRIs. Serotonin has varying effects on the dopaminergic system. In many cases, extrapyramidal related symptoms such as dystonic reactions, akathisia, dyskinesia, hypokinesia, and parkinsonian symptoms have been reported in association with SSRI therapy.[10] Consequently, SSRIs should be used cautiously with antipsychotic agents because SSRIs can potentiate antidopaminergic activity. Gastrointestinal complaints such as nausea, diarrhea, constipation, vomiting, and anorexia are commonly reported by patients taking SSRIs. Other adverse effects less commonly reported include dry mouth, increased sweating, blurred vision, hyponatremia, and hypoglycemia. Hyponatremia is believed to be secondary to inappropriate secretion of antidiuretic hormone (syndrome of inappropriate antidiuretic hormone or SIADH). Sexual dysfunction (e.g., anorgasmia) is a relatively common SSRI-related adverse effect and is reversible with drug discontinuation. Priapism has been reported but is extremely rare. A withdrawal syndrome consisting of nonspecific neurologic, psychiatric, and gastrointestinal symptoms has been described in conjuncture with abrupt SSRI discontinuation. It is less likely to occur with fluoxetine, since it has a long-acting metabolite.

Acute Overdose Toxicity

Despite the tremendous popularity of SSRIs, there is limited information on their toxicity in overdose. The greatest amount of human overdose experience has been with fluoxetine.[11] The information from case series involving the other SSRIs is consistent with the information accumulated on fluoxetine.[12–15] However, important differences may exist between the different SSRIs that will become evident only with greater exposure of patients to individual SSRIs. Fortunately, all of the SSRIs are characterized by a high toxic to therapeutic ratio, and fatalities are uncommon with pure SSRI overdoses. Approximately one-half of all adult patients and 75 percent of pediatric patients remain asymptomatic following SSRI overdose. The most common symptoms seen in SSRI overdose include nausea, vomiting, sedation, tremor, and sinus tachycardia. These symptoms are almost identical to the adverse effect profile of SSRIs except for sinus tachycardia, which is more common in overdose and rarely reported as an adverse effect. Less frequently observed symptoms include mydriasis, seizures, diarrhea, agitation, hallucinations, hypertension, and hypotension. Sertraline may produce mild CNS stimulation in pediatric patients.[13] Sinus bradycardia was observed more frequently in fluvoxamine overdoses than with other SSRIs. Citalopram produced QRS widening in approximately one-third of cases when more than 600 mg was ingested.[15] In another case series, prolongation of the QT interval has been reported in association with significant citalopram ingestions. Other SSRIs have rarely been reported to produce similar electrocardiographic abnormalities. It most cases, the electrocardiographic abnormalities gradually resolve over 24 h. Tachycardia, mild hypotension, and lethargy are more commonly seen when SSRIs are combined with ethanol. Mixed-drug ingestions can produce a wide variety of additional symptoms, depending on the coingestant toxicity. Serotonin syndrome can occur as a consequence of acute SSRI overdose. The results of laboratory tests are usually normal in SSRI overdoses. As previously mentioned, SSRI therapy has been associated with drug-induced SIADH secretion, which may result in symptomatic hyponatremia.

Treatment

Patients who intentionally overdose with SSRI require immediate attention, establishment of a peripheral intravenous line, and cardiac monitoring. Overall, pure SSRI overdoses are associated with limited toxicity except for the infrequent development of life-threatening complications such as generalized seizures and serotonin syndrome. The optimal method of gastrointestinal decontamination in SSRI poisoning remains undetermined. Based on the high therapeutic index and unlikelihood of serious toxicity, single-dose activated charcoal (1 g/kg) is logical for most ingestions, and gastric lavage is probably unnecessary in the majority of SSRI overdoses. However, gastric lavage may have greater utility in the setting of mixed-drug overdoses or if extremely large doses of SSRIs have been recently ingested. Due to the potential for seizures and CNS sedation, syrup of ipecac is contraindicated in adult intentional ingestions.

All patients should be observed for at least 6 h, during which supportive care is generally all that is required. Psychiatric evaluation is warranted for intentional ingestions. Hospital admission is recommended for all patients who remain tachycardic or lethargic 6 h after ingestion. Patients at higher risk for complications include those with underlying seizure disorders, symptoms of serotonin syndrome, or mixed-drug overdoses that have the potential for additional or delayed toxicity. Sodium bicarbonate therapy is indicated in cases of SSRI-induced QRS prolongation, primarily seen after citalopram ingestions of greater than 600 mg, and is administered in an identical manner as described in Chapter 152. Other SSRIs have only rarely been associated with QRS widening. Benzodiazepines are recommended as initial anticonvulsant therapy. Barbiturates are probably equally as effective as benzodiazepines but are more sedating. Rare reports of delayed seizures, up to 16 h after ingestion, have been reported. Delayed onset of serotonin syndrome or extrapyramidal reactions are theoretic possibilities that should be considered in all patients.

VENLAFAXINE

Venlafaxine (Effexor), a bicyclic compound that is structurally different from other antidepressants, was released in 1994 for the treatment of depression. In contrast to the SSRIs, venlafaxine is a nonselective inhibitor of serotonin, norepinephrine, and dopamine reuptake.[16] Whether this nonselectivity offers any advantage over SSRIs, bupropion, trazodone, nefazodone, or mirtazapine is currently unknown. Venlafaxine has no significant direct effect on presynaptic or postsynaptic neurotransmitter receptors and does not inhibit MAO activity. It is available in 25-mg, 37.5-mg, 50-mg, 75-mg, and 100-mg tablets. The recommended starting dose is 75 mg/day, which can be gradually increased up to a maximum daily dose of 375 mg. It has a category C rating in pregnancy.

Peak levels occur 2 h after ingestion. It is poorly protein bound (27 percent), and it has volume of distribution of 6 to 7 L/kg and a half-life of approximately 5 h. The majority of venlafaxine undergoes hepatic P-450 oxidation, but it is a weak inhibitor of P-450 enzyme activity. To date, no significant pharmacokinetic drug interactions have been reported. It has one active metabolite, *O*-desmethylvenlafaxine, which is pharmacologically similar to its parent drug, except for a longer half-life of 11 h. The adverse effect profile for venlafaxine is similar to the aforementioned one for SSRIs. The only notable exception is the occurrence of mild to moderate hypertension when doses exceed 225 mg/day, which is probably secondary to inhibition of norepinephrine reuptake. Venlafaxine has the same potential as other serotonin agonists to produce serotonin syndrome. Therefore, it should not be combined with MAOIs or other serotonin agonists. Because of its shorter half-life, venlafaxine requires only a 1-week abstinence period before initiating MAOI therapy. However, a 2-week abstinence period is still required after MAOI discontinuation before starting venlafaxine therapy.

Acute Overdose Toxicity

Information regarding venlafaxine toxicity in overdose is limited to isolated case reports. Unfortunately, most of these cases also include significant coingestants, confounding the interpretation of "pure" venlafaxine toxicity. Sympathetic nervous system stimulation, via inhibition of norepinephrine reuptake, predisposes patients to tachycardia, hypertension, diaphoresis, tremor, and mydriasis. These symptoms are frequently seen in venlafaxine overdoses. Severe hypotension, requiring vasopressors, was reported one case. Otherwise, most vital sign abnormalities are of moderate severity and do not require specific pharmacologic therapy. CNS sedation is also commonly reported and occasionally progresses to coma requiring endotracheal intubation and ventilatory support. Generalized seizures are frequently reported and tend to occur early after ingestion. Electrocardiographic abnormalities include sinus tachycardia, QRS widening, and QTc interval prolongation. In most cases, symptoms completely resolve gradually over 36 h with supportive care alone.

Treatment

There are no established guidelines for treating venlafaxine overdoses. All patients require at least 6 h of observation. Venlafaxine toxicity is often precipitous and should be anticipated in all intentional overdoses. These patients require immediate emergency physician evaluation, establishment of a peripheral intravenous line, and cardiac monitoring. Venlafaxine appears to have greater toxicity in overdose than SSRIs and probably deserves more aggressive gastric decontamination. Gastric lavage should be strongly considered for most intentional ingestions with early presentation. Accidental ingestions can be treated with single-dose activated charcoal alone. Benzodiazepines are the anticonvulsants of choice. Hypertension and sinus tachycardia rarely require specific pharmacologic therapy. β Blockers have the theoretical disadvantage of allowing unopposed α-adrenergic receptor stimulation. Sodium bicarbonate therapy should be considered in venlafaxine overdoses associated with QRS widening greater than 100 ms. All symptomatic patients should be admitted to a monitored bed.

SEROTONIN SYNDROME

Serotonin syndrome is a rare but important idiosyncratic drug-induced complication of antidepressant therapy.[17] It can be produced by any drug or, more commonly, by a combination of drugs that increase central serotonin neurotransmission (Table 153-1). The stimulation of specific postsynaptic serotonin receptors (5-HT_{1A} and 5-HT_2) is required for full expression of this syndrome. Drugs (like ondansetron) that block serotonin postsynaptic receptors are incapable of inducing this syndrome. The majority of cases occur at therapeutic levels, with fewer than 13 percent of cases being associated with drug overdose. Serotonin syndrome is characterized by alterations in cognition and behavior, autonomic nervous system function, and neuromuscular activity. The degree of abnormality in any one area is highly variable. Serotonin syndrome usually occurs either relatively soon after the dose of a potent serotonin agonist (MAOI or SSRI) has been increased or shortly after a second serotonergic agent (e.g., dextromethorphan) has been added. The importance of serotonin syndrome in emergency practice is twofold. First, the diagnosis of serotonin syndrome is very challenging due to its nonspecific symptomatology. Mild cases of serotonin syndrome are frequently attributed to other psychiatric and medical disorders. Severe cases are often misdiagnosed as neuroleptic malignant syndrome. Second, without proper recognition of patients at risk for serotonin syndrome, emergency physicians may inadvertently precipitate serotonin syndrome by administering serotonergic agents (e.g., meperidine). Therefore, emergency physicians should exercise the same drug-interaction precautions in treating patients taking newer antidepressants as those listed in Chapter 154, "Monoamine Oxidase Inhibitors."

The true incidence and severity of serotonin syndrome are unknown. Prospective studies on serotonin syndrome tend to overesti-

TABLE 153-1 Serotonergic Potential of Various Drugs

Extreme Potency	Moderate Potency	Low Potency	None
Amitriptyline	Amphetamine	Amantadine	Acetaminophen
Citalopram	Buspirone	Bromocriptine	Granisetron
Clomipramine	Cocaine	Bupropion	Metoclopramide
Dexfenfluramine	Desipramine	Carbamazepine	Morphine
Dextromethorphan	Doxepin	Cisapride	NSAIDs
Fenfluramine	Levodopa	Codeine	Ondansetron
Fluoxetine	LSD	Pentazocine	Salicylates
Fluvoxamine	Mescaline	Pergolide	
Imipramine	Mirtazapine	Reserpine	
Isocarboxazid	Nefazodone		
L-Tryptophan	Nortriptyline		
5-Hydroxytryptophan (5-HTP)‡	St. John's wort‡		
Lithium	Sumatriptan		
MDMA	Trazodone		
Meperidine			
Moclobemide*			
Pargyline†			
Paroxetine			
Phenelzine			
Selegiline			
Sertraline			
Tramadol			
Tranylcypromine			
Venlafaxine			

*Not available in the United States.
†No longer manufactured in the United States.
‡Over-the-counter herbal product.
Note: The serotonergic potential of the drugs listed was determined by both objective and subjective criteria and can be influenced by different doses and formulations.
Abbreviations: LSD, lysergic acid diethylamide; MDMA, 3,4-methylenedioxymethamphetamine; NSAIDs, nonsteroidal anti-inflammatory drugs.

mate its incidence and underestimate its severity. Conversely, case reports are often associated with incomplete documentation and tend to overestimate the severity and underestimate the incidence of serotonin syndrome. The most commonly reported signs and symptoms associated with serotonin syndrome are listed in Table 153-2. Interestingly, muscle rigidity, when present, is especially prominent in the lower extremities. This finding can serve as a valuable clinical marker for serotonin syndrome. Patients with ataxia should be carefully examined for lower extremity hypertonia. Unilateral muscle rigidity or focal neurologic findings have not been reported. Seizures are always generalized and usually short-lived. Hyperthermia is usually of moderate severity, but temperatures greater than 106°F (41°C) are not rare. Hypertension is twice as common as hypotension and is associated with a more favorable prognosis.

There are no confirmatory laboratory tests for serotonin syndrome. Therefore, the diagnosis of serotonin syndrome is based entirely on clinical suspicion and exclusion of other psychiatric and medical conditions. Serum chemistry tests, drug levels, cerebral spinal fluid analysis, and brain computed tomographic scan results are usually within normal limits. The differential diagnosis for serotonin syndrome is identical to those conditions listed in Chap. 154, "Monoamine Oxidase Inhibitors," Table 154-3.

The initial treatment of serotonin syndrome includes discontinuing all serotonergic drugs and providing appropriate supportive care. All patients with serotonin syndrome should be admitted to the hospital until their symptoms have completely resolved. The more severely ill patients require admission to an intensive care unit. Approximately 25 percent of patients require endotracheal intubation and ventilatory support. Most patients will show dramatic improvement within 24 h after symptom onset. However, fatalities have been reported. There is an estimated 11 percent mortality rate associated with serotonin syndrome.

TABLE 153-2 Clinical Presentation of Serotonin Syndrome*

Cognitive-Behavioral	%	Autonomic Dysfunction	%	Neuromuscular Dysfunction	%
Confusion/disorientation	54	Hyperthermia	46	Myoclonus	57
Agitation	35	Diaphoresis	46	Hyperreflexia	55
Coma	28	Sinus tachycardia	41	Muscle rigidity	49
Anxiety	16	Hypertension	33	Tremor	49
Hypomania	15	Tachypnea	28	Hyperactivity	43
Lethargy	15	Dilated pupils	26	Ataxia	38
Seizures	14	Unreactive pupils	18	Shivering	25
Insomnia	10	Flushed skin	14	Babinski sign	14
Hallucinations	6	Hypotension	14	Nystagmus	13
Dizziness	6	Diarrhea	12	Teeth chattering	6
		Abdominal cramps	5	Opisthotonus	6
		Salivation	5	Trismus	6

*Percentages are based on a retrospective study of 127 cases of serotonin syndrome.
Source: Adapted from Mills,[17] with permission.

At present, there are no accepted guidelines for the use of serotonin antagonists in the treatment of serotonin syndrome. Isolated human case reports suggest that cyproheptadine, methysergide, and propranolol have the potential to be effective antiserotonergic agents. Benzodiazepines are nonspecific serotonin antagonists and can be used to decrease patient discomfort and promote muscle relaxation. Cyproheptadine (Periactin) appears to be the most effective antiserotonergic agent in humans.[17,18] It should be on most hospital formularies. The initial dose is 4 to 8 mg PO. This dose can be repeated in 2 h if no response is noted to the initial dose. Cyproheptadine therapy should be discontinued if no response is noted after 16 mg has been administered. Patients who respond to cyproheptadine are usually given 4 mg every 6 h for 48 h to prevent recurrences. The use of dopamine agonists (e.g., bromocriptine) have no accepted role in managing patients with serotonin syndrome. Dantrolene (0.5 to 2.5 mg/kg IV q6h, maximum 10 mg/kg/24 h or 50 to 100 mg bid PO) is a nonspecific muscle relaxant that is occasionally used in serotonin syndrome, but it should be primarily restricted for the treatment of malignant hyperthermia. Patients with muscle rigidity, seizures, or hyperthermia should be closely monitored for rhabdomyolysis and/or metabolic acidosis. Once a patient recovers from serotonin syndrome, it is best to avoid future exposure to serotonergic drugs (Table 153-1), although the risk of recurrence is unknown.

REFERENCES

1. Litovitz TI, Klein-Schwartz W, Dyer KS, et al: 1997 Annual report of the American Association of Poison Control Centers Toxic Exposure Surveillance System. *Am J Emerg Med* 16:443, 1998.
2. Haria M, Fitton A, McTavich D: Trazodone: A review of its pharmacology, therapeutic use in depression, and therapeutic potential in other disorders. *Drugs Aging* 4:331, 1994.
3. Cyr M, Brown CS: Nefazodone: Its place among antidepressants. *Ann Pharmacother* 30:1006, 1996.
4. Goodnick PJ: Pharmacokinetics of second generation antidepressants: Bupropion. *Psychopharmacol Bull* 27:513, 1991.
5. Spiller HA, Ramoska EA, Krenzelok EP: Bupropion overdose: A 3-year multi-center retrospective analysis. *Am J Emerg Med* 12:43, 1994.
6. Puzantian T: Mirtazapine, an antidepressant. *Am J Health System Pharm* 55:44, 1998.
7. Bremmer JD, Wingard P, Walshe TA: Safety of mirtazapine in overdose. *J Clin Psychiatry* 59:233, 1998.
8. Mourilhe P, Stokes PE: Risks and benefits of selective serotonin reuptake inhibitors in the treatment of depression. *Drug Saf* 18:57, 1998.
9. Mitchell PB: Drug interactions of clinical significance with selective serotonin reuptake inhibitors. *Drug Saf* 17: 390, 1997.
10. Caley CF: Extrapyramidal reactions and the selective serotonin-reuptake inhibitors. *Ann Pharmacother* 31:1481, 1997.
11. Borys DJ, Setzer SC, Ling LJ, et al.: Acute fluoxetine overdose: A report of 234 cases. *Am J Emerg Med* 10:115, 1992.
12. Klein-Schwartz W, Anderson B: Analysis of sertraline-only overdoses. *Am J Emerg Med* 14:456, 1996.
13. Lau GT, Horowitz BZ: Sertraline overdose. *Acad Emerg Med* 3:132, 1996.
14. Myers L, Krenzelok EP: Paroxetine (Paxil) overdose: A pediatric focus. *Vet Hum Toxicol* 39:86, 1997.
15. Personne M, Sjoberg G, Persson H: Citalopram overdose: Review of cases treated in Swedish Hospitals. *Clin Toxicol* 35:237, 1997.
16. Ellingrod VL, Perry PJ: Venlafaxine: A heterocyclic antidepressant. *Am J Hosp Pharm* 51:3033, 1994.
17. Mills KC: Serotonin syndrome: A clinical update. *Crit Care Clin* 13:763, 1997.
18. Graudins A, Stearman A, Chan B: Treatment of the serotonin syndrome with cyproheptadine. *J Emerg Med* 16:615, 1998.

154 MONOAMINE OXIDASE INHIBITORS

Kirk C. Mills

EPIDEMIOLOGY

Monoamine oxidase inhibitors (MAOIs) have been in clinical use for over 40 years; they were the first effective agents in the treatment of major depression. However, because of their inherent toxicity and the development of safer antidepressants, MAOIs are now generally reserved for atypical or refractory cases. Despite their decreasing popularity, MAOIs still pose one of the most complex pharmacologic and toxicologic challenges faced by emergency medicine physicians. They are associated with a narrow therapeutic index, potential for fatal food (e.g., tyramine reaction) and drug (e.g., serotonin syndrome) interactions as well as severe toxicity in overdose. Currently, three MAOIs are used as antidepressants in the United States: phenelzine (Nardil), tranylcypromine (Parnate), and isocarboxazid (Marplan). Approximately 14 million tablets of tranylcypromine were sold during 1997 and 40,000 prescriptions for phenelzine were filled during the first quarter of 1998 (personal communication: Parke-Davis and SmithKline Beecham Pharmaceuticals). The American Association of Poison Control Centers Toxic Exposure Surveillance System recorded 2325 exposures to MAOIs between 1997 and 1993.[1] Of these exposures, 75 percent occurred in adults, 40 percent were intentional ingestions, and 80 percent of patients developed symptoms. There were also 21 reported MAOI-related deaths during the same 5-year period, averaging 1 death for every 100 exposures. Mortality rates of up to 33 percent have been reported.[2] In contrast, trazodone (an atypical antidepressant) averaged 1 death for every 1200 exposures.[1] This comparison underscores the greater toxicity of MAOIs as compared with newer antidepressant agents.

The only federally approved indication for MAOI antidepressant therapy is for the treatment of nonendogenous depression (i.e., atypical depression or depression refractory to other antidepressants). Other conditions that have shown positive responses to MAOI antidepressant therapy include social phobia disorders, panic disorders, posttraumatic stress syndrome, obsessive-compulsive disorder, bulimia, and narcolepsy. MAOIs inhibitors are not approved for use in children below 16 years of age. Several newer MAOI antidepressants with improved safety and tolerability have been developed, but they are available only outside the United States. Conceivably, some of these newer MAOI antidepressants may gain future approval for domestic release and marketing.

St. John's wort (*Hypericum perforatum*) is a popular over-the-counter herbal treatment for depression and has been reported to demonstrate slight MAOI activity.[3] A specific history of herb use should be sought, since most patients do not consider St. John's wort a "drug." Although generally safe, St. John's wort should still be viewed with caution, since even mild MAOI activity may become more clinically significant in overdose or with certain drug interactions.

Selegiline (Eldepryl) is a MAOI that is devoid of antidepressant activity but is used as an adjunct to the treatment of Parkinson disease.[4] However, at increasing doses, it has activity similar to that of traditional MAOI antidepressants (see below). Some drugs have MAOI activity as an unrelated action, which may predispose patients using them to experience drug interactions. Examples include procarbazine (Matulane), a chemotherapeutic agent for severe Hodgkin lymphoma, and furazolidone (Furoxone), a synthetic nitrofuran with antimicrobial and antiprotozoan activity. Pargyline (Eutonyl) has been discontinued for over a decade but was an antihypertensive agent whose primary mechanism of action was MAO inhibition. Although the information in this chapter has relevance to all drugs with MAOI activity, it focuses primarily on phenelzine, tranylcypromine, isocarboxazid, and selegiline toxicity.

PATHOPHYSIOLOGY

Monoamine oxidase (MAO) is an intracellular enzyme bound to the outer mitochondrial membrane.[5] It has been identified in most human cells. A notable exception is erythrocytes, which do not contain mitochondria. MAO removes amine groups from both endogenous and exogenous biogenic amines. This oxidation deamination process is the primary mechanism by which endogenous biogenic amines such as norepinephrine (NE), dopamine (DA), and 5-hydroxytryptamine (serotonin or 5-HT) become inactivated. A second important function of MAO is to decrease the systemic availability of absorbed dietary biogenic amines (e.g., tyramine) via hepatic and intestinal metabolism. Therefore, inhibition of MAO leads to the accumulation of neurotransmitters in presynaptic nerve terminals (both centrally and peripherally) and allows for increased systemic availability of dietary amines. Monoamine oxidase has a negligible role in metabolizing circulating catecholamines, which are either secreted endogenously (e.g., by the adrenal gland) or administered intravenously (e.g., epinephrine). This function is accomplished by a different enzyme, catechol-O-methyl transferase (COMT), which is located extraneuronally and is not affected by MAOIs.

MAO is actually two separate isoenzymes, designated MAO-A and MAO-B. Each isoenzyme has its own relative preference for different neurotransmitters, dietary amines, and MAOIs. These substrate preferences are entirely dose-dependent and can be overcome at higher substrate concentrations or MAOI doses (e.g., selegiline). For example, MAO-A has a 1000 times greater affinity for serotonin than MAO-B, but the ability of MAO-B to metabolize serotonin increases at higher serotonin concentrations. Norepinephrine is primarily metabolized by MAO-A, whereas MAO-A and MAO-B have equal ability to metabolize dopamine and tyramine. Overall, the human brain contains more MAO-B than MAO-A, with MAO-B predominance increasing with advancing age. Dopamine neurons appear to lack MAO-B activity and have limited MAO-A activity.[6] Significant MAO-B activity has been detected in surrounding astrocytes and glial cells. Thus, dopamine inactivation may be dependent on astrocyte and glial-cell metabolism. Interestingly, MAO-B is the exclusive isoenzyme found in serotonergic neurons. This paradox may be explained by simple conservation of energy, where the MAO-B isoenzyme has a lower affinity for 5-HT and allows for more 5-HT to become recycled. It also allows for increased metabolism of nonserotonin bioamines, thus keeping the neuron free of false neurotransmitters. Intestinal MAO activity is mostly secondary to MAO-A, whereas approximately equal proportions of both isoenzymes are found in the liver. The dual representation of both isoenzymes in the intestines and liver affords greater protection against the tyramine reaction if only one isoenzyme is inhibited (i.e., selective inhibitors).

MAOIs share structural similarities with endogenous amines (e.g., NE, 5-HT, DA), and this allows them to act as potential substrates for MAO. The antidepressant activity of phenelzine, tranylcypromine, and isocarboxazid has generally been attributed to their ability to increase NE and 5-HT neurotransmission by increasing presynaptic concentrations of serotonin and norepinephrine. The actual mechanism by which they exert their therapeutic effects remains unproved but is probably related to delayed postsynaptic receptor modifications (e.g., downregulation). Other potential mechanisms of action include indirect release of neurotransmitters and inhibition of neurotransmitter reuptake. MAOIs also inhibit other enzyme systems (e.g., pyridoxal phosphokinase, diamine oxidase, etc.), but this finding is of uncertain clinical significance. Selegiline has limited effects on NE and 5-HT metabolism at therapeutic doses (10 mg/day). The therapeutic benefit of selegiline in Parkinson disease is thought to be related to increased striatal dopamine neurotransmission and protecting against neuronal damage from oxidative stress.[4,6] However, at doses greater than 30 mg/day, selegiline is capable of increasing presynaptic NE and 5-HT concentrations and thus has the potential to produce drug-related toxicity similar to that of phenelzine and tranylcypromine.

All of the currently available MAOI antidepressants are irreversible and nonselective (MAO-A, MAO-B) in their enzyme inhibition. MAOIs form irreversible covalent bonds with the MAO enzymes, and this renders the enzyme permanently inactive. Once an irreversible MAOI has been discontinued, it takes approximately 2 weeks before new enzyme synthesis has returned MAO activity to 50 percent of normal. MAOIs do not affect enzyme production. At therapeutic doses, selegiline primarily inhibits MAO-B, but this selectivity is lost at higher doses. Reversible MAOIs do not form irreversible covalent bonds with MAO. Thus, new enzyme synthesis is not necessary to restore MAO activity and MAO activity will gradually return to normal over a period of hours as the drug-enzyme complex spontaneously dissociates. As previously mentioned, reversible MAOIs are currently not available in the United States but are commonly utilized in other countries. Examples of reversible MAOIs include moclobemide, toloxatone, brofaromine, and cimoxatone.

All MAOIs are rapidly and completely absorbed from the gastrointestinal tract.[8] They have relatively low bioavailability because of a large first-pass effect of hepatic metabolism. Their dependence on hepatic metabolism predisposes them to potential drug interactions with other drugs requiring hepatic oxidation. Peak drug levels usually occur 1 to 3 h after ingestion. They have relatively large volumes of distribution (1 to 5 L/kg) and are highly protein-bound. Elimination half-life averages between 2 and 3 h. It is important to recognize that clinical toxicity is usually delayed well after most of the MAOI has already been metabolized. Thus, blood MAOI levels do not correlate with clinical toxicity. Selegiline has many active metabolites, such as desmethylselegiline, amphetamine, and methamphetamine. Tranylcypromine has long been suspected of having amphetamine as a metabolite, but this has rarely been detected. Phenelzine metabolism results in multiple active metabolites such as B-phenylethylamine, which also serves as a substrate for MAO-B.[7] The pharmacokinetic profile of most MAOIs suggests that attempts at extracorporeal removal (e.g., hemodialysis) or administering repeat doses of activated charcoal would be unsuccessful in significantly reducing MAOI plasma levels.

TYRAMINE REACTION

Tyramine is an exogenous dietary amine that is normally metabolized by intestinal and hepatic MAO enzymes.[8] In patients taking a nonselective MAOI, a greater amount of tyramine is able to reach the systemic circulation. Tranylcypromine is more frequently associated with tyramine reactions than phenelzine or isocarboxazid. Selegiline (MAO-B selective) is unlikely to produce a tyramine reaction if taken at therapeutic doses. Tyramine is classified as an indirect sympathomimetic and is structurally similar to amphetamine. Like most indirect sympathomimetics, tyramine enters the presynaptic neuron through amine uptake pumps. Once inside the neuron, indirect sympathomimetics are capable of releasing presynaptic stores of norepinephrine and to a lesser degree serotonin and dopamine. Tyramine can also displace epinephrine from the adrenal gland. This action produces the "cheese" reaction since aged cheese contains a large amount of tyramine. In similar fashion, broad (fava) beans contains large quantities of dopamine.

Tyramine is found in over 70 foods and beverages, and any one of these sources may trigger such a reaction.[9] It has been reported that less than 30 percent of patients comply with a MAOI-restrictive diet. In addition, approximately 4 to 8 percent of compliant patients will experience a tyramine reaction during their course of therapy. Nonetheless, newer guidelines call for avoiding only a few high-risk food groups such as meat or fish that is not fresh, sauerkraut, aged meats and cheeses, alcohol (Chianti wine and vermouth), pickled fish (herring), concentrated yeast extracts, and broad beans.

The tyramine reaction is typically of rapid onset, occurring within 15 to 90 min after the dietary amine is ingested. The severity of this reaction is highly variable and partially related to the total amount of tyramine ingested. The hallmark symptom of the tyramine reaction is a severe occipital or temporal headache. Other associated symptoms include hypertension, diaphoresis, mydriasis, neck stiffness, pallor, neuromuscular excitation, palpitations, and/or chest pain. Most symptoms gradually resolve over 6 h without specific therapy but fatalities have been rarely reported, usually due to intracranial hemorrhage or myocardial infarction. Therefore, an electrocardiogram should be obtained on all patients with tyramine-associated chest pain. Focal neurologic findings or a persistent severe headache warrants investigation with a computed tomography (CT) scan of the head.

In cases of severe hypertension the drug of choice remains phentolamine (Regitine), which is given intravenously in 2.5- to 5-mg doses every 5 to 15 min until the blood pressure is controlled. The half-life of phentolamine is approximately 20 min, and its duration of action less than 1 h. Nitroprusside (Nipride) is another rapidly acting direct vasodilator, which is always administered as a continuous infusion (1 to 4 μg/kg per minute). In cases of moderate hypertension, nifedipine (Procardia) and prazosin (Minipress) have been reported to be effective. Newer recommendations for the treatment of accelerated chronic hypertension discourage the use of nifedipine due to concerns of excessive blood pressure reduction. These concerns may not apply to the acute hypertension seen in tyramine reactions. Beta-adrenergic blockers should be considered contraindicated due to unopposed alpha-receptor stimulation. Hospital admission should be strongly considered for patients whose symptoms do not completely resolve within 6 h after onset.

DRUG INTERACTIONS

Chronic MAOI drug therapy predisposes to many potentially significant drug interactions (Table 154-1). However, documentation of human MAOI drug interactions is often limited to single case reports or case series.[10] Controlled human studies are impractical due to the life-threatening nature of these reactions. Animal studies often have limited applicability to human toxicity. Most importantly, emergency physicians should never administer medications to patients taking MAOIs unless absolutely necessary. Drug compatibility with monoamine oxidase inhibitors should always be confirmed prior to drug administration.

Drug interactions involving MAOIs can be grouped into three categories: pharmacodynamic, pharmacokinetic, and idiosyncratic. The most common pharmacodynamic reaction involves indirect-acting sympathomimetics. They have the potential to produce a hyperadrenergic condition similar to the tyramine reaction (see above) and can be found in over-the-counter preparations, drugs of abuse, and some prescription products. Pharmacokinetic drug interactions have been noted with MAOIs because they are metabolized through the cytochrome oxidase enzyme system and thus can inhibit the metabolism of other drugs. The potentiation of opiate and sedative-hypnotic drugs is an example of this type of enzyme inhibition. Tranylcypromine and phenelzine have been shown to increase insulin release and predispose to hypoglycemia, especially in patients taking oral sulfonylureas agents. Insulin dosage may also warrant reduction. Serotonin syndrome is a rare, potentially life-threatening idiosyncratic reaction. It most commonly occurs when MAOIs are combined with other serotonergic agents. A complete description of serotonin syndrome as well as a listing of serotonergic medications can be found in Chap. 153, on newer antidepressants. However, specific emphasis pertaining to emergency physicians is placed on the avoidance of using meperidine (Demerol),[11] dextromethorphan, or tramadol (Ultram) in combination with MAOIs. Even after a patient discontinues MAOI therapy, it still takes 2 weeks before 50 percent of MAO enzyme activity returns. Consequently, there should always be at least a 2-week abstinence period between the time of MAOI discontinuation and the time that any contraindicated drug is administered. This recommendation is particularly important to prevent the development of serotonin syndrome.

It is also important to note which medications are generally considered safe in patients on MAOIs (Table 154-2). Aspirin, acetaminophen, ibuprofen, and morphine have been used in combination with MAOIs without complications. Morphine should be given in decreased doses due to impaired morphine metabolism and enhanced opiate effects. Direct-acting sympathomimetic agents (e.g., norepinephrine) can be used with caution, utilizing the lowest possible effective dose. Direct sympathomimetics do not rely on the release of neurotransmitters for their activity and they are inactivated by the enzyme COMT, which is unaffected by MAOIs.

TABLE 154-1 Drugs Contraindicated with MAOIs*

Indirect Sympathomimetics	Miscellaneous Drugs
Benzphetamine	Beta blockers
Bretylium	Bupropion
Cocaine	Buspirone
Dexfenfluramine	Caffeine
Diethylpropion	Carbamazepine
Dopamine	Cyclobenzaprine
Ephedrine	Dextromethorphan
Fenfluramine	Disulfiram
Guanethidine	Ergot alkaloids
Isometheptene	Fentanyl
Mephentermine	Furazolidone
Metaraminol	Ketamine
Methamphetamine	Levodopa (L-dopa)
3,4-methylenedioxymethamphetamine (MDMA)	Lithium
Methyldopa	Meperidine
Methylphenidate	Mirtazapine
Pemoline	Oral hypoglycemic agents
Phentermine	Phenothiazines
Phencyclidine	Procarbazine
Phenylpropanolamine	St. John's wort
Propylhexedrine	Sumatriptan
Pseudoephedrine	Theophylline
Reserpine	Tramadol
Ritodrine	Tricyclic antidepressants
Tyramine	

*See additional list of drugs causing serotonin syndrome in Chap. 153, on newer antidepressants, Table 153-3.

CLINICAL FEATURES (ACUTE OVERDOSE)

MAOIs have a dangerously low toxic-to-therapeutic ratio. Ingestions of greater than 2 to 3 mg/kg of body weight can be life-threatening, and doses that are less than 2 mg/kg may still produce mild to moderate toxicity. The lethal dose of irreversible MAOI toxicity is reported to be between 4 and 6 mg/kg.[12] Deaths have been reported in adults with as little as 170 mg of tranylcypromine and 375 mg of phenelzine. Selegiline overdoses have not been reported but should be assumed to produce toxicity similar to that of the traditional MAOI antidepressants until determined otherwise. The average therapeutic dose of tranylcypromine ranges from 20 to 40 mg/day, with a maximum daily dose of 60 mg/day. It is available as a small, round, red 10-mg tablet. Therapeutic doses of phenelzine range between 45 and 75 mg/day, with a maximum of 90 mg/day. The drug comes as a small, round, orange 15-mg tablet. Isocarboxazid is manufactured as a 10-mg peach-colored tablet with therapeutic doses ranging between 10 and 30 mg/day. Selegiline has a standard dose of 10 mg/day and comes as an aqua 5-mg capsule.

An important clinical aspect of MAOI overdoses is that symptoms are characteristically delayed between 6 to 12 h postingestion but can be delayed as long as 24 h. The delayed onset of toxicity is believed to be secondary to the gradual accumulation of NE and 5-HT levels in the brain and in peripheral sympathetic neurons. Symptoms of MAOI overdose are most consistent with a hyperadrenergic state secondary to excessive stimulation of alpha- and beta-adrenergic receptors, but symptoms related to excessive serotonin receptor activity are also seen. Patients on chronic MAOI therapy may show earlier signs of toxicity due to preexisting enzyme inhibition. In severe cases, the hyperadrenergic state can be rapidly followed by hypotension and central nervous system depression resembling a sympatholytic condition. Toxicity usually persists for 1 to 4 days after ingestion.

The signs and symptoms of MAOI toxicity are often nonspecific. Even in its most severe form, it can resemble numerous other conditions (see below). Most clinical overdose information has come from single case reports or case series, with tremendous variation in presentation. Hence, there is no "typical" presentation to MAOI toxicity nor is there an orderly progression of symptoms. The clinician should anticipate the rapid development of life-threatening symptoms in all MAOI overdose patients. The initial symptoms of MAOI overdose are reported to include headache, agitation, irritability, nausea, palpitations, and tremor. The earliest signs of MAOI toxicity include sinus tachycardia, hyperreflexia, hyperactivity, fasciculations, mydriasis, hyperventilation, nystagmus, and generalized flushing. In cases of moderate toxicity, opisthotonus, muscle rigidity, diaphoresis, chest pain, hypertension, diarrhea, hallucinations, combativeness, confusion, marked hyperthermia, and trismus may become evident. A peculiar ocular finding has been observed with some cases of MAOI toxicity and is described as a "ping-pong" gaze because of the bilateral, wandering horizontal eye movements. The mechanism of this gaze

TABLE 154-2 Drugs Considered Safe with MAOIs*

Direct sympathomimetics
Albuterol aerosol
Dobutamine
Epinephrine
Isoproterenol
Methoxamine
Norepinephrine
Terbutaline
Miscellaneous drugs
Acetaminophen
Aspirin
Barbiturates
Benzodiazepines
Calcium channel blockers
Cephalosporins
Corticosteroids
Granisetron
Inhalation anesthetics
Lidocaine
Morphine
Nitroglycerin
Nitroprusside
Nonsteroidal anti-inflammatory drugs
Ondansetron
Penicillins
Phentolamine
Procainamide
Tropisetron

*Always use the lowest effective dose.

TABLE 154-3 Differential Diagnosis of Monoamine Oxidase Inhibitor Overdose

Intoxications	Medical conditions	Adverse drug reactions
Amphetamines	Heat stroke	Dystonic reactions
Antimuscarinics	Hypoglycemia	Malignant hyperthermia
Cathinone	Hyperthyroidism	Serotonin syndrome
Clonidine (early)	Pheochromocytoma	Tyramine reaction
Cocaine		Spontaneous hypertensive crisis
Lysergic acid diethylamide (LSD)		Neuroleptic malignant syndrome
Methylphenidate		
MDMA*		
Nicotine (early)		
Phencyclidine		
Phenylpropanolamine		
Strychnine		
Theophylline		
Tricyclic antidepressants (early)		
Withdrawal states	**Infectious diseases**	**Psychaitric**
Ethanol (delirium tremens)	Encephalitis	Lethal catatonia
Sedative-hypnotics	Meningitis	
Clonidine	Rabies	
Beta blockers	Sepsis	
	Tetanus	

*3,4-Methylenedioxymethamphetamine.

disorder is unknown. In all cases, it gradually resolves as the patient improves. Severe toxicity is accomplished by bradycardia, cardiac arrest, hypoxia, papilledema, hypotension, seizures, coma, and worsening hyperthermia. Hypotension is an ominous finding that commonly remains resistant to therapeutic attempts at correction. Fetal demise, cerebral edema, pulmonary edema, and intracranial hemorrhage have all been reported in association with MAOI overdoses. The most common electrocardiographic abnormality seen in MAOI toxicity is sinus tachycardia, but T-wave abnormalities are not uncommon. Deaths are usually secondary to multiple organ failure.

DIAGNOSIS

MAOI poisoning is not associated with any confirmatory laboratory tests. It remains a clinical diagnosis based solely on the history of excessive MAOI ingestion. Plasma MAOI levels and drug screens cannot be relied upon to assist in making the diagnosis of MAOI toxicity for two reasons. First, all commonly used drug screens are qualitatively unable to detect MAOIs. Second, specific quantitative plasma MAOI levels are not routinely available in most hospitals, nor do they correlate with observed clinical toxicity. Selegiline is likely to produce amphetamine metabolites, which can be detected on most urine drug screens. Tranylcypromine has the potential to produce amphetamine metabolites, but these have rarely been detected. The best use of laboratory tests is to assist in the differential diagnosis of MAOI toxicity and to identify possible complications of MAOI overdose, which include hypoxia, rhabdomyolysis, renal failure, hyperkalemia, metabolic acidosis, hemolysis, and disseminated intravascular coagulation. Leukocytosis and thrombocytopenia are commonly seen with MAOI toxicity.

The differential diagnosis of a MAOI overdose includes all drugs and medical conditions capable of producing a hyperadrenergic state, altered mental status, and/or muscle rigidity. As evidenced by the extensive number of conditions listed in Table 154-3, the differential diagnosis of the unknown MAOI ingestion is extremely challenging. In addition, MAOI toxicity can also be associated with a sympatholytic presentation, thus broadening the differential possibilities even further. In reality, without a history of exposure to MAOIs, it is highly unlikely that the correct diagnosis will be made in the emergency department (ED), since no confirmatory tests are available.

An interesting diagnostic dilemma exists when a patient on chronic MAOI therapy presents with elevated blood pressure. At therapeutic doses, hypertension can result from tyramine reactions, spontaneous hypertensive crisis, and serotonin syndrome. Tyramine reactions are likely to occur in close relation to food or drug ingestions containing indirect sympathomimetics. Spontaneous hypertensive crisis is a rare condition usually occurring in relation to recent MAOI dosing.[13] Serotonin syndrome most commonly occurs shortly after exposure to other serotonergic agents and is usually associated with significant cognitive-behavioral and neuromuscular abnormalities.

MANAGEMENT

General Emergency Department Care

All MAOI overdose patients require immediate emergency physician evaluation, establishment of at least one preferably large-base peripheral intravenous line, cardiac monitoring, supplemental oxygen, and gastric decontamination. General laboratory tests should be ordered on all patients, with particular emphasis on identifying early hyperkalemia, metabolic acidosis, and rhabdomyolysis. There are no known antidotes for MAOI toxicity. ED management is therefore directed toward supportive care and early treatment of complications. Onset of toxicity is usually gradual and delayed, sometimes up to 24 h postingestion. However, the abrupt development of seizures, coma, respiratory insufficiency, hyperadrenergic storm, and cardiovascular collapse is entirely possible. Greater toxicity for any given dose of MAOI is predicted in the setting of significant underlying medical problems, pediatric patients, geriatric patients, or coingested drugs.

The best method of gastric decontamination in the setting of MAOI overdose has never been studied. Therefore, the following recommendations are general guidelines based on the pharmacokinetic profile of MAOIs as well as results of human case reports. Syrup of ipecac is contraindicated in the setting of MAOI overdose because of the significant potential for cardiovascular collapse and loss of consciousness. Activated charcoal should be administered as a single dose of 1 g/kg as soon as possible. Multiple-dose administration of activated charcoal is not expected to be advantageous. Gastric lavage is recommended in all significant ingestions and should be performed within the first 2 h after ingestion to maximize drug removal. Since MAOIs are rapidly absorbed, delayed gastric lavage or whole-bowel irrigation is unlikely to be of any clinical benefit. Hemodialysis, hemoperfusion, and peritoneal dialysis have no established role in the treatment of MAOI poisoning. Urinary acidification is not recommended because it is ineffective at enhancing MAOI elimination and predisposes to acute renal failure secondary to myoglobin precipitation within renal tubules.

Management of Specific Conditions

HYPERTENSION The acutely hypertensive patient should be treated only with short-acting intravenous antihypertensive agents because of the potential to develop precipitous hypotension. In most cases, an intraarterial catheter is required for accurate blood pressure monitoring. The traditional antihypertensive agents of choice are phentolamine (Regitine) and nitroprusside (Nipride). Phentolamine is a nonspecific alpha-adrenergic receptor blocker usually administered in 2.5- to 5.0-mg boluses every 10 to 15 min until blood pressure elevation is controlled. It can also be given as a continuous infusion (0.2 to 0.5 mg/min) for maintenance therapy. Phentolamine use is commonly associated with reflex tachycardia. Nitroprusside is as effective as phentolamine. It is given as a continuous infusion with an initial rate of 1 μg/kg per minute and then titrated according to blood pressure response. Prolonged high doses of nitroprusside can predispose to cyanide toxicity, but this potential complication is rarely noted in the ED. The addition of thiosulfate to nitroprusside infusions eliminates the possibility of cyanide toxicity. Nitroglycerin is indicated for the relief of anginal chest pain and in patients with signs of myocardial ischemia. Fenoldopam (Corlopam) is a recently approved short-acting parenteral antihypertensive agent.[14] Its mechanism of action is secondary to peripheral dopamine (D_1) receptor stimulation. It reportedly does not cross the blood-brain barrier. There are no known contraindications to its use in MAOI-induced hypertension. Fenoldopam is administered as a titratable infusion with a suggested starting dose of 0.05 to 0.1 μg/kg per minute. Intravenous diltiazem (Cardizem) is expected to be an effective antihypertensive agent, but its long duration of action makes it less desirable than the previously mentioned shorter-acting agents. Beta blockers pose a theoretical risk of increasing the blood pressure through unopposed vasoconstriction and would appear to be contraindicated. Despite this concern, beta blockers have occasionally been used to treat hyperadrenergic symptoms in MAOI overdose without serious complications. At best, beta blockers should be used with great caution in the setting of MAOI toxicity. Labetalol is a beta blocker with slight alpha-receptor blocking ability. The theoretical benefit of its alpha-blocking capacity must be balanced against its beta-blocking activity, which is seven times greater.

HYPOTENSION Hypotension carries a poor prognosis in MAOI overdose. Isotonic intravenous fluid boluses of 10 to 20 mL/kg are the initial treatment of hypotension. When vasopressors are required, it is important to avoid all indirect-acting agents (see Table 154-1). Norepinephrine is the vasopressor of choice, with epinephrine as the second choice. MAOI patients usually demonstrate an increased sensitivity to vasopressors, and lower initial doses are recommended.

DYSRHYTHMIAS Sinus tachycardia rarely calls for specific drug therapy unless it is producing cardiac ischemia. Lidocaine and procainamide are the most effective antiarrhythmics in treating MAOI-induced ventricular dysrhythmias. Bradycardia may quickly degrade into asystole in the later stages of the overdose and require pacemaker placement. Pharmacologic treatment of bradycardia includes atropine, isoproterenol, and dobutamine. Bretylium should be avoided due to its indirect sympathomimetic activity (see Chap. 18).

SEIZURES Benzodiazepines are the anticonvulsants of choice in treating MAOI-induced seizures. Barbiturates are as effective as benzodiazepines but may cause hypotension, especially at higher doses. Phenytoin is generally ineffective in stopping drug-induced seizures. General anesthesia and/or muscle paralysis may be necessary in cases of status epilepticus to prevent the metabolic acidosis, hyperthermia, and rhabdomyolysis that commonly accompany persistent seizure activity. Muscle paralysis is best accomplished using nondepolarizing neuromuscular blocking agents. The action of succinylcholine may be enhanced by MAOIs. Pancuronium is probably less desirable than other nondepolarizing agents because of its propensity to produce elevations in heart rate and blood pressure. Vecuronium in doses of 0.25 mg/kg may produce paralysis in 90 s although its use with succinylcholine is relatively contraindicated in this setting. Tachycardia and histamine release do not occur. Electroencephalographic monitoring is required when muscle paralysis is used to control the peripheral manifestations of seizure activity. See Chap. 224 for details of treating seizures.

HYPERTHERMIA Antipyretics are generally ineffective at lowering drug-induced fever. Benzodiazepines are useful first-line agents by reducing muscle hyperactivity and thus decreasing secondary heat production. Increasing evaporative and conductive heat loss is essential for the successful treatment of hyperthermia. This is best accomplished by using cool mist spray, evaporative fans, and ice baths. Hyperthermia is often resilient in the setting of persistent muscle rigidity. Muscle paralysis (nondepolarizing agents) should be considered when diffuse rigidity is refractory to benzodiazepine therapy. Dantrolene has been successfully used as a muscle relaxant in resistant cases of muscle rigidity. The intravenous dose of dantrolene ranges from 0.5 to 2.5 mg/kg every 6 h. Dantrolene is associated with hepatotoxicity and should be used only when other measures have failed. Older reports of MAOI-induced hyperthermia cited successful treatment with phenothiazines (chlorpromazine). However, these agents are not currently recommended owing to their potential to lower the seizure threshold, worsen hypotension, and produce extrapyramidal reactions.

ADMISSION CRITERIA

All intentional MAOI overdoses and accidental exposures of greater than 1.0 mg/kg require admission to an intensive care unit. Accidental exposures of less than 1.0 mg/kg still require hospital admission but are unlikely to develop life-threatening complications. Therefore, these patients can be admitted to a less acutely monitored bed. It is important to remember that even a single MAOI pill may produce life-threatening drug interactions, such as serotonin syndrome, under the right circumstances. Therefore, emergency physicians should have a very low threshold to admit all MAOI exposures. Asymptomatic patients should be monitored for at least 24 h before medical clearance. Vital sign abnormalities should be recognized early and treated appropriately. Dietary and medication restrictions should be meticulously followed during the hospitalization. All patients should be instructed to avoid contraindicated foods and medications for a minimum of 2 weeks. Consultation with a medical toxicologist through the nearest regional poison control center is strongly recommended. Patients who require transfer to hospitals with intensive care units should be transferred as soon as possible to avoid the problems anticipated with delayed onset of toxicity. All patients being transferred should be accompanied by medical personnel capable of performing advanced cardiac life support and endotracheal intubation.

REFERENCES

1. Litovitz TI, Klein-Schwartz W, Dyer KS, et al: 1997 Annual report of the American Association of Poison Control Centers Toxic Exposure Surveillance System. *Am J Emerg Med* 16:443, 1998.
2. Meredith TJ, Vale JA: Poisoning due to psychotropic agents. *Adverse Drug React Ac Pois Rev* 4:83, 1985.

In addition to neurologic changes, renal dysfunction is common. Due to diabetes insipidus, patients complain of polyuria and polydipsia. Fluid losses may exacerbate toxicity. Acute renal failure may develop, particularly in patients with preexisting renal impairment, advanced age, diabetes, hypertension, or dehydration.

GI symptoms are common in both acute and chronic toxicity. Patients present with gastroenteritis, nausea, vomiting, diarrhea, bloating, or generalized abdominal pain. Leukocytosis can occur. Cardiac abnormalities are more common in acute toxicity, with hypotension, conduction abnormalities, and ventricular dysrhythmias. Electrocardiographic changes with transient ST depression and T-wave inversion are seen in some patients. Less common effects include hyperthermia, hypothermia, peripheral neuropathy, and severe leukopenia.

Up to 10 percent of patients die, generally of respiratory failure or cardiovascular collapse.[8] Most patients who recover will have no long-term sequelae. Chronic renal failure occasionally develops. Permanent cerebellar damage may develop and progress over several weeks following the toxic episode.[9,10] Patients have truncal ataxia, ataxic gait, scanning speech, and diffuse incoordination. Short-term memory loss, dementia, and a tremor of the hands and head accompany the cerebellar signs. Most patients improve over several months, but symptoms are permanent in some cases. Permanent seizure disorder has been reported.

TREATMENT

As in all toxicities, initial stabilization of patients must include protection of the airway, ventilatory support, and hemodynamic support. Intravenous access, cardiac monitoring (including 12-lead electrocardiogram), and laboratory analysis of blood and urine, including renal function, fluid/electrolytes, calcium, magnesium, complete blood count, urine specific gravity, and drug levels for lithium, acetaminophen, and other possible ingestants should be obtained. A complete medical history, including an assessment of baseline neurologic function, must be documented. Search for precipitating factors such as volume depletion or electrolyte imbalance. A complete listing of medications (prescription, over-the-counter, and herbal agents) taken in the previous week should be obtained. A thorough physical and neurologic examination is necessary.

Seizures should be treated with intravenous benzodiazepines. Refractory seizures may require phenobarbital or general anesthesia. Phenytoin decreases renal excretion of lithium and is often ineffective in drug-induced seizures.

GI decontamination is difficult in lithium toxicity. Activated charcoal is ineffective at adsorbing lithium at gastric pH.[11] Its use is not contraindicated, however, because it may be effective in cases of polydrug toxicity. Gastric emptying is as effective in lithium overdose as in other drug overdoses, and if it is done early after ingestion, some drug can be removed. Since lithium tablets are often quite large, small-bore tubing may be ineffective in removing the drug. Whole bowel irrigation (polyethylene glycol, 2 L/h in adults and 500 mL/h in children) is helpful, especially in cases where sustained-release medications have been ingested. Whole bowel irrigation initiated in the first hour can remove 60 percent of the drug.[12]

Aggressive hydration with normal saline is important. Nearly all patients with significant toxicity have some sodium and volume deficit. Sodium and water depletion impairs lithium elimination, and this increases and prolongs toxicity. In fact, in volume-depletion states, lithium may be preferentially resorbed by the kidney in an attempt to counter sodium loss. Volume repletion reestablishes normal elimination kinetics. Forced diuresis does not enhance lithium elimination once fluid losses have been replaced. In fact, loop and thiazide diuretics can be dangerous, because they further sodium and water loss.[13]

Although nearly all toxicologists agree that hemodialysis should be used for severely toxic patients, the threshold for initiating this treatment is still debated. Patients with levels greater than 3.5 meq/L (4.0 meq/L in acute ingestion), patients with little change in their lithium level of 1.5 to 3.5 meq/L after 6 h of hydration, or patients with sustained levels more than 1.0 meq/L after 36 h will benefit from hemodialysis.[14] In addition, patients with renal failure, those with rapidly increasing levels, or those who have ingested sustained-release preparations should be considered for treatment. Bicarbonate dialysate leads to greater intracellular extraction of lithium.[15]

TABLE 156-5 Comparison of Half-Life of Lithium with Treatment

Therapy	Serum Half-Life, h	Clearance, mL/min
No treatment	14–54	15
Saline		15
Peritoneal dialysis		10–15
Hemodialysis	4–6	50
Sodium polystyrene sulfonate	12	
Charcoal hemoperfusion		20

The goal of hemodialysis is to reduce the serum lithium level to less than 1 meq/L. Because of the cellular concentration of lithium, an increase in serum levels following termination of dialysis is common.[16] Drug levels must be monitored for up to 8 h following dialysis. If levels rise to greater than 1 meq/L, hemodialysis should be reinstituted. Because of the intracellular concentration of lithium in the CNS, neurologic symptoms may persist and even worsen during treatment.

Peritoneal dialysis and charcoal hemoperfusion have been used but are less effective than hemodialysis (Table 156-5).

In less severe toxicity, sodium polystyrene sulfonate (SPS, or Kayexalate; 15 g qid PO or 30 g rectal) is useful in decreasing serum half-life of lithium.[17,18] Approximately 75 percent of lithium is bound to SPS in vitro compared with less than 25 percent when activated charcoal is used. Although experience with SPS is limited, it may be useful for mild to moderate toxicity. Because SPS is an exchange resin, large electrolyte shifts may occur during its use, and electrolyte level must be monitored and derangements treated aggressively.

Treatments mentioned in anecdotal case reports, such as sodium bicarbonate and acetazolamide (both in urinary alkalinization) and aminophylline, cannot be recommended at this time. Among treatments found to be ineffective or harmful are water loading, diuretics (furosemide, thiazide, ethacrynic acid, or spironolactone), and ammonium chloride.

DISPOSITION

Admission decisions must be weighted by the presence and persistence of factors predisposing the patient to toxicity, the acuity of the toxicity, and the circumstances that led to the toxicity. Acute ingestions must be treated as already described, and patients should be monitored for 4 to 6 h, even if asymptomatic, and receive psychiatric consultation. Remember that drug levels are less likely to correlate with symptoms in acute ingestion. Any patient with acute ingestion of a sustained-release preparation should be admitted. Patients with levels of greater than 1.5 meq need admission.

Patients with grade 1 chronic toxicity without additional risk factors may be managed with hydration for 4 to 6 h. Once levels return to the normal range (less than 1.5 meq), there is clinical improvement and usually, after psychiatric evaluation, the patient may be discharged. Repeat values obtained within 24 h by home health services can be considered.

Patients with grade 2 or 3 chronic toxicity require admission.

REFERENCES

1. Amdisen A: Clinical features and management of lithium poisoning. *Med Toxicol Adverse Drug Reactions* 3:18, 1988.
2. Litovitz TL, Klein Schwartz W, Dyer KS, et al: 1997 Annual report of the American Association of Poison Control Centers Toxic Exposure Surveillance System. *Am J Emerg Med* 16:443, 1998.
3. Kofman O, Belmaker RH: Biochemical behavior and clinical studies of inositol in lithium treatment and depression. *Biol Psychiatry* 34:839, 1989.
4. Baldessarini RJ, Vogt M: Release of ^{3}H-dopamine and analogous monoamines from rat striatal tissue. *Cell Mol Neurobiol* 8:205, 1988.
5. Treiser SL, Cascio CS, O'Donohue TL, et al: Lithium increases serotonin release and decreases serotonin receptors in the hippocampus. *Science* 213:1529, 1981.
6. Gelenberg AJ, Jefferson JW: Lithium tremor. *J Clin Psychiatry* 56:283, 1995.
7. Bendz H, Aurell M, Balldin J, et al: Kidney damage in long-term lithium patients: A cross-sectional study of patients with 15 years or more on lithium. *Nephrol Dial Transplant* 9:1250, 1994.
8. Sheean GL: Lithium neurotoxicity. *Clin Exp Neurol* 28:112, 1991.
9. Manto M, Godaux E, Jacquy J, Hildebrand JG: Analysis of cerebellar dysmetria associated with lithium intoxication. *Neurol Res* 18:416, 1996.
10. Kores B, Lader MH: Irreversible lithium neurotoxicity: An overview. *Clin Neuropharmacol* 20:283, 1997.
11. Favin FD, Klein-Schwartz W, Oderda GM, Rose SR: In vitro study of lithium carbonate adsorption by activated charcoal. *Clin Toxicol* 26:443, 1988.
12. Smith SW, Ling LH, Halstenson CE: Whole bowel irrigation as treatment for acute lithium overdose. *Ann Emerg Med* 20:536, 1991.
13. Finley PR, Warner MD, Peabody CA: Clinical relevance of drug interactions with lithium. *Clin Pharmacokinet* 29:172, 1995.
14. Jaeger A, Sauder P, Kopferschmitt J, et al: When should dialysis be performed in lithium poisoning? A kinetic study in 14 cases of lithium poisoning. *Clin Toxicol* 31:429, 1993.
15. Szerlip HM, Heeger P, Feldman GM: Comparison between acetate and bicarbonate dialysis for the treatment of lithium intoxication. *Am J Nephrol* 12:116, 1992.
16. Jacobsen D, Aasen G, Grederichsen P, Eisenga B: Lithium intoxication: Pharmacokinetics during and after terminated hemodialysis in acute intoxications. *Clin Toxicol* 25:81, 1987.
17. Linakis JG, Lacouture PG, Eisenberg MS, et al: Administration of activated charcoal or sodium polystyrene sulfonate (Kayexalate) as gastric decontamination for lithium intoxication: An animal model. *Pharmacol Toxicol* 65:387, 1989.
18. Roberge RJ, Martin TM, Schneider SM: Use of sodium polystyrene sulfonate in a lithium overdose. *Ann Emerg Med* 22:1911, 1993.

BARBITURATES

Raquel M. Schears

Barbiturates have been in common clinical use since 1903. These agents possess sedative properties used to reduce anxiety and hypnotic properties used to induce sleep—hence their classification as sedative-hypnotics. The therapeutic efficacy of these agents is best illustrated in their use as anticonvulsants in the treatment of seizure disorders, as induction agents in rapid-sequence intubation, and as antihypertensives in the management of increased intracranial pressure.[1]

Barbiturates abuse, both prescription and illicit, peaked in the 1970s. The availability, as measured by sales and by the accidental death rate, was significantly correlated with their use for suicide.[2] In the last two decades, the number of toxic exposures involving barbiturates and the incidence of overall barbiturate-related deaths have declined dramatically. This has been attributed to the advent and popularity of safer sedative-hypnotics such as the benzodiazepines and other major tranquilizers, rescheduling of barbiturates to class II, III, and IV drugs, and improvements in supportive care in overdose

*S may replace O

FIG. 157-1. Chemical structure of barbituric acid.

settings.[3] Nonetheless, illicit barbiturate use has again increased steadily in the United States since 1990, especially in adolescent populations. Reasons for this include youth perceptions that barbiturates are not very harmful and may be useful when taken in tandem with cocaine and methamphetamine to mitigate the unpleasant extremes of the stimulant effects.[4,5] Also worrisome is the featured prominence of barbiturates used in recent mass suicide rituals and recommended in prescriptions for suicide published in the popular press and on the Internet.[6] According to the 1997 Annual Report of the American Association of Poison Control Centers, barbiturates were involved in 5628 reported poisonings, with one-half of these captured as intentional overdoses that resulted in 54 deaths.[7] Clearly, barbiturates continue to rank among the most toxic classes of sedative-hypnotic agents that can pose life-threatening management problems for clinicians.

PHARMACOLOGY

The parent compound, barbituric acid (2,4,6-trioxohexahydropyrimidine), itself has no central depressant activity. R-group substitutions primarily at position 5 give these compounds their sedative-hypnotic properties. Substituting a sulfur for the oxygen at position 2 creates a thiobarbiturate, which is more lipid soluble than an oxybarbiturate (Fig. 157-1). High lipid solubility allows an agent to rapidly transit the blood-brain barrier and confers a shorter duration of action and greater degree of hypnotic activity.[5] Traditionally, barbiturates have been classified according to their duration of action (Table 157-1).

Long-acting barbiturates tend to be weaker acids (lower pK_a values), less lipid soluble, and less protein bound than shorter-acting barbiturates. This translates to a delayed onset of action, decreased volume of distribution, and longer duration of action when compared with short-, ultrashort-, and intermediate-acting compounds. Furthermore, tissue permeability of long-acting barbiturates is uniquely affected by body fluid pH changes. Only nonionized drug is membrane permeable. Phenobarbital has a pK_a of 7.24 and is 95 percent ionized at pH 7.4. Ionization will increase in a basic medium, and permeability will decrease. Conversely, an acidic medium will facilitate phenobarbital permeability by maintaining more drug in a nonionized state. This principle underpins the therapeutic usefulness of alkaline diuresis in long-acting barbiturates overdose.

Short-, ultrashort-, and intermediate-acting barbiturates are not affected by body pH changes. Secobarbital, for example, has a pK_a of 7.9 and is 98 percent nonionized at pH 7.4. Rate of barbiturate delivery to the membrane determines tissue permeability with these classes. These compounds are stronger acids (higher pK_a values), more lipid soluble, and more protein bound, enabling a more rapid onset of action, greater volume of distribution, and shorter duration of action compared with the long-acting barbiturates.[5]

Bulk absorption of barbiturates occurs in the stomach and small intestine, where most of the drug exists in a nonionized state. Overall, barbiturates readily diffuse into the body tissues and cross the blood-brain barrier, with highest concentrations occurring in the brain, liver, kidney, and adipose tissue. Barbiturates are excreted in breast milk and easily cross the placenta. Fetal blood barbiturate concentrations

TABLE 157-1 Selected Properties and Classification of Commonly Used Barbiturates

	Long Acting*		Intermediate Acting*		Short Acting*		Ultrashort Acting*	
Generic name	Barbital†	Phenobarbital†	Amobarbital	Amobarbital plus secobarbital	Pentobarbital	Secobarbital	Thiopental	Methohexital
Trade name	Veronal	Luminal	Amytal	Tuinal	Nembutal	Seconal	Pentothal	Brevital
Street name‡	Carbutol	Purple hearts, goof balls, phennies	Blue heavens, downers	Gorilla pills, F-66's, rainbows, double trouble	Yellow jackets, Abbotts, Mexican yellows	Reds, red devils/birds, lilly, pinks, pink ladies		
pK_a	7.4	7.24	7.75	7.85	7.96	7.90	7.6	7.9
Major route of detoxification	Renal (33%)	Renal (30%)	Hepatic	Hepatic	Hepatic	Hepatic	Hepatic	Hepatic
Plasma protein binding (%)	5	20	ND	ND	35	44	65	73
Volume of distribution V_D (L/kg)	ND	0.7	1.05	1.0	1.0	1.5	1.4–6.7	1.1
Hypnotic dose (mg)	300–500	100–200	50–200	100	50–100	100–200	50–100	50–120 IV
Duration of action (h)	>6	>6	3–6	3–6	<3	<3	0.3	0.3
Plasma half-life (h)	ND	24–96	14–42	16–40	21–42	20–28	6–46	1–2
Fatal dose (g)§	10	5	ND	ND	30	30	ND	ND

ND = no data.
*This classification scheme is a convention only; it preceded the discovery that the elimination half-lives do not conform to the apparent duration of action.
†Only drugs responsive to alkaline diuresis.
‡Barbituates possessing street names are relatively common drugs of abuse.
§In nontolerant individuals.
Source: Adapted from Robinson RR: Treatment of acute barbiturate intoxication. *Mod Treat* 8:561, 1971; and Osborn H: Sedative-hypnotic agents, in LR Goldfrank, NE Flomenbaum (eds): *Goldfrank's Toxicologic Emergencies*, 5th ed. Norwalk, CT: Appleton and Lange, 1994, pp 787–810.

closely reflect maternal plasma levels.[4] Interestingly, in utero exposure to phenobarbital has been significantly linked to verbal intelligence deficits in adult men.[8] Tolerance develops with chronic barbiturate use, and higher doses are required to produce the same effects. Most barbiturates are metabolized by the liver to inactive by-products. Hepatic biotransformation occurs primarily through routes involving the cytochrome P-450 microsomal enzyme system. All barbiturates are capable of inducing the activity of this enzyme system. Increased rates of metabolism for many drugs, including oral contraceptives, anticoagulants, and corticosteroids, have been observed in patients with chronic barbiturate use. Depending on the degree of hepatic biotransformation, variable amounts of barbiturates are excreted unchanged in the urine. Barbital and phenobarbital are less protein bound and thus most dependent on the renal excretion pathway.[9] Elimination half-life of barbiturates can be greatly accelerated in infants and children and very prolonged in the elderly and in patients with liver or renal disease.[4,5]

The main action of barbiturates is to depress activity in nerve and muscle tissues. In the central nervous system (CNS) this is accomplished by enhancing the action of the primary inhibitory neurotransmitter γ-aminobutyric acid (GABA) at the postsynaptic membrane. Additionally, barbiturates may act by inhibiting calcium-mediated excitatory neurotransmitter release at the presynaptic junction.[1,4,5]

CLINICAL FEATURES

Mild to moderate barbiturate intoxication closely resembles the drug "high" produced by alcohol. Drowsiness, disinhibition, ataxia, slurred speech, and mental confusion are common features that escalate with increasing dose. The progressive CNS depression seen with severe barbiturate intoxication predictably manifests as a range from stupor to coma to complete neurologic unresponsiveness. Scales gauging the depth of coma are useful in describing patient presentation and monitoring interval changes in the level of consciousness during treatment in overdose settings.[10] The most common vital sign abnormalities seen in overdose are hypothermia, respiratory depression, and hypotension. The abnormal temperature control and respiratory depression are centrally mediated phenomena, whereas hypotension is due primarily to increased vascular capacitance and venous pooling. The end product of these derangements can be a patient who is cold, apneic, and in shock. Pulse rate is not diagnostic; pupil size, light reactivity, nystagmus, and deep tendon reflexes are variable. Gastrointestinal tract motility is slowed, resulting in delayed gastric emptying and ileus. Skin bullae, referred to as barbiturate blisters, are uncommon and may indicate nothing more than the effects of local skin pressure.[5,10] Even when it is known that a barbiturate was ingested, it is prudent to consider coingestions and alternate explanations for the observed symptom complex.

Early deaths in barbiturate overdose result from cardiovascular collapse and respiratory arrest. Most common complications are hypoglycemia, followed by the delayed pulmonary problems of aspiration pneumonia, noncardiogenic pulmonary edema, and adult respiratory distress syndrome. Current mortality rates range between 1 and 3 percent and are more often the result of multiple organ system failure. Lethal dose is uncertain, but severe poisoning can be assumed if more than 10 times the hypnotic dose has been ingested in a single exposure.[10]

Laboratory evaluation in barbiturate overdose should include determination of glucose levels, blood chemistries, complete blood count, arterial blood gas measurement, toxicology screen, chest radiograph, and an electrocardiogram. Barbiturate serum levels are useful in establishing the diagnosis of a comatose patient and should be obtained and used to distinguish long- from short-acting agents because treatment approaches differ. As a rule of thumb, patients presenting with a serum concentration of more than 10 mg/dL for a long-acting barbiturate, more than 7 mg/dL for an intermediate-acting barbiturate, and more than 3 mg/dL for a short-acting barbiturate, left untreated, have a greater risk of death from the exposure. These measurements are not reliable in predicting clinical course in overdose because they do not reflect brain barbiturate concentrations and may underestimate the clinical condition of a patient in the setting of polydrug exposure. Such levels are also invalid in chronic barbiturate abusers who have developed physiologic tolerance and in patients with renal or hepatic disease who have decreased clearance.[4,5,10]

TREATMENT

In barbiturate overdose, reaching a treatment center predicts favorable outcome largely because supportive management alone is effective over a broad range of serum concentrations.

Airway Assessment and Stabilization

Airway assessment and stabilization are the first management priorities. Intubation in severe sedative-hypnotic overdose is often required and should precede any attempt at gastrointestinal evacuation. Standard monitoring of vital signs, cardiac electrical activity, and pulse oxymetry should be instituted, as should IV access and supplemental O_2.

Volume Expansion

Volume expansion is the mainstay of circulatory support in barbiturate-induced shock. In the absence of cardiac failure, rapid infusion of 1 to 2 L of isotonic intravenous fluid is indicated; administration of bolus therapy, e.g., 200-cc aliquots, is prudent in the elderly, those with cardiac decompensation, or in the face of renal impairment. If fluid resuscitation fails to correct hypotension, vasopressors such as dopamine and norepinephrine should be initiated.[11]

Gastric Emptying

Gastric lavage accomplished within 4 to 6 h of ingestion effectively decreases absorption of barbiturates. However, there are no data that gastric lavage is superior to activated charcoal alone. Given the CNS depression associated with this overdose, ipecac should not be used, and induction of emesis should be avoided.

Oral activated charcoal augments drug extraction by adsorbing drugs from the gastrointestinal tract. Multiple-dose activated charcoal (MDAC) is beneficial in reducing serum phenobarbital concentrations; however, no significant difference in clinical outcome has yet been demonstrated.[12,13] Still, most studies suggest that activated charcoal is at least as effective as lavage and may be better, given its immediate functional effectiveness. Loading dose of activated charcoal is 50 to 100 g, and this may be followed by a single dose of cathartic agent; standard MDAC is 20 to 50 g every 4 h.[14]

Forced Diuresis

Forced diuresis with fluid loading and diuretic therapy is most effective for phenobarbital. Intravenous furosemide should be titrated to effect a urinary flow of 4 to 6 mL/kg/h. Diuresis is contraindicated in the setting of hypotension or shock. Iatrogenic congestive heart failure and fluid overload preclude the usefulness of this therapy for other barbiturates that have limited renal excretion.[5,10]

Urinary Alkalinization

Urinary alkalinization will promote the excretion of long-acting barbiturates only, as explained earlier. The reasons for this singular application are pharmacologically based. Long-acting barbiturates tend to be weaker acids (lower pK_a values), less lipid soluble, less protein bound, and are appreciably excreted in the urine compared with shorter-acting barbiturates. In basic solutions, long-acting barbiturates (weak acids) are relatively more ionized. Since only nonionized drug forms can cross cell membranes, these barbiturates will be trapped in the tubular fluid and excreted if the urinary pH favors the ionized form. Alkalinizing the urine is not effective for shorter-acting barbiturates because these drugs have higher pK_a values (stronger acids), are more protein bound, and are metabolized primarily by the liver. The 5- to 10-fold increase in basal excretion rate is best accomplished by giving a 1 to 2 meq/kg sodium bicarbonate intravenous bolus, followed by 50 to 100 meq in 500 mL of 5% D/W. Drip rate is sufficient if it maintains an arterial pH of 7.45 to 7.50, urinary pH of 8.0, and urinary output of 2 mL/kg/h. Serum potassium must remain at least 4 meq/L to achieve continuous urinary alkalinization. Adequacy of therapy should be monitored every 2 to 4 h.[3,5]

Hemodialysis and Hemoperfusion

Hemodialysis and hemoperfusion are techniques used to maximize barbiturate elimination that are reserved for patients who are deteriorating despite institution of aggressive supportive care. Effectiveness of these modalities is limited by drug characteristics and potential complications.

DISPOSITION

Mild to moderate barbiturate intoxication responds well to general supportive care and MDAC. Frequent reassessment of neurologic status and vital sign parameters indicating improvement over 6 to 8 h allow eventual patient transfer to psychiatric services. Severe overdose with previously described historical and clinical features will require admission, ongoing medical stabilization, and psychiatric intervention. Early poison center contact and specialty service consultation is recommended.

BARBITURATE ABSTINENCE SYNDROME

Abrupt discontinuation of barbiturates in a chronically dependent user will produce minor withdrawal symptoms within 24 h and major life-threatening symptoms within 2 to 8 days. The severity of the withdrawal reflects the degree of physical dependence and drug half-life. Cessation of short-acting barbiturates results in more severe abstinence symptoms than stopping long-acting barbiturates. This is consistent with the clinical observation that the brain has more time to adapt to declining drug concentrations that are gradual. Clinical manifestations of abstinence mimic those described for alcohol withdrawal. Minor symptoms include anxiety, restlessness, depression, insomnia, anorexia, nausea, vomiting, muscle twitching, abdominal cramping, and sweating. Major symptoms include psychosis, hallucinations, delirium, generalized seizures, hyperthermia, and cardiovascular collapse.[3,4,15]

Priorities in the treatment of major abstinence symptoms are cardiovascular stabilization and seizure control. Intravenous benzodiazepines usually are effective in treating seizures, although intravenous barbiturates may be required. Due to the mortality associated with sedative-hypnotic abstinence, gradual in-hospital withdrawal of the addicting agent is recommended.[4,15]

REFERENCES

1. Ho IK, Harris RA: Mechanism of action of barbiturates. *Annu Rev Pharmacol Toxicol* 21:83, 1981.
2. Lester D: Barbiturate sales and their use for suicide. *Percept Mot Skills* 69:442,1989.
3. Stern TA, Mulley AG, Thibault GE: Life-threatening drug overdose. *JAMA* 251:1983, 1984.
4. Coupey SM: Barbiturates. *Pediatr Rev* 18:260, 1997.
5. Bertino JJ, Reed MD: Barbiturate and nonbarbiturate sedative hypnotic intoxication in children. *Pediatr Clin North Am* 33:703, 1986.
6. Humphry D: *Final Exit.* Secaucus, NJ: Carol Publishing, 1991.
7. Litovitz TL, Klein-Schwartz W, Dyer KS, et al: 1997 Annual Report of the American Association of Poison Control Centers National Data Collection System. *Am J Emerg Med* 16:445, 1998.
8. Reinisch JM, Sanders SA, Mortensen EL, et al: In utero exposure to phenobarbital and intelligence deficits in men. *JAMA* 274:1518, 1995.
9. Sampson I: Barbiturates. *Mt Sinai J Med* 50:283, 1983.
10. McCarron MM, Schulze BW, Walberg CB, et al: Short-acting barbiturate overdosage: Correlation of intoxication score with serum barbiturate concentration. *JAMA* 248:51, 1982.
11. Shubin H, Well MH: Shock associated with barbiturate intoxication. *JAMA* 215:263, 1971.
12. Berg M, Berlinger W, Goldberg M, et al: Acceleration of the body clearance of phenobarbital by oral activated charcoal. *N Engl J Med* 307:647, 1982.
13. Levy G: Gastrointestinal clearance of drugs with activated charcoal. *N Engl J Med* 307:676, 1982.
14. Pond S, Olson K, Osterloh J, et al: Randomized study of the treatment of phenobarbital overdose with repeated doses of activated charcoal. *JAMA* 251:3104, 1984.
15. Khantzian EJ, McKenna GJ: Acute toxic and withdrawal reactions associated with drug use and abuse. *Ann Intern Med* 90:351, 1979.

BENZODIAZEPINES

George M. Bosse

Benzodiazepines are pharmacologic agents commonly used for the treatment of anxiety, insomnia, seizures, and alcohol withdrawal. They also are used in conscious sedation as well as general anesthesia. Fourteen generic benzodiazepines are currently approved for use in the United States (Table 158-1).

TABLE 158-1 Benzodiazepines Approved for Use in the United States

Generic Name	Brand Name	Half-life, h*	Metabolite Characteristics†
Alprazolam	Xanax	6–26	Inactive
Chlorazepate dipotassium	Tranxene	1.1–2.9	Active
Chlordiazepoxide	Librium	5–30	Active
Clonazepam	Klonopin	39	Inactive
Diazepam	Valium	20–70	Active
Estazolam	Prosom	10–24	Inactive
Flurazepam	Dalmane	2–3	Active
Halazepam	Paxipam	14	Active
Lorazepam	Ativan	9–19	Inactive
Midazolam	Versed	2–5	Inactive
Oxazepam	Serax	5.4–9.8	Inactive
Quazepam	Doral	25–41	Active
Temazepam	Restoril	10–16	Inactive
Triazolam	Halcion	1.6–5.4	Inactive

*Elimination of half-life of parent compound.
†Some of the derivatives listed as having inactive metabolites actually are converted to active compounds. However, rapid metabolism results in no appreciable accumulation of active intermediates.

Benzodiazepines are frequently agents of accidental and intentional overdose. In the 1996 Annual Report of the American Association of Poison Control Centers Toxic Exposure Surveillance System, benzodiazepines accounted for 39,029 exposures, both as single agents and in combination with other drugs.[1] Although the ingestion of benzodiazepines alone appears to result in relatively few deaths, increased rates of morbidity and mortality do result from mixed overdose. Parenteral administration of benzodiazepines may also result in significant complications, particularly respiratory depression and hypotension.

PHARMACOLOGY

A specific benzodiazepine receptor has been identified in the central nervous system (CNS).[2] Specific peripheral receptor sites also have been identified, but the predominant clinical effects of benzodiazepines are mediated through the CNS receptors. Although the receptor has not been fully characterized, research supports the existence of a neuronal cell-surface protein complex containing a benzodiazepine receptor, a gamma-aminobutyric acid (GABA) receptor, and a chloride channel. GABA is an inhibitory neurotransmitter. Effects of stimulation of GABA pathways include sedation, anxiolysis, and striated muscle relaxation. Stimulation of the benzodiazepine receptor appears to increase the sensitivity of the GABA receptor complex to stimulation by GABA. The enhancement of GABA transmission by the administration of benzodiazepines is thought to occur by either increasing the affinity of the GABA receptor for its ligand or improving coupling between the GABA receptor and its associated chloride channel. Increased GABA output leads to inhibitory effects throughout the neuroaxis and the resultant typical clinical effects of benzodiazepines. The presence of an endogenous ligand for the benzodiazepine receptor has been proposed, but such a ligand has not been conclusively identified.

In general, benzodiazepines are well absorbed from the gastrointestinal tract. The onset of action after oral ingestion is limited more by the rate of absorption from the gastrointestinal tract than by the relatively rapid passage from the bloodstream into the brain. With the exception of lorazepam and midazolam, intramuscular injection of benzodiazepines results in unpredictable absorption.

Benzodiazepines are all relatively lipid soluble, with some variation among the agents. Increased lipid solubility is associated with more rapid diffusion across the blood-brain barrier. After single doses, the more highly lipophilic benzodiazepines have a shorter onset of action but also a shorter duration of activity. This short duration of activity occurs because of rapid egress of the drug from the brain and bloodstream into inactive tissue storage sites. For this reason, the half-life may not be a good indicator of the duration of action in an acute ingestion. For example, diazepam is a derivative with a long elimination half-life but a relatively short duration of action.

Benzodiazepine derivatives undergo metabolism by hepatic biotransformation through either oxidation or conjugation. Several derivatives are metabolized by both oxidative and conjugative processes. Oxidation often produces active metabolites, which prolong the biologic half-life of the parent compounds. Conjugation is a rapid process that produces inactive metabolites. Oxidation is more susceptible to impairment by such factors as disease states (e.g., chronic liver disease), demographic characteristics (e.g., old age), and concurrent treatment with drugs that impair oxidizing capacity (e.g., cimetidine, estrogen, isoniazid, ethanol, and phenytoin). Examples of agents that undergo conjugation primarily include oxazepam, lorazepam, and temazepam. Administration of benzodiazepines that undergo conjugation may be safer in susceptible groups.

Selection of a benzodiazepine for use by a physician depends on the clinical properties of the particular derivative. Although individual drugs are marketed for specific conditions, there is considerable overlap of activity. For this reason, some hospital formulary commitees have limited the number of available agents.

CLINICAL FEATURES

Isolated benzodiazepine overdose is notable for the relative lack of significant rates of morbidity and mortality.[3] Most reported cases of serious toxicity have occurred in the setting of coingestion of other agents or with parenteral administration. However, deaths in isolated overdose have been reported and appear to be more likely with short-acting derivatives, such as triazolam, alprazolam, and temazepam.

The clinical presentation of benzodiazepine intoxication is nonspecific. Clinical assessment also may be difficult because of the frequent coingestion of other agents. Except for additive effects, drug interactions of benzodiazepines with other sedative-hypnotics are unusual.

The nonspecific presentation of benzodiazepine toxicity is similar to that of other sedative-hypnotics. However, other agents can have at least a few distinguishing features. Chloral hydrate is known to precipitate cardiac dysrhythmias. Ethchlorvynol can produce prolonged coma and may be suspected by the presence of a vinyl-like odor. Glutethimide may give rise to fluctuating levels of CNS impairment and anticholinergic signs. Barbiturates are more likely than benzodiazepines to produce coma and depressant myocardial effects.

The predominant manifestations of benzodiazepines are neurologic. CNS effects include drowsiness, dizziness, slurred speech, confusion, ataxia, and impairment of intellectual function. Coma, particularly if prolonged, is atypical and should prompt suspicion of intoxication with other agents or a nontoxin-related medical condition. The elderly are more prone to manifest the CNS effects of benzodiazepines.

Paradoxical reactions, including excitement, anxiety, aggression, hostile behavior, rage, and delirium, have been reported but are uncommon. Although unclear, the etiology of such effects is probably not idiosyncratic. Benzodiazepines may have a disinhibiting effect, which, in the presence of various extrinsic factors, can lead to such actions as aggressive or hostile behavior. Other effects that have been reported and that have unclear etiologies include headache, nausea, vomiting, chest pain, joint pain, diarrhea, and incontinence.

Uncommonly, respiratory depression and hypotension may occur, generally with either parenteral administration or in the presence of coingestants. Intravenous administration is more likely to cause serious cardiorespiratory effects with rapid administration of large doses. In addition, the elderly and those with underlying cardiorespiratory disease are more susceptible to adverse effects of intravenous administration. The use of propylene glycol as a diluent in parenteral preparations of diazepam has also been implicated as a factor in cardiorespiratory arrest.

Extrapyramidal reactions have been associated with the use of benzodiazepines. Various allergic, hepatotoxic, and hematologic reactions also have been reported, but they are infrequent. In general, benzodiazepines have no long-term organ-system toxicity other than that which can be ascribed to indirect effects from CNS or cardiorespiratory depression.

Laboratory data in benzodiazepine ingestion are of limited value. Determination of serum benzodiazepine levels is not indicated routinely because they do not correlate well with the clinical state. Qualitative testing may be helpful, but the laboratory may not test routinely for all available derivatives. Familiarity with laboratory capabilities at a given institution is essential.

TREATMENT

Benzodiazepines often are ingested with other agents, and the history frequently is inaccurate. Therefore, administration of concentrated dextrose, thiamine, and naloxone should be considered in such patients when depressed or altered mental status is present. Induction of emesis should be avoided in benzodiazepine overdose because CNS depression may ensue. Gastric lavage is safer and is recommended if the amount ingested is large or in coingestions with toxic agents. Activated charcoal binds benzodiazepines effectively and should be administered in most situations. Elimination enhancement by forced diuresis, hemodialysis, or hemoperfusion is not effective, and most patients do not manifest toxicity serious enough to warrant consideration of such measures. The patient should be monitored closely for CNS and respiratory depression. Indications for hospital admission include significant alterations in mental status, respiratory depression, and hypotension. If CNS depression persists or is profound, other agents or conditions must be considered.

Flumazenil is a unique selective antagonist of the central effects of benzodiazepines.[4] Clinical applications include the management of benzodiazepine overdose and reversal of benzodiazepine-induced conscious sedation. Its use in benzodiazepine toxicity may obviate the need for tracheal intubation and respiratory support. As a diagnostic aid in obscure alterations of mental status, flumazenil may reduce the need for expensive and invasive procedures, such as computed tomography or lumbar puncture.

In the emergency department, flumazenil is useful mainly in reversing the effects of benzodiazepines administered for diagnostic and therapeutic procedures. The plasma elimination half-life of flumazenil is approximately 1 h. Its duration of action is variable and depends on the dose of flumazenil and the benzodiazepine administered. Recurrent benzodiazepine toxicity may result once the effects of flumazenil have worn off. This is less likely for an agent with a short duration of action, such as midazolam. The dose of flumazenil is 0.2 mg intravenously every minute to response or to a total of 3 mg.

Several considerations should limit the empirical administration of flumazenil to a poisoned patient. Generalized seizures have occurred in patients given flumazenil after coingestions of benzodiazepines and seizure-inducing agents, particularly cyclic antidepressants.[5,6] Seizure activity after flumazenil administration has also occurred in patients physically dependent on benzodiazepines and in patients receiving benzodiazepines for control of a seizure disorder. The putative explanation for this convulsive activity is either the reversal of the cerebroprotective and anticonvulsive effects of benzodiazepines or the precipitation of a benzodiazepine withdrawal syndrome. Another reason to avoid empirical administration of flumazenil in overdose patients is that the history is often unreliable or unavailable. Flumazenil is also contraindicated in patients with a suspected elevation of intracranial pressure, such as in severe head injury. This contraindication is due to its effects on cerebral hemodynamics. In all cases of benzodiazepine toxicity, supportive care is the cornerstone of treatment.

BENZODIAZEPINE ABUSE AND DEPENDENCE

Genuine physiologic addiction to benzodiazepines may occur, particularly with prolonged and high doses.[3,7] However, the abuse potential of benzodiazepines appears to be low in comparison with that of agents such as alcohol, cocaine, opiates, and barbiturates.[8,9] Benzodiazepine abuse usually occurs in individuals with a history of abuse of other psychoactive drugs. Primary drug abuse with benzodiazepines is not common.

Benzodiazepine withdrawal may occur on abrupt discontinuation and is more likely in patients with prolonged use and high doses. Because of the long biologic half-life of several derivatives, withdrawal manifestations may not occur for several days to over 1 week after the benzodiazepine has been discontinued. Unfortunately, it is often difficult to distinguish between withdrawal and underlying symptoms for which the drugs were prescribed initially.

Reported withdrawal manifestations include anxiety, irritability, insomnia, nausea, vomiting, tremor, sweating, and anorexia. Serious manifestations, including confusion, disorientation, psychosis, and seizures, also have been reported. For patients with an acute organic brain syndrome, a history of possible benzodiazepine withdrawal should always be pursued. Withdrawal reactions may be avoided by dose tapering. Treatment of withdrawal reactions may be accomplished by drug substitution or by reintroduction of a benzodiazepine and subsequent tapering.

REFERENCES

1. Litovitz TL, Smilkstein M, Felberg L, et al: 1996 Annual Report of the American Association of Poison Control Centers Toxic Exposure Surveillance System. *Am J Emerg Med* 15:447, 1997.
2. Mohler H, Okada T: Benzodiazepine receptor: Demonstration in the central nervous system. *Science* 198:849, 1977.
3. Guadreault P, Guay J, Thivierge RL, Verdy I: Benzodiazepine poisoning: Clinical and pharmacologic considerations and treatment. *Drug Safety* 6:247, 1991.
4. Votey SR, Bosse GM, Bayer MJ, Hoffman JR: Flumazenil: A new benzodiazepine antagonist. *Ann Emerg Med* 20:181, 1991.
5. Spivey WH, Roberts JR, Derlet RW: A clinical trial of escalating doses of flumazenil for reversal of suspected benzodiazepine overdose in the emergency department. *Ann Emerg Med* 22:1813, 1993.
6. Spivey WH: Flumazenil and seizures: An analysis of 43 cases. *Clin Ther* 14:292, 1992.
7. Marriott S, Tyrer P: Benzodiazepine dependence: Avoidance and withdrawal. *Drug Safety* 9:93, 1993.
8. Warneke LB: Benzodiazepines: Abuse and new use. *Can J Psychiatry* 36:194, 1991.
9. Woods JH, Katz JL, Winger G: Use and abuse of benzodiazepines: Issues relevant to prescribing. *JAMA* 260:3476, 1988.

NONBENZODIAZEPINE SEDATIVE-HYPNOTICS

Raquel M. Schears

The term *nonbenzodiazepine sedative-hypnotic* is currently used to refer to a diverse group of agents that share the ability to allay anxiety and promote sleep, categorically exclusive of the benzodiazepines. Several of these chemical entities, such as ethchlorvynol, meprobamate, glutethimide, and methaqualone, are rarely encountered in clinical use, yet toxic exposures continued to be reported. Newer agents such as buspirone and zolpidem are used commonly, making toxicity and overdose characteristics important to recognize and treat in the emergency department (Tables 159-1 and 159-2).

Some chemical compounds possess sedative-hypnotic properties but were marketed as health food products and until recently escaped Food and Drug Administration (FDA) regulation. Among these drugs, gamma-hydroxybutyrate (GHB) is gaining notoriety as a product to illicitly inflict the harm of involuntary intoxication or chemical submission, commonly referred to as "date rape." GHB has no legitimate clinical purpose in the United States and is being cited increasingly as a toxic and dangerous agent. Despite this irony, it remains readily available via recipes on the Internet and stovetop component mixes by mail order. Certainly, patients presenting with complaints of drug-induced physical and sexual assault will pose novel diagnostic, medical, and legal problems to challenge emergency physicians.[1]

Agents in this chapter share certain pharmacologic and clinical similarities. These drugs tend to be highly lipophilic and concentrate in the central nervous system (CNS), causing varying degrees of CNS depression with gradual redistribution and eventual hepatic degradation. Clinically, mild intoxication manifests as sedation and incoordination that progresses to lethargy, worsening ataxia, and deepening coma in overdose.

It is recognized that reaching a treatment center predicts a favorable outcome in all types of nonbenzodiazepine sedative-hypnotic overdoses. Improvements in general supportive care underpin declining trends seen in mortality associated with these agents over broad dose ranges. Therefore, general treatment guidelines take precedence in management of all these agents in overdose.

TABLE 159-1 Selected Properties and Characteristic Overdose Features of Nonbenzodiazepine Sedative-Hypnotic Drugs

Drug Class	Alcohol	Carbinols	Piperidinediones	Carbonated Propandiol	Quinazolines	Azapirones	Imidazopyridines	Neurotransmitter
Generic name	**Chloral Hydrate***	**Ethchlorvynol***	**Glutethimide***	**Meprobamate***	**Methaqualone***	**Buspirone**	**Zolpidem**	**Gamma/hydroxybutyrate**
Trade name	**Noctec**	**Placidyl**	**Doriden**	**Miltown, Equanil**	**Qualude, Parest, Mequin, Sopor†**	**BuSpar**	**Ambien, Stilnox, Niotal, Bikalm**	**ND**
Street name	**(+Ethanol ≫ knockout drops, Mickey Finn)**	**Pickles, Jelly beans, Mr. Green Jeans**	**(+Codeine ≫ sets, hits, packs, loads, threes and eights, four doors)**	**ND**	**Quads, ludes, soapers, mandies, love-drug, wall banger**	**ND**	**ND**	**Grievous Bodily Harm, Georgia Home Boy, Liquid Ecstacy, Liquid X or E, GHB, GBH, Soap, Scoop, Easy Lay, Salty Water, Cherry Menth, organic qualude**
Detoxification	Hepatic, renal 10%	Hepatic, renal 10%	Hepatic	Hepatic, renal 10%	Hepatic	Hepatic, fecal 30%	Hepatic	Pulmonary
Plasma protein binding (%)	35–40	50–60	47–59	20	70–90	95	92	ND
V_d (L/kg)	6–1.6	3–4	2–7	0.65	5.8–6.0	433	54	4–58
Hypnotic dose (mg)‡	500–1000	500–1000	250–500	400	150–300	15–30	10–20	3000
Plasma half-life (h)§	8 (M)	10–20	12 (M)	11	19	2–3 (M)	2–5	0.3
Fatal dose (g)	5–10	10	10–20	12	8	ND	ND	ND
Lethal blood level (mg/dL)	25	15	3–10	20	10–15	ND	ND	ND
Overdose clues	Pearlike breath odor Ventricular dysrhythmias Gastrointestinal bleeding	Vinyl-like breath odor Prolonged coma Hypothermia ARDS	Anticholinergic symptoms Fluctuating prolonged coma	Gastric concretions Severe hypotension Fluctuating prolonged coma	Hyperacusis Hypertonicity, seizures Bleeding diathesis	Drowsiness Dysphoria	Drowsiness Vomiting	Athletic physique, seizures Agitation, apnea Sudden reversible coma
Extracorporeal methods	HP > HD	HP > HD	HP	HP > HD	HP	ND	ND	ND

*Agent causes significant life-threatening abstinence syndrome requiring hospital admission.
†Legal synthesis in USA terminated 1984.
‡All agents have both sedative and hypnotic properties; maximum adult hypnotic dose listed can be given in divided doses to that total dose/day for sedative purposes.
§Half-life given at therapeutic dose; generally half-life in overdose is considerably longer. M = active metabolites. Fatal dose is an estimate complicated by history of tolerance, coingestion, and patient reliability. Extracorporeal methods: HP = hemoperfusion, HD = hemodialysis, > denotes preferred method; ND, no data; Va, volume of distribution.
Source: Adapted from Osborn H: Sedative-hypnotic agents, in LR Goldfrank and NE Flomenbaum (eds): *Goldfrank's Toxicologic Emergencies,* 5th ed. Norwalk, CT: Appleton and Lange, 1994, pp 787–810 with permission.

TABLE 159-2 Reported Toxic Exposures to Nonbenzodiazepine Sedative-Hypnotic Agents in 1996

Substance	No. of Exposures	Deaths
Chloral hydrate	510	1
Ethchlorvynol	124	1
Glutethimide	15	0
Meprobamate	254	1
Methaqualone	45	0
Buspirone	Unknown	0
Zolpidem	Unknown	0
Gamma-hydroxybutyrate	2	0

Source: From Litovitz et al.[11]

This chapter reviews current drugs implicated and reported as toxic exposures of the nonbenzodiazepine sedative-hypnotic variety. Departures from general clinical presentation, complications, and management of overdose unique to a specific agent correspondingly will be highlighted in the discussion of that agent.

GAMMA-HYDROXYBUTYRATE (GHB)

GHB is an endogenous metabolite of gamma-aminobutyric acid (GABA), the major inhibitory neurotransmitter in the CNS. GHB is a putative neurotransmitter capable of inducing profound CNS depression. Abroad, it is used primarily as an anesthetic and in the treatment of narcolepsy and substance withdrawal. In the United States, it is only used for investigational research and is not approved for any clinical use. In the 1980s it was sold to bodybuilders as a health food product. GHB was touted as an effortless means to diet and build muscles during sleep by enhancing fat metabolism and the release of growth hormone. Within the last few years, it has become more prevalent as a drug of abuse for its reported euphoric and aphrodisiac effects in ''rave'' clubs and on college campuses. Despite a 1990 ban by the FDA on manufacture and sales, possession of GHB remains legal under federal law.[1]

The substance is considered an alternative to ''ecstasy'' or methamphetamine and is often coingested with alcohol. At least five fatalities related to GHB overdose have been reported. Data from the Drug Abuse Warning Network (DAWN) strongly suggest that there has been an increase in the abuse of GHB. The data indicate that GHB-related hospital emergency department (ED) visits increased from 20 in 1992 to 629 in 1996. Two-thirds of the episodes occurred among those aged 18 to 25 years, and 79 percent of patients were Caucasian males. Nearly 60 percent of episodes involved multiple drugs. Among episodes involving GHB for which a motive was reported, 91 percent reported ''recreational use'' as the reason for drug use. In those episodes in which a reason for the ED visit was documented, ''overdose'' was listed in 65 percent of the episodes and ''unexpected reaction'' in 33 percent.[2]

More recently, GHB has been cited as an agent of choice for substance-induced rape along with flunitrazepam (Rohypnol). These drugs are favored because of their abrupt coma-inducing effects, ready accessibility, and ease of administration. GHB is available as an odorless, colorless, and nearly tasteless liquid, powder, or capsule. Concerns regarding such illicit use, compounded by the growing popularity of GHB, prompted passage of a 1996 federal law, the Drug-Induced Rape Prevention and Punishment Act, which sets prison terms of up to 20 years for anyone convicted of using any controlled substance with the intent to commit a violent crime, including sexual assault. GHB case reports continue to demonstrate it to be a potentially life-threatening substance, especially when combined with other drugs of abuse. Furthermore, the unique difficulties posed by alleged substance-induced rape and assault require special consideration.

GHB is rapidly absorbed from the gastrointestinal (GI) tract, with peak plasma concentrations occurring 20 to 60 min after ingestion. The drug freely diffuses across the blood-brain barrier and concentrates in the CNS, kidney, heart, and muscle tissue. GHB is a CNS depressant capable of increasing dopamine levels and altering endogenous opioid systems, and it may have effects through other independent receptor-dependent mechanisms that are not well understood. GHB has a half-life of 20 min, and degradation generates no active metabolites. It is almost completely oxidized to carbon dioxide and water in the lungs and then expired.[1,3]

Clinical effects primarily involve the CNS system and are dose-related. Low doses produce euphoria, nystagmus, ataxia, and dizziness; moderate doses produce sedation; and high doses produce coma, respiratory depression, apnea, and rarely, death. Under controlled conditions, 10 mg/kg results in amnesia, hypotonia, and ataxia; 30 mg/kg induces euphoria, drowsiness, and dizziness. Doses of 50 mg/kg produce unconsciousness. Doses above 50 mg/kg causes bradycardia, respiratory depression, and seizure-like activity. Since most GHB is ''home brewed,'' dose uncertainty is guaranteed, and patients may present anywhere along this clinical spectrum. Additional symptoms reported in GHB overdose are vomiting, emergence delirium, and Cheyne-Stokes respirations. Characteristic clinical clues to GHB toxicity include marked agitation on stimulation despite periods of prolonged apnea and hypoxia. Historical features common in GHB intoxication include an abrupt onset of uncharacteristic aggressive behavior followed by sudden drowsiness, dizziness, euphoria, or coma with rapid reawakening and amnesia.[4]

Treatment is supportive for isolated GHB ingestion; aspiration precautions are recommended because of the potential for sudden changes in mental status. Bradycardia responds to atropine if simple stimulation fails to suffice. Neither naloxone nor flumazenil has been effective in treating CNS depression induced by GHB. Lavage or charcoal is of limited value because of the small amounts ingested and the drug's rapid absorption. The drug is undetectable in the urine after 12 h and missed by most routine toxicologic screens. Patients with symptoms of mild intoxication who improve rapidly (6 h of observation) and clear completely can be discharged from the ED; all others should be admitted for observation. Serious GHB intoxication complicated by coingestion of alcohol or other CNS depressants often will require emergent airway stabilization and cardiovascular support. Because GHB functions as an anesthetic induction agent, rapid-sequence intubation can proceed with paralytic agents alone. Once the airway is secured, routine gastric decontamination for coingestants is indicated. Extracorporeal elimination methods have not been evaluated in GHB overdose. A small case series indicates that dependence liability and a non-life-threatening withdrawal syndrome may exist with abrupt cessation of GHB in chronic use.[5]

When patients present to the ED seeking evaluation for possible substance-induced rape and/or assault, the best recommendation is compassionate advocacy. Currently, this is accomplished by collecting evidence, including urine samples that can be submitted for testing according to strict chain-of-custody procedures, which will be critical if the case is prosecuted. Even if the patient chooses not to report the incident to law enforcement authorities, drug testing can be important in identifying substances used. A free drug testing service has been made available to hospital EDs and rape crisis centers by Hoffmann-LaRoche, the manufacturer of Rohypnol. This testing program, accessed by calling (800) 608-6540, uses an independent forensic toxicology laboratory certified by the U.S. Department of Health and Human Services that follows strict chain-of-custody procedures. Testing for GHB and alcohol in addition to a wide range of other abused drugs was initiated in March of 1997. Results are returned in 10 days to the submitting agency to facilitate patient counseling.[6]

CHLORAL HYDRATE

Introduced in 1869, chloral hydrate was used as a popular sedative in clinical medicine until the advent of barbiturates largely supplanted their use in the early 1900s. Chloral hydrate is still used effectively for promoting sedation in children because in therapeutic doses it does not depress respiratory drive or circulatory function. Drawbacks include its narrow margin of safety, minimal analgesic activity, and propensity to develop tolerance and physical dependence. Withdrawal symptoms mimic those of alcohol abstinence. Toxic doses produce severe CNS, respiratory, and cardiovascular depression. Ethanol potentiates the sedative effects of chloral hydrate when taken in combination. This observation led to the street use of the two substances for malicious intent, as in slipping someone a "Mickey (Finn)" or "knockout drops." Chloral hydrate is a schedule III drug with recognized abuse potential.

Chloral hydrate absorption occurs rapidly and completely from the GI tract. It is a well-known mucous membrane irritant, especially when taken in quantity or undiluted. Development of GI bleeding is a useful clue in overdose. Chloral hydrate is lipid-soluble and easily transits all cell membranes. Volume of distribution and protein-binding properties are moderate. Metabolism occurs in the liver via alcohol dehydrogenanse and results in the generation of a longer-acting active metabolite, trichloroethanol, thought to be responsible for most of the drug's sedative action. Neither the parent drug nor the metabolite induces hepatic enzyme activity.

Chloral hydrate is a CNS depressant, with an unknown mechanism of action. Toxic doses also depress myocardial contractility, shorten the refractory period, and sensitize the myocardium to catecholamines. These factors create the substrate for resistant ventricular dysrhythmias that are the leading cause of mortality overdose.[7]

Clinical clues to the ingestion of chloral hydrate are a pearlike breath odor, hypotension, and cardiac dysrhythmias. Because chloral hydrate is radiopaque, abdominal x-rays may help narrow the differential diagnosis and guide decontamination. Serum levels are rarely helpful in guiding clinical management.[7]

Barring evidence of caustic injury causing perforation, gastric lavage should be considered and activated charcoal administered. Cardiac monitoring is mandatory, but treatment of ventricular dysrhythmia may prove difficult. There are anecdotal reports of successes using lidocaine and propanolol. Overdrive pacing in the setting of ventricular tachycardia may prove necessary. Avoid β-adrenergic drugs such as epinephrine, isoproterenol, and dopamine, which can potentiate dysrhythmias in the catecholamine-sensitized myocardium. If hypotension does not respond to volume loading, α-acting pressors such as norepinephrine should be used. Hemodialysis and hemoperfusion have been shown to be beneficial in severe overdose.

ETHCHORVYNOL

Ethchlorvynol, a schedule IV drug, was marketed initially in 1955 as an alternative to barbiturates, possessing a more rapid onset and shorter duration of action. However, the drug's high abuse potential, coupled with its tendency toward tolerance, physical dependence, and life-threatening withdrawal, overshadowed any claim of superior efficacy. The drug is available as a liquid-filled capsule, allowing both intravenous and oral abuse.

Ethchlorvynol is absorbed rapidly from the GI tract. It is highly lipophilic, concentrates in the CNS, and possesses a large volume of distribution. Its biphasic distribution is characterized by an initial period of adipose tissue deposition, 3 to 5 h after ingestion, with sedative effects disappearing only to resurface 7 to 10 h later when the drug redistributes from fat stores. Ethchlorvynol is moderately protein-bound and hepatically metabolized but does not induce microsomal enzymes. It also crosses the placenta and causes neonatal withdrawal symptoms. Mechanisms of CNS sedative action and hepatic degradation are unknown. Ethanol potentiates CNS depressant effects.

Distinguishing clinical clues in oral and intravenous overdose are a vinyl-like breath odor (although the patient may report a mintlike taste in the mouth), dypsnea, and dry cough. CNS effects include nystagmus, lethargy, and extremely prolonged coma. Isoelectric electroencephalographic (EEG) tracings have been reported but do not preclude full recovery. Hypothermia, hypotension, and relative bradycardia signal hemodynamic instability. Noncardiogenic pulmonary edema can be seen in massive oral overdose, although it is more characteristic of intravenous overdose. Polydrug exposures that potentiate CNS depression can result in respiratory arrest and cardiovascular collapse. Psychological and physical dependence develop rapidly. Chronic abusers may present with a variety of neurologic symptoms: ataxia, dysarthria, tremors, facial numbness, confusion, weakness, and visual disturbances (e.g., toxic amblyopia and central scotomata). Abstinence symptoms resembling those seen with alcohol withdrawal include states reminiscent of delirium tremens, with psychotic hallucinations, seizures, agitation, confusion, hypertension and tachycardia.

Successful treatment of ethchlorvynol overdose centers on the usual attention to supportive care and general decontamination. Serum levels of ethchlorvynol are not helpful in guiding management except to confirm diagnosis or trigger use of an extracorporeal elimination method in refractory cases. Charcoal hemoperfusion is superior to hemodialysis because of the drug's degree of protein binding and redistribution characteristics. Forced diuresis is not recommended because the risk of inducing pulmonary edema outweighs the minimal enhancement of drug cleared by the kidney.

GLUTETHIMIDE

Glutethimide was introduced in 1954 as a safe, nonaddicting sedative-hypnotic drug substitute for barbiturates. However, its clinical usefulness was quickly eclipsed by recognition of its potential adverse effects, which closely resembled those of barbiturates. Similarities include its ability to induce prolonged coma, addiction, tolerance, and severe withdrawal. In large overdose, several complications (e.g., cerebral and pulmonary edema, hypotension, seizures, and sudden apnea) make treatment of this schedule II substance more difficult. Illicit abuse centers on street combinations of codeine and glutethimide that reportedly produce a similar but longer-acting euphoria than can be obtained with intravenous heroin use. Side effects with chronic use include "hangover," headaches, blurred vision, rash, bone marrow suppression, hypocalcemia, and osteomalacia.[8,9]

Poor water solubility causes glutethimide to be slowly and erratically absorbed from the GI tract. However, coingestion of alcohol markedly enhances drug dissolution and absorption. The drug is lipophilic and initially concentrates in the CNS and adipose tissue, with eventual redistribution. Drug half-lives up to 40 h have been observed in overdose. Glutethimide has a large volume of distribution, is moderately protein-bound, and is capable of inducing hepatic microsomal enzymes. Hepatic degradation results in several active metabolites that may play a role in the prolonged fluctuating coma seen in overdose. Glutethemide crosses the placenta, and fetal blood concentrations equal those of the mother. Minimal amounts of unchanged drug are excreted in breast milk.[9]

Clinical manifestations of glutethimide overdose mirror those seen with barbiturate toxicity with two exceptions. Anticholinergic symptoms are prominent, and the unique fluctuating nature of the prolonged coma complicates management. Mydriasis, dry mucous membranes, tenacious secretions, tachycardia, hypertension, ileus, urinary retention, hyperpyrexia, delirium, seizures, and agitation may be observed.[8]

Serum levels of one of the active metabolites, 4-HG, may correlate better with toxicity than do levels of the parent compound. As with ethchlorvynol, complete clinical recovery is possible despite an isoelectric EEG if the patient has been spared the insults of cerebral hypoxia and/or ischemia. Coingestion of other sedative-hypnotic drugs, prolonged coma, and age over 60 years are predictive of negative outcomes in glutethimide overdose.[10]

Late gastric lavage (12 h after ingestion) has been shown to be beneficial in obtunded patients whose overdose has resulted in delayed gastric emptying due to anticholinergic effects. In asymptomatic patients presenting 4 h or more after ingestion, the poor water solubility of glutethimide limits the effectiveness of lavage. Activated charcoal and cathartics are recommended in all patients, but the utility of multiple-dose activated charcoal (MDAC) remains unproven. The use of physostigmine to reverse anticholinergic CNS toxicity is not recommended. Forced diuresis is not effective and can precipitate the development of pulmonary edema. Improvement in clinical outcomes for the elderly and those patients with severe intoxications (serum glutethimide levels > 40 mg/L) has been documented using extracorporeal techniques to increase drug clearance. Hemoperfusion is the preferred method, but efficacy remains controversial, so hemoperfusion should be limited to patients not responding to supportive measures alone. Given the potential for delayed, erratic absorption and characteristic fluctuating mental status, admission and prolonged observation of patients with significant overdose are indicated.[8-10]

MEPROBAMATE

Meprobamate has been in clinical use as a schedule IV drug with anxiolytic and sedative-hypnotic properties since 1955. Several combination products remain available, but prescription practices have changed in recent years, favoring the safer benzodiazepine derivatives. Nonetheless, toxic exposures continue to be reported, with intentional overdose commonly implicated as the rationale. Also notable, carisoprodol (Soma), a structurally related muscle relaxant that is metabolized to meprobamate, is emerging as a street drug of abuse. Carisoprodol often is combined with Tylenol and codeine. The combination is known as "Soma-Do" and "Soma-Coma." According to the 1996 Annual Report of the American Association of Poison Control Centers, carisoprodol has a similar number of deaths due to overdose as meprobamate. However, the actual number of exposures is unknown.[11]

Absorption of meprobamate occurs in the small intestine. The compound is poorly water-soluble, stable in acidic environments, and able to decrease gastric motility. These characteristics lend themselves to the development of gastric concretions. Meprobamate has a large volume of distribution, is poorly protein-bound, and is metabolized primarily in the liver, where it can induce microsomal enzymes. Approximately 10 percent of the drug is excreted unchanged in the urine. Meprobamate crosses the placenta, and fetal blood levels approximate those of the mother. It is also excreted in breast milk.[12]

Meprobamate depresses the CNS by reducing sensory transmission, particularly in the thalamus. In overdose, meprobamate also concentrates in myocardial tissue, causing direct cardiotoxicity, manifesting as depressed contractility and hypotension often in the absence of respiratory depression.[12]

Clinical features of meprobamate toxicity are similar to those of other sedative-hypnotic agents. CNS symptoms range in mild exposures from nystagmus and dysarthria to ataxia, confusion, and deep coma in overdose. In contrast to barbiturates, hypotension may be an early sign of toxicity occurring in lesser stages of coma. Prolonged and fluctuating coma is due to continued drug absorption from concretions. Hypotension is the hallmark of serious meprobamate overdose. Seizures, cardiac dysrhythmias, and pulmonary edema have been reported rarely. Abstinence syndromes reflective of the degree of physical dependence and tolerance develop quickly, usually within 1 to 2 days of drug discontinuation, and can be severe.[12]

Utility of serum levels of meprobamate is limited but confirmative of ingestion. It may guide the need for extracorporeal removal. The treatment approach after stabilization of the airway and circulation centers on gastric decontamination given meprobamate's propensity to form concretions. Delayed gastric lavage and whole-bowel irrigation using a polyethylene glycol solution until rectal effluent is clear is advocated but not well studied. Multiple-dose activated charcoal (MDAC) also appears to be safe and effective in increasing the clearance of meprobamate, although solid clinical outcome data are lacking.[13] Gastrostomy and endoscopic removal of concretions have been reported anecdotally as successful. Hemoperfusion is the preferred extracorporeal method to enhance drug elimination when usual intensive supportive measures fail or serum levels dictate. Forced diuresis is controversial. Given the limited renal elimination of meprobamate and the risk of inducing pulmonary edema, it is not recommended. Management of hypotension should include the early use of vasopressors and inotropes to avoid fluid overload.[13]

METHAQUALONE

One of the more ubiquitous sedative-hypnotic barbiturate substitutes, methaqualone was introduced in 1965 and withdrawn from the U.S. market in 1984 because promotions of safety and nonaddictiveness proved false. High abuse potential owed to methaqualone's popularity as a street aphrodisiac. The college pastime of "luding out," slang for a standard combination of 300 mg methaqualone ingested with wine, was used for attainment of characteristic deep relaxation, disinhibition, and euphoria.[14] In the 1980s the drug was used increasingly to mitigate the unpleasant side effects of popular stimulants as a "cocaine downer." Even though the drug continues to be clandestinely manufactured abroad and smuggled into the United States, actual reports of toxicity and mortality are becoming rare. Cessation of legal synthesis and readily available benzodiazepine alternatives explain this trend.

Methaqualone is rapidly absorbed from the GI tract, is highly lipophilic, and concentrates in the brain, adipose tissue, and liver. It exists as a weak base with a large volume of distribution and is highly protein-bound. The majority of its metabolism occurs in the liver; no active metabolites are generated, and microsomal enzymes are moderately induced.

The drug is a CNS depressant like all the other sedative-hypnotics; however, its mechanism of action is more of a mystery. In contrast to other sedative-hypnotics that depress muscle tone and reflexes, methaqualone increases muscle tone and motor activity by selectively depressing polysynaptic spinal reflexes at high dose. Clinically, hypertonicity, clonus, hyperreflexia, and muscle twitching are seen along with the usual sedative-hypnotic symptom profile of lethargy, ataxia, dysarthria, seizures, and coma at escalating dose.[15] Hyperacusis is also reported and may be a helpful diagnostic clue to ingestion. More often the drug-induced dissociative "high," poor judgment, and impulsive behavior result in death due to trauma rather than from the direct toxic effects of overdose.[16]

Cardiopulmonary symptoms include hypotension due to decreased myocardial contractility and respiratory depression. However, such symptoms occur less commonly than with other sedative-hypnotics, even in comatose patients. Coingestion of other CNS depressants can lead to severe respiratory depression and sudden apnea. Pulmonary edema can be seen as a result of increased capillary permeability, a risk common to most sedative-hypnotics.

GI distress and hemorrhage have been noted in methaqualone overdose. Drug-induced platelet aggregation inhibition, prolonged prothrombin and partial thromboplastin times, and decreased factors V and VII are causative.[17] As with other sedative-hypnotic agents, decontamination and supportive care remain the mainstays of therapy. Specific management considerations for methaqualone overdose include early use of benzodiazepines to control hypertonicity and seizures along with administration of blood products (i.e., platelets, vitamin

K, fresh-frozen plasma) in the setting of hemorrhage. Charcoal hemoperfusion is more effective than hemodialysis in clearing methaqualone but is reserved for patients who fail to respond to maximal supportive therapy or whose serum methaqualone levels are greater than 10 to 15 mg/dL. Severe abstinence symptoms occur in chronic users when this drug is stopped abruptly and require hospital admission for gradual withdrawal.

BUSPIRONE

Buspirone is a prototype anxiolytic drug from the azapirone family introduced in 1984. The agent is not chemically or pharmacologically related to the other sedative-hypnotics, although its efficacy profile is comparable with that of the benzodiazepines. Clinical indications for buspirone are not fully delineated; however, it appears most useful in the treatment of conditions such as chronic anxiety, especially in the elderly, and mixed anxiety-depression states. It does not affect GABA or benzodiazepine receptors and therefore produces less sedation, euphoria, psychomotor impairment, and ethanol potentiation. It does affect CNS serotonergic, dopaminergic, and noradrenergic neurotransmission, but the mechanisms are not fully understood. Buspirone appears to have several merits when compared with the other sedative-hypnotics. It exhibits a virtual absence of potential for addiction, a wide margin of therapeutic safety, and no documented delayed toxicity or withdrawal reactions with abrupt discontinuation of chronic use.[18]

Buspirone is rapidly absorbed, highly protein-bound, and widely distributed to the tissues. Metabolism occurs in the liver, with at least one active metabolite generated. Fecal elimination accounts for 20 to 40 percent of drug clearance.

Experience in overdose may be limited by the drug's wide margin of safety. Patients have taken up to 3 g (which is 150 times the average anxiolytic dose) in overdose without lasting ill effects. Most common clinical symptoms in overdose are nonspecific drowsiness and dysphoria. Rarely, hypotension, bradycardia, seizures, GI upset, dystonia, and priapism also have been described. Spontaneous acute hypertensive reactions have developed in patients coprescribed buspirone and monoamine oxidase inhibitors. No other adverse drug interactions or unexpected toxicities have emerged with buspirone use.[18]

Treatment is supportive. Serum levels are not useful clinically, and extracorporeal methods of elimination enhancement have not been evaluated.

ZOLPIDEM

Zolpidem is a new short-acting hypnotic agent introduced in 1988 for the treatment of insomnia. It is an imidazopyridine derivative, structurally different from benzodiazepines and other sedative-hypnotics. It binds preferentially to one of the benzodiazepine receptor subtypes (omega-1, benzodiazepine-1) in the CNS. The drug is rapidly absorbed, has an onset of action within 30 min, and is effective for up to 6 h. Zolpidem is metabolized in the liver to inactive metabolites that are excreted in the urine and feces. Its advantage over the benzodiazepines is the absence of reported addiction, tolerance, or withdrawal symptoms.[19] Experience in overdose is limited.

Signs of acute overdose in larger series commonly include drowsiness and vomiting and, rarely, coma and respiratory depression. These symptoms escalate with dose and are complicated by coingestion of other psychotropic drugs and ethanol. In most cases, symptoms of intoxication remit rapidly, and therapy is usually limited to general supportive measures.[20]

Treatment is not aided by obtaining serum zolpidem levels; the utility of multidose activated charcoal and extracorporeal elimination enhancement methods has not been evaluated in overdose. Anecdotally, flumazenil has been effective in reversing the CNS and respiratory actions of zolpidem.[21] The recommended initial dose is 0.2 mg IV over 30 s. If no improvement in consciousness is observed within 30 s, an additional dose of 0.3 mg may be administered over 30 s. This dosing regimen (0.2 mg followed by 0.3 mg) can be repeated one more time, to a total dose of 1 mg, at an interval of 1 min if adequate consciousness is not obtained. Flumazenil at a total dose of 1 mg or less IV leaves 50 percent of the benzodiazepine receptors unoccupied and therefore should limit the risk of acute withdrawal so long as this dose is not exceeded. Flumazenil is best avoided in overdose settings where there is evidence that a drug capable of causing seizures has been ingested. Furthermore, the presence of any of the following contraindications would obviate the use of flumazenil in overdose: (1) suspected tricyclic overdose and/or clinical signs that could be related to tricyclic activity, (2) overdose of unknown agents, (3) known seizure disorder, and (4) history of prescribed benzodiazepines or chronic benzodiazepine dependence. In the event of a flumazenil-induced seizure, a therapeutic dose of benzodiazepine should be effective.

TABLE 159-3 General Management of Nonbenzodiazepine Sedative-Hypnotics in Overdose

General treatment remains the same for all agents:

1. Ensure airway patency in all patients prior to gastric decontamination or charcoal administration.
2. Use pulse oximetry and/or arterial blood gas sampling to monitor the adequacy of oxygenation and ventilation.
3. Monitor cardiac status.
4. Provide intravenous access and initiate crystalloid fluid resuscitation, up to 2 L in adults or to a systolic blood pressure of 100 mmHg. The early use of vasopressors is indicated because most sedative-hypnotics have the propensity to cause pulmonary edema.
5. Administer glucose, naloxone, and thiamine intravenously to all patients with an altered mental status.
6. Ipecac is contraindicated given the CNS depression associated with these agents in overdose. Gastric lavage should be considered and may be required for certain ingestions. Charcoal (1 g/kg) and sorbitol (1 g/kg) should be administered. MDAC (20–50 g q4h) may be useful in profoundly comatose patients or in special cases such as glutethimide. Neither whole-bowel irrigation nor MDAC is recommended in patients with an ileus. Forced diuresis is not useful with these agents due to limited renal excretion.
7. Laboratory evaluation should include glucose levels, blood chemistries, creatine phosphokinase, complete blood count, arterial blood gas measurement, toxicologic screen, chest radiograph, and electrocardiogram. Serum levels generally are not helpful clinically except to establish diagnosis and in nonresponders may guide decisions regarding extracorporeal elimination.
8. Avoid CNS stimulants or physostigmine to reverse coma. The contraindications to flumazenil use should be reviewed prior to its administration, and its efficacy in reversing sedation with most of the preceding agents has not been well studied.
9. In general, hemoperfusion is superior to hemodialysis in enhancing drug elimination because these drugs tend to be highly lipophilic and protein-bound.
10. Most patients will recover with meticulous supportive care. Anticipate clinical complications of abstinence states during admission and take precautions in the ED for seizures, aspiration pneumonia, ARDS, and rhabdomyolysis to limit associated overdose morbidity.

GENERAL TREATMENT GUIDELINES

The agents discussed in this chapter share certain generalities useful in guiding management (Table 159-3). Most overdoses of nonbenzodiazepine sedative-hypnotics are taken orally and often involve coingestants. Therefore, a diligent search for other treatable substances (e.g., acetaminophen and salicylates) is mandatory. Coingestants also may obscure expected toxidrome features or potentiate symptoms, complicating management. All the agents discussed, with the possible exceptions of buspirone, zolpidem, and GHB, cause physical dependence and tolerance in chronic use. Thus hospitalized patients who have been treated for acute toxicity subsequently may develop life-threatening abstinence states that are best anticipated from the ED.

REFERENCES

1. Centers for Disease Control and Prevention: Gamma-hydroxybutyrate use. *MMWR* 46:281, 1997.
2. Office of Applied Studies, Substance Abuse and Mental Health Services Administration: Drug Abuse Warning Network 1992-1996. Rockville, MD: U.S. Department of Health and Human Services (unpublished data).
3. Tunnicliff G: Sites of action of gamma-hydroxybutyrate (GHB): A neuroactive drug with abuse potential. *Clin Toxicol* 35:581, 1997.
4. Li J, Stokes SA, Woeckener A: A tale of novel intoxication: A review of the effects of gamma-hydroxybutyric acid with recommendations for management. *Ann Emerg Med* 31:729, 1998.
5. Galloway GP, Frederick SL, Staggers FE Jr, et al: Gamma-hydroxybutyrate: An emerging drug of abuse that causes physical dependence. *Addiction* 92:89, 1997.
6. Armstrong R: When drugs are used for rape. *J Emerg Nurs* 23:378, 1997.
7. Bowyer K, Glasser SP: Chloral hydrate overdose and cardiac arrhythmias. *Chest* 77:232, 1980.
8. Maher JF, Schreiner GE, Westervett FB Jr: Acute glutethimide intoxication: Clinical experience (22 patients) compared to acute barbiturate intoxication (63 patients). *Am J Med* 33:70, 1962.
9. Bender FH, Cooper JV, Dreyfus R: Fatalities associated with acute overdose of glutethimide (Doriden) and codeine. *Vet Hum Toxicol* 30:332, 1988.
10. Hansen AR, Kennedy KA, Ambre JJ, et al: Glutethimide poisoning: A metabolite contributes to morbidity and mortality. *N Engl J Med* 292:251, 1975.
11. Litovitz TL, Smilkstein M, Felberg L, et al: 1996 Annual report of the American Association of Poison Control Centers National Data Collection System. *Am J Emerg Med* 15:447, 1997.
12. Dennison J, Edwards JN, Volans GN: Meprobamate overdosage. *Hum Toxicol* 4:215, 1985.
13. Hassan E: Treatment of meprobamate overdose with repeated oral doses of activated charcoal. *Ann Emerg Med* 15:73, 1986.
14. Agar SA: Luding out. *N Engl J Med* 287:51, 1972.
15. Abboud PT, Freedman MT, Rogers RM, et al: Methaqualone poisoning with muscular hyperactivity necessitating the use of curare. *Chest* 65:204, 1974.
16. Wetli CV: Changing patterns of methaqualone abuse: A survey of 246 fatalities. *JAMA* 249:621, 1983.
17. Mills DG: Effects of methaqualone on blood platelet function. *Clin Pharmacol Ther* 23:685, 1978.
18. Napoliello MJ, Domantay AG: Buspirone: A worldwide update. *Br J Psychiatry* 159:40, 1991.
19. Roger M, Attali P, Coquelin JP: Multicenter, double-blind, controlled comparison of zolpidem and triazolam in elderly patients with insomnia. *Clin Ther* 15:127, 1993.
20. Garnier R, Guerault E, Muzard D, et al: Acute zolpidem poisoning: Analysis of 344 cases. *Clin Toxicol* 32:391, 1994.
21. Lheureux P, Debailleul G, DeWitte O, et al: Zolpidem intoxication mimicking narcotic overdose: Response to flumazenil. *Hum Exp Toxicol* 9:105, 1990.

160 ALCOHOLS

William A. Berk
Wilma V. Henderson

ETHANOL

Ethanol is the most frequently used and abused intoxicant in the United States[1] and most other societies, including those where it is proscribed.

TABLE 160-1 Substances That Contribute to the Serum Osmolality*

Substance	Molecular Weight	mOsm/L at 100 mg/dL	Correction Factor
Ethanol	46	22	4.6
Isopropanol	60	17	6.0
Methanol	32	31	3.2
Ethylene glycol	62	16	6.2

*Molecular weight and contribution of alcohols to serum osmolality. To estimate concentration of an alcohol in mg/dL, use the following formula: (osmolal gap-10) × correction factor. This estimation is valid only if the alcohol is the only unmeasured abnormal contributor to osmolality.

Nearly three-quarters of adult Americans consume at least one alcoholic drink each year, compared with only 36 percent who smoke at least one cigarette. Beer ranks as the fourth most popular beverage in terms of volume consumed, after soft drinks, milk, and coffee. Adult consumption of beverages containing ethanol peaked in 1980–1981 at 2.77 gallons per person of pure ethanol, but by 1993 this had declined to 2.25 gallons.[1] In recent years wine coolers have accounted for up to 25 percent of all U.S. ethanol consumption.

Distilled spirits typically contain ethanol volumes of 40 to 50 percent (80 to 100 proof), although brands with volumes of 75 percent or more exist. Wines have an ethanol volume of 10 to 20 percent, while beers range from 2 to 6 percent. Ethanol is also a constituent of mouthwashes (up to 75 percent volume), colognes (40 to 60 percent), and medicinal preparations (0.4 to 65 percent).

The medical, psychiatric, social, legal, and public health implications of ethanol use are well known to emergency physicians. Emergency departments (EDs) are expected to provide a safe haven for intoxicated individuals. Ethanol has been detected in the blood of 15 to 40 percent of unselected ED patients, depending on locale.[2] Yet emergency physicians and inpatient specialists fail to recognize 50 percent of patients with ethanol dependence.[3] The formal diagnosis of alcoholism has rested on instruments such as CAGE (see Chap. 287) and the Michigan Alcohol Screening Test. In the clinical setting, pointed questioning, when appropriate, about quantity of ethanol intake, medical complications usually caused by drinking, and whether the patient or others has ever felt he or she had a drinking problem will usually uncover such problems. There is growing evidence that the manner in which questions are understood by the patient may be culture- and gender-specific and thus may need to be specifically tailored. See Chap. 287 for a discussion of identification and referral issues.

Pathophysiology

Ethanol is a central nervous system depressant which inhibits neuronal activity, probably through its effects on cell membranes. Behavioral stimulation is often observed at low blood concentrations. Cross-tolerance exists between ethanol and other sedative-hypnotic agents, including benzodiazepines and barbiturates. Absorption occurs from the mouth and esophagus to a small extent, from the stomach and large bowel to a moderate extent, but chiefly from the proximal portion of the small bowel.

Gender-related differences in the metabolism of ethanol explain the considerably higher blood ethanol levels in women versus men after similar dosing on a gram-per-kilogram basis. Women have a smaller volume of distribution (0.6 L/kg) for ethanol than men (0.7 L/kg) and have decreased first-pass metabolism of ethanol because their gastric walls contain less alcohol dehydrogenase than do those of men.[4]

Approximately 2 to 10 percent of ethanol may be excreted by the lungs, in urine, or in sweat, the proportion being dependent on blood concentration. The remainder is metabolized to acetaldehyde in the liver by one of two pathways. In the cell, cytosol alcohol dehydrogenase with nicotinamide adenine dinucleotide as a cofactor produces acetaldehyde, which in turn is metabolized by aldehyde dehydrogenase. The second pathway, which is clinically significant at high blood ethanol concentrations and has increased activity with repeated exposures to ethanol, is a microsomal alcohol oxidizing system.

Clinical Features

Symptoms and signs of ethanol intoxication include slurred speech, nystagmus, disinhibited behavior, central nervous system depression, and decreased motor coordination and control. A lowering of usual blood pressure or even hypotension may occur secondary to ethanol-mediated decrease in total peripheral resistance or as a result of volume loss. Reflex tachycardia may also be observed. When hypotension is present, causes other than ethanol intoxication must be considered. Morbidity and mortality in association with acute intoxication are predominantly the result of accidental injuries, often motor vehicle collisions, related to ethanol-induced deficits in judgment or physical capabilities.

Because of the phenomenon of tolerance, blood alcohol levels correlate poorly with degree of intoxication. While death from respiratory depression may occur in unhabituated individuals at concentrations of 400 to 500 mg/dL, it is not uncommon for some alcoholics to appear minimally intoxicated if at all at blood concentrations as high as 400 mg/dL.[5] Although most states have adopted 100 or 80 mg/dL as the legal definition of intoxication for the purposes of driving a motor vehicle, there is considerable evidence to suggest that impairment may be seen with levels as low as 5 mg/dL, especially in unhabituated individuals.

Treatment

Management of acute ethanol intoxication consists of observation until clinical sobriety is attained and attending to associated injuries or medical illness. A careful examination should be performed to evaluate for complicating injuries or medical conditions. Ethanol levels are not necessarily required for mild or moderate intoxication where no other abnormality is suspected, but many institutions offer a blood alcohol screening panel that tests for ethanol, methanol, and isopropanol. One advantage of the alcohol screening panel is the detection of otherwise unsuspected isopropanol or methanol. The assays for each alcohol are specific and do not cross-react with each other. Hypoglycemia should be excluded by a bedside glucose determination. Ethanol does not bind to activated charcoal, so it is not needed unless other adsorbable substances have been ingested. Any alcoholic with severe CNS depression, even if apparently attributable to intoxication, should receive thiamine. Because nutritional status is often wanting, folate and other vitamin supplements are often added to the intravenous solution. Patients with mild to moderate intoxication do not necessarily require intravenous line placement, treatment with vitamin supplements other than thiamine, or intravenous fluid administration unless clinical signs of volume depletion are present. The IV solution should be 5% D/0.9% NaCl since alcoholics are often glycogen depleted. Careful and serial observation is crucial, as deterioration in mental status should be considered secondary to causes other than ethanol and managed accordingly. Unhabituated patients eliminate ethanol from the bloodstream at a rate of 15 to 20 mg/dL per hour, while alcoholics average 25 to 35 mg/dL per hour. Most patients with central nervous system depression secondary to ethanol ingestion improve within a few hours of emergency department arrival at the ED. Respiratory depression may result in hypoventilation and carbon dioxide retention, which, if severe, may rarely require advanced airway management.

Alcoholics should be questioned about concomitant drug use. In the past, ethylene glycol or methanol was occasionally substituted for or combined with ethanol. Today cocaine has clearly become the most common concomitant drug used by alcoholics. The attraction of abusing these drugs together may relate to the formation of a metabolite, cocaethylene, which has 40 times the affinity for cocaine receptors of cocaine itself[6] and is thus an extremely potent intoxicant. The risk of sudden death among users of both drugs simultaneously may be as high as 20 times that with cocaine alone. Ethanol is the most common cause of an osmolal gap (Table 160-1), which also characterizes isopropanol, methanol, and ethylene glycol poisoning. However, a distinguishing feature of methanol and ethylene glycol is the wide-anion-gap metabolic acidosis. It is seductive to attribute the metabolic acidosis to the presence of ethanol. This can lead to missing or a significantly delay in establishing the correct diagnosis. Indeed, metabolism of alcohol in the liver leads to the formation of ketoacids, relatively depleting NAD while increasing NADH. As a consequence, high NADH diverts pyruvate, destined for glucose formation, to lactate, resulting in acidosis and hypoglycemia. However, the presence of significant acidosis should never be ascribed to alcohol intoxication alone. An alternate cause must be sought expeditiously and will invariably be found. For a discussion on other issues related to the ethanol-intoxicated patient, see Chap. 299.

Disposition

Patients with acute ethanol intoxication rarely require hospital admission for treatment of this problem alone. However, questions frequently arise over alcoholics who appear clinically sober while still having considerable blood ethanol concentrations. Medical judgment of mental competence should not be confused with any particular blood alcohol (BAC) level. Patients whose intoxication has resolved to the extent that they do not constitute a danger to themselves or others *and* who will not be responsible for their own transport, may be discharged on their own recognizance or preferably in the company of friends or relatives who can assist them and take some responsibility for their care.

ISOPROPANOL

Isopropanol ($CH_3CHOHCH_3$), also known as isopropyl alcohol and 2-propanol, is commonly found in the home as rubbing alcohol. It is also used widely in industry as a solvent and disinfectant and is a component of a variety of skin and hair products, jewelry cleaners, detergents, paint thinners, and antifreeze. Poisoning usually results from ingestion but may also occur after inhalation in poorly ventilated areas—for example, during alcohol sponge bathing. Toxicity occurring after administration of an isopropanol enema has also been reported. Its principal metabolite, acetone, does not cause the eye, kidney, cardiac, or metabolic toxicity caused by the metabolites of methanol and ethylene glycol.

Isopropanol is approximately twice as potent as ethanol in causing central nervous system depression and has a duration of two to four times that of ethanol. As a result it is on occasion utilized as a substitute intoxicant by alcoholics as well as in suicide attempts. After ethanol, it is the second most commonly ingested alcohol. It is more toxic than ethanol, though considerably less so than methanol or ethylene glycol.

Pathophysiology

Isopropanol is a clear, volatile liquid with a bitter, burning taste and an aromatic odor. It is rapidly absorbed after being ingested, with 80 percent of an oral dose being absorbed after 30 min and complete absorption within 2 h. The substance has a volume of distribution of

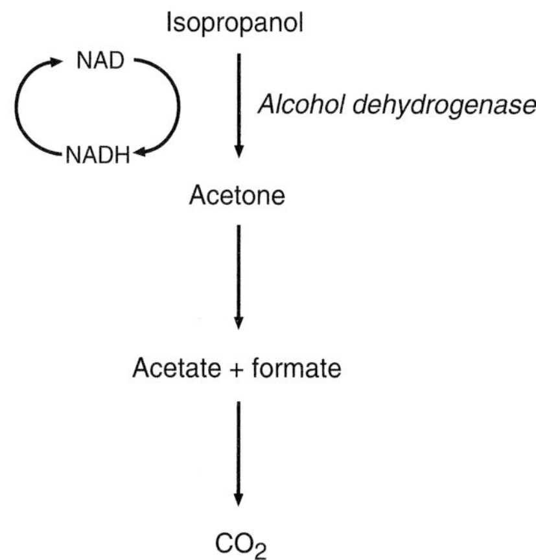

FIG. 160-1. Metabolic pathway of isopropanol in the liver.

0.6 to 0.7 L/kg. Small and clinically insignificant amounts are resecreted by the salivary glands and stomach.

The kidneys excrete 20 to 50 percent of an absorbed dose unchanged. However, the major pathway for metabolism of isopropanol is in the liver, where it is oxidized to acetone by alcohol dehydrogenase (Fig. 160-1). Acetone is further metabolized to acetate, to formate, and then finally to carbon dioxide. Mild acidosis may result from the conversion of acetone to acetic acid and formic acid. However, unlike methanol and ethylene glycol, significant acidoses directly ascribed to isopropanol or its metabolites is not seen. A hallmark of isopropanol toxicity is ketonemia and ketonuria, but without elevated blood glucose or glycosuria. This feature helps differentiate isopropanol ingestion from poisoning with ethylene glycol or methanol.

Isopropanol most closely follows concentration-dependent (first-order) kinetics. The half-life of isopropanol in the absence of ethanol is 6 to 7 h, while the half-life of acetone is 22 to 28 h. The long half-life of acetone may be the cause of the prolonged symptomatology often associated with isopropanol poisoning. Ethanol administration has not been used clinically to inhibit isopropanol metabolism to acetone.

The toxic dose of 70% isopropanol is approximately 1 mL/kg, with the lethal dose in an adult approximately 2 to 4 mL/kg. As little as 0.5 mL/kg may cause symptoms, but survival has been reported following ingestions of up to 1 L. Children are especially susceptible to toxic effects and may develop symptoms with as little as three swallows of 70% isopropanol.

Clinical Features

The clinical features of isopropanol intoxication are similar to those seen with ethanol intoxication except that the duration of symptoms and signs is longer and central nervous system depression may be more profound because of the formation of acetone. Onset of symptoms occurs within 30 to 60 min, with peak effects in a few hours. Nystagmus is usually present. Severe poisoning is marked by early onset of coma, respiratory depression, and hypotension.[7]

Massive ingestion may cause hypotension secondary to peripheral vasodilatation, with contributions possible from hemorrhagic gastritis. Serious dysrhythmias are rare.[7]

Hemorrhagic gastritis secondary to gastric irritation appears early and is a striking feature of isopropanol ingestions, resulting in nausea, vomiting, abdominal pain, and upper gastrointestinal hemorrhage.[7]

Hypoglycemia may occur secondary to depressed gluconeogenesis. Less common complications include hepatic dysfunction, acute tubular necrosis, myoglobinuria, hemolytic anemia, rhabdomyolysis, and myopathy.[7]

Isopropanol poisoning should be suspected when the smell of rubbing alcohol is present on the breath, when there is acidosis associated with ketonuria and ketonemia without glycosuria or hyperglycemia, and in the presence of an elevated osmolal gap.[7] Acidosis, if present, is mild. The use of alcohol screening panels helps detect unsuspected isopropanolism.

As previously mentioned, isopropanol has approximately twice the intoxicating effect of ethanol at the same blood concentration. Although isopropanol levels of 50 mg/dL are associated with mild intoxication in individuals who are not habituated to ethanol, alcoholic patients may be considerably more resistant to the central nervous system effects of isopropanol.

Treatment

If there is suspicion of isopropanol poisoning, intravenous access should be established with bedside testing for blood glucose, and administration of thiamine and naloxone if indicated. Patients should be monitored for central nervous system or respiratory depression. Because of the rapid absorption of isopropanol, there is no utility to performing gastric lavage. Activated charcoal binds isopropanol poorly and is not necessary in the absence of ingestion of adsorbable substances. Laboratory studies are guided by the results of examination and clinical condition. Serum electrolytes, CBC, glucose, and acetone are generally needed as a minimum.

In severely obtunded patients, airway management may require intubation and ventilatory support. Hypotension usually responds to intravenous fluids. In severe cases, support with pressors may be indicated. Patients with severe hemorrhagic gastritis may require blood transfusion. The acidosis associated with isopropanol poisoning is usually mild. If acidosis is significant, vigorous investigation for another cause must be made. For example, if the patient is hypotensive, consider lactic acidosis. Hemodialysis is indicated when hypotension is refractory to conventional therapy, resulting in hemodynamic instability, or when the predicted peak isopropanol level is greater than 400 mg/dL. Hemodialysis is effective in eliminating both isopropanol and acetone. Peritoneal dialysis is less effective.

Patients with lethargy or prolonged central nervous system depression should be admitted to the hospital. Those who remain asymptomatic for 6 to 8 h may be discharged or referred for substance abuse counseling or psychiatric evaluation.

METHANOL

Methanol (CH_3OH)—also referred to as methyl alcohol, wood spirits, or wood alcohol—is used widely in commercial, industrial, and marine solvents. It is a component of many paint removers, varnishes, shellacs, windshield washing fluids, and antifreeze formulations. It is a product of wood distillation. Methanol poisoning has resulted from the consumption of contaminated whiskey, accidental ingestion by desperate alcoholics, or intentional ingestion during suicide attempts. Methanol's toxicity is due to the formation of two toxic metabolites, formaldehyde and formic acid. Therapeutic strategies are therefore based on prevention of the formation of these metabolites or their removal from the body.

Pathophysiology

Methanol is a colorless, volatile liquid with a distinctive odor. It is well absorbed from the gastrointestinal tract, with peak levels attained 30 to 90 min after ingestion. Most incidents of toxicity occur after oral ingestion, but significant absorption may also occur through the lungs or skin. The serum half-life after mild toxicity is 14 to 20 h. With severe toxicity, this increases to 24 to 30 h. Methanol has a volume of distribution of 0.6 to 0.7 L/kg.

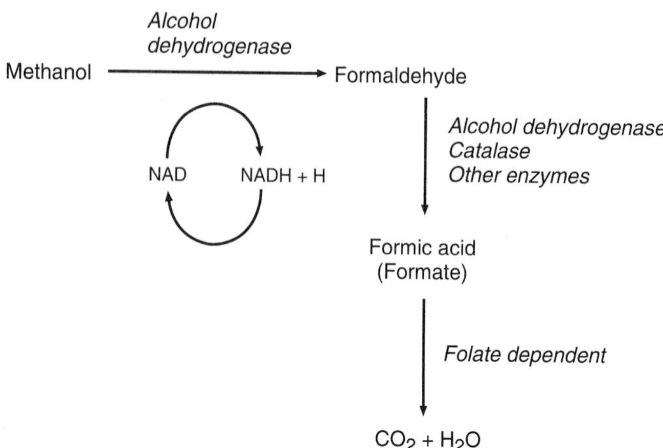

FIG. 160-2. Metabolism of methanol in the liver.

Following ingestion, highest concentrations are found in the kidney, liver, and gastrointestinal tract, but high levels are also found in the vitreous humor and optic nerve. Most methanol—90 to 95 percent—is eliminated by the liver, while renal excretion accounts for 2 to 5 percent; pulmonary excretion is minimal. In overdose situations, elimination follows saturation (zero-order) kinetics.

Toxicity from methanol poisoning results from the metabolism by hepatic alcohol dehydrogenase of methanol to formaldehyde and formic acid (Fig. 160-2). The accumulation of formic acid is associated with the onset of clinical symptoms. Lactate is produced from formate-induced inhibition of mitochondrial respiration, as a result of tissue hypoxia, and to a lesser extent as a result of a decrease in the intracellular NAD/NADH ratio caused by the oxidation of methanol and thus stimulation of anaerobic glycolysis and lactate production. Formaldehyde production in the retina causes optic papillitis and retinal edema, in severe cases resulting in blindness; hence the term "blind drunk." Since folate is a cofactor in the breakdown of formic acid to carbon dioxide and water, alcoholics who are folate-deficient may be especially susceptible to methanol toxicity.

The amount of methanol required to cause toxicity varies; death has been reported after ingestion of a dose as small as 15 mL of a 40% solution. Although 30 mL of a 40% solution is considered the minimal lethal dose, amounts as large as 500 to 600 mL have been ingested with survival reported.

Clinical Features

The symptoms of methanol poisoning may not appear for up to 12 to 18 h after ingestion because of the time it takes for methanol to be metabolized to its toxic metabolites. The delay in symptoms may be even longer if ethanol has been ingested. The cardinal clinical manifestations of methanol poisoning are central nervous system depression similar to that of ethanol, visual disturbances, abdominal pain, nausea and vomiting, and wide-anion-gap metabolic acidosis. As with isopropanol, the early phase of elation commonly seen in ethanol intoxication is absent.

On arrival at the hospital, the victim may be confused or, in severe cases, comatose. There may be complaints of headache or vertigo, and seizures may occur. Visual disturbances are seen in approximately 50 percent of patients. These include diplopia, blurred vision, decreased visual acuity, photophobia, descriptions of "looking into a snow field," constricted visual fields, and blindness. The clinician may find nystagmus, fixed and dilated pupils, retinal edema, and optic atrophy or hyperemia of the optic disk. Computed tomography of the brain may reveal basal ganglia infarcts consistent with the parkinsonian syndrome, which has been reported after methanol poisoning.[7] Methanol is a potent mucosal irritant and causes severe abdominal pain as well as nausea and vomiting in over one half the cases; pancreatitis has also been commonly reported. However, serious ingestions may occur without subsequent gastrointestinal symptoms. Although an increased osmolal gap is usually present with serious methanol ingestion, methanol poisoning with a normal osmolal gap has been reported. This is due to complete metabolism of the methanol itself, while resultant toxic metabolites are exerting their effect.

Hypotension and bradycardia are late findings and suggest a poor prognosis.[7] Outcome is best correlated with the severity of the acidosis rather than serum methanol concentration.

Diagnosis of methanol poisoning rests on history, the presence of the characteristic clinical features outlined above, and the presence of a wide-anion-gap metabolic acidosis and osmolal gap. While confirmation of a tentative diagnosis depends on identification of the substance in the bloodstream, treatment should be initiated based on compatible clinical presentation to avoid morbidity resulting from delay. In any case, serum methanol determinations at many institutions depend on outside laboratories and may not be available for several hours. However if the ethanol level is known, the methanol level can be estimated from the osmolal gap (Table 160-1).

Normal methanol blood concentration from endogenous sources is 0.05 mg/dL. Asymptomatic individuals usually have peak levels below 20 mg/dL, while levels above 50 mg/dL indicate serious poisoning. Central nervous system symptoms usually appear when levels rise above 20 mg/dL; eye problems are associated with levels greater than 50 mg/dL, and the risk of fatality rises with levels greater than 150 to 200 mg/dL.

The differential diagnosis should include other potential causes of a wide-anion-gap metabolic acidosis—i.e., ethylene glycol, diabetic ketoacidosis, paraldehyde, isoniazid, salicylates, iron, lactic acidosis, phenformin, and uremia.

Treatment

Intravenous access should be established, with immediate bedside testing for blood glucose and administration of thiamine and naloxone if indicated. The general measures involved in treatment are (1) supportive care, (2) correction of acidosis, (3) administration of fomepizole (or ethanol) to decrease conversion to toxic metabolites, and (4) dialysis to eliminate the methanol. Unless the patient presents immediately after the ingestion, gastric lavage is unlikely to be of benefit. Activated charcoal has been shown to bind methanol poorly and therefore is not necessary in the absence of ingestion of other, adsorbable substances. Care should be taken to maintain an adequate airway with intubation if necessary for proper ventilatory support. Sodium bicarbonate should be administered with the goal of maintaining a near normal pH, since correction of metabolic acidosis moderates some of the toxic effects of methanol poisoning, including visual impairment.

4-Methylpyrazole (fomepizole) has been used successfully for initial treatment of methanol intoxication,[8] although case experience is not as great as that for its administration in cases of ethylene glycol ingestions (see below). A competitive inhibitor of alcohol dehydrogenase, fomepizole blocks the metabolism of methanol to its toxic metabolites. Unlike ethanol, it does not cause central nervous system depression. Many authorities recommend its use as a substitute for ethanol in initial treatment of adult methanol ingestions—specifically when methanol poisoning is suspected, in cases of high anion gap metabolic acidosis with an osmolal gap, if methanol concentration is found to be greater than 20 mg/dL, when the quantity of methanol ingested is calculated to be 0.4 mL/kg or more, or when symptoms consistent with methanol poisoning are present. Its use does not change the indications for dialysis. Some clinicians, however, still advocate the use of ethanol as the initial treatment of adult methanol intoxication. There is a lack of data on the use of fomepizole in children.

Fomepizole is administered in a loading dose of 15 mg/kg, followed by doses of 10 mg/kg every 12 h for four doses. Each dose is given by slow intravenous infusion over 30 min. More frequent dosing is required for patients requiring hemodialysis because fomepizole is removed during the procedure.

Ethanol, the traditional initial treatment of methanol intoxication, competitively inhibits the metabolism by alcohol dehydrogenase. Ethanol's affinity for the enzyme is 10 to 20 times that of methanol and its presence largely inhibits the formation of the toxic metabolites. Blood ethanol level should be maintained between 100 and 150 mg/dL to completely inhibit formation of toxic metabolites. Blood concentrations below 100 mg/dL are considerably less effective and therefore increase the risk of severe toxicity.

Ethanol may be administered intravenously, orally, or by nasogastric tube. Intravenous administration is preferred, though it may result in superficial thrombophlebitis. The intravenous solution should contain 10% ethanol in 5% D/W. A 20 to 30% ethanol concentration can be used for oral dosing. Higher concentrations have been used, but they can cause gastritis. To maintain an ethanol level of 100 to 150 mg/dL, a loading dose of 0.6 to 0.8 g/kg should be given intravenously or by mouth, with maintenance doses at approximately 0.11 g/kg per hour. If the recommended solution of 10% ethanol in 5% D/W is utilized, the loading dose is 10 mL/kg and maintenance is 1.6 mL/kg per hour. If the patient is habituated to ethanol, with enhanced hepatic elimination, the maintenance infusion should be started at 15 g/kg. When intravenous ethanol is not immediately available, oral therapy can be initiated with commercial distilled spirits. To calculate the ethanol content of distilled spirits, the following formula may be used:

$$\text{Ethanol (g)} = \text{vol of beverage (mL)} \times 0.9 \times (\text{proof}/200)$$

Ethanol levels should be assayed on a frequent basis, with the dose adjusted to maintain a concentration of 100 to 150 mg/dL. Administration should continue until the methanol level is zero. If dialysis is initiated, a higher maintenance infusion starting at 0.24 g/kg per hour will be necessary, as ethanol is dialyzable. As hypoglycemia may occur with ethanol administration, especially in children, blood glucose levels should be monitored closely.

Dialysis should be performed for methanol poisoning if there are signs of visual or central nervous system dysfunction, if peak methanol levels are greater than 25 mg/dL, if severe metabolic acidosis develops regardless of levels, and if there is a history of ingesting more than 30 mL. Hemodialysis is considerably more effective than peritoneal dialysis, but peritoneal dialysis may be utilized if hemodialysis is unavailable. Dialysis eliminates both the parent compound and its toxic metabolites. The indications for dialysis are unchanged for patients who receive treatment with fomepizole.

Folate is a cofactor for the conversion of formic acid to carbon dioxide. It is especially important to provide supplements to alcoholic patients who may be folate-deficient. Administration of folic acid 50 mg intravenously q4h for several days to all patients is recommended.

Disposition decisions are based on criteria identical to those used for ethylene glycol poisoning (see below). It should be emphasized that asymptomatic patients with history of significant ingestion should be admitted and treatment initiated, even if no acidosis is evident.

ETHYLENE GLYCOL

Ethylene glycol has many commercial uses as a coolant (antifreeze), preservative, and glycerine substitute; it has also been used in lacquers, cosmetics, polishes, and detergents. It may be ingested as an alcohol substitute by alcoholics, in suicide attempts, and accidentally by children. Ethylene glycol's toxicity is the result of the formation of two toxic metabolites, formaldehyde and formic acid. As with methanol, therapeutic strategies are based on prevention of formation of these metabolites or their removal from the body.

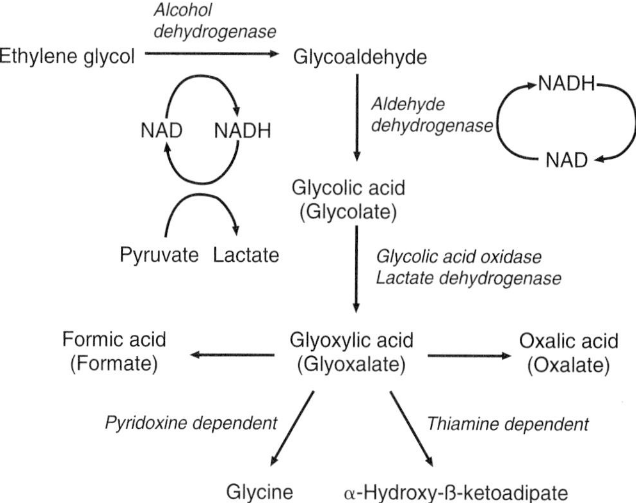

FIG. 160-3. Metabolic pathway of ethylene glycol.

Pathophysiology

Ethylene glycol is a colorless, odorless, sweet-tasting substance. It is highly water-soluble and rapidly absorbed when ingested orally, but not by the lungs or skin. Peak blood levels occur within 1 to 4 h of an ingestion. The volume of distribution is 0.83 L/kg and the plasma half-life is 3 to 5 h. Ethanol at a concentration of 100 to 200 mg/dL has an increased half-life of 17 h. Ethylene glycol is metabolized in the liver and kidneys to toxic metabolites—aldehydes, glycolate, oxalate, and lactate—which, in turn, cause toxicity to the lungs, heart, and kidneys. These metabolites also cause the metabolic acidosis associated with ethylene glycol poisoning.[7]

Ethylene glycol is metabolized to glycoaldehyde by the alcohol dehydrogenase (Fig. 160-3). This conversion involves the reduction of NAD+ to NADH, which causes inhibition of the citric acid cycle and formation of lactic acid. Glycoaldehyde is further metabolized to glycolic acid and to glyoxylic acid, which, in turn, are converted to several new compounds. Pyridoxal phosphate is a cofactor in the conversion of glyoxylic acid to glycine, which is nontoxic, while thiamine pyrophosphate is the cofactor in the conversion of glyoxylic acid to another nontoxic compound called α-hydroxy-β-ketoddipate. A deficiency of either pyridoxal phosphate or thiamine may shift the metabolism of ethylene glycol to the production of toxic metabolites.

Glyoxylic acid is also metabolized to formic acid and oxalic acid. Glycolic acid contributes to the metabolic acidosis observed in ethylene glycol poisoning. Oxalate crystalluria is a striking feature caused by calcium oxalate salt deposition. Oxalate crystals are present in the urine in only about 50 percent of cases.

The potentially lethal dose in adults is 2 mL/kg, although survival has been reported after ingestions ranging from 240 to 970 mL.

Clinical Features

Ethylene glycol poisoning often exhibits three distinct clinical phases, the severity and progression of which depends on the amount ingested. The initial phase is characterized by central nervous system depression, usually within 1 to 12 h after ingestion. Patients may appear inebriated, with slurred speech and ataxia but without the odor of ethanol on their breath. Hallucinations, coma, seizures, and death may also occur during this initial phase. These central nervous system symptoms correlate with peak glycoaldehyde production. The optic fundus is usually normal, differentiating the syndrome from methanol poisoning, although nystagmus and ophthalmoplegia may be observed: Lumbar puncture may demonstrate elevated CSF pressure and protein, and a few polymorphonuclear cells.

The second, cardiopulmonary phase develops 12 to 24 h after ingestion. Tachycardia, mild hypertension, and tachypnea are the most common symptoms; congestive heart failure, adult respiratory distress syndrome, cardiomegaly, and circulatory collapse are also observed. Myositis has also been reported less commonly during this phase.

The third phase, marked by nephrotoxicity, occurs 24 to 72 h after ingestion. Early symptoms consist of flank pain and costovertebral angle tenderness. Oliguric renal failure and acute tubular necrosis ensue. Complete anuria may occur, but most patients recover without renal damage if they receive appropriate therapy. Nephrotoxicity is caused by aldehyde metabolites and oxalic acid. Two forms of urinary calcium oxalate crystals may be identified on microscopic evaluation of the urine. The dihydrate form (octahedral crystals) shows tent-shaped crystals and the monohydrate form (monclinic crystals) shows crystals that are dumbbell- or prism-shaped. The monohydrate form was at one time felt to represent a salt of hippurate, explaining previous reports of hippurate crystals in the urine.

Hypocalcemia may develop secondary to precipitation of calcium as calcium oxalate and may be severe enough to cause tetany and prolongation of the QT interval. Elevated serum creatine phosphokinase levels may accompany and explain the generalized myalgias experienced by some patients.

Ethylene glycol intoxication should be considered when a patient presents with inebriation and no ethanol scent on the breath, a wide-anion-gap metabolic acidosis with osmolal gap, and calcium oxalate crystalluria. The mechanisms of anion-gap metabolic acidosis and osmolal gap are similar to those observed with methanol.

Tentative diagnosis and initiation of treatment should be based on history and characteristic clinical presentation. As with methanol poisoning, confirmation of a tentative diagnosis depends on identification of the substance in the bloodstream, but treatment should be initiated based on compatible clinical presentation to avoid morbidity resulting from delay. Serum levels greater than 20 mg/dL are likely to result in toxicity. Survival has been reported with levels up to 650 mg/dL, while fatality has been associated with levels between 98 and 775 mg/dL.

Leukocytosis is common and should not be considered a manifestation of infection unless clinical signs are present. One-third of patients may have hypocalcemia, with shortening of the QT interval present on the electrocardiogram. Serious intoxication has been reported in the absence of an osmolal gap or calcium oxalate crystalluria. The mechanism for the absence of an osmolal gap is based on the same explanation as given for methanol (above).

As with methanol, the differential diagnosis should include other potential causes of a wide-anion-gap metabolic acidosis.

Treatment

The management of ethylene glycol poisoning is similar to that of methanol. For indications for gastric lavage and guidelines for administration of sodium bicarbonate, refer to instructions given for methanol, above. If the patient is hypocalcemic, 10 mL of calcium gluconate 10% should be given intravenously. Pyridoxine 100 mg and thiamine 100 mg intramuscularly or intravenously should be administered daily to facilitate metabolism of ethylene glycol by nontoxic pathways. Magnesium has also been shown to be a cofactor in the metabolism of toxic metabolites and should be given if patients are hypomagnesemic, as is often the case with alcoholics. Laboratory tests that may be useful in evaluating patients suspected of ethylene glycol ingestion include complete blood count, serum electrolytes, acetone, alcohol toxicology panel with ethanol, isopropanol, and methanol determinations, electrolytes, blood urea nitrogen, creatinine, salicylate level, arterial blood gases, urinalysis, serum ethylene glycol level, calcium, creatine phosphokinase (CPK), and magnesium levels. Lactate levels should also be determined if the reason for the severe acidosis is unclear.

Fomepizole has supplanted ethanol as the initial treatment of choice for adults with ethylene glycol intoxication.[9,10] Fomepizole is a potent inhibitor of alcohol dehydrogenase and has an affinity for the enzyme which is 8000 times greater than that of ethanol. Headache, nausea, and dizziness are the most common adverse effects. It has fewer side effects than ethanol, especially in regard to central nervous system depression. Fomepizole should be administered if there is strong suspicion of ethylene glycol intoxication based on clinical presentation, if ethylene glycol level is more than 20 mg/dL, or if acidosis is present. Administration and dose is described in the section on methanol. If fomepizole is not readily available, ethanol should be administered immediately in suspected cases of ethylene glycol ingestion. There is a paucity of experience with fomepizole in children. Hemodialysis is still indicated for those patients with ethylene glycol concentrations greater than 50 mg/dL and for severe metabolic acidosis or anuria.

If fomepizole is not readily available, ethanol should be administered as soon as the diagnosis is suspected.[7] Ethanol's affinity for alcohol dehydrogenase is 100 times that of ethylene glycol, resulting in a prolongation of the half-life of ethylene glycol to 17 h. Oral and intravenous dosing guidelines for ethanol are identical to those outlined for methanol, above.

Dialysis should be initiated if a history, clinical presentation, or laboratory results consistent with ethylene glycol or poisoning is present, when serum concentration of ethylene glycol is greater than 20 to 25 mg/dL, when there are signs of nephrotoxicity, or when metabolic acidosis is present.[7] Treatment with fomepizole does not change the indications for dialysis. As with methanol, hemodialysis has been shown to be considerably more effective, but peritoneal dialysis can be used if hemodialysis is unavailable.

Disposition

Any patient with the serious signs and symptoms associated with ethylene glycol or methanol intoxication or a history of significant ingestion even in absence of symptoms should be admitted to an intensive care setting. Fomepizole or ethanol administration and dialysis should be continued until serum blood levels are zero and acidosis has resolved. Suicidal patients should receive a psychiatric evaluation when their condition improves and prior to discharge from any facility.

Patients seen at facilities unable to provide hemodialysis or intensive care should be transferred (if sufficiently stable) to institutions capable of providing such care. Because the symptoms of ethylene glycol and methanol intoxication may be delayed, patients who have ingested these substances should be admitted to the hospital for observation and laboratory testing even if they are asymptomatic initially.

REFERENCES

1. Secretary of Health and Human Services: *Ninth Special Report to the U.S. Congress on Alcohol and Health.* Washington, DC: U.S. Department of Health and Human Services, 1997.
2. Stephens Cherpitel CJ: Breath analysis and self-reports as measures of alcohol-related emergency room admissions. *J Stud Alcohol* 50:155, 1989.
3. Lowenstein SR, Weissberg MP, Terry D: Alcohol intoxication, injuries and dangerous behaviors—And the revolving emergency department door. *J Trauma* 30:1252, 1990.
4. Frezza M, Di Padova C, et al: The role of decreased gastric alcohol dehydrogenase activity and first-pass metabolism. *N Engl J Med* 322:95, 1990.
5. Sullivan JB, Hauptman M, Bronstein AC: Lack of observable intoxication in humans with high blood alcohol concentrations. *J Forens Sci* 32:1660, 1987.
6. Farre M, de la Torre R, Gonzalez ML, et al: Cocaine and alcohol interactions in humans: Neuroendocrine effects and cocaethylene metabolism. *J Pharmacol Exp Ther* 283:164, 1997.
7. Burkhart KK, Kulig KW: The other alcohols: Methanol, ethylene glycol and isopropanol. *Emerg Med Clin North Am* 8:913, 1990.

8. Burns MJ, Graudins A, Aaron CK, et al: Treatment of methanol poisoning with intravenous 4-methylpyrazole. *Ann Emerg Med* 30:829, 1997.
9. Baud FJ, Galliot M, Astier A, et al: Treatment of ethylene glycol poisoning with 4-methylpyrazole. *N Engl J Med* 319:97, 1988.
10. Jobard E, Harry P, Turcant A, et al: 4-Methylpyrazole and hemodialysis in ethylene glycol poisoning. *Toxicol Clin Toxicol* 34:373, 1996.

OPIOIDS

Suzanne Doyon

The term *opioids* is an all-inclusive term for antagonists, endogenous and exogenous substances that possess morphine-like activity. Opioids are classified as natural, semisynthetic or synthetic (Table 161-1). The most commonly abused opioids are heroin and methadone. The National Institute of Drug Abuse estimates that approximately 2.5 million people have a history of heroin abuse in the United States. Heroin abuse has significantly increased over the last decade because of lower street costs and easy availability. Also, street purity has increased from about 10 percent in the past to 70 percent or greater today, making nasal insufflation rather than injection a viable method. Thus, heroin has seen increased popularity on college campuses and among the afluent, rising to the status of a glamour drug. The public perception of addiction is that heroin use occurs predominantly among impoverished minorities. Heroin addiction does affects minorities disproportionately; however, its use among Caucasians is widespread. From 1990 through 1995, heroin-related emergency department (ED) visits more than doubled to 76,000, as did the rate per 100,000 population (from 15 to 33), according to data from the Drug Abuse Warning Network (DAWN).

PHARMACOLOGY

Opioids modulate nociception in the terminals of afferent nerves in the central nervous system (CNS), peripheral nervous system, and gastrointestinal tract. They are agonists at the mu1, mu2, kappa, delta, sigma, and epsilon receptors in these tissues. The opioids with a preference for the mu receptors are the more potent analgesics, but delta and kappa agonists are effective analgesics as well.[1] Opioids bind to the receptor sites and either decrease neurotransmitter release or open potassium channels, resulting in hyperpolarization of the neuronal membranes. Specific binding at different receptor sites located within the locus ceruleus activate the "pleasure pathway" and result in dependence and craving. The endogenous opioids—enkephalins, endorphins, and dynorphins—are the natural ligands at all the receptor sites mentioned above.

PHARMACOKINETICS

A detailed discussion of the absorption, distribution, and elimination of opioids is beyond the scope of this chapter. However, when clinically relevant, details of absorption and elimination of specific opioids are given. Knowledge of duration of action and elimination half-life is useful and is provided in Table 161-1.

Most opioids are more effective when given parenterally than orally, owing to variable but significant first-pass effect. Opioids with good oral potency are codeine, oxycodone, levorphanol, and methadone.

The metabolism of codeine, morphine, propoxyphene, oxycodone, meperidine, and methadone is mostly hepatic. The hepatic metabolites may be pharmacologically active. Concurrent use of benzodiazepines, barbiturates, and alcohol is common in the opioid abuser either because of their additive effect or their capacity to inhibit hepatic metabolism, especially the metabolism of methadone. Cyclic antidepressants and propoxyphene also decrease methadone metabolism.

CLINICAL FEATURES

Patients present to the emergency department in one of two states: intoxication with opioids or acute withdrawal from them.

The opioid toxidrome can encompass a wide variety of signs and symptoms. Opioids cause respiratory depression, mental status depression, analgesia, miosis, orthostatic hypotension, and nausea and vomiting, histamine release resulting in localized urticaria and occasionally bronchospasm, decreased gastrointestinal motility, and urinary retention secondary to increased vesical sphincter tone. The mental status depression can be variable but may be extremely profound. The respiratory depression may also be variable. One should look for shallow respirations, cyanosis, bradypnea, hypercarbia, and hypoxia. Miosis is not universally present. In fact, normal or even enlarged pupils have been documented secondary to exposure to meperidine, morphine,

TABLE 161-1 Classification and Characteristics of Major Opioids

	Analgesic Dose Equivalent to 10 mg of Morphine, mg	Analgesic Duration of Action, hours	Elimination Half-Life, hours
Natural			
Codeine	120	4–5	2.2–3.6
Morphine	10	4–5	1.4–2.4
Semisynthetic			
Heroin	5	4–5	0.5
Hydromorphone (Dilaudid)	1.3	4–5	2–3
Oxycodone (Percodan)	10–15	4–5	—
Oxymorphone (Numorphan)	1	4–6	2–3
Synthetic			
Diphenoxylate (Lomotil)	40–60	?	—
Fentanyl (Sublimaze)	0.125	1	3.3–4.1
Levorphanol (Levo-dromoran)	2	4–5	12–16
Meperidine (Demerol)	75–100	2–4	2.4–4.0
Methadone (Dolophine)	10	4–5	24–48
Propoxyphene (Darvon)	240	4–6	6–12

Source: Adapted from Goldfrank LR, Weisman RS: Opioids, in Goldfrank LR (ed): *Goldfrank's Toxicological Emergencies,* 6th ed. Stamford, CT: Appleton & Lange, 1998.

propoxyphene, pentazocine, and diphenoxylate; this sign may be secondary to severe cerebral hypoxia and it may also be attributable to coingestants.

The abrupt withdrawal of an opioid causes a host of other clinical signs and symptoms. It usually starts with feelings of anxiety, insomnia, yawning, lacrimation, diaphoresis, rhinorrhea, diffuse myalgias, piloerection, mydriasis, nausea and profuse vomiting, diarrhea, and abdominal cramping.

DIAGNOSIS

The diagnosis of opioid overdose or withdrawal is clinical.

The classic triad of coma, miosis, and respiratory depression strongly suggests chronic or acute opioid intoxication. Hoffman and coworkers attempted to determine clinical criteria predictive of the presence of opioid overdose. Their criteria of respirations $\leq$12 breaths per minute, presence of miosis, and circumstantial evidence of opioid use (drug paraphernalia, needle marks, presence of a tourniquet, bystander corroboration) were highly sensitive in predicting response to naloxone (92 percent), hence establishing the diagnosis of exposure to opioids. Unfortunately in this study, a respiratory rate only was used as a measure of respiratory depression—not an assessment of depth or quality of the respirations nor a pulse oximetry or blood gas measurement. Examination of the urine for opioids may aid in the diagnosis of opioid intoxication, but the results have a high false-negative rate and are not available to the clinician prior to the need to initiate prescriptive therapy.[2]

The diagnosis of opioid withdrawal is established when a constellation of withdrawal symptoms is temporally related to the abrupt cessation of an opioid.

Differential Diagnosis

The differential diagnosis of opioid overdose includes toxic or depressant effects of clonidine, organophosphates and carbamates, phenothiazines, sedative-hypnotic agents, and carbon monoxide. Gamma hydroxybutyrate (GHB), known as a ''date rape'' drug, may cause CNS depression, apnea, and occasionally miosis. Based on animal studies, GHB can potentially respond to naloxone, although this has not been shown clinically. There are no ancillary tests that will help the ED physician to differentiate GHB from opioids. Similarly, olanzapine in at least one case has caused CNS depression and miosis. Again, there is no ancillary test available to differentiate olanzapine from opioids except that olanzapine will not respond to naloxone. Clonidine overdoses are characterized by periods of apnea that respond to tactile or auditory stimulation. Organophosphate and carbamate overdoses cause muscle fasciculations, profuse vomiting and diarrhea and sweating. Phenothiazines cause intraventricular conduction delays and a partial anticholinergic toxidrome due to decreased alpha-adrenergic tone overriding anticholinergic effects, thus leading to miosis instead of mydriasis. Sedative-hypnotic agent and carbon monoxide cause profound CNS depression but are not usually associated with miosis. Hypoglycemia, hypoxia, CNS infections, postictal states, and pontine hemorrhages should also be considered in the differential diagnosis.

TREATMENT

When minute ventilation is depressed, appropriate airway measures should be undertaken. Once the airway is assured, the administration of naloxone may follow.

Naloxone was introduced in 1976. It is a specific ''pure'' antagonist at mu, kappa, and delta receptors. Naloxone can fully reverse the opioid-induced respiratory depression, mental status changes, and analgesia. It can be used as a diagnostic or therapeutic tool.

Naloxone can be administered intravenously, intratracheally, intramuscularly, subcutaneously, and even intralingually. The intravenous route is the most rapid and is preferred.

When the establishment of an intravenous line is difficult, these other routes are options. A recent study suggests that subcutanous (SQ) injection of 0.8 mg naloxone will have the desired effect. However, the slower absorption with SQ or intramuscular (IM) injection will likely offset the delay in establishing intravenous (IV) access.[3] Unless delay is anticipated to be inordinate and the patient's circumstances dictate immediate reversal, it is preferable to wait for IV access, even if femoral or other central venous access is required.

In the prehospital setting, there is no indication to rush reversal of the opioid's pharmacologic effects in a patient who is hemodynamically stable. In fact, early reversal may complicate transport. There are many reports of patients who regain consciousness in ambulances and become combative, rendering transport difficult and placing prehospital providers at physical risk. Patients who have regained their faculties have even invoked their ''right'' to decline treatment, demanding release from the ambulance, and placing prehospital providers at further risk.

A positive response to the naloxone establishes the diagnosis of opioid intoxication, acute or chronic. The recommended diagnostic dose is 0.1 to 2.0 mg IV in adults and children and 0.01 mg/kg in neonates. A full 2.0 mg IV should be administered to the patient presenting with respiratory depression. If the effect is minimal or absent, repeated doses of 2 mg every 3 min are recommended until a maximum of 10 mg IV has been reached or an effect is noted. Exposures to propoxyphene, fentanyl, pentazocine, or dextromethorphan may require these larger doses. If there is no response to 10 mg of naloxone IV, it is unlikely that an isolated opioid intoxication is the cause of the patient's altered mental status.

A smaller dose, for example, 0.1 to 0.4 mg IV, is advocated in overdose patients with a history of opioid dependence and little or no respiratory depression to avoid precipitation of withdrawal. The dose can be added to in small increments of 0.1 to 0.4 mg IV until a desired maximum or effect has been noted. The technique is to titrate 0.1 mg aliquots to effect. This particular regimen can be useful in treating the patient with chronic pain as well as chronic addicts.

The therapeutic dose of naloxone varies somewhat from the diagnostic dose. Reversal of opioid toxicity with naloxone will last 20 to 60 min. Repeated IV boluses or naloxone infusions are occasionally required in order to maintain respirations. This is especially true if the ingested opioid has a prolonged duration of action, at least more prolonged than that of naloxone. An infusion should be considered only if the patient has responded to the initial naloxone bolus and is not meant to be used in lieu of the bolus. To calculate the infusion rate and dose, first establish what initial bolus dose was successful in reversing the respiratory depression. Administer approximately two-thirds of that dose per hour by IV infusion. For example, two-thirds of a 1-mg dose is about 0.6 mg. Mix 6 mg of naloxone into 1 L of 5% D/W and run at 100 mL/h.[4] Adjustments in infusion rates may be required if the patient develops respiratory depression (renew the bolus and increase infusion rates) or withdrawal symptoms (decrease infusion rates). Patients requiring naloxone infusions should be admitted to a monitored setting capable of rapid airway intervention.

Recent literature suggests that the number of opioid receptors is similar in adults and children. Thus, the same therapeutic/diagnostic approach can be used with children as described above for adults. The traditional dose of 0.01 mg/kg of naloxone IV is probably appropriate for the neonate in the peripartum period but is inappropriate in treating the toddler with an accidental exposure to an opioid.

The most adverse effect associated with the administration of naloxone is precipitation of opioid withdrawal: anxiety, nausea, vomiting, diarrhea, abdominal cramps, piloerection, yawning, and rhinorrhea. The incidence of withdrawal can be minimized by judicious dosing. A small body of literature from the 1970s reported cases of cardiac dysrhythmias and death following the administration of naloxone IV. In most of these cases, the patients experienced a deteriorating course before naloxone was administered. Widespread clinical experience during the last 25 years suggests naloxone is one of the safest antidotes for toxicity diagnosis and reversal. Of note, large doses and rapid administration of naloxone to the neonate may induce seizure activity. In short, the administration of naloxone remains safe in the vast majority of clinical settings.[4,5]

Endotracheal intubation may be necessary for severe respiratory depression where adequate ventilation cannot be achieved by bag-valve-mask or if there is no response to naloxone.

For ingested opioids, gastric decontamination should not be performed routinely. Lavage may be considered on a patient who has ingested a potentially life-threatening amount of opioid within the previous hour.[6] Syrup of ipecac is not recommended due to the potential risk of aspiration of stomach contents in patients with altered mental status.

Administration of activated charcoal is of value: 50 g of activated charcoal orally followed by a cathartic such as sorbitol 0.5 to 1.0 g orally are standard doses. Multiple-dose activated charcoal is particularly useful in diphenoxylate and propoxyphene overdoses because of their large enterohepatic circulation.

An acetaminophen level should be obtained in cases of propoxyphene, oxycodone, or codeine overdose.

Approximately one-third of naloxone responders will relapse into opioid toxicity within 30 to 120 min. Hence, the minimum observation period is 2 h. The author recommends an observation period of 4 to 6 h in the ED for most cases of opioid intoxication. Although not a standard of care, this conservative approach is recommended to allow complete recovery and allow recognition of potential coingestants with delayed effects. Except in certain cases, illustrated below, it is acceptable to discharge the opioid-intoxicated patient after a reasonable period of observation and resolution of symptoms and signs. The moderately to severely methadone-intoxicated patient usually requires a 24 to 48 h hospital admission due to the prolonged elimination half-life of methadone. A psychiatric evaluation is mandatory in all cases of suicidal intent.[7]

SPECIAL CONSIDERATIONS

Meperidine and its metabolite, normeperidine, are proconvulsive agents. Normeperidine is reported to have twice the convulsant activity of meperidine. Use of these agents may result in seizures without underlying hypoxia. A wide range of seizure activity from multifocal myoclonus to generalized tonic-clonic seizures is reported. Normeperidine is almost entirely renally excreted. It accumulates in patients whose renal function is diminished: e.g., dialysis patients, those with cancer, the elderly, and sickle cell patients. Orally administered meperidine is more likely to lead to an accumulation of the toxic metabolite than parenterally administered meperidine because of a large first-pass effect. Therefore, patients with underlying renal dysfunction who receive oral meperidine, especially repeated oral doses, are at increased risk of seizures. Patients with new meperidine-induced seizures should receive a full diagnostic evaluation for seizures. The proconvulsive effects of meperidine and normeperidine are long lasting. Clusters of seizures over 24 h can be seen. Accordingly, patients exhibiting seizure should be admitted. Naloxone will not be useful in the treatment of meperidine induced seizures. Treatment of acute seizures is with benzodiazepines.

The combination of meperidine or dextromethophan with monoamine oxidase inhibitors can result in an increase in the amount of serotonin in the neuronal terminals in the CNS. The clinical syndrome is characterized by disorientation, severe hyperthermia, hypo/hypertension, and muscle rigidity. Deaths have been reported. Naloxone should have no effect and thus it is not indicated. Its administration could potentially complicate the patient's course by precipitating withdrawal. Treatment involves the administration of benzodiazepines and aggressive cooling (see Chap. 153).

Propoxyphene and its metabolite, norpropoxyphene, are particularly cardiotoxic and neurotoxic. Propoxyphene overdoses have been associated with intraventricular conduction disturbances, heart block, a prolonged QT interval, and ventricular bigeminy. Seizures have also been reported. Naloxone cannot reverse these effects. Treatment includes cardiac monitoring for about 6 h in the ED. If the patient remains asymptomatic and a repeat electrocardiogram is normal, discharge is appropriate. Otherwise, the patient should be admitted for continued cardiac monitoring for 24 h. The administration of hyperosmolar sodium bicarbonate, 1 mEq/kg IV, may reverse the cardiotoxic effects of propoxyphene.

The mixed agonists-antagonists include pentazocine (Talwin), butorphanol (Stadol), buprenorphine (Buprenex), and nalbuphine (Nubain). They have variable but mostly antagonist activity at the mu receptor and are agonists at the kappa receptors. They may cause significant respiratory depression in overdose situations, especially buprenorphine. Naloxone should be effective in reversing the respiratory depression. Mixed agonists-antagonists usually precipitate withdrawal when taken in excess by an opioid-dependent individual, hence reducing their potential for abuse.

Diphenoxylate is a frequently prescribed antidiarrheal agent. The medication is manufactured in a pill form containing a combination of diphenoxylate 2.5 mg and atropine 0.025 mg and is called Lomotil. It is a schedule IV drug. Anticholinergic effects predominate initially due to atropinic effects: flushing, tachycardia, hyperthermia, hallucinations, dry mucous membranes, and urinary retention. These signs and symptoms regress as the patient enters the second phase of the intoxication. Phase 2 is characterized by a predominantly opioid-like picture due to the effects of diphenoxylate. Naloxone is marginally effective in reversing the effects of diphenoxylate. There are two important clinical points to remember: first, children can be particularly sensitive to diphenoxylate; second, absorption can be delayed, up to 6 to 12 h. Current recommendations are to admit all pediatric exposures and monitor for respiratory depression. Multiple-dose activated charcoal is recommended in all cases of moderate to severe Lomotil intoxication.

Tramadol (Ultram) overdoses are associated with agitation, hypertension, respiratory depression, and seizures, especially at doses exceeding 500 mg orally in an adult. Treatment remains supportive. Naloxone is ineffective in reversing the seizures.

"Designer" opioids have included fentanyl and methylfentanyl, which are 100 and 2000 times more potent than morphine. They require large doses of naloxone, up to 10 mg IV, in order to reverse the respiratory depression. They remain undetectable in urine toxicology assays.

Recent clinical experience with heroin-cocaine (i.e., Speedball) and heroin-scopolamine (e.g., Polo, Homicide, Sting, and others) mixtures has raised issues regarding the blind administration of naloxone. Often naloxone "unmasks" the underlying cocaine or scopolamine intoxication. Cocaine has a relatively short duration of action, but the same is not true of scopolamine. Unmasked scopolamine overdoses often require control with benzodiazepines. Administration of physostigmine, to reverse scopolamine toxicity, can be considered but is best left to experienced physicians familiar with the use of this antidote.[8]

Retained drug packets pose special challenges to the clinician. Current literature supports the use of a polyethylene glycol solution (Go-Lytely) via NG tube at a rate of 2 L/h until the rectal effluent is clear. Multiple dose activated charcoal is also recommended. Large doses of naloxone may be required to reverse the respiratory depression associated with the leakage or breakage of the packets.

Special mention must be made of opioid-induced noncardiogenic pulmonary edema, a rare complication associated with heroin and methadone abuse. Acute lung injury (formerly referred to as noncardiogenic pulmonary edema) can occur immediately or be delayed up to

24 h in profoundly comatose patients and should be suspected in any patient who develops tachypnea, rales, or decreased oxygen saturation. Up to 50 percent of heroin users may experience noncardiogenic pulmonary edema at some time in their lives. Its occurrence is independent of route of exposure. The pathophysiology is poorly understood but some degree of direct capillary injury is present. Treatment includes oxygenation, consideration of airway intervention with possible use of positive end-expiratory pressure, and possible placement of a of Swan-Ganz catheter for appropriate monitoring. Diuretics and digoxin are usually not indicated. Naloxone will not reverse this complication.

Hospitalized Patients

The management of opioid dependent individuals hospitalized for medical or surgical reasons remains controversial. It is generally agreed that detoxification from opioids during the acute course of a medical illness is usually unsuccessful. Alleviation of withdrawal symptoms should be the goal of therapy. Daily administration of a verified dose of methadone orally (or half the verified dose intramuscularly if the patient is to take nothing by mouth) is recommended to inhibit withdrawal symptoms and reduce craving. This applies only to individuals who are actively enrolled in a methadone maintenance program and in whom the dose can be verified externally. The habitual user who is not on methadone maintenance therapy can receive methadone 20 mg by mouth (PO) or 10 mg IM. These dosages should inhibit withdrawal symptoms but not induce euphoria. No methadone should be administered to the habitual user until the appearance of withdrawal symptoms.

Occasionally, patients will present to the ED requesting methadone because they missed their outpatient or community program appointment. Unless the provider or clinic can be contacted and they indicate that the request is appropriate and valid, it should not be honored. Indiscriminate dispensing of methadone undermines methadone maintenance programs. Similarly, it is difficult to think of any valid rationale to prescribe methadone for outpatient use from the ED. In fact, pharmacies will generally not honor methadone prescriptions written on standard ED prescription pads. The Drug Enforcement Administration (DEA) rigidly controls how methadone is prescribed. Methadone prescriptions for detoxification programs (maximum 3 days) and maintenance therapy (longer than 3 days), can be filled only at methadone clinics sanctioned by the DEA. Reprimand and even loss of license to practice medicine has occurred for violations.

Withdrawal States

Downregulation of endogenous endorphins and dynorphins occurs from chronic usage, as does downregulation of opioid receptors. Abrupt cessation of opioid use does not allow time for upregulation of these endogenous ligands or receptors and results in increased neuronal firing and their withdrawal symptoms. Classic opioid withdrawal includes anxiety, craving, yawning, lacrimation, rhinorrhea, diaphoresis, mydriasis, nausea and vomiting, diarrhea, abdominal cramps, and diffuse myalgias. Onset of withdrawal is usually within 12 h of last heroin usage and within 30 h of last methadone exposure. It can be precipitated by the administration of naloxone or naltrexone.

Opioid withdrawal states are rarely life-threatening. They can be rendered more tolerable by the administration of the central alpha2 agonist clonidine, antiemetics, and antidiarrheal agents. Clonidine may be used at doses of 5 μg/kg PO if the blood pressure is above 90 mmHg systolic. Clonidine can be prescribed in a 0.1- or 0.2-mg oral dose tid. It is medically sound to discharge patients from the ED with a 3-day prescription until counseling can be obtained. The only concern is that some addicts abuse clonidine, as it enhances the opioid ''high.'' One option that has merit in many situations is to discharge patients with a clonidine patch. This is the best option for patients who are not in a position to take a medication three times daily, such as those returning to a jail. The patch is effective for 7 days and has no resale value.

Contaminants

Intravenous heroin continues to contain many adulterants: strychnine, quinine, lactose, and talc. The actual role of many adulterants in the etiology of medical illnesses attributable to intravenous drug usage remains largely unknown. An exception to this statement must be made in the case of MPTP (N-methyl-4-phenyl-1,2,3,6-tetrahydropyridine). A meperidine analogue synthesized in the 1980s contained MPTP as a contaminant. When used intravenously, MPTP caused a severe form of movement disorder similar to parkinsonism. It is metabolized by monoamine oxidase B in the substantia nigra to MPP^+, which is directly neurotoxic.[9]

Medical Complications

Medical complications from intravenous drug use include bacterial endocarditis, septic pulmonary emboli, aspiration pneumonia, tuberculosis, venous thrombosis, nephropathy, pulmonary talcosis, tetanus, hepatitis, human immunodeficiency virus (HIV) and other blood-borne infections, pneumothorax, pseudoaneurysms, mycotic aneurysms, multiple skin abscesses, cellulitis, septic arthritis, osteomyelitis, and intestinal pseudoobstruction secondary to fecal impaction. Given the risk, a thorough history of tetanus immunization should be sought.

REFERENCES

1. Stein C: The control of pain in peripheral tissues by opioids. *N Engl J Med* 332:1685, 1995.
2. Hoffman JR, Schriger DL, Luo J: The empiric use of naloxone in patients with altered mental status: A reappraisal. *Ann Emerg Med* 20:246, 1991.
3. Wagner K, Brough L, MacMillan I: Intravenous vs subcutaneous naloxone for out-to hospital management of presumed opioid overdose. *Acad Emerg Med* 5:283, 1998.
4. Schug SA, Zech D, Grond S: Adverse effects of systemic opioid analgesics. *Drug Safety* 7:200, 1992.
5. Michaelis LL, Hickey PR, Clark TA, et al: Ventricular irritability associated with the use of naloxone hydrochloride. *Ann Thorac Surg* 18:608, 1984.
6. Position statement: Gastric lavage. *Clin Toxicol* 35:711, 1997.
7. Smith DA, Leake L, Loffin JR, Yealy DM: Is admission after intravenous heroin overdose necessary? *Ann Emerg Med* 21:1326, 1992.
8. Perrone JM, Hamilton RH, Nelson L, et al: Scopolamine poisoning among heroin users—New York City, Philadelphia and Baltimore 1995 and 1996. *MMWR* 45:392, 1996.
9. Burns RS, Lewitt PA, Ebert MH, et al: The clinical syndrome of striatal dopamine deficiency: Parkinsonism induced by MPTP. *N Engl J Med* 312:1418, 1985.

STIMULANTS, COCAINE, AND AMPHETAMINES

Jeanmarie Perrone
Robert S. Hoffman

OVERVIEW

Cocaine, amphetamines, and other stimulants produce toxicity by activating the sympathetic nervous system. Although cocaine abuse is most prevalent and has dominated reports of stimulant toxicity, amphetamines and other substances that resemble cocaine produce unique toxic complications as well. The regional prevalence of each of these drugs of abuse may help the clinician decide which agent is present in a patient with sympathomimetic findings. The scope of toxicity is broad and includes chest pain following use of cocaine or amphetamines, blunt or penetrating trauma related to cocaine trafficking, and depression associated with chronic cocaine or amphetamine abuse.[1] This chapter focuses on cocaine abuse and its multiorgan toxic effects; it highlights unique toxicities associated with amphetamines and other stimulants.

Epidemiology

Cocaine abuse is widespread, but few data sources can provide an accurate estimate of its use. The 1996 National Household Survey on Drug Abuse reported that 71.7 million Americans were current cocaine users. Approximately 40 percent of these patients were crack users in urban areas. Cocaine use is highest among young persons aged 18 to 25 years and appears to be increasing in this age group. The National Center for Alcohol and Drug Abuse Interventions reports that there are greater than half a million new cocaine users each year (1998). Correspondingly, the Drug Abuse Warning Network (DAWN) reports that emergency department ED visits by cocaine-abusing patients tripled since 1988. Fatal injuries (homicides, suicides, falls, and overdoses) following cocaine use are a leading cause of death among young adults in New York City and probably in many other urban environments as well.[2] A recent 3-year study demonstrated cocaine metabolites in 26 percent and free cocaine in 18 percent of all patients with fatal injuries. Methamphetamine use was recently reported as a frequent cause of drug-related ED visits in the western United States, and its use is increasing in eastern states as well.

Pathophysiology

Cocaine is the naturally occurring alkaloidal extract of *Erythroxylon coca*, a plant indigenous to South America. The water-soluble hydrochloride salt is absorbed across all mucosal surfaces, including the oral, nasal, gastrointestinal, and vaginal epithelium; thus cocaine can be applied topically, swallowed, or injected intravenously. Although the hydrochloride form is most often insufflated (snorted) or injected intravenously, ether extraction yields crack cocaine, a form that is stable to pyrolysis and can be smoked, producing the popping sound that characterizes its name. The onset and duration of action vary with the route of administration. When cocaine is insufflated nasally, the peak effect occurs within 30 min and the duration of effect is 1 to 3 h. The delayed and prolonged effect is due to vasoconstrictive properties that limit mucosal absorption. A fraction of insufflated cocaine is swallowed and thus absorbed from the stomach as well. Gastrointestinal absorption is also slowed by vasoconstriction, producing a peak effect at 90 min and a duration of effect as long as 3 h. Both the intravenous and the inhalational routes produce a rapid peak effect (within 30 s to 2 min), with a duration of effect of 15 to 30 min. This rapid onset but short duration property helps explain why more crime and increased risk of human immunodeficiency virus (HIV) and other blood-borne infections are associated with the highly addictive drug. Frequent use is required to maintain the ''high.'' Cocaine is primarily metabolized to ecgonine methyl ester by plasma cholinesterase. Relative deficiency of this enzyme may predispose affected patients to life-threatening toxicity.[3] Benzoylecgonine is the other major metabolite excreted in the urine and is the one routinely sought by most urine toxicology screens.

Cocaine is both a local anesthetic and a central nervous system (CNS) stimulant. Like other local anesthetics, cocaine inhibits conduction of nerve impulses by blocking fast sodium channels in the cell membrane. In vivo, cocaine has been demonstrated to have quinidine-like effects on conduction causing QRS widening and QTc prolongation. Thus in large doses, cocaine may exert a direct toxic effect on the myocardium resulting in negative inotropy, wide complex dysrhythmia, bradycardia, and hypotension. Central effects are mediated through activation of the sympathetic nervous system via enhanced effects of excitatory amino acids and blockade of presynaptic reuptake of norepinephrine, dopamine, and serotonin. The resultant excess of neurotransmitters at postsynaptic receptor sites leads to sympathetic activation, producing the characteristic physical findings of mydriasis, tachycardia, hypertension, and diaphoresis and predisposing the user to dysrrhythmias, seizures, and hyperthermia. Cocaine use produces a euphoria associated with enhanced alertness and a general sense of well-being. It is thought that the psychological addiction, drug craving, and withdrawal effects are mediated through interference with dopamine and serotonin balance in the central nervous system. Subsequent dopamine depletion at the nerve terminals may account for the dysphoria and depression associated with long-term abuse. Many of ED visits attributed to cocaine are for the depression associated with chronic abuse.

Amphetamines

Amphetamines comprise a broad class of structurally similar derivatives of phenylethylamine. The derivative methamphetamine, also known as ''ice,'' is abused by ingestion, intravenous injection, inhalation, or insufflation. As with cocaine, amphetamine's absorption and peak effects occur rapidly with inhalation, insufflation, and intravenous injection. However, the effects of some amphetamines such as methamphetamine (MDA) and methylenedioxymethamphetamine (MDMA) may persist for 12 h.

Amphetamines enhance the release and block the reuptake of catecholamines and may also directly stimulate catecholamine receptors. Some amphetamine metabolites inhibit monoamine oxidase, thus also increasing cytoplasmic concentrations of norepinephrine. Certain amphetamine derivatives can also induce release of serotonin and affect central serotonin receptors. The serotonergic effects account for the hallucinogenic properties of some amphetamine derivatives such as MDA, MDMA, and methylenedioxyethamphetamine (MDEA, or mescaline). Dopamine receptor activity may contribute to the withdrawal phenomenon. Mortality from amphetamine toxicity, like that from cocaine, is due to dysrhythmias, seizures, hyperthermia, hypertension (intracranial hemorrhage or infarction), and encephalopathy.

The stimulants ephedrine and phenylpropanolamine produce toxic syndromes similar to those caused by cocaine and amphetamines, although there are some distinguishing features. Phenylpropanolamine is abused as a stimulant and anorectic agent and is found in many over-the-counter diet aids and decongestants. It is primarily a peripheral alpha agonist that causes significant vasoconstriction resulting in hypertension and, often, a marked reflex bradycardia. Hypertensive encephalopathy and intracranial hemorrhage are associated with overdose. Ephedrine is a plant-derived indirect-acting sympathomimetic with both alpha- and beta-adrenergic activity due to the release of dopamine and norepinephrine from neuronal stores. Although used therapeutically for asthma in the past, it is currently promoted as a ''natural'' stimulant and anorectic. Significant cardiovascular and neurologic toxicity, psychosis, mania, and severe hypertension have been reported, including several deaths.[4]

CLINICAL FEATURES

Cardiac

Cocaine induces dysrhythmias, myocarditis, cardiomyopathy and myocardial ischemia and infarction. Other vascular complications include aortic rupture and aortic and coronary artery dissection. Evidence in both animal and human experimental trials demonstrates that even at relatively low doses cocaine induces vasoconstriction in coronary arteries.[5] Vasoconstriction is one of the proposed mechanisms of cocaine-induced myocardial ischemia and infarction. Coronary vasoconstriction is exacerbated by β-adrenergic blockade and antagonized by phentolamine, suggesting that it is mediated through the stimulation of α-adrenergic receptors.[6] This effect is further potentiated by cigarette smoking. Myocardial ischemia has been demonstrated in chronic abusers undergoing cocaine withdrawal. It is thought that cocaine withdrawal is a dopamine-depleted state, resulting in intermittent coronary spasm. Animal data demonstrate increased platelet aggregation and thrombogenesis, accelerated atherosclerosis, direct myocardial toxicity, and increased myocardial oxygen demand.

A profile of the patient at risk for myocardial ischemia can be elucidated from a compilation of 91 case reports of patients with cocaine-induced myocardial infarction and a prospective evaluation of patients with cocaine-associated chest pain.[7,8] The average patient with cocaine-associated myocardial infarction was young and male (mean age 32.8, range 18 to 52; male-to-female ratio, 7:1) and most (83 to 89 percent) were cigarette smokers and regular cocaine users. Two-thirds of patients presented within 3 h of cocaine use and all routes of cocaine administration were reported. Of the patients with follow-up cardiac catheterization, coronary artery disease was present in 31 percent. Electrocardiographic (ECG) abnormalities were variably present, and both Q-wave and non-Q-wave infarctions occurred. Many studies have reported myocardial infarction in patients with atypical histories and unremarkable ECGs.

Myocardial ischemia and infarction and aortic dissection are also reported in association with ephedrine, phenylpropanolamine, or amphetamine use. Additionally, reports of mitral and aortic valve abnormalities associated with use of the amphetamine combination phentermine-fenfluramine prompted a voluntary recall of these drugs. Cardiopulmonary toxicity from other amphetamine diet aids has also been reported.

Central Nervous System

An array of neurologic syndromes are described in association with cocaine abuse, most commonly seizures, intracranial infarctions, and hemorrhages. Pathology results from the hyperadrenergic tone, inducing severe transient hypertension, hemorrhage, or focal vasospasm and sometimes, exacerbation of underlying abnormalities of cerebral blood vessels. In their studies using a dog model, Catravas and Waters demonstrated that lethal doses of intravenous cocaine initially induced seizures, lactic acidosis, hyperthermia, and death.[9] Progression of toxicity could be prevented by sedation and cooling. These authors also demonstrated that diazepam was an optimal sedative because it prevented hyperthermia and seizures in the cocaine-poisoned dog and thereby improved survival. Although coronary vasospasm has been well documented in humans exposed to cocaine, a recent study using magnetic resonance angiography also demonstrated cerebral vasoconstriction following cocaine administration. Other CNS manifestations reported include spinal cord infarctions, cerebral vasculitis, and intracranial abscesses. Acute dystonic reactions following cocaine use and withdrawal are both reported. Choreoathetosis and other repetitive movements are associated with cocaine and amphetamine intoxication, and all seem to be related to dopamine dysregulation. An interesting syndrome termed ''cocaine washout'' occurs in patients following a prolonged crack binge. Patients have a depressed level of consciousness but can be aroused to normal with stimulation. Resolution of lethargy can take up to 24 h. Unilateral blindness occurs secondary to central retinal artery occlusion and bilateral blindness from diffuse vasospasm. A syndrome of corneal abrasions and ulcerations secondary to smoke and irritation is known as ''crack eye.'' Keratitis due to methamphetamine use is described as well.

Amphetamines, phenylpropanolamine, and ephedrine are also associated with intracranial hemorrhages, infarctions, encephalopathy, and seizures. Amphetamines also cause a CNS vasculitis resulting in focal neurologic deficits. A profound paranoid psychosis occurs with chronic amphetamine abuse and withdrawal.

Pulmonary

Respiratory effects of cocaine use have become more prevalent with the epidemic of crack cocaine, which is smoked. Pulmonary hemorrhage, barotrauma, pneumonitis, asthma, and pulmonary edema are described. Pneumomediastinum, pneumothorax, and pneumopericardium result from barotrauma secondary to the Valsalva maneuvers performed following inhalation or insufflation in an attempt to enhance drug effect. Pneumonitis, asthma, and bronchiolitis may be immunologic phenomena or the result of the numerous adulterants known to be present in cocaine. A recent case control study in an urban ED examined the association between bronchospasm and cocaine use.[11] The authors demonstrated a higher incidence of recent cocaine use in patients presenting with new-onset bronchospasm as compared with age- and sex-matched ED patients. Another study demonstrated bronchoconstriction following the inhalation of crack but not following intravenous injection of cocaine.[12] This suggests that such bronchospasm may be due to local airway irritation. Pulmonary edema may be catecholamine-mediated, in view of a similar syndrome described in patients with adrenergic excess from pheochromocytoma and intracranial hemorrhage. Upper airway irritation and a presumed thermal uvulitis occurs in patients smoking crack cocaine.

Gastrointestinal

Patients who are thought to have swallowed poorly packaged cocaine following police pursuit are called ''body stuffers.'' Such patients are often brought to the hospital by police and may or may not show signs of cocaine intoxication. In contrast, the ''body packer'' swallows a large number of well-sealed packages of cocaine in order to smuggle drugs into this country. Because of the large quantities of relatively pure drug contained in these packages, toxicity and death can occur if even a single bag ruptures.

Cocaine-induced mesenteric vasospasm may contribute to the many reported cases of intestinal ischemia, bowel necrosis, ischemic colitis, and splenic infarctions. In addition, gastrointestinal bleeding and perforation occur in association with cocaine use.

Renal

Traumatic and nontraumatic rhabdomyolysis occurs secondary to cocaine or amphetamine use. In one series of cocaine-induced rhabdomyolysis, one-third of patients developed acute renal failure and half of those died. Risks for developing rhabdomyolysis include altered mental status, seizures, dysrhythmias, and hemodynamic instability including cardiac arrest.[13] Patients whose initial serum CK is less than 1000 U/L with normal creatinine, white blood cell count, and only one or no risks in addition to cocaine itself are unlikely to develop complications[13] and need not necessarily be admitted for this alone. In addition to renal failure resulting from rhabdomyolysis, stimulants may further exacerbate renal injury through hyperthermia, vasoconstriction, hypotension, and hypovolemia. One must be aware of this potential late complication and augment fluid resuscitation to maintain a urine output of 1 to 3 mL/kg per hour. Renal infarction has been described following intravenous cocaine use.

The Pregnant Patient

Cocaine is a potent vasoconstrictor and has been shown to alter uteroplacental blood flow. An increased incidence of spontaneous abortions, abruptio placentae, fetal prematurity, and intrauterine growth retardation results from cocaine abuse in pregnancy.[14] Both spontaneous abortions and abruptio placentae appear to occur from placental vasoconstriction and increased uterine contractility, with concomitant maternal hypertension. Intoxication of a breast-fed infant secondary to maternal cocaine use has been reported as well. Methamphetamine abuse during pregnancy has similar detrimental effects on fetal growth.

DIAGNOSIS

The cocaine- or amphetamine-intoxicated patient can often be identified initially by vital signs. Adrenergic stimulation may produce tachycardia, tachypnea, hypertension, and possibly hyperthermia. The patient's mental status can range from normal to paranoid or severely agitated to coma. Organ-system involvement may be suspected from symptoms such as chest pain, palpitations, dyspnea, headache, or focal neurologic complaints. The patient may be postictal or may present with seizures. Other physical findings may include mydriasis and diaphoresis. In the absence of an adequate history, it may be difficult to distinguish this presentation from other conditions of catecholamine excess, such as withdrawal from alcohol or sedative-hypnotics. Metabolic acidosis may be present following seizures or as a result of vasoconstriction and hypoperfusion. As with all intoxicated patients, occult trauma and hypoglycemia must be excluded.

Concomitant use of alcohol and other drugs frequently alters the clinical presentation. For example, a patient ingesting both opioids and stimulants may present with a decreased level of consciousness and few if any other revealing findings. When the opioid is reversed with naloxone, the stimulant effects are unmasked, sometimes in dramatic fashion.

Laboratory

Laboratory studies may be helpful in diagnosing complications of cocaine or amphetamine abuse. Any patient with significant agitation or elevated temperature should have a chemistry panel and CPK obtained to screen for a metabolic acidosis, renal failure, or rhabdomyolysis. Hyponatremia of unknown etiology sometimes occurs following the use of hallucinogenic amphetamines (MDMA). Cardiac enzymes including CPK-MB or troponin are appropriate to screen for cardiac injury. A urine sample may be helpful in detecting rhabdomyolysis as well, since it may dip positive for hemoglobin with only few or no red blood cells by microscopy. Patients with hyperthermia should have baseline coagulation and liver function studies, since these values increase dramatically in the first 24 h. Most patients with altered mental status not responding to standard measures should undergo computed tomography of the head, since associated neurovascular injuries are common. A chest radiograph and ECG are fundamental to the evaluation. Laboratory confirmation of cocaine or amphetamine use is readily available but must be interpreted with caution. Urine drug screening for the cocaine metabolite benzoylecgonine is sensitive to 200 to 300 ng/mL; cocaine use within the past 24 to 72 h will typically be detected depending on dose and chronicity of cocaine use. Cocaine can be detected in chronic users by more sensitive techniques (radioimmunoassay, gas chromatography) for up to 2 weeks after last use. Although these qualitative drug screens will be positive for cocaine in the presence of the drug, they may be misleading in the chronic cocaine abuser who used the drug in the preceding several days, but now presents with a nontoxicologic condition. While most of the rapid screening tests for cocaine are fairly specific for cocaine metabolites and exhibit little cross-reactivity, the opposite is true for the amphetamine immunoassays. Interfering substances as well as false positives due to other phenylethylamine compounds may produce erroneus results. In addition, excessive use of certain nasal inhalers that contain stimulant-class drugs may cross-react with immunoassay methods and yield false-positive tests.

TREATMENT

The basic protocol specific to stimulants outlined in Chapter 151 should be followed. Charcoal may be given if appropriate. Intravenous access should be obtained in most patients and supplemental oxygen delivered to those with potential ischemia. The cornerstone of therapy is adequate sedation and close assessment of vital signs. The patient with hypertension and tachycardia will often respond to treatment with benzodiazepines, which decrease central sympathetic outflow. Lorazepam 2 mg or diazepam 5 mg can be administered intravenously and titrated with repeated doses to decrease the autonomic excess and CNS stimulation. Haloperidol and chlorpromazine should be avoided as these lower the seizure threshold. A core temperature should be measured in the evaluation of an agitated patient. Hyperthermia is potentially lethal and patients must be cooled rapidly to decrease subsequent morbidity and mortality. Ice-bath immersion produces the most rapid cooling; however, it is sometimes difficult to accomplish quickly. Cool mist spray to the skin and fans to increase heat loss by convection and evaporation may decrease temperature adequately. Application of ice packs and cooling blankets is insufficient to cool a hyperthermic poisoned patient. Aggressive fluid resuscitation is critical to maintain urine output.

Seizures may be treated with benzodiazepines as well; however, in status epilepticus, phenobarbital loading or neuromuscular blockade may be necessary to control motor activity and prevent hyperthermia, acidosis, and rhabdomyolysis. Computed tomography is recommended in all cases of stimulant-induced seizures because the finding of intracranial pathology creating a seizure focus is common.

The patient complaining of chest pain should be evaluated for possible myocardial ischemia as well as the common pulmonary etiologies mentioned in this population. Cocaine use should be considered an additional risk factor in reevaluation of any patient with chest pain. Patients suspected of myocardial ischemia should be managed with nitrates, morphine, benzodiazepines and aspirin.[15] β-adrenergic antagonist therapy is absolutely contraindicated because unopposed stimulation of α-adrenergic receptors may worsen coronary and peripheral vasoconstriction, hypertension, and possibly ischemia.[6] Although labetalol (a mixed α- and β-adrenergic antagonist) has been suggested, labetalol increased seizures and mortality in an animal model of cocaine toxicity and does not decrease cocaine-induced coronary vasoconstriction in humans. Furthermore, it has predominant β-adrenergic antagonist effects and may still lead to predominant α-adrenergic activity, thus worsening peripheral vasoconstriction and hypertension. Consultation may be helpful before administering thrombolytic therapy in cocaine-associated myocardial infarction. Despite the increased incidence of coronary atherosclerosis, vasospasm, coronary artery dissection, and severe hypertension would all be contraindications to its use.[16,17]

Wide complex tachydysrhythmias and QRS prolongation secondary to the quinidine-like effects of cocaine may be treated by alkalinizing the serum to a pH of 7.45 to 7.5 with a sodium bicarbonate infusion.[18] Although lidocaine has been used safely in this setting, some animal studies and theoretical evidence suggest that lidocaine may potentiate cocaine neurotoxicity and should be used with caution in patients with dysrhythmias who are not responsive to sodium bicarbonate.

Severe hypertension not responding to sedation may require treatment with nitroprusside infusion or phentolamine (phentolamine starting dose: 2.5 to 5 mg IV). Blood pressure may be lowered aggressively provided that the patient does not have chronic hypertensive disease. Treatment for refractory hypertension would be similar to that for hypertensive emergencies of any etiology (see Chap. 53).

The treatment of patients with cardiovascular or neurologic sequelae of amphetamine or other stimulant use is comparable to that outlined for cocaine. Acidification of the urine to increase amphetamine excretion was previously recommended but should not be done because of the increased risk of renal tubular precipitation of myoglobin in the presence of rhabdomyolysis. Dialysis is not of value.

The management of an asymptomatic cocaine "body packer" brought in by police or customs officials constitutes a new dilemma for the emergency physician. If the patient shows no signs of toxicity, we recommend a dose of activated charcoal followed by whole bowel irrigation with polyethylene glycol electrolyte lavage solution (GoLYTELY or Colyte) to gently hasten elimination of the potentially lethal packets. If the patient begins to show signs of intoxication, such as agitation, hypertension, or tachycardia, benzodiazepines should be administered while immediate surgical consultation for emergent laparatomy and packet removal is made. Neither upper nor lower endoscopy should be attempted because both routes have been associated with packet rupture. Following passage of the ''last'' packet, a radiologic imaging procedure (a Gastrografin upper gastrointestinal series with small bowel follow-through or abdominal CT with contrast) should be performed to ensure that the gut has been purged of all containers. In contrast to ''body packers,'' ''body stuffers'' are more likely to be seen in the ED. These patients can be given a dose of activated charcoal, sedated (if indicated), and given supportive care if intoxicated, since it is known the toxicity should be shorter-lived and often involves smaller amounts of drug.

Drug Interactions

There are a few potential drug interactions to be aware of in the treatment of the stimulant poisoned patient. Since cocaine is metabolized by plasma cholinesterase, coadministration of other drugs such as succinylcholine and mivacurium, which are metabolized by plasma cholinesterase, may have a prolonged duration of effect due to decreased metabolism. This may have significant implications during a failed rapid-sequence intubation with these agents.

Both lidocaine and cocaine are local anesthetics and act as sodium channel antagonists. It is thought that neurotoxic effects from both occur by similar mechanisms. Animal studies examining cocaine and lidocaine together are inconclusive, demonstrating both synergistic neurotoxicity as well as protective effects of lidocaine pretreatment on cocaine-induced lethality. Although there may be some theoretical risk of treating cocaine-induced dysrhythmias with lidocaine, it has been used safely to date in patients with cocaine-associated myocardial infarction.

Monoamine oxidase inhibitors block the degradation of catecholamines and lead to increased levels of presynaptic catecholamines. Amphetamines are indirect-acting sympathomimetic amines and weak inhibitors of monoamine oxidase as well. Thus, patients taking monoamine oxidase inhibitors who subsequently use amphetamines or phenylpropanolamine (and to a lesser extent cocaine) may precipitate an acute syndrome of excessive catecholamine release, resulting in severe hypertension, tachycardia, hyperthermia, agitation, tremors, and possible severe neurotoxicity.

Withdrawal

Cocaine withdrawal is characterized by irritability, paranoid ideation, and delayed depression. Symptoms are generally milder than for amphetamines. Psychological addiction may be particularly strong. Amphetamine withdrawal is characterized by drowsiness, lethargy, hunger, tremor, and chills. There is considerable potential for long-term depression and suicide.

DISPOSITION

Patient disposition depends on initial patient presentation, response to therapy, the particular stimulant involved, and expected duration of effect. Patients who present with adrenergic excess following recent cocaine use and who respond to sedation may be expected to improve completely during a period of observation in the ED secondary to the relatively limited duration of cocaine effect. In contrast, amphetamines have a longer duration of effect and may be expected to produce more prolonged toxicity, necessitating hospital admission or prolonged observation in some cases. Patients demonstrating resolution of toxicity and clear sensorium in the absence of focal complaints or end-organ damage should be advised of the medical risks of their drug abuse and referred to appropriate detoxification, counseling, and social support services. In general, patients with significantly increased creatine phosphokinase levels, hyperthermia, myoglobinuria, or ECG changes consistent with myocardial ischemia should be hospitalized in an intensive care setting.[13]

Disposition of patients who present with cocaine-associated chest pain and normal electrocardiograms may be difficult. Although several studies have examined risk factors associated with myocardial ischemia in this population, clinical parameters were not helpful in identifying those patients who subsequently did have myocardial infarctions. The incidence of myocardial ischemia in a large cohort of patients with cocaine-associated chest pain was approximately 6 percent. Admission to a telemetry or ED observation unit for serial cardiac enzymes and ECGs is sufficient, since the complication rate in stable patients is quite low. Young patients who ''rule out'' do not need a follow-up stress test unless there are other indications. Patients with unremitting chest pain, dysrhythmias, congestive heart failure, or evolving ECGs require hospital admission.

REFERENCES

1. Rich JA, Singer DE: Cocaine related symptoms in patients presenting to an urban emergency department. *Ann Emerg Med* 20:616, 1991.
2. Marzuk PM, Tardiff K, Leon AC, et al: Fatal injuries after cocaine use as a leading cause of death among young adults in New York City. *N Engl J Med* 332:1753, 1995.
3. Hoffman RS, Henry GC, Howland MA, et al: Association between life-threatening cocaine toxicity and plasma cholinesterase activity. *Ann Emerg Med* 21:247, 1992.
4. Perrotta DM, Coody G, Culmo C: Adverse events associated with ephedrine-containing products–Texas, December 1993–September 1995. *MMWR* 45:689, 1996.
5. Lange RA, Cigarroa RG, Yancy CW, et al: Cocaine-induced coronary artery vasoconstriction. *N Engl J Med* 321:1557, 1989.
6. Lange RA, Cigarroa RG, Flores ED, et al: Potentiation of cocaine-induced coronary vasoconstriction by beta-adrenergic blockade. *Ann Intern Med* 112:897, 1990.
7. Hollander JE, Hoffman RS: Cocaine induced myocardial infarction: An analysis and review of the literature. *J Emerg Med* 10:169, 1992.
8. Hollander JE, Hoffman RS, Gennis P, et al: Prospective multicenter evaluation of cocaine associated chest pain. *Acad Emerg Med* 1:330, 1994.
9. Catravas JD, Waters IW: Acute cocaine intoxication in the conscious dog: Studies on the mechanism of lethality. *J Pharmacol Exp Ther* 217:350, 1981.
10. Kaufman MJ, Levin JM, Ross MH, et al: Cocaine induced cerebral vasoconstriction detected in humans with magnetic resonance angiography. *JAMA* 279:376, 1998.
11. Osborn HH, Tang M, Bradley K, et al: New onset bronchospasm or recrudescence of asthma associated with cocaine abuse. *Acad Emerg Med* 4:689, 1997.
12. Tashkin DP, Kleerup EC, Koyal SN, et al: Acute effects of inhaled and intravenous cocaine on airway dynamics. *Chest* 110:904, 1996.
13. Brody SL, Wrenn KD, Wilber MM, Slovis CM: Predicting the severity of cocaine associated rhabdomyolysis. *Ann Emerg Med* 19:1137, 1990.
14. Plessinger MA, Woods JR: Cocaine in pregnancy: Recent data on maternal and fetal risks. *Obstet Gynecol Clin North Am* 25:99, 1998.
15. Hollander JE: The management of cocaine associated myocardial ischemia. *N Engl J Med* 333:1267, 1995.
16. Hollander JE, Burstein JL, Hoffman RS, et al: Cocaine-associated myocardial infarction: Clinical safety of thrombolytic therapy. *Chest* 107: 1237,1995.
17. Hollander JE, Wilson LD, Leo PJ, Shih RD: Complications from the use of thrombolytic agents in patients with cocaine associated chest pain. *J Emerg Med* 14:731, 1996.
18. Beckman KJ, Parker RB, Hariman RJ, et al: Hemodynamic and electrophysiological actions of cocaine: Effects of sodium bicarbonate as an antidote in dogs. *Circulation* 83:1799, 1991.

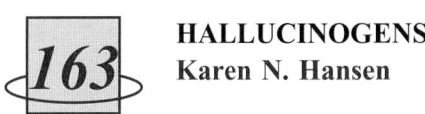

HALLUCINOGENS

Karen N. Hansen

EPIDEMIOLOGY

Modern interest in hallucinogenic drugs dates from Albert Hofman's 1943 discovery of the properties of lysergic acid diethylamide (LSD) through inadvertent ingestion.[1]

The popularity of hallucinogens as recreational drugs peaked in the 1960s, and is currently undergoing a resurgence among adolescents and young adults.[2] In the United States in 1995, 8.4 percent of high school seniors, and 6.8 percent of college students used LSD.[2] In the same year, marijuana was used by 34.7 percent of high school seniors and 31.2 percent of college students.[2] Of particular concern is the current popularity of the psychoactive amphetamine-derivative MDMA (''ecstasy'' or ''Adam'') among college students.[3] Encouragingly, the incidence of emergency department (ED) visits due to phencyclidine (PCP) has decreased sharply in the past decade.[4] In 1995, annual prevalence of PCP use among high school seniors was 1.8 percent, and among young adults was only 0.3 percent.[2]

Terms such as ''psychedelic'' are sometimes preferred to ''hallucinogen.'' Many of the drugs within this group rarely produce true hallucinations, which are sensory perceptions occurring in the absence of any external stimulus. Perceptual alterations based on some environmental cue are termed illusions, and are far more common. These effects may involve any sensory modality, but are most often visual. Users may also experience distortions of body image, and a distorted sensation of the passage of time. Alterations in mood and heightened suggestibility are common.

The ''classical'' hallucinogens include agents from the indole alkylamine (LSD, psilocybin), and phenylethylamine (mescaline and others) chemical families (Table 163-1). These drugs share a common proposed mechanism of action, and are capable of producing the profound psychological effects and sensory distortions characteristic of the psychedelic ''trip.'' In addition to classical hallucinogens, a number of other drugs, such as MDMA (''ecstasy''), phencyclidine (PCP), and marijuana, possess the ability to alter sensory perceptions, and can be placed within the broader category of hallucinogens.

DIAGNOSIS

LSD

LSD (lysergic acid diethylamide) can be chemically synthesized or obtained by hydrolysis of ergot alkaloids from the fungus *Claviceps purpurea*. It is one of the most potent psychoactive compounds known. Evidence suggests that the psychedelic effects of LSD are mediated through serotonergic (5-HT) systems, and that LSD acts as an agonist at 5-HT_2 receptors.[5]

The typical LSD dose of 50 to 300 μg is most commonly delivered through ingestion of a small square of dried ''blotter'' paper that has been saturated with a solution of the compound. Blotter acid is often imprinted with fanciful designs or cartoons which may serve as trademarks for the manufacturer. Other forms of LSD, including ''microdots'' (tiny tablets), ''windowpane'' (gelatin sheets), and liquid LSD, are currently uncommon. LSD is relatively inexpensive; a dose costs the user less than $15.

LSD is rapidly absorbed following ingestion. Onset of psychedelic effects occurs after about 30 minutes, peak effects occur within the first 4 hours, and the total duration of an LSD ''trip'' is between 8 and 12 h. The serum half-life of LSD is approximately 3 h. The physiological effects of LSD usually precede the psychedelic effects, and are dominated by sympathomimetic symptoms. These include marked mydriasis, and mild elevations of pulse, blood pressure, and temperature. Facial flushing, mild gastric distress, piloerection, increased muscle tension, and hyperreflexia may be seen. Severe or life-threatening complications are extremely uncommon. Seizures have been reported rarely. Massive overdose of LSD may produce coma, respiratory arrest, hyperthermia, and coagulopathy.[6]

The psychedelic effects of LSD may be perceived as pleasurable or horrifying, depending on the user's prevailing mood and expectations (''set''), and external environmental factors (''setting''). Acute adverse psychological effects (''bad trip'') include panic attacks, extreme paranoia, acute psychotic reactions, and depressive reactions. Potential physical trauma as a consequence of dangerous or impulsive behavior is a serious hazard. Occasional suicides have been reported. Prolonged and sometimes permanent psychosis following LSD use has been well described, and affects between 0.08 percent and 4.6 percent of users.[7] The term ''flashback'' has been replaced by Hallucinogen Persisting Perception Disorder,[7,8] a debilitating malady in which patients experience chronic perceptual distortions reminiscent of the drug-induced state, often accompanied by anxiety or panic.

Patients who present to the ED due to effects of LSD will usually be able to give a history of the drug ingestion. In most ED settings, the available routine toxicology screen will not detect LSD, but toxicological screening may be indicated if other intoxicants are suspected. If the history is clear, and in the absence of medical complications or possible co-ingestants, observation in a quiet, safe environment, with reassurance and emotional support, are generally the only interventions required to manage a patient experiencing a ''bad trip.'' Oral or parenteral benzodiazepines may be given if the patient is extremely agitated. Haloperidol may be used as a second choice if additional sedation is required. Patients who are lucid and medically stable may be released into the custody of family or friends. Patients with paranoid or psychotic symptoms lasting longer than 8 to 12 h may require hospital admission. Rarely do patients with medical complications due to massive overdose require hospital admission; they can be expected to recover quickly with supportive management.[6]

Psilocybin

Psilocybin and the related compound psilocin are hallucinogens of the indole alkylamine class, and are structurally related to LSD. Psilocybin and psilocin are believed to act as 5-HT_2 agonists in a manner similar to LSD. They occur naturally in mushrooms of the *Psilocybe* genus, most notably *P. semilanceata* (liberty cap), and *P. cubensis*. Psilocybin-containing mushrooms grow naturally in many areas of the United States and Europe, and kits containing spores and the ingredients necessary for propagation are advertised in drug-oriented publications. Hallucinogenic mushrooms purchased on the street are often nonpsychoactive mushrooms that have been adulterated with LSD or PCP.[9] Psilocybin-containing mushrooms may be dried or cooked without losing potency. Because the size of the mushrooms and the concentration of psychoactive compounds varies, there is little correlation between the number of mushrooms ingested and the hallucinogenic effects. A user may ingest as few as 5 or as many as 100 mushrooms for a single ''dose.''

Symptom onset occurs about 30 min after ingestion of psilocybin-containing mushrooms, and the total duration of hallucinogenic effects is about 4 to 6 h. The hallucinogenic effects are similar to, although less powerful than, those produced by LSD. Other common effects include mydriasis, mild tachycardia, hyperreflexia, and nausea and vomiting. Serious medical side effects are extremely rare, but seizures and hyperthermia have occurred, and the death of a small child has been reported.

ED management of patients presenting with isolated hallucinogenic mushroom ingestion is largely supportive. Routine drug screens do not detect psilocybin or psilocin. However, a drug screen may indicate whether the ingested mushrooms were adulterated with PCP. If the patient's symptoms are not consistent with psilocybin, the possibility

TABLE 163-1 Characteristics of Hallucinogens

Drug	Chemical Classification	Mechanism of Action	Typical Dose	Duration of Action	Clinical Features	Complications	Specific Treatment
LSD	Indole Alkylamine	5-HT_2 agonist	50–300 μg	8–12 h	Mydriasis, Sympathominetic symptoms, Nausea, Muscle tension	Persistent psychosis, Hallucinogen persisting perception disorder	Supportive, Benzodiazepines
Psilocybin	Indole Alkylamine	5-HT_2 agonist	5–100 mushrooms, 4–6 mg of psilocybin	4–6 h	Mydriasis, Sympathomimetic symptoms, Nausea	Seizures (rare), Hyperthermia (rare)	Supportive, Benzodiazepines
Mescaline	Phenyl-ethylamine	5-HT_2 agonist	3–12 ''buttons,'' 200–500 mg of mescaline	6–12 h	Mydriasis, Abdominal pain, Vomiting, Dizziness, Sympathomimetic symptoms	Rare	Supportive, Benzodiazepines
MDMA (''Ecstasy'')	Phenyl-ethylamine	5-HT release	50–200 mg	4–6 h	Mydriasis, Sympathomimetic symptoms, Bruxism, Jaw tension, Ataxia	Dysrhythmias, Hypertension, Seizures, Hyperthermia, Rhabdomyolysis, DIC	Benzodiazepines, Hydration, Active cooling, ?Dantrolene,* ?5-HT antagonists†
Phencyclidine (PCP)	Piperidine Derivative	Glutamate agonist at NMDA receptor	1–9 mg	4–6 h	Miois or midsize pupils, Nystagmus, Hypertension, Sympathomimetic, Anticholinergic, and Cholinergic symptoms	Coma, Seizures, Hyperthermia, Rhabdomyolysis, Hypertension, Hypoglycemia	Benzodiazepines, Hydration, Multiple-doses of activated charcoal, Active cooling, ?Dantrolene,* ?Alkalinize urine‡
Marijuana	Cannabinoid	Binds Canna-binoid receptor	5–15 mg of THC	2–4 h	Tachycardia, Conjunctival injection	Rare	Supportive, Benzodiazepines

*Dantrolene possibly indicated for severe hyperthermia.
†Experimental treatment.
‡Urinary alkalinization for rhabdomyolysis.

that the mushrooms ingested were of another more toxic variety should be considered.

Mescaline

Mescaline (3,4,5-trimethoxyphenylethylamine) is the hallucinogenic alkaloid found in the Mexican peyote cactus *Lophophora williamsii*. It is a member of the phenylethylamine class of hallucinogens, and is structurally related to amphetamines. As for LSD, the hallucinogenic action of mescaline is believed to result from HT_2 agonist properties.[10] Mescaline, however, is a much weaker hallucinogen than LSD.

The small 8-mm crowns of the peyote cactus are dried and sold as peyote ''buttons,'' each containing approximately 45 mg of mescaline. A typical dose of 200 to 500 mg will require 3 to 12 of these ''buttons.'' Mescaline can be extracted from peyote or be chemically synthesized, but these methods are expensive. Pills or capsules sold on the street as ''mescaline'' are unlikely to be genuine,[9] and may instead contain LSD or PCP.

Peyote is bitter tasting, and causes significant uncomfortable physical side effects within an hour of ingestion. Initial signs and symptoms, which often include nausea and vomiting, abdominal discomfort, diaphoresis, dizziness, nystagmus, ataxia, and headache, generally resolve after about 2 h. Adrenergic stimulation causes mydriasis, and mild elevations in pulse, blood pressure, and temperature. The hallucinogenic effects, which are very similar to those produced by LSD, begin several hours after ingestion and persist for 6 to 12 hours. Death due to aberrant behavior while under the influence of the drug has occurred, but reports of significant morbidity or mortality due to physiological effects of mescaline are absent from the literature. Patients presenting to the ED due to peyote ingestion can generally be managed supportively. Mescaline is not detected by routine drug screens.

MDMA

MDMA (3,4-methylenedioxymethamphetamine; ''Ecstasy'' or ''Adam'') is a synthetic phenylethylamine derivative that is structurally related to both amphetamines and mescaline. MDA (3,4-methylenedioxyamphetamine) and MDEA (3,4-methylenedioxymethamphetamine; ''Eve'') are related compounds with similar properties. The effects of MDMA are believed to result from stimulation of 5-HT release from central serotonergic nerve terminals.[11]

MDMA is usually ingested in doses of 50 to 200 mg. Tablets are typically round and white, often imprinted with bird motifs. Acute effects last about 4 to 6 hours. MDMA rarely causes actual hallucinations, but can produce sensory effects such as alterations in the intensity of colors or sensation of textures. Users often report feelings of euphoria, enhanced sociability, verbosity, and heightened sexual interest. Common physical manifestations of MDMA include sympathomimetic effects, particularly mydriasis and mild elevations of pulse and blood pressure, as well as nausea, jaw tension, bruxism, dry mouth, muscle aches, and ataxia.

The increase in popularity of MDMA has been accompanied by an increase in reports of serious complications and death related to its use. Fatal dysrhythmias and death due to cardiac effects have been reported in patients with and without underlying cardiac disease.[12] Severe hypertension and intracranial hemorrhage have been reported.[12] A pattern of toxicity manifested by hyperthermia, seizures, disseminated intravascular coagulation (DIC), rhabdomyolysis, and renal failure has been increasingly recognized.[13] This pattern shares many features of the serotonin syndrome.[14] Hepatic toxicity and possibly long-term damage to serotonergic neurons may result from chronic MDMA use.[15]

Patients presenting to the ED with complications due to MDMA should receive activated charcoal if the ingestion was recent. Dysrhythmias are managed with standard therapy. Hypertension and tachycardia will often respond to benzodiazepines alone, but if hypertension is severe, phentolamine or nitroprusside can be used. β-Blockers, such as propranolol, should probably be avoided due to the risk of possible unopposed α stimulation. Hyperthermia should be managed aggressively with active cooling measures and hydration. Dantrolene has been recommended for treatment of hyperthermia,[13] and has been used successfully in sporadic cases. Because of the similarity of the hyperthermic MDMA syndrome and the serotonin syndrome, the use of 5-HT antagonists such as methysergide or cyproheptadine has been suggested.[14]

Phencyclidine

Phencyclidine is a synthetic piperidine derivative. It is a dissociative anesthetic agent structurally related to ketamine. PCP is unlike the classic hallucinogens in that it causes clouding of the sensorium rather than heightened sensory awareness. PCP is believed to act as a glutamate antagonist at the NMDA (*N*-methyl-*d*-aspartate) receptor.[16]

PCP can be easily and inexpensively synthesized. Powdered drug ("angel dust") is most often combined with tobacco, marijuana, or other vegetable matter and smoked, but PCP can be ingested orally, sniffed intranasally, or injected intravenously. Unfortunately, PCP is often sold as another drug, or used to adulterate another drug, and thus may be unknowingly ingested.[9] The onset of action depends on the mode of administration; onset of action is about five min if PCP is smoked. Acute effects generally last 4 to 6 h, but can persist much longer. The half-life is very variable, possibly due to the significant enterohepatic circulation and high lipid solubility of the drug. PCP is a weak base, and is concentrated in acidic environments. It is largely metabolized by the liver, and metabolites are excreted in the urine.

Because of the remarkable variability of clinical effects produced, recognition of PCP intoxication can be challenging. Patients may present with CNS stimulation or depression, and may be physically violent, catatonic, or comatose. A combination of cholinergic, anticholinergic, and sympathomimetic effects may be present. Many patients have taken a combination of drugs, compounding the clinical picture.[17] In a series of 1000 PCP-intoxicated patients, nystagmus and hypertension were the most common findings, each occurring in 57 percent of patients.[17] Hypertension was generally mild. Other prevalent manifestations were: acute brain syndrome (37 percent); violent (35 percent), agitated (34 percent), or bizarre (29 percent) behavior; hallucinations or delusions (19 percent); and tachycardia (30 percent).[17] Diaphoresis, muscle rigidity, dystonic reactions, ataxia, and a decreased response to painful stimuli have also been described. Pupil size is variable; unlike classic hallucinogens, widely dilated pupils are not common.[17]

Medical complications due to PCP use occur frequently. Coma has been seen in 10.6 percent,[18] and seizures in 3.1 percent,[17] of PCP-intoxicated patients. Elevated serum creatinine phosphokinase (CPK), due to increased muscle activity and/or a possible direct toxic effect of PCP, was found in 70 percent of patients in one study.[17] Frank rhabdomyolysis may occur, and sometimes results in renal failure requiring dialysis.[18] Hypoglycemia, sometimes severe, was found in 22 percent of PCP-intoxicated patients.[17] Hypertension causing intracerebral hemorrhage, and hyperthermia causing hepatic necrosis, have also been reported. In addition, significant traumatic injury, and sometimes death, may occur as a result of the violent or aberrant behavior characteristic of PCP use.

The ED evaluation of a patient with known or suspected PCP intoxication should include examination for occult trauma and evaluation for the possibility of hypoglycemia or rhabdomyolysis. If the urine dipstick is positive for occult blood, but microscopic urinalysis shows no red blood cells, myoglobinuria should be suspected, and a total CPK level obtained. Results of toxicological screening for PCP can be misleading. Tests can be falsely negative due to fluctuations in serum and urine drug levels. Conversely, chronic PCP users may test positive for weeks following their last use,[19] so a positive test does not necessarily indicate acute PCP intoxication.

Violence and agitation are common features of PCP intoxication, and sedation or physical restraints are frequently required to prevent patients from harming themselves and to protect ED personnel. Pharmaceutical intervention is preferable to physical measures because the muscular activity a patient expends while fighting against restraints may contribute to the development of rhabdomyolysis. Parenteral benzodiazepines are recommended, but haloperidol can also be used.

Gastric lavage is only indicated for patients with very recent oral ingestions of large amounts of PCP, or who may have significant co-ingestions. Patients who are comatose should be endotracheally intubated for airway control prior to gastric lavage. Regardless of the original mode of drug administration, circulating PCP is secreted into the stomach, and becomes trapped in the acidic environment. Therefore, continuous gastric suction or multiple-dose charcoal administration can help facilitate drug removal; either is recommended for patients with significant PCP intoxication. Administration of multiple doses of charcoal is probably preferred to continuous gastric suction, as it is likely to be easier and safer to accomplish in this patient population. Urinary acidification is of theoretical benefit, but is contraindicated because it may exacerbate myoglobin precipitation in the kidneys. Due to the large volume of distribution of PCP, hemodialysis is not effective.

Management of patients with PCP intoxication is generally supportive, but patients with severe CNS toxicity, or who have specific medical complications, require appropriate intervention. Patients in coma require endotracheal intubation and evaluation for other causes of altered consciousness, including hypoglycemia and head injury. Seizures should be treated with benzodiazepines, and patients in status epilepticus may require endotracheal intubation and neuromuscular blockade. Hyperthermia is treated with rapid cooling, and possibly dantrolene. Hypertension usually responds to sedation, but severe hypertension can be treated with nitroprusside. Treatment of rhabdomyolysis includes aggressive hydration. Administering intravenous sodium bicarbonate to alkalinize the urine may help prevent acute tubular necrosis in this setting.

Based on a large study of patients presenting with acute PCP intoxication, four major and five minor clinical patterns of PCP intoxication have been described.[18] The major clinical patterns are coma, catatonia, toxic psychosis, and acute brain syndrome. Most patients presenting with one of the major patterns of PCP intoxication require hospital admission for medical or psychiatric reasons. Patients exhibiting one of the minor clinical patterns of PCP intoxication (lethargy, bizarre behavior, violent behavior, or agitation) can often be discharged if their condition improves after observation.[18]

Marijuana

Dried leaves and flowers from the hemp plant *Cannabis sativa* are called marijuana, and dried resin from the flower tops of this plant is known as hashish. The psychoactive ingredient of marijuana is δ^9-tetrahydrocannabinol (δ^9-THC). δ^9-THC binds to a specific brain receptor for which an endogenous ligand has been discovered.[20]

Marijuana is usually smoked, but it can be ingested. Symptoms persist for 2 to 4 hours, or longer if ingested. Drowsiness, euphoria, heightened sensory awareness, paranoia, distortions of time and space, and feelings of unreality are described. Hallucinations do not normally occur at usual doses. Common physiological effects of marijuana are mild tachycardia, injected conjunctiva, bronchodilation, orthostatic hypotension, and impaired motor coordination. Although significant medical complications occur rarely, if at all, users may experience panic reactions, or even brief toxic psychoses due to δ^9-THC.

Acute psychiatric symptoms due to marijuana use can usually be managed with reassurance alone, but benzodiazepines can be used if medication is warranted. Urine tests are unreliable indicators of acute marijuana intoxication because it is detectable for days after use in novice users, and for weeks after the last use in chronic users.[21]

Other Hallucinogens

Seeds of the morning glory plant (*Ipomoea violacea, Ipomoea tricolor,* and others) contain lysergic acid amide (ergine), a compound closely related to LSD. They are sometimes intentionally ingested for the hallucinogenic effects. Several hundred seeds may be taken as a "dose." Physical and psychological manifestations closely resemble effects of LSD, and patients can be managed similarly.

Accidental or intentional ingestion of large amounts of nutmeg can cause delirium with hallucinations. Nutmeg is the dried seed from the tropical *Myristica fragrans* tree. The hallucinogenic properties of nutmeg may be due to a component, myristicin, but the mechanism is not well understood. Ingestion of 1 to 3 nutmegs or 5 to 15 g of the ground spice produces psychological effects, which begin 3 to 6 h later and last for 6 to 24 h. Uncomfortable physical symptoms are prominent, and may include tachycardia, flushing, dry mouth, nausea, and abdominal pain. Signs and symptoms may resemble anticholinergic poisoning, but pupils are usually small or midsize. Management is generally supportive.

Jimson weed (*Datura stramonium*) and angel's trumpet (*Datura candida*) plants grow naturally in the United States, and contain the anticholinergic alkaloids atropine, scopolamine, and hyoscyamine. Seeds or other parts of the plant can be ingested or smoked, and cause the anticholinergic toxic syndrome. Delirium, hallucinations, and seizures can occur, along with other classic anticholinergic effects, such as mydriasis, tachycardia, dry mouth and skin, blurred vision, urinary retention, and hyperthermia. Gastric emptying can be delayed, so gastric decontamination is an important part of the management of such patients. Medications with anticholinergic properties, such as phenothiazine, should be avoided. Use of physostigmine should be reserved for patients with severe anticholinergic toxicity who do not respond to supportive measures.

TREATMENT

The initial ED management of a patient presenting with hallucinations, bizarre behavior, or altered thought processes should concentrate on assessing the patient's general medical condition and stabilizing the patient's airway, breathing, and circulation. Hypoglycemia should be considered in all patients with altered mental status. Among the many conditions that can mimic hallucinogen intoxication are alcohol or benzodiazepine withdrawal, anticholinergic poisoning, thyrotoxicosis, and acute psychosis. Numerous prescription and nonprescription medications can also cause hallucinations.

Hallucinogens are usually taken intentionally, so in most cases a history of what was taken and the mode of administration is available. Because the identity of street drugs is often misrepresented,[9] the possibility that the substance used was adulterated or substituted by another, more toxic drug, particularly PCP, should be considered. Drug testing is of limited utility because most hallucinogens will not be detected by routinely available drug screens. In addition, a positive test for PCP or marijuana can be misleading, as it may be indicative of use days or weeks prior to testing.

Patients under the influence of hallucinogens may present with severe anxiety, agitation, or violent behavior. In many cases, calm reassurance in a supportive environment is sufficient to soothe the patient. In other cases, pharmacological intervention, and possibly physical restraints, may be necessary to ensure the safety of the patient and the ED staff, and to facilitate evaluation and treatment of the patient. Benzodiazepines are considered the mainstay of treatment. Diazepam, 5 mg po or IV, or lorazepam, 1 to 2 mg po, IM, or IV, can be given depending on the severity of symptoms and the clinical situation. Repeated doses can be given as needed, provided the patient is monitored for the possibility of respiratory depression. Phenothiazine should not be used. Use of haloperidol, a butyrophenone, or droperidol may be considered in the unlikely event that a second sedating agent is required. Haloperidol and droperidol, however, lower the seizure threshold, have anticholinergic properties, and can cause dystonias. They should be used with caution, and should be avoided completely if the patient is exhibiting significant anticholinergic symptoms. Haloperidol or droperidol can be administered IM or IV in 5 mg increments. Physical restraints are sometimes necessary. Physical restraints may cause injury, may exacerbate paranoia and agitation, and may contribute to the development of rhabdomyolysis in patients who struggle against them.

Most hallucinogens are rapidly absorbed. Patients experiencing adverse effects usually present several hours after the drug was administered. Therefore, gastric decontamination is of limited utility in most cases. Gastric lavage should only be considered for very recent large ingestions, or if significant toxic co-ingestions are suspected. Administration of oral activated charcoal is sufficient in the majority of cases. PCP is secreted into the stomach from the systemic circulation, so continuous gastric suction or, preferably, multiple doses of activated charcoal are recommended for patients exhibiting significant toxicity from PCP.

Hemodialysis is not indicated, as it does not effectively remove hallucinogens from the body. Although urinary acidification would theoretically enhance elimination of PCP and the hallucinogenic amphetamines, it can also cause renal injury due to myoglobin precipitation, and is therefore contraindicated.

The management of patients with hallucinogen intoxication is largely supportive, but medical complications can occur, and should be treated appropriately. Tachycardia and hypertension often respond to sedation with benzodiazepines alone. Significant dysrhythmias are treated using standard protocols. Severe hypertension can be treated with nitroprusside. The dose of a nitroprusside infusion starts at 0.5 μg/kg per minute, and can be titrated to a maximum of 10 μg/kg per minute as needed. Propranolol should probably be avoided because many of the hallucinogens cause significant adrenergic stimulation, and use of a β-blocker may lead to paradoxical hypertension due to unopposed α stimulation. Rapid cooling measures should be initiated for patients with significant hyperthermia. Treatment of severe hyperthermia may require neuromuscular paralysis with endotracheal intubation and possibly the administration of dantrolene. Seizures are treated with benzodiazepines and standard anticonvulsants. Patients with rhabdomyolysis require aggressive IV hydration and IV sodium bicarbonate to achieve a urinary pH of 7 to 8.

DISPOSITION

Most patients seen in the ED due to adverse reactions from hallucinogen use can be discharged into the custody of family or friends if they are lucid and medically stable after a period of observation. Patients with persistent psychotic symptoms or other significant psychiatric disturbance may require psychiatric evaluation and possible hospital admission. Patients with significant medical complications of hallucinogen use, such as severe hypertension, hyperthermia, seizures, or rhabdomyolysis, should be admitted to the hospital for continued treatment and observation. All patients should be assessed for suicide wish.

REFERENCES

1. Hoffman AA: *LSD: My Problem Child.* Los Angeles, JP Tarcher, 1983.
2. Johnston LD, O'Malley PM, Bachman JG (eds): *National Survey Results from the Monitoring the Future Study, 1975–1995.* Washington, DC, U.S. Department of Health and Human Services, 1996.
3. Cuomo MJ, Dyment PG, Gammino VM: Increasing use of "ecstasy" (MDMA) and other hallucinogens on a college campus. *J Am Coll Health* 42:271, 1994
4. Substance Abuse and Mental Health Administration: *Year End Preliminary Estimates from the 1996 Drug Abuse Warning Network (DAWN).* Washington, DC, US Department of Health and Human Services, 1997.
5. Glennon RA: Do hallucinogens act as 5-HT_2 agonists or antagonists? *Neuropsychopharmacology* 3:509, 1990.
6. Klock JC, Boerner U, Becker CE: Coma, hyperthermia, and bleeding associated with massive LSD overdose: a report of eight cases. *Clin Toxicol* 8:191, 1975.
7. Abraham HD, Aldridge AM: Adverse consequences of lysergic acid diethylamide. *Addiction* 88:1327, 1993.
8. American Psychiatric Association: *Diagnostic and Statistical Manual of Mental Disorders,* 4th ed. Washington, DC, American Psychiatric Association, 1994.
9. Renfroe CL, Messinger TA: Street drug analysis: An eleven year perspective on illicit drug alteration. *Semin Adolesc Med* 1:247, 1985.
10. Davis M: Mescaline: Excitatory effects on acoustic startle are blocked by $serotonin_2$ antagonists. *Psychopharmacology* 93:286, 1987.
11. Johnson MP, Hoffman AJ, Nichols DE: Effects of the enantiomers of MDA, MDMA, and related analogues on [3H]serotonin and [3H]dopamine release from superfused rat brain slices. *Eur J Pharmacol* 132:269, 1986.
12. Dowling GP, McDonough ET, Bost RO: 'Eve' and 'ecstasy': A report of five deaths associated with the use of MDEA and MDMA. *JAMA* 257:1615, 1987.
13. Henry JA, Jeffreys KJ, Dawling S: Toxicity and deaths from 3,4 methylenedioxymethamphetamine ("ecstasy"). *Lancet* 340:384, 1992.
14. Mueller PD, Korey WS: Death by "ecstasy": the serotonin syndrome? *Ann Emerg Med* 32:377, 1998.
15. McCann UD, Rideroun A, Shaham Y, et al: Isolation and structure of a brain constituent that binds to the cannabinoid receptor. *Science* 258:1946, 1992.
16. Javitt DC, Zukin SR: Recent advances in the phencyclidine model of schizophrenia. *Am J Psychiatry* 148:1301, 1991.
17. McCaron MM, Schulze BW, Thompson GA, et al: Acute phencyclidine intoxication: incidence of clinical findings in 1,000 cases. *Ann Emerg Med* 10:237, 1981.
18. McCarron MM, Schulze BW, Thompson GA, et al: Acute phencyclidine intoxication: clinical patterns, complications, and treatment. *Ann Emerg Med* 10:290, 1981.
19. Simpson GM, Khajawall AM, Alatorre E et al: Urinary phencyclidine excretion in chronic abusers. *J Toxicol Clin Toxicol* 19:1051, 1982.
20. Devane WA, Hanus L, Breuer A, et al: Isolation and structure of a brain constituent that binds to the cannabinoid receptor. *Science* 258:1946, 1992.
21. Dackis CA, Pottash ALC, Annitto W, et al: Persistence of urinary marijuana levels after supervised abstinence. *Am J Psychiatry* 139:1196, 1982.

SALICYLATES

Luke Yip
Richard C. Dart

EPIDEMIOLOGY

The widespread availability of aspirin (acetylsalicylic acid, or ASA) in prescription and over-the-counter preparations, confusion between product names and brand names, and the ease with which incremental chronic dosing can cause toxicity make salicylism a common and sometimes fatal occurrence. Data from the American Association of Poison Control Centers Toxic Exposures Surveillance System showed that, in 1996, aspirin was implicated in 25,281 exposures, with 12,385 cases (49 percent) treated in a health care facility; 48 deaths (0.2 percent of cases) were attributed to salicylate toxicity.[1]

Many people use over-the-counter medications without realizing that they may contain significant amounts of salicylate. For example, Pepto Bismol (261 mg of salicylate per 30 mL) will deliver large amounts of salicylate in patients who overuse the product. Children may become salicylate toxic from extensive application of keratolytic agents or other agents containing oil of wintergreen (methyl salicylate). One milliliter of a 98% methyl salicylate contains 1400 mg of salicylate. Liniments and products used in hot vaporizers have high concentrations of methyl salicylate, and an ingestion of 5 to 10 mL can be lethal for an infant or a toddler.

PATHOPHYSIOLOGY

Absorption of salicylate may be delayed or erratic, depending on the product. After ingestion of large amounts of non-enteric-coated ASA, absorption from the gastrointestinal (GI) tract may be slowed because of the inhibitory effect of ASA on gastric emptying and the impaired dissolution of tablets in gastric fluids at high concentrations. Peak serum salicylate levels may not be reached for 18 to 24 h, although toxic levels are usually evident within 6 h. Methyl salicylate is a liquid that produces peak levels earlier, whereas peak levels following enteric-coated or sustained-release ASA overdose have been reported to occur 10 to 60 h after ingestion.[2] Some formulations of ASA may coalesce to form a gelatinous gastric mass, and significant amounts of ASA may remain in the stomach long after an intentional overdose, providing a source for continued absorption.

After absorption, ASA is hydrolyzed to salicylic acid (salicylate) and is distributed throughout body tissues. The severity of toxicity depends on the cellular salicylate concentration. Salicylate is responsible for both the therapeutic and the toxic effects of ASA. At higher salicylate concentrations, a lesser percentage of the drug is protein bound and more free drug is available to diffuse into tissues and cause toxicity. The pK_a of salicylate is 3.0 and, at physiologic pH (7.40), almost all salicylate molecules are ionized. If the systemic pH decreases, the change in equilibrium will form a greater portion of nonionized molecules. This is an important concept because nonionized molecules will cross cellular membranes, such as the blood-brain barrier. Thus, for a given salicylate level, brain salicylate levels will be substantially higher in the presence of acidemia.[3] Although the precise mechanism remains to be determined, the concentration of salicylate in the brain is correlated directly with mortality rate.[3]

The ionized state of salicylate can be used to enhance its elimination. If the urine pH is above 8.0, more salicylate molecules in the urine will be ionized compared with the renal tubular cell pH of 7.4 and reabsorption across the urinary tubule will be reduced.[4]

Acute salicylate overdose may produce nausea and vomiting as a result of local gastric irritation and stimulation of the chemoreceptor trigger zone.[5] Vomiting may result in volume depletion, which reduces renal perfusion and urine flow, adversely affecting renal salicylate elimination and contributing to acid-base and electrolyte disturbances.

Salicylate initially increases respiratory rate through a direct stimulatory effect on the medullary respiratory center in the central nervous system (CNS),[6] but very high levels of salicylate depress respiration, a finding usually seen later in the course. Salicylate also stimulates skeletal muscle metabolism, which causes an increase in oxygen consumption and carbon dioxide production.[6] The clinical manifestation of the initial respiratory center stimulation (the dominant component) and the increase in carbon dioxide production causes an increased respiratory rate resulting in respiratory alkalosis.[6] Initially, this will counter the enduring metabolic acidosis. If ventilatory compensation fails to keep pace with increased carbon dioxide production, respiratory acidosis will develop and will compound the metabolic acidosis.

The loss of the respiratory buffering effect is very dangerous, because the kidneys, even under ideal conditions, cannot react with sufficient rapidity to counter the acidosis meaningfully. Also, the critical alkalemia seen early when respiratory alkalosis predominates causes the kidneys to increase bicarbonate and potassium excretion. The urinary bicarbonate loss will eventually decrease the body's bicarbonate stores and impair compensation for the metabolic acidosis of salicylism.

Salicylate enhances lipolysis, uncouples oxidative phosphorylation, and inhibits various Krebs cycle enzymes involved in energy production and amino acid metabolism, resulting in (1) increased catabolism that leads to increased carbon dioxide production, (2) increased heat production, (3) increased glycolysis and peripheral demand for glucose, and (4) production of metabolic intermediaries (organic acids, lactate, pyruvate, and keto acids), which contribute to the metabolic acidosis of salicylate toxicity.[7] Overall, the acid-base disturbance associated with salicylate poisoning is mixed and includes respiratory alkalosis, metabolic alkalosis (due to volume contraction) and a wide-anion-gap type metabolic acidosis.

Salicylate-induced noncardiogenic pulmonary edema has been observed in humans[8–11] and studied in animals. Salicylate toxicity causes increased pulmonary vascular permeability, whereas pulmonary vascular pressures and cardiac performance are unaffected. This vascular injury may also involve the kidneys. Proteinuria is a prominent early finding in salicylate toxicity, starting at a serum salicylate level greater than 30 mg/dL, and it is directly related to salicylate levels.[9]

Salicylate also affects both central and peripheral glucose homeostasis. Salicylate causes mobilization of glycogen stores, resulting in hyperglycemia. However, salicylate is also a potent inhibitor of gluconeogenesis. Therefore, normoglycemia, hyperglycemia, or hypoglycemia may occur in salicylate toxicity. The brain involves a unique problem with glucose delivery. Animal studies demonstrate that toxic doses of salicylate produce a profound decrease in brain glucose concentration despite normal serum glucose levels.[12] This finding suggests that the supply of glucose to the brain in salicylate poisoning may be inadequate, even though serum glucose levels are normal.

Antiplatelet activity is a well-known effect of ASA, but hemorrhage is a rare complication of acute, single, massive overdose of salicylate. Salicylate has a molecular structure similar to both vitamin K and dicumarol. *Chronic* administration of large doses of salicylate may cause significant hypoprothrombinemia when the serum salicylate concentration exceeds 60 mg/dL.[13] This is presumably due to salicylate's competitive inhibition of the vitamin K effect.

Salicylate ototoxicity is characterized by a reversible sensorineuronal hearing loss, which is not idiosyncratic; it is related to serum salicylate concentrations.[14] When serum salicylate concentrations exceed 40 mg/dL, hearing loss reaches its maximum of 40 decibels.[14]

CLINICAL FEATURES AND DIAGNOSIS

Clinical manifestations of salicylism depend on the dose of salicylate ingested, duration of exposure, and age of the patient. In general, acute ingestion of less than 150 mg/kg may produce "mild" toxicity, with nausea, vomiting, and GI irritation, but significant toxicity is not expected. Acute ingestion of 150 to 300 mg/kg may produce "mild to moderate" toxicity, with vomiting, hyperpnea, diaphoresis, tinnitus, and acid-base disturbances. Acute ingestion of more than 300 mg/kg may produce "severe" toxicity.

The features of pediatric and adult salicylate intoxication differ. *Acute* pediatric salicylate intoxication is characterized by a known history of ingestion and onset of symptoms within a few hours of ingestion. Patients usually present soon after the ingestion. Symptoms are usually mild and the intoxication well tolerated.[15] The acid-base disturbance on presentation may be related to the patient's age. When the duration of salicylate intoxication is between 12 to 24 h, metabolic acidosis and acidemia (pH < 7.38) occur primarily in children younger than age 4, and nearly all children younger than age 1 have acidosis.[16] The acid-base disturbance in older children (age 4 or older) changes to a mixed disturbance with respiratory alkalosis, and increased anion-gap metabolic acidosis; alkalemia (pH > 7.42) tends to be observed.

Chronic or "therapeutic" (repeated dose) pediatric salicylate poisonings are generally more serious and are fatal more frequently than are acute ingestions.[15,17] Often, several days elapse between the initial administration of salicylate and the onset of symptoms.[17] There is often a coincidental illness that prompted the salicylate administration, and children usually appear more ill than those with acute intoxication. The presenting signs are hyperventilation, volume depletion, acidosis, severe hypokalemia, and CNS disturbances.[15] Chronic salicylism is often mistaken for an infectious process. Young children are prone to develop hyperpyrexia, which indicates a worse prognosis.[17] Renal failure may be a significant complication, but pulmonary edema is unusual in the pediatric population.[17] The delay in diagnosis may account for the more severe clinical picture with "therapeutic" salicylism.

Acute salicylate intoxication in adults is usually due to intentional ingestion, most often occurs in young women, and the patient frequently has a psychiatric or drug overdose history.[18] The typical clinical presentation includes nausea, vomiting, tinnitus, sweating, and hyperventilation, which are reported to occur when the serum salicylate concentration is above 30 mg/dL.[19] However, tinnitus may develop when the serum salicylate concentration exceeds 19.6 mg/dL.[19] Most patients have a mixed acid-base disturbance of respiratory alkalosis and metabolic acidosis.[20] However, when patients have also ingested sedative drugs that impair the hyperpneic response associated with salicylate toxicity, their acid-base profile is altered. Respiratory acidosis, rather than respiratory alkalosis, is more likely to occur.[20] Patients with mixed ingestions had a normal anion-gap metabolic acidosis 40 percent of the time compared with patients who had a larger mean anion gap when salicylate was ingested alone.[20] Therefore, salicylate intoxication in adults who present with a normal anion-gap metabolic acidosis should raise the suspicion that a coingestion including a CNS depressant has occurred. A normal anion gap does not rule out salicylate toxicity in patients with an unknown ingestion.

The complex triple-mixed acid-base disturbance of wide-anion-gap acidosis, metabolic alkalosis, and respiratory alkalosis may not be seen frequently in salicylate toxicity but, when it is noted, the differential diagnosis is quite limited. The only other wide-anion-gap acidosis seen with the other two components is sepsis (lactic acidosis, contraction metabolic alkalosis, and respiratory alkalosis). The main contribution to the metabolic acidosis in sepsis is lactate. In contrast, any lactic acidosis associated with salicylate poisoning should be mild unless there is significant hypotension and impaired tissue perfusion. The presence of significant lactic acidosis should always prompt a search for an alternate etiology (see Chap. 21).

Uncommon features of acute adult salicylism include fever, neurologic dysfunction, renal failure, adult respiratory distress syndrome (ARDS), noncardiogenic pulmonary edema, and hypoglycemia. Each of these uncommon manifestations indicates more severe poisoning, with associated greater morbidity and mortality rates. Hyperpyrexia appears to be an adverse prognostic indicator, and death is usually preceded by a predominant metabolic acidosis and neurologic deficits.[18,20] Other rare complications may include rhabdomyolysis, gastric perforation, and GI hemorrhage. Risk factors for death from acute salicylate toxicity include unconsciousness on presentation, fever, severe acidosis, seizures, cardiac dysrhythmias, and advanced age. The development of respiratory acidosis is usually a premorbid event.

The diagnosis of chronic salicylate intoxication (supratherapeutic misadventures or chronic excessive dosing) in adults is different, particularly in the elderly. These patients are more likely to have underlying medical conditions that they are treating with salicylates.[18] Signs and symptoms of chronic intoxication include hyperventilation, tremor, papilledema, agitation, paranoia, bizarre behavior, memory deficits, confusion, and stupor.[21] Neurologic abnormalities are much more common in chronic salicylate poisoning and often mislead physicians.[18] Chronic salicylism should be considered in any patient with unexplained CNS dysfunction, especially in the presence of a mixed acid-base disturbance, tachypnea or dyspnea, unexplained noncardiogenic pulmonary edema, or nonfocal neurologic or behavioral abnormalities. Adults with chronic salicylate toxicity have a higher morbidity rate, including pulmonary edema, seizures, and renal failure, as well as higher mortality rate.[18]

The distinction between acute and chronic salicylate toxicity may not always be clear. A patient may present many hours after an acute severe salicylate overdose, when altered mental status, acidosis, elevated prothrombin time, and serious toxicity with a ''therapeutic'' serum salicylate level are signs consistent with a chronically poisoned patient. Significant toxicity may be evident despite ''therapeutic'' or declining salicylate levels. In these situations, the patient's clinical status is the most important parameter in the assessment of the severity of toxicity.

Chronic salicylism may develop in patients taking carbonic anhydrase inhibitors for treatment of glaucoma.[22] The non-wide-anion-gap (hyperchloremic) metabolic acidosis produced by carbonic anhydrase inhibitors increases the volume of distribution for salicylate and facilitates its entry into the CNS, causing toxicity at a ''therapeutic'' salicylate blood level.

SPECIFIC ISSUES

The Done nomogram was created to assist in clarifying the level of salicylate intoxication that should prompt intervention: ''This (nomogram) provides only a rough guide to a single criterion of severity in previously well patients . . . it obviously does not supplant clinical judgement.''[23] Although widely taught and used for almost 40 years, the Done nomogram is typically misunderstood and often misused. Thus, it is strongly recommended that the patient's clinical condition and early course, rather than the nomogram, guide clinical therapy. The nomogram was based primarily on previously healthy pediatric patients with acute single salicylate ingestion.[23] The patients' presentations were clinically graded. The initial serum salicylate concentration was extrapolated based on toxicokinetic data. The clinical grade was then correlated to the extrapolated initial salicylate concentration. The potential usefulness of the nomogram is to assist in predicting the degree of toxicity after an acute, single ingestion of ASA in patients who have not been taking salicylate recently. However, there are severe limitations to the usefulness of the Done nomogram. The nomogram is *not* useful when (1) salicylate has been ingested over several hours or days, (2) the preparation is an enteric-coated or a sustained-release tablet, (3) the compound is oil of wintergreen, which is rapidly absorbed, (4) the patient has renal insufficiency or failure, (5) the time of ingestion is unknown or uncertain, (6) the patient is acidemic, or (7) a salicylate level drawn before 6 h after ingestion returns nontoxic. In such situations, the clinical condition of the patient should be considered paramount and not the salicylate level. The degree of toxicity is determined by serial evaluation of a patient's clinical condition and serial salicylate levels. Evolution of a ''nontoxic'' salicylate level into severe salicylate intoxication has surprised many physicians. Failure to anticipate worsening intoxication is generally due to reliance on a single salicylate level, without regard to the formulation or the time of ingestion. If the level was drawn before 6 h, it may underestimate the severity. It is prudent in most patients to draw serial serum salicylate levels every 1 to 2 h until the levels are declining and the patient's clinical status stabilizes. Acidemia must alter estimation of the severity of the intoxication. Due to its limitations and deceptive utility, use of the Done nomogram is not recommended and, as such, a description of its use is not provided in this text.

The presence of salicylate may be determined with the ferric chloride test, which uses several drops of 10% ferric chloride added to 1 mL of urine. A purple color will be seen in the presence of salicylic acid, acetoacetic acid, or phenylpyruvic acid. This test is very sensitive to small quantities of salicylic acid, and a positive test result does not indicate salicylate poisoning or toxicity. False-negative results have not been reported. However, false-positive results may occur when a small quantity of urine that has been used for dipstick analysis with the N-multistix or Bili Labstix is then used for ferric chloride testing. Presumably, some impregnated chemical from the dipstick dissolves in the urine and causes a false-positive reaction. Another bedside test for salicylic acid utilizes the Ames Phenistix, which turns brown when either salicylic acid or phenothiazines are present in the urine or serum. Adding one drop of 20 *N* sulfuric acid to the strip bleaches out the color in the case of phenothiazines but not in the case of salicylic acid. The color change is often difficult to interpret. Both the ferric chloride and Ames Phenistix tests are qualitative tests. All positive urine results must be confirmed with serum salicylate level. There are severe limitations associated with bedside detection techniques for salicylic acid, and we do not advocate their use in the clinical setting.

Assessing the condition of patients who have ingested enteric-coated or a sustained-release aspirin preparation is difficult. These products are formulated to remain intact in the acidic gastric environment, but to dissolve in the alkaline intestinal fluids. Drug release is therefore primarily a function of gastric emptying, and peak levels may not be apparent until 10 to 60 h after ingestion.[2]

Another problem with enteric-coated and sustained-release tablets is their large size, which makes them difficult to remove from the stomach even through a 40-French gastric lavage tube. A plain radiograph of the abdomen has been recommended for enteric-coated medications, but not all are radiopaque.[24] Thus, a positive radiograph can confirm that pills are present, but a negative radiograph does not rule out an enteric-coated or sustained-release ASA in the GI tract. If a potentially lethal number of enteric-coated or sustained-release tablets have been ingested, the patient should be observed for a minimum of 24 h and serial serum salicylate levels obtained until a declining level is assured.[2]

Many standard texts assert that urinary alkalinization is impossible until hypokalemia has been corrected.[16,25,26] The kidneys will attempt to excrete H^+ in order to retain potassium, leading to paradoxical aciduria despite alkalemia. However, there seem to be little or no clinical data specifically regarding the role of potassium replacement in alkalinization of urine during salicylate intoxication. In one human study, no correlation was found between serum potassium levels and urinary pH, and the patients' urines remained acidic in spite of alkalemia and normokalemia.[27] Although it is important to administer supplemental potassium to hypokalemic patients, it is inappropriate to delay the administration of sodium bicarbonate until normokalemia is achieved. Potassium and sodium bicarbonate should be administered simultaneously.

When aggressive management for ARDS with endotracheal intubation, mechanical ventilation, and sedation becomes necessary, hyperventilation must be maintained or acute deterioration may occur as a result of iatrogenic respiratory acidosis, causing a rapid shift of salicylate into the CNS.

TREATMENT

There is no specific antidote for salicylate toxicity. The main goals of therapy are immediate resuscitation; maintenance of airway, breathing, and circulation; correction of volume depletion and metabolic derangements; GI decontamination; and reduction in body salicylate burden.

The first step is to determine that clinically significant salicylate toxicity exists. This decision is made based on serial clinical assessment of the patient and serial serum salicylate concentrations. Recommended laboratory tests include serum electrolytes, glucose, blood urea nitrogen, creatinine, liver function tests, complete blood count, chest x-ray, electrocardiogram, and urinalysis with urine pH determination.

Reducing a patient's salicylate burden involves minimizing further absorption of salicylate from the GI tract and hastening elimination of salicylate already absorbed. Salicylate absorption is effectively reduced by the administration of activated charcoal (AC) both for regular and for sustained-release forms.[28] AC, 1 to 2 g/kg, should be administered to patients who have ingested potentially toxic amounts of salicylate. In contrast, no convincing data support the use of repeated doses or multiple doses of AC. Evidence supports the use of whole bowel irrigation as a more effective means of GI decontamination when dealing with enteric-coated or sustained-release ASA in the GI tract.[29]

Patients with severe salicylate intoxication are usually volume depleted and have acid-base disturbances that require general supportive and specific measures to enhance elimination. Careful assessment of a patient's volume and electrolyte status is important particularly in the elderly and in patients with a history of cardiac disease. Fluid replacement of volume deficits should be undertaken while preparations are made for other measures. A glucose-containing crystalloid (e.g., 5% D/0.9% NaCl) should be used in most patients because hypoglycemia has been implicated in the pathophysiology of salicylate CNS injury.[12] When hypokalemia is evident, potassium should be added to the intravenous fluids after urine output has been established. Note that correction of acidemia might further exacerbate hyopkalemia due to a shift of potassium into cells.

Urinary salicylate clearance is directly proportional to urine flow rate, but, more importantly, it is logarithmically proportional to urine pH.[30] Urine alkalinization is more effective than forced diuresis or forced alkaline diuresis, and it avoids the potential complication of fluid overload that may result from forced diuresis, especially in those with marginal cardiac reserve or cardiac performance.[30]

Opinions differ on the approach to initial fluid resuscitation and alkalinization of the urine. In practice, often both hydration and urine alkalinization are initiated simultaneously. Our approach has been to volume replete patients with normal saline with a target urine output of 1 to 2 mL/kg/h. Concurrently, in a second intravenous line, administer an intravenous bolus of sodium bicarbonate (1 to 2 meq/kg), followed by a continuous infusion of 5% D/W, to which 3 ampules (either 44 or 50 meq/ampule) of sodium bicarbonate have been added, starting at 1.5 to 2.0 times the maintenance rate and then adjusted to maintain the urine pH above 7.5. Except for the fluids used for hydration, all intravenous fluids administered should contain a minimum of 50 g/L glucose (5% D/W).[31] When hypoglycemia or neurologic symptoms are present, a minimum of 100 g/L glucose (10% D/W) has been suggested.[31] It is important to monitor the patient's clinical course diligently. The patient's urine pH, and serum salicylate concentration, as well as volume, acid-base and electrolyte status, and cardiopulmonary and neurologic status should be evaluated at least every hour. Potassium (40 meq/L) should be supplemented in the normal saline after adequate urine output has been established.

Patients with salicylate-induced (noncardiogenic) pulmonary edema should be managed as are patients with ARDS from other causes. Pulmonary edema begins to improve concomitantly with the lowering of serum salicylate levels.[8,18] This would suggest that aggressive efforts toward rapid elimination by hemodialysis may be beneficial in this subset of patients. In addition, early hemodialysis enables removal of salicylate without the volume challenge that accompanies sodium bicarbonate administration, and it avoids the possibility of aggravating pulmonary edema.

Although bleeding diathesis is frequently mentioned in texts, hemorrhagic complications are rarely seen in single massive salicylate overdoses. Salicylate has a molecular structure similar to both vitamin K and dicumarol. Chronic administration of large doses does cause significant hypoprothrombinemia when serum salicylate concentration exceeds 60 mg/dL.[13] Hemorrhage, even under this scenario, however, is rarely seen in clinical practice or in animal experiments. When bleeding does occur, it rarely appears to be a contributing factor in death from salicylate poisoning. Patients who are actively bleeding should have judicious administration of fresh-frozen plasma and vitamin K_1. Observations in animals and humans indicate that administering large doses of vitamin K after the development of hypoprothrombinemia has little or no effect on the plasma prothrombin time when salicylate concentration is high. After discontinuing salicylate, the prothrombin time rapidly returns to normal.

Hemodialysis is considered the extracorporeal technique of choice for the treatment of serious salicylate toxicity, because hemodialysis can normalize acid-base and electrolyte abnormalities while rapidly reducing the salicylate burden.[32] Indications for hemodialysis include (1) clinical deterioration despite intensive supportive care and an alkaline diuresis, (2) unsuccessful attempts to detect clinical deterioration and an alkaline urine, (3) renal insufficiency or renal failure, (4) severe acid-base disturbance, (5) altered mental status, and (6) patients with ARDS.

Determination of the serum salicylate concentration may be helpful but should not be the sole determinant in the decision to initiate hemodialysis. A level of 100 mg/dL after an acute ingestion in a healthy patient may not require hemodialysis, whereas a patient with a level of 30 mg/dL in a chronic ingestion may be moribund. One should err on the side of hemodialysis in patients who are elderly, have ingested ASA chronically, have altered mental status, have acidemia, or have a severe underlying disease (e.g., coronary artery disease or chronic obstructive pulmonary disease).

In significant ingestions, serum salicylate levels should be monitored at least every 2 h until a peak has been reached and then every 4 to 6 h until the peak falls into the nontoxic range. In severe ingestions, serum salicylate levels should be determined hourly and clinical decisions should be based on the trend of the serum salicylate levels as well as the patient's clinical status.

DISPOSITION

A patient may be discharged following adequate GI decontamination, if there is progressive clinical improvement, no significant acid-base disturbance, and a documented serial decline in serum salicylate levels toward the therapeutic range. If there is any doubt, the patient should be admitted to an appropriate setting.

In the management of salicylism, "knee jerk" responses should be avoided when assessing salicylate level. Therapeutic decisions should not be based solely on the serum salicylate concentration. Although the determination of serial salicylate levels offers valuable information regarding the effectiveness of the treatment implemented, it is a poor substitute for clinical evaluation of a patient. The final decision when considering management options should be individualized according to the clinical condition of the patient and not depend on a particular salicylate level. Early consultation with a clinical toxicologist is prudent.

REFERENCES

1. Litovitz TL, Smilkstein M, Felberg L, et al: 1996 Annual report of the American Association of Poison Control Centers Toxic Exposure Surveillance System. *Am J Emerg Med* 14:447, 1997.
2. Wortzman DJ, Grunfeld A: Delayed absorption following enteric-coated aspirin overdose. *Ann Emerg Med* 16:434, 1987.
3. Hill JB: Salicylate intoxication. *N Engl J Med* 288:1110, 1973.
4. Smith PK, Gleason HL, Stoll CG, et al: Studies on the pharmacology of salicylates. *J Pharmacol Exp Ther* 87:237, 1946.
5. Smith MJH: The metabolic basis of the major symptoms in acute salicylate intoxication. *Clin Toxicol* 1:387, 1968.
6. Tenny SM, Miller RM: The respiratory and circulatory actions of salicylate. *Am J Med* 19:498, 1955.
7. Schwartz R, Landy G: Organic acid excretion in salicylate intoxication. *J Pediatr* 66:658, 1965.
8. Heffner JE, Starkey T, Anthony P: Salicylate-induced noncardiogenic pulmonary edema. *West J Med* 130:263, 1979.
9. Hormaechea E, Carlson BW, Rogove H, et al: Hypovolemia, pulmonary edema and protein changes in severe salicylate poisoning. *Am J Med* 66:1046, 1979.
10. Walters JS, Woodring JH, Stelling CB, et al: Salicylate-induced pulmonary edema. *Radiology* 146:289, 1983.
11. Fisher CJ, Albertson TE, Foulke GE: Salicylate-induced pulmonary edema: Clinical characteristics in children. *Am J Emerg Med* 3:33, 1985.
12. Thurston JH, Pollock PG, Warren SK, et al: Reduced brain glucose with normal plasma glucose in salicylate poisoning. *J Clin Invest* 49:2139, 1970.
13. Clausen FW, Jager BV: The relation of the plasma salicylate level to the degree of hypoprothrombinemia. *J Lab Clin Med* 31:428, 1946.
14. Myers EN, Bernstein JM, Fostiropolous G: Salicylate ototoxicity a clinical study. *N Engl J Med* 11:587, 1965.
15. Gaudreault P, Temple AR, Lovejoy FH: The relative severity of acute versus chronic salicylate poisoning in children: A clinical comparison. *Pediatrics* 70:566, 1982.
16. Done AK: Treatment of salicylate poisoning: Review of personal and published experiences. *Clin Toxicol* 1:451, 1968.
17. Snodgrass W: Salicylate toxicity following therapeutic doses in young children. *Clin Toxicol* 18:247, 1981.
18. Anderson RJ, Potts DE, Gabow PA, et al: Unrecognized adult salicylate intoxication. *Ann Intern Med* 85:745, 1976.
19. Mongan E, Kelly P, Nies K, et al: Tinnitus as an indication of therapeutic serum salicylate levels. *JAMA* 226:142, 1973.
20. Gabow PA, Anderson RJ, Potts DE, et al: Acid-base disturbances in the salicylate-intoxicated adult. *Arch Intern Med* 138:1481, 1978.
21. Greer HD III, Ward HP, Corbin KB: Chronic salicylate intoxication in adults. *JAMA* 193:555, 1965.
22. Anderson CJ, Kaufman PL, Sturm RJ: Toxicity of combined therapy with carbonic anhydrase inhibitors and aspirin. *Am J Ophthalmol* 86:516, 1978.
23. Done AK: Significance of measurements of salicylate in blood in cases of acute ingestion. *Pediatrics* 26:800, 1960.
24. Savitt DL, Hawkins HH, Roberts JR: The radiopacity of ingested medications. *Ann Emerg Med* 16:331, 1987.
25. Goldfrank LR, Bresnitz EA, Hartnett L, et al: Salicylates, in Goldfrank LR, Flomenbaum NE, Lewin NA, et al (eds): *Goldfrank's Toxicologic Emergencies,* 4th ed. Norwalk, CT, Appleton and Lange, 1990, pp 261–269.
26. Rumack BH: Salicylates, in Behrman RE, Kliegman RM, Nelson WE, Vaughan VC III (eds): *Nelson Textbook of Pediatrics,* 14th ed. Philadelphia, WB Saunders, 1992, 1778–1779.
27. Prescott LF, Critchley JAJH, Proudfoot AT: Diuresis or urinary alkalinisation for salicylate poisoning? *BMJ* 286:147, 1983.
28. Levy G, Tsuchiya T: Effect of activated charcoal on aspirin absorption in man. *Clin Pharmacol Ther* 13:317, 1972.
29. Kirshenbaum LA, Mathews SC, Sitar DS, et al: Whole-bowel irrigation versus activated charcoal in sorbitol for the ingestion of modified-release pharmaceuticals. *Clin Pharmacol Ther* 46:264, 1989.
30. Prescott LF, Balali-Mood M, Critchley JAJH, et al: Diuresis or urinary alkalinisation for salicylate poisoning? *BMJ* 285:1383, 1982.
31. Pierce AW: Salicylate poisoning. *Pediatrics* 54:342, 1974.
32. Jacobsen D, Wiik-Larsen E, Bredesen JE: Haemodialysis or haemoperfusion in severe salicylate poisoning? *Hum Toxicol* 7:161, 1988.

ACETAMINOPHEN

Oliver Hung
Lewis S. Nelson

Acetaminophen (*N*-acetyl-*p*-aminophenol, or APAP) is the most popular over-the-counter analgesic used in the United States. As an ingredient found in a wide variety of prescription and over-the-counter remedies, acetaminophen is one of the most common toxic exposures reported to poison centers nationwide. Because of its ubiquitous presence, acetaminophen poisonings often occur because of the erroneous belief that this medication is benign or because the victim was unaware that it was an ingredient in the ingested preparation. According to the Toxic Exposure Surveillance System in 1996, acetaminophen accounted for 5 percent of all toxic exposures, but also accounted for 11 percent of reported fatalities.[1]

PHARMACOLOGY

The recommended dosing of acetaminophen is 650 mg every 4 to 6 h up to 4 g a day in adults and 10 to 15 mg/kg every 4 to 6 h in children. After ingestion, acetaminophen is rapidly absorbed from the gastrointestinal (GI) tract. In therapeutic doses, peak serum levels are usually achieved within 30 min to 2 h. Even in overdose, peak serum levels are usually achieved within 2 h. However, delayed absorption of acetaminophen has been reported with overdoses of acetaminophen propoxyphene preparations and overdose of a new acetaminophen preparation, Tylenol Extended Relief.

Acetaminophen is primarily metabolized by the liver through sulfation (20 to 46 percent) and glucuronidation (40 to 67 percent). A small percentage (less than 5 percent) of acetaminophen undergoes direct renal elimination. A small percentage is also oxidized by cytochrome P-450 to a toxic metabolite, *n*-acetyl-*p*-benzoquinoneimine (NAPQI), which is quickly detoxified by hepatic stores of glutathione to a nontoxic acetaminophen-mercaptate compound that can be eliminated through renal excretion (Fig. 165-1A).

However, during acetaminophen overdose, hepatic metabolism through glucuronidation and sulfation is quickly saturated. A larger proportion of acetaminophen is metabolized by cytochrome P-450 to NAPQI, depleting glutathione. When hepatic stores of glutathione decrease to less than 30 percent of normal, hepatic toxicity occurs. A reactive metabolite, NAPQI readily binds to other sulfur containing amino acids, primarily hepatic proteins and enzymes (Fig. 165-1B). Within the hepatic lobule, cytochrome P-450 is concentrated within hepatocytes surrounding the terminal hepatic vein and least concentrated within hepatocytes surrounding the portal triad. As a result, acetaminophen-induced hepatic injury results in the characteristic feature of hepatic centrilobular necrosis (Fig. 165-2).

Although the clinical manifestations of acetaminophen toxicity are classically delayed, hepatic injury actually occurs very early. In an animal model of acetaminophen hepatic toxicity, early signs of hepatic necrosis occurred within 12 h of exposure.[2] This was based on microscopic evidence of hepatic cellular necrosis and immunofluorescent staining of NAPQI-hepatic protein adducts (3-Cys-A) within hepatocytes. Hepatic necrosis continues to progress until day 2, when cell lysis occur, releasing hepatic enzymes such as transaminases and NAPQI-hepatic protein adducts into the circulation where they can be detected in the serum. This corresponds to the development of clinical toxicity in humans (Fig. 165-3).

CLINICAL PRESENTATION

The clinical presentation of human acetaminophen toxicity can be roughly divided into four stages. During the first 24 h after exposure (stage 1), patients often have minimal signs and symptoms of toxicity. Many patients may be asymptomatic and appear normal. Some may

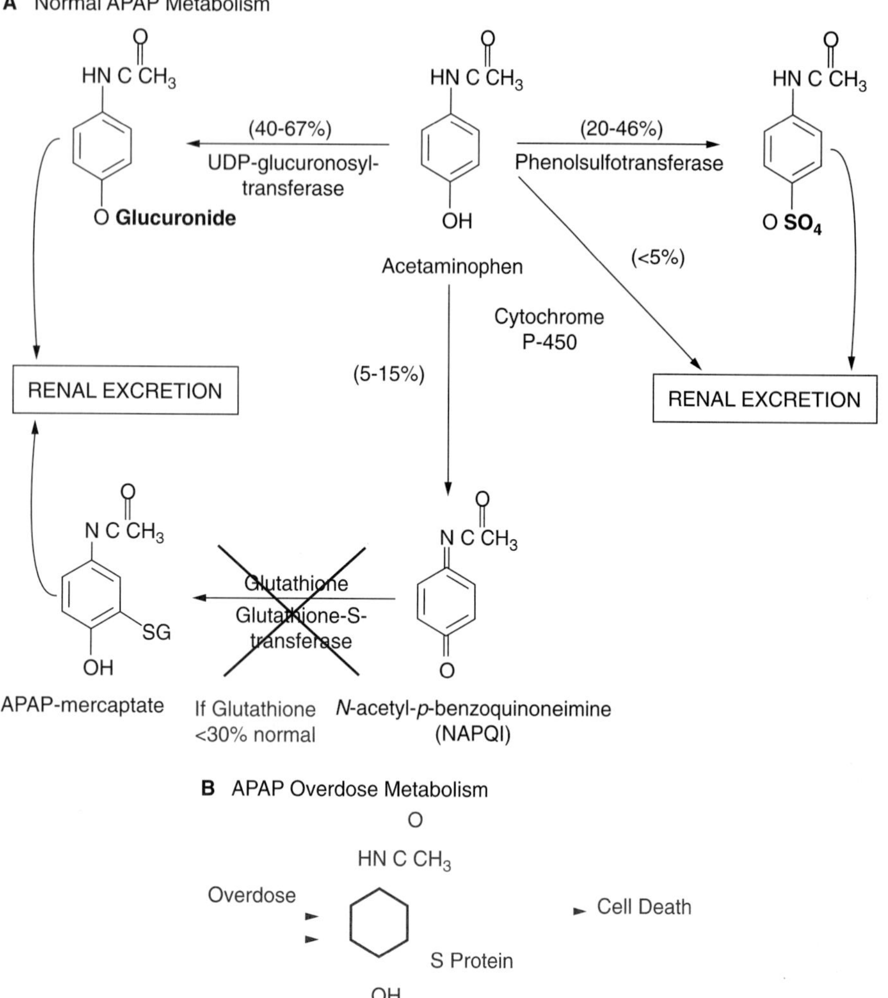

FIG. 165-1A and B. Acetaminophen (*N*-acetyl-*p*-aminophenol, or APAP) metabolism.

have minor, nonspecific GI signs and symptoms, such as anorexia, nausea, vomiting, and malaise. By days 2 to 3 (stage 2), clinical signs of hepatotoxicity that may be discerned in hepatotoxic patients include right upper quadrant abdominal pain and tenderness, and abnormal laboratory test results, such as elevated serum aspartate aminotransferase (AST), alanine aminotransferase (ALT), and bilirubin. Even without treatment, most of these patients will recover without sequelae. By days 3 to 4 (stage 3), however, the condition of some patients will progress to fulminant hepatic failure. Characteristic findings include metabolic lactic acidosis, coagulopathy, renal failure, encephalopathy, and recurrent GI symptoms. Those patients who survive the complications of fulminant hepatic failure will begin to recover over the next week (stage 4), with complete resolution of hepatic dysfunction in survivors.

Patients with insufficient glutathione stores (alcoholics and AIDS patients) and patients with induced cytochrome P450 enzymatic activity (alcoholics and those taking concurrent anticonvulsant or antituberculous medications) may be at greater risk for developing acetaminophen-induced hepatotoxicity following overdose. In contrast, children, because of their greater ability to metabolize acetaminophen through hepatic sulfation, may be at decreased risk for developing hepatotoxicity when compared with adults.[3]

Acetaminophen may also cause acute, extrahepatic toxic effects, presumably due to the presence of cytochrome P-450 present in other organs. Ingestion of massive doses of acetaminophen (4-h acetaminophen level greater than 800 μg/mL) has been associated with the acute development of altered sensorium (coma or agitation) and metabolic acidosis.[4] Acetaminophen overdose has also been infrequently associated with the direct development of renal insufficiency. In rare cases, cardiac toxicity and pancreatitis have also been reported.

DIAGNOSIS

A toxic exposure to acetaminophen is possible when more than 140 mg/kg is ingested in a single dose or when more than 7.5 g is ingested within a 24-h period. Unlike other types of poisoning, the diagnosis of acetaminophen toxicity depends on laboratory testing, because the initial clinical presentation is unhelpful and nonspecific. Also, the initial manifestations of toxicity (GI signs and symptoms) are usually delayed.

The diagnosis of acetaminophen toxicity depends solely on obtaining a serum acetaminophen level and estimating the time of ingestion. The acetaminophen level should be determined for all patients arriving at the emergency department (ED) with overdose of any drug. Acetaminophen is widely available in many single and multidrug over-the-counter and prescription medications. Consequently, many patients are unaware of their ingestion of acetaminophen. In one study, one in 500 patients arriving at the ED after an overdose and denying a history of acetaminophen ingestion was determined to have potentially toxic acetaminophen levels.[5] In economic terms, empirical testing of all patients with intentional overdoses may be cost effective. The cost of treatment of one patient for complications of acetaminophen-induced hepatotoxicity is commonly estimated to outweigh the cost of laboratory testing for 500 patients with nontoxic acetaminophen levels.

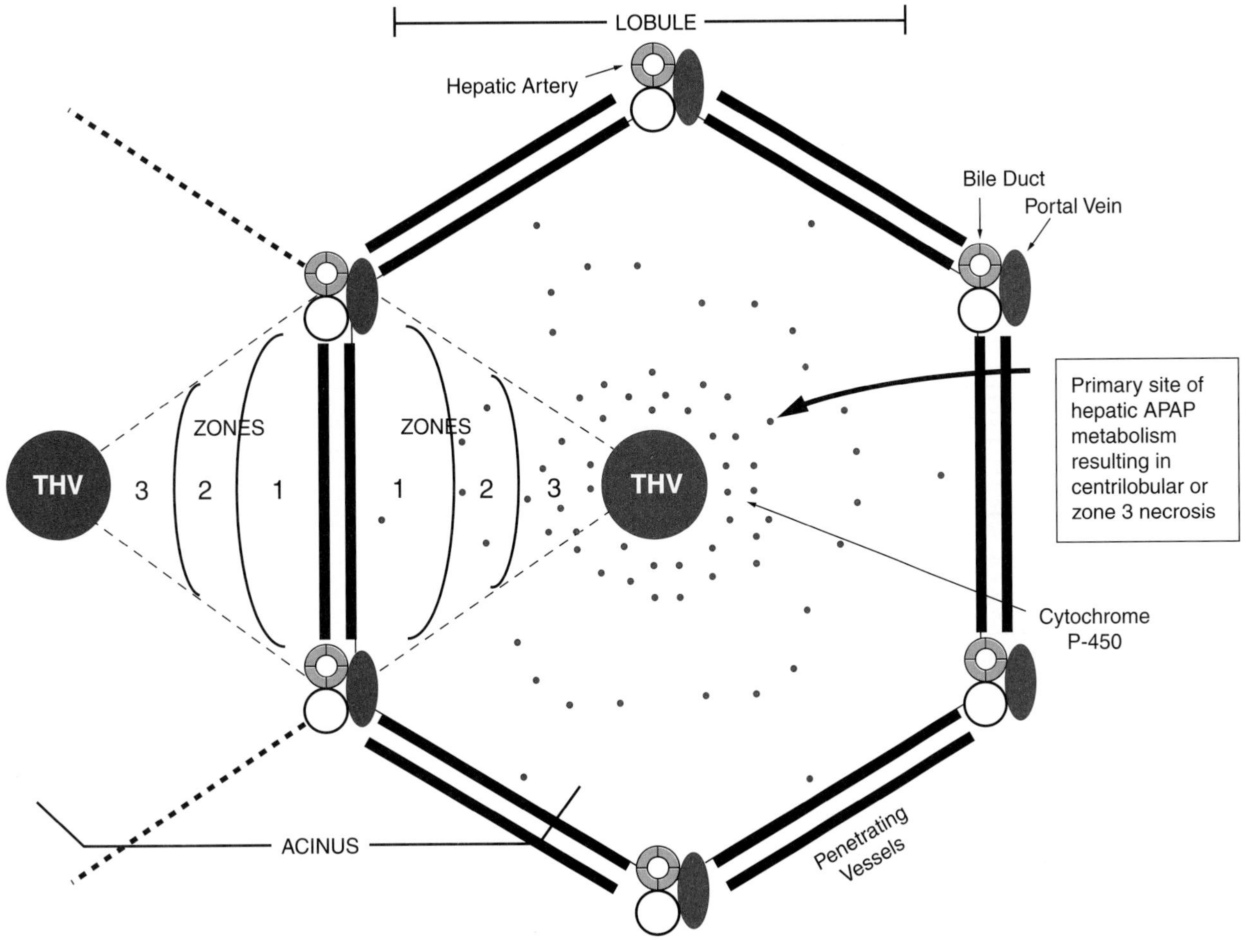

LOBULE
Hepatic Artery
Bile Duct
Portal Vein
THV
3
2
1
ZONES
ZONES
1
2
3
THV
Primary site of hepatic APAP metabolism resulting in centrilobular or zone 3 necrosis
Cytochrome P-450
ACINUS
Penetrating Vessels

FIG. 165-2. Hepatic centrilobular necrosis. THV, terminal hepatic vein.

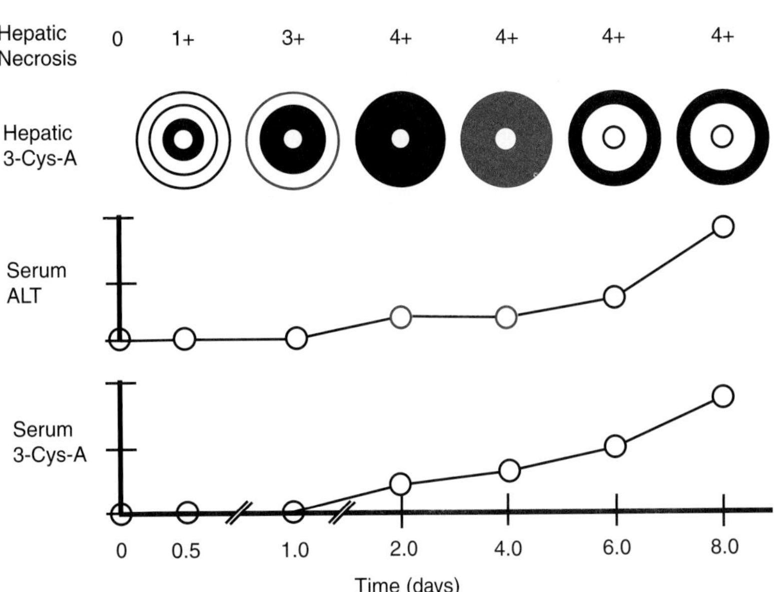

FIG. 165-3. Acetaminophen (APAP) toxicity time course. *Abbreviations:* 3-Cys-A, APAP-hepatic protein adduct; ALT, alanine aminotransferase. From Roberts et al,[2] with permission.

Hepatic Necrosis
0
1+
3+
4+
4+
4+
4+
Hepatic 3-Cys-A
Serum ALT
Serum 3-Cys-A
0
0.5
1.0
2.0
4.0
6.0
8.0
Time (days)

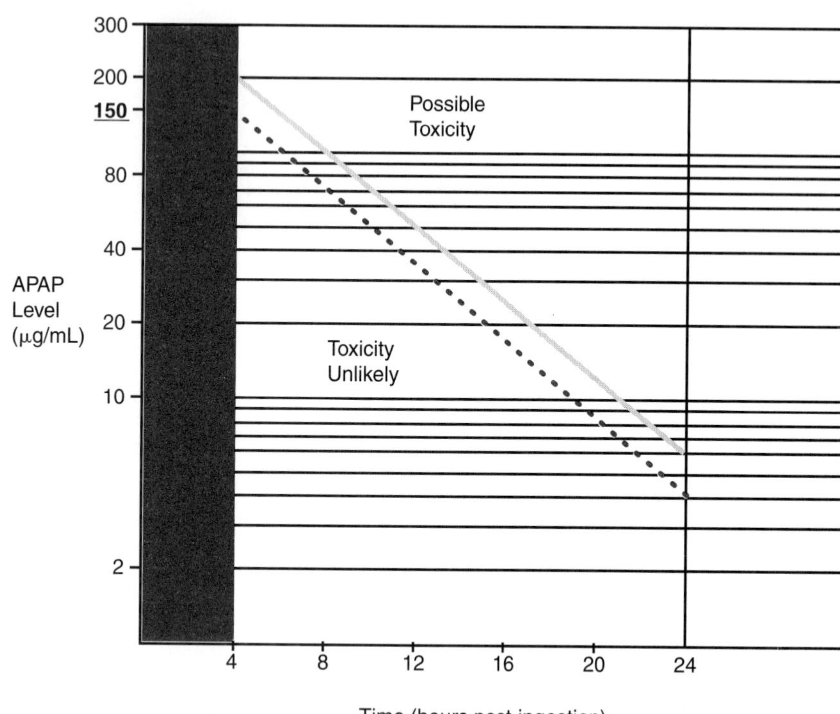

FIG. 165-4. Rumack-Matthew nomogram. *Abbreviation:* APAP, *N*-acetyl-*p*-aminophenol (acetaminophen). From Rumack and Matthew,[6] with permission.

The interpretation of a measured acetaminophen level depends on plotting the level on the Rumack-Matthew nomogram[6] (Fig. 165-4). This nomogram was empirically based on a retrospective analysis of previous acetaminophen overdose patients and their clinical outcomes. The original nomogram line was based on a 4-h acetaminophen level of 200 μg/mL, but was subsequently modified in the United States by the FDA to increase the safety margin by moving the line to a 4-h acetaminophen level of 150 μg/mL. More importantly, the nomogram only applies to an acetaminophen level measured after 4 h following ingestion and before 24 h after ingestion. It cannot be applied to acetaminophen levels determined outside of that 20-h period.

Measuring multiple acetaminophen levels is not indicated. The nomogram cannot interpret multiple levels because it is not based on acetaminophen kinetics. In addition, the calculation of acetaminophen kinetics by measuring multiple levels over a short period is usually mathematically inaccurate because of the intrinsic laboratory error present in the acetaminophen assay.

Based on historical data before the widespread use of antidotal therapy, patients with serum acetaminophen levels above the original 200 μg/mL nomogram were observed to have a 60 percent risk of developing hepatotoxicity (AST >1000 IU/mL), 1 percent risk of renal failure, and a 5 percent risk of death.[7] In addition, patients with extremely high serum acetaminophen levels (above a parallel line coinciding with a 300 μg/mL 4-h level) were observed to have a greater risk (90 percent) of developing hepatotoxicity (Fig. 165-5). The safety level below the US nomogram line (4-h level corresponding to 150 μg/mL) was confirmed in a prospective study involving 11,195 patients.[8] The risk of hepatotoxicity in patients with acetaminophen levels below the nomogram was 1 percent. No patients received antidotal therapy, and all recovered without any complications (Fig. 165-6).

TREATMENT

Treatment for acetaminophen toxicity consists of GI decontamination, the timely use of the antidote—*N*-acetylcysteine (NAC)—and supportive care. For most cases of acetaminophen poisoning, adequate GI decontamination consists of the early administration of activated charcoal orally or through nasogastric tube. Emesis induced by administering syrup of ipecac is undesirable because it delays the administration of the antidote, NAC. In addition, more aggressive forms of decontamination such as orogastric lavage or whole bowel irrigation, are unnecessary because of the rapid GI absorption of acetaminophen and the great success of treating acetaminophen poisoning with NAC. However, aggressive GI decontamination should be considered in cases of polydrug overdose in which a coingestant is likely to be life-threatening (e.g., a cyclic antidepressant or a sustained-release calcium-channel blocker).

The mainstay of treatment for acetaminophen toxicity is the administration of the antidote, NAC. Although its mechanisms of action are not fully understood, NAC is thought to have two important beneficial effects. In early acetaminophen toxicity (less than 8 h after ingestion), NAC prevents toxicity by inhibiting the binding of the toxic metabolite NAPQI to hepatic proteins. NAC may act as a glutathione precursor or substitute, act as a sulfate precursor, or it may directly reduce NAPQI back to acetaminophen. In late acetaminophen toxicity (more than 24 h after ingestion), NAC diminishes hepatic necrosis by nonspecific mechanisms. NAC may act as an antioxidant, decrease neutrophil proliferation, improve microcirculatory blood flow, and increase tissue oxygen delivery and extraction.

The standard 72-h oral NAC regimen used in the United States is a loading dose of 140 mg/kg followed by maintenance doses 70 mg/kg every 4 h for 17 doses. If treatment is initiated within 8 h of acetaminophen ingestion, NAC is nearly 100 percent effective in preventing the development of hepatotoxicity, as defined by an AST level of greater than 1000.[8] The longer NAC therapy is delayed past 8 h after ingestion, the greater is the risk of developing hepatotoxicity. Even by 24 h after acetaminophen ingestion, however, NAC treatment is associated with a lower risk of hepatotoxicity than are historical controls[7] (Fig. 165-6).

The major complications of oral NAC therapy are nausea and vomiting due to its foul odor and taste of rotten eggs. To hide these disagreeable characteristics, the standard 10% or 20% NAC solution should be diluted to a 5% concentration in a chilled beverage such as

FIG. 165-5. Outcomes of acetaminophen overdose (no antidote treatment). *Abbreviations:* APAP, *N*-acetyl-*p*-aminophenol (acetaminophen); AST, aspartate aminotransferase. Adapted from (1) from Prescott[7] and (2) Smilkstein et al,[8] with permission.

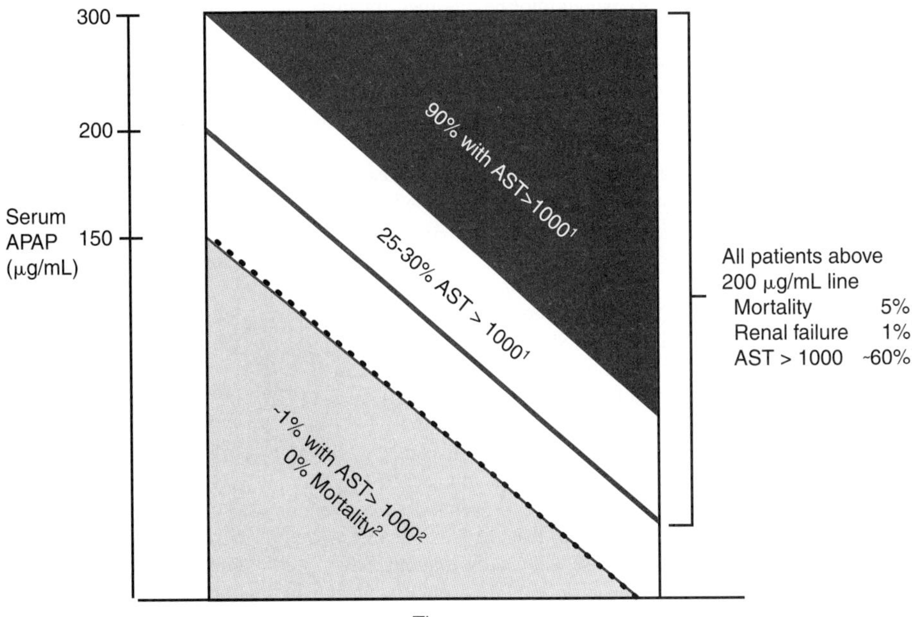

fruit juice or a soft drink prior to administration. NAC's disagreeable odor may be further minimized by having the patient sip the drink through a straw from a covered cup or by administering the dose by nasogastric or duodenal tube. Some patients with persistent nausea and vomiting may require concomitant antiemetic treatment with intravenous (IV) metoclopramide (Reglan), 0.1 mg/kg up to 1.0 mg/kg, ondansetron (Zofran), 0.15 mg/kg, or granisetron (Kytril), 0.01 mg/kg, to prevent vomiting and to administer NAC successfully.

Alternative IV NAC regimens have been used successfully in other countries for over 20 years but remain experimental in the United States.[9,10] These regimens possess potential limitations. IV NAC administration may be less effective for the treatment of acetaminophen overdoses in patients arriving more than 10 h after ingestion and is also associated with anaphylactoid reactions.[11] At this time, the clinical experience of IV NAC usage in the United States remains too limited to recommend it as a replacement for the traditional oral NAC regimen used for early acetaminophen poisoning. However, IV administration of NAC may be required for patients with refractory vomiting and for patients with contraindications to oral therapy (e.g., caustic ingestions). IV NAC may also be preferable to oral NAC for the treatment of acetaminophen-induced fulminant hepatic failure.[12]

Currently, there is no IV NAC formulation available in the United States. If it is to be used, the oral NAC formulation, which is sterile, can be made into an IV formulation. Clinical experience suggests that patients with poor glutathione reserves have similar excellent clinical outcomes when the standard treatment guidelines are applied to their

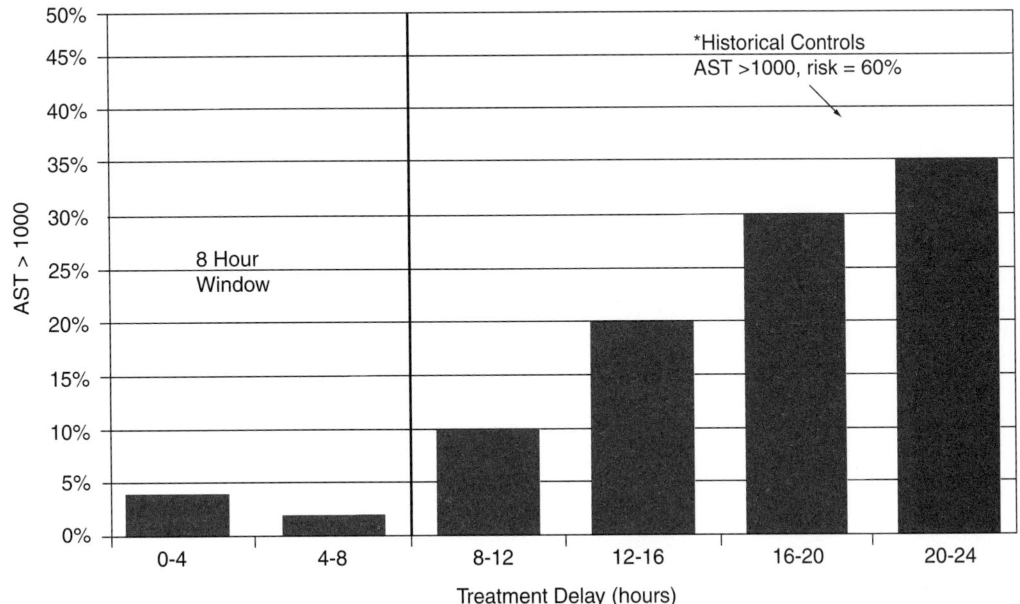

FIG. 165-6. Hepatotoxicity: acetaminophen and *N*-acetylcysteine (n = 11,195 cases). *Abbreviation:* AST, aspartate aminotransferase. From Smilkstein et al,[8] with permission.

care. Thus, the dosage of NAC should not be modified for these patients.

In many clinical situations, NAC therapy is often started in close temporal proximity to the administration of activated charcoal. Although NAC is adsorbed by activated charcoal, there is no evidence that activated charcoal inhibits the clinical effectiveness of NAC.[13] Most authorities believe that NAC dosing is probably excessive. NAC dosing is based on a patient's weight and bears no relationship to the dose of acetaminophen ingested. In addition, NAC appears to be equally effective in preventing hepatotoxicity following the largest acetaminophen overdose.[14] Separating the first dose of NAC and activated charcoal by 1 to 2 h, when possible, is a reasonable method to minimize potential NAC and activated charcoal interaction.

There are no data on which order is superior, and there is no evidence that administration of activated charcoal and NAC in a closer time frame is a problem.

Finally, the weight of clinical evidence suggests that NAC therapy is safe to use during pregnancy and that the approach to treating a pregnant patient following an acetaminophen overdose should remain the same. An ovine model demonstrated that NAC was unable to cross the placenta.[15] Finally, fetal demise and malformations have been described when NAC treatment was delayed for acetaminophen overdose in first-trimester pregnant women.[15]

TREATMENT GUIDELINES

Treatment guidelines for acetaminophen poisoning are based on the time to presentation to the ED after ingestion: acetaminophen ingestions less than 4 h prior to presentation, acetaminophen ingestions longer than 4 h but less than 24 h ago, and acetaminophen ingestions of unknown time or longer than 24 h prior to presentation (Fig. 165-7). No further acetaminophen serum measurements are necessary once the need for NAC therapy has been determined. Treatment with NAC should continue for the full 72-h course (18 doses).

For patients with acetaminophen ingestions who present within less than 4 h to the ED, treatment begins with GI decontamination (usually activated charcoal) and awaiting the determination of a 4-h postingestion acetaminophen level. If the hospital laboratory can determine the acetaminophen level within 8 h after ingestion, the clinician should wait for that measurement and plot it on the nomogram to determine whether NAC therapy is necessary. If the hospital laboratory cannot determine the acetaminophen level within 8 h, the clinician should empirically administer the first dose of NAC (within 8 h of acetaminophen ingestion) without waiting for the measurement. Subsequently, when the acetaminophen level is determined, it should be plotted on the nomogram to determine whether additional NAC therapy is necessary.

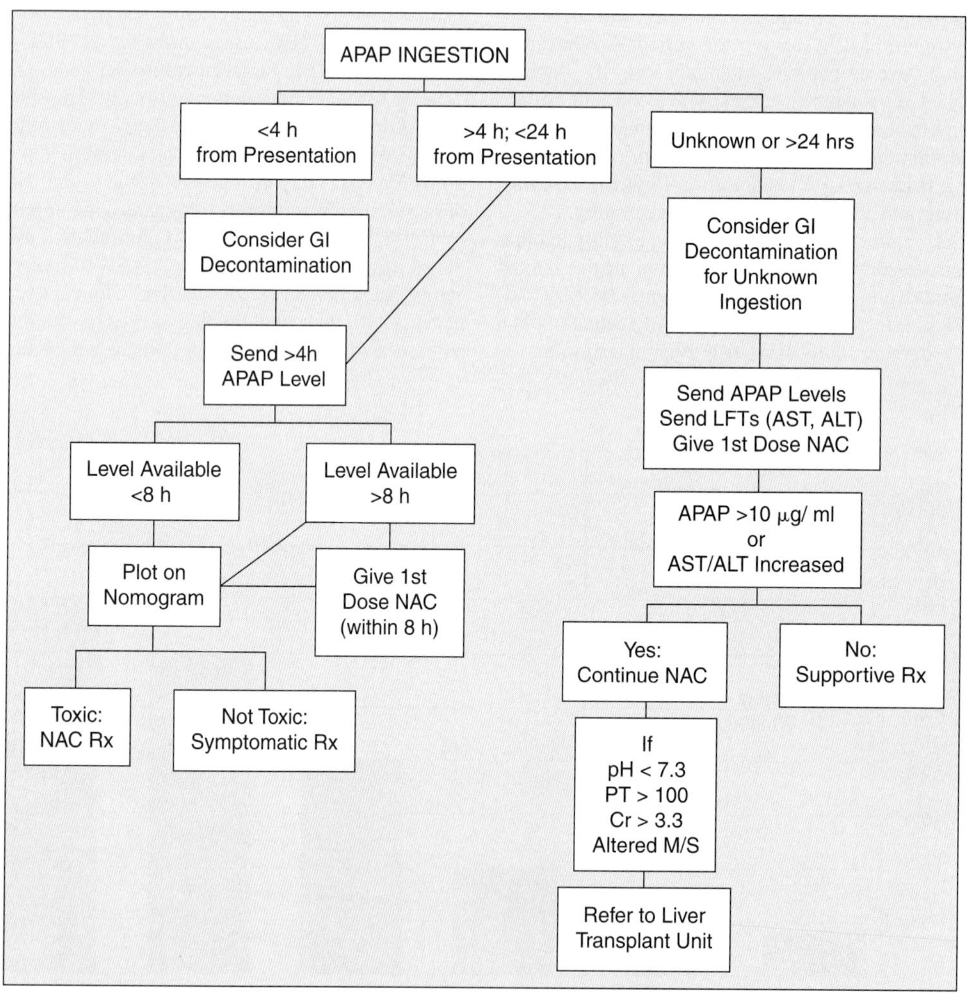

FIG. 165-7. Treatment guidelines for acetaminophen ingestion. *Abbreviations:* ALT, alanine aminotransferase; APAP, *N*-acetyl-*p*-aminophenol (acetaminophen); AST, aspartate aminotransferase; GI, gastrointestinal; LFTs, liver function tests; M/S ; NAC, *N*-acetylcysteine; PT, prothrombin time; Rx, treatment.

For patients with acetaminophen ingestions who present longer than 4 h but less than 24 h to the ED, the serum acetaminophen level should be determined by the laboratory as soon as possible. GI decontamination may be performed, but it may have limited effectiveness because of the delay in presentation. It should be considered more in light of possible coingestions. Similarly, if the hospital laboratory can determine the acetaminophen level within 8 h after ingestion, the clinician should wait for the serum acetaminophen level and plot it on the nomogram to determine whether NAC therapy is necessary. Otherwise, the first dose of NAC (within 8 h of acetaminophen ingestion, if possible) should be administered without waiting for the measurement. When the acetaminophen level is determined, it should be plotted on the nomogram to determine whether additional NAC therapy is necessary.

Finally, for acetaminophen ingestions of unknown time or longer than 24 h ago, the clinician should consider whether GI decontamination is required. A serum acetaminophen level should be determined and liver function tests (AST and ALT) should be performed by the hospital laboratory. In addition, the first dose of NAC therapy should be started as soon as possible. In this scenario, a detectable acetaminophen level (>10 μg/mL) suggests that the patient may be at risk for developing hepatotoxicity. Similarly, elevated AST and ALT enzymes suggest the possibility of ongoing hepatic toxicity. Therefore, continued NAC therapy is indicated if the acetaminophen level is measurable or if the serum AST or ALT is elevated.

Supportive therapy for acetaminophen poisoning, as in all overdose presentations to the ED, should include obtaining early IV access and a 12-lead electrocardiogram interpretation to exclude cardiac toxins (e.g., cyclic antidepressants, digoxin, β blockers, and calcium-channel blockers). Hypoglycemia and hypoxemia should be quickly considered and excluded for all patients presenting with altered sensorium. All patients requiring NAC therapy should be admitted to the hospital until the completion of the therapy. In general, admission to an unmonitored hospital bed is adequate unless a patient is hemodynamically unstable or a patient is suicidal and 24 h direct observation cannot be arranged. Patients who are not at risk for developing acetaminophen-induced hepatotoxicity (acetaminophen level below the nomogram, unmeasurable acetaminophen level with normal liver function test results) should be observed in the ED for a minimum of a 4 to 6-h period to exclude potentially toxic coingestants. This observation period is sufficient to exclude untoward events. Psychiatric evaluation should be considered for all patients with intentional acetaminophen overdose.

FULMINANT HEPATIC FAILURE

Unfortunately, a small percentage of patients with toxic acetaminophen ingestions will develop fulminant hepatic failure. The mortality rate for these patients (without NAC therapy) is estimated to be 58 to 80 percent. Most fatalities occur on days 3 to 5 after overdose and are attributed to hepatic complications such as cerebral edema, hemorrhage, shock, acute respiratory distress syndrome, sepsis, and multiorgan failure. Patients who eventually survive fulminant hepatic failure generally begin to show evidence of their recovery by days 5 to 7. Eventually, all survivors will develop complete hepatic regeneration without any persistence of hepatic impairment.

NAC also appears to be beneficial in the treatment of acetaminophen-induced fulminant hepatic failure. When compared with controls, NAC therapy was associated with increased survival (48 vs 20 percent), decreased cerebral edema (40 vs 68 percent), and decreased vasopressor requirements (40 vs 80 percent).[12] NAC appears to be beneficial in the treatment of other forms of hepatic failure, too, including viral hepatitis and alcoholic cirrhosis.[16]

Prognostic indicators have been developed to determine those patients with the highest risk of mortality from acetaminophen-induced fulminant hepatic failure. As a result, they also serve as early predictors of patients who will subsequently require liver transplantation. A variety of laboratory and clinical markers have been used, including serum pH, prothrombin time (PT), serum creatinine, and mental status evaluation. The presence of a metabolic acidosis, pH $<$ 7.3, despite fluid and hemodynamic resucitation, or a combination of coagulopathy (PT $>$ 100), renal failure (creatinine $>$ 3.3 mg/dL), and encephalopathy (grade III or IV) is extremely useful in predicting patients who will die without liver transplantation.[17]

Treatment for acetaminophen-induced fulminant hepatic failure includes NAC therapy, aggressive correction of coagulopathy and acidosis, monitoring for and aggressive treatment for cerebral edema, and early patient referral to a liver transplant center. Unlike the treatment of early acetaminophen toxicity, NAC therapy should be continued past the 72-h standard regimen until the patient recovers, receives a liver transplant, or dies. Since all clinical studies supporting the use of NAC to treat fulminant hepatic failure utilized the IV administration of NAC, IV NAC therapy may be preferable to oral NAC. IV NAC should be administered at the same dosage as oral NAC. Because of the risk of anaphylactoid reaction, IV NAC infusions should be administered slowly and adjusted based on repeated blood pressure measurements to prevent hypotension.

SPECIAL CONSIDERATIONS: MULTIPLE-DOSE ACETAMINOPHEN INGESTIONS AND TYLENOL EXTENDED RELIEF

Multiple-dose acetaminophen ingestions and Tylenol Extended Relief ingestions represent two unique aspects of acetaminophen poisoning since the Rumack-Matthew nomogram does not apply to these two scenarios. In addition, since there is little clinical data regarding multiple-dose acetaminophen ingestions and Tylenol Extended Relief, treatment guidelines remain conservative.

The scenario of multiple ingestions of acetaminophen over a period of time is problematic because the acetaminophen level measured cannot be interpreted by the nomogram since a specific single time of ingestion cannot be determined. Theoretically, an ingestion of multiple doses of acetaminophen over a period of time should be less toxic than a single ingestion of the same total dose of acetaminophen. In the case of multiple doses, the liver may be able to regenerate glutathione stores between ingestions to lessen the possibility or severity of hepatic toxicity. However, the approach to multiple acetaminophen ingestions remains conservative. A single ingestion is assumed to occur at the earliest possible time stated by the patient. Based on this artificial time, an acetaminophen level is plotted on the Rumack-Matthew nomogram and treatment decisions are made accordingly. For example, if a patient ingests five doses of 50 mg/kg of acetaminophen over a 4-h period beginning 8 h earlier, a single acetaminophen ingestion is assumed to have occurred 8 h earlier and the serum level is plotted on the nomogram.

Tylenol Extended Relief (Tylenol ER) represents a new acetaminophen formulation by McNeil Pharmaceuticals.[18] These caplets consist of a bilayered formulation containing a total of 650 mg acetaminophen. One side of the caplet contains 325 mg of ''regular'' immediate-release acetaminophen. The other side consists of 325 mg acetaminophen placed within a slowly releasing matrix. Ingestion of these caplets results in prolonged GI absorption that may delay peak acetaminophen levels when compared with the original formulation. In addition, there are case reports describing Tylenol ER ingestions in which the initial acetaminophen level was below the nomogram line, but a second acetaminophen level was found to ''cross the nomogram line.''[19] These reports should be interpreted with caution since the Rumack-Matthew nomogram was not meant to apply and cannot be applied to ingestions of Tylenol ER.

Currently, no data suggest that Tylenol ER is more toxic than regular acetaminophen. Theoretically, Tylenol ER could be less toxic than an equivalent amount of regular acetaminophen since the prolonged GI absorption may allow additional time for hepatic regeneration of glutathione. Because of the continued uncertainty, however, the approach remains conservative. Two additional hours are added to the estimated time of ingestion to increase the safety margin and to account for potential ingestions that might "cross the nomogram" (i.e., the 6-h postingestion level is read as a 4-h postingestion level). The acetaminophen level and the "revised" time of ingestion are plotted on the nomogram to determine risk of toxicity.

REFERENCES

1. Litovitz TL, Smilkstein M, Felberg L, et al: 1996 annual report of the American Association of Poison Control Centers Toxic Exposure Surveillance System. *Am J Emerg Med* 15:447, 1997.
2. Roberts DW, Bucci TJ, Benson RW, et al: Immunohistochemical localization and quantification of the 3-(cystein-S-*yl*)-acetaminophen protein adduct in acetaminophen hepatotoxicity. *Am J Pathol* 138:350, 1991.
3. Lieh-Lai MW, Sarnaik AP, Newton JF, et al: Metabolism and pharmacokinetics of acetaminophen in a severely poisoned young child. *J Pediatr* 105:125, 1984.
4. Flanagan RJ, Mant TGK: Coma and metabolic acidosis early in severe acute paracetamol poisoning. *Hum Toxicol* 5:179, 1986.
5. Ashbourne JF, Olson KR, Khayam-Bashi H: Value of rapid screening for acetaminophen in all patients with intentional drug overdose. *Ann Emerg Med* 18:1035, 1989.
6. Rumack BH, Matthew H: Acetaminophen poisoning and toxicity. *Pediatrics* 55:871, 1975.
7. Prescott LF: Paracetamol overdosage. *Drugs* 25:290, 1983.
8. Smilkstein MJ, Knapp GL, Kulig KW, et al: Efficacy of oral *N*-acetylcysteine in the treatment of acetaminophen overdose. *N Engl J Med* 319:1557, 1988.
9. Prescott LF: Treatment of severe acetaminophen poisoning with intravenous acetylcysteine. *Arch Intern Med* 141:386, 1981.
10. Smilkstein MJ, Bronstein AC, Linden C, et al: Acetaminophen overdose: A 48 hour intravenous *N*-acetylcysteine treatment protocol. *Ann Emerg Med* 30:1058, 1991.
11. Mann TG, Tempowski JH, Volons GN, et al: Adverse reactions to acetylcysteine and effect of overdose. *BMJ* 289:217, 1984.
12. Keays R, Harrison PM, Wendon JA, et al: Intravenous acetylcysteine in paracetamol induced fulminant hepatic failure: A prospective controlled trial. *BMJ* 303:1026, 1991.
13. Spiller HA, Krenzolak EP, Grande GA, et al: A prospective evaluation of the effect of activated charcoal before *N*-acetylcysteine in acetaminophen overdose. *Ann Emerg Med* 23:519, 1994.
14. Kobrinsky NL, Hartfield D, Horner H, et al: Treatment of advanced malignancies with high-dose acetaminophen and *N*-acetylcysteine rescue. *Cancer Invest* 14:202, 1996.
15. Riggs BS, Bronstein AC, Kulig K, et al: Acute acetaminophen overdose during pregnancy. *Obstet Gynecol* 74:247, 1989.
16. Harrison PM, Wendon JA, Gimson AES, et al: Improvement by acetylcysteine of hemodynamics and oxygen transport in fulminant hepatic failure. *N Engl J Med* 324:1852, 1991.
17. O'Grady JG, Alexander GJM, Hayllar KM, et al: Early indicators of prognosis in fulminant hepatic failure. *Gastroenterology* 87:439, 1988.
18. Temple AR, Mrazik TJ: More on extended-release acetaminophen. *N Engl J Med* 333:1508, 1995.
19. Graudins A, Aaron CK, Linden CH: Overdose of extended-release acetaminophen. *N Engl J Med* 333:196, 1995.

166 NONSTEROIDAL ANTI-INFLAMMATORY DRUGS

G. Richard Bruno
Wallace A. Carter

Nonsteroidal anti-inflammatory drugs (NSAIDs) are among the most widely used and prescribed drugs in the United States. They are effective antipyretics, nonnarcotic analgesics, and anti-inflammatory agents. There are between 35 and 70 million NSAID prescriptions written in United States each year, and several agents are now available over the counter.[1] The world market for NSAIDs is reported to be a 6 billion dollars per year industry. Given the tremendous use and easy availability of NSAIDs, they are relatively safe agents with respect to acute ingestion and overdose. The American Association of Poison Control Centers (AAPCC) reports 261,795 NSAID exposures resulting in 2130 major outcomes (life-threatening signs and symptoms or significant residual disability) and 26 deaths between 1992 and 1996. These cumulative data compare favorably to aspirin and acetaminophen, with fewer major outcomes and deaths per exposure (Table 166-1). The morbidity from NSAIDs in acute overdose is far overshadowed by complications of NSAIDs at therapeutic doses. It is estimated that NSAID-related gastrointestinal (GI) bleeding accounts for 7500 deaths and 75,000 hospitalizations annually in the United States.[2] NSAIDs have also be reported to account for a substantial proportion of drug-induced renal failure. This chapter reviews basic pharmacology of NSAIDs, significant interactions of NSAIDs with other drugs, side effects of chronic NSAIDs use, clinical presentation of acute overdose, and management of overdose.

TABLE 166-1 Major Outcomes and Deaths

5-Year Cumulative AAPCC Data, 1992–1996	NSAIDs	Acetaminophen	Aspirin
Number of exposures	261,795	357,866	79,754
Major outcomes*	634	2,130	721
Deaths	26	248	213

*Major outcomes are defined as signs or symptoms that are life threatening or result in significant disability.
Abbreviations: AAPCC, American Association of Poison Control Centers; NSAIDs, nonsteroidal anti-inflammatory drugs.

PHARMACODYNAMICS

NSAIDs are a structurally varied group of compounds with common therapeutic effects (Table 166-2). NSAIDs inhibit the enzyme cyclooxygenase (COX), which is responsible for the production of prostaglandins from arachidonic acid. NSAIDs mediate inflammation through inhibition of prostaglandin production but may also inhibit neutrophils via nonprostaglandin mechanisms. NSAIDs work as antipyretics through inhibition of prostaglandin E_2 (PGE_2) in the hypothalamus. The mechanism of NSAID-mediated analgesia is less clear than anti-inflammatory and antipyretic effects, but NSAIDs appear to attenuate prostaglandin-mediated hyperalgesia and local pain-fiber stimulus.

There are at least two forms of cyclooxygenase: COX I and II. COX I is found predominately in blood vessels, stomach, and kidneys at steady levels. COX II is not usually found at significant levels in human tissue; rather, production of the enzyme is induced by local inflammatory mediators. Most NSAIDs inhibit both COX I and COX II. Inhibition of COX I is believed to be responsible for much of the unwanted side effects of NSAIDs. Work is currently under way to develop selective inhibitors of COX II, which may be better anti-inflammatory agents and have fewer ill effects on the renal/GI and vascular system.

PHARMACOKINETICS

All NSAIDs are rapidly absorbed from the GI tract and are highly protein bound in the plasma. Most NSAIDs undergo at least partial metabolism in the liver via glucuronic acid conjugation or oxidation in the microsomal enzyme system before elimination in the urine or feces. Plasma half-lives of NSAIDs range from 2 to 4 h for ibuprofen to longer than 50 h for the long-acting agents piroxicam and phenylbutazone.

SIGNIFICANT DRUG-DRUG INTERACTION

Warfarin

Warfarin and NSAIDs have important interactions. Two NSAIDs (phenylbutazone and naproxen) have been reported to displace warfarin from plasma proteins, leading to increased warfarin levels in serum and elevated prothrombin times. Phenylbutazone has also been shown to decrease elimination of warfarin. Other NSAIDs have not been reported to change warfarin protein binding or elimination, but the use of any NSAID is contraindicated in warfarin users because NSAID inhibition of platelet aggregation may significantly increase the risk for bleeding.

Diuretics and Other Antihypertension Agents

NSAIDs may decrease the effectiveness of some antihypertensives, including diuretics, α-adrenergic blockers, angiotensin-converting enzyme inhibitors, and β-adrenergic blockers. The blood pressure change when both NSAIDs and antihypertensives are used ranges from little effect to hypertensive urgencies. Inhibition of prostaglandin synthesis is believed to be central to the attenuation of antihypertensive effects. Lower prostaglandin levels result in decreased renal sodium clearance, water retention, changes in vascular tone, and alterations in the renin-angiotensin system, all which may attenuate the effectiveness of antihypertensive agents.[3]

Decrease Renal Clearance of Drugs

NSAIDs may also decrease the renal clearance and elimination of certain drugs. NSAID use inhibits renal clearance of lithium and leads to elevated serum lithium levels. Methotrexate elimination is also decreased with coadministration of NSAIDs and has resulted in fatal toxicity.

TABLE 166-2 Classes of Nonsteroidal Agents Available in the United States

Salicylates
Aspirin
Salsalate (Salflex, Disalcid)
Diflusinal (Dolobid)
Acetic acids
Tolmetin (Tolectin)
Ketorolac (Toradol)
Diclofenac (Voltaren)
Indomethacin (Indocin)
Sulindac (Clinoril)
Nabumetone (Relafen)
Etodolac (Lodine)
Fenamic acids
Mefenamic acid (Ponstel)
Meclofenamate (Meclomen)
Propionic acids
Ibuprofen (Advil, Motrin, Nuprin)
Naproxen (Naprosyn, Aleve)
Ketoprofen (Orudis)
Fenoprofen (Nalfon)
Flurbiprofen (Ansaid)
Oxaprozin (Daypro)
Pyrazolones
Phenylbutazone
Oxicams
Piroxicam (Feldene)

CLINICAL PRESENTATION OF TOXICITY

Toxicity of NSAIDs at Therapeutic Doses

NSAIDs are relatively safe drugs that have a number of well-documented side effects at therapeutic doses. Given the huge number of NSAID prescriptions written by emergency department physicians, it is important to be aware of common side effects. Morbidity and death from renal insufficiency and GI bleeding with chronic NSAID use far overshadow that of acute NSAID overdose. Other organ systems that may show toxicity at therapeutic doses include the central nervous system (CNS), cardiovascular, respiratory, hepatic, and dermatologic. It is generally believed that indomethacin and the long-acting agents phenylbutazone and piroxicam are responsible for a greater proportion of side effects, and that the propionic acid agents such as ibuprofen are responsible for fewer side effects.

Central Nervous System

Toxic CNS side effects of NSAIDs are far less frequent than GI or renal toxicity; however, various CNS effects include headache, cognitive difficulties, behavioral change, and aseptic meningitis. Acute psychosis has been reported with indomethacin and sulindac use and is hypothesized to result from the structural similarity of these NSAIDs to serotonin.

One of the most interesting side effects of NSAID use is aseptic meningitis. The literature reports cases in which patients repeatedly present with symptoms of headache, fever, neck stiffness, and fever within hours of taking NSAIDs. Cerebrospinal fluid analysis in these patients reveals elevated white blood cell, elevated protein, and normal or decreased glucose levels. Symptoms resolve after NSAID use is stopped and can be elicited with repeat NSAID challenges. This phenomenon is most often seen with patients who have underlying autoimmune diseases, such as systemic lupus erythematosus. The phenomenon is thought to be a hypersensitivity reaction. A complete workup to rule out infectious meningitis must be undertaken before the diagnosis of NSAID-induced aseptic meningitis is entertained.[4]

Pulmonary System

NSAIDs have been responsible for various adverse pulmonary reactions, including hypersensitivity pneumonitis, bronchospasm in asthmatics, and pulmonary edema. Patients with NSAID-related hypersensitivity pneumonitis present with symptoms of fever, cough, shortness of breath, pulmonary infiltrates on chest x-ray, leukocytosis, and often-peripheral eosinophilia. Cessation of NSAIDs results in the resolution of symptoms, whereas readministration causes a recurrence of symptoms. NSAIDs implicated in hypersensitivity pneumonitis include naproxen, diflunisal, piroxicam, sulindac, and diclofenac. The mechanism of NSAID-mediated pneumonitis is believed to be an immune-mediated hypersensitivity reaction.

NSAID-induced bronchospasm is a well-described phenomena in patients with reactive airway disease. The spectrum of hypersensitivity reaction varies from rhinitis to severe bronchospasm with laryngeal edema. Patients with underlying reactive airway disease and nasal polyps appear to be at greater risk for these complications. Aspirin is most often involved in hypersensitivity reactions. Aspirin-induced bronchospasm occurs in 8 to 20 percent of all asthmatics and in 14 to 23 percent of asthmatics with nasal polyps.[5] Cross-sensitivity between aspirin and other NSAIDs is believed to be as high as 90 percent.[6] The mechanism of this hypersensitivity to NSAIDs in asthmatics has not been identified but does not appear to be an immunoglobulin E-mediated event.

Gastrointestinal-Hepatic System

Perhaps the greatest morbidity from NSAID use is bleeding from the GI tract. At therapeutic doses, NSAIDs inhibition of cytoprotective gastric prostaglandins (PGI_2 and PGE_2) increases the risk of gastric erosion, gastritis, and GI bleeding. There is a two- to fivefold increased risk of perforation or hemorrhage in NSAID users over the non-NSAID-using population. Data suggest that the risk for life-threatening bleeding is between 1.3 and 4 percent per year among NSAID users. It is estimated that NSAID-related GI bleeding contributes to 7500 deaths and 75,000 hospitalizations annually in the United States. The prostaglandin analogue misoprostol is effective at preventing NSAID-related gastric erosions at doses of 200 μg qid. Recently, the proton-pump inhibitor omeprazole has been shown to be effective at treating NSAID-related ulcers, but its role in prophylactic therapy is less clear.[7]

Hepatic System

NSAIDs may cause a spectrum of hepatic dysfunction from asymptomatic elevation of transaminases to fulminant hepatic failure. NSAIDs that have caused idiosyncratic fulminant hepatic failure include diclofenac, bromfenac, ibuprofen, sulindac, naproxen, phenylbutazone, and oxaprozin. Hepatic toxicity can occur at any time during NSAID administration and is most common in patients with underlying liver disease, in the elderly, and in patients with preexisting autoimmune diseases.

Renal System

The inhibition of prostaglandin synthesis by NSAIDs has specific effects on the kidneys. These effects range from mild changes in fluid and electrolyte homeostasis to acute renal insufficiency. NSAIDs promote sodium and water retention by attenuating prostaglandin-mediated inhibition of chloride reabsorption. NSAIDs may lead to hyperkalemia either by increased potassium reabsorption secondary to decreased sodium concentration at the distal tubule or by decreased secretion of renin. There is at least one report in the literature of cardiac arrest secondary to NSAID-induced hyperkalemia.[8]

Prostaglandins have a vasodilatory effect on the renal vasculature. The most important of these renal vasodilatory prostaglandins are PGI_2 and PGE_2. Prostaglandin-mediated vasodilatation is probably of little importance in euvolemic patients with normally functioning kidneys. However, prostaglandins appear to attenuate the vasoconstricting affects of the renin-angiotensin system and sympathetic nervous system during times of stress, during periods of decreased intravascular volume (sepsis, hemorrhage, and diuretic therapy),[9] and in disease states that predispose patients to sodium retention (congestive heart failure, cirrhosis, and nephrotic syndrome).[9] The lack of these vasodilatory prostaglandins, due to COX inhibition by NSAIDs, may put stressed kidneys at risk for azotemia and renal insufficiency. The aforementioned comorbid states are speculated to contribute to the risk of NSAID-mediated renal insufficiency.

Hematologic System

NSAIDs inhibit platelet formation of thromboxane A_2, a potent stimulator of platelet aggregation. This leads to qualitative platelet deficiencies. Most NSAIDs decrease platelet aggregation only when significant concentrations of the drug are present. Increased bleeding tendencies secondary to NSAIDs are not widely reported in the literature. However, patients taking aspirin are at risk for increased bleeding during surgery and patients maintained on coumadin are advised to avoid all NSAIDs.

NSAIDs may cause other blood disorders. Bone marrow suppression is a rare but reported hematological complication with use of NSAIDs. Aplastic anemia has been reported with almost all classes of NSAIDs, but phenylbutazone, indomethacin, and diclofenac are responsible for most cases.[10] NSAID use has also resulted in agranulocytosis, red cell aplasia, thrombocytopenia, and hemolytic anemia.

Dermatologic System

NSAIDs account for approximately 10 percent of cutaneous drug reactions.[11] Agents most frequently involved in dermatologic complications include phenylbutazone, piroxicam, and benoxaprofen.[12] Drug reactions to NSAIDs range from benign maculopapular rashes to the severe Stevens-Johnson syndrome and toxic epidermal necrolysis. NSAIDs are some of the most often-implicated drugs in cases of toxic epidermal necrolysis, accounting for up to one-third of drug-related cases in one series.[13] NSAIDs of all types (oral and topical) can cause photosensitivity reactions, including increased sensitivity to sun exposure (phototoxic) and true photoallergic reactions. Piroxicam and ketoprofen are the NSAIDs most frequently involved in photoallergic reactions. One NSAID of the oxicam family, isoxicam, was removed from the US market after fatal skin reactions.

Pregnancy

Prostaglandins are found in high concentration in the term uterus and have a stimulatory effect on normal labor. NSAIDs inhibit uterine motility through COX-mediated inhibition of prostaglandin synthesis. Indomethacin is sufficiently effective at slowing uterine contractions that it has been used to treat preterm labor. Although NSAIDs are not believed to be teratogenic in humans, they do cross the placenta later in pregnancy. One of the most significant effects of fetal exposure to NSAIDs is premature constriction of the ductus arteriosus, which may result in pulmonary hypertension. Other reported effects of in utero exposure to NSAIDs include oligohydramnios, renal dysfunction, necrotizing enterocolitis, and CNS hemorrhage.

NSAID-induced inhibition of platelet aggregation may place the fetus and the mother at increased risk for bleeding. Mothers who take NSAIDs during the latter part of pregnancy appear to be at risk for increased peripartum hemorrhage. The safest recommendation is to avoid NSAID use during pregnancy, especially during the third trimester.

PRESENTATION OF ACUTE OVERDOSE

Most patients with acute overdoses suffer little morbidity, but patients with significant overdoses may present with CNS, metabolic, hemodynamic, GI, or renal dysfunction.[14] It is generally accepted that patients taking NSAIDs of the pyrazolone (phenylbutazone and oxyphenylbutazone) and the fenamic acid (mefenamic acid) families may present with the most severe clinical symptoms. It does not appear that NSAID metabolism is changed after acute overdose, and symptoms of acute overdose are usually apparent within 4 h of ingestion.

Central Nervous System

CNS manifestation of acute NSAID overdose is usually minimal, but patients with significant overdose may present with altered mental status. Other CNS manifestations of acute overdose have included diplopia, nystagmus, and headache. Seizures have been reported after large overdoses and appear to be of special concern after ingestion of mefenamic acid.

Cardiovascular System

Acute NSAID overdose has resulted in hypotension and bradydysrhythmia. NSAIDs are not known to be primary causes of dysrhythmias, but fluid and electrolyte abnormalities may place patients at risk for cardiac dysrhythmias. Cardiovascular dysfunction is responsive to conventional critical care management.

Electrolytes

Electrolyte and acid-base abnormalities have been reported in acute NSAID overdoses. Alterations in serum electrolytes may occur secondary to decreased prostaglandin synthesis or from NSAID-induced renal failure. Sodium and water retention may lead to volume overload, with patients having preexisting renal failure, cirrhosis, or congestive heart failure. Hyperkalemia, hypocalcemia, and hypomagnesemia have been reported in NSAID overdoses complicated by acute renal failure.[15]

Increased anion-gap acidosis has been observed in large overdoses of the propionic acid NSAIDs ibuprofen and naproxen. Prostaglandin inhibition is not directly responsible for the anion-gap acidosis; rather, acidosis is likely to be related to lactic acidosis. Case reports of large overdoses suggest that the acidosis is related to large quantities of these mildly acidic NSAIDs and their metabolites in serum.[16] However, these studies neither measured nor considered lactate as the possible mechanism. Concurrent lactic acidosis in the setting of NSAID-induced seizures may worsen the acidosis in some cases.

Gastrointestinal-Hepatic System

Patients presenting after acute NSAID overdose may have abdominal pain, nausea, and vomiting. Life-threatening GI hemorrhage is not a typical finding after acute overdoses. Overdose may also result in hepatic injury, as witnessed by elevated transaminase level and cholestasis.

Renal Failure

Acute renal failure is rare after NSAID overdose, but NSAID overdose may place a stressed renal system at risk for failure. Clinical presentation may include hematuria, elevations in blood urea nitrogen/creatine, and oliguria. The mechanism of renal insufficiency in acute overdose is believed to be renal vascular changes secondary to COX-mediated prostaglandin inhibition. Patients with underlying renal insufficiency appear to be at greatest risk for acute renal failure. Most patients have recovery of renal function, but the need for long-term dialysis has been reported.

TREATMENT

Most patients who present with NSAID overdose will be asymptomatic. Patients who present with symptomatic ingestions (altered mental status, seizure, electrolyte disturbances, anion-gap acidosis, or renal insufficiencies) should be treated with supportive care using emergency medicine and toxicology principles (Fig. 166-1). Airway management should be initiated in obtunded or apneic patients, hypotension should be managed with fluid boluses or vasopressor agents when refractory,

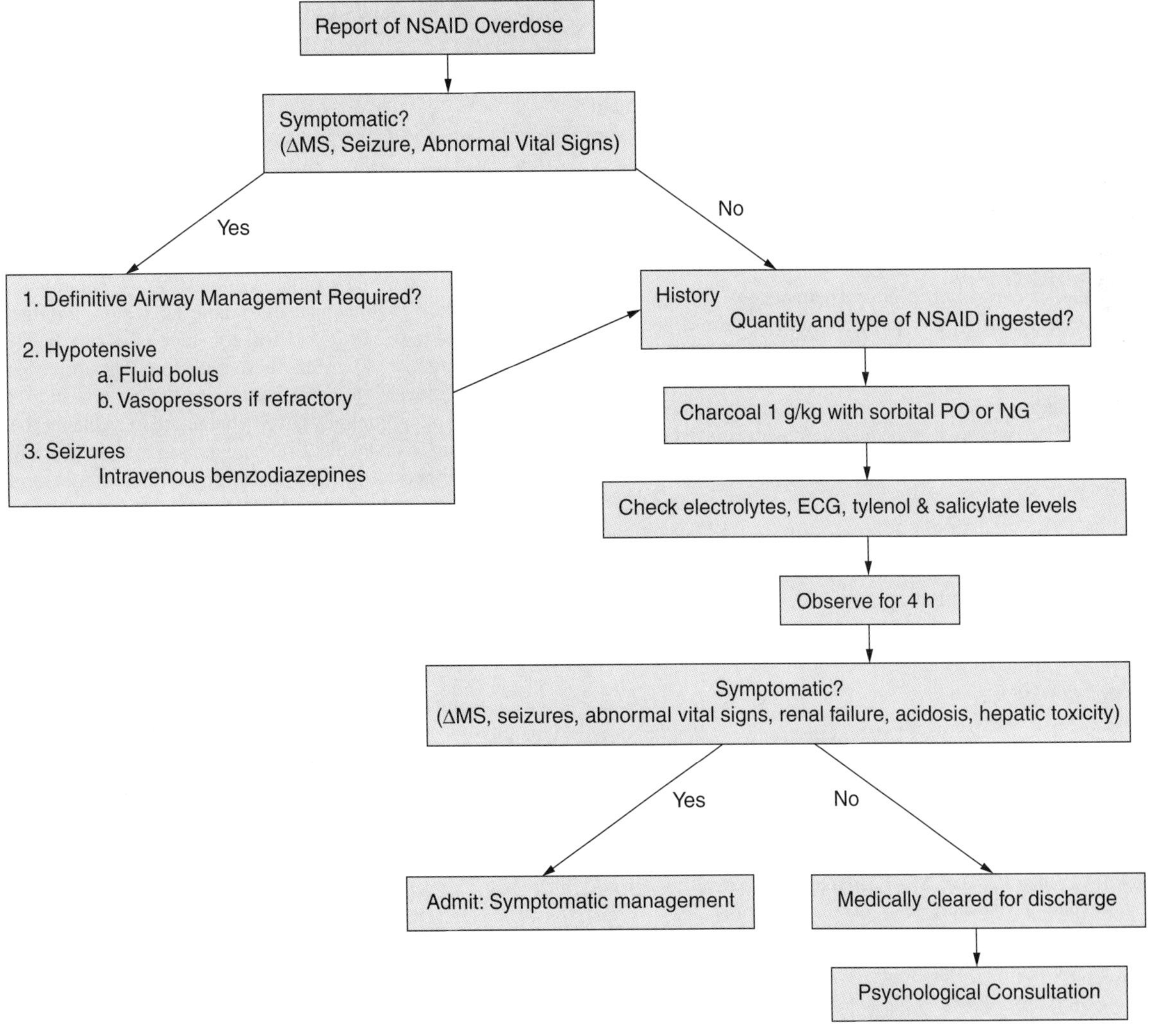

FIG. 166-1. Approach to treatment of acute NSAID overdose. *Abbreviation:* ΔMS, change in mental status.

and seizures should be treated initially with intravenous benzodiazepines.

Patients who present as hemodynamically stable with a report of acute ingestion should have a directed history and physical examination with attention focused on mental status, GI symptoms, and any signs of renal dysfunction (Fig. 166-1). The history should include amount and type NSAID ingested and questions about coingestants. Ibuprofen is the most common NSAID encountered in acute ingestion, and it is generally accepted that an ingestion of less than 100 mg/kg is unlikely to result in toxicity and that greater than 400 mg/kg places the patient at greatest risk for toxicity. Most authorities believe that patients with acute ingestions will show symptoms within 4 h.

Laboratory Evaluation

Laboratory evaluation of patients with acute ingestions should focus on acid-base status, electrolyte level, and renal function. Electrolyte panel, determination of hepatic profile, complete blood count, coagulation profile, and aspirin and acetaminophen levels should also be sent. Evaluation of drug levels for specific NSAIDs are not indicated. A nomogram for ibuprofen intoxication does exist but is not clinically useful. NSAID levels do not correlate well with observed toxicity or outcomes.[17]

Decontamination and Enhanced Elimination

Gastric decontamination should be initiated in all patients with suspected NSAID overdoses. Activated charcoal with the cathartic sorbitol should be given orally or through a nasogastric tube. Repeated doses of activated charcoal without sorbitol are indicated in symptomatic patients. Dialysis and charcoal hemoperfusion are not effective in enhancing elimination, because NSAIDs are highly protein bound. Manipulation of serum and urine pH through alkalinization is not helpful in enhancing elimination.

DISPOSITION OF PATIENTS WITH ACUTE OVERDOSES

Most patients with asymptomatic NSAID ingestions can be safely discharged after screening for coingestants and a 4- to 6-h period of observation. Any patient with symptomatic overdose (altered mental status, abnormal vital signs, electrolyte abnormalities, or acute renal failure) should be admitted for observation and supportive care. The psychosocial situation within which the overdose occurred requires careful evaluation.

Prognosis

The majority of NSAID overdoses will not cause significant sequelae. Even patients with major symptoms have a good prognosis if they overcome the initial insult (Table 166-1).

REFERENCES

1. Singh G, Ramey DR, Morfeld D, Fries JF: Comparative toxicity of nonsteroidal anti-inflammatory agents. *Pharmacol Ther* 62:175, 1994.
2. Grahman DY: Nonsteroidal anti-inflammatory drugs, Helicobacter pylori, and ulcers: Where we stand. *Am J Gastroenterol* 91:2080, 1996.
3. Houston MC: Nonsteroidal anti-inflammatory drugs and antihypertensives. *Am J Med* 90(5A):42S, 1991.
4. Hoppmann RA, Peden JG, Ober SK: Central nervous system side effects of nonsteroidal anti-inflammatory drugs. *Arch Intern Med* 151:1309, 1991.
5. Camu F, Lauwers MH, Vanlersberghe C: Side effects of NSAIDs and dosing recommendations for ketorolac. *Acta Anaesthesiol Belg* 47:143, 1996.
6. Mathison DA, Stevenson DD, Simon RA: Precipitating factors in asthma: Aspirin, sulfites, and other drugs and chemicals. *Chest* 87(suppl 1):50S, 1985.
7. Hawkey CJ, Karrasch JA, Szczepanski L, et al: Omeprazole compared with misoprostol for ulcers with nonsteroidal antiinflammatory drugs. *N Engl J Med* 338:727, 1998.
8. Kharasch MS, Johnson KM, Strange GR: Cardiac arrest secondary to indomethacin-induced renal failure: A case report. *J Emerg Med* 8:51, 1990.
9. Kleinknecht D: Interstitial nephritis, the nephrotic syndrome, and chronic renal failure secondary to nonsteroidal anti-inflammatory drugs. *Semin Nephrol* 15:228, 1995.
10. Storti E, Molinari E: Blood disorders secondary to the use of non-steroidal anti-inflammatory drugs. *Haematologica (Pavia)* 73:239, 1988.
11. Roujeau JC, Stern RS: Severe adverse cutaneous reactions to drugs. *N Engl J Med* 331:1272, 1994.
12. Alhava E: Reported adverse drug reactions and consumption of non-steroidal anti-inflammatory drugs. *Pharmacol Toxicol* 75(suppl 2):37, 1994.
13. Roujeau JC, Kelly JP, Naldi L, et al: Medication use and the risk of Stevens-Johnson syndrome or toxic epidermal necrolysis. *N Engl J Med* 333:1600, 1995.
14. Hall AH, Smolinske SC, Conrad FL, et al: Ibuprofen overdose: 126 cases. *Ann Emerg Med* 15:1308, 1986.
15. Al-Harbi NN, Somnuek D, Lirenman DS: Hypocalcemia and hypomagnesemia after ibuprofen overdose. *Ann Pharma Fr* 31:432, 1997.
16. Martinez R, Smith DW, Frankel LR: Severe metabolic acidosis after acute naproxen sodium ingestion. *Ann Emerg Med* 18:1102, 1989.
17. McElwee NE, Veltri JC, Bradford DC, et al: A prospective, population-based study of acute ibuprofen overdose: Complications are rare and routine serum levels not warranted. *Ann Emerg Med* 19:657, 1990.

XANTHINES

Daniel J. Kranitz
Charles L. Emerman

Theophylline use is complicated by its narrow therapeutic window, with a metabolism that depends on the patient's coincident medical problems and use of other medications. The 1996 Annual Report of the American Association of Poison Control Centers Toxic Exposure Surveillance System reported 3100 exposures to aminophylline or theophylline, resulting in major toxicity in 76 patients and death in 11. There were 7316 exposures to caffeine, resulting in major toxicity in 16 patients with 2 deaths.[1] Most consider a theophylline level greater than 20 μg/mL (110 μmol/L) toxic, although side effects may be seen at lower levels.[2] Recent changes in the US Food and Drug Administration dosing guidelines have been aimed at reducing the likelihood of developing toxic levels. Life-threatening toxicity from theophylline poisoning can result in significant cardiac, neurologic, and metabolic abnormalities.[3] Toxic side effects of caffeine have many similarities to those of theophylline, but serious side effects are rare. Several modalities are available for treating theophylline toxicity, but indications for their use in patients without life-threatening symptoms is controversial.

PHARMACOLOGY

Theophylline and related products (Table 167-1) have a complex mechanism of action that has not been entirely elucidated.[4] Although tradi-

TABLE 167-1 Theophylline Content of Related Drugs

Drug	Theophylline Content, %
Aminophylline	80–85
Oxtriphylline	65
Dyphylline	50

tional teaching is that theophylline acts by inhibiting the action of phosphodiesterase, the concentration required for effective in vivo inhibition far exceeds the concentration usually produced by clinical dosages. Others have suggested that theophylline may act by affecting the binding of cyclic adenosine monophosphate, cyclic glucose monophosphate phosphodiesterase inhibition, prostaglandin antagonism, modification of intracellular calcium, stimulation of catecholamine release, or adenosine antagonism. In addition to its bronchodilatory effect, theophylline affects both the immune and inflammatory mechanisms.[5]

Theophylline is readily absorbed after oral administration, with peak levels occurring 90 to 120 min after ingestion. Oral absorption is enhanced by fasting or ingestion of large volumes of fluid and is decreased following ingestion of certain foods. Enteric-coated tablets and sustained-released preparations reach peak plasma levels between 6 and 8 h. The newer, once-daily preparations have an erratic absorption rate, particularly after eating, which may lead to drug ''dumping'' (rapid absorption) and elevated theophylline levels. Peak levels are reached within 30 min after intravenous administration of aminophylline. The absorption of intramuscularly and rectally administered drug is erratic and unpredictable. Consequently, these routes should not be used.

Theophylline is approximately 60 percent protein bound, with less binding in neonates and patients with cirrhosis. The volume of distribution ranges from 0.3 to 0.7 L/kg, with an average of 0.5 L/kg. Theophylline is primarily (85 to 90 percent) eliminated by the hepatic P450 cytochrome system, and the remaining 10 to 15 percent is eliminated by urinary excretion. Metabolism generally follows first-order elimination. The half-life is 4 to 8 h in young, healthy, nonsmoking adults and shorter in children and smokers. Some authors have recommended a lowering of the target serum concentration from 20 to 15 μg/mL, since most bronchodilation occurs by that level.

A number of factors affect theophylline's half-life, including cigarette use, diet, cardiac and liver disease, and medications that interfere with the cytochrome P450 pathway (Table 167-2). Theophylline acts as an adenosine antagonist. It markedly inhibits the coronary vasodilating effects of adenosine and may interfere with the usefulness of pharmacologic stress tests. Theophylline has been reported to reverse adenosine-induced bronchoconstriction. Few studies have examined the effects of theophylline on the therapeutic use of adenosine to reverse supraventricular tachycardia. One study reported on the successful conversion from supraventricular tachycardia in two patients with therapeutic theophylline levels. A few case reports describe the use of adenosine in theophylline-induced dysrhythmias, but experience on which to base recommendations is inadequate.

Caffeine is probably the most commonly used drug in the world. It is readily absorbed after oral administration, with an onset of action of 30 min and peak effect at 60 to 120 min (Table 167-3). Caffeine is also metabolized by demethylation in the liver, forming L-methyluric acid and L-methyl xanthine, the active agents. As with theophylline, about 10 percent of the drug is eliminated by urinary excretion. Many of the factors that affect the half-life of theophylline, such as severe liver disease, also affect that of caffeine.

TOXIC EFFECTS

Theophylline has a range of toxic effects from minor gastrointestinal symptoms to life-threatening dysrhythmias. Although it is commonly thought that symptom severity is serum-level dependent, in fact, life-threatening adverse effects may occur with little warning and before minor symptoms are evident.

Cardiovascular

Even at therapeutic levels (10 to 20 μg/mL), theophylline can cause cardiac side effects. Sinus tachycardia may occur after administration, and increased atrial automaticity, with premature atrial contractions, atrial tachycardia, multifocal atrial tachycardia, atrial fibrillation, and atrial flutter, occurs more frequently with levels above 20 μg/mL. Ventricular dysrhythmias with premature ventricular contractions and self-limited runs of ventricular tachycardia may also occur. Sustained ventricular tachycardia may occur in older patients with chronic overdose at levels of around 40 to 60 μg/mL. Younger patients with acute intentional overdose may tolerate levels above 100 μg/mL without developing life-threatening cardiac effects.[6] Patients with a history of dysrhythmias may experience a recurrence of dysrhythmias with levels

TABLE 167-2 Factors Affecting Theophylline Half-Life

Decreased Half-life	Increased Half-life
DRUGS	
Carbamazepine	Cimetidine
Phenobarbital	Allopurinol
Phenytoin	Zileuton
Rifampin	Ticlopidine
	Interferon
	Methotrexate
	Estrogens
ANTIBIOTICS	
Sulfinpyrazone	Erythromycin
	Clarithromycin
	Quinolones
	Thiabendazole
ANTIDYSRHYTHMICS	
	Mexiletine
	Propranolol
	Verapamil
	Tocainide
	Propafenone
CONDITIONS AND OTHER FACTORS	
Smoking	Cirrhosis
Charcoal-broiled foods	Congestive heart failure
Children	Pneumonia
Hyperthyroidism	Severe COPD
	Viral illness in children
	Obesity
	Neonates

TABLE 167-3 Caffeine Content of Various Products

Product	Caffeine Content, mg
No Doz Maximum, Vivarin	200
Espresso coffee	120
Regular coffee	103
No Doz	100
Jolt Cola	72
Aspirin-free Excedrin	65
Excedrin ES	65
Instant coffee	57
Black tea	53
Most sodas	35–55

less than 40 μg/mL. Hypotension has also been associated with acute ingestion but may also occur with chronic overmedication.

Neurologic

Even with therapeutic levels, theophylline use can be associated with agitation, headache, irritability, sleeplessness, tremors, and muscular twitching. Seizures, including both generalized tonic-clonic and focal motor, have been reported in patients with therapeutic levels. Patients with a history of epilepsy are particularly susceptible to aminophylline-induced seizures. The incidence of seizures increases as toxic levels increase.[7] Status epilepticus resistant to treatment can occur as the level rises above 25 μg/mL. When seizures occur at only mildly elevated levels, there are usually underlying neurologic deficits. The occurrence of seizures does not appear to correlate with prognosis. Theophylline toxicity has also been associated with hallucinations and psychosis.

Metabolic

Theophylline produces a dose-dependent increase in circulating catecholamines. There is a concomitant increase in glucose, free fatty acid, and insulin levels and white blood cell count. Hypokalemia may occur, with the fall in serum potassium level inversely related to the theophylline concentration. Hypokalemia appears to be a particular problem in patients with acute overdose or acute overdose superimposed on chronic use. Administration of a β agonist may also be associated with hypokalemia and, with the hypokalemia produced by theophylline overdose, may lead to cardiac dysrhythmias. Lactic acidosis (tissue ischemia) may also be present.

Gastrointestinal

TOXIC EFFECTS OF THEOPHYLLINE Theophylline has a direct central nervous system effect, leading to nausea and vomiting. In addition, theophylline increases gastric acid secretion. Nausea and vomiting can be seen with therapeutic levels, although the incidence of nausea and vomiting increases markedly with levels above 15 μg/mL. Approximately 25 percent of patients with levels greater than 20 μg/mL have nausea or vomiting. Gastrointestinal bleeding, with epigastric pain, may also occur. Esophageal reflux has also been reported.

TOXIC EFFECTS OF CAFFEINE Caffeine shares many effects with theophylline. Gastrointestinal symptoms generally occur with overdose and include abdominal pain, vomiting, and occasional hematemesis. Central nervous system effects include agitation, seizures, and coma. Ventricular dysrhythmias other than premature ventricular contractions are rare, but paroxysmal atrial tachycardia may occur. Rhabdomyolysis, hyperglycemia, leukocytosis, and metabolic acidosis have been reported. Toxicity is seen after 1-g doses in adults. Doses of around 80 mg/kg may lead to symptoms in children.

TREATMENT

Following acute ingestion (2 to 4 h) of potentially toxic doses of aminophylline or theophylline, gastric emptying with gastric lavage should be considered. Gastric lavage is probably not indicated for patients whose dose is calculated to have raised their levels to less than 30 μg/mL (approximately 15 mg/kg), unless coingestion of other medications is suspected. Ipecac may complicate the use of other therapies for enhancing the elimination of theophylline and, given the seizure potentiation, should not be used. In addition, vomiting is usually a prominent symptom in theophylline toxicity.

Cathartics should be administered to enhance the passage of ingested theophylline through the gastrointestinal tract. Some investigators have found magnesium citrate not to be effective in lowering the theophylline level. Further, there have been reports of magnesium toxicity after the use of magnesium cathartics.

Sorbitol may be a better choice. A 70% sorbitol solution (100 mL) can be used either alone or in combination with activated charcoal for patients with potentially toxic ingestions. There have been reports of the successful use of whole-bowel irrigation with polyethylene glycol, but this treatment is controversial.

Theophylline undergoes hepatobiliary enteric circulation. Administration of repeated doses of activated charcoal at 2- to 4-h intervals significantly decreases the half-life of theophylline.[8] Doses of 30 to 60 g should be used in adults. Charcoal may also be administered as a continuous nasogastric infusion at rates of 0.25 to 0.5 g/kg/h. In patients with markedly elevated theophylline levels, the administration of charcoal is complicated by repeated episodes of emesis. In one study, patients with levels greater than 50 μg/mL could not tolerate any of their charcoal doses because of repeated episodes of emesis. Patients who cannot tolerate oral administration of activated charcoal should be pretreated with ranitidine.

Treatment of theophylline toxicity is hindered by the recurrent nausea and vomiting produced by toxic levels. Administration of ranitidine, 50 mg intravenously, is useful when nausea and vomiting are present. It permits the use of repeated doses of activated charcoal to enhance drug elimination.

Diazepam, phenobarbital, and phenytoin have been used in the treatment of theophylline-induced seizures. Unfortunately, status epilepticus may be resistant to those drugs. The airway should be protected in patients with theophylline-induced status epileticus, particularly after administration of oral activated charcoal. Patients with status epilepticus resistant to traditional therapy may require general anesthesia for more aggressive measures to lower the serum theophylline level.

Although it is less effective at drug removal than hemoperfusion, hemodialysis may be used for patients with toxicity.[9] The clearance rate induced by hemodialysis is approximately 200 mL/kg/h. Charcoal hemoperfusion with resin or charcoal filters produces extraction ratios above 0.85 with clearance rates of up to 300 mL/kg/h. Recent prospective studies, however, indicate that hemoperfusion is associated with a higher complication rate without any signficant increase in clinical efficacy over hemodialysis.[10] The indications for hemoperfusion or hemodialysis are controversial (Table 167-4). In the view of some investigators, hemoperfusion or hemodialysis is not absolutely indicated at any theophylline level in the absence of life-threatening symptoms, such as status epilepticus or resistant ventricular dysrhythmias. Others have felt that patients with increased half-lives, advanced age, or theophylline levels above 40 μg/mL may be candidates for hemoperfusion or hemodialysis. Young, healthy patients with an acute ingestion may be able to tolerate levels over 100 μg/mL without

TABLE 167-4 Indications for Hemoperfusion

Clinical Conditions	Recommendation
Life-threatening toxicity (i.e., seizures, tachydysrhythmias) not responsive to other therapy	Hemoperfusion or dialysis indicated
Acute overdose with level >100 μg/mL	Hemoperfusion or dialysis possibly indicated
Chronic overdose with level >60 μg/mL	Hemoperfusion or dialysis possibly indicated
Elderly patient with prolonged half-life, severe liver or severe cardiac disease, or level >40 μg/mL	Hemoperfusion or dialysis controversial
Theophylline level <30 μg/mL	Hemoperfusion or dialysis not indicated

adverse incident. The decision to use hemoperfusion or hemodialysis should be made considering the potential for life-threatening toxicity.

Hypotension or life-threatening cardiac dysrhythmias may be an indication for β-blocker therapy when symptoms do not respond to other therapy. The use of β blockers may be complicated by further cardiac depression or exacerbation of airway obstruction. They should be administered cautiously in low doses and monitored for adverse effect. Propanolol may be used, given in 1-mg doses up to a total of 10 mg. Alternatively, one of the newer β-blocker agents, such as labetalol or the short-acting esmolol, may be used.

In addition to being treated with β blockade, cardiac dysrhythmias may be treated with other antiarrhythmics. Verapamil has been effective in animal studies. The use of digoxin, lidocaine, and phenytoin has been reported for treatment of venticular dysrhythmias. Adenosine may be considered for supraventricular dysrhythmias, but it may induce bronchospasm. The contributory effect of hypokalemia should be considered in treating patients with resistant ventricular dysrhythmias, and correction of serum electrolyte abnormalities may be effective in terminating recurrent dysrhythmias.

INDICATIONS FOR TREATMENT AND ADMISSION

Although theophylline toxicity can lead to life-threatening side effects, toxic theophylline levels are common, and most patients tolerate them with only minor toxic manifestations.[11] Serum theophylline concentrations do not correlate well with severity of toxicity in chronic exposures. However, serum levels for acute exposures are more valuable in predicting toxicity and clinical course. No well-conducted studies have demonstrated that prophylactic use of antiarrhythmics or antiepileptics decreases morbidity or mortality rates. Similarly, while hemodialysis, hemoperfusion, and oral activated charcoal therapy enhance theophylline clearance, there is no compelling evidence that their use lowers morbidity or mortality rates for patients with only mild toxic symptoms or minimally elevated levels.

On the other hand, ventricular dysrhythmias or seizures may occur in patients before the manifestation of other minor toxic effects, leading some authors to advocate aggressive therapy. Older patients with concomitant medical problems are more susceptible to life-threatening theophylline toxicity following chronic overmedication than are younger patients with an acute overdose.[12] Prophylactic use of hemoperfusion has been reported to decrease rates of major morbidity in elderly patients.

In general, patients with a history of seizures or ventricular dysrhythmias should be monitored until their theophylline level returns to normal. Patients with levels below 25 μg/mL and minor symptoms do not require specific therapy other than discontinuation or modification of theophylline administration. Such patients generally do not require hospitalization. Patients with levels above 30 μg/mL should be treated with oral activated charcoal (repeated) and monitored for toxic side effects. Hemoperfusion or hemodialysis use is controversial but may be indicated for older patients with levels above 30 μg/mL or for younger patients with acute intentional overdose with levels above 100 μg/mL.

PREVENTION

Theophylline toxicity is only rarely a result of intentional overdose. Physician prescribing errors, patient self-overmedication, and variations in plasma clearance due to deteriorating cardiac or hepatic status, smoking cessation, or concomitant administration of drugs that affect theophylline clearance all may lead to elevated levels. Aminophylline infusions should be started using standard guidelines with close monitoring of serum levels. Because the history of outpatient theophylline use has been found to be a poor guide to the serum concentration, loading doses of aminophylline should be calculated using the initial theophylline level. As a rough approximation, each milligram per kilogram of aminophylline will raise the theophylline level by 2 μg/mL. The initial dose of oral theophylline should not exceed 900 mg/day. Patients should be started at a much lower dose (400 mg/day) to avoid the nausea and vomiting frequently accompanying initial theophylline use. Levels should be determined in order to monitor therapy. The presence or absence of mild side effects is not a good predictor of drug levels.[13] Patients should be cautioned not to alter their medication regimen without physician guidance. Patients being started on erythromycin or cimetidine should have their theophylline dose decreased by approximately 25 percent, with monitoring of the effect on levels.

REFERENCES

1. Livotitz T, Smilkstein M, Felberg MA, et al: 1996 Annual Report of the American Association of Poison Control Centers Toxic Exposure Surveillance System. *Am J Emerg Med* 15:447, 1997.
2. Bertino JS, Walker JW: Reassessment of theophylline toxicity: Serum concentrations, clinical course, and treatment. *Arch Intern Med* 147:757, 1987.
3. Baker MD: Theophylline toxicity in children. *J Pediatr* 109:538, 1986.
4. Hendeles L, Weinberger M, Szefler S, et al: Safety and efficacy of theophylline in children with asthma. *J Pediatr* 120:177, 1992.
5. Weinberger M, Hendeles L: Theophylline in asthma. *N Engl J Med* 334:1380, 1996.
6. Olson KR, Benowitz NL, Woo OF, et al: Theophylline overdose: Acute single ingestion vs chronic repeated overmedication. *Ann Emerg Med* 3:386, 1985.
7. Sessler CN: Theophylline toxicity: Clinical features of 116 consecutive cases. *Am J Med* 88:567, 1990.
8. Goldberg MJ, Park GD, Berlinger WG: Treatment of theophylline intoxication. *J Allergy Clin Immunol* 78:811, 1986.
9. Greenberg A, Piraino BH, Kroboth PC, et al: Role of conservative measures, anti-arrhythmic agents, and charcoal hemoperfusion. *Am J Med* 76:854, 1984.
10. Shannon MW: Comparative efficacy of hemodialysis and hemoperfusion in severe theophylline intoxication. *Acad Emerg Med* 4:674, 1997.
11. Emerman CL, Devlin C, Connors AF: Risk of toxicity in patients with elevated theophylline levels. *Ann Emerg Med* 19:643, 1990.
12. Shannon M: Predictors of major toxicity after theophylline overdose. *Ann Intern Med* 119:1161, 1993.
13. Melamed J, Beaucher WN: Minor symptoms are not predictive of elevated theophylline levels in adults on chronic therapy. *Ann Allergy Asthma Immunol* 75:516, 1995.

DIGITALIS GLYCOSIDES

William H. Dribben
Mark A. Kirk

EPIDEMIOLOGY

For centuries, digitalis glycosides have been recognized for their medicinal benefits and potential toxicity. Digitalis preparations are used most commonly in the treatment of supraventricular tachydysrhythmias and congestive heart failure. In addition to their availability as pharmaceuticals, cardiac glycosides are also found in plants such as foxglove, oleander, and lily of the valley. It is important that physicians recognize digitalis toxicity because potentially fatal cardiac dysrhythmias can be reversed with prompt administration of a highly specific antidote, digoxin specific Fab fragments.[1] According to the American Association of Poison Control Centers, 2963 exposures to cardiac glycosides were reported in 1997. Of these exposures, 416 (34 percent) patients demonstrated moderate or major morbidity with 12 (1 percent) deaths.[2] Even though digitalis use has declined due to newer modes of therapy, reported exposures and morbidity and mortality have remained constant over the past 5 years.

PHARMACOLOGY AND PATHOPHYSIOLOGY

Digoxin is currently the most widely used digitalis preparation. It is rapidly absorbed from the gastrointestinal tract and is primarily eliminated through renal excretion. It has a volume of distribution of 6 L/kg. The half-life of a therapeutic dose is 36 to 48 hours.

Digitalis has a narrow therapeutic-toxic margin. Toxicity results from an exaggeration of its therapeutic actions. Digitalis binds to a specific receptor site on the cardiac cell membrane, inactivating the sodium-potassium adenosine triphosphate pump (Na-K ATPase).[3] This pump concentrates sodium extracellularly and potassium intracellularly to maintain the electrochemical membrane potential vital to conduction tissues. When Na-K ATPase is inhibited, the sodium-calcium exchanger removes accumulated intracellular sodium in exchange for calcium. This exchange increases sarcoplasmic calcium and is the mechanism thought to be responsible for the positive inotropic effect of digitalis. Inhibition of the Na-K ATPase pump also results in an increase in extracellular potassium.[3] Digitalis increases vagal tone and decreases conduction through the AV node. In toxic doses, these effects result in various bradydysrhythmias. Automaticity is increased due to slowing of conduction in the electrical system along with a shortened refractory period in the myocardium. Intracellular calcium overload can create delayed after-depolarizations, causing electrical oscillations in cell membranes that give rise to triggered dysrhythmias.[4]

CLINICAL FEATURES

When a poisoned patient presents to the emergency department, the clinician should determine if toxicity is due to an accidental ingestion, massive intentional ingestion, or chronic toxicity from therapeutic use of digitalis. If the ingestion is intentional, historical information may be inaccurate or incomplete, and coingestants should be suspected. The time of ingestion is extremely helpful in interpreting laboratory information. Because various plants contain digitalis glycosides and cause similar toxicity to medicinal forms, an attempt should be made to accurately identify any ingested plants.

Preexisting medical conditions and current medications may identify risk factors that potentiate digitalis toxicity. Increased susceptibility is seen in patients who are elderly, have coexisting diseases (heart disease, renal dysfunction, hepatic dysfunction, hypothyroidism, and chronic obstructive pulmonary disease), electrolyte disturbances (hypokalemia, hypomagnesemia, and hypercalcemia), and hypoxia.[5] Drug interactions, most notably class IA antidysrhythmics, calcium channel blockers, and β blockers, potentiate digitalis toxicity. Carefully evaluate the cardiac, neurologic, and gastrointestinal systems for clues of developing toxicity.

Cardiac dysrhythmias in digitalis toxicity are nonspecific and may be life-threatening. Suspect digitalis toxicity in patients with any dysrhythmia or junctional escape rhythms and AV block. The most common dysrhythmia is frequent premature ventricular beats, especially in a diseased heart. Bidirectional ventricular tachycardia, a narrow complex tachycardia with right bundle branch morphology, is rare but specific for digitalis toxicity.[6]

In addition to cardiac manifestations, gastrointestinal distress, dizziness, headache, weakness, syncope, and seizures may occur. Reported psychiatric symptoms include confusion, disorientation, delirium, and hallucinations. Any elderly patient taking digitalis presents with mental status changes should be evaluated for toxicity. Patients with toxicity have reported seeing yellow-green halos around objects.[7] No single clinical feature or laboratory value is diagnostic of digitalis toxicity.

DIAGNOSIS

Digitalis glycoside toxicity is determined by evaluating the entire clinical presentation. The history, physical examination, and laboratory studies provide important clues, with no single element that excludes or confirms the diagnosis.

Laboratory Evaluation

Serum potassium and digoxin levels will assist in providing information necessary to make adequate therapeutic decisions. Acute poisoning of the Na-K ATPase pump may result in markedly elevated serum potassium levels.[3] A high incidence of hyperkalemia has been noted in patients with severe acute poisoning. The serum potassium may be a better indicator of end organ toxicity and a better prognostic indicator than the serum digoxin level in the acutely poisoned patient. Hyperkalemia is less common in chronically poisoned patients. Potassium status may be less predictive in patients with renal insufficiency or dehydration, or who are receiving diuretic therapy.

Accepted therapeutic digoxin levels are 0.5 to 2.0 ng/mL. In most laboratories, the serum digoxin level is not part of the routine toxicologic screen and must be specifically requested.

Serum digoxin levels in both acute and chronic toxicity should be interpreted in the overall clinical context, and not relied upon as the sole indicator of the presence or absence of toxicity. In acute exposures, digoxin is absorbed into the plasma compartment and then redistributed slowly into the tissue compartment. Hence, high digoxin levels are not always associated with clinical signs and symptoms of poisoning. Serum levels are most reliable when obtained six hours after ingestion, when distribution is complete. In patients with clinical evidence of chronic digitalis toxicity, a "therapeutic" level does not exclude toxicity, especially when predisposing factors are present. Conversely, levels above the upper limits of normal do not always cause symptoms. Given the above limitations, it is still most common that the higher the serum level, the greater the likelihood of toxicity.[8]

A positive serum assay is diagnostic of acute ingestion if the patient has not received digitalis glycosides therapeutically. The rare exception is in the presence of digoxin-like immunoreactive substance that has been detected in neonates and patients with renal insufficiency or hepatic dysfunction. In addition, naturally occurring digitalis glycosides from plants and animals may cross-react with the digoxin assay. The degree of cross-reactivity is unknown and no correlation has been established between serum levels of these glycosides and toxicity.

Additional laboratory evaluation includes the determination of adequate oxygenation, renal and hepatic function, and electrolyte determinations in addition to potassium. Continuous electrocardiographic monitoring is essential to detect dysrhythmias and evidence of hyperkalemia.

Differences in the Presentation of Acute and Chronic Toxicity

A distinct clinical presentation exists for both acute and chronic digitalis glycoside toxicity (Table 168-1). Acute poisoning most often results from accidental or intentional ingestion. There may be an asymptomatic period of several hours prior to development of symptoms. Gastrointestinal symptoms are often the earliest manifestation of toxicity. In the early period of toxicity, increased central vagal tone produces cardiac dysrhythmias that are typically bradydysrhythmias, or supraventricular dysrhythmias with AV block; however, life-threatening ventricular dysrhythmias may develop at any stage in an acute massive ingestion.[6] Acute toxicity most closely correlates with hyperkalemia, and correlates poorly with the serum digoxin level.[9]

Chronic toxicity occurs most typically in the elderly cardiac patient taking digoxin and diuretics. Signs and symptoms may mimic more common illnesses such as influenza and gastroenteritis. An altered mental status or psychiatric symptoms may not be recognized as signs of digitalis toxicity. Almost any cardiac dysrhythmia may be seen, but ventricular dysrhythmias occur more frequently in chronic than in acute poisonings.[6] The serum digoxin level is not an accurate predictor of toxicity, and the serum potassium is usually decreased, normal, or may even be elevated in the setting of renal failure.

TABLE 168-1 Clinical Presentation of Digitalis Toxicity

Acute Toxicity
- Clinical History: Intentional or accidental ingestion
  - GI Effects: Nausea and vomiting
  - CNS Effects: Headache, dizziness, confusion, coma

Cardia effects: Predominately supraventricular tachydysrhythmias with AV block; bradydysrhythmias
  - Electrolyte Abnormalities: Hyperkalemia
  - Digoxin Level: Marked elevation

Chronic Toxicity
- Clinical History: Typically an elderly cardiac patient taking diuretics. May have renal insufficiency
- GI Effects: Nausea, vomiting, diarrhea, abdominal pain
- CNS Effects: Fatigue, weakness, confusion, delirium, coma
- Cardiac Effects: Ventricular dysrhythmias are common. Almost any ventricular or supraventricular dysrhythmia can occur.
- Electrolyte Abnormalities: Hypokalemia or normal serum K hypomagnesemia
- Digoxin Level: Minimally elevated or therapeutic range

Differential Diagnosis

Other toxins and medical illnesses may present with a clinical picture similar to digitalis toxicity. Other toxins causing bradydysrhythmias include calcium and β-blocker overdoses, class IA antidysrhythmics (procainamide and quinidine) overdoses, clonidine overdoses, organophosphate insecticide poisoning, and cardiotoxic plants (e.g., rhododendron, monkshood, tobacco, false hellebore, and yew berry). Sinus node disease can also mimic digitalis toxicity.

Factors Enhancing Toxicity

A variety of factors increase susceptibility to digitalis toxicity. True end organ sensitivity is seen with myocardial disease or ischemia, and metabolic or electrolyte abnormalities. Hypokalemia, hypomagnesemia, and hypercalcemia all predispose to increased toxicity.[3] The elderly are more susceptible to toxicity. Decreased renal function, hepatic disease, hypothyroidism, chronic obstructive pulmonary disease, and drug interactions can all augment toxic effects.[5] Drug interactions potentially resulting in digitalis toxicity include quinidine, procainamide, β blockers, calcium channel blockers, amiodarone, spironolactone, indomethacin, clarithromycin, and erythromycin.

EMERGENCY DEPARTMENT CARE

The basic emergency department management of any poisoned patient includes general supportive care, treatment of specific complications of toxicity, prevention of further drug absorption, enhanced drug elimination, antidote administration, and safe disposition (Table 168-2). Patients with intentional or accidental ingestions may present with no symptoms. Still, life-threatening complications of toxicity should be anticipated. The management of the asymptomatic patient should focus on preventing drug absorption and closely monitoring for development of toxicity. Continuous cardiac monitoring, intravenous access, and frequent reevaluations should be provided for any patient with a potentially toxic ingestion of digitalis. Toxicity may not develop for several hours after an acute ingestion; therefore, extended observation (12 h) is required for anyone with a confirmed ingestion.[8] Admission to the intensive care unit and frequent reassessment is required for any patient developing signs of toxicity.

Treatment of Life-Threatening Conditions

Approach the symptomatic patient methodically. Ensure a patent airway, adequate ventilation, and effective circulation. Rapidly correct conditions such as hypoxia, hypoglycemia, hypovolemia, and electrolyte abnormalities.

Conventional and antidote therapies are available to treat digitalis-induced dysrhythmias. Atropine and cardiac pacing (external and transvenous) have been used successfully in treating bradydysrhythmias. Both phenytoin and lidocaine depress ventricular automaticity and increase the fibrillation threshold. Because of phenytoin's ability to accelerate conduction at the AV node, it has been considered the antidysrhythmic of choice by some for digitalis-induced ventricular dysrhythmias. Bretylium has effectively suppressed dysrhythmias in the clinical setting, although in a digitalis-toxic animal model, it was found to enhance dysrhythmias.[10] IA antidysrhythmics, such as quinidine and procainamide, are contraindicated because they depress AV nodal conduction, which in turn may enhance digitalis-induced cardiac toxicity. Intravenous magnesium has been reported to counteract ventricular irritability in digitalis toxicity.[11] Electrocardioversion may induce intractable ventricular fibrillation and should be considered only as a last resort. If necessary, use a low setting (10 to 25 W-s) and

TABLE 168-2 Treatment of Digitalis Glycoside Poisoning

Asymptomatic patients
- Obtain accurate history
- Continuous cardiac monitoring
- Intravenous access
- Gastrointestinal decontamination:
  - Activated charcoal (1 g/kg)
  - ±Gastric lavage
- Frequent reevaluation
- Fab fragments at bedside (Calculate dose required for emergent use)

Symptomatic Patients
- ABCs
  - Intravenous access
  - Continuous cardiac monitoring
- Treat altered mental status
  - Oxygen
  - Dextrose (if indicated)
  - Naloxone (if indicated)
- Dysrhythmias
  - Bradydysrhythmias
    - Atropine (0.5–2.0 mg IV)
    - Pacemaker (external or transvenous)
    - Fab fragments (IV infusion)
  - Ventricular dysrhythmias
    - Fab fragments (IV infusion or bolus)
    - Lidocaine (1 mg/kg) or Phenytoin (15 mg/kg: infuse no faster than 25 mg/min)
    - Magnesium sulfate (2–4 g IV)
    - Electrocardioversion (10–25 W-s; last resort)
  - Cardiac arrest
    - CPR
    - ACLS protocols
    - Fab fragments (IV bolus; give 10–20 vials if amount ingested is unknown)
- Electrolyte abnornalities
  - Hyperkalemia
    - Avoid calcium chloride
    - Glucose-insulin
    - Sodium bicarbonate
    - Fab fragments (IV infusion or bolus)
    - Potassium resin binder
    - Hemodialysis
  - Hypomagnesemia
    - Evaluate renal status prior replacement
    - Magnesium sulfate (2–4 g IV)
- Gastrointestinal decontamination
  - Activated charcoal (1 g/kg then 0.5 g/kg every 4–6 h)
  - ±Gastric lavage

prepare to treat resulting ventricular fibrillation. In severe toxicity, conventional treatment may be unsuccessful. When available, digoxin-specific Fab fragments are the treatment of choice for those dysrhythmias that are life-threatening and do not respond immediately to conventional therapy.[12]

Hyperkalemia may be life-threatening and needs immediate treatment. Treatment includes intravenous administration of dextrose, insulin, sodium bicarbonate, and enteral administration of a potassium-binding resin.[12] Calcium chloride administration in the face of digitalis-induced hyperkalemia may promote cardiac toxicity and should be avoided. If digitalis-induced hyperkalemia is not rapidly corrected by conventional therapy, then Fab fragments are indicated for reversal (see below).[12]

Gastrointestinal Decontamination and Enhanced Elimination

Ipecac clearly has no role in the emergency department management of digitalis glycoside poisoning. After initial stabilization, administer activated charcoal to prevent further drug absorption.[13] The use of gastric lavage is controversial. Because activated charcoal is so effective, lavage has a minimal role, if any. Asystole has been reported in a digoxin-toxic patient presumably from vagal stimulation during lavage. If lavage is contemplated, pretreatment with atropine prior to performing gastric lavage has been suggested. Forced diuresis, hemodialysis, or hemoperfusion have no role in enhancing elimination of digitalis.

Antidote Therapy

Digoxin specific Fab (Digibind, Burroughs-Wellcome) is derived from the IgG fragment of sheep antidigoxin antibodies. Fab fragments distribute widely throughout tissues and remove digitalis from tissue binding sites.[12] In a series of 150 severely poisoned patients, 90 percent showed reversal or significant improvement in life-threatening dysrhythmias and hyperkalemia after Fab fragment administration.[12] In most cases, clinical improvement in cardiac rhythm occurs within one hour of antidote administration. Those patients developing cardiac arrest prior to Fab administration had a 50 percent survival, which is significantly improved from survival by treatment with conventional therapies.[12] Fab fragments have also been reported to be beneficial in treating digitoxin and oleander poisonings.[14]

Indications for digitalis specific Fab fragments are: ventricular dysrhythmias; hemodynamically significant bradydysrhythmias unresponsive to standard therapy; and hyperkalemia in excess of 5.5 mEq/L[12] associated with a toxic digitalis level or a presumptive diagnosis of overdose. Elevated serum digoxin levels should not be the sole indication for Fab fragment administration.

Fab fragment administration has resulted in few adverse effects.[12] Cardiogenic shock has been reported in patients dependent upon digoxin for inotropic support.[15] In addition, ventricular response to atrial fibrillation may be increased. Hypokalemia may develop rapidly as digitalis toxicity is reversed. Only mild, acute hypersensitivity reactions including rash, flushing, and facial swelling have been reported. No incidences of serum sickness or anaphylaxis have been observed, even in patients with repeated administration.[15] Because Fab is derived from sheep protein, skin testing should be considered in patients with a strong history of allergies, especially to antibiotics, or those with asthma. If cardiac arrest is imminent, Fab fragment infusion should not be delayed for skin testing. Failures to Fab fragment therapy have been attributed to inadequate dosing, moribund state prior to administration, and incorrect diagnosis of digitalis toxicity.[15]

The Fab fragment dosage is based on an estimation of total body load of digoxin.[12] This can be determined from the serum digoxin level or based on the estimated dose ingested (Table 168-3). Clinical series have reported that an average of 200 to 480 mg (5 to 12 vials) were required to effectively treat severely digitalis toxic patients.[12] When the ingested dose is unknown, 5 to 10 vials are recommended as initial treatment in life-threatening situations. Fab fragments are administered intravenously through a 0.22-μm filter over 30 minutes, except in a cardiac arrest, where it may be given as a bolus.

TABLE 168-3 Calculating Digoxin-Specific Fab Fragment Dosage

1) Calculate total body load

Based on history of amount ingested:

Total body load = amount ingested (mg) × 0.80 (bioavailability)

Based on serum digoxin concentration:

$$\text{Total body load} = \frac{\text{serum digoxin level} \times 5.6\ \text{L/kg} \times \text{Patient's weight (kg)}}{1000}$$

2) Calculate number of vials of digoxin-specific Fab fragments needed to neutralize the calculated total body load:

It is assumed that an equimolar dose of Fab fragments is required for neutralization.

One vial (40 mg) of Fab fragments binds 0.6 mg of digoxin.

$$\text{Number of vials required} = \frac{\text{Total body load}}{0.6}$$

A simple and accurate variation of the above calculations:

$$\text{Number of vials of Fab} = \frac{\text{serum digoxin level} \times \text{Patient's weight (kg)}}{100}$$

The serum digoxin level has no correlation with clinical toxicity following Fab administration because most laboratories use assays that measure both bound and unbound digoxin, although there are some laboratories that measure only free digoxin levels. Minutes after Fab fragment administration, the free digoxin level falls to zero, but the total serum digoxin level (bound to Fab fragments) increases 10- to 20-fold.[12] The Fab-digoxin complex is eliminated by renal excretion.[16] In the case of renal failure, the complex may persist in the circulation for prolonged periods. Recurrent toxicity can occur up to 10 days after Fab fragment administration in patients with renal failure. Hemodialysis does not enhance the elimination of the digoxin-Fab complex.[16]

DISPOSITION

Patients with signs of toxicity or a history of a large, ingested dose, especially if coexisting risk factors increase susceptibility to digitalis toxicity should be admitted to a monitored unit. Contacting the local poison center and medical toxicologist can facilitate difficult management and treatment decisions regarding when to administer Digibind. Any patient receiving Fab fragments requires ICU observation for at least 24 h. All suspected suicidal patients should have a psychiatric evaluation prior to discharge. Accidental exposures with no signs of toxicity after 12 h can be discharged home.

REFERENCES

1. Woolf AD, Wenger T, Smith TW, et al: The use of digoxin-specific Fab fragments for severe digitalis intoxication in children. *N Engl J Med* 326:1739, 1992.
2. Litovitz TL, Klein-Schwartz W, Dyer KS, Shannon M, Lee S, Powers M: 1997 Annual Report of the American Association of Poison Control Centers Toxic Exposure Surveillance System. *Am J Emerg Med* 16:443, 1997.
3. Smith TW: Digitalis: Mechanisms of action and clinical use. *N Engl J Med* 318:358, 1988.
4. Rosen MR: Cellular electrophysiology of digitalis toxicity. *J Am Coll Cardiol* 5:22A, 1985.
5. Wofford JL, Ettinger WH: Risk factors and manifestations of digoxin toxicity in the elderly. *Am J Emerg Med* 9:11, 1991.

6. Moorman JR, Pritchett EL: The arrhythmias of digitalis intoxication. *Arch Intern Med* 145:1289, 1985.
7. Piltz JR, Wertenbaker C, Lance SE, et al: Digoxin toxicity: Recognizing the varied visual presentations. *J Clin Neuro-ophthalmol* 13:275, 1993.
8. Seltzer A: Role of serum digoxin assay in patient management. *J Am Coll Cardiol* 5:106A, 1985.
9. Bismuth C, Gaultier M, Conso F, et al: Hyperkalemia in acute digitalis poisoning: Prognostic significance and therapeutic implications. *Clin Toxicol* 6:153, 1973.
10. Vincent JL, Dufaye P, Berre J, et al: Bretylium in severe ventricular arrhythmias associated with digitalis intoxication. *Am J Emerg Med* 2:504, 1984.
11. French JH, Thomas RG, Siskind AP, et al: Magnesium therapy in massive digoxin intoxication. *Ann Emerg Med* 13:562, 1984.
12. Antman EM, Wenger TL, Butler VP, et al: Treatment of 150 cases of life-threatening digitalis intoxication with digoxin-specific Fab antibody fragments: Final report of a multicenter study. *Circulation* 81:1744, 1990.
13. Lalonde RL, Deshpande R, Hamilton PP, et al: Acceleration of digoxin clearance by activated charcoal. *Clin Pharmacol Ther* 37:367, 1985.
14. Shumaik GM, Wu AW, Ping AC: Oleander poisoning: Treatment with digoxin-specific Fab antibody fragments. *Ann Emerg Med* 17:732, 1988.
15. Hickey AR, Wenger TL, Carpenter VP, et al: Digoxin immune Fab therapy in the management of digitalis intoxication: Safety and efficacy results of an observational surveillance study. *J Am Coll Cardiol* 17:590, 1991.
16. Clinton GD, McIntyre WJ, Zannikos PN, et al: Free and total serum digoxin concentrations in a renal failure patient after treatment with digoxin immune Fab. *Clin Pharm* 8:441, 1989.

TABLE 169-1 β-Blocker Pharmacologic Profile

Agent	β_1 Selective	Partial Agonist	Na^+ Channel Blockage
Acebutolol	Yes	Yes	Yes
Atenolol	Yes	No	No
Esmolol	Yes	No	No
Labetolol	No	Yes	No
Metoprolol	Yes	No	No
Nadolol	No	No	No
Oxprenolol	No	Yes	Yes
Pindolol	No	Yes	Yes
Propranolol	No	No	Yes
Sotalol	No	No	No
Timolol	No	No	No

Source: Adapted from Frishman WH, Jacob H, Eisenberg E: *Am Heart J* 98:798, 1979, with permission.

β-BLOCKER TOXICITY

William P. Kerns II

β-adrenergic receptor antagonists, or β-blockers, alleviate such manifestations of cardiovascular disease as hypertension, tachydysrhythmias, and myocardial infarction. Considering the high prevalence of cardiovascular disease and the widespread use of β-blockers, it is not surprising that accidental and intentional poisoning is common. Poison control center data from 1996 demonstrate over 7200 exposures to β blockers. Of these, 134 were serious poisonings, resulting in 16 deaths.[1] These data probably underestimate the true prevalence of β-blocker toxicity due to underreporting of poisonings.

PHYSIOLOGY

The β receptor is a glycoprotein within the cell membrane whose stimulation ultimately results in increased cytosolic calcium, which is integral for excitation-contraction coupling. The β receptor is coupled to an intracellular second messenger, cyclic adenosine monophosphate (cAMP), by a regulatory protein within the cell membrane called the G protein. Upon β-receptor stimulation, the G protein undergoes a conformational change that activates adenyl cyclase, increasing intracellular cAMP. Cyclic AMP stimulates protein kinase, which phosphorylates calcium channels, leading to calcium entry into the cell. Calcium entry into the cell triggers additional calcium release from storage organelles. Phosphodiesterase then hydrolyzes cAMP.

Three β-receptor subtypes have been identified: the β_1 subunit in the myocardium, kidney, and eye; the β_2 subunit in adipose tissue, pancreas, liver, and muscle; and the β_3 subunit in adipose tissue. Stimulation of each subunit serves a unique function. For example, β_1 stimulation increases the force and rate of myocardial contraction. β_2 stimulation relaxes vascular smooth muscle. β_2 activation also increases metabolic substrate availability needed for stress by stimulating lipolysis and glycogenolysis. The β_3 subunit alters lipid metabolism.

TOXICOPHYSIOLOGY

Excessive β-receptor blockade predictably decreases inotropy, chronotropy, and metabolic effects that are expected from subunit stimulation, resulting in hallmark bradycardia and hypotension.

Other mechanisms may contribute to β-blocker toxicity. Several β-blocker drugs antagonize myocardial sodium channels (Table 169-1) in a manner similar to the effects of quinidine or cyclic antidepressants. Impedance of sodium entry slows phase zero of the action potential, resulting in prolonged QRS duration and myocardial depression. Thus, patients may present with wide-complex bradycardia.

Experimental evidence implicates altered calcium and potassium homeostasis as a contributing mechanism of toxicity.[2]

PHARMACOLOGY AND PHARMACOKINETICS

Many β blockers are available. They differ slightly in pharmacologic (Table 169-1) and pharmacokinetic (Table 169-2) properties. Pharmacologic differences among drugs influence expression of toxicity. Highly lipid-soluble agents penetrate the blood-brain barrier to a greater extent than do water-soluble β blockers, resulting in more central nervous system toxicity. Propranolol, acebutolol, labetolol, oxprenolol, and pindolol inhibit myocardial sodium channels, making these drugs potentially more cardiotoxic. Several β blockers have partial agonist activity, and thus weak stimulation of the β receptor occurs concurrently with blockade. Thus, partial agonist activity may have a protective effect in overdose. Labetolol has the potential to cause profound hypotension due to combined α_1- and β-receptor antagonism.

Clinically relevant pharmacokinetic characteristics include drug formulation (regular versus sustained release), rate of drug absorption, lipid solubility, and volume of distribution (Vd). Absorption of normal-release β blockers occurs rapidly, with peak effect in 1 to 4 h. For this reason, toxic symptoms begin soon after ingestion. The high degree of protein binding, the large Vd, and lipid solubility predict that extracorporeal drug removal will not be useful for most β blockers. Hemodialysis may be beneficial for atenolol, nadolol, and sotalol because these agents have lower protein binding, are hydrophilic, and have Vds similar to that of water.

TABLE 169-2 β-Blocker Pharmacokinetics

Agent	Absorption, %	Protein Binding, %	Onset of Action, h*	Volume of Distribution, L/kg	Metabolism and Half-Life, h	Lipophilic
Acebutolol	70	25	1–3	3	Renal, 3–4	Moderate
Atenolol	50	<5	2–4	0.6–1.1	Renal, 6–9	Weak
Esmolol	NA	55	5 min	3.4	Blood esterase, 9 min	Weak
Labetolol	90	50	1–3	5.1–9.4	Hepatic, 3–4	Weak
Metoprolol	90	12	1–2	5.6	Hepatic, 3–4	Moderate
Nadolol	30	30	3–4	1.8–2	Renal, 14–24	Weak
Oxprenolol	90	80	1–2	1.2	Hepatic, 2–3	Moderate
Pindolol	90	57	1¼	1.2–2	Renal, 3–4	Moderate
Propranolol	90	93	1–1½	3.4–6	Hepatic, 3–4	High
Sotalol	70	0	2–3	0.23–0.7	Renal, 9–10	Weak
Timolol	90	10	1–2	1.3–3.6	Renal, 4–5	Weak

*Regular-release preparations.
Abbreviation: NA, not applicable.
Source: Compiled from Weinstein RS: *Ann Emerg Med* 13:1123, 1984; Frishman WH, Jacob H, Eisenberg E: *Am Heart J* 98:798, 1979; and Hoffman BB, Lefkowitz RJ, in Hardman JG, Limbird LE, Molinoff PB, et al (eds): *Goodman and Gilman's: The Pharmacological Basis of Therapeutics,* 9th ed. New York, McGraw-Hill, 1996.

CLINICAL PRESENTATION

Patients who ingest β blockers manifest a spectrum of clinical presentations ranging from minimal symptoms to profound bradycardia, hypotension, and cardiogenic shock. The majority of serious cases result from ingestion of propranolol.[3] Symptoms typically develop within 1 to 3 h after acute ingestion, but the onset may range from 15 min to 10 h. Delays are expected following ingestion of sustained-release formulations. Systemic toxicity has been reported following instillation of ophthalmic preparations.[4]

Slowing of the heart due to sinus node suppression or conduction abnormalities occur in all significant β-blocker intoxications except overdoses of β blockers that have partial agonist activity, in which case bradycardia may not be present. QRS widening may occur with β blockers that antagonize sodium channels, such as propranolol, pindolol, and acebutolol.

Ventricular dysrhythmias are common with sotalol poisoning. Sotalol has properties consistent with the Vaughan Williams class III antidysrhythmic drugs that prolong action potential duration in His-Purkinje tissue, resulting in a prolonged Q-T interval. Premature ventricular contractions, bigeminy, ventricular tachycardia, ventricular fibrillation, and torsades de pointes have been reported.

Hypotension results from poor contractility. Together, bradycardia and depressed contractility may produce severe cardiac failure.

Depressed consciousness, seizures, and psychosis may occur due to poor perfusion or direct neuronal toxicity. Lipophilic agents are more likely to cause coma and seizures. Seizures are generalized and tend to be brief, lasting seconds to minutes. Status seizures are rare but may be refractory to treatment.[5] Acute psychosis preceded myocardial manifestations in a case of propranolol overdose.[6] When patients survive, neurologic recovery appears to be complete.

Bronchospasm following overdose is infrequent despite potential β_2 antagonism but has been reported with atenolol, metoprolol, oxprenolol, and propranolol poisoning.

Hypoglycemia is rare, despite potential for altered glucose homeostasis.

Rare complications of poisoning include esophageal spasm, mesenteric ischemia, and acute renal failure.

DIAGNOSIS

A limited number of other medications, chemicals, and natural toxins potentially result in bradycardia and hypotension. Common drugs include calcium channel antagonists, centrally acting α-agonists, and digoxin. Many plants (e.g., oleander, digitalis, and rhododendron) contain cardiac glycosides that may cause symptoms following ingestion of plant parts or consumption of teas brewed from the plant. Chinese medicinal preparations and aphrodisiacs often contain animal-derived cardiac glycosides (e.g., bufotoxin) that may cause bradycardia and hypotension. Such chemicals as organophosphate insecticides, cyanide, or hydrogen sulfide cause bradycardia.

Diagnostic Studies

A twelve-lead electrocardiogram and continuous rhythm monitoring are essential in evaluation and ongoing assessment. Laboratory testing is directed at supportive monitoring of renal function, glucose level, oxygenation, and acid-base status. Specific drug levels may be determined to confirm an exposure, but the results will not alter acute management, since symptoms do not necessarily correlate with levels and levels are not rapidly available. Radiographs to detect β-blocker pills in the gastrointestinal tract are not useful, since these drugs are not radiopaque.[7]

TREATMENT

Initially, all β-blocker exposures should be evaluated in a high-acuity area of the emergency department. For serious cases, treatment begins by establishing adequate airway patency, ventilation, and oxygenation. Multiple intravenous access sites, as well as central venous access, may be required.

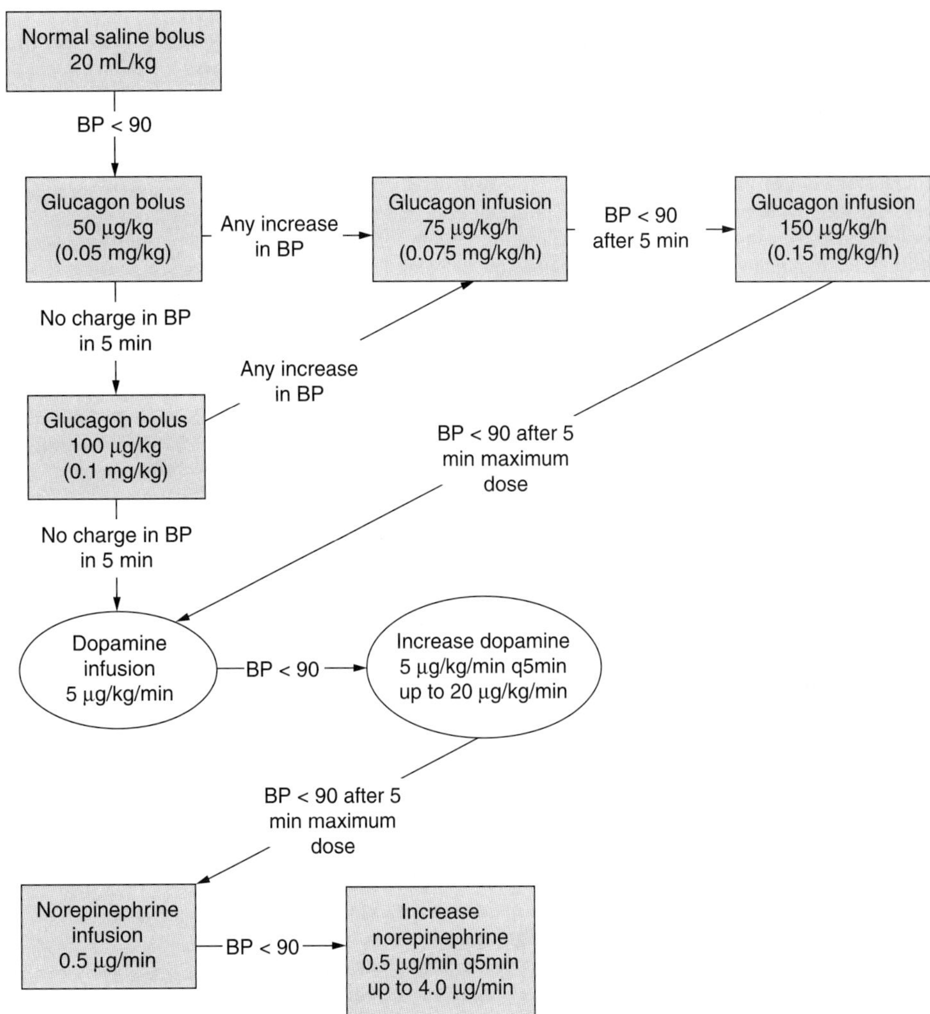

FIG. 169-1. Algorithm for drug therapy for β-blocker overdose.

The goal of specific cardiovascular drug therapy is to restore perfusion to critical organ systems by improving myocardial contractility, increasing heart rate, or both. Current therapy is derived principally from reports of case studies and includes glucagon, adrenergic agonists, atropine, and phosphodiesterase inhibitors. Overall, these therapies have met with variable success. Figure 169-1 is an algorithm for use of these drugs based on review of available human cases and limited experimental studies.

Glucagon is widely accepted as first-line therapy. It enhances myocardial performance by increasing cAMP concentrations in a manner identical to that of catecholamines but is thought to act via its own receptor.[8] Thus, glucagon may bypass the blocked β receptor. Clinical experience with this antidote has generally produced favorable results, often after other treatments have failed. However, only two cases report glucagon as the sole pharmacologic agent to resuscitate severely toxic propranolol overdoses.[9] In several instances, glucagon failed to reverse toxicity.[10,11] A limited number of animal models directly comparing glucagon to other therapies support the use of glucagon.[12]

The initial glucagon dose is 50 to 150 μg/kg intravenous bolus. For a 70-kg patient, this represents 3.5 to 10 mg. The bolus may be repeated as needed. Because the duration of action of glucagon is 15 min, a constant infusion of 1 to 10 mg/h may be necessary to sustain its effect. There is no defined maximum therapeutic dose of glucagon. Cumulative bolus doses ranged from 1 to 30 mg.[13,14] Infusions have been continued for up to 26 h.[15]

Compared to the potential benefits of increasing heart rate and blood pressure, the adverse effects of glucagon are minimal. Nausea and vomiting may occur due to esophageal sphincter relaxation. Mild, transient hyperglycemia may develop. When using large amounts of glucagon, excessive exposure to phenol, the manufacturer's diluent, may occur, resulting in seizures, hypotension, or dysrhythmias.[16] To avoid these unwanted effects, discard the supplied diluent and reconstitute glucagon with normal saline solution.

Unfortunately, sufficient amounts of glucagon are frequently unavailable in hospital pharmacies.[17] If glucagon is not available or fails to restore organ perfusion, the next step is to add a catecholamine.

β-adrenergic receptor agonists (catecholamines) are a logical therapy for β-blocker toxicity. Nevertheless, their use has met with disappointing results, restoring heart rate in only two-thirds of cases and blood pressure in only half. Results may not have been optimal because of inadequate dosing. For example, in humans, the dose of isoproterenol required to maintain heart rate and blood pressure had to be increased 26-fold following an infusion of labetolol.[18] In canines, isoproterenol and dopamine had to be increased 15 and 5 times, respectively, to overcome the depressant effects of propranolol.[19]

When faced with significant β-blocker toxicity, dopamine or norepinephrine are the catecholamines of choice. These agents may be preferable to epinephrine for two reasons. First, in animal models of propranolol toxicity, epinephrine had no effect on mortality rates.[20] Second, in similar calcium channel blocker toxicity models, epinephrine failed to provide optimal myocardial energy substrates needed during shock.[21] Dopamine or norepinephrine is administered as a constant infusion. Dopamine is more likely to work for mildly toxic cases. For severe toxicity, one may need to start with norepinephrine. Potential adverse effects of catecholamines include dysrhythmia, tissue necrosis, and increased myocardial oxygen demand.

Phosphodiesterase inhibitors have been used to treat β-blocker toxicity. In theory, they inhibit cAMP breakdown, thereby facilitating maintenance of intracellular calcium levels. In propranolol-induced heart failure, amrinone demonstrated positive inotropic effects without increasing myocardial oxygen demands.[22] However, other animal studies are not encouraging. Amrinone and milrinone increased cardiac output but had no appreciable effect on heart rate.[12] When administered with glucagon, neither amrinone or milrinone provided any additional benefit over that of glucagon.[23] Thus, phosphodiesterase inhibitors have no advantage over glucagon. However, if glucagon is not available, phosphodiesterase inhibitors can be reasonable alternatives.

Atropine is unlikely to be effective in the management of bradycardia and hypotension.

Treatment of ventricular dysrhythmias due to sotalol requires pharmacologic measures different from those required for other β blockers. Isoproterenol, lidocaine, and overdrive pacing have been successfully used. Magnesium may also be of benefit.[24]

Extrinsic pacing may be required to maintain heart rate. However, electrical capture is not always successful, and, if capture does occur, blood pressure is not always restored. Cardiac pacing may be most beneficial in treating torsades de pointes associated with sotalol.[24]

Occasionally, extreme means of resuscitation, including extracorporeal circulation[25] and aortic balloon pump,[26] have been successful. Insulin-dextrose was superior to standard antidotes in animals[19] and was used successfully in a combined amlodipine and atenolol overdose.[27]

Gastrointestinal decontamination with 1.0 g/kg plain activated charcoal should be initiated unless oral intake is contraindicated. Gastric lavage may be beneficial prior to instillation of charcoal if it can be accomplished within 1 to 2 h of ingestion. Syrup of ipecac is contraindicated, since β-blocker intoxicated patients may experience a rapid decline in mental status, with risk of aspiration during vomiting.

Based on previously described pharmacokinetic properties, hemodialysis would not be expected to effectively remove lipophilic β-blocker drugs that have a large volume of distribution or extensive protein binding. Hemodialysis may be useful for atenolol, nadolol, and sotalol overdose because these drugs have a lower volume of distribution and less protein binding than do other β blockers.

DISPOSITION

Patients who develop altered mental status, bradycardia, conduction delays, or hypotension should be managed in the intensive care unit. Overdose patients who present initially without symptoms can be safely discharged to psychiatric care after an observation period of 8 to 10 h provided they remain asymptomatic with normal vital signs and electrocardiogram, receive gastrointestinal decontamination, and are not expected to develop delayed complications from sustained-release formulation or coingested drugs.

REFERENCES

1. Litovitz TL, Smilkstein M, Felberg L: 1996 annual report of the American Association of Poison Control Centers toxic exposure surveillance system. *Am J Emerg Med* 15:447, 1997.
2. Kerns W, Ransom M, Tomaszewski C, et al: The effects of extracellular ions on β-blocker cardiotoxicity. *Toxicol Appl Pharmacol* 137:1, 1996.
3. Reith DM, Dawson AH, Epid D, et al: Relative toxicity of beta-blockers in overdose. *J Toxicol Clin Toxicol* 34:273, 1996.
4. Adverse Drug Reaction Advisory Committee: Systemic adverse reactions with betoxalol eye drops. *Med J Aust* 162:84,1995.
5. Smith RC, Wilkinson J, Hull RL: Glucagon for propranolol overdose. *JAMA* 254:2412, 1985.
6. Love JN, Handler JA, : Toxic psychosis: An unusual presentation of propranolol intoxication. *Am J Emerg Med* 13:536, 1995.
7. Savitt DL, Hawkins HH, Roberts JR: The radiopacity of ingested medications. *Ann Emerg Med* 16:331, 1987.
8. Levy GS, Fletcher MA, Klein I, et al: Characterization of ^{125}I-glucagon binding in a solubilized preparation of cat myocardial adenylate cyclase. *J Biol Chem* 249:2665, 1974.
9. Wilkinson J: Beta blocker overdose. *Ann Emerg Med* 15:982, 1986.
10. Hurwitz MD, Kallenbach JM, Pincus PS: Massive propranolol overdose. *Am J Med* 81:118, 1986.
11. Freestone S, Thomas HM, Bhamra RK: Severe atenolol poisoning: Treatment with prenalterol. *Hum Toxicol* 5:343, 1986.
12. Love JN, Leasure JA, Mundt DJ, et al: A comparison of amrinone and glucagon therapy for cardiovascular depression associated with propranolol toxicity in a canine model. *J Toxicol Clin Toxicol* 30:399, 1992.
13. Lewis M, Kallenbach J, Germond C, et al: Survival following massive overdose of adrenergic blocking agents (acebutolol and labetolol). *Eur Heart J* 4:328, 1983.
14. Adlerfliegel F, Leeman M, Demaeyer P, et al: Sotalol poisoning associated with asystole. *Intensive Care Med* 19:57, 1993.
15. Kenyon CJ, Aldinger GE, Joshipura P, et al: Successful resuscitation using external cardiac pacing in β-adrenergic antagonist-induced bradysystolic arrest. *Ann Emerg Med* 17:711, 1988.
16. Mofenson HC, Caraccio TR, Laudano J: Glucagon for propranolol overdose. *JAMA* 255:2025, 1986.
17. Love JN, Tandy TK: β-Adrenoreceptor antagonist toxicity: A survey of glucagon availability. *Ann Emerg Med* 22:267, 1993.
18. Richards DA, Prichard BNC, Boakes AJ, et al: Pharmacological basis for antihypertensive effects of intravenous labetolol. *Br Heart J* 39:99, 1977.
19. Avery GJ II, Spotnitz HM, Rose EA, et al: Pharmacological antagonism of β-adrenergic blockade in dogs: I. Hemodynamic effects of isoproterenol, dopamine, and epinephrine in acute propranolol administration. *J Thorac Cardiovasc Surg* 77:267, 1979.
20. Kerns W, Schroeder D, Williams C, et al: Insulin improves survival in a canine model of acute β-blocker toxicity. *Ann Emerg Med* 29:748, 1997.
21. Kline JA, Raymond RM, Leonova E, et al: Insulin improves heart function and metabolism during nonischemic cardiogenic shock in awake canines. *Cardiovasc Res* 34:289, 1997.
22. Alousi AA, Canter JM, Fort DJ: The beneficial effect of amrinone on acute drug-induced heart failure in the anesthetized dog. *Cardiovasc Res* 19:483, 1985.
23. Love JN, Leasure JA, Mundt DJ: A comparison of combined amrinone and glucagon therapy to glucagon alone for cardiovascular depression associated with propranolol toxicity in a canine model. *Am J Emerg Med* 11:360, 1993.
24. Leatham EW, Holt DW, McKenna WJ: Class III antiarrythmics in overdose: Presenting features and management principles. *Drug Safety* 9:450, 1993.
25. McVey FK, Corke CF: Extracorporeal circulation in the management of massive propranolol overdose. *Anaesthesia* 46:744, 1991.
26. Lane AS, Woodward AC, Goldman MR: Massive propranolol overdose poorly responsive to pharmacologic therapy: Use of an intra-aortic balloon pump. *Ann Emerg Med* 16:1381, 1987.
27. Litovitz TL, Bailey KM, Schmitz BF: 1990 annual report of the American Association of Poison Control Centers national data collection system. *Am J Emerg Med* 9:461, 1991.

CALCIUM CHANNEL BLOCKERS

Jeffrey A. Kline

EPIDEMIOLOGY

Each year for the past decade, calcium channel blocker poisoning required hospital treatment for over 5000 persons and caused 30 to 50 mortalities in the United States.[1] Calcium channel blockers (CCBs) are one of the most commonly prescribed classes of cardiovascular drugs. It is likely that toxicity from these drugs will increase in the next decade.

PATHOPHYSIOLOGY AND PHARMACOLOGY

Intracellular calcium is the primary stimulus for smooth and cardiac muscle contraction and for impulse formation in sinoatrial pacemaker

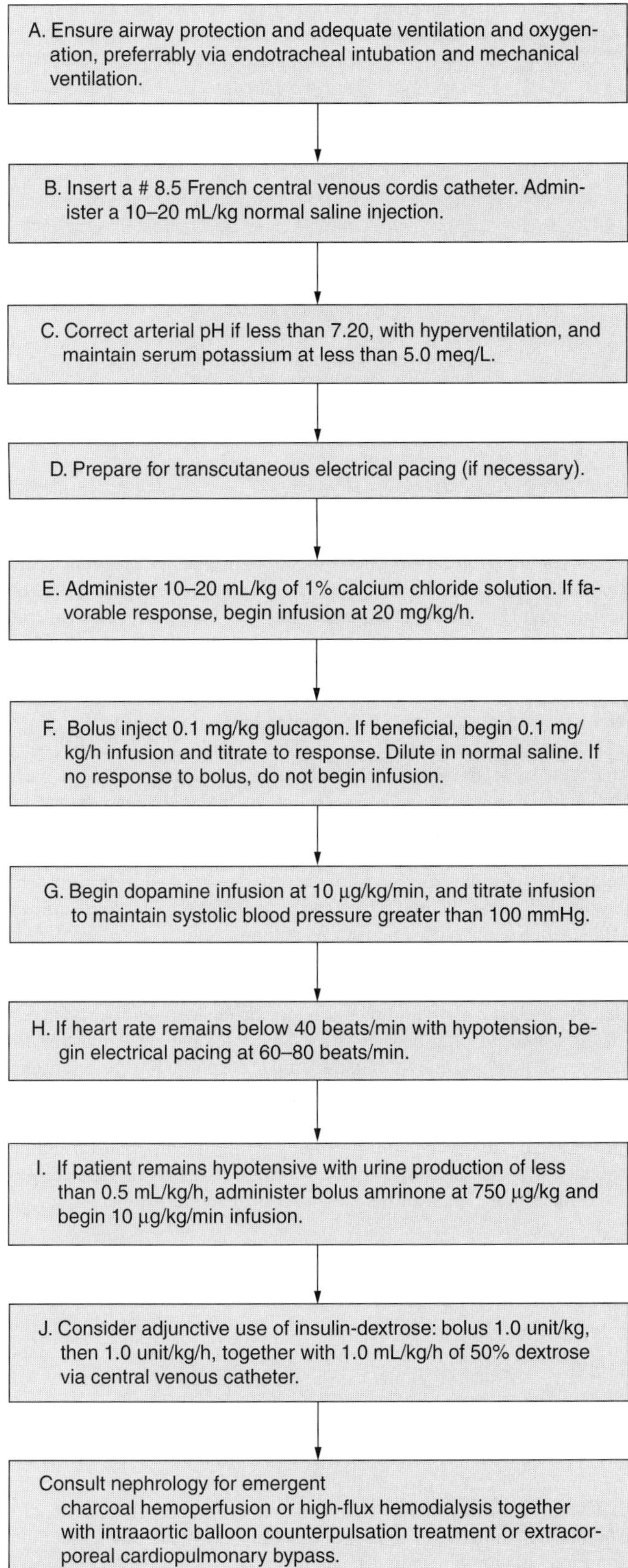

A. Ensure airway protection and adequate ventilation and oxygenation, preferrably via endotracheal intubation and mechanical ventilation.
B. Insert a # 8.5 French central venous cordis catheter. Administer a 10–20 mL/kg normal saline injection.
C. Correct arterial pH if less than 7.20, with hyperventilation, and maintain serum potassium at less than 5.0 meq/L.
D. Prepare for transcutaneous electrical pacing (if necessary).
E. Administer 10–20 mL/kg of 1% calcium chloride solution. If favorable response, begin infusion at 20 mg/kg/h.
F. Bolus inject 0.1 mg/kg glucagon. If beneficial, begin 0.1 mg/kg/h infusion and titrate to response. Dilute in normal saline. If no response to bolus, do not begin infusion.
G. Begin dopamine infusion at 10 μg/kg/min, and titrate infusion to maintain systolic blood pressure greater than 100 mmHg.
H. If heart rate remains below 40 beats/min with hypotension, begin electrical pacing at 60–80 beats/min.
I. If patient remains hypotensive with urine production of less than 0.5 mL/kg/h, administer bolus amrinone at 750 μg/kg and begin 10 μg/kg/min infusion.
J. Consider adjunctive use of insulin-dextrose: bolus 1.0 unit/kg, then 1.0 unit/kg/h, together with 1.0 mL/kg/h of 50% dextrose via central venous catheter.
Consult nephrology for emergent charcoal hemoperfusion or high-flux hemodialysis together with intraaortic balloon counterpulsation treatment or extracorporeal cardiopulmonary bypass.

FIG. 170-1. Treatment guidelines for severe CCB ingestion.

rhythm with normal blood pressure, with severe poisoning, treatment goals should focus on *stabilization* rather than on normalization of heart rate, arterial blood pressure, urine output, arterial base deficit, and cardiac output (if available) or left ventricular ejection fraction. There are no reports of perminant cardiomyopathy or central nervous system (CNS) dysfunction from direct CCB effect.

Calcium

Calcium salts are recommended by many toxicologists for the first-line treatment of CCB overdose. As a guideline, calcium chloride should be initiated as a 10 to 20 mg/kg bolus injection. Calcium chloride may be preferable to gluconate preparations because it produces more reliable plasma ionized calcium concentrations. Calcium chloride is available in a 10-mL 10% solution, which may be diluted to 100 mL in normal saline and infused over 5 min via central venous catheter as a test bolus in adults. If this infusion improves heart rate or conduction on ECG or increases the arterial blood pressure, then a constant infusion at 20 to 50 mg/kg/h $CaCl_2$ should be initiated. As a general end point, ionized plasma calcium concentrations should be maintained between 2.0 and 3.0 meq/L. The elevated plasma calcium concentration improves cardiac conduction and contraction simply by increasing the driving force of the calcium ion's entry through L-type channels that are not closed. If the calcium channels are uniformly saturated by a CCB (in particular, verapamil), then the proportion of L-channels that are closed will be nearly 100 percent. In this situation, even the highest of plasma calcium concentrations will not improve cardiac function. Calcium infusion also may cause vomiting, acute rhythm disturbances including asystole, and local irritative effects that may result in serious sequelae, including upper extremity compartment syndromes.

Glucagon

If calcium infusion provides inadequate clinical response, glucagon should be tested next. Glucagon is capable of inducing an immediate and remarkable positive chronotropic and inotropic response in mild to moderate toxicity. Glucagon binds to at least one specific membrane receptor, which is distinct from the β-adrenergic receptor. The glucagon receptor activates the stimulatory G-protein, leading to an elevation in cytosolic cyclic adenosine monophosphate (cAMP). The increased cAMP signals for the activation of protein kinases that phosphorylate the cytosolic domain of the L-channel. Channel phosphorylation increases the probability of channel opening, even if an organic CCB is bound to the channel. However, the degree of recruitment in channel opening is entirely dependent on the proportion of channels that have CCB bound to them. If binding is widespread, then the net increase in channel opening will be very low, even with maximal cAMP–protein kinase stimulation. Thus, with severe CCB poisoning, glucagon may be ineffective.

Glucagon should be diluted in normal saline, as opposed to using the phenol provided in the package, and a 0.1 mg/kg intravenous test bolus should be administered. In general, one of two responses occurs with glucagon injection with CCB overdose. The patient may show immediate evidence of improvement, both on ECG and in blood pressure. Alternatively, the patient may vomit, and deteriorate.[13–15] If a benefit is observed, a constant infusion of glucagon should be initiated, starting at 0.1 mg/kg/h. The infusion rate should be minimized to maintain sinus rhythm or a systolic blood pressure above 100 mmHg with urine production above 1 mL/kg/h. Note that wholesale cost of glucagon is about $20/mg.

Catecholamines

Catecholamines should be tested as the next step for refractory CCB overdose. The predominant mechanism by which all catecholamines increase cardiac function and systemic vascular resistance is through binding to two membrane receptors. Activation of the β_1 adrenoreceptor increases cardiac cAMP in a postreceptor manner identical to glucagon and causes increased heart rate and force of cardiac contraction. Activation of the α_1 receptor causes an increase in vascular smooth muscle tone and increases cardiac inotropy via a mechanism separate from the cAMP–protein kinase pathway. Dopamine is the most commonly used agent and can be given in doses standard for cardiogenic shock (1–20 μg/kg/h).[16] Other catecholamines such as dobutamine, norepinephrine, and isoproterenol have been used in patients and animal studies with variable success. Epinephrine also has shown benefit in CCB-intoxicated humans and animals.[17–19] However, in one clinically relevant dog model of verapamil toxicity, epinephrine tended to worsen heart function and did not improve survival compared with saline treatment.[20] If epinephrine is used, a trial of 0.1 μg/kg/min can be titrated to a maximum of 1.0 μg/kg/min. If there is no satisfactory improvement within 5 min of the maximum infusion rate, then epinephrine should be discontinued in favor of an alternative agent.

Other Cardioactive Agents

Amrinone also has been reported to be successful in treating refractory CCB overdose. Amrinone inhibits the action of the cardiac phosphodiesterase (known as the peak III PDE), which leads to an elevation in cytosolic cAMP. Amrinone's main benefit is its positive inotropic action. Amrinone requires a loading bolus of 750 μg/kg, followed by a constant infusion at 1 to 20 μg/kg/h.

Atropine also is used frequently for treating CCB overdose.[16] Although atropine probably has no adverse effects in this setting, it seldom produces any benefit as a sole treatment.

Insulin

High-dose insulin infusion also has provided benefit in two models of verapamil toxicity.[18,20] Insulin appears to improve myocardial mechanical efficiency and contractility by accelerating carbohydrate oxidation. Insulin is also potent a positive inotrope that operates through a mechanism similar to the postreceptor action of the α_1 adrenoreceptor. Insulin does not produce a sharp improvement in hemodynamic indexes when bolus infused. Instead, insulin slowly but steadily improves heart contractility. Insulin has no direct effect on cardiac conduction but may lower plasma potassium concentrations and indirectly improve automaticity and conduction. Perhaps the best role of insulin is as an adjunctive therapy for suspected massive overdose, and it is more effective in humans when administered before profound hypodynamic shock supervenes.[21] A suggested infusion dose is 1.0 unit/kg/h for the first hour, followed by 0.5 unit/kg/h.[21] Depending on the severity of overdose, resistance to insulin-mediated glucose clearance may be significant; in general, adults require 20 to 30 g of glucose per hour to maintain euglycemia with a high-dose insulin infusion. The concomitant use of catecholamines should not deter the use of insulin. When insulin infusion is added to catecholamine infusion, an additional positive inotropic effect is observed, even in the depressed heart.[22]

RESCUE TREATMENTS

For patients with cardiogenic shock that is refractory to the preceding treatments, several options remain open. Electrical cardiac pacing may help restore heart rate and should be considered for patients with shock and a heart rate below 40 beats/min. At the level of the heart cell, CCBs delay both systolic calcium transients and diastolic calcium reuptake. The heart cell cannot be forced into normal rhythmicity and electrical depolarization. In fact, ventricular stroke volume tends to be maximized at a heart rate of 45 to 50 beats/min. Electrical pacing faster than this rate actually may reduce stroke volume. As a result, electrical pacing at too rapid a rate may not improve cardiac output.

4-Aminopyridine (4-AP) is a potassium channel blocking agent that is now available for the treatment of multiple sclerosis. Based on several animal studies of verapamil toxicity, (4-AP) can be considered for a patient who is dying despite all efforts.[23,24] 4-Aminopyridine should be infused in doses of 10 to 50 μg/kg/h.

Venovenous hemodialysis or venovenous charcoal hemoperfusion can lower the plasma concentration of verapamil and diltiazem. However, these procedures should be considered with caution. Both require insertion of a large-bore dialysis catheter, and both require heparin anticoagulation. Hemodialysis—and to a lesser extent hemoperfusion—can worsen cardiovascular instability in a patient already suffering hypodynamic shock. First, to achieve adequate drug removal, relatively high rates of blood flow across the artificial kidney may be required. Second, hemodialysis can remove plasma catecholamines. Third, approximately 10 percent of patients develop an idiosyncratic hypotensive response to the polysulphone membrane used in most hemodialysis and hemoperfusion circuits. Thus, when the pump is started, the patient's blood pressure may drop. Also, with large ingestions, a mass of drug usually is present in the patient's intestine for at least 12 h, which allows ongoing drug absorption. For these reasons, continuous hemoperfusion is advised over episodic dialysis.

Intraaortic balloon counterpulsation also has been reported to improve shock from verapamil poisoning.[25,26] Extracorporeal cardiopulmonary bypass also may provide a bridge to survival, especially if used in conjunction with hemodialysis or hemoperfusion.

TABLE 170-3 Pharmacokinetics of Generic versus Long-Acting Calcium Channel Antagonist Overdose[27–34]

Drug	Peak Toxicity (h)	$t_{1/2}$ (h)
Verapamil	1–2	5–7
Verelan SR	6–7	>12
Calan SR	2–3	7–12
Diltiazem	1–2	8–9
SR, CD, XR	3–5	5
Nifedipine	1	3
Adalat retard	3–10	20–25
Procardia XL	3–5	12–18
Amlodipine	6–12	>24
Felodipine	6–12	>12

DISPOSITION

Patients with trivial ingestions (<3 mg/kg of a first-generation dihydropyridine, <0.2 mg/kg of a second-generation dihydropyridine, or <5 mg/kg of diltiazem or verapamil), a normal heart rate and blood pressure, and no symptoms can be observed for approximately 6 h and discharged. Patients who report a large overdose of a sustained-release preparation (>10 mg/kg of verapamil or diltiazem) or a dihydropyridine derivative with a half-life over 12 h (Table 170-3) should be admitted for ECG monitoring for at least 12 h, even if they exhibit no symptoms. All patients with signs and symptoms of CCB toxicity should be admitted to an appropriate setting. Any patient who requires inotropic support (including bolus doses of calcium salts) should be admitted to an intensive care unit.

REFERENCES

1. Litovitz TL, Smilkstein M, Klein-Schwartz W, et al: 1996 Annual Report of the American Association of Poison Control Centers toxic exposure surveillance system. *Am J Emerg Med* 15:447, 1997.

2. Devis G, Somers G, Ban Obberghen E, Malaisse WJ: Calcium antagonists and islet function: I. Inhibition of insulin release by verapamil. *Diabetes* 24:547, 1975.
3. Kline JA, Raymond RM, Schroeder JD, Watts JA: The diabetogenic effects of acute verapamil poisoning. *Toxicol Appl Pharmacol* 145:357, 1997.
4. Jolly SR, Keaton N, Movahed A, et al: Effect of hyperkalemia on experimental myocardial depression by verapamil. *Am Heart J* 121:517, 1991.
5. Nugent M, Tinker JH, Moyer TP: Verapamil worsens rate of development in hemodynamic effects of acute hyperkalemia in halothane-anesthetized dogs: Effects of calcium therapy. *Anesthesiology* 60:435, 1984.
6. Kline JA, Leonova E, Williams TC, et al: Myocardial metabolism during graded intraportal verapamil infusion in awake canines. *J Cardiovasc Pharmacol* 27:719, 1995.
7. Howarth DM, Dawson AH, Smith AJ, et al: Calcium channel blocking drug overdose: An Australian series. *Hum Exp Toxicol* 13:161, 1994.
8. Buckley N, Dawson AH, Howarth D, et al: Slow-release verapamil poisoning: Use of polyethylene glycol whole-bowel lavage and high-dose calcium. *Med J Aust* 158:202, 1993.
9. Cienki JJ, Akhtar J, Burkhart KK, Donovan JW: Cardiovascular parameters in calcium-channel blocker. *Acad Emerg Med* 3:420, 1996.
10. Kuo MJ, Tseng YZ, Chen TF, et al: Verapamil overdose and severe hypocalcemia. *J Toxicol Clin Toxicol* 30:309, 1992.
11. Anthony T, Jastremski M, Elliot W: Charcoal hemoperfusion for the treatment of a combined diltiazem and metoprolol overdose. *Ann Emerg Med* 15:1344, 1986.
12. Rosansky SJ: Verapamil toxicity—Treatment with hemoperfusion. *Ann Intern Med* 114:340, 1991.
13. Doyon S, Roberts JR: The use of glucagon in a case of calcium channel blocker overdose. *Ann Emerg Med* 22:1229, 1993.
14. Walter FG, Frye G, Mullen JT, et al: Amelioration of nifedipine poisoning associated with glucagon therapy. *Ann Emerg Med* 22:1234, 1993.
15. Wolf LR, Spadafora MP, Otten EJ: Use of amrinone and glucagon in a case of calcium channel blocker overdose. *Ann Emerg Med* 22:1225, 1993.
16. Ramoska EA, Spiller HA, Wilter M, Borys D: A one-year evaluation of calcium channel blocker overdose: Toxicity and treatment. *Ann Emerg Med* 22:196, 1993.
17. Schramm M, Thomas G, Towart R, et al: Novel dihydropyridines with positive inotropic action through activation of Ca^{++} channels. *Nature* 303:535, 1983.
18. Kline JA, Tomeszewski CA, Schroeder JD, et al: Insulin is a superior antidote for cardiovascular toxicity induced by verapamil in the anesthetized canine. *J Pharmacol Exp Ther* 267:744, 1993.
19. Gay RG, Alego S, Lee R, et al: Treatment of verapamil toxicity in intact dogs. *J Clin Invest* 77:1805, 1986.
20. Kline JA, Raymond RM, Leonova ED, et al: Myocardial metabolism during treatment of non-ischemic cardiogenic shock in awake canines. *Cardiovasc Res* 34:289, 1997.
21. Yuan TH, Kerns WP, Tomaszewski CA, et al: Insulin-glucose as adjunctive therapy for severe calcium channel antagonist poisoning. *J Toxicol Clin Toxicol.* In press, 1999.
22. Reikeras O, Gunnes P, Sorlie D, et al: Hemodynamic and metabolic effects of dopamine infusion during acute left ventricular failure in dogs. *J Cardiovasc Pharmacol* 8:303, 1986.
23. Agoston S, Maestrone E, van Hezik EJ, et al: Effective treatment of verapamil intoxication with 4-aminopyridine in the cat. *J Clin Invest* 73:1291, 1984.
24. ter Wee PM, Kremer Hovinga TK, Uges DRA, van der Geest S: 4-Aminopyridine and hemodialysis in the treatment of verapamil intoxication. *Hum Toxicol* 4:327, 1985.
25. Melanson P, Shir RD, DeRoos F, et al: Intra-aortic balloon counterpulsation in calcium channel blocker overdose. *Vet Hum Toxicol* 35:345, 1993.
26. Welch CD, Knoerzer RE, Lewis GS: Verapamil and acebutolol overdose results in asystole: Intra-aortic balloon pump provides mechanical support. *J Extracorpor Tech* 24:36, 1992.
27. Abramowicz M: Amlodipine—A new calcium channel blocker. *Med Lett* 34:99, 1992.
28. Ferner RE, Odemuyia O, Field AB, et al: Pharmacokinetics and toxic effects of diltiazem in massive overdose. *Hum Toxicol* 8:497, 1989.
29. Ferner RE, Monkman S, Riley J, et al: Pharmacokinetics and toxic effects of nifedipine in massive overdose. *Hum Exp Toxicol* 9:309, 1990.
30. Edgar B, Regardh CG, Johnsson G, et al: Felodipine kinetics in healthy men. *Clin Pharmacol Ther* 38:205, 1985.
31. Roberts D, Honcharik N, Sitar DS, et al: Diltiazem overdose: Pharmacokinetics of diltiazem and its metabolites and effect of multiple dose charcoal therapy. *Clin Toxicol* 29:45, 1991.
32. Krick SE, Gums JG, Grauer K, Cooper GR: Severe verapamil (sustained release) overdose. *Ann Pharmacother* 24:705, 1990.
33. Hermann P, Rodger SD, Remones G, et al: Pharmacokinetics of diltiazem after intravenous and oral administration. *Eur J Clin Pharmacol* 24:349, 1983.
34. Malcom N, Callegari P, Goldberg P, Strauss H: Massive diltiazem overdosage: Clinical and pharmacokinetic observations. *Drug Intell Clin Pharmacol* 20:888, 1993.

ANTIHYPERTENSIVES

Arjun Chanmugam

Hypertension is one of the most common diseases in the United States, affecting almost 24 percent of the population.[1] Medications used to control hypertension are among the most commonly prescribed drugs. As a result, the potential for overdose, inadvertent or intentional, is quite high. In 1997, according to the Toxic Exposure Surveillance System, cardiovascular drugs, including antihypertensive medications, accounted for nearly 3 percent of all adult toxic exposures.[2]

There are many classes of antihypertensive medications available for use, with new agents introduced into the market routinely. The initial management of patients with an acute overdose of antihypertensive medication remains relatively uniform. Airway, breathing, and circulation remain the initial priorities, so oxygen, cardiac monitoring, and intravenous access remain the key initial interventions. If mental status changes are present glucose and naloxone should be also be considered as initial interventions. If no contraindications are present, antihypertensive-induced hypotension should be treated initially with volume expansion, using normal saline or an equivalent crystalloid solution (such as Ringer lactate solution). In most adults, initial fluid therapy should consist of bolus challenges of 500 mL or 10 to 20 mL/kg over 10 to 15 min. If hypotension persists despite fluid challenges, the use of a vasopressor may be warranted. In most cases, dopamine is the vasopressor of choice, with infusion rates started at 2 to 5 μg/kg/min and increased as necessary.

Supportive measures and appropriate monitoring should be instituted as early as possible. The use of activated charcoal is indicated in most overdose situations, but gastric decontamination should be considered only in appropriate patients. The management of patients with antihypertensive poisonings rarely depends on serum levels of medications but instead depends on symptoms. However, a key to managing these patients is to determine the medication involved and target interventions specific for that class of antihypertensive agent (Table 171-1). In the following discussion, antihypertensive toxicology is divided into sections based on the class of medications. β Blockers, monoamine oxidase inhibitors, and calcium-channel blockers are discussed in separate chapters.

DIURETICS

Diuretics are among the most commonly prescribed of all antihypertensives because they are recommended as a first-line medication in the treatment of hypertension.[1] Depending on their mechanism of action, diuretics can be subdivided into several groups.

Thiazides and Loop Diuretics

Thiazides and loop diuretics are two classes of diuretics commonly used. The classic thiazide diuretic is hydrochlorothiazide, which can be used as single-drug therapy or as part of a multidrug regimen.

TABLE 171-1 Specific Antihypertensive Medications

Name of Drug	Mechanism of Action	Therapeutic Range	LD_{50}	Dialysis	Maximum Tolerated Exposure	Therapeutic Interventions and Comments
Hydrochlorothiazide	Inhibits reabsorption of Na^+ and Cl^- in the distal convoluted tubule of the kidney	12.5–100 mg qd (in divided doses)	10 g/kg in mice/rats	Partially	1 g	IV fluids, correct electrolytes, vasopressor (dopamine) if necessary
Furosemide	Decreases reabsorption of Na^+ and Cl^- in the loop of Henle	20–600 mg qd	1000 mg/kg in rats/dogs	No	Not established	IV fluids, correct electrolytes, vasopressor (dopamine) if necessary
Spironolactone	Specific antagonist of aldosterone	25–400 mg qd		Yes	Not established	IV fluids, correct electrolytes
Triamterene	Inhibits the reabsorption of sodium ions in exchange for potassium and hydrogen ions at the distal tubule	100–150 mg bid	380 mg/kg mice	Yes	Not established	IV fluids, correct electrolytes, vasopressor (dopamine) if necessary
Acetazolamide	Inhibits carbonic anhydrase in the kidney	Up to 1000 mg qd	No deaths reported	Possibly	Not established	IV fluids, correct electrolytes, pH vasopressor (dopamine) if necessary
Mannitol	Osmotic diuresis	0.5 g/kg to 2 g/kg	Not known	Yes	Not established	IV fluids, correct electrolytes, vasopressor (dopamine) if necessary
Clonidine	Central α_2 agonist	0.1–2.4 mg/day	Oral LD_{50} rats, 465 mg/kg	No	11.25 mg	IV fluids, vasopressors (dopamine), nalaxone, Tolazoline
Captopril	Angiotensin-converting enzyme	6.25–150 mg tid	No deaths reported	Yes	7.5 g	IV fluids, vasopressors (dopamine), nalaxone
Enalapril	Angiotensin-converting enzyme	5–40 mg qd	Oral LD_{50}, 2000 mg/kg in mice/rats	Yes	300 mg	IV fluids, vasopressors (dopamine), nalaxone
Methyldopa	Central inhibitory α-adrenergic receptors, false neurotransmission, and/or reduction of plasma renin activity	250–3000 mg qd	Oral LD_{50}, >1.5 g/kg in mice/rats	Yes	Not established	IV fluids, vasopressors (dopamine)
Hydralazine	Directly relaxes arteriolar smooth muscle	10–50 mg qid	Oral LD_{50}, 173 mg/kg in rats	No	Not established	IV fluids; vasopressors should be avoided secondary to dysrhythmias
Minoxidil	Direct peripheral vasodilator	5–100 mg/day	Oral LD_{50}, 1321–3492 mg/kg in rats	Partially	Not established	IV fluids, dopamine; epinephrine and norepinephrine should be avoided
Sodium nitroprusside	Relaxes arteriolar and venous smooth muscle	0.5–10 μg/kg/min	LD_{50}, rabbits and dogs, 2.8 and 5.0 mg/kg	Yes, for thiocyanate toxicity	Unknown	Prolonged use can cause cyanide and/or thiocyanate toxicity; for cyanide toxicity, use cyanide antidote protocol
Prazosin	Arteriolar dilator, competitive blockade of postsynaptic α_1-adrenergic receptors	1 mg bid to 20 mg qd	Not known	No	200 mg	IV fluids, vasopressors (dopamine)

Combination products are becoming more common in the treatment of hypertension, and hydrochlorothiazide is often used as a component of these fixed-combination medications. In general, toxicity associated with thiazides is rare.

The diuretic action of thiazides is due to its ability to inhibit reabsorption of sodium and chloride at the distal convoluted tubule. This results in a greater excretion of water and other essential electrolytes, including potassium and bicarbonate. At higher doses, thiazides can act as carbonic anhydrous inhibitors. Calcium regulation is also affected by thiazides by two separate mechanisms: (1) They inhibit synthesis of vitamin D to decrease calcium absorption from the gastrointestinal tract. (2) They inhibit renal excretion of calcium.

Loop diuretics include such drugs as furosemide, bumetanide, and ethacrynic acid. These drugs act on the ascending limb of the loop of Henle to decrease reabsorption of sodium, chloride, and water. They act similarly to the thiazides in that they alter the regulation of other essential electrolytes, particularly potassium and calcium. Loop diuretics also increase venous capacitance and are used in acute situations with elevated cardiac filling pressures.

The toxicity associated with thiazides and loop diuretics involves two basic processes: volume contraction and electrolyte derangements. Symptoms associated with intravascular volume depletion include hypotension, tachycardia, and altered mental status. Common electrolyte derangements include hyponatremia, hypokalemia, hypocalcemia, hypomagnesemia, and hypochloremic metabolic alkalosis. Other adverse reactions from thiazides and loop diuretics may include rash, pruritis, hearing loss, leukopenia, and thrombocytopenia.

Normal saline administration is the preferred therapy for hypovolemia, hyponatremia, and alkalosis. The use of vasopressors is rarely indicated for hypotension. Potassium replacement should be instituted early, although renal function should be assessed and monitored during therapy to avoid inducing iatrogenic hyperkalemia in acute or chronic renal failure. In general, if comorbid conditions are not present, most asymptomatic individuals can be medically cleared after therapy and observation. Poisonings sufficient to cause significant electrolyte abnormalities are likely to be associated with total body deficits of various elements and may require prolonged therapy. Elderly patients and individuals at suicide risk need to be monitored carefully.

Potassium-Sparing Diuretics

The most common medications of this subclass are spironolactone, triamterene, and amiloride. Spironolactone, a competitive inhibitor of aldosterone, acts to allow potassium retention while inducing sodium and water excretion. Triamterene has direct effects on the renal tubule to inhibit sodium exchange for potassium and hydrogen. Amiloride's mechanism of action, also independent of aldosterone, is to promote potassium retention in exchange of sodium and water. Volume depletion, hyperkalemia, hyponatremia, and hypochloremia are common manifestations of toxicity for this class of medication. Treatment for potassium-sparing diuretic toxicity is directed at maintaining intravascular volume, repleting sodium, and reversing the hyperkalemia. Hypotension is best initially treated with intravenous fluids, usually normal saline. If hypotension is persistent, a vasopressor such as dopamine is warranted. The most serious manifestations of hyperkalemia include neurologic and cardiovascular dysfunction. Treatment of hyperkalemia should remain a priority, and can be serious enough to warrant dialysis.

Carbonic Anhydrase Inhibitors

The prototype for this subclass of diuretic is acetazolamide, which is a nonbacteriostatic sulfonamide whose adverse reactions include severe allergic reaction and Stevens-Johnson syndrome. The primary action of this class of diuretic is to inhibit carbonic anhydrase in the kidney to prevent the reversible reaction of carbon dioxide and water to form carbonic acid. This results in loss of bicarbonate ions in the urine, along with sodium, potassium, and water. Overdose with this class of medication can lead to volume depletion and electrolyte disturbances, as well as non-anion-gap metabolic acidosis. Treatment is directed at reversing volume depletion, monitoring electrolytes, and restoring normal pH balance.

Osmotic Agents

Osmotic agents, such as mannitol, are not absorbed by the nephron. Rather, they induce diuresis by raising the osmolarity of the glomerular filtrate, thereby attracting more water in the tubules to increase urine volume. The main effect of osmotic agents is to decrease intravascular volume, but toxicity can result in pulmonary edema, anaphylaxis, and acute renal failure. Overdoses can cause profound volume loss, accompanied by electrolyte imbalances. Treatment is aimed at repleting the intravascular volume and correcting any electrolyte imbalances. Other adverse reactions—such as pulmonary congestion, acidosis, electrolyte loss, dryness of mouth, thirst, marked diuresis, urinary retention, edema, headache, blurred vision, convulsions, nausea, vomiting, rhinitis, skin necrosis, thrombophlebitis, chills, dizziness, urticaria, dehydration, fever and angina-like chest pains—have been reported during or following mannitol infusion.

CLONIDINE

This centrally acting antihypertensive has long been a favorite for the acute management of hypertension. Two forms of clonidine are commonly prescribed, including an oral version and a transdermal patch. Clonidine has gained prominence in recent years because of its ability to mitigate opiate and alcohol withdrawal symptoms. Although it has not been approved by the Food and Drug Administration for this use, clonidine has been used as standard clinical practice for the treatment of narcotic withdrawal for almost 2 decades.[3] With the advent of the clonidine patch in 1986, drug delivery could be reliably maintained for 7 days at a variety of doses, which increased its attractiveness for prescribers. However, plasma concentrations of clonidine remain high enough to maintain a hypotensive effect for approximately 8 h after the removal of the patch. Regardless of the route of administration, clonidine's most common adverse effects are dry mouth and drowsiness.

Clonidine is an imidazoline whose principle site of action is on the α_2 receptors in the lower brainstem. Stimulation of the central α_2-receptor decreases norepinephrine release in the central nervous system (CNS), resulting in a lower heart rate and blood pressure. Although clonidine acts as a central α_2 agonist, it has other effects. For example, it reduces noradrenergic output in the locus ceruleus, which is stimulated by the cessation of narcotic use, thereby mitigating the symptoms of opioid withdrawal. At higher doses, clonidine can act as a partial peripheral α agonist, resulting in a paradoxical increase in blood pressure and heart rate. However, this effect is relatively short-lived and the antihypertensive effects usually predominate.

The primary symptoms associated with clonidine toxicity include hypotension and bradycardia, which can lead to cardiac ischemia and congestive heart failure. Mental status changes range from agitation and hallucinations to sedation and coma. Respiratory depression and recurrent apnea can occur, especially in children. The other symptoms of clonidine toxicity include seizures, diarrhea, hypothermia, and miosis.

Treatment of clonidine overdoses is centered on maintaining adequate blood pressures. In the acute phase of toxicity, a brief blood pressure elevation may occur. This paradoxical hypertensive response is due to peripheral adrenergic stimulation but usually evolves rapidly into hypotension as central α_2-agonist stimulation predominates. Treatment is rarely indicated for transient blood pressure elevation, but if aggressive intervention is warranted, nitroprusside is the drug of choice due to its rapid onset and dissipation. The peak effects of clonidine usually occur in 1 to 3 h. Intravenous fluids are usually adequate for the treatment of hypotension, but in cases of persistent hypotension, a dopamine infusion beginning at a midlevel (dose) rate of 2 to 5 μg/kg/min can be initiated.

The other serious cardiovascular condition caused by clonidine toxicity—sinus bradycardia—must be monitored closely. Symptomatic bradycardia should be treated with repeated doses of atropine sulfate. The other toxic effects of clonidine occur less commonly but may be serious. Respiratory depression is rare, but recurrent apnea, especially in children, may require intubation. Seizures require supportive measures and usually respond to standard anticonvulsant therapy. Hypothermia associated with clonidine toxicity also responds to standard interventions.

In cases of severe refractory hypotension or CNS depression, the use of naloxone has been suggested, although its mechanism of action is not well understood. Tolazoline, 10 mg intravenously titrated every 30 min, is only recommended after intravenous fluids, dopamine, atropine, and naloxone have failed to reverse the cardiovascular effects of clonidine. There is also a single case report of clonidine toxicity being successfully treated with yohimbine, a CNS α_2-adrenergic antagonist.[4]

Clonidine's range of toxicity has not been well established. Severe toxicity has been reported in children at doses as low as 0.1 mg, whereas adults have survived with levels exceeding 15 mg. Symptoms of clonidine toxicity can persist for up to 72 h, so admission should be considered for any patient suspected of clonidine overdose.

Abrupt cessation of clonidine therapy can result in withdrawal. Signs and symptoms range from hypertensive encephalopathy to jitteriness and headache. This rebound hypertensive state results from elevated catecholamine concentrations in the plasma and, in rare cases, has been reported to be fatal. However, clonidine-related rebound hypertensive states are usually associated with high-dose therapy. If end-organ damage results, clonidine withdrawal should be managed as a hypertensive emergency (see Chap. 53). If no evidence of hypertensive emergency is found, resumption of clonidine therapy or the administration of labetolol, 200 mg orally, is adequate intervention. The use of other β blockers should be avoided in clonidine withdrawal states, as the unopposed α-adrenergic effects may worsen the hypertension.

ANGIOTENSIN-CONVERTING ENZYME INHIBITORS

Angiotensin-converting enzyme (ACE) inhibitors come in two basic forms: an active drug form, best represented by captoril, and a prodrug form, represented by enalapril. Recently, enalaprilat, the active form of enalapril, became available for intravenous use. However, there are many ACE inhibitors available today, and all work to inhibit the conversion of the prohormone, angiotensin I, to the potent endogenous vasoconstrictor, angiotensin II. Besides being a vasoconstrictor, angiotensin II stimulates aldosterone release to increase sodium and water retention. Aside from these two effects, ACE inhibitors have other mechanisms of action to decrease total peripheral resistance without increasing heart rate or cardiac output. For example, by inhibiting ACE (also known as bradykininase), the degradation of the vasodilator peptide, bradykinin, is prevented.

Adverse effects of ACE inhibitors include hypotension, angioedema, rash, anaphylactoid reactions, cough, drug fever, proteinuria, glomerulopathy, neutropenia, and agranulocytosis. With overdoses of ACE inhibitors, the most important concern is hypotension, which can be profound. The preferred therapy to reverse the hypotension is the administration of normal saline, and, if necessary, vasopressors, such as intermediate or high-dose dopamine, can be added. Although ACE inhibitors are dialyzable, peritoneal dialysis and hemodialysis are not recommended at this time. Naloxone has been reported to be useful in reversing the hypotension induced by captopril, although its mechanism is unclear.

ANGIOTENSIN II RECEPTOR ANTAGONIST

The antihypertensive medications of this relatively new class are reversible, competitive inhibitors of the angiotensin II receptor. Losartan, the first drug of this class to be approved, has no effect on ACE but is a selective blocker of the AT_1 receptor found in vascular smooth muscle. Experience is limited with losartan, but adverse effects have been reported to be minimal. Toxicity includes hypotension and bradycardia. Supportive measures, including intravenous normal saline, adequate monitoring, and close observation is indicated for anyone who may have ingested an overdose of an angiotensin II receptor antagonist.

OTHER CENTRALLY ACTING ANTIHYPERTENSIVES

Centrally acting antihypertensives all work by decreasing sympathetic outflow in the CNS. The importance of many of these medications has decreased as other classes of medications have gained in prominence. Two medications in particular are considered in this section: guanabenz and methyldopa. Overdoses of these medications result in similar effects, including hypotension, symptomatic bradycardia, dry mouth, and potential mental status changes. Hypotension should be treated with intravenous fluids; if necessary, vasopressors such as norepinephrine or dopamine should be considered. Bradycardia can be treated with atropine. Methyldopa can be dialyzed, but there is no clear evidence that guanabenz can be dialyzed. A rebound hypertensive condition, similar to that of clonidine withdrawal, may occur with the abrupt cessation of any centrally acting antihypertensive medication.

PERIPHERAL VASODILATORS AND GANGLIONIC BLOCKERS

The toxic manifestations of these classes of medications include hypotension and bradycardia. Hypotension is best treated with intravenous fluids and, if necessary, vasopressors. If symptomatic bradycardia develops, atropine should be used. Seizures are a potential complication and should be treated with standard anticonvulsant therapy.

In addition to hypotension, α-adrenergic antagonists such as phentolamine may also cause CNS effects. No deaths have been attributed to the acute toxicity of phentolamine or to the ganglionic blocker trimethaphan. Other specific vasodilators are discussed below.

Prazosin

Prazosin is an arteriolar dilator whose mechanism of action involves competitive blockade of postsynaptic α_1-adrenergic receptors. Reported toxicity associated with this drug is uncommon. A first-dose phenomenon has been reported with prazosin use that results in an unanticipated sudden hypotensive episode potentially leading to syncope. Inadvertent hypotension generally occurs within 30 to 60 min after the first dose has been given and is usually preceded by tachycardia. The first-dose phenomenon usually occurs in individuals with impaired hepatic function or congestive heart failure.

Other toxic symptoms include headache, vertigo, paresthesias, gastrointestinal discomfort, and weakness. Case reports have indicated that priapism, pulmonary edema, and acidosis can also occur as a result of overdose with prazosin. However, the most common manifestation of prazosin overdose remains hypotension and tachycardia. Treatment is supportive with intravenous fluids, careful monitoring, and vasopressors, if necessary.

Hydralazine

Hydralazine, a smooth muscle vasodilator whose mechanism of action is poorly understood, is available both in tablet form and in parental form. Acute toxicity with hydralazine is uncommon, and no fatalities due to acute poisoning have been reported. Chronic use does lead to a hydralazine-induced systemic lupus erythematosus syndrome, but this generally occurs in individuals who have slow hepatic acetylation. Treatment is supportive; the hypotension associated with hydralazine responds well to intravenous fluids. Vasopressors should be used with caution in order to avoid precipitating dysrhythmias. Dopamine should be used judiciously if a vasopressor is necessary. Symptomatic tachycardia can be cautiously treated with β blockers.

Minoxidil

Minoxidil is a direct-acting peripheral vasodilator that lowers systolic and diastolic blood pressure without much affect on the CNS. It also has the advantage of not interfering with vasomotor reflexes and therefore does not induce orthostatic hypotension.

Minoxidil, in tablet form, is usually reserved for the treatment of severe or refractory hypertension, and reported toxicity has been rare. A common side effect of minoxidil is hirsuitism. In 1988, a 2% topical solution of minoxidil was approved for the treatment of baldness. At least one case report exists involving ingestion of the topical solution. Regardless of the preparation, the most common symptoms of toxicity include hypotension and tachycardia. In patients with renal failure, fluid retention and pericardial effusion have been reported. Treatment is supportive and includes intravenous fluids. If the hypotension is persistent, dopamine or phenylephrine should be considered. Vasopressors with β-adrenergic activity, such as epinephrine, should be avoided because of the potential for excessive cardiac stimulation. β blockers can be used for symptomatic tachycardia.

Sodium Nitroprusside

This is the drug of choice for hypertensive emergencies. It is a rapidly absorbed and rapidly dissipated drug whose principle action is to lower blood pressure by relaxing smooth muscle in arteries and veins. Sodium nitroprusside causes toxicity by three primary mechanisms: (1) The most common adverse effect is direct vasodilation resulting in hypotension and dysrhythmias. (2) Thiocyanate toxicity occurs infrequently, resulting in tinnitus, altered mental status changes, nausea, and abdominal pain. (3) In rare cases, cyanide toxicity can occur, resulting in coma, metabolic acidosis, or respiratory arrest. In very rare cases and in susceptible patients, methemoglobinemia can occur, which, if levels reach greater than 15 percent, can result in symptomatic cellular hypoxia. Toxicity associated with sodium nitroprusside is usually related to prolonged administration or occurs in patients with renal or hepatic failure.

Nitroprusside reacts with hemoglobin to form cyanomethemoglobin and cyanide. Methemoglobin is derived from hemoglobin and will bind cyanide until the intraerythrocyte methemoglobin has been saturated. Thiosulfate will react with the remaining cyanide to form thiocyanate, which is excreted in the urine. A limiting factor in cyanide metabolism is the amount of thiosulfate in the body, and that limit is usually achieved at a nitroprusside infusion rate of 5 μg/kg/min.

The direct vasodilatation effects of nitroprusside can result in excessive hypotension, resulting in mental status changes and dysrhythmias. Thiocyanate toxicity causes anorexia, fatigue, and mental status changes, including psychosis, weakness, seizures, tinnitus, and hyperreflexia. Cyanide toxicity is often associated with the odor of almonds on breath and can result in acidosis, tachycardia, mental status changes, and death.

Excessive hypotension secondary to nitroprusside administration can be avoided by careful monitoring using an arterial line and frequent clinical evaluations. In general, blood pressure reduction should not exceed a 25 percent reduction in mean arterial pressure. Thiocyanate toxicity can be minimized by avoiding prolonged administration of nitroprusside and by limiting drug use in patients with renal insufficiency. If necessary, thiocyanate can be removed by dialysis. Cyanide toxicity can be avoided by the coadministration of sodium thiosulfate or by limiting the administration of nitroprusside. Details of the treatment of cyanide toxicity are discussed in Chapter 182, "Cyanide."

REFERENCES

1. Joint National Committee on Detection, Evaluation, and Treatment of High Blood Pressure: The sixth report of the Joint National Committee on Detection, Evaluation, and Treatment of High Blood Pressure. *Arch Intern Med* 157:2413, 1997.
2. Litovitz TL: Annual report of the American Association of Poison Control Centers Toxic Exposure Surveillance System. *Am J Emerg Med* 16:443, 1997.
3. Center for Substance Abuse Treatment: *Treatment Improvement Protocol Series January 1, 1995*. Washington, DC, US Department of Health and Human Services, Public Health Service, 1995; Copyright 8.
4. Roberge RJ: Yohimbine as an antidote for clonidine overdose. *Am J Emerg Med* 14:678, 1996.

PHENYTOIN AND FOSPHENYTOIN TOXICITY

Harold H. Osborn

It is estimated that over 2 million Americans suffer from epilepsy, and as many as 10 percent of the population may suffer at least one seizure in their lifetime. Phenytoin is a primary anticonvulsant for all types of epilepsy except absence. It is useful in the treatment of status epilepticus in conjunction with other more rapidly acting anticonvulsants.[1] Phenytoin has been used prophylactically in a variety of settings (head trauma, alcohol withdrawal, and drug overdose) but has so far only proven useful in the setting of head trauma.

Phenytoin has been employed in the management of chronic pain syndromes. Historically, it has also been used as an antidysrhythmic agent, especially in the setting of digoxin toxicity, but it is no longer considered a first-line agent. Morbidity or mortality is unusual following intentional phenytoin overdose if good supportive care is provided. Most phenytoin-related deaths have been caused by rapid intravenous administration or hypersensitivity reactions.

Data from the American Association of Poison Control Centers (AAPCC) regarding exposures are almost certainly underestimates, in that major toxicity related to oral preparations is more likely to be reported from parenteral adverse events and minor drug reactions related to oral preparations. Still, in 1997, a total of 4630 exposures were reported, of which 56 percent were unintentional, 32 percent intentional, 8 percent adverse reactions, and the rest "other." Among these exposures, 25 percent were considered inconsequential, 22 percent minor, 13 percent moderate, and less than 2 percent major. Only two deaths were reported.[2]

MECHANISM OF ACTION

Phenytoin exerts its anticonvulsant effect by blocking voltage-sensitive and frequency-dependent sodium channels in the neurons. Phenytoin stabilizes sodium channels in an inactive state, and this inhibitory effect, similar to the action of local anesthetics, is dependent on the voltage and frequency of firing of the neuron. Phenytoin has no effect on the amplitude or duration of the action potential. Rather, it limits the ability of the neuron to fire trains of action potentials at high frequency by delaying recovery. In this fashion, it suppresses repetitive neuronal activity and prevents the spread of a seizure focus. At higher concentrations, phenytoin delays activation of outward potassium currents in nerves and prolongs the neuronal refractory period. It may also exert an anticonvulsant effect by influencing calcium channels or γ-aminobutyric acid (GABA) receptors, although this is not yet fully established.

PATHOPHYSIOLOGY

The toxic effects of phenytoin vary with route administration, duration of exposure, and dosage used. Of these determinants of toxicity, the most important is the route of administration. The intravenous administration of phenytoin carries the greatest risk, in large part due to the other constituents of the parenteral vehicle (see the section "Effects of Propylene Glycol and Ethanol Diluents"). The most serious reactions following intravenous administration are cardiovascular (bradycardia, hypotension, and asystole), although tissue necrosis and sloughing following extravasation have been described.[3] Major cardiac toxicity occurs only following parenteral administration; in general, oral overdose does not lead to cardiovascular morbidity.[4] It is more common in the elderly and those with underlying cardiac disease but has been described in young healthy patients, as well.

Many of the side effects of the oral preparation are dose related and are predictable at higher plasma concentrations. Still, different people have differing tolerance profiles, and adverse effects can be evident in some at seemingly therapeutic doses, whereas others may display untoward effects well beyond the therapeutic range. Early toxicity is manifested by vestibular/ocular/cerebellar signs: nystagmus, dysdiadochokinesia, and ataxia. At higher levels, central nervous system (CNS) depression and other cognitive effects (confusion, dizziness, and loss of concentration and memory) are seen. Only two areas of the brain normally exhibit spontaneous neuronal burst discharge: the hippocampus and the cerebellum. Phenytoin's ability to suppress these areas may result in impaired memory and balance, respectively. Paradoxically, very high levels of phenytoin may be associated with seizures. Acute oral overdose is usually manifested by nystagmus, nausea and vomiting, ataxia, dysarthria, choreoathetosis, opisthotonos, and CNS depression or excitation.[5] Deaths from oral ingestion of phenytoin are extremely rare and occur in association with ingestion of other substances.[6] The chronic administration of phenytoin is associated with numerous side effects that involve a variety of organ systems. Many of these are dose and duration dependent, but some are idiosyncratic. Hypersensitivity reactions to phenytoin usually occur within the first few months of therapy and include fever, skin rashes, blood dyscrasia, and, rarely, hepatitis. Deaths due to Stevens-Johnson syndrome have occurred, and anyone with this syndrome should never receive phenytoin again.

PHARMACOKINETICS

Phenytoin is a weak acid with a pKa of 8.3. Thus, in the acid milieu of the stomach, and even at physiologic pH, its aqueous solubility is limited. The parenteral form of phenytoin is adjusted to pH 12 to keep the drug in solution, but it is very irritating to the tissues, and intramuscular injections result in local precipitation of phenytoin with erratic absorption and is, therefore, not recommended. Absorption after oral ingestion is slow, variable, and often incomplete, especially following an overdose. Consequently, it is necessary to obtain serial levels in suspected overdose, to determine peak levels. Significant differences in bioavailability exist among different phenytoin preparations. Peak levels typically occur anywhere from 3 to 12 h after a *single* oral dose.

Following absorption, phenytoin is distributed throughout the body with a volume of distribution of 0.6 L/kg. Brain tissue concentrations equal those in plasma within about 10 min of intravenous infusion and correlate with therapeutic effects, whereas cerebrospinal fluid and myocardium equilibrate within 30 to 60 min. At steady state, concentrations are higher in neural tissue than in the serum. Within the CNS, concentrations are higher in the brainstem and cerebellum than in the cerebral cortex.

PROTEIN BINDING AND FREE PHENYTOIN FRACTIONS

Phenytoin is extensively (90 percent) bound to plasma proteins, especially albumin. The free, unbound, form is the biologically active moiety responsible for the drug's clinical effect and toxicity. The free phenytoin fraction normally constitutes 10 percent of the plasma level. The unbound fraction of the drug is greater in the following groups of patients: neonates; the elderly; pregnant women; individuals with uremia, hypoalbuminemia (cirrhosis, nephrosis, malnutrition, burns, trauma, or cystic fibrosis), and hyperbilirubinemia; and individuals taking drugs that displace phenytoin from binding sites (salicylate, valproate, phenylbutazone, tolbutamide, and sulfisoxazole).

Although patients with decreased protein binding may have higher levels of free phenytoin and a greater biologic effect, they may have lower levels of total phenytoin, since more of the drug is available for metabolism. Theoretically, such patients may become toxic with total phenytoin levels in the therapeutic range. Patients who exhibit toxic signs in the therapeutic range and those with decreased protein binding should have free phenytoin levels measured.

Phenytoin concentrations are most commonly measured by an enzyme-mediated immunoassay (EMIT) technique, which is specific and sensitive to less than 1 μg/mL. If available, free phenytoin concentrations are more useful to predict toxicity. Corrected serum phenytoin levels can be calculated in hypoproteinemic patients with a known serum albumin level. To calculate the phenytoin concentration (C_{normal}) that would be present if a patient's serum albumin were normal, the following equation is used:

$$C_{normal} = \frac{C_{measured} \times 4.4}{\text{albumin concentration}}$$

where phenytoin concentrations are in micrograms per milliliter and albumin concentration is in grams per deciliter.

METABOLISM

Following absorption and distribution, only 4 to 5 percent of phenytoin is excreted unchanged in the urine. The remainder is metabolized by hepatic microsomal enzymes. The drug is primarily hydroxylated to a series of inactive compounds. The major (60 to 70 percent) metabolite is the parahydroxyphenyl derivative. It is glucuronidated, secreted in the bile, reabsorbed, and subsequently excreted in the urine. Phenytoin is not appreciably removed by hemodialysis or hemoperfusion. The metabolism of phenytoin is capacity limited (dose dependent). At plasma concentrations below 10 μg/mL, elimination is first order (a fixed percentage of drug metabolized per unit of time). However, at higher concentrations, including those in the therapeutic range (10 to 20 μg/mL), the metabolic pathways may become saturated, and the elimination may change to zero-order kinetics (a fixed amount metabolized per unit of time). This change in kinetics can markedly prolong the half-life of phenytoin, which is normally 6 to 24 h. An understanding of capacity-limited kinetics is essential to the proper dosing of phenytoin, the avoidance of side effects with chronic therapy, and the management of overdoses. At higher levels in the therapeutic range, any increase in the daily dose may result in a disproportionate increase in the plasma level. Thus, incremental doses should be limited to 30 mg and levels should be carefully monitored when it is necessary to raise phenytoin doses above 300 mg (about 5 mg/kg) per day.

Because phenytoin's half-life is 24 h or less, once-a-day regimens may result in erratic levels and become problematic for patients requiring tight control. Only one phenytoin preparation (Phenytoin Kapseals)

TABLE 172-1 Phenytoin-Drug Interactions

Phenytoin *increases* serum level of	
Acetaminophen	
Oral anticoagulants	
Primidone	
Phenytoin *decreases* serum level of	
Amiodarone	Disopyramide
Carbamazepine	Mexiletine
Levodopa	Doxycycline
Methadone	Furosemide
Contraceptives	Quinidine
Glucocorticoids	Theophylline
Cyclosporine	Valproic acid
Phenytoin levels are *increased* by	
Amiodarone	Fluconazole
Oral anticoagulants	Phenylbutazone*
Chloramphenicol	Sulfonamides*
Isoniazid	Valproic acid*
Cimetidine	High-dose salicylate*
Disulfiram	Tolbutamide*
Trimethoprim	
Phenytoin levels are *decreased* by	
Antineoplastic drugs	Theophylline
Diazoxide	Phenobarbital
Folic acid	Diazepam
Rifampin	Ethanol
Sucralfate	Calcium

*These drugs displace phenytoin from its protein-binding sites, thus increasing the free phenytoin fraction, although the total phenytoin level may *decrease.*

is approved by the Food and Drug Administration for once-a-day use. Concomitant use of drugs that either inhibit or enhance hepatic microsomal activity may result in an increase or decrease of phenytoin level, respectively. Phenytoin also affects the metabolism of various other agents (Table 172-1).

EFFECTS OF PROPYLENE GLYCOL AND ETHANOL DILUENTS

The acute cardiovascular toxicity seen with intravenous phenytoin infusion has frequently been ascribed to its diluent. The vehicle for the older parenteral formulation of phenytoin (Dilantin) is 40% propylene glycol and 10% ethanol, adjusted to a pH of 12 with sodium hydroxide. The glycol component has been shown to cause coma, seizures, circulatory collapse, ventricular dysrhythmias, atrioventricular (AV) node depression, and hypotension in human and animals.[7] Propylene glycol is a strong myocardial depressant and vasodilator and increases vagal tone. Other toxic effects of propylene glycol include hyperosmolality, hemolysis, and lactate-associated metabolic acidosis. Louis and colleagues compared the acute toxicities of intravenous phenytoin and propylene glycol both alone and in combination in a feline model. Phenytoin alone did cause hypotension but did not cause significant electrocardiographic effects and instead partially reversed the toxic effects that occurred when propylene glycol was given.[8] Acute toxic effects of propylene glycol are also strongly related to the rate of infusion. This is further evidence for its role in intravenous phenytoin toxicity, a phenomenon that is almost always related to infusion rate. The ethanol diluent fraction of parenteral phenytoin may also precipitate a reaction in patients taking disulfiram. The preparation with glycol is still available in the United States (although the original manufacturer no longer makes it). With intravenous infusion pumps controlling rate of administration, adverse effects are not as common, and phenytoin is less expensive compared with the alternative (see below).

The limitations of this parenteral form of phenytoin (incomplete aqueous solubility, irritating nature of the vehicle, and tendency to precipitate in intravenous solutions) have prompted a search for a more suitable preparation. Recently, a prodrug of phenytoin (fosphenytoin) has been synthesized that is more soluble and less irritating to the tissues. Fosphenytoin is the disodium phosphate ester of phenytoin. It is freely soluble in aqueous solutions and is formulated with TRIS buffer only at a pH of 8.8. Fosphenytoin is converted to phenytoin by phosphatases in the blood and various organs. For simplicity, the concentration and dose of fosphenytoin are expressed in phenytoin equivalents (PEs). The conversion half-life is 10 to 15 min.[9] Fosphenytoin is tolerated intravenously and intramuscularly, and patients can be successfully loaded within 30 min with one or more intramuscular injections without significant side effects.[10]

Given intravenously, fosphenytoin can cause pruritis and hypotension. It is not clear whether fosphenytoin administered intravenously can result in therapeutic levels more quickly and with fewer side effects than intravenous phenytoin. Blood pressure and cardiac monitoring are recommended when loading with fosphenytoin intravenously but not intramuscularly. The adverse and toxic effects of fosphenytoin are the same as with phenytoin, except that the effects of glycol and ethanol are not present with fosphenytoin.

SERUM LEVELS AND RANGE OF TOXICITY

Therapeutic phenytoin levels are described as being 10 to 20 μg/mL (40 to 80 μmol/L), with a free phenytoin level of 1 to 2 μg/mL.[11] Although 50 percent of seizure patients achieve reduction of seizure frequency with amounts below these levels, some patients require levels above 20 μg/mL for adequate seizure control. The therapeutic range for phenytoin is rather narrow. However, some patients have a greater propensity for side effects than others. Individual variation in toxicity is a function of baseline neurologic status, individual response to the drug, and free drug fraction. Patients with underlying brain disease are predisposed to toxicity and may become toxic at low levels. Long-term therapy must be individualized and based on clinical response, drug levels, and signs of toxicity. In general, toxicity correlates fairly well with increasing plasma levels (Table 173-2), but this is not a universal tenet as some patients tolerate levels above 40 μg/mL quite well. Nystagmus usually appears first at a phenytoin level of 20 μg/mL but may occur at lower or higher levels. Almost all patients with phenytoin-induced seizures will have levels well above 30 μg/mL. Signs of toxicity occur at free phenytoin levels of 2.0 μg/mL and are consistently severe above 5.0 μg/mL.

TABLE 172-2 Correlation of Plasma Phenytoin Level and Side Effects

Plasma Level (μ/mL)	Side Effects
<10	Usually none
10–20	Occasional mild nystagmus
20–30	Nystagmus
30–40	Ataxia, slurred speech, nausea and vomiting
40–50	Lethargy, confusion
>50	Coma, seizures

CLINICAL FEATURES

Central Nervous System Toxicity

As toxic phenytoin levels are reached, both inhibitory cortical and excitatory cerebellar-vestibular effects begin to occur. The usual initial sign of toxicity is nystagmus, which is seen first on forced lateral gaze and then becomes spontaneous. Vertical, bidirectional, or alternating nystagmus may occur with severe intoxication. A decreased level of consciousness is common with initial sedation, lethargy, ataxic gait, and dysarthria progressing to confusion, coma, and even apnea in large overdose. Chronically impaired cognitive function or acute encephalopathy may occur. Nystagmus may disappear at levels sufficient to cause coma and complete ophthalmoplegia and loss of corneal reflexes may occur. Therefore, absence of nystagmus does not exclude severe phenytoin toxicity. Nystagmus then returns as serum drug levels decrease and coma lightens.

Phenytoin-induced seizures are usually brief and are usually generalized. They are quite rare and almost always preceded by other signs of toxicity, especially in acute overdose.[12] Cerebellar stimulation and alteration in dopaminergic and serotonergic activity may be responsible for acute dystonias and movement disorders such as opisthotonos and choreoathetosis. Either depressed or hyperactive deep tendon reflexes, clonus, and extensor toe responses may also be elicited. Some signs of neurologic toxicity may outlast the presence of drug by months, especially mild peripheral neuropathy or acute reversible cerebellar degeneration with ataxia.

Cardiovascular Toxicity

Cardiac toxicity after oral phenytoin overdose in an otherwise healthy patient has not been reported and, if observed, requires assessment for other causes (e.g., hypoxia and other drugs). Cardiovascular complications have been almost entirely limited to cases of intravenous administration. Complications include hypotension with decreased peripheral vascular resistance, bradycardia, conduction delays progressing to complete AV nodal block, ventricular tachycardia, primary ventricular fibrillation, and asystole. Electrocardiographic changes include increased PR interval, widened QRS interval, and altered ST-segments and T-waves. Bradycardia, hypotension, and syncope in healthy volunteers have been reported even after small undiluted intravenous doses. Some of these complications can be attributed to rapid intravenous administration of the preparation containing propylene glycol and are avoidable with cautious administration (Table 172-3). Even slowly administered intravenous phenytoin (less than 25 mg/min) has also been reported to cause arrest in critically ill patients receiving dopamine infusions to support blood pressure.

Vascular, Extravasation, and Soft Tissue Toxicity

Intramuscular injection of phenytoin results in localized crystallization of the drug, and hematoma, sterile abscess, and myonecrosis at the injection site. Complications after intravenous infusion have included skin and soft tissue necrosis requiring skin grafting, and compartment syndrome, gangrene, amputation, and death. A syndrome of delayed bluish discoloration of the affected extremity, followed by erythema, edema, vesicles, bullae, and local tissue ischemia, has also been described.[13] The propylene glycol diluent, strong alkalinity of the intravenous solution, and crystallization of the drug contribute. Fosphenytoin by contrast, is well tolerated when given IV or IM.

Hypersensitivity Reactions

Hypersensitivity reactions usually occur within 1 to 6 weeks of beginning phenytoin therapy and can include fever, systemic lupus erythematosus, erythema multiforme, toxic epidermal neurolysis, Stevens-Johnson syndrome, hepatitis, rhabdomyolysis, acute interstitial pneumonitis, lymphadenopathy, leukopenia, disseminated intravascular coagulation, and renal failure. One should always ask about a history of previous hypersensitivity reactions before deciding to restart phenytoin in the emergency department setting.

Miscellaneous Effects

Other side effects from phenytoin include gingival hyperplasia, hirsutism, hypocalcemia, megaloblastic anemia responsive to folate administration, lymphoma, and hemorrhagic disease of the newborn responsive to vitamin K (Table 172-4). Gingival hyperplasia is so common, its absence should suggest poor compliance. Another clinically significant effect in some is hyperglycemia, felt to be secondary to inhibition of insulin release. This can lead to diabetic ketoacidosis or nonketotic hyperosmolar coma in diabetics. The teratogenic fetal hydantoin syndrome is well described, so oral phenytoin therapy in a pregnant patient should never be initiated or continued by an emergency physician without consultation and close follow-up from an attending neurologist and obstetrician.

DIFFERENTIAL DIAGNOSIS

Intoxication with almost any CNS-active or sedative-hypnotic drug may mimic early phenytoin intoxication, especially ethanol, carbamazepine, benzodiazepines, barbiturates, and lithium. Disease states resembling phenytoin toxicity include hypoglycemia, Wernicke encephalopathy, and posterior fossa hemorrhage or tumor. Although seizures may be caused by phenytoin at toxic levels, other epileptogenic drug overdoses and seizures due to trauma and to drug and alcohol withdrawal should be considered first.

TREATMENT

Initial general treatment of severe oral phenytoin overdose, including intravenous access and airway management, is similar to that for other ingested drugs. Respiratory acidosis due to ventilatory insufficiency or metabolic acidosis from any cause should be corrected to decrease the active free phenytoin fraction. Multiple doses of oral activated

TABLE 172-3 Guidelines for Safe Phenytoin Loading

Intravenous
- Loading dose is 18 mg/kg phenytoin or phenytoin equivalents (PEs)
- Mix total dose in 150–200 mL of normal saline (keep concentration ≤6.7 mg/mL)
- Administer phenytoin through Millipore filter using an infusion pump
- Rate of administration should not exceed 30 mg/min (less in patients with cardiovascular disease)
- Monitor the blood pressure and cardiac rhythm continually during the infusion
- In the event of complications, immediately stop the infusion and administer isotonic crystalloid and other treatment as indicated

Intramuscular
- Administer 15 mg/kg PEs of the fosphenytoin preparation in either one or multiple intramuscular sites

Oral*
- Loading dose is 20 mg/kg
- Phenytoin tablets or suspension may be used
- Patient must be conscious with an intact gag reflex and not actively seizing or vomiting
- Administer the total amount in one dose

*Unlike intravenous loading, not all patients orally loaded will reach a therapeutic level.

TABLE 172-4 Toxicity of Phenytoin

Central nervous system Dizziness, tremor (intention), visual disturbance, horizontal and vertical nystagmus, diplopia, miosis or mydriasis, ophthalmoplegia, abnormal gait (bradykinesia, truncal ataxia), choreoathetoid movements, vomiting, dysphagia, respiratory distress, irritability, agitation, confusion, hallucinations, fatigue coma, death (rare), encephalopathy, pseudodegenerative disease, dysarthria, meningeal irritation with pleocytosis, seizures (rare)
Peripheral nervous system Peripheral neuropathy, urinary incontinence
Hypersensitivity reactions Eosinophilia, rash, pseudolymphoma (diffuse lymphadenopathy), systemic lupus erythematosus, pancytopenia
Gastrointestinal Nausea and vomiting, hepatotoxicity
Skin Hirsutism, acne, rashes (including Stevens-Johnson syndrome)
Other Fetal hydantoin syndrome, gingival hyperplasia, coarsening of facial features
Parenteral preparations May cause hypotension, bradycardia, conduction disturbances, myocardial depression, ventricular fibrillation, asystole, and sloughing of tissues

charcoal (1 g/kg) within the first 24 h may be of benefit, given the known poor solubility and resultant extended absorptive phase of oral phenytoin in overdose.[14] Hemodialysis and hemoperfusion are of no clinical benefit in phenytoin poisoning. Seizures may be treated with intravenous benzodiazepines or phenobarbital, again with the caution that seizures are not common in phenytoin overdose and other causes must be ruled out. Cardiovascular toxicity is extremely rare in oral overdose and should suggest other etiologies.

Prolonged cardiac monitoring after oral ingestion is unnecessary. Atropine and temporary cardiac pacing may be used for symptomatic bradydysrhythmias associated with intravenous phenytoin. Hypotension that occurs during intravenous administration of phenytoin usually responds to discontinuation of the infusion and the administration of isotonic crystalloid. Hospital admission and appropriate orthopedic or plastic surgery consultation should be obtained for patients with any significant extravasation of intravenous phenytoin or other signs of local vascular or tissue toxicity after infusion. To minimize complications due to infusion, intravenous phenytoin and fosphenytoin should be administered under close observation, with constant cardiac and blood pressure monitoring. The infused solution should be given slowly (less than 30 mg phenytoin or 150 mg fosphenytoin PEs/min) through a large, well-positioned catheter.

ADMISSION CONSIDERATIONS

Patients with serious complications following an oral ingestion (seizures, coma, altered mental status, ataxia, etc.) should be admitted for further evaluation and treatment. Others with only mild symptoms may be treated with activated charcoal in the emergency department and discharged after their levels have returned to normal, provided they are not actively suicidal. Prolonged observation and frequent assessment of levels is not practical in many emergency departments. Thus, patients with continuing symptoms may need to be admitted or their case followed in an observation unit. Given the long and erratic absorption phase of phenytoin after oral overdose, the decision to discharge or medically clear a patient for psychiatric evaluation cannot be based on a single serum level. Patients with symptomatic chronic intoxication should be admitted for observation unless signs are minimal, adequate care can be obtained at home, and they are 8 to 12 h from their last therapeutic dose. Phenytoin therapy should be stopped in all cases and, if toxicity continues to resolve, a serum level may be reassessed in 2 to 3 days to guide resumption of therapy.

Patients with significant or persistent complications following the intravenous administration of phenytoin should be admitted. Those with transient effects need not be.

REFERENCES

1. Working Group on Status Epilepticus: Treatment of convulsive status. *JAMA* 270:854, 1993.
2. Litovitz TL, Klein-Schwarz W, Dyer KS, et al: 1997 Annual report of the American Association of Poison Control Centers Toxic Exposure Surveillance System. *Am J Emerg Med* 16:443, 1998.
3. Earnest MP, Mark JA, Drury LR: Complications of intravenous phenytoin for acute treatment of seizures. *JAMA* 249:762, 1983.
4. Wyte CD, Berk WA: Severe oral phenytoin overdose does not cause cardiovascular morbidity. *Ann Emerg Med* 20:508, 1991.
5. Mellick LB, Morgan JA, Mellick GA: Presentations of acute phenytoin overdose. *Am J Emerg Med* 7:61, 1989.
6. Berry DJ, Wiseman HM, Volans GN: A survey of non-barbiturate anticonvulsant drug overdose. *Hum Toxicol* 2:357, 1983.
7. Gross DR, Kitzman JV, Adams HR: Cardiovascular effects of intravenous administration of propylene glycol in calves. *Am J Vet Res* 40:783, 1979.
8. Louis S, Kutt H: The cardiocirculatory changes caused by intravenous Dilantin and its solvent. *Am Heart J* 74:523, 1967.
9. Eldon MA, Loewen GR, Voigtman RE: Pharmacokinetics and tolerance of fosphenytoin and phenytoin administered intravenously to healthy subjects. *Can J Neurol Sci* 20(suppl):180, 1993.
10. Dean JC, Smith KR: Safety, tolerance, and pharmacokinetics of intramuscular fosphenytoin in neurosurgery patients. *Epilepsia* 34(suppl 6):111, 1993.
11. McNamara JO: Drugs effective in the therapy of epilepsies, in Hardman JG, Limbird LE (eds): *Goodman and Gilman's The Pharmacological Basis of Therapeutics,* 9th ed. New York, McGraw-Hill, 1996, pp 461–486.
12. Osorio I, Burnstein TH, Pemler B: Phenytoin induced seizures: A paradoxical effect at toxic concentrations in phenytoin patients. *Epilepsia* 30:230, 1989.
13. Hanna DR: Purple glove syndrome: A complication of intravenous phenytoin. *J Neurosci Nurs* 24:340, 1992.
14. Howard CE, Roberts S, Ely DS: Use of multiple-dose activated charcoal in phenytoin toxicity. *Ann Pharmacother* 28:201, 1994.

IRON

Joseph G. Rella
Lewis S. Nelson

PHYSIOLOGY

Iron is essential to life for humans. Iron is incorporated into red cells, hemoglobin, myoglobin, cytochromes, and other enzymes and cofactors. Since excess iron is toxic, the body utilizes several mechanisms to maintain appropriate iron availability while preventing toxicity. These mechanisms include serum protein binding, intracellular storage and, most importantly, regulation of gastrointestinal (GI) absorption.

The oral bioavailability of inorganic iron is less than 10 percent, and ferrous iron (Fe^{+2}) is better absorbed than ferric (Fe^{+3}) iron. Chelated iron, most readily found in heme, is best absorbed, accounting for one beneficial effect of eating meat. In the duodenum and jejunum, a mucosal carrier protein takes up iron and immediately stores it as ferritin. In times of iron need, the body produces transferrin, which removes iron from the cells. Alternatively, the iron is stored in the intestinal cell and is eventually eliminated from the body when the mucosa is sloughed. This is the principle mechanism for limiting absorption, and failure of this mechanism is critical following iron overdose.

Transferrin, the carrier protein that binds ferric iron, is the major mechanism for safe iron transport through the body. The total iron-binding capacity (TIBC) primarily measures the amount of serum transferrin. The TIBC is generally two to three times the normal iron concentration.

Ferritin is a large intracellular storage protein that can reversibly bind as many as 4500 molecules of iron. When an iron deficit exists, iron is transported from ferritin and the GI tract to the liver, spleen, and bone marrow, where it is incorporated into appropriate molecules.[1]

PATHOPHYSIOLOGY

Iron is a direct GI irritant and causes vomiting, diarrhea, and abdominal pain soon after a significant ingestion. Mucosal ulceration and bleeding, as well as intestinal perforation, may also occur. Hypovolemia from GI losses may produce hypotension, tissue hypoperfusion, and metabolic acidosis (based on tissue ischemia). As the mucosal surface is injured, iron passes unimpeded into the blood. When the ability of transferrin to combine with iron is exhausted, *free iron* becomes available. Free iron enters the mitochondria and inhibits oxidative phosphorylation to produce metabolic acidosis. Iron also participates in the production of toxic hydroxyl free radicals and subsequent membrane lipid peroxidation. Other systemic findings of iron poisoning include coagulopathy through inhibition of serum proteases,[2] myocardial dysfunction,[3] and encephalopathy. Coagulopathy may be biphasic, with prolonged prothrombin time and partial thromboplastin time within the first 24 h[2] that appear reversible with chelation therapy as free iron initially interferes with the activity of factors in the coagulation cascade. Later, as iron poisoning causes hepatic injury, factor production decreases, potentially worsening the coagulopathy.

TOXIC DOSE

Similar to most exposures, larger ingestions are more likely associated with greater toxicity. However, it is the amount of ingested elemental iron that determines a patient's potential for experiencing toxicity. Since the fraction of elemental iron varies with different preparations, it is important to determine which of these was ingested. These fractions may range from 12 to 33 percent, with ferrous sulfate containing 20 percent elemental iron (e.g., a 325-mg tablet of ferrous sulfate contains 60 mg of elemental iron). Pediatric multivitamins may contain from 10 to 18 mg of elemental iron per tablet. Toxic effects have been reported following oral doses as low as 10 and 20 mg/kg elemental iron.

In general, moderate toxicity occurs at doses of 20 to 60 mg/kg, and severe toxicity can be expected following doses of greater than 60 mg/kg.[4] These guidelines can be useful in predicting potential toxicity based on the history of ingestion. The majority of exposures, however, involve children under age 6, who mostly remain asymptomatic or develop only minimal toxicity.

LABORATORY ASSESSMENT

Serum iron levels have been used to determine toxicity and to direct management, but this use is limited, since excess iron is toxic intracellularly and not in the blood. In general, serum iron levels between 300 and 500 μg/dL correlate with significant GI toxicity, and mild systemic toxicity and serum iron levels between 500 and 1000 μg/dL correlate with moderate systemic toxicity. Levels greater than 1000 μg/dL are associated with significant morbidity. Although high serum iron levels support the potential for toxicity, low levels do not connote its absence. Other potential pitfalls in utilizing serum iron levels to predict toxicity include variable times to peak level following ingestion of different iron preparations[5,6] and artifactually lower measured iron levels in the presence of deferoxamine.

Leukocytosis and hyperglycemia have also been examined for their ability to predict iron toxicity. One early study found that a white blood cell count (WBC) of greater than 15,000/μL with glucose level of greater than 150 mg/dL correlated with an iron level of more than 300 μg/dL.[7] This study, however, assumed that a serum iron level of greater than 300 μg/dL denoted toxicity, which is not true in all cases. Subsequent studies were unable to validate the association between these laboratory values and also did not correlate these laboratory values with clinical illness.[8,9]

It was previously accepted that toxicity was not likely when the serum iron level did not exceed the TIBC. Although conceptually valid, TIBC has little value in the assessment of iron-poisoned patients, because it becomes falsely elevated in the presence of elevated serum iron levels or deferoxamine.[10] Additionally, in conditions of chronic iron overload (e.g., thalassemia and hemochromatosis), significant organ pathology occurs despite the TIBC remaining higher than serum iron level.

Use of radiographic studies can lead to diagnostic problems, as well. Radiopaque iron tablets are visible on x-ray and can guide GI decontamination when visualized. However, many iron preparations are not routinely detected, including pediatric chewable and liquid preparations, and negative radiographs do not exclude iron ingestion.[9]

CLINICAL FEATURES

Clinically, five stages of toxicity have been described corresponding to the pathophysiology of iron poisoning although, more practically, acute iron toxicity manifests in two clinical stages: local GI toxicity and systemic toxicity.

Abdominal pain, vomiting, and diarrhea characterize stage 1 of iron poisoning. Iron is directly irritating and corrosive to the GI tract and typically induces vomiting within the first few hours following ingestion. The absence of these symptoms within 6 h of ingestion essentially excludes a diagnosis of significant iron ingestion. Vomiting is the clinical sign most consistently associated with acute iron toxicity.[7–9]

Stage 2, or the ''latent'' stage, of iron poisoning is not always seen. Occurring within the 6- to 24-h period following ingestion, GI symptoms may resolve, so a patient may have few, if any, symptoms, which may falsely reassure a physician. However, this is not a truly quiescent phase. Patients who have significant toxicity will have ongoing and perhaps progressive systemic deterioration due to volume loss and worsening metabolic acidosis, despite the absence of GI symptoms. Patients may not vomit but will still be clinically ill, and may have abnormal vital signs and evidence of poor tissue perfusion. Patients with large ingestions may progress directly from GI distress (stage 1) to signs of systemic toxicity (stage 3). Alternatively, symptoms in patients with limited ingestions may resolve completely prior to this phase. These latter patients will have normal vital signs and normal findings on physical examination.

Systemic toxicity characterizes stage 3 of iron toxicity. During this stage, intracellular iron disrupts cellular metabolism with resultant shock and (lactic) acidosis. Iron-induced coagulopathy may worsen bleeding and hypovolemia. Hepatic dysfunction, renal failure, and cardiomyopathy may also occur.

The hepatic stage of iron poisoning (stage 4) develops 2 to 5 days after ingestion. Thought to result from iron uptake by the reticuloendothelial system, it manifests as elevation of aminotransferases and may progress to frank hepatic failure.

Stage 5 of iron poisoning refers to delayed sequelae, including gastric outlet obstruction secondary to the corrosive effects of iron on the mucosa. These changes present only rarely and are seen 4 to 6 weeks after ingestion.

TREATMENT

Evaluation and Supportive Care

Iron poisoning is a clinical diagnosis. Patients who arrive at an emergency department asymptomatic and with normal findings on physical examination, and who remain so for 6 h following ingestion, do not require specific medical treatment for iron poisoning. Patients who are symptomatic from their ingestion should first be stabilized with attention to airway, breathing, and circulation, after which GI decontamination and chelation therapy may proceed. Dialysis is not effective in clearing iron.

In general, patients whose vomiting resolves after two or three episodes, and who have normal vital signs, are mildly iron toxic and require only supportive care. Patients who continue to vomit (i.e., five to six or more times), or who have moderately abnormal vital signs, have moderate iron toxicity, and deferoxamine therapy may be indicated. Those patients with persistent vomiting and severely abnormal vital signs or other signs of poor perfusion or shock should be aggressively fluid resuscitated and treated with deferoxamine.

Intravenous (IV) fluid resuscitation and medication, as appropriate, should be initiated in those patients who are symptomatic or show signs of hypoperfusion or shock. Coagulopathy should be addressed with parenteral vitamin K_1 (5 to 25 mg) and fresh-frozen plasma (10 to 25 mL/kg in adults; 10 mL/kg in pediatric patients). Significant blood loss may require transfusion.

Laboratory tests should include complete blood cell count and determination of serum electrolyte level, blood urea nitrogen, and coagulation parameters, as well as serum glucose and serum iron levels, with the understanding that the importance of these values may be limited.

Arterial blood-gas (ABG) determination is usually unnecessary in mild cases because determination of serum electrolytes will yield all important information. However, in the moderately to severely toxic patient, or in those with respiratory compromise, ABG determination, often more rapidly available, will yield vital information regarding the patient's acid-base status. Typing, screening, and crossmatching should be requested from the blood bank in anticipation of potential need.

Gastrointestinal Decontamination

In general, syrup of ipecac is not used, because it may obscure the initial signs of clinical toxicity. Additionally, ipecac-induced vomiting is not thought to be more effective at gastric emptying than is iron-induced vomiting. Activated charcoal does not adsorb significantly to iron, and its use is not recommended in cases of isolated iron ingestion. Its use may also complicate endoscopy, should that be necessary. Cathartics should not be used. Orogastric lavage may not be effective if the ingested tablets are large or if several hours have elapsed since ingestion, but it may be used early after ingestion. Instillation of bicarbonate solution following gastric lavage has been advocated on the basis that free ferrous salt is converted into poorly absorbed ferrous carbonate. There are no data to support the efficacy of sodium bicarbonate or phosphosoda instillation during lavage to prevent iron absorption. Pills located on radiograph may indicate a potential for progressive toxicity and may guide decontamination.

Whole bowel irrigation with a polyethylene glycol solution has demonstrated efficacy in several pediatric patients with large iron ingestions. Administration of 250 to 500 mL/h in children and 2 L/h in adults via nasogastric tube may clear the GI tract of iron pills before absorption can occur. Endoscopy has been used to remove large iron loads but may not be practical where there are large numbers of pills requiring multiple endoscope insertions. Gastrotomy may also be an option where other measures are unsuccessful or impractical.[11] Antiemetics such as metoclopramide or ondansetron can be used to treat nausea and vomiting.

Deferoxamine

Deferoxamine is a specific chelating agent derived from *Streptomyces pilosus* and has been used to treat iron toxicity since the 1960s. Deferoxamine binds directly to free iron and indirectly to iron from ferritin, hemosiderin, and non-protein-bound ferric salts, as well as to intracytoplasmic and mitochondrial free iron to form the complex ferrioxamine, which is renally excreted. It is safely administered to children and pregnant women. Complete complexation of ingested iron is not the goal of therapy. Indeed, only a small fraction of the total amount of ingested iron is found in the urine following chelation. Deferoxamine administration may be a clinically effective treatment by removing a critical amount of intracellular iron from its target, restoring cellular function.

Deferoxamine can be administered by various routes. Oral deferoxamine is not recommended due to the risk of increased GI absorption of iron-deferoxamine complex and enhanced toxicity. Deferoxamine may be administered subcutaneously but only in cases of chronic iron overload. Patients with mild iron toxicity from an acute ingestion may be treated with intramuscular (IM) administration of deferoxamine 90 mg/kg up to 1 g in children and 2 g in adults. The dose may be repeated every 4 to 6 h as clinically indicated (see below). This route of administration, however, can become difficult due to the volume of injected material required when used in children.

In patients with severe iron poisoning, fluid loss and hypovolemia may become significant. Since these patients require aggressive fluid resuscitation and since more consistent absorption of deferoxamine is achieved parenterally, therapy should be given IV, because this addresses both issues at once. Additionally, IM deferoxamine is not reliably absorbed in hypotensive patients. Hypotension is the rate-limiting factor in IV administration, and it is recommended to begin the infusion slowly (5 mg/kg/h). A second IV access will likely be required so as not to impede simple volume resuscitation. Deferoxamine can be increased to 15 mg/kg/h within the first hour of treatment, as tolerated. In fact, much higher doses have been used safely to achieve appropriate chelant excess before systemic toxicity occurred. However, it is generally not recommended to exceed a total daily dose of 6 to 8 g, although there are no specific data supporting this limit in acutely iron-poisoned patients. Administering deferoxamine at this rate will achieve a total of 6 g in about 6 h in an average-sized adult. Once this amount is reached, it is prudent to decrease the rate of deferoxamine administration, because of several associated risks. Adverse effects may include mucormycosis infection,[12] renal insufficiency,[13] pulmonary toxicity,[14] and sepsis from *Yersinia enterocolitica,* which may be related to duration of therapy.

The determination of the efficacy and duration of deferoxamine therapy involves acquisition of serial urine samples. As ferrioxamine is excreted, the urine color changes to what is classically called *vin rosé* but may actually appear brown or rusty. Theoretically, the disappearance of the *vin rosé* means that a patient no longer has a significant toxicity. It is important to obtain a urine sample prior to initiating treatment, because patients who are hypovolemic will likely produce concentrated urine, which may also be somewhat dark and may be confused with the *vin rosé* appearance. False negatives, color-change latency, and difficulty visualizing a color change can limit the utility of this test.

There is some controversy surrounding how long deferoxamine therapy should continue. Recommended end points range from clinical recovery and normal iron levels, to measurement of iron-to-creatinine ratios,[15] to clinical recovery with normal iron level in conjunction with normal urine color.[4] Since measured iron levels are artificially depressed by the presence of deferoxamine and urine color change can be unreliable, and since iron toxicity is a clinical diagnosis, clinical recovery of the patient is probably the most important factor in terminating therapy. For patients who continue to exhibit severe iron toxicity after 24 h of deferoxamine therapy, the therapy should continue carefully at a decreased dose, for reasons mentioned earlier.

Previously advocated was the *deferoxamine challenge test,* a *half-dose* of 50-mg/kg IM injection of deferoxamine followed by examination of urine samples for change in color that would indicate the presence of chelated free iron and therefore confirm iron toxicity. More recently, a *first dose* of 90 mg/kg IM has been used, also utilizing change in urine color to verify toxicity. There may be several problems with this management strategy. Single-dose deferoxamine can be unreliable in eliciting a visible color change in urine, especially if a pre-deferoxamine urine sample was not obtained, and should not be the sole factor in deciding toxicity.[4] Additionally, IM therapy does not address the issue of fluid resuscitation, which these patients very frequently require even if they do not require the antidote.

Pitfalls

Common errors in managing iron-toxic patients are many. The traditionally accepted indication of significant poisoning included a WBC of greater than 15,000/μL glucose level of more than 150 mg/dL, a 4-h serum iron level of more than 300 μg/dL, a serum iron level greater than TIBC, a positive deferoxamine challenge test, and a history of significant ingestion. However, reliance on iron levels and TIBC, WBC, serum glucose levels, and negative radiographs can lead physicians away from the proper diagnosis and increase time to treatment. Equating the so-called latent stage with clinical recovery when vital signs and clinical appearance are abnormal is an error in assessment and may lead to morbidity. Waiting for iron levels before beginning deferoxamine therapy is a misuse of time better spent aggressively caring for the patient. Withholding chelation therapy from a pregnant patient for fear of fetal toxicity from deferoxamine is not supported in the literature and should not occur.

PROGNOSIS

Patients who ingest small amounts and remain asymptomatic through the first 6 h after ingestion generally will recovery fully. Symptomatic patients are at higher risk for morbidity. Coma or shock is indicative of a grave prognosis, with approximately a 10 percent mortality rate. Most patients with shock or coma should survive with appropriate care. Generally, prognosis is improved with early recognition and initiation of treatment. Long-term sequelae include strictures, which may occur in patients with minimal symptoms.

DISPOSITION

Only those patients without a history of significant ingestion, and not symptomatic after at least 6 h of observation, can be considered for discharge. Patients in whom deferoxamine treatment is initiated should be admitted to an intensive care unit–type setting. All patients should be assessed for suicide risk, and child abuse or neglect should at least be considered in pediatric cases.

REFERENCES

1. Finch CA, Huebers H: Perspectives in iron metabolism. *N Engl J Med* 306:1520, 1982.
2. Tenenbein M, Israels SJ: Early coagulopathy in severe iron poisoning. *J Pediatr* 113:695, 1988.
3. Tenenbein M, Kopelow ML, deSa DJ: Myocardial failure and shock in iron poisoning. *Human Toxicol* 7:281, 1988.
4. Schauben JL, Augenstein WL, Cox J, Sato R: Iron poisoning: Report of three cases and a review of therapeutic intervention. *J Emerg Med* 8:309, 1990.
5. Burkhart KK, Kulig KW, Hammond KB, et al: The rise in the total iron-binding capacity after iron overdose. *Ann Emerg Med* 20:532, 1991.
6. Ling LJ, Hornfeldt CS, Winter JP: Absorption of iron after experimental overdose of chewable vitamins. *Am J Emerg Med* 9:24, 1991.
7. Lacouture PG, Wason S, Temple AR, et al: Emergency assessment of severity in iron overdose by clinical and laboratory methods. *J Pediatr* 99:89, 1981.
8. Chyka PA, Butler AY: Assessment of acute iron poisoning by laboratory and clinical observations. *Am J Emerg Med* 11:99, 1993.
9. Palatnick W, Tenenbein M: Leukocytosis, hyperglycemia, vomiting, and positive x-rays are not indicators of severity of iron poisoning. *Am J Emerg Med* 14:454, 1996.
10. Bentur Y, St Louis P, Klein J, Koren G: Misinterpretation of iron-binding capacity in the presence of deferoxamine. *J Pediatr* 118:139, 1991.
11. Foxford R, Goldfrank LR: Gastrotomy: A surgical approach to iron overdose. *Ann Emerg Med* 14:1223, 1985.
12. Daly AL, Velazquez LA, Bradley SF, Kauffman CA: Mucormycosis: Association with deferoxamine therapy. *Am J Med* 87:468, 1989.
13. Koren G, Bentur Y, Strong D, et al: Acute changes in renal function associated with deferoxamine therapy. *Am J Dis Child* 143:1077, 1989.
14. Tenenbein M, Kowalski S, Sienko A, et al: Pulmonary toxic effects of continuous desferrioxamine administration in acute iron poisoning. *Lancet* 339:699, 1992.
15. Yatscoff RW, Wayne EA, Tenenbein M: An objective criterion for the cessation of deferoxamine therapy in the acutely iron poisoned patient. *Clin Toxicol* 29:1, 1991.

HYDROCARBONS AND VOLATILE SUBSTANCES

Paul M. Wax

INTRODUCTION

Hydrocarbons are a diverse group of organic compounds consisting primarily of carbon and hydrogen atoms arranged in various aliphatic and aromatic configurations. Products containing hydrocarbons are found in many household and occupational settings. Examples include fuels, lighter fluids, lamp oil, paints, paint removers, cleaning and polishing agents, spot removers, degreasers, lubricants, and solvents. Volatile liquid chemicals or gases are substances sometimes abused for their euphoric effects. Examples of commonly abused volatiles include many hydrocarbon-containing substances such as glue (which contains toluene), propellants (e.g., butane, trichloroethylene, Freon), and gasoline. Other volatile chemicals not generally classified as hydrocarbons, such as nitrites (e.g., isobutyl nitrite) and nitrous oxide, are also subject to abuse. Hydrocarbon and volatile substance exposure may cause life-threatening toxicity and, in some cases, sudden death.

Classification

Most hydrocarbons are produced from petroleum distillation, which results in predominantly aliphatic (open-chain) mixtures of hydrocarbons of different chain lengths. Gasoline, for instance, consists of approximately 80 percent saturated and unsaturated aliphatic hydrocarbons of chain length C_4 to C_{10} and 20 percent aromatic hydrocarbons. Chain length determines the phase of the hydrocarbon at room temperature. Short-chain aliphatic compounds, such as methane, propane, or butane, are gases; long-chain aliphatic compounds, such as tar, are solids. Intermediate-chain (C_5 to C_{15}) aliphatic compounds are in liquid form and account for most hydrocarbon exposures seen in the emer-

TABLE 174-1 Substances that Predominantly Contain Aliphatics

Substance	Commercial Use
Gasoline	Motor fuel
Kerosene	Stove and lamp fuel
Mineral seal oil	Furniture polish
Naphtha (petroleum ether)	Lighter fluid
Diesel oil	Lubricant
N-Hexane	Plastic cement, rubber cement
Methane, butane, propane	Fuel

TABLE 174-3 Common Halogenated Hydrocarbons

Substance	Commercial Use
Carbon tetrachloride	Solvent, refrigerant, aerosol propellant
Chloroform	Solvent, chemical intermediate
Methylene chloride	Paint stripper, varnish remover, aerosol paint, degreaser
Trichloroethylene (TCE)	Spot remover, degreaser, typewriter correction fluid
Trichloroethane (TCA)	Spot remover, degreaser, typewriter correction fluid
Tetrachloroethylene (perchloroethylene)	Dry cleaning agent, degreaser

gency department (Table 174-1). Pulmonary toxicity secondary to aspiration is the most common complication from ingesting liquid aliphatic hydrocarbons.

The wood distillates (e.g., turpentine and pine oil) are derived from pine, consist mainly of cyclic terpene derivatives, and comprise another class of hydrocarbons. Gastrointestinal (GI) absorption of wood distillates tends to be greater than that of aliphatic petroleum distillates, increasing the risk for central nervous system (CNS) depression.

Aromatic hydrocarbons (containing a benzene ring; Table 174-2) and halogenated hydrocarbons (aliphatics with at least one substituted halogen group; Table 174-3) are widely used industrial solvents. Freon is the trade name for a group of halogenated hydrocarbons that contain fluoride such as dichlorodifluoromethane and bromochlorodifluoromethane. Although many of these chlorofluorocarbons (CFCs) are thought to cause atmospheric ozone changes and are being replaced by more environmentally friendly compounds, Freon may still be found as a refrigerant gas and component of fire extinguishing systems. Inhalational exposure is the usual route of toxicity for aromatic and halogenated hydrocarbons, although ingestion of these chemicals may also be problematic. Substance abusers and workers in certain occupational settings are most often affected. Such exposures may result in significant systemic toxicity.[1] Along with their potent CNS effects, specific cardiovascular, hepatic, renal, and hematologic toxicity are attributed to aromatic and halogenated hydrocarbons. Finally, some hydrocarbons have toxicity related to an additive, such as lead in gasoline and pesticides. With these, the toxic additive usually dictates the clinical approach.

Epidemiology

Exposures to hydrocarbons and volatiles most commonly occur in one of two settings: ingestion or inhalation. Hydrocarbon ingestions account for approximately 3 to 10 percent of all unintentional childhood poisonings in the United States. Ingestions of gasoline, kerosene, lighter fluid, mineral seal oil, and turpentine are most frequent. In less-developed countries kerosene ingestion accounts for 33 to 59 percent of unintentional childhood poisonings.[2] It is estimated that 3.5 to 10 percent of young people have experimented with volatile substance inhalation to produce inebriation.[3]

TABLE 174-2 Common Aromatic Hydrocarbons

Substance	Commercial Use
Benzene	Chemical intermediate, gasoline (small amount; average 0.8%)
Toluene	Airplane glue, plastic cement, acrylic paint
Xylene	Solvent, cleaning agent, degreaser

Most hydrocarbon exposures have a benign clinical course. The 1997 American Association of Poison Control Centers Toxic Exposure Surveillance System revealed that 66,645 potential hydrocarbon exposures were reported to poison control centers (3 percent of all reported exposures). Of these, 3.6 percent involved aromatic hydrocarbons and 12.2 percent involved halogenated hydrocarbons and/or propellants. Three thousand and fifty-eight (4.6 percent) developed moderate to severe toxicity, and 12 died.[4] Nine of the 12 deaths followed inhalational exposure; 8 involved intentional inhalational abuse and 7 occurred in teenagers. Two of the other fatalities were in toddlers who ingested and aspirated gasoline and paint thinner. An epidemiologic study of volatile substance abuse in the United Kingdom revealed that 605 people under age 18 years died from volatile substance abuse during the period 1981 to 1990.[5] The most commonly implicated volatiles were butane (39 percent), aerosols (26 percent), cleaners (16 percent), and glue (10 percent).

PATHOPHYSIOLOGY AND CLINICAL FEATURES

Determinants of Toxicity

The toxic potential of hydrocarbons depends on physical characteristics (volatility, viscosity, and surface tension), chemical characteristics (aliphatic, aromatic, or halogenated), presence of toxic additives such as pesticides or heavy metals, route of exposure, concentration, and dose. Viscosity, defined as the resistance to flow, and surface tension, denoting ''creeping'' ability, both play a major role in determining the aspiration potential. Viscosity is measured in Saybolt Seconds Universal (SSU). Patients ingesting substances with viscosities less than 60 SSU (e.g., gasoline, kerosene, mineral seal oil, turpentine, and aromatic and halogenated hydrocarbons) are at greater risk for aspiration than those ingesting substances with viscosities greater than 100 SSU (e.g., diesel oil, grease, mineral oil, paraffin wax, and petroleum jelly). Low surface tension also increases the risk of aspiration. Volatility denotes the ability of a substance to vaporize. Inhalation of highly volatile agents, such as aromatic hydrocarbons, halogenated hydrocarbons, or gasoline, results in systemic absorption and the potential for significant toxicity.

Dermal exposure to hydrocarbons causes local toxicity, and occasionally leads to systemic absorption. Dermal toxicity secondary to intravenous administration of hydrocarbons has also been reported. When used intravenously, hydrocarbons may cause pulmonary toxicity by their first-pass exposure through the lungs.

Toxicity from hydrocarbon exposure can be divided into different clinical syndromes based on the organ system(s) predominately affected. Characteristic presentations usually affect one or more of the following systems: pulmonary, neurologic (central and/or peripheral), GI, cardiac, hepatic, renal, hematologic, or dermal.

Pulmonary Toxicity

Pulmonary complications, especially aspiration, are the most frequent adverse effects of hydrocarbon exposure. Typically, this involves the unintentional childhood ingestion of small amounts of aliphatic hydrocarbon mixtures commonly stored in the household. Aliphatic hydrocarbons have a limited GI absorption; toxicity usually results from aspiration of the low-viscosity compounds or inhalation (intentional or inadvertent) of compounds with high volatility. Although ingestion of aromatic or halogenated hydrocarbons may also result in aspiration, GI absorption is greater. Hence, CNS and other systemic toxicity secondary to GI absorption often predominate after aromatic and halogenated hydrocarbon ingestion.

Aspiration is not dependent on volume ingested. Experimentally in rats, as little as 0.2 mL instilled intratracheally has caused pneumonitis. Pulmonary toxicity does not result from GI absorption but occurs from direct aspiration of the hydrocarbon into the pulmonary tree. This occurs at the time of ingestion when the hydrocarbon migrates from the hypopharynx into the airway. There is no evidence that hydrocarbons reflux from the stomach into the airway. Spontaneous vomiting, however, does increase the risk of aspiration.[6] Pulmonary toxicity manifested as acute bilateral pneumonitis has also been reported from the inhalation of an aerosolized aliphatic hydrocarbon such as gasoline or kerosene.

Hydrocarbon aspiration causes chemical pneumonitis by direct toxic injury to the pulmonary parenchyma and altered surfactant function. Destruction of alveolar and capillary membranes results in increased vascular permeability and edema. Early distal airway closure and alveolar collapse produces clinical bronchospasm and ventilation/perfusion mismatch. The CNS manifestations seen after ingestion of a poorly GI-absorbed aliphatic hydrocarbon are thought to be from hypoxia secondary to the hydrocarbon induced pneumonitis and/or direct CNS toxicity following the pulmonary absorption of a volatile hydrocarbon. Studies performed in animals in which hydrocarbons were instilled into the stomach after ligation of the esophagus demonstrate negligible absorption of aliphatic compounds from the GI tract with no evidence of subsequent pneumonitis.[7] Pneumatoceles, pneumothoraces, and/or pneumomediastinum are occasionally associated with hydrocarbon aspiration. Other complications include bacterial superinfection, acute respiratory distress syndrome, and death. Long-term pulmonary dysfunction may occur.

In one study of 950 children who ingested products containing hydrocarbons and who were brought to the hospital, 19 percent had clinical or radiographic evidence of pulmonary aspiration.[8] In another study of 184 pediatric hydrocarbon ingestions called to a poison center, 35 percent had initial symptoms, but only 3 percent had progressive pulmonary symptoms.[9] The clinical manifestations of pulmonary aspiration are usually apparent almost immediately on ingestion. The early effects result from irritation of the oral mucosa and tracheobronchial tree. Symptoms include coughing, choking, gasping, dyspnea, and burning of the mouth. Patients with these symptoms should be assumed to have aspirated until proven otherwise. Physical examination may reveal grunting respirations, retractions, tachypnea, tachycardia, and cyanosis. An odor of the hydrocarbon may be noted on the patient's breath. An elevated temperature of 39°C (102.2°F) or greater is common and may occur upon initial presentation or be delayed for 6 to 8 h.

Auscultation may be normal, or reveal wheezing, and decreased, or absent breath sounds. Arterial blood gas analysis may demonstrate a widened alveolar-arterial oxygen gradient or frank hypoxemia. The development of a necrotizing pneumonitis and hemorrhagic pulmonary edema usually occurs within hours in severe aspiration.

Most fatalities from these complications occur within 24 to 48 h. With less severe damage, symptoms usually subside within two to five days, except with pneumatoceles and lipoid pneumonias whose symptoms may persist for weeks to months.

Although most patients with clinically significant aspiration have abnormal chest x-rays, the time course of radiographic changes varies and correlation with physical examination may be poor. Changes may be seen as early as 30 min after aspiration, but the initial radiograph in the symptomatic patient may be deceptively clear. Radiographic changes usually appear by 2 to 6 h and are almost always present by 18 to 24 h if they are to occur. The infiltrates range in appearance from streaking to flocculent to homogeneous, and are usually located in the dependent lobes. Multilobar involvement is more common than single-lobe involvement and right-sided involvement is more common than left-sided involvement. Radiographic changes limited to bilateral perihilar regions with clear lung bases are also common.

High-viscosity compounds such as lubricants, mineral oil, or tar, are not aspirated readily and tend to be less toxic when ingested. Occasionally, however, aspiration occurs that results in the development of lipoid pneumonia. Deaths from hydrocarbon lipoid pneumonia have been reported.

Central Nervous System Toxicity

Central nervous system toxicity may result from either a direct toxic response to the systemic absorption of the hydrocarbon, as an indirect result of severe hypoxia secondary to aspiration, or as a result of simple asphyxiation. Systemic absorption usually occurs through the inhalation of highly volatile petroleum distillates, which may be absorbed inadvertently, for example as an occupational risk, or deliberately associated with solvent abuse.

Volatile solvent abuse most often occurs in teenagers and younger adults, especially from lower socioeconomic backgrounds and in particular cultures (e.g., Native Americans).[10] These patients are described as "huffers" or "baggers" depending on whether they inhale through a rag soaked with the hydrocarbon held to the mouth or rebreathe into a plastic bag containing the hydrocarbon. The act of rebreathing to facilitate inhalation may also contribute to toxicity by producing significant hypercarbia and hypoxia. Many of the most commonly abused volatiles are listed in Table 174-4.

Many of the hydrocarbons that affect the CNS are organic solvents and have a natural affinity for the lipid-rich neural tissue. They behave similarly to the inhalational anesthetic agents. Hydrocarbon intoxication may be confused with ethanol inebriation. CNS depression ranges in severity from dizziness, slurred speech, ataxia, and lethargy to obtundation and coma. Depression of the central ventilatory drive may also occur. These effects are usually dose-dependent. Although hydrocarbons are CNS depressants, they often have an initial excitatory effect manifested as euphoria, exhilaration, and giddiness, effects sought by those who abuse them. More severe excitatory features include tremor, agitation, and convulsions. Perceptual changes, such as confusion, hallucinations, and psychosis, may occur.

Chronic CNS sequelae may result from recurrent inhalational exposure to hydrocarbons in the workplace or with solvent abuse.[11] These sequelae are seen among house painters and solvent abusers exposed to toluene-containing substances. Recurrent headaches, cerebellar ataxia, and a chronic encephalopathy consisting of tremors, emotional lability, mental status changes, cognitive impairment, and psychomotor impairment, characterize the syndrome. These effects may be transitory or permanent. The development of encephalopathy, ataxia, tremor, chorea, and myoclonus also is associated with the habitual sniffing of leaded gasoline. In this case, symptoms are thought to be secondary to the effects of tetraethyl lead and its toxic metabolites.

TABLE 174-4 Commonly Abused Volatile Substances

Product	Volatile Agent
Acrylic spray paint	Toluene
Adhesives/glue	Toluene, trichloroethylene
Aerosol propellants	Propellants and butane
Cigarette lighter refills	Butane
Degreasing agents	Trichloroethylene
Dry-cleaning agents	Tetrachloroethylene
Fire extinguishers	Bromochlorodifluoromethane
Inhalational anesthetics	Nitrous oxide, halothane
Lighter fluid	Naphtha
Nitrites (poppers)	Isobutyl nitrite, amyl nitrite
Paint stripper	Methylene chloride
Petrol	Gasoline
Plastic modeling cement	Methyl ethyl ketone, toluene
Spot removers	Trichloroethylene, trichloroethane
Typewriter correction fluid	Trichloroethane, trichloroethylene

Peripheral Nervous System Toxicity

Exposure to *n*-hexane, methyl *n*-butyl ketone, and other six-carbon aliphatic hydrocarbons is associated with the development of a characteristic peripheral polyneuropathy caused by demyelinization and retrograde axonal degeneration.[12] Onset of symptoms may be delayed for months to years after initial exposure. Toxicity is attributed to a metabolite, 2,5-hexanedione, produced by the cytochrome P-450-mediated biotransformation of the parent compounds. This neurotoxic metabolite is thought to inhibit glutaraldehyde-3-phosphate dehydrogenase, which supplies energy for axonal transport. Long, distal nerves seem to be most vulnerable, characteristically producing foot and wrist drop with numbness and paresthesias. The electromyelogram typically shows a decrease in nerve conduction velocity.

Gastrointestinal Toxicity

Most hydrocarbons act as intestinal irritants, resulting in burning in the mouth and throat, abdominal pain, belching, nausea, vomiting, and diarrhea. Vomiting, which occurs in about one-third of the patients with aliphatic hydrocarbon ingestions, is particularly troublesome because of the increased risk of pulmonary aspiration.

Cardiac Toxicity

Life-threatening dysrhythmias, such as ventricular tachycardia and ventricular fibrillation, may occur with systemic absorption (gastrointestinal or inhalational) of a variety of hydrocarbon compounds.[13] Most commonly, dysrhythmias occur after exposure to halogenated hydrocarbons and aromatic hydrocarbons. Exposures to predominantly aliphatic mixtures, such as gasoline or mineral spirits, and exposure to butane have also been reported to cause dysrhythmias and sudden death.[14] The mechanism of toxicity is believed to be secondary to a sensitization of the heart to catecholamines. The term ''sudden sniffing death'' describes solvent abusers who die suddenly after exertion, panic, or fright.[13] The sudden release of catecholamines in these situations is thought to induce these fatal dysrhythmias.[14] Cardiac dysrhythmias as a consequence of industrial exposure to volatile hydrocarbons have also been described. Other mechanisms for sudden death include asphyxia, respiratory depression, and vagal inhibition. The use of exogenous catecholamines, such as epinephrine, may precipitate sudden dysrhythmias and should be avoided except if required for cardiac resuscitation. Decreases in myocardial contractility and peripheral vascular resistance as well as bradycardia and atrioventricular conduction blocks have also been associated with volatile solvent abuse.

Hepatic Toxicity

Hydrocarbon-induced hepatic damage resulting from halogenated hydrocarbons is well described.[15] Carbon tetrachloride toxicity has been used as a model for toxin-induced hepatic dysfunction. As little as 3 mL of carbon tetrachloride has been associated with the development of fatal liver injury.[16] Other halogenated hydrocarbons, such as chloroform, are also associated with liver dysfunction. Free-radical metabolites of these agents that cause lipid peroxidation are apparently responsible for hepatocellular destruction.

Pathologic examination reveals acute fatty degeneration of the liver with areas of centrilobular necrosis. Phenobarbital, ethanol, and other agents that induce cytochrome P-450 enzymes are contraindicated because of the propensity to increase the production of the toxic metabolites. The time-course of hepatic dysfunction with acute exposures appears similar to acetaminophen hepatotoxicity. Liver function tests may be elevated within 24 h after ingestion, with the development of liver tenderness and jaundice in 48 to 96 h. Chronic exposure to carbon tetrachloride may be associated with the development of cirrhosis and hepatomas.

Renal and Metabolic Toxicity

Solvent abuse and occupational exposure to hydrocarbons may result in renal dysfunction. Exposure to hepatotoxic halogenated hydrocarbons, such as carbon tetrachloride and trichloroethylene, has caused acute renal failure as well as centrilobular hepatic necrosis.[15] Occupational hydrocarbon exposures have been associated with a variety of glomerulonephritides including Goodpasture's syndrome.[17,18]

Renal tubular acidosis may occur in patients who abuse toluene-containing substances.[1] Patients present with a non-anion gap metabolic acidosis, hypokalemia, and hypophosphatemia. The serum potassium may be so low (<2 meq/L) that severe muscle weakness develops, occasionally resulting in quadriparesis. Significant rhabdomyolysis may also result. Toluene toxicity may also cause a high anion gap metabolic acidosis as a result of the accumulation of hippuric acid and benzoic acid metabolites. Proteinuria and renal insufficiency can occur in patients who abuse toluene.

Hematologic Toxicity

Chronic exposure to benzene, the prototypical aromatic hydrocarbon, is associated with an increased incidence of hematologic disorders including aplastic anemia, acute myelogenous leukemia, and multiple myeloma.[19] This association has received much attention because of the extensive use of benzene in the workplace. The etiology of these blood dyscrasias is probably not benzene itself but rather a toxic metabolite. Although aplastic anemia is associated with glue sniffing, this is most likely due to the benzene fraction of the glue and not the toluene. Hydrocarbon-induced hemolysis has occurred following the acute ingestion of gasoline, kerosene, and tetrachloroethylene, and inhalation of mineral spirits.[20] Consumptive coagulopathy has also been reported.

A peculiar complication of methylene chloride exposure is the endogenous production of carbon monoxide.[21] This is unlike ordinary carbon monoxide exposure from exogenous sources where maximum carboxyhemoglobin level occurs at the time of the exposure. With methylene chloride exposure, carbon monoxide formation may continue after cessation of exposure due to slow release of methylene chloride from the tissues prior to its metabolism to carbon monoxide. When patients exposed to methylene chloride present with CNS and cardiac symptoms, impairment due to significant carbon monoxide production must be considered.

Dermal Toxicity

Dermal exposure to hydrocarbons may also result in toxicity. Cutaneous injury is most often associated with the short-chain aliphatic, aromatic, and halogenated hydrocarbons. These agents act as primary irritants and as sensitizers. Clinically, skin findings can range from local erythema, papules, and vesicles to a generalized scarlatiniform eruption and an exfoliative dermatitis. A ''huffer's rash'' may be noted over the face of patients who chronically abuse the volatile hydrocarbons. Pruritus may also be present. A defatting dermatitis, similar to a chronic eczematoid dermatitis, may occur. Frostbite of the face may develop during the inhalational abuse of fluorinated agents. Cellulitis and sterile abscesses have been associated with the injection of hydrocarbons. Extensive partial-thickness and full-thickness bums following immersion in hydrocarbons may also occur.

Exposure to heated high-viscosity, long-chain aliphatics, such as tar, asphalt, or bitumen, present a particularly challenging problem because of their association with burns and hyperthermia, and difficulty with decontamination.[22]

TREATMENT

Prehospital

Not all patients who have ingested hydrocarbons require emergency department evaluation. In a retrospective study of 211 patients with hydrocarbon ingestions called to a poison center, fewer than one percent required physician intervention.[9] This data suggests that patients who are asymptomatic or quickly become asymptomatic after ingestion can be watched safely at home. This approach of home observation for asymptomatic patients can be supported when the ingestion is accidental, the ingredients are known and do not cause significant systemic toxicity when ingested, and reliable follow-up can be ensured. All symptomatic patients and intentional exposures should be referred to the hospital for further evaluation. Patients who ingest hydrocarbons that may cause significant systemic toxicity (e.g., aromatic, halogenated hydrocarbons, or toxic additives), whether or not symptomatic, should also be referred to the hospital. Volatile substance abusers and others exposed to volatiles should have immediate cardiac monitoring and advanced life support transport, if available, due to the potential for life-threatening dysrhythmias.

TABLE 174-5 ED Management of Hydrocarbon Exposures

Find out what type of hydrocarbon and route of exposure
- Utilize MSDS (material safety data sheets) and Regional Poison Control Center as resources

Ingestion: aliphatic mixtures (gasoline, kerosene, lamp oil, etc.; see Table 174-1)
- GI decontamination: usually unnecessary
- Skin decontamination: if spilled on clothes or skin, soap and water
- Diagnostic: observe for evidence of aspiration and CNS symptoms (CXR, pulse oximetry)
- Treatment
  - If evidence of aspiration-respiratory support (oxygen, inhaled β agonists, ventilatory support)
  - No need for steroids, no need for antibiotics unless documented infection
  - Disposition: admit if symptomatic, discharge home if unintentional ingestion and asymptomatic after 6 h

Ingestion: aromatics, halogenated, other volatiles (see Tables 174-2, 174-3, 174-4)
- GI decontamination: consider activated charcoal, gastric aspiration if highly toxic (e.g., CCl_4, chloroform, benzene)
- Skin decontamination: if spilled on clothes or skin, soap and water
- Diagnostic adjuncts
  - Observe for evidence of aspiration and CNS symptoms (CXR, pulse oximetry)
  - Continuous cardiac monitoring for dysrhythmias
  - Abdominal radiographs to evaluate suspected chlorinated hydrocarbon ingestions
  - Methylene chloride: check COHb level, serial levels may be necessary, O_2
  - Toluene: check potassium, anion gap, CPK
  - Benzene: follow CBC
  - Potent halogenated hydrocarbons (CCL_4, chloroform, TCE, TCA) follow LFTs
  - Nitrites: check methemoglobin level
- Treatment
  - Oxygen
  - Avoid exogenous catecholamines if possible (dopamine, norepinephrine)
  - Consider β-adrenergic antagonists to treat dysrhythmias
  - Consider NAC therapy for potent halogenated hydrocarbon exposure
  - Consider HBO if markedly elevated COHb level from methylene chloride
  - Disposition: admit symptomatic exposures or hydrocarbons with delayed toxicity (CCl_4)

Inhalation: aliphatic mixtures, aromatics, halogenated, other volatiles
- Treat as #3 but no need for GI decontamination

Dermal: tar and asphalt
- Immediate cooling with water
- Debridement of blistered skin
- Remove adherent substance with petroleum based solvent (e.g., De-Solv-It, Tween 80, Polysporin)

Emergency Department

General principles of poison management apply to the initial approach to patients once they reach the hospital. Establishing the airway and maintaining ventilation is the critical first maneuver in any patient who presents with respiratory depression and/or significant CNS depression. The detection of a sweet odor may be associated with certain halogenated hydrocarbon exposures (especially chloroform or trichloroethylene) while a petrol odor suggests gasoline or some other petroleum derivative. The patient should be connected to a continuous cardiac monitor and an electrocardiogram should be obtained. Hydrocarbon-induced dysrhythmias, if present, would generally occur shortly after the exposure, especially with inhalational use. Hypotension should be treated with aggressive fluid resuscitation. Catecholamines, such as dopamine, norepinephrine, or epinephrine, should be avoided to prevent precipitating dysrhythmias, especially following exposure to halogenated hydrocarbons and aromatic hydrocarbons. The administration of glucose, thiamine, and naloxone should be considered in cases of altered mental status. (See Table 174-5.)

The patient needs to be fully undressed to prevent ongoing contamination from hydrocarbon-soaked clothes. Dermal decontamination with soap and water, and eye decontamination with saline irrigation, should be performed. Pre-hospital decontamination is preferable. The staff should wear protective gloves and aprons to prevent possible secondary exposure. Specific antidotal treatment directed at the complications of toxic additives, such as organophosphates or heavy metals, may also be needed.

Useful diagnostic tests include the chest x-ray and arterial blood gas to detect pulmonary aspiration and hypoxemia. Abdominal radiographs may show evidence of chlorinated hydrocarbon ingestions, such as carbon tetrachloride, because of the radiopaque nature of these substances.[23] Tests of liver and renal function should be obtained in all aromatic and halogenated hydrocarbon exposures to check for the development of hepatic and renal injury. A blood lead level may be helpful when evaluating patients with chronic gasoline exposure. A carboxyhemoglobin level is useful to evaluate the extent of endogenous carbon monoxide production following methylene chloride exposure. Pulse oximetry will not differentiate between oxyhemoglobin and carboxyhemoglobin. Routine drug screens are not useful for the detection of hydrocarbons, but as in all intentional ingestions, an acetaminophen level, ethanol level, anion gap, and osmolality may be helpful in assessing for the presence of other coingestants.

Gastrointestinal Decontamination

For most hydrocarbon ingestions, gastrointestinal decontamination would provide little benefit; supportive care and appropriate treatment of coexisting ingestions are all that is required. The necessity for GI decontamination depends on the type of hydrocarbon and route of exposure. The risk of systemic toxicity by intestinal absorption has to be weighed against the risks of aspiration associated with gastric emptying. The majority of hydrocarbon ingestions, which consist of aliphatic hydrocarbons mixtures (see Table 174-1), do not require GI decontamination. These agents have poor GI absorption and their toxicity is limited primarily to pulmonary aspiration. In the typical childhood accidental ingestion, the actual amount ingested is usually one swallow or about 5 mL. Suicidal ingestions, which involve larger amounts of hydrocarbons, frequently are associated with spontaneous emesis, and further decontamination is usually not required. Some recommend GI decontamination if emesis has not occurred and the dose is greater than 1 to 2 mL/kg, although this strategy has not been studied.

GI decontamination may be warranted when the ingested hydrocarbon is known to have good GI absorption and may cause significant systemic toxicity (e.g., toluene, chloroform, wood distillates) or an additive in the toxic agent (e.g., organophosphate pesticides are often mixed in petroleum distillates). The CHAMP mnemonic (camphor, halogenated hydrocarbons, aromatic hydrocarbons, metals, pesticides) is helpful in remembering most situations where GI decontamination should be considered. Unfortunately, little data is available that evaluates the clinical benefits of gastrointestinal decontamination in these settings.

If the patient presents to the ED shortly after the ingestion of these toxic hydrocarbons, aspiration with a small nasogastric tube may be useful. In patients who present with an altered mental status, the airway should be protected with a cuffed endotracheal tube, although in smaller children under eight years of age, the cuff should be kept inflated only during the period of lavage because of cuff-related injury from prolonged inflation. Ipecac-induced emesis has been advocated in the past but its risks appear to outweigh any potential benefits.

Although activated charcoal may adsorb some hydrocarbon compounds, its use is not recommended for most hydrocarbon ingestions. Charcoal instillation may distend the stomach increasing the risk for vomiting and aspiration. The use of charcoal should only be considered if one of the CHAMP-type hydrocarbons has been ingested.

The use of cathartics to hasten GI transit and facilitate decontamination has no proven efficacy in hydrocarbon ingestions. Many patients will already have diarrhea from the hydrocarbon, and further catharsis is not required. Oil-based cathartics, which had been used in the past to thicken the ingested hydrocarbon to increase its viscosity and decrease the subsequent risk of aspiration, are contraindicated. They may actually increase GI absorption and are associated with an increased risk of lipoid pneumonia when aspirated.

Pulmonary Treatment

Nebulized oxygen is helpful in the treatment of pulmonary aspiration. Inhaled β_2 agonists may also be useful, especially in the setting of bronchospasm, but their role in the treatment of hydrocarbon pneumonitis has not been studied. Positive end-expiratory pressure (PEEP) or continuous positive-airway pressure (CPAP) may sometimes be required, but because of the potential for further injury from barotrauma, one should observe for the development of pneumatoceles or pneumothoraces. In cases of severe pulmonary aspiration resulting in refractory hypoxemia, treatment with extracorporeal membrane oxygenation (EMCO) and high frequency jet ventilation (HFJV) has proved successful.[24,25] Consensus remains that corticosteroids are contraindicated because they impair the cellular immune response and increase the chance of bacterial superinfection.[26] Antibiotics have no proven role in prophylaxis and are usually not required except in cases of continued pulmonary deterioration because of the risk of a superimposed bacterial pneumonitis.

Other

There are few antidotes to counteract the actions of hydrocarbons. *N*-Acetyl cysteine[16] and hyperbaric oxygen[27] may have a role in preventing hepatic toxicity after carbon tetrachloride (and possibly chloroform) exposure, but more studies are needed. Hyperbaric oxygen therapy is indicated for patients who develop significant carbon monoxide toxicity after exposure to methylene chloride. β blockers may be useful in the treatment of hydrocarbon-induced malignant dysrhythmias.[28] Although extracorporeal removal with hemodialysis, hemoperfusion, or peritoneal dialysis has been attempted for severe intoxications, clinically controlled evidence of efficacy is lacking.

The treatment of tar and asphalt injuries is a particular problem because of the difficulty in removing these substances without causing further tissue injury. Immediate cooling with cold water for at least 30 min is critical. Debridement of blistered skin can aid in the removal of adherent substances. De-Solv-It, a surface-active petroleum-based solvent, has proven both nonirritating and effective in removing these agents.[29] Polyoxyethylene sorbitan-containing ointments, such as Polysorbate 80 or Tween 80, have also proven useful. Petrolatum-containing preparations, such as Neosporin (although occasionally sensitizing) or Polysporin, may also work and are readily available. In some instances, early excision and skin grafting are required to treat the more significant hot tar burns.

Undoubtedly, the best therapy begins with preventive measures to reduce accessibility of these compounds to young children. Proper labeling of containers that store hydrocarbons, mandatory use of safety closures, and public education on the risks of hydrocarbons also limit the potential for inadvertent hydrocarbon toxicity.

DISPOSITION

A medical toxicologist or regional poison control center should be consulted on most symptomatic hydrocarbon exposures and asymptomatic exposures that involve halogenated, aromatic, and hydrocarbon exposures with toxic additives. Hospitalization is required for patients who have ingested aliphatic hydrocarbons who are symptomatic at the time of evaluation. After a six-hour observation period, asymptomatic patients with a normal chest x-ray may be discharged home.[8] Similar disposition of asymptomatic patients, with abnormal chest x-rays has also been suggested if reliable follow-up can be ensured. However some physicians prefer to watch these patients for 24 h in the hospital. Hospitalization is advisable for those who ingest hydrocarbons capable of producing delayed complications (e.g., halogenated hydrocarbons causing hepatic toxicity) and those with toxic additives (organophosphates). All patients taking ingestions with suicidal intent or presenting with complications of solvent abuse should have psychiatric evaluation following medical clearance.

REFERENCES

1. Streicher HZ, Gabow PA, Moss AH, et al: Syndromes of toluene sniffing in adults. *Ann Intern Med* 94:758, 1981.
2. Gupta P, Singh RP, Murali MV, et al: Kerosene oil poisonings childhood menace. *Indian Pediatr* 29:979, 1992.
3. Ramsey J, Anderson HR, Bloor K, et al: An introduction to the practice, prevalence and chemical toxicology of volatile substance abuse. *Hum Toxicol* 8:261, 1989.
4. Litovitz TL, Klein-Schwartz WK, Dyer KS, et al: 1997 annual report of the American Association of Poison Control Centers Toxic Exposure Surveillance System. *Am J Emerg Med* 16:443, 1998.
5. Esmail A, Meyer L, Pottier A, et al: Deaths from volatile substance abuse in those under 18 years: Results from a national epidemiological study. *Arch Disease Child* 69:356, 1993.
6. Press E: Cooperative kerosene poisoning study: Evaluation of gastric lavage and other factors in the treatment of accidental ingestion of petroleum distillate products. *Pediatrics* 29:648, 1962.
7. Dice WH, Ward G, Kelley J, et al: Pulmonary toxicity following gastrointestinal ingestion of kerosene. *Ann Emerg Med* 11:138, 1982.
8. Anas N, Namasonthi V, Ginsburg CM: Criteria for hospitalizing children who have ingested products containing hydrocarbons. *JAMA* 246:840, 1981.
9. Machado B, Cross K, Snodgrass WR: Accidental hydrocarbon ingestion cases telephoned to a regional poison center. *Ann Emerg Med* 17:804, 1988.
10. Coulehan JL, Hirsch W, Brillman J, et al: Gasoline sniffing and lead toxicity in Navajo adolescents. *Pediatrics* 71:113, 1983.
11. Goodheart RS, Dunne JW: Petrol sniffer's encephalopathy: A study of 25 patients. *Med J Australia* 160:178, 1994.
12. Herskowitz A, Ishii N, Schaumburg H: N-Hexane neuropathy: A syndrome occurring as a result of industrial exposure. *N Engl J Med* 285:82, 1971.
13. Bass M: Sudden sniffing death. *JAMA* 212:2075, 1970.
14. Shepherd RT: Mechanism of death associated with volatile substance abuse. *Hum Toxicol* 8:289, 1989.
15. Baerg RD, Kimberg DV: Centrilobular hepatic necrosis and acute renal failure in "solvent sniffers." *Ann Intern Med* 73:713, 1970.
16. Ruprah M, Mant TGK, Flanagan RJ: Acute carbon tetrachloride poisoning in 19 patients: Implications for diagnosis and treatment. *Lancet* 1:1027, 1985.
17. Bombassei GJ, Kaplan AA: The association between hydrocarbon exposure and anti-glomerular basement membrane antibody-mediated disease (Goodpasture's syndrome). *Am J Indust Med* 21:141, 1992.
18. Mutti A, Alinovi R, Bergamaschi E, et al: Nephropathies and exposure to perchloroethylene in dry-cleaners. *Lancet* 340:189, 1992.
19. Rinsky RA, Smith AB, Hornung R, et al: Benzene and leukemia: An epidemiologic risk assessment. *N Engl J Med* 316:1044, 1987.
20. Algren JT, Rodgers CYC: Intravascular hemolysis associated with hydrocarbon poisoning. *Pediatr Emerg Care* 8: 34, 1992.
21. Leikin JB, Kaufman D, Lipscomb JW, et al: Methylene chloride: Report of five exposures and two deaths. *Am J Emerg Med* 8:534, 1990.
22. James NK, Moss AL: Review of burns caused by bitumen and the problems of its removal. *Burns* 16:214, 1990.
23. Dally S, Garnier R, Bismuth C: Diagnosis of chlorinated hydrocarbon poisoning by X-ray examination. *Br J Ind Med* 44:424, 1987.
24. Chyka PA: Benefits of extracorporeal membrane oxygenation for hydrocarbon pneumonitis. *J Toxicol Clin Toxicol* 34:357, 1996.
25. Bysani GK, Rucoba RJ, Noah ZL: Treatment of hydrocarbon pneumonitis: high frequency jet ventilation as an alternative to extracorporeal membrane oxygenation. *Chest* 106:300, 1994.
26. Marks MI, Chicoine L, Legere G, et al: Adrenocorticosteroid treatment of hydrocarbon pneumonia in children: A cooperative study. *J Pediatr* 81:366, 1972.
27. Burk RF, Reiter R, Lane JM: Hyperbaric oxygen protection against carbon tetrachloride hepatotoxicity in the rat. *Gastroenterology* 90:812, 1986.
28. Kobayashi H, Hobara T, Kawamoto T, et al: Effect of 1,1,1-trichloroethane inhalation on heart rate and its mechanism: A role of the autonomic nervous system. *Arch Environ Health* 42:140, 1987.
29. Stratta RJ, Saffle JR, Kravitz M, et al: Management of tar and asphalt injuries. *Am J Surg* 146:766, 1983.

175 CAUSTICS

G. Richard Bruno
Wallace A. Carter

The American Association of Poison Control Centers (AAPCC) reports approximately 100,000 potentially caustic exposures in the United States annually (Table 175-1).[1] Caustic exposures include dermal, ocular, and oral ingestions. Most exposures are unintentional, with a large portion occurring in children younger than age 6. In 1996, there were approximately 167 exposures that resulted in significant morbidity and 16 in death. Intentional adult ingestions with suicide intent account for a greater percentage of serious injuries than unintentional oral ingestions by curious children.

Many chemicals used in industry have caustic potential. Alkali substances used in industry include sodium hydroxide and potassium hydroxide in cleaning fluids, calcium hydroxide in concrete, lithium hydroxide in photography, and ammonium hydroxide in fertilizers (Table 175-2). Common acids used in industry include hydrochloric acid and sulfuric acids as cleaners, hydrofluoric acid in etching and metal cleaning, chromic acid in metal plating, and formic acid in leather/textile tanning. Industrial strength cleaners and chemicals accounted for approximately 8000 alkali exposures and 12,000 acid exposures in the 1996 AAPCC data (Table 175-1).[1]

Household caustics are common, and many are less concentrated forms of industrial strength cleansers. Alkali caustics found in the home include sodium hydroxide in drain cleaners, oven cleaners, and Clinitest tablets (Table 175-2). Caustic ammonium compounds are found in glass, tub, and tile cleaners. Household bleach (sodium hypochlorite) is the most common alkali exposure reported in AAPCC data, accounting for more than 50,000 exposures per year. Most bleach exposures are benign, but 44 patients reported in the 1996 data suffered major morbidity. Common household acids include sulfuric acid in drain cleaners and automobile batteries, hydrochloric acid in cleaners, formic acid in airplane glue, and hydrofluoric acid in rust removers.

PATHOPHYSIOLOGY OF CAUSTIC INJURIES

Alkali

Alkali injuries can induce deep tissue injury from liquefaction necrosis. After caustic alkali exposures, proteins are rapidly denatured and lipids undergo saponification. Initially, there is direct cellular destruction from contact with the alkali. This is followed by thrombosis of local microvasculature that leads to further tissue necrosis. Solid or granular alkali caustics often injure the oropharynx and proximal esophagus. Liquid alkali ingestions are characterized by esophageal injuries. Severe intentional alkali ingestion may cause multisystem organ injuries, including gastric perforation, and necrosis of abdominal viscera. Severe injuries to the pancreas, gallbladder, and small intestine after intentional ingestion have been reported.[2]

The most common household alkali is bleach, a 3% to 6% sodium hypochlorite solution with a pH of approximately 11. Household liquid bleach is not corrosive to the esophagus, but ingestion may cause emesis secondary to gastric irritation or pulmonary irritation related to chlorine gas production in the stomach or when mixed with other substances.[3] Other injuries reported with bleach include pneumonitis after aspiration and sight-limiting ocular injuries. Industrial strength bleach may contain much higher concentrations of sodium hypochlorite, and ingestion may result in esophageal necrosis.

Solid alkali ingestions may have greater potential for proximal esophageal tract injury and less for distal injury.

Acids

Injuries by strong acids produce coagulation necrosis. Tissue destruction and cell death result in eschar formation, which is believed to

TABLE 175-1 Epidemiology of Caustic Ingestions Reported to the American Association of Poison Control Centers, 1996

	No. Exposures	Age <6	Unintentional	Intentional	Major Outcome*	Death
Alkalis						
Chemicals	5,355	1,210	5,201	85	32	0
Household cleaners	23,906	10,205	22,924	706	88	5
Industrial cleaners	3,101	691	2,962	87	23	0
Total alkali exposures	32,362	12,823	31,087	878	143	5
Acids						
Chemicals	10,522	1,044	10,193	211	72	5
Household cleaners	8,549	3,195	8,229	271	35	4
Rust remover	2,054	308	1,992	160	22	2
Industrial cleaner	1,583	435	1,529	42	6	0
Total acid exposures	22,708	4,982	21,943	546	120	11
Disc batteries	1,982	1,255	1,940	38	4	0
Bleach	54,075	22,498	51,508	1,926	44	0

*Major outcomes are defined as signs or symptoms that are life threatening or result in significant disability.
Source: Litovitz et al,[1] with permission.

protect against deeper injury. Ingested acids settle in the stomach, where gastric necrosis, perforation, and hemorrhage may result. It was previously thought that acids were esophagus sparing, with most tissue injury concentrated in the stomach, but a study by Zargar and colleagues[4] reported a similar incidence of gastric and esophageal injury (85.4 percent gastric and 87.8 percent esophageal) after acid ingestion. Despite relatively less tissue destruction, strong acid ingestion results in a higher mortality rate than does strong alkali ingestion. This higher mortality rate after acid ingestion is hypothesized to result from complications of systemic absorption of acid (metabolic acidosis, hemolysis, and renal failure).

CLINICAL FEATURES

Patients who present after caustic ingestion may have severe pain, odynophagia, dysphonia, oral/facial burns, respiratory distress, and/or abdominal pain, and be drooling, coughing, or vomiting. Dysphonia, stridor, and respiratory distress may indicate laryngotracheal injury, whereas dysphagia, odynophagia, epigastric pain, and vomiting may indicate esophageal and gastrointestinal (GI) injury.

Conflicting data exist on the reliability of presenting signs and symptoms to predict upper GI injuries. An early retrospective study of caustic ingestions by Gaudreault and colleagues[5] reported 12 percent of patients who presented without initial signs or symptoms of upper GI injury were subsequently found to have serious esophageal injuries of grade 2 or higher (Table 175-3). A subsequent prospective study by Gorman and coworkers found that no single symptom, or group of symptoms, had 100 percent positive or negative predictive value for esophageal injury.[6] All patients with serious esophageal injuries (grade 2 or 3) in the study by Gorman and colleagues[5] had some initial sign or symptom (drooling, abdominal pain, etc.).

TABLE 175-2 Common Caustic Compounds

	Found in
Alkali	
Sodium hydroxide	Industrial chemical, Clinitest tablets, drain cleaners, oven cleaners
Potassium hydroxide	Drain cleaners, batteries
Calcium hydroxide	Cement
Ammonium hydroxide	Hair straighteners, skin peels, toilet cleaners, glass cleaners, fertilizers
Lithium hydroxide	Photography developer, batteries
Sodium tripolyphosphate	Detergents
Sodium hypochlorite	Bleach
Acids	
Sulfuric acid	Automobile batteries, drain cleaners, explosives, fertilizer
Acetic acid	Printing and photography, disinfectants, hair neutralizer
Hydrochloric acid	Cleaning agents, metal cleaning, chemical production
Hydrofluoric acids	Rust remover, petroleum industry, glass etching, jewelry cleaners
Formic acid	Model glue, leather and textile manufacturing, tissue preservation
Chromic acid	Metal plating, photography
Nitric acid	Fertilizer, engraving, electroplating
Phosphoric acid	Rust proofing, metal cleaners, disinfectants

MANAGEMENT

Initial Assessment

During the initial and subsequent evaluations, the emergency department (ED) staff should take precautions to prevent personal injury secondary to caustic exposure (Fig. 175-1).

The first step is immediate airway evaluation. Patients with respiratory distress may have significant oral, pharyngeal, and/or laryngotracheal injury, and may require emergency airway management. Ideally, patients with potential airway injuries should have fiber-optic evalua-

TABLE 175-3 Endoscopic Grading of Upper Gastrointestinal Caustic Injuries

Grade 0	Normal examination findings
Grade 1	Edema and hyperemia of mucosa
Grade 2a	Friability, hemorrhages, erosions, blisters, whitish membrane, exudates, and superficial ulcerations
Grade 2b	Grade 2a plus deep discrete or circumferential ulceration
Grade 3a	Small scattered necrosis
Grade 3b	Extensive necrosis

Source: From Zargar et al,[23] with permission.

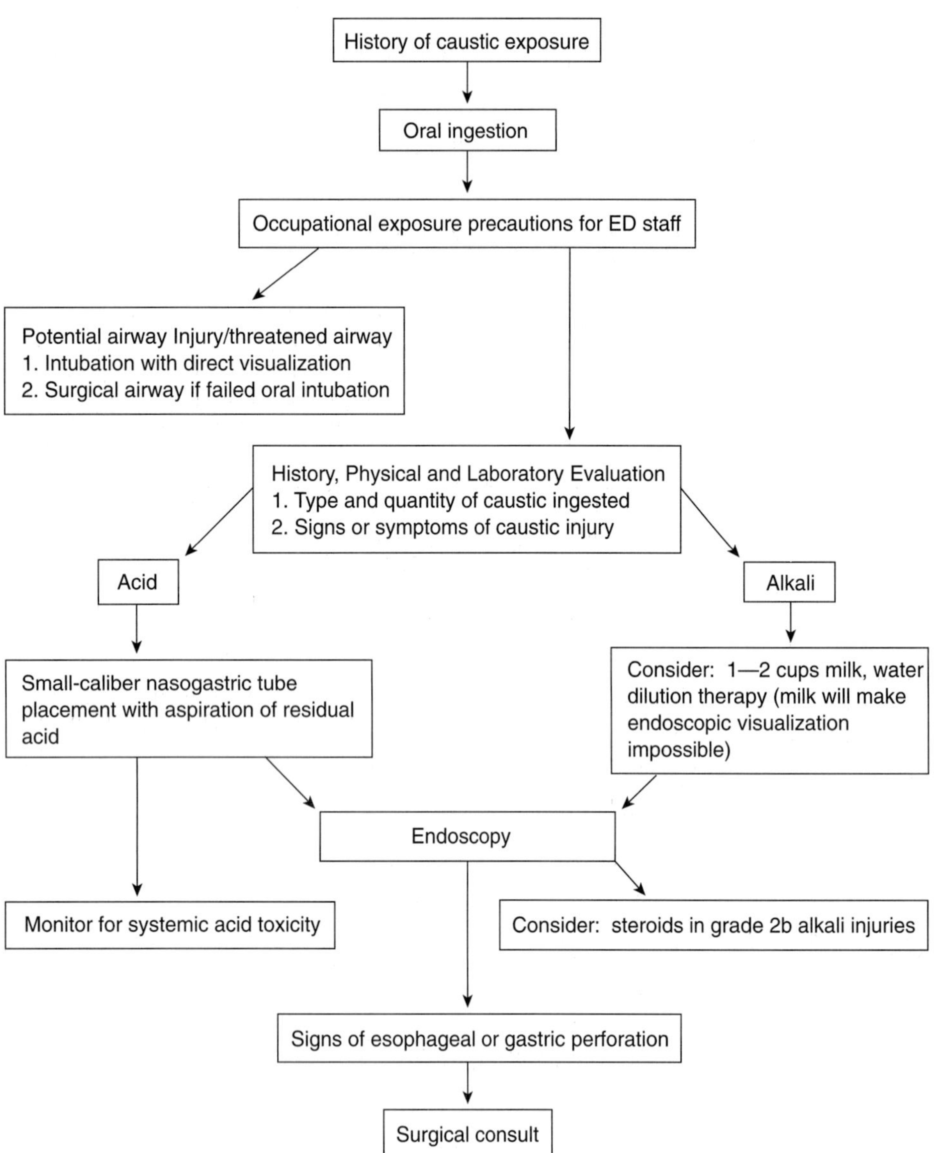

FIG. 175-1. Guidelines for treatment of caustic exposures.

tion of the airway prior to intubation to determine the extent of the damage, but this may not always be possible. Blind nasotracheal intubation is contraindicated secondary to the potential for exacerbating airway injuries. Oral intubation with direct visualization is the first choice for definitive airway management, but surgical cricothyrotomy may be required if oral intubation is not possible. When in doubt, it is prudent to establish an airway early rather than risk greater difficulty later as secondary effects of injury, such as edema, complicate the situation.

A directed history and physical examination should be performed to determine the type and amount of caustic ingested. It should also be determined whether the ingestion was intentional or unintentional. Patients should be assessed for hemodynamic instability. Etiologies for shock in these patients include GI bleeding, complications of GI perforation, and volume depletion. Patients should be examined for peritoneal signs from hollow viscous perforation, and mediastinitis should be considered in patients complaining of chest discomfort. Examinations should be performed to detect dermal and ocular caustic exposures.

Laboratory/Ancillary Test

Laboratory evaluation should include arterial blood-gas level, electrolyte panel, hepatic profile, complete blood count, and coagulation profile. Strong acid ingestions may cause severe acid-base disorders, and an arterial line may be indicated if serial blood-gas determinations are required. Special attention should be given to serum calcium and magnesium levels after hydrofluoric acid exposures (vide infra). All patients should have an upright chest radiograph to screen for peritoneal and mediastinal air. After intentional ingestions, electrocardiography should be done and aspirin and acetaminophen levels should be obtained to screen for potential coingestants.

Gastric Decontamination

Gastric decontamination is a difficult issue because much of the morbidity and death related to caustic ingestion is secondary to destruction of the GI tract. Caustics do not bind well to activated charcoal, and charcoal is not useful in either alkali or acid ingestions. Gastric lavage and ipecac are also not used. They may increase the risk for repeat exposure to the ingested caustics secondary to vomiting. Nasogastric (NG) tube placement is also controversial. The use of an NG tube is contraindicated in obvious gastric or esophageal perforation. An NG tube is also not used after alkali ingestions, because the risk of GI perforation is considered too great. In cases of strong acid ingestion, the risk for perforation is considered lower because coagulation necrosis may protect deeper tissue from injury. Placement of a small NG tube under endoscopic guidance has been recommended by some to aspirate residual acid from the stomach.

Neutralization and Dilution

Recommendations about dilution and or neutralization therapy after caustic ingestions vary. Dilution of caustic alkalis with water or milk has been shown to decrease tissue destruction in animal models.[7] The literature generally recommends dilution therapy with 1 to 2 cups of water or milk early after alkali exposures. The toxicology literature suggests a greater theoretical benefit to dilution in treating solid alkali ingestions, because dilution might wash off adherent particles. Potential dangers of such therapy include vomiting, which may lead to further exposure of the esophagus and airway to caustic material and/or aspiration. Dilution therapy is contraindicated with patients who have obvious signs of perforation or airway injury. Most sources do not recommend dilution therapy for the treatment of acid ingestion. Rather, placement of a small NG tube with aspiration of gastric contents appears to be the chief means of gastric decontamination.

Neutralization therapy has long been considered contraindicated in caustic ingestions, because neutralization of strong bases with acids (and the reverse) are exothermic reactions. It is feared that the heat generated during neutralization could worsen injuries. Recently, a series of animal studies by Homan and colleagues[8] has questioned the significance of heat generated during neutralization therapy. Currently, the best recommendation with respect to dilution or neutralization therapy is small volumes of water or milk in alkali ingestions without signs of perforation. Neutralization of alkali with weak acids is contraindicated until further study and data are available.

Endoscopy

Endoscopy is an important tool used to evaluate the location and severity of injury to the esophagus, stomach, and duodenum after caustic ingestion. Indications for endoscopy vary. Some authorities recommend endoscopy in all cases of caustic ingestions, whereas others advocate endoscopy based on signs and symptoms.[9] Endoscopy is generally indicated in the presence of any signs or symptoms of serious injury (vomiting, drooling, dyspnea, or stridor), in the presence of oral-pharyngeal burns, and after intentional ingestions.

Zargar and colleagues[4] developed the most commonly referenced system for endoscopic staging of upper GI tract caustic injuries and prospectively demonstrated the safety of using the endoscope in caustic ingestions. Injuries are divided into four grades (Table 175-3). Patients with grade 2b and 3 injuries are at risk of long-term sequelae, including stricture formation. Patients with grade 3 lesions are at greatest risk of perforation, fistula, and hemorrhage.

Traditionally, endoscopists terminated their examination at the first sign of severe esophageal injury (grade 2b or 3). However, a more complete exam to document all injuries to the esophagus, stomach, and duodenum may outweigh the risk of perforation. Most experts agree that the timing of the endoscopy should be within the first several hours of ingestions and that follow-up exams should be avoided between days 5 and 15. Other noninvasive diagnostic means to evaluate and follow caustic GI injuries include abdominal computed tomography (CT) and ultrasonography. For patients not requiring emergent laparotomy, CT may be used to screen for intraabdominal necrosis outside the GI tract or in areas not reachable with the endoscope. Sonographic evaluation, both transabdominal and endoscopic, has been advocated for evaluation and follow-up of gastric injury after caustic ingestion.[10]

Steroids

One of the most controversial aspects of caustic ingestion management is the use of steroids to potentially decrease the risk of stricture formation. The ability of steroids to inhibit the inflammatory response led to the hypothesis that steroids may decrease stricture formation after caustic ingestion. The largest study of steroid use in human caustic ingestions was not able to demonstrate a benefit from steroid use.[11] Opponents of steroid use believe that steroids may increase the risk of infection, perforation, and hemorrhage. However, no compelling data support these fears in caustic ingestions.[12,13] Steroid use has never been recommended in acid ingestions, because the risk of esophageal stricture formation is believed to be lower. Recommendations vary for steroid use after alkali caustic ingestions from not using steroids at all to using them only in endoscopic grade 2b lesions (circumferential deep ulcerated lesions). Steroids are not indicated in grade 1 and grade 2a lesions because these lesions do not form strictures and grade 3 lesions are probably best handled by surgical resection. Steroids, if used, should be used early, within the first 6 h, at a dose approximately equivalent to 2 mg/kg/24 h of prednisolone for 3 weeks, followed by a taper.

Antibiotics

Most caustic ingestions do not require prophylactic antibiotics. If steroids are to be used after caustic ingestion, some evidence indicates that antibiotics may help to reduce rates of infection. Antibiotics used in these cases are penicillin, ampicillin, or clindamycin in penicillin-allergic patients.

Systemic Toxicity

Morbidity or death from alkali injuries usually results from the complications of direct tissue necrosis, but acid ingestions may result in systemic toxicity from absorption of the acid in addition to local tissue destruction. Significant acid-base disorders, hemolysis, and renal failure may result. In cases of systemic toxicity, traditional critical care principles should be applied to optimize the patient's hemodynamics. Manipulation of serum pH with sodium bicarbonate may be required if the serum pH is consistently below 7.10.

Ocular Exposures

Ocular injuries after caustic exposures can be devastating to vision. The Eye Bank Association of America reports that 300 of the 1000 corneal transplants in the United States in 1995 were secondary to eye injuries caused by chemicals.[14] Caustic alkali injuries to the eye are generally more severe than acid-related eye injuries. Alkali injuries penetrate deep into ocular tissue and continue to be destructive after superficial removal, whereas acidic injuries are usually superficial. The coagulation necrosis after acid injury limits the penetration of acid into ocular tissue.

Ocular injuries should be immediately treated with copious irrigation (Fig. 175-2). Patients should have continuous irrigation with at least 2 L of normal saline per affected eye. Nitrazine (pH) paper should be utilized to ensure that the offending acid or base is eliminated. The expected pH after irrigation should be between 7.5 and 8.0, and irrigation should continue until this pH range is achieved. A waiting period of 10 min before checking the pH will more accurately reflect the pH of the eye and not the irrigation fluid. After irrigation, all patients should have a complete eye exam, including fluorescein staining, and all except the most superficial exposures should have ED ophthalmology consultation.

A recently reported ocular injury that ED clinicians should be aware of is alkali keratitis after deployment of motor vehicle airbags. A small amount of aerosolized sodium hydroxide and sodium carbonate is released during airbag deployment. These caustic alkalis may enter the eye and cause significant injury. The recommendation is to treat these injuries as other caustic ocular exposures, with copious irrigation, pH testing, and ophthalmology consultation.[15,16]

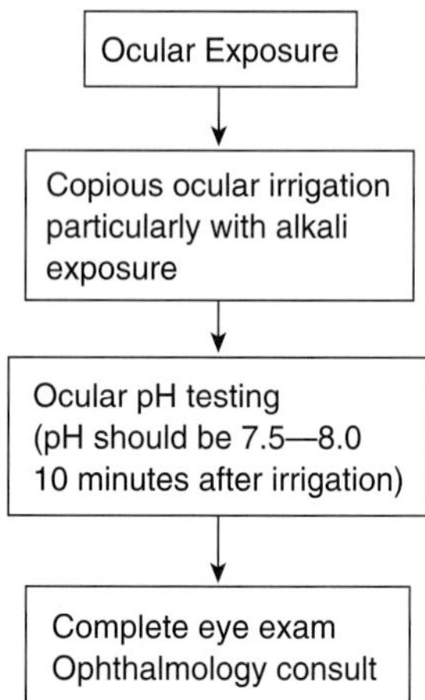

FIG. 175-2. Guidelines for treatment of caustic ocular exposures.

Treatment of Dermal Exposures

Caustic injuries to the skin most frequently occur on the extremities. Most acid injuries, excluding hydrofluoric acid, respond well to local copious saline irrigation. Alkali dermal exposures may appear deceptively superficial, yet burn more deeply and for extended periods.[17] Management of these injuries should include copious irrigation and local wound debridement to remove residual compound (Fig. 175-3). In cases of lime exposure and other caustic powders, patients should brush off the dry compound and remove contaminated clothing before irrigating.

Portland or ready-mix cement is an alkali mixture of lime that warrants special mention. When water is added to the dry mixture, calcium, sodium, and potassium hydroxide are produced. Patients may initially present with severe pain without obvious injury but eventually develop blisters and skin necrosis if the affected area is not irrigated early. All cutaneous caustic injuries require close follow-up or early referral to a plastic surgeon to ensure the injuries are not progressing.

Experimental Therapies

Many different therapies have been tried to decrease the toxic effects of caustic ingestions. Most experiential therapies have been aimed at preventing esophageal strictures after caustic alkali ingestion. Animal data have showed decreased stricture formation with drugs that affect collagen deposition, including β-aminopropionitrile, *N*-acetylcysteine, and D-penicillamine. Pentoxifylline, a local inflammatory and microcirculation mediator, has also been used experimentally. Oral agents to coat and protect the GI tract from insult, including sulcrafate, bismuth subsalicylate, and sodium polyacrylate, have been tried experimentally with some success. None of these agents have been evaluated in controlled clinical trials in humans, and more data are needed before a recommendation with respect to their use can be made.

Surgery/Stents/Dilation

Major ingestions of caustic agents may result in immediate perforation of the GI tract and require emergency surgery. The indications for emergency laparotomy include peritoneal signs or free intraperitoneal air. Esophageal perforation diagnosed by mediastinal air on plain films or by endoscopy is also an indication for emergent surgery. More controversial is the management of severe esophageal injuries, grade

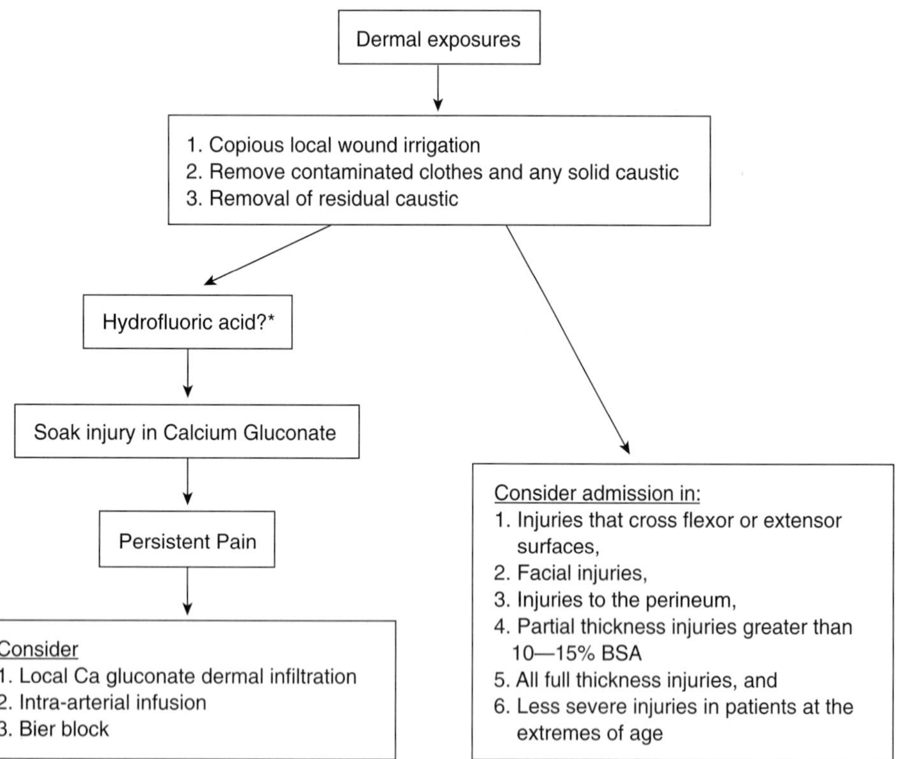

FIG. 175-3. Guidelines for treatment of caustic dermal exposures.

2b and 3, without obvious perforation. Some authorities recommend early dilation therapy (in the first 3 weeks) with or without stenting, whereas others report good results with early surgical resection.[18,19]

DISPOSITION

All patients with symptomatic caustic ingestions should be admitted to the hospital. Patients with grade 1 and 2a lesions will do well but warrant hospitalization to ensure that symptoms do not progress. The majority of ocular injuries will require ED ophthalmology consultation and follow-up. Mild to moderate dermal injuries can be safely discharged after local wound irrigation, aseptic dressings, and close follow-up. The following dermal exposures may warrant admission: injuries that cross flexor or extensor surfaces, facial injuries, injuries to the perineum, partial-thickness injuries greater than 10 to 15 percent of body surface area, all full-thickness injuries, and less severe injuries in patients at the extremes of age.

SPECIAL CASES

Disc Batteries

Disc batteries are a common, potentially caustic ingestant. Each year, there are approximately 2000 disc battery ingestions in the United States, mostly by children younger than age 6 (Table 175-1). Batteries may contain manganese dioxide, zinc, mercuric acid, silver oxide, or lithium in an alkaline medium. Most disc batteries pass through the GI tract without incident. Batteries have the potential for alkali injury if they leak secondary to casing damage or from hydroxide production related to external current from intact batteries. Pressure necrosis may also play a role in injury if the disc battery becomes lodged in the GI tract. Heavy-metal toxicities, while a theoretical consideration in disc battery ingestion, have not been documented.[20]

With patients who present after disc battery ingestion, chest and abdominal radiographs should be obtained to determine the position of the battery. Batteries in the airway or esophagus should be removed by endoscopy/bronchoscopy immediately. If a battery has passed the gastroesophageal junction and appears to be in the stomach, then a follow-up film should be obtained in 24 to 48 h to ensure that the battery has passed through the pylorus. Batteries in the intestines should pass without difficulty, but checking the stools and follow-up film are used to ensure passage.

Hydrofluoric Acid

Hydrofluoric acid is a relatively weak acid ($pK_a = 3.8$) used in industry for glass etching, metal cleaning, and petroleum processing. It may also be found in household products such as chrome wheel cleaner and rust remover. Despite being a relatively weak acid, hydrofluoric acid has great potential for causing morbidity and death. The major mechanism of injury with hydrofluoric acid is not coagulation necrosis; rather, the free fluoride ion complexes with body calcium and magnesium, resulting in cellular death. Most injuries are to the upper extremities. Patients often present with benign-appearing wounds but complain of a tremendous amount of pain. These wounds often have a slight white discoloration but may become black and necrotic as cellular damage results. Severe injuries may result in hypocalcemia, hypomagnesemia, hyperkalemia, acidosis, and ventricular dysrhythmias. Ventricular fibrillation and death have been reported with dermal exposure of between 2.5 and 22 percent of body surface area.

Treatment of minor hydrofluoric acid injuries consists of first thoroughly irrigating the affected area with water and then placing the area in a paste of calcium gluconate or benzalkonium chloride solution. Paste can be made with surgical lubrication and calcium gluconate powder (2.5 percent wt/vol) or alternately with a commercial preparation of benzalkonium chloride (Zephiran) is available. The affected area is soaked in the gel, with pain relief being used as end point for therapy. Other effective treatments include intradermal injections of 5% calcium gluconate or magnesium sulfate around the affected area (not to exceed 0.5 mL/cm^2). For distal upper extremity injuries that do not respond to the aforementioned treatments, intraarterial infusion of calcium gluconate has been used. It is recommended that 10 mL of 10% calcium gluconate diluted in 40 mL of normal saline be infused over 4 h or until pain resolves. The use of calcium chloride should be avoided for fear of skin necrosis if extravasation occurs. The use of calcium gluconate with a Bier block has been advocated for treating serious hydrofluoric injuries.[21]

Oral ingestion of hydrofluoric acid has a high mortality rate. NG tube placement and gastric lavage with normal saline are recommended. Oral magnesium or calcium should be given in hydrofluoric ingestions on a milliequivalent-for-milliequivalent basis. If the amount of hydrofluoric acid ingested is not known, then 300 mL of magnesium citrate or calcium salts should be given. In serious exposures of any type, attention should be focused on hemodynamic monitoring for dysrhythmias. Serum calcium and magnesium levels should also be followed closely. Intravenous supplementation with large amounts of calcium and magnesium may be required.

LONG-TERM MORBIDITY

Most long-term sequelae from caustic exposure are related to injuries to the GI tract. Acid ingestions may scar the pylorus and result in gastric outlet obstruction. Caustic alkali ingestions may result in esophageal strictures, which may result in dysphagia, odynophagia, and malnutrition. Controversy exists on the appropriate treatment—long-term dilation therapy versus surgery—for strictures.[22]

Patients with caustic injuries to the esophagus are at risk for cancer of the esophagus. Increased risked for esophageal malignancy is up to 1000 times greater in patients with a history of caustic ingestion and is often seen decades after the initial ingestion and resulting esophageal injury. Some authorities advocate prophylactic esophagectomy in grade 3 lesions to decrease risk of potential future malignancy.

REFERENCES

1. Litovitz TL, Smilkstein M, Feldberg L, et al: 1996 Annual report of the American Association of Poison Control Centers toxic exposure suveillance system. *Am J Emerg Med* 15:447, 1997.
2. Losanoff J, Kjossev K: Multivisceral injury after liquid caustic ingestion. *Surgery* 119:720, 1996.
3. Karnak I, Tanyel FC, Bukupamukcu N, Hicsonmez A: Pulmonary effects of household bleach ingestions in children. *Clin Pediatr* 35:471, 1996.
4. Zargar SA, Kochhar R, Nagi B, et al: Ingestion of corrosive acids: Spectrum of injury to the upper gastrointestinal tract and natural history. *Gastroenterology* 97:702, 1989.
5. Gaudreault P, Parent M, McGuigan M, et al: Predictability of esophageal injury from signs and symptoms: A study of caustic ingestion in 378 children. *Pediatrics* 71:767, 1983.
6. Gorman RL, Khin-Maung-Gyi MT, Klein-Schwartz W, et al: Initial symptoms as a predictors of esophageal injury in alkaline corrosive ingestions. *Am J Emerg Med* 10:189, 1992.
7. Homan CS, Maitra SR, Lane B, et al: Therapeutic effects of water and milk for acute injury of the esophagus. *Ann Emerg Med* 24:14, 1994.
8. Homan CS, Singer AJ, Henry MC, Thode HC: Thermal effects of neutralization and water dilution for acute alkali exposures in canines. *Acad Emerg Med* 4:27, 1997.
9. Christesen HB: Prediction of complications following unintentional caustic ingestion in children. Is endoscopy always necessary? *Acta Paediatr Scand* 84:1177, 1995.
10. Aviram G, Kessler A, Reif S, et al: Corrosive gastritis: Sonographic findings in the acute phase and follow-up. *Pediatr Radiol* 27:805, 1997.
11. Anderson KD, Rouse T, Randolph JG: A controlled trial of corticosteroids in children with corrosive injury of the esophagus. *N Engl J Med* 323:637, 1990.

12. Howell JM, Dalsey WC, Hartsell FW, Butzin CA: Steroids for the treatment of corrosive esophageal injury: A statistical analysis of past studies. *Am J Emerg Med* 10:421, 1992.
13. Oakes DD: Reconsidering the diagnosis and treatment of patients following ingestion of liquid lye. *J Clin Gastroenterol* 21:85, 1995.
14. Blais BR: Treating chemical eye injuries. *Occup Health Saf* 65:23, 1996.
15. Hallock GG: Mechanisms of burn injuries secondary to airbag deployment. *Ann Plast Surg* 39:111, 1997.
16. White JE, McClafferty K, Orton RB, et al: Ocular alkali burn associated with automobile air-bag activation. *CMAJ* 153:933, 1995.
17. O'Donoghue JM, Al-Ghazal SK, McCann JJ: Caustic soda burns to the extremities: Difficulties in management. *Br J Clin Pract* 50:108, 1996.
18. Berthert B, Castellani P, Brioche MI, et al: Early operation for corrosive injury to the upper gastrointestinal tract. *Eur J Surg* 162:951, 1996.
19. Ochi K, Ohashi T, Santo S, et al: Surgical treatment for caustic ingestion injury of the pharynx, larynx, and esophagus. *Acta Otolaryngol (Stockh)* 522:116–9, 1996.
20. Litovitz T, Schnitz BF: Ingestion of cylindrical and button batteries: An analysis of 2382 cases. *Pediatrics* 89:747, 1992.
21. Graundis A, Burns MJ, Aaron CK: Regional intravenous infusion of calcium gluconate for hydrofluoric acid burns of the upper extremities. *Ann Emerg Med* 30:604, 1997.
22. Berkovits RN, Bos CE, Wijburg FA, Holzki J: Caustic injury of the oesophagus: Sixteen years experience, and introduction of a new model oesophageal stent. *J Laryngol Otol* 110:1041, 1996.
23. Zargar SA, Kochhar R, Mehta SK: The role of fiberoptic endoscopy in the management of corrosive ingestion and modified endoscopic classification of burns. *Gastrointest Endosc* 37:165, 1991.

176 INSECTICIDES, HERBICIDES, RODENTICIDES

Walter C. Robey III
William J. Meggs

Pesticides are used to kill pests but also can be harmful or deadly to humans. Compounds considered to be pesticides include insecticides, herbicides, and rodenticides. In the United States, over 85,225 pesticide exposures were reported to poison centers in 1997.[1] About 45,390 of these involved children under 6 years of age. There were 14 deaths.

Pesticide intoxication results from intentional, accidental, and occupational exposures. Because of the number of chemical compounds marketed as multiple formulations and brand names and the complex clinical syndromes that result from exposure to their active ingredients, management often necessitates consultation with a poison center. Many pesticides contain inactive ingredients, such as petroleum distillates, that also can have harmful effects and modify management. Each class of pesticides has specific toxicologic properties that may produce predictable clinical findings after excessive exposure. However, there may be very nonspecific, subtle syndromes early on or in the case of chronic exposure. Many of the pesticides are responsible for both local and systemic effects. Supportive measures play an important role in most toxic exposures, even though specific antidotal therapy occasionally may be available. Broad-spectrum insecticides are responsible for most human pesticide intoxications.

INSECTICIDES

Chemical insecticides exert their toxic action by affecting the nervous system. Toxicity may include acute, chronic, and delayed sequelae of acute exposure. The four major classes of insecticides in use today are the organophosphates, carbamates, organochlorines, and pyrethroids. Organophosphate and carbamate cholinesterase inhibitors have replaced organochlorine insecticides because of their improved effectiveness and lack of persistence in the environment and human tissues. In 1997, 70,739 insecticide exposures were reported by the American Association of Poison Control Centers.[1] Children younger than 6 years of age were involved in 30,317 of these. Of the total, 66,217 were unintentional, 13,249 were treated in health care facilities, and 2365 patients had moderate to major clinical toxicity associated with exposure. Insecticide poisoning is worldwide. In a Jordanean study of 52 patients with insecticide poisoning, mixed organophosphate and carbamate exposure was responsible in 34.5 percent and isolated organophosphate or carbamate each was responsible for 25 percent.[2]

Organophosphates

Commonly used organophosphates include diazinon, orthene, malathion, parathion, and chlorpyrifos. In addition to their use as insecticides, organophosphates have been used as chemical warfare agents since World War II. Most recently, the organophosphate sarin was used in the terrorist attack on the Tokyo subway in 1995.[3] Organophosphates and carbamates are the most common insecticides associated with systemic illness. Potency does vary, however. Highly potent compounds such as parathion are used primarily in agriculture. Those of intermediate potency include coumaphos and trichlorfon, which are used in animal care. Low-potency products used in the household and on golf courses include diazinon and malathion. These compounds are very toxic at higher exposures. Poisoning results primarily from accidental exposure in the home, in agriculture, in industry (in workers involved in the manufacture and transport of these products), and in areas of insect control. Exposure to flea-dip products has been reported in pet groomers and children. Widespread food contamination and the potential for mass toxic exposure are always a risk. In addition, these chemicals are involved in intentional poisonings and occasionally in homicides. Systemic absorption of organophosphates occurs by inhalational, transdermal, transconjunctival, and gastrointestinal exposure.

PATHOPHYSIOLOGY The mechanism of action of organophosphates involves the inhibition of the enzyme cholinesterase in the nervous system. Acetylcholinesterase (true or red blood cell acetylcholinesterase) is found primarily in erythrocytes and in nervous tissue. Plasma cholinesterase (pseudocholinesterase) is found in the serum, liver, heart, pancreas, and brain. Acetylcholine is a major neurotransmitter in the central, autonomic, and somatic nervous systems. The role of the cholinesterases is to hydrolyze acetylcholine into the inactive components choline and acetic acid after neurochemical transmission. Inhibition of cholinesterase leads to acetylcholine accumulation at nerve synapses and neuromuscular junctions, resulting in overstimulation of acetylcholine receptors. This initial overstimulation is followed by paralysis of cholinergic synaptic transmission in the central nervous system (CNS), in autonomic ganglia, at parasympathetic and some sympathetic nerve endings (e.g., sweat glands), and in somatic nerves. A *cholinergic crisis* results in a central and peripheral clinical toxidrome.

Organophosphates bind irreversibly to cholinesterase, thus inactivating the enzyme through the process of phosphorylation. A concept known as "aging" is used to describe the latency of permanent, irreversible binding of the organophosphate to the cholinesterase. This takes approximately 24 to 48 h to occur. The organophosphate-cholinesterase bond is irreversible without pharmacologic intervention. This time period of 24 to 48 h after exposure is therefore the critical interval during which administration of an antidote can reverse the process. Once "aging" occurs, however, the enzymatic activity of cholinesterase is permanently destroyed, and new enzyme must be resynthesized over a period of weeks before clinical symptoms resolve and normal enzymatic function returns. Therapeutic agents that remove the organophosphate and reactivate the cholinesterases are ineffective after "aging" is complete.

CLINICAL FEATURES Clinical presentations depend on the specific agent involved, the quantity absorbed, and the type of exposure. A number of organophosphates are associated with local irritation of the skin and respiratory tract with resulting dermatitis and wheezing, respectively, without evidence of systemic absorption. A few cases of persistent reactive airway disease independent of cholinesterase inhibition have been reported.[4]

Acute systemic organophosphate poisoning results in a variety of clinical CNS, muscarinic, nicotinic, and somatic motor manifestations. In mild to moderate poisoning, symptoms occur in various combinations. Time to onset varies with route and chemical but usually occurs within 12 to 24 h. Onset is most rapid with inhalation and least rapid with transdermal absorption; however, dermatitis or skin excoriation may hasten this. Symptoms can occur within minutes with massive ingestion.

CNS symptoms of cholinergic excess include anxiety, restlessness, emotional lability, tremor, headache, dizziness, mental confusion, delirium, hallucinations, and seizures. Coma with depression of respiratory and circulatory centers may result. Aggressive behavior has been described.

Muscarinic receptor stimulation by acetylcholine is usually predominant and leads to salivation, lacrimation/sweating, urinary incontinence, diarrhea, gastrointestinal distress, emesis (SLUDGE), and bradycardia. Bradycardia is usually predominant, but tachycardia may occur.[5] Bradycardia may present as rate-related dizziness or syncope. Bronchospasm and bronchorrhea resulting from acetylcholine excess can lead to hypoxia and tachycardia. Miotic pupils and blurred vision are due to cholinergic effects on the pupillary constrictors and ciliary body.

Acetylcholine is the presynaptic neurotransmitter that stimulates nicotinic receptors in the sympathetic ganglia and adrenal medulla. Overstimulation results in pallor, mydriasis, tachycardia, and hypertension. Parasympathetic stimulation usually dominates, but sympathetic domination with tachycardia and hypertension are seen. Nicotinic stimulation at neuromuscular junctions results in muscle fasciculations, cramps, and muscle weakness. This syndrome may progress to paralysis and areflexia. Respiratory muscle paralysis results in acute respiratory failure and death. Miosis and muscle fasciculations are considered by some as reliable clinical signs of toxicity.

An intermediate syndrome may occur 1 to 4 days following an acute organophosphate poisoning.[6] The patient appears to be recovering from an acute poisoning when this manifests. Clinically, there is paralysis of neck flexor muscles, muscles innervated by the cranial nerves, and proximal limb and respiratory muscles to the extent that some patients may require respiratory support. Electromyography (EMG) may assist in making the diagnosis by indicating a problem at the neuromuscular junction. Aggressive, early antidote therapy and supportive measures may prevent this syndrome. Symptoms usually resolve within 4 to 18 days.

A non-cholinesterase-related neurotoxic syndrome known as *organophosphate-induced delayed neuropathy* (OPIDN) may occur 2 to 3 weeks after acute poisoning with a flaccid paralysis of the lower limbs. This is thought to be due to the inhibition of a neuropathy target enzyme. Delayed bilateral recurrent laryngeal nerve paralysis has been reported as a manifestation of this syndrome.

Chronic neurologic and neurobehavioral sequelae after acute organophosphate poisoning include neuropsychiatric deficits and paralysis.[7] More lipid-soluble organophosphates may not produce immediate symptoms of toxicity, and symptoms may persist for several weeks. Low-grade chronic organophosphate exposures occur among farm workers, pesticide manufacturing plant workers, and exterminators. Symptoms and signs are often less dramatic and nonspecific, with varying degrees of headache, nausea, weakness, or fatigue and a subtle cholinergic syndrome. Neuropsychological effects have been described with chronic exposure.

Special Considerations Organophosphates are the principal toxins found in nerve gases. Chemical warfare nerve agents referred to as *G agents* were synthesized in search of better insecticides. Their mechanism involves the inactivation of acetylcholinesterase. These chemicals, however, produce "aging" within minutes, thus making them particularly toxic. They are rapid acting and extremely potent, and death occurs within minutes of inhalation or dermal exposure. Accordingly, those exposed are unlikely to present to the emergency department (ED) alive.

DIAGNOSIS Suspicion of exposure to organophosphates is based on the history, the presence of a suggestive toxidrome, and laboratory cholinesterase assays. Diagnosis is often difficult owing to a constellation of clinical findings that may be vague in both acute and chronic poisonings. Toxicity may masquerade as a nonspecific flulike syndrome. Degree of toxicity may be based on the presence of specific signs and symptoms. Mild, moderate, and severe toxicities are described.

Clinically, noting a characteristic petroleum or garlic-like odor may assist in diagnosis. The cholinergic toxidrome may vary depending on the predominance of muscarinic, nicotinic, and CNS manifestations of the toxin and the severity of the intoxication. An initial test dose of intravenous atropine that does not result in the expected improvement in signs and symptoms in the case of poisoning may assist in making a diagnosis. Differential diagnosis of CNS alterations includes all nontoxic causes of mental status changes, coma, and seizures. Muscarinic manifestations may imitate asthma, exacerbation of chronic obstructive pulmonary disease, cardiogenic pulmonary edema, acute gastroenteritis, and primary cardiac brachycardia or hypotension. Miosis may appear late, whereas the presence of mydriasis may indicate hypoxia. Ocular exposure may cause persistent miosis. Nicotinic manifestations may imitate other causes of striated muscle dysfunction and respiratory failure. Sympathomimetic toxins and other causes of sympathetic hyperactivity should be considered when signs and symptoms of nicotinic stimulation predominate.

Functional assays of plasma and red blood cell (RBC) cholinesterases are helpful for diagnosis and as a guide for therapy but may not be readily available. Clinical toxicity is predominately due to the toxic effect of the organophosphate on RBC acetylcholinesterase; therefore, this enzyme assay is a more accurate indicator of synaptic cholinesterase inhibition. However, plasma cholinesterase is easier to assay and more available. The degree of cholinesterase inhibition necessary to produce symptomatic illness is variable, with symptoms generally occurring only after more than 50 percent inhibition from baseline determinations. Although there is patient variability, a high-normal cholinesterase level excludes acute systemic poisoning. The degree of depression from baseline cholinesterase levels is thought to correlate with toxicity. A patient may show mild clinical toxicity with normal levels. With a 60 percent decrease in cholinesterase level, headache and parasympathetic stimulation develop. Moderate symptoms develop, including muscle weakness, tremor, and neuropsychiatric symptoms, with a 60 to 90 percent decrease. After a 90 percent decrease, severe symptoms include seizures, cyanosis, pulmonary edema, respiratory failure due to muscle weakness, and coma, and death may occur.

Without treatment, plasma cholinesterase takes up to 4 to 6 weeks and RBC acetylcholinesterase as long as 90 to 120 days to return to baseline after exposure. Plasma cholinesterase levels have poor prognostic value in patients with acute organophosphate poisoning. Levels do not correlate with the amount of atropine required or the need for mechanical ventilation.[8] When the rate of cholinesterase falls gradually, as in chronic exposure, clinical symptoms may be minimal. Plasma cholinesterase levels may be depressed in genetic variants, chronic disease states, liver dysfunction, cirrhosis, malnutrition and low serum albumin states, neoplasia, infection, and pregnancy. RBC acetylcholinesterase is affected by factors that influence the circulating life of erythrocytes such as hemoglobinopathies.

Routine laboratory test abnormalities are nondiagnostic but may include evidence of pancreatitis, hypo- or hyperglycemia, and liver function abnormalities. A chest radiograph may show pulmonary edema in severe cases.

The electrocardiogram (ECG) may be abnormal and correlate with degree of toxicity and outcome. Common abnormalities include ventricular dysrhythmias, torsade de pointes, and idioventricular rhythms. Heart blocks and prolongation of the QT_c interval are common.[9]

TREATMENT Treatment consists of intensive respiratory support, general supportive measures, decontamination, and prevention of absorption. Therapy includes the administration of antidotes and is based on the degree of toxicity. Therapy should not be withheld pending determination of cholinesterase levels.

Secondary contamination of health care workers must be prevented during patient resuscitation. Protective gloves and gowns must be worn. Patients with suspected exposure must be removed from the contaminated environment. All clothes and accessories must be removed completely and placed in plastic bags for disposal. The patient is immediately decontaminated externally with copious amounts of soapy water and possibly a second washing with dilute ethanol. Decontamination must include the scalp, hair, fingernails, skin, and conjunctivae. Abrasion or irritation of the skin should be avoided. Contaminated runoff water should be drained and discarded separately and safely.

The patient is placed on 100% oxygen, a cardiac monitor, and pulse oximeter. A 100 percent non-rebreather mask will optimize oxygenation in the patient with excessive airway secretions and bronchospasm and may reduce the chance of ventricular dysrhythmias during antidote therapy. Gentle suction will assist in clearing airway secretions from hypersalivation, bronchorrhea, or emesis. Coma, seizures, respiratory failure, excessive respiratory secretions, or severe bronchospasm may necessitate endotracheal intubation. A nondepolarizing agent should be used when neuromuscular blockade is needed. An intravenous line is established, and baseline blood sampling and determination of cholinesterase levels should be done. Hypotension may necessitate initial fluid boluses of normal saline. Substrates such as dextrose and naloxone should be considered. In a recent or large ingestion, gastric lavage may be of value. Activated charcoal is recommended. Protection of the airway must be ensured before lavage in the event a hydrocarbon vehicle is involved. When there is significant diarrhea due to cholinergic effects, catharsis is withheld. Hemodialysis and hemoperfusion are of no proven value.

Pharmacologic intervention consists of concomitant atropine and pralidoxime (2-PAM) therapy in significant poisonings. Atropine, a competitive antagonist of acetylcholine at CNS and peripheral muscarinic receptors, is used to reverse muscarinic and central effects secondary to excessive parasympathetic stimulation. The dose is titrated to dry copious tracheobronchial secretions. Pupillary dilatation is not a therapeutic end point. Atropine should not be withheld in the face of a tachycardia that may be the result of hypoxia due to secretions, respiratory muscle paralysis, or ganglionic stimulation. In moderate to severe poisoning, atropine is administered in a dose of 2 to 4 mg intravenously in the adult and 0.05 mg/kg in children as a test dose. Intramuscular administration is possible, if not ideal. Failure to respond to a trial dose of atropine is indicative of organophosphate poisoning. If no effect is noted, this dose is doubled every 5 to 10 min until muscarinic symptoms are relieved. The dose necessary to dry secretions may be on the order of hundreds of milligrams in massive overdoses, and prolonged therapy may be necessary. Atropine infusion for as long as several weeks has been reported.[10] The most common cause of treatment failure is inadequate atropinization.

Compounds called *oximes* are used to displace organophosphates from the cholinesterases. Pralidoxime, or 2-PAM, is a specific antidote available in the United States. This antidote restores acetylcholinesterase activity by regenerating phosphorylated acetylcholinesterase and appears to prevent toxicity by detoxifying the remaining organophosphate molecules. Clinically, this compound ameliorates muscarinic, nicotinic, and CNS symptoms and can reverse organophosphate-related muscle paralysis. The cholinergic nicotinic effects not reversed by atropine are reversed by pralidoxime. After blood samples are obtained for determination of cholinesterase levels, it is important that pralidoxime is administered early before permanent and irreversible binding or ''aging'' occurs. It is ideal to administer this within 24 to 36 h of acute exposure. If there is a strong clinical suspicion of organophosphate toxicity, administration of 2-PAM should not be delayed. It is more effective in acute than in chronic intoxications. The recommended dose is 1 g for adults and 20 to 40 mg/kg up to 1 g for children. It should be infused in normal saline over 30 min. This may be repeated in 1 h, and multiple doses may be needed. Administration of 2-PAM should occur every 6 to 8 h for 24 to 48 h, or until signs and symptoms resolve. A continuous infusion may be administered. Combination therapy does reduce atropine requirements. This antidote is not administered to asymptomatic patients or to patients with known carbamate exposures presenting with minimal symptoms.

Response to 2-PAM therapy with a decrease in muscle weakness and fasciculation and relief of muscarinic effects with atropine usually occurs within 10 to 40 min of administration. Use of 2-PAM may prevent later subacute or chronic sequelae.[11]

Seizures are treated with airway manipulation, oxygen, benzodiazepines, and antidotal therapy. Pulmonary edema and bronchospasm are treated with oxygen, intubation, positive-pressure ventilation, atropine, and 2-PAM. Altered heart rate is treated with supportive therapy and antidotes. Management of dysrhythmias follows advanced cardiac life support guidelines. Succinylcholine, ester anesthetics, and beta blockers may potentiate poisoning and should be avoided.

DISPOSITION Mild exposure may require only decontamination and 6 to 8 h of observation in the ED. Reexposure must be avoided until cholinesterase activity returns to baseline. Patients may return to work if it does not involve reexposure risk. Admission to the intensive care unit is necessary for all significant exposures. Most patients respond to 2-PAM therapy within 48 h. If toxins are fat soluble, the patient may be symptomatic for prolonged periods of time and dependent on 2-PAM.[12] During a period of weeks while awaiting resynthesis of new enzyme, supportive care and respiratory support may be needed. The end point of therapy is determined by the absence of signs and symptoms on withholding 2-PAM therapy. Following an acute exposure, the patient may have a variety of neurologic sequelae and nonspecific symptoms lasting days to months. Chronic exposure may necessitate serial enzyme determinations to identify a trend. Death from organophosphate poisoning usually occurs in 24 h in untreated patients. If there is no posthypoxic brain damage, and if the patient is treated early, symptomatic recovery occurs in 10 days. Respiratory failure secondary to paralysis of respiratory muscles or CNS depression and bronchorrhea is the usual cause of death.

Carbamates

EPIDEMIOLOGY *N*-Methyl carbamates are cholinesterase inhibitors that are structurally related to the organophosphates. Commonly used carbamates are Sevin, Baygon, Lannate, and Aldicarb.

PATHOPHYSIOLOGY Carbamates transiently and reversibly inhibit the cholinesterase enzyme through carbamoylation. Regeneration of enzyme activity by dissociation of the carbamyl-cholinesterase complex occurs within minutes to a few hours. This involves rapid, spontaneous hydrolysis of the carbamate from the cholinesterase enzymatic site. Unlike organophosphate poisoning, it is not necessary for new enzyme to be synthesized for normal function to be restored.

CLINICAL FEATURES Symptoms of acute intoxication are similar to the cholinergic crisis observed with organophosphates but are of shorter duration. Because carbamates do not effectively penetrate the

CNS, less central toxicity is seen, and seizures do not occur. Presentation of carbamate poisoning in childhood with a predominance of CNS depression and nicotinic effects differs clinically from that of adults.[13]

DIAGNOSIS Cholinesterase levels and thus enzymatic activity may return to normal spontaneously 4 to 8 h after exposure. Measurement of RBC cholinesterase activity is therefore not useful unless done shortly after poisoning.

TREATMENT Initial treatment is the same as for organophosphates. Atropine is the antidote of choice and is administered for muscarinic symptoms. This is usually all that is necessary while waiting for the carbamoylated acetylcholinesterase complex to dissociate and recover function. Therapy is usually not needed for more than 6 to 12 h. The use of 2-PAM in carbamate poisoning is controversial. The carbamate-binding half-life to cholinesterase is approximately 30 min, and irreversible binding does not occur; therefore, there is little need for 2-PAM. The older literature suggests that 2-PAM may potentiate toxicity of the carbamate carbaryl, but a recent study found benefit.[14] Thus, it should not be avoided in severe carbamate poisonings. 2-PAM is indicated in mixed poisonings with an organophosphate and a carbamate or if the type of insecticide is unknown.

DISPOSITION Morbidity and mortality are limited because of the transient cholinesterase inhibition and rapid enzyme reactivation. These are less toxic and the clinical course more benign. Most patients recover completely within 24 h. In mild poisonings, observation suffices, and the patient may be discharged with follow-up. Moderate poisonings necessitate 24-h observation that includes ruling out concomitant exposure to or toxicity from inactive ingredients or vehicles such as hydrocarbons.

Chlorinated Hydrocarbons

EPIDEMIOLOGY Dichlordiphenyltrichloroethane (DDT) is the prototype pesticide of the chlorinated hydrocarbons. Chlordane is an example of an organochlorine that was used for termite and roach control. Most have been restricted or banned in the United States because of their persistence in the environment, long half-life in the human body, and moderate toxicity. Hexachlorocyclohexane (lindane) is a general garden insecticide that is used commonly to control ticks, scabies, and lice. This compound is well absorbed on ingestion, by inhalation, and to a minimal extent transdermally unless the skin is abraded or repeated applications are used. Children and the elderly are prone to developing CNS toxicity and seizures with therapeutic use of 1% lindane.

PATHOPHYSIOLOGY These agents are CNS stimulants absorbed primarily by the transdermal route, but they can be ingested or inhaled. The physical state, whether a liquid or solid, and the type of vehicle affects the transdermal absorption of organochlorines. Toxicity results from a decrease in permeability of membrane sodium channels following the action potential, which causes repetitive neuronal discharges. These agents are highly lipid soluble and are stored indefinitively in human tissues, and most are capable of inducing the hepatic microsomal enzyme system. Therefore, therapeutic efficacy of other chemicals and drugs that use this system is reduced in the presence of organochlorines.

CLINICAL FEATURES Neurologic symptoms predominate in the acute intoxication. Mild poisoning presents with dizziness, fatigue, malaise, headache, neurologic stimulation with hyperexcitability, irritability, and delirium, apprehension, tremulousness, myoclonus, and facial paresthesias. Fever is common. More severe exposure may result in seizures that occur occasionally without prodromal symptoms, coma, respiratory failure, and death. Respiratory findings may indicate aspiration of an inactive hydrocarbon ingredient. In addition, these agents may induce myocardial irritability with ventricular fibrillation. Chronic neurotoxic effects associated with low-level exposure to the organochlorine compound chlordane have been noted to include deficits in tests of balance, reaction time, and verbal recall.[15]

DIAGNOSIS History is important, and valuable information can be obtained from the package label regarding the product and vehicle involved. Laboratory evaluation is generally not helpful, but these agents can be detected in the serum and urine.

TREATMENT Treatment includes administration of oxygen, with intubation indicated to treat hypoxia secondary to seizures, aspiration, and respiratory failure. Benzodiazepines are indicated for seizure control. Dysrhythmia control may be indicated, but atropine and epinephrine should be avoided in the organochlorine-sensitized myocardium. Hyperthermia must be managed. Skin decontaminated with soap and water is important. Avoid using oils on skin because they promote absorption. Activated charcoal and possibly gastric lavage are indicated for ingestions. The exchange resin cholestyramine should be administered to symptomatic patients exposed to Chlordecone.

DISPOSITION Patients are observed for 6 h and admitted to the hospital if signs of significant toxicity develop or if ingestion involved a hydrocarbon.

Pyrethrins

EPIDEMIOLOGY Pyrethins are naturally occurring botanic substances found in the chrysanthemum plant. They have potential insecticidal activity but are less toxic than other insecticides. Pyrethroids are synthetic analogues of pyrethrins. These agents are used commonly as aerosols in automated insect sprays in public areas; therefore, inhalation is the most common source of exposure. These agents are available as dusts and liquids in a hydrocarbon base.

PATHOPHYSIOLOGY Pyrethrins block the sodium channel at the neuronal cell membrane, causing repetitive neuronal discharge. There is an additional effect on gamma-aminobutyric acid receptors. Other effects include increased nicotinic cholinergic transmission, norepinephrine release, and interference with sodium-calcium exchange across membranes.

CLINICAL FEATURES These compounds are responsible for dermal, pulmonary, gastrointestinal, and neurologic findings. Allergy, however, is their most common effect. Allergic reactions manifest as dermatitis, asthma, allergic rhinitis, hypersensitivity pneumonitis, and anaphylaxis. Dermal absorption is minimal, but these compounds are well absorbed from the gastrointestinal tract. Skin contact may lead to tingling and burning within 30 min of exposure and persisting up to 8 h. Contact dermatitis syndromes and allergic rhinitis result from both compounds. Allergic reactions including fatal asthma attacks have been reported. Upper and lower airway irritation occurs with local inhalation exposure. When absorbed, these compounds are metabolized rapidly in the liver, thus resulting in minimal systemic toxicity. These compounds are responsible for occasional systemic occupational poisonings. Systemic symptoms of paresthesias, hyperexcitability, tremors, incoordination, seizures, muscle weakness, respiratory failure, dizziness, headache, and nonspecific nausea, vomiting, diarrhea, and fatigue are seen with significant intentional ingestions. Alteration of consciousness, muscle fasciculations, pulmonary edema, and seizures may occur in severe poisonings.

DIAGNOSIS Differential diagnosis includes asthma-like and neurologic diseases. Laboratory tests are of little assistance clinically.

TREATMENT Treatment includes removal from exposure, decontamination, treatment of allergic manifestations, and supportive care.

DISPOSITION Disposition is usually related to the severity of asthmatic and allergic manifestations. The clinical course is usually benign and hospitalization not necessary.

HERBICIDES

Herbicides are pesticides used to kill weeds. There are several classes in general use that pose a health hazard to humans despite their low acute toxicity in mammals. Toxicity in plants is due to inhibition of photosynthesis, respiration, protein synthesis, or growth stimulation mimicking plant hormones called *auxins*. Herbicides may be classified as chlorophenoxy, bipyridyl, and urea-substituted compounds. There were 10,379 exposures to herbicides reported by the American Association of Poison Control Centers in 1997.[1] Of these, 139 were intentional, with 2820 occurring in children under 6 years of age. About 2300 patients were treated in health care facilities, and 339 exposures resulted in moderate to major morbidity, including 5 deaths.

Chlorophenoxy Herbicides

EPIDEMIOLOGY *Dioxins* and *furans* are the common names of these chemicals. The most commonly used compounds are 2,4-dichlorophenoxyacetic acid (2,4-D) and 4-chloro-2-methylphenoxyacetic acid (MCPA). 2,4,5-Trichlorophenoxy acetic acid (2,4,5-T) has been banned because of its contamination with 2,3,7,8,-tetrachlorodibenzo-*p*-dioxin (TCDD). The aerially applied defoliant Agent Orange used during the Viet Nam war was a mixture of 2,4-D and 2,4,5-T. These compounds are effective against broadleaf plants and are used as weed killers on lawns and grain crops.

PATHOPHYSIOLOGY The metabolic pathway or mechanism related to toxicity is unknown. Skeletal muscle toxicity can result in respiratory failure or rhabdomyolysis.[16] Toxicity results from dermal contact, inhalation, or ingestion. Local exposure results in dermal and gastrointestinal irritation.

CLINICAL FEATURES Local exposure leads to eye and mucous membrane irritation. After ingestion, nausea, vomiting, and diarrhea occur. Tachypnea may indicate pulmonary edema. Cardiovascular findings include hypotension, tachycardia, and dysrhythmias. Muscle toxicity manifests by muscle tenderness, fasciculations, and myotonia with resulting rhabdomyolysis. The patient may become hyperthermic. Peripheral neuropathy has been described in the recovery phase and in chronic exposure.

DIAGNOSIS Diagnosis is based on the history of exposure. Ancillary tests generally are nonspecific but may demonstrate a metabolic acidosis and evidence of hepatorenal dysfunction. Toxin levels are not immediately available. Myoglobinuria and an elevated creatine phosphate level indicate rhabdomyolysis. Differential diagnosis includes other causes of acute myopathy.

TREATMENT Treatment is supportive, including decontamination measures and respiratory support for myopathic-related respiratory failure. Alkalinization is suggested but not proven to increase the elimination of these compounds. Rhabdomyolysis should be monitored and treated.

DISPOSITION Severe toxicity and serious complications are not common. Since toxic effects usually appear within 4 to 6 h, patients with mild symptoms can be observed and discharged after that time. Significant toxicity warrants admission.

Bipyridyl Herbicides

These compounds, paraquat and diquat, are nonselective contact herbicides. Both are still widely used and are responsible for significant morbidity.

PARAQUAT **Epidemiology** Paraquat is manufactured as a liquid, granules, or an aerosol and is commonly combined with diquat and other herbicides. Most products contain an emetic. Ingestion is responsible for the majority of paraquat deaths.[17] Deaths have been reported after transdermal exposure, ingestion, and inhalation. The inhalation of sprays is unlikely to cause systemic toxicity.

Pathophysiology There is minimal transdermal absorption of paraquat in the absence of preexisting skin lesions that increase systemic absorption. Ingested paraquat is absorbed, rapidly, particularly if the stomach is empty. Plasma concentration peaks within minutes to 2 to 4 h after ingestion. Paraquat is then distributed to most organs, with the highest concentration found in the kidneys and lungs. Acute exposure causes liver and renal necrosis that is followed within a few weeks by pulmonary fibrosis.

Paraquat actively accumulates in the alveolar cells of the lungs, where it is transformed into a reactive oxygen species, the superoxide anion. This anion is responsible for lipid peroxidation that leads to degradation of cell membranes, cell dysfunction, and death. A redox reaction results in two phases of lung injury. An initial destructive phase is characterized by loss of type I and type II alveolar cells, infiltration by inflammatory cells, and hemorrhage. These changes may be reversible initially. The later, proliferative phase is characterized by fibrosis in the interstitium and alveolar spaces. Paraquat and oxygen enhance each other's toxicity by sustaining the redox cycle. Myocardial injury and necrosis of the adrenal glands may occur.

Clinical Features Paraquat's caustic effects produce local skin irritation and ulceration of epithelial surfaces. Severe corrosive corneal injury may result from eye exposure. Upper respiratory tract exposure may result in mucosal injury and epistaxis. Inhalation may lead to cough, dyspnea, chest pain, pulmonary edema, and hemoptysis.

Ingestion causes gastrointestinal mucosal lesions and ulcerations. An acute burning sensation of the lips or mouth may be followed by ulceration 1 to 2 days later. Buccopharyngeal, esophageal, and abdominal pain and vomiting occur. Caustic lesions of lips, oral cavity, and gastrointestinal tract can occur within a few minutes to hours. Hypovolemia occurs from gastrointestinal fluid losses and decreased oral intake. Cardiovascular collapse may occur early in intoxication. Multisystem effects then result, including gastrointestinal tract corrosion, acute tubular necrosis, and extensive pulmonary injury. Ingestion of greater than 30 mg/kg leads to pulmonary edema, congestive heart failure, and renal failure within hours. Seizures, gastrointestinal perforation and hemorrhage, and hepatic failure may occur. Massive ingestion may lead to multisystem failure with death within a few days. Clinical manifestations of renal failure and hepatocellular necrosis develop between the second and fifth days, with pulmonary fibrosis leading to refractory hypoxemia 5 days to several weeks later. Metabolic (lactic) acidosis is common as a result of pulmonary effects (hypoxemia) and multisystem failure.

Diagnosis Early diagnosis and therapy are important. The history may be indicative of an accidental or intentional poisoning and of the route of exposure. The differential diagnosis includes exposure to other corrosive agents and herbicides. Qualitative and quantitative analyses for paraquat in urine and blood can assist in the diagnosis.[18] Nomograms have been presented for predicting survival based on plasma paraquat concentration and time of ingestion.[18–20] A 10-h level greater than 0.4 mg/L carries a high probability of death. Serial pulmonary function tests, chest radiographs, and arterial blood gas determinations, including alveolar-arterial gradient, may be used to monitor toxicity.

Chemistry abnormalities reflect multiorgan necrosis. Hypokalemia may be present. Chest radiographs may show pneumomediastinum or pneumothorax in the case of corrosive rupture of the esophagus. Radiographic abnormalities of diffuse consolidation indicating parenchymal injury on the chest radiograph may not parallel the severity of clinical symptoms. Upper gastrointestinal endoscopy should be performed to identify the extent and severity of mucosal lesions.

Treatment The goal of early and vigorous decontamination is to prevent pulmonary toxicity. Any exposure to paraquat is a medical emergency, with hospitalization indicated even if the patient is asymptomatic. Early treatment is mainly supportive but is an important determinant of survival. An attempt should be made to prevent superoxide radical formation by using low inspired oxygen to produce a therapeutic hypoxemia with the goal of reducing pulmonary injury. The use of low oxygen mixtures ($F_iO_2 < 21$ percent) with positive-pressure ventilation reduces pulmonary toxicity in experimental models and may be of therapeutic benefit. It is suggested that the fraction of inspired oxygen should be maintained at greater than 21 percent only when arterial oxygen pressure is less than 40 mmHg. The skin should be decontaminated with soap and water without causing abrasions that may increase absorption. Ocular irrigation with copious amounts of water or saline must take place. Fluid and electrolytic losses from gastrointestinal tract damage, vomiting, and cathartics need to be replaced. Maintaining intravascular volume and urine output is important in preventing prerenal failure. Pain associated with oropharyngeal lesions should be treated with opioids. Gastric lavage via orogastric tube is recommended despite the risk of perforation.

Immediate gut decontamination with absorbants that bind paraquat is indicated. Activated charcoal (1–2 g/kg), diatomaceous Fuller's earth (1–2 g/kg in 15% aqueous suspension), or bentonite (1–2 g/kg in a 7% aqueous slurry) may be used. Subsequent doses every 4 h may be administered. A 70% sorbitol 2 cc/kg cathartic should be administered initially. Early charcoal hemoperfusion, preferably within 12 h of ingestion, offers better clearance than hemodialysis and has been associated with some successful clinical outcomes when levels were low to moderate. Multiple other therapies have been proposed to decrease the toxic effects on the lungs, but none are of proven efficacy. Corticosteroids have been used traditionally and should be considered.

Supportive care includes airway protection, maintaining intravascular volume, monitoring of vital signs and arterial blood gases, pain relief, treatment of renal failure and complications, and treatment of infection. Maintaining renal function will assist in avoiding toxic accumulation in other tissues.

Disposition An attempt to determine prognosis should be made. The mortality rate from ingestion is as high as 75 percent.[17] Outcome is determined by the amount ingested; therefore, intentional ingestions tend to have a worse prognosis. A poor prognosis is seen when paraquat is ingested in a highly concentrated formulation,[18] on an empty stomach thus increasing absorption, and when ingestion results in upper gastrointestinal ulcerations and renal failure.[21] Ingestion of a concentrated liquid solution is usually fatal. Dilute solid formulations rarely cause death. Three categories of toxicity have been described.[22] Ingestion of less than 20 mg/kg of paraquat ion or 28 mg/kg of paraquat dichloride produces no or only moderate gastrointestinal symptoms. Recovery is usually without sequelae. Ingestion of 20 to 40 mg/kg usually results in death 5 days to several weeks after ingestion. Early development of gastrointestinal corrosion, acute renal tubular necrosis, and symptoms of systemic toxicity predominates, with subsequent extensive pulmonary injury and pulmonary fibrosis causing death in most patients. Death may be delayed 2 to 3 weeks. Patients who ingest more than 40 mg/kg of paraquat usually die in 1 to 5 days. Mortality from multiorgan failure and corrosive gastrointestinal effects is 100 percent in this group.

If more than a mouthful (50 mg/kg) is ingested, death occurs within 72 h and is due to multiorgan failure, renal tubular necrosis, myocarditis, liver necrosis, adrenal necrosis, and corrosive lesions of the gastrointestinal tract. If less than a mouthful (20–50 mg/kg) is ingested, death may be delayed up to 70 days and usually results from pulmonary fibrosis.[23] Cardiogenic shock is the usual cause of death in patients with very high plasma concentrations. Death from lower levels is due to pulmonary fibrosis and respiratory failure.

DIQUAT Diquat has a similar structure and mechanism as paraquat but is less toxic. For identification purposes, formulations containing diquat do not contain the dye, stenching agent, or emetic added to paraquat. The lethal dose is similar to that of paraquat, but severe poisoning and death are less common. The extent of pulmonary injury and fibrosis is less due to diquat's lower affinity for pulmonary tissue. Diquat is caustic to the skin and gastrointestinal tract, and primary effects result in renal and liver necrosis. Treatment is similar to that for paraquat poisoning. Mortality approaches 50 percent despite diquat's lower toxicity.

Urea-Substituted Herbicides

These compounds, such as chlorimuron, diuron, fluometron, and isopturon, are inhibitors of photosynthesis and have low systemic toxicity. In humans, methemoglobinuria may occur with ingestion. Treatment includes decontamination, supportive care, and treatment with methylene blue.

RODENTICIDES

Epidemiology

Several classes of compounds are used as rodenticides or rat poisons. Because these compounds are accessible in the home, young children are at risk. According to the American Association of Poison Control Centers, in 1997 there were 17,562 reported exposures to rodenticides in the United States. Of these, 16,562 were unintentional exposures, and 15,065 of the total exposures involved children under 6 years of age. Nearly 6000 patients were treated in a health care facility. There were 6 deaths, and 3 involved long-acting warfarins. About 150 exposures resulted in moderate to major morbidity. Individuals at risk are suicide victims, attempted homicide or abuse victims, exterminators, the intoxicated, the impaired elderly, and psychiatric patients. Intentional ingestions are often associated with significant morbidity and mortality. Most accidental exposures occur in children under 6 years of age and result in minimal or no toxicity.[1,24]

Most commonly used rodenticides are the anticoagulants, derivatives of fluoroacetic acid, alpha-methyl-thiourea, and various inorganic compounds (Table 176-1). The toxic mechanisms and degree of toxicity vary depending on the specific compound. Rodenticides may be classified according to the type of compound, time of onset of signs and symptoms, and degree of toxicity. Common rodenticides will be grouped and discussed by degree of toxicity. The pathophysiology, clinical features, diagnosis, and treatment will be described for each entity.

High Toxicity

Highly toxic compounds include *sodium monofluoroacetate* (SMFA) and its derivatives, fluoroacetamide (compound 1081) and *N*-methyl-*N*-(1-naphtyl-fluoroacetamide), or MNFA. SMFA is a white crystalline, odorless, tasteless, water-soluble powder licensed only by commercial exterminators. It is toxic when absorbed through broken skin,

TABLE 176-1 Examples of Rodenticides

Sodium monofluoroacetate
Strychnine
Thallium
Zinc phosphide
Phosphorus
Arsenic
α-Naphthylthiourea
Cholecalciferol
Red squill
Warfarin
Superwarfarins

ingested, or inhaled. The active component, fluoroacetate, is converted to fluorocitrate, which interferes with the Krebs cycle. Aerobic glycolysis is thus blocked. As a result, glucose metabolism, cellular respiration, and energy production are blocked, resulting in anaerobic metabolism and lactic acidosis. Onset of toxicity is usually delayed from 2 to 20 h after ingestion. This lag time results from the delay in conversion to fluorocitrate. Signs of toxicity are nausea, apprehension, and then lactic acidosis, seizures, coma, respiratory depression, cardiac dysrhythmias, and pulmonary edema. ECG abnormalities such as ST-T wave changes, tachycardia, premature ventricular contractions, ventricular tachycardia, and fibrillation are seen. Hyperkalemia and hypocalcemia are common. Hypotension, an elevated serum creatinine level, and decreased blood pH are prognostic indicators of death.[25]

Treatment includes activated charcoal, sorbitol cathartic, seizure and dysrhythmia control, and supportive care. Experimental regimens include glycerol monoacetate and ethanol loading, which necessitates consultation with a toxicologist.

Strychnine is a highly toxic, naturally occurring alkaloid that comes from the seeds of the tree *Strychnis nux-vomica*. Strychnine is rarely used as a rodenticide today. It is an odorless, colorless crystal or white, bitter-tasting powder that can be absorbed through the gastrointestinal tract or nasal mucosa. Toxicity results from its competitive antagonism of the inhibitory neurotransmitter glycine at the postsynaptic spinal cord motor neuron. Signs and symptoms of CNS stimulation begin approximately 15 to 20 min after ingestion. Toxicity manifests by muscle twitching, painful extensor spasms, opisthotonos, trismus, and facial grimacing. Of diagnostic importance is that the patient remains conscious during episodes of painful muscle spasm and convulsions and that there is no postictal phase. Medullary paralysis and death can follow. Ancillary testing is not useful for diagnosis. Treatment includes aggressive airway control, a quiet environment (because any noise or manipulation may precipitate contractures), and activated charcoal. Gastric lavage may precipitate convulsions. Benzodiazepines and pain medications are administered to control painful spasms, but barbiturates and neuromuscular blocking agents may be needed. Recovery is usually complete if therapy is aggressive.

Thallium sulfate is a heavy metal with moderate to high acute toxicity that is used by industry and found in homeopathic remedies. It is a white, crystalline, odorless, and tasteless powder. It is a cumulative poison that distributes in almost every tissue of the body. Thallium combines with mitochondrial sulfhydryl groups, interfering with oxidative phosphorylation. It is readily absorbed through the skin, by inhalation, and through the gastrointestinal tract.

Gastrointestinal symptoms including hemorrhage develop acutely within 12 to 48 h. A latent period with constipation is then followed in 2 to 5 days by neurologic sequelae, painful paresthesias of the lower extremities, myalgias, headache, lethargy, tremors, ataxia, delirium, coma, and seizures. Respiratory failure and dysrhythmias may cause death in severe cases. Chronic sequelae include various neurologic syndromes, neuropathies, and alopecia. Urine sediment may be of diagnostic value, showing RBCs and protein. Liver function tests may be abnormal. Thallium can be measured in the hair, serum, and urine.

Thallium ingestion is treated by multiple doses of activated charcoal, sorbitol initially, and supportive care. Potassium chloride infusion increases renal secretion but also may facilitate entry into cells. Multiple doses of activated charcoal or Prussian blue (ferric ferrocyanide) may interrupt enterohepatic circulation and increase secretion in stool.

Zinc phosphide is a dark-gray, crystalline, water-insoluble powder that is present in multiple products (Acme Mole and Gopher Killer). It has a characteristic ''phosphorus'' or ''rotten fish'' odor. Zinc and phosphine gas are released on contact with water and acid. Toxicity is due to the phosphine formed following hydrolysis in the stomach. This gas may be inhaled and absorbed secondarily. Exposure causes cellular toxicity to the gastrointestinal tract, kidney, and liver if ingested and to the lungs if inhaled. The exact mechanism is unclear, but the toxin appears to block oxidative phosphorylation.

Onset of clinical syndromes begins within hours of ingestion but may be delayed following inhalation. Nausea, vomiting, and epigastric pain may ensue within 10 to 15 min. Signs and symptoms include a ''phosphorous'' or ''fishy'' breath, black vomitus, and signs of gastrointestinal irritation or ulceration. There is myocardial toxicity, shock, and noncardiogenic pulmonary edema with nonprominent CNS manifestations such as agitation, coma, and seizures. Hepatorenal injury is common. Metabolic acidosis and hypocalcemic tetany may occur.

Treatment includes preventing gastric conversion to toxic substances by intragastric alkalinization with sodium bicarbonate, milk, or water, activated charcoal, a cathartic, and supportive therapy. Those who survive 3 days usually recover.

Elemental or yellow phosphorus (Stearn's Electric Brand Paste) is a yellow, waxy, fat-soluble rat or roach paste that has a ''garlicky'' odor. It is easily mixed with molasses or peanut butter or spread on bread for rodents to eat. It ignites on contact with moisture. Skin contact causes local irritation and severe burns within minutes to hours. Toxicity is related to its ability to uncouple oxidative phosphorylation. It appears to have direct toxic effects on the myocardium and peripheral vessels. Clinically, toxicity may manifest by jaundice, cardiovascular collapse, dysrhythmias, coma, delirium, seizures, or cardiac arrest.

Three stages of clinical manifestations after ingestion consist of an initial stage of oral burns, abdominal pain, hemetemesis, ''smoking'' phosphorescent vomitus and stool, a garlicky odor, and possible early death from cardiovascular collapse. The second stage is relatively asymptomatic. Finally, CNS depression with multisystem toxicity including a hepatorenal syndrome may occur.

Gastric lavage with dilute potassium permanganate or hydrogen peroxide solution may convert phosphorus to harmless oxides. Activated charcoal and sorbitol catharsis, with aggressive supportive care and monitoring, are needed. Emesis should be avoided. Early cardiac and CNS toxicity are poor prognostic signs.

Arsenic is a heavy metal in the form of a white crystalline powder. It is no longer used because of its high toxicity. After ingestion, this compound combines with sulfhydryl groups and interferes with a variety of enzymatic reactions. Symptoms may occur as early as 1 h after ingestion, with death from cardiovascular collapse occurring within 24 h. Clinical presentation includes dysphagia, nausea and vomiting, bloody diarrhea, altered mental status, seizures, and late peripheral neuropathies. Treatment consists of lavage, activated charcoal, and catharsis and chelation therapy using dimercaptosuccinic acid (DMSA, succimer), dimercaprol, or penicillamine.

Moderate Toxicity

α-Naphthyl-thiourea (ANTU) is a moderately toxic rodenticide. It is very selective for target species, with humans being relatively resistant. This compound is a fine, blue-gray powder that is odorless, water-insoluble, and slightly bitter. The mechanism of action is unknown, but this toxin does appear to increase alveolar capillary permeability, causing pulmonary edema. Patients present clinically with dyspnea, cough, pleuritic chest pain, noncardiogenic pulmonary edema, and pleural effusion. Treatment is supportive and includes activated charcoal and catharsis.

Cholecalciferol (vitamin D_3) is used widely by professional exterminators and the general public. This compound is marketed as Quintox, Rampage, or Ortho Mouse-B-Gon. In rodents, toxic doses result in the mobilization of calcium from bones, producing hypercalcemia, osteomalacia, and systemic metastatic calcifications. No severe human toxicity or deaths have been reported. Small amounts are probably nontoxic and do not require therapy.

Signs and symptoms are those associated with vitamin D intoxication and hypercalcemia. Clinically, patients present with nausea, vomiting, abdominal pain, constipation, and CNS depression. Nerve and muscle dysfunction and dysrhythmias may be seen. Serum calcium, magnesium and electrolyte levels should be monitored. Normal levels obtained 48 h after acute ingestion probably exclude significant toxicity. Therapy after acute massive ingestion includes activated charcoal and sorbitol. Treatment of moderate to severe hypercalcemia involves intravenous infusion of normal saline, furosemide, steroids, and calcitonin (see Chap. 23).

Low Toxicity

Red squill is a botanic cardiac glycoside derived from the plant *Urginea maritima*, or sea onion. It is marketed as Deathdiet, Rat Snax, Rat Nip and has a very bitter taste. Toxicity is related to the ability to block sodium-potassium adenosine triphosphatase. Duration of onset is from 30 min to 6 h. Because of its potent emetic properties, patients present with nausea, protracted vomiting, diarrhea, and abdominal pain. Massive ingestion causes hyperkalemia, ventricular irritability with dysrhythmias, and death.

Treatment is similar to that for digoxin toxicity using antiarrhythmics and atropine as indicated. In severe poisoning, an infusion of 10 vials of digitalis-specific antibody (Fab) is recommended. Activated charcoal should be given.

Warfarin-type (3α-acetonylbenzyl-4-hydroxy-coumarin) anticoagulants (Kill-Ko, Rat Busters) were the first rodenticides. They are commonly disguised as yellow corn meal or rolled oats and are among the most commonly ingested substances in the United States. It is important to differentiate these from the more toxic superwarfarins. Most warfarin ingestions are insignificant accidental poisonings and do not cause any bleeding problems.

A single acute exposure results in virtually no bleeding in children or adults. Toxicity requires large amounts in a single exposure or a repetitive exposure over several days. Lipid solubility of the individual anticoagulant determines its elimination half-life. Warfarin's biologic half-life is approximately 42 h. These anticoagulants inhibit, almost immediately, the synthesis of Vitamin K_1–dependent clotting factors II, VII, IX, and X. Coagulopathy develops when the level of at least one critical coagulation factor falls to 25 percent of normal.[26] This time interval is approximately 12 to 18 h.

Ingestion of a single mouthful is usually nontoxic, and therapy is not necessary. If potential toxicity is suspected, therapy consists of activated charcoal and a cathartic, with baseline prothrombin time (PT) and partial thromboplastin time (PTT) determinations to be repeated in 12 to 24 h. If the PT is greater than twice normal and the risk of bleeding exists, vitamin K_1 (phytonadione) administration is indicated. The suggested oral dose is 1 to 5 mg in children and 20 mg in adults administered two to four times daily due to its short half-life and a PT is checked every 4 h initially, then every 24 h until stable.

Second-generation superwarfarins and the indandione derivatives were introduced when rodent resistance to warfarin began to appear. They are responsible for approximately 80 percent of human rodenticide exposures reported in the United States.[1] Their mechanisms are the same as those of the warfarins, but they are more potent, have more prolonged anticoagulant activity, and therefore have the potential to be highly toxic. Poisonings involving the indandione derivatives pindone, diphacinone, and chlorophacinone have toxic and clinical characteristics similar to those of the superwarfarins.

The superwarfarins include the 4-hydroxy-coumarins brodifacoum, diphenacoum, and bromadiolone. These are readily available over the counter as grain-based bait. Since the biologic half-life of brodifacoum is approximately 120 days, a single ingestion may result in marked anticoagulation effects from weeks to months. Acute intentional or repeated ingestions can cause severe bleeding. After intentional ingestions, adults often develop a coagulopathy within 24 to 48 h.[24]

A single ingestion usually does not result in immediate toxic effects, and an ingestion may or may not be identified by history. Small children and depressed patients having an unexplained coagulopathy should elevate the index of suspicion. Clinical findings of toxicity consist of ecchymoses, hematuria, uterine or gastrointestinal bleeding, gingival hemorrhage and epistaxis, hematomas, and hemoptysis. Their onset, however, may be delayed for several days, and they may persist for several days.

An abnormal PT may identify chronic ingestions or patients who present hours or days after exposure to a long-acting warfarin. Specific serum assays for superwarfarins are available in reference laboratories. Superwarfarins are not detected by warfarin assays. Initial differential diagnosis in the patient with an elevated PT and PTT includes disseminated intravascular coagulation, liver failure, pathologic inhibitors of coagulation, acquired vitamin K deficiency, or ingestion of a vitamin K antagonist. Warfarin abuse must be suspected when no other cause of vitamin K deficiency can be found.

Resuscitation of acute hemorrhage consists of oxygen administration and repletion of volume losses with normal saline or transfusion. Fresh-frozen plasma should be used if bleeding is severe or unresponsive to vitamin therapy. Vitamin K_1 can be diluted and administered by slow intravenous infusion, less than 1 mg per minute, to minimize the risk of an anaphylactoid reaction and cardiovascular collapse. Oral absorption takes approximately 2 to 3 h. Because of the extended half-life of the anticoagulant, prolonged therapy with high doses of vitamin K_1 may be required to maintain hemostasis. Doses of vitamin K_1 should be titrated to effect. Initial doses of 1 to 5 mg in children and 20 mg in adults have been recommended, but doses up to 100 mg per day for 10 months have been reported.[27] The PT is followed every 4 h and then every 24 h.

Treatment of acute ingestion consists of gastrointestinal decontamination. Recent ingestion of amounts greater than 0.1 mg/kg necessitates activated charcoal and a cathartic. Of 110 children having ingested long-acting anticoagulants, only 8 were found to have an elevated PT, but history was not predictive.[24] Hence any patient with a superwarfarin exposure needs PT determinations at 24 and 48 h. If the PT is elevated, high-dose vitamin K_1 is initiated for at least 6 weeks. Discontinuation of vitamin K_1 therapy is followed by serial PT determinations to ensure that further therapy is not needed. After initial parenteral therapy, prolonged oral administration for several months may be required as the PT normalizes.

Clinical Approach

A number of agents with distinct toxicities are used as rodenticides. The clinical approach to rodenticide exposure is determined by whether the nature of the toxin is known or unknown or whether delayed toxicity is suspected. Identifying product name is essential for appropriate management, but actual active ingredients need to be known over the commercial name. It must be recognized that similar brand names are used for more than one agent and that some agents are no longer on the market but remain on consumers' shelves. The time of ingestion and onset of clinical symptoms should be elicited. If a specific agent is identified, evaluation and treatment are determined. It must be recognized that chemicals can be mistakenly termed rodenticides when obtaining a history and that ingestion may involve coingestants.

If a clinician only knows that a rodenticide was ingested, specific odors or CNS, cardiopulmonary, gastrointestinal, skeletal muscle, metabolic, or hemorrhagic signs and symptoms may suggest a specific toxin. A metabolic acidosis suggests sodium monofluoroacetate or its derivatives. Painful paresthesias and metallic densities on abdominal radiographs suggest thallium ingestion. Emesis and cardiac dysrythmias suggest red squill poisoning. An abnormally high PT suggests superwarfarin ingestions, but the PT may be normal initially.

Initial assessment includes immediate identification and resuscitation of any airway compromise, respiratory failure, or cardiovascular collapse. Vital signs including an accurate core temperature should be obtained immediately. Administration of diagnostic/therapeutic substrates should be considered. Orogastric lavage may be indicated if ingestion took place within 1 h, followed by activated charcoal and a cathartic. Specific antidotes are considered. Blood chemistries other than an initial PT are not particularly helpful unless the patient is clinically symptomatic.

Disposition

Disposition depends on the toxin ingested. When exposure is suspected, given the low frequency of individual physician experience with these types of exposures, poison center consultation may assist in recommending a plan for managing the patient based on the presentation and toxin. When a patient has been exposed to a rodenticide having a rapid effect, symptoms usually manifest within 4 to 6 h of ingestion. Patients who have ingested a highly toxic rodenticide and are symptomatic are admitted after initial ED therapy. Symptoms related to agents with delayed onset typically begin 12 h or more after exposure. Therefore, if there is historical evidence of an acute ingestion and there are no signs or symptoms within 4 to 6 h, rodenticides with delayed effects are then considered, the patient is discharged after initial therapy, and reevaluation with coagulation studies is done in 24 and 48 h. The threshold for hospital admission should be low for intentional ingestions. In accidental ingestions, the patient can be treated with decontamination, observed in the ED for 6 h, and, if asymptomatic, discharged with follow-up. For asymptomatic patients who have accidentally ingested a superwarfarin, baseline PT and PTT determinations are done, follow-up is ensured, and coagulation studies are repeated at 24 and 48 h. Prevention measures should be emphasized.

REFERENCES

1. Litovitz TL, Klein-Schwartz W, Dyer KS, et al: Annual report of the American Association of Poison Control Centers Toxic Exposure Surveillance System. *Am J Emerg Med* 16:443, 1998.
2. Saadeh AM, Al-Ali MK, Farsakh NA: Clinical and sociodemographic features of acute carbamate and organophosphate poisoning: A study of 70 adult patients in North Jordan. *Clin Toxicol* 34:45, 1996.
3. Okumura T, Takasu N, Ishimatsu S, et al: Report of 640 victims of the Tokyo subway Sarin attack. *Ann Emerg Med* 28:129, 1996.
4. Deschamps D, Questel F, Baud FJ, et al: Persistent asthma after acute inhalation of organophosphate insecticide. *Lancet* 344:1712, 1994.
5. Agarwal SB: A clinical, biochemical, neurobehavioral, and sociopsychological study of 190 patients admitted to hospital as a result of acute organophosphorus poisoning. *Environ Res* 62:63, 1993.
6. Senanayake N, Karalliedde L: Neurotoxic effects of organophosphorus insecticides: An intermediate syndrome. *N Engl J Med* 316:761, 1987.
7. Steenland K, Jenkins B, Ames RG, et al: Chronic neurological sequela to organophosphate pesticide poisoning. *Am J Public Health* 84:731, 1994.
8. Nouira S, Abroug F, Elatrous S, et al: Prognostic value of serum cholinesterase in acute organophosphate poisoning. *Chest* 106:1811, 1994.
9. Chuang FR, Jang SW, Lin JL, et al: QTc prolongation indicates a poor prognosis in patients with organophosphate poisoning. *Am J Emerg Med* 14:451, 1996.
10. Beards SC, Kraus P, Lipman J: Paralytic ileus as a complication of atropine therapy following severe organophosphate poisoning. *Anaesthesia* 49:791, 1994.
11. Grob D, Johns RJ: Use of oximes in the treatment of intoxication by anticholinesterase compounds in normal subjects. *Am J Med* 24:497, 1958.
12. Merril DG, Mihn FG: Prolonged toxicity of organophosphate poisoning. *Crit Care Med* 10:550, 1982.
13. Lifshitz M, Rotenberg M, Sofer S, et al: Carbamate poisoning and oxime treatment in children: A clinical and laboratory study. *Pediatrics* 93:652, 1994.
14. Mercurio-Zuppala M, Hack J, Salvador A, Hoffman RS: Carbaryl poisoning: Two PAM or not two-PAM. *J Toxicol Clin Toxicol* 5:428, 1998.
15. Kilburn KH, Thornton JC: Protracted neurotoxicity from chlordane sprayed to kill termites. *Environ Health Perspect* 103:691, 1995.
16. Suskind RR, Hertzberg VS: Human health effects of 2,4,5-T and its toxic contaminants. *JAMA* 251:2372, 1984.
17. Onyon LJ, Volans GN: The epidemiology and prevention of paraquat poisoning. *Hum Toxicol* 6:19, 1987.
18. Hart TB, Nevitt A, Whitehead A: A new statistical approach to the prognostic significance of plasma paraquat concentrations. *Lancet* 2:1222, 1984.
19. Proudfoot AT, Stewart MS, Levitt T, et al: Paraquat poisoning: Significance of plasma paraquat concentrations. *Lancet* 2:330, 1979.
20. Scherrmann JM, Houze P, Bismuth C, Bourdon R: Prognostic value of plasma and urine paraquat concentrations. *Hum Toxicol* 6:91, 1987.
21. Bismuth C, Garnier R, Dally S, et al: Prognosis and treatment of paraquat poisoning: A review of 28 cases. *J Toxicol Clin Toxicol* 19:46, 1982.
22. Vale JA, Meredith TJ, Buckley BM: Paraquat poisoning: Clinical features and immediate general management. *Hum Toxicol* 6:41, 1987.
23. Bismuth C, Baud FJ, Barnier R, et al: Paraquat poisoning: Biological presentation. *J Toxicol Clin Exp* 8:211, 1988.
24. Smolinske SC, Scherger DL, Kearns PC, et al: Superwarfarin poisoning in children: A prospective study. *Pediatrics* 84:490, 1989.
25. Chi CH, Chen KW, Chan SH, et al: Clinical presentation and prognostic factors in sodium monofluoroacetate intoxication. *J Toxicol Clin Toxicol* 34:707, 1996.
26. Freedman MD: Oral anticoagulants: Pharmacodynamics, clinical indications, and adverse effects. *J Clin Pharmacol* 32:196, 1992.
27. Lipton RA, Klass EM: Human ingestion of ''superwarfarin'' rodenticide resulting in prolonged anticoagulant effect. *JAMA* 252:3004, 1988.

ANTICHOLINERGIC TOXICITY

Leslie R. Wolf

Because of the frequent use of tricyclic antidepressants, phenothiazines, antihistamines, and antiparkinsonian drugs, anticholinergic toxicity is commonly seen in the emergency department. Anticholinergic medications are commonly prescribed for elderly patients, often resulting in drug-induced delirium. Many drugs have anticholinergic properties (Table 177-1) that may be mild at therapeutic doses but are life-threatening in overdose.[1] The use and abuse of some plants and mushrooms also may result in anticholinergic toxicity.

PHARMACOLOGIC PROPERTIES

Drug absorption can occur after ingestion, smoking, or ocular use. The rate of absorption varies depending on the drug and the route of exposure. Because cholinergic blockade delays gastric emptying and decreases intestinal motility, absorption and peak clinical effects are often delayed.[2]

TABLE 177-1 Anticholinergic Substances

Antihistamines	**Belladonna alkaloids, synthetic cogeners**
Ethanolamines	Atropine (Hyoscyamine)
Dimenhydrinate (Dramamine)	Belladonna alkaloid mixtures
Diphenhydramine (Benadryl)	Glycopyrrolate (Robinul)
Ethylenediamines	Homatropine (Dia-Quel, Malcotran)
Tripelennamine (Pyribenzamine)	Methscopolamine bromide (Pamine)
Alkylamines	Scopolamine hydrobromide (Hyoscine)
Chlorpheniramine (Teldrin)	**Cyclic antidepressants**
Piperazines	Amitryptyline hydrochloride (Elavil, Amitril, Endep)
Astemizole (Hismanal)	Desipramine hydrochloride (Norpramin, Pertofrane)
Terfenadine (Seldane)	Doxepin hydrochloride (Sinequan, Adapin)
Loratadine (Claritin)	Imipramine hydrochloride (Tofranil, Pramine)
Cyclizine (Marezine)	Nortriptyline hydrochloride (Aventyl, Pamelor)
Meclizine (Antivert)	Protriptyline hydrochloride (Vivactil)
Phenothiazines	Trimipramine (Surmontil)
Prochlorperazine (Compazine)	Maprotiline hydrochloride (Ludiomil)
Promethazine (Phenergan)	Zimelidine hydrochloride
Antiparkinsonian drugs	Fluoxetine (Prozac)
Benztropine mesylate (Cogentin)	Amoxapine (Asendin)
Biperiden (Akineton)	**Ophthalmic products**
Ethopropazine (Parsidol)	Atropine and scopolamine solutions
Trihexyphenidyl (Artane)	Cyclopentolate hydrochloride (Cyclogyl)
Procyclidine (Kemadrin)	Tropicamide (Mydriacyl)
Antipsychotics	**OTC medications (including antihistamines and belladonna alkaloids)**
Phenothiazines	Analgesics: Excedrin PM, Percogesic
Chlorpromazine (Thorazine)	Cold remedies: Actifed, Allerest, Coricidin, Dristan, Flavihist, Romex, Sine-Off
Thioridazine (Mellaril)	Hypnotics: Compoz, Sleep-Eze, Sominex
Perphenazine (Trilafon)	Menstrual products: Pamprin, Premesyn PMS
Nonphenothiazines	**Skeletal muscle relaxants**
Clozaril (Clozapine)	Orphenadrine citrate (Norflex)
Molindone (Moban)	Cyclobenzaprine hydrochloride (Flexeril)
Loxapine (Loxitane)	**Mushrooms**
Antispasmodics	*Amanita muscaria*
Clidinium bromide (Quarzan, Librax)	*Amanita pantherina*
Dicyclomine (Bentyl)	**Other**
Methantheline bromide (Banthine)	Diphenidol (Cephadol, Vontrol)
Propantheline bromide (Pro-Banthine)	
Tridihexethyl chloride (Pathilon)	
Plants	
Deadly nightshade	
Mandrake	
Jimsonweed	

Source: Adapted from Goldfrank et al,[1] with permission.

The signs and symptoms of anticholinergic toxicity are a result of both central and peripheral cholinergic blockade. Muscarinic acetylcholine receptors predominate in the brain, while nicotinic receptors predominate in the spinal cord. Depending on the drug involved, antagonism of muscarinic, nicotinic, or both receptors may occur.[2] The central effects of cholinergic blockade include agitation, amnesia, anxiety, ataxia, coma, confusion, delirium, disorientation, dysarthria, hallucinations, hyperactivity, lethargy, somnolence, seizures, circulatory collapse, mydriasis, and respiratory failure. The peripheral effects include dysrhythmias, tachycardia, decreased bronchial secretions, dysphagia, decreased gastrointestinal motility, hyperthermia, hypo- or hypertension, decreased salivation, decreased sweating, urinary retention, and vasodilation.[1,3,4]

CLINICAL PRESENTATION

The classic presentation of patients with anticholinergic toxicity can be remembered as

Hot as Hades
Blind as a Bat
Dry as a Bone
Red as a Beet
Mad as a Hatter

Clinical characteristics include unreactive mydriasis, hypo- or hypertension, absent bowel sounds, tachycardia, flushed skin, disorientation, urinary retention, hyperthermia, dry skin and mucous membranes, and auditory and visual hallucinations. Patients also can present with seizures or coma. Cardiogenic pulmonary edema may occur secondary to depression of myocardial contraction.[1,3,4]

The diagnosis of anticholinergic toxicity must be based on clinical presentation. The diagnosis may be confused with delirium tremens or an acute psychiatric disorder. Anticholinergic toxicity can be differentiated from delirium tremens and sympathomimetic toxicity by the presence of dry skin and the absence of bowel sounds. Acute psychiatric disorders may have associated tachycardia and tachypnea, but usually the physical examination is normal. Complications from anticholinergic toxicity occur secondary to hyperthermia, dysrhythmias, seizures, and circulatory collapse.[1,4]

Electrocardiographic abnormalities may include QRS prolongation, abnormal conduction, bundle branch block, AV dissociation, and atrial and ventricular tachycardias. Sinus tachycardia is the most common

TABLE 177-2 Treatment of Anticholinergic Toxicity

General	Seizures	Hypotension	Dysrhythmias
ABC's	Benzodiazepines	Fluids	Standard therapy
Cardiac monitor	Barbiturates	Sodium bicarbonate	Avoid Class Ia antidysrhythmics
Intravenous line			Sodium bicarbonate (agents that cause channel blockade)
Gastric lavage (within 1 h)			
Whole-bowel irrigation (jimsonweed seeds)			
Treat agitation with benzodiazepines			

abnormality.[1,4] Routine laboratory evaluations, including measurement of electrolytes, glucose, and arterial blood gases, should be checked in the presence of abnormal mental status but should be normal in isolated anticholinergic toxicity. Comprehensive toxicologic screens are of little value in the acute setting, and some anticholinergic agents (e.g., scopolamine) may not be detected. The screen can be used for confirmation, but the diagnosis should be based on clinical findings.

TREATMENT

Conservative, supportive therapy is the mainstay of treatment of anticholinergic toxicity (Table 177-2). Evaluation of the airway, breathing, and circulation is a priority. An intravenous line should be established and an ECG monitor placed in any patient with significant symptoms. Gastric lavage may be useful in patients presenting within 1 h of ingestion.[5] Activated charcoal may be useful to decrease drug absorption, particularly with agents that undergo enterohepatic circulation or when the agents ingested are unknown.

Hyperthermia should be controlled with conventional therapy. Seizures can be treated with benzodiazepines and barbiturates. Hypertension usually does not require treatment, but conventional therapy should be used if necessary. The treatment of dysrhythmias depends on the type and on the causative agent. Standard antiarrhythmics are usually effective, but class Ia agents should be avoided due to the quinidine-like effect of many anticholinergic drugs. Dysrhythmias, including a widened QRS, and hypotension associated with agents that cause sodium channel blockade can be treated with intravenous sodium bicarbonate (Table 177-2).[1] Agitation can be treated with benzodiazepines. Because of their anticholinergic effects, phenothiazines should be avoided.

The most controversial topic surrounding anticholinergic toxicity is the use of physostigmine. Physostigmine is a tertiary ammonium compound that is a reversible acetylcholinesterase inhibitor that crosses the blood-brain barrier and reverses both central and peripheral anticholinergic effects.[2] Physostigmine may aggravate dysrhythmias and seizures and must be used with extreme caution.[7] The indications for its use include the presence of peripheral anticholinergic signs and seizures unresponsive to conventional therapy, uncontrollable agitation, hemodynamically unstable dysrhythmias unresponsive to conventional therapy, coma with respiratory depression, malignant hypertension, or refractory hypotension. Physostigmine should be avoided in cyclic antidepressant overdose because it may potentiate toxicity and increase mortality.[7] The initial dose of physostigmine is 0.5 to 2.0 mg IV over 5 min. Improvement of central signs usually occurs within 5 to 15 min. The minimal effective dose should be used. Due to rapid elimination, repeat doses may be necessary every 30 to 60 min. Physostigmine use is contraindicated in patients with cardiovascular disease, bronchospasm, intestinal obstruction, heart block, peripheral vascular disease, and bladder obstruction. Patients receiving physostigmine should be on a cardiac monitor and observed for cholinergic symptoms (salivation, lacrimation, urination, and defecation).

Patients with mild symptoms of anticholinergic toxicity can be discharged after 6 h of observation if their symptoms are improving. Patients receiving physostigmine usually require admission for at least 24 h.

JIMSONWEED

Many plants have anticholinergic effects, including deadly nightshade, henbane, mandrake, burdock root, jimsonweed, and others. They are often used for medicinal purposes or brewed in teas. *Datura stramonium*, also known as jimsonweed, is a member of the Solanaceae family. It is a common weed that grows to be 3 to 6 ft high and can be found throughout the United States.[1,4] Its leaves are large, jagged, and have a bitter taste and foul odor. The plant has large white or purple trumpet-shaped flowers that bloom in the late spring and become thorny quadripartite capsules in the fall, filled with black seeds. The entire plant is toxic and contains atropine, hyoscyamine, and scopolamine in various amounts. In the past, jimsonweed was marked and sold in health food stores in a preparation for the treatment of asthma. Many accidental childhood poisonings from jimsonweed have been reported. Over the past 20 to 30 years, jimsonweed has been involved in inadvertent overdoses in persons experimenting with mind-altering drugs. The plant can be smoked or ingested. Fifty to one hundred seeds contain the equivalent of 3 to 6 mg atropine.[1,4]

Symptoms of anticholinergic toxicity occur within 2 to 6 hr after the ingestion of jimsonweed. As with other agents causing anticholinergic toxicity, patients present with fever, erythema, mydriasis, delirium, hallucinations, tachycardia, and amnesia. The treatment is the same as that described earlier. Because the seeds may remain in the stomach for prolonged periods, whole-bowel irrigation is recommended up to 12 to 24 h after the ingestion of seeds. The most persistent symptom of jimsonweed toxicity is blurred vision, since mydriasis can persist for up to 1 week. Mydriasis also can occur from isolated local contact of jimsonweed with the eye (''cornpicker's pupil'').[8]

REFERENCES

1. Goldfrank LR, (ed): *Goldfrank's Toxicologic Emergencies,* 6th ed. Stanford, CT, Appleton & Lange, 1998.
2. Goodman LS, Gilman A: *The Pharmacologic Basis of Therapeutics*, 8th ed. Elmsford, NY, Pergamon, 1990.
3. Goldfrank LR, Flomenbaum NE, Lewin NA: Anticholinergic poisoning. *J Toxicol Clin Toxicol* 19:17, 1982.
4. Ellenhorn MJ: *Ellenhorn's Medical Toxicology, Diagnosis and Treatment of Human Poisoning*, 2d ed. Baltimore, Williams & Wilkins, 1997.

5. American Academy of Clinical Toxicology; European Association of Poisons Centres and Clinical Toxicologists: Position Statement: Gastric Lavage. *Clin Toxicol* 35(7):711–719, 1997.
6. American Academy of Clinical Toxicology; European Association of Poisons Centres and Clinical Toxicologists: Position Statement: Single-Dose Activated Charcoal. *Clin Toxicol* 35(7):721–741, 1997.
7. Shannon M: Toxicology reviews: Physostigmine. *Pediatr Emerg Care* 14:224, 1998.
8. Savitt DL, Roberts JR, Siegel EG: Anisocoria from jimsonweed. *JAMA* 255:1439, 1986.

METALS AND METALLOIDS

Marsha D. Ford

Acute metal and metalloid toxicity is an uncommon clinical entity that can be a cause of significant morbidity and mortality if unrecognized and inappropriately treated. Because of their effects on numerous enzymatic systems in the body, the metals and metalloids often present with protean manifestations primarily affecting four systems: neurologic, gastrointestinal, hematologic, and renal. Effects on the endocrine and reproductive systems are less clinically apparent. One should be familiar with the toxic manifestations of the most common metals and metalloids—lead, arsenic, and mercury—in order to appropriately diagnose poisoned patients. It is important to recognize an initial "index case" in order to prevent others from being poisoned when the metal source is environmental or industrial (Table 178-1).

LEAD

Epidemiology

Lead is the most common cause of chronic metal poisoning and remains a major environmental contaminant. Elevated blood levels in children aged 1 to 5 years have been linked with these community characteristics: urban dwellings, dwellings built before 1974 (especially those built prior to 1946), poverty, non-Hispanic black race/ethnicity, and higher population density.[1,2] Data from phase 2 of the National Health and Nutritional Survey III (NHANS III) for children aged 1 to 5 years indicate that an estimated 890,000 children have blood lead levels of 10 μg/dL or more; this represents a substantial decline in the prevalence of elevated blood lead levels since 1976.[3] This decline is attributed to bans on lead in household paints, gasoline, plumbing systems, and food and drink cans, as well as lead abatement programs and the promulgation of standards for industrial use of lead.[1]

Elevated lead levels may have detrimental effects on intellectual development,[4] and thus lead toxicity remains a significant public health problem. Both inorganic and organic forms of lead produce clinical toxicity. Inorganic lead affects the central and peripheral nervous systems, hematopoietic system, kidney, gastrointestinal tract, liver, myocardium, and reproductive capacity. With organic lead intoxication, central nervous system (CNS) effects predominate.

Inorganic Lead

PHARMACOLOGY Absorption is by the respiratory and gastrointestinal tracts, whereas skin absorption is negligible. Dietary deficiencies in calcium, iron, copper, and zinc may contribute to increased gastrointestinal absorption in children. Absorption also occurs when retained lead bullets or shot are in contact with body fluids such as synovial fluid. Lead can be transferred placentally to the fetus of a mother with an elevated blood lead level, which can be further exacerbated by increased bone turnover during pregnancy. In the body, lead distributes into the blood, soft tissues, and bone. Greater than 90 percent of the total-body lead is stored in bone, where it easily exchanges with the blood. Excretion of lead occurs slowly; the biologic half-life of lead in bone has been estimated to be 30 years.

PATHOPHYSIOLOGY In the CNS lead injures astrocytes, with secondary damage to the microvasculature and resulting disruption of the blood-brain barrier,[5] cerebral edema, and seizures; decreases cyclic adenosine monophosphate (CAMP) and protein phosphorylation, which contribute to memory and learning deficits; and alters calcium homeostasis, which leads to spontaneous neurotransmitter release. In

TABLE 178-1 Sources of Heavy Metals

Heavy Metal	Source
Lead	
Inorganic	Soldering; battery burning/reclamation, bronzing; brassmaking; glassmaking; ingesting ceramic lead glaze; stripping old paint, "deleading" homes; "moonshine" whiskey; liquids in improperly glazed pottery; contaminated herbal medications; indoor shooting ranges; ingestion of paint chips, lead-laden floor dust, lead foreign bodies; lead bullets in abdomen or joint spaces.
	Workers at risk: jewelers, painters, lead burners and smelters, pipe cutters, pigment makers, printers, welders, pottery makers, radiator repair personnel, battery reclamation workers, construction workers
Organic	Leaded gasoline
Arsenic	
Inorganic [arsenite (As^{3+}), arsenate (As^{5+}), elemental]	Insecticides, rodenticides, herbicides, mining, smelting/refining, homeopathic medicines, kelp.
Organic	Parasitical medicines (veterinary)
Gas (arsine)	Mining smelting/refining, semiconductor industry; made by mixing acids with arsenic-containing insecticides.
Mercury	
Elemental	Battery and thermometer manufacture; sphygmomanometer repair; dentistry; jewelry and lamp manufacture; photography; mercury mining; manufacture of scientific instruments.
Salts	Taxidermy; fur processing; tannery work; chemical laboratories; manufacture of explosives, fireworks, disinfectants, button batteries, inks, and vinyl chloride.
Organic (methylmercury, ethylmercury, phenylmercury)	Contaminated seafood; embalming; manufacture of drugs, fungicides, bactericides, handling of insecticides; pesticides, coated seeds; manufacture of chloralkali; working with wood preservatives.

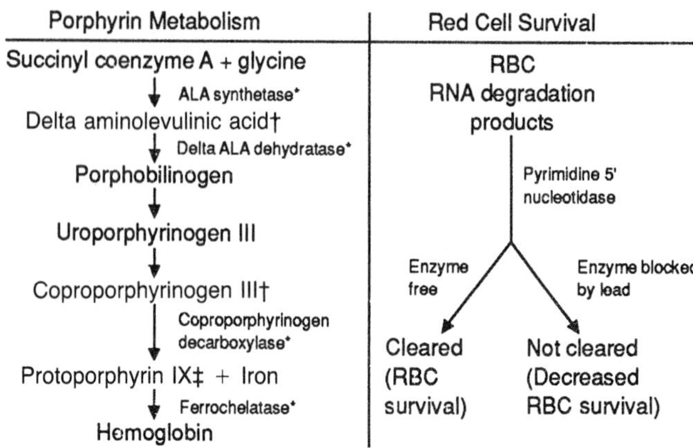

FIG. 178-1. Effects of lead on the hematopoietic system. *Enzymes affected by lead.†Levels elevated in urine.‡Level elevated in RBCs.

the peripheral nervous system (PNS), nerves undergo primary segmental demyelination, followed by secondary axonal degeneration, primarily of the motor nerves. In the hematopoietic system, lead interferes with porphyrin metabolism, which may contribute to lead-induced anemia (Fig. 178-1). The two enzymes chiefly affected are D-aminolevulinic acid dehydratase and ferrochelatase, the latter being the enzyme that catalyzes the transfer of iron from ferritin to protoporphyrin to form hemoglobin. Coexisting iron deficiency may act synergistically with lead toxicity to produce a more profound anemia and, in children, may be more important than lead as the cause of a microcytic anemia. Hemolytic anemia also occurs as a result of inhibition of red blood cell (RBC) pyrimidine 5′-nucleotidase, an enzyme responsible for clearing cellular RNA degradation products. On a blood peripheral smear, these products produce the RBC basophilic stippling sometimes seen in lead-poisoned patients.

In the kidney, acute lead toxicity affects the proximal tubule, producing a Fanconi syndrome with aminoaciduria, glycosuria, phosphaturia, and renal tubular acidosis. Chronic effects include persistence of a partial Fanconi syndrome for 13 years or longer,[6] interstitial nephritis, and increased uric acid levels due to increased tubular reabsorption of urate. Chronic lead toxicity has been linked with gout, hypertension, and chronic renal failure.

Toxic hepatitis with mildly elevated transaminases, normal bilirubin, and normal alkaline phosphatase can occur. Lead-induced adverse effects on the reproductive system include increased fetal wastage, premature membrane rupture, depressed sperm counts, abnormal/nonmotile sperm, and sterility. Chronic lead toxicity can depress free thyroxine levels without producing clinical hypothyroidism.

CLINICAL FEATURES The common signs and symptoms of acute, chronic, and delayed toxicity are listed in Table 178-2. Young children are more susceptible than adults to the effects of lead. Encephalopathy, a major cause of morbidity and mortality, may begin dramatically with seizures and coma or develop indolently over weeks to months with decreased alertness and memory progressing to mania, delirium, and cerebral edema.[7] It has developed in infants with blood lead levels of 70 μg/dL or less. Gastrointestinal and hematologic manifestations occur more frequently with acute than with chronic poisoning, and the colicky abdominal pains may be associated with concurrent hemolysis. Patients may complain of a metallic taste and, with long-term exposure, have bluish-gray gingival lead lines. Delayed cognitive development can occur in infants and children whose cord and blood lead (PbB) levels are 10 μg/dL or more. Finally, adult and pediatric patients may be asymptomatic in the face of significantly elevated PbB levels.

DIAGNOSIS History of an exposure—occupational, hobby, environmental, or related to retained lead bullets—is the most important

TABLE 178-2 Clinical Effects of Inorganic Lead Toxicity

System	Acute	Chronic	Late
Central nervous system	Encephalopathy (more common in children), seizures (focal or generalized), confusion, obtundation, coma, papilledema, optic neuritis, vomiting, ataxia May have complaints listed under chronic Normal cerebellar and cranial nerve function	Headache, irritability, depression, fatigue, behavioral change, memory deficit, apathy, sleep disturbances, attention deficit disorder	
Peripheral nervous system	Paresthesias May have some or all findings listed under chronic	Motor weakness, including classic wrist drip (peripheral neuropathy rare in children), depressed/absent DTRs, normal sensory function	
Hematologic	Hypoproliferative and/or hemolytic anemias Basophilic stippling (uncommon and nonspecific)	Same as in acute	
Gastrointestinal	Abdominal pain (colicky)	Abdominal pain (usually not severe, often absent), constipation, diarrhea	
Renal	Fanconi syndrome: aminoaciduria, glucosuria, phosphaturia, renal tubular acidosis	Interstitial nephritis, persistent partial Fanconi syndrome	Hypertension, gout, chronic renal insufficiency
Reproductive		Decreased libido, impotence, sterility, abortions, premature births, insufficient and abnormal sperm production	
Other	Bone pain	Arthralgias, weakness, weight loss	

clue to making the diagnosis. The physician should focus on symptoms, developmental and dietary histories (in children), pica, any house or day-care remodeling, previous serum iron and blood lead levels, and possible lead toxicity in other family members. Occupational and hobby histories should be elicited, both for adults being evaluated and for children who may be exposed to lead secondarily from these adult activities.

The combination of abdominal or neurologic dysfunction with a hemolytic anemia should raise the suspicion of lead toxicity. Emergency physicians should consider the diagnosis in all children presenting with encephalopathy. Toxicity due to retained lead bullets has manifested in patients as long as several decades after being shot. Hyperthyroidism, pregnancy, fever, reinjury, or immobilization of the affected extremity can promote lead release after years of dormancy.

Laboratory studies in the emergency department (ED) should focus on evaluation for anemia and examination of bone radiographs in children for ''lead bands'' and abdominal radiographs for radiopaque material consistent with lead in the gastrointestinal tract. The anemia can be normocytic or microcytic, possibly with evidence of hemolysis such as an elevated reticulocyte count and increased serum free hemoglobin.

The peripheral smear may show basophilic stippling of the RBCs. Both anemia and basophilic stippling occur variably, and their absence does not rule out lead toxicity. Basophilic stippling of RBCs is nonspecific for lead toxicity, since it is also found in arsenic toxicity, sideroblastic anemia, and the thalassemias. In children, radiographs of long bones, especially of the knee, may reveal horizontal, metaphyseal lead bands, which represent failure of bone remodeling rather than deposition of lead.

The definitive diagnosis rests on finding an elevated PbB level, with or without symptoms. The PbB level is the best single test for evaluating lead toxicity, and levels of 10 μg/dL or more are considered toxic. Screening levels may be performed on fingerstick capillary blood, but because of the potential for environmental lead contamination, elevated levels always should be confirmed on a venous blood sample.[8] Previously, a calcium disodium versenate ($CaNa_2$-EDTA) provocation test was used to evaluate total-body lead stores and the need for chelation therapy when PbB levels were between 25 and 55 μg/dL. However, animal data demonstrating that one dose of $CaNa_2$-EDTA redistributes lead to the brain, the technical difficulties in performing the test, the lowering of the toxic PbB level to 10 μg/dL or more, and the advent of dimercaptosuccinic acid (DMSA) as a safe and effective oral chelator raise concerns about the utility of the provocation test. Some major lead treatment centers have abandoned its use. Also, with the lowering of the toxic PbB level to 10 μg/dL or more, the erythrocyte protoporphyrin (EP) test can no longer be used to screen for lead toxicity because of its unacceptably low sensitivity at these lower PbB levels.[9]

DIFFERENTIAL DIAGNOSIS The differential diagnosis of lead toxicity includes causes of encephalopathy such as Wernicke's encephalopathy, withdrawal from ethanol and other sedative-hypnotic drugs, meningitis, encephalitis, human immunodeficiency virus (HIV) infection, intracerebral hemorrhage, hypoglycemia, severe fluid and electrolyte imbalances, hypoxia, arsenic, thallium, and mercury toxicity, and poisoning with cyclic antidepressants, anticholinergic drugs, ethylene glycol, or carbon monoxide. The abdominal pains can mimic sickle cell crisis or the hepatic porphyrias. Chronic lead toxicity can masquerade as depression, neurosis, hypothyroidism, polyneuritis, gout, iron deficiency anemia, and learning disability.

TREATMENT All patients with appropriate symptoms and an elevated PbB level are classified as lead toxic and should be treated.

Severe Toxicity Lead-induced encephalopathy rarely occurs now, but it remains a major cause of serious morbidity and mortality in lead-poisoned patients. In severely toxic patients, standard life support measures should be instituted and seizures treated with benzodiazepines, phenobarbital, phenytoin, and general anesthesia, if necessary. If abdominal films demonstrate radiopaque flecks consistent with lead, whole-bowel irrigation with a polyethylene glycol electrolyte solution should be instituted. The solution should be administered continuously at a rate of 500 to 2000 mL/h for adults and 100 to 500 mL/h for children until the abdominal radiograph is clear. It will not alter fluid or electrolyte balance in the patient. Larger lead bodies such as fishing sinkers may require surgical removal. Fluid administration should be controlled carefully to avoid worsening cerebral edema. Lumbar puncture may precipitate cerebral herniation and should be performed carefully, if at all, with the removal of a small amount of cerebrospinal fluid (CSF) only.

Chelation therapy should be instituted immediately (i.e. in the ED) prior to obtaining laboratory verification of the diagnosis. All chelating agents supply sulfhydryl groups to which the lead attaches. Dimercaprol (British anti-Lewisite, or BAL), 75 mg/m^2, should be administered intramuscularly first, followed 4 h later by $CaNa_2$-EDTA, 1500 mg/m^2 per 24 h, in a continuous intravenous infusion. BAL administration is continued every 4 h. BAL chelates intracellular as well as extracellular lead and may be administered to patients in renal failure because it is also excreted in the bile. It is mixed in peanut oil and must be given intramuscularly. $CaNa_2$-EDTA chelates extracellular lead only and may exacerbate lead-induced CNS toxicity in patients with high PbB levels unless preceded by BAL therapy. Continuous intravenous infusion is the preferred method of delivery. $CaNa_2$-EDTA can cause renal toxicity, and patients should be adequately hydrated to promote diuresis and minimize the risk of this complication. It should not be used in patients with renal failure. Adverse effects of the chelating agents are listed in Table 178-3.

TABLE 178-3 Adverse Effects of Chelating Agents

Chelating Agent	Adverse Effects
BAL (dimercaprol)	Hypertension Febrile reaction, diaphoresis Painful injection Nausea/vomiting, salivation Headache Lacrimation, rhinorrhea Hemolysis in G-6-PD deficient patients
$CaNa_2$-EDTA	Renal toxicity (especially if dehydrated) Can increase CNS levels of lead if given prior to BAL Chelates essential metals (e.g., copper, zinc, iron) Dermatitis Minor: Headache, chills, fever, myalgias, fatigue
D-Penicillamine	Nausea/vomiting Fever Rash Leukopenia, thrombocytopenia Eosinophilia Hemolytic anemia Stevens-Johnson syndrome (Probably safe in penicillin-allergic patients)
DMSA	Nausea, vomiting, diarrhea Abdominal gas, pain Transient elevated AST, alkaline phosphatase Rash, pruritus Sore throat, rhinorrhea Drowsiness, paresthesia Thrombocytosis, eosinophilia

For symptomatic patients without encephalopathy, and for asymptomatic patients with elevated PbB levels requiring chelation, the use of BAL or DMSA (see discussion below) with or without $CaNa_2$-EDTA and the dosing schedules are determined by the PbB levels, the presence or absence of symptoms, and changing practice as more experience with DMSA is obtained. Treatment may be initiated in the ED. Children who are symptomatic but not encephalopathic can be treated as discussed earlier, except with doses of BAL, 50 mg/m^2, and $CaNa_2$-EDTA, 1000 mg/m^2 per 24 h, or with DMSA plus EDTA. A retrospective study of 45 children with lead levels of 45 μg/dL or more treated either with BAL plus EDTA or DMSA plus EDTA found comparable reductions in lead levels, with fewer side effects in the DMSA group.[10] The Centers for Disease Control and Prevention (CDC) recommend immediate chelation therapy for children with blood lead levels of 70 μg/dL or more.[8] Symptomatic, nonencephalopathic adults may be treated with BAL and $CaNa_2$-EDTA, with $CaNa_2$-EDTA alone, or with DMSA.

In asymptomatic patients, the standards for determining lead toxicity and the need for treatment differ for children and adults. In asymptomatic children, chelation therapy should be performed if the PbB level is 45 μg/dL or more. As indicated earlier, chelation therapy should begin immediately (i.e., in the ED) if the PbB lead level is 70 μg/dL or more. If the PbB level is 20 to 44 μg/dL, treatment strategies include environmental and nutritional evaluation, medical examination, and possibly chelation therapy, either with DMSA, $CaNa_2$-EDTA, or D-penicillamine. For children with PbB levels between 10 and 19 μg/dL, interventions include nutritional and medical evaluation, repeat screening PbB levels, and environmental investigation for persistently high levels. In asymptomatic adults, the guidelines are less rigorous. In asymptomatic workers, a PbB level of less than 40 μg/dL is accepted as normal, levels of 40 to 50 μg/dL require increased job surveillance, and levels greater than 50 μg/dL require temporary removal from the job until the PbB level drops below 40 μg/dL. Details on therapy for these various groups can be found in standard toxicology references.

In patients in whom the lead level is elevated on a capillary stick sample, it is best to await verification on blood, unless the clinical presentation strongly supports lead toxicity. Capillary samples may give false-positive results, as noted earlier.

Two oral chelating agents are being used in lead toxicity. DMSA, an analogue of dimercaprol, effectively chelates lead in adults and children.[11,12] Its advantages include oral administration without increasing lead absorption from the gastrointestinal tract, no serious adverse effects, and minimal chelation of essential metals. High cost is its main disadvantage. The dose is 10 mg/kg every 8 h for 5 days, followed by the same dose every 12 h for 14 days. Repeat treatment may be necessary after a 2-week drug-free period. D-Penicillamine is a less effective chelating agent but has the advantage of being inexpensive. It has been used for outpatient therapy in both asymptomatic children and adults with mild PbB elevations.

DISPOSITION Removal of the source of lead is mandatory for all patients. Patients should not be discharged to their former environments until appropriate deleading and decontamination measures have been accomplished. Family members and coworkers should be evaluated for occult lead toxicity.

A guide for hospitalization includes

1. All children with symptoms or with a PbB level of 70 μg/dL or more
2. All adults with CNS symptoms
3. All patients with suspected toxicity when returning to the environment is considered dangerous

PROGNOSIS Approximately 85 percent of patients who suffer encephalopathy develop permanent CNS damage, including seizures, mental retardation in children, and cognitive deficits in adults. Abdominal colic usually subsides within days after beginning chelation therapy, and other acute manifestations clear within 1 to 16 weeks with therapy. Lead-induced nephropathy may be partially reversible with chelation therapy.

Organic Lead

Exposure to tetraethyl lead (TEL), found in leaded gasoline, can occur with gasoline sniffing or in the occupational setting. TEL is metabolized to inorganic lead and triethyl lead. Triethyl lead is the primary toxic product that produces predominantly CNS toxicity. Symptoms range from behavioral changes with irritability, insomnia, restlessness, and nausea and vomiting to tremor, chorea, convulsions, and mania. Muscle, hepatic, and renal damage can occur. Anemia and elevated erythrocyte protoporphyrin levels are usually not found. PbB levels may be normal or elevated. Therapy consists of removal from the source, symptomatic treatment, and chelation only if the PbB level is elevated. Sequelae include dementia, mental status alterations, and persistent organic psychosis.

ARSENIC

Arsenic is a nearly tasteless, odorless metal; it is the most common cause of acute metal poisoning and the second leading source of chronic metal toxicity. Arsenicals are found in a variety of compounds and industries (see Table 178-1) and continue to be used as tools for homicides and suicides.

Elemental, inorganic and organic salts, and gaseous forms exist. Elemental and organic forms have little to no toxicity and will not be discussed further. Inorganic compounds include arsenite (As^{3+}) and arsenate (As^{5+}). These compounds are the most toxic forms, and the discussion below will focus on inorganic arsenic toxicity. Arsine, a gaseous form, has toxicopathologic mechanisms and treatment that differ from those of other arsenical compounds. It will be discussed under a separate heading.

Pharmacology

Arsenic is well absorbed via the gastrointestinal, respiratory, and parenteral routes and may be absorbed through damaged skin. Owing to its water solubility, pentavalent arsenic (arsenate) is more readily absorbed through mucous membranes, e.g., the gastrointestinal tract, than trivalent arsenic (arsenite). Arsenite penetrates the skin more readily due to its increased lipid solubility. After absorption, arsenic localizes in erythrocytes and leukocytes or binds to serum proteins. Within 24 h, redistribution into the liver, kidney, spleen, lung, gastrointestinal tract, muscle, and nervous tissues occurs with subsequent integration into hair, nails, and bone. Metabolism of inorganic arsenic occurs via methylation. Elimination from the blood is rapid, and excretion is predominantly renal.[13] Toxicity of the various forms is partially determined by excretory rates, with the more toxic arsenite being excreted at a slower rate than arsenate or the organic arsenical compounds. Arsenic crosses the placenta and has produced teratogenicity in both animals and humans.

Pathophysiology

Arsenic reversibly binds with sulfhydryl groups found in many tissues and enzyme systems. The mechanisms of toxicity for inorganic arsenic are as follows:

1. For arsenite, inhibition of the pyruvate dehydrogenase complex is the primary biochemical lesion. This inhibition results in diminished adenosine triphosphate (ATP) production and, indirectly, in decreased gluconeogenesis, possibly leading to hypoglycemia. Arsenic also interferes with insulin-dependent cellular glucose uptake.[14]

2. For arsenate, uncoupling of oxidative phosphorylation and loss of ATP occur when As^{5+} substitutes for inorganic phosphate in one step of the glycolysis reaction.

Pathologically, acute exposure produces dilation and increased permeability of small blood vessels, resulting in gastrointestinal mucosal and submucosal inflammation and necrosis, cerebral edema and hemorrhage, myocardial tissue destruction, and fatty degeneration of the liver and kidneys. Subacute or chronic exposure can cause a primary peripheral axonal neuropathy with secondary demyelination.

Clinical Features

The signs and symptoms of toxicity vary with the form, amount, and concentration ingested and the rates of absorption and excretion of the various arsenical compounds. Arsenite (trivalent) is more toxic than arsenate (pentavalent). Symptoms usually occur within 30 min to several hours of ingestion. Severe gastroenteritis with nausea, vomiting, and cholera-like diarrhea is the hallmark of acute poisoning and may last several days to weeks, frequently necessitating hospitalization. Patients may complain of a metallic taste. Hypotension and tachycardia secondary to volume depletion, capillary leak, and myocardial dysfunction occur in moderate to severe cases. The electrocardiogram (ECG) may demonstrate nonspecific ST-segment and T-wave changes with a prolonged QT_c, although these findings are more common in chronic intoxication. Ventricular tachycardia with a torsade de pointes morphology has been reported.[15] Secondary myocardial ischemia may occur, leading to an erroneous diagnosis of primary myocardial infarction. Acute encephalopathy with delirium, seizures, and coma, pulmonary edema, acute renal failure, rhabdomyolysis, and death may ensue.

Patients with subacute or chronic toxicity typically present with complaints of peripheral neuropathy, skin rash, or a nonspecific malaise and weakness, often with a history of gastroenteritis occurring 1 to 6 weeks earlier. Survivors of acute poisonings can develop the same problems. The peripheral neuropathy develops in a stocking-glove distribution and is initially sensory, with later motor symptoms. Patients with severe poisonings can develop an ascending paralysis mimicking Guillain-Barré syndrome. The dermatologic manifestations vary. Hyperpigmentation, hyperkeratosis of the palms and soles, morbilliform rash, and epidermoid cancer have been reported. Mee lines (1- to 2-mm-wide transverse white lines in the nails) may be seen 4 to 6 weeks after an acute ingestion, whereas nasal septal perforation has been found in workers exposed occupationally to arsenic. Patients may complain of weakness, muscular aching, abdominal pain, memory loss, personality changes, periorbital and extremity edema, or decreased hearing secondary to sensorineural damage. Chronic encephalopathy with delirium, hallucinations, disorientation, agitation, and confabulation resembling Korsakoff syndrome has been reported.[16] Chronic exposure to arsenic has been linked with the development of squamous cell and basal skin carcinomas, respiratory tract cancer, hepatic angiosarcoma, and possibly with leukemia (Table 178-4).

Diagnosis

Without a history of known exposure to arsenic, the diagnosis must be based on the presenting signs and symptoms and a strong index of clinical suspicion. Physicians rarely encounter arsenic toxicity, and unfortunately, criminal poisonings often go undetected. The diagnosis of acute arsenic poisoning should be considered in any patient with hypotension of unknown etiology that was preceded by a severe gastroenteritis. The diagnosis of chronic arsenic toxicity should be considered in a patient with a peripheral neuropathy, typical skin manifestations, or recurrent bouts of unexplained gastroenteritis.

An abdominal radiograph may demonstrate intestinal radiopaque metallic flecks in cases of arsenic ingestions.[17] The complete blood count (CBC) may reveal either a normocytic, normochromic, or megaloblastic anemia and/or a thrombocytopenia. The white blood cell (WBC) count may be elevated in acute toxicity and decreased in chronic toxicity. A relative eosinophilia, up to 21 percent, and basophilic stippling of the RBCs have been reported. Elevated reticulocyte counts are found in cases with a component of hemolytic anemia. The ECG often reveals a prolonged QT_c interval, especially in chronic poisoning.

Definitive diagnosis of acute poisoning depends on finding elevated arsenic levels in a 24-h urine collection. All urinary measurements of metals should be collected in metal-free containers. Normal urinary arsenic level is less than 0.05 mg/L, and total urinary arsenic excretion in an unexposed patient should not exceed 0.1 mg/24 h. If the baseline urinary level is within normal limits and arsenic intoxication is still suspected, hair and nail clippings should be harvested for laboratory analysis. Owing to the rapid distribution of arsenic in tissues, blood arsenic levels are unreliable. Toxicologic texts provide a detailed discussion of laboratory testing and interpretation of results in arsenic toxicity.[18]

Arsenic toxicity should be included in the differential diagnosis for septic shock, encephalopathy, peripheral neuropathy (including Guillain-Barré syndrome), Addison's disease, hypo- and hyperthyroidism, patients with the previously mentioned dermatologic manifestations, Korsakoff syndrome, persistent gastroenteritis and/or cholera-like diarrhea, porphyria, other metal toxicities such as thallium and mercury, and unexplained, prolonged malaise and weakness.

Treatment

Acute arsenical toxicity is a life-threatening illness requiring aggressive management. The first task is to ensure adequate respiratory and circulatory function. Hypotension and dysrhythmias are the chief causes of death. Hypotension, usually due to volume depletion, should be managed initially with crystalloid volume replacement. Invasive hemodynamic monitoring followed by further crystalloid and pressor therapy with dopamine or norepinephrine may be required. Overhydration should be avoided because pulmonary and cerebral edema can occur. Cardiac monitoring should be instituted. Ventricular tachycardia and fibrillation may be treated with lidocaine, bretylium, and electrical defibrillation as necessary. Isoproterenol, magnesium, and overdrive pacing therapies should be considered for torsade de pointes dysrhythmias. Drugs that prolong the QT_c, including classes IA (procainamide, quinidine, disopyramide), IC, and III antidysrhythmics should be avoided. Potassium, calcium, and magnesium levels should be monitored and corrected as necessary to prevent further prolongation of the QT_c with possible exacerbation of torsade de pointes dysrhythmias.

Gastric lavage with a large-bore orogastric tube should be performed in all cases of acute ingestion, and activated charcoal (1 g/kg of body weight) and a cathartic should be instilled. Activated charcoal poorly adsorbs arsenic but may be effective if coingestants were taken. Whole-bowel irrigation should be considered if abdominal radiographs reveal intestinal radiopaque materials consistent with arsenic. Seizures can be treated with benzodiazepines, phenobarbital, phenytoin, and general anesthesia as necessary.

Initial management of chronic toxicity should be directed toward prevention of further arsenic absorption and gastrointestinal decontamination, if appropriate. In cases of suspected homicidal intent, patients should be advised to avoid food and drinks prepared by others, and visitor contact with hospitalized patients should be monitored carefully.

Chelation therapy with BAL should be instituted immediately in all cases of known or suspected acute arsenical poisoning. BAL doses range 3 to 5 mg/kg intramuscularly every 4 h for 2 days followed by 3 to 5 mg/kg every 6 to 12 h. In severe, life-threatening toxicity, BAL therapy should be continued until the clinical condition stabilizes and

TABLE 178-4 Signs and Symptoms of Arsenic Toxicity

System	Acute	Subacute	Chronic
Central nervous system	Encephalopathy, delirium, seizures, coma	Encephalopathy, irritableness, confusion, decreased memory, hallucinations, (VI) cranial nerve palsy	Encephalopathy
Peripheral nervous system	Subacute symptoms can develop early	Sensory symptoms, early: diminished/absent vibration, DTRs, pinprick, light touch Motor weakness, ascending paralysis Severe extremity pain with light touch	Sensorimotor neuropathy
Cardiovascular	Dysrhythmias: prolonged QT_c, torsade de pointes Pulmonary edema Myocarditis Hypotension	Dysrhythmias: prolonged QT_c, torsade de pointes	
Gastrointestinal	Nausea, vomiting Diarrhea Abdominal pain Toxic hepatitis	Persistence of acute symptoms Anorexia Weight loss	May be absent Nausea, diarrhea Colicky abdominal pain
Pulmonary	Pulmonary edema Respiratory failure	Cough, rales, hemoptysis Chest pain Interstitial lung infiltrates	Cough
Hematologic	Hemolytic anemia	Pancytopenia	Anemia Aplastic anemia Agranulocytosis
Renal	Acute tubular necrosis Cortical necrosis		
Otolaryngologic	Metallic taste Mucous membrane irritation		
Dermatologic		Alopecia Macular pruritic rash Brawny desquamation Mee's lines Facial/peripheral edema	Hypopigmentation/hyperpigmentation Palmoplantar keratoses Papular keratoses Ulcerative lesions Facial/peripheral edema Skin carcinomas: basal-cell, squamous, Bowen's disease
Other	Fever Rhabdomyolysis, acute myopathy	Fever Diaphoresis Fatigue	Fatigue Cancer: lung, hemangiosarcoma Cirrhosis Noncirrhotic portal hypertension Blackfoot's disease

Source: Reprinted with permission from Ford M: Arsenic, in LR Goldfrank, NE Flomenbaum, NA Lewin, et al (eds): *Goldfrank's Toxicologic Emergencies,* 5th ed. Norwalk, CT: Appleton and Lange, 1994, pp 1011–1025.

DMSA, the less toxic oral chelating agent, can be substituted. In cases of suspected chronic toxicity with stable symptoms, therapy may be withheld pending diagnosis. DMSA is the preferred chelating agent in these patients.[19] It is given according to the dosing regimen for lead, but therapy may be required beyond the initial 19-day regimen. D-Penicillamine does not effectively chelate arsenic and should no longer be used.[20] During chelation, intermittent 24-h urinary arsenic levels should be measured and therapy continued until the urine level falls below 0.05 mg/L per 24 h. Hemodialysis can remove small amounts of arsenic (2 to 4.5 mg) in patients with acute renal failure but is not indicated otherwise.[21]

Hospitalization Guidelines

1. All patients with acute or life-threatening known or suspected arsenic poisoning
2. All chronically poisoned patients requiring BAL therapy
3. All patients in whom suicidal or homicidal intent is suspected

Disposition

In acute toxicity, prognosis may be influenced favorably by the rapid institution of BAL therapy. Recovery from arsenical neuropathy appears to be related more to initial severity of symptoms than to institution of chelation therapy, although in those patients who do recover, BAL appears to significantly shorten the duration of illness. Often, neurologic recovery occurs slowly over months to years. Normalization of hematologic values can occur in the absence of any specific therapy. BAL has a variable effect on the dermatologic manifestations; hyperpigmentation is unresponsive to this therapy.

Arsine

Arsine is a colorless, nonirritating gas encountered in the semiconductor industry, ore smelting, and refining processes and is also produced when arsenic-containing insecticides are mixed with acids. Arsine attaches to sulfhydryl groups of hemoglobin, producing an acute hemolytic anemia with resulting jaundice, abdominal pain, and hemoglobinuria-induced acute renal failure. Acute poisonings are managed with blood transfusions, exchange transfusion to remove the nondialyzable arsine, and hemodialysis for the acute renal failure. BAL therapy has no role in the management of arsine toxicity.

MERCURY

Mercury occurs in both inorganic and organic forms. Inorganic compounds are divided further into elemental mercury and mercurous and mercuric salts. Organic mercurials exist as short- and long-chained alkyl and aryl compounds. The short-chained alkyls, such as methyl mercury and ethyl mercury, are more toxic to humans, with dimethylmercury being lethal in small amounts.[22] All forms of mercury are toxic but differ in the routes of absorption, constellations of clinical findings, and responses to therapy. Sources are listed in Table 178-1.

Pharmacology

Elemental mercury is primarily absorbed via inhalation of its vapor but also may be absorbed dermally. Absorption by the gastrointestinal tract is usually negligible. Intramuscular injections of mercury can induce abscess and granuloma formation; delayed systemic toxicity can occur.[23] Intravenous injections have produced mercury pulmonary and systemic emboli. Both mercuric salts and organic mercury are absorbed primarily through the gastrointestinal tract, with the short-chained alkyl organic compounds being better absorbed than the aryl organic compounds. Elemental mercury crosses the blood-brain barrier, where it is ionized and trapped in the CNS. Mercuric salts are deposited in the ionized form primarily in the kidney, as well as in the liver and spleen. The salts do not enter the CNS in consequential amounts.

With organic mercury compounds, the highly lipid-soluble short-chained alkyls easily cross membranes, accumulating in RBCs, the CNS, liver, kidney, and the fetus. Longer-chained alkyl and the aryl compounds are biotransformed into inorganic mercuric ions in the body. Therefore, toxicity with these compounds more closely resembles inorganic mercury toxicity.

Inorganic and the aryl organic mercurials are eliminated in the urine and feces. The short-chained alkyl compounds are primarily excreted in the bile, where they undergo significant enterohepatic circulation.

Pathophysiology

Mercury binds with sulfhydryl groups, affecting a diverse number of enzyme and protein systems. Methyl mercury also inhibits choline acetyl transferase, which catalyzes the final step in the production of acetylcholine, and may produce an acetylcholine deficiency. Mercuric salts produce proximal renal tubular necrosis.

Clinical Features

The clinical effects of mercury poisoning depend on the form and, in some cases, the route of administration. In general, the neurologic, gastrointestinal, and renal systems are predominantly affected. The short-chained alkyl compounds, methyl, dimethyl, and ethyl mercury, have the most devastating effects on the CNS,[24] followed by elemental mercury, whose primary toxicity is neurologic. Both forms of mercury produce erethism, a constellation of neuropsychiatric abnormalities including anxiety, depression, irritability, mania, sleep disturbances, excessive shyness, and memory loss. Tremor, either intention or nonintention, is a common physical finding.[25] The short-chained alkyls produce paresthesias (early sign), ataxia, muscular rigidity or spasticity, and visual and hearing impairment and induce CNS teratogenic effects. Gastrointestinal effects of both elemental and short-chained alkyl compounds are mild. In cases of severe, chronic poisoning with elemental mercury, stomatitis, gingivitis, and excessive salivation are seen. Chronic toxicity of elemental and organic forms may cause renal glomerular and tubular damage. Acute mercury inhalation can produce pneumonitis, adult respiratory distress syndrome, and progressive pulmonary fibrosis with death.[26]

In contrast, the mercury salts have little to no effect on the CNS but produce a severe corrosive gastroenteritis with abdominal pain that may be followed rapidly by cardiovascular collapse. Renal effects are typical, including acute tubular necrosis within 24 h. Children exposed to all forms of mercury except the short-chained alkyls can develop acrodynia, an immune-mediated condition characterized by a generalized rash, fever, irritability, splenomegaly, and generalized hypotonia with particular weakness of the pelvic and pectoral muscles. Further details of clinical findings are listed in Table 178-5.

Swallowing mercury contained in a glass thermometer usually does not produce adverse effects because the mercury is not absorbed from the gastrointestinal tract unless the tract is damaged or contains fistulas.

Diagnosis

A thorough history, including occupational exposures, and typical physical findings, especially tremor or a constellation of signs and symptoms suggesting erethism or acrodynia, may alert the emergency physician to mercury toxicity. Ingestion of mercuric chloride can produce a rapidly fatal course and should be considered in any patient presenting with a corrosive gastroenteritis. Often, however, the diagnosis of mercury toxicity is subtle, arrived at only after many other diagnoses have been investigated.

For all forms of mercury except short-chained alkyls, a 24-h urinary measurement of mercury should be performed. Most unexposed individuals will have levels of 10 to 15 μg/L or less. A level of greater than 20 μg/dL either before or after therapy indicates meaningful exposure. In cases of chronic toxicity, this measurement may be falsely low. Whole-blood mercury levels are less reliable diagnostically. A seafood meal (contaminated with mercury) can temporarily elevate the blood level to the toxic range until the mercury is eliminated.

Short-chained alkyl mercury compounds are predominantly excreted via the bile, rendering urinary measurements invalid. Laboratory diagnosis rests on finding elevated whole-blood mercury levels, since these compounds concentrate in erythrocytes. Whole-blood mercury levels are normally less than 1.5 μg/dL.

Magnetic resonance imaging (MRI) findings in methyl mercury toxicity from ingestion of contaminated seafood include marked atropy of the visual cortex, cerebellar vermis and hemispheres, and the post-central cortex.[27]

The differential diagnosis of mercury toxicity depends on the form ingested. Hypothyroidism, apathetic hyperthryroidism, metabolic encephalopathy, senile dementia, adverse effects of therapeutic drugs (such as lithium, theophylline, phenytoin), Parkinson disease, delayed neuropsychiatric sequelae of carbon monoxide poisoning, lacunar infarction, cerebellar degenerative disease or tumor, and ethanol or sedative-hypnotic drug withdrawal may produce behavioral changes or tremor similar to those caused by elemental mercury. Causes of corrosive gastroenteritis such as iron, arsenic, phosphorus, acids, or alkalis should be considered in the differential diagnosis for mercury salts. Many of the differential diagnoses for elemental mercury also apply to the organic mercury compounds. Cerebral palsy, intrauterine hypoxia, and teratogenic effects of therapeutic and illicit drugs and environmental contaminants should be considered when evaluating an infant thought to be affected in utero by the short-chained alkyl mercury compounds.

TABLE 178-5 Clinical Effects of Mercury Toxicity

Organic System Elemental	Inorganic Salts	Long-Chained Short-Chained Alkyls*	Alkyls, Aryls
Neurologic	Tremor intention and (-) nonintention, peripheral neuropathy (sensorimotor) Seizures (vapor inhalation)	Paresthesias (early sign); ataxia; sensory and hearing impairment; constricted visual fields; dysarthria; muscular rigidity or spasticity; seizures (rare); muscle tenderness; and optic atrophy (EM only)	MM; sensorimotor neuropathy
Erethism‡	+	−	+
GI	Stomatitis, gingivitis, excessive salivation (severe chronic poisoning); blue gum line Similar to elemental stomatitis, proctitis, colitis	Severe gastroenteritis, may be hemorrhagic; abdominal pain, EM: Nausea/vomiting, abdominal cramps	MM: Rarely symptoms
Renal	Glomerular and tubular damage (chronic) (severe poisoning); proteinuria, hematuria and casts (mild poisoning) Nephrotic syndrome	Acute tubular MM-necrosis	Similar to elemental EM: Polyuria, proteinuria
Pulmonary (inhaled)	Pneumonitis, pulmonary edema, ARDS, progressive fibrosis, pneumothorax, pneumomediastinum	Same as elemental	Same as elemental
Skin	Slate-gray pigmentation Brownish-yellow discoloration of anterior capsule of eye Allergic dermatitis	Urticaria, vesication, allergic dermatitis	Erythroderma, pruritus
Teratogenicity	Cerebral palsy, mental retardation, micrognathia, microcephaly, cleft palate, blindness, chorea, ataxia		
Acrodynia†	+	+	+
Other	Rapid cardiovascular collapse with mercuric chloride	EM: Severe musculoskeletal pain	

*MM, methyl mercury; EM, ethyl mercury.
†Generalized rash with erythema and desquamation of hands, feet, and nose; fever, diaphoresis, splenomegaly; hypotonia, irritability, weakness of pelvic/pectoral muscles. Does not occur in newborns or adults.
‡Systemic or organ specific irritability.

Treatment

General therapeutic measures include removal from exposure and supportive therapy. Ingestion of mercury salts should be treated with aggressive gastrointestinal decontamination, including instillation of milk or egg whites to bind the mercury, lavage, and activated charcoal. Given the profuse diarrhea that may ensue, a cathartic may not be indicated. A polythiolated resin (commercially unavailable) has been used to bind intestinal methyl mercury and interrupt the enterohepatic circulation. Neostigmine may improve motor function in methyl mercury–poisoned patients by improving acetylcholine levels.

BAL is the preferred chelator for mercury salts and is administered in a regimen of 3 to 5 mg/kg per dose intramuscularly every 4 h for 2 days and then every 6 h for 2 days, followed by every 12 h for 7 days. BAL is contraindicated in methyl mercury poisoning owing to exacerbation of CNS symptoms. The BAL-mercury complex is dialyzable, and hemodialysis may be helpful in patients receiving BAL who have diminished renal function. Plasma exchange transfusion also was beneficial in a case of mercuric chloride ingestion.[28] D-Penicillamine is used in elemental mercury and less severe cases of mercury salt toxicities. The dose is 100 mg/kg per day, to a maximum of 1 g in four divided doses for 3 to 10 days. D-Penicillamine has been used with variable results in organic mercury poisoning. DMSA has demonstrated efficacy in binding mercury, including organic forms and may become the treatment of choice for the short-chained alkyl compounds.[29]

Hospitalization Guidelines

1. All patients known or suspected of ingesting mercury salts
2. All patients known to have or suspected to have inhaled elemental mercury vapor with pulmonary injury
3. All patients requiring BAL therapy.

Disposition

Outcome depends on the form of mercury and the severity of toxicity. Mild cases of elemental and mercury salt poisoning and very mild cases of organic mercury toxicity may result in complete recovery. Death can occur in severe cases of mercuric chloride poisoning and with dimethyl mercury exposure. Most patients with organic mercury poisoning are left with residual neurologic deficits.

REFERENCES

1. Update: Blood lead levels—United States, 1991–1994. *MMWR* 46:141, 1997.
2. Lanphear BP, Roghmann KJ: Pathways of lead exposure in urban children. *Environ Res* 74:67, 1997.
3. Pirkle JL, Brody DJ, Gunter EW, et al: The decline of blood lead levels in the United States: The National Health and Nutrition Examination Surveys. *JAMA* 272:284, 1994.
4. Tong S, Baghurst P, McMichael A, et al: Lifetime exposure to environmental lead and children's intelligence at 11–13 years: The Port Pirie cohort study. *Br Med J* 312:1569, 1996.
5. Finkelstein Y, Markowitz ME, Rosen JF: Low-level lead-induced neurotoxicity in children: An update on central nervous system effects. *Brain Res Brain Res Rev* 27:168, 1998.
6. Loghman-Adham M: Aminoaciduria and glycosuria following severe childhood lead poisoning. *Pediatr Nephrol* 12:218, 1998.
7. al Khayat A, Menon NS, Alidina MR: Acute lead encephalopathy in early infancy: Clinical presentation and outcome. *Ann Trop Paediatr* 17:39, 1997.
8. Centers for Disease Control and Prevention: *Screening Young Children for Lead Poisoning: Guidance for State and Local Public Health Officials.* Atlanta: CDC, 1997.
9. McElvaine MD, Orbach HG, Binder S, et al: Evaluation of the erythrocyte protoporphyrin test as a screen for elevated blood lead levels. *J Pediatr* 119:548, 1991.
10. Besunder JB, Super DM, Anderson RL: Comparison of dimercaptosuccinic acid and calcium disodium ethylene diaminetetraacetic acid versus dimercaptopropanol and ethylene diaminetetraacetic acid in children with lead poisoning. *J Pediatr* 130:966, 1997.
11. Graziano JH, Lolacono NJ, Moulton T: Controlled study of meso-2, 3-dimercaptosuccinic acid for the management of childhood lead intoxication. *J Pediatr* 120:133, 1992.
12. Lifshitz M, Hashkanazi R, Phillip M: The effect of 2,3-dimercaptosuccinic acid in the treatment of lead poisoning in adults. *Ann Med* 29:83, 1997.
13. McKinney JD: Metabolism and disposition of inorganic arsenic in laboratory animals and humans. *Environ Geochem Health* 14:43, 1992.
14. Leibl B, Muckter H, Doklea E, et al: Reversal of oxophenylarsine-induced inhibition of glucose uptake in MDCK cells. *Fund Appl Toxicol* 27:1, 1995.
15. Beckman KJ, Bauman JL, Pimental PA, et al: Arsenic-induced torsades de pointes. *Crit Care Med* 19:290, 1991.
16. Park MJ, Currier M: Arsenic exposures in Mississippi: A review of cases. *South Med J* 84:461, 1991.
17. Hilfer RJ, Mandel A: Acute arsenic intoxication diagnosed by roentgenograms. *N Engl J Med* 266:663, 1962.
18. Ford M: Arsenic, in LR Goldfrank, NE Flomenbaum, NA Lewin, et al (eds): *Goldfrank's Toxicologic Emergencies,* 6th ed. Stamford, CT: Appleton & Lange, 1998, pp 1261–1273.
19. Muckter H, Liebl B, Reichl FX, et al: Are we ready to replace dimercaprol (BAL) as an arsenic antidote? *Hum Exp Toxicol* 16:460, 1997.
20. Kreppel H, Reichl FX, Forth W, Fichtl B: Lack of effectiveness of D-penicillamine in experimental arsenic poisoning. *Vet Hum Toxicol* 31:1, 1989.
21. Mathieu D, Mathieu-Nolf M, Germain-Alonso M, et al: Massive arsenic poisoning: Effect of hemodialysis and dimercaprol on arsenic kinetics. *Intensive Care Med* 18:47, 1992.
22. Nierenberg DW, Nordgren RE, Chang MB, et al: Delayed cerebellar disease and death after accidental exposure to dimethylmercury. *N Engl J Med* 338:1672, 1998.
23. Dell-Omo M, Muzi G, Bernard A, et al: Long-term pulmonary and systemic toxicity following intravenous mercury injection. *Arch Toxicol* 72:59, 1997.
24. Eto K: Pathology of Minamata disease. *Toxicol Pathol* 25:614, 1997.
25. Taueg C, Sanfilippo DJ, Rowens B, et al: Acute and chronic poisoning from residential exposures to elemental mercury—Michigan 1989–1990. *J Toxicol Clin Toxicol* 30:63, 1992.
26. Lim HE, Shim JJ, Lee SY, et al: Mercury inhalation poisoning and acute lung injury. *Korean J Intern Med* 13:127, 1998.
27. Korogi Y, Takahashi M, Okajima T, Eto K: MR findings of Minamata disease: Organic mercury poisoning. *J Magn Reson Imaging* 8:308, 1998.
28. Yoshida M, Satoh H, Igarashi M, et al: Acute mercury poisoning by intentional ingestion of mercuric chloride. *Tohoku J Exp Med* 182:347, 1997.
29. Roels HA, Boeckx M, Ceulemans E, et al: Urinary excretion of mercury after occupational exposure to mercury vapour and influence of the chelating agent meso-2,3-dimercaptosuccinic acid (DMSA). *Br J Ind Med* 48:247, 1991.

HERBALS AND VITAMINS

G. Richard Braen

Vitamins and herbal preparations, particularly those sold in health food stores, have been considered by many to be innocuous, but several have tremendous potential as toxins. This chapter covers most of the available vitamins and selected herbals. Agents compounded with vitamins, such as iron, are covered in other chapters.

VITAMIN A

Vitamin A has two primary preformed types: retinol (vitamin A_1 alcohol) and 3-dehydroretinol (vitamin A_2). Yellow carotenoid plant pigments contain a number of forms of provitamin A, but β-carotene has the highest biologic activity of these forms. There are two molecules of vitamin A per molecule of β-carotene.

The retinyl esters of dietary vitamin A are hydrolyzed into retinol in the gastrointestinal tract. Retinol is then absorbed into intestinal mucosal cells where it combines with a fatty acid to again become a retinyl ester. The retinyl ester then travels through the lymphatic system and bloodstream to storage sites in the liver. The liver contains about 95 percent of the vitamin A of the entire body.

Vitamin A forms part of the visual pigments of the retina (rhodopsin and iodopsin), is important for the formation of mucus-secreting cells of the columnar epithelium, maintains bone growth, and maintains cellular membrane stability. The daily adult recommended doses range from 4000 IU for women to 5000 IU for men.

Hypervitaminosis A generally occurs when children are given excessive amounts of a high-potency supplement and when their capacity to store vitamin A in the liver is exceeded. In the liver, retinol is bound to a liver protein (retinol-binding protein) and is stored in this bound form. As the liver binding and storing capacity is exceeded, blood levels of a retinyl ester loosely bound to low-density lipoproteins increase. This loosely bound vitamin is believed to be toxic to cell membranes. Members of Mawson's Antarctic expedition (1911–1913) are said to have died from hypervitaminosis A after eating the livers of their dogs to try to avoid starvation.

When the total dosage is similar, water-miscible preparations are more toxic than oily preparations because of better absorption. High doses of preformed vitamin A must be ingested for long periods before signs and symptoms of hypervitaminosis A develop. There is a high degree of variability among patients in the amounts necessary to develop hypervitaminosis. Dialysis patients can be at risk of developing a type of vitamin A toxicity in which resorption of bone causes hypercalcemia.

Symptoms of hypervitaminosis A include blurred vision, appetite loss, abnormal skin pigmentation, loss of hair, dry skin, pruritis, long-bone pain, and an increased incidence of bone fractures. Massive doses can additionally cause pseudotumor cerebri.

The treatment of hypervitaminosis A depends on the condition of the patient. Generally, when vitamin A is discontinued, the symptoms resolve over a period of time and no additional treatment is needed.[1] Treatment of hypercalcemia is outlined in Chap. 23, ''Fluid and Electrolyte Problems.'' β-Carotene intoxication is very rare and does not generally cause hypervitaminosis A. In diabetics and patients with hypothyroidism, however, large doses of β-carotene can cause a yellowish discoloration of the skin, which fades once β-carotene is stopped.

VITAMIN D

Vitamin D function comes from two major compounds: calciferol (vitamin D_3) and ergocalciferol (vitamin D_2). The naturally occurring provitamin forms of each of these two compounds (7-dehydrocholesterol for D_3 and ergosterol for D_2) convert to the active forms following irradiation by ultraviolet light. Most studies in humans have been made on vitamin D_3 (cholecalciferol), which is converted in the body to 1,25-dihydroxycholecalciferol, the physiologically active form of vitamin D.

Absorption of vitamin D is aided by bile and takes place in the jejunum. From there it is transported via lymph chylomicrons to the bloodstream.[1] When it reaches the liver, it is hydroxylated to 25-hydroxycholecalciferol. From the liver, it travels to the kidney, where it is again hydroxylated to 1,25-dihydroxycholecalciferol. The major function of 1,25-dihydroxyhydrocalciferol is to elevate the plasma calcium and phosphorus levels to enable normal bone mineralization.

The average daily adult requirement of vitamin D is about 400 IU, and therapeutic doses sometimes exceed 5000 IU. Infants may develop hypercalcemia from doses as low as 2000 IU, but adults require much higher doses before toxicity develops. The toxicity results from the hypercalcemia and includes anorexia, nausea, abdominal pain, lethargy, weight loss, polyuria, constipation, confusion, and coma.[1] Symptoms from massive doses (1000 to 3000 IU/kg) develop in 2 to 8 days. Persistently elevated levels of calcium can cause soft tissue calcification and renal failure.

Treatment of hypervitaminosis D includes discontinuation of vitamin D, reduction of the calcium intake, and reduction of serum calcium levels.

VITAMIN E

Vitamin E activity is not limited to one compound alone. Eight different fat-soluble, naturally occurring alcohols (called tocopherols and tocotrienols) have vitamin E activity, but α-tocopherol is the most active form. Because of its ability to be rapidly oxidized, α-tocopherol protects other foods from being oxidized, and thus is termed an *antioxidant*.[2] Foods high in vitamin E include wheat germ, corn, soybean, sunflower seed, cod liver, and others.

Vitamin E is absorbed and distributed through the body just as any fat-soluble vitamin, through the intestines and then through lymphatic chylomicrons. Between 30 and 90 percent of available vitamin E in the diet is absorbed. Normal tocopherol levels in adults range from 0.5 mg to 2.0 mg/dL. The minimum daily requirement for women is about 8 mg α-tocopherol and for men is 10 mg α-tocopherol. An IU is the activity of 1 mg of α-tocopherol. Vitamin E needs for children increase with increasing body weight and increase for pregnant or lactating women.

Vitamin E is felt to be nontoxic at daily doses of up to 600 IU. At doses higher than 600 IU/day, taken on a long-term basis, a metabolite of vitamin E acts as a competitive inhibitor of vitamin K-dependent γ-carboxylation, increasing the daily vitamin K requirements. Additionally, through the production of thromboxane, high levels of vitamin E inhibit platelet aggregation. People ingesting large amounts of vitamin E who are on anticoagulants should be observed closely for bleeding tendencies, but those not on anticoagulants rarely have coagulation difficulties, except for neonates, who are more sensitive to the effects of vitamin E. Other effects in adults who take large doses for a long period of time include nausea, fatigue, headache, weakness, and blurred vision. These symptoms resolve weeks after discontinuation of the vitamin.

VITAMIN K

Vitamin K is represented by several compounds that have antihemorrhagic activity: the parent compound called menadione; vitamin K_1, which is a naturally occurring phylloquinone from plant sources; and vitamin K_2, which is a naturally occurring menaquinone from microbial sources. Vitamin K forms are generally heat resistant but are broken down by alkali, strong acids, light, and some oxidizing agents. High levels of dietary vitamin A inhibit the absorption of vitamin K. Vitamin E at high levels acts as a vitamin K–antagonist in its liver production of clotting factors.

Vitamin K is absorbed in different sites and by different mechanisms, depending on the type of compound. Phylloquinones are absorbed from the proximal intestine through an energy-requiring process. Menadione and menaquinones are absorbed from the lower intestine and colon through a passive mechanism. Both mechanisms require the presence of bile and pancreatic juice. Between 10 and 80 percent is absorbed. Once absorbed, it is carried by the lymph chylomicrons and then transferred in the blood to β-lipoproteins. About 50 percent of the vitamin comes from the diet and 50 percent from bacterial synthesis in the intestines. The total dietary requirement of vitamin K is about 2 μg/kg body weight. Since most adults ingest a diet that contains 300 to 500 μg vitamin K, deficiency states are uncommon. In contrast to the other fat-soluble vitamins, vitamin K is not stored in the body to any significant extent. About 70 percent of menadione is excreted in the urine. Phylloquinone is excreted mainly in bile.

Vitamin K is required for the maintenance of normal prothrombin tines through its effect on factor II (prothrombin), factor VII (proconvertin), factor IX (Christmas factor), and factor X (Stuart-Prower factor). These factors are part of the extrinsic, intrinsic, and common pathways for blood clotting. Coumarin compounds work on the clotting-factor synthesis sites in the liver to stop prothrombin synthesis and to reduce the levels of all vitamin K–dependent clotting factors.

Megadoses of menadione can be toxic. Toxic effects include hemolytic anemia, kernicterus, and hemoglobinuria in premature infants and renal tubular degeneration, liver damage, hypoprothrombinemia, and petechial hemorrhages in adults. Large doses can also paradoxically inhibit the effects of oral anticoagulants. Treatment includes stopping vitamin K, monitoring prothrombin times, and monitoring liver function studies. Additionally, doses exceeding 500 μg daily have been associated with skin rashes. Fatalities from overingestion of vitamin K are rare.

VITAMIN B_1 (THIAMINE)

Vitamin B_1 is converted to thiamine pyrophosphate which acts as a cofactor for several metabolic reactions, including transketolations. Measurement of erythrocyte transketolase activity is used to reflect the availability of thiamine pyrophosphate in the tissues. Food sources of thiamine include fruits, grain, meats, fish, and milk, among others. The highest levels are found in pork products (0.63 mg/serving). The average daily adult requirement is 1.5 mg.[1]

Intestinal absorption of thiamine seems to be greatest in the jejunum. An active carrier-mediated absorption process occurs at normal levels of dietary thiamine, but passive diffusion is the major means of thiamine absorption at higher levels.

Thiamine is not stored in the body to any significant extent. At low dietary levels renal excretion decreases, whereas, at high levels of ingestion, renal excretion increases proportionately. Because of the renal excretion of thiamine, there is no toxicity to the ingestion of large doses of vitamin B_1 over prolonged periods.

VITAMIN B_2 (RIBOFLAVIN)

Vitamin B_2 (riboflavin) works as an antioxidant through its activity in the formation of glutathione reductase and glutathione. As a part of the group of enzymes called flavoproteins, it is involved in the metabolism of fats, proteins, and carbohydrates. It is not stored in appreciable quantities in the body and must be replenished daily. Vigorous exercise increases the daily requirement of riboflavin, and a deficiency results in cracked lips, reddened tongue, and eczema of the face and genitals. The average daily adult requirement is 1.7 mg.[1]

Riboflavin is excreted through the urine, and toxicity is rare regardless of the amount ingested. No adverse effects result from overdosage.

VITAMIN B_3 (NIACIN)

There are two active forms of niacin—nicotinic acid and nicotinamide—which, in conjunction with thiamine and riboflavin, have antipellagra activity. Niacin, thiamine, and riboflavin all function as a coenzyme in energy metabolism. Niacin becomes part of the coenzymes nicotinamide adenine dinucleotide (NAD) and nicotinamide adenine dinucleotide phosphate (NADP). NAD is required in all major metabolic pathways in which there is oxidative breakdown of amino acids, fatty acids, and other compounds. It also acts in the oxidation of ethanol.

Niacin is found in poultry, meat, and fish, with less found in plants. Niacin deficiency causes changes first in cells of the skin, nervous system, and gastrointestinal tract. Deficiency states create symptoms such as anorexia, anxiety, depression, irritability, and weakness.

Whereas doses of nicotinic acid in the range of 100 to 200 times the recommended allowance of 20 mg daily will lower serum cholesterol and β-lipoprotein, nicotinamide does not. Large doses can also deplete cardiac muscle glycogen and can cause liver toxicity. Some patients experience a frightening "niacin flush" when taking a dose of more than 100 mg. The niacin flush, caused by histamine release and vasodilation, is characterized by face, neck, and chest burning, itching, and reddening.[1] It generally resolves within an hour. Antihistamines can provide symptomatic relief. Higher doses may additionally cause nausea, abdominal cramping, diarrhea, and headache. Even higher doses (2000 mg and above) over a prolonged period can produce abnormalities of liver function, impaired glucose tolerance, hyperuricemia, and skin changes such as dryness and discoloration. Subacute and chronic symptoms resolve within days to weeks.

VITAMIN B_6 (PYRIDOXINE)

Vitamin B_6 is a complex of three physiologically active compounds, the most active being pyridoxine. Pyridoxine is converted to pyridoxal-5-phosphate, which is a coenzyme in the transamination of amino acids that is required for the utilization of most amino acids for energy and for the synthesis of nonessential amino acids. A deficiency in vitamin B_6 in infants results in convulsive seizures (due to a reduced synthesis of γ-aminobutyric acid), anemia (due to impaired synthesis of heme), xanthurenic aciduria (due to reduced formation of hydroxyanthranilic acid), cystathionuria (due to decreased cleavage of cystathionine to cysteine) and homoserine), and homocystinuria (due to impaired formation of cystathionine). Deficiency states can be induced through ingestion of antagonists to vitamin B_6, such as isoniazid, cycloserine, and penicillamine.

Vitamin B_6 deficiency in infants may lead to growth retardation, weight loss, hyperirritability, convulsions, and anemia. Vitamin B_6 deficiency in adults may result in depression, convulsions, seborrheic dermatitis, and cheilosis. The daily requirement is 2.2 mg/day for men and 2.0 mg/day for women with increased requirements during pregnancy and lactation. Many animal and vegetable sources contain vitamin B_6 (especially pork and glandular meats, legumes, potatoes, oatmeal, wheat germ, and bananas), but there is considerable loss of the vitamin during cooking.

In high doses, particularly over a long period of time, vitamin B_6 excess will cause nerve damage. Most people can tolerate 20 mg/day without difficulty, but 5 g/day or more over several weeks will produce an unstable gait and numbness of the feet. This is followed by similar symptoms in the hands and arms. There may be a marked loss of position and vibration senses. After withdrawal of the vitamin, recovery occurs within several months. Some patients, however, have residual neurologic losses.

Vitamin B_6 also can cause intestinal inactivation of levodopa in patients receiving that medication for Parkinson's disease. Patients should be instructed not to take the vitamin at the same time as the medication.

VITAMIN B_{12}

Vitamin B_{12} deficiency causes pernicious anemia identified by macrocytosis (high mean corpuscular volume) and intramedullary hemolysis (very high lactate dehydrogenase level). Associated neurologic problems include symmetric paresthesias of the hands and feet, and decreased position and vibratory senses. Vitamin B_{12} is a very potent vitamin (relatively small amounts are needed to treat patients with pernicious anemia) that takes several forms: cyanocobalamin (vitamin B_{12}), hydroxocobalamin (vitamin B_{12a}) aquocobalamin (vitamin B_{12b}), nitritocobalamin (vitamin B_{12c}), 5′-deoxyadenosylcobalamin (coenzyme B_{12}), and methylcobalamin (methyl B_{12}). All are complex nitrogenous compounds associated with cobalamin that participate in metabolic reactions necessary for the formation of amino acids, protein, and DNA.

Partially because of the size and complexity of the vitamin B_{12} molecules, deficiencies of this water-soluble vitamin result more from absorption problems than from dietary insufficiencies.[2] Absorption depends on the production of intrinsic factor (IF) by the parietal cells of the stomach. Vitamin B_{12}–IF complexes are formed in the stomach. The complexes pass to the ileum, where IF attaches to the intestinal epithelium, facilitating the absorption of the vitamin B_{12}. Once absorbed, the cobalamin portion of the molecule attaches to the protein transcobalamin II which carries the B_{12} through the bloodstream to various tissues. Vitamin B_{12} is stored in the liver in such quantities that it takes several years for pernicious anemia to develop in an individual who is a strict vegetarian and ingests little B_{12} or in someone unable to produce IF. Meat, eggs, dairy products, and seafood contain vitamin B_{12}.

Health food enthusiasts believe that supplemental vitamin B_{12} will energize the body, prevent mental deterioration, and protect against cancer, toxins, and infections. Because of the rate limited fashion in which vitamin B_{12} is absorbed, there is no toxicity to the ingestion of large amounts of vitamin B_{12}. Overdosage from injection is rare and results primarily in a variety of skin changes that clear over 1 to 2 weeks.

BIOTIN

Biotin is produced in the intestines by bacterial action and is a cofactor in fatty acid synthesis. Deficiencies of biotin result in baldness and dry skin, lassitude, anorexia, depression, and hypercholesterolemia. Those taking chronic antibiotics and those on extremely low-calorie diets are at risk of developing a biotin deficiency. For such individuals, 100 to 300 μg of biotin per day are recommended. There is no known toxicity to biotin overdosage.

FOLIC ACID

Folic acid is essential for the production of DNA, RNA, and proteins. Although folic acid may reverse the megaloblastic red blood cell aspects of pernicious anemia, it will not reverse the neurologic changes associated with pernicious anemia. It is found in fresh leafy green vegetables, yeasts, and liver. Folic acid is absorbed in the small and large intestines in the form of polyglutamates. At the brush border of the intestinal cells, excess glutamates are removed from the folate molecule, making a functioning intestinal mucosa necessary for absorption.

The adult daily recommended dosage of folic acid is 400 μg/day.[2] Dietary supplementation of 100 μg/day will reverse the red cell changes of pernicious anemia but will not reverse the neurologic effects; therefore, preparations with more than 100 μg are available only through prescription. Except for the problem with masking of the hematologic changes of pernicious anemia, there are no known adverse effects to the ingestion of large doses of folic acid.

VITAMIN C

The major form of vitamin C, L-ascorbic acid, is a strong reducing agent that participates in hydroxylation reactions such as that necessary for the formation of collagen. Scurvy results from vitamin C deficiency and results in collagen, protein, and lipid metabolism abnormalities. Additionally, the presence of vitamin C in the intestines increases the absorption rate of iron. Those with a vitamin C deficiency will also be iron depleted.

Vitamin C, which is found primarily in fruits and vegetables,[2] is absorbed through the jejunum and ileum. The absorption rates decrease with increasing intraluminal quantities of vitamin C. For example, 90 percent of a 100-mg dose might be absorbed, whereas only 20 percent of a 10-g dose might be absorbed. The daily recommended dose for adults is 60 mg. Vitamin C levels, although high in fruits and vegetables, are reduced by heat, drying, and storage.

Large doses of vitamin C can produce attacks of gout and nephrolithiasis in individuals with these conditions. Others may develop diarrhea and abdominal cramps, which subside with discontinuation. Megadoses of vitamin C may result in false negative guaiac testing of feces, and may give falsely elevated glucose levels on dipstick testing.

HERBAL AGENTS

In 1997 sales of over-the-counter herbal preparations exceeded $1.5 billion in the United States. Between 1994 and 1998, the sales of herbal supplements will have increased about 105 percent. According to the New York Times, July 23, 1998, between 1995 and 1997, the sales of St. John's wort have increased by 1900 percent.[3] Many other home grown and imported herbal preparations add to the total amount of herbal agents ingested, inhaled, and rubbed on. The list is staggering and this review will encompass only some of the more common herbals used. Herbal agents can be classified as generally safe, potentially toxic, and toxic. Some generally safe herbal agents are listed in Table 179-1.

TABLE 179-1 Some Generally Safe Herbal Agents

Agent	General Use	Rare Adverse Effect
Chamomile	Antispasmodic	Anaphylaxis if patient allergic to ragweed
Echinacea	To cure URIs and UTIs	Anaphylaxis if patient allergic to daisies May deplete vitamin stores
Feverfew[5]	To cure migraines	Suddenly discontinuing may precipitate migraine If chewed, can cause mouth ulcers and dermatitis
Garlic	For hypertension, colic, hyperlipidemia	Hypotension, rash, nausea, vomiting, diarrhea; death has been reported in massive doses in children
Ginko	For dementia, vertigo, Raynaud's disease	May inhibit platelet aggregation and interact with warfarin May cause gastrointestinal upset
Ginseng[6,7]	For impotence, fatigue, ulcers, stress	May interact with warfarin Lowers blood glucose May cause insomnia, nervousness
St. John's wort	As antidepressant	Phototoxicity May interact with serotonin reuptake inhibitors; avoid tyramine-containing foods
Valerian	For sedation	Interacts with other sedating drugs May have paradoxical stimulant effect

Abbreviations: URIs, upper respiratory infections; UTIs, urinary tract infections.

Some of the moderately unsafe herbal preparations include absinthe (wormwood), black cohosh, comfrey, juniper, and lobelia. *Absinthe* (wormwood)—which is popular in Europe and is being produced there in clandestine laboratories—is a toxic liquor that contains volatile oils that produce psychosis, intellectual deterioration, ataxia, headache, vomiting, and diarrhea. Absinthe is used as a flavoring in alcoholic drinks.

Black (or blue) cohosh contains an estrogen-like compound and has been used to delay or treat menopause. It may cause nausea, vomiting, dizziness, and weakness.

Comfrey is used as a digestive stimulant in teas. It has, however, been linked to liver toxicity and hepatic carcinoma. The toxic action comes from the formation of pyrroles that act on DNA.

Juniper is used as a diuretic but may also be hallucinogenic. Toxicity also includes renal toxicity, nausea, and vomiting.

Lobelia is used for asthma and as an expectorant. Other uses include smoking it as a marijuana substitute for its mild euphoric effect. The active ingredients include lobeline, atropine, and scopolomine, which can produce anticholinergic symptoms.

Some herbs that are unsafe but are commonly found on store shelves include chaparral, ephedra, nutmeg, and yohimbine.

Chaparral is derived from the leaves of the creosote bush and is used for its antioxidant effects as a potential cancer preventative. It is also felt to be effective in pain control but is felt to be hepatotoxic.

Ephedra is used in weight loss and has been implicated in multiple toxic deaths. This herbal agent is contraindicated for patients with hypertension, diabetes, or glaucoma.

Nutmeg is used for dyspepsia, muscle aches, and arthritis. It contains terpines, ethers, and myristicin. Myristicin can produce hallucinations (at about 2 to 4 teaspoonfuls of ground nutmeg). At various dosages, it can also produce gastrointestinal upset, agitation, coma, miosis, and hypertension.

Yohimbine is thought to be an aphrodisiac. Toxic effects include hallucinations, weakness, hypertension and paralysis. Yohimbine, if combined with pheopropanolamine, can lead to a stroke through marked elevation of the blood pressure.

REFERENCES

1. Cushing C, Anderson AC: Hypervitaminosis, in Viccellio P, Bania T, Brent J, et al (eds): *Emergency Toxicology*, 2d ed. New York, Lippincott-Raven, 1998, pp 607–625.
2. Vitamin supplements. *Med Lett* 40:75, 1998.
3. Canedy D: Real medicine or the medicine show. *New York Times* 23 July 1998, p C1.
4. Poisoning associated with herbal teas: Arizona, Washington. *MMWR* 26:257, 1977.
5. Perharic L, Shaw D, Murray V: Toxic effects of herbal medicines and food supplements. *Lancet* 342:180, 1993.
6. Keji C: The effect and abuse syndrome of ginseng. *J Tradit Chin Med* 1:69, 1981.
7. Punnonen R, Lukola A: Oestrogen-like effect of ginseng. *Br J Med* 1:69, 1981.

ANTIMICROBIALS

G. Richard Bruno
Wallace A. Carter

Antimicrobial agents are estimated to account for 15 to 30 percent of the world medical drug expenditure.[1] Most adverse reactions to antibiotics occur at therapeutic doses. The most common adverse effects of antimicrobial use include hypersensitivity reactions, alterations in body microbial flora, interactions with other drugs, and cutaneous drug reactions. Data from the American Association of Poison Control Centers (AAPCC) suggest that antimicrobial exposures are a frequent source of inquiry to poison control centers but rarely result in life-threatening outcomes. During the 5 years from 1992 through 1996, the AAPCC reported 316,653 exposures, which resulted in significant morbidity in 768 cases (0.24 percent) and 23 fatalities (less than 0.01 percent). Emergency physicians must be familiar with the common adverse effects of antimicrobial agents at therapeutic doses (Table 180-1), any significant interactions with other drugs, effects on pregnancy (Table 180-2), and the clinical presentation and management of acute antimicrobial overdose. Hypersensitivity reactions account for the highest morbidity and mortality rates related to the use of antimicrobial agents. Most patients who present after antimicrobial overdose will be asymptomatic. Observation and screening for coingestants are adequate before medical clearance in most cases. The poison control center should be contacted to assist in patient management and to aid in accurate statistical tracking of toxin exposures.

COMMON ADVERSE EFFECTS OF ANTIMICROBIAL AGENTS

Almost all antimicrobial agents have resulted in immunoglobulin E-mediated anaphylaxis in sensitized individuals. Antibiotics, led by penicillins, account for the largest number of anaphylactic deaths in the United States annually.[2] In addition to immediate hypersensitivity reactions, antibiotics may cause delayed hypersensitivity reactions (Table 180-3). A comprehensive review of the presentation and management of hypersensitivity reactions is beyond the scope of this chapter, but they are important considerations when prescribing and caring for patients on antibiotics.

The normal body microbial flora is altered with use of antimicrobial agents. Patients taking antimicrobial agents are at risk for infection

TABLE 180-1 Adverse Effects of Common Antimicrobial Agents at Therapeutic Doses

Antimicrobial Agents	Adverse Effects
Penicillins/cephalosporins	Seizures Impaired hemostasis Interstitial nephritis Dermatologic reactions
Aminoglycosides	Ototoxicity Nephrotoxicity Neuromuscular blockade
Sulfonamides	Gastrointestinal irritation Dermatologic reactions Hematologic abnormalities
Macrolides	Gastrointestinal irritation Dysrhythmias*
Fluoroquinolones	Potential cartilage abnormalities in children Seizures and mild central nervous system dysfunction Photosensitivity
Tetracyclines	Dental discoloration in children Gastrointestinal irritation
Vancomycin	Ototoxicity Nephrotoxicity Redman syndrome
Chloramphenicol	Bone marrow suppression Gray baby syndrome

*Possible when erythromycin is taken with astemizole or terfenadine.

TABLE 180-2 Antimicrobials in Pregnancy

FDA Classification of Drugs in Pregnancy		Antimicrobials
A	Controlled studies in humans demonstrate no risk to fetus	
B	No evidence of risk in humans	Penicillins Cephalosporins Erythromycin* Azithromycin Clindamycin Nitrofurantoin Metronidazole†
C	Animal studies show fetal risk and no human data, or data lacking in animals and humans	Sulfonamides Clarithromycin Fluoroquinolones Mefloquine Dapsone INH Chloramphenicol Vancomycin Rifampin
D	Positive evidence of human risk exists, but benefit may outweigh risk in some situations	Aminoglycosides Tetracyclines
X	Fetal risk outweighs any possible benefit	Quinine

*Erythromycin estolate preparations are contraindicated in pregnancy.
†Metronidazole should not be used in first trimester of pregnancy due to concerns for teratogenicity.
Abbreviations: FDA, Food and Drug Administration; INH, isonicotinoylhydrazine (isoniazid).

TABLE 180-3 Classification of Hypersensitivity Reactions

Type	Immunologic Mechanism	Antimicrobial Examples
I	IgE mediated immediate, anaphylaxis	Almost all antimicrobial agents
II	IgG mediated, cytotoxic antibody	Hemolytic anemia Penicillin
III	Antigen-antibody mediated, "serum sickness"	Serum sickness Cefaclor Penicillin Sulfonamides Streptomycin
IV	T-cell mediated, delayed hypersensitivity reactions	Contact dermatitis Neomycin Nitrofurantoin Penicillin Sulfonamides

Abbreviation: Ig, immunoglobulin.

with a number of resistant pathogens. The oral and other mucosal surfaces may become infected with *Candida albicans.* Alteration of the gastrointestinal flora may result in pseudomembranous colitis from superinfection by *Clostridium difficile.* The antibiotics most commonly associated with pseudomembranous colitis are cephalosporins, penicillins, and clindamycin.

Antibiotics account for the greatest number of adverse dermatologic drug reactions. Ampicillin and trimethoprim-sulfamethoxazole (TMP-SMX) are reported to be the most common offending agents.[3] The mechanisms of these cutaneous reactions are not well understood but appear to be mediated immunologically. Most benign skin reactions begin within 1 to 2 weeks of exposure to the drug. Rashes are often pruritic erythematous, morbilliform, or macular eruptions, which typically resolve within several days after administration of the offending drug has been stopped.

Serious drug reactions are rare. Sulfonamides were recently implicated in a large case-control study as the drugs with the highest relative rate for development of the severe drug eruptions of Stevens-Johnson syndrome (SJS) and toxic epidermal necrolysis (TEN). The sulfonamides are estimated to account for 4.5 cases of SJS and TEN per million users of the drug per week.[4] Other antibiotics significantly associated with SJS and TEN include cephalosporins, fluoroquinolones, tetracyclines, and aminopenicillins.

SPECIFIC AGENTS AND ADVERSE EFFECTS AT THERAPEUTIC DOSES

Penicillins/Cephalosporins/β Lactams

The penicillins and cephalosporins are among the most widely used antimicrobial agents. They share a common β-lactam ring and are bactericidal through inhibition of bacterial cell wall synthesis. Potential adverse effects associated with therapeutic use of penicillin and β lactams include hypersensitivity reactions, central nervous system (CNS) disturbances, impaired hemostasis, interstitial nephritis, and hepatitis.

Penicillin and β lactams have been implicated in all types of hypersensitivity reactions (types I to IV). Hypersensitivity reactions are believed to develop in 0.6 to 10 percent of patients who use these agents. Immediate hypersensitivity reactions are believed to occur less frequently and result in less morbidity with oral penicillin than with parenteral administration of penicillin. There are four reported fatalities related to oral penicillin use compared with approximately 100 to 300 deaths per year from parenteral penicillin.

The risk of hypersensitivity reactions to cephalosporins in patients with known penicillin allergies is an issue of clinical importance. The overall incidence of adverse reactions to cephalosporins is low (between 1 and 10 percent) and mostly limited to dermatologic reactions. Adverse reactions to cephalosporins occur in approximately 4 percent of non-penicillin-allergic patients and 8 percent of patients with penicillin allergies. Severe hypersensitivity reactions are reported to have an incidence of less than 0.02 percent in the general population and less than 0.04 percent in patients with penicillin allergies. A recent review concludes that cross-reactivity between penicillins and cephalosporins is low (approximately a twofold increase over the general population) and probably only significant between first-generation cephalosporins and penicillin.[5] Administration of cephalosporins to penicillin-sensitive patients is possible but should be done with caution and avoided in patients with a history of severe penicillin hypersensitivity reaction (airway compromise, bronchospasm, or hypotension).

Hoingne's syndrome, which is another ''reaction'' seen with use of penicillin, is believed to be related to rapid absorption of procaine. The syndrome consists of behavioral abnormalities, including headache, hallucinations, sensation of impending doom, acute psychosis and, rarely, seizure after intramuscular injection of procaine penicillin. Most symptoms are self-limited and resolve within 30 min.

Penicillins and the β-lactam agents may result in significant adverse CNS effects. Confusion, agitation, myoclonic jerking, and seizures have been reported with high-dose penicillin G (more than 20 to 30 million U/day), cephalosporins, and imipenem. Encephalopathy, agitation, and absence seizures have been reported with ceftazidime. CNS effects of penicillins and β-lactam agents are believed to result from antagonism of the γ-aminobutyric acid (GABA) receptor. Patients most at risk for adverse CNS effects during β-lactam therapy are those with renal failure, with underlying CNS abnormalities, or receiving high-dose therapy.

Penicillins and β-lactam agents have the potential to impair hemostasis. Hypoprothrombinemia has been reported with several β-lactam agents (cephalothin, cephazolin, moxalactam, cefoperazone, and cefotetan).[6] These agents may decrease the production of the vitamin K-dependent coagulation factors by decreasing vitamin K absorption from the gastrointestinal tract, by interfering with vitamin K metabolism, and/or through direct enzymatic inhibition of coagulation factor activation. Qualitative and quantitative platelet disorders have also been reported with β-lactam agents. Penicillin, ampicillin, moxalactam, carbenicillin, ticarcillin, piperacillin, mezlocillin, and nafcillin have all been reported to decrease platelet aggregation and increase bleeding time in a dose-dependent manner. The absolute risk for clinically important bleeding with penicillins and β-lactam agents is not well established, but patients with renal failure and preexisting coagulopathy appear to be at greatest risk.

Dermatologic reactions are common with penicillins and include mild and severe eruptions. Cephalosporins and aminopenicillins (ampicillin and amoxicillin) are the β-lactam agents that account for most cases of the severe skin eruptions (i.e., SJS and TEN). An interesting but not well-understood erythematous, maculopapular rash is associated with ampicillin use in infectious mononucleosis. The rash has been reported in 69 to 100 percent of infectious mononucleosis cases treated with ampicillin. Typically, the rash appears 5 to 14 days into therapy and resolves with cessation of ampicillin. Recently, a similar rash has been reported with cephalexin use in a patient with mononucleosis.[7]

Aminoglycosides

Animoglycosides are bactericidal agents that bind to the 30 S bacterial ribosome and inhibit protein synthesis. Agents include gentamicin, tobramycin, amikacin, kanamycin, streptomycin, spectinomycin, and netilmicin. Aminoglycosides have a low therapeutic to toxic ratio, with ototoxicity and nephrotoxicity being common adverse effects. All aminoglycosides have the potential to damage vestibular and cochlear sensory cells, but neomycin is by far the most ototoxic. The incidence of hearing loss related to aminoglycoside has been reported to be between 2 and 25 percent. Hearing loss correlates closely with high-dose or prolonged therapy. Nephrotoxicity results from damage to the proximal renal tubules and correlates with drug dose, therapy duration, volume status, and extremes of age. Mild renal insufficiency may result in 10 to 25 percent of patients using aminoglycosides, as reflected in elevations in serum creatine. Renal damage is largely reversible with cessation of therapy, but renal function should be monitored closely during therapy.

An interesting adverse effect of aminoglycoside use is possible neuromuscular blockade. The aminoglycosides are believed to inhibit the release of acetylcholine presynaptically and block binding postsynaptically. Myasthenia gravis patients appear to be at greatest risk for weakness related to aminoglycoside usage due to a potential curare-like effect, but apnea has been reported in neurologically normal individuals after they have received intraperitoneal neomycin. Aminoglycosides may also prolong the effects of the non-depolarizing paralytic agents.

Sulfonamides/Bactrim

The sulfonamides are bactericidal agents that inhibit folic acid synthesis in bacteria. Sulfonamides are para-aminobenzoic acid (PABA) analogues and competitively inhibit the enzyme dihydropteroate synthetase in the folate synthesis pathway. Available sulfonamides include sulfisoxazole and sulfamethoxazole. Sulfonamides have a high incidence of bacterial resistance, and today the most widely used sulfonamide is sulfamethoxazole in combination with trimethoprim (Bactrim, Septra, Sulfatrim, or Cotrim). Trimethoprim also inhibits folate synthesis by inhibiting the activity of bacterial dihydrofolate reductase and produces a synergistic bactericidal effect with sulfonamides.[8] TMP-SMX has become one of the most important drugs in preventing opportunistic infections in HIV-positive individuals.

Sulfonamides have a relatively high incidence of adverse drug reactions, including immediate hypersensitivity, serum sickness, gastrointestinal irritation, dermatologic reactions, photosensitivity reactions, and hematologic abnormalities. Adverse drug reactions related to TMP-SMX are more common in HIV-positive individuals, with an incidence reported to be as high as 40 to 60 percent. Cutaneous reactions to sulfonamides and TMP-SMX are placed at approximately 3.4 percent in hospitalized patients. As previously stated, sulfonamides and TMP-SMX account for the greatest incidence of drug-related SJS and toxic epidermal necrolysis (4.5 cases per million users of the drug per week). Hematologic disorders seen with sulfonamides include aplastic anemia, agranulocytosis, hemolytic anemia, and thrombocytopenia. Patients with glucose-6-phosphate dehydrogenase (G6PD) deficiency should not receive sulfonamides or TMP-SMX secondary to an increased risk for hemolytic anemias. TMP-SMX should be used with caution in patients with impaired renal function, because trimethoprim interferes with potassium excretion from the kidney.

Macrolides

Macrolides are bacteriostatic agents that bind to the 50 S ribosome and inhibit bacterial protein synthesis. Available agents include erythromycin, azithromycin, clarithromycin, and dirithromycin. Macrolides rarely cause hypersensitivity reactions, but adverse effects of macrolide use include gastrointestinal irritation, reversible ototoxicities, pancreatitis, and cholestatic hepatitis.

The most important adverse reaction reported with macrolide use is cardiac dysrhythmias associated with erythromycin and possibly clarithromycin. Erythromycin-related polymorphic ventricular tachycardia (torsades de pointes) has been well documented in two clinical situations: (1) after intravenous erythromycin administration and (2) when oral erythromycin is taken with specific drugs (astemizole, terfenadine, and cisapride).

Erythromycin can prolong action potential duration and delay repolarization. Clinically, this is witnessed by prolongation of the QT interval. The mechanism of this QT prolongation is believed to be erythromycin blockade of the selective delayed rectifier potassium current in Purkinje fibers. Recently, prolongation of the QT interval and torsades de pointes was also reported with clarithromycin.[9]

Erythromycin and clarithromycin inhibit cytochrome P-450, which can lead to increased serum levels of astemizole, carbamazepine, cisapride, corticosteroids, cyclosporine, digoxin, terfenadine, theophylline, warfarin, valproate, and ergot alkaloids. Cases of torsades de pointes have occurred with coadministration of erythromycin and the antihistamines astemizole and terfenadine. It is believed that increased drug level of these antihistamines is responsible for prolongation of the QT interval. Recently, prolonged QT interval and ventricular dysrhythmias have also been reported with coadministration of clarithromycin and with cisapride.[10] Azithromycin does not inhibit the P-450 system and, to date, has not been linked to ventricular dysrhythmias.

Fluoroquinolones

The fluoroquinolones are bactericidal agents that inhibit bacterial DNA gyrases. Available agents include ciprofloxacin, enoxacin, levofloxacin, lomefloxacin, norfloxacin, ofloxacin, sparafloxacin, and trovafloxacin. Children under the age of 18 and pregnant women should not use fluoroquinolones, because of the potential for cartilage abnormalities. The fluoroquinolones are generally considered safe, with gastrointestinal irritation being the most commonly reported side effect. Fluoroquinolones are weak GABA inhibitors, and adverse CNS effects may include behavioral abnormalities, visual changes, dizziness, and seizures.[11] Photosensitivity reactions have been reported, and rarely fluoroquinolone use may result in renal insufficiency or hepatic toxicity.

Tetracyclines

Tetracyclines are bacteriostatic agents that inhibit bacterial protein synthesis through binding to the 30 S ribosome subunit in bacteria. Available agents include demeclocycline, doxycycline, minocycline, and tetracycline. Tetracycline use may result in adverse reactions that include photosensitivity reactions, discoloration of dentition in children, gastrointestinal irritation, lupus-like syndromes, renal insufficiency, and hepatic toxicity.[12] Tetracyclines are among the most frequent causes of phototoxic drug reactions. The phototoxic potential is greatest with demeclocycline and doxycycline, and least with minocycline.[13]

Tetracycline complexes with calcium and is deposited in teeth and bones. Children are at risk for permanent dental discoloration from tetracycline up to the age of 8, with the highest incidence occurring before 6 months of age. The degree of discoloration appears to be dose related. Tetracyclines should not be used in pregnancy, because they cross the placenta and permanent dental discoloration may result in children born to tetracycline-treated mothers.

Vancomycin

Vancomycin is a bactericidal agent that interferes with bacterial cell wall synthesis. In addition to hypersensitivity reactions, vancomycin use may result in an urticarial, erythematous, flushed rash termed redman syndrome. The rash is typically on the face but may also involve the trunk and extremities. Transient tachycardia and hypotension have also been noted in some cases. Red-man syndrome is most often related to rapid infusion of parenteral vancomycin, but there are case reports with oral and intraperitoneal vancomycin.[14] The reaction is believed to result from histamine release. Termination of vancomycin infusion, fluids, and H_1 antagonist may help in the acute episodes, and extending the time of vancomycin infusion or H_1 blockers can help prevent this reaction with future vancomycin doses.

Vancomycin may also result in nephrotoxicity and ototoxicity. Patients with renal insufficiency or who are using other nephrotoxic drugs (e.g., aminoglycosides or amphotericin B) are at increased risk for vancomycin-induced renal damage. Ototoxicity is rare at therapeutic doses of vancomycin, but hearing defects may result at high doses and in patients with renal insufficiency.

Chloramphenicol

Chloramphenicol is a bacteriostatic agent that binds to the 50 S ribosome of bacteria and inhibits protein synthesis. Despite broad antimicrobial activity, chloramphenicol is rarely used in the United States secondary to potential adverse effects at therapeutic doses. Chloramphenicol may result in hypersensitivity reactions, neurologic abnormalities, and hematologic toxicity. The most notorious is a symptom complex of vomiting, poor sucking, cyanosis, and diarrhea in neonates and children. The syndrome (gray baby syndrome) is seen after several days of high-dose chloramphenicol administration and often progresses to obtundation, palor, hypotension, hypothermia, and death. The toxicity of chloramphenicol in neonates is believed to result from inability to metabolize the drug.

Chloramphenicol is responsible for two types of hematologic toxicity: the most common is reversible myelosuppression, and the second is aplastic anemia. Reversible bone marrow suppression appears to be related to mitochondria injury in bone marrow. This inhibition is reversed with cessation of use of the drug. Aplastic anemia is a rare complication, occurring in from 1:24,000 to 1:40,500 recipients of the drug. The mechanism of toxicity is hypothesized to be a toxic metabolite resulting in stem cell damage.[15] Aplastic anemia with chloramphenicol is not dose related and does not typically resolve with cessation of the drug.

Antimycobacterial Drugs

Infection with *Mycobacterium tuberculosis* (tuberculosis or TB) is common in developing countries, and during 1990s there was an increased incidence of TB in the United States. Patients being treated for active TB as well as patients taking chemoprophylaxis for positive purified protein derivative (PPD) skin tests are now commonplace in many urban emergency departments. First-line therapy for TB includes isoniazid (isonicotinylhydrazide or INH), rifampin, pyrazinamide, ethambutol, and streptomycin.

Antimycobacterials may have adverse effects at therapeutic doses. Rifampin may result in gastrointestinal distress, flulike symptoms, hepatic toxicity, renal toxicity, and various dermatologic reactions. Rifampin is also noted for a nontoxic orange-red discoloration of skin, mucous membranes, urine, semen, and tears. Pyrazinamide is the most hepatotoxic of the first-line TB medications and also inhibits the excretion of urate, with acute episodes of gout possible secondary to therapy. Adverse effects of ethambutol include gastrointestinal irritation, optic neuritis, headache, behavioral changes, pruritis, and joint pain. Optic neuritis is manifested by the loss of green-red differentiation and is usually reversible with termination of therapy.

INH In addition to treating active TB, INH is also used for chemoprophylaxis in patients with positive PPD tests. INH has important adverse effects, including hepatic toxicity and neurotoxicity, at therapeutic doses. Approximately 10 to 20 percent of patients who use INH for chemoprophylaxis will have elevation in serum transaminases and 1 percent will develop overt hepatitis.[16] Patients should have the serum transaminase level evaluated frequently, and therapy should be terminated if the level is elevated two to three times above normal.

Neurotoxicity includes paresthesias, ataxia, obtundation, optic neuritis, behavioral abnormalities, peripheral neuropathies, and seizures. INH inhibits production of the neurotransmitter GABA. Seizures related to INH are believed to result from decreased levels of GABA and are most commonly seen after acute overdoses or in patients who have underlying seizure disorders. INH forms hydrazones with pyridoxine (vitamin B_6), which causes pyridoxine deficiencies. Peripheral neuropathies are believed to result from pyridoxine deficiencies, and supplementation with pyridoxine may relieve symptoms.

Acute INH ingestion of more than 20 to 30 mg/kg may cause seizures that are refractory to standard anticonvulsive therapy (benzodiazepines, barbiturates, etc.). Most INH-induced seizures occur within 2 h of overdose, and patients who remain asymptomatic for 6 h are safe for medical clearance. INH ingestion should be entertained in any patient presenting with refractory seizures. INH seizures are treated with pyridoxine (vitamin B_6). The dose is a gram-for-gram equivalent to the amount of INH ingested. For patients who ingest an unknown quantity of INH, the recommended dose of pyridoxine is 5 g intravenously over 3 to 5 min.

Antimalarial Drugs

Antimalarials are not used in the United States as frequently as other antimicrobials; however, they are among the agents with the greatest potential for toxic effects. Common agents include quinine, chloroquine, mefloquine, and primaquine. Adverse effects associated with quinine at therapeutic doses include *cinchonism,* which is the symptom complex of ringing in ears, headache, visual disturbance, and nausea. Chloroquine, quinine and, to lesser extent, primaquine may be associated with ventricular dysrhythmias. Primaquine and chloroquine have been associated with methemoglobinemia. Hemolytic anemia is also reported with quinine, primaquine, and chloroquine in patients with G6PD deficiency. CNS effects associated with the antimalarials include headache, visual disturbances, dizziness, seizures, and behavioral changes. Mefloquine use results in greater neuropsychiatric reactions than the other antimalarials and has been associated with acute psychotic reactions.

Quinine and chloroquine may both result in severe CNS and cardiac abnormalities in acute overdose. CNS manifestation of toxicity includes obtundation, headache, and seizures. Quinine also has significant ocular toxicity in acute overdose, and blindness may result with serum levels of greater than 10 to 15 μg/mL. Possible electrolyte abnormalities include hypoglycemia with quinine and hypokalemia with chloroquine. Both drugs have cardiac effects and may lead to PR, QT, or QRS prolongation. Patients may be hypotensive, with early cardiovascular collapse. Aggressive supportive care is used for overdose.[17] A decreased mortality rate has been demonstrated in chloroquine overdose treated with early intubation, gastric lavage, deep sedation with benzodiazepines, and vasoactive pressor support with epinephrine to maintain a systolic blood pressure of 100 mmHg.[18] Sodium bicarbonate (to adjust serum pH of 7.45 to 7.50) may be helpful in treating dysrhythmias related to the sodium-channel blockade from quinine and chloroquine, although good data do not exist to support its use.

Metronidazole

Metronidazole is effective for treating anaerobic bacteria, *Trichomonas,* and anaerobic protozoal parasites. Adverse effects of metronidazole use include gastrointestinal distress, CNS toxicities, stomatitis, and disulfiram-like reactions. CNS toxicities include headache, paresthesias, behavioral changes, vertigo, and seizures. Disulfiram-like reactions are common with metronidazole, and all patients should be warned not to drink alcohol.

Antiviral and Common HIV Medications

Current treatment for human immunodeficiency virus (HIV) and the resulting acquired immune deficiency syndrome (AIDS) requires patients to take multidrug regimens to prevent progression of their disease and to treat opportunistic infections. HIV therapy has grown complex over the past several years with the introduction of new therapeutic agents and evolving recommendations for prophylaxis against opportunistic infections. Drugs used to decrease the HIV load in the body include nucleoside analogues (zidovudine, lamivudine, etc.), nonnucleoside reverse transcriptase inhibitors (nevirapine and delaviridine), and protease inhibitors (indinavir, ritonavir, etc.). Adverse effects seen with the antivirals include nausea, malaise, gastrointestinal irritation, myalgias, neurologic abnormalities, and bone marrow suppression. Neurologic abnormalities include headache, peripheral neuropathy, and seizure. In acute overdose, there is little experience with many of the new antiviral agents. Zidovudine (AZT) overdose has resulted in seizure, but major morbidity or deaths have not been reported.

Antimicrobial agents used against opportunistic infections are numerous and a comprehensive review is beyond the scope of this chapter; however, several agents warrant mention. TMP-SMX to treat and prevent *Pneumocystis carinii* pneumonia (PCP) has a 40 to 60 percent incidence of cutaneous reactions in HIV-positive patients. Parenteral pentamidine also used against PCP may result in nephrotoxicity, hepatic toxicity, hypoglycemia secondary to pancreatic necrosis, hypotension, and ventricular tachycardia at therapeutic doses.[19] Dapsone, a second-line agent for PCP and toxoplasmosis, may have significant adverse effects at therapeutic doses and in overdose: its use may result in headache, nausea, rash, neuropathy, and seizures. The two most important adverse effects of dapsone use are methemoglobinemia and hemolysis. Hemolysis is most common with patients who have G6PD deficiency.[20]

EVALUATION AND TREATMENT OF ANTIMICROBIAL OVERDOSE

Most antimicrobial overdoses will be asymptomatic; however, significant ingestions of agents such as INH, chloroquine, and quinine can result in severe toxicities. Patients who present with symptomatic ingestions (altered mental status, seizure, electrolyte disturbances, anion-gap acidosis, or renal failure) should be treated with supportive care using emergency medicine principles. The history should include the amount and type of antimicrobial ingested. Patients should also be asked about possible coingestants. Suicide potential should be assessed.

Asymptomatic antimicrobial ingestions require minimal laboratory evaluation. As is common in all cases of possible overdose, patients should have acetaminophen levels determined and an electrocardiogram performed to screen for coingestants. Emergency medicine and critical care principles should guide laboratory evaluation in symptomatic overdoses. The electrolyte level should be determined to evaluate potential anion-gap acidosis in cases of suspected INH overdose. Methemoglobin levels should be determined in dapsone, chloroquine, and primaquine overdoses. Drug levels are not helpful in the management in the acute antimicrobial overdose but may be confirmatory and are available for several antibiotics (INH, quinine, and chloroquine).

Gastric decontamination should be initiated in all patients with suspected antimicrobial overdoses. Activated charcoal with the cathartic sorbitol should be given orally or through a nasogastric tube. Repeat-dose activated charcoal without sorbitol is indicated in symptomatic patients. Dialysis and charcoal hemoperfusion are effective at eliminating aminoglycosides and possibly pentamidine but are not highly effective at removing other antimicrobial agents.

REFERENCES

1. Blanca M: Allergic reactions to penicillins: A changing world? *Allergy* 50:777, 1995.
2. Bochner BS, Lichtenstein LM: Anaphylaxis. *N Engl J Med* 324:1785, 1991.
3. Stren RS, Steinberg LA: Epidemiology of adverse cutaneous reactions to drugs. *Dermatol Clin* 13:681, 1995.
4. Roujeau JC, Kelly JP, Naldi LN, et al: Medication use and the risk of Steven-Johnson syndrome or toxic epidermal necrolysis. *N Engl J Med* 333:1600, 1995.
5. Anne S, Reisman R: Risk of administering cephalosporin antibiotics to patients with histories of penicillin allergy. *Ann Allergy Asthma Immunol* 74:167, 1995.
6. Sattler FR, Weitekamp MR, Ballard JO: Potential for bleeding with the new beta-lactam antibiotics. *Ann Intern Med* 105:924, 1986.
7. McCloskey GL, Massa MC: Cephalexin rash in infectious mononucleosis. *Cutis* 59:251, 1997.
8. Cockerill FR, Edson RS: Trimethoprim-sulfamethoxazole. *Mayo Clin Proc* 66:1260, 1991.
9. Lee KL, Jim MH, Tang SC, Tai YT: QT prolongation and torsades de pointes associated with clarithromycin. *Am J Med* 104:395, 1998.
10. Sekkarie MA: Torsades de pointes in two chronic renal failure patients treated with cisapride and clarithromycin. *Am J Kidney Dis* 30:437, 1997.
11. Walker RC, Wright AJ: The fluoroquinolones. *Mayo Clin Proc* 66:1249, 1991.
12. Shapiro LE, Knowles SR, Shear NH: Comparative safety of tetracycline, minocycline, and doxycycline. *Arch Dermatol* 133:1224, 1997.
13. Gould JW, Mercurio MG, Elmets CA: Cutaneous photosensitivity diseases induced by exogenous agents. *J Am Acad Dermatol* 33:551, 1995.
14. Bergeron L, Boucher FD: Possible red-man syndrome associated with systemic absorption of oral vancomycin in a child with normal renal function. *Ann Pharmacother* 28:581, 1994.
15. Yunis AA: Chloramphenicol toxicity: 25 years of research. *Am J Med* 87:44N, 1989.
16. Chan-Tompkins NH: Toxic effects and drug interactions of antimycobacterial therapy. *Clin Dermatol* 13:223, 1995.
17. Clemessy JL, Taboulet P, Hoffman JR, et al: Treatment of acute chloroquine poisoning: A 5 year experience. *Crit Care Med* 24:1189, 1996.
18. Riou B, Barriot P, Rimailho A, et al: Treatment of severe chloroquine poisoning. *N Engl J Med* 318:1, 1988.
19. Watts RG, Conte JE, Zurlinde E, Waldo B: Effect of charcoal hemoperfusion on clearance of pentamidine isethionate after accidental overdose. *J Toxicol Clin Toxicol* 35:89, 1997.
20. Sin DD, Shafran SD: Dapsone and primaquine induced methemoglobinemia in HIV infected individuals. *J Acquir Immune Defic Syndr Hum Retrovirol* 12:477, 1996.

HAZARDOUS MATERIALS EXPOSURE

Suzanne R. White

Col. Edward M. Eitzen, Jr.

A *hazardous material* can be defined as any substance (chemical, nuclear, or biologic) that may pose a risk to health, safety, property, or the environment. There are currently over 500,000 potentially toxic chemicals and compounds listed in the most commonly used poisoning database, Poisindex, and it is estimated that 600 new chemicals are introduced yearly into the workplace. Given the quantity (1.5 billion tons per year) and frequency of transport (500,000 shipments per day) of hazardous substances throughout the United States, it seems inevitable that the practicing emergency physician will be faced with the management of a chemically exposed or contaminated patient.[1]

The Hazardous Substances Emergency Events Surveillance (HSEES) database registered 5531 hazardous chemical accidents during 1997.[2] Petroleum products, which account for approximately 50 percent of hazardous materials spills, were not included, and this reporting included only 13 states. Similar registries such as Chemtrec and the National Response Center logged over 13,000 and 25,000 hazardous oil and chemical incidents, respectively, during that same time period.[3] Eighty percent of events occur at fixed facilities, while 20 percent are transportation-related, and over 10 percent occur within hospitals and schools. Seventy percent of hazardous materials accidents occur Monday through Friday 6 A.M. to 6 P.M.[4] Incidents typically result in one or two victims, usually employees and less frequently the general public and first responders. Of the 10 to 30 percent of incidents that involve victims, traumatic injury is common.[5,6] Nontraumatic injuries most commonly include respiratory and eye irritation, nausea, vomiting, headache, dizziness, or other neurologic effects. Sixty-five percent of fatalities following a hazardous materials incident result from trauma, 22 percent from burns, and 10 percent are attributed to respiratory compromise. Most injuries and deaths are associated with exposure to chlorine, ammonia, nitrogen fertilizer, or hydrochloric acid. Other commonly involved chemicals include petroleum products, pesticides, corrosives, metals, and volatile organics. Unknown or unclassified chemicals constitute a full 25 percent of events.[7]

As indicated by the recent World Trade Center, Oklahoma City, 1996 Summer Olympics site, and abortion clinic bombings, along with the use of *Salmonella, Shigella,* and cyanide to taint food and pharmaceuticals in this country, state-sponsored or terrorist use of readily available hazardous substances has become a reality. Materials used in a terrorist event may be nuclear, biologic, or chemical and are referred to as *NBC agents* or *weapons of mass destruction* (WMD). During the 1995 release of sarin in the Tokyo subway system, 5510 people sought medical attention. Six hundred and forty chemically contaminated patients arrived by private conveyance within the first few hours of the incident to a single health care facility. Twenty-three percent of emergency department (ED) staff at that hospital became secondarily poisoned as the nerve agent was transported via contaminated victims from the scene.[8,9]

Chemical disasters, whether they be at industrial fixed-facility sites, transportation-related, or terrorist-mediated, share many features. They may involve mass casualties with serious concomitant injuries, such as trauma, burns, or smoke inhalation, that outstrip medical resources. Communication breakdown is prevalent, as is chaos among medical personnel who are unfamiliar with the agents involved, unaware of available resources, or have become secondarily contaminated. The need for emergency community and medical preparedness to mitigate the adverse consequences of such hazardous materials accidents cannot be overly stressed.

PLANNING

The hospital and ED have the following responsibilities when planning for hazardous materials exposure: (1) identify any potential local hazards, (2) recognize that a hazardous material is involved, (3) identify the agent involved, (4) obtain information about the toxicity and secondary contamination potential of the agent, (5) protect hospital personnel, other patients, and the facility itself from secondary contamination and loss of serviceability to other patients, (6) triage and decontaminate victims, (7) stabilize and treat the injured, and (8) protect the community from secondary contamination. One excellent resource for designing such procedures is the ATSDR *Medical Management Guidelines for Acute Chemical Exposures*.[10] Chapter 5, Disaster Medical Services, covers planning in detail.

ADVANCE INFORMATION RETRIEVAL

Detailed information about the involved chemical(s) is most helpful if received prior to patient arrival. Regional poison control centers (PCCs) are already integrated into the emergency medical, HazMat, and Metropolitan Medical Response Systems (MMRS).[11,12] Another information resource is the Material Safety Data Sheet (MSDS), a document that identifies health and safety information for any product containing hazardous chemicals. MSDSs may be obtained by facsimile from the work-site employer or safety officer, regional PCCs, Chemtrec, NRC, the Internet, and computer databases such as Safetydex™. Included are chemical and physical hazard data as well as information regarding safe use, handling, and storage. Basic first aid procedures are outlined, but advanced medical information usually is not included. While the merit of MSDSs has been questioned,[13] at the least they will assist with correct identification and spelling of the chemical agent(s) involved. Limitations of MSDSs use are that they may not exist for all toxic substances, they are not always comprehensive with regard to ingredient listing or toxicity data, they may not be up to date, ingredients listed as "inert" may be toxic, and "trade secret" ingredients may be deleted (although trade secret toxicity data must be listed, and the treating physician is entitled to immediate identity on request). Other resources that may assist with hazard identification determination of toxicity are listed in Table 181-1.

DECONTAMINATION ZONES

Patient decontamination should occur outside the hospital. Hot, warm, and cold zones should be established and cordoned off with brightly colored tape. The hot zone is the area of the spill or chemical release (at the scene) or the hospital area where arriving patients with no prior decontamination are held. Therefore, only those trained and properly attired may enter. Only the most immediate life threats are addressed in the hot zone (opening of the airway, cervical spine immobilization, brushing off of gross contaminants, and applying pressure to stop arterial bleeding). The warm zone is an area where thorough decontamination and further medical stabilization occur. Theoretically, this area poses no risk of primary contamination (direct exposure to the toxin), but secondary contamination (transfer of the toxic material from the victim to personnel or equipment) may still occur. Access, therefore, is also restricted, and the use of protective clothing is required. The cold zone is the area to which fully decontaminated patients are transferred. There is no personnel flow between hot/warm or warm/cold areas.

Personal Protection

The various levels of personal protection are levels A through D. Level A attire [fully encapsulating chemical-resistant suit and self-contained breathing apparatus (SCBA)] is recommended when the highest level of eye, mucous membrane, skin, and respiratory protection is needed. Lower levels of protection include level B (splash protection with chemical-resistant clothing and a SCBA) and level C (splash protection with chemical-resistant clothing and a full-faced air-purifying respirator). Level D protection is a standard work uniform and includes firefighter bunker gear. Military mission-oriented protective posture (MOPP) level IV gear, comprised of an air-purifying respirator, protective mask, hood, charcoal-impregnated suit, and butyl rubber gloves and boots, affords effective protection against the biochemical weapons of mass destruction.

While level A protection is recommended by National Institute of Occupational Safety and Health (NIOSH) and the Environmental Protection Agency (EPA) in situations where the concentration or identity of toxins involved is unknown (i.e., most hazardous materials incidents), there is no consensus regarding the level of protection needed for the hospital decontamination of patients. This is particularly controversial with regard to nontraditional hazardous threats such as WMD. Only limited patient care can be rendered while wearing level A gear, and air availability restricts its use to only short periods of time. Furthermore, specialized protective gear is only recommended for those with prior training and fitting, given the added level of physical and heat stress and false sense of security that its use may render. Despite these limitations, if level A protection is to be used by the emergency staff, it is recommended that the hospital coordinate equipment acquisition with the local fire departments or HazMat team so that regulator fittings (replacement air bottles) are interchangeable. Practically speaking, most hospitals have only level C protection available to employees. Ideally, persons responsible for selecting the personal protective equipment and decontamination process should be trained to the first responder operations level under OSHA 29 CFR 1910.120.

TRIAGE

The first wave of minimally exposed victims arrives within 30 min of the incident, overwhelming the ED and impeding the care of patients who will arrive later.[14] ED triage must be efficient and should occur outdoors. *First and foremost, the patient should not be allowed to enter the ED.* Second, those personnel who are not in an appropriate level of protective gear should not be allowed in the triage/decontamination area. The incoming ambulance or ambulatory patients should be met by a triage officer, an individual in appropriate level of personal

TABLE 181-1 Aids in Chemical Identification and Hazard Determination

Department of Transportation (DOT) placards: diamond-shaped placards on tank trucks or rail cars		
United Nations classification numbering system on vehicles: at bottom of placards or on shipping papers, defines hazard		
Bill of lading (cargo manifest in cab of truck)		
Waybill (with train conductor)		
Shipping papers		
National Fire Protection Association (NFPA) marking system labels on containers		
Material Safety Data Sheet (MSDS)		
On-scene chemical analysis (by fire department or HazMat team)		
Regional Poison Control Centers		
Chemtrec	24-h assistance to emergency responders regarding chemical spills	1-800-424-9300
REAC/TS	24-h emergency consultative assistance for radiation accidents	423-576-3131
	(after business hours)	423-481-1000
Motherisk program	Teratology information service	416-813-6780
	(after business hours)	416-813-5900
ATSDR/CDC emergency response 24-h hotline		404-639-0615
EPA environmental response hotline		201-321-6660
National Response Center		1-800-424-8802
Local emergency planning committee (LEPC)		
Company records or company safety officer		
Metropolitan Medical Response System or technical support team (local expertise in weapons of mass destruction identification and management)		
Local FBI representative		
Local health department		
Local government agencies		
U.S. Army Medical Research Institute of Infectious Diseases (USAMRIID), Fort Detrick, Maryland		1-888-872-7443
Centers for Disease Control and Prevention (CDC)		404-639-3311
National Pesticide Telecommunication Network		1-800-858-7378
Computer databases: Poisindex, Safetydex, Tomes Plus, ToxNet, others		

Other references:
- ATSDR *Managing Hazardous Materials Incidents,* Vol. III (obtain by calling 404-639-6360).
- DOT *Emergency Response Guidebook,* 1996 (obtain by calling 1-800-327-6868).
- Sullivan's *Hazardous Materials Toxicology: Clinical Principles of Environmental Health.* Baltimore: Williams & Wilkins, 1992.
- *Medical Management of Biological Casualties Handbook,* 3rd ed. U.S. Army Medical Research Institute of Infectious Diseases, Fort Detrick, Frederick, Maryland, 1998.
- *Medical Management of Chemical Casualties Handbook,* 2d ed. U.S. Army Medical Research Institute of Chemical Defense, Aberdeen Proving Ground, Maryland, 1995.
- Biological agents as weapons. *JAMA* 278(5), 1997.

protective gear, to determine whether decontamination has been performed and, if so, its adequacy. The most difficult situations involve those victims who are seriously injured and who have bypassed the field decontamination procedure. A management dilemma is created between immediate medical treatment and decontamination. While the appropriate response varies depending on the chemical(s) involved, many situations involve unknown chemicals and therefore unknown risk to personnel. It is always prudent to err on the side of decontamination before treatment in unknown situations. Examples of those substances with little or no risk of secondary contamination include gases, vapors, and substances with no serious toxicity or skin absorption. Patients exposed to gases or vapors only, with no symptoms other than respiratory irritation and no signs of condensation of vapor on the clothing, do not require decontamination beyond clothing removal. This may not hold true, however, for large numbers of victims exposed to nerve agent vapor or for those in confined spaces. Substances with high risk of secondary contamination include highly toxic substances that are readily absorbed dermally, radioactive agents, and certain biologic agents.

DECONTAMINATION

Outside portable decontamination systems include portable showers, large inflatable heated tents, or a series of kiddy pools with privacy screens. Effluent must be contained, and disposable equipment should be used wherever feasible. Suggested equipment for outdoor hospital

TABLE 181-2 Suggested Equipment for Outdoor Hospital Decontamination

Biohazard/radiation hazard tape
Decontamination stretcher (alternative fiberglass backboard with sawhorses)
Hose with warm water and soft-stream shower head
Disposable butyl rubber, nitrile rubber, and neoprene rubber gloves in various sizes
Disposable chemical-resistant jump suits (Tyvek or Saranex) with hoods and boots
Rubber aprons
Mild soap/shampoo
Splash protective goggles
Plastic bags for clothing and waste container liners
Multiple wading pools for ambulatory patients (to contain runoff)
Adsorbent materials (for diking of waste water)
Oxygen tanks with delivery supplies
Disposable towels and gauze
Blankets and sheets for patient privacy
Portable privacy barriers

Source: Modified from ATSDR *Managing Hazardous Materials Incidents, Vol 3: Medical Guidelines for Acute Chemical Exposures.* Washington: U.S. Department of Health and Human Services, Agency for Toxic Substances and Disease Registry, 1991.

decontamination is listed in Table 181-2. Decontamination inside the hospital should only be done in a designated room with a separate entrance, separate ventilation, and separate water drainage systems.

The goal of decontamination is to decrease the absorbed dose for the victim and prevent secondary contamination of health care providers. Clothing should be removed quickly because this is thought to accomplish 80 percent of the decontamination. Those covered with particulate or radioactive matter should remove clothing very carefully by the roll-down method. Further particulate matter should be brushed away prior to showering, since interaction of some dry chemicals with water may produce heat. All clothing should be double bagged and treated as toxic waste. All patients' belongings and waste must be accounted for by a tracking log. Jewelry and valuables should be bagged separately from clothing, which may require disposal.

While undergoing decontamination, the nonambulatory patient should have a patent airway ensured, the cervical spine immobilized, oxygen administered, ventilation assisted, and pressure maintained on arterial bleeding. Further medical care, such as intubation or intravenous line insertion, is delayed until gross decontamination has been completed and the patient has been transferred to the cold zone. Ocular exposures take precedence and should be treated first with immediate eye irrigation. Ideally, this should have begun in the prehospital phase. Wounds are the next decontamination priority and should be irrigated, debrided of gross contaminants, and then covered with a water-occlusive dressing to prevent recontamination during subsequent showering. Whole-body decontamination should begin with the head and proceed downward. Along with the hands, the face and head generally are the most heavily contaminated areas and should be washed or shampooed in the head-back position to avoid runoff onto other body parts and incorporation of toxic material. This may best be accomplished initially in the sitting position, prior to showering. Most agents are readily removed with copious amounts of water and a mild soap, shampoo, or detergent. Tincture of green soap has been recommended by some based on its small concentration of ethanol that enhances dissolution of certain agents such as hydrocarbons. Typically, 3 to 5 min of showering is recommended, although 15 min may be required for concentrated, strongly alkaline materials or oily, adherent substances. The use of abrasives, such as corn meal or scrub brushes, is generally not advised, since abrading the skin may increase toxin absorption. New amphoteric decontamination solutions, such as Diphoterine, for specific acid, base, solvent, oxidizer, and reducing agent exposures are under investigation. Water temperature should be tepid, since heat potentially will increase dermal absorption of some toxins.

Certain agents may be removed more effectively with the use of specific decontamination solutions. Dilute household bleach solutions (9 parts water to 1 part bleach) will inactivate nerve agents and most biologic agents. The use of neutralizing solutions for acid or alkaline corrosives is controversial. Other agents requiring targeted decontamination solutions include phenol and hydrofluoric acid and are discussed below. One should not delay decontamination if such solutions are not readily available but rather begin washing with deluge volumes of water in an attempt to prevent toxin absorption through massive dilution.

Certain metals such as sodium, lithium, and potassium react violently with water, releasing heat, hydroxide ion, and hydrogen gas and potentially causing thermal burns. Proper treatment of alkali metal burns involves clothing removal, covering the affected area with mineral or cooking oil, followed by removal of any remaining metal with dry forceps. Only then can wounds be copiously irrigated with water. Burning fragments should be extinguished by smothering or with a class D fire extinguisher. Again, in the absence of proper solutions, decontamination with deluge volumes of water may be considered. Other water-reactive chemicals are listed in Table 181-3. In contrast to water-reactive chemicals, white phosphorus ignites spontaneously on exposure to air. Burns from this agent must be kept continuously moist with water or saline dressings until adequate debridement is accomplished. Each phosphorus particle must be removed. The application of copper sulfate solution blackens the phosphorus, aids in visualization, and provides neutralization. Alternatively, a Wood's lamp may be used. Some adherent toxins are extremely difficult to remove from the skin. Epoxy resins and cyanoacrylates (glues) may be removed by swabbing with acetone. Use of vegetable or mineral oil or saline-soaked gauze pads for the eyes and mucous membranes is safe. Hot tar, typically inflicting burns to the face and upper extremities, should be allowed to cool prior to removal. Effective tar removal has then been reported using Neosporin cream, Tween 80, plain Vaseline,

TABLE 181-3 Water-Reactive Substances

Acetic anhydride, acetyl chloride
Alkali metals: lithium, sodium, potassium (also form caustic sodium and potassium hydroxides)
Calcium
Chlorosulfonic acid
Concentrated sulfuric acid (oleum), concentrated muriatic acid
Dry lime (calcium oxide), calcium carbide
Hydrides: boranes, silanes
Inorganic chlorides (some): titanium tetrachloride peroxides
Organometallics: alkylaluminums
Zinc phosphide

Shur Clens, Desolv-It, or mayonnaise. No attempt should be made to remove tar by mechanical means, since this may increase tissue destruction and result in hair follicle loss.

Nausea and vomiting are common following chemical exposures. These symptoms may indicate toxin ingestion with gastrointestinal irritation or, more commonly, systemic toxin effect or hysteria. Regardless of the cause, secondary contamination by toxic vomitus may occur, and the need for its containment should be anticipated. Furthermore, some materials may react with stomach acid to produce secondary poisoning through toxic gas formation (sodium azide→hydrazoic acid, cyanide salts→hydrogen cyanide gas). Suction with outdoor venting should be available. If spontaneous emesis has not occurred already, gastric emptying or the administration of charcoal may be considered for large ingestions. Induction of vomiting is not recommended. Following the accidental ingestion of a corrosive material, 4 to 8 oz of water may be administered, if the patient is conscious. Decisions regarding gastrointestinal tract decontamination may be guided by the regional PCC.

Following decontamination, zipping patients into body bags or placing them into hooded Tyvek suits prior to transport to the support zone is no longer recommended. This technique is not effective in minimizing the transfer of toxin to hospital staff and poses the risk of increased toxin absorption by the patient. The patient simply should be wrapped in clean blankets or sheets prior to transfer to the cold zone.[10]

Complete medical assessment and specific medical treatment can be carried out in the support zone (cold zone). ED personnel in this area should maintain protective gear (chemical-resistant gowns, latex gloves, eye protection) until the chemical has been definitively identified and the risk of secondary contamination is known.

SPECIFIC MEDICAL MANAGEMENT

Inhaled Toxins

Gases, mists, aerosols, fumes, or dusts may be inhaled. Determinants of airborne agent toxicity include many factors such as concentration of the inhaled toxin, duration of exposure, and whether the exposure occurred in an enclosed space. Other influencing factors include vapor density, allergic or nonallergic bronchospastic response, exertional state or metabolic rate of the victim, and unique host susceptibility such as the underlying reactive airways disease, history of smoking, or extreme age. Aspiration of gastric contents may cause further pulmonary insult.

Other primary determinants of injury pattern include toxin particle size and solubility in water. Those agents with particles diameters greater than 10 μm or that are highly water soluble are deposited primarily in the upper airways. Examples of water-soluble chemicals include ammonia, sulfur dioxide, and acid gases such as hydrochloric acid and sulfuric acid. Following exposure, signs of upper airway irritation develop rapidly and are accompanied by eye and mucous membrane irritation. Coughing, wheezing, or stridor may progress to upper airway obstruction in severe exposures. Those inhaled toxins of smaller particle size or lower water solubility such as phosgene, ozone, or nitrogen oxides will reach the lower respiratory tract and may result in delayed symptom onset. Gases with intermediate water solubility, such as chlorine, may cause early irritative symptoms following mild exposure or delayed pulmonary edema after massive exposure.

The presence of fire or explosion complicates the ability to predict patterns of illness following toxin inhalation. Because it is particulate, smoke carries adherent products of combustion such as acrolein, ammonia, acids, and diisocyanates deeper into the lungs than normally would be expected. Thermal physical damage to respiratory tract also may occur, particularly in the presence of steam. General management of the patient with toxic inhalation injury involves removal from the source, application of 100% oxygen, humidification if irritative symptoms are present, and inhaled bronchodilators for bronchospasm. A detailed examination should include inspection of the upper airway for evidence of singed nasal hair, soot in the oropharynx, facial or oropharyngeal burns, erythema or parching of the mucous membranes, stridor, hoarseness, dysphagia, cough, carbonaceous sputum, tachypnea, retractions, accessory muscle use, wheezing, rales, diaphoresis, or cyanosis. Early intubation should be considered for patients with upper airway edema. Pertinent laboratory studies include arterial blood gas analysis with carboxyhemoglobin, methemoglobin, and lactate levels; red blood cell (RBC) cyanide levels for persistent acidosis; electrocardiographic (ECG) monitoring; and chest x-ray. The role for diagnostic or therapeutic bronchoscopy in inhaled toxin exposure is controversial. Administration of sodium thiosulfate to victims of smoke inhalation with persistent acidosis who are suspected to have cyanide toxicity is indicated. Management of noncardiogenic pulmonary edema may involve the use of positive end-expiratory pressure or BiPAP, but diuretics generally are not indicated. The use of prophylactic steroids with antibiotics is reserved for nitrogen oxide exposures. Systemic toxicity from products of combustion such as cyanide or carbon monoxide is common and is reviewed in Chaps. 182 and 198.

Many highly toxic gases produced in large quantities in the industrial sector are potential agents for malicious use. Those with a history of previous battlefield use or stockpiling, such as phosgene, chlorine, or ammonia, are of particular concern. Their toxicology has been reviewed extensively elsewhere[15] and is summarized below.

Phosgene (CG, carbonyl chloride, D-Stoff, or green cross) is a gas with a density four times that of air. Once released, it forms a white cloud with a characteristic odor of newly mown hay. It is relatively water insoluble and therefore reaches the alveoli, where hydrolysis forms carbon dioxide and hydrochloric acid. Acylation of alveolar capillary membranes results in diffuse capillary leak and noncardiogenic pulmonary edema, which is delayed for up to 24 h. If the exposure is massive, immediate dyspnea and mucous membrane and eye irritation may occur. The onset of dyspnea or pulmonary edema within 4 h of exposure suggests a very poor prognosis. Those who become symptomatic greater than 6 h after exposure generally survive if intensive medical care is available. Recovery occurs in 3 to 4 days with respiratory supportive care and management of noncardiogenic pulmonary edema. Since exertion is known to increase pulmonary edema from phosgene, rest is mandatory for those exposed. Furthermore, a 24-h observation period with frequent reassessments is indicated, even if the patient is asymptomatic.

Chlorine is also widely available in the industrial sector, in the setting of paper manufacture, swimming pool chemical distribution, and municipal water treatment. This dense green-yellow gas has an acrid, pungent odor and is of intermediate water solubility. The formation of acids and oxidants on contact with moist membranes causes inflammation. Immediate ocular and upper airway irritation along with nausea and vomiting are seen following mild exposures. More significant exposure results in coughing, hoarseness, and pulmonary edema, usually within 12 to 24 h. Permanent reactive airways disease has been described following significant chlorine gas inhalation. Care is primarily supportive with the use of humidified oxygen and bronchodilators as needed. The role of nebulized sodium bicarbonate as a neutralizing therapy is controversial.

Nitrogen oxides are encountered in the form of silo gas, as products of fire combustion, in industrial processes, or as military smokes and obscurants. These oxides have limited water solubility and generally result in lower airway toxicity. Slow conversion of nitrogen oxide to nitric acid in the alveoli results in delayed alveolar injury and pulmonary edema. A triphasic illness typically is seen with initial dyspnea and flulike symptoms, transient improvement, and then worsening dyspnea, which heralds the onset of pulmonary edema 24 to 72 h after exposure. Methemoglobinemia also may occur. Bronchiolitis obliterans, a potential late complication, may be prevented by the use of steroids.

Ammonia is a highly water-soluble alkaline corrosive gas that rapidly reacts with wet surfaces to form ammonium hydroxide. The presence of ammonia is usually obvious based on its characteristic pungent odor and immediate induction of symptoms of mucous membrane, eye, and throat irritation. Bronchospasm, pulmonary edema, and residual reactive airways disease have all been described following massive exposures. Treatment is supportive with humidified oxygen and bronchodilators. Anhydrous ammonia is extremely hazardous to the eyes and can penetrate the anterior chamber within 1 min of exposure. Prolonged irrigation and a careful ophthalmologic examination are warranted, as outlined below under "Ocular Toxins."

Riot control agents (CS, CN or "mace," capsaicin or "pepper spray") are a group of compounds that cause transient noxious effects on exposure. Although generally considered to be only briefly incapacitating, fatalities from pulmonary edema have occurred following large exposures in confined spaces. Typically, symptoms include immediate irritation of the eyes and respiratory tract, blepharospasm, lacrimation, coughing, sneezing, and rhinorrhea, followed by a burning sensation of exposed skin and mucous membranes. Nausea, vomiting, headache, and photophobia may be seen. These symptoms usually disappear within a few hours after cessation of the exposure. Burns and sensitization of the skin have been described, especially if contact with the agent is prolonged. Long-term corneal damage is more likely to occur with CN than CS. Management includes removal of the patient from the area, copious irrigation of the eyes with normal saline, and skin decontamination with soap and water as indicated. Contact with water can briefly exacerbate skin symptoms from CS. The use of bleach solutions to decontaminate the skin may increase irritation or trigger blister formation from some agents. Patients with preexisting lung disease should be observed carefully for bronchospasm.[16]

Neurotoxins

Hydrocarbon inhalation results in early stimulatory effect followed by headache, dizziness, confusion, lethargy, stupor, or coma. Central nervous system (CNS) stimulants such as organophosphates or nitrophenols may cause seizures, agitation, excessive muscular activity, and hyperthermia. Simple asphyxiants such as nitrogen, carbon dioxide, natural gas, and argon also may produce dramatic CNS effect, especially if encountered in confined-space situations. High concentrations of these gases may displace oxygen and result in symptoms of hypoxia such as headache, dizziness, giddiness, nausea, confusion, collapse, hyperventilation, seizures, or even death. Treatment consists of the administration of 100% oxygen and removal from the environment. Large acute exposures to some substances may harbor long-term neurotoxicity. Examples include metals, carbon monoxide, hydrogen sulfide, methanol, ethylene glycol, and pesticides. Patients exposed to these agents will require close follow-up.

The most likely neurotoxins to be used maliciously are the nerve agents. Their toxicologic profiles have been reviewed extensively by Sidell[17] and are summarized below. Currently the most toxic chemical threats known, nerve agents were developed by the Germans around the time of World War II, placed in munitions, yet never employed on the battlefield. Despite the cessation of chemical synthesis for military use, precursors are commonly found in industry. Five organophosphorus compounds are recognized as nerve agents: tabun (GA), sarin (GB), soman (GD), GF, VX. GF is believed to be obsolete. Properties of these liquids vary in terms of vapor pressure, persistence in the environment, and potency, with VX being the most potent and persistent and sarin (GB) the most volatile. A potentially fatal exposure to VX involves a skin area of only 2 to 3 mm in diameter. The agents are mildly irritating with odors variably described as fruity (tabun), odorless (sarin, VX), or fruity/camphorous (soman).

The nerve agents are powerful inhibitors of acetylcholinesterase (AChE), found in nerve, skeletal muscle, and other tissues innervated by cholinergic neurons. Likewise, RBC cholinesterase and plasma pseudocholinesterase, found in RBCs and plasma, are inhibited and serve as laboratory markers of toxicity. The ability of nerve agents to interfere with normal acetylcholine hydrolysis at cholinergic synapses causes accumulation of this neurotransmitter and greatly enhanced neurotransmission. Excess acetylcholine at brain synapses, for example, results in seizures, coma and respiratory depression, and apnea. Acetylcholine accumulation at the motor endplate causes initial fasciculations with progression to weakness and paralysis. Overstimulation of sympathetic and parasympathetic ganglia of the peripheral nervous system results in tachycardia, hypertension, diaphoresis, miosis, lacrimation, salivation, bronchorrhea, bronchospasm, bradycardia, vomiting, diarrhea, and urination. Extremely high risk of secondary contamination is posed to physicians caring for exposed patients because these agents are readily absorbed by all routes.

The onset and type of symptoms are determined by both concentration and route of exposure to nerve agents. Following sarin vapor inhalation, death may occur within minutes. Likewise VX dermal exposure may cause death within minutes if the exposure is massive, but symptoms may be delayed for up to 18 h following milder dermal exposures. Vital sign abnormalities may result from stimulation of both the sympathetic and parasympathetic ganglia. While bradycardia is expected from stimulation of the parasympathetic nervous system, 90 percent of patients exposed to nerve agents have normal heart rates or are tachycardic. Vapor exposure typically creates a triad of ocular, nasal, and respiratory symptoms. The eyes and nose are most sensitive, with miosis, conjunctival injection, pain, and rhinorrhea developing at low doses. Respiratory effects such as chest tightness, dyspnea, and copious secretions are seen at higher concentrations. Neurologic findings such as giddiness, collapse, convulsions, fasciculations, and flaccid paralysis develop with severe exposures. Apnea resulting from central respiratory depression is a predominant cause of death. In contrast to vapor exposure, dermal exposure results in a unique pattern of early symptoms. Miosis may not be seen initially, but localized sweating and fasciculations will be noted surrounding the exposed area. Nausea, vomiting, diarrhea, and fatigue manifest with increasing dose. As with vapor exposure, respiratory and neurologic symptoms indicate severe toxicity.

Once a nerve agent release has been recognized, self-protection and patient decontamination take precedence over other medical treatment. The use of self-contained breathing apparatus is suggested, since neither surgical nor HEPA masks render protection from these agents. Even double latex gloves will be ineffective in preventing dermal exposure, and butyl rubber gloves are preferred. As stressed earlier, removal of patient clothing alone may provide significant decontamination. In addition, a 0.5% sodium hypochlorite solution (9:1 household bleach to water) will effectively inactivate these agents and should be followed with copious water irrigation. A considerable amount of VX may remain on the skin even after decontamination, and precautions should be taken to avoid secondary contamination.

Following decontamination, restoring oxygenation is the single most critical step in medical management. Succinylcholine, if used to facilitate intubation, may have prolonged effect because the plasma cholinesterase level is inhibited. Cardiac monitoring for dysrhythmias should be instituted. Specific antidote therapy with atropine and pralidoxime should be anticipated. Atropine blocks muscarinic receptors and reverses the parasympathetic findings of lacrimation, bronchorrhea, bronchoconstriction, salivation, and gastrointestinal spasm, along with some CNS manifestations. It does not affect the motor endplate or symptoms of fasciculations or weakness. The dose is best determined by signs, symptoms, and route of exposure (Table 181-4). The endpoint for dosing of atropine is drying of pulmonary secretions. Miosis is not a useful therapeutic endpoint, and tachycardia is not a contraindication to use of atropine. In contrast to organophosphate

TABLE 181-4 Nerve Agent Symptoms, Severity, and Treatment Summary

Exposure Route	Category	Signs and Symptoms	Drug Therapy
Inhalation (vapor)	Minimal	Miosis ± rhinorrhea Visual complaints	Observation Consider homatropine eye drops for intractable eye pain
	Mild	Miosis, rhinorrhea, and mild dyspnea	Atropine 2 mg* 2-PAMCl 600 mg†
	Moderate	Miosis, rhinorrhea, moderate to severe dyspnea, N&V	Atropine 4 mg 2-PAMCl 1200 mg
	Severe	Severe dyspnea, copious secretions, N&V, diarrhea, LOC, seizures, flaccid paralysis, apnea	Atropine 6 mg 2-PAMCl 1800 mg, consider benzodiazepines
Dermal (liquid)	Mild	Localized sweating, fasciculations	Atropine 2 mg* 2-PAMCl 600 mg†
	Moderate	Above plus GI symptoms	Atropine 2 mg* 2-PAMCl 600 mg†
	Severe	Above plus respiratory or neuromuscular signs (same as "severe inhalational" above)	Atropine 6 mg 2-PAMCl 1800 mg, consider benzodiazepines

*May be given IM or IV. Pediatric dose = 0.02 mg/kg. Initial doses may be repeated every 10–15 min or administered by continuous infusion at 0.02–0.08 mg/kg/h. Higher doses (5 mg in adults or 0.05 mg/kg in children) may be needed to treat severe exposures.
†2-PAMCl is most effective if given intravenously, although the IM route is an acceptable alternative. Adult doses begin at 600 mg. The pediatric dose is 25–50 mg/kg and may be repeated in 1 h if symptoms are worsening.
Source: Modified from Sidell FR: Nerve agents, in *Textbook of Military Medicine, Medical Aspects of Chemical and Biological Warfare.* Washington: Office of the Surgeon General, United States Army, 1997, pp 129–171.

poisoning, continued atropine therapy generally is not necessary beyond 2 to 3 h following nerve agent exposure. Pralidoxime (2-PAMCl) also has antidotal efficacy against certain nerve agents via nucleophilic attack on those molecules phosphorylated to AChE. Subsequent liberation of the enzyme occurs along with detoxification of the nerve agent. This ameliorates nicotinic, muscarinic, and CNS effects. Whereas atropine is not effective in treating neuromuscular findings such as weakness or fasciculations, 2-PAMCl will reverse these symptoms so long as "aging" of the enzyme has not occurred. Aging is the process whereby permanent inhibition of AChE activity occurs due to nerve agent alkyl group hydrolysis and covalent binding. This reaction, which occurs within 2 min of soman exposure and within 5 h of sarin exposure, provides a rationale for early 2-PAMCl therapy. Like atropine, PAMCl dosing in adults is determined by route of exposure and signs and symptoms (see Table 181-4). Unlike pesticide exposures, long-term or continuous infusions of 2-PAMCl have not been required. Seizures generally do not continue after ventilatory support, atropine, and 2-PAMCl therapy are instituted. If present, they should be treated aggressively with benzodiazepines, which have been shown to decrease neuropathologic lesions in animals exposed to nerve agents. Military Mark I autoinjector kits contain 2 mg atropine and 600 mg 2-PAMCl for immediate intramuscular administration in the field. The emergency physician should be familiar with this form of these antidotes, since these kits may be stockpiled for civilian use by MMRS throughout the United States. Symptomatic patients or those with dermal exposures should be kept under close observation for 24 h.

Dermal Toxins

Factors that enhance the dermal absorption of toxins include the presence of wounds, defatting properties of the chemical (solvents), temperature (heat increases absorption), and high lipid solubility of the agent (organophosphate or organochlorine pesticides). Commonly encountered agents that may cause systemic toxicity via dermal absorption are listed in Table 181-5.

CORROSIVES Local dermal injury from corrosive agents may be obvious immediately after exposure to mineral acids or may be delayed following exposure to alkaline corrosives or hydrofluoric acid. Alkaline burns (sodium hydroxide, cement) are most common. These agents tend to penetrate tissues and cause liquefaction necrosis. In general, injury to the skin is more extensive than that from acids, which coagulate proteins and do not penetrate tissues deeply. Acids may cause desiccation of the skin and form darkened areas or eshcars. Treatment may involve prolonged irrigation or hydrotherapy of the area. The use of nitrazine paper to monitor pH may guide therapy. Contact with other substances may cause frostbite or freezing injuries to the skin, including liquid forms of phosphine, phosgene, ammonia, chlorine, ethylene oxide, hydrogen sulfide, and propane. Hydrocarbons such as gasoline may cause dermal burns or a defatting dermatitis.

PHENOL Phenol and its derivatives, creosol, carboxylic acid, and the polycyclic phenols, cause intense cutaneous destruction. They are then rapidly absorbed through the skin and may produce CNS depression, hypotension, intravascular hemolysis, pulmonary edema, and hepatic and renal dysfunction. Theoretically, phenol absorption may be enhanced by small volumes of water. Deluge volumes of water, however, should remove the toxin safely. The burn area may then be lavaged or soaked for 5 to 10 min with gauze impregnated with polyethylene glycol (PEG 300 or 400). Glycerol or isopropanol may be substituted if PEG solutions are not available. Because phenol acts as a local anesthetic, pain may not be an appropriate indicator of ongoing tissue destruction.

HYDROFLUORIC ACID Hydrofluoric acid is an aggressive substance commonly used in the semiconductor or glass-etching industry and also marketed for household use as a metal or brick cleaner, wheel brightener, and rust remover. Dermal contact with concentrations greater than 50% cause immediate throbbing pain, blanching, and blistering. Contact with lower concentrations causes no immediate symptoms but results in delayed pain, swelling, and potentially serious injury 8 to 24 h later. Accidents involving only 2.5 percent surface area exposure to concentrated forms may be fatal. Systemic absorption may result in malignant cardiac dysrhythmias, seizures, local tissue destruction, bone demineralization, hypocalcemia, hyperkalemia, and hypomagnesemia. Inhalation of hydrofluoric acid vapor is rare but may result in delayed fatal pulmonary edema. Overall management involves cardiac monitoring, intravenous calcium or magnesium administration as indicated, skin decontamination, topical application of calcium gluconate gel to the affected area, and narcotics for pain.

TABLE 181-5 Dermally Absorbed Agents Through Intact Skin Resulting in Systemic Toxicity

Acrylamide
Acrylonitrile, acetonitrile, propionitrile
Aniline
Chlordane
Dinitrophenol
Hydrocarbons: benzene, gasoline, toluene, toluene diisocyanate, xylene (all slowly absorbed)
Hydrogen cyanide, cyanide salts
Hydrogen fluoride (hydrofluoric acid)
Metals (organic mercury, thallium)
Methyl bromide
Methylene chloride (slow)
Nerve agents
Nitrates
Nitrobenzene
Pesticides
Phenol
T2 toxin
Others: may be absorbed through abraded skin

Injection of calcium gluconate (never calcium chloride) into the affected area at a maximum of 0.5 mL/cm^2 of tissue may be considered for intractable pain to neutralize the fluoride ion. Since such infiltration may cause fingertip ischemia, intraarterial calcium through a radial arterial line has been recommended for digital burns (10 mL 10% calcium gluconate in 50 mL D_5W infused over 4 h). Hydrofluoric acid burns are often much more painful than the appearance of the wound would indicate, and persistent pain represents continuous injury. Newer decontamination solutions such as Hexafluorine are currently under evaluation. There is little data to support the instillation of calcium or magnesium solutions into the eyes.

Vesicants

The terrorist use of vesicants, or agents that produce blisters, would overwhelm the ED with patients presenting with severe dermal complaints. The toxicology of these agents has been reviewed extensively elsewhere and is summarized below.[18] Mustards are the most likely threat among this group, since over a dozen countries have mustard in their arsenals and they are the easiest of the chemical agents to synthesize. Mustards caused more casualties than all other chemical agents combined during World War I and were used again during the recent Iran-Iraq war. Sulfur mustard (H, HS, HD) is an oily liquid with an odor of garlic or mustard. The LD_{50} is approximately 1.5 teaspoons, which can result in a 20 percent body surface area (BSA) burn. Mustards are alkylating agents that are highly reactive and electrophilic. They induce toxicity through immediate combination with peptides, proteins, RNA, DNA, and cell membranes. At low doses vesication occurs, whereas at higher doses systemic cytotoxicity is seen. Clinical effects are delayed for 4 to 8 h. Skin erythema progresses to blister formation over the next day. Warm, moist areas are affected most. Ocular findings are similarly delayed and include edema of the lid, conjunctival injection, and corneal ulceration in the most severe exposures. Respiratory involvement is delayed for 4 to 6 h and manifests as a dry, barking cough and hoarseness. Tachypnea or dyspnea indicates exposure to a lethal amount of mustard. In such cases, bronchospasm, bronchiolar obstruction by sloughed pseudomembranous bronchial epithelium, and hemorrhagic pulmonary edema ensue over 1 to 2 days. Systemic absorption is seen with massive exposures and results in hematopoietic, gastrointestinal tract, and CNS involvement. Mortality is approximately 3 percent in those reaching medical facilities.

Lewisite (L) is an oily colorless liquid with the odor of geraniums. It has a potency similar to that of mustard. Known stockpiles of a Lewisite-mustard mixture are possessed by Russia. While its active ingredient, trivalent arsenic, inhibits various enzymes throughout the body and interferes with glycolysis, the mechanism for vesication is not clear. Unlike mustard, skin irritation from Lewisite exposure occurs within 15 to 30 min. Blister formation also occurs more quickly (within 2 h) and is followed by cessation of pain. Resulting lesions heal more quickly and have less secondary infection and scarring than those caused by mustard. Ocular pain and irritation also occur within minutes, and in most cases, reflex blepharospasm seems to prevent the severe injury seen with mustard exposure. Immediate upper airway irritation progresses to pulmonary edema only in the most severe cases. Hypotension and hemolytic anemia are seen rarely and result from systemic arsenic toxicity.

Phosgene oxime (CX), an agent that causes extensive tissue damage, is considered here even though it is not a true vesicant. Its mechanism of action is unknown. Following exposure, instantaneous irritation of skin, eyes, and airways occurs, after which the affected skin blanches, turns grayish, and becomes urticarial, erythematous, and edematous. Necrosis of the area may penetrate to the muscle layers and results in eschar formation. Prolonged hospitalization is usually needed.

Immediate skin and eye decontamination, ideally within 1 to 2 min of exposure, is the only effective way of preventing tissue damage from the vesicants. Late decontamination is recommended, however, because spread to uninvolved areas of the skin or to other personnel may be prevented. A dilute hypochlorite solution is recommended for skin decontamination of mustards and Lewisite, which are relatively water insoluble. Water alone is the preferred decontamination solution for phosgene oxime. BAL (British anti-Lewisite, or dimercaprol) is an arsenic chelator that will prevent or greatly decrease the severity of skin and eye lesions if applied topically within minutes of Lewisite exposure, but the topical form is not widely available. Given intramuscularly, BAL reduces the mortality from systemic effects of Lewisite. There are no antidotes for mustard poisoning, although mustard scavengers, antioxidants, nicotinamide-adenine dinucleotide (NAD) precursors, polymerase inhibitor, and corticosteroids are investigational.

As with thermal burns, aggressive airway, fluid, electrolyte, and pain management, along with prevention of secondary infection with topical antibiotics and sterile dressing changes, is the mainstay of therapy for chemical burns. All burns resulting from caustic chemical agents are classified as ''major'' by the American Burn Association and require referral to a burn surgeon.

Ocular Toxins

Symptoms following ocular chemical burns include blepharospasm, clouding of the cornea, and conjunctival injection. In severe exposures, corneal ulceration or globe perforation may be evident. Cessation of pain may not necessarily be an indicator of cessation of ocular damage, particularly with penetrating toxins such as alkaline corrosives or hydrofluoric acid. Three grades of corneal involvement are described. Grade I involves irritation only; grade II includes corneal erosion, congestion, or chemosis; and grade III includes corneal stromal damage or conjunctival and scleral necrosis or both.[19] In pure ocular exposures, prehospital irrigation of the eyes for 15 to 20 min at the scene prior to transport is recommended. Contact lenses should be removed. Eye hydrotherapy can continue during transport with the use of a large water-filled container in which the patient intermittently submerges the face and blinks the eyes open and closed. In the ED, irrigation should continue until the pH of the conjunctival sac returns to 7.4. Visual acuity, fluorescein staining, and slit-lamp evaluation are indicated. Consultation with an ophthalmologist is warranted in all but the most trivial of exposures, especially for chemically induced disruption of the cornea, anterior chamber reaction, hyphema, or obvious globe perforation.

Metabolic Toxins

Hydrogen sulfide is a colorless flammable gas that may be encountered in industry or as a natural product of organic decomposition, such as sewer or manure gas. The ability to detect its characteristic rotten egg odor is lost at high concentrations or with lengthy exposures to low concentrations. Its mechanism of toxicity is similar to that of cyanide, with disruption of oxidative phosphorylation through inhibition of cytochrome oxidase aa3. Cellular asphyxia and impaired ATP production promote anaerobic metabolism with lactate accumulation and metabolic acidosis. It is one of the few chemical asphyxiants that also possesses irritative properties, and respiratory and ocular irritation occur following exposure. In high concentrations, rapid loss of consciousness, seizures, and death may occur after only a few breaths. Delayed pulmonary edema and corneal destruction should be anticipated with massive exposures. Treatment involves decontamination of the skin and eyes as appropriate. Administration of the nitrite component of the cyanide antidote kit to promote low-level methemoglobin formation may result in conversion of sulfide to less toxic sulfmethemoglobin. Other treatments include 100% oxygen and possibly hyperbaric oxygen therapy. Other metabolic poisons such as carbon monoxide and cyanide are discussed in depth in Chaps. 182 and 198.

Myocardial Toxins

Certain solvents such as halogenated hydrocarbons, Freons, and aromatic hydrocarbons may sensitize the myocardium to the dysrhythmic effect of catecholamines. Myocardial irritability may persist for several hours following exposure. Avoidance of physical activity or sympathomimetic drugs, other than selective β_2 agonists, for the treatment of bronchospasm is warranted. Furthermore, dc countershock cannot be administered to patients soaked with flammable chemicals until decontamination has been carried out due to fire and explosion risk. Hydrofluoric acid exposures may result in cardiac dysrhythmias as a result of hypocalcemia, hypomagnesemia, or hyperkalemia. In this setting, the administration of intravenous calcium may be lifesaving.

Hematologic Toxins

Hematologic toxicity may be caused by many chemical exposures. Both hemolysis and methemoglobinemia (oxidation of the iron of heme) may result from exposure to chemical oxidants or drugs. Derivatives of aniline or nitrites are the industrial chemicals most frequently associated with RBC oxidant stress. Other workplace agents include chlorates, benzene, acetanilid, nitrogen oxides, nitrophenols, *para*-toluidine, phenols, and sulfonamides.

Pediatric Exposures

Children are uniquely sensitive to chemical exposures. The child's thinner stratum corneum results in increased skin permeability. A relatively greater surface area (approximately 2.5 times larger than that of adults on a pound-per-pound basis), greater fluid intake per body weight, and increased minute volume provide greater dermal, oral, and respiratory uptake of chemicals. Children are at greater risk than adults to develop methemoglobinemia when exposed to oxidant stresses based on low NADH methemoglobin reductase activity. Other factors rendering them more susceptible to toxins include lower oxygen-carrying capacity, owing to lower baseline hematocrits, and greater susceptibility to bronchospasm following exposure to inhaled toxins.[20] When wet, infants develop rapid hypothermia; therefore, special consideration for decontamination will need to be made with use of warm liquids and control of ambient temperature. Finally, ocular irrigation is difficult in children. One method involves the use of a "papoose" followed by flooding the bridge of the nose with normal saline rather than the eyes directly.

BIOLOGIC HAZARDS

Biologic weapons (BWs) are microorganisms or biologic toxins that are used to produce death or disease in humans, animals, or plants (Table 181-6). Some are more deadly per weight than chemical agents, including nerve agents and cyanide. Recent awareness of proliferating offensive programs, stockpiles of munitions containing botulinum toxin and anthrax by countries like Iraq hostile to the United States, and terrorist threats surrounding their use suggest that a large-scale incident involving bioagents is now more likely than at any point in history. Aspects of a biologic release have been completely reviewed by military experts,[21,22] as summarized below.

Desirable BW agents must be stable, deliverable as an aerosol with particle diameter size of 1 to 5 μm, and highly infectious, without an effective vaccine to counter the threat. These agents could be disseminated by missile warheads loaded with bomblets, by aerosol generators either through line sources (airplanes, boats) or point sources (fixed aerosol device), through contamination of food or water, or less likely, percutaneously. The covertness of these agents comes from their variable incubation period and the fact that they are essentially undetectable at the time of exposure. The most likely route of transmission is respiratory. Those agents felt to be significant threats are discussed below.

Anthrax

In 1979, an accident involving aerosolized anthrax spores at a Soviet bioweapons military compound resulted in fever, respiratory difficulty, and over 60 fatalities in civilians living downwind from the facility. Anthrax has been weaponized by other countries as well. A recent hoax involving the delivery of a leaking package to the B'nai B'rith Center in Washington, D.C., labeled "Anthrachs" resulted in temporary yet serious disruption of that city's activities. This incident has been followed by numerous similar threats in many areas of the United States such that anthrax threats have become the "bomb scares" of the late 1990s. The problem is that such threats must be taken seriously, at least initially, since this organism is potentially so deadly. Early expert consultation is critical in such situations to assess whether a legitimate threat to health exists (i.e., biologic agents are nonvolatile and generally not dermally active, so if there is no aerosol generated, then there usually is no credible threat). Soap and water decontamination generally is adequate in this type of scenario, and postexposure antibiotic therapy usually can be delayed for up to 24 h to allow time for determining whether a lethal agent is indeed present.

Anthrax spores are stable and relatively easy to cultivate. Dispersion by a line source of 50 kg of spores over a population of 500,000 has been estimated to result in up to 220,000 people killed or seriously incapacitated. Infectious spores germinate and elaborate toxins that result in tissue edema and necrosis. Various forms of this zoonosis exist in nature. Most commonly, human illness is acquired by handling animal fluids or pelts. Following skin inoculation, the developing "malignant pustule" has an untreated mortality of 25 percent and a

TABLE 181-6 Summary of Biological Warfare Agents*

Agent	Infective Dose (Aerosol)	Incubation Period	Diagnostic Samples (BSL)	Diagnostic Assay	Patient Isolation Precautions	Chemotherapy (Rx)	Chemoprophylaxis (Px)	Vaccine Availability	Comments
Anthrax	8000 to 50,000	1–5 d	Blood (BSL-2)	Gram stain Ag-ELISA, Serology: ELISA	Standard precautions	Ciprofloxacin 400 mg IV q 8–12 h Doxycycline 200 mg IV, then 100 mg IV q 8–12 h Penicillin 2 million units IV q 2 h plus streptomycin 30 mg/kg IM qd (or gentamicin)	Ciprofloxacin 500 mg PO bid × 4 wk; if unvaccinated, begin initial doses of vaccine Doxycycline 100 mg PO bid × 4 wk plus vaccination	Michigan Biological Products Institute vaccine (licensed): 0.5 mL SC at 0, 2, 4 wk and 6, 12, 18 mo, then annual boosters	Vaccine: boost at-risk annually Alternates for Rx: gentamicin, erythromycin, and chloramphenicol
Brucellosis	10–100 organisms	5–60 d (occasionally months)	Blood, bone marrow, acute and convalescent sera (BSL-3)	Serology: agglutination Culture	Standard precautions Contact isolation if draining lesions present	Doxycycline 200 mg/d PO plus rifampin 600–900 mg/d PO × 6 wk	Doxycycline and rifampin for 3 wk in inadvertently inoculated persons	No vaccine available for human use	Trimethoprim-sulfamethoxazole may be substituted for rifampin; however, relapse rate with this drug may be up to 30%
Plague	100–500 organisms	2–3 d	Blood, sputum, lymph node aspirate (BSL-2/3)	Gram or Wright-Giemsa Stain Ag-ELISA, Culture, Serology: ELISA, IFA	Pneumonic: droplet precautions until patient treated for 3 d	Streptomycin 30 mg/kg IM qd in 2 divided doses × 10 d (or gentamicin) Doxycycline 200 mg IV then 100 mg IV q 12 h × 10–14 d Chloramphenicol 1 g IV q 6 h × 10–14 d	Tetracycline 500 mg PO qid × 7 d Doxycycline 100 mg PO q 12 h × 7 d	Greer inactivated vaccine (licensed): 1.0 mL, then 0.2 mL boost at 1–3 and 3–6 mo	Boost at-risk 12, 18 mo & yearly. Plague vaccine not protective against aerosol in animal studies Alternate Rx: chloramphenicol or trimethoprim-sulfamethoxazole Rx: chloramphenicol for plague meningitis
Q fever	1–10 organisms	10–40 d	Serum (BSL-2/3)	Serology: ELISA, IFA	Standard precautions	Tetracycline 500 mg PO q 6 h × 5–7 d Doxycycline 100 mg PO q 12h × 5–7 d	Tetracycline start 8–12 d postexposure × 5 d Doxycycline start 8–12 d postexposure × 5 d	IND 610-inactivated whole cell vaccine given as single 0.5 mL SC	Recommend skin test before vaccination
Tularemia	10–50 organisms	2–10 d	Blood, sputum, serum EM of tissue (BSL-2/3)	Culture Serology: agglutination	Standard precautions	Streptomycin 30 mg/kg IM qd × 10–14 d Gentamicin 3–5 mg/kg/d × 10–14 d	Doxycycline 100 mg PO q 12 h × 14 d Tetracycline 2 g/d PO × 14 d	Live attenuated vaccine (IND): scarification	Culture difficult and potentially dangerous
Smallpox	Assumed low (10–100 organisms)	7–17 d	Pharyngeal swab, scab material (BSL-4)	ELISA, PCR, virus isolation	Airborne precautions	Cidofovir (effective in vitro)	Vaccinia immune globulin 0.6 mL/kg IM (within 3 d of exposure; best within 24 h	Wyeth calf lymph vaccinia vaccine (licensed) DOD cell-culture derived vaccinia vaccine (IND): scarification	Preexposure and postexposure vaccination recommended if >3 y since last vaccination

Viral encephalitides	10–100 organisms	VEE, 2–6 d EEE/WEE, 7–14 d	Serum VEE (BSL-3) EEE (BSL-2) WEE (BSL-2)	Viral isolation Serology: ELISA or hemagglutination inhibition	Standard precautions (mosquito control)	Supportive therapy analgesics anticonvulsants as needed	NA	VEE DOD TC-83 live attenuated vaccine (IND): 0.5 mL SC × 1 dose VEE DOD C-84 (formalin inactivated TC-83) (IND): 0.5 mL SC for up to 3 doses EEE inactivated (IND): 0.5 mL SC at 0 & 28 d WEE inactivated (IND): 0.5 mL SC at 0, 7, and 28 d	TC-83 reactogenic in 20% No seroconversion in 20% Only effective against subtypes 1A, 1B, and 1C Vaccine used for nonresponders to TC-83 EEE and WEE inactivated vaccines are poorly immunogenic, and multiple immunizations are required
Viral hemorrhagic fevers	1–10 organisms	4–21 d	Serum, blood Most viral hemorrhagic fevers (BSL-4) RVF, KHF, and YF (BSL-3)	Viral isolation Ag-ELISA RT-PCR Serology: Ab-ELISA	Contact precautions Consider additional precautions if massive hemorrhage	Supportive therapy Ribavirin (CCHF/arenaviruses) 30 mg/kg IV initial dose 15 mg/kg IV q 6 h × 4 d 7.5 mg/kg IV q 8 h × 6 d Antibody passive for AHF, BHF, Lassa fever, and CCHF	NA	AHF Candid #1 vaccine (x-protection for BHF) (IND) RVF inactivated vaccine (IND)	Aggressive management of secondary infections and hypotension is important
Botulinum	0.001 μg/kg (type A)	1–5 d	Nasal swab (possibly) (BSL-2)	Ag-ELISA, Mouse neutral	Standard precautions	DOD heptavalent antitoxin for Serotypes A–G) (IND): equine despeciated 1 vial (10 mL) IV CDC Trivalent equine antitoxin for Serotypes A, B, E (licensed)	NA	DOD pentavalent Toxoid for serotypes A–E (IND): SC at 0, 2, & 12 wk, then yearly boosters	Skin testing for hypersensitivity before equine antitoxin administration Ventilatory assistance
Staphylococcal enterotoxin B	30 ng/person (incapacitating); 1.7 μg/person (lethal)	1–6 h	Nasal swab, serum, urine (BSL-2)	Ag-ELISA Serology: Ab-ELISA	Standard precautions	Ventilatory support and supportive care	NA	No vaccine available	Vomiting and diarrhea may occur if toxin is swallowed

*Information on diagnostics, medical management, and vaccines is available by contacting Commander, USAMRIID, at 301-619-2833 (phone) or 301-619-4625 (fax). Readers are advised to consult product literature before administering drugs or vaccines. BSL indicates biosafety level; Rx, chemotherapy; Px, chemoprophylaxis; Ag, antigen; ELISA, enzyme-linked immunosorbent assay; IV, intravenously; q, every; IM, intramuscular; qd, each day; bid, twice a day; PO, by mouth; IFA, immunofluorescent assay; IND, Investigational New Drug; SC, subcutaneous; EM, electron microscopy; PCR, polymerase chain reaction; VIG, vaccinia immune globulin; DOD, Department of Defense; VEE, Venezuelan equine encephalitis; EEE, eastern equine encephalitis; WEE, western equine encephalitis; NA, not available; RVF, Rift Valley fever; KHF, Korean hemorrhagic fever; YF, yellow fever; RT-PCR, reverse transcriptase polymerase chain reaction; Ab, antibody; CCHF, Congo-Crimean hemorrhagic fever; AHF, Argentine hemorrhagic fever; BHF, Bolivian hemorrhagic fever; CDC, Centers for Disease Control and Prevention.

treated mortality of less than 1 percent. Gastrointestinal and inhalational forms of illness, as in an aerosol attack, have nearly 100 percent mortality if not treated within 24 to 48 h.

A WMD attack would likely result from inhalation of anthrax spores or "Woolsorter's disease." An incubation period of 1 to 6 days is seen, followed by fever, myalgia, cough, chest pain, and fatigue. Transient improvement may be noted after 1 to 2 days of symptoms but is followed by abrupt onset of sepsis, hypotension, and death in 24 to 36 h. Hemorrhagic meningitis occurs in 50 percent of patients. The disease does not involve the lung parenchyma but instead causes a necrotizing hemorrhagic mediastinitis. The chest x-ray in late stages is characteristic, with significant mediastinal widening, pleural effusion, but no infiltrates. The diagnosis in most laboratories rests on Gram stain and blood cultures for the bacillus (not spores) late in the illness. Other methods of confirmation are available in some laboratories. Treatment involves ciprofloxacin 400 mg IV every 8 to 12 h or doxycycline 100 mg IV every 12 h. Others exposed, even if asymptomatic, should be started on either of the preceding antibiotics orally for 4 weeks while being immunized with three doses of vaccine after exposure. A licensed vaccine exists and is currently administered to U.S. soldiers. It is safe (side effects are local and self-limited) and is extremely effective in animal studies, providing protection against high-dose aerosol exposures to virulent strains. Standard precautions in caring for a patient with anthrax are recommended. There are no known cases of human-to-human transmission of inhalation anthrax. Iodine or hypochlorite at disinfectant strengths is required to destroy spores on equipment, although a dilute (1:9) household bleach solution is recommended to decontaminate victims immediately after exposure. Soap and water are probably adequate decontamination for human skin as well.

Plague

Plague, transmitted by *Yersinia pestis,* is a rodent zoonosis passed in nature from fleas to humans. In nature, the illness occurs following skin inoculation, transport of the organism to regional lymph nodes, and subsequent dissemination through blood. This bubonic form, characterized by one or more tender lymph nodes, hepatosplenomegaly, skin lesions, and septicemia, has a 50 percent mortality. A WMD attack likely would involve inhalation of the aerosolized organisms. The resulting illness, pneumonic plague, has an untreated mortality of 80 to 100 percent. Two to three days following inhalation, a fulminant illness involving malaise, fever, headache, cough, bloody sputum, shock, and a bleeding diathesis develops. Cardiopulmonary collapse ensues. Laboratory features include patchy infiltrates on chest x-ray, leukocytosis with a left shift, disseminated intravascular coagulation (DIC), and elevated transaminases. The diagnosis is confirmed by Gram stain and culture of lymph node aspirate, blood, sputum, or cerebrospinal fluid (CSF). ELISA or serology is confirmatory. Treatment must be started within 24 h of symptom onset to affect survival. Streptomycin 30 mg/kg per day IM bid for 10 days (or gentamicin if streptomycin is unavailable) or doxycycline 100 mg IV bid for 10 to 14 days is recommended. Chloramphenicol is the antibiotic of choice for patients with meningitis. Prophylaxis of those exposed includes oral ciprofloxacin or doxycycline for 7 days. Secondary transmission is possible for pneumonic plague. Respiratory isolation and droplet precautions are necessary for at least 48 h until sputum cultures are documented as negative.

Tularemia

Tularemia is a zoonosis that most commonly causes an ulceroglandular disease in humans exposed to diseased animal fluids or bites from infected deerflies, mosquitoes, or ticks. Typhoidal or septicemic forms can occur following inhalation of the inciting organism, *Francisella tularensis.* While not highly fatal, both its extremely high infectivity and ability to escape laboratory detection make this a likely terrorist agent. Infectivity by the inhalation route approaches 100 percent, with an untreated mortality of 35 percent. Only 10 to 50 organisms are required for an infection. Following a 2- to 10-day incubation period, fever, prostration, chest pain, and dry cough develop. Patchy infiltrates and hilar adenopathy may be seen on chest x-ray. The diagnosis is confirmed by serology. Antibiotic treatment includes streptomycin 1 g IM every 12 h for 14 days (30 mg/kg per day) or gentamicin 3 to 5 mg/kg per day. Prophylaxis with oral tetracycline or doxycycline for 14 days is recommended for those exposed. Immunity following tularemia is permanent. Person-to-person transmission does not occur, and respiratory isolation is not required. Standard precautions should be sufficient in protecting health care professionals.

Q Fever

Q fever is a zoonotic illness spread in nature by contact with animal secretions. Its extremely high infectivity by the aerosol route and persistence in the environment make it a biologic threat. Following inhalation, a long incubation period of 10 to 20 days is seen. Subsequently, a self-limiting febrile illness characterized by chills, sweats, severe headache, cough, and myalgias develops. Patchy infiltrates are seen on chest x-ray, along with leukocytosis, and elevated transaminases. The illness is generally incapacitating but self-limited. Laboratory culture of the agent should not be attempted because only one organism is needed to cause infection. Specimens should be sent to U.S. Army Medical Research Institute of Infectious Diseases (USAMRIID) or the Centers for Disease Control and Prevention (CDC) for serologic testing (see Table 181-1). The antibiotic of choice is tetracycline or doxycycline for 5 to 7 days. Prophylactic antibiotic therapy should not be initiated until 8 to 12 days after exposure and should be given for 5 days. Tetracycline or doxycycline is currently recommended. Secondary transmission does not occur.

Smallpox

The last documented case of endemic smallpox occurred in Somalia in 1977. While repositories of the virus currently are held by the United States and Russia, it is possible that others exist. An outbreak of smallpox would be an international emergency, given the high rate of person-to-person transmission and the termination of public vaccination programs that has rendered civilian and military populations now susceptible. Desirable properties of this virus in terms of weaponization are its relative ease of cultivation and stability on freeze-drying. Mortality of variola major is 3 to 30 percent depending on immune status. Following an incubation period averaging 12 days, abrupt onset of fever, rigors, vomiting, headache, backache, and in severe cases, delirium occurs. Two to three days later, an enanthem appears, along with a centrifugal rash on the face, hands, and forearms. The lower extremities and trunk become involved over the next week as lesions progress from macules to papules to pustules and then scab over. All lesions are in the same stage of eruption, unlike chickenpox. The diagnosis is clinical and may be confirmed by polymerase chain reaction or electron microscopy. Treatment is primarily supportive, although there are antiviral drugs that are investigational. Strict quarantine of the patient until all lesions scab over or for 17 days for all those in contact with the index case is recommended. Vaccination of all exposed within 5 days and administration of vaccinia-immune globulin (VIG), if available, should be carried out as well. Supplies of vaccine and VIG are unfortunately limited.

Viral Encephalitis

Viral encephalitides such as Eastern equine encephalitis (EEE), Western equine encephalitis (WEE), and Venezuelan equine encephalitis (VEE) caused by the alphaviruses are naturally transmitted by mosquitoes. These agents, stable for delivery by aerosol, are highly infectious, with nearly 100 percent of persons exposed to such aerosols developing illness. Children are affected most severely. Neurologic symptoms suggestive of viral encephalitis include headache, confusion, obtundation, dysphasia, seizures, paresis, ataxia, myoclonus, and cranial nerve palsies. Fever, photophobia, sore throat, myalgia, and vomiting are common prodromal symptoms. EEE is most severe, with a 75 percent case fatality and a 35 percent incidence of neurologic sequelae. Other forms are milder, resulting in neurologic symptoms in 0.5 to 4 percent and complete recovery in survivors; however, inhaled VEE may be much more severe clinically than what is seen with natural vector-borne disease. Laboratory studies may show leukopenia, elevated transaminases, and CSF lymphocytic pleocytosis. The diagnosis is made through viral isolation or serology. Magnetic resonance imaging (MRI) is a sensitive technique in identifying early, characteristic findings. Treatment is supportive, and respiratory isolation may be recommended, since person-to-person transmission may occur, although it has not been seen clinically. Patients' rooms should be treated with a residual insecticide to prevent mosquito-borne transmission.

Hemorrhagic Fever

Viruses causing viral hemorrhagic fever (VHF) are highly infectious by the aerosol route, cause high morbidity, and are easily grown in cell culture. RNA viruses causing Ebola and Marburg (filoviruses), Lassa, Argentine, Bolivian, Venezuelan, Brazilian, Rift Valley, and Congo-Crimean hemmorhagic fevers are felt to be possible threats. Common to all these illnesses is an acute febrile illness, characterized by malaise, prostration, and signs of vascular permeability. Findings of conjunctival injection, hypotension, flushing, petechial hemorrhages, and mucous membrane, neurologic, pulmonary, and hematopoietic involvement are seen. Some unique differences among these agents exist. Lassa fever, for example, is characterized by fewer hemorrhagic and neurologic complications. RVF classically presents with retinitis and hepatitis. Congo-Crimean hemorrhagic fever and Marburg/Ebola may cause profound DIC and hemorrhage. The diagnosis is made at a diagnostic laboratory with highest level (BL-4) containment possible (USAMRIID or CDC) using ELISA, reverse transcriptase polymerase chain reaction, cell culture, or the characteristic "shepherd's crook" appearance of the filoviruses on electron microscopy. Treatment involves supportive care, blood product replacement, and convalescent plasma for AHF. Ribavirin may be considered if within 7 days of symptom onset but is not effective against the filoviruses.

Botulism

Botulism, the most potent toxin known, has been weaponized by several countries. In 1995, an Iraqi defector revealed Iraqi research into and deployment of over 100 munitions containing the toxin. Both aerosol delivery and food supply contamination are possible methods of attack. The toxin exerts its effect through entering presynaptic cholinergic neurons and blocking acetylcholine release. Failed acetylcholine transmission results throughout the nervous system. This causes a clinical picture that is physiologically the opposite of nerve agent intoxication (too much acetylcholine in synapses). Following an incubation period of 3 to 8 days (ingestion) or 24 to 36 h (inhalation), bulbar palsies, diplopia, ptosis, mydriasis, dysarthria, dysphonia, and dysphagia develop. A classic descending, symmetric skeletal muscle paralysis ensues. Death is usually related to respiratory failure. The diagnosis is clinical and is confirmed by cultures of food, stool, and gastric contents. ELISA nasal mucosa swabs may be helpful within 24 h of inhaled botulinum toxin exposure. Treatment is directed primarily at providing respiratory support. Antitoxin is available through the CDC or USAMRIID (see Table 181-1). The CDC-licensed antitoxin is trivalent (effective against three toxin types) and is a horse IgG product, with attendant risks of anaphylaxis and serum sickness. The USAMRIID product is heptavalent (effective against toxin types A through G), and although also equine derived, it is a FAB-fragment product with a theoretically lower risk of anaphylaxis and serum sickness. It is only available for use under an IND protocol. An investigational pentavalent vaccine also exists for high-risk groups.

Staphylococcus

Staphylococcal enterotoxin B (SEB) is a heat-stable toxin, commonly associated with food poisoning. Less well recognized is the ability of this bacterial superantigen to incapacitate those who inhale it through stimulation of cytokine production and other mechanisms. The toxin therefore could be delivered either by aerosols or in sabotaged food or water supplies. It is expected that patients would present in large numbers over a very short period of time. Early symptoms include fever, headache, chills, myalgia, cough, and chest pain, beginning 3 to 12 h following inhalation. Nausea, vomiting, or diarrhea may be seen if the toxin is ingested. Massive exposures may cause pulmonary edema. Victims of inhalation exposure may develop an incapacitating fever and cough that may last for up to 4 weeks. The physical examination is generally unremarkable, except for mild conjunctival injection immediately following exposure to the aerosolized form. The diagnosis is made clinically or possibly by nasal swabs or urine samples for SEB metabolites during the first 24 h. Treatment is supportive.

Ricin

Ricin is a potent cytotoxin derived from castor bean mash. Over a million tons of mash are processed each year into industrial fluids. Traditionally, toxicity occurs following the ingestion of masticated castor beans. Hemorrhagic gastroenteritis, vascular collapse, and multisystem organ failure result from inhibition of protein synthesis. Following exposure to aerosolized ricin, airway necrosis is seen. Fever, chest tightness, cough, dyspnea, arthralgias, and profuse sweating begin within 4 to 8 h. Over the next 2 to 3 days, severe lung inflammation manifests as a progressive cough and hemorrhagic pulmonary edema. The diagnosis is difficult but may be confirmed by ELISA testing of serum or tissue. Treatment is supportive. If ricin is ingested, aggressive gut decontamination including the administration of activated charcoal may be considered.

Trichothecene

Trichothecene (T2) mycotoxins are nonvolatile fungal products that are extremely stable agents. Their use is suspected to have caused widespread toxicity in Laos, Kampuchea, and Afghanistan in the late 1970s and early 1980s, although this is still an issue of much debate. Russia realized these mycotoxins' potential as BW agents following the accidental contamination of flour resulting in a severe illness known as *alimentary toxic aleukia* (ATA) in civilians. These potent toxins exert their effects through bone marrow suppression and protein synthesis inhibition. Unique among biologic toxins are the mycotoxins' strong irritant effect and capacity for dermal absorption. These agents also may be inhaled or swallowed following an aerosol release. Symptoms include intense burning of the skin, eye pain, and tearing within minutes of exposure. Progression to skin blistering, necrosis, epistaxis, rhinorrhea, cough, wheezing, nausea and vomiting, bloody diarrhea, and death may occur over minutes to days depending on dose. Blood and environmental samples may be analyzed by gas chromatography–mass spectroscopy to confirm or support the diagnosis.

Detectors for biowarfare agents are being fielded in the military, but realistically, the first indication of a terrorist-mediated biologic agent release will be ill patients. Critical management points for all biologic agents include mandatory standard precautions for all health care providers and containment of all bodily fluids. Additionally, airborne precautions are necessary for smallpox, droplet precautions for plague, and contact precautions for VHFs. A dilute household bleach solution will effectively neutralize most biohazardous materials and should be used for patient decontamination. Full-strength bleach solution should be used to clean up body fluids and blood. Respiratory isolation should be maintained for those agents known or suspected of causing secondary transmission (smallpox, pneumonic plague, and possibly viral hemorrhagic fevers). Initiation of antibiotic therapy for treatable agents should be expedient and not delayed for definitive diagnosis. Persons exposed to anthrax but not yet ill should be immunized with three doses of anthrax vaccine over 30 days in addition to receiving antibiotics. Persons exposed to smallpox patients should be immunized within 3 to 5 days to prevent secondary cases. Personnel familiar with infection control and biologic waste disposal should be contacted to provide cleanup services.

POSTINCIDENT RESPONSE

Prolonged observation should be considered following significant exposures to those agents listed in Table 181-7.

Patients with chemical contamination may require special medical follow-up, depending on the nature of the contaminant. About 30 percent of those who were symptomatic will have persistent symptoms at 2 weeks after exposure.[23] Medical resources such as the company's occupational physician or medical toxicologist should be involved.

TABLE 181-7 Toxins with Delayed Onset of Symptoms or Requiring Prolonged Monitoring

Acrylonitrile, acetonitrile, propionitrile	Cyanide toxicity
Aniline	Methemoglobinemia
Arsine	Hemolysis
Benzene	Bone marrow suppression and leukemia
Chlorine	Pulmonary edema (high doses)
Ethylene oxide	Pulmonary edema and neurotoxicity
Halogenated solvents	Hepatorenal toxicity
Hydrofluoric acid	Pulmonary edema, burns, electrolyte changes
Hydrogen sulfide	Pulmonary edema
Metals	Hepatorenal, neurotoxicity
Methanol	Neurologic, acid-base disturbance
Methyl bromide	Pulmonary edema
Methylene chloride	Carbon monoxide toxicity, dysrhythmias
Organophosphates (highly lipid soluble, or dermal exposure to nerve agents)	Cholinergic toxicity
Nitrogen oxides	Pulmonary edema, methemoglobinemia
Ozone (rare)	Pulmonary edema
Paraquat	Pulmonary edema/fibrosis
Phosgene	Pulmonary edema
Phosphine	Pulmonary edema
Zinc phosphide	Pulmonary edema

This allows for continuity of care and provides the patient with a common medical provider knowledgeable in the area of toxic exposures. Counseling may be needed in the areas of carcinogenesis or reproductive or developmental effects. Follow-up liver and renal function tests several days to 1 week after exposure may be warranted.

Psychological factors affect health after toxicologic disasters. Victims of a hazardous materials incident may experience a post-traumatic stress disorder consisting of anxiety, depression, insomnia, amplification of symptoms, and somatization. This is estimated to occur in 25 percent of victims, as evidenced by abnormal psychological test scores.[24] Early psychological debriefing and interviews with patients and personnel can help prevent postexposure stress syndrome.

All medical equipment used during outdoor or indoor decontamination remains in the area used until it can be decontaminated adequately. An industrial hygienist or environmental cleanup company must be involved to determine the extent of cleanup that is needed. It should be determined in advance what agencies will be involved in the decontamination of facility and ALS vehicles. Contaminated departments or vehicles will be taken out of service until decontaminated. Contaminated clothing or other items should not be released to the patient. Contact the ATSDR/CDC emergency response 24-h hotline or EPA environmental response for advice on the disposal of contaminated equipment and clothing.

The requirements for reporting of work-related hazardous materials accidents vary by state. Advance determination of regional requirements can be made by contacting local or state health departments and governmental agencies. Patients should be advised to contact regional Occupational Health and Safety Administration (OSHA) offices to report a suspected violation of safe work practices. Reporting of a suspected terrorist event should begin with local government and health departments. Ultimately, the FBI has jurisdiction over such situations in terms of crisis management, with jurisdiction being passed to Federal Emergency Management Administration (FEMA) under the federal response plan for consequence management. Local public health officials should be involved as early as possible in a biologic incident.

ACKNOWLEDGMENT

We would like to thank Dr. Constance Doyle, who contributed to this chapter in the previous edition.

The views, opinions, assertions, and findings contained herein are those of the authors and should not be construed as official U.S. Department of Defense or Department of the Army positions, policies, or decisions unless so designated by other documentation.

REFERENCES

1. Couturier AM, McCuney RJ: Physicians' work in emergency response. *Occup Health Safety* 66(2):46, 1997.
2. Hazardous Substances Emergency Events Surveillance (HSEES), Annual Report 1997, Dept. of Health and Human Services, Agency for Toxic Substances and Disease Registry, Atlanta, GA.
3. Chemical Manufacturer's Association, FAX Back Document Number 104.
4. Kaye W: Hazardous Substances Emergency Events Surveillance 1993–1996, Agency for Toxic Substance and Disease Registry.
5. Kales SN, Polyhronpoulos GN, Castro MJ, et al: Injuries caused by hazardous materials accidents. *Ann Emerg Med* 30(5):598, 1997.
6. Hall HI, Dhara VR, Price-Green PA, Kaye WE: Surveillance for emergency events involving hazardous substances: United States, 1990–1992. *MMWR, CDC Surveillance Summaries* 43(2):1, 1994.
7. Phelps AM, Morris P, Giguere M: Emergency events involving hazardous substances in North Carolina, 1993–1994. *N Carolina Med J* 59(2):120, 1998.
8. Okumura T, Takasu N, Ishimatsu S: Report on 640 victims of the Tokyo subway sarin attack. *Ann Emerg Med* 28:129, 1996.

9. Okumura T, Suzuki K, Fukuda A, et al: The Tokyo subway sarin attack: Disaster management, Part 2: Hospital response. *Acad Emerg Med* 5:618, 1998.
10. *Medical Guidelines for Acute Chemical Exposures, Managing Hazardous Materials Incidents*, Vol. III. U.S. Department of Health and Human Services, Agency for Toxic Substance and Disease Registry, 1991.
11. Burgess JL, Keifer MC, Barnhart S, et al: Hazardous materials exposure information service: Development, analysis, and medical implications. *Ann Emerg Med* 29(2):248, 1997.
12. Tong TG: Role of the regional poison center in hazardous materials accidents, in Sullivan JB, Kreiger GR (eds): *Hazardous Materials Toxicology: Clinical Principles of Environmental Health*. Baltimore: Williams & Wilkins, 1992, pp 396–401.
13. Greenberg MI, Cone DC, Roberts JR: Material Safety Data Sheet: A useful resource for the emergency physician. *Ann Emerg Med* 27(3):347, 1996.
14. Waeckerle JF: Disaster planning and response. *N Engl J Med* 324(12):815, 1991.
15. Urbanetti JS: Toxic inhalation injury, in Sidell FR, Takafuji ET, Franz DR (eds): *Medical Aspects of Chemical and Biological Warfare*. Washington: Office of the Surgeon General, TMM Publications, 1997, pp 247–270.
16. Hu H, Fine J, Epstein P, et al: Tear gas: Harassing agent or toxic chemical weapon? *JAMA* 262:660, 1989.
17. Sidell FR: Nerve agents, in Sidell FR, Takafuji ET, Franz DR (eds): *Medical Aspects of Chemical and Biological Warfare*. Washington: Office of the Surgeon General, TMM Publications, 1997, pp 129–179.
18. Sidell FR, Urbanetti JS, Smith WJ, Hurst CG: Vesicants, in Sidell FR, Takafuji ET, Franz DR (eds): *Medical Aspects of Chemical and Biological Warfare*. Washington: Office of the Surgeon General, TMM Publications, 1997, pp 197–228.
19. Saari KM, Leinonen J, Aine E: Management of chemical eye injuries with prolonged irrigation. *Acta Ophthalmol Suppl* 161:52, 1984.
20. Healthy Children, Toxic Environments. Report to the Child Health Workgroup Board of Scientific Counselors, U.S. Department of Health and Human Services, Agency for Toxic Substances and Disease Registry, 1997, pp 2–7.
21. Medical Management of Biological Casualties Handbook, 3d ed. US Army Medical Research Institute of Infectious Diseases, Fort Detrick, Frederick, MD, 1998.
22. Eitzen EM: Use of biological weapons, in Sidell FR, Takafuji ET, Franz DR (eds): *Medical Aspects of Chemical and Biological Warfare*. Washington: Office of the Surgeon General, TMM Publications, 1997, pp 437–466.
23. Burgess JL: Hospital preparedness of hazardous materials incidents and treatment of contaminated patients. *West J Med* 167:387, 1997.
24. Burgess JL: Poison center response to hazardous materials incidents: The Washington State experience (in press).

CYANIDE

Kathleen A. Delaney

Cyanide is a potent cellular toxin with an infamous history. The ability of extracts of bitter almonds and cherry laurel leaves to cause rapid death has been known for centuries, although the causative agent was not identified as cyanide until the end of the eighteenth century. Cyanide was used in state executions by the ancient Greeks and Romans and, until recently, by the state of California. The first chemist to synthesize hydrogen cyanide gas succumbed dramatically in 1786 when a vial of the gas broke on his laboratory floor. In 1978, hundreds of people died in Jonestown, British Guiana, following a mass suicidal cyanide ingestion.

Cyanide is a simple, highly reactive compound of carbon and nitrogen that has many uses in industry and the chemical laboratory. Its wide availability was emphasized by the experience of investigators who found 65 legitimate sources of cyanide in the Chicago area during attempts to trace the source of cyanide used in the infamous Tylenol-substitution poisonings.[1] In nature it is found in large amounts in certain nuts, plants, and fruit pits in the form of cyanogenic glycosides.[2] Tobacco smoke has been estimated to contain from 100 to 1600 parts per million (ppm) of cyanide, and smokers have been shown to have higher levels of cyanide and thiocyanate, a "detoxified" form of cyanide.[3] The antihypertensive agent, sodium nitroprusside contains cyanide.

Since it is so ubiquitous in nature, animals have evolved biochemical means of detoxifying cyanide. In humans and many other mammals, the enzyme rhodanese detoxifies cyanide by converting it to thiocyanate, a less toxic form that is excreted by the kidneys.[4,5]

SOURCES OF EXPOSURE

Acute cyanide poisoning occurs in a number of settings: (1) inadvertent occupational poisonings, (2) inadvertent, suicidal, or homicidal ingestions of cyanide or chemicals metabolized to cyanide, (3) iatrogenic toxicity due to infusion of sodium nitroprusside,[6] (4) ingestion of plant products containing naturally occurring cyanogenic glycosides,[2] and (5) inhalation of smoke from burning plastics in closed-space fires.[7,8]

Industrial Exposure

Cyanide compounds are both precursors and incidental by-products in the production of plastics, solvents, enamels, high-strength paper, paints, glues, wrinkle-resistant fabrics, herbicides, pesticides, and fertilizers.[9] The affinity of cyanide for metals makes it useful in the extraction of ores, in metal polishing, and in electroplating.[9] It is also used to strip hair from hides in the leather industry. The once widespread use of cyanide as a fumigant resulted in many poisonings.[5] Cyanide is produced in industry by combining ammonia (NH_3) and methane (CH_4) to form hydrogen cyanide gas (HCN). Commercial quantities of water-soluble salts such as sodium cyanide (NaCN) and potassium cyanide (KCN) are synthesized from hydrogen cyanide gas.[9] HCN is readily liberated when cyanide salts are exposed to acid. Industrial exposures occur most commonly through inhalation; however, skin exposure to solutions of cyanide salts also has resulted in poisoning. Inadvertent ingestion of cyanide salts while eating in a contaminated work setting also has been proposed as a cause of accidental subacute poisoning in the workplace.[10]

Smoke Inhalation

Large amounts of hydrogen cyanide may be released when natural and synthetic nitrogen-containing polymers such as wool, silk, polyurethane, or vinyl are burned. Elevated cyanide levels have been reported frequently in victims of smoke inhalation, most often in association with elevated carbon monoxide levels, and have been implicated in fire-related fatalities.[7,8]

Chronic Exposure

Adverse physiologic effects due to chronic subacute cyanide exposure have been proposed but are poorly defined. Studies of workers chronically exposed to cyanide have demonstrated a higher incidence of thyroid disease and vitamin B_{12} deficiency.[10] Linamarin is a cyanogenic glycoside found in the cassava plant, a significant source of carbohydrate in many developing countries. In areas of the world where cassava ingestion is high, goiter and tropical ataxic neuropathy are endemic, and plasma and urinary levels of cyanide are elevated. A recent epidemiologic survey in Cuba of patients with optic neuropathy showed that poorly nourished smokers were at greatest risk and implicated an etiologic association between elevated levels of cyanide found in cigarette smokers and dietary deficiency of the natural cyanide scavengers vitamin B_{12} and β carotene.[4]

BIOCHEMICAL TOXICOLOGY

The avidity with which cyanide binds to metals accounts for its serious physiologic effects in poisoning. Cyanide disrupts metabolism by inhibiting the function of a number of important metal-containing enzymes. Its most dramatic physiologic effects are produced by the disruption of mitochondrial oxidative phosphorylation through the inhibition of cytochrome A_3.[4,11] Cytochrome A_3 uses trivalent ferric (Fe^{3+}) to catalyse the reduction of molecular oxygen to water, which is the final step in electron transport. Inhibition at this step blocks the ability of body tissues to use oxygen so that only anaerobic metabolism occurs. This inhibitory binding of cyanide to the cytochrome ferric ion is labile and readily reversible.[4]

CLINICAL TIME COURSE OF POISONING: ROUTES OF EXPOSURE

The time course and severity of the clinical effects of cyanide are a function of the nature of the cyanide-containing compound, the route of exposure, and the concentration of cyanide to which the patient is exposed. The onset of symptoms of poisoning following inhalational exposure to hydrogen cyanide gas is virtually immediate. Symptoms depend on the concentration of inspired gas. Several hours of exposure to low concentrations of gas (<50 ppm) cause restlessness, anxiety, palpitations, dyspnea, and headache.[12] Death may occur following prolonged exposure at these levels. Inhalational exposure to higher levels of hydrogen cyanide gas leads to severe dyspnea, loss of consciousness, seizures, and cardiac dysrhythmias. Coma, cardiovascular collapse, and death may occur immediately on exposure to very high levels. The LD_{50} for humans has been estimated at 200 ppm for a 30-min exposure and 680 ppm for a 5-min exposure.[12]

Although in most industrial accidents it has been difficult to separate the effects of inhalational absorption from percutaneous absorption, animal studies and studies of human skin have shown clearly that absorption of both cyanide ion (CN^-) and HCN vapor occur through intact skin.[10]

The onset of symptoms following ingestion of a cyanide salt may occur within minutes, depending on the amount of cyanide ingested and the rate of absorption. Deaths have occurred in adults following the ingestion of as little as 50 mg of cyanide salt, and survival has been reported in much larger ingestions with aggressive resuscitation and use of antidotes. The median lethal dose of the potassium or sodium salt of cyanide in an untreated adult is 140 to 250 mg.[12]

Symptoms of poisoning are delayed following the ingestion of compounds that require metabolic activation to release free cyanide. Acetonitrile, a solvent sold commercially as a cosmetic nail remover, undergoes hepatic oxidative metabolism that results in the release of hydrogen cyanide. Severe poisonings and deaths attributed to cyanide poisoning have been reported following latency periods as long as 24 h after ingestion.[13] Amygdalin is a cyanogenic glycoside that is found in particularly high concentrations in apricot pits and bitter almonds. It is the principal constituent of Laetrile, a compound popular for nontraditional cancer therapies in the late 1970s. Because the release of cyanide requires hydrolysis of the glycoside by enzymes in the small intestine, the progression of symptoms following these ingestions is characteristically slow, with a latency of onset of several hours. Amygdalin does not produce cyanide poisoning when given intravenously.[2]

CLINICAL FEATURES

Symptoms of Poisoning

The symptoms are somewhat dose-dependent (Table 182-1). At the onset of poisoning, there is an inspiratory gasp followed by hyperventilation. Patients complain of breathlessness and feel anxious. Symptoms related to anxiety about the exposure also may mimic these initial symptoms of toxicity. During inhalational exposure, these symptoms will resolve following removal from the toxic exposure. In significant exposures, cerebral function is affected rapidly. Loss of consciousness occurs, often associated with seizures.[14]

TABLE 182-1 Signs and Symptoms of Acute Cyanide Toxicity

Cardiovascular:	
Tachycardia	Mild
Hypertension	↓
Bradycardia	↓
Hypotension	↓
Cardiovascular collapse	↓
Asystole	Severe
Central nervous system:	
Headache	Mild
Drowsiness	↓
Seizures	↓
Coma	Severe
Pulmonary:	
Dyspnea	Mild
Tachypnea	↓
Apnea	Severe

Early cardiac effects include sinus tachycardia, atrial dysrhythmias, and premature ventricular contractions. This progresses to bradycardia and asystolic arrest. As with hypoxia, ventricular tachycardia and fibrillation are uncommon.

Pathophysiology

The clinical signs and symptoms of cyanide poisoning mimic those of hypoxia, with one exception: Unless respiratory arrest has occurred, patients are not cyanotic. Although small amounts of cyanide bind to the ferrous (Fe^{2+}) form of hemoglobin, there is no significant interference with the ability of hemoglobin to bind oxygen.[15] The clinical manifestations of cyanide poisoning are readily understood based on the effect of cyanide on cytochrome oxidase activity. Blockade of the ability of mitochondria to use oxygen produces a state of severe hypoxia despite the presence of oxygen. The resulting anaerobic metabolism generates large amounts of lactic acid.[4,11] Unexplained lactic acidosis is an important, albeit nonspecific clinical clue to the timely diagnosis of cyanide poisoning in case of an "unknown" exposure.

The inability to use oxygen leads to decreased oxygen extraction by tissues with a concomitant increase in the oxygen content of venous blood. This results in a decrease in the normal arteriolar-venous oxygen [(A-V) O_2] difference, a measure of the amount of oxygen extracted by the tissues.[6] Although discussion of these concepts facilitates understanding of the cellular effects of cyanide, it is difficult to detect this underutilization of oxygen in an emergency setting. A reliable estimation of the (A-V) O_2 difference requires that the venous sample be taken from the pulmonary artery. This is most practical in the invasively monitored intensive care unit patient who has suspected cyanide toxicity due to a nitroprusside infusion.[6,16] Anticipated laboratory abnormalities are shown in Table 182-2.

Some authors suggest measurement of the oxygen saturation of venous blood drawn from the femoral vein, which is about 40 mmHg in normal patients on room air.[12] The oxygen saturation from an antecubital vein reported in one cyanide poisoned patient on 100% O_2 was 95 percent.[16] Unfortunately, the range of normal values for peripheral venous oxygen saturation and the effects of oxygen administration on these values have not been well studied. Thus, little useful information is likely to be gained.[17] An indirect but potentially useful finding related to this phenomenon is due to increased "arterialization" of veins on funduscopic examination due to increased Po_2.[16]

TABLE 182-2 Anticipated Laboratory Abnormalities in Cyanide

Test	Result	Cause
Serum electrolytes	Elevated anion gap	Lactic acidosis from increased anaerobic metabolism
Arterial blood gas	Metabolic acidosis Normal Po_2	As above
Measured % O_2 saturation	Normal	Hemoglobin has normal O_2 binding capacity
(A-V) O_2 difference	Decreased	Decreased tissue O_2 utilization
Serum cyanide level		
Toxic	>0.5 mg/L	
Fatal	>3.0 mg/L	
Erythrocyte cyanide level		
Normal	<1.9 μM/L (50 μg/L)	
Fatal	>40 μM/L (1 mg/L)	
Whole-blood cyanide level	Not useful	

The Unknown Exposure

A brief occupational history may provide a clue to the diagnosis of cyanide poisoning in an acutely ill adult. In patients with work-related industrial poisoning, the diagnosis is suggested by the patient's occupation and circumstances. Often, multiple exposures result from the same incident. Suicidal ingestions of cyanide often occur in patients whose occupations provide access to cyanide salts. These include industrial and research chemists, laboratory technicians, science students, and jewelers. A history of use of nontraditional cancer therapies would provide a clue to the ingestion of Laetrile or other cyanogen-containing preparations. Victims of homicide do not provide a history of exposure. Accidental or suicidal ingestions of cyanide-containing commercial products, such as metal polishes or acetonitrile-containing solvents, have been associated with severe cyanide toxicity.[13] Careful identification of ingestants in asymptomatic patients will prevent the mistaken discharge of a patient who has ingested a compound with delayed toxicity.[13]

Cyanide-poisoned patients frequently present to emergency departments without any history of exposure. Although isolated individual poisonings with cyanide are relatively rare, it is important that emergency physicians recognize signs of serious poisoning because specific antidotal treatment is available and effective. Rapid onset of symptoms is an important clue. Cyanide salts are caustic and may cause oral burns when concentrated solutions or undiluted salts are ingested. A deeply comatose, acidotic patient without evidence of cyanosis or hypoxia on arterial blood gas examination should cause the clinician to think of cyanide. The finding of bright red retinal vessels, an elevated venous oxygen saturation, oral burns, or the smell of bitter almonds supports the diagnosis, although clues of this nature are elusive. It is estimated that only 20 to 40 percent of the population can detect the characteristic almond odor of cyanide.

Nitroprusside Therapy

Sodium nitroprusside contains 40 percent cyanide by weight. Cyanide is released by the deterioration of sodium nitroprusside in aqueous solutions, especially when exposed to bright sunlight. The rate of rise of cyanide levels in patients on a nitroprusside infusion is proportional to the infusion rate and increases at infusion rates greater than 1 to 2 μg/kg/min.[6] The onset of poisoning occurs after several days of therapy, so the emergency physician will see this problem only if called to the intensive care unit to evaluate a deteriorating patient. Cyanide poisoning should be suspected in patients receiving nitroprusside infusions who develop mental state disturbances or unexplained metabolic acidosis. In patients in whom a Swan-Ganz catheter is used for monitoring, a narrow (A-V) O_2 difference, especially in the setting of an unchanged or declining cardiac output, suggests cyanide toxicity.[6]

DIFFERENTIAL DIAGNOSIS

Cyanide poisoning always should be considered in the poisoned patient with metabolic acidosis. The differential diagnosis of acidosis in the setting of inhalational exposure includes other cellular toxins such as hydrogen sulfide and carbon monoxide and simple asphyxiants. Hydrogen sulfide is a product of organic decomposition encountered in septic tanks and sewers, petroleum production, and a number of other occupational settings. The characteristic odor of "rotten eggs" is frequently detectable. Carbon monoxide poisoning is readily confirmed by measurement of a carboxyhemoglobin level. The differential diagnosis of (increased anion-gap type metabolic) acidosis in patients with suspected ingestions includes methanol, ethylene glycol, metformin, salicylates, and iron. The slower time course of deterioration and the variable depth of mental status depression frequently help to distinguish the effects of these agents from those of cyanide. Severe isoniazid and cocaine poisoning are also associated with significant acidosis that occurs in the setting of seizures. The initial manifestations of severe intoxication with these agents may be indistinguishable clinically from cyanide intoxication.

The diagnosis of thiocyanate toxicity should be considered in the patient receiving a sodium nitroprusside infusion who becomes encephalopathic. Thiocyanate, the product of metabolic detoxification of cyanide, accumulates in patients with renal insufficiency and results in encephalopathy without the development of lactic acidosis or impaired oxygen utilization.[6] Levels of thiocyanate greater than 100 mg/L support the diagnosis of toxicity.[6]

PHARMACOLOGIC PRINCIPLES OF TREATMENT

Standard accepted therapy for cyanide poisoning in the United States is based on experimental and chemical principles developed in 1933.[5] The antidotes are contained in a kit now provided by Taylor Pharmaceuticals. The kit contains nitrites in two forms, an ampule of amyl nitrite for inhalation and 10 cc of a 3% solution of sodium nitrite for intravenous infusion. It also contains 50 cc of a 25% solution of sodium thiosulfate. The usual adult dose of sodium nitrite is 300 mg (10 mL of the 3% solution), followed by 12.5 g (50 mL of the 25% solution) of sodium thiosulfate. The pediatric dose is 0.33 mL/kg of 10% sodium nitrite and 1.65 mL/kg of 25% sodium thiosulfate.[18] A case report of the death of a child who succumbed to methemoglobinemia following aggressive treatment of a nonlethal ingestion of cyanide has led to the standard practice of adjusting the pediatric dose of sodium nitrite according to the patient's hemoglobin level, as illustrated in Table 182-3.[19] Inhaled amyl nitrite is used to temporize in the prehospital setting or until intravenous access can be obtained and does not need to be administered when sodium nitrite is readily available.

The initial rationale for using nitrites was based on their capacity to form methemoglobin. Methemoglobin binds avidly to cyanide and prevents its binding to cytochrome oxidase. Although the antidotal efficacy of nitrites is not disputed, their actual mechanism of action has been questioned recently.[4] The formation of methemoglobin is a slow process relative to the rapidity of the therapeutic response to nitrites. In addition, the reversal of cyanide toxicity in animals by nitrites has been demonstrated to occur in the presence of methylene

TABLE 182-3 Treatment of Cyanide Poisoning

Adults
1. 100% oxygen.
2. Amyl nitrite inhaler; crack vial and inhale 30 s.*
3. Sodium nitrite: 10 mL IV (10-mL ampule 3% $NaNO_2$ = 300 mg).†
4. Sodium thiosulfate: 50 mL IV (50-mL ampule 25% $Na_2S_2O_3$ = 12.5 g).
5. Repeat at half dose if symptoms persist.

Children (adapted from recommendations by Berlin[19] and Isom and Johnson[18])
1. 100% oxygen.
2. IV sodium nitrite and sodium thiosulfate:

Hb (g/100 mL)	3% $NaNO_2$* (mL/kg)	25% $Na_2S_2O_3$ (mL/kg)
7	0.19	1.65
8	0.22	1.65
9	0.25	1.65
10	0.27	1.65
11	0.30	1.65
12	0.33	1.65
13	0.36	1.65
14	0.39	1.65

3. Repeat once at half dose if symptoms persist.
4. Monitor methemoglobin to keep level less than 30 percent.

*Not necessary if IV is in place.
†Avoid nitrites in the presence of severe hypotension if diagnosis is unclear.

blue, which prevents the formation of methemoglobin.[4] Rapid methemoglobin formers, such as dimethyl-4-aminophenol, which is now used in Germany to treat cyanide poisoning, do not appear to have a more rapid effect than sodium nitrite.[4] Many papers imply that a level of methemoglobin of at least 25 percent should be a goal of therapy. This is based on work in dogs, who are much more sensitive to the methemoglobin-forming effects of nitrites than humans.[5] It has been demonstrated repeatedly that the rapid clinical reversal of cyanide toxicity occurs despite the demonstration of only very small amounts of methemoglobin.[20]

It should be noted that nitrites have a potential to cause serious side effects. Their vasodilatory properties can exacerbate hypotension. Death has been reported secondary to massive methemoglobinemia in an asymptomatic child with an inconsequential cyanide ingestion.[19]

Following the administration of sodium nitrite, sodium thiosulfate is given. Studies of the cyanide LD_{50} in animals demonstrate that the therapeutic effect of the combination of sodium nitrite and sodium thiosulfate is greater than the additive effects of both agents alone.[4,5] Sodium thiosulfate enhances the activity of the body's own detoxification enzyme, rhodanese, by acting as a sulfur donor. Rhodanese catalyzes the transfer of a sulfur molecule from thiosulfate to cyanide, forming thiocyanate, which is excreted by the kidneys. The rate of this detoxification reaction in humans is limited by the availability of sulfur.[4] There are limited data on the efficacy of sodium thiosulfate as sole therapy for cyanide poisoning in humans, although anecdotal reports suggest that it may be very effective as sole therapy.[21] This may be an important finding because sodium thiosulfate has very limited toxicity in comparison with nitrites and is a safer empirical therapy when the diagnosis is not clear.[8,18]

If the only mechanism of toxicity of cyanide were binding to cytochrome A_3, then oxygen would not be expected to have any therapeutic effect. However, administration of 100% oxygen has been shown in animal studies clearly to enhance the therapeutic efficacy of antidotal therapy of cyanide poisoning.[4] It has been proposed that oxygen may affect the binding of cyanide to cytochrome oxidase or the ability to form methemoglobin. Hyperbaric oxygen has not been shown to offer any benefit over 100% oxygen in animal studies of cyanide poisoning.[4] Hyperbaric oxygen is very useful in the management of patients with suspected cyanide poisoning who have concomitant carbon monoxide poisoning.[8]

Because of the potential side effects of the nitrites, a great deal of effort has been made to develop equally efficacious but less toxic therapies. Many agents bind cyanide and render it nontoxic. Cobalt compounds have a high affinity for cyanide and are less toxic than cobalt salts, which injure the myocardium.[4] Hydroxocobalamin (vitamin B_{12a}) has been shown to reverse cyanide toxicity but can cause anaphylactoid reactions. In addition, the large amounts (in the range of 5 g) of the agent needed to neutralize cyanide require large-volume infusions in the concentrations (1 mg/μL) currently available in the United States.[4,8,12] Hydroxocobalamin in combination with sodium thiosulfate is used widely in France to treat cyanide poisoning. The concurrent use of sodium thiosulfate is thought to "recycle" the hydroxocobalamin binding sites, allowing administration of a smaller dose of hydroxocobalamin. When only hydroxocobalamin is administered, cyanide is held in the form of cyanocobalamin. When sodium thiosulfate is added, cyanide appears in the form of thiocyanate. This effect has been termed *antidotal synergy*.[12]

Dicobalt edetate (Kelocyanor) is the therapeutic agent used as first-line treatment of cyanide poisoning in the United Kingdom. It is highly effective as a cyanide antidote but is not devoid of toxicity. Metabolic acidosis and hypotension have occurred in animals, and massive edema and ventricular tachycardia have been attributed to its administration to humans. The toxicity of dicobalt edetate is greater when cyanide is not present, limiting its use as an empirical therapy.[4]

4-Dimethylaminophenol (DMAP) is an agent developed in Germany for the treatment of cyanide poisoning. It rapidly produces methemoglobinemia but has not been demonstrated to be more clinically efficacious than sodium nitrite. It does not cause the same degree of hypotension but has been associated with renal failure in experimental animals. Unlike dicobalt edetate, it does not have greater side effects in the absence of cyanide.[4] In practice, most of these agents are used in combination with sodium thiosulfate.

MANAGEMENT DECISIONS: USE OF SPECIFIC ANTIDOTES

Severely poisoned patients have survived with supportive care, although survival in cases of massive exposure undoubtedly has been facilitated by antidotal therapy. The largest reported ingestion where survival occurred with supportive care alone was 600 mg. Patients have survived following much larger ingestions with use of specific antidotes. All patients with known or suspected cyanide poisoning should receive 100% oxygen by mask, be put on a cardiac monitor, and have an intravenous line in place. Patients with a history of ingestion should have careful gastric lavage, followed by endoscopic inspection of the esophagus to exclude caustic injury once the danger of death from the toxin is past. Ipecac is absolutely contraindicated because of the expected rapid onset of symptoms. Gastric decontamination should never take priority over resuscitation of the symptomatic patient. Superactivated charcoal has been shown to bind small amounts of cyanide and may be useful in decreasing the significance of an ingestion. Patients with inhalational exposures do not require gastric decontamination. Extensive decontamination of the skin with water should be accomplished in patients with cutaneous exposure, with adequate precautions to protect the staff from skin contamination. Patients with inhalational exposures often recover following their rescue from the toxic exposure. They do not require antidotal treatment if significant recovery has occurred prior to reaching medical attention.[14]

The decision to administer the sodium nitrite–thiosulfate antidote is straightforward when faced with a comatose, bradycardic patient with a clear history of cyanide exposure. Hypotension is not a contraindication to sodium nitrite therapy in this setting. Due to the potential toxicity of the nitrites, it is never appropriate to treat an asymptomatic patient. A patient with mild to moderate symptoms may be observed closely for more serious signs prior to the initiation of treatment. More difficult management decisions arise in (1) patients with smoke inhalation who have or may have carbon monoxide exposure as well as suspected cyanide exposure and (2) patients who are critically ill and acidotic without any history of cyanide exposure. In these patients, an antidote that is effective and has no toxicity obviously would be useful as empirical therapy for cyanide poisoning. The empirical administration of nitrites is problematic for two reasons. First, it may induce significant hypotension, and second, it may induce methemoglobinemia. Empirical administration of nitrites to patients who have or may have elevated carboxyhemoglobin levels has been considered to be contraindicated by some authors because of the decreased oxygen-carrying capacity caused by simultaneous induction of methemoglobinemia.[7,8] A limited study of seven patients with smoke inhalation and elevated cyanide and carboxyhemoglobin who were treated empirically with both sodium nitrite and sodium thiosulfate demonstrated that the measured decrease in oxygen-carrying capacity accounted for by combined carboxyhemoglobin and methemoglobin ranged from 10 to 21 percent and was not clinically significant. The maximum elevation of the methemoglobin level was 13 percent 1 h after treatment with sodium nitrite. None of these patients had initial carbon monoxide levels greater than 38 percent.[7] Due to limitations of this study, the safety of administering both agents in this setting remains unclear. The clinical detection of cyanide poisoning in victims of smoke inhalation also has been problematic because lactic acidosis may be the result of cyanide, carbon monoxide, hypoxia, severe burns, shock, or any state that induces anaerobic metabolism. A recent study of smoke inhalation victims showed a significant correlation between toxic cyanide levels and plasma lactate levels greater than 10 mM/L. This association was independent of the carbon monoxide concentration.[8] For the critically ill victim of smoke inhalation with significant lactic acidosis, the safest immediate empirical therapy that avoids the hypotensive effects of nitrites and the concerns about decreased oxygen-carrying capacity due to methemoglobin formation is the administration of sodium thiosulfate in addition to 100% oxygen.[8] The institution of hyperbaric oxygen therapy for patients with carbon monoxide poisoning obviates concern about induction of methemoglobinemia in the smoke inhalation victim with carbon monoxide poisoning.

The differential diagnosis of the comatose patient with metabolic acidosis is extensive. Empirical therapy in the unknown patient with suspected poisoning who is critically ill should include 100% oxygen, 50% dextrose, and naloxone, in addition to aggressive supportive care. When cyanide poisoning is considered, anecdotal reports support the utility of the empirical administration of sodium thiosulfate.[21] Significant hypotension is a contraindication to the empirical administration of sodium nitrite. Following the demonstration of adequate oxygenation and the absence of an elevated carboxyhemoglobin level, sodium nitrite may be administered after the sodium thiosulfate if the diagnosis is strongly entertained. A summary of nitrite and thiosulfate therapy is given in Table 182-3.

LABORATORY EVALUATION

In order to be effective, treatment of cyanide poisoning must be instituted long before confirmatory laboratory studies can be accomplished. Cyanide levels are useful to confirm a clinical diagnosis in retrospect or for forensic purposes. They cannot be obtained in time to make the diagnosis at the bedside. Because cyanide is sequestered in erythrocytes, erythrocyte and plasma cyanide levels should be obtained. Whole-blood cyanide levels are not useful. Cyanide levels do not correlate well with toxicity but will support a diagnosis. Normal erythrocyte cyanide levels are less than 1.9 μM/L (50 μg/L), while death from cyanide is associated with erythrocyte levels greater than 40 μM/L (1 mg/L). Toxicity is seen with serum cyanide levels ranging from 0.5 mg/L (anxiety, confusion, tachypnea) to more than 3 mg/L (apnea, cardiovascular collaspse).[6] The arterial blood gas is a rapid and useful test, as noted earlier. The absence of a metabolic acidosis is inconsistent with the diagnosis of acute cyanide poisoning (Table 182-2). Recently, the demonstration of a serum lactate level greater than 10 mM/L was shown to have a significant correlation with toxic cyanide levels in victims of smoke inhalation.[8] The measurement of carboxyhemoglobin levels by use of a cooximeter is important in the assessment of smoke inhalation victims. Table 182-2 summarizes laboratory findings anticipated in cyanide poisoning.

DISPOSITION

Full recovery is anticipated in many cases of severe poisoning where treatment is initiated rapidly and cardiac arrest has not yet occurred. Recovery despite cardiac arrest also has been reported. Most patients who survive do not suffer neurologic injury, although anoxic encephalopathy may ensue.

REFERENCES

1. Wolnick KA, Fricke FL, Bonnin E, et al: The Tylenol tampering incident: Tracing the source. *Anal Chem* 56:466, 1984.
2. Braico KT, Humbert JR, Terplan KL, et al: Laetrile intoxication. *N Engl J Med* 300:238, 1979.
3. CNFIT (Cuba Neuropathy Field Investigation Team): Epidemic optic neuropathy in Cuba: Clinical characterization and risk factors. *N Engl J Med* 333:1176, 1995.
4. Way JL, Leung P, Cannon E, et al: The mechanisms of cyanide intoxication and its antagonism. *Ciba Found Symp* 140:232, 1988.
5. Chen KK, Rose CL: Nitrite and thiosulfate therapy in cyanide poisoning. *JAMA* 149:113, 1952.
6. Curry SC, Arnold-Capell P: Toxic effects of drugs used in the ICU: Nitroprusside, nitroglycerin, and angiotensin-converting enzyme inhibitors. *Crit Care Clin* 7:555, 1991.
7. Kirk MA, Gerace R, Kulig KW: Cyanide and methemoglobin kinetics in smoke inhalation victims treated with the cyanide antidote kit. *Ann Emerg Med* 22:1413, 1993.
8. Kulig K: Cyanide antidotes and fire toxicology. *N Engl J Med* 325 (25):1801, 1991.
9. Homan ERJ: Reactions, processes and materials with potential for cyanide exposure, in Ballantyne B, Marrs TC (eds): *Clinical and Experimental Toxicology of Cyanide*. Bristol, England: Wright, 1987.
10. Blanc P, Hogan M., Mallin K, et al: Cyanide intoxication among silver-reclaiming workers. *JAMA* 253:367, 1985.
11. Baud FJ, Borron SW, Bavoux E., et al: Relation between plasma lactate and blood cyanide concentrations in acute cyanide poisoning. *Br Med J* 312:26, 1996.
12. Hall AH, Rumack, BH: Clinical toxicology of cyanide. *Ann Emerg Med* 15:1067, 1986.
13. Caravati EM, Litovitz TL: Pediatric cyanide intoxication and death from an acetonitrile-containing cosmetic. *JAMA* 260:3470, 1988.
14. Peden NR, Taha A, McSorley PD, et al: Industrial exposure to hydrogen cyanide: Implications for treatment. *Br Med J* 293:538, 1986.
15. Curry SC, Patrick HC: Lack of evidence for a percent saturation gap in cyanide poisoning. *Ann Emerg Med* 20:523, 1991.
16. Johnson RP, Mellors JW: Arterialization of venous blood gases: A clue to the diagnosis of cyanide poisoning. *J Emerg Med* 6:401, 1988.
17. Yeh MM, Becker CE, Arieff AI: Is measurement of venous oxygen saturation useful in the diagnosis of cyanide poisoning? *Am J Med* 93 (5):582, 1992.
18. Isom GE, Johnson JD: Sulphur donors in cyanide intoxication, in Ballantyne Br, Marrs TC (eds): *Clinical and Experimental Toxicology of Cyanide*. Bristol, England: Wright, 1987, pp 413–425.

19. Berlin CM: The treatment of cyanide poisoning in children. *Pediatrics* 46:793, 1970.
20. Johnson WS, Hall AH, Rumack BH: Cyanide poisoning successfully treated without "therapeutic methemoglobin levels." *Am J Emerg Med* 7:437, 1989.
21. El-Harasis A, Panlasigul L, Lee M: Collapse and coma. *Hosp Pract* 25:16, 1990.

DYSHEMOGLOBINEMIAS

Sean M. Rees
Lewis S. Nelson

The dyshemoglobinemias are a constellation of disorders in which the hemoglobin molecule is structurally altered and prevented from carrying oxygen. The most clinically relevant dyshemoglobinemias are carboxyhemoglobin, methemoglobin, and sulfhemoglobin. Carboxyhemoglobin develops following carbon monoxide exposure and due to its unique importance and prevalence is discussed in Chap. 198. This section of the text reviews methemoglobinemia and sulfhemoglobinemia. Although the exact prevalence of these disorders remains undefined, the American Association of Poison Control Centers database reports thousands of exposures to drugs and chemicals capable of producing methemoglobinemia, but unfortunately, cases in which methemoglobinemia actually occurred are not tallied.[1]

METHEMOGLOBINEMIA

Pathophysiology

Under normal circumstances, the iron moiety within deoxyhemoglobin exists in the ferrous (Fe^{2+}) form. Iron in this oxidation state avidly interacts with compounds seeking electrons, such as oxygen, and in the process is oxidized to the ferric (Fe^{3+}) state. On exposure to a nonoxygen oxidizing agent, iron donates an electron and transforms oxidation states from Fe^{2+} to Fe^{3+}. The ferric iron that remains is unreactive, and the hemoglobin that contains the ferric iron is termed *methemoglobin.* Methemoglobin, therefore, is unable to bind oxygen. Under normal circumstances, a small amount of methemoglobin exists in the blood (<1 percent). An elevated level of methemoglobin defines methemoglobinemia, although this is somewhat of a misnomer as the hemoglobin is contained within the erythrocyte and not free within the blood. The accumulation of methemoglobin is normally limited by enzymatic reduction of the ferric iron back to the ferrous form as rapidly as it forms. The enzyme NADH-methemoglobin reductase (also referred to as NADH cytochrome-b_5 reductase) is primarily responsible for this reduction, in which NADH (reduced nicotine adenine dinucleotide) donates its electrons to cytochrome-b_5, which subsequently reduces methemoglobin to hemoglobin.[2] In this process, NAD+ (oxidized NAD) is regenerated (Fig. 183-1). This pathway is responsible for reducing nearly 95 percent of the methemoglobin. A second enzymatic pathway utilizes NADPH and NADPH-methemoglobin reductase to effect methemoglobin reduction analogous to the NADH-linked enzyme system. This enzyme is of limited importance normally (<5 percent total reduction) due to the lack of a suitable molecule to shuttle electrons in a manner similar to cytochrome-b_5. However, this enzyme is crucial for the antidotal effect of methylene blue, which performs this function when administered exogenously (Fig. 183-1). To a very limited extent, nonenzymatic reduction systems, such as vitamin C and glutathione, may participate in the reduction of methemoglobin to hemoglobin. This limited effect of glutathione explains why patients with glucose-6-phosphate dehydrogenase deficiency, who are deficient in reduced glutathione, are not at increased risk of developing methemoglobinemia.

The primary clinical effect of methemoglobin is to reduce the oxygen content of the blood. Because the hemoglobin-bound oxygen accounts for the vast majority of an individual's oxygen-carrying capacity, as the methemoglobin level rises, oxygen delivery to the tissues fall. However, patients with methemoglobinemia are more symptomatic than patients who suffer from a simple anemia that produces an equivalent reduction in their oxygen-carrying capacity. This is due to a leftward shift in the oxyhemoglobin dissociation curve, the consequence of which is a reduced release of oxygen from the erythrocyte to the tissue at a given partial pressure of oxygen (Fig. 183-2).

Acquired Methemoglobinemia

Methemoglobinemia is acquired when the normal mechanisms responsible for the elimination of methemoglobin are overwhelmed by an exogenous oxidant stress, such as a drug or chemical agent (Table 183-1). Drugs rarely produce clinically significant methemoglobinemia in conventional doses, although subclinical methemoglobinemia may go unrecognized. Currently, most cases of methemoglobinemia are due to phenazopyridine (a commonly used agent for the symptomatic treatment of urinary tract infections), benzocaine (a topical anesthetic), and dapsone (an antibiotic often used in HIV-related therapy) (Table 183-1). Many of these compounds require metabolism to the "active" oxidant, and a substantial time delay until toxicity may occur. Methemoglobinemia can affect any age group and, due to undeveloped methemoglobin reduction mechanisms, the perinatal and infant age groups are more susceptible than older age groups. This

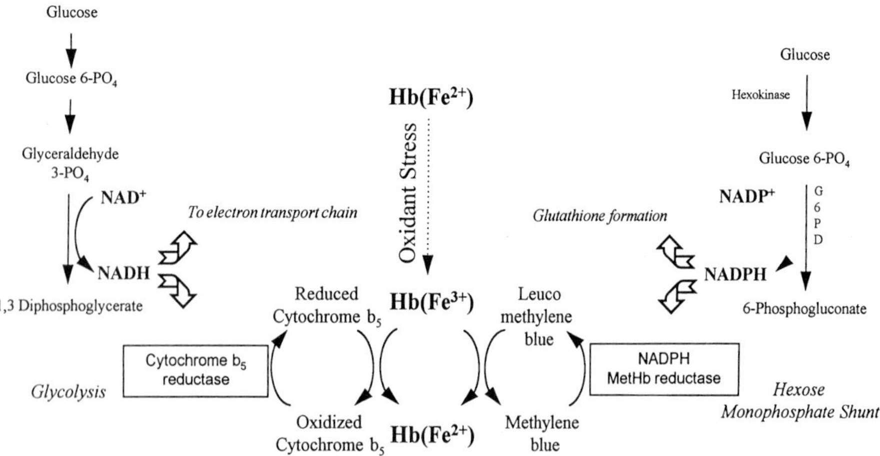

FIG. 183-1. Pathophysiology of methemoglobin formation and mechanism of action of methylene blue.

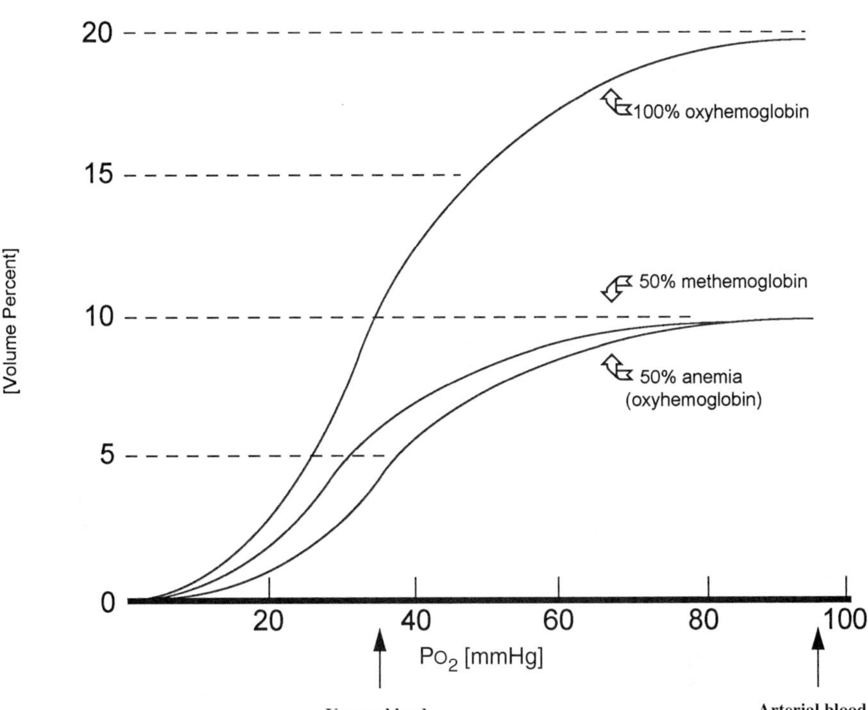

FIG. 183-2. The oxyhemoglobin dissociation curve describes the change in oxygen binding to hemoglobin as the dissolved oxygen (pO_2) varies. The oxyhemoglobin dissociation curve of blood with a 50 percent reduction in erythrocytes (anemia) follows a curve similar to that of nonanemic blood, although the oxygen content is lower to start; i.e., unbinding of half of the oxygen occurs at the same pO_2. The oxygen dissociation curve of blood with 50 percent methemoglobin is shifted to the left so that it is less willing to give up its oxygen despite a similar reduction in oxygen binding sites as the anemic blood.

explains the relatively common development of methemoglobinemia in infants given certain nitrogenous vegetables (e.g., spinach) or well-water that contains high nitrate levels. Bacteria within the gastrointestinal flora are capable of converting nitrates to the nitrite form, accounting for the toxicity of nitrates in well water and vegetables. Another common cause of acquired infantile methemoglobinemia is gastroenteritis, although the exact cause remains undefined.[3]

Epidemics of methemoglobinemia continue to occur and most commonly are related to nitrogenous chemicals that inadvertently admix with water or food.[4] Methemoglobin induction with sodium nitrite is a therapeutic goal in the management of patients suffering from cyanide poisoning.

Hereditary Methemoglobinemia

Although not usually diagnosed in the emergency department, patients may present with profound cyanosis that is related to a genetic abnormality. Hereditary methemoglobinemia results from either an enzymatic deficiency (i.e., NADH cytochrome-b_5 reductase) or from the presence of an amino acid substitution within the hemoglobin molecule itself (i.e., Hb M). Patients with NADH cytochrome-b_5 reductase deficiency develop methemoglobin levels of 20 to 40 percent, but these are easily reduced by the administration of daily oral doses of methylene blue or vitamin C.[4] Cyanosis in these individuals begins at birth, but they remain asymptomatic and develop normally. Hemoglobin M is an abnormal form of hemoglobin in which it's tertiary structure is altered and the heme iron exists in an environment favoring the ferric form. This disease only occurs in the heterozygous form, as the homozygous form is incompatible with life. Currently there is no treatment for this form of methemoglobin. As with NADH cytochrome-b_5 reductase deficiency, patients develop profound cyanosis, but tolerate the elevated methemoglobin concentrations extremely well.

TABLE 183-1 Agents Commonly Implicated in Patients with Methemoglobin

Nitrates/nitrites	Dapsone
Amyl nitrite	Phenazopyridine
Isobutyl nitrite	Local anesthetics
Sodium nitrite	Benzocaine
Ammonium nitrate	Lidocaine
Silver nitrate	Prilocaine
Well water	Dibucaine
Nitroglycerin	

Clinical Features

Patients with normal hemoglobin concentrations do not develop clinically significant effects until the methemoglobin levels rise above 15 percent of the total hemoglobin. However, patients may seek evaluation for the profound cyanosis that occurs when the methemoglobin concentration reaches about 1.5 g/dL, which is about 10 percent of the total hemoglobin in normal individuals. At levels between 15 and 30 percent, symptoms, including anxiety, headache, weakness, and lightheadedness develop, and patients may exhibit tachypnea and sinus tachycardia. Methemoglobin levels of 50 to 60 percent impair oxygen delivery to vital tissues, resulting in myocardial ischemia, dysrhythmias, depressed mental status (including coma), seizures, and lactate-associated metabolic acidosis. Levels above 70 percent are largely incompatible with life. Anemic patients may not exhibit cyanosis until the methemoglobin level rises dramatically above 10 percent, because it is the absolute concentration (i.e., 1.5 g/dL), not the percentage of methemoglobin that determines cyanosis. Anemic patients may likewise suffer significant symptoms at lower methemoglobin concentrations because the relative percentage of hemoglobin in the oxidized form is greater. Patients with preexisting diseases that impair oxygen delivery to the red blood cells (e.g., COPD, CHF) will also manifest symptoms with less significant elevations in their methemoglobin levels.

On the other hand, conditions that shift the oxyhemoglobin dissociation curve to the right such as acidosis or elevated 2,3-DPG, may result in somewhat better toleration of methemoglobin.

Diagnosis

The diagnosis of methemoglobinemia should be considered in all patients who present with cyanosis, and is particularly suspect in those whose cyanosis does not improve with supplemental oxygen. The blood of these patients has a characteristic ''chocolate brown'' color, analogous to that seen in the chocolate agar used to plate gonococcus (which contains methemoglobin). The ability to detect this discoloration is improved when compared directly to normal blood.[5] Pulse oximetry should be used cautiously in patients with methemoglobinemia. Because the pulse oximeter cannot properly differentiate oxyhemoglobin from methemoglobin, it may read an inappropriately normal value in patients with moderate methemoglobinemia, and it trends toward 85 percent in patients with severe methemoglobinemia.[6] Definitive identification of this abnormal hemoglobin species relies on co-oximetry, which is an in vitro spectrophotometric method that is capable of differentiating among oxy-, deoxy-, met- and carboxyhemoglobin species. This widely available test requires only a venous specimen, although arterial blood may be used if arterial puncture is indicated for another reason. The oxygen saturation obtained from a conventional arterial blood gas analyzer will also be falsely normal, because it is calculated from the dissolved oxygen tension, which is appropriately normal.

Treatment

Patients with methemoglobinemia require optimal supportive measures to ensure oxygen delivery and the administration of appropriate antidotal therapy if indicated. In general, gastric decontamination is limited, because there often is a substantial time interval between exposure to the toxic agent and the development of methemoglobin. If a source of continuing exposure exists, decontamination is indicated, and in most stable patients a single dose of activated charcoal is likely sufficient. Antidotal therapy with methylene blue is reserved for patients with documented methemoglobinemia or a high clinical likelihood of the disease. Highly unstable patients should receive methylene blue, but may require transfusion or exchange transfusion to produce an immediate enhancement of oxygen delivery.

Methylene blue serves to indirectly accelerate the enzymatic reduction of methemoglobin by NADPH-methemoglobin reductase, a normally minor enzymatic pathway. In this capacity, methylene blue is reduced to leucomethylene blue, which itself is capable of directly reducing the oxidized iron back to its oxygen carrying form (Fig. 183-1). The initial dose of methylene blue is 1 to 2 mg/kg intravenously (0.1 mL/kg of the 1% solution, about 7 mL in an adult) and its effect should be seen with 20 min. As the methemoglobin concentration falls, the most severe signs and symptoms will resolve first. Resolution of the cyanosis is a late finding, occurring only after the concentration of methemoglobin falls below 1.5 g/dL. Repeat dosing of methylene blue may be acceptable if needed, but high doses of methylene blue (<7 mg/kg) may actually induce methemoglobin formation. Treatment failures may result if the patient is deficient in glucose-6-phosphate dehydrogenase (G6PD), because this enzyme is critical in the production of NADPH within the hexose monophosphate shunt (see Fig. 183-1).[7] Because this group of patients does not lack NADH cytochrome-b_5 reductase, they are not at increased risk of developing methemoglobinemia, and they only lack the ability to respond to methylene blue. The concomitant occurrence of methemoglobinemia and hemolysis is not unexpected because both occur through similar oxidative mechanisms, and it is the rule for some agents such as chlorates. However, hemolysis may impede a response to methylene blue, which requires an intact erythrocyte to be effective. Oxidant drugs with long serum half-lives, such as dapsone ($T\frac{1}{2}$ ~50 h) produce prolonged oxidant stress to the red blood cell. Although not a true treatment failure, exposed patients may require repetitive dosing of methylene blue. In rare instances, patients may be deficient in NADPH-methemoglobin reductase, the required enzyme for methylene blue activation. Lastly, treatment failure may occur in patients with sulfhemoglobinemia, which is clinically indistinguishable from methemoglobinemia, but which is not responsive to methylene blue (see below). Patients that do not respond to methylene blue should be treated supportively. If clinically unstable, the use of blood transfusions or exchange transfusions is indicated. In the event that the newly administered red blood cell hemoglobin undergoes oxidation, it will likely respond appropriately to methylene blue.

SULFHEMOGLOBINEMIA

Sulfhemoglobinemia is less common than methemoglobinemia. Although patients with sulfhemoglobinemia have a clinical presentation similar to those with methemoglobinemia, the disease process itself is substantially less concerning.[8] Although the reduction in the patients oxygen carrying capacity is quantitatively similar, the patient's oxygen dissociation curve is shifted rightward, not leftward as in methemoglobinemia, favoring the release of hemoglobin-bound oxygen to the tissue. Because the pigmentation of the blood by sulfhemoglobin is substantially more intense than other colored hemoglobin species, only 0.5 g/dL of sulfhemoglobin is needed to produce a cyanosis equivalent to that produced by 1.5 g/dL of methemoglobin. At the level of the hemoglobin molecule, sulfhemoglobin occurs by oxidation of the porphyrin ring. Many of the responsible agents are identical to those that induce methemoglobin, and the agents do not need to contain sulfur. The diagnosis is difficult to confirm, because standard co-oximetry does not differentiate sulfhemoglobin from methemoglobin because of similar spectral absorbances. The addition of cyanide to the laboratory sample differentiates the two hemoglobin species, because cyanide binds to methemoglobin and changes its spectrophotometric pattern. Thus, if the addition of cyanide to this sample fails to eliminate the methemoglobin peak, the diagnosis of sulfhemoglobinemia is confirmed. Sulfhemoglobin is not reduced by treatment with methylene blue, and generally patients require only supportive care, although transfusions may be necessary for severe toxicity.

REFERENCES

1. Litovitz TL, Smilkstein M, Felberg L, et al: 1996 Annual report of the American Association of Poison Control Centers Toxic Exposure Surveillance System. *Am J Emerg Med* 15:447–500, 1997.
2. Hulquist DE, Passon PG: Catalysis of methemoglobinemia reduction by erythrocyte cytochrome-b_5 reductase. *Nature* 229:252, 1971.
3. Pollack ES, Pollack CV: Incidence of subclinical methemoglobinemia in infants with diarrhea. *Ann Emerg Med* 24:652–656, 1994.
4. Shih RD, Marcus SM, Genese CA, et al: Methemoglobinemia attributable to nitrite contamination of potable water through boiler fluid additives—New Jersey, 1992 and 1996. *MMWR* 46:202–203, 1997.
5. Henretig RM, Gribetz B, Kearney T, Lacouture P, Lovejoy FH: Interpretation of color change in blood with varying degree of methemoglobinemia. *J Toxicol Clin Toxicol* 26:293–301, 1988.
6. Barker SJ, Tremper KK, Hyatt J: Effects of methemoglobinemia on pulse oximetry and mixed venous oximetry. *Anesthesiology* 70:112–117, 1989.
7. Rosen PJ, Johnson C, McGehee WG, Beutler E: Failure of methylene blue treatment in toxic methemoglobinemia: Association with glucose-6-phosphate dehydrogenase deficiency. *Ann Intern Med* 75:83, 1971.
8. Park CM, Nagel RL: Sulfhemoglobinemia: Clinical and molecular aspects. *N Engl J Med* 310:1579–1584, 1984.

HYPOGLYCEMIC AGENTS

Joseph G. Rella
Lewis S. Nelson

Diabetes mellitus is the most common endocrine disorder in the United States, and the mainstay of pharmacotherapy includes the hypoglyce-

TABLE 184-1 Manifestations of Hypoglycemia

Signs of Neuroglycopenia	Signs of Autonomic Response to Hypoglycemia
Dizziness	Diaphoresis
Confusion	Anxiety
Dysarthria	Nausea
Decreased ability to concentrate	Tremor
Headache	Palpitations
Diplopia	Tachycardia
Lethargy, coma	Dry mouth
Focal or generalized seizures	Pallor

TABLE 184-2 Characteristics of Hypoglycemic Agents

Class and Name	Duration of Action, h	Metabolism
	INSULIN	
Ultra–short acting		
Lispro	<5	Hepatic
Short acting		
Regular	6–8	Hepatic
Semilente	12–16	Hepatic
Intermediate acting		
Lente	24	Hepatic
NPH	24	Hepatic
Mixtard	24	Hepatic
Long acting		
PZI	24–36	Hepatic
Ultralente	>36	Hepatic
	SULFONYLUREAS	
First generation		
Acetohexamide	12–24	Renal
Chlorpropamide	24–72	Renal
Tolazamide	12–24	Renal
Tolbutamide	6–12	Renal
Second generation		
Glipizide	10–16	Renal
Glyburide	24	Renal, hepatic

mic agents. Poisoning by hypoglycemic agents may be the result of unintentional therapeutic misadventures, intentional self-poisoning, or homicidal intent. Many factors contribute to unintentional poisoning, including prescription errors, dosing errors, and the onset of complicating metabolic factors.

It is difficult to ascertain an accurate rate of overdose among diabetics. Generally, up to 20 percent of patients with diabetes using insulin or oral hypoglycemic agents experience hypoglycemic symptoms sufficient to visit an emergency department sometime during their lives. The 1997 annual report of the American Association of Poison Control Centers recorded 3846 exposures to oral hypoglycemics, 1619 of them in children under 6 years of age. There were 4 reported deaths.[1] Among oral hypoglycemic agents, severe hypoglycemia occurs in 1 percent of the populations using tolbutamide and tolazamide, 2 to 4 percent of glipizide users, and 4 to 6 percent of chlorpropamide users.[2]

Hypoglycemia, the failure to maintain a blood glucose above 60 mg/dL, is perhaps the most common endocrine emergency. However, the presenting clinical findings in patients with hypoglycemia may be quite varied (Table 184-1).[3] Neuroglycopenia, or insufficient glucose supply to the brain, can be manifested as dizziness, confusion, dysarthria, decreased concentrating ability, headache, diplopia, lethargy, coma, focal or generalized seizures, and status epilepticus. Hypoglycemia typically precipitates a physiologic attempt to try to correct the deficiency in blood glucose. This response includes an autonomic-nervous-system–mediated release of catecholamines, which produces the most common symptoms in hypoglycemic patients, including diaphoresis, anxiety, nausea, tremor, and palpitations.[4]

In healthy persons, complex regulatory systems maintain a constant level of glucose in the blood. Unfortunately, certain medical conditions may impair the ability of the body to maintain glucose levels, and hypoglycemia results. Chronic ethanol users are at increased risk for hypoglycemia due to diminished glycogen supply and impaired gluconeogenesis. Persons at extremes of age are also potentially at increased risk for hypoglycemia. Young children have a disproportionately higher brain requirement for glucose as well as smaller glycogen reserves. The elderly may have health problems that alter the normal counterregulatory response to hypoglycemia as well as contribute to hypoglycemia (e.g., hepatic or renal disease). Older patients are also more likely to be taking medications that may exacerbate hypoglycemia or blunt the normal response to hypoglycemia (e.g., β-adrenergic antagonists).

INSULIN

Insulin is the agent most commonly associated with severe hypoglycemia in patients evaluated in the emergency department. The hypoglycemic effects of excessive use of insulin may exceed the patient's caloric intake and precipitate hypoglycemia. The Diabetic Control and Complications Trial research group demonstrated that, although tighter glycemic control delayed the onset and progression of microvascular and neurologic complications in patients with type 1 diabetes, there were at least 120 episodes of treatment-requiring hypoglycemia per 100 patient years.[5,6] Therefore, intensive therapy directed at maintaining euglycemia increases the risk of hypoglycemia.

The pharmacokinetics of the various forms of insulin weigh heavily in management decisions. The rapidly acting but short-lived regular insulin produces relatively predictable hypoglycemia, whereas the long-acting insulins, such as NPH, have less predictable kinetic characteristics. Following large parenteral overdose, regular insulin manifests the unpredictable kinetics characteristic of the long-acting forms of insulin (Table 184-2).

SULFONYLUREAS

Sulfonylureas stimulate the β-islet cells of the pancreas to release insulin through inhibition of potassium channels and changes in membrane potential.[7] First-generation sulfonylureas, such as chlorpropamide, reduce hepatic clearance of insulin and have active metabolites. These agents are renally excreted, complicating glycemic control in diabetics with intrinsic renal disease. Second-generation sulfonylureas, such as glyburide and glipizide, have half-lives that exceed 24 h and are therefore associated with frequent episodes of hypoglycemia. Sulfonylureas represent about 1 percent of all prescriptions in the United States and are therefore a prevalent cause of hypoglycemia.[2] In addition, the onset of hypoglycemia is unpredictable and commonly does not occur for 12 to16 h following ingestion.

BIGUANIDES

The biguanides include metformin and phenformin, both of which are derivatives of guanidine. Metformin acts to increase the peripheral sensitivity to insulin and to suppress endogenous glucose output. Metformin also inhibits gluconeogenesis, which reduces glucose production, and while it stimulates glucose uptake by cells, it does not stimulate insulin secretion.[8] Metformin lowers blood glucose levels only in diabetic patients and is more appropriately termed an antihyperglycemic than a hypoglycemic agent.

Phenformin was withdrawn from the US marketplace in 1976 due to its association with fatal lactic acidosis. Although not completely clear, the mechanism appears to be an enhanced production and inhibited metabolism of lactic acid, with a resultant fall in serum pH and cardiovascular collapse. Although metformin has not been demonstrated to alter lactate metabolism, lactic acidosis occurs in about 3 cases per 100,000 patient-years of therapy.[9] The risk of adverse reactions from metformin also rises with coexisting medical conditions, such as liver disease, congestive heart failure, and renal insufficiency. Phenformin toxicity is occasionally seen in the United States, since it is still available in other countries.

α-GLUCOSIDASE INHIBITORS

Acarbose acts to decrease postprandial glucose concentrations by decreasing gastrointestinal absorption of carbohydrates. Acarbose inhibits the brush-border enzyme α-glucosidase, thereby preventing the metabolism of polysaccharides into smaller units for absorption. By itself, acarbose does not cause hypoglycemia. To date, experience with acarbose overdose is limited. However, flatulence, bloating, and malabsorption can complicate use of this medication and should be expected in overdose.

THIAZOLIDINEDIONES

Troglitazone, a thiazolidinedione, offers the theoretical advantage of reducing hyperglycemia without increasing insulin secretion. Troglitazone effectively reduces plasma glucose concentrations both when given alone and in combination with either a sulfonylurea or insulin.[10] Troglitazone reduces insulin resistance as well as decreasing endogenous glucose production, and its effects are evident in both the liver and the skeletal muscle. Troglitazone exerts its antihyperglycemic effect only in the presence of insulin and does not cause hypoglycemia in nondiabetics. Troglitazone has been demonstrated to improve glycemic control in patients with type 2 diabetes mellitus.[11]

To date, the package insert of troglitazone has been altered three times since its release. Each version suggests closer monitoring of hepatic function due to the risk of potential hepatic failure.

MISCELLANEOUS SOURCES OF HYPOGLYCEMIA

The ackee tree is native to Jamaica, where it produces a fruit that is commonly eaten. The unripened fruit contains hypoglycins, a group of toxins that produce vomiting (Jamaican vomiting sickness), central nervous system sedation, and seizures. In addition, hypoglycins inhibit hepatic gluconeogenesis and may contribute to hypoglycemia. Epidemics of hypoglycin-mediated hypoglycemia have occurred only during times of famine, when poor nutrition and the increased eating of unripened fruit are perhaps more commonplace. Ackee is available in the United States in canned form, but only the unripe, fresh fruit is associated with hypoglycemia.

The sympathetic nervous system mediates glucose autoregulation partly through the release of epinephrine, which prevents the release of insulin and elevates blood glucose levels. This mechanism explains the role of epinephrine in the counterregulatory response to hypoglycemia. β-adrenergic antagonists interfere with both of these effects, potentially resulting in hypoglycemia through excessive insulin release while preventing the development of the typical autonomic response to hypoglycemia.[12–14] In addition, caffeine has been demonstrated to enhance patients' awareness of hypoglycemic events, theoretically because of its ability to induce neuroglycopenia.[15]

An increased incidence of neonatal hypoglycemia during the first day of life has been reported many times in those whose mothers had received β-adrenergic antagonists.[16] Neonates may also demonstrate characteristic radiographic findings on computed tomography resulting from hypoglycemia (Table 184-3).[17]

TABLE 184-3 Drugs or Toxins Associated with Hypoglycemia

Angiotensin-converting enzyme inhibitors	Pentamidine
Acetaminophen	Phenylbutazone
Ackee	Propoxyphene
β-adrenergic antagonists	Quinine
Chloramphenicol	Salicylates
Disopyramide	Streptozocin
Ethanol	Sulfonamide
Haloperidol	Trimethoprim-sulfamethoxazole
Monoamine oxidase inhibitors	Pyriminil
Para-aminobenzoic acid	

TREATMENT

Hypoglycemia should be considered part of the differential diagnosis for all patients with either gross or subtle alterations in mental status. Initial management includes rapid blood glucose determination with a reagent strip or glucometer, followed by administration of 1 g/kg body weight dextrose using 50% dextrose in water in adults. Since approximately 3 percent of hypoglycemic patients present with a new focal neurologic deficit as the chief complaint,[3] rapid glucose assessment prior to further care, such as computed tomography scan or thrombolytic therapy, is critical in patients with presumed cerebrovascular accidents. For children, 25% or 10% dextrose in water is used, since the hypertonicity of the dextrose preparation may damage their smaller blood vessels.

It is critical that, after the initial serum glucose correction has been made, therapy continues to prevent recurrence. Although the pharmacokinetics of intravenous dextrose is not completely defined, it has been demonstrated that the duration of hyperglycemia following its administration is transient and lasts only about 30 min. In normal subjects, intravenous glucose induces a rebound hypoglycemia 1 to 2 h following the bolus, presumably due to pancreatic insulin release.

Once the patient is awake and alert, 10% dextrose should be infused at a rate sufficient to maintain euglycemia (100 to 250 mg/dL). The blood glucose level should be closely monitored during the initial stages of therapy. In addition to a continuous infusion, repeat boluses of dextrose may be necessary initially to maintain euglycemia. Iatrogenic hypokalemia may result from repetitive boluses of dextrose, as may dilutional hyponatremia following exceedingly large infusions of dextrose-containing solutions.

Food is the best medicine for awake hypoglycemic patients. At least 300 g of carbohydrates should be provided to replete stores of glycogen and maintain euglycemia. This goal may be achieved by a variety of food sources, such as soda, chocolate, orange juice, or apple juice. More substantial food may also be available in the emergency department, such as sandwiches or snacks, as additional sources of carbohydrates. A single bolus of 50 mL of 50% dextrose in water contains only 100 calories, none of which may persist to be stored as glycogen, whereas a sandwich may contain significantly more calories and produce more favorable glucose pharmacokinetics.

Glucagon should not be used as empiric therapy for hypoglycemia except in specific cases. Since the action of glucagon is to mobilize glycogen stores, those patients who are glycogen-depleted (e.g., alcoholics, children, the malnourished, or the elderly) may not improve with glucagon. This may mislead the caretaker from establishing the diagnosis of hypoglycemia. For this reason, glucagon is better utilized in patients known to be diabetic or for whom intravenous access is not easily obtained. In such patients, glucagon 1 mg intramuscularly or intravenously in adults and children over 10 kg body weight may be administered. In children who weigh less than 10 kg, 0.1 mg/kg up to a maximum dose of 1 mg may be given. Glucagon requires several minutes for effect, and intravenous administration of hypertonic dextrose should never be delayed while waiting for glucagon to work. Glucagon is available as a 1-mg unit dose in lyophilized powder, accompanied by 10 mL of diluent that contains 2 mg/mL of phenol. As a precaution against systemic phenol toxicity, it is recommended that sterile water, rather than the accompanying diluent, be used for injection. Since emesis is common following glucagon administration, precautions should be taken to assure airway patency.

Diazoxide, formerly used as an antihypertensive agent, directly inhibits insulin secretion by opening potassium channels in β-islet cells. Hypoglycemia secondary to insulin-secreting tumors or refractory to oral hypoglycemic agents may require diazoxide, but diazoxide does not improve hypoglycemia from insulin overdose.[18] Oral and intravenous preparations of diazoxide are available. Diazoxide 300 mg is administered intravenously over 30 min, and dosing may be repeated every 4 h. Diazoxide may cause hypotension and sodium retention. Oral diazoxide may be given at a dose of 200 to 300 mg every 4 h but is rarely needed.

Octreotide, a somatostatin analogue, has been demonstrated to inhibit glucose-stimulated insulin release through a mechanism utilizing a G protein within the pancreatic β-islet cells.[19] In healthy subjects, octreotide has a half-life of 72 h following intravenous administration, which directly contributes to its success in treating hypoglycemia from oral hypoglycemic agents, insulinomas, and quinine-induced hypoglycemia. Octreotide may be given in a dose of 50 μg subcutaneously every 12 h and is not expected to be useful in cases of insulin overdose.

The cornerstone of management of most poisoned patients is gastrointestinal decontamination to prevent absorption into the body, and this is equally true of patients who have overdosed with oral hypoglycemic agents. Several oral hypoglycemic agents have been demonstrated to adsorb well to activated charcoal in vitro, and there is no reason to suspect that the rest are not adsorbed as well.[20] A single dose, and perhaps several doses, of activated charcoal may be beneficial for such patients.

Emesis has not been demonstrated to produce consistent evacuation of the stomach contents and may be complicated should altered consciousness or seizure activity develop abruptly from the hypoglycemia. Gastric lavage with a large-bore tube may evacuate pill fragments and allow administration of activated charcoal but is associated with aspiration, esophageal injury, and vagal complications. Whole-bowel irrigation with a polyethylene glycol-based electrolyte solution may specifically benefit patients who have ingested sustained-release preparations. Since large pills may not be evacuated by a lavage tube and supplying adequate doses of activated charcoal may be difficult, whole-bowel irrigation may be the only effective means of preventing profound and prolonged hypoglycemia.

Following large subcutaneous deposition of insulin, toxicity may be reduced by removal of the reservoir. Percutaneous aspiration or excision may reduce the extent and duration of hypoglycemia, although this therapy is not commonly recommended.[21]

The half-life of chlorpropamide may be reduced from 49 to 13 h by alkalinization of the urine through ion trapping, in a fashion analogous to treatment of salicylate toxicity.[22] However, this effect may be limited to this agent. Alkalinization may be accomplished by adding three ampules (135 to 150 meq) of hypertonic sodium bicarbonate (7.5 to 8.4%) to a liter of 5% D/W for intravenous administration and infusing this solution, which is near isotonic, at a rate of twice maintenance. The ideal urine pH is 7.5 to 8 for maximal excretion, and difficulty in obtaining this pH is often related to inadequate serum potassium levels. Potential complications include excessive alkalinization and fluid overload.

The management of metformin-associated lactic acidosis must be aggressive to reduce the 50 percent mortality rate.[23] In addition to discontinuation of the drug, supportive care is critical. Hemodialysis appears to be the most beneficial therapy and should be instituted early.[24]

DISPOSITION

Patients with hypoglycemia resulting from nonintentional overdose of a short- or intermediate-acting insulin may not require admission if their condition is corrected and a normal blood glucose level is maintained prior to discharge. Those with hypoglycemia resulting from long-acting insulin should be admitted, as should those with underlying diseases, such as liver or renal insufficiency or starvation. Patients with serious complications of hypoglycemia, such as seizures, and those with refractory hypoglycemia should be closely monitored. Patients who are hypoglycemic due to attempted suicide, attempted homicide, or abuse should be admitted.

Hypoglycemia may occur in a delayed fashion after the ingestion of an oral hypoglycemic agent, particularly in children. Therefore, adults who have deliberately overdosed with oral hypoglycemics and children who have ingested even a single pill should be admitted for 24 h of observation, even though they may demonstrate euglycemia for many hours. Investigations of child abuse may arise from the unindicated administration of insulin to children.

REFERENCES

1. Litovitz TL, Klein-Schwartz W, Dyer KS, et al: 1997 annual report of the American Association of Poison Control Centers toxic surveillance system. *Am J Emerg Med* 16:468, 1998.
2. Gerich JE: Oral hypoglycemic agents. *N Engl J Med* 321:1231, 1989.
3. Malouf R, Brust JC: Hypoglycemia: Causes, neurological manifestations, and outcome. *Ann Neurol* 17:421, 1985.
4. Service FJ: Hypoglycemic disorders. *N Engl J Med* 332:1144, 1995.
5. Diabetic Control and Complications Trial (DCCT) Research Group: Epidemiology of severe hypoglycemia in diabetes control and complications trial. *Am J Med* 90:450, 1991.
6. Davis EA, Keating B, Byrne GC, et al: Impact of improved glycaemic control on rates of hypoglycaemia in insulin dependent diabetes mellitus. *Arch Dis Child* 78:111, 1998.
7. Eliasson L, Renström E, Ämmälä C, et al: PKC-dependent stimulation of exocytosis by sulfonylureas in pancreatic β cells. *Science* 271:813, 1996.
8. Bailey CJ, Turner RC: Metformin. *N Engl J Med* 334:574, 1996.
9. Crofford OB: Metformin. *N Engl J Med* 333:588, 1995.
10. Inzucchi SE, Maggs DG, Spollett GR, et al: Efficacy and metabolic effects of metformin and troglitazone in type 2 diabetes mellitus. *N Engl J Med* 338:867, 1998.
11. Schwartz S, Raskin P, Fonesca V, Graveline JF: Effect of troglitazone in insulin-treated patients with type 2 diabetes mellitus. *N Engl J Med* 338:861, 1998.
12. Shorr RI, Ray WA, Daugherty JR, Griffin MR: Antihypertensives and the risk of serious hypoglycemia in older persons using insulin or sulfonylureas. *JAMA* 278:40, 1997.
13. Burge MR, Schmitz-Fiorentino K, Fischette C, et al: A prospective trial of risk factors for sulfonylurea-induced hypoglycemia in type 2 diabetes mellitus. *JAMA* 279:137, 1998.
14. Boyle PJ, Kempers SF, O'Connor AM, Nagy RJ: Brain glucose uptake and unawareness of hypoglycemia in patients with insulin-dependent diabetes mellitus. *N Engl J Med* 333:1726, 1995.
15. Kerr D, Sherwin RS, Pavalkis F, et al: Effect of caffeine on the recognition of and responses to hypoglycemia in humans. *Ann Intern Med* 119:799, 1993.
16. Fox RE, Marx C, Stark AR: Neonatal effects of maternal nadolol therapy. *Am J Obstet Gynecol* 152:1045, 1985.
17. Barkovich AJ, Ali FA, Rowley HA, Bass N: Imaging patterns of neonatal hypoglycemia. *Am J Neuroradiol* 19:523, 1998.
18. Palatnick W, Meatherall RC, Tenenbein M: Clinical spectrum of sulfonylurea overdose and experience with diazoxide therapy. *Arch Intern Med* 151:1859, 1991.
19. Boyle PJ, Justice K, Krentz AJ, et al: Octreotide reverses hyperinsulinemia

and prevents hypoglycemia induced by sulfonylurea overdoses. *J Clin Endocrinol Metab* 76:752, 1993.

20. Kannisto H, Neuvonen PJ: Adsorption of sulfonylureas onto activated charcoal in vitro. *J Pharm Sci* 73:253, 1984.

21. Campbell IW, Ratcliffe JG: Suicidal insulin overdose managed by excision of insulin injection site. *BMJ* 285:408, 1982.

22. Neuvonen PJ, Kärkkäinen S: Effects of charcoal, sodium bicarbonate and ammonium chloride on chlorpropamide kinetics. *Clin Pharmacol Ther* 33:386, 1983.

23. Luft D, Schmulling RM, Eggstein M: Lactic acidosis in biguanide-treated diabetics: A review of 330 cases. *Diabetologia* 14:75, 1978.

24. Lalau JD, Westeel PF, Debussche X, et al: Bicarbonate hemodialysis: An adequate treatment for lactic acidosis in diabetics treated by metformin. *Intensive Care Med* 13:383, 1987.

ENVIRONMENTAL INJURIES

FROSTBITE AND OTHER LOCALIZED COLD-RELATED INJURIES

Mark B. Rabold

Throughout history the most celebrated and extreme reports of cold-related injuries have been in the field of military endeavor. From Hannibal's losing half his 46,000-man army crossing the Pyrenean Alps to frostbite and hypothermia, to the tens of thousands of cases of trench foot during World War I, we have learned much. Perhaps the most famous cold-injury mass-casualty incident was Napoleon's retreat from Moscow during the dreadful winter of 1812–1813. This first authoritative account, as described by Napoleon's surgeon-in-chief, Baron de Larrey, described how each evening thousands of French soldiers thawed, and often inadvertently burned, their frozen extremities over campfires, only to refreeze them again on the next day's march. Combined heat and cold injury coupled with refreezing and forced ambulation resulted in abysmal outcomes. In addition, thousands died from the tetanus sustained from their frostbite wounds. It was from this experience that Larrey recommended rubbing frostbitten extremities with snow. This destructive therapy was the standard of care until the 1950s and is still used occasionally by the lay public. It was not until 1956 that rapid rewarming of frozen extremities was studied by a Public Health Service medical officer in Tanana, Alaska, which laid the foundation of modern therapy.[1]

PATHOPHYSIOLOGY

It is the inability to physiologically compensate for cold that produces injury. However, cold itself is not the only factor in determining whether injury will occur. Duration of contact, humidity, wind, altitude, clothing, medical conditions, behavior, and individual variability all contribute to the picture.

Cold-induced injury may be instantaneous, as with contact frostbite after touching a cold metal bottle of fuel, or more chronic, as in chilblains. Humidity is also important because it contributes to evaporative heat loss. Wet skin is more conducive to both subcutaneous ice crystal formation and trench foot. Wind velocity and cold, the wind-chill factor, have a synergistic effect on heat loss. For example, an ambient temperature of −7°C (19.4°F), when combined with a wind of 72.5 kph (45 mph), will feel equivalent to −40°C (−40°F) on a windless day. The rigors of travel at high altitude may also predispose to cold injury. Although the lower barometric pressure has not been shown to directly influence susceptibility to cold injury, a variety of factors associated with high altitude travel have. The fatigue, dehydration, and hypoxia often seen in climbers or trekkers, coupled with the sometimes extreme weather conditions and remote locations, all contribute to the incidence and severity of cold-related injuries at high altitude.[1]

Inadequate clothing is probably the most avoidable cause of cold-related injuries. Constrictive clothing and boots can reduce circulation to extremities and predispose to frostbite. An exposed head and neck can account for 80 percent of body heat loss. Natural-fiber clothing, such as wool and cotton, when compared to modern synthetics, such as polypropylene, have poorer wicking ability and greater thermal conductance and moisture retention.[1] Simply changing out of cold, wet clothes into dry ones can also be preventive. During World War I, the British decreased the number of trench foot cases from 29,172 in 1915 to a total of only 443 in 1916–1918 by frequent foot drying and sock changing.[2,3]

Certain disease states, such as atherosclerosis, arteritis, hypovolemia, diabetes, vascular injury secondary to trauma or infection, and previous cold-related injuries, may predispose to cold-related injury.

Individual behavior is extremely important as well. In fact, alcohol- or drug-intoxicated persons, combined with psychiatric patients, account for the majority of frostbite cases in the United States. Impaired judgment and lack of self-preservation instincts prevent these populations from dressing adequately and making rational decisions about exposure to the cold. Alcohol consumption also increases peripheral vasodilatation and heat loss, which increases the risk for hypothermia. In addition, many of these patients smoke, which results in peripheral vasoconstriction and increases the risk of frostbite.[1] Other examples of the precipitation of cold injury by individual behavior can be seen in recent case reports of significant facial frostbite by inhalation abuse of fluorinated hydrocarbons (e.g., Freon) and nitrous oxide.[4,5] There have also been case reports of full-thickness frostbite resulting from inappropiate use of dry ice as a first-aid cold pack.[6]

Military studies suggest that dark-skinned soldiers and those from warmer climatic regions are more susceptible to frostbite. Conversely, peoples indigenous to frigid climates, such as Eskimos, Tibetans, and Laplanders, are often "acclimated" to the cold and are less prone to injury.[1]

Local cold-related injuries are classified into nonfreezing and freezing injuries.

NONFREEZING COLD INJURIES: CHILBLAINS AND TRENCH FOOT

Clinical Features

Chilblains, or pernio, is characterized by usually mild but uncomfortable inflammatory lesions of the skin of bared extremities caused by chronic intermittent exposure to damp, nonfreezing ambient temperatures. It is precipitated by acute exposure to cold. The hands, ears, lower legs, and feet are most commonly involved. The cutaneous manifestations, which appear up to 12 h after acute exposure, include localized edema, erythema, cyanosis, plaques, nodules, and, in rare cases, ulcerations, vesicles, and bullae. Patients may complain of pruritus and burning paresthesias. Rewarming may result in the formation of tender blue nodules, which may persist for several days. This is primarily a disease of women and children, and, although rare in the United States, chilblains is common in the United Kingdom and other countries with a cold or temperate, damp climate. Also, it appears that young females with Raynaud phenomenon are at greatest risk, as well as those in households with inadequate heating and lack of warm clothing.[7]

Trench foot was given its current name after it was frequently found among World War I troops who had been confined for long periods in trenches filled with standing cold water. Significant numbers of cases were also seen in the Falkland and Vietnam wars. Immersion foot describes a more severe variant of trench foot seen in downed pilots and shipwrecked sailors exposed for extended periods in life rafts in the North Atlantic Ocean. Although they are a significant problem in military operations, trench foot and immersion foot are rarely seen in the civilian population.

The pathophysiology is multifactorial but involves direct injury to soft tissue sustained from prolonged cooling, and it is accelerated by wet conditions. The peripheral nerves seem to be the most sensitive to this form of injury. Trench foot develops slowly over hours to days and is initially reversible but if allowed to progress will become irreversible. Early symptoms progress from tingling to numbness of the affected tissues. On initial examination, the foot is pale, mottled, anesthetic, pulseless, and immobile, which initially does not change after rewarming. A hyperemic phase begins within hours and is associated with severe burning pain and reappearance of proximal sensation. As perfusion returns to the foot over 2 to 3 days, edema and bullae form, and the hyperemia may worsen. Anesthesia frequently persists for weeks but may be permanent. In more severe cases, tissue sloughing and gangrene may develop. Hyperhidrosis and cold sensitivity are common late features and may persist for months to years. Severe cases may be associated with prolonged convalescence and permanent disability.

Treatment

Management of chilblains is supportive. The affected skin should be rewarmed, gently bandaged, and elevated. Some European studies support the use of nifedipine (Procardia), at a dose of 20 mg tid, as both prophylactic and therapeutic. Topical corticosteroids (.025% fluocinolone cream) or even a brief burst of oral corticosteroids, such as prednisone, have been shown to be useful. Affected areas are more prone to reinjury.

Effective prophylaxis for trench foot includes keeping warm, ensuring good boot fit, changing out of wet socks several times a day, never sleeping in wet socks and boots, and, once early symptoms are identified, maximizing efforts to warm, dry, and elevate the feet. Once injury has occurred, treatment is supportive. Currently there is no specific therapy. Feet should be kept clean, warm, dryly bandaged, and elevated. Signs of early infection should be monitored.[1–3]

FREEZING COLD INJURIES: FROSTNIP AND FROSTBITE

Pathophysiology

Cutaneous vascular tone can be altered by direct heating (e.g., warming hands over a fire) and indirect heating (e.g., putting on a hat to increase core temperature), and is modulated by sympathetic adrenergic vasoconstrictive fibers. In a euthermic 70-kg male, the total basal cutaneous blood flow is 200 to 500 mL/min. However, as the skin temperature drops to 14°C (57.2°F), the flow falls to 20 to 50 mL/min. As cooling continues to 10°C (50°F), cutaneous blood flow becomes negligible, and 5- to 10-min cycles of vasodilatation and vasoconstriction, known as the hunter's response, or cold-induced vasoconstriction, occur. For individuals who are well acclimated to the cold, such as Eskimos, the intervals between cycles are often much shorter. As the vasodilatory phases carry cooled blood back from the extremities, the core temperature begins to fall. These cycles continue until the core temperature is threatened. The body attempts to maintain thermal integrity by completely shutting down flow to the coldest extremities. This begins phase I of frostbite, and irreversible tissue damage commences. As skin temperatures fall well below 0°C (32°F), ice crystals form in the extracellular space. Crystals exert an osmotic force and pull fluid from the intracellular space, resulting in cellular dehydration and hyperosmolarity. The intracellular NaCl concentration may rise ten fold. As the damage continues, proteins are denatured, enzymes are destroyed, and the cellular membranes are altered. Theoretically, intracellular ice crystals then form, especially in rapid freeze and refreeze injuries, and may be even more lethal to the cell. Actual structural damage from the ice crystals may result.

Phase II is characterized by reperfusion injury as the involved extremity is rewarmed and some initial blood flow returns. Over a period of several hours to days, the damaged endothelium-lined capillaries allow leakage of fluid into the interstitium, intracellular swelling occurs, and oxygen free radicals are generated, which furthers endothelial damage. An arachidonic acid cascade forms, which liberates prostaglandin and thromboxane. This cascade promotes vasoconstriction, platelet aggregation, and leukocyte sludging, which results in venule and arterial thrombosis and subsequent ischemia, necrosis, and dry gangrene. Profound vasoconstriction and arteriovenous shunting occur at the margin between injured and noninjured tissue. Phase II is remarkably similar to the dynamics of a burn injury.[8]

TABLE 185-1 Frostbite Pathophysiology Summary

PREFREEZE STATE
Tissue cooling
Increased viscosity
Capillary constriction-dilatation cycle
FROZEN STATE
Extracellular ice crystal formation
Intracellular dehydration and hyperosmolarity
Fluid crossing cell membrane
ISCHEMIC AND VASCULAR COMPLICATIONS
Reperfusion injury
Endothelium leaky
Coagulation from stasis
Leakage of destructive prostaglandins and oxygen free radicals
Vasoconstriction and arteriovenous shunting
Necrosis demarcation and gangrene

Frostbite injury can be divided into three zones. The zone of coagulation is the most severe, distal region of damage and is irreversible. The zone of hyperemia is the more superficial, proximal region with the least cellular damage and generally recovers without treatment in less than 10 days. The zone of stasis is the middle ground and is characterized by severe, but possibly reversible, cell damage. It is here that treatment is directed.[9]

Table 185-1 summarizes the pathophysiology of frostbite.

Clinical Features

Frostbite can occur on any skin surface but is generally limited to the nose, ears, face, hands, and feet. Frostbite has been reported in the penis and scrotum of joggers and in burn patients after prolonged treatment with ice. Also, a freezing keratitis of the cornea has been reported in snowmobilers and skiers who did not wear protective goggles.

Frostnip is on a continuum with frostbite and is a superficial freeze injury characterized by lack of extracellular ice crystal formation and absence of progressive tissue loss. The involved extremity appears pale from intense vasoconstriction and is associated with some discomfort. Symptoms resolve on rewarming, and tissue loss does not occur.

There has been much debate over the proper classification of the severity of frostbite.[10] One may classify frostbite into degrees of injury or into superficial and deep groups (Table 185-2). First- and second-degree injuries are classified as superficial, whereas third- and fourth-degree injuries are classified as deep. The initial clinical appearance is often deceiving, especially if some warming has not occurred. Most patients present after some warming has occurred and are in phase II of the injury. Frostbite classification is based on the time of presentation.

First-degree injury is characterized by partial skin freezing, erythema, mild edema, lack of blisters, and occasional skin desquamation several days later. The patient may complain of transient stinging and burning, followed by throbbing. Prognosis is excellent.

Second-degree injury is characterized by full-thickness skin freezing, formation of substantial edema over 3 to 4 h, erythema, and formation of clear blisters rich in thromboxane and prostaglandins. The blisters form within 6 to 24 h, extend to the end of the digit, and usually desquamate and form black, hard eschars over several days. The patient complains of numbness, followed later by aching and throbbing. Prognosis is good.

Third-degree injury is characterized by damage that extends into the subdermal plexus. Hemorrhagic blisters form and are associated with skin necrosis and a blue-gray discoloration of the skin. The patient may complain that the involved extremity feels like a ''block of wood,'' followed later by burning, throbbing, and shooting pains. Prognosis is often poor.

Fourth-degree injury is characterized by extension into subcutaneous tissues, muscle, bone, and tendon. There is little edema. The skin is mottled, with nonblanching cyanosis, and eventually forms a deep, dry, black, mummified eschar. Vesicles often present late, if at all, and may be small, bloody blebs that do not extend to the digit tips. The patient may complain of a deep, aching joint pain. Prognosis is extremely poor.[1,10–14]

Treatment

FIELD MANAGEMENT Field management of frostbite by emergency medical service personnel is simple. The hypothermia and dehydration associated with frostbite should be addressed. Wet and constrictive clothing should be removed. The involved extremities should be elevated and carefully wrapped in dry sterile gauze, with affected fingers and toes separated. Further cold injury should be avoided. In most cases, more aggressive wound management should be avoided and the patient transported to the emergency department. However, in some cases the patient may be several days away from evacuation and medical services and more complex management might be indicated before arrival to the hospital (Table 185-3).

There is a correlation between the length of time tissue is frozen and the degree of cellular damage. Rapid rewarming is the single most effective therapy for frostbite. However, rewarming in the field is often impractical and is sometimes dangerous. In fact, in some unusual circumstances, it is best to endeavor to keep the affected part frozen until definitive care can be administered. For instance, if the victim has frozen feet and the only avenue to evacuation is prolonged ambulation, then rewarming can significantly complicate matters. The risk of refreezing the feet and causing even more severe damage is a real concern. Also, if adequate analgesia is not available, the rewarming process itself can be excessively painful. Ambulation on edematous and blistered feet may not be possible because of pain. In extreme situations such as this, it may be wise to keep the feet frozen and ambulate the patient to a location where more advanced evacuation can occur. If rewarming is attempted in the field, only clean water warmed to 40° to 42°C (104° to 107.6°F), as measured by thermometer, should be used. The use of hot, untested tap water should be avoided because the 50° to 60°C (122° to 140°F) temperatures will cause a destructive thermal injury and worsen the prognosis. Attempts to directly warm with dry air, such as campfires and heaters, should be avoided. Dry heat tends to desiccate damaged tissue, and temperature cannot be adequately measured. Adding a thermal injury to frostbite will worsen the outcome. Rubbing snow on frostbitten tissue to stimulate circulation is ineffective, destructive, and absolutely contraindicated.

Controversy surrounds management of the blisters associated with frostbite. Clear blisters are rich in tissue-injurious thromboxane and prostaglandins. Common sense suggests that blister débridement or aspiration would limit contact with these chemicals and allow direct contract with aloe vera (Dermaide Aloe Cream) to countereact their injurious effects. Also, tense blisters, which tend to only worsen when immobilization is not possible, are painful. Débridement or aspiration can bring some pain relief. When the patient is ambulating on rewarmed, frostbitten feet, the associated blisters often rupture anyway. Field débridement of clear blisters is controversial, but adequate research is lacking to support or condemn this practice. Hemorrhagic blisters should not be drained in the field.

One possible complication of field aspiration or débridement is the theoretical increased risk of infection. Prophylactic use of penicillin might be wise in the field setting to combat any potential wound infection. Wounds should be cleansed daily, and, if feet are involved, socks should be clean and changed at least once or twice per day. Affected digits should be covered with aloe vera and separated by dry, sterile cotton and dressings should be changed daily. Pain management

TABLE 185-2 Classification of Cold Injury According to Severity

Classification	Symptoms
SUPERFICIAL	
First degree: partial skin freezing	Transient stinging and burning
Erythema, edema, hyperemia	Throbbing and aching possible
No blisters or necrosis	May have hyperhidrosis
Occasional skin desquamation (5–10 d later)	
Second degree: full-thickness injury	Numbness
Erythema, substantial edema, vesicles with clear fluid	Vasomotor disturbances in severe cases
Blisters that desquamate and form blackened eschar	
DEEP	
Third degree: full-thickness skin and subcutaneous freezing	Initially, no sensation
Violaceous or hemorrhagic blisters	Tissue feels like ''block of wood''
Skin necrosis	Later, shooting pains, burning, throbbing, aching
Blue-gray discoloration	
Fourth degree: full-thickness skin, subcutaneous tissue, muscle, tendon, and bone freezing	Possible joint discomfort
Little edema	
Initially mottled, deep red, or cyanotic	
Eventually dry, black, mummified	

Source: From Britt LD, Dascombe W, Rodriquez A: *Surg Clin North Am* 71:359, 1991, with permission.

TABLE 185-3 Frostbite Treatment Summary

THAW

Give thermometer bath at 40–42°C (104–107.6°F) for 10–30 min with active motion.
Give parenteral analgesics (morphine 0.1 mg/kg, meperidine 1–1.5 mg/kg) as needed.

POSTTHAW

Débride clear blisters.
Leave hemorrhagic vesicles intact.
Dress all with aloe vera (Dermaide Aloe Cream).
Give tetanus prohylaxis as needed.
Give ibuprofen 400 mg orally q12h.
Consider penicillin G 500,000 U q6h for 48–72 h.
Begin daily hydrotherapy.

should begin with nonsteroidal anti-inflammatory drugs, such as ibuprofen 12 mg/kg/day in divided doses, to counteract the arachidonic acid cascade and should be continued even if opioids analgesics are required as well. The victim should be discouraged from smoking because it exacerbates vasoconstriction and tissue damage.[1,10–14]

EMERGENCY DEPARTMENT MANAGEMENT In taking the patient's history, it is important to determine as many prognostic factors as possible. What was the temperature and wind velocity? How long was the extremity frozen, and, if it was thawed, did any refreezing occur? Was there any self-treatment, such as rubbing with snow or use of aloe vera or ibuprofen? Were recreational drugs, alcohol, or tobacco involved? Are there any predisposing medical conditions?

Frostbite is often associated with systemic hypothermia and dehydration, both of which can have a negative impact on the prognosis for tissue salvage. Rehydration and general warming are important adjuncts to therapy when indicated.

Frostbitten patients often present to the emergency department subacutely (>24 h after injury) and with the involved extremity in a partially thawed state. This more prolonged injury and slow, partial thawing usually translates to significantly longer hospital stays and greater tissue loss. However, this should not mean the patient is treated any less aggressively than the acute patient. The target of treatment remains minimizing tissue loss by focusing on the zone of stasis, where damaged but potentially salvageable tissue exists.

Rapid rewarming is the core of frostbite therapy and should be initiated as soon as possible. The injured extremity should be placed in gently circulating water at a temperature of 40° to 42°C (104° to 107.6°F) for approximately 10 to 30 min, until the distal extremity is pliable and erythematous. Frostbitten faces can be thawed using moistened compresses soaked in warm water. Some patients may tolerate immersion of their ears in a bowl or pool of warmed water. Anticipate severe pain during rewarming and titrate with parenteral narcotics. The patient will probably require daily hydrotherapy and physical therapy during the inpatient phase.

Blister management is somewhat controversial, as is the use of prophylactic antibiotics. The current consensus is that clear blisters should be débrided or at least aspirated. The blister fluid is rich in destructive thromboxane and prostaglandins. Removal limits damage from these chemicals and enables access to the underlying tissue for topical therapy. Hemorrhagic blisters should not be débrided because this often results in tissue desiccation and worsened outcome. However, there is some controversy as to whether aspiration is helpful. Both blister types should be treated with topical aloe vera (Dermaide Aloe Cream) q6h, which helps to combat the arachidonic acid cascade. Affected digits should be separated with cotton and wrapped with sterile, dry gauze. Elevation of the involved extremities helps decrease edema and pain.

The role of prophylactic antibiotics is unclear. The edema associated with the first several days after injury does appear to predispose to infection. *Staphylococcus aureus, Staphylococcus epidermidis,* and β-hemolytic streptococci account for nearly half of infections, but anaerobes, *Pseudomonas,* and *Enterococcus* are important pathogens as well. Therapy with penicillin G 500,000 U intravenously q6h, for 48 to 72 h, is recommended in several successful protocols and seems to be beneficial. One study, however, demonstrated better infection prophylaxis using topical bacitracin. Silver sulfadiazine (Silvadene) cream has also been advocated by some, but it has not been shown to be consistently beneficial. One disadvantage of using topical antibiotics is that it complicates the concurrent use of aloe vera (Dermaide Aloe Cream). It is important to address tetanus status and administer appropriate vaccination, if needed, because frostbite is a tetanus-prone wound.

Several agents besides aloe vera (Dermaide Aloe Cream) have been advocated to battle the arachidonic acid cascade and thereby limit tissue damage. The most commonly advocated oral medication is ibuprofen at a daily dose of 12 mg/kg. Animal studies suggest possible future roles for oral methimazole, a thromboxane synthetase inhibitor, and topical 1% methylprednisolone acetate, which acts as a phospholipase A_2 inhibitor, preventing the formation of arachidonic acid.

Another controversial area is the use of sympathectomy to relieve vasospasm and edema. The treatment may be medical, as in the use of intraarterial reserpine, or surgical. There is no role for early sympathectomy, and the controversy is beyond the scope of emergency department management.

Heparin, and hyperbaric oxygen therapy have been studied and appear to be of little value. To date; frostbite treatment with intravenous low-molecular-weight dextran has not been studied clinically in human, but anecdotal reports have been encouraging. Some preliminary data from a study using intraarterial recombinant tissue plasminogen activator in patients with third-degree frostbite suggest that it may hold some promise in decreasing the rate of amputation.[15] A recent limited study suggests that the prostaglandin E_1 analogue limaprost may be an effective prophylactic and therapeutic vasodilator for local cold injuries at high altitudes.[16]

Early surgical intervention is not indicated in the management of frostbite. Premature surgery has been an important contributor to necessary tissue loss and poor results in the past. This is primarily due to the inability to assess the depth of frostbite at early stages and the fact that the blackened, mummified carapace is protective of the underlying regenerating tissue. Limited, early escharotomy may be indicated if the eschar is preventing adequate range of motion or circulation. Fasciotomy is rarely, if ever, indicated. Amputation may be unavoidable, however, if wet gangrene or infection complicates recovery. It usually takes at least 3 to 4 weeks for full demarcation to occur. Most amputations and grafts occur during the third week. The mean length of hospital stay for all degrees of frostbite is reported to be 8.5 days to 33.2 days. To minimize extended hospital stays, some have advocated the early use of radionuclide angiography with bone scan at 7 to 14 days to assess tissue viability and possible early surgical débridement.[17,18] However, a recent case report suggests that the use of magnetic resonance imaging with magnetic resonance angiography may prove to be more helpful in the early determination of the degree of tissue damage and the eventual prognosis.[19]

Disposition

Since it is difficult to determine the extent of frostbite on initial examination, it is best to be conservative when contemplating admission. It has been the standard of care in the past to admit all but the most isolated and superficial frostbite cases. It is important to consider the associated social factors as well. The homeless or elderly, especially when unable to care for themselves adequately, should never be discharged into subfreezing temperatures. If the frostbite is extensive and the hospital and staff are not equipped to treat the degree of severity, transfer to a tertiary hospital should be considered after initial rewarming and treatment. Patients who are discharged from the emergency department should be treated with topical aloe vera (Dermaide Aloe Cream) and oral ibuprofen and encouraged not to smoke. Close surgical follow-up should be arranged.

Sequelae

The sequelae of frostbite can be significant and prolonged. Permanent cold sensitivity, pain, tingling, and hyperhidrosis are common. Skin color changes may occur. When deep frostbite involves bones or joints, arthritis may result. In pediatric patients, growth plate damage may result in digit shortening and radial deviation. Infection is a possible complication and often results in a poor outcome. Deep frostbite often results in amputation.

REFERENCES

1. Smith DJ, Robson MC, Heggers JP: Frostbite and other cold-related injuries, in Auerbach PS, Geehr EC (eds): *Management of Wilderness and Environmental Injuries,* 3d ed. St Louis, Mosby, 1995, pp 129–145.
2. Burr RE: Trench foot. *J Wilderness Med* 4:348, 1993.
3. Tek DT, Mackey S: Non-freezing injury in a Marine infantry battalion. *J Wilderness Med* 4:353, 1993.
4. Hwang JCF, Himel HN, Edlich RF: Frostbite of the face after recreational misuse of nitrous oxide. *Burns* 22:4, 1996.
5. Kurbat RS, Pollack VP: Facial injury and airway threat from inhalant abuse: A case report. *J Emerg Med* 16:2, 1998.
6. Gamble WB, Bonnecarre ER: Coffee, tea, or frostbite? *Aviation, Space Environ Med* 67:9, 1996.
7. Carruthers R: Chilblains (pernosis). *Aust Fam Physician* 17: 968, 1988.
8. Vogel EJ, Dellon AL: Frostbite injuries of the hand. *Clin Plast Surg* 16:565, 1989.
9. Jackson D: The diagnosis of the depth of burning. *Br J Surg* 40:588, 1953.
10. Heggers JP, Phillips LG, McCauley RL, Robson MC: Frostbite: Experimental and clinical evaluations of treatment. *J Wilderness Med* 1:27, 1990.
11. Heggers JP, Robson MC, Manaualen K, et al: Experimental and clinical observations on frostbite. *Ann Emerg Med* 16:1056, 1987.
12. McCauley RL, Heggers JP, Robson MC: Frostbite: Methods to minimize tissue loss. *Postgrad Med* 88:8, 1990.
13. McCauley RL, Hing DN, Robson MC, Heggers JP: Frostbite injuries: A rational approach based on the pathophysiology. *J Trauma* 23:143, 1983.
14. Valnicek SM, Chasmar LR, Clapson JB: Frostbite on the prairies: A 12-year review. *Plast Reconstr Surg* 92:4, 1993.
15. Skolnick AA: Early data suggest clot-dissolving drug may help save frostbite limbs from amputation. *JAMA* 267:2008, 1992.
16. Saito S, Shimada H: Effect of prostaglandin E_1, analogue administration on peripheral skin temperature at high altitude. *Angiology* 45:455, 1994.
17. Mehta RC, Wilson MA: Frostbite injury: Prediction of tissue viability with triple-phase bone scanning. *Radiology* 170:511, 1989.
18. Salini Z, Vas W, Tang-Barton P, et al: Assessment of tissue in frostbite by 99m-Tc pertechnetate scintigraphy. *AJR* 42:415,1984.
19. Barker JR, Haws MJ, Brown RE, et al: Magnetic resonance imaging of severe frostbite injuries. *Ann Plast Surg* 38:275, 1997.

HYPOTHERMIA

Howard A. Bessen

EPIDEMIOLOGY

Hypothermia is defined as a core temperature less than 35°C (95°F). While most commonly seen in cold climates, it may develop without exposure to extreme environmental conditions. Hypothermia is not uncommon in temperate regions and may even develop indoors during the summer. In the United States, more than 700 people die from hypothermia each year. Half of those who die from hypothermia are older than 65 years.[1]

Individuals at the extremes of age and those with an altered sensorium for any reason are particularly susceptible to developing hypothermia. The elderly may lose their ability to sense cold; neonates easily become hypothermic because of their large surface area to volume ratio. Both groups have a limited ability to increase heat production and to conserve body heat. Individuals with an altered sensorium, if unable to carry out the appropriate behavioral responses to cold stress, may develop hypothermia despite otherwise intact thermoregulatory mechanisms.

PHYSIOLOGY OF TEMPERATURE HOMEOSTASIS

Body temperature may fall as a result of heat loss by conduction, convection, radiation, or evaporation. *Conduction* is the transfer of heat by direct contact, down a temperature gradient, e.g., from a warm body to the cold environment. Since the thermal conductivity of water is approximately 30 times that of air, the body loses heat rapidly when immersed in water, producing a rapid decline in body temperature.

Convection is the transfer of heat by the actual movement of heated material, e.g., wind disrupting the layer of warm air surrounding the body. Convective heat loss increases in windy conditions, a particular hazard for outdoors enthusiasts.

Heat also may be lost by *radiation* to the environment (primarily from noninsulated body areas) and by *evaporation of water*. Evaporation of the water contained in exhaled, water-saturated air occurs over a wide range of ambient temperatures and may be prevented by inhalation of warmed, humidified air.

Opposing the loss of body heat are the mechanisms of heat conservation and gain. In general, these are controlled by the hypothalamus; thus hypothalamic dysfunction may cause an impairment in temperature homeostasis. Heat is conserved by peripheral vasoconstriction and, importantly, by behavioral responses. If behavioral responses such as putting on clothing or coming indoors from a cold environment are impaired for any reason (e.g., drug intoxication or trauma), the risk of hypothermia is increased.

Heat gain is effected by shivering and by "nonshivering thermogenesis." The nonshivering component of heat production consists of an increase in metabolic rate brought about by increased output from the thyroid and adrenal glands.

ETIOLOGY

Although there are other, more unusual etiologies of hypothermia, nearly all patients seen in the emergency department will have hypothermia due to one or more of the causes noted in Table 186-1.

"Accidental" hypothermia may be divided into immersion and nonimmersion cold exposure. Exposure to cold environmental conditions may lead to hypothermia even in healthy subjects, especially in wind and rain. Inadequate clothing and physical exhaustion contribute to the loss of body heat. The high thermal conductivity of water leads to the rapid development of immersion hypothermia. Though the rate of heat loss is determined by water temperature, immersion in any water less than 16 to 21°C (60.8–69.8°F) may lead to hypothermia.

Metabolic causes of hypothermia include various hypoendocrine states (hypothyroidism, hypoadrenalism, hypopituitarism), which lead to a decrease in metabolic rate. Hypoglycemia also may lead to hypothermia; the probable mechanism is hypothalamic dysfunction secondary to glucopenia.

Other causes of hypothalamic and CNS dysfunction (e.g., head trauma, tumor, stroke) may interfere with mechanisms of temperature regulation. Wernicke's disease may involve the hypothalamus; this is a rare but important cause of hypothermia, since it is potentially reversible with parenteral thiamine.

TABLE 186-1 Causes of Hypothermia: Clinical Settings

"Accidental" (environmental)
Metabolic
Hypothalamic and CNS dysfunction
Drug-induced
Sepsis
Dermal disease
Acute incapacitating illness
Iatrogenic (fluid resuscitation)

In the United States, the majority of hypothermic patients are intoxicated with ethanol or other drugs. Ethanol is a vasodilator, and because of its anesthetic and CNS depressant effects, intoxicated subjects neither feel the cold nor respond to it appropriately. Other drugs commonly implicated in the development of hypothermia include sedative-hypnotics, phenothiazines, and occasionally insulin.

Sepsis may alter the hypothalamic temperature set point and is a well-known cause of hypothermia. Subnormal body temperature is a poor prognostic factor in patients with bacteremia.[2]

Severe dermal disease may impair the skin's thermoregulatory functions. Significant burns or severe exfoliative dermatitis may prevent cutaneous vasoconstriction and increase transcutaneous water loss, predisposing to the development of hypothermia.

Hypothermia may develop in anyone with an acute incapacitating illness. Thus patients with severe infections, diabetic ketoacidosis, immobilizing injuries, and various other conditions may have impaired thermoregulatory function, including altered behavioral responses.

Hypothermia also may be induced by resuscitation with room-temperature fluid or cold blood. This is a particular risk in patients undergoing massive volume replacement, such as trauma patients.

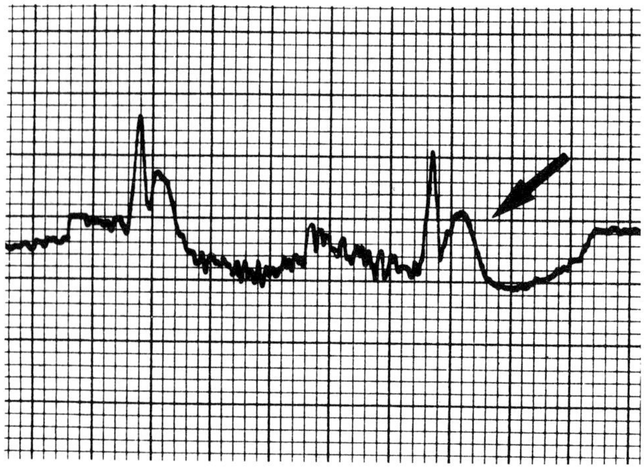

FIG. 186-1. Rhythm strip from patient with temperature of 25°C (77°F) showing atrial fibrillation with a slow ventricular response, muscle tremor artifact, and Osborn (J) wave (*arrow*).

PATHOPHYSIOLOGY AND CLINICAL FEATURES

The response of various organ systems to lowered temperature varies widely among individuals.[3–5] In general, however, body temperatures from 32 to 35°C (89.6–95°F) constitute ''mild'' hypothermia. In this temperature range, the patient is in an excitation (responsive) stage, in which physiologic adjustments attempt to retain and generate heat.

When temperature drops below 32°C (89.6°F), general excitation gives way to the slowing (adynamic) stage, in which there is a progressive slowdown of bodily functions. Metabolism slows, causing a decrease in both oxygen utilization and CO_2 production. Shivering ceases when body temperature falls below 30 to 32°C (86–89.6°F).

In the initial excitation phase, heart rate, cardiac output, and blood pressure all rise. With decreasing temperature, these all decline. Cardiac output and blood pressure may be markedly depressed by the negative inotropic and chronotropic effects of hypothermia and further depressed by concomitant hypovolemia.

Hypothermia causes characteristic ECG changes and may induce life-threatening dysrhythmias (Table 186-2). The Osborn (J) wave, a slow, positive deflection at the end of the QRS complex (Fig. 186-1), is characteristic, though not pathognomic, of hypothermia.

Patients are at risk for dysrhythmias at body temperatures below 30°C (86°F); the risk increases as body temperature decreases. Although various dysrhythmias may occur at any time, the typical sequence is a progression from sinus bradycardia to atrial fibrillation with a slow ventricular response, to ventricular fibrillation, and ultimately, to asystole. The hypothermic myocardium is extremely irritable, and ventricular fibrillation may be induced by a variety of manipulations and interventions that stimulate the heart, including rough handling of the patient.[4,6]

TABLE 186-2 ECG Changes in Hypothermia

T-wave inversions
PR, QRS, QT prolongation
Muscle tremor artifact
Osborn (J) wave
Dysrhythmias:
Sinus bradycardia
Atrial fibrillation or flutter
Nodal rhythms
AV block
PVCs
Ventricular fibrillation
Asystole

Pulmonary effects include initial tachypnea, followed by a progressive decrease in respiratory rate and tidal volume. Cold-induced bronchorrhea, along with a depression of cough and gag reflexes, makes aspiration pneumonia a common complication.

Much attention has been paid to the temperature correction of arterial blood gases in the hypothermic patient. Since the blood gas analyzer warms the blood to 37°C (98.6°F), thus increasing the partial pressure of dissolved gases, the machine will report a higher P_{O_2} and P_{CO_2} and lower pH than the actual values at the patient's body temperature. Correction factors and nomograms are available to determine the actual values in the patient's body; however, the optimal or ''normal'' values in hypothermia are not known. The simplest solution is to use the uncorrected values as if the patient were normothermic; studies suggest that this approach is the most physiologically sound.[7,8] P_{CO_2} is often quite low secondary to depressed metabolism and decreased CO_2 production, and iatrogenic hyperventilation may lead to marked respiratory alkalosis.

Hypothermia causes a leftward shift of the oxyhemoglobin dissociation curve, potentially impairing oxygen release to tissues. Patients may have minimal oxygen reserves despite diminished oxygen requirements, warranting the administration of supplemental oxygen.

The CNS is affected by hypothermia, with a progressive depression of consciousness with decreasing temperature. Mild incoordination is followed by confusion, lethargy, and coma; pupils may be dilated and unreactive. These changes are associated with a decrease in cerebral blood flow. An even greater decrease in cerebral oxygen requirements may protect the brain against anoxic or ischemic damage.

Hypothermia impairs renal concentrating abilities and induces a ''cold diuresis,'' leading to significant volume losses. Because of this concentrating defect, urine flow and specific gravity are unreliable indicators of intravascular volume and circulatory status. The immobile hypothermic patient is prone to rhabdomyolysis, and acute tubular necrosis may occur because of myoglobinuria and renal hypoperfusion.

Intravascular volume is also lost due to a plasma shift to the extravascular space. The combination of hemoconcentration, cold-induced increase in blood viscosity, and poor circulation may lead to intravascular thrombosis and subsequent embolic complications. Disseminated intravascular coagulation may occur because of release of tissue thromboplastins into the bloodstream, especially when circulation is restored during rewarming.

Because cold inhibits both platelet function and the enzymatic reactions of the coagulation cascade, hypothermic patients are prone to bleeding. The coagulopathy may be evident clinically but not detected with routine coagulation tests, which are performed at 37°C (98.6°F).

Endocrine function is fairly well preserved at low body temperatures. Plasma cortisol and thyroid hormone levels are usually normal or elevated unless the patient has a preexisting deficiency. Glucose levels may be normal, low, or elevated. Though hyperglycemia is common due to decreased insulin release as well as decreased glucose utilization, hypoglycemia may occur in up to 40 percent of patients.[9]

Acid-base disturbances are common in hypothermia but follow no uniform pattern. Acidosis may occur due to severe respiratory depression and CO_2 retention and to lactic acid production from shivering and poor tissue perfusion. Alkalosis may result from diminished CO_2 production with low metabolic rates or from iatrogenic hyperventilation or sodium bicarbonate administration.

Pancreatitis (not only hyperamylasemia but true pancreatic necrosis) may occur in hypothermia. Hepatic function is depressed by cold, so drugs normally metabolized, conjugated, or detoxified by the liver (e.g., lidocaine) may rapidly accumulate to toxic levels.

Finally, local cold injury and frostbite may occur in the hypothermic patient.

DIAGNOSIS

The diagnosis of hypothermia is often not obvious; exposure to profound cold is *not* necessary to produce hypothermia. Since many standard clinical thermometers record only to 34.4°C (94°F), low-reading glass or electronic thermometers are required to accurately measure the temperature of hypothermic patients. Electronic thermometers with flexible probes can be used to continuously monitor rectal or esophageal temperatures.

TREATMENT

Treatment includes both general supportive measures and specific rewarming techniques.[3–6] Therapy begins with careful, gentle handling, since manipulation can precipitate ventricular fibrillation in the irritable hypothermic myocardium.

Controversy has arisen regarding the performance of CPR on an unmonitored patient who appears to be profoundly hypothermic and in cardiopulmonary arrest. Opponents of CPR argue that pulses may be difficult to detect in this setting and that chest compressions may precipitate ventricular fibrillation. They recommend withholding CPR until the presence of an arrested rhythm (ventricular fibrillation or asystole) is confirmed. Alternatively, withholding CPR in the patient who is truly in cardiac arrest may unnecessarily subject the brain and other organs to prolonged ischemia. This CPR controversy applies only to patients with severe hypothermia, with core temperatures less than 28°C (82.4°F); practically, it may be difficult to confirm this diagnosis in the field. To avoid inappropriate chest compressions, prehospital care personnel should examine the patient for 30 to 60 s before diagnosing pulselessness. If no pulses are detected, most physicians recommend initiating CPR. The optimal rate of chest compressions and ventilations has not been determined.

Similar considerations apply to monitored patients. Some authors recommend avoiding chest compressions in severely hypothermic patients with "nonarrested rhythms" (sinus bradycardia, artrial fibrillation with slow ventricular response, junctional rhythms), even without a palpable pulse. Most, however, recommend full CPR in patients with pulseless electrical activity, even with profound hypothermia.

Oxygen and intravenous fluids should be warmed, and patients should have constant monitoring of their core temperature, cardiac rhythm, and oxygen saturation. Pulse oximetry is usually accurate in hypothermic patients,[10] although unreliable data may be obtained with profound vasoconstriction or a very low cardiac output. If central venous lines are placed, care should be taken to avoid entering and irritating the heart. In general, indications for endotracheal intubation are the same as in the normothermic patient. Concern has been raised regarding induction of dysrhythmias during intubation; however, there is a very low complication rate with careful intubation after oxygenation.[11]

Although dysrhythmias in the hypothermic patient may represent an immediate threat to life, most rhythm disturbances (e.g., sinus bradycardia, atrial fibrillation or flutter) require no therapy and revert spontaneously with rewarming. In addition, the activity of antiarrhythmic and cardioactive drugs is unpredictable in hypothermia, and the hypothermic heart is relatively resistant to atropine, pacing, and countershock.

Ventricular fibrillation may be refractory to therapy until the patient is rewarmed. The American Heart Association's 1992 guidelines suggest initial defibrillation attempts with up to three shocks. If this is unsuccessful, CPR should be instituted and rapid rewarming begun. Defibrillation should be reattempted as the core temperature rises. Bretylium has been suggested as the drug of choice for the prophylaxis or treatment of ventricular fibrillation in hypothermic patients, although data concerning its efficacy are conflicting.[12,13]

Drug Therapy

Because many hypothermic patients are thiamine-depleted alcoholics (and because Wernicke's disease may cause hypothermia), patients should be given intravenous thiamine. Fifty to 100 mL of 50% dextrose should be administered if a dipstick serum glucose measurement is low or if a rapid test is unavailable.

Administration of antibiotics, steroids, and thyroid hormone must be individualized. Serious, often occult, infections may either precipitate or complicate hypothermia, and a thorough search for infection is indicated. Routine steroid therapy is generally not indicated, but hydrocortisone (100 mg) should be given to the patient with a history of adrenal suppression or insufficiency preceding the hypothermic episode, as well as to the patient with myxedema coma.

Hypothermia and hypothyroidism share many clinical features. While the majority of patients with myxedema coma are hypothermic, only a small minority of hypothermic patients are hypothyroid; thyroid hormone levels are most often normal or elevated. Thyroxine in large doses is necessary for the patient in myxedema coma but could potentially cause dysrhythmias or cardiac ischemia in other hypothermic patients. Therefore, thyroid hormone replacement is indicated only in patients with a known history of hypothyroidism, a thyroidectomy scar, or other strong clinical evidence of myxedema coma.

Rewarming Techniques

Modalities available for rewarming are listed in Table 186-3. The choice of method is a matter of controversy. There are no prospective, controlled studies comparing rewarming methods in humans, and each method has advantages and disadvantages.

Passive rewarming allows patients to rewarm on their own, using endogenous heat produced by metabolism. Since patients often become hypothermic over a period of hours to days, slow, passive rewarming is physiologically sound, avoiding rapid changes in cardiovascular status and the complications associated with active rewarming methods.

Patients must have intact thermoregulatory mechanisms and be capable of metabolic heat production for successful passive rewarming. With severe hypothermia or hypothermia secondary to an underlying illness (see Table 186-1), patients may fail to rewarm passively; active rewarming is then indicated. In addition, since temperature rises slowly with passive rewarming, it is inappropriate for patients with cardiovascular compromise.

TABLE 186-3 Rewarming Techniques

Passive rewarming:
Removal from cold environment
Insulation
Active external rewarming:
Warm water immersion
Heating blankets
Heated objects (water bottles, etc.)
Radiant heat
Forced air
Active core rewarming:
Inhalation rewarming
Heated IV fluids
GI tract lavage
Bladder lavage
Peritoneal lavage
Pleural lavage
Extracorporeal rewarming
Mediastinal lavage via thoracotomy

Active external rewarming (application of exogenous heat to the body) is often very effective in raising body temperature. Most of the methods listed in Table 186-3 are easily instituted, although some, especially warm water immersion, make resuscitation and monitoring difficult. Rewarming with heated air forced through slits in commercially available plastic or paper blankets appears very promising; this method has been used successfully in moderately to severely hypothermic patients.[14,15]

External rewarming does have disadvantages. It may be ineffective with poor perfusion of the periphery, especially in patients in cardiac arrest. Application of external heat may cause peripheral vasodilation and venous pooling, leading to relative hypovolemia and hypotension (rewarming shock). Washout of lactic acid from the peripheral tissues may lead to ''rewarming acidosis,'' and an increase in metabolic demands of the periphery before the hypothermic heart can provide adequate tissue perfusion may lead to further tissue hypoxia and acidosis.

The core temperature may continue to decline after rewarming has begun. This ''core temperature afterdrop'' was previously ascribed to the return of cold blood to the core induced by external warming and peripheral vasodilation. This mechanism is unlikely; afterdrop can be explained by the continued conduction of heat from the relatively warmer core to the colder peripheral tissues. The incidence and magnitude of afterdrop are unclear, and it is probably of little clinical significance.[6]

Active core rewarming has several theoretical advantages. Internal organs including the heart are preferentially rewarmed, decreasing myocardial irritability and returning cardiac function. Peripheral vasodilation is avoided, decreasing the incidence and magnitude of rewarming shock and acidosis. However, some internal rewarming techniques are invasive and may be difficult to institute.

Inhalation rewarming—administration of warmed, humidified oxygen via mask or endotracheal tube—provides a fairly small heat gain and is not effective for rapid rewarming. This is an important modality, however, because it minimizes heat loss from the lungs, a potential loss of up to 30 percent of the total metabolic heat production. Similarly, intravenous fluids should be warmed to avoid further cooling by the administration of fluids at room temperature. Heat gain is usually fairly small, although warming of infused fluid and blood can contribute significant amounts of heat to patients receiving massive fluid resuscitation. Commercial fluid warmers allow the temperature of infused fluids to be precisely controlled. Inhalation rewarming and warm intravenous fluids should be used in all but mild cases of hypothermia, since these are simple, noninvasive techniques with minimal risk of complications.

Gastrointestinal tract (gastric or colonic) lavage with warmed saline is technically simple, and patients can be lavaged with large volumes of fluid in a short time period. The obtunded hypothermic patient may develop pulmonary aspiration if lavaged with an unprotected airway. In a manner similar to gastrointestinal tract lavage, the bladder can be lavaged with warm saline solution using a Foley catheter.

Peritoneal lavage affords relatively rapid rewarming.[16] It is widely available, may be instituted rapidly and with little technical difficulty, and has been shown to be effective in both animal studies and human applications. Potassium-free dialysis solution is warmed to 40 to 45°C (104–113°F), instilled, and then removed; the use of two catheters (one for fluid instillation and one for removal) may increase the rewarming rate.

Pleural lavage using thoracostomy tubes has provided effective rewarming in animal studies and a few human cases.[17] Lavaging the left thoracic cavity delivers heated fluid in close proximity to the heart, potentially allowing rapid cardiac warming. Two thoracostomy tubes (for fluid inflow and outflow) have generally been employed. If this technique is chosen, care must be taken to monitor the net fluid infusion, as increased intrathoracic pressure and tension hydrothorax may complicate the procedure. The risk of precipitating dysrhythmias during chest tube insertion is unknown.

Rapid internal rewarming also can be accomplished through an extracorporeal circuit.[18,19] This consists of an arteriovenous shunt in which blood is routed to a warming device and then returned to the patient. Pump-assisted cardiopulmonary bypass using the femoral vessels for access is the most commonly used extracorporeal technique; right atrial-aortic bypass using a median sternotomy and heated hemodialysis also have been employed. Continuous arteriovenous rewarming using a countercurrent heat exchanger (a modified commercial fluid warmer) interposed between catheters placed in the femoral vessels, with flow driven by the patient's blood pressure, also has been reported.[20] This technique obviates the need for pump support and systemic heparinization but is ineffective in hypotensive patients.

Profoundly hypothermic patients may be rewarmed in a very short time period with these methods.[18,19] In addition to allowing rapid rewarming, pump-driven partial (femoral-femoral) or complete cardiopulmonary bypass provides circulatory support and oxygenation of blood, a great advantage in the management of patients in cardiac arrest or with severe cardiovascular compromise. Specialized equipment and personnel are required, however, and lack of immediate availability often precludes the use of this technique. In addition, the heparinization required for some extracorporeal techniques may cause complications in hypothermic trauma patients.

Various diathermy and radiowave techniques, although promising, have had limited use in hypothermic humans.

Finally, mediastinal irrigation using open thoracotomy has been used successfully as a rewarming technique in a few patients. It is possible that these patients could have been resuscitated using less invasive modalities. Thoracotomy has many potential complications and should only be considered in arrested patients. Even then, indications for this procedure are unclear.

Approach to Rewarming

No prospective, controlled studies comparing the various rewarming modalities have been done in humans. Therefore, firm guidelines for therapy cannot be given.

Patients with mild hypothermia, who are still in the ''excitation'' stage, generally improve spontaneously, as long as endogenous heat production mechanisms are functional. In addition, at temperatures above 30°C (86°F), the incidence of dysrhythmias is low, and rapid rewarming is rarely necessary.

By far the most important consideration is the patient's cardiovascular status; a secondary consideration is the presenting temperature. Some feel that patients with a stable cardiac rhythm (including sinus bradycardia and atrial fibrillation) and stable vital signs do not need rapid rewarming, even if the temperature is very low. They recommend passive rewarming and noninvasive internal modalities (e.g., warm moist oxygen and warm intravenous fluids) in this setting. Others argue that profoundly hypothermic patients, even if currently "stable," are at risk of developing life-threatening dysrhythmias. They recommend rapid rewarming until the temperature has reached 30 to 32°C (86–89.6°F) to minimize the time period during which dysrhythmias may develop. The relative merits of each approach have not been studied.

Patients with cardiovascular insufficiency or instability, including persistent hypotension and life-threatening dysrhythmias, need to be rewarmed rapidly. The best method remains to be definitively determined. Extracorporeal techniques offer many advantages but are often unavailable. If extracorporeal rewarming is not available, multiple other rewarming modalities can be used simultaneously.

PROGNOSIS

Many hypothermic patients have severe infections or other life-threatening illnesses. Patients with "uncomplicated" hypothermia (often purely due to cold exposure) have a fairly low mortality rate; patients with significant associated diseases have a much worse prognosis.[21] In terms of ultimate outcome, the underlying disease process is far more important than the initial temperature or the rewarming method chosen. Therefore, evaluation and treatment of these patients must include a search for associated diseases as well as treatment of the hypothermia itself.

The protective effect of hypothermia may have an important influence on prognosis; decreased oxygen requirements can protect the brain and other organs against anoxic and ischemic damage. This means that the usual criteria indicating death or irreversibility of disease are not valid in the hypothermic patient, who may even survive prolonged cardiac arrest without neurologic sequelae.

Hypothermic patients may recover completely after presenting in a rigid, apneic state with fixed and dilated pupils. Recovery has been documented with core temperatures as low as 14.2°C (57.6°F),[22] and with cardiac arrest for 6.5 h.[23] Death in hypothermia must be defined as a failure to revive with rewarming; unless there is strong evidence that the patient is not viable, resuscitative efforts should be continued until core temperature is at least 30 to 32°C (86–89.6°F).

DISPOSITION

Patients with mild accidental hypothermia caused purely by environmental exposure may be discharged after rewarming in the emergency department, provided that they are asymptomatic and can return to a warm environment. Most other hypothermic patients require hospital admission, both for the management of hypothermia and for the evaluation and management of underlying diseases.

REFERENCES

1. Centers for Disease Control and Prevention: Hypothermia-related deaths—Georgia, January 1996–December 1997, and United States, 1979–1995. *MMWR* 47:1037, 1998.
2. Clemmer TP, Fisher CJ, Bone RC, et al: Hypothermia in the sepsis syndrome and clinical outcome. *Crit Care Med* 20:1395, 1992.
3. Danzl DF, Pozos RF: Accidental hypothermia. *N Engl J Med* 331:1756, 1994.
4. Weinberg AD: Hypothermia. *Ann Emerg Med* 22(part2):370, 1993.
5. Corneli HM: Accidental hypothermia. *J Pediatr* 120:671, 1992.
6. Lloyd EL: Accidental hypothermia. *Resuscitation* 32:111, 1996.
7. Delaney KA, Howland MA, Vassallo S, et al: Assessment of acid-base disturbances in hypothermia and their physiologic consequences. *Ann Emerg Med* 18:72, 1989.
8. Ream AK, Reitz BA, Silverberg G: Temperature correction of P_{CO_2} and pH in estimating acid-base status: An example of the emperor's new clothes? *Anesthesiology* 56:41, 1982.
9. Fitzgerald FT: Hypoglycemia and accidental hypothermia in an alcoholic population. *West J Med* 133:105, 1980.
10. Palve H, Vuori A: Pulse oximetry during low cardiac output and hypothermia states immediately after open heart surgery. *Crit Care Med* 17:66, 1989.
11. Danzl DF, Pozos RS, Auerbach PS, et al: Multicenter hypothermia survey. *Ann Emerg Med* 16:1042, 1987.
12. Elenbaas RM, Mattson K, Cole H, et al: Bretylium in hypothermia-induced ventricular fibrillation in dogs. *Ann Emerg Med* 13:994, 1984.
13. Murphy K, Nowak RM, Tomlanovich MC: Use of bretylium tosylate as prophylaxis and treatment in hypothermic ventricular fibrillation in the canine model. *Ann Emerg Med* 15:1160, 1986.
14. Koller R, Schnider TW, Neidhart P: Deep accidental hypothermia and cardiac arrest—Rewarming with forced air. *Acta Anaesthesiol Scand* 41:1359, 1997.
15. Steele MT, Nelson MJ, Sessler DI, et al: Forced air speeds rewarming in accidental hypothermia. *Ann Emerg Med* 27:479, 1996.
16. Otto RJ, Metzler MH: Rewarming from experimental hypothermia: Comparison of heated aerosol inhalation, peritoneal lavage, and pleural lavage. *Crit Care Med* 16:869, 1988.
17. Barr GL: Correction of hypothermia by continuous pleural perfusion. *Surgery* 103:553, 1988.
18. Walpoth BH, Walpoth-Aslan BN, Mattle HP, et al: Outcome of survivors of accidental deep hypothermia and circulatory arrest treated with extracorporeal blood warming. *N Engl J Med* 337:1500, 1997.
19. Lazar HL: The treatment of hypothermia. *N Engl J Med* 337:1545, 1997.
20. Gentilello LM, Cobean RA, Offner PJ, et al: Continuous arteriovenous rewarming: Rapid reversal of hypothermia in critically ill patients. *J Trauma* 32:316, 1992.
21. Miller JW, Danzl DF, Thomas DM: Urban accidental hypothermia: 135 cases. *Ann Emerg Med* 9:456, 1980.
22. Dobson JA, Burgess JJ: Resuscitation of severe hypothermia by extracorporeal rewarming in a child. *J Trauma* 40:483, 1996.
23. Lexow K: Severe accidental hypothermia: Survival after 6 hours 30 minutes of cardiopulmonary resuscitation. *Arctic Med Res* 50(Suppl 6):112, 1991.

HEAT EMERGENCIES

James S. Walker
S. Brent Barnes

Humankind has developed an amazing ability to acclimatize and adapt to environmental heat. Despite these adaptations, history is filled with the accounts of the devastating effects of heat on humans. Heat-related illnesses are not simply an interesting historical footnote but are still commonly seen today.

EPIDEMIOLOGY

Between 1979 and 1995, a total of 6615 deaths (about 390 per year) in the United States were considered to be caused by the effects of heat and excessive heat exposure.[1] Because many of those who died were elderly, with underlying cardiopulmonary illnesses, there is a general acknowledgment that deaths caused by heat are underreported.[2] Estimations of the number of heat-related deaths per year have been as high as 4000 in the United States. The annual rate of heat-related deaths is highest among the elderly: fewer than 1 per million in the 5- to 44-year age group and increasing to about 5 per million in the over-85-year age group.[1] The young are also at increased risk, with attack rates of 0.3 per million among those younger than age 4 versus 0.05 among those older than age 4.[1] Heat-related illness is the second leading cause of death among young athletes. For patients with heatstroke, the most severe heat-related illness syndrome, mortality rates range from 10 to 75 percent. Heat-related illness and deaths are clearly related to high environmental temperature, and increased numbers have been seen in urban heat waves in the United States and elsewhere.[3,4] Although heat-related illness occurs in healthy individuals exposed to extremes of heat and humidity, it is especially dangerous for those impaired by chronic illness, drugs, and age.

PATHOPHYSIOLOGY

Body temperature is dependent on the balance between heat production from metabolism and heat loss (or gain) to the environment. The heat-balance equation is

$$\text{Body heat} = \text{metabolism} + [+\ \text{conduction} + \text{radiation} + \text{convection} - \text{evaporation}]$$

$$\text{Body heat} = M + [+K + R + C - E]$$

Through the four mechanisms of radiation, convection, conduction, and evaporation, the body is able to maintain core temperature within a very narrow range. Radiation, conduction, and convection are considered sensible or ''dry'' heat-exchange mechanisms. Heat can be transferred in either direction by these three methods: heat can be gained or lost, depending on the environment and the body. Radiation, which is heat transferred by electromagnetic waves, is the primary mechanism of heat loss when the air temperature is lower than body temperature, accounting for 65 percent of cooling in such an environment. Convection is heat exchange between a surface and a medium, usually the air water molecules circulating around the body, and is usually a minor mechanism of heat loss, accounting for only 10 to 15 percent. Once environmental air temperature exceeds body temperature, however, convection can be a source of heat gain. Convection is greatly affected by winds: as wind speed increases, the amount of heat loss through convection also increases. Conduction, which is heat exchange between two surfaces in direct contact with each other, accounts for only 2 percent of heat loss under normal circumstances. However, the conductivity of water is 25 percent times greater than air; thus, heat can be lost very quickly with immersion in cool water.

Evaporation is considered insensible or ''wet'' heat exchange. Unlike the ''dry'' or sensible heat exchanges in which heat can be gained or lost, evaporation can only result in heat loss. Evaporation is the conversion of liquid to a gaseous phase at the expense of energy. Humans primarily disperse heat by evaporation through the mechanism of sweating; the respiratory component of evaporation does not contribute significantly to heat loss. Sweating can dissipate a tremendous amount of heat, and in an environment in which the air temperature is greater than the body temperature, sensible exchange mechanisms cease to become a source of heat gain, and evaporation becomes the only means of heat dispersal. Sweat that drips to the ground or is wiped off does not result in significant heat loss. Actual evaporation must take place for heat loss to occur. Conditions of high humidity block evaporation, and conditions of both high humidity and high ambient temperatures are particularly hazardous.

PHYSIOLOGIC RESPONSE TO HEAT

The body shows a rapid and remarkable response to heat stress. As the core temperature rises, afferent receptors stimulate the anterior hypothalamus, causing multiple physiologic responses that result in heat loss. The hypothalamus stimulates the autonomic nervous system, resulting in a decrease in vasomotor tone and increased blood flow to the skin. This can cause a marked increase in cutaneous blood flow, from 0.2 to 0.5 L/min in cool temperature to 7 to 8 L/min in hot temperature. Sweating is stimulated by parasympathetic fibers, with the recruitment of more sweat glands followed by an increase in sweating rate of each gland. Sweating can increase dramatically, from less than 0.5 L/day in a temperate environment to 10 to 15 L/day in a trained individual exercising in a warm environment. Sweating is an efficient means of cooling. Evaporation of 1 L of sweat consumes 600 kcal of heat. For this reason, dehydration can predispose individuals to heat illness by inhibiting their sweating.[5] The tremendous peripheral vasodilation results in significant stress on the heart; cardiac output rises approximately 3 L/min for each 1°C (1.8°F) rise in core body temperature.[6] Since stroke volume is reduced by peripheral vasodilation, a compensatory rise in heart rate is required in order to maintain cardiac output. Patients with preexisting cardiac disease or on medications that blunt an increased heart rate are at significant risk for heat injury.

Acclimatization

Through acclimatization, the body adapts to a more efficient response to intense heat exposure. Acclimatization results from repeated bouts of moderate exercise in a hot environment. During acclimatization, physiologic changes occur that result in sweating at lower temperatures, a higher sweat rate, an increase in peripheral blood flow, and a decreased sodium chloride concentration in sweat and urine, due to increased aldosterone secretion. The end result of these physiologic changes includes a decreased heart rate, a decreased core body temperature, increased plasma volume, increased exercise tolerance time, and decreased perceived exertion.[7,8] Acclimatization requires repeated exposures to heat: usually 1 to 4 h/day for 14 days. The results of acclimatization are transient and are lost if heat exposure does not continue.

Factors Predisposing to Heat Injury

Serious heat injury does not occur at random: heat-injury victims almost always have one or more identifiable risk factors. The three factors that influence the temperature regulation of the body are (1) increased internal heat production, (2) increased external heat gain, and (3) decreased ability to disperse heat. Conditions that produce increased heat gain or decreased heat dispersal can quickly overwhelm the body's physiologic adaptive systems and lead to serious heat injury.

INCREASED INTERNAL HEAT PRODUCTION The three most common causes of increased heat production are physical activity, febrile illnesses, and pharmacologic agents. Any form of vigorous physical activity can quickly produce temperature elevation through internal heat production. Exercise is the most common cause of internal heat production from physical activity. Highly trained athletes have been shown to generate heat in excess of 1033 kcal/h, which can lead to an increase in body temperature of 0.3°C/min (0.54°F/min).[9] Other forms of activity that involve skeletal muscle contraction, such as seizures, neuroleptic malignant syndrome, combative behavior, and drug-withdrawal states, can also markedly increase internal heat production.

A febrile illness is the most common cause of an increased core body temperature. Hyperthermia due to fever has a completely different pathophysiologic cause than does environmental hyperthermia. Fever results from pyrogens derived from activated immune system cells that ''reset'' the thermoregulatory center in the hypothalamus. The body will actually utilize heat-producing mechanisms, such as shivering, to maintain this new set point. Treatment of simple fever differs drastically from treatment of environmental hyperthermia. Attempts at cooling the body of a patient with fever will result in shivering and an attempt to maintain the increased set-point temperature. Fever is treated with antipyretics, which block the molecular interaction that leads to fever. Antipyretics are not useful in environmental hyperthermia. A febrile illness is a risk factor for heat injury, because the body will use autonomic mechanisms to increase body temperature. Hyperthyroidism and pheochromocytoma also lead to increased endogenous heat production.

Many pharmacologic agents can increase internal heat production through various mechanisms. Amphetamines and cocaine cause increased muscle activity and lead to heat production. Lysergic acid diethylamide (LSD) and phencyclidine (PCP) act on the central nervous system (CNS) to induce a hypermetabolic state. Salicylates uncouple oxidative phosphorylation, causing cellular energy generated by the oxidation of facts and glucose to be released as heat rather than stored as ATP.

INCREASED EXTERNAL HEAT GAIN Exposures to high ambient temperatures and high humidity can lead to rapid exogenous heat gain. During heat waves, direct exposure to sunlight, living on higher floors of multistory buildings, and lack of air conditioners have been shown to increase the risk of heatstroke markedly.[3,4,10] Interestingly, the use of fans has not been shown to decrease the risk of heatstroke.[11] During the heat wave of 1980, the risk of heatstroke was 49 times greater for people without home air-conditioning than for those with continuous home air-conditioning, making the lower socioeconomic class with poorer living conditions at increased risk. It has also been reported than simply spending 2 h/day in an air-conditioned environment such as a shopping mall significantly decreases the risk of heat injury for those not living in an air-conditioned environment.

Several measurements of environmental heat stress have been developed to help assess the risk of heat injury. Simple temperature measurement alone is not adequate in predicting risk of heat injury, because humidity and direct radiation must also be considered. The wet-bulb globe temperature (WBGT) index was developed to provide an indication of thermal load on military troops training in the field. The WBGT measures air temperature through a dry-bulb thermometer, humidity through a wet-bulb thermometer, and the radiant heat with a black-globe thermometer. Many agencies, including the military, use the WBGT as a guide for recommended outdoor activity levels:

$$\text{WBGT} = 0.7\ T_{wb} + 0.2\ T_{bg} + 0.1\ T_{db}$$

where T_{wb} is the wet-bulb temperature of ambient air measured in the shade, T_{bg} is black-globe temperature, and T_{db} is dry-bulb temperature. A WBGT greater than 33°C (91.4°F) has been shown to increase the incidence of heat injury and heatstroke significantly. The wet-bulb temperature is the most significant variable in the WBGT equation, emphasizing the importance of humidity in heat injury.

Another measurement of heat stress that is commonly reported in the weather segment of television newscasts is the heat index, which is determined by a complicated formula developed by the National Weather Service using the air temperature and relative humidity (Table 187-1). The heat index, often referred to as ''apparent temperature,'' is a measurement of how hot it actually feels when relative humidity is combined with the effects of air temperature. The heat index is calculated for shady, light-wind conditions. If there is exposure to direct sunlight, the heat index should be adjusted by adding 15°F.[6] The National Weather Service has reported that increasingly severe heat illnesses are seen with prolonged exposure or activity when the heat index is 105°F or greater. For this reason, the National Weather Service has identified specific procedures that will be followed when the heat index is expected to exceed 105° to 110°F for at least 2 consecutive days in a geographic region:

1. Heat index values will be included in zone and city weather forecasts
2. Special weather statements and public information statements will be released with a detailed discussion of the extent of the hazard including heat-index values, who will be most at risk for heat injury, and safety rules for reducing the risk of heat injury
3. Assistance will be given to state and local health officials in preparing Civil Emergency Messages in severe heat waves which will include detailed medical information and names and telephone numbers of health officials
4. All of the above information will be released to the media and over the National Oceanic and Atmospheric Administration's Weather Radio.

FACTORS THAT DECREASE ABILITY TO DISPERSE HEAT Several factors can lead to a decreased ability to disperse heat (Table 187-2). One of the most important of these is dehydration, which can develop

TABLE 187-1 Heat-Index Chart

Air temperature (°F)*										
120°	116	130	148							
115°	111	120	135	151						
110°	105	112	123	137	150					
105°	100	105	113	123	135	149				
100°	95	99	104	110	120	132	144			
95°	90	93	96	101	107	114	124	136		
90°	85	87	90	93	96	100	106	113	122	
85°	80	82	84	86	88	90	93	97	102	108
80°	75	77	78	79	81	82	85	86	88	91
75°	70	72	73	74	75	76	77	78	79	80
Relative humidity	10%	20%	30%	40%	50%	60%	70%	80%	90%	100%

*Add 15° to heat index if in direct sunlight.

Heat Index (°F)	Possible Heat Injuries with Prolonged Exposure
80–89	Fatigue possible
90–104	Heat cramps and heat exhaustion possible
105–129	Heat cramps, heat exhaustion likely, heatstroke possible
≥130	Heatstroke likely

Source: National Weather Service, Silver Spring, MD.

TABLE 187-2 Risk Factors for Serious Heat Injury/Heatstroke

Dehydration
Obesity
Heavy or impermeable clothing
Poor physical fitness
Lack of acclimatization
Cardiovascular disease
Skin diseases Burns Scleroderma Eczema Psoriasis Sweat gland disorders
Extreme ranges of age
Lack of mobility
Febrile illnesses
Hyperthyroidism
Alcoholism
Drug use Cocaine Amphetamines Opiates LSD PCP
Poor socioeconomic conditions Lack of air-conditioning Living on upper floor of multistory building
Prolonged exertion in heat Athletes Military recruits Miners Steelmill workers Firefighters Disaster relief workers
Medications Antipsychotics Anticholinergics Calcium-channel blockers β Blockers Diuretics α Agonists Sympathomimetics

quickly under intense heat stress. Even mild dehydration (as little as 1 percent) can impair physiologic and performance responses.[12] It is estimated that every 1 percent decrease in body weight from dehydration results in a body temperature increase of 0.1 to 0.3°C (0.18° to 0.54°F). Dehydration impairs cardiovascular and thermoregulatory function by decreasing skin blood flow and sweating rate, leading to a decreased ability to disperse heat. Even when fluid is available, the human body is not able to assess fluid losses accurately and compensate by oral rehydration. Even when fluid is readily available to athletes during exercise, they will voluntarily ingest only 50 percent of their sweat loss and can rapidly become dehydrated.[5]

Extremes of age are risk factors for heat illness. Infants and children are at increased risk of heat illness due to a greater surface area-mass ratio, the production of more metabolic heat per mass unit, and a decreased sweating capacity as compared with adults. The elderly are generally unable to disperse heat as well as younger people due to the frequent presence of neurovascular and cardiovascular disease, the use of multiple drugs that affect heat dispersal, increased obesity, decreased cutaneous blood supply, poorer physical conditioning, and reduced sweat production.

Cardiovascular disease is also a risk factor for heat illness, because the cardiovascular system is one of the primary systems that disperse heat. Patients with chronic cardiovascular diseases such as cardiomyopathies, congestive heart failure, valvular disease, and coronary artery disease may be unable to compensate for the increased stress that heat exposure causes on the cardiovascular system. This increased stress can lead to arrhythmias, myocardial infarction, congestive heart failure exacerbation, or heatstroke.

Obese people are at increased risk for heat illness. Adipose tissue has decreased vascularity and inhibits heat dispersal by decreasing blood flow to the skin. Obesity makes less area available for heat exchange, and the lower water content of adipose tissue leads to a higher elevation of body temperatures with exertion. In essence, adipose insulates the body.

By diminishing sweating ability, many skin diseases can decrease the ability to disperse heat. Scleroderma, cystic fibrosis, eczema, psoriasis, and burns decrease sweating ability. Congenital diseases, such as ectodermal dysplasia, involving the sweat glands increase risk of heat injury. Interestingly, even the presence of simple heat rash has been shown to decrease sweating. Histologic studies of skin with heat rash have demonstrated obstruction of sweat gland ducts by keratin debris, resulting in significantly lower sweating rates and decreased tolerance time in a hot environment.[13]

Clothing can act as a major deterrent to heat dispersal. Thick clothing has less thermal conductance, a lower evaporative capability, and less wind resistance and thus can significantly impair heat loss. The evaporative rate of water loss from wet skin depends on skin-clothing–ambient air vapor pressure gradient.[14] Clothing that interferes with evaporation of sweat from skin causes an increase in skin temperature and lower cooling efficiency.

Many medications decrease the body's ability to disperse heat. The most notable agents include the anticholinergic agents, diuretics, phenothiazines, cardiovascular drugs, and sympathomimetic agents (this can be remembered by the mnemonic All Desert People Capitulate Sweat). All anticholinergic agents impair the sweating response. Diuretics lead to volume depletion and a decreased cardiac output, resulting in diminished sweating. Phenothiazines deplete the central stores of dopamine and interfere with the thermoregulatory center of the hypothalamus. They also have anticholinergic properties. Cardiovascular medications such as β blockers, calcium-channel blockers, or α agonists decrease the cardiovascular response to heat and reduce peripheral blood flow and the ability to sweat. Sympathomimetics lead to cutaneous vasoconstriction, which decreases sweating.

Alcohol and drug abuse can lead to decreased heat dispersal. Alcohol inhibits antidiuretic hormone and leads to a relative dehydration that can contribute to heat illness. The influence of alcohol can also blunt the stimulation to leave a hot area and seek a cooler environment. Other drugs such as heroin and cocaine can predispose individuals to heat injury. Endogenous endorphins and adrenocorticotropic hormone are likely involved in the body's adaptation to heat. Chronic abusers of heroin, cocaine, or alcohol have disruption of the endorphin response to thermal stress, predisposing them to heat injury.[15]

CLINICAL FEATURES

Heat-related illnesses are usually divided into minor syndromes (e.g., heat edema, prickly heat, heat syncope, heat cramps, and heat exhaustion) and major syndromes (e.g., heatstroke).

Heat Edema

This is a self-limited process manifested by mild swelling and tightening of the hands and feet that appears within the first few days of exposure to a hot environment. Heat edema is due to cutaneous vasodilatation and orthostatic pooling of interstitial fluid in the extremities. Some authorities feel increased secretion of aldosterone and antidiuretic hormone also plays a role. It is found most commonly in elderly nonacclimatized individuals who are physically active after a prolonged period of sitting in a car, bus, or plane. To a lesser extent, it is seen in healthy travelers just arriving from a colder climate. Edema is usually mild and does not restrict normal activities. Rarely, pitting edema of the ankles may develop, but heat edema does not progress to the pretibial region. A typical history and thorough physical examination are sufficient to exclude systemic causes of edema. Heat edema usually resolves spontaneously in a few days but may take up to 6 weeks. No special treatment is necessary. If a patient is insistent on treatment, elevation of the legs and the use of support hose will facilitate the removal of the interstitial fluid. Diuretics are not effective and can predispose patients to electrolyte abnormalities, volume depletion, or a more serious heat illness.

Prickly Heat

This is a pruritic, maculopapular, erythematous rash over clothed areas of the body. Also known as lichen tropicus, miliaria rubra, or heat rash, it is an acute inflammation of the sweat ducts caused by blockage of the sweat pores by macerated stratum corneum. The ducts become dilated under pressure and ultimately rupture, producing superficial vesicles in the malpighian layer of the skin on a red base. Itching is the predominant clinical feature during this phase and is treated successfully with antihistamines. Prickly heat can be prevented by wearing clean, light, and loose-fitting clothing and avoiding sweat-generating situations. The use of talc or baby power is of no benefit. Sometimes, ducts become secondarily infected with *Staphylococcus aureus*. Chlorhexidine in a light cream or lotion is the treatment of choice in the acute phase.

With prolonged heat exposure, a keratin plug fills the duct, causing obstruction in the stratum malpighian layer. When the duct ruptures a second time, the resultant vesicle will be driven deeper into the dermis. This rash simulates the white papules of piloerection and is not pruritic. This is known as the profunda stage of prickly heat and can readily advance into a chronic dermatitis. Infection with *S. aureus* is a common complication and requires the use of dicloxacillin or erythromycin. The skin can be desquamated by applying 1% salicylic acid to the affected area three times a day. Caution should be used to avoid salicylate toxicity.

Heat Syncope

This is a variant of postural hypotension resulting from the cumulative effect of peripheral vasodilation, decreased vasomotor tone, and relative volume depletion. It occurs most commonly in nonacclimatized individuals during the early stages of heat exposure. It does not necessarily represent a state of significant volume depletion.

Evaluation of patients with heat syncope requires the usual exclusion of neurologic, metabolic, and cardiovascular disorders. Patients should also be examined for any injuries acquired as a result of the syncopal episode and subsequent fall. Treatment consists of removal from the heat source, oral or intravenous rehydration, and rest. Hospitalization is usually not necessary. Most patients with heat syncope recover promptly with fluids.

Heat Cramps

These are painful, involuntary, spasmodic contractions of skeletal muscles, usually those of the calves, although they may involve the thighs and shoulders. Heat cramps usually occur in individuals who are sweating liberally and replace fluid loss with water or other hypotonic solutions. Cramps may occur during exercise or after a latent period of several hours. Unconditioned or nonacclimatized individuals who are just starting manual labor in a hot environment are at high risk for developing heat cramps. Although heat cramps usually do not cause significant morbidity and are considered to be self-limiting, the pain associated with them can readily result in an emergency department visit. In fact, the pain is commonly recalcitrant to the effects of narcotics alone.

The exact pathogenesis of heat cramps is not known but is generally accepted to be a relative deficiency of sodium, potassium, and fluid at the cellular level. The production of large amounts of sweat, which has a high sodium content, coupled with inadequate sodium replacement results in hyponatremia. This in turn produces muscle cramps by interfering with calcium-dependent muscle relaxation. Hypokalemia from hyperventilation and dehydration may also play a contributing role.

Treatment consists of rest in a cool environment and fluid and salt replacement, either orally or intravenously. For mild cases, or if an overwhelming number of patients require treatment, a 0.1% to 0.2% saline solution can be given orally. Many electrolyte drinks are commercially available. More severe cases of heat cramps will respond to intravenous rehydration with normal saline. Rarely, rhabdomyolysis occurs secondary to protracted and diffuse muscle spasm.

Heat cramps can be prevented by maintaining adequate dietary salt intake or by drinking commercial electrolyte beverages. Salt tablets by themselves should not be used because (1) the tablets are a gastric irritant and often result in nausea and vomiting and (2) they do not replace volume.

Heat Tetany

This is characterized by hyperventilation resulting in respiratory alkalosis, paresthesia, and carpopedal spasm, and is usually associated with short periods of intense heat stress. Treatment consists of removal from heat and decreasing the respiratory rate. Generally, concomitant heat cramps are not present.

Heat Exhaustion

This is an obscure syndrome characterized by nonspecific symptoms such as dizziness, weakness, malaise, light-headedness, fatigue, nausea, vomiting, headache, and myalgias. Clinical manifestations include syncope, orthostatic hypotension, sinus tachycardia, tachypnea, diaphoresis, and hyperthermia. The core temperature is variable, however, and can range from normal to 40°C (104°F). Mental status remains normal. Because of the ill-defined and nonspecific symptoms, heat exhaustion is a diagnosis of exclusion. Physiologically, heat exhaustion is characterized by a combination of salt depletion and water depletion. Heat cramps may also be present on rare occasions.

Laboratory studies will almost universally demonstrate hemoconcentration, although specific electrolyte abnormalities depend on the ratio of fluid and electrolyte losses to intake. Patients who have virtually no fluid intake of any kind will usually develop hypernatremia, whereas those who partially rehydrate with salt-containing fluids may develop isotonic dehydration with normal sodium and chloride levels. Serum potassium and magnesium levels are variable.

Heat exhaustion is treated by rest and volume and electrolyte replacement. Rapid administration of moderate amounts of intravenous fluids (1 to 2 L of saline solution) may be necessary in some patients who demonstrate significant tissue hypoperfusion. The choice of solution is guided by laboratory determinations, but balanced salt solutions may be used until specific electrolyte abnormalities are determined to be present. Generally, these patients do not require hospitalization.

The signs and symptoms of early heatstroke may be difficult to differentiate from heat exhaustion. Patients with heat exhaustion will have normal findings on neurologic examination and normal mental status, although they may complain of headache, dizziness, weakness, or blurring of vision. Any patient with altered mental status in this situation has heatstroke.

Heatstroke

Classically, heatstroke is defined as the triad of a core temperature greater than 40.5°C (104.9°F), CNS dysfunction, and anhidrosis. However, anhidrosis, or a lack of sweating may not be present for a variety of reasons and is not considered to be an absolute diagnostic criterion. Subsequently, anyone with hyperpyrexia and CNS dysfunction should be considered to have a heatstroke, which is a medical emergency with multiple organ system involvement and a high mortality rate and requires immediate intervention.

The CNS is particularly vulnerable in heatstroke, manifesting with such symptoms as irritability, bizarre behavior, combativeness, hallucinations, seizures, or coma. The cerebellum is highly sensitive to heat, and ataxia can be an early finding. Virtually any neurologic abnormality may be present in heatstroke, including plantar responses, decorticate and decerebrate posturing, hemiplegia, status epilepticus, and coma. Cerebral edema is a common finding. CNS dysfunction is universal at core temperatures higher than 42°C (107.6°F). However, there is no arbitrary core temperature threshold for heatstroke. Cellular injury is a function of both the maximum temperature reached and the time of exposure. Patients with lower temperatures for longer periods may do worse than patients with higher temperatures for shorter periods.

The presence or absence of sweating has traditionally been one of the important distinctions between true heatstroke and other heat emergencies. The presence of sweating does not exclude the diagnosis of heatstroke. Patients with early heatstroke typically demonstrate marked sweating but eventually develop anhidrosis due to profound volume depletion or sweat gland dysfunction.

Heatstroke is a total breakdown of thermoregulation. Traditionally, two forms of heatstroke have been described: nonexertional and exertional. Nonexertional or ''classic'' heatstroke usually occurs during summer heat waves. Since physical exertion is not a major component of heat production in classic heatstroke, it tends to be more insidious in onset. Because of this slow evolution, there is sufficient time for fluid and electrolyte abnormalities to develop. The poor, the elderly, infants, and the chronically ill are a greatest risk. The pathophysiology is increased exogenous heat gain and diminished heat dispersion. The specific stressors are lack of air-conditioning, presence of cardiovascular disease, older age, and use of cardiovascular or anticholinergic drugs. Small children are at risk because of the immaturity of their thermoregulatory systems, as well as their dependence on others for fluids.

Exertional heatstroke usually strikes a younger segment of the population as a consequence of vigorous physical activity. The primary cause is increased endogenous heat production. Individuals who perform physical labor or exercise in a hot, humid climate are especially prone to develop exertional heatstroke. The distinction between exertional and nonexertional heatstroke is moot, because signs, symptoms, and management are the same. The primary factor that contributes to the morbidity and mortality of heat illness is the severity of underlying disease and not the absolute height of the core temperature.

The definitive diagnosis of environmental heatstroke is a diagnosis of exclusion. The differential diagnosis for fever and altered mental status is varied and lengthy (Table 187-3). However, once heatstroke is suspected, efforts to lower the body temperature must be initiated immediately by whatever means available, whether in the prehospital or emergency department setting. A delay in cooling represents a primary reason for the high potential mortality rate associated with heatstroke.

TABLE 187-3 Differential Diagnosis of Heatstroke

Alcohol withdrawal syndrome	Meningitis
Neuroleptic malignant syndrome	Brain abscess
Malignant hyperthermia	Malaria (cerebral falciparum)
Anticholinergic toxicity	Typhoid fever
Salicylate toxicity	Status epilepticus
PCP, cocaine, or amphetamine toxicity	Cerebral hemorrhage
Tetanus	Diabetic ketoacidosis
Sepsis	Thyroid storm
Encephalitis	

TREATMENT OF HEATSTROKE

Initial Resuscitation

Initial attention must be paid to the ABCs, with the initiation of high-flow supplemental oxygen, continuous pulse oximetry and cardiac monitoring, and intravenous access (we recommend the initial infusion of normal saline or lactated Ringer's solution at 250 mL/h). If a patient is elderly or has cardiovascular disease, it is wise to monitor cardiac filling pressures (central venous pressure or pulmonary artery occlusion pressure) to guide fluid therapy. A Foley catheter should be inserted. Of paramount importance is the serial monitoring of the patient's core temperature. This is best accomplished by inserting an electronic rectal thermistor probe or a temperature probe equipped Foley catheter. Another option, especially in intubated patients, is the use of an esophageal thermometer.

Diagnostic studies necessary to detect the end-organ sequelae of heatstroke include a complete blood cell count, comprehensive metabolic profile, hepatic panel, coagulation profile (prothrombin time, partial thromboplastin time, and international normalized ratio), creatine kinase, urinalysis, toxicology screen, ECG, and chest radiograph. Computed tomography of the head and lumbar puncture may also be indicated as part of the evaluation of altered mental status.

Cooling Techniques

Rapid reduction of core temperature to 40°C (104°F) is the primary goal of treatment and is accomplished by physical cooling techniques. Antipyretics are not effective. The fastest cooling techniques reported in the literature are usually implemented in a structured research laboratory environment, using animal models and equipment and techniques that are not universally available. In clinical practice, a technique that allows easy patient access and is readily available is preferable to a technique that may be faster but is difficult to perform or does not permit easy access to the patient (Table 187-4). Many of the techniques may be used in combination. Although effective and reported to be widely used, immersion cooling is relatively contraindicated if the patient may require cardiac monitoring and defibrillation. Also, the efficiency of immersion has been primarily documented in young, healthy patients without comorbid diseases. The safety and efficacy of immersion in classic heatstroke victims has not been established. Special considerations should be taken for invasive cooling techniques. Iced gastric lavage should not be used unless the airway is protected.

TABLE 187-4 Comparison of Cooling Techniques

Technique	Advantages	Disadvantages
Evaporative	Simple, readily available Noninvasive Easy monitoring and patient access Relatively more rapid	Constant moistening of skin surface required to maximize heat loss
Immersion	Noninvasive Relatively more rapid	Cumbersome Patient monitoring and access difficult Shivering Poorly tolerated by conscious patients
Ice packing	Noninvasive Readily available	Shivering Poorly tolerated by conscious patients
Strategic ice packs	Noninvasive Readily available Can be combined with other techniques	Relatively slower Shivering Poorly tolerated by conscious patients
Cold gastric lavage	Can be combined with other techniques	Relatively slower Invasive May require airway protection Human experience limited
Cold peritoneal lavage	Very rapid	Invasive Human experience limited

Iced peritoneal lavage is relatively contraindicated if the patient is pregnant or has had previous abdominal surgery.

We favor evaporative cooling as the technique of choice: it is simple and the fastest noninvasive cooling technique in humans. Other simple measures include ice packs placed at the groin and axillae to cool blood in the axillary and femoral vessels. Gastric lavage is safe if a patient is intubated. Cooling with peritoneal lavage is an effective and rapid central cooling technique. Immersion cooling should be limited to situations where evaporative cooling is not possible.

Evaporative cooling is performed by positioning fan(s) close to the completely undressed patient and then sponging the skin or spraying tepid water on the patient. Inexpensive plastic spray bottles work the best. We avoid covering the patient with sheets and then wetting the sheets, because this impairs evaporation of heat from the skin. Only one person is needed to monitor and continue cooling the patient.

An extremely effective means of evaporative cooling reported in the literature is the Makkah body cooling unit (BCU).[16] Patients are placed undressed on a modified hammock or litter, sprayed with lukewarm water, and room temperature air is blown over them with powerful fans. This is the method of field treatment for pilgrims traveling to Mecca who succumb to heatstroke. The BCU is very effective in treating patients who are vasodilated and in a dry environment. This mode of therapy would not be ideal for patients in shock or in a humid environment. Also, it may be difficult to reproduce these physical conditions in conventional clinical practice.

Two problems associated with complications of evaporative cooling are shivering and inability of cardiac electrodes to adhere to the skin. Shivering is treated primarily with intravenous benzodiazepines and secondarily with phenothiazines. Phenothiazines, however, lower the seizure threshold. Cardiac electrodes can be applied to a patient's back.

Immersion cooling is performed by placing an undressed patient into a tub of water deep enough to cover the trunk and extremities. The head must be kept out of the water. Cardiac monitoring electrodes and rectal temperature probes must be secured to the patient. Problems associated with immersion cooling include shivering, displacement of monitoring leads, and inability to perform defibrillation or resuscitative procedures.

The most rapid method of cooling a heatstroke victim is cardiopulmonary bypass. Although the logistics and availability are major drawbacks, it may be required if a patient's condition is recalcitrant to all other measures.

Regardless of the cooling technique chosen, cooling efforts should be discontinued when the rectal temperature reaches 40°C (104°F). Continued cooling below this temperature will lead to "overshoot hypothermia."

Treatment of Complications

Some of the complications associated with heatstroke occur early as opposed to late (Table 187-5). In patients with a relatively intact cardiovascular system, heat stress causes an increase in heart rate and cardiac index. Most heatstroke victims have a high cardiac index, elevated central venous pressure, and a low peripheral resistance. However, heart failure, pulmonary edema, and cardiovascular collapse can occur even in young healthy individuals. In any age group, the presence of hypotension, decreased cardiac output, and a falling cardiac index indicates a particularly poor prognosis. A pulmonary artery catheter may be necessary in the assessment of appropriate volume replacement.

Centrilobular necrosis due to direct thermal injury results in abnormal liver functions, although jaundice is unusual. Recovery is to be expected. Renal injury is manifested by microscopic hematuria, proteinuria, and hyaline and granular casts. Patients with hypovolemic complications and decreased renal blood flow may develop acute tubular necrosis. Exercise-induced heatstroke is often complicated by rhabdomyolysis, sometimes with massive myoglobinuria and renal failure. This complication may not develop until several days after the initial injury, so that careful monitoring of creatine kinase levels and renal function is necessary. Occasionally, a patient may present to the emergency department with the dark urine of myoglobinuria and should be questioned about recent heat exposure or heavy exertion.

Widespread hematologic disorders may be apparent both clinically and on laboratory evaluation. Purpura, conjunctival hemorrhages, petechiae, pulmonary, gastrointestinal, and renal hemorrhages may be present. Coagulation studies may show thrombocytopenia, hypopro-

TABLE 187-5 Complications of Heatstroke

Initial	Delayed
Hypotension	Hyperkalemia
Shivering	Hypocalcemia
Seizures	Hyperuricemia
Coma	Renal failure
Hypothermia, overshoot	Cerebral edema
Hyperthermic rebound	Hyperosmolar coma
Electrocardiographic changes	Persistent neurologic deficit
Pulmonary edema (cardiogenic)	Thrombocytopenia
Congestive heart failure	Disseminated intravascular coagulation
Hypokalemia	Hepatic failure
Hypernatremia	Adult respiratory distress syndrome
Rhabdomyolysis	Gastrointestinal hemorrhage
Diarrhea	

Source: Adapted from Tek and Olshaker,[8] with permission.

thrombinemia, and hypofibrinogenemia. Thermal injury to the vascular endothelium causes increased platelet aggregation, changes in capillary permeability, thermal deactivation of plasma proteins resulting in a decreased level of clotting factors, and, rarely, disseminated intravascular coagulation or fibrinolysis.

As expected, the fluid and electrolyte abnormalities vary with the onset and duration of the disorder, underlying disease (especially cardiovascular disease), and prior use of medications such as diuretics. The most important consideration with respect to fluid and electrolyte abnormalities in heatstroke is that dehydration and volume depletion may not occur in classic heatstroke, whereas they are common signs in heat exhaustion. Vigorous fluid administration may produce pulmonary edema, especially in the elderly. A myriad of blood-gas abnormalities may be encountered, from respiratory alkalosis to severe metabolic acidosis.

Disposition

All of the minor heat illnesses except for heat exhaustion can be managed totally in the emergency department, and then patients can be safely discharged to home care and for outpatient follow-up. Patients with heat exhaustion who are at the extremes of age and have substantial volume depletion, comorbid diseases, or heat-induced end-organ damage should be admitted to the hospital.

Heatstroke is a true medical emergency, and all patients with this diagnosis should be admitted. The issue of whether to admit to the floor as opposed to the intensive care unit depends on the level of service that will be required as an inpatient. Patients who are hemodynamically labile, those who need continued cooling, or those who require invasive hemodynamic monitoring should be admitted to the intensive care unit. If the original health care facility is unable to provide the services needed for quality care, then the patient should be referred to a higher-level facility.

Prevention

Serious heat-related illness is predictable and preventable. The incidence of heatstroke can be reduced by (1) attention to environmental conditions, (2) social service care for the chronically ill and the elderly, (3) access to air-conditioning for individuals at risk, (4) acclimatization for workers, athletes, and the military, (5) paced work schedules for those who need to work under adverse conditions, and (6) adequate hydration.[17–19]

REFERENCES

1. Centers for Disease Control and Prevention: Heat-related mortality: United States, 1997. *MMWR* 47:473, 1998.
2. Shen T, Howe HL, Alo C, Moolenaar RL: Toward a broader definition of heat-related death: A comparison of mortality estimates from medical examiners' classification with those from total death differentials during the July 1995 heat wave in Chicago, Illinois. *Am J Forensic Med Pathol* 19:113, 1998.
3. Semenza JC, Rubin CH, Falter KH, et al: Heat-related deaths during the July 1995 heat wave in Chicago. *N Engl J Med* 335:84, 1996.
4. Faunt JD, Wilkinson TJ, Aplin P, et al: The effete in the heat: Heat-related hospital presentations during a ten day heat wave. *Aust NZ J Med* 25:117121, 1995.
5. Noakes TD, Adams BA, Myburgh C, et al: The danger of an inadequate water intake during prolonged exercise. *Eur J Appl Physiol* 57:210, 1988.
6. Bross MH, Nash BT, Carlton FB Jr: Heat emergencies. *Am Fam Physician* 50:389, 1994.
7. Barrow MW, Clark KA: Heat-related illnesses. *Am Fam Physician* 58:749, 1998.
8. Tek D, Olshaker JS: Heat illness. *Emerg Med Clin North Am* 10:299, 1992.
9. Hubbard RW: The role of exercise in the etiology of exertional heatstroke. *Med Sci Sports Exerc* 22:2, 1990.
10. *Heat wave: A Major Summer Killer*. Washington, DC, US Department of Commerce, National Oceanic and Atmospheric Administration, 1985; publication NOAA/PA 85001.
11. Khogali M: Heat-related illnesses. *Middle East J Anesthesiol* 12:531, 1994.
12. Sawka MN, Pandolf KB: Effect of body water loss on physiological function and exercise performance, in Gisolfi CV, Lamb DR (eds): *Perspectives in Exercise Science and Sports Medicine*, vol 3. Indianapolis, IN, Benchmark, 1990, pp 1–38
13. Pandolf KB, Griffin TB, Munro EH, Goldman RF: Persistence of impaired heat tolerance from artificially induced miliaria rubra. *Am J Physiol* 2393:R226, 1980.
14. Pascoe DD, Bellingar TA, McCluskey BS: Clothing and exercise: Influence of clothing during exercise/work in environmental extremes. *Sports Med* 18:94, 1994.
15. Vescovi PP, Coiro V: Hyperthermia and endorphins. *Biomed Parmacother* 47:301, 1993.
16. Khogali M: Makkah body cooling unit, in Khogali M, Hales JR S (eds): *Heat Stroke and Temperature Regulation*. Sydney, Academic, 1983, pp 139–148.
17. Armstrong LE, Maresh CM: The induction and decay of heat acclimatization in trained athletes. *Sports Med* 12:302, 1991.
18. Dellinger AM, Kachur SP, Sternberg E, Russell J: Risk of heat-related injury to disaster relief workers in a slow-onset flood disaster. *J Occup Environ Med* 38:689, 1996.
19. Dickinson JG: Heat illness in the services. *J R Army Med Corps* 140:7, 1994.

ARTHROPOD BITES AND STINGS

Richard F. Clark

The phylum Arthropoda is the largest division of the animal kingdom. The American Association of Poison Control Centers reported 79,378 cases of exposures to arthropods in 1997.[1] Just over 100 of these were listed as resulting in major or severe reactions, including severe pain, neurotoxicity, or other signs and symptoms. Only two fatalities were listed from contact with arthropods—both from Hymenoptera stings. Clearly, these number are the tip of the iceberg. Toxic reactions to multiple stings by members of the order of Hymenoptera and severe systemic allergic reactions to one or more stings or bites of other insects such as deerflies, blackflies, horseflies, and kissing bugs can all present as emergency, life-threatening situations (Table 188-1). Other arthropod envenomations merit review either for causing various organ system toxicities or as infectious disease vectors. This chapter will review the most common arthropod envenomations encountered by emergency physicians in the United States.

HYMENOPTERA (WASPS, BEES, AND ANTS)

The Hymenoptera are the most important venomous insects known to humans, and more fatalities result from stings by these insects than any other arthropod. There are three major subgroups or superfamilies of medical importance: (1) Apidae, including the honeybee and bumblebee, (2) Vespidae, including the yellow jackets, hornets, and wasps, and (3) Formicidae, or ants (Fig. 188-1).

Bees and Wasps (Apidae and Vespidae)

Apids, such as honeybees and bumblebees, are docile and tend to sting only when provoked. Bees are capable of stinging only once since its stinger has multiple barbs that cause the sting apparatus to detach from its body. Africanized honeybees, or so-called killer bees, are now found in Texas, Arizona, California, and some other southeastern states. These bees are hybrids of African bees that escaped from laboratories in Brazil during the 1950s and have spread successfully northward along the coasts and temperate regions of the continent.[2] Their venom is no more toxic than that of the American counterpart, but African honeybees are very aggressive and a hive can respond to

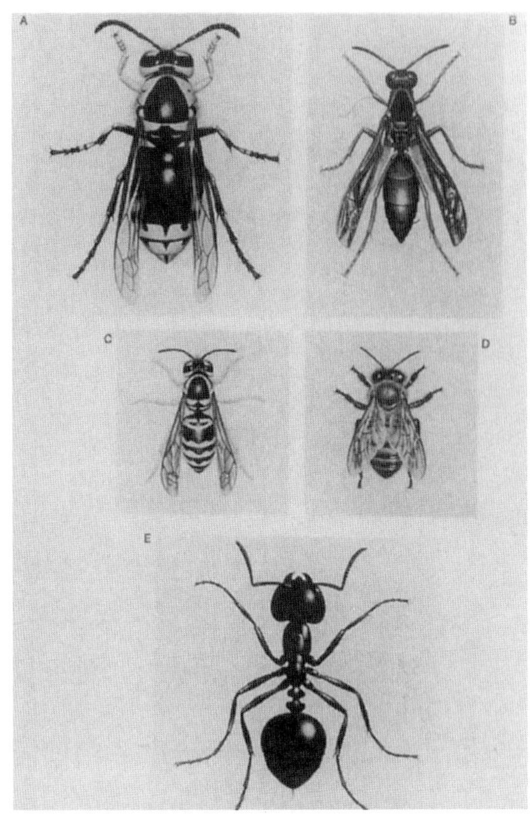

FIG. 188-1. Representative venomous hymenoptera. **A.** Hornet (*Vespula maculata*). **B.** Wasp (*Chlorion ichneumerea*). **C.** Yellow jacket (*Vespula maculiforma*). **D.** Honey bee (*Apis mellifera*). **E.** Fire ant (*Solenopsis invicta*). (Reproduced by permission of Merck, Sharp & Dohme, Division of Merck & Co., Inc.)

TABLE 188-1 Harmful Arthropods of the United States

Class and Order	Common Name	Bite	Sting
Hexapoda (Insecta)			
Hymenoptera	Bumblebees		×
	Sweat bees		×
	Honey bees		×
	Wasps		×
	Hornets		×
	Yellow jackets		×
	Fire ants		×
	Harvester ants		×
Diptera	Mosquitoes	×	
	Deerflies	×	
	Horseflies	×	
	Stable flies	×	
	Blackflies	×	
	Biting midges	×	
Hemiptera	Bedbugs	×	
	Kissing bugs	×	
Coleoptera	Blister beetles		×
Lepidoptera	Puss caterpillars		×
	Browntail caterpillars		×
	Buck mouth caterpillars		×
Siphonaptera	Fleas	×	
Anoplura	Lice	×	
Arachnida			
Araneida	Black widow	×	
	Brown recluse	×	
	Hobo spider	×	
	Tarantula	×	
Acarina	Chiggers (mite larvae)	×	
	Ticks	×	
Scorpionida	Scorpions		×

Source: Frazier CA: *Insect Allergy*. St. Louis: WH Green, 1987, p 421. Used by permission.

a perceived threat with 10 or more times the number of bees as a typical North American bee response. An attack from Africanized bees can lead to massive stinging resulting in multisystem damage and death from severe venom toxicity.[3] With no natural predators, it is predicted that Africanized bees eventually will inhabit much of the Southeast and Southwest of the United States.

Most of the allergic reactions reported each year from Hymenoptera occur from vespid (wasp, hornet, and yellow jacket) stings. These arthropods nest in the ground or in walls, have volatile tempers, and may be disturbed by work around the yard, including mowing, gardening, and outdoor sports. As with bees, only the females have stingers, adapted from the ovipositor on the posterior aspect of the abdomen. Although some vespids possess barbed stingers, all have adapted the ability to withdraw their stingers from the victim, enabling multiple stings.

VENOM Hymenoptera venom contains several components. Although histamine is one of those components and was once thought to be responsible for most of the reactions observed following envenomation, other substances have now been recognized as more important. Mellitin, a known membrane-active polypeptide, constitutes over 50 percent of the dry weight of bee venom. Since all Hymenoptera share many of these components, cross-sensitization may occur in individuals allergic to one species. Yellow jacket venom is perhaps the most potent sensitizer.

CLINICAL FEATURES The most common response to Hymenoptera venom consists of pain, slight erythema, edema, and pruritus at the

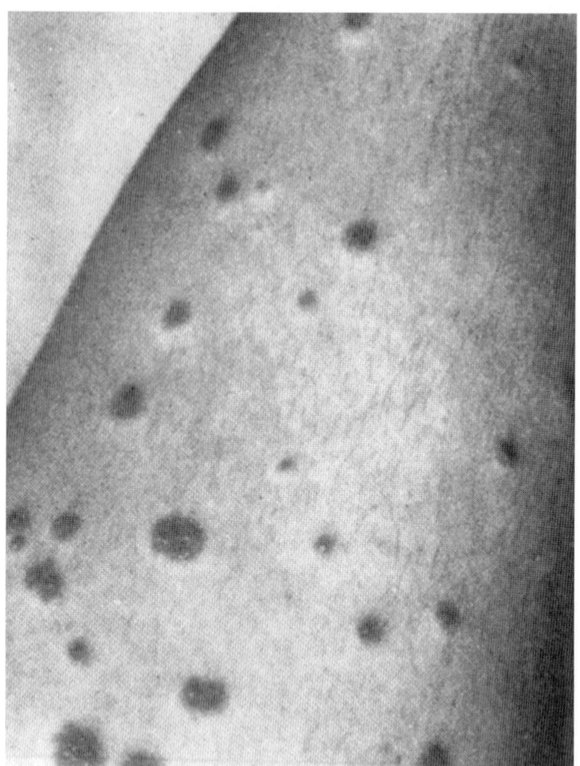

FIG. 188-2. Inflamed nodular reaction to insect bites. (From Moschella SL, Hurley HJ, eds: Dermatology, 2d ed. Philadelphia: Saunders, 1985, with permission.)

sting site. In addition to this response, more significant reactions may occur.[4,5]

Local Reaction A local reaction consists of marked and prolonged edema contiguous with the sting site (Fig. 188-2). Although there are no systemic signs or symptoms, a severe local reaction may involve one or more neighboring joints. A local reaction occurring in the mouth or throat can produce airway obstruction. Stings around the eye or on the lid may result in the development of an anterior capsule cataract, atrophy of the iris, lens abscess, perforation of the globe, glaucoma, or refractive changes. When local reactions become increasingly severe, the likelihood of future systemic reactions appears to increase and, if skin tests are positive, may warrant immunotherapy.

Toxic Reaction When there is a history of multiple stings, such as in an Africanized bee attack, a systemic toxic reaction from venom may occur. Symptoms of a toxic reaction may resemble anaphylaxis, but there is generally a greater frequency of nausea, vomiting, and diarrhea. Light-headedness and syncope are common signs. There also may be headache, fever, drowsiness, involuntary muscle spasms, edema without urticaria, and occasionally seizures. Urticaria and bronchospasm are not present, although respiratory insufficiency and arrest may occur. Renal and hepatic failure also has been reported, as well as disseminated intravascular coagulation (DIC). Symptoms usually subside within 48 h, but may last for several days in severe cases. Toxic reactions are believed to occur from a direct multisystem effect of the venom.

Anaphylactic Reaction A generalized systemic allergic or anaphylactic reaction, whether in response to a single sting or multiple stings, may range from mild to fatal, and death can occur within minutes. The majority of such reactions occur within the first 15 min, and nearly all occur within 6 h. There is no correlation between systemic reactions and the number of stings. In general, the shorter the interval between the sting and the onset of symptoms, the more severe is the reaction. Fatalities that occur within the first hour of the sting usually result from airway obstruction or hypotension. Initial symptoms usually consist of itching eyes, facial flushing, generalized urticaria, and dry cough. Symptoms may intensify rapidly with chest or throat constriction, wheezing, dyspnea, cyanosis, abdominal cramps, diarrhea, nausea, vomiting, vertigo, chills and fever, laryngeal stridor, shock, syncope, involuntary bowel or bladder action, and bloody, frothy sputum. Initial mild symptoms may progress swiftly to anaphylactic shock.

Generalized systemic allergic reactions to Hymenoptera venom are thought to be immunoglobulin E (IgE)-mediated. When an individual predisposed to allergy to bees is stung, there is usually an increase in the production of IgE antibodies, which become attached to the mast cells and basophils. This sensitizes the individual so that a subsequent sting may result in an antigen-antibody interaction releasing pharmacologically active mediators such as histamine, the slow-reacting substance of anaphylaxis (SRS-A) and eosinophil chemotactic factors of anaphylaxis (ECF-A). It is these mediators that actually cause tissue damage and systemic symptoms.

Delayed Reaction A delayed reaction, appearing 10 to 14 days after a sting, consists of serum sickness-like signs and symptoms of fever, malaise, headache, urticaria, lymphadenopathy, and polyarthritis. Frequently, the patient has forgotten about the encounter and is puzzled by the sudden appearance of symptoms. This reaction is likely immune complex–mediated.

Unusual Reactions Infrequently, a reaction to Hymenoptera venom produces neurologic, cardiovascular, and urologic symptoms, with signs of encephalopathy, neuritis, vasculitis, and nephrosis. A case of Guillain-Barré syndrome has been reported as a possible consequence of a Hymenoptera sting.

DIAGNOSIS Identification of the offending insect can be difficult, except for the honeybee, which almost invariably leaves its stinger with venom sac attached in the lesion. In general, definitive identification is unnecessary because signs and symptoms of envenomation are similar among all Hymenoptera. A careful history is often necessary to distinguish members of Vespidae from each other, and slides or pictures of the various species can aid the patient in recall. Skin tests are of little value in the identification process.

If edema persists at the sting site, secondary infection, such as cellulitis, must be considered. Severe local reactions on the foot or ankle can be misdiagnosed as gout if the insect sting is not visible.

TREATMENT If the bee stinger is present in the wound, try to remove it. Although conventional teaching suggested scraping the stinger out to avoid squeezing remaining venom from the retained venom gland into the victim, involuntary muscle contraction of the gland continues after evisceration and the venom contents are quickly exhausted. Immediate removal is the important principle and the method of removal is irrelevant.[6] As a general rule, the sting site should be washed thoroughly with soap and water to minimize the possibility of infection. For local reactions, ice packs at the site will diminish swelling and delay the absorption of venom while limiting edema. Oral antihistamines and analgesics may limit discomfort and pruritus. Nonsteroidal anti-inflammatory drugs (NSAIDs) can be effective in relieving pain. Standard doses of opioid analgesics also can be administered. If edema is significant, elevation and rest of the affected limb should limit swelling unless secondary infection develops, in which case antibiotics will be necessary. In local tissue reactions, there is often significant inflammatory erythema and swelling, making it difficult to distinguish from infection; as a general rule, infection is only present in a minority of cases.

TABLE 188-2 Long-Term Management for Patients with Reactions to Hymenoptera Stings

Type of Reaction	Risk of Systemic Reaction on Subsequent Stings	Should Skin Testing Be Performed	Results of Skin Testing	Recommended Treatment
Never stung	Minimal	No		None
Local reaction				
Minor local reaction: immediate pain, swelling and itching at sting site, resolves in 1 day	Minimal	No		None
Extensive local reaction: swelling develops 24–48 h after sting and resolves in 3–7 d	Less than 10 percent	No		Epinephrine syringe
Systemic reaction				
Adult (urticaria, angioedema, anaphylaxis)	High	Yes	+	Venom immunotherapy
			−	Epinephrine syringe
Child (urticaria and mild angioedema)	Low	Yes	+	Venom immunotherapy or epinephrine syringe
			−	Epinephrine syringe
Child (anaphylaxis)	Moderate	Yes	+	Venom immunotherapy
			−	Epinephrine syringe

While the initial signs and symptoms of a systemic reaction may be mild, victims can deteriorate rapidly in a matter of minutes. Treatment regimen is that for anaphylaxis and the most important agent to administer is epinephrine hydrochloride 0.3 to 0.5 mg (0.3–0.5 mL of 1:1000) in adults and 0.01 mg/kg in children (never more than 0.3 mg). It should be injected subcutaneously and the injection site massaged to hasten absorption of the drug. The patient should then be observed for several hours to ensure that symptoms do not intensify or relapse. Parenteral administration of standard antihistamines (diphenhydramine 25–50 mg) and H_2 receptor antagonists (ranitidine 50 mg) is recommended. While steroids (methylprednisolone 125 mg) are of little help in combating the immediate effects, their administration tends to limit urticaria and edema and may potentiate the effects of other measures. Bronchospasm is treated with β-agonist nebulization. Hypotension may require massive crystalloid infusion, and central venous pressure monitoring may be helpful in some patients. Persistent hypotension after massive volume replacement may require dopamine. If dopamine is ineffective, an intravenous infusion of epinephrine can be used. The patient who suffers a severe systemic reaction should be admitted and monitored for potential cardiac, bleeding, renal, or neurologic complications.

LONG-TERM MANAGEMENT AND PREVENTIVE CARE Skin tests and radioallergosorbent tests (RAST) are not fully reliable in determining which patients are at risk for systemic reaction during future encounters with Hymenoptera (Table 188-2). Patients with negative results may have been sensitized by the skin tests themselves. Every patient who has had a systemic reaction should be provided with an insect sting kit containing premeasured epinephrine and be carefully instructed in its use. The Ana-Kit (Hollister-Stier, Spokane, WA) contains a sterile syringe preloaded with two doses of epinephrine (1:1000, 0.5 mL in each dose with a stop between) and several antihistamine tablets. The Epi-Pen (Dey Laboratories, Napa, CA) contains a single self-injecting, spring-loaded syringe of epinephrine 1:1000. Its advantage is the ease of injection; its disadvantages are that to be on the safe side, the patient should carry two kits, and there is no way to measure proper dosage for children. The physician should stress that the patient must inject the epinephrine subcutaneously at the first sign of a systemic reaction.

Physicians should, as a matter of course, advise their patients who are allergic to insects to wear Medic Alert tags, and they should provide such patients with a list of avoidance measures to prevent being stung (see Table 188-3).

Ants (Formicidae)

There are five known species of fire ants (*Solenopsis*) in the United States: *S. aurea, S. geminata, S. xyloni,* and the two imported species, *S. invicta* and *S. richteri.* The two imported species entered the United

TABLE 188-3 Prevention of Insect Stings

1. Seek and destroy Hymenoptera nests that may be in the vicinity of the home, outbuildings, and yard. Begin with the advent of warm weather and conduct the searches periodically until the first hard frost. This task, however, should not be undertaken by the insect-allergic individual, but rather by a nonallergic person or a professional exterminator.
2. Avoid going barefoot or wearing sandals outdoors.
3. When outdoors, wear light colors such as white, tan, khaki, or light green. Do not wear bright colors or flowery prints.
4. Do not use perfumed lotions, aftershaves, or shampoos during the warm months.
5. Cover up with long sleeves and long pants and wear gloves when working outdoors; refrain from wearing floppy clothing that could entangle an irate stinging insect and from wearing bright jewelry that could attract one. Suede and leather articles may not only attract but also irritate Hymenoptera.
6. Anyone severely allergic to insects should not mow lawns, pick flowers, or clip hedges. Such an individual should be wary when eating outdoors, especially sugary food or drinks, and should avoid areas near garbage cans, littered picnic grounds, or fruit trees where fruit lies rotting on the ground.
7. If confronted by a member or members of Hymenoptera, remain calm, never swat or move hastily, but rather retreat as slowly and calmly as possible. If retreat seems impossible, lie on the ground and cover your head with your arms.

Source: Fraizer CA: *Insect Allergy.* St. Louis: WH Green, 1969.

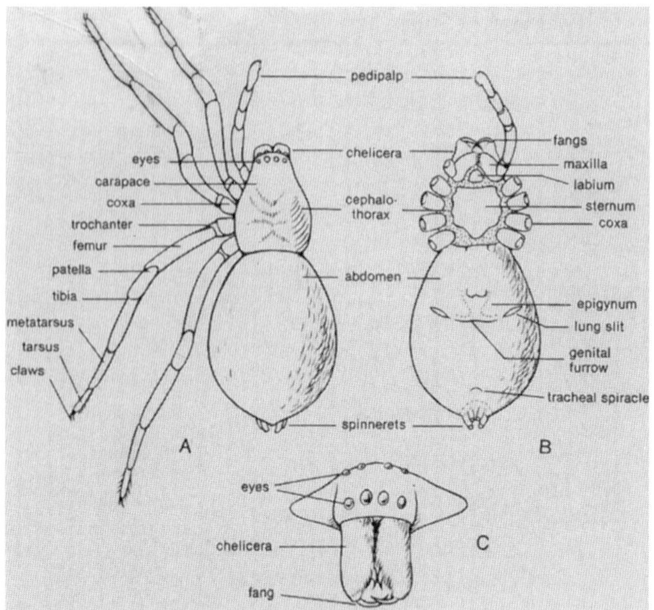

FIG. 188-3. External anatomy of a spider. **A.** Dorsal. **B.** Ventral. **C.** Frontal. (Reproduced with permission from Management of Wilderness and Environmental Emergencies. St. Louis: Mosby, 1989.)

States through Mobile, Alabama, in the 1930s and have now spread throughout the Gulf Coast states and are pushing westward.[7] The fire ant inhabits a loose amount of dirt and breeds 9 to 10 months of the year. One mature nest can produce 200,000 ants during a 3-year period, which accounts for the rapid spread of this arthropod. The venom of the fire ant is almost entirely an insoluble alkaloid. There is potential cross-reactivity between the venoms of fire ants and other Hymenoptera, and individual stings may produce systemic toxicity in sensitized individuals.

Fire ants are characterized by their tendency to swarm when provoked and they may attack in great numbers. Most often fire ants in a swarm position themselves on their victim and sting simultaneously in response to an alarm pheromone released by one or several individuals. Each sting usually results in a papule, which becomes a sterile pustule in 6 to 24 h. Localized necrosis, scarring, and secondary infection can result.[8] There may be a systemic reaction manifested by urticaria and angioedema.

One study has estimated a hypersensitivity rate to the fire ant of 16 percent in the general population.[8] Treatment of fire ant stings consists of local wound care. If there is evidence of systemic reaction, give the usual treatment for anaphylaxis. Desensitization should be directed to any person exhibiting a potentially life-threatening reaction to these arthropods.

ARACHNIDA

Spiders (Araneae)

There are over 30,000 species of spiders worldwide, of which approximately 50 species in the United States have been implicated in medically significant envenomations. All spiders are carnivores utilizing venom to paralyze their prey prior to ingestion (Fig. 188-3).

Loxosceles and Necrotic Arachnidism

Loxosceles spiders have a worldwide distribution. There are 18 species in the genus *Loxosceles* in North America, with 13 of these found in the United States. Five of these, *L. reclusa, L. laeta, L. refuscens, L. arizona,* and *L. unicolor,* have been associated with ulcers and necrotic skin lesions. *L. reclusa* (the brown recluse spider) is one of the most common species found in the United States and has been reported in over 20 states, particularly those in the region of the Missouri, Ohio, and Mississippi river basins, but also in several southwestern, southern, and midwestern states. *L. reclusa* prefers warm dry areas such as abandoned buildings, wood piles, and cellars and is generally nocturnal in activity. It is difficult to find the exact incidence of severe bites from these spiders, although one U.S. study of 460 deaths from venomous bites attributed 63 (14 percent) to *L. reclusa.* Loxoscelism is the reaction to the envenomation by species of the brown spider.

CLINICAL FEATURES Bites by *Loxosceles* spiders are initially painless, prohibiting definitive identification of the spider. The most common manifestation of a *Loxosceles* bite consists of a mild erythematous lesion that may become firm and heal with little or no scar over several days to weeks.[9] Occasionally, a more severe reaction occurs, with mild to severe pain several hours after the bite. There may be erythema and blister formation and bluish discoloration within the first 24 h (Fig. 188-4). This lesion may become necrotic over the next 3 to 4 days (Fig. 188-5), with eschar formation by the end of the first week. These lesions may vary in size from 1 to 30 cm.

The necrosis is caused by aggregation of leukocytes and platelets forming a hemostatic plug in venules and arterioles. The bite of the brown recluse spider also may cause systemic involvement, which generally occurs within 48 h of the bite. The patient may experience fever, chills, nausea, vomiting, myalgias, arthralgias, petechiae, and hemolysis. Hemolysis is apparently mediated by direct effect of the spider venom on red blood cell membranes and may be severe, causing hemoglobinuria, renal failure, DIC, and rarely, death. Systemic reaction is more common in children and almost all deaths are reported in children under 7 years of age. There may be little correlation between systemic symptoms of *Loxosceles* envenomation and the severity of the skin lesions.

The venom of *Loxosceles* consists of multiple proteases, alkaline phosphatase, lipase, anaronidase, and other substances that involve the complement system. It is still unclear which of these substances is the major factor related to the necrosis-producing activity of the spider.

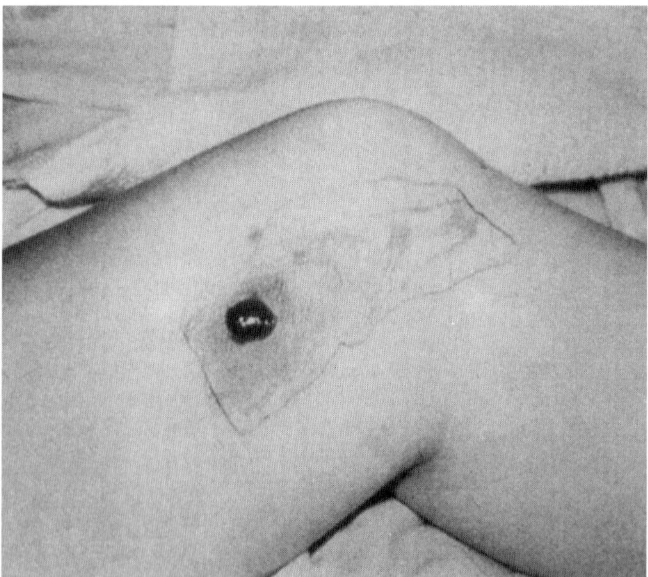

FIG. 188-4. Brown recluse spider bite approximately 12 h old. Note central hemorrhagic vesicle with surrounding spread of toxin. (Reproduced by permission from Management of Wilderness and Environmental Emergencies. St. Louis: Mosby, 1989.)

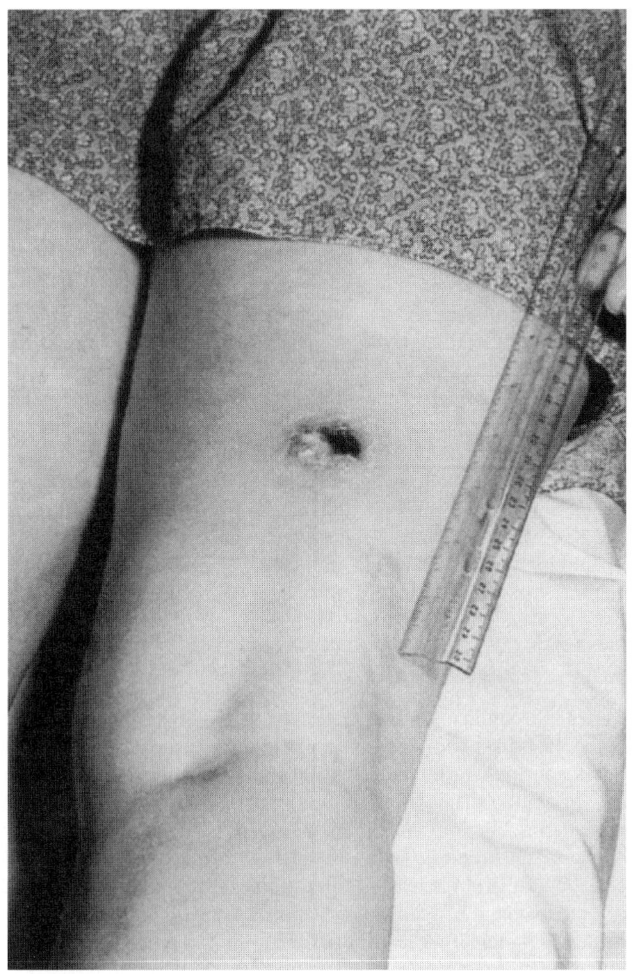

FIG. 188-5. Brown spider bite 4 days after injury. (Reproduced with permission from Emergency Medicine, June 1988.)

DIAGNOSIS In the United States, *L. argiope, L. atrax, L. chiracanthium, L. lycosa, Tegenaria agrestis* and numerous other varieties can all cause bites similar to that of *L. reclusa.*[10] Although the brown recluse spider is the most renowned biting spider to produce necrotic lesions in humans, the most common biting spider in the United States is the so-called jumping spider, one of the *Phidippus* species. These small, furry, and relatively aggressive spiders are sometimes confused with the black widow spider because of their black and red markings. Although jumping spiders bite and tend to hang onto the victim and can lead to a necrotic lesion, they generally only produce a local reaction, which may take hours to days to subside.

In patients suspected of having a bite from *L. reclusa* and exhibiting signs and symptoms of envenomation, a complete blood count (CBC), creatinine, blood urea nitrogen (BUN), and coagulation profile should be ordered, as well as an urinalysis for hemoglobinuria. No laboratory tests yet exist to confirm bites of *Loxosceles.*

TREATMENT Treatment of a brown recluse or any necrotic spider bite should include the usual supportive measures. No antivenom is available commercially. For those bites with cytotoxic reactions and necrosis, tetanus prophylaxis and daily wound care should be given. Antibiotics should be used if evidence of infection exists. In some cases, analgesic therapy will be required. In general, surgery should not be done until the necrotic ulcers are greater than 2 cm in diameter and the borders of the ulcers are well established, usually 2 to 3 weeks after the bite.

Dapsone has been suggested by some clinicians to prevent ongoing necrosis from *L. reclusa* bites by inhibiting local infiltration by polymorphonuclear leukocytes, although there are no controlled data to substantiate this claim. More recently, hyperbaric oxygen has been proposed as treatment for severely necrotic *Loxosceles* bites based on case reports. However, controlled trials in animals failed to demonstrate superiority of this treatment over simple supportive wound management.[11]

Adults and children with evidence of a significant systemic reaction to a brown recluse spider bite warrant hospitalization and close observation. If hemolysis occurs, appropriate hydration, red blood cell transfusion, and monitoring of renal function are important to avoid complications such as acute renal failure.

Hobo Spider (*Tegenaria agrestis*)

The hobo spider is a venomous spider found in the Pacific Northwest and its bite is often misattributed to the brown recluse spider, which is not found in that region.[10] Originally native to Europe, the hobo spider entered the Pacific Northwest and has spread as far as central Utah and southern Alaksa. Hobo spiders are brown with gray markings and 7 to 14 mm in body size with 27- to 45-mm leg span. These spiders live in dark areas close to the ground in wood piles or basements.

CLINICAL FEATURES, DIAGNOSIS, AND TREATMENT Local reaction to *T. agrestis* bite is similar to that of the brown recluse spider. The bite is initially painless, followed by induration and expanding erythma. Blisters eventually develop that rupture, leaving an encrusted, cratered wound. Healing occurs gradually over 45 days, often with a permanent scar. Severe headache is the most common systemic symptom, followed by nausea, vomiting, diarrhea, and lethargy. Aplastic anemia has been reported rarely as a severe complication.

The hobo spider is rarely seen by the victim because the bite is painless, the bite occurs in dark areas where the spider lives, and the spider moves quickly away (up to 1 m/s) after the bite. No diagnostic test exists for hobo spider envenomation.

No proven treatment exists for *T. agrestis* local or systemic reactions.[10] Surgical excision and grafting eventually may be required for severe wounds. Corticosteroids may be of some benefit for aplastic anemia.

Black Widow (*Latrodectus*)

Latrodectus or ''widow'' spiders are found throughout the United States. Of the estimated 30,000 species of spiders, the black widow is probably the most well known, although of the five species found commonly in the United States, only three (*L. mactans, L. variolus,* and *L. hesperus*) are actually black. Other varieties may be predominantly brown or red (*L. geometricus,* or brown widow, and *L. bishopi,* or red widow). The classic orange-red hourglass-shaped marking is noted only in *L. mactans.* Female spiders are relatively large, with a body size ranging up to 1.5 cm in length and leg spans of 4 to 5 cm. The male spider is approximately one-third the size of the female, lighter in color, and his bite can not penetrate human skin. Black widow spiders are found most often in wood piles, basements, garages, or sheds. *Latrodectus* will aggressively defend her web, particularly when guarding her eggs. Most black widow bites occur between April and October and usually are seen on the hands and forearms.

The black widow spider injures its victim by secretion of one of the most potent neurotoxic venoms produced by any animal, producing release of acetylcholine, norepinephrine, and other neurotransmitters at the neurosynaptic junction.

CLINICAL FEATURES Most *Latrodectus* bites are almost immediately mild to moderately painful. The pain often begins as a pinprick sensation at the bite site but may spread quickly to include the entire bitten

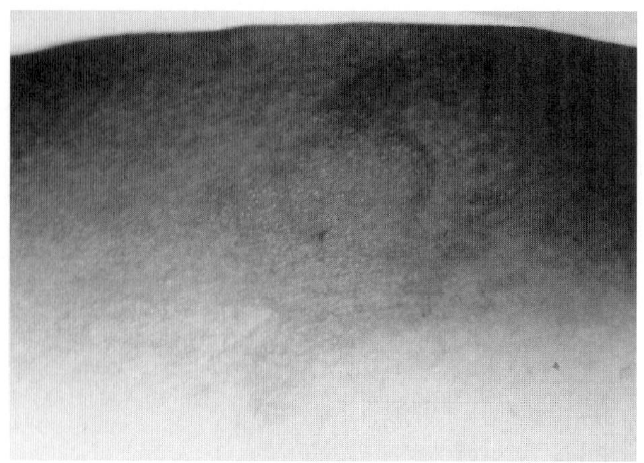

FIG. 188-6. Classic "target lesion" from patient bitten by a black widow spider.

extremity.[12] Erythema appears approximately 20 to 60 min after the bite. In over 50 percent of cases, the initial erythema evolves into a lesion resembling a "target," with a diameter of about 1 to 2 cm (Fig. 188-6). Victims frequently complain of muscle cramp-like spasms in large muscle groups, although physical examination of the "cramping" extremity rarely exhibits rigidity, and serum creatine kinase concentrations do not appear to be significantly elevated. The pain often increases progressively, becomes generalized, and can involve the trunk, back, and abdomen. Involvement of the abdominal wall musculature with severe pain and cramping has been mistaken for peritonitis.

Latrodectus bite victims may experience severe pain for 24 h or more that can be intermittent in course. Rarely, pain may persist for several days, whereas muscle weakness may continue for weeks to months. The most serious complications include hypertension, which is reported in 10 to 30 percent of envenomations and is likely the result of catecholamine release. In addition, severe envenomation also may cause shock, coma, and respiratory failure secondary to muscle paralysis.

DIAGNOSIS AND TREATMENT Since an immediate pinprick sensation is almost always reported with *Latrodectus* bites, it is rare for victims not to see the offending spider. There are no confirmatory laboratory tests, but the presence of the typical target lesion along with pain, muscle spasms, and toxic appearance is virtually pathognomonic of the diagnosis.

The initial therapy is supportive care of the airway, breathing, and circulation. Wound care should consist of routine cleansing of the bite site and tetanus prophylaxis, if indicated.

Patients should be given appropriate opioid analgesics and benzodiazepines for pain relief and muscle relaxation. Intravenous calcium gluconate has been advocated to relieve pain and muscle spasms from the black widow bite, although controlled data are lacking, and a review of 163 patients with *Latrodectus* envenomation found ineffective relief of muscle spasm and pain with calcium treatment.[12] Most severe bites will require parenteral opioids for extended periods, necessitating admission for observation. Antivenom is reserved only for severe envenomation refractory to the measures indicated earlier.[12] The usual dose is one to two vials infused over 20 to 30 min. Since antivenom is a horse-serum preparation, anaphylaxis can occur, particularly in patients with a history of allergy to horse-serum products or those who have been sensitized by prior antivenom treatment.[12] Skin testing should be performed before antivenom administration. Serum sickness, while a theoretical possibility, was not observed in 58 patients treated with 1 or 2 vials of antivenom.[12]

Tarantula

The term *tarantula* is used for several species of large spiders such as the desert tarantula, which is found in the southwest region of the United States and is a member of the family Theraphosidae. Despite their large size (up to 7 cm), their venom is very mild and usually does not produce systemic reactions. The typical tarantula bite causes local swelling and pain at the bite site often resembling a Hymenoptera sting that may last for a few hours and is treated successfully with local wound care.[13]

Perhaps the most common problem with tarantulas involves the hairs on their abdomen. When threatened, these spiders can use their hind legs to flick these hairs a distance of 1 to 2 m. The body of their hair follicle is studded with what appears to be spurs when viewed with a dissecting microscope and can become imbedded in skin. The hairs are quite irritating and can lead to a significant contact dermatitis. Cases have been reported of these hairs being impaled in the cornea of a victim, necessitating surgical removal.

The South American tarantula, also known as the *banana spider,* is aggressive and frequently bites when threatened. This spider also has a potent venom and its bite may cause both necrotic and systemic reactions. An antitoxin is available.

Scabies (*Sarcoptes scabiei*)

Scabies infestation resembles that of lice but is generally concentrated around the hands and feet, especially in the web spaces between the fingers and toes. In children, the face and scalp may be infested as well. In adults, scabies frequently affect the nipples in females and the penis in males.

The scabies mite is a universal pest that appears to follow a 30-year cycle of proliferation. During the past several years, there has been an epidemic of scabies infestation in the United States. Scabies infestation is more likely to occur by direct contact between the infested individual and the non-infested individual than by indirect contact with clothing and personal articles.

Diagnostically, pruritus is the dominant symptom, although it takes up to a month for sensitization to develop and itching to begin. In patients who become infested and are already sensitized, inflammation and pruritus may develop within a few hours of contact.

The distinctive feature of scabies infestation is the burrow that the female mite digs into the skin to lay her eggs. Vesicles and papules form at the surface of these zigzag, whitish, threadlike channels that may contain small gray spots at the closed ends where the parasite rests. Burrows tend to enlarge and be more visible in children. The burrows can be traced with a hand lens and the female mite scraped out with a needle or razor blade. A thin shaving of skin containing both burrow and mite can be examined under a microscope to formally establish the diagnosis. Unfortunately, burrows are often disguised by excoriations, crusting, eczematization, and secondary infection.

Treatment for scabies infestation consists of a thorough application of a scabicide. Although lindane is usually effective, scabies mites have developed immunity to the compound in many areas, and less toxic alternatives are available. Permethrins (Nix, Warmer-Lambert; Elimite, Allergan, Inc.) and pyrethrins (RID, Pfizer) are effective scabicides with little human toxicity, some of which are available in pharmacies over the counter. These agents are usually applied from the neck down, following a warm bath with liberal use of soap. The patient should be cautioned to keep the substance from the eyes and mucous membranes and to avoid inhaling the vapors. The scabicide is left on for 8 to 12 h and then is washed off.

Even after the scabies mites have been destroyed, lesions and pruritus can persist. No further use of scabicide is needed, but calamine lotion, oral antipruritic agents, and analgesics will help alleviate discomfort. Antibiotics are only necessary where secondary infection occurs.

Ticks (*Ixodes, Dermacentor,* and Others)

Ticks are found throughout the world, mostly in rural areas. Their bodies consist of a fused abdomen and thorax in an oval shape and vary from a millimeter or less in length to over a centimeter when engorged with blood. Ticks attach to humans painlessly with strong jaws and cement-like adhesive. Granulomas may develop at the site of a tick bite and require several months to heal.

The main concern with ticks is that they are disease vectors. Typhus, tularemia, Colorado tick fever, Rocky Mountain spotted fever, viral encephalitis, and Lyme disease (*Borrelia burgdorferi*) all can be transmitted through tick bites. Tick paralysis, a symmetric ascending paralysis, occurs from the secretion of a neurotoxin by some species and may lead to respiratory failure in humans. It is treated by removing the tick.

Insect repellants and tight-fitting clothing can be helpful in preventing tick bites in infested areas. Although organic solvents, heat, and other methods have been advocated to aid in dislodging a tick so as not to leave its mouth parts beneath the skin surface and to prevent further toxin release, no technique has definitively proven superior.[14] The often insidious presentation of tick-borne illnesses such as Lyme disease has prompted some physicians to prophylactically administer antibiotics following tick bites. However, less than 5 percent of tick bites in highly endemic areas result in *B. burgdorferi* infection. In addition, most people remove the tick before it has been attached for the 36 to 48 h required to transmit an infectious dose of *B. burgdorferi.* For these reasons, routine prophylaxis of tick bites to prevent Lyme disease is neither cost effective nor recommended.[15]

Chiggers (Trombiculidae)

Chigger infestations are caused by mite larvae that feed on host skin cells. European varieties of these arachnids are called *harvest mites.* The combination of the effect of digestive enzymes secreted by the mite and an immune response of the host produces the typical pruritic lesions. Although the usual response is intense pruritus at the bite site, more severe systemic reactions and chigger-borne diseases also may occur. Mites live comfortably in warm and cold climates. There are approximately 2500 species of chigger mites, with *Trombicula alfreddugèsi* the most common. Mites are quite small, 0.3 to 1.0 mm in length, and attach themselves to the host skin with their mandibular structures, known as *chelicerae.* Once attached they release digestive enzymes to liquefy epidermal cells, leading to an immune response in the victim and subsequent symptomotology.

Itching usually begins a few hours after the chigger bite, with a papule developing initially that ultimately enlarges over 24 to 48 h to form a nodule. Pruritus usually peaks on the second day, and the nodules can persist for up to 14 days. Children who play or sit on the grass are prone to chigger bites in the genital area. Bites can manifest in some patients as impressive soft tissue edema (Fig. 188-7). Mite infestations may be associated with fever and an erythema multiforme–like rash. The diagnosis of chigger infestation usually can be made on the basis of known outdoor exposure and typical skin lesions.

The treatment of chigger bites consists largely of symptomatic measures to control the itching. Chiggers may be killed with lindane 1% topical lotion or crotamiton 10% topical lotion (Eurax, Westwood-Squibb Pharmaceuticals). For moderate to severe cases, topical steroid creams and oral antihistamines may provide some relief. There have been reports of systemic steroids providing relief for severe pruritus. If secondary infection occurs, antibiotic therapy is indicated. Clothes fitting snugly at the neck, wrists, and ankles, supplemented with insect repellent, can help prevent chigger infestation.

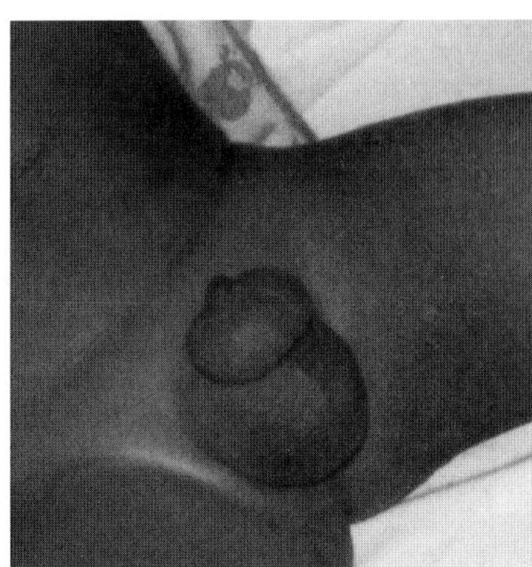

FIG. 188-7. Chigger bites. Edema of the foreskin, scrotum, and penis is dramatic. There is no meatal obstruction.

Scorpions (Scorpionidae)

Several species of scorpions are found in the warmer parts of the southern United States. All are generally nocturnal and capable of stinging humans. Most species found in this country cause little more than localized pain similar to that following Hymenoptera stings. Cytotoxicity or inflammation does not occur from North American scorpion venom, and the exact site of the sting may not be readily apparent. Only *Centruroides exilicauda,* or the bark scorpion, found throughout Arizona, New Mexico, and parts of Texas and California, possesses venom potent enough to cause systemic toxicity.

C. exilicauda venom can open sodium channels on neurons, causing prolonged and excessive firing of axons, and may lead to abnormal activity along motor, sensory, and autonomic fibers. Systemic symptoms following envenomation by this scorpion can be pronounced and variable. Immediate onset of pain and paresthesias in the stung extremity is usually noted and may become generalized. In severe cases, cranial nerve and somatic motor dysfunction can develop, resulting in abnormal roving eye movements, blurred vision, pharyngeal muscle incoordination, and drooling, occasionally leading to respiratory compromise. Excessive motor activity may present as restlessness or uncontrollable jerking of the extremities, appearing to be seizure-like activity. Nausea, vomiting, and tachycardia can be present in significant envenomations. Symptoms usually last 24 to 48 h. Cardiac dysfunction, pulmonary edema, pancreatitis, bleeding disorders, skin necrosis, and occasionally death can be seen with stings from Asian and African scorpions such as *Buthus, Tityus,* and *Androctonus* but are not found following envenomation by scorpions native to the United States.[16]

Diagnosis of a scorpion sting is clinical. Stings can be confused initially with anything that causes local pain, especially in children. As the syndrome progresses in moderate to severe cases to include autonomic and motor findings, the diagnosis becomes more apparent. Treatment is supportive and should include liberal use of analgesics and sedatives. A *Centruroides*-specific antivenom is available only in the state of Arizona and is produced from goat serum. Like all partially purified animal-derived serum products, both immediate and delayed allergic reactions and serum sickness occur with administration of *Centruroides* antivenom, and it therefore should be used only in severe cases.[17] One to two vials are generally enough to provide a resolution of symptoms. The patient should be skin tested prior to administration of the antivenom.

MOSQUITOS, FLIES, FLEAS, AND LICE (DIPTERA)

Mosquitoes

Mosquitoes are aquatic breeding arthropods found in all parts of the world. Like other members of this group, they possess one pair of wings, the second pair having evolved into smaller structures used as stabilizers.

Mosquitoes penetrate skin with a piercing motion of a bayonet-like proboscis. The actual puncturing of the skin surface causes minimal trauma and is frequently not felt by the host. A type of local anesthetic is injected into the wound that causes local tissue damage and local hypersensitivity. Bites can lead to both immediate and delayed reactions. An immediate skin reaction includes redness, a wheal, and itching. A delayed reaction usually consists of edema and a burning pruritus. The immediate reaction tends to be of short duration, whereas a delayed reaction may persist for hours, days, and even weeks. Severe local reactions with skin necrosis occur occasionally. The history of an allergy to mosquito saliva constituents consists of an increasing reaction to seasonal exposures with more and more pronounced edematous and pruritic lesions, accompanied sometimes by complications such as fever, malaise, generalized edema, severe nausea and vomiting, and necrosis with resulting scarring. Treatment is symptomatic, with antihistamines and NSAIDs.

The greatest dangers from mosquitos in other countries is their function as disease vectors. Even with extensive pest control programs, arboviruses and malaria are epidemic in some parts of the world. Japanese B encephalitis, yellow fever, dengue hemorrhagic fever, and various types of equine encephalitis are among the many viruses transmitted by mosquitos. Malaria is encountered frequently in patients in the United States after travel and in immigrant populations from areas where malaria is endemic.

Flies

Bloodsucking flies range in size from the tiny sand fly, about 1 to 3 mm in length, to horse flies that can be over 2 cm. All members stab and pierce the skin, causing some degree of pain and, commonly, subsequent pruritus. Several species, such as deerflies, blackflies, horseflies, and sand flies, can produce allergic reactions, although rarely as severe as those produced by Hymenoptera venom. There is also the possibility of myiasis with fly bites, but this, too, is rare in the United States.

The diagnosis of fly bites depends chiefly on the patient's history and a knowledge of the arthropods that frequent the area of encounter. Treatment for most local reactions to Diptera bites is symptomatic, whereas treatment of systemic reactions is the same as it is for Hymenoptera venom. Cold compresses may alleviate localized edema. Secondary infection from Diptera bites can occur, and antibiotics may be necessary in some cases. Oral antihistamines such as diphenhydramine and hydroxyzine may be helpful in relieving pruritus in these cases, but, topical steroids can be used when local reactions are severe, and oral steroids are indicated when systemic hypersensitivity symptoms are present.

Fleas (Siphonaptera)

Bites of fleas, lice, and scabies produce lesions so similar that diagnosis is often difficult. Flea bites are frequently found in zigzag lines, especially on the legs and in the waist area. The lesions have hemorrhagic puncta surrounded by erythematous and urticarial patches. Pruritus is intense, and often, even after the lesions clear, dull red spots persist.

The main concern in the treatment of flea bites is the possibility of secondary infection. Children may develop impetigo as a complication. The lesions should be washed thoroughly with soap and water. Children with flea bites should have their fingernails cut short to prevent scratching. To relieve discomfort and itching, starch baths at bedtime (about 1 kg starch to a tubful of water), local application of calamine, cool soaks, and oral antihistamines may be helpful. For severe discomfort, application of a topical steroid cream or spray may be necessary. If secondary infection develops, topical or oral antibiotics may be needed.

Lice (Anoplura)

Body lice concentrate about the waist, shoulders, axillae, and neck. The lice and their eggs often can be found in the seams of clothing. The lesions produced from bites of these arthropods begin as small, noninflammatory red spots that quickly become papular wheals. They are so intensely pruritic that their linear scratch marks are diagnostically suggestive of infestation. The white ova of head lice can be mistaken for dandruff, but unlike dandruff, they cannot be brushed out because they are glued to the hair itself (''nits'').

Pubic lice leave bluish spots in the abdomen and thighs, and ova are evident on the shafts of pubic hairs. If sensitization to lice saliva and feces components occurs, delayed allergic reactions may develop, leading to fever and malaise. Secondary infection may produce enlarged lymph glands or cellulitis. Long periods of infestation may bring a decrease in pruritus and often impart a thick, dry, scaly appearance to the skin.

Treatment for body lice infestation is similar to that for scabies. Permethrin or pyrethrin shampoos and creams are usually effective in eliminating body and hair infestations, but sterilization of clothing, bedding, and personal articles also must occur. Lice and eggs are destroyed by temperatures in excess of 52°C, necessitating hot water washing. Storage of articles in plastic bags for 2 weeks also can eliminate infestations.

KISSING BUGS AND BED BUGS (HEMIPTERA)

Triatoma species, commonly known as *conenose, reduviid,* or *kissing bugs,* are found mainly in the southeastern and Pacific Coast regions of the United States. They feed on the blood of vertebrate animals, including humans. Their common name derives from their habit of feeding at night on any exposed surface of a sleeping victim, which is commonly the face. Since their bite is relatively painless, the victim is rarely aware of the attack. Bed bugs (*Cimex lectularis*) cause a similar pattern of envenomation in humans at night, and can be found throughout the United States. These arthropods are adapted to domestic environments, living in baseboards, between cracks in walls and floors, and in furniture.

Bites are usually multiple and consist of hemorrhagic papules or bullae if they occur on the hands or feet and large wheals if they are on the trunk. Diagnostically, kissing bug bites can be differentiated from bedbug bites in that they often do not appear in a linear formation and usually are not accompanied by telltale brown or black patterns of excrement on the bed linen characteristic of bed bugs.

Treatment of Hemiptera bites is symptomatic, with cool compress applications and antihistamines to relieve pruritus. Some individuals become highly sensitive to kissing bugs and react with systemic allergic symptoms following a bite. These individuals should be treated as previously outlined for Hymenoptera envenomation.

CATERPILLARS AND MOTHS (LEPIDOPTERA)

There are at least 10 families of venomous caterpillars and moths. Stinging moths are found in the southern United States that can cause an illness termed *lepidoterism.* Some caterpillars possess hollow spines among their hairs that contain urticating poisons that can cause symptoms ranging from local dermatitis to generalized systemic reactions. The puss caterpillar or woolly slug, larval stage of the moth *Megalopyge opercularis,* is perhaps the most toxic variety in the United States and is especially hazardous for children who tend to find it intriguing and thus handle it.[18] Puss caterpillars are found primarily in the southeastern states and especially in Texas and Florida. The venom of the puss caterpillar can induce hemolysis and increase vascular permeability. The venom of the flannel moth caterpillar (*L. crispata*), saddleback caterpillar (*Sibine stimulae*), range caterpillar (*A. io*), and oak slug (*E. delphinii*) is not as toxic, tending to produce only urticaria. The gypsy moth caterpillar (*Porthetria dispas*) may produce a delayed hypersensitivity type of dermatitis in some individuals.

Stings from the hairs of the puss caterpillar most often cause skin irritation with a pruritic erythematous lesion at the site on contact. In severe cases, the victim may complain of immediate intense pain, often rhythmic or cyclic. The characteristic lesions consist of white or red papules and vesicles, frequently forming a gridlike pattern where the caterpillar made contact. Systemic symptoms occur commonly, with fever and muscle cramps. Shocklike symptoms also have been reported. Within several hours or days, local desquamation may develop. Lymphadenopathy has been described.

Treatment should begin with thorough washing of the affected area. Broken-off spines can be removed by placing cellophane tape over the sting site. Calcium gluconate, 10 mL of a 10% solution intravenously, has been reported to provide analgesia in some severe cases of caterpillar stings, whereas oral antihistamines usually bring relief in milder cases. Generalized symptoms are treated supportively.

BLISTER BEETLES (COLEOPTERA)

Although there are more members of the Coleoptera or beetle family than any other arthropod, the only ones with clinical significance for envenomation in humans are blister beetles. Blister beetles (families Staphylindae and Meloidae) are found throughout the United States, and include beetles known as Spanish fly (*Lytta vesicatoria*).[19] When disturbed or crushed on the skin, they exude a vesicating agent called *cantharidin* from the joints of their legs or from their bodies that can penetrate the epidermis to produce irritation and blistering within a few hours of contact. If ingested, cantharidin can produce intense gastrointestinal disturbances with symptoms of nausea, vomiting, diarrhea, and abdominal cramps.[20] Initial contact with the beetle produces a burning, tingling sensation and a mild rash. Within a few hours, flaccid, elongated vesicles and bullae develop from a few millimeters to several centimeters in diameter. Blebs erupt 2 to 5 h after contact and can be hemorrhagic and painful. A severe chemical conjunctivitis can occur if cantharidin contacts the eyes from contaminated hands.

Treatment consists of protecting the bullae from secondary infection with an occlusive dressing. Large bullae should be drained and an antibiotic ointment applied. Bullae occurring on the feet should be managed with wet dressings applied for 24 to 48 h. Application of steroid creams to blebs may be helpful. Lesions usually resolve in 2 to 3 days.

REFERENCES

1. Litovitz TL, Klein-Schwartz W, Dyer KS, et al.: 1997 Annual report of the American Association of Poison Control Centers Toxic Exposure Surveillance System. *Am J Emerg Med* 16:443, 1998.
2. Tunget CL, Clark RF: Invasion of the ''killer'' bees: Separating fact from fiction. *Postgrad Med* 94:92, 1993.
3. Franca FOS, Benvenuti LA, Fan HW, et al: Severe and fatal mass attacks by ''killer'' bees (Africanized honey bees—*Apis mellifera scutellata*) in Brazil: Clinicopathological studies with measurement of serum venom concentrations. *Q J Med* 87:269, 1994.
4. Reisman RE: Natural history of insect sting allergy: Relationship of severity of symptoms of initial sting anaphylaxis to re-sting reactions. *J Allergy Clin Immunol* 90:335, 1992.
5. Reisman RE: Current concepts: Insect stings. *N Engl J Med* 331:523, 1994.
6. Visscher PK, Vetter RS, Camazine S: Removing bee stings. *Lancet* 348:301, 1996.
7. Stafford CT, Hutto LS, Rhoades RB, et al: Imported fire ants as a health hazard. *South Med J* 82:1515, 1989.
8. DeShazo RD, Butcher BT, Banks WA: Reactions to the stings of the imported fire ant. *N Engl J Med* 323:462, 1990.
9. Wright SW, Wrenn KD, Murray L, Seger D: Clinical presentation and outcome of brown recluse spider bite. *Ann Emerg Med* 30:28, 1997.
10. Centers for Disease Control and Prevention: Necrotic arachnidism—Pacific Northwest, 1988–1996. *MMWR* 45:433, 1996.
11. Phillips S, Kohn M, Baker D, et al: Therapy of brown spider envenomation: A controlled trial of hyperbaric oxygen, dapsone, and ciproheptadine. *Ann Emerg Med* 25:363, 1995.
12. Clark RF, Wethern-Kestner S, Vance MV, Gerkin R: Clinical presentation and treatment of black widow spider envenomation: A review of 163 cases. *Ann Emerg Med* 21:782, 1992.
13. de Haro L, Jouglard J: The dangers of pet tarantulas: Experience of the Marseilles Poison Center. *Clin Toxicol* 36:51, 1988.
14. Needham GR: Evaluation of five popular methods for tick removal. *Pediatrics* 75:997, 1985.
15. Dennis DT, Meltzer MI: Antibiotic prophylaxis after tick bites. *Lancet* 350:1191, 1997.
16. Gueron M, Ilia R, Sofer S: The cardiovascular system after scorpion envenomation: A review. *Clin Toxicol* 30:245, 1992.
17. Gateau T, Bloom M, Clark RF: Response to specific *Centruroides sculpturatus* antivenom in 151 cases of scorpion stings. *Clin Toxicol* 32:165, 1994.
18. Neustater BR, Stollman NH, Manten HD: Sting of the puss caterpillar: An unusual cause of acute abdominal pain. *South Med J* 89:826, 1996.
19. Nicholls DSH, Med DG-U, Christmas TI, Greig DE: Oedemerid blister beetle dermatosis: A review. *J Am Acad Dermatol* 22:815, 1990.
20. Karras DJ, Farrell SE, Harrigan RA, et al: Poisoning from ''Spanish fly'' (cantharidin). *Am J Emerg Med* 14:478, 1996.

189 REPTILE BITES

Richard C. Dart
Hernan F. Gomez
Frank F. S. Daly

RATTLESNAKE BITES

Approximately 19 of the 115 snake species in the United States are venomous. Snakes inflict about 45,000 bites each year in the United States, of which 8000 are inflicted by venomous snakes. Most bites occur in the warm summer months, when snakes and victims are most active. In the past, it was estimated that mortality from venomous snakebite approached 25 percent. Because of the availability of antivenom and advances in emergency and critical care, mortality rates today are below 0.5 percent. Approximately 5 to 10 deaths occur per year.[1]

Except for bites by imported species, North American venomous snakebite involves the pit vipers (Crotalidae family) or coral snakes (Elapidae family). The crotalids are represented by the rattlesnakes (*Crotalus* species), pygmy rattlesnakes and massasauga (*Sistrurus* species), and the copperheads and water moccasins (*Agkistrodon* species).

Poisonous snakebites from imported exotic species are infrequent but may occur in zoo personnel as well as in amateur herpetologists. A regional poison center can provide information on snake identification, expected toxicity, and location of antivenom.

The crotalid snakes are called pit vipers because of bilateral depressions or pits located midway between and below the level of the eye and the nostril (Fig. 189-1). The pit is a heat receptor that guides strikes against warm-blooded prey or predators. Crotalid snakes are also distinguished by two fangs that can be folded against the roof of the mouth, in contrast to the coral snakes, which have shorter, fixed, and erect fangs. Within the pit vipers, the rattle distinguishes the rattlesnake from other crotalids. The mistaken belief that rattlesnakes always rattle before striking has persisted for centuries. In truth, many strikes occur without a warning rattle.[2]

Pathophysiology

Crotalid venom is a complex enzyme mixture that causes local tissue injury, systemic vascular damage, hemolysis, fibrinolysis, and neuromuscular dysfunction, resulting in a combination of local and systemic effects. Crotalid venom quickly alters blood vessel permeability, lead-

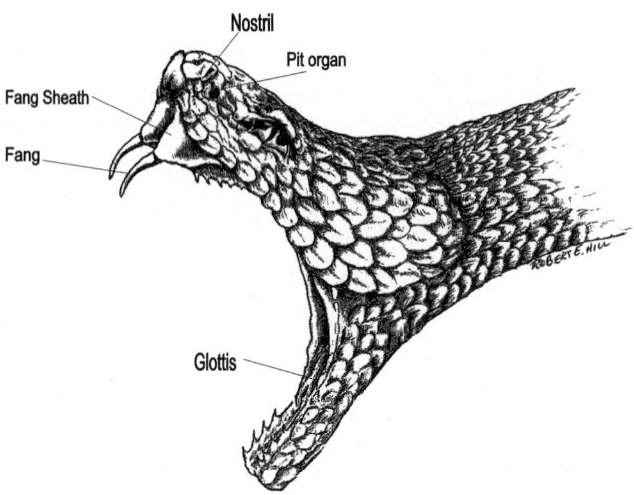

FIG. 189-1. Rattlesnake surface anatomy. (Reprinted with permission from Robert E. Hill.)

ing to loss of plasma and blood into the surrounding tissue and causing hypovolemia. It also consumes fibrinogen and platelets, causing a coagulopathy. In some species, specific venom fractions block neuromuscular transmission, leading to ptosis, respiratory failure, and other neurologic effects.

TABLE 189-1 Grading of Envenomation by Crotalid Snakes

Minimal envenomation
Swelling, erythema, or ecchymosis limited to immediate area of the bite site.
Systemic signs and symptoms not present or minimal.
Coagulation parameters all normal. No other significant laboratory abnormalities.
Moderate envenomation
Swelling, erythema, or ecchymosis present, may involve most of an extremity, and may be spreading slowly.
Systemic signs and symptoms present, but not life-threatening. These may include nausea, vomiting, oral paresthesia or unusual tastes, mild hypotension (systolic blood pressure >80 mmHg), mild tachycardia, and tachypnea.
Coagulation parameters may be abnormal, but no clinically significant bleeding is present. Severe abnormalities of other laboratory tests are not present.
Severe envenomation
Swelling or ecchymosis involve the entire extremity and are spreading rapidly.
Systemic signs and symptoms are markedly abnormal, including severe alteration of mental status, nausea and vomiting, hypotension (systolic blood pressure <80 mmHg), severe tachycardia, tachypnea, or other respiratory compromise.
Coagulation parameters abnormal with serious bleeding present or threat of spontaneous bleeding, including prothrombin time unmeasurable, partial thromboplastin time unmeasurable, platelets <20,000/μL, or fibrinogen undetectable. Severe abnormalities of other laboratory values should also be considered severe envenomations.

Clinical Features

Up to 25 percent of crotalid snakebites are termed dry: venom effects do not develop. The manifestations of crotalid venom poisoning involve a complex interaction of the venom and the victim. The species and size of the snake, the age and size of the victim, the time elapsed since the bite, and characteristics of the bite (location, depth, and number, the amount of venom injected) all affect the clinical appearance. The severity of poisoning following a crotalid bite is therefore variable. Crotalid bites are generally classified as *minimal, moderate,* or *severe,* depending on the degree of local and systemic injury (Table 189-1). An initially minimal bite may evolve into a moderate or severe bite and require large amounts of antivenom.

The cardinal manifestations of crotalid venom poisoning are the presence of one or more fang marks, localized pain, and progressive edema extending from the bite site.[3] Other early symptoms and signs of rattlesnake venom poisoning are nausea and vomiting, weakness, oral numbness or tingling of tongue and mouth, tachycardia, dizziness, hematemesis, hematuria, thrombocytopenia, and fasciculations. In general, swelling becomes apparent within 15 to 30 min, but in some cases it may not start for several hours. In severe cases, edema may progress to involve an entire limb within an hour. In less severe cases, edema may progress over a 1- to 2-day period. Edema near an airway or in a muscle compartment may threaten life or limb without the presence of systemic effects.

Progressive ecchymosis may also occur because of leakage of blood into subcutaneous tissue. Ecchymoses may appear within minutes or hours in the area of the snakebite. Hemorrhagic blebs may occur within several hours for similar reasons. Hemoconcentration often develops as a result of fluid loss into subcutaneous tissue, followed by a decrease in hemoglobin over several days from blood loss secondary to coagulopathy.

Diagnosis

The diagnosis of snakebite is based on the presence of fang marks and a history consistent with exposure to a snake (walking through a field, etc.). Snake envenomation involves the presence of a snake bite plus evidence of tissue injury. Clinically, the injury may be manifest in three ways: local injury (swelling, pain, ecchymosis), coagulopathy (thrombocytopenia, elevated prothrombin time, hypofibrinoginemia), or systemic effects (oral swelling or paresthesias, metallic or rubbery taste in the mouth, hypotension, tachycardia, etc.). Abnormalities in any one of these areas indicate that venom effect is developing. The absence of all three manifestations for a period of 8 to 12 h following the bite indicates that no venom was injected.

Treatment

FIRST AID First aid measures should never substitute for definitive medical care or delay the administration of antivenom. All patients bitten by a pit viper should be taken to a health care facility. Table 189-2 lists one prudent approach to first aid. Several first aid products are marketed. The Coghlan's Snake Bite Kit (Coghlan's Ltd.) or similar products should not be used because it contains cups that produce little suction and seal poorly on digits. The blade in the kit or any method of incision can injure digital nerves, arteries, and tendons; incision is not recommended. The Sawyer Extractor (Sawyer Products) suction pump removes venom without incision, producing up to 750 mmHg of suction over a puncture site. The usefulness of

TABLE 189-2 Recommended First Aid Measures

Retreat well beyond striking range. Many victims are bitten again while trying to capture the snake.
Remain calm. Movement will increase venom absorption.
Immobilize the extremity in a neutral position below the level of the heart.
Keep physical activity minimal.
Promptly transport the victim to a medical facility regardless of whether overt signs of envenomation are quickly apparent. Signs and symptoms of snakebite may be delayed.

this device is unknown, although it has been shown to remove some venom in one animal study. Other useless or dangerous techniques are electric shock and ice. Electric shock treatment of the bite site is mentioned only to be condemned. This dangerous procedure is not effective and has resulted in electrical injuries. Ice-water immersion worsens the injury.

Tourniquets are contraindicated because they obstruct arterial flow and cause ischemia. Constriction bands may be of some use, especially when immediate medical care is not available. A constriction band is an elastic bandage or Penrose drain, rope, or piece of clothing wrapped circumferentially above the bite, applied with tension that restricts superficial venous and lymphatic flow while maintaining distal pulses and capillary fill. The band should be snug but loose enough to easily slide a finger underneath. In theory, a constriction band retards venom absorption. This should increase local tissue injury but reduce the severity of systemic effects. Anecdotal human reports and animal studies suggest that constriction band use delays venom absorption without causing increased swelling.[4] Additional controlled studies are needed to better define the clinical indications for constriction band use.

TABLE 189-3 Management of Compartment Syndrome*†

1. Determine intracompartmental pressure.
2. If not elevated, continue standard management.
3. If signs of compartment syndrome are present and compartment pressure is >30 mmHg:
   - Elevate limb.
   - Administer mannitol 1–2 g/kg IV over 30 min.
   - Simultaneously administer *additional* Antivenin (Crotalidae) polyvalent, 10 to 15 vials IV over 60 min.
   - If elevated compartment pressure persists another 60 min, consider fasciotomy.

*Elevated compartment pressure is caused by the action of the venom on the tissues; thus, the most effective treatment is to neutralize the venom, which may reduce the compartment pressure.

†This protocol delivers a high osmotic load and should not be used when contraindicated. The protocol must be completed promptly so that, if ever needed, fasciotomy may be performed as early as possible.

Emergency Management

In the prehospital phase, personnel should be directed to immobilize the limb, establish intravenous access in another limb, administer oxygen, and transport the victim to a medical facility. Previously placed tourniquets and constriction bands should not be removed until intravenous access is established.

As in any emergency, initial snakebite management should include advanced life support. If the patient is hypotensive, initial treatment should include rapid intravenous isotonic fluid infusion. Other supportive care measures should include limb immobilization to reduce further venom absorption. Consultation with a physician or poison center familiar with the management of snake envenomation is recommended for all but the simplest of cases.

Antivenin (Crotalidae) polyvalent is the mainstay of therapy for poisonous snakebite.[4] It is the name for a refined and concentrated preparation of polyclonal equine immunoglobulins capable of neutralizing the venoms (an ''antivenom'') of North, Central, and South American pit vipers. All crotalid bites that show evidence of progressive signs and symptoms should immediately receive the antivenom. Progression is defined as worsening of local injury (e.g., pain, ecchymosis, or swelling), laboratory abnormalities (e.g., worsening platelet count, prolonged coagulation times, decreased fibrinogen), or systemic manifestations (e.g., unstable vital signs or abnormal mental status).

Because Antivenin (Crotalidae) polyvalent is derived from horse serum, it is common for patients to develop an allergic reaction during infusion. An intradermal skin test should be applied before antivenom is given, but only when a definite decision to administer the antivenom has been made. This is to prevent unnecessary sensitization. A positive test (wheal >10 mm in diameter) indicates that the patient may develop an allergic reaction, whereas a negative result usually indicates that the patient will tolerate the infusion. Some patients with negative skin tests will develop acute allergic reactions; likewise, some patients with positive skin tests tolerate antivenom infusion without difficulty. The skin test is a guide and antivenom decisions should be based on a risk-benefit analysis of the patient's condition. To prevent a delay while waiting for the skin test results, the antivenom should be mixed simultaneously with placement of the skin test. Because the antivenom takes 15 to 45 min to enter solution, it will be ready when the skin test is interpreted.

The recommended dose of antivenom has increased over the years. The use of at least 10 vials is recommended as the initial dose in rattlesnake bites. In rapidly progressive envenomations or hemodynamically unstable cases, an initial dose of at least 20 vials of antivenom is recommended in addition to aggressive supportive care. Poisoning by water moccasins usually requires lesser doses, whereas in copperhead bites, antivenom may not be required except for severe cases, children, and the elderly. Under no circumstances should antivenom be injected directly into finger or toes. Intramuscular injection is also not recommended because venom-induced hypovolemia may retard absorption of antivenom. Hospital pharmacies in those regions of the United States where poisonous snakes are prevalent should maintain adequate stocks of antivenom. Unfortunately, many hospitals stock insufficient amounts of antivenom, even in endemic areas.[5]

The package insert may be used as a guide for antivenom preparation. Antivenom should be administered only in a critical care facility such as an emergency department or intensive care unit. After reconstitution, the antivenom should be diluted in 250 to 500 mL of crystalloid and infused slowly, until it is evident that anaphylaxis will not occur. If a reaction does not develop, the rate should be increased in a stepwise manner until the infusion is complete, usually in 1 h. Infusion of antivenom should be done under the direct supervision of a physician. If an acute allergic reaction occurs, the infusion should be stopped immediately and antihistamines administered (both H_1- and H_2-receptor blockers). Epinephrine should be added depending on the severity of the reaction.

The end point of antivenom therapy is arrest of progression or improvement of clinical findings. One infusion of 10 to 20 vials is often sufficient. It is extremely important, however, that observation for progression of edema and systemic signs of envenomation be continued even after antivenom infusion. Limb circumference should be measured at several sites above and below the bite, and the advancing border of edema should be outlined with a pen every 30 to 60 min. This serves as an index of the progression as well as a guide for antivenom administration. Laboratory determinations are repeated q4h or after each course of antivenom therapy, whichever is more frequent. Additional antivenom therapy may be warranted if the patient's condition worsens.

The value of aggressive supportive care cannot be overemphasized. Isotonic fluid resuscitation followed by pressor agents is appropriate for hypotension. Antivenom is the best treatment for coagulopathy, but if active bleeding occurs, blood component replacement may be necessary. Another complication of snakebite is compartment syndrome. Increased compartment pressure may occur when venom is injected into a compartment during a bite. This is usually manifest by severe pain, localized to a compartment, that is resistant to narcotic analgesia. The use of fasciotomy is controversial. Recommended management is shown in Table 189-3.

The wound area should be cleaned and the need for tetanus booster determined. Cultures and antibiotic therapy should be initiated only if signs of infection are present. Although recommended by some authors, no objective evidence supports the use of prophylactic antibiotics.[6] The use of steroids is also controversial. Several studies suggest lack of efficacy or even deleterious effects. Without evidence of efficacy, steroids should be reserved for the treatment of allergic reactions or the treatment of serum sickness.

Disposition

Patients are ready for discharge when swelling begins to resolve, the coagulopathy has been reversed, and the patient is ambulatory. During recovery, the bitten part (particularly the hand) should be regularly exercised to preserve as much function and strength as possible. Outpatient follow-up is necessary to monitor for infection and serum sickness.

It cannot be overemphasized that one can easily be deceived by a bite that initially appears innocuous. An unremarkable physical and laboratory examination at presentation does not reliably indicate an insignificant envenomation. We recommended that physicians observe patients for at least 8 h. Patients with severe or life-threatening bites and patients receiving antivenom should be admitted to an intensive care unit. The general ward is appropriate for patients with mild or moderate envenomations who have completed or do not require further antivenom therapy.

Patients with dry bites who have been observed for at least 8 h may be discharged. They should return if pain, swelling, or bleeding develops.

CORAL SNAKE BITE

North American coral snakes include the eastern coral snake (*Micrurus fulvius fulvius*), the Texas coral snake (*Micrurus fulvius tenere*), and the Arizona (Sonoran) coral snake (*Micruroides euryxanthus*). The eastern coral snake is found primarily in the southeast United States. The Texas and Arizona coral snakes are found primarily in the states that bear their names. Coral snakes account for 20 to 25 bites a year.

All coral snakes are brightly colored with black, red, and yellow rings. The red and yellow rings touch in coral snakes, but they are separated by black rings in nonpoisonous snakes, creating the well known rhyme: ''Red on yellow, kill a fellow; red on black, venom lack.'' This rule is *not* true outside of the United States.

Coral snake venom is primarily composed of neurotoxic components that do not cause marked local injury. Elapid bites produce primarily neurologic effects: tremors, salivation, dysarthria, diplopia, bulbar paralysis with ptosis, fixed and contracted pupils, dysphagia, dyspnea, and seizures. The immediate cause of death is paralysis of respiratory muscles. Signs and symptoms may be delayed up to 12 h.

The potential coral snake victim should be admitted to the hospital for 24 to 48 h of observation. Coral snake venom effects may develop hours after a bite and are not easily reversed. It is suggested that 3 vials of the Antivenin (*Micrurus fulvius*) be administered to patients who have definitely been bitten because it may not be possible to prevent further effects or reverse effects that have already developed.[7] Additional coral snake antivenom is reserved for the appearance of symptoms or signs of coral snake envenomation. However, because respiratory failure may result from clinical effects of the neurotoxin, baseline and serial pulmonary function parameters (such as inspiratory pressure and vital capacity) in addition to intensive care observation may be useful. Prolonged ventilatory support may be required in severe cases. The patient must be observed closely for signs of respiratory muscle weakness and hypoventilation. Bites by the Sonoran coral snake are mild. Medical care is not usually needed.

GILA MONSTER BITE

Gila monsters are slow-moving lizards that inhabit the desert in the southwestern United States. They possess a venom as potent as rattlesnake venom but lack the apparatus to effectively inject it. Instead of fangs, they simply have short, grooved teeth down which their venom flows. Therefore, envenomation requires a prolonged bite. Gila monsters bite tenaciously and may be difficult to remove from the bitten extremity.

Most bites result in local pain and swelling only, which worsens over several hours and then subsides over several more hours. Dislodged teeth often contaminate the wound. Occasionally, a more severe syndrome of systemic toxicity develops, including weakness, lightheadedness, paresthesia, and diaphoresis. Severe hypertension may occur, which also resolves over several hours. There are few if any documented deaths from gila monster bite.

First aid involves removal of the reptile from the bite site without sustaining another bite. This may require force. It helps to place the animal on a solid surface; like other animals, it will often loosen its grip when it is no longer suspended in midair. Otherwise, standard local wound care is sufficient, taking care to remove any teeth in the wound. The usefulness of prophylactic antibiotics is unknown and tetanus status should be determined.

AUSTRALIAN ELAPIDS

About 3000 people are bitten by snakes each year in Australia, of whom at least 200 receive antivenom.[8] In the decade up to 1992, there was an average fatality rate of 1.8 per year, but in the years 1992–1994, the rate was 3.7 deaths per year (the Australian population is approximately 18.5 million). Half of all Australian snakebite deaths are caused by the brown snake (genus *Pseudonaja*).[9]

Biology

The venomous snakes of Australia are members of the family Elapidae, of which the cobras are also members. In contrast to North American Crotalidae, the Elapidae possess a relatively unsophisticated venom delivery apparatus with nonretractile small- to medium-sized paired fangs that have grooved venom channels rather than hollow venom ducts. It is thought that the Elapidae exert voluntary control over the injection of venom, hence the occurrence of the ''dry bite,'' without envenomation.[9]

The venom of the Australian elapids contains several important components.[9] Neurotoxins (tiger snake, taipan, and death adder) act at the neuromuscular junction and cause paralysis. Signs may become apparent 2 to 4 h after the bite and may include ptosis, partial ophthalmoplegia (diplopia), dysarthria, loss of facial expression, and loss of airway control as well as respiratory paralysis in severe cases. Myolysins are structurally related to the neurotoxins but instead produce rhabdomyolysis, which may result in muscle pain, weakness, myoglobinuria, renal failure, and hyperkalemia. The procoagulant toxins (brown snake, tiger snake, taipan) act as prothrombin converters, leading to fibrinogen consumption and resulting in a coagulopathy. Intracranial hemorrhage is a recognized complication. Renal impairment or failure may also result from snakebite. The mechanisms are poorly understood and may include hypotension, myoglobinuria, coagulopathy, and direct renal toxicity (the brown snake).[10] Local tissue destruction is uncommon with any Australian species, although mild to moderate ecchymosis and swelling may occur.

The brown snakes are capable of inflicting bites that cause rapid collapse and death.[4] Brown snake venom has been found to cause severe cardiovascular depression in anesthetized dogs, and these effects may account for the sudden deaths described.

Clinical Presentation

Patients typically present with a myriad of symptoms including nausea, vomiting, headache, diplopia, dysphonia, progressive muscle weakness, neck stiffness, discoloration of urine, collapse, and seizures. Young children may not provide a history of snakebite; therefore a high index of suspicion is required in this group. The absence of signs or symptoms at presentation does not exclude significant systemic envenomation.

First Aid

The aim of first aid is to delay absorption of venom from the bite site until the patient is in a facility that can administer antivenom if required.[8] The pressure-immobilization method described below is used for elapid bites because they do not manifest much local soft tissue swelling. This technique is not recommended for crotalid bites because the immobilization dressing causes severe pain when swelling develops.[12,13] All patients should immediately have the bitten extremity wrapped in a snug elastic bandage from either the ankle to the hip or the wrist to shoulder. The bandage should be applied as if to a sprained joint; if it is too loose or too tight, it will be ineffective.[13] The idea is to contain the venom and prevent systemic absorption. The limb is splinted to prevent motion. The patient should rest until help arrives. Examination of lymphatic flow rates with simulated venom has demonstrated that even if the upper or lower limb is appropriately bandaged and immobilized, walking will hasten systemic envenomation.[13] Tourniquets are an outmoded therapy and are contraindicated because they obstruct arterial flow and add ischemia injury to venom injury. In the rare circumstance that a bite is inflicted on the trunk, firm pressure should be applied without restricting breathing.

Management

Any history suggestive of snakebite should prompt the initiation of first aid, investigation, and observation, as detailed below. The pressure bandage should remain in place until the patient can receive antivenom. Once in a suitable facility, bandages and splints should not be left on for prolonged periods, as venom is then not available for interaction with circulating antivenom. In addition, there is no evidence that venom is inactivated by being trapped at the bite site.[8] If the patient's condition deteriorates immediately after bandage removal, the bandages may be reapplied while antivenom is given. Snakebite cases often present a number of complex clinical problems; therefore early consultation with an expert is recommended.

The Commonwealth Serum Laboratory (CSL) Snake Venom Detection Kit (SVDK) detects snake venom in the urine or at the bite site, identifies the type of snake involved, and provides guidance in antivenom selection if antivenom is needed. Positive SVDK identification of venom at the bite site or in the urine is not an indication for antivenom therapy without other evidence of systemic venom effect. False-positive and false-negative results have been described for blood testing by the SDVK and so should not be used.[8]

Antivenom should be given only in cases when there is clear clinical or laboratory evidence of systemic venom effect. Clinical indications for immediate antivenom therapy include vomiting and severe headache; neurotoxic effects such as ptosis, cranial nerve involvement, progressive muscle weakness, or diaphragmatic involvement; or evidence of coagulopathy. Pertinent investigations include full blood count, serum electrolytes, renal function, creatine kinase levels, and urine testing for hematuria or myoglobinuria.[9] Abnormal renal or coagulation studies may provide laboratory evidence of systemic venom effect before neurotoxic effects are apparent. If prothrombin time or activated partial thromboplastin time are prolonged, then levels of fibrinogen and fibrin degradation products should be obtained.

In the absence of clinical or laboratory evidence of venom effect, the elastic bandage should be removed and the patient observed for 12 h. Delayed envenomation after benign presentation has been documented. If significant envenomation has occurred, most patients will develop clinical or laboratory evidence of envenomation within 2 h of removing a bandage.[8] Therefore, coagulation studies should be repeated 2 h after bandage removal and at intervals thereafter, depending on the patient's condition.

Five antivenom products, derived from equine IgG, are produced by the CSL to treat envenomation by certain groups of Australian snakes. These are termed *monovalent antivenoms*. A polyvalent antivenom, also equine IgG, neutralizes the venom of all five major groups of dangerous Australian snakes. The reader is directed to more detailed sources or CSL product information for the species covered by each antivenom product.[2]

If indicated, antivenom should be given immediately in sufficient doses to improve coagulation studies. A child should receive the same dose as an adult.[8] Pregnancy is not a contraindication to antivenom therapy. Skin testing before antivenom administration is not routinely recommended.[8] If the type of snake cannot be identified, one or two appropriate monovalent antivenoms, specific for a known group of snakes, may be selected using knowledge of snakes found in the geographic area. Polyvalent antivenom is used in the following circumstances: (1) monovalent antivenom is not available; (2) the SVDK is not available or has failed to identify the type of snake and the range of possible snakes would require the mixing of three or more monovalent antivenoms; (3) the patient is severely envenomated, there is insufficient time to wait for SVDK results, and the range of possible snakes would require the mixing of three or more monovalent antivenoms; or (4) stocks of appropriate monovalent antivenom have been exhausted and the patient requires further antivenom treatment.[9]

In contrast to experience around the world, anaphylaxis appears to be a rare complication of antivenom therapy in Australia.[8,14] Nevertheless, patients should be treated in a setting where anaphylaxis can be managed. Premedication with a subcutaneous dose of 0.3 mL of 1:1000 epinephrine (adrenaline) in an adult or 0.1 mL in a child along with a parenteral antihistamine is recommended by some authors.[8,15] Although prospective data are lacking, corticosteroids may have a role in premedication and prevention of serum sickness. Most treatment protocols dictate that patients with a history of allergy to equine proteins should receive corticosteroids. In addition, a 5-day course of prednisolone may be prescribed in an attempt to reduce the incidence of serum sickness in those patients who receive large doses of monovalent antivenom or polyvalent antivenom.[8]

REFERENCES

1. Langley RL, Morrow WE: Deaths resulting from animal attacks in the United States. *Wild Environ Med* 8:8, 1997.
2. Klauber LM: *Rattlesnakes: Their Habits, Life, Histories and Influence on Mankind,* vol 2, 2d ed. San Diego, CA: University of California Press, Zoological Society of San Diego, 1972.
3. Russell FE: *Snake Venom Poisoning,* 3d ed. Great Neck, NY: Scholium International, 1983.
4. Burgess JL, Dart RC, Egen NB, Mayersohn M: The effects of constriction bands on rattlesnake venom absorption: A pharmacokinetic study. *Ann Emerg Med* 21:1086, 1992.
5. Dart RC, Stark Y, Fulton B, et al: Insufficient stocking of poisoning antidotes in hospital emergency departments. *JAMA* 276:1508, 1996.
6. Clark RF, Selden BS, Furbee B: The incidence of wound infection following crotalid envenomation. *J Emerg Med* 11:583, 1993.
7. Kitchens CS, Van Mierop LHS: Envenomation by the eastern coral snake (*Micrurus fulvius fulvius*): A study of 39 victims. *JAMA* 258:1615, 1987.
8. Sutherland SK, Leonard RL: Snakebite deaths in Australia 1992–1994 and a management update. *Med J Aust* 163:616, 1995.
9. White J: *CSL Antivenom Handbook.* Melbourne: CSL Ltd, 1995.
10. Acott CJ: Acute renal failure after envenomation by the common brown snake. *Med J Aust* 149:709, 1988.
11. Sutherland SK: Deaths from snake bite in Australia, 1981–1991. *Med J Aust* 157:740, 1992.
12. Sutherland SK, Coulter AR, Harris RD: Rationalisation of first-aid measures for elapid snake bite. *Lancet* 1:183, 1979.

13. Howath DM, Southee AE, Whyte IM: Lymphatic flow rates and first-aid in simulated peripheral snake or spider envenomation. *Med J Aust* 161:695, 1994.
14. Corrigan P, Russell FE, Wainschel J: Clinical reactions to antivenene. *Toxicon* 16(suppl 1):457, 1978.
15. Tibballs J: Premedication for snake antivenom. *Med J Aust* 160:4, 1994.

TRAUMA AND ENVENOMATIONS FROM MARINE FAUNA

Paul S. Auerbach

Although encounters with noxious marine organisms occur predominantly in warm temperatures and tropical seas, dangerous marine animals are found to a significant degree as far north as 50° N latitude. Because of increasing numbers of recreational divers and private saltwater aquariums, as well as the ease of international travel, emergency physicians everywhere should be familiar with treatment for injuries and illnesses associated with the marine environment. Included among these dangers are injuries from traumatizing and envenoming animals. Exposure to these creatures may occur while walking on the beach, wading in tidal pools, deep-water diving, or simply changing the water in a home aquarium. The infections that may occur after marine trauma are sometimes unique and can be debilitating.

MARINE TRAUMA

The notoriety of shark attacks seems undeserved when the statistics are examined.[1] Fewer than 100 attacks are reported annually worldwide, with 10 or fewer fatalities. Of approximately 370 shark species, only 32 have been definitely implicated in human attacks, the majority by the tiger, great white, blue, mako, hammerhead, bull, and grey reef sharks.

Two general attack behaviors have been described: feeding and agonistic. Feeding attacks appear to be the result of mistaking a human for a pinniped or other common shark prey. Such attacks often terminate as soon as the shark realizes the mistake. Agonistic attacks seem to be defensive or territorial-protective.

Shark attack wounds range from severe dermal abrasions (due to sharkskin denticles) following a ''bumping'' to massive tissue loss with fractures and hemorrhage. Such injuries occur from razor-sharp teeth on jaws brought together with an estimated force approaching 18 tons/in^2 tooth to tooth. ''Hit-and-run'' attacks occur in the majority of instances, and 70 percent of victims are bitten only once or twice. The lower extremity is most frequently injured, followed by the upper extremity. Death is usually the result of hemorrhagic shock or drowning.

As with other resuscitative endeavors, the ABCs are fundamental, with special attention to hemorrhage control, volume resuscitation, and rewarming as needed. Tetanus toxoid and tetanus immunoglobulin should be administered as indicated. Prophylactic intravenous antibiotics are empirically recommended to counter a potential *Vibrio* species infection. Third-generation cephalosporins, trimethoprim-sulfamethoxazole, chloramphenicol, ciprofloxacin, norfloxacin, or an aminoglycoside may be given. Meticulous wound care is most appropriately performed in the operating room for adequate surgical exploration, irrigation, and débridement of wounds. To minimize tissue destruction associated with an infection, wounds may be packed open for delayed primary closure or closed around drainage systems.

It has been suggested that most shark attacks could be prevented if a few precautionary measures were taken: (1) avoid swimming in river mouths, low-visibility waters, or shark-infested waters; (2) avoid wearing bright or shiny clothing, jewelry, or equipment; (3) avoid swimming with an open (bleeding) wound; and (4) obey beach authorities and posted warnings.

The great barracuda (*Sphyraena barracuda*) is the only barracuda species implicated in human attacks. Attacks are generally by solitary fish and occur only in tropical climes. Moray eels, found in tropical-to-temperate waters, can inflict severe puncture wounds or lacerations, commonly to the hands of inquisitive divers. Other marine vertebrates known to cause traumatic injuries to humans include giant groupers, sea lions, seals, crocodiles, alligators, needlefish, wahoos, piranas, and triggerfish. Wounds resulting from interactions with such creatures are a combination of crush injury, abrasion, puncture, and laceration. Treatment of such injuries is analogous to that of shark bites, with an emphasis on irrigation, removal of foreign bodies (e.g., teeth), and allowing adequate wound drainage (e.g., leaving puncture wounds open).

Coral cuts are probably the most common injuries sustained underwater. The initial reactions to a coral cut are stinging pain, erythema, and pruritus, most commonly on the hands, forearms, elbows, and knees. Within minutes, a break in the skin may be surrounded by an erythematous wheal, which fades over 1 to 2 h.

With or without treatment, the local reaction of red, raised welts and local pruritus may progress to cellulitis with ulceration and tissue sloughing. The wounds heal slowly over 3 to 6 weeks. In extreme cases, the victim develops cellulitis with lymphangitis, reactive bursitis, local ulceration, and wound necrosis. *Coral poisoning* usually refers to systemic malaise, fever, diarrhea, and general inanition associated with a wound from coral.

Coral cuts should be promptly and vigorously irrigated to remove all foreign matter. Any fragments that remain can become embedded and increase the risk of infection or foreign-body granuloma. If stinging is a major symptom, there may be envenomation by nematocysts. A brief rinse with dilute acetic acid (vinegar) or papain solution may diminish the discomfort. If a coral-induced laceration is severe, it should be closed with adhesive strips, rather than sutures, if possible. Sharp débridement each day for 3 to 4 days is preferable if the wound is deep. For superficial (no fat showing) wounds, utilize daily saline solution or dilute povidone-iodine wet-to-dry dressing changes, or apply a topical antiseptic under a nonadherent dressing.

Bacteriology of the Marine Environment and Antibiotic Therapy

Ocean water provides a rich saline milieu for microbes.[2] Although the greatest number and variety of bacteria are found near the ocean surface, diverse bacteria and fungi are found in marine silts, sediments, and sand. Microbes, including bacteria, microalgae, protozoa, yeasts, and viruses, are most abundant in areas with the greatest number of life forms. Marine bacteria are generally gram-negative rods. Bacteria isolated from the marine environment or from marine-acquired wounds of greatest concern to humans include *Aeromonas hydrophila, Bacteroides fragilis, Chromobacterium violaceum, Clostridium perfringens, Erysipelothrix rhusopathiae, Escherichia coli, Mycobacterium marinum, Pseudomonas aeruginosa, Salmonella enteritidis, Staphylococcus aureus, Streptococcus* species, and *Vibrio* species.

There is no substitute for meticulous wound care, including irrigation and débridement of devitalized tissue, with particular attention to retained foreign bodies, such as teeth, vegetable matter, and spines. Quantitative wound culture prior to the appearance of clinically evident wound infection has not been shown to be useful. The issue of prophylactic antibiotics in the treatment of marine wounds has not been well studied. Pending a prospective study of prophylactic antibiotics in this setting, the following recommendations are generally advised, based on the morbidity of soft-tissue infections caused by *Vibrio* species:[3]

- Minor abrasions and lacerations of the normal, immunocompetent patient do not require prophylactic antibiotics.
- Minor abrasions and lacerations of immunocompromised or chronically ill patients require initiation of therapy with trimethoprim-sulfamethoxazole, tetracycline, cefuroxime axetil, norfloxacin, or ciprofloxacin.

- High-risk wounds (e.g., extensive lacerations or burns; deep puncture wounds, particularly involving the joint space; or grossly contaminated wounds) require initiation of parenteral trimethoprim-sulfamethoxazole, a third-generation cephalosporin, an aminoglycoside, chloramphenicol, or one of the oral agents mentioned above.

The objectives for the management of infections from marine microorganisms are to recognize the clinical condition, culture the organism, and provide antimicrobial therapy. The appearance of an infection indicates the need for prompt débridement and search for a retained foreign body. Infected wounds should be cultured for aerobes and anaerobes. Since special media may be necessary for culture and sensitivity testing, the clinician should alert the microbiology laboratory that a marine-acquired organism might be present. Empirical antibiotic therapy should be initiated based on the clinical condition.

Management of marine-acquired infections must include coverage against *Vibrio* species with a third-generation cephalosporin, trimethoprim-sulfamethoxazole, tetracycline, norfloxacin, ciprofloxacin, or cefuroxime. Freshwater infections may be treated with the abovementioned agents, imipenem, or an aminoglycoside, to cover *Aeromonas* species. Appropriate antibiotic coverage against staphylococcal and streptococcal species is mandatory, since they remain the most common infecting organisms. Imipenem-cilastatin is reserved for established wound infections and/or sepsis.

Several special clinical conditions are of note. A patient with rapidly progressive cellulitis, myositis, or necrotizing fasciitis warrants consideration of *Vibrio parahaemolyticus* or *Vibrio vulnificus* infection. *Vibrio vulnificus* can also cause primary septicemia in chronically ill individuals, particularly those with hepatic disease. Mortality rates for such patients approach 60 percent. *Erysipelothrix rhusopathiae* is the infectious agent in "fish-handler's disease" and causes sharply marginated, painful, expanding plaques on the fingers or hands following cutaneous inoculation. It responds to penicillin, ampicillin, cephalexin, β-lactam antimicrobials, ciprofloxacin, and clindamycin. Resistance has been noted to vancomycin, the aminoglycosides, trimethoprim-sulfamethoxazole, tetracycline, and erythromycin. *M. marinum* is an acid-fast bacillus that causes "swimming-pool granuloma" or "aquarium granuloma." Some 3 to 4 weeks following an abrasion or puncture wound, the patient develops a red papule, which progresses to a cutaneous granuloma. Excision or antibiotics (minocycline, trimethoprim-sulfamethoxazole, rifampin, or ethambutol) are the treatments of choice, although spontaneous resolution typically occurs over 2 to 3 years. *Aeromonas hydrophila* is a gram-negative bacterium found in marine and freshwater environments; it causes wound infections that can rapidly become cellulitic and progress to necrotizing myositis.

MARINE ENVENOMATIONS

Marine venoms are large-molecular-weight compounds of vasoactive and proteolytic enzymes with diffuse effects on the circulatory, neurologic, immunologic, and respiratory systems.[4–7] They require a specialized delivery system, are commonly heat and gastric-acid labile, show nonseasonal toxicity, and can be released in varying amounts. Conversely, poisons are usually metabolic byproducts of lower molecular weight. They are ingested (thereby requiring no delivery system), are usually heat and gastric-acid stable, and carry some seasonal toxicity.

Venoms are produced in specialized glands and are broadly classified as parenteral toxins, which are injected mechanically, or crinotoxins, which are delivered topically as slimes (mucous or gastric secretions). Practically, venoms are used offensively or defensively. An offensive venom is employed to kill prey and is typically located near the mouth or on the tentacles. Defensive venoms are used to protect the animal and are usually located near the tail. A human's reaction to an envenomation can be allergic or toxic.

Invertebrate Envenomations

Envenoming invertebrates are found in five phyla: Cnidaria (Coelenterates), Porifera, Echinodermata, Mollusca, and Annelida.[4]

CNIDARIA (COELENTERATES) The phylum Cnidaria is an enormous group of approximately 9000 species, at least 100 of which are dangerous to humans. The phylum contains three classes: Hydrozoa, Scyphozoa, and Anthozoa. Cnidariae, from *cnid,* the stem of the Greek word "nettle," are known for their specialized venom-containing stinging cells, called cnidocytes. The cnidocytes are located near the mouth or on the outer surfaces of tentacles. A physical or chemical stimulus causes the release of a hollow, sharply pointed threadlike tube from the contained nematocyst.[8] This tube penetrates the victim's skin, allowing injection of the venom, with diffusion into the general circulation.[8,9] Detached, moistened tentacles carry live nematocysts capable of discharging for months. Air-dried nematocysts may retain considerable potency for weeks.

The class Hydrozoa includes the hydroids, milleporina (fire corals), and siphonophores (Portuguese man-of-war and bluebottle jellyfish). Hydroids are the most numerous of the hydrozoans. The feather hydroids are plumelike animals that sting the victim who brushes against or handles them.[10] Coastal storms can break off feather hydroid branches and infest a local swimming area.

Contact with the nematocysts of a feather hydroid induces a mild reaction, which consists of instantaneous burning, itching, and urticaria. If the exposure is brief, the skin rash may not be noticeable or may consist of a faintly erythematous morbilliform eruption. A second variety of envenomation consists of a delayed papular, hemorrhagic, or zosteriform reaction occurring 4 to 12 h after contact. Rarely, erythema multiforme or a desquamative eruption may develop. Systemic manifestations are rarely reported.

The *Millepora* species, or fire corals, are not true corals. The fire coral *Millepora alcicornis* probably accounts for the majority of coelenterate envenomations. Fire corals are widely distributed in shallow tropical waters and often mistaken for seaweed. Tiny nematocyst-bearing tentacles protrude from numerous minute surface gastropores. Immediately following contact with fire coral, the victim notices burning or stinging pain, with rare proximal radiation. Over the course of 5 to 30 min, pruritic urticarial lesions develop. The pain generally resolves without treatment in 30 to 90 min. In the case of multiple stings, regional lymph nodes may become inflamed. Skin lesions resolve over 3 to 7 days, occasionally resulting in postinflammatory hyperpigmentation, which may take months to disappear.

The Atlantic Portuguese man-of-war (*Physalia physalis*) inhabits the surface of the ocean.[10] It is constructed of a floating sail (pneumatophore) from which are suspended multiple nematocyst-bearing tentacles measuring up to 30 m in length. The smaller Pacific bluebottle (*Physalia utriculus*) usually has a single fishing tentacle that attains lengths of up to 15 m. Each tentacle in a larger specimen may carry more than 750,000 nematocysts. Nematocysts from fractured tentacles may remain active for months. The most common reaction from contact is an immediate, toxic dermal reaction with linearly arranged urticarial lesions.[11] Respiratory distress and death have been reported following *P. physalis* envenomation.

The class Scyphozoa, or jellyfish, includes the Indo-Pacific box jellyfish (*Chironex fleckeri*), the sea nettle (*Chrysaora quinquecirrha*), and the thimble jellyfish (*Linuche unguiculata*).[11] The Indo-Pacific chirodropids are armed with some of the most potent venoms in existence. An extreme example of envenomation occurs with the Indo-Pacific box jellyfish. Found along the northern coast of Australia, *C. fleckeri* has killed at least 65 people in the past century. Death is attributed to hypotension, profound muscle spasm, muscular and respiratory paralysis, and subsequent cardiac arrest. The overall mortality rate following box jellyfish stings approaches 15 to 20 percent. Most stings are minor, but severe reactions or death can follow skin contact with tentacles in excess of 6 to 7 m. The sting is instantly and intensely painful, and the victim may struggle purposefully for only a minute or two prior to collapse. The toxic skin reaction may be quite intense, with rapid formation of wheals, vesicles, and a darkened reddish-brown or purple whiplike flare pattern with stripes of 8 to 10 mm in width. Major stings show skin blistering within 6 h, with superficial necrosis in 12 to 18 h. On occasion, a pathognomonic "frosted" appearance with a transverse crosshatched pattern may be present.

Sea nettles (*Chrysaora* and *Cyanea* species) are found in tropical and temperate waters, particularly the Chesapeake Bay, and are far less dangerous. Sea nettle envenomation presents similarly to that from *Physalia* species.

Seabather's eruption, commonly referred to by the misnomer "sea lice," is a vesicular or morbilliform pruritic dermatitis.[12] It occurs a few minutes to 12 h after saltwater exposure. The eruption primarily involves skin surfaces covered by bathing suits, swim caps, or fins. Divers may be afflicted on the neck when floating in water churned by boat propellers that have ground floating jellyfish into fragments. Dermatitis persists for 2 to 14 days and resolves spontaneously. Other symptoms include headache, chills, pronounced nocturnal pruritus, malaise, conjunctivitis, and urethritis. The 0.5-mm larval form of the thimble jellyfish *Linuche unguiculata* has been recently identified as the cause of outbreaks in southern Florida and the Caribbean. The planula form of the sea anemone *Edwardsiella lineata* has been implicated in outbreaks off the coast of Long Island, New York.

The class Anthozoa includes the sea anemones, stony (true) corals, and the soft corals. Anemones are attractive creatures often found in tidal pools, where the unwary may brush up against them or inquisitively touch them. Like other coelenterates, they possess tentacles loaded with nematocysts. The dermatitis resulting from contact is identical to that produced by fire coral. If the envenomation is severe, hemorrhagic bullae with necrosis and ulceration may occur.

Due to considerable phylogenetic resemblance among *Cnidaria* species, the clinical features of *Cnidaria* envenomation are similar across a wide spectrum of severity. The toxicity of envenomation depends on the venom dose, the marine species, and the victim. Mild envenomation results in bothersome dermatitides that resolve spontaneously over 1 to 2 weeks, with occasional postinflammatory hyperpigmentation. Anemones, *Physalia* species, and scyphozoans may cause moderate-to-severe envenomations compounded by systemic symptoms. These symptoms may appear immediately or within several hours.

Therapy is directed at the ABCs, detoxifying the venom, and providing symptomatic and pain relief. Nematocysts still attached to the patient need to be deactivated and removed to prevent continued envenomation. All victims with systemic signs or symptoms should be observed for at least 8 h, since rebound of symptoms can occur. *Chironex fleckeri* produces the only venom for which there is a specific topical antidote, 5% acetic acid (vinegar). While the venoms are heat labile, this fact does not appear to be of clinical significance, and hot water immersion is not recommended.

Deactivation of attached nematocysts is important but controversial, due to locale-dependent variations in therapy.[13] A generally accepted method is to immediately apply a topical decontaminant (see below), if available, to putatively inactivate undischarged nematocysts. Freshwater rinsing is not recommended because the hypotonic solution is felt to stimulate nematocyst discharge. However, some lifeguards in Florida report that a victim of a *Physalia* sting may find relief from being showered with a forceful stream of water, which implies that the mechanical removal of nematocysts supercedes the deleterious effect of hypotonicity. Gentle application of fresh water is prohibited. After decontamination, visible tentacles can be removed with forceps or a double-gloved hand.

As a decontaminant, 5% acetic acid (vinegar) is the treatment of choice to inactivate most venoms. It is absolutely indicated in the event of a sting from *Chironex*. An alternative therapy is isopropyl alcohol (40 to 70%), which is not recommended for *Chironex*. For *Chrysaora* or *Cyanea*, a slurry of baking soda (sodium bicarbonate) is effective. Vinegar is not very effective for seabather's eruption, for which papain solution may be much more effective. The detoxicant should be applied continuously for at least 30 min or until there is no further pain. Once the nematocysts have been inactivated, the easiest way to remove them is to apply shaving cream or a paste of baking soda, flour, or talc and then shave the area with a razor or similar instrument. Topical anesthetics, antihistamines, or steroids may be of benefit. Prophylactic antibiotics are not needed, but standard antitetanus prophylaxis and diligent wound care should be carried out.

In general, only severe *Physalia* and box jellyfish stings will result in rapid decompensation. Other than the usual resuscitative measures and sheep-derived antivenom specific for *Chironex* envenomation (Commonwealth Serum Laboratories, Melbourne, Australia), there are no new therapies on the horizon. Pain can be excruciating and requires narcotic analgesia. For such severe envenomations, it may be useful to apply the pressure-immobilization technique to the envenomed extremity. This is done by wrapping the limb with a venous-lymphatic occlusive bandage and then applying a splint. The wrap is maintained until the victim is brought to a medical facility where intensive care and antivenom can be provided. Corneal envenomations can be irrigated with an isotonic solution and treated judiciously with topical steroids.

PORIFERA The phylum *Porifera* contains approximately 4000 species of sponges that are composed of horny but elastic skeletons.[10] Embedded in the connective tissue matrices are spicules of silicon dioxide or calcium carbonate. Secondary coelenterate inhabitants are responsible for the dermatitis and local necrotic skin reaction termed *sponge diver's disease.* A number of sponges produce crinotoxins that may be direct dermal irritants.

Two general syndromes are induced by contact with sponges. The first is a pruritic dermatitis similar to plant-induced allergic dermatitis. Within a few hours after skin contact, itching and burning develop, which may then progress to local joint swelling and stiffness, soft-tissue edema, and vesiculation, particularly if small pieces of broken sponge are retained in the skin near the interphalangeal or metacarpophalangeal joints. The skin may become mottled or purpuric. Untreated mild reactions will subside within 3 to 7 days. With large-surface-area exposure, the victim may complain of fever, chills, malaise, dizziness, nausea, and muscle cramps. Bullae may become purulent. Erythema multiforme or an anaphylactoid reaction may develop 1 to 2 weeks after a severe exposure.

The second syndrome induced by contact with sponges is an irritant dermatitis and follows the penetration of small spicules of silica or calcium carbonate into the skin. Crinotoxins enter microtraumatic lesions caused by the spicules. In severe cases, superficial desquamation of the skin may follow in 10 days to 2 months. There is no medical intervention that can prevent this process. Recurrent eczema and persistent arthralgias are rare complications.

Because it is usually impossible to distinguish clinically between the allergic and spicule-induced reactions, it is safest to treat for both. The skin should be gently dried. Spicules should be removed, if possible, using adhesive tape, a thin application of rubber cement, or a facial peel. Beginning as soon as possible, 5% acetic acid (vinegar) soaks should be applied for 10 to 30 min three to four times daily to affected areas. Isopropyl alcohol (40 to 70%) is a reasonable second choice. Although topical steroids may help to relieve the secondary inflammation, they are of no initial value. If steroids are applied before the vinegar soaks, they appear to worsen the primary reaction. Delayed primary therapy or inadequate decontamination may result in the persistence of bullae. Erythema multiforme may require supportive care, including intravenous hydration, particularly if mucosal surfaces are involved, and topical steroids for symptomatic relief. The use of systemic steroids for erythema multiforme is controversial. If the allergic component is severe, systemic glucocorticoids (prednisone 40 to 80 mg per day tapered over 2 weeks) may be beneficial. Severe itching may be controlled with an antihistamine.

ECHINODERMATA The phylum Echinodermata has five classes: sea lilies, brittle stars, starfish, sea urchins, and sea cucumbers.[10] Only the latter three are of emergency medical interest. The venom apparatuses of sea urchins consist of the sharp, brittle, venom-filled spines and the triple-jawed globiferous pedicellariae. Venomous spines cause immediate, intense pain. Burning pain rapidly evolves into severe local muscle aching, with erythema and swelling of the skin surrounding the puncture sites. Frequently, spines break off and lodge in the victim. If a spine enters a joint, it may rapidly induce severe synovitis. If multiple spines have penetrated the skin, particularly if they are deeply embedded, the victim may rapidly develop systemic symptoms, including nausea, vomiting, paresthesias, muscular paralysis, abdominal pain, syncope, hypotension, and respiratory distress. Pedicellariae can cause more severe symptoms, which are predominantly neurologic.

Starfish (Asteroidea) are covered with thorny spines that deliver a slimy venom produced in special glandular tissue. The crown-of-thorns sea star, *Acanthaster planci,* is a particularly venomous species. The sharp, rigid, venomous aboral spines of this animal may grow to 4 to 6 cm. As the spines enter the skin, they carry venom into the wound, causing immediate pain, copious bleeding, and mild edema. The wound may become dusky or discolored. Multiple puncture wounds may result in acute systemic reactions, including paresthesias, nausea, vomiting, lymphadenopathy, and muscular paralysis.

Sea cucumbers (Holothuroidea) produce a toxin that is concentrated in the tentacular organs. Direct contact may induce a contact dermatitis, which is usually mild, since the venom is diluted in seawater. The greater risk is to the corneas and conjunctivae, which may become intensely inflamed.

Treatment of echinoderm wounds consists of immediate immersion in hot water to tolerance [45°C (113°F)] for 30 to 90 min or until there is significant pain relief. Prompt removal of pedicellariae and spines, especially those in intraarticular areas, is necessary. Soft-tissue radiographs or magnetic resonance imaging are helpful in locating retained spines. Treatment of systemic symptoms is supportive, and analgesia may be needed. Granuloma formation occurs and may require excision. Sequelae that reflect an immune response, such as erythema nodosum or tenosynovitis, may require therapy with glucocorticoids. Since sea cucumbers dine on coelenterates and secrete the nematocyst venom, topical vinegar or isopropyl alcohol may provide some symptomatic relief.

ANNELIDA The phylum Annelida contains the fireworms, or bristleworms, which are segmented worms covered with cactuslike bristles that can penetrate the skin.[10] These bristles easily detach in the skin and can be difficult to remove. Envenomation causes intense inflammation with a burning sensation and erythema. Untreated, the pain generally resolves within a few hours, but erythema may last for 2 to 3 days. Bristles should be removed with forceps, a thin application of rubber cement, a facial peel, or adhesive tape, and topical vinegar or isopropyl alcohol may be applied. The inflammatory response may require a course of glucocorticoids.

MOLLUSCA The phylum Mollusca contains two potentially envenoming classes: the gastropods (cone shells and nudibranchs) and the cephalopods (octopuses).[10] Cone shells are beautiful, univalve creatures found in shallow Indo-Pacific waters. They are predators that feed by injecting a potent neurotoxin via detachable, dartlike, radular teeth. Mild stings resemble hymenopteran envenomations. More severe reactions include local and then generalized paresthesias and muscular paralysis, with ventilatory failure.

The Australian blue-ringed octopus produces the neurotoxin tetrodotoxin. Octopus bites typically occur on the upper extremity and consist of two small puncture wounds. Local reactions are often absent, and generalized paresthesias may be the first indication of an envenomation. Further neurologic symptoms may develop, with flaccid paralysis and ensuing ventilatory failure. Treatment is supportive, with mechanical ventilation as needed, and full recovery is expected. No antivenom is available. Wide excision of the bite wound has been done to remove sequestered venom. However, there is no scientific evidence of speedier recovery to support this practice.

For both cone shell and paralytic octopus envenomations, the most commonly recommended field first aid technique is pressure-immobilization, described above.

Vertebrate Envenomations

Stingrays are the most common group of fish to inflict human envenomations. The venom organ of stingrays consists of one to four venomous spines on the dorsum of a whiplike tail.[10] When an unwary human handles, corners, or steps on a ray, the tail reflexively whips upward and accurately thrusts the spines into the victim, producing a puncture wound or jagged laceration in addition to an envenomation. On occasion, the entire spine tip is broken off and remains in the wound. Envenomation causes immediate local intense pain, edema, and variable bleeding. The pain, which may radiate centrally, peaks at 30 to 60 min and may last for up to 48 h. The wound is initially dusky or cyanotic and rapidly progresses to become erythematous and hemorrhagic, with fat and muscle involvement and possible necrosis. Systemic manifestations include weakness, nausea, vomiting, diarrhea, diaphoresis, vertigo, headache, syncope, seizures, muscle cramps, fasciculations, generalized edema (with truncal wounds), paralysis, hypotension, arrhythmias, and death.

Scorpionfish are found in tropical and, less commonly, temperate oceans and, unfortunately, in private aquariums.[10] They can be grouped according to the severity of their envenomation in ascending order from the beautifully ornate lionfish (mild) to the camouflaged scorpionfish (moderate to severe) to the motionless stonefish (severe to life-threatening). The venom organs consist of 12 or 13 dorsal, 2 pelvic, and 3 anal spines with associated venom glands. Although they are frequently large, plumelike, and ornate, the pectoral spines are not associated with venom glands.

Scorpionfish venom has been likened in potency to cobra venom. Its principal action appears to be direct muscle toxicity, resulting in paralysis of cardiac, involuntary, and skeletal muscles. The presentation of injury is similar to stingray envenomation. Pain is immediate and intense, with radiation centrally. Untreated, the pain peaks at 60 to 90 min and persists for 6 to 12 h. In the case of the stonefish, the pain may be severe enough to cause delirium and may persist at high levels for days. The wound and surrounding area are initially ischemic and then cyanotic, with surrounding areas of erythema, edema, and warmth. Vesicles may form, and rapid tissue sloughing, with surrounding areas of cellulitis, may develop within 48 h. Systemic effects are similar to those of coelenterate envenomation.

Other venomous fish that sting in a manner similar to scorpionfish include catfish, weeverfish, surgeonfish, homed sharks, toadfish, ratfish, rabbitfish, stargazers, and leatherbacks. Approximately 1000 species of catfish inhabit both fresh- and saltwater. Catfish venom apparatus consists of a single dorsal and two pectoral fin spines and the axillary venom glands. Catfish also produce a crinotoxin that can be introduced into the wound during envenomation. The sting of the marine catfish is usually more severe than that of its freshwater counterpart. The weeverfish, the most venomous fish in the temperate zone, is found in the Mediterranean and European coastal areas. Weeverfish are bottom dwellers that sting when stepped on. The five to seven envenoming dorsal spines can penetrate a leather boot and create a substantial puncture wound.

The success of therapy for stings from marine animal spines depends on rapid initiation. Treatment is directed at combating the effects of the venom, alleviating pain, and preventing infection. The wound should be irrigated immediately, and any visible pieces of the spine or integumentary sheath should be removed. As soon as possible, the wound should be immersed in hot water to tolerance [45°C (113°F)] for 30 to 90 min or until there is pain relief. During the hot-water soak, the wound should be explored and foreign material removed.

Narcotics may be necessary for pain control. Local infiltration of the wound with lidocaine without epinephrine or a regional nerve block may be very useful.

After the soaking procedure, the wound should be prepared in an aseptic fashion, reexplored, and thoroughly débrided. Soft-tissue radiography should be employed to visualize calcified matter. Wounds should remain open for delayed primary closure or sutured loosely, ensuring adequate drainage. Prophylactic antibiotics are recommended because of the high incidence of ulceration and necrosis with subsequent secondary infection. If a victim is to be treated and released, he or she should be observed for at least 4 h for systemic side effects. A stonefish antivenom is available for severe systemic reactions to stonefish or other scorpionfish.

Sea snakes (family Hydrophidae) are the most abundant venomous reptiles.[10] There are 52 species of sea snakes, all of which are venomous. The snakes are distributed in the tropical and warm temperate Pacific and Indian Oceans. None are found in the Atlantic Ocean, the Caribbean, or North American coastal waters. Hawaii is the only US state that has sea snakes.

Most sea snakes are 3 to 4 ft (about 1 m) long, although some attain lengths of up to 9 ft (3 m). They can be distinguished from land snakes by their flat tails and valvelike nostril flaps and from eels by the presence of scales and the absence of gills and fins. Sea snakes swim in an undulating fashion and can move backward or forward in the water with equal speed. The venom apparatus consists of two to four hollow maxillary fangs and a pair of associated venom glands. The fangs are short and easily detached. Approximately 80 percent of bites do not result in significant envenomations.

Sea snake venom contains a peripherally acting neurotoxin that causes paralysis and a myotoxin that causes muscle necrosis. Due to the lack of an immediate local reaction, the bite often goes unnoticed. Symptoms typically become apparent 2 h after the bite but may begin as soon as 5 min or as late as 8 h afterward. The first complaint may be of euphoria, malaise, or anxiety. Classic muscle aches then develop, along with a ''thick tongue'' and sialorrhea. Ascending flaccid or spastic paralysis follows shortly and is accompanied by other neurologic signs and symptoms, such as ophthalmoplegia, ptosis, facial paralysis, and pupillary changes. Death is most commonly due to ventilatory failure.

Diagnosis of a sea snake bite is based on the combination of snake identification and the presence of a multiple-puncture bite wound that

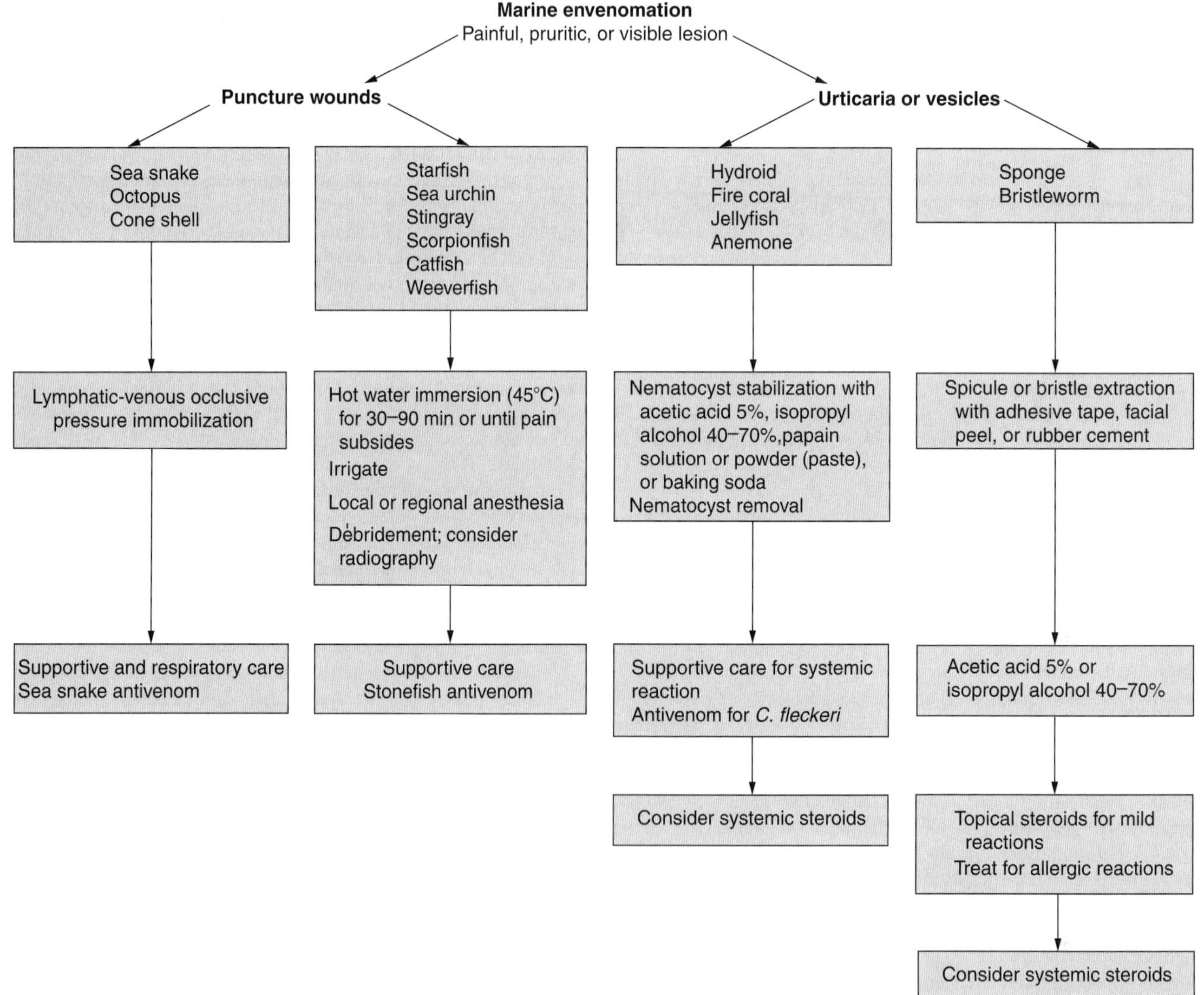

FIG. 190-1. Algorithmic approach to marine envenomation. (Adapted from Auerbach PS: Marine envenomations. *N Engl J Med* 325:490, 1991, with permission.)

was initially painless and occurred in the water. Envenomation should be suspected if the characteristic symptoms, primarily myalgias, develop. The presence of myoglobinuria and elevated hepatic enzyme levels is also typical. Neurotoxic symptoms are rapid in onset and usually appear within 2 to 3 h. If no symptoms develop by 6 to 8 h, envenomation did not occur.

Treatment of a sea snake bite involves pressure-immobilization of the affected limb to provide venom sequestration. Incision and suction therapy are not recommended. Supportive measures are necessary but are not an adequate substitute for sea snake antivenom, which is absolutely indicated. With any clinical evidence of envenomation, polyvalent sea snake antivenom should be administered after skin testing. Tiger snake (*Notechis scutatus*) antivenom is also available as a second choice. If neither of these is available, Crotalidae polyvalent antivenin can be used.

The administration of antivenom should begin as soon as possible but remains useful up to 36 h after envenomation. Intensive supportive care and monitoring of renal, metabolic, and respiratory function are critical. Since the relatively small molecular weight of sea snake neurotoxin makes it dialyzable, hemodialysis may be of benefit. Figure 190-1 provides an algorithmic approach to unidentified marine envenomation.

REFERENCES

1. Auerbach PS, Halstead BW: Injuries from nonvenomous aquatic animals, in Auerbach PS (ed): *Wilderness Medicine: Management of Wilderness and Environmental Emergencies,* 3d ed. St. Louis, Mosby, 1995, pp 1303–1326.
2. Auerbach PS, Yaijko DM, Nassos PS, et al: Bacteriology of the marine environment: Implications for clinical therapy. *Ann Emerg Med* 16:643, 1987.
3. McLaughlin JC: *Vibrio*, in Murray PR (ed): *Manual of Clinical Microbiology,* 6th ed. Washington, ASM Press, 1995, pp 465–476.
4. Auerbach PS: Marine envenomation, in Auerbach PS (ed): *Wilderness Medicine: Management of Wilderness and Environmental Emergencies,* 3d ed. St. Louis, Mosby, 1995, pp 1327–1374.
5. Halstead BW: *Poisonous and Venomous Marine Animals.* Princeton, Darwin, 1988.
6. Williamson JA: Current challenges in marine envenomation: An overview. *J Wild Med* 3:422, 1992.
7. Williamson JA, Fenner PJ, Burnett JW, Rifkin JF (eds): *Venomous and Poisonous Marine Animals.* Sydney, Australia, University of New South Wales Press, 1996.
8. Hessinger DA, Lenhoff HM (eds): *The Biology of Nematocysts.* San Diego, Academic, 1989.
9. Lotan A, Fishman L, Loya Y, Zlotkin E: Delivery of a nematocyst toxin. *Nature* 375:456, 1995.
10. Halstead BW, Auerbach PS: *Dangerous Aquatic Animals of the World: A Color Atlas.* Princeton, Darwin, 1992.
11. Burnett JW, Calton CJ: Jellyfish envenomation syndromes updated. *Ann Emerg Med* 16:1000, 1987.
12. Tomchik RS, Russell MT, Szmant AM, Black NA: Clinical perspectives: Seabather's eruption, also known as "sea lice." *JAMA* 269:1669, 1993.
13. Rifkin JF, Fenner PJ, Williamson JAH: First aid treatment of the sting from the hydroid *Lytocarpus philippinus*: The structure of and in vitro discharge experiments with its nematocysts. *J Wild Med* 4:252, 1993.
14. Tu AT: Biotoxicology of sea snake venoms. *Ann Emerg Med* 16:1023, 1987. http://www.wch.sa.gov.au/paedm/clintox/cslavh_marine.htm/

HIGH ALTITUDE MEDICAL PROBLEMS

Peter H. Hackett
Mark B. Rabold

Many millions of visitors annually visit the mountainous areas of the western United States at altitudes over 8000 feet (2440 meters). In addition, tens of thousands travel to high altitude regions in other parts of the world.

Physicians working or traveling in or near these locations are increasingly likely to encounter persons ill with a high altitude illness or suffering an untoward effect of altitude on a preexisting condition. Although the focus of this chapter is hypoxia-related problems, patients in the mountain environment also may require care for associated illnesses such as hypothermia, frostbite, trauma, ultraviolet keratitis, dehydration, and lightning injury, which are covered elsewhere in this text.

High altitude is a hypoxic environment. Because the concentration of oxygen in the troposphere remains constant at 21 percent, the partial pressure of oxygen decreases as a function of the barometric pressure. In Denver (1610 m), air pressure is 17 percent less than at sea level and therefore contains 17 percent less oxygen. The air of Aspen, Colorado (2438 m) has 26 percent less oxygen, and the barometric pressure on top of Mt. Everest is merely one-third that of sea level. Paul Bert, in his classic experiments of the late nineteenth century, showed that supplemental oxygen prevented symptoms of altitude illness during hypobaric exposure and concluded that hypoxia, not hypobaria, was responsible for illness.

For the purposes of discussion, altitude may be divided into stages according to physiologic effects. *Intermediate altitude,* 5000 to 8000 feet (1500 to 2440 meters), produces decreased exercise performance and increased alveolar ventilation, without major impairment in arterial oxygen transport. Medical sickness due to altitude is rare in this range, although mild illness may develop in individuals with decreased cardiopulmonary reserve. *High altitude,* 8000 to 14,000 feet (2440 to 4270 meters), is associated with a decrease in arterial oxygen saturation, and hypoxemia may occur during exercise and sleep. Most cases of medical problems associated with altitude occur in this range because of the availability of overnight tourist facilities located at these heights. *Very high altitude,* 14,000 to 18,000 feet (4260 to 5490 meters), is difficult to find in the United States, but is encountered by visitors to the mountainous regions of South America and the Himalayas. Abrupt ascent can be dangerous and a period of acclimatization is required to prevent illness. *Extreme altitude,* over 18,000 feet (5490 meters), is available to only mountain climbers and accompanied by severe hypoxemia and hypocapnia. At this height, progressive physiologic deterioration eventually outstrips acclimatization and sustained human habitation is impossible.

ACCLIMATIZATION TO HIGH ALTITUDE

Persons rendered acutely hypoxic become dizzy, faint, and rapidly unconscious if hypoxic stress is sufficient ($Sa_{O_2} < 65\%$). These same individuals, given days to weeks to develop the exact same degree of hypoxia, are able to function quite well. While the fundamental process of this acclimatization takes place in the metabolic machinery of cells and mitochondria, acute "struggle" responses are critical while allowing the cells time to adjust.

Ventilation

Defense of alveolar Pa_{O_2} through increased ventilation is the primary initial adaptation. The hypoxic ventilatory response (HVR) is effected by the carotid body, which senses a decrease in arterial oxygenation and inputs to the central respiratory center in the medulla to increase ventilation. The vigor of this inborn response is related to successful acclimatization and increased performance. Respiratory depressants or stimulants may affect HVR, as does chronic hypoxia, which eventually blunts the response. A low hypoxic drive may allow extreme hypoxemia to develop during sleep. The initial hyperventilation is quickly attenuated by respiratory alkalosis, which acts as a brake on the respiratory center. As renal excretion of bicarbonate compensates for the respiratory alkalosis, pH returns toward normal, and ventilation continues to increase. This process of maximizing ventilation, termed ventila-

TABLE 191-1 Blood Gases and Altitude

Altitude (meters)	Pa_{O_2} (mmHg)	Sa_{O_2}%	Pa_{CO_2} (mmHg)
Sea level	90–95	96	40
1524 (5000 ft)	75–81	95	35.6
2286 (7500 ft)	69–74	92–93	31–33
4572 (15,000 ft)	48–53	86	25
6096 (20,000 ft)	37–45	76	20
7620 (25,000 ft)	32–39	68	13
8848 (29,029 ft)	26–33	58	9.5–13.8

tory acclimatization, culminates after four to seven days at a given altitude. With continuing ascent to higher altitudes, the central chemoreceptors reset to progressively lower P_{CO_2} values, and the completeness of acclimatization can be gauged by the arterial P_{CO_2}. Acetazolamide, which forces a bicarbonate diuresis, greatly facilitates this process. An appreciation of the normal values for blood gases and acid-base status with acclimatization at various altitudes is necessary in order to distinguish abnormalities (Table 191-1).

Blood

The hematopoietic response to altitude was first observed in 1890 by Viault. We now know that within two hours of ascent to altitude, erythropoietin is increased in plasma and, over days to weeks, results in increased red cell mass. This adaptation has no importance during initial acclimatization when altitude illness develops and, when excessive, results in chronic mountain polycythemia. Shifts in the oxyhemoglobin dissociation curve are thought to be minimal in vivo at altitude, because the increase in 2,3-diphosphoglyceric acid, which is proportional to the severity of hypoxia and shifts the curve to the right, is offset by the respiratory alkalosis, which shifts the curve to the left. Naturally occurring left-shifted hemoglobin is an advantage at high altitude.

Fluid Balance

Peripheral venous constriction on ascent to altitude causes an increase in central blood volume, which triggers baroreceptors to suppress antidiuretic hormone (ADH) and aldosterone and induce a diuresis. Combined with the bicarbonate diuresis from the respiratory alkalosis, this can result in decreased plasma volume and hyperosmolality (serum osmolality of 290 to 300 mOsm/L), which the body appears to permit by a reset of the osmol center of the brain. Clinically, diuresis and hemoconcentration is considered a healthy response. Antidiuresis is a hallmark of acute mountain sickness.

Cardiovascular

Stroke volume is decreased initially, and an increased heart rate maintains cardiac output. Maximum exercising heart rate declines at altitude proportional to the decrease in maximum oxygen consumption (V_{O_2} max). Cardiac muscle in healthy persons is able to withstand extreme levels of hypoxemia (Pa_{O_2} < 30 mmHg) without evidence of ST segment changes or ischemic events. Blood pressure is mildly elevated on ascent secondary to increased sympathetic tone.

The pulmonary circulation constricts with exposure to hypoxia. This is an advantage during regional alveolar hypoxia, such as pneumonia, but is a disadvantage during the global hypoxia of altitude exposure. As a result, pulmonary pressure increases. This degree of hypertension is quite variable, with those having a hyperreactive response much more susceptible to high altitude pulmonary edema.

Cerebral blood flow transiently increases on ascent to altitude (despite the hypocapnic alkalosis), which increases oxygen delivery to the brain. This response, however, is limited by the increase in cerebral blood volume, which may increase intracranial pressure and aggravate symptoms of altitude illness.

Effects on Exercise

Exercise capacity, as measured by V_{O_2} max, drops dramatically on ascent to altitude, approximately 10 percent for each 1000-m altitude gain above 1500 m. During acclimatization, submaximal endurance increases appreciably after 10 days, but V_{O_2} max does not. The mechanism of this decrement might be lack of adequate oxygen supply to the muscle cells due to the low driving pressure for diffusion of oxygen from the capillary. Another theory suggests that the CNS limits muscle activity to preserve its own oxygenation.

Limitations

There are limits to acclimatization. Even those who are by nature good acclimatizers cannot tolerate the hypoxia of extreme altitude for long. Miners from South America report that they cannot live at altitudes above 5800 m because of weight loss, increasing lethargy, poor quality sleep, weakness, and headache. High altitude mountaineers cannot survive for more than a few days above 8000 m without supplemental oxygen because of more acute deterioration in physiologic functioning. Considerable weight loss, both of fat and lean body mass, are unavoidable at extreme altitude, and help contribute to demise. Other factors limiting ability to acclimatize to extreme altitude include right ventricular strain from excessive pulmonary hypertension, intestinal malabsorption, impaired renal function, polycythemia and microcirculatory sludging, and prolonged cerebral hypoxia. Even at more modest altitudes, some individuals are very slow or poor acclimatizers for reasons not entirely known but, at least in part, due to poor carotid body function and inadequate ventilation.

Sleep at High Altitude

Sleep stages III and IV are reduced at altitude, while sleep stage I is increased. More time is spent awake, with a significant increase in arousals, but with only slightly less rapid eye movement (REM) time. The frequent arousals are a common source of bitter complaints from skiers and others, but they are innocuous and improve with time at altitude. The typical periodic breathing (Cheyne-Stokes) in those sleeping above 2700 m (9000 ft) consists of 6- to 12-s apneic pauses interspersed with cycles of vigorous ventilation. Interestingly, the frequent awakenings are not necessarily related to the sleep periodic breathing, and neither are they related to acute mountain sickness. Presumably, the mechanism of the lighter sleep is related to cerebral hypoxia. Quality of sleep and arterial oxygenation during sleep improves with acclimatization and with acetazolamide.

HIGH ALTITUDE SYNDROMES

High altitude syndromes of primary concern are those attributed directly to the hypoxia: acute hypoxia; acute mountain sickness; pulmonary edema; cerebral edema; retinopathy; peripheral edema; sleeping problems; and a group of neurologic syndromes. The other syndromes, not necessarily related to hypoxia, include thromboembolic events (which may be attributable to dehydration, prolonged incapacitation, polycythemia, and cold), high altitude pharyngitis and bronchitis, and ultraviolet keratitis. Although the different hypoxic clinical syndromes overlap, all share a fundamental mechanism, all are seen in the same setting of rapid ascent in unacclimatized persons, and all respond to the same essential therapy: descent and oxygen.

Acute Hypoxia

The syndrome of acute hypoxia occurs in the setting of sudden and severe hypoxic insult, such as accidental decompression of a pressurized aircraft cabin or a failed oxygen system in a pilot or high altitude mountaineer. Sudden overexertion precipitating arterial desaturation, acute onset of pulmonary edema, carbon monoxide poisoning, and sleep apnea may result in relatively acute hypoxia as well. Unacclimatized persons become unconscious at an arterial oxygen saturation of 50 to 60 percent, an arterial Pa_{O_2} of less than about 30 mmHg, or a jugular venous Pa_{O_2} less than 15 mmHg. Acute hypoxia is reversed by immediate administration of oxygen, rapid descent, and correction of the underlying cause, such as removal of the carbon monoxide source or repair of the oxygen delivery system. Symptoms of acute hypoxia reflect the sensitivity of the CNS to this insult: dizziness, lightheadedness, and dimmed vision progressing to loss of consciousness. Hyperventilation has been shown to increase the time of useful consciousness during acute alveolar hypoxia.

Acute Mountain Sickness (AMS)

INCIDENCE AMS occurs in the setting of more gradual and less severe hypoxic insult than with acute hypoxic syndrome. Its incidence varies by location, depending on ease of access, rate of ascent, and sleeping altitude reached. A recent study at 2100 m (6900 ft) found a 25 percent incidence of AMS in physicians attending a continuing-education meeting in Colorado. Other studies at resorts between 2220 and 2700 m (7200 and 9000 ft, respectively) claimed an incidence between 17 and 40 percent, and a sleeping altitude of 2750 m (9000 ft) seemed to be a threshold for increased attack rate.[1] Approximately 40 percent of trekkers in Nepal on the path to Mt. Everest suffer AMS, while climbers on Mt. Rainier have the very-high incidence of 70 percent because of the rapidity of ascent.

SUSCEPTIBILITY In addition to rate of ascent and sleeping altitude, inherent factors determine individual susceptibility to acute mountain sickness. Factors identified so far are low hypoxic ventilatory response and low vital capacity. Age has little influence on incidence, with children being as susceptible as adults. Women are just as likely, if not more so, to develop mountain sickness but appear to have less pulmonary edema. Susceptibility to AMS is generally reproducible in an individual on repeated exposures. Persons living at intermediate altitudes of 1000 to 2000 m already are acclimatized partially and do much better than lowlanders upon ascent to higher altitudes. There is no relationship of susceptibility to AMS and physical fitness.

CLINICAL PRESENTATION The diagnosis of AMS is based on the setting, symptoms, and physical findings. The setting is rapid ascent of an unacclimatized person to 2000 m (6600 ft) or higher. Typically, the person on arrival feels lightheaded and slightly breathless, especially with exercise. One to six hours later, but sometimes delayed for one day or more (and especially after a night's sleep), the typical symptoms of mild AMS develop; they are similar to an alcohol hangover. The headache usually is described as bifrontal and worsened with bending over and the Valsalva maneuver. Gastrointestinal symptoms include anorexia, nausea, and sometimes vomiting, and the chief constitutional symptoms are lassitude and weakness. The person with AMS is often irritable and wants to be left alone. Sleepiness and a deep inner chill, also are common. If the illness progresses, the headache becomes more severe, and vomiting, oliguria, and increased dyspnea develop. Lassitude may progress to the victim requiring assistance for eating and dressing. The most severe form of AMS, high altitude cerebral edema (HACE), is heralded by onset of ataxia and altered level of consciousness; coma may ensue within 12 h if treatment is delayed. The diagnosis can be difficult in preverbal children.[2]

Physical findings in mild AMS are nonspecific. Heart rate and blood pressure are variable, and usually in the normal range, although postural hypotension may be present. Localized rales are detectable in up to 20 percent of persons with AMS. Body temperature may be slightly elevated (up to 38.5°C) in AMS, and more so in high altitude pulmonary edema (HAPE) and HACE.[3] Funduscopy reveals venous tortuosity and dilatation, and retinal hemorrhages are common over 5000 m or in those with pulmonary and cerebral edema. Fluid retention is a hallmark of AMS, in contrast to the usual diuresis of acclimatization, and may result in peripheral edema, especially of the face. Differential diagnosis in this setting includes hypothermia, carbon monoxide poisoning, pulmonary or CNS infection, dehydration, and exhaustion.

The natural history of AMS at a Colorado resort (3000 m or 10,000 ft) recently was documented. Mean duration of symptoms was 15 h, with a range to 94 h, despite the fact that one-half of those with symptoms self-medicated.[4] At higher sleeping altitudes, the illness may last much longer, even weeks if untreated, and is more likely to progress to pulmonary or cerebral edema. Eight percent of those with AMS at 4243 m (14,000 ft) in Nepal developed cerebral or pulmonary edema, or both.

PATHOPHYSIOLOGY AMS is due to hypobaric hypoxia, but the exact sequence of events leading to illness is unclear. Figure 191-1 offers a schema for the pathophysiology. The symptoms indicate a neurologic etiology; scans confirming cerebral edema have been obtained in persons severely ill. Whether the more common mild illness of headache, anorexia, and malaise is due to mild cerebral edema has yet to be confirmed, but seems likely. Two types of cerebral edema have been proposed. One is cytotoxic edema, due to failure of the sodium-potassium pump with subsequent intracellular accumulation of sodium and water. The other is a vasogenic edema, due to a leaky blood-brain barrier.

No direct evidence for cytotoxic edema in humans at altitude has been reported, but a large shift of fluid into the total intracellular space, presumably including the brain, was demonstrated to take place over the first three days at altitude, when AMS occurs. The time required for fluid shift and overhydration of the brain may explain the time lag in onset of symptoms, which distinguishes AMS from acute hypoxia. In support of the vasogenic theory, white-matter brain edema on magnetic resonance imaging (MRI) recently was demonstrated in persons with high altitude cerebral edema, and it may also occur in AMS.[5] The leaky blood-brain barrier is due either to loss of autoregulation and overperfusion or to hypoxia-induced increased permeability. The fact that corticosteroids so effectively treat AMS also supports the notion of vasogenic edema, since this is the only type of cerebral edema responsive to steroids. Further research is likely to reveal that brain swelling is due to both cytotoxic and vasogenic mechanisms.

The cerebral edema, interstitial pulmonary edema, peripheral edema, and the antidiuresis observed in AMS all point to an abnormality of water handling by the body. The mechanism is thought to be increased renin-angiotensin, aldosterone, and ADH in contrast to the normal ADH and aldosterone suppression at high altitude, and usual diuresis. A decrease in glomerular filtration also has been observed. The effectiveness of diuretics in prevention and treatment of AMS reinforces the importance of fluid retention in the pathophysiology. Increased sympathetic activation is thought to play a role in the pulmonary and renal circulations contributing to the pathophysiology[6] (see Fig. 191-1).

Relative hypoventilation due to a sluggish hypoxic ventilatory response is a characteristic of AMS-susceptible individuals and has been linked to fluid retention. Hypoventilation, of course, results in greater hypoxic stress and is equivalent to being at a higher altitude. Higher Pa_{CO_2} and lower Pa_{O_2} also increases cerebral blood flow and aggravates

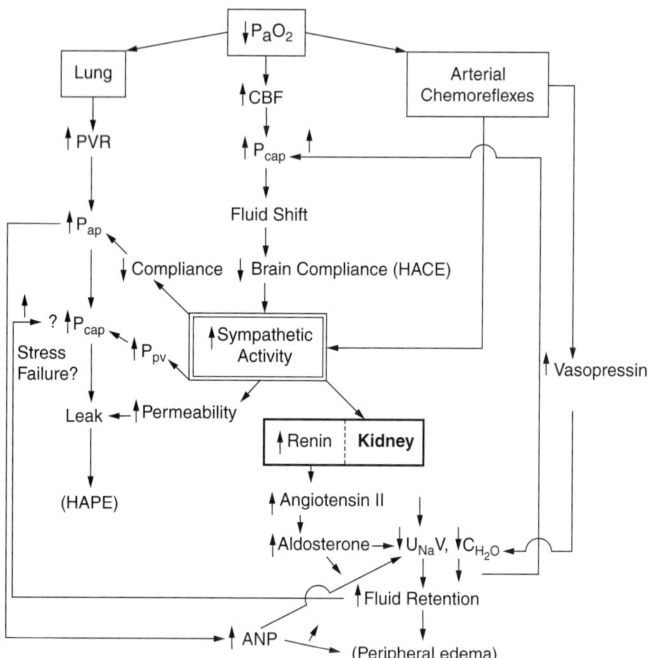

FIG. 191-1. High altitude illnesses. Central role of elevated sympathetic activity in the edemas of altitude: Hypoxemia (↓ Pa_{O_2}) elevates cerebral blood flow (CBF), which in turn raises cerebral capillary hydrostatic pressure (P_{cap}) such that a transcapillary fluid shift occurs. The resulting high-altitude cerebral edema (or AMS) reduces brain compliance. Elevated intracranial pressure and distortion of CNS structures provokes elevation of peripheral sympathetic activity above levels normally produced by stimulation of peripheral chemoreflexes. Hypoxia raises pulmonary vascular resistance, which raises pulmonary artery pressure (P_{ap}). Elevated sympathetic activity to the lungs decreases compliance of pulmonary arteries and provokes pulmonary venous constriction and increased capillary permeability. The precise influence of hypoxic pulmonary vascular responses combined with increased pulmonary sympathetic activity on pulmonary hydrostatic pressure is unclear. The relative importance of pulmonary capillary stress failure is uncertain (?). Only small elevations of P_{cap} are required to cause large fluid fluxes if permeability is increased such that HAPE occurs. Increased sympathetic activity is associated with a neurogenic anti-natriuresis such that fluid retention and peripheral edema occur. Increased aldosterone from sympathetic stimulation of renin or from ACTH, and increased vasopressin from stimulation of chemoreflexes add to the tubular α-adrenergic antinatriuresis and opposes natriuretic effects from atrial natriuretic peptide (ANP) released by elevated central blood volume. However, ANP could contribute to peripheral edema, HAPE, or HACE. Renal fluid retention contributes to elevated P_{cap} in lung, brain, and peripheral tissues. (From Krasney JA: A neurogenic basis for acute altitude illness. *Med Sci Sport Exerc* 26:195, 1994.)

brain swelling. Less hypocapnia also may reduce the stimulus for bicarbonate diuresis and aggravate fluid retention.

TREATMENT (Table 191-2) **Descent and Oxygen** The goals of treatment are to prevent progression, abort the illness, and improve acclimatization; early diagnosis is essential. Initial clinical presentation does not predict eventual severity, and all persons with AMS must be observed carefully for progression. The three principles of treatment are: (1) to not proceed to a higher sleeping altitude in the presence of symptoms; (2) to descend if symptoms do not abate or become worse despite treatment; and (3) to descend and treat immediately in the presence of a change in consciousness, ataxia, or pulmonary edema. Mild AMS is self-limited and generally improves with an extra 12 to 36 h of acclimatization if ascent is halted. Descent is the definitive treatment for all forms of altitude illness, although it is not always an option, nor always necessary. Remarkably, a drop in altitude of only 500 to 1000 m usually is effective promptly. Evacuation to a hospital or to sea level is unnecessary except in the most severe cases. To simulate descent, portable hyperbaric bags are being used in various locations to treat AMS. The patient is inserted into the fabric chamber, and a pressure of 2 psi is achieved by means of a manual or automated pump; the pressure is equivalent to a drop in altitude of 1500 m (5000 ft). A valve system creates sufficient ventilation to avoid CO_2 accumulation or O_2 depletion.

Oxygen effectively relieves symptoms, but it often is unavailable in the field and generally reserved for moderate to severe AMS in order to conserve supplies. Oxygen promptly relieves headache, dizziness, and most other symptoms, although ataxia may resolve more slowly. Nocturnal low flow oxygen (0.5 to 1 L/min) is particularly helpful and efficient. The combination of oxygen and descent provides optimal therapy, especially in more severe cases.

Medical Therapy Pharmacologic treatment offers an alternative to descent or oxygen in mild to moderately severe AMS. Acetazolamide is very helpful in speeding acclimatization and aborting illness, especially when used early. The drug acts by inhibiting the enzyme carbonic anhydrase, slowing the hydration of carbon dioxide to hydrogen and bicarbonate ions. In the kidney, acetazolamide reduces reabsorption of bicarbonate, causing a bicarbonate diuresis and metabolic acidosis, which stimulates ventilation. The drug essentially mimics the process of ventilatory acclimatization. As a result, arterial P_{O_2} is higher, and sleep oxygenation remains high and stable, without periods of apnea. The drug also maintains cerebral blood flow despite greater hypocapnia, and because of its diuretic action, it counteracts the fluid retention of AMS. Many trials have shown its value for prevention; and recently treatment.[7] Current indications for acetazolamide are: (1) a history of altitude illness; (2) abrupt ascent to over 3000 m (10,000 ft); (3) for treatment of AMS; and (4) bothersome sleep periodic breathing. The dosage regimen varies; 5 mg/kg per day in two or three divided doses is sufficient, whether for prevention or treatment; or 125 mg bid,

TABLE 191-2 Suggested Treatment of High Altitude Illness

Mild AMS	Stop ascent Descend to lower altitude or acclimatize at same altitude Acetazolamide 125–250 mg bid to speed acclimatization Symptomatic treatment as necessary with analgesics and antiemetics
Moderate AMS	Immediate descent for worsening symptoms Low flow oxygen if available Acetazolamide 250 mg bid and/or dexamethasone 4 mg q6h Hyperbaric therapy
HACE	Immediate descent or evacuation Oxygen 2–4 L/min or titrated to Sa_{O_2} >90% Dexamethasone 8 mg po, IM, or IV, then 4 mg q6h Hyperbaric therapy if cannot descend
HAPE	Immediate descent or evacuation to medical facility Oxygen 4 L/min or titrated to Sa_{O_2} >90% Nifedipine 10 mg po q4–6h or 30 mg extended release q12h if no oxygen or descent Hyperbaric therapy if cannot descend Continuous positive airway pressure Minimize exertion and keep warm
Periodic breathing	Acetazolamide 125 mg at bedtime as needed

which is empirically effective.[8] Treatment should be continued until symptoms of AMS resolve, and then the drug should be restarted if symptoms return. Because the drug acts by improving acclimatization, fear of masking serious illness is unwarranted. Common side effects of acetazolamide include peripheral paresthesias and sometimes nausea or drowsiness, and the usual precautions of sulfa drugs apply to acetazolamide because of the sulfhydryl moiety. Because the drug inhibits the instant hydration of CO_2 on the tongue, the carbon dioxide in carbonated beverages can be tasted, ruining the flavor of beer and other drinks.

Symptomatic treatment of AMS is sometimes sufficient. Aspirin 650 mg, acetaminophen 650 to 1000 mg (with or without codeine), or ibuprofen 600 to 800 mg can be given for headache. Aspirin also effective for prevention of headache.[9] Prochlorperazine 5 to 10 mg intramuscularly is useful for nausea and vomiting, and has the advantage of augmenting the hypoxic ventilatory response. The short-acting benzodiazepines such as triazolam 0.25 mg and temazepam 15 mg also can be used to treat the complaint of frequent wakening, but they are potentially dangerous in ill persons because of respiratory depression and may decrease oxygenation even in persons acclimatizing well. A combination of acetazolamide and benzodiazepine may work very well for bothersome insomnia.

Dexamethasone 4 mg PO, IM, or IV every six hours is quite effective therapy for mountain sickness, but it is best reserved for moderate to severe AMS, because it may be associated with significant side effects and does not aid acclimatization, sometimes resulting in rebound symptoms when discontinued. A short taper period may prevent this rebound phenomenon. The mechanism of action of dexamethasone may be to reduce vasogenic edema, to lower intracranial pressure, or to act as an antiemetic and mood elevator. The use of acetazolamide to speed acclimatization and a brief course of dexamethasone to treat illness can be a useful combination. The use of diuretics is reasonable because of the fluid retention associated with mountain sickness. Furosemide 20 to 40 mg every 12 h until improved was reported effective by the Indian army, although other investigators have not been enthusiastic about its use because of concerns for avoiding hypovolemia, hypotension, and incapacitation.

PREVENTION Graded ascent with adequate time for acclimatization is the best prevention. A recommendation for those visiting medium altitude resorts in the western United States is to spend a night at an intermediate altitude of 1500 to 2000 m (Denver or Salt Lake City) before sleeping at altitudes above 2500 m (8200 ft). Mountaineers and trekkers should avoid abrupt ascent to sleeping altitudes over 3000 m and then allow two nights for each 1000-m altitude gain in camp altitude, starting at 3000 m. Other preventative measures include avoiding overexertion, alcohol, and respiratory depressants, and eating a high-carbohydrate diet. Acetazolamide is a useful prophylactic agent for those with a history of AMS or for forced abrupt ascent without acclimatization stages. The drug should be started 24 h before the ascent and continued for the first 2 days at altitude. The medication then can be discontinued and started again if illness develops. Acetazolamide can be expected to reduce the symptoms of AMS by approximately 75 percent in persons ascending rapidly to sleeping altitudes of over 2500 m. An alternative for those allergic to sulfa is dexamethasone 4 mg every 12 h starting the day of ascent and continuing for the first 2 days at altitude.

Neurologic Syndromes of High Altitude

Until recently, most neurologic events at high altitude were attributed to HACE or AMS. Clearly, this has been a diagnostic oversimplification. Other syndromes now recognized as related to high altitude include altitude syncope, cerebrovascular spasm (migraine equivalent), cerebral arterial or venous thrombosis (infarct), transient ischemic attack, and cerebral hemorrhage. These syndromes are characterized by more focal neurologic findings than in cerebral edema, though differentiation in the field may be impossible.

Other problems may be due to exacerbation or unmasking of underlying disease, such as previously asymptomatic brain tumors and epilepsy. Presumably, space-occupying lesions become symptomatic because of increased brain volume at altitude. Hyperventilation (hypocapnic alkalosis), which is commonly used to induce seizure activity on electroencephalography, may explain unmasking of a seizure disorder at altitude, while changes in cerebral blood flow may exacerbate vascular lesions.

High Altitude Cerebral Edema

HACE is defined clinically as the presence of progressive neurologic deterioration in someone with AMS or HAPE. It is characterized by altered mental status, ataxia, stupor, and progression to coma if untreated. Headache, nausea, and vomiting are not always present. Because of raised intracranial pressure, focal neurologic signs such as third and sixth cranial nerve palsies may result from distortion of brain structures or by extraxial compression.

HACE is usually associated with pulmonary edema. Pathologically, necropsies have described severe, diffuse cerebral edema with multiple small hemorrhages and sometimes thrombosis.

The treatment of HACE is the same as for severe AMS: oxygen, descent, and steroids (Table 191-2). Descent is the highest priority. Acetazolamide may be an adjunct, but immediate reversal of the illness is the goal; improving acclimatization comes later. In acutely ill patients who cannot descend, the combination of steroids, supplemental oxygen, and a hyperbaric bag is optimal therapy, but rarely available. Persons remaining ataxic or confused after descent should be admitted to the hospital. Comatose patients require additional airway management, bladder drainage, and other coma care. For coma, the use of hyperventilation to decrease intracranial pressure is a reasonable approach, keeping in mind that the Pa_{CO_2} is already low and pH high in these individuals. Additional acute hyperventilation could produce cerebral ischemia; monitoring of arterial blood gases and, if available, cerebral blood velocities by transcranial Doppler ultrasonography may be advisable. Loop diuretics such as furosemide 40 to 80 mg or bumetanide 1 to 2 mg may help reduce brain overhydration, but hypoperfusion must be avoided. Hypertonic solutions of saline, mannitol, or urea have been used too infrequently to establish clinical guidelines. In the hospital setting, mannitol in a patient who does not respond immediately is worth considering. Coma may persist for days, even for weeks after evacuation to lower altitude, and the patient may still recover, only sometimes with permanent sequelae. Persistent coma is unusual, however, and mandates exclusion of other possible etiologies.

Cerebrovascular Syndromes of Altitude

Strokes, due both to infarct and hemorrhage in the arterial circulation, as well as venous thrombosis have been reported in young healthy persons at altitude who otherwise would not be considered at risk for such conditions. Transient ischemic attack, cortical blindness, and various focal neurologic signs, such as hemiparesis or hemiplegia of a transient nature, also occur. Because these latter events are reversible, they suggest etiologies such as vasospasm, watershed hypoxia between arterial zones, or transient ischemic attack.

Differentiation of the various neurologic syndromes may be impossible in the field, and treating as if cerebral edema were present may be reasonable, with a rapid descent to lower altitude, oxygen, and steroids, and evacuation to a hospital if symptoms persist despite treatment. Fortunately, focal neurologic signs usually resolve spontaneously and do not recur upon reascent. However, a thorough cerebrovascular evaluation before advising reascent may be prudent.

TABLE 191-3 Severity Classification of HAPE

Grade	Symptoms	Signs	Chest Radiograph
1 Mild	Dyspnea on exertion, dry cough, fatigue while moving uphill	Resting HR <100, resting RR <20, dusky nailbeds, localized rales, if any	Minor exudate involving less than one-fourth of one lung field
2 Moderate	Dyspnea, weakness, fatigue on level walking, raspy cough, headache, anorexia	HR 90–100, RR 16–30, cyanotic nailbeds, rales present, ataxia may be present	Some infiltrate involving 50% of one lung or smaller area of both lungs
3 Severe	Dyspnea at rest, productive cough, orthopnea, extreme weakness, stupor, coma, blood-tinged sputum	Bilateral rales, HR >110, RR >30, facial and nailbed cyanosis, ataxia	Bilateral infiltrates >50% each lung

Source: Hultgren HN: High altitude pulmonary edema, in Staub NC (ed): *Lung Water and Solute Exchange.* New York, Marcel Dekker, 1978, pp 437–469.

High Altitude Pulmonary Edema

HAPE is the most lethal of the altitude illnesses. Because the condition is easily reversible with descent and oxygen, the cause of death is usually lack of early recognition, misdiagnosis, or inability to descend to a lower altitude. Litigation commonly results from HAPE deaths, a fact worth considering for physicians involved in such cases.

EPIDEMIOLOGY The incidence of HAPE varies from less than 1 in 10,000 skiers in Colorado to 2 to 3 percent of climbers on Mt. McKinley, and was reported as high as 15 percent in some regiments in the Indian army who were airlifted to high altitude during the Indian/Chinese war. Women appear less susceptible than men. Risk factors include heavy exertion, rapid ascent, cold, excessive salt ingestion, use of sleeping medication, and a previous history indicating inherent individual susceptibility. Such susceptibility was recently related to immunogenetic factors,[10] as well as to physiologic factors.[11] Preexisting respiratory infection predisposes children to HAPE.[12]

CLINICAL PRESENTATION (Table 191-3) Early in the course of illness, when the edema is still interstitial or localized, the victim develops a dry cough, decreased exercise performance, dyspnea on exertion, increased recovery time from exercise, and localized rales, usually in the right midlung field. Late in the course of the illness, there develops tachycardia, tachypnea, and dyspnea at rest, marked weakness, productive cough, cyanosis, and more generalized rales. As hypoxemia worsens, consciousness becomes impaired. Victims usually become comatose and then die. Early diagnosis is critical, and decreased exercise performance and dry cough is enough to raise the suspicion of early HAPE. The typical victim is strong and fit and may or may not have symptoms of AMS before onset of HAPE. The condition typically worsens at night and is noticed most commonly on the second night at a new altitude. Unfortunately, rales may not be audible in 30 percent of persons with HAPE at rest but can be elicited immediately after a short bout of exercise. Fever up to 38.5°C is common, and tachycardia and tachypnea generally correlate with the severity of illness. On cardiac auscultation, a prominent P2 and right ventricular heave may be appreciated. ECG generally reveals right axis deviation and a right ventricular strain pattern consistent with acute pulmonary hypertension. Chest x-ray findings progress from interstitial to localized alveolar to generalized alveolar infiltrates as the illness progresses from mild to severe.[13]

PATHOPHYSIOLOGY The pioneering work of Hultgren established HAPE as a noncardiogenic edema. Left ventricular function is normal. Left ventricular end diastolic pressure, wedge pressures, and left atrial pressures are low to normal, cardiac output is low, and pulmonary vascular resistance and pulmonary artery pressure are markedly elevated. The exact cause of the edema is still unclear. Pulmonary hypertension is an essential component, and persons with a history of HAPE have been shown to have exaggerated pulmonary pressor responses to hypoxia. Whether this represents one end of a normal distribution or a pathologic subpopulation is unknown. However, not all persons with pulmonary hypertension develop HAPE; another factor must also be present, which induces a change in capillary membrane permeability. Pulmonary venous constriction, fibrin and platelet thrombi, and uneven arterial vasoconstriction leading to overperfusion of some areas of the vasculature have all been proposed. Predisposed individuals have a low hypoxic ventilatory response, an abnormal pulmonary circulation, and tend to suffer HAPE on repeated exposures.

TREATMENT The key to successful treatment of HAPE (Table 191-2) is early recognition, because the condition in its early stage is easily reversible. The optimal therapy depends upon the environmental setting, evacuation options, availability of oxygen or hyperbaric units, and ease of descent. Immediate descent is the treatment of choice, but this is not always possible. During descent, exertion by the victim must be minimized. Reports of victims dying during descent probably are related to overexertion offsetting the benefit of lower altitude. With descent, oxygen is unnecessary except in severe cases. Oxygen provides excellent results and can completely resolve pulmonary edema without descent to a lower altitude, but may require 36 to 72 h to do so. Such quantities of oxygen rarely are available to trekking, mountaineering, and skiing groups, but they may be available at ski resorts or medical facilities. Oxygen immediately lowers pulmonary artery pressure and improves arterial oxygenation. Its use is life saving when descent is not an option; in such cases, rescue groups should make delivery of oxygen to the victim the highest priority. As in the treatment of AMS and HACE, the portable hyperbaric bag is a very useful adjunct to therapy when immediate descent is not possible.

Bedrest may be adequate for very mild cases, and bedrest with supplemental oxygen may suffice for moderate illness, as long as the safety of the patient can be assured by the presence of a medical facility, adequate oxygen, or immediate descent capability should the patient's condition deteriorate.[14] Because cold stress elevates pulmonary artery pressure, the patient should be kept warm. The use of an expiratory positive airway pressure (EPAP) mask has been shown to increase arterial oxygen saturation by 10 to 20 percent in HAPE patients by enhancing alveolar recruitment. The mask is lightweight, well tolerated, and may be a useful adjunct to descent.

Because oxygen and descent are so effective, experience with drugs has been limited. Morphine and furosemide were used with good results by the Indian army, and both seem physiologically reasonable because they augment venous pooling, reduce pulmonary blood flow, and therefore reduce hydrostatic force for fluid extravasation in the lung. However, patients with HAPE often are dehydrated intravascularly, and caution must be exercised to avoid hypotension. Several studies have demonstrated that nifedipine, either 10-mg capsule or 30-mg extended-release formulation, orally, was of clinical benefit in reducing pulmonary artery pressure by 30 to 50 percent, and in increasing arterial oxygen saturation. Nifedipine, at a dose of 20 mg slow-release preparation every eight hours while ascending, has also been shown to be an effective prophylactic agent in those who have had previous episodes of HAPE.[15] Other vasodilators, such as hydralazine and phentolamine, show promise, as well, in the treatment of HAPE.[16] The mechanism presumably is by lowering pulmonary pressure and, therefore, the pressure gradient for flux of fluid across the membrane. Nitric oxide also lowers pulmonary artery pressure, and redistributes blood away from edematous areas.[17] Hypotension is a potential problem with nifedipine, and the results are not nearly as dramatic as with oxygen or descent, which still remain the treatments of choice.

Hospitalization may be warranted for severe cases that do not respond immediately to descent, especially if cerebral edema is present. Intubation, high $F_{I_{O_2}}$, and positive end-expiratory pressure ventilation are rarely required. Antibiotics are indicated for coexisting infection when present. Occasionally pulmonary artery catheterization is useful to exclude a cardiac component to the edema in persons with heart disease. The patient with HAPE who does not make the usual rapid improvement (or develops HAPE at altitudes <2500 m [8200 ft]) should be evaluated for pulmonary emboli, mediastinal pulmonary artery obstruction, or other pulmonary circulatory abnormalities, such as congenital absence of a pulmonary artery. Echocardiography can assess presence or absence of shunting from a patent foramen ovale or other cardiac abnormality. Adequate discharge criteria are progressive clinical and radiographic improvement, and an arterial Pa_{O_2} of 60 mmHg or arterial oxygen saturation greater than 90 percent. Residua such as fibrosis and impaired pulmonary function tests have not been reported. Patients are advised to resume activities gradually and are warned that they may feel weak for one to two weeks. An episode of HAPE is not a contraindication to subsequent ascent, but patients should be advised on staged ascent, acetazolamide and/or nifedipine prophylaxis, and recognition of early signs and symptoms.

Peripheral Edema

Swelling of the face and distal extremities is common at high altitude. Peripheral edema was reported in 18 percent of trekkers at 4200 m in Nepal and was twice as likely in women. It was often associated with AMS, but not necessarily. The presence of peripheral edema should raise suspicion of altitude illness and prompt a thorough examination for pulmonary and cerebral edema. The problem can be treated with diuretics, but if left untreated, it will resolve spontaneously with descent. The mechanism is presumably similar to that of the fluid retention of AMS but with edema formation peripherally rather than in the brain and lung.

High Altitude Retinopathy

Retinal abnormalities described at high altitude include retinal edema, tortuosity and dilatation of retinal veins, disc hyperemia, retinal hemorrhages, and, rarely, cotton-wool exudates. Retinal hemorrhages are asymptomatic, except for rarely occurring macular hemorrhages, and are not considered an indication for descent unless visual changes are present. They resolve spontaneously in 10 to 14 days. Hemorrhages are common above a sleeping altitude of 5000 m and occur at lower altitudes in persons with altitude illness.

High Altitude Pharyngitis and Bronchitis

Most unacclimatized persons exercising at altitudes over 2500 m develop a dry, hacking cough. With exposure to extreme altitudes for prolonged periods of time, a purulent bronchitis and a painful pharyngitis become nearly universal. These problems may not be of an infectious nature; high volumes of dry, cold air through the lungs may induce respiratory heat loss and cause purulent secretions on that basis alone. Bronchospasm may also be triggered by respiratory heat loss. Severe coughing spasms can result in cough fracture of the ribs.

Pharyngeal membranes become dry, painful, and cracked because of the dehydration and high ventilation. Mucosal cracks may be an entry for pathogens, or the erythema and dryness may cause discomfort strictly on a mechanical basis. Antibiotics generally are not helpful, supporting the concept of a noninfectious etiology. Breathing of steam, ingesting hard candies or lozenges to increase salivation, and forcing hydration may provide some benefit with systemic analgesics as necessary. A silk Balaclava or similar material across the nose and mouth that is sufficiently porous to allow large volume ventilation but trap some moisture and heat helps ameliorate these bothersome high altitude conditions.

Chronic Mountain Polycythemia (CMP)

Monge's disease, also called chronic mountain sickness or CMP, has now been recognized in all high altitude locations of the world. Both long-term high altitude residents and lowlanders who relocate to high altitude may develop this condition after variable length of residence. The incidence is much higher in males and increases with age. The disease is characterized by excessive polycythemia for a given altitude, which causes symptoms such as headache, muddled thinking, difficulty sleeping, impaired peripheral circulation, drowsiness, and chest congestion. The diagnosis is made by the characteristic symptoms and a hemoglobin value greater than expected for the altitude, generally over 20 to 22 g/dL. Any problem causing hypoxemia at sea level causes greater hypoxemia at altitude, and the etiology of CMP can be traced to problems such as chronic obstructive pulmonary disease (COPD) and sleep apnea in 50 percent of patients. The etiology of pure CMP is attributed to idiopathic hypoventilation on the basis of diminished respiratory drive.

Therapy includes phlebotomy, relocation to lower altitude, or home oxygen use. Respiratory stimulants such as acetazolamide (250 mg twice a day) and medroxyprogesterone acetate (20 to 60 mg/day) have also been employed successfully. The response to respiratory stimulants supports the role of hypoventilation in this disorder.

Ultraviolet Keratitis (Snow Blindness)

Ultraviolet light (UVA and UVB) penetrates the atmosphere to a greater degree at high altitude because of less cloud cover, less water vapor, and less particulate matter in the air. Radiation increases roughly 5 percent for every 300 m (1000 ft) gained, and it is exacerbated by reflection back from snow. UV radiation below 300 nm (UVB) is absorbed by the cornea, and high exposure levels can cause corneal burns in 1 h, although symptoms do not become apparent for 6 to 12 h. The typical symptoms of photokeratitis are severe pain, a foreign body or gritty sensation, photophobia, tearing, marked conjunctival erythema, chemosis, and eyelid swelling. UV keratitis generally is self-limited and heals within 24 h, but the condition is sufficiently painful to warrant systemic analgesics. Cold compresses may also provide some relief, and eye patches may be necessary for comfort. Prevention is obviously of great importance, since this condition can be disabling, especially in hazardous terrain. Adequate sunglasses should transmit less than 10 percent of UVB light. Side shields are necessary if traveling on snow, and polarizing lenses help by absorbing glare. Makeshift protection can be fashioned by cutting narrow horizontal slits in cardboard, foam, or any available material (Eskimo sunglasses).

ILLNESSES AGGRAVATED BY HIGH ALTITUDE

Chronic Lung Disease

COPD patients ascending to altitude often report increased dyspnea and reduced exercise ability. Those with hypoxemia, pulmonary hypertension, disordered control of ventilation, and sleep-disordered breathing at sea level might have greater problems at altitude because of the greater alveolar hypoxia. Such patients may require supplemental oxygen at altitude when they do not at sea level (and avoid having to descend), and oxygen-dependent patients at sea level may need to increase the $F_{I_{O_2}}$. The required $F_{I_{O_2}}$ can be calculated by multiplying low-altitude $F_{I_{O_2}}$ by the ratio of low altitude barometric pressure divided by high altitude barometric pressure. This will ensure the delivery of the same partial pressure of oxygen as at low altitude. There are no data to suggest that persons with COPD are more likely to develop AMS or HAPE, although such persons may be self-selected to avoid travel to high altitude locations. In fact, persons with mild to moderate COPD already are partially acclimatized and may do well at modest altitude, as suggested by Graham and Houston. High altitude per se does not exacerbate asthma, and persons with chronic bronchospasm often report easier breathing at high altitude, due to lower air density and/or cleaner air.

Arteriosclerotic Heart Disease (ASHD)

The healthy heart and cardiovascular system tolerates even extreme hypoxia very well. Numerous ECG studies, echocardiograms, heart catheterizations and exercise tests do not demonstrate cardiac ischemia or cardiac dysfunction in healthy persons at high altitude, even when arterial Pa_{O_2} was less than 30 mmHg. Those with arteriosclerotic disease may not have the same adaptive capabilities and intuitively seem more likely to suffer from acute cardiac events. Epidemiologic data, however, do not support this supposition. Morbidity and mortality from arteriosclerotic heart disease is reduced in persons with long-term residence at high altitude, and visitors apparently do not have increased risk of acute myocardial infarction. Recent work, however, suggested earlier onset of angina at high altitude compared with sea level during the first few days at 2500 m. After five days, an elderly group with CAD acclimatized well, and performed at sea-level exercise capacity without increased or early-onset angina.[18] Even men with coronary artery disease and low LV ejection fraction (mean = 39%) but without overt heart failure tolerated exercise at 2500 m as well as at low altitude.[19] Congestive heart failure (CHF) may worsen in tourists arriving at the medium altitude of ski resorts, and it is related apparently to fluid retention rather than depressed ventricular function from hypoxia. Patients with CHF should therefore maintain or increase their diuretic regimen during travel to high altitude, and clinicians may want to consider low flow oxygen during sleep for CHF patients, at least for the first few nights. Patient status-post coronary artery bypass grafting have trekked to altitudes over 5000 m without problems, the issue of safety having generated much debate. Overall, high altitude does not impose as much stress on the heart as would seem intuitively obvious. Further study will more clearly define subcategories of cardiac patients at risk.

Ascent to altitude produces a mild increase in blood pressure in normotensive persons, secondary to increased sympathetic tone; the same was found in hypertensives. However, blood pressure response was quite variable, with a large increase in some patients' blood pressure. Patients should continue hypertensive medications at altitude. No data suggest that hypertensives are more likely to succumb to any of the altitude illnesses, and in general, hypertension would not seem to be a contraindication to altitude exposure.[20]

Sickle Cell Disease

Even the modest simulated altitude of a pressurized aircraft (1500 to 2000 m) may cause persons with hemoglobin SC and sickle-thalassemia to have a vasoocclusive crisis. High altitude exposure without supplemental oxygen is considered a contraindication in these persons. Sickle cell trait is not considered an increased risk, although splenic infarction syndrome during heavy exercise at altitude has been reported in those with trait.

Pregnancy

Pregnant residents of high altitude have an increased prevalence of hypertension, low-birthweight infants, and neonatal hyperbilirubinemia. However, an increased incidence of pregnancy complications in lowlanders who visit high altitude has not been reported. The normal Pa_{O_2} of the fetus is 29 to 33 mmHg, and the mild maternal hypoxia induced by traveling to resort-type altitudes does not generate significantly more hypoxic stress. The few studies available suggest that exercise in pregnant women at altitudes of 2500 m is safe for mother and fetus.[20] Until more data become available, pregnant patients should not be advised to curtail reasonable activities they wish to undertake. Perhaps of more concern than mild hypoxia is the fact that high altitude locations are often remote from medical facilities, and patients need to be aware that without access to sophisticated medical care, complications could have more serious consequences than at home.

REFERENCES

1. Honigman B, Theis MK, Koziol-McLain J, et al: Acute mountain sickness in a general tourist population at moderate altitudes. *Ann Intern Med* 118:587, 1993.
2. Yaron M, Waldman N, Niermeyer S, et al: The diagnosis of acute mountain sickness in pre-verbal children. *Arch Pediatr Adolesc Med* 152: 683, 1998.
3. Maggiorini M, Bartsch P, Oelz O: Association between raised body temperature and acute mountain sickness: cross sectional study. *BMJ* 315:403, 1997.
4. Dean AG, Yip R, Horrmann RE: High incidence of mild acute mountain sickness in conference attendees at 10,000 foot altitude. *J Wilderness Med* 1:86, 1990.
5. Hackett PH, Yarnell PR, Hill R, et al.: High altitude cerebral edema evaluated with magnetic resonance imaging: Clinical correlation and pathophysiology. *J Am Med Assoc* 280:1920, 1998.
6. Krasney JA: A neurogenic basis for acute altitude illness. *Med Sci Sport Exerc* 26:195, 1994.
7. Grissom CK, Roach RC, Sarnquist FH, et al: Acetazolamide in the treatment of acute mountain sickness: Clinical efficacy and effect on gas exchange. *Ann Intern Med* 116:461, 1992.
8. Hackett PH, Roach RC: High-altitude medicine, in Auerbach PA (ed): *Wilderness Medicine,* 3rd ed. St. Louis: CV Mosby, 1995, pp 1–37.
9. Burtscher M, Likar R, Nachbauer W, et al: Aspirin for prophylaxis against headache at high altitudes: randomised, double-blind, placebo-controlled trial *BMJ* 316:1057, 1998.
10. Hanaoka M, Kubo K, Yamazaki Y, et al: Association of high-altitude pulmonary edema with the major histocompatibility complex. *Circulation* 97:1124, 1998.
11. Steinacker J, Tobias P, Menold E, et al: Lung diffusing capacity and exercise in subjects with previous high altitude pulmonary edema. *Eur Respir J* 11:643, 1998.
12. Durmowicz A, Noordeweir E, Nicholas R, et al: Inflammatory processes may predispose children to high-altitude pulmonary edema. *J Pediatr* 130:838, 1997.
13. Hultgren H: High altitude pulmonary edema: Current concepts. *Ann Rev Med* 47:267, 1996.
14. Hultgren H, Honigman B, Theis K, et al: High-altitude pulmonary edema at a ski resort. *West J Med* 164:222, 1996.
15. Bärtsch P, Maggiorini M, Ritter M, et al: Prevention of high-altitude pulmonary edema by nifedipine. *N Engl J Med* 325:1284, 1991.
16. Hackett PH, Roach RC, Hartig GS, et al: The effect of vasodilators on pulmonary hemodynamics in high altitude pulmonary edema: A comparison. *Intl J Sport Med* 13:S68, 1992.
17. Scherrer U, Vollenweider L, Delabays A, et al: Inhaled nitric oxide for high-altitude pulmonary edema. *N Engl J Med* 334:624, 1996.

18. Levine B, Zuckerman J, deFilippi C: Effect of high-altitude exposure in the elderly: The Tenth Mountain Division study. *Circulation* 96:1224, 1997.
19. Erdmann J, Sun K, Masar P, et al: Effects of exposure to altitude on men with coronary artery disease and impaired left ventricular function. *Am J Cardiol* 81:266, 1998.
20. Hackett P: High altitude and common medical conditions, in Hornbein T, Schoene R (eds): *High Altitude.* New York, Marcel Dekker, 1999.

DYSBARISM

Kenneth W. Kizer

DYSBARIC DIVING CASUALTIES

There are now over 4 million recreational scuba[1] divers in the United States, and over 400,000 new sport divers are certified each year. In addition, diving is an integral part of many commercial and scientific activities (Table 192-1).

The health problems associated with diving are due to the hazards of the aquatic environment and the breathing of compressed gases at higher than normal atmospheric pressure. Table 192-2 categorizes the majority of diving-related medical problems.

Physical Principles

Many adverse physical conditions are encountered in the underwater environment. These include cold, wetness, changes in light and sound conduction, increased density of the surrounding environment, and increased atmospheric pressure. Of these, the indirect or direct effects of pressure account for the majority of serious diving medical problems.

PRESSURE Pressure is force per unit area and is measured in a number of different units (Table 192-3). The weight of air at sea level is equal to 14.7 lbs/in^2 (psi) or 1 atm absolute (ATA). Under water, pressure increases because of the weight of the water. Because water is much denser than air, large changes in pressure will accompany small fluctuations in depth. Thus, at a depth of 33 ft of seawater (fsw) the pressure is 2 ATA, and at 165 fsw it is 6 ATA (Table 192-4).[2] The proportionate change in pressure per unit depth is greatest near the surface and progressively diminishes with increasing depth. Because fresh water is less dense than saltwater, it takes a depth change of 34 ft of fresh water (ffw) to change the pressure 1 ATA. Scuba diving is generally done at pressure of less than 6 ATA, with the overwhelming majority in the 2- to 4-ATA range.

Because body tissues are composed mostly of water, which is not compressible, they are not directly affected by pressure changes. However, gases are compressible, and, consequently, gas-filled organs of the body are directly affected by pressure changes.

GAS LAWS Diving physiology is largely explained by three gas laws.

The first is *Boyle's law,* which states that the volume of a gas is inversely proportional to its pressure at a constant temperature. This is expressed by the equation.

$$PV = K$$

where P is pressure, V is volume, and K is a constant. Thus, as shown (see Table 192-4), when the pressure is doubled the volume of a unit of gas is halved, and conversely when the pressure is decreased in half, the volume doubles. Boyle's law explains the basic mechanism of all types of barotrauma.

The second is *Dalton's law,* which states that the pressure exerted by each gas in a mixture of gases is the same as each gas would exert if it alone occupied the same volume, or, alternatively, the total pressure of mixture of gases is equal to the sum of the partial pressures of the component gases. This is mathematically stated as

[1] *Scuba* is an acronym for *s*elf-*c*ontained *u*nderwater *b*reathing *a*pparatus.

[2] In diving and hyperbaric medicine, the most commonly used units of pressure and depth are ATA and fsw.

TABLE 192-1 Types of Commercial and Scientific Diving

Recovery of natural resources	Construction
Oil and natural gas	Piers and harbors
Minerals	Bridges and tunnels
Fish and shellfish	Dams
Pearls, corals, and shells	Underwater photography and motion picture production
Algae (e.g., kelp)	Marine studies
Wood (logging)	Biology
Aquaculture	Geology
Salvage and recovery operations	Archeology
Maintenance and repair work	Other sciences
Ship hulls	Law enforcement
Nuclear power plants	Rescue and recovery operations
Bridges and tunnels	Sport diving instructors and tour guides
Piers and harbors	
Aquariums	
Water treatment plants	

TABLE 192-2 Medical Problems of Scuba Divers

Environmental exposure problems
Motion sickness
Near drowning
Hypothermia
Heat illness
Sunburn
Phototoxic and photoallergic reactions
Irritant dermatitides
Infectious diseases
Mechanical trauma
Dysbarism
Barotrauma
Dysbaric air embolism (arterial gas embolism)
Decompression sickness (DCS)
Dysbaric osteonecrosis
Dysbaric retinopathy
Hyperbaric cephalgia
Breathing gas-related problems
Nitrogen narcosis
Hypoxia
Oxygen toxicity
Hypo- or hypercarbia
Carbon monoxide poisoning
Nitrogen oxide toxicity
Lipoid pneumonitis
Hazardous marine life
Envenomations
Animals that inflict trauma (e.g., bites)
Toxic ingestions
Miscellaneous
Hearing loss
Carotogenic blackout
Panic and other psychological problems

Source: Adapted from Kizer KW: Management of dysbaric diving casualties. *Emerg Med Clin North Am* 1:659, 1983. Used by permission.

TABLE 192-3 Pressure Equivalents

1 atmosphere absolute (ATA)	= 33 ft seawater (fsw)*
	= 5.5 fathoms seawater
	= 34 ft fresh water (ffw)
	= 14.7 pounds per square inch (psi)
	= 760 mm Hg
	= 29.9 in Hg
	= 1.033 kg/cm^2
	= 1.013 bar
	= 10.06 m
	= 0 atm gauge

*1 fsw = 0.445 psi = 0.0303 atm.
Source: From Kizer KW: Management of dysbaric diving casualties. *Emerg Med Clin North Am* 1:659, 1983. Used by permission.

$$P_t = P_{O_2} + P_{N_2} + P_x$$

where P_t is the total pressure, P_{O_2} is the partial pressure of oxygen, P_{N_2} is the partial pressure of nitrogen, and P_x is the partial pressure of the remaining gases in the mixture. This law explains why the partial pressures of component gases in a mixture change proportionately to changes in ambient pressure even though their absolute concentrations remain constant. This law is fundamental to the understanding of decompression sickness and other breathing gas-related problems.

Henry's law states that the amount of gas dissolved in a given volume of fluid is proportional to the pressure of the gas with which it is in equilibrium. The formula is

$$C_X = P_X \times \text{solubility}$$

where C_X is the concentration of gas dissolved in a liquid and P_X is the partial pressure of gas *X*. This law explains why more inert gas (e.g., nitrogen) dissolves in the diver's body as ambient pressure is increased with descent and, conversely, is released from tissue with ascent.

Direct Effects of Pressure—Barotrauma

The pressure-related diving syndromes can be divided into problems caused by the mechanical effects of pressure (i.e., barotrauma) and problems caused by breathing gases at elevated partial pressures (i.e., gas toxicities and decompression sickness [DCS]).

Barotrauma is the most common affliction of divers. It is defined as tissue damage resulting from contraction or expansion of gas spaces that occurs when the gas pressure in the body, or its compartments, is not equal to ambient pressure. For purposes of discussion, barotrauma can be viewed according to whether it occurs during descent or ascent.

TABLE 192-4 Pressure-Volume Relationships According to Boyle's Law

	Depth, fsw	Gauge Pressure, atm*	Absolute Pressure, atm	Gas Volume, %	Bubble Diameter,† %
Air	0	0	1	100	100
Seawater	33	1	2	50	79
	66	2	3	33	69
	99	3	4	25	63
	132	4	5	20	58
	165	5	6	17	54

*Gauge pressure is always 1 atm less than absolute pressure.
†Bubble diameter is probably more important than volume in consideration of the ability of recompression to restore circulation to a gas-embolized blood vessel.
Source: Adapted from Kizer KW: Management of dysbaric diving casualties. *Emerg Med Clin North Am* 1:659, 1983. Used by permission.

BAROTRAUMA OF DESCENT Barotrauma of descent, or "squeeze," as it is known in common diving parlance, results from the compression of gas in enclosed spaces as ambient pressure increases with underwater descent. Gas pressure in the various air-filled spaces of the body is normally in equilibrium with the environment; however, if something obstructs the portals of gas exchange, pressure equalization is precluded. If the air-filled space is not collapsible, the resulting pressure imbalance will cause tissue distortion, vascular engorgement and mucosal edema, hemorrhage, and other tissue damage. The ears and paranasal sinuses are most likely to be affected by such a process.

Aural barotrauma is the most common type of barotrauma and is a major cause of morbidity among divers, experienced by essentially all divers at one time or another. There are three main types of aural barotrauma, depending on which part of the ear is affected, and they may occur singly or in combination.

The first type involves the external auditory canal and is generally referred to as *external ear squeeze,* or *barotitis externa.* The external ear canal normally communicates with the environment and, consequently, the air in the canal is replaced by water when a diver is submerged. However, if the external ear canal is occluded (e.g., by cerumen, foreign bodies, exostoses, or earplugs), water entry is prevented, and compression of the enclosed air with descent will have to be compensated for by tissue collapse, outward bulging of the tympanic membrane, or hemorrhage. This is typically manifested by pain or bloody otorrhea. Physical examination may reveal petechiae or blood-filled cutaneous blebs along the canal, along with erythema or rupture of the tympanic membrane. Treatment involves keeping the canal dry, prohibiting swimming or diving until healed, and, in special cases, taking antibiotics and analgesics.

The next, and by far the most common, type of aural barotrauma is *middle ear squeeze,* or *barotitis media.* This results from a failure to equalize the middle ear and environmental pressures because of occlusion or dysfunction of the eustachian tube.

The eustachian tubes normally open and allow equalization of middle ear pressure when the pressure difference between the middle ear and pharynx reaches about 20 mmHg. This can be facilitated by yawning, swallowing, or using various autoinflation techniques (e.g., the Valsalva or Frenzel maneuvers). If middle ear pressure equalization is not achieved, the diver will notice discomfort or pain when the pressure differential reaches 100 to 150 mmHg or, roughly, when there has been a 20 percent reduction in middle ear gas volume. As the pressure differential is increased, mucosal engorgement and edema, hemorrhage, and inward bulging of the tympanic membrane develop. Eventually, these will be inadequate to compensate for the gas volume contraction, and the tympanic membrane ruptures. Fortunately, this is uncommon.

A number of factors may cause eustachian tube blockage or dysfunction—mucosal congestion secondary to upper respiratory infection, allergies, or smoking; mucosal polyps; excessively vigorous autoinflation maneuvers; and previous maxillofacial trauma. Persons with such conditions are at increased risk of middle ear barotrauma.

Divers having a middle ear squeeze usually complain of ear fullness or pain. As would be expected from the way that pressure changes with depth (Table 192-4), most problems occur near the surface. The pain is substantial and usually causes the diver to abort the dive. If not, it will continue to worsen until the eardrum ruptures, at which time the diver may feel air bubbles escaping from the ear and experience disorientation, nausea, and vertigo secondary to the caloric stimulation of cold water entering the middle ear. This sequence has been responsible for cases of panic and near drowning.

The otoscopic appearance of the tympanic membrane in cases of middle ear squeeze varies according to the severity of the injury and can be graded according to the amount of hemorrhage in the eardrum, with grades running from 0 (symptoms only) to 5 (gross hemorrhage and rupture). Physical examination may also disclose blood around the nose or mouth and a mild conductive hearing loss, which is usually only temporary.

Treatment of middle ear squeeze involves abstinence from diving until the condition has resolved and use of decongestants, which may be combined with antihistamines if there is an allergic component to the eustachian tube dysfunction. A combination of oral and long-acting spray decongestants is usually most efficacious. Antibiotics should be used when there is a tympanic membrane rupture or a preexisting infection. No diving should be done until a perforated eardrum has healed. Oral analgesics or topical aural anesthetics may be needed for a couple of days. In general, eardrops should not be used when there is a tympanic membrane perforation. Ideally, an audiogram should be obtained in anyone having more than a trivial middle ear squeeze, and serial audiograms should be obtained in patients having hearing loss. Most middle ear squeezes will resolve without complication in three to seven days. Prevention is preferable; a diver should refrain from diving when unable to easily equalize pressure in the ears and should always heed warning signs of ear pain.

Although less common, the third type of aural barotrauma, *inner ear barotrauma,* is much more serious than middle ear barotrauma because of possible permanently disabling injury to the cochleovestibular system. Inner ear barotrauma typically results from the sudden or rapid development of markedly different pressures between the middle and inner ear, such as may occur as a result of an overly forceful Valsalva maneuver intended to equalize the pressure in the middle ear or an exceptionally rapid descent during which the middle ear pressure is not equalized.

Patients with inner ear barotrauma typically are quite symptomatic, having a feeling of fullness or "blockage" of the affected ear, nausea, vomiting, nystagmus, diaphoresis, disorientation, or ataxia. The classic triad of symptoms indicating inner ear barotrauma is tinnitus, vertigo, and deafness. The onset of these symptoms may occur soon after the injury or may be delayed many hours, depending on the specific type of inner ear injury and the diver's activities during and after the dive. Findings on physical examination may be normal or may reveal signs of middle ear barotrauma or vestibular dysfunction, and audiometry may demonstrate a mild to severe sensorineural hearing loss. Any scuba diver with a hearing loss or vestibular symptoms following a nondecompression dive should be considered to have inner ear barotrauma until shown otherwise.

Clinically, there appear to be four categories or mechanisms for these injuries: hemorrhage within the inner ear (especially in the basal turn of the cochlea); rupture of Reissner's membrane, resulting in the mixing of endolymph and perilymph; fistulation of the round or oval window; and a mixed injury involving a combination of any or all of the other three. Injury to the membranous labyrinth may be either implosive or explosive.

Hemorrhage within the inner ear usually is associated with findings of middle ear barotrauma, no (or transient) vestibular symptoms, and a diffuse mild to severe sensorineural hearing loss (SNHL). Treatment of these patients should consist of bed rest with head elevated, avoidance of strain or strenuous activities, and symptomatic measures, as needed. The potential for full recovery is excellent, with the hearing loss usually completely resolved in three weeks to three months.

Manifestations of a tear in Reissner's membrane are similar to those of inner ear hemorrhage, although a persistent localized SNHL remains commensurate with the area of membrane tear. Treatment is similar to that of inner ear hemorrhage.

Inner ear fistulas typically present with a mild high-frequency SNHL or a marked cochleovestibular deficit and no or little evidence of middle ear barotrauma. Initially, these should be treated with bedrest, avoidance of strain, and other symptomatic measures, as needed. Worsening of hearing or vestibular symptoms or persistence of significant vestibular symptoms after a few days indicates the need for surgical exploration and repair. Some authorities, however, recommend immediate tympanotomy if severe symptoms are present initially. Importantly, recompression is contraindicated unless DCS or air embolism is also suspected to be present.

Any of the paranasal sinuses may fail to equalize pressure during descent. Manifestations of sinus squeeze include a sensation of fullness or pressure in the affected sinus, pain, or hemorrhage. Predisposing conditions for barosinusitis include upper respiratory infections, sinusitis, nasal polyps, or anything else that impairs the free flow of air from sinus cavity to nose. The maxillary and frontal sinuses are most often affected. Treatment for sinus squeeze is much the same as for middle ear squeeze, although antibiotics are usually indicated in cases involving the frontal sinuses.

Squeeze can also affect any other gas space that does not equilibrate with ambient pressure. For example, conjunctival, scleral, and periorbital hemorrhage may result if the diver fails to exhale into the mask during descent, resulting in telltale erythema, ecchymosis, and petechiae of the part of the face enclosed by the face mask—"face mask squeeze." If an area of skin is tightly enclosed by a dry diving suit a "suit squeeze" may occur. Although the appearance of these injuries may be spectacular, no special treatment is required, and they usually resolve in a few days.

Another special kind of squeeze may occur in divers who, while holding their breath, descend below the depth at which their total lung volume is reduced to less than residual volume. As occurs in other types of barotrauma of descent, the underventilated lung air spaces fill with tissue fluids and blood in an attempt to relieve the negative pressure. Clinical manifestations include chest pain, cough, hemoptysis, dyspnea, and pulmonary edema. Treatment includes administration of 100% oxygen, fluid replacement, and other supportive measures as clinically indicated. Because of the intrinsic lung injury and consequent potential for gas embolism, positive-pressure breathing (e.g., positive end-expiratory pressure or continuous positive airway pressure) should be avoided if possible. Very few divers attempt to free dive to depths likely to cause lung squeeze, and it is rare.

BAROTRAUMA OF ASCENT If there has been adequate equilibration of the pressure in the body's air-filled spaces during descent, the gas in those spaces will expand according to Boyle's law as ambient pressure decreases with ascent. The resulting excess gas is normally vented to the atmosphere. However, if this is prevented by obstruction of the air passages, the expanding gases will distend the tissues surrounding them; the resulting damage is known as *barotrauma of ascent* and is the reverse process of squeeze.

Although the ears and sinuses may be affected by barotrauma of ascent, this is unusual, because impediment of air egress is highly unlikely if pressure equalization is achieved with descent. However, middle ear and sinus barotrauma of ascent, or *reverse squeeze,* can occur, especially in divers having upper respiratory congestion treated with a short-acting nasal spray whose vasoconstrictive effect wears off while the diver is submerged. Similarly, *alternobaric vertigo* (ABV) resulting from unequal vestibular stimulation due to asymmetric middle ear pressure may occur during ascent. Although usually only transient, ABV may be severe enough to cause panic. Rarely, it may last for several hours, or even a day or two, after a dive.

Three other types of barotrauma of ascent should be discussed. The first may occur with either ascent or descent, although more commonly with ascent, and is known as *barodontalgia,* or, less accu-

TABLE 192-5 Manifestations of Pulmonary Barotrauma

Pneumomediastinum
Subcutaneous emphysema
Pneumopericardium
Pneumothorax
Pulmonary interstitial emphysema
Pneumoperitoneum
Diffuse alveolar hemorrhage
Arterial gas embolism Brain Heart Viscera

rately, ''tooth squeeze.'' Several specific conditions are associated with this problem (e.g., pulp decay, peridontal infections, or recent extraction sockets or fillings), but it may be due to anything that causes a pressure disequilibrium in an air-filled space in or about a tooth. Although rare and usually self-limited, anyone presenting with a toothache after diving should be referred for dental evaluation after maxillary sinus squeeze has been excluded.

Another unusual type of barotrauma of ascent is gastrointestinal (GI) barotrauma, which is also known as *aerogastralgia,* or ''gas in the gut.'' This occurs most commonly in novice scuba divers, who are more prone to aerophagia, and is caused by expansion of intraluminal bowel gas as ambient pressure is decreased during ascent. Other predisposing conditions include repeated performance of the Valsalva maneuver in the head-down position (which forces air into the stomach), drinking carbonated beverages or eating a heavy meal before diving (especially one containing legumes or other flatogenic substances), or chewing gum while diving. Symptoms of gastrointestinal barotrauma include abdominal fullness, colicky abdominal pain, belching, and flatulence. It is rarely severe because most divers will readily vent any excess bowel gas during ascent; however, it has been know to cause syncope and shocklike states. Actual gastric rupture from GI barotrauma has occurred, but this is exceedingly rare.

The last and most serious type of barotrauma of ascent is pulmonary barotrauma (PBT). Several different injuries can result from PBT of ascent, and these are collectively referred to as the pulmonary overpressurization syndrome (POPS) or ''burst lung'' (Table 192-5).

Diving equipment is designed to deliver compressed gas to the diver at the same pressure as the surrounding environment (e.g., at 33 fsw the diver breathes gas at a pressure of 2 ATA). Consequently, the compressed gas will expand during ascent according to Boyle's law, and the diver must allow the expanding gas to escape from the lungs, or it will rupture and dissect into the surrounding tissue. The resultant injury will depend on the location and amount of escaped gas. Symptoms of PBT sustained during ascent can appear immediately on surfacing or develop later.

Mediastinal and subcutaneous emphysema are the most common forms of the POPS. The patient usually presents with gradually increasing hoarseness, neck fullness, and substernal chest pain several hours after diving. Dyspnea, dysphagia, syncope, and other symptoms may be present as well. The history is usually diagnostic, although radiographs are indicated to verify the location of gas and exclude the presence of a pneumothorax.

The development of a pneumothorax as a result of PBT is uncommon but especially serious, for intrapleural gas cannot be released to the environment and is likely to progress to tension pneumothorax during ascent, leading to syncope, shock, or unconsciousness on surfacing.

Except for pneumothorax, which may require needle aspiration or tube thoracostomy, treatment of uncomplicated POPS typically requires only observation, rest, and, sometimes, supplemental oxygen. Recompression is necessary only in extremely severe cases.

Arterial Gas Embolism

The most feared complication of PBT is air embolism. Indeed, dysbaric air embolism (DAE), or arterial gas embolism (AGE), is one of the most dramatic and serious injuries associated with diving and is a major cause of death and disability among sport divers.

AGE results from the entry of gas bubbles into the systemic circulation through ruptured pulmonary veins. This usually occurs at the alveolar or terminal bronchiole level. After passing through the heart, bubbles lodge in small arteries, occluding the more distal circulation. The resulting manifestations will depend on the location of the occlusion. Depending on the site, even minute quantities of gas can have disastrous consequences. AGE can occur at depths as shallow as 1 m.

AGE usually presents immediately after a diver surfaces, at which time the high intrapulmonic pressure resulting from lung overexpansion is relieved, which allows air bubble-laden blood to return to the heart. Although the classic history is that the diver ascends rapidly because of running out of air, panic, or some similar circumstance, this is not always the case. Localized overinflation also may result from focally increased elastic recoil of the lungs in some divers. It is axiomatic that symptoms of AGE develop within 10 min of surfacing from a dive, although most often they are clearly evident within 2 min.

The presenting manifestations of AGE are sudden, dramatic, and often life-threatening. Coronary occlusion and cardiac arrest or arrhythmias may occur, although the brain is by far the most often affected organ. The neurologic manifestations are typical of an acute stroke, such as mono- or multiplegia, focal paralysis, sensory disturbance, blindness, deafness, vertigo, dizziness, confusion, convulsions, or aphasia. Asymmetric multiplegias are the most common presentation, and the differentiation of AGE from severe neurologic DCS is sometimes impossible. *Sudden loss of consciousness on surfacing should always be assumed to be due to gas embolism until proved otherwise.* Other reported clinical findings such as visualization of bubbles in the retinal arteries or Liebermeister's sign (a sharply circumscribed area of glossal pallor) are exceedingly rare. Patients with diving-related AGE may be intravascularly volume depleted and have similar laboratory abnormalities as seen with decompression sickness; except for hemoconcentration, the clinical significance of these abnormalities is unclear.

All cases of suspected AGE must be referred for recompression treatment—hyperbaric oxygen treatment—as quickly as possible. This is the primary and essential treatment for this condition, as is discussed later. Hyperbaric oxygen should also be used for cases of delayed AGE; it may be effective even up to 10 days after the event.

Some patients with very severe initial neurologic symptoms may improve spontaneously. The mechanism of spontaneous recovery is not clear. Nonetheless, such patients should still be referred for recompression because even subtle dysbaric injuries may become irreversible without definitive care. Before recompression, pneumothorax should be ruled out.

Indirect Effects of Pressure

Nitrogen narcosis and DCS sickness may develop as a result of breathing gases at higher-than-normal atmospheric pressure.

NITROGEN NARCOSIS Nitrogen and other lipid-soluble inert gases have an anesthetic effect at elevated partial pressures. The narcotic effects are similar to those of alcohol and become evident in most divers between 90 and 100 fsw. Many divers are so impaired at 200 fsw that they can do no useful work, and at depths over 300 to 350 fsw unconsciousness ensues. Although narcotic effects are reversed as the P_{N_2} decreases with ascent, nitrogen narcosis is not an uncommon precipitating factor in diving accidents and may impair a diver's memory of the circumstances leading up to the accident.

DECOMPRESSION SICKNESS Decompression sickness is a multisystem disorder resulting from the liberation of inert gas from solution with the formation of gas bubbles in blood and body tissues when ambient pressure is decreased. The critical factor in its pathogenesis is increased tissue absorption of inert gas, which in most diving situations is nitrogen.

As an air-breathing diver descends, ambient pressure increases, and the diving equipment delivers air to the lungs at increasing pressure, giving rise to a positive pressure gradient of nitrogen from alveoli to blood to tissue. After a time at depth this gradient will diminish, eventually becoming zero as a new equilibrium is reached. The time that it takes for the new equilibrium to be achieved will depend on the alveolar-to-tissue inert gas gradient, the tissue blood flow, and the ratio of blood-to-tissue inert gas solubility. Consequently, the rate at which a diver reaches a new inert gas equilibrium will be an exponential function of the diffusion and perfusion characteristics of the different tissues.

The tissue absorption of inert gas is the first step toward DCS, but it is only when ambient pressure is, in turn, decreased too rapidly to allow the diffusion of inert gas from tissues that DCS occurs.

The pathophysiology of decompression sickness results from both the mechanical and biophysical effects of bubbles (Fig. 192-1). The major mechanical effect of bubbles in DCS is vascular occlusion. Of note, the bubbles in DCS form primarily in the venous circulation and thus impair venous return, in contrast to the more usual arterial occlusion that occurs in most other conditions. However, the bubbles in DCS can form anywhere, such as in lymphatics, or intracellularly or extravascularly. Lymphedema, cellular distension and rupture, and intercellular dislocation can all compound the effects of vascular occlusion. Also, venous gas emboli may cause paradoxical arterial embolization via intrapulmonic and intracardiac shunts. Indeed, it is now clear that some dysbaric cerebral injuries are due to paradoxical embolization through previously unrecognized right-to-left intracardiac shunts that may only be open during abnormal pressure conditions found during diving. Since a patent foramen ovale (PFO) has been shown to be present in about 30 percent of the normal population, it can be assumed that about 30 percent of divers are likely to have a PFO. The presence of a PFO has been reported to produce a 2.5 times increase in the odds ratio for developing serious DCS. Such paradoxical embolization may help explain the high frequency of apparent combined DCS/air embolism noted in some series.

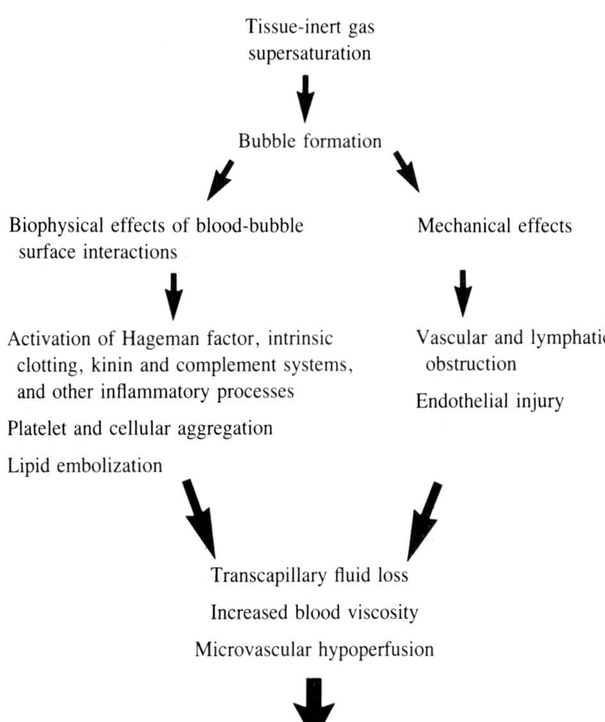

FIG. 192-1. Schematic representation of the pathogenesis of decompression sickness. (Adapted from Kizer KW: Management of dysbaric diving casualties. *Emerg Med Clin North Am* 1:659, 1983. Used by permission.)

TABLE 192-6 Clinical Forms of Decompression Sickness

Cutaneous ("skin bends")
Lymphatic
Musculoskeletal (the "bends" or pain-only bends)
Neurologic
Spinal cord
Cerebral
Cerebellar (the "staggers")
Inner ear
Peripheral nerves
Pulmonary (the "chokes")
Cardiovascular (decompression shock)
Visceral

Bubbles also exert a variety of biophysical effects due to blood-bubble surface interaction. In essence, bubbles are viewed by the immune system as foreign matter, and they incite an inflammatory reaction. The key step in the process is activation of Hageman factor, which, in turn, activates the intrinsic clotting mechanisms and kinin and complement systems, which results in platelet activation, cellular clumping, lipid embolization, increased vascular permeability, interstitial edema, and microvascular sludging. The net effect of all these processes is decreased tissue perfusion and ischemic injury.

The clinical manifestations of DCS are protean (Table 192-6), but the joints and spinal cord are most often affected. Technically, the term *bends* refers only to the musculoskeletal form of DCS, but it is commonly used in a generic sense to mean any type of DCS. The various forms of DCS have also been arbitrarily categorized as either types I or II, with type I referring to the mild forms of DCS (skin, lymphatic, and musculoskeletal systems) and type II including the neurologic and other serious types. Although this latter categorization is firmly entrenched in the literature, it is clinically more meaningful to refer to the systems affected when discussing patients with DCS.

In recent years, approximately 30 percent of DCS cases reported to the Divers Alert Network (DAN), have been Type I, and about 70 percent have been Type II.

Cutaneous manifestations of DCS include pruritus, subcutaneous emphysema, and scarlatiniform, erysipeloid, or mottled rashes. Localized swelling or peau d'orange may result from lymphatic obstruction.

Periarticular joint pain is typically described as a deep, dull ache, although it may be throbbing or sharp. There may be a vague area of numbness or dysesthesia around the affected joint. Movement of the affected extremity usually aggravates the pain, but inflation of a blood pressure cuff around the involved joint may relieve the pain for as long as the cuff is inflated. The shoulders and elbows are the joints most often affected in scuba divers, although essentially any joint may be involved.

Neurologic DCS may be manifested by a vast array of symptoms and signs. In fact, essentially any symptom is compatible with neurologic DCS. Classically, however, neurologic DCS involves the lower thoracic, lumbar, and sacral portions of the spinal cord and produces paraplegia or paraparesis, lower extremity paresthesias, and bladder dysfunction. Historically, urinary retention was such a frequent manifestation of spinal cord DCS that a urethral catheter used to be part of the diver's standard equipment. Hallenbeck and colleagues have convincingly demonstrated that at least some cases of spinal cord DCS result from venous infarction of the cord due to obstruction of venous drainage in the epidural vertebral venous plexus.

Pulmonary DCS results from massive venous air embolization and usually does not become symptomatic until at least 10 percent of the pulmonary vascular bed is obstructed. Signs and symptoms include chest pain, cough, dyspnea, shock, and pulmonary edema. The clinical course is often fulminantly downhill.

Many divers develop intravascular bubbles but no apparent illness; these have been called "silent bubbles" and their clinical significance is unclear.

A variety of laboratory abnormalities may be demonstrated in DCS, but most of them have little clinical relevance to acute care. Two tests that may be useful, though, are the urine specific gravity and hematocrit, because intravascular volume depletion and hemoconcentration are common in serious DCS. (This hemoconcentration may exacerbate the increased erythrocyte aggregation that has been demonstrated to occur at mild increased ambient pressure.) These two tests can help guide fluid replacement, which is an integral part of therapy.

Dysbaric casualties should be rapidly referred for hyperbaric treatment. However, the patient should also be evaluated for life-threatening nondysbaric injuries and, if present, resuscitation commenced.

Treatment of Diving Casualties

THE DIVING ACCIDENT HISTORY Most diving problems can be properly diagnosed by history and physical examination alone. The specific diving accident history should encompass these key points:

1. The type of diving engaged in and the equipment used. Some kinds of diving or certain types of equipment are associated with specific problems (e.g., hypercarbia or oxygen toxicity with rebreathing apparatus). Nitrox diving (aka enriched air nitrox or oxygen-enriched air diving) has become quite popular in recent years and requires special equipment and decompression tables.
2. The number, depth, bottom time, and surface interval between repetitive dives for all dives in the 72 h preceding symptom onset. Even if this information is not especially meaningful to you, having it available will facilitate communication with the diving medicine consultant who will want to ascertain whether required decompression was omitted.
3. In-water decompression. Again, this is relevant to the determination of the likelihood of the diver having DCS.
4. In-water recompression. Except in very unusual situations using 100% oxygen, full face mask, and other specialized support, in-water recompression should never be attempted. Recompression with compressed air should not be done, for it almost always leaves the diver in worse condition than originally and is fraught with other hazards.
5. Site of diving (e.g., ocean, lake, or quarry) and environmental conditions (e.g., water temperature, amount of current) associated with the dive. Other things being equal, DCS is more likely to occur after diving into very cold water, but nondysbaric problems related to the environment (e.g., motion sickness) must be excluded.
6. Primary diving activity (e.g., spearfishing, photography). DCS is more likely after an arduous dive.
7. Presence of predisposing factors. A number of factors have been anecdotally related to the development of DCS. These include advanced age (decreased tissue perfusion), obesity (increased absorption of inert gas), dehydration, recent alcohol intoxication, cold water (decreased peripheral perfusion), vigorous underwater exercise (increased gas uptake), local physical injury (decreased local perfusion), and multiple repetitive dives in unacclimatized individuals (gradual buildup of inert gas).
8. Dive complications. These include running out of air, marine animal envenomation, mechanical trauma, or some other unexpected event. Musculoskeletal pain may be due to overexertion or muscle strain, and numbness in an extremity may be from a jellyfish sting rather than DCS.
9. Predive and postdive activities. Activities such as jogging and unpressurized airplane travel after diving may precipitate DCS. Likewise, trivial dysbaric symptoms may become severe after similar activities.
10. Onset of symptoms. Certain conditions are more likely to occur at given times in the dive profile, and a differential scheme can be derived on the basis of time of symptom onset.

DIFFERENTIAL DIAGNOSIS OF DIVING ACCIDENTS Classically, a scuba dive is divisible into five stages, each of which is associated with characteristic problems.

The Predive Surface Phase The predive surface phase includes all activities prior to going underwater and beginning to breathe compressed air. This often involves considerable surface swimming to the dive site. The most often encountered problems during this phase of the dive are motion sickness, hyperventilation, mechanical trauma, near drowning, and untoward marine animal encounters.

Descent Phase The primary problems associated with descent are the squeeze syndromes, especially aural barotrauma, although inner ear barotrauma and ABV may also occur. Similarly, carbon monoxide poisoning, hypoxia, or other breathing gas problems may develop early in the dive.

At-Depth or Bottom Phase Overall, few problems occur "on the bottom," and the most likely ones are mechanical trauma or encounters with dangerous marine life. Nitrogen narcosis may contribute to an underwater accident. Inner ear barotrauma or gas mixture problems may first become symptomatic at this time even though they occurred earlier.

Ascent Phase Again, barotrauma is the problem most often encountered with ascent although much less frequently than during descent. The relationship of POPS, AGE, and inner ear barotrauma with ascent have already been discussed. Gas mixture problems may become manifest at this time, and hypercarbia can be experienced toward the end of a dive. DCS rarely occurs while a diver is still submerged; if this happens, it usually implies a very serious problem.

Postdive Surface Phase The postdive surface phase is divided into immediate (within 10 min of surfacing) and delayed (after 10 min). Any symptom occurring in the immediate postdive phase should be considered an air embolism until shown otherwise. Any symptom that begins more than 10 min after the dive should be viewed as DCS until otherwise explained. More than half of all DCS patients will become symptomatic in the first hour after surfacing, with most of the rest experiencing symptoms within six hours. A few patients (1 to 2 percent) may first note their symptoms 24 to 48 h after diving. Other problems that may be first noted in the delayed postdive phase include mild forms of the POPS, sequelae of barotrauma, inner ear barotrauma, motion sickness, exhaustion, irritant or venomous dermatoses, and nondysbaric conditions related to physical activity.

Of note, in sport diving, relatively few divers follow this classical dive profile; instead, they are much more likely to be repeatedly ascending and descending during the dive.

IMMEDIATE MANAGEMENT The victim should be rescued from the water and life support measures begun as needed. Hypothermia should be considered an aggravating factor in every aquatic accident victim.

If AGE is suspected, it is recommended that the patient be maintained supine in the field and during transport. Placement in the Trendelenburg or Durant positions is no longer recommended because of the uncertain benefit of such maneuvers and concerns about causing or aggravating cerebral edema (especially if left in the head-down position for longer than 30 to 60 min) and the increased respiratory difficulty attendant to being in such positions.

Supplemental 100% oxygen should always be given as soon as possible, being best administered by mask at 6 to 8 L/min. This facilitates offgassing of the nitrogen bubbles and improves oxygenation of damaged tissues.

Depending on local circumstances, patients with suspected AGE or DCS may be taken directly to the recompression chamber or may need emergency department intervention. Whichever is the case, transportation should be as expeditious as possible. If air transportation is used, the patient should be subjected to the least possible pressure reduction so as not to cause any further gas expansion. Either a low-flying helicopter or light airplane capable of flight at 1000 ft (300 m) or less should be used. Alternatively, aircraft that can be pressurized to 1 ATA (e.g., Lear jet, Cessna Citation, or C-130 Hercules) can be used.

Advanced life support drugs should be administered according to the victim's condition and standard protocols. In general, most DCS victims are at least mildly volume depleted, so parenteral and oral (if the patient is alert) fluids should be given at a brisk rate unless they are contraindicated for other reasons.

Although high-dose parenteral corticosteroids have been widely recommended and used in the past as an adjunct to recompression treatment of both neurologic DCS and AGE, little objective evidence supports their benefit. The use of glucocorticoids became prevalent based on the belief that they were beneficial in the treatment of cerebral edema, shock, and other conditions pertinent to DCS, but their benefit in many of these other conditions is now questioned. A few anecdotal cases suggesting that steroids are beneficial, either alone or with other pharmacologic interventions combined with standard recompression therapy, have been reported, but there have been no published clinical series or controlled trials demonstrating their efficacy. In contrast, controlled studies of high-dose parenteral dexamethasone or methyl prednisolone in DCS-affected dogs showed that the use of glucocorticoids as an adjunct to conventional hyperbaric oxygen treatment produced no benefit.

If the need for recompression or the location of the nearest hyperbaric treatment facility is uncertain, assistance is available 24 h a day through the Divers Alert Network (DAN) at Duke University, Durham, NC, (919) 684-8111.

HYPERBARIC TREATMENT Pressure and oxygen are the keystones of treatment for DCS and AGE and are administered according to well-established protocols. Various types of hyperbaric chambers may be used for treatment, and the relative merits of one type or another need not be recounted here.

The outcome of recompression treatment will, of course, depend on the severity of the disease, the delay in commencing hyperbaric treatment, and the victim's health prior to the accident. Overall, 80 to 90 percent success rates have been reported from a variety of sources, and even though recompression is generally believed to be more likely beneficial the sooner that it is commenced after the onset of symptoms, it should not be refused to someone who presents 2, 3, or more days after an accident, for dramatic recoveries have been reported after treatment delays of 10 days or longer. It is not possible to determine in advance what the effect of a delay in recompression will be for any individual patient.

POSTRECOMPRESSION EVALUATION Because recompression treatment does not always result in complete resolution of dysbaric neurologic injury and because occasional situations arise when the differential diagnosis of acute diving-related neurologic dysfunction includes intracranial hemorrhage, trauma, or other nondysbaric injury, it is sometimes important to characterize the site, extent, and origin of central nervous system (CNS), lesions beyond what can be achieved by the traditional means of history and physical examination.

Both computed tomography (CT) and magnetic resonance imaging (MRI) have been used in this regard. Regrettably, conventional CT has not been found to be an efficient investigative tool for the posttreatment evaluation of DCS, and CT imaging of spinal cord lesions (which constitute the majority of neurologic DCS) is not feasible. In contrast, limited clinical data support the feasibility and efficacy of MRI of these conditions, especially when intracranial injury is present.

In contrast, CT of the chest, and especially spiral volumetric CT, is very helpful in demonstrating bullae, including subpleural blebs or cysts, as the cause of pulmonary barotrauma.

BLAST INJURY

The phenomenon of blast injury has been recognized for as long as human beings have used explosives although it has been mainly a wartime concern. However, in the past few decades there has been a dramatic increase in the incidence of peacetime civilian explosive blast injuries because of the popularity of the homemade bomb as a vehicle of social protest or terrorist activity, and the continued hazard of explosions in mining, grain storage, and other industries. In addition, blast injuries remain a prominent cause of fire-related morbidity.

Blast Physics and Terminology

Explosives are materials that are rapidly converted into gases when detonated. *Blast* and *blast injury* are, respectively, general terms used to describe this gaseous decomposition and the damage occurring in an organism subjected to the pressure field produced by an explosion.

Blasts are characterized by the release of large quantities of energy in the form of pressure and heat, with the exact amount depending on the type and amount of explosive. If the explosion is confined within some sort of casing (e.g., a bomb), the pressure will rupture the housing and eject the resulting fragments at high velocity. The remaining energy is transmitted to the surrounding environment in the form of a blast wave, blast winds, ground shock, and fire.

The *blast wave* begins as a single pulse of increased pressure that rises to peak levels within a few milliseconds and then rapidly falls to a minimum pressure that is lower than the original atmospheric pressure (Fig. 192-2). It is propagated outward radially from the explosion, with the sharply marginated periphery of the sphere becoming the blast, overpressure, or shock wave, as it has been variously called. The duration and level of the high-pressure peak depends on the nature of the explosive, the conducting medium, and the distance from the detonation point. This blast wave pressure peak determines the *overpressure* that an object in its path is subjected to and is the main determinant of primary blast injury. Conversely, the negative pressure wave, or suction of the blast wave, lasts several times longer than the high-pressure wave but can never be greater than −760 mmHg (−14.7 psi). Representative pressure effects are listed in Table 192-7.

The rapidly expanding gases from an explosion also displace air, causing it to move away at very high velocity and produce transient

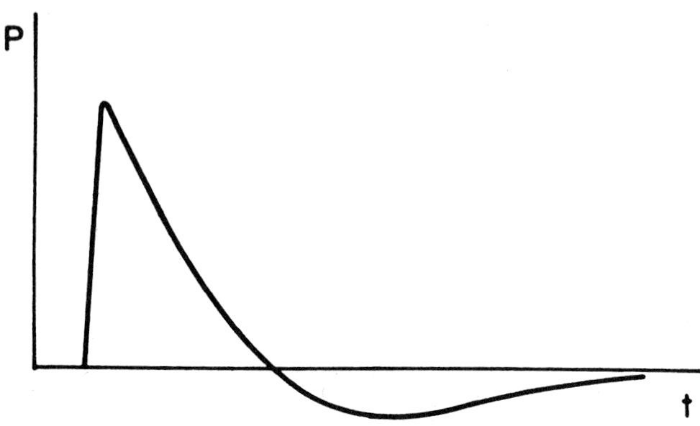

FIG. 192-2. The general form of a blast wave. (From Stapczynski JS: Blast injuries, in Edlich RF, Spyker DA (eds): *Current Emergency Therapy '85*. Rockville, MD, Aspen Systems Corporation, 1985, p 294.)

TABLE 192-8 Categories of Blast Injury

Category	Injury Caused by	Primary Target Organs
I. Primary blast injury	Blast wave	Ears, lungs, GI tract, CNS
II. Secondary blast injury	Victim struck by flying debris	Integument, CNS, eyes, musculoskeletal system
III. Tertiary blast injury	Bodily displacement, i.e., victim impact with stationary objects	Abdominal viscera, CNS, lungs, integument, musculoskeletal system
IV. Miscellaneous	Inhalation of dust or toxic gases, thermal burns, radiation, other	Lungs, integument, eyes

blast winds that travel immediately behind the shock front of the blast wave. The blast wave may also accelerate loose objects (e.g., people) through the air, causing acceleration-deceleration injuries. In the immediate vicinity of an explosion, this *windage* can cause atomization, or total disintegration, of a body, evisceration, or traumatic amputations, depending on the force of the explosion. Illustrative of the force of such winds, an overpressure of about 5200 mmHg (100 psi) produces a blast wind having a velocity of about 2400 kph (1500 mph).

In addition to the amount and duration of overpressure caused by an explosion, the overall effect of the blast wave also depends on the exact waveform of the overpressure (i.e., its rise time), the victim's body mass and orientation to the explosion, the presence of deflecting and reflecting surfaces in the environment, and the medium through which the shock wave is conducted. For example, because of the greater density of water and its relative incompressibility, blast waves produced by underwater explosions travel much faster and farther than those produced by terrestrial explosions. Consequently, blast injuries in water occur at greater distances from the detonation point and tend to be more severe. Underwater blast injury has other peculiarities, too, but these are beyond the scope of this discussion.

Categories and Manifestations of Blast Injury

Explosive blast injuries can be divided into four categories (Table 192-8).

PRIMARY BLAST INJURY *Type I,* or *primary, blast injury* results directly from the sudden changes in environmental pressure caused by the blast wave. Tissues vary in their susceptibility to primary blast injury, with homogeneous or solid tissues being at least risk because they are essentially noncompressible and merely vibrate as a whole when subjected to a blast wave. Conversely, gas-filled organs are compressible and have tissue-gas interfaces, which means that displacement occurs wherever tissues of different densities interface, resulting in tissue distortion and tearing. Thus, primary blast injury mainly affects organs containing air and causes the most severe damage at the junctions between tissues, where loose, poorly supported tissue is displaced beyond its elastic limit.

TABLE 192-7 Selected Effects from Blast Waves

Pressure, psi*	Effect
5	Possible tympanic membrane rupture
15	50% incidence of tympanic membrane rupture
30	Possible lung injury
75	50% incidence of lung injury
100	Possible fatal injuries
200	Death more likely than not

*1 psi = 51.7 mmHg.

There are three general mechanisms whereby a blast shock wave can damage living tissue. The first of these is known as *spalling* and occurs when a shock wave traveling through a medium of higher density (e.g., liquid) passes into a medium of lower density (e.g., gas), creating a negative reflection at the interface and, thus, fragmenting the surface of the heavier medium. This is analogous to hitting the outside of a rusty bucket with a hammer, which causes flakes to come off inside the bucket.

The second mechanism is implosion of gas-filled spaces as the high pressure in the surrounding fluid or solid compresses these spaces. Similarly, because there is a pressure differential between the air-filled and vascular spaces, blood and fluid are forced into the air-filled spaces. This mechanism is of particular importance in the lungs, where it contributes to pulmonary hemorrhage. In addition, as the negative pressure wave follows the initial positive pressure, smaller internal secondary explosions occur as the compressed gas reexpands.

Third, tissues of different densities will be accelerated and decelerated at different rates relative to each other, producing shearing forces that can tear or otherwise damage the tissue.

The organs most vulnerable to primary blast injuries are the ears, lungs, CNS, and gastrointestinal tract. Abdominal visceral injury is relatively rare in air blast casualties but is of considerable concern in persons exposed to underwater blasts.

Otolaryngologic Manifestations The ears are most often affected by explosive blasts, with hearing loss being the primary manifestation. Hearing can be damaged in one of three ways. First, the tympanic membranes may rupture. This usually occurs in adults at a pressure differential between the middle and external ears of around 360 mmHg (7 psi), and most often presents as a linear perforation of the pars tensa. The second way is dislocation of the ossicles, which may accompany tympanic membrane rupture or occur as the sole injury. Finally, deafness may result from blast effects on the inner ear, causing perilymph fistula and other damage. In addition to hearing loss, primary symptoms of inner ear damage include vertigo and tinnitus.

The paranasal sinuses are also susceptible to blast injury, usually manifesting barotraumatic damage similar to the squeeze syndromes that occur with compressed air diving.

Pulmonary Manifestations The lungs are generally the organs most severely affected by blast injury, and these injuries are likely to present a threat to life. (Of course, the severe injuries resulting from windage in the immediate vicinity of the explosion are also life-threatening). The blast wave causes widespread alveolar damage because of its effects on tissue-gas interfaces, producing interstitial and intra-alveolar hemorrhage and edema, parenchymal and pleural lacerations, and alveolar-venous fistulas. Because of the widespread nature of this damage a variety of specific injuries may be found, including pulmonary edema, pneumothorax and other extra-alveolar air syndromes, and air embolism. Similarly, pulmonary contusions result from compression of the lung between the spine, thoracic wall, and rising diaphragm, as well as from being thrown against solid objects in the environment.

The actual symptoms experienced by victims of blast lung injury will vary with the severity and nature of their specific injuries, but, in general, they will present with dyspnea, shortness of breath, chest pain, hemoptysis, rales, rhonchi and signs of pulmonary edema or hemorrhage, as well as symptoms of the POPS.

Gastrointestinal Manifestations Blast injuries to the stomach and bowels are due to damage at tissue-gas interfaces, producing hemorrhage into the wall and lumen along with perforations, which tend to be multifocal. Because the large bowel usually contains more gas than the small bowel, it tends to be more severely affected. Common clinical manifestations include abdominal pain, melena, signs of peritonitis, and free air in the abdomen. Evisceration and other gross damage may be found in victims who were very close to the detonation site, but these types of injury are nearly always fatal.

Neurologic Manifestations Blast injuries of the CNS are of two main types. First are the direct shock wave effects, which produce a concussion syndrome and various types of intra- and extra-axial hemorrhage, and second are the effects of cerebral air embolism. As with dysbaric diving casualties, the specific neurologic manifestations of air embolism are myriad.

OTHER CATEGORIES OF BLAST INJURY *Type II,* or *secondary, blast injuries* are due largely to the blast wind and result from the victim being struck by flying debris. Conversely, *type III,* or *tertiary, blast injuries* are those that result from the victim being displaced through space by the blast wind and impacting a stationary object; this sudden deceleration usually causes more harm than the acceleration through space. *Type IV blast injuries* include a wide variety of injuries resulting from inhalation of dust and toxic gases, exposure to radiation, thermal burns, and so on.

The myriad number of bodily insults that can result from these latter types of blast injury are far too numerous to list here. Of particular concern, though, are the traumatic amputations, occurring in about 25 percent of severely wounded victims, and liver, spleen, or other visceral injuries produced from the acceleration-deceleration forces of the blast wind. Likewise, bomb-casing fragments or missiles, such as nails, nuts and bolts, screws, ball bearings, etc., can cause high-velocity missile injuries.

Management of Blast Casualties

Analysis of urban bomb blast injuries from Israel, Ireland, and the United Kingdom have identified common patterns:

1. Most victims are far enough from the explosion that they sustain only minor injuries, usually from flying debris.
2. Injuries most often affect the face, neck, and exposed extremities, indicating the protective role of ordinary clothing.
3. Injuries to the chest and abdomen are uncommon, but are associated with increased morbidity and mortality.
4. Injuries to the head are associated with the highest mortality.
5. While tympanic membrane rupture is common, primary blast injuries to other organs are unusual.

Blast injury victims should be managed in the same manner as any multiple trauma victim, except that particular attention should be directed to the respiratory system. This includes giving special attention to maintenance of a patent airway (especially when maxillofacial, cervical spine, or other head and neck injuries are present); administering supplemental oxygen; judiciously using intravenous fluids and analgesics; evacuating pneumo- and hemothoraces; and promptly implementing mechanical ventilation if signs of respiratory failure or inadequate oxygenation are present. Although positive pressure ventilation may be necessary to maintain adequate oxygenation, its use is fraught with hazard because the diffuse alveolar-capillary damage present in blast lung greatly increases the risk of causing extra-alveolar extravasation of air, including air embolism.

Systemic air embolization presents particular problems in the management of blast casualties, because the effects on the brain, heart, and viscera caused by air emboli may be indistinguishable from other types of injury. Yet, the preferred therapy for air embolism is hyperbaric oxygen treatment, which may not be readily available or may be impractical because of coexistent injuries or other logistical problems. Whenever possible, though, hyperbaric oxygen treatment should be implemented as expeditiously as possible, being given in a manner similar to the treatment of dysbaric diving casualties, because of its potential to reverse cerebral or coronary injuries if administered soon after the injury.

Tympanic membrane rupture and other otolaryngologic trauma, as well as most other types of blast injury, should be treated essentially the same as they are treated when due to other causes. Closed abdominal injuries are always of particular concern and should be treated according to the patient's signs and symptoms, with prompt surgical exploration being undertaken whenever there are signs of peritonitis or peritoneal free air. Abdominal visceral injuries should be especially looked for in victims of underwater explosion. Lacerations, fractures, amputations, and missile wounds should be treated in the usual manner, except for delayed primary closure being the generally preferred method of wound management.

Explosions in closed spaces produce greater injury and death than those occurring in the open. Primary blast injuries are especially common. Closed-space explosions also expose the victim to dust, smoke, and toxic gases, increasing the incidence of inhalation injury. Again, though, the inhalation injury is treated essentially the same as that resulting from other circumstances.

Because primary blast injuries may not always be present when the victim is first evaluated, all blast-injured patients should be closely observed for at least 6 to 12 h after the accident. This is particularly true if there is perforation of the eardrums, which is generally an indication of significant exposure to high pressure.

BIBLIOGRAPHY

Diving Injuries

Azimuddin K, Porter J: Survival after cardiac arrest from documented venous air embolism. *J Trauma* 44:398, 1998.

Ball R: Effect of severity, time to recompression with oxygen, and re-treatment on outcome in forty-nine cases of spinal cord decompression sickness. *Undersea Hyperb Med* 20:133, 1993.

Bitterman H, Melamed Y: Delayed hyperbaric treatment of cerebral air embolism. *Isr J Med Sci* 29:22, 1993.

Boussuges A, Carturan D, Ambrosi P, et al: Decompression induced venous gas emboli in sport diving: Detection with 2D echocardiography and pulses Doppler. *Int J Sports Med* 19:7, 1998.

Hardy KR: Diving-related emergencies. *Emerg Med Clin North Am* 15:223, 1997.

Madsen J, Hink J, Hyldegaard O: Diving physiology and pathophysiology. *Clin Physiol* 14:597, 1994.

Maoloff AL: Delayed onset of arterial gas embolism. *Aviat Space Environ Med* 64:1040, 1993.
Neuman TS, Jacoby I, Bove AA: Fatal pulmonary barotrauma due to obstruction of the central circulation with air. *J Emerg Med* 16:413, 1998.
Reuter M, Tetzlaff K, Warninghoff V, et al: Computed tomography of the chest in diving-related pulmonary barotrauma. *Br J Radiol* 70:440, 1997.
Smith RM, Neuman TS: Elevation of serum creatine kinase in divers with arterial gas embolism. *N Engl J Med* 330:19, 1994.
Smith RM, Van Hoesen KB, Neuman TS: Arterial gas embolism and hemoconcentration. *J Emerg Med* 12:147, 1994.
Tetzlaff K, Reuter M, Leplow B, et al: Risk factors for pulmonary barotrauma in divers. *Chest* 112:654, 1997.
Tibbles PM, Edelsberg JS: Hyperbaric-oxygen therapy. *N Engl J Med* 334:1642, 1996.
Tomassoni AJ: Cardiac problems associated with dysbarism. *Cardiol Clin* 13:266, 1995.

Blast Injuries

Argyros GJ: Management of primary blast injury. *Toxicology* 121:105, 1997.
Boffard KD, MacFarlane C: Urban bomb blast injuries: Patterns of injury and treatment. *Surg Annu* 25(part 1):29, 1993.
Coupland RM: Hand grenade injuries among civilians. *JAMA* 270:624, 1993.
Garth RJ: Blast injury of the ear: An overview and guide to management. *Injury* 26:363, 1995.
Hull JB, Cooper GJ: Pattern and mechanism of traumatic amputation in explosive blast. *J Trauma* 40(suppl 3):S198, 1996.
Karmy-Jones R, Kissinger D, Golocovsky M, et al: Bomb-related injuries. *Mil Med* 159:536, 1994.
Kozuka M, Nakashima T, Fukuta S, Yanagita N: Inner ear disorders due to pressure change. *Clin Otolaryngol* 22:106, 1997.
Liebovici D, Gofrit ON, Stein M, et al: Blast injuries: Bus versus open-air bombings—A comparative study of injuries in survivors of open-air versus confined-space explosions. *J Trauma* 41:1030, 1996.
Mallonee S, Shariat S, Stennies G, et al: Physical injuries and fatalities resulting from the Oklahoma City bombing. *JAMA* 276:382, 1996.
Mayorga MA: The pathology of primary blast overpressure injury. *Toxicology* 121:17, 1997.
Quintana DA, Parker JR, Jordan FB, et al: The spectrum of pediatric injuries after a bomb blast. *J Pediatr Surg* 32:307, 1997.
Sorkin P, Szold O, Kluger Y, et al: Permissive hypercapnia ventilation in patients with severe pulmonary blast injury. *J Trauma* 45:35, 1998.
Stuhmiller JH: Biological response to blast overpressure: A summary of modeling. *Toxicology* 121:91, 1997.

NEAR DROWNING

Bruce E. Haynes

Drowning, like other causes of accidental death, often strikes young, otherwise healthy individuals, and prevention is the most important way to reduce these unnecessary deaths. The patient's prognosis after near drowning depends on the speed of rescue and resuscitation, emphasizing the role of emergency medical care.

DEFINITIONS

Almost as many definitions of drowning exist as authors in the field. One approach is to define *drowning* as death from suffocation after submersion, while those who suffer *near drowning* survive, at least temporarily, after suffocation by submersion. A few use the more generic term *immersion syndrome* to highlight the blurred margins between the two entities, although this term also has been used to refer to sudden death after immersion in cold water. *Postimmersion syndrome,* or *secondary drowning,* refers to the deterioration of a seemingly well patient after immersion.

EPIDEMIOLOGY

Drowning is the third leading cause of accidental death in the United States, killing about 4500 people each year. Although the exact number is uncertain, many more individuals survive serious near-drowning episodes.

Freshwater drowning, especially in pools, is more common than saltwater drowning, even in coastal areas. There is a bimodal age distribution, with large numbers of deaths among children under age 4 and then later among teenagers, although risk climbs again in the elderly from bathtub drowning. Young children are also at risk for drowning in a bathtub, even in the presence of siblings, and neglect or intentional injury should be considered in such cases.[1] Responses to a careful history may change over time and reveal inconsistencies, especially in regard to developmental age. Caretakers must ensure constant attention by an individual of appropriate age.

Alcohol or drug use by victims or even by supervising adults often plays a role in drowning and boating accidents. Consistent use of personal flotation devices by adults and children when boating is crucial. Children may be oblivious to potentially dangerous situations, especially in rivers and lakes. Some cases follow traumatic injury in or around the water, including spinal injury. Hypothermia is a factor in some drownings, while causes of syncope, including hyperventilation before underwater swimming, are responsible for a few cases. Patients with seizure disorders must receive careful supervision if swimming and should, depending on seizure control, probably bathe in showers or tubs with open drains and plastic stalls. This patient education is important when first-time seizure patients are discharged from emergency departments.

Drowning deaths may be prevented by adequate, well-maintained fencing with self-locking gates that surrounds pools themselves, rather than simply isolating the backyard, leaving access to the pool from the house and yard. However, fencing is not a complete answer.[2] Childhood pool drowning occurs rapidly and silently, and caretakers must not be diverted by chores, socializing, telephone calls, or other seemingly momentary distractions. Cardiopulmonary resuscitation (CPR) is frequently not started by rescuers, and pool owners should be encouraged to learn CPR and have telephones in the pool area. Swimming lessons for young children are controversial. Toddlers cannot understand their true skill level, nor the danger posed by water, nor do they have the strength to exit a pool. Swimming lessons, or more accurately, floating lessons, may induce a dangerous false sense of security among caretakers, putting the child at even more risk. On the other hand, there is evidence that trained children entering the water accidentally may have the skill to remain on the surface longer.[3]

PATHOPHYSIOLOGY

Respiratory failure and ischemic neurologic injury are the threats to life after submersion although associated injuries are occasionally present. Older victims who are not immediately unconscious may panic, struggle in the water, hold their breath, or hyperventilate. Once under water, involuntary breathing resumes at a break point determined by the Pa_{O_2} or Pa_{CO_2}. This soon leads to vomiting and aspiration of water and emesis. "Dry drowning" without aspiration results from laryngospasm and glottal closure. Whatever the mechanism, the final common pathway is profound hypoxemia.

Initial hypoxemia results from flooding of alveoli and impairment of gas exchange. Although both seawater and fresh water wash surfactant out of alveoli, fresh water also changes the surface tension properties of surfactant. Surfactant loss leads to atelectasis, ventilation perfusion mismatch, and breakdown of the alveolar capillary membrane.[4] Hypoxemia follows aspiration of small amounts of water and is seen experimentally with aspiration of 2.2 mL/kg of either fresh water or saltwater. Contributing to pulmonary injury may be aspiration of bacteria, algae, sand, particulate matter, emesis, and chemical irritants.

Noncardiogenic pulmonary edema results from direct pulmonary injury, surfactant loss, inflammatory contaminants, and cerebral hypoxia.

Poor perfusion and hypoxemia lead to metabolic acidosis in a majority of patients, yet perhaps as a result of the young age of most victims, the cardiovascular status is remarkably stable. Blood volume shifts depend on the nature and quantity of the fluid aspirated, although life-threatening changes are unusual in resuscitated patients, because most human drowning victims aspirate quantities of water below those which produce significant disturbances. Electrolyte abnormalities in near-drowning patients are seldom significant, and hematologic values are usually normal, although the clinician occasionally will see hemoconcentration or hemolysis that results in anemia. Rarely, disseminated intravascular coagulation will occur.

Renal function is usually adequate, although proteinuria may occur, and hemoglobinuria can follow hemolysis. Acute tubular necrosis can result from hypoxia or myoglobinuria.

TREATMENT

Prehospital Care

Treatment of near drowning begins at the scene with rapid, cautious removal of the victim from the water (Table 193-1). Spinal precautions should be observed if the mechanism of injury, such as diving or surfing, raises suspicion of such injury. The vast majority of spinal injuries are to the lower cervical spine after diving. Clues to spinal injury may be paradoxical respiration (abdominal breathing without movement of intercostal muscles), flaccidity, priapism, or unexplained hypotension or bradycardia. Lifeguards and emergency medical technicians should maintain spinal precautions during rescue if possible. Initial history may be unreliable, and the physician should have a low threshold for obtaining cervical spine x-rays.

A patent airway must be maintained and ventilation assisted as needed; patients should receive supplemental oxygen. CPR should be started on any arrested patient with even a remote possibility of success. Sodium bicarbonate may be considered in hemodynamically unstable patients. Any patient with a significant episode, including those asymptomatic at the scene, should be transported to the hospital for evaluation.

In-water CPR is generally ineffective and dangerous for the rescuer and should not be attempted unless a firm, stable surface is available. Human near-drowning victims aspirate small quantities of water; postural drainage or the abdominal thrust (Heimlich maneuver) is of unproven efficacy in removing water from the lungs or improving oxygenation. No drainage procedure appears to significantly affect oxygenation in experimental preparations. Field limitations to postural drainage include the danger of aspiration from an uncontrolled airway, interruption of ventilation or CPR, the danger of spinal injury, and the possibility of aggravating other undiagnosed injuries. An appropriate maneuver for airway obstruction should be used only if ventilation is obstructed.

TABLE 193-1 Prehospital Care of Near-Drowning Victims

Rapid, cautious rescue
Spinal precautions
Cardiopulmonary resuscitation
Supplemental oxygen on all patients
Transport all patients

TABLE 193-2 Hospital Care of Near-Drowning Victims

Clear spine
Laboratory studies: CBC, electrolytes, glucose, PT/PTT, urinalysis Arterial blood gases, pulse oximetry Chest x-ray Electrocardiogram
Pulmonary support: Supplemental oxygen on all patients High-flow O_2 as needed Intubation and positive pressure (PEEP, CPAP)
Nasogastric tube
Foley catheter
Monitor: Oxygenation Acid-base balance Temperature Volume status
Evaluate and treat: Associated injuries Specific conditions: hypovolemia, hypothermia, hypoglycemia, etc.

Abbreviations: PT = prothrombin time, PTT = partial thromboplastin time.

Hospital Care

Hospital evaluation and care of drowning victims emphasizes initial resuscitation, treatment of respiratory failure, and evaluation of associated injuries (Table 193-2).

Although patient survival in a persistent vegetative state is a concern, substantial numbers of patients, predominantly children, requiring CPR on emergency department arrival have survived with good outcomes, and physicians should err on the side of providing resuscitation.[4–6] The physician should gather sufficient history to allow an estimate of prognosis and gauge the patient's response to resuscitative efforts.

On the victim's arrival in the emergency department, adequate oxygenation should be ensured, the integrity of the patient's spine should be confirmed if necessary, and associated injuries should be sought. Pulmonary insufficiency may be indicated by dyspnea, tachypnea, or use of accessory muscles of respiration. Physical examination may reveal wheezing, rales, or rhonchi, although the chest may be normal to auscultation after aspiration.

All patients should receive supplemental oxygen during evaluation, and those with more than mild symptoms should be on 100% oxygen until adequate oxygenation is documented. If high-flow oxygen (40% to 50%) cannot maintain the arterial P_{O_2} greater than 60 mmHg in adults or 80 mmHg in children, the patient should be intubated and mechanical ventilation used.

Intubated patients generally require positive end-expiratory pressure (PEEP) or continuous positive airway pressure (CPAP). Occasionally, a patient may require only increased oxygenation and CPAP without mechanical ventilation. Only patients who are alert and unlikely to vomit are candidates for mask or nasal CPAP or other noninvasive ventilation.

All patients need an accurate temperature that reflects core temperature, since resuscitation may be impossible until hypothermia is treated. Hypothermia can immobilize a swimmer, resulting in drowning, may cause ventricular fibrillation, or may be responsible for a variety of adverse metabolic effects. Hypothermic patients have body temperatures less than 30°C (86°F), after submersion in water less than 20°C (68°F). Severe hypothermia often indicates prolonged submersion and

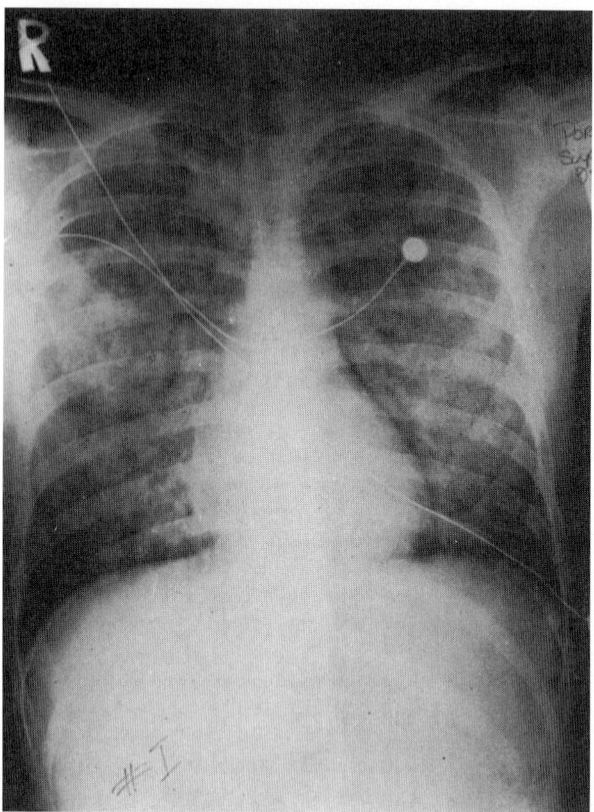

FIG. 193-1. Chest roentgenogram of near-drowning patient demonstrating diffuse noncardiogenic pulmonary edema.

is a bad prognostic sign. Despite this, individuals have survived after prolonged submersion (more than 60 min) in cold or icy water. Aspiration of cold water in concert with intact circulation for several minutes rapidly cools the body to low temperatures.[7] The nature of the protective effect of hypothermia is unclear. It is most likely generalized slowing of metabolism, but preferential shunting of blood to the brain, heart, and lungs (diving reflex) may play some role. Hypothermic near-drowning victims in whom resuscitation is attempted should be warmed to at least 30 to 32.5°C (86°–90.5°F) before resuscitation efforts are abandoned. In selected cases of submersion in extremely cold water, extracorporeal rewarming may be helpful.[8]

Appropriate laboratory data should be obtained (see Table 193-2). Direct measurement of oxygenation and acid-base status by arterial blood gas analysis and pulse oximetry guide pulmonary therapy and the need for sodium bicarbonate.

Roentgenograms of the chest may be normal after a significant near-drowning incident or may show generalized pulmonary edema (Fig. 193-1), perihilar infiltrates, or other patterns. Chest films do not necessarily correlate with arterial Pa_{O_2}, making direct measurement of oxygen saturation important, although many patients with significantly abnormal films will require intubation.

Standard treatment of hypothermia, hypotension and hypovolemia, bronchospasm, electrolyte imbalance (including hypoglycemia), seizures, and arrhythmias should be undertaken. Some patients may need fluid resuscitation in the face of noncardiogenic pulmonary edema. To avoid inducing arrhythmias, central venous catheters, if used, should not enter the heart in hypothermic patients. A nasogastric tube will empty the stomach and help prevent vomiting, and a Foley catheter will help to monitor urine output. Neither antibiotics nor steroids alter the course of aspiration pneumonia or pulmonary edema in drowning, and they should not be given prophylactically.

PROGNOSIS AND CEREBRAL RESUSCITATION

Statistics on survival and the incidence of severe neurologic deficits after near drowning are difficult to interpret. They vary with regard to definitions, patient age, water temperature, treatment regimens, and many other variables.[9–11] Almost all patients who are alert and fully conscious will survive without sequelae, as will the vast majority of victims who are obtunded but have a purposeful response to pain. As many as 24 percent of children admitted to intensive care units who required full CPR and had an initial Glasgow Coma Scale score of 3 in the referring emergency department have survived with intact neurologic function.[5] CPR, requiring cardiotonic medications, or unreactive pupils all indicate a poor prognosis, but no one indicator or scoring system fully differentiates survivors with acceptable neurologic outcome from children who die. Quan and Kinder have suggested resuscitation is indicated if the time of submersion is likely to be 10 min or less, and that patients not responding to advanced life support measures within 25 min will not live.[12]

Life support can be withdrawn in the intensive care unit once the patient's condition is stable, the likely outcome more clear, and the family has had time to consider treatment options.[6]

Outcome depends primarily on the duration of submersion but also on the amount of time until resuscitative efforts begin.

DISPOSITION

Most older reports on drowning recommend admission and monitoring of all near-drowning victims. This recommendation arose from descriptions of "secondary drowning" in which 2 to 25 percent of near-drowning patients deteriorated significantly or died after a seemingly successful rescue or resuscitation. Most of the patients in these reports, however, simply had pulmonary insufficiency that progressed and symptoms or signs that today would be discovered easily by an adequate evaluation.[13,14] The decision of whom to admit must focus on those at risk for pulmonary insufficiency or other complications.

Patients at risk have undergone a "significant" episode and display symptoms such as coughing, dyspnea tachypnea, or have historical factors such as unconsciousness in the water. Occasionally, patients who suffered transient severe hypoxia or who have underlying cardiovascular disease will fall into the same group.

The physician's approach should depend on the patient's symptoms and the results of screening examinations. For convenience, patients may be separated into four groups, although one should take particular care in evaluating young children. One group will have no evidence of significant submersion and may be discharged quickly. Chest roentgenograms and arterial blood gas determinations are unnecessary in the face of a benign history, but the studies or pulse oximetry may lend weight to the decision to discharge.

A second group will be asymptomatic or have mild symptoms after a significant episode. They can frequently be observed in the emergency department for several hours and then discharged if their social situation allows adequate follow-up. The third group will have mild to moderate hypoxemia corrected by oxygen therapy. These patients are admitted and then discharged when the hypoxemia resolves if no complications ensue.

The final group is composed of patients who require intubation and mechanical ventilation whose prognosis usually depends more on their neurologic status than on pulmonary injury, unless they develop serious aspiration pneumonia or progressive, irreversible lung injury.

REFERENCES

1. Lavelle JM, Shaw KN, Seidl T, Ludwig S: Ten-year review of pediatric bathtub near drownings: Evaluation for child abuse and neglect. *Ann Emerg Med* 25:344, 1995.
2. Logan P, Branche CM, Sacks JJ, et al: Childhood drownings and fencing of outdoor pools in the United States, 1994. *Pediatrics* 101:E3, 1998.

3. Asher KN, Rivara FP, Felix D, et al: Water safety training as a potential means of reducing risk of young children's drowning. *Inj Prev* 1:228, 1995.
4. Modell JH: Drowning. *N Engl J Med* 328:253, 1993.
5. Allman FD, Nelson WB, Pacentine GA, et al: Outcome following cardiopulmonary resuscitation in severe pediatric near-drowning. *Am J Dis Child* 140:571, 1986.
6. Christensen DW, Jansen P, Perkin RM: Outcome and acute care hospital costs after warm water near drowning in children. *Pediatrics* 99:715, 1997.
7. Conn AW, Miyasaka K, Katayama M, et al: A canine study of cold water drowning in fresh versus salt water. *Crit Care Med* 23:2029, 1995.
8. Bolte RG, Black PG, Bowers RS, et al: The use of extracorporeal rewarming in a child submerged for 66 minutes. *JAMA* 260:377, 1988.
9. Nussbaum E, Maggi JC: Pentobarbital therapy does not improve neurologic outcome in nearly drowned, flaccid-comatose children. *Pediatrics* 81:630, 1988.
10. Zuckerman GB, Gregory PM, Santos-Damiani SM: Predictors of death and neurologic impairment in pediatric submersion injuries. *Arch Pediatr Adolesc Med* 152:134, 1998.
11. Spack L, Gedeit R, Splaingard M, et al: Failure of aggressive therapy to alter outcome in pediatric near-drowning. *Pediatr Emerg Care* 13:98, 1997.
12. Quan L, Kinder D: Pediatric submersions: Prehospital predictors of outcome. *Pediatrics* 90:909, 1992.
13. Pratt FD, Haynes BE: Incidence of "secondary drowning" after saltwater submersion. *Ann Emerg Med* 15:1084, 1986.
14. Szpilman D: Near-drowning and drowning classification: A proposal to stratify mortality based on the analysis of 1,831 cases. *Chest* 112:660, 1997.

THERMAL BURNS

Lawrence R. Schwartz
Chenicheri Balakrishnan

EPIDEMIOLOGY

Approximately 1.25 million patients present to the emergency department (ED) with burn injuries in the United States each year and about 50,000 are hospitalized.[1] The majority of burn patients are treated and discharged from the ED to be followed as outpatients.

The risk of burns is highest in the 18- to 35-year-old age group. There is a male to female ratio of 2:1 for both injury and death. There is higher incidence of scalds from hot liquids in children 1 to 5 years of age and in the elderly. The death rate in patients over 65 years of age is much higher than that in the overall burn population.[2]

Significant strides have been made in the overall care of the burn patient during the last two decades.[3] These advances are reflected in a decreased mortality rate among patients with major thermal injury; only about 4 percent of those treated in specialized burn treatment centers die from their injuries or associated complications.[4] The incidence of inpatient admissions has decreased over time owing to improvements in outpatient care both in the ED and in the burn unit.[1,3]

PATHOPHYSIOLOGY

Skin consists of two layers: the epidermis and dermis. In the very young and the elderly, the skin thickness is less than that of a person in the prime of life. Skin thickness also varies significantly throughout the body. The skin is very thick in the palm of the hand and the sole of the foot. The upper part of the back is thicker than other parts of the body. Thus exposure to same temperature for same duration will lead to different depths of injury in different parts of the body.

Skin functions as a semipermeable barrier to evaporative water loss. Other functions of the skin include protection from the adversities of the environment, control of body temperature, sensation, and excretion. Partial-thickness thermal injury can result in disruption of the barrier function and contribute to free water deficits. The effect may be significant in moderate to large burns.

Thermal injury results in a spectrum of local and systemic homeostatic derangements that contribute to burn shock. These include disruption of normal cell membrane function, hormonal alterations, changes in tissue acid-base balance, hemodynamic changes, and hematologic derangement.[5]

Fluid and electrolyte abnormalities seen in burn shock are largely the result of alterations of cell membrane potentials with intracellular flux of water and sodium and extracellular migration of potassium secondary to dysfunction of the sodium pump. In burns of greater than 60 percent of body surface area, depression of cardiac output is frequently observed with lack of response to aggressive volume resuscitation. Although disputed by others, Baxter and Shires have explained this phenomenon on the basis of circulating myocardial depressants.[6] Also, there is increased systemic vascular resistance. A significant metabolic acidosis may be present in early stages of a large burn injury.

Hematologic derangements associated with massive thermal injury vary from an increase in hematocrit with increased blood viscosity during the early phase followed by anemia from erythrocyte extravasation and destruction. However, transfusion is infrequently required for patients with isolated burn injury.[3]

Thermal injury is a progressive injury. Local effects of thermal injury include liberation of vasoactive substances, disruption of cellular function, and edema formation. The systemic response consists of responses by the neurohormonal axis and profound alterations of all organ systems. Substances implicated in these events are histamine, kinin, serotonin, arachidonic acid metabolites, and free oxygen radicals. These substances exert their primary effects at the local level and cause progression of the burn wound. Preservation of the blood supply by decreasing the inflammatory response has been attempted with pharmacologic manipulations using drugs such as nonsteroidal anti-inflammatories.[5]

Although many factors may influence prognosis, the severity of the burn, presence of inhalation injury, associated injuries, patient's age, preexisting disease, and acute organ system failure are most important.[2] The burn's size and depth are functions of the burning agent, its temperature, and the duration of exposure. Cell damage occurs at a temperature greater than 45°C (113°F) owing to denaturation of cellular protein. The burn wound is described as having three zones: the zone of coagulation, where tissue is irreversibly destroyed with thrombosis of blood vessels; the zone of stasis, where there is stagnation of the microcirculation; and the zone of hyperemia, where there is increased blood flow. The zone of stasis can become progressively more hypoxemic and ischemic if resuscitation is not adequate. In the zone of hyperemia, there is minimal damage to the cells and spontaneous recovery is likely.

CLINICAL FEATURES

Burn Size

The size of a burn injury is quantified as the percentage of body surface area (BSA) involved.[7] One method of calculating the percentage of BSA burned is to use the rule of nines (Fig. 194-1). This method divides the body into segments that are approximately 9 percent or multiples of 9 percent, with the perineum forming the remaining 1 percent. In infants and children, this method must be modified because of their larger heads and smaller legs.

Another method is based on the fact that the area of the back of a patient's hand is approximately 1 percent BSA. The number of "hands" that equal the area of the burn can approximate the percentage of BSA burned.

A more precise estimation of the percentage of BSA burned is obtained by using a Lund and Browder burn diagram (Fig. 194-2). This allows for accurate determination of the size and depth. These

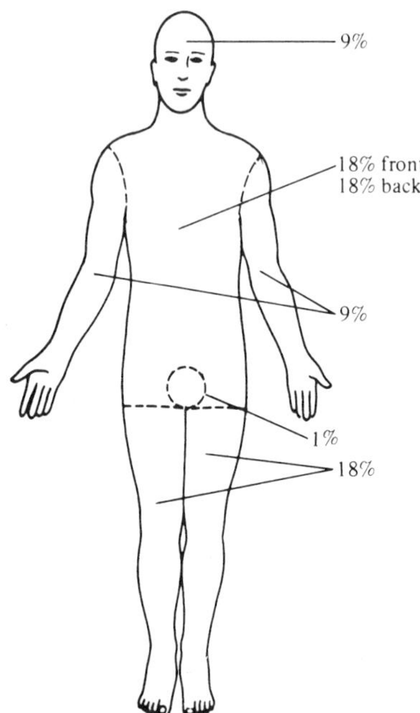

FIG. 194-1. Rule of nines to estimate percentage of burn.

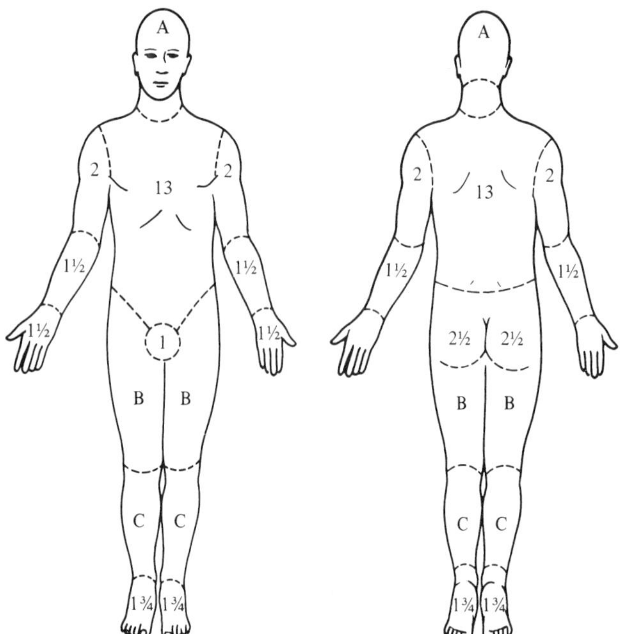

Relative Percentages of Areas Affected by Growth (Age in Years)

	0	1	5	10	15	Adult
A: half of head	9½	8½	6½	5½	4½	3½
B: half of thigh	2¾	3¼	4	4¼	4½	4¾
C: half of leg	2½	2½	2¾	3	3¼	3½

Second degree ____________ and

Third degree ____________ =

Total percent burned ___

FIG. 194-2. Lund and Browder diagram to estimate percentage of pediatric burn.

charts are age-adjusted, hence allowing for changes in children at different ages.

Experienced burn-care nurses and physicians are reliable in estimating burn size regardless of the method used.[8] However, it is common for inexperienced individuals to estimate burn size incorrectly when patients are first assessed in the ED.

Burn Depth

The depth of a burn has been historically described in degrees: first, second and third.[9] However, a classification of burn depth according to the need for surgical intervention has become the accepted approach in burn treatment centers: superficial partial-thickness, deep partial-thickness, and full-thickness burns.[3] Determination of burn depth requires judgment, using the commonly seen clinical features; there is no objective method of measuring burn depth, and burn wound biopsy has not become routine practice.

A first-degree burn involves only the epidermal layer of skin. Sunburn is usually given as a common example of a first-degree burn, although sunburn is caused by ultraviolet light instead of thermal injury.[9] The burned skin is red, painful, and tender without blister formation. First-degree burns usually heal in about 7 days without scarring and require only symptomatic treatment.

Second-degree burns extend into the dermis and are divided into superficial partial-thickness and deep partial-thickness burns.

In superficial partial-thickness burns, the epidermis and the superficial (papillary layer) dermis are injured. The deeper layers of the dermis, hair follicles, and sweat and sebaceous glands are spared. Superficial partial-thickness burns are often caused by hot water. There is blistering of the skin and the exposed dermis is red and moist at the blister's base. These burns are very painful to touch. There is good perfusion of the dermis with intact capillary refill. Superficial partial-thickness burns heal in 14 to 21 days, scarring is usually minimal, and there is full return of function.

Deep partial-thickness burns extend into the deep (reticular layer) of the dermis. There is damage to hair follicles as well as sweat and sebaceous glands, but their deeper portions usually survive. Hot liquids, steam, grease, or flame usually causes deep partial-thickness burns. The skin may be blistered and the exposed dermis is pale white to yellow in color. The burned area does not blanch; it has absent capillary refill and absent pain sensation. Deep partial-thickness burns may be difficult to distinguish from full-thickness burns. Healing takes 3 weeks to 2 months. Scarring is common; it is related to the depth of the dermal injury. Surgical debridement and skin grafting may be necessary to obtain maximum function.

Third-degree or full-thickness burns involve the entire thickness of the skin. All epidermal and dermal structures are destroyed. Full-thickness burns are usually caused by flame, hot oil, steam, and contact with hot objects. The skin is charred, pale, painless, and leathery. These injuries will not heal spontaneously, as all dermal elements are destroyed. Surgical repair and skin grafting are necessary and there will be significant scarring.

Fourth-degree burns are those that extend through the skin to the subcutaneous fat, muscle, and even bone. These are devastating, life-threatening injuries. Amputation or extensive reconstruction is required.

SPECIFIC ISSUES

The American Burn Association has devised a classification of burns, dividing them into major, moderate, and minor.[7] Criteria for burn unit transfer are listed in Table 194-1. Children younger than 10 years of age and adults above age 50 are considered high-risk patients. Patients with underlying medical illnesses such as heart disease, diabetes, or chronic pulmonary problems are considered poor-risk.

TABLE 194-1 American Burn Association Criteria for Transfer to a Burn Unit

1. Partial- or full-thickness burns involving greater than 10 percent of body surface area (BSA) in patients under 10 or over 50 years of age.
2. Partial- or full-thickness burns of greater than 20 percent of BSA in other age groups.
3. Partial- or full-thickness burns with the threat of functional or cosmetic impairment that involve face, hands, feet, genitalia, perineum, or major joints
4. Full-thickness burns of greater than 5 percent of BSA in any age group.
5. Electrical burns, including lightning injury.
6. Chemical burns with the threat of functional or cosmetic importance.
7. Inhalation injury with burns.
8. Circumferential burns of the extremities or chest.
9. Burn injury in patients with preexisting medical disorders that could complicate management, prolong recovery, or affect mortality.
10. Any burn patient with concomitant trauma, such as fracture.
11. Hospitals without qualified personnel or equipment for the care of children should transfer burned children to a burn center with these capabilities.

Source: From American Burn Association,[10] with permission.

Major Burns

Major burns are defined as (1) partial-thickness burns greater than 25 percent BSA in the 10- to 50-year-old age group; (2) partial-thickness burns greater than 20 percent BSA in children under 10 or adults over 50; (3) full-thickness burns of greater than 10 percent BSA in anyone; (4) burns involving the hands, face, feet, or perineum; (5) burns crossing major joints; (6) circumferential burns of an extremity; (7) burns complicated by inhalation injury; (8) electrical burns; (9) burns complicated by fractures or other trauma; (10) burns in infants and the elderly; and (11) and burns in poor-risk patients.

Moderate Burns

Moderate burns are (1) partial-thickness burns of 15 to 25 percent BSA in the 10- to 50-year-old age group; (2) partial-thickness burns of 10 to 20 percent BSA in children under 10 or adults over 50; and (3) full-thickness burns of less than 10 percent BSA in anyone. Partial-thickness burns of the hands, face, feet, or perineum or circumferential burns of an extremity are excluded.

Minor Burns

Minor burns include (1) partial-thickness burn of less than 15 percent BSA in the 10- to 50-year-old age group; (2) partial-thickness burn of less than 10 percent BSA in children under 10 or adults over 50; and (3) full-thickness burns of less than 2 percent BSA in anyone without associated injuries. These burns imply outpatient treatment.

Inhalation Injury

With improvements in the treatment of burn shock and sepsis, inhalation injury has emerged as the main cause of mortality in the burn patient.[2,4] Despite advances in respiratory support, smoke inhalation injury significantly increases mortality; half of all fire-related deaths are due to smoke inhalation. Inhalation injuries are associated with closed-space fires, and conditions that decrease mentation—such as overdose, alcohol intoxication, drug abuse, and head injury. Exposure to smoke includes exposure to heat, particulate matter, and toxic gases.[11]

There is general consensus that direct thermal injury is limited to the upper airway. Thermal injuries below the vocal cords occur only in cases of steam inhalation.

Smoke contains particulate matter, usually less than 0.5 μm in size, which is formed from incomplete combustion of organic material. Small particles may reach the terminal bronchioles, where they can initiate an inflammatory reaction leading to bronchospasm and edema.

Toxic inhalants are divided into three large groups: tissue asphyxiants, pulmonary irritants, and systemic toxins. The two major tissue asphyxiants are carbon monoxide and hydrogen cyanide.

Carbon monoxide poisoning is a well-known consequence of smoke inhalation injury.[11] Severe carbon monoxide poisoning will produce brain hypoxia and coma. Comatose patients lose airway protective mechanisms, which may result in aspiration, thus further exacerbating the pulmonary injury from smoke inhalation. All patients with suspected carbon monoxide exposure should be started on 100% oxygen by non-rebreathing mask. Further details of treatment of carbon dioxide poisoning are discussed in Chap. 198.

Hydrogen cyanide is formed when nitrogen-containing polymers—such as wool, silk, polyurethane, or vinyl—are burned. Cyanide binds to and disrupts mitochrondrial oxidative phosphorylation, leading to profound tissue hypoxia. Further discussion of management of cyanide poisoning is discussed in Chap. 182.

Inhalation injury damages endothelial cells, produces mucosal edema of the small airways, and decreases alveolar surfactant activity leading to bronchospasm, airflow obstruction, and atelectasis. With time, tracheal and bronchial epithelial sloughing occurs. As these patients are resuscitated with large quantities of fluid for their burn injury, pulmonary edema develops. Hence, the potential for adult respiratory distress syndrome (ARDS) from inhalation injury should be recognized and careful fluid management instituted with emphasis on hemodynamic monitoring.

Bronchospasm may occur early, but lower airway edema is usually not clinically evident for up to 24 h. Upper airway edema, however, can occur rapidly. Although the injury is mainly to the airways, pulmonary vascular changes do occur. There is no single method capable of demonstrating the extent of inhalation injury. Diagnosis of smoke inhalation is made from the history of a fire in an enclosed space and physical signs that include facial burns, singed nasal hair, soot in the mouth or nose, hoarseness, carbonaceous sputum, and expiratory wheezing. Carboxyhemoglobin levels are useful to document prolonged exposure within an enclosed space with incomplete combustion. The chest radiograph may be normal initially; bronchoscopy and radionuclide scanning are useful in determining the full extent of injury.

Treatment of suspected inhalation injury should be instituted prior to definitive diagnosis. Humidified oxygen (100%) should be administered by mask. Arterial blood gases including carboxyhemoglobin levels should be obtained. In suspected cases, control of upper airway is achieved by prompt endotracheal intubation. Indications for intubation include (1) full-thickness burns of the face or perioral region, (2) circumferential neck burns, (3) acute respiratory distress, (4) progressive hoarseness or air hunger, (5) respiratory depression or altered mental status, and (6) supraglottic edema and inflammation on bronchoscopy.

TREATMENT

The management of patients with *moderate to major* burns can be divided into three phases: (1) prehospital care, (2) emergency department resuscitation and stabilization, and (3) admission or transfer to a specialized burn center.

Prehospital Care

The following principles are the basis of prehospital care for burn patients: (1) stop the burning process, (2) establish the airway, (3) initiate fluid resuscitation, (4) relieve pain, (5) protect the burn wound, and (6) transport the patient to an appropriate facility.

On-site assessment of a burned patient is divided into primary and secondary surveys. In the primary survey, immediate life-threatening conditions are quickly identified and treated. Initial management of the burned patient should be the same as for any other trauma patient, with emphasis on airway, breathing, circulation, and cervical spine immobilization. During the secondary survey, a thorough head-to-toe evaluation is carried out.

The patient must be removed from the burning process and burning clothing must be immediately removed and the remainder of the clothing removed after the airway, breathing, and circulation (ABCs) are secured. All rings, watches, jewelry, and belts should be removed, as they can retain heat and produce a tourniquet-like effect on the extremity causing ischemia. A 100% oxygen mask should be applied. Thought should be given to an airway that has potential to swell rapidly, even though initial assessment may be acceptable. Prophylactic intubation should be considered in burns about the face sustained in a closed-space fire. Intravenous fluids are started with isotonic crystalloid: usually Ringer's lactate solution. The patient should be covered with clean sheets to protect the wound. Early cooling can reduce the depth of burn and reduce pain, but uncontrolled cooling will result in hypothermia. Analgesia can be given upon direction of the on-line medical control physician. The patient should be transported to the nearest hospital capable of caring for a burn patient, or, if none is available, the nearest hospital for stabilization.

Emergency Department Management

Upon arrival at the ED, a directed history should be obtained from the patient and emergency medical services (EMS) personnel. What was the burning agent? Were chemicals involved? What was the duration of exposure? Was the fire in an open or enclosed space? If the fire was in an enclosed area, what substances were burned? Was there an explosion causing the patient to suffer a blast injury? Was there any contact with electricity? Was there any other trauma or loss of consciousness? A general history including past medical and surgical illnesses, chronic disease, allergies, medications, and tetanus immunization status should be obtained from the patient or family.

The ABCs should be reassessed and stabilized. The adequacy of or need for cervical immobilization should also be reassessed. The patient should be examined for signs of inhalation injury, evidence of facial burn, carbonaceous sputum, singed nasal hair, and soot in the mouth. If there is any evidence of airway compromise with swelling of the neck, burns inside the mouth, or wheezing, endotracheal intubation should be performed.

The adequacy of circulation is initially assessed by the blood pressure, pulse rate, capillary refill time, mental status, and urinary output. Intravenous lines can be inserted though a burned area if required and resuscitation started according to the burn resuscitation formula.

During the secondary examination, the patient needs a head-to-toe assessment. The eyes should be examined for corneal burns. The size of the burn and its depth should be estimated and recorded. Patients with a greater than 20 percent partial-thickness burn routinely require a nasogastric tube, as ileus frequently occurs. A Foley catheter should be inserted to measure urinary output and prevent urinary retention in patients with perineal burns.

Routine laboratory tests including a CBC, electrolytes, BUN, creatinine, and glucose should be obtained. In patients with suspected inhalation injury, arterial blood gases, carboxyhemoglobin, chest radiograph, and ECG should be obtained. Fiberoptic bronchoscopy is indicated where there is a suspicion of inhalation injury and in intubated patients, as this is both diagnostic and therapeutic in clearing the airways. A urinalysis, urine for mycoglobin and creatine kinase (CK) levels are obtained along with an electrocardiogram (ECG) in patients with electrical injury to assess muscle or cardiac injury. Additional radiographs should be taken as indicated for other suspected trauma.

TABLE 194-2 Parkland Formula

Adults
Lactated Ringer's 4 mL × weight (kg) × % BSA over initial 24 h
Half over the first 8 h from the time of burn
Other half over the subsequent 16 h
Example 70 kg adult with 40% burn
4 mL × 70 kg × 40 = 11200 mL over 24 h
Children
Lactated Ringer's 3 mL × weight (kg) × % BSA over initial 24 h plus maintenance
Half over the first 8 h from the time of burn
Other half over the subsequent 16 h

The burn shock resuscitation formulas in use today are based on laboratory studies of burn shock and resuscitation. The purpose of these formulas is to provide a *guide* for fluid resuscitation. The Baxter or Parkland formula is probably the most widely used thermal injury resuscitation regimen in North America.[3] This formula calls for 4 mL of lactated Ringer's solution multiplied by the percent BSA burned multiplied by body weight in kilograms. Half of this total is given in the first 8 h after injury and the rest during the next 16 h (Table 194-2). The amounts may be large and hemodynamic monitoring techniques are now commonly used to protect against inadvertent volume overload.

Electrical injuries, incineration burns, and associated crush injuries may produce rhabdomyolysis and myoglobinuria, leading to renal failure. See Chap. 271 for further discussion.

Thermal injury in the presence of concomitant multisystem trauma generally requires fluids in excess of calculated needs. Inhalation injuries have been shown to increase total fluid needs. Burn patients with preexisting cardiac or pulmonary disease require much greater attention to fluid management. Fluid resuscitation should be monitored closely by frequent assessment of the patient's vital signs, signs of cerebral and skin perfusion, and urinary output as well as hemodynamic monitoring. The urinary output should be 0.5 to 1.0 mL/kg per hour.

There are several methods of calculating fluid resuscitation for infants and children. One method is to use the Parkland formula and modify it to maintain urinary output of 1 mL/kg per hour. Alternatively, a pediatric maintenance rate for 24 h can be calculated plus an additional amount of 2 to 4 mL/kg multiplied by percent of BSA burned, with the entire amount infused over the first 24 h. In children weighing less than 25 kg, a urine output of 1.0 ml/kg per hour is necessary.

It is possible for patients with major burns to receive excessive intravenous fluids during the prehospital and ED phases, particularly if two large-bore peripheral catheters are in place with fluid infusing wide open. Total fluids infused should be documented and titrated to the patient's response.

Two additions or modifications to isotonic crystalloid resuscitation have been studied—adjuvant colloid and hypertonic saline. However, neither improves patient outcome. Adjuvant colloid given along with isotonic crystalloid resuscitation has not proven beneficial and is associated with increased accumulation of water in the lungs and decreased glomerular filtration rate.[12] Hypertonic saline has produced an increased rate of renal failure and death.[13]

Routine tetanus toxoid prophylaxis should be administered based on the patient's immunization history. Tetanus immune globulin should be administered in patients without a history of primary immunization. The use of systemic prophylactic antibiotics is inappropriate.

Treatment of inhalation injury includes humidified oxygen, intubation and ventilation, bronchodilators, pulmonary toilet, and hyperbaric oxygen for severe carbon monoxide poisoning.

Burns to a pregnant patient are associated with significant morbidity to mother and child. The outcome of the pregnancy is determined by the extent of mother's injury; spontaneous termination of pregnancy is the common outcome in large-BSA burns. Fluid requirements may exceed the estimated formula. Fetal monitoring and early consultation with the obstetrician is mandatory.

Wound Care

After evaluation and resuscitation, the burn wounds are addressed.[14] Initially in the ED, the wound is best covered with a clean, dry sheet. Later, small burns can be covered with a moist saline-soaked dressing while the patient is awaiting admission or transfer. The soothing effect of cooling on burns is most likely due to local vasoconstriction. Studies have shown that cooling stabilizes mast cells and reduces histamine release, kinin formation, and thromboxane B_2 production. In large burns, sterile drapes are better, as saline-soaked dressings applied to a large area can cause hypothermia. The admitting service should be consulted early. The use of antiseptic dressing should be avoided in the ED as the admitting service will need to assess the wound. If the patient is going to be transferred, the accepting burn unit should be contacted for specific instructions regarding burn care. Do not delay transfer for debridement of the wound. The transferring facility should utilize the regional burn center's treatment protocol.

Patients with circumferential deep burns of the limbs may develop compromise of the distal circulation. Distal pulses need to be monitored closely; a Doppler flow probe may be very helpful. If there is compromise to the circulation, escharotomy will be needed. The eschar needs to be incised on the midlateral side of the limb, allowing the fat to bulge through. This may be extended to the hand and fingers (Fig. 194-3). Escharotomy may provoke substantial soft tissue bleeding, often calling for electrocautery.

If there are circumferential burns of the chest and neck, the eschar may cause mechanical restriction to ventilation. An escharotomy of the chest wall needs to be done to allow adequate ventilation. Incisions need to be made at the anterior axillary line from the level of the second rib to the level of the twelfth rib. These two incisions should be joined transversely so that the chest wall can expand (Fig. 194-4).

Pain Control

All burns are painful and superficial partial-thickness burns are most painful. Burn injury not only makes an injured area and surrounding

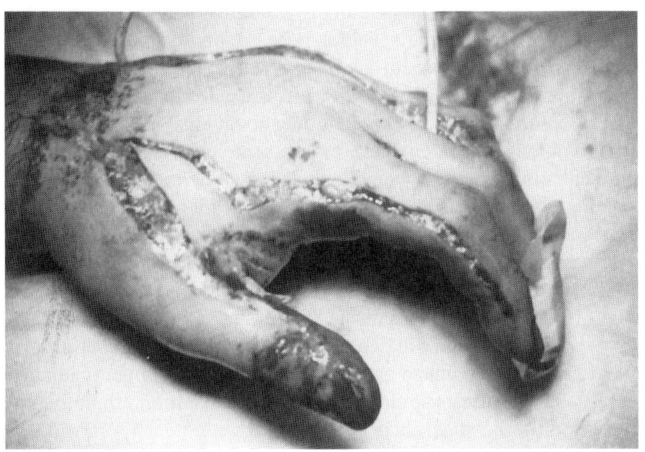

FIG. 194-3. Escharotomy of the hand.

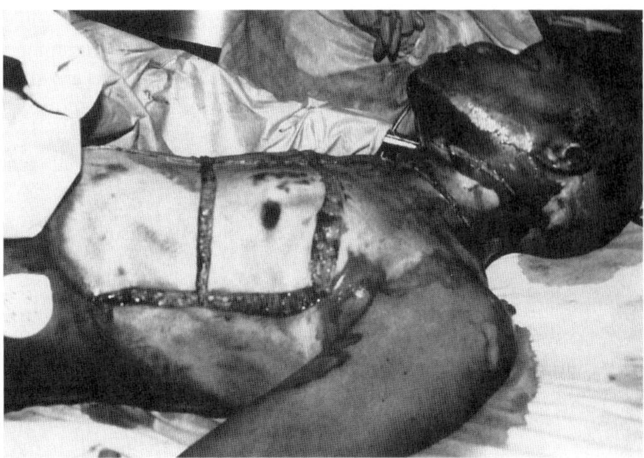

FIG. 194-4. Escharotomy of the chest wall.

tissue more painful but also causes hyperalgesia, chiefly due to the A fibers. Pain management should not be neglected.

During the emergency phase, the preferred route for most medication is intravenous, because of the potential problems with absorption from the muscle and gastrointestinal tract related to decreased perfusion. Morphine is the most widely used drug for relief of pain, and relatively large doses may be required. Anxiolytic agents should be used as adjuvants in pain management.

During the acute phase and for ambulatory patients treated in the ED, narcotic analgesics are required for procedural pain. Oral analgesics like codeine, hydrocodone, oxycodone, or nonsteroidal anti-inflammatory drugs may be used for the background pain.

CARE OF MINOR BURNS IN THE EMERGENCY DEPARTMENT

The American Burn Association has defined minor burns that can be treated on an outpatient basis.[7] To qualify as a minor burn, the injury should be isolated and not involve hands, face, feet, or perineum. The burn should not cross major joints or be circumferential. In treating a minor burn, the patient's social and medical situation should be considered. An elderly patient or one with medical problems is best treated as an inpatient even though the burn involves less than 10 percent of the BSA. The patient's reliability should be considered as an important factor for outpatient treatment. Care of minor burns requires coordination between the ED and the referral specialist who will see the patient in follow-up.[14]

As burns are painful, appropriate analgesia is required. After appropriate analgesia, the burn wound is cleaned with mild soap and water or dilute antiseptic solution. Blisters may be left intact or drained, or the overlying epithelium may be debrided; the decision depends on size and location. Large blisters or those over very mobile joints should be debrided. Small blisters on nonmobile areas should be left intact. Where compliance is questionable, patients should have the blisters debrided, because an intact or spontaneously collapsed blister may serve as a nidus for wound infection. The patient's tetanus immunization status should be assessed and tetanus toxoid and/or immunoglobulin should be administered as needed.

Topical antimicrobials have an important role in reducing bacterial colonization and enhancing the rate of healing in burns.[3,15] A wide variety of topical agents are commonly used for minor burns. The most common is 1% silver sulfadiazine because it is easy to apply and has relatively little toxicity. The usual practice is to apply a thin layer of silver sulfadiazine cream to the burn and then cover it with gauze dressing. Silver sulfadiazine should not be used in patients with sulfa allergy or on the face because of potential staining. Alternative topical agents to use in these circumstances are bacitracin or triple-antibiotic (neomycin, polymixin B, and bacitracin zinc) ointments. Although 11.1% mefanide acetate and 2% furacin ointments are available for topical use, these should be used with caution if applied to large burns in an outpatient setting. Mafenide is a carbonic anhydrase inhibitor and can cause metabolic acidosis. Furacin is in a polyethylene glycol vehicle which can be toxic if absorbed in patients with compromised renal function. Mafenide penetrates the eschar well and has utility in treating patients with invasive infections. Dressings are ideally changed twice daily as long as the wounds continue to weep; then they are changed daily until the burn is healed.

Synthetic occlusive dressing is an alternative method of managing partial-thickness burns in outpatients. The wounds are cleansed and debrided prior to application of these dressings (e.g., Biobrane, Dow Hickan Pharmaceuticals; Tegaderm, 3M Health Care). This method is most successful for clean burns on flat surfaces. The goal is to have the dressing adherent to the wound so that it acts as artificial skin. Adherence is important, as most of the bacteria causing infection produce fibrinolytic agents. Wounds are checked at 24 to 48 h for adherence and the dressing is left in place until spontaneous separation occurs.

Patients must be given discharge instructions that explain home burn care and symptoms and signs of infection. The patient should be advised to return to the ED immediately if there are any signs or symptoms of infection. Extremity burns should be elevated for 24 to 48 h to prevent edema. All burn wounds should be reassessed at 24 h for depth and extent of burn. The follow-up visit schedule should be clearly explained and analgesics prescribed. Deep partial-thickness, full-thickness, and mixed-thickness burns should be referred to a plastic surgeon or burn-care specialist in 2 to 4 days for reevaluation and consideration of skin grafting.

REFERENCES

1. Brigham PA, McLoughlin E: Burn incidence and medical care use in the United States: Estimate, trends, and data sources. *J Burn Care Rehabil* 17:95, 1996.
2. Ryan CM, Schoenfeld DA, Thorpe WP, et al: Objective estimates of the probability of death from burn injuries. *N Engl J Med* 338:362, 1998.
3. Manafo W: Initial management of burns. *N Engl J Med* 335:1581, 1996.
4. Saffle JR, Davis B, Williams P, American Burn Association Registry Participant Group: Recent outcomes in the treatment of burn injury in the United States: A report from the American Burn Association Patient Registry. *J Burn Care Rehabil* 16:219, 1995.
5. Arturson G: Pathophysiology of the burn wound and pharmacological treatment: The Rudi Hermans Lecture. *Burns* 22:255, 1996.
6. Baxter CR, Shires T: Physiological response to crystalloid resuscitation of severe burns. *Ann NY Acad Sci* 150:874, 1968.
7. American Burn Association: *Guidelines for Service Standards and Severity Classification in the Treatment of Burn Injury.* Chicago, American Burn Association, 1984.
8. Miller SF, Finley RK, Waltman M, Lincks J: Burn size estimate reliability: A study. *J Burn Care Rehabil* 12:546, 1991.
9. Hendricks WM: The classification of burns. *J Am Acad Dermatol.* 22:838, 1998.
10. American Burn Association: Hospital and prehospital resources for optimal care of patients with burn injury: Guidelines for development and operation of burn centers. *J Burn Care Rehab* 11:98, 1990.
11. Harrigan R: Smoke inhalation and fire toxicology. *Emerg Med Rep* 15:203, 1994.
12. Gore DC, Dalton JM, Gehr TW: Colloid infusions reduce glomerular filtration in resuscitated burn victims. *J Trauma* 40:356, 1996.
13. Huang PP, Stucky FS, Dimick AR, et al: Hypertonic sodium resuscitation is associated with renal failure and death. *Ann Surg* 221:543, 1995.
14. Smith S, Duncan M, Mobley J, et al: Emergency room management of minor burn injuries: A quality management evaluation. *J Burn Care Rehabil* 18:76, 1997.
15. Nguyen TT, Gilpin DA, Meyer NA, Herndon DN: Current treatment of severely burned patients. *Ann Surg* 223:14, 1996.

CHEMICAL BURNS

Fred P. Harchelroad, Jr.
J. Michael Ballester

Chemical burns occur in the home, industrial, agriculture, and military settings, school and research laboratories, and as a result of civilian assaults, hobby accidents, and other accidents. Chemical burns also occur as a result of innocent application of products for medical purposes and for hair, skin, and nail care.

More than 25,000 products are capable of producing chemical burns. Both occupational exposure and contact with numerous chemicals during daily life contribute to the large number of chemical injuries to the skin. There are no good epidemiologic data on the incidence of toxic cutaneous exposure in the nonoccupational setting. However, about 40 percent of all occupationally related diseases reported concern the skin, and about 25 percent of these are due to chemical burns.

Common household chemical burns are caused by lye (drain cleaners, paint removers, urine sugar reagent test tablets), phenols (deodorizers, sanitizers, disinfectants), sodium hypochlorite (disinfectants, bleaches), methacrylic acid (artificial nail products), and sulfuric acid (toilet bowl cleaners). In industries, chemicals are used for cleaning, tanning, curing, extracting, preserving, soldering, and other functions. The most commonly used industrial acids are tungstic, picric, sulfosalicylic, tannic, formic, sulfuric, acetic, cresylic, trichloroacetic, chromic, hydrochloric, and hydrofluoric. Widely used alkalis are the hydroxide salts of sodium, potassium, ammonium, lithium, barium, and calcium. White phosphorus used in munitions was the most common cause of chemical burns to military personnel during times of armed conflict in the 1960s. White phosphorus is also found in rodenticides, pesticides, and fireworks.

The body sites most often burned by chemicals are the face, eyes, and extremities. Fewer than 5 percent of patients admitted to major burn centers suffer from chemical burns. In general, chemical burn average sizes are small, and the mortality rate is lower than for thermal burns, but wound healing and hospital stay times are higher.

PATHOPHYSIOLOGY

The skin interfaces with the external environment and constitutes a barrier and transition zone between the internal and external milieus. The outer stratum corneum layer of the skin functions as an excellent barrier against certain chemical agents, whereas others may penetrate readily. The skin contains three main layers: an outer layer of epithelial tissue (epidermis), a loose connective tissue layer (dermis), and a variable-thickness inner layer containing adipose and connective tissue (hypodermis or panniculus adiposus).

Chemicals can produce burns, dermatitis, allergic reaction, thermal injury, or systemic toxicity. Pathophysiologically, burns produced by all chemicals are similar.[1] The skin has a limited variety of toxic responses, corresponding to the major patterns of possible structural or functional changes. Toxic reactions are described mainly on the basis of morphologic rather than functional responses.[2] There are morphologic, physiologic, and biochemical protective mechanisms and elements in the skin which include the epidermal barrier, eccrine sweating, phagocytic cells, metabolic detoxification, immunologic processes, and melanin pigmentation. However, these vary on a phenotypic basis and may be affected by systemic or local disease.

Skin damage by chemicals may demonstrate the classic manifestations of thermal injury (erythema, blistering, or full-thickness loss); however, an acute injury may be deceptively mild, only to be followed by extensive skin damage and systemic toxicity. A superficial (first-degree) burn causes capillary and arterial dilatation. Initially, this involves only the superficial vessels, but then extends to the deeper subcutaneous vessels by both direct and reflex action. Tissue hyperemia and congestion results in symptoms of itching, burning, or pain.

More extensive inflammatory reactions result in an outpouring of fluid into the extracellular space, causing edema and vesicle or bulla formation characteristic of partial-thickness (second-degree) burns. Continued chemical damage through the dermis or into the hypodermis results in a full-thickness (third-degree) burn. Tissue damage is determined by

- Strength/concentration of the agent
- Manner of contact
- Quantity of agent
- Duration of contact
- Mechanism of action
- Extent of penetration

Factors enhancing percutaneous absorption of chemical are body site (areas of thin skin, i.e., genitalia, face; chemical contact between skinfolds; amount of surface area exposed); integrity of skin (traumatized skin, elderly skin, decreased lipid, dehydration, inflammation); nature of the chemical (lipid solubility, pH, concentration); and occlusion (garments, occlusive dressings).

The majority of chemical burns are caused by acids or alkalis. At similar volumes and manner of contact, alkalis usually produce far more tissue damage than acids. Acids in general cause coagulation necrosis with protein precipitation. Tough leathery eschar may form with development of underlying ulcers. The eschar limits spread of the agent. Heat may be released during reaction of acid with skin. Alkalis produce liquefaction necrosis with loosening of material that allows deeper penetration of the unattached chemical into tissue. Not all chemicals causing burns can be considered acid or alkali. A useful classification by Jelenko groups chemicals by the manner in which they damage protein:[3]

1. Oxidizing agents: Damage is produced when a chemical becomes oxidized in contact with tissue. Often a toxic moiety is released during this reaction.
2. Corrosives: Extensive protein denaturation is produced, resulting in soft eschar and shallow, indolent ulcers.
3. Reducing agents: Protein denaturation is produced by binding of free electrons in tissue protein.
4. Desiccants: Severe cellular dehydration is produced, and thermal injury occurs due to exothermic reaction.
5. Vesicant: Blisters are produced, tissue amines are liberated, local ischemia and anoxic tissue damage and pandermic inflammation occurs.
6. Protoplasmic poisons: Protein is denatured by salt formation or by metabolic competition/inhibition (i.e., binding calcium or other inorganic ions necessary for tissue viability and function).

GENERAL APPROACH

The goal of treatment is to minimize any area of irreversible injury and maximize salvage of the zone of reversible damage. With few exceptions, hydrotherapy is the cornerstone of initial treatment for chemical burns. Chemical agents may continue to damage tissue until they are removed or inactivated. The first priority is to stop the burning process. Immediate removal from the offending chemical, removal of garments, and counteraction of the chemical remaining on the body by dilution, debridement, or neutralization are important measures. Dry chemical particles such as lime should be brushed away before irrigation. Initially sodium metal and related compounds should be covered with mineral oil or excised, since water can cause a severe exothermic reaction. Dilution of phenol (carbolic acid) with water may enhance penetration. For the most part, however, use of water or saline to irrigate a chemical burn should not be delayed while searching for a neutralizing agent and should begin at the scene of the accident. In general, the earlier the irrigation, the better is the prognosis.

The amount of elapsed time to initiate dilution or removal of chemical agents relates to the depth and degree of injury. Wounds irrigated 3 min after contact with some chemicals have a twofold greater chance of becoming full-thickness burns than wounds irrigated within 1 min of chemical contact. When using agents to neutralize a chemical burn, additional tissue injury may occur through heat production. In some cases, heat of dilution may be produced using water irrigation, but copious amounts will decrease the rate and amount of chemical reaction and dissipate the heat. Irrigation should be maintained at a gentle flow to avoid driving the chemical deeper into tissue or splashing chemical into the victim's or rescuer's eyes. The time required for irrigation varies; irrigation may need to be continued for hours in the case of alkali burns. Use of pH litmus paper may help determine continued presence of alkali or acid in burn wounds. A more accurate pH result will be obtained if the test is performed 10 to 15 min after completion of irrigation. This will allow residual chemical in the deeper areas to diffuse to the surface.

After irrigation and debridement of remaining particles and devitalized tissue, topical antimicrobial agents should be used and tetanus immunization should be updated as needed. Other than measures specific for a particular chemical burn, treatment following initial therapy is basically the same as for thermal burns. Patients sustaining chemical burns require the same aggressive fluid replacement as those with thermal burns. Analgesics may be needed, and, in the case of allergic responses to chemicals, antihistamines, steroids, and epinephrine may be required. Hemodialysis may be required in cases of severe systemic toxicity and renal failure. Autografts, heterografts, homografts, or synthetic material may be necessary for full-thickness burns. Hyperbaric oxygen may be utilized to assist healing of resistant burn wounds.

SPECIFIC CHEMICALS

Acids

With the exception of hydrofluoric acid, strong acids produce coagulation necrosis from the desiccating action of the acid on proteins in the superficial tissue. Injury severity is related to the physical characteristics of the acid. Most substances with a pH less than 2 are strong corrosives. Other important tissue-damaging properties of acids include concentration, molarity, and complexing affinity for hydroxy ions. The higher each of these factors is, the greater is the tissue damage. Contact time with the skin is the most important chemical burn feature that health care professionals may alter. Instantaneous skin decontamination of 18 *M* sulfuric acid will cause no burn; however, a 1-min exposure can cause full-thickness skin damage. Examination of a patient with a significant chemical burn from these acids should not be limited to observation of the skin, because several of these acids are respiratory and mucous membrane irritants as well. Furthermore, skin absorption of some compounds may occur and result in systemic signs and symptoms. The most commonly used chemicals that cause burns are listed in Table 195-1.

ACETIC ACID The dilute (<40%) acetic acid solution found in hair-wave neutralizer solutions is perhaps the most common cause of chemical burns to the scalp in women. Prolonged contact, especially with an already damaged scalp, may cause a partial-thickness burn that heals slowly because of the constant bacterial flora on the hair. Initial treatment is copious water irrigation. As trimming the hair is not a viable option in these patients, oral antibiotics are often given if the entire scalp is involved.

PHENOL Phenol (carbolic acid), a corrosive organic acid used widely in industry and medicine, denatures proteins and causes chemical burns characterized by a white or brown coagulum that is relatively painless. Systemic absorption may result in life-threatening complications. Its unpleasant, acrid odor, detectable in air at 0.047 parts per million, and its low volatility help prevent airborne exposure. Though

TABLE 195-1 Chemicals That Cause Burns

Agent	Use	Initial Treatment
Acetic acid	Permanent-wave neutralizers, printing, dyeing, hatmaking	Water irrigation
Alkyl mercury compounds	Disinfectants, fungicides, wood preservatives	Water irrigation and prompt removal of blister fluid and overlying skin to prevent intoxication
Cantharides ("Spanish fly")	Veterinary aphrodisiac	Water irrigation
Chromic acid	Microelectronics/microinstruments, photography, metal cleaning and plating, leather tanning, cement manufacture	Water irrigation
Cresol (Lysol)	Disinfectant	Water irrigation
Creosote	Fungicides, wood preservative	Water irrigation
Cresylic acid	Industry	Water irrigation
Dimethyl sulfoxide (DMSO)	Topical treatment for sprains, arthritis	Water irrigation
Diquat dibromide	Herbicides	Water irrigation
Formic acid	Acrylate-glue making	Water irrigation
Hydrocarbons	Industry, commerce, paint removers	Water irrigation
Hydrochloric acid (muriatic acid)	Bleaching agents, metal cleaning, chemistry laboratories, fireproofing material, semiconductor industry	Water irrigation
Hydrofluoric acid	Microelectronics/microinstruments, petroleum refining, glass etching/frosting, metal etching, rust removal, dyes, plastics, germicides, leather tanning	Water irrigation Calcium gluconate
Lime	Agriculture, cement	Brush off, water irrigation
Lyes (alkalis) KOH, NaOH, NH_4OH, LiOH, $Ba(OH)_2$, $Ca(OH)_2$	Industrial cleansers, washing powders, drain cleaners, paint removers, urine sugar reagent tablets, portland cement	Water irrigation
Metals	Industry	Cover with mineral oil, excision
Mustard gas	Chemical warfare	Water irrigation/mineral oil/adsorbent powders/M258A1 kit
Nitric acid	Electroplating, engraving, fertilizer manufacturing, casting iron/steel	Water irrigation
Oxalic acid	Leather tanning, blueprint paper	Water irrigation, IV calcium gluconate
Phenols (carbolic acid)	Dyes, deodorizers, sanitizers, disinfectants, cosmetics, plastics manufacture, agriculture	Water irrigation, PEG-IMS or glycerol, or isopropyl alcohol
Phosphoric acid	Metal cleaning, disinfectants, rustproofing	Water irrigation
Picric acid	Industry	Water irrigation
Potassium permanganate	Disinfectants, bleach, deodorizers, medical	Water irrigation
Sodium hypochlorite (Clorox)	Cleanser	Water irrigation
Sulfosalicylic acid	Industry	Water irrigation
Sulfuric acid	Casting iron/steel, chemistry laboratories	Water irrigation
Tannic acid	Industry	Water irrigation
Trichloroacetic acid	Industry	Water irrigation
Tungstic acid	Industry	Water irrigation
White phosphorus	Warfare incendiary, insecticides, rodent poison, fertilizers	Water irrigation, 1% copper sulfate irrigation

Source: From Jelenko C: Chemicals that "burn." *J Trauma* 14:65, 1974, with permission.

commercially available in concentrations of 1 to 90%, even dilute solutions of 1 to 2% phenol may cause a burn if contact is prolonged. Hexylresorcinol is a bactericidal phenol derivative. Chemically related phenolic compounds that induce skin damage include cresol, creosote, and cresylic acid.

Coagulation necrosis of the involved area is common. Necrotic tissue may delay absorption temporarily, but phenol may become entrapped under the eschar. Contaminated clothing should be removed and water lavage begun immediately. Water lavage alone may be ineffective, presumably because the necrotic coagulum inhibits water penetration to the deeper layers. Paradoxically, dilute phenol penetrates tissue more readily than when concentrated.

More effective decontamination has been demonstrated with a 5- to 10-min swab with a combination of polyethylene glycol 300 (PEG 300) and industrial methylated spirits (IMS) in a 2:1 mixture. This should not only reduce the extent of cutaneous corrosion but also decrease systemic toxicity. The PEG 300 is mixed with the IMS for a more liquid (and therefore easier to use) formulation. However, the viscous PEG 300 or PEG 400 may be used alone, and, indeed, glycerol is an acceptable substitute if the PEG-IMS mixture is not available. The use of an isopropyl alcohol rinse appears to be equal to PEG-IMS in removing phenol.[4] The advantage of isopropyl alcohol is its easy availability.

CHROMIC ACID The toxicity of chromium compounds is related to the powerful oxidizing action of the hexavalent compounds (Cr^{6+}). The chromate ion in chromic acid will produce a chronic penetrating ulcerating lesion of the skin. Associated signs and symptoms are conjunctivitis, lacrimation, ulceration of the nasal septum, and systemic chromium toxicity. A 10-percent total body surface area cutaneous burn caused by chromic acid can be fatal due to systemic toxicity. Any acute skin exposure to chromic acid should be treated with copious water irrigation and observation for systemic effects.

FORMIC ACID Formic acid in 60% solution is used by acrylate-glue makers, cellulose formate workers, and tanning workers. Formic acid produces coagulation necrosis of the skin. Systemic effects including decreased respirations and an anion-gap metabolic acidosis have been reported.[5] Treatment includes immediate decontamination and irrigation with water. Open lesions should be treated like any damaged skin: with debridement of devitalized tissue, prevention of further damage and infection, and skin grafting if the defect is full thickness and of a size requiring closure.

HYDROCHLORIC AND SULFURIC ACIDS The dermal toxicity of hydrochloric acid and sulfuric acid is so well recognized that early decontamination and water irrigation usually prevent severe burns to the skin. These acids can burn the skin dark brown or black. Toilet bowl cleaners may contain 80% solutions of sulfuric acid. Some drain cleaners may be 95 to 99% sulfuric acid solutions. Munitions, chemical, and fertilizer manufacturers commonly use 95 to 98% sulfuric acid solutions in their industrial processes. Automobile battery fluid is 25% sulfuric acid. Most household bleaches are only 3 to 6% hypochlorite solutions, which, though acidic, cause little damage unless they are in contact with skin for a prolonged time. Treatment is the same as for formic acid burns.

HYDROFLUORIC ACID Hydrofluoric acid (HF) is unique among the corrosives in its mechanism of action and degree of toxicity. HF acts like alkalis and will cause progressive tissue loss, including bony destruction. HF, considered a protoplasmic poison, penetrates the skin, dissociates, and releases fluoride ions. Fluoride ions immobilize intracellular calcium and magnesium and poison cellular enzymatic reactions. Potassium permeability is increased and results in spontaneous depolarization of nerve tissue and pain.

Industrial applications include use in production of high-octane fuel, etching and frosting glass, semiconductors, microelectronics/microinstruments, germicides, dyes, plastics, tanning, and fireproofing material and use in cleaning stone and brick buildings. It is also a very effective rust remover.

HF rapidly penetrates the skin and causes both local and systemic toxicity. Its systemic effects include hypocalcemia, hypomagnesemia, and hyperkalemia. The dermal effects may not be immediately noted and appear to be more related to the concentration of HF than to the duration of exposure. Solutions greater than 50% produce immediate pain and tissue destruction; solutions less than 20% may not produce signs and symptoms until 12 to 24 h after exposure. The skin may develop a blue-gray appearance with a surrounding region of erythema.

Unlike the treatment of dermal injury caused by other acids, the treatment of HF burns consists of two phases. The first, which should be immediate, is copious water irrigation of the affected skin for 15 to 30 min. This may be the only treatment that is needed if the HF solution is less than 20% concentrated, the duration of exposure was very brief, and decontamination is begun immediately. Unfortunately, this is rarely the case. Severe, persistent pain denotes a more serious injury requiring the second phase of treatment.

The second phase of treatment is aimed at detoxifying the enzyme-poisoning fluoride ion. Two ions—calcium (Ca^{2+}) and magnesium (Mg^{2+})—have been shown to be beneficial in binding the fluoride and curtailing its toxic effects. However, the overwhelming clinical experience to date has been with the use of calcium gluconate, and it should be considered the agent of choice at present. Several therapeutic modalities are available for using calcium gluconate: topical, subcutaneous/intradermal injection, or intraarterial infusion. An intravenous regional perfusion technique based on Bier's method has been described and reported effective.[6] High-dose intravenous magnesium sulfate appears to be effective in animal models, but human data are lacking.[7]

A calcium gluconate gel made of either Surgilube (E. Fougera & Co.) or dimethyl sulfoxide (DMSO) in a 2.5 to 10% concentration may be applied directly to the affected area.[8] The main limitation of topical therapy is the impermeability of the skin to calcium. Penetration into the dermis and subcutaneous tissues may be enhanced if the formulation with DMSO is used. The topical therapy can be used in the outpatient setting, and industries utilizing HF should keep this topical formulation on hand for emergency use.

Subcutaneous and intradermal injection of a 5 to 10% calcium gluconate solution through a 30-gauge needle into the HF-burned skin is the most widely used treatment. A maximum dose of 0.5 mL of 10% calcium gluconate per square centimeter of burned skin is recommended. Pain relief is nearly immediate, and indeed, the elimination of pain may be used as a guide for further therapy. Recurrence of pain indicates the need for further therapy. Unfortunately, injection therapy has several disadvantages: (1) only limited amounts of calcium are delivered to the tissue; (2) hyperosmolarity and inherent toxicity of free calcium ions cause more pain initially, and more tissue damage is possible if calcium is not bound to fluoride; (3) vascular compromise can result if too much fluid is injected, especially into digits; and (4) rapid penetration of HF beneath the nail requires nail removal to administer the calcium gluconate into the nailbed adequately.

Intraarterial infusion of calcium gluconate may be used to prevent tissue necrosis and stop the pain associated with HF burns. This should be performed as soon as possible after the initial burn, preferably within 6 h of insult. An intraarterial catheter should be placed in the appropriate vascular supply (the brachial artery if the entire hand is affected) and connected to a three-way stopcock to which is attached an arterial pressure-monitoring device and the infusion syringe of calcium gluconate. A 50-mL syringe may be filled with 10 mL of a 10% calcium gluconate solution and 40 mL of 5% dextrose. This should be infused over 2 to 4 h. The arterial pressure-monitoring device ensures that the catheter has not dislodged from the lumen of the cannulated artery. Infusion of the calcium solution into the deep tissues may cause further tissue damage. Repeat infusion may be needed if pain recurs within 4 h. This intraarterial infusion avoids the disadvantages of local infiltration therapy; however, it has its own disadvantages: an invasive vascular procedure (1) may result in arterial spasm or thrombosis and (2) requires more time and resources, including hospital admission.

Nebulized calcium gluconate is a recognized treatment for inhalational exposures to HF. Ocular exposure to HF requires water irrigation for at least 30 min. Treatment with calcium chloride or magnesium chloride by subconjunctival injection or irrigation may increase corneal damage. There is a reported case, however, of complete and quick recovery by utilizing 1% calcium carbonate eyedrops in a patient who had sustained a large corneal erosion due to a 49% HF burn.

Systemic toxicity related to dermal HF exposure has resulted in death. This appears to be related to myocardial irritability and subsequent ventricular fibrillation as a result of systemic acidosis, hyperkalemia, hypomagnesemia, and hypocalcemia. Cardiac monitoring, intravenous access, and electrolyte monitoring should be performed in cases of all significant HF dermal burns.

NITRIC ACID Nitric acid is used in industry for casting iron and steel, electroplating, engraving, and fertilizer manufacturing. Upon contact with skin, nitric acid can produce tissue damage by oxidation and may turn the skin yellowish as it is burned.

OXALIC ACID Oxalic acid is used for leather tanning and blueprint paper. Like hydrofluoric acid, it poisons enzymatic processes. Oxalic acid binds calcium and prevents muscle contraction. The burn wounds should be irrigated with water, intravenous calcium may be required. Serum electrolytes and renal function should be checked, and cardiac monitoring should be performed after serious dermal exposure.

METHACRYLIC ACID Methacrylic acid found in many artificial nail cosmetic products can produce severe dermal burns, usually in preschoolers.[9]

Alkalis

Alkalis penetrate skin much more deeply and longer than acids, causing liquefaction necrosis of tissue, with danger of toxicity from systemic absorption. Wounds may look superficial and in 2 to 3 days become full-thickness burns. Alkalis combine with protein and lipids in tissue to form soluble protein complexes and soaps that permit passage of hydroxyl ions deep into tissue. Soft, gelatinous, friable, brownish eschars are often produced. Strong alkalis have a pH $\geq$12.

LYES Strong, corrosive alkalis (''lyes'') include ammonium, barium, calcium, lithium, potassium (caustic potash), and sodium (caustic soda) hydroxides. Lyes are widely used in industry and found in home products (drain and toilet cleaners, washing powders, and paint removers). The urine sugar reagent tablet Clinitest (Bayer) contains anhydrous sodium hydroxide. As a mode of assault, lyes have a lower mortality rate than gunshot wounds or stabbings, but victims often suffer long-term pain, scarring, and blindness.[10] Lyes are extremely corrosive and penetrating, and burns require copious irrigation for long periods. Suicidal ingestion of lye requires aggressive airway management. Early death results from upper airway occlusion. Late morbidity related to esophageal and gastric necrosis may be minimized by early surgical intervention with esophagogastrectomy.

LIME Lime (calcium oxide) is found in agriculture products and cements. It is converted by water to the alkali calcium hydroxide. Contact with lime draws water out of the skin. All dry particles should be brushed away prior to irrigation. Paradoxically, a small amount of water may generate an exothermic reaction with tissue injury secondary to calcium hydroxide formation. A large amount and strong stream of water (taking care to avoid splashing in eyes) should be used and will permit dissipation of heat. There is considerable variability of lime content in different grades of cement, with fine to textured masonry cement having more than concrete.

PORTLAND CEMENT Portland cement, which accounts for a major proportion of the cement used in the United States, is a mixture of sand, lime, and other metal oxides. In the presence of water, calcium hydroxide, sodium hydroxide, and potassium hydroxide may all be formed. Workers who kneel in wet cement or get cement in their boots may discover burns hours after initial contact. In addition, skin may become irritated from gritty material, and a contact dermatitis may develop in individuals sensitive to the chromate contained in the material.

Metals

Foundry workers are sometimes burned by molten metal, which may spill or splash on body parts and run down into the boots. Elemental metals, sodium, lithium, potassium, magnesium, aluminum, and calcium may all cause burns. When exposed to air, some elemental metals spontaneously ignite. Water is generally contraindicated in extinguishing burning metal fragments embedded in the skin, because the explosive exothermic reaction that may result can lead to significant tissue injury. Burning metal may be extinguished with a class D fire extinguisher or smothered with sand. Covering metal fragments with mineral oil, however, appears to be the favored treatment method. Wound debridement should include excision of metal fragments that cannot be wiped away. Metal fragments should be placed in mineral oil to prevent further accidents.

Others

HYDROCARBONS Hydrocarbons will cause a fat-dissolving corrosive injury to the skin. In our present petroleum-dependent society, gasoline is a common agent of burns. Patients sustaining gasoline immersion burns usually have undergone some other traumatic insult (e.g., a motor vehicle accident). Gasoline is a complex mixture of alkanes, cycloalkanes, and aromatic hydrocarbons. A hydrocarbon chemical burn resembles either a thermal scald or a partial-thickness burn.[11] Full-thickness burns secondary to prolonged contact with gasoline have been reported. Topical gasoline exposure in cold weather can result in frostbite of the digits due to rapid evaporation of gasoline resulting in heat loss from the skin. Any potential for systemic effects of the involved hydrocarbon (or what it was a solvent for) must be recognized, as this may expose the patient to greater morbidity than the skin damage. Dehydration of the skin associated with solvent contact contributes to injury. Treatment involves decontamination; otherwise, management is as for a thermal burn.

Hot tar is derived from long-chain petroleum and coal hydrocarbons. Roofing tars and asphalt are heated to temperatures in excess of 500°F (260°C) and the burns sustained are usually thought of more as thermal than chemical. Liquefaction injury to tissue can occur. Though the surface area size of the burn is usually small, solidified material stuck to skin and hair is hard to remove. The tar should be cooled to prevent continued thermal injury. Manual mechanical debridement can be painful and destructive to skin structures. Polyoxylene sorbitan (polysorbate) contained in Neosporin is an emulsifying agent that can be used to remove tar. De-solv-it, a citrus and petroleum distillate, is also reported effective in tar removal. Mayonnaise has been reported as a home remedy used topically in a similar fashion.

DMSO, CANTHARIDES, AND MUSTARD GAS DMSO, cantharides, and mustard gas are considered to be vesicant agents. Skin burns with edema and blister formation can occur due to production of ischemia and anoxic necrosis at the site of contact. DMSO is a water-soluble organic solvent that has been used industrially since the 1940s.

General therapeutic interest in DMSO began in the 1960s, when it was used topically by thousands of patients for sprains, bruises, minor burns, and arthritis. Its use has declined substantially because of eye toxicity, although it is still used for research and some clinical problems. Cantharides (''Spanish fly'') is used as a veterinary aphrodisiac and occasionally by human beings as well for its supposed aphrodisiac effects. Mustard gas is a war gas that is unlikely to be seen in civilian practice. Historically, the most important of these agents, and still used in battle most often, is sulfur mustard.[12] Burns resulting from vesicants should be irrigated copiously with water or saline. Skin can be decontaminated by using adsorbent powders (flour, talcum powder, Fuller's earth) if the supply of water is limited. The powder adsorbs the mustard from the skin and should be wiped away with a moist towel. The military uses M258A1 kits for skin decontamination. These kits contain three sets of towelettes, one for each containing phenol, hydroxide, and chloramine. Chloramine produces ''free'' chlorine, which inactivates sulfur mustard. Mineral oil is also recommended for treatment of mustard gas burns.

POTASSIUM PERMANGANATE Potassium permanganate is an oxidizing agent that is mildly irritating in dilute solution but in concentrated solution can produce dermal burns with a thick, brownish purple eschar of coagulated protein. Burns should be copiously irrigated.

ALKYL MERCURY COMPOUNDS Alkyl mercury compounds, which are reducing agents used in disinfectants, fungicides, and wood preservatives, can produce dermatitis or burn lesions. Lesions typically are erythematous with blister formation. The blister fluid is high in metallic mercury content. The burning process continues as long as the agent remains in contact with skin. Partial-thickness burns deepen if the blister fluid is allowed to remain. The treatment is to debride, remove blister fluid, and irrigate copiously.

DIQUAT DIBROMIDE Full-thickness skin burns have been reported to occur after prolonged exposure to the herbicide diquat dibromide. These burns were treated with skin grafting. It is unknown whether earlier therapy would have prevented the chain of events.

LACRIMATORS (CHLOROACETOPHENONE, CHLOROBENZYLIDENEMALONITRILE, AND DIBENZOXAPINE) Lacrimators (tear gas) such as chloroacetophenone (CN), chlorobenzylidenemalonitrile (CS) and dibenzoxazepine (CR) cause skin and mucosal irritation and contact dermatitis. The epidermal injury is limited, in contrast to the possible pulmonary parenchymal damage. Burns to the skin are treated with standard water irrigation. Ocular irritation is treated with copious water irrigation, followed by slit-lamp exam for corneal damage. Structural damage to the cornea occurs at high concentrations of these lacrimators. Pepper gas (trichloronitromethane), so named because of its pepper-like odor and propensity to induce sneezing, is used in some areas by law enforcement agencies. As with the other lacrimators, it will cause mucous membrane, occular, and upper airway irritation (as well as bronchospasm in susceptible patients). Treatment is copious irrigation with saline and removal of the patient from the offending agent.

WHITE PHOSPHORUS White phosphorus is a chemical used as an incendiary and in insecticides, rodenticides, and fertilizers. It can ignite spontaneously when exposed to air and is rapidly oxidized to phosphorus pentoxide. White phosphorus is commonly found in hand grenades and other warfare munitions and thus is implicated in wartime and accidental burns to military personnel. In munitions, white phosphorus is solid, but some of it may liquefy with detonation. Burns may be caused by liquid or solid forms. White phosphorus burns may be complicated by multiple traumatic injuries as a result of shell fragments and the force of weapon explosions. Because of its many uses, white phosphorus burns also occur in civilians.

Flaming droplets of inorganic phosphorus may embed beneath the skin. The heat of reaction can be directly destructive to tissue. Particles continue to oxidize slowly until either debrided, neutralized, or completely oxidized. Contaminated clothing should be removed. Debride visible particles and irrigate the burns copiously with normal saline or water. A brief rinse with 1% copper sulfate solution may be helpful. Copper sulfate combines with phosphorus to form a dark-copper phosphide coating on the particles that makes them easier to see and debride and also impedes further oxidation. After copper sulfate use, the burn should be irrigated again to remove copper and prevent systemic copper toxicity. Some investigators have found copper sulfate ineffective in preventing death and also toxic in animal studies.

Airbag Burns

Approximately 8 percent of individuals suffering injuries related to airbag deployment are burned. Airbags deploy by ignition of a solid propellant—sodium azide—that creates an exothermic reaction leading to quick inflation of the airbag. Many other gases are created during activation, including corrosives such as sodium hydroxide, nitric oxide, ammonia, and multiple hydrocarbons. An airbag is deflated within 2 s of inflation through exhaust side ports on the bag. Burns associated with airbags include friction, thermal, and chemical.[13] Sodium hydroxide has been implicated in the chemical keratitis reported after airbag deployment. Sodium azide may cause cutaneous burns in addition to severe systemic effects, but its contribution to airbag chemical burns is limited. Treatment of airbag chemical burns is similar to any alkali burn: immediate and copious water irrigation.

OCULAR BURNS

Chemical burns to the eyes are common and considered true ocular emergencies requiring immediate treatment.[14] Typically, chemical burns to the eye occur in the industrial setting, in laboratories, or as a result of accidents such as battery explosion and intentional assaults. Rupture of automobile airbags with spillage of chemicals onto the face represents a new potential for ocular as well as skin burns. Early signs and symptoms of eye burns include tearing, rubbing, redness, pain, and blepharospasm. Conjunctivas, if severely injured, may appear pale due to ischemia. Swelling of the corneal epithelium, clouding of the anterior chamber, pupillary dilatation, and corneal ulceration may all occur.

If the nature of the chemical is not known, pH paper should be used to determine the presence of acid or alkali. Acid quickly precipitates the superficial tissue proteins of the eye, producing the typical ''ground glass'' appearance of the cornea. Penetration is limited by local buffering and barrier effects of the precipitated proteins. The damage sustained secondary to acid burns in most cases is immediate and limited to the area of contact. The posterior segment of the eye rarely suffers injury, and there are usually no late effects such as cell disruption or tissue softening.

Alkali burns are much more serious, and results are frequently unsightly and disastrous. In general, the higher the pH of the alkali, the more damage occurs. In a short period, strong alkali can penetrate the cornea, anterior chamber, and the retina, with destruction of all sensory elements, thus causing complete blindness. Alkali combines with cellular membrane lipids, resulting in cell disruption and tissue softening. The stromal mucopolysaccharides of the cornea are severely disrupted. The penetration of alkali can continue for hours to days. An opaque, marbled appearance of the cornea and even perforation may occur with deep injury. Conjunctival and scleral blood vessels and collecting veins of the anterior chamber may be destroyed, leading to secondary glaucoma.

Chronic inflammation of the iris and ciliary body (iridocyclitis) and adhesions between lens and iris (posterior synechiae) are complications. Other complications of eye burns include ectropion (lid deformity), cataract formation, scarring and marked revascularization of the cornea, and scarring of both palpebral and bulbar conjunctiva with resulting adhesions between the lids and globe (symblepharon).

Treatment of eye burns should begin immediately, with the rare exception of burns from chemicals that react violently with water. Immediate treatment is copious and continuous irrigation at the scene, in transport, and at the hospital. Time should not be wasted in search for a neutralizing substance. Special eye-irrigating kits may be used, but in general intravenous tubing set up using 1 to 2 L of normal saline for 30-min continuous irrigation is the minimum treatment, particularly for alkali burns.

Acid burns may not require as much volume or treatment time. For treatment of alkali burns, 24 h or more of continuous irrigation has been recommended by some. Checking the pH in the conjunctival sac to see whether it has returned to normal may be helpful in determining need for further irrigation (tears have a pH between 7.3 to 7.7). The eyelid may have to be held open manually or with retractors, due to severe orbicularis spasm. The eyelids should be everted if they are not too edematous. All particulate matter should be removed by using a moistened cotton applicator or forceps.

Pain control with topical anesthetics initially and subsequently; systemic analgesics may be necessary. Cycloplegics, mydriatics, and antibiotics should be used, and the use of an eye patch may encourage corneal reepithelialization. The patient should be hospitalized and ophthalmology consultation obtained for severe burns.

Another treatment modality is the use of collagenase inhibitors such as cysteine and acetylcysteine (Mucomyst) to prevent loss of corneal stroma, which occurs with liberation of collagenase from injured corneal and conjunctival epithelium. Topical steroids may reduce iridocyclitis but may also exacerbate collagenase-induced corneal ulceration. Use of scleral contact lens may reduce adhesions and scarring. Agents to reduce intraocular pressure should be used if glaucoma develops. Paracentesis may be required in severe alkali burns to introduce sterile phosphate buffer solution into the anterior chamber in attempt to reduce the pH of the inner eye. Surgery to the eye is usually not indicated during the early phase of burn management unless for corneal grafting following corneal perforation. Blepharoplasty, keratoplasty, or keratoprosthesis may be eventually required.

IATROGENIC CHEMICAL BURNS

Iatrogenic chemical burns have been caused by the use of potassium permanganate for dermatologic problems at an inappropriately high concentration. DMSO used as a transcutaneous vehicle for minor sprains has caused burns. Patients in the operating room may develop burns from skin-prep solutions. Thimerosal, which has a high mercury content, is the most common agent implicated. Mechanical abrasion of the skin from scrubbing and from pooling of the skin-prep agent under the torso or tourniquet predisposes patients to burns. Blister formation, skin sloughing, and eschar development have been reported in neonates when isopropyl alcohol pledgets were substituted for conducting paste beneath limb electrocardiograph electrodes. Silver nitrate utilized to cauterize umbilical granulomas in infants reportedly has caused periumbilical burns.

SYSTEMIC TOXICITY

Death early after severe chemical burns is usually related to hypotension, acute tubular necrosis, and shock as a result of fluid loss. However, systemic toxicity and subsequent morbidity and mortality may also occur with some chemicals that are absorbed through denuded dermis. Acidosis, hypotension, and shock can occur with significant absorption of acids. Hypocalcemia has been reported with both oxalic acid and hydrofluoric acid burns. Profound hypocalcemia and hypomagnesemia may be accompanied by hyperkalemia, cardiac arrhythmias, and sudden death. Tannic acid, chromic acid, formic acid, picric acid, and phosphorus may cause hepatic necrosis and nephrotoxicity. Cresol can cause methemoglobinemia, massive hemolysis, and multiple organ failure. Gasoline immersion with large surface area exposure and absorption of hydrocarbon aromatic components may result in severe pulmonary, cardiovascular, neurologic, renal, and hepatic complications. The gasoline lead additives such as tetraethyl and tetramethyl can cause lead encephalopathy. Carburetor-cleaning solvent containing phenol and methylene chloride may cause renal and hepatic failure. Phenol (carbolic acid) when absorbed can lead to intravascular hemolysis, cardiovascular, pulmonary, and central nervous system toxicity. The use of phenolkin disinfectant by medical personnel in the 1800s caused chronic toxicity (carbolic marasmus) characterized by weight loss, vertigo, salivation, and increased skin and scleral pigmentation.

Sodium nitrate and potassium nitrate can cause a severe toxic methemoglobinemia from absorption with refractory cyanosis. Significant absorption of dichromate solution can result in liver failure and acute tubular necrosis and death despite hemodialysis.

Just as with thermal burns, overwhelming sepsis can be a systemic complication with chemical burns.

REFERENCES

1. Luterman A, Curreri PW: Chemical burn injury, in Boswick JA (ed): *The Art and Science of Burn Care*. Rockville, MD, Aspen, 1987, pp 233–239.
2. Rice RH, Cohen DE: Toxic responses of the skin, in Klaassen CD, Amdur MO, Doull J (eds): *Cassaret and Doull's Toxicology: The Basic Science of Poisons*. New York, McGraw-Hill, 1996, pp 529–546.
3. Jelenko C: Chemicals that "burn." *J Trauma* 14:65, 1974
4. Hunter DM, Timerding BL, Leonard RB, et al: Effects of isopropyl alcohol, ethanol, and polyethylene glycol/industrial methylated spirits in treatment of acute phenol burns. *Ann Emerg Med* 21:1303, 1992.
5. Chan TC, Williams SR, Clark RF: Formic acid skin burns resulting in systemic toxicity. *Ann Emerg Med* 26:383, 1995.
6. Graudins A, Burns MJ, Aaron CK: Regional intravenous infusion of calcium gluconate for hydrofluoric acid burns of the upper extremity. *Ann Emerg Med* 30:604, 1997.
7. Williams JM, Hammad A, Cottington EC, Harchelroad FP: Intravenous magnesium in the treatment of hydrofluoric acid burns in rats. *Ann Emerg Med* 23:464, 1994.
8. Borkhart KK, Brent J, Kirk MA, et al: Comparison of topical magnesium and calcium treatment for dermal hydrofluoric acid burns. *Ann Emerg Med* 24:9, 1994.
9. Woolf A, Shaw J: Childhood injuries from artificial nail primer cosmetic products. *Arch Pediatr Adolesc Med* 152:41, 1998.
10. Yeong EK, Ming CT, Mann R, et al: Facial mutilation after an assault with chemicals: 15 cases and literature review. *J Burn Care Rehabil* 18:234, 1997.
11. Hansbrough JF, Zapata-Sirvent R, Dominic W, et al: Hydrocarbon contact injuries. *J Trauma* 25:250, 1985.
12. Borak J, Sidell FR: Agents of chemical warfare: Sulfur mustard. *Ann Emerg Med* 21:303, 1992.
13. Hallock GG: Mechanisms of burn injury secondary to airbag deployment. *Ann Plast Surg* 39:111, 1997.
14. Wagoner MD: Chemical injuries of the eye: Current concepts in pathophysiology and therapy. *Surv Ophthalmol* 41:275, 1997.

ELECTRICAL INJURIES

Ann S. Chinnis
Janet M. Williams
Kimberly N. Treat

The spectrum of electrical injuries ranges from local cutaneous burns secondary to household current to severe, deep, and extensive muscle, nerve, and vascular injury or even death from high-voltage sources. The evaluation and treatment of electrical injuries require an understanding of the unique pathophysiology of this type of injury.

TABLE 196-1 Body Tissue Resistance

Most	Bone Fat Tendon
Intermediate	Dry skin
Least	Muscle Blood vessels Nerves

TABLE 196-2 Skin Resistance

Callused skin	1,000,000 ohms
Normal dry skin	40,000 ohms
Sweaty skin	300 ohms
Wet skin (pool or bathtub)	150 ohms

EPIDEMIOLOGY

There are no precise figures on the number of electrical injuries treated in US emergency departments each year, but estimates are as high as 17,000 victims per year who require emergency treatment. Electrocution accounts for 3 to 6 percent of admissions to burn centers and, since an estimated 50,000 patients are admitted to US burn centers each year, about 1500 to 3000 individuals sustain electrical injuries severe enough to require specialized care. Three distinct populations are at highest risk for electrical injury. The first trimodal injury peak occurs in toddlers who sustain electrical injuries from household electrical sockets and cords, accounting for about 20 percent of electrical injuries. The second peak is in adolescents who engage in risky behavior or have motor vehicle collisions involving high-voltage wires, accounting for an estimated 25 percent of electrical injuries. The third peak occurs in those who work with electricity for a living, accounting for about 25 percent of electrical injuries.

Unintentional electrocution caused 560 deaths in the United States in 1995: 144 were related to generating plants and transmission lines, 84 to domestic wiring and appliances, 42 to industrial wiring and machines, and 291 to unspecified electrical events.[1] The annual occupational death rate from electrocution is approximately 1 per 100,000, with utility workers having the highest death rate (10 per 100,000), followed by miners (5.9 per 100,000) and construction workers (2.5 per 100,000).[2] Fatal unintentional household electrocutions are most commonly related to unsafe hair dryer use in bathtubs.

PATHOPHYSIOLOGY

Electrical *current* is the movement of electrical charge from one location to another; this flow is measured as amperes (A) (defined as 1 coulomb per second). Current flows when there is a *potential difference* between two locations; this potential difference is measured as volts (V). The intervening material resists the flow of electrical current; this resistance is measured as ohms. Ohm's law describes the relation between potential difference (V), current (I), and resistance (R) for simple materials: $V = I \times R$.

Materials that allow electrical current to flow easily with low resistance are called *conductors.* Conductors include the metals copper and aluminum and electrolyte solutions such as normal saline. Materials that do not allow electrical current flow are called *insulators.* Most biologic materials conduct electricity to some extent and can be classified as having low, moderate, or high resistance (Table 196-1). Tissues with a high fluid and electrolyte content conduct electricity better than tissues with less fluid and electrolyte content. Bone is the biologic tissue most resistant to the passage of electricity. Skin resistance varies widely (Table 196-2). Moist skin has reduced resistance that, according to Ohm's law, enables more current to flow such that voltages that ordinarily would not cause much damage can now become fatal.

As current flows through a resistor, energy is deposited into the material in the form of heat. The amount energy can be calculated according to Joule's law: energy $= I^2 \times R \times$ time.

High voltage is usually defined in the medical literature as greater than 1000 V. However, there is evidence that the risk for serious and fatal electrical injury increases significantly with voltages above 600 V; therefore, for medical decision making, a value of 600 V is a more appropriate threshold to separate low from high voltage.[3] Interestingly, the National Electric Code defines high voltage as greater than 600 V. Power lines in US residential areas are typically 7620 V that is stepped down by transformers to 220 V as they enter a home (Table 196-3). The voltage in US household circuits is 110 V. Clothes dryers, electric ranges, heavy-duty appliances, and many air conditioners operate on special circuits that carry 220 V. Although high voltage is more dangerous than low voltage, because low voltage is more accessible to the population, 40 to 60 percent of electrical injuries and 50 percent of the deaths are due to low-voltage electricity.

Contact with electrical current causes injury through thermal heating, induced muscle contraction, thermal burns, and blunt trauma (Table 196-4). Direct tissue heating, predicted by Joule's law, has been generally implicated as the direct etiology of tissue damage from electricity, although that concept has been challenged when contact time is brief.[4] Regardless, current intensity is the most critical determinant of tissue damage, but from a practical standpoint, while voltage is frequently known in an electrical exposure, current is not. Thus, voltage is usually used as a proxy for current in predicting the potential damage from an electrical shock.

As high current passes through the body, the tissues through which it passes are heated. This heating produces neural injury, vasospasm, vascular thrombosis, and myonecrosis. Current flow through a body region with a small cross-sectional diameter (e.g., a finger) may result in more tissue destruction than current flow through a body portion with a large cross-sectional diameter (e.g., the thorax).

Contact burns occur at entry and exist points where the victim makes contact with the electrical source. These lesions are typically charred in the center and surrounded by a zone of grayish-white necrosis, with only mild damage in the periphery of these wounds. Extensive contact burns usually indicate severe underlying pathology. However, not all serious injuries display cutaneous injury. A patient with low skin resistance (e.g., sitting in the bathtub) may sustain a low-voltage injury (e.g., radio falls in the bathtub) and not have a contact lesion.

Arc burns cause the most destructive indirect injury. An electrical arc is a spark of high-voltage current through the air between objects

TABLE 196-3 Levels of Electrical Exposure

Long-distance communication lines	24 V
Telephone Lines	65 V
Household circuits and appliances	110 V
Electrical range or dryer	220 V
House power lines	220 V
Subway third rails	600 V
Residential trunk lines	7620 V

TABLE 196-4 Mechanisms of Electrical Injury

Contact burns (entry and exit)
Thermal heating
Flash burns
Arc burns
Ignition and flame thermal burn
Blunt trauma
Prolonged muscular tetany

of differing electrical potential that are not in contact with one another. Usually a typical arc burn is from an electrical source through the air to the patient. Arcs can extend through the air for distances of approximately 25 cm per 100,000 V of potential difference. The temperature of an arc ranges from 500° to 2500°C. The arc may ignite clothes, causing thermal burns. Such high voltages produce falls and tetanic musculoskeletal injuries.

In addition to current flow, other factors affect the injury severity from electrical exposure (Table 196-5). Prolonged contact leads to more severe injury secondary to heat production and the concomitant thermal burn. The type of current, whether alternating or direct, contributes to the duration of the exposure. Electric current can be either continuous in one direction (direct current or DC) or with a periodic reversal of the direction of current flow (alternating current or AC). DC is used in medical devices such as defibrillators and pacemakers. AC is found in electricity supplied to homes and businesses. The frequency of the AC is the time during which the current cycles through both positive and negative voltages. In the United States, most AC (including standard home current) is 60 cycles per second (hertz or Hz). At 60 Hz, household current has the same frequency response as skeletal muscle and can produce tetany beginning at 10 mA (Table 196-6). With muscular tetany in an extremity, the flexors overpower the extensors and the patient is drawn closer to the electrical source. This tetanic phenomenon can cause injuries such as scapular fractures and shoulder dislocations. In contrast, a high-voltage AC or DC injury usually produces a single violent skeletal muscle contraction that tends to throw the victim away from the source.

The pathway that the current takes through the body also determines the nature of injury. Current that traverses the body vertically is more likely to induce cardiac damage or produce respiratory arrest than is current that transverses horizontally.[5]

TABLE 196-5 Factors Associated with Severity of Electrical Injuries

Current intensity (A)
Electrical potential (V)
Type of current (AC or DC)
Tissue resistance (skin and internal)
Duration of contact (instantaneous versus prolonged)
Area of contact (localized versus diffuse)
Current pathway—vertical (''hand to foot'' or ''head to toe'') more dangerous than horizontal (''hand to hand'' or ''foot to foot'')
Multisystem involvement (cardiac and neurologic)
Environmental circumstances (water immersion)

TABLE 196-6 Effects of Electricity

Current Intensity	Effect
1–5 mA	Tingling sensation
5–10 mA	Painful sensation
10–20 mA	If contacted by hand, induces tetanic muscle contraction and prevents voluntary release of grip from current source
30–50 mA	Respiratory arrest secondary to diaphragmatic and thoracic muscle tetany
30–90 mA	Respiratory arrest if current directed through medulla
50–100 mA	Ventricular fibrillation
2–5 A	Cutaneous burns
5–10 A	Asystole

Electric weapons, such as the stun gun and Taser, produce a series of damped sinusoidal electrical pulses, typically 10 to 15/s, designed to induce involuntary muscle contraction and incapacitation in the victim.[6,7] The amount of current delivered depends on the device output (typically 50,000 V for a Taser) and the nature of the electrical contact. Although most patients do not sustain demonstrable injury from electric weapons, several individuals have died within minutes of their use, presumably from cardiac arrhythmias. Most deaths were associated with concomitant drug use (usually phencyclidine), trauma due to struggling, or preexisting cardiac disease.[8]

CLINICAL FEATURES

Cardiac arrest is the primary cause of death caused by electrocution. The specific fatal arrhythmia varies according to the type (either AC or DC) and intensity (as predicted by the voltage) of the electrical current (Table 196-7). Low-voltage AC generally produces ventricular fibrillation. High-voltage AC that causes greater current intensity is more likely to produce asystole. DC is also more likely to cause asystole. The most common arrhythmia encountered in victims who sustain cardiac arrest from electrical injury is ventricular fibrillation. Electricity may also produce cardiac rhythm disturbances, although this is unlikely if the voltage is 120 or less and if water contact is not involved.[9] Arrhythmias are seen in 20 to 30 percent of high-voltage injuries. The most common disturbances are sinus tachycardia, but premature atrial contractions, premature ventricular contractions, supraventricular tachycardia, atrial fibrillation, and first- or second-degree atrioventricular block can be seen.

Acute myocardial infarction is an uncommon complication of electrical injuries.[9] Those patients most at risk have sustained major cutaneous burns and a transthoracic current circuit.[5] Because of spurious elevation from extensive skeletal muscle damage, the CK-MB (MB isoenzyme of creatine kinase) fraction has limited value to detect myocardial damage.

Neurologic injury is reported in approximately 50 percent of patients with high-voltage electrical injuries. Transient loss of consciousness is common, and other behavioral manifestations include agitation, confusion, or prolonged coma, from which recovery may occur. Central nervous system manifestations include seizures, headaches, quadriplegia, hemiparesis, aphasia, tinnitus, and visual disturbances. High-voltage current that passes through the skull may cause subdural and epidural hematomas, as well as intraventricular hemorrhage.

Peripheral nerve injuries may be immediate in onset or delayed. The median nerve is the most common peripheral nerve affected. The

TABLE 196-7 Complications of Electrical Injury

Type of Involvement	Complications
Cardiovascular	Sudden death (ventricular fibrillation, asystole), chest pain, dysrhythmias, ST-T-segment abnormalities, bundle branch block, myocardial damage, ventricular dysfunction, myocardial infarction (rare), hypotension (secondary to volume depletion), hypertension (secondary to endogenous catecholamine release)
Neurologic	Altered level of consciousness, confusion, agitation, amnesia, coma, seizures, cerebral edema, hypoxic encephalopathy, headache, aphasia, quadriplegia, paraplegic, focal motor weakness, spinal cord dysfunction (may be delayed), peripheral neuropathy, cognitive impairment, insomnia, emotional lability
Cutaneous	Electrothermal contact injuries; noncontact arc burns and "flash" burns, secondary thermal burns (clothing ignition, heating of metal objects, e.g., rings or belt buckles)
Vascular	Vascular thrombosis, intravascular hemolysis, delayed vessel rupture, compartment syndrome
Pulmonary	Respiratory arrest, aspiration pneumonia, pulmonary edema, pulmonary contusion (rare)
Renal/metabolic	Acute renal failure (secondary to heme pigment deposition and hypovolemia), myoglobinuria, metabolic (lactic) acidosis, hypokalemia, hypocalcemia, hyperglycemia
Gastrointestinal (GI)	Paralytic ileus ("electroileus"), intestinal perforation, intramural esophageal hemorrhage, hepatic necrosis, pancreatic necrosis, stress ulceration (Curling ulcers), GI bleeding, GI tract dysfunction
Muscular	Myonecrosis, compartment syndrome, clostridial myositis, muscle fibrosis
Skeletal	Vertebral compression fractures, long bone fractures, shoulder dislocations (anterior and posterior), scapular fractures, aseptic necrosis, periosteal burns, bony matrix destruction, osteomyelitis
Infectious	Sepsis, local wound infection, clostridial myonecrosis, cellulitis, pneumonia, osteomyelitis
Ophthalmologic	Corneal burns, delayed cataract formation, intraocular hemorrhage or thrombosis, uveitis, retinal detachment, orbital fracture
Auditory	Hearing loss, tinnitus, tympanic membrane perforation (rare)
Oral burns	Delayed labial artery hemorrhage, scarring and facial deformity, delayed speech development, hypoplastic mandible growth, impaired dentition development
Fetal	Spontaneous abortion, fetal death, oligohydramnios, intrauterine growth retardation, hyperbilirubinemia

peripheral neuropathies range from transient paresthesias to delayed, profound, permanent loss of sensory and/or motor function. Spinal cord injuries range from the immediate caused by direct trauma to delayed patterns of pathology that cause sclerosis, ascending paralysis, complete and incomplete cord syndromes, acute spasticity, transverse myelitis, and amyotropic lateral sclerosis.

Contact with electrical current produces cutaneous burns at the point of entry and exit of the current. The majority of entrance burns are on the upper extremity or the skull, and most exit burns are on the heels. These burns are painless, gray to yellow depressed areas of skin. It cannot be overemphasized that the underlying tissue damage is massive, and attempts to predict injury and gauge therapy by applying the thermal burn rules using percent of body surface area burned will grossly underestimate internal damage, morbidity, mortality, and fluid resuscitation needs.

Flexor crease burns occur as current arcs across the flexor creases of the knees, elbows, and axilla. These arc burns in a "kissing pattern" usually indicate extensive underlying tissue damage. Flash burns can cause metallic particles to become volatilized and may cause the skin to become discolored with a metallic sheen from the impregnation of tiny metallic particles. Thermal burns may occur from the combustion of clothing and heated materials on the skin.

Electrical current passing along peripheral arteries may cause arterial spasm, arterial thrombosis, or aneurysm formation. Whereas spasm may be apparently early, thrombosis and aneurysm formation are typically delayed. Extensive vascular damage may cause compartment syndromes with massive myonecrosis. Detection of an evolving compartment syndrome may be difficult in an extremity that has sustained an electrical burn and has insensate skin. Measurement of compartment pressures is usually necessary to detect a compartment syndrome and ensure timely fasciotomy. Delayed arterial thrombosis can convert partial-thickness cutaneous burns into full-thickness ones. Massive areas of deep tissue necrosis may result in clostridial infection, including tetanus and gas gangrene.

Blunt trauma is common in the setting of electrical injuries occurring from either the forcible thrust back away from a high-voltage AC or DC blast, from the tetanic contractions associated with an AC injury, or from a fall due to a loss of consciousness or balance. Tetanic contractions may produce compression fractures of the thoracic spine, long-bone fractures, and dislocations of the shoulder (particularly posterior).

An oral injury may occur when a child chews through the insulation on an electrical cord. The salivary electrolytes complete the electrical circuit and allow the propagation of current throughout the tissues of the lip. Current arcing can produce temperatures as high as 2500°C. Injuries may extend more than 2 cm from the vermilion border of the lip. Most injury sites are unilateral and involve the commissure, the tongue, and the alveolar ridge. Vascular injury to the labial artery is not immediately apparent due to vascular spasm, thrombosis, and the overlying eschar. Delayed hemorrhage may occur, usually after 5 days, as the thrombus lyses and the eschar separates.

Cataracts may develop within 4 to 6 months following electrical injury to the head, neck, and upper chest. Retinal detachment, corneal burns, intraocular hemorrhage, and intraocular thrombosis may be seen after high-voltage injury.

Renal consequences of electrical injuries are secondary to myoglobinuria from massive muscle destruction. Abdominal injuries such as hollow viscous perforation or necrosis may occur after current traverses the abdominal wall. Parenchymal damage to the liver and pancreas, paralytic ileus, and stress ulcers of the stomach have been reported.

DIAGNOSIS

The diagnosis of an electrical injury is usually made based on history provided by the patient, bystanders, or emergency medical services. Occasionally, the history may be unclear if the patient is found unconscious in a bathtub or is amnestic to the event. If available, a history should be obtained as to the voltage, the type of current, the duration of contact, the likely pathway of the current, any skin resistance modifying factors (e.g., water or sweating), and any symptoms suggestive of the aforementioned complications. The presence of underlying disease, such as coronary artery disease, diabetes, and neurologic disease, should be determined.

The physical examination should assess tissue damage and identify associated complications. Airway, respiratory, and cardiovascular status should first be stabilized, followed by evaluation for cutaneous burns and secondary trauma. A careful vascular examination of injured extremities must be performed along with a detailed examination of peripheral nerve function. As noted above, occult and delayed injuries occur, and clinicians must be wary that the absence of physical findings does not exclude serious injury.

An electrocardiogram (ECG) and a period of cardiac monitoring is recommended for (1) all patients who have been exposed to high-voltage electricity (more than 600 V) and (2) all patients exposed to low-voltage electricity with suggestive symptoms or signs (loss of consciousness, amnesia, altered mental status, other neurologic symptoms, palpitations, chest pain, or irregular pulse).

Patients with high-voltage injury, extensive cutaneous burns, or evidence of systemic injury require laboratory investigation including a complete blood count and determination of electrolyte, calcium, blood urea nitrogen, creatinine, creatine kinase (CK), and serum myoglobin levels. Urinalysis and determination of the urine myoglobin level should be performed. Urine that tests positive for blood by urine dipstick but has no red blood cells on the microscopic examination is suggestive of myoglobin consistent with muscle damage. Liver function tests and an amylase evaluation should be obtained in those patients who are suspected of having an intraabdominal injury.

Cervical spine films must be obtained in patients who have altered levels of consciousness, neurologic deficits, neck pain or tenderness, or significant distracting injuries. Cranial computed tomography should be performed for those patients who show altered levels of consciousness. Additional studies such as plain films, arteriography for suspected vascular injury, and radionuclide scan to detect cardiac muscle damage should be ordered as needed.

SPECIAL PATIENTS

Electrical shock during pregnancy is felt to be associated with potential fetal demise, as amniotic fluid is an excellent conductor of electricity. This belief was substantiated in a review of 15 published cases of electrical injury during pregnancy, with 11 resulting in fetal death.[10] However, this summation of published cases may represent publication bias. In a recent prospective observational study of 31 pregnant women who sustained electrical shock (28 to household current), 28 gave birth to normal healthy infants and only one sustained a spontaneous abortion.[11] Thus, although the risk may be low, it is advisable to observe pregnant patients for a short period after an electrical shock. In patients with a fetus that is over 24 weeks of gestational age, fetal monitoring should be performed during this observation. Auscultation of fetal heart tones and ultrasound evaluation of a fetus less than 24 weeks of age is recommended. In general, obstetric consultation should be obtained for an electrical shock involving household current.

MANAGEMENT

When providing medical control of prehospital personnel, scene safety is paramount. Emergency medical service providers need to ensure that electrical power has been shut off by authorized personnel. The insulating material surrounding the wire should not be considered protective to rescuers; it merely protects the wire from the elements. ''Insulated'' objects such as rubber mats and ropes should not be used to extricate the patient from the power source, as these may be damaged or wet and may conduct high-voltage electricity.

TABLE 196-8 High-Risk Patients with Low-Voltage Exposure

Wet skin
Tetany
Current traverses the thorax (vertical pathway)
220-V exposure

The initial stabilization of an electrically injured patient should focus on the airway, breathing, and circulation. Respiratory arrest caused by current traversing the medulla or the chest wall is treated with immediate intubation and assisted ventilation. Electrical injuries alone do not usually cause upper airway edema, but thermal burns or inhalation injuries may cause airway obstruction. Spinal immobilization must be maintained if the possibility of cervical spine trauma exists. High-flow oxygen via face mask and continuous pulse oximetry should be provided. Cardiac arrhythmias should be treated with the advanced cardiac life support (ACLS) protocol, including standard doses of electrical shock. Cardiac monitoring should be instituted for all high-voltage patients, all symptomatic, and all high-risk low-voltage patients (Table 196-8).

Fluid resuscitation should be commenced with two large-bore intravenous lines (IVs) infusing Ringer's lactate or normal saline. If possible, an IV should not be started on an extremity that was part of the current pathway, because delayed thrombosis may occlude the infusion line. Fluid requirements for victims of electrical burns are higher than the fluid requirements for victims of thermal burns, and formulas based on percent of body surface area involved will not provide enough volume to avert rhabdomyolysis and maintain tissue perfusion. An initial fluid challenge of 20 to 40 mL/kg over the first hour is appropriate for most patients. Further fluid requirements are guided by clinical and hemodynamic assessment. Central venous or pulmonary artery pressure monitoring may be necessary to guide fluid replacement and avoid volume overload in patients at risk for congestive heart failure.

Rhabdomyolysis with myoglobinuria should be treated with urinary alkalization; 44 to 50 meq of sodium bicarbonate added to each liter of intravenous (IV) fluid. Blood pH should be maintained 7.45 or greater and urine output at 1.5 to 2.0 mL/kg/h. IV mannitol may be administered to encourage urine flow at an initial dose of 25 g in adults and 0.5 to 1 g/kg in children. Mannitol infusions may be given until the urine is free of myoglobin, but it is very important that patients not become hypovolemic. If thermal burns are also present, mannitol should not be given, due to the risk of hypovolemia. (See Chap. 271, ''Rhabdomyolysis.'')

Wound care for minor localized and partial-thickness wounds consists of cleansing and application of silver sulfadiazine. Full-thickness burns with an eschar are better treated with mafenide acetate, because it penetrates eschar well. Side effects from mafenide are metabolic acidosis and pain with application. Tetanus prophylaxis should be administered as indicated. For patients with extensive muscle damage and soil contamination, the risk of tetanus is such that tetanus immune globulin should be considered even if the patient's tetanus immunizations are up to date. There is no scientific evidence to support the prophylactic administration of parenteral antibiotics (e.g., high-dose penicillin) to prevent clostridial infection in patients with extensive devitalized tissue.

DISPOSITION

All patients with high-voltage exposure (more than 600 V) should be admitted for observation even if there is no apparent injury. Patients

TABLE 196-9 Indications for Admission

High voltage >600 V
Symptoms suggestive of systemic injury Cardiovascular: chest pain, palpitations Neurologic: loss of consciousness, confusion, weakness, headache, paresthesias Respiratory: dyspnea Gastrointestinal: abdominal pain, vomiting
Evidence of neurologic or vascular injury to a digit or extremity
Burns with evidence of subcutaneous tissue damage
Arrhythmia or abnormal ECG
Suspected foul play, abuse, or suicidal intent
High-risk exposures
Associated injuries requiring admission
Comorbid diseases (cardiac, renal, neurologic)

with serious high-voltage injuries (neurologic, cardiac, vascular, or muscle damage) should be admitted to a specialized burn center. Routine cardiac rhythm monitoring is not required for patients admitted with high-voltage injuries unless there is an initial abnormal ECG or arrhythmia.[12] Disposition of patients with a low-voltage injury is more problematic (Table 196-9).

Adults with low-voltage injury (less than 600 V) and evidence of complications should be admitted. Multiple studies have substantiated the negligible risk of delayed arrhythmias in asymptomatic patients with a 110-V exposure and no tetany, wet skin, or vertical current flow. Asymptomatic adults who sustain a household shock may be discharged home if they have a normal ECG on presentation and normal examination findings.[9] Exposure to 220 V probably carries little risk for occult or delayed cardiac injury, although the published literature is less than definite. Two studies totaling 90 patients from Australia where household current is single-phase AC at 50 Hz with voltage varying between 220 and 260 V found that only one patient sustained an arrhythmia, and that was present on admission.[13,14]

Children with exposure or injury to 110-V household current usually sustain oral burns or minor hand burns and rarely develop cardiac or significant deep injury.[15–17] Children with an electrical cutaneous burn and a loss of consciousness, vertical current path, tetany, or wet skin should be admitted for a period of cardiac monitoring.[16,17] Likewise, a child with a home situation of equivocal safety or reliability should also be admitted, although cardiac monitoring is not routinely required for these ''social'' admissions. Children with minor hand burns from outlet injuries and no initial evidence of cardiac or neurovascular injury can also be sent home with local wound care.[18]

Oral electrical burns in children have been extensively studied.[19] Because of the risk of wound contracture and delayed hemorrhage, such children were formerly commonly admitted to the hospital for observation and the initiation of splinting. More recent series indicate that most children with oral electrical burns do not require admission, provided (1) there is no history of loss of consciousness, (2) there are no other injuries that require admission, (3) the ECG is normal, (4) the child is able to drink fluids, and (5) the parents are reliable.[17] These children can be discharged home with instructions to apply pressure should the oral burn bleed, return in 24 h for a wound check, and arrange follow-up with a plastic or oral surgeon. The risk of cardiac or muscle damage is so low that urinalysis, CK, and myoglobin testing is not required.[16] Prolonged cardiac rhythm monitoring is not necessary, provided the initial ECG is normal. Splinting for a minimum of 4 months is beneficial to control wound contracture and reduce the need for commissuroplasty.[20]

Since a large percentage of electrical injuries involve tort claims against employers, power companies, or manufacturers, the medical record must meticulously detail the history, clinical findings, and treatment.

PREVENTION

Kennelly proposed one of the most effective precautions against electrical injury in 1927 when he suggested keeping one hand in the pocket when visiting an electrical plant.[21] Household precautions include the education of parents about the hazards of unused sockets, including the use of plastic caps and two-step sockets, the hazards of extension cords, and restricting access to small metallic objects that can be inserted into the outlet.[22] A visit to the emergency department for a benign low-voltage injury in the toddler is a fertile time to provide safety education to parents.

Ground fault interrupters (GFIs) should be installed in circuits around water in the home (e.g., the bathroom or kitchen). These are fast-acting circuit breakers that electronically detect current leaks before they become a danger. A GFI will trip when it senses a 0.005-A difference in the current flowing into an appliance on the hot leg as compared with the current leaving the appliance on the neutral leg—thus assuring protection against a shock. Other measures that home handymen can take are to use double-insulated power tools, inspect cords and insulation on tools, and make sure that screw connections and contacts are tight and free from corrosion to prevent arcing.

REFERENCES

1. Hoskin AF, Fearn KT, Miller T, et al: *Accident Facts.* Itasca, IL, National Safety Council, 1997.
2. Ore T, Casini V: Electrical fatalities among US construction workers. *J Occup Environ Med* 38:587, 1996.
3. Rabban J, Adler J, Rosen C, et al: Electrical injury from subway third rails: Serious injury associated with intermediate voltage contact. *Burns* 23:515, 1997.
4. Lee C: Injury by electrical forces: Pathophysiology, manifestations, and therapy. *Curr Probl Surg* 34:677, 1997.
5. Chandra NC, Siu CO, Munster AM: Clinical predictors of myocardial damage after high voltage electrical injury. *J Trauma* 18:293, 1990.
6. O'Brien DJ: Electronic weaponry: A question of safety. *Ann Emerg Med* 20:583, 1991.
7. Burdett-Smith P: Stun gun injury. *J Accid Emerg Med* 14:402, 1997.
8. Fish R: Electric shock: I, II, and III. *J Emerg Med* 11:309, 457, and 599, 1993.
9. Arrowsmith J, Usgaocar RP, Dickson WA: Electrical injury and the frequency of cardiac complications. *Burns* 23:576, 1997.
10. Fatovich DM: Electric shock in pregnancy. *J Emerg Med* 11:175, 1993.
11. Einarson A, Bailey B, Inocencion G, et al.: Accidental electric shock in pregnancy: A prospective cohort study. *Am J Obstet Gynecol* 176:678, 1997.
12. Purdue GF, Hunt JL: Electrocardiographic monitoring after (high-voltage) electrical injury: Necessity or luxury. *J Trauma* 26:166, 1986.
13. Cunningham P: The need for cardiac monitoring after electrical injury. *Med J Aust* 154:765, 1991.
14. Fatovich DM, Lee KY: Household electric shocks: Who should be monitored? *Med J Aust* 155:301, 1991.
15. Zubair M, Besner GE: Pediatric electrical burns: Management strategies. *Burns* 23:413, 1997.
16. Garcia CT, Smith GA, Cohen DM, Fernandez K: Electrical injuries in a pediatric emergency department. *Ann Emerg Med* 26:604, 1995.
17. Bailey B, Gaudreault P, Thivierge RL, Turgeon JP: Cardiac monitoring of children with household electrical injuries. *Ann Emerg Med* 25:612, 1996.
18. Wallace BH, Cone JB, Vanderpool RD, et al: Retrospective evaluation of admission criteria for pediatric electrical injuries. *Burns* 21:590, 1995.
19. Canady JW, Thompson SA, Bardach J: Oral commissure burns in children. *Plast Reconstr Surg* 97:738, 1996.

20. Al-Qattan MM, Gillett D, Thomson HG: Electrical burns to the oral commissure: Does splinting obviate the need for commissuroplasty? *Burns* 22:555, 1996.
21. Hussmann J, Kucan JO, Russell RC, et al: Electrical injuries—Morbidity, outcome and treatment rationale. *Burns* 21:530, 1995.
22. Rabban JT, Blair JA, Rosen CL, et al: Mechanisms of pediatric electrical injury: New implications for product safety and injury prevention. *Arch Pediatr Adolesc Med* 151:696, 1997

LIGHTNING INJURIES

Kimberly N. Treat
Janet M. Williams
Ann S. Chinnis

Lightning injury is one of the most frequent injuries by natural phenomenon and, although accurate data is lacking, is likely to result in several hundred deaths per year in the United States.[1,2] Mortality rates associated with lightning have been estimated to range from 20 to 30 percent but are thought to be overestimated, because medical databases are biased toward collecting information on only the most severe and fatal cases and exclude the many less severe injuries that occur.[1] Nonfatal lightning injuries are more common, with estimates of several hundred to several thousand cases per year.[1,3,4] As many as 75 percent of survivors sustain significant morbidity and permanent sequelae.

A significant number of lightning injuries are associated with transportation.[5] The majority of transportation-related lightning injuries occur when victims are struck while standing near a vehicle. Aircraft are at risk for lightning strike that injures or kills the occupants. Between 1963 and 1985, the National Transportation Safety Board recorded 40 lightning-related aircraft accidents (10 commercial and 30 private aircraft), with 290 fatalities and 74 serious injuries.[6]

Sports are associated with increased risk of lightning injury. Among all outdoor activities, the largest number of injuries and fatalities have occurred during water sports.[7]

Even though lightning is electrical energy, lightning injuries differ substantially from high-voltage electrical injuries seen from human-generated sources: different injury patterns, different injury severity, and different emergency treatment.

PATHOPHYSIOLOGY

Unlike conventional electricity in which the alternating current tends to fix a victim to the current source by tetanic muscle contraction creating a longer contact time, lightning is direct current that imparts an instantaneous but extremely high-voltage discharge of electricity to the body. The pattern of injury seen with lightning differs from that of injury caused by both high-voltage and low-voltage alternating current (Table 197-1). Unlike conventional electricity, lightning current tends to flow over the body in a phenomenon called *flashover*, thus sparing injury to the deeper vital organs and explaining how victims are able to survive exposure to tremendous magnitudes of current. Less commonly, lightning current may enter victims and suddenly disrupt cardiac, respiratory, or neurologic function.

Injuries from lightning relate to its potential to impart electrical as well as mechanical, thermal, acoustic, and photic forces to victims. Lighting creates mechanical energy in two ways: through the direct force of the strike or as a result of the rapid expansion of the surrounding air, which may cause victims to fall or be struck by flying debris. Blunt injury has been reported in 32 percent of lightning victims.[8] Lightning may inflict thermal injury as moisture on the victim's skin is transformed into steam, reaching temperatures between 8000° and 30,000°C. An individual found dead with tattered clothing nearby might even be mistaken for a crime victim when, in reality, the rapidly expanding steam blew clothing and shoes off. Lightning can also heat metal objects such as jewelry, watches, and coins in pockets and cause burns through direct skin contact. Sound waves caused by the thunderclap may rupture tympanic membranes and lead to other acoustic injuries. Photic injury caused by the bright flash may cause retinal damage and cataracts.

The nature and severity of injury also vary according to the type of lightning strike. There are five basic types of lightning strikes. A *direct strike* occurs when a victim is struck directly by a lightning discharge; this is the most serious form of lightning injury. The risk of a direct strike increases when individuals carry a metal object such as an umbrella or golf club or wear metal accessories such as hairpins, jewelry, hearing aids, or shoes with metal cleats. The *side flash* occurs when a nearby object is struck and current then traverses through the air to strike a victim. A side flash may injure multiple victims simultaneously, such as a softball team in a huddle near a structure that is struck. A *contact strike* occurs when lightning strikes an object that an individual is touching and current is directly transferred to the person. A *ground current* occurs when the lightning hits the ground and is transferred to a person standing near the strike site. The amount of current reaching a victim decreases as the radius between the victim and the strike point increases. A *stride potential* or *step voltage* occurs when lightning strikes the ground and encounters a potential difference between the legs of a person. The current enters the closer leg, traverses the lower body, and exits through the farther leg. This may result in *keraunoparalysis*, which is characterized by temporarily paretic, cold, insensate, and pulseless legs.

CLINICAL FEATURES

Although lightning injuries may involve all organ systems, injuries to the cardiovascular system and central nervous system (CNS) are usually the most devastating[9] (Table 197-2).

Cardiovascular Injury

The immediate cause of death due to a lightning strike is usually direct current depolarization of the myocardium and sustained cardiac asystole. Although cardiac automaticity may spontaneously return, concomitant respiratory arrest due to medullary respiratory center paralysis may outlast cardiac arrest and ultimately lead to a hypoxic cardiac arrest. The duration of apnea, rather than the duration of asystole, appears to be a critical prognostic factor. Patients may suffer a variety of other cardiovascular effects, including direct myocardial damage, coronary artery spasm, cardiac contusion from blunt trauma, acute global cardiac dysfunction, atrial and ventricular dysrhythmias, pericardial effusion, and transient hypertension and tachycardia. The electrocardiogram (ECG) may show acute injury with ST-segment elevation and a prolonged QT interval. T-wave changes may be seen especially in the presence of cerebrovascular injuries. Although creatine kinase (CK) and CK-MB (isoenzyme) fraction elevations are common, myocardial infarction is not, occurring in only 7 percent of victims.

Neurologic Injury

The nervous system is particularly vulnerable to lightning injury, since resistance to current flow is lowest in nerve tissue. In addition to direct electrical trauma, CNS injuries may result from hypoxia secondary to cardiac arrest or to blunt trauma.[10] The most lethal CNS injuries involve heat-induced coagulation of the cortex (as current passes through the brain parenchyma), formation of epidural or subdural hematomas, paralysis of the medullary respiratory centers, and intraventricular hemorrhage. When lightning victims present with coma, the differential diagnosis may include prolonged hypoxia, acute cerebral edema, closed head injury, ischemia, and hemorrhage, as well as other less

TABLE 197-1 Comparison of Lightning and Electrical Injuries

Factor	Lightning	High-Voltage AC	Low-Voltage AC
Current duration	1–3 ms	Generally brief (1–2 s), but may be prolonged	Prolonged
Energy level: voltage current	10 million to 2 billion V; 20,000–200,000 A	600–70,000 V; <1000 A	<600 V; usually <20–30 A
Current characteristics	Unidirectional (DC)	Alternating (AC)	Alternating (AC)
Current pathway	Skin flashover	Horizontal (hand to hand), vertical (hand to foot)	Horizontal (hand to hand), vertical (hand to foot)
Burn characteristics	Superficial, minor	Deep tissue destruction	Somtimes deep tissue destruction
Initial rhythm in cardiac arrest	Asystole	Asystole greater than ventricular fibrillation	Ventricular fibrillation
Renal involvement	Rare	Myoglobinuria and renal failure common	Myoglobinuria and renal failure occasionally
Fasciotomy and amputation	Rarely necessary	Relatively common	Sometimes necessary
Blunt injury	Explosive effect with shockwave	Being thrown from current source or falls	Tetanic contraction or falls
Immediate cause of death	Prolonged apnea	Apnea	Ventricular fibrillation

Abbreviations: AC, alternating current; DC, direct current.

TABLE 197-2 Complications Associated with Lightning Strikes

System Affected	Early Injury	Late Injury
Cardiovascular	Dysrhythmias (asystole, ventricular fibrillation, premature ventricular contractions, ventricular tachycardia), electrocardiogram changes	Myocardial infarction
Pulmonary	Respiratory arrest, pulmonary edema, contusion, hemorrhage	Pulmonary infarction, pneumonia
Central nervous	Loss of consciousness, confusion, amnesia, intracranial hemorrhage, respiratory center paralysis, cerebral edema, cerebral infarction	Hemiplegia, amnesia, neuritis, decreased reflexes, seizures, parkinsonian syndrome, progressive muscular atrophy, amyotrophic lateral sclerosis, progressive cerebellar syndrome, myelopathy
Peripheral nerves	Transient paralysis, paresthesias, mottling, intense vasomotor spasm	Neuritis, neuralgia
Cutaneous	Burns (first to third degree)	Scars and contractures
Ophthalmologic	Corneal lesions, uveitis, iridocyclitis, vitreous hemorrhage, diplopia, chorioretinitis, retinal detachment, hyphema	Cataracts, macular degeneration, optic atrophy
Otologic	Tympanic membrane rupture, cerebrospinal fluid otorrhea, hemotympanum, temporary deafness	Hearing loss, chronic otitis
Renal	Myoglobinuria, hemoglobinuria, renal failure (rare)	None
Gastrointestinal	Gastric atony, ileus, intestinal perforation	None
Psychiatric	Hysteria, anxiety	Sleep disturbance, depression, anxiety, storm phobia, cognitive dysfunction
Miscellaneous	Secondary blunt trauma, muscular compartment syndrome, disseminated intravascular coagulation	

TABLE 197-3 Assessment and Treatment Essentials

History	Physical Examination	Diagnostic Studies	Admission Criteria
History of thunderstorm	ABCs	Electrocardiogram and cardiac rhythm monitoring	Cardiorespiratory arrest
Outdoor occurrence	Cervical spine immobilization	Urinalysis, urine myoglobin	Cranial burns
Evidence of charred marks at the scene	Secondary survey	Complete blood count, electrolytes, blood urea nitrogen, creatinine, creatine kinase (CK), and CK-MB	Leg burns
Location of patient versus site of strike	Neurologic examination	Computed tomography of head and abdomen as indicated	Any loss of consciousness
Clothing disintegration	Hearing acuity	Radiographs as indicated	Unresolved neurologic deficits
	Visual acuity and slit-lamp examination	Fetal monitoring (pregnancy)	Pregnancy

obvious etiologies such as hypoglycemia, drug toxicity, and hypothermia (Table 197-3). Autonomic dysfunction caused by the lightning strike may manifest as pupillary dilation, areflexia, anisocoria, or Horner's syndrome. These pupillary abnormalities are not related to CNS injury and have no relation to prognosis in comatose lightning-strike victims.

Neurologic symptoms are typically classified either as immediate but transient or as delayed and usually progressive. However, some neurologic injuries can be severe, immediate, and permanent.[11] Immediate but transient symptoms include confusion and amnesia, loss of consciousness, temporary lower extremity paralysis, and temporary upper extremity paralysis.[10] Lower extremity paralysis (keraunoparalysis) is often a consequence of step-voltage injury and is usually associated with paleness, sensory loss, loss of pulses, and vasomotor changes.[12] These immediate but transient symptoms typically resolve within 24 h. Delayed and usually progressive disorders include seizures, spinal muscular atrophy, amyotrophic lateral sclerosis, parkinsonian syndromes, progressive cerebellar ataxia, myelopathy and neuropathy, paraplegia and quadriplegia, paresthesias, and chronic pain syndromes.

Respiratory Injury

Paralysis of the brainstem respiratory center may result in apnea, but this central apnea may be temporary and a patient may survive if ventilated until cardiac and respiratory activity return. Other respiratory injuries include immediate and delayed pulmonary edema, pulmonary contusion, adult respiratory distress syndrome, and pulmonary hemorrhage.

Peripheral Vascular Effects

Lightning that traverses the lower extremities during a stride potential pathway may cause vasomotor instability and the aforementioned phenomenon of keraunoparalysis. Paresis, blue, cold, and pulseless lower extremities characterize this transient form of paralysis.[12] Keraunoparalysis is thought to be caused by endogenous catecholamines and does not usually require surgical intervention. Some victims will develop permanent paralysis and paresthesias due to prolonged vasospasm. Initially, keraunoparalysis may be difficult to distinguish from acute spinal cord injury.

Dermatologic Injury

The six main dermatologic manifestations of lighting injury are feathering burns (Lichtenberg figures), flash burns, punctate burns, contact burns, erythema, and blistering, and linear streaking. The pathognomonic skin finding for lightning is the *Lichtenberg figure*, which results from electron showering over the skin surface, which is not a true burn.[13] Lichtenberg figures are superficial, appear in a fern pattern, and resolve within 24 h (Fig. 197-1). A comatose patient exhibiting Lichtenberg figures should be treated as a victim of lightning injury. *Flash burns* are similar to those found in welders, appear as mild erythema, and may involve the cornea. *Punctate burns* look similar to cigarette burns in that they are usually smaller than 1 cm and are full-thickness burns. *Contact burns* occur when metal worn close to

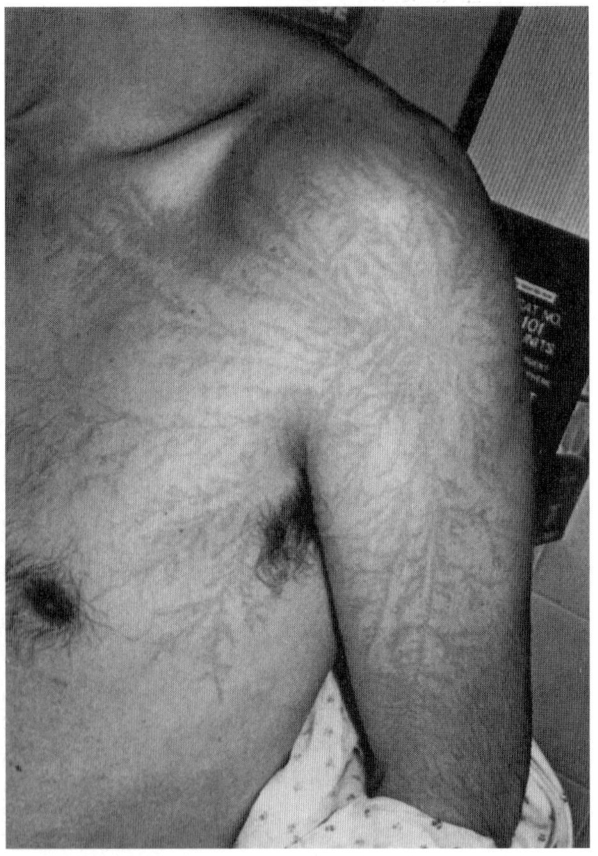

FIG. 197-1. Lichtenberg figures demonstrating the superficial ferning pattern.

the skin, such as coins, zippers, and belts, is heated by the lightning current. *Erythema* and *blistering* are usually transient, and superficial skin loss may occur. *Linear burns* may be seen in areas of sweat, such as the axilla or groin, and are full-thickness burns usually less than 5 cm wide. Less common burns found on lightning victims include those associated with ignition of clothing. Entrance and exit wounds, characteristic of nonlightning electrical injuries, are not commonly seen in lightning victims.

Ocular Injury

Half of all lightning victims will have ocular injuries, including optic nerve atrophy, papilledema, retinal hemorrhage, retinal detachment, corneal abrasion, hyphema, uveitis, vitreous hemorrhage, and cataracts. Cataracts are the most common single injury and may develop immediately or as late as 2 years after a strike. Pupillary findings may include iridocyclitis, mydriasis, anisocoria, and Horner's syndrome. Dilated unresponsive pupils may be due to transient autonomic dysfunction and should not be used as a sign of brain death.

Otologic Injury

Otologic injuries range from transient hearing loss and vertigo to complete disruption of the auditory system. Tympanic membrane rupture is seen in more than 50 percent of lightning victims and may result from the explosive forces of the strike, basilar skull fracture, direct trauma to the ear canal, or direct lightning burn to the canal. Victims who were using a conventional corded telephone at the time of the lighting strike are at higher risk for these injuries. Long-term complications may include chronic otitis media and hearing loss.

Gastrointestinal Injury

Gastrointestinal complications include paralytic ileus, gastric dilatation, stress ulcers, and upper gastrointestinal bleeding. Blunt abdominal trauma may result in a ruptured viscus or solid organ injury.

Renal Injury

Permanent renal damage is rare but may occur from prolonged hypotension. Myoglobinuria occurs less commonly than in electrical burns and is seen in only 6 percent of lightning victims.[14] Routine forced diuresis and alkalinization of the urine is not recommended in lightning victims, due to the risk of volume overload and cerebral edema.

Musculoskeletal Injury

A variety of musculoskeletal injuries may result, including fractures and soft tissue injuries due to blunt forces, compartment syndromes, muscular rupture, and posterior shoulder dislocations, and cervical spine fractures from intense myotonic contractions.

Psychosocial Problems

Lightning victims may suffer from long-term cognitive dysfunction, depression, and anxiety. Posttraumatic stress disorder and storm phobias are known to develop. Children are more prone to anxiety, storm phobias, and recurrent nightmares.

Pregnancy

Although maternal outcomes are generally good, there is a 50 percent rate of fetal death in pregnant women struck by lightning, because amniotic fluid serves as a preferential path for the electrical current flow. Fetal monitoring should be performed on all pregnant women with lightning injuries.

TABLE 197-4 Common Misdiagnoses of Lightning Injuries

Cerebrovascular accidents
Seizure disorders
Cerebral, spinal cord, or other neurologic trauma
Stokes-Adams attacks
Toxic ingestion or envenomation
Myocardial infarction
Cardiac dysrhythmias
Hypertensive crisis with intracranial hemorrhage
Physical assault

DIAGNOSIS

All patients with lightning injury should have a 12-lead ECG performed to evaluate for arrhythmias and injury patterns (Table 197-3). Laboratory tests that should be conducted in most patients with moderate to severe injuries include determination of serum electrolytes, calcium, magnesium, blood urea nitrogen, creatinine, CK, CK-MB, arterial blood gas, and urine myoglobin levels; coagulation studies; a complete blood count; and urinalysis. A chest x-ray should be obtained to evaluate for aspiration, pulmonary edema, pulmonary contusion, rib fractures, and pneumothorax. Cervical spine films should be obtained in patients with suspected spinal injuries or trauma secondary to falls, and in obtunded patients in whom a history of trauma is uncertain. Computed tomography of the head should be performed in patients with an altered or deteriorating level of consciousness or evidence of a head injury. Additional studies may be indicated based on clinical findings.

The differential diagnosis of an unwitnessed victim of lightning strike is quite broad and includes trauma, metabolic disturbance, toxic exposure, and other causes of an altered mental status (Table 197-4). Lightning injuries can be suspected when the environmental setting is compatible and a victim displays physical findings unique to such injuries. For example, an unconscious rain-soaked patient with perforated tympanic membranes and Lichtenberg figures (fernlike skin markings) who is found in a field near a tractor is almost definitely a lightning victim.

TREATMENT

Prehospital Treatment

Emergency medical service personnel and bystander safety must be the first priority, since lightning can and does frequently strike twice in the same place. The standard airway, breathing, circulation, disability, and exposure protocols with advanced life support (ALS) protocols are required. Reverse triage (care for the apparently dead first) is appropriate in the case of multiple victims, because (a) most victims who are not in cardiopulmonary arrest survive without the need for ALS and (b) victims in cardiac arrest may survive if ventilated until cardiac and respiratory activity resumes.[15] Thus, concentrating limited ALS resources on apparently dead victims in a multicasualty lightning-strike event is appropriate. Due to the unusual neurologic manifestations of lightning injuries, patients with fixed and dilated pupils may survive and live a normal life. Patients who are blue, with mottled extremities, in whom it may be difficult to find a pulse or a blood pressure, may recover without sequelae. Aggressive fluid resuscitation is rarely required. Victims of a lightning strike should be transported in full spinal immobilization, due to the possibility of traumatic injuries.

Emergency Department Treatment

Standard ALS and trauma treatment principles should be followed. Intravenous access, supplemental oxygen, and continuous cardiac monitoring should be initiated immediately. Lightning victims in cardiac arrest have a better prognosis than do victims in arrest due to trauma or acute myocardial infarction.[16] For this reason, aggressive resuscitative efforts should be taken even after a prolonged anoxic period. Hypotension warrants a search for occult hemorrhage, such as intraabdominal or intrathoracic hemorrhage, and pelvic or long-bone fractures.

Once the primary survey is completed, a careful head-to-toe examination should be performed to identify occult injuries. The cutaneous examination may disclose burns and may help determine the path of the current and locate potential organ injuries. Care for a superficial lightning burn includes cleansing, debridement, application of a topical antimicrobial agent, and administration of tetanus prophylaxis, if indicated. Fasciotomy is rarely indicated, since circulatory disorders are frequently consequences of vasospasm and resolve spontaneously. A careful neurologic examination should be performed to detect motor and sensory deficits. Ophthalmologic (including slit-lamp examination) and otologic examinations should be done to rule out visual and hearing disturbances, as well as tympanic membrane rupture. Abdominal distention due to ileus should be treated with gastric decompression. An acute abdomen may be due to blunt injury and intraperitoneal injury.

DISPOSITION

The majority of patients with lightning strike injuries require admission to a center with appropriate capabilities for providing specialized, comprehensive care. Conditions associated with serious mortality and morbidity include cardiorespiratory arrest, cranial burns, leg burns, ECG changes and dysrhythmias, any CNS lesions or loss of consciousness, any neurologic injuries without rapid resolution, and myoglobinuria.[14] Consultation with trauma surgery, neurosurgery, cardiology, and neurology services may be indicated. All pregnant patients require admission for fetal monitoring and ultrasound fetal assessment.

Those with minor injuries who show improvement within the first several hours after a strike may benefit from admission for careful monitoring of neurologic and cardiovascular status, due to the potential for delayed sequelae. Patients who have no neurologic deficits and only minor abnormalities found on a thorough examination may be monitored in the emergency department and discharged with adequate follow-up. Consider neurologic; ear, nose, and throat; and ophthamologic referral for evaluation of potential long-term sequelae in all victims.

PREVENTION

The risk factors and recommendations for the prevention of lightning injuries are well described.[17] Lightning is more likely to occur on hot, humid days. Static on a local radio station may indicate high electrical activity in the atmosphere. In anticipation of a thunder and lightning storm, individuals should remain indoors or seek shelter in a vehicle. Individuals should avoid open doorways or open windows, stay clear of metallic objects (stoves, water pipes, sinks, and bathtubs), and not use plug-in electrical appliances such as radios, televisions, and telephones. Campers should avoid placing tents under tall trees, near bodies of water, or on the highest hill in an area. If caught outside during a storm, all metal objects (fishing rods, golf clubs, umbrellas, and jewelry) should be discarded. If no shelter is possible, individuals should head for dense woods or lie on the ground in a ditch. Groups of people should separate to avoid all becoming victims. All machinery work outside should be stopped; for example, tractors are often struck by lightning. Individuals should get out of water and off small boats. A lightning strike is imminent when an individual's hair stands on end (due to surrounding electrical charge). The individual should squat (much like the position of a baseball catcher) with hands on knees and feet close together to decrease strike potential.

ACKNOWLEDGMENT

Special thanks to John E. Gastineau, Ph.D (physicist) for his assistance with the creation of this chapter.

REFERENCES

1. Lopez RE, Holle RL: Demographics of lightning casualties. *Semin Neurol* 15:286, 1995.
2. Centers for Disease Control and Prevention: Lightning-associated deaths: United States, 1980–1995. *MMWR* 22:391, 1998.
3. Cooper MA: Electrical and lightning injuries. *Emerg Med Clin North Am* 2:489, 1984.
4. Brigham PA: Lightning injuries revisited. *Ann Emerg Med* 26:528, 1994.
5. Cherington M: Lightning and transportation. *Semin Neurol* 15:362, 1995.
6. Cherington M, Mathys K: Deaths and injuries as a result of lightning strikes to aircraft. *Aviat Space Environ Med* 66:687, 1995.
7. Cherington M, Vervalin C: Lightning injuries: Who is at greatest risk? *Phys Sports Med* 15(8):59, 1990.
8. Blount BW: Lightning injuries. *Am Fam Physician* 42:405, 1990.
9. Cherington M: Lightning injuries. *Ann Emerg Med* 25:517, 1995.
10. Kleinschmidt-DeMasters BK: Neuropathology of lightning-strike injuries. *Semin Neurol* 15:323, 1995.
11. Cherington M, Yarnell P, Lammereste D: Lightning strikes: Nature of neurologic damage in patients evaluated in hospital emergency departments. *Ann Emerg Med* 21:575, 1992.
12. Ten Duis HJ, Klasen HJ, Reenalda PE: Keraunoparalysis, a 'specific' lightning injury. *Burns Incl Therm Inj* 12:54, 1985.
13. Resnik BI, Wetli CV: Lichtenberg figures. *Am J Forensic Med Pathol* 17:99, 1996.
14. Cooper MA: Lightning injuries: Prognostic signs for death. *Ann Emerg Med* 9:134, 1980.
15. Graber J, Ummenhofer W, Herion H: Lightning accident with eight victims: Case report and brief review of the literature. *J Trauma* 40:288, 1996.
16. Fontanarosa PB: Electrical shock and lightning strike. *Ann Emerg Med* 22(part 2):378, 1993.
17. Holle RL, Lopez RE, Howard KW, et al: Safety in the presence of lightning. *Semin Neurol* 15:375, 1995.

CARBON MONOXIDE POISONING

Keith W. Van Meter

Carbon monoxide (CO) exposure and toxicity is a potentially lethal disorder with immediate and delayed side effects.

EPIDEMIOLOGY

In the United States and most industrialized countries, CO is the single toxin responsible for more mortality and morbidity than any other.[1,2] Industrial sources of CO include fossil fuel engine exhaust, gas- or coal-heater emissions, smoke from accidental fires, and fumes from cupolas of steel foundries, pulp paper mills, or formaldehyde-producing plants. Indoor burning of charcoal—particularly in some countries such as Korea, with a tradition of charcoal subfloor home heating—produces a disproportionate level of accidental CO intoxication.[3] Unintentional CO toxicity and deaths are more common in northern climates and during the winter months.[4]

Interestingly, industrial sources produce slightly less environmental CO per land area as compared with CO produced from the burning of tropical forests.[5] Little is known about the impact these low atmospheric levels have on health. It is known that regular cigarette smoking can produce carboxyhemoglobin (HbCO) levels of 5 to 10 percent, and this chronic CO exposure is implicated in the acceleration of atherosclerosis seen in smokers. Truck drivers sitting in the cabs of their vehicles in heavy traffic can reach similar levels of HbCO as tobacco smokers. Besides combustion, CO toxicity can develop when inhaled methylene chloride vapor in paint strippers or from leaking "bubble" electric Christmas tree lights is slowly metabolized to produce CO.[6]

PATHOPHYSIOLOGY

CO is an odorless, clear gas (in extremely high concentrations, it has a lavender odor), with a density of 0.97 that of air. In most instances, CO mixes evenly in turbulent air. A small amount of CO is endogenously produced from the metabolism of hemoglobin to bilirubin and HbCO levels rise in hemolytic anemia. CO may function as an endogenous central nervous system (CNS) neurotransmitter.[7]

CO forms a ligand with respiratory pigments and enzymes such as hemoglobin, myoglobin, cytochrome P-450, and cytochrome aa_3. In fact, cytochrome P-450 was named after the *peak* (p) absorption of light at 450 μm when the enzyme is 50% saturated with CO. Respiratory enzymes have varying binding affinities for CO compared to oxygen. For example, CO bonds with hemoglobin 210 to 280 times as tenaciously as oxygen, but CO has only one-ninth the affinity of oxygen for cytochrome aa_3.[8] When CO competes with oxygen for binding sites, it prevents utilization of oxygen by that enzyme or pigment. Thus, HbCO will carry less oxygen according to the number of binding sites occupied by CO.

In addition, the binding of CO to hemoglobin also transforms the oxyhemoglobin dissociation curve from a sigmoid shape to an asymptotic shape, increasing the ability of HbCO to hold on to oxygen at the remaining heme moiety sites (Fig. 198-1). In CO toxicity, both the reduced oxygen carriage and the transformation of oxyhemoglobin dissociation curve impair tissue oxygen delivery. In effect, high HbCO imposes the equivalent of a sudden "chemical" anemia in the patient. The tolerance of the patient to this sudden chemical anemia may be worse than its hemorrhagic equivalent because of the toxic effects of CO on other respiratory pigments and enzymes. While tissue oxygen delivery is decreased, CO delivery still occurs by the dissolved CO in the circulating plasma. Experimental exchange transfusion in dogs of autologous red blood cells (RBCs) exposed extracorporeally to CO before transfusion, resulting in HbCO 60%, demonstrated no signs of CO toxicity. Thus, while impairment of O_2 delivery by reduction of O_2 carriage is a part of CO toxicity, it may be that delivery of CO contributes more to the toxic effects of CO. In fact, hemoglobin may provide a protective buffer, preferentially binding CO and preventing binding to other respiratory pigments and mitochondrial cytochromes.

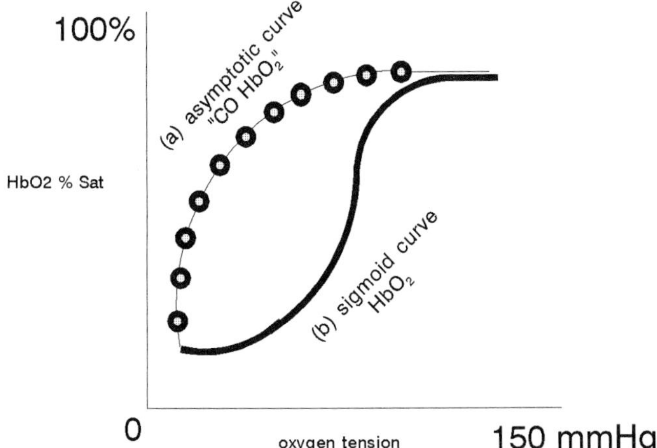

FIG. 198-1. HbCO "shift to the left" by reshaping of the Hbo_2 dissociation curve [(a) hyperbaric oxygen (Hbo_2) asymptotic and (b) Hbo_2 sigmoid]. (Remember, decrements in temperature, H^+ concentration, CO_2 and DPG levels also "shift to the left" of the Hbo_2 dissociation curve in a similar fashion.)

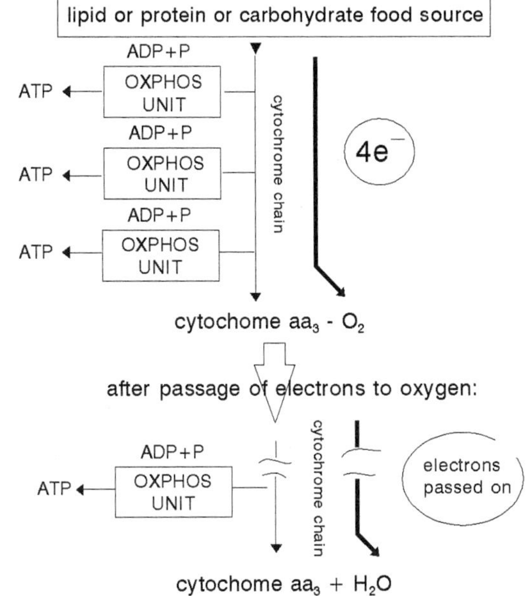

FIG. 198-2. Nascent oxygen can attach to cytochrome aa_3. Oxygen, with its electron-deficient shell, becomes an electron sink (electrophile). Oxygen attached to cytochrome aa_3 in this manner prevents the formation of intermediate destructive oxygen free radicals ($O^{\bar{\cdot}}$, OH^-, and H_2O_2). Water is the end product instead.

CO binding to mitochondrial cytochromes stops electrons—derived from aerobic metabolism of lipids, protein and carbohydrates—from flowing through the cytochrome chain. The cytochrome chain "encases" the fall in energy level of the electrons, allowing a four-electron reduction of nascent O_2 attached to cytochrome aa_3 at the end of the mitochondrial cytochrome chain. Thus, oxygen gets reduced to H_2O without formation of potentially destructive oxygen free radical intermediates, such as $O^{\bar{\cdot}}$, OH^-, and H_2O_2[8] (Fig. 198-2). As electrons pass down the cytochrome chain, energy is captured and stored by the generation of ATP in a process called *oxidative phosphorylation.* CO binding to cytochrome aa_3 prevents the attachment of O_2, preventing the reduction of O_2 to H_2O. The cessation of cytochrome oxidative phosphorylation causes CO to "wreck the machine," as Haldane so aptly described the role of CO toxicity in aerobic metabolism.

CO binds strongly to intracellular pigments, such as myoglobin. In muscle with high oxygen utilization, such as the heart, the binding of CO to myoglobin markedly reduces the availability of oxygen for aerobic metabolism. CO poisoning of myocardial myoglobin reduces myocardial contractility, diminishes cardiac output, and further decreases tissue oxygen delivery.

CO toxicity, by imposing ischemic damage, causes white blood cells to become adherent to endothelial surfaces of tissue microvasculature on reperfusion of ischemic tissue.[9] Immediately after reperfusion of ischemic CO-poisoned tissue, products from these adherent white cells accelerate cell membrane lipid peroxidation, a process termed *reperfusion injury.*[10]

CLINICAL FEATURES

High-oxygen-extracting organs like the brain and the heart easily become dysfunctional from CO intoxication. Neurologic symptoms and signs include fatigue, malaise or flulike symptoms, nausea, difficulty in thinking, emotional lability, dizziness, paresthesias, weakness, vomiting, lethargy, somnolence, stroke, coma, seizure, or respiratory arrest. Cardiovascular symptoms and signs include chest pain from myocardial ischemia, palpitations from dysrhythmias, mildly to severely mottled skin from diminished circulation, poor capillary refill, hypotension, or cardiac arrest. In a pattern of secondary injury from ischemia imposed by CO poisoning, the following clinical injury syndromes may occur[11]:

1. Rhabdomyolysis
2. Noncardiogenic pulmonary edema (NCPE)
3. Multiorgan failure (MOF)
4. Disseminated intravascular coagulation
5. Dermal blistering or increased dermal susceptibility to dermal pressure wounding
6. ''Interval CO syndrome'' of leukoencephalopathy of the centrum ovale (cerebral subcortical white matter) along with ischemic damage to basal ganglia and hippocampus
7. Acute tubular necrosis

It has been observed that the symptoms and signs of CO toxicity are exacerbated by circumstances that increase neurologic and myocardial oxygen demand. It is common that patients will describe the onset of symptoms while at rest and a marked increase after physical exertion. One example would be a patient who develops toxicity from using an internal combustion engine in a closed space. Starting to feel ill, the patient walks or runs outside to fresh air, only to collapse as his or her brain and heart are not able to utilize oxygen to meet the increased metabolic demands. It has also been observed that CO intoxication is more severe in patients who have increased oxygen demands from the comorbidity of trauma, concurrent drug ingestion, burns, myocardial ischemia, cerebrovascular disease, and smoke inhalation.[12]

DIAGNOSIS

Signs and symptoms of CO injury correlate reasonably well with on-the-scene co-oximetry determination of HbCO. However, by the time the patient gets to the ED after breathing air and with prehospital oxygen administration, the positive predictive value (PPV) of HbCO levels falls considerably. A very careful history, coupled with a careful screening neurologic examination that includes a CO neuropsychometric screening battery (CONSB), is a sensitive but not specific assay for CO intoxication. The CONSB has a good PPV for discerning neurologic dysfunction or injury from CO intoxication.[13,14] The CONSB should be done with the patient breathing room air to be most sensitive.

Patients with CO exposure and only mild symptoms (no loss of consciousness, no cardiopulmonary symptoms, awake and cooperative) require minimal ancillary testing: a measure of HbCO and possibly an electrocardiogram (ECG) to detect silent myocardial ischemia. Patients with moderate to severe exposures should have additional studies done to assess the extent of ischemic injury.

1. Co-oximetry determination of HbCO measures actual levels. Pulse oximetry confuses HbCO for oxyhemoglobin and gives spuriously high values for percent of oxygen saturation.[15]
2. The extent of metabolic acidosis—as measured by the serum pH, serum bicarbonate level, or serum lactate level—is a measure of the ischemic damage. CO, by blocking the cytochrome chain, reduces pyruvate utilization by the Krebs cycle, and the excess pyruvate is metabolized to lactate (Fig. 198-3). The arterial blood gases (ABG), serum electrolytes, and serum lactate are used to detect metabolic acidosis.
3. A complete blood count (CBC) will help in evaluating hemoglobin level to estimate arterial oxygen content (Cao_2).
4. The ECG is indicated if the patient has chest pain, palpitations, or dysrhythmia on the monitoring lead. The ECG should also be used in older patients who may have silent myocardial ischemia.
5. The extent of myocardial injury can be measured by serum CK isoenzyme (CK-MB) and troponin levels.
6. The extent of skeletal muscle injury (e.g., rhabdomyolysis) can be measured by serum CK, serum myoglobin, and urine myoglobin.
7. For patients short of breath, with abnormal ausculatory findings, or with multiple trauma, the chest radiograph is indicated.
8. Urine toxicologic screens can be useful when concurrent drug ingestion is suspected.
9. Computed tomography (CT) and magnetic resonance imaging (MRI) of the brain are modestly sensitive but nonspecific in documenting CNS ischemic injury 6 h after CO exposure.[16] Diffusion-weighted MRI brain scanning is being investigated for its utility in defining brain injury from CO intoxication.
10. Single-photon-emission computed tomography (SPECT) with radiolabeled hexamethylpropylene amine oxime (HMPAO–technetium 99m) is immediately sensitive but not specific for acute ischemic CNS injury in CO poisoning.[17] The brain HMPAO/SPECT scan has the advantage that the radionuclide may be initially injected as the patient arrives in the emergency department without interrupting the resuscitation effort. The patient can be scanned later after stabilization, with a lasting ''snapshot'' of pre-resuscitation brain metabolism and perfusion. The bulk of HMPAO is taken up by the brain on first pass as it crosses the blood-brain barrier. Accordingly, the HMPAO ''locks'' into CNS tissue without much redistribution during the successive half-lives of the HMPAO radionuclide. The positron emission tomography (PET) brain scan may be helpful in illustrating CNS ischemic injury, but the scanner is rarely available and hard to have on-line for critically injured patients.

SPECIFIC ISSUES

CO intoxication is especially harsh on the very old and very young. It does not differentiate as to gender. Pregnant patients with CO intoxication have no greater risk, but the fetus is at greater risk than the mother for ischemic injury due the greater affinity of fetal hemoglobin than adult hemoglobin for CO.[18]

CO intoxication is more severe in patients with the comorbidity of multiple trauma, thermal or chemical burns, smoke inhalation, cerebral ischemia, or myocardial ischemia. CO intoxication coupled with drug intoxicants increases the risk of failure at self-evacuation from a toxic atmosphere. Further, concurrent inhalation of inert gas (natural gas), carbon dioxide, or chemical asphyxiants (NO, H_2S, HCN) can augment ischemic insult in a CO patient.

Missed diagnosis of CO intoxication is a potential malpractice liability for the emergency physician. The return of a patient to a yet unidentified toxic environment must be prevented. In particular, the failure to understand that serious CO intoxication with residual ischemic injury may exist in a patient even with low HbCO levels has led to malpractice judgments against the emergency physician. In addition, the failure to identify, in a CO-injured patient, nonresponse to normobaric oxygen treatment and hence the failure to access hyperbaric oxygen treatment has resulted in large awards to the patient.

TREATMENT

The ABCs (airway, breathing, and circulation) of resuscitation apply to the seriously ill or injured victim with presumed CO intoxication. Normobaric oxygen (NBO) therapy should be administered as soon as possible with 100% oxygen by mask [nonrebreathing mask with reservoir (NRMR)]. Patients who require ventilatory assistance should

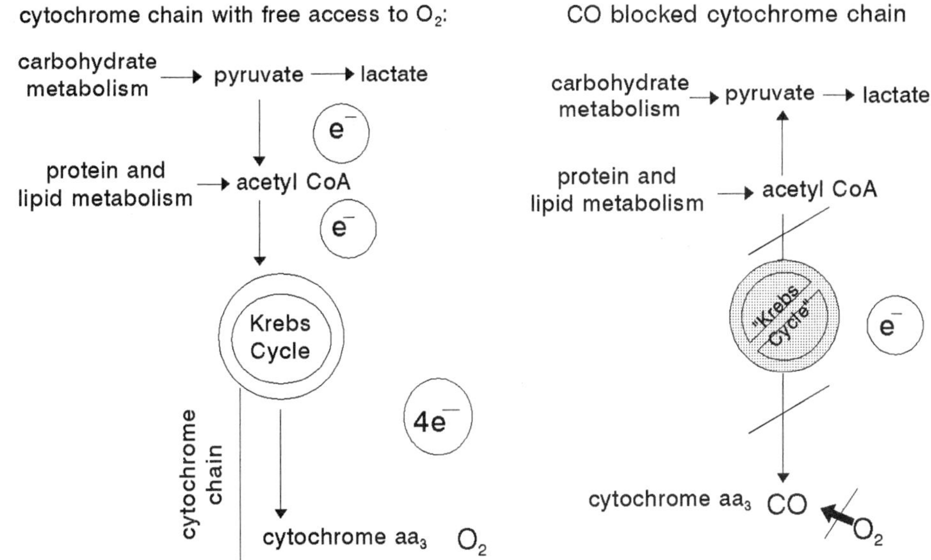

FIG. 198-3. In mitochondria, the cytochrome aa_3 CO ligand brings to a halt the orderly flow of electrons from food sources to oxygen. As a result, pyruvate stops its entry into the Krebs cycle and redirects its metabolic route to formation of lactate.

have bag-valve-mask (BVM) ventilation with 100% oxygen until spontaneous ventilation recovery or endotracheal intubation can be performed in the field or the ED.

Once the patient reaches the ED, decisions about further treatment are guided by the clinical evaluation (Table 198-1). Patients with only mild symptoms (nausea, headache, weakness, or flulike malaise) should receive 100% NBO for a period of about 4 h, with periodic reassessment. The ability of oxygen treatment to eliminate CO from the body has often been estimated using the half-life of HbCO with different treatment regimens. As noted above, HbCO may be a poor marker of the severity of CO poisoning. The half-life of HbCO is about 320 min by breathing room air, 60 min by breathing 100% NBO, and 23 min with 100% hyperbaric oxygen (HBO) at 2.8 atmospheres of pressure (2.8 ATA). Failure of mild symptoms to resolve after 4 h of NBO administration, if no other likely cause for the symptoms can be found, should lower the emergency clinician's threshold for the use of HBO therapy.

Major symptoms (any history of loss of consciousness, amnesia, or myocardial ischemia) have traditionally been an indication for initial HBO treatment.[1,14] While dramatic improvement in symptoms and signs is generally seen, there is continued debate as to whether HBO is better than NBO with regard to short- and long-term outcomes.[19]

TABLE 198-1 Treatment Recommendations for CO Toxicity

Mild CO Toxicity	Serious CO Toxicity
Weakness Nausea Dizziness Headache Mildly abnormal CONSB (with patient on room air while testing)	Loss of consciousness or near syncope Confusion (moderately abnormal CONSB) Focal neurologic changes Myocardial ischemia Persisting hypotension Persisting acidosis Pregnant mother with HbCO >15% Concurrent injury or intoxication
100% NBO for 4 h	HBO 90-min treatment session
Reassess; if symptoms persist, consider HBO versus continued NBO	Reassess after first treatment; if symptoms persist, repeat HBO in 3–6 h

Key: CONSB, CO neuropsychometric screening battery; NBO, normobaric oxygen; HBO, hyperbaric oxygen.

Prospective, randomized studies comparing HBO and NBO have yielded conflicting results, possibly due to different entry criteria, the intensity of the outcome measure, and the duration of follow-up.[20–22] There appears to be some benefit to HBO in reducing neurophysiologic sequelae, but that difference may be detectable only with specific testing and the benefit may disappear after 12 months of follow-up.

While the patient is being prepared for referral to a hyperbaric chamber, he or she should be maintained on 100% NBO. Traditional recommendations for HBO treatment for CO poisoning have sometimes stressed the use of HbCO criteria. This approach is no longer advocated because of the poor correlation between clinical symptoms, morbidity, mortality, and ED HbCO levels. In addition, there is no evidence that HBO treatment based on HbCO level alone is beneficial.

The added mortality or morbidity incurred by transport to an HBO treatment facility has been established to occur in less than 5 percent of cases so handled. Both monoplace and multiplace hyperbaric chambers have critical care capability for ventilator support of endotracheally intubated patients, blood pressure monitoring, central venous manometry, and cardiac monitoring. U.S. emergency physicians can find the location of the nearest hyperbaric chamber by calling the Divers Alert Network (DAN), Duke University, Durham, NC, at 1-919-684-8111.

Standard HBO treatment for CO intoxication uses 100% oxygen at 2.4 to 2.8 ATA for 90 min. Most patients with moderate symptoms respond to one treatment, although some may have persistent symptoms that require one or two more treatments during the first 24 h to fully resolve. Treatment costs for HBO are approximately $500 per session, in comparison to about $150 to $200 for 4 h of NBO in an ED.

In addition to enhancing the elimination of CO from the body, HBO treatment has several theoretical advantages over NBO treatment. HBO improves oxygen delivery to ischemic tissue and CO elimination from hemoglobin. HBO, not NBO, lessens CO-induced reperfusion injury by truncating lipid peroxidation and lessening leukocyte endothelial adherence in microvasculature.[9,10]

Complications of HBO treatment include a very low incidence of oxygen-induced seizures (approximately 1 per 1000 patients), ear and sinus barotrauma, pulmonary barotrauma, and vascular gas embolism. Pregnancy is not a contraindication to HBO treatment. The only absolute contraindication to HBO treatment is an untreated pneumothorax.

DISPOSITION

CO-intoxicated patients with mild symptoms (headache, nausea, flulike symptoms, weakness, and dizziness) that remit after 4 h of 100% NBO may be discharged with the proviso that they return for evaluation if symptoms return. Patients should be reevaluated in about 24 to 48 h. If patients with minor symptoms do not improve after 4 h of NBO therapy but the symptoms remit after a single HBO treatment, then the patient can be discharged with the same instructions. If symptoms do not remit, the patient should be admitted with appropriate neurologic consultation.

CO-intoxicated patients with the history of loss of consciousness, amnesia, or seizure should be admitted even if symptoms improve with HBO treatment. CO-intoxicated pregnant patients should be admitted for fetal monitoring. CO-intoxicated patients with evidence of myocardial ischemia should be admitted for evaluation and management.

A subset of CO patients have ''interval CO injury'' or delayed development of neurologic symptomatology from 2 days to 1 month after initial improvement. Discharge instructions should include this information.

Amelioration of neurologic residual injury with delayed treatment has occurred up to at least 20 days postinjury with HBO treatment. A short series of daily ''tailing'' low-dose HBO treatments has been anecdotally used to resolve or ameliorate lingering residual neurologic injury.

REFERENCES

1. Merridith T, Vale A: Carbon monoxide poisoning, *Br Med J* 296:77, 1988.
2. National Center for Health Statistics: *Vital Statistics for the United States, 1990: II. Mortality. Part A.* DHHS publication number 95-1101. Washington DC: NCHS, 1994.
3. Hampson NB, Kramer CC, Dunford RG, Norkool DM: Carbon monoxide poisoning from indoor burning of charcoal briquettes. *JAMA* 271:52, 1994.
4. Centers for Disease Control and Prevention: Deaths from motor-vehicle-related unintentional carbon monoxide poisoning. *MMWR* 45:1029, 1996.
5. Newell RE, Rachle HG, Seiler W: Carbon monoxide and the burning earth. *Sci Am* 261(4):82, 1989.
6. Rioux JP, Myers RAM: Methylene chloride poisoning: A paradigmatic view. *J Emerg Med* 6:227, 1988.
7. Dawson TM, Snyder SH: Gases as biological messengers: Nitric oxide and carbon monoxide in the brain. *J Neurosci* 14:5147, 1994.
8. Piantadosi CA: Carbon monoxide, oxygen transport and oxygen metabolism. *J Hyperbar Med* 2:27, 1987.
9. Thom SR: Functional inhibition of leukocyte B2 integrins by hyperbaric oxygen in carbon monoxide-mediated brain injury in rats. *Toxicol Appl Pharmacol* 123:248, 1993.
10. Thom SR, Elbuken ME: Oxygen-dependent antagonism of lipid peroxidation. *Free Radic Biol Med* 10:413, 1991.
11. Gorman DF, Clayton D, Gilligan JE, Webb RK: A longitudinal study of 100 consecutive admissions for carbon monoxide poisoning to the Royal Adelaide Hospital. *Anesth Intens Care* 20:311, 1992.
12. Goulon M, Barois A, Rapin M, et al: Carbon monoxide poisoning and acute anoxia due to breathing coal gas and hydrocarbons. *J Hyperbar Med* 1:23, 1992.
13. Messeir LD, Myers RAM: A neuropsychological screening battery for emergency assessment of carbon monoxide-poisoned patients. *J Clin Psychol* 47:675, 1991.
14. Thom SR, Keim L: Carbon monoxide poisoning, a review: Epidemiology, pathophysiology, clinical findings and treatment options including hyperbaric oxygen therapy. *Clin Toxicol* 27:141, 1989.
15. Bozeman WP, Myers RAM, Barish RA: Confirmation of the pulse oximetry gap in carbon monoxide poisoning. *Ann Emerg Med* 30:608, 1997.
16. Pracyk JB, Stolp BW, Fife CE, et al: Brain computerized tomography after hyperbaric oxygen therapy for carbon monoxide poisoning. *Undersea Hyperbar Med* 22:1, 1995.
17. Choi IS, Soon KK, Lee SS, Choi YC: Evaluation of outcome of delayed neurologic sequelae after carbon monoxide poisoning by technetium-99m hexamethylpropylene amine oxime brain single photon emission computed tomography. *Eur Neurol* 35:137, 1995.
18. Caravati EM, Adams CJ, Joyce SM, Schafer NC: Fetal toxicity associated with maternal carbon monoxide poisoning. *Ann Emerg Med* 17:714, 1988.
19. Tibbles PM, Perrotta PL: Treatment of carbon monoxide poisoning: A critical review of human outcome studies comparing normobaric oxygen with hyperbaric oxygen. *Ann Emerg Med* 24:269, 1994.
20. Thom SR, Taber RL, Mendiguren II, et al: Delayed neuropsychologic sequelae after carbon monoxide poisoning: prevention by treatment with hyperbaric oxygen. *Ann Emerg Med* 25:474, 1995.
21. Scheinkestel CD, Jones K, Cooper DJ, et al: Interim analysis—controlled clinical trial of hyperbaric oxygen in acute carbon monoxide (CO) poisoning. *Undersea Hyperbar Med* 23(suppl):7, 1996.
22. Mathieu D, Wattel F, Mathieu-Nolf M, et al: Randomized prospective study comparing the effect of HBO versus 12 hours NBO in noncomatose CO poisoned patients: Results of the interim analysis. *Undersea Hyperbar Med* 23(suppl):7, 1996.

RADIATION INJURIES

Pamela L. Piggott

INTRODUCTION

Since 1978, the US Joint Commission on Accreditation of Healthcare Organizations (JCAHO) has required that all hospitals have an active plan to manage radiation accidents. Casualties from radiation accidents are rare events in comparison with other types of hazardous material accidents. However, with today's widespread use of radiation technology in medicine, research, industry, power production, and national defense, there is a growing potential for radiation injuries. Of further importance is the potential of large numbers of casualties from a terrorist attack employing nuclear weapons. An understanding of basic radiation physics and pathogenesis of injury will aid the emergency physician in the triage and initial management of radiation injuries.

The emergency physician must also be prepared for the potential situation in which an individual has gained possession of a radiation source without being aware of its hazard and the individual develops injury. A significant case of this occurred in 1987 in Guiana, Brazil, when a teletherapy source of Cs-137 was released into the public domain. Two weeks elapsed before the radiation accident was fully discovered. Patients with gastrointestinal symptoms were initially misdiagnosed as having a food allergy. One patient with severe radiation skin injury was referred to a specialty center for suspected tropical disease infection. This incident resulted in over 200 contaminations, 20 significant exposures, and 4 deaths. The ability to recognize signs and symptoms of radiation injury will enable the physician to deliver more prompt and effective treatment to these types of patients.

INCIDENCE OF RADIATION ACCIDENTS

The most recognized and comprehensive record of radiation accidents is the registry maintained by an asset of the US Department of Energy, the Radiation Emergency Assistance Center/Training Site (REACTS). Since the inception of the registry in 1944, 403 radiation accidents have been recorded worldwide with victims totaling 133,617 individuals; 2965 with significant exposure and 120 fatalities (Table 199-1). The 1986 Chernobyl accident accounts for 116,500 individuals and 28 acute fatalities. The most frequent radiation accident is one of high-dose local exposure, usually to the hands, from a radiation device. The majority of these accidents have occurred in the industrial setting with inadvertent exposure from radiation devices used in radiography to verify integrity of metals such a pipe welds.[1]

FUNDAMENTALS OF RADIATION PHYSICS

Nonionizing and Ionizing Radiation

The electromagnetic radiation spectrum includes long wavelength, low frequency, low-energy forms of nonionizing radiation and progresses

TABLE 199-1 Major Radiation Accidents Worldwide. Human Experiences 1944–March 1999

Location	Number of Accidents	Persons Involved	Significant Exposures*	Fatalities
US	241	1339	786	30
Outside US	162	132,278	2179	90
	403	133,617	2965	120

*A significant radiation exposure is one in which an individual receives one or more of the following: whole body dose of 0.25 Sv (25 rem) of more, skin dose of 6 Sv (600 rem) or more, other tissue dose of 0.75 Sv (75 rem) or more, or internal contamination level equal to or greater than half of the maximum permissible body burden.
Source: Adapted from Radiation Emergency Assistance Center/Training Site (REACTS) Radiation Accident Registry.

to short wavelength, high frequency, high-energy forms of ionizing radiation. ''Ionizing'' refers to the ability of high-energy radiation to displace electrons from atoms and cause matter through which it passes to become electrically charged. Nonionizing forms include ultraviolet rays, visible rays, infrared rays, microwaves, and radio waves. Lasers, ultrasound, and nuclear magnetic resonance systems are other examples of nonionizing radiation used in the medical field. X-rays and gamma waves are ionizing forms of electromagnetic radiation.

Ionizing radiation is emitted from unstable forms of elements called radioisotopes. An isotope is a variation of an element with a different number of neutrons in the nucleus. Because its number of protons identifies an element, all isotopes of an element have the same number of protons and thus the same atomic number. However, the different numbers of neutrons give isotopes of the same element different atomic weights.

Some isotopes are unstable and spontaneously transform in order to reach a more stable configuration. This transformation is a process called decay or disintegration and may involve the release of ionizing radiation. An isotope that emits ionizing radiation during its decay is referred to as a radioisotope. Radioisotope is a general term for radioactive isotopes of any element and radionuclide is a term that refers to a radioactive isotope of a specific element.

Biological Effect of Ionizing Radiation

The biological effect of ionizing radiation occurs at the cellular level. DNA and other macromolecules of the cell may be directly ionized by radiation or indirectly damaged by highly reactive free radicals created by ionization of cellular water. High levels of radiation exposure may cause direct cell death. More commonly, lower levels of radiation interrupt the cell's reproductive process by damaging the cell's mitotic capability, making it unable to divide. Injury occurs at the time of exposure but the onset of clinical manifestation of radiation injury varies among cell type. Short-lived cells, such as blood cells, are quickly depleted and injury may become evident before new cells are generated. Longer-lived cells, such as the lens of the eye, regenerate slowly and thus injury may not become apparent for years after the exposure.

Radiosensitivity is the response of cells to acute manifestations of radiation injury. In general, poorly differentiated cells and cells with a short life span and high turnover rate are most vulnerable to the detrimental effects of radiation. Rapidly proliferating cells, such as those of the hematopoietic, gastrointestinal, and reproductive systems are more radiosensitive than the more slowly dividing cells of the nervous system and musculoskeletal system.

Types of Ionizing Radiation

Radiation is emitted as either particles or waves. Particulate radiation includes alpha, beta, and neutrons, whereas gamma and x-rays are electromagnetic waves (Table 199-2).

The biological effect of these forms of radiation is a function of the mass, charge, and energy that the type of radiation possesses. Linear Energy Transfer (LET) describes the rate at which radiation deposits its energy as it travels through matter. In general, particulate radiation has a high LET and electromagnetic radiation has a low LET. High LET radiation interacts readily with matter, creating a dense number of ionizations in the matter through which it passes. Thus, high LET radiation dissipates its energy quickly and does not penetrate deeply. This intense ionization in a concentrated area creates a potential for significant biological damage when high LET radiation is deposited internally. Conversely, low LET radiation interacts less readily with matter, creating less ionization along its traveled path. These properties enable low LET radiation to penetrate deeply into body tissue. Exposure to an external source of low LET radiation creates a potential for significant biological damage.

TABLE 199-2 Types of Radiation

Type (Symbol)	Mass*	Charge	Penetration	Shield	Hazard	Source
Alpha (α)	4	+2	Few cm in air	Paper, Keratin layer of skin	Internal contamination only	Transuranic elements, i.e., plutonium found in nuclear weapons and isotope production facilities
Beta (β)	1/200	−1	~8 mm into skin	Clothing	Skin and internal contamination	Most radioisotopes decay by β usually following by γ emission
Neutron (N)	1	0	Variable	Material of high hydrogen content	Whole-body irradiation	Criticality accidents around nuclear power production facilities or nuclear weapons
Gamma (γ)	0	0	Several cm in tissue	Concrete Lead	Whole-body irradiation	Most radioisotopes emit γ following β decay

*Approximate measurement in atomic mass units (AMU).

ALPHA PARTICLES Alpha radiation is a heavy, highly charged particle composed of 2 protons and 2 neutrons. Because of its large mass and charge, alpha particles travel at a low velocity and interact readily with matter. Alpha particles have the highest LET of the different types of radiation and therefore deposit a large amount of energy in a small volume of tissue. However, an alpha particle dissipates its energy quickly, traveling only a few centimeters in air. Alpha radiation is easily shielded and cannot penetrate paper. The keratin layer of skin also blocks alpha particles. Thus alpha radiation possesses a significant biological hazard only when internalized. Heavy radioisotopes with an atomic number above 82, such as uranium and plutonium, are sources of alpha particle emission.

BETA PARTICLES Beta particles have a smaller mass and charge and generally have a greater velocity than alpha particles. When compared to alpha, beta particles have a lower LET, interacting with matter to a lesser extent and creating less ionization along the path it travels. These properties enable beta radiation to travel further and penetrate deeper than alpha radiation. Beta radiation penetrates approximately 8 mm into exposed skin and can cause serious burns. Like alpha, beta is also a hazard if internally deposited but to a lesser extent. Most radioisotopes decay by beta radiation followed by gamma emission.

NEUTRONS Neutrons are electrically neutral particles with a wide range of energy, velocity, and penetration power. Exposure to neutrons is unique. Unlike irradiation by other forms, high-level neutron exposure can induce radioactivity. That is, neutron irradiation can cause previously stable atoms of the absorbing material to become radioactive. In human tissue, the induced radioactive isotope is primarily Na-24, which can be detected in blood and urine specimens. In peacetime, neutron exposure is unlikely and sources of neutrons are limited primarily to nuclear power plants, particle accelerators, and weapon assembly sites.

GAMMA AND X-RAYS Gamma and x-rays are electromagnetic waves with no mass and no charge that travel at the speed of light. These rays have a low LET, creating sparse ion pairs as they travel through tissue. X-rays are generated by excitation of the orbital electrons while gamma is a photon emitted from the nucleus. X-rays have longer wavelengths, lower frequency, and lower energy than gamma rays. Gamma rays are the most penetrating type of ionizing radiation and travel several meters in air and many centimeters into tissue. Exposure to an external source of gamma or high-energy x-rays presents a significant whole-body radiation hazard and high doses may result in acute radiation syndrome.

Units of Measure

Radiation can be measured as activity, exposure, or dose (Table 199-3). Conventional units include the curie, roentgen, rad, and rem. The International System (SI), is now more widely used and includes the becquerel, gray, and sievert.

The curie (Ci) and becquerel (Bq) are units of activity and describe the amount of radioactivity present. A radioisotope's activity is a function of its rate of decay or number of disintegrations per second. The roentgen (R) is a unit of exposure and measures the amount of x or gamma radiation that produces a given number of ionizations in air. The roentgen is not applicable to particulate types of radiation. Many radiation survey instruments record exposure rate per hour of x or gamma radiation. The SI equivalent of roentgen is coulomb per kilogram (coul/kg). The rad (r) and gray (Gy) are units of absorbed dose and reflect the amount of energy that the radiation imparts to matter through which it passes. These units are used for photon as well as particulate radiation and are not restricted to measurement in air.

Because the different types of radiation have different magnitudes of biological effect on man, units of dose-equivalent are used to provide a common scale of measurement for the different types of radiation. The rem and sievert (Sv) are units of dose-equivalent and are obtained by multiplying the absorbed dose by modifying factors. Differentiation between units of absorbed dose and dose equivalent is most important with high LET radiation, particularly alpha radiation. Because of the large amount of energy that alpha particles deposit in a concentrated area, alpha's potential for biological damage is greater. The dose equivalent of alpha radiation is approximately 20 times the absorbed dose. In other words, one rad (or gray) of alpha radiation is approximately equivalent to 20 rem (or sievert).

For beta, x, and gamma radiation, the dose equivalent is essentially equal to the absorbed dose. In simplified terms, a rad (or gray) of beta, x, or gamma radiation is roughly equivalent to a rem (or sievert). For these types of low LET radiation, units of absorbed dose and dose-equivalent are often used interchangeably.

TABLE 199-3 Radiation Units of Measure

Description	Conventional Units	SI Unit	Conversion
Activity Units of activity describe the amount of radioactivity present. These units reflect the rate of decay or the number of disintegrations occurring per second (dps). 1 Ci = 3.7×10^{10} dps. 1 Bq = 1 dps.	Curie (Ci)	Becquerel (Bq)	1 Bq ~ 2.7×10^{-11} Ci 1 Ci ~ 3.7×10^{10} Bq
Exposure Units of exposure measure the amount of X or gamma radiation that produces a given number of ionizations in air.	Roentgen (R)	coul/kg	1 R = 2.58×10^{-4} coul/kg
Adsorbed Dose Units of absorbed dose can be applied to any type of radiation and reflects the energy imparted to matter	Rad (r)	Gray (Gy)	1 rad = 0.01 Gy 1 Gy = 100 rad
Dose Equivalent Units that provide a common scale of measure for the different types or radiation. These units are calculated by multiplying the absorbed dose by modifying factors that take into account the different biological effect of different radiation types.	Rem	Sievert (Sv)	1 rem = 0.01 Sv 1 Sv = 100 rem
Internalized Radiation Term that reflects the amount of radiation that will be delivered to the body from internally deposited radioisotopes.	Body burden	N/A	

TABLE 199-4 Radiation Monitoring Equipment

Equipment Type	Device	Common Type of Measurement	Units Commonly Recorded
Dosimeter	TLD or film badge	Cumulative dose of beta, x, and gamma	Rem or Sievert
Dosimeter	Pocket dosimeter	Cumulative exposure to x and gamma	mR
Survey meter	GM tube	Low exposure rates of x, gamma, and beta	cpm*
Survey meter	Ion chamber	Higher exposure rates of x and gamma	mR/h

*2500 cpm is approximately 1 mR/h.

Body burden is used in reference to internally deposited radioactive material. Different radionuclides will deliver varying amounts of radiation to the body when internalized. The amount of radioactivity that may be present in the body for a working lifetime and pose no reasonable expectation of health risk is referred to as the Maximum Permissible Body Burden (MPBB). The amount of internally deposited radioactive material is quantified as a percentage of the MPBB that has been established for the particular radionuclide. The MPBB is based on continuous exposure in a working lifetime, thus the MPBB must be interpreted with caution in an accident setting involving acute exposure. Annual Limit of Intake (ALI) is a newer term that is also used to quantify internally deposited radioactive material.

Radiation Monitoring Equipment

Common radiation monitoring equipment includes dosimeter and survey meters (Table 199-4). Dosimeters are small devices that are typically worn on the upper torso to record the cumulative amount of radiation an individual receives while wearing the device. Survey instruments are rate meters that record the amount of radiation detected in an area per unit of time.

PERSONAL DOSIMETERS A thermoluminescent dosimeter (TLD), or film badge, is used to provide permanent records of cumulative-dose received. Most of these devices measure beta, x, and gamma radiation. The dose is recorded in rem or sievert. Dose measurements are not immediately available to the wearer because both of these devices require processing. Self-reading pocket dosimeters may be used in addition to TLDs. These devices provide immediate estimates of cumulative exposure of x and gamma radiation. Most pocket dosimeters can be directly read when held up to a light source. Estimates are typically recorded in milliroentgen (mR).

RADIATION SURVEY METERS Ion chambers are common types of survey meters for recording exposure rates of x and gamma radiation. Some types of ion chambers are equipped to also detect beta radiation with a Mylar (Dupont) window beneath a removable shield. These instruments are usually calibrated in mR/h. Geiger-Müeller (GM) instruments are commonly used to perform surveys for external contamination. These instruments detect lower exposure rates of x and gamma radiation, as well as beta radiation. With special instrument probes, alpha radiation can also be detected. The units recorded are typically counts per minute (cpm). For comparison, 2500 cpm is approximately equal to 1 mR/h.

RADIATION ACCIDENT PREPARATION

Every EMS system should have a prehospital plan for the evacuation of victims from a radiation disaster. The scene is first evaluated for safety and containment of contamination, and radiation counters provided for prehospital personnel. HAZMAT is often the responsible agency. Scene safety must be assured before evacuation begins. Every hospital should have a written protocol detailing instructions for receiving and treating radiation accident victims. The initial medical evaluation and treatment of the victims often falls under the purview of the emergency physician, so that the emergency physician should take an active role in the development of the hospital's radiation accident plan. Several publications are available to provide specific detailed guidance for the development of an Emergency Department Radiation Accident Protocol, as well as prehospital management of radiation accident victims.[2,3]

Emergency Department Notification

Local facilities that may potentially refer a radiation accident victim to the emergency department should be identified in advance and instructed to provide as much advance notification of potential incidents as possible to allow adequate time for mobilization of resources and the physical preparation of the emergency department. When receiving notification of a radiation accident, the emergency physician should request information that will facilitate the necessary preparation for receiving and treating the patient. Useful information to obtain includes:

1. Circumstances of the accident
2. Number of victims
3. Medical condition and physical injuries of the victims
4. Type and extent of radiological insult: irradiated, externally contaminated, or internally contaminated
5. Identification of the radioactive material
6. Exposure to other hazardous material that may be chemically toxic or corrosive.

This notification should serve to activate the Emergency Department Radiation Accident Protocol. The protocol should clearly identify the members and individual responsibilities of the radiation emergency response team as well as the location and contents of the radiation emergency supply kit. Additionally, the protocol should include specific details for the physical preparation of the emergency department and staff that is necessary to safely receive and treat a radiation accident victim. Such preparations, outlined in Table 199-5, are time-consuming and should be initiated prior to the patient's arrival.

Initial activation of the protocol should include requesting assistance from predetermined local radiation specialists and, ideally, health physics professionals. Radiation specialists may assist by monitoring radiation dose of personnel, surveying personnel and areas for contamination, directing contamination control and decontamination efforts, and disposing of contaminated wastes. If faced with a severe or extensive radiological accident, additional sources of assistance are provided at the end of this chapter.

Triage and Treatment Philosophies

Managing hazardous material accidents of *any* type requires health care providers to perform the following initial key actions:

TABLE 199-5 Key Contamination Control Principles

Emergency Department Preparation

1. A separate and controlled entrance into the hospital is established in advance.
2. An area for decontamination and treatment of victims is identified in advance. This is often referred to as the Radiation Emergency Area (REA) and should be located apart from the usual flow of hospital traffic.
3. Pregnant women, nonessential personnel and equipment are removed from the area.
4. Equipment and supplies are obtained from preassembled emergency kits that are stored in or nearby the REA. Kits should contain supplies for REA set-up and decontamination, personal dosimeters, radiation survey meters, and specimen collection containers.
5. Boundaries are established that clearly demarcate "clean" from potentially contaminated areas.
   a. Radiation warning signs are posted.
   b. The pathway from the ambulance entrance to the REA is marked off with rope boundaries.
   c. Floors of the pathway and REA are covered with nonskid plastic. Floor coverings are secured with tape.
   d. Control point is established for entering and exiting the REA.
6. If airborne contamination is a possibility, the area ventilation system is turned off.

Patient Arrival and Evaluation

1. Emergency Response Team members don protective clothing and dosimeters.
   a. Standard emergency protective equipment is adequate and should include water-repellent coveralls or aprons and shoe covers, surgical cap and mask, eye protection, and double pair of latex gloves.
   b. Inner gloves are taped in place and outer pair is changed after handling contaminated items.
   c. Dosimeters are attached on the torso to the outside of the outermost clothing.
2. Emergency Response Team meets the ambulance outside the ED to assess the patient. If medically stable, the patient is transferred onto a clean stretcher prior to transporting into the hospital.
3. All potentially contaminated clothing or items are placed in plastic bags or plastic lined waste containers and labeled.
4. No persons, equipment, or material should leave the REA until monitored and cleared by Health Physics personnel or the Radiation Safety Officer.
5. If emergency intervention or treatment is required outside the REA, i.e., CT scans or surgery, this should not be delayed because of contamination. Covering the patient and gurney with sheets prior to transporting can minimize contamination spread.

- secure the safety of the accident scene
- provide lifesaving emergency care
- limit exposure to the hazardous substance
- contain the spread of the hazardous substance

Additional precautions are required when managing radiation accidents because, unlike hazardous material of other types, radiation can be detected only by monitoring devices. After scene safety is secured and emergent resuscitation and stabilization is provided, medical management of these patients must employ the use of protective equipment and monitoring devices. Practices of dose reduction, contamination control, and decontamination are necessary in order to protect the safety of patients, health care providers, and the environment.

Radiation accidents can be most effectively managed if the patients are separated into one of the following three situations: (1) externally contaminated patients, (2) internally contaminated patients, or (3) externally irradiated patients. Each patient type requires specific treatment considerations, which are discussed below and illustrated in Table 199-6. If there are multiple casualties, triage is based on the patient's acute medical condition. If all patients are medically stable, the order listed above is the suggested priority for providing treatment.

CLINICAL PRESENTATION AND MANAGEMENT

Externally Contaminated Patients

A patient is externally contaminated when radioactive materials are physically deposited onto the patient's skin or clothing. All victims of radiation accidents should be handled as if contaminated until known otherwise. Upon arrival to the hospital, all patients should be surveyed for contamination. If radiation-monitoring devices are not available, patients should be routinely decontaminated and then surveyed for contamination when monitoring equipment is obtained.

The dose from external contamination to either the patient or the attending medical staff is rarely significant. Spreading the contamination in the environment and the potential of internalization are the main hazards with external contamination. Thus special precautions are required for receiving and treating these patients. The hospital's radiation response team should be trained in radiation monitoring and decontamination techniques. Specific contamination control principles and physical decontamination techniques are required for the care of these patients (Tables 199-5 and 199-7).

It is not immediately crucial to know the identity of the radionuclide, however it is important to determine whether the nuclide emits beta-gamma radiation and/or alpha radiation. Commonly used radiation survey meters easily detect beta and gamma radiation. Detection of alpha radiation requires special instrument probes and careful monitoring techniques. Alpha radiation is shielded by any moisture, including perspiration and blood. Therefore, only trained individuals should perform surveys for alpha-emitting contamination.

Internally Contaminated Patients

Radioactive material gains entry into the body by three principal routes: inhalation, ingestion, or absorption from contaminated mucous membranes or abraded skin. Misadministration of a radiopharmaceutical is a potential source of internal contamination that can occur in the hospital setting. Internal contamination becomes a major concern of the population if large amounts of radioactive material are released into the atmosphere as a result of nuclear weapon detonation, large-scale nuclear power plant accident, or even a volcanic eruption. Such events may result in inhalation of airborne radioactive material or ingestion of radioactive material deposited onto agricultural land with subsequent transfer into the food chain.

Internal contamination is medically significant because internally deposited radioactive material will continue to irradiate tissues until it decays to a stable isotope or is biologically eliminated. As with other types of radiation exposure, the dose received depends on the amount and energy of the radioactive material and the time exposed. Additionally, the route of intake into the body, the biochemical form, and the physical and biological half-life of the particular radionuclide affect the dose received from internal contamination. The biochemical nature of the radionuclide determines if it is disseminated throughout the body or concentrated in a specific organ. The term critical organ is used to describe the organ that receives the highest dose of radiation or is the site of the most significant biological damage.

IDENTIFICATION AND MEASUREMENT In contrast to external contamination, identification of the specific radionuclides that become internalized is important for determining the method of treatment. When the substance is not known, laboratory identification is possible. Internally deposited radionuclides are identified by radioanalysis of substances excreted from the body. Radiochemistry laboratories identify and quantify the specific radionuclides by analyzing swabs from nares, oropharynx, and wounds, as well as sputum, urine, and fecal specimens. This technique of internal dose assessment is referred to as an excretion method or bioassay measurement. Internal dose assessment by this method requires that all body excreta from internally

TABLE 199-6 Initial Medical Management of Radiation Accident Victims

Radiological Insult	Key Actions
Prior to Patient Arrival	• Contact radiation specialists for assistance. • Assemble the hospital's Radiation Emergency Response Team and supply kit. • Establish the Radiation Emergency Treatment Area as outlined in Table 199-5. • Provide all team members with personal dosimetry and appropriate protective clothing.
For All Cases of Radiation Injury	• Perform resuscitation and stabilization of medical conditions. • Obtain complete history to determine the type of radiological insult. • Survey the body for possible external contamination. • Obtain swabs of nares, oropharynx, and wounds, as well as urine specimens for evaluation of possible internal uptake of contamination. • Obtain baseline CBC and differential. • Contact radiation specialists for assistance.
External Contamination	• Initiate contamination control practices and decontaminate techniques described in Tables 199-5 and 199-7.
Internal Contamination	• After swabs have been obtained, irrigate wounds with normal saline. • Begin collection of body excreta (sputum, urine, feces, emesis) for bioassay to identify and quantify radioisotopes. • Continue collection of urine and feces for 4 days to monitor excretion rate. • If ingestion is suspected, begin gut decontamination methods. • If high levels of contamination are suspected, particularly radioiodine or alpha-emitting radiation, obtain expert consultation for assistance with decorporation procedures.
Irradiation	• Obtain blood specimens for dose estimation and for cell and HLA typing. • Document time of onset of all symptoms, i.e., anorexia, nausea, vomiting. • Symptomatic treatment, i.e., antiemetics, pain management, anxiolytics. • Supportive treatment, i.e., IV fluids, blood products, TPN • Consider prophylactic measures, i.e., reverse isolation, prophylactic antibiotics and antifungals. • If severe bone marrow suppression is anticipated, consider administration of hematopoietic growth factors. • If neutron irradiation is a concern, obtain blood and urine specimens and monitor for induced radioactivity of Na-24. Monitor all metals on the patient's body for induced radioactivity.

contaminated patients be collected. The collection should continue for several days because repeated measurements are used to monitor the excretion rates of the contamination.

Radioactivity within the body can also be measured in vivo by a device called a whole-body counter. These detectors predominately measure gamma-emitting radiation and some high-energy beta radiation. Internalized alpha and lower-energy beta-emitting radiation do not escape from the body and are not detected by these devices. Whole-body counters are very sensitive and give false measurements if external contamination is present on the body. For this reason and because these detectors are not readily accessible, whole body counters are generally not practical in the acute setting of a radiation accident.

TABLE 199-7 Key Decontamination Techniques

1. Remove patient's clothing. This may remove as much as 90% of external contamination. Ideally, this is done at the accident scene prior to transport.
2. Place patient on a table allowing for washing and drainage with collection of wash fluid.
3. Monitor the patient for contamination and document the level and body location of contamination.
4. Wounds and body orifices are the first priority of decontamination because of the potential for systemic absorption. Intact skin with the highest level of surface contamination follows, progressing to the area of lowest contamination.
5. Obtain swab samples from wounds, nares, and oropharynx. If contaminated, suspect absorption, inhalation, or ingestion of radioactive material and initiate irrigation with normal saline. If significant uptake is suspected, request assistance from expert consultants for management of internal contamination.
6. The majority of skin contamination is removed with copious but gentle irrigation. Showering is not recommended unless contamination is extensive.
7. Resurvey the patient after each decontamination attempt. Remaining contamination may be removed with mild detergent and gentle scrubbing. Vigorous decontamination may damage the skin and thus facilitate absorption. Debridement or excision may be necessary if contamination is embedded in a wound.

GENERAL TREATMENT When the contaminating radionuclide is not known, radiochemical laboratory identification of radioisotopes may take several days. Prior to obtaining identification, methods can be initiated for removal of the most commonly encountered radionuclides that are suspected for the particular accident type. As with other hazardous material, treatment is aimed at reducing absorption or hastening elimination. After all swabs have been obtained, wounds should be irrigated with physiological saline.

Pulmonary clearance of inhaled radioactive particles is not effectively enhanced by medications. If large quantities of insoluble radioactive material have been inhaled, bronchopulmonary lavage may be considered. This treatment carries the associated risk of general anesthesia and is performed more commonly in Britain than in this country.

Reduction in gastrointestinal absorption may be accomplished with gastric lavage, emetics, and purgatives. Additionally, antacids containing aluminum cause many metals to precipitate as insoluble hydroxides. Cathartics can then be administered to decrease the transit time of these precipitants.

DECORPORATION TREATMENT Once the radioactive material crosses into the extracellular fluid, incorporation has occurred and elimination is more difficult. Methods of decorporation include blocking agents, isotopic dilution, displacement, mobilizing agents, and chelation. Treatment with blocking agents reduces the uptake of a radioisotope at an organ or metabolic site by saturating the site with a stable form of the isotope. Isotopic dilution therapy involves

TABLE 199-8 Commonly Treated Forms of Internal Contamination

Radionuclide	Primary Route of Intake	Principal Hazard	Treatment Mechanism	Agent	Usual Administration*
I-131	Inhalation Ingestion Percutaneous absorption	Thyroid	Block thyroid uptake	KI	Oral: 390 mg a day for 7 to 14 days
Pu-239	Inhalation Ingestion Absorption through wounds	Bone Liver Lung	Chelation Increase excretion	DTPA	1 g/day for 5 days IV: 1 g in 250 mL NS or 5% dextrose in H_2O over 30 min Aerosol: 1 g in nebulizer; inhale over 15 to 20 min
H-3	Inhalation Ingestion Percutaneous absorption	Whole-body dose	Isotopic dilution Increase excretion	Water	Oral: 3–4 liters a day for 2 wks
Cs-137	Inhalation Ingestion	Whole-body dose	Mobilization Decrease GI uptake	Ferric Ferrocyanide (Prussian blue)	Oral: 1 g in 100–200 mL water tid for several days

*Duration of therapy is based on dose estimations from radiochemical measurements of urine and fecal samples.

administering large quantities of a stable form of the isotope, thus diluting the concentration of the radioisotope. In displacement treatment, a different but similar stable element is administered that will act as a competitor with the radioisotope for an uptake site. Mobilizing agents induce body tissues to release radioisotopes by increasing the natural turnover process. Chelating agents are organic compounds that provide an ion exchange matrix. The exchanging of inorganic ions results in stable nonionized ring complexes that can be excreted.

Frequently treated causes of internal contamination are radioactive forms of iodine, plutonium, cesium, and hydrogen (Table 199-8). Of particular importance and effectiveness are the treatments discussed below for radioiodine and alpha-emitting contamination such as plutonium.

RADIOIODINE Inhalation or ingestion of radioiodine is particularly hazardous to the thyroid with a potential risk of causing hypothyroidism or thyroid cancer. I-131 is the predominant internal contaminate resulting from incidents that involve the release of nuclear fission products such as a nuclear reactor accident or nuclear weapons test. Studies on the health effects of the Chernobyl accident have shown that populations in heavily contaminated areas have an increase in thyroid cancer presumed to have resulted from radioiodine exposure. The number of thyroid cancers reported in these areas continues to increase, with the highest prevalence in individuals who were under the age of 10 years at the time of the accident.[4]

Rapid detection of radioiodine uptake is essential because treatment is most beneficial when administered within 12 hours. Radioiodine is a soluble nuclide that is detected in the urine immediately after exposure. Thus urine excretion measurements are used to provide early identification of radioiodine uptake. A more rapid, but less sensitive, method is direct measurement with a survey meter held over the thyroid gland.

Early administration of stable potassium iodine (KI) is recommended for high levels of accidental radioiodine exposure. Oral administration of 300 mg of stable iodine (390 mg of KI) within one hour of exposure is approximately 90 percent effective at blocking the thyroid uptake of radioiodine. KI administered six hours after exposure reduces thyroid uptake by approximately 50 percent. Little protective effect is seen when KI is given after 12 h of exposure. KI should be continued daily for 7 to 14 days to prevent recycling of radioiodine.[5] Administration of antithyroid medications, such as propylthiouracil or methimazole, may be considered if the time since exposure is more than 12 h.[6] In the event of widespread release of radioiodine, the FDA has approved the use of nonprescription KI. State and local officials are responsible for the procurement and distribution of KI to the general public.

ALPHA CONTAMINATION Early treatment is recommended for contamination with alpha-emitting radionuclides such as Pu-239. Alpha radiation has a high LET with potential for significant damage when internally deposited. This internal contamination hazard is a result of alpha's deposition of large amounts of energy in a short range and thus causing intense ionization in a concentrated area. This potential damage is made worse by the fact that many of the radioisotopes that emit alpha radiation have very long half-lives.

Chelating agents such as calcium and zinc salts of diethylenetriamine pentaacetic acid (Ca-DTPA and Zn-DTPA, respectively) are effective treatments for contamination with heavy metals and rare earths that emit alpha radiation. If alpha-emitting contamination is detected in wounds or in the nares or oropharynx, treatment with DTPA should be initiated promptly, ideally within 1 to 2 h after contamination has occurred. Potential contraindications for the use of DTPA are severe renal dysfunction, thrombocytopenia, or leukopenia. DTPA is administered systemically by slow IV push or by aerosol administration. Ca-DTPA has been shown to be more effective in animal studies and is the preferred form of drug for the initial one to two days of treatment. Zn-DTPA is less toxic and recommended for treatments of longer duration and of pregnant females. For aerosol administration, Ca-DTPA is preferred because of the metallic taste associated with Zn-DTPA. Most DTPA solutions in nuclear medicine departments are a too dilute concentration for effective decorporation. DTPA for this purpose can be obtained from Oak Ridge Associated Universities, REACTS, Oak Ridge, TN 37831.

The success of decorporation techniques depends on early administration. The risks associated with therapy must be weighed against the risk of untreated internal radiation exposure. Assistance from expert consultants should be requested prior to beginning decorporation therapy.

Externally Irradiated Patients

Several general concepts are essential for understanding the radiation injury resulting from exposure to an external source:

1. An acute dose of radiation results in more biological damage than the same radiation dose delivered over a more protracted period of time.

TABLE 199-9 Acute Radiation Syndrome

Approximate Dose	Onset of Prodrome	Duration of Latent Phase	Manifest Illness
>2 Gy (200 rad)	Within 2 days	1–3 weeks	Hematopoietic syndrome with pancytopenia, infection, and hemorrhage.
>6 Gy (600 rad)	Within hours	<1 week	GI syndrome with dehydration, electrolyte abnormalities, GI bleeding, and fulminant enterocolitis.
>30 Gy (3000 rad)	Within minutes	None	CV/CNS syndrome with refractory hypotension and circulatory collapse. Fatal within 24–72 h.

2. Biological injury from radiation occurs at the time of exposure and the clinical signs and symptoms manifest over time.
3. The elapsed time from exposure to the onset of symptoms is inversely related to the radiation dose received.
4. Exposure to penetrating types of radiation (gamma, x-ray, and neutron) results in a whole-body dose. Acute high-level irradiation to a significant portion of the body may result in acute radiation syndrome. Partial-body irradiation may result in local radiation injury.
5. Nonpenetrating types of radiation, alpha and beta, do not deliver a whole-body dose.

Whole-Body Irradiation/Acute Radiation Syndrome

Characteristic and relatively predictable signs and symptoms develop when a significant portion of the body is exposed to a high level of penetrating radiation over a short period of time, typically less that 24 hours.[7] These signs and symptoms are collectively referred to as acute radiation syndrome (ARS) (Table 199-9). A whole-body gamma dose in excess of 2 Gy (200 rad) is the primary cause of acute radiation syndrome. Alpha and low-energy beta radiation lack sufficient energy to penetrate the skin and deliver a whole-body radiation dose. Neutron exposure is rare, but high-level neutron irradiation is also capable of producing ARS. Additionally, there are a few reports of ARS following significant amounts of internal radioactive contamination.

Four distinct phases are seen in the unfolding of ARS: prodromal phase; latent phase; manifested illness phase; and recovery phase or death. The prodromal phase is a transient period of self-limiting symptoms that may occur within minutes, hours, or days after exposure. The acuity of onset and the duration of this phase are directly related to the dose received. The prodromal phase is an autonomic nervous system response that initiates gastrointestinal symptoms such as anorexia, nausea, vomiting, and, with high doses, diarrhea. In addition, neuromuscular symptoms often accompany the autonomic response and may include hypotension, pyrexia, diaphoresis, cephalgia, and fatigue. The latent phase is a symptom-free interval that follows the resolution of the prodromal phase. Shorter latent phases correspond to higher levels of dose received. The latent period may last 1 to 3 weeks with a dose of less than 4 Gy (400 rad), but the latent period may last only a few hours when a dose above 15 Gy (1500 rads) is received.

The manifest illness phase is often divided into three dose-dependent subsyndromes. In ascending order of severity, these syndromes are clinically related to injury of the hematopoietic, gastrointestinal, and cardiovascular/central nervous systems. The toxic effects to these organ systems are not discrete. There is considerable overlap as well as additive detrimental effects among these syndromes.

HEMATOPOIETIC SYNDROME The hematopoietic system is the first organ system to manifest injury from whole-body irradiation and symptoms are seen from doses above 1.5 to 2 Gy (150 to 200 rad). Self-limiting prodromal symptoms begin within several hours or days and typically resolve within 48 hours. An asymptomatic latent period follows and typically lasts for one to three weeks. Radiation destroys circulating lymphocytes and damages stem cells in the bone marrow and lymphatic system. The rapid decline in lymphocytes is a hallmark of the hematopoietic syndrome and is one of the best early indicators of the extent of radiation injury. Granulocytes, and to a lesser extent, platelet counts, display an initial rise followed by an accelerated decrease reaching a nadir at about 30 days. The red blood cell population also decreases in concentration with resultant mild anemia, but to a lesser extent than other blood cell lines. The kinetics of blood cells are discussed below in more detail in reference to dose estimation. The effects of this syndrome result in pancytopenia and immunosuppression with subsequent hemorrhage and infection as the principal causes of morbidity and mortality. Survival is possible with extensive medical intervention.

GASTROINTESTINAL SYNDROME At doses higher than those resulting in the hematopoietic syndrome, toxicity to the gastrointestinal tract occurs. Gastrointestinal syndrome is the second subsyndrome of the manifest illness phase of ARS and may occur after doses above 6 to 7 Gy (600 to 700 rad) are received. This syndrome is distinguished from the hematopoietic syndrome by the onset of nausea, vomiting, and, often, diarrhea within hours after exposure. These prodromal symptoms are followed by a short latent period of one week or less. Reappearance of gastrointestinal symptoms then occurs with severe nausea, vomiting, diarrhea, and abdominal pain. There is damage of the intestinal mucosal barrier with massive fluid losses resulting in profound dehydration and electrolyte disturbances. The denuded gastrointestinal mucosa allows enteric flora to disseminate into the bloodstream. Declines in blood cell populations are similar to that which occurs with the hematopoietic syndrome, but abnormalities occur sooner and with greater magnitude. With the concurrent immunocompromised state, a fulminating enterocolitis follows. There are few documented cases of gastrointestinal syndrome in humans, all of which resulted in fatalities.

CARDIOVASCULAR AND CENTRAL NERVOUS SYSTEM SYNDROME The cardiovascular and central nervous system syndrome is the third subsyndrome of the manifest illness phase of ARS that occurs after doses above 20 to 30 Gy (2000 to 3000 rad) are received. This syndrome presents with immediate prostration, nausea, vomiting, explosive, bloody diarrhea as well as hypotension. Alterations in consciousness including lethargy, disorientation, ataxia, tremors and convulsions occur within hours after exposure. Hypotension is persistent and refractory to treatment. This syndrome is universally fatal with death occurring within 24 to 72 hours, predominately due to circulatory collapse. The lymphocyte count promptly falls to near-zero levels. Granulocytosis develops early and persists until death.

In addition to these organ system injuries of the manifest illness syndromes, radiation doses above 8 to 9 Gy (800 to 900 rad), may damage the pulmonary system with resulting pneumonitis, fibrosis, and interstitial edema.[8]

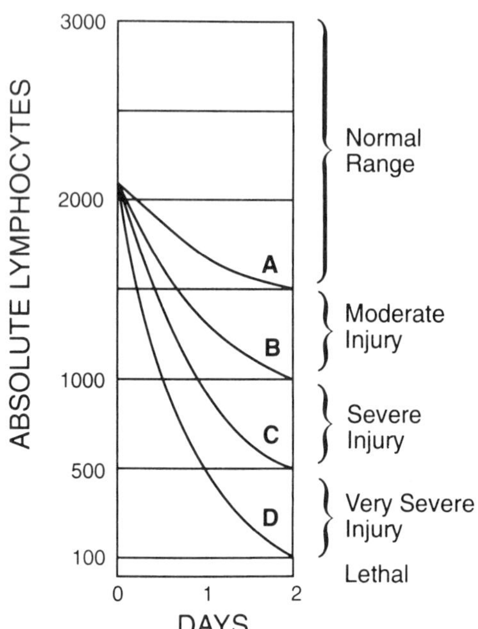

FIG. 199-1. Estimated radiation dose and degree of injury from early changes in lymphocyte counts. Approximate whole-body dose: Curve A—3.1 Gy (310 rad); Curve B—4.4 Gy (440 rad); Curve C—5.6 Gy (560 rad); Curve D—7.1 Gy (710 rad). (Reproduced from *Health Physics* 72:514, 1997 with permission from the Health Physics Society. Figure has been modified from its original version.)

DOSE ESTIMATION If the patient was not wearing a personal dose monitor (dosimeter) at the time of the accident, estimations of dose can be calculated from the circumstances of the accident. The dose received is a function of the individual's proximity to the source, the type and energy of the particular source, as well as the duration of exposure and extent of shielding. This information may not be available at the time of the patient's presentation to the emergency department and estimates of the radiation injury received must be obtained by assessing physical symptoms and laboratory data.

Hematological Data for Estimating Radiation Injury The earliest laboratory indicator of biological damage from radiation is a marked decrease in peripheral lymphocytes, often within eight hours postexposure. The more precipitous the decline in lymphocytes, the greater the dose received. (Fig. 199-1). The lymphocyte count 24 hours postexposure is useful in predicting the patient's clinical course. If the lymphocyte count is maintained above 1200/μL, no clinical support is required. If the count falls below 500/μL, a severe clinical course can be anticipated. If the entire lymphocyte count is depleted within six hours, a fatal outcome is likely.

Because circulating lymphocytes are very radiosensitive, dose estimation by lymphocyte count is less reliable with doses above 3 Gy (300 rad) and more accurate estimates can be obtained from the granulocyte pattern. In contrast to lymphocytes, circulating granulocytes are not directly killed by radiation. However, damage to blood progenitor cells in bone marrow results in a later decline in the granulocyte population. A transient increase in peripheral granulocytes is seen immediately after exposure due to a stress-related release of granulocytes from the bone marrow stores into the peripheral circulation. Granulocytopenia occurs after these stores are mobilized and then localize in radiation damaged tissues, reaching a nadir at about 30 days after exposure. Granulocytes may show a transient rise about 10 to 15 days postexposure when damaged stem cells begin proliferation but die before reaching their full reproductive capability. Absence of this transient rise in granulocyte numbers indicates exposure above 5 Gy (500 rad) and is a poor prognostic sign.[9]

Platelet counts may slightly increase in the first few days after exposure and then fall to a nadir at about 30 days. The red blood cell population shows a milder decrease in concentration with resultant mild anemia. The decrease in the red cell line is less pronounced than other hematopoietic cells and reflects the red cells' longer life span in the peripheral circulation (Fig. 199-2).

Dose Estimation by Cytogenetic Analysis Cytogenetic analysis of circulating lymphocytes is another method of dose estimation. Radiation induces some characteristic chromosome aberrations, particularly rings and dicentrics, in a dose-dependent manner. The frequency of these abnormalities can be scored in cytogenetic laboratories to obtain estimates of radiation dose received. This process is technically challenging, time-consuming, and expensive but is the most sensitive biological measurement for quantifying dose from whole-body irradiation.[9]

Clinical Symptoms for Estimating Radiation Injury The absence or time of onset of nausea and vomiting are useful for assessing the injury severity. Diarrhea is a less useful symptom unless there is prompt, explosive, bloody diarrhea, which indicates a likely fatal outcome. Individuals who have received doses less than 1 Gy (100 rad) seldom experience nausea or vomiting. Less than 1 Gy is a reliable dose estimate for individuals who remain asymptomatic 24 hours postexposure; hospital admission for these individuals is generally unnecessary.[10]

LETHAL DOSE The LD50/60 from exposure to ionizing radiation is defined as the dose of penetrating ionizing radiation that will result in the deaths of 50 percent of the exposed population within 60 days. Three values are commonly cited for human survival. The most commonly cited value is LD50/60 of approximately 4.5 Gy (450 rad). This value assumes intensive medical therapy is provided, including antibiotics, blood products, and reverse isolation. With only minimal treatment, such as basic first aid, the LD50/60 falls to approximately 3.4 Gy (340 rad). Victims of the Chernobyl nuclear accident have demonstrated that humans can survive radiation doses greater than anticipated. Intensive medical support to Chernobyl victims provided a high survival rate in individuals receiving less than 6 Gy (600 rad). With newer advances in medical treatment, such as stem cell transplantation and cytokine administration, it may be possible to raise the LD50/60 to 11 Gy (1100 rad).[11]

TREATMENT OF WHOLE-BODY IRRADIATION The patient who has only been exposed to an external source of penetrating radiation is not radioactive or contaminated and therefore requires no special precautions for handling or treating. A rare exception is exposure to high-level neutron irradiation, which can induce radioactivity. In the unlikely event of a criticality accident, neutron exposure becomes a concern. Patient specimens of blood and urine should be collected and assayed for induced radioactivity in the body, predominately Na-24. In addition, all metal objects on the patient's body or clothing should be monitored for potential radioactivity, including jewelry, coins, dental fillings, wristwatches, and buttons.

Initial treatment of the irradiated patient is directed toward alleviating the symptoms of the prodromal phase and may include the use of antiemetics and anxiolytics. Pain management may be required if there is associated trauma. Medical treatment has been unsuccessful in the few documented cases of high radiation doses that cause major damage to the GI or CV/CNS systems. Survival is possible for individuals with lower radiation doses resulting in the hematopoietic form of ARS.

The ultimate treatment goal is to provide support during the period of deficient defenses against infection and hemorrhage until marrow recovery occurs. Supportive treatment may include IV fluids, blood products, and total parenteral nutrition, as well as reverse isolation, prophylactic antibiotics, and antifungal medications. The

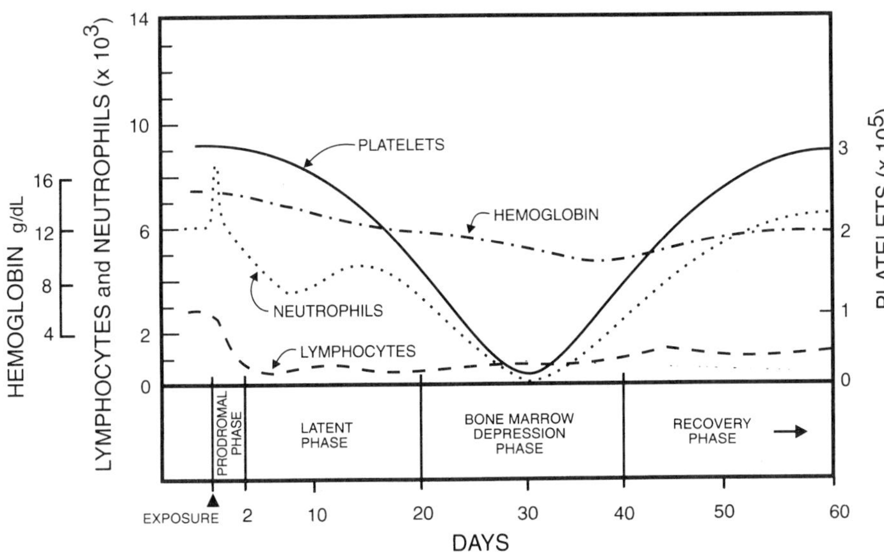

FIG. 199-2. Typical hematological course and clinical stages after sublethal (~300 rad) exposure to total body irradiation. (Reprinted with permission from *Radiobiological Factors in Manned Space Flight,* copyright 1965 by the National Academy of Sciences. Washington, DC, National Academy Press, 1965.)

patient, as well as family members who may be potential blood donors, should undergo HLA typing in preparation of white cell and platelet transfusions if marrow suppression becomes severe. The most severe marrow depression occurs at two to three weeks after exposure. Spontaneous recovery of granulocytes and platelets is quite rapid after the fifth week.

Bone marrow transplantation may be considered for patients who have received doses above 8 or 9 Gy (800 to 900 rad).[12] Bone marrow transplantation is advocated only for patients who are likely to die from radiation-induced myelosuppression if they have a well-matched donor and do not have irreversible damage to other major organ systems. Transplantation was provided for 13 victims of the Chernobyl accident who had received a dose greater than 5.6 Gy (560 rad). Within the following 3 months, 11 of these 13 patients died. The causes of these deaths were multifactorial and included graft-versus-host disease, burns, traumatic injury, radiation pneumonitis, ARDS, and renal and hepatic failure.

Other treatment modalities for myelosuppression that do not carry a risk of graft-versus-host disease are being studied. The administration of hematopoietic growth factors is currently under intense clinical investigation. Hematopoietic growth factors are cytokines such as erythropoietin, interleukins, and colony-stimulating factors. These proteins have been shown to stimulate the proliferation and differentiation of the surviving stem cells and thus accelerate reconstitution of the bone marrow. These growth factors are most efficacious in animal models when administered immediately after irradiation and demonstrates the importance of early dose estimation. Patients in whom the estimated dose is high enough to cause severe marrow damage may benefit from prompt administration of these growth factors.

Obtaining data and specimens for dose estimation is therefore a crucial aspect of planning therapy and predicting the patient's clinical course. The time of onset of all clinical symptoms should be carefully observed and documented. Serial blood specimens should be obtained for hematological and cytogenetic dose assessment.

If significant radiation dose was received, the patient should have long-term periodic follow-up for potential delayed effects of radiation damage such as cataracts, infertility, thyroid dysfunction, leukemia, or other neoplasms.

Local Radiation Injury

The majority of radiation accidents in the United States result in local radiation injury from partial-body exposure. In contrast to whole-body irradiation, partial-body irradiation rarely causes systemic manifestations. A rare exception is the development of ARS following partial-body irradiation that affects a significant amount of the bone marrow. Most commonly, a portion of the extremities is affected and the clinical picture consists of cutaneous changes.

Local radiation injury from doses above 2 to 3 Gy (200 to 300 rad) may result in erythema with associated hyperesthesia and itching. These signs occur within hours after exposure and are transient. Depending on the dose received, the erythema may reappear. Early onset of the initial erythema and quick reappearance of erythema correspond to higher doses. With doses below 3 Gy (300 rad), the erythema may not reappear. Doses of 6 Gy (600 rad) result in reoccurrence of significant erythema in 1 to 3 weeks. Much higher doses may result in prompt and persistent erythema.[10]

Other cutaneous changes resulting from local radiation injury include epilation, desquamation, and necrosis. Epilation or alopecia begins within 2 to 3 weeks after doses of 3 Gy (300 rad) are received. Epilation may be complete after doses above 5 Gy (5 rad) and may be permanent after doses above 6 Gy (600 rad). Doses of 12 to 15 Gy (1200 to 1500 rad) result in dry desquamation within 2 to 3 weeks. Doses in excess of 25 Gy (2500 rad) result in wet desquamation, blistering bulla, and ulceration within 3 to 5 weeks. Radionecrosis is seen after doses above 50 Gy (5000 rad).[13]

These skin manifestations may appear similar to thermal burns. However, unlike thermal burns, cutaneous radiation injury may be associated with waves of transient erythema described above, as well as with a delayed onset of pain, followed by a more prolonged and severe pain. Another important distinction of radiation injury is that the clinical changes evolved over a more prolonged time period. The exception is very high doses on the order of 50 Gy (5000 rad) that result in prompt transdermal injury resembling a thermal third-degree burn. The pain is immediate and excruciating. Surgical resection and grafting may be required.

Emergency department care of cutaneous radiation injury is limited to analgesics, routine burn care, and, if indicated, surgical referral. Physical therapy and splinting may be useful for preventing contractures and preserving joint range of motion. These patients must be carefully monitored for hemorrhage, infection and necrosis. In addition, prolonged observation is needed for later neoplastic changes of the skin.

Prenatal Exposures

When a pregnant female is exposed to ionizing radiation special consideration must be given to the radiosensitive unborn child.[14,15] Fetal cells are largely undifferentiated and highly proliferative and thus have

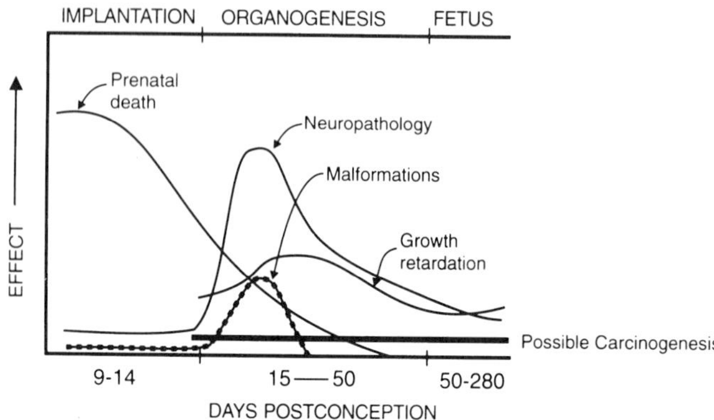

FIG. 199-3. The various adverse effects associated with radiation and their relative incidence at different stages of gestation. (Reprinted with permission from *Medical Effects of Ionizing Radiation,* 2d ed. Philadelphia, WB Saunders, 1995.)

increased radiosensitivity depending on the phase of gestation (Fig. 199-3). At 0 to 2 weeks postconception, there is an all-or-none phenomenon. Irradiation during this time usually results in death with resorption of the conceptus or no observable damage. This phenomenon is a result of the pluripotential of the early blastomeres that allows injured cells to be replaced by remaining cells when the damage is not extensive. After two weeks gestation, organogenesis begins and the embryo is at risk of congenital malformations. The risk of injury is greatest for the particular organ system that is under development at the time of radiation exposure. After seven weeks, the fetal period begins. Major organogenesis is complete, with the exception of the CNS. The CNS has continued susceptibility to radiation injury during the early fetal period.[15]

Data of radiation-induced anomalies in humans has been derived from Japanese atomic bomb survivors who received radiation exposure in utero. The most common injuries are related to the CNS, particularly microcephaly and mental retardation. Other malformations, such as growth retardation and ocular defects, have been reported less frequently. Radiation exposure during 8 to 15 weeks' gestation correlates with the most significant CNS injury. This increased radiosensitivity is due to the extensive proliferation and migration of neuronal cells at this time.[15] Both human and animal studies indicate that a minimum fetal exposure of 0.1 to 0.2 Gy (10 to 20 rad) is required for injury.[15] Official agencies, including the National Council on Radiation Protection (NCRP), recommend that the dose to an unborn child be limited to 500 millirem (5 milliSv).[16] Below this limit, the risks to the unborn child exposed with radiation do not exceed the baseline rate of birth defects seen in infants not exposed to radiation.[17]

If a fetal dose is above 500 millirem (5 milliSv), particularly during the vulnerable period of 8 to 15 weeks' gestation, risks such as CNS damage or growth defects, must be considered. In such a case, a physician with expertise in radiation injury should be consulted to provide counseling to the expecting parents.

	Regional Coordinating Office	Post Office Address	Telephone for Assistance
①	Brookhaven Area Office	Upton, L.I., New York 11973	(516) 344-2200
②	Oak Ridge Operations Office	PO Box E, Oak Ridge Tennessee, 37830	(423) 576-1005
③	Savannah River Operations Office	PO Box A, Aiken, SC 29801	(803) 725-3333
④	Albuquerque Operations Office	PO Box 5400, Albuquerque New Mexico 87185	(505) 845-4667
⑤	Chicago Operations Office	9800 S. Cass Ave., Argonne, Illinois 60439	(630) 252-4800
⑥	Idaho Operations Office	785 DOE PL, Idaho Falls, Idaho 83402	(208) 526-1515
⑦	San Fransico Operations Office	1301 Clay Street MS 700-N, Oakland, CA 94612	(510) 637-1794
⑧	Richland Operations Office	PO Box 550, Richland, Washington 99352	(509) 373-3800

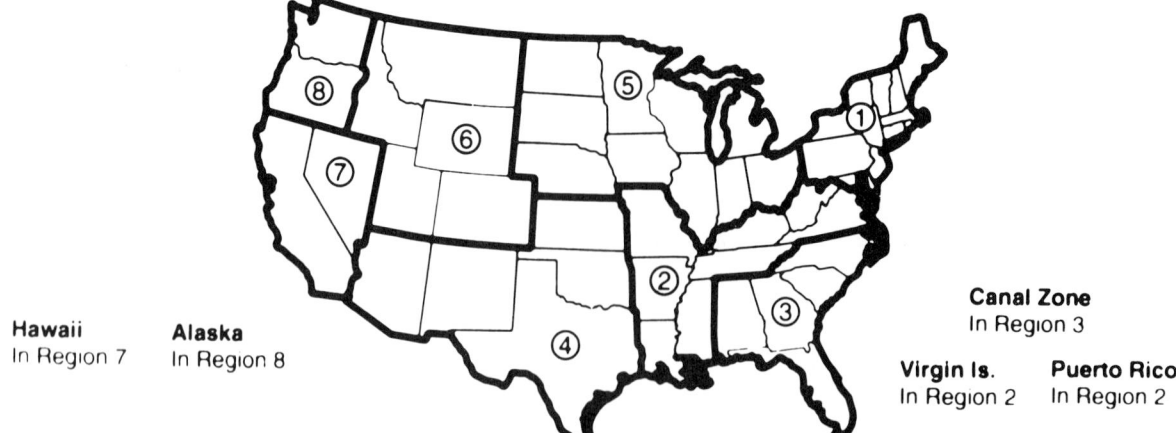

FIG. 199-4. Regional coordinating offices for Department of Energy Radiological Assistance Program. (Courtesy of the United States Department of Energy Regional Coordinating Offices.)

DOSE REDUCTION TECHNIQUES

When working in a radiation area, the dose received is decreased by three principal means: shielding the radiation source, minimizing the time in the radiation area, and increasing the distance from the radiation source. The exposure rate in an area decreases by the square of the distance from the source. This concept is referred to as the inverse square law and is a very effective technique of dose reduction. For example, increasing the distance from the source by a factor of 4 decreased the exposure rate by a factor of 16.

SOURCES OF ASSISTANCE

Emergency department personnel should be familiar with authorities that can provide advice and assistance when radiation accidents occur. Radiation emergency call lists may be prepared in advance and include the following contacts:

1. Local facilities which staff medical and health physics professionals trained in radiation accidents.
2. Local civil defense or disaster offices.
3. State radiological health office (title may vary by state).
4. Federal Emergency Management Agency (FEMA)
5. US Department of Energy (DOE). Seven assets of DOE are dedicated to radiological emergency response: Aerial Measuring System (AMS), Atmospheric Release Advisory Capability (ARAC), Accident Response Group (ARG), Federal Radiological Monitoring and Assessment Center (FRMAC), Nuclear Emergency Search Team (NEST), Radiological Assistance Program (RAP), and Radiation Emergency Assistance Center/Training Site (REACTS). These assets provide expert technical support throughout the U.S. in response to radiation accidents, nuclear weapons incidents, lost or stolen radioactive materials, or acts of nuclear terrorism.

RAP has 8 regional coordinating offices that provide assistance in preparing for radiological emergencies and provide radiological assessments of accidents (Fig. 199-4).

REACTS is the medical asset of DOE Radiological Emergency Response that provides training programs, consultation assistance, and treatment capabilities. REACTS has the capability to dispatch an emergency response team of health professionals to assist at an accident site. After initial treatment and decontamination actions are complete, REACTS may also accept severely contaminated or irradiated patients for transfer to its facilities for more definitive care. REACTS daytime phone is (423) 576-3131. REACTS 24-hour emergency number is (423) 481-1000.

ACKNOWLEDGMENT

The author wishes to acknowledge John T. Meredith, M.D., F.A.C.E.P., Faculty Advisor, Assistant Professor, Department of Emergency Medicine, East Carolina University, School of Medicine and Ronald E. Goans, Ph.D., M.D., Section Leader, Medical Director, Radiation Emergency Assistance Center/Training Site, Oak Ridge Institute of National Science for their support and assistance in the preparation of this chapter.

REFERENCES

1. Mettler FA Jr: Assessment and Management of Local Radiation Injury, in Mettler FA Jr, Kelsey CA, Ricks RC (eds): *Medical Management of Radiation Accidents,* Boca Raton, FL, CRC Press, 1990, p 128.
2. Leonard RB, Ricks RC: Emergency department radiation accident protocol. *Ann Emerg Med* 9:462-470, 1980.
3. Mettler FA, Kelsey CA, Ricks RC (eds): *Medical Management of Radiation Accidents.* Boca Raton, FL, CRC Press, 1990.
4. McCarthy PL Jr: A perspective on clinical disorders of radiation accident victims. *Stem Cells* 15(Suppl 2):122, 1997.
5. Voelz GL, Bushberg JT: Medical management of internal contamination accidents, in Raabe O (ed): *Internal Radiation Dosimetry,* Proceedings of the Health Physics Society, Madison, WI, Medical Physics Publishers, 1994, pp 602–605.
6. Voelz GL: Evaluation and treatment of persons exposed to internally deposited radionuclides, in Mettler FA Jr, Kelsey CA, Ricks RC (eds): *Medical Management of Radiation Accidents,* Boca Raton, FL, CRC Press, 1990, p 164.
7. Mettler FA Jr: Effects of whole body irradiation, in Mettler FA Jr, Kelsey CA, Ricks RC (eds): *Medical Management of Radiation Accidents,* Boca Raton, FL, CRC Press, 1990, p 82.
8. Wald N: Acute radiation injury and their medical management, in Mossman KL, Mills WA (eds): *The Biological Basis of Radiation Protection Practice,* Health Physics Society, Baltimore, MD, William & Wilkins, 1992, p 188.
9. Kastengerg WE: Principal issues and future projects of nuclear energy, in Champlin RE (ed): Radiation accidents and nuclear energy: Medical consequences and therapy. *Ann Intern Med* 109:739, 1998.
10. American Medical Association: *A Guide to the Hospital Management of Injuries Arising from Exposure to or Involving Ionizing Radiation,* Chicago, IL, AMA, 1984.
11. Gale RP: Immediate medical consequences of nuclear accidents. Lessons from Chernobyl. *JAMA* 285:627, 1987.
12. Berger ME, Ricks RC: Management of emergency care for radiation accident victims, in Miller KL (ed): *CRC Handbook of Management of Radiation Protection Programs,* 2d ed. Boca Raton, FL, CRC Press, 1992, p 106.
13. Ricks RC: *Hospital Emergency Department Management of Radiation Accidents,* Oak Ridge, TN, Oak Ridge Associated Universities, 1984, p 6.
14. Streffer C, Lake JV, Bock GR, Cardew G (eds): Biological effects of prenatal irradiation, in Lake JV, Bock GR, Cardew G (eds): *Health Impacts of Large Releases of Radionuclides.* Ciba Foundation Symposium 203, New York, John Wiley, 1997, pp 155–163.
15. Mettler FA Jr, Upton AC (eds): Radiation exposure in utero, in Mettler FA Jr, Upton AC (eds): *Medical Effects of Ionizing Radiation*, 2d ed. Philadelphia, PA, WB Saunders, 1995, pp 322–325.
16. US Nuclear Regulatory Commission: *Instructions Concerning Prenatal Radiation Exposure,* Washington, DC, US Nuclear Regulatory Commission, 1987. US Nuclear Regulatory Guide 8.13, Rev. 2.
17. Brent RL: Protocols: Ionizing radiation. *Contemp Obstet Gynecol* 8:25, 1987.

MUSHROOM POISONING

Sandra M. Schneider
Anne Brayer

Mushrooms are one of the more common toxic exposures, with over 12,000 mushroom exposures reported to poison centers in 1996, or roughly 5 for every 100,000 population.[1] Over 95 percent of these ingestions were unintentional, with nearly 70 percent occurring in children under the age of 6. Most ingestions resulted in little or no gastrointestinal (GI) toxicity.

Depending on the type of mushroom, adverse effects from ingestion range from mild GI symptoms to major cytotoxic effects resulting in organ failure and death. Toxicity may also vary based on the amount ingested, the age of the mushroom, the season, the geographic location, and the way in which the mushroom has been prepared prior to ingestion. Individuals also vary in their response to any given mushroom ingestion, so that one person may show significant effects while others may be asymptomatic ingesting the same mushroom (Table 200-1).

Mushroom toxicity is divided into early toxicity (within 1 h after ingestion) and delayed toxicity (6 h to 20 days). In general, if toxicity begins within 2 h of ingestion of a mushroom, the clinical course will most likely be benign. If symptoms begin 6 h or later after ingestion, however, in general the clinical course will be more serious and potentially fatal. Nearly all fatalities in the United States occur from the ingestion of the *Amanita* species (*Amanita phalloides, Amanita virosa,* and *Amanita verna*).

Mushroom poisoning occurs among four main groups of individuals: young children who ingest mushrooms inadvertently, wild-mush-

TABLE 200-1 Mushrooms: Symptoms, Toxicity, and Treatment

Symptoms	Mushrooms	Toxicity	Treatment
Gastrointestinal symptoms			
Onset <2 h	*Chlorophyllum molybdites* *Omphalotus illudens* *Cantharellus cibarius* *Amanita caesarea*	Nausea, vomiting, diarrhea (occasional bloody) Initial: nausea, vomiting, diarrhea	IV hydration Antiemetics IV hydration, glucose, monitor, AST, ALT, PT, PTT, bilirubin, BUN, creatinine
Onset 6–24 h	*Gyromitra esculenta:* fall season *Amanita phalloides, Amanita verna,* and *Amanita virosa:* spring season	Day 2: rise in AST, ALT Day 3: hepatic failure	For *Amanita:* activated charcoal Penicillin G 300,000–1,000,000 U/kg/day. Silymarin 20–40 mg/kg/day. Consider cimetidine 4–10 g/day. Hyperbaric oxygen
Muscarinic (SLUDGE) syndrome Onset <30 min	*Inocybe* *Clitocybe*	Salivation, lacrimation, diarrhea, gastrointestinal distress, emesis	Supportive atropine 0.01 mg/kg repeated as needed for severe secretions
CNS excitement Onset <30 min	*Amanita muscaria* *Amanita pantherina*	Intoxication, dizziness, ataxia, visual disturbances, seizures, tachycardia, hypertension, warm dry skin, dry mouth, mydriasis (anticholinergic effects)	Supportive sedation with phenobarbital 30 mg IV or diazepam 2–5 mg IV as needed for adults
Hallucinations Onset <30 min	*Psilocybe* *Gymnopilus*	Visual hallucinations, ataxia	Supportive sedation with phenobarbital 0.5 mg/kg or, for adults, 30–60 mg IV, or diazepam 0.1 mg/kg or 5-mg IV for adults
Disulfiram 2–72 h after mushroom, and <30 min after alcohol	*Coprinus*	Headache, flushing, tachycardia, hyperventilation, shortness of breath, palpitations	Supportive IV hydration Propranolol for supraventricular tachycardia Norepinephrine for refractory hypotension

Abbreviation: ALT, alanine amino transferase; AST, aspartate amino transferase; BUN, blood urea nitrogen; CNS, central nervous system; PT, prothrombin time; PTT, partial thromboplastin time; SLUDGE syndrome, salivation, lacrimation, urination, defecation, gastrointestinal hypermotility, and emesis.

room foragers, individuals attempting suicide or homicide, and individuals looking for a hallucinatory ''high.'' Identification of the mushroom ingested may be difficult and time consuming. In all cases, treatment should be directed by a patient's symptoms rather than by attempts at mushroom identification. Very often, foragers will mix different species of mushrooms together, so it is not always clear that the species being identified is the same one that was ingested. Treatment of the patients should always be based on presenting symptoms.

Identification of the *Amanita* species may be helpful; however, there are many *Amanita* mushrooms that are nontoxic. *Amanita* species generally have warts on the cap (remnants of the membrane covering the emerging mushroom), which often give it a spotted appearance. The gills are ''free,'' ending before the stem begins. The stem characteristically has a membrane ring around it and widens as it enters the soil. In most cases, the stem of the mushroom is contained in a cup or volva, which may be underground.

This chapter deals with each of the major toxic groups separately, as their toxicity, clinical features, and treatment vary significantly.

EARLY-ONSET GASTROINTESTINAL SYMPTOMS

Pathophysiology

The most commonly ingested toxic mushrooms are those that cause GI irritation. These mushrooms can be of many types. In North America, *Chlorophyllum molybdites* is particularly common and is sometimes mistaken for an *Amanita.* Many of the so-called little brown mushrooms (LBMs) found commonly in lawns, and often accidentally ingested by children, are in this category. The actual toxin varies with the species of mushroom, but most toxins are poorly described.

Clinical Features

Typically, patients will present with acute onset of vomiting and diarrhea less than 2 h after ingesting the mushroom. There may be intestinal cramping, chills, headaches, and myalgias. The diarrhea is usually watery, but occasionally may be bloody, with fecal leukocytes. Most commonly, symptoms are mild and self-limited. Infrequently, the vomiting and diarrhea may lead to significant dehydration and electrolyte imbalance. The history of ingestion is frequently offered by the patient, but in cases where it is not, the presentation may be confused with acute gastroenteritis or acute food poisoning.

Treatment

General treatment for toxic mushroom ingestion includes GI decontamination. Activated charcoal (0.5 to 1.0 g/kg orally or via nasogastric tube) is indicated for all ingestions unless toxic species can be ruled out. Treatment for ingestion of GI irritants is largely supportive, including IV fluid and electrolyte replacement when necessary. Judicious use of antiemetics is probably justified, but antidiarrheal agents are best withheld, because they may prolong the exposure to the toxin.

In most cases, the illness is self-limited, with symptoms resolving within 12 to 24 h. Rarely, symptoms may persist and hospitalization may be indicated for fluid and electrolyte replacement.

EARLY-ONSET NEUROLOGIC SYMPTOMS

Pathophysiology

There are several classes of mushrooms that can cause neurologic symptoms. These include the hallucinogenic mushrooms (''magic'' mushrooms) that are intentionally ingested for their mind-altering qualities. These mushrooms contain psilocybin or psilocin toxins, which are neuroactive chemicals similar to lysergic acid diethylamide (LSD). They act on serotonin-dependent neurons in the central nervous system (CNS), causing effects similar to those of LSD. Mushrooms from the *Psilocybe* genus, which are the most commonly ingested in this class, are small brown mushrooms that commonly grow on dung in warmer climates and often turn a greenish blue when bruised or cut. They may also be cultivated at home from purchased spores. Nontoxic mushrooms may also be laced with phencyclidine (PCP) or LSD and sold as hallucinogenic mushrooms.

Clinical Features

The clinical symptoms usually present within 2 h of ingestion, with euphoria, a heightened imagination, a loss of time sensation, and visual distortions or hallucinations. There may be tachycardia and hypertension. Fever and seizures have rarely been reported. Symptoms typically last 4 to 6 h. There are infrequent reports of patients suffering from flashbacks for up to 4 months after ingestion.

Treatment

Treatment should be largely supportive. Placing the patient in a darkened quiet room, devoid of visual stimuli, and providing reassurance are often sufficient. If sedation is required, benzodiazepines such as diazepam (0.1 mg/kg for children and 5 mg for adults, administered intravenously) are preferred to phenothiazine derivatives because the latter can lower seizure threshold.

EARLY-ONSET ANTICHOLINERGIC SYMPTOMS

Pathophysiology

Mushrooms containing the isoxazole derivatives, ibotenic acid and muscimol, are known for their neurologic effects. *Amanita muscaria* is an easily identified member of this group. It has an orange or red cap with white warts (remnants of the universal veil present in young specimens) as well as a ring (annulus) and cup (volva) on the stem. *Amanita pantherina,* another member of the group, is 5 to 14 cm in length and diameter, with a white to brown cap and with the ring and cup on the stem. Both specimens grow under trees in woodlands throughout North America.

Clinical Features

Patients ingesting these mushrooms usually present with symptoms within 30 min of ingestion. Most commonly, the symptoms are anticholinergic, including tachycardia, hypertension, warm, dry skin and mucous membranes, and mydriasis. Dizziness, mild intoxication, ataxia, and difficulty with size, time, and place perceptions are common. Much less commonly, patients may present with cholinergic symptoms, including salivation, lacrimation, urination, defecation, GI hypermotility, and emesis. Seizures have been reported in children. Symptoms are typically self-limited, resolving within 3 to 4 h after ingestion.

Treatment

Treatment begins with GI decontamination. Syrup of ipecac may be appropriate if it can be administered within 30 to 60 min of ingestion, but caution is advised due to the potential for CNS depression and seizures. Activated charcoal administration is advised in most cases. In patients with significant vomiting and diarrhea, fluid and electrolyte replacement may be necessary. Patients who are agitated should be appropriately restrained. Sedation may be provided as necessary with benzodiazepines (diazepam or lorazepam) or phenobarbital. Seizures have been successfully treated with benzodiazepines.

For patients with severe anticholinergic symptoms, treatment with physostigmine may be considered. Physostigmine has been known to produce bradycardia, hypotension, and seizures, so administration should be reserved for severely symptomatic patients. The dosage is 1 to 2 mg IV slowly in adults and 0.5 mg in children. Patients should have continuous cardiorespiratory and blood pressure monitoring during administration. In the rare patients with cholinergic symptoms, administration of IV atropine may be considered (0.5 to 1 mg for adults and 0.01 mg/kg for children). Dosage should be titrated to clinical effect, using drying of pulmonary secretions as the end point. Atropine has been shown to cause worsening of CNS symptoms in patients who ingest isoxazole derivatives, so administration should be reserved for patients with severe cholinergic symptoms.

EARLY-ONSET MUSCARINIC SYMPTOMS

Pathophysiology

Mushrooms containing muscarine cause neurologic symptoms and muscarinic or cholinergic effects. The symptoms are characterized by the SLUDGE syndrome, with salivation, lacrimation, urination, defecation, GI hypermotility, and emesis. Mushrooms of the *Inocybe* and *Clitocybe* genus are common causes of muscarinic poisoning. The *Inocybe* mushrooms are small brown mushrooms with conical caps, typically found under hardwoods and conifers. The *Clitocybe* mushrooms are usually found individually on lawns and in parks, and are white to gray, with a cup-shaped cap. *Amanita muscaria,* despite its name, contains far less muscarine than these other families and only rarely causes cholinergic poisoning symptoms.

Clinical Features

In addition to the SLUDGE syndrome, patients with muscarine ingestions can present with diaphoresis, muscle fasciculations, miosis, bradycardia, and bronchorrhea. Symptoms typically present within 30 min of ingestion and spontaneously resolve in 4 to 12 h.

Treatment

In most cases, symptoms are mild and self-limited. Supportive care is often sufficient. Because emesis is a common presenting symptom, activated charcoal administration is often difficult. Patients with severe vomiting may require IV fluid and electrolyte replacement.

Atropine is an antidote for muscarinic symptoms and can be administered in severe cases. It can be effective in treating bradycardia and hypotension unresponsive to IV fluids. Atropine is helpful in the treatment of diaphoresis, increased oral secretions, and bronchorrhea. It may also help reduce GI cramping, emesis, and diarrhea. The dose is 0.5 to 1.0 mg for adults and 0.01 mg/kg for children, administered intravenously. The dose can be repeated as necessary to control bronchorrhea, bradycardia, or hypotension. Large doses may be necessary to treat severe toxicity. Patients should be carefully monitored during administration. Oxygen and inhaled β agonists (albuterol or metaproterenol) are recommended for the treatment of patients with increased pulmonary secretions and bronchospasm.

DELAYED GASTROINTESTINAL SYMPTOMS

Pathophysiology

Two different mushrooms, *Gyromitra* and *Amanita,* cause significant toxicity, which characteristically presents several hours after ingestion. *Gyromitra esculenta* (the false morel) grows primarily in the spring in North America and is found in several other European countries. It has a brown convoluted top resembling a brain and is often mistaken for the tasty morel mushroom. Gyromitrin (*N*-methyl-*N*-formylhydrazone) is a volatile heat-labile toxin and primarily responsible for symptoms. Parboiling the mushroom can partially eliminate the toxin. Gyromitrin is hydrolyzed in the stomach to form *N*-methyl-*N*-formylhydrazine (MFH) and *N*-methylhydrazine (MH). MH is chemically identical to rocket fuel, and workers exposed to MH develop CNS toxicity. MH binds to pyridoxine and thus interferes with enzymes that require pyridoxine as a cofactor. γ-Aminobutyric acid (GABA) is lowered in the CNS, which may be a possible etiology for the seizures. MFH is converted into a free radical in the liver and causes local hepatic necrosis by blocking the activity of the P-450 system, glutathione, and other hepatic enzyme systems.[2] These two chemicals explain the CNS and hepatic dysfunction characteristic of gyromitrin toxicity. The etiology of the initial GI symptoms remains obscure.

Amanita phalloides, Amanita virosa, and *Amanita verna* commonly occur in the Northern Hemisphere and are particularly common in North Central Europe. Mushrooms of this species are found throughout the West Coast, Midwest, and in parts of the Northeast. Immigrants may mistake these mushrooms for edible varieties common in Eastern Asia. Mushrooms of the *Amanita* species are responsible for 95 percent of deaths associated with mushrooms.

Amanita phalloides contains several amatoxins and phallotoxins. Phallotoxins are bicyclic peptides that inactivate F-actin. Although this action has been of interest to basic scientists, phallotoxins do not appear to be active in human toxicity. Amatoxins are bicyclic octapeptides that are rapidly absorbed through the intestinal mucosa, carried to the liver, and undergo enterohepatic circulation. Recent human kinetic data show that α amanitin is cleared from the plasma within 48 h.[3] Concentrations in the plasma are quite small; amatoxins are not protein bound but actively transported into hepatocytes where they bind to RNA polymerase II and inhibit the formation of messenger RNA.[4] Some literature regarding studies with animals suggests that free radical formation may also be involved in toxicity.[5] Pathologic evidence of nuclear fragmentation and condensation of chromatin occur within 24 h.

Amanita virosa also contains five distinct virotoxins, which like phallotoxins do not appear to have clinical significance in humans because they are not absorbed from the GI tract. *Lepiota* mushrooms contain a high concentration of amatoxin (higher than *Amanita phalloides*) and have recently been described as causing symptoms identical to those seen with *Amanita phalloides.*[6]

The diagnosis of gyromitrin toxicity is generally assumed from the clinical features and the identification of the mushroom, either by the patient or from samples. Identification of *Amanita* species generally requires a trained mycologist. The Meixner colorimetric test is used to look for the presence of amatoxin. Although it is sensitive, it is not very specific, as other nontoxic mushrooms may test positive. Thin-layer chromatography, high-performance liquid chromatography, and radioimmunoassay have been developed to detect amatoxin. Amatoxin can be detected in plasma, urine, GI contents, and feces. However, its presence merely confirms amatoxin poisoning. Levels do not appear to correlate with clinical severity, and many patients do not have amatoxin detected, presumably because of rapid clearance.

Clinical Features

The distinct characteristic of these mushrooms is the onset of intense GI symptoms (nausea, vomiting, and diarrhea) 6 to 24 h after ingestion. At least with the *Amanita* species, the later the onset of the GI symptoms, the milder is the disease. After resolution of the initial GI symptoms, patients may develop hepatic injury.

Patients who ingest a gyromitrin-containing mushroom typically have a delayed onset of GI symptoms, which appear 6 to 8 h after ingestion. Initial GI symptoms are accompanied by neurologic symptoms, including dizziness and headache. In a mild ingestion, patients will have neurologic symptoms for several days and recover without difficulty. In severe cases, however, hepatic failure becomes symptomatic on day 3 and may result in death by as soon as day 7. Hypovolemia is common in the first phase of toxicity. Hypoglycemia occurs during the GI phase and again in the acute hepatic failure phase. Seizures, lack of coordination, and muscle cramps may occur.

Patients who ingest amatoxin-containing mushrooms also have delayed onset of GI symptoms (6 to 24 h). The gastroenteritis is intense, often requiring fluid and electrolyte replacement. Hypovolemia and hypoglycemia are quite common during the early GI phase. The gastroenteritis generally subsides after 12 h, and patients may again feel well. Hepatic failure becomes symptomatic on day 3 or 4, and death may follow as soon as day 7. Patients rapidly develop jaundice and right upper quadrant pain, and may develop a decreased level of consciousness, an elevated ammonia level, and cerebral edema. Liver enzymes, bilirubin, and prothrombin time rapidly become abnormal. Renal failure occurs either as a direct result of the toxin or as part of the hepatorenal syndrome.

In both toxicities, serum transaminases begin to increase 36 to 72 h after ingestion. Levels may be quite elevated. Prothrombin time may be elevated and unresponsive to vitamin K or fresh frozen plasma replacement. Amylase and lipase elevation suggests acute pancreatitis, although symptomatic pancreatitis is rare. Abnormal laboratory test findings in amatoxin poisoning include a decrease in neutrophils, lymphocytes, and platelets, and abnormal thyroid function. Hypophosphatemia (primarily noted in children), hypocalcemia, and elevated insulin levels occur. None of these laboratory abnormalities correlate with clinical disease, and their cause is unknown.

Pathologic changes are well described. Patients who ingest gyromitrin show diffuse hepatocellular damage and interstitial nephritis. Patients who ingest amatoxins show fatty degeneration of the liver, with intranuclear collection of lipids and extensive hepatic necrosis. Electron microscopy shows vacuolization of the mitochondria and clumping of the chromatin in the nucleoli. There are extensive lipid peroxidation changes in both the nucleus and the cytoplasm.

Several cases of mushroom toxicity during pregnancy have been reported. Aside from a slightly lower birth weight, compared with normal controls, all of these pregnancies have been completed without difficulty.[7] The babies appeared to be healthy and neurologically normal. This is in keeping with the findings that amatoxin do not cross the placental barrier.

The mortality rate from *Gyromitra* ingestion is estimated at 15 to 35 percent. Although, historically amatoxin hepatic failure had a mortality rate as high as 50 percent, more recently mortality has been reduced to 10 to 15 percent, based on improved care for hepatic failure. Liver transplant is often successful in patients with fulminant hepatic failure.

Patients who survive severe hepatic failure from amatoxin may develop signs of chronic active hepatitis with persistent elevation in liver transaminases, development of anti-smooth muscle antibodies, and cryoglobulins; the long-term consequences are unclear. No prolonged effects from gyromitrin toxicity have been reported.

Treatment

Most patients present with GI symptoms. Initial symptoms are severe vomiting and diarrhea. If a patient presents within a few hours of ingestion, gastric decontamination is indicated. Repeated doses of charcoal may be effective, particularly in the presence of amatoxin (as it undergoes enterohepatic circulation), at least for the first 24 h, but no clinical studies have shown the efficacy of charcoal for gyromitrin or amatoxin. Fluid and electrolyte replacement is mandatory. Glucose should be monitored and replaced, if necessary. Hypoglycemia still represents one of the most common causes of death in early mushroom toxicity.

All patients who have ingested amatoxin- or gyromitrin-containing mushrooms should be closely monitored for 48 h for the development of hepatic failure. Liver enzymes and prothrombin time should be monitored several times a day. Patients should be treated with a low-protein diet and receive standard supportive therapy for hepatic failure. Fresh frozen plasma and vitamin K can be used for the treatment of prolonged prothrombin time; in many cases, however, coagulopathy does not respond to treatment.

Patients who develop hepatic failure should be monitored closely and, in severe cases, preparations made for liver transplant. Although, no firm criteria exist to determine which patients will require liver transplant, clinical studies of amatoxin suggest aspartate aminotransferase (AST) levels greater than 2000 IU, grade 2 hepatic encephalopathy, and prothrombin time greater than 50 s despite therapy are indicative of the need for emergency liver transplant.[8] Many patients have met this criteria and survived without a hepatic transplant, and many patients have died without achieving these "target" values. Liver transplant, however, does provide the only option for patients in fulminant hepatic failure and has been quite successful. Recently, a child was given a temporary liver transplant, which allowed time for her own liver to regenerate. The transplanted liver was then removed.

Gyromitrin-Specific Treatment

The neurologic symptoms associated with gyromitrin are successfully treated with high-dose pyridoxine. Pyridoxine provides the cofactor required for the regeneration of GABA. High doses of pyridoxine (25 mg/kg up to a maximum of 25 g/day) are recommended, but doses of pyridoxine in excess of 40 g have been associated with severe peripheral neuropathy.[9] Pyridoxine does not affect the development or course of hepatic failure, and there is no specific therapy for gyromitrin-induced hepatic failure.

Amatoxin-Specific Treatment

Historically, there have been many anecdotal and largely ineffective treatments used to counteract this deadly toxin. Because 80 percent of the toxin is eliminated in the urine, forced diuresis may have some theoretical basis, but no clinical trials have shown efficacy. Amatoxins are dialyzable, and both hemodialysis and hemoperfusion had been a standard for therapy. However, because of the small plasma concentration, early binding in the liver, and rapid clearance from the plasma (within 48 h), hemodialysis and hemoperfusion are of limited usefulness. Many patients who receive hemodialysis actually do worse than patients treated with other forms of therapy. Attempts to interrupt enterohepatic circulation have also been tried but are of limited usefulness. Although high concentrations of amatoxin are excreted into bile, the small amount of liquid produced does not yield a large amount of the amatoxin extracted.

Thioctic acid, which has been used for many years in Europe, is a known free radical scavenger and may be effective in the treatment of acute hepatic failure of undifferentiated cause. Thioctic acid and glutathione appear to protect against microsomal lipid peroxidation and therefore may be of theoretical use in amatoxin poisoning. Animal and human studies, however, have not shown thioctic acid to be effective.

For patients in the United States, penicillin appears to be the most effective therapy. High doses of penicillin appear to block the uptake of amatoxin into the liver by its shared active transport system.[10] In addition, penicillin increases renal excretion of the toxin. Other antibiotics, such as rifampin and cephalosporins, have a similar effect in animal studies. Huge doses of penicillin G [300,000 to 1,000,000 U/kg/day] are required to decrease toxicity. Such doses are associated with seizures, and patients should be appropriately monitored. Penicillin should be started very soon after ingestion, if amatoxin ingestion is suspected. Penicillin-allergic patients either should not be treated with penicillin or should undergo desensitization.

Silymarin (silybinin), which has been used successfully in Europe to treat amatoxin ingestion, acts as a free radical scavenger and may interrupt the enterohepatic circulation of amatoxin when given orally. It is not available in the United States, but a recent study in Europe showed success in patients with amatoxin poisoning.[11]

Hyperbaric oxygen, which has been used in Europe as a treatment for amatoxin poisoning,[12] has been shown to be beneficial in other cases of hepatic failure, perhaps by increasing hepatic regeneration and interfering with free radical formation as well. No controlled studies exist, and animal studies have produced conflicting results.

There have been animal studies of other therapies that have not been yet definitively tested in humans. High-dose cimetidine (10 g/day) has been shown to be effective in animals and recently has been used successfully in humans.[5] Vitamin C, zinc, and thiol compounds have also been useful in animal models. Fab monoclonal antibodies have been developed against amatoxin.[13] Although successful in reducing hepatic failure, severe renal toxicity has developed. Theoretically, such Fab antibodies could be used with plasmapheresis to remove the antibody-antigen complexes.

DELAYED-ONSET RENAL FAILURE

Pathophysiology

Orellanine and ortinarin A and B are nephrotoxic compounds found in species of *Cortinarius* (*C. orellanus, C. speciosissimus,* and *C. gentilis*). These toxins are heat stable, and their mechanisms of action are unknown. Mushrooms of this species are found primarily in Europe and do not represent a significant problem in the United States. Recently, a similar delayed onset of renal toxicity was reported following the ingestion of *Amanita smithiana.*[14] This mushroom is commonly mistaken for pine mushrooms and grows commonly in the Pacific Northwest. Nephrotoxins in this mushroom are norleucine (aminohexadrenoic acid) and chlorocrotylglycine.

Clinical Features

Patients who ingest mushrooms containing nephrotoxins are generally asymptomatic. Occasionally, paresthesias, abnormal taste, and cognitive dysfunction are reported. Symptoms of renal failure begin between 3 and 20 days following ingestion. There is some evidence to suggest that patients who ingest *Amanita smithiana* may develop renal failure earlier. Many patients who ingest these mushrooms have no evidence of renal dysfunction, suggesting host variability. Supportive hemodialysis may be required in as many as 30 to 50 percent of patients, but 50 percent of patients will have spontaneous return of normal renal function.[15,16]

Ultrasonography shows enlarged kidneys. Renal biopsy shows mononuclear inflammatory infiltrate and signs of acute tubular damage with cell necrosis, cell shedding into the lumen, and de-differentiation of the proximal tubular epithelia. Electron microscopy show mitochondrial swelling, apical cytoplastic vacuolization, and a distortion of the brush border. These findings are consistent in both human and animal models.[16] The toxin appears to bind to tubular cells and can be detected in biopsy specimens as late as 180 days after ingestion.

Treatment

There is no specific treatment for patients who develop renal failure from *Cortinarius* or *Amanita smithiana.* Urine output and electrolyte, calcium, magnesium, blood urea nitrogen, and creatinine levels should be monitored. Hemodialysis support is indicated for refractory hyperkalemia, refractory acidosis, uremic symptoms, or severe renal dysfunction. As spontaneous improvement is reported, renal transplant should be withheld for several months to monitor patient response. Renal transplant has been used in several patients with good success.

DELAYED ONSET ACCOMPANYING ALCOHOL INGESTION

Pathophysiology

Perhaps the most interesting, but clinically least important, is a mushroom toxin contained in the *Coprinus* genus. This mushroom, which is very common in North America, is known as the "inky-cap" or "shaggy mane." It is a tall, white, thin mushroom with a shaggy cap. As the mushroom ages, the cap liquefies and blackens, and black liquid drips from the necrosing cap. The mushroom contains coprine, which is chemically related to disulfiram. Coprine inhibits alcohol dehydrogenase with the onset of activity 2 h after ingestion, and activity may last up to 72 h. If alcohol is consumed during this "sensitive" period, patients will develop a typical disulfiram reaction. Mushrooms ingested at the same time as alcohol produce no toxicity.

Clinical Features

Because of the delay between mushroom consumption and alcohol consumption, few patients will link their symptoms to the ingestion of a mushroom. Patients present with facial flushing, diaphoresis, headache, tachycardia, nausea, and vomiting. Most symptoms are mild.

Treatment

Because alcohol is readily absorbed from the GI tract, GI decontamination has no role. Likewise, charcoal would not be expected to have great benefit. Patients occasionally become hypotensive and respond to IV fluids or, in refractory cases, norepinephrine. Supraventricular tachycardia is rare but responds to propranolol. Patients should be educated about the link between the alcohol and mushroom ingestion.

REFERENCES

1. Litovitz TL, Smilkstein M, Felberg L, et al: Annual report of the American Association of Poison Control Centers Toxic Exposure Surveillance System. *Am J Emerg Med* 15:447, 1997.
2. Michelot S, Toth B: Poisoning by *Gyromitra esculenta:* A review. *J Appl Toxicol* 11:235, 1991.
3. Jaeger A, Jehl F, Flesch F, et al: Kinetics of amatoxins in human poisonings: Therapeutic implications. *J Toxicol Clin Toxicol* 31:63, 1993.
4. Lindell TJ, Weinberg F, Morris PW, et al: Specific inhibition of nuclear RNA polymerase II by alpha-amanitin. *Science* 170:447, 1970.
5. Schneider SM, Borochovitz D, Krenzelok EP: Cimetidine protection against α amanitin hepatoxicity in mice: A potential model for the treatment of *Amanita phalloides* poisoning. *Ann Emerg Med* 16:1136, 1987.
6. Meunier BC, Camus CM, Houssein DP, et al: Liver transplantation after severe poisoning due to amatoxin-containing *Lepiota*: Report of 3 cases. *J Toxicol Clin Toxicol* 33:165, 1995.
7. Timar L, Czeizel AE: Birth weight and congenital anomalies following poisonous mushroom intoxication during pregnancy. *Reprod Toxicol* 11:861, 1977.
8. Fanatozzi R, Ledda F, Caramelli L, et al: Clinical findings and follow-up evaluation of an outbreak of mushroom poisoning: Survey of *Amanita phalloides* poisoning. *Klin Wochenschr* 64:38, 1986.
9. Albin RL, Albers JW, Greenberg HS, et al: Acute sensory neuropathy-neuronopathy from pyridoxine overdose. *Neurology* 37:1729, 1987.
10. Floersheim GL, Schneeberger J, Buscher K: Curative potencies of penicillin in experimental *Amanita phalloides* poisoning. *Agents Actions* 2:138, 1971.
11. Carducci R, Armellino MF, Volpe C, et al: Silibinin and acute poisoning with *Amanita phalloides*. *Minerva Anesthesiol* 62:187, 1996.
12. Parish RC, Doering PL: Treatment of *Amanita* mushroom poisoning: A review. *Vet Hum Toxicol* 28:318, 1986.
13. Faulstich H, Kirshner K, Derenzini M: Strongly enhanced toxicity of mushroom toxin α-amanitin by an amatoxin-specific FAB or monoclonal antibody. *Toxicon* 26:491, 1988.
14. Warden CR, Benjamin DR: Acute renal failure associated with suspected *Amanita smithiana* mushroom ingestion: A case series. *Acad Emerg Med* 5:808, 1998.
15. Bouget J, Bousser J, Pats B, et al: Acute renal failure following collective intoxication by *Cortinarius orellanus*. *Intensive Care Med* 16:506, 1990.
16. Holzl B, Regele H, Kirchmair M, Sandhofer F: Acute renal failure after ingestion of *Cortinarius speciocissimens*. *Clin Nephrol* 48:260, 1997.

POISONOUS PLANTS

Mark A. Hostetler
Sandra M. Schneider

Poisonous and injurious plants number in the hundreds and have a wide variety of toxicities. Rather than attempting a comprehensive listing, this chapter focuses on the most important plant-related encounters clinically relevant to emergency medicine. It includes descriptions of the most prevalent and poisonous plants (Tables 201-1 and 201-2), those plants most commonly mistaken for being poisonous (Table 201-3), the most severely poisonous plants, and those most frequently encountered during the holiday season.[1–3] Individual plants are discussed in terms of their pathophysiology, clinical features, and treatment.

EPIDEMIOLOGY

According to statistics gathered by the American Association of Poison Control Centers (AAPCC), plants are the fourth most common reason for poison center notification and account for 5 to 10 percent of all calls received.[3] This high rank is a reflection of their wide availability rather than any unusually high level of innate toxicity. Children under 6 years of age account for 70 to 80 percent of all plant-related exposures, the vast majority of which (96 percent) are unintentional. The most common plant-related call received by a poison control center is for completely nontoxic plants (21 percent) and, on average, fewer than 10 percent of patients require treatment in a health care facility. Of those suffering any sequelae, minimally bothersome effects are most common and occur in 10 percent of all ingestions. Dermatitis and gastrointestinal irritation are most common and occur in approximately 20 percent of patients. Moderate effects of a more systemic nature occur in 1 percent. Severe effects associated with life-threatening or disabling injuries are extremely uncommon and occur in only 0.04 percent. Death due to plant-related exposures are rare, and occur at a rate of less than 0.001 percent.

Toddlers experience the world by first putting it into their mouth. Since 80 percent of the exposures occur among toddlers younger than age 6 years, and most within the home, prevention is paramount. All poisonous and injurious plants must be kept out the reach of toddlers and preschoolers. Homes should be purged of all potentially toxic plants just as they are for medications and cleaning supplies, and children should be specifically instructed never to eat plants or wild berries.

TREATMENT

Most plant-related exposures require no treatment, and those that do often can be managed by simple decontamination procedures. Those patients with a potentially serious exposure who are asymptomatic should be observed in the emergency department for at least 4 to 6 h. If they remain asymptomatic, they may be discharged with appropriate instructions and follow-up. Symptomatic patients require ongoing

TABLE 201-1 Most Commonly Encountered Plants (in Descending Order)

Philodendron species
Dieffenbachia
Poinsettia (*Euphorbia* species)
Peppers (*Capsicum* species)
Holly (*Ilex* species)
Jade plant (*Crassula* species)*
Ficus (*Ficus* species)*
Poison ivy (*Toxicodendron* species)
Pokeweed (*Phytolacca* species)
Umbrella plant (*Schefflera* species)*
Nightshade (*Solanum* species)
Pothos (*Epipremnum* species)
Pyracantha species*
Yew (*Taxus* species)
Azalea (*Rhododendron* species)
Spider plant (*Chlorophytum* species)*
Aloe species
Oleander (*Nerium oleander*)
Caladium species
Dracaena species*
Cactus species
Lily of the Valley (*Convallaria* species)
Jimsonweed (*Datura* species)
Mistletoe (*Phoradendron*)
Coleus species*

*Denotes nonpoisonous plants
Source: Adapted from Krenzelok and Jacobsen,[2] with permission.

monitoring and care and should be admitted to the hospital, because toxicity may continue to evolve. Few plants have specific antidotes.

It is recommended that all exposures be reported to the regional poison control center, which is the only national organization currently tracking all poisonous and injurious plants, and their input is invaluable. Poison centers are also helpful with plant identification. All exposures are potential toxicologic emergencies and should be treated accordingly, with appropriate consultation.

TABLE 201-2 Most Toxic Plants

Castor bean (*Ricinus communis*)
Foxglove (*Digitalis purpurea*)
Jequirity bean (*Abrus precatorius*)
Oleander (*Nerium oleander*)
Poison hemlock (*Conium maculatum*)
Water hemlock (*Cicuta maculata*)
Yew (*Taxus* species)

TABLE 201-3 Nonpoisonous Plants Commonly Mistaken for Being Poisonous

African violet (*Episcia reptans*)
Coleus (*Coleus X hydrus*)
Dracaena species
Ficus species (climbing or weeping fig)
Jade plant (*Crassula argentea*)
Honeysuckle (*Lonicera* species)
Pyracantha species
Rubber tree plant (*Ficus elasticus*)
Schefflera species (*Brassaia actinophylla,* umbrella plant)
Spider plant (*Chlorophytum comosum*)
Wandering jew (*Tradescantia albiflora*)

SEVERELY POISONOUS PLANTS

Castor Bean (*Ricinus communis*)

Ricin is a potent toxalbumin that inhibits protein synthesis and causes severe cytotoxic effects on multiple organ systems. It may be one of the most poisonous naturally occurring substances known.[4,5] Although present in all parts of the plant, it is concentrated most in the seeds. Beans are covered by a hard, relatively impervious outer shell that must be chewed or in some way broken in order for the ricin to result in toxicity.

Symptoms include delayed gastroenteritis, which may be severe and hemorrhagic, followed by delirium, seizures, coma, and death. Beans are particularly antigenic and may cause severe hypersensitivity and cutaneous and systemic allergic reactions.

Whole bowel irrigation (WBI) has been advocated to ensure rapid and complete decontamination of the GI tract. Rapid elimination of the bean before erosion of the outer shell occurs may decrease or prevent the release of potent toxins. Beans should be counted to assure complete recovery. Patients should be observed for at least 8 to 12 h. Once symptomatic, supportive care involves attention to fluid, glucose, and electrolyte replacement.

Foxglove (*Digitalis purpurea*)

Foxglove contains cardiac glycosides similar in structure and action to digitalis. Its toxicity lies somewhere between lily of the valley and oleander (see *oleander* below).

Jequirity Bean (*Abrus precatorius*)

Jequirity beans contain the toxalbumin abrin, one of the most lethal naturally occurring toxins known.[5] Children have died as a result of chewing alone (without swallowing) the beans. Chewing and swallowing just one bean may be lethal to an adult. Symptoms include a delayed gastroenteritis, which may be severe and hemorrhagic, followed by delirium, seizures, coma, and death. Like castor bean, recovery of the intact bean by WBI is preferred. Patients should be observed for at least 8 to 12 h. Treatment is otherwise supportive, with attention to fluid replacement and monitoring of electrolytes.

Oleander (*Nerium oleander*)

Similar in structure and effect to digitalis, all parts of the plant contain the cardiac glycosides oleandrin, oleandroside, nerioside, and digitoxigenin. Cardiac glycosides act by inhibiting the Na, K-ATPase pump and lead to hyperkalemia and a variety of dysrhythmias. Of all plants containing cardiac glycosides (lily of the valley, foxglove, and oleander), oleander is the most toxic.

These glycosides cross-react sufficiently such that a positive serum digoxin level will qualitatively confirm an ingestion. Quantitative levels are not accurate, however, and should not be used to quantify the amount of ingestion or potential toxicity. Effects include nausea, vomiting, diarrhea, abdominal pain, confusion, and cardiac dysrhythmias.

Potassium levels should be closely monitored. Hyperkalemia may be severe and refractory to the usual treatments (insulin, dextrose, bicarbonate), and may require hemodialysis.[6] Calcium is generally not recommended, as it may exacerbate the digitalis toxicity. In addition to GI decontamination and routine antidysrhythmic therapy, digoxin-specific Fab antibody fragments are recommended for patients with significant symptoms.[7]

Poison Hemlock (*Conium maculatum*)

All parts contain conine alkaloids similar in structure and effect to nicotine. Symptoms occur rapidly in 15 min to 1 h and begin with complaints of burning and dryness of the mouth. Tachycardia, tremors, diaphoresis, mydriasis, profound muscle weakness, and seizures may develop. In severe cases, ascending paralysis, bradycardia, coma, and death occur. Although most cases are unintentional, there are some case reports of toxicity resulting from the intentional use by patients for a presumed narcotic-like effect.[8] Treatment consists of GI decontamination, activated charcoal, and supportive care which may include IV fluids, antidysrhythmics, and anticonvulsants.

Water Hemlock (*Cicuta maculata*)

Cicutoxin, a highly unsaturated higher alcohol, is found in highest concentrations in the root, but all parts contain the poison. Its exact mechanism of action is unknown. One mouthful may be fatal in as soon as 15 min. Initial symptoms include nausea, vomiting, and abdominal pain, followed by delirium, seizures, and death. Seizures may be severe and refractory to conventional anticonvulsant therapy. The mortality rate may be as high as 30 percent.[9] GI decontamination is paramount. Treatment is otherwise supportive, with IV fluids, anticonvulsants, and bicarbonate if necessary for acidosis.

Yew (*Taxus* Species)

Yew contains taxine alkaloids in the leaves and seeds. Symptoms include nausea, vomiting, and abdominal pain, followed by seizures, cardiac dysrhythmias, coma, and occasionally death. Treatment consists of GI decontamination, activated charcoal, fluids, and antidysrhythmics as necessary.

COMMON POISONOUS AND INJURIOUS PLANTS

Aloe (*Aloe barbadensis*)

Sap from this common succulent house plant contains an anthraquinone that acts as a cathartic. Symptoms include abdominal pain and diarrhea within 6 to 12 h of ingestion. It may occasionally turn the urine red, and large doses may cause nephritis. There is no specific antidote. Intravenous (IV) fluids may be necessary to support GI fluid losses.

Azalea (*Rhododendron* Species)

Andromedotoxins are found in the leaves, flowers, and nectar. Symptoms produced include salivation, lacrimation, bradycardia, hypotension, progressive paralysis, and potentially (but rarely) death. Most cases display minimal toxicity. In addition to gastrointestinal (GI) decontamination, treatment consists of atropine for symptomatic bradycardia and fluids or pressors for hypotension.

Cactus

Needles or spines may embed in the skin and cause direct mechanical injury.[10] Patients complain of pain and irritation at the site. Unlike other foreign bodies such as glass that are inert, spines contain proteinaceous material and should be removed if possible. They may be removed by applying a thin layer of rubber cement or other similar type substance. The substance is allowed to dry and then gently peeled off removing the spines. Complications such as infection and granuloma formation occur, but are uncommon.[10]

Caladium

Toxicity is similar to dieffenbachia (calcium oxalate raphides), but less severe.

Crocus (Autumn Crocus)

Colchicine is contained in all parts of the autumn crocus and glory lily. Colchicine causes a gastroenteritis that is delayed and severe, and is followed by severe multisystem organ failure. Common effects include coagulopathy, bone marrow suppression with granulocytopenia and thrombocytopenia, cardiac dysrhythmias, cardiogenic shock, adult respiratory distress syndrome, hepatic insufficiency, delirium, seizures, coma, and death. In addition to GI decontamination, treatment usually requires aggressive fluid resuscitation. Colchicine-specific Fab fragments are commercially available for severe poisonings.

Dieffenbachia (Dumbcane)

Plants contain calcium oxalate crystals packaged into bundles known as raphides. In addition to the calcium oxalate crystals, these plants also contain preoteolytic enzymes with antitrypsin-like activity that stimulate the release of histamine and bradykinin. It remains unclear why some plants such as schefflera, which also contain calcium oxalate crystals, are completely nontoxic. Children who chew the leaves develop immediate burning and irritation of the oral mucosa. Cases of severe swelling, drooling, dysphagia, and respiratory compromise have been reported, but are not common. In a large retrospective study of 188 patients suffering oxalate exposure, all cases were minor and resolved with little or no treatment.[11] Demulcifying agents such as cold milk or ice cream may help. Analgesics may be necessary. Steroids may be beneficial for severe cases, although there have been no controlled trials.

Fava Beans

There are limited examples of genetic predispositions being associated with increased potential for toxicity. Among persons affected by glucose-6-phosphate dehydrogenase deficiency, 10 to 20 percent develop favism after consuming fava beans. Symptoms include GI upset, fever, and headache. Patients may develop hemolytic anemia, hemoglobinuria, and jaundice.[12] There is no specific antidote.

Jimsonweed (*Datura* Species)

Jimsonweed (also known as thorn apple, devil's trumpet, or locoweed) is a wildly occurring weed infamous for its hallucinatory properties.

Exposures most commonly are intentional and occur through experimentation.[13] All parts of the plant are toxic and contain atropine-like alkaloids (hyoscyamine, atropine, and scopalamine) capable of precipitating acute anticholinergic crises by competitive inhibition of cholinergic muscarinic receptors.[14]

Symptoms occur within 30 to 60 min and may last for up to 48 h because of delayed gastric motility. Symptoms include hyperthermia (''hot as a hare''), flushed skin (''red as a beet''), dry skin and mucus membranes (''dry as a bone''), mydriasis (''blind as a bat''), and hallucinations or delirium (''mad as a hatter''). Tachycardia and urinary retention are also common.

Treatment includes GI decontamination with emesis or lavage, activated charcoal, and supportive care (IV fluids, external cooling, and restraints for patient protection). GI decontamination may be useful for up to 48 h after ingestion if the patient remains symptomatic.[14] Physostigmine, a cholinesterase inhibitor, antagonizes both the central and peripheral effects and may be required in 30 to 40 percent of cases.[13] It should be considered for severe cases exhibiting hyperthermia, seizures, or frank psychosis. An initial dose of 0.5 mg for children or 1.0 to 2.0 mg for adults is given slowly IV over 5 min. Repeat doses may be required.[13] See Chapter 177, ''Anticholinergic and Antihistaminic Toxicity,'' for more discussion.

Lily of the Valley (*Convallaria majalis*)

In addition to ingestion of the plant itself, toxicity has been reported from drinking of water in which the freshly cut flowers were kept (see the *oleander* section).

Nettle (Stinging Nettle, Bull Nettle)

Nettles contain a specialized system for injecting their toxins. Stinging hairs are connected to a bladder filled with various irritants (histamine, acetylcholine, 5-hydroxytryptamine). Handling of the plant stimulates the injection of these substances via the hair tube. An immediate burning response may last for hours. Treatment is symptomatic.

Nightshade, Common or Woody (*Solanum* species, Nightshade)

The glycoalkaloid solanine is present in all parts of the plant. Ingestion results in nausea, vomiting, diarrhea, and abdominal pain. Delirium, hallucinations and coma may also occur with larger doses. There is no specific treatment.

Nightshade, Deadly (*Atropa belladonna*)

This contains atropine-like substances with anticholinergic properties (see the *jimsonweed* section).

Peach, Apricot, Pear, Crab Apple, and *Hydrangea*

Amygdalin, a cyanogenic glycoside, is metabolized by the enzyme emulsin to hydrocyanic acid. In sufficient quantities, hydrocyanic acid may lead to acute cyanide toxicity. The requisite enzyme (emulsin) is present in the pits or seeds listed above and may be present to some degree in intestinal bacteria. Ingestion of large amounts of seeds or pits results in diaphoresis, nausea, vomiting, abdominal pain, and lethargy. Symptoms develop over hours. GI decontamination is needed. If symptomatic, antidotal therapy may be needed for cyanide toxicity (amyl nitrate, sodium nitrate, and sodium triosulfate). See Chapter 182, ''Cyanide,'' for further discussion.

Pepper (*Capsicum*)

Capsicum causes irritation, burning, and pain upon contact with mucous membranes as a result of depletion of substance P from terminal nerve endings. There is intense burning of the mucous membranes with contact. Patients typically self-innoculate their eyes while preparing peppers. Police use pepper sprays to subdue combative individuals. In addition to cutaneous decontamination with copious amounts of water and a gentle hand soap, demulcifying agents such as cold milk or ice cream may help. Analgesics may be necessary.

Philodendron (Elephant's Ear)

All parts contain oxalate raphides and may produce symptoms similar to dieffenbachia, although less severe.

Pokeweed (*Phytolacca americana*)

All parts of the plant are toxic, but especially the roots, unripe berries, and seeds. Phytotoxins (phytolaccotoxin and phytolaccine) cause direct mucosal irritation and GI symptoms. Patients complain of burning in the mouth and throat, with abdominal pain, nausea, vomiting, and profuse diarrhea that may be foamy.[15] Severe intoxications may result in coma and death. Although their safety remains somewhat controversial, ripe berries are occasionally used in pies and the leaves boiled for greens. Treatment is GI decontamination with emesis or lavage, charcoal, and supportive care consisting of fluid-electrolyte replacement.

Pothos (Devil's Ivy, *Epipremnum*)

This plant has toxicity similar to dieffenbachia, but less severe.

Red/Yellow Sage (*Lantana*)

Leaves and unripe fruit contain the toxin lantadene. Patients develop dilated pupils, vomiting, diarrhea, weakness, and coma. Symptoms may be delayed for 2 to 6 h. Treatment is GI contamination and fluids for dehydration.

Solanum Species (Potato, Eggplant, Common Nightshade)

Solanine is contained in green potatoes and in the sprouts, and is destroyed by cooking. Delayed gastroenteritis may be seen (see *common nightshade* above).

Toxicodendron Species (Poison Ivy, Oak, and Sumac)

Plants contain the antigenic resin, urushiol. Once exposed, most, but not all, individuals develop sensitization as the antigenic resin binds with skin proteins and forms a complete antigen. Reexposure then stimulates a T-cell-mediated immune response. Reactions begin with itching, burning and redness developing over 12 to 48 h, and may progress to include varying degrees of vesiculobullous formation. Resin may remain after the plant has dried and may be aerosolized during burning. Antipruritic and topical therapies (oatmeal baths and topical steroids) are commonly used. Facial, genital or widespread involvement requires systemic steroids for 10 to 14 days. Patients should be advised to clean under their fingernails and wash all contaminated clothing. IvyBlock, a new product recently approved by the Food and Drug Administration, contains bentoquatam and binds urushiol to prevent absorption. Skin cleansers (such as Tecnu, Oak-N-Ivy Brand) may be used after the rash has begun to develop, up to 8 h after exposure, to decontaminate the skin. (See Chap. 239 for further discussion.)

COMMON HOLIDAY OR SEASONAL PLANTS (POISONOUS AND NONPOISONOUS)

Holly (*Ilex* Species)

The leaves are nontoxic, whereas the berries contain a variety of toxins known as saponins. Gastroenteritis is most common and may occur with as few as two or three berries, whereas 20 to 30 berries may be fatal. Treatment is GI decontamination followed by IV fluids to prevent dehydration.

Poinsettia (*Euphorbia pulcherrima*)

Poinsettia is a much maligned plant ubiquitous during the Christmas holidays. Originally implicated as being toxic, recent evidence suggests that at most it may occasionally cause some local irritation to skin, mouth, or conjunctiva.[16]

Mistletoe (*Phoradendron*)

All parts are poisonous and contain phoratoxin, a toxalbumin. Gastroenteritis may occur following ingestion of a large number of berries. Treatment is GI decontamination with fluid and electrolyte monitoring.

Easter Lily (*Lilium longiflorum*)

Toxicity has not been reported in humans.

REFERENCES

1. Borys DJ, Setzer SC, Hornfeldt CS: A retrospective review of plant exposures as reported to the Hennepin Regional Poison Center in 1985. *Vet Hum Toxicol* 29:83, 1987.
2. Krenzelok EP, Jacobsen TD: Plant exposures . . . A national profile of the most common plant genera. *Vet Hum Toxicol* 39:248, 1997.
3. Litovitz TL, Klein-Schwartz W, Dyer KJ: 1997 annual report of the American Association of Poison Control Centers national data collection system. *Am J Emerg Med* 16:443, 1998.
4. Challoner KR, McCarron MM: Castor bean intoxication. *Ann Emerg Med* 19:1177, 1990.
5. Kinamore PA, Jaeger RW, Castro FJ: Abrus and ricinus ingestion. *Clin Toxicol* 17:401, 1980.
6. Haynes BE, Bessen HA, Wightman WD: Oleander tea: Herbal draught of death. *Ann Emerg Med* 14:350, 1985.
7. Shumaik GM, Wu AW, Ping AC: Oleander poisoning: Treatment with digoxin-specific Fab antibody fragments. *Ann Emerg Med* 17:732, 1988.
8. Drummer OH, Roberts AN, Bedford PJ, et al: Three deaths from hemlock poisoning. *Med J Austr* 162:592, 1995.
9. Starreveld E, Hope E: Cicutoxin poisoning. *Neurology* 25:730, 1975.
10. Lindsey D, Lindsey WE: Cactus spine injuries. *Am J Emerg Med* 6:362, 1988.
11. Mrvos R, Dean BS, Krenzelok EP: Philodendron/dieffenbachia ingestions: Are they a problem? *Clin Toxicol* 29:485, 1991.
12. Wong W, Powars D, Williams WD: Yewdow-induced anemia. *West J Med* 15:459, 1989.
13. Klein-Schwartz W, Oderda GM: Jimsonweed intoxication in adolescents and young adults. *JAMA* 138:737, 1984.
14. Hanna JP, Schmidley JW, Braselton WE: Datura delirium. *Clin Neuropharmacol* 15:109, 1992.
15. Roberge R, Brader E, Martin ML, et al: The root of evil: Pokeweed intoxication. *Ann Emerg Med* 15:470, 1986.
16. Krenzelok EP, Jacobsen TD, Aronis JM: Poinsettia exposures have good outcomes . . . Just as we thought. *Am J Emerg Med* 14:671, 1996.

ENDOCRINE EMERGENCIES

HYPOGLYCEMIA

William J. Brady
Richard A. Harrigan

Although there is no universally accepted definition of hypoglycemia, it is generally defined as (1) a serum glucose level of less than 50 mg/dL, (2) symptoms consistent with the diagnosis; and (3) resolution of symptoms following glucose administration. Up to 20 percent of patients with diabetes mellitus using insulin or oral hypoglycemic agents (OHAs) will experience symptoms of hypoglycemia in their lifetime, requiring emergency department (ED) evaluation and therapy.[1-3] If one considers all patients with altered mentation arriving at the ED, hypoglycemia is the underlying process in approximately 7 percent. In addition to diabetes, other clinical settings associated with hypoglycemia include sepsis, liver disease, alcohol intoxication, starvation, and certain toxic ingestions. Hypoglycemia should be considered in the differential diagnosis in any patient with altered mental status or focal neurologic signs.[4,5]

PATHOPHYSIOLOGY

Blood glucose homeostasis involves complex neural, metabolic, and hormonal interactions. The central nervous system (CNS) requires a continuous supply of carbohydrate fuel for normal function and utilizes about 150 g/day of glucose. The CNS has a small reservoir of glucose that is sufficient for only a few minutes of normal brain function. Despite these stringent demands, the body normally functions quite well in maintaining plasma glucose levels within a narrow range despite constant changes in glucose intake and/or utilization.

The primary glucoregulatory organs are the liver, the pancreas, adrenals, and pituitary gland. These organs maintain glucose control by the release and interaction of various hormonal agents, including insulin, glucagon, the catecholamines epinephrine and norepinephrine, cortisol and other glucocorticoids, and growth hormone. Insulin is the major metabolic regulatory factor, acting predominantly on the liver, skeletal muscle, and adipose tissue. Insulin suppresses endogenous glucose production, stimulates glucose utilization, and increases glucose storage in the form of glycogen, thus lowering the plasma glucose concentration.

The first defense against the development of hypoglycemia is a decrease in insulin secretion, but both glucagon and epinephrine are also important for the acute protection against hypoglycemia. Both of these counterregulatory hormones are the only agents capable of stimulating hepatic glucose production within minutes of their release into circulation, primarily via glycogenolysis—the release of glucose from its intracellular storage-depot glycogen. The effect of these two hormones beyond the immediate period after their release—ranging from several hours to several days—is felt predominantly through their effect on gluconeogenesis—the de novo production of glucose from other metabolic substrates. Glucagon is felt to be the major counterregulatory hormone while epinephrine is important under certain conditions, especially during glucagon deficiency and in the generation of warning symptoms of hypoglycemia. Epinephrine also stimulates hepatic glucose production as well and also limits glucose utilization. In contrast to glucagon and epinephrine, glucocorticoid and growth hormone responses are largely involved in the protection against prolonged hypoglycemia over days to weeks.

Hormonal responses are largely determined by glucose intake and vary between the fed and the fasting states. The fed state extends for up to 3 h after the ingestion of food. In the fed state, glucose absorption from the gut stimulates the release of insulin from the pancreas, causing a shift of carbohydrate from the circulation into the various tissues for either consumption or storage. In certain cases, after entry into the cell, glucose is immediately used for energy production via glycolysis, with the glycolytic products proceeding on to the tricarboxcylic acid (TCA) cycle and down the electron transport chain, generating additional ATP. If the glucose is destined for fuel storage, it may take various forms, depending on the host tissue location: glycogen in the liver, triglycerides in adipose tissue, and protein in muscle. Insulin also acts on the liver to decrease glucose output by inhibiting glycogenolysis and gluconeogenesis. It inhibits lipolysis and promotes lipogenesis in adipose cells, and encourages the uptake of amino acids and inhibits proteolysis.

The fasting period is the interval between feedings, beginning approximately 4 h after eating and extending up to the next meal. In fasted individuals, the maintenance of normal blood glucose levels depends on an adequate supply of endogenous gluconeogenic substrates (amino acids, glycerol, and lactate), functionally intact hepatic glycogenolytic and gluconeogenic enzymatic systems, and normal endocrinologic function for integrating and modulating these processes. Hypoglycemia may result if any part of this system is disrupted. During fasting, relatively low insulin levels initiate the mobilization of these various stored fuels from host tissue sources. The most readily and rapidly available source of glucose is hepatic glycogen. Glucose is formed by glycogenolysis, which is potentiated in the liver by glucagon and epinephrine. The glycogen reserve is limited and will be depleted after 24 to 48 h of fasting in healthy patients and possibly earlier in malnourished individuals. With continuation of fasting (approximately 4 to 6 h), gluconeogenesis becomes the primary source of blood glucose required for CNS metabolism and other bodily processes. Gluconeogenesis, occurring primarily in the liver, uses various metabolic substrates to generate an additional glucose supply. Amino acids are mobilized from muscle tissue via proteolysis, which is facilitated by low insulin levels and mediated by cortisol and glucagon. Lactate, from recycled glucose, and glycerol, from lipolysis, are minor yet important substrates for gluconeogenesis. During nonprolonged overnight fasting, 90 percent of gluconeogenesis occurs via proteolysis with conversion of amino acids to glucose.

If fasting is prolonged beyond the functional capabilities of both gluconeogenesis and glycogenolysis, the mobilization of other fuel stores is initiated with a decline in plasma insulin levels, thus removing the insulin-mediated inhibitory action on lipolysis and proteolysis; alternative fuel stores are then mobilized. Fat stores in the form of triglycerides are a major source of energy. Lipolysis, potentiated by a relative decline in serum insulin levels and the presence of both epinephrine and growth hormone, produces free fatty acids (FFAs) and glycerol. Most tissues, except the CNS and cellular blood elements, use FFAs as a source of energy, simultaneously allowing the body to conserve glucose for brain metabolism and sparing protein from catabolism for gluconeogenesis. The released glycerol may also be converted to glucose in the liver.

Hypoglycemia unawareness—the development of low serum sugar values without the physiologic ability to react—places individuals at greater risk for coma and other neurologic sequelae. Extremes of age, comorbidity, medications, autonomic neuropathy, and the degree of serum sugar control are some factors affecting awareness of hypoglycemia. It has been suggested that elderly patients are more likely to experience hypoglycemia without an awareness of the event. As an example, the presence of previous stroke in older patients could increase the chance of unrecognized hypoglycemia. β-Adrenergic receptor antagonists block the effects of epinephrine, therefore contributing to patient unawareness of hypoglycemia. Further, patients with diabetes mellitus and autonomic neuropathy demonstrate blunted counterregulatory responses to hypoglycemia.[6] With increasingly rigid control of the serum glucose, patients with diabetes mellitus without neuropathy may also have reduced responsiveness of the counterregulatory hormones, potentiating an unawareness of hypoglycemia.[7] Such a clinical unawareness may result from either a lack of CNS recognition of hypoglycemia or impaired autonomic response to low serum sugar.

CLINICAL FEATURES

Table 202-1 lists common causes of hypoglycemia in adults. The most common causes treated in an urban ED were diabetic medical therapy, 54 percent; ethanol use, 48 percent; and sepsis, 12 percent.[4]

Common scenarios in diabetic patients include inadequate food intake, increased physical exertion, incorrect medication dosing, or drug interactions. The characteristics of diabetic patients who are more likely to experience hypoglycemia include male gender, adolescent and very elderly age groups, African American heritage, a past history of hypoglycemia, ''intensive'' diabetic medical therapy, insulin use (compared with OHA therapy), polypharmacy (more than five agents), and recent hospitalization.[1–3]

The introduction of metformin, a biguanide, has added another medication to the list of agents encountered in diabetic patients. Metformin improves the end-organ sensitivity to insulin and acts via a number of mechanisms in diabetic patients, including a reduction in hepatic glucose output and enhanced peripheral glucose uptake. Metformin is considered an antihyperglycemia drug rather than a hypoglycemic agent such as the sulfonylureas and insulin. Hypoglycemia is rarely encountered in patients using only metformin.

The nonselective β-blocker agents impair glycogenolysis and the hyperepinephrinemic response to lowered serum sugar levels, thus predisposing individuals to hypoglycemia. Hypoglycemia resulting from the sole ingestion of such adrenergic-blocking agents is rare.[5]

Approximately 50 percent of patients treated for hypoglycemia in an urban ED were acutely intoxicated with ethanol or were chronic alcohol abusers.[4] Alcohol inhibits hepatic gluconeogenesis, which becomes problematic when a patient has not eaten for a prolonged period and the glycogen stores have been depleted by glycogenolysis. A 12-h fast is often sufficient for severely malnourished alcoholics to become hypoglycemic. Hypoglycemia has also been produced in healthy adults by infusing 75 g of alcohol after a 36-h fast. Rapid bedside serum glucose determinations should be performed on all patients with any mental status abnormality or evidence of alcohol use.

TABLE 202-1 Potential Etiologies of Hypoglycemia in Adults

Cause/Syndrome
Sepsis
Medication/toxin effect
Alcohol
Salicylates
Barbiturates
Insulin
Oral hypoglycemic agents
β Blockers
Endocrinopathies
Hypothyroidism
Adrenal insufficiency
Insulinoma
Malnutrition/fasting
Suicide attempt

Source: Reprinted from Luber et al,[22] with permission.

TABLE 202-2 Frequency of Presenting Signs and Symptoms in Hypoglycemia

Clinical Presentation	Frequency (%)
Depressed sensorium	52
Other mental status changes	30
Hyperepinephrinemic findings	8
Seizure	7
Focal neurologic findings	2

Source: From Malouf and Brust,[4] with permission.

Sepsis may cause hypoglycemia by inhibition of gluconeogenesis and by increased responsiveness to insulin. Systemic hypoperfusion, often associated with sepsis, increases peripheral glucose utilization while metabolic acidosis decreases gluconeogenesis. The multiorgan failure associated with the sepsis syndrome not infrequently includes hepatic dysfunction and an increased potential for hypoglycemia.

Patients with hypoglycemia may have a wide array of symptoms and signs (Table 202-2). The clinical manifestations of hypoglycemia are divided into two broad categories: neuroglycopenic and hyperepinephrinemic (also known as the autonomic or sympathomimetic findings). As glucose is the main energy source for CNS function, it is not surprising that most episodes of symptomatic hypoglycemia include neurologic dysfunction. With a decline in serum sugar, the brain quickly exhausts its reserve supply of carbohydrate fuel, resulting in CNS dysfunction. This manifests most commonly by alterations in consciousness, such as lethargy, confusion, combativeness, agitation, and unresponsiveness. Other neuroglycopenic manifestations include seizures and focal neurologic deficits. A review of 125 cases of hypoglycemia in an urban ED showed that the neuroglycopenic findings predominated.[4] A depressed sensorium was noted in 52 percent of cases, with other mental status changes—agitation and combativeness—found in 30 percent of patients. Described less frequently, seizure activity and focal neurologic findings were encountered in 7 percent and 2 percent, respectively.[4]

A rapid fall in blood glucose levels or the hypothalamic sensing of neuroglycopenia causes the release of the counterregulatory hormones, primarily the catecholamines epinephrine and norepinephrine. The release of the latter is responsible for the hyperepinephrinemic findings, including anxiety, nervousness, irritability, nausea, vomiting, palpitations, and tremor. Such signs and symptoms were noted in 8 percent of ED patients with hypoglycemia.[4]

The term ''hyperepinephrinemic'' is a misnomer in that cholinergic factors resulting from autonomic nervous system stimulation are also noted in certain patients. Stimulation of the cholinergic nervous system also occurs and may result in manifestations such as sweating, changes in pupillary size, bradycardia, and salivation.

The rapidity of onset of the hypoglycemic event determines in part the presentation. A gradual onset of hypoglycemia results from a relatively slow decrease in the serum glucose and the development of the neuroglycopenic signs and symptoms. Conversely, a sudden drop in the blood sugar level will produce anxiety, diaphoresis, tremor, and the other hyperepinephrinemic findings. In most cases of hypoglycemia, however, CNS dysfunction predominates with some degree of alteration in the level of awareness, accompanied by diaphoresis and tachycardia.

Hypoglycemia has been misdiagnosed as stroke, transient ischemic attack, seizure disorder, traumatic head injury, brain tumor, narcolepsy, multiple sclerosis, psychosis, sympathomimetic drug ingestion, hysteria, altered sleep patterns and nightmares, and depression.[6–11] Although uncommon, bradycardia has also been reported.[12]

DIAGNOSIS

Failure to determine the blood glucose level early in the evaluation can result in a delayed or missed diagnosis with associated morbidity due to CNS injury or unnecessary invasive procedures and therapies.[13] Always consider hypoglycemia as a potential cause of altered mentation and rapidly screen for it at the bedside, followed by replacement therapy, regardless of the presumed reason for a patient's condition. The use of bedside testing is preferred in that the result is immediately available to the clinician and its result may alter therapeutic and diagnostic plans.[13] The accuracy of bedside reflectance tests is acceptable though less reliable at extremely low and high glucose levels.

If possible, immediately prior to intravenous (IV) dextrose therapy, a serum sample should be obtained and sent to the lab for confirmation. Glucose values of whole blood are approximately 15 percent less than serum or plasma. This discrepancy is due to the relatively low glucose concentration in red blood cells—with storage, equilibration occurs. Venous blood has a 10 percent lower glucose concentration when compared with either capillary or arterial blood. Finally, the collecting tube should contain fluoride to inhibit glycolysis in vitro before the sample is assayed.

TREATMENT

Initial management is the administration of 1 g/kg body weight dextrose, as 50% dextrose in water (D_{50}/W) in adults. This can be followed by the infusion of 10% dextrose at a rate to maintain the serum glucose above 100 mg/dL. Repeat bedside glucose determination should be done every 30 min for the first 2 h, to detect rebound hypoglycemia. The best replacement is oral, however. A total of 300 g (1200 cal) of carbohydrate should be given orally, as sodas, juices, sandwiches, or snacks. A total of 50 mL of 10_{50} W contains only 100 cal. Whereas some suggest that each ampule of glucose (50 g of a 50% dextrose solution) will raise the serum glucose by 60 mg/dL,[14] others feel that prediction of posttreatment levels is impossible.[15]

Glucagon, 1 mg intramuscularly or IV, can be used in diabetics or in those in whom IV access is unobtainable. Response to glucagon therapy is generally slower when compared with IV dextrose, requiring 7 to 10 min prior to normalization of mental status; additionally, the response to glucagon administration may be short-lived. The condition of alcoholics, the elderly, and others with depleted glycogen stores will generally not improve with glucagon. Fructose and other complex carbohydrates should not be used to correct hypoglycemia in that these sugars do not cross the blood-brain barrier effectively or require extensive metabolic conversion.

Persistent hyperglycemia, maintained by slow administration of dextrose, indicates that the infusion may be reduced and eventually withdrawn. Failure to respond to parenteral glucose administration should prompt consideration of other causes of hypoglycemia.

A total of 100 mg parenteral thiamine should be given in conjunction with glucose, because, historically, the administration of glucose without thiamine in severe nutritional deficiency states could precipitate Wernicke's encephalopathy.[16] Today, this is rare. Thiamine acts as a coenzyme in several reactions in intermediary metabolism, specifically in the conversions of pyruvate to acetyl coenzyme A (linking glycolysis to the TCA cycle) and α-ketoglutarate to succinate (a reaction in the TCA cycle). As thiamine reserves disappear, the reactions halt, removing the CNS's main source of ATP and causing the acute development of Wernicke's syndrome.

Steroid administration should be considered for hypoglycemia that is either resistant to aggressive glucose replacement therapy or associated with the signs of adrenal insufficiency (see Chap. 208). The dose is 100 to 200 mg hydrocortisone IV in adults.

Studies in the early 1980s suggested that hyperglycemia at the time of hospital admission is associated with poor neurologic recovery in stroke patients[17] and survivors of out-of-hospital cardiopulmonary arrest.[18] More recently, similar concern has been voiced regarding the association of worsened neurologic outcome and hyperglycemia in patients with acute head injury.[19,20] It is theorized that hyperglycemia accentuates local tissue damage by continued or increased anaerobic metabolism, lactate production, and intracellular acidosis. Acidosis may trigger a cascade that includes calcium entry into cells, lipolysis, and cytotoxic fatty acid release, culminating in neuronal death. The clinical significance has not been demonstrated, and this information should not alter the clinical management of hypoglycemia at this time.

DISPOSITION

Factors affecting disposition include (1) the patient's current mental status as well as the level of consciousness during observation in the ED, (2) serial determinations of the serum glucose, (3) both the timing and extent of the response to resuscitative therapy, (4) the need for additional replacement therapy, (5) etiology of the hypoglycemic event, (6) comorbidity, (7) the patient's social situation, (8) any psychiatric issues, and (9) the agent ingested.

Either continued or recurrent mental status alteration, recurrent hypoglycemia, or a downward trend in serial glucose values during ED observation despite adequate replacement therapy demands admission to the hospital. Also, any patient requiring large doses of dextrose as both bolus and infusion should be admitted. An inpatient disposition in a critical care setting is likely warranted in cases involving the following etiologies: massive insulin or OHA ingestion, marked malnutrition, sepsis, acute liver failure, or any other event associated with the tendency toward profound hypoglycemia. Further, patients without proper outpatient supervision should be admitted for observation. The case suitable for outpatient observation is characterized by a responsible adult who will monitor the patient's mental status every 3 h, coupled with a motivated patient who will perform serum glucose determinations frequently and who can maintain oral feeding. The suspected or known intentional ingestion of either insulin or OHA must be admitted for ongoing medical and psychiatric care.

The particular medication agent ingested must be strongly weighed in disposition decisions. Short-acting insulin preparations do not always demand hospitalization, whereas intermediate and long-acting preparations likely will require admission for ongoing observation and, at times, continued supportive care. Care must be exercised in large short-acting insulin exposures in that the pharmacodynamics of such insulin preparations are altered with massive doses. The expected short half-life may not be encountered. OHAs also represent an indication for hospitalization due to relatively long serum half-life with a prolonged tendency toward the development of hypoglycemia. Low serum glucose may develop as long as 16 h after ingestion, though the majority of patients will become symptomatic within 8 h of exposure.[21] A single tablet ingestion by a child can produce significant hypoglycemia. Finally, if any doubt exists as to the need for inpatient observation, admission for short-term observation is justified. If a patient is discharged, follow-up should be provided in 24 h with the primary care physician.

REFERENCES

1. Hayward RA, Manning WG, Kaplan SH, et al: Starting insulin therapy in patients with type 2 diabetes: Effectiveness, complications, and resource utilization. *JAMA* 278:1663, 1997.
2. Anonymous: Hypoglycemia in the Diabetes Control and Complications Trial: The Diabetes Control and Complications Trial Research Group. *Diabetes* 46:271, 1997.

3. Shorr RI, Ray WA, Daugherty JR, Griffin MR: Incidence and risk factors for serious hypoglycemia in older persons using insulin or sulfonylureas. *Arch Intern Med* 157:1681, 1997.
4. Malouf R, Brust JCM: Hypoglycemia: Causes, neurological manifestations, and outcome. *Ann Neurol* 17:421, 1985.
5. Seltzer HS: Drug-induced hypoglycemia: A review based on 473 cases. *Diabetes* 21:955, 1972.
6. Fanelli C, Pampanelli S, Lalli C, et al: Long-term intensive therapy of IDDM patients with clinically overt autonomic neuropathy: Effects on hypoglycemia awareness and counterregulation. *Diabetes* 46:1172, 1997.
7. Boyle PJ, Kempers SF, O'Connor AM, Nagy RJ: Brain glucose uptake and unawareness of hypoglycemia in patients with insulin-dependent diabetes mellitus. *N Engl J Med* 333:1726, 1995.
8. Wallis WE, Donaldson I, Scott RS, Wilson J: Hypoglycemia masquerading as cerebrovascular disease (hypoglycemic hemiplegia). *Ann Neurol* 18:510, 1985.
9. Foster JW, Hart RG: Hypoglycemic hemiplegia: Two cases and a clinical review. *Stroke* 18:944, 1987.
10. Brady WJ, Duncan CW: Hypoglycemia masquerading as acute psychosis and acute cocaine intoxication. *Am J Emerg Med* 17:318, 1999.
11. Luber S, Brady W, Brand A, et al: Acute hypoglycemia masquerading as head trauma: A report of four cases. *Am J Emerg Med* 14:543, 1996.
12. Pollock G, Brady WJ, Hargarten S, et al: Hypoglycemia manifested by sinus bradycardia: A report of three cases. *Acad Emerg Med* 3:700, 1996.
13. Brady WJ, Butler K, Fines R, Young J: Hypoglycemia in multiple trauma victims. *Am J Emerg Med* 17:4, 1999.
14. Hoffman RS, Goldfrank LR: The poisoned patient with altered consciousness: Controversies in the use of a "coma cocktail." *JAMA* 274:562, 1995.
15. Balentine JR, Gaeta TJ, Kessler D, et al: Effect of 50 milliliters of 50% dextrose in water administration on the blood sugar of euglycemic volunteers. *Acad Emerg Med* 5:691, 1998.
16. Watson AJS, Walker GH, Tomkin MMR, et al: Acute Wernicke's encephalopathy precipitated by glucose loading. *Ir J Med Sci* 150:301, 1981.
17. Pulsinelli WA, Levy DE, Sigsbee B, et al: Increased damage after ischemic stroke in patients with hyperglycemia with or without established diabetes mellitus. *Am J Med* 74:540, 1983.
18. Longstreth WT, Inui TS: High blood glucose level on hospital admission and poor neurological recovery after cardiac arrest. *Ann Neurol* 15:59, 1984.
19. Lam AM, Winn HR, Cullen BF, et al: Hyperglycemia and neurologic outcome in patients with head injury. *J Neurosurg* 75:545, 1991.
20. Young B, Ott L, Dempsey R, et al: Relationship between admission hyperglycemia and neurologic outcome of severely brain-injured patients. *Ann Surg* 210:466, 1989.
21. Quadrani DA, Spiller HA, Widder P: Five year retrospective evaluation of sulfonylurea ingestion in children. *J Toxicol Clin Toxicol* 34:267, 1996.
22. Luber S, Meldon S, Brady W: Hypoglycemia presenting as acute respiratory failure in an infant. *Am J Emerg Med* 16:281, 1998.

203 DIABETIC KETOACIDOSIS

Michael E. Chansky
Cary L. Lubkin

INTRODUCTION

Diabetic ketoacidosis (DKA) is an acute, life-threatening complication of diabetes mellitus. DKA occurs predominately in patients with type I or insulin-dependent diabetes mellitus, but is also well described in type II or non-insulin-dependent diabetes mellitus.[1] DKA accounts for 8 to 28 percent of all diabetic admissions, and has an incidence among diabetics in the United States of 3 to 8 episodes per 1000 patients.[2] Europe has a comparable incidence. Twenty to 30 percent of cases occur in patients with new-onset diabetes. There was a decline in mortality from DKA in the 1960s and 1970s because of early recognition, improved patient education, and advances in management. Better understanding of pathophysiology and an aggressive, uniform approach to diagnosis and management has reduced mortality to less than 5 percent of reported episodes.[3] However, mortality is higher in the elderly due to underlying renal disease or coexisting infection.[4]

PATHOPHYSIOLOGY

In simplest terms, DKA represents the body's response to cellular starvation, brought on by relative insulin deficiency and counterregulatory or catabolic hormone excess (Fig. 203-1).[5] Insulin is the only anabolic hormone and is responsible for the metabolism and storage of carbohydrates, fat, and protein. Counterregulatory hormones include glucagon, catecholamines, cortisol, and growth hormone. This lack of insulin and excess counterregulatory hormones results in hyperglycemia (due to excess production and underutilization of glucose, the resultant osmotic diuresis and decreased glomerular filtration rate),[2] ketone formation, and an anion gap metabolic acidosis.

Insulin

Ingested glucose is the primary stimulant of insulin release from the β cells of the pancreas. Insulin's main action occurs at the three principal tissues of energy storage and metabolism (i.e., liver, adipose tissue, and skeletal muscle). Insulin acts on the liver to facilitate the uptake of glucose and its conversion to glycogen while inhibiting glycogen breakdown (glycogenolysis) and suppressing gluconeogenesis. The net effect of these actions is to promote the storage of glucose in the form of glycogen. Insulin's effect on lipid metabolism is to increase lipogenesis in the liver and adipose cells by the production of triglycerides from free fatty acids and glycerol while inhibiting the breakdown of triglycerides. Insulin stimulates the uptake of amino acids into muscle cells with subsequent incorporation into muscle protein while preventing the release of amino acids from muscle and hepatic protein sources.

Deficiency in insulin secretion is the predominant lesion in diabetes mellitus and it may be partial or total. In the initial stages of diabetes mellitus, the secretory failure of β cells impairs fuel storage and may only be evident during a glucose-tolerance test. As the disease progresses and levels of insulin decrease, fuel stores are mobilized during fasting, resulting in hyperglycemia. When pancreatic β-cell reserve is present, hyperglycemia may trigger an increase in insulin and a return to normal glucose concentration. With further disease progression, hyperglycemia can no longer trigger an increase in insulin activity. Despite the presence of elevated intravascular glucose, in the absence of insulin the cells are unable to utilize glucose as a fuel source. The body responds by breakdown of protein and adipose stores to try and produce a usable intracellular fuel. Loss of the normal physiologic effects of insulin leads to secretion of catabolic hormones and resultant hyperglycemia and ketonemia.

Counterregulatory Hormones

The response to cellular starvation seen with insulin insufficiency is increased levels of glucagon, catecholamines, cortisone, and growth hormone. Glucagon is the primary counterregulatory hormone. The catabolic effects of these hormones includes increased gluconeogenesis and glycogenolysis, breakdown of fats into free fatty acids and glycerol, and proteolysis with increased levels of amino acids. Increased levels of glucogenic precursors, such as glycerol and amino acids, facilitate gluconeogenesis, worsening hyperglycemia.

Free fatty acids released in the periphery are bound to albumin and transported to the liver where they undergo conversion to ketone bodies. The primary ketone bodies β-hydroxybutyric acid (βHB) and acetoacetic acid (AcAc) account for the metabolic acidosis seen in DKA. The two are in equilibrium: AcAc + NADH $\rightleftharpoons$ βHB + NAD. AcAc is metabolized to acetone, another major ketone body. Depletion of baseline hepatic glycogen stores tends to favor ketogenesis. Low insulin levels decrease the ability of the brain, cardiac, and skeletal muscle to use ketones as an energy source, also increasing ketonemia. Persistently elevated serum glucose eventually causes an osmotic diuresis. The resulting volume depletion worsens hyperglycemia and

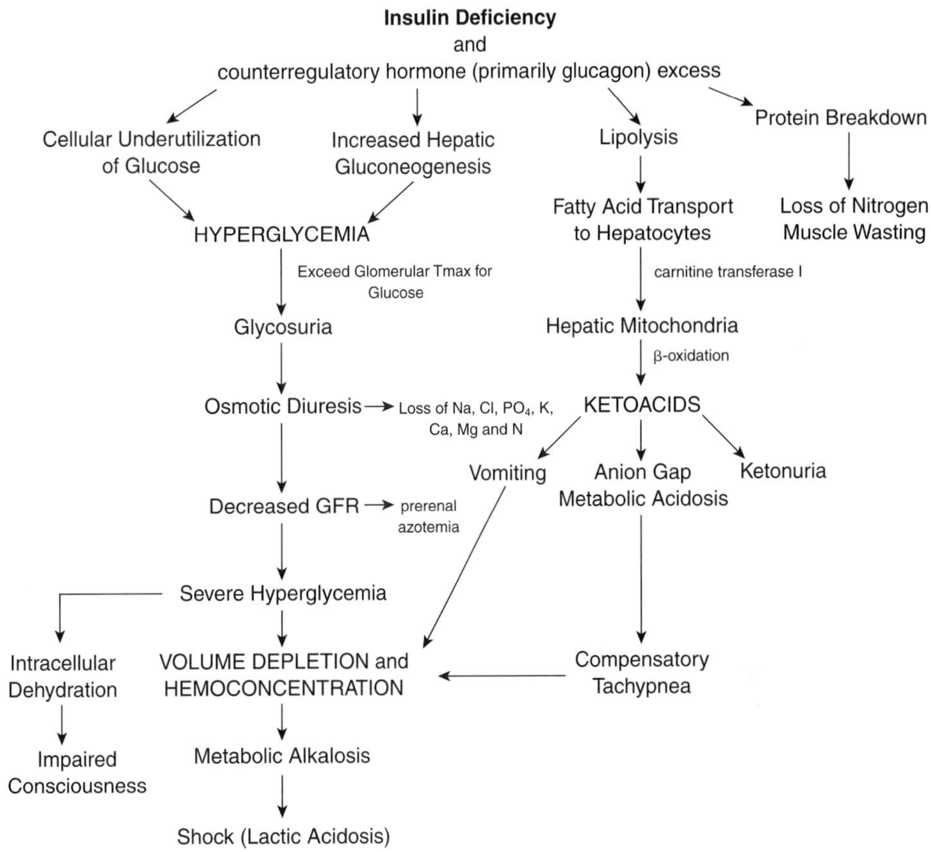

FIG. 203-1. Pathogenesis of DKA, secondary to relative insulin deficiency and counterregulatory hormone excess.

ketonemia. The renin angiotensin aldosterone system, activated by volume depletion, exacerbates renal potassium losses already occurring from osmotic diuresis. In the kidney, chloride is retained in exchange for the ketoanions being excreted. This loss of ketoanions represents a loss of potential bicarbonate. In the face of marked ketonuria a superimposed hyperchloremic acidosis is also present. The presence of a concurrent hyperchlorene acidosis can be detected by noting a $[HCO_3^-]$ lower than explainable by the amount the anion gap has increased (see Chap. 21). As adipose tissue is broken down, prostaglandins PGI_2 and PGE_2 are produced. Both account for the paradoxical vasodilation that occurs despite profound levels of volume depletion. They may be responsible for the fact that acute renal failure and extremity gangrene rarely develop in DKA despite depletion volume.

DKA IN PREGNANCY

Several physiologic changes in pregnant patients make them more prone to DKA. Maternal fasting serum glucoses are normally lower, which leads to relative insulin deficiency and an increase in baseline free fatty acid levels in the blood. Pregnant patients normally have increased levels of counterregulatory hormones. In addition, the chronic respiratory alkalosis seen in pregnancy leads to decreased bicarbonate levels due to a compensatory renal response resulting in a decrease in buffering capacity. Pregnant patients also have an increased incidence of vomiting and infections (e.g., urinary tract infections, sinusitis, otitis media), which are frequent precipitants of DKA. In addition, DKA is triggered at lower sugar levels in the pregnant population.[6] Maternal acidosis causes fetal acidosis and also decreases uterine blood flow and fetal oxygenation. Maternal hypokalemia can also lead to fetal dysrhythmias and death.

CAUSES OF DIABETIC KETOACIDOSIS

Factors known to precipitate DKA include omission of daily insulin injections and a variety of stressful events, such as infection, stroke, myocardial infarction, trauma, pregnancy, hyperthyroidism, pancreatitis, pulmonary embolism, surgery, and steroid usage. Recent studies have shown that errors in insulin usage are a much more common precipitant than previously thought, especially in the younger population.[7] In approximately 25 percent of patients, no clear precipitating cause is found.[8]

CLINICAL PRESENTATION

The clinical manifestations of DKA are directly related to the three primary metabolic derangements—hyperglycemia, volume depletion, and acidosis. Hyperglycemia causes an increased osmotic load with movement of intracellular water into the vascular compartment. The ensuing osmotic diuresis gradually leads to volume loss in addition to renal losses of sodium, chloride, potassium, phosphorous, calcium, and magnesium. Initially, patients may compensate by increasing their fluid intake. In this initial period, polyuria and polydipsia are usually the only symptoms until ketonemia and acidosis develop. As the acidosis progresses, the patient develops a compensatory augmented ventilatory response. Increased ventilation is physiologically stimulated by acidemia to diminish the P_{CO_2} and thus counter the metabolic acidosis. The acidosis combined with the effects of prostaglandin I_2 and E_2 lead to the peripheral vasodilation despite profound levels of volume depletion. Prostaglandin release is also felt to play a role in the often unexplained nausea, vomiting, and abdominal pain that are frequently seen at presentation, especially in children. Vomiting, which may be a maladaptive physiologic response to diminish the acid load, unfortunately exacerbates the renal potassium losses and contributes to rapidly progressive volume loss, weakness, and weight loss. As volume depletion progresses, poor absorption of subcutaneous insulin renders it ineffective. Mental confusion or coma may be present at the time of presentation; these symptoms are much more likely with serum osmolarity >340 mOsm/L. If the serum osmolarity is <340 mOsm/L in a comatose patient, another cause of the coma should be sought.

Abnormal vital signs may be the only significant physical findings at the time of presentation. Tachycardia and either significant orthostasis or hypotension are usually present. Poor skin turgor denotes significant volume depletion. With severe acidemia, both the rate and depth of respirations are elevated secondary to compensatory hyperventilation (Kussmaul respirations). Acetone produces the characteristic fruity odor on the breath found in some patients. The absence of fever does not exclude infection as a source of the patient's ketoacidosis. Hypothermia is occasionally present.

Abdominal pain and tenderness can be due to gastric dilatation, ileus, or pancreatitis. Due to the frequency of abdominal pain and the presence of an elevated serum amylase in both DKA and pancreatitis, distinguishing the diagnoses may be difficult. Elevated serum lipase is more specific to pancreatitis and should be used to differentiate the two conditions.

LABORATORY

Almost all patients with DKA present with blood glucose greater than 300 mg/dL. Patients who present just after receiving insulin or who have impaired gluconeogenesis (e.g., in alcohol abuse or liver failure) may have lower initial serum glucose levels.[2] Elevated serum levels of βHB and AcAc cause acidosis and ketonuria. The nitroprusside reagent normally used to detect urine and serum ketones only detects AcAc. Acetone is only weekly reactive and βHB not at all. NADH accumulation in mitochondria, as may occur with lactic acidosis or alcohol metabolism, favors the βHB side of the equation noted earlier. The enzymatic test for βHB is reliable but not widely available. Paradoxically, ketone levels will increase as the patient is being treated and improve as the body converts the more acidic βHB to AcAc. Therefore, ketones need only be checked initially. Serum electrolytes should be carefully examined for multiple metabolic abnormalities. Elevated serum ketones lead to a high anion gap metabolic acidosis. Hyperchloremic acidosis also occurs on the basis of ketoanion exchange for chloride in the urine; this is especially true in patients who maintain good hydration status and thus their glomerular filtration rate despite ketoacidosis. Metabolic alkalosis also can occur due to vomiting, osmotic diuresis, and concomitant diuretic use. Some patients with DKA may present with "normal" appearing [HCO_3^-] or even alkalemia if these other processes are severe enough to mask the acidosis. In such situations, an elevated anion gap may be the only clue to the presence of an underlying metabolic acidosis otherwise masked by the concomitant volume contraction-related metabolic alkalosis.

Arterial blood gases (ABG) have traditionally been used to help determine precise acid-base status in order to direct treatment. A very low P_{CO_2} usually reflects respiratory compensation for metabolic acidosis, but may also reflect a primary respiratory alkalosis, which may be an early indication of pulmonary disease (e.g., pneumonia, pulmonary embolus) as a possible trigger of the DKA. Chapter 21 details how compensatory changes in P_{CO_2} can be distinguished from a primary respiratory alkalosis. Recent studies have shown a strong correlation between venous and arterial pH in patients with DKA.[9] Venous pH obtained during routine phlebotomy can potentially be used to avoid ABGs, which are painful and may cause arterial vascular complications.

Total body potassium is depleted by renal losses. However, measured serum potassium is normal or elevated in most patients[10] because of two important factors: extracellular shift of potassium secondary to acidemia and increased intravascular osmolarity caused by hyperglycemia.[11] Prerenal azotemia also contributes by interfering with kaliuresis. Osmotic diuresis leads to excessive renal losses of sodium chloride in the urine. However, the presence of hyperglycemia tends to artificially lower the serum sodium levels. The standard correction is by adding 1.6 meq to the reported sodium value for every 100 mg of glucose over 100 mg/dL. Osmotic diuresis also causes urinary losses and total body depletion of phosphorous, calcium, and magnesium. Be aware that hemoconcentration frequently leads to initial artificially elevated levels. As therapy progresses lower serum levels of each will be evident.

Serum creatinine will frequently be artificially elevated because AcAc interferes with the laboratory assay. Liver function studies may be elevated because of fatty infiltration of the liver, which corrects as the acidosis is treated. CPK and amylase are also frequently elevated at the time of presentation. Leukocytosis is often present because of hemoconcentration and stress. However, an elevated band count of 10 or more has been shown to reliably predict infection in this population.[12]

Electrocardiographic changes of hyperkalemia or hypokalemia may be seen. These changes are often very transient because of the rapidly changing metabolic status. The cardiogram should also be evaluated for ischemia as myocardial infarction may precipitate DKA. The underlying rhythm is usually sinus tachycardia.

DIFFERENTIAL DIAGNOSIS

Although the exact definition of DKA is variable, most experts agree that a blood glucose greater than 250 mg/dL, bicarbonate level less than 15 meq/L, and an arterial pH of less than 7.3 with moderate ketonemia constitute the disease.[2]

The differential diagnosis of metabolic coma in a diabetic patient includes hypoglycemia, nonketotic hyperosmotic coma, alcoholic ketoacidosis, lactic acidosis, and other causes of wide anion gap acidosis. A rapid differentiation can be made in the emergency department using glucose reagent strips, urine dipsticks for ketones, and blood gas analysis. As an initial rapid diagnostic step, the finding of elevated glucose with the concomitant detection of ketones by near-patient testing methods, and the presence of metabolic acidosis on venous or arterial blood gas analysis, has few rival diagnoses other than DKA. However, evaluation of the anion gap is usually superior to pH or [HCO_3^-] determination alone, because any "widening" of the anion gap is independent of potentially masking effects of concurrent other acid/base disturbances. The clinician who is not well acquainted with the nuances of blood gas interpretation (Chap. 21), will be confused when the pH and [HCO_3^-] are not much altered from normal. Although the pH and [HCO_3^-] are usually examined to determine the presence of an acidosis, both can be affected by concurrent acid/base disturbances as may occur when metabolic alkalosis is also present (pH and [HCO_3^-] affected) or when respiratory alkalosis is also present (pH affected). Patients with hyperosmolar, nonketotic coma tend to be older, have a more prolonged course, and have prominent mental status changes. Their serum glucose levels are generally much higher (>1000 mg/dL), and they have little to no anion gap metabolic acidosis.

The differential diagnosis of DKA includes any entity that causes a high anion gap metabolic acidosis. These include alcoholic or starvation ketoacidosis, uremia, lactic acidosis, and various ingestions (e.g., methanol, ethylene glycol, and aspirin). The ketosis in alcoholic ketoacidosis and starvation ketosis tends to be milder and glucose is usually low or normal. βHB predominates in alcoholic ketoacidosis so the urinary ketone test may be negative. If an ingestion is suspected, serum osmolarity or drug-level testing is required. Depending on the hemodynamic status, lactic acidosis (poor perfusion) may occur simultaneously with DKA; in these cases, serum lactate levels are indicated. The absence of, or presence of, only moderate ketonemia should elicit a search for lactic acidosis, as its presence favors the undetected βHOB as the predominant ketone.

TREATMENT

The diagnosis of DKA should be suspected at triage, and aggressive fluid therapy initiated prior to lab results (Fig. 203-2).[13] Patients should immediately be placed on a monitor in an acute care room and have at least one large-bore (16- to 18-gauge) intravenous line of 0.9% saline (NS) running, a second intravenous line of 0.45% normal saline at KVO (keep vein open), and have a rapid finger stick blood sugar, urine dipstick, and EKG performed. A CBC, electrolytes, phosphate, magnesium, calcium, blood cultures, and other laboratory tests should be sent as indicated. Arterial blood gases are optional, and are only required for the diagnosis and monitoring of critically ill patients. Consider utilizing venous pH (approximately 0.03 lower then arterial pH)[9] for monitoring. The goals of therapy include volume repletion, reversal of the metabolic consequences of insulin insufficiency, correction of electrolyte and acid-base imbalance, recognition and treatment of precipitating causes, and avoidance of complications. Metabolic disturbances should be corrected at the rate of occurrence, or over 24 to 36 h.

A variety of therapeutic approaches have been advocated in the literature. Meeting the goals of safely replacing deficits and supplying missing insulin requires frequent (every one to two hours) monitoring of electrolytes (glucose, potassium, anion gap), vital signs, level of consciousness, and volume input/output until recovery is well established. Resolving hyperglycemia alone is not the end point of therapy. Concomitant resolution of the metabolic acidosis (or inhibition of ketoacid production) signifies resolution of DKA. Normalization of the anion gap usually requires 8 to 16 h, and reflects clearance of ketoacids. The order of therapeutic priorities is fluid, insulin, potassium, phosphate, magnesium, and bicarbonate.

Fluid Administration

Rapid fluid administration is the single most important initial step in the treatment of DKA.[3] Fluid helps restore intravascular volume and normal tonicity, perfuse vital organs, improve glomerular filtration rate (GFR), and lower serum glucose and ketones. The average adult patient has a water deficit of 100 mL/kg (5 to 10 L) and a sodium deficit of 7 to 10 meq/kg.[3] NS is the most frequently recommended fluid for initial rehydration even though the extracellular fluid of the patient is initially hypertonic. NS does not provide "free water" to correct intracellular dehydration, but it does prevent an excessively rapid fall in extracellular osmolarity and excessive transfer of water into the central nervous system (CNS). After initial resuscitation with NS, most authors favor alternating the administration of NS with half-normal saline, or utilizing two intravenous lines—one NS and one-half NS.

Based on clinical suspicion alone and prior to initial electrolyte results, the first liter of NS should be administered well within the first 30 min unless there are mitigating circumstances. In general, the first 2 L are administered rapidly over 0 to 2 h, the next 2 L over 2 to 6 h, and 2 L more over 6 to 12 h. This replaces approximately 50 percent of the total water deficit over the first 12 h, with the remaining 50 percent water deficit to be replaced over the subsequent 12 h. The blood glucose and ketone body concentration begin to fall after fluid administration and before implementation of any other therapeutic modality.[13] Hydration alone will reduce the glucose concentration by 17 to 80 percent over 12 to 14 h.[14] Tissue perfusion is restored with rehydration, improving the effectiveness of insulin. The subsequent rise in GFR allows for glucose and ketone body clearance, lowering serum glucose concentration and osmolarity. The patient's blood glucose needs to be carefully monitored, and 5% dextrose added to the rehydration solution when the glucose is 250 to 300 mg/dL.

The fluid should be changed to a hypotonic solution after the initial replacement of intravascular volume with normal saline. Patients presenting without extreme volume depletion can be safely managed with a modest fluid replacement regimen (500 cc/h for 4 h).[15] Monitoring central venous pressure or pulmonary artery wedge pressure should be considered during fluid replacement in elderly patients or in those with heart disease. Although the most common pitfall is failure to give adequate volume replacement,[3] excess fluid may contribute to the development of adult respiratory distress syndrome and cerebral edema.

Insulin

Initial hydration reduces the level of counterregulatory hormones, replaces vital fluid and electrolytes, and importantly, makes cells more responsive to insulin. In the early 1970s the dose, rate, and method of insulin administration in DKA was studied extensively. It is generally accepted that the "ideal way" to administer insulin is by continuous infusion of small doses of regular insulin through an infusion pump.[5,13,14,16] This approach appears to be more physiologic, helps produce a more linear fall in serum glucose and ketone bodies, and is associated with less-severe metabolic complications (hypoglycemia, hypokalemia, and hypophosphatemia).

Low-dose insulin administration by an infusion pump is simple, safe, and effective. Continuous insulin administration ensures that a steady blood concentration is maintained, and this technique allows flexibility in adjusting the insulin dose. Insulin inhibits gluconeogenesis, lipolysis, catabolic hormone secretion, and the production of ketoacids, in addition to promoting potassium, glucose, and phosphate uptake in tissues. After the initial fluid bolus, insulin is administered at 0.1 U/kg/h. Recent reviews have different recommendations regarding the use of an insulin-loading or -priming dose.[2,3,8] The effect of insulin begins almost immediately after the initiation of the infusion, and a loading dose has not been proven necessary. An intravenous loading dose of 0.1 U/kg is optional. The half-life of insulin given intravenously is 4 to 5 min, with an effective biologic half-life at the tissue level of approximately 20 to 30 min. Because insulin binds to plastic tubing, the first 25 mL of a prepared insulin solution (100 U of regular insulin in 100 mL of normal saline) should be wasted, and the drip plugged into an established intravenous line on an infusion pump at the port closest to the skin. Serious complications with continuous intravenous low-dose insulin infusions are minimal. Frequent monitoring is required to ensure that insulin is being administered in the desired amount.

Intramuscular or subcutaneous administration of regular insulin in DKA is to be discouraged.[5] Insulin absorption may be erratic in the volume-depleted, vasoconstricted patient, delaying the achievement of adequate insulin levels. Furthermore delayed absorption can produce deposits of insulin that may be later absorbed, causing hypoglycemia.

The incidence of nonresponders to low-dose continuous intravenous insulin administration is 1 to 2 percent. Infection is the primary reason for failure to respond. If the patient fails to respond to low-dose insulin therapy in the first hour (assuming adequate hydration), the infusion rate should be doubled or an intravenous bolus (0.2 to 0.4 U/kg) administered.

The insulin infusion should continue until ketonemia has cleared,[5] and the anion gap has normalized. As previously noted, there is conversion from βHB to AcAc, with "increasing ketones" measurable in the serum and urine. Therefore, the anion gap is the more accurate determinant of ongoing recovery. Resolution of hyperglycemia usually occurs earlier than the anion gap[14] and it may be necessary to administer glucose from the beginning of insulin therapy, or shortly after its institution. In most patients, continuous intravenous insulin therapy should continue for at least 12 h (or until resolution of the anion gap),

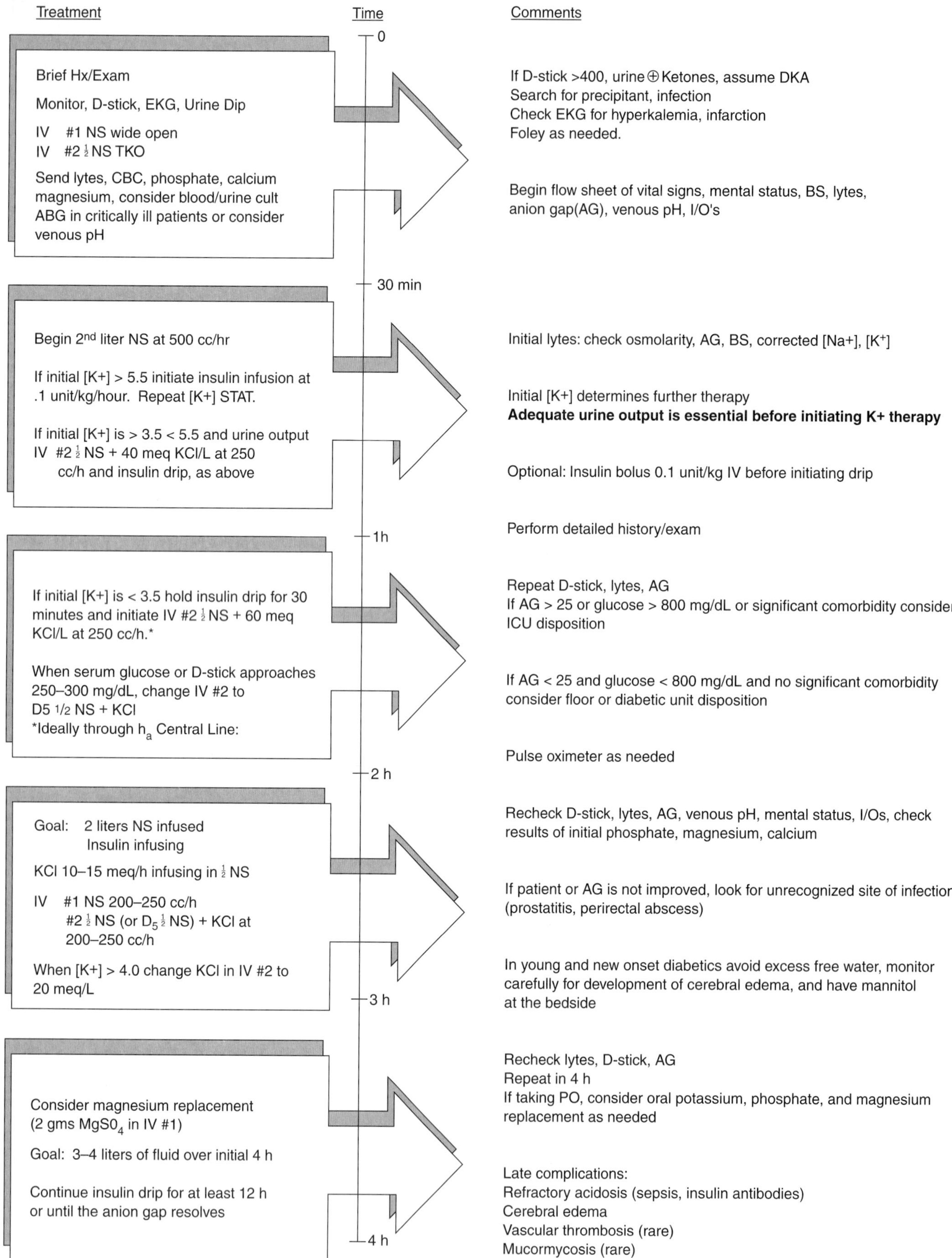

Treatment
Time
Comments
0
Brief Hx/Exam
Monitor, D-stick, EKG, Urine Dip
IV #1 NS wide open
IV #2 ½ NS TKO
Send lytes, CBC, phosphate, calcium magnesium, consider blood/urine cult ABG in critically ill patients or consider venous pH
If D-stick >400, urine ⊕ Ketones, assume DKA
Search for precipitant, infection
Check EKG for hyperkalemia, infarction
Foley as needed.
Begin flow sheet of vital signs, mental status, BS, lytes, anion gap(AG), venous pH, I/O's
30 min
Begin 2nd liter NS at 500 cc/hr
If initial [K+] > 5.5 initiate insulin infusion at .1 unit/kg/hour. Repeat [K+] STAT.
If initial [K+] is > 3.5 < 5.5 and urine output IV #2 ½ NS + 40 meq KCl/L at 250 cc/h and insulin drip, as above
Initial lytes: check osmolarity, AG, BS, corrected [Na+], [K+]
Initial [K+] determines further therapy
Adequate urine output is essential before initiating K+ therapy
Optional: Insulin bolus 0.1 unit/kg IV before initiating drip
1h
Perform detailed history/exam
If initial [K+] is < 3.5 hold insulin drip for 30 minutes and initiate IV #2 ½ NS + 60 meq KCl/L at 250 cc/h.*
When serum glucose or D-stick approaches 250–300 mg/dL, change IV #2 to D5 1/2 NS + KCl
*Ideally through ha Central Line:
Repeat D-stick, lytes, AG
If AG > 25 or glucose > 800 mg/dL or significant comorbidity consider ICU disposition
If AG < 25 and glucose < 800 mg/dL and no significant comorbidity consider floor or diabetic unit disposition
Pulse oximeter as needed
2 h
Goal: 2 liters NS infused
Insulin infusing
KCl 10–15 meq/h infusing in ½ NS
IV #1 NS 200–250 cc/h
#2 ½ NS (or D5 ½ NS) + KCl at 200–250 cc/h
When [K+] > 4.0 change KCl in IV #2 to 20 meq/L
Recheck D-stick, lytes, AG, venous pH, mental status, I/Os, check results of initial phosphate, magnesium, calcium
If patient or AG is not improved, look for unrecognized site of infection (prostatitis, perirectal abscess)
In young and new onset diabetics avoid excess free water, monitor carefully for development of cerebral edema, and have mannitol at the bedside
3 h
Consider magnesium replacement (2 gms MgSO4 in IV #1)
Goal: 3–4 liters of fluid over initial 4 h
Continue insulin drip for at least 12 h or until the anion gap resolves
Recheck lytes, D-stick, AG
Repeat in 4 h
If taking PO, consider oral potassium, phosphate, and magnesium replacement as needed
Late complications:
Refractory acidosis (sepsis, insulin antibodies)
Cerebral edema
Vascular thrombosis (rare)
Mucormycosis (rare)
4 h

FIG. 203-2. Time line for the typical adult patient with suspected DKA.

and an overlap period in which subcutaneous insulin is given should precede discontinuation of the insulin infusion. In the rare patient with initial hypokalemia (<3.5 meq), insulin can precipitate life-threatening hypokalemic effects.[14] Parenteral potassium should be started in these patients (10 to 15 meq/h) for at least 30 min prior to insulin.

Potassium

Patients in DKA usually present with profound total body potassium deficits in the range of 3 to 5 meq/kg.[3] This deficiency is created by insulin deficiency, metabolic acidosis, osmotic diuresis, and frequent vomiting. Only 2 percent of total body potassium is intravascular, and the initial serum concentration is usually normal or high because of the intracellular exchange of potassium for hydrogen ions during acidosis, total body fluid deficit, and diminished renal function. Initial hypokalemia indicates severe total body potassium depletion, and large amounts of potassium are necessary for replacement in the first 24 to 36 h.

The goals of potassium replacement are to maintain a normal extracellular potassium concentration during the acute phases of therapy and to replace the intracellular deficit over a period of days. During initial therapy for DKA, the serum potassium concentration may fall rapidly, primarily due to the action of insulin promoting reentry of potassium into cells and, to a lesser degree, to the dilution of extracellular fluid, correction of acidosis, and increased urinary loss of potassium. If these changes occur too rapidly, precipitous hypokalemia may result in fatal cardiac arrhythmias, respiratory paralysis, paralytic ileus, and rhabdomyolysis. The development of severe hypokalemia is potentially the most life-threatening electrolyte derangement during the treatment of DKA.[3] This complication is avoidable if the pathophysiology is understood and the effects of therapy frequently monitored.

Early potassium replacement is now a standard modality of care. Potassium is not added blindly to the first liter of NS administered to restore circulation, because giving potassium rapidly to a patient in a hyperkalemic potentiating state (i.e., acidemia, insulin deficiency) may dangerously increase extracellular potassium and precipitate fatal ventricular tachycardia or fibrillation. The patient's initial EKG often provides early evidence of hyperkalemia, progressively manifested by peaked T waves, prolonged PR interval, absent P wave, increasing QRS interval, and, lastly, a sine-wave pattern. The initial measurement of serum electrolytes and presence of urine output determine initial potassium therapy. As a general guideline, initial serum potassium greater than 3.5 meq/L and less than 5.5 meq/L (prior to fluid resuscitation and insulin) coupled with urine output calls for 10 meq KCl/h replacement in intravenous fluid for at least four hours. Because the most rapid changes occur during the first few hours of therapy, plasma potassium is initially measured every one to two hours. If oliguria is present (fortunately this is rare secondary to the protective osmotic diuresis) renal function must be evaluated and potassium replacement must be decreased. An initial serum potassium greater than 5.5 meq/L usually reflects a more profound acidemia. Intravenous potassium replacement is withheld until the serum potassium is documented to be below 5.5 meq/L and urine output is established. Fluid and insulin therapy alone will usually lower the serum potassium rapidly. Initial hypokalemia (<3.5 meq/L) necessitates more aggressive replacement prior to insulin therapy. Intravenous potassium should be given at 15 to 20 meq/h, with insulin initiated 30 min later. There is no documented advantage using potassium phosphate over potassium chloride; excessive use of potassium phosphate may result in metastatic precipitation of calcium phosphate in tissues.

The goal is to maintain serum potassium levels within the normal range of 4 to 5 meq/L and avoid life-threatening hyper- or hypokalemia. Oral potassium replacement is safe and effective, and should be utilized as soon as the patient can tolerate oral fluids. During the first 24 h, potassium chloride 100 to 200 meq is usually required. Occasionally, as much as 500 meq is necessary.

Phosphate

Phosphate plays an integral role in the conversion of energy from adenosine triphosphate (ATP) and in the delivery of oxygen at the tissue level through 2,3-diphosphoglyceric acid (2,3-DPG). In addition, many important enzymes, cofactors, and biochemical intermediates depend upon phosphate. Phosphate is primarily intracellular, and shifts to the extracellular compartment during DKA. Serum levels are often normal or increased upon presentation, and do not reflect the total body phosphate deficits secondary to enhanced urinary losses.[8] Phosphate (similar to glucose and potassium) reenters the intracellular space during insulin therapy, resulting in low phosphate concentrations. Hypophosphatemia is usually most severe 24 to 48 h after the start of insulin therapy. Acute phosphate deficiency (<1.0 mg/dL) has been associated with a variety of clinical disorders, including hypoxia, rhabdomyolysis, hemolysis, respiratory failure, and cardiac dysfunction. Fortunately, all are extremely rare during therapy of DKA.[5]

The role of phosphate replacement during the treatment of DKA remains controversial. No clinical trial has demonstrated significant benefits from routine intravenous phosphate therapy.[8,14] In general, intravenous therapy should be withheld unless the serum phosphate concentration is less than 1 mg/dL. Hypophosphatemia can be corrected safely and effectively with oral replenishment, which may cause diarrhea.

There is no established role for initiating intravenous potassium phosphate in the ED. Significant hypophosphatemia tends to develop only many hours into therapy, after the patient is already admitted. Several undesirable side effects from intravenous phosphate administration have been reported. These include hyperphosphatemia, hypocalcemia, hypomagnesemia, metastatic soft tissue calcifications, and hypernatremia and volume loss from osmotic diuresis. If deemed necessary (phosphate <1.0 mg/dL early in therapy and/or patient vomiting), intravenous phosphate replacement should be done by, or in consult with, experienced physicians in an ICU setting. Serum phosphate, calcium, and magnesium levels should be monitored during therapy of DKA; but, again, the case for routine early parenteral phosphate replacement has not been made.

Magnesium

Ongoing osmotic diuresis may cause significant depletion of magnesium stores (from bone) and hypomagnesemia. Hypomagnesemia may inhibit parathyroid hormone secretion, causing hypocalcemia and hyperphosphatemia. Symptomatic hypomagnesemia in DKA (hyperreflexia, positive Chvostek or Trousseau signs) is rare, as is the need for intravenous therapy. If serum magnesium is <1.2 mg/dL or symptoms are suggestive of hypomagnesemia, magnesium can be given orally in the form of magnesium oxide or parenterally as magnesium sulfate. It is recommended to monitor serum magnesium and calcium on presentation and 24 h into therapy unless symptoms suggestive of hypomagnesemia or hypocalcemia occur.

Bicarbonate

The role of bicarbonate in DKA has been debated for decades. Arbitrary initial pH levels to utilize bicarbonate are still currently recommended in many texts. To date, not a single study clearly demonstrates improved clinical outcome using bicarbonate in the treatment of DKA. Acidotic patients routinely recover from DKA without alkali therapy. Routine use of supplemental bicarbonate in the treatment of DKA is not recommended.[8,17,18]

Severe metabolic acidosis is associated with numerous cardiovascular (impaired contractility, vasodilation, hypotension) and neurologic (cerebral vasodilation and coma) complications.[14] Theoretical advantages of bicarbonate include improved myocardial contractility, elevated ventricular fibrillation threshold, improved catecholamine tissue response and decreased work of breathing.[17] These theoretical advantages appear outweighed by the possible disadvantages of bicarbonate administration in DKA of severe and worsening hypokalemia; paradoxical central nervous system acidosis; worsening intracellular acidosis; impaired oxyhemoglobin dissociation; rebound alkalosis; hypertonicity and sodium overload; delayed recovery from ketosis;[18] elevation of lactate levels;[17] and possible precipitation of cerebral edema.[14] During routine therapy of DKA hydrogen ion production ceases when ketogenesis stops; excessive hydrogen ions are eliminated through the urine and respiratory tract. Ketone body metabolism results in the endogenous production of alkali. Children with initial pH values as low as 6.73 have been shown to promptly recover from DKA without bicarbonate.[17]

Severe acidosis (pH <7.0) and worsening pH despite aggressive therapy for DKA should prompt the clinician to rule out other causes of metabolic acidosis (i.e., lactate from sepsis or bowel infarction, methanol ingestion, etc.). The potential benefits of bicarbonate in the elderly with cardiovascular instability and DKA must be balanced against the potential disadvantages.[8]

COMPLICATIONS AND MORTALITY

Complications can be categorized as those occurring secondary to the acute disease, early complications related to therapy, and late complications. A critically ill, lethargic patient is at risk for aspiration, and airway protection and evacuation of gastric contents may be indicated. In general, the greater the presenting serum osmolarity, blood urea nitrogen, and blood glucose concentration, the greater the mortality. There is also increased mortality for patients presenting with a serum bicarbonate level of less than 10 mEq/L.

Of the factors responsible for precipitating DKA, infection and myocardial infarction are the main contributors to high mortality. Half the patients with DKA die when myocardial infarction is the precipitating event. Additional factors that reduce the chances of survival include old age, severe hypotension, prolonged and severe coma, and underlying renal and cardiovascular disease. Severe volume depletion leaves the elderly at risk for vascular stasis and deep vein thrombosis. Prophylactic heparin should be instituted in high-risk patients as inpatients.

Major complications related to therapy of DKA include hypoglycemia, hypokalemia, hypophosphatemia, ARDS, and cerebral edema. The goal of therapy is to produce a gradual return to normal metabolic balance. Rapid shifts of water, electrolytes and other solutes can be avoided by using isotonic saline as the initial intravenous fluid, using continuous intravenous low-dose insulin, replacing potassium early, and avoiding bicarbonate. Above all, a basic understanding of the pathophysiology of DKA, constant monitoring of the patient, and attention to detail are essential to prevent complications of therapy.

ARDS is a rare complication of therapy. Aggressive fluid therapy decreases plasma oncotic pressure and raises left atrial end diastolic pressure, favoring a shift of fluid across the pulmonary capillary membrane. Fortunately, widening of the alveolar arterial gradient, hypoxia, and chest radiograph changes are very rare. Elderly patients who present with rales on chest exam may be at increased risk and should be monitored closely for this complication with continuous pulse oximetry and serial exams; they should also receive lower rates of fluid.[3]

The development of cerebral edema during the treatment of DKA, especially in young patients, is a potentially catastrophic complication.[13] Cerebral edema tends to occur during the first 24 h of therapy when the patient appears to be improving clinically and biochemically.[8] The true incidence of clinically apparent cerebral edema is unknown, but estimated to be 0.7 to 1.0 per 100 episodes of DKA in children.[8] Cerebral edema complicating DKA has a reported mortality of 70 percent. One hypothesis is that the osmotic diuresis promotes loss of water and sodium from both intra- and extracellular spaces. Hyperglycemia leads to a hyperosmolar extracellular state. Brain cells enzymatically produce osmotically active particles, or idiogenic osmoles that protect cells from further loss of water and shrinkage. During therapy with intravenous fluid and insulin, water moves into brain cells faster then idiogenic osmoles can dissipate, promoting cellular swelling.[8,14] Subclinical brain swelling has been reported in asymptomatic children during treatment of DKA.[14]

Multiple studies and reviews have found no specific presentation or treatment variables that predict or contribute to the development of cerebral edema.[14] Young age and new-onset diabetes are the only identified potential risk factors. Excessive initial fluid administration of greater than 4 L/m^2 body surface area per day has been associated with cerebral edema.[14] Initial "corrected" hypernatremia may be a risk factor in children as well. Recent data suggests that children who develop cerebral edema initially may have a relatively normal serum osmolarity and subsequently develop progressive hyponatremia and/or a trend of declining serum sodium before developing cerebral edema.[19] Approximately one-half of the patients who developed cerebral edema had premonitory symptoms of severe headache; incontinence; change in arousal or behavior; pupillary changes; blood pressure changes; seizures; bradycardia; or disturbed temperature regulation. Any change in neurologic function early in therapy should prompt the clinician to immediately administer mannitol at 1 to 2 g/kg body weight, which should be at the bedside of high-risk patients. Mannitol should be given prior to obtaining confirmatory CT scans,[8] as serious morbidity and mortality may be prevented. Other aggressive measures such as intubation, hyperventilation, and fluid restriction may be necessary. Gradual replacement of water and sodium deficits and slow correction of hyperglycemia may lessen the risk.

It is important to monitor for late complications of DKA. Metabolic acidosis refractory to routine therapy may be secondary to unrecognized infection (lactic acidosis), insulin antibodies, or improper preparation or administration of the insulin drip. Shock, unresponsive to aggressive fluid therapy suggests gram-negative bacteremia or silent myocardial infarction. Hyperchloremic non-anion gap metabolic acidosis develops in virtually every patient during therapy due to rapid volume expansion in the face of reduced HCO_3^- content. Also, bicarbonate equivalents are excreted in the urine as ketones and replaced with chloride provided by the normal saline. This emphasizes the importance of monitoring the anion gap during therapy, not the bicarbonate concentration. The non-anion gap metabolic acidosis (should it be present) resolves during recovery as bicarbonate is regenerated and excess chloride excreted in the urine.

Late vascular thrombosis may occur in any muscular artery, though cerebral vessels appear to be most susceptible.[5] Volume depletion, low cardiac output, increased blood viscosity, and underlying atherosclerosis may predispose the elderly to this rare complication. Thrombosis may occur several hours or days after institution of therapy, and after resolution of ketoacidosis.[13]

Mortality in DKA results mainly from sepsis or pulmonary and cardiovascular complications in the elderly, and fatal cerebral edema in children and young adults (<28 years old).[8] Age-adjusted death rates per 100,000 diabetic population for DKA and DKA-related deaths declined between 1980 and 1987, increased in 1988 and 1989, and then began decreasing again in 1990. Overall, both the age-adjusted DKA death rate and the DKA-related death rate were 34 percent lower in 1994 than in 1980. The highest death rates were among persons aged >75 years, followed by persons aged <45 years. Among race-sex groups, DKA death rates were highest among black males, followed by black females, and then by whites. In 1994, the age-adjusted DKA death rate for black males was almost twice that for white males.[20]

DISPOSITION

The great majority of patients require hospitalization in a monitored setting, where there is nursing experience with insulin drips. In most institutions patients are initially cared for in an intensive care or intermediate intensive care unit. A select group of patients with an initial anion gap <25, glucose <800 mg/dL, and no comorbidity may be safely managed on an inpatient unit with nursing expertise utilizing insulin drips and managing diabetic patients. Patients presenting early in the course of their illness, who can tolerate oral liquids may be safely managed in the ED or observation unit and discharged after four to six hours of therapy.[3]

REFERENCES

1. Westphal SA: The occurrence of diabetic ketoacidosis in non-insulin-dependent diabetes and newly diagnosed diabetes and newly diagnosed diabetic adults. *Am J Med* 101:19, 1996.
2. Umpierrez GE, Khajavi M, Kitabchi AE: Review: Diabetic ketoacidosis and hyperglycemic hyperosmolar nonketotic syndrome. *Am J Med Sci* 310(5):225, 1996.
3. Kitabchi AE, Wall BM: Diabetic ketoacidosis. *Med Clin North Am* 79(1):9, 1995.
4. Malone ML, Gennis V, Goodwin JS: Characteristics of diabetic ketoacidosis in older versus younger adults. *J Am Geriatr Soc* 40(11):1100, 1992.
5. Foster DW, McGarry JD: The metabolic derangements and treatment of diabetic ketoacidosis. *N Engl J Med* 309:159, 1989.
6. Chauhan SP, Perry KG, Jr: Management of diabetic ketoacidosis in the obstetric patient. *Obstet Gynecol Clin North Am* 22(1):143, 1995.
7. Thompson CJ, Cummings F, Chalmers J, et al: Abnormal insulin treatment behavior: A major cause of ketoacidosis in the young adult. *Diabet Med* 12:429, 1995.
8. Lebovitz HE: Diabetic ketoacidosis. *Lancet* 345:767, 1995.
9. Brandenburg MA, Dire DJ: Comparison of arterial and venous blood gas values in the initial emergency department evaluation of patients with diabetic ketoacidosis. *Ann Emerg Med* 31(4):459, 1998.
10. Johnson DD, Palumbo PJ, Chu CP: Diabetic ketoacidosis in a community-based population. *Mayo Clin Proc* 55:83, 1980.
11. Adrohue HJ, Lederer ED, Suki WN, et al: Determinants of plasma potassium levels in diabetic ketoacidosis. *Medicine* 65(3):163, 1986.
12. Slovis CM, Mork BGC, Slovis RJ, et al: Diabetic ketoacidosis and infection: Leukocyte count and differential as early predictors of serious infection. *Am J Emerg Med* 5(1):1, 1987.
13. Clements RS, Vourganti B: Fatal diabetic ketoacidosis: Major causes and approaches to their prevention. *Diabetes Care* 1:314, 1978.
14. Krane EJ, Rockoff MA, Wallman JK, et al: Subclinical brain swelling in children during treatment of diabetic ketoacidosis. *N Engl J Med* 312:1147, 1985.
15. Adrogue HJ, Barrero J, Eknoyan G: Salutary effects of modest fluid replacement in the treatment of adults with diabetic ketoacidosis. *JAMA* 262(15):2108, 1989.
16. Butkiewicz EK, Leibson CL, O'Brien PC, et al: Insulin therapy for diabetic ketoacidosis. *Diabetes Care* 18(8):1187, 1995.
17. Green SM, Rothrock SG, Ho JD, et al: Failure of adjunctive bicarbonate to improve outcome in severe pediatric diabetic ketoacidosis. *Emerg Med* 31:41, 1998.
18. Okuda Y, Adrogue HJ, Field JB, et al: Counterproductive effects of sodium bicarbonate in diabetic ketoacidosis. *J Clin Endocrinol Metab* 81:314, 1996.
19. Hale PM, Rezvani I, Braunstein AW, et al: Factors predicting cerebral edema in young children with diabetic ketoacidosis and new onset type I diabetes. *Acta Paediatr* 86:626, 1997.
20. Centers for Disease Control and Prevention: *Diabetes Surveillance, 1997: Diabetic Ketoacidosis.* Atlanta, GA, US Department of Health and Human Services, 1997, pp 6-7.

ALCOHOLIC KETOACIDOSIS

William A. Woods
Debra G. Perina

Alcoholic ketoacidosis (AKA) is a wide anion-gap acidosis most often associated with acute cessation of alcohol consumption after chronic alcohol abuse. The metabolism of alcohol with little or no glucose sources results in the elevated levels of ketoacids that typically produce the metabolic acidosis present in this illness. Although usually seen in chronic alcoholics, ketoacidosis has been described in first-time drinkers who binge drink, particularly in association with volume depletion from poor oral intake and vomiting.

PATHOPHYSIOLOGY

AKA occurs in the setting of a large quantity of alcohol ingestion and relative starvation. Starvation decreases glycogen and insulin stores and increases catecholamines, glucagon, growth hormone, and cortisol. As glycogen stores decrease, insulin production is retarded, resulting in increased lipolysis, increased hepatic ketogenesis, and peripheral use of ketones. Elevated levels of catecholamines, glucagon, growth hormone, and cortisol also stimulate lipolysis and hepatic ketogenesis. Both of these metabolic pathways lead to ketoacidosis.

Three types of ketones are produced in varying amounts: β-hydroxybutyrate (βHB), acetoacetate, and acetone (Fig. 204-1). Acetone, a metabolite of acetoacetate and a nonacidotic ketone, is rapidly excreted in urine. βHB and acetoacetate are the predominant primary ketones producing the acidosis seen in this illness, with βHB usually in greater concentration. The usual ratio of these ketones in healthy patients is 1:1. The ratio of these ketones is 5:1 to 10:1 in patients with AKA. The lack of nicotinamide adenosine dinucleotide (NAD), a necessary cofactor used to form acetoacetate from βHB, is thought to be the principle cause of this disparity.

The enzyme alcohol dehydrogenase metabolizes alcohol to acetaldehyde and acetate. Acetaldehyde is metabolized by the enzyme aldehyde dehydrogenase to acetyl coenzyme A, which forms free fatty acids, ketone bodies, and enters the Krebs cycle for glucose metabolism (Fig. 204-1). Under normal metabolic conditions, the majority of acetyl coenzyme A enters the Krebs cycle, and few ketone bodies are produced. NAD is a necessary cofactor for this step and is continually renewed through mitochondrial oxidation.

Under conditions of relative starvation, as seen in AKA, there is a relative insulin deficiency, whose release is further inhibited by the α-adrenergic response to volume contraction. Thus, glucose is not available for utilization in the Krebs cycle and the equation shifts to production of ketone bodies. In addition, the rate of NAD oxygenation by mitochondria also declines, resulting in a deficiency of this cofactor to metabolize alcohol and acetaldehyde, which further stimulates ketone body production (Fig. 204-1). The resulting deficiency of NAD can persist for several days after alcohol consumption has ceased. Hepatic gluconeogenesis is also decreased, due to the lack of available NAD cofactor for metabolism, along with decreased glycogen stores. Thus, AKA occurs in the setting of increased ketone production and an increased ratio of NADH (the reduced form of NAD) to NAD.

Additional mechanisms that contribute to ketone production include alcohol-induced mitochondrial structural changes and mitochondrial phosphorus depletion. Hypophosphatemia also inhibits the utilization of NADH and increases ketone body formation. Finally, acute vomiting and starvation superimposed on chronic malnutrition also contributes to the ketoacidosis state.

EPIDEMIOLOGY

There are no gender differences. The age of presentation is variable but usually between 20 to 60 years. Patients often experience repeated episodes of ketoacidosis, with 23 percent of patients having more than one episode of AKA in one series. The true incidence of this illness is unknown, but most likely mirrors the incidence of alcoholism in the population.[1] This illness may be more prevalent than previously suspected. One study indicated that analysis of serum chemistries of alcoholics arriving at emergency departments with complaints related to excessive alcohol intake incidentally found ketoacidosis in 25 per-

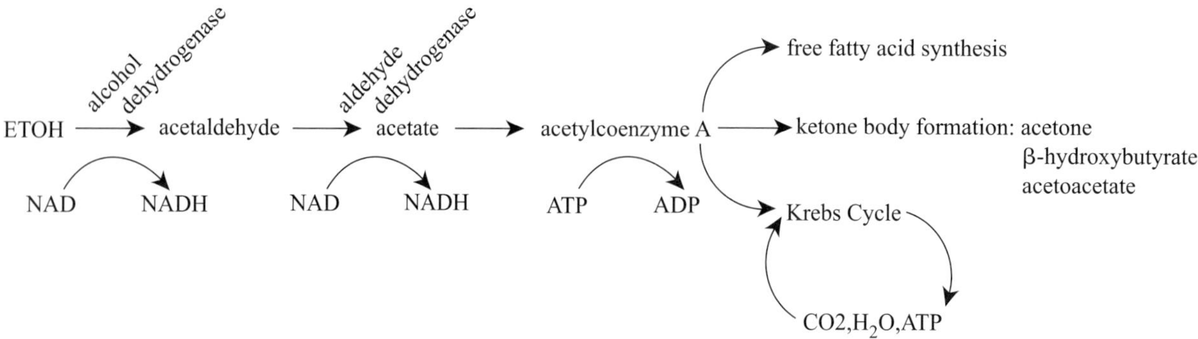

FIG. 204-1. Ethanol metabolism.

cent of patients. Although with proper treatment this illness is self-limited, poor outcomes can occur. Medical examiner literature notes that 10 percent of deaths in known alcoholics are from AKA.[2]

CLINICAL FEATURES

AKA typically occurs after an acute decrease in alcohol intake in association with several days of poor food intake or vomiting. It is most commonly seen after a patient has had an episode of heavy drinking followed by decreases in alcohol and food intake. The nausea, vomiting, and abdominal pain that may be associated with gastritis or pancreatitis may exacerbate the progression of the illness. As anorexia continues, the symptoms worsen, leading the patient to seek health care. Symptoms, listed in Table 204-1, are nonspecific, making diagnosis difficult without laboratory studies as confirmation.

There are no specific physical findings associated solely with AKA. The most common findings are tachycardia, tachypnea, and diffuse, mild to moderate abdominal tenderness. Volume depletion resulting from anorexia, diaphoresis, and vomiting causes the frequently seen tachycardia and hypotension. Most patients are awake at presentation. Mental status changes in patients with ketoacidosis should alert clinicians to other potential causes, such as toxic ingestion, hypoglycemia, alcohol-withdrawal seizures, postictal state, or unrecognized head injury.

LABORATORY

Alcohol levels are usually low or undetectable at the time of presentation, but some patients may present with an elevated blood alcohol level, making diagnosis more challenging. An elevated anion gap caused by ketones is essential for diagnosing AKA. As βHB predominates, the degree of ketonemia may not be appreciated, depending on the method of ketone detection (see Chap. 203 for a complete discussion). The initial anion gap is usually 16 to 33, with a mean of 21. Patients frequently have mild hypophosphatemia, hyponatremia, and/or hypokalemia. Most patients will also have elevated bilirubin and liver enzymes due to a long history of chronic ethanol use. Blood urea nitrogen and creatinine kinase levels are frequently elevated due to relative volume depletion. Serum lactate levels can be mildly elevated. Glucose levels are most often only mildly elevated, but a subset of patients will have hypoglycemia. On rare occasions, the glucose level may be greater than 200 mg/dL.

TABLE 204-1 Common Symptoms and Signs in Alcoholic Ketoacidosis

Symptoms,	%	Signs/Anion Gap,	%
Nausea	76	Tachycardia	56
Vomiting	73	Tachypnea	49
Abdominal pain	62	Abdominal tenderness	43
Shortness of breath	20	Heme-positive stool	18
Tremulousness	20	Hepatomegaly	18
Hematemesis	19	Altered mental status	15
Dizziness	19	Hypotension	12

Source: From Wrenn et al[1] and Soffer and Hamburger,[4] with permission.

Acid-Base Balance

Serum pH is typically acidemic, but the pH may be normal or even alkalemic early in the course of the illness. In one study, 15 percent of patients were alkalemic, 30 percent had normal pH, and 55 percent had acidemia.[1] The degree of acidosis is typically less than that seen in patients with diabetic ketoacidosis. If the acidosis is mild and the patient also has a primary respiratory alkalosis (i.e., due to fever, sepsis, or alcohol withdrawal), then the pH may be normal or even alkalemic. Similarly, contraction metabolic alkalosis may mask the presence of a concurrent wide anion-gap acidosis and result in a "normal" or even elevated [$HCO3^-$], rendering the pH normal or alkalemic. Since volume loss, whether due to poor volume intake or vomiting, is virtually always present in AKA, some degree of metabolic alkalosis is sure to exist.

Without routine evaluation of the anion gap in every patient at risk for AKA, the diagnosis can be easily missed. An anion gap greater than the patient's baseline (or greater than 15 in any case) signifies the presence of a wide anion-gap acidosis regardless of the actual [$HCO3^-$] concentration or the pH, even if the patient is alkalemic. For example, a common serum chemistry result in a patient with AKA may be along the following lines: [Na^+], 145, [Cl], 95, [K^+], 4.1, and [$HCO3^-$], 25. In this example, the anion gap (25, excluding [K^+]) is elevated by at least 10, yet the [$HCO3^-$] and electrolyte levels are normal. The only explanation is that a mixed acid-base abnormality of approximately equal but opposing magnitudes exists. Arterial blood-gas determination is not needed to arrive at the correct diagnosis for this relatively complicated acid-base disturbance. (For a more detailed discussion, the reader is referred to Chap. 21, "Acid-Base Disorders.")

Ketones

Ketone bodies may be detected by the serum and urine nitroprusside test, which is the standard test for ketone detection. While βHB is the predominant ketone present in AKA, acetoacetate is the ketone normally detected by the nitroprusside test. As patients with AKA may have elevated acetoacetate levels, it is important not to develop a false sense of security with a negative or only weakly positive test. As treatment progresses and NAD levels increase, the acetoacetate levels may actually increase and the nitroprusside test will reflect an increasingly positive reaction. This natural progression should be expected and does not indicate a worsening of the patient's condition. The clinical application of this test is thus quite variable. Most authors suggest measuring βHB and acetoacetate levels only if the diagnosis is unclear or other ways are not available to follow the patient's response to therapy.[3]

DIAGNOSIS

The diagnosis is established in the classic presentation of the chronic alcoholic, with recent anorexia, vomiting, abdominal pain, unexplained metabolic acidosis with a positive nitroprusside test, elevated anion gap, and a low or mildly elevated serum glucose level. However, this presentation is uncommon. Establishing this diagnosis can be difficult for several reasons. First, the blood alcohol level may be zero, and the patient may not voluntarily provide the history of alcohol consumption. Second, urine nitroprusside testing may be negative or weakly positive, despite significant ketoacidosis. Third, the pH may vary from reflecting significant acidemia to mild alkalemia, depending on how advanced the pathophysiology is and the degree of ketone body production, as explained above.

Initial laboratory studies usually include determination of electrolyte, blood urea nitrogen, creatinine, white blood cell, hematocrit, hepatic and pancreatic enzyme levels, and urinalysis. The anion gap should be calculated. Determination of serum lactic acid level and serum osmolarity may also be helpful. Further laboratory studies may be needed to delineate the cause of the increased anion-gap acidosis if other ingestions besides ethanol are suspected (see the following section on differential diagnosis). An arterial blood-gas determination is unnecessary unless a primary respiratory acid-base disturbance is suspected (Table 204-2).

Differential Diagnosis

The differential diagnosis for AKA is very broad. It is essentially the differential diagnosis of wide anion-gap metabolic acidosis. Lactic acidosis, uremia, and ingestants (particularly methanol and ethylene glycol) should be considered. A mild lactic acidosis is occasionally present in AKA related to ethanol metabolism, but it is comparatively inconsequential. A significant lactic acidosis always stems from another cause. Lactic acidosis related to anaerobic metabolism (e.g., hypotension, sepsis, or tissue ischemia) or associated with methanol, ethylene glycol, and salicylic acid are usually markedly more severe and less readily masked by concurrent metabolic alkalosis. Both salicylic acid poisoning and sepsis (related lactic acidosis) often present with triple acid-base disturbances (metabolic acidosis, metabolic alkalosis, and primary respiratory alkalosis). Renal failure as a potential etiology can be ascertained from the serum chemistries. Diabetic ketoacidosis has a blood sugar level greater than 300 mg/dL. Finally, a differentiation from starvation ketosis is an academic exercise and unimportant, because underlying pathophysiology, treatment, and implications are similar. Isopropyl alcohol ingestion results in production of ketones and is on occasion associated with a mild lactic acidosis on a similar basis as is found in AKA. The presence of an osmolal gap (which is also a feature of methanol and ethylene glycol poisoning) may be differentiating. However, ethanol is osmotically active and, if present, will also contribute to an osmolal gap. If the blood alcohol level is known, then its contribution to any osmolal gap can be calculated. If the entire osmolal gap cannot be attributed to the ethanol level, then isopropyl alcohol (mild or no acidosis), methanol, or ethylene glycol (severe acidosis) may well be the explanation. Each 100 mg/dL of ethanol raises the osmolal gap by 22. (A full discussion on the diagnostic approach to distinguish various wide anion-gap type acidosis is found in Chap. 21, "Acid-Base Disorders." Details of osmolal gap are discussed in Chap. 23, "Fluids and Electrolyte Problems.")

TABLE 204-2 Diagnostic Criteria for Alcoholic Ketoacidosis

Glucose level less than 300 mg/dL
Vomiting
Recent ethanol intake, with decline over 1 to 3 days
Wide anion-gap metabolic acidosis without alternate explanation

Source: From Soffer and Hamburger,[4] with permission.

Patients with AKA often have concurrent illnesses that may have promoted the alcohol cessation and anorexia. Thus, a thorough investigation for underlying illnesses should be performed. Common concurrent illnesses are pancreatitis, gastritis or upper gastrointestinal bleeding, seizures, alcohol withdrawal, sepsis, and hepatitis.

TREATMENT

Treatment of AKA is symptomatic. Therapy is aimed at both glucose administration and volume repletion. Ketoacidosis can be treated with only saline administration, but the addition of glucose hastens recovery. Glucose stimulates insulin production, which stops lipolysis and halts the further formation of ketones. Glucose also increases the oxidation of NADH to NAD, thereby further stopping ketone production. Patients with AKA are not hyperosmolar, and cerebral edema is of less concern with large volumes of fluid resuscitation. Even with vigorous fluid resuscitation, no cases of cerebral edema have been reported among those being treated for AKA.

Insulin is of no proven benefit and can be dangerous because patients often have depleted glycogen stores and normal glucose levels. Sodium bicarbonate is not indicated unless patients are severely acidemic, with a pH of 7.1 or lower. As noted, this level of acidemia is unlikely to be explained by AKA alone. A vigorous search for an alternate explanation must be undertaken. Hypophosphatemia is frequently seen in chronic alcoholic patients and can retard the resolution of acidosis, as phosphorus is necessary for mitochondrial utilization of glucose to produce NADH oxidation. However, phosphate replacement is generally unwarranted as part of this treatment in the ED, unless very low levels are encountered (less than 1.0 mg/dL). Oral replenishment is safe and effective. Nitroprusside tests correlated with clinical status may be used to help guide therapy, as an increasingly positive reaction signifies improvement. To prevent precipitation of Wernicke disease, all patients should receive 50 to 100 mg of thiamine prior to the administration of glucose. Concomitant administration of magnesium sulfate and multivitamins should be considered and guided by laboratory results. Acidosis may clear within 12 to 24 h. Patients whose course is uncomplicated may be safely discharged home if there is resolution of acidosis over time and the patient is able to tolerate oral fluids. Those patients with a complicated course, underlying illnesses, or persistent acidosis should be admitted for further evaluation and treatment.

REFERENCES

1. Wrenn KD, Slovis CM, Minion GE, Rutkowski R: The syndrome of alcoholic ketoacidosis. *Am J Med* 91:119, 1991.

2. Thomsen JL, Simonsen KW, Felby S, Frohlich B: A prospective toxicology analysis in alcoholics. *Forensic Sci Int* 90:33, 1997.
3. Elisaf M, Merkouropoulos M, Tsianos EV, Siamopoulos KC: Acid-base and electrolyte abnormalities in alcoholic patients. *Miner Electrolyte Metab* 20:274, 1994.
4. Soffer A, Hamburger S: Alcoholic ketoacidosis: A review of 30 cases. *J Am Med Women's Assoc* 37:106, 1982.

205 HYPEROSMOLAR HYPERGLYCEMIC NONKETOTIC SYNDROME

Charles S. Graffeo

The disease process discussed in this chapter is frequently referred to as *nonketotic hyperosmolar coma* to characterize the syndrome of severe hyperglycemia, hyperosmolarity, and a relative lack of ketonemia in patients with poorly controlled or undiagnosed type 2 diabetes mellitus. The literature is replete with a score of other acronyms for this syndrome. The nomenclature used by the American Diabetes Association, *hyperosmolar nonketotic state* (HNS) and *hyperosmolar hyperglycemic nonketotic syndrome* (HHNS) are both commonly used and more appropriate. This chapter uses the HHNS designation. Placing emphasis on the presence or lack of coma, is likely to underestimate the severity of disease, and thus ''coma'' should be excluded from the nomenclature. In fact, although patients may present with a host of symptoms referable to the central nervous system, less than ten percent actually present with coma.[1] What is more typical, is a broad range of clinical presentations that correlate with the degree of serum osmolarity, volume depletion, underlying medical illness and severity of precipitating factors such as acute infection.

In general, HHNS is ''defined'' by extreme hyperglycemia with serum glucose usually greater than 400 mg/dL, an elevated calculated plasma osmolality of greater than 315 mosm/kg, serum bicarbonate greater than 15, an arterial ph of >7.3, and serum negative for ketones in a 1:2 dilution. These values, however, are fairly arbitrary and, depending on the severity of disease, serum glucose measurements may be well over a thousand. A profound metabolic acidosis and even mild degrees of ketonemia may both be found in HHNS. The importance of recognizing the potential for a variety mixed acid-base patterns in patients presenting with HHNS cannot be overemphasized.

Many authors propose that HHNS and diabetic ketoacidosis (DKA) should be viewed as similar disease processes with the fundamental difference being in the metabolism of lipids during a period of relative insulin deficiency. Shared features of both include hyperglycemia, hyperosmolarity, severe volume depletion, electrolyte disturbances and, sometimes, acidosis. The acidosis associated with HHNS may be due to tissue hypoperfusion (lactic acidosis), a mild starvation ketosis, and azotemia, in various combinations. In contrast, patients with DKA at similar levels of tissue perfusion also have much higher levels of circulating ketone bodies, which contribute additional anions, resulting in a more profound acidosis.

Early identification is the most effective means of preventing serious diabetes complications, including HHNS. Mild elevations of serum glucose identified on emergency department laboratory panels should not be ignored. Patients with evidence of hyperglycemia should be made aware of this potentially significant finding and referred for evaluation. The diagnostic criteria for diabetes should be used for the identification of undiagnosed diabetes (Table 205-1).[2]

EPIDEMIOLOGY

The basic epidemiology of diabetes is discussed in Chap. 209. Although HHNS occurs much less frequently than DKA, mortality rates are much higher. Reported range of mortality in HHNS is 15 to 35 percent versus approximately 5 percent in DKA.[3]

TABLE 205-1 American Diabetes Association Diagnostic Criteria for Diabetes and Impaired Fasting Glucose

1. Symptoms of diabetes plus a casual plasma glucose concentration > 200 mg/dL. *Casual* is defined as any time of day without regard to the time since last meal. Symptoms include polyuria, polydipsia, and unexplained weight loss.
2. Fasting plasma glucose ≥ 126 mg/dL. *Fasting* is defined as no caloric intake for at least 8 h.
3. 2-h postglucose (PG) tolerance test, 2-hPG value of ≥ 200.

Impaired fasting glucose
1. Fasting plasma glucose ≥ 110 and < 126 mg/dL.
2. 2-hPG ≥ 140 and < 200 mg/dL = impaired glucose tolerance.

Source: Adapted from Report of the Expert Committee on the Diagnosis and Classification of Diabetes Mellitus,[2] with permission.

PATHOPHYSIOLOGY

The basic pathophysiology of diabetes is discussed in Chap. 209. The development of HHNS is attributed to three main factors: (1) decreased insulin utilization, (2) increased hepatic gluconeogenesis and glycogenolysis, and (3) impaired renal excretion of glucose.

During a state of poorly controlled type 2 diabetes mellitus, inadequate tissue utilization of glucose caused by insulin resistance results in hyperglycemia. In the absence of an adequate peripheral response to insulin, hepatic glycogenolysis and gluconeogenesis occurs, further elevating serum glucose. As serum glucose concentration increases, it creates an osmotic gradient that draws water out of the intracellular space and into the intravascular compartment. This initial increase in intravascular volume is accompanied by a temporary increase in the glomerular filtration rate (GFR). As serum glucose concentration exceeds approximately 180 mg/dL, the renal reabsorbtive capacity for glucose is exceeded, and glucosuria and a profound osmotic diuresis occur.

Patients with free access to water are often able to prevent profound volume depletion by replacing lost water with large free water intake. If this water requirement is not met (as may occur in a nonambulatory nursing home patient), volume depletion occurs. During osmotic diuresis, urine produced is markedly hypotonic. Still significant urinary loss of sodium and potassium, as well as more modest loss of calcium, phosphate, magnesium, and urea, also occur. As volume concentration progresses, renal perfusion decreases and the GFR is reduced. Renal tubular excretion of glucose is consequently impaired, which further worsens the hyperglycemia. A sustained osmotic diuresis may result in total body water losses that often exceed 20 percent of total body weight or approximately 9 L in a 70-kg patient.

The reason for the absence of ketoacidosis in HHNS is not clearly understood. Though some degree of a starvation ketosis does occur, clinically significant ketoacidosis does not. This lack of ketoacidosis in HHNS has been attributed to three possible mechanisms: (1) lower levels of counterregulatory hormones, (2) higher levels of endogenous insulin, which strongly inhibits lipolysis, and (3) inhibition of lipolysis by the hyperosmolar state.

There is controversy about the role that counterregulatory hormones glucagon, cortisol, growth hormone, and epinephrine play in HHNS. When compared with DKA, glucagon and growth hormone levels have been shown to be lower, which may help prevent lipolysis. When compared with DKA, significantly higher levels of insulin are found in the peripheral and portal circulation in HHNS. Though these levels of insulin are insufficient to overcome hyperglycemia, they appear to be sufficient to inhibit lipolysis.[4] Finally, there have also been limited experimental animal studies that have shown that both the hyperosmolar state and severe hyperglycemia inhibit lipolysis in adipose tissue.[5]

TABLE 205-2 Conditions That May Precipitate Hyperglycemic Hyperosmolar Nonketotic Syndrome

Diabetes	Infection
Parental or enteral alimentation	Myocardial infarction
Gastrointestinal hemorrhage	Severe burns
Pulmonary emboli	Renal insufficiency
Pancreatitis	Peritoneal or hemodialysis
Heat related illness	Cerebrovascular events
Mesenteric ischemia	Rhabdomyolysis

CLINICAL FEATURES

The typical patient with HHNS is usually elderly, who is often referred by a caretaker for abnormalities in vital signs and or mental status; with complaints which include weakness, anorexia, or fatigue. Many will have either undiagnosed or poorly controlled type 2 diabetes. These patients often have some level of baseline cognitive impairment, and self-referral for medical treatment is rare. In general, any patient with hyperglycemia, an impaired means of communication, and limited access to unassisted free water intake is at risk for HHNS. The presence of renal insufficiency or cardiovascular disease is common to this patient population. The medications such as diuretics that are commonly used to treat these underlying chronic problems, predisposes to the development of HHNS.

Usually some precipitating event causes a patient to develop an insidious state of progressive hyperglycemia and hyperosmolarity, which goes unchecked. By far, acute infection is the most common precipitating cause of HHNS. Urinary tract infection and pneumonia are most common, though uremia, viral illness, and a host of metabolic and iatrogenic causes have been identified (Table 205-2). Similarly, several drugs may predispose or contribute to hyperglycemia, volume depletion, or other effects leading to HHNS (Table 205-3).

Physical Findings

The physical manifestations associated with HHNS are nonspecific. Generally, clinical signs of volume depletion such as poor skin turgor, dry mucous membranes, sunken eyeballs, and orthostatic hypotension, will correlate with degree of hyperglycemia and hyperosmolality and duration of physiologic imbalance.

A wide range of findings from subtle changes in vital signs and cognition to clear evidence of profound shock and coma may occur. HHNS may unexpectedly be found in patients who present with concurrent medical insults such as an acute cerebrovascular accident (CVA), severe burns, myocardial infarction, infection, pancreatitis, or other acute illness (Table 205-3). Up to 15 percent may present with seizures. These are typically focal, though generalized seizures, which are often resistant to anticonvulsants, may occur.[6]

TABLE 205-3 Drugs That May Predispose Individuals to the Development of HHNS

Diuretics	Glucocorticoids
Lithium	Neuroleptics
β Blockers	Phenytoin
Mannitol	Didanosine
	Calcium-channel blockers

Other central nervous system (CNS) symptoms may include tremor, clonus, hyperreflexia or hyporeflexia, a positive plantar response, reversible hemiplegia, or hemisensory defects (without CVA or structural intracerebral lesion). The degree of lethargy and coma is proportional to the level of osmolality.[7,8] Those with coma tend to have higher osmolarity, hyperglycemia, and greater volume contraction. In view of the age of the patient population, it is not surprising that the misdiagnosis of stroke or organic brain disease is common.

Laboratory

The laboratory parameters used to define HHNS—glucose >400, osmolarity >315, ph >7.3, and negative serum ketones—are fairly arbitrary. Those values are found in the American Diabetes Association position statement for Hospital Admission Guidelines for Diabetes Mellitus.[9] Depending on concurrent illness and duration of disease, a "mixed disorder" with metabolic acidosis may be found. Essential laboratory tests should include serum glucose, electrolytes, calculated and measured serum osmolality, blood urea nitrogen (BUN), ketones, and creatinine, as well as cell blood count. In view of the frequency of precipitating causes and underlying medical conditions associated with HHNS, a broad range of ancillary studies should be considered. These should include blood cultures, sputum collection, urinalysis and culture, liver and pancreatic enzyme determinations, cardiac enzymes, thyroid function, and coagulation profiles. Other ancillary studies such as chest x-ray, electrocardiogram, computed tomography, and lumbar puncture and toxicologic studies should be considered. Arterial blood-gas determination is of added value only if there is suspicion of a respiratory component to the acid-base abnormality, as both P_{CO_2} and pH can be predicted from HCO_3^- concentration obtained in venous electrolytes (see Chap. 21, "Acid-Base Disorders").

In general, electrolyte abnormalities reflect a contraction alkalosis with varying degrees of wide-anion-gap metabolic acidosis. Initial serum electrolyte determinations can be reported as seemingly normal because the metabolic alkalosis and acidosis may largely cancel out each other's effect. A lack of careful analysis of serum chemistries may lead to a delayed appreciation of the severity of the underlying abnormalities, including volume loss. The only clue to a serious derangement may be the widened anion gap. Serum sodium is suggestive but not a reliable indicator of degree of volume contraction. Although the patient is certainly total body sodium depleted, the serum sodium (even corrected for the glucose elevation) may be low, normal, or elevated. Measured serum sodium, however, is often reported as low due to the dilutional effect of hyperglycemia. It is important to correct for this effect. Serum sodium decreases by approximately 1.6 meq per every 100 mg/dL increase in serum glucose above 100 mg/dL or

$$\text{corrected }[\text{Na}^+] = \text{measured }[\text{Na}^+] + \frac{1.6 \times [\text{glucose} - 100]}{100}$$

Elevated corrected serum sodium during severe hyperglycemia is usually explainable only by significant volume contraction. Normal sodium level or hyponatremia usually (but not invariably) suggests modest dehydration.

Serum osmolality has also been shown to correlate with severity of disease as well as neurologic impairment and coma. A calculated effective serum osmolality excludes osmotically inactive urea, which is usually included in laboratory measures of osmolarity. The formula for calculated effective osmolality is

$$2([\text{Na}^+] + [\text{K}^+]) = \frac{\text{glucose}}{18}$$

Normal serum osmolality range is approximately 275 to 295 mosm/kg. Values above 300 mosm are usually clinically indicative of significant hyperosmolality.

Hypokalemia probably poses the most immediate electrolyte-based risk and should be anticipated. Losses of 300 to 600 meq are not uncommon. Initial values may be reported as normal during a period of severe volume contraction. Again, the patient is surely total body potassium depleted, but acid-base abnormalities may conspire to mask or augment the deficit. As intravascular volume is replaced, potassium losses become more apparent. Patients who have low serum $[K^+]$ during the period of severe volume contraction are at greatest risk for dysrhythmia. The importance of K^+ replacement during periods of rehydration and insulin therapy cannot be overemphasized.

Both prerenal azotemia and renal azotemia are common with plasma BUN-creatinine ratios often exceeding 30:1. Leukocytosis is variable and, when present, is usually due to infection or hemoconcentration. Hypophosphatemia may occur during periods of prolonged hyperglycemia. Acute consequences such as CNS abnormalities, cardiac dysfunction, and rhabdomyolysis are rare and usually associated with serum phosphate levels below 1.0 mg/dL. Routine replacement of phosphate or magnesium, unless severe, is usually unnecessary. Both electrolytes tend to normalize as the metabolic derangement is addressed. When necessary, gradual replacement minimizes the risks of complications such as renal failure. Metabolic acidosis is a wide-anion-gap type often due to poor tissue perfusion resulting in lactic acidosis, uremia, mild starvation ketosis, or all three.

TREATMENT

The treatment of HHNS consists of correction of hypovolemia, treatment of precipitating causes, correction of electrolyte abnormalities, and correction of hyperglycemia. Rapid treatment is reserved only for potentially life-threatening electrolyte abnormalities. Hydration and restoration of euglycemia should be done slowly.

Fluid Resuscitation

Initial fluid resuscitation should be aimed at reestablishing adequate tissue perfusion and decreasing serum glucose. Replacement of intravascular fluid losses alone can account for reductions in serum glucose on average 35–70 mg/h or up to 80 percent initial values. The expansion of intravascular volume decreases serum osmolarity, inhibits counterregulatory hormones, and improves renal excretion of glucose.

The average fluid deficit in HHNS is in the range of 20 to 25 percent of total body water (TBW) or 8 to 12 L. In the elderly, about 50 percent of body weight is due to TBW. By using patient's usual current weight in kilograms, normal TBW and water deficit can be calculated. One-half of the fluid deficit should be replaced over the initial 12 h and the balance over the next 24 h. The actual rate of fluid administration should be individualized for each patient based on the presence of renal and cardiac impairment. Initial rates of 500 to 1500 mL/h during the first 2 h, followed by rates of 250 to 500 mL/h are usually well tolerated. In fact, the initial liter of fluid can usually be infused ''wide open'' without risk of adverse sequelae in almost all patients. Patients with cardiac disease may require the more conservative rate of volume repletion. Renal and cardiovascular function should be carefully monitored. Central venous and urinary tract catheterization should be considered in patients with preexisting renal or cardiac disease.

Most authors agree that the use of isotonic saline (0.9% NaCl) is the most appropriate initial crystalloid for the replacement of intravascular volume. It is hypotonic to the patient's serum osmolarity and will more rapidly restore plasma volume. Once hypotension, tachycardia, and urinary output improve, half-normal saline (0.45% NaCl) can be used to replace the remaining free water deficit.

A limited number of reports of cerebral edema occurring during or soon after the resuscitation phase of patients with both DKA and HHNS have been described.[10,11] Most cases have occurred in children, and the mechanism is unclear. If changes in mental status occur during treatment, fluid should be stopped and head computed tomography obtained. Mannitol (1 g/kg IV bolus) can be given but effectiveness is unclear.

Electrolytes

Potassium deficits and shifts by far pose the most immediate electrolyte-based risk. On average, potassium losses range from 3 to 5 meq/kg, though deficits as high as 10 meq/kg body weight have been reported. Despite these total body deficits, initial serum laboratory measurements may be normal. Serum potassium may even be high in the presence of acidemia. Patients whose initial serum potassium measurements are low are at highest risk for cardiac dysrhythmia and respiratory arrest and should be treated with urgency. Insulin therapy will likely correct acidemia while increasing renal potassium losses as GFR is restored. Also, insulin therapy may cause precipitous shift of potassium into the cell. Usually well within the first 12 h of therapy, most patients will be hypokalemic if replacement therapy has not begun.

With adequate urinary output, potassium replacement should begin at serum $[K^+]$ of 4.5 to 5.0 meq/L. In general, potassium should be replaced at a rate of 10 to 20 meq/h, though life-threatening hypokalemia may warrant utilizing infusion rates of up to 60 meq/h. Some authors feel that potassium infusion through a central venous catheter poses risk for conduction defects and should be avoided. If properly diluted, peripheral infusions of potassium through two peripheral intravenous lines are well tolerated. Monitoring of serum potassium should occur every hour until a steady state has been achieved.

Sodium deficits are replenished fairly rapidly, considering the amount of normal saline and half-normal saline given during fluid replacement. Phosphate and magnesium levels should be measured. In cases of severe hypophosphatemia or hypomagnesemia, replacement therapy is indicated.

Insulin

The absorption of insulin by intramuscular or subcutaneous route is unreliable in patients with HHNS, and a continuous infusion of regular insulin should be given. Infusion rates should begin at 0.1 (units/kg)/h after an initial bolus of 0.1 units/kg. Insulin for infusion should be mixed in a 1:1 ratio (e.g., 250 units or regular insulin in 250 mL of 0.9% NaCl). Pump infusion rates will thus correlate exactly to hourly rate of units of insulin. Steady states utilizing infusion pumps occur within 30 min of infusion. This usually results in a decrease in the plasma concentration of glucose of 80 to 150 (mg/dL)/h. Some patients will demonstrate insulin resistance and require higher doses of insulin. Once serum glucose decreases to less than 300 mg/dL, the intravenous solution should be changed to D_5W 0.45 percent NaCl and the insulin infusion should be reduced to half or 0.05 (units/kg)/h.

Initial volume replacement should always precede the initiation of an insulin drip in HHNS. If insulin is utilized prior to rehydration, intravascular volume may be further depleted. Insulin will cause a shift of osmotically active glucose into the intracellular space, bringing free water with it. This will further deplete the intravascular compartment and may precipitate vascular collapse. Another relative contraindication to the early use of insulin in HHNS is hypokalemia. Insulin promotes transport of potassium into cells and it should be withheld until the potassium level is known and hypokalemia has been treated.

DISPOSITION

Most patients with HHNS require intensive care monitoring for the first 24 h. Patients requiring ongoing replacement of potassium should have continuous cardiac monitoring until those losses are replenished and serum potassium has stabilized.

Some patients may actually meet the criteria for HHNS, have mild symptoms, and have a negative evaluation for comorbidity. In cases when a reliable discharge plan can be arranged, outpatient treatment may be acceptable following appropriate emergency department care. If there is any doubt, the patient should be admitted.

REFERENCES

1. Lorber DL: Nonketotic hypertonicity in diabetes. *Endocrinologist* 3:29, 1993.
2. Report of the Expert Committee on the Diagnosis and Classification of Diabetes Mellitus: *Diabetes Care* 20:1183, 1997.
3. Centers for Disease Control and Prevention: *National Diabetes Fact Sheet: National Estimates and General Information on Diabetes in the United States.* Atlanta, US Department of Health and Human Services, Centers for Disease Control and Prevention, 1997.
4. Chaupin M, Charbonnel B, Chaupin F: C-peptide blood levels in ketoacidosis and in hyperosmolar non-ketotic diabetic coma. *Acta Diabet Lat* 18:123, 1981.
5. Turpin BP, Duckworth WC, Solomon SS: Simulated hyperglycemic hyperosmolar syndrome: Impaired insulin and epinephrine effects upon lipolysis in the isolated rat fat cell. *J Clin Invest* 63:403, 1979.
6. Wachtel TJ, Tetu-Mouradjian LM, Goldman DL, et al: Hyperosmolarity and acidosis in diabetes mellitus: A three year experience in Rhode Island. *J Gen Intern Med* 6:495, 1991.
7. Fulop M, Rosenblatt A, Kreitzer SM: Hyperosmolar nature of diabetic coma. *Diabetes* 24:594, 1975.
8. Arnett AI: Cerebral edema complicating nonketotic hyperosmolar coma. *Miner Electrol Metab* 12:383, 1986.
9. American Diabetes Association: Clinical Practice Recommendations 1998: Position Statement—Hospital Admission Guidelines for Diabetes Mellitus. *Diabetes Care* 21(suppl), 1998.
10. Rosenblum AL: Intracerebral crisis during treatment of diabetic ketoacidosis. *Diabetes Care* 13:22, 1990.
11. Silver SM, Clark EL, Schroeder BM, Sterns RH: Pathogenesis of cerebral edema after treatment of diabetic ketoacidosis. *Kidney Int* 51:1237, 1997.

HYPERTHYROIDISM AND THYROID STORM

Horace K. Liang

Hyperthyroid states may result from various disorders. Manifestations of disease may range from subtle, nonspecific complaints to life-threatening emergencies. Recognition and appropriate empiric treatment of thyroid storm is life saving.

NORMAL THYROID STATE

Regulation of synthesis and release of thyroid hormone is under the control of the anterior pituitary gland via thyroid-stiumulating hormone (TSH), or thyrotropin. Regulation of TSH in turn is by hypothalamic thyrotropin-releasing hormone (TRH) and also by means of a feedback loop to the pituitary gland by circulating thyroxine (T_4) and triiodothyrinine (T_3) levels. Thyroid hormone production depends on adequate iodine intake and synthesis of thyroglobulin. Following release from the thyroid, thyroid hormones are reversibly bound to various circulating plasma proteins, of which thyronine-binding globulin (TBG) is the major constituent. The free, unbound portions of the hormone are biologically active. Normally, T_4 is the predominant circulating hormone. T_4 is peripherally deiodinated to T_3 and is responsible for producing 80 percent of the circulating T_3 hormone. Free T_3 is biologically more active than T_4 but has a shorter half-life (1 day versus 1 week).

Thyroid hormone exerts its action on a wide host of metabolic processes. It appears that thyroid hormone is active mainly at the cellular level and mediated by nuclear receptors for T_3. Binding of these receptors modulates expression of specific target genes and subsequent protein synthesis.[1] Thyroid hormone may also mediate cellular metabolism.

HYPERTHYROIDISM

Hyperthyroidism occurs at all ages but is less common under the age of 15. It is 10 times more common in women than in men, with an annual incidence of about 1 per 1000 women.[2] Causes of hyperthyroidism are shown in Table 206-1. Graves disease is by far the most common cause, accounting for more than 80 percent of cases of hyperthyroidism in the United States.[3] Toxic multinodular and toxic (adenoma) nodular goiters are the next most frequent causes. Graves' disease is common in the third and fourth decades of life. It is characterized by hyperthyroidism due to an autoimmune activation of TSH, diffuse goiter, ophthalmopathy, and dermopathy. In contrast, toxic multinodular goiter usually occurs in a somewhat older population, commonly with a previous history of simple goiter.[2] Often, these patients have milder symptoms of thyrotoxicosis. Less common causes of hyperthyroidism are thyroiditis, pituitary tumors, metastatic thyroid cancer, and dermoid tumors or teratomas of the ovary. Medication-induced hyperthyroidism may be due to iodine ingestion, lithium therapy, or thyroid medication (thyrotoxicosis facticia). Amiodarone-induced thyrotoxicosis has been reported to be between 1 and 23 percent.[4]

Classically, patients with hyperthyroidism may complain of heat intolerance, palpitations, weight loss, sweating, tremor, nervousness, weakness, and fatigue (Table 206-2). An individual with hyperthyroidism who is exhibiting only mild symptoms may be safely referred for further evaluation as an outpatient. Clinical suspicion of hyperthyroidism is confirmed by thyroid function tests. An elevated free T_4 and a low or undetectable TSH level is consistent with a diagnosis of hyperthyroidism. In some cases of Graves' disease, the T_4 level may be normal and the TSH level decreased but the patient appears to be thyrotoxic. A T_3 level should be determined to rule out T_3 toxicosis. Patients with hyperthyroidism secondary to pituitary adenomas will have elevated TSH.

Palliative treatment for mild hyperthyroidism can be accomplished by using various β-blocker medications, the most common of which is propranolol. The goals of therapy include decreased heart rate,

TABLE 206-1 Causes of Thyrotoxicosis

Primary hyperthyroidism
Graves' disease (toxic diffuse goiter)
Toxic multinodular goiter
Toxic nodular (adenoma) goiter
Iodine intake (jodbasedow disease)
Central hyperthyroidism
Pituitary adenoma
Thyroiditis
Subacute painful (de Quervain's disease)
Silent subacute
Postpartum
Radiation thyroiditis
Nonthyroidal disease
Ectopic thyroid tissue (struma ovarii)
Metastatic thyroid cancer
Drug induced
Lithium
Iodine (including radiographic contrast material)
Amiodurone
Excessive thyroid hormone ingestion (thyrotoxicosis facticia)

TABLE 206-2 Signs and Symptoms of Symptoms of Hyperthyroidism

Symptoms	Signs
Weakness	Goiter or thyroid bruit
Fatigue	Hyperkinesis
Heat intolerance	Ophthalmopathy
Nervousness	Lid retraction or stare
Increased sweating	Lid lag
Tremor	Tremor
Palpitation	Warm, moist skin
Increased appetite	Muscle weakness
Weight loss	Hyperreflexia
Hyperdefecation	Tachycardia or arrhythmia
Dyspnea	Systolic hypertension
Menstrual abnormalities	Widened pulse pressure

Source: From Tietgens and Leinung,[12] with permission.

decreased tremor, increased muscle strength, and overall improvement in the patient's sense of well-being.[5] Treatment of Graves' disease may include long-term antithyroid medication, propylthiouracil or methimazole (MMI), radioiodine (iodine 131), or surgical ablation (subtotal thyroidectomy). Toxic multinodular goiter and solitary adenomas may also be treated with radioiodine. Hyperthyroidism due to thyroiditis is usually self-limited, and specific therapy is rarely needed. Common causes of thyroidtis are subacute (painful) thyroiditis (due to viral causes), silent thyroiditis (lymphocytic infiltrate), and postpartum thyroiditis (transient immune destruction). Thyrotoxicosis factitia may be suspected with the absence of thyromegaly, low serum thyroglobulin levels, and decreased or absent radioactive uptake with thyroid scanning. Hyperthyroidism during pregnancy is almost always due to Graves' disease. Often, Graves' disease improves with progression of gestation. The lowest dose of medication should be used in order to maintain a euthyroid state. Treatment options include propylthiouracil (PTU) (it causes fewer fetal anomalies than does MMI), but neonatal goiter has been reported with its use. The use of β blockers has been controversial.[6] Administration of radioiodine is contraindicated in pregnant women.[7]

TABLE 206-3 Differential Diagnosis for Thyroid Storm

Sepsis
Sympathomimetic ingestion (e.g., cocaine, amphetamine)
Heat stroke
Delirium tremens
Malignant hyperthermia
Malignant neuroleptic syndrome
Hypothalamic stroke
Pheochromocytosis
Medication withdrawal

TABLE 206-4 Precipitants of Thyroid Storm

Infection
Trauma
Diabetic ketoacidosis
Myocardial infarction
Cerebrovascular accident
Pulmonary thromboembolic disease
General surgery
Withdrawal of thyroid medication
Iodine administration
Palpation of the thyroid gland
Ingestion of thyroid hormone
Unknown cause (20–25% of cases)

THYROID STORM

The life-threatening hypermetabolic state due to hyperthyroidism is termed thyroid storm. It is a rare occurrence but constitutes a medical emergency. The presentation is usually dramatic. The diagnosis is based on clinical suspicion, treatment is empirically initiated, and the patient is admitted to an appropriately monitored setting. The differential diagnosis is listed in Table 206-3. Classically, thyroid storm occurs as a result of previously unrecognized or poorly treated hyperthyroidism. Etiologies that precipitate thyroid storm are often recognized (Table 206-4), but the pathophysiology is not clearly understood. Most studies have not demonstrated differences in thyroid hormone levels between patients with symptomatic, uncomplicated hyperthyroidism and those with thyroid storm. Some studies have noted higher levels of free T_4 in individuals who have presented with thyroid storm. Enhanced sympathetic nervous system activity explains many of the presenting clinical findings of thyroid storm. Despite treatment, mortality rates are high (20 to 50 percent). The signs and symptoms of thyroid storm are listed in Table 206-5. The hallmarks of this disease are fever, tachycardia out of proportion to the fever, and changes in normal mental status (confusion, delirium, seizure, or coma). Burch has described a diagnostic point scale based on clinical

TABLE 206-5 Presenting Signs and Symptoms of Thyroid Storm

Fever
Tachycardia
Dysrhythmia
Congestive heart failure
Central nervous system dysfunction Agitation Confusion Delirium Stupor Coma Seizure
Volume depletion
Exhaustion

presentation in order to distinguish among uncomplicated thyrotoxicosis, impending thyroid storm, and established thyrotoxic storm.[8]

Laboratory analysis is usually not helpful. Thyroid function tests are not routinely readily available to emergency physicians. Nonspecific laboratory findings may include leukocytosis, hyperglycemia, increased transaminase levels, and increased bilirubin levels.

Treatment

Initial treatment of thyroid storm consists of stabilization, airway protection, oxygenation, intravenous fluids, and monitoring. Specific therapy is outlined in Table 206-6. β blockers are used to treat the severe adrenergic symptoms. Utilizing propranolol has the additional benefit of inhibiting peripheral conversion of T_4 to T_3. If there is a contraindication to propranolol administration (e.g., asthma, congestive heart failure, or chronic obstructive pulmonary disease), a selective β_1 medication (e.g., esmolol) may be substituted. Guanethidine (inhibits norepinephrine release at the sympathetic junction) or reserpine (depletes stored catecholamines both centrally and peripherally including the adrenal medulla) may be considered as alternative therapy. An additional treatment goal is to decrease synthesis of hormone by the administration of PTU or MMI. PTU also decreases T_4 to T_3 conversion. After PTU administration has been initiated, treatment is directed toward decreasing the release of preformed thyroid hormone by the administration of iodine. It is important to not administer iodine until the synthetic pathway has been blocked. Otherwise, the addition of iodine will promote further hormone production. Various iodine-containing preparations, including iodine-containing radiographic contrast material (iopodate [Oragrafin] and ipanoate [Telepaque]) have been utilized for this purpose. Administration of lithium should be considered in patients with a prior history of iodine allergies. Note that many of the drugs used to treat thyroid storm are oral preparations and subsequently may need to be administered via orogastric tube. In cases where clinical deterioration occurs despite appropriate therapy, direct removal of circulating thyroid hormone has been accomplished by exchange transfusion,[9] plasma transfusion,[10] plasmapheresis, and charcoal plasmaperfusion.[11] Other therapeutic goals include treatment of hyperthermia with cooling blankets, ice packs, and antipyretics (acetaminophen). Avoidance of salicylates has been recommended because of displacement of T_4 from TBG, thereby increasing free T_4 levels. The empiric use of corticosteroids has been suggested to treat the potential adrenal insufficiency that may occur with such a hypermetabolic state.

Comorbid factors that may have precipitated thyroid storm must also be treated. Electrocardiograms, chest radiographs, urinalysis, blood cultures, and administration of empiric antibiotics should always be considered in patients presenting in thyroid storm. Standard therapy for heart failure due to ischemic or hypertensive heart disease may be utilized. All patients should be admitted to an appropriately monitored setting for further evaluation and care. Definitive therapy is usually via radioiodine administration once the patient is stable and euthyroid.

TABLE 206-6 Treatment of Thyroid Storm

Clinical suspicion and stabilization
Airway protection
Oxygen
IV fluids
Monitoring
Decreasing de novo synthesis
Propylthiouracil 600–1000 mg PO initially, then 200–250 mg q4h
Methimazole 40 mg PO initial dose, then 25 mg PO q6h
Preventing release of hormone (after synthesis blockade initiated)
Iodine
Potassium iodide (SSKI) 5 drops PO q6h
Sodium iodide 0.5–1.0 g IV q12h
Lugol solution 8–10 drops PO q6h
Lithium carbonate 800–1200 mg/d PO
Preventing peripheral effects
β blockade
Popranolol (IV) titrate 1–2 mg q-5min prn (may need 240–480 mg/d PO)
Esmolol (IV) 500 μg/kg IV bolus, then 50–200 (μg/kg)/min maintenance
Guanethidine 30–40 mg PO q6h
Reserpine 2.5–5 mg IM q4–6h
Other considerations
Corticosteroids
Hydrocortisone 100 mg IV q8h
Dexamethasone 2 mg IV q6h
Antipyretics
Cooling blanket
Acetaminophen 650 mg PO q4h
Treatment of precipitating cause
Admission to appropriately monitored setting

Abbreviations: IM, intramuscular; IV, intravenous; PO, by mouth; prn, as needed; q, every; SSK1, supersaturated potassium iodide.

REFERENCES

1. Brent GA: The molecular basis of thyroid hormone action. *N Engl J Med* 331:847, 1994.
2. Lazarus JH: Hyperthyroidism. *Lancet* 349:339, 1997.
3. Ron E, Doody MM, Becker DV, et al: Cancer mortality following treatment for adult hyperthyroidism. *JAMA* 280:347, 1998.
4. Harjai KJ, Licata AA: Effects of amiodarone on thyroid function. *Ann Intern Med* 126:63, 1997.
5. Klein I, Becker DV, Levey GS: Treatment of hyperthyroid disease. *Ann Intern Med* 121:281, 1994.
6. Burrow GN: The management of thyrotoxicosis in pregnancy. *N Engl J Med* 313:562, 1985.
7. Roti E, Minelli R, Salvi M: The management of hyperthyroid and hypothyroidism in the pregnant woman. *J Clin Endocrinol Metab* 81:1679, 1996.
8. Burch HB, Wartofsky L: Life-threatening thyrotoxicosis: Thyroid storm. *Endocrinol Metab Clin North Am* 22:263, 1993.
9. Ashkar FS, Katims RB, Smoak WM, et al: Thyroid storm treatment with blood exchange and plasmapheresis. *JAMA* 214:1275, 1970.
10. Tajri J, Katsuya H, Kiyokawa T, et al: Successful treatment of thyrotoxic crisis with plasma exchange. *Crit Care Med* 12:536, 1984.
11. Candrina R, DiStefano O, Spandrio S, et al: Treatment of thyrotoxic storm by charcoal plasmaperfusion. *J Endocrinol Invest* 12:133, 1989.
12. Tietgens ST, Leinung MC: Thyroid storm. *Med Clin North Am* 79:169, 1995.

HYPOTHYROIDISM AND MYXEDEMA COMA

Horace K. Liang

Hypothyroidism arises from many etiologies. The severe manifestation of extreme hypothyroidism—myxedema coma—is a rare, potentially life-threatening illness. Correct diagnosis requires a high degree of clinical suspicion, and initiation of treatment is an empiric decision.

HYPOTHYROIDISM

Normal thyroid physiology is discussed in Chapter 206, "Hyperthyroidism and Thyroid Storm." Hypothyroidism occurs when there is insufficient hormone production or secretion. A general hypometabolic

TABLE 207-1 Etiologies of Hypothyroidism

Primary
Autoimmune etiologies (Hashimoto thyroiditis)
Idiopathic
Postablation (surgical, radioiodine)
Postexternal radiation
Iodine deficiency
Thyroiditis (subacute, silent, postpartum)*
Infiltrative disease (lymphoma, sarcoid, amyloidosis, tuberculosis)
Congenital
Secondary (pituitary)
Panhypopituitarism
Tertiary (hypothalamic)
Neoplasms
Infiltrative
Drugs
Amiodarone
Lithium
Iodine (in patients with preexisting autoimmune disease)
Antithyroid medication

*Self-limited etiologies, often preceded by a hyperthyroid phase.

state is the principle feature of this disease. Hypothyroidism occurs more frequently among women than men. The prevalence of hypothyroidism among women ranges from 0.6 to 5.9 percent.[1] The most common etiologies of hypothyroidism are primary thyroid failure due to autoimmune diseases (of which Hashimoto thyroiditis is most common), idiopathic causes, postablative therapy, and iodine deficiency.[2] Hypothyroidism may be transient as in some cases of thyroiditis. The pathophysiology of this entity is unclear but may be viral in origin. Postpartum thyroiditis occurs within 3 to 6 months postpartum and reportedly occurs in 2 to 16 percent of women.[1] Secondary (due to pituitary tumors, infiltrative disease, or hemorrhage) or tertiary (hypothalamic disease) etiologies of hypothyroidism are less common (Table 207-1). Several medications have been reported to induce hypothyroidism. Amiodarone-associated hypothyroidism has been reported to occur in from 1 percent to as many as 32 percent of patients.[3] The mechanism is probably due to the large amount of iodine that is released by the metabolism of the drug, which then inhibits thyroid hormone synthesis and release. Lithium acts similarly to iodine and decreases thyroid hormone release.[4] When initiating lithium therapy, especially in patients with prior hypothyroidism, thyroid function must be carefully monitored.

Primary hypothyroidism usually has an insidious onset. Clinical signs and symptoms of hypothyroid patients are listed in Table 207-2. Individuals with suspected uncomplicated hypothyroidism may be evaluated as outpatients. Typical laboratory findings in primary hypothyroidism include low thyroxine (T_4) and high thyrotropin (thyroid-stimulating hormone or TSH). Triiodothyronine (T_3) is an unreliable indicator of hypothyroidism and is not routinely measured. There is little urgent need for performing thyroid function tests, and typically they are not available during an emergency department visit. However, obtaining blood for testing in the emergency department may be helpful to a patient's health provider in follow-up care. In many cases, elderly patients with hypothyroidism may exhibit a paucity of symptoms. Because of the high prevalence of hypothyroidism in women over age 60, it is recommended that they be routinely screened with a serum TSH measurement.[5,6]

Primary uncomplicated hypothyroidism is treated with T_4 administration. Initiation of oral therapy begins at a dose of 50 to 100 μg/day and is gradually increased. The average daily adult dose is 75 to 150 μg. Elderly patients with underlying heart disease are treated with lower initial dosages. Therapy is monitored to ensure that appropriate serum thyrotropin levels are achieved after 6 to 8 weeks following initiation of therapy. If hypothyroidism is due to less common secondary etiologies, initiation of thyroid hormone replacement may exacerbate preexisting adrenal insufficiency. Therefore, the etiology of hypothyroidism (primary versus secondary failure) should be determined prior to initiating T_4 replacement. Initiation of therapy in the emergency department is rarely warranted for simple hypothyroidism. Clinical clues that may differentiate primary and secondary hypothyroidism are listed in Table 207-3.

TABLE 207-2 Symptoms and Signs of Hypothyroidism

Fatigue	Hoarseness
Weight gain	Hypothermia
Cold intolerance	Periorbital puffiness
Depression	Delayed relaxation of ankle jerks
Menstrual irregularities	Loss of outer third of eyebrow
Constipation	Cool, rough, dry skin
Joint pain	Nonpitting edema
Muscle cramps	Bradycardia
Infertility	Peripheral neuropathy

MYXEDEMA COMA

Myxedema coma describes a rare, clinical state in which an individual with long-standing preexisting hypothyroidism presents with life-threatening decompensation.[7] In reality, few patients present comatose with severe myxedema. Affected patients are commonly in the geriatric population. Various etiologies may be a precipitant to this syndrome

TABLE 207-3 Differentiation of Primary and Secondary Hypothyroidism[7]

Primary	Secondary
Previous thyroid operation	No prior thyroid operation
Obese	Less obese
Goiter present	No goiter present
Hypothermia more common	Hypothermia less common
Voice coarse	Voice less coarse
Pubic hair present	Pubic hair absent
Skin dry and coarse	Skin fine and soft
Heart increased in size	Heart usually normal
Normal menses and lactation	Traumatic delivery, no lactation, amenorrhea
Sella turcica normal	Sella turcica may be increased in size
Serum TSH increased	Serum TSH decreased
Plasma cortisol normal	Plasma cortisol decreased
No response to TSH	Good response to TSH
Good response to levothyroxine without steroids	Poor response to levothyroxine without steroids

Abbreviation: TSH, thyroid-stimulating hormone.

TABLE 207-4 Precipitants of Myxedema Coma

Infection
Cold exposure
Drugs (sedatives, lithium, amiodarone)
Trauma
Stroke
Congestive heart failure
Inadequate thyroid hormone replacement
Previously undiagnosed hypothyroidism

(Table 207-4). The clinical presentation is one of a severe decompensated metabolic state that may include an alteration in mental status, hypothermia, bradycardia, hypoventilation, and even cardiovascular collapse (Table 207-5). These findings are not only secondary to a decline in metabolic function but also due to neurovascular and cardiovascular adaptations. Some of these adaptations are similar to those that occur in euthyroid patients exposed to a cold environment (decline in oxygen consumption and heat generation, and redistribution of blood flow centrally). In addition, there is a change in end-organ responsiveness to catecholamines and a decline in cardiac performance. This is due to an absolute diminution in β-adrenergic receptors (decreased inotrope and chronotrope activity). There is also relatively increased α-adrenergic responsiveness resulting in mild diastolic hypertension.[8] Increased CO_2 retention occurs because of decreased respiratory muscle strength and diminished ventilatory drive in response to hypercapnia. There is also decreased free-water clearance resulting in a dilutional hyponatremia, impaired gluconeogenesis, and decreased drug clearance that predisposes patients to drug toxicity from medication.[9]

Diagnosis of myxedema coma requires high clinical suspicion. A patient suspected of presenting with myxedema coma commonly has a prior history of primary hypothyroidism or previous thyroid surgery. Medication noncompliance or coexisting stressors such as cold exposure, severe infection, or the addition of new medications may precipitate the onset of myxedema coma. The decline in function is usually gradual and insidious in onset. The physical examination may confirm a history of long-standing hypothyroidism. In addition, there may be clinical findings of hypothermia, hypoventilation, hypotension, bradycardia, and alteration or deterioration of the patient's mental status.

Laboratory evaluation of patients with suspected myxedema coma may reveal anemia; hyponatremia; hypoglycemia; elevated transaminases, creatine phosphokinase, and lactate dehydrogenase levels; hypercholesterolemia; and arterial blood-gas abnormalities (decreased Po_2 and increased Pco_2). The electrocardiogram may demonstrate sinus bradycardia, prolongation of the QT interval, and low voltage with flattening or inversion of T waves. A chest radiograph may demonstrate an enlarged cardiac contour caused by a pericardial effusion.[9,10]

TABLE 207-5 Clinical Presentation of Myxedema Coma

Decreased mental status
Hypothermia
Bradycardia
Hypoventilation
Periorbital edema
Nonpitting edema
Delayed deep tendon reflexes
Hypoglycemia
Hyponatremia

TABLE 207-6 Treatment of Myxedema Coma

Recognition
Supportive measures, including ventilatory support
Thyroid replacement Levothyroxine (300 to 500 μg slow IV initial dose and then 50 to 100 μg IV per day) T_3 (25 μg IV or PO q8h) Combination of T_4 plus T_3
Glucocorticoid Hydrocortisone (100 mg IV q8h)
Hypothermia Prevent additional loss Passive external rewarming
Electrolyte correction Gentle fluid restriction for dilutional hyponatremia Hypertonic saline for severe hyponatremia
Hypoglycemia Dextrose containing IV solution Monitoring
Aggressive treatment of precipitating cause
Admit patients to a monitored setting

Abbreviations: T_3, triiodothyronine; T_4, thyroxine.

Treatment

There are no prospective studies on the optimum therapy for patients in myxedema coma; therefore, treatment recommendations are not uniform. However, initial therapy is directed toward stabilization. Patients may require endotracheal intubation and mechanical ventilation for airway protection and correction of hypoventilation, hypercapnia, and hypoxia. Indications for airway intervention are the same as for other conditions (see Chap. 15, "Tracheal Intubation and Mechanical Ventilation"). Correction of hypothermia is directed toward decreasing further heat loss. Cautious use of gentle passive external rewarming should be initiated but care should be taken to avoid hypotension from reversal of a patient's hypothermic vasoconstriction.

Specific therapy includes intravenous levothyroxine, which is recommended by most authors.[11] An initial intravenous bolus of levothyroxine (Table 207-6) is administered, followed by a reduced daily dose until the patient can take oral medication. This has the advantage of repleting the T_4 pool and allowing the hormone to enter tissues slowly. Other authors suggest that there may be decreased T_4 to T_3 conversion and subsequently recommend T_3 as the initial replacement hormone.

Routine administration of glucocorticoid is recommended to avoid the potential of precipitating adrenal crisis in patients with unrecognized adrenal insufficiency or hypothyroidism secondary to hypopituitarism. If possible, a baseline cortisol level should be drawn prior to initiating therapy. Correction of hyponatremia is by means of fluid restriction. Severe hyponatremia has been successfully treated with hypertonic saline administration (see Chap. 23, "Fluids and Electrolyte Problems").

A search for a precipitating etiology must be initiated and aggressively treated. Infection is a common precipitant of myxedema coma. If possible, appropriate cultures should be obtained prior to initiating empiric antibiotic therapy.

All patients with a suspected diagnosis of myxedema coma should be admitted to an appropriately monitored inpatient bed for further evaluation and treatment.

REFERENCES

1. Mulder JE: Thyroid disease in women. *Med Clin North Am* 82:103, 1998.
2. Lindsay RS, Toft AD: Hypothyroidism. *Lancet* 349:413, 1997.
3. Harja KJ, Licata AA: Effects of amiodarone on thyroid function. *Ann Intern Med* 126:63, 1997.
4. Waldman SA, Park D: Myxedema coma associated with lithium therapy. *Am J Med* 87:355, 1989.
5. Sawin CT: Thyroid dysfunction in older persons. *Adv Intern Med* 37:223, 1991.
6. Helfand M, Redfern CC: Screening for thyroid disease: An update. Position papers: Clinical guideline, Part 2. *Ann Int Med* 129:144, 1998.
7. Senior RM, Birge SJ, Wessler S, et al: The recognition and management of myxedema coma. *JAMA* 217:61, 1971.
8. Jordan RM: Myxedema coma: Pathophysiology, therapy and factors affecting prognosis. *Med Clin North Am* 79:185, 1995.
9. Nicoloff JT, LoPresti JS: Myxedema coma: A form of decompensated hypothyroidism. *Endocrinol Metab Clin North Am* 22:279, 1993.
10. Tsitouras PD: Myxedema coma. *Clin Geriatr Med* 11:251, 1995.
11. Singer PA, Cooper DS, Levy EG, et al: Treatment guidelines for patients with hyperthyroidism and hypothyroidism. *JAMA* 273:808, 1995.

208 ADRENAL INSUFFICIENCY AND ADRENAL CRISIS

Gene Ragland

Adrenal insufficiency consists of decreased levels or absence of hormones produced by the adrenal glands and results from structural or functional lesions of the adrenal cortex, the anterior pituitary gland, or the hypothalamus. Deficit of adrenal hormones may manifest clinically as a chronic, insidious disorder, or as an acute, life-threatening emergency. Therapy of adrenal insufficiency is specific and includes replacement of the deficient hormones.

Chronic adrenal insufficiency is due to a variety of causes. It may be primary (Addison's disease), due to failure of the adrenal glands. It also may occur secondarily because of failure of the pituitary gland (hypopituitarism) or as a tertiary insufficiency due to hypothalamic dysfunction. Iatrogenic adrenal suppression from chronic steroid use is termed iatrogenic tertiary adrenal insufficiency. Acute adrenal insufficiency (adrenal crisis) may result from certain acute events, or when a person with chronic adrenal insufficiency is subjected to stress and exhausts reserve adrenal hormones, or when replacement hormone medication is discontinued.

PATHOPHYSIOLOGY OF THE ADRENAL GLANDS

The adrenal glands are divisible into the cortex and medulla. The adrenal cortex is essential for life and produces glucocorticoid, mineralocorticoid, and androgenic steroid hormones. The medulla secretes the catecholamines epinephrine and norepinephrine, largely under neural control. No definite clinical condition has been ascribed to hypofunction of the adrenal medulla. Most of the manifestations of adrenal insufficiency occur when the physiologic requirement for glucocorticoid and mineralocorticoid hormones exceeds the capacity of the adrenal glands to produce them.

Cortisol

The major glucocorticoid is cortisol, which is secreted in response to direct stimulation by adrenocorticotropic hormone (ACTH) from the anterior pituitary gland. Secretion of ACTH is governed by the hormone corticotropin-releasing factor (CRF) from the hypothalamus. This normally occurs with a diurnal rhythm, with the highest levels in the morning and the lowest levels in the late evening. On stimulation by ACTH, the adrenal glands respond in minutes to secrete cortisol in direct proportion to the ACTH concentration. Cortisol is normally secreted at the rate of 20 to 25 mg/day. Through negative feedback inhibition, the plasma cortisol level acts to suppress ACTH release.

By an undefined mechanism, stress factors such as anoxia, trauma, infections, and hypoglycemia also can trigger CRF and ACTH release and produce cortisol levels several times normal. The release of CRF in response to stress is resistant to suppression through negative feedback inhibition.

Cortisol is a potent hormone and affects the metabolism of most body tissues. In general, cortisol acts to maintain blood glucose levels by decreasing glucose uptake at extrahepatic sites and by providing precursors for gluconeogenesis via protein and fat breakdown. Cortisol governs the distribution of water between extracellular and intracellular compartments and possesses a minor sodium-retaining effect. It also acts to enhance the pressor effects of catecholamines on heart muscle and arterioles. In supraphysiologic amounts, cortisol inhibits inflammatory and allergic reactions. Finally, through negative feedback inhibition, cortisol suppresses the secretion of ACTH and melanocyte-stimulating hormone (MSH) from the anterior pituitary gland.

Aldosterone

The major mineralocorticoid is aldosterone. The renin-angiotensin system and plasma potassium concentration regulate aldosterone through negative feedback loops. These mechanisms are probably of equal importance and far more important than the minor aldosterone-stimulating effect of ACTH.

Aldosterone acts to increase sodium reabsorption and potassium excretion, primarily in the distal tubules of the kidneys. Other tissue effects of aldosterone are minor in comparison with its regulation of sodium and potassium levels.

Androgens

Androgenic hormone production by the adrenal glands is regulated by ACTH and is trivial in men in comparison with the production of these hormones by the gonads. In women, however, androgens from the adrenal glands *do* contribute a significant proportion to androgen metabolism.

PRIMARY ADRENAL INSUFFICIENCY

Idiopathic

Primary adrenal insufficiency, or Addison's disease, is due to disease or destruction of the adrenal cortex and has a wide variety of causes (Table 208-1). Approximately 90 percent of the adrenal cortex must be involved before clinical manifestations of adrenal failure result. Idiopathic atrophy of the adrenal glands is the leading cause of chronic adrenal insufficiency. Idiopathic adrenal insufficiency has been further divided into autoimmune (70–75 percent) and truly idiopathic (25–30 percent).

There is an overwhelming association between idiopathic adrenal insufficiency and other autoimmune diseases. Associated diseases include diabetes mellitus, Hashimoto's thyroiditis, pernicious anemia, and primary ovarian failure. Other investigators have reported frequent

TABLE 208-1 Pathogenesis of Primary Adrenal Insufficiency

Primary, chronic
Idiopathic (autoimmune)
Infiltrative or infectious
Tuberculosis
Fungal infections
Sarcoidosis
Amyloidosis
Hemochromatosis
Acquired immunodeficiency syndrome (AIDS)
Neoplastic (metastatic) disease
Adrenoleukodystrophy
Hemorrhage or infarction
Bilateral adrenalectomy
Drugs
Congenital adrenal hyperplasia
Congenital unresponsiveness to ACTH
Primary, acute
Hemorrhage (adrenal apoplexy)
Fulminant septicemia
Newborn
Anticoagulants
Discontinuation of replacement steroids

association with hypoparathyroidism, chronic active hepatitis, malabsorption, chronic mucocutaneous candidiasis, alopecia, and vitiligo.

Infiltrative or Infectious

Adrenal tuberculosis has declined in frequency as a cause of Addison's disease but is still reported to be a cause in 17 to 21 percent of the cases. Fungal infections and other infiltrative processes are infrequent causes of adrenal insufficiency during active, disseminated disease. Adrenal insufficiency as a complication of the acquired immunodeficiency syndrome (AIDS) has been reported. Infectious infiltration of the adrenal glands with *Mycobacterium avium* or *M. intracellular* or with cytomegalovirus may have caused the adrenal failure. Metastatic carcinoma in the adrenal glands is a relatively frequent finding at autopsy in patients with certain carcinomas, but it rarely causes adrenal insufficiency.

Bilateral Adrenal Hemorrhage

Bilateral adrenal gland hemorrhage is rare. In general, patients with a serious underlying condition whose adrenal glands are stressed are at risk for this complication. Stress-stimulated adrenal glands are hemorrhage prone. The association between adrenal hemorrhage and anticoagulant therapy with heparin and dicumarol is well established. Adrenal hemorrhage in this setting is most likely to occur between the third and eighteenth day of anticoagulation. Sudden deterioration with hypotension and pain in the flank, costovertebral angle, or epigastrium should suggest this disastrous event. Associated findings may include fever, nausea, vomiting, and disturbed sensorium. Computed tomography (CT) and ultrasound can assist in establishing this diagnosis. Other stressful events that have been associated with adrenal hemorrhage include surgery, trauma, burns, convulsions, pregnancy, and adrenal vein thrombosis.

Adrenal crisis as a consequence of adrenal hemorrhage also occurs with overwhelming septicemia and in the newborn. Fulminant septicemia with meningococcus, pneumococcus, staphylococcus, streptococcus, *Haemophilus influenzae,* and gram-negative organisms has been reported to cause adrenal hemorrhage. The Waterhouse-Friderichsen syndrome is a life-threatening disorder resulting from overwhelming septicemia due to meningococcemia. The patient is acutely ill and has shaking chills, severe headache, and a petechial rash that may progress to extensive purpura. Bilateral adrenal gland hemorrhage frequently occurs with this disorder. Vascular collapse and death may result unless the patient is promptly treated.

Miscellaneous

Another cause of primary adrenal failure is bilateral adrenalectomy for metastatic breast or prostate cancer or for Cushing's syndrome. Following such a procedure, the patient is totally dependent upon replacement corticosteroids for life. Chemotherapeutic agents such as mitotane (*o,p'*-DDD) used in treatment of Cushing's disease can produce adrenal failure. Other drugs such as methadone, rifampin, and ketoconazole have been reported to cause adrenal insufficiency. Finally, rare congenital and inherited disorders can cause adrenal insufficiency.

In children, adrenal insufficiency is due to rare congenital causes or to acquired lesions of the hypothalamus, pituitary or adrenal cortex. By far, the most common cause of acquired chronic adrenal insufficiency is autoimmune destruction of the adrenal glands. Type I autoimmune polyendocrinopathy manifests with chronic mucocutaneous candidiasis, hypoparathyroidism and Addison's disease. Type II autoimmune disease presents with adrenal failure in association with thyroid disorder or insulin dependent diabetes mellitus.

Infections account for approximately 20 percent of the cases of pediatric adrenal insufficiency. Among those are infiltrative destruction of the gland by fungal infections and tuberculosis. Hemorrhage into the adrenal glands may occur in the neonatal period as a consequence of a complicated labor or asphyxia. Another cause of adrenal gland hemorrhage is the Waterhouse-Friderichsen syndrome resulting from meningococcemia and producing shock. Finally, about one-third of patients with adrenoleukodystrophy will develop adrenal insufficiency, usually after 4 years of age.

Clinical Features

The clinical manifestations of chronic adrenal insufficiency develop gradually with subtle signs and symptoms that provide a diagnostic challenge. The clinical presentation of Addison's disease can be explained on the basis of a deficiency of cortisol and aldosterone and a lack of feedback suppression of ACTH and MSH.

Cortisol deficiency manifests clinically with anorexia, nausea, vomiting, lethargy, hypoglycemia with fasting, and inability to withstand even minor stresses without shock. The ability to excrete a free water load is also impaired and can lead to water intoxication. Lack of aldosterone results in impaired ability to conserve sodium and excrete potassium. The patient with aldosterone deficiency presents with sodium depletion, dehydration, hypotension, postural syncope, and decreased cardiac size and output. Renal blood flow is decreased, and azotemia may develop. Hyperkalemia is commonly seen but rarely is severe. Lack of suppression of ACTH and MSH secretion occurs because of deficient cortisol levels and results in increased pigmentation.

The overall clinical picture of a patient with Addison's disease is that of one who is weak and lethargic, with loss of vigor, and fatigue on exertion. The patient may have a feeble tachycardic pulse. Postural hypotension and syncope are common. In spite of hypotension, the extremities usually remain warm. Heart sounds may be soft or almost inaudible on auscultation.

Gastrointestinal symptoms are a prominent feature of chronic adrenal insufficiency and include anorexia, nausea, vomiting, weight loss, abdominal pain, and sometimes diarrhea.

Cutaneous manifestations of Addison's disease include increased brownish pigmentation over exposed body areas such as the face, neck, arms, and dorsum of the hands, and over friction or pressure points such as the elbows, knees, fingers, toes, and nipples. Pigmentation of mucous membranes, darkening of nevi and hair, and longitudinal pigmented bands in the nails may be seen. Vitiligo, mucocutaneous candidiasis, and alopecia may occur with Addison's disease that has an autoimmune cause. Women with Addison's disease may exhibit decreased growth of axillary and pubic hair because of adrenal androgen deficiency. This is not seen in men because of adequate testicular androgen.

Mentally these patients vary from alert to confused. Unconsciousness is rare unless the condition is preterminal. The sensory modalities of taste, olfaction, and hearing may be increased. Hyperkalemic paralysis is a rare, emergent complication of adrenal insufficiency; the patient presents with a rapidly ascending muscular weakness which leads to flaccid quadriplegia. Treatment of this complication consists of the intravenous administration of glucose and insulin or bicarbonate.

LABORATORY The usual laboratory findings in patients with primary adrenal insufficiency include hyponatremia, hyperkalemia, hypoglycemia, and azotemia. Hyponatremia is usually mild to moderate, and severe hyponatremia (<120 mEq/L) is rare. Hyperkalemia is usually mild, and the potassium level rarely exceeds 7 mEq/L. Initial potassium levels may be normal or low if protracted vomiting has occurred. Rarely, hyperkalemia may be severe and cause cardiac dysrhythmia or paralysis.

Hypoglycemia is infrequent in adults with chronic adrenal insufficiency in the absence of infection, fever or alcohol ingestion. Moderate elevation of the blood urea nitrogen (BUN) level may occur because of dehydration secondary to aldosterone deficiency. Azotemia is usually reversible with rehydration.

Electrocardiographic changes include flat or inverted T waves, a prolonged QT interval, low voltage, a prolonged PR or QRS interval, and a depressed ST segment. The ECG changes reflective of hyperkalemia may also be present. The chest x-ray film may show a small, narrow cardiac silhouette due to decreased intravascular volume. A flat plate film of the abdomen may show adrenal calcification, which is most commonly due to tuberculosis but may occur with infection or hemorrhage.

SECONDARY AND TERTIARY ADRENAL INSUFFICIENCY

Secondary adrenal insufficiency may be due to disease or destruction of the pituitary gland, and tertiary insufficiency due to hypothalamic dysfunction, resulting in impaired capacity of the pituitary to secrete ACTH. Those disorders responsible for secondary or tertiary adrenal failure are listed in Table 208-2.

TABLE 208-2 Pathogenesis of Secondary or Tertiary Adrenal Insufficiency

Secondary
- Pituitary tumor (chromophobe adenoma, craniopharyngioma, hamartoma, meningioma, glioma)
- Pituitary hemorrhage or vascular accident
- Postpartum pituitary infarction (Sheehan's syndrome)
- Infiltrative and granulomatous disease
  - Sarcoidosis
  - Hemochromatosis
  - Histiocytosis X
- Internal carotid artery aneurysm
- Head trauma (basilar skull fracture)
- Infection (meningitis, cavernous sinus thrombosis)
- Hypophysectomy
- Pituitary gland irradiation
- Isolated ACTH deficiency

Tertiary
- Iatrogenic HPA suppression due to steroid therapy
- Discontinuation of replacement steroids

The most common cause of tertiary adrenal insufficiency and adrenal crisis is iatrogenic adrenal suppression from prolonged steroid use. Rapid withdrawal of steroids from patients with adrenal atrophy secondary to chronic steroid use may result in collapse and death, especially under circumstances of increased stress. Exogenous administration of glucocorticoids may cause hypothalamic-pituitary-adrenal (HPA) suppression and subsequent adrenal atrophy. This complication has been reported to occur not only with oral steroids but also with those given by the intrathecal, topical, and inhalant routes.

The mechanism of continued adrenal atrophy following discontinuation of exogenous steroids may be a failure of normal diurnal release of CRF. Stress-induced release of ACTH may remain intact, but the atrophic adrenal glands are unable to secrete sufficient cortisol to meet the physiologic requirements in response to stress. The shortest time interval or the smallest dose at which HPA suppression occurs is unknown. As a general rule, there is no suppression regardless of the dose if its duration of use is less than three weeks. In addition, there is no suppression if the dose is <10 mg of prednisone regardless of the duration unless it is given on an h.s. timetable. Any patient who is on more than 20 mg of prednisone for greater than three weeks is suppressed and should have the necessary precautions taken.

Following prolonged supraphysiologic dosages of steroids, it may take up to 6 to 12 months for recovery of HPA function when steroids are withdrawn completely. Until complete recovery has occurred, it is wise to assume the patient will need basal steroid therapy and supplementary therapy during intercurrent illness or stress. Adrenal suppression must be suspected based upon the history of prior steroid use. When in doubt about the HPA status of a seriously ill or deteriorating patient, steroids should be given.

Clinical Features

Significant clinical and laboratory differences exist between patients with primary and those with secondary adrenal insufficiency. With secondary adrenal failure, the capacity of the pituitary to secrete ACTH is impaired. The level of aldosterone is largely unaffected because of its regulation by the renin-angiotensin system and the plasma potassium concentration. The clinical manifestations of secondary adrenal failure are due to insufficiency of cortisol and adrenal androgens. In addition, insufficiency of other anterior pituitary hormones such as growth hormone, thyroid hormone, and gonadotropic hormone may cause clinical abnormalities.

Patients with secondary adrenal insufficiency are better able to tolerate sodium deprivation without developing shock. This is true because of intact aldosterone secretion. Hyponatremia, hyperkalemia, and azotemia are not prominent features of secondary failure. Hypoglycemia, however, may be more common in patients with hypopituitarism because of concomitant growth hormone deficiency. Hyperpigmentation does not occur with secondary failure because ACTH and MSH are eliminated at their source, the pituitary gland. Finally, with secondary failure, men as well as women may exhibit signs of androgen deficiency because of insufficient gonadotopic hormone from the pituitary.

DIAGNOSIS

Primary adrenal insufficiency is diagnosed by demonstrating a low baseline plasma cortisol level and failure to increase this level in response to exogenous administration of ACTH. Any patient who has cortisol level of >20 μg/dL does not have adrenal insufficiency of any type. Failure to respond to ACTH stimulation occurs because the adrenal cortex is damaged or destroyed and has no functional capacity to respond. Secondary adrenal insufficiency is diagnosed by demonstrating low plasma cortisol and urinary metabolite levels that increase in a stepwise fashion with repetitive ACTH stimulation over a period of days. A variety of tests to assess the integrity of the HPA axis are available.

A rapid screening test can reliably distinguish patients with normal adrenal function from those with adrenal insufficiency. This test is based on the fact that adrenal response to a single injection of ACTH is maximal within 1 h. Plasma for measurement of baseline cortisol level is drawn, and then 25 units of corticotropin (synthetic ACTH) is administered subcutaneously, intramuscularly, or intravenously. Another plasma cortisol level is obtained 30 to 60 min later. Normal persons should respond with a doubling of the baseline cortisol level, unless the patient has an already existing high basal level due to stress or some other factor. In this instance, the cortisol level would not double but the patient could still have normal physiology. Patients with primary adrenal insufficiency show no increase in plasma cortisol levels, whereas those with secondary adrenal failure may show no, or a slight, response to corticotropin. A normal response is defined by a peak cortisol value of greater than or equal to 20 μg/dL. However, both falsely normal and abnormal rapid ACTH test results have been reported. This test should be used as a screening test, or to assess adrenal reserve in patients previously receiving steroids, but not as a diagnostic test for adrenocortical failure. A more prolonged period of ACTH stimulation is necessary to confirm adrenal failure and to reliably distinguish primary from secondary adrenal insufficiency. However, measurement of ACTH will also help clarify this differential and will be less labor-intensive.

TREATMENT

Glucocorticoid

Therapy of primary adrenal insufficiency consists of replacement of cortisol and aldosterone, and, on occasion, supplemental androgen therapy in the female patient. The usual maintenance dosage for glucocorticoid replacement varies from 20 to 37.5 mg of cortisol per day. Various preparations may be used (see Table 208-3 for steroid equivalents). A generally accepted dosage schedule is 5 mg of prednisone in the morning followed by 2.5 mg of prednisone in the afternoon. This simulates the normal diurnal variation of cortisol secretion. A few patients, especially large active men, may require a total daily dose of 10 mg of prednisone for optimum response.

Another treatment alternative is 5 mg of prednisone h.s. or 15 to 20 mg of hydrocortisone on awakening and 5 to 10 mg in the early afternoon. Finally, once a day dosing for prednisone is sufficient.

TABLE 208-3 Steroid Equivalents

Drug	Equivalent Dose, mg	Na^+ Retention
Short-acting		
Cortisone	25	2+
Hydrocortisone (cortisol)	20	2+
Prednisone	5	1+
Prednisolone	5	1+
Methylprednisolone	4	0
Intermediate-acting		
Triamcinolone	4	0
Long-acting		
Dexamethasone	0.75	0
Betamethasone	0.6	0

Mineralocorticoid

Mineralocorticoid replacement in patients with primary adrenal insufficiency can be achieved by administration of the synthetic mineralocorticoid fludrocortisone acetate (Florinef), 0.05 to 0.2 mg/day orally. This dosage should be appropriately reduced in patients in whom hypertension develops. It is also important for the patient with Addison's disease to maintain an adequate dietary salt intake.

Androgen

The woman with primary adrenal insufficiency may show signs of androgen deficiency such as decreased growth of axillary and pubic hair. Supplemental androgen therapy can be achieved with 2 to 5 mg of fluoxymesterone (Halotestin) orally per day.

Secondary Insufficiency

Treatment of secondary adrenal insufficiency differs from that of primary adrenal insufficiency with regard to mineralocorticoid and androgen replacement. Patients with secondary adrenal failure usually do not require mineralocorticoid therapy and can maintain salt and fluid balance with a diet generous in sodium chloride. In the presence of hypotension, however, supplementary fludrocortisone acetate, 0.05 to 0.1 mg/day, is indicated. Evidence of androgen insufficiency may occur with male and female patients with hypopituitarism. Sufficient androgen in the female patient can be achieved with 2 to 5 mg of fluoxymesterone orally per day. Larger dosages of this preparation or long-acting testosterone (Depo-Testosterone) can be used in the male patient. Patients with secondary insufficiency will also require thyroid hormone replacement.

ADRENAL CRISIS

Adrenal crisis is an acute, life-threatening emergency that must be suspected and treated based upon clinical impression. It is due primarily to cortisol insufficiency and to a lesser extent, aldosterone insufficiency, and occurs when the physiologic demand for these hormones exceeds the capacity of the adrenal glands to produce them.

Adrenal reserve may be exhausted in patients with chronic adrenal insufficiency when they are subjected to intercurrent illness or stress. These patients should be taught to respond to minor febrile illness or stress by increasing their glucocorticoid dose by 2 to 3 times the usual dose for a few days during the illness. Mineralocorticoid dose does not need to be changed. During an emergency from severe trauma or stress, dexamethasone 4 mg IM can be self-administered. A variety of conditions may precipitate crisis; these include major or minor infections, trauma, surgery, burns, pregnancy, hypermetabolic states such as hyperthyroidism, and drugs, especially hypnotics or general anesthetics. Adrenal crisis may also occur in patients with chronic adrenal failure if the patient fails to or is unable to take replacement steroid medication. The most common cause of adrenal crisis is abrupt withdrawal of steroids from a patient with iatrogenic adrenal suppression due to prolonged steroid use. Finally, bilateral adrenal gland hemorrhage from fulminant septicemia or other causes can produce adrenal crisis.

Clinical Features

The clinical manifestations of adrenal crisis are due primarily to insufficiency of cortisol and, to a lesser extent, insufficiency of aldosterone. Patients appear acutely ill. They are profoundly weak and may be confused. Hypotension, especially postural hypotension, is usual. Circulatory collapse may be profound. The pulse is feeble and rapid, and heart sounds may be soft. Temperature elevation is common but may be due to underlying infection. Anorexia, nausea, vomiting, and abdominal pain are almost universal. The abdominal pain may be severe, simulating an acute abdomen. Patients in crisis may exhibit increased motor activity which can progress to delirium or seizures.

Laboratory findings vary. The serum sodium level is usually moderately decreased but may be normal. Potassium levels may be normal or slightly increased. Rarely the potassium concentration may be markedly increased, and this can cause cardiac dysrhythmias or hyperkalemic paralysis. Hypoglycemia is characteristic and can be severe.

Treatment

Treatment must be instituted promptly based on clinical impression and should not be delayed for confirmatory testing of adrenal function. Therapeutic measures in treatment of adrenal crisis include replacement of fluids and sodium, administration of glucocorticoid, correction of hypotension and hypoglycemia, reduction of hyperkalemia, and identification and treatment of a precipitating cause of the crisis.

Fluids

A rapid infusion of 5% dextrose and isotonic saline should be started immediately. This acts to correct dehydration, hypotension, hyponatremia, and hypoglycemia. The extracellular volume deficit in the average adult in adrenal crisis is approximately 20 percent, or 3 L. The first liter should be given over 1 h, and 2 or 3 L may be required during the first 8 h of therapy. The functional capacity of the cardiovascular system is reduced with adrenal insufficiency, and the usual precautions with the rapid administration of saline should be observed.

Steroids

A water-soluble glucocorticoid should be administered promptly. As soon as the diagnosis of adrenal crisis is entertained, 100 mg of hydrocortisone sodium succinate (Solu-Cortef) or phosphate should be given in an intravenous bolus. In addition, 100 mg of hydrocortisone should be added to the intravenous solution. Usually, 200 mg of hydrocortisone is given every 6 h during the first 24 h of therapy. Glucocorticoid therapy acts to correct hypotension, hyponatremia, hyperkalemia, and hypoglycemia.

Mineralcorticoid therapy is not required during initial treatment of adrenal crisis. High dosages of hydrocortisone provide sufficient mineralocorticoid effect. As the total dosage of glucocorticoid is reduced below 100 mg/24 h, many patients need supplementary mineralocorticoid, which can be provided as desoxycorticosterone acetate (Percorten), 2.5 to 5.0 mg intramuscularly one or twice daily. If hypotension persists despite adequate volume and corticosteroid replacement, additional corticosteroid can be given and other causes of hypotension should be investigated. Vasopressors may be needed to correct hypotension. Adrenal hemorrhage should be considered, especially if the patient is receiving anticoagulants.

Simultaneous Treatment and Testing

It is possible to treat adrenal crisis and to perform simultaneous, confirmatory diagnostic testing for adrenal insufficiency. Physiologic saline is administered, but instead of hydrocortisone, 4 mg of dexamethasone is added to the infusion. Additionally, 25 units of corticotropin is added to the solution, and this liter is infused in the first hour. Blood for plasma cortisol assay is obtained before and at the completion of the infusion. A 24-h urine collection for measurement of 17-hydroxycorticosteroid (17-OHCS) is collected. Additional corticotropin is added to subsequent intravenous solutions so that at least 3 units is infused each hour for 8 h. A third blood specimen for cortisol assay is obtained between the sixth and eighth hours of intravenous therapy.

If the patient has primary adrenal insufficiency, all plasma cortisol levels are low (<15 μg/dL), and the urinary 17-OHCS is also low, confirming the inability of the adrenals to respond to ACTH stimulation. An adequate rise in the plasma cortisol level excludes the diagnosis of adrenal insufficiency. A response indicative of partially intact adrenocortical reserve excludes the diagnosis of primary adrenal failure in favor of secondary adrenal insufficiency, but further testing is required to confirm this diagnosis. Other methods for simultaneous diagnosis and treatment have been described.

The adrenal crisis should begin to resolve favorably within a few hours after initiation of appropriate therapy. Intensive treatment and monitoring should continue for 24 to 48 h. Once the patient's condition has stabilized, the transition to an oral maintenance program can begin. Usually, 7 to 10 days are required for this transition.

The main causes of death during adrenal crisis are circulatory collapse and hyperkalemia-induced dysrhythmias. Hypoglycemia may contribute to demise in some cases. With prompt recognition and appropriate treatment, most patients in adrenal crisis should do well.

BIBLIOGRAPHY

DeGroot LJ (ed): *Endocrinology,* 3d ed. Philadelphia, Saunders, 1994.
James VHT (ed): *The Adrenal Gland,* 2d ed. New York, Raven Press, 1992.

209 DIABETES MELLITUS

Micheal D. Rush
Sonia Winslett
Kimberley Dawn Wisdom

Diabetes mellitus is a group of metabolic diseases characterized by deficiency of insulin production, deficiency of insulin action, or a combination of the two deficiencies resulting in hyperglycemia. Chronic hyperglycemia is a final common pathway leading to long-term complications involving the eye, the nervous system, the kidneys, and the immune system that collectively can be grouped as microvascular complications. These complications are leading causes of blindness, chronic renal failure, and lower extremity amputation. Diabetes mellitus also predisposes individuals to accelerated atherogenesis, and the resultant hypertension leads to macrovascular complications of atherosclerotic cardiovascular, cerebrovascular, and peripheral vascular disease. Emergency physicians are frequently called on to evaluate and treat the complications of diabetes, and may in some cases make the initial diagnosis of diabetes. Early diagnosis and treatment are essential in preventing long-term complications of the disease.

This chapter focuses on the classification, epidemiology, pathophysiology, clinical features, and diagnosis of diabetes; management of acute hyperglycemia; and indications for hospital admission. This chapter also presents overviews on therapy for chronic hyperglycemia and the diagnosis and management of the microvascular complications of diabetes. Chapters on common diabetic emergencies, such as diabetic ketoacidosis (DKA), hyperosmolar nonketotic coma [newer terminology: hyperglycemic, hyperosmolar, nonketotic syndrome (HHNS)], and hypoglycemia, as well as individual chapters on stroke, myocardial ischemia and infarction, and peripheral vascular disease, common macrovascular complications of diabetes, are presented elsewhere in this text.

CLASSIFICATION

Diabetes can be grouped into four major categories (Table 209-1).[1] *Type 1 diabetes* [older terminology: insulin-dependent diabetes mellitus (IDDM) or juvenile-onset diabetes mellitus (JODM)] is characterized by an absolute deficiency of insulin secretion. The disease is believed to be primarily autoimmune in nature with a genetic predispo-

TABLE 209-1 Etiologic Classification of Diabetes Mellitus

Type 1 diabetes* (β-cell destruction, usually leading to absolute insulin deficiency)
- Immune mediated
- Idiopathic

Type 2 diabetes* (may range from predominantly insulin resistance with relative insulin deficiency to a predominantly secretory defect with insulin resistance)

Secondary Causes of Diabetes
- Genetic defects of B-cell function
  - Chromosome 12, HNF-1α (formerly MODY3)
  - Chromosome 7, glucokinase (formerly MODY2)
  - Chromosome 20, HNF-4α (formerly MODY1)
  - Mitochondrial DNA
- Genetic defects in insulin action
  - Type A insulin resistance
  - Leprechaunism
  - Rabson-Mendenhall syndrome
  - Lipoatrophic diabetes
- Diseases of the exocrine pancreas
  - Pancreatitis
  - Trauma/pancreatectomy
  - Neoplasia
  - Cystic fibrosis
  - Hemochromatosis
  - Fibrocalculous pancreatopathy
- Endocrinopathies
  - Acromegaly
  - Cushing's syndrome
  - Glucagonoma
  - Pheochromocytoma
  - Hyperthyroidism
  - Somatostatinoma
  - Aldosteronoma
- Drug or chemical induced
  - Vacor
  - Pentamidine
  - Nicotinic acid
  - Glucocorticoids
  - Thyroid hormone
  - Diazoxide
  - β-Adrenergic agonists
  - Thiazides
  - Dilantin
  - Interferon α
- Infections
  - Congenital rubella
  - Cytomegalovirus
- Uncommon forms of immune-mediated diabetes
  - "Stiff-man" syndrome
  - Anti-insulin receptor antibodies
- Other genetic syndromes sometimes associated with diabetes
  - Down's syndrome
  - Klinefelter's syndrome
  - Turner's syndrome
  - Wolfram syndrome
  - Friedreich's ataxia
  - Huntington's chorea
  - Laurence-Moon-Biedl syndrome
  - Myotonic dystrophy
  - Porphyria
  - Prader-Willi syndrome

Gestational diabetes mellitus

*Patients with any form of diabetes may require insulin treatment at some stage of their disease. Such use of insulin does not, of itself, classify the patient.
Source: Reproduced from the Expert Committee on the Diagnosis and Classification of Diabetes Mellitus,[1] with permission.

sition and a possible link with viral infections or other environmental factors (such as absence of breast-feeding, diet, and factors related to low socioeconomic status) as possible triggers. Individuals with type 1 diabetes require insulin therapy to sustain life and are prone to DKA.

Type 2 diabetes [older terminology: non-insulin-dependent diabetes mellitus (NIDDM) or adult-onset diabetes mellitus (AODM)] represents a combination of resistance to the action of insulin by the target organs and tissues with a relative inadequacy of compensatory insulin secretion. Type 2 diabetes is also believed to have a strong genetic predisposition, although it is clear that lifestyle issues such as diet and exercise can impact the development and severity of the disease. Patients with type 2 diabetes can have a variety of initial presentations ranging from life-threatening HHNS, or complications related to hyperglycemia alone, for years prior to having clinical symptoms of diabetes. Type 2 diabetics often require insulin at some point in their course for adequate glycemic control. The likelihood of insulin requirement increases with duration of disease, with 22 percent needing insulin in the first 4 years to about 60 percent after 20 years.

The third group represents *secondary* causes for diabetes. Collectively, patients with secondary diabetes represent only about 1 percent of all diabetes cases. The fourth group, *gestational diabetes mellitus* (GDM), is present only during pregnancy, and complicates about 4 percent of pregnancies in the United States annually (or about 135,000 cases). Excellent glycemic control is essential in preventing fetal cardiac and central nervous system abnormalities, as well as fetal macrosomia.[1]

EPIDEMIOLOGY

It is estimated that 100 million people worldwide have diabetes, with 85 percent of cases being type 2. It is projected that by the year 2010 this number will increase to 215 million. In most developed countries, diabetes is one of the five leading causes of death.[2]

From 1990 to 1992 data, according to the National Health Information Survey (NHIS), approximately 7.8 million Americans, or 3.1 percent of the total US population, had been diagnosed with diabetes mellitus, with the majority, more than 90 percent of cases, classified as type 2 (NIDDM). The prevalence of diabetes in the United States is increasing over time—from 0.37 percent in 1935 to 0.91 percent in 1960 to 3.1 percent in 1993. Approximately 625,000 new cases of diabetes of all types were diagnosed each year in the United States from 1990 to 1992, or 2.42 cases per thousand of population, with more than 90 percent of cases diagnosed as type 2 diabetes. This incidence rate has been stable over the last 20 years. The increased prevalence is accounted for by an increase in the population older than age 65, the group with highest diabetes prevalence.[3]

Incidence rates for type 1 diabetes worldwide range from less than 1 per thousand population in Shanghai, China, Mexico City, Mexico, and the Republic of Korea to a high of 35 per thousand population in Finland. Scandinavian countries tend to have much higher incidence rates for type 1 diabetes, whereas Asian countries tend to have much lower incidence rates. The incidence for type 1 diabetes is about 30,000 new cases diagnosed each year. It is reasonable to assume that Americans with ancestry in these ethnic groups would exhibit a similar epidemiologic trend.[4]

For type 1 diabetes in the United States, the prevalence is slightly higher among men than women, whereas the prevalence among type 2 diabetes is roughly equal between men and women. For type 1 diabetes, non-Hispanic whites are most commonly affected, followed by African Americans and Hispanic Americans. Type 2 diabetes is more common among African Americans, Mexican Americans, Japanese Americans, and Native Americans than among non-Hispanic whites.

In 1986, type 2 diabetes was estimated to account for 17.2 percent of all deaths in the United States, ranging from 1 percent in the 25 to 44-year age bracket to 13.7 percent among those aged 75 years or older. Among the total diabetic population aged 25 years or older, diabetes accounted for 5.4 percent of all deaths. Approximately 40 percent of deaths are due to ischemic cardiovascular disease. Generally, a middle-aged person with type 2 diabetes can expect 5 to 10 years of decreased life expectancy because of the disease. African Americans, Hispanics, and Native Americans are more likely to die of diabetes than are non-Hispanic whites. Individuals with type 1 diabetes are twice as likely to have diabetes listed as their underlying cause of death than are type 2 diabetics. Among type 1 diabetics, 15 percent will die before age 40, which is 20 times as likely as a person of similar age in the general population. DKA and coma are the most common causes of death in the early years of type 1 diabetes. Renal disease becomes the most common up to age 30, and cardiovascular disease is the most common after age 30. Although diabetes is listed relatively infrequently as the primary cause of death, diabetes ranks seventh in the leading underlying causes of death in the United States.[5,6]

RISK FACTORS

Type 1 Diabetes

Genetic and immunologic risk factors for type 1 diabetes include having a parent with type 1 disease, especially the father (three times more likely than if the mother has type 1). Certain HLA antigens (HLA-DR3 and HLA-DR4) located on chromosome 6 are present in 95 percent of type 1 diabetics. Type 1 diabetics also have a higher prevalence of islet cell cytoplasmic antibodies (ICAs), antibodies to insulin, and antibodies to the enzyme glutamic acid decarboxylase (GAD). Since concordance of type 1 diabetes occurs in only about 36 percent of monozygous twins, environmental factors must also play a role in the development of type 1 disease.

Dietary factors—such as breast-feeding for less than 3 months or not breast-feeding at all; exposure to cow's milk proteins, casein, and bovine serum albumin at age younger than 3 months; and exposure to food additives such as nitrates and nitrosamines—have also been associated with increased risk for development of type 1 diabetes.

Viral infections, especially Coxsackie B group, are strongly associated with type 1 disease, because these viruses are routinely isolated from the sera of patients newly diagnosed with type 1 disease. Other viral infections with possible epidemiologic associations with type 1 diabetes include congenital rubella, cytomegalovirus (CMV), and mumps.

Older maternal age, birth order, and lower socioeconomic status may also contribute to development of type 1 diabetes, but the results of studies are conflicting.

Type 2 Diabetes

Twin studies in type 2 diabetes establish a strong genetic link to development of the disease, with concordance rates of 34 to 100 percent for monozygous twins. Several candidate genes and defects in these genes are being studied as being associated with the development of type 2 disease. As previously noted, either background is associated with type 2 disease. Persons having a history of impaired fasting glucose (IFG) or impaired glucose tolerance (IGT) constitute a high-risk group for developing diabetes. Women with a history of gestational diabetes are much more likely to develop type 2 diabetes. Hypertension and hypertriglyceridemia are also risk factors for the development of diabetes.

Environmental risk factors for type 2 diabetes include a high-fat diet, increased alcohol intake, sedentary lifestyle, and obesity; particularly, increased abdominal girth, low birth weight, and lower socioeconomic status.[7,8]

PATHOPHYSIOLOGY

Type 1 diabetes results from destruction of insulin producing pancreatic β cells and absolute insulin deficiency. Type 2 diabetes begins with insulin resistance and increased insulin production.

The organs and tissues that are most affected by diabetes—the retina, the kidney, and the nerves—all readily take up glucose, leading to its intracellular accumulation and subsequent metabolic end products. Two major mechanisms leading to microvascular complications from hyperglycemia are the increased formation and accumulation of sorbitol and other polyols via the aldose reductase pathway and the formation of advanced glycosylation end products (AGEs) due to reactions of excess glucose with various cellular proteins.

Sorbitol formed from glucose through the aldose reductase pathway competitively inhibits *myo*-inositol formation, which causes a decrease in uptake of phosphoinositides into cell membranes, which subsequently decreases Na^+K^+-ATPase activity, with the ultimate clinical effect being slowed nerve conduction. This decrease in the synthesis of *myo*-inositol may be the common metabolic link to membrane damage in neuropathy, retinopathy, and nephropathy. Clinical trials with aldose reductase inhibitors in the prevention and treatment of microvascular complications of diabetes are ongoing.

Glycosylation and the subsequent formation of AGEs is another major explanation for diabetic microvascular pathology. Chemical crosslinks form between excess glucose and various cellular proteins, altering their structure and function; most notable of these is glycosylated hemoglobin ($HgbA_{1c}$), which forms proportional to glucose concentrations in the blood over time and is now used as a measure of glucose control in diabetes therapy. AGEs are thought to play a role in diabetic microvascular complications via effects on the structure and function of extracellular matrix and its interaction with the cell. An example of this is AGE formation on collagen, which, by trapping low-density lipoproteins, may be the etiology of accelerated atherogenesis seen in diabetes clinically.[9] A second potential mechanism for the pathogenesis of AGE formation from hyperglycemia is via action on AGE-specific receptors, which alters levels of various hormones and cytokines, such as nitric oxide, ultimately leading to vascular proliferation and decreased elasticity in existing vessels. Intracellularly, AGE formation on DNA molecules leads to subsequent mutations and other harmful effects on gene expression in mammalian cell cultures in vitro. Ongoing clinical trials using aminoguanidine, an inhibitor of AGE formation, show promise in the prevention and treatment of microvascular complications of diabetes.

Accelerated atherogenesis in diabetes is multifactorial and is related to microalbuminuria, insulin resistance, formation of AGE, modification/oxidation of lipoproteins, and endothelial injury (Table 209-2).

CLINICAL FEATURES

Type 1 diabetes nearly always presents as DKA, often associated with an acute infection or other significant physiologic stress, in adolescents or in young adults. Type 2 diabetes can be present for years prior to the onset of clinical symptoms. It may present suddenly with HHNS.

TABLE 209-2 Classification of Diabetic Vascular Disease

Type	Findings	Location
Nonspecific	Atherosclerosis	Large vessels of extremities, heart, and brain
Specific	Microangiopathic or endothelial proliferative changes of arterioles	Basement membranes of small vessels, i.e., retina, renal glomeruli, brain, and myocardium

Frequently, type 2 diabetes is only diagnosed concurrently with the initial presentation of a macrovascular or microvascular complication of the disease.

Classic diabetes signs and symptoms include polyuria, polydipsia, fatigue, polyphagia, unexplained weight loss, poor wound healing, blurred vision, and a higher prevalence of certain infections, especially candidal vaginitis and balanitis, recurrent skin and skin structure infections, and malignant otitis externa. The presence of any of these symptoms or infections should lead an emergency clinician to check the patient's blood glucose level.

Documentation of the medical history of diabetic patients in the emergency department should be complaint directed but generally should also include questions on access to and frequency of home blood glucose monitoring, frequency and causes, if known, of recent hyperglycemia or hypoglycemia, recent glycosylated hemoglobin ($HgbA_{1c}$) values, presence of and therapy for microvascular and macrovascular complications of diabetes, recent adjustments by the patient or the patient's physician in their glycemic control regimen, any problems with adherence to therapy, and symptomatology suggestive of complications. Symptoms suggestive of potential complications or poor glucose control include visual changes, neurologic symptoms (especially numbness, dizziness, and weakness), chest pain, gastrointestinal symptoms, and genitourinary symptoms (especially overflow incontinence, changes in amount of urine, and sexual dysfunction). A thorough history of any recent or concurrent chronic medical illness, injury, or infection should be obtained. Current medications, diet and exercise history, and social history are also important components of the evaluation of diabetic patients. Medications such as diuretics or β blockers may affect glycemic control. Socioeconomic issues may be present, such as living conditions or the inability to afford home blood glucose monitoring or medications. Symptoms of depression and social history factors, including alcohol, tobacco, or illicit drug use, should be considered. Finally, diabetic patients should be fed according to schedule and they should receive their diabetic medication while being evaluated in the emergency department.

The physical examination of diabetics should be tailored to the patient's chief complaint. However, it should generally include blood pressure measurement, funduscopy (to look for hemorrhage or proliferative retinopathy), cardiovascular exam (including ausculation of the carotids and abdomen for bruits and assessment of peripheral pulses), extremity exam (especially the feet, for signs of skin breakdown and vascular disease), skin exam (including intertriginous areas, to assess for irritations and infections, especially around peripheral insulin injection sites and in the hands, assessing lancet puncture sites), and a neurologic exam (to screen for neuropathy). In children, measurements of height, weight, and sexual maturity should be obtained and compared with normals for age.[10]

DIAGNOSIS

The diagnostic criteria for diabetes have recently been revised, lowering the serum glucose values at which the diagnosis can be made, and include an intermediate category for patients whose glucose levels do not meet criteria for diagnosis of diabetes but are significantly abnormal. These changes reflect advances in knowledge of what levels constitute abnormality significant enough to produce the complications of diabetes. Replacing the old term of "borderline" diabetes are IFG ($\geq$110 to <126 mg/dL) and IGT, which constitute a group of patients who are generally euglycemic in everyday life but manifest hyperglycemia on oral glucose tolerance tests (>126 but <200 mg/dL) 2 h after an oral 75-g glucose load. In nonpregnant patients, these categories are not diagnostic entities in themselves but represent a group of patients at high risk of developing diabetes. An additional 12 million to 14 million Americans are thought to be glucose intolerant.

Diabetes can be diagnosed in three ways. Two of these may be feasible for emergency department physicians (Table 209-3). The criteria are based on symptoms of diabetes and a random or nonfasting plasma glucose level of 200 mg/dL or more, fasting plasma glucose level (no caloric intake for at least 8 h) of 126 mg/dL or more, or a 2-h post-75-g oral glucose challenge plasma glucose level of 200 mg/dL or more. Unless a patient is showing unequivocal hyperglycemia (300 mg/dL or more in the setting of acute metabolic decompensation such as DKA or HHNS), these values should be reproducible on at least one separate occasion to confirm the diagnosis.[1]

TABLE 209-3 Criteria for the Diagnosis of Diabetes Mellitus

Symptoms of diabetes plus casual plasma glucose concentration $\geq$ 200 mg/dL (11.1 mmol/L). Casual is defined as any time of day without regard to time since last meal. The classic symptoms of diabetes include polyuria, polydipsia, and unexplained weight loss. *or*
FPG $\geq$ 126 mg/dL (7.0 mmol/L). Fasting is defined as no caloric intake for at least 8 h. *or*
2hPG $\geq$ 200 mg/dL during an OGTT. The test should be performed as described by the World Health Organization,[2] using a glucose load containing the equivalent of 75-g anhydrous glucose dissolved in water.
In the absence of unequivocal hyperglycemia with acute metabolic decompensation, these criteria should be confirmed by repeat testing on a different day. The third measure (OGTT) is not recommended for routine clinical use.

Abbreviations: FPG, fasting plasma glucose level; 2hPG, 2 hr plasma glucose level; OGTT, oral glucose tolerance test.
Source: Reproduced from the Expert Committee on the Diagnosis and Classification of Diabetes Mellitus,[1] with permission.

THERAPY

Therapy for diabetes can best be divided into acute therapy of severe hyperglycemia and life-threatening metabolic decompensation and the day-to-day prevention of hyperglycemia through insulin or oral hypoglycemic agent therapy.

DKA and HHNS are the acute life-threatening entities involving metabolic decompensation, with primarily type 1 diabetics in the case of DKA and type 2 diabetics with HHNS. Some overlap of DKA and HHNS can be seen in either type of diabetes. Acute hyperglycemia and chronic hyperglycemia represent intermediates between good glycemic control and the development of life-threatening metabolic decompensation as well as macrovascular and microvascular complications of diabetes. DKA and HHNS are discussed elsewhere in this book (Chaps. 203 and 205, respectively).

ACUTE HYPERGLYCEMIA

Acute hyperglycemia, defined as a blood glucose level of greater than 300 mg/dL, can represent impending metabolic decompensation. High glucose levels, if present chronically, represent high risk for development of both macrovascular and microvascular complications of diabetes. Acute hyperglycemia should be treated aggressively in terms of seeking out and treating precipitating causes as well as correcting the glucose and other associated electrolyte abnormalities.

Clinical Features

Noncompliance with insulin or oral hypoglycemic therapeutic regimen should be a diagnosis of exclusion in patients with known diabetes. The history and physical examination should focus on finding an underlying cause for the hyperglycemia and include a thorough medication history to ascertain the potential contributions of glucose-altering medications, most commonly corticosteroids, sympathomimetics, diuretics, anticonvulsants, salicylates, and β-adrenergic receptor agonists or antagonists. A thorough evaluation for infections is indicated, with pneumonia, urinary tract, and foot/skin structure infections being most commonly associated with acute disturbances in glucose metabolism. Acute coronary or central nervous system ischemia is also a common cause of acute hyperglycemia. Finally, changes in or noncompliance with insulin or oral hypoglycemic therapy may be the etiology for the hyperglycemia.

Symptomatically, younger adults may have only polyuria and/or polydipsia as symptoms, whereas elderly diabetics may be severely volume depleted, with acute mental status changes, hypovolemic shock, and acute renal insufficiency or failure.

Determination of serum electrolyte, blood urea nitrogen, and serum creatinine levels is indicated in the clinical assessment of acute hyperglycemia. Clinicians experienced in acid-base interpretation should be able to diagnose abnormalities based on venous electrolyte levels only, using respiratory rate and pulse oximetry to guide the rare need for ABG determination. Capillary blood glucose measurement is indicated every 1 to 2 h during therapy, with the caveat that capillary blood glucose (glucometer) determination may be inaccurate at low (less than 30 mg/dL) or high (more than 400 mg/dL) levels and may even be incorrect within this range. Coefficients of analytic variation within glucometer systems have been found to range from 4 to 33 percent. Ideally, analytic and user error would be no more than 10 percent.[11] Serum osmolality can be estimated from readily available blood chemistries by using the formula

$$\text{OSM} - 2 \times [\text{Na}^{+}] + \frac{\text{glu}}{18} + \frac{\text{BUN}}{2.8}$$

Diagnosis of Underlying Causes

New-onset diabetes should be a diagnosis of exclusion as a cause of acute hyperglycemia. In the presence of a previously established diagnosis of diabetes, poor compliance may be a factor, particularly among youth but, again, it should be reserved as an etiology of exclusion for the adult presentation. A thorough history documentation and physical examination should guide the evaluation and, based on history or clinical findings, might include electrocardiogram and determination of the levels of cardiac enzymes, such as CK-MB and troponin I or T, to rule out ischemic heart disease or myocardial infarction; complete neurologic exam and computed axial tomography (CAT) of the head to exclude cerebral vascular accident; chest radiograph to assess for pneumonia; and urinalysis to rule out infection or rhabdomyolysis. Cellular and skin abscess should be sought. In sexually active females, the pelvis should be examined to rule out cervicitis or pelvic inflammatory disease as an occult precipitating factor.

Therapy

Therapy for simple acute hyperglycemia is similar to that for DKA and HHNS and includes volume repletion, intravenous (IV) regular insulin therapy, correction of electrolyte imbalance, and specific therapies directed toward any identified underlying cause of hyperglycemia.

The cornerstone of therapy for acute hyperglycemia is restoration of intravascular volume and reperfusion of vital organs, especially the kidneys. Infusion of normal saline (NS) 0.9% NaCl solution at a rate of 500 to 1000 mL/h should be initiated as soon as possible unless specific entities such as myocardial infarction with cardiogenic shock, acute renal failure, or stroke with cerebral edema contraindicate aggressive volume resuscitation. The use of two IV lines, 18 gauge or larger, are advisable to facilitate fluid resuscitation and correction of electrolyte imbalance. Aggressive volume resuscitation should be geared to the end point of lowering the serum glucose, restoring organ perfusion, and replacing extracellular volume depletion. Use caution with aggressive volume resuscitation in patients with a history of congestive heart failure or chronic renal insufficiency and reassess for further therapy frequently (approximately every hour or every 500 mL of IV fluid). Once improvement is noted in vital signs, hyperglycemia (200 mg/dL or less), and adequate urine output ensured, IV fluids may be reduced to maintenance levels or discontinued if the patient is taking oral fluids well.

Depending on the assessment of the degree of extracellular volume depletion, insulin therapy should generally be accomplished with regular human insulin intravenously since absorption of subcutaneous insulin in a volume-depleted patient can be erratic and unpredictable. Typically, an initial bolus of 0.1 U/kg IV regular human insulin is given, which may be repeated in 1 to 2 h. While the addition of a bolus priming dose of insulin may speed the onset of ketone body metabolism, no advantage in the outcome of patients with DKA has been demonstrated. Thus, a patient may simply be started on a regular insulin infusion of 0.1 U/kg ideal body weight per hour, with hourly capillary blood glucose monitoring to assess therapy. The blood glucose level will generally decrease much more rapidly in patients with type 2 diabetes than in those with type 1. If a patient is judged not to have clinical evidence of extracellular volume depletion, subcutaneous insulin administration at a 0.1 U regular insulin per kilogram dose is also acceptable. Once the capillary blood glucose level reaches 250 mg/dL or less, with resolution of symptoms and effective treatment of any underlying cause for hyperglycemia, patients are at low risk for acute metabolic decompensation.

The most prominent and generally most clinically significant electrolyte disorder in acute hyperglycemia is hypokalemia. There is frequently a total body deficit of potassium secondary to severe extracellular volume loss. A mild metabolic acidosis and hyperosmolar state may lead to nearly normal serum potassium levels initially. However, potassium replacement should remain a priority as soon as the potassium level is at or below 5.5 meq/L if renal function is assured. Potassium levels of less than 3.0 meq/L represent severe deficit and mandate emergent supplementation to prevent lethal dysrhythmias. This can be accomplished by adding 20 to 40 meq potassium chloride (KCl) per liter to the IV infusion. Potassium can also be replaced orally with multiple doses of 20 meq KCl. Phosphate therapy is not without complications and there is no indication for routine phosphate supplementation in the treatment of acute hyperglycemia, DKA, or HHNS. Patients with hyperglycemia refractory to therapy, severe electrolyte disturbance, significant prerenal azotemia or increase in baseline blood urea nitrogen and creatinine, or with serious underlying cause, should be admitted to the hospital for further workup and therapy.[12]

CHRONIC THERAPY FOR HYPERGLYCEMIA

The general guiding principal of diabetes therapy is to lower glucose levels on a consistent basis to normal or near normal. Keeping glucose levels at or near normal in type 1 diabetics ($\text{HgbA}_{1c} \leq 7.0$ percent; normal, 4.0 to 6.0 percent) through intensive insulin therapy as practiced in the Diabetes Control and Complications Trial (DCCT) dramatically reduces the risk of developing both the microvascular and the macrovascular complications of diabetes.[13]

Several preliminary studies affirm the association of good glycemic control with fewer complications in type 2 diabetes. However, more study is needed to define the population of type 2 patients that will receive the most benefit, given the increased risk of hypoglycemia involved with intensive insulin therapy.[14]

Intensive insulin therapy (2 h postprandial and an occasional middle of the night check) is indicated for well-motivated patients who administer multiple daily injections, and who can adjust doses and caloric intake appropriately. Target glucose values for therapy should be tailored to the individual. However, generally the goal is to keep blood

TABLE 209-4 Pharmacology of Commonly Available Insulin Preparations

Insulin	Onset (h)	Peak (h)	Duration (h)
Lispro	$\frac{1}{4}$–$\frac{1}{2}$	$\frac{1}{2}$–$1\frac{1}{2}$	2–4
Regular	$\frac{1}{2}$–1	2–4	5–7
NPH	1–2	6–14	24+
Lente	1–3	6–14	24+
Ultralente	6	18–24	36+

Source: Adapted from Koda-Kimble and Carlisle,[15] with permission.

glucose at 140 mg/dL or less in intensive-therapy candidates and 180 to 200 mg/dL or less in diabetics who do not meet criteria for intensive therapy. Target $HgbA_{1c}$ of 7.0 percent or less in intensive-therapy patients and 8.0 percent or less in non-intensive-therapy patients is a reasonable goal to prevent, delay the onset of, and delay progression of complications. Intensive therapy is generally not indicated for patients with autonomic insufficiency, adrenal or pituitary insufficiency, atherosclerotic coronary or cerebrovascular disease; for patients taking β-blocker medication; for patients with counterregulatory hormone deficiency; for the elderly or small children; for patients with psychiatric disorders; and for unreliable, chronically noncompliant patients.

Euglycemia reduces the chance of developing DKA or HHNS. Lowering blood glucose reduces the clinical signs and symptoms of diabetes, such as polyuria, polydipsia, blurred vision, weight loss, and poor wound healing. Consistently near-normal glucose values reduce the risk of microvascular complications of diabetes (specifically, neuropathy, retinopathy, and nephropathy). Excellent glycemic control is also associated with a more favorable and less atherogenic lipid profile, leading to fewer macrovascular complications.

Glycemic control in type 1 diabetes is accomplished primarily with multiple daily insulin injections, whereas glycemic control in type 2 patients is staged. Stage 1 is diet modification and weight reduction. Stage 2 includes oral hypoglycemics. Stage 3 represents insulin requirement, alone or in addition to oral hypoglycemic agents. Table 209-4 presents the various forms of insulin commonly prescribed, time to onset of action, time to peak effect, and their durations of action when given subcutaneously.[15] Insulin preparations available today are extremely pure and represent genetically engineered forms of human insulin produced by bacteria or yeast. Immunogenicity is rare. Table 209-5 presents frequently prescribed oral hypoglycemic agents with their usual dose, half-life, and duration of activity. Caution should be used in prescribing these agents to the elderly or to patients with impaired renal or hepatic function due to serious complications of hypoglycemia. Once the symptoms of acute hyperglycemia are controlled, and underlying causes or exacerbating factors are sought out and treated, initiation of oral hypoglycemic and/or insulin therapy in new-onset type 2 diabetics can usually be left to the primary care provider at 24 to 48-h follow-up if admission was not warranted. Finding new-onset type 1 diabetes in the absence of serious precipitating illness or metabolic disorder is rare. An excellent review on initiating insulin and/or oral hypoglycemic therapy is presented in *Applied Therapeutics: The Clinical Use of Drugs,* 6th edition.[15]

Insulin can also be administered as a continuous subcutaneous insulin infusion (CSII), by means of a small pump that delivers insulin subcutaneously into the abdominal wall through a butterfly needle. Insulin is usually infused at a continuous basal rate with preprogrammed boluses just before meals. Both hypoglycemia and ketoacidosis are more frequent in patients with CSII. For emergency department patients with CSII who develop hypoglycemia, marked hyperglycemia, or DKA, it is best to shut off the pump in the emergency department while standard glucose or insulin therapy is administered.

A working knowledge of the pharmacology, including time to peak effect and duration of action of the various insulin and oral hypoglycemic preparations, should enable the emergency physician to make adjustments in a patient's usual insulin or oral hypoglycemic regimen, especially if the patient arrives with a home blood glucose diary. It is a good general rule not to change the total number of units of insulin by more than a 10 percent increase or decrease in a single day. Adjustment of oral agent dosage can generally be left to the primary care provider because it requires careful and close monitoring. If that option is not readily available, oral hypoglycemic agent dosing should generally not exceed a 20 percent increase or decrease. If the patient is not doing regular home glucose monitoring, be sure that he or she has the equipment and the knowledge to test regularly during

TABLE 209-5 Pharmacology of Commonly Available Oral Hypoglycemic Agents

Drug	Dosing Range (Min–Max Daily Dose)/Div of Dose	Half-Life (h)	Duration (h)
Sulfonylureas			
1st Generation			
Acetohexamide	0.25–1.5 g qd or bid	6	12–18
Chlorpropamide	0.1–0.5 g qd	35+	24–72
Toluzamide	0.2–1.0 g qd or bid	7	12–14
Tolbutamide	0.5–3.0 g bid or tid	7	6–12
2nd Generation			
Glipizide	2.5–40 mg qd or bid	3	12–24
Glipizide extended release	5–20 mg qd	4–13	24
Glyburide	1.25–20 mg qd or bid	4–13	12–24
Micronized glyburide	1.0–12 mg qd	4	24
Insulin resistance			
Reduction agent			
Troqlitazone	200–600 mg qd		16–34
Biquanides			
Metformin	0.5–2.5 g bid or tid	3	6–12

Note: These drugs should be used with great caution, if at all, in the treatment of patients with hepatic and renal insufficiency.
Source: Adapted from Koda-Kimble et al,[15] with permission.

the adjustment period to avoid severe hypoglycemia or hyperglycemia. When the availability of a primary physician is in question, some emergency departments are able to send a home health nurse to the patient's home for teaching and assessment.

A good home blood glucose-testing regimen is to take measurements prior to meals and at bedtime. Less than four home-monitored glucose values per day has been associated with poor glycemic control.[11] The "intensive therapy" was described earlier.

An alternate rotating testing regimen of taking measurements (before breakfast, 3 days; before lunch, 3 days; before the evening meal, 3 days; and before bedtime, 3 days) decreases the number of fingersticks per day. It is less useful, however, when adjusting insulin or oral agent dosages, but may increase compliance. If a patient is unwilling or unable to test his or her blood glucose regularly during an adjustment and is not at high risk for metabolic decompensation, any adjustment of regimen and further education should be left to a primary care provider or endocrinologist.

COMPLICATIONS OF DIABETES MELLITUS

Cardiovascular Complications

The heart is a major target organ for insulin, and marked changes in cardiac function occur in patients with diabetes mellitus.[16] Whether type 1 or type 2, coronary artery disease accounts for more than half of deaths in diabetics.[16] Factors contributing to the diabetic cardiac dysfunction are increased incidence of atherosclerosis of the coronary arteries, autonomic neuropathy, and microvascular disease (associated with hypertension and renal disease). Diabetics are prone to "silent" myocardial infarction, or infarction associated with atypical symptoms, such as weakness. Even in the absence of vascular disease and hypertension, some diabetics develop cardiomegaly, with systolic and diastolic ventricular dysfunction that may evolve into congestive heart failure.[17] Diabetic cardiomyopathy may be a direct effect of insulin deficiency or resistance on myocardial cell function. The detrimental effects of diabetes mellitus on the heart are more prominent in young diabetics and women.[17] Women usually have a lower risk of coronary artery disease but diabetes renders them more vulnerable to reinfarction and death after myocardial infarction and congestive heart failure. Vascular disease in diabetics may be either nonspecific (atherosclerosis of large vessels) or specific (microangiopathic disease in small vessels) for diabetes.

Most standard emergency department treatments for hypertension and cardiac disease can be utilized in diabetics with appropriate precautions. Moderate to severely elevated glucose levels should be decreased by utilizing small intravenous doses of regular insulin, but the glucose level should not be tightly controlled; the patient is undergoing a stressful event and the added stress and consequences of hypoglycemia should be avoided. There is a risk for intraocular bleed from thrombolytic administration to a diabetic with proliferative retinopathy. Even though the risk of intraocular bleed is low, *proliferative retinopathy is an absolute contraindication to thrombolytic therapy*. The challenge to the emergency physician is expedient evaluation for proliferative retinopathy while simultaneously evaluating the need for thrombolytics.

Retinopathy

Diabetic retinopathy is the leading cause in new cases of blindness in patients aged 25 to 74 in the United States. Patients with this complication are 29 times more likely to become blind than those without retinopathy. Glaucoma and cataracts, also more common in diabetics, can contribute to new cases of blindness in diabetic patients. Blindness due to diabetes is estimated to account for more than 500 million dollars in lost income and public expense annually. An estimated 97 percent of diabetics taking insulin (types 1 and 2), and 80 percent of diabetics who do not take insulin (type 2 only) who have had their diabetes for 15 years or longer have some diabetic retinopathy. Among those with this complication, 40 percent of insulin-using and 5 percent of non-insulin-using diabetics have the most severe form—proliferative retinopathy—that frequently leads to blindness.[18] In the DCCT, type 1 patients who had no retinopathy at baseline had their risk of developing sustained retinopathy lowered by 76 percent over patients who did not practice intensive glucose control. In those patients with mild retinopathy at the start of the study, intensive therapy reduced their risk for sustained retinopathy by 54 percent, the progression to proliferative retinopathy by 47 percent, and the need for laser photocoagulation treatment by 56 percent.[13]

Obtain a history of any visual changes from diabetic patients. On examination, low visual acuity and the presence of visual field defects should arouse suspicion for retinopathy. Dilated funduscopy is often not practical in the emergency department, but a nondilated retinal exam can frequently reveal "cotton wool" exudates, microaneurysms, and vascular proliferation consistent with diabetic retinopathy (Table 209-6). A red and/or painful eye in association with headache or simply unexplained headache in diabetics should prompt measurement of intracocular pressures to rule out acute glaucoma. The presence of these findings should prompt a referral to an ophthalmologist for further examination and therapy.

Laser photocoagulation of proliferative retinopathy has been proven to be efficacious in preventing blindness from proliferative retinopathy, particularly in patients with macular edema. Vitrectomy may be necessary to preserve vision in cases of severe proliferative retinopathy with vision loss secondary to retinal hemorrhage and detachment or vitreous hemorrhage.[19] Experimental trials involving aldose reductase inhibitors and aminoguanidine in the treatment of diabetic retinopathy are ongoing.

Nephropathy

Diabetic nephropathy is one of the leading causes of end-stage renal disease. Approximately one-third of new cases of renal failure each year are due to diabetic nephropathy. Incidence approaches 40 percent lifetime in type 1 diabetes and 4 to 20 percent in type 2 diabetes. Since the overwhelming majority of diabetics are type 2, most patients with nephropathy will have this form of the disease. Hyperglycemia leads to glomerular hypertension and hyperfiltration, which in turn lead to deposition of protein in the mesangium. These protein deposits ultimately lead to sclerosis of the glomerulus and to renal failure. Intensive insulin therapy as practiced in the DCCT reduced by 60 percent the frequency of microalbuminuria, the clinical herald of diabetic nephropathy. In addition to being a marker for nephropathy,

TABLE 209-6 Changes in the Diabetic Retina

Background (Simple)	Proliferative
Increased capillary permeability	New vessels
Capillary closure and dilation	Scars (retinitis proliferans)
Microaneurysms	Vitreal hemorrhage
Arteriovenous shunts	Retinal detachment
Dilated veins	
Hemorrhages	
Cotton-wool spots	
Hard exudates	

albuminuria has also been shown to correlate with high risk for coronary ischemic events. Angiotensin-converting enzyme (ACE) inhibitors have been shown to delay both the onset and progression of diabetic nephropathy. The effect of ACE inhibitors appears to be independent of their effect on controlling blood pressure. Overall prevention of nephropathy involves a combination of glycemic control, effective treatment of hypertension, restriction of dietary protein, and avoidance of nephrotoxic drugs or dyes.

The most useful clinical marker for nephropathy is the presence and degree of microalbuminuria. Patients with albumin excretion rates of as little as 30 mg/day are at high risk for developing diabetic nephropathy and subsequent renal failure. Unfortunately, standard urine dipsticks do not give positive results until the urinary excretion of albumin is greater than 360 mg/day. The 24-h albumin excretion can be estimated from quantitative analysis of single-voided, early-morning urine specimens, but the gold standard is measurement of albumin in a 24-h urine collection. Albumin excretion can vary and should not be measured during urinary infections, DKA, HHNS, or after exercise.

Blood pressure control, ideally 130/85 mmHg or lower, is crucial to slowing the progression of nephropathy. Calcium-channel blockers and ACE inhibitors are the best agents to begin therapy with in diabetic patients. Thiazide diuretics have side effects such as hyperglycemia, hypokalemia, and hyperlipidemia that make them unattractive. Patients with nephropathy should also be encouraged to eat a lower-protein diet (0.8 g/kg ideal body weight per day; consult a dietician) and avoid nephrotoxic drugs such as the nonsteroidal anti-inflammatory drugs (NSAIDs).

Neuropathy

Neuropathy can be divided into peripheral neuropathy and autonomic neuropathy. The degree of functional and structural abnormalities in nerves can be correlated directly with the degree and duration of hyperglycemia.

Symptomatic peripheral neuropathy results from loss of both myelinated and unmyelinated nerve fibers and blunted nerve fiber reproduction, resulting in abnormal firing of sensory neurons. Usually bilateral, it often consists of symmetrical stocking–glove loss in the distal extremities. Symptoms run a spectrum from numbness to paresthesias to constant burning pain. Physical examination may also demonstrate loss of vibratory sense and deep tendon reflexes. Intensive glycemic control as practiced in the DCCT reduced the incidence of clinical neuropathy by 60 percent. Drugs that have been proven effective in treating the pain associated with diabetic neuropathy include tricyclic antidepressants, especially amitriptyline, topical capsaicin, phenytoin, and carbamazepine. Narcotic analgesics have a high abuse potential in this setting, so their use should be avoided. The use of NSAIDs should also be avoided secondary to potential nephrotoxicity. Sensory nylon monofilament testing (Semmes-Weinstein) is a useful screening tool for early neuropathy.[20] Diabetic patients with depressed or absent Achilles' reflex or loss of vibratory sensation in the foot are at high risk for developing foot ulcers. Pain often subsides with time as neurons become destroyed.

Diabetic mononeuropathy usually affects a large peripheral nerve (femoral, obturator, sciatic, median, or ulnar) or an isolated cranial nerve (usually the third, fourth, or sixth). Patients present with sudden onset of symptoms related to the involved nerve. Mononeuritis multiplex, a rare form of mononeuropathy, involves several isolated nerves simultaneously. The symptoms of mononeuropathy usually resolve spontaneously after a few days to weeks. It may be difficult in the emergency department to differentiate the signs and symptoms of diabetic mononeuropathy from a transient ischemic attack or cerebrovascular accident.

Autonomic neuropathy represents the clinical entities of gastroesophageal reflux disease (GERD), gastroparesis, neurogenic bladder, impotence and sexual dysfunction, autonomic diarrhea (nocturnal, often with incontinence), and orthostatic hypotension. Symptoms of GERD include dysphagia, chest pain, and heartburn. Distinction from myocardial ischemia in the emergency department is often impossible, unless GERD has been previously diagnosed. Gastroparesis is the nonprogressive and nonrhythmic contraction of the gastric antrum, often with pylorospasm. Symptoms include epigastric pain, bloating, anorexia, nausea, early satiety, or vomiting.[21] Gastroparesis has been shown to respond to erythromycin, cisapride, and metoclopramide, all of which decrease gastric emptying time. Severe cases may not respond to medication.

Theories on the etiology of diarrhea in diabetics include (1) generalized autonomic neuropathy in poorly controlled type 1 diabetes; (2) small bowel dysmotility and abnormal intraluminal pressures; and (3) dysfunction of the α_2-adrenergic receptors of the small and large intestine that are responsible for stimulating sodium absorption and bicarbonate secretion. Infection, inflammatory bowel disease, irritable bowel syndrome, bacterial overgrowth due to small bowel stasis, or pancreatic exocrine deficiency can mimic the diarrhea associated with diabetes. Chronic diarrhea of diabetes is defined as increased frequency or liquidity of bowel movements of greater than three weeks duration. Incompetence of the internal anal sphincter may also mimic diabetic diarrhea and asymptomatic sensorimotor deficit commonly exists in the anal canal of diabetic patients. Rectal examination is always necessary to exclude fecal impaction as a cause of diarrhea.

Constipation is probably the most common gastrointestinal symptom in diabetics and is associated with autonomic neuropathy. The diet should include 30 mg of dietary fiber per day. Digital examination and sigmoidoscopy should exclude other anal and rectal diseases. Treatment with bethanechol may cause constipation. Autonomic diarrhea may respond to tetracycline therapy 1 to 2 doses orally (250 to 500 mg) early in the attack.[22] Clonidine has also been used successfully in treating diabetic diarrhea. The diarrhea usually will also respond to traditional antidiarrheal medicines. Neurogenic bladder may respond to bethanechol therapy. Erectile dysfunction may be successfully treated with the new oral agent, sildenafil, but this drug is contraindicated in patients using any form of organic nitrate therapy and should be used with caution in patients with known coronary artery disease. Symptomatic orthostasis can be treated by judicious increases of salt intake (in the absense of hypertension) or by using elastic stockings (which should be fitted by a specialist), or the symptoms may respond to fludrocortisone, which increases arterial tone and expands intravascular volume.[22]

Infections

Diabetics who achieve and maintain excellent glycemic control ($HgbA_{1c} < 7$ percent) are probably not at any greater risk from infection than the general population. A variety of factors, both those related to associated defects in immunity and disease-related effects, may account for the increased prevalence of certain infections in the diabetic population and poor wound healing in general.

There are possible epidemiologic associations between diabetes and urinary tract infections, candidal vulvovaginits, cystitis, and balanitis, pneumonia, influenza, chronic bronchitis, bacteremia, primary and reactivation tuberculosis, mucormycosis, malignant otitis externa, lower extremity skin and soft tissue structure infections, surgical wound infections, and Fournier gangrene.[23] However, only a few of these conditions have been shown to be more frequent in diabetics than in a nondiabetic control group in controlled studies.

There are several impairments seen in polymorphonuclear leukocytes in diabetic patients, including impaired migration, phagocytosis, intracellular killing, and chemotaxis that lead to an intrinsic decrease in immunity and in the ability to heal wounds properly. Disease-specific factors such as neuropathy, impairments in bladder emptying, and poor local circulation may further impair the immune response.

Urostasis and increased glucosuria facilitate bacterial colonization in the urinary tracts of diabetics. Poor sensation may lead patients to ignore a minor wound on the lower extremities that subsequently becomes a serious infection. Atherosclerotic vascular disease may limit local circulation that is essential to proper wound healing. Even though there are few controlled outcome studies comparing diabetics with nondiabetics, it is probably prudent based on the known defects in the immune response to have a low threshold for hospitalization of diabetic patients with upper urinary tract, lower respiratory tract, or skin/skin structure infections for initial intravenous antibiotic therapy. However, the availability of home intravenous infusion therapy, and the development of oral antibiotics with excellent antimicrobial coverage, provide outpatient alternatives for the management of mild to moderate infectious complications.

There is little in the literature to guide the emergency physician when confronted with a febrile diabetic patient without an obvious source of infection. Given the potential for problems with host defects in immunity in patients with poor glycemic control, and given that many infections associated with diabetes can be catastrophic, fever without a clear source is a good reason to admit the patient. Some serious diabetic infectious complications are discussed below.

RHINOCEREBRAL MUCORMYCOSIS Rhinocerebral mucormycosis is an invasive fungal infection of the nasal and paranasal sinuses, cometimes involving the palate and adjacent tissues. An estimated 70 percent of these infections occur in diabetic patients with ketoacidosis; the other 30 percent usually present in immunocompromised nondiabetic patients. The onset is sudden and rapidly progressive; patients present with periorbital or perinasal pain; blood-tinged nasal discharge; unilateral headache; increased tearing; swelling of eyelids and conjunctiva; and decreased vision. Physical signs can include black eschar on the nasal mucosa or hard palate due to ischemia, proptosis, and if the infection progresses, cranial nerve involvement or seizures. The organism has a propensity for vascular occlusion, therefore cavernous sinus thrombosis, as well as brain abscesses, can occur.[23]

Untreated patients usually die within a week, therefore prompt diagnosis and immediate, aggressive therapy must be initiated. Acidosis must be corrected and a surgeon consulted for extensive debridement of necrotic tissue and drainage of sinuses or abscesses. Computed tomography and/or magnetic resonance imaging should be obtained to both determine the extent of the infection and rule out an intracranial process. Amphotericin B is the drug of choice. Even with aggressive therapy, only 50 to 85 percent of patients are cured.

MALIGNANT OTITIS EXTERNA This infection almost exclusively occurs in elderly diabetic patients without ketoacidosis. Unlike other serious infections in patients with diabetes mellitus, well-controlled glucose levels are present in up to half and systemic toxicity is often absent. Microangiopathies in the external auditory canal of diabetics is thought to be a predisposing factor for this infection. Patients present with unilateral otalgia, purulent discharge, and sometimes fever. Examination finds a tender, inflamed external auditory canal, and almost all have a mass of granular-appearing tissue. Neuropathies, usually of the seventh, ninth, tenth, or eleventh cranial nerves, occur in about one-half of patients and signals a poor prognosis; 50 percent of patients with cranial nerve paralysis die and the rest have some persistent paralysis.[24] The infection can progress to osteomyelitis of the mastoid,

TABLE 209-7 Empiric Antibiotic Therapy for Diabetic Lower Extremity Infections

Classification	Therapy
Non-limb-threatening	
Less than 2 cm of cellulitis/inflammation	1st-Generation cephalosporin orally such as cephalexin 250–500 mg qid
No deep structure involvement	*or*
Well-perfused limb	Clindamycin 300 mg orally qid
Limb-threatening	
More than 2 cm of cellulitis/inflammation	2nd-Generation cephalosporin such as cefoxitin 2 g IV q8h
Ascending lymphangitis	*or*
Deep ulceration or abscess	Ciprofloxacin 400 mg IV q12h + clindamycin 450–900 mg IV q8h
Large necrotic areas	*or*
Involvement of deep structures	Metronidazole 500 mg IV q8h
Gangrene	*or*
Lower extremity ischemia, decreased or absent pulses	Trovafloxicin 200 mg IV qd
Life-threatening	
High fever or hypothermia	Imepenem 500 mg IV q6h
Leukocytosis	*or*
Hypotension	Meropenem 1 g IV q8h
Tachycardia	*or*
Tachypnea	Ampicillin-sulbactam 3 g IV q8h
Altered mental status	*or*
DKA or HHNS	Ticarcillin-clavulinic acid 3.1 g IV q8h
	or
	Trovafloxicin 200 mg IV qd
	or
	Piperacillin (PID)-Tazobactam 3.375 g IV q8°
	or
	Penicillinase-resistant synthetic penicillin + antipseudomonal aminoglycoside 5.1 mg/kg qd
	or
	Aztreonam 2 g IV q8°

Abbreviations: DKA, diabetic ketoacidosis, HHNS, hyperglycemic, hyperosmolar, nonketotic syndrome.
Source: Adapted from Gilbert et al,[25] with permission.

temporal bone, or base of skull, and meningitis, venous sinus thrombosis, or subdural emphysema. Magnetic resonance imaging or computed tomography can define the extent of anatomic involvement.

Infection is almost always due to *Pseudomonas aeruginosa* but staphylococci, fungi, and other gram-negative organisms have been isolated. Hence, recommended therapy parenteral antibiotics is imipenem, meropenem, ciprofloxacin, or the combination of a third-generation cephalosporin (ceftazidime) plus an antipseudomonal penicillin (ticarcillin) for four to six weeks.[24] Early surgical debridement and frequent cleansing are critically important.

CHOLECYSTITIS Diabetics have a predisposition to cholelithiasis and acute cholecystitis has a higher morbidity and mortality rates, higher incidence of perforation, and greater chance (up to 25 percent) of developing emphysematous cholecystitis. Diabetics with unexplained fever, with or without abdominal pain, should be evaluated with ultrasound for cholecystitis. Emphysematous cholecystitis is a rare gas-producing infection that occurs more frequently in male diabetic patients, is associated with higher incidence of gangrenous gallbladders, and is more likely to perforate. Patients present with symptoms similar to acute cholecystitis and abdominal radiographs can reveal gas in the gallbladder and biliary tree. The causative agents are most frequently a clostridium species in addition to streptococci, *Escherichia coli,* and pseudomonas. Despite prompt treatment and surgery, the mortality rate (15 percent) is 3 to 10 times higher than ordinary cholecystitis.

PYELONEPHRITIS, PERINEPHRIC ABSCESS, AND PAPILLARY NECROSIS Diabetics are at increased risk for two serious renal infections: emphysematous pyelonephritis and perinephric abscess. Emphysematous pyelonephritis is a rare, life-threatening infection with gas production in and around the kidney. Over 70 percent of these patients are diabetic. Patients with emphysematous pyelonephritis are ill with fever, flank pain, and sometimes a palpable mass. Bacteremia is often present. Aggressive treatment with parenteral antibiotics and nephrectomy is required. Even then, the mortality rate is still about 40 percent. Diabetics account for 35 percent of patients with perinephric abscess. Patients usually do not respond completely to parenteral antibiotics and surgical drainage is usually required. Even with surgical drainage, mortality is about 20 percent.

About 50 percent of patients who develop renal papillary necrosis have diabetes. Patients may be asymptomatic and not notice the sloughed papillary tissue excreted in their urine, or they may present with symptoms similar to acute pyelonephritis. Renal infection with ureteral obstruction may develop into sepsis and septic shock in these diabetic patients. Necrotic tissue fragments, red and white blood cells, and bacteria may be seen in the urine. Ureteral obstruction can be detected with ultrasound, computed tomography, and retrograde pyelography. Intravenous pyelogram should be avoided, especially if preexisting renal disease exists. Patients presumed to have pyelonephritis, but who appear to fail to respond to parenteral antibiotics, should be evaluated for renal papillary necrosis and perinephric abscess. Likewise, symptoms of flank pain suggesting renal colic should always be evaluated fully to exclude infection or papillary necrosis. Treatment still consists of aggressive intravenous antibiotics, urinary drainage, and, if severe, surgery to remove necrotic tissue.

TABLE 209-8 Cutaneous Disorders and Infections Associated with Diabetes Mellitus

Name	Features
Diabetic dermopathy	Also called "skin spots." Small rounded plaques with raised borders, may have central ulceration and crusting at the edge. Linear pattern. Over anterior tibial surface. Patient usually >30 years. Healing results in depressed scar with diffuse brown discoloration
Acanthosis nigricans	Not specific to diabetes but seen 2° to insulin resistance. Brown to black velvety hyperpigmentation, usually on posterior and and latent folds of neck, also axilla, groin, and umbilicus. Can also signal internal malignancy.
Bullosis diabeticorum	Superficial bullae with clear serum or mildly hemorrhagic.
Scleroderma	Benign and common in diabetes. Thickened skin over shoulders and upper back.
Necrobiosis lipoidica diabeticorum	Round, firm, reddish brown to yellow translucent plaques; usually on legs but can occur on hands, arms, abdomen, and head. Usually within the first year of onset of diabetes.
Furuncles and carbuncles	Fluctuant pustular masses of various sizes; usually due to *S. aureus.*
Erythrasma	Pink to red to brown lesions of stratum corneum; well-demarcated borders; results in dry, scaling, often puritic patches in inguinal, genital, perineal regions; may affect axillae; interdigital spaces, intertriginous areas.
Necrotizing fasciitis	Subcutaneous infection that advances along facial planes; resembles cellulitis; can follow trauma to extremities or perineum; crepitus, cutaneous signs occur late as the infection spreads rapidly; mixed aerobic and anaerobic etiology.
Synergistic necrotizing cellulitis	Resembles necrotizing fasciitis, but is distinguished by muscle involvement in addition to fascial involvement.
Gas gangrene (clostridial myonecrosis)	Clostridial infection of skeletal muscle; usually follows trauma; 6 h to 3 days incubation period; systemic toxicity; bacteremia in 15%; crepitus and gas bubbles with foul-smelling discharge.
Nonclostridial gas gangrene	Favored targets are muscles of ischemic lower extremities; gas present; less pain and toxicity than clostridial myonecrosis and slower spread.
Phycomycotic gangrenous cellulitis	Fungal; central black necrotic ulcer with purple, edematious margin; often follows trauma to skin and subcutaneous tissue; slow or rapid progression; uncommon.
Group B streptococcal (*S. agalactiae*)	Cellulitis, necrotizing fasciitis, postoperative wound infections, and pneumonia

Diabetic Foot Ulcers

Foot and lower extremity ulcers and associated infections are a major source of morbidity in the diabetic population, affecting some 15 percent of diabetics during their lifetime and accounting for 20 percent of diabetic admissions and nearly 50 percent of all lower extremity amputations in the United States. Direct costs each year for diabetic lower extremity ulcers and their complications exceed 500 million dollars annually. A pathologic triad of neuropathy, premature atherosclerotic vascular disease, and impaired immunity combine to make diabetic foot ulcers a multidisciplinary treatment challenge.

Peripheral neuropathy predisposes diabetic feet to ulceration, infection, and joint degeneration (Charcot joints) through the mechanisms of lack of sensation, diminished or absent proprioception, anhidrosis, and poor circulatory and thermal regulation. Risk factors for foot and lower extremity ulcers include high $HgbA_{1c}$ levels, older age, longer duration of diabetes, foot deformities, smoking, retinopathy, peripheral neuropathy, albuminuria, and low diastolic blood pressure. Preventing foot ulcers involves education on foot care and proper fitting of footwear, combined with good glycemic control to limit development of neuropathy and premature vascular disease.

A thorough clinical examination of the diabetic patient's feet should be performed during all emergency department visits even for unrelated complaints. Hair and nail growth, calluses, corns, deformities, erythema, swelling, sensation, and vascular function should be assessed. Any ulcerations found should be unroofed surgically and probed using a blunt-ended rigid probe to determine the depth and possible bone, joint, or tendon involvement. The ability to probe to bone through the ulcer suggests the strong possibility of osteomyelitis and deep space soft tissue infection.

Based on the initial patient evaluation and foot examination, foot ulcers can be classified into non-limb-threatening, limb-threatening, and life-threatening infections. *Non-limb-threatening infection* is defined as small (under 2 cm of cellulitis or inflammation), does not involve deep structures or bone, and is the result of recent injury to a well-perfused limb. *Limb-threatening infection* (more than 2 cm of cellulitis or inflammation) with associated ascending lymphangitis, deep ulceration or abscess, large area of necrotic tissue, involvement of deep structures or bone, gangrene, or critical lower extremity ischemia defined by absence of palpable pulses. *Life-threatening infection* has clinical signs of sepsis, including fever, leukocytosis, hypotension, tachycardia, tachypnea, altered mental status, and metabolic abnormalities ranging from hypoglycemia to DKA and HHNS.

Generally, it is suggested that the debridement of foot and leg ulcers be just sufficient to judge the depth and extent of the ulcer and to rule out deep abscess. Management of foot ulcers that do not appear infected and do not expand to the deep structures or bone on exploration should include topical antibiotics and nonadherent padded dressings. Follow-up referral with a specialist in diabetic foot care should occur within a few days. Constrictive dressings, such as Unna paste boot (alkaline methylene blue), and tight-fitting shoes should be avoided. Avoidance of weight bearing on the affected limb is critical to avoid progression to infection and for proper healing.

Radiographs of the foot are indicated to exclude subcutaneous gas, foreign bodies, osteomyelitis, and Charcot joints. Swab cultures of foot ulcers may provide misleading results. Culture of tissue excised from the base of the ulcer provides the most accurate identification of the bacteria involved. Commonly isolated organisms include *Bacteroides* species, *Staphylococcus aureus, Staphylococcus epidermidis, Enterococcus, Escherichia coli, Proteus mirabilis,* and *Pseudomonas aeruginosa*. Empiric antibiotic therapy should be directed against these organisms.

In choosing antibiotic therapy for these infections, severity should be taken into account (Table 209-7). The use of aminoglycosides should generally be avoided because of their associated nephrotoxicity. For limb-threatening and life-threatening infections, immediate surgical consultation is indicated for incision and debridement, possible revascularization, or amputation.

TABLE 209-9 Disposition/Guidelines for Hospital Admission

Inpatient care for the diabetic patient is generally appropriate for the following clinical situations:
• Life-threatening metabolic decompensation such as diabetic ketoacidosis or hyperglycemic, hyperosmolar, nonketotic syndrome.
• Newly diagnosed diabetes in children or adolescents.
• Chronic, poor metabolic control that necessitates close monitoring to determine the cause of the poor control, with subsequent modification of the therapeutic plan.
• Severe chronic complications of diabetes, such as chronic renal insufficiency or failure, atherosclerotic cardiovascular disease, infected lower extremity ulcers, retinopathy with acute loss of vision, neuropathy with intractable pain or affecting ability to ambulate, and autonomic neuropathy, i.e., gastroparesis with intractable nausea and vomiting that require admission for intensive therapy or to prevent metabolic decompensation.
• Conditions that impact adversely on diabetes control or are complicated by the presence of diabetes, such as acute asthma or chronic obstructive pulmonary disease exacerbations requiring high doses of corticosteroids as therapy.
• Uncontrolled or newly discovered diabetes during pregnancy.
• Institution of insulin pump or other intensive insulin regimens for glycemic control.
• Hyperglycemia (>400 mg/dL) associated with severe volume depletion.
• Hyperglycemia that does not respond to appropriate interventions or with associated metabolic deterioration.
• Hypoglycemia with neuroglycopenia (altered level of consciousness, altered behavior, coma, seizure) that does not rapidly resolve with correction of hypoglycemia.
• Hypoglycemia resulting from long-acting oral hypoglycemic agents.
• Hypoglycemia with adequate resolution of symptoms but no responsible adult to be with the patient for the next 12 h.
• Recurrence of hypoglycemia despite interventions.
• Admissions for complications of diabetes should be driven by the appropriate care for the particular diagnostic entity, such as infected lower extremity ulcer, renal failure, congestive heart failure, or unstable angina.
• Admissions for other medical conditions should be considered if rapid initiation of glucose control can improve outcome, such as in pregnancy, infections, or surgery. Also, consider admission if the medical illness can lead to acute onset of retinal, renal, neurologic, or cardiovascular complications of diabetes, for example, hypertensive urgency/emergency. These guidelines may result in admissions for diabetic patients for conditions that may be treated on an outpatient basis in the nondiabetic population.
• Fever without an obvious source in patients with poorly controlled diabetes.

Source: Adapted from the American Diabetes Association,[19] with permission.

Skin and Soft Tissue Complications

Several cutaneous disorders and infections are more common in diabetics (Table 209-8). Serious infections usually develop due to the combination of poorly controlled serum glucose, vascular insufficiency, and tissue hypoxia. These infections may spread rapidly with dramatic skin changes. The most common sites are lower extremities, but such

TABLE 209-10 Discharge Instructions and Follow-Up Care

- Follow a healthy diet.
- Self-monitor blood glucose regularly.
- Take insulin or oral hypoglycemics as directed.
- Reduce weight where appropriate.
- Cease smoking where appropriate.
- Exercise regularly in the absence of contraindications, such as foot ulcers.
- Practice good general foot care (check regularly for minor trauma and hot spots, keep nails trimmed properly, and wear well-fitted shoes).
- Wearing a Medic-alert bracelet or necklace.
- Be able to recognize symptoms of high blood sugar, such as frequent urination, thirst, dizziness, headache, nausea or vomiting, abdominal pain, lethargy, or blurry vision.
- Be able to recognize symptoms of low blood sugar, including fatigue, headache, drowsiness, agitation, pale or moist, visual changes, or loss of consciousness.
- Know how to help yourself or others with low blood sugar by self-administering or giving an awake person (who can swallow without gagging or choking) candy, fruit juice, or sugar or by calling an emergency phone number (e.g., 911) if the affected person is not able to respond.

infections may occur on the peritoneum, scrotum, and abdominal wall (especially at sites of penetrating trauma or surgery). They all require emergent, aggressive medical and surgical treatment. Hemodynamic support and correction of ketoacidosis and/or hyperglycemia is often required.

DISPOSITION AND INDICATIONS FOR HOSPITAL ADMISSION

Guidelines for admission considerations are listed in Table 209-9. These guidelines may result in admissions for diabetic patients for conditions that may be treated on an outpatient basis in the nondiabetic population.[26]

Patients who present with new-onset type 2 diabetes, type 1 diabetes without evidence of metabolic decompensation, acute hypoglycemia or hyperglycemia, and do not meet the aforementioned criteria for admission should see their primary care provider within 24 to 48 h as a general rule to arrange for general education and dietary evaluation and to initiate appropriate therapy for glycemic control. General discharge instructions for all diabetics, new or established, are detailed in Table 209-10.

REFERENCES

1. Expert Committee on the Diagnosis and Classification of Diabetes Mellitus: Report of the Expert Committee on the Diagnosis and Classification of Diabetes Mellitus. *Diabetes Care* 20:1183, 1997.
2. Zimmet PZ, McCarty DJ, de Courten MP: The global epidemiology of non-insulin dependent diabetes mellitus and the metabolic syndrome. *J Diabetes Complications* 11:60, 1997.
3. Kenny SJ, Aubert RE, Geiss LS: Prevalence and incidence of non-insulin dependent diabetes, in Harris MI, Cowie CC, Stern MP, et al (eds): *Diabetes in America*, 2d ed. Washington, DC, US Government Printing Office, NIH publication 95-1468, 1995, pp 47–68.
4. LaPorte RE, Matsushima M, Chang Y-F: Prevalence and incidence of insulin-dependent diabetes, in Harris MI, Cowie CC, Stern MP, et al (eds): *Diabetes in America*, 2d ed. Washington, DC, US Government Printing Office, NIH publication 95-1468, 1995, pp 37–46.
5. Portuese E, Orchard T: Mortality in non-insulin-dependent diabetes, in Harris MI, Cowie CC, Stern MP, et al (eds): *Diabetes in America*, 2d ed. Washington, DC, US Government Printing Office, NIH publication 95-1468, 1995, pp 221–232.
6. Geiss LS, Herman WH, Smith PJ: Mortality in non-insulin-dependent diabetes, in Harris MI, Cowie CC, Stern MP, et al (eds): *Diabetes in America*, 2d ed. Washington, DC, US Government Printing office, NIH publication 95-1468, 1995, pp 233–258.
7. Rewers M, Hamman RF: Risk factors for non-insulin-dependent diabetes, in Harris MI, Cowie CC, Stern MP, et al (eds): *Diabetes in America*, 2d ed. Washington, DC, US Government Printing Office, NIH Publication 95-1468, 1995, pp 179–220.
8. Rubin RJ, Altman WM, Mendelson DN: Health care expenditures for people with diabetes mellitus. *J Clin Endocrinol Metab* 78:809A, 1992.
9. Brownlee M, Vlassara H, Cerami A: Non-enzymatic glycolysation products on collagen covalently trap low-density lipoproteins. *Diabetes* 34:938, 1985.
10. American Diabetes Association: Standards of medical care for patients with diabetes mellitus [position statement]. *Diabetes Care* 20(suppl):S5, 1997.
11. American Diabetes Association: Self-monitoring of blood glucose [consensus statement]. *Diabetes Care* 19(suppl 1):S62, 1996.
12. Umpierrez GE, Khajavi M, Kitabachi AE: Review: Diabetic ketoacidosis and hyperglycemic hyperosmolar nonketotic syndrome. *Am J Med Sci* 311:225, 1996.
13. Diabetes Control and Complications Trial (DCCT) Research Group: The effect of intensive treatment of diabetes on the development and progression of long-term complications in insulin-dependent diabetes mellitus. *N Engl J Med* 329:977, 1993.
14. Andersson DKG, Svardsudd K: Long term glycemic control relates to mortality in type II diabetes. *Diabetes Care* 18:1534, 1995.
15. Koda-Kimble MA, Carlisle BA: Diabetes mellitus, in Young LY, Koda-Kimble MA, Kradjan WA, Guglielmo BJ (eds): *Applied Therapeutics: The Clinical Use of Drugs*, 6th ed. Vancouver, WA, Applied Therapeutics, 1995, vol 48, pp 1–62.
16. Paulson DJ: The diabetic heart is more sensitive to ischemic injury. *Cardiovasc Res* 34:104, 1997.
17. Limball TR, Daniels SR: Cardiovascular status in young patients with insulin-dependent diabetes mellitus. *Circulation* 90:357, 1994.
18. Klein R, Klein BEK: Vision disorders in diabetes, in Harris MI, Cowie CC, Stern MP, et al (eds): *Diabetes in America*, 2d ed. Washington, DC, US Government Printing Office, NIH Publication 95-1468, 1995, pp 293–338.
19. Early Treatment Diabetic Retinopathy Study Research Group: Early photocoagulation for diabetic retinopathy: ETDRS report number 9. *Ophthalmology* 98(suppl):766, 1991.
20. Armstrong DG, Lavery LA, Vela SA, et al: Choosing a practical screening instrument to identify patients at risk for diabetic foot ulceration. *Arch Intern Med* 158:289, 1998.
21. Sninsky CA: Gastrointestinal complications of diabetes mellitus. *Curr Ther Endocrinal Metab* 5:420, 1994.
22. Nathan DM: Long-term complications of diabetes mellitus. *N Engl J Med* 328:1676, 1993.
23. File TM, Tan JS: Infections complications in diabetic patients. *Curr Ther Endocrinol Metab* 6:491, 1997.
24. Smitneuman KO, Peacock JE: Infections emergencies in patients with diabetes mellitus. *Med Clin North Am* 79:53, 1995.
25. Gilbert DN, Moellering Jr RC, Şande MA (eds): *The Sanford Guide to Antimicrobial Therapy 1998*, 28th ed. Vienna, VA, Antimicrobial Therapy, 1998, p 11.
26. American Diabetes Association: Hospital admission guidelines for diabetes mellitus [position statement]. *Diabetes Care* 20(suppl 1):S52, 1997.

HEMATOLOGIC AND ONCOLOGIC EMERGENCIES

EVALUATION OF ANEMIA AND THE BLEEDING PATIENT

Mary E. Eberst

EVALUATION OF THE PATIENT WITH ANEMIA

Emergency physicians encounter patients with anemia on a daily basis. Some of these patients have an acute anemia as a result of blood loss from trauma, gastrointestinal bleeding, or other acute hemorrhage. Many emergency department (ED) patients have chronic anemia that may or may not be related to the complaint that brought them to the ED.

Pathophysiology

Anemia is defined as a reduced concentration of red blood cells (RBCs). In healthy persons, normal erythropoiesis (RBC production) ensures that the number of RBCs present is adequate to meet the body's demand for oxygen and that RBC destruction equals production in order to maintain a stable RBC concentration. Anemia results when RBC production cannot keep up with RBC loss resulting from blood loss, hemolysis, or normal RBC senescence. Quantification of the RBC concentration is reflected in the RBC count per μL, hemoglobin concentration, or hematocrit (percentage of RBC mass to blood volume). Normal RBC values for adults are slightly different for males and females (Table 210-1). Based on pathophysiologic mechanisms, there are three categories of anemia (Table 210-2).

Clinical Features

Regardless of the cause of anemia, the clinical manifestations are the same. The severity of symptoms and signs related to anemia depend on several factors: the rate of development of anemia, the extent of anemia that is present, and the adequacy of cardiopulmonary adaptation. The symptoms of anemia are reflective of the cardiovascular compensation that occurs in an attempt to maintain tissue oxygenation in the face of decreased oxygen-carrying capacity in the blood. These compensatory mechanisms are increased cardiac output and the centralization of blood flow to provide oxygen to the most sensitive tissues. Symptoms such as palpitations, dizziness, feeling of postural faintness, exertional intolerance, and tinnitus are reflective of increased cardiac output. Clinical signs of increased cardiac output are tachycardia, a hyperdynamic precordium, and systolic murmurs. Pallor of the conjunctivae, skin, and nail beds reflects centralization of blood flow. Tachypnea at rest and hypotension are late signs and are ominous. Decreased tissue perfusion occurs long before hypotension. Coronary artery blood flow usually is not limited until the hemoglobin is 50 percent or less of normal, although it can occur at lesser levels of anemia in patients with restriction of coronary blood flow. In an otherwise healthy patient, the symptoms and signs of anemia resulting from increased cardiac output may not occur at rest until the hemoglobin concentration is below about 7g/dL, although tissue perfusion may be impaired. The emergency physician must keep in mind that the hemodynamic response to anemia may be altered by the use of ethanol, prescription drugs, or recreational drugs.

TABLE 210-1 Normal RBC Values for Adults

	Male	Female
RBC count (million/μL)	4.5–6.0	4.0–5.5
Hemoglobin (g/dL)	14–17	12–15
Hematocrit (%)	42.0–49.0	38.5–46.0

Diagnosis

The diagnosis of anemia is established by the finding of a decreased RBC count, hemoglobin, and hematocrit on the routine complete blood count (CBC). Other than in patients who are acutely hemorrhaging, it is often not essential that a specific cause of anemia be established in the ED. Further workup can be initiated in the ED and should be started before the transfusion of packed red blood cells (PRBCs).

The basic evaluation of a patient newly diagnosed with anemia includes the following: Hemocult (Smith-Kline Diagnostics, Inc.) examination if not already performed, review of the RBC indices provided with the CBC, reticulocyte count, and review of the peripheral blood smear (Table 210-3). The mean cellular volume (MCV) is the most useful guide to the possible etiology of an anemia. The reticulocyte count reflects activity in the bone marrow and, along with the MCV, can help classify an anemia quickly and provides a differential diagnosis and further course of action (Table 210-4).

TABLE 210-2 Pathophysiologic Classification of Anemia

I. Loss of RBCs by hemorrhage
- As a result of acute or chronic blood loss.
- In the setting of acute blood loss, the bone marrow has not had sufficient time to increase erythropoiesis to replace the lost RBCs.
- In chronic blood loss, erythropoiesis may not be adequate to replace the lost RBCs.

II. Increased destruction of RBCs—hemolytic anemias
- Hereditary hemolytic anemias
- Acquired hemolytic anemias

III. Impaired production of RBCs

A. Hypochromic anemias
- The RBCs have a decreased amount of hemoglobin in each cell (hypochromic), and the cells typically are small (microcytic).
- Results from impaired hemoglobin synthesis.
- Examples are iron deficiency, anemia of chronic disease, thalassemias, sideroblastic anemias.

B. Aplastic/myelodysplastic anemias
- The RBCs are of normal size (normochromic) or large (macrocytic).
- Results from marrow stem cell failure.
- Caused by chemicals (including ethanol), radiation, infections (including HIV, human parovirus B_{19}), chronic renal failure, marrow infiltration, myelodysplastic syndromes, idiopathic.

C. Megaloblastic anemias
- The RBCs are large (macrocytic).
- Results from impaired DNA synthesis.
- Caused by deficiency of vitamin B_{12} or folate, drugs (chemotherapeutics, HIV drugs)

Note: RBC, red blood cells; HIV, human immunodeficiency virus; DNA, deoxyribonucleic acid.

TABLE 210-3 Initial Laboratory Evaluation of Anemia

Test	Interpretation	Normal Value	Clinical Correlation
RBC indices:			
MCV, mean cellular volume	Reflects average RBC size	80–95 fL	*Decreased MCV* (microcytosis)—chronic iron deficiency, thalassemia, anemia of chronic disease *Increased MCV* (macrocytosis)—decreased level of vitamin B_{12} or folate, chronic ethanol ingestion, chronic liver disease, reticulocytosis, phenytoin, HIV drugs
MCH, mean cellular hemoglobin	Reflects weight of hemoglobin in average RBC	28–32 pg	The MCH and MCHC do not provide much additional information for the classification of anemia.
MCHC, mean cellular hemoglobin concentration	Reflects concentration of hemoglobin in average RBC	32–36%	
Reticulocyte count	These RBCs of intermediate maturity are an index of the production of mature RBCs by the bone marrow, reported as a percent of total RBCs	0.5–1.5%	*Decreased reticulocyte count* reflects impaired RBC production; seen with low levels of iron, vitamin B_{12}, folate, bone marrow failure *Elevated reticulocyte count* reflects accelerated erythropoisis, the normal marrow response to anemia; seen with blood loss and hemolytic anemias
Peripheral blood smear	Used for the evaluation of: 1. Overall size of the RBCs; example: normocytic, microcytic, macrocytic 2. Amount of hemoglobin in the RBCs; example: hypochromic 3. Look for abnormal shapes such as sickled cells or schistocytes (evidence of hemolysis) 4. Examination of white blood cells and platelets		

TABLE 210-4 An Approach to the Patient with Anemia

Diagnosis of anemia (low RBC count, low hemoglobin, low hematocrit):
- Do rectal exam and Hemocult if not already done.
- Add reticulocyte count to laboratory work.
- Review of RBC indices and peripheral blood smear.

To initiate workup in the ED:
1. Anemia with low MCV and low reticulocyte count:
   - Differential diagnosis includes iron deficiency, anemia of chronic disease, thalassemia, sideroblastic anemia.
   - Additional labs to order: serum iron, iron-binding capacity, ferritin.
   - Further evaluation may include hemoglobin electrophoresis to diagnose thalassemia, bone marrow aspiration/biopsy to assess iron stores.
2. Anemia with elevated MCV and low reticulocyte count:
   - Differential diagnosis includes vitamin B_{12} or folate deficiency, myelodysplastic syndrome, liver disease, hypothyroidism.
   - Additional labs to order: serum vitamin B_{12}, serum folate.
   - Further evaluation may include thyroid function tests, liver function tests, bone marrow aspiration/biopsy.
3. Anemia with normal MCV and low reticulocyte count:
   - Differential diagnosis includes aplastic anemia, anemia of chronic disease, chronic renal failure, marrow infiltration, infection, myelodysplastic syndromes.
   - Additional labs to order: serum iron, iron-binding capacity, ferritin, creatinine, liver function tests, thyroid function tests.
   - Further evaluation may include erythropoietin level, bone marrow aspiration/biopsy.
4. Anemia with increased reticulocyte count:
   - Differential diagnosis includes acute blood loss, splenic sequestration, hemolytic anemias.
   - Additional labs to order: direct and indirect Coombs' tests, total and indirect bilirubin, LDH, haptoglobin.
   - Further evaluation may include hemoglobin electrophoresis.

Note: RBC, red blood cell; MCV, mean cellular volume; LDH, lactate dehydrogenase.

Treatment

The treatment of anemia depends on the etiology of the anemia and the symptoms and clinical status of the patient. In the ED setting, one is faced most commonly with the management of anemia resulting from acute blood loss. All patients who have ongoing blood loss and anemia should have blood typed and crossmatched so that it is available for transfusion if needed. The decision to transfuse PRBCs has to be individualized for each patient with consideration of clinical symptoms, objective signs, age of the patient, presence of comorbid disease, and the likelihood of further blood loss. In general, patients who are symptomatic and hemodynamically unstable and have evidence of tissue hypoxia and/or limited cardiopulmonary reserve should have PRBCs transfused. In most settings, patients with anemia resulting from acute blood loss are transfused at hemoglobin levels of 7g/dL, if not at higher levels, as dictated by patient considerations discussed earlier.

ED patients with chronic anemia or a newly diagnosed anemia of uncertain etiology not caused by acute blood loss may not require immediate transfusion unless they are hemodynamically unstable, hypoxic, or have acidosis or ongoing cardiac ischemia. In a patient with newly diagnosed anemia of uncertain etiology, it is important that laboratory studies that may be required for hematologic evaluation are obtained prior to transfusion. Consultation with a hematologist may be beneficial to guide this evaluation. The condition of some patients with chronic anemias or anemias of uncertain etiology can be made worse by transfusion, so transfusion should not be undertaken unless specifically indicated.

Disposition

Any patient with anemia from ongoing blood loss should be admitted to the hospital for further evaluation and treatment. Patients with isolated anemia that is chronic or newly diagnosed and not related to blood loss do not necessarily require admission if they are asymptomatic, hemodynamically stable, have minimal comorbid disease, and close follow-up can be arranged. Patients newly diagnosed with anemia who also have abnormalities in the white blood cell or platelet count should have immediate hematologic consultation and probable admission.

THE BLEEDING PATIENT

Most bleeding that is seen in the ED is normal—the result of local wounds, lacerations, or other structural lesions. The majority occurs in patients with normal hemostasis. With careful attention to the history and physical findings, patients with pathologic bleeding often can be readily identified. Generally speaking, patients who manifest spontaneous bleeding from multiple sites, bleeding from untraumatized sites, delayed bleeding several hours after trauma, and bleeding into deep tissues or joints should be considered to possibly have a bleeding disorder.

Important historical data for the presence of a congenital bleeding disorder include the presence or absence of unusual or abnormal bleeding in the patient and other family members and the possible occurrence of excessive bleeding after dental extractions, surgical procedures, or trauma. Many patients with abnormal bleeding have an acquired disorder. Questioning about liver disease and drug use (particularly ethanol, aspirin, nonsteroidal anti-inflammatory drugs, warfarin, antibiotics, and other aspirin-containing products) may be helpful.

The site(s) of bleeding may provide an indication of the hemostatic abnormality. Mucocutaneous bleeding, including petechiae, ecchymoses, epistaxis, gastrointestinal, genitourinary, or heavy menstrual bleeding is characteristic of qualitative or quantitative platelet disorders. Purpura often are associated with thrombocytopenia and commonly indicate systemic illness. Bleeding into joints and potential spaces, such as between fascial planes and into the retroperitoneum, as well as delayed bleeding, is most commonly associated with coagulation factor deficiencies. Patients who demonstrate both mucocutaneous bleeding and bleeding in deep spaces often have disorders such as disseminated intravascular coagulation, where both platelet abnormalities and coagulation factor abnormalities are present.

Review of Normal Coagulation

The normal hemostatic system consists of a complex process that limits blood loss by the formation of a platelet plug (primary hemostasis) and the production of cross-linked fibrin (secondary hemostasis), which strengthens the platelet plug. These reactions are counterregulated by the fibrinolytic system, which limits the size of fibrin clot that is formed, thereby preventing excessive clot formation. Congenital and acquired abnormalities occur in all these systems. The affected patients may have excessive hemorrhage, excessive thrombus formation, or both.

PRIMARY HEMOSTASIS *Primary hemostasis* is the platelet interaction with the vascular subendothelium that results in the formation of a platelet plug at the site of injury. Required components for this to occur are normal vascular subendothelium (collagen), functional platelets, normal von Willebrand factor (connects the platelet to the endothelium via glycoprotein Ib), and normal fibrinogen (connects the platelets to each other via glycoprotein IIB-IIIA). Figure 210-1 depicts primary hemostasis.

SECONDARY HEMOSTASIS *Secondary hemostasis* describes the reactions of the plasma coagulation proteins by a tightly regulated mechanism. The final product is cross-linked fibrin, which is insoluble and strengthens the platelet plug formed in primary hemostasis. Figure 210-2 diagrams the reactions of secondary hemostasis.

THE FIBRINOLYTIC SYSTEM This complex system regulates the hemostatic mechanism by limiting the size of fibrin clots that are formed. A simplified schema is depicted in Fig. 210-3. The principal physiologic activator is tissue plasminogen activator (tPA), which is released from endothelial cells. tPA converts plasminogen, which is synthesized in the liver and adsorbed in the fibrin clot, to plasmin. Plasmin degrades fibrinogen and fibrin monomer into low-molecular-weight fragments known as *fibrin degradation products* (FDPs) and cross-linked fibrin into D-dimers.

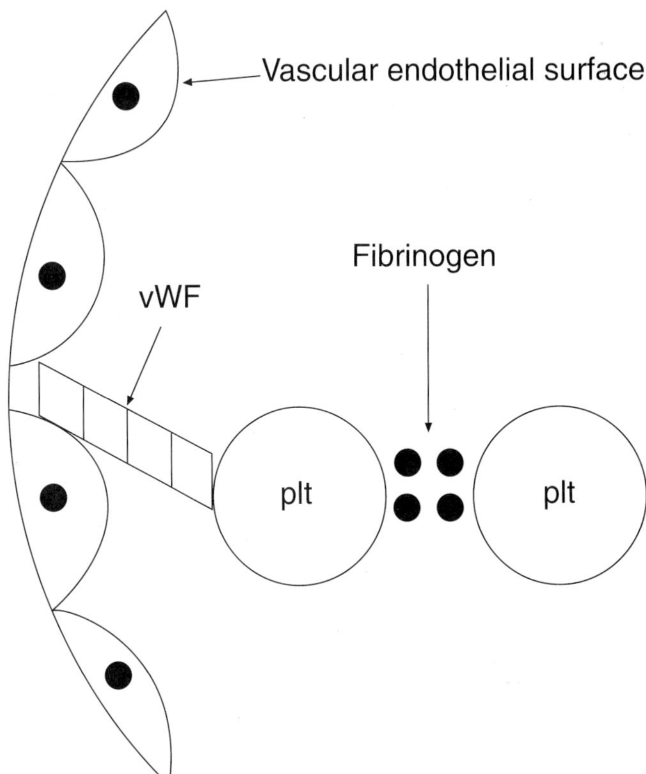

FIG. 210-1. Primary hemostasis. See text for details. vWF, von Willebrand factor; plt, platelet.

Other physiologic inhibitors of hemostasis with prevalent clinical applicability include antithrombin III and the protein C–protein S system. Antithrombin III is a protein that forms complexes with all the serine protease coagulation factors (factors XII_a, XI_a, IX_a, and thrombin), thereby inhibiting their function. Heparin potentiates this interaction, and this is the basis for its use as an anticoagulant. Protein C, which requires the presence of protein S for activation, is capable of inactivating the two plasma cofactors, factors V and VIII, and inhibiting their participation in the coagulation cascade.

Tests of Hemostasis

Table 210-5 outlines the screening tests of primary and secondary hemostasis as well as other commonly used coagulation tests. Table 210-6 lists many commonly used drugs that are associated with thrombocytopenia.

LABORATORY INVESTIGATION The basic laboratory parameters that should be obtained in a patient with a suspected bleeding disorder are a complete blood count and platelet count, prothrombin time, and activated partial thromboplastin time. The results of these tests coupled with clinical evaluation should enable one to formulate a differential diagnosis. Further hematologic evaluation, using the tables provided in the chapter, can then follow. Hematologic consulation should be sought if the differential diagnosis or the laboratory approach is unclear.

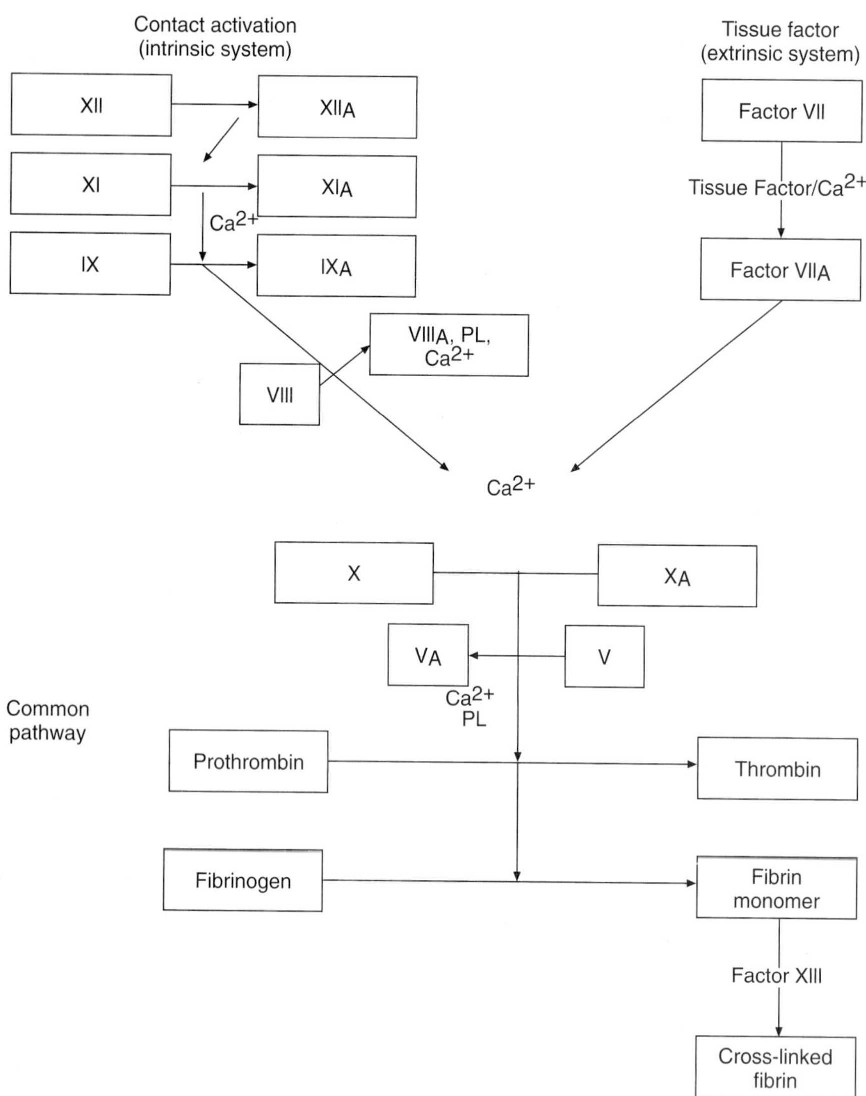

FIG. 210-2. Secondary hemostasis, also known as the coagulation cascade. The unactivated coagulation proteins (factors) are indicated by roman numerals; after the reaction occurs, the factor is activated and designated by subscript A. There are two independent activation pathways. The contact system is known as the *intrinsic pathway,* and the tissue factor system is known as the *extrinsic pathway.* The pathways merge at the point of activation of factor X. This begins the common pathway that generates the final product, cross-linked fibrin. Ca^{2+}, calcium; fibrinogen is factor I; PL, phospholipid surface (often platelets); prothrombin is factor II.

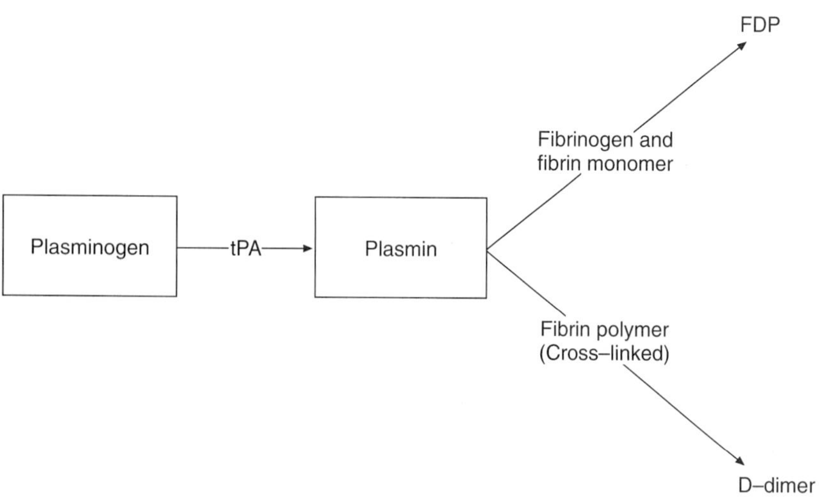

FIG. 210-3. The fibrinolytic pathway. See text for details. FDP, fibrin degradation product; tPA, tissue plasminogen activator.

TABLE 210-5 Tests of Hemostasis

Screening Tests	Normal Value	Measures	Clinical Correlations
		PRIMARY HEMOSTASIS	
Platelet count	150,000–300,000/μL	Number of platelets per μL	Decreased platelet count (thrombocytopenia) Bleeding usually not a problem until platelet count <50,000/μL; high risk of spontaneous bleeding including CNS with count <10,000/μL. Causes Decreased production—viral infections (measles); marrow infiltration; drugs (thiazides, ethanol, estrogens, interferon-α) (see Table 210-6) Increased destruction—viral infections (mumps, varicella, EBV, HIV); ITP, TTP, DIC, HUS; drugs (heparin, protamine) (see Table 210-6) Splenic sequestration (hypersplenism, hypothermia) Loss of platelets (hemorrhage, hemodialysis, extracorporeal circulation) Pseudothrombocytopenia—platelets are clumped but not truly decreased in number; examine blood smear to recognize this Elevated platelet count (thrombocytosis)—commonly reactive to inflammation or malignancy, or in polycythemia vera; can be associated with hemorrhage or thrombosis
Bleeding time (BT)	2.5–10 min (template BT)	Interaction between platelets and the subendothelium	Prolonged BT caused by: Thrombocytopenia (platelet count <50,000/μL) Abnormal platelet function (vWD, ASA, NSAIDs, uremia, liver disease) Collagen abnormalities (congenital abnormality or prolonged use of steroids)
		SECONDARY HEMOSTASIS	
Prothrombin time (PT)	10–12 s, but laboratory variation	Extrinsic system and common pathway—factors VII, X, V, prothrombin, and fibrinogen	*Prolonged PT*—most commonly caused by: Use of warfarin (inhibits vitamin K–dependent factors II, VII, IX, and X) Liver disease with decreased factor synthesis Antibiotics, some cephalosporins, (moxalactam, cefamandole, cefotaxime, cefoperazone) that inhibit vitamin K–dependent factors
Activated partial thromboplastin time (aPTT)	Depends on type of thromboplastin used; "activated" with Kaolin	Intrinsic system and common pathway including factors XII, XI, IX, VIII, X, V, prothrombin, and fibrinogen	*Prolongation of aPTT* most commonly caused by: Heparin therapy Factor deficiencies; factor levels have to be <30% of normal to cause prolongation **Note:** high doses of heparin or warfarin can cause prolongation of both the PT and aPTT due to their activity in the common pathway.
Thrombin clotting time (TCT)	10–12 s	Conversion of fibrinogen to fibrin monomer	*Prolonged TCT* caused by: Low fibrinogen level (DIC) Abnormal fibrinogen molecule (liver disease) Presence of heparin, FDPs or a paraprotein (multiple myeloma); these interfere with the conversion Very high fibrinogen level (acute phase reactant)
"Mixes"	Variable	Performed when one or more of the above screening tests is prolonged; the patients plasma ("abnormal") is mixed with "normal" plasma and the screening test is repeated	*If the "mix" corrects* the screening test, one or more factor deficiencies are present. *If the "mix" does not correct the screening test,* an inhibitor is present.
		OTHER HEMOSTATIC TESTS	
Fibrin degradation products and D-dimer (evaluate fibrinolysis)	Variable	*FDPs* measure breakdown products from fibrinogen and fibrin monomer; *D-Dimer* measures breakdown products of cross-linked fibrin	Levels of these are elevated in DIC, thrombosis, pulmonary embolus, liver disease.
Factor level assays	60–130% (0.60–1.30 units/mL)	Measures the percent activity of a specified factor compared to normal	Used to identify specific factor deficiencies and in therapeutic management of patients with deficiencies
Inhibitor screens	Variable	Verifies the presence or absence of antibodies directed against one or more of the coagulation factors	*Specific inhibitors*—directed against one coagulation factor, most commonly against factor VIII; can be in patients with congenital or acquired deficiency. *Nonspecific inhibitors*—directed against more than one of the coagulation factors; example is lupus-type anticoagulant

Note: ASA, aspirin; CNS, central nervous system; DIC, disseminated intravascular coagulation; EBV, Epstein-Barr virus; FDPs, fibrin degradation products; HIV, human immunodeficiency virus; HUS, hemolytic uremic syndrome; ITP, idiopathic thrombocytopenic purpura; NSAIDs, nonsteroidal anti-inflammatory drugs; TTP, thrombotic thrombocytopenic purpura; vWD, von Willebrand disease.

TABLE 210-6 Drugs Associated with Thrombocytopenia

	Relative Incidence		Relative Incidence
Heparin	4+	Thiazides	2+
Gold salts	4+	Furosemide	2+
Sulfa-containing antibiotics	4+	Procainamide	2+
Quinine/quinidine	4+	Digoxin/digitoxin	2+
Amrinone	3+	Cimetidine/ranitidine	2+
Ethanol (chronic use)	3+	Phenytoin	1+
Aspirin	3+	Penicillins/cephalosporins	1+
Indomethacin	3+	Estrogens	1+
Valproic acid	3+	Protamine sulfate	1+
Heroin	3+	Interferon-α	1+

Note: Relative incidence based on number of case reports: 4+ equivalent to at least 50–100 reports; 3+ is 20 or more reports; 2+ is 10–20 reports; 1+ is 10 or less case reports.

BIBLIOGRAPHY

Baron BJ, Scalea TM: Acute blood loss. *Emerg Med Clin North Am* 14(1):35, 1996.

Berliner N, Duffy TP, Abelson HT: Approach to the adult and child with anemia, in Hoffman R, Benz EJ Jr, Shattil SJ, et al (eds): *Hematology, Basic Principles and Practice,* 2d ed. New York: Churchill Livingstone, 1995, p 468.

Bockenstedt PL: Laboratory methods in hemostasis, in Loscalzo J, Schafer AI (eds): *Thrombosis and Hemorrhage,* 2d ed. Baltimore: Williams & Wilkins, 1998, p 517.

Coller BS, Schneiderman PI: Clinical evaluation of hemorrhagic disorders: Bleeding history and differential diagnosis of purpura, in Hoffman R, Benz EJ Jr, Shattil SJ, et al (eds): *Hematology, Basic Principles and Practice,* 2d ed. New York: Churchill Livingstone, 1995, p 1606.

Thurer RL: Evaluating transfusion triggers. *JAMA* 279(3):238, 1998.

ACQUIRED BLEEDING DISORDERS

Mary E. Eberst

PLATELET ABNORMALITIES

Acquired platelet abnormalities include both quantitative and qualitative defects. Quantitative problems are usually associated with bleeding complications at a platelet level of less than 50,000/μL with spontaneous bleeding, including central nervous system (CNS) hemorrhage, likely at a level below 10,000/μL. Table 211-1 depicts the causes of acquired thrombocytopenia; Table 210-6 displays the drugs most commonly associated with thrombocytopenia. Platelet counts above 400,000/μL are encountered most commonly in inflammatory reactions, patients with malignancy, splenectomized patients, and those with polycythemia vera. Thrombocytosis can be associated with bleeding or thrombosis and is considered an emergency when platelet levels exceed 1 million/μL or are associated with evidence of CNS dysfunction or acute thrombosis or hemorrhage.

Acquired qualitative platelet abnormalities, characterized by abnormal platelet function, occur in many disease states (Table 211-2). When present, functional abnormalities can be associated with excessive bleeding regardless of the platelet count. Table 211-3 outlines some commonly used drugs that can cause platelet dysfunction.

The emergency management of patients with thrombocytopenia is based on the control of acute hemorrhage and maintenance of an adequate intravascular volume to maintain normal hemodynamics. Most patients with active bleeding and platelet counts less than 50,000/μL should receive platelet transfusion. Each unit of platelets infused should raise the platelet count by 10,000/μL. Patients with platelet antibodies, such as those with idiopathic thrombocytopenic purpura (ITP) or hypersplenism, are unlikely to respond to platelet transfusions. Some disease states, such as disseminated intravascular coagulation

TABLE 211-1 Pathophysiologic Mechanisms of Acquired Thrombocytopenia

Mechanism	Associated Clinical Conditions
Decreased platelet production	Marrow infiltration (tumor or infection) Aplastic anemia Viral infections (measles) Drugs (thiazides, estrogens, ethanol, interferon-α, chemotherapeutic agents) Radiation Vitamin B_{12} and/or folate deficiency
Increased platelet destruction	Idiopathic thrombocytopenic purpura Thrombotic thrombocytopenic purpura Hemolytic uremic syndrome Disseminated intravascular coagulation Viral infections (HIV, mumps, varicella, EBV) Drugs (heparin, protamine)
Splenic sequestration	Hypersplenism Hypothermia
Platelet loss	Excessive hemorrhage Hemodialysis Extracorporeal circulation
Pseudothrombocytopenia	Not a disease state, laboratory phenomenon

Note: EBV, Epstein-Barr virus; HIV, human immunodeficiency virus.

TABLE 211-2 Clinical Conditions Associated with Qualitative Platelet Abnormalities

Uremia
Liver disease
Disseminated intravascular coagulation
Drugs (see Table 211-3)
Antiplatelet antibodies (ITP, SLE)
Cardiopulmonary bypass
Myeloproliferative disorders (PCV, CML)
Dysproteinemias (multiple myeloma, Waldenström's macroglobulinemia)
Preleukemias, AML, ALL
von Willebrand disease (congenital or acquired)

Note: ALL, acute lymphocytic leukemia; AML, acute myelogenous leukemia; CML, chronic myelogenous leukemia; ITP, idiopathic thrombocytopenic purpura; PCV, polycythemia vera; SLE, systemic lupus erythematosus.

TABLE 211-3 Commonly Used Drugs Associated with Platelet Dysfunction

Aspirin, NSAIDs	Calcium channel blockers
Heparin and thrombolytics	Propranolol
Penicillins and cephalosporins	Nitroprusside
Nitrofurantoin	Nitroglycerin
Prostaglandins	Tricyclic antidepressants
Dextran	Phenothiazines
Chemotherapeutics	Antihistamines

Note: NSAIDs, nonsteroidal anti-inflammatory drugs.

(DIC) and thrombotic thrombocytopenic purpura (TTP), actually may be exacerbated by platelet transfusion; hematologic consultation should be obtained. All patients with platelet counts less than 10,000/μL should receive immediate platelet transfusion, regardless of the underlying etiology, because of the high risk of spontaneous hemorrhage. Nonemergency therapies for thrombocytopenia with which the emergency physician should be familiar include antithymocyte globulin (ATG) for aplastic anemia; prednisone, intravenous gamma globulin, and splenectomy for ITP; prednisone, aspirin (ASA), plasma infusion, and plasma exchange for TTP and hemolytic uremic syndrome (HUS); as well as other immunosuppressive and chemotherapeutic agents with direct effect on the bone marrow or peripheral antibody production.

The long-term management of qualitative platelet abnormalities that result from underlying disease is directed at treatment of the underlying problem. Acute hemorrhage in these patients sometimes can be controlled with platelet transfusion, but often this is only a temporary solution because the transfused platelets soon acquire the same functional defect. Other management options in patients with the more common acquired types of platelet dysfunction, such as liver disease, uremia, and DIC, are discussed below.

WARFARIN AND VITAMIN K DEFICIENCY

Prothrombin (factor II) is a vitamin K–dependent coagulation factor, as are factors VII, IX, and X, protein C, and protein S. In the liver, reduced vitamin K is required as a cofactor for the carboxylation of glutamic acid residues in the precursors of these coagulation proteins. Deficiency of vitamin K or inhibition of this process by an antagonist such as warfarin results in decreased levels of these factors in the plasma. In the United States, all hospital-born infants are prophylactically treated with intramuscular vitamin K_1. Nutritional deficiency of vitamin K is rare in adults; however, it does occur as a result of poor nutrition and malabsorption in patients with liver disease.

Sodium warfarin, a vitamin K antagonist, is widely used as an oral anticoagulant. Even in those who are closely monitored, as many as 25 percent of patients taking warfarin develop hemorrhagic complications due to severe coagulation factor deficiencies. Routinely monitored by the prothrombin time (PT), large doses of warfarin also can cause prolongation of the activated partial thromboplastin time (aPTT). The treatment of overdosage of warfarin depends on the severity of clinical manifestations, not the degree of prolongation of the PT. If there is no evidence of bleeding, temporary discontinuation of the warfarin may be all that is needed. Warfarin has a half-life of 2.5 days in patients with normal hepatic function. Patients who manifest bleeding complications can be treated with fresh frozen plasma (FFP) or vitamin K_1 (intravenous, intramuscular, or subcutaneous)—each has advantages and disadvantages. Infusion of FFP can result in the rapid repletion of coagulation factors and control of hemorrhage. FFP, however, carries some risk of viral transmission and the risk of volume overload. Parenteral administration of vitamin K_1 will reverse the warfarin effect in 12 to 24 h. Some do not advise intravenous administration of vitamin K_1 because of the risk of hypersensitive anaphylactic reactions, although usually 1 mg can be given intravenously safely. Intramuscular or subcutaneous vitamin K_1 is typically given in doses of 5 to 10 mg daily in states of coagulation factor deficiency. The use of oral vitamin K_1 for the treatment of acute bleeding is not recommended. Its absorption is erratic and the effect may not be observed for several days to weeks. In addition to the risk of intravenous administration of vitamin K_1, the major disadvantage to its use is that its effect may last up to 2 weeks, making it difficult or impossible to anticoagulate the patient using warfarin during that time.

Drug-induced deficiency of the vitamin K–dependent factors also can be seen in patients receiving some antibiotics, particularly the third-generation cephalosporins that contain the *N*-methylthiotetrazole side chain (moxalactam, cefamandole, cefotaxime, cefoperazone).

Warfarin has long been used as a rodenticide; however, resistance has developed in the animals, and new products known as *superwarfarins* are now used. Brodifacoum is the most widely available of these agents. Many case reports now in the literature describe intentional and accidental ingestion of these products. Such patients present with a severe coagulopathy; major mucosal bleeding and internal bleeding are common and can be fatal. Treatment with high doses of vitamin K_1, up to 50 to 100 mg/day for several weeks, is often required to correct this coagulopathy because of the long half-life of these products.

LIVER DISEASE

Acute and chronic diseases of the liver can be associated with many hemostatic abnormalities of clinical significance. Parenchymal diseases such as cirrhosis and hepatitis, and infiltrative diseases, such as metastatic neoplasms, cause a variety of coagulation problems (Table 211-4).

Decreased Protein Synthesis The hepatocytes are the site of synthesis of all the coagulation factors except factor VIII. Diseases affecting the hepatic parenchyma result in decreased synthesis of coagulation factors.

Vitamin K Deficiency The synthesis of factors II (prothrombin), VII, IX, and X depends on vitamin K carboxylation. Vitamin K deficiency in patients with liver disease results from nutritional deficiency, malabsorption, and cholestasis, which prevents the absorption of this fat-soluble vitamin.

Thrombocytopenia This is most often due to portal hypertension, which leads to hypersplenism and splenic sequestration. Ethanol causes direct bone marrow suppression and reduced production of all hematopoietic cells including platelets.

TABLE 211-4 Hemostatic Abnormalities in Patients with Liver Disease

Coagulation factor deficiency due to decreased protein synthesis
Vitamin K deficiency
Thrombocytopenia
Increased fibrinolysis
Anemia

TABLE 211-5 Treatment Options for Patients with Liver Disease and Bleeding

Packed red blood cells to maintain hemodynamic stability
Vitamin K_1
Fresh frozen plasma
Platelet transfusions
Desmopressin (DDAVP)

Increased Fibrinolysis Several findings indicate that patients with significant liver disease have increased fibrinolysis and, according to some, a compensated, low-grade DIC. Fibrinogen levels are often low, and abnormal fibrinogen molecules are synthesized (dysfibrinogenemia). Fibrin and fibrinogen degradation products (FDPs and D-dimers) are often elevated due to poor hepatic clearance. The inactivator of plasmin, α_2-plasmin inhibitor, is synthesized in the liver. Decreased synthetic capability reduces the amount of this enzyme that is present and can lead to unregulated plasmin activity and increased fibrinolysis.

Anemia Although not directly a result of the liver disease, anemia is common in patients with liver disease, particularly those whose hepatic dysfunction results from the use of ethanol. Ethanol causes direct bone marrow suppression and is commonly associated with folate and iron deficiency.

Patients with mild or moderate hepatic dysfunction most often have subclinical hemostatic abnormalities. Those with severe liver disease may have life-threatening bleeding. Laboratory studies that should be obtained include hemoglobin/hematocrit, PT, aPTT, thrombin clotting time (TCT), and platelet count. Fibrinogen levels and measurement of FDPs or D-dimers may not be readily available. In general, prolongation of the PT is a poor prognostic sign in patients with liver disease.

The management of patients with liver disease and a coagulopathy depends on the presence or absence of active bleeding and the need to do invasive procedures (Table 211-5). If there is no evidence of bleeding and no need for invasive procedures, treatment is not mandatory. When treatment is indicated, the following should be used. *Packed red blood cells* should be transfused if there is significant bleeding or blood loss to maintain hemodynamic stability. *Vitamin K_1* should be given to all patients with liver disease and bleeding. A trial dose of 10 to 15 mg given subcutaneously or intramuscularly may take up to 24 h to have an effect. In most patients with significant liver disease, vitamin K_1 alone will not totally correct the prolonged PT. *FFP* can be given to temporarily replace coagulation factors. Its use is limited by the potential for volume overload; often the patient cannot tolerate the volume that would be required to completely replete the coagulation factors. Each unit is 200 to 250 mL and contains 200 to 250 units of each coagulation factor. *Platelet transfusions* may be used in severe bleeding situations, but in general, this will have a transient effect before the transfused platelets are sequestered in the spleen. *Desmopressin (DDAVP),* a synthetic analog of vasopressin, shortens the prolonged bleeding time in some patients with liver disease. There are no controlled trials to support its use, but generally its side effects are mild and there are few adverse effects from a trial administration. The dose is 0.3 μg/kg subcutaneously or intravenously every 12 h up to three doses.

RENAL DISEASE

Hemostatic abnormalities are encountered commonly in patients with renal disease. Bleeding can be a complication of acute or chronic renal failure. Spontaneous bleeding commonly occurs involving the skin (purpura), mucous membranes (epistaxis and menorrhagia), and gastrointestinal and urinary systems. Less common is bleeding involving the central nervous system, retroperitoneum, pericardium, and other internal bleeding. Surgery or trauma can lead to fatal hemorrhage, even with aggressive management.

The bleeding tendency in patients with renal disease is related to the degree and duration of uremia. The bleeding time is the clinical test most often prolonged in uremia, although it cannot be used directly to predict hemorrhage. In patients with uremia, a number of factors contribute to the bleeding diathesis: uremic retention products, chronic anemia, platelet dysfunction, deficiency of coagulation factors, and thrombocytopenia. Anemia contributes to the bleeding by making it difficult for the platelets to adhere to the subendothelium at sites of damage. Platelet function is optimized when the hematocrit is maintained between 26 and 30 percent. Acquired deficiencies of clotting factors are common in patients with the nephrotic syndrome. Mild thrombocytopenia is common in patients with renal failure; the etiology is multifactorial, but the platelet count is generally above 100,000/μL.

Management of these hemostatic defects is both preventive and directed at acute bleeding episodes (Table 211-6). *Dialysis* improves platelet function transiently, lasting for 1 to 2 days. Optimally, patients are well dialyzed three times per week. *Partial correction of the anemia* of chronic renal disease also improves platelet function. This can be accomplished by the use of recombinant human erythropoietin on a chronic basis or transfusion of packed red blood cells in the acute setting. Desmopressin is a synthetic analog of vasopressin. In uremic patients with prolonged bleeding times, 50 to 75 percent will have shortening or normalization of the bleeding time when treated with desmopressin. The usual dose is 0.3 μg/kg body weight given subcutaneously or intravenously. This dose is given every 12 h up to three or four doses before transient tachyphylaxis develops. Intranasal desmopressin may also be effective in this setting. Side effects associated with desmopressin are generally mild and include headache, flushing, minor hypotension, tachycardia, nausea, abdominal cramps, and local site reaction. Severe complications—hyponatremia and thrombosis—rarely occur. Although the mechanism is unknown, *conjugated estrogens* also improve the bleeding time and clinical bleeding in more than 80 percent of uremic patients treated. *Cryoprecipitate infusion* is one of the older treatments for bleeding associated with renal failure. Its use has largely been replaced by the use of desmopressin, which has no risk of viral transmission because it is not a blood product. *Platelet transfusions* are not routinely used in this setting and are not effective because the infused platelets quickly acquire the uremic defect. Infusions of cryoprecipitate and platelets are only indicated for life-threatening bleeding used in combination with packed red blood cells, desmopressin, and conjugated estrogens.

DISSEMINATED INTRAVASCULAR COAGULATION

Disseminated intravascular coagulation (DIC) is a loosely defined syndrome that is reflective of serious underlying disease. Patients who

TABLE 211-6 Treatment Options for Patients with Uremia and Excessive Bleeding

Dialysis
Optimize hematocrit (recombinant human erythropoietin or transfusion of PRBCs)
Desmopressin (DDAVP)
Conjugated estrogens
Cryoprecipitate infusion*
Platelet transfusion*

Note: PRBCs, packed red blood cells.
*Only in life-threatening bleeding situation.

TABLE 211-7 Common Causes of Disseminated Intravascular Coagulation

Clinical Setting	Comments
Infection: Bacterial Viral Fungal	Probably the most common cause of DIC; 10–20% of patients with gram-negative sepsis have DIC; endotoxins stimulate monocytes and endothelial cells to express tissue factor; Rocky Mountain Spotted Fever causes direct endothelial damage; DIC more likely to develop in asplenic patients or those with cirrhosis; septic patients are more likely to have thrombosis than bleeding.
Carcinoma: Adenocarcinoma Lymphoma	Malignant cells may cause endothelial damage and allow the expression of tissue factor as well as other procoagulant materials; most adenocarcinomas tend to have thrombosis (Trousseau's syndrome), except prostate cancer tends to have more bleeding; DIC is often chronic and compensated.
Acute leukemia	DIC most common with promyelocytic leukemia (M_3); blast cells release procoagulant enzymes, there is excessive release at time of cell lysis (chemotherapy); more likely to have bleeding than thrombosis.
Trauma	DIC especially with brain injury, crush injury, burns, hypothermia, hyperthermia, rhabdomyolysis, fat embolism, hypoxia.
Shock	
Liver disease	May have chronic compensated DIC; have acute DIC in the setting of acute hepatic failure, tissue factor is released from the injured hepatocytes.
Pregnancy	Placental abruption, amniotic fluid embolus, septic abortion, intrauterine fetal death (can be chronic DIC); can get DIC in HELLP syndrome (hemolysis, elevated liver enzymes, low platelets).
Vascular disease	Large aortic aneurysms (chronic DIC can become acute at time of surgery), giant hemangiomas, vasculitis, multiple telangiectasias.
Envenomation	DIC can develop with bites of rattlesnakes and other vipers; the venom damages the endothelial cells; bleeding is not as bad as expected from laboratory values.
ARDS	Microthrombi are deposited in the small pulmonary vessels, the pulmonary capillary endothelium is damaged; 20% of patients with ARDS develop DIC and 20% of patients with DIC develop ARDS.
Transfusion reactions: Acute hemolytic reaction Massive transfusion	DIC with severe bleeding, shock, and acute renal failure.
Surgical procedures: Liver transplantation Vascular surgery	

have severe DIC have a mortality rate of up to 85 percent. DIC can be triggered by a wide variety of disorders (Table 211-7) and can be acute and life-threatening or chronic and compensated. The most common trigger of DIC is the liberation of tissue factor. Tissue factor is usually confined within the extravascular space; when it is released, the coagulation system is activated (Fig. 211-1). Small fibrin clots are formed and deposited as thrombi or emboli in the microcirculation. Fibrinolysis then occurs and can be massive. FDPs are released and further inhibit hemostasis. The usually tightly regulated system of coagulation and fibrinolysis becomes unbalanced. Because of clot formation, coagulation factors and platelets are consumed. Microthrombi in the circulation can lead to tissue hypoxia, and the red

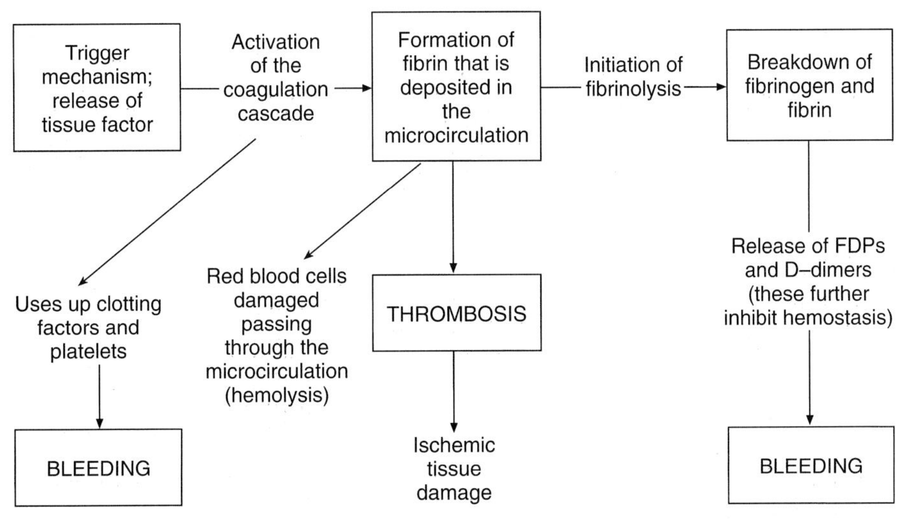

FIG. 211-1. Pathophysiology of disseminated intravascular coagulation. Refer to text for details. FDPs, fibrin/fibrinogen degradation products.

blood cells are damaged trying to pass through the microcirculation. The severity of DIC that develops depends on the synthetic function of the liver, the integrity of the vascular endothelium, and the capacity of the bone marrow to replace platelets. Chronic, compensated DIC occurs when the rate of consumption of clotting factors and platelets does not exceed their rate of production.

Table 211-7 lists the more common causes of DIC, particularly as encountered in the emergency setting. The reader is referred to a standard text for a complete list of causes. DIC occurs in its most extreme form in *Neisseria meningitidis* sepsis and acute myelogenous leukemia, promyelocytic (M3) type.

The clinical complications of DIC are bleeding, thrombosis, and purpura fulminans. Although hemorrhage and thrombosis may occur simultaneously, in an individual patient, one may predominate. Bleeding occurs in up to 75 percent of patients with DIC. Bleeding from the skin and mucous membranes is most common; usually there is bleeding from several sites, including venipuncture sites, surgical wounds, epistaxis, petechiae, and ecchymoses. Hematuria and gastrointestinal bleeding are seen; intracerebral bleeding carries a very poor prognosis. Thromboses (usually microthrombi) predominate in some patients. Clinical signs of this include mental status changes, focal ischemia or gangrene, oliguria, renal cortical necrosis, and adult respiratory distress syndrome (ARDS). Purpura fulminans occurs when there are widespread arterial and venous thromboses. Gangrene develops in the digits or extremities and there is hemorrhagic infarction of the skin. Purpura fulminans is most commonly seen with high-grade bacteremia (*Streptococcus pneumoniae* or *N. meningitidis*).

The diagnosis of DIC is based on the clinical setting and characteristic laboratory abnormalities. The typical laboratory results in DIC are outlined in Table 211-8. Patients with chronic DIC have laboratory evidence of the disorder but no clinical evidence of hemorrhage or thrombosis.

TABLE 211-8 Laboratory Abnormalities Characteristic of Disseminated Intravascular Coagulation

Studies	Result
	MOST USEFUL
Prothrombin time	Prolonged
Platelet count[a]	Usually low
Fibrinogen level[b]	Low
	HELPFUL
Activated partial thromboplastin time	Usually prolonged
Thrombin clot time[c]	Prolonged
Fragmented red blood cells[d]	Should be present
FDPs and D-dimers[e]	Elevated
Specific factor assays[f]	
Factor II	Low
Factor V	Low
Factor VII[g]	Low
Factor VIII[h]	Low, normal, high
Factor IX	Low (decreases later than other factors)
Factor X	Low

Note: FDP, fibrin degradation products.
[a]Platelet count usually low, most important that it is falling if it started at an elevated level.
[b]Fibrinogen level correlates best with bleeding complications; it is an acute phase reactant so it may actually start out at an elevated level; fibrinogen level <100 mg/dL correlates with severe DIC.
[c]Not a sensitive test, prolonged by many abnormalities.
[d]Fragmented red blood cells and schistocytes are not specific for DIC.
[e]Levels may be chronically elevated in patients with liver or renal disease.
[f]The factors in the extrinsic pathway are most affected (VII, X, V, and II).
[g]Factor VII is usually low early because it has the shortest half-life.
[h]Factor VIII is an acute phase reactant so its level may be normal, low, or elevated in DIC.

The management of acute DIC is based on the symptoms demonstrated by the patient and the underlying disease state. Many patients with DIC require no specific therapy if there is no evidence of bleeding or thrombosis and laboratory studies are not deteriorating. The first principle of management is to stabilize the patient hemodynamically, providing oxygen, fluids, and life support as needed. If possible, the primary cause of the DIC needs to be treated. The high mortality rate in severe DIC is primarily due to the underlying disorder. Antibiotics can be given and the fetus or retained uterine products removed; however, in many circumstances, little can be done rapidly. Further management depends on the predominant symptoms of the patient—bleeding or thrombosis.

Bleeding requires replacement therapy based on the amount of bleeding, risk of bleeding (i.e., postoperative), and the extent of depletion of coagulation factors and platelets. The PT is the best indicator of clotting factor depletion. If the PT is prolonged by more than 2 to 3 s and there is bleeding, replacement is indicated. Factor levels also can be used to guide therapy if they are readily available. The fibrinogen level should be maintained above 100 to 150 mg/dL and the other factor levels at or above 50 percent of normal. FFP is used to replace clotting factors; each unit contains 200 to 250 units of each factor. Usually given 2 units at a time, there are 200 to 250 mL of fluid per unit, making volume overload a potential problem. Cryoprecipitate is used to replace fibrinogen. There are 100 to 250 mg fibrinogen per bag of cryoprecipitate; 10 bags are typically given at one time. Platelet replacement is indicated if the count is less than 50,000/μL and there is bleeding or if it is less than 20,000/μL regardless of bleeding. Each unit of platelets transfused should raise the platelet count 10,000/μL; typically, 6 units of random donor platelets (or one apheresis unit) are given at a time. As with the use of any blood products, there is a small risk of viral transmission. Patients with DIC also should be given vitamin K_1 and folate.

The treatment of microthromboses in DIC with systemic heparinization is controversial. Its use has not been conclusively shown to improve survival and may make the overall clinical situation worse. Heparin should be considered and may be beneficial for some patients with DIC if the underlying condition is carcinoma, acute promyelocytic leukemia, or retained uterine products. Patients with purpura fulminans may also benefit from anticoagulation. In this setting, the continuous infusion of low-dose heparin (5–10 units/kg/h) is recommended. Patients with large thromboses, such as seen with Trousseau's syndrome, should receive full-dose heparinization. Antifibrinolytic agents such as ε-aminocaproic acid (EACA) and tranexamic acid are used in DIC with great caution. Although these drugs may reduce bleeding and fibrinogen consumption, they may convert a bleeding disorder into a thrombotic disorder. When used, these antifibrinolytic agents usually are given in conjunction with low-dose heparin infusion to minimize the potential for thrombosis. They are occasionally used in DIC patients with acute promyelocytic leukemia or prostate cancer.

HEPARIN AND THROMBOLYTIC THERAPY

Heparin

Heparin is an anticoagulant widely used for the treatment and prevention of venous thrombotic and thromboembolic disease. Administered intravenously or subcutaneously, heparin prevents thrombus formation and the extension and propagation of the preformed thrombus. Heparin reduces the ability of blood to clot by enhancing the ability of antithrombin III to form complexes with the activated serene protease coagulation factors (XII_a, XI_a, IX_a, and thrombin), thereby inhibiting their activity in the coagulation cascade. Heparin also may have an anti-inflammatory effect. Because it does not cross the placenta, heparin is the drug of choice when anticoagulation is needed during pregnancy. The dosing of heparin depends on the clinical setting (see Chapter 216). Heparin therapy is generally monitored by the aPTT, with variable goals depending on the clinical setting and laboratory standards. As with any drug, there are risks when heparin is used; these risks need to be weighed against the risk of not using heparin. The fatality rate is up to 15 percent for untreated venous thromboses.

Bleeding is the major complication of heparin therapy, occurring in up to 33 percent of all treated patients, with 1 to 7 percent of these episodes considered serious or life-threatening (requiring transfusion of blood). Some patients are at higher risk of developing bleeding complications, particularly those with a history of renal failure, gastrointestinal bleeding, head injury, heavy alcohol use, malignancy, recent surgery or trauma, or hemorrhagic disorders. Concomitant use of medications such as aspirin, warfarin, steroids, or nonsteroidal anti-inflammatory drugs (NSAIDs) also places patients at higher risk of bleeding complications. If significant bleeding complications develop, the heparin should be immediately stopped. The half-life of heparin is 60 to 90 min but can be longer if high levels are present. Protamine sulfate can be used to neutralize heparin; 1 mg protamine sulfate neutralizes 100 units of standard molecular weight heparin.

Thrombocytopenia is the other major complication of heparin therapy. Two types of thrombocytopenia can occur. The more common type of thrombocytopenia develops in up to 25 percent of patients treated with heparin. This is a benign, transient decrease in platelets; the platelet count usually remains greater than 100,000/μL and is thought to be due to platelet aggregation and sequestration in the spleen. Heparin therapy generally does not have to be discontinued, and the platelet count rises spontaneously. The second type of thrombocytopenia, known as *heparin-induced thrombocytopenia,* occurs in 1 to 5 percent of patients treated with heparin and can be life-threatening. Heparin-induced thrombocytopenia occurs when antibodies are formed against the platelets. This can occur immediately in patients who have received heparin previously, but it takes 6 to 10 days for the antibodies to form in previously untreated patients. Severe thrombocytopenia results; platelet counts less than 50,000/μL and arterial thromboses can occur. In this setting, the heparin must be completely eliminated, and other anticoagulants can be used if necessary (warfarin, dextran). Lepirudin (recombinant hirudin) is a new anticoagulant recently approved for use in patients with heparin-induced thrombocytopenia who require anticoagulation. The platelet count usually will return to normal 4 to 6 days after the heparin is stopped. It is controversial whether these patients should ever be treated with heparin again. Long-term use of heparin, for greater than 1 month, is associated with accelerated osteoporosis.

Low-molecular-weight heparins (LMWHs) were introduced into clinical practice in the early and middle 1990s. These compounds are made by chemical or enzymatic hydrolysis of unfractionated heparin and have about one-third the molecular weight of unfractionated heparin. The mechanism of anticoagulant activity of the LMWHs is not completely understood. Like unfractionated heparin, they have inhibitory effect against factor X_a, but other mechanisms are also postulated.

The indications for use of LMWHs are currently being evaluated in clinical trials. At this time, LMWHs are frequently used for the prophylaxis of deep venous thrombosis (DVT) after orthopedic surgery and treatment of patients with acute DVT. In patients with acute, proximal DVT, there is sufficient evidence that LMWHs are an effective and safe alternative to treatment with intravenous unfractionated heparin. Other clinical settings where LMWHs have been used are currently being further studied: treatment of malignancy-associated thromboembolic disorders, acute pulmonary embolus, unstable angina, thrombotic and ischemic stroke, after interventional cardiac procedures, for maintenance of the patency of arterial grafts, and for prevention of DVT during pregnancy and the postpartum period.

The advantages of LMWHs compared with unfractionated heparin are the following: increased bioavailability, longer half-life that allows for once- or twice-daily subcutaneous administration, a more predictable anticoagulant response; they are generally safe and effective for home treatment, and there are fewer complications with bleeding and heparin-induced thrombocytopenia. Reported side effects of LMWHs include bleeding, heparin-induced thrombocytopenia, local skin reaction, pruritus, and rare skin necrosis.

Enoxaparin, dalteparin, and ardeparin are the most widely available of the LMWH products. Compared with unfractionated heparin, LMWHs have a lower anticoagulant potency but a more predictable anticoagulant effect. Because of their weaker anticoagulant effect, the LMWHs usually do not prolong the aPTT, so their effect is not monitored by the aPTT. In general, treatment with LMWH is not monitored by laboratory testing. If needed, monitoring could be done by anti-factor X_a assay. With long-term therapy, platelet counts should be monitored periodically. It is important to note that the different LMWHs are given according to a dose specific for that preparation.

TABLE 211-9 Currently Available Thrombolytic Agents

Agent	Abbreviation
Streptokinase	SK
Urokinase	UK or uPA
Alteplase (recombinant tissue plasmogen activator)	tPA
Anistreplase (anisoylated plasminogen streptokinase activator complex)	APSAC
Reteplase (recombinant deletion mutation of tissue plasmogen activator)	rPA

Thrombolytics

Thrombolytic agents are able to dissolve preformed arterial and venous thrombi and emboli and restore blood flow to anoxic tissue. Currently available thrombolytics are listed in Table 211-9. These products work by inducing a systemic fibrinolytic state. This fibrinolytic state is not limited to the thrombus; it occurs throughout the circulation. This results in the potential for major hemorrhagic complications, which occur in about 9 percent of patients treated with thrombolytics compared with an average of 4 percent significant bleeding complications in patients treated with heparin. Because of this risk, the diagnosis of thrombus or embolus should be firmly established before treatment begins. Although theoretically more thrombus specific, major and minor bleeding complications are as common with recombinant tissue plasminogen activator (r-tPA) as with streptokinase.

Clinical indications for consideration of the use of thrombolytic therapy are as follows:

Deep venous thrombosis—Thrombolytics have been used for the treatment of acute, large DVTs; thrombolytics produce complete or near-complete lysis of clots, superior to that seen when heparin is used alone. There is a decreased incidence of postphlebitic syndrome and lower extremity ulcers. Some studies show an increased risk of hemorrhagic complications up to three times that seen with heparin alone, so patients must be selected carefully.

Acute myocardial infarction—Vascular reperfusion is the major determinant of improved clinical outcome and mortality reduction. The best results are found in patients with recent onset of chest pain (less than 6 h). Thrombolytics are administered systemically or by intracoronary injection.

Pulmonary embolism—The role of thrombolytic therapy in patients with pulmonary embolism is not clearly defined; however, it should be considered in patients with acute onset of symptoms (<48 h), evidence of hemodynamic compromise, presence of massive emboli,

TABLE 211-10 Contraindications to Thrombolytic Therapy

Absolute contraindications:
Active bleeding from any site
Hemorrhagic stroke at any time, CVA in the previous 6 months
Intracranial neoplasm
Intracranial trauma or surgery within 1 to 2 months
Suspected aortic dissection
Relative contraindications:
Surgical procedures or other invasive procedures within 3 weeks
History of gastrointestinal bleeding
Baseline coagulopathy or thrombocytopenia
Severe arterial hypertension, diastolic blood pressure >120 mmHg
Pregnancy or first ten days postpartum
Prolonged cardiopulmonary resuscitation
Major trauma within 4 weeks
Known active cavitary lung disease
Known allergy to agent

or the presence of submassive emboli superimposed on chronic cardiopulmonary disease. Patients with pulmonary embolism who receive thrombolytic therapy have greater reperfusion, earlier normalization of the perfusion scan, and decreased pulmonary artery pressures, although no clinical trial has confirmed improved survival.

Peripheral arterial occlusion—Acute peripheral arterial occlusions as well as those in some central sites are commonly treated with systemic or intra-arterial infusion of thrombolytic agents. In this setting, urokinase may be superior to streptokinase.

Acute ischemic stroke—Until recently, no clinically effective therapy for acute ischemic stroke has been available. Several multicenter randomized clinical trials have studied the use of r-tPA for the treatment of acute ischemic stroke in progress. The best outcome occurs when treatment is initiated within 3 h of the onset of symptoms in carefully selected patients. Patients treated with r-tPA have an improved neurologic outcome at 3 months, although there is an increased risk (three to nine times compared with placebo) of intracranial hemorrhage.

Specific recommendations for the use of thrombolytic agents in various clinical settings are available in Chapter 216. Many institutions have protocols for the use of thrombolytic agents. Contraindications to use the thrombolytic therapy are outlined in Table 211-10.

Bleeding is the major complication of thrombolytic therapy. Less common complications include fever, embolization of thrombi, and allergic reactions. Bleeding complications are primarily due to the dissolution of hemostatic plugs at sites of recent vascular injury. Superficial bleeding is usually not a major problem and can be controlled with local measures. Thrombolytic agents are discontinued at the first indication of major bleeding. Although the half-life of the thrombolytics is short, the systemic fibrinolytic state remains for 12 to 36 h after the infusion is stopped because it takes that long for fibrinogen to replenish itself. Cryoprecipitate can be given to replete fibrinogen and reverse the lytic state. EACA can also be given to inhibit the fibrinolytic state.

INFECTION WITH HUMAN IMMUNODEFICIENCY VIRUS

The current use of combination therapy, including the use of protease inhibitors, for the treatment of HIV-1 infection has improved the morbidity and mortality associated with HIV-1 infection significantly. These therapies, however, have not yet had a significant impact on the hemostatic abnormalities commonly seen in patients infected with HIV-1. The most common hemostatic abnormalities observed in patients infected with HIV-1 are thrombocytopenia and acquired circulating anticoagulants—lupus-type anticoagulants and anticardiolipin antibodies.

Thrombocytopenia is one of the earliest findings in asymptomatic HIV-1-infected individuals. Three to 60 percent of all HIV-1-infected patients will have thrombocytopenia at some time during the course of their illness. Both increased peripheral platelet destruction and decreased platelet production occur. Patients infected with HIV-1 have an increased incidence of immune platelet destruction, such as ITP. HIV-1 also can directly infect bone marrow megakaryocytes, resulting in decreased thrombopoiesis. The use of zidovudine (AZT) may result in improved platelet counts and rarely causes thrombocytopenia.

After thrombocytopenia, the most common hemostatic abnormality in HIV-1-infected patients is prolongation of the aPTT. This is usually due to the presence of a lupus-type anticoagulant. Often a transient defect, the lupus-type anticoagulant may appear with an acute opportunistic infection and disappear when the infection is treated. Anticardiolipin antibodies, which are detected by enzyme-linked immunosorbent assay (ELISA) and do not affect the basic hemostatic screening tests, are also more common in HIV-1-infected patients. One or both of these antibodies occur in 22 to 82 percent of patients with HIV-1 infection. These antibodies themselves do not predispose to clinical bleeding, but they result in an increased risk of thrombosis. However, concomitant hemostatic abnormalities such as platelet dysfunction or hypoprothrombinemia (associated with lupus-type anticoagulant) may lead to bleeding manifestations.

Another hemostatic complication of HIV-1-infection is anemia, which occurs in the majority of patients at some time in the course of their disease. Etiologies include ineffective erythropoiesis, the effect of HIV-1 and opportunistic infections on the bone marrow, and the use of AZT, which causes significant anemia in at least one third of patients. TTP is an uncommon but well-described complication of HIV-1 infection. TTP may be the initial manifestation of the infection and is characterized by the pentad of fever, thrombocytopenia, neurologic symptoms, renal insufficiency, and microangiopathic hemolytic anemia (see Chap. 214). Many patients infected with HIV-1 are also infected with the hepatitis viruses and have significant liver disease with resultant coagulation abnormalities.

USE OF ASPIRIN AND NONSTEROIDAL ANTI-INFLAMMATORY DRUGS

Table 211-3 depicts many of the commonly used drugs that can affect platelet function. Of these, the most commonly used are aspirin and the NSAIDs, which will be discussed in more detail.

Aspirin inhibits platelet function by acetylating and irreversibly inactivating platelet cyclooxygenase. Normally, platelet cyclooxygenase allows the formation of endoperoxides and thromboxanes, which stimulate platelet aggregation. This effect can be seen with as little as 80 mg aspirin per day and can continue for as long as 7 to 10 days after the aspirin is stopped, until the affected platelets are replaced by new platelets. The clinical significance of aspirin ingestion and bleeding is usually minimal except in some surgeries, cardiothoracic, plastic, and neurosurgery, where small amounts of blood loss are crucial, and in patients with underlying bleeding disorders (congenital or acquired) such as von Willebrand's disease, hemophilia, liver disease, uremia, or heavy ethanol ingestion. Chronic aspirin ingestion can lead to gastrointestinal blood loss; however, this is primarily from the direct effect of aspirin on the gastric mucosa. Platelet transfusion is the only acute treatment to overcome the platelet dysfunction induced by aspirin but this is rarely required.

The NSAIDs such as ibuprofen, indomethacin, and naproxen reversibly inhibit platelet cyclooxygenase. Inhibition of platelet cyclooxygenase occurs only as long as there is active drug in the circulation. The transient defect in platelet aggregation usually lasts less than 24 h. An exception is the drug piroxicam, which has a 2-day half-life;

the resultant platelet dysfunction may be present for days. NSAIDs can be safely used in patients with hemophilia.

CIRCULATING ANTICOAGULANTS

Acquired inhibitors of blood coagulation, also known as *circulating anticoagulants,* can have serious clinical consequences or only be laboratory phenomena that have little clinical impact. These inhibitors are antibodies directed against one or more of the coagulation factors. Although inhibitors have been described against most of the coagulation factors, the two most common are discussed here. Factor VIII inhibitors are a type of ''specific'' inhibitor, directed only against factor VIII. The lupus anticoagulant is a ''nonspecific'' inhibitor that is directed against several of the coagulation factors.

Factor VIII Inhibitors

Factor VIII inhibitors most commonly occur in patients with congenital factor VIII deficiency, hemophilia A (see Chap. 212). Factor VIII inhibitors also can develop in patients with previously normal hemostasis; the incidence is estimated at 0.2 to 1.0 per million persons per year. Although uncommon, this is an important clinical entity to recognize because the mortality rate approaches 50 percent. About one-half the affected patients are otherwise healthy individuals, usually older than age 65. The other patients have underlying associated conditions such as autoimmune disorders [systemic lupus erythematosus (SLE), rheumatoid arthritis, ulcerative colitis], lymphoproliferative disorders (multiple myeloma, Waldenström's macroglobulinemia, benign monoclonal gammopathy of uncertain significance), women in pregnancy and the postpartum period, and patients with allergic drug reactions (penicillins, sulfonamides, phenytoin). Clinically, these patients without a prior bleeding history present with massive spontaneous bruises, ecchymoses, and hematomas. Laboratory studies classically show a normal PT, normal TCT, and greatly prolonged aPTT that does not correct with ''mixing.'' A factor VIII–specific assay will show that the factor VIII activity is very low or absent. The other specific factor assays should be normal or only slightly decreased. Quantitative measurement of the inhibitor by the Bethesda inhibitor assay is important for the emergency management of bleeding episodes. Long-term management is directed at the suppression of antibody production by steroids, intravenous gamma globulin, or cytotoxic agents. The management of acute, often life-threatening bleeding episodes should be directed by a hematologist or coagulation specialist. Treatment options include high doses of factor VIII concentrates, the use of unactivated or activated prothrombin complex concentrates, porcine factor VIII, and potentially recombinant factor VII_a.

Lupus Anticoagulant

The lupus anticoagulant is an antiphospholipid antibody that interferes in vitro with many of the coagulation reactions. Its name is a misnomer because the majority of affected patients do not have lupus and very few have a clinical bleeding disorder. The lupus anticoagulant is identified in 5 to 15 percent of patients with SLE. Associated conditions include other autoimmune disorders, drug reactions (procainamide and phenothiazines), malignancies, and patients with HIV-1 infection in the setting of acute opportunistic infections. Many affected patients have no underlying disease state. Clinically, many patients are asymptomatic, with the abnormality discovered on routine coagulation screening tests. Arterial or venous thromboses occur in 23 to 58 percent of patients. Recurrent fetal loss, thought to be due to thrombosis of placental vessels and placental infarction, is also common. Some patients have thrombocytopenia, but they also may have ITP. Bleeding abnormalities are uncommon in patients with the lupus anticoagulant unless they have associated hypoprothrombinemia (usually patients with SLE), significant thrombocytopenia, or other underlying abnormality predisposing them to hemorrhage, such as uremia.

Laboratory studies of patients with the lupus anticoagulant typically show a normal or slightly prolonged PT, mild to moderate prolongation of the aPTT (not usually more than 10–15 s prolonged), and a normal TCT. The prolonged aPTT will not correct with ''mixing.'' If the PT is prolonged by more than 3 s, the patient should be evaluated for concomitant hypoprothrombinemia (factor II). Factor-specific assays done in this setting will show a decrease in all the factor levels, although none are extremely low. Various tests can be done to verify the presence of the lupus anticoagulant. These are the dilute Russell viper venom time, kaolin clot time, platelet neutralization procedure, and tissue thromboplastin inhibition test. Asymptomatic patients found to have the lupus anticoagulant require no treatment. If there is an associated underlying disorder, it should be treated, and with resolution, the lupus anticoagulant may disappear. Patients who suffer thrombotic events are managed with long-term anticoagulation (those with venous thrombosis) or low-dose aspirin (those with arterial thrombosis). Patients with the lupus anticoagulant can often be managed through a successful pregnancy when treated with prednisone and ASA.

BIBLIOGRAPHY

Eberst ME, Berkowitz LR: Hemostasis in renal disease: Pathophysiology and management. *Am J Med* 96:168, 1994.

Goodnight SH, Feinstein DI: Update in hematology. *Ann Intern Med* 128(7):545, 1998.

Jeske W, Messmore HL Jr, Fareed J: Pharmacology of heparin and oral anticoagulants, in Loscalzo J, Schafer AI (eds): *Thrombosis and Hemorrhage,* 2d ed. Baltimore: Williams & Wilkins, 1998, p 1193.

Koopman MM, Buller HR: Low-molecular-weight heparins in the treatment of venous thromboembolism. *Ann Intern Med* 128(12 pt 1):1037, 1998.

Kothari R, Pancioli A, Brott T, Broderick J: Thrombolytic therapy for cerebral infarction. *Acad Emerg Med* 3(9):881, 1996.

Leopold JA, Keaney JF Jr, Loscalzo J: Pharmacology of thrombolytic agents, in Loscalzo J, Schafer AI (eds): *Thrombosis and Hemorrhage,* 2d ed. Baltimore: Williams & Wilkins, 1998, p 1215.

Levine JD, Groopman JE: Hemostatic complications of HIV infection, in Loscalzo J, Schafer AI (eds): *Thrombosis and Hemorrhage,* 2d ed. Baltimore: Williams & Wilkins, 1998, p 1065.

National Institute of Neurologic Disorders and Stroke r-TPA Stroke Study Group: Tissue plasminogen activator for acute ischemic stroke. *N Engl J Med* 333:1581, 1995.

Rao RB, Palmer M, Touger M: Thrombocytopenia after rattlesnake envenomation. *Ann Emerg Med* 31(1):139, 1998.

Williams E: Disseminated intravascular coagulation, in Loscalzo J, Shafer AI (eds): *Thrombosis and Hemorrhage,* 2d ed. Baltimore: Williams & Wilkins, 1998, p 963.

HEMOPHILIAS AND VON WILLEBRAND'S DISEASE

Mary E. Eberst

Hemophilias are hereditary bleeding disorders due to deficiency of factor VIII (hemophilia A, classic hemophilia) or factor IX (hemophilia B, Christmas disease). Von Willebrand's disease is a related hereditary deficiency of a portion of the factor VIII complex. These disorders are discussed below.

HEMOPHILIA

Patients with hemophilia A, factor VIII deficiency, account for 85 percent of patients with hemophilia. This X-linked, recessive disorder occurs in 1 in 10,000 live male births. Hemophilia B, factor IX deficiency, is also an X-linked recessive disorder and occurs in 1 in 25,000 to 30,000 live male births. Thirty percent of affected patients have no family history of hemophilia; spontaneous mutations are believed to be responsible. Females are generally carriers of hemophilia A or B, have 50 percent of normal factor VIII or factor IX activity, and are asymptomatic. On occasion, due to extreme lyonization, a female carrier can have lower factor VIII or factor IX levels and have clinical manifestations of the disease.

Classification

The clinical classification of the hemophilias is based on the severity of deficiency. Patients classified as mildly deficient have 6 to 60 percent of normal factor VIII or factor IX activity; moderate disease is 1 to 5 percent of normal; severe hemophilia describes patients with less than 1 percent of normal factor activity and accounts for 60 percent of all patients. The most common bleeding manifestations are outlined in Table 212-1. Unless there is other underlying disease, patients with hemophilia do not have problems with minor cuts and abrasions. Bleeding in hemophiliacs is characterized by deep hematomas and hemathroses that occur spontaneously or with minimal trauma; the bleeding is often delayed several hours after minor injury.

Unfortunately, bleeding is not the only problem facing patients with hemophilia. Many hemophiliacs also have chronic hepatitis and are infected with the human immunodeficiency virus type 1 (HIV-1) as a result of their exposure to blood products. In hemophilic patients who received plasma products prior to the mid-1980s, 90 percent have serologic evidence of hepatitis B, 85 to 100 percent have hepatitis C antibodies, and 60 to 90 percent have HIV-1 infection. Those most likely to be infected with HIV-1 are patients with severe hemophilia A without an inhibitor. Hemophilia B patients are less likely to be infected with HIV-1 as a result of the products they receive for treatment—about 50 percent are infected. Since 1985, acquired immunodeficiency syndrome (AIDS) has become the leading cause of death in patients with hemophilia. Hemophilic patients with AIDS account for 1 percent of the total U.S. AIDS population. Since 1986, as a result of new viral inactivation procedures, there have been few seroconversions resulting from the use of currently available factor replacement products.

Patients with hemophilia are usually identified in childhood or adolescence; however, those with a mild deficiency may go undetected until there is a major hemostatic challenge. Occasionally, an emergency physician will encounter a patient with acute bleeding who may have an undiagnosed coagulopathy. Table 212-2 lists some historical and clinical findings that might be indicative of the presence of a bleeding disorder. Hematologic consultation should be obtained for these patients.

TABLE 212-1 Common Bleeding Manifestations in Patients with Hemophilia

Site	Comments
Hemarthroses	Leads to joint destruction and chronic arthropathy if not treated aggressively
Hematomas	Bleeding into soft tissues or muscle; this bleeding can dissect along fascial planes; most dangerous near in the neck (airway compromise), limbs (compartment syndromes) and retroperitoneum (massive blood loss)
Mucocutaneous bleeding	Bleeding in the oropharynx, gastrointestinal tract, epistaxis, hemoptysis, bleeding after dental extractions
Central nervous system	Intracranial bleeding is the most common cause of bleeding death in hemophiliacs, has a 34% mortality; subdural hematomas—occur spontaneously or with minimal trauma
Hematuria	Common, usually not serious, and the source is rarely found
Pseudotumor	Bone cysts that result from unresolved hematomas; usually have to be removed surgically

TABLE 212-2 Historical and Clinical Findings Suggestive of an Underlying Coagulopathy

History of easy bruising, epistaxis, menorrhagia, or gastrointestinal bleeding
History of the development of hematomas following minor trauma
History of excessive bleeding after dental extractions or minor surgery
Family history of any of the preceding
Apparent excessive bleeding from minor wounds in the absence of aspirin or nonsteroidal anti-inflammatory therapy
Abnormal coagulation studies not previously known to be abnormal

Testing

Coagulation screening tests in patients with hemophilia typically show a normal prothrombin time (PT), normal thrombin clot time (TCT), and prolonged activated partial thromboplastin time (aPTT), reflective of the abnormality in the intrinsic pathway. However, if the factor VIII level in hemophilia A or factor IX level in hemophilia B is greater than 30 percent of normal activity (mild hemophilia), the aPTT can be normal. The only way to distinguish hemophilia A and hemophilia B is by specific factor assays of factors VIII and IX. Inhibitors are circulating antibodies, usually IgG, that are directed against factor VIII or factor IX, whichever factor the patient is lacking. Inhibitors occur in 10 to 15 percent of patients with severe hemophilia A and in about 10 percent of patients with severe hemophilia B. Inhibitors develop in response to exposure to the ''missing factor'' through replacement therapy. Most of these develop early in life. An inhibitor is diagnosed in the laboratory when the plasma of a patient with hemophilia with a prolonged aPTT is ''mixed'' 50-50 with the plasma of a ''normal'' control. If the aPTT corrects to normal with this ''mix,'' no inhibitor is present, just a factor deficiency. If, however, the mix does not correct, an inhibitor is present. Further testing can be done to determine which coagulation factor the inhibitor is directed against, although in patients with known hemophilia, it is against the missing factor. The quantity of inhibitor that is present is measured most commonly by the Bethesda inhibitor assay (BIA) and is reported in BIA units. This quantitation is important in determining what type of factor replacement therapy the patient will require.

Bleeding Complications

The emergency physician needs to be aware of major bleeding emergencies that can develop in patients with hemophilia. These patients require emergent factor replacement therapy and management by hemophilia specialists. Air transport to specialized centers should be considered for intracranial, intrathoracic, or intraabdominal bleeding, even if the patient appears ''stable.'' Bleeding into the *central nervous system* (CNS) can occur spontaneously as well as with trauma. Any patient with hemophilia who complains of a new headache or any neurologic symptoms requires immediate factor replacement therapy followed by immediate computed tomographic (CT) scanning of the head. Spontaneous or traumatic bleeding into *the neck, retropharynx, or pharynx* has a high potential for airway compromise. Such bleeding can be spontaneous or precipitated by successful or unsuccessful placement of external jugular lines or other trauma. These patients require immediate factor replacement and immediate CT scanning to define the bleeding area. Airway management, including oral intubation, takes priority. If not preceded by factor replacement therapy, intubation must be followed immediately by factor replacement. Hemophilic patients with complaints of back, thigh, groin, or abdominal pain may have bleeding into the *retroperitoneum.* Bleeding into this potential space can be life-threatening because of the large potential area and the ability of the bleeding to dissect along fascial planes. Immediate factor replacement and CT scanning are indicated. *Compartment syndromes* result from muscle bleeds within the fascial compartments of the extremities. Complaints of pain and paresthesias and the findings of sensory, motor, or vascular deficits raise this possibility. After factor replacement therapy is initiated, the compartment pressure can be measured. Surgical fasciotomy may be required and needs to be done within 8 h after the onset of symptoms for best chance of full neurovascular recovery. The most common manifestation of hemophilia that will be encountered is the hemarthrosis. There may or may not be clinical evidence of an acute problem with the joint, but the patient can reliably report when bleeding is occurring. Prompt treatment of hemarthroses can prevent or reduce the long-term sequelae of hemophilic arthropathy. Patients with hemophilia should never receive intramuscular injections unless factor replacement is given and maintained for several days. Central lines, including femoral lines and external jugular lines, should not be placed in patients with hemophilia prior to factor replacement therapy; life-threatening bleeding can result. Arterial blood gases or lumbar puncture should not be performed on patients with hemophilia without coverage of factor replacement therapy. A compartment syndrome can result in the extremity, or epidural bleeding in the spinal canal.

The management of hemophilic bleeding depends on the type of hemophilia that is present, the severity of deficiency, the presence or absence of an inhibitor, and the location of bleeding. Each of these will be discussed separately.

Management of Factor VIII Deficiency (Hemophilia A) without an Inhibitor

Patients with mild or moderate hemophilia A may respond to treatment with desmopressin (1-desamino-8-D-arginine vasopressin, desmopressin). It is helpful to know if the patient has been treated previously with desmopressin successfully. In patients who respond, desmopressin can raise the factor VIII activity level up to threefold. Its mechanism of action is not entirely understood, but desmopressin is believed to cause release of von Willebrand factor (vWF) from storage sites in the endothelial cells; the increased amount of vWF is then capable of carrying additional amounts of factor VIII in the plasma. The usual dose of desmopressin is 0.3 μg/kg of body weight administered intravenously or subcutaneously every 12 h. Some authors suggest 30 μg as a maximum dose. A concentrated form of desmopressin can be administered intranasally. The dose is 150 μg (one metered dose) for patients weighing less than 50 kg and 300 μg for patients weighing 50 kg or more. A response in the factor VIII level should be seen in 1 h. This dose can be repeated three or four times before temporary tachyphylaxis develops. The advantages of desmopressin are that it is not a blood product and therefore carries no risk of viral transmission, and it is easily administered in the hospital or home setting. Serious side effects are uncommon. Common reactions include facial flushing and headache, and mild hyponatremia can develop, especially in pediatric patients.

Patients with moderate or severe hemophilia A and significant bleeding will require treatment with factor VIII concentrates. In settings where virally safe factor VIII concentrates are not available and life-threatening bleeding requires treatment, cryoprecipitate or fresh-frozen plasma (FFP) can be used temporarily; however, these products carry a risk of viral transmission, so they should be administered for this purpose only in true emergencies. Each bag of cryoprecipitate contains about 100 units of factor VIII. FFP contains 1 unit of factor VIII per milliliter of FFP. Most patients with hemophilia A without an inhibitor are treated with factor VIII products made by recombinant DNA technology. Table 212-3 outlines the currently available factor VIII concentrates. Other products of lesser purity, which carry some small risk of hepatitis transmission (but not HIV-1), may still be available and used electively by some patients who are already infected, because of their lower price. These products should not be given to patients with negative or uncertain infection status unless it is a true emergency. Factor VIII concentrates are dosed by units; 1 unit is the amount of factor VIII activity in 1 mL of normal plasma. One unit of factor VIII per kilogram should raise the circulating factor VIII level by 2 percent. The amount of factor VIII needed to raise a patient with hemophilia to a desired circulating level of factor VIII can be calculated by

$$\text{Factor VIII (units)} = \text{weight in kg}/2 \times (\% \text{ activity desired} - \% \text{ intrinsic activity})$$

TABLE 212-3 Currently Available Factor VIII Concentrates

Recombinant products:	Monoclonal antibody purified:
Recombinate	Koate
Kogenate	Monoclate-P
Bioclate	Hemofil-M
Helixate	Monarc-M

Typical dose: One unit of factor VIII per kilogram should raise the circulating factor VIII level by 2%; products are typically dosed every 8–12 h for moderate or life-threatening bleeding events and every 12–24 h for minor bleeding events; dosing depends on patient response and postinfusion factor VIII levels.

Table 212-4 outlines specific treatment recommendations for factor VIII replacement therapy in patients with hemophilia A. After the loading dose, subsequent doses of factor VIII should be adjusted based on factor VIII level assays.

Ancillary therapies in the management of bleeding episodes include rest, potential immobilization, analgesia, and the use of antifibrinolytic agents, which are most commonly used in patients undergoing dental or oral surgery. ε-Aminocaproic acid (EACA) and tranexamic acid are examples. These can be used alone in some cases or in conjunction with factor VIII concentrates. These agents are contraindicated in patients with hematuria.

Management of Factor VIII Deficiency (Hemophilia A) with Inhibitor Present

The use of factor replacement therapy in hemophilic patients with inhibitors is guided by the inhibitor titer (number of BIA units) and the type of response the patient has to factor VIII concentrates. This anamnestic response is usually either a rapid increase in the inhibitor titer within 2 to 3 days (high responders) or a low response where the inhibitor increases little or none (low responders). Table 212-5 outlines the treatment options available for treatment of hemophilia A patients with inhibitors.

Management of Factor IX Deficiency (Hemophilia B) without an Inhibitor

Table 212-6 outlines the goals of replacement therapy for patients with hemophilia B. The products that are available for replacement therapy are listed in Table 212-7. The highly purified factor IX concentrates are the treatment of choice if available. One unit of factor IX

TABLE 212-4 Factor VIII Replacement Therapy for Patients with Hemophilia A (No Inhibitor)

Type of Hemorrhage	Factor VIII Level Required for Hemostasis, % of Normal	Factor VIII Dose in Units/kg (Initial Dose)	Dosing Interval, h*	Duration of Therapy, Days
Minor				
Hemarthroses	30–50	15–25	24	1–2
Superficial muscular or soft tissue	30–50	15–25	24	1–2
Moderate				
Epistaxis	30–50	15–25	12	Until resolved
Dental extractions	50	25	12–24	1–2
Muscular or soft tissue with dissection	50–100	25–50	12	Variable
GI bleeding	50–100	25–50	12	7–10
Hematuria	50–100	25–50	12	Until resolved
Life threatening				
Central nervous system	75–100	50	12	10–14
Retropharynx/pharnyx	75–100	50	12	10–14
Retroperitoneum	75–100	50	12	10–14
Surgery	75–100	50	12	Variable

Note: GI, gastrointestinal.
*Continuous infusion of factor VIII concentrate may be used in hospitalized patients; a typical dose after the loading dose is 150 units/h; this is adjusted based on factor VIII levels.

per kilogram should raise the circulating factor IX level by 1 percent. This amount can be calculated by

Factor IX (units) = kg × (% activity desired − % intrinsic activity)

If it is necessary to raise the factor IX level to 75 to 100 percent (e.g., life-threatening situations), this should be done with the highly purified concentrates because they carry essentially no risk of thrombogenicity. In settings where factor IX concentrates are not available, FFP can be used to raise the factor IX level. The use of FFP in this setting should be limited to emergency treatment because of the small risk of viral transmission and the inability to raise the factor IX levels adequately because of volume constraints. One unit of FFP will raise the factor IX level by 3 percent in an average-sized person.

TABLE 212-5 Replacement Therapy for Hemophilia A Patients with Inhibitors

Type of Product (Trade Names)	Used For	Dose	Frequency, h	Comments
Factor VIII concentrates	Inhibitor titer less than 5–10 BIA units	5000–10,000 unit bolus	Continuous infusion at about 1000 units/h	If patient is a "high responder," in about 3 days the inhibitor titer will rise
Prothrombin complex concentrates (PCCs)				
PCCs contain factors II, VII, IX, X (Bebulin VH, Proplex T, Profilnine HT, and Konyne-80)	Inhibitor titer >10 units; known good response to these products	75–100 units/kg of body-weight	Repeat dose q8–12h	Complications of use include development of thromboembolic disease, DIC, very low risk of hepatitis transmission
Activated prothrombin complex concentrates				
aPPCs contain factors II, VII, IX, and X with variable amounts of activated factors VII_a, IX_a, and X_a (Autoplex, FEIBA)	Patients who do not respond to PCCs	Same as with PCCs	Repeat dose q12–24h	Same as with PCCs
Porcine factor VIII	Patients with high inhibitor titers not responsive to the above products	Variable	Variable	Patients will often develop an inhibitor to the procine product
Recombinant factor VII_a	Not yet commercially available	Variable	Variable	Less thrombogenic risk than PCCs and no risk of viral transmission

TABLE 212-6 Factor IX Replacement Therapy for Patients with Hemophilia B

Type of Hemorrhage	Factor IX Level Required for Hemostasis, % of Normal	Initial Factor IX Dose in Units/kg	Duration of Therapy, Days
Minor			
Hemarthroses	20–30	20–30	1–2
Superficial muscular or soft tissue	20–30	20–30	1–2
Moderate			
Epistaxis	25–50	25–50	Until resolved
Dental extractions	25–50	25–50	2–7
Muscular or soft tissue bleeds with dissection	25–50	25–50	Until resolved
Hematuria	25–50	25–50	Until resolved
GI bleeding	50	50	5–10
Life-threatening*			
Central nervous system	50	50	7–10
Retropharynx/pharynx	50	50	7–10
Retroperitoneum	50	50	7–10
Surgery	50	50	7–10

*Factor IX levels higher than 50% may be necessary and are safely obtained using the highly purified factor IX concentrates.

Management of Factor IX Deficiency (Hemophilia B) with Inhibitor Present

The products available for the treatment of hemophilia B patients with inhibitors are outlined in Table 212-8 along with treatment guidelines. The treatment of each patient must be individualized based on the clinical response.

Indications for Hospital Admission

Hemophilic patients with bleeding episodes will require hospital admission in these situations:

TABLE 212-7 Products used for Replacement Therapy in Patients with Hemophilia B

Highly purified factor IX concentrates:	**Typical dose:**
• Benefix (recombinant factor IX)	One to two units of factor IX per kilogram should raise the circulating factor IX level by 1%; usually dosed every 12–24 h based on patient response and postinfusion factor IX levels.
• Mononine	One unit of factor IX per kilogram should raise the circulating factor IX level by 1%; usually dosed every 18–30 h based on patient response and postinfusion factor IX levels.
Prothrombin complex concentrates:	**Typical dose:**
• Bebulin VH • Proplex T • Profilnine HT • Konyne-80	One unit of factor IX per kilogram raises the factor IX level by 1%; subsequent doses are typically given every 12 h based on patient response.

TABLE 212-8 Products Used for Replacement Therapy in Patients with Hemophilia B with Inhibitors

Type of Product	Used for	Initial Dose
Highly purified factor IX concentrates	Bethesda inhibitor titer <10 units	Variable
Prothrombin complex concentrates (PCCs)	Bethesda inhibitor titer <10 units	75 units/kg
Activated prothrombin complex concentrates (aPCCs)	Bethesda inhibitor titers >10 units or unresponsive to the above	Variable, about 75 units/kg
Recombinant factor VII_a	Not yet commercially available	Variable

- The patient has potentially life-threatening bleeding involving the CNS, neck, pharynx, retropharynx or retroperitoneum, or potential compartment syndrome.
- The patient is not capable of administering factor replacement therapy at home.
- The patient requires treatment for several days.
- The patient needs close monitoring.
- The patient requires parenteral pain control.

VON WILLEBRAND'S DISEASE

Von Willebrand's disease, which is caused by a deficiency or abnormality of vWF, is the most common inherited bleeding disorder. The vWF is a glycoprotein that is synthesized, stored, and secreted by vascular endothelial cells; it is also found in plasma and platelets. vWF has two functions: (1) in primary hemostasis, vWF allows platelets to adhere to the damaged endothelium; and (2) vWF carries factor VIII in the plasma.

It is estimated that 1 in 100 persons has a gene defective for vWF, which is inherited in an autosomal dominant pattern. However, only 1 in 10,000 manifests a clinically significant bleeding disorder. The most severe type of von Willebrand's disease (vWD), known as type III, is very rare, occurring in 1 in 1 million persons; it results from an autosomal recessive defect.

Testing

A variety of tests are used to establish the diagnosis of vWD. Coagulation screening tests will show a normal PT, normal TCT, and usually normal aPTT, although it may be prolonged in moderate or severe vWD due to the decreased factor VIII activity. The other tests used in the evaluation of vWD are outlined in Table 212-9. The diagnosis of vWD can be difficult to establish because of variability in test results. Oftentimes, patients have to be tested repeatedly when there is a high index of suspicion in order to establish the diagnosis. The tests can be affected by estrogens, progesterones, oral contraceptive agents, thyroid disease, infections, and exercise.

Based on the results of testing, patients with vWD can be classified into three main types, outlined in Table 212-10. There are many subtypes that are clinically unimportant.

Von Willebrand's disease can be difficult to distinguish from mild hemophilia A. The bleeding time should be normal in hemophilia, although it is also often normal in patients with vWD. The von Willebrand antigen and activity should be normal or elevated in patients with hemophilia. The factor VIII activity level will be low in patients with hemophilia and may be normal or slightly low in patients with

TABLE 212-9 Laboratory Evaluation of Patients with von Willebrand's Disease*

Test	Typical Result in vWD	Comments
Bleeding time	Prolonged	Measures platelet and vessel wall interaction (primary hemostasis); this test has high variability—if prolonged, it is important data; if normal, does not rule out vWD
vWF antigen	Low or normal	Is an acute phase reactant, increased in stress and pregnancy
vWF activity	Low	Evaluates the function of vWF by measuring the ability of vWF to agglutinate platelets in the presence of the antibiotic ristocetin
Factor VIII activity	Low or normal	May be normal or slightly decreased in vWD, except very low or absent in type III vWD
Multimeric analysis	Variable	Separates the vWF molecule into its subunits (multimers) based on molecular weight; needed to distinguish types of vWD

Note: vWF, von Willebrand's factor; vWD, von Willebrand's disease.

vWD. In some cases, it is nearly impossible to distinguish type I vWD and mild hemophilia A.

Bleeding Complications

The hemorrhagic tendency in patients with vWD is highly variable among patients with the same type of vWD, even among patients from the same family who have an identical genetic defect. Most characteristics are mild bleeding symptoms from mucocutaneous surfaces (such as epistaxis), easy bruising, bleeding after dental extractions, menorrhagia, and gastrointestinal bleeding. Patients with type III vWD have a severe bleeding diathesis with spontaneous hematomas and hemarthroses similar to patients with severe hemophilia.

Treatment

The treatment of vWD depends on the type of disease that is present and the severity of bleeding. Table 212-11 shows the recommended therapy for patients with vWD. Desmopressin is the mainstay of therapy for patients with type I vWD; plasma products that contain vWF are used for types II and III. Desmopressin can be administered subcutaneously or intravenously at a dose of 0.3 μg/kg of body weight. This dose is given every 12 h to a total of three or four doses before temporary tachyphylaxis develops. A concentrated form of desmopressin can be administered intranasally. The dose is 150 μg (one metered dose) for patients weighing less than 50 kg and 300 μg for patients weighing 50 kg, more. In a setting where treatment is essential and desmopressin or the specifically recommended factor VIII concentrates are not available, cryoprecipitate can be used to replace the vWF that is needed for hemostasis. Each bag of cryoprecipitate contains about 100 units of vWF activity. Cryoprecipitate should only be used in emergencies because there is a small risk of viral transmission. Women with vWD are often treated with hormonal agents (estrogens and/or progesterones), which cause an increase in the vWF activity. Bleeding associated with dental procedures can often be managed with fibrinolytic inhibitor agents such as EACA and tranexamic acid.

TABLE 212-10 Classification of von Willebrand's Disease

Type	Occurrence	Defect
I	70–80% of patients with vWD	All multimeric forms are present but their quantity is diminished
II	10–15%	The vWF molecule is abnormal, missing some of the multimers
III	<10%	Essentially no vWF is present

Note: vWD, von Willebrand's disease; vWF, von Willebrand's factor.

TABLE 212-11 Suggested Treatment for Patients with von Willebrand's Disease

Type I	Desmopressin (DDAVP)
Type II	Factor VIII concentrates (Humate-P or Koate-HS) or cryoprecipitate
Type III	Factor VIII concentrates (Humate-P or Koate-HS) or cryoprecipitate

BIBLIOGRAPHY

DiMichele DM, Green D: Hemophilia: Factor VIII deficiency, in Loscalzo J, Schafer AI (eds): *Thrombosis and Hemorrhage,* 2d ed. Baltimore: Williams & Wilkins, 1998, p 757.

Lusher JM, Sarnaik S: Hematology. *JAMA* 275 (23):1814, 1996.

Nichols WC, Cooney KA, Ginsburg D, Ruggeri ZM: Von Willebrand disease, in Loscalzo J, Schafer AI (eds): *Thrombosis and Hemorrhage,* 2d ed. Baltimore: Williams & Wilkins, 1998, p 729.

Roberts HR, Bingham MD: Other coagulation factor deficiencies, in Loscalzo J, Schafer AI (eds): *Thrombosis and Hemorrhage,* 2d ed. Baltimore: Williams & Wilkins, 1998, p 773.

Seremetis SV, Aledort LM: Desmopressin nasal spray for hemophilia A and type I van Willebrand disease. *Ann Intern Med* 126(9):744, 1997.

Triemstra M, Rosendaal FR, Smit C, et al: Mortality in patients with hemophilia: Changes in a Dutch population from 1986 to 1992 and 1973 to 1986. *Ann Intern Med* 123(11):823, 1995.

Voelker R: New focus placed on von Willebrand disease. *JAMA* 278(14):1137, 1997.

HEREDITARY HEMOLYTIC ANEMIAS

Mary E. Eberst

This chapter discusses the most common inherited hemolytic anemias including the hemoglobinopathies, sickle cell anemia and its variants, glucose-6-phosphate dehydrogenase deficiency (which is a red blood cell enzymatic defect) and hereditary spherocytosis (a defect in the red blood cell membrane).

SICKLE CELL ANEMIA

Pathophysiology

A hemoglobinopathy is an inherited disease resulting from the presence of one or more abnormal hemoglobins. More than 400 hemoglobin variants have been described. Normal human hemoglobin consists of four polypeptide chains and four heme groups. The four polypeptide chains consist of two alpha chains and two nonalpha chains, which are most commonly beta. The majority of hemoglobin in a normal adult consists of two alpha chains and two beta chains and is called *hemoglobin A* (HbA, $\alpha_2\beta_2$). Other normal nonalpha chains are gamma (hemoglobin F) and delta (hemoglobin A_2) (Table 213-1).

The most common hemoglobin variant, known as *hemoglobin S* (HbS), results from a single point mutation on the beta chain: Valine is substituted for glutamic acid in the sixth position. Hemoglobin S is little problem when it is carrying oxygen (oxyhemoglobin form), but when it is deoxygenated, HbS polymerizes within the red blood cell causing the sickle shape. Sickled red blood cells increase the viscosity of the blood, leading to sludging or obstruction in the microcirculation. Eventually, the cells may become irreversibly sickled. Conditions that increase the amount of sickling include acidosis and increased 2,3-diphosphoglycerate (both cause the oxygen dissociation curve to shift to the right, which favors the formation of the deoxyhemoglobin form), vascular stasis, dehydration, the presence of higher levels of HbS in the cells, and low oxygen tension. The presence of hemoglobin F (HbF) has a protective role; higher HbF levels are associated with less sickling phenomena. Sickled red blood cells are rapidly hemolyzed resulting in a red blood cell survival of 10 to 20 days, compared with the normal red blood cell lifespan of 120 days.

In the US African-American population, about 8 percent carry the sickle cell gene; these persons have HbAS ($\alpha_2\beta S$, sickle cell trait). Inherited in an autosomal codominant pattern, sickle cell disease (SCD) results when the patient inherits the sickle gene from both parents. This is hemoglobin SS ($\alpha_2 S_2$) and occurs in 0.14 to 0.20 percent of the US African-American population, resulting in about 50,000 patients with SCD. When the sickle cell gene is inherited from one parent and another abnormal beta-chain gene is inherited from the other parent, heterozygous hemoglobinopathies result, such as hemoglobin SC disease and sickle–β thalassemia (see below).

Clinical Features

The clinical manifestations of SCD are variable between patients, but all are related to chronic hemolytic anemia, and virtually every organ system can be affected by recurrent vasooclusive events. First, we will review the common clinical findings in patients with SCD; then we will discuss the problems that are likely to bring the patient to the emergency department (Table 213-2).

Patients with SCD have a chronic hemolytic anemia with a baseline hemoglobin of 6 to 9 g/dL and a reticulocyte count of 5 to 15 percent. These patients commonly have cardiopulmonary disease, including decreased pulmonary function and reserve, decreased resting arterial oxygen tension, systolic and diastolic flow murmurs, congestive heart failure, cardiomegaly, and cor pulmonale. Myocardial infarction is rare in patients with SCD. Icterus is the rule as a result of chronic hemolysis. Bilirubin gallstones are found in up to 75 percent of patients with SCD. Hepatomegaly and liver function test abnormalities are common. Splenomegaly is seen in children with SCD; however, by adulthood, the spleen is usually small as a result of recurrent infarction. Renal abnormalities including isosthenuria (inability to concentrate urine) and papillary necrosis occur commonly because of sickling phenomena in the hypertonic, acidic renal medulla. Bony abnormalities, resulting from expansion of the marrow space, and bony infarcts are typical. Radiographs of the bones show thinning of the cortices and sparseness of the trabecular pattern; the biconcave "fishmouth" changes in the vertebrae are pathognomonic of SCD. Skin ulcerations occur over the distal lower extremities. Ophthalmologic problems primarily involving the retinae are common. Chronic disabilities resulting from central nervous system vasoocclusive events are seen.

TABLE 213-1 Composition of Normal Human Hemoglobin and the Sickle Hemoglobin Variants

Phenotype	Types of Hemoglobin Present	Percent	Genotype
Normal adult	HbA	96–98	2 alpha 2 beta
	HbF	0.5–0.8	2 alpha 2 gamma
	HbA_2	1.5–3.2	2 alpha 2 delta
Sickle cell trait (heterozygous)	HbAS	A 60–65 S 35–40	2 alpha 1 beta 1 sickle
Sickle cell disease (homozygous)	HbSS	S 80–90	2 alpha 2 sickle
	HbF	F 2–20	2 alpha 2 gamma
	HbA_2	A_2 2–4	2 alpha 2 delta

TABLE 213-2 Clinical Emergencies in Patients with Sickle Cell Anemia

Vasoocclusive Crises	Hematologic Crises	Infectious Crises
Musculoskeletal pain	Splenic sequestration	Pneumonia
Abdominal pain	Aplastic crisis	Meningitis
Pulmonary crisis		Osteomyelitis
Central nervous system crisis		Urinary tract infection
Priapism		Sepsis
Hand and foot syndrome		
Renal crisis		

Since the mid-1990s, many patients with SCD have been treated with hydroxyurea. Hydroxyurea can significantly decrease the clinical manifestations of SCD in many patients. Hydroxyurea is believed to work by increasing the concentration of HbF and results in decreased sickling phenomena.

Table 213-2 outlines the types of crises that occur in patients with SCD. Frequently, a patient will have more than one type of crisis at a time.

VASOOCCLUSIVE CRISES Painful vasoocclusive crises are the most common reason for visits to the emergency department (ED) by patients with SCD. These crises account for the greatest morbidity and mortality among these patients. The average adult sickle cell patient has four severe attacks per year; however, some patients experience crises daily. Vasoocclusive events are more common in adult patients with higher hemoglobin levels and lower amounts of HbF. The underlying pathophysiology is sludging of sickled red blood cells in the microcirculation with infarction. This event can be precipitated by infection, exposure to cold, dehydration, and high altitude. In children, up to 80 percent of the vasoocclusive events are infection-related. In adults, up to one-third of vasoocclusive crises are related to bacterial or viral infections, but the majority of crises are unexplained. Patients can have "typical" crises with pain in the same location recurrently, but the pain can be anywhere.

Musculoskeletal Pain Vasoocclusive crisis with pain involving the bones, joints, and muscles is the most prominent manifestation of SCD. This pain can be anywhere but most often involves the humerus, tibia, femur, and low back area. Examination may reveal local tenderness, but often there are no physical findings. The differential diagnosis includes osteomyelitis and acute arthritides such as gout and rheumatoid arthritis. Pain in the hip with difficulty walking raises the possibility of avascular necrosis (AVN) of the femoral head. If there is local tenderness or an effusion, an aspirate should be obtained for culture or the joint fluid evaluated for signs of infection. Plain radiographs may show changes of osteomyelitis or AVN but are of little value in detecting bony infarction. Magnetic resonance imaging (MRI) can be used to document infarction. Bone scans and gallium scans can differentiate infarction from osteomyelitis and may show osteomyelitis in the early stages before plain radiographs will show abnormalities.

Abdominal Pain This is the second most common type of vasoocclusive crisis experienced by patients with SCD. Abdominal pain due to vasoocclusive crisis typically is of relatively acute onset, diffuse, poorly localized, and often recurrent. These patients have diffuse pain without peritoneal signs; bowel sounds should be present. Pain in the right upper quadrant (RUQ) raises the possibility of cholecystitis and the RUQ syndrome. At least 75 percent of patients with SCD have bilirubin gallstones; however, only 10 percent are ever symptomatic. The RUQ syndrome involves the sudden onset of RUQ pain, progressive hepatomegaly, and extreme hyperbilirubinemia (>50 mg/dL). Resulting from intrahepatic cholestasis, the outcome of the RUQ syndrome is usually benign in pediatric patients, but some adult patients progress to liver failure. The remainder of the differential diagnosis of sickle cell patients with abdominal pain suspected of having vasoocclusive crisis includes pancreatitis, mesenteric infarction, hepatitis, hepatic infarction, appendicitis, perforated viscus, and pelvic inflammatory disease. Ultrasound examination and computed tomographic (CT) scanning of the abdomen and pelvis may be helpful. Surgical consultation is indicated if the diagnosis remains uncertain.

Pulmonary Crisis This problem occurs in up to 30 percent of patients with SCD and accounts for 15 percent of adult deaths. The presentation of pleuritic chest pain, fever, leukocytosis, and possible pulmonary infiltrate raises the differential diagnosis of pulmonary infarction, acute chest syndrome, bacterial or viral pneumonia, and pulmonary thromboembolus. The acute chest syndrome occurs when a pulmonary infarct becomes secondarily infected. This is a major cause of death in patients with SCD above age 10. Such patients often have a precipitous decrease in pulmonary function and severe hypoxia. The chest radiograph may not show an infiltrate for up to 2 days. Arterial blood gas analysis, complete blood count (CBC), and the presence of sputum may be helpful. Ventilation-perfusion ($\dot{V}/\dot{Q}$) scan of the lung may be helpful, especially if a baseline study for comparison is available. Pulmonary angiography should be avoided, if possible, because the contrast material can induce more pulmonary sickling. Sickle cell patients with significant pulmonary signs or symptoms should be admitted to the hospital. Empiric antibiotics are often given until the diagnosis becomes clear.

Central Nervous System Crisis This is the only type of vasoocclusive crisis that is painless. Overall, neurologic complications occur in 15 to 25 percent of patients with SCD. The most common problems are cerebral infarction in children and cerebral hemorrhage in adults. Other complications of central nervous system (CNS) vasoocclusive events are transient ischemic attacks, seizures, headache, dizziness, cranial nerve palsies, unexplained coma, paresthesia, meningitis, vestibular dysfunction, and sensory hearing loss. There is an increased incidence of subarachnoid hemorrhage (SAH) in patients with SCD. Evaluation of patients with CNS complaints should include a CT scan of the head and a lumbar puncture to rule out SAH and meningitis. MRI is better than CT scanning for demonstrating the CNS effects of vasoocclusive phenomena.

Priapism This complication occurs in up to 30 percent of males with SCD. The persistent, painful erection results from the sickling of cells in the corpus cavernosum, which prevents the emptying of blood from the penis. Surgical decompression may be required, and permanent impotence may result.

Hand and Foot Syndrome (Dactylitis) This complication of SCD usually occurs in the first 2 years of life and may be the first sign that a child has SCD. The patient presents with swelling of the hands and/or feet (one to four extremities involved) that is the result of vasoocclusion of the nutrient arteries to the metacarpals and/or metatarsals. Avascular necrosis of the bone marrow in the involved bones occurs.

Renal Crisis Vasoocclusive events involving the kidneys are very common but often asymptomatic. Infarction in the renal medulla may cause flank pain, renal colic-type pain, and costovertebral angle tenderness. Patients may have gross or microscopic hematuria and may pass tissue resulting from papillary necrosis. Pyelonephritis and urinary tract infection must be excluded, and adequate/stable renal function should be documented.

HEMATOLOGIC CRISES Heralded by an acute drop in the hemoglobin level, patients with hematologic crisis will present with weakness, shortness of breath, fatigue, worsening of congestive heart failure, or shock. There are two types of hematologic crisis.

Acute Splenic Sequestration This occurs primarily in children and is the second most common cause of death in children with SCD under the age of 5. Often preceded by viral infections, sickled cells block the splenic outflow, causing pooling of peripheral blood and sickled cells in the spleen. Such patients present in hypovolemic shock with an enlarged spleen. These crises are divided into major and minor. In a major sequestration crisis, the spleen enlarges rapidly and the hemoglobin drops to <6 g/dL or >3 g/dL from baseline. A minor sequestration crisis is specified by an enlarging spleen and a hemoglobin >6 g/dL. These patients will have a higher than usual reticulocyte count reflective of normal compensatory bone marrow activity. Such patients are managed with transfusion of red blood cells and exchange transfusions; splenectomy may be considered.

Aplastic Crisis This life-threatening complication of SCD occurs when bone marrow erythropoiesis is slowed or stopped. The hematocrit falls to as low as 10 percent, and the reticulocyte count falls to as low as 0.5 percent. The white blood cell count and platelet counts usually remain stable. Aplastic crises can be precipitated by viral infections (particularly parvovirus B_{19}), folic acid deficiency, or the ingestion of bone marrow toxins such as phenylbutazone. This is usually a self-limited problem, but red blood cell transfusions may be required for severe anemia or cardiopulmonary compromise.

INFECTIOUS CRISES Infection is a common contributor to death in patients of all ages with SCD, especially children under the age of 5. Functionally asplenic after early childhood and with impaired phagocyte functioning, patients with SCD are and should be treated as immunocompromised hosts. Sickle cell patients who present with an unexplained fever of 38.3°C (101°F) or higher require evaluation for a source of bacterial infection and consideration for early treatment with broad-spectrum antibiotics. Sickle cell patients can be rapidly overwhelmed by bacterial sepsis, particularly with encapsulated organisms, such as *Hemophilus influenzae* and *Streptococcus pneumoniae.* Other common diseases are pneumonia caused by these organisms as well as *Mycoplasma pneumoniae,* meningitis, and osteomyelitis due to *Salmonella typhimurium, Staphylococcus aureus,* and *Escherichia coli.* Patients with iron overload from frequent transfusions who are treated with the chelating agent deferoxamine are at risk for infection with *Yersinia enterocolitica.*

Diagnosis

The diagnosis of SCD is usually established in early life based on the family history, ideally before the child begins to develop complications. The diagnosis is made by documenting the presence of sickle hemoglobin. Sickled red blood cells should be seen on the peripheral smear. Quick tests to determine the presence of sickle hemoglobin are the metabisulfite test and the Sickledex (Ortho-Clinical Diagnostics) test. Hemoglobin electrophoresis is required to distinguish homozygous SS disease from sickle cell trait and the other heterozygous sickle syndromes.

LABORATORY STUDIES The laboratory evaluation required for an individual patient who presents to the ED can be tailored to the symptoms of the patient and the physical findings. Commonly obtained studies include the following evaluations.

Complete Blood Count A complete blood count (CBC) should be obtained in most sickle cell patients with severe crisis. The "normal" white blood cell count in patients with SCD ranges from 12,000/μL to 18,000/μL but usually has a normal differential. Elevations higher than the patient's baseline or the presence of a left shift are notable. The baseline hemoglobin in sickle cell patients is typically 6 to 9 g/dL. A fall in the hemoglobin by 2 g/dL or a fall in the hematocrit by 4 to 6 percent may reflect hematologic crisis or blood loss. The platelet count is often elevated at baseline. The peripheral smear should show sickled cells and Howell-Jolly bodies, which indicate the loss of splenic function.

Reticulocyte Count A reticulocyte count should be obtained if the hemoglobin has fallen by 2 g/dL or more. The baseline reticulocyte count is typically 5 to 15 percent; lower values may reflect aplastic crisis.

Electrolytes Electrolytes should be obtained in any patient who appears significantly dehydrated, because imbalances occur readily due to isosthenuria.

Liver Function Tests Liver function tests should be obtained in sickle cell patients who present with abdominal pain. These patients often have baseline abnormalities and a chronically elevated indirect bilirubin due to chronic hemolysis.

Erythrocyte Sedimentation Rate The erythrocyte sedimentation rate (ESR) is not a reliable indicator of inflammation or infection in patients with SCD because sickled cells cannot form rouleaux, which is the basis for the test. The ESR is helpful only if it is elevated, since a normal value does not rule out infection or inflammation.

Arterial Blood Gas An arterial blood gas should be obtained in any patient with SCD who presents with respiratory complaints. It is very helpful to know a baseline value because adults may have chronic mild to moderate hypoxia. A Pa_{O_2} of less than 60 mmHg in adults or less than 70 mmHg in children usually indicates an acute problem.

Urinalysis A urinalysis should be obtained in any sickle cell patient with urinary symptoms or fever.

RADIOLOGIC STUDIES **Chest X-ray** A chest x-ray should be obtained in any patient with pulmonary signs or symptoms. In the acute chest syndrome, the chest x-ray may be normal for 2 days, so a normal radiograph does not exclude a problem.

Bone Films Bone films should be considered for the patient who presents with localized bone tenderness. Plain radiographs will not show infarction and will only show osteomyelitis after about 10 days. A bone scan or MRI can show changes of osteomyelitis within 24 h.

Abdominal Ultrasound or CT Scan An abdominal ultrasound or CT scan may be helpful in patients with abdominal pain. The presence of vasoocclusive crisis will not alter these studies; however, they may show changes of cholecystitis, pancreatitis, bowel infarction, abscesses, or appendicitis.

Computed Tomography of Head or MRI Scan Computed tomography of the head (head CT) or an MRI scan should be obtained in any sickle cell patient who presents with neurologic symptoms or signs. MRI is a more sensitive study in this setting.

General Management

General recommendations will be reviewed here as well as some specific guidelines for the initial treatment of complications. Additional suggestions are included above under the types of crises and laboratory and radiologic evaluation.

The general management of patients with sickle cell disease who present to the ED is primarily supportive. Patients with unstable vital signs or neurologic compromise need emergency care. The basic care of patients who present with "crisis" include the following:

Hydration. Any type of crisis may be precipitated or exacerbated by dehydration. Oral rehydration can be attempted if the patient can tolerate fluids and the episode is relatively mild. Intravenous rehydration will be needed for patients who are orthostatic or in severe pain. Fluid overload needs to be avoided in light of potential underlying cardiopulmonary disease. One-half normal saline at a rate of one to one and a half times maintenance dose is a reasonable fluid choice.

Analgesia. Sickle cell patients need prompt pain relief with adequate analgesia. The presence of narcotic addiction or the potential for its development should not alter what is prescribed in the ED. Sickle cell patients who frequently seek help in the ED will benefit from a protocol treatment plan so they know what to expect and manipulative behavior is minimized. The emergency staff should have a consistent approach to the use of narcotics in these patients. It is reasonable to administer up to two doses of narcotics in the ED over a 4- to 6-h period; if patients still have significant pain, they should be admitted to the hospital. Nonnarcotic analgesics such as acetaminophen or ibuprofen can be used for mild pain, although most sickle cell patients do not come to the ED for mild pain. Although ketorolac will not manage the pain of a severe crisis, some have found it helpful as an adjunctive treatment. Oral narcotics such as acetaminophen-codeine or oxycodone may be adequate for moderate pain. Parenteral narcotics are necessary for severe pain. A combination of meperidine and promethazine is commonly used. A typical dose would be 100 mg of meperidine and 25 mg of promethazine intravenously or intramuscularly. Some patients will have developed tolerance to narcotics and require larger doses. Intravenous morphine, sometimes via patient-controlled analgesia is useful in selected patients.

Supplemental oxygen. Supplemental oxygen is only beneficial if the patient is hypoxemic.

Cardiac monitoring. Cardiac monitoring should be considered if the patient has a history of cardiopulmonary compromise or any acute complaints referable to those systems.

Specific Recommendations for Complications

INFECTIONS Sickle cell patients with infectious symptoms or a temperature greater than 38.3°C (101°F) should be presumed to have a bacterial infection. Basic laboratory studies should be obtained as well as cultures of blood, sputum, and urine as indicated. Radiographs should be obtained. There should be a low threshold for lumbar puncture. In most patients, parenteral antibiotics should be administered for 48 h or until the cultures are finalized. Intravenous cephalosporins such as cefuroxime or ceftriaxone are generally used. Suggested oral or outpatient regimens would be cefprozil or amoxicillin/clavulanate.

Sickle cell patients need to be vaccinated in childhood against *S. pneumoniae, H. influenzae,* and hepatitis B. Children with SCD generally receive prophylactic daily oral penicillin up to age 6; this practice is not known to be helpful in adults.

PULMONARY CRISIS Sickle cell patients with pulmonary crisis need aggressive management including hospitalization until the diagnosis becomes apparent. Since the differential diagnosis includes pneumonia, empirical antibiotics such as cefuroxime and erythromycin are often given. Oxygen is administered for hypoxemia, and close monitoring is needed for possible decompensation. Pulmonary thromboembolism is also in this differential diagnosis. If significant $\dot{V}/\dot{Q}$ mismatch is demonstrated on $\dot{V}/\dot{Q}$ scan or large vessel occlusion on pulmonary angiography, heparinization is indicated. Patients with significant cardiopulmonary decompensation may be treated with exchange transfusion.

CNS CRISIS Sickle cell patients with signs or symptoms of neurologic compromise need emergent care and close monitoring. After the patient is stabilized, a head CT or MRI should be obtained. If there is no contraindication, a lumbar puncture should be performed to rule out SAH and meningitis. Seizures and cerebral edema are managed conventionally. These patients require admission to an intensive care unit. When there is an acute CNS event, exchange transfusion is used to lower the HbS concentration to less than 30 percent.

LOCALIZED BONE PAIN This finding, especially when accompanied by fever and leukocytosis, raises the possibility of osteomyelitis. Radiographs, bone scan, or MRI may not be immediately helpful or available. The site should be directly aspirated for culture, and the patient started on parenteral antibiotics to cover *S. aureus* and *S. typhimurium,* such as fluoroquinolone or third-generation cephalosporin.

PRIAPISM When a patient with sickle cell disease presents with priapism, urologic consultation should be obtained. The patient should receive analgesia and hydration, and the bladder should be emptied by catheterization, if possible. Exchange transfusions may be instituted, but if not successful, surgical intervention will be necessary.

Disposition

After evaluation in the ED (including physical examination and laboratory and radiographic studies as indicated), conservative supportive therapy, and observation, a diagnosis usually can be established that will dictate the disposition of the patient.

The following are some guidelines for hospital admission for sickle cell patients:

1. Patients with pulmonary, neurologic, or infectious crisis
2. Patients with splenic sequestration or aplastic crisis
3. Patients with other types of vasoocclusive crises who do not have adequate pain control after analgesics in the ED, the determination to be made after 4 to 6 h and no more than 2 doses of narcotic analgesics.
4. Patients who are unable to maintain adequate hydration
5. Patients in whom the diagnosis is uncertain

Patients with SCD who are discharged from the ED need to have the following:

1. The ability to maintain adequate oral hydration
2. A 2- or 3-day supply of oral analgesics that provide adequate pain relief
3. Instructions to return to the ED for increased pain, fever greater than 38°C (100.4°F), or a change in their symptoms
4. Follow-up, preferably with their primary care physician, in 12 to 24 h for children or 24 to 48 h for adults.

VARIANTS OF SICKLE CELL DISEASE

Sickle Cell Trait

This carrier state for SCD is the most frequently encountered sickle hemoglobin variant; it is *not* a mild form of sickle cell disease. Approximately 8 percent of the US African-American population, or 2.5 million people, carry the gene for sickle hemoglobin. This heterozygous state is a result of autosomal dominant inheritance and results in HbAS. Each red blood cell contains both normal HbA (60 percent) and HbS (40 percent). The abundance of normal HbA prevents sickling under most physiologic circumstances. Hematologically, these patients are normal. Their red blood cells have a normal life span, so they are not anemic. Sickled red blood cells should not be seen on peripheral blood smear except under extreme hypoxia; if seen under normal circumstances, the diagnosis is incorrect.

Clinically, patients with sickle cell trait have minimal complications. The kidney is the most frequently affected organ. Microinfarcts occur in the medulla, leading to papillary necrosis and impaired concentrating ability. Hematuria can be found in 1 percent of patients with sickle cell trait. Exposure to high altitude has been associated with splenic infarction and cerebrovascular complications. Women with sickle cell trait have an increased incidence of urinary tract infections and hematuria during pregnancy. Persons with sickle cell trait have an increased incidence of sudden death during physical training, presumably due to increased sickling with extreme exertion. However, the majority of patients with sickle cell trait are asymptomatic, lead normal lives, and overall have a normal life expectancy.

Sickle Cell–Hemoglobin C Disease (HbSC Disease)

This heterozygous sickle cell variant results when the gene for HbS is inherited from one parent and the gene for HbC is inherited from the other parent. Hemoglobin C results from a single point mutation in the beta-chain gene; lysine is substituted for glutamic acid at the sixth position. About 2.4 percent of US African-Americans carry the gene for HbC. This gene frequency is one-fourth that for HbS, but the prevalence among adults of SC and SS disease is almost the same because those with HbC have a near-normal life expectancy. The red blood cells of these patients contain 50 percent HbS and 50 percent HbC. Because HbC does not polymerize as readily as HbS, the disease generally has less severe clinical consequences. These patients have a mild to moderate hemolytic anemia and mild reticulocytosis. The peripheral smear shows abundant target cells and a few sickle cells, and HbC may be seen precipitated as a rhomboid crystal in the red blood cells. Splenomegaly is a feature of HbSC disease and persists into adulthood in 60 percent of patients. Overall, patients with HbSC disease have few clinical complications, although some have profound medical problems as complex as those seen in patients with SCD. Patients with HbSC disease can have painful crises and organ infarcts. They are at higher-than-normal risk for bacterial infections. Ocular complications and visual loss occur, as well as infarcts in the renal medulla and avascular necrosis of the femoral heads. Women with HbSC disease have an increased incidence of complications in pregnancy.

Sickle Cell–Beta (β) Thalassemia Disease

This heterozygous sickle cell variant occurs when the gene for sickle hemoglobin is inherited from one parent and the gene for β thalassemia is inherited from the other parent. In US African-Americans, the gene frequency for β thalassemia is 0.8 to 1.0 percent. The frequency of sickle cell–β-thalassemia disease is 2 per 3200 births. The severity of the disease that results, including the degree of anemia and frequency of clinical complications, depends on the type of β-thalassemia gene that is inherited. Between 80 and 90 percent of affected individuals have a β-thalassemia gene that results in the production of some normal beta chains; thus some normal HbA is made. These patients have a mild hemolytic anemia with near-normal hemoglobin levels, few crises, and minimal organ damage. Those 10 to 20 percent of patients who inherit a β-thalassemia gene that produces no beta chains, and therefore no normal hemoglobin, have severe hemolytic anemia and vasoocclusive symptoms comparable with patients with SCD. Splenomegaly is found in 70 percent of patients with sickle cell–β thalassemia disease.

DEFICIENCY OF GLUCOSE-6-PHOSPHATE DEHYDROGENASE

Deficiency of the red blood cell (RBC) enzyme glucose-6-phosphate dehydrogenase (G-6-PD) is the most common human enzyme defect, affecting nearly one-tenth of the world's population. In this inherited abnormality, the activity of this enzyme is markedly diminished. As a result, the RBC is unable to protect itself against oxidant stress. Normally, reduced glutathione is generated to protect the sulfhydryl groups of hemoglobin and the red cell membrane from oxidation. When the enzyme is deficient, the hemoglobin sulfhydryl groups become oxidized and the hemoglobin precipitates within the RBC, forming Heinz bodies that are readily removed from the circulation.

Clinically, the resulting hemolytic anemia varies greatly in severity. It is an X-linked disorder, and clinical manifestations are seen in male heterozygotes and female homozygotes. In the United States, 15 percent of African-American males have a mild form of this deficiency. Acute hemolytic crises occur that are incited by bacterial and viral infections, exposure to oxidant drugs, metabolic acidosis (such as diabetic ketoacidosis), and ingestion of fava beans in some patients. Within 1 to 3 days following oxidant stress, the patient can develop hemoglobinuria and the potential for vascular collapse. These hemolytic crises are generally well tolerated and self-limited because only the older RBCs will hemolyze. In more severe but less common variants of this disease, the patient can have severe chronic hemolytic anemia. The diagnosis of G-6-PD deficiency can be established by the demonstration of decreased enzyme activity through quantitative assay. There is no specific treatment for this disease. Prevention of hemolytic episodes is crucial, with prompt treatment of infections and the avoidance of oxidant drugs. The drugs most commonly associated with oxidant stress are sulfa drugs, antimalarials, pyridium, and nitrofurantoin. HIV-positive patients are commonly screened for this defect because of the common use of the sulfa drugs for the treatment and prophylaxis of *Pneumocystis carinii* pneumonia.

HEREDITARY SPHEROCYTOSIS

Hereditary spherocytosis (HS) is the most prevalent hereditary hemolytic anemia among people of northern European descent. An estmated 1 in 4500 persons is affected. The disease is typically inherited in an autosomal dominant pattern, but in up to 20 percent of patients it is the result of an apparent spontaneous mutation. The abnormal shape of the RBCs results from molecular abnormalities in the cytoskeleton of the RBC membrane, most commonly with the proteins spectrin and ankyrin. Because of their abnormal shape, the RBCs are caught in the spleen and destroyed. As a result of the typically mild symptoms, the diagnosis may not be established until adulthood. Clinically, HS is characterized by a hemolytic anemia that is usually mild (a small minority of patients have severe anemia), splenomegaly, and intermittent jaundice from indirect bilirubin (due to hemolysis). Pigment gallstones are common.

Patients with HS have a mild anemia, and the peripheral blood smear shows spherocytes with a normal mean corpuscular volume and increased mean corpuscular hemoglobin concentration (>36 percent). The diagnosis of HS is established by the osmotic fragility test. Splenectomy is the treatment for patients with HS. This cures the anemia, although the spherocytes are still present.

BIBLIOGRAPHY

Charache S, Terrin ML, Moore D, et al: Effect of hydroxyurea on the frequency of painful crises in sickle cell anemia. *N Engl J Med* 332:1317, 1995.

Kerle KK, Runkle GP: Sickle cell trait and sudden death in athletes. *JAMA* 276(18): 1472, 1996.

Krachman SL, Lodato RF, D'Alonzo GE: Managing the acute chest syndrome in sickle cell patients. *J Crit Illness* 9:375, 1994.

Martin JJ, Moore GP: Pearls, pitfalls and updates for pain management. *Emerg Med Clin North Am* 15(2):399, 1997.

Platt OS, Brambilla DJ, Rosse WF, et al: Mortality in sickle cell disease, life expectancy and risk factors for early death. *N Engl J Med* 330:1639, 1994.

Pollack CV Jr: Emergencies in sickle cell disease. *Emerg Med Clin North Am* 11:365, 1993.

Pollack CV Jr: Usefulness of empiric chest radiography and urinalysis testing in adults with acute sickle cell pain crisis. *Ann Emerg Med* 20:1210, 1991.

ACQUIRED HEMOLYTIC ANEMIAS

Mary E. Eberst

This chapter reviews some of the anemias that result from hemolysis that is precipitated by an acquired or extrinsic abnormality. Table 214-1 outlines these conditions, which include antibody-mediated (immune) hemolytic anemias; fragmentation hemolysis, either microvascular or macrovascular; anemias resulting from direct toxic effects; anemias resulting from mechanical injury; and anemia that is the result of abnormal splenic function (hypersplenism).

The general laboratory evaluation of patients with suspected hemolysis is reviewed here; the characteristic results for each type of anemia

TABLE 214-1 Classification of Acquired Hemolytic Anemias

I. Autoimmune hemolytic anemia (antibody-mediated)
  A. Warm antibodies
  B. Cold antibodies
    1. Cold agglutin disease
    2. Paroxysmal cold hemoglobinuria
  C. Drug-induced

II. Fragmentation hemolysis
  A. Microangiopathic hemolytic anemia (MAHA)
    1. Thrombotic thrombocytopenic purpura (TTP)/hemolytic uremic syndrome (HUS)
    2. Pregnancy-associated hemolysis (HELLP)
    3. Disseminated intravascular coagulation (DIC)
    4. Malignancy-associated hemolysis
    5. Hemolysis in vasculitis
    6. Hemolysis in malignant hypertension
  B. Macrovascular hemolysis
    1. Due to abnormal cardiac valves

III. Direct toxic effects causing hemolysis
  A. Infections
  B. Other toxins—bites, copper
  C. Drug-induced oxidative hemolysis—methemoglobinemia

IV. Mechanical damage causing hemolysis
  A. Heat denaturation
  B. March hemoglobinuria
  C. Cardiopulmonary bypass

V. Anemia due to abnormal splenic function (hypersplenism)

will be discussed below. Patients newly diagnosed with or suspected of having any of these hemolytic anemias should have immediate hematologic consultation and be admitted to the hospital.

LABORATORY EVALUATION OF HEMOLYTIC ANEMIA

1. *Complete blood count* (CBC). The anemia that occurs may be mild or severe; verify normal/abnormal white blood cell count and platelet count.
2. *Reticulocyte count.* This is the single most useful test in ascertaining the presence of hemolysis and a normal bone marrow response; this should be elevated and can be as high as 30 to 40 percent.
3. *Review of the peripheral blood smear.* Most hemolytic disorders are associated with changes in the morphology of the red blood cells (RBCs); typical changes may include
   a. *Spherocytes.* These are the most common morphologic abnormality in hemolytic diseases; they will be most abundant in patients with warm antibody immune hemolysis and those with hereditary spherocytosis (Chap. 213).
   b. *Schistocytes.* These are fragmented RBCs that result from direct trauma within the vasculature, most often in the microvasculature (known as *microangiopathic hemolytic anemia,* MAHA), but also can occur in the macrovasculature; schistocytes are markers of nonimmune hemolysis.
4. *Unconjugated (indirect) bilirubin.* This should be elevated in the presence of hemolysis as a result of heme catabolism; the direct (conjugated) bilirubin should be normal unless there is concomitant hepatic or biliary dysfunction.
5. *Haptoglobin.* This binds to the protein globin that is released when hemoglobin is catabolized, so this should be low or absent in the presence of significant hemolysis. Haptoglobin is an acute-phase reactant that may be increased in conditions such as severe infection, tissue destruction, myocardial infarction, and burns and in some cancer patients; in these settings, the haptoglobin level may be increased, despite the presence of hemolytic anemia.
6. *Plasma free hemoglobin.* This should be elevated in hemolysis.
7. *Lactic dehydrogenase* (LDH). This should be elevated in hemolysis; it can be a relatively sensitive marker used to follow the course of a hemolytic disease.

AUTOIMMUNE HEMOLYTIC ANEMIAS

There are three types of antibody-mediated, so-called immune, hemolytic anemias:

1. Warm antibody hemolytic anemia. These antibodies are reactive at body temperature.
2. Cold antibody hemolytic anemia. These antibodies react with the patient's RBCs at temperatures below normal body temperature.
3. Drug-induced immune hemolytic anemia. Certain drugs can cause an immune reaction in some patients that results in destruction of their RBCs.

Immune hemolytic anemias are characterized in the laboratory by the Coombs antiglobulin test, also known as the *direct Coombs' test* or *direct antiglobulin test* (DAT). This test demonstrates the presence of immunoglobulin (IgG) or complement (C3) on the surface of the RBC. It is only positive in immune-mediated hemolytic anemias. The indirect Coombs' test is used primarily for pretransfusion screening for antibodies; it demonstrates the presence of free antibodies in the patient's serum. Immune hemolysis is typified by abundant spherocytes on the peripheral blood smear.

Warm Antibody Hemolytic Anemia

This disease is characterized by the presence of antibodies directed against IgG and/or C3 that are deposited on the surface of the RBC. It comprises 70 percent of all cases of immune hemolytic anemia. These antibodies react with the RBCs at 37°C. After the antibody-RBC interaction, the RBCs are trapped and destroyed in the spleen.

Patients of any age may be affected, but warm antibody hemolytic anemia is most likely to occur in older adults, women more often than men. Most often it is idiopathic; however, up to 25 percent of affected patients have an underlying disease that affects the immune system such as chronic lymphocytic leukemia, Hodgkin's or non-Hodgkin's lymphoma, or systemic lupus erythematosus (SLE). In adults, the disease is typically relapsing. In young children, it often follows an acute infection or immunizations and is unlikely to recur.

The clinical presentation and course of disease are highly variable depending on the severity of the anemia and how rapidly it develops. Many patients will have a mild anemia with splenomegaly. In this setting, the Coombs' test will be positive for IgG but not C3, and the indirect Coombs' test will be negative. Life-threatening anemia also can occur with hemoglobin levels less than 7 g/dL and a reticulocyte count greater than 30 percent. These patients may have marked splenomegaly, pulmonary edema, and mental status changes. Venous thrombosis also can occur. Patients with severe hemolysis generally have a Coombs' test that is positive for both IgG and C3, and the indirect Coombs' test is also often positive. Rare patients have Evans's syndrome, where there is coexistent immune destruction both of RBCs and platelets by different antibodies.

The treatment of warm antibody hemolytic anemia depends on the degree of anemia that develops and the ability of the patient to hemodynamically tolerate anemia. When there is only mild anemia, no treatment is necessary. When significant hemolysis is present, the first-line treatment is prednisone, 1.0 mg/kg per day. About 75 percent of patients will respond to steroid therapy, but up to one-half of these will relapse after the steroids are tapered. Transfusion of red blood cells is difficult in these patients because they will be impossible to crossmatch. Transfusion is indicated for symptoms of angina, congestive heart failure, mental status changes, orthostasis, or hypoxia. In this setting, the patient is slowly transfused with the best match available; acute transfusion reactions can occur. Splenectomy is the second-choice treatment for patients who fail or cannot tolerate steroids. Immunosuppressive drugs such as azathioprine and cyclophosphamide are used occasionally. Treatment of any underlying immunologic disease also may help control the hemolytic anemia. Death in these patients results from severe anemia that cannot be corrected, immunosuppression, venous thrombosis, or underlying immunologic disease.

Cold Antibody Hemolytic Anemia

Cold-reactive antibodies, those which react maximally at temperatures between 4 and 20°C and not usually above 32°C, account for 10 to 20 percent of patients with immune hemolytic anemia. There are two types of diseases where this occurs: cold agglutinin disease and paroxysmal cold hemoglobinuria. These antibodies react with the RBCs in the superficial microcirculation where it is cool, then the hemolysis occurs when the red blood cells reenter the central circulation and are warmed.

COLD AGGLUTININ DISEASE This can be an acute, transient disease mostly seen in younger people or a chronic disease primarily in older patients. It is typically caused by an IgM antibody, and the Coombs' test will only be positive for C3, because the IgM will not be attached to the RBCs at warmer temperature. The acute form of this disease is mostly seen in patients with *Mycoplasma* pneumonia or infectious mononucleosis; the IgM antibodies are directed against the I antigen or i antigen on the RBC surface, respectively. Only rare patients develop significant hemolysis, but severe anemia and renal failure can occur. The acute form of this disease is self-limited. Chronic cold agglutinin disease is more common than the acute form and primarily occurs in patients with underlying lymphoid neoplasms.

These patients typically have a mild to moderate anemia that results from hemolysis occurring in portions of the body exposed to lower temperatures (acrocyanosis). These patients should be kept in a warm environment, and treatment is directed against the underlying disease. Some of the hemolysis may respond to treatment with prednisone.

PAROXYSMAL COLD HEMOGLOBINEMIA This disease is characterized by acute episodes of hemolysis following exposure to cold. Two groups of patients can be affected by this disease: (1) those with congenital or tertiary syphilis that is untreated and (2) patients with viral illnesses such as mumps or measles. In this disease, the immune hemolysis is caused by an IgG antibody called the *Donath-Landsteiner antibody,* which is directed against the P-antigen complex on the RBC surface. Clinically, after exposure to cold, affected patients will have hemoglobinuria, chills, fever, and pain involving the back, legs, and abdomen. The direct Coombs test is only positive during an acute attack. When associated with syphilis, this disease goes away after appropriate antibiotic therapy. Now most commonly seen in patients with viral infections, the hemolysis is self-limited but can cause transient severe anemia.

Drug-Induced Hemolytic Anemia

Many drugs have been directly linked to immune hemolytic anemia. There are three types of reactions that can occur and result in hemolysis.

AUTOANTIBODY INDUCTION α-Methyldopa is the prototype drug of this reaction, and 10 to 20 percent of patients taking moderate-to-high doses will develop a positive direct Coombs' test. In this drug reaction, the RBCs become coated with an IgG that is directed against the Rh complex. Other drugs that can cause this are L-dopa, procainamide, ibuprofen, diclofenac, and thioridazine. Generally, it takes an extended period of drug exposure to develop the positive Coombs' test, and only a small number of those patients will develop severe hemolysis. The hemolysis ceases after the drug is stopped, but the Coombs' test may remain positive for a year or more.

HAPTEN-INDUCED IMMUNE HEMOLYSIS Penicillin is the classic drug associated with this reaction. Immune hemolysis can develop in patients receiving large intravenous doses of penicillin or penicillin-type antibiotics and usually starts 1 to 2 weeks after the therapy begins. The patient forms an antibody against the offending drug; then the antibody combines with the drug-RBC complex and causes hemolysis. Other drugs that can cause hemolysis by this mechanism include oxacillin, ampicillin, carbenicillin, and some cephalosporins. The hemolysis stops when the drug is discontinued.

INNOCENT BYSTANDER IMMUNE HEMOLYSIS Quinidine is the prototype drug for this reaction. Antibodies (IgG or IgM) are formed against the drug; then the drug-antibody complex binds to the RBC and hemolyzes it. Other drugs linked to this mechanism include quinine, isoniazid, sulfonamides, hydrochlorothiazide, antihistamines, insulin, chlorpromazine, tetracycline, acetaminophen, hydralazine, cephalosporins, fenoprofen, and sulindac. Even a small dose of the drug can cause hemolysis; however, these drugs are very commonly prescribed and the associated hemolysis is very rare.

FRAGMENTATION HEMOLYSIS

Microangiopathic Hemolytic Anemia (MAHA)

This type of hemolytic anemia is associated with a variety of disorders; however, the mechanism leading to hemolysis is consistent. The fragmentation of RBCs results from their passage through abnormal arterioles: usually there is damage to the vessel wall or endothelial surface or fibrin has been deposited in the arteriole. Schistocytes are characteristically found on the peripheral blood smear.

THROMBOTIC THROMBOCYTOPENIC PURPURA (TTP) AND HEMOLYTIC UREMIC SYNDROME (HUS) These diseases will be discussed separately; however, TTP and HUS may well represent variant clinical presentations of a single disease. In selected patients, the specific diagnosis may be impossible to establish.

Thrombotic Thrombocytopenic Purpura TTP is a heterogeneous clinical syndrome characterized by this pentad of symptoms and signs:

1. Microangiopathic hemolytic anemia (MAHA) with characteristic schistocytes on the peripheral blood smear and a reticulocytosis
2. Thrombocytopenia with platelet counts ranging from 5000 to 100,000/μL
3. Renal abnormalities including renal insufficiency, azotemia, proteinuria, or hematuria
4. Fever
5. Neurologic abnormalities including headache, confusion, cranial nerve palsies, seizures, or coma

TTP has been diagnosed in patients of all ages but occurs most commonly between the ages 10 and 60. Women are affected more commonly than men. The course of the disease is typically acute and fulminant, lasting days to months, but it can be chronic and relapsing in 10 percent of patients. The overall survival rate is 80 percent, but the course is rapidly fatal in some patients. The majority of patients diagnosed with TTP have no apparent predisposing condition. In a small number of patients, TTP has been linked to genetic predisposition, pregnancy, immunologic diseases (SLE, rheumatoid arthritis, Sjögren's syndrome), or infections (viral, *Mycoplasma* pneumonia, subacute bacterial endocarditis, human immunodeficiency virus).

The pathogenesis of TTP is uncertain, but the presence of one or more platelet aggregating agents is likely responsible. Several abnormalities of the vascular endothelium and endothelial cell function have been implicated, including the release and presence of large von Willebrand multimers, decreased production of prostacyclin, inadequate fibrinolysis as a result of deficient tissue plasminogen activator (tPA) production, the presence of a platelet agglutinating protein, and deficient production of IgG molecules. Whatever the etiology, the result is the deposition of hyaline material within the lumina of capillaries and arterioles. These microthrombi are made of platelets and a small amount of fibrinlike material. These deposits may be found in any tissue but occur most frequently in the heart, brain, kidneys, pancreas, and adrenal glands.

The diagnosis of TTP is established clinically by the presence of the signs and symptoms listed above. Treatment should begin immediately based on these clinical and laboratory features. Biopsies are sometimes done of the gingiva, kidney, or bone marrow but are not essential to establish the diagnosis and should not delay therapy.

Clinically, the neurologic abnormalities are the most common presenting complaint, but hemorrhagic signs and symptoms and those referable to anemia are also common presentations. Laboratory studies will reflect the presence of MAHA with an anemia of variable degree (the hemoglobin will be less than 6 g/dL in one out of three patients), reticulocytosis, elevated indirect bilirubin, elevated LDH, negative Coombs' test, and the presence of schistocytes on the peripheral smear (the diagnosis of TTP is doubtful without schistocytes). Thrombocytopenia, reflective of the intravascular microthrombi, is often severe with the count less than 20,000/μL in 50 percent of patients. A mild leukocytosis with a left shift is common. The blood urea nitrogen (BUN) and creatinine are typically elevated to a mild to moderate degree. Urinalysis usually shows some degree of proteinuria and may show microscopic hematuria. Coagulation screening tests should be normal.

TABLE 214-2 Characteristics of Acquired Hemolytic Anemias*

	Evans Syndrome	TTP	HUS	DIC	HELLP
Autoimmune hemolytic anemia	Present	No	No	No	No
Microangiopathic hemolytic anemia (MAHA)	No	Prominent	Prominent	Often present	Present
Coombs test	Positive	Negative	Negative	Negative	Negative
Thrombocytopenia	Present	Prominent	Present	Present	Present
Renal abnormalities	No	Mild	Prominent	No	No
Neurologic abnormalities	No	Prominent	No or mild	No	No
Hepatic dysfunction	No	May have	May have	May have	Prominent
Fever	No	Present	Present	May have	No
Coagulation studies	Normal	Normal	Normal	Abnormal	Normal
Pregnancy-associated	No	Can be	Can be	Can be	Always

Note: TTP, thrombotic thrombocytopenic purpura; HUS, hemolytic uremic syndrome; DIC, disseminated intravascular coagulation; HELLP, hemolysis, elevated liver functions, low platelets.
*Disease descriptions here are based on presence of isolated disease without complications; individual patients often have other problems that make syndromes less readily identified.

The salient features in the differential diagnosis of TTP are outlined in Table 214-2.

The diagnosis of TTP represents a medical emergency. Patients should be treated by experienced hematologists. Rapid transport to a tertiary care center is indicated. Some centers have a policy of initially admitting all TTP patients to an intensive care unit. When the diagnosis of TTP is established or suspected, fresh-frozen plasma should be infused immediately. The foundation of therapy for TTP is plasma exchange transfusion (PLEX). Some patients will respond favorably to plasma infusions alone, and these can be given until the exchanges can be initiated. The plasma exchange uses fresh-frozen plasma (FFP) or fresh unfrozen plasma (FUP). The plasma is thought to provide a substance that the patient is lacking or remove an unknown toxic substance. These exchanges may be required daily for a period of several months. TTP patients are also treated with prednisone (or methylprednisolone), 1 mg/kg per day, and antiplatelet therapy consisting of aspirin or dipyridamole. Refractory patients may receive immunosuppressive therapy such as vincristine, azathioprine, or cyclophosphamide. Splenectomy is sometimes done but has little correlation with clinical improvement. Supportive care includes the transfusion of packed red blood cells as needed and hemodialysis if indicated. Platelet transfusions should be avoided, unless there is uncontrolled hemorrhage, because they can aggravate the thrombotic process. Clinical and hematologic progress in patients with TTP is assessed by improvement in neurologic and renal function, decrease in the reticulocyte count, decrease in the LDH, and increase in the platelet count.

Hemolytic Uremic Syndrome HUS is a disease mainly of infancy and early childhood, with a peak incidence between 6 months and 4 years of age. An adult form also exists (see below). The overall mortality rate is 5 to 15 percent, and the prognosis is worse in older children and adults. HUS is one of the most common causes of acute renal failure in childhood. HUS is characterized by acute renal failure, microangiopathic hemolytic anemia, fever, and thrombocytopenia.

In children, the development of HUS often follows a prodromal infectious disease, usually diarrhea or an upper respiratory infection. Diarrhea, particularly that associated with *Escherichia coli* serotype 0157:H7, as well as with *Shigella, Yersinia, Campylobacter,* and *Salmonella,* may be antecedent. Other implicated bacteria and viruses include *Streptococcus pneumoniae,* varicella, echovirus, and coxsackie A and B. Some cases of HUS are familial, with a genetic or HLA-type predisposition.

As noted earlier, HUS and TTP actually may be clinical variations of the same disease. Like TTP, HUS is pathologically identified by microthrombi, consisting of platelet aggregates, that occlude the arterioles and capillaries. In HUS, the microthrombi are confined mostly to the kidneys; in TTP, they occur throughout the microcirculation. The platelet-fibrin hyaline material is found in the afferent arterioles and glomerular capillaries. A defect in the vascular endothelium is thought to cause these platelet aggregates. It is not precisely known how the endothelial damage occurs, but the toxins released from bacteria or viruses have been implicated. The damaged endothelial cells are then thought to release large and ultralarge vonWillebrand factor multimers that lead to platelet aggregation.

Like TTP, HUS is primarily a clinical and laboratory diagnosis. The signs and symptoms of acute renal failure predominate. Although neurologic dysfunction is not a key feature of HUS, it does occur in up to one-third of HUS patients at some point in the course of their disease. Laboratory studies reflect the presence of MAHA. Thrombocytopenia is present but generally not to the degree seen in TTP. The BUN and creatinine will be markedly elevated, and urine, if present, will contain protein and red blood cells. Coagulation studies are usually normal.

The treatment of HUS primarily consists of early dialysis for management of renal failure and general supportive care. Up to 90 percent of HUS patients with acute renal failure will eventually regain normal renal function. Plasma exchange or infusion is not usually used in the treatment of childhood HUS. HUS is rarely a recurrent disease, but it has been known to recur in patients who have undergone renal transplantation.

Adult HUS When HUS occurs in adult patients, it can be difficult or impossible to differentiate between HUS and TTP. HUS is diagnosed when there is prominent renal failure and minimal neurologic dysfunction. Of adults diagnosed with HUS, two-thirds are women. Associated factors are the use of oral contraceptive agents, preeclampsia, eclampsia, other obstetric complications, and the postpartum period. HUS also rarely occurs in association with the chemotherapeutic drug mitomycin C and in other cancer patients who may or may not have received chemotherapy. The renal failure in adults with HUS may be reversible, even after as long as 1 year.

PREGNANCY-ASSOCIATED HEMOLYSIS Microangiopathic hemolytic anemia (MAHA) can occur in pregnancy as a complication of preeclampsia, eclampsia, or placental abruption. The presence of preeclampsia, hemolysis, elevated liver enzymes, and low platelet counts is known as the *HELLP syndrome.* The HELLP syndrome can occur with minimal signs or symptoms of preeclampsia. The pathogenesis is not entirely known, but preeclampsia can be associated with microvesicular fatty infiltration of the liver and with localized or systemic endothelial damage that can lead to MAHA. Untreated, HELLP can result in hepatic failure or rupture, disseminated intravascular coagulation (DIC), or congestive heart failure. Treatment begins with prompt delivery of the infant followed by supportive care.

DISSEMINATED INTRAVASCULAR COAGULATION DIC is discussed in Chap. 211. MAHA occurs in about 25 percent of patients with DIC. The degree of hemolysis that occurs in DIC is much less than that seen in TTP or HUS. The basic pathology in DIC is the deposition of fibrin in the microvasculature. Fragmentation and hemolysis of the RBCs occur as they pass through the microcirculation. Schistocytes, reflective of MAHA, are often found on the peripheral smear of patients with DIC, but their absence does not rule out DIC. Along with the factor replacement therapy required in DIC, patients with significant hemolysis and anemia will require transfusion of packed red blood cells to maintain adequate circulation and oxygenation.

MALIGNANCY-ASSOCIATED HEMOLYSIS MAHA can be seen in patients with widely disseminated cancer. Gastric adenocarcinoma is the malignancy most frequently associated with MAHA, although it also occurs with adenocarcinomas of the lung, breast, and of unknown primary. The pathogenesis is uncertain, but hypotheses include the following: vessels that supply malignant tumors may be structurally abnormal; circulating tumor cells may damage the endothelial surface; or tumor cells may give off factors that promote platelet aggregation and microvascular changes. Patients with MAHA due to widespread malignancy have a very poor prognosis.

HEMOLYSIS IN VASCULITIS MAHA can be seen in vascular diseases such as SLE, polyarteritis nodosa, Wegener's granulomatosis, and scleroderma. In this setting, damage to the endothelial surface is thought to result from deposition of immune complexes and fibrin in the microcirculation.

HEMOLYSIS IN MALIGNANT HYPERTENSION Patients with malignant or accelerated hypertension can develop MAHA as a result of narrowing and hardening of the afferent arterioles and swelling of the endothelial cells. This hemolysis subsides after normalization of the blood pressure.

Macrovascular Hemolysis

Traumatic hemolysis can occur in patients with artificial heart valves or severe calcific aortic stenosis. Some degree of hemolysis occurs in up to 10 percent of patients with aortic prostheses; mechanical valves are more likely to cause hemolysis than porcine valves. Mitral valve replacements cause less hemolysis because of the lower pressure gradient. Hemolysis also can occur in patients with prosthetic patches in the heart and, rarely, in patients who have undergone aortofemoral bypass. The hemolysis that occurs in this setting is generally mild and well tolerated. These patients should receive supplemental iron and folate. If the hemolysis is severe, the defective valve may have to be replaced.

DIRECT TOXIC EFFECTS CAUSING HEMOLYSIS

Infections

Destruction of RBCs occurs commonly in the course of many infectious diseases. Those diseases with the most profound effect on RBCs will be reviewed here.

Transmitted by mosquitoes, malaria is the world's most common cause of hemolytic anemia. RBC hemolysis results from direct parasitization of the RBCs. Hemolysis also results from direct parasitization of RBCs in babesiosis, which is transmitted by ticks or blood transfusions. Infection with *Bartonella* is also associated with direct parasitization of RBCs and resultant hemolysis.

Hemophilus influenzae type B infection can produce hemolysis by altering the RBC surface. The capsular polysaccharide of the bacterium binds to the RBC surface and then antibodies destroy the bacterium as well as the RBC. Those with *H. influenzae* meningitis have the greatest potential to develop severe hemolysis.

Clostridium perfringens (welchii) infection can result in severe hemolysis by direct lysis of red blood cells. The organism releases enzymes that acutely degrade the phospholipids of the RBC membrane bilayer and the proteins in the structural membrane. This infection is seen most commonly in patients with acute cholecystitis, after surgery involving the biliary tree, after abortions, and in uterine infections. Clinically, the patient may have acute hemodynamic collapse and profound intravascular hemolysis. *Clostridium* septicemia has a mortality rate over 50 percent.

Mycoplasma pneumoniae and infectious mononucleosis are associated with cold agglutin disease, as described earlier.

Many viral infections can be accompanied by hemolytic anemia, including measles, cytomegalovirus, varicella, herpes simplex, coxsackie, and human immunodeficiency virus.

Other Toxins that Cause Hemolysis

Insect, Spider, and Snake Bites Acute intravascular hemolysis can occur following bites/stings of bees, wasps, the southern black widow spider, and the brown recluse spider. The bites of American snakes, pit vipers and coral snakes, are known to cause coagulation abnormalities but rarely cause hemolysis. The bite of the cobra snake does cause intravascular hemolysis.

Copper Copper has a direct hemolytic effect on red blood cells. Copper sulfate contamination from copper pipes can taint hemodialysis fluid, and copper sulfate is sometimes used in suicide attempts. Patients with Wilson's disease experience transient episodes of hemolysis as a result of their elevated copper levels.

Drug-Induced Oxidative Hemolysis

Oxidative hemolysis of RBCs can result from exposure to a number of drugs that cause the formation of methemoglobin. These drugs oxidize ferrous hemoglobin (+2) to ferric hemoglobin (+3), which is methemoglobin. Methemoglobin cannot bind oxygen, so the oxygen-carrying capacity of the blood is decreased. A large number of commonly used drugs can cause methemoglobinemia, but not at therapeutic doses (Table 214-3). Toxic methemoglobinemia occurs when more than 10 percent of the hemoglobin has been oxidized to the ferric form. Clinically, methemoglobinemia should be suspected in patients who are cyanotic without cardiopulmonary disease. This cyanosis is not relieved by oxygen. The venous blood appears chocolate brown. The arterial blood gas will reflect a normal Pa_{O_2}, but decreased measured oxygen saturation. Table 214-4 shows the clinical effects of acute methemoglobinemia. Levels of methemoglobin greater than 20 to 30 percent of the total hemoglobin should be treated. Methylene

TABLE 214-3 Drugs That Cause Oxidative Hemolysis

Benzocaine, lidocaine
Nitrates, nitrites
Sulfonamides
Phenacetin
Azulfidine
Pyridium
Dapsone and other antimalarials

blue is given intravenously at a dose of 1 to 2 mg/kg in a 1% solution over 5 min. Methylene blue reduces methemoglobin back to oxygen-carrying hemoglobin through a series of reactions.

MECHANICAL DAMAGE CAUSING HEMOLYSIS

Heat Denaturation Temperatures above 47°C cause direct damage to erythrocytes by denaturation of the cytoskeletal protein, spectrin. This can occur in patients with extensive burns. Within 24 h of the burns, acute hemolytic anemia can develop with gross hemoglobinuria and spherocytes and schistocytes on the peripheral blood smear.

March Hemoglobinuria This type of hemolysis can occur in soldiers and joggers and in karate and conga-drumming enthusiasts. Red blood cell destruction is the result of direct trauma to the cells in the vessels of the feet or hands. These patients rarely become anemic but do have hemoglobinuria after strenuous exercise or activity.

Cardiopulmonary Bypass Patients who have been on cardiopulmonary bypass can develop a *postperfusion syndrome* that consists of acute intravascular hemolysis, leukopenia, and fever. This hemolysis is thought to result from the activation of complement as blood passes through the oxygenator.

ANEMIA DUE TO ABNORMAL SPLENIC FUNCTION

There are many disease states that result in splenic enlargement (Table 214-5). The main function of the normal spleen is to filter defective red blood cells and foreign particles and to participate in antigen processing and antibody synthesis. When the spleen is enlarged, its activity is increased, a condition known as hypersplenism. Hypersplenism results in the sequestration of red blood cells as well as platelets and white blood cells. Unlike the platelets and white blood cells, which can survive within the spleen and be released back into the circulation, the sequestered red blood cells are not metabolically self-sufficient and are prematurely destroyed within the spleen. Hemolysis within the spleen is greatest when the splenomegaly is caused by inflammatory states or splenic congestion due to elevated portal pressure.

TABLE 214-4 Clinical Effect of Acute Methemoglobinemia

Percent of Total Hemoglobin that Is Methemoglobin	Clinical Effects
10–15	Peripheral cyanosis
30–35	Headache, weakness, breathlessness
55	Dyspnea, bradycardia, seizures, arrhythmias
60–70	Vascular collapse, coma
80 or more	Incompatible with life

TABLE 214-5 Disease States Associated with Hypersplenism and Hemolysis

Cause of Splenic Enlargement	Disease Example(s)
Splenic congestion due to elevated portal pressure	Cirrhosis, portal vein thrombosis, splenic vein obstruction, congestive heart failure, Budd-Chiari syndrome
Infiltrative disease	Leukemia, lymphoma, amyloidosis, polycythemia vera
Inflammatory states	Rheumatoid arthritis, SLE, sarcoidosis
Infections	Bacterial endocarditis, infectious mononucleosis, miliary tuberculosis, malaria, schistosomiasis
Hereditary hemolytic anemias	Sickle cell anemia
Acquired hemolytic anemias	Autoimmune hemolytic anemia

Note: SLE, systemic lupus erythematosus.

BIBLIOGRAPHY

Bridgman J, Witting M: Thrombotic thrombocytopenic purpura presenting as a sudden headache with focal neurologic findings. *Ann Emerg Med* 27(1):95, 1996.

Leo PL, Cooper C, Songco C: Hemolytic uremic syndrome: Just another case of gastroenteritis? *Am J Emerg Med* 12:358, 1994.

Moake JL: Thrombotic microangiopathies: Thrombotic thrombocytopenic purpura and the hemolytic-uremic syndrome, in Loscalzo J, Schafer AI (eds): *Thrombosis and Hemorrhage,* 2d ed. Baltimore: Williams & Wilkins, 1998, p 583.

Schwartz RS, Silberstein LE, Berkman EM: Autoimmune hemolytic anemias, in Hoffman R, Benz EJ Jr, Shattil SJ, et al (eds): *Hematology, Basic Principles and Practice,* 2d ed. New York: Churchill-Livingstone, 1995, p 710.

Sibai BM, Ramadan MK, Usta I, et al: Maternal morbidity and mortality in 442 pregnancies with hemolysis, elevated liver enzymes, and low patients (HELLP syndrome). *Am J Obstet Gynecol* 169:1000, 1993.

Williams E: Disseminated intravascular coagulation, in Loscalzo J, Schafer AI (eds): *Thrombosis and Hemorrhage,* 2d ed. Baltimore: Williams & Wilkins, 1998, p 963.

BLOOD TRANSFUSIONS AND COMPONENT THERAPY

Mary E. Eberst

Since the time of the first blood transfusions in the late 1600s and recognition of the ABO blood grouping system by Landsteiner in 1900, transfusion medicine has become a complex medical specialty. It is not important that all practitioners be familiar with the intricacies of blood banking, but any physician who is responsible for the transfusion of blood products to patients needs to have a basic understanding of what products are available, what product is appropriate in a given clinical situation, and what are the potential complications of the transfusion.

This chapter reviews the different types of blood products that are available, with an emphasis on component therapy. The potential complications of transfusions, immediate and delayed, are reviewed. Two topics of particular importance in emergency medicine, emergency transfusion and massive transfusion, are briefly discussed.

AVAILABLE BLOOD PRODUCTS

Whole Blood

Modern transfusion medicine recommends that it is preferable to give patients only the specific portions of blood they require. This is achieved by the use of component therapy. Therefore, whole blood is rarely used in current practice, except for exchange transfusions for neonates. A unit of whole blood contains 435 to 500 mL of blood plus a preservative-anticoagulant solution. CPDA-1 (citrate phosphate dextrose adenine) is the additive in current use. With proper collection and storage of the blood at 2° to 6°C, in the presence of this additive, whole blood has a shelf life of 35 days. The *shelf life* is defined as viability of at least 70 percent of the red blood cells 24 h after infusion. Whole blood is not entirely ''whole'' at the time of administration because during storage, beginning 24 h after collection, there is a loss of platelets and some coagulation factors. By 72 h after collection, there are virtually no viable platelets and negligible factor VIII activity in ''whole'' blood. Experts suggest that fewer than 10 percent of all patients requiring transfusions actually require all the components of whole blood. Whole blood has the advantage of simultaneously providing volume and oxygen-carrying capacity. This is also accomplished by the use of packed red blood cells and crystalloid solution, and this is the preferred procedure. Disadvantages to the use of whole blood transfusion are that it is rarely available in the United States; clotting factors are present in low levels; whole blood often contains elevated levels of potassium, hydrogen ion, and ammonia; the patient is exposed to a large number of antigens; and volume overload can occur before the needed components are replenished.

Component Therapy

A unit of donated blood contains about 450 mL of whole blood. In current practice, shortly after collection this blood is separated into its components: red blood cells, platelets, plasma, and cryoprecipitate. This method allows for the widest usage of available blood and optimal storage for each component.

Packed Red Blood Cells

Packed red blood cells (PRBCs) are prepared from whole blood by centrifugation followed by the removal of 80 to 90 percent of the plasma. A preservative solution, such as Adsol (dextrose, adenine, and mannitol), is added, resulting in a storage time of up to 42 days. PRBCs are stored at 4°C. Each unit of PRBCs transfused should raise the hemoglobin by 1 g/dL or the hematocrit by 3 percent. The advantages to the use of PRBCs compared with whole blood include reduced risk of volume overload; decreased infusion of citrate, ammonia, and organic acids; and the decreased risk of alloimmunization because the patient is exposed to fewer antigens. PRBCs provide rapid restoration of oxygen-carrying capacity in patients with acute or chronic blood loss.

It is impossible to set specific criteria for the transfusion of PRBCs, although general guidelines can be used and adapted to each clinical setting. The decision to transfuse must be individualized for each patient. The impact of blood loss is variable among patients, depending on the underlying cause, the rate of blood loss, the patient's underlying health status, the cardiopulmonary reserve, and the activity level of the patient. There are three common settings where the transfusion of PRBCs should be considered:

1. *Acute hemorrhage.* Acute hemorrhage, as seen in patients with trauma, bleeding from the gastrointestional (GI) tract, or from a ruptured aortic aneurysm, often requires emergency transfusion of PRBCs. In otherwise healthy patients, the loss of up to about 1500 mL of blood (about 25 to 30 percent of the blood volume in a 70-kg person) can be replaced entirely with crystalloid solutions. Blood losses greater than this usually require the transfusion of PRBCs to replace oxygen-carrying capacity and crystalloid solution to replace volume.
2. *Surgical blood loss.* Otherwise healthy surgical patients usually do not require preoperative transfusion of PRBCs unless the hemoglobin is less than 7 g/dL or large amounts of blood loss are expected. Intraoperative blood loss of 1500 to 2000 mL can often be replaced with just crystalloid if the patient initially had a normal hemogram. Most patients will require transfusion of PRBCs and crystalloid when blood loss exceeds 2 L.
3. *Chronic anemia.* Patients with chronic stable anemia probably only require transfusion of PRBCs if the hemoglobin falls to less than 7 g/dL or if they are symptomatic or have underlying cardiopulmonary disease.

Some general guidelines for patients in the emergency department (ED) whose blood should be typed and crossmatched for potential transfusion include those with (1) evidence of shock from whatever cause, since early on it may not be clear what the etiology is; (2) known blood loss of more than 1000 mL; (3) ongoing gross bleeding; (4) those with a hemoglobin less than 10 g/dL or hematocrit less than 30 percent; or (5) patients who are potentially going for surgery where blood may be lost (laparotomy after trauma or for ectopic pregnancy).

Other patients who may need blood products but do not meet these criteria should have blood sent to the blood bank for typing and antibody screening. Many institutions have criteria for the number of units to be crossmatched in a particular clinical setting. Many clinicians believe that it is not worth the risks of transfusion to transfuse just one unit of PRBCs; i.e., do not transfuse until the patient requires 2 or more units to be transfused.

In addition to PRBCs, red blood cells are available as leukocyte-poor, frozen, or washed, when required for certain patients. *Leukocyte-poor RBCs* have 70 to 85 percent of the leukocytes removed by centrifugation, filters, or ultraviolet irradiation. This preparation is indicated for patients who are transplant recipients or transplant candidates (bone marrow or solid organ) in order to prevent immunization against leukocytes and in patients who have a history of previous febrile nonhemolytic transfusion reactions. *Frozen RBCs* are prepared by adding a cryoprotective agent and then storing the cells for as long as several years at below freezing temperatures. The freezing process destroys the other blood constituents except for a small number of immunocompetent lymphocytes. Prior to transfusion, the cells are thawed and washed with a solution that removes 99.9 percent of the plasma and cellular debris. This process is expensive but can provide a supply of rare blood types, provides metabolically superior RBCs, and results in reduced antigen exposure for transplant candidates. *Washed RBCs* are prepared from whole blood or PRBCs. Isotonic saline is used to wash the RBCs, resulting in the removal of plasma proteins, some leukocytes, and some platelets. Washed RBCs must be infused within 24 h because of the risk of bacterial contamination during processing. Washed RBCs are used for patients who have hypersensitive reactions to plasma (usually IgA-deficient patients), neonatal transfusions, and in patients with paroxysmal nocturnal hemoglobinuria in order to avoid the precipitation of hemolytic episodes.

Platelets

Platelets for transfusion are obtained through whole blood donations or by plateletpheresis of a single donor. Platelets can be stored for up to 5 days at 20° to 24°C with agitation, although platelet recovery and survival is sometimes better with shorter storage periods. Generally, random donor units are given six at a time (6-pack), or the patient is given one plateletpheresis pack. Each of these totals 250 to 350 mL and contains about 4×10^{11} platelets. Six random donor packs or one plateletpheresis pack should raise the platelet count by 50,000 to 60,000/μL in an average-size adult. The posttransfusion platelet count should be checked 1 and 24 h after platelet infusion. Transfused platelets should survive 3 to 5 days unless there is platelet consumption or refractoriness. Patients with fever, certain infections, disseminated intravascular coagulation (DIC), excessive bleeding, splenomegaly, or antibodies against the transfused platelets may be refractory to platelet transfusion. It is preferable to use ABO-compatible platelets whenever possible to avoid the passive administration of ABO-incompatible plasma. This is particularly true in patients weighing less than 40 kg and patients who receive numerous transfusions. A small amount of RBCs contaminate the platelets, so Rh-negative women of childbearing age should receive Rh-negative platelets.

The clinical indications for the transfusion of platelets depend on the underlying etiology of the thrombocytopenia, the presence or absence of active bleeding, the presence of other disease states that may cause platelet dysfunction, and the need for surgical or invasive procedures. When the patient has thrombocytopenia due to the presence of antiplatelet antibodies, platelet transfusion is generally futile. General guidelines for platelet transfusion in adults include the following:

1. When the platelet count is above 50,000/μL, excessive bleeding due to thrombocytopenia is unlikely unless there is platelet dysfunction present.
2. The platelet count should be maintained at 50,000/μL or greater in patients undergoing major surgery or in those with ongoing significant bleeding.
3. When the platelet count is between 10,000 and 50,000/μL, there is an increased risk of bleeding with trauma or invasive procedures; bleeding that develops spontaneously or as a result of invasion should be treated with platelet transfusions; patients with concurrent disease (renal or liver) causing platelet dysfunction can bleed spontaneously with these counts.
4. When the platelet count is below 10,000/μL, there is a high risk of spontaneous hemorrhage and platelets should be transfused prophylactically, although in patients with immune thrombocytopenia, there may be little or no effect to platelet transfusion.

Special platelet preparations are indicated for some patients. Those who become refractory after multiple transfusions may need HLA-matched platelets. Immunosuppressed patients should receive irradiated platelets to prevent the alloimmunization that can occur as a result of leukocyte contamination.

Fresh-Frozen Plasma

Fresh-frozen plasma (FFP) is plasma that is obtained after the separation of whole blood donations into its plasma and cellular (RBCs and platelets) components. Frozen within 6 h of the collection, FFP is stored at −18°C for up to 1 year. Each bag of FFP contains 200 to 250 mL and, by definition, contains 1 unit of each coagulation factor per milliliter of FFP and 1 to 2 mg of fibrinogen per milliliter of FFP. Transfused FFP should be ABO-compatible. The desired dose to be transfused can be estimated from the plasma volume and the desired incremental increase in factor activity. A typical starting dose is 8 to 10 mL/kg, or approximately two to four bags of FFP. After infusion, the patient should be reevaluated for clinical bleeding and posttransfusion coagulation studies obtained.

The indications for transfusion of FFP are as follows:

1. The presence of a coagulopathy due to acquired factor(s) deficiency with active bleeding or prior to invasive procedures; the patient should have significant (1.5×) prolongation of the prothrombin time (PT) and/or activated partial thromboplastin time (aPTT), or a specific coagulation factor assay less than 25 percent of normal; patients in this category include those with liver disease, DIC, and those taking warfarin.
2. Patients with congenital isolated factor deficiencies when specific virally safe replacement products are not available (see below); those with isolated deficiencies of fibrinogen, factor VIII, or factor XIII are probably better treated with cryoprecipitate.
3. Patients with thrombotic thrombocytopenic purpura (TTP) in the process of plasma exchange (see Chap. 214).
4. Some patients who receive massive transfusion and have evidence of a coagulopathy and active bleeding (see below).
5. Patients with antithrombin III deficiency when antithrombin III concentrates are not available.

FFP is *not* indicated for patients who require volume expansion.

TABLE 215-1 The Contents of Cryoprecipitate (per Bag)

Factor VIIIC	80–120 units
von Willebrand Factor	80 units
Fibrinogen	200–300 mg
Factor XIII	40–60 units
Fibronectin	Variable

Cryoprecipitate

Cryoprecipitate is the cold precipitable protein fraction derived from FFP thawed at 1° to 6°C; it can be stored frozen for up to 1 year. The contents of a bag of cryoprecipitate are outlined in Table 215-1. The typical dose of cryoprecipitate given is two to four bags per 10 kg—usually 10 to 20 bags at a time. When given in large volumes, it is preferable to use ABO-compatible cryoprecipitate.

The indications for transfusion of cryoprecipitate are as follows. Keep in mind that it should not be used to treat hemophilia unless virally safe (recombinant or monoclonal-antibody purified) factors are not available and the patient has an immediately life-threatening bleed (see Chap. 212).

1. For patients with hypofibrinogenemia. In patients with congenital deficiency of fibrinogen or those with consumptive coagulopathy such as DIC, transfusion is indicated when the fibrinogen level is less than 100 mg/dL.
2. For patients with von Willebrand disease and active bleeding, cryoprecipitate should only be used when desmopressin (DDAVP) is not available or does not work and factor VIII concentrates containing von Willebrand factor are not available.
3. For patients with hemophilia A, only when virally inactivated factor VIII concentrates are not available.
4. For use as fibrin glue surgical adhesives.
5. For fibronectin replacement, which may be beneficial to promote healing in patients with trauma, severe burns, or sepsis.

Albumin

Albumin accounts for about 50 percent of the circulating protein and 75 percent of the plasma oncotic pressure. Albumin replacement products are available as 5% or 25% solutions in saline. Plasma protein fraction (PPF) is a similar product; it is a 5% solution containing 88 percent albumin and 12 percent globulins. These products undergo heat inactivation for 10 h at 60°C and are not known to transmit viral diseases.

The clinical indications for albumin infusion are controversial but may include the following:

1. As colloid replacement to replace or maintain oncotic pressure. Most clinical experimental studies suggest that there is no advantage to colloid solutions over crystalloid in the acute management of hemorrhagic shock. Infused albumin solutions rapidly distribute to the extravascular space and are expensive.
2. In conjunction with large volume paracentesis in patients with refractory ascites.
3. In patients with severe burns. Most centers are moving away from this practice.

Immunoglobulins

Intravenous immunoglobulins, commonly referred to as *IVIg*, are being increasingly used for a variety of medical conditions. There are six preparations currently available in the United States. Several incidences of transmission of the hepatitis C virus have been documented with use of these products. The current indications for use are as follows:

1. Primary and secondary immunodeficiency, such as in patients with congenital immunodeficiency or chronic lymphocytic leukemia, bone marrow transplant patients, pediatric patients infected with the human immunodeficiency virus (HIV-1), and for the prevention of sepsis in premature infants and of infection in patients in intensive care settings.
2. Patients with immune or inflammatory disorders such as immune thrombocytopenic purpura or Kawasaki syndrome.

Two notable and interesting complications that may occur with the infusion of immunoglobulins are (1) anaphylaxis, which can occur in patients with IgA deficiency; these patients need to be given the IgA-depleted product; and (2) development of transient positive serologies in some patients due to the passive transfer of antibodies against hepatitis C and cytomegalovirus (CMV)

Antithrombin III (ATIII)

Antithrombin III is a serum protein that has inhibitory effects on coagulation factors, activated factor II (thrombin), as well as activated factors IX, X, XI, and XII. Deficiency of ATIII can be congenital or acquired. Replacement ATIII is available in two preparations obtained by heparin-affinity chromatography. The products undergo viral inactivation for 10 h at 60°C, which inactivates HIV-1. There are ever-expanding uses for ATIII replacement, but currently its main use is for patients with hereditary deficiency of ATIII with acute thromboembolism or the prophylaxis of thrombosis in these patients. It is also being used experimentally for the prevention of thrombosis in surgical patients, for obstetric emergencies, and for shock and DIC.

Specific Factor Replacement Therapy

The most common congenital factor deficiencies, hemophilia A, hemophilia B, and von Willebrand disease, are discussed in Chap. 212. Other congenital factor deficiencies are rare and unlikely to be encountered, but the emergency physician needs to be aware of their existence and have a basic knowledge of what products are used for the management of acute bleeding episodes. Table 215-2 outlines the recommended therapy for congenital factor deficiencies.

TABLE 215-2 Replacement Therapy for Congenital Factor Deficiencies

Coagulation Factor	Incidence*	Replacement Therapy
Factor I (fibrinogen)	150 cases	Cryoprecipitate
Factor II (prothrombin)	>30 cases	FFP for minor bleeding episodes Prothrombin complex concentrate† for major bleeding
Factor V	150 cases	FFP
Factor VII	150 cases	FFP for minor bleeding episodes Prothrombin complex concentrates for major bleeding Recombinant factor VII_A (experimental)
Factor VIII‡	1 in 10,000 males	Factor VIII concentrates (cryoprecipitate or FFP if not available) Desmopressin for those with mild hemophilia
von Willebrand disease	up to 1 in 100 persons	Desmopressin (or some factor VIII concentrates or cryoprecipitate)
Factor IX‡	1 in 30,000 males	Factor IX concentrates
Factor X	1 in 500,000	FFP for minor bleeding episodes Prothrombin complex concentrates for major bleeding
Factor XI§	3 in 10,000 Ashkenazi Jews 1 in 1,000,000 in general	FFP
Factor XII	Several hundred cases	Replacement not required
Factor XIII	>100 cases	FFP or cryoprecipitate

*Incidence as of 1998.
†See Chap. 212 for details concerning prothrombin complex concentrates.
‡See Chap. 212 for detailed management recommendations for patients with hemophilia A and hemophilia B.
§Factor XI levels correlate poorly with bleeding complications; many patients have low levels, but no bleeding complications.

COMPLICATIONS OF TRANSFUSIONS

Up to 20 percent of all transfusions may lead to some type of adverse reaction. Fortunately, most of these reactions are mild and not of long-term consequence to the patient. Transfusion reactions can occur while the transfusion is in process (immediate reactions) or the adverse result may not become apparent for hours to years (delayed reactions). Table 215-3 outlines the types of acute transfusion reactions and their management and evaluation.

Immediate Transfusion Reactions

ACUTE HEMOLYTIC TRANSFUSION REACTION This is a medical emergency that occurs when incompatible RBCs are transfused. Most often this is an intravascular event resulting from incompatibility in the ABO blood group system. Table 215-4 reviews compatibility in the ABO blood group system. An acute hemolytic reaction occurs when the incompatible transfused cells are immediately destroyed by antibodies. The overall incidence of acute hemolytic transfusion reactions is estimated at 1 in 21,000 to 1 in 250,000 units transfused, but the outcome is fatal in 1 in 100,000 transfusions.

Clinically, a transfusion reaction should be suspected when the patient complains of fever, chills, low back pain, breathlessness, or a

TABLE 215-3 Acute Transfusion Reactions: Recognition, Management, Evaluation

Reaction Type	Signs and Symptoms	Management	Evaluation
Acute intravascular hemolytic reaction	Fever, chills, low back pain, flushing dyspnea, tachycardia, shock, hemoglobinuria	Immediately stop transfusion IV hydration to maintain diuresis; diuretics may be necessary Cardiorespiratory support as indicated Can be life threatening	Retype and crossmatch Direct and indirect Coombs tests CBC, creatinine, PT, aPTT Haptoglobin, indirect bilirubin, LDH, plasma free hemoglobin Urine for hemoglobin
Acute extravascular hemolytic reaction	Often have low-grade fever but may be entirely asymptomatic	Stop transfusion Rarely causes clinical instability	Hemolytic workup as above to rule out the possibility of intravascular hemolysis
Febrile nonhemolytic transfusion reaction	Fever, chills	Stop transfusion Manage as in intravascular hemolytic reaction (above) because cannot initially distinguish between the two Can treat fever and chills with acetaminophen and meperidine Usually mild but can be life threatening in patients with tenuous cardiopulmonary status Consider infectious work-up	Hemolytic workup as above because initially cannot distinguish the etiology
Allergic reaction	If mild, urticaria, pruritus If severe, dyspnea, bronchospasm, hypotension, tachycardia, shock	Stop transfusion If mild, reaction can treat with diphenhydramine; if symptoms resolve, can restart transfusion If severe, may require cardiopulmonary support; do not restart transfusion	For mild symptoms that resolve with diphenhydramine, no further workup is necessary, although blood bank should be notified For severe reaction, do hemolytic workup as above because initially will be indistinguishable from a hemolytic reaction
Hypervolemic	Dyspnea, tachycardia, hypertension, headache, jugular venous distention, pulmonary rales, hypoxia	Stop transfusion or decrease rate to 1 mL/kg/h Diuresis Can be difficult to distinguish from a hemolytic reaction; if cannot distinguish, stop transfusion and treat as if intravascular hemolytic reaction	If clearly hypervolemic, no further evaluation is needed; CXR may be helpful If hemolytic reaction is a possibility, do hemolytic workup as above

Note: IV, intravenous; CBC, complete blood count; PT, prothrombin time; aPTT, activated partial thromboplastin time; LDH, lactate dehydrogenase; CXR, chest radiograph.

burning sensation at the site of infusion. If the reaction progresses, the patient may develop hypotension, bleeding, respiratory failure, and acute tubular necrosis. More severe reactions occur in anesthesized or unconscious patients because of their inability to alert the staff that something is amiss. The management of a patient with a possible transfusion reaction begins with the immediate discontinuation of the transfusion. While the transfusion workup is in progress, the patient should be aggressively hydrated in order to maintain a brisk diuresis (at least 100 mL/h) for at least 24 h. Furosemide may be required to maintain the diuresis. Cardiorespiratory support may be needed. The laboratory evaluation of a possible hemolytic transfusion reaction includes the finding of hemoglobinemia (elevated plasma free hemoglobin) and hemoglobinuria. Other tests for hemolysis should be performed including haptoglobin and bilirubin. Direct and indirect Coombs test should be performed on pre- and posttransfusion blood samples. A complete blood count, creatinine, and coagulation tests will also be helpful.

TABLE 215-4 ABO Blood Group System Compatibility

Phenotype	Antigens on RBCs	Antibodies in Serum	Can Receive RBCs of Type
A	A	anti-B	A, O
B	B	anti-A	B, O
AB	A and B	None	A, B, O
O	None	anti-A; anti-B	O

A less common and less serious type of acute hemolytic transfusion reaction is extravascular hemolysis (in the spleen), usually caused by transfusion of incomplete Rh cells. These patients may be asymptomatic and only rarely have hemoglobinemia and hemoglobinuria. Laboratory studies in this situation will show a positive Coombs test, elevated level of indirect bilirubin, and a poor response to the transfusion—the hemoglobin and hematocrit do not rise as expected. This type of hemolytic reaction usually does not require any treatment.

FEBRILE NONHEMOLYTIC TRANSFUSION REACTION This reaction is estimated to occur once for every 200 units transfused. During the transfusion or within a few hours after its completion, the patient has a temperature elevation of at least 1°C and usually has chills. The usual cause of this febrile reaction is an antigen-antibody reaction involving the plasma, platelets, or white blood cells that are passively transfused to the recipient along with the RBCs. Such a reaction occurs most commonly in patients who have been multiply transfused or in multiparous women. Febrile reactions not involving hemolysis are

TABLE 215-5 Tests Performed on Donated Blood

ABO, Rh determination	Hepatitis B surface antigen
Antibody to HIV-1	Hepatitis B core antibody
Antigen to HIV-1 p24	Antibody to hepatitis C
Antibody to HIV-2	ALT
Antibody to HTLV-I/II	Serology for syphilis

Note: HIV, human immunodeficiency virus; HTLV, human T-cell leukemia virus; ALT, alanine transaminase.

usually mild but can be life threatening in patients with tenuous cardiopulmonary status or in those who are already critically ill. As in the acute hemolytic transfusion reaction, the first step in management is to stop the transfusion. Clinically, it is impossible to distinguish initially between a febrile nonhemolytic reaction and the more serious acute hemolytic transfusion reaction. The hemolytic transfusion must be ruled out by repeat crossmatching of the blood and repeat Coombs testing. Infections that could potentially be responsible for the fever and chills should be considered. Patients with a known history of febrile reactions to transfusions can be pretreated with acetaminophen or aspirin and meperidine can be given to treat the chills, or the patient can be given leukocyte-depleted blood components.

ALLERGIC TRANSFUSION REACTION Allergic reactions to the transfused products occur in about 1 percent of all transfusions. The reaction is thought to be due to exposure to plasma proteins. Such reactions most commonly occur in IgA-deficient patients. Typical allergic symptoms such as skin erythema, urticaria, pruritus, bronchospasm, vasomotor instability, and, rarely, anaphylaxis occur. True anaphylaxis occurs only once in 20,000 transfusions. Such reactions are rarely serious. The severity of the reaction is not dose-related—the transfusion often can be completed. When an apparent allergic transfusion reaction occurs, the infusion should be discontinued while the patient is evaluated and treated with diphenhydramine. If the patient improves with this therapy, the transfusion can be restarted. Some clinicians routinely premedicate patients who have a history of allergic transfusion reactions.

Delayed Reactions

INFECTIONS Since HIV-1 was identified in the U.S. blood supply in the mid-1980s, several screening methods have been instituted to ensure the safety of the blood products in current use. The majority of blood products available in the United States today are collected from volunteer donors who reliably provide a safer product than that obtained from paid donors. There are two levels of screening of the donors and blood: (1) donor prescreening by a questionnaire that excludes persons with a high risk of viral exposure and (2) serologic testing of the donor blood. The tests typically performed on donor blood are outlined in Table 215-5. Some component products, factor replacement products in particular, undergo further treatment to ensure viral inactivation. The risks of transmission of various infections by transfused blood products are listed in Table 215-6. These risks are averages; the actual risk may be higher or lower depending on the incidence of infection in the area the blood is collected. Rarely, blood products become contaminated with bacteria during preparation or bacterial infection can come from an infected donor. This should be considered when a patient develops fever during or shortly after the transfusion of blood products.

DELAYED HEMOLYTIC REACTION This reaction occurs 7 to 10 days after transfusion as a result of an antigen-antibody reaction that develops after the transfusion. Laboratory studies reflect a slowly falling hemoglobin, and a previously negative Coombs test becomes positive. The patient is generally asymptomatic. Further blood bank workup is needed to detect the causative antibody.

HYPERVOLEMIA The transfusion of PRBCs or plasma results in the rapid expansion of intravascular volume. Such expansion may not be well tolerated by patients with limited cardiovascular reserve, particularly infants and elderly patients. Patients may complain of headaches and shortness of breath; on examination, they will have signs of congestive heart failure. Treatment consists of slowing the rate of infusion and diuresis of the patient. As a general guide, infusions in adults are at a rate of 2 to 4 mL/kg/h. This can be slowed to 1 mL/kg/h in patients at risk of fluid overload.

HYPOTHERMIA Hypothermia may develop in patients who receive rapid infusion of large quantities of refrigerated blood. This is generally only a problem if three or more units are given rapidly. PRBCs are stored at 4°C, platelets at 20° to 24°C, and FFP at −18°C. Rapid infusers/warmers may be used but should not raise the temperature to more than 40°C, or hemolysis can occur. The easiest method for warming blood is to infuse it along with warmed (39° to 43°C) normal saline, which will warm and dilute the blood.

NONCARDIOGENIC PULMONARY EDEMA Noncardiogenic pulmonary edema occurs in approximately 1 in 5000 transfusions. Believed to be due to incompatibility of passively transferred leukocyte antibodies, the problem usually develops within 4 h of the transfusion. Clinically, the patient has respiratory distress, fever, chills, and tachycardia, and a chest radiograph shows diffuse patchy infiltrates without cardiomegaly. There is no evidence of fluid overload or congestive heart failure. In the majority of cases, the pulmonary infiltrates resolve over a few days and only supportive care is needed. This reaction can, however, be fatal in patients who are already critically ill.

ELECTROLYTE IMBALANCE Citrate is a component of the preservative solution used in blood storage; it functions as an anticoagulant by chelating calcium. Significant hypocalcemia rarely occurs as a result of transfusion-related citrate exposure because patients with normal hepatic function readily metabolize citrate to bicarbonate. Even with massive transfusion, calcium replacement is rarely needed.

Hypokalemia can be a problem when large amounts of blood are transfused. When the citrate is metabolized to bicarbonate, the blood becomes alkalotic and potassium is driven to the intracellular compartment.

Hyperkalemia rarely is a problem after blood transfusions even though the potassium content increases in stored blood. This may be a problem for patients with renal failure or neonates.

GRAFT-VERSUS-HOST DISEASE This unfortunate reaction, which is fatal in more than 90 percent of cases, can occur after the transfusion of nonirradiated cellular blood components into an immunocompromised host. Graft-versus-host disease occurs when immunologically competent lymphocytes are passively transferred to an immunoincompetent host who is unable to destroy the donor lymphocytes. The donor lymphocytes engraft, recognize the host as foreign, then attack the host tissues. Bone marrow aplasia commonly results.

EMERGENCY TRANSFUSIONS

In the ED, the administration of type O blood or type-specific incompletely crossmatched blood may be lifesaving; however, it carries the risk of severe, life-threatening transfusion reactions. Massive, uncontrolled hemorrhage from any cause may necessitate transfusion with uncrossmatched type O blood. Its use is limited to the early resuscitative phase of patients with shock from exsanguinating hemorrhage

TABLE 215-6 Estimated Risk of Infection Transmission via Blood Products, 1998

Virus	Risk per Units Transfused	Infection	Risk per Units Transfused
HIV-1[a]	1 in 680,000 units	Epstein-Barr virus (EBV)[d]	Rare[e]
Hepatitis B	1 in 63,000 units	Syphilis	Rare
Hepatitis C	1 in 100,000 units	Malaria	1 in 250,000 units
HTLV I/II[b]	1 in 641,000 units	Babesiosis	1 in 1 million units
CMV[c]	1 in 2 units	Toxoplasmosis	Rare
Parvovirus	1 in 10,000 units	Trypanosomiasis[f]	1 in 50,000

[a]HIV-2 is rarely found in the United States; data not available for its transmission.
[b]HTLV-I/II cause adult T-cell leukemia and myelopathy; only transmitted by RBCs, not plasma or cryoprecipitate.
[c]CMV is transmitted by RBCs, not by plasma or cryoprecipitate; CMV-negative blood products should be considered for immunosuppressed patients and bone marrow or solid organ transplant candidates or recipients.
[d]EBV is only transmitted by RBCs, not plasma or cryoprecipitate.
[e]"Rare"—specific incidence not available or unknown but of minimal clinical significance.
[f]Trypanosomiasis is a parasite that causes Chagas' disease.
Note: HIV, human immunodeficiency virus; HTLV, human T-cell leukemia virus; CMV, cytomegalovirus.

and insufficient response to infused crystalloid solutions. Patients with trauma, massive GI bleeding, ruptured aortic aneurysm, or unexpected intraoperative hemorrhage may be candidates to receive emergency transfusions. Before any transfusions are given, baseline laboratory studies should be done, including blood for typing and crossmatching. Current practice limits the use of uncrossmatched type O blood to the initial resuscitation of patients with massive hemorrhage. Type-specific blood often can be obtained from the blood bank in 10 to 15 min after the sample is received and will avoid the majority of transfusion reactions. Fully crossmatched blood typically can be obtained in 30 to 60 min. Most hospitals use Rh-negative blood when it has not been fully crossmatched. PRBCs are the only blood product that can be given for emergency transfusion. Plasma products contain too many antibodies and should not have a role in the early phase of treatment of massive hemorrhage. As soon as type-specific crossmatched PRBCs are available, they should be given. Subsequent crossmatching will become more difficult as increasing amounts of uncrossmatched blood are transfused.

MASSIVE TRANSFUSION

Massive transfusion is defined as the replacement of a volume equivalent to the patient's normal blood volume within a 24-h period. Potential complications of this procedure are bleeding, citrate toxicity, and hypothermia. Bleeding is the most frequent complication and is related to platelet and factor deficiencies. Actual thrombocytopenia does not regularly occur in this setting because even after the replacement of one blood volume, most patients still have about 35 to 40 percent of their original platelet count, about 100,000/μL. Bleeding is the result of mild thrombocytopenia combined with platelet dysfunction from renal or liver disease or DIC, and coagulation factor deficiencies. Coagulation factor deficiencies can develop in the setting of massive transfusion because stored blood has low levels of coagulation factors, especially factors V and VIII. The coagulopathy may be worsened by hypothermia, shock, sepsis, underlying liver disease, or DIC. In current practice, the routine use of platelet transfusions and FFP in massive transfusion is unwarranted, costly, and dangerous. Platelet transfusions should be given only if there is thrombocytopenia with oozing or excess bleeding. FFP should be given only when there is a documented coagulopathy and bleeding.

In modern blood banking, citrate toxicity is rarely a problem unless whole blood is being transfused. Patients receiving more than five units of whole blood, neonates, or patients with liver disease are at risk of hypocalcemia. An ionized calcium level should be obtained. The QT interval is not a reliable indicator of hypocalcemia in this setting. If calcium needs to be repleted, 5 to 10 mL of calcium gluconate given slowly IV is recommended.

Hypothermia is a potential risk when the patient receives three or more units of blood rapidly. When giving large quantities of blood rapidly, the blood itself needs to be warmed or it can be administered with warm saline (see above) in order to prevent iatrogenic hypothermia.

BLOOD ADMINISTRATION

The administration of blood products begins with the absolute identification of the patient and the unit to be transfused. Blood products are generally infused through large bore intravenous tubing (16 gauge or greater) to prevent hemolysis and permit rapid infusion if needed. Normal saline is the only crystalloid fluid compatible with PRBCs. Saline is usually given with the blood to dilute it and facilitate infusion. If multiple units of blood are to be given or are being given rapidly, warmed saline can be given concurrently (warmed to 39° to 43°C) or the blood itself can be warmed in an electric blood warmer. Blood will hemolyze if warmed to more than 40°C. Except in emergency settings, the infusion of blood is started slowly over the first 30 min, when reactions are most likely to occur. Patients without cardiovascular disease can be given a unit of PRBCs over 1 to 2 h. Those with a risk of hypervolemia should receive each unit over 3 to 4 h. Micropore filters should be used when giving any blood product in order to filter microaggregates of platelets, fibrin, and leukocytes. Rapid infusion of blood in the emergency setting may be facilitated by the use of pressure infusion devices that apply pneumatic pressure (up to 300 mmHg) to the blood unit.

BIBLIOGRAPHY

AuBuchon JP, Birkmeyer JD, Busch MP: Safety of the blood supply in the United States: Opportunities and controversies. *Ann Intern Med* 127(10):904, 1997.

Baron BJ, Scalea TM: Acute blood loss. *Emerg Med Clin North Am* 14(1):35, 1996.

Brugnara C, Churchill WH: Plasma and component therapy, in Loscalzo J, Schafer AI (eds): *Thrombosis and Hemorrhage,* 2d ed. Baltimore: Williams & Wilkins, 1998, p 1135.

Lungberg GD: Practice parameter for the use of fresh frozen plasma, cryoprecipitate, and platelets. *JAMA* 271:777, 1994.

Ness PM, Rothko K: Principles of red blood cell transfusion, in Hoffman R, Benz EJ Jr, Shattil SJ, et al (eds): *Hematology, Basic Principles and Practice,* 2d ed. New York: Churchill-Livingstone, 1995, p 1981.

Roberts HR, Bingham MD: Other coagulation factor deficiencies, in Loscalzo J, Schafer AI (eds): *Thrombosis and Hemorrhage,* 2d ed. Baltimore: Williams & Wilkins, 1998, p 773.

EXOGENOUS ANTICOAGULANTS AND ANTIPLATELET AGENTS

Stephen D. Emond
John R. Cooke
J. Stephan Stapczynski

Antithrombotic therapy is standard for numerous arterial and venous thromboembolic conditions, including acute myocardial infarction (AMI), unstable angina pectoris, deep venous thrombosis (DVT), pulmonary embolism (PE), and stroke or cerebrovascular accident (CVA). Moreover, antithrombotic agents help prevent occlusive vascular disease in patients at risk for thrombosis. These agents, however, also have the potential to cause life-threatening complications, primarily uncontrolled hemorrhage. This chapter provides an overview of antithrombotic agents, including mechanisms, indications, contraindications, and therapies, as well as evaluation and management of acute bleeding complications. Detailed management of thromboembolic disorders is discussed in their respective chapters.

PATHOPHYSIOLOGY OF THROMBOSIS

The clotting cascade is discussed in detail in Chap. 210. Arterial thrombi, composed primarily of platelets bound by thin fibrin strands, develop under high-flow conditions, especially at sites of ruptured atherosclerotic plaques. Both anticoagulants and platelet-inhibiting drugs effectively prevent and treat arterial thrombosis. In contrast, venous thrombi form in areas of sluggish blood flow, and are composed mainly of red blood cells and large fibrin strands. Anticoagulant drugs are effective in preventing and treating venous thromboembolism, while platelet-suppressing agents are less important.[1]

AGENTS

Both arterial and venous thrombi may result in local vascular obstruction or distant embolization. Antithrombotic agents interfere with these processes by (1) preventing formation of the platelet-fibrin net (blocking thrombin activation or platelet function) or (2) accelerating clot breakdown (fibrinolysis). Antithrombotic agents are grouped by mechanism of action.[2] Anticoagulants block synthesis and activation of clotting factors. Antiplatelet agents interfere with platelet activation or aggregation. Fibrinolytics (inaccurately referred to as thrombolytics) dissolve the fibrin component of thrombi.

Oral Anticoagulants

Oral anticoagulants are used for prophylaxis of thromboembolic CVAs (in patients with atrial fibrillation, left ventricular thrombus, or cardiac valvular abnormalities or prostheses), DVT, and PE, as well as for certain peripheral arterial diseases (Table 216-1).

Sodium warfarin, a hydroxycoumarin compound, is the most widely used oral anticoagulant in North America. Readily absorbed from the gut, it reaches peak blood concentrations in 90 min and has a circulating half-life of 36 to 42 h. Warfarin blocks activation of vitamin K and thereby interferes with hepatic carboxylation of coagulation factors II, VII, IX, and X (Fig. 216-1). Without these vitamin K–dependent cofactors, the extrinsic pathway of thrombus formation is blocked. Warfarin also blocks the synthesis of proteins C and S, which work together to inhibit the function of factors V and VII in the coagulation cascade. Warfarin dosing is guided by the international normalized ratio (INR), a standardized measurement of prothrombin time (PT), with a desired therapeutic range of 2.0 to 2.5 in most cases.[3] Drugs and food that interfere with warfarin absorption or hepatic metabolism can have a profound effect on warfarin activity (Table 216-2).[4]

The pharmacologic effect of warfarin is to inhibit the synthesis of the four coagulation factors and protein C and S, resulting in a decrease in their plasma levels according to their half-life. Protein C has the shortest half-life (8 h), and its plasma level falls the most quickly. Factor VII has the shortest half-life of the coagulation factors, about 7 h, and plasma levels fall thereafter. Factor II has the longest half-life, about 60 h, and its plasma levels fall the most slowly after the start of warfarin therapy. The phase delay between the fall in protein C (an antithrombotic protein) and the fall in the affected four coagulation factors (thrombotic proteins) results in a transient state of increased thrombogenesis that lasts for about 24 to 36 h. This potential hypercoagulable state is reduced but not eliminated by initiating warfarin therapy with 5-mg/d doses.[5] For patients in whom sudden intravascular thrombosis can be fatal (e.g., those with a prosthetic heart valve), anticogulation should be ensured with heparin [or perhaps a low-molecular-weight (LMW) product] before starting oral warfarin. Thus, a noncompliant patient with a prosthetic heart valve who has stopped oral anticoagulants should not simply be discharged with instructions to restart warfarin.

There also appears to be rebound during warfarin withdrawal. During the first 4 days, factors VII and IX increase more rapidly than proteins C and S, resulting in an imbalance between provokers and inhibitors of coagulation.[6] This potential hypercoagulable condition appears to exist biochemically for about 4 days during warfarin withdrawal. However, prospective studies have shown no increased incidence of clinical episodes of thrombosis with sudden termination of warfarin therapy compared to gradual tapering. The thromboembolic events that occur in patients after warfarin discontinuation are related more to the underlying condition than to the method of termination.

The two major complications of warfarin therapy are major bleeding episodes and skin necrosis. Bleeding is usually related to the degree of anticoagulation and can be prevented by laboratory monitoring with dose adjustments. Reversal with vitamin K_1 or factor replacement may be necessary for major hemorrhage. Skin necrosis occurs primarily in patients with protein C deficiency. This complication usually develops 3 to 8 days after starting treatment and is due to thrombosis of small cutaneous vessels. Warfarin in contraindicated in pregnancy because it is teratogenic and causes fetal hemorrhage.

Parenteral Anticoagulants

UNFRACTIONATED HEPARIN A mixture of glycosaminoglycan chains of varying lengths, unfractionated heparin contains a unique subunit that binds antithrombin III (AT-III). The heparin–AT-III complex binds to and inhibits coagulation factors IX_a and X_a, of the intrinsic pathway, and, most important, thrombin. Heparin is not an anticogulant by itself, and AT-III deficiency is a rare but important cause of heparin resistance. Unfractionated heparin must be given parenterally (intravenously or subcutaneously). Its half-life (30 to 150 min) depends on the dose and route. Weight-based intravenous heparin dosing protocols are the most reliable approach for rapidly achieving a therapeutic response and preventing further thrombosis during acute thromboembolic events. The subcutaneous method is less reliable for the treatment of acute thromboembolic disease because the bioavailability of subcutaneous unfractionated heparin ranges from 10 to 90 percent, depending on the dose. However, the subcutaneous route may be acceptable for prophylaxis, as opposed to treatment of thrombosis. One

TABLE 216-1 Antithrombotic Therapy Guidelines

Clinical Indication	Comments
TREATMENT OF DEEP VENOUS THROMBOSIS OR PULMONARY EMBOLISM	
Heparin: 70–80 U/kg IV bolus, then 15–18 U/kg/h continuous infusion, with the aPTT checked after 6 h and the infusion adjusted to maintain the aPTT 1.5–2.5 times control *with* concurrent institution of warfarin	In most cases, heparin and warfarin can be started simultaneously, with an overlap of 3–5 days. Warfarin should be continued for at least 3 months.
Enoxaparin: 1 mg/kg SC bid	Caval interruption if anticoagulant therapy contraindicated
Dalteparin: 100 IU/kg SC bid	
SK: 250,000 U IV bolus, then 100,000 U/h continuous infusion for 1–3 d	
tPA: front-loaded regimen (up to 100 total dose) over the first 90 min	
Urokinase: 4400 U/kg IV bolus, then 4400 U/kg/h continuous infusion for 1–3 d	
ATRIAL FIBRILLATION	
High-risk patients: warfarin (INR 2.0–3.0)	High risk: increasing age, left ventricular dysfunction, female gender, hypertension, valvular heart disease, previous thromboembolism
Low-risk patients: aspirin 325 mg/d	Low risk: ''lone'' AF (no structural heart disease)
Before elective cardioversion: heparin, then long-term warfarin (INR 2.0–3.0)	In new AF (>2d): IV heparin, then short-term warfarin (4 wk) *if* stable sinus rhythm persists and no atrial thrombus on transesophageal echocardiogram
RHEUMATIC VALVULAR HEART DISEASE	
History of embolism or atrial fibrillation: warfarin (INR 2.0–3.0)	Rheumatic aortic valve disease without history of embolism, AF, or concomitant mitral disease should *not* receive warfarin prophylaxis.
Mitral valve disease and left atrium >5.5 cm: warfarin (INR 2.0–3.0)	
MITRAL VALVE PROLAPSE	
TIA: aspirin 81 mg/d	
TIA with aspirin *or* embolism or AF: warfarin (INR 2.0–3.0)	
TIA with aspirin *and* warfarin contraindication: ticlopidine 250 mg bid	
MITRAL ANNULAR CALCIFICATION	
History of embolism or AF: warfarin (INR 2.0–3.0)	
INFECTIVE ENDOCARDITIS (PROPHYLAXIS *AFTER* INFECTION)	
Uncomplicated, native or bioprosthetic valve: *no* prophylaxis	Indications for prophylaxis *during* acute endocarditis are uncertain and depend on comorbid factors, evidence and size of vegetations, and severity of embolism.
Mechanical prosthetic valve: warfarin (INR 2.5–3.5)	
PROSTHETIC HEART VALVES	
Mechanical prosthetic valves: warfarin (INR 2.5–3.5)	
With systemic embolism: warfarin plus aspirin 81–160 mg/d *or* warfarin plus dipyridamole 400 mg/d	
With high risk of bleeding: warfarin (INR 2.0–3.0) ± aspirin 81–160 mg/d	
Bioprosthetic heart valves	
Mitral: warfarin for 3 months (INR 2.0–3.0)	
Aortic: aspirin 325 mg/d	
With history of embolism, AF, or atrial thrombus (high-risk patients): warfarin (INR 2.0–3.0) plus aspirin 81 mg/d	

disadvantage of unfractionated heparin is that it interferes with most laboratory investigations for hypercoagulable states. However, functional assays for protein C and S can be performed if heparin is removed from the plasma by an absorbent column or by heparinase.[7] Both unfractionated heparin and the newer LMW derivatives do not cross the placenta and are safe to use in pregnancy.

The two major complications of unfractioned heparin are major bleeding episodes and heparin-induced thrombocytopenia. Bleeding is related to the degree of anticoagulation and can be prevented by laboratory monitoring with dose adjustment. In the event of major hemorrhage, the infusion can be stopped, and the anticoagulant effect will be greatly diminished in a few hours. Heparin-induced thrombocytopenia (HIT) is due to an antibody, usually IgG, that attaches to and stimulates platelets. This platelet activation produces both thrombocytopenia and a tendency for thrombosis. The incidence of HIT is between 1 and 3 percent in patients treated with unfractionated heparin but significantly less in patients treated with LMW products. The onset of HIT is usually 5 to 12 days after heparin treatment is started but may be sooner for patients who developed the antibody from a previous exposure. The platelet count nadir is often modest, typically 20,000 to 150,000 per μL. Thrombosis may involve the skin (similar to warfarin-induced cutaneous necrosis), the arteries (e.g., femoral artery thrombosis), or the veins (e.g., recurrent DVT or PE).

The anticoagulant effect of heparin has been traditionally monitored with the activated partial thromboplastin time (aPTT), which is widely available from clinical laboratories (Table 216-1).[2,8] However, the reagents used in the aPTT vary significantly in their sensitivity to unfractionated heparin, and the therapeutic range must be defined for each brand of aPTT reagent. In addition, there is not a linear relationship between heparin concentration, the anticoagulant activity of hepa-

TABLE 216-1 Antithrombotic Therapy Guidelines *(Continued)*

Clinical Indication	Comments
ACUTE MYOCARDIAL INFARCTION	
Antiplatelet therapy: aspirin (nonenteric coated) for all patients with suspected AMI 160–325 mg/d	All post-myocardial-infarction patients should receive aspirin 160–325 mg/d for an indefinite period (unless contraindicated or if on warfarin).
Heparin: most experts recommend use of heparin after tPA treatment (75–80 U/kg IV bolus, then 15–18 U/kg/h IV adjusted to keep aPTT 1.5–2.5 times control *or* 17,500 U SC bid	
Patients with AMI: *low-dose* heparin for DVT prophylaxis (e.g., 5000 U SC bid until ambulatory)	
Patients at high risk for mural thrombosis or systemic embolism: heparin, then warfarin for 1–3 months (INR 2.0–3.0)	
Fibrinolytic therapy	Optimal strategies are unclear. Research is evolving rapidly.
Streptokinase: 1–1.5 million U IV over 60 min	
tPA: 15 mg bolus, then 0.75 mg/kg over 30 min (maximum, 50 mg), then 0.50 mg/kg over 60 min (maximum, 35 mg)	See Table 216-3 for contraindications to fibrinolytic therapy.
Reteplase: 10 U IV bolus, then a second dose at 30 min (ongoing trials)	
UNSTABLE ANGINA PECTORIS	
Aspirin: 162 mg/d	
Heparin: 75–80 U/kg IV bolus, then 15–18 U/kg/h IV to keep aPTT 1.5–2.5 times control	
Glycoprotein IIb-IIIa receptor blockers: eptifibatide 180 μg/kg bolus IV, then 2.0 μg/kg/min for 72 h plus heparin (emergency department use controversial)	
PERIPHERAL VASCULAR DISEASE	
Aspirin: 160–325 mg/d for all patients with peripheral vascular disease (high risk for AMI or CVA)	
CEREBROVASCULAR DISEASE	
Acute CVA within 3 h of symptom onset and no intracranial hemorrhage on brain CT: tPA 90 mg over 1 h, with 0.9 mg/kg as initial bolus	Use of fibrinolytics in acute CVA requires *strict* adherence to national guidelines and should be done with informed consent (see text). Adjunctive use of anticoagulants must be avoided for 48 h.
Acute cardioembolic stroke	
Small-to-moderate size, no hemorrhage on CT or MRI: IV heparin, then warfarin (INR 2.0–3.0)	Some evidence suggests that ticlopidine may be the preferred agent in patients with completed stroke.
Large size *or* poorly controlled hypertension: delay anticoagulation for 5–14 d	
Completed stroke: aspirin 81–325 mg/d or ticlopidine if aspirin allergic or intolerant	
TIA: aspirin 81–325 mg/d or ticlopidine if aspirin allergic or intolerant	
Asymptomatic carotid bruit or symptomatic carotid stenosis: aspirin 81–325 mg/d	

Abbreviations: AF, atrial fibrillation; aPTT, activated partial thromboplastin time; AMI, acute myocardial infarction; bid, twice a day; CT, computed tomography; CVA, cerebrovascular accident; DVT, deep venous thrombosis; INR, international normalized ratio; IV, intravenous; MRI, magnetic resonance imaging; SC, subcutaneous; SK, streptokinase; TIA, transient ischemic attack; and tPA, tissue plasminogen activator.

rin (as measured by its anti-factor X_a activity), and the aPTT. For most purposes, a therapeutic range for heparin can be either an aPTT of 1.5 to 2.5 the "normal" value, or a heparin level of 0.2 to 0.4 U/mL when assayed by protamine titration or 0.3 to 0.7 U/mL when assayed for anti-Xa activity.[8] Unfractionated heparin can increase the PT and INR by a variable amount, depending on the heparin concentration and the thromboplastin reagent used in the assay. Typically, therapeutic concentrations of heparin increase the PT by approximately 1 to 5 s.

LOW-MOLECULAR-WEIGHT HEPARIN FRACTIONS Enoxaparin, dalteparin, and ardeparin are prepared from unfractionated heparin and contain almost solely short (<18 saccharide units) chains. LMW heparin binds to AT-III, but the short saccharide chains of LMW are not adequate for binding to thrombin. However, the LMW/AT-III complex can bind to and inhibit factor X_a, accounting for the anticoagulant effect.[9] Compared to unfractionated heparin, LMW heparin is highly bioavailable (90 percent) and has a longer circulating half-life (3 to 4 h), allowing once- or twice-daily subcutaneous dosing. LMW heparin is used primarily for DVT prophylaxis, and enoxaparin can be used in unstable angina and non-Q wave AMI.[10] Compared to unfractionated heparin, the dose-response curve of LMW heparin is much more predictable, and laboratory monitoring is not routinely required in clinically stable patients, particularly those receiving prophylactic treatment for venous thrombosis or higher doses for treatment of venous thromboembolism.[11] LMW heparin is cleared by the kidneys, and, in patients with significant renal impairment, therapy may be monitored by anti-X_a activity.[9,11] The therapeutic level is not precisely known. An anti-X_a activity of 0.6 to 1.0 IU/mL obtained 4 h after a twice-daily subcutaneous treatment of venous thromboembolism appears to be a conservative therapeutic range. The LMW heparins produce small, dose-related elevations in the PT, INR, and aPTT. Compared to unfractionated heparin, LMW heparin has the advantage that therapy does not affect the laboratory investigation of potential hypercoagulable states.

DANAPAROID Danaparoid is a mixture of LMW glycosaminoglycans that produces predominately anti-X_a activity. The bioavailability

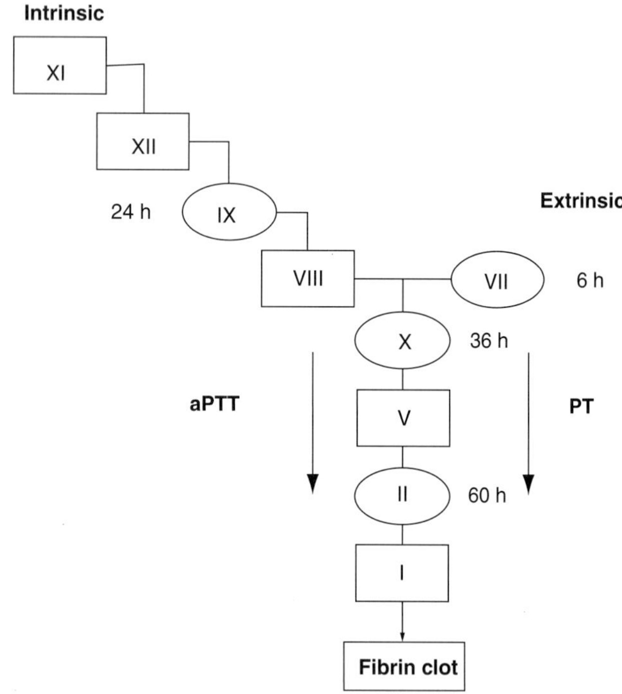

FIG. 216-1. Clotting factors and tests of coagulation.

of danaparoid is nearly 100 percent, and it has an antithrombotic half-life of about 8 h. Danaparoid is currently recommended only for DVT prophylaxis at doses of 750 U (1250 U for patients >90 kg) twice daily by subcutaneous injection. Laboratory monitoring is not routinely required for this prophylactic regimen.[11] Like other LMW heparins, danaparoid produces minimal elevation in PT, INR, or aPTT. Intravenous danaparoid can also be used for systemic anticoagulation, but this approach is not currently approved by the US Food and Drug Administration (FDA).

HIRUDIN Derived from the medicinal leech, hirudin exerts its anticoagulant activity by binding tightly to thrombin, blocking both the active and the substrate binding sites.[11] Hirudin produces its anticoagulant activity independently of AT-III and, unlike heparin, is not affected by plasma and platelet proteins. Hirudin is prepared by recombinant technology and differs slightly from the natural substance. Recombinant hirudin has been modified into a number of available analogues such as lepirudin and bivalirudin. Hirudin and its analogues are currently FDA-approved for anticoagulation in patients with heparin-associated thrombocytopenia. Administered intravenously, hirudin has a half-life of 50 min. Administered subcutaneously, the bioavailability is 90 percent, and the half-life is 2 to 3 h. Intravenous hirudin is monitored using the aPTT, generally maintaining a target range of 1.5 to 2.5 times the "normal" value. In theory, hirudin should both prevent new clot formation and dissolve existing thrombus. However, clinical trials of hirudin versus heparin in AMI or unstable angina demonstrated excess bleeding complications with no long-lasting benefits.[12] While a recent study showed benefit when hirudin was administered after reperfusion with streptokinase, hirudin is not currently approved for this indication.[13]

TABLE 216-2 Warfarin Interactions

Consideration	Prothrombin Time (PT)*
MAJOR	
Vitamin K malabsorption or dietary deficiency	↑
Excess vitamin K	↓
Reduced gut bacteria (antibiotics)	↑
Decreased warfarin absorption	↓
Altered warfarin metabolism (cytochrome P-450)	↑ or ↓
Drug effects	↑ or ↓
OTHER	
Decreased clotting factor production (liver disease)	↑
Increased metabolism of clotting factors (fever)	↑
Confounding technical or laboratory factors (e.g., phlebotomy, handling in transport, thromboplastin reagents)	↑ or ↓

* ↑ = PT prolonged; ↓ = PT decreased.

Blockers of Platelet Activation

Aspirin irreversibly blocks cyclooxygenase, an enzyme that in the platelet stimulates arachidonic acid conversion to thromboxane A_2 and in the blood vessel wall promotes prostacyclin synthesis. The net effect of aspirin in ischemic arterial beds depends on the balance between thromboxane A_2, a potent vasoconstrictor and platelet-aggregation agent, and prostacyclin, a vasodilator and platelet-aggregation inhibitor. Since prostacyclin synthesis is stimulated at lower aspirin levels than is thromboxane A_2 conversion, treatment plans often use low-dose strategies (e.g., 81 mg/day). For more rapid antiplatelet effect, a medium or higher dose (e.g., 162 mg) is indicated (Table 216-1).[14]

Aspirin is quickly absorbed in the upper gastrointestinal tract, reaches peak blood concentrations in 15 to 20 min, and circulates with a half-life of 30 to 60 min. However, its inhibitory effect is irreversible and lasts for the life span of the platelet (about 10 days). The bleeding time (BT) has been sometimes used to detect the antiplatelet activity of aspirin, but virtually all recognize that BT has poor reproducibility, sensitivity, and specificity when used to measure platelet-aggregation abnormalities.

Side effects are mainly gastrointestinal and dose related, and may be reduced with concomitant use of antacids, enteric coating, and buffering agents. Aspirin should be avoided in patients with known hypersensitivity and used cautiously in those with bleeding disorders or severe hepatic disease. Active gastrointestinal hemorrhage (e.g., bleeding peptic ulcer) is a contraindication to aspirin use. However, in AMI and unstable angina with occult gastrointestinal bleeding (e.g., guaiac-positive stool), most experts favor aspirin use with careful monitoring.[14] Aspirin therapy is also associated with a slightly increased risk of hemorrhagic stroke (12 per 10,000 over 3 years), but this risk is more than counterbalanced by a tenfold reduction in the risk of myocardial infarction and a threefold reduction in the risk of ischemic stroke.[15]

Blockers of Platelet Aggregation

During platelet aggregation, fibrinogen forms a bridge between adjacent platelets by binding to the platelet-surface receptor, glycoprotein IIb-IIIa. A variety of agents that interfere with the platelet membrane and the glycoprotein IIb-IIIa receptor have been introduced into clinical practice during the past few years.

PLATELET MEMBRANE ALTERING AGENTS Ticlopidine and clopidogrel deform the region of the platelet membrane next to its fibrinogen receptor and render it ineffective. Both of these agents have little utility in the acute setting. Ticlopidine (250 mg twice daily) improves outcomes in unstable angina but has a 24- to 28-h delay in its onset of action and is associated with reversible neutropenia. Ticlopidine is currently approved for use in patients with cerebrovascular diseases for whom aspirin therapy fails or who are aspirin-intolerant or allergic.[16] Clopidogrel (75 mg per day), a similar agent, has been approved for secondary prevention of AMI and CVA and in established peripheral artery disease. Its side effects include gastrointestinal upset and possible interactions with other medications.[17]

GLYCOPROTEIN IIB-IIIA RECEPTOR INHIBITORS Abciximab, eptifibatide, and tirofiban, glycoprotein IIb-IIIa receptor inhibitors, have been studied in AMI, unstable angina, and high-risk patients undergoing percutaneous angioplasty (PCTA).[18] Benefit has been consistently found when these agents are used in combination with other antithrombotic (aspirin, ticlodipine, or heparin) and reperfusion (fibrinolytics or PCTA) therapy.[18,19] Patients receiving glycoprotein IIb-IIIa inhibitors are more likely to have bleeding complications (particularly if heparin is also used and usually related to catheterization or coronary artery bypass surgery) but have no increased risk of intracranial hemorrhage. However, there is no clear evidence that glycoprotein IIb-IIIa inhibitors need to be started in the emergency department, as opposed to waiting until the patient reaches the catheterization laboratory or coronary care unit.[20]

Fibrinolytic Agents

Although mechanisms vary, each fibrinolytic agent eventually activates plasminogen to plasmin, which then dissolves the fibrin component of thrombi. Fibrinolytics currently approved in the United States include streptokinase (SK); anisoylated plasminogen-streptokinase activator complex (APSAC), or anistreplase; recombinant tissue plasminogen activator (tPA), or alteplase; reteplase; and urokinase.

STREPTOKINASE AND ANISTREPLASE SK, derived from β-hemolytic streptococci, binds to and activates plasminogen, producing plasmin, which in turn catalyzes fibrin lysis and thrombus dissolution. Circulating fibrinogen also undergoes plasmin-induced lysis, producing a state of "systemic fibrinolysis." SK is administered as a slow infusion (usually 1.0 to 1.5 million U intravenously over 60 min) and has a serum half-life of about 23 min, but in most patients systemic effects persist for up to 24 h. Because of the prolonged fibrinolytic state and increased risk of hemorrhage, anticoagulation with heparin is usually delayed following treatment with SK. SK is the least expensive fibrinolytic; typical wholesale costs approximate $300 per dose. Anistreplase, a modified active plasminogen-streptokinase complex, has an effect similar to that of SK, but its chief advantage is that it can be administered as a slow bolus (usually 30 mg intravenously over 5 min) and has a serum half-life of about 90 min. Anistreplase is costly ($1700 per dose) and has produced no improvement in outcome when compared to SK. Both SK and anistreplase are antigenic. In the Global Utilization of Streptokinase and Tissue Plasminogen Activator for Occluded Coronary Arteries (GUSTO) trial, allergic reactions occurred in about 6 percent of patients treated with SK and subcutaneous heparin.[21] Antibodies to SK develop approximately 5 days after treatment and persist for 6 months; retreatment with SK or anistreplase is not advised during this interval. In addition, SK or anistreplase should not be administered within 12 months of a streptococcal infection.

TISSUE PLASMINOGEN ACTIVATOR AND RETEPLASE tPA is a naturally occurring enzyme in vascular endothelial cells that directly cleaves a specific peptide bond in plasminogen, converting it to active plasmin, with subsequent fibrinolysis. tPA has binding sites for fibrin, which would suggest specificity for activity in the thrombus and less systemic fibrinolysis. Despite the in vitro clot specificity of tPA, its clinical side-effect profile is comparable to that of other fibrinolytics. The serum half-life of tPA is less than 5 min, and it produces a shorter fibrinolytic state that does SK. Heparin is commonly administered shortly after the completion of tPA infusion. Unlike SK and anistreplase, tPA is not antigenic. In the GUSTO trial utilizing front-loaded tPA and intravenous heparin, the rate of allergic reactions was under 2 percent.[21] Currently, tPA is commonly used for AMI, for which it is administered in a front-loaded format: 15-mg bolus, then 0.75 mg/kg over 30 min (maximum 50 mg), and then 0.50 mg/kg over 60 min (maximum 35 mg; Table 216-1). Reteplase, a derivative of tPA, is dosed as a double bolus (10-U bolus followed by a second dose at 30 minutes).[22] Both tPA and reteplase are expensive, approximately $3000 per treatment.

UROKINASE Urokinase has become nearly obsolete in acute management of thromboembolic disease, except for dissolution of indwelling-catheter-associated fibrin sheath and thrombosis, for which it is given as a local infusion starting at 500 U/kg/h (without a bolus) delivered directly into the catheter or into the affected vessel.[23] Systemic and other bleeding complications are infrequent with low-dose local therapy.

INDICATIONS FOR ANTITHROMBOTIC THERAPY

Acute Myocardial Infarction

The National Heart Lung and Blood Institute has established the principle that routine AMI patients should receive emergency reperfusion therapy, either fibrinolytic therapy initiated within 30 min or angioplasty within 60 min after arrival in the emergency department. There are four general criteria for emergent fibrinolytic therapy in AMI: (1) clinical presentation consistent with AMI within 12 h of symptom onset, (2) an electrocardiogram showing ST-segment elevation in two or more contiguous leads or new-onset left bundle branch block, (3) absence of contraindications (Table 216-3), and (4) absence of cardiogenic shock. Angioplasty, if available within 60 min of presentation, are preferred over peripheral fibrinolytic therapy for AMI with cardiogenic shock. Important additional considerations, however, include patient age, location of the infarct, relative contraindications to fibrinolysis, and duration of symptoms within the 12-hour criterion.

The decision to administer a fibrinolytic agent for a routine AMI should be made by the emergency physician. Specialty consultation may only delay treatment under such circumstances and is not necessary before initiating fibrinolysis. Patients who do *not* meet all four eligibility criteria (e.g., because symptoms have been present for >12

TABLE 216-3 Contraindications to Fibrinolytic Therapy

ABSOLUTE
Active or recent internal bleeding (≤14 d)
CVA <2–6 months or hemorrhagic CVA
Intracranial or intraspinal surgery or trauma <2 months
Intracranial or intraspinal neoplasm, aneurysm, or arteriovenous malformation
Known severe bleeding diathesis
On anticoagulants (warfarin, PT >15 s, heparin, increased aPTT)
Uncontrolled hypertension (i.e., blood pressure >185/100 mmHg)
Suspected aortic dissection or pericarditis
Pregnancy
RELATIVE
Active peptic ulcer disease
Cardiopulmonary resuscitation >10 min
Hemorrhagic ophthalmic conditions
Puncture of noncompressible vessel <10 d
Advanced age >75 years
Significant trauma or major surgery >2 weeks and <2 months
Advanced kidney or liver disease

*Concurrent menses is *not* a contraindication.
†In ischemic CVA, symptoms >3 h, severe hemispheric stroke, platelets <100/mL, and glucose <50 or >400 mg/dL are additional contraindications.

h or relative contraindications to fibrinolytic therapy are present) may still derive benefit from fibrinolytic therapy provided that no absolute contraindications are present and the differential diagnosis does not include disorders in which fibrinolytic therapy is harmful (e.g., aortic dissection). Under such circumstances, consultation with the physician who will assume continued definitive care of the patient (e.g., a cardiologist or internist) is reasonable and appropriate before initiating fibrinolysis.

The rapid administration of fibrinolytic therapy is of greater importance than the specific agent used. After this general principle, there is great debate concerning the differential benefit, if any, of particular agents. For example, in the GUSTO trial, the 30-day overall mortality rate with front-loaded tPA and intravenous heparin was 6.3 percent compared to SK and subcutaneous heparin, with a 7.2 percent mortality rate, or SK and intravenous heparin, with a 7.4 percent mortality rate.[21] This approximately 1 percent difference in absolute mortality rates translates into the observation that approximately 100 patients need to be treated with tPA for one additional life to be saved compared to treatment with SK. Further subgroup analysis revealed that the benefits of tPA over SK were less or nonexistent for patients with inferior myocardial infarction, those over 75 years of age, or those in whom fibrinolysis was not initiated until more than 4 h after symptom onset. While SK can be used in most cases, tPA is the agent of choice for patients with any of the following: (1) known allergy to SK or anistreplase, (2) prior administration of SK in the previous 6 months or anistreplase in the previous 12 months, (3) prior streptococcal infection in the previous 12 months, or (4) hemodynamic instability.[14]

Trials of prehospital fibrinolysis for AMI using bolus therapy (anistreplase) suggests that paramedic-initiated fibrinolytic therapy might be delivered earlier than hospital-initiated fibrinolysis without increased complications.[24] However, no mortality rate difference has been demonstrated. Very early fibrinolytic therapy (i.e., within 70 min of symptom onset), whether paramedic- or hospital-initiated, resulted in markedly diminished in-hospital mortality rates and infarct size. The American College of Emergency Physicians has stated that prehospital fibrinolytic therapy for AMI is still investigational, but in rural and remote communities, such therapy seems medically reasonable when excessive delays (>30 min) until arrival at the hospital may occur.[25] Special paramedic training in the clinical evaluation and treatment of AMI must be done on a continuing basis.

Immediate administration of aspirin alone results in a 23 percent reduction in rates from AMI, an effect that is even more pronounced when aspirin is used in combination with a fibrinolytic agent.[14] Aspirin should be given at a dose of 160 to 325 mg (chewed). Intravenous heparin is generally given to patients who receive tPA and is continued for at least 72 h. Intravenous heparin is usually started simultaneously with tPA at a dose of 70 to 80 U/kg intravenous bolus, followed by a continuous infusion of 15 to 18 U/kg/h. As noted above, heparin therapy is usually monitored with the aPTT, which should be first checked 6 h after the bolus dose and every 6 h thereafter during the first 24 h of therapy. Heparin is of uncertain benefit with SK and anistreplase, since it may increase bleeding complications and thus is not recommended if these fibrinolytic agents are used.[14]

Deep Venous Thrombosis or Pulmonary Embolism

Treatment for acute DVT or PE can be accomplished with unfractionated heparin using a weight-based intravenous regimen with monitoring by the aPTT and subsequent adjustments guided by the results. Alternatively, acute PE or DVT can be treated with LMW heparin, either enoxaparin 1 mg/kg or dalteparin 100 IU/kg, administered subcutaneously twice a day. The advantages of LMW heparin are a more predictable anticoagulant effect, easier administration, no requirement for laboratory monitoring, and a decreased risk of complications (major bleeding and heparin-induced thrombocytopenia). LMW heparin appears to be as effective as unfractionated heparin in the treatment of acute DVT or PE and, with the abovementioned advantages, has much to recommend it. The major disincentive to using LMW heparin is greater cost than for unfractionated heparin.

Fibrinolytic therapy offers significant advantages over conventional anticoagulant therapy in DVT and may result in prompt resolution of symptoms, prevention of PE, restoration of normal venous circulation, preservation of venous valvular function, and prevention of the postphlebitic syndrome.[26] Fibrinolytic therapy does not prevent clot propagation, rethrombosis, or subsequent embolization. Heparin therapy and oral anticoagulant therapy must always follow a course of fibrinolysis.

Unfortunately, patients with DVT may have absolute contraindications to fibrinolytic therapy. Fibrinolytic therapy is also not effective once the thrombus is adherent and begins to organize. Venous thrombi in the legs are often large and associated with complete venous occlusion. Theoretically, fibrinolytics, which act on the surface of the clot, may not be able to penetrate and lyse the entire thrombus. In such cases, catheter-directed fibrinolytic therapy is useful. Nevertheless, in selected patients, fibrinolytic therapy is more effective than heparin in achieving vein patency and reduces by half the incidence of postphlebitic syndrome at 3 years.

The hemorrhagic complications of fibrinolytic therapy are formidable (about three times higher than with heparin), including the small, but potentially fatal, risk of intracerebral hemorrhage. Currently, fibrinolytic therapy is not recommended in routine cases of DVT but may be considered for patients with massive iliofemoral vein thrombosis or young patients with acute onset of extensive DVT.

Ischemic Stroke

Prompt restoration of cerebral blood flow in acute ischemic stroke leads to improvement or resolution of neurologic deficits, but at the risk of intracranial hemorrhage. Only tPA has been shown to benefit carefully selected patients with acute ischemic stroke if given within 3 h of the onset of stroke symptoms.[27]

At the time of publication, three large randomized, double-blind, placebo-controlled studies—the National Institute of Neurologic Disorders and Stroke (NINDS) tPA Stroke Trial, the European Cooperative Acute Stroke Study (ECASS I), and the Second European-Australasian Acute Stroke Study (ECASS II)—had evaluated the efficacy of tPA for ischemic CVA.[28–30] Only the NINDS trial found statistical benefit in the primary end points for patients seen within 3 h of stroke symptom onset.[28] Eligibility criteria were strict: only 4 percent of the patients screened in NINDS were eligible for treatment. ECASS I patients were enrolled within 6 h of symptom onset and had no improvement in the primary end points but had some improvement in secondary functional measures and neurologic outcomes.[29] In ECASS II, patients again enrolled within 6 h after symptom onset had no statistical benefit with tPA in the primary end points, although post hoc analysis showed some benefit.[30] All three studies found that fibrinolytic treatment increased the incidence of intracranial hemorrhage from three to ten times, partially reducing the potential benefit of cerebral reperfusion.

In NINDS, patients in the tPA group were given 0.9 mg/kg, up to 90 mg total, over 1 h (10 percent of the total was given as an initial bolus). Antiplatelet and anticoagulation agents were withheld for the first 24 h following treatment. On the basis of these studies, tPA is contraindicated in patients with rapidly improving neurologic signs or minor symptoms, significant pretreatment hypertension (blood pressure > 185/110 mmHg or requiring aggressive therapy to control), seizure at onset, or symptoms suggestive of subarachnoid hemorrhage (Table 216-4). Currently, tPA can be recommended only if the protocol used in the NINDS stroke trial is strictly followed. Physicians are advised to obtain informed consent from patients or their proxies in all cases. It is best to have an emergency department policy developed in cooperation with neurologists concerning the administration of tPA for acute CVA.

TABLE 216-4 Inclusion and Exclusion Criteria for Fibrinolytic Therapy in Acute Ischemic Stroke

INCLUSION CRITERIA
Age >18 years
Clinical diagnosis of ischemic stroke
Symptom onset <3 h before treatment, CT (noncontrast) with no evidence of hemorrhage
EXCLUSION CRITERIA
History
Stroke or head trauma in previous 3 months
History of prior intracranial hemorrhage
Major surgery or recent serious trauma <14 d
Gastrointestinal or genitourinary bleeding <21 d
Arterial puncture at noncompressible site <7 d
Lumbar puncture <7 d
Pregnant or lactating female
Clinical
Rapidly improving symptoms
Seizure at onset of stroke
Symptoms of subarachnoid hemorrhage (even with normal CT)
Persistent systolic blood pressure >185 or diastolic >110 mmHg, or requiring aggressive therapy for control
Clinical evidence for AMI or pericarditis
Radiographic
CT evidence of hemorrhage
CT evidence of hypodensity and/or effacement of cerebral sulci in over one-third of middle cerebral artery territory
Laboratory
Glucose <50 or >400 mg/dL
Platelets <100,000/μL
On warfarin and PT >15 s
On heparin within 48 h and elevated aPTT

COMPLICATIONS OF ANTICOAGULATION AND ANTITHROMBOTIC THERAPY

The presentation and management of clinically important bleeding varies by agent. Effective management requires prompt identification of bleeding, supportive care, and agent-specific remedies (see Table 216-5). Major bleeding complications include intracranial hemorrhage or any bleeding requiring transfusion.

Warfarin

Risk of warfarin-induced bleeding is related to the intensity of therapy. For most purposes, the target INR is 2.0 to 2.5, except with mechanical valves, which require more intense anticoagulation (Table 216-1). The INR should be checked regularly, and special care should be paid to patients of extreme age (>80), with low–vitamin K diets, or on antibiotics or other medications with warfarin interactions (Table 216-2).

While melena or unexplained hematomas may be obvious signs of warfarin complications, less obvious presentations should also prompt investigation. Subtle confusion in an elderly patient on warfarin may suggest a subdural hematoma, and tachycardia with back pain may occur with retroperitoneal bleeding. An episode of gastrointestinal bleeding or hematuria may be a marker for underlying pathology and mandates further investigation.

Warfarin excess is confirmed by measuring the PT (INR). In patients with a high PT (INR) *without* clinically evident bleeding, cessation of warfarin, careful observation, and periodic monitoring is the safest course.[31] With clinically significant bleeding, however, reversal may be required, but the speed and extent of reversal must be balanced against the risk of recurrent thromboembolism in patients who require therapeutic anticoagulation. For example, an overanticoagulated patient with a prosthetic mitral valve may develop fatal thrombosis if rapidly and fully reversed. Five methods are available for reversal of warfarin: oral vitamin K_1, subcutaneous vitamin K_1, intravenous vitamin K_1, fresh-frozen plasma (FFP), and coagulation factor concentrates.

One mg of oral vitamin K_1 reliably reverses warfarin overanticoagulation in patients with INRs between 4.5 and 9.5.[32,33] Reversal is significant by 16 h, and the INR is within the therapeutic range by the second day. Subcutaneous vitamin K_1 (1 to 2 mg) reverses warfarin, with a measurable effect on the INR by 8 to 12 h.[34] Additional doses are often required up to a mean total dose of 4 to 5 mg to return the INR to 3 or less. Both oral and subcutaneous vitamin K_1 are given as warfarin doses are withheld, and both approaches require normal liver function to be effective. Low-dose oral and subcutaneous vitamin K_1 carry a small risk for patients who require therapeutic anticoagulation, and it is recommended that the emergency physician consult an appropriate specialist before using either approach.

Intravenous vitamin K_1 carries a rare but serious risk of anaphylaxis and should not be used for routine reversal of therapeutic overanticoagulation. For patients who require continued anticoagulation, intravenous administration carries the risk of overcorrection not associated with oral or subcutaneous use.[35] For patients with INRs between 6 and 12, the intravenous dose of vitamin K_1 should be 0.5 mg.[36] Intravenous vitamin K_1 should be used for patients poisoned by an ingestion of warfarin (suicidal overdose) or a rodentcide (superwarfarin).[37] Generally, such patients do not require therapeutic anticoagulation, and reversal does not carry the risk of recurrent thrombosis. Since the theapeutic half-life of vitamin K_1 is short (2 h) and that of warfarin is long (up to 4 days), significantly poisoned patients require continued doses until the therapeutic effect of warfarin is depleted.

From the standpoint of the risk of recurrent thrombosis, the safest method of reversing therapeutic overanticoagulation is with coagulation factor infusion using either FFP or factor concentrates. A dose of FFP 15 mL/kg (typically 3 U) will acutely restore coagulation factor levels to at least 30 percent of normal and control most bleeding without undue risk. Reversal of anticoagulation with FFP is usually safe for short periods, regardless of indication for anticoagulant therapy.[38] For patients with life-threatening hemorrhage and who require rapid, complete reversal, coagulation factor concentrates are more reliable and preferred.[39]

Heparin

Heparin-induced bleeding is treated according to the clinical severity and aPTT level.[40] Up to one-third of patients receiving heparin develop some form of bleeding complication, with a 2 to 6 percent risk for major bleeding. An increased risk (up to 20 percent) for major bleeding is associated with a number of comorbid conditions, including recent surgery or trauma, renal failure, alcoholism, malignancy, liver failure, and gastrointestinal bleeding as well as the concurrent use of warfarin, fibrinolytics, steroids, or antiplatelet drugs. Unfortunately, heparin-associated bleeding is not always reflected by a supratherapeutic aPTT. Other complications of brief heparin use include a benign transient thrombocytopenia (due to splenic sequestration and platelet aggregation), and allergic reactions.

A more serious problem is HIT. Heparin therapy must be stopped as soon as the condition is recognized. Protamine is not effective against this immune-mediated response. The platelet count generally returns to normal in 4 to 6 days. During the recovery phase, however, the risk of arterial or venous thrombosis is substantially elevated, and the potential complications include gangrene, stroke, and death. It is unclear whether such patients should ever be exposed to heparin again. LMW heparin preparations do not eliminate the risk of HIT, because of potential cross-reactivity.

If bleeding develops during heparin therapy, heparin administration should be stopped immediately. While heparin's half-life is dose de-

TABLE 216-5 Emergency Treatment of Bleeding Complications of Antithrombotic Therapy

Agent	Management
WARFARIN	
Elevated PT/INR without clinically evident bleeding	Cessation of warfarin administration and observation with serial PT/INR
Clinically significant bleeding	FFP to acutely restore coagulation factors to ≥30% of normal Oral vitamin K_1 1–2 mg Parenteral vitamin K_1 1–2 mg SC (preferred) or 0.5 mg IV Requires 12–24 h for full effect May require >1 treatment May induce unwanted thrombosis and/or overcorrection
HEPARIN	
Clinically significant bleeding	Immediate cessation of heparin administration in every case Supratherapeutic aPTT not always present Anticoagulation effect lasts up to 3 h from last dose
Minor bleeding	Observation with serial aPTT may be sufficient
Major bleeding	Protamine (1 mg per 100 U heparin) IV given slowly over 1–3 min to a maximum of 50 mg over any 10-min period May need to be repeated Anaphylaxis risk Does not reverse all LMW heparins (e.g., enoxaparin)
ASPIRIN	
Clinically significant bleeding: correlates poorly with BT	Cessation of aspirin administration and platelet transfusion to increase count by 50,000/μL Typically requires at least 6 U Multiple transfusions may be necessary Aspirin inhibition lasts for life of affected platelets
FIBRINOLYTICS	
Minor external bleeding	Manual pressure
Significant internal bleeding	Immediate cessation of fibrinolytic agent, aspirin, heparin Reversal of heparin with protamine as above Typed and crossmatched blood ordered with verification of aPPT, complete blood count, TCT, and fibrinogen level, volume replacement with crystalloid and blood as necessary
Massive bleeding with hemodynamic compromise	All measures listed for significant internal bleeding, above, and 10 U cryoprecipitate If fibrinogen level <1 g/L, repeat cryoprecipitate. If bleeding remains after cryoprecipitate or despite fibrinogen level >1 g/L, administer 2 U of FFP. If bleeding continues after FFP, check BT. If BT <9 min, give ε-aminocaproic acid 5 g IV over 60 min, then 1 g/h infusion for 8 h or until bleeding stops or tranexamic acid (10 mg/kg q6–8h) If BT >9 min, give ε-aminocaproic acid or tranexamic acid as above with 10 U transfusion of platelets
Intracranial hemorrhage	All measures listed for significant internal and massive bleeding, above, with immediate neurosurgery consultation

Abbreviations: BT, bleeding time; LMW, low-molecular weight; FFP, fresh-frozen plasma; TCT, thrombin clotting time.

pendent (30 to 150 min), its anticoagulation effect can last up to 3 h. Thus, observation may be appropriate in less severe cases, with serial aPTTs used to determine when therapy may be resumed. While protamine can reverse the anticoagulant effect of heparin (a ratio of 1 mg intravenous protamine neutralizes 100 U of heparin administered in the prior 4 h), the adverse effects of protamine are significant. Protamine should be given slowly intravenously over 1 to 3 min and not exceed 50 mg in any 10-min period. However, because the half-life of protamine is short, a heparin rebound may occur, requiring a second treatment. Allergic reactions are possible, and about 0.2 percent of patients receiving protamine develop anaphylaxis (which has a 30 percent mortality rate). Thus, protamine should be reserved for major bleeding complications.

In general, LMW heparin preparations cause less bleeding than does unfractionated heparin. The effectiveness of protamine in reversing LMW heparin effects is compound specific; for example, protamine does not completely reverse the actions of enoxaparin.

Aspirin

Upper gastrointestinal irritation is the most common side effect of aspirin therapy, while life-threatening gastrointestinal bleeding is uncommon.[41] As noted above, intracranial hemorrhage, the most feared complication of anticoagulation and antithrombotic therapy, appears to occur rarely with aspirin alone.[15] Some patients are markedly sensitive to aspirin such that even low doses lead to markedly prolonged bleeding times and risk of severe clinical hemorrhage, particularly related to surgery or trauma. Uremic patients are especially sensitive to bleeding induced by aspirin. The combination of alcohol and aspirin can also prolong a patient's bleeding time.

Unfortunately, the BT is a poor test to confirm bleeding complications of aspirin. If aspirin-associated bleeding is suspected [e.g., persistent oozing after tooth extraction despite normal platelet count (>100,000/μL) and coagulation studies], further workup should include obtaining a careful history for ingestion (significant unintentional ingestion may occur, since some 300 over-the-counter medications contain aspirin), and a salicylate level. Management of acute aspirin-induced hemorrhage involves the transfusion of enough normal platelets to increase the platelet count by 50,000/μL (e.g., 6 U). Because of the irreversible effect of aspirin on platelets, the hemostatic compromise might last for 4 to 5 days after aspirin has been discontinued, and platelet transfusions may have to be repeated daily.

Fibrinolytics

The most significant complications of fibrinolytic therapy are hemorrhagic, and the most catastrophic complication is intracranial hemorrhage, seen in at least 1 to 3 percent of patients.[42] In the GUSTO trial, the incidence of "moderate or worse" bleeding was highest in the front-loaded tPA plus heparin arm.[21] Fibrinolytics should not be given to any patient with an absolute contraindication (Tables 216-3 and 216-4). In patients with a relative contraindication, careful weighing of potential risks and benefits of fibrinolysis in consultation with the physician who will assume in-hospital care of the patient is indicated.

Allergic reactions and anaphylaxis from SK and anistreplase should be treated with 50 mg diphenhydramine and 125 mg methylprednisolone intravenously. Hypotension occurs in up to 10 percent of patients treated with either SK or tPA, and is treated by slowing the fibrinolytic infusion rate and administering intravenous crystalloid, paying close attention to the patient's volume status.

To minimize the bleeding risks associated with fibrinolytic therapy, the following precautions should be observed: (1) avoid all unnecessary needle sticks, (2) avoid any arterial punctures, (3) limit venous access to easily compressible sites (e.g., avoid central lines, especially the jugular or subclavian veins), and (4) avoid both nasogastric tubes and nasotracheal intubation.

Careful monitoring of the patient is crucial. The hematocrit should be checked every 4 to 6 h after fibrinolytic therapy is initiated. A fall in hematocrit of greater than 2 percent should prompt a search for the source of blood loss. Most bleeding episodes (more than 70 percent) occur at vascular puncture sites, but intracranial, intrathoracic, retroperitoneal, gastrointestinal, genitourinary, or soft-tissue extremity hemorrhage may occur.

External bleeding at any site should be controlled with prolonged manual pressure. Significant bleeding, especially from an internal site, mandates discontinuation of the fibrinolytic agent, aspirin, and heparin. Volume replacement using normal saline or lactated Ringer's solution should be provided as necessary and supplemented with red blood cell transfusions if clinically indicated. The thrombin time, aPTT, platelet count, and fibrinogen level should be checked. Heparin administered within 4 h of the onset of bleeding can be reversed with protamine (1 mg of protamine for every 100 U heparin).

Massive bleeding with hemodynamic compromise necessitates coagulation factor replacement in addition to the interventions recommended above. Ten units of cryoprecipitate (rich in fibrogen) should be administered and the fibrinogen level rechecked. If the fibrinogen level is less than 100 mg/dL, the dose of cryoprecipitate should be repeated. If bleeding continues after cryoprecipitate or if bleeding persists despite a fibrinogen level above 100 mg/dL, 2 U of FFP should be given. If bleeding persists after appropriate cryoprecipitate and FFP treatments, a BT should be checked. If it is less than 9 min, 10 U of platelets should be administered, followed by an antifibrinolytic agent (e.g., ε-aminocaproic acid or tranexamic acid); if the BT time is less than 9 min, platelets are not necessary, but an antifibrinolytic agent should still be administered for continuing hemorrhage. The dose of ε-aminocaproic acid is 5 g intravenously over 60 min, followed by a continuous infusion of 1.0 g/h for 8 h or until bleeding stops. The dose of tranexamic acid is 10 mg/kg intravenously every 6 to 8 h.

Fibrinolytic-associated intracranial hemorrhage requires an aggressive and rapid approach. Immediately discontinue the fibrinolytic agent, aspirin, and heparin. Administer protamine in the dose outlined above if the patient received heparin. The patient should also receive cryoprecipitate, FFP, platelet transfusion, and an antifibrinolytic agent (e.g., ε-aminocaproic acid or tranexamic acid). A neurosurgeon should be consulted immediately.

REFERENCES

1. White H: Unmet therapeutic needs in the management of acute ischemia. *Am J Cardiol* 80:2B, 1997.
2. Becker RC, Ansell J: Antithrombotic therapy: An abbreviated reference for clinicians. *Arch Intern Med* 155:149, 1995.
3. Fairweather RB, Ansell J, Van den Besselaar AM, et al: College of American Pathologists Conference XXXI on Laboratory Monitoring of Anticoagulant Therapy: Laboratory monitoring of oral anticoagulant therapy. *Arch Pathol Lab Med* 122:768, 1998.
4. Wells PS, Holbrooke AM, Crowther NR, Hirsh J: Interactions of warfarin with drugs and food. *Ann Intern Med* 121:676, 1994.
5. Crowther MA, Ginsberg JB, Kearon C, et al: A randomized trial comparing 5-mg and 10-mg warfarin loading doses. *Arch Intern Med* 159:48, 1999.
6. Grip L, Blomback M, Schulman S: Hypercoagulable state and thromboembolism following warfarin withdrawal in post-myocardial-infarction patients. *Eur Heart J* 12:1225, 1991.
7. Jones MP, Alving B: Laboratory testing for hypercoagulable disorders. *Curr Opin Hematol* 3:365, 1996.
8. Olson JD, Arkin CF, Brandt JT, et al: College of American Pathologists Conference XXXI on Laboratory Monitoring of Anticoagulant Therapy: Laboratory monitoring of unfractioned heparin therapy. *Arch Pathol Lab Med* 122:782, 1998.
9. Pineo GF, Hull RD: Unfractionated and low-molecular-weight heparin: Comparisons and current recommendations. *Med Clin North Am* 82:587, 1998.
10. Spinler SA, Nawarskas JJ: Low-molecular-weight heparins for acute coronary syndromes. *Ann Pharmacother* 32:103, 1998.
11. Laposata M, Green D, Van Cott EM, et al: College of American Pathologists Conference XXXI on Laboratory Monitoring of Anticoagulant Therapy: The clinical use and laboratory monitoring of low-molecular-weight heparin, danaparoid, hirudin and related compounds, and argatroban. *Arch Pathol Lab Med* 122:799, 1998.
12. The Global Use of Strategies to Open Occluded Coronary Arteries (GUSTO) IIb investigators: A comparison of recombinant hirudin with heparin for the treatment of acute coronary syndromes. *N Engl J Med* 335:775, 1996.
13. Metz BK, White HD, Granger CB, et al: Randomized comparison of direct thrombin inhibition versus heparin in conjunction with fibrinolytic therapy for acute myocardial infarction: Results from the GUSTO-IIb Trial. *J Am Coll Cardiol* 31:1493, 1998.
14. Collins R, Peto R, Baigent C, Sleight P: Aspirin, heparin, and fibrinolytic therapy in suspected acute myocardial infarction. *N Engl J Med* 336:847, 1997.
15. He J, Whelton PK, Vu B, Klag MJ: Aspirin and risk of hemorrhagic stroke: A meta-analysis of randomized controlled trials. *JAMA* 280:1930, 1998.
16. Ryan TJ, Anderson JL, Antman EM, et al: ACC/AHA guidelines for the management of patients with acute myocardial infarction: Executive summary, a report of the American College of Cardiology/American Heart Association Task Force on Practice Guidelines (Committee on Management of Acute Myocardial Infarction). *Circulation* 94:2341, 1996.
17. CAPRIE Steering Committee: A randomised, blinded, trial of clopidogrel versus aspirin in patients at risk of ischaemic events (CAPRIE). *Lancet* 348:1329, 1996.
18. The PURSUIT trial investigators: Inhibition of platelet glycoprotein IIb/IIIa with eptifibatide in patients with acute coronary syndromes. *N Engl J Med* 339:436, 1998.

19. PRISIM-PLUS investigators: The Platelet Reception Inhibition in Ischemic Syndrome Study: Inhibition of the platelet glycoprotein IIb/IIIa receptor with tirofiban in unstable angina and non-Q wave myocardial infarction. *N Engl J Med* 338:1488, 1998.
20. Gibler WB, Wilcox RG, Bode C, et al: Prospective use of glycoprotein IIb/IIIa receptor blockers in the emergency department setting. *Ann Emerg Med* 32:712, 1998.
21. The GUSTO investigators: An international randomized trial comparing four thrombolytic strategies for acute myocardial infarction. *N Engl J Med* 329:673, 1993.
22. Bode C, Smalling RW, Berg G, et al: Randomized comparison of coronary thrombolysis achieved with double- bolus reteplase (recombinant plasminogen activator) and front-loaded, accelerated alteplase (recombinant tissue plasminogen activator) in patients with acute myocardial infarction. *Circulation* 94:891, 1996.
23. Meers C, Toffelmire EB: Urokinase efficacy in the restoration of hemodialysis catheter function. *J Cannt* 8:17, 1998.
24. Brouwer MA, Martin JS, Maynard C, et al: Influence of early prehospital thrombolysis on mortality and event-free survival (the Myocardial Infarction Triage and Intervention [MITI] Randomized Trial). *Am J Cardiol* 78:497, 1996.
25. Benson NH, Maningas PA, Krohmer JR, et al: Guidelines for the prehospital use of thrombolytic agents. *Ann Emerg Med* 23:1047, 1994.
26. Goldhaber SZ: Thrombolytic therapy in venous thromboembolism: Clinical trials and current indications. *Clin Chest Med* 16:307, 1995.
27. Kasner SE, Grotta JC: Emergency identification and treatment of acute ischemic stroke. *Ann Emerg Med* 30:642, 1997.
28. The National Institute of Neurological Disorders and Stroke rt-PA Stroke Study Group: Tissue plasminogen activator for acute ischemic stroke. *N Engl J Med* 333:1581, 1995.
29. Hacke W, Kaste M, Fieschi C, et al: Intravenous thrombolysis with recombinant tissue plasminogen activator for acute hemispheric stroke: The European Cooperative Acute Stroke Study (ECASS). *JAMA* 274:1017, 1995.
30. Hecke W, Kaste M, Fieschi C, et al: Randomized double-blind placebo-controlled trial of thrombolytic therapy with intravenous alteplase in acute ischemic stroke (ECASS II): Second European-Australasian Acute Stroke Study. *Lancet* 352:1245, 1998.
31. Glover JJ, Morrill GB: Conservative management of overanticoagulated patients. *Chest* 108:987, 1995.
32. Weibert RT, Le DT, Kayser Sr, Rapaport SI: Correction of excessive anticoagulation with low-dose oral vitamin K_1. *Ann Intern Med* 126:959-962, 1997.
33. Crowther MA, Donovan D, Harrison L, et al: Low-dose oral vitamin K reliably reverses over-anticoagulation due to warfarin. *Thromb Haemostat* 79:1116, 1998.
34. Fetrow CW, Overlock T, Leff L: Antagonism of warfarin-induced hypoprothrombinemia with use of low-dose subcutaneous vitamin K_1. *J Clin Pharmacol* 37:751, 1997.
35. Whitling AM, Bussey HI, Lyons RM: Comparing different routes and doses of phytonadione for reversing excessive anticoagulation. *Arch Intern Med* 158:2136, 1998.
36. Shetty HGM, Backhouse G, Bentley DP, Routledge PA: Effective reversal of warfarin-induced excessive anticoagulation with low dose vitamin K. *Thromb Haemostat* 67:13, 1992.
37. Baglin T: Management of warfarin (coumarin) overdose. *Blood Rev* 12:91, 1998.
38. Makris M, Greaves M, Phillips WS, et al: Emegency oral anticoagulant reversal: The relative efficacy of infusions of fresh frozen plasma and clotting factor concentrate on correction of the coagulopathy. *Thromb Haemostat* 77:477, 1997.
39. Levine MN, Raskob G, Landefeld S, Hirsh J: Hemorrhagic complications of anticoagulant treatment. *Chest* 108:276S, 1995.
40. Hirsh J, Raschke R, Warkentin TE, et al: Heparin: Mechanism of action, pharmacokinetics, dosing considerations, monitoring, efficacy, and safety. *Chest* 108:258S, 1995.
41. Hirsh J, Dalen JE, Fuster V, et al: Aspirin and other platelet-active drugs: The relationship among dose, effectiveness, and side effects. *Chest* 108:247S, 1995.
42. Levine MN, Goldhaber SZ, Gore JM, et al: Hemorrhagic complications of thrombolytic therapy in the treatment of myocardial infarction and venous thromboembolism. *Chest* 108:291S, 1995.

EMERGENCY COMPLICATIONS OF MALIGNANCY

John J. Sverha
Marc Borenstein

The approach to patients with potential emergency complications of malignancy can be hindered by many factors. Patients may be uncomfortable or have insufficient knowledge to candidly discuss the extent of their malignancy in the emergency department (ED). The emergency physician may be unfamiliar with the large and frequently changing number of chemotherapeutic agents as well as the complex classification and staging of malignancies. Both patients and physicians may have the false impression that aggressive diagnostic and therapeutic interventions are futile in the presence of advanced malignancy.

Changing trends in the management of cancer-related emergencies include an increasing number of older patients receiving chemotherapy, more aggressive chemotherapy regimens, broader use of chemotherapy particularly with solid tumors (nonhematologic malignancies), and an increasing use of bone marrow transplantation. This, coupled with an increasing prevalence of malignant disease, longer patient survival, and increased complications of treatment, demands from emergency physicians the ability to recognize and treat a wide spectrum of oncologic emergencies.

Myelosuppression from chemotherapy and radiotherapy can result in coagulopathies and infection. Tumor growth can produce signs and symptoms of local compression on the spinal cord or airway, and certain tumors are associated with unique complications, such as hyperviscosity syndromes from tumor-related gammopathies. Table 217-1 lists the most important life-threatening oncologic emergencies. Table 217-2 lists common chemotherapeutic agents, their indications, and toxicities associated with their use.

ACUTE SPINAL CORD COMPRESSION

Multiple myeloma
Non-Hodgkin's and Hodgkin's lymphomas
Lung carcinoma
Prostate carcinoma
Breast carcinoma

Spinal cord compression can result from bleeding, infection, or fracture. It may be the first sign of a neoplasm or can complicate preexisting metastatic disease. The incidence is estimated at greater than 5 percent, and repeated occurrences in the same patient have been

TABLE 217-1 Emergency Complications of Malignancy

Related to local tumor compression
Acute spinal cord compression
Upper airway obstruction
Malignant pericardial effusion with tamponade
Superior vena cava syndrome
Related to biochemical derangement and systemic collapse
Hypercalcemia of malignancy
Syndrome of inappropriate ADH (SIADH)
Hyperviscosity syndrome
Adrenocortical insufficiency with shock
Related to myelosuppression
Granulocytopenia and sepsis
Immunosuppression and opportunistic infections
Thrombocytopenia and hemorrhage
Anaphylaxis and transfusion reactions

TABLE 217-2 Chemotherapeutic Agents: Toxicities and Therapeutic Uses

Agent	Toxicity	Type of Cancer Treated
	ALKYLATING AGENTS	
Cyclophosphamide (Cytoxan)	Nausea and vomiting, diarrhea, hemorrhagic cystitis, interstitial pneumonitis/fibrosis, bone marrow suppression, alopecia, congestive heart failure, hemorrhagic myocarditis	Lymphoma, breast cancer, bladder cancer, lung cancer, ovarian cancer, solid tumors of children
Ifosfamide (Ifex)	Nausea and vomiting, hemorrhagic cystitis, CNS toxicity, bone marrow suppression	Lymphoma, ovarian cancer, testicular cancer, sarcomas
Melphalan (Alkeran)	Interstitial pneumonitis, bone marrow suppression	Multiple myeloma
Chlorambucil (Leukeran)	Interstitial pneumonitis/fibrosis, bone marrow suppression	Chronic lymphocytic leukemia, low-grade lymphoma
Thiotepa (Thioplex)	Bone marrow suppression, mucositis	Bladder cancer
Triethylenemelamine (TEM)	Bone marrow suppression, mucositis	High-dose regimen with autologous bone marrow transplant
Busulfan (Myleran)	Endocardial fibrosis, bronchopulmonary dysplasia/fibrosis, bone marrow suppression, skin pigmentation, gynecomastia	Chronic myelocytic leukemia
Carmustine (BCNU)	Nausea and vomiting, nephrotoxicity, interstitial pneumonitis/fibrosis, bone marrow suppression	Lymphoma, brain tumors
Lomustine (CCNU) Semustine (methyl-CCNU)	Nausea and vomiting, bone marrow suppression, nephrotoxicity, pulmonary fibrosis	Lymphoma, brain tumors, melanoma, GI tumors
Dacarbazine	Nausea and vomiting, hepatotoxicity, flulike syndrome, bone marrow suppression	Hodgkin's disease, sarcoma, melanoma
Cisplatin (Platinol)	Nausea and vomiting, mild bone marrow suppression, myocardial ischemia, nephrotoxicity, peripheral neuropathy, ototoxicity	Ovarian cancer, testicular cancer, lung cancer, head and neck cancer, bladder cancer
Carboplatin (Paraplatin)	Nausea and vomiting, bone marrow suppression, nephrotoxicity	Ovarian cancer
	ANTIMETABOLITES	
Methotrexate (amethopterin, Folex)	Nausea and vomiting, mucositis, bone marrow suppression, hepatic fibrosis, interstitial pneumonitis, skin rash, nephrotoxicity	Acute lymphocytic leukemia, breast cancer, choriocarcinoma, head and neck cancer
Fluorouracil (5-FU, Adrucil)	Nausea and vomiting, mucositis, diarrhea, bone marrow suppression, myocardial infarction, acute cerebellar syndrome	Breast cancer, colon cancer, head and neck cancer
Floxuridine (fluorodeoxyuridine, FUDR)	Nausea and vomiting, bone marrow suppression, hepatotoxicity, neurotoxicity	Colon cancer metastatic to liver
Cytarabine (ara-C, Cytosar-U)	Nausea, diarrhea, mucositis, bone marrow suppression, hepatotoxicity, neurotoxicity, pulmonary edema	Acute leukemia, lymphoma
Mercaptopurine (6-MP, Purinethol)	Nausea and vomiting, bone marrow suppression with high doses only, hepatotoxicity	Acute leukemia
Thioguanine (6-TG)	Nausea and vomiting, bone marrow suppression with high doses only	Acute leukemia
Fludarabine (Fludara)	Bone marrow suppression, neurotoxicity, interstitial pneumonitis	Chronic lymphocytic leukemia
Pentostatin (Nipent)	Nausea and vomiting, bone marrow suppression, skin rash, neurotoxicity, acute renal failure	T-cell lymphoma, hairy cell leukemia
Cladribine (Leustatin)	Bone marrow suppression	Hairy cell leukemia, low-grade lymphoma
	ANTIMITOTIC DRUGS	
Vinblastine (Velban, Velsar)	Nausea and vomiting, bone marrow suppression, myocardial infarction	Hodgkin's disease
Vincristine (Oncovin)	Abdominal cramping, constipation, mild bone marrow suppression, myocardial infarction, neuropathies	Hodgkin's disease, lymphoma
Paclitaxel (Taxol)	Nausea and vomiting, bone marrow suppression, bradycardia, neuropathies	Ovarian cancer, breast cancer
	TOPOISOMERASE INHIBITORS	
Etoposide (VP-16, VePesid)	Nausea and vomiting, hypotension, bone marrow suppression, alopecia, secondary leukemia	Testicular cancer, lung cancer, lymphoma, acute leukemia, breast cancer, Kaposi's sarcoma
Dactinomycin (actinomycin D, Cosmegen)	Nausea and vomiting, stomatitis, bone marrow suppression, alopecia	Rhabdomyosarcoma, Wilms' tumor, choriosarcoma
Daunorubicin (daunomycin, Cerubidine)	Bone marrow suppression, stomatitis, cardiotoxicity, alopecia	Acute leukemia
Doxorubicin (Adriamycin)	Bone marrow suppression, mucositis, cardiotoxicity, alopecia	Acute leukemia, lymphoma, breast cancer
Idarubicin (Idamycin)	Bone marrow suppression, stomatitis, cardiotoxicity, alopecia	Acute leukemia
Bleomycin (Blenoxane)	Interstitial pneumonitis/fibrosis, skin ulcers, rare hyperthermia with cardiovascular collapse	Lymphoma, epidermoid carcinoma, testicular cancer
Plicamycin (mithramycin, Mithracin)	Bone marrow suppression, nephrotoxicity, hepatotoxicity, bleeding diathesis	Testicular cancer
Mitomycin (Mutamycin)	Bone marrow suppression, stomatitis, myocardial damage, nephrotoxicity, hemolytic uremic syndrome, interstitial pneumonitis	Cervical cancer, colorectal cancer, breast cancer, bladder cancer, head and neck cancer, lung cancer

reported. Spinal cord compression occurs most commonly as a complication of breast or lung carcinoma and lymphoma. In at least 95 percent of patients, a long history of back pain, often several weeks to several months, elapses prior to diagnosis. The pain is progressive in severity and duration, typically continuous, and requires analgesics. It may be radicular, and when affecting the thoracic spine, radicular pain is characteristically bilateral. Symptoms and signs of myelopathy are late findings. Once neurologic deficits from spinal cord compression are present, the tempo of deterioration increases dramatically, with some patients progressing from weakness to complete paralysis in a matter of hours. Once ambulatory function is seriously impaired or lost, less than 10 percent of patients recover the ability to ambulate despite aggressive management.

The single most important approach to the diagnosis of spinal cord compression is for the emergency physician to recognize the significance of persistent, progressive unexplained back or neck pain in a patient with known malignancy. Symptoms suggestive of cord compression include decreased sensation, urinary retention, lower extremity weakness, and difficulty with walking. Pain of involved vertebrae may be localized and/or intensified with percussion during physical examination. The neurologic examination should assess reflexes, motor and sensory function, rectal sphincter tone, and gait. A major exception to the nearly routine presence of pain is in lymphoma; if lytic bony metastases are absent, the patient may have a diminished sensory level or flaccid paralysis with absent or minimal pain.

Plain radiographs should be obtained in any patient having a history of malignancy who presents with persistent, progressive back or neck pain. In the absence of prior disk or degenerative disease associated with chronic back pain or acute trauma, this principle may be applied to all adult patients presenting with unexplained persistent, progressive back pain of 1 to 6 months' duration, particularly in patients over age 50. Discovery of bony metastases on radiographs *even in the absence of any neurologic deficits* requires either magnetic resonance imaging (MRI) or myelography. Although still the "gold standard" in many institutions, myelography is being supplanted by MRI.

If spinal cord compression is suspected, dexamethasone 100 mg/day IV in four divided doses should be initiated in the ED and typically is tapered over 4 to 5 days. The patient's overall status should be assessed with hematologic, electrolyte, and other laboratory studies. Further treatment decisions, including candidacy for emergency surgery, is assessed by a team approach using neurosurgery, oncology, radiology, and radiation oncology. Radiation therapy is the definitive treatment for most patients. Surgical laminectomy and decompression are indicated if there is architectural instability, tissue confirmation of cancer is required, maximal radiation therapy has been given previously, or the tumor is particularly radioresistant.

UPPER AIRWAY OBSTRUCTION

Laryngeal carcinoma
Thyroid carcinoma
Lymphoma
Metastatic lung carcinoma

Acute upper airway obstruction is generally associated with aspiration of foreign bodies or food, with epiglottitis, or with other oropharyngeal infections. Malignancy-related obstruction to airflow is more insidious and often attended by voice change. This is generally a late manifestation of tumors arising in the oropharynx, neck, and superior mediastinum. Acute compromise is uncommon unless infection, hemorrhage, or inspissated secretions supervene. Rapidly growing tumors such as Burkitt's lymphoma and anaplastic carcinoma of the thyroid are capable of compromising airflow within weeks and should be suspected in afebrile individuals with stridor and palpable anterior neck masses.

Fiberoptic laryngoscopy is usually necessary to evaluate airway lumen size, because local anatomy is generally greatly distorted. Lateral soft-tissue x-rays are of value in assessing laryngotracheal patency. Establishment of an effective airway is crucial, and surgical tracheostomy may be required prior to the intitiation of radiotherapy.

MALIGNANT PERICARDIAL EFFUSION WITH TAMPONADE

Malignant melanoma
Hodgkin's lymphoma
Lung carcinoma
Breast carcinoma
Ovarian carcinoma

Malignant melanoma has special predilection for the heart, but the most common cause of malignant pericardial effusion is carcinoma of the lung and breast. Pericardial disease also can result from mediastinal irradiation, infection, or drugs such as cyclophosphamide, granulocyte-macrophage colony-stimulating factor (GM-CSF), and cytarabine.

The hemodynamic consequences of malignant pericardial effusions are a function of the volume and speed of accumulation. Even collections greater than 500 mL may be well tolerated if development is slow. Sudden intrapericardial bleeding is associated with dyspnea, chest pain, and hypotension. If the myocardium is also involved with metastatic disease, cardiac dysfunction will result in a decrease in cardiac output as well.

The classic clinical features of cardiac tamponade are (1) hypotension and a narrowed pulse pressure, (2) jugular venous distention, (3) diminished heart sounds, (4) pulsus paradoxus greater than 10 mmHg, (5) low QRS voltage on electrocardiography, and (6) cardiomegaly without evidence of congestive heart failure on chest radiograph. Diagnosis is confirmed by echocardiography. Emergency percutaneous pericardiocentesis may be life-saving. It can be done blindly, if extreme haste is needed, or under fluoroscopic guidance.

The care of patients with malignant pericardial effusions who are not in extremis should be discussed with an oncologist. The patient's tumor type, symptom severity, and prognosis are all considered in determining a treatment plan that may include systemic chemotherapy, intrapericardial chemotherapy, elective pericardiocentesis, creation of a pleuropericardial window, or other surgical techniques.

CORONARY ARTERY DISEASE

Many cancer patients also have coronary artery disease. Anemia from bone marrow suppression or malignant infiltration can result in decreased myocardial oxygen supply. Interferon and interleukin 2 (IL-2) can increase cardiac output, resulting in an increased myocardial oxygen demand. Several chemotherapeutic agents have been associated with cardiac ischemia, including 5-fluorouracil, vinblastine, and IL-2. Sternal pain mimicking angina has been associated with GM-CSF.

Many agents have been associated with tachyarrhythmias, bradyarrhythmias, and atrioventricular conduction blocks. These include the anthracyclines, 5-fluorouracil, interferon, IL-2, GM-CSF, and paclitaxel. Myocarditis has been reported in association with anthracyclines and cyclophosphamide. Anthracyclines are directly toxic to myocardial cells, while cyclophosphamide toxicity appears to be vascular. Anthracycline-induced cardiomyopathy may occur months to years after cessation of treatment and is related to the total cumulative dose. It is irreversible. It is evaluated and managed in the same manner as any dilated, congestive cardiomyopathy.

SUPERIOR VENA CAVA SYNDROME

Small-cell (oat-cell) lung carcinoma
Squamous cell lung carcinoma
Lymphoma
Breast carcinoma

The superior vena cava syndrome is frequently a de novo diagnosis first established in the ED. A history of previously documented malignancy is often lacking, and patients may seek medical attention because of the insidious and progressive nature of their symptoms. Obstruction to blood flow in the superior vena cava elevates venous pressure in the arms, neck, face, and cerebrum. Patients with moderate obstruction complain of headache, edema of the face and arms, or a nondescript feeling of head congestion and fullness in the neck and face. As venous pressure rises, intracranial pressure also rises, and syncope may ensue. Critical intracranial pressure elevations associated with bilateral papilledema are rare but represent a true medical emergency.

On physical examination, neck vein and upper chest vein distention may be apparent. Facial plethora and telangiectasia often are prominent, but edema of the face and arms is generally subtle. Papilledema on funduscopic examination indicates critical intracranial pressure and justifies early diuretic therapy. A palpable supraclavicular mass due to direct tumor extension occasionally can be noted with tumors of the superior mediastinum. Chest radiography will demonstrate an enlarged mediastinum and possibly an isolated primary lesion in the lung parenchyma.

Prompt administration of diuretics and glucocorticoids may help reduce venous pressure. Furosemide 40 mg intravenously, methylprednisolone 120 mg intravenously, or dexamethazone 16 to 20 mg intravenously is frequently used.

Superior vena cava compression is generally not life-threatening. In most cases, it is very important to obtain tissue diagnosis prior to initiation of therapy because treatment with chemotherapeutic agents may be used exclusively or combined with radiation therapy depending on specific tumor type. Tissue sampling can be done safely by a number of approaches, including fiberoptic bronchoscopy with transbronchial biopsy, lymph node biopsy, pleural fluid cytology, needle biopsy, or limited thoracotomy.

HYPERCALCEMIA OF MALIGNANCY

Renal cell carcinoma
Multiple myeloma
Squamous cell lung carcinoma
Breast carcinoma
Lymphoma

Mild elevations of serum calcium are well tolerated and produce little in the way of symptoms. However, when serum calcium levels rise rapidly or exceed ionic thresholds, cardiac, neural, and muscular electrophysiology may be greatly altered. A number of mechanisms have been identified that promote release of bony calcium into the circulation. Bony involvement with myeloma, carcinoma of the breast, or carcinoma of the lung will release calcium by local matrix destruction. Squamous cell carcinoma of the lung may produce a parathormone-like substance, and an osteoclast-activating factor has been associated with lymphoma.

Approximately 40 percent of patients with multiple myeloma will have hypercalcemia, often accompanying the clinical triad of back pain, anemia, and lethargy. Hypercalcemia from any cause may produce nausea, vomiting, anorexia, and constipation. Altered mental status, confusion, and coma are consistent with rapid and/or high levels of hypercalcemia. Elevated ionized calcium is responsible for neuromuscular dysfunction, and therefore, serum calcium levels should be interpreted in conjunction with serum phosphorus, albumin, and blood pH determinations. The QT interval of the electrocardiogram may shorten as the serum calcium rises.

The majority of patients with malignancy-induced hypercalcemia will improve with saline infusion and intravenous furosemide (1–2 L saline load and 80 mg of IV furosemide). This will promote renal calcium excretion but depends on adequate renal function and glomerular filtration. Because renal insufficiency is a common accompaniment in myeloma, assessment of blood urea nitrogen and creatinine levels is important to ensure both adequacy of response and avoidance of iatrogenic fluid overload. Hemoconcentration and dehydration additionally may aggravate hypercalcemia. For severe hypercalcemia, hemodialysis or peritoneal dialysis against a low- or no-calcium dialysate may be necessary.

Other measures are part of the overall management of hypercalcemia but have an onset of action that is too slow to be effective in the ED. The intravenous administration of inorganic phosphate is a rapid and effective method for decreasing blood calcium level but should not be used in most patients because it may produce metastatic tissue calcification leading to hypotension, renal failure, and death. Oral phosphate, given as 1 g of sodium acid phosphate daily, produces a maximal effect after several days. Glucocorticoids should not be given prior to oncology consultation because they may become part of the patient's chemotherapy regimen. The effect of glucocorticoids is greatest in the hematologic malignancies, lymphomas, and breast cancer but may take several days to develop. Mithromycin acts by inhibiting bone resorption. The dose is 25 μg/kg delivered as an IV infusion, and its effect is usually evident in 24 to 48 h.

SYNDROME OF INAPPROPRIATE ADH

Primary and metastatic malignancy of the brain
Small cell lung carcinoma
Pancreatic adenocarcinoma
Prostate carcinoma

Ectopic secretion of antidiuretic hormone (ADH) may come from a variety of malignancies. In addition, excessive endogenous secretion of ADH may be caused by chemotherapy (*Vinca* alkaloids, cyclophosphamide), narcotics, phenothiazines, antidepressants, and head trauma. Regardless of etiology, the syndrome of inappropriate ADH (SIADH) consists of serum hyponatremia, less than maximally dilute urine, excessive urine sodium excretion ($U_{Na} > 30$ meq/L), and decreased serum osmolarity, all in the presence of euvolemia, absence of diuretic therapy, and normal renal, adrenal, and thyroid function.

Symptoms of hyponatremia range from anorexia, nausea, vomiting, and weakness to confusion, decreased mental status, seizures, and coma. Patients with a serum sodium level above 125 mEq/L generally are asymptomatic or mildly symptomatic and usually can be controlled with water restriction of 500 mL/day along with close follow-up. Demeclocyline, a tetracycline derivative, can be given at a dose of 250 mg qid, and this raises the serum sodium by producing a nephrogenic diabetes insipidus. Patients with serum sodium concentrations below 115 mEq/L may present with severe, life-threatening manifestations requiring acute care monitoring, meticulous attention to intake and output measurements, and frequent electrolyte determinations. Furosemide 0.5 to 1.0 mg/kg is given with normal saline supplementation to maintain euvolemia and effect a net free water clearance. In addition, 3% hypertonic saline may be used, but the amount must be calculated carefully to avoid volume overload and congestive heart failure. Hemodynamic monitoring may be necessary for patients with associated cardiopulmonary disease. Seizures, when present, are typically tonic-clonic and may be recurrent. Treatment is with standard loading doses of phenytoin. Focal seizure or the development of neurologic deficits requires head computed tomographic (CT) imaging. To avoid the development of central pontine myelinolysis, the rate of rise in serum sodium should not exceed 1 mEq/L per hour.

HYPERVISCOSITY SYNDROME

Multiple myeloma
Waldenström's macroglobulinemia
Chronic myelocytic leukemia

Viscosity is the flow-resisting characteristic of fluids. Marked elevations in certain serum proteins will produce sludging and a reduction in microcirculatory perfusion. IgA myeloma components and IgG subtype 3 proteins have a tendency to polymerize, leading to symptomatic hyperviscosity. Macroglobulinemia is the most common cause for hyperviscosity by virtue of the high molecular weight and high intrinsic viscosity of IgM proteins. Serum viscosity relative to water is normally 1.4 to 1.8, and symptoms develop at viscosities greater than five times that of water.

Fatigue, headache, anorexia, and somnolence are early nonspecific symptoms. As blood flow slows, microthromboses may occur, with the advent of local symptoms such as deafness, visual disturbances, and jacksonian or generalized seizures. The diagnosis of hyperviscosity must be considered in the emergency department when patients with unexplained stupor or coma are found to have anemia, with rouleau formation on the peripheral blood smear. The most readily appreciated physical findings are in the ocular fundi and include "sausage-linked" retinal vessels, hemorrhages, and exudates. Laboratory evaluation should include coagulation, renal, and electrolyte profiles. Hypercalcemia can coincide, and when M-component protein concentrations are high, "factitious" hyponatremia may also be present. A clue to the presence of hyperviscosity may be the laboratory's inability to perform chemical tests because of the serum stasis in the analyzers, undoubtedly due to "too thick" blood. Serum viscosity and protein electrophoresis determinations are diagnostic.

The emergency physician's role is predominantly suspicion and recognition of the syndrome in patients with unexplained stupor and coma. Hyperviscosity is generally a presenting manifestation of certain plasma cell dyscrasias, and a history of previously documented disease is often lacking. Initial therapy is rehydration followed by hematology consultation and emergency plasmapheresis. When coma is present and the diagnosis rapidly established, a temporizing measure may be a two-unit phlebotomy with saline infusion and replacement of the patient's red cells.

ADRENAL INSUFFICIENCY AND SHOCK

Lung carcinoma
Breast carcinoma
Malignant melanoma
Retroperitoneal malignancies
Withdrawal of chronic steroid therapy

Adrenal insufficiency may be related to adrenal gland replacement by metastatic tumors or to adrenocortical suppression by therapeutic glucocorticoid administration. In either case, maximal adrenal function may be inadequate to support the individual when stressed by infection, dehydration, surgery, or trauma. Adrenal crisis and shock with vasomotor collapse may be sudden and fatal. The differential diagnosis of cancer patients with fever, dehydration, hypotension, and shock would more frequently include sepsis and hemorrhagic shock. Adrenal crisis is less common than bleeding and sepsis, but the steroid-dependent patient should be empirically given intravenous steroids with both glucocorticoid and mineralocorticoid effect.

Laboratory clues to the possible concomitant presence of adrenal insufficiency may be mild hypoglycemia, hyponatremia, hyperkalemia, and eosinophilia. Azotemia is, however, nonspecific and is often present in dehydration from any cause. In suspected cases, a serum cortisol should be drawn prior to steroid treatment.

Normal adrenal glands maximally produce approximately 300 mg per day of hydrocortisone when stressed. This has served as a guideline for replacement therapy. Adrenalectomized individuals are maintained on average doses of 35 to 40 mg of hydrocortisone per day, and this is increased during potential stress. Appropriate emergency doses of hydrocortisone hemisuccinate (Solucortef) would be 250 to 500 mg intravenously.

GRANULOCYTOPENIA, IMMUNOSUPPRESSION, AND INFECTION

Overwhelming infection is a common cause of death in the immunocompromised host. A variety of factors may contribute to increased susceptibility to infection in cancer patients. Important factors include

1. Malnutrition and cachexia
2. CNS dysfunction
3. Granulocytopenia
4. Impaired humoral immunity and antibody production, as in chronic lymphocytic leukemia or multiple myeloma
5. Altered cellular immunity, as in Hodgkin and other lymphomas
6. Postsplenectomy susceptibility to serious pneumococcal infections
7. Reactivation tuberculosis with concurrent glucocorticoid therapy
8. Polymicrobial enteric sepsis from bowel organism entry; carcinoma of colon or mucosal damage from chemotherapy
9. Nosocomial infections transmitted through blood transfusion and blood products
10. Immunosuppression and myelosuppression of chemotherapy
11. Indwelling catheters

Both the frequency of infection and the mortality rate increase significantly when the circulating granulocyte pool is below 1000 to 1500/μL. Cancer patients are at risk for a variety of bacterial, viral, and fungal infections. Frequently encountered infections include pneumococcal sepsis and pneumonia; *Staphylococcus aureus* infection; enteric gram-negative pneumonia or sepsis, including *Pseudomonas* infections; and localized or disseminated varicella-zoster viral and cytomegalovirus infections. Immunosuppression predisposes to invasion by organisms that are normally held at bay by host defenses and biocompetition from normal body flora. Such opportunistic infections include *Pneumocystis carinii* pneumonia (protozoal), disseminated candidiasis, aspergillosis, cryptococcal meningitis, pulmonary nocardiosis, and histoplasmosis. Recent trends include a decreasing incidence of *Pseudomonas* and an increasing incidence of methicillin-resistant staphylococci and the emergence of gram-positive corynebacteria.

Patients with an absolute neutrophil count of 500 or less and a fever greater than 38.5°C on one occasion or greater than 38°C on two to three occasions constitute a true medical emergency. Although only 60 to 80 percent of neutropenic patients with fever are culture proven or clinically documented to have an infectious etiology (the others presumably have fever secondary to the malignant process itself or its treatment), the emergency physician must assume an infectious etiology and act accordingly, rapidly obtaining cultures and initiating appropriate antibiotics. Life-threatening sepsis, regardless of specific antimicrobial etiology, may progress rapidly, producing shock and irreversible end-organ damage. Restoration of euvolemia and the use of broad-spectrum bactericidal antibiotics are recommended. Attention to local institutional bacterial sensitivities is very important in making specific antibiotic choices. Frequently used combinations include an aminoglycoside (gentamicin or tobramicin) with an extended-spectrum penicillin (ticarcillin) or an aminoglycoside (gentamicin or tobramicin) with an third-generation cephalosporin (ceftazidime or ceftriaxone). Amikacin should be reserved for bacterial resistance documented on culture and not initiated as part of an initial regimen. Empirical use of vancomycin for methicillin-resistant staphlococci generally depends on the degree to which these organisms are encountered at one's institution. Aztreonam or the new fluoroquinolones may be substituted for an extended-spectrum penicillin or a third-generation cephalosporin if a patient is highly penicillin allergic with a history of serious systemic reaction or anaphylaxis. Anaerobic coverage may be obtained by the addition of clindamycin or metronidazole.

BONE MARROW TRANSPLANTS

Emergency physicians can expect to care for increasing numbers of bone marrow transplant patients due to the rising prevalence and survivability of this procedure. Bone marrow transplants are currently performed for malignant conditions such as leukemia, lymphoma, and selected solid tumors as well as for nonmalignant conditions such as aplastic anemia, thalassemia, and sickle cell anemia.

Bone marrow transplants can be categorized as either allogeneic or autologous. In an allogeneic transplant, bone marrow is first obtained from an HLA-matched donor, preferably a sibling. The patient then receives high-dose chemotherapy or radiotherapy to eliminate native bone marrow and destroy residual cancer cells. The donor marrow is then administered to the recipient intravenously. The recipient is profoundly myelosuppressed for a period of 1 to 3 weeks until the transplanted cells assume their place in the recipient's bone marrow by a process known as *engraftment.* Autologous transplantation is performed in a similar manner, although a sample of a patient's own marrow is taken before high-dose chemotherapy, and it is this sample that is used to reestablish hematopoetic cell function.

Emergency physicians are unlikely to encounter the acute complications of bone marrow transplantation because these patients often are kept in the hospital for several weeks following their transplant until engraftment occurs. However, emergency physicians should be aware of the long-term complications and consequences of bone marrow transplantation. Like solid-organ transplant recipients, bone marrow recipients are at increased risk of infection. This risk is not just confined to the period of granulocytopenia preceding engraftment. Even with a normal neutrophil count, bone marrow transplant patients have a residual cellular and humoral immunodeficency that persists for 12 to 24 months after transplantation. Return of immune function generally is slower in allogeneic transplant recipients than in autologous transplant recipients. Bone marrow transplant patients are at particular risk of infection from encapsulated bacteria, *Pneumocystis carinii,* cytomegalovirus (CMV), varicella-zoster virus, *Candida,* and *Aspergillus.* CMV pneumonitis is the most common infectious cause of death after bone marrow transplantation and typically occurs 1 to 6 months following the transplant. To decrease the risk of opportunistic infection, bone marrow transplant patients are often prophylactically administered penicillin, trimethoprim-sulfamethoxazole, and ganciclovir for the first 3 to 6 months following their transplant. A fever or other sign of infection should be taken very seriously in a bone marrow transplant patient (even if the neutrophil count is normal), and a treatment plan should be developed in conjunction with the patient's hematologist.

A complication unique to bone marrow transplant patients is graft-versus-host disease. This disorder occurs only in allogeneic transplant patients. It is caused by immunologically competent donor cells attacking target antigens in the recipient. Patients develop rash, diarrhea, and an elevated serum bilirubin level. The diagnosis is confirmed histologically by appropriate biopsy. Without treatment, the condition is often fatal. Treatment with prednisone, cyclosporine, antithymocyte globulin, or thalidomide improves the long-term prognosis of these patients. Unfortunately, these drugs also delay immunologic recovery and increase the risk of opportunistic infection.

Another unusual complication of bone marrow transplantation is hepatic venoocclusive disease. This condition usually occurs within 30 days of transplantation and is caused by thrombotic obstruction of small intrahepatic venules with resulting damage to the surrounding centrilobular hepatocytes. The exact precipitant of this disease is unknown. The diagnosis should be considered in patients with jaundice, tender hepatomegaly, and ascites. Up to 20 percent of all bone marrow transplant recipients have some degree of hepatic venoocclusive disease. In severe cases, progressive hepatic and renal failure occur. Treatment is largely supportive, although thrombolytic therapy has shown some promise.

HEMATOLOGIC SYNDROMES

Thromboembolism is not uncommon in cancer patients and is due to a number of factors such as a hypercoagulable state; decreased proteins C, S, and antithrombin III; and the effect of metastases on activation of the coagulation pathway. Cancer patients are at increased risk for both deep venous thrombosis and pulmonary embolism. However, anticoagulation may result in bleeding at sites of metastatic disease, so that treatment options are more complex and may include placement of a filter in the inferior vena cava.

Polycythemia is enhanced production of red cells due to increases in sensitivity of erythropoietin. Any organ system can be affected by resulting thrombosis, bleeding, or hyperviscosity, but CNS effects are the most devastating. Celiac or mesenteric vessel ischemia, or Budd-Chiari syndrome, is seen when gastrointestinal vessels are involved. If the hematocrit is greater than 60 percent and symptoms are present, emergency phlebotomy is necessary.

Either acute or chronic leukemias can result in white blood cell counts greater than $100,000/\mu L$. A leukocrit of greater than 10 percent is often associated with clinically significant hyperviscosity, and CNS dysfunction and respiratory distress can occur from capillary leukostasis. Diuretics worsen symptoms because they will increase the leukocrit. Treatment is directed at the underlying malignancy, and allopurinol should also be administered in anticipation of massive tumor lysis, to prevent acute gouty arthropathy and renal failure.

GASTROINTESTINAL SYNDROMES

Acute gastrointestinal complications may or may not be related to the underlying malignancy. In patients with cancer, even gastric cancer, the major causes of gastrointestinal bleeding are still hemorrhagic gastritis and peptic ulcer disease. Intraarterial hepatic chemotherapy infusions have been associated with gastrointestinal bleeding, especially from the duodenum. Chemotherapy or radiotherapy can cause vomiting, resulting in Mallory-Weiss tears or reflux esophagitis.

Cancer patients with acute abdominal processes present with typical signs and symptoms unless they are receiving exogenous steroids. Acute appendicitis has been reported to occur in up to 4 percent of patients with leukemia.

RENAL AND UROLOGIC SYNDROMES

Renal insufficiency in the cancer patient often has multiple etiologies. Prerenal azotemia is common due to vomiting, anorexia, or diuretic use. Hepatic and peritoneal disease also may cause sequestration of fluid in the peritoneal cavity, leading to intravascular volume depletion. Multiple myeloma and lymphoma can cause rapidly progressive renal failure by intraglomerular amyloid deposition. In addition, several chemotherapeutic agents (i.e., carmustine, cisplatin, and mitomycin) are directly nephrotoxic.

Urologic emergencies in the cancer patient include urinary tract hemorrhage, urinary tract obstruction, and priapism. Gross hematuria is often the presenting symptom of urinary tract cancers but also can be caused by local invasion of the urinary tract by colonic or gynecologic tumors. Hemorrhagic cystitis occurs after cyclophosphamide administration in about 5 percent of patients. Hemorrhage can be life-threatening, with up to 20 percent requiring blood transfusion. Hemorrhagic cystitis also occurs after radiation therapy of gynecologic, genitourinary, and rectal cancers. Bleeding can occur months to years after radiation treatment, and while bleeding is usually minor, rarely serious bleeding can occur.

Ureteral obstruction in the cancer patient can be caused by direct tumor compression or uric acid nephropathy during chemotherapy or may be secondary to retroperitoneal fibrosis following radiation therapy. Acute ureteral obstruction presents with flank pain similar to urolithiasis. Chronic ureteral obstruction is often painless and, if unilateral, is often only detected incidentally. Chronic bilateral ureteral obstruction eventually will cause renal failure with patients presenting with symptoms of uremia. Urinary retention at the level of the bladder is also seen in cancer patients. It can be caused by mechanical bladder outlet obstruction, brain or spinal cord metastases, or as a side effect of medications.

Priapism in cancer patients may be caused by a primary hematologic malignancy (i.e., leukemia, myeloma), metastases to the corporal bodies of the penis, or secondary to disruption of venous outflow by pelvic tumor. Corporal shunting procedures used for idiopathic priapism usually are not effective in priapsim caused by malignancy.

BIBLIOGRAPHY

DeAngelis LM, Posner JB: Neurologic complications in patients with cancer, in Holland JF, Frei E III, Bast RC, et al (eds): *Cancer Medicine,* 4th ed. Baltimore: Williams & Wilkins, 1997.

Friefeld AG, Pizzo PA, Walsh TJ: Infections in the cancer patient, in DeVita VT, Hellman S, Rosenberg SA (eds): *Cancer: Principles and Practice of Oncology,* 5th ed. Philadelphia: Lippincott-Raven, 1997.

Fuller BG, Heise J, Oldfield EH: Spinal cord compression, in DeVita VT, Hellman S, Rosenberg SA (eds): *Cancer: Principles and Practice of Oncology,* 5th ed. Philadelphia: Lippincott-Raven, 1997.

Moore GP, Jorden RC (eds): Hematologic/oncologic emergencies. *Emerg Med Clin North Am* 11:2, 1993.

Morris JC, Holland JF: Oncologic emergencies, in Holland JF, Frei E III, Bast RC, et al (eds): *Cancer Medicine,* 4th ed. Baltimore: Williams & Wilkins, 1997.

Rolston KV, Bodey GP: Infections in patients with cancer, in Holland JF, Frei E III, Bast RC, et al (eds): *Cancer Medicine,* 4th ed. Baltimore: Williams & Wilkins, 1997.

Warrell RP Jr: Metabolic emergencies, in DeVita VT, Hellman S, Rosenberg SA (ed): *Cancer: Principles and Practice of Oncology,* 5th ed. Philadelphia: Lippincott-Raven, 1997.

Yahalom J: Superior vena cava syndrome, in DeVita VT, Hellman S, Rosenberg SA (eds): *Cancer: Principles and Practice of Oncology,* 5th ed. Philadelphia: Lippincott-Raven, 1997.

THE NEUROLOGIC EXAMINATION IN THE EMERGENCY SETTING

Hubert S. Mickel

The *emergency* neurologic assessment is focused on obtaining the information that is needed to make rapid management decisions, establish the priorities in examination and management, and assist in making a decision regarding intervention, further examination, and disposition. Stated simplistically, the emergency physician's responsibility, once any immediate threat to life has been addressed, is primarily to determine *that* a neurologic problem potentially exists and *that* the critical conditions associated with that problem are identified or excluded; the neurologist or neurosurgeon often subsequently determines *what* the problem is. This chapter describes the elements of the basic *neurologic examination* appropriate to the emergency department.

ASSESSMENT OF THE NEUROLOGIC EXAMINATION

Overview

A quick assessment of the normal nervous system is provided by finding a normal gait with normal associated movements, a normal speech process and content, and a normal mental status. Conversely, many neurologic deficits can be quickly ascertained by simply looking at the patient. There may be a dense hemiparesis, or there may be neglect of one side. A conversation with the patient may demonstrate a significant mental status abnormality or speech deficit.

There is no universally accepted neurologic screening examination for the emergency setting. However, the brief neurologic screening examination should include as a minimum these components:

1. Mental Status	Orientation, affect, speech (content and process)
2. Cranial Nerves	Pupillary response, fundoscopy, extraocular movements, facial muscle strength, visual fields as appropriate
3. Motor System	Strength in basic muscle groups, resistance to passive movement (tone), pronator drift
4. Sensation	Light touch, proprioception, pain, as appropriate
5. Coordination	Gait, finger-to-nose or other cerebellar testing, Romberg
6. Reflexes	Deep tendon reflexes (biceps, triceps, knees, ankles), plantar reflexes

Mental Status Examination

The goal of the mental status examination is to determine if an abnormality of mental status exists and whether it points to a structural, metabolic, toxic, or infectious etiology.

An alteration of mental status requires a deficit in alertness or awareness or both. Alertness requires the normal functioning of the ascending reticular activating system (ARAS), which passes through the midline of the brainstem up through the thalamus, resulting in arousal of the cerebral hemispheres. Awareness, tested as orientation, requires alertness plus the normal functioning of the cerebral hemispheres. The obtunded patient responds to voices, but there is an abnormality in alertness. Because the ARAS passes through the pontine tegmentum in proximity to the medial longitudinal fasciculus, one needs to examine for focal brainstem deficits, especially pupillary or gaze abnormalities, in the obtunded patient. The drowsy patient may have a decreased level of alertness or awareness, so that one needs to examine for cortical and brainstem deficits. The alert patient may have deficits in awareness but no brainstem lesions that affect the ascending reticular activating system. Deficits in awareness point to abnormalities in cortical function. Questions to assess awareness center on orientation to time, place, person, and situation, as well as the ability to follow simple commands. Determining the digit span (normally seven numbers forward and five numbers backwards) can provide a quick assessment of the mental ability impaired in dementia. Confusion of right and left and the inability to calculate (subtracting 7 serially from 100 or 3 serially from 20) are abnormalities resulting from a dominant parietal lobe lesion. Having the patient recall three objects after a five-minute interval assesses recent memory.

Reversible causes of altered mental status such as hypoglycemia, narcotic overdose, hypoxia, or hypercarbia should be quickly investigated and treated. If a structural etiology of altered mental status is indicated by history or associated neurologic findings, a noncontrast head CT or possibly other neuroimaging study is needed emergently.

Delirium is a distinctly abnormal mental state characterized by disorientation, fear, irritability, misperception of sensory stimuli, and, often, visual hallucinations. Delirium accompanies diffuse metabolic and multifocal cerebral illness, and its presence implies a generalized impairment of brain functions or at least a bilateral involvement of limbic structure. In the elderly patient presenting with delirium from a nursing facility, a diagnosis of high frequency is urosepsis.

Psychiatric causes of altered mental status produce abnormalities of affect, behavior, and content of consciousness, but not of alertness and awareness. In psychosis, there is a defect in reality testing, so that hallucinations and delusions are accepted many times as real. Psychiatry uses *organic brain syndrome* to denote a dementia, which is an impairment of awareness due to various pathological lesions usually scattered throughout the cerebral hemispheres.

Speech

If a speech problem exists, a key question is whether *dysarthria,* a disorder of the motor mechanism of articulation, may result from either cerebellar dysfunction or from primary motor dysfunction. The character of the dysarthria is different, and dependent upon the cause. Cerebellar disease may produce an abnormality in cadence of speech, while motor dysfunction produces abnormalities in enunciation. Examples of words or phrases that when rapidly spoken demonstrate a subtle dysarthria are: "Seventy-Seven Register Street" and "Methodist Episcopal." Alert, aware, dysarthric patients may be able to tell you that their speech is different than usual.

Dysphasia is a disorder of the normal cerebral processing of speech by which meanings are comprehended and expressed. The defect may be in finding words or names, with or without difficulty in writing, but without defect in comprehension (expressive dysphasia); or a difficulty in understanding spoken or written speech (receptive dysphasia); or a more diffuse difficulty in the appreciation of word sounds and grammatical construction, with or without a defect in manipulating numbers, with or without a jumbling of spoken words (jargon speech). In expressive dysphasia, the abnormality lies in executing speech and may be obvious. Asking the patient to name several objects, or to tell the name of parts of a watch or articles of clothing, may elucidate a mild dysnomia. On the other hand, the receptive dysphasic patient does not understand speech and may not understand written language.

Many dysphasic patients have abnormality in both executing (expressive dysphasia) and understanding speech (receptive dysphasia).

Cranial Nerves

Generally speaking, if cranial nerves II to VIII are intact, it is less likely that the lower cranial nerves are involved in isolation. Cranial nerve I abnormality can be found in isolation, but when it occurs is often related to injury or tumor (e.g., olfactory groove meningioma).

CRANIAL NERVE I There are occasions when testing olfactory perception is of value. In testing olfaction, the patient needs to be able to identify an odor or to distinguish between two odors, neither pungent (which may test cranial nerve (cranial nerve) V more than cranial nerve I). One cause for loss of olfactory perception is distraction of the olfactory nerves from the cribriform plate, as may occur with fracture through the cribriform plate or from falls onto the occiput.

CRANIAL NERVE II Examination of the visual fields by confrontation is important whenever a CNS hemispheral lesion is suspected or whenever the patient complains of a visual deficit. Visual field testing can be done at the bedside by comparing the patient's visual perception of moving fingers, or a moving small, white object, to your own perception in all four quadrants of the visual fields. Rapid screening of visual field deficit can be done with both eyes, but, customarily, the visual field of each eye should be tested alone.

The physiologic blind spot, increased in papilledema and inflammation of the optic nerve, can be measured using a small, white object and bisecting the distance between you and the patient. When the patient looks with one eye at your eye, find your own physiologic blind spot in the temporal field lateral to the point of fixation, by determining where the white object disappears. Measure the size of the patient's physiologic blind spot to yours, with the assumption that yours is normal.

Lesions posterior to the optic chiasm produce a homonymous visual field defect that may be complete, e.g., hemianopsia, or partial, e.g., quadrantanopsia. Lesions affecting the crossing fibers of the optic chiasm produce a bitemporal defect, which requires testing the visual field of each eye alone for recognition. Visual fields may constrict as a consequence of glaucoma, papilledema, or retinitis pigmentosa.

In nondominant parietal lobe dysfunction, bedside testing may also demonstrate visual inattention to double simultaneous stimulation. The patient perceives the visual stimulus when tested singly in the abnormal visual field but is inattentive to the stimulus when both visual fields are stimulated simultaneously. The consultant generally does more complex visual field testing.

Fundoscopic examination is an important part of the examination in conditions such as hypertensive urgencies, visual loss or visual complaints, ocular pathology, and suspected increased intracranial pressure (ICP).

The use of mydriatics for fundoscopic examination in altered mental status is problematic, because another examiner may mistake the pupillary dilatation for evidence of herniation. Furthermore, pupillary size as a finding of value in assessing clinical changes is lost.

Papilledema develops rapidly in the child (unless the fontanelles are still open), but it is not likely to be found in the adult within the first 24 h following an acute CNS lesion that results in ICP. Instead of papilledema, the early fundoscopic findings of increased ICP are:

1. The ratio of the diameter of retinal venules to arterioles increases from the normal 3:2 ratio to as high as 4:1;
2. Capillary engorgement occurs that makes the optic disc pinker;
3. The physiologic cup fills in from the bottom and all sides, obscuring the white lamina cribrosa at its depth;
4. Venous pulsations disappear, which, when seen in the upright patient, are normally at the edge of the physiologic cup. Venous pulsations are difficult for many examiners to identify; but, when seen, they may be abated by pressure on the globe. This phenomenon can be used to confirm that venous pulsations are indeed present;
5. The optic disc begins to elevate. Initially the elevation of the disc is nasal, superior, and inferior, and lastly, temporal. To determine if slight elevation of the optic disc exists, one focuses on a vessel that traverses the disc and then focuses on the same vessel on the retina. If the vessel is seen 1 diopter more positive on the disc, the disc is elevated.

Increased ICP occurring acutely many times results in an alteration of the sensorium due to involvement at a midbrain level. However, one cannot use this association to prove the presence or absence of increased ICP. Patients with pseudotumor cerebri may have increased ICP with papilledema but without demonstrable alteration of mental status.

CRANIAL NERVES III, IV, AND VI Extraocular muscle function and pupillary function are a basic part of the examination with all CNS complaints. First, one observes the pupils, their size, shape, and equality, then their reaction to light. Is there a consensual reaction to light? Is there a reaction to convergence? Table 218-1 describes common pupillary abnormalities.

The extraocular muscle (EOM) function can be assessed by having the patient follow your finger through upward, downward, lateral, superolateral, and inferolateral gaze. The examiner looks for dysconjugate movements or for the patient's report of diplopia. An optimal way to examine EOM function is to use a red lens over one eye and test with a small flashlight. If diplopia exists, the patient perceives both a red and a white light, separated horizontally, vertically, or on an angle. Because diplopia is the result of weakness of movement of the affected eye, the visual image of light in that eye is further away from the macula, so that the image is perceived as further away in the direction the eye is tested; for example, further to the right on testing right lateral gaze. The eye with the visual image furthest from the center is the abnormal one.

Abnormality in EOM function result from lesions affecting cranial nerve nuclei III, IV, and VI within the brainstem; the medial longitudinal fasciculus that extends between the cranial nerve VI nucleus caudally to the opposite cranial nerve III nucleus rostrally, passing throughout the midline of the pontine tegmentum; as well as the cranial nerves themselves after exiting the pons. A lesion of the medial longitudinal fasciculus, most commonly from demyelination or ischemia, results in an internuclear ophthalmoplegia.

A lesion of the cranial nerve III or nucleus results in pupillary dilation as well as weakness to paralysis of ocular motion medially, inferiorly, and superiorly. A lesion of cranial nerve VI or nucleus results in impaired ability to move the eye laterally past the midline. Function of the cranial nerve IV nerve is seldom tested in the presence of normal cranial nerve III and cranial nerve VI function.

Normal functioning to look to the side starts with a signal to the abducens nerve (cranial nerve VI) from the parabducens nucleus. The signal is then sent upwards over the medial longitudinal fasciculus (MLF) to cranial nerve III. With an internuclear ophthalmoplegia, a lesion of the MLF prevents the signal from arriving. The result is that the ipsilateral eye looks lateral (abducts), but the contralateral one continues to look straight-ahead (failure to adduct).

Uncal herniation does not occur without altering the function of the ascending reticular activating system. Uncal herniation characteristically occurs when expanding lesions within the temporal lobe or within the temporal fossa shift the inner, basal edge of the uncus and hippocampal gyrus toward the midline so that they bulge over the incisural edge of the tentorium. The midbrain becomes flattened against the opposite incisural edge. If forceful enough, a notching of the cerebellar peduncle on the side contralateral to the lesion (Kernohan's notch) occurs with resulting hemiparesis contralateral to the herniating

TABLE 218-1 Common Pupillary Abnormalities

ABNORMALITY	SIZE	DESCRIPTION AND REACTIVITY	CAUSE
Argyll Robertson	Constricted	Reacts to accommodation but not light	Tertiary syphilis
Hippus phenomenon	Variable	Alternating constriction and dilatation of pupil when light shined into the eye	Midbrain dysfunction
Adie's	Dilated	Minimal reaction to light, greater for accommodation	Developmental
Horner's syndrome	Constricted	Pupil dilates poorly in dim illumination. Miosis, ptosis, and anhydrosis	Sympathetic denervation
Iritis	Constricted	Photophobia. Posterior synechiae (adhesions) occur	Inflammation of the iris
Marcus Gunn	Variable	Deafferented eye. Constricts to light stimulus in other eye	Any total lesion of cranial nerve II
Narcotic overdose	Markedly constricted	Pin point pupils. Light reflex is difficult to elicit but present	Heroin most frequent cause
Anticholinergic syndrome	Widely dilated	Minimally to non-reactive	Anticholinergic overdose
Anoxia or ischemia	Widely dilated	Fixed	Cardiac arrest good example
Hypothermia	Dilated	Fixed	Hypothermia
Metabolic encephalopathies	Small to midposition	Pupillary light reflex is preserved	Endogenous metabolic disturbance
Midbrain damage	Midposition	Fixed to light. Hippus phenomenon	Herniation Vascular lesions
Pontine hemorrhage	Markedly constricted	Pin point pupils, irregular in shape. Light reflex very minimal	Pontine bleed into tegmentum
Uncal herniation	Widely dilated	Fixed	Compression of cranial nerve III
Cranial nerve III lesion	Widely dilated	Fixed. Associated weakness of upward, medial, and lateral gaze	Diabetes, Herniation, Trauma

side. The ipsilateral third nerve, as well as the posterior cerebral artery, becomes compressed against the free edge of the tentorium, or cranial nerve III is caught between stretched branches of the posterior cerebral artery, producing a scissors-like compression of cranial nerve III. The pupillomotor fibers that are carried on the outside of the nerve are first affected, producing dilation of the pupil, initially with a sluggish reaction to light. Later, fibers for extraocular movements are involved, producing the fixed, blown pupil. Decorticate posture is likely at this point. As the opposite pupil begins to dilate, the functioning level becomes still lower in the brainstem, so that decerebrate posturing may begin to become evident. As function progressively deteriorates, the clinical findings become identical to those of the lower stages of central transtentorial herniation.

Central transtentorial herniation results from both hemispheres herniating through the tentorium somewhat symmetrically, compressing the midbrain and diencephalon. In the early diencephalic stage of central transtentorial herniation, pupils show a small range of contraction to light, and patients make appropriate motor responses to orbital roof pressure, In the later diencephalic stage, the motor response to stimulation is stiffening of the legs and arms (decerebrate rigidity). In the midbrain-upper pons stage, the pupils are midposition and fixed, with the patient assuming a decerebrate posture. In the lower pons-upper midbrain stage, eyes are fixed, EOMs are motionless, and the patient is flaccid.

EOM testing alone may point to a diagnosis. In myasthenia gravis, diplopia or ptosis worsens on sustained effort. In acute Wernicke's encephalopathy, there is an inability to look laterally to either side as a result of involvement of periaqueductal gray matter in the upper brainstem. Upon the parenteral administration of thiamine, the abnormality may correct itself within several minutes.

CRANIAL NERVE V The corneal reflex requires the first division of the trigeminal nerve for sensory input and the facial nerve (cranial nerve VII) for the motor response. The corneal reflex may be abnormal in cerebellopontine angle lesions, which may involve cranial nerve V, VII, and VII, making it important to perform the test in patients presenting with auditory, labyrinthine, or cerebellar complaints. The nasociliary reflex involves the same sensory input as the corneal reflex, but the motor response lies with cranial nerve III. Hence, the two reflexes do not test the same level of motor response, although they do involve similar testing of cranial nerve V's sensory input and provide alternatives for testing facial sensation in the unresponsive patient. The trigeminal nerve also provides innervation to the masseter muscles. Masseter muscle testing should also be performed when checking the trigeminal nerve.

CRANIAL NERVE VII Check for facial asymmetry by looking at the palpebral fissure width as well as the depth of the nasolabial fold. If asymmetry is present, be certain that there is no bony asymmetry of the face, where the larger side looks flatter. If facial weakness is suspected, test willed movement such as showing the teeth, shutting the eyes, frowning, and smiling. Significant asymmetry of strength in wrinkling the forehead suggests a peripheral motor lesion, whereas maintenance of forehead movement and loss of the lower half of facial muscle strength suggest an upper motor neuron lesion. The tympanic membranes should always be examined in the presence of a facial palsy to look for vesicles associated with herpes zoster and Ramsey-Hunt syndrome, as well as to identify a purulent otitis media, which can affect the chorda tympani nerve. Testing taste is important in peripheral facial lesions. Sense of *taste* on the anterior two-thirds of the tongue may be lost from a lesion of the facial nerve proximal to the chorda tympani branch.

CRANIAL NERVE VIII Auditory acuity can be assessed by rubbing fingers together or by whispered voice. If one uses a tuning fork, lateralization of the sound to one side, when the tuning fork is placed in the midline towards the vertex of the skull, is an abnormal finding (Weber test). Sound is lateralized to the side of a conduction-hearing deficit and away from the side of a neural- or sensory-hearing deficit. A conduction hearing loss is present if the sound perceived is louder or heard longer when the tuning fork is placed on the bone behind the external pinna as compared with in front of the ear (Rinne test). The tuning fork most frequently used for testing is 128 cps, or C. A higher-frequency tuning fork is more easily drowned out by background noise. Also, patients with high-frequency hearing loss may provide a different test result with tuning forks of high frequency. A lower-frequency tuning fork has the disadvantage of increased size. Given the loudness of background noise in most emergency departments, subtle differences are not likely to be detected.

Labyrinthine dysfunction is suspected in the presence of nystagmus or a history of vertigo. Formal testing of labyrinthine function should be reserved for the patient with vertigo. There is a note of caution, however. Maximal turning of the head to one side may compress the ipsilateral vertebral artery. Extension of the neck, as in looking at the ceiling, may compress both vertebral arteries. It is possible that the vertigo elicited by these maneuvers results from vertebrobasilar disease rather than from labyrinthine disturbance, especially in the elderly patient.

One may test for positional vertigo with the Barany maneuver. One should be hesitant to perform this test on the elderly vertiginous patient, given the possibility of vertebrobasilar disease. The patient should sit close enough to one end of the stretcher so that the head would be over the edge if the patient were lying down. The patient keeps the eyes open during the maneuver and reports any nausea or vertigo. The patient's head is turned 45° to one side. The examiner supports the head and shoulders and brings the patient quickly to a reclining position with the head still rotated and hanging over the edge of the stretcher. The position is maintained for 20 s. The examiner observes the eyes for nystagmus, noting the time of onset from the change in position, direction of eye movement, the nature of associated symptoms, whether the nystagmus disappears while maintaining the same head position, and whether the response fatigues on repeated testing. The head is turned to the other side and the same maneuver and observations are done. A peripheral lesion produces predominantly horizontal, sometimes rotatory nystagmus, with the fast component away from the side of the lesion, and the response can be suppressed by visual fixation. A central lesion within the brainstem or cerebellum produces nystagmus in any direction and is sometimes vertical. When horizontal, the fast component is towards the side of the lesion, and the response cannot be suppressed by visual fixation.

Ice water calorics are not customarily a high priority in the emergency department, but may be valuable in selected circumstances of significant brainstem dysfunction or suspected brain death. To attempt to elicit doll's eyes movement in the emergency department in a comatose patient who may have fallen is hazardous in view of possible cervical fracture. Further, neither maneuver is likely to alter the need for imaging studies.

CRANIAL NERVES IX AND X The gag reflex should be assessed in any patient in which there is a question of handling secretions appropriately. Absence of or asymmetry in eliciting the gag reflex suggests a brainstem lesion. (Presence or abscence of the gag reflex should never be used to determine the necessity of airway intervention.)

CRANIAL NERVE XI The trapezius and sternocleidomastoid muscles should be tested by elevating the shoulders against resistance and turning the head to each side against resistance when adjacent cranial nerves are affected and in patients with motor weakness.

CRANIAL NERVE XII It is important to test tongue movements if lower cranial nerves are affected, or in the presence of generalized or lateralized weakness. The tongue may deviate to one side when protruded. Placing the tip of the tongue against the adjacent cheek tests for strength of the tongue muscles.

Finding atrophy indicates a chronic lower motor neuron lesion. Fasciculations of the tongue occur frequently in amyotrophic lateral sclerosis.

Motor System

POSTURE *Decorticate posture* consists of abnormal flexor response in the arm at the elbow and wrist with extension of the leg. Fully developed, this pattern is referred to as decorticate rigidity. The arms are brought up over the chest with both the elbows and wrists flexed. *Decerebrate posture* consists of abnormal extensor response in the arm and the leg. Fully developed, this pattern is referred to as decerebrate rigidity and consists of opisthosthotonus with the teeth clenched, arms stiffly extended, adducted, and hyperpronated. The legs are stiffly

TABLE 218-2 Segmental Innervation of Muscles

Neck:	Trapezius	C2, C3*, C4
	Sternomastoid	C1, C2
	Diaphragm	C4
Shoulder:	Deltoid	C5
	Supra- and infraspinatus	C5, C6
	Serratus magnus	C5, C6, C7
Arm:	Biceps, brachialis anticus and brachioradialis	C5, C6
	Triceps	C6, C7*, C8
Forearm:	Extensors of wrist	C6, C7*, C8
	Extensors of metacarpophalangeal joints	C6, C7, C8
	Flexors of wrist	C7, C8*, CT1
	Radial deviation of wrist	C6, C7*
	Ulnar deviation of wrist	C7, C8*, CT1
	Supination	C5*, C6
	Pronation	C6, C7*, C8
Hand:	Lumbricals, interossei, opposition of thumb	C8, CT1*
	Abductor and flexor pollicis brevis	C7, C8*
Pelvic Girdle:	Iliopsoas	T12, L1*, L2*, L3
	Glutei	L4, L5*, LS1
Thigh:	Quadriceps	L2, L3*, L4
	Adductors	L2, L3, L4
	Semitendinosus and semimembranosus	L4, L5, LS1
	Biceps femoris	L5*, LS1, L2
Leg:	Gastrocnemius and soleus	L5, LS1*, L2
	Tibialis anticus	L4, L5
	Peronei	L5, LS1
Foot:	Short plantar muscles	S1, S2
Bladder:	(Smooth muscle)	S2, S3
Anus:	Levator ani and associated peroneal muscles	S3, S4

*Where innervation is chiefly from one motor root, the number is starred.

TABLE 218-3 Features of Tremor Types

	PARKINSONIAN (*RESTING*)	ESSENTIAL (*POSTURAL*)	CEREBELLAR (*INTENTION*)
History			
Age at onset	60 or older	All ages More common >60	All ages
Family history	Negative	Frequently positive (Autosomal dominant)	Rarely positive
Response to ETOH	No effect	Often suppresses tremor	No effect
Examination			
Frequency	3–6/s	6–12/s	3–5/s
Symmetry	Almost always begins unilaterally	Symmetrical	Either symmetrical or asymmetrical
Body affected	Arms > legs	Hand > head	Arms > legs, trunk or head
Associated signs	Rigidity, postural instability, bradykinesia	None	Dysarthria, broad-based gait, nystagmus

extended and the feet are plantar flexed. Early in the development of an acute cerebral lesion, an abnormal posture may occur only in response to a noxious stimulus. Hemiparesis alone results in external rotation of the leg and foot on the affected side. The finding is not dissimilar to that seen with hip fracture, except that the leg is not foreshortened, and there is neither hip tenderness nor pain on hip movement. Seeing abnormalities in posture should be part of the initial observation of a patient. If a hemiparetic posture is suspected, one should look for evidence of facial flattening on the same side: wider palpebral fissure and flatter nasolabial fold, as well as an extensor plantar response or other indications of hemiparesis.

STRENGTH Motor strength is usually tested when focal or generalized weakness is either the presenting complaint or suspected by history or examination. (Table 218-2). Strength should be assessed in all four extremities. The earliest upper motor neuron weakness occurs in the dorsiflexors of the wrist and ankle. An adequate screening motor examination includes abduction of the shoulder, extension and flexion of the elbow, extension of the wrist and fingers, grip (testing with two fingers), flexion of the hip, extension of the knee, and dorsiflexion of the foot.

The following rating scale may be used for documentation:

0 = No movement
1 = Flicker
2 = Able to move when gravity eliminated
3 = Able to move against gravity
4 = Able to move against resistance
5 = Normal strength

Apart from determining the existence of a deficit, the initial examination is important to note further evolution or improvement.

The greatest concern in patients presenting with generalized weakness is whether the patient has the strength to breathe and ventilate adequately. Forced vital capacity and a peak negative inspiratory force should be obtained. Abnormal results can be followed to determine a trend, or, if markedly abnormal, can indicate the need for intubation.

RESISTANCE TO PASSIVE MOVEMENT The early parkinsonian patient may present with *rigidity* or with a *cogwheel phenomenon*. Alteration in resistance to passive movement may occur in some demented patients where the amount of resistance is proportional to the amount of force applied (*gegenhalten*). The *spastic catch,* with a "clasp-knife" character from spasticity, is seldom present in an acutely developing lesion. *Flaccidity* results from denervation, which may be peripheral, as well as from deep coma.

ATROPHY One should examine the bulk of the muscles and the relationship of atrophy to loss of power of contraction. This may give important information on how long the deficit may have been present. In amyotrophic lateral sclerosis, the area of the first dorsal interosseus, between the metacarpal bones of the thumb and index finger, is frequently atrophic. In the presence of atrophy, one should look for fasciculations and consider amyotrophic lateral sclerosis. The tongue is also a place where fasciculations are commonly found.

TREMOR AND INVOLUNTARY MOVEMENTS Involuntary movements are usually seen when the limbs are at rest, such as the rhythmic tremor of parkinsonism, but may be more obvious during movement, as in chorea or the distal, rhythmic, sometimes rotatory, essential tremor (Table 218-3). Most involuntary movements represent slowly developing neurologic disorders and do not require emergent intervention. An exception is the abrupt, constant while awake, proximal, swinging movements of hemiballismus, a violent form of hemichorea, caused by a lesion (infarct, hemorrhage, metastasis) of the subthalamic nucleus.

PRONATOR DRIFT The *pronator drift* is tested by having the patient hold the arms outstretched with the palms upwards and the eyes closed. A positive finding results from turning or pronating the hand while the arm drift downwards. The pronator drift is a valuable screening tool for determining the presence of a subtle neurologic deficit and should be incorporated in the emergency examination of a conscious patient when any hemispheric lesion is suspected. A normal finding requires normal strength and motor functioning as well as normal proprioception mediated through the sensory fibers of the posterior columns.

GAIT AND STANCE Gait testing is an essential part of every neurologic examination. If the patient cannot stand, try to determine whether it is the result of weakness or of unsteadiness. If the patient can stand but is unsteady, note whether the patient tends to consistently fall in one direction, and whether the unsteadiness is increased with the eyes closed (Romberg's test).

The characteristic disorders of gait are:

1. Hemiplegic gait—circumduction of the leg with a stiff knee, scraping the floor.
2. Spastic paraplegic gait—slow, stiff movements, tilting of the pelvis and delayed flexion of hips.
3. Steppage gait—flopping feet, lifted too high, as with a foot drop.
4. Sensory ataxia—wide base, uneven steps, stamping.
5. Cerebellar—wide base, with irregularity, deviation or reeling, staggering or turning.
6. Parkinsonism (festinating)—stooped, with short steps, may accelerate, chasing center of gravity, or may have some degree of retropulsion, finding it difficult to stop when stepping backwards.

Chronic gait abnormalities can be detected by examining the soles of shoes for asymmetrical wear. Spasticity from hemiparesis results

TABLE 218-4 Cerebellar and Proprioceptive Incoordination

EXAMINATION	CEREBELLAR	PROPRIOCEPTIVE
Influence of vision	Darkness or closing eyes does not affect symptoms or signs	Darkness or closing eyes markedly increases symptoms and signs
Sensory changes	Sensory problems not integral part but may be superimposed as in sensory neuropathy and alcoholic cerebellar degeneration	Impaired position and vibratory sense are integral to diagnosis
Finger-to-nose and heel-to-shin tests	Marked intention tremor with dysmetria may be present Present with eyes open	Inaccuracy in tests, most marked in legs, aggravated by eye closure
Gait	Wide-based with asynchronous limb movements. Difficulty in mounting curbs while crossing streets	Wide-based, steppage (high-stepping, foot-slapping) gait (often from foot drop from motor neuropathy)
Romberg test	Patient equally unsteady with eyes open or closed	Patient may be stable with eyes open but becomes markedly unsteady with eyes closed (positive Romberg)

in increased wear of the toe of the shoe on the affected side. Midline cerebellar disease produces a widened stance and a wide-based gait. For cerebellar hemispheric lesions, the initial subtle finding may only be a difficulty in turning rapidly, especially if asymmetrical. Walking heel-to-toe may accentuate a subtle abnormality in coordination. Standing with the eyes closed and the feet together (Romberg test) requires normal position sense functioning as well as adequate strength in both legs. If a patient can stand with the feet together with the eyes opened but cannot do so with the eyes closed, this suggests a difficulty in proprioception or position sense (posterior columns). If this is not accomplished with the eyes opened or there is tendency to veer to one side on walking, the lesion is likely cerebellar or labyrinthinc. When walking successively forwards and backwards with the eyes closed, movement in a direction perpendicular to the line of walking occurs in cerebellar hemispheric lesions. A progressive turning clockwise or counterclockwise (compass gait) occurs in labyrinthine lesions.

COORDINATION When possible, gait testing and performance of the Romberg test are important to assess complaints of incoordination. The finger-to-nose test, heel-to-shin test, and testing rapid alternating movements are valuable in assessing cerebellar function. In finger-to-nose and heel-to-shin testing, cerebellar lesions produce movements perpendicular to the line of movement. The rapid rhythmic cadence is disrupted in rapid alternating movements (Table 218-4).

TABLE 218-5 Common Motor Reflexes Tested in Neurologic Examination

SPINAL ROOTS	REFLEX
C5 to T1	Pectoralis
C5/C6	Biceps, brachioradialis
C6/C7	Pronator reflex
C7/C8	Triceps
T8/T9	Upper abdominal reflex*
T11/T12	Lower abdominal reflex*
L2 to L4	Quadriceps (knee jerk, patellar reflex)
L5	Achilles (ankle jerk)
S1/S2	Plantar reflex*
S3/S4	Superficial anal*

*Reflex arc receptors are in the skin rather than stretch receptors in muscle fibers.

Reflexes

DEEP TENDON REFLEXES The deep tendon reflexes (DTRs) (Table 218-5) can be pathologic by being asymmetric, absent, or hyperactive. Hyperactivity is generally associated with upper motor neuron dysfunction and is manifested by clonus, i.e., repetitive jerking of the reflex, or by pathologic spread, i.e., muscles that are innervated by adjacent motor nerve roots contract. Examples of pathologic spread

TABLE 218-6 Methods to Overcome Voluntary Patient Movements and Feigned Deficits

OCCURRENCE	PROCEDURE
Feigned weakness in leg	Patient is instructed to lift the weak leg up off the bed. Your hand under the heel of the opposite foot should experience downward pressure if a real attempt is made. Procedure is not of value with bilateral weakness.
Feigned weakness in arm or feigned unconsciousness	Lifting the hand above the face and dropping it should result in the hand striking the face in real weakness or unconsciousness. When feigned, the hand will slip to the side, not striking the face.
Feigned unconsciousness	Painful, noxious stimulus can be produced without much force by pressure on the supraorbital nerve above the pupil in the eyebrow.
Plantar reflex contaminated by withdrawal	External rotation of the leg with flexion of the knee decreases the amplitude of withdrawal.
Feigned continuous seizure	No lactic acidosis in serum chemistries. Prolactin is not elevated. Behavior is sometimes suggestible.
Feigned blindness	A cloth or wheel with stripes or repeating pattern is moved across the visual field from left to right and right to left. The presence of nystagmus demonstrates that there is visual perception (opticokinetic nystagmus).

are adductor spread when eliciting a knee jerk or finding a positive Hoffmann reflex, with the thumb flexing on flicking the tip of the middle finger. Hypoactive reflexes in the lower extremities can be recruited by the Jendrassik maneuver: locking the finger tips together and pulling. This maneuver decreases the inhibition of the reflex arc by internuncial neurons within the spinal cord. The major value of the maneuver lies in assisting in determining whether a weak reflex is present or not. Finding abnormality in DTRs can help in the assessment of spinal cord lesions, radicular lesions, and peripheral nerve lesions.

PLANTAR REFLEX This reflex, described by Babinski originally as an up-going large toe and fanning of the other toes, was elicited using a goose quill. After a 10-year dispute with Sherrington and the English neurophysiologists, Babinski settled for motion of the large toe alone but supposedly still carried the goose quill. Observing the movement of the other toes can occasionally prove helpful, however, when the response of the large toe is in doubt. Asymmetry of the plantar reflexes should be observed and recorded.

A strong or painful stimulus is not needed to elicit the plantar reflex. A gentle sensory stimulus from the heel towards the toes in the distribution of S1 in the lateral foot will suffice. If the plantar response is contaminated by withdrawal, externally rotating the leg, so that the lateral knee lies on the stretcher, does much toward minimizing the effects of withdrawal.

ABDOMINAL REFLEX The abdominal reflex is obtained by gentle scratching as with a broken Q-tip stick in all four abdominal quadrants. The normal response is contraction of the abdominal musculature in that quadrant. The reflex is normally present in people with strong abdominal musculature, but may be absent in older persons or those with abdominal surgery or multiple pregnancies. The normal finding

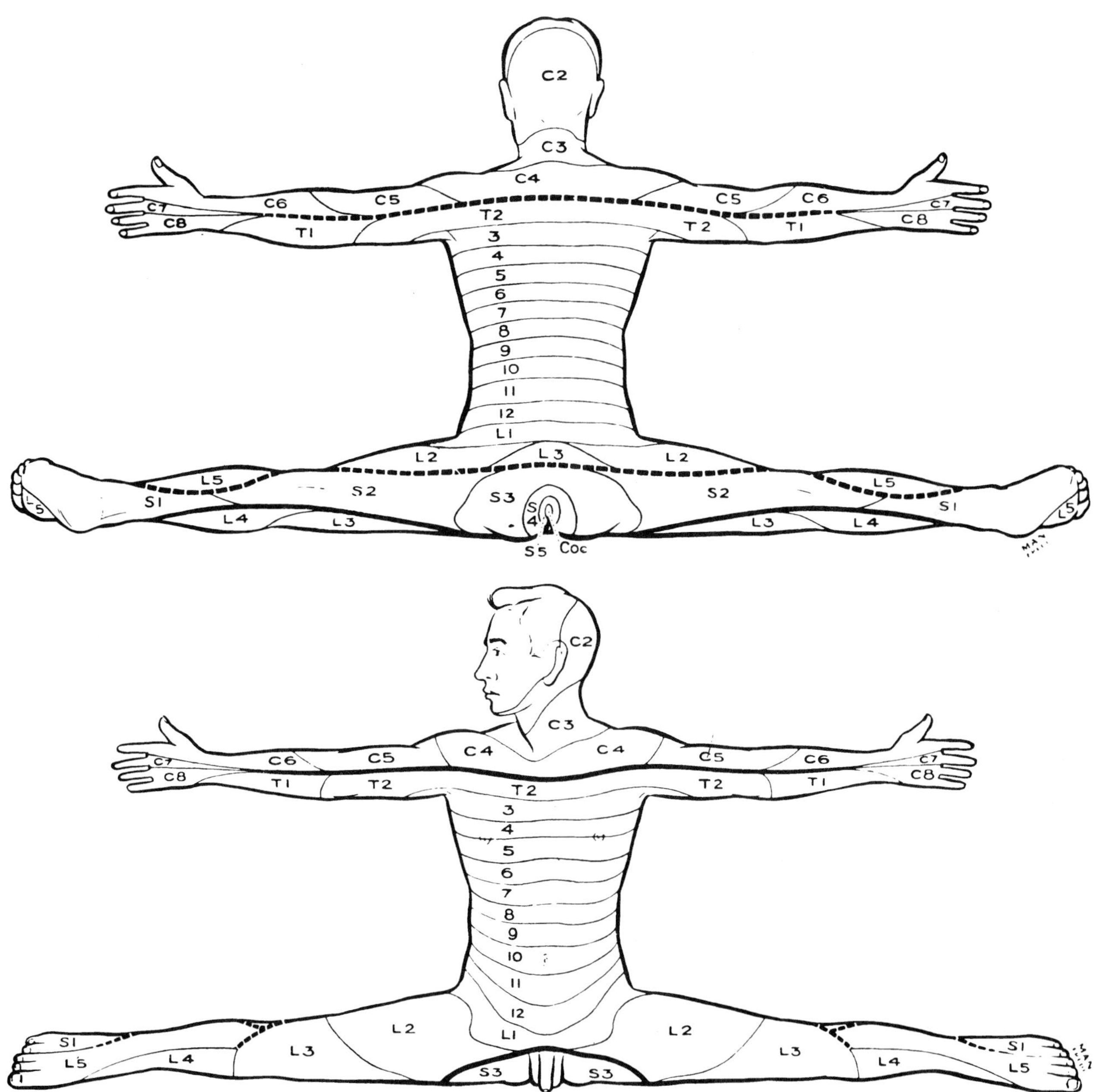

FIG. 218-1. Nerve root origin of various reflexes. (From Haymaker W, Woodhall B: *Peripheral Nerve Injuries: Principles of Diagnosis.* Philadelphia: WB Saunders, 1945, p. 16. Used by permission.)

is similar in relevance to a normal plantar response. The chief value of the reflex is when there is asymmetry or loss below a certain level. Finding normal abdominal reflexes in the face of asymmetrical plantar reflexes decreases some concern over the asymmetrical plantar reflexes.

ANAL REFLEX The superficial anal reflex results from a contraction of the levator ani and associated peroneal muscles when perianal skin is scratched on either side. It is lost with damage to S3-S4, segments of the spinal cord or their nerve roots. This reflex, as well as rectal sphincter tone, is important to assess following spinal cord trauma.

Sensory Examination

The sensory examination (Fig. 218-1) is the least reliable part of the neurologic examination. It is also very time-consuming to test systematically touch, pain, temperature, position, and vibratory sensations. Situations where a careful sensory examination is needed include:

1. Pain syndrome, especially on the trunk, looking for a dermatomal pattern as in preeruptive herpes zoster, or in the leg, looking for discogenic radiculopathy.
2. Localized atrophy or weakness.
3. Numbness, pins and needles, tingling, coldness or pain in any part.
4. Trophic changes, especially painless ulcers, blisters, and joint lesions, should lead to careful testing for loss of pain sense.
5. Presence of ataxia should always lead to careful evaluation of position and vibratory sense.
6. Visual inattention suggesting a non-dominant parietal lobe lesion.
7. Recurrent paroxysms of pain, suggesting a thalamic syndrome.
8. Spinal cord trauma or other causes of a sensory level or dissociated sensory loss.
9. Perianal sensation in suspected spinal cord dysfunction.
10. Following trauma to an extremity with motor or sensory complaints.
11. Following stroke with finding of a hemiparesis or hemianopia.

If sensory abnormalities exist related to the median, ulnar, or peroneal nerves, examination for Tinel's sign should be performed, if feasible, over the carpal ligament, the ulnar groove, and distal to the head of the fibula, respectively.

Two-point discrimination has utility, particularly for peripheral nerve lesions. There is normal variation when regions are compared. In the tongue, normal two-point discrimination is 1 mm, while the finger tip is 2 to 6 mm, the forearm and chest are 40 mm, and the thigh and upper arm are 75 mm.

Patients will on occasion attempt to influence the examiner to make a diagnosis that does not exist. A few counter maneuvers may be helpful to determine if lesions are real (Table 218-6).

219 HEADACHE AND FACIAL PAIN

Michael Schull

HEADACHE

Headache represents up to 4 percent of all emergency department (ED) visits.[1] ED physicians are generally concerned with identifying those patients whose headaches are caused by life-threatening conditions. Most patients, however, have benign primary headache syndromes and are concerned with receiving rapid and effective treatment for their headaches. Both of these priorities need to be kept in mind.

Epidemiology

Migraine headaches have prevalence rates of approximately 17 percent in women and 5 percent in men.[2] Most ED patients have benign primary headache syndromes, but approximately 3.8 percent have serious or secondary pathology.[1]

Classification

Detailed headache classification criteria were published by the International Headache Society in 1988.[3] For practical purposes, headaches are generally divided into primary headache syndromes, including migraine, tension-type, and cluster headaches, and secondary causes. The most common secondary causes are listed in Table 219-1.

TABLE 219-1 Primary and Secondary Causes of Headache

PRIMARY HEADACHE SYNDROMES
Migraine
Tension type
Cluster
SECONDARY CAUSES OF HEADACHE
Vascular
Subarachnoid hemorrhage
Intraparenchymal hemorrhage
Subdural or epidural hematoma
Ischemia (stroke, TIA)
Cavernous sinus thrombosis
Arteriovenous malformation
Temporal arteritis
Carotid or vertebral artery dissection
CNS Infection
Meningitis (bacterial, viral, other)
Encephalitis
Cerebral abscess
Non-CNS Infection
Focal or systemic
Sinusitis
Herpes zoster of face or scalp
Other CNS
Tumor (benign or malignant)
Pseudotumour cerebri
Ophthalmic
Glaucoma
Iritis
Optic neuritis
Drug-Related and Toxic or Metabolic
Nitrates and nitrites
MAOI drugs
Chronic analgesic use and abuse
Hypoxia or high altitude
Hypercapnia
Hypoglycemia
Monosodium glutamate
Carbon monoxide poisoning
Alcohol withdrawal
Miscellaneous
Malignant hypertension
Preeclampsia
Pheochromocytoma
Fever
Post-lumbar puncture
Dental (referred)
Otic (referred)

Abbreviations: CNS, central nervous system; MAOI, monoamine oxidase inhibitor; TIA, transient ischemic attack.

TABLE 219-2 ACEP Headache Categories

Headache Category	Examples
I. Critical secondary causes requiring emergent identification and treatment	Subarachnoid hemorrhage, meningitis, brain tumor with raised ICP
II. Critical secondary causes not necessarily requiring emergent identification or treatment	Brain tumor without raised ICP
III. Generally benign and reversible secondary causes	Sinusitis, hypertension, post-lumbar puncture headache
IV. Primary headache syndromes	Migraine, tension type, or cluster

Abbreviation: ICP, intracranial pressure.

Approach to Patients with Headache in the Emergency Department

The American College of Emergency Physicians (ACEP) clinical policy for adults with headache[4] groups all causes of headache into four broad categories (Table 219-2). Evaluation of the headache patient has four essential objectives:

1. To appropriately select patients for emergency investigation and treatment of suspected critical secondary headache causes
2. To diagnose and effectively treat patients with generally benign and reversible secondary headache causes
3. To provide effective treatment for primary headache syndromes
4. To provide appropriate disposition and follow-up (including outpatient investigations and referral as necessary) for all discharged patients

The central role played by the history in the evaluation of the headache patient is emphasized in the guidelines published by ACEP and those of other groups.[2,4,5] Patients with an atypical history, a substantial change from the previous headache pattern, or certain high-risk features, as summarized below, need to be investigated in the ED.[2,4,5]

HISTORY **Headache Pattern** Atypical features include first severe headache or worst headache ever. Headaches that began days earlier and steadily worsen should be considered atypical. Patients with a long-standing history of headaches should be investigated emergently if their headache is significantly different from prior ones in terms of its duration, severity, or associated symptoms.[2,4]

Onset Sudden-onset headache, especially if is begins during exertion, is an independent predictor of intracranial pathology,[1] and up to 25 percent of such headaches are caused by subarachnoid hemorrhages (SAHs).[6]

Headache Location The location of the headache is nonspecific and should not be relied upon for diagnosis. Migraines are most commonly unilateral and tension-type headaches bilateral, but the reverse may also be true.[7] Occipito-nuchal location of headache among ED patients is an independent predictor of intracranial pathology, though, its positive predictive value is only 16 percent.[1] It is, however, the most common location for the headache of an acute SAH.[8]

Associated Symptoms Other atypical features include a history of syncope, altered level of consciousness, confusion, neck pain or stiffness, persistent visual disturbance, fever, or seizures.[2,4] The history should also include a search for symptoms of nonneurologic conditions causing headache, such as visual change and eye pain from glaucoma or iritis; jaw claudication, suggestive of temporal arteritis; or congestion and facial pain, suggestive of sinusitis.[4]

Other History Medications [e.g., nitroglycerin, chronic analgesic use, monoamine oxidase inhibitors (MAOIs), or anticoagulants], a remote history of trauma, or toxic exposures (e.g., carbon monoxide) may be important risk factors. Inquire also about prior headache history, the results of any previous neuroimaging, and comorbid conditions, such as malignancies, AIDS or HIV seroconversion, coagulopathy, and hypertension.[4]

Family History Migraine headaches occur more commonly in patients with a family history of migraines or motion sickness.[9] Headache patients should be asked about relatives with SAH, since the risk of ruptured intracranial aneurysm in first- and second-degree relatives is up to four times higher than in the general population.[10]

PHYSICAL EXAMINATION Vital sign abnormalities are warning signs of a possible serious cause. Fever suggests infection, such as meningitis or sinusitis, but can also occur in SAH. Marked hypertension should raise suspicion of a hypertensive urgency or emergency.

A focused examination looking for important nonneurologic causes of headache is then carried out. In the head and neck, the sinuses should be examined for evidence of sinusitis, the temporal arteries palpated for tenderness or reduced pulsation, suggestive of temporal arteritis, and the dentition and temporomandibular joints examined for tenderness.[4] An eye examination should be carried out to exclude acute glaucoma or iritis. Fundoscopy may reveal papilledema or the absence of venous pulsations, both signs of raised intracranial pressure (ICP), or subhyaloid hemorrhage (gravity-dependent venous hemorrhage between the retina and vitreous membrane, convex at the bottom and flat at the top when the patient is examined sitting), which is highly suggestive of SAH.

Finally, a careful neurologic examination is mandatory, focusing on the mental status, cranial nerves, motor and sensory exams, reflexes, gait, and cerebellar testing. The patient should also be examined for papilledema, visual field defects, or meningial signs. Abnormalities in the setting of headache require emergent investigation,[2,4,5] since focal or nonfocal neurologic findings in an ED headache patient have a 39 percent positive predictive value for intracranial pathology.[1]

SPECIAL CONSIDERATIONS **Women** Migraine headaches are more common in women and are influenced by hormonal factors. Menarche, menstruation, oral contraceptive use, pregnancy, and menopause may all affect migraine. Higher estrogen levels are generally associated with improved symptoms.[11]

Pregnancy Preeclampsia should be ruled out in pregnant women. Pregnancy improves migraine symptoms in 60 to 70 percent of patients.[11]

Older Age Headaches that begin in patients over 50 years of age are worrisome and may herald the presence of a secondary cause.[1] However, one study of new-onset headache in older patients still found primary headache syndromes to be the commonest diagnosis.[12]

Children The basic approach to headaches in the pediatric population is the same as in adults but somewhat modified in recognition of different likelihoods among the causes (Fig. 219-1). Classification of pediatric headaches is shown in Table 219-3. Most children presenting to the ED have headache related to an underlying febrile illness, such as an upper respiratory or other viral infection, or trauma. Dental causes may be a common source. Migraines are possible but not frequent, and only rarely does the first headache result in ED presentation. There is usually a family history of migraines or motion sickness.

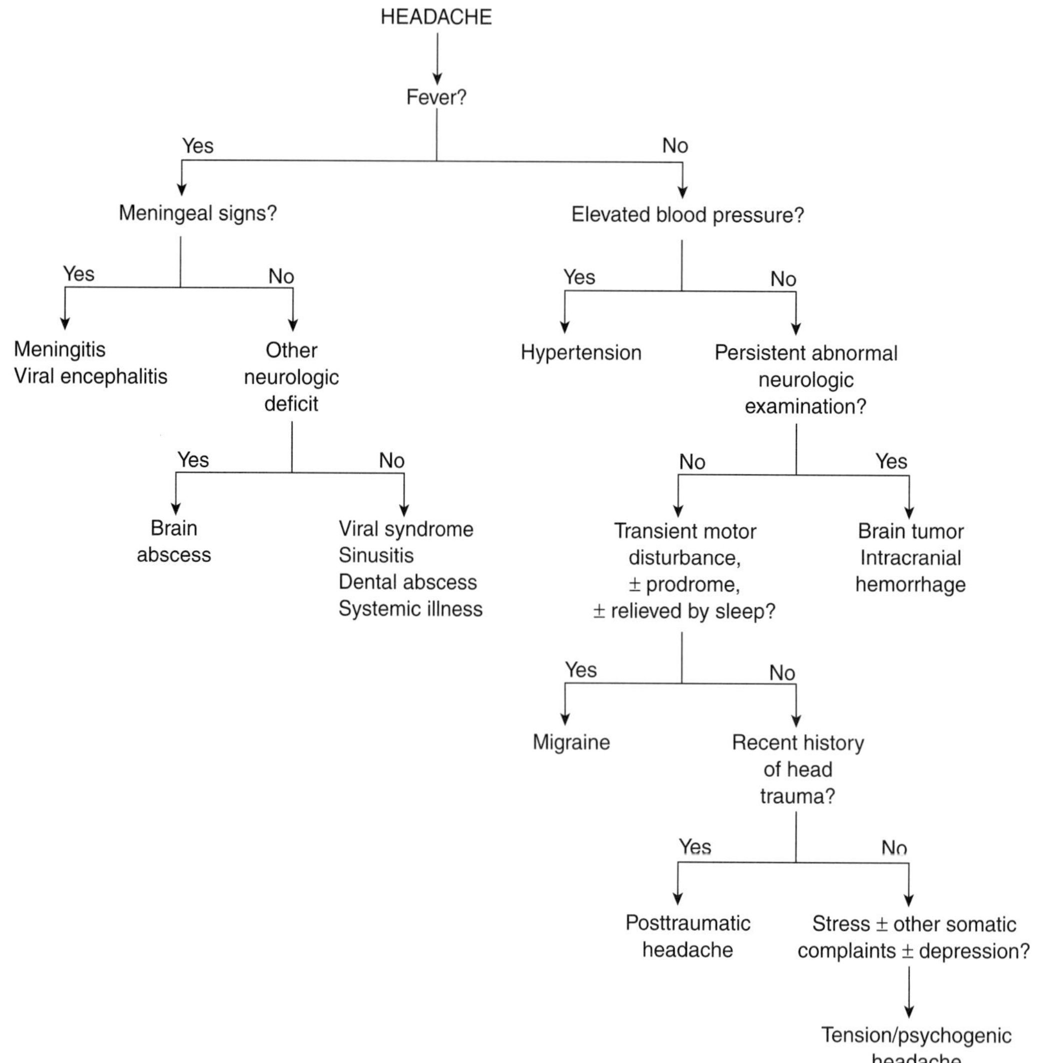

FIG. 219-1. Diagnostic approach to headache in the pediatric population. (From Charney E: Headache, in Ludwig S, Fleisher G (eds): *Pediatric Emergency Medicine.* Baltimore, Williams & Wilkins, 1993, p 375, with permission.)

Transient neurologic deficits may accompany migraines. Life-threatening causes of headache include meningitis or encephalitis, mass lesions and increased ICP, and hypertension. Absence of fever in particular should prompt accurate assessment of blood pressure. Inadvertent or intentional poisonings should also be considered. For example, headache may be the presenting (and only) complaint of carbon monoxide poisoning. Shunt malfunction in children with hydocephalus often presents with headache as a major component.

Children with chronic headaches do not usually present to the ED with headache as their primary complaint, and, although vigilance is required, such headaches are usually due to nonacute causes, such as muscle tension, vision disturbance, or psychogenic causes.

If a thorough examination does not reveal a life-threatening condition, symptomatic treatment with simple analgesics and antipyretics is sufficient, and patients should be referred to their primary care physician for follow-up and further evaluation.

Using Clinical Data to Guide Decision-Making

With the clinical data compiled in the history and physical examination, patients may be classified according to the ACEP groupings (Table 219-2). Patients suspected of having critical secondary causes of headache should undergo emergent investigations, as outlined below, and have appropriate treatment initiated. Those suspected of benign and reversible secondary causes should undergo diagnostic tests if required and have treatment initiated, generally as outpatients. The largest group of ED headache patients have assessments that suggest a benign primary headache syndrome, and the objective for these patients is to provide effective therapy.

Appropriate follow-up should be ensured for all discharged patients. Outpatient investigation and referral may be required, especially in cases such as poorly controlled primary headache syndromes or occasionally a patient with a suspected critical secondary cause not needing emergent investigation (e.g., suspected brain tumor without raised ICP). In cases such as the latter, outpatient workup is appropriate only if the physician is confident that the patient will not be lost to follow-up.

Investigation of the ED Headache Patient

COMPUTED TOMOGRAPHY SCANNING The ED patient whose headache requires emergent investigation usually begins with a noncontrast computed tomography (CT) scan.[4] The use of contrast material

TABLE 219-3 Classification of Headaches in the Pediatric Population

Common	Life-Threatening
INFLAMMATORY	
Dental infection	Intracranial
Sinus infection	Meningitis
	Encephalitis
TRACTION	
Neoplasm	Increased intracranial pressure
Post-lumbar puncture	Cerebral edema
	Hydrocephalus
	Intracranial hemorrhage or hematoma
	Brain abscess
VASCULAR	
Febrile illness	Hypertension
Migraine	Vascular anomalies
	Seizures
	Hypoxia
	Poisoning
MUSCLE CONTRACTION	
Tension	
Fatigue	
OTHER	
Traumatic and posttraumatic	
Psychogenic	
Ocular	

Source: Adapted from Charney E, in Ludwig S, Fleisher G (eds): *Pediatric Emergency Medicine.* Baltimore, Williams & Wilkins, 1993, with permission.

increases the time, expense, and risk of adverse effects (minor 10 percent, severe 0.1 percent),[5] and the noncontrast CT scan usually adequately excludes critical lesions or mass effects requiring emergent interventions. In particular, the noncontrast CT scan is the best neuroimaging test for diagnosing an acute SAH, but CT scan cannot rule it out. When there is strong suspicion of small lesions likely to be missed without contrast (e.g., in an AIDS patient suspected of cerebral toxoplasmosis or suspected small brain mass), then a CT with contrast material may be needed.[5]

LUMBAR PUNCTURE Lumbar puncture (LP) is required in cases such as suspected meningitis, or suspected SAH with a normal CT scan. Contraindications to LP include the suspicion of raised ICP, which can be excluded by the absence of papilledema, normal level of consciousness, and normal findings on neurologic examination. Venous pulsations seen at the disc margins on fundoscopic examination with the patient upright effectively rule out ICP. Venous pulsations may be terminated temporarily with pressure on the globe. If these conditions are met, then a CT scan need not necessarily be carried out prior to LP, especially if the CT is likely to be delayed. In cases of suspected meningitis without evidence of raised ICP, LP may be done without prior CT in order to avoid any delay in starting antibiotics.[4]

MAGNETIC RESONANCE IMAGING The cost and restricted availability of magnetic resonance imaging (MRI) limit its utility in the emergency investigation of headache. MRI is more sensitive than CT in evaluating brain injuries, such as diffuse axonal injuries, small parenchymal contusions, or isodense subdural hemorrhages, and most tumors.[5] In acute SAH, however, MRI is no more sensitive than CT in the first few days following a bleed.[13] CT scanning and LP are adequate for the large majority of ED headache patients requiring emergent investigation.

Primary Headache Syndromes

The term "primary headache" includes all forms of migraine, tension-type, and cluster headaches. There is considerable clinical overlap in primary headache syndromes, and it has been suggested that they share a pathophysiology and represent different ends of a clinical spectrum.[7]

MIGRAINE **Epidemiology** Migraine headaches are common, with onset usually in the early teens or even younger. Prevalence is estimated at approximately 5 percent for males and 15 to 17 percent for females.[2] Prevalence peaks in both sexes at around 40 years of age and then gradually declines.

Pathophysiology Early theories postulated abnormal vasculature as the root cause of migraine headaches, with vasoconstriction being responsible for the aura and rebound vasodilatation the cause of the pounding headache. It now seems clear that migraines are a primary response of brain tissue to some trigger, while the disordered activity of blood vessels is secondary.

Auras are thought to be due to primary neuronal dysfunction. The neurologic symptoms of auras are believed to result from a slowly spreading wave of neuronal hypoactivity traveling across brain tissue. There is a corresponding decrease in local blood flow where neuronal activity is reduced. This reduction in blood flow does not follow vascular territories, which makes it unlikely to be vasospastic in origin.[9]

Pain-sensitive intracranial structures, such as blood vessels and the dural matter, are largely supplied by sensory axons of the trigeminal ganglion in the supratentorium, while the upper cervical roots innervate the posterior fossa. Animal models suggest that the headache of migraine is related to activation of these sensory axons, leading to the release of various peptides. This causes sterile neurogenic inflammation in pain-sensitive arteries, the dura, and meningial tissues, and promotes local vasodilatation. The release of these peptides and the resulting inflammation and plasma extravasation can be blocked by sumatriptan, a selective agonist of 5-HT_{1D} (serotonin) receptors, as well as by ergots, indomethacin, and others. Sumatriptan also has direct vasoconstricting effects. Both mechanisms may explain its efficacy at revealing migraine headache. The neurophysiologic pathways linking auras and headaches are still poorly understood.

What actually triggers these complex mechanisms for migraines? Enhanced excitability of occipital cortex neurons in migraine patients has been proposed as a possible trigger, but no clear answer has yet emerged.[9]

Clinical Features Migraine without aura accounts for about 80 percent of migraines. The headache generally is slow in onset and lasts from 4 to 72 h. It is typically unilateral and pulsating, and worsened by physical activity. Nausea, vomiting, and photo- or phonophobia frequently accompany the headache.[3] The scalp may or may not be tender. These features, however, are not entirely sensitive (migraines need not be unilateral or pulsating) or specific (the same features can be present in tension-type headaches).[7] Suspicion should be raised when a patient presents with a "migraine" that is significantly different from prior headaches. The headache in migraine with aura is similar but is preceded or accompanied by an aura that develops gradually over minutes, lasts no more than 60 min, and is fully reversible.

Visual auras are the commonest, usually consisting of scintillating scotomata (i.e., dark spots) or flashing lights, but virtually any neurologic symptom or sign can occur. Other "typical" auras include hemiparesthesia, hemiparesis, aphasia, or other speech difficulties. Rarer types of aura include those with brainstem symptoms (basilar migraine), those lasting longer than 60 min (migraine with prolonged aura), and aura without accompanying headache (migraine aura without headache). Auras should be distinguished from migraine prodromes, which occur many hours prior to the headache and can consist of lethargy, hyperactivity, yawning, depression, food craving, polyuria, or fluid retention.[9]

Other, less common forms of migraine include ophthalmoplegic migraine, in which headache overlaps with paresis of one or more of cranial nerves III, IV, and VI, or retinal migraine, with sudden monocular scotoma or blindness associated with headache. Childhood periodic syndromes (previously known as migraine equivalents) are ill-defined childhood syndromes thought to be associated with migraine, in which symptoms such as abdominal pain or vomiting are prominent while headache may be absent.[3] Rarely, migrainous infarction may occur (previously called complicated migraine), characterized by an aura lasting more than 7 days or neuroimaging evidence of cerebral infarction.[3]

Clearly, in a patient who presents with a focal neurologic deficit and headache, migraine of any sort must be a diagnosis of exclusion unless the patient has a clear history of previous similar migraines, including the neurologic deficit, and normal results of prior investigations. Given that they rarely last more than 60 min, the aura and deficits would be expected to resolve in migraine patients prior to discharge from the ED.

Treatment Advances in the understanding of the pathophysiology of migraine have been paralleled by much improved ED treatment options for severe migraine. Yet, while an impressive array of medications has been studied and virtually every route of administration has been tried, there remains a wide spectrum of clinical practice and no clear consensus on the best therapy. This reflects the fact that, to date, no migraine treatment has been shown to be superior in all respects.[14]

Physicians choosing a medication should consider several factors besides efficacy in relieving headache in the ED, including the ability to *abort* migraine (i.e., prevent recurrence after relief of symptoms), contraindications, relief of other symptoms, side effects, cost, ease of administration, and time to return to normal activities. Patients should also be asked about their previous experience with a drug and whether they are willing to accept the same treatment again. Unfortunately, many migraine studies do not adequately assess these outcomes and suffer from other limitations.

At present, several effective options are available for the ED management of acute severe migraine headache, based on a review of ED randomized controlled trials (RCTs) and consensus guidelines prepared by the Canadian Headache Society.[2] Dihydroergotamine (DHE), a 5-HT_{1D} (serotonin) receptor agonist, is highly effective in relieving headaches and is an appropriate first-line therapy for migraine.[2,15] However, DHE causes vomiting in a significant proportion of patients, probably due to its affinity for other serotonin and dopamine receptors. Patients should therefore be pretreated with an antiemetic, such as metoclopramide or prochlorperazine.[2] Sumatriptan, a more selective 5-HT_{1D} agonist than DHE, is effective in relieving headache in the ED and causes less nausea and vomiting.[14,16] However, ED-based studies have shown that subcutaneous sumatriptan results in frequent but short-lived minor adverse effects (e.g., sensations of heat, tingling, chest discomfort, and injection site reactions), is more costly, and has a higher 24-h recurrence rate than DHE.[16] While sumatriptan may still be useful for migraines unresponsive to other medications, it should not be given within 24 h of the administration of DHE or other ergots, since both cause vasoconstriction.[2]

Other migraine drugs studied in ED-based RCTs and shown to be effective include metoclopramide,[17] chlorpromazine,[15,18] prochlorperazine,[17] and ketorolac.[18] Table 219-4 summarizes dosing, contraindications and precautions for each drug. Regardless of medication chosen, patients should be placed in a darkened, quiet area in order to lessen the associated phono- and photophobic symptoms. Given that patients may have been vomiting and had poor oral intake for hours or days prior to their arrival in the ED, intravenous rehydration is also frequently of benefit.[2]

Dexamethasone has been touted as effective in reducing the rate of recurrent migraine following standard treatment.[2] In one ED-based RCT, patients received either 20 mg intravenous dexamethasone or placebo after standard migraine therapy. A significant reduction in the rate of 48- to 72-h recurrent migraine was found in the dexamethasone group as compared to the placebo group.[19]

Special mention is reserved for the use of opioid analgesics in migraine. Meperidine is still used as an acute migraine treatment despite several studies that have shown it to be less effective than other agents.[20] The frequent use of opioids in chronic and recurrent headache conditions may lead to adverse effects, and may even exacerbate headaches.[20] While some patients may require opioid analgesics, the preferred treatment is one of the numerous, more effective alternatives to opioids.[2]

Pregnant Women Migraines generally improve during pregnancy, especially after the first trimester. Nonpharmacologic therapy, such as rest and ice, should be tried first, but in patients with intractable headache or nausea and vomiting, medications may be used.[11] Acetaminophen and nonsteroidal anti-inflammatory drugs (NSAIDs) are considered class B by the US Food and Drug Administration (i.e., no evidence of risk in pregnant women, but there are no controlled trials) and can be used. However, NSAIDs should be used very cautiously, if at all, in the third trimester, since they inhibit labor and decrease amniotic fluid volume. Metoclopramide, another class B drug, can be very useful, especially if there is significant nausea and vomiting.[11]

Prophylaxis Patients with frequent recurrent migraines may benefit from prophylactic medications, such as β blockers without intrinsic sympathomimetic activity (atenolol, metoprolol, nadolol, propanolol), calcium–channel blockers, tricyclic antidepressants, or NSAIDs. However, obstetric or neurologic consultation should be obtained before starting these drugs in the ED. In patients already on prophylaxis and experiencing breakthrough migraines, drugs should be titrated up to maximally tolerated doses for several months before concluding that a given medication is ineffective. They also must be withdrawn slowly to prevent rebound headaches.[2]

TENSION-TYPE HEADACHES Previously, extracranial muscle tension was thought to be a causative factor in tension-type headaches. However, this relationship has been questioned, given the problem of demonstrating muscle tension and the difficulty of determining whether it is a cause or merely an epiphenomenon. More recent theories suggest that tension-type headaches and migraines may share a common pathophysiology and that they represent different ends of a clinical spectrum.[7]

Tension-type headaches are defined in such a way as to distinguish them from migraines. Therefore, they are described as bilateral, nonpulsating, not worsened by exertion, and not associated with nausea or vomiting.[3] However, patients with severe tension-type headaches may indeed have nausea and vomiting, and mild migraine might easily fit the description of a tension-type headache.[7]

Treatment for mild headaches consists of simple analgesics or NSAIDs. For severe tension-type headaches, treatment is the same as for migraines, given the difficulty of distinguishing between the two entities.

CLUSTER HEADACHES Cluster headaches are generally rare (prevalence rates of 0.4 percent of the general population), and they are very short-lived even without treatment. Unlike other primary headaches, they are more common in men, and onset is usually after 20 years of age.

TABLE 219-4 Emergency Department Treatment Options for Migraine Headache

Treatment Options	Recommended Dosing and Adjuncts	Contraindications, Precautions, and Notes
DHE	Pretreat with metoclopramide or prochlorperazine to reduce nausea and vomiting 1 mg IV DHE over 3 min; if inadequate relief, may repeat once after 60 min	Contraindications: pregnancy, uncontrolled hypertension, coronary artery disease, peripheral vascular disease, recent sumatriptan use Precautions: may cause nausea and vomiting, diarrhea, abdominal pain, leg cramps
CPZ	Pretreat with IV normal saline bolus to reduce risk of hypotension 7.5 mg IV CPZ q15min to maximum of 25–35 mg or headache relief	Precautions: class C in pregnancy,* may cause hypotension, drowsiness, dystonic reactions Notes: effective antiemetic
Prochlorperazine	5–10 mg IV or PR	Precautions: class C in pregnancy,* may cause drowsiness, dystonic reactions Notes: effective antiemetic
Metoclopramide	10 mg IV	Precautions: class B in pregnancy,* may cause drowsiness, dystonic reactions. Notes: effective antiemetic
Ketorolac	IV 30 mg or IM 60 mg	Contraindications: gastric intolerance to NSAIDs or history of peptic ulcers, especially in the elderly Precautions: class B in pregnancy,* but avoid in the third trimester
Sumatriptan	6 mg SC May repeat 6 mg SC after 1 h if not improved, but studies suggest little benefit of repeat dosing	Contraindications: pregnancy, uncontrolled hypertension, coronary artery disease, ergot use in previous 24 h, MAOI use Precautions: high rate of minor adverse effects; rarely, coronary artery spasm, myocardial infarction, dysrhythmias Notes: good relief of nausea, vomiting, and photophobia; costly; high 24-h recurrence rate

*US Food and Drug Administration drug safety ratings in pregnancy (class A, no risk to fetus; class B, no evidence of risk in humans, but no controlled trials; class C, risk to humans has not been ruled out).
Abbreviations: CPZ, chlorpromazine; DHE, dihydroergotamine; IM, intramuscular; IV, intravenous; MAOI, monoamine oxidase inhibitor; NSAID, nonsteroidal anti-inflammatory drug; PR, per rectum; and SC, subcutaneous.

Dysfunction of the trigeminal nerve is believed to cause cluster headaches, and the fact that they respond to 5-HT_{1D} agonists suggests a common mechanism with migraines.[21]

Cluster headaches are characterized by very severe, unilateral orbital, supraorbital, or temporal pain lasting 15 to 180 min. The pain is such that patients can rarely lie still, and most are pacing and restless. The headaches are associated with at least one of the following signs on the ipsilateral side: conjunctival injection, lacrimation, nasal congestion, rhinorrhea, facial swelling, miosis, or ptosis. They tend to occur in ''clusters,'' that is, daily on the same side of the face for several weeks, before remitting for anywhere from weeks to years.[3]

Given the short duration of cluster headaches, any medication used in their treatment must act very rapidly. Oxygen is effective in up to 70 percent of patients, and DHE and sumatriptan have also been shown to be rapidly effective. Oral agents are unlikely to be effective for acute attacks, given the long time for absorption and the short duration of cluster headaches, but NSAIDs may be useful in reducing the frequency and severity of future attacks.[21]

DISPOSITION OF PATIENTS WITH PRIMARY HEADACHE SYNDROMES Regardless of the type of primary headache, poor response to treatment should heighten suspicion of a secondary cause and prompt emergent investigations. However, improvement of a presumed primary headache as a result of treatment does not rule out secondary causes.[4] Patients who respond well to ED management may usually be discharged with appropriate follow-up. Occasionally, a patient with intractable migraine may require admission for more aggressive pain control.

Secondary Causes of Headache

More complete discussions of most of these entities are found elsewhere in this text.

SUBARACHNOID HEMORRHAGE **Epidemiology** SAH has an annual incidence of approximately 1 per 10,000 in the United States[10] and represents 1 percent of all nontraumatic headaches seen in the ED.[1] However, SAH accounts for up to a quarter of all sudden severe headaches.[6] SAH occurs in young people, with a median age of 50 years. Mortality rates from SAH are high; 50 percent of patients die within 6 months, and only 58 percent of survivors regain their premorbid neurologic state.[22]

Clinical Features At the time of presentation, almost half of patients with SAH have normal findings on neurologic examination, including normal vital signs, normal level of consciousness, and no neck stiffness.[22] The headache of SAH is most commonly severe and of sudden onset, but it may also be more subtle. The most common location for the headache is occipitonuchal.[8] Many presentations are atypical and may mislead the clinician. For example, sudden-onset intense neck pain may be mistakenly attributed to radiculopathy. Also, resolution of the pain even without treatment does not exclude the diagnosis. Beware of radiation of pain down along the spine, since this suggests tracking of subarachnoid blood down the spinal canal.

Diagnosis Investigation of suspected SAH usually begins with a plain CT scan of the head. Retrospective studies suggest sensitivity of newer generation CT may be in excess of 93 percent for the detection of SAH when symptom presentation is within 24 h and may be even higher if performed within 12 h of symptom onset.[23] However, no study has convincingly shown that CT alone can rule-out SAH, even within 12 h.[24] CT sensitivity falls to slightly over 80 percent after 24 h and decays rapidly thereafter. Older generation CT scanners were less sensitive among patients who were alert compared to those with altered sensorium.[25] It remains unclear whether this finding holds with new generation scanners.[26]

Most authorities consider an LP to be mandatory following a negative CT. An alternate view suggests that LP may be unnecessary when the pretest probability is very low.[27] However, this view has itself been challenged on the basis that so-called low-probability patients (isolated severe headache and absence of neurologic findings) may still have up to a 12 percent chance of SAH and that CT may be less sensitive in these patients.[28] Thus, given the potential for catastrophic outcome, it remains prudent to perform an LP on all patients suspected of SAH in whom the CT scan was negative. In fact, restricting investigations to only an LP has been proposed for patients meeting ''lone acute sudden headache'' criteria (acute sudden headache without neck stiffness and normal neurologic examination, vital signs and level of consciousness). However, the utility of this protocol has not been proven in clinical studies.[28]

The gold standard for the diagnosis of SAH is the presence of xanthochromia in the cerebrospinal fluid supernatant. If LP is performed 12 h or longer after headache onset (sufficient time for xanthochromia to develop) and spectrophotometry is used for the cerebrospinal fluid analysis, xanthochromia is virtually 100 percent sensitive for up to 2 weeks following a bleed. Naked-eye detection of xanthochromia may lead to false-negative results in up to 50 percent of cases.[10]

MENINGITIS All forms of meningitis can cause headache. In viral or bacterial meningitis, the headache may be severe and of rapid onset, and is usually accompanied by fever and meningismus. Opportunistic infections in immunocompromised patients, such as cryptococcal meningitis, may present with a more insidious onset of headache, and fever and neck stiffness may be absent. An LP is required if there is any suspicion of meningitis, and it need not be preceded by a CT scan in patients with normal findings on neurologic examination, a normal level of consciousness, and no papilledema. If the LP must be delayed for any reason and bacterial meningitis is suspected, antibiotics should be started immediately.[4]

INTRAPARENCHYMAL HEMORRHAGE AND CEREBRAL ISCHEMIA About 55 percent of patients with intraparenchymal hemorrhage report headaches at the onset of their symptoms. Only 17 percent of ischemic stroke patients and 6 percent of patients with transient ischemic attacks (TIAs) complain of headache. Other neurologic signs and symptoms are present in most patients.

SUBDURAL HEMATOMA A history of remote trauma in a patient with a headache should raise suspicion of a subacute or chronic subdural hematoma. A low threshold for initiating investigations is appropriate for high-risk patients, including patients on anticoagulants, chronic alcoholics, and the elderly, in whom there may be no clear history of trauma.[4]

BRAIN TUMOR Up to 70 percent of patients with brain tumors complain of headache at the time of diagnosis, and only about 8 percent have normal findings on neurologic examination.[12] The headache may be unilateral or bilateral, intermittent or continuous. The classic headache of brain tumors (worse in the morning, associated with position and nausea and vomiting) occurs in only a few. If headache is suspected of being due to a tumor and 24-h follow-up can be ensured, a reliable patient with normal findings on neurologic examination, including no papilledema, can be investigated as an outpatient.[4,12]

TEMPORAL ARTERITIS **Epidemiology** Temporal arteritis (TA) occurs almost exclusively in patients over 50 years of age. In this age group, there is an annual incidence rate of 15 to 30 cases per 100,000 persons, and it occurs more commonly in women.[29]

Pathophysiology TA is a systemic panarteritis that selectively involves arterial walls with significant amounts of elastin.[12]

Clinical Features Headache is the most common symptom of TA, reported in 60 to 90 percent of patients. The headache is most often severe, throbbing, and usually located over the frontotemporal region. Other strongly suggestive features include jaw claudication or evidence of polymyalgia rheumatica, with which TA is strongly associated. The involved temporal artery may be nonpulsatile or tender, or have a diminished pulse. The most serious complication is loss of vision, usually due to ischemic optic neuritis.[12,29]

Diagnosis The diagnosis is established by fulfilling three of the five following criteria: age over 50 years, new-onset localized headache, temporal artery tenderness or decreased pulse, erythrocyte sedimentation rate over 50 mm/h, and abnormal arterial biopsy findings.[29]

Treatment In order to prevent loss of vision, treatment should begin immediately with 40 to 60 mg/day prednisone when TA is clinically suspected. Patients should be referred urgently for definitive diagnosis and follow-up.[29]

OPHTHALMIC DISORDERS Acute glaucoma may present with headache, and in other eye disorders, such as iritis or optic neuritis, some patients may describe eye or supraciliary pain as headache. These conditions can usually be distinguished by a careful history and eye examination, including measurement of intraocular pressure when necessary.[4]

HYPERTENSION Hypertension may cause headaches, with higher diastolic pressures generally associated with more severe headaches. Physicians should be cautious prior to making this diagnosis, however, since hypertension may also occur as a sign of other secondary headache conditions (e.g., stroke, pheochromocytoma, or preeclampsia) or may simply be secondary to the pain and anxiety associated with a primary headache syndrome.[4] When other secondary causes of headache, including hypertensive emergency (see Chap. 53), have been ruled out, reduction of the blood pressure should result in improvement or resolution of the headache. While some consider isolated headache associated with hypertension as evidence of possible end-organ involvement, most such patients can be discharged following complete resolution of symptoms and blood pressure reduction if follow-up in the next 24 to 48 h can be arranged.

SINUSITIS Infection of the sinuses may result facial pain or headache. Maxillary sinusitis, by far the commonest type, causes pain over the anterior aspect of the face, rather than headache. Involvement of other sinuses can cause headache: frontal sinusitis over the forehead, ethmoid sinusitis behind and between the eyes, and sphenoid sinusitis a diffuse headache. The headache frequently varies with head position. Symptoms predictive of sinusitis include colored nasal discharge, maxillary toothache, and poor response to decongestants, while reliable signs include purulent nasal discharge and abnormal transillumination (not easy to do properly in the ED). Regardless of plain sinus x-ray findings, patients with four or more of the abovementioned features have a very high likelihood of sinusitis, while those with fewer than two features are very unlikely to have sinusitis.

DRUG-RELATED AND TOXIC OR METABOLIC HEADACHES Various drugs, such as nitrates, MAOIs, or chronically used analgesics, may cause headache. Such metabolic conditions as hypoxia, hypercapnia, and hypoglycemia and such toxins as monosodium glutamate and carbon monoxide may cause headache as well. Withdrawal from alcohol may also result in headache. Such headaches can be identified either in the history or through appropriate laboratory testing.[4]

BENIGN INTRACRANIAL HYPERTENSION (PSEUDOTUMOUR CEREBRI) A rare entity, benign intracranial hypertension (BIH) should be considered in a young, obese patient presenting with long-standing headaches. Nausea, vomiting, and visual disturbance may also be present. While its cause is unknown, BIH has been linked to the use of oral contraceptives, vitamin A, and tetracycline and to thyroid disorders. BIH is characterized by papilledema, a normal level of consciousness, normal CT scan findings, and markedly elevated cerebrospinal fluid pressure on LP. The only serious adverse outcome is the potential for visual loss. Initial treatment is usually with acetazolamide or steroids. When these fail, repeated LPs to drain cerebrospinal fluid or surgery (cerebrospinal fluid shunts or optic nerve sheath fenestration) may be tried.

INTERNAL CAROTID AND VERTEBRAL ARTERY DISSECTION While rare, dissection of the internal carotid or vertebral artery is frequently associated with headache. Dissection may be spontaneous or the result of trauma and generally occurs in younger patients (median age, 40 years). Internal carotid artery dissection may be suspected in a patient with unilateral anterior neck pain or headache, usually around the eye or frontal area. Most patients present with or eventually develop neurologic signs, such as TIA, stroke, Horner syndrome, transient monocular blindness, or cranial nerve palsies. Vertebral artery dissection typically presents with marked occipital or posterior neck pain associated with signs of a brainstem TIA or stroke. Diagnosis is usually made by angiography. Duplex scanning and MRI may also identify vessel abnormalities. SAH may be caused by dissection through the adventitia of the vessel, and this must be ruled out prior to initiating anticoagulant therapy.

POST–LUMBAR PUNCTURE HEADACHE Between 10 and 36 percent of patients who undergo LP develop a headache within 24 to 48 h due to a persistent cerebrospinal fluid leak from the dura. The incidence of post-LP headaches can be minimized through the use of smaller-bore needles with noncutting tips in order to spread, rather than cut, dural fibers.[30] Patients who present to the ED with a post-LP headache may respond to simple analgesics, but, if this treatment fails, a blood patch may be required. This procedure involves an epidural injection of autologous blood at the level of the LP in order to ''patch'' the cerebrospinal leak.[31]

CRANIAL AND FACIAL PAIN DISORDERS

Temporomandibular Disorder

Temporomandibular disorder (TMD) refers to persistent discomfort due to dysfunction of the temporomandibular joint (TMJ), surrounding muscles, and ligaments. Symptoms include TMJ noise and pain on movement, limited jaw movements, locking of the jaw on opening, bruxism, and tongue, lip, or cheek biting. Headache may be associated with TMD as well, but in patients with headache and bruxism, it is often not clear which is cause and which is effect. Patients with TMD can usually locate their pain in the TMJ area. It is usually acute and associated with jaw movement. More diffuse symptoms may be the result of dysfunction of the muscles and ligaments used for mastication. Effective management of TMD often requires a multidisciplinary team, and improvement usually occurs with conservative measures. Simple radiographs of the TMJs are of little use in the ED, since the diagnosis of TMD frequently requires more sophisticated imaging techniques. Simple analgesics or NSAIDs can be tried as an initial treatment.

Trigeminal Neuralgia (Tic Douloureux)

Trigeminal neuralgia is characterized by paroxysms of severe unilateral pain in the trigeminal nerve distribution lasting only seconds, with normal findings on neurologic examination. There is no pain between paroxysms. Treatment can be medical or surgical. Carbamazepine is a very effective treatment. If it fails, the patient is unlikely to have trigeminal neuralgia. Patients with trigeminal neuralgia may present to the ED because symptoms are of recent onset or recurrent, and they should be started or restarted on carbamazepine. Pain control is rarely an issue, since the paroxysms are so brief. Patients with intractable symptoms despite medical therapy should be referred to a neurologist or neurosurgeon.

REFERENCES

1. Ramirez-Lassepas M, Espinosa CE, Cicero JJ, et al: Predictors of intracranial pathologic findings in patients who seek emergency care because of headache. *Arch Neurol* 54:1506, 1997.
2. Pryse-Phillips WE, Dodick DW, Edmeads JG, et al: Guidelines for the diagnosis and management of migraine in clinical practice. *Can Med Assoc J* 156:1273, 1997.
3. International Headache Society: Classification and diagnostic criteria for headache disorders, cranial neuralgias and facial pain. *Cephalagia* 8(suppl 7):10, 1988.
4. American College of Emergency Physicians: Clinical policy for the initial approach to adolescents and adults presenting to the emergency department with a chief complaint of headache. *Ann Emerg Med* 27:821, 1996.
5. Frishberg BM: The utility of neuroimaging in the evaluation of headache in patients with normal neurological examinations. *Neurology* 44:1191, 1994.
6. Linn FH, Wijdicks EFM, van der Graaf Y, et al: Prospective study of sentinel headache in aneurysmal subarachnoid hemorrhage. *Lancet* 344:590, 1994.
7. Solomon S: Diagnosis of primary headache disorders: Validity of the International Headache Society criteria in clinical practice. *Neurol Clin* 15:15, 1997.
8. Weir B: Headaches from aneurysms. *Cephalagia* 14:79, 1994.
9. Goadsby PJ: Current concepts on the pathophysiology of migraine. *Neurol Clin* 15:27, 1997.
10. Schievink WI: Intracranial aneurysms. *N Engl J Med* 336:28, 1997.
11. Silberstein SD: Migraine and pregnancy. *Neurol Clin* 15:209, 1997.
12. Evans RW: Diagnostic testing for the evaluation of headaches. *Neurol Clin* 14:1, 1996.
13. Atlas SW: MR imaging is highly sensitive for acute subarachnoid hemorrhage . . . not! *Radiology* 186:319, 1993.
14. The Subcutaneous Sumatriptan International Study Group: Treatment of migraine attacks with sumatriptan. *N Engl J Med* 325:316, 1991.
15. Bell R, Montoya D, Shuaib A, Lee MA: A comparative trial of three agents in the treatment of acute migraine headache. *Ann Emerg Med* 19:1079, 1990.
16. Akpunonu BE, Mutgi AB, Federman DJ, et al: Subcutaneous sumatriptan for the treatment of acute migraine in patients admitted to the emergency department: A multicenter study. *Ann Emerg Med* 25:464, 1995.
17. Coppola M: Randomized, placebo-controlled evaluation of prochlorperazine versus metoclopramide for emergency department treatment of migraine headache. *Ann Emerg Med* 26:541, 1995.
18. Shrestha M, Singh R, Moreden J, Hayes JE: Ketorolac vs chlorpromazine in the treatment of acute migraine without aura. *Arch Intern Med* 156:1725, 1996.
19. Innes GD, MacPhail I, Dillon EC, et al: Dexamethasone prevents relapse after emergency department treatment of acute migraine: A randomized clinical trial. *Can J Emerg Med* 1:26, 1999.
20. Lane PL, McLellan BA, Baggoley CJ: Comparative efficacy of chlorpromazine and meperidine with dimenhydrinate in migraine headache. *Ann Emerg Med* 18:360, 1989.
21. The Sumatriptan Cluster Headache Study Group: Treatment of acute cluster headache with sumatriptan. *N Engl J Med* 325:322, 1991.
22. Kassel NF, Torner JC, Haley EC, et al: The international cooperative study on the timing of aneurysm surgery: I. Overall management results. *J Neurosurg* 73:18, 1990.
23. Sidman R, Connolly E, Lemke T: Subarachnoid hemorrhage diagnosis: Lumbar puncture is still needed when the computed tomography scan is normal. *Acad Emerg Med* 3:827, 1996.

24. Morgenstern LB, Luna-Gonzales H, Huber JC: Worst headache and subarachnoid hemorrhage: Prospective, modern computed tomography and spinal fluid analysis. *Ann Emerg Med* 32:297, 1998.
25. Adams HP, Kassel NF, Torner JC, et al: CT and clinical correlations in recent aneurysmal subarachnoid hemorrhage: A preliminary report of the cooperative aneurysm study. *Neurol* 33:981, 1983.
26. Sames TA, Storrow AB, Finkelstein JA, Magoon MR: Sensitivity of new generation computed tomography in subarachnoid hemorrhage. *Acad Emerg Med* 3:16, 1996.
27. Signal BM: A tap in time? *Acad Emerg Med* 3:823, 1996.
28. Schull MJ: Lumbar puncture first: An alternative model for the investigation of lone acute sudden headache. *Acad Emerg Med* 6:131, 1999.
29. Hunder GG: The American College of Rheumatology 1990 criteria for the classification of giant cell arteritis. *Arthritis Rheum* 33:1122, 1990.
30. Carson D, Serpell M: Choosing the best needle for diagnostic lumbar puncture. *Neurology* 47:33, 1996.
31. Serpell MG, Haldane GJ, Jamieson DRS, Carson D: Prevention of headache after lumbar puncture: Questionnaire survey of neurologists and neurosurgeons in the United Kingdom. *BMJ* 316:1709, 1998.

220 STROKE, TRANSIENT ISCHEMIC ATTACK, AND OTHER CENTRAL FOCAL CONDITIONS

Phillip A. Scott
William G. Barsan

Stroke is the third leading cause of death and the leading cause of disability in the United States. Over 700,000 Americans are afflicted yearly; of these, almost 20 percent will die within the first year. Those who survive are often socially and financially devastated, losing their ability to walk, speak, or care for themselves. Stroke-related costs, including physician and nursing services, hospital and nursing-home care, and lost wages, currently exceed $30 billion a year. These figures are expected to increase with the aging US population, as the incidence of stroke doubles each decade after age 55. Research suggests that early accurate diagnosis and management of patients arriving with stroke at the emergency department may lessen the impact of this disease.[1]

The use of tissue plasminogen activator for select patients with ischemic stroke requires a high level of involvement by emergency physicians. The etiology of stroke is diverse, ranging from cardiac emboli to a rupture of a congenital berry aneurysm. Effective treatment for one stroke type may be disastrous when applied to another stroke type. The anatomic location of the lesion and the mechanism of the stroke must be determined before effective treatment can be administered.

STROKE TYPE

A stroke results from any disease process that disrupts vascular blood flow to a distinct region of the brain. Injury in stroke occurs from (1) ischemia due to vessel occlusion, which deprives neurons of needed oxygen and substrate; or (2) hemorrhage due to vessel rupture, with resultant injury by direct cellular trauma, mass effect, elevated intracranial pressure, and/or the release of deleterious biochemical substances. From 80 to 85 percent of all strokes are ischemic, whereas 15 to 20 percent are hemorrhagic.

Ischemic Stroke

Ischemic stroke can be subdivided into three major categories: thrombotic, embolic, and hypoperfusion. The majority of all strokes are caused by vessel thrombosis, which occurs when clot formation is superimposed upon gradual vessel narrowing or alterations in the luminal lining of the vessel. Atherosclerotic disease is the most common cause of thrombotic stroke in the United States. Atherosclerosis primarily affects the larger intracranial and extracranial arteries and causes hyperplasia and fibrous deposition in the subintimal area with plaque formation. Plaques cause luminal narrowing and platelet adhesion, which lead to vessel thrombosis. Other causes of thrombosis include vasculitis, dissection, polycythemia, and hypercoagulable states. Less common causes are infectious diseases, such as HIV, syphilis, tuberculosis, aspergillosis, and trichinosis, that lead to vessel wall injury. The signs and symptoms of a thrombotic stroke usually develop gradually over minutes to hours and may wax and wane in severity. Upon questioning, patients often give a history of similar but transient symptoms that have occurred in the past, suggesting a transient ischemic attack (TIA) in the same vascular distribution.

One-fifth of all strokes are embolic in nature. In embolism, intravascular material from a proximal source is released and then occludes a distal vessel. In contrast to thrombotic stroke, there is no intrinsic vascular disease in the occluded vessel. Thus, emboli are less adherent to the vessel walls and are more likely to fragment and move distally than are clots due to thrombosis. The most common sources of emboli are the heart and major vessels (aorta, carotid arteries, and vertebral arteries). Cardiac sources of emboli include valvular vegetations, mural thrombi (due to atrial fibrillation, myocardial infarction, or dysrhythmia), paradoxical emboli (due to an atrial or ventricular septal defect), or cardiac tumors (myxomas). Artery-to-artery emboli usually occur when a platelet-fibrin clump is dislodged from a tight stenotic lesion or from a large vessel atherosclerotic plaque. Rarer causes of embolic stroke include fat emboli, particulate emboli from intravenous drug injection, or septic emboli.

Systemic hypoperfusion is a less common mechanism of ischemic stroke than thrombosis or embolism. It is most commonly due to cardiac pump failure (myocardial infarction or dysrhythmias). Hypoperfusion leads to a more generalized or diffuse injury pattern than thrombosis or emboli. It is most evident in border zones or so-called watershed regions at the periphery of the major vascular-supply territories. Patients often have diffuse findings that wax and wane according to their hemodynamic status.

Hemorrhagic Stroke

Although hemorrhagic strokes comprise only one of every five strokes, they have a 30-day mortality rate of 30 to 50 percent and occur in a younger population of patients. Hemorrhagic strokes can be divided into two subtypes: intracerebral hemorrhage (ICH) and subarachnoid hemorrhage (SAH).

The majority of hemorrhagic strokes are intracerebral hemorrhages. In ICH, bleeding occurs directly into the brain parenchyma. Increasing age and a history of prior stroke are the leading risk factors for developing an ICH. Race also plays a prominent role, with Asians and blacks having a higher incidence relative to whites. Tobacco and alcohol abuse are additional risk factors. The majority of ICHs are associated with chronic hypertension. In hypertensive ICH, blood is thought to leak from small intracerebral arterioles damaged by chronically elevated blood pressure. Amyloidosis is another major cause of ICH, especially among elderly patients with lobar or multiple hemorrhages. Other causes of ICH include bleeding diathesis due to iatrogenic anticoagulation or thrombolytic use, vascular malformations, and cocaine use.

SAH is half as common as ICH. In SAH, blood leaks from a cerebral vessel into the subarachnoid space. Blood from a ruptured artery is released at near systemic arterial pressure, in contrast to ICH, in which arteriolar rupture occurs more gradually at lower pressures. The sudden release of blood under high pressure leads to direct cellular trauma as well as a rapid increase in intracranial pressure. Half of all SAHs are due to berry aneurysm rupture, most commonly occurring at arterial bifurcations. Arteriovenous malformations make up another 6 percent of all SAHs.

PATHOPHYSIOLOGY

Basic knowledge of the anatomy and pathophysiology of the brain can assist physicians in identifying the location of a lesion and in understanding the rationale behind various therapeutic interventions.

Anatomy

The vascular supply to the brain is derived from two sources: the anterior and posterior circulations, which supply blood to different regions of the brain. Hypoperfusion of specific areas of the brain leads to typical neurologic findings that can help clinically differentiate the location of the lesion and the vessels that may be involved.

The anterior circulation, which supplies blood to four-fifths of the brain, originates from the carotid system. The common carotid arteries divide into the right and left internal and external carotid arteries at the level of the angle of the mandible. The internal carotid arteries then course intracranially along the sella turcica within the cavernous sinus. The first branch off the internal carotid artery is the ophthalmic artery, which supplies the optic nerve and retina. Sudden onset of painless monocular blindness (amaurosis fugax) identifies the stroke as involving the anterior circulation (specifically, the carotid artery) at or below the level of the ophthalmic artery. The internal carotid arteries terminate by branching into the anterior and middle cerebral arteries at the circle of Willis. The anterior circulation supplies blood to the optic nerve, retina, and frontoparietal and anterotemporal lobes of the brain.

Although the posterior circulation is smaller (supplying blood to only one-fifth of the brain), it supplies the brainstem, which is critical for normal consciousness, movement, and sensation. The posterior circulation is derived from the two vertebral arteries that ascend through the transverse processes of the cervical vertebrae. The vertebral arteries enter the cranium through the foramen magnum, supplying the cerebellum via the posteroinferior cerebellar arteries. They join to form the basilar artery, which branches to form the posterior cerebral arteries. The posterior circulation supplies the brainstem, cerebellum, thalamus, auditory and vestibular functions of the ear, medial temporal lobe, and the visual occipital cortex.

The extent of stroke also depends on the presence of collateral blood flow distal to the vessel occlusion. A patient with excellent collateral blood flow from the contralateral hemisphere may have minimal clinical deficits despite a complete carotid occlusion. In contrast, a patient with poor collateral flow may be hemiplegic with the same lesion.

Ischemic Stroke

Neurons are very sensitive to changes in cerebral blood flow. Brain cells die within a few minutes of complete cessation of blood flow. However, despite complete occlusion of a cerebral vessel during an acute ischemic stroke, some perfusion remains even in the center of the ischemic brain region, due to collateral flow and variations in local tissue pressure gradients. Cells vary from irreversibly injured neurons in the center of the ischemic region to reversibly injured neurons in the periphery (the penumbra). The degree and duration of occlusion determine the viability of the cells in the penumbra. Theoretically, the earlier reperfusion occurs, the greater is the chance of cell survival. The use of intravenous and intraarterial thrombolytic therapy for ischemic stroke is based on this rationale as well as on investigative trials involving the use of neuroprotectant drugs.

Hemorrhagic Stroke

In intracerebral and SAH, a cerebral blood vessel ruptures, with a dramatic increase in intracranial pressure and a decrease in global cerebral perfusion that can last for minutes. After these immediate changes, intracranial pressure and perfusion gradually improve, although not back to baseline. A marked reduction in cerebral perfusion occurs near the hematoma and is probably due to local compression. Areas of the brain remote from the bleed also have alterations in perfusion, which are thought to be due to vasoconstriction caused either by chemical release from blood breakdown products or by neuronal mediation (diaschisis).

CLINICAL FEATURES

The clinical presentation of stroke is often subtle and varied. Physicians must approach patients systematically and logically. Armed with the basic knowledge of the various stroke types and anatomy, the history taking and physical examination should be aimed at determining the underlying cause of the stroke and the location of the lesion.

History

A review of the patient's demographics and past medical history can often suggest the etiology of the stroke. A 40-year-old patient with a stroke syndrome is more likely to have a hemorrhagic stroke (rather than a thrombotic stroke) than a 65-year-old patient. A history of hypertension, coronary artery disease, and diabetes mellitus are all suggestive of underlying atherosclerotic disease and vessel thrombosis. In contrast, atrial fibrillation, valvular replacement, or recent myocardial infarction suggests a cardioembolic source of infarction.

Patients should be thoroughly questioned regarding recent history of TIAs, since this can help differentiate stroke types. A transient neurologic deficit in the same vascular distribution is suggestive of underlying vascular disease consistent with a thrombotic stroke, in contrast to multiple TIAs involving different vascular distributions, which suggest emboli.

Accurate and detailed histories of the presenting illness can further direct physicians to the cause of stroke. Initial onset of symptoms and any fluctuations in symptoms should be documented, since diagnostic studies and inpatient management may differ depending on this history. Sudden onset of symptoms suggests an embolic or hemorrhagic stroke, whereas a stuttering or waxing and waning deficit suggests a thrombotic stroke or a stroke due to hypoperfusion. Concomitant complaints such as headache, vomiting, or recent trauma should be recorded. Headache occurs in the majority of patients with hemorrhage but in only 10 to 20 percent of those with ischemic stroke. A recent history of neck injury, such as in a motor vehicle accident or a sports-related injury, suggests a carotid dissection.

Physical Examination

Prior to initiating a neurologic examination, a general physical examination should be completed. If a patient is febrile, the source of infection should be identified. An infection may be the cause of a patient's deterioration or may be a complication of the stroke (e.g., aspiration pneumonia). The skin should be examined for signs of emboli (e.g., Janeway lesions and Osler nodes) or bleeding dyscrasia (e.g., ecchymosis or petechiae). A funduscopic examination should be completed to identify signs of papilledema (suggesting a mass lesion or hypertensive crisis), preretinal hemorrhage (consistent with an SAH), or evidence of extensive hypertensive retinopathy. A history suggestive of possible cardiac disease such as myocardial infarction, angina, dysrhythmias, palpitation, or worsening of congestive heart failure should be investigated. Physical findings such as rales, an S3 gallop, or carotid bruit should be recorded.

Neurologic Examination

The goal of the neurologic examination is to localize the brain lesion and rule out other neurologic disease processes. The National Institutes of Health (NIH) stroke scale is a 15-item neurologic evaluation that is reproducible, correlates to infarct volume, and can be performed in less than 7 min (see Table 220-1). This allows a serial, standardized neurologic evaluation of a patient over time by either a nurse or a physician.[2] The neurologic examination can be broken down into six major areas: (1) level of consciousness, (2) visual assessment, (3) motor function, (4) sensation and neglect, (5) cerebellar function, and (6) cranial nerves.

TABLE 220-1 National Institute of Health Stroke Scale: A Rapid, Reproducible Neurologic Evaluation of Patients with Stroke

Category	Patient Response	Score
1a. Level of consciousness (LOC)	Alert	0
	Drowsy	1
	Stuporous	2
	Coma	3
1b. LOC questions	Answers both correctly	0
	Answers one correctly	1
	Answers none correctly	2
1c. LOC commands	Obeys both correctly	0
	Obeys one correctly	1
	Obeys none correctly	2
2. Best gaze	Normal	0
	Partial gaze palsy	1
	Forced deviation	2
3. Best visual	No visual loss	0
	Partial hemianopsia	1
	Complete hemianopsia	2
4. Facial palsy	Normal	0
	Minor facial weakness	1
	Partial facial weakness	2
	No facial movement	3
5. Best motor arm	No drift after 10 s	0
	Drift	1
	Cannot resist gravity	2
	No effort against gravity	3
6. Best motor leg	No drift after 5 s	0
	Drift	1
	Cannot resist gravity	2
	No effort against gravity	3
7. Limb ataxia	Absent	0
	Present in upper or lower extremities	1
	Present in both upper and lower extremities	2
8. Sensory	Normal	0
	Partial loss	1
	Dense loss	2
9. Neglect	No neglect	0
	Partial neglect	1
	Complete neglect	2
10. Dysarthria	Normal articulation	0
	Mild to moderate dysarthria	1
	Near unintelligible or worse	2
11. Best language	No aphasia	0
	Mild to moderate aphasia	1
	Severe aphasia	2
	Mute	3

LEVEL OF CONSCIOUSNESS A patient's level of alertness should be evaluated by asking simple questions (birth date or month of the year) and by having the patient follow simple commands (close their eyes, make a fist). Patients may be alert, drowsy (requiring minor stimulation to answer or obey), lethargic (requiring repeated or painful stimulation to respond), or obtunded (postures or is totally unresponsive). Several assessments are available for the mental status examination, such as the mini-mental, or the brief mini-mental, exam. Many of the elements are contained in the NIH stroke scale.

VISUAL ASSESSMENT Evaluation of visual fields and extraocular movements can provide information regarding occipital lobe or brainstem lesions. Visual fields can be tested by confrontation, using finger counting or visual threat as appropriate. Gaze palsy can be assessed by evaluating both voluntary and reflex (by turning the patient's head) horizontal eye movements.

MOTOR FUNCTION Upper extremity motor weakness is best determined by testing for pronator drift. Patients close their eyes and extend their arms with palms facing the ceiling. The test is positive if one arm pronates or drifts lower than the other within 10 s. Lower extremity strength can be similarly evaluated by a patient's ability to elevate each leg 45 degrees individually for 5 s while lying in bed. For subtle signs of lower extremity weakness, observe the patient's gait or have patients walk on their toes and then on their heels. Facial motor weakness (facial droop) due to a central nervous system (CNS) lesion can be distinguished from a peripheral seventh nerve palsy (e.g., Bell palsy) by a patient's ability to wrinkle the forehead on the affected side.

CEREBELLAR FUNCTION Cerebellar function can be tested by observing a patient's gait, finger-to-nose testing, heel-to-shin testing, and by having patients stand with arms outstretched forward, palms up (Romberg test). These tests are all performed with the patient's eyes open and then closed to differentiate from posterior column disease (see Chap. 221, ''Altered Mental Status and Coma'').

SENSATION AND NEGLECT Sensory deficits and neglect should be evaluated by pinprick testing, having the patient identify numbers gently written on the palm (graphesthesia), and by double-simultaneous extinction (the physician touches the patient's right and left limbs individually and then simultaneously). The double-simultaneous extinction test is positive if the patient feels the sensation in either limb individually but only on one side when touched simultaneously, and it suggests neglect. Neglect can be further confirmed by having the patient draw a box or house. Patients with neglect will often omit figures on one side of the drawing.

LANGUAGE The terms dysarthria and aphasia are often erroneously interchanged. *Dysarthria* is a disturbance in articulation and is due to paralysis or incoordination of muscles used for speech. Dysarthric speech is often slurred. Having a patient repeat simple nursery rhymes can identify subtle cases. In contrast, *aphasia* is due to a disturbance in processing language (either written or spoken) and can be receptive (difficulty in comprehension), expressive (difficulty in communicating thoughts), or both. Receptive aphasia can be tested by having patients follow simple commands (either vocal or written). Having patients identify simple objects or describe what is happening in a magazine picture assists in evaluating an expressive aphasia. Patients with expressive aphasia will use inappropriate words or use nonfluent sentences, whereas the words of patients with dysarthria will be slurred.

CRANIAL NERVES Cranial nerves should be individually tested in all patients to identify possible brainstem involvement. Unlike anterior circulation strokes, which cause contralateral motor deficits, brainstem involvement causes ipsilateral cranial nerve deficits with contralateral motor weakness.

STROKE SYNDROMES

After recording a complete medical history and performing a physical examination, the physician must integrate physical findings with brain anatomy and function to determine the anatomic location of the lesion and the possible vessels that may be involved. Physical findings often follow classic patterns that can assist a physician in localizing the lesion.

Transient Ischemic Attack

A TIA is a neurologic deficit that resolves within 24 h (although more than 80 percent resolve within 30 min) and is most commonly associated with thrombotic strokes. The incidence of prior TIAs is 50 to 75 percent in patients with subsequent thrombotic, extracranial carotid artery strokes, but only 10 percent in all other stroke types. TIAs have been thought to cause reversible brain injury; however, recent studies indicate that over 60 percent may be associated with computed tomography (CT) findings of infarction. The true significance of TIAs is their associated 5 to 6 percent risk of stroke per year.

Ischemic Stroke Syndromes

ANTERIOR CEREBRAL ARTERY INFARCT Lesions of the anterior cerebral artery cause contralateral leg weakness greater than arm weakness with mild cortical sensory deficits. Patients may perseverate with speech or motor actions and respond slowly. Anarthria (speechlessness) with paraplegia may occur in a bilateral parasagittal infarct if the anterior cerebral arteries originate from an occluded common trunk.

MIDDLE CEREBRAL ARTERY INFARCT A stroke involving the middle cerebral artery (MCA) territory is the most common and presents with contralateral weakness and numbness variably affecting the face and arm greater than the leg. If the dominant hemisphere is involved, aphasia (receptive, expressive, or both) is often present. Inattention, neglect, or extinction on double-simultaneous stimulation localizes the lesion to the nondominant hemisphere. Constructional apraxia in these patients can be demonstrated by the inability to draw a clock and fill in the appropriate numbers. Patients may be dysarthric but typically are not aphasic. In right-handed patients, and up to 80 percent of left-handed patients, the left hemisphere is the dominant hemisphere. A homonymous hemianopsia and gaze preference toward the side of the infarct may also be found.

POSTERIOR CEREBRAL ARTERY INFARCT Patients with posterior cerebral artery (PCA) infarcts may be unaware of their deficits until formally tested. Motor involvement is minimal, and visual cortex abnormalities may go unrecognized. Light-touch and pinprick sensory modalities, however, may be significantly reduced. The anastomoses of branches of the PCA with arteries from the anterior cerebral artery and MCA territories are common locations of watershed infarcts in hypotensive states.

VERTEBROBASILAR SYNDROME The posterior circulation supplies blood to the brainstem, cerebellum, and visual cortex. Signs and symptoms attributable to a stroke in this distribution may be subtle. They include findings such as dizziness, vertigo, diplopia, dysphagia, ataxia, cranial nerve palsies, and bilateral limb weakness, singly or in combination. The hallmark of posterior circulation stroke is crossed neurologic deficits (i.e., ipsilateral cranial nerve deficits with contralateral motor weakness).

The lateral medullary (Wallenberg's) syndrome is a specific posterior circulation infarct involving the vertebrobasilar arteries and/or the posterior inferior cerebellar artery and in its pure form has a good prognosis. Presenting signs include ipsilateral loss of facial pain and temperature sensation with contralateral loss of these senses over the body, gait and limb ataxia, and an ipsilateral Horner syndrome (typically incomplete, with ptosis and miosis commonly found and anhidrosis absent).

BASILAR ARTERY OCCLUSION Occlusion of the basilar artery causes severe quadriplegia, coma, and the locked-in syndrome. The locked-in syndrome occurs with lesions in the pontine tectum and causes complete muscle paralysis except for upward gaze.

CEREBELLAR INFARCT An important subset of posterior circulation strokes involve the cerebellum. Patients commonly present following a ''drop attack'' with the sudden onset of inability to walk or stand. This is often accompanied by central vertigo, headache, nausea, vomiting, and neck pain. Cranial nerve abnormalities are often present. Bone artifact on CT imaging of the posterior fossa can obscure initial identification, and a high index of suspicion should be maintained in patients with appropriate findings. Typically, after a delay of 6 to 12 h, one-third of patients will develop significant edema with subsequent increased brainstem pressure and decreased level of consciousness. Surgical decompression, and diuretic and corticosteroid use for relief of pressure and/or edema prevention, may be lifesaving.

LACUNAR INFARCT Lacunar infarcts are pure motor or sensory deficits that are due to infarction of small penetrating arteries and are commonly associated with chronic hypertension. Lesions are primarily located in the pons and the basal ganglia.

ARTERIAL DISSECTION Dissections are often associated with severe trauma but can occur from such mild events as turning the head sharply. Patients may complain of severe neck pain or headache hours to days prior to onset of neurologic deficits. Dissections may occur in the carotid or vertebral circulation.

Hemorrhagic Stroke Syndromes

INTRACEREBRAL HEMORRHAGE ICH may be clinically indistinguishable from cerebral infarction and also presents with contralateral hemiplegia, hemianesthesia, hemianopsia, and aphasia or neglect (depending on the hemisphere involved). The presentation may differ from infarction in that the patients are more commonly lethargic and may have marked hypertension. Headache, nausea, and vomiting often precede the neurologic deficit. The condition of patients can quickly deteriorate and require emergent intubation. Bleeding is usually localized to the putamen, thalamus, pons, or cerebellum (in decreasing frequency) in patients with hypertensive ICH. Lobar hemorrhages are suggestive of amyloid angiopathy and are associated with a better prognosis than are deep hypertensive bleeds.[3]

CEREBELLAR HEMORRHAGE A patient presenting with sudden onset of dizziness, vomiting, marked truncal ataxia, and inability to walk must be immediately suspected of having a cerebellar infarction or hemorrhage. These findings may be associated with gaze palsies and increasing stupor. Patients may rapidly progress to coma and herniation unless surgical decompression and/or hematoma evacuation are quickly initiated.

SUBARACHNOID HEMORRHAGE SAH occurs more commonly in women, but men dominate among patients younger than age 40. Pa-

TABLE 220-2 Hunt and Hess Classification of Subarachnoid Hemorrhage

Classification	Symptoms
Grade I	Asymptomatic or minimal headache and mild nuchal rigidity
Grade II	Moderate to severe headache, nuchal rigidity, and no neurologic deficit other than cranial nerve palsy
Grade III	Drowsiness, confusion, or mild focal deficit
Grade IV	Stupor, moderate to severe hemiparesis, possible early decerebrate rigidity, and vegetative disturbance
Grade V	Deep coma, decerebrate rigidity, and moribund appearance

tients present with sudden onset of a severe constant headache that is often occipital or nuchal. A recent history suggestive of a ''sentinel hemorrhage'' with a severe headache lasting for days can be obtained in 15 to 31 percent of cases. Vomiting often presents with the onset of headache, and patients may be noted to have a decreased level of consciousness. Presentation is usually sudden, and a carefully recorded history may reveal activities such as defecation or coughing at onset. Occasionally, the pain is only nuchal, misleading clinicians to consider only local C-spine etiologies. Neurologic deficits may be present due to the aneurysm compressing adjacent brain tissue or cranial nerves. A grading classification based on neurologic condition can aid in determining prognosis and eligibility for surgery (see Table 220-2).

DIAGNOSIS

Differential Diagnosis: Other Central Focal Conditions

Although strokes are the most common cause of unilateral weakness, other causes must be considered (see Table 220-3). All patients with neurologic deficits should have the blood glucose checked for hypoglycemia. Bell's palsy (peripheral seventh cranial nerve palsy) usually occurs in younger patients, is associated with upper and lower facial paralysis, and does not involve the extremities. Evidence of trauma should be sought, since an epidural or subdural hematoma can mimic an acute stroke. Although stroke can present with marked hypertension, one can usually differentiate stroke from hypertensive encephalopathy by history and physical examination. Unlike stroke, the onset of hypertensive encephalopathy is more gradual, and focal neurologic deficits, if present, are superimposed upon global cerebral dysfunction (e.g., decreased level of consciousness) rather than isolated to one brain region. Papilledema, flame-shaped retinal hemorrhages, and acute renal failure may be seen with hypertensive encephalopathy but are not invariable findings. Other diseases that may mimic the mental status changes of stroke include diabetic ketoacidosis, hyperosmotic coma, and meningoencephalitis. Another mimicker of stroke is Wernicke's encephalopathy, with its triad of ataxia, ophthalmoplegia, and confusion, typically found in chronic alcoholics. Multiple sclerosis, presenting commonly in the third and fourth decades of life, with a female predominance, may present with focal deficits, depending on the area of demyelination. The onset of symptoms, however, is more gradual than those in acute stroke. Meniere's disease may be distinguished by its paroxysmal course of vertigo, tinnitus, and deafness. Drug toxicity may also masquerade as acute stroke, with lithium toxicity inducing dysarthria, cranial nerve deficits, and confusion. Phenytoin and carbamazepine toxicity may present with ataxia, vertigo, nausea, and abnormal reflexes.

TABLE 220-3 Differential Diagnosis of Acute Stroke

Hypoglycemia
Postictal paralysis (Todd paralysis)
Bell palsy
Hypertensive encephalopathy
Epidural/subdural hematoma
Brain tumor/abscess
Complicated migraine
Meningitis/encephalitis
Diabetic ketoacidosis
Hyperosmotic coma
Wernicke's encephalopathy
Labyrinthitis
Meniere's disease
Demyelinating disease (multiple sclerosis)
Drug toxicity (lithium, phenytoin, carbamazepine)

Diagnostic Tests

Although clinical data can direct physicians toward the diagnosis of stroke, including the cause and location of a lesion, diagnostic tests are often required to confirm these suspicions and to rule out other etiologies. Tests that may require immediate emergency department interventions include a glucose determination, CT, and an electrocardiogram. The blood glucose level should be determined early (by prehospital providers, if possible) to rule out hypoglycemia as the cause of the neurologic deficit, and 50% dextrose should be administered immediately to any patients with neurologic deficit and hypoglycemia.

An emergent noncontrast CT of the head is essential because it can quickly differentiate ischemic infarction from hemorrhage particularly if the scan is obtained after 12 h of symptom onset. This information is crucial for subsequent therapeutic decisions. CT can identify almost all parenchymal bleeds greater than 1 cm and up to 95 percent of all SAHs. A lumbar puncture is required in all patients strongly suspected of having SAH when the CT scan is normal. Most ischemic strokes will not be visualized by routine CT for at least 6 h and often considerably longer, depending on the size of the infarct. In addition to distinguishing ischemia from hemorrhage, CT can also rule out other life-threatening processes, such as abscess, tumor, and subdural or epidural hematoma.

An electrocardiogram should be obtained to rule out an associated cardiac cause of the stroke. Atrial fibrillation and acute myocardial infarction are associated with up to 60 percent of all cardioembolic strokes. Untreated chronic atrial fibrillation may increase the risk of stroke up to 6 percent yearly. In addition, stroke occurrence is 2.5 percent among patients with acute myocardial infarction within the first 4 weeks of their cardiac event.

Blood tests that may be helpful include a complete blood count (CBC) with platelet count, coagulation studies, toxicologic screen, and cardiac enzymes. A hematocrit can identify polycythemia, which can affect blood flow by increasing viscosity. A platelet count can identify thrombocytosis or thrombocytopenia that may precipitate thrombosis or hemorrhage. Coagulation studies are especially helpful in patients with hemorrhagic stroke to rule out coagulopathy or excessive anticoagulation with warfarin. A toxicologic screen to rule out cocaine or amphetamine use should be obtained in patients with either ischemic or hemorrhagic stroke in which substance abuse is suspected, particularly young adults with stroke. Although of minimal use in the emergency department, determination of cardiac enzymes will assist inpatient evaluation for a possible myocardial infarction.

Other diagnostic tests that may be of assistance, depending on the circumstances, include an echocardiogram, carotid duplex scanning, angiogram, and magnetic resonance imaging (MRI) or magnetic resonance imaging angiography (MRA). An echocardiogram can identify a mural thrombus, tumor, or valvular vegetation in patients with a suspected cardioembolic stroke. Carotid duplex scanning may be helpful in patients with worsening neurologic deficit or crescendo TIAs with known or suspected high-grade carotid stenosis. Such patients may be candidates for emergent carotid endarterectomy or heparinization. Carotid duplex scanning can accurately identify carotid stenosis of greater than 60 percent, but an angiogram is required to distinguish 95 percent stenosis from complete occlusion.

Angiography is the definitive test to demonstrate stenosis or occlusion of both large and small blood vessels of the head and neck. It can detect subtle arterial abnormalities, such as dissection, which may be missed with other imaging techniques. Angiography is the "gold standard" for demonstrating the cause of SAH and for defining the anatomic relationships of aneurysms. Cost, availability, and invasiveness have limited its use.

MRI currently has a marginal role in the emergency department evaluation of stroke. MRI will visualize ischemic infarcts earlier than CT and is more effective than CT at identifying acute posterior circulation strokes. However, it is less accurate at differentiating ischemia from hemorrhage. Emergent MRI should be considered when a dural sinus thrombosis is suspected or confirmation of a brainstem lesion is required. MRA enables demonstration of large vessel occlusions at the base of the skull, but small intracranial vascular occlusion may not be readily apparent. Improvement in MRA speed and resolution may allow greater use of this technology, and MRAs may replace the need for angiograms in the future.

SPECIFIC ISSUES THAT IMPACT EVALUATION AND TREATMENT

Sickle Cell Disease

Stroke occurs by age 20 in over 10 percent of patients with sickle cell anemia and is the most common cause of ischemic stroke in children. The risk is inversely proportional to age, with the highest incidence noted between ages 2 and 5. Symptoms are similar to those in patients without sickle cell disease and range from brief TIAs to hemiparesis, depending on the vascular territory involved and duration of ischemia. Cerebral aneurysms also occur with increased frequency in patients with sickle cell anemia, and careful evaluation for SAH is mandated for patients presenting with headache and neurologic findings.

Emergent management of stroke in patients with sickle cell anemia includes supportive care with oxygen, intravenous fluids, and immediate CT scanning to evaluate for ruptured cerebral aneurysm or ICH. Initial laboratory studies should include CBC, reticulocyte count, and type and crossmatch for transfusion. Lumbar puncture is indicated in patients with suspected SAH and a nondiagnostic CT. If SAH is established, it is recommended delaying arteriography until hemoglobin-S levels are below 30 percent of the total hemoglobin concentration and generous hydration is established. This may avoid increased sickling as a result of vasospasm from hyperosmolar contrast media.

In sickle cell patients with ischemic stroke, emergent simple or exchange transfusion should begin as soon as blood is available to reduce hemoglobin S to less than 30 percent. This is targeted toward improving blood flow and oxygen delivery to the infarct zone. The same therapy is indicated in hemorrhagic stroke in order to reduce vasospasm and secondary ischemic infarction. Regular transfusion therapy reduces the rate of first-ever stroke in children with abnormal transcranial Doppler results and is recommended for patients following ischemic stroke, so as to reduce the risk of recurrence. The efficacy of the use of aspirin or warfarin sodium therapy following ischemic stroke in this population has not been established. Early consultation with a patient's hematologist and the neurology department are in order, and admission to an intensive care unit (ICU) setting is indicated for close neurologic monitoring for increased intracranial pressure. Patients with TIA should also undergo exchange transfusion to the above hemoglobin-S levels.[4]

Young Adults with Stroke

Particular care should be exercised when evaluating the young adult (ages 15 to 50) with acute stroke. In this group, arterial dissection accounts for 20 percent of all ischemic strokes and may often be preceded by only minor trauma. The young adult with a cardioembolic event may have mitral valve prolapse, rheumatic heart disease, or paradoxical embolism as the originating cause. Migrainous stroke in this age group is a potential, with a female predominance. Air embolism should be considered in patients with a history of recent scuba diving or an invasive medical procedure. Such patients should be placed in a left lateral decubitus position and also placed on 100% oxygen. Emergent recompression in a hyperbaric chamber should be arranged. Finally, this population is at risk for ischemic stroke from substance abuse, with heroin, cocaine, and amphetamines often implicated. Any drug with sympathomimetic effects increases the risk of hemorrhagic stroke.

Pregnancy

While early pregnancy itself has not been associated with an increased risk of stroke, the peripartum and postpartum periods (up to 6 weeks after birth) have been identified as having an increased incidence of both ischemic and hemorrhagic stroke. Potential contributors to this increased risk include the presence of preeclampsia/eclampsia and the decrease in blood volume and alterations in hormonal status following birth.[5] Treatment should be targeted toward the underlying etiology.

The Elderly

The fastest growing population in the United States are those aged 85 and over. The Census Bureau estimates a doubling in the size of this group from its current 3.6 million by the year 2025 and a fivefold increase to 18.2 million by 2050. There is no limitation on the basis of age on the use of intravenous recombinant tissue plasminogen activator (rt-PA) in patients meeting treatment criteria. In elderly patients with ICH, particular consideration should be given to amyloid angiopathy as a pathologic cause due to its increased incidence in the elderly.

Medicolegal Issues

Failure to record a complete history and perform a complete physical examination, with documentation of the necessary elements of the neurologic examination, is a common shortcoming in emergency departments. The chart note "Neuro: nonfocal" is insufficient in a patient in whom a focal CNS event is being sought. Nor should the diagnostic process end with the diagnosis of "stroke." A consideration of the probable etiology is in order. If a cerebellar infarct or hemorrhage is identified, early neurosurgical evaluation is warranted. Timing of initiation of anticoagulation in ischemic stroke or TIA is without a solid scientific basis and consultation with a neurologist is recommended, particularly in a patient with a stuttering deficit.

With US Food and Drug Administration (FDA) approval of tissue plasminogen activator for the treatment of acute (0 to 3 h from symptom onset) ischemic stroke, the need for early identification of stroke in the emergency department has assumed increased importance. Delays in patient evaluation may prevent use of thrombolytic therapy when appropriate and place the physician at potential medicolegal risk.

TREATMENT

General Approach to Treatment of Ischemic Stroke

Upon entry of patients with ischemic stroke into the emergency medical service (EMS) or emergency department setting, priority should be given to airway management and oxygenation. Patients should be placed on oxygen, the head of the bed slightly elevated, and a monitor and intravenous line established. Unless there is hypotension, fluids should be administered judiciously to prevent cerebral edema. Volume depletion in patients with ischemic stroke deserves prompt treatment, because it may contribute to decreased cerebral blood flow in the ischemic region. Avoidance of dextrose-containing solutions is warranted except in those with proven hypoglycemia. Hyperglycemia has been associated with an increase in infarct volume and poor long-term outcome.[6,7] Patients with fever should have antipyretics promptly administered. Experimental studies suggest that hyperthermia increases CNS metabolic demands, whereas hypothermia has demonstrated neuroprotective effects.

The use of anticonvulsants is not recommended for seizure prophylaxis in ischemic stroke. If seizures occur, the patient should be treated acutely with benzodiazepines and then given a loading dose of phenytoin (20 mg/kg IV at 25 mg/min).

EMS protocols should be established to provide early notification to receiving hospitals of patients with new neurologic deficits. This facilitates early activation of acute stroke systems and preparations for rapid patient assessment. A proposed "out-of-hospital NIH stroke scale" uses an abbreviated three-item test (facial palsy, arm weakness, and abnormal speech) to identify stroke patients, and early evaluations have demonstrated a sensitivity of 100 percent and specificity of 88 percent in identifying stroke patients.[8]

A cautious approach to the management of elevated blood pressure is recommended in patients with acute ischemic stroke. In general, frequent monitoring of blood pressure in hypertensive stroke patients is indicated and only persistent, severe hypertension (greater than 220 mmHg systolic or more than 130 mmHg mean arterial pressure) should be considered for treatment. Pharmacologic lowering of systemic blood pressure may reduce perfusion to the penumbra, converting an area with reversible injury to an area of infarction. Recommended agents include parenteral drugs that are easily titrated and that have minimal effects on cerebral blood vessels, such as labetalol or enalapril. Sublingual use of calcium-channel antagonists should be avoided.[9] Numerous clinical case series have reported neurologic deterioration immediately following iatrogenic reduction of blood pressure. In contrast, elevating blood pressure by means of vasopressors may be indicated in patients with ischemic stroke and relative hypotension.

In hypertensive patients being considered for thrombolytic stroke therapy, the use of one or two doses of nitroglycerin paste or labetalol is acceptable to reduce blood pressure below 185/115 mmHg to allow treatment. Requirements for more aggressive treatment for blood pressure reduction below 185/115 mmHg exclude the use of tissue plasminogen activator in stroke patients. Following the use of rt-PA in acute stroke, however, aggressive treatment with the aforementioned agents or, if control is inadequate, nitroprusside is warranted to maintain the blood pressure below 185/115 mmHg. Hypertension is a significant cofactor in the risk of ICH in patients treated with thrombolytics.[10]

Thrombolysis in Acute Ischemic Stroke

BACKGROUND Significant progress has been achieved in the last 10 years toward identifying potential therapies for ischemic stroke. The most important single step, however, has been the 1995 publication of the results of the NIH National Institute of Neurologic Disorders and Stroke (NINDS) trial evaluating the use of intravenous recombinant rt-PA. This trial demonstrated, for the first time, that stroke was a treatable disease in carefully selected patients who received rt-PA within 3 h of symptom onset. The time-critical nature of thrombolytic therapy highlights the need for the involvement of emergency medicine in a coordinated, multidisciplinary approach to the treatment of stroke patients.

The NIH/NINDS study was a randomized, double-blind, placebo-controlled trial conducted at 40 geographically diverse hospitals (30 community and 10 university settings) comparing intravenous rt-PA (0.9 mg/kg; maximum dose, 90 mg) against placebo in 624 patients meeting specific enrollment criteria. Neurologists in private practice treated many patients in the trial, and some were evaluated and treated by emergency physicians. At 3 months, patients treated with rt-PA were at least 30 percent more likely to have minimal or no disability as measured by four different neurologic outcome scales, with an absolute increase in favorable outcome of 11 to 13 percent. The odds ratio for a favorable outcome with rt-PA was 1.7 (95 percent CI, 1.2–2.6). Benefit was found regardless of ischemic stroke subtype and has been demonstrated to continue for up to 1 year following therapy. Symptomatic ICH attributable to drug occurred in 6.4 percent of treated patients compared with 0.6 percent in the placebo group. Despite this, the mortality rate at 3 months was not significantly different between treatment and placebo groups (17 percent, rt-PA patients; 21 percent, placebo; $p = 0.3$), and the percentage of patients left severely disabled was lower in those receiving rt-PA.[11]

Four other trials of intravenous thrombolysis have been published, and their conflicting results have generated reasoned debated within the medical community over the role of thrombolysis in stroke. One of these, the European Cooperative Acute Stroke Study (ECASS), also evaluated the use of rt-PA, though at a higher dosage (1.1 mg/kg; maximum dose, 100 mg) and longer time window (0 to 6 h). Though this was a negative study in that it failed to demonstrate a difference in its primary end points between treatment and placebo groups, it must be considered that 109 of the 620 enrolled patients had major protocol violations. After excluding protocol violators, neurologic recovery at 3 months was significantly better for patients treated with rt-PA.[12] The three trials of intravenous streptokinase in ischemic stroke were all halted prematurely for safety considerations. Potential explanations of the increased risk include the use of streptokinase itself, the high dosage used (1.5 million units), the allowance of concurrent heparin and aspirin use, and the time to treatment (the majority of patients were treated within 3 to 6 h).[13–15]

The use of intraarterial delivery of thrombolytics remains investigational. Advantages include specific evaluation of the occluded vascular territory, use of lower total doses of thrombolytic drugs, and the possibility of mechanical clot disruption. Early studies evaluating pro-urokinase given within 6 h of symptom onset found superior recanalization compared with placebo but with high rates of hemorrhagic complications.[16] Intraarterial thrombolysis may have a role in the treatment of patients with acute brainstem infarcts, as this tissue may tolerate longer periods of ischemia, compared with the cerebral cortex.

The US FDA approved the use of intravenous rt-PA in acute ischemic stroke in 1996 and approval was granted in Canada in 1999. The American Heart Association (grade A recommendation)[17] and the American Academy of Neurology[18] support its use under specified conditions. The American College of Emergency Physicians was invited to coendorse the aforementioned policies but issued a lower level of acceptance "Agree with Reservations."[19]

TABLE 220-4 Criteria for Intravenous Thrombolysis in Ischemic Stroke[14]

Inclusion	Exclusion*
1. Age 18 or over	1. Minor stroke symptoms
2. Clinical diagnosis of ischemic stroke	2. Rapidly improving neurologic signs
3. Time since onset well established to be less than 3 h	3. Prior intracranial hemorrhage
	4. Blood glucose <50 or >400 mg/dL
	5. Seizure at onset of stroke
	6. Gastrointestinal or genitourinary bleeding within preceding 21 days
	7. Recent myocardial infarction
	8. Major surgery within preceding 14 days
	9. Pretreatment systolic blood pressure > 185 mmHg or diastolic blood pressure > 110 mmHg
	10. Previous stroke within preceding 90 days
	11. Previous head injury within preceding 90 days
	12. Current use of oral anticoagulants or prothrombin time > 15 s or international normalized ratio > 1.7
	13. Use of heparin within preceding 48 h and a prolonged partial thromboplastin time
	14. Platelet count < 100,000/mm^3
	15. Other: suspected aortic or vascular dissection as a cause of stroke; acute lumbar puncture
	16. Proliferative diabetic retinopathy

*Caution is advised before giving recombinant tissue plasminogen actuator (rt-PA) to persons with severe stroke (National Institutes of Health stroke scale score > 22).

ROLE OF THE EMERGENCY DEPARTMENT Specific critical pathways similar to those used for AMI (Door, Data, Decision, Drug) should be used to speed the evaluation of patients with acute stroke. Triage personnel should be educated to identify patients with symptoms of acute stroke and instructed to immediately place such patients in a monitored bed and initiate the aforementioned general recommendations. Automatic studies include a CBC with platelet count, coagulation profile, type and screen, bedside glucose determination, and an electrocardiogram. The emergency physician should be notified of a potential acute stroke, and an acute stroke system, if in place, should be activated.

Carefully identify the time of symptom onset, as this is the most difficult historical element to establish and no recommendation exists for the use of intravenous rt-PA beyond 3 h (Table 220-4). Exclusion and inclusion criteria based on CT findings are shown in Table 229-2 in Chap. 229. Taking the patient and family chronologically through the events immediately prior to the stroke is of particular help in unclear cases. Often families can utilize the timing of television or radio programming to identify time of onset accurately. Thrombolytic use in stroke is not recommended when the time of onset cannot be ascertained reliably. Strokes recognized upon awakening should be timed from when the patient was last known to be without symptoms. A focused neurologic examination should be completed; the NIH stroke scale is a useful tool for rapid evaluation. A review of rt-PA inclusion and exclusion criteria (Table 220-4) should be completed and an emergent noncontrast head CT and neurologic consultation arranged. The use of a preprinted informed consent document (where required) and/or patient education materials may assist the family's decision-making process.

DOSING, ADMISSION, AND COMPLICATIONS The total dose of rt-PA is 0.9 mg/kg, with a maximum dose of 90 mg; 10 percent of the dose is administered as a bolus, with the remaining amount infused over 60 min. Blood pressure and neurologic checks should be assessed every 15 min for 2 h after starting the infusion. Table 220-5 outlines the emergent management of hypertension following thrombolytic administration. No aspirin or heparin is given in the initial 24 h following treatment. Patients should be admitted to an ICU setting familiar with the use of thrombolytic drugs and neurologic monitoring. Intracerebral bleeding should be suspected as the cause of any neurologic worsening until repeat CT imaging is obtained. If bleeding is suspected, a CBC with platelet count, coagulation studies, fibrinogen and type and crossmatch for 4 units (U) packed red blood cells, 4 U cryoprecipitate or fresh-frozen plasma, and 1 U single-donor platelets should be obtained. An emergent hematology and neurosurgical consultation, as necessary, is appropriate. Patients may be cared for at hospitals without in-house neurosurgical availability as long as access, or transport, to neurosurgical care can be arranged while a patient is stabilized.

Subacute Ischemic Stroke

EMBOLIC STROKE Patients with embolic stroke who have minor deficits should undergo anticoagulation. Older studies, which included patients with mechanical valves, found that 12 to 14 percent of stroke patients had recurrent emboli within 2 weeks of the initial event, some within 24 h. More recent trials found that only 1.5 percent of patients had recurrent embolism in the first 7 days,[20] suggesting immediate

TABLE 220-5 Emergent Management of Hypertension Following the Use of rt-PA in Acute Stroke*

Monitor arterial blood pressure during the first 24 h after starting treatment.

- Every 15 min for 2 h after starting the infusion, then every 30 min for 6 h, and then every 60 min for 24 h total.

If SBP is 180–230 mmHg or DBP is 105–120 mmHg for two or more readings 5–10 min apart:

- Give IV labetalol 10 mg over 1–2 min. The dose may be repeated or doubled every 10–20 min up to a total dose of 150 mg.
- Monitor blood pressure every 15 min during labetalol treatment and observe for hypotension.

If SBP is >230 mmHg or if DBP is 121–140 mmHg for two or more readings 5–10 min apart:

- Give IV labetalol 10 mg over 1–2 min. The dose may be repeated or doubled every 10–20 min up to a total dose of 150 mg.
- Monitor blood pressure every 15 min during labetalol treatment and observe for hypotension.
- If no satisfactory response, infuse sodium nitroprusside [0.5–1.0 (μg/kg)/min], continuous arterial monitor advised.

If DBP is >140 mmHg for two or more readings 5–10 min apart:

- Infuse sodium nitroprusside [0.5–1.0 (μg/kg)/min], continuous arterial monitor advised.

*From the American Heart Association, with permission.
Abbreviations: DBP, diastolic blood pressure; IV, intravenous; SBP, systolic blood pressure.[14]

administration of anticoagulants is unnecessary. The exact timing, method, and degree of anticoagulation following a stroke remain controversial, with little clear data guiding its use. Consultation and/or locally approved specific protocols on its use are recommended. Anticoagulation with heparin should be withheld for 3 to 4 days following large cardioembolic stroke, because of the increased risk of spontaneous hemorrhagic changes associated with heparin in these types of strokes. The use of low-molecular-weight heparin and heparinoids in improving outcome remains to be proven.

THROMBOTIC STROKE Treatment for stable completed thrombotic stroke is largely supportive. Anticoagulation has not proven beneficial and should not be used in patients with completed strokes. The use of aspirin (300 mg/day) significantly reduces the risk of recurrent ischemic stroke and death.[21] Large randomized stroke trials studying the efficacy of thrombolytic therapy within 3 to 6 h of symptom onset are currently under way. Consultation concerning heparinization should be considered in patients with stuttering or progressively worsening symptoms. Glycoprotein IIb/IIIa inhibitors, potent inhibitors of platelet aggregation, may have a future role in the treatment of subacute thrombotic stroke and are currently in clinical trials.

Emergency thrombectomy or endarterectomy in patients with persistent neurologic deficit due to cerebral ischemia is controversial and unproven. Some authors suggest that emergency surgery should be considered for progressive stroke in the extracranial anterior circulation where there are favorable angiographic findings such as stenosis greater than 90 percent, carotid dissection or aortic aneurysm, or intraluminal clot attached to a plaque.

VERTEBROBASILAR INFARCTION Unfortunately, no study definitively establishes the advantages or disadvantages of a specific therapy for patients with acute, well-defined, occlusive vascular disease within the posterior circulation presenting later than 3 h after onset. Published studies are either small or not randomized. Most authors suggest the use of heparin in patients with posterior circulation TIAs or progressive vertebrobasilar strokes. The use of intraarterial thrombolysis may be of benefit beyond the 3-h treatment window recommended for intravenous thrombolysis.

CEREBELLAR INFARCTION Early neurosurgical consultation is needed in the treatment of all patients with cerebellar infarction. Cerebellar swelling can lead to rapid deterioration with herniation, and consultation is required to determine the need for emergency posterior fossa decompression in these patients.

Secondary Stroke Prevention/Transient Ischemic Attacks

Although limited proven pharmacologic interventions exist to reverse an acute ischemic stroke, considerable options have been identified with regard to secondary stroke prevention in patients with a completed stroke or TIA.

Agents preventing platelet aggregation form the cornerstone of secondary prevention of stroke in those patients without atrial fibrillation or high-grade carotid stenosis as a contributing factor. The use of acetylsalicylic acid (aspirin) is associated with a stroke risk reduction of 20 to 25 percent compared with placebo. Aspirin decreases the synthesis of thromboxane A_2 by irreversibly inhibiting cyclooxygenase for the life of the platelet, causing decreased platelet aggregation. No dose-effect response has been identified between high (1000 to 1500 mg/day), medium (250 to 500 mg/day), and low (50 to 100 mg/day) doses,[22] suggesting that lower doses may be as effective and better tolerated.

Dipyridamole, another antiplatelet agent, acts via phosphodiesterase inhibition, thereby increasing cyclic AMP and inhibiting platelet function. Three small, early trials failed to establish the superiority of combination therapy of dipyridamole with aspirin over aspirin alone. A larger (6602 patients), more recent trial evaluating dipyridamole alone (200 mg bid), aspirin alone (50 mg/day), dipyridamole with aspirin, and placebo found that dipyridamole alone reduced the risk of stroke or death by 15 percent compared with placebo in patients with prior stroke or TIA. Importantly, this reduction appeared additive, such that dipyridamole combined with aspirin resulted in a 37 percent relative risk reduction compared with placebo.[23]

Ticlopidine (250 mg bid) acts via inhibition of ADP-dependent platelet activation and release and is marginally superior to aspirin in the prevention of secondary vascular events, but its use is limited by the frequency of adverse events, including diarrhea, nausea, skin rash, and neutropenia. Clopidogrel is pharmacologically related to ticlopidine and has similar efficacy, with few side effects. The use of clopidogrel (75 mg/day) in patients with atherosclerotic vascular disease resulted in a statistically significant 0.5 percent absolute reduction in the annual risk of ischemic stoke, myocardial infarction, or vascular death when compared with aspirin (325 mg/day).[24] No combination studies have been reported. The use of clopidogrel is ideal for those patients who cannot tolerate, or fail, aspirin therapy.

The effectiveness of heparin is unproven in the management of acute stroke and is not recommended as routine therapy, either acutely or long term, for patients with TIAs. Its use should be considered, though, in patients with recent TIAs who are at high risk for recurrence. These include patients with (1) known high-grade stenosis in the appropriate vascular distribution for the symptoms, (2) a cardioembolic source (except infective endocarditis), (3) TIAs of increasing frequency (crescendo TIAs), and (4) TIAs despite antiplatelet therapy. Urgent carotid endarterectomy should be considered for TIAs that resolve within the first 6 h and are associated with 70 to 99 percent stenosis of the appropriate carotid artery. Endarterectomy has been shown to reduce the risk of future strokes significantly in these patients with anterior circulation TIAs.[25] The role of endarterectomy in patients with moderate-grade stenosis is currently under investigation. The role of angioplasty and cerebral artery stenting are unclear and they should be considered within the conduct of appropriately designed clinical trials.

General Approach to Hemorrhagic Stroke

After appropriate attention to the ABCs, early management of hemorrhagic stroke should focus on regulation of blood pressure, control of brain edema, and prompt neurosurgical evaluation.

INTRACEREBRAL HEMORRHAGE To date, there are no large randomized studies evaluating the appropriate management of blood pressure in ICH. Current published recommendations are that only severe hypertension (i.e., greater than 220 mmHg systolic or more than 120 mmHg diastolic) be treated.[26] When treated, blood pressure should be lowered gradually to prehemorrhage levels by using either labetalol or nitroprusside. The exceptions to this rule are cases of ICH associated with cardiac failure or arterial dissection, in which more rapid reduction is required. If a patient is known to have chronic hypertension, the blood pressure should not be lowered to normotensive levels but rather to an approximation of the patient's usual hypertensive blood pressure.

The use of hyperventilation, mannitol, and furosemide (standard doses) is recommended in patients with evidence of increased intracranial pressure with features such as mass effect, midline shift, or herniation.

The role of acute surgical intervention remains controversial and depends on the neurologic status of the patient as well as the size and location of the hemorrhage. Surgical decompression and hematoma evacuation are strongly recommended in patients with cerebellar hematomas greater than 3 cm in diameter or those near the brainstem.

SUBARACHNOID HEMORRHAGE Rebleeding and vasospasm are the major morbid complications in SAH. Risk of rebleeding is greatest in the first 24 h. Lowering systolic blood pressure to 160 mmHg and/or maintaining a mean arterial pressure of 110 mmHg has been associated with lower risk of rebleeding and a decreased mortality rate. Current recommendations are that blood pressure should be maintained at prehemorrhage levels.

Cerebral ischemia due to vasospasm occurs from 2 days to 3 weeks after aneurysm rupture. Nimodipine, given orally 60 mg every 6 h, has been found to reduce the incidence and severity of vasospasm and should be given to all patients with SAH who are in good neurologic condition (grades I to III). Preliminary studies indicate that tirilazad mesylate may also be beneficial in patients with SAH.

Seizures and persistent vomiting can cause elevations in systemic and intracranial pressure. Phenytoin loading is recommended as prophylaxis against seizures. Nausea and vomiting should be promptly treated with antiemetics. Pain should be appropriately managed.

Usually, candidates for early angiography and surgical intervention are stable patients with good neurologic condition (Hunt and Hess grades 1 to 3). However, there is little published evidence that this regimen reduces the long-term morbidity or mortality rates. Alternative approaches for patients with appropriate aneurysms include endovascular obliteration through the use of intraluminal platinum coils or detachable balloon embolization.

ADMISSION GUIDELINES

All patients with new-onset strokes should be admitted for further evaluation, education, and early rehabilitation. Patients with anterior circulation strokes should be evaluated for surgically correctable lesions and observed for any progression in their symptoms. Patients with vertebrobasilar strokes should be admitted for observation and possible heparinization.

Patients with new-onset TIAs should be evaluated for possible cardiac sources of TIAs or high-grade stenosis in the carotid arteries. The incidence of stroke after TIA in high-risk patients may be as high as 20 to 25 percent in the first year, with the greatest incidence in the first month. Because of the proven efficacy of carotid endarterectomy, patients should be admitted unless high-grade stenosis of the carotid artery can be ruled out in the emergency department. Patients without high-grade stenosis may be safely discharged on antiplatelet therapy with close follow-up.

Patients with a prior history of an anterior circulation stroke who have been previously studied, who present with a minor, completed (less than 24 h old), recurrent stroke or TIA, and who have a reliable support system may be discharged home after an appropriate emergency department workup. The use of aspirin, ticlopidine, or clopidogrel should be discussed with the family physician or neurologist, and follow-up within 48 h should be arranged. The patient and family members should be given clear instructions to return for further medical treatment if the patient experiences worsening of symptoms.

ACKNOWLEDGMENT

The authors thank Dr. Rashmi U. Kothari for his previous contributions to this chapter in the 4th edition of this book, *Emergency Medicine: A Comprehensive Study Guide.*

REFERENCES

1. American Heart Association: *1998 Heart and Stroke Facts Statistical Update.* Dallas, American Heart Association, 1997.
2. Brott T, Adams HP, Olinger CP, et al: Measurements of acute cerebral infarction: A clinical examination scale. *Stroke* 20:864, 1989.
3. Brott T, Broderick JP: Intracerebral hemorrhage. *Heart Dis Stroke* 2:59, 1993.
4. Reid CD, Charache S, Lubov B, et al (eds): *Management and Therapy of Sickle Cell Disease.* National Heart, Lung and Blood Institute; NIH Publication 96-2117, revised December 1995, 3d ed.
5. Kittner SJ, Stern BJ, Feeser BR, et al: Pregnancy and the risk of stroke. *N Engl J Med* 335:768, 1996.
6. Pulsinelli WA, Levy DA, Sigsbee B, et al: Increased damage after ischemic stroke in patients with hyperglycemia with or without established diabetes mellitus. *Am J Med* 74:540, 1983.
7. Auer RN: Insulin, blood glucose levels, and ischemic brain damage. *Neurology* 51(suppl 3):S39, 1998.
8. Kothari R, Hall K, Brott T, Broderick J: Early stroke recognition: Developing and out-of-hospital NIH stroke scale. *Acad Emerg Med* 4:986, 1997.
9. Adams HP Jr, Brott TG, Furlan AJ, et al, from the Special Writing Group of the Stroke Council, American Heart Association: *Guidelines for the Management of Patients with Acute Ischemic Stroke: American Heart Association Medical/Scientific Statement 1994.* Dallas, TX, American Heart Association, 1994.
10. Gebel JM, Sila CA, Sloan MA, et al, for the GUSTO-1 Investigators: Thrombolysis-related intracerebral hemorrhage: A radiographic analysis of 244 cases from the GUSTO-1 trial with clinical correlation. *Stroke* 29:563, 1998.
11. National Institute of Neurological Disorders and Stroke rt-PA Stroke Study Group: Tissue plasminogen activator for acute ischemic stroke. *N Engl J Med* 333:1581, 1995.
12. Hacke W, Kaste M, Fieschi C, et al, for the ECASS Study Group: Intravenous thrombolysis with recombinant tissue plasminogen activator for acute hemispheric stroke: The European Cooperative Acute Stroke Study (ECASS). *JAMA* 274:1017, 1995.
13. Multicenter Acute Stroke Trial–Europe Study Group: Thrombolytic therapy with streptokinase in acute ischemic stroke. *N Engl J Med* 335:145, 1996.
14. Multicentre Acute Stroke Trial–Italy (MAST-I) Group: Randomised controlled trial of streptokinase, aspirin, and combination of both in treatment of acute ischaemic stroke. *Lancet* 346:1509, 1995.
15. Donnan GA, Davis SM, Chambers BR, et al, for the Australian Streptokinase (ASK) Trial Study Group: Streptokinase for acute ischemic stroke with relationship to time of administration. *JAMA* 276:961, 1996.
16. del Zoppo GJ, Higashida RT, Furlan AJ, et al, and the PROACT Investigators: PROACT: A phase II randomized trial of recombinant pro-urokinase by direct arterial delivery in acute middle cerebral artery stroke. *Stroke* 29:4, 1998.
17. Adams HP Jr, Brott TG, Furlan AJ, et al, from the Special Writing Group of the Stroke Council, American Heart Association: Guidelines for thrombolytic therapy for acute stroke: A supplement to the guidelines for the management of patients with acute ischemic stroke. *Circulation* 94:1167, 1996.
18. Report of the Quality Standards Subcommittee of the American Academy of Neurology: Practice advisory: Thrombolytic therapy for acute ischemic stroke—Summary statement. *Neurology* 47:835, 1996.

19. Anonymous: ACEP "agrees with reservations" to new stroke guidelines. *ACEP News* 3:3, October 1996.
20. Publications Committee for the Trial of ORG 10172 in Acute Stroke Treatment (TOAST) Investigators: Low molecular weight heparinoid, ORG 10172 (Danapaoid), and outcome after acute ischemic stroke—A randomized controlled trial. *JAMA* 279:1265, 1998.
21. International Stroke Trial Collaborative Group: The International Stroke Trial (IST): A randomised trial of aspirin, subcutaneous heparin, both, or neither among 19,435 patients with acute ischaemic stroke. *Lancet* 349:1569, 1997.
22. Tijssen JGP: Low-dose and high-dose acetylsalicylic acid, with and without dipyridamole: A review of clinical trial results. *Neurology* 51(suppl 3):S15, 1998.
23. Diener HC, Cunha L, Forbes C, et al: European Stroke Prevention Study: 2. Dipyridamole and acetylsalicylic acid in the secondary prevention of stroke. *J Neurol Sci* 143:1, 1996.
24. CAPRIE Steering Committee: A randomised, blinded trial of clopidogrel versus aspirin in patients at risk of ischaemic events (CAPRIE). *Lancet* 348:1329, 1996.
25. Feinberg WM, Albers GW, Barnett HJM, et al, from the Ad Hoc Committee on Guidelines for the Management of Transient Ischemic Attacks of the Stroke Council of the American Heart Association: *Guidelines for the Management of Transient Ischemic Attacks. American Heart Association Medical/Scientific Statement, 1994.* Dallas, TX, American Heart Association, 1994.
26. Brott TG, Goldstein M, Grotta JC, et al: National Stroke Association Consensus Statement: Stroke: The first six hours, emergency evaluation and treatment. *Stroke Clin Updates* 4:1, 1993.

ALTERED MENTAL STATUS AND COMA

J. Stephen Huff

ALTERED MENTAL STATUS

Introduction and Definition

Consciousness has long been a perplexing subject for philosophers and physicians, and it may be argued that human consciousness is still poorly understood. However, emergency physicians need an operational definition for the disorders of consciousness that are frequently encountered in emergency departments. Dementia is a chronic state of reduced cognitive ability. The individual once was able to function but has lost intellectual skills and memory so that normal functioning has become impaired. The onset of dementia is typically difficult to pinpoint. Delirium or acute confusional state is typically of brief duration, and the degree of intellectual impairment often fluctuates rapidly. Thinking is disorganized and the ability to sustain attention is diminished. Psychosis indicates impairment of reality testing with delusions, hallucinations, disorganized behavior, or loosened associations (Table 221-1).

One useful scheme is to divide consciousness into arousal and content functions. Arousal functions include wakefulness and basic eyes-open alerting functions. Anatomically, neurons responsible for these arousal functions reside in the reticular activating system, a collection of neurons scattered through the midbrain, pons, and medulla. The neuronal structures responsible for the content of consciousness reside in the cerebral cortex. Content of consciousness includes self-awareness, language, reasoning, spatial relationship integration, emotions, and the myriad complex integration functions that we regard basic to being human.

Following this model, disorders of consciousness may be divided into processes that affect either arousal functions, content of consciousness functions, or combinations of both functions. Dementia may be thought of as failure of the content portions of consciousness with relatively preserved alerting functions. Predominant arousal system dysfunction describes delirium, although content of consciousness is affected as well. Coma represents one extreme with failure of both arousal and content functions. Psychiatric disorders and altered mental states may share features such as hallucinations or delusion; some distinctions between the different states are summarized in Table 221-1.[1]

TABLE 221-1 Features of Delirium, Dementia, and Psychiatric Psychosis

Delirium	Dementia	Psychiatric (psychoses)
	ONSET	
Sudden	Insidious	Sudden
	COURSE OVER 24 H	
Fluctuating	Stable	Stable
	CONSCIOUSNESS	
Reduced or clouded	Alert	Alert
	ATTENTION	
Disordered	Normal	May be disordered
	COGNITION	
Disordered	Impaired	May be impaired
	ORIENTATION	
Impaired	Often impaired	May be impaired
	HALLUCINATIONS	
Usually visual	Often absent	Usually auditory
	DELUSIONS	
Transient, poorly organized	Usually absent	Sustained
	MOVEMENTS	
Asterixis, tremor may be present	Often absent, if present usually unrelated	Absent

Source: Modified from Lipowski Z: Delirium in the elderly patient. *N Engl J Med* 320:578, 1989.

Mental status is the clinical state of emotional and intellectual functioning of the individual. Testing the mental status is done both formally and informally during patient evaluation. The higher mental or cognitive functions need specific tests for assessment; screening tests are described in the following section.

DELIRIUM

Introduction and Definition

Delirium, acute confusional state, acute cognitive impairment, acute encephalopathy, and other synonyms refer to a transient disorder where attention and cognition are impaired. Delirium represents a form of brain failure, but the patient is more alert than in coma. Alerting functions are working, perhaps overworking. The patient may have difficulty in focusing, shifting, or sustaining attention. The formal definition also includes disturbed wake-sleep cycles and a fluctuating waxing and waning course of confusion.

Epidemiology

The incidence of delirium in the ED population is not clear. One study showed that 5 percent of EMS transports in one system were for the sole reason of acute cognitive impairment in the elderly.[2] This would seem to underestimate the problem if fever or respiratory distress, for example, were listed as a chief reason for transport. It is estimated that 10 to 25 percent of elderly hospitalized patients have delirium at time of admission.[3]

Pathophysiology

The functions of intellect as well as arousal are disordered in the central nervous system in delirium. Pathologic mechanisms are complex and are thought to involve widespread neuronal or neurotransmitter dysfunction. Four groups encompass most patients: primary intracranial disease; systemic diseases that secondarily affected the CNS; exogenous toxins; and drug withdrawal.[1] Delirium implies the presence of an acute reversible organic cause, unlike dementia, which is usually stable or slowly progressive and only sometimes amenable to treatment. Differentiation from acute psychosis on a pathophysiologic basis may be more problematic in that the psychosis may occur related to medical conditions in addition to psychiatric or functional conditions. Clinically, psychosis is less likely to have a waxing and waning pattern, and while reality perception is impaired, consciousness is not clouded (Table 221-1).

Clinical Features

Delirium, or acute confusional state, is acute in the sense that it is present over days to weeks; by definition less than 1 month, although rapid onset may be noted. Attention and the cognitive functions of perception, thinking, and memory are all distorted to varying degrees. Alertness (but not necessarily consciousness) is reduced. The patient may appear quite awake but attention is impaired. Activity levels may be increased with agitation or decreased in a quiet delirium. Three variants are described: a hypoalert-hypoactive type, a hyperalert-hyperactive type, and a mixed type. The patient with the mixed variety may fluctuate rapidly between hypoactive and hyperactive states. Symptoms may be intermittent, and it is not unusual for different caregivers to witness completely different behaviors within a brief time span.[3] The sleep-wake cycles are often disrupted with increased somnolence during the day and agitation at night. The increased nocturnal agitation is commonly referred to as "sundowning." Tremor or asterixis may be present in some patients. Associated symptoms may be present, such as tachycardia, sweating, hypertension, or emotional outbursts.

Hallucination, delusions, and illusions may be present in up to 40 percent of cases of delirium.[1] Hallucinations tend to be visual, though auditory hallucinations may occur.

Diagnosis

Both history and physical findings are necessary to confirm the diagnosis of delirium. The history is needed to confirm the acuity of the change in behavior and reveal the fluctuating confusion consistent with the delirium. The history from caregivers, spouse, or other family members is the primary mechanism for diagnosing delirium.[3] General physical examination is directed at discovering an underlying process such as an infection. Ancillary testing should include basic chemistries, urinalysis, and blood count, and a chest radiograph. Cranial CT and CSF analysis should be considered on an individual basis. The physician must decide if an identified acute illness is sufficient to cause the delirium or if further diagnostic workup is necessary; this is often not an easy decision. In absence of a definitive explanation, CT and CSF analysis are advised but, depending on the acuity of onset, could be deferred as part of a continuing inpatient workup.

TABLE 221-2 Six Elements of Mental Status Evaluation

Appearance, behavior, and attitude
Is dress appropriate?
Is motor behavior at rest appropriate?
Is the speech pattern normal?
Disorders of thought
Are the thoughts logical and realistic?
Are false beliefs or delusions present?
Are suicidal or homicidal thoughts present?
Disorders of perception
Are hallucinations present?
Mood and affect
What is the prevailing mood?
Is the emotional content appropriate for the setting?
Insight and judgement
Does the patient understand the circumstances surrounding the visit?
Sensorium and intelligence
Is the level of consciousness normal?
Is cognition or intellectual functioning impaired?

Source: Modified from Zun L, Howes DS: The mental status evaluation: Application in the emergency department. *Am J Emerg Med* 6:165, 1988.

One key feature of examination is the mental status examination. The standard mental status evaluation may be divided into six categories: appearance, behavior, and attitude; disorders of thought; disorders of perception; mood and affect; insight and judgement; and sensorium and intelligence (Table 221-2). The "standard" mental status examination is useful particularly to determine potential for a psychiatric condition. The emergency physician is unlikely to have time to perform the same detailed evaluation as a general psychiatrist or neurologist. However, the assessment of mood, affect, dress, situational behavior, and, in particular, speech content and process are key aspects in uncovering a psychiatric condition. While the standard mental status examination may not be as useful in the ED for assessment of cognitive function as the other approaches that are discussed later, assessment of orientation and level of consciousness are still helpful as initial screens, as these are usually unimpaired in pure psychiatric conditions, except possibly when the condition is severe. Thus, impairments in cognitive function uncovered with this examination suggest the presence of delirium or other organic mental disorder, and further evaluation along these lines is warranted.

The mini-mental state examination (MMSE) (Table 221-3) has withstood the test of time[4] and is perhaps the most familiar to consultants in neurology and psychiatry should they become involved. It is, for all intents and purposes, a subset of the "standard" mental status examination (Table 221-2), with a focus on determining the level of cognitive impairment. This test is valuable in directing the physician to study aspects of attention and memory that might not otherwise be formally tested. A score of 23 or less may indicate the presence of dementia or other cognitive dysfunction and, in an acute setting, indicates the need for further evaluation.[5] Age, education, and verbal abilities may all affect scores.

Several other shorter evaluation systems have been proposed. However, the brief mental status examination (BMSE) was developed specifically for emergency settings (Table 221-4)[6] but may not yet be widely practiced and may in fact be unknown to potential consultants. It also concentrates on determining level of cognitive impairment. It is simpler and requires less time to complete than the well accepted MMSE (see Table 221-3). The score attained on the BMSE (see Table 221-4) is indicative of the level of impairment.

TABLE 221-3 The Mini-Mental State Examination

Maximum Score	Score	
		ORIENTATION
5	( )	What is the: (year) (season) (date) (day) (month)?
5	( )	Where are we: (state) (county) (town) (hospital) (floor)?
		REGISTRATION
3	( )	Name 3 objects; ask patient to repeat.
		ATTENTION AND CALCULATION
5	( )	The serial 7 test; 1 point for each correct. Stop after 5 answers. Option: spell ''world'' backwards.
		RECALL
3	( )	Ask for the 3 objects repeated above. 1 point scored for each correct object recalled.
		LANGUAGE
9	( )	Name a pencil and watch (2 points) Repeat the following, ''No ifs, ands, or buts.'' (1 point) Follow 3-stage command: ''Take a paper in your right hand, fold it in half, and put it on the floor.'' (3 points) Read and follow the following printed command: ''Close your eyes'' (1 point) Write a sentence (1 point) Copy design (1 point)

SCORING: A score of 23 or less may indicate the presence of dementia or another cognitive disorder and suggests the need for further testing and evaluation.

Instructions for administering the Mini-Mental State Examination

Orientation: Ask for the date. Specifically ask for any omitted information. One point for each correct answer.

Registration: Ask permission to test memory. Name 3 unrelated objects clearly and slowly about 1 s apart. After you have said all 3, ask the patient to repeat. The first repetition determines the score. In order to test recall (discussed below) the examiner should repeat the items in order up to 6 times, until the patient can repeat all 3. If the patient is unable to do this, recall can't be tested.

Attention and calculation: Ask the patient to begin with 100 and count backward by 7. Stop after 5 subtractions and score correct answers. If the patient cannot calculate, ask him or her to spell ''world'' backwards. The score is the number of letters in correct order.

Recall: Ask the patient if he or she can recall the 3 words previously asked to remember. Score 0–3.

Language: Naming: Show the patient a wristwatch and pencil and ask name. Score 0–2.
Repetition: Ask the patient to repeat a sentence. Allow one trial. Score 0 or 1.
3-stage command: Give the patient a piece of paper and repeat the command. Score 1 point for each portion of the command correctly performed.
Reading: Print clearly on a piece of paper in large letters the command, ''Close your eyes.'' Ask the patient to read and perform the command. Score 1 point if the eyes are closed.
Writing: Give the patient a blank piece of paper and ask him or her to write a sentence of his or her own choosing. It must contain a subject and a verb to be scored 1 point. Punctuation does not matter for scoring purposes.
Copying: On a clean piece of paper, draw intersecting pentagons, each side 1 in, and ask the patient to copy exactly. All 10 angles must be present and the 2 figures must intersect to score 1 point. Any rotation of the figures or tremor is ignored.

Source: Modified from Folstein MF, Folstein SE: ''Mini-mental state'': A practical method for grading the cognitive state of patients for the clinician. *J Psychiatr Res* 12:189, 1975.

Independent of these tests, the acute onset of attention deficits and cognitive abnormalities with fluctuating severity through the day and worsening at night is practically diagnostic of delirium.[7]

Specific Issues

The diagnosis of delirium prompts the search for an underlying disease process. The point that must be remembered is that delirium is secondary to another process that might or might not be related to the central nervous system. Making the diagnostic task more difficult is that chronic cognitive impairment may also be present in the individual patient, therefore making the assessment of the acuity of the mental status change difficult. The main features differentiating delirium from dementia and psychiatric conditions are the relative acute onset of the process (not a feature of dementia) and its fluctuating nature (not a feature of either dementia or psychosis).

Depression can resemble a hypoactive delirium with withdrawal, slowed speech, and poor results in cognitive testing being present in both conditions. Rapid fluctuation of the symptoms, however, is common in delirium but absent in depression. Additionally, clouding of consciousness is absent in patients with depression; usually testing finds them oriented and able to perform commands.[3] Table 221-5 lists common etiologies of altered sensorium (although not all cause delirium).

Treatment

Treatment is directed at the underlying cause of the delirium. The patient must be protected while diagnostic workup is in progress. Delirium in the elderly is associated with a mortality rate of roughly 20 to 30 percent related to the underlying medical condition.

TABLE 221-4 The Brief Mental Status Examination

ITEM	SCORE (number of errors)	×	(weight)	=	(Total)
What year is it now?	0 or 1	×	4	=	________
What month is it?	0 or 1	×	3	=	________
Present memory phrase: ''Repeat this phrase after me and remember it: *John Brown, 42 Market Street, New York.*''					
About what time is it? (Answer correct if within 1 h.)	0 or 1	×	3	=	________
Count backward from 20 to 1.	0, 1, or 2	×	2	=	________
Say the months in reverse.	0, 1, or 2	×	2	=	________
Repeat memory phrase (each underlined portion is worth 1 point).	0, 1, 2, 3, 4, or 5	×	2	=	________
FINAL SCORE IS THE SUM OF THE TOTALS					

The score represents the sum of the weighted errors. The lowest possible score with no errors is 0. The highest possible score is 28. For this screening examination, scores of 0 to 8 are normal, 9 to 19 implies mild impairment, and 20 to 28 implies severe impairment.
Source: After Kaufman DM, Zun L: A quantifiable, brief mental status examination for emergency patients. *J Emerg Med* 13:449, 1995.

Medication history, including over-the-counter medications, should be examined in detail. In the elderly, medication side effects or toxicity may be observed in what are ordinarily regarded as therapeutic and safe doses.

Recognition, identification, and stabilization are the issues. The identification of a relatively common etiology does not necessarily exclude the possibility of a CNS infection (see Table 221-5). Hypoxia may also be present. Again, in the face of what appears to be adequate cause for the delirium, the physician must decide if further investigation is needed.

TABLE 221-5 Common Medical Causes of Altered Mental Status

Infection*	Meningitis/encephalitis Sepsis Urinary tract infection Pneumonia
Toxic	Drug toxicity (including alcohol) Drug withdrawal (e.g., alcohol) Environmental exposure (e.g., carbon monoxide)
Metabolic	Electrolyte disturbance (e.g., hyper/hyponatremia, hypercalcemia) Endocrine disorders (e.g., hyper/hypo: -glycemia, -adrenal, -thyroid) Hepatic encephalopathy Uremia Environmental exposure (e.g., hypothermia)
Hypoxemia/hypercarbia	e.g., CHF, PE, COPD
Cerebrovascular	Trauma-related (e.g., subdural hematoma) CVA (bland, hemorrhagic) CNS vasculitis Hypertensive encephalopathy
CNS (other)	Trauma (diffuse injury with increased ICP) Space occupying lesions Seizure and postictal states
Psychiatric†	Functional psychosis Severe depression

*Seemingly minor infections (urinary tract, pneumonia) may alter sensorium in the elderly.
†Other etiologies should be considered before a psychiatric etiology becomes the working diagnosis.

Environmental manipulations such as adequate lighting and psychosocial support may be helpful in enhancing the patient's ability to interpret the surroundings correctly.[3] Sedation may be needed to relieve severe agitation. Haloperidol at an initial dose of 1 to 5 mg may be given orally or parenterally. This may be repeated at 20- to 30-min intervals as the clinical situation indicates. It should be avoided if the underlying cause is seizure promoting or potentiates hypotension. Benzodiazepines such as lorazepam may be used in combination with haloperidol in doses of 1 to 2 mg, the dose varying widely because of the age and size of the patient and the degree of agitation. Any institutional confinement or restraint policies should be appropriately addressed. Sedation or restraint is no substitute for diagnostic activities and specific illness-targeted therapy.

Disposition

Unless a readily reversible cause for the acute mental status change is discovered, treatment initiated, and improvement and stability evident, the majority of patients will be hospitalized for further treatment and possibly additional diagnostic testing. This decision is individualized to the patient, the resources in the home or health care facility, and the individual risk profile of the patient.

DEMENTIA

Introduction and Definition

Dementia implies a loss of mental capacity; the individual who once functioned at a certain psychosocial level with certain cognitive abilities is now failing or behavioral problems have developed. The majority of dementias are idiopathic and are termed Alzheimer's disease (AD). The other large category is vascular dementia. However, many other disorders more treatable than Alzheimer's disease or vascular dementia may also cause dementia or simulate dementia. The largely untreatable dementias are thus to a degree diagnoses of exclusion; the physician must take care that a treatable dementia is not being overlooked (Tables 221-6 and 221-7).

TABLE 221-6 Classification of Dementia by Cause

Degenerative
Alzheimer's disease
Huntington's disease
Parkinson's disease, others
Vascular
Multiple infarcts
Hypoperfusion (cardiac arrest, profound hypotension, others)
Subdural hematoma
Subarachnoid hemorrhage
Infectious
Meningitis (sequelae of bacterial meningitis, fungal, TB)
Neurosyphilis
Viral encephalitis (herpes, HIV), Creutzfeldt-Jakob disease
Inflammatory
Lupus
Demyelinating disease, others
Neoplastic
Primary tumors and metastatic disease
Carcinomatous meningitis
Paraneoplastic syndromes
Traumatic
Traumatic brain injury
Subdural hematoma
Toxic
Alcohol (chronic effect)
Medications (anticholinergics, polypharmacy)
Metabolic
B_{12} or folate deficiency
Thyroid disease
Uremia, others
Psychiatric
Depression
Hydrocephalus
Normal pressure hydrocephalus (communicating hydrocephalus)
Noncommunicating hydrocephalus

Source: Modified from Fleming KC, Adams AC, Petersen RC: Dementia: Diagnosis and evaluation. *Mayo Clin Proc* 70:1093, 1995.

TABLE 221-7 Mnemonic for Potentially Treatable/Reversible Causes of Dementia

D	Drugs (anticholinergic, narcotic, sedatives, phenothiazines, others)
E	Electrolytes, eye or ear problems (partial blindness or deafness)
M	Metabolic disturbances (thyroid disease, hepatic failure, others)
E	Emotional (depression, schizophrenia)
N	Nutritional (B_{12}, folate deficiency, Wernicke-Korsakoff), Normal pressure hydrocephalus
T	Trauma, tumor (includes subdural hematoma)
I	Inflammation (SLE, others) Infections (chronic meningitis, syphilis, Lyme, HIV)
A	Alcohol*

*Chronic effects of alcohol are not easily reversible; however, with abstinence and proper nutrition, even severely affected (ex-) alcoholics may show improvement.
Source: Modified from Tueth MJ: Dementia: Diagnosis and emergency behavioral complications. *J Emerg Med* 13:519, 1995.

The typical course of dementia is slow with insidious symptom onset; the abrupt onset of symptoms or rapidly progressing symptoms should prompt a search for another process simulating a dementia or a comorbid problem. The physician must look for compounding factors that may be exacerbating symptoms. Some sentinel occurrence or event usually precipitates presentation to the ED. Attention should be directed to discovering any comorbid process as well as discovering any treatable causes of dementia or dementia imitators.

Epidemiology

Dementia is found in all populations and is largely a disorder of the elderly. It is estimated that 1 percent of the U.S. population suffers from dementia at age 60, but by age 85, 50 percent may be affected.[8] Estimates are similar in other industrialized countries. Vascular disease may be the most common cause of dementia in Japan and Scandinavia. The frequency of the types of dementia is to some degree dependent on the age of the population.[9]

Pathophysiology

The majority of cases of dementia in the United States are due to Alzheimer's disease, with estimates up to 70 percent. Alzheimer's is a neurodegenerative disorder of unknown etiology. Pathophysiology of Alzheimer's disease is complex, with a reduction of neurons in the cerebral cortex as well as increased amyloid deposition into plaques and the production of neurofibrillary tangles. Other neurodegenerative diseases have their own unique pathology.

Vascular dementia accounts for the next largest number of individuals with dementia, with estimates of 10 to 20 percent. The pathology is that of cerebrovascular disease with multiple infarctions.

Clinical Features

Impairment of memory, particularly recent memory, is gradual and progressive. Remote memories are often preserved. Impairment of memory and orientation with preservation of motor and speech abilities is said to be characteristic of the onset of Alzheimer's disease.[10] Degenerative dementias, such as Alzheimer's disease, may be divided into early, middle, and late stages.[11] Early in the disease, complaints of memory loss, naming problems, or forgetting items are common. The middle stage shows progression of these problems plus loss of reading, decreased performance in social situations, and losing directions. Late stage of the illness may include extreme disorientation, inability to dress and perform self-care, and personality change. Typically, the onset of symptoms is slow and gradual; if the onset of symptoms is acute the possibility of a reversible process (Table 221-7) is increased. Clinical features of Alzheimer's disease or other dementias may include affective symptoms such as depression and anxiety, behavioral disorders, and speech difficulties.

Vascular or multi-infarct dementia has symptoms similar to AD but may have findings on physical examination of exaggerated or asymmetric deep tendon reflexes, gait abnormalities, or weakness of an extremity.[11]

Diagnosis

The history of memory problems is usually one of slow progression without landmark occurrences. If specific dates of worsening are noted, the possibility of a vascular dementia increases. Family history may be significant. One inherited dementia, Huntington's disease, has a clear autosomal dominant pattern of inheritance.

General physical examination does not determine the diagnosis of dementia as findings are largely nonspecific or normal.[9,12] The presence of focal neurologic signs may suggest vascular dementia or a mass lesion. Increased motor tone and other extrapyramidal signs such as rigidity or a movement disorder may suggest Parkinson's disease. Mental status testing should be performed as outlined previously (Tables 221-2, 221-3, and 221-4).

Controversy exists about diagnostic testing in patients with typical features of Alzheimer's type dementia. Again, about 10 to 20 percent of patients may have a treatable form of dementia (see Table 221-7). The American Academy of Neurology has published a practice parameter that recommends complete blood count; serum electrolytes; calcium, glucose, BUN, creatinine, and liver function tests; thyroid function tests; serum B_{12}; and serology for syphilis. Other laboratory tests that are optional, but that may be helpful in certain circumstances, include sedimentation rate, serum folate level, HIV testing, chest x-ray, and urinalysis.[9] Neuroimaging such as CT or MR should be considered in every patient. CSF analysis is not recommended in every case but should be performed if clinical suspicion of a condition with an inflammatory CSF exists. Local practice patterns and the patient's social support will influence whether tests are done as inpatient or in the ED or other outpatient setting.

Diagnosis of probable vascular dementia not only requires cognitive dysfunction but also signs of cerebrovascular disease upon neurologic examination. The relationship between stroke and cognitive decline must be temporally related with dementia within 3 months of the stroke or abrupt deterioration of memory and other cognitive abilities. A fluctuating stepped course suggests vascular dementia.[13]

Specific Issues

The possibility of a comorbid condition suddenly worsening cognitive functioning should be strongly considered and often is the thrust of investigation in the ED. Urinary tract infection, congestive heart failure, or hypothyroidism are just a few of the conditions that may cause a mildly demented but functioning individual to rapidly deteriorate. The condition blurs with that of delirium as discussed above. The differential diagnosis is important particularly for consideration of depression imitators, the so-called treatable causes of dementia (Table 221-7).

Depression may coexist with dementia; however, depression-imitating dementia (pseudodementia) should be considered. Appropriate inpatient or outpatient follow-up may be arranged for further psychiatric evaluation. If the patient is thought to be seriously depressed, consideration should be given to admission.

Treatment

All types of dementia are treatable at least to some degree by environmental or psychosocial interventions. Treatments for Alzheimer's disease are an intense area of research. Recently, tacrine, a cholinesterase inhibitor, was shown to improve cognitive function in patients with Alzheimer's disease. Tacrine has been approved by the FDA for AD treatment. It does not slow progression of the disease. This therapy is best initiated and monitored by caregivers that will follow the patient through the course of the disease. Other treatments are under active investigation with goals of reducing oxidative stress and inflammation, modifying protein processing, and prolonging neuronal life.[14]

The behavioral symptoms of patients with Alzheimer's may be disruptive to the home environment and distressing to the patient and caregivers. Hallucinations, delusions, repetitive behaviors, and depression are all common. Patients may misidentify other people and family members may be regarded as strangers, sometimes with apparent great fear. Antipsychotic drugs have been used for management of the psychotic and nonpsychotic behaviors, but treatment remains problematic because of adverse drug effects. Use of these drugs should be selective and reserved for patients with persistent psychotic features or those with extreme disruptive or dangerous behaviors.[15] Again, treatment is best coordinated with caregivers that are in a position to monitor the patient's behavior patterns over time.

Treatment of vascular dementia is limited to treatment of risk factors including hypertension.

If a treatable form of dementia is suspected or discovered during evaluation, efforts should be directed toward that underlying cause. Even so, treatments must be individualized. For example, the discovery of chronic subdural hematomas and subsequent evacuation may lead to improvement of a dementia for one patient, but at times an underlying dementia will remain unchanged for another.

The diagnosis of normal pressure hydrocephalus (NPH) is problematic. Excessively large ventricles discovered on CT may prompt consideration of a trial of ventricular shunting. The clinical suspicion of NPH should be increased with the presence of urinary incontinence and gait disturbance at a relatively early point in the disease.[16] Improvement in some individuals may be striking, but controversies remain on patient selection and the duration of improvement.[16,17]

Disposition

A new diagnosis of dementia may be entertained in the emergency department but the decision-making and depth of the workup usually exceeds the time available during the ED stay. A decision to admit or arrange an outpatient diagnostic plan is the usual course in the ED after the differential diagnosis has been considered. Attention should be directed to the possible presence of delirium or a treatable cause of dementia. After investigations have largely excluded any comorbid process acutely worsening symptoms, the patient who is functioning at baseline may be discharged to a safe home environment if caretakers are available. The existence of comorbid medical problems, a rapidly progressive or atypical clinical course, or an unsafe or uncertain home situation should prompt consideration for admission.

COMA

Introduction and Definition

Coma is difficult to define because brain failure exists along a spectrum of unresponsiveness. Both the alerting and the content portions of consciousness are impaired in coma. The definition of an eyes-closed state with inappropriate responses to environmental stimuli is still a useful one. A variety of terms are used to describe patients with lowered levels of consciousness; delirium is discussed in some detail above. Stupor, obtundation, and lethargy are so inexactly used that they have little meaning. A description of the patient's responses to stimuli at one moment in time is still the best assessment of level of consciousness. Though originally designed for statistical analysis of head-injured patients, the Glasgow coma scale is widely used in many clinical situations. Its advantages include a simple scoring system and assessment of separate verbal, motor, and eye-opening functions. Its disadvantages include lack of assessment of hemiparesis or other focal motor signs and lack of testing of higher cognitive functions.

Epidemiology

The epidemiology of coma in emergency departments has been little studied. Current estimate is that acute unresponsiveness is present in 0.5 to 1 percent of ED admissions, but that may vary depending on referral patterns, trauma volume, and toxicology volume of different institutions. The only paper addressing frequency of coma in the ED dates from 1934 and is of historic interest because it predates modern

TABLE 221-8 Differential Diagnosis of Coma

COMA FROM CAUSES AFFECTING THE BRAIN DIFFUSELY
Encephalopathies
Hypoxic
Metabolic
Hypoglycemia
Diabetic ketoacidosis
Hyperosmolar state
Other electrolyte abnormalities
Organ system failure
Hepatic encephalopathy
Uremia/renal failure
Endocrine
Hypertensive encephalopathy
Toxins and drug reactions
CNS sedatives
Alcohol
Carbon monoxide, other inhalants
Neuroleptic malignant syndrome
Environmental causes—hypothermia, hyperthermia
Deficiency state: Wernicke's encephalopathy
COMA FROM PRIMARY CNS DISEASE OR TRAUMA
Direct CNS trauma
Vascular disease
Intraparenchymal hemorrhage
Hemispheric
Basal ganglia
Brainstem
Cerebellar
Infarction
Hemispheric
Brainstem
Subarachnoid hemorrhage
CNS infections
Neoplasms
Seizures
Nonconvulsive status epilepticus
Postictal state

EMS and advanced life support procedures. In that 1934 study, 3 percent of the patients presented to the hospital in coma.[18] Some of the common causes of coma then as now were alcohol intoxication, trauma, cerebrovascular disease, poisoning, meningitis, and cardiopulmonary failure (Table 221-8). One striking difference was the lack of hypoglycemia; insulin therapy was not in widespread use at that time.

Pathophysiology

The pathophysiology of coma is complex, but simplification is possible. As with delirium, deficiency of substrates needed for neuronal function may occur as with hypoglycemia or hypoxia secondary to many different causes. Coma may occur from processes primary to the CNS or from systemic causes (Table 221-8). With systemic causes, the brain is usually globally affected and signs that localize dysfunction to a specific area of the brainstem or cortex are usually lacking. In primary CNS causes, the coma may result from brainstem disease such as hemorrhage, herniation, vertebrobasilar artery thrombosis, or from bilateral cortical dysfunction. Signs localizing to specific areas of CNS dysfunction, such as hemiparesis or cranial nerve abnormalities, may be concomitantly present. A useful concept is that unilateral hemispheric disease, such as stroke, should not by itself result in coma. The function of either the brainstem and/or both hemispheres must be impaired for unresponsiveness.

A traditional view of reduced consciousness from mass lesions involves secondary compression of the brainstem by physical shifting of brain tissue.[19] In the uncal herniation syndrome, the most common of the herniation syndromes, the medial temporal lobe shifts to compress the upper brainstem, resulting in progressive drowsiness and then unresponsiveness. Usually, the pupillary light reaction on the same side of the mass is sluggish and the pupil may enlarge, eventually becoming widely dilated and nonreactive. The anatomic correlate of these events is suspected compression of the ipsilateral third cranial nerve by the medial temporal lobe herniating over the tentorium. In this scenario, the pupil ipsilateral to the mass first enlarges, then other signs of third nerve dysfunction progress with loss of extraocular movements. Hemiparesis may develop contralateral to the mass from compression of the descending motor tracts in the ipsilateral cerebral peduncle, reflecting dysfunction of the descending motor tracts prior to their decussation in the medulla. The above is the usual presentation of temporal lobe or uncal herniation; that is, ipsilateral third nerve palsy with contralateral hemiparesis. Less commonly, so-called falsely localizing signs are present with third nerve dysfunction contralateral, or hemiparesis ipsilateral, to the herniating temporal lobe. This is referred to as Kernohan's phenomenon and is thought to reflect compression of third nerve and midbrain structures against the tentorium contralateral to the mass. A central herniation syndrome is also described. These models spring from postmortem examination of brains from patients with expanding mass lesions.

The herniation syndromes serve as models, but their exact mechanism has been questioned. The fact that herniation syndromes may be reversed by interventions is evidence against simple physical displacement of the tissues and physical distortion of the brainstem. Additionally, the amount of midline shift of structures as evaluated by neuroimaging seemingly correlates with the level of consciousness without invoking physical herniation. In the patient with an acute lesion, the patient may be awake with up to 3 to 4 mm of pineal shift, with unresponsiveness deepening as the pineal shift increases to 10 mm.[20] The perimesencephalic cisterns are invariably diminished in patients with pineal shift of about 9 mm.[20] The shift is in true dimensions as adjusted from the CT scan, which typically displays a miniaturized image. Less correlation of midline shift and consciousness has been noted with more anterior structures such as the septum.

Ischemia from compression of vessels is undoubtedly a factor in cerebral edema and effects of increased intracranial pressure. Increased intracranial pressure (ICP) may occur within regions of the brain, perhaps initiating a herniation syndrome or midline shift as described above. Increased ICP may also occur diffusely resulting in widely distributed CNS dysfunction. Cerebral blood flow (CBF) is usually constant between mean arterial blood pressures (MAP) of approximately 50 to 100 mmHg through the process of cerebral autoregulation. At MAP outside this range, CBF is reduced and ischemia may develop. Cerebral perfusion pressure (CPP) is equal to the MAP minus the intracranial pressure (CPP = MAP − ICP). It follows that in extreme uncontrolled elevation of the ICP, cerebral perfusion pressure is inadequate or lost as ICP approaches the MAP, and ischemia develops. Some authorities suggest that the upper range of MAP that allows constant CBF is about 150 mmHg, at least in the uninjured brain. There are many opinions, but little data to substantiate the exact range. (See Chap. 247 for a more detailed discussion.)

Clinical Features

The clinical features of coma vary both with the depth of coma and the etiology of coma. Coma speaks to the unresponsive state. However, there is a spectrum of signs within unresponsiveness that may point toward an etiology.

A variety of abnormal breathing patterns may be seen in the comatose patient. They are of interest but offer little information in the acute setting. Pupillary findings, the results of other cranial nerve evaluations, hemiparesis, and response to stimulation are all part of the clinical picture that needs to be assessed. These findings help the clinician sort the cause of the coma into a likely etiology—diffuse

CNS dysfunction (toxic-metabolic coma) or structural coma. A further division of structural coma into hemispheric (supratentorial) and posterior fossa (hemispheric) coma is often possible at the bedside.

Toxic and metabolic causes of coma result from a wide range of clinical conditions. In general, the diffuse nature of the CNS dysfunction is reflected by the lack of physical examination findings that might point to a specific region of dysfunction within the brain. For example, in toxic-metabolic coma, if the patient is having either spontaneous movements or reflex posturing, the movements are symmetric without evidence of hemiparesis. Reflexes are symmetric. Pupillary response is generally preserved in toxic-metabolic coma, unless the toxin specifically affects pupillary function. Typically the pupils are small but reactive in nonspecific toxic-metabolic coma. If extraocular movements are present, again they are symmetric. However, if extraocular movements are absent, it is of no value in differentiating toxic-metabolic from structural coma. A notable exception is severe sedative poisoning as with barbiturates; the pupils may be large, extraocular movements absent, muscle tone flaccid, and the patient apneic, simulating the appearance of brain death.

Coma from lesions of the hemispheres, or supratentorial masses, may present with progressive hemiparesis; asymmetric muscle tone and reflexes may also be present. A patient in coma with a hemispheric hemorrhage may still have some muscle tone; careful examination may allow detection of decreased muscle tone on the side of the hemiparesis. The hemiparesis may be suspected with asymmetric responses to stimuli or asymmetric extensor or flexor postures. Additionally, there may be ocular signs of the eyes conjugately deviated toward the side of the hemorrhage. With expansion of the hemorrhage and surrounding edema, and increase in intracranial pressure or brainstem compression, the unresponsiveness may progress to a complete loss of motor tone, as well as loss of the ocular findings. Frequently, large acute supratentorial lesions are seen without the features consistent with temporal lobe herniation. Coma without lateralizing signs may result from decreased cerebral perfusion secondary to increased intracranial pressure. Reflex changes in blood pressure and heart rate may be observed with increased ICP or brainstem compression. Hypertension and bradycardia in a comatose patient may represent the Cushing reflex from increased ICP.

Posterior fossa or infratentorial lesions comprise another coma syndrome. An expanding mass, such as cerebellar hemorrhage or infarction, may cause abrupt coma, abnormal extensor posturing, loss of pupillary reflexes, and loss of extraocular movements. The anatomy of the posterior fossa leaves little room for accommodating an expanding mass. Early brainstem compression with loss of brainstem reflexes may develop rapidly. Another infratentorial cause of coma is pontine hemorrhage, which may present with the unique signs of pinpoint-sized, seemingly unreactive pupils. If magnification is used, these pinpoint pupils may be seen to be reactive.

Vertebrobasilar occlusion by thrombosis or embolism may cause the ''locked-in'' syndrome, which may readily be confused with coma. These patients have lost voluntary movement, except perhaps for vertical eye movements. Consciousness and understanding may well be intact; the patient cannot move, speak, or interact with the environment except, again, by vertical eye movements.[21]

Pseudocoma or psychogenic coma is occasionally encountered and may present a perplexing clinical problem. Adequate history and observation of responses to stimulation will reveal findings that differ from the syndromes described above. Pupillary responses, extraocular movements, muscle tone, and reflexes will be shown to be intact on careful examination. Tests of particular value are observing the response of the patient to manual eye opening (there should be little or no resistance in the truly unresponsive patient) and extraocular movements. Specifically, if avoidance of gaze is consistently seen with the patient always looking away from the examiner, or nystagmus is demonstrated on caloric testing, this is strong evidence for nonphysiologic or feigned unresponsiveness.

Diagnosis

In the approach to the comatose patient, stabilization, diagnosis, and treatment actions overlap and are often performed simultaneously. Examination, laboratory procedures, and neuroimaging allow determination of the cause of coma in almost all patients in the ED. As with any patient, airway, breathing, and circulation issues need to be immediately addressed. Reversible causes of coma should always be considered. Hypoxia, hypoglycemia, hypo- and hypertension, and hyperthermia are readily diagnosed entities. Hypoglycemia is a frequent cause of acute coma. Rapid bedside determination of glucose may obviate the empiric administration of intravenous dextrose.

The paradox in evaluation of the comatose patient is that history often holds the key to diagnosis but the patient cannot verbally relate that history. Exploit all possible historical sources. EMS personnel frequently have valuable information about the scene including medication history or the possibility of poisoning or trauma. Caregivers, family, or witnesses may provide valuable information. Medical records may be of immense value if promptly available.

Knowing the tempo of onset of the coma is of great value. Abrupt coma suggests abrupt CNS failure with possible causes of trauma, catastrophic stroke, or seizures. Cardiac causes may also cause abrupt loss of consciousness. A slowly progressive onset of coma may suggest a progressive CNS lesion such as tumor or subdural hematoma. Metabolic causes such as hyperglycemia may also develop over several days.

The physical examination of the comatose patient presents other challenges. General examination and vital signs (including oxygen saturation and temperature) should receive special attention following stabilization and resuscitation. General examination may reveal signs of trauma or suggest other diagnostic possibilities of the unresponsiveness. For example, a toxidrome may be present that suggests diagnosis and therapy, such as the hypoventilation and small pupils found with opioid overdose.

Neurologic testing deviates from the standard examination. Fine tests of weakness in the alert patient, such as testing for pronator drift of the outstretched upper extremities, are not possible in the unresponsive patient. However, assessment of cranial nerves through pupillary examination, corneal reflexes, and oculovestibular reflexes may suggest focal CNS lesions. Abnormal extensor or flexor postures are nonspecific for localization or etiology of coma but suggest profound CNS dysfunction. Again, asymmetric muscle tone or reflexes raise the suspicion of a focal lesion. The goal of the physician is to rapidly determine if the CNS dysfunction is from diffuse impairment of the brain or if signs point to a focal (and perhaps surgically treatable) region of CNS dysfunction.

CT scanning is the neuroimaging procedure of choice. Acute hemorrhage is readily identified, as are midline shifts. No clear high-yield criteria for ordering CT scanning have been developed for the comatose patient. Because exceptions to the guideline for clinical assignment of patients to structural or nonstructural coma are frequent, CT is often obtained even in situations where the pretest probability is low. For example, detection of a clinically occult subdural hematoma might radically change management from supportive medical care to aggressive surgical intervention.

The medical community expects the emergency physician to stabilize the patient and to take initial diagnostic and therapeutic steps. The etiology of coma is discovered or strongly suspected in most patients during the ED evaluation. The system depends on the emergency physician to distribute the comatose patient to appropriate specialty services.

Specific Issues

Airway issues of importance in the comatose patient include concerns for cervical spine injury and increased intracranial pressure. If trauma is suspected, stabilization of the cervical spine during the diagnostic process must be maintained. Issues of intubation in the head-injured patient, or in a comatose patient with suspected increased intracranial pressure who needs modification of rapid sequence intubation techniques, are discussed at length in Chaps. 15 and 247.

In the pediatric patient, causes of coma differ from the adult. Toxic ingestions, infections, and child abuse all assume a greater frequency.

Nonconvulsive status epilepticus, or subtle status epilepticus, is an area of increasing interest. Patients who have had generalized seizures and remain unresponsive may have a prolonged postictal state or be in a continuing state of electrical seizures without corresponding motor movements. This has been termed *electromechanical dissociation of the brain and body.* If the motor activity of the seizure has been stopped and the patient's level of consciousness has not lightened within 30 min, the existence of this subtle status epilepticus should be considered and urgent EEG or neurologic consultation sought.

Treatment

Treatment of coma involves identification of the etiology of the brain failure and initiation of specific therapy directed at the underlying cause. Brain-saving procedures must be performed while diagnostic steps are taking place. Again, stabilization with attention to airway, ventilation, and circulation assume priority. Attention should be paid to readily reversible causes of coma such as hypoglycemia and opioid toxicity. Management steps are summarized in Table 221-9.

The "coma cocktail" that was routinely given to all comatose patients has come under scrutiny. Certainly, hypoglycemia is common, but with rapid glucose determinations, empiric administration of dextrose is not always necessary. It has been axiomatic that thiamine should be administered before glucose administration. This may remain reasonable in a patient with a suspected history of alcohol abuse or malnutrition, but there is no empiric evidence that the administration of thiamine must precede glucose administration in any acute setting. Naloxone, an opiate antagonist, should be given with known or suspected opiate overdose. While administration of opiate antagonists need not be routine, anecdotal reports of opiate reversal when the condition was masked or unsuspected abound. Routine use of flumazenil in unknown coma is not recommended.[22]

Several rapid decisions face the emergency physician. An early decision involves assigning the patients to probable traumatic or structural coma etiology or to a toxic-metabolic etiology. History and physical examination allow that initial categorization with many patients but maintaining a low threshold for CT scanning is encouraged because exceptions to the tentative clinical diagnosis are frequent. Further, consultants will invariably request this investigative modality except when the emergency clinician misses an obvious reversible cause. However, patients should be stable prior to obtaining this test, and causes such as carboxyhemoglobinemia and hypothermia, conditions easy to overlook at times, should also be sought.

If history, physical, or neuroimaging suggests increased intracranial pressure, specific steps may be indicated to reduce or ameliorate any further rise in ICP. In the intubated patient, hyperventilation with reduction of $Paco_2$ to roughly 30 mmHg will reduce cerebral blood volume and transiently lower ICP. Any noxious stimulus including "bucking" the ventilator will increase ICP. Paralysis and sedation should be readily used. Osmotic diuretics such as mannitol (0.5 to 1 g/kg) will decrease intravascular volume and brain water and may transiently reduce ICP. In cases of brain edema associated with tumor, steroids such as dexamethasone will reduce edema over several hours. Data to recommend specific therapy is lacking, and preferences among individuals and institutions vary greatly; early communication is encouraged with consultants and admitting physicians. Management of ICP is discussed in detail in Chap. 247.

TABLE 221-9 Management Steps for the Comatose Patient

I. History-utilize all resources

II. Initial assessment
- A. Primary survey
  1. Establish unresponsiveness/protect cervical spine
  2. *A*-manage airway, *B*-assess breathing, *C*-circulation
- B. Resuscitation/life-saving intervention
  1. Oxygen supplementation
  2. Establish intravenous access/draw initial blood sample
  3. Cardiac monitor
  4. Pulse oximetry monitor
  5. Thiamine: 100 mg IV (adults only)
  6. Glucose: 50 mL of 50% dextrose solution or glucose test
  7. Naloxone: administer 2 mg IV or SQ (or more)
- C. Secondary assessment
  1. Complete vital signs and general physical examination
  2. Neurologic examination
     - a. Respiratory pattern
     - b. Observation of posture and movements
     - c. Verbal and motor response to stimulation
     - d. Cranial nerve examination
     - e. Reflexes
     - f. Assignment to rating system/serial examinations
  3. Other monitoring
     - a. Arterial blood gas analysis
     - b. ECG monitor

III. Laboratory evaluation
- A. Routine labs: electrolytes, CBC, ABG
- B. Additional labs in selected patients
  1. COHgb, toxicologic screen, hepatic, CSF, thyroid, cortisol

IV. Radiologic evaluation tailored to patient. C-spine, CXR, cranial CT

V. Definitive care
- A. Supportive, monitoring
- B. Treatment
  1. Specific treatment if possible in emergency department
  2. Nonspecific treatment in selected cases
     - a. Osmotic agents or loop diuretics
     - b. Steroids
     - c. Hyperventilation, head position
- C. Appropriate consultation

Disposition

Patients with readily reversible causes of coma, such as insulin-induced hypoglycemia, may be discharged if home care and follow-up care is adequate and a clear cause for the episode is suspected. For patients with enduring altered consciousness, admission is necessary. Most systems depend on emergency physicians to stabilize the patient and correctly assign a tentative diagnosis so that the patient may be admitted to the proper specialty service. For example, neurosurgery at most institutions will admit patients with isolated cranial trauma or intracranial hemorrhage. Medical intensivists commonly care for patients with toxic or systemic etiologies of coma. Neurologists may admit patients with primary CNS causes of coma. Patterns of admission vary among institutions. If the appropriate intensive care unit is not available, transfer should be considered after stabilization.

REFERENCES

1. Lipowski Z: Delirium in the elderly patient. *N Engl J Med* 320:578, 1989.
2. Wofford L, Loehr LR, Schwartz E: Acute cognitive impairment in elderly ED patients: Etiologies and outcomes. *Am J Emerg Med* 14:649, 1996.
3. Rummans TA, Evans JM, Krahn LE, Fleming KC: Delirium in elderly patients: Evaluation and management. *Mayo Clin Proc* 70:989, 1995.

4. Folstein MF, Folstein SE: ''Mini-mental state'': A practical method for grading the cognitive state of patients for the clinician. *J Psychiatr Res* 12:189, 1975.
5. Tonglos EG, Smith GE, Ivnik RJ, et al: The mini-mental state examination in general medical practice: Clinical utility and acceptance. *Mayo Clin Proc* 71:829, 1996.
6. Kaufman DM, Zun L: A quantifiable, brief mental status examination for emergency patients. *J Emerg Med* 13:449, 1995.
7. Lipowski ZJ: Delirium (acute confusional states). *JAMA* 258:1789, 1987.
8. Geldmacher DS, Whitehouse PJ: Evaluation of dementia. *N Engl J Med* 335:330, 1996.
9. Corey-Bloom J, Thal LJ, Galasko D, et al: Diagnosis and evaluation of dementia. *Neurology* 4:211, 1995.
10. Friedland RP: Alzheimer's disease: Clinical features and differential diagnosis. *Neurology* 43(suppl 4):S45, 1993.
11. Tueth MJ: Dementia: Diagnosis and emergency behavioral complications. *J Emerg Med* 13:519, 1995.
12. Fleming KC, Adams AC, Petersen RC: Dementia: Diagnosis and evaluation. *Mayo Clin Proc* 70:1093, 1995.
13. Gold G, Giannakopoulos P, Montes-Paixao C, et al: Sensitivity and specificity of newly proposed clinical criteria for possible vascular dementia. *Neurology* 49:690, 1997.
14. Aisen PS, Davis KL: The search for disease-modifying treatment for Alzheimer's disease. *Neurology* 48(suppl 6):S36, 1997.
15. Borson S, Raskind MA: Clinical features and pharmacologic treatment of behavioral symptoms of Alzheimer's disease. *Neurology* 48(suppl 6):S17, 1997.
16. Friedland RP: ''Normal''-pressure hydrocephalus and the saga of the treatable dementias. *JAMA* 262:2577, 1989.
17. Clarfield AM: Normal-pressure hydrocephalus: Saga or swamp? (editorial). *JAMA* 262:2592, 1989.
18. Solomon P, Aring CD: The causes of coma in patients entering a general hospital. *Am J Med Sci* 188:805, 1934.
19. Plum F, Posner JB: The pathologic physiology of signs and symptoms of coma, in Plum F, Posner J (eds): *The Diagnosis of Stupor and Coma.* Philadelphia, FA Davis, 1980, pp 1–86.
20. Ropper AH: Transtentorial herniation, in Young GB, Ropper AH, Bolton CF (eds): *Coma and Impaired Consciousness: A Clinical Perspective.* New York, McGraw-Hill, 1998, pp 119–130.
21. Becker KJ, Purcell LL, Hocke N, et al: Vertebrobasilar thrombosis: Diagnosis, management, and the use of intra-arterial thrombolytics. *Crit Care Med* 24:1729, 1996.
22. Hoffman RS, Goldfrank LR: The poisoned patient with altered consciousness: Controversies in the use of a ''coma cocktail.'' *JAMA* 274:562, 1994.

ATAXIA AND GAIT DISTURBANCES

J. Stephen Huff

Ataxia and gait disturbances are symptoms of a variety of disease processes and generally are not themselves diagnoses. Ataxia is the failure to produce smooth intentional movements. Gait disorders include ataxic gait, as well as a variety of other conditions. The presenting complaint may be articulated by the patient or family as weakness, dizziness, stroke, falling, or another nonspecific or even inaccurate chief complaint. These symptoms do not exist in isolation from the nervous system and must always be viewed in the context of the patient's overall clinical picture. For example, a patient with an acute intracerebral hemorrhage may be aphasic and hemiplegic with the inability to walk, yet no one would consider this primarily a gait disturbance. However, if the intraparenchymal hemorrhage were in the cerebellum, the inability to walk may be one of the dominating signs and symptoms. This chapter focuses on an approach to patients with ataxia or gait disturbance, the generation of a differential diagnosis, and diagnostic options. Acute ataxia are emphasized; chronic or progressive forms such as those associated with some inherited disorders are covered only in a list.

PATHOPHYSIOLOGY

Ataxia or gait disturbances may result from many conditions that affect different elements of the central and peripheral nervous systems (Table 222-1). Clinicians tend to think that these disorders result primarily from cerebellar lesions. Cerebellar lesions do cause ataxia, but isolated lesions of the cerebellum are not the most common cause of these complaints.

The summation and integration of proprioceptive information from the joints and tendons, visual information, and vestibular inputs while the head, body, or limbs are moving, and the production of a smooth, steady muscular movement is a complex process involving different areas of the central nervous system (CNS) and elements of the peripheral nervous system. Transmission of proprioceptive information from the peripheral nervous system into the CNS is required, as well as integration and processing that does occur mainly in the cerebellum. Conscious and unconscious input from the cortex is also thought to occur. Visual input is involved in compensation of abnormal movements. The entire process is complex, intricate, and occurs continuously during voluntary and involuntary movements.

Ataxia may be roughly categorized into two types. Motor ataxias are usually due to disorders of the cerebellum; the sensory receptors and afferent pathways are intact, but integration of the proprioceptive information is faulty. Involvement of the lateral cerebellum (the cerebellar hemispheres) may lead to a motor ataxia of the ipsilateral limb. Lesions affecting primarily the midline portion of the cerebellum often cause problems with axial muscle coordination reflected in difficulty maintaining a steady upright standing or sitting posture. Motor ataxia is also referred to in the literature as cerebellar ataxia.

There are reports of lesions in what would seem to be unexpected locations producing motor ataxia. Supratentorial infarctions, particu-

TABLE 222-1 Common Etiologies of Acute Ataxia and Gait Disturbances

I. Systemic conditions
  A. Intoxications with diminished alertness
    1. Ethanol
    2. Sedative-hypnotics
  B. Intoxications with relatively preserved alertness (diminished alertness at higher levels)
    1. Phenytoin
    2. Carbamazepine
    3. Valproic acid
    4. Heavy metals—lead, organic mercurials
  C. Other metabolic disorders
    1. Hyponatremia
    2. Inborn errors of metabolism
II. Disorders predominantly of the nervous system
  A. Conditions affecting predominantly one region of the central nervous system
    1. Cerebellum
      a. Hemorrhage
      b. Infarction
      c. Degenerative changes
      d. Abscess
    2. Cortex
      a. Frontal tumor, hemorrhage, or trauma
      b. Hydrocephalus
    3. Subcortical
      a. Thalamic infarction or hemorrhage
      b. Parkinson's disease
    4. Spinal cord
      a. Cervical spondylosis
      b. Posterior column disorders
  B. Conditions affecting predominantly the peripheral nervous system
    1. Peripheral neuropathy
    2. Vestibulopathy

larly small deep infarctions or lacunes of the posterior limb of the internal capsule, have been reported to cause isolated hemiataxia. It is postulated that interruption of either ascending or descending cerebellar to cortical pathways are the cause of this motor-type ataxia.[1] Small infarctions or hemorrhages in thalamic nuclei may produce a clinical picture of motor or cerebellar like ataxia with hemisensory loss. These effects are seen contralateral to the lesion.[2] Lesions affecting the frontal lobe, such as tumor or hydrocephalus, may cause a motor ataxia of the contralateral extremities through poorly understood mechanisms.[3]

Sensory ataxia occurs with a failure in transmission of proprioception or position sense information to the CNS. This may occur in the peripheral nerves, spinal cord, or cerebellar input tracts. Coordinated motor performance is faulty even though motor systems and the cerebellum are intact. Sensory ataxia may be compensated to a degree consciously with visual sensory information. Loss of this visual information leads to the observation that sensory ataxia often worsens in poor lighting conditions and may by brought out during examination (see below).

CLINICAL FEATURES

Historical information should be collected about the entire symptom constellation in addition to complaints of headache, nausea, fever, weakness, or numbness. A history of febrile illness, medication history, or family history may be the key element leading to a correct diagnosis in individual cases. The nature of onset of symptoms and the time course of the process guide the pace of investigations. For example, abrupt onset of gait difficulty in a patient with severe headache, drowsiness, nausea, and vomiting should suggest an acute process within the CNS, possibly a hemorrhage into the cerebellum. The possible complications of that diagnosis are severe and require immediate attention. On the other extreme, a patient without significant medical history who is brought to the emergency department with a stumbling gait after an episode of binge drinking requires examination but may need nothing other than observation unless history or physical examination suggests trauma or some alternative cause for the symptoms.

The following discussion of the neurologic examination assumes that the gait disorder is the dominating abnormality, but a complete examination including testing of cranial nerves, mental status, or the motor system is always necessary and may yield findings that lead to an unanticipated diagnosis.

Gait testing is one of the most important parts of the directed neurologic examination. Observing the patient sit upright in the stretcher, rise, stand, walk, and turn gives information about many parts of the nervous system. The patient should be asked to walk at a normal speed, then walk on the heels, and then toes. Tandem gait is toe-to-toe walking and also tests many elements of the nervous system. Do not assume a normal examination without specifically testing gait or ambulation.

Cerebellar functions are tested by asking the patient to perform smooth voluntary movements and rapidly alternating movements; dyssynergia (breakdown of movements into parts), dysmetria (inaccurate fine movements), or dysdiadochokinesia (clumsy rapid movements) may be indicative of a problem in the lateral cerebellum. The thigh-patting test particularly examines rapidly alternating movements. This is correctly performed by patting the thigh with the palm then the back of the same hand in alternating fashion, making a sound with each rapid slap. The maneuver is performed with each hand in turn. The familiar finger-to-nose test (dyssynergia) may be helpful in distinguishing between cerebellar and posterior column lesions. Performing this test with the eyes closed tests proprioception in the upper extremity. A test for cerebellar function that emphasizes the lower extremities (and another part of the cerebellum) is the familiar heel-to-shin test (also dyssynergia). In cerebellar disease, the knee may be initially overshot. In posterior column disease, there may be difficulty locating the knee but the ride down the shin weaves from side to side or falls off. Other tests commonly used for cerebellar function in the Stewart-Holme rebound sign (sudden release of the flexed forearm may rebound back and forth in several cycles).

The Romberg test is a test of sensation and, if positive, distinguishes sensory from motor ataxia. With the patient standing with arms outstretched and the eyes open, the patient is observed for signs of unsteadiness. The feet should be narrowly spaced, and the posture should be easily maintained. The inability to maintain a steady standing posture (or in extreme cases, a seated position) confirms that an ataxia is present but does not yet give any information about the type of ataxia. The patient is then asked to close the eyes with resulting loss of visual orienting information. If the ataxia worsens with this loss of visual input, then the Romberg sign is present or positive, suggesting a sensory ataxia with a problem of proprioceptive (posterior column) or vestibular function. In patients who show little or no change in their unsteadiness with eye closure (Romberg test negative), a motor ataxia is suggested with possible localization of that problem to the cerebellum. Note that many normal individuals will have some increase in unsteadiness with eye closure. Further neurologic examination is indicated to confirm the suspicion of sensory etiology of the ataxia.

In the last century, tabes dorsalis (neurosyphilis) was a common cause of sensory ataxia. The neuropathologic descriptions of this disorder and correlation with the physical examination were the foundation of modern principles of anatomic localization of neurologic function.[4] In tabes dorsalis, the posterior columns and posterior spinal roots degenerate, primarily in the lumbosacral region. The loss of proprioceptive information from the lower extremities renders the patient dependent on visual cues for correct gait. The classic description paints the picture of a patient who walks slowly with wide gait while staring at the ground. In darkness or with interruption of vision, the patient is unable to walk. The gait in this condition is peculiar with the foot first raised and then slapped to the ground with each step. These abnormalities reflect the loss of proprioceptive information from the posterior root and posterior column degeneration. The possibility of vitamin B_{12} deficiency should always be a consideration in patients with evidence of posterior column disease. If left untreated, an initial unsteady gait progresses to weakness, spasticity, and ataxia. The finding of a megaloblastic anemia may be a clue, but it is not always present.

Sensory examination in a patient with unsteady movements should include position or vibration testing (posterior columns), as well as testing sensation to pinprick. Testing of the deep tendon reflexes will serve largely to discover asymmetry or spasticity that might suggest an alternative diagnosis. Acute cerebellar injury may result in muscle hypotonia for a few days or weeks.[5]

Nystagmus is seen in many different disorders due to lesions in a variety of different locations of the CNS, but this does suggest that the pathologic process is intracranial, and not in the spinal cord or peripheral nervous system (see Chap. 223, ''Vertigo and Dizziness).

No organized classification scheme exists for gait disorders, and different authors categorize abnormal gaits largely in descriptive terms. A brief summary of some of more commonly used terms follows. A *cerebellar* or *motor ataxic* gait is wide-based with unsteady and irregular steps; compensation to barriers in the environment may be lacking. The gait of sensory ataxia resulting from loss of proprioception is notable for abrupt movement of the legs and slapping impact of the feet with each step.

An *apraxic* gait is one in which the patient seemingly has lost the ability to initiate the process of walking, a sort of ''ignition failure.'' Apraxia describes the inability of a patient to perform a voluntary act even though the motor system and understanding are intact. This may occur with right or nondominant hemispheric lesions. Frontal lobe dysfunction may result in a similar gait. This may be seen in normal pressure hydrocephalus.

Foot drop from peroneal muscle weakness will be reflected in an *equine* (high stepping) gait. The high stepping from hip flexion is necessary for the foot to clear the ground.

The term *festinating* gait is used to describe narrow-based miniature shuffling steps. Once the walk begins, the steps may become more rapid. This is common in Parkinson's disease and may be accompanied by other elements of Parkinson's disease, such as increased muscle tone, lack of facial expression, slow movements (bradykinesia), and tremor.

An unusual gait with outward swinging or circumabduction of the leg suggests a mild hemiparesis reflecting the asymmetric weakness of the proximal lower extremity muscles. The examination should then be directed to find other signs of hemiparesis. This weakness of the trunk and pelvic girdle muscles may result in a waddling gait from failure to maintain the normal position of the pelvis relative to the lower extremities.

A *functional* gait disorder is one in which the patient is unable to walk normally though all motor pathways, sensory pathways, and cerebellar functions may be demonstrated to be functioning normally. The underlying problem is often a conversion disorder. These gaits may be bizarre, resembling a person wildly balancing on a tightrope and seemingly threatening to fall but not falling. The wildness of flailing movements without falling actually demonstrates that the strength, balance, and coordination are intact. This dramatic functional gait is termed *atasia-abasia.*

A unifying concept defines gait disorders according to the level of processing of neurologic information (Table 222-2).[6] Low-level gait disturbance refers to disorders of proprioception or dysfunction of the musculoskeletal system. Middle-level gait disturbance causes distortion of appropriate interaction of postural and motor processes or synergies. This might include stroke with paralysis, cerebellar dysfunction, or diseases of the basal ganglia such as Parkinson's disease. On examination, patients might have findings of spasticity, muscular tone, paralysis, or abnormal movements. High-level gait disturbances seemingly involve structures or processes that choose the appropriate responses for the support surface, body position in space, and intention of the patient. Cautious gait, apraxic gait, and the frontal gait disorder conceptually fall into this group with pathology that correlates with lesions in the frontal cortex or thalamus. This latter group is the least understood and the source of clinical confusion. This classification scheme is not ideal but does allow a thoughtful approach to patient diagnosis.

TABLE 222-2 Classification of Gait Disorders

I. Low-level gait disorders
A. Musculoskeletal problems
1. Arthritic gait or other joint or skeletal problems
2. Muscle weakness
B. Peripheral sensory problems
1. Sensory ataxic gait
2. Vestibular problems
II. Middle-level gait disorders
A. Hemiplegia
B. Paraplegia
C. Motor or cerebellar ataxia
D. Parkinson's disease
E. Dystonia, chorea, other movement disorders
III. High-level gait disorders
A. Senile gait (cautious gait)
B. Frontal ataxic gait
C. Apraxic gait (gait ignition failure)
D. Frontal disequilibrium

Note: "Level" refers to the level of processing of sensorimotor information.
Source: Modified from Nutt et al,[6] with permission.

DIAGNOSIS

History and physical examination remain the key in evaluation of ataxia and gait disorders. If other symptoms or signs are present in addition to ataxia or gait disturbance, then the diagnostic approach might follow that clinical pathway. When the predominant complaint is ataxia or gait disturbance, determine whether ataxia is sensory or motor. Attempt to determine whether the primary process is systemic or within the nervous system. If within the nervous system, the next question is one of localization to the peripheral nervous system versus the CNS and perhaps to a more specific anatomic location. Finally, the tempo of the illness, comorbid diseases, and other clinical findings guide investigations and may allow a disease-specific diagnosis.

A patient with acute gait failure over hours to days needs thorough evaluation in the emergency department, consultation if available, and possible admission, in contrast to a patient with gradual loss of abilities over weeks or months, where outpatient referral and evaluation may be appropriate.

SPECIFIC ISSUES THAT IMPACT EVALUATION AND TREATMENT

Geriatric Issues

The gait changes with advancing age. A typical constellation includes gait slowing, shortening of the stride, and widening of the base. This results in the appearance of a guarded gait, that is, the gait of someone about to slip and fall. Many patients are aware of the loss of speed and adaptive balance and acknowledge the need to be careful. The nature of this *senile* gait is not fully understood but may represent a mild degree of neuronal loss, failing proprioception, slowing of corrective responses, or weakness of the lower extremities. Senile gait disorder is thought to exist in up to one-quarter of the elderly population. Some authorities divide this disorder into components of gait ataxia with mild truncal instability and widened gait, and gait slowing with diminished spontaneous arm swing and bradykinesia.[7] However elements of the senile gait are also found in neurodegenerative diseases, and caution is urged to consider the possible presence of a neurodegenerative disorder such as Parkinson's disease in elderly patients with gait impairment.[7]

Pediatric Issues

In evaluating children with acute ataxia or gait disorder, examination must exclude weakness and musculoskeletal disorders. The child may be awake, alert, and playful but is visibly unsteady or wobbly sitting on a stretcher. The differential diagnosis is long (Table 222-3).

Intoxications are a cause of ataxia in children, and the ingestion may be surreptitious. Though ethanol may be suspected by odor, other drugs such as phenytoin or carbamazepine will not be detected in that manner. History should include queries about any medications in the household.

Unusual metabolic disorders such as pyruvate decarboxylase complex deficiency may present with ataxia. Family history may or may not suggest a metabolic disorder. Typically, the onset is gradual, but abrupt decompensations may occur. Other systemic or CNS abnormalities will be present.

Posterior fossa mass lesions and other CNS masses may present with ataxia, though usually some abnormality of cranial nerves or strength will be discovered with careful examination. Attention is needed to exclude abnormalities on physical examination that might suggest problems not localized to the cerebellum. Abnormal ocular movements should increase the suspicion of a mass lesion.

TABLE 222-3 Causes of Acute Ataxia in Children Roughly in Order of Frequency

Cause	Example
Drug intoxication	Ethanol Isopropyl alcohol Phenytoin Carbamazepine Sedatives Lead, mercury Others
Acute viral infection, postinfectious inflammatory causes, and postimmunization	Varicella Coxsackievirus A and B Mycoplasma Echovirus
Neoplasm	Neuroblastoma Other central nervous system tumors
Trauma	Subdural or epidural posterior fossa hematoma
Congenital or hereditary	Pyruvate decarboxylase deficiency Friedreich's ataxia Hartnup's disease Others
Hydrocephalus	
Cerebellar abscess	
Labyrinthitis/vestibular neuronitis	
Meningoencephalitis	
Idiopathic	

Source: Modified from Belcher[8] and Chutorian and Pavlakis,[11] with permission.

Rarely, ataxia can follow immunizations, viral illnesses, or varicella but also has been rarely reported in the preeruptive phase of varicella.[8] Most children are in the 2- to 4-year-old range. The onset of gait ataxia is abrupt, and only occasionally is fever present at the time ataxia begins. The latency from the prodromal illness to the onset of ataxia is from 2 days to 2 weeks. Other neurologic findings encountered included truncal ataxia, dysmetria and, uncommonly, cranial nerve abnormalities. Varicella patients appear to have uniform excellent recovery compared with patients with acute cerebellar ataxia from other causes that may have some residual problems.[9] Little workup is needed if the ataxia occurs in the convalescent phase of varicella, and antiviral medications are not indicated. Otherwise, neuroimaging, lumbar puncture, and consultation are advisable. One study showed that while roughly half of the patients had cerebrospinal fluid inflammatory changes with pleocytosis or elevated immunoglobulin G index, magnetic resonance imaging (MRI) identified inflammatory changes in the cerebellum in only a minority of cases.[9] Another small report noted MRI abnormalities not only in the cerebellum but in other areas of the CNS. This ''syndrome'' may in fact consist of several subgroups, some of which involve transient demyelination.[10]

TREATMENT AND DISPOSITION

The underlying cause must be identified and any available therapy directed toward the primary disease process.

Disposition depends on the final diagnostic formulation and a risk assessment of likely progression of process and patient safety. At most centers, a suspicion of a mass lesion will have been addressed by the performance of a neuroimaging study, likely computed tomography because of availability, prior to any disposition decision.

Gait failure in the elderly is of specific concern, and the safety of patients must always be considered. Patients unable to walk or care for themselves should be admitted for supportive care. If the clinical course is one of slowly progressive impairment of gait or ataxia, then outpatient referral to the primary care physician or neurologist may be the proper course.

REFERENCES

1. Luijckx GJ, Baiten J, Lodder J, et al: Isolated hemiataxia after supratentorial brain infarction. *J Neurol Neurosurg Psychiatry* 57:742, 1994.
2. Solomon DH, Barohn RJ, Bazan C, Grissom J: The thalamic ataxia syndrome. *Neurology* 44:810, 1994.
3. Terry JB, Rosenberg RN: Frontal lobe ataxia. *Surg Neurol* 44:583, 1995.
4. Schiller F: Staggering gait in medical history. *Ann Neurol* 37:127, 1995.
5. Diener H-C, Dichgans J: Pathophysiology of cerebellar ataxia. *Move Disord* 7:95, 1992.
6. Nutt JG, Marsden CD, Thompson PD: Human walking and higher-level gait disorders, particularly in the elderly. *Neurology* 43:268, 1993.
7. Waite LM, Broe GA, Creasy H, et al: Neurologic signs, aging, and the neurodegenerative syndromes. *Arch Neurol* 53:498, 1996.
8. Belcher RS: Preeruptive cerebellar ataxia in varicella. *Ann Emerg Med* 27:511, 1996.
9. Connolly AM, Dodson WE, Prensky AL, Rust RS: Course and outcome of acute cerebellar ataxia. *Ann Neurol* 35:673, 1994.
10. Maggi G, Varone A, Aliverti F: Acute cerebellar ataxia in children. *Child Nerv Syst* 13:542, 1997.
11. Chutorian AM, Pavlakis SG: Acute ataxia, in Pellock JM, Myer EC (eds): *Neuroligc Emergencies in Infancy and Childhood.* Boston, Butterworth-Heinemann, 1993, pp 208–219.

223 VERTIGO AND DIZZINESS

Brian Goldman

As many as 0.5 percent of the population consult their physician each year regarding vertigo, and 1 percent report dizziness.[1] The evaluation of dizziness can test the diagnostic skill of most emergency physicians. The difficulties begin with the patient's chief complaint. The term *dizziness* is nonstandardized and ambiguous. Dizziness may mean vertigo, syncope, presyncope, weakness, giddiness or anxiety, or a disturbance in mentation. The patient's symptoms should therefore be clarified as much as possible.

Vertigo is the perception of movement where no movement exists. Patients may describe themselves as moving or may describe the environment as moving in relation to themselves. The type of movement may be described as rotatory or vertical; alternatively, the patient may describe a sense of staggering, swaying, or being pulled or hurled to the side or onto the ground.

Syncope is a transient loss of consciousness that is accompanied by loss of postural tone with spontaneous recovery. It is associated with a transient reduction of cerebral blood flow, oxygen, and glucose to the reticular activating system. To meet the definition of syncope, no exogenous electrical or chemical cardioversion should be required to regain consciousness. Syncope accounts for 3 percent of emergency department (ED) visits and 1 to 6 percent of hospital admissions. Near-syncope is defined as light-headedness signifying an impending loss of consciousness without loss of consciousness actually occurring.

Psychiatric dizziness has recently been defined as a sensation of dizziness not related to vestibular dysfunction that occurs exclusively in combination with other symptoms as part of a recognized psychiatric symptom cluster.[2] In dizziness clinics, the frequency of this category can range between 20 and 50 percent of patients.

Disequilibrium is another term that is sometimes used to describe a feeling of unsteadiness or imbalance while walking. Some patients describe a sensation of feeling as if they were "floating." It is often due to decreases in visual acuity or proprioception.

PATHOPHYSIOLOGY

Equilibrium and spatial orientation are determined by a sophisticated network of complex interactions within the central nervous system (CNS). The CNS coordinates and integrates sensory input from the visual, vestibular, and proprioceptive systems. The three streams of information are combined in the brain to form an impression of the orientation of the head and body as well as of motion. Vertigo arises from a mismatch of information from two or more of the involved senses, which, in turn, is caused by dysfunction in the sensory organ or its corresponding pathway.

Visual inputs arise from the eyes, the optic pathways, and the visual cortex, providing spatial orientation. Proprioceptors that are located primarily in the joints and muscles of the limbs, neck, and trunk help convey a sense of movement and body position; they relate movements and indicate the position of the head relative to that of the body. In the vestibular system, the otoliths produce an orientation to gravity. The cupulae contain sensors that track rotary motion. The presence of embedded otoconia or particles on the cupulae may transform them into linear motion sensors capable of sensing gravity. There are three semicircular canals that sense orientation to movement and head tilts. The semicircular canals are filled with a fluid called endolymph, the water component of which derives from the perilymph. The striae vascularis are important in maintaining the ionic composition of the fluid. The endolymphatic sac produces glycoproteins that create an osmotic sink necessary to maintain flow. The movement of fluid in the semicircular canals causes specialized hair cells inside the canals to move, causing afferent vestibular impulses to fire. Sensory input from the vestibular apparatus travels to the nucleus of the eighth cranial nerve (Fig. 223-1).

The CNS structures involved in integrating sensory input from all three sensory modalities include the medial longitudinal fasciculus, the red nuclei, the cerebellum, and the parietal lobes and superior temporal gyrus of the cerebral cortex. Connections between these structures and the oculomotor nuclei that drive the vestibuloocular reflex (VOR) complete the system. The VOR prevents retinal slip and thus visual blurring that would otherwise result from head movements and body sway.

Several neurotransmitters are involved in vestibular transmission. Glutamate is a major neurotransmitter of vestibular nerve impulses. Muscarinic cholinergic receptors involved in this system (chiefly the M2-type) have been found in the pons and medulla. Gamma-aminobutyric acid (GABA) is an inhibitory neurotransmitter found in connections between central vestibular and oculomotor neurons. Histaminergic receptors are located pre- and postsynaptically on vestibular cells. Both noradrenaline and dopamine have been found to have a modulating effect on the vestibular system.[3]

In the presence of balanced input from the vestibular apparatus on both sides, there is no perception of motion. Altering the symmetry of input from both sides produces vertigo. Thus, any unilateral lesion of the vestibular apparatus may produce vertigo. In addition, the apparatus on either side may be induced to fire excessively due to abnormal motion of the endolymph. Unlike the preceding example, although vertigo is produced, there is no other clinical evidence of damage to the vestibular apparatus. Rapid head movements induce vertigo by accentuating the imbalance. Damage to or dysfunction of any of the central structures mentioned previously can also lead to vertigo. Bilateral damage does not usually produce vertigo but may lead to truncal or gait instability.

The most striking clinical sign associated with vertigo is nystagmus. Nystagmus is a rhythmic movement of the eyes that has both a fast and a slow component. The direction of nystagmus is named by its fast component. The slow component is due to the vestibuloocular reflex and is generated by the excitation of the semicircular canal, producing eye movement away from that canal. The fast component of nystagmus is caused by the cortex, which exerts a quick corrective movement in the opposite direction. With disorders of the vestibular apparatus, the sensation of vertigo is usually associated with nystagmus. The nystagmus of vestibular injury or dysfunction is provoked when the affected side is in the dependent position, and the characteristic pattern is vertical and rotational or horizontal. When horizontal nystagmus is present, its slow-beating component points to the injured labyrinthe. Vertical nystagmus by itself (and not associated with a rotational component) usually indicates a brainstem abnormality.

The likelihood of vertigo and other forms of dizziness increases as people age. Decreases in visual acuity, proprioception, and vestibular input may occur. These may manifest as vertigo or unsteady gait that is reported as "dizziness" by the patient. The risk of near-syncope also increases due to causes such as dysrhythmias, orthostatic hypotension, and autonomic dysfunction. In addition, as people age, they are more likely to have free-floating otoconia within the semicircular canals. Otoconia are particles made of calcium carbonate that become displaced from the utricular maculae by aging, head trauma, and diseases of the labyrinth. The particles are heavier than the surrounding endolymph and tend to collect in the most dependent part of the endolymph system, where they tend to clump. It is unknown what percentage of people without symptoms have such particles.[4]

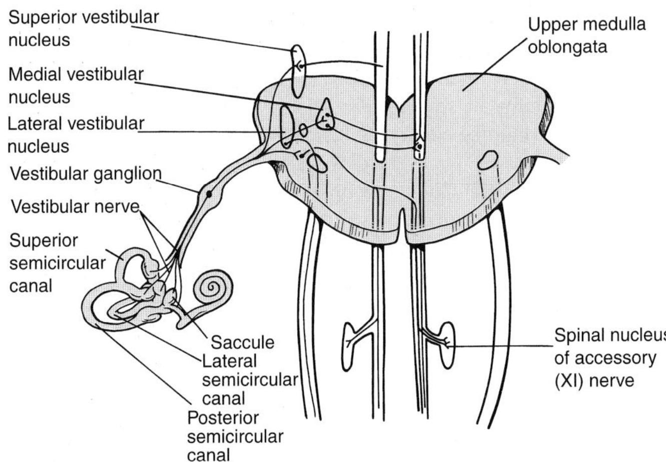

FIG. 223-1. Vestibular innervation.

CLINICAL FEATURES

The conditions that cause vertigo are summarized in (Table 223-1). Vertigo is typically subdivided into peripheral and central causes. Unfortunately, clinical abilities to distinguish the severity of vertigo are limited since there is no measurement scale for vertigo. While the discussion below does classify vertigo somewhat by severity, the clinician must also use information such as age, comorbidity, and vascular disease to stratify the probability of central versus peripheral vertigo. Peripheral vertigo is caused by disorders affecting the vestibular apparatus and the eighth cranial nerve, while central vertigo is caused by disorders affecting central structures, such as the brainstem and the cerebellum. The characteristics distinguishing peripheral and central vertigo are found in Table 223-2. Figure 223-2 shows how the nystagmus pattern itself may help to differentiate peripheral and central vertigo.

Although disorders causing peripheral vertigo tend to produce more distressing symptoms, they are seldom life-threatening. Disorders

TABLE 223-1 An Etiologic Classification of Vertigo

Vestibular/otologic	Benign paroxysmal positional vertigo Traumatic: after head injury Infection: labyrinthitis, vestibular neuronitis, Ramsay Hunt syndrome
Syndrome	Ménière syndrome Neoplastic Vascular Otosclerosis Paget disease Toxic or drug-induced: aminoglycosides
Neurologic	Vertebrobasillar insufficiency Lateral Wallenburg syndrome Anterior inferior cerebellar artery syndrome Neoplastic: cerebellopontine angle tumors Cerebellar disorders: hemorrhage, degeneration Basal ganglion diseases Multiple sclerosis Infections: neurosyphilis, tuberculosis Epilepsy Migraine headaches Cerebrovascular disease
General	Hematologic: anemia, polycythemia, hyperviscosity syndrome Toxic: alcohol Chronic renal failure Metabolic: thyroid disease, hypoglycemia

TABLE 223-2 Classification of Vertigo

	Peripheral	Central
Onset	Sudden	Slow
Severity of vertigo	Intense spinning	Ill defined, less intense
Pattern	Paroxysmal, intermittent	Constant
Aggravated by position/movement	Yes	No
Associated nausea/diaphoresis	Frequent	Infrequent
Nystagmus	Rotatory-vertical, horizontal	Vertical
Fatigue of symptoms/signs	Yes	No
Hearing loss/tinnitus	May occur	Does not occur
Abnormal tympanic membrane	May occur	Does not occur
CNS symptoms/signs	Absent	Usually present

causing central vertigo may produce less distressing symptoms and have a slower onset than those due to peripheral vertigo, but they are generally of a more serious nature, requiring urgent or semiurgent diagnostic imaging or consultation with a neurologist or neurosurgeon. Unfortunately, these clinical features of vertigo are not always sufficient or specific enough to clearly classify the disorder as central or peripheral.

DISORDERS CAUSING PERIPHERAL VERTIGO

Peripheral vertigo is noted for its abrupt (often explosive) onset. Peripheral vertigo produces an intense sensation of spinning or hurtling toward the ground or surrounding walls. It is typically worsened by rapid movement and by changes in head position. Peripheral vertigo is frequently associated with nausea, often severe vomiting, and diaphoresis; it may be associated with signs of increased vagal tone such as bradycardia and hypotension.

Benign Paroxysmal Peripheral Vertigo

Benign paroxysmal peripheral vertigo (BPPV) is one of the most common causes of peripheral vertigo, accounting for as many as 17 to 22 percent of patients presenting to dizziness clinics.[5] The incidence of BPPV has been estimated as being as high as 64 per 100,000 per year.[6] This estimate was derived from patients seen only by ear/nose/throat (ENT) specialists, omitting those seen only by primary care physicians. Thus, the incidence may be underestimated. BPPV is defined as a mechanical disorder of the inner ear causing transient vertigo (with autonomic symptoms) and associated nystagmus that is precipitated by certain head movements. The condition was first described by Barany in 1921, and most of the essential clinical features were described by Dix and Hallpike in 1952.[7]

The most widely accepted hypothesis to explain BPPV is known as *canalolithiasis.* According to this hypothesis, BPPV is caused by inappropriate activation of the posterior semicircular canal (typically unilateral) by the presence of free-floating particles or otoconia. The otoconia become displaced from the utricular macula by aging, head trauma, or labyrinthine disease. Because the particles are heavier than the surrounding endolymph, they tend to collect in the long arm of the posterior semicircular canal, the most dependent part of the endolymph system. Once the particles clump in sufficient mass, changes in head position cause gravitation of the particles, which creates a hydrodynamic drag (or plunger effect) on the endolymph, causing the cupula to be displaced. This results in aberrant neural firing, causing both vertigo and nystagmus.

BPPV can occur at any age, but the average age of onset is in the mid-fifties. Women are twice as likely to be affected as men. The onset is sudden, and an attack is typically precipitated by rolling over in bed, assuming a supine position, leaning forward, looking up at the sky or ceiling, or turning the head. Nausea is often present, although vomiting is unlikely because of the transient nature of the symptoms. Because the symptoms fatigue, they tend to be worse in the morning and become less pronounced as the day progresses. Patients may eliminate the offending activities. There is no associated hearing loss or tinnitus and no physical findings on examination of the external auditory canal.

Several findings support a diagnosis of BPPV (Table 223-3). There is a latency period of 1 to 5 s between assuming the offending head position and onset of vertigo and nystagmus. Both the vertigo and nystagmus crescendo to a peak of intensity, then subside within 5 to 40 s. BPPV is diagnosed using the Dix Hallpike position test. Although Nylen and Barany are sometimes credited with discovering the maneuver, Dix and Hallpike clearly published the first description of the test in wide use today.[8] When the head is rotated 30 to 45° toward the affected side and the patient is brought to the supine position with the head lying 30° below the level of the examining table, this brings the affected ear into the dependent position. After a latency of 1 to 5 s, this causes rotatory nystagmus with a fast-beating component toward the undermost ear. The nystagmus may reverse direction as the head is returned to the erect position. The response to repeated provocative testing fatigues, causing the vertigo and nystagmus to disappear.[8]

Meniere's Disease

Meniere's disease is a disorder associated with an increased volume of endolymph within the cochlea and labyrinth. It occurs equally in

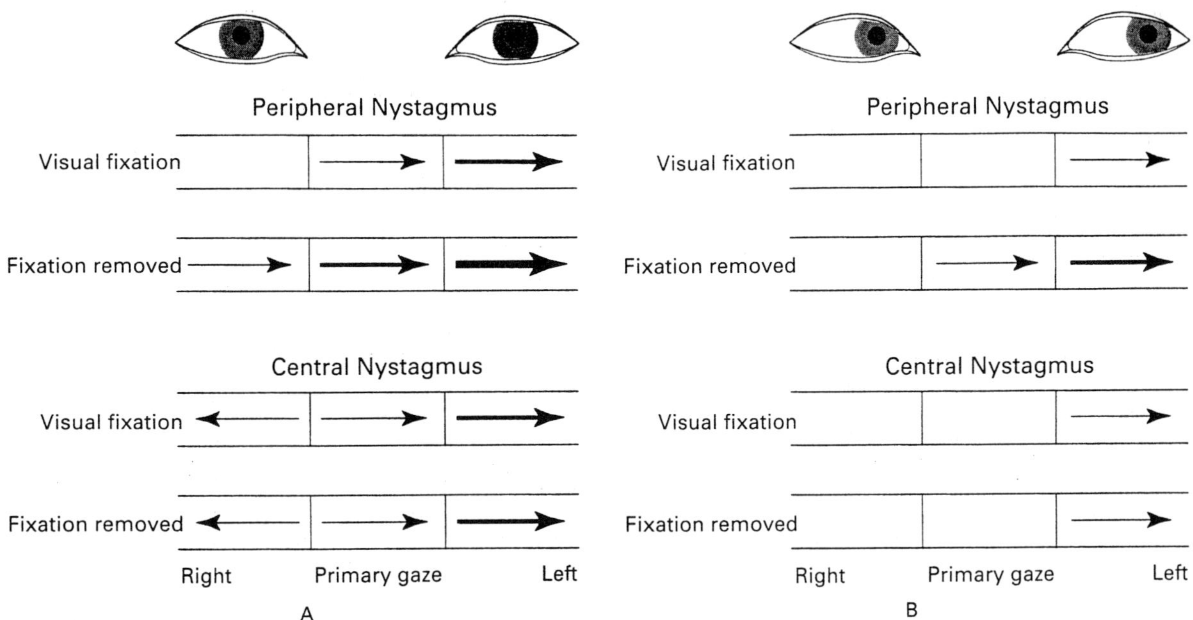

FIG. 223-2. Schematic drawing of peripheral and central vestibular nystagmus with and without visual fixation. The direction of the arrows indicates the horizontal direction of the fast phase of the nystagmus (a torsional component is not shown). The thickness of the arrows represents the relative intensity of the nystagmus. Panel A shows findings typical of peripheral nystagmus, which remains in the same direction when the direction of gaze changes, and central nystagmus, which changes direction when the direction of gaze changes. Removal of visual fixation increases the intensity of peripheral nystagmus but not of central nystagmus. Panel B illustrates how removal of fixation helps to differentiate peripheral from central nystagmus when the nystagmus is predominantly in one direction of gaze during fixation. With removal of fixation, peripheral nystagmus may increase in intensity and become apparent in more than one direction of gaze. (Reprinted by permission.)

men and women, with onset in middle age. The disease is usually unilateral to begin with and often becomes bilateral over time. The precise pathogenesis is unknown, but evidence suggests that patients have difficulty regulating the volume, flow, and composition of endolymph. Histologic studies have demonstrated that the endolymphatic sac contains immunologically active tissue, raising the possibility of an autoimmune mechanism. As with BPPV, the onset of vertigo is usually sudden. However, the duration of vertigo ranges from 20 min to 12 h (typically 2 to 8 h). It is associated with nausea, vomiting, and diaphoresis. The frequency of attacks can vary from several times per week to several times per month. Between attacks, the patient is usually well, although deafness may persist. Other hallmarks of the diagnosis include associated symptoms such as roaring tinnitus, diminished hearing, and fullness in one ear. Current treatments offer symptomatic relief without altering the course of the disease.

TABLE 223-3 Supportive Findings in Benign Paroxysmal Peripheral Vertigo

1. There is a latency period of 1–5 s between the provocative head position and onset of nystagmus.
2. The intensity of nystagmus increases to a peak before slowly resolving.
3. The duration of vertigo and nystagmus ranges from 5–40 s.
4. If nystagmus is produced in one direction by placing the head down, then the nystagmus reverses direction when the head is returned to the sitting position.
5. Repeated head positioning causes both the vertigo and accompanying nystagmus to fatigue and subside.

Perilymph Fistula

A perilymph fistula is an opening in the round or oval window, permitting pneumatic changes in the middle ear to be transmitted to the vestibular apparatus. Trauma, infection, or a sudden change in the pressure inside the cerebrospinal fluid may cause the tear. The diagnosis is suggested by the sudden onset of vertigo associated with flying, scuba diving, severe straining, heavy lifting, coughing, or sneezing. The diagnosis is confirmed by nystagmus elicited by pneumatic otoscopy (Hennebert sign).

Vestibular Neuronitis

Vestibular neuronitis is a disorder of suspected viral etiology that causes intense peripheral vertigo. The location of the viral infection is unknown, although inflammation of the eighth cranial nerve or brainstem has been suspected. Unlike BPPV and Ménière disease, vestibular neuronitis typically lasts several days and does not recur. The onset is usually sudden, and the patient is otherwise well except for possible symptoms of an upper respiratory infection. The vertigo is often so intense that the patient requires several days of bed rest; it then usually decreases dramatically, resolving completely over several weeks. Elderly patients may have persistent unsteadiness of gait. Unilateral loss of hearing and tinnitus may occur. Positional nystagmus is evident in up to one-third of cases.

Labyrinthitis

Labyrinthitis is an infection of the labyrinth that produces peripheral vertigo associated with hearing loss. The precise etiology is often unknown. The infection may be viral, in which case the clinical course is similar to that of vestibular neuronitis. Cases have reportedly been associated with measles and mumps. Bacteria may also cause labyrinthitis. Although unusual, an infection within the labyrinth can develop from otitis media, in which bacteria and toxins diffuse across the membrane of the round window. A cholesteatoma can erode into the inner ear, creating a portal of entry for bacteria. Other possible antecedents for bacterial labyrinthitis include otitis media with fistula, meningitis, mastoiditis, and dermoid tumor. The hallmarks of this disease include sudden onset of vertigo with associated hearing loss and middle ear findings. Serous labyrinthitis may occasionally produce vertigo.

Ototoxicity

Aminoglycoside antibiotics produce hearing loss and peripheral vestibular dysfunction by accumulating inside the endolymph, where they cause the death of cochlear and vestibular hair cells. However, since both inner ears are affected, vertigo is uncommon. Typical clinical manifestations include ataxia and oscillopsia, which is defined as an inability to maintain visual fixation while moving. The damage is irreversible, although the degree of toxicity depends on the dose and duration of treatment with antibiotics. Loop diuretics (furosemide and ethacrynic acid) also cause irreversible vestibular and ototoxicity. Cytotoxic agents associated with vestibular damage include vinblastine and cisplatin. The antiarrhythmic drug quinidine and antimalarial drugs derived from quinine, such as chloroquine and mefloquine, can also cause vestibular symptoms that may be irreversible (Table 223-4).

Reversible causes of vestibular damage and ototoxicity include minocycline, erythromycin, and some quinolones. Isolated cases of unsteady gait have been observed with antiviral and antiparasitic agents. Acetyl salicylic acid (ASA) in toxic doses causes tinnitus and hearing loss but is unlikely to cause vertigo. Other nonsteroidal anti-inflammatory drugs such as indomethacin, ibuprofen, and naproxen may cause the same symptoms. The lesion is metabolic rather than destructive and readily resolves with discontinuation of therapy.

Numerous solvents and other chemicals can cause both peripheral as well as central vestibular symptoms. These include propylene glycol, mercury, and hydrocarbons. Drugs that induce a central vestibular syndrome include anticonvulsants, tricyclic antidepressants, neuroleptics, opiates, and alcohol. Phencyclidine is a prominent example of a recreational drug that causes central vestibular symptoms, including nystagmus and ataxia. Drugs causing irreversible cerebellar toxicity include phenytoin and toluene as well as cancer chemotherapeutic agents. In general, most patients adapt to vertigo that is chronic by relying on increased sensory input from unaffected modalities such as proprioception and vision. However, certain drugs that are used as antivertigo therapy may exacerbate preexisting chronic vertigo by delaying or inhibiting such compensation. These drugs include alcohol, benzodiazepines, barbiturates, and neuroleptics. Thus, with chronic vertigo, antivertigo therapy should not be used on a long-term basis.

TABLE 223-4 Ototoxic and Vestibulotoxic Agents

Agent	Dose Dependent	Reversible
Aminoglycosides	Yes	No
Erythromycin	No	Yes
Minocycline	No	Yes
Quinolones	No	Yes
NSAIDs	Yes	Yes
Loop diuretics	No	Can be irreversible
Cytostatic drugs	Yes	No
Antimalarials	No	Yes

Benign Paroxysmal Vertigo of Childhood

This disorder is so named because it causes severe yet brief attacks of vertigo in children less than 3 years of age. This is now generally recognized as a phenomenon related to migraine headaches. The vertigo tend to be self-limited and to resolve within childhood, sometimes giving rise to migraine headaches. Since vertigo may represent the aura of a seizure, referral to a pediatric neurologist for an assessment and an electroencephalogram (EEG) might be warranted in some cases.

Eighth-Nerve Lesions

Lesions of the eighth cranial nerve may produce vertigo. Meningiomas and acoustic schwannomas are typical causes. The onset of vertigo is usually gradual, remaining constant until central compensation can take place. It is seldom as intense, and may manifest only as unsteadiness. The vertigo is usually preceded by hearing loss. Tumors involving the cerebellopontine angle may also cause symptoms such as ipsilateral facial weakness, impaired corneal reflex, and cerebellar signs.

Herpes zoster oticus, also known as the Ramsay Hunt syndrome, is a neuropathic disorder characterized by deafness, vertigo, and facial nerve palsy. The diagnosis is made by the presence of grouped vesicles on an erythematous base inside the external auditory canal.

Cerebellopontine Angle Tumors

Vertigo is sometimes associated with tumors of the cerebellopontine angle. Such tumors include acoustic neuromas, meningiomas, and dermoids. They usually present with a cluster of findings including deafness and ataxia as well as ipsilateral facial weakness, loss of the corneal reflex, and cerebellar signs.

Posttraumatic Vertigo

Closed head injuries account for a significant percentage of patients with vertigo. Vertigo or gait unsteadiness is a common complaint following a head injury. Acute posttraumatic vertigo is caused by a direct injury to the labyrinthine membranes. Its onset is immediate following the head injury, and it produces constant vertigo, nausea, and vomiting. Such patients may have sustained a concomitant fracture of the temporal bone. Vertigo immediately associated with a closed head injury warrants computed tomography (CT) or magnetic resonance imaging (MRI) to rule out an extradural or intradural hematoma. Vertigo due to direct labyrinthine trauma tends to resolve within several weeks. Closed head trauma can also displace otoconia from the utricular maculae, precipitating an attack of BPPV. Some patients with a history of a closed head injury develop a postconcussive syndrome. Although true vertigo is uncommon with this disorder, gait unsteadiness or a vague sense of dizziness are quite common. Such patients should be referred to a neurosurgeon or neurologist for special imaging and neuropsychiatric testing.

DISORDERS CAUSING CENTRAL VERTIGO

Central vertigo is caused by disorders affecting the cerebellum and the brainstem. It can produce a strikingly different clinical picture from that of peripheral vertigo. The onset is usually gradual, the sensation less intense, and symptoms are not provoked by changes in position. Central vertigo is unlikely to be associated with nausea, vomiting, or diaphoresis. Unlike conditions causing peripheral vertigo, both tinnitus and hearing impairment are unlikely. Nystagmus is more likely to be vertical than horizontal or rotatory and may be present in the absence of vertigo. Oscillopsia is a common finding. Central vertigo tends to be accompanied by other signs of brainstem disease, such as ataxia, blurred vision, long tract signs, dysphagia, dysarthria, and diplopia.

Cerebellar Hemorrhage and Infarction

Cerebellar hemorrhage typically manifests symptoms such as acute vertigo and ataxia. Headache, nausea, and vomiting may or may not be present. The vertigo is not as intense and is not similar to the sense of hurtling that characterizes peripheral vertigo. Instead, the patient may complain of a sense of side-to-side or front-to-back motion. He or she will have truncal ataxia and may not be able to sit without support. Romberg testing and tandem gait will be abnormal. Occasionally, there may be a sixth cranial nerve palsy, or conjugate eye deviation away from the side with the hemorrhage. Cerebellar infarction has a similar clinical presentation.

Wallenberg Syndrome

A lateral medullary infarction (Wallenberg syndrome) of the brainstem can cause vertigo as part of its clinical presentation. Classic ipsilateral findings include facial numbness, loss of corneal reflex, Horner syndrome, and paralysis or paresis of the soft palate, pharynx, and larynx (causing dysphagia and dysphonia). Contralateral findings include loss of pain and temperature sensation in the trunk and limbs. Occasionally, lesions of the sixth, seventh, and eighth cranial nerves can occur, causing vertigo, nausea, vomiting, and nystagmus.

Vertebrobasilar Insufficiency

Transient ischemic attacks (TIAs) of the brainstem due to vertebrobasilar insufficiency (VBI) can produce vertigo. Such patients should present with the usual risk factors for cerebrovascular disease. As with other symptoms of a TIA, the vertigo may be of sudden onset and typically lasts minutes to hours. By definition, it should completely resolve within 24 h. VBI-induced vertigo can be accompanied by other manifestations such as diplopia, dysphagia, dysarthria, bilateral long-tract signs, and bilateral loss of vision. As diagnostic modalities improve, it is becoming clear that VBI may present without these additional symptoms. Unlike other causes of central vertigo, VBI may be provoked by position. Turning the head partially occludes the ipsilateral vertebral artery. If the contralateral artery is stenotic, head turning could cause transient ischemia to the brainstem, causing VBI. A sufficient loss of brainstem circulation caused by a head turn could affect the reticular activating system, causing near-syncope or syncope.

Multiple Sclerosis

Demyelinating disease may cause isolated areas of demyelination in the brainstem, causing vertigo. The vertigo tends to occur as a discrete episode lasting several hours to several days or weeks. It is usually nonrecurrent. Other manifestations of multiple sclerosis such as ataxia or optic neuritis may be present or may have occurred previously. The vertigo is less intense than that experienced in peripheral conditions and is accompanied by nystagmus. The nystagmus may be more prominent than the vertigo reported by the patient.

Neoplasms

Neoplasms of the fourth ventricle can cause brainstem signs and symptoms, including vertigo. Such tumors include ependymomas in younger patients and metastases in older patients.

TABLE 223-5 Diagnostic Criteria for Basilar Migraine*

Bilateral visual symptoms in both the nasal and temporal fields
Vertigo
Tinnitus
Decreased hearing
Diplopia
Dysarthria
Ataxia
Bilateral paresis
Bilateral paresthesias
Decreased level of consciousness

*Fulfills criteria for migraine with aura (two or more of the above aura symptoms).

Migraine-Related Dizziness and Vertigo

Vertigo can be a symptom of an aura, an analogue or equivalent of the headache phase itself, or as an associated symptom to the migraine prodromes. Basilar migraine is a migraine headache in which the aura is associated with clinical manifestations similar to those of VBI. The International Headache Society's diagnostic criteria for basilar migraine[9] are shown in Table 223-5. These include vertigo, decreased hearing, tinnitus, bilateral long-tract signs, bilateral visual disturbances, dysarthria, diplopia, and decreased level of consciousness. Vertigo as an aura should develop over 5 to 20 min and should subside within 60 min. Vertigo as a symptom of a migraine aura may precede the headache or may occur in the absence of a headache. The headache is typically occipital in location, throbbing in character, and associated with nausea and vomiting.

Aside from basilar migraine, a strong association has been found between migraine and cochleovestibular disturbances. True episodic vertigo has been shown to occur in 26 to 33 percent of unselected migraine patients seen in large head clinics. Such patients may complain of episodes of constant vertigo, positional vertigo, or nonvertiginous dizziness. In cases of true vertigo, the vertigo may accompany the headache or may occur independently. Such episodes of vertigo are of two typical durations. Some patients complain of vertigo lasting from several minutes to 2 h, while others experience vertigo lasting longer than 24 h. The pathogenesis of migraine-related dizziness has not been determined, but probably relates to a centrally mediated excess sensitivity to vestibular stimuli. The diagnostic criteria for migraine-related vertigo include a history of vertigo not attributable to other known conditions, along with a present or past history of migraine or a strong family history. Successful treatment has been reported with pharmacologic agents used to treat migraine, such as tricyclic antidepressants, calcium channel blockers, β blockers, and clonazepam.

Physiologic Vertigo

Physiologic vertigo is vertigo not caused by disease of the cochleovestibular system. It results from a mismatch between visual, proprioceptive, and vestibular input. This may be the pathogenesis of motion sickness as well as the transient vertigo associated with watching a film that captures the visual sensation of motion without the corresponding vestibular or proprioceptive input (''visual vertigo''). Visual vertigo is triggered by complex visual environments such as shopping malls and by viewing complex floor or wallpaper patterns.

OTHER CONDITIONS

Disequilibrium of Aging

Disequilibrium of aging is a condition manifesting as ill-defined dizziness and gait unsteadiness. Loss of hearing and balance occur normally with age. Patients over the age of 70 may have a 20 to 40 percent loss of vestibular hair cells. In addition, elderly patients often experience a decrease in visual as well as proprioceptive input, a decline in central integration and processing, as well as a decrease in motor responses. Approximately 50 percent of individuals over the age of 70 experience imbalance; of those, more than half report falls.[10] The disequilibrium of aging may be precipitated or exacerbated by diminished ambient light (with worsening of symptoms at night), unfamiliar surroundings, and the use of benzodiazepines and drugs with anticholinergic effects such as tricyclic antidepressants and neuroleptic agents. The concomitant presence of near syncope or risk factors for near syncope may complicate the diagnosis.

Near Syncope

Near syncope is a feeling of light-headedness, which, in its most severe form, leads to loss of consciousness (syncope). Some patients with near syncope may refer to the sensation of light-headedness as dizziness. Syncope and near syncope differ only in their severity. The most common categories of near syncope are vasovagal, situational, orthostatic hypotension, and drug-induced syncope. Cardiac causes such as valvular heart disease as well as cardiac dysrhythmias are also significant causes. The cause of near syncope is not determined in a significant percentage of patients. Recent evidence suggests that the majority of patients with unexplained presyncope may have vasovagal presyncope. Sole reliance on the typical clinical presentation of vasovagal presyncope may lead to underdiagnosis. Positive upright tilt testing, in which the patient is placed in the passive upright position at 60° for 45 min, is generally recommended.[12] Some protocols involve the use of isoproterenol. The end points of a positive tilt test include the development of syncope or presyncope associated with hypotension, bradycardia, or both. In normal subjects, tachycardia usually results from a passive tilt test.[11]

Syncope and near syncope in the elderly are associated with daily events, including micturition, defecation, postural changes, meals, laughing, coughing, and swallowing. Orthostatic hypotension is extremely common in the elderly and is associated with volume depletion, venous insufficiency, poor conditioning, polyneuropathy, preganglionic autonomic dysfunction (Shy-Drager syndrome), as well as the use of medications including vasodilating drugs, diuretics, other antihypertensive agents, and antiparkinsonian and anticholinergic medications. According to a position paper by the American College of Physicians, syncope in the elderly often results from polypharmacy and abnormal responses to daily events.

A new diagnostic entity has emerged called postural orthostatic tachycardia syndrome. This is a relatively mild disorder associated with a fall in blood pressure in which patients experience near-syncope, nonvertiginous dizziness, and symptoms suggestive of TIA. This condition may involve less dramatic falls in blood pressure than those seen in syncope. The pathogenesis is thought to be mild autonomic dysfunction. Findings on tilt testing include an increase in heart rate of 30 beats per minute over baseline within the first 10 min of testing (unassociated with profound hypotension), along with recurrence of the symptom complex.[12]

Convulsive Disorders

Nonconvulsive status epilepticus (NCSE) is characterized by altered mental status without loss of consciousness or tonic-clonic phenomena associated with electroencephalographic (EEG) evidence of seizure activity. The incidence is unknown because some cases may either go undetected or be attributed to other causes of altered mental status. With NCSE, patients have vague or nonspecific changes in mentation and behavior, although they may be able to answer questions and complete complex tasks. Some will complain of nonvertiginous dizziness. Symptoms may last for hours to days. The diagnosis is made by EEG as well as by determining the underlying mechanism for the seizure.[13] In addition, some patients presenting to the emergency department with nonvertiginous dizziness may be postictal.

Hyperventilation Syndrome

Patients with primary hyperventilation may experience nonvertiginous dizziness or near syncope during an episode. However, such symptoms can usually be reproduced by asking the patient to hyperventilate.

Psychiatric Dizziness

Psychiatric dizziness is defined as dizziness that occurs in combination with other symptoms as part of a recognized psychiatric disorder or symptom complex that is not related to known vestibular disorders. Although such dizziness has been characterized as nonvertiginous dizziness in the past, it is now recognized that patients with certain psychiatric disorders can present with true vertigo as part of their presenting symptoms. Dizziness is the second most common symptom reported by patients with panic disorder. In addition, a large percentage of patients with dizziness meet the criteria for panic or mood disorder. A majority of patients with panic disorder have objective abnormalities on testing of vestibular function. The strongest correlation is with patients who suffer from agoraphobia. Such patients suffer from what is known as ''space and motion discomfort'' (SMD). SMD is defined as comprising uncomfortable symptoms such as dizziness, imbalance, and anxiety occurring in situations delineated by certain spatial or motion characteristics. Generally, these are complex visual environments such as shopping malls. Agoraphobia may develop as a way to combat the symptoms.[13]

Psychiatric dizziness should not be confused with the phenomenon of psychogenic overlay. In the latter, the patient may manifest some symptoms of neurootologic disease, but illness behavior is augmented by the presence of psychiatric conditions. These include hypochondriasis and personality disorders. Patients who are withdrawn from serotonin reuptake inhibitors used on a long-term basis may experience nonvertiginous dizziness, along with gastrointestinal and flu-like symptoms, sleep deprivation, altered sensations, anxiety, and irritability.[14]

DIAGNOSIS

History

The diagnosis of vertigo or nonvertiginous dizziness rests largely upon a detailed history and physical examination, including provocative testing (Fig. 223-3). Determine early whether the patient is suffering from vertigo, near syncope, loss of consciousness, or less worrisome symptoms such as nonvertiginous dizziness or mild unsteadiness. Thus, the key purpose of history taking is to obtain an accurate unprompted description of what the patient means by dizziness. It is important to avoid leading questions, as they may bias the patient's responses. If the patient has difficulty describing the dizziness, it is useful to ask him or her to describe the initial episode in detail. Often this is the most vivid episode, and the patient is more likely to recall key

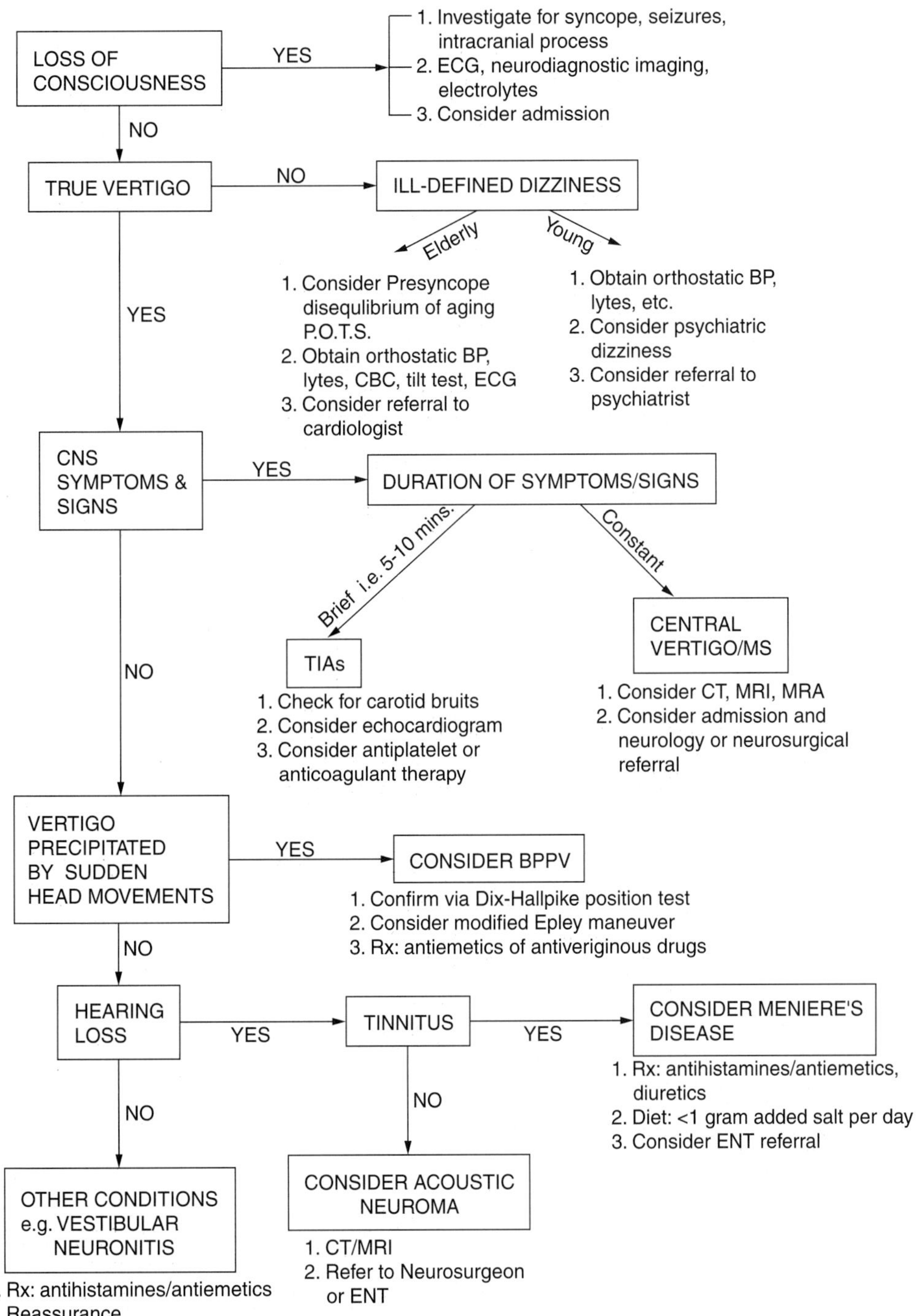

FIG. 223-3. Guideline approach to vertigo.

precipitants. Further history taking depends on how the dizziness is categorized.

If the patient has experienced true vertigo, the next step is to determine whether the vertigo is of peripheral or central origin. Although the symptoms of central vertigo may not be severe, they are more likely to represent potentially life-threatening disorders. The temporal pattern and precipitating causes can help to distinguish the different etiologies of vertigo (Tables 223-6 and 223-7). Peripheral vertigo is more likely than central vertigo to be intense and to be associated with nausea, vomiting, diaphoresis, tinnitus, hearing loss, and photophobia. Central vertigo is more likely to be associated with neurological symptoms and signs such as diplopia, dysarthria, and bilateral visual and sensory abnormalities. An associated headache or history of headache suggests migraine or a space-occupying lesion. Inquiry into history of head trauma and medications is required, as these can precipitate episodes of dizziness or interfere with central adaptation.

Because of central adaptation, true vertigo is unlikely to be constant. Thus, constant symptoms are more likely to represent nonvertiginous dizziness and psychogenic complaints. A history of numerous chronic somatic complaints increases this possibility. When such a pattern emerges, it is prudent to obtain a psychiatric history and to ask about panic disorder and agoraphobia. However, the diagnosis of psychogenic symptomatology should only be entertained after other poten-

TABLE 223-6 Temporal Patterns Seen in Vertigo

Pattern	Conditions
Seconds	BPPV,* postural hypotension
Minutes	TIAs†
Hours	Ménière disease
Days	Viral labyrinthitis
Constant	Nonspecific dizziness

*Benign paroxysmal peripheral vertigo.
†Transient ischemic attacks.

tial causes have been ruled out, and thus it is rarely if ever appropriate to entertain in the ED. Constant oscillopsia suggests a central neurologic diagnosis.

Physical Examination

The physical examination is directed by the history obtained. General physical examination should include vital signs, orthostatic blood pressure measurements where appropriate, plus cardiac and chest examinations. In elderly patients, the carotids and vertebrobasilar system should be auscultated. Carefully check the deep tendon reflexes and sensation in the lower extremities to identify peripheral neuropathy. Always check gait and tandem gait, and perform the Romberg test. Observe whether the patient can sit up and get off the stretcher unaided. Truncal ataxia will often be precipitated during such actions.

Patients with vertigo should have ear, neurologic and vestibular examinations. The external auditory canal and tympanic membrane should be examined for evidence of otitis media, cholesteatoma, and other pathology. Insufflation of air by use of a pneumatic otoscope that precipitates a burst of vertigo with nystagmus is diagnostic of an inner ear fistula. Hearing should be screened by whispering questions to the patient in one ear while lightly covering or rubbing one's fingers in front of the contralateral ear. Patients with decreased hearing should have Webber and Rinne testing to distinguish between conductive and sensorineural hearing loss.

Neurologic and vestibular examinations overlap. The cranial nerves should be examined in detail, especially the eighth cranial nerve. Where central vertigo is considered, note abnormalities such as absent corneal reflex, facial paresis, difficulty swallowing, dysphonia, and depressed gag reflex. Test cerebellar function by rapid alternating movement. The vestibulospinal system and cerebellum are tested by tandem gait and Romberg testing. Proprioception and vibration should also be tested.

TABLE 223-7 Precipitants of Dizziness

Precipitant	Conditions
Head movements	BPPV*
Ingestion of salty foods	Ménière disease
Assuming a supine position	BPPV
Assuming a standing position	Orthostatic hypotension
Coughing, straining	Perilymph fistula
Specific environment	Visual vertigo, panic disorder, agoraphobia

*Benign paroxysmal peripheral vertigo.

Nystagmus is the principal objective sign of vertigo. The eyes should be examined for spontaneous nystagmus, and the direction of such nystagmus should be noted. Because visual fixation can suppress nystagmus, the patient should ideally be wearing a pair of Frenzel glasses, which are high-diopter lenses in a frame equipped with a light source. Examine for nystagmus while testing extraocular movements to 40° from the midline. Note that several beats of nystagmus at the extremes of lateral gaze is a normal finding. Nystagmus on gaze testing suggests peripheral or central vertigo. The nystagmus pattern and behavior can assist in determining whether the lesion is central or peripheral (Fig. 223-2).

To diagnose BPPV, perform a Dix-Hallpike position test. This test should not be performed on patients with carotid bruits. It may be performed on patients with cervical spondylosis provided that the neck is not hyperextended. The patient should be cautioned that the test might provoke vertigo. Pretreatment with dimenhydrinate 50 mg IM or IV may make the test more tolerable but will not obliterate nystagmus. Patients should keep their eyes open at all times and stare at the examiner's nose or forehead. The initial position of the patient on an examining table is upright and seated, close enough to the head of the table so that when the patient lies down, the head will be able to extend backward an additional 30 to 45°. To test the right posterior semicircular canal, the head is initially rotated 30 to 45° to the right. Keeping the head in this position, the patient is rapidly brought to the recumbent position until the head is 30 to 45° below the level of the stretcher or examining table. A positive test is indicated by rotatory nystagmus following a latency of 1 to 5 s; the nystagmus exhibits rapid eye torsions toward the affected ear and lasts for 10 to 40 s. The patient is then returned to the upright sitting position and the test is repeated on the left side. The side exhibiting the positive test is the side of the lesion.

Patients with suspected near-syncope should have a detailed cardiovascular examination. Orthostatic hypotension is defined as a drop in systolic blood pressure of greater than 20 mmHg with reproduction of symptoms for up to 2 min upon standing. Orthostatic blood pressure measurements are notoriously unreliable, especially in elderly patients and even in patients with documented blood pressure changes. A study of elderly patients demonstrated that blood pressure readings tended to be more reliable when taken in the morning.[15] On cardiac examination, note the heart rate and rhythm and evaluate the patient for evidence of valvular disease.

ANCILLARY TESTS

Laboratory investigations should be used as confirmatory tests. Most patients with peripheral vertigo do not require emergent laboratory investigations. If bacterial labyrinthitis is within the differential diagnosis, blood for a complete blood count (CBC) and blood cultures should be obtained. Vertigo associated with a closed head injury warrants a CT scan or MRI to rule out intracranial bleeding. Patients with near syncope should have an electrocardiogram (ECG) and cardiac monitoring as well as a CBC if anemia is suspected. Ambulatory Holter monitoring may be indicated if an dysrhythmia is suspected. Emergent echocardiography is not generally indicated unless symptomatic valvular heart disease (such as aortic stenosis) or conditions causing compromised cardiac output are suspected. Electrolytes, glucose, and renal function tests are occasionally of value in patients with nonvertiginous dizziness, such as disequilibrium of aging. Thyroid testing may be of use if anxiety due to thyrotoxicosis is suspected.

Patients with suspected central vertigo may require more urgent investigations. If a cerebellar hemorrhage or infarction is suspected, a CT scan should be obtained immediately. If a cerebellopontine angle tumor is suspected, an immediate CT scan or MRI is not required unless the patient has signs and symptoms of increased intracranial pressure. Patients with suspected VBI require an ECG, cardiac monitoring and echocardiography if cardiac emboli are suspected. With

VBI, it is sufficient to leave investigations such as duplex ultrasound of the cartotids and MRI with MRA to the consulting neurologist. A psychiatric assessment for consideration of panic and/or mood disorders might be warranted in patients with persistent unexplained dizziness. In addition, patients with agoraphobia suggestive of SMD might warrant a full neurologic assessment.

Detailed testing of cochleovestibular function such as electronystagmography, posturography, and rotating chair tests are not necessary in the emergency management of peripheral vertigo. They can be left to the otologist or ENT specialist.

TREATMENT

The key principle guiding therapy is to determine the nature of the patient's dizziness. In general, short-term treatment with pharmacotherapy is the mainstay for patients with peripheral vertigo (see Table 223-8). However, such medications may exacerbate symptoms in patients with nonvertiginous dizziness. Specific treatment varies somewhat with the etiology of peripheral vertigo.

Drug Therapy

The goals of pharmacotherapy are the reduction or elimination of vertigo, the enhancement or noncompromise of vestibular compensation, and the reduction of accompanying symptoms such as nausea, vomiting, and anxiety. Many of the agents used in the treatment of vertigo may suppress both vertigo and vestibular compensatory mechanisms.

Drugs with anticholinergic effects can be quite effective in the treatment of vertigo. The current agent of choice is transdermal scopolamine. Antihistamines are the most commonly prescribed drugs for the treatment of vertigo. Their mechanism of action is not precisely known. Although they have prominent anticholinergic effects, some antihistamines such as astemizole have antivertigo properties without appreciable anticholinergic effects. A separate central action is also postulated. H_1 antihistamines are considered effective against vertigo, but H_2 antihistamines are not. The calcium channel blocker flunarizine is useful in the treatment of vertigo. Its mechanism of action remains unknown, but flunarizine does possess significant antihistaminic activity. Antidopaminergic (neuroleptic) agents such as promethazine have also been shown to be effective in the treatment of vertigo. Such agents reduce neurovegetative symptoms such as nausea and vomiting by blocking dopaminergic receptors in the area postrema of the brainstem. They also possess antihistamine and anticholinergic effects. Prochlorperazine and chlorpromazine should not be used in the management of vertigo as they tend to cause excesive orthostatic hypotension, which can exacerbate the underlying dizziness.[3] Case reports

TABLE 223-8 Pharmacotherapy of Acute Peripheral Vertigo

Anticholinergics	Scopolamine	0.5 mg transdermal patch q 3–4 days (behind ear)
Antihistamines	Dimenhydrinate	50–100 mg IM or PO q 4 h
	Diphenhydramine	25–50 mg IM or PO q 6 h
	Cyclizine	50 mg PO q 4 h (not to exceed 200 mg/24 h)
	Meclizine	25 mg PO q 8–12 h
Antiemetics	Hydroxyzine	25–50 mg q 6 h
	Promethazine	25–50 mg q 6–8 h
Benzodiazepines	Diazepam	2 mg PO q 8–12 h
	Clonazepam	0.5 mg q 12 h
Calcium antagonists	Cinnarizine	15 mg PO q 8 h
	Flunarizine	10 mg PO qd

have indicated that ondansetron, a serotonin 5-HT_3 receptor antagonist, may be useful in the treatment of intractable vertigo accompanying brainstem disorders. The lack of controlled data and its high cost make it difficult to recommend this drug for use in emergency management.[16]

Despite lack of evidence for efficacy, benzodiazepines continue to be used widely in the United States. By binding to GABA receptors in the brainstem, benzodiazepines may act centrally to suppress vestibular responses. They may also impair vestibular compensation. Their only indication should be in the relief of severe anxiety accompanying vertigo. Small doses of medium-duration benzodiazepines such as diazepam and clonazepam are recommended.

There are several recognized complications of symptomatic therapy. Antihistamines can cause sedation and anticholinergic adverse effects. Antidopaminergic neuroleptic agents can induce or exacerbate orthostatic hypotension. These drugs can also cause somnolence and acute dystonia and can exacerbate anticholinergic adverse effects. Because of overlapping anticholinergic and antidopaminergic effects, anticholinergic, antihistaminic, and neuroleptic drugs should never be used in combination. Benzodiazepines may interfere with central compensatory mechanisms.

Vestibular neuronitis is treated symptomatically. Antihistamines and antinausea drugs should be used at the outset and withdrawn after several days if possible. Patients with bacterial labyrinthitis may benefit from symptomatic treatment but also require antibiotics and referral to an otologist or ENT specialist for likely admission and possible surgical drainage. Meniere's disease is managed symptomatically, as current drug therapy does not alter the degenerative process. Standard antihistamines and antinausea agents have been shown to be more effective than placebo in relieving acute symptoms. Treatment with a combination of the diuretics triamterene and hydrochlorthiazide has been shown to be effective in controlling vertigo. Betahistine, a histadine analogue, has been widely used in Europe for the treatment of vertigo due to Meniere's disease. The dosage of betahistine is 8 to 16 mg PO tid. None of these drug treatments improves hearing. A salt-restricted diet (less than 1 g/day of added salt) continues to be recommended. Invasive treatments for patients with Meniere's disease include surgical intervention and intratympanic applications of aminoglycosides such as gentamicin or streptomycin. Perilymph fistula is managed with symptomatic treatment and bed rest, with referral to an ENT specialist for surgical repair.

Patients with vertiginous migraine headaches should be referred to a neurologist for outpatient assessment. Initial management is symptomatic, with antivertigo therapy; migraine prophylactic agents such as β blockers and calcium channel antagonists may be instituted. Patients with nonvertiginous dizziness and disequilibrium of aging should not be treated with antivertigo medication. Patients with psychiatric dizziness related to panic disorder may be treated with a brief course of benzodiazepines. The long-term use of benzodiazepines and tricyclic antidepressants in the treatment of panic and mood disorders can worsen ataxia and further compromise central compensatory mechanisms in maintaining balance.

Vestibular Rehabilitation Exercises

Vestibular exercises are indicated for patients with BPPV, chronic vertigo, and psychiatric dizziness.[17] They are relatively simple to teach and can be quite helpful in giving patients a measure of control over their own symptoms. The principle behind vestibular exercises is the fatiguing response observed with Dix-Hallpike testing. Exercises developed by Brandt and Daroff have been shown to be efficacious. (1) The patient sits in the middle of the examining table with legs over the side. (2) The patient is then instructed to lie to one side of the table and to remain in that position until the vertigo has subsided. He or she is then asked to sit up, waiting again for any symptoms to subside. (3) The patient repeats the same maneuver, this time by lying down on the opposite side of the examining table. (4) These exercises are repeated in one session until no further vertigo is provoked. Brandt-Daroff exercises can be repeated at 3-hourly intervals at home.

Particle Repositioning Maneuver

The development of the "canalolithiasis" hypothesis for BPPV has led to a new form of treatment. The principle behind the particle repositioning maneuver is to use gravity to induce the particles to move along the semicircular canals until they end up inside the utricle, where they are unlikely to exert a plunger effect and cause vertigo. The maneuver is also known as the canalith repositioning maneuver or "Epley" maneuver.[18]

A modified form of the Epley maneuver is as follows. The affected ear is determined by Dix-Hallpike position test. An antihistamine or antiemetic may be administered prior to the maneuver for the patient's comfort. (1) The patient is seated as in the Dix-Hallpike position test and the head is turned 45° toward the affected ear. (2) The patient is gently brought to the recumbent position with the head hanging 30 to 45° below the examining table. (3) The head is gently rotated 45° to the midline. (4) The head is then rotated a further 45° to the unaffected side. (5) The patient rolls onto the shoulder of the unaffected side, at the same time rotating the head a further 45°. (6) The patient is returned to the sitting position and the head is returned to the midline.

Each portion of the maneuver should be done slowly and evenly to permit the particles to traverse their intended course. If the maneuver is done correctly, nystagmus in the same direction as that observed during Dix-Hallpike position testing may be observed. If nystagmus in the opposite direction is observed, then the particles have moved back toward the cupula; this portends an unsuccessful maneuver. The maneuver is repeated several times until both the vertigo and accompanying nystagmus have disappeared. To prevent the particles from traveling retrograde to the semicircular canal, some authors recommend that patients sleep upright for 48 h following successful treatment and avoid provocative head movements. Several randomized trials have demonstrated subjective improvement as well as objective improvement as evidenced by Dix-Hallpike testing. Although spontaneous recovery from BPPV is the usual outcome, the Epley maneuver appears to hasten complete recovery.

The Epley maneuver should not be performed on patients with cervical spondylosis or back pain that might be exacerbated. The maneuver has several potential adverse effects. As many as 20 percent of patients may experience light-headedness or mild imbalance for 1 or 2 days following treatment. In addition, a small number of patients may experience exacerbation of their vertigo accompanied by a change in the precipitating movements. The mechanism is a movement of the particles from the posterior to the anterior or horizontal canals, which resolves upon further treatment. This underscores the need for careful follow up by an ENT specialist or physician familiar with the maneuver and its potential complications.[19]

DISPOSITION

The disposition of the patient depends on the cause of the dizziness. Inability to classify the disorder as either peripheral or central is an indication for neurologic consultation. Patients with peripheral vertigo may in general be safely discharged from the ED. The criteria for admission for peripheral vertigo include vertigo with intractable nausea and vomiting as well as bacterial labyrinthitis. An accompanying fever that is unexplained should increase suspicion of a more serious process and may warrant admission. All patients with a first episode of peripheral vertigo should follow up with their primary care physician or be referred directly to an otologist or ENT specialist for further testing. It would be helpful for the emergency physician to convey the results of Dix-Hallpike position testing (paying close attention to the type and direction of nystagmus on testing) as well as caloric testing if done. Patients with BPPV who have had a particle repositioning maneuver should be referred to an otologist or ENT specialist for follow-up. The specialist should be notified that the maneuver has been carried out and given the results of follow-up Dix-Hallpike testing.

Patients with central vertigo require a consultation with a neurologist or a neurosurgeon. Patients suspected of having cerebrovascular disease (including VBI, lateral medullary syndrome, and cerebellar infarction) should be referred for neurologic consultation and possible admission. Patients suspected of having a seizure should be referred to a neurologist and possibly be admitted. On the other hand, patients suspected of having less urgent causes of central vertigo such as multiple sclerosis and migraine headache may be referred to a neurologist as outpatients. Patients suspected of having a cerebellopontine angle tumor or cerebellar hematoma should have an emergent CT scan or MRI or be referred to a neurosurgeon immediately if such imaging is unavailable. The presence of cranial nerve abnormalities should be mentioned to the consultant, as well as the presence or absence of vertical nystagmus.

Patients with near-syncope should be referred on an outpatient basis to a cardiologist for tilt testing, an echocardiogram, and Holter monitoring. Elderly patients should be referred for admission to a cardiologist if they have symptomatic coronary artery or valvular disease, exhibit a potentially life-threatening dysrhythmia, or have a past history of syncopal episodes.

In general, psychiatric consultation should only be considered once organic causes of vertigo have been ruled out. This can rarely if ever be accomplished in the ED. Psychiatric consultation may be considered for patients with dizziness not related to vestibular dysfunction that occurs exclusively in combination with other symptoms as part of a recognized psychiatric symptom cluster or for patients in whom dizziness appears to be amplified by psychogenic overlay. In addition, patients with SMD and other symptoms suggestive of panic disorder with or without agoraphobia should also be referred for outpatient psychiatric consultation.

REFERENCES

1. Yardley L, Luxon LM: Treating dizziness with vestibular rehabilitation. *Br Med J* 308:1252, 1994.
2. Furman JM, Jacob RG: Psychiatric dizziness. *Neurology* 48:1161, 1997.
3. Rascol O, Hain TC, Brefel C, et al: Antivertigo medications and drug-induced vertigo: A pharmacological review. *Drugs* 50:777, 1995.
4. Parnes LS, McClure J: Free-floating endolymph particles: A new operative finding during posterior semicircular canal occlusion. *Laryngoscope* 102:988, 1992.
5. Nedzelski JM, Barber HO, McIlmoyl L: Diagnoses in a dizziness unit. *J Otolaryngol* 15:101, 1986.
6. Froehling DA, Silverstein MD, Mohr DN, et al: Benign positional vertigo: Incidence and prognosis in a population-based study in Olmsted County, Minnesota. *Mayo Clin Proc* 66:596, 1991.
7. Lanska DJ, Remler B: Benign paroxysmal positioning vertigo: Classic descriptions, origins of the provocative positioning technique, and conceptual developments. *Neurology* 48:1167, 1997.
8. Hughes CA, Proctor L: Benign paroxysmal peripheral vertigo. *Laryngoscope* 107:607, 1997.
9. Headache Classification Committee of the International Headache Society: Classification and diagnostic criteria for headache disorders, cranial neuralgias and facial pain. *Cephalagia* 8:19, 1988.
10. Sixt E, Landahl S: Postural disturbances in a 75-year-old population. I: Prevalence and functional consequences. *Age Aging* 16:393-398, 1987.
11. Kapoor WN: Workup and management of patients with syncope. *Med Clin North Am* 79:1153, 1995.
12. Grubb BP, Kosinski DJ, Boehm K, Kip K: The postural orthostatic tachycardia syndrome: A neurocardiogenic variant identified during head-up tilt table testing. *Pacing Clin Electrophysiol* 20:2205, 1997.
13. Asmundson GJG, Larsen DK, Stein MB: Panic disorder and vestibular disturbance: An overview of empirical findings and clinical implications. *J Psychosom Res* 44:107, 1998.

14. Schatzberg AF, Haddad P, Kaplan EM, et al: Serotonin reuptake inhibitor discontinuation syndrome: A hypothetical definition. Discontinuation consensus panel. *J Clin Psychiatry* 58(suppl):5, 1997.
15. Ward C, Kenny RA: Reproducibility of orthostatic hypotension in symptomatic elderly. *Am J Med* 100:418, 1996.
16. Milne RJ, Heel RC: Ondansetron: therapeutic use as an antiemetic. *Drugs* 41:574, 1991.
17. Beynon GJ: A review of management of benign paroxysmal positional vertigo by exercise therapy and by repositioning maneuvers. *Br J Audiol* 31:11, 1997.
18. Epley JM: The canalith repositioning manoeuvre: For treatment of benign paroxysmal positional vertigo. *Otolaryngol Head Neck Surg* 107:399, 1992.
19. Herdman SJ, Tusa RJ: Complications of the canalith repositioning procedure. *Arch Otolaryngol Head Neck Surg* 122:281, 1996.

SEIZURES AND STATUS EPILEPTICUS IN ADULTS

Christina Catlett Viola

INTRODUCTION

A seizure is an episode of abnormal neurologic function caused by an abnormal electrical discharge of brain neurons. The seizure is the clinical attack experienced by the patient; some patients with "epileptic" electroencephalographic (EEG) discharges may not experience any clinical symptoms. Conversely, some seizure-like clinical episodes may be due to causes other than abnormal brain electrical activity; such attacks, however impressive, are not true seizures (see below).

Epilepsy is a clinical condition in which an individual is subject to recurrent seizures; it implies a more or less fixed condition of the brain responsible for the seizures. Ordinarily, the term *epileptic* is not used to refer to an individual with recurrent seizures caused by reversible conditions such as alcohol withdrawal, hypoglycemia, or other metabolic derangements.

The occurrence of one or more seizures indicates abnormal function of cerebral neurons. When this occurs in patients who are otherwise normal and in whom no evident cause for the attacks can be discerned, the seizures are referred to as *primary* or *idiopathic*. Seizures that occur as a consequence of some other identifiable neurologic condition, such as a mass lesion, are referred to as *secondary* or *symptomatic*. Any individual can have a seizure under appropriate conditions. Electrical stimulation of the brain, convulsant potentiating drugs, profound metabolic disturbances, or a sharp blow to the head may induce seizures (termed *reactive seizures*) in otherwise normal individuals. Such attacks are generally self-limited, and such persons are not considered to have a seizure disorder or epilepsy.

Seizures are very common. There are approximately 100,000 new cases diagnosed in the United States each year. An estimated 6 to 10 percent of individuals will experience at least one seizure during their lives, and 1 to 2 percent of persons are subject to recurrent seizures. Hauser and Hesdorffer[1] from the Epilepsy Foundation of America analyzed reports of incidence and prevalence of seizures and epilepsy worldwide and deduced an overall age-adjusted incidence of 30.9 to 56.8 per 100,000. Incidence rates are highest among people less than 20 years old, with a second peak in incidence in those older than 60 years, reflecting a difference in seizure etiology between these two groups. There is a slightly higher male predominance (estimated 1.1 to 1.7 greater incidence).

The mechanisms involved in generating clinical seizures appear to be multifactorial, requiring intense and prolonged neuronal electrical discharges, and failure or inhibition of normal protective mechanisms. Scars from previous insults, such as penetrating head trauma or stroke, can act as epileptogenic foci. Factors such as medical noncompliance, fever, sleep deprivation, convulsant drugs, alcohol withdrawal, and infection can lower the seizure threshold.

SEIZURE CLASSIFICATION

Many attempts have been made to provide a clinically useful classification of seizure types, both to facilitate communication among physicians and to provide a basis for treatment decisions. Formerly, seizures were identified using the terms grand mal, petit mal, and psychomotor. The International League Against Epilepsy[2] recommends dividing seizures into two major groups: *generalized seizures* and *partial seizures* (Table 224-1). When there is inadequate data to categorize the seizure, the seizure is called *unclassified.*

Generalized Seizures

Generalized seizures are thought to be caused by a nearly simultaneous activation of the entire cerebral cortex, perhaps caused by an electrical discharge originating deep in the brain and spreading outward. The attacks begin with abrupt loss of consciousness. This may be the only clinical manifestation of the seizures (as in absence attacks), or there may be a variety of motor manifestations (myoclonic jerks, tonic posturing, clonic jerking of the body and extremities, etc.).

Generalized tonic-clonic seizures (*grand mal*) are the most familiar and dramatic of the generalized seizures. They begin with abrupt loss of consciousness; there is usually no warning or aura. In a typical attack, the patient suddenly becomes rigid, trunk and extremities are extended, and the patient falls to the ground. Patients are often apneic during this period and may be deeply cyanotic. They often urinate and may vomit. As the rigid (tonic) phase subsides, there is increasing coarse trembling that evolves into a symmetrical rhythmic (clonic) jerking of the trunk and extremities. As the attack ends, the patient is left flaccid and unconscious, often with deep, rapid breathing. Typical attacks last from 60 to 90 s (occasionally longer). Bystanders generally overestimate the duration of the seizure. Consciousness returns gradually, and postictal confusion and fatigue may persist for several hours or longer.

Absence seizures (*petit mal*) are very brief, generally lasting only a few seconds. The patients suddenly lose consciousness without losing postural tone. They appear confused, detached, or withdrawn, and current activity ceases. They may stare and have twitching of their eyelids. They do not respond to voice or to other stimulation, exhibit voluntary movements, or lose continence. The attack ceases abruptly, and the patients are able to resume their previous activity with no postictal symptoms. Both the patients and witnesses may be unaware that anything has happened. Classic absence seizures are limited to school-aged children and are often attributed by parents and teachers to daydreaming or not paying attention. The attacks may be very frequent, sometimes occurring 100 or more times daily, and may result

TABLE 224-1 Classification of Seizures

Generalized seizures (consciousness always lost)
Tonic-clonic seizures (grand mal)
Absence seizures (petit mal)
Myoclonic seizures
Tonic seizures
Clonic seizures
Atonic seizures
Partial (focal) seizures
Simple partial (no alteration of consciousness)
Complex partial (consciousness impaired)
Partial seizures (simple or complex) with secondary generalization
Unclassified (due to inadequate information)

in poor school performance. Petit mal attacks may occur alone or in association with other kinds of seizures. They usually resolve as the child matures. Similar attacks in adults are more likely to be minor complex partial seizures and should not be called absence. The distinction is important, because the causes and treatment of the two seizures are quite different.

There are four less-common seizure classifications with which the clinician should be familiar. *Myoclonic seizures* are characterized by brief, "shock-like" muscular contractions that may be generalized or limited to one or more extremities. *Clonic seizures* involve repetitive clonic jerks without the tonic element. *Tonic seizures* have a prolonged, strained, contraction of the body with deviation of the head and eyes. The patient becomes pale, flushed, then cyanotic, and the body may rotate around in position. *Atonic seizures* are characterized by a sudden loss of postural tone in the head, trunk, and/or limbs, which may be associated with a brief loss of consciousness.

Partial (Focal) Seizures

Partial seizures are due to electrical discharges, which begin in a localized region of the cerebral cortex; the discharge may remain localized or may spread to involve nearby cortical regions or the entire cortex. Focal seizures are generally thought to be *secondary* seizures, their occurrence implying a localized structural lesion of the brain.

In ***simple partial focal seizures***, the seizure remains localized, and consciousness and mentation are not affected. It is possible to deduce the likely location of the initial cortical discharge from the clinical features at the onset of the attack. Unilateral tonic or clonic movements, often limited to one extremity, suggest a focus in the motor cortex, while tonic deviation of the head and eyes suggests a frontal lobe focus. Sensory hallucinations (e.g., paresthesias or numbness) suggest a discharge in the sensory cortex. Visual symptoms, especially flashing lights or distortions of vision, suggest an occipital focus. Bizarre olfactory or gustatory hallucinations suggest a focus in the medial temporal lobe. Such sensory phenomena, known as *auras*, are often the initial symptoms of attacks that then become more widespread, and that are termed *secondary generalization.*

Complex partial seizures are focal seizures in which consciousness and/or mentation *are* affected. They are often caused by a focal discharge originating in the temporal lobe and are sometimes referred to as *temporal lobe seizures.* Because of their alterations of thinking and behavior, they are occasionally called *psychomotor seizures.* As such seizures may originate from brain regions other than the temporal lobes, and to avoid any confusion with psychiatric illness, the term complex partial seizures is preferred. Often thought to be rare, they are, in fact, quite common.

Because of their frequently bizarre symptoms, complex partial seizures are commonly misdiagnosed as psychiatric problems. Their symptoms may include automatisms, visceral symptoms, hallucinations, memory disturbances, distorted perception, and affective disorders. Automatisms are typically simple, repetitive, purposeless movements such as lip smacking, fiddling with clothing or buttons, or repeating short phrases. More complex behaviors may occur, but well-organized, purposeful activity is unlikely. Visceral symptoms often consist of a sensation of "butterflys" rising up from the epigastrium. Hallucinations may be olfactory, gustatory, visual, or auditory. There may be complex distortions of visual perception, time, and memory. Affective symptoms may include intense sensations of fear, paranoia, depression, or, rarely, elation or ecstasy.

As noted, a focal seizure discharge may spread to involve both hemispheres, mimicking a typical generalized seizure. This is termed *secondary generalization.* For the purpose of classification, diagnosis, and treatment, such attacks are regarded as focal seizures. In some patients, the discharge may spread so rapidly that no focal symptoms are evident, and the correct diagnosis may depend on demonstration of the focal discharge on an EEG recording.

CLINICAL EVALUATION OF SEIZURE PATIENTS

The first step is to determine whether the attack was truly a seizure. The physician should take a detailed history and perform a careful physical. Laboratory tests, radiologic studies, and consultations may be obtained if clinically indicated.

History

A careful history of the details of the attack should be obtained from the patient, if possible, and from any bystanders who actually witnessed the attack. Only a physical description of the attack should be sought as witnesses, even physicians, may mislabel the activity or even mistake nonseizure activity as a seizure.

Important avenues of inquiry include preceding aura, abrupt or gradual onset, progression of motor activity, loss of bowel or bladder control, and whether the activity was local or generalized, symmetrical or not. Finally, the duration of the attack and any postictal confusion or lethargy should be sought. The patient should be asked whether he or she has any recollection of the attack.

Next, the clinical context in which the attack occurred should be determined. If the patient is a known epileptic, the baseline seizure pattern should be established. In patients presenting with an attack consistent with their previously documented seizures, the history should be directed toward factors that may have precipitated epileptic activity. Missed doses of antiepileptics or recent alterations in medication, including dosage change or conversion from brand name to generic formulation, may be the inciting element. Other possible factors that might provoke a seizure include sleep deprivation, alcohol withdrawal, infection, and use or cessation of other drugs.

If there is no previous history of seizures, a more detailed history is needed. Symptoms that might suggest previous unwitnessed or unrecognized seizures, such as blank or staring spells in school, involuntary movements, unexplained injuries, nocturnal tongue biting, and enuresis, may be clues to a more long-standing problem. A history of recent or remote head injury should be sought. Persistent, severe, or sudden headache should prompt a search for intracranial pathology. Concurrent pregnancy or recent delivery suggests the possibility of eclampsia. A history of metabolic derangements or electrolyte abnormalities, hypoxia, systemic illness (especially cancer), coagulopathy or anticoagulation, drug ingestion or withdrawal (licit and illicit), and alcohol use, may help identify factors that predispose patients to seizures (Table 224-2).

Physical Examination

The general physical examination should be directed toward discovering any injuries, especially head or spine, that might have resulted from the seizure. Seizures may cause injuries such as fractures, sprains, and bruises; posterior dislocations of the shoulder are common and may be overlooked. Tongue lacerations and aspiration are frequent sequelae. A search for any systemic illness that may have caused the attack should be undertaken. Temperature should be noted, and a bedside glucose determination should be obtained.

A directed neurologic examination should be performed with follow-up serial exams. Level of consciousness and mentation should be followed closely. Profound obtundation that improves steadily is likely benign; however, progressive deterioration requires prompt intervention. Signs of increased intracranial pressure should be sought. Any focal neurologic deficit should be noted. A transient focal deficit following a simple or complex focal seizure is referred to as *Todd's paralysis,* and should resolve within 48 hours.

Differential Diagnosis

Many episodic disturbances of neurologic function may be mistaken for seizures (Table 224-3). A complete review of these conditions is

TABLE 224-2 Causes of Secondary Seizures

Intracranial hemorrhage (subdural, epidural, subarachnoid, intraparenchymal)
Structural abnormalities Vascular lesion (aneurism, arteriovenous malformation) Mass lesions (primary or metastatic neoplasms) Degenerative diseases Congenital abnormalities
Trauma (recent or remote)
Infection (meningitis, encephalitis, abscess)
Metabolic disturbances Hypo- or hyperglycemia Hypo- or hypernatremia Hyperosmolar states Uremia Hepatic failure Hypocalcemia, hypomagnesemia (rare)
Toxins and drugs (many) Cocaine, lidocaine Antidepressants Theophylline Alcohol withdrawal Drug withdrawal
Eclampsia of pregnancy (may occur up to eight weeks postpartum)
Hypertensive encephalopathy
Anoxic-ischemic injury (cardiac arrest, severe hypoxemia)

too lengthy for inclusion here, but several of the more important entities should be mentioned.

Syncope usually is attended by premonitory symptoms such as dizziness, diaphoresis, nausea, and "tunnel vision." Patients often are aware that they are going to faint and can clearly describe the onset of the attacks. Cardiac syncope, however, may occur suddenly without any warning. Injury or incontinence may attend syncope; in addition, some patients may experience brief tonic-clonic activity, especially if they are prevented from falling. Recovery is usually rapid, with few or no postictal-like symptoms.

Psychogenic seizures, or *pseudoseizures,* are common and may be extremely difficult to distinguish from true seizures in the emergency department. They may occur, as well, in a patient who has a documented seizure disorder. They are psychiatric, rather than neurogenic, in origin, and are not accompanied by an alteration in brain activity. They are often associated with a conversion disorder, panic disorder, psychosis, impulse control disorder, Munchausen's syndrome, or malingering. The patients are usually female, and there may be a history of physical or sexual abuse. The diagnosis of pseudoseizures should be suspected when seizures occur regularly in response to emotional upset or when seizures only occur with witnesses present. The attacks are often very bizarre and highly variable. Patients often are able to protect themselves from noxious stimuli during the attack. Characteristic movements include side-to-side head thrashing, rhythmic pelvic thrusting, and clonic extremity motions that are alternating rather than symmetric. Incontinence and injury are uncommon, and there is usually no postictal confusion.

TABLE 224-3 Paroxysmal Disorders: Differential Diagnosis

Seizures
Syncope
Pseudoseizures
Hyperventilation syndrome
Migraines
Movement disorders
Narcolepsy/cataplexy

Accurate diagnosis of pseudoseizures may require prolonged EEG or video monitoring to demonstrate the presence of normal EEG activity during an attack. The lack of lactic acidosis, as evidenced by the presence of an anion gap acidosis on serum electrolytes drawn within 10 to 15 min of the cessation of seizure-like activity, makes generalized seizures unlikely.

Hyperventilation syndrome is common and is often misdiagnosed as a seizure disorder. A careful history will reveal the gradual onset of the attacks with shortness of breath, anxiety, and perioral numbness. Such attacks may progress to involuntary spasm of the extremities and even loss of consciousness. The episodes often are reproduced easily by asking the patient to hyperventilate.

Movement disorders, such as dystonia, chorea, myoclonic jerks, tremors, or tics, may occur in a variety of neurologic conditions. Consciousness is always preserved during these movements. Though involuntary, the movements can often be temporarily suppressed by the patient.

Migraines may be preceded by an aura similar to that seen in some partial seizures. The most common migraine aura is the scintillating scotoma. Migraines may also be accompanied by focal neurologic symptoms such as homonymous hemianopsia and hemiparesis.

Narcolepsy is characterized by brief attacks of uncontrollable daytime sleepiness. Patients are able to feel their attacks coming on and can sometimes control them with judiciously timed naps. Other symptoms of narcolepsy include vivid dreams, often at the onset of sleep or immediately upon awakening, and attacks of sleep paralysis. An associated symptom is *cataplexy,* characterized by a sudden brief loss of postural muscle tone that is often triggered by emotional upset, laughter, or crying. The patient collapses but remains fully conscious; there are no involuntary movements.

Clinical features that help to distinguish seizures from other kinds of mimicking attacks include:

1. Abrupt onset and termination. Although some focal seizures are preceded by auras that last 20 to 30 s (or more), most attacks begin abruptly. Attacks that develop over several minutes, or longer, should be regarded with suspicion. Most seizures last only one or two minutes, unless the patient is in status epilepticus.
2. Lack of recall. Except for simple partial seizures, patients usually cannot recall the details of an attack, the responses and acts of bystanders, and so forth.
3. Movements or behavior during the attack generally are purposeless or inappropriate. Rare exceptions have been described.
4. Most seizures, except for simple absence attacks (petit mal) or simple partial seizures, are followed by a period of postictal confusion and lethargy.

Although a clinical diagnosis of seizures often can be made with a high degree of certainty, there are occasions when the presentation is not convincing. In such cases, it is better to admit uncertainty and provide follow-up for exact diagnosis, not to use the term seizure, or to begin inappropriate and potentially hazardous treatment. Multiple EEG recordings, prolonged EEG monitoring, and neurologic evaluation may be necessary.

Laboratory Examination

The need for laboratory studies must be assessed on an individual basis. In a patient with a well-documented seizure disorder who has had a single unprovoked seizure, the only test that may be needed is an anticonvulsant level.

In the case of a patient with a first seizure or when the history is unclear, more extensive studies may be helpful. A serum glucose should be obtained, and serum electrolytes, blood urea nitrogen (BUN), and creatinine, calcium, and magnesium, a pregnancy test, and a toxicology screen may be indicated depending on the clinical context. If the patient's urine is positive for hemoglobin, but there are no red cells in the urine, a CPK should be done to rule out rhabdomyolysis.

The patient should demonstrate a wide anion gap metabolic (lactic) acidosis following a major seizure, which should correct spontaneously within one hour.[3] The majority will clear within 30 min. If the diagnosis is in doubt, serum lactate can be drawn within 15 min of the episode. The blood prolactin level may also be elevated for a brief period (15 to 60 min) immediately following a seizure and may be helpful in distinguishing a true seizure from a pseudoseizure;[4] a normal prolactin level, however, is not helpful.

The presence of anticonvulsant drugs in the blood of a patient from whom no history is available suggests (but does not prove) the presence of a seizure disorder. Anticonvulsant drug levels must be interpreted with caution, as the time the last dose was taken needs to be known to properly interpret levels. The usual therapeutic and toxic levels indicated in laboratory reports are helpful only as rough guides. The therapeutic level of a drug is that level that provides adequate seizure control without unacceptable side effects. A phenytoin level of 15 mg/mL may be toxic in a given patient; conversely, a phenytoin level of 24 mg/mL may result in excellent seizure control and be well tolerated. A marked change in previously stable drug levels may indicate noncompliance, a change in medication (e.g., from one brand name or generic to another), malabsorption of a drug (as in severe diarrhea or vomiting), or ingestion of a potentiating or competing drug.

Radiographic Studies

The issue of neuroimaging following seizures remains controversial. In 1996, the American College of Emergency Physicians (ACEP)[5] in conjunction with a panel of neurologists, neurosurgeons, and neuroradiologists, developed a practice parameter outlining the role and timing of neuroimaging following seizures. In patients with a febrile seizure or seizure typical of their documented epilepsy, radiographic studies usually are not indicated. However, for patients with a first seizure or a change in their established seizure pattern, CT scanning of the head is appropriate to identify a structural lesion. Table 224-4 lists guidelines for emergent CT scanning following a seizure. Noncontrast CT is an appropriate screening tool.[6]

If the patient does not meet the above criteria, has recovered from the seizure, and no metabolic cause for the seizure has been identified, a head CT may be obtained later as part of the disposition in conjunction with follow up with a neurologist.

TABLE 224-4 ACEP Recommendations for Obtaining Emergent Neuroimaging Following a Seizure[5]

New focal deficits
Persistent altered mental status
Recent head trauma
Fever
Anticoagulation therapy
Known or suspected HIV-positive
History of cancer
Persistent or severe headache
Change in seizure pattern

Because many important processes, such as metastatic or primary tumors or vascular anomalies, may not be evident on noncontrast studies, a follow-up enhanced CT or MRI may be arranged. MRI is more sensitive than CT in detecting subtle alterations of brain structure and is often the study of choice in the evaluation of patients with seizures. In patients with uncomplicated first seizures, it is reasonable to omit the CT scan and obtain an MRI instead. Consultation with a neurologist or radiologist may be helpful in choosing the best approach and avoiding unnecessary examinations.

Other radiographic studies may be indicated in some cases. Radiographs of the cervical spine or neck should be obtained if there is suspicion for head trauma. Chest x-rays may reveal primary or metastatic tumors. There may be evidence of aspiration, although related radiographic findings are usually delayed. Skull x-rays are generally not indicated. Special examinations, such as angiography, are rarely part of the emergency department evaluation.

ELECTROENCEPHALOGRAPHY

While EEG may be very helpful, it is not readily available in most emergency departments. Emergency EEG can be considered in the evaluation of a patient with persistent, unexplained, altered mental status to rule out nonconvulsive status epilepticus; to evaluate a paroxysmal attack when a seizure is suspected; or in status epilepticus to detect ongoing seizures after paralysis for intubation, or induction of general anesthesia.[7]

In the outpatient setting, the EEG may be used to distinguish generalized from focal seizures and to identify specific epileptic syndromes. The diagnostic yield of EEG recordings can be increased by appropriate patient preparation (especially sleep deprivation) or by activation techniques such as hyperventilation, photic stimulation, and sleep recordings. More elaborate examinations, such as 24-h recordings or video-EEG recordings, may also be used. Consultation with a neurologist ensures that the appropriate studies are chosen.

TREATMENT

Certain general measures should be taken for any seizure patient. A patent airway must be assured and vital signs should stabilized. Initial interventions should include an IV, oxygen, pulse oximetry, bedside glucose determination, and a cardiac monitor, if warranted. Intubation should be considered for prolonged seizures, persons that require GI decontamination, and patients who may need to be transferred offsite. In and of themselves, simple seizures do not usually warrant intubation. Standard measures for management of any unconscious patient should be employed. The likelihood of trauma should be assessed. Care should be taken to identify and treat any underlying metabolic disorder.

The first objective is to make an accurate diagnosis; only in patients with status epilepticus is it necessary to initiate specific treatment before diagnostic evaluation has been completed.

Specific management is reviewed of these four clinical situations: the patient who is actively seizing; the patient with previous epilepsy who has a seizure; the patient with a first seizure; and status epilepticus.

The Active Seizure

There is little to be done during the course of an actual seizure other than to protect the patient from injury. Gentle but firm restraint should be used to prevent falls. If possible, the patient should be turned to one side to reduce the risk of aspiration. It is usually not possible to insert a bite block between the teeth without using considerable force and risking damage to teeth. If a bite block is used, be certain that it cannot be aspirated or swallowed. It is usually not necessary or even possible to ventilate a patient effectively during a seizure, but once the attack subsides, ensure a clear airway. Suction and airway adjuncts should be readily available. There is no indication for intravenous anticonvulsant medications during the course of an uncomplicated seizure. Expectant treatment is best. Seizure activity should be observed to determine if it is focal. Unnecessary sedation at this point will complicate evaluation and result in a prolonged decrease in level of consciousness. Seizures that fail to abate are considered status epilepticus (see below).

Patients with Previous Seizures

Proper management of a patient with a well-documented seizure disorder who presents after one or more seizures depends on the particular circumstance of the case. Potential precipitants that may lower seizure threshold should be sought. Many such seizures occur because of failure to take anticonvulsant medication as prescribed. Some anticonvulsants have short serum half-lives (Table 224-5), and missing even a single dose may result in a sharp drop in serum levels.

If anticonvulsant levels are very low, supplemental doses may be given and the patient restarted on his or her regular regimen. Without a loading dose, the patient may not achieve anticonvulsant effects for two days to three weeks (see Table 224-5). An oral loading-dose of phenytoin (usually 18 mg/kg po, that is often divided into 3 doses given q2h) will achieve therapeutic serum concentrations in 2 to 24 h. Alternatively, the same loading dose of IV phenytoin (no faster than 50 mg/min) achieves anticonvulsant effects in 1 to 2 h. Carbamazepine can be loaded using the oral suspension at a dose of 8 mg/kg.

If anticonvulsant levels are adequate and the patient has had a single attack, specific treatment may not be needed if the pattern and frequency of occurrence falls within the expected range for the patient. Even well-controlled patients may have occasional breakthrough seizures. Any precipitants that have lowered the seizure threshold should be identified. If there has been a recent change in the frequency or pattern of breakthrough seizures, a change in, or adjustment of, medication may be needed. These include factors such as infection, sleep deprivation, stress, or injury. The primary care physician or neurologist should make this decision. If a medication's maintenance dose is increased, only very small increments should be made, and follow-up within one to three days should be provided, because even small dose changes may result in dramatic increases in serum levels. If the problem is noncompliance or missed medication, the patient's primary care physician or neurologist should be made aware of the situation and participate in decision making.

TABLE 224-5 Properties of Commonly Used Anticonvulsant Drugs

Drug	Oral Dose, mg/day*	Therapeutic Level, μg/mL†	Days to Reach Steady State‡	Serum Half-life, h
Phenytoin	300–600	10–20	5–10	7–42
Carbamazepine	400–1200	3–14	2–4	12–17
Phenobarbital	100–300	10–40	14–21	48–144
Primidone	750–2000	5–12	4–7	10–21
Valproic acid	750–2000	50–150	2–4	12–18
Ethosuximide	500–1500	40–100	5–10	40–60
Clonazepam	1.5–20	20–80	?	19–39

*Average therapeutic dose. Initiation dosing may be different. Daily dose must be individualized for each patient. Drug-drug interactions may dramatically change daily doses in patients receiving multiple drugs.
†See text for definition of therapeutic and toxic levels.
‡Indicates time required to establish stable serum levels after any change in dose.
Information obtained from McEvoy GK (ed): *American Hospital Formulary Service Drug Information.* Bethesda, MD, Society of Health-Systems Pharmacists, 1998.

The Patient with a First Seizure

There has been considerable controversy about the appropriate management of a patient who has experienced an apparent first seizure. The decision to begin outpatient treatment with antiepileptics depends on the risk of recurrent seizures weighed against the risk/benefit ratio of anticonvulsant therapy. Until recently, reliable data on these questions have been unavailable. Previous studies have suggested rates of recurrence ranging from 23 to 71 percent. Some studies have found no benefit from treatment, while others have reported a 50 percent reduction in the risk of recurrence.

A careful analysis[8] found that in patients with an apparent first seizure, the most important predictors of the risk of recurrence were the etiology of the seizure and the results of the EEG. In patients with idiopathic seizures and a normal neurologic exam, the risk of a recurrent seizure within two years was 24 percent if the EEG was normal and 48 percent if the EEG was abnormal. In patients with previous neurologic injury or illness or an abnormal neurologic exam, the risk was 48 percent if the EEG was normal, and 65 percent if the EEG was abnormal. Neither family history, age, sex, nor the presence of status epilepticus at the time of the first seizure was a strong predictor of the risk of recurrence. Unfortunately, EEG results are often not available to the emergency physician who must make a treatment decision.

A randomized multicenter clinical trial of 397 patients demonstrated that treatment of first unprovoked seizures appears to reduce the risk of recurrent seizures from 51 to 25 percent during two years of follow-up.[9] Given these two studies, some general recommendations can be made. Patients with secondary seizures due to an identifiable neurologic condition should generally be treated, as their risk of recurrence is quite high (48 to 65 percent). In patients with idiopathic seizures, the decision is less clear. Their risk of recurrence may be as low as 24 percent if the EEG is normal. Given the expense, inconvenience, and potential side effects of treatment, some patients may wish to defer a decision about treatment until an EEG and neurologic consultation are obtained. In these patients, the only realistic approach is a full discussion of the risks and benefits of treatment. Often, a decision need not be made in the emergency department and patients can be referred to their regular physicians within one week for further evaluation and management.

The ideal antiepileptic regimen is a single-drug therapy that controls seizures with minimum toxicity. If treatment is initiated, drug selection is based on the type of seizure (Table 224-6). For generalized tonic-clonic or focal seizures, either phenytoin or carbamazepine would be an appropriate choice for most adults (see above for loading information), both drugs are equally as efficacious and have similar side effect profiles. Valproate, phenobarbital, and primidone may also be used. For absence seizures, ethosuximide or valproate may be used (see Table 224-5 for dosing). Gabapentin (900 mg to 1.8 g daily) and lamotrigine (300 to 500 mg daily) are newly approved drugs useful as adjunctive therapy.

Determining Need for Consultation and Admission

ACEP guidelines[6] recommend *neurologic consultation* for patients with first-time seizures, seizures with persistent altered mental status, new focal neurologic deficits, and new intracranial lesions (Table 224-7). Pregnant patients and those with a marked change in seizure pattern

TABLE 224-6 Anticonvulsant Drugs: Indications

Seizure Category	Drug of Choice	Alternatives
I. Generalized seizures		
Tonic-clonic seizures:	Carbamazepine Phenytoin Valproic acid	Phenobarbital Primidone
Absence seizures:	Ethosuximide Valproic acid	Clonazepam
Myoclonic seizures:	Valproic acid	Clonazepam
Atonic seizures	Valproic acid	Clonazepam *Felbamate
II. Partial seizures: (simple or complex, with or without generalization)	Carbamazepine Phenytoin Valproic acid	Phenobarbital Primidone *Gabapentin *Lamotrigine

*Adjunctive therapy.

TABLE 224-8 ACEP Guidelines for Hospital Admission of Patients with New-Onset Seizure[6]

Persistent altered mental status
CNS infection
New intracranial lesion
Underlying correctable medical problem Significant hypoxia Hypoglycemia Hyponatremia Dysrhythmia Significant alcohol withdrawal
Acute head trauma
Status epilepticus
Eclampsia

or poorly controlled seizures may also warrant consultation. *Hospital admission* is recommended for patients with persistently altered mental status, and for patients with seizures due to CNS infections, new intracranial lesions, or clinically significant hypoxia, hypoglycemia, hyponatremia, or dysrhythmias (Table 224-8). Patients with status epilepticus or seizures in the setting of eclampsia or head trauma should also be admitted. Alcohol or drug-related seizures do not necessarily require admission, although detoxification or withdrawal should be addressed.

Disposition

There are no evidence-based rules for how long a patient must be observed prior to discharge. Some clinicians discharge patients with nontherapeutic anticonvulsant levels after administration of a loading dose of an anticonvulsant, if vital signs are normal and the mental status is at baseline. As previously discussed, therapeutic serum concentrations can be achieved as early as one hour after IV-loading of phenytoin. Patients given oral loading doses should be warned of continued risk for seizures until anticonvulsant effect has been achieved. If possible, the patient should be discharged with a reliable family member or friend, with imperative medical follow-up arranged in a week.

Patients should be instructed to take precautions to minimize the risks for injury from further seizures. Swimming should be avoided. Working with hazardous tools or machines and working at heights should be avoided. The emergency physician should be familiar with driving regulations and reporting requirements, which vary from state to state. Regardless of local laws, it is prudent to advise patients against driving and other hazardous activity until they have stabilized and have been seen in follow-up. The emergency department record should reflect the precise instructions given to the patient.

TABLE 224-7 ACEP Guidelines for Obtaining Neurology Consultation[6]

New onset seizures
Focal neurologic exam
Persistent altered mental status
New intracranial lesion
Marked change in seizure pattern
Poorly controlled seizures
Pregnant patient

SPECIAL CONSIDERATIONS

Seizures in the HIV-Positive Patient

Seizures are a common manifestation of CNS disease in patients infected with HIV, although the etiology of seizures in this population differs somewhat from immunocompetent patients (Table 224-9). Mass lesions, HIV encephalopathy, and meningitis are seen more frequently.[10,11] The most common mass lesion is caused by toxoplasmosis, followed by lymphoma. Cryptococcal, bacterial, or aseptic meningitis, or encephalitis due to herpes simplex, varicella zoster, or cytomegalovirus may cause seizures. HIV encephalopathy or AIDS dementia complex is an under-recognized etiology of seizures for HIV-infected patients. Other etiologies to consider are progressive multifocal leukoencephalopathy, CNS tuberculosis, and neurosyphilis.

While the evaluation of seizures in HIV-positive patients should include a search for metabolic or toxicologic causes, the high incidence of space-occupying lesions mandates a thorough ED evaluation. If no space-occupying lesion is identified on noncontrast head CT scan, and there is no evidence of increased intracranial pressure, a lumbar puncture should be performed to rule out meningitis. Finally, if the initial head CT scan is negative or no other explanation for seizures

TABLE 224-9 Causes of Seizures in the HIV Patient

Mass lesion Toxoplasmosis Lymphoma
Meningitis/Encephalitis Cryptococcal Bacterial/aseptic Herpes zoster Cytomegalovirus
HIV encephalopathy/AIDS dementia complex
Progressive multifocal leukoencephalopathy
CNS tuberculosis
Neurosyphilis

is found, a contrast-enhanced head CT or an MRI may be obtained in the ED, or arranged by the primary physician as part of the disposition. Some HIV patients will have no discernible cause for seizures after a thorough evaluation, particularly if the neurologic examination in the interictal period is normal.

Treatment of the first-time seizure in the HIV patient is controversial. Most authorities recommend treatment with phenytoin or phenobarbital because the seizure recurrence rate in this population is high, but there is a 10 percent incidence of hypersensitivity reactions to phenytoin in patients with HIV.

Seizures in Pregnancy

The management of seizures during pregnancy requires a multidisciplinary approach. Antiepileptic drugs have been associated with neural tube defects, fetal facial dysmorphism, cleft lip and palate, heart defects, and digital defects. Despite the potentially teratogenic effects of anticonvulsants, the risks of uncontrolled seizures to the mother and fetus warrant continuation of seizure medications in the known epileptic during pregnancy. Ideally, counseling of the mother regarding risks and benefits should begin prior to conception.

Efforts can be made to reduce the risk to the fetus. For example, single-drug regimens are preferred to multidrug regimens, dosing can be split to avoid high peak levels of drugs, and supplementation of folic acid and vitamin K may be given to reduce the risk of neural tube defects and neonatal hemorrhage. Compliance can be a problem during pregnancy, often due to the mother's concern for drug toxicity.

Initial evaluation of a pregnant woman with a seizure is generally as discussed above, with some important distinctions. An obstetrical evaluation is needed to determine gestational age and fetal well-being. Since pregnancy is a hypercoagulable state, stroke as an etiology for the seizure should be considered. Head CT scan may be performed with lead shielding of the abdomen. MRI is also considered safe in pregnancy, although this has not been well studied.

When a woman beyond 20 weeks of gestation develops seizures in the setting of hypertension, edema, and proteinuria, her condition is referred to as *eclampsia.* Attention should be paid to signs and symptoms associated with eclampsia such as headache, blurry vision, confusion, hyperreflexia, and epigastric pain. Rarely, eclampsia may occur up to eight weeks postpartum.

The decision to initiate treatment for a first-time seizure in a pregnant female is complex and should involve the obstetrician and neurologist. The emergency physician should not make definitive treatment decisions alone. There are many factors involved, including cause and type of seizure, risk of recurrence, and gestational age of the fetus.

Although a healthy fetus should tolerate a single generalized seizure, there are two situations, eclampsia and status epilepticus, which can be life-threatening to both the mother and the fetus. Although not an anticonvulsant per se, magnesium sulfate (4 to 6 g IV followed by 1 to 2 g/h IV drip) has been used to treat eclampsia with good results since 1925. An international multicenter, randomized, clinical trial involving 1687 eclamptic women compared magnesium sulfate to diazepam and phenytoin. The study demonstrated a 52 percent lower risk of recurrence of seizures in women allocated magnesium sulfate rather than diazepam. Furthermore, the women allocated magnesium sulfate had a 67 percent lower risk of recurrence than those given phenytoin. The women administered magnesium sulfate also had a lower incidence of pneumonia, ICU admission, and assisted ventilation than those administered phenytoin.[12] A review of randomized, controlled trials of eclamptic women derived a seizure recurrence rate following phenytoin of 23.1 percent, whereas the recurrence rate following magnesium sulfate was 9.4 percent.[13] The definitive treatment of eclampsia is delivery of the fetus. This topic is discussed in greater detail in Chap. 101.

Status epilepticus may occur in both epileptics and nonepileptics. Treatment should proceed as for any nonpregnant patient, but should include fetal monitoring as well as assistance from an obstetrician and neonatologist if delivery is a possibility. Lorazepam and diazepam are the two benzodiazepines of choice; phenytoin or phenobarbital may be used as second-line choices (see Fig. 224-1 for doses). EEG should be used to confirm seizure cessation. Because both the seizure and the treatments can cause respiratory depression or hypotension, close monitoring is necessary.

	Time Frame
Establish/maintain airway ↓ IV, oxygen, monitor ↓	
Dextrose 25–50 g IV if indicated	0–5 min
↓ Consider Thiamine 100 mg IV and Magnesium 1–2 g IV for alcoholic or malnourished patients ↓ Lorazepam 2 mg/min IV up to 0.1 mg/kg (*or* diazepam 5 mg IV q5 min up to 20 mg) ↓	10–20 min
Phenytoin 20 mg/kg IV at 50 mg/min *or* fosphenytoin 20 mg/kg PE IV at 150 mg/min ↓ Additional phenytoin 5–10 mg/kg IV *or* additional fosphenytoin 5–10 mg/kg PE IV ↓ Phenobarbital up to 20 mg/kg IV at 50–75 mg/min IV ↓	
Additional phenobarbital 5–10 mg/kg IV	30 min
↓ General anesthesia with Midazolam 0.2 mg/kg slow IVP then 0.75–10 μg/kg/min *or* propofol 1–2 mg/kg IV then 1–15 mg/kg/h *or* pentobarbital 10–15 mg/kg IV over 1 h then 0.5–1.0 mg/kg/h	

FIG. 224-1. Guidelines for management of status epilepticus. (Adapted from Lowenstein and Alldredge.[14])

Seizures in the Alcohol Abuser

Seizures and alcohol are associated through missed doses of medication; sleep deprivation as an epileptogenic trigger; propensity for head injury; toxic coingestions; electrolyte abnormalities; alcohol withdrawal seizures; and alcohol-related seizures. *Alcohol-related seizures* are precipitated by alcohol intake.

The *alcohol withdrawal syndrome* involves a spectrum of symptoms that follow reduction or cessation of alcohol. Minor symptoms of alcohol withdrawal, which can begin within 24 h of cessation of drinking, include tremulousness, nausea, anxiety, tachycardia, hypertension, and insomnia. When autonomic hyperactivity becomes more pronounced, disorientation, visual hallucinations, paranoid ideation, or delirium may occur, in the symptom complex of *delirium tremens.*

Classic *alcohol withdrawal seizures* usually occur within 6 to 48 h after reduction or cessation of alcohol, but may occur up to 1 week later. The seizures are generalized, and the interval EEG is usually normal. There may be several seizures occurring over several hours.

The alcohol-abusing patient with a first seizure should be evaluated and treated as any patient with a first-time seizure (see previous discussion), with additional evaluation for toxic-metabolic abnormalities, and intracranial bleeding. For suspected head injury, focal findings on neurologic exam, deteriorating mental status, or prolonged postictal state, head CT scan is needed. Cervical spine precautions should be taken as appropriate.

Most authorities agree that patients with alcohol withdrawal seizures usually do not require chronic anticonvulsant therapy. Acute or chronic treatment with phenytoin is neither necessary nor effective.[15]

Use of benzodiazepines such as chlordiazepoxide, diazepam, oxazepam, and lorazepam, in doses sufficient to manage withdrawal will usually afford adequate protection from acute seizures. The exception is withdrawal that is complicated by status epilepticus, which requires prompt treatment. Patients with epilepsy exacerbated by alcohol withdrawal should be managed as any other seizure patient with recurrent seizures.

If the clinical presentation and evaluation are consistent with alcohol withdrawal seizures, and the patient remains stable and seizure-free for several hours, the patient may be discharged and referred for detoxification. Outpatient detoxification with a benzodiazepine regimen is most appropriate for patients with mild to moderate withdrawal symptoms, no significant medical or psychiatric problems, no concurrent drug use, and no history of DTs. Patients with more than two seizures should be admitted.

STATUS EPILEPTICUS

There are an estimated 100,000 to 150,000 cases of status epilepticus per year in the United States, with 55,000 deaths. In 12 to 30 percent of these, status is the first epileptic event.[14,16] Estimations of acute mortality range from 1 to 10 percent.

Status epilepticus is defined as either continuous seizure activity 30 min or more, or two or more seizures that occur without full recovery of consciousness between the attacks. It remains unclear how long a seizure can occur before permanent neurologic sequelae ensue. Although this question has never been satisfactorily answered, it does appear that permanent CNS injury is more likely to occur the longer seizures are allowed to progress.[17,18] Thus treatment should be initiated as soon as possible in all patients with continuous seizure activity lasting more than 10 min. The longer the seizure is allowed to continue the more difficult it will be to control.[19]

The diagnosis of status epilepticus is usually obvious in patients with continuous tonic-clonic movements. However, convulsive activity may gradually lessen over time or with partial treatment, giving the impression that the seizures have been controlled, with continued subtle signs such as nystagmus, or twitching of the face, hands, or feet. Correct diagnosis requires a high index of suspicion, a perceptive physician, and sometimes an EEG. Any type of seizure may occur continuously or in rapid succession, fulfilling the criteria for status epilepticus. *Epilepsia partialis continua* is repeated partial seizures without loss of consciousness and often with one's ability to follow simple commands retained. Altered mentation, diminished responsiveness, confusion, amnesia, or dream-like states without motor symptoms suggest continuous absence seizures.

Treatment

The goal of treatment of convulsive status epilepticus and epilepsia partialis continua is seizure control within 30 min of presentation (Fig. 224-1). Morbidity is due hypoxemia, hyperthermia, circulatory collapse, and eventual neuronal injury.

A brief history and physical examination should be directed toward discovery of the cause of the seizures and to any injury that may have resulted. Any of the causes of seizures (see Table 224-2) may result in status epilepticus; in many patients, no specific etiology is found.

A large-bore IV line should be established and a bedside glucose determination made. Use of an IV fluid without glucose will facilitate administration of anticonvulsant drugs (glucose is not compatible with phenytoin). The patient should be placed on oxygen, a cardiac monitor, and pulse oximeter.

Despite periods of apnea and cyanosis, which can occur during seizure activity, most patients can be maintained on nasal cannula or oxygen mask with a nasopharyngeal device if the gag reflex and airway are intact. Endotracheal intubation should be performed if there is any concern about the adequacy of ventilation or safety of the airway. Many prefer orotracheal intubation because the patient is likely to undergo diagnostic imaging and may require procedures. If a paralytic agent is used to assist with intubation, a short-acting agent, such as vecuronium, should be used as the physician will be unable to monitor ongoing seizure activity during the period of paralysis.

Initial laboratory evaluation should include blood glucose, metabolic panel including calcium and magnesium, and, if appropriate, a pregnancy test, a toxicology screen, and anticonvulsant levels.

Thiamine (100 mg) and glucose (25 to 50 g) should be given IV if hypoglycemia is suspected or confirmed. There is no benefit to giving additional glucose to normoglycemic patients. Rectal temperature should be monitored, and hyperthermia should be treated with passive cooling. A Foley catheter should be placed to monitor urine output and a nasogastric tube to minimize aspiration.

If ingestion is suspected as the cause of seizures, GI decontamination should ensue. Emergency lumbar puncture should not be attempted during status epilepticus. If bacterial meningitis is suspected, empiric antibiotic therapy should be started. Status epilepticus can induce a brief peripheral leukocytosis as well as a mild CSF pleocytosis. Radiographic studies (such as a CT scan) will usually need to be delayed until the seizures are controlled.

Anticonvulsant Drugs in Status Epilepticus

The drugs most often used in the therapy of status epilepticus are the benzodiazepines (diazepam or lorazepam), phenytoin or fosphenytoin, and phenobarbital (Fig. 224-1).

Benzodiazepines are used in patients with continuous or very frequent seizures to temporarily control the seizures until more specific agents can be given. A double-blind, randomized, controlled study of IV lorazepam (4 to 8 mg) and IV diazepam (10 to 20 mg) demonstrated equal efficacy in controlling status epilepticus.[20] Although diazepam has a slightly faster onset than lorazepam (2 min vs. 3 min), lorazepam has a significantly longer duration of action (12 to 24 h) as compared to diazepam (15 to 30 min), and is considered the agent of choice. Lorazepam is also more effective than phenytoin or phenobarbital as the initial drug.[21] Respiratory depression and hypotension may occur when benzodiazepines are used, especially in young children and in patients who have taken alcohol, barbiturates, narcotics, or other sedatives. Although diazepam enters the brain readily, it is redistributed quickly to fatty tissues, so serum concentrations fall rapidly. Therefore, a longer-acting agent such as phenytoin should follow diazepam.

Phenytoin is the most important drug used in the management of status epilepticus. It may be given immediately after a benzodiazepine or may be used as primary therapy in patients whose seizures are less frequent. The recommended loading dose is 18 to 20 mg/kg IV; note that doses well in excess of the usual 1000 mg are required for many adults. A smaller loading dose (15 mg/kg) may be used in the elderly, but the loading dose is not reduced in patients with renal or hepatic disease. Due to the myocardial depression and the effects of ethylene glycol, the diluent, phenytoin should be infused at a rate not greater than 50 mg/min; a rate of 25 mg/min is safer in the elderly. Phenytoin should not be mixed with any glucose-containing IV fluid and should not be given intramuscularly due to erratic absorption. The drug is contraindicated in the presence of second- or third-degree AV block, or during a MI or CHF. Adverse effects include significant infusion-site reactions, hypotension, and cardiac dysrhythmias, so continuous cardiac monitoring is needed. If side effects develop, the infusion should be stopped and may be restarted at a lower rate when the side effects have resolved; in some cases, patients are unable to tolerate the drug.

Fosphenytoin is a water-soluble pro-drug of phenytoin that is rapidly converted to phenytoin in the plasma. In status epilepticus, fosphenytoin has similar time of onset, effectiveness, and cardiac effects as phenytoin. Its advantages include fewer infusion-site reactions due to the lack of propylene glycol and ethanol as the diluents. Secondly, fosphenytoin may be infused at a faster rate. Fosphenytoin dosing is expressed as ''phenytoin equivalents (PE)'' to prevent confusion. The loading dose is 15 to 20 mg PE per kg, which can be infused at 100 to 150 mg PE per minute. Unlike phenytoin, fosphenytoin can be given intramuscularly, which is useful if the patient is not in status epilepticus. The only apparent drawback is the cost. Fosphenytoin can cost 10 to 60 times more than phenytoin.

Phenobarbital (up to 20 mg/kg IV) is usually used as a second-line drug in patients who are unable to tolerate phenytoin or in patients whose seizures are not controlled despite full loading doses of benzodiazepines and phenytoin. Respiratory depression and hypotension are common, especially at higher doses or when diazepam or lorazepam is also given. Because of very slow elimination, large doses of phenobarbital may result in prolonged obtundation.

In a few patients, seizure control is not obtained with these regimens and further treatment is needed.

Refractory Status Epilepticus

The standard regimens of benzodiazepines, phenytoin, and phenobarbital suffice to control status epilepticus within 30 min of presentation in most patients. In a few cases (generally patients with structural lesions or CNS infections), seizures continue even after such treatment. Various approaches have been advocated, including IV infusions of midazolam, propofol, or barbiturates to induce anesthesia (see Fig. 224-1). These modalities are best used in an intensive care setting, as advanced respiratory and cardiovascular support, as well as continuous EEG and invasive hemodynamic monitoring, may be needed. Consultation from an anesthesiologist and neurologist should be obtained.

Anesthesia may be induced to treat refractory status epilepticus by administering infusions of midazolam or propofol for 12 to 24 h.[22–25] General anesthesia may also be obtained with IV barbiturates such as thiopental and pentobarbital. Midazolam and propofol have the advantage over barbiturates of having a short half-life and rapid clearance, allowing for earlier extubation and earlier clinical assessment; midazolam also causes less hypotension.

Neuromuscular blocking agents (usually pancuronium or vecuronium) are sometimes helpful. These drugs will abolish tonic-clonic movements and may facilitate ventilation and other measures; they have no effect on abnormal neuronal activity. EEG monitoring is necessary to assess the effectiveness of anticonvulsant therapy when neuromuscular blockers are utilized.

REFERENCES

1. Hauser WA, Hesdorffer DC: *Epilepsy Frequency, Causes and Consequences.* New York, Demos, 1990.
2. Commission on Classification and Terminology of the International League against Epilepsy: Proposal for revised clinical and electroencephalographic classification of epileptic seizures. *Epilepsia* 22:489, 1981.
3. Orringer LE, Eustace JC, Wunsch CD, Gardner LB: Natural history of lactic acidosis after grand mal seizures; A model for the study of an anion gap acidosis not associated with hyperkalemia. *N Engl J Med* 297:796, 1977.
4. Rao ML, Stefan H, Bauer BJ: Epileptic but not psychogenic seizures are accompanied by simultaneous elevation of serum pituitary hormones and cortisol levels. *Neuroendocrinology* 49:33, 1989.
5. American College of Emergency Physicians, American Academy of Neurology, American Association of Neurologic Surgeons, and American Society of Neurology. Practice parameter: Neuroimaging in the emergency patient presenting with seizure (summary statement). *Ann Emerg Med* 28:114, 1996.
6. American College of Emergency Physicians: Clinical policy for the initial approach to patients presenting with a chief complaint of seizure who are not in status epilepticus. *Ann Emerg Med* 29(5):706, 1997.
7. Privitera MC, Strawsburg RH: Electroencephalographic monitoring in the emergency department. *Emerg Med Clin North Am* 12:1089, 1994.
8. Berg AT, Shinnar S: The risk of seizure recurrence following a first unprovoked seizure: A quantitative review. *Neurology* 41:965, 1991.
9. First Seizure Trial Group: A randomized clinical trial on the efficacy of antiepileptic drugs in reducing the risk of relapse after a first unprovoked tonic-clonic seizure. *Neurology* 43:478, 1993.
10. Holtzman DM, Kaku DA, So YT: New-onset seizures associated with human immunodeficiency virus infection: Causation and clinical features in 100 cases. *Am J Med* 87:173, 1989.
11. Pesola GR, Westfal RE: New-onset generalized seizures in patients with AIDS presenting to an emergency department. *Acad Emerg Med* 5(9): 905, 1998.
12. The Eclampsia Trial Collaborative Group: Which anticonvulsant for women with eclampsia? Evidence from the Collaborative Eclampsia Trial. *Lancet* 345:1455, 1995.
13. Witlin AG, Sibai BM: Magnesium sulfate therapy in preeclampsia and eclampsia. *Obstet Gynecol* 92(5):883, 1998.
14. Lowenstein DH, Alldredge BK: Status epilepticus. *N Engl J Med* 338(14):970, 1998.
15. Rathler NK, D'Onofrio G, Fish SS, et al: The lack of efficacy of phenytoin in the prevention of alcohol-related seizures. *Ann Emerg Med* 23:513, 1994.
16. Hauser WA: Status epilepticus: Epidemiologic considerations. *Neurology* 40(suppl 2):9, 1990.
17. Meldrum BS, Brierley JB: Prolonged epileptic seizures in primates, ischemic cell change and its relation to ictal physiological events. *Arch Neurol* 28:10, 1973.
18. Bleck TP: Convulsive disorders: Status epilepticus. *Clin Neuropharmacol* 14(3):191, 1991.
19. Lothman E: The biochemical basis and pathophysiology of status epilepticus. *Neurology* 40(suppl 2):13, 1990.
20. Leppik IE, Derivan AT, Homan RW, et al: Double-blind study of lorazepam and diazepam in status epilepticus. *JAMA* 249:1452, 1983.
21. Treiman DM, Meyers PD, Walton NY, et al: A comparison of Four treatments for generalized convulsive status epilepticus. *N Engl J Med* 339:792, 1998.
22. Kumar A, Bleck TP: Intravenous midazolam for the treatment of refractory status epilepticus. *Crit Care Med* 20(4):483, 1992.
23. Parent JM, Lowenstein DH: Treatment of refractory generalized status epilepticus with continuous infusion of midazolam. *Neurology* 44:1837, 1994.
24. Stecker MM, Kramer TH, Raps EC, et al: Treatment of refractory status epilepticus with propofol: clinical and pharmacokinetic findings. *Epilepsia* 39(1):18, 1998.
25. Dichter MA, Brodie MJ: New antiepileptic drugs. *N Engl J Med* 334:1583, 1996.

ACUTE PERIPHERAL NEUROLOGIC LESIONS

Michael M. Wang

When confronted with a patient with neurologic complaints, one should first localize the problem anatomically based on the history and physical examination. In the process of localization, one of the initial distinctions that should be made is whether the pathologic process involves the peripheral or central nervous system. Sometimes the distinction is not clear. The purpose of this chapter is to focus on the diagnosis of peripheral nervous system disease and to discuss the approach and management in the emergency setting. Myasthenia gravis is discussed in Chap. 226.

HALLMARKS OF PERIPHERAL NERVOUS SYSTEM DISORDERS

The peripheral nervous system serves sensory, motor, and autonomic functions. The patient with a peripheral nerve problem thus may have symptoms reflecting disorder of any or a combination of these functions. Sensory symptoms may include numbness, tingling, dysesthesias, pain, and ataxia due to proprioceptive dysfunction. Motor symptoms are predominantly weakness. Autonomic disability can include orthostatic symptoms, bowel or bladder dysfunction, gastroparesis, and sexual dysfunction.

On physical examination, the most important finding in a peripheral nerve process is reduction or absence of reflexes. The sensory examination, which includes tests of proprioception, vibratory sensation, and pain and temperature sensibility, is also often abnormal. When the motor system is involved, in addition to weakness, wasting and fasciculations may be seen. Autonomic dysfunction can cause hair loss, anhidrosis, pupillary dysfunction, orthostatic hypotension, and tachy- and bradyarrhythmias.

Similar symptoms and signs may be seen in disorders of the central nervous system (CNS). Weakness and numbness can be seen in both peripheral and central disorders. Hyporeflexia sometimes occurs with acute central lesions, but hyperreflexia and spasticity invariably develop later. Peripheral nervous system disorders, like CNS diseases, affect bulbar structures, resulting in diplopia, dysarthria, or dysphagia. Nevertheless, CNS disorders frequently have other features that are not seen in peripheral diseases. For example, aphasia, apraxia, and visual loss are hallmarks of cortical disease. Signs on examination such as hyperreflexia and clear lateralization of weakness should prompt evaluation for CNS disorders.

LOCALIZATION OF NEUROLOGIC DISEASE

Once a peripheral disorder has been established, it is necessary to determine which part of the peripheral nervous system is involved. A localized process, such as numbness and tingling of the fifth and half of the fourth digits of one hand, strongly suggests a focal lesion (ulnar nerve). The lesion may involve the nervous system at a number of locations: the nerve, plexus, or root. Basic knowledge or the aid of an anatomy text or neurology handbook should be sufficient to accurately localize focal lesions of these types. Figure 225-1 shows a schematized view of the peripheral nervous system and illustrates the signs associated with disease of specific parts of the neuromuscular system. Most muscle-related processes result in weakness of large proximal muscles, and patients may have a difficult time lifting their arms over their heads or arising from a seated position. Pain and tenderness of the muscles occur commonly (although usually these are not predominant symptoms and if not accompanied by weakness rarely indicate myopathy), and creatine phosphokinase (CPK) is usually elevated, sometimes dramatically. Diseases that affect other components of the peripheral nervous system seldom cause muscle tenderness and elevations in CPK. Neuromuscular junction processes also affect large proximal muscles and frequently affect the bulbar musculature, resulting in pupillary dysfunction, diplopia, dysarthria, or dysphagia. Unlike muscle and neuromuscular junction disorders, neuropathies frequently affect both the motor and sensory systems; because these diseases most severely affect longer nerves, distal power is reduced most dramatically. Polyradiculopathy, which frequently follows a progressive and stepwise course, usually results in electrical pain sensations, assorted sensory abnormalities, areflexia, and weakness.

Once localization of the peripheral problem is accomplished, efforts should be made to pinpoint the etiology. Specific historical points that always should be addressed include the time course of the illness, whether there are diurnal fluctuations in the symptoms, other systemic symptoms or conditions, a review of medications, and antecedent illnesses. A serum chemistry and metabolic profile and creatine kinase are frequently useful blood tests in the emergency department (ED) setting. Further testing is usually deferred in the acute setting but may include a variety of blood tests, nerve conduction studies, electromyography, lumbar puncture, and nerve/muscle biopsy.

TREATMENT: GENERAL CONSIDERATIONS

Management of peripheral nervous system disorders depends on the specific diagnosis. However, a few general remarks about care should be made. When a peripheral disorder is suspected or diagnosed in the ED, one should arrange for neurologic consultation for further specific treatments. Many neuromuscular disorders are difficult to diagnose and require complex treatments such as immunomodulation with intravenous immunoglobulin, immunosuppressive drugs, and plasmapheresis. Given potential morbidity from the therapies themselves, it is prudent to refer the patient to a neurologist and have the diagnosis confirmed with contemporary diagnostic tools.

Careful supportive care is mandatory for severe, life-threatening neuromuscular diseases and should begin in the ED. Patients with the potential to experience respiratory failure, aspiration, and lethal cardiac dysrhythmias should be monitored appropriately. Where the presentation warrants, baseline forced vital capacity or negative inspiratory pressure should be measured in the ED to assess whether there is need for imminent respiratory support or admission to an intensive care unit.

With few exceptions, admission to the hospital is generally required for acute peripheral neurologic conditions in which there is danger of respiratory or autonomic compromise or in cases of debilitating or rapidly progressing weakness. Admission allows rapid initiation of the diagnostic workup and treatment and intensive rehabilitation, which is frequently delayed in the outpatient setting. Specific indications for hospital admission are discussed below for individual disease entities.

SPECIFIC NEUROMUSCULAR DISORDERS

The number of neuromuscular disorders is extensive and cannot be discussed fully in this text; this section thus covers the most common and most important disorders to recognize and the diseases that have acute therapies available.

Myopathies

Polymyositis is an inflammatory myopathy that affects individuals over the age of 30, with a slight propensity for women.[1] Usually, patients present with chronic complaints of proximal symmetric weakness, although the disorder occasionally presents subacutely. Some patients will have dysphagia, and a few will progress to respiratory failure. There may be muscle pain and tenderness. On examination, there is reduced proximal strength, which may best be tested by asking the patient to arise from a chair with his or her arms crossed or to lift a light object over his or her head. There is no sensory loss, and unless weakness is profound, reflexes should be intact. If deep tendon reflexes are diminished, neuropathy should be considered. Laboratory testing may reveal an elevated erythrocyte sedimentation rate (ESR), leukocytosis, and creatine kinase. The differential diagnosis includes Lambert-Eaton myasthenic syndrome, inclusion body myositis, toxic myopathies, dermatomyositis, endocrinopathies, and an assortment of muscular dystrophies.

Patients with newly suspected polymyositis should be assessed for potential respiratory compromise and aspiration risk in the ED. Admission is usually warranted in cases of newly suspected polymyositis to monitor progress, rapidly work up the patient, and begin treatment. Further diagnostic studies likely pursued under the direction or consultative advice of a neurologist typically include electromyography (EMG) and muscle biopsy. Long-term treatment consists of immunosuppressive agents such as steroids and methotrexate.

Dermatomyositis, unlike polymyositis, can affect children and, like polymyositis, affects mostly women.[1] The clinical manifestations of dermatomyositis are similar to those of polymyositis, except for the usual appearance of a violaceous rash typically over the face and hands. The neurologic examination shows a myopathic distribution of weakness without sensory or reflex abnormalities in most cases. The laboratory findings are also similar, with an elevated ESR and CPK in most instances. Despite similarities in the clinical presentation compared with polymyositis, the pathology and pathophysiology of the two disorders are quite distinct.[1] Treatment is aimed at immunosuppression.

Other Myopathies A large number of substances, including environmental (alcohol), occupational, and pharmacologic agents (steroids, cholesterol-lowering drugs, AZT), can cause myopathy. Several important medication-induced myopathies are summarized in Table

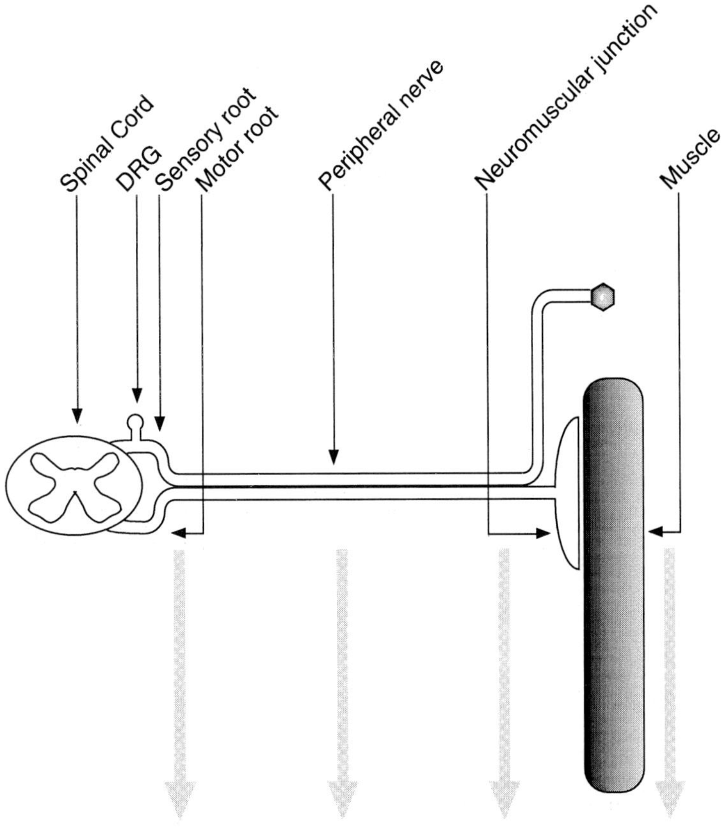

	Radiculopathy	Neuropathy	NMJ disease	Myopathy
Motor involvement	+	+	+	+
Sensory involvement	+	+	−	−
Autonomic involvement	−	+/−	+/−	−
Bulbar involvement	+/−	+/−	+	+/−
Proximal prominence	+/−	−	+	+
Reflexes	↓	↓	↔	↔

FIG. 225-1. Schematic view of the neuromuscular system and typical findings with disease of each component of the system. *Abbreviations:* DRG, dorsal root ganglion; NMJ, neuromuscular junction.

225-1. Although usually chronic, some present subacutely and cause a predominantly proximal pattern of weakness with normal sensation and preserved tendon reflexes (except with severe weakness). CPK is usually elevated. Viral myositis causes an acute myopathy, occasionally involving the heart, and is usually associated with a febrile illness, myalgia, and elevated CPK levels. Trichinosis should be suspected in patients with myalgias, bulbar and proximal muscle weakness, facial edema, and eosinophilia; symptoms occur within days of ingesting undercooked pork. Definitive diagnosis is made on visualization of parasitic cysts on muscle biopsy.

Disorders of the Neuromuscular Junction

Myasthenia gravis is discussed in Chap. 226.

Botulism Ingestion of foods contaminated with *Clostridium botulinum* toxin causes botulism, an acute disease marked by weakness and gastrointestinal slowing. Adults whose disease is caused not by bacterial infestation but by ingestion of botulinum toxin may report exposure to foods such as home-canned vegetables in the preceding 1 to 2 days. Unlike adults, infants, whose guts are not colonized fully, are susceptible to infection with viable bacteria that elaborate toxin. Parents of infants should be questioned for possible ingestion of *C. botulinum* spores, commonly transmitted by feeding honey. Infants may present with poor sucking. Botulism caused by infection through a wound is rare. On examination, mentation is normal, but there may be bulbar weakness. The extraocular movements are sometimes abnormal, and an important diagnostic clue is the absence of the pupillary light reflex, which distinguishes this disorder from myasthe-

TABLE 225-1 Drugs That Cause Myopathy

Chloroquine	ε-Amino-caproic acid	Thiazides
Emetine	D-Penicillamine	Amphotericin
Corticosteroids	Chlorpromazine	Amphetamines
Amiodarone	Zidovudine	Toluene
Adriamycin	Colchicine	Ethanol
Procainamide	Vincristine	Phencyclidine
Perhexilene	Clofibrate	
Imipramine	Lovastatin	

Source: Kuncl RW, Wiggins WW: Toxic myopathies. *Neurol Clin* 6:593, 1988.

nia gravis. There is proximal limb weakness, sensation is intact, and reflexes generally are normal except in the case of severe weakness.

Botulism is treated with antibiotics (infants only) and immune serum, which is obtained from the Centers for Disease Control and Prevention (Atlanta). The serum, derived from immunized horses, is first used in skin tests to rule out hypersensitivity. For adults, 10,000 units is administered the first day, and thereafter, the patient is given 50,000 units daily until improvement is seen.[2] Patients should be admitted to the hospital for treatment, monitoring, and testing. In cases where the diagnosis is not clear, treatment with immune serum, which has potential morbidity, should be withheld until electrodiagnostic studies are performed. Nerve conduction studies show an incremental response on repetitive nerve stimulation.

Acute Peripheral Neuropathies

Guillain-Barré syndrome (GBS) affects individuals of all ages and is the most common form of acute generalized neuropathy. Frequently, patients report an antecedent viral illness, especially gastroenteritis. There is an association between acute *Campylobacter jejuni* infection and development of GBS. Sometimes the patient first notices numbness and tingling of the lower extremities. This is followed by weakness of thighs, legs, and then arms. There are numerous variants of the syndrome, and some patients may experience facial weakness, which can mimic Bell's palsy, ophthalmoparesis, severe shooting pains, or ataxia caused by proprioceptive difficulty. In most, but not all, cases, GBS is caused by an autoimmune attack on myelinated motor nerves.

In classic cases, there is symmetric extremity weakness, more pronounced in the legs. Despite subjective sensory disturbances, sensation on examination is usually normal. The hallmark finding in GBS is the lack of deep tendon reflexes. In variant cases, there may be ophthalmoplegia and pupillary disturbances. Occasionally, there may be facial weakness involving the forehead. Autonomic instability, marked by brady- and tachycardia or blood pressure fluctuation, may be apparent in a few cases. Where ophthalmoparesis is present, there may be a marked limb ataxia, and the patient may not be able to walk or stand despite reasonable strength. In all forms of the disease, there is a chance of developing respiratory failure and lethal autonomic fluctuations.

Lumbar puncture should be performed when acute disease is suspected. The classic laboratory finding in GBS is a high cerebrospinal fluid (CSF) protein with normal glucose and cell count. However, the protein will not be elevated until after the first week of symptoms and may not be present even after 1 week. Though many patients will have a modest CSF pleocytosis (up to 100 lymphocytes/mm^3), the presence of cells in the CSF should prompt consideration of other systemic diseases sometimes associated with GBS, such as HIV infection, lupus, and lymphoma. Lyme disease can present with a clinical picture similar to GBS and would be suggested by a CSF pleocytosis in combination with a history of tick bites or the presence of CSF Lyme antibodies. Carcinomatous meningitis also can present with similar symptoms but will be evident with malignant cells in the CSF or extremely high protein or low glucose levels. Tick paralysis mimics GBS, and all patients with suspected GBS should be examined thoroughly for ticks. Acute intermittent porphyria (discussed below) and spinal cord compression should be considered in the differential diagnosis; the presence of upper motor neuron signs and bowel and bladder incontinence would suggest the latter.

Patients with GBS should be admitted to the hospital for monitoring and treatment. When forced vital capacity (FVC) is under 1 L, the patient should be intubated. No specific treatment is warranted in the ED; treatment is composed of plasma exchange or intravenous immunoglobulin, which both have been shown in controlled studies to shorten the duration of the illness.[2]

Acute intermittent porphyria is a rare autosomal dominant condition in which patients suddenly experience the symptom triad of weakness, psychosis, and abdominal pain. Seizures can occur. The three occasionally occur together, but in many cases occur independently. The disease activates acutely in flares that are usually precipitated by medications such as barbiturates, phenytoin, sulfonamides, and estrogen.

The major neurologic findings are weakness and diminished reflexes, particularly of the lower extremities, which are the direct consequence of an acute peripheral neuropathy. There may be sensory findings such as diminished pain and temperature sensation, although these signs are usually outweighed by motor deficits. In the acute setting, basic ancillary laboratory studies may be normal. Further testing reveals elevation in urine δ-aminolevulonic acid and porphobilinogen.

The key management issue is recognition of the disorder and identification and discontinuation of the offending drug. Care also must be taken to avoid overtreatment of symptoms such as pain and seizures with medications that may exacerbate the illness. Other treatment modalities include supportive care, glucose infusions to prevent heme biosynthesis, vitamin B_6, and hematin (4 mg/kg daily for 1 to 2 weeks). The differential diagnosis includes other disorders that cause pain and lower extremity weakness. Spinal cord compression causes back pain, which frequently radiates around the trunk and is followed by lower extremity weakness, but reflexes in this situation are brisk with upgoing toes (positive Babinski's reflex). An aortic aneurysm or dissection also can cause abdominal pain and lower extremity weakness if spinal arteries are occluded by the expanding aneurysm.

Entrapment Neuropathies

The most common entrapment neuropathies are discussed below. For the most part, the nerve damage is reversible, and referral to the appropriate specialist for relief on entrapment is necessary.

Carpal tunnel syndrome (CTS) is the most commonly seen entrapment neuropathy. Patients describe intermittent pain and/or numbness in the thumb and first two fingers, prominently at night. Symptoms frequently awaken the patient from sleep, occur in both hands independently, and may be poorly localized (i.e., numbness is often described going up to the elbow). The symptoms usually can be reproduced by compression of the nerve over the carpal tunnel or by tapping on the nerve, although these signs are neither sensitive nor specific. Occasionally, these symptoms are mistaken for cerebrovascular disease until a history of bilateral, repeated, and stereotypical nocturnal occurrence is obtained. When symptoms become long-standing and severe, weakness of the thenar musculature develops. Wrist splints worn at night are useful in the conservative management of CTS. Patients should be referred to a hand surgeon as an outpatient for further diagnostics and management. A carpal tunnel release may be performed in patients who fail to respond to conservative management.

Ulnar nerve entrapment, usually occurring at the elbow, produces numbness in the fifth digit and medial half of the fourth finger, but symptoms are frequently poorly localized. Weakness and wasting of the hypothenar muscles occur very late in the course. The patient should be referred to a specialist for electrodiagnostic confirmation because occasionally C8 radiculopathy can mimic this common condition. Severe cases are treated surgically with ulnar nerve transposition.

Entrapment of the deep peroneal nerve at the fibular head can cause footdrop and numbness of the web between the great and second toes. This condition occurs in the setting of injury to the leg, rapid weight loss, or habitual crossing of the legs. Peroneal entrapment should be confirmed by EMG to be differentiated from lumbar root disease or motor neuron disease. Almost all cases are treated conservatively and improve without specific therapy.

Meralgia paresthetica is entrapment of the lateral cutaneous nerve of the thigh. The diagnosis is often overlooked in the ED, being mistaken for a hip-related orthopedic disorder. Patients describe numbness and dysesthesias of the lateral aspect of the upper leg. This occurs after weight loss and notably following pelvic surgery or obstetric procedures where the legs are abducted and flexed for a prolonged period of time. Tricyclic antidepressants (TCA) are useful in the management of the dysesthesias associated with meralgia paresthetica. The condition resolves without sequelae and requires no specific therapy.

Mononeuritis multiplex is a syndrome of multiple nerve dysfunctions caused by a vasculitis. Patients experience multiple deficits in a stepwise fashion, usually involving both sides of the body. For example, a patient may experience wristdrop on the right, followed by footdrop on the left, and then footdrop on the opposite side a few weeks later. This condition requires urgent referral to a neurologist to determine the etiology and initiate treatment, usually in collaboration with a rheumatologist. Frequently this disorder is caused by a systemic vasculitis, and a thorough serologic examination and nerve biopsy are required to establish specific treatment plans. The condition must be differentiated from multiple compression neuropathies and from multifocal motor neuropathy.

Bell's palsy should be viewed as a diagnosis of exclusion. It is the most common cause of acute facial paralysis but is similar to other processes that are important to recognize. Patients with Bell's palsy complain of sudden facial weakness, difficulty with articulation, problems keeping an eye closed, or inability to keep food in the mouth on one side. Because the seventh cranial nerve also serves other functions, the patient may have variable degrees of dry eye, metallic taste of the mouth, and facial pain, commonly around the ear. The examination is notable for one-sided weakness of the face involving the forehead. There may be decreased sensation along the external acoustic meatus (Hitselberger's sign). Other cranial nerves are normal. Diminished reflexes suggest a different diagnosis.

Several alternative diagnoses should be considered. Stroke can lead to sudden facial weakness that involves only the lower face but also leads to neurologic involvement below the neck or other cranial neuropathies. Lyme disease and GBS can cause facial paralysis, as discussed elsewhere in this chapter. In patients with cancer, facial weakness may herald the metastatic spread of malignancy. The ear should be inspected carefully to rule out ulcerations caused by cranial herpes-zoster activation (Ramsay Hunt syndrome), which should be treated with oral acyclovir. Facial paralysis also can be seen in sarcoidosis, collagen vascular disease, and polio. All patients with facial weakness should be screened for HIV risk factors, since seventh nerve palsy can occur at the time of seroconversion.

The treatment of Bell's palsy with steroids is controversial. While some believe that they have no role, most neurologists argue in favor of a short course of prednisone in individuals with low risk for complications from corticosteroids. The recommended dose is 50 mg per day for 7 days. More recent studies[3] have suggested that steroids in combination with acyclovir (200 mg five times a day for 10 days) leads to better outcomes. If the patient is seen more than a week after paresis began, steroids generally are not given.

Eye care must be meticulous to avoid corneal abrasions. Patients are instructed to tape the affected eye so that the palpebral fissure is narrowed to prevent drying of the cornea. Patients should apply Lacrilube and patch the eye before sleeping.

Lyme disease affects individuals exposed to the tick-born pathogen *Borrelia burgdorferi*. Although its neurologic manifestations are multiple, one of the most common sites of involvement is the peripheral nervous system.[4] Patients often, but not always, report prior tick exposure and have spent time in areas known to have deer ticks. Initial manifestations of Lyme disease include arthralgias and fatigue. Neurologic complications ensue in the following weeks. A common neurologic sign of Lyme infection is seventh nerve palsy, which should not be confused with Bell's palsy. Lyme disease affects the peripheral nerves and the nerve roots. The patient may describe the acute or subacute progression of weakness and sensory loss, sometimes associated with radicular pain. On examination, the patient will have one of several signs. Unless there is encephalitis (a rare complication of Lyme disease), mental status will be normal. Apart from seventh nerve involvement, there may be weakness in the limbs, and if there is localized radicular inflammation, there will be a patchy myotomal pattern. Similarly, depending on the regional involvement of the disease, selected deep tendon reflexes will be diminished. Laboratory features suggestive of Lyme disease include serum and CSF Lyme antibodies. A CSF pleocytosis and increased protein with a normal glucose is the most common abnormality. When the diagnosis is made with confidence and other entities such as syphilis, carcinomatous meningitis, and sarcoidosis excluded, a 3-week course of intravenous antibiotics, either ceftriaxone or doxycycline, is given. Further discussion and treatment of Lyme disease are found in Chap. 145.

Plexopathies

Brachial neuritis is an acute condition that tends to affect younger individuals with a slight male predominance. Patients report excruciating shoulder, back, or arm pain followed by weakness of the arm or shoulder girdle. In a third of cases, it is bilateral. The cause is idiopathic, but cases have been reported following immunizations or viral infections. On examination, the patient has weakness in various distributions of the brachial plexus. The upper trunk is the preferred site of involvement, affecting strength of proximal arm and shoulder musculature. The anterior interosseous nerve is also affected preferentially, causing inability to form a pincer with the index finger and thumb. Sensory abnormalities are found but are not as profound as the motor dysfunction. Reflexes are diminished in the affected limb.

The differential diagnosis includes multiple cervical radiculopathies, Pancoast tumors, and neoplastic or inflammatory infiltration of the plexus. The diagnosis is usually clear, since a history of pain followed by weakness that plateaus in a week or two makes other diagnoses unlikely. A chest x-ray should be performed to look for mass lesions involving the brachial plexus. CSF analysis is required if there is a suspicion of other etiologies. Spine imaging and EMG may be performed outside the ED setting.

The management of brachial plexitis is conservative, and no therapies have been shown to affect the course of the illness. The prognosis is good, with most patients experiencing full recovery in months. If careful follow-up with a neurologist can be arranged and other causes or symptoms are excluded, admission to the hospital is elective.

Lumbar plexopathy, or diabetic amyotrophy, occurs in diabetic patients and presents with back pain followed by weakness. Patients report the acute onset of ipsilateral back pain, followed within days by progressive leg weakness. Sensory findings are absent. The examination reveals decreased leg power in a variety of patterns reflecting impairment of plexus function with relatively symmetric sensation. There may be muscle wasting in affected limbs in long-standing dis-

TABLE 225-2 A Framework to Approach Chronic Neuropathies

	PREDOMINANT SYMPTOMS			
Etiologies	Sensory	Motor	Sensory and Motor	Autonomic
Infectious	HIV Leprosy	Lyme	Syphilis Lyme	Chagas' disease
Medications	Cisplatin	Dapsone	INH	Vincristine
Toxins	Arsenic Alcohol	Lead	Alcohol	
Nutritional	Beriberi		B_{12} deficiency	
Metabolic	Diabetes		Uremia	Diabetes
Neoplastic	Paraneoplastic ganglionopathy		Paraneoplastic polyneuropathy	
Hereditary	Hereditary sensory neuropathy		Charcot-Marie-Tooth	Amyloidosis Riley-Day
Inflammatory	Sjögren's disease	CIDP	Mononeuritis multiplex	
Paraproteinemias, dysproteinemias	Anti-MAG sensory neuropathy	Anti-G_{M1} motor neuropathy	Waldenstrom's macroglobulinemia	Amyloidosis

Note: Examples of a variety of causes of chronic neuropathy. This table is meant to illustrate the major classes of etiologies and the usefulness of classifying neuropathy by symptom complex. Syndromes of pure symptomatology (e.g., pure motor neuropathy) are rare but suggest a small number of potential causes. Note that the table is incomplete and does not necessarily list the most common neuropathies in each class. Many neuropathies present with distinct symptoms from those described above. Para- and dysproteinemias are assumed, but have not been proven, to be causative etiologies of nerve dysfunction.

ease. Deep tendon reflexes may be diminished on the affected side. Bowel and bladder functions are not affected.

Laboratory studies are generally not helpful in the emergency setting. In the ED, routine plain films of the lumbar spine are useful to screen for spine compression from degenerative or neoplastic disease, and MRI is usually ultimately needed. The differential diagnosis also includes the cauda equina and conus medullaris syndromes and compression from arteriovenous malformations. CT scanning of the abdomen is useful to rule out aortic aneurysm and psoas muscle masses, which also lead to asymmetric lower extremity weakness. Patients with acute weakness from lumbar plexopathy should be admitted to the hospital for testing and rehabilitation to definitely determine the cause of weakness.

HIV-Associated Peripheral Neurologic Disease

HIV infection, its complications, and its pharmacologic treatments are associated with a number of peripheral neurologic disorders. Fortunately, the most common of these, HIV neuropathy and drug-induced neuropathy, are chronic processes that do not cause sudden disability or symptoms. HIV-infected patients also have a higher rate of *mononeuritis multiplex* and an inflammatory myopathy resembling *polymyositis*.

Occasionally, patients will complain of weakness that progresses over the course of days. Patients in the early stages of HIV infection have greater susceptibility to GBS. The presentation is similar to that of the non-HIV-infected patient, except that a CSF pleocytosis is seen commonly. Such patients should be treated as discussed earlier.

Cytomegalovirus (CMV) Radiculitis In the latter stages of AIDS, patients may suffer from an acute radiculitis caused by CMV infection. These patients almost always have evidence of CMV infection elsewhere in the body and may have ongoing CMV retinitis. Patients become acutely weak, with primarily lower extremity involvement, and may have variable degrees of bowel and bladder dysfunction. The examination shows primarily lower extremity weakness and hyporeflexia, with decreased sensation in the lower extremities and groin. Rectal tone may be impaired. Lumbar puncture reveals a pleocytosis with predominantly polymorphonuclear cells and modestly increased protein; viral DNA is detected by polymerase chain reaction in most patients and is highly specific. MRI of the lumbosacral spine demonstrates swelling and clumping of the cauda equina. Imaging of these patients is mandatory to rule out mass lesions of the lower spine or nerve roots. The treatment of CMV radiculitis is intravenous ganciclovir, started at 5 mg/kg every 12 h for 14 days, which may be initiated prior to definitive diagnosis.

CHRONIC CONDITIONS

Patients with some frequency present to the ED with neuropathy associated with an underlying condition. Many are of a chronic nature, and a few are subacute. Most of these do not present acute management issues. However, conditions such as syphilis, Lyme disease, and vitamin B_{12} deficiency benefit from early detection. A detailed discussion of neuropathies associated with underlying medical illness is worthy of an entire text. The interested reader is referred to standard neurology texts.[5] Table 225-2 shows the expected presentations for some diseases associated with peripheral neuropathies.

REFERENCES

1. Dalakas M: Polymyositis, dermatomyositis, and inclusion body myositis. *N Engl J Med* 325:1487, 1991.
2. van der Meche FGA, Schmitz PIM, and the Dutch Guillain-Barré Study Group: A randomized trial comparing intravenous immune globulin and plasma exchange in Guillain-Barré syndrome. *N Engl J Med* 326:1123, 1992.
3. Adour KK, Ruboyianes JM, Von Doersten PG, et al: Bell's palsy treatment with acyclovir and prednisone compared with prednisone alone: A double-blind, randomized, controlled trial. *Ann Otol Rhinol Laryngol* 105:371, 1996.
4. Logigian EL: Peripheral nervous system Lyme borreliosis. *Semin Neurol* 17:25, 1997.
5. Adams RD, Victor M: *Principles of Neurology*, 5th ed. New York, McGraw-Hill, 1993.

CHRONIC NEUROLOGIC DISORDERS

Edward P. Sloan

The chronic neurologic disorders discussed in this chapter include amyotrophic lateral sclerosis (ALS), multiple sclerosis (MS), myasthenia gravis (MG), Parkinson's disease (PD), and poliomyelitis and its late sequelae, postpolio syndrome. A knowledge of these diseases and their treatments is necessary in order to address complications, especially acute respiratory failure.

AMYOTROPHIC LATERAL SCLEROSIS

Amyotrophic lateral sclerosis (ALS) is characterized by rapidly progressive muscle wasting and weakness resulting from the degeneration of both upper and lower motor neurons. ALS causes varying degrees of spasticity, hyperreflexia, and muscle paralysis, eventually leading to pulmonary complications and the need for mechanical ventilatory support. Because there is no curative therapy for this disease, symptomatic management is directed at prevention of deaths caused by respiratory failure and pulmonary infections.

Epidemiology

There are three forms of ALS, the most common, sporadic ALS (sALS); familial ALS (fALS), which is genetically present in only 149 patients from 53 families worldwide (including a rare juvenile form); and an endemic focus of ALS in the western Pacific.[1] The worldwide annual incidence rate for sALS is 0.6 to 2.0 per 100,000, and the prevalence is 4 to 6 per 100,000.[2] The mean age of onset for sALS is 56 years, with no gender differences noted. The incidence of fALS is only 10 percent of that of sALS, with a 1.5-fold higher disease rate for men. There are no race differences with either form of ALS. There is a higher prevalence of ALS in individuals older than 60 years, and the annual worldwide ALS mortality rate is 1 per 100,000.

Pathophysiology

Current theories for cell death include excitotoxins (glutamate), free radicals, heavy metals, viral agents, and autoimmune reactions against such tissues as spinal cord collagen.[3] Programmed cell death due to apoptosis is also being studied as a possible etiology. The most likely cause of ALS is genetic superoxide dismutase dysfunction related to a variety of environmental insults.[4]

Gross central nervous system (CNS) pathology includes frontal cortical atrophy, degeneration of the corticospinal and spinocerebellar tracts, a reduction in large cervical and lumbar motor neurons, and cranial nerve nuclei degeneration. Both motor and sensory peripheral nerves are noted to undergo axonal degeneration and segmental demyelination, including motor end plate and axon terminal involvement.

Clinical Presentation

Upper motor neuron dysfunction causes limb spasticity, hyperreflexia (including Babinski's sign and a brisk jaw-jerk reflex), and emotional lability. Lower motor neuron dysfunction causes limb muscle weakness, atrophy, cramps, and fasiculations, as well as dysarthria, dysphagia, and difficulty in mastication. At the time of initial presentation, extremity cramping, fatigue, and weakness are seen, as well as muscle fasciculations and atrophy.[5] These symptoms are more prominent in the upper extremities, with asymmetric weakness seen commonly. Regardless of the initial symptomatology, widespread motor and respiratory dysfunction progresses within weeks to months. Atrophic, fasciculating, hyperreflexic extremities are seen, as well as foot drop and claw deformity of the hand. Patients also may present with an atrophic fasciculating tongue and monotonous speech, with relative sparing of facial and eye movements. Patients with fALS more often present with isolated lower extremity weakness and atrophy at the time of diagnosis. Some patients eventually diagnosed as having ALS present initially with cervical or back pain consistent with an acute compressive radiculopathy, leading to surgery. Despite successful operative intervention, these patients develop significant muscle wasting consistent with motor neuron dysfunction shortly after the procedure.[6]

Progressive respiratory muscle weakness causes dyspnea with mild activity, until dyspnea at rest occurs. Dementia and parkinsonism also may be seen in up to 15 percent of patients, especially those with fALS. Other cognitive problems such as apathy, poor attention and motivation, and altered social skills may be noted in patient with ALS.

Clinical Diagnosis

The clinical diagnosis of ALS is suggested when there are signs of both upper and lower motor neuron dysfunction without other CNS dysfunction. ALS-like symptoms can be seen with other systemic illnesses such as diabetes, dysproteinemia, thyroid dysfunction, vitamin B_{12} deficiency, lead toxicity, and vasculitis, as well as CNS and spinal cord tumors. The diagnosis of ALS also requires that other inflammatory neuropathies such as myasthenia gravis be excluded. Established criteria for the diagnosis of ALS, the El Escorial criteria, have been developed by the World Federation of Neurology.[7]

Electromyography (EMG) is the most useful diagnostic tool, showing decreased muscle action potential amplitude and decremental responses to repetitive nerve stimulation

Disease Management

Therapy is designed to enhance muscle function, especially those which support breathing, swallowing, and speech, in order to avoid malnutrition, recurrent aspiration, or choking. Two drugs that may delay disease progression include riluzone and gabapentin, both of which prevent cell toxicity through modulation of the excitotoxin glutamate. Respiratory insufficiency is suggested by atrophy of the deltoids and trapezii, and a decrease in forced vital capacity by 50 percent increases the risk of respiratory failure. Pulmonary function testing, respiratory therapy, incentive spirometry, and intermittent positive-pressure breathing, intermittent negative-pressure (external) ventilation, and long-term assisted ventilation all can enhance the quality of life as diaphragm weakness progresses.

Emergency Diagnosis and Management

Patients with ALS most often will not present to the emergency department (ED) undiagnosed unless there is extremely rapid disease progression or a long period without medical care. Emergency management usually is required for acute respiratory failure, aspiration pneumonia, choking episodes, or trauma related to extremity weakness. A vital capacity drop below 25 mL/kg increases the risk of aspiration pneumonia and respiratory failure. Blood gas determination does not reliably predict impending respiratory failure, since mild hypoxia and hypercarbia may exist throughout the disease course. Although no acute therapies exist for worsening ALS, therapies that optimize pulmonary function (e.g., nebulized medications, steroids, antibiotics, intubation) are indicated. Because the need for long-term ventilatory assistance rarely reverses, it is important to establish the patient's preference regarding intubation via a living will or the power of attorney for health care. Hospitalization is indicated with impending respiratory failure, pneumonia, the inability to control secretions, or a worsening overall status that requires social service intervention for long-term placement.

Long-Term Outcome

ALS causes a consistent, predictable deterioration in motor function, leading to tracheostomy in most patients within 2 to 4 years.[8] ALS leads to complete respiratory failure in 80 percent and complete limb paralysis in 45 percent of patients. Although early diagnosis and aggressive management have increased the median survival of sALS, 50 percent of patients die within 3 years of diagnosis, and only 10 percent survive beyond 10 years. Patient diagnosed prior to age 40 may live up to four times longer than those diagnosed after age 60, especially if swallowing and airway control are spared. Survival in fALS is shorter, with a median survival of 2 years and a 23 percent 5-year survival rate. Long-term outcome is currently being followed in a longitudinal European survey termed the European ALS Health Profile Study.

MULTIPLE SCLEROSIS

Multiple sclerosis (MS) is a neurologic disorder that causes variable motor, sensory, visual, and cerebellar dysfunction due to multifocal areas of CNS myelin destruction. Paresthesias, gait difficulty, extremity weakness, poor coordination, and visual disturbances occur most often with a relapsing and remitting clinical course. Despite the lack of a definitive cure, immunosuppression and immunomodulation provide adequate symptomatic therapy in the majority of patients. Most patients with MS sustain only mild to moderate lifetime morbidity without a reduction in overall life expectancy.

Epidemiology

Three clinical courses are noted in patients with MS. Roughly two-thirds have a relapsing and remitting course, with relapses lasting weeks to months. The remaining one-third of patients have either a relapsing and progressive course or a chronically progressive clinical course, which is more common with advanced age. The incidence of MS is 4.5 to 8 per 100,000, and the prevalence is greater than 50 per 100,000.[9] In the United States, the peak age of onset for either sex is during the third decade of life. Females are two to three times more likely to contract MS, and they do so at a younger age than men. Males, however, are more likely to have a chronically progressive disease course from the onset of symptoms. MS is two times more likely in whites than in blacks, and it is rare in Asian populations. There is a geographic MS distribution, with temperate climates of economically developed countries experiencing a higher prevalence. Communities of northern Europe and the United States have prevalence rates of up to 173 per 100,000 in the white population. In the northern hemisphere there is a diminishing MS prevalence gradient that runs from north to south, while the opposite is true in the southern hemisphere. In general, 5 to 10 percent of MS patients will sustain a malignant course, and 20 to 35 percent will have a very benign disease course. Pregnancy reduces by 50 percent the MS relapse rate, but relapse risk increases up to sixfold during the postpartum period.

Pathophysiology

Although the etiology of MS is unknown, it is best described as an inflammatory disorder resulting in scattered neuron demyelination. The most frequently postulated theory for MS is a genetic predisposition triggered by a virus (such as herpes or HTLV-1) or environmental toxins that induce an immune-mediated neuronal inflammation and demyelinization.[10] MS causes a dysfunction in oligodendrocytes such that the axonal myelin sheaths are damaged, slowing nerve impulse conduction. These scattered cerebral and spinal plaques cause gliosis primarily in the white matter, with relative axon sparing.

These plaques occur in multiple areas, including the cerebrum, brainstem, spinal cord, and cranial nerves. The brain may have variable amounts of atrophy and ventricular dilatation. Nerves in the corticospinal tracts, posterior columns, and spinothalamic tracts will cause upper motor neuron, proprioception/vibration, and pain/temperature dysfunction, respectively. Cranial nerve dysfunction most often causes optic neuritis, but facial motor and sensory deficits are also common.

Clinical Presentation

MS is suggested when a young person presents multiple times with neurologic symptoms that suggest different areas of pathology, often with resolution of the prior symptoms. Most MS patients will have more severe lower extremities symptoms as compared with the upper extremities. For example, a young person might complain of an inability to walk on a street without tripping over a curb or uneven sections of pavement.

The physical examination may reveal decreased strength, increased tone, hyperreflexia, clonus, Babinski's reflex, a decrease in vibration sense and joint proprioception, as well as a reduction in pain and temperature sense. Although sensory and motor deficits are present initially in only one-third of patients, all patients will experience a deficit at some point during the disease course. Patients describe these deficits as a heaviness, weakness, stiffness, or extremity numbness. Lhermitt's sign is commonly experienced during the course of MS and is described as an electric shock sensation, a vibration, or dysesthetic pain radiating down the back and often into the arms or legs resulting from the flexion of the neck.

Rarely, patients with established MS may present with complete or near-complete loss of motor function, termed *acute transverse myelitis* (ATM). Cerebellar lesions may cause a kinetic tremor, saccadic dysmetria, and/or truncal ataxia. Vertigo also may be seen as a result of brainstem MS lesions.

Optic neuritis, which usually causes a subacute or acute central vision loss, may be the initial sign of MS in up to 30 percent of patients. The loss, which occurs over several days and is usually unilateral, often is preceded by retrobulbar pain or extraocular muscle pain that may be reproduced with periorbital palpation. Optic neuritis may cause an afferent pupillary defect, or Marcus Gunn pupil. Although funduscopy is most often normal in the acute setting, the optic disk may be noted to have pallor due to axonal loss and gliosis. Although the ocular pain most often resolves over several days, it may take up to months for the visual disturbances to resolve. Most MS patients at some time experience blurred vision, compromised color vision, and/or eye pain due to optic neuritis. In fact, visual acuity may worsen due to increases in body temperature, known as *Uhthoff's phenomenon*. Nystagmus and diplopia are often seen in MS, as is internuclear ophthalmoplegia (INO). INO causes abnormal adduction and horizontal nystagmus, usually bilaterally. When bilateral INO is seen acutely in an otherwise healthy young person, it is highly suggestive of MS.

Dysautonomias can cause vesicourethral, gastrointestinal tract, and sexual dysfunction. Vesicourethral dysfunction results in urinary retention, urgency, frequency, detrusor-external sphincter dyssynergia (DESD), and stress or overflow incontinence. Constipation and fecal incontinence both can occur often with MS. Sexual dysfunction, especially in males, may be the presenting MS symptom and is correlated with other types of urologic dysfunction.

Cognitive and emotional changes, including dementia, decreased motivation, and/or mood disorders (depression, bipolar), occur in most MS patients. Cerebral MS, which affects only 5 percent of MS patients, can cause a severe, disabling decrease in intellect as well as focal seizures.

MS symptoms often will worsen with increases in body temperatures, as seen with exercise, fever, or even hot baths. Most initial MS attacks or exacerbations will progress over several days, peaking at about 1 week, with resolution over several weeks to months. Complete recovery from an acute attack or exacerbation is more common early in the course of the disease.

Clinical Diagnosis

The diagnosis of MS is clinically based, relying heavily on the neurologic history and physical examination. The diagnosis is suggested when a patient has either two or more prolonged (days to weeks) episodes with neurologic dysfunction that suggests distinct white matter pathology or spinal cord dysfunction that worsens over several months.[11] Optic findings, lack of focal pathology, clinical remissions, cerebrospinal fluid (CSF) findings, and typical features such as dysautonomias all suggest the diagnosis of MS.[12] Symptoms that mimic MS are seen with systemic lupus erythematosus (SLE), Lyme disease, neurosyphilis, and HIV disease. The clinical features of these other diseases, as well as the presence of consistent laboratory and neuroimaging findings in MS, can help to confirm the diagnosis of MS.

Nearly all MS patients will demonstrate some CNS pathology using magnetic resonance imaging (MRI). T2-weighted scans demonstrate either discrete lesions in the supratentorial white matter or homogeneous borders surrounding the ventricles. Although computed tomography (CT) is not as sensitive as MRI, it may show cerebral atrophy, ventricular enlargement, and low-density focal lesions in the cerebrum, brainstem, or optic nerves.

CSF protein and gamma-globulin concentrations are elevated in many MS patients. A slight increase in CSF white blood cells (up to 25/hpf) is also seen, most of which are T lymphocytes. Evoked potentials (EP) demonstrate scattered slowing in CNS pathway conduction in the majority of MS patients.

Disease Management

The long-term management of MS is directed at slowing the progression of the disease and providing symptomatic relief during exacerbations. In order to modify the disease and its exacerbations, immunomodulation with adrenocorticotropic hormone (ACTH), corticosteroids, interferon, and other immunosuppressive drugs has been studied. High-dose methylprednisolone therapy may shorten the duration of exacerbations, especially early in the disease course. Several weeks of oral prednisone therapy can be added to the initial IV steroid therapy, but the effect on the disease is unclear. Alternatively, ACTH can be given. Diets high in fruits, vegetables, and grains may protect against the development of MS symptoms.[13] Intravenous immunoglobulins are probably not effective in the treatment of MS.[14]

Emergency Diagnosis and Management

Emergency therapy is directed at minimizing the complications of acute MS exacerbations. Fever must be reduced in order to minimize the weakness caused by elevated temperature. Seizures can be treated with the standard benzodiazepine, phenytoin, and barbiturate regimen. Optic neuritis, severe constipation, and worsening muscle weakness also may complicate an MS exacerbation.

Respiratory infections and distress must be managed aggressively. Endotracheal intubation should proceed with caution, using the Sellick maneuver, because of an increased aspiration risk due to decreased gastric motility. Respiratory function in MS patients who require emergent surgery should be assessed and stabilized. Also, because many MS patients have labile autonomic nervous system function, they are at greater risk of developing hypotension with both emergent intubation and surgical anesthesia.

Urinary tract infections (UTIs) and pyelonephritis must be excluded during any MS exacerbation, especially those associated with a residual urine greater than 100 cc.[15] A postvoid residual urine determination should be made whenever there is clinical evidence of a UTI or significant bacteriuria. A urine culture should be performed, and antibiotic therapy initiated. When possible, discharged patients should manage elevated residual urine volumes with intermittent sterile catheterization as opposed to placement of a Foley catheter.

Hospitalization is indicated for any exacerbation that puts the MS patient at risk of further complications or when IV antibiotic or steroid therapy needs to be initiated. Admission is also indicated when depression and a significant risk of suicide require inpatient management.

Long-Term Outcome

Staging of the severity and progression of MS is characterized using a neurologic impairment scale, the Expanded Disability Status Scale (EDSS).[16] Up to one-third of MS patients can live a relatively unencumbered life despite having MS. Generally, sensory and cranial nerve symptoms predict a more favorable outcome than those caused by motor nerve or cerebellar dysfunction. Exacerbations are to be expected in the face of significant physical and emotional stress, with disease progression occurring over decades. For those with the most severe progression, severe disability can occur over months to years. In these patients, the risk of suicide is over seven times greater than for the population as a whole. Regardless of the rate of progression, most significant complications and mortality are due either to suicide or to neurologic, pulmonary, and renal dysfunction seen with advanced disease and age. Mean life expectancy exceeds 30 to 40 years after the time of initial diagnosis.

MYASTHENIA GRAVIS

Myasthenia gravis (MG) is an autoimmune disease characterized by muscle weakness and fatigue, seen especially with repetitive use of voluntary muscles. Acetylcholine receptor (AChR) antibodies impair the function of the AChR at the neuromuscular junction, causing variable amounts of muscle weakness. The muscle weakness is seen most often in proximal muscles, generally is relieved by rest, and requires long-term immunotherapy. Because the mechanism and optimal therapies for MG are well understood, much of the morbidity and mortality associated with the disease can be avoided. Aggressive management of respiratory complications associated with a myasthenic crisis is the most important issue for MG patients and emergency physicians.

Epidemiology

The incidence of MG is less than 1 case per 100,000, and the prevalence is 10 to 15 per 100,000.[17] There are about 25,000 cases in the United States and 100 million cases worldwide. The most common age of onset for females is in the second and third decades. In males, the peak onset age is in the seventh and eighth decades. Although females were believed to have up to a 4-fold higher disease prevalence, with aging of the population, the higher prevalence has shifted to males. There is a slightly higher prevalence in the African-American population. Although family members of patients with MG are much more likely to develop MG, the disease is not transmitted by traditional Mendelian inheritance.

Pathophysiology

In the normal neuromuscular junction, acetylcholine (ACh) release by the nerve fiber causes a localized end-plate potential that leads to muscle fiber contraction. In MG there is a marked decrease in the number and function of the muscle fiber ACh receptors (AChR) despite normal nerve anatomy and function. Failure to respond to ACh stimulation causes decreased muscle fiber potential amplitudes, causing some fibers to fail to function and leading to decreased muscle strength.

The autoimmune etiology of MG is demonstrated by the consistent presence of AChR autoantibodies in nearly all MG patients. These antibodies react to the AChR, can be transferred passively (causing the disease), and can be induced by immunization with the AChR proteins, and disease severity can be correlated with AChR autoantibody levels. These autoantibodies cause accelerated AChR degradation and blockade and also cause receptor dysfunction through complement activation.

The etiology of the pathologic autoimmune response is believed to be due to dysfunction of either the thymus gland or the immune response to exogenous infectious antigens. The thymus is found to be abnormal in 75 percent of MG patients, most often with hyperplasia or the presence of a thymoma. Thymectomy resolves or improves the symptoms in most MG patients. It is possible that the AChR autoantibodies arise following exposure to similar antigens, such as those caused by herpes simplex virus or bacteria infection. These antigens, because of their resemblance to the AChR, cause a pathologic attack on the ACh proteins.

Clinical Presentation

The symptoms of MG can mimic the symptoms seen in many other chronic neurologic disorders, such that some call it "the great imitator." Prior to the establishment of a definitive diagnosis, most MG patients have general weakness, especially of the proximal extremities muscle groups, neck extensors, and facial or bulbar muscles. Ptosis and diplopia are the most common presenting symptoms, but oropharyngeal symptoms (dysphagia and dysarthria) and limb weakness also can be seen. Although 10 percent of patients will have weakness that is restricted only to the ocular muscles, most MS patients subsequently will develop weakness in the oropharyngeal and limb muscles. The maximum extent of this weakness usually becomes manifest within the first year of diagnosis. These symptoms can fluctuate throughout the day, usually worsening as the day progresses or with prolonged muscle group use, such as with prolonged reading or prolonged chewing during a meal. Despite the presence of profound muscle weakness, there usually is no deficit in sensory, reflex, or cerebellar functioning. There may be a coexistent endocrine disorder, and the disease is often associated with thymoma.

MG in elderly patients can be misdiagnosed as ischemic stroke, especially when new-onset facial weakness is seen.[18] In very rare instances, undiagnosed MG patients may present with extreme weakness in the muscles of respiration, resulting in respiratory failure. This life-threatening situation, termed *myasthenic crisis,* can be seen prior to MG diagnosis or as a result of inadequate drug therapy or drug tolerance. The complications associated with the respiratory failure seen in acute myasthenic crisis are the leading cause of death in MG patients.

Clinical Diagnosis

The diagnosis of MG should be considered in any patient who complains specifically of ocular disturbances or proximal limb muscle weakness not associated with systemic causes of generalized fatigue. Involvement of the facial muscles, muscles of mastication, and those which facilitate swallowing all may suggest MG, as well as the observations that the symptoms worsen as the day progresses and that rest alleviates the symptoms. MG is graded as being either focal, generalized with mild to severe weakness, or myasthenic crisis, which may require ventilatory support.

Other causes of symptoms that suggest MG include congenital MG, Lambert-Eaton syndrome (seen with oat cell lung tumors), drug-induced myasthenia (e.g., penicillamine, procainamide, quinines, aminoglycosides), botulism, thyroid disorders, and other causes of ocular disorders, such as progressive external ophthalmoplegia or intracranial mass lesions.

The diagnosis of MG is established through the administration of edrophonium chloride (an acetylcholinesterase inhibitor), EMG, and serologic testing for AChR antibodies. In the presence of abnormal neuromuscular transmission, edrophonium or neostigmine is expected to improve muscle strength in objectively weak limb muscles and in weak ocular and pharyngeal muscles. Because these drugs also can cause profound weakness in the presence of other disorders that impair neuromuscular transmission, one must be ready to provide ventilatory support or intubation as a complication of testing. EMG testing with repetitive nerve stimulation demonstrates a rapid reduction in the size of the muscle action potential, a finding that correlates with the clinical observation of enhanced weakness with prolonged or repetitive muscle use. AChR antibody testing is the most specific test for MG, but up to 15 percent of MG patients may have undetectable AChR antibody titers, especially those who have isolated ocular disturbances.

Other tests that may be necessary to confirm the diagnosis of MG or exclude other etiologies of muscle weakness include mediastinum imaging, laboratory testing for lupus and thyroid disorders as well as tuberculosis, and pulmonary function testing.

Disease Management

The management of MG includes the administration of acetlycholinesterase inhibitors, thymectomy, chronic immune suppression, and acute immune modulation (plasma exchange, IV immune globulin), when indicated. Muscle weakness usually does not return to normal with the use of these modalities, and there can be great temporal variability in the nature and amount of muscle weakness. Under- or overdosing can cause significant complications. Variability in the amount of muscle weakness can be seen in response to asthma exacerbations, infections, menstruation, pregnancy, emotional stress, hot weather, and other disorders that alter the response to medication, such as renal and gastrointestinal disease.

Most MG patients show a favorable response to thymectomy. Most show improvement with oral corticosteroids, although some patients initially become weaker prior to symptom improvement when high-dose steroids are administered. Severe MG symptoms often require the use of IV immunoglobulins or a combination of high-dose steroids and plasma exchange.

Emergency Management and Diagnosis

Respiratory failure is usually precipitated by infection, surgery, or the rapid tapering of immunosuppressive drugs. Otherwise minor illnesses, such gastroenteritis or upper respiratory infections, can worsen MG. The neurologist always should be consulted before making a disposition.

Several drugs are known to affect neuromuscular function, and caution must be exercised with their use in MG patients. Drugs that should be avoided are listed in Table 226-1. If a drug is absolutely necessary, such as steroids for status asthmaticus, equipment for emergency endotracheal intubation should be immediately available because respiratory failure can develop rapidly.

Myasthenic patients being treated in the ED for other conditions should receive their usual dose of cholinergic inhibitors such as pyridostigmine (Mestinon). The dose is often 60 to 90 mg PO every 4 h. If a dose has been missed, the next dose is usually doubled. If the patient is NPO or intubated, one-thirtieth the oral dose of pyridostigmine is given by slow intravenous infusion. Neurology consultation generally is needed to determine the optimal intravenous dose, rate of infusion, and timing of repeat doses.

The most feared complication of MG in the ED is respiratory failure. Intubation should be considered in patients with a forced vital capacity of less than 1 L. Blood gases have a poor predictive value for intubation. Because of the increased sensitivity of MG patients to neuromuscular junction inhibitors, if avoidable, patients preferably should not receive either depolarizing or nondepolarizing paralytic agents in preparation for intubation. Even small doses may have profound effects. Short-acting agents such as etomidate or fentanyl can be used instead and in smaller doses.[19] Propofol is an alternative agent

TABLE 226-1 Drugs That Should Be Used With Caution in Myasthenia Gravis

Steroids	Kanamycin*	Amitriptyline	Lidocaine	**Others**
ACTH*	Gentamicin	Droperidol	Dilantin	Amantadine
Methylprednisolone*	Tobramycin	Haloperidol	Trimethaphan	Diphenhydramine
Prednisone*	Dihydrostreptomycin*	Imipramine	**Local Anesthetic**	Emetine
Anticonvulsants	Amikacin	Paraldehyde	Lidocaine*	Diuretics
Dilantin	Polymyxin A	Trichlorethanol	Procaine*	Muscle relaxants
Ethosuximide	Polymyxin B	**Antirheumatics**	**Analgesics**	CNS depressants
Trimethadione	Bacitracin	D-Penicillamine	Narcotics	Respiratory depressants
Paraldehyde	Sulfonamides	Colchicine	Morphine	Sedatives
Magnesium sulfate	Viomycin	Chloroquine	Dilaudid	Procaine*
Barbiturates	Colistin	**Cardiovascular**	Codeine	Tranquilizers
Antimalarials	Colistimethate*	Quinidine*	Pantopon	**Neuromuscular blocking agents**
Chloroquine*	Lincomycin	Procainamide*	Meperidine	Tubocurarine
Quinine*	Clindamycin	Beta blockers	**Endocrine**	Pancuronium
IV Fluids	Tetracycline	Propranolol	Thyroid replacement*	Gallamine
Na lactate solution	Oxytetracycline	Oxprenolol	**Eyedrops**	Dimethyl tubocurarine
Antibiotics	Rolitetracycline	Practolol	Timolol*	Succinylcholine
Aminoglycosides	**Psychotropics**	Pindolol	Ecothiopate	Decamethonium
Neomycin*	Chlorpromazine*	Sotalol		
Streptomycin*	Lithium carbonate*			

*Case reports implicate drugs in exacerbations of MG.
Source: This table is a modified version of the table from Adams SL, Matthews J, Grammer LC: Drugs that may exacerbate myasthenia gravis. *Ann Emerg Med* 13:532, 1984. Used with permission.

in the operating suite. Patients with myasthenia are extremely sensitive to both depolarizing and non-depolarizing paralytic agents. Paralytic effects can be expected to persist at least 2–3 times longer than in normal patients.

Fortunately, the need for paralytic agents for emerging intubation of myasthenic patients is rare. If etomidate or fentanyl are ineffective and paralytic agents are necessary, some have recommended utilizing one-half the dose of paralytic agents, although there are no clinical studies supporting this recommendation.

Differentiation of myasthenic crisis (disease exacerbation or inadequate drug therapy) from cholinergic crisis (excessive drug delivery) is by means of the Tensilon test. Edrophonium chloride (Tensilon) is used because of its rapid onset (30 s) and the short duration (approximately 5 to 10 min) of its effects. A positive result, one that suggests that the symptoms are due to a myasthenia exacerbation, is characterized by the resolution of muscle weakness within a few minutes.

In order to establish that the patient does not react adversely to edrophonium, suggesting that the symptoms are due to excessive cholinergic effects, 1 to 2 mg IV should first be injected. The occurrence of muscle fasiculations and respiratory depression within a few minutes suggests that the muscle weakness is related to a cholinergic crisis, and further edrophonium administration is contraindicated. If there is no evidence of a cholinergic crisis, up to 10 mg of edrophonium should be administered in order to demonstrate benefit in the face of a presumed myesthenic crisis.

If the Tensilon test is positive, indicating a myasthenic crisis, neostigmine can be given parenterally or orally. IM or SC neostigmine is given in 0.5 to 2 mg doses, with clinical effectiveness by 30 minutes, lasting for up to 4 h. Alternatively, 15 mg neostigmine tablets can be given, each having a clinical effect comparable with that of a 0.5 mg parenteral injection.

In children, the total edrophonium IV dose is 0.15 mg/kg, not to exceed 10 mg. To test hypersensitivity in children, an initial IV edrophonium dose one-tenth that of the total dose can be given. For children weighing up to 75 lb (34 kg), a test dose of 1 mg is appropriate, and a total dose of 5 mg can be used in 1 mg increments. In infants, or when IV access is not available in children up to 75 lb, IM edrophonium at 0.5 to 2 mg can be given as a test dose.

Caution should be exercised when administering edrophonium to patients with cardiac disease, since it rarely may cause bradycardia, atrioventricular (AV) block, and cardiac arrest. Although atropine will counteract these muscarinic effects of edrophonium, it is ineffective in reversing the nicotinic effects, such as skeletal muscle paralysis, that can occur in the face of a cholinergic crisis.

Acute respiratory failure can result from either acute myasthenic or acute cholinergic crisis. Cholinergic crisis patients who fail the Tensilon test may require immediate intubation and management of excessive secretions and acute bronchospasm. Other complications of muscle weakness, such as impaired swallowing, aspiration pneumonia, dehydration, and decubitus ulcers, also must be considered.

LAMBERT-EATON MYASTHENIC SYNDROME

Lambert-Eaton Myasthenic Syndrome (LEMS) is predominantly a disease associated with lung cancer, affecting mostly older men. Patients complain of chronic weakness and fatigue along with autonomic symptoms (e.g. dry mouth and impotence), and the examination shows signs of proximal muscle weakness. Repeated examination of the same limb can sometimes elicit improved strength initially. Eye movements are unaffected except for the pupillary reaction in some cases. Reflexes are diminished. The sensory examination can be normal, but because LEMS is associated with cancer, paraneoplastic or chemotherapy induced neuropathy can lead to a superimposed sensory deficit. Routine laboratory testing may be normal. The differential diagnosis includes myopathies and neuromuscular junction disorders listed above.

The acute treatment of LEMS is supportive. Only in rare cases does this disease progress to respiratory or bulbar failure. Chronic treatment includes eradication of neoplasia, steroids, 3,4-aminopyridine, and anticholinesterases. Hospital admission is reserved for the most severe cases of debilitating weakness or where there is a danger of respiratory compromise.

PARKINSON'S DISEASE

Parkinson's disease (PD) is the most common of the chronic neurodegenerative diseases, affecting many older patients to varying degrees. It is an extrapyramidal movement disorder characterized by the presence of a resting tremor, cogwheel rigidity, bradykinesias or akinesias, and impaired postural reflexes. Although the etiology of the disease is unknown, PD patients consistently are seen to have a reduced number of functional dopaminergic receptors in the substantia nigra. Drug therapy enhances central dopaminergic activity and decreases the relative excess in central cholinergic activity. The availability of multiple drug therapies has improved the symptoms associated with PD, although the disease still progresses without symptom remission in most patients.

Epidemiology

Although the etiology of PD is unknown, epidemiologic studies suggest that it is caused primarily by environmental factors in patients who possibly may have a genetic predisposition to the disease. The overall U.S. incidence is 16 cases per 100,000 persons and is as high as 200 per 100,000 in patients in their seventh and eighth decades of life. The average onset age is between 55 and 60 years, with the peak age of onset between 70 to 79 years.

Pathophysiology

Although the etiology of PD is unknown, the disease is characterized by consistent CNS neuropathology. Cellular changes include the presence of cytoplasmic inclusions termed *Lewy bodies*. There are also extracellular pigment granules that stimulate macrophage activity. A disturbance in oxidative phosphorylation that causes the formation of free radicals is thought to be one possible mechanism for these changes.[20]

In the pigmented areas of the midbrain, especially the substantia nigra, there is depigmentation, dopaminergic neuron loss, and gliosis. These cellular changes result in the loss of functional dopaminergic receptors, causing a decrease in the overall level of striatal dopamine.

Clinical Presentation

The clinical diagnosis of PD is based on the presence of one or more of four hallmark neurologic signs, including resting tremor, cogwheel rigidity, bradykinesia or akinesia, and impairment in posture and equilibrium. Besides these signs, identified in the mnemonic *TRAP,* there also may be other signs, including facial and postural changes, voice and speech abnormalities, depression, and muscle fatigue. Prior to the diagnosis of PD, most patients will have symptoms for months to years, including a general feeling of slowness or stiffness and/or difficulties with handwriting and other skills that require manual dexterity.

Most often patients will complain initially of a unilateral arm resting tremor. The tremor is a repetitive movement of low amplitude that occurs five or more times per minute. This alternating movement is described as ''pill rolling'' because it involves repetitive movements of the fingers and thumb. These tremors also can be seen in the legs or face and most often dissipate when intentional movement is performed. The resting tremor of PD can be differentiated from the kinetic tremor of other neurologic disorders by asking the patient to perform the finger-to-nose maneuver. The resting tremor of PD will become less prominent with the performance of this test and resume once the purposeful movement is ended and the limb is supported and at rest.

Cogwheel rigidity is elicited by causing passive movement of the limb through a full range of motion. As the limb is moved, the muscles will develop an increased tone, and a ratchet-like movement is noted. Bradykinesia, the general sense of slowness of voluntary movement, is often felt to be the most debilitating symptom of PD. In its most extreme form, PD causes akinesia, the inability to perform the movements necessary for daily living, such as turning over in bed, rising from a seated position, or walking. When PD impairs postural reflexes, patients may have an impaired ability to turn or change direction while walking or may lose their balance and fall.

Clinical Diagnosis

The clinical diagnosis of PD is easy to recognize, given the presence of the TRAP symptoms. Once noted, the patient should be questioned about any family history of neurologic disorders, a prior history of encephalitis or other CNS infections, concurrent drug use, and any exposure to toxins or street drugs. The symptoms of PD also can be seen in postencephalitis patients and those with other infections such as neurosyphilis, subacute spongiform encephalopathy, and AIDS. Parkinsonism also can occur as a result of street drugs, toxins, neuroleptic drugs, hydrocephalus, head trauma, and with more rare and complex neurologic disorders such as progressive supranuclear palsy, striatonigral degeneration, and corticobasal ganglionic degeneration. Although thought to be a common cause of parkinsonism, cerebral infarction is now considered an unusual cause of these symptoms.

In drug-induced PD, akinesia is the most common sign, with resting tremor less commonly observed. Other characteristics of drug-induced parkinsonism include a history of drug ingestion known to interfere with central dopamine activity, short interval between symptom onset and maximal disability, bilateral presentation of motor dysfunction, and the presence of other drug-related motor abnormalities.

There is no definitive laboratory or neuroimaging study that is pathognomonic for PD. Although positron emission tomographic (PET) scans may be useful in demonstrating this CNS pathology, CT and MRI most often only show CNS atrophy.

Disease Management

Although currently available therapies do not change the underlying pathology of PD, their use can significantly reduce symptoms. These drugs include anticholinergics such as trihexyphenidyl and benztropine; drugs that increase central dopamine levels such as amantadine, levodopa, and carbidopa; and dopamine receptor drugs such as bromocriptine and pergolide. When PD symptoms cause severe motor dysfunction, the monoamine oxidase (MAO) inhibitor selegiline HCl and the COMT inhibitors entacapone and tolcapone may be effective through the prevention of dopamine metabolism.

Levodopa, which is converted into dopamine by decarboxylases that are present peripherally, can cause symptoms such as anorexia, nausea, and vomiting due to excess peripheral dopamine levels. When levodopa is combined with carbidopa, a peripheral decarboxylase inhibitor, smaller doses of levodopa are required for effectiveness, and side effects are reduced. Over time, the effectiveness of levodopa will diminish, requiring the additional use of dopamine receptor agonist therapy. PD patients who are fully mobile, in the ''on'' state, can suddenly convert to the ''off'' state and become akinetic, especially in the morning shortly after rising and prior to taking the initial daily dose. This ''on-off'' phenomenon is treated by the use of controlled-release preparations of the combined carbidopa-levodopa therapy.

When drug therapy effectiveness diminishes over time, or when significant motor or psychiatric complications occur, a ''drug holiday'' lasting about 1 week is often attempted. Despite the fact that withdrawal of dopaminergic therapy can worsen PD symptoms, functioning actually can improve once therapy is resumed, lasting weeks to months. Patients who are refractory to optimal medical management may benefit from posteroventral pallidotomy, a sterotactic neurosurgical procedure that maintains medical therapy benefit and reduces overall symptom severity.[21,22]

The treatment for drug-induced parkinsonism, which most often presents with akinesia, is termination of the causative agent, which presumably either acts to block central dopamine receptors (neuroleptics, metoclopramide) or reduces central dopamine levels (reserpine).

Emergency Diagnosis and Management

Although most PD patients present to the ED already diagnosed, some might present undiagnosed with motor or sensory symptoms that may not be related immediately to the diagnosis of PD. Patients may experience motor symptoms such as freezing episodes, dysphagia, or abnormalities of whole-body movement. Sensory complaints may include akathesias, paresthesias, muscles aches, or extremity pain. Although severe pain is usually related to the loss of medication efficacy, it can be the prominent symptom of undiagnosed PD.

Complications related to the motor, gait, and truncal disability of PD include deep venous thrombosis, pulmonary embolism, aspiration pneumonia, and compressive neuropathies. Trauma related to falls is common. Autonomic disturbances such as orthostatic hypotension, intestinal motility disorders, and bladder dysfunction can occur. Facial seborrhea also is common. Behavior abnormalities caused by frontal lobe dysfunction and dementia also are seen.

Dyspnea, respiratory distress, and pneumonia are more likely during the ''off'' periods, when drug efficacy is reduced. The most common cause of death in severe PD is respiratory failure.

Dopaminergic therapy toxicities can include psychiatric and sleep disturbances, cardiac dysrhythmias, orthostatic hypotension, dyskinesias, and dystonias. Patients may manifest lingual, facial, or bucchal dystonias and can demonstrate choreic movements similar to those seen with Huntington's chorea or tardive dyskinesia. These drug effects unfortunately are relatively common but can be alleviated with a drug holiday or a decrease in levadopa dosage. Depression and panic attacks are also common, independent of dopaminergic therapy.

Psychiatric complication can occur with dopaminergic therapy, including sleep disturbances, vivid nightmares, auditory and visual hallucinations, paranoia, and frank psychosis. The severity of psychiatric side effects, especially visual hallucinations, is related to the treatment dose and duration and can be improved by a drug holiday or a reduction in drug dosage. Psychotropes that are known to cause tardive dyskenesia, such as haloperidol, must be used cautiously in patients with PD due to an increased risk of this complication.

Adjustment of chronic PD therapies should be done in consultation with the patient's primary care physician, who can help determine which symptoms reflect dopaminergic excess and whether prior drug holidays have improved the patient's symptoms.

POLIO MYELITIS AND POSTPOLIO SYNDROME

Poliomyelitis is a neurotropic enterovirus that causes paralysis through motor neuron destruction and muscle denervation and atrophy. Despite the eradication of most polio cases through effective use of the polio vaccine in the United States, there are still cases that occur in children who are immunized and in populations that are not immunized. An important sequelae of acute poliomyelitis is postpolio syndrome, also termed *postpoliomyelitis progressive muscular atrophy* (PPMA). This disorder is characterized by the recurrence of motor symptoms following a latent period of several decades after the resolution of the motor symptoms caused by the initial infection.

Epidemiology

Poliomyelitis, an infection caused by a group of enteroviruses, leads to significant striated muscle paralysis in less than 5 percent of infected patients.[23] Prior to mass immunization, virtually all children were exposed to and developed antibodies to this enterovirus infection by age 4 years. A 1952 polio epidemic caused 14 new cases of paralytic polio per 100,000 persons, a rate similar to that seen in developing countries that are unable to provide mass immunization. Polio rates as high as 600 cases per 100,000 were seen as recently as the early 1980s in India. Mass immunization with the inactivated poliovirus vaccine (IPV) or attenuated oral poliovirus (OPV) has dramatically reduced the incidence of polio, which was 0.003 cases per 100,000 persons in the United States in 1981. Polio outbreaks still occur in populations that are not consistently immunized, such as was seen in the 1979 U.S. Amish epidemic, which was caused by the wild poliovirus type 1. Outbreaks also have been seen in association with inadequate immunization with modified poliovirus type 3, as was seen in the Finland outbreak in 1984–1985. With the use of OPV, some immunized children will develop polio, as will some young adults who are exposed to children who have been vaccinated with the OPV vaccine. Immunocompromised patients are at greater risk for contracting polio after exposure to children who were vaccinated with the OPV vaccine. In developing countries, recent IM injections, tonsillectomy, and strenuous exercise all have been associated with increased polio infection severity.

The prognosis for most enteroviral CNS infections is favorable with the exception of paralytic poliomyelitis and those enteroviral infections which occur during the first year of life.

The postpolio syndrome (PPMA) is expected to afflict up to 100,000 of the 250,000 U.S. adults with a prior history of polio. Since the majority of these polio cases occurred prior to mass immunization, these patients most likely will be older than age 50. There in no gender predisposition for PPMA. Although PPMA most often occurs after a stable, disease-free period of 20 to 30 years, there are risk factors that predict an earlier onset of postpolio syndrome. These include greater age at the time of initial polio infection, greater residual motor disability, residual bulbar or respiratory signs, and the occurrence of recent injuries that require limb immobilization.

Pathophysiology

In developed countries the viral transmission is oral to oral, whereas in developing countries where the sanitation is poor the transmission is fecal to oral. Acutely, the polio enterovirus enters the body via the gastrointestinal tract and reproduces in the gastrointestinal lymphoid tissue, termed *gut-associated lymphoid tissue* (GALT). Oral secretion of the virus takes place for several days and stool excretion for several weeks.

At a critical concentration, the virus spreads to the large motor nuclei of the spinal cord, the brainstem, and the reticular formation. The vestibular and brainstem motor nuclei, hypothalamus, thalamus, cerebellum, and the precentral motor cerebral cortex also can be infected by the poliovirus. The infected neurons, because of Nissl granule dissolution, are phagocytosed by inflammatory cells, causing neuronal loss and gliosis. Most affected neurons have an altered morphology, and half are destroyed during the first week of acute paralysis. Neuron loss then causes a cycle of muscle denervation and reinnervation, resulting in muscle loss of function.

The pathology of the postpolio syndrome remains unclear. It is suggested that postpolio fatigue is similar to that seen in chronic fatigue syndrome, both of which may cause fatigue by causing a relative depletion of central dopamine.[24] This theory is supported by preliminary data that suggest a decrease in postpolio symptoms with the use of bromocriptine, the same drug used for relief of PD symptoms.[25]

Clinical Presentation

Polio infection remains asymptomatic in over 90 percent of cases. The majority a symptomatic polio infections involve only a minor viral illness that causes no paralysis, termed *abortive polio.* After an incubation period of a few days, symptoms may include fever, malaise, headache, sore throat, and gastrointestinal symptoms. Some of the patients who experience the minor viral illness, especially young children, may develop aseptic meningitis as the infection resolves. Only 1 to 2 percent of all poliovirus infections result in the major illness associated with neurologic involvement. Often there is resolution of the minor viral illness symptoms prior to development of neurologic symptoms, such that it is difficult to identify the preceding minor viral illness. Muscle pain, stiffness, and weakness during the early viral syndrome may suggest the later occurrence of paralysis. Because exercise can exacerbate the severity of the subsequent paralysis, patients with these symptoms suspected of having polio should be advised to avoid exercise.

When the major illness occurs, most commonly the spinal cord anterior horn cells are affected, causing asymmetric proximal limb weakness, especially in the legs. Spinal polio is characterized by flaccid and weak muscles, absent tendon reflexes, and fasciculations. Although pain, paresthesias, and transient sensory abnormalities are noted by polio patients, sensory deficits are usually not found on clinical examination. Maximal paralysis usually occurs within 5 days, and muscle wasting then occurs over several weeks. Autonomic dysfunction, including sweating disturbances, urine retention, delayed gastric emptying, and constipation, is commonly found. Nearly all spinal polio patients will demonstrate improved motor function, with paralysis resolution occurring within the first year after the acute infection.

Up to 20 percent of polio patients with paralysis will develop bulbar polio, which causes speech, swallowing, facial muscle, and rarely extraocular muscle dysfunction. Acute polio infection also can cause encephalitis and can disturb the reticular formation, resulting in cardiac dysrhythmias, blood pressure alterations, hypoxia, and hypercarbia. Patients who survive the acute episode of encephalitis normally will recover without residual affects.

Patients who present with postpolio syndrome complain of muscle fatigue, joint pain, worsening of skeletal deformities, or weakness in muscles that were spared during the initial viral infection.[26] These complaints can occur decades after maximal resolution of the neurologic symptoms caused by the initial polio infection. When muscle weakness is observed, atrophy, pain, and fasciculations may be noted both in previously unaffected muscle groups and in those previously involved. Patients with PPMA also may present with new bulbar, respiratory, or sleep difficulties. For example, laryngeal muscle weakness can cause progressive dyspnea, dysphagia, and/or hoarseness. Some patients complain of abnormal movements in sleep that disturb normal sleep, requiring therapy with benzodiazepines or dopaminergic drugs.[27] These symptoms occur independent of any concurrent neurologic, orthopedic, psychiatric, or systemic medical illness.

Clinical Diagnosis

Acute paralytic poliomyelitis should be considered whenever an at-risk patient presents with an acute febrile illness, aseptic meningitis, and asymmetric flaccid paralysis associated with the loss of deep tendon reflexes and normal sensation. As with other causes of aseptic meningitis, the CSF reveals pleocytosis during the first week after paralysis onset. The CSF white cell count can elevate into the hundreds, with a predominance of neutrophils early in the disease course. These cells allow noninflammatory causes of paralysis to be excluded from the differential diagnosis. Although the poliovirus can be cultured from the CSF early in the disease course, throat and rectal swabs will provide a greater yield. When a particular viral serotype is identified, serial serum antibody titers can be used to verify the cultures.

The most important cause of paralysis that must be excluded is Guillain-Barré syndrome, which, unlike the acute polio infection, causes more symmetric muscle weakness. Acute paralysis can result from peripheral neuropathies caused by infectious mononucleosis, Lyme disease, or porphyria. Paralysis also can result from inflammatory myopathies, electrolyte abnormalities, toxins, or other viruses, such as Coxsackie, mumps, echoviruses, and nonpolio enteroviruses. Paralysis also can result from acute spinal cord compression, vascular lesions, and myelitis, all of which should produce a sensory level and sphincter disturbances. In children, it is necessary to rule out spinal muscular atrophy, which can be undiagnosed until it is manifested by dramatic limb weakness caused by an acute febrile illness.

In order to diagnose postpolio syndrome, the patient should have a history of acute paralytic poliomyelitis with stable recovery of motor function associated with residual muscle atrophy, weakness, and areflexia with normal sensation in at least one limb. Additionally, there should be new muscle symptoms or weakness not attributable to an acute injury, neuropathy, radiculopathy, or systemic, neurologic, or psychiatric illness.

Disease Management

Treatment of the new muscle weakness seen with PPMA is primarily symptomatic, with analgesic and anti-inflammatory medications. Dyspnea, respiratory dysfunction, sleep disorders, and psychiatric disorders all must be addressed in patients with worsening PPMA.[28]

ACKNOWLEDGMENT

The author would like to thank Justin Macariola-Coad for his assistance in collecting information for this chapter.

REFERENCES

1. Tandan R: Disorders of the upper and lower motor neurons, in Bradley WG et al (eds): *Neurology in Clinical Practice: The Neurological Disorders.* Boston, Butterworth-Heinemann, 1996, pp 1843–1852.
2. Brooks BR: Clinical epidemiology of amyotrophic lateral sclerosis. *Neurol Clin* 14:399, 1996.
3. Ono S, Imai T, Munakata S, et al: Collagen abnormalities in the spinal cord from patients with amyotrophic lateral sclerosis. *J Neurol Sci* 160:140, 1998.
4. Liu R, Althaus JS, Ellerbrock BR, et al: Enhanced oxygen radical production in a transgenic mouse model of familial amyotrophic lateral sclerosis. *Ann Neurol* 44:763, 1998.
5. Swash M: Early diagnosis of ALS/MND. *J Neurol Sci* 160(suppl 1):S33, 1998.
6. Sostarko M, Vranjes D, Brinar V, Zovic Z: Severe progression of ALS/MND after intervertebral discectomy. *J Neurol Sci* 160(suppl 1):S42, 1998.
7. Wilbourn AJ: Clinical neurophysiology in the diagnosis of amyotrophic lateral sclerosis: The Lambert and the El Escorial criteria. *J Neurol Sci* 160(suppl 1):S25, 1998.
8. Pradas J, Finison L, Andres PL, et al: The natural history of amyotrophic lateral sclerosis and the use of natural history controls in therapeutic trials. *Neurology* 43:751, 1993.
9. Weinshenker BG: Epidemiology of multiple sclerosis. *Neurol Clin* 14:291, 1996.
10. Sobel RA: The pathology of multiple sclerosis. *Neurol Clin* 13:1, 1998.
11. Poser CM, Paty DW, Scheinberg L, et al: New diagnostic criteria for multiple sclerosis: Guidelines for research protocols. *Ann Neurol* 13:227, 1983.
12. Swanson JW: Multiple sclerosis: Update in diagnosis and review of prognostic factors. *Mayo Clin Proc* 64:577, 1989.
13. Ghadirian P, Jain M, Ducic S, et al: Nutritional factors in the aetiology of multiple sclerosis: A case-control study in Montreal, Canada. *Int J Epidemiol* 27:845, 1998.
14. Lisak RP: Intravenous immunoglobulins in multiple sclerosis. *Neurology* 51:S25, 1998.
15. Metz LM, McGuinness SD, Harris C: Urinary tract infections may trigger relapse in multiple sclerosis. *Axone* 19:67, 1998.
16. Kurtzke JF: Rating neurological impairment in multiple sclerosis: An expanded disability status scale (EDSS). *Neurology* 33:1444, 1983.
17. Robertson NP, Deans J, Compston DA: Myasthenia gravis: A population-based epidemiological study in Cambridgeshire, England. *J Neurol Neurosurg Psychiatry* 65:492, 1998.
18. Kleiner-Fisman G, Kott HS: Myasthenia gravis mimicking stroke in elderly patients. *Mayo Clin Proc* 73:1077, 1998.
19. Barrows RW: Drug-induced neuromuscular blockade and myasthenia gravis. *Pharmacotherapy* 17:1220, 1997.
20. Tanner CM, Goldman SM: Epidemiology of Parkinson's disease. *Neurol Clin* 14:317, 1996.
21. Uitti RJ, Wharen REJ, Turk MF: Efficacy of levodopa therapy on motor function after posteroventral pallidotomy for Parkinson's disease. *Neurology* 51:1755, 1998.

22. Volkmann J, Sturm V: Indication and results of stereotactic surgery for advanced Parkinson's disease. *Crit Rev Neurosurg* 8:209, 1998.
23. Jubelt B: Enterovirus and mumps virus infections of the nervous system. *Neurol Clin* 2:187, 1984.
24. Bruno RL, Creange SJ, Frick NM: Parallels between post-polio fatigue and chronic fatigue syndrome: A common pathophysiology? *Am J Med* 105:66S, 1998.
25. Bruno RL, Zimmerman JR, Creange SJ, et al: Bromocriptine in the treatment of post-polio fatigue: A pilot study with implications for the pathophysiology of fatigue. *Am J Phys Med Rehabil* 75:340, 1996.
26. Wekre LL, Stanghelle JK, Lobben B, Oyhaugen S: The Norwegian polio study 1994: A nationwide survey of problems in long-standing poliomyelitis. *Spinal Cord* 36:280, 1998.
27. Bruno RL: Abnormal movements in sleep as a post-polio sequelae. *Am J Phys Med Rehabil* 77:339, 1998.
28. Stanghelle JK, Festvag LV: Postpolio syndrome: A 5 year follow-up. *Spinal Cord* 35:503, 1997.

MENINGITIS, ENCEPHALITIS, AND BRAIN ABSCESS

Keith E. Loring
David C. Anderson
Alan J. Kozak

In cases of bacterial meningitis, the two most critical actions in the emergency department are to suspect it and begin empirical treatment promptly. It is often impossible to distinguish with certainty meningitides due to viruses, fungi, and other organisms or those due to neoplastic, toxic, and autoimmune processes from bacterial meningitis on the basis of clinical findings and even lumbar puncture (LP) results. Although obtaining appropriate studies, particularly cultures, is enormously helpful in eventually arriving at an appropriate diagnosis, the prompt initiation of therapy must take priority over all diagnostic maneuvers when bacterial meningitis is part of the differential diagnosis. If the clinical situation and the emergency physician's practice environment permit, the diagnostic groundwork can be laid for establishing alternative diagnoses, but never at the expense of initiating timely therapy against likely bacterial pathogens.

Epidemiology

Approximately 25,000 cases of bacterial meningitis occur yearly in the United States. Attack rates are age specific, ranging from almost 400 per 100,000 in neonates to 1 to 2 per 100,000 in adults. Two-thirds of cases are in children. The mortality rate is about 5 percent in children beyond infancy, 25 percent in neonates, and 25 percent in adults.[1,2] Long-term complications, such as cognitive deficits, epilepsy, hydrocephalus, and hearing loss, affect about a quarter of survivors. Prior to 1985, three species accounted for the majority of bacterial meningitis: *Haemophilus influenzae* (45 percent), *Streptococcus pneumoniae* (18 percent), and *Neisseria meningitidis* (14 percent). However, the specific cause of bacterial meningitis has changed in the era of vaccination against *H. influenzae* type b. From 1985 to 1991, the incidence of *H. influenzae* meningitis dropped 82 percent in children under 5 years old. Hence, *S. pneumoniae* and *N. meningitidis* have become the predominant causes of meningitis in children 1 month of age or older.[3] Antibiotic resistance of *S. pneumoniae* to penicillins and ceftriaxone is becoming more prevalent in the United States. While such resistance has been encountered to date mostly in children, the clinician should consider modifying antibiotic selection for both children and adults with suspected pneumococcal meningitis (Table 227-1). The following discussion focuses on bacterial meningitis in adults.

Pathophysiology

Bacterial meningitis begins with the entry of organisms into the well-defended subarachnoid space. The ability to infect the subarachnoid space is not shared equally by all bacteria. The dominance of three organisms—*S. pneumoniae, H. influenzae* type b, and *N. meningitidis*—which cause over two-thirds of bacterial meningitis, is no accident. These encapsulated organisms share the ability to invade the host through the upper airway, survive dissemination through the bloodstream, and then gain access to the subarachnoid space. The subcapsular constituents of these organisms are a strong trigger of inflammatory cascades in the host. Inflammation produces the clinical picture of fever, meningismus, and eventually altered mental status, which are the hallmarks of the disease.[4]

Stimulation of pain-sensitive structures in meninges and posterior spinal roots leads to headache and meningeal signs. The brain and meninges, encased in the fixed-volume skull, become edematous. Cerebrospinal fluid (CSF) drainage is reduced by interference with its flow in the subarachnoid pathways as well as its absorption by the arachnoid granulations. Hence, the quantity of CSF increases, causing communicating or noncommunicating hydrocephalus. Intracranial blood vessels initially expand, increasing the volume occupied by that compartment. The brain itself swells by several mechanisms. Disruption of the blood-brain barrier allows entry of protein and ultimately water (vasogenic edema), while hydrocephalus forces CSF into the periventricular parenchyma (interstitial edema). Eventually, cell membrane homeostasis may be compromised, leading to increased intracellular water (cytotoxic edema).

The sum of these expanded volumes overwhelms the compensatory displacement of CSF into the more compliant spinal compartment, and intracranial pressure rises as a result. Since brain perfusion depends on arterial pressure's exceeding tissue pressure (in this case intracranial pressure), ischemia may develop. Diminished perfusion is all the more likely, since the vascular supply is burdened with an inflammatory infiltrate whose functional and structural consequences include faulty autoregulation, inflammatory narrowing, and a prothrombotic milieu. There are some variations on the pathophysiologic themes described above. For example, organisms sometimes gain entry to the CSF, not by hematogenous seeding, but through direct contiguity. Such direct spread may be from infected parameningeal structures (e.g., brain abscess, otitis media, and sinusitis), traumatic or congenital communications with the exterior, or neurosurgery. The bacteriologic characteristics of these infections may vary. Immunologic deficiency states are increasingly common and predispose to yet other organisms. The clinical and pathophysiologic effects of organisms other than *S. pneumoniae, H. influenzae* type b, and *N. meningitidis* depend on their capacity to stimulate the host's immune processes and the host's response.[5]

Clinical Features

SIGNS AND SYMPTOMS Definitive diagnosis is based on demonstrating bacterial organisms in the subarachnoid space along with a corresponding inflammatory response. The possibility of meningitis must be considered if the diagnosis is to be made. In classic and fulminant cases, about 25 percent of adult cases, there is little diagnostic challenge. The patient presents with rapidly developing fever, headache, stiff neck, photophobia, and altered mental status. Seizures occur in 25 percent of adults and at least that many children. In some patients, typically the very young and the elderly, the clinical features are nonspecific.

Certain historic data should increase the suspicion of meningitis and suggest specific pathogens. Several areas deserve special attention:

TABLE 227-1 Guidelines for Empiric Treatment of Bacterial Meningitis* with No Organisms on Gram Stain

Patient Category	Potential Pathogens	Empiric Therapy
	AGE	
18–50 years	*S. pneumoniae, N. meningitidis*	Ceftriaxone 2 g IV q12h plus vancomycin or rifampin if *S. pneumoniae* resistance possible
Older than 50 years	*S. pneumoniae, N. meningitidis, L. monocytogenes,* aerobic gram-negative bacilli	Ceftriaxone 2 g IV q12h plus ampicillin 2 g IV q4h plus vancomycin or rifampin if *S. pneumoniae* resistance possible
	SPECIAL CIRCUMSTANCES	
CSF leak with history of closed head trauma	*S. pneumoniae, H. influenzae,* group B streptococcus	Ceftriaxone 2 g IV q12h
History of recent penetrating head injury, neurosurgery, CSF shunt	*S. aureus, S. epidermidis,* diphtheroids, aerobic gram-negative bacilli	Vancomycin 25 mg/kg IV load (not >500 mg/h infused), then 19 mg/kg at intervals dictated by Matzke nomogram plus ceftazidime 2 g IV q8h
Immunocompromised host	*S. pneumoniae, N. meningitidis, L. monocytogenes,* aerobic gram-negative bacilli	Vancomycin 25 mg/kg IV load (not >500 mg/h infused), then 19 mg/kg at intervals dictated by Matzke nomogram plus ampicillin 2 g IV q4h plus ceftazidime 2 g IV q8h

*For pediatric meningitis treatment, see Chap. 118.
Source: From Quagliarello and Scheld,[1] with permission.

living conditions, trauma, immunocompetence, immunization history, and antibiotic use. Army barracks and college dormitories are typical environments in which clusters of cases due to *N. meningitidis* occur. Day-care centers may become a source for multiple cases due to *H. influenzae* type b. A history of head trauma (*S. pneumoniae*) or neurosurgery (staphylococcal species or gram-negative rods) may be significant. Conditions that affect immunocompetence (e.g., history of surgical or functional splenectomy, glucocorticoid therapy, and HIV) should be sought. On the other hand, a history of immunization to *H. influenzae* type b in the past will make meningitis due to this organism unlikely. It is important to inquire about recent exposure to antibiotics, which may influence the clinical course, and CSF findings.

Examination must include assessment for meningeal irritation with resistance to passive neck flexion, Brudzinski sign (flexion of hips and knees in response to passive neck flexion), and Kernig sign (contraction of hamstrings in response to knee extension while hip is flexed). Examination of the skin is also crucial for seeking the purpuric rash characteristic of meningococcemia and, less commonly, other pathogens. Cutaneous stigmata suggesting microembolization (e.g., petechiae, splinter hemorrhages, and pustular lesions) should be aspirated when possible for Gram stain and culture. Paranasal sinuses should be percussed, and ears examined for evidence of primary infection. Fundi must be assessed for papilledema or absence of venous pulsation, indicating increased intracranial pressure. Neurologic examination should seek evidence of focal neurologic dysfunction, such as disordered eye movements, homonymous visual field deficits, facial asymmetry, and hemiparesis.[4,5]

LUMBAR PUNCTURE Blood cultures (two specimens drawn 15 min apart) yield the responsible organism in about 50 percent of cases of bacterial meningitis, but CSF analysis is paramount. Appropriate sequencing of LP, cranial imaging studies, and initiation of empirical antibiotics are further discussed below. However, LP should be carried out as quickly as possible.

LP should be performed if intracranial mass lesions and coagulopathy are unlikely on historical or clinical grounds. Specifically, patients with coma, papilledema, or focal neurologic findings require cranial imaging before LP. Prior to imaging, blood cultures should be obtained and empiric antibiotic therapy should be instituted. LP can then proceed if no intracranial mass lesion or mass effect exists. Antibiotic therapy given up to 2 h prior to lumbar puncture will not decrease the diagnostic sensitivity if CSF bacterial antigens assays are obtained along with CSF culture.[6]

Local anesthetic should be used to improve patient comfort, relaxation, and cooperation. Anxiolitics such as benzodiazapines, which are helpful adjuncts in the performance of painful procedures, can cloud the patient's sensorium and confuse subsequent clinical assessment. The L3–L4 interspace should be punctured (L4–L5 in newborn infants) while the patient is curled as tightly as possible in a fetal position. In adults, a line drawn between the iliac crests crosses the spine at the L3–L4 interspace. Alternatively, the patient may be seated on the edge of a bed or cart leaning over a tray stand. The latter technique is particularly useful when landmarks are uncertain, as they may be in an obese patient. The site should be prepared with povidone-iodine and allowed to dry thoroughly to avoid introduction by puncture and the production of chemical arachnoiditis. A $2\frac{1}{2}$-in. 22-gauge needle should be used in children and a $3\frac{1}{2}$-in. 20-gauge needle in adults. Although useful, the opening pressure is not critical for interpretation of the procedure. To obtain meaningful results, the pressure must be measured with the patient lying extended on his or her side. Pressures measured with the patient still curled in extreme flexion or while sitting will be artificially elevated. Normal pressure is less than 170 mm-H_2O. Careful repositioning (straightening the curled patient or helping the seated patient to a lying position on his or her side) is safely performed with the needle in situ.

Four tubes, each containing at least 1 mL of CSF, are typically obtained. More volume —up to 5 mL—may be preferable in patients who are immunocompromised. Red and white blood cell counts with differential counts are requested for tubes 1 and 4. The two-tube assessment helps detect a traumatic tap because the rate of bleeding changes rapidly, causing a difference in red blood cell count between the two tubes. Tube 4 may also be used for culture and Gram stain. Tube 2 is sent for determination of protein and glucose levels. Tube 3 should be saved for other studies, discussed below, if necessary. Closing pressure is not necessary.[7]

Diagnosis

The differential diagnoses may be categorized into parenchymal or meningeal disorders. When fever and focal neurologic symptoms and signs predominate, parenchymal central nervous system infections are concerns (e.g., brain abscess, viral encephalitis, cerebral toxoplasmosis, and other parenchymal processes). When meningeal signs predominate, other infectious meningitides, meningeal neoplasm, and subarachnoid hemorrhage are possible.

TABLE 227-2 Typical Spinal Fluid Results for Meningeal Processes

Parameter (Normal)	Bacterial	Viral	Neoplastic	Fungal
OP (<170 mmCSF)	>300 mm	200 mm	200 mm	300 mm
WBC (<5 mononuclear)	>1000/μL	<1000/μL	<500/μL	<500/μL
% PMNs (0)	>80%	1–50%	1–50%	1–50%
Glucose (>40 mg/dL)	<40 mg/dL	>40 mg/dL	<40 mg/dL	<40 mg/dL
Protein (<50 mg/dL)	>200 mg/dL	<200 mg/dL	>200 mg/dL	>200 mg/dL
Gram stain (−)	+	−	−	−
Cytology (−)	−	−	+	+

Abbreviations: OP, opening pressure; PMNs, polymorphonuclear cells; and WBC, white blood cells.
Source: From Greenlee JE.[8]

For evaluation of parenchymal brain infections, LP is unhelpful and potentially dangerous, since it can lead to transtentorial or tonsillar herniation. A cranial computed tomography (CT) scan should be done first if the patient exhibits papilledema or focal neurologic signs. A cranial CT scan is also the preferred mode in diagnosing subarachnoid hemorrhage.

For meningeal disorders other than subarachnoid hemorrhage, CSF examination is most helpful. Typical CSF findings for bacterial, viral, neoplastic, and fungal meningitides are displayed in Table 227-2, but there is considerable overlap in findings. Some bacteria (e.g., *Mycoplasma, Listeria,* spirochetes, syphilis, *Leptospira,* and *Borrelia*) produce CSF alterations that in Table 227-2. An aseptic profile, suggesting viral infection, is typical of partially treated bacterial infections (one-third or more of pediatric cases have received antimicrobial treatment before presenting with meningitis). The same is true of untreated bacterial infections adjacent to but not communicating with the subarachnoid space, such as abscesses of the brain and subdural or epidural spaces. The percentage of polymorphonuclear cells may be higher in early viral meningitis, and glucose levels may be reduced in some viral cases.

Additional helpful tests may include viral cultures in suspected viral meningitis, tests for *Borrelia* antibodies in patients with possible Lyme disease, india ink and latex agglutination assay for fungal antigen in cryptococcal meningitis (serum cryptococcal antigen, if available, obviates this CSF analysis), acid-fast stain and culture for mycobacteria in tuberculous meningitis, and latex agglutination or counterimmune electrophoresis for bacterial antigens in potentially partially treated bacterial cases. Assays are most widely available for *S. pneumoniae,* other group *B streptococci, H. influenzae* type b, and *N. meningitidis.* Rarely, CSF may be normal or nearly so in very early bacterial meningitis, especially during meningococcemia. Empiric antibiotic treatment, admission, and repeated LP are appropriate if clinical suspicion is great despite negative initial CSF results.[8]

Treatment

Ideal management has several goals. The first priority is the rapid administration of a bactericidal antibiotic that gains rapid entry to the subarachnoid space. A secondary priority in some cases is use of an anti-inflammatory agent to suppress the normal inflammatory processes, which are amplified by antibiotic-induced bacteriolysis. A tertiary concern is to counter the adverse effects of increased intracranial pressure and vasculopathy, which may lead to brain ischemia. Finally, when several options that accomplish these goals are available, those with the lowest expense and rates of treatment morbidity should be employed.

Agents to which local bacterial resistance has developed should be avoided. Currently, for example, about 30 percent of *H. influenzae* type b isolates are resistant to ampicillin. Bacteriostatic agents should not be used alone or in combination with a bactericidal agent, since they are antagonistic. Agents of current choice for given bacterial meningitides are indicated in Table 227-1. Empiric therapy in cases warranting antibiotics before LP or when results of Gram stain are negative (about 30 percent of untreated cases, 50 percent of those receiving antibiotics before LP) is based on the patient's age and should also take risk factors into consideration.[9]

Empiric treatment for bacterial meningitis is based on the likelihood of certain pathogens (Table 227-1) and results of CSF Gram stain. For patients aged 18 to 50 with no organisms evident on Gram stain, ceftriaxone 2 g intravenously every 12 h is the current recommendation. For patients with Gram stain suggesative of *S. pneumoniae* (gram-positive cocci in clusters), a broad-spectrum cephalosporin and vancomycin should be given to ensure coverage of resistant organisms. For gram-negative cocci, presumed *N. meningitidis,* penicillin G is still effective. For gram-ppositive rods, *Listeria monocytogenes* is the presumed agent, and the recommended regimen is ampicillin and gentamicin. For gram-negative rods, the recommendation is ceftazidime and an aminoglycoside.

A variety of inflammation suppressants have been shown to improve outcome in experimental bacterial meningitis. Only glucocorticoids, and specifically dexamethasone, have been tested in clinical trials. Evidence is persuasive that dexamethasone given before or at the time of the first antibiotic dose most effectively reduces morbidity rates of bacterial meningitis due to *H. influenzae* type b. Many authorities now recommend intravenous dexamethasone, 0.15 mg/kg, as adjunctive therapy in children with this infection. A lower but clear efficacy has been shown in children with *S. pneumoniae* meningitis, and dexamethasone is thus recommended in these cases as well. Some would extrapolate the favorable results noted in children to adults, especially those with a heavy burden of organisms (reflected by a positive CSF Gram stain results) or evidence of increased intracranial pressure. Dexamethasone at the same dosage would seem to be the glucocorticoid of choice for these patients as well, but no adequate studies of efficacy and safety exist to date, and therefore it is not recommended.[10–12]

Also important in management is surveillance for and correction of complications, including seizures, hyponatremia, hydrocephalus, and cerebrovascular accidents. General treatment measures include maintenance of normal blood volume. Hypotonic fluids should be avoided. The serum sodium level should be monitored serially to detect a syndrome of inappropriate antidiuretic hormone or cerebral salt wasting. Hyperpyrexia should be treated. Coagulopathies should be corrected using specific replacement therapies. Phenytoin loading is indicated in patients who develop seizures. For marked cerebral edema, as evidenced by clinical or CT findings, the following are indicated: head elevation, hyperventilation to a P_{CO_2} of 25 to 30 mmHg, and use of mannitol. Measurement of intracranial and systemic arterial pressure is useful in severe cases to enable monitoring of cerebral perfusion pressure.

Chemoprophylaxis is indicated for high-risk contacts of patients with documented *N. meningitidis* or *H. influenzae* type b, including household contacts; school or day-care contacts in the previous 7 days; those who have had direct exposure to the patient's secretions through kissing, shared utensils, or shared toothbrushes; and those who have performed mouth-to-mouth resuscitation or have intubated the patient while unprotected with a face mask. First-line treatment is with rifampin 10 mg/kg (to a maximum of 600 mg per dose) every 12 h for four doses. Alternatives are ceftriaxone, ciprofloxacin, and sulfisoxasole. High-risk contacts should be instructed to return at once if they develop symptoms.[13]

VIRAL MENINGITIS

A number of viruses can cause aseptic meningitis, including nonpolio enteroviruses, mumps, cytomegalovirus, herpes simplex virus, lymphocytic choriomeningitis, adenovirus, and HIV. Specific diagnosis depends on isolation of the virus or positive results on immunoassay of the CSF. Nonpolio enteroviruses (echovirus, coxsackievirus, and enterovirus) account for about 85 percent of all cases of viral meningitis in the United States.

While the diagnosis of viral meningitis is often straightforward (Table 227-2), there can be overlap of CSF findings with early bacterial meningitis and partially treated bacterial meningitis, making specific diagnosis for some cases difficult in the emergency department. Neutrophils may predominate in the CSF for the first 24 h in viral meningitis. Standard references report up to a 10 percent incidence of lymphocytic predominance in CSF with bacterial meningitis, more common with *L. monocytogenes* and in neonatal meningitis. Depending on clinical diagnostic certainty, a range of approaches can be employed in the management of presumed viral meningitis, from admission with empiric antibiotic therapy until culture results return, to discharge from the emergency department with follow-up in 24 h.

VIRAL ENCEPHALITIS

Viral encephalitis is a viral infection of brain parenchyma that produces an inflammatory response. It is distinct from, although often coexists with, viral meningitis, in which the infectious agent and inflammatory response are in the subarachnoid space. Clinically the distinction is made by the presence of neurologic abnormality in encephalitis, whereas only meningeal symptoms and signs (e.g., photophobia, headache, and stiff neck) occur in meningitis. The true incidence of viral encephalitis is difficult to estimate because of the variability of clinical expression, ranging from profound neurologic involvement to clinically silent cases, as well as variability in reporting policies. Several thousand cases are reported yearly in the United States.

Epidemiology

The incidence of the various types of viral encephalitis varies from year to year, depending on whether sporadic or epidemic outbreaks occur. In relative terms, the incidence is about one-tenth that of bacterial meningitis. Arboviruses account for 10 percent of cases during times of sporadic, isolated cases but can account for up to 50 percent of cases during epidemic outbreaks. The four most common arboviral encephalitides in the United States are the California encephalitis serogroup, St. Louis equine encephalitis, western equine encephalitis, and eastern equine encephalitis. California encephalitis is reported most often, with 76 cases reported in 1994. It is seen in the midwestern and eastern United States exclusively, despite its name. Ninety percent of reported cases occur in children. St. Louis encephalitis is seen throughout the United States in periodic outbreaks, with the yearly incidence ranging from 20 reported cases to 2000. It is seen primarily in young children and the elderly and has a 20 percent mortality rate in the latter. Western equine encephalitis prevails in the western United States and Canada. Disease is most severe in the very young, causing seizures in 90 percent of affected infants and permanent neurologic deficits in 50 percent. Eastern equine encephalitis is prevalent in the Atlantic and Gulf coast regions and accounts for the most severe cases of arboviral encephalitis. It tends to occur in sporadic epidemics and has a mortality rate of nearly 70 percent.

Herpes simplex virus type 1 (HSV-1) and herpes simplex virus type 2 (HSV-2) encephalitis occurs in 1 in 250,000 to 1 in 500,000 cases annually in the United States. HSV-1 is typically seen in older children and adults as reactivation disease, while HSV-2 is seen in neonates as a result of perinatal transmission and generally leads to devastating neurologic outcomes.

Pathophysiology

In North America, viruses that cause encephalitis include the arboviruses, HSV-1, herpes zoster, Epstein-Barr virus (EBV), and rabies. Entry portals are highly virus specific for the encephalitis-producing viruses. The arboviruses (*arbo* meaning "arthropod borne") are transmitted by mosquitoes and ticks, and rabies is transferred by the bite of an infected animal. Impaired immune status may play a role in herpes zoster and cytomegalovirus (CMV) encephalitis. Common to all is preliminary viral invasion of the host at a site where replication takes place that is outside the central nervous system. Most viruses then reach the nervous system hematogenously during viremia. However, at least three important viruses—rabies, herpes simplex virus (HSV), and herpes zoster—reach the spinal cord and eventually the brain by traveling backward within axons from a distal site where they have gained access to nerve endings.

Once in the brain, the virus enters neural cells. Neurologic dysfunction and damage are caused by the disruption of neural cell functions by the virus and by the effects of the host's inflammatory responses. Gray matter is predominantly affected, resulting in cognitive and psychiatric signs, lethargy, and seizures. Multifocal white matter damage occurs predominantly in postinfectious encephalomyelitis and rarely during acute encephalitis. Sensorimotor deficits referable to one hemisphere or to the spinal cord are more typical of this immune-mediated pathologic process, which may follow viral encephalitis and meningitis of any type.

Clinical Features

Encephalitis should be considered in patients presenting with the following clinical features singly or in combination: new psychiatric symptoms, cognitive deficits (e.g., aphasia, amnestic syndrome, or acute confusional state), seizures, and movement disorders. Features of meningeal involvement, such as headache and photophobia, are usually, but not invariably, present. The same is true for fever.

Patients with herpes zoster (shingles or chickenpox), EBV, or CMV encephalitis (lymphadenopathy and hepatosplenomegaly) may have a history and signs typical of clinical syndromes caused outside the central nervous system by these viruses. Other circumstances of the case may suggest both the broad diagnosis of encephalitis and a specific viral cause (Table 227-3). For example, a late-summer encephalopathy suggests the possibility of an arbovirus encephalitis, and an animal bite for which no antirabies treatment was obtained has obvious relevance.

Signs of meningeal irritation and increased intracranial pressure should be sought. Neurologic findings reflect the areas of involvement. A careful assessment of cognition is crucial. Sensorimotor deficits are

TABLE 227-3 Viral Pathogens Causing Encephalitis in North America

Virus	Clinical Clues	Diagnosis	Prognosis
HSV-1	"Psychiatric" presentation	MRI, EEG, PCR of CSF, biopsy	30% die, 30% have deficits
Herpes zoster	Shingles, chickenpox, immunosuppressed state	Skin vesicle or CSF culture, serology	Mortality 10–20%
EBV	Mononucleosis	Serology	5–10% die
Rabies	Animal bite	Saliva or CSF culture, biopsy, serology	90% die
Arboviruses	Seasonal		
California	Midwest, children	CSF or blood culture, serology	Good
St. Louis	Midwest, older urban dwellers	As above	5–10% die
Western equine	West, outside workers	As above	5–10% die
Eastern equine	Southeast, outside workers	As above	50% die

Source: From Bale JF Jr.[14]

not typical. Encephalitides may show special regional tropism. Herpes simplex virus (HSV) involves limbic structures of the temporal and frontal lobes, with prominent psychiatric features, memory disturbance, and aphasia. Some arboviruses predominantly affect the basal ganglia, causing choreoathetosis and parkinsonism. Involvement of the brainstem nuclei that control swallowing leads to the hydrophobic choking response characteristic of rabies encephalitis.[14,15]

Diagnosis

Diagnosis rests on imaging studies using magnetic resonance imaging (MRI) or CT if MRI is not reasonably available, electroencephalography (EEG), and LP. Imaging not only excludes other potential lesions, such as brain abscess, but also may display findings that are highly suggestive of HSV encephalitis, a treatable infection, with involvement of medial temporal and inferior frontal gray matter. MRI is more sensitive than CT in this regard. EEG is quite useful in establishing the broad diagnosis as well. Almost by definition, the EEG findings are abnormal in encephalitis, in contrast to isolated viral meningitis or to a primary psychiatric disorder. Furthermore, HSV produces an almost pathognomonic picture in the setting of acute febrile encephalopathy, with the EEG showing periodic, usually asymmetric sharp waves. These findings can be present before any abnormality is visible on MRI. Realistically, LP is the most useful diagnostic procedure in the emergency department once imaging studies, if clinically indicated and available, rule out the risk of uncal herniation. Findings of aseptic meningitis are typical on CSF examination. It is at least theoretically possible to have encephalitis without meningitis, but it is quite rare.

The differential diagnosis depends on the nature of the presentation. When fever and meningeal symptoms predominate, bacterial meningitis is suspected. In less fulminant meningeal cases, Lyme disease; tuberculous, fungal, and neoplastic meningitis; and subacute subarachnoid hemorrhage are part of the differential diagnosis. When parenchymal features are prominent, brain abscess, bacterial endocarditis, postinfectious encephalomyelitis, and toxic or metabolic encephalopathies should be considered.

The clear diagnostic imperative in the emergency department is to exclude the most immediately life-threatening alternative processes requiring immediate treatment. The two most important are bacterial meningitis and acute subarachnoid hemorrhage. Once that is satisfactorily accomplished, the mandate is less definite. Of the viruses causing encephalitis, only HSV has been shown by clinical trial to be responsive to antiviral therapy. HSV can be isolated in as many as 50 percent of neonatal infections but is rarely found in older children and adults. The polymerase chain reaction (PCR) analysis of CSF has 95 percent sensitivity and 100 percent specificity in the diagnosis of HSV infection with respect to brain biopsy. Regardless of diagnostic approach, because current antiviral treatment is relatively risk and side effect free, empiric therapy is recommended in cases of clinical encephalitis.[16] Of the other viral encephalitides, CSF culture results are positive for 50 to 70 percent of patients with enteroviral meningitis but for a much smaller percentage of those with isolated enteroviral encephalitis. The use of PCR techniques for the enteroviruses is also showing promise for central nervous system diagnosis in the future.

Treatment

The agent of choice for HSV is acyclovir 10 mg/kg every 8 h for 14 to 21 days. Based on anecdotal data, patients with herpes zoster and CMV encephalitis may also benefit from antiviral therapy: acyclovir for herpes zoster and ganciclovir for CMV encephalitis.

Prognosis depends on the virus and host. Rabies encephalitis, while rare, continues to be neurologically devastating and usually fatal. Eastern equine encephalitis and HSV also have high mortality rates and frequently produce residual deficits. For the others, adverse outcome is seen mainly in elderly patients or in those with compromising preexisting systemic or neurologic conditions.

Disposition

Patients with encephalitis should in general be admitted. The outcome in cases of HSV encephalitis is related to the neurologic condition at the time that antiviral therapy is initiated. Patients who are already in coma do very poorly, making timely diagnosis and therapy a priority for this form of encephalitis. Empiric initiation of acyclovir 10 mg/kg in the emergency department in encephalitis suspects should be highly considered.[14,15]

BRAIN ABSCESS

A brain abscess is a focal pyogenic infection. When fully developed, it is composed of a central pus-filled cavity, ringed by a layer of granulation tissue and an outer fibrous capsule. Surrounding this is edematous brain tissue infiltrated with inflammatory cells. It is a pathologic response typical of a relatively competent immune system against a bacterial invader. Focal brain infections due to other organisms, such as granulomas due to tuberculosis, necrotic lesions of toxoplasmosis in immunocompromised patients, or cystic lesions of cysticercosis, are not abscesses in the pathologic sense. These nonpurulent focal lesions are not considered here.

Epidemiology

Brain abscess is rather uncommon, accounting for 1 in 10,000 hospitalizations. This incidence is much less than that of bacterial meningitis and is only 2 percent that of brain tumors. The rate has gradually fallen over the past century, probably reflecting the effect of antibiotics on predisposing conditions, such as otitis media. Mortality rates for diagnosed cases have also fallen, from about 50 percent in the early twentieth century to a current level of 10 to 20 percent. Long-term sequelae are seen in about a third of survivors.

Age distribution corresponds to the various predisposing conditions. Most patients with brain abscess related to a paranasal sinus focus are in the 10- to 30-year-old range. When the source is otic, a bimodal incidence occurs in ages less than 20 and greater than 40 years. Twenty-five percent of cases occur in children under 15 years old, with the majority occuring in the 4- to 7-year-old range. Pockets of higher incidence occur along the lines of age, origin of initial infection, and, in some cases, gender.

Pathophysiology

Organisms reach the brain by one of three known routes: hematogenously (one-third of cases); from contiguous infections of middle ear, sinus, or teeth (one-third of cases); or by direct implantation by neurosurgery or penetrating trauma (about 10 percent of cases). The route is unknown in about 20 percent. Circumstances that reduce oxygenation of brain parenchyma are important predisposing factors for bacterial invasion. For example, spread from a contiguous infection usually involves intervening cerebral thrombophlebitis, with congestive ischemic hypoxemia of tissue destined to become infected. Hematogenous seeding is facilitated by systemic hypoxemia, as in congenital heart diseases with right-to-left shunt and chronic pulmonary suppuration. This is demonstrated by the prominent role of anaerobic bacteria in brain abscesses. The source of brain abscess should be identified for the dual purpose of eliminating the source itself and gaining insight into the probable bacteriologic characteristics of the abscess. For example, gram-negative rods, especially *Bacteroides*, are the usual pathogens in otogenic brain abscesses, which are typically single and located in the adjacent temporal lobe or cerebellum. Anaerobic and microaerophilic streptococci are the most common pathogens in sinogenic and odontogenic abscesses and are more typically located in the frontal lobes. Abscesses formed from hematogenous spread are often multiple and polymicrobial, with anaerobic and microaerophilic streptococci commonly represented. Staphylococci are typical pathogens in abscesses due to direct implantation. Gram-negative rods are also suspected in cases related to a neurosurgical procedure.

Clinical Features

Presenting features of brain abscess are notoriously nonspecific. Patients rarely appear acutely ill, and the classic triad of headache, fever, and focal neurologic deficit is present in less than one-third of all patients. As a result, the diagnosis is often delayed. Symptoms reflect the infectious and neurologic (focal and mass effect–producing) aspects of the disease. The most common symptom is headache, which is a complaint in almost all cases. Fever is present in about half of all cases, and neck stiffness in fewer than half. Toxic appearance is rare until late in the disease process. Focal neurologic symptoms, such as hemiparesis or seizures, are present in about a third. Other symptoms of increased intracranial pressure, such as vomiting, confusion, or obtundation, are present in about half of cases. The presentation may be dominated by the origin of the infection (e.g., ear or sinus pain).

Meningeal signs are present in less than half of cases on examination. Papilledema is noted on funduscopy in about a third of patients. Focal neurologic signs reflecting the site of the lesion (e.g., frontal lobes, hemiparesis; temporal lobes, homonymous superior quadrant visual field deficits or aphasia; or cerebellum, limb incoordination or nystagmus) are present in about 60 percent of patients on careful examination. Discovery of potential sites of origin may raise suspicion of brain abscess when the presentation is otherwise nonspecific (e.g., otitis media, sinus tenderness, evidence of pulmonary suppuration, or right-to-left shunting) in a patient with subacute headache and lethargy.

Diagnosis

Brain abscess is diagnosed by imaging studies. CT with contrast infusion classically demonstrates one or several thin, smoothly contoured rings of enhancement surrounding a low-density center and surrounded by white matter edema. Early in the course, a ring may be thicker and less well defined, with the only CT finding being an area of focal hypodensity. Suspected brain abscess is one of the rare instances in the emergency department when a contrast-enhanced study is preferred over a noncontrast study. MRI usually demonstrates a ring, even without gadolinium enhancement. Both types of studies are highly sensitive, and one imaging modality has no real advantage over the other except that CT is usually more readily available in the emergency department. Other studies, such as blood analysis, EEG, and CSF examination, are too nonspecific for definitive diagnosis, and LP is contraindicated when suspicion is high and when focal neurologic signs are present. Cultures of blood or other sites of infection may guide future management and should always be obtained.

Differential diagnosis of the clinical presentation is broad because of its nonspecific and variable nature. A sudden onset with focal features may suggest cerebrovascular disease. Prominent fever, stiff neck, and confusion may suggest meningitis. A protracted course with features of increased intracranial pressure may suggest neoplasm. Brain neoplasm, subacute brain hemorrhage, other focal lesions, and other focal brain infections, such as toxoplasmosis, may mimic the imaging findings of brain abscess. Biopsy or aspiration for confirmation of diagnosis as well as for bacteriologic studies is necessary in most cases.

Treatment

The cornerstone of early ED treatment of brain abscess is antibiosis. The susceptibility of the likely pathogen and the penetration of the agent into the lesion should be considered when choosing an antibiotic. The bacteriologic characteristics of the lesion may be inferred if the origin is obvious. Initial empiric antibiotic choice should take advantage of such information. Initial treatment in a suspected otogenic case is with a third-generation cephalosporin, such as cefotaxime, or trimethoprim-sulfamethoxazole with metronidazole or chloramphenicol. For presumed abscess of sinogenic or odontogenic origin, high-dose penicillin is a good choice. Penicillin is also appropriate for an abscess of hematogenous origin. Chloramphenicol or metronidazole, which by virtue of their lipophilic nature penetrate abscesses very well, is usually added to these penicillin regimes. When communication with the exterior is suspected, as in penetrating trauma or after neurosurgery, nafcillin or vancomycin are indicated. Addition of ceftazidime may be required if gram-negative aerobes are suspected. For patients in whom no mechanism is apparent or suspected, the combination of a third-generation cephalosporin, such as cefotaxime, and metronidazole provides good coverage.

Most cases require neurosurgery for diagnosis and bacteriologic analysis, if not for definitive treatment. Total excision has become necessary less often with the availability of imaging techniques for following the course of abscesses treated medically after surgical aspiration. In cases in which intracranial pressure is high, excision is still carried out. The role of glucocorticoids is controversial. Steroids may produce temporary improvement of increased intracranial pressure.[17,18]

REFERENCES

1. Quagliarello VJ, Scheld WM: Bacterial meningitis: Pathogenesis, pathophysiology, and progress. *N Engl J Med* 327:864, 1992.

2. Feigin RD, McCracken GH Jr, Klein JO: Diagnosis and management of meningitis. *Pediatr Infect Dis J* 11:785, 1992.
3. Adams WG, Deaver KA, Cochi SL, et al: Decline of childhood *Haemophilus influenzae* type b (Hib) disease in the Hib vaccine era. *JAMA* 269:221, 1993.
4. Durand ML, Calderwood SB, Weber DJ, et al: Acute bacterial meningitis in adults: A review of 493 episodes. *N Engl J Med* 328:21, 1993.
5. Ashwal S, Tomasi L, Schneider S, et al: Bacterial meningitis in children: Pathophysiology and treatment. *Neurology* 42:739, 1992.
6. Talan DA, Zibulewsky J: Relationship of clinical presentation to time to antibiotics for the emergency department management of suspected bacterial meningitis.*Ann Emerg Med* 22:1733, 1993.
7. American Academy of Neurology Quality Standards Subcommittee, Daube JR, Frishber BM, et al: 1992: *Practice Parameters: Lumbar Puncture.* Minneapolis, American Academy of Neurology, 1992.
8. Greenlee JE: Approach to diagnosis of meningitis: Cerebrospinal fluid evaluation. *Infect Dis Clin North Am* 4:583, 1990.
9. Quagliarello VJ, Scheld WM: Treatment of bacterial meningitis. *N Engl J Med* 336:708, 1997.
10. Wald ER, Kaplan SI, Mason EO Jr, et al: Dexamethasone therapy for children with bacterial meningitis. *Pediatrics* 95:21, 1995.
11. Geiman BJ, Smith AL: Dexamethasone and bacterial meningitis: A meta-analysis of randomized controlled trials. *West J Med* 157:27, 1992.
12. Talan DA, Hoffman JR, Yoshikawa TT, Overturf GD: Role of empiric parenteral antibiotics prior to lumbar puncture in suspected bacterial meningitis: State of the art. *Rev Infect Dis* 10:365, 1988.
13. Tauber MG, Sande MA: General principles of therapy of pyogenic meningitis. *Infect Dis Clin North Am* 4:661, 1990.
14. Bale JF Jr: Viral encephalitis. *Med Clin North Am* 77:25, 1993.
15. Johnson RT: Acute encephalitis. *Clin Infect Dis* 23:219, 1996.
16. Rowley AH, Whitley RJ, Lakeman FD, et al: Rapid detection of herpes simplex-virus DNA in cerebrospinal fluid of patients with herpes simplex encephalitis. *Lancet* 335:440, 1990.
17. Heilpern KL, Lorber B: Focal intracranial infections. *Infect Dis Clin North Am* 10:879, 1996.
18. Seydoux C, Francioli P: Bacterial brain abscesses: Factors influencing mortality and sequelae. *Clin Infect Dis* 15:394, 1992.

COMPLICATIONS OF CNS DEVICES

Joseph Pagane

CEREBROSPINAL FLUID SHUNTS

The shunting of cerebrospinal fluid (CSF) was first described in 1895, but it was not until the 1950s that shunting ventricular CSF became a routine procedure.[1,2] Hydrocephalus has an incidence of 3 cases per 1000 live births. Mechanical shunting is the primary treatment as there is usually no alternative corrective surgical or medical therapy for this disorder. Each year there are approximately 18,000 CSF shunts inserted, making it the most common pediatric neurosurgical procedure performed in the United States.[1] The CSF shunt is also the neurosurgical procedure with the highest incidence of postoperative complications.[1,2]

Many types of CSF shunt systems exist. Most systems consist of three components beginning with a silastic tube passed into the ventricle via a burr hole. This tubing is tunneled subcutaneously to a valve chamber. The valve chamber, the second component, establishes a pressure gradient that ensures drainage of fluid away from the ventricle. The valve chamber, or in some cases a separate reservoir, allows access to the shunt system for patency testing, pressure measurement, CSF sampling, medication injection (e.g., chemotherapy, antibiotics), or contrast administration. Distal tubing, which is the third component, connects the valve chamber to a drainage point. The most common drainage site is the peritoneal cavity. Other drainage sites include the right atrium, gallbladder, pleural cavity, and ureter.

Shunt Malfunction

Shunt malfunctions are the most common complications encountered with CSF shunts, occurring in up to 67 percent of patients during their lifetime. Obstruction is the most common type of shunt malfunction and most commonly occurs in the proximal tubing followed by the distal tubing, and, finally, the valve chamber. Proximal obstructions usually occur within the first two years after shunt insertion. Causes include tissue debris, chorioid plexus, clot, infection, catheter-tip migration, or following a localized immune response to the tubing. Kinking or disconnection of the tube, pseudocyst formation, or infection can cause distal obstruction. Distal obstruction is the most frequently encountered obstruction in shunts in place for longer than two years.[1,2]

SLIT VENTRICLE SYNDROME Overdrainage and the slit-ventricle syndrome are seen in approximately 5 percent of shunted patients. Due to overdrainage, the tissues actually occlude the orifices of the proximal shunt apparatus. As ICP increases, the same occluding tissue is disengaged, allowing drainage to resume. This phenomenon is cyclical and is responsible for the episode or waxing and waning aspect of the presenting complaint. Patients present with episodes of elevated intracranial pressure caused by a transient obstruction of the ventricular catheter from a collapsed ventricle. Decreased cerebral compliance may prevent the ventricles from fully expanding as intracranial pressure and volume increase, further contributing to ventricular collapse. Newer shunt systems with antisiphon devices and improved shunt valves have a lower rate of this complication.[1,2]

CLINICAL PRESENTATION Symptoms of shunt malfunction usually develop over several days although rapid deterioration within 24 h has been reported. Clinical features include mental status changes; headache; nausea; vomiting; abdominal pain; lethargy; decreased intellectual performance; ataxia; coma; and autonomic instability. Often the presenting complaint is vague. As intracranial pressure increases, paralysis of upward gaze or sundowning, dilated pupils and papilledema may develop. ''Sundowning'' is due to impingement of the brainstem by the third ventricle as it engorges. Symptoms of slit ventricle syndrome are exacerbated or precipitated by standing or exercise due to excessive CSF drainage and relieved by lying down or the Trendelenburg position.

SHUNT EVALUATION Identification of shunt type is important although frequently difficult. Many different types exist and appropriate assessment is dependent on the apparatus implanted. Shunt function is evaluated by manual testing and radiologic studies. Palpation of the shunt allows the physician to locate the valve chamber. Shunt patency is evaluated somewhat differently for each type of device depending on such features as valves, dome or cylinder-shaped reservoirs. Generally, testing follows intuitive expectations but may yet prove perplexing to inexperienced clinicians. For a simple device, once the chamber is located, it is gently compressed and observed for refill. Difficulty compressing the chamber indicates distal flow obstruction, while slow refill, defined as greater than 3 s following compression, indicates a proximal obstruction. Clinicians should realize that compression is inaccurate in identifying shunt obstruction as up to 40 percent of obstructed shunts have normal refill during manual palpation.[2] In any case, further evaluation is required.

A shunt series of plain films includes an AP and lateral radiographs of the skull, and an AP view of the chest and abdomen (for ventriculoperitoneal shunts). While plain radiography will identify kinking, migration or disconnection of the shunt system, CT is required to evaluate ventricular size. Comparison to previous CT scans is needed as many shunted patients have an abnormal baseline ventricular size. In one series, using CT, or both CT and plain films, 25 percent of patients with documented shunt malfunction had no radiologic evidence of shunt malfunction.[3] Therefore, in patients with suggestive clinical features, unimpressive CT and/or shunt series cannot be relied on to exclude shunt obstruction. In this instance, obtain neurosurgical consultation whenever shunt malfunction is suspected.

A shunt tap may need to be performed to make the diagnosis of shunt malfunction, rule out infection, or to alleviate life threatening increased intracranial pressure. The shunt tap should be performed by a neurosurgeon if available. Emergency physicians should be prepared to perform a shunt tap if a neurosurgeon is unavailable or if a shunt tap is needed to control life threatening increased intracranial pressure.

To perform a shunt tap, locate and sterilely prepare the site over the valve system or reservoir. The scalp should be shaved. A 23-g needle or butterfly attached to a manometer is inserted into the reservoir. If no fluid returns or flow ceases, a proximal obstruction is likely. The opening pressure should be measured while occluding the reservoir outflow. An opening pressure of 20 cm or greater indicates a distal obstruction while low pressures indicate a proximal obstruction. The normal basal intracranial pressure is around 12 ± 2 cm.

MANAGEMENT Surgical intervention is generally required for shunt obstruction. As a temporizing measure intracranial pressure can be lowered by standard methods—hyperventilation and osmotic diuresis (mannitol). If these measures fail and surgical intervention is not immediately available, the emergency physician can lower intracranial pressure when the malfunction is distal by removing CSF via the reservoir as previously described. To prevent choroid plexus bleeding, CSF is removed slowly, and the process is discontinued when intracranial pressure reaches 10 to 20 cm. Stable patients with suspected obstruction require admission and neurosurgical consultation. These patients should be observed for any neurologic changes, abdominal complaints, or development of fever.

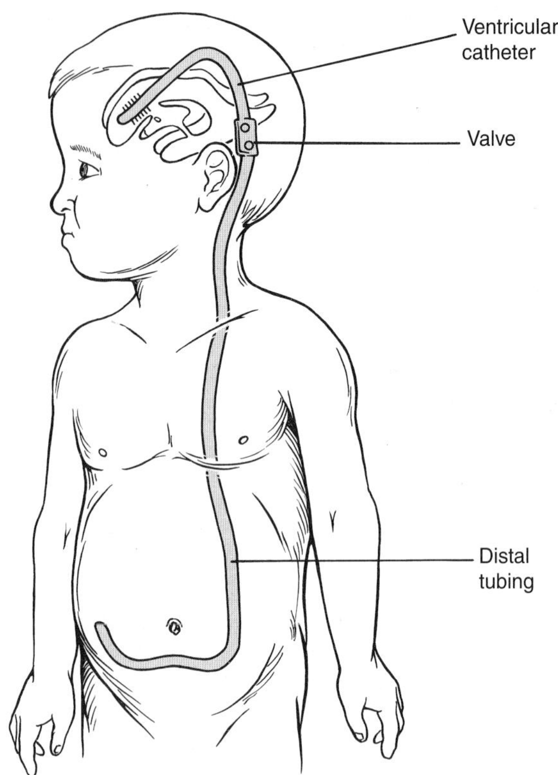

FIG. 228-1. Ventriculoperitoneal shunt system.

Shunt Infection

Infection was a common complication of CSF shunts, occurring in up to one-third of shunted patients. With improved techniques and shunts, infection rates have decreased to 5 to 8 percent per procedure.[2] The highest rates of infection are found in the very young and old, and in patients who have had multiple shunt revisions. There is no association between shunt type and infection rates.

Half of all shunt infections present within the first two weeks of placement, 70 percent present within two months of placement, and 80 percent of shunt infections present within six months of placement. CSF shunt infection can be categorized into internal and external infections. An internal infection involves the shunt and the CSF contained within that shunt. External infections involve the subcutaneous tract around the shunt, which is usually tender and there is often an associated fluid collection within the skin. If diagnosed and treated in a timely fashion, mortality from shunt infections is low. However, if ventriculitis develops, mortality is 30 to 40 percent, underscoring the need for prompt diagnosis and aggressive management.[1,2]

BACTERIOLOGY CSF shunt infections are typically caused by low-virulence organisms. The most commonly cultured agent is *Staplylococcus epidermidis,* which accounts 50 percent of all shunt infections; *Staplycococcus aureus,* the next most commonly cultured agent, accounts for 25 percent of all shunt infections. Gram-negative, anaerobic and mixed infections account for approximately 5 to 10 percent of shunt infections. Gram-negative infections are associated with the highest mortality. Patients with CSF shunts have a higher risk of developing meningitis from typical pathogens (e.g., *Haemophilus influenzae, Streptococcus pneumoniae,* and *Neisseria meningitidis*) compared to the general population. This increased risk may be due to disruption of the blood-brain barrier by foreign material.

CLINICAL FEATURES The clinical presentation varies with the virulence of the organism and the severity of the infection. Typically, patients will present with obstructive and possibly meningeal symptoms, including mental status changes, headache, nausea, vomiting, and irritability. Fever, meningismus and abdominal pain may also be present. Unfortunately, these signs are not universally present. In fact, the finding of fever is highly variable and meningismus may only be present in only a third of patients with shunt infection.[2] Abdominal pain may be the predominant symptom in patients with ventriculoperitoneal shunts. Swelling, erythema, and tenderness along the site of the shunt tubing are highly suggestive of external shunt infection.

EVALUATION To exclude CSF shunt infection, a shunt tap is required (Fig. 228-1) (see evaluation of shunt malfunction). This procedure should be performed by a neurosurgeon or by an emergency physician only after consultation with a neurosurgeon. A traditional lumbar puncture often misses CSF shunt infection and has no meaningful role in the evaluation when infection is suspected.

The cell count of patients with infected CSF shunts usually reveals an elevated leukocyte count, elevated protein, and normal glucose levels. Almost one-fifth of patients evaluated for shunt malfunction may have positive CSF culture despite normal CSF analysis. Non-CSF lab values are rarely helpful in diagnosing CSF shunt infection. CT scan and plain radiographs of the shunt (shunt series) are required to exclude mechanical shunt malfunction, which often coexists with shunt infection.[3] Abdominal ultrasound or CT scan are indicated if an abdominal fluid collection, pseudocyst, or abscess is suspected.

MANAGEMENT All patients with CSF shunt infection or suspected shunt infection require emergent neurosurgical consultation and admission. Most neurosurgeons advocate replacement of the infected shunt, external CSF drainage and administration of intravenous and intrathecal antibiotics. This combination of therapy has a 96 percent success rate. Until the infecting agent is identified, broad-spectrum antibiotics effective against typical pathogens are recommended (e.g., intravenous third-generation cephalosporin and aminoglycoside, plus intravenous or intrathecal vancomycin). Meningitis caused from typical pathogens has been successfully treated with antibiotics alone.

HALO DEVICES

The Halo vest provides one of the most rigid types of cervical immobilization available. The Halo consists of a lightweight radiolucent ring attached to a lightweight adjustable vest. Current vests allow adjustment of the cervical spine in multiple planes. Titanium pins that do not interfere with MRI images, are stronger, lighter, and more expensive than older stainless steel pins. Pins are usually tightened to 6 to 8 in lb.[4,5]

INDICATIONS Halo devices are indicated for stabilization of an unstable cervical spine, including fractures, dislocations, subluxations, and alignment of severe kyphotic and scoliotic spines. A halo is not applied if there is a sensory deficit that extends beneath the Halo vest as this leads to a higher risk of skin breakdown and infection. Pin sites are chosen to avoid nerve vessels and muscle while attempting to place the pins in the thickest area of calvarium possible. Four pins are usually used. The anterior pins are placed in the frontal or temporal regions. Posterior pins are placed relatively opposite to the anterior pin sites.

COMPLICATIONS Pin loosening is the most common complication encountered in the emergency department. It occurs in 36 to 60 percent of patients with halo devices.[5,6] Neurosurgical consultation should be obtained, and infection of the pin site ruled out. If resistance is met within the first rotations, the pin can usually be retightened to 6 to 8 in lb. If no resistance is met, the pin has to be removed. This is usually done by the neurosurgeon after placement of a new pin is completed to avoid any loss of stability in the halo device.

If pin loosening has caused movement of the Halo device, assume that the cervical spine is unstable, immobilize the cervical spine using an alternate technique, and obtain plain radiographs to assess for proper alignment. Tangential plain radiographs, CT, or MRI can be used to rule out penetration of a pin through the inner table of the skull.

Pin-site infection is second most frequently encountered complication. It occurs in about 20 to 22 percent of patients with halo devices.[5,6] Careful examination is required to differentiate a localized pin-site infection from less common, more serious infection, such as cellulitis, osteomyelitis, and abscess formation. Patients with cellulitis usually have fever, and systemic signs and symptoms of infection. Patients with osteomyelitis usually have a prolonged infection, pin-site loosening, and radiologic abnormalities. Patients who develop an abscess usually have neurologic changes and evidence of inter-table penetration (CSF leak, trauma). Local pin-site infections are commonly managed with local wound care. The skin around the pin site must be pulled away to allow thorough cleaning of the skin beneath the pin and skin-pin interface with soap and water four times a day. Culture the wound site. If antibiotics are administered, agents effective against skin pathogens (e.g., staphylococcus and streptococcus species) are used. If local infection does not respond to treatment, or if cellulitis, osteomyelitis, or abscess is suspected, neurosurgical consultation is required for admission, IV antibiotics, and possible surgical intervention.

Pin-site discomfort occurs in 18 percent of patients.[5,6] It is most commonly a result of local inflammation. Examine the patient to exclude a localized or systemic infection, or other local complication. Sensory and motor deficits or paresthesias indicate nerve damage or pressure, while painful mastication indicates temporalis muscle inflammation. After excluding infection a short course of analgesics is recommended. Neurosurgical consultation is required if pain continues or a serious complication is suspected.

Ring migration and/or loss of immobilization occurs in 10 to 13 percent of patients.[5,6] Suspect loss of immobilization in patients complaining of neck pain and or mobility, and change in fit or position of the ring or vest. Immediately immobilize the cervical spine using an alternative technique (e.g., hard collar plus backboard). Obtain plain films to assess for changes in alignment and neurosurgical consultation for reapplication of the Halo.

Skin breakdown and pressure sores occur in 4 to 11 percent of patients.[5,6] If these are present, inspect the vest for adequate padding and strap position. Urgent referral to a neurosurgeon for refitting may be required.

Dysphagia occurs in 2 percent of patients.[5,6] Immobilization holding the head in exaggerated extension is the usual cause of the dysphagia. Halo adjustment will remedy this problem. Alternatively, dysphagia can occur following anterior displacement of a bone graft. This diagnosis can be made by plain films and/or a swallowing study and will require emergency surgical intervention.

Dural punctures occur in 1 percent of patients and are due to halo system trauma.[5,6] Symptoms include headache, malaise, or visual changes. Physical exam may reveal a CSF leak or evidence of skull fracture. All patients require admission and neurosurgical consultation. Treatment includes elevation of head, IV antibiotics, and pin removal.

Rarely, CPR is required in patients with Halo devices. To perform chest compressions, remove the anterior portion of the vest. Instructions for removing the halo vest are printed on the front of most vests. Perform intubation with the Halo in place. If orotracheal intubation is unsuccessful, attempt nasotracheal intubation (if respirations are present) or cricothyrotomy.

OTHER CENTRAL NERVOUS SYSTEM DEVICES

Intrathecal Baclofen Infusions

Generalized dystonia occurs in 15 to 25 percent of patients with cerebral palsy. These patients typically respond poorly to medical and surgical treatment plans aimed at controlling their dystonia. Baclofen, a γ-aminobutyric acid agonist that acts at the level of the spinal cord by impeding the release of excitatory neurotransmitters, decreases spasticity. Oral baclofen offers patients only mild relief because of its inability to cross the blood-brain barrier, because it is poorly lipid soluble. Intrathecal administration is more effective, requires lower doses, and leads to higher CSF levels. Intrathecal baclofen reduces spasticity, improves gait, sitting ability, and upper extremity function in most patients.[7,10] Complications observed in patients receiving continuous intrathecal baclofen include hypotension, bradycardia, apnea, oversedation, respiratory depression, local infection, meningitis, and CSF fistula formation. Newly available intrathecal catheters cause fewer complications compared to original catheters. More experience is needed with continuous intrathecal baclofen to determine the long-term benefits and complications. Currently, it appears that complication occurs in approximately 20 percent of cases, while infection requiring removal occurs in about 5 percent of cases.[7–10]

Implantable CNS Stimulators

The pathogenesis of Parkinson's disease is thought to involve unregulated activity of the subthalamic nucleus and globus pallidus intermedius. Neurophysiologists have shown that high-frequency stimulation can reversibly inactivate nerve conduction in these areas.[11,12]

High-frequency stimulation with implantable CNS devices are being used for suppression of parkinsonian and essential tremors. This neurostimulation is typically used if drug therapy has failed to control tremors. Neurostimulation is as efficient at controlling tremors as classic thalamotomy, but is less invasive.

Little has been reported about complication rates for these neurostimulators and there is little ED experience related to complications to date. Limited studies suggest that neurostimulation has a lower risk of physical or cognitive impairment compared to thalamotomy. Patients may present to the emergency department with varied complaints including problems related to the subcutaneous pulse generator, temporary or permanent paresthesias, dysarthria, dysequilibrium, or failure of the neurostimulator to suppress tremors. Neurosurgical consultation is needed as these complaints may represent lead displacement or migration requiring surgical correction or replacement. If the diagnosis remains uncertain, observation may be required with the stimulator in the off position to help differentiate mechanical failure from an acute neurologic deficit.[11,12]

REFERENCES

1. Blount JP, Campbell JA: Complications in ventricular cerebrospinal fluid shunting. *Neurosurg Clin N Am* 4:633, 1993.
2. Key CB, Rothrock SG: Cerebrospinal fluid shunt complications: An emergency medicine perspective. *Pediatr Emerg Care* 11:265, 1995.
3. Iskandad BD, McLaughlin C: Pitfalls in the diagnosis of ventricular shunt dysfunction: Radiology reports and ventricular size. *Pediatrics* 101:1031, 1998.
4. Manthey DE: Halo traction device. *Emerg Med Clin North Am* 12:771, 1994.
5. Botte MS, Bynne TP: The halo skeletal fixator: Current concepts of application and maintenance. *Orthopedics* 18:463, 1995.
6. Glaser JN, Whitehall R: Complications associated with the halo vest. *J Neurosurg* 65:762, 1986.
7. Albright AL, Barry MJ: Infusion of intrathecal baclofen for generalized dystonia in cerebral palsy. *J Neurosurg* 88:73, 1998.
8. Armstrong RW, Steinbok P: Intrathecally administered baclofen for treatment of children with spasticity of cerebral origin. *J Neurosurg* 87:409, 1997.
9. Albright AL: Intrathecal baclofen in cerebral palsy movement disorders. *J Child Neurol* 11:29, 1996.
10. Albright AL: Baclofen in the treatment of cerebral palsy. *J Child Neurol* 11:77, 1996.
11. Krack P, Pollack P: Opposite motor effects of pallidal stimulation in Parkinson's disease. *Ann Neurol* 43:180, 1998.
12. Benabid AL, Pollack P: Acute and long-term effects of subthalamic nucleus stimulation in Parkinson's disease. *Sterotact Funct Neurosurg* 62:76, 1994.

APPROACH TO NEUROIMAGING IN THE EMERGENCY DEPARTMENT

Norman J. Beauchamp, Jr.

GENERAL OVERVIEW OF COMMON TECHNIQUES

Although a more thorough discussion of techniques is provided in other chapters of this textbook, a brief introduction to the more common techniques will be beneficial to understanding the optimal approach to cranial neuroimaging. Plain films are an essential tool. X-rays generate two-dimensional images based on attenuation of a collimated beam. The attenuation is proportional to the electron density of the structures through which it passes with the final image reflective of tissue density. This results in high spatial resolution and thus sensitivity for the detection of fractures. However, detection of abnormalities requires that there be no obscuration of the region of interest by overlying bone or other dense material. Thus, whereas a skull fracture of the calvarium is often readily detected, a fracture involving the skull base is typically obscured due to overlying bone. Plain films also provide a coarse view of the extracranial soft tissues, but intracranial soft tissues are obscured. Because the primary goal of ED neuroimaging is the detection of intracranial soft tissue abnormalities, the role of plain films is largely limited to the primary assessment of spinal trauma, the assessment of some facial fractures, assessment of some subtle, linear skull fractures oriented in the axial plane of acquisition, or as part of the skeletal survey for child abuse.

Computed tomography (CT) has largely supplanted plain films for neuroimaging. CT images are generated using a rotating x-ray tube that projects a collimated beam through the brain with resultant attenuation of the beam proportional to the electron density (tissue density) of the tissue through which it passes. Thus, rather than interrogating the tissue of interest from one direction (as in conventional x-rays), computerized processing of the circumferentially projected attenuated rays enables reconstruction of tissue maps largely unobscured by overlying tissues. Differentiation of adjacent tissues such as bone, gray and white matter, and cerebrospinal fluid (CSF) is possible due to perceivable differences in tissue density. Vasogenic and cytotoxic edema and hemorrhage alter the density of the tissue effected, making CT highly sensitive in the detection of disease. Further, the fine anatomic detail enables detection of morphologic alterations such as fractures and parenchymal swelling.

Magnetic resonance imaging (MRI) involves placing a patient inside an externally applied magnetic field. Due to its odd number of nuclides, hydrogen will align with this magnetic field. These "magnetized" hydrogen atoms are then "energized" by the input of an applied radiofrequency pulse and the pattern of energy release provides information about the biophysical properties of the tissue being evaluated. The shifts in water (hydrogen) distribution that characterize all pathologic processes alter these biophysical properties. Detectable changes occur prior to a detectable change in tissue density. Thus, MRI is more sensitive than CT in detecting parenchymal pathologic processes such as cerebral ischemia, infection, or metastases. Equally important is that the presence of certain blood products (deoxy- and methemoglobin, hemosiderin) develops over time postbleeding. These cause a detectable alteration in local magnetic field. MRI is thus nearly equivalent to CT in the detection of fresh bleeding, but is much more sensitive in the detection of staid blood. Blood becomes CT "normal" in density 7 to 10 days postbleed, but can generate an abnormal magnetic field for months to years. Lastly, MRI enables multiplanar acquisition while the patient remains supine. In CT, imaging requires patient positioning specific for the plane of interest. This can be difficult for the very young, the elderly, and for trauma patients.

Notably, cortical bone is relatively depleted of hydrogen. Thus, the cortex of bone is nearly invisible on MRI. Although this is of benefit in that parenchyma can be assessed without compromise from adjacent dense bone (e.g., infratemporal region and posterior fossa assessment is slightly limited in CT due to artifact from the adjacent skull base) (Figs. 229-1*A* and *B*), MRI is inadequate for the assessment of bony integrity. Compared to CT, MRI is frequently less (or even not) available in many Emergency Departments; is contraindicated in the presence of devices such as pacemakers, cochlear implants, and metallic foreign matter near vital structures; requires greater patient cooperation; and impedes monitoring of critically ill patients. As a result, despite its superior sensitivity to most pathological processes, MRI plays an important but more limited role in the ED.

Ultrasound generates images based upon transmittance of sound waves. In general, sonographic imaging enables evaluation of soft tissue structures provided that air or bone does not obscure the area of interest. In neuroimaging, most of the structures of interest are obscured by the calvarium. However, in infants, patency of the fontanel provides an adequate sonographic window enabling high sensitivity for the detection of intracranial masses, hemorrhages, or hydrocephalus. In infants and very young children, ultrasound is the study of choice for intracranial assessment.

Ultrasound can also be used to assess for traumatic globe injury or masses. However, this technique is highly operator-dependent, is limited in the assessment of the orbital apex, and is typically performed by an ophthalmologist.

Ultrasound images can be generated in which flowing blood produces color images scaled to flow velocity. These images give information on lumen caliber and hemodynamic alterations (such as occur with a distal occlusion or proximal stenosis). Ultrasound has become

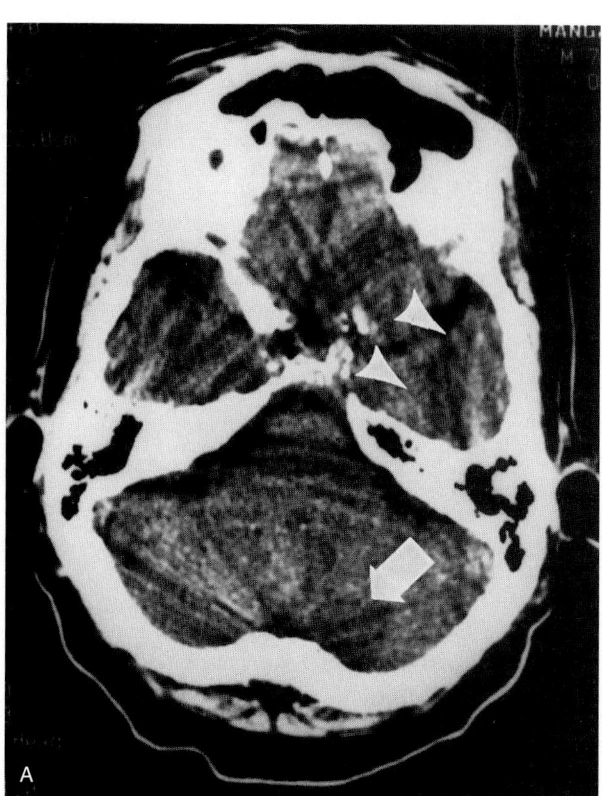

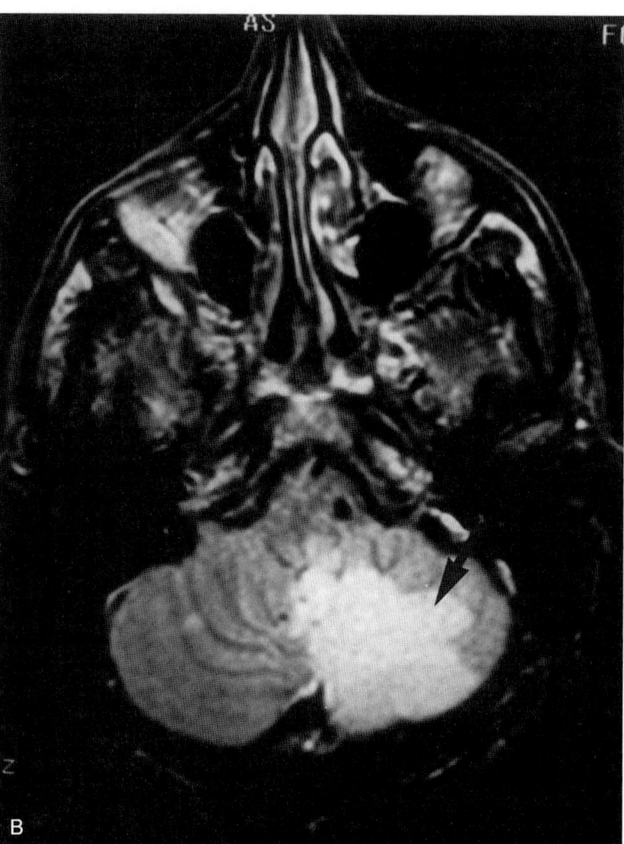

FIG. 229-1. A. Axial CT obtained in a patient presenting with a left cerebellar infarct. Initial CT demonstrates a focal area of decreased attenuation in the left cerebellar hemisphere difficult to detect due to artifact generated by adjacent bone (*arrow*). Incidental note is made of similar obscuration of the inferior temporal lobe by artifact (*arrowheads*). **B.** Axial MRI clearly demonstrates an area of infarction in the left cerebellum. Visualization is clear with no artifact generated despite proximity to bone.

the screening technique of choice in assessing for common carotid bifurcation atherosclerotic disease. Transcranial Doppler and power Doppler ultrasound enables assessment of the distal most aspects of the internal carotid arteries, the proximal cerebral arteries, the circle of Willis, and the superficial parenchyma. Assessment of the posterior circulation and deeper parenchyma remains limited.

The vasculature can also be assessed noninvasively with CT angiography (CTA) or MR angiography (MRA). CTA and MRA are appealing techniques because they are noninvasive and can be incorporated into a comprehensive CT or MR examination with minimal additional time or difficulty (Fig. 229-2*A* and *B*). MRA utilizes a gradient echo pulse sequence that results in increased intravascular signal intensity with normal flow. CTA is performed following the peripheral venous administration of iodinated contrast. An image similar to a conventional arteriogram can be reconstructed from the axial images. Both are sensitive to large vessel occlusion or narrowing in the internal carotid, vertebral, basilar, and first and second segments of the anterior, middle, and posterior cerebral arteries. Furthermore, both techniques can be modified to look at venous structures (i.e., CTV or MRV). CTA requires less patient cooperation with an assessment of the vasculature complete in approximately 30 s. However, vascular detail is limited when vessels are in direct apposition to bone. Vascular assessment with MRA is not limited in the presence of bone. It is useful for assessing the vertebral arteries as they course through the bony transverse foramina and skull base, and in assessing the cephalad course of the internal carotid artery.

Both CTA and MRA techniques have resolution inferior to catheter angiography. For example, neither CTA nor MRA can reliably detect intracranial aneurysms less than 3 mm. The primary use of both techniques is as a screening tool for vascular occlusion and generally should be supplemented with catheter angiography when clinical suspicion remains. Catheter angiography utilizes plain x-rays in conjunction with administration of intra-arterial contrast through a catheter placed from a femoral artery approach and positioned proximal to the vasculature to be assessed. The intra-arterial contrast delineates vascular anatomy and detects pathologic changes such as narrowing and occlusion. It is the definitive procedure for assessment of the intra- and extracranial vasculature. However, there is a 1 to 2 percent risk of stroke associated with catheter angiography.

Near infrared spectroscopy (NIRS) measures changes in absorbance of an infrared light beam projected transcranially. Specifically, near infrared light (700 to 1000 nm) has relatively good transcranial penetration and hemoglobin (Hb) has characteristic absorption spectra. The absorbance of light is dependent on the presence of Hb and the oxygen content of the Hb. Thus, this technology can be used to assess for the presence of hemorrhage and to assess the oxygen state of the superficial microcirculation. For example, in one investigation, 24 of 27 patients with delayed traumatic intracranial hemorrhages demonstrated increases in the NIRS absorbance.[1] NIRS units are portable and relatively inexpensive, but the role for NIRS remains to be determined.

Radioisotope scans are performed following the administration of radioisotopes that emit photons. Photon imaging studies can be used to assess ventriculoperitoneal shunt patency, CSF leaks, hydrocephalus, Ommaya reservoirs, and brain death. Anatomic scans can also be performed that enable detection of space-occupying lesions. In general, nuclear medicine neuroimaging studies are infrequently utilized in the ED setting due to the superior resolution, increased availability, and expedience of CT and MR.

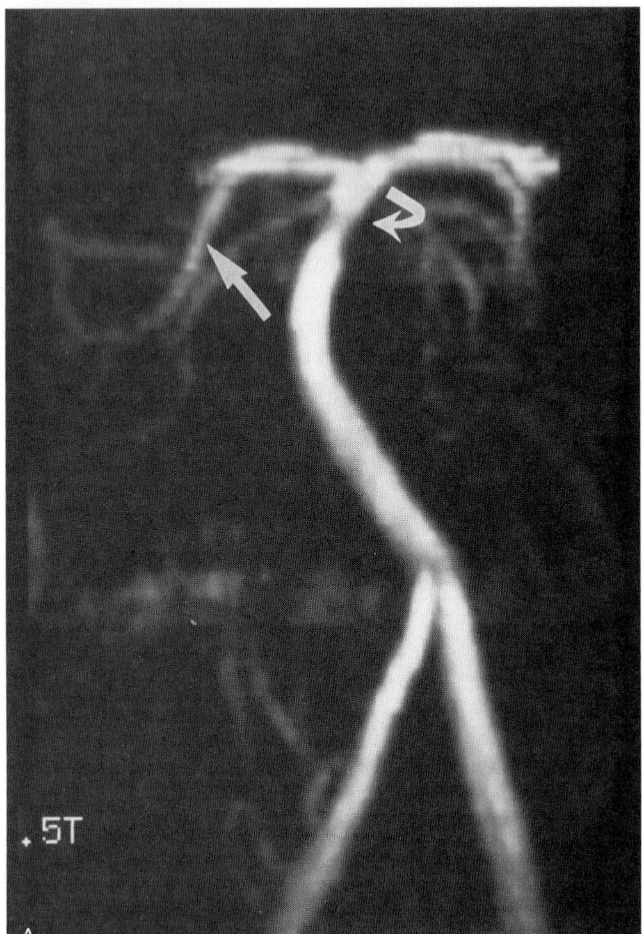

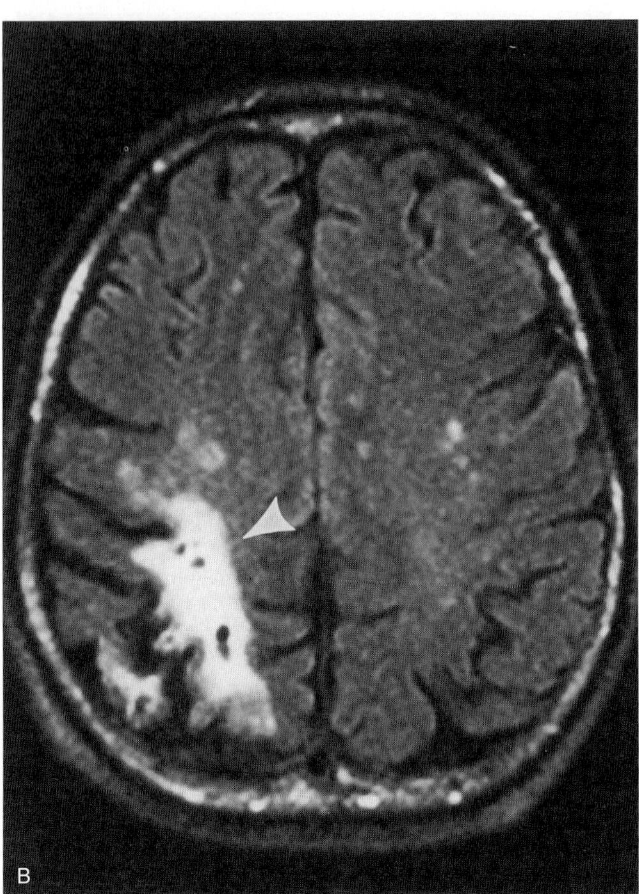

FIG. 229-2. A. MR angiogram demonstrates an area of focal stenosis involving the basilar artery (*curved arrow*). However, the right posterior cerebral artery is clearly demonstrated excluding large vessel occlusion (*straight arrow*). **B.** MR axial FLAIR image demonstrates and area of hyperintensity corresponding to an acute right parietal infarct (*arrowhead*).

There are numerous available neuroimaging techniques for cranial imaging. Fortunately, the majority of imaging can be performed with plain films, CT, or MR. The choice of modality varies depending on the clinical question to be answered, the availability of the modality, and the ability of the patient to tolerate the examination. Although a consensus is often difficult to attain, some guiding principles exist. The remainder of this review focuses on guiding principles for the assessment of the most common emergency neurologic complaints.

HEADACHE

Recommendations for which subset of patients with acute headache requires some form of neuroimaging are as varied as they are numerous. However, neuroimaging has been accepted as the standard of care in specific clinical situations (Table 229-1). In addition to atypical headache (associated with neurologic signs), severity of headache is an indicator for imaging. Specifically, acute onset of the ''worst headache of my life'' raises concern for subarachnoid hemorrhage. Identification is essential because rupture of an intracranial aneurysm is the most common cause of nontraumatic subarachnoid hemorrhage. Furthermore, if subarachnoid hemorrhage (SAH) remains undetected, there is a 50 percent two-week risk of rebleeding with an associated 50 percent mortality. In this instance, nonenhanced head CT is the recommended study (Fig. 229-3). Its sensitivity in the detection of SAH is within 93 to 100 percent if performed within 12 to 24 h of the event.[2] In addition to the demonstration of high-density acute blood in the subarachnoid spaces, it also demonstrates other manifestations of SAH, including intraventricular and intraparenchymal hemorrhage and hydrocephalus. With small amounts of acute hemorrhage, SAH can be overlooked and the sensitivity of CT decreases to about 80 percent after 24 h,[2] and continues to diminish significantly over time to less than 30 percent 3 days postrupture. Thus, if the CT is negative, lumbar puncture is necessary. A positive CT or LP requires conventional angiography.

Headache associated with unexplained fever is also an indication for neuroimaging, particularly when there is associated meningismus and photophobia. Although diagnosis is made by lumbar puncture, imaging is typically recommended to exclude hydrocephalus. Despite

TABLE 229-1 Considerations for Nonenhanced Head CT for Headache

Unexplained mental status change or focal neurological signs
''Worst headache of life'' of sudden onset
Unexplained fever
Meningismus
Extremes of vital signs (blood pressure, bradycardia or respiratory rate, although seldom an isolated finding)

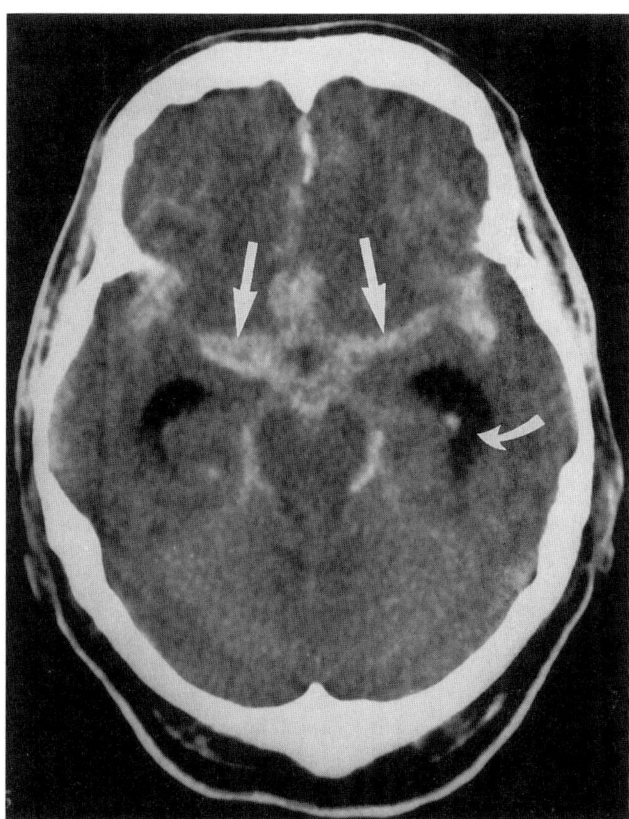

FIG. 229-3. Axial CT demonstrates areas of increased density compatible with subarachnoid hemorrhage (SAH) (*straight arrows*). There is also early hydrocephalus with the temporal horns dilated (*curved arrow*).

the absence of scientific validation, it has become the standard of care to precede lumbar puncture with nonenhanced head CT (NECT). Secondary hydrocephalus tends not to obviate performing lumbar puncture, but it will lead the physician to performing a low-volume lumbar puncture. Further, it can alert the physician to the possible need for shunt placement.

Acute or recurrent hydrocephalus can present with headache as well as nausea, incontinence, and ataxia. There is generally an increase in the intraventricular volume. Hydrocephalus can be caused by a number of processes including prior subarachnoid hemorrhage, prior trauma, meningitis, masses obstructing the ventricular system, or masses external to the ventricles but causing obstructing compression due to size or edema. In the evaluation of patients with suspected hydrocephalus, NECT is an adequate evaluation. It will enable detection of patients requiring emergency placement of intraventricular shunt catheters. If hydrocephalus is identified and the etiology remains undefined, a contrast-enhanced MRI examination with its superior ability to image in multiple planes should be performed. Lastly, in examining patients with an intraventricular shunt catheter and suspected recurrent hydrocephalus, the NECT should be accompanied with a plain film shunt series. The latter will detect possible kinks or disruptions of the catheter (see Chap. 228 for detailed discussion).

Generally an intraparenchymal mass, large enough to cause headache will be associated with neurologic signs prior to, or concurrent with, the development of headache. Thus, in instances where tumors are associated with headache, they are large and readily detectable on NECT; indirect effects, such as obstruction to CSF outflow, will also be evident on NECT.

MENTAL STATUS CHANGE

The issue of whether to image patients under the influence of alcohol or other substances to also consider other etiologies as a possible explanation for mental status change frequently arises in ED practice. The approach is discussed in detail in Chaps. 221 and 247. Generally, patients with Glasgow Coma Score (GCS) of 13 or less, those that fail to improve with time, or those in whom alcohol or drug levels are not in keeping with the clinical findings, require imaging.

An initial NECT can be performed in patients with mental status changes who also have a known primary tumor, or who have a suspected metastases or primary brain tumor. This will suffice in detecting lesions resulting in mental status change, such as marked cerebral edema, herniation, and intracranial hemorrhage, that require emergent intervention. However, the optimal choice of imaging is based on the availability of imaging resources as well as the clinical suspicion. For example, contrast MRI is the more sensitive test and is typically required for patients in which clinical concern persists, even if the initial CT is normal. However, if MRI resources were immediately available, it would be more appropriate in instances of high suspicion to proceed directly to MRI and avoid unnecessary time delay and additional imaging costs to the patient. Contrast-enhanced CT subjects patients to the small, but unnecessary, risk of iodinated contrast, and is less sensitive than MRI.

Proceeding directly to imaging with MRI when available, is also indicated with certain cerebral infections. Encephalitis presents as acute mental status change and fever. Herpes type 2 encephalitis is a particularly devastating form, but can have a good clinical outcome if diagnosed and treated early in the course of the disease. Herpes often has a characteristic appearance in which the temporal lobes are first effected (Fig. 229-4). Due to the difficulties assessing parenchyma in direct apposition to bone structures, detection of the subtle early findings of cytotoxic edema involving the temporal lobes can be difficult when utilizing NECT in the first three days. Sensitivity is not increased by the addition of intravenous contrast. Conversely, MR is highly sensitive to the early manifestations of encephalitis. It is often positive in the first 24 h and can be helpful in expeditious diagnosis.

The approach to imaging the HIV-positive patient with mental status change is greatly debated (see Chap. 139). There is a tendency to provide an emergent screening examination with NECT followed by nonemergent performance of contrast-enhanced MRI as indicated. Using this approach, processes creating vasogenic edema and those requiring immediate intervention, such as toxoplasmosis and lymphoma, will undoubtedly be detected. However, further investigation using contrast MRI is often requested to better characterize these lesions and for the detection of HIV encephalopathy and progressive multifocal leukoencephalopathy. A cost-effective approach of proceeding directly to MRI has also been recommended. This largely depends on the institutional availability of MRI and the management practices of clinicians.

SEIZURES

In recurrent seizures, determination of a sole cause such as noncompliance typically eliminates the need for imaging. Similarly, neuroimaging is not indicated for the evaluation of children with simple febrile seizures. However, the optimal approach for the evaluation of first-time seizures is debated. The American College of Emergency Physicians Special Panel suggests CT scanning for first-time seizures.[3]

CT is nearly 100 percent sensitive for etiologies of seizures that require emergent intervention such as brain abscesses, hemorrhage, or other space-occupying lesions. However, the neurologist may additionally request multiplanar MRI emergently or electively depending on the clinical situation, although not necessarily while the patient is in the ED.

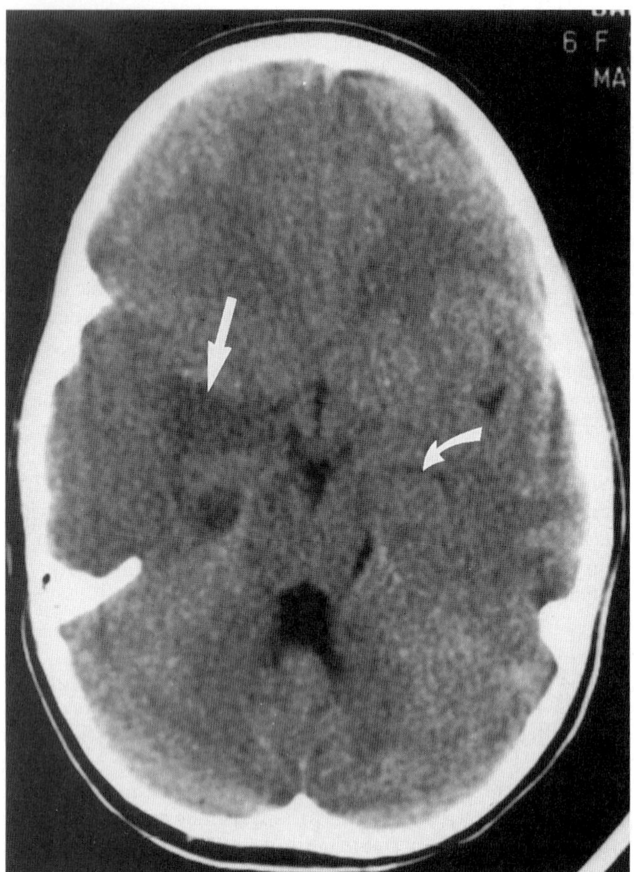

FIG. 229-4. Axial CT scan demonstrates decreased attenuation in the right temporal lobe (*straight arrow*). In a young patient with acute onset mental status change, this is highly suggestive of herpes encephalitis. Note the normal left temporal horn (*curved arrow*) as compared to the effaced right temporal horn.

STROKE

Although presented elsewhere in this textbook (Chap. 220), determining the optimal approach to imaging cerebral infarction is becoming increasingly complex and is thus relevant to the discussion of modality selection in neuroimaging.

FDA guidelines require performance of a NECT prior to the institution of thrombolytic therapy. Intravenous contrast administration is of limited value in the CT evaluation of acute stroke. Contrast enhancement is generally not seen during the first three days. Experience from the European Cooperative Acute Stroke Trial (ECASS) has demonstrated that efficacy of treatment is contingent on accurate CT interpretation.[4] Specifically, treated patients who had evidence of extensive infarction on CT had a worsened outcome. These patients should be excluded from treatment. However, this can be challenging because the signs of infarction initially are quite subtle. For example, trained readers did not detect 12 percent of areas of advanced infarction in the ECASS study.[4] Optimal treatment is most likely to occur when all members of the treatment team are familiar with the early signs of infarction (Table 229-2). Briefly, the presence of hemorrhage or evidence of progressive infarct are contraindications to treatment (Fig. 229-5). The sensitivity of CT for the detection of hemorrhage has been previously discussed. An important sign of acute stroke is the hyperdense middle cerebral artery (HMCAS) sign. This corresponds to a thrombus (angiographically) and is demonstrable at the time of ictus. The early CT findings of infarction are due to cytotoxic edema—cellular injury with influx of fluid in the intracellular space.

TABLE 229-2 CT Appearance Exclusion and Inclusion Criteria for the Administration of rt-PA in Patients Presenting Within 3 H of Ictus. Based on Recommendations by the American Heart Association and Experience from the NINDS and ECASS Trials

Grade 0—Normal CT
Grade 1—Possible early signs of infarction: May still give rt-PA depending on the clinician's judgement Vague blurring of gray-white boundaries Slight attenuation of the insular ribbon Slight indistinctness of basal ganglia gray matter Suggestion of crowding of sulci
Grade 2—Subtle but definite signs of early infarction: likely will not treat Same as above except findings are distinct
Grade 3—Prominent signs of early infarction: contraindication to treatment Mass effect—i.e., ventricular effacement, subfalcine or uncal herniation Clearly demonstrated hypodensity Intracranial hemorrhage Note: In the ECASS study, the major early signs of infarction included: diffuse swelling of the affected hemisphere and effacement of the cerebral sulci in more than 33% of the MCA territory.

The four CT signs that can be seen in the acute period are: (1) blurring of the clarity of the internal capsule; (2) loss of distinctness of the insular ribbon cortex; (3) loss of differentiation between the cortical gray and the subjacent white matter; and (4) swelling of the cortical gray matter resulting in effacement of interposed sulci. In addition to the attenuation changes, morphologic changes occur due to the

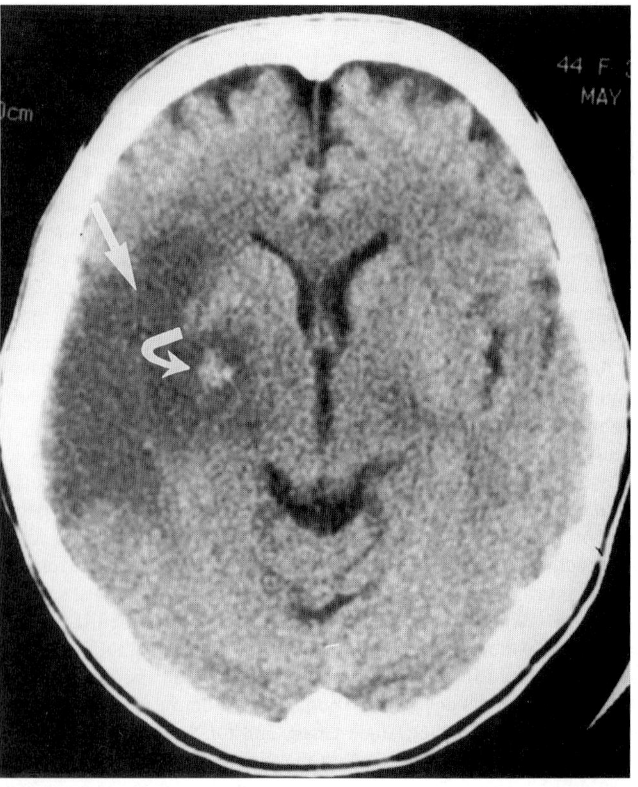

FIG. 229-5. Axial CT demonstrating clear evidence of decreased attenuation compatible with infarction (*straight arrow*). Additional, there is a focal area of hemorrhage (*curved arrow*), which further obviates thrombolysis.

accumulation of intracellular fluid causing *swelling* of the cortical gyri. This results in effacement of the spaces demarcated by the gyral infoldings (sulci) and is referred to as ''sulcal effacement.'' The extent of these changes determines whether treatment with thrombolysis is indicated.

MR has a greater sensitivity and specificity than CT for the acute changes of stroke. In the first 24 h, over 80 percent of MR scans are positive as compared to 60 percent of CT scans. MR is particularly superior for the detection of stroke in the posterior fossa where CT is limited due to a beam-hardening artifact from the adjacent skull base (Fig. 229-1). The earliest MR changes are morphologic swelling of the gray matter, increased signal intensity on the T2W and SDW (referred to as T2 hyperintensity), and loss of normal intravascular flow voids (see Chap. 297 for details on the physics of MR). More importantly, MRI can be combined with MRA for the detection of large vessel occlusion.

Although superior to CT, conventional MRI remains incapable of demonstrating the parenchymal changes of infarction during the first three hours. A recently developed advanced MR technique known as MR diffusion imaging utilizes pulse sequences sensitive to small-scale water-molecule motion (i.e., diffusion).[5] Alterations in water motion indicative of infarction can be detected within four minutes of vascular occlusion. This sensitivity dramatically improves that ability to determine extent of infarction and thus should improve the safety profile of rt-PA administration.

Neither clinical examination, CT, nor conventional MR imaging techniques provides information on the ischemic penumbra. Two advanced MR imaging techniques, MR perfusion and MR spectroscopic imaging, appear capable of providing this information (see Chap. 297). Perfusion imaging is performed following the bolus administration of intravascular contrast that result in changes in signal intensity proportional to regional cerebral blood volume and relative cerebral blood flow.[6] When ischemia is present, perfusion imaging shows a delay in peak signal loss in the affected distribution. MRS generates maps of hydrogen spectra containing major resonances from N-acetyl aspartate (NAA) and lactate.[7] Signals from lactate are not normally detected, but are demonstrated in the presence of ischemia and acute infarction. NAA is thought to be a marker of neuronal viability with decreased NAA a marker for cell death. Clinical MRS has demonstrated central areas of infarction with decreased NAA that corresponded to areas of T2W signal increase. Peripheral areas with elevated lactate, but normal NAA is felt to correspond to the ischemic region at risk for infarction. Future studies are needed to validate these findings and to determine which, if any, interventions may improve outcome in the penumbral region and when intervention is indicated. As the logistic difficulties associated with MRI are resolved, the ability to detect regions of infarction and ischemia suggest that CT will eventually be replaced in the evaluation of acute ischemia.

HEAD TRAUMA

Debate remains whether imaging is required for GCS of 15. Clear indications for neuroimaging include GCS less than 15; unexplained transient or persistent loss of consciousness; other forms of altered sensorium; focal neurologic signs; depressed skull fractures; seizure; persistent variations; progressive headache; and penetrating injuries.[8,9] In these instances, NECT plays an essential role for diagnosis and for detecting processes that require emergent intervention, such as epidural and subdural hematomas, increased intracranial pressure, and depressed skull fractures. Although discussed elsewhere, a number of points related to optimal imaging are worthy of emphasis.

The differential density of blood facilitates the detection of intraparenchymal and extraaxial hemorrhage. Density is displayed on a relative scale referred to in Hounsfield Units (HU). For example, water or CSF is assigned a value of zero, bone or metal varies between 100 and 1000 HU (hyperdense), fat is approximately −100 HU (hypodense), and air is −1000 HU. Further, acute blood has a density of 60 to 100 HU, and normal brain parenchyma has a density of approximately 35 (white matter) to 40 HU (gray matter). This differential density enables the increased density of blood or the decreasing density with accumulating edema to be detectable. Images are filmed in a manner that accentuates differences in the parenchymal range of densities. To optimize sensitivity for detecting parenchymal injuries, a gray scale is assigned such that regions of higher density are not easily differentiable. As such, blood in proximity to bone can be difficult to detect using parenchymal windows (Fig. 229-6*A* and *B*).

When evaluating for the presence of subdural and epidural collections it is important that images are formatted in a fashion so that the high densities are also distinguishable (i.e., blood windows). At many institutions it may not be routine to print these windows due to associated added film costs, but at a minimum, images should be reviewed on the CT console to exclude small blood collections. This is particularly true in the pediatric population where subdural hematomas can be a marker of intentional trauma. Detection is also facilitated by attention to the subtle secondary signs of extra-axial blood including loss of sulcal demarcation, mass effect on a ventricle, or displacement of the gray white junction from the inner table (Fig. 229-6*A*). These secondary signs are also important because not all acute blood is hyperdense. In anemic patients (hemoglobin level 8 to 10 g/dL) or patients with a coagulopathy, acute blood may be isodense and thus difficult to visualize.

Occasionally, MRI can be of value in assessing trauma patients. For example, in assessing for small acute subdural hematomas or for subacute/chronic hematomas, CT may be limited due to the hematomas' proximity to bone or because over time the density of blood becomes isodense to normal brain (subacute) or to normal CSF (chronic) (Fig. 229-6*B*). However, these blood products will remain abnormal with MRI for months to years. This can be of value in children when new and old coexistent extra-axial hematomas are essentially pathognomonic for child abuse.

MRI is also more sensitive in detecting diffuse axonal injury in which differential movement of parenchyma results in neuronal shearing. Diffuse axonal injury should be suspected when coma occurs immediately after severe injury and the degree of compromise is out of proportion to the CT findings. MR may be beneficial in that it will show multiple punctate areas of blood products below the threshold of CT detection. Specific anatomic structures that tend to be involved include the corpus callosum, adjacent to the superior cerebellar peduncle, the internal capsule, and gray-white matter junction.

Intra- or extracranial arterial dissection may be the result of trivial trauma, blunt trauma, or penetrating injury. MR can detect the presence of an acute dissection with T1 hyperintense blood seen in the vessel wall. In combination with MR angiography, it provides a fairly sensitive screening for a dissection. It enables an adequately sensitive but noninvasive method for vascular assessment and simultaneous assessment of the brain parenchyma and the extra-axial spaces. Other vascular lesions associated with trauma are pseudoaneurysms, which may occur in any dissected vessel, both intracranially and extracranially, and are prone to bleed. Catheter angiography remains the gold standard, but should be restricted to those patients with equivocal or abnormal MRA findings or a high-level of clinical suspicion.

Catheter angiography is also recommended in all patients with penetrating injuries to zone 1 and zone 3 of the neck, although assessment of zone 3 injuries is slightly more equivocal.[10] This is imperative for evaluating vessels of the thoracic inlet and above the mandible, respectively, because they are not accessible to visual inspection. Further, surgical exploration when indicated will require a vascular road map. Zone 2 injuries can be observed without angiography, which is recommended for expanding hematomas or where there is the development of respiratory or neurologic compromise.[11]

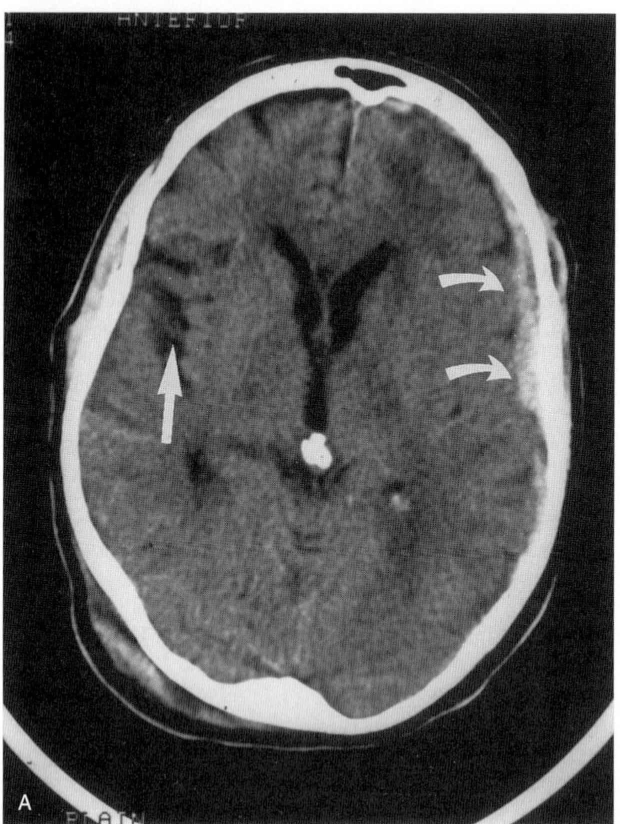

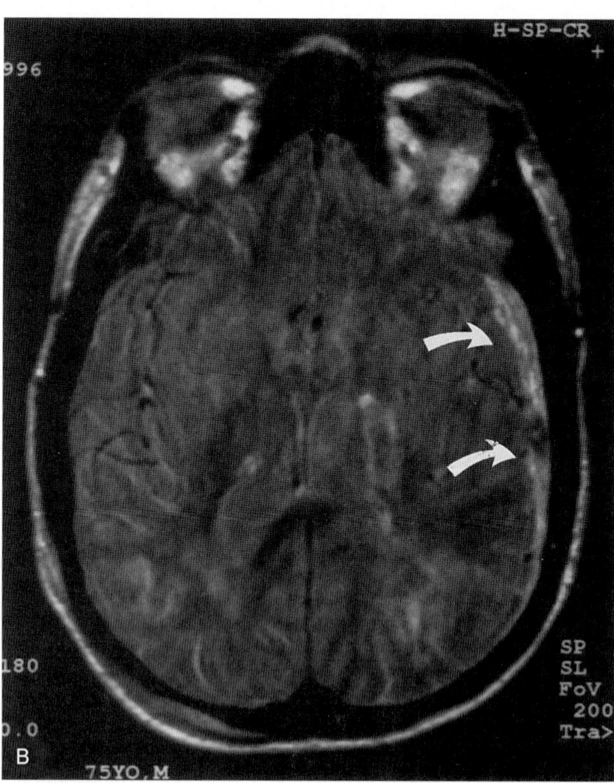

FIG. 229-6. A. Axial CT demonstrates a somewhat subtle left subdural hematoma (*curved arrows*). Note secondary signs of mass effect with the contralateral sylvian fissure detectable but compressed on the side of the subdural hematoma (*straight arrow*). **B.** Axial MR demonstrating the increased conspicuity of blood due to the lack of obscuration by adjacent bone.

REFERENCES

1. Gopinath SP, Robertson CS, Contant CF, et al: Early detection of delayed traumatic intracranial hematomas using near infrared spectroscopy. *J Neurosurg* 83:438, 1995.
2. Sedman R, Connolly E, Lemke T: Subarachnoid hemorrhage diagnosis: Lumbar puncture is still needed when the computed tomography scan is normal. *Acad Emerg Med* 3:827, 1996.
3. American College of Emergency Physicians, American Academy of Neurology, Association of Neurologic Surgeons and American Society of Neurology Practice Parameters: Neuroimaging in the emergency patient presenting with seizure (summary statement). *Ann Emerg Med* 28:114, 1996.
4. Hacke W, Kaste M, Fieschi C, et al: For the ECASS Study Group: Intravenous thrombolysis with recombinant tissue plasminogen activator for acute hemispheric stroke: The European cooperative acute stroke study. *JAMA* 274:1017, 1995.
5. Moseley ME, Cohen Y, Mintorovitch J, et al: Early detection of regional cerebral ischemia in cats: Comparison of diffusion and T2W MRI and spectroscopy. *Magn Reson Med* 14:330, 1990.
6. Detre JA, Leigh JS, Williams DS, Koretsky AP: Perfusion imaging. *Magn Reson Med* 23:37, 1992.
7. van der Toorn A, Verheul HB, van der Sprenkel JW, et al: Changes in metabolites and tissue water status after focal ischemia in cat brain assessed with localized proton MR spectroscopy. *Magn Reson Med* 32:685,1994.
8. Feuerman T, Wackym PA, Gade GF, et al: Value of skull radiography, head CT scanning and admission for observation in cases of minor head trauma. *Neurosurgery* 22:449, 1988.
9. Stein SC, Ross SE: The value of CT scans in patients with low-risk head injuries. *Neurosurgery* 26;638, 1990.
10. Jurkovich GH, Zingarelli W, Wallace J: Penetrating neck trauma: Diagnostic studies in the asymptomatic patient. *J Trauma* 25:819, 1985.
11. Golueke PJ, Goldstein AS, Sclafani SJA, et al: Routine versus selective exploration of penetrating neck injuries: A randomized prospective study. *J Trauma* 24:1010, 1984.

EYE, EAR, NOSE, THROAT, AND ORAL SURGERY

OCULAR EMERGENCIES

John D. Mitchell

A wide range of ocular emergencies, conditions, and manifestations of systemic illness are regularly encountered in the emergency department (ED). The recognition of these conditions and comfort in diagnosing and treating them are important to both the patient and the physician. As with any other part of the body, proper and early intervention can significantly enhance recovery and outcome. The ED physician should be comfortable with the use of a slit lamp, Tonopen and/or Schiøtz tonometer, and direct ophthalmoscope and be familiar with ocular anatomy (Figs. 230-1, 230-2) and neuro-ophthalmology. The approach to the patient should proceed in typical fashion with a good history and physical examination, with treatment of life-threatening conditions taking priority.

EYE EXAMINATION

History

A detailed history of the chief complaint and circumstances surrounding the onset should be obtained. The past ocular and medical history will provide additional information and help you arrive at a differential diagnosis. With this information you can then focus your physical examination and enhance your opportunity to correctly diagnose and treat the condition. A history of sudden, painless monocular visual loss associated with a history of atrial fibrillation or carotid stenosis would suggest a central retinal artery occlusion, while a history of eye pain occurring while hammering metal on metal would suggest a projectile corneal or intraocular foreign body. Past visual acuity and presence of a refractive error (need for glasses or contact lenses) provides information on acuity testing expectations. Use of soft contact lenses, especially the extended-wear type, is associated with a higher incidence of corneal ulceration from microbial infection. Flashing lights and a ''curtain or veil'' obstructing a portion of the visual field suggests a retinal detachment. A history of diabetes or chronic hypertension and acute isolated sixth-nerve palsy suggests an ischemic cranial neuropathy. A careful medical history and history of present illness (HPI) will guide you toward an accurate differential diagnosis in the majority of cases.

Physical Examination

The physical examination typically proceeds in a sequential fashion unless the circumstances require otherwise (i.e., chemical ocular injuries require intervention *prior* to assessment of visual acuity). The glossary of terms and abbreviations below is useful in documenting the findings. The typical eye examination sequence is as follows.

VISUAL ACUITY An attempt should be made to obtain an assessment of visual acuity in each eye in all consciously alert patients. Each eye should be tested individually. If the patient uses glasses or contacts but the glasses are not available, pinhole testing can be performed to obtain an estimate of corrected visual acuity. Distance charts are preferable but are not practical with patients confined to a stretcher. Nearsighted patients and those under age 45 can use a near card to test their visual acuity. Patients in their midforties or older may require reading glasses or bifocals to read a near card because of presbyopia. If these patients do not have their glasses available, a pinhole occluder, again, can be used with a near card. The patient with a corneal abrasion or foreign body is frequently experiencing significant photophobia, pain, and tearing; here, a drop of a topical anesthetic will often reduce the patient's discomfort sufficiently to allow a more accurate assessment of visual acuity. Documentation of best acuity in each eye and whether prosthetic devices were used (glasses, pinhole) should be noted. If the patient cannot read the chart or near card, try asking him or her to count how many fingers you are holding up and record the furthest distance at which the fingers can be counted correctly (e.g., at 4 ft). If the patient is unable to count fingers, assess his or her ability to detect hand motion 1 to 2 ft in front of the eye. If the patient is unable to detect hand motion, turn off all the lights in the room, fully occlude the contralateral eye, and test for light perception. In recording the results of visual acuity testing, refer to the glossary of abbreviations, terms, and notations below.

EXTERNAL EYE Examine the periorbital skin and lids for trauma, infection, dysfunction, or deformity. Proptosis should be recognized and recorded. Subcutaneous emphysema can be found with blowout fractures of the medial orbital wall (ethmoid). The orbital rims should be palpated for step-off deformities in trauma cases.

CONFRONTATION VISUAL FIELDS Testing of the gross confrontation visual field of each eye can provide additional supportive diagnostic information if the history suggests a process that typically causes a field loss [i.e., bitemporal hemianopia in pituitary adenoma, homonymous hemianopia associated with some cerebrovascular accidents (CVAs), and monocular field cuts sometimes seen with significant retinal detachments].

PUPILS Pupil assessment should be performed under slightly dim lighting conditions in testing for an afferent pupillary defect (Fig. 230-3). A positive afferent pupillary defect (APD) is indicative of an optic nerve disorder, and it is important to note that the pupils will be equal in size *prior* to testing because of the consensual light response. Therefore an APD does not cause a baseline anisocoria and will be discovered only if it is specifically tested for. Causes of unequal pupils (anisocoria) can range from an acute emergency [posterior communicating artery (PCA) aneurysm], to chronic baseline conditions such as previous intraocular trauma or surgery. A careful history is important to determine whether the anisocoria is preexistent. Ocular medications such as pilocarpine can cause extreme miosis, resulting in small, nonreactive pupils. Some patients with uveitis will be using a cycloplegic agent (scopolamine, cyclopentolate, or atropine) and have a chemically dilated, unreactive pupil. It is not worthwhile to attempt to ''reverse'' a chemically altered pupil in the ED, as the results are variable and unreliable.

OCULAR MOTILITY Eye movements are controlled by the six extraocular muscles attached to each eye (Figs. 230-4 and 230-5). These muscles are innervated by cranial nerves III, IV, and VI. Cranial nerve IV controls the superior oblique muscle, cranial nerve VI controls the lateral rectus muscle, all other extraocular muscles are controlled by cranial nerve III. Ocular motility can be impaired by restriction, interrupted or decreased innervation, or trauma. Examples of restriction include thyroid orbitopathy, myositis, and mechanical entrapment of a muscle secondary to an orbital blowout fracture. Cranial nerve palsies or paresis may be caused by CVAs, myasthenia gravis, diabetes, hypertension, tumors, aneurysms, infections, and trauma. Penetrating

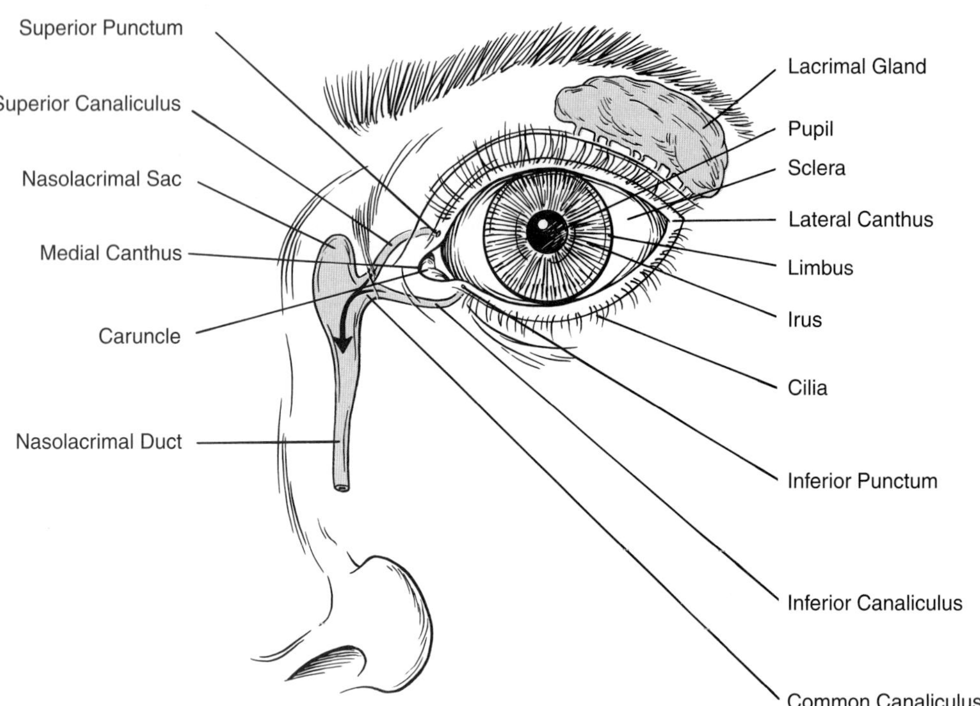

FIG. 230-1. Anatomic diagram of eye and adnexa.

or blunt traumatic injury to an extraocular muscle can also result in motility disturbance. Diplopia may develop, especially when the patient is attempting to look in the direction of the malfunctioning muscle. Ocular alignment should be evaluated in primary gaze initially (looking straight ahead), followed by testing in all fields of gaze.

ANTERIOR SEGMENT The conjunctiva, cornea, anterior chamber, iris, lens, and ciliary body make up the anterior segment. All of these structures except the ciliary body can be inspected directly on slit-lamp examination. A slit lamp is a biomicroscope that affords an excellent view of these structures and should be used whenever possi-

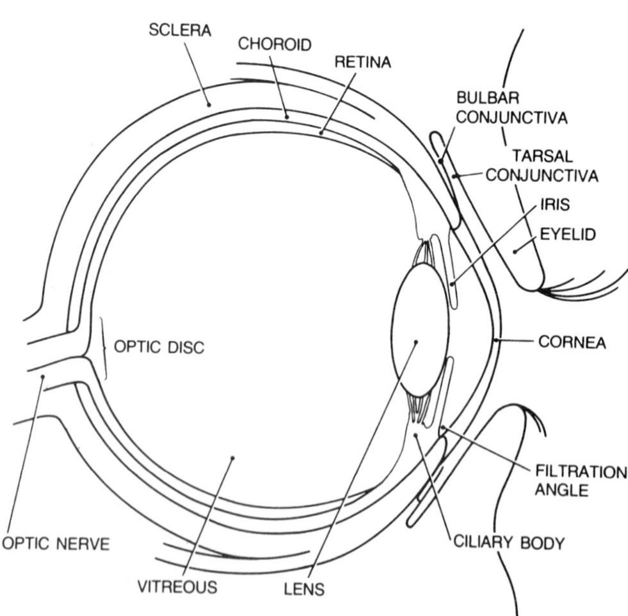

FIG. 230-2. Horizontal cross-sectional diagram of eye.

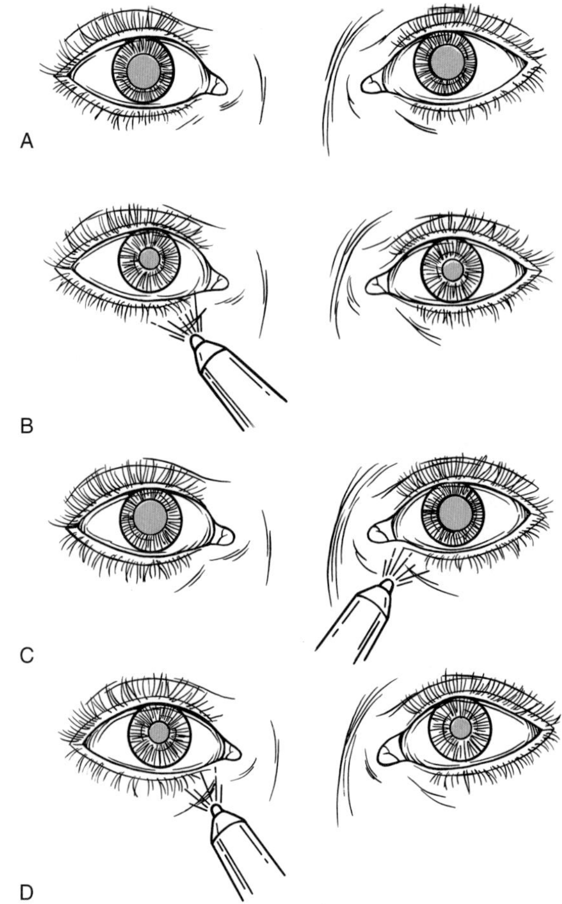

FIG. 230-3. ''Swinging flashlight test'' revealing an afferent pupillary defect (Marcus-Gunn pupil) of the left eye. **B.** The test is positive when the affected pupil dilates in response to light.

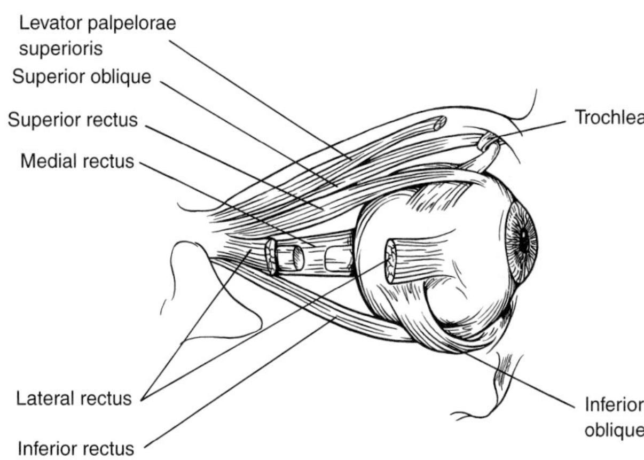

FIG. 230-4. Extraocular muscles of the eye.

ble. The conjunctiva should be inspected for hemorrhages, discharge, inflammation, trauma, and foreign bodies. The upper lid should always be everted anytime a foreign-body sensation or abrasion is present. The cornea should be assessed by narrowing the light source to produce a slit beam and optically sectioning the cornea (Fig. 230-6), which allows an oblique section to be seen and facilitates evaluation of the entire corneal thickness. This is a particularly important technique when one is trying to determine if a corneal foreign body has caused a full-thickness penetration. Fluorescein dye should be instilled and the cobalt-blue filter used to identify corneal abrasions, dendrites, and perforations. The modified Seidel test is useful in identifying corneal perforations. The eye is anesthetized and held open and the cobalt-blue filter is used to observe the eye while a moistened fluorescein strip is ''painted'' across the suspicious site. Leakage of aqueous through a penetrating wound will appear as a lime-green fluid oozing onto the dark violet corneal surface (Fig. 230-7, Plate 9). The anterior chamber should be checked for clarity and the presence of a hyphema (Fig. 230-8, Plate 10) or hypopyon (Fig. 230-9, Plate 11). Cell and flare may be present in acute injuries or in chronic uveitis/iritis conditions and should be checked for as follows: The slit beam should be shortened to about 1 mm and all of the room lights should be out. The high-magnification position should be selected. The incident light source should create an angle of 45 to 60° with the objective (similar to optical sectioning). The light beam should be focused on the pupillary margin, then pull back on the joy stick to focus on the cornea, then move the focus inward halfway between the iris and cornea, with the pupillary aperture as a dark backdrop. This will place your focus in the center of the aqueous, and the light beam will illuminate cells slowly drifting up and down in the aqueous convection currents. Flare is typically described as the appearance of ''headlights in a fog'' and represents the ability to see the course of the normally transparent light beam through the aqueous. This is caused by increased aqueous protein content, which is commonly seen with inflammatory conditions. The iris should be inspected for tears and foreign bodies if trauma occurred. The lens should likewise be inspected for injury, subluxation, and foreign bodies.

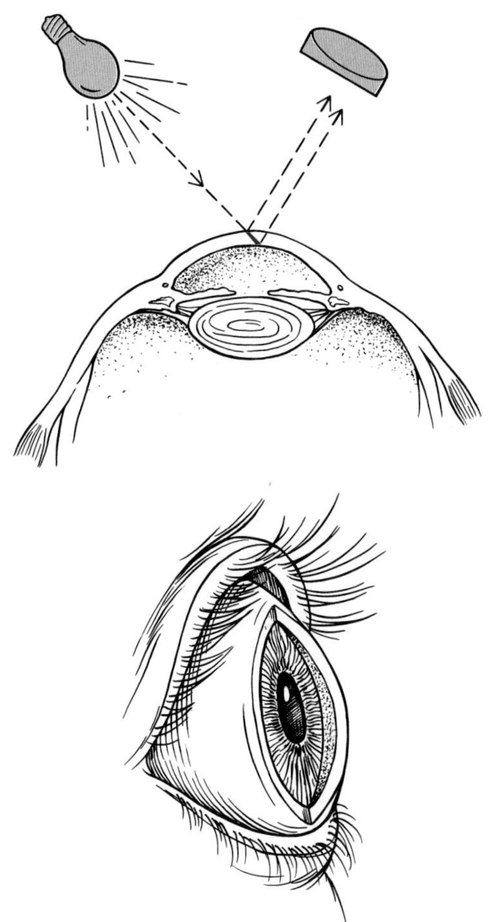

FIG. 230-6. Optical sectioning: By creating an angle of 45 to 60° between the slit-beam light source and the observer's biomicroscope objective, the cornea can be optically ''scctioned'' obliquely. This allows a cross-sectional view of the cornea and is helpful in ascertaining depth of penetration of corneal foreign bodies and injuries.

FUNDUS The optic nerve, macula, and retina can be viewed with a direct ophthalmoscope in the ED. A dilated pupil makes it easier to see these structures, and unless the patient has a rare contraindication (narrow angles without a previous peripheral iridectomy), dilation can be performed if a posterior segment view is needed. Dilation can be achieved by using one drop of 1% tropicamide (Mydriacyl) in Caucasians and one drop each of 1% tropicamide and 2.5% phenylephrine (Neo-Synephrine) in all others. A dilated examination is particularly important if an intraocular foreign body, central retinal artery occlusion (CRAO), or retinal detachment is suspected. A vitreous hemorrhage from diabetes or trauma can obscure or significantly reduce the view of the posterior pole. In these patients an ophthalmologist may need

FIG. 230-5. Cranial nerve IV, superior oblique muscle; cranial nerve VI, lateral rectus muscle; cranial nerve III, superior rectus, inferior rectus, inferior oblique, and medial rectus muscles.

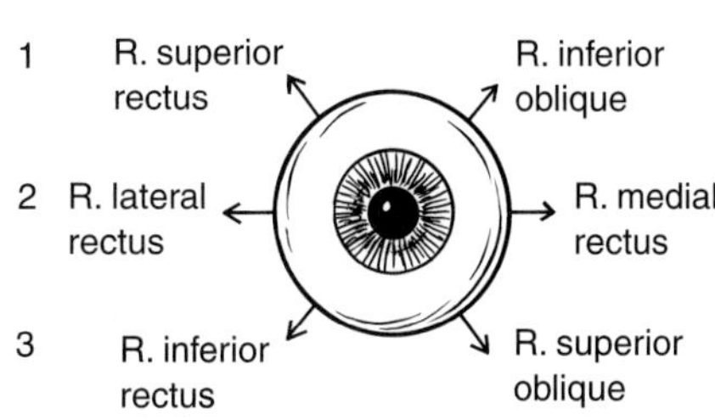

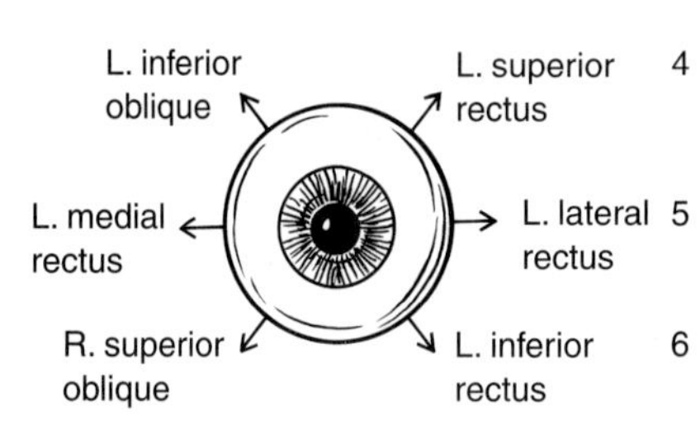

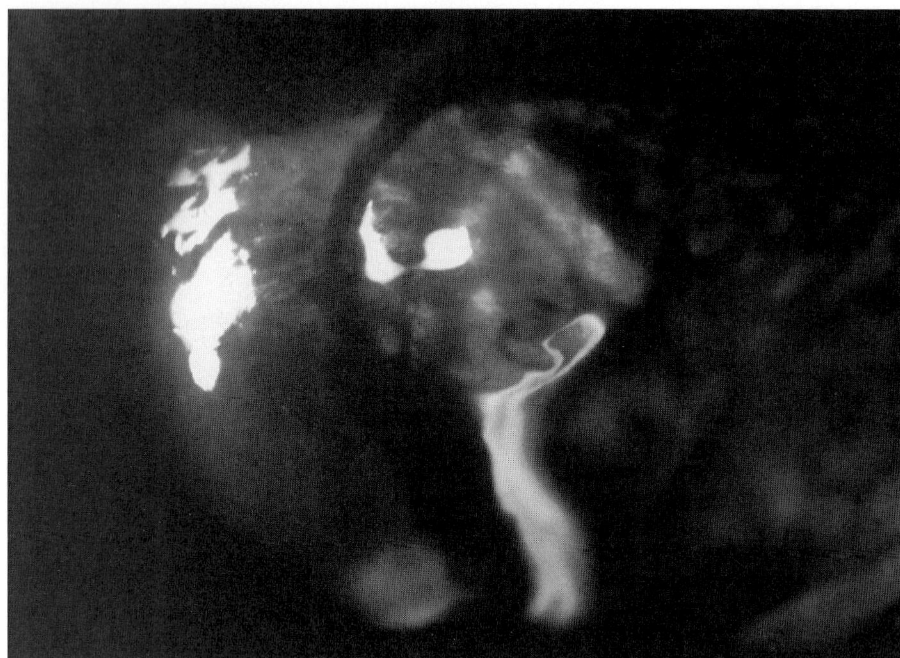

FIG. 230-7 (Plate 9). Positive Seidel test showing aqueous leaking through a full-thickness corneal wound. Aqueous will turn fluorescein lime-green under a cobalt-blue light as it oozes through the wound while being observed at the slit lamp.

to perform an ultrasound-B scan to evaluate the posterior segment. An indirect ophthalmoscope provides an excellent three-dimensional view of the optic nerve and retina but requires extensive practice to use and generally is not a tool for the nonophthalmologist.

INTRAOCULAR PRESSURE The eye remains consistently ''inflated'' because of a delicate balance between intraocular aqueous fluid production and outflow. Intraocular pressure [(IOP)/tension] can decrease due to reduced ciliary body production (some cases of iritis and uveitis) or loss of globe integrity (perforating injury). An increase in IOP occurs when intraocular fluid production exceeds outflow (glaucoma, hyphema). The normal IOP is 10 to 21 mmHg, and three main methods are used to achieve a measurement. Applanation tonometry is the preferred method by ophthalmologists and physicians trained in using this slit-lamp attachment. Practice and previous experience is recommended, however. The Tonopen, a handheld instrument for measuring intraocular pressure, has gained popularity because it is easier for a nonophthalmologist to use and has reasonable accuracy on edematous corneas owing to high intraocular pressure (attacks of acute angle closure). The Schiøtz tonometer is another instrument that can be readily used if a Tonopen is not available. All methods require an anesthetized cornea and a cooperative patient. Care must be taken to avoid any pressure on the globe with your fingers when holding the lids open, as this will cause a falsely high reading. The lids should be held open, with the fingers compressing the lids against the bony rims of the orbit. The method used should always be recorded. In

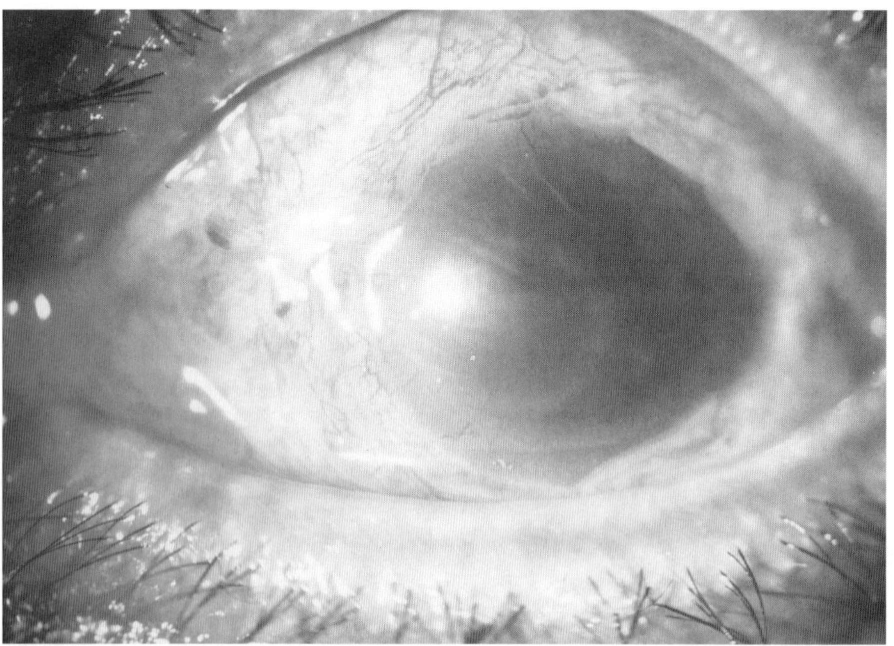

FIG. 230-8 (Plate 10). Hyphema secondary to blunt trauma. Note the blood filling the lower half of the anterior chamber and hazy appearance of cornea suggesting increased IOP.

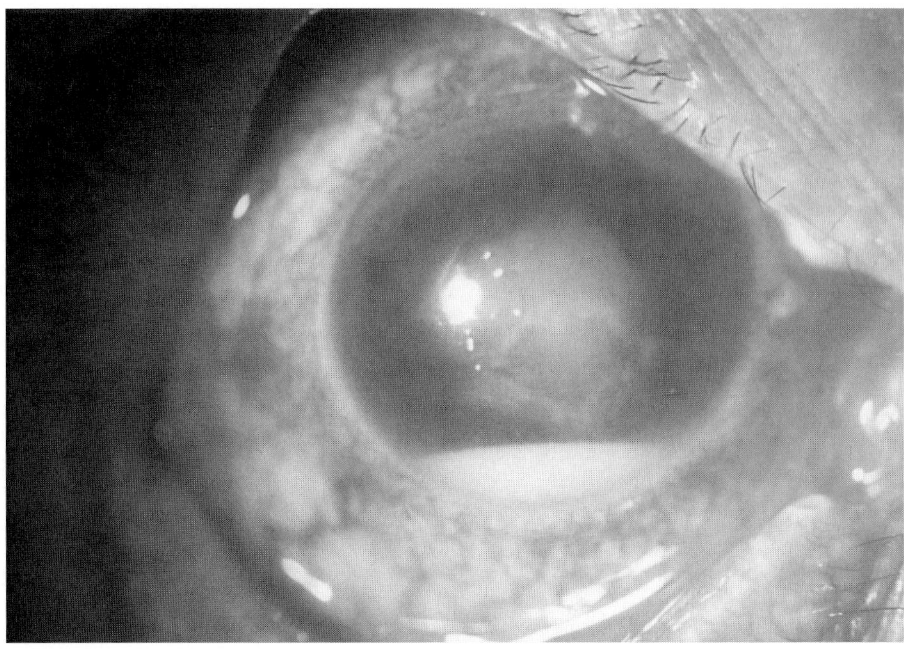

FIG. 230-9 (Plate 11). Corneal ulcer with hypopyon. The ulcer is seen as a shaggy white corneal infiltrate surrounding the borders of the epithelial defect. The hypopyon represents the accumulation of white cells layering out in the lower one-sixth of the anterior chamber.

recording the IOP, refer to the glossary of terms, abbreviations, and notations.

GLOSSARY OF TERMS, ABBREVIATIONS, AND NOTATIONS

It is important to understand the terms and abbreviations used in ophthalmology, not only to be more effective and precise when interacting with consultants but also to aid you in interpreting their written consultations.

AC: Anterior chamber, the first portion of the anterior segment
Anisocoria: Unequal pupil size under equal lighting conditions
Anterior segment: Consists of the anterior chamber and posterior chamber. Aqueous is produced in the posterior chamber of the anterior segment and circulates through the pupil into the anterior chamber of the anterior segment.
APD: Afferent pupillary defect (Fig. 230-3)
CF: counting fingers (visual acuity assessment)
CVF: Confrontation visual fields
EOM: Extraocular muscle
HM: hand motion (visual acuity assessment)
Hyphema: Red blood cells in the anterior chamber
Hypopyon: White blood cells in the anterior chamber
INO: Internuclear ophthalmoplegia
IOFB: Intraocular foreign body
IOP: Intraocular pressure (mmHg)
Limbus: Circumferential border where clear cornea ends and white sclera begins
NLP: no light perception (blind)
OD: Oculus dexter (right eye)
OS: Oculus sinister (left eye)
OU: Oculus uterque (each eye)
PH: pinhole visual acuity
RD: Retinal detachment
Tonopen: a handheld, pen-shaped device for measuring intraocular pressure
T_{tono}: Tension (IOP) with subscript representing method used (tono = Tonopen, S = Schiøtz, A = applanation).
V_{Ac}: visual acuity with correction (glasses or contact lenses)
V_{As}: visual acuity without correction

By convention, in documenting the visual acuity (V_A) or IOP, the right eye is listed above the left, as follows:

$$V_{Ac} < \begin{matrix} 20/20 \\ 20/30 \end{matrix}$$

This represents a visual acuity *with* glasses/contacts of 20/20 right eye and 20/30 left eye.

$$V_{As} < \begin{matrix} 20/400 \rightarrow 20/30 \\ \text{CF at 8 ft} \rightarrow 20/40 \end{matrix}$$

This represents a visual acuity *without* glasses/contacts of 20/400 in the right eye, improving to 20/30 with pinhole testing; counting fingers at 8 ft in the left eye, improving to 20/40 with pinhole testing.

Pinhole testing is helpful in assessing the visual acuity of someone who has a refractive error but does not have corrective lenses available. The pinhole allows only parallel rays (collimated light) to fall on the macula, thereby reducing the refractive error and allowing an estimate of the person's corrected visual acuity.

$$T_{tono} < \begin{matrix} 14 \\ 15 \end{matrix}$$

This represents an intraocular pressure of 14 mmHg in the right eye and 15 mmHg in the left eye measured by Tonopen.

INFECTIONS

Lids

STYE (EXTERNAL HORDEOLUM) A stye is an acute staphylococcal infection of an oil gland associated with an eyelash. It is located at the lash line and has the appearance of a small pustule. It can be either ruptured or left alone. Warm compresses and erythromycin ophthalmic ointment bid for 7 to 10 days is usually sufficient treatment.

CHALAZION (INTERNAL HORDEOLUM) A chalazion is an acute or chronic inflammation of the eyelid secondary to blockage of one of the meibomian oil glands in the tarsal plate. A reddened, tender lump develops in the lid or at the lid margin. Initial conservative treatment consists of warm, moist compresses three or four times a day and erythromycin ophthalmic ointment applied to the eyelid margin qid. Some ophthalmologists will also add a 14- to 21-day course of doxycycline (tetracycline derivatives are secreted in the oil glands). The patient should follow up with an ophthalmologist in about 6 weeks or less if any worsening occurs. Chronic inflammation will induce a cystic wall, and a discrete lump develops that is usually both palpable and visible in the lid. Chalazions can cycle between being quiet or acutely inflamed. The patient with a chronic, recurrent chalazion should be referred to an ophthalmologist for surgical excision and curettage, which is the definitive procedure.

Treatment:

1. Warm moist compresses three to four times a day.
2. Erythromycin ophthalmic ointment applied to lid margins qid.
3. Consider doxycycline 100 mg PO bid for 14 to 21 days if chronic and recurrent.
4. Ophthalmology referral 4 to 6 weeks.

Conjunctivitis

BACTERIAL CONJUNCTIVITIS Bacterial conjunctivitis generally presents with a mucopurulent discharge and inflammation of the conjunctiva. Often the eyelids are stuck together upon awakening. The condition can be monocular or binocular. The cornea is clear *without* fluorescein staining. Frequently there is a history of recent exposure to someone with ''pink eye.'' Treatment consists of a topical ocular antibiotic for 5 to 7 days qid. Treatment with a broad-spectrum agent is safe for patients 2 months of age and older; Polytrim (trimethoprim and polymyxin B), for example, is very effective and avoids potential allergies to sulfa and neomycin preparations. Wearers of soft contact lenses should be treated with a fluoroquinolone (Ciloxan, Ocuflox) or aminoglycoside (Tobrex) to cover for *Pseudomonas.* With the expanding choices of well-tolerated topical antibiotic drops, gentamicin is now seldom used by ophthalmologists because of the high incidence of ocular irritation associated with it.

Treatment:

1. Fluorescein stain cornea (especially infants) to avoid missing a corneal abrasion, ulcer, or dendrite.
2. Non-contact-lens wearer: broad-spectrum topical antibiotic (Polytrim), one drop qid for 5 to 7 days.
3. Contact-lens wearer: fluoroquinolone (Ciloxan or Ocuflox) or aminoglycoside (Tobrex), one drop qid for 5 to 7 days.

VIRAL CONJUNCTIVITIS Viral conjunctivitis tends to follow an antecedent upper respiratory infection and often will have a palpable preauricular node, which aids in confirming the diagnosis. Generally one eye will be involved initially, with the other eye becoming involved within days. The discharge tends to be watery and the conjunctiva is reddened and edematous (chemosis). The cornea is clear, with occasional punctate staining with fluorescein dye (multiple tiny dots of stain uptake seen only on slit-lamp examination). It is important to stain the cornea to avoid missing a herpes dendritic keratitis. Treatment consists of cool compresses; Naphcon-A, one drop tid as needed for redness and conjunctival congestion; and artificial tears five or six times a day. Viral conjunctivitis can take 1 to 3 weeks to run its course and is highly contagious. The physician examining a patient with possible conjunctivitis should wear gloves in order to avoid self-contamination. If, after a history and physical examination, it is still uncertain if the conjunctivitis is viral or bacterial, it is not unreasonable to add an antibiotic eyedrop until the patient can be reexamined by an ophthalmologist.

Treatment:

1. Fluorescein stain the cornea to avoid missing a herpes dendrite.
2. Cool compresses qid.
3. Naphcon-A one drop tid or qid as needed for conjunctival congestion/itching.
4. Consider a topical antibiotic if there is uncertainty as to whether an infection is viral or bacterial.
5. Ophthalmology follow-up in 7 to 10 days if cornea is clear.

ALLERGIC CONJUNCTIVITIS Allergens can cause ocular discharge, redness, and itching. Itching is a very common and consistent symptom seen with allergic conjunctivitis. Treatment consists of cool compresses qid, antihistamine/decongestant drops (Patanol bid or Naphcon-A qid), and artificial tears as needed.

NEONATAL CONJUNCTIVITIS (OPHTHALMIA NEONATORUM) Newborns with conjunctivitis require a careful history to elicit exposure to herpesvirus, *Chlamydia,* or *Neisseria gonorrhoeae* in the maternal birth canal. Conjunctivitis occurring in the first 28 days needs to be cultured with immediate Gram staining followed by the institution of both topical and systemic antibiotics. A careful examination to rule out systemic infection is essential. Infection with *N. gonorrhoeae* and herpes simplex virus (HSV) II can occur in the first 3 days of life; the former can cause rapid corneal ulceration and perforation if not treated. HSV II can occur in the first 3 to 15 days, and concomitant systemic involvement can be devastating. *Chlamydia, Haemophilus, Staphylococcus aureus,* and *Streptococcus pneumoniae* usually present 5 to 10 days after delivery. Treatment for *N. gonorrhoeae* consists of topical erythromycin ointment qid and systemic ceftriaxone (1 g IM or 30 to 50 mg/kg per day IV). HSV II requires topical Viroptic q 2 h and pediatric consultation for systemic evaluation and consideration of systemic acyclovir. *Chlamydia* requires topical and oral erythromycin treatment and awareness that the neonate is at increased risk for concomitant chlamydial pneumonia. *Haemophilus* should be treated with topical erythromycin and a systemic cephalosporin. Staph and strep can be treated with topical erythromycin. A typical standard treatment approach to the neonate with conjunctivitis is as follows:

Treatment:

1. Obtain cultures, Gram stain.
2. Institute topical erythromycin ointment and systemic ceftriaxone.
3. Assess neonate for possible systemic involvement and consult pediatrics for possible admission/septic workup.

Herpes Simplex Virus

HSV can affect the eyelids, conjunctiva, and cornea. Skin involvement has typical vesicular eruptions and the conjunctiva can also become inflamed. Ocular HSV can alternately present with only corneal findings on physical examination. The ''dendrite'' of herpes keratitis is an epithelial defect that can be seen with fluorescein staining and has a linear branching pattern with terminal bulbs (Fig. 230-10, Plate 12). An initial outbreak of HSV involving the lids and conjunctiva can be treated with an oral acyclovir derivative such as Zovirax or Famvir and topical antiviral drops (Viroptic five times a day without corneal involvement, nine times a day with corneal involvement). Erythromycin ophthalmic ointment can be added to prevent secondary infection of the vesicular eruption. HSV keratitis can progress to corneal scarring and requires prompt treatment with topical antiviral agents. Viroptic—one drop nine times a day—represents standard treatment, and Vira-A ointment five times a day or Stoxil can be substituted for those who are allergic to Viroptic. Topical steroids should be strictly avoided, and all patients should be referred to an ophthalmologist for outpatient follow-up.

Treatment:

1. If the initial outbreak lasts longer than 3 to 4 days, consider oral acyclovir-class medications.
2. Erythromycin ophthalmic ointment qid to skin and conjunctival lesions to avoid secondary bacterial infection.

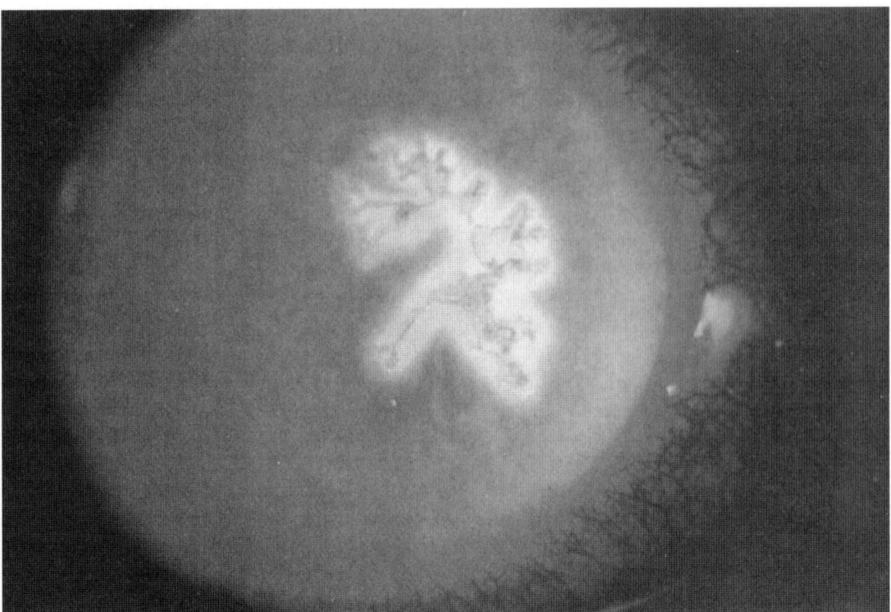

FIG. 230-10 (Plate 12). Herpes simplex corneal dendrite seen with fluorescein staining and cobalt-blue light.

3. HSV *without* corneal involvement: Viroptic one drop five times a day.
4. HSV *with* corneal involvement: Viroptic one drop nine times a day.
5. Ophthalmology follow-up in 1 to 3 days.

Herpes Zoster Ophthalmicus

Herpes zoster ophthalmicus (HZO) represents shingles in the trigeminal nerve distribution with ocular involvement. When the cutaneous lesions include the tip of the nose (Hutchinson sign), the nasociliary nerve is involved and the eye frequently becomes inflamed. An iritis can occur with photophobia and pain. Cutaneous lesions and conjunctival involvement is treated with erythromycin ointment to prevent secondary bacterial infection. The cornea can have a ''pseudodendrite,'' which is a poorly staining mucous plaque with no epithelial erosion (unlike HSV, which has a true dendrite with epithelial erosion and staining). The anterior chamber on slit-lamp examination can show manifestations of iritis (cell and flare). Iritis can be treated with topical steroids prednisolone acetate 1% (Pred Forte), one drop four to five times a day, and pain reduction can be achieved with topical cycloplegic agents (scopolamine 0.25% one drop tid or cyclopentolate 1% one drop tid). If HZO is diagnosed, admission and intravenous acyclovir should be considered, especially if any intracranial symptoms are present.

Treatment:

1. Erythromycin ophthalmic ointment to lesions to prevent secondary infection.
2. Oral narcotic analgesia if necessary.
3. Pred Forte one drop five times a day if iritis present and *no corneal epithelial defect* is seen on fluorescein staining and slit-lamp examination.
4. Cycloplegic pain reduction with 0.25% scopolamine or 1% cyclopentolate one drop tid.
5. Consideration for admission and intravenous acyclovir—dosage 30 mg/kg per day divided tid if creatinine is below 2.

Preseptal Cellulitis (Periorbital Cellulitis)

Preseptal cellulitis is a periocular superficial cellulitis that has not breached the orbital septum. The eyelids become edematous, warm, and red. The eye itself is not involved, with *acuity and pupillary reaction maintained* and *full ocular motility preserved*. The majority of cases occurring in children and adults are the result of inoculation secondary to skin infection or trauma (see Chap. 117, ''Skin and Soft Tissue Infections''). The offending agent is usually *Staph. aureus*. These patients can frequently be treated with oral antibiotics, but if orbital involvement becomes evident, then intravenous antibiotics, CT scanning, and possible admission should be considered.

Preseptal cellulitis in children under 5 years of age is a special circumstance due to the association with bacteremia, septicemia, and meningitis and warrants a complete workup, including blood cultures and intravenous antibiotics. Although *Staph. aureus* is still the most common organism, often these children will have bacteremic spread of *H. influenzae* from otitis media or pneumonia. The incidence of *H. influenzae* preseptal cellulitis has been decreasing with the advent of the *H. influenzae* type b vaccine. Consultation with a pediatrician is recommended for consideration of admission.

Treatment:

1. Ascertain no restriction of ocular motility, no proptosis, no pain with eye movement, and preserved pupillary response and acuity.
2. Regarding those above 5 years of age:
   Children: Augmentin 20 to 40 mg/kg per day PO divided tid.
   Adults: Augmentin 500 mg PO tid.
3. Regarding those below 5 years of age or in severe cases, admit for intravenous antibiotics and systemic workup.
   Children: Ceftriaxone 100 mg/kg per day IV divided bid plus vancomycin 40 mg/kg per day IV divided tid.
   Adults: Ceftriaxone 1 to 2 g IV q 12 h plus vancomycin 0.5 to 1.0 g IV q 12 h.

Orbital Cellulitis (Postseptal Cellulitis)

Orbital cellulitis is an *orbital* infection; therefore it is deep to the orbital septum. This is a serious ocular infection that has the potential to be life-threatening. *Staph. aureus* is the most common pathogen; however, *H. influenzae* flu should be considered in young children and mucormycosis in diabetics and immunocompromised patients. Polymicrobial infection is common. Orbital extension of paranasal sinus infection (especially ethmoid sinusitis) is the most frequent source. Orbital and sinus computed tomography (CT) scans should be performed in the ED. If the CT is negative, an enhanced CT should be performed looking for a subperiosteal abscess. Diagnostic clinical findings that help distinguish this infection from preseptal cellulitis include EOM motility impairment, pain, fever, and occasionally proptosis. Decreased visual acuity is a late finding. Cavernous sinus thrombosis can also occur. These patients require a full workup, admission, and intravenous antibiotics.

Treatment:

1. Intravenous cefuroxime alone, or intravenous penicillin plus nafcillin, or chloramphenicol plus nafcillin. In penicillin-allergic patients vancomycin or a cephalosporin can be substituted.
2. CT scanning of orbits and paranasal sinuses; if CT is negative, then CT with contrast should be ordered to identify subperiosteal abscess.
3. Admission

Corneal Ulcer

A corneal ulcer is a serious infection involving multiple layers of the cornea. Corneal ulcers develop secondary to breaks in the epithelial barrier, allowing infectious agents to gain access to the underlying corneal stroma. The initial disruption of the epithelial layer can be due to desquamation, trauma, or direct microbial invasion. Exposure keratitis from incomplete lid closure secondary to Bell palsy can cause corneal desiccation and sloughing of the epithelium, allowing bacteria to gain access to the underlying stroma and create an ulcer. Trauma can also breach the epithelium and inoculate the cornea. Wearing of soft contact lenses is a very common cause of corneal ulcers, and the incidence increases dramatically in those who use extended-wear lenses and wearers who sleep with them in place.

Typically the patient will have a painful red eye, with tearing and occasionally photophobia. Examination reveals a staining epithelial defect and a white, hazy infiltrate underlying the defect and spreading into adjacent stroma. Occasionally a hypopyon is also present on slit-lamp examination (see Fig. 230-7), signifying an intraocular inflammatory response. Corneal ulcers need to be treated aggressively with topical antibiotics. A fluoroquinolone such as ciprofloxacin (Ciloxan) or ofloxacin (Ocuflox), one drop every hour in the affected eye, is the recommended treatment. A topical cycloplegic agent such as cyclopentolate 1% (Cyclogyl), one drop tid, can also help with pain control. The eye *should not be patched* because of risk of *Pseudomonas* infection, which can cause rapid, aggressive ulceration, with corneal melting and perforation. All corneal ulcers should be referred to an ophthalmologist to be seen within 12 to 24 h.

Treatment:

1. Ciloxan or Ocuflox, one drop every hour.
2. No patching.
3. Topical cycloplegic (1% cyclopentolate or 0.25% scopolamine tid).
4. Ophthalmology referral within 24 h.

TRAUMA

Superficial Trauma

SUBCONJUNCTIVAL HEMORRHAGE The fragile conjunctival vessels can rupture from trauma, sudden Valsalva pressure spikes (sneezing, coughing, vomiting, straining), hypertension, or spontaneously with no discernible etiology. No treatment is necessary, and the hemorrhage usually resolves within 2 weeks. If multiple recurrent episodes occur, coagulation studies and further investigation are warranted.

CONJUNCTIVAL ABRASION Superficial conjunctival abrasions without any other associated ocular injury only requires erythromycin ointment bid for 2 to 3 days or no treatment if very small. The lid should be everted and the fornix inspected under magnification for any residual particulate matter or organic debris.

CORNEAL ABRASION Abrasions of the cornea are associated with pain, photophobia, and tearing. They can be the result of trauma or contact-lens wear. Visual acuity assessment can be difficult because of the patient's extreme discomfort. A drop of a topical anesthetic will often reduce the discomfort temporarily and facilitate visual acuity testing. A corneal epithelial defect will be present and is best seen with fluorescein staining and examination with a cobalt-blue light. The eyelid should be everted and inspected for foreign bodies. Examine the cornea for possible full-thickness injury (optical sectioning) and assess the anterior chamber with the slit lamp, looking for any associated injury. Adequate and persistent cycloplegia is essential to controlling pain. Reduction of ciliary spasm contributes significantly to pain relief and in most cases eliminates the need for narcotic pain medication. By the same token, inadequate cycloplegia almost mandates the need for oral analgesics. If an abrasion is larger than 2 mm or very painful, consider having the patient instill a cycloplegic agent (cyclopentolate 1%, homatropine 5%, or scopolamine 0.25%), one drop every 6 to 8 h at home to help control discomfort. Scopolamine dilates the pupil for several days and is usually reserved for very large, painful abrasions. Cyclopentolate 1% (Cyclogyl) one drop tid does an excellent job of providing cycloplegia and wears off within 24 h of discontinuation. Erythromycin ophthalmic ointment should be instilled and an eye patch may be placed, if desired, provided that the abrasion was not from an organic source or from the wearing of soft contact lenses. Abrasions will heal with or without a patch and ophthalmologists will treat patients either way. Some patients appear to be more comfortable with an eye patch for the first 12 to 18 h, but this is not uniform and the physician can make an individual decision with the patient. Abrasions from organic sources have fungal potential and should not be patched. Abrasions related to the wearing of soft contact lenses pose a risk of *Pseudomonas* infection and likewise should not be patched. These patients should be treated with tobramycin ointment qid, followed by a fluoroquinolone (Ciloxan, Ocuflox) drop or tobramycin drop qid once the epithelial defect starts to close. Do not prescribe a topical anesthetic for pain relief, most anesthetics cause corneal toxicity when recurrently dosed and can lead to blinding complications.

Documenting the Dimensions of a Corneal Abrasion Some slit lamps (Haag-Streit) have a measuring dial attached to the mechanism that varies the length of the slit beam (Fig. 230-11, Plate 13). If your slit lamp is equipped with this feature, you can vary the length of the slit beam on the cornea until it corresponds to the length or width of the abrasion. The reading on the wheel equals the length of the slit beam in millimeters. This additional feature allows you to document the dimensions of the abrasion precisely, thereby enabling subsequent examiners to evaluate the wound's healing response objectively.

Treatment:

1. Identify source of abrasion if possible.
2. Cycloplegia (cyclopentolate 1%, or homatropine 5%) one drop now and repeat q 6–8 h as needed for pain. Warn patient that the pupil will dilate, lose its ability to focus at near, and that the drop will burn for 10 to 15 s when placed in the eye.
3. Not related to contact-lens wear: Erythryomycin ophthalmic ointment and eye patch, or no patch and erythromycin ointment qid.
4. Related to contact-lens wear: Tobramycin ophthalmic ointment qid. *No patch.*
5. Organic source: Erythromycin ophthalmic ointment qid. *No patch.*
6. Ophthalmology referral or reexamine next day.

CONJUNCTIVAL FOREIGN BODIES Conjunctival foreign bodies can usually be removed with a moistened, cotton-tipped applicator after anesthetizing the eye with a topical anesthetic. The upper eyelid should be everted and inspected under the highest magnification available to avoid missing any additional foreign bodies. Frequently small

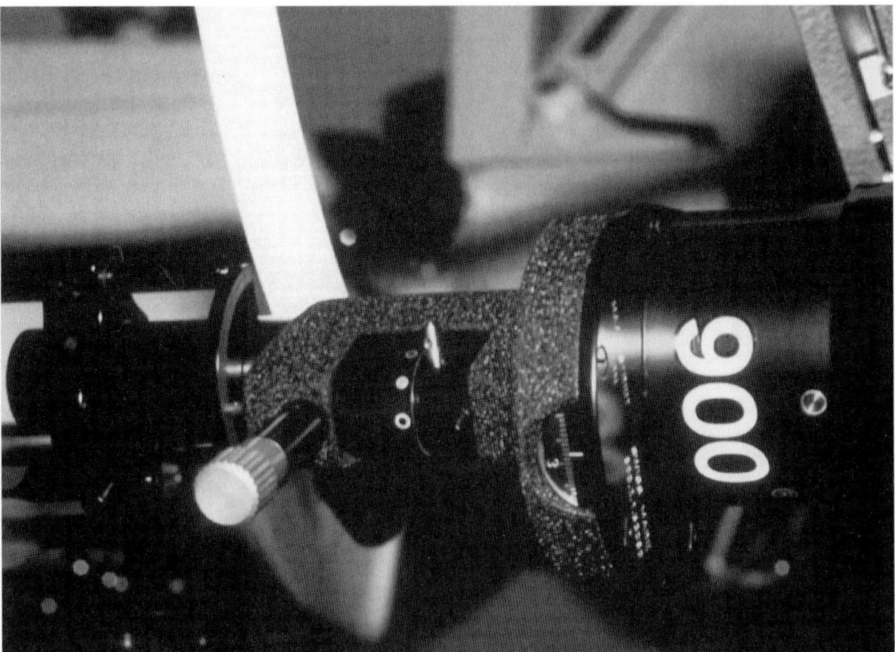

FIG. 230-11 (Plate 13). Slit-lamp measuring wheel. The length of the light beam on the cornea can be varied and the reading on the dial represents the length in millimeters. Useful in measuring corneal abrasion dimensions.

wooden particles such as sawdust will blend into the conjunctiva when moistened by the tears and be difficult to find without slit-lamp magnification. Small, fine vertical corneal abrasions seen only with fluorescein staining will often alert the physician to the presence of a foreign body embedded in the tarsal conjunctiva of the upper lid.

CORNEAL FOREIGN BODIES Foreign bodies should be removed carefully under the best magnification available. The slit lamp provides sufficient magnification and allows both hands to be free for use. A history consistent with high-velocity ocular impact (i.e., hammering metal on metal) should alert you to the possibility of a penetrating injury. The cornea should be inspected using "optical sectioning" (see Fig. 230-11) to assess depth of penetration *prior* to removal. Full-thickness foreign bodies should not be removed in the ED and require an ophthalmology consult. Fortunately most corneal foreign bodies are superficial and can be removed easily and safely. A "golf-club spud" is a handy tool for this task, but a small 30- to 25-gauge needle under slit lamp magnification, or moistened, cotton-tipped applicator will work most of the time. A topical anesthetic should be instilled prior to removal, and it is helpful to also instill an anesthetic drop in the unaffected eye to suppress reflex blinking during removal. Many slit lamps have an attached "fixation light" that is mobile and can be moved in front of the unaffected eye to give the patient a steady target to concentrate on. This reduces the random movements that can occur when you are trying to remove the foreign body. The eyelids can be held open with your fingers, or a wire eyelid speculum can provide excellent support during the procedure. Metallic foreign bodies can create rust rings that are toxic to the corneal tissue. If a rust ring is present, the spud or an ophthalmic burr can be used to remove most of the rust. Even if a thorough job is done initially, the next day more rust can often be seen, requiring additional burring. It is therefore not necessary to go after all the rust aggressively in the ED if the patient can be seen by an ophthalmologist the next day. The rust-ring area can soften overnight and be removed in the office the next day. The deeper the stromal involvement, the higher the risk of corneal scarring; therefore, only a superficial burring should take place in the ED. No ED drill burring should take place if the rust ring is located in the visual axis (pupil) owing to the risk of causing visually significant scarring. These patients should have an ophthalmologist remove the stromal rust in the office within 24 h. As with any foreign body of the eye, the lid should be everted and inspected under magnification to ensure that no additional foreign bodies are present. The corneal abrasion that will be present after the removal of a foreign body should be treated as previously discussed, with adequate cycloplegia, antibiotic ointment, and optional patching.

Treatment:

1. Instill topical anesthetic in both eyes to suppress the blink reflex.
2. Test visual acuity (sometimes easier after an anesthetic drop is administered).
3. Assess if this is a full-thickness or penetrating injury.
4. Remove the foreign body under slit-lamp magnification and remove superficial rust if possible. Use burr if available, but avoid burring in visual axis.
5. Evert lid to rule out additional foreign bodies.
6. Treat resultant corneal abrasion with topical cycloplegia, erythromycin ointment, and optional patching (see "Conjunctival Abrasion," above).
7. Referral to ophthalmologist, to be seen the next day.

Lid Lacerations

Full-thickness lid lacerations should be repaired by an ophthalmologist, if at all possible, within 24 h. Proper alignment of the lid margin during repair under magnification (loupes or microscope) is essential to preserve proper lid function and even corneal wetting with each blink. Improper lid closure can result in notching of the lid and create a functional deformity. If there is no opportunity for the patient to see an ophthalmologist, repair should be performed as in Fig. 230-12. One 6-0 silk vertical mattress suture, using the meibomian gland orifices as a landmark, or two 6-0 silk sutures (one approximating the anterior and the other the posterior lamella) are used to repair the lid margin. The ends of the silk sutures should be left long enough to tuck under the more distal skin sutures to avoid corneal irritation. The tarsus should be repaired with 5-0 Vicryl from the external side so as to approximate the wound without the need for sutures on the conjunctival side of the lid (which would abrade the cornea with each blink). Skin closure can be performed with 6-0 or 7-0 monofilament or silk

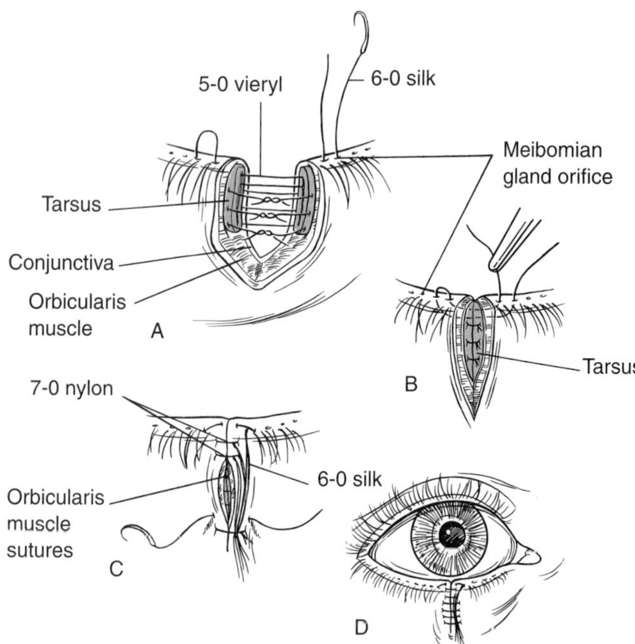

FIG. 230-12. Full-thickness lid repair. 6-0 silk used for lid margin. 5-0 Vicryl used to approximate tarsal plate. The Vicryl sutures should not pass through the conjunctiva on the inside of the eyelid to avoid mechanical abrasion of the cornea during blinking. 7-0 nylon is used for skin closure, and the lid margin silk suture tail can be incorporated into these sutures to avoid corneal irritation.

suture. Deep lacerations medial to the punctum can potentially transect the canalicular system. These patients need to be seen by an ophthalmologist for evaluation of the nasolacrimal duct system's integrity. If a canalicular laceration is discovered, the patient will need to go to the operating room within 24 to 36 h for repair and Silastic tube stenting (Fig. 230-13, Plate 14). Because a meticulous repair by an experienced eye surgery team is preferable, it is not unreasonable for the ophthalmologist to discharge a patient seen late in the evening or on the weekend with arrangements for surgical repair to take place within the next 36 h. Patients discharged pending repair should be placed on oral and topical antibiotics and told to use cold compresses. Oral cephalexin (Keflex) 500 mg bid or qid and topical erythromycin ophthalmic ointment qid are reasonable choices.

Partial-thickness lid lacerations can usually be repaired in the ED with referral for ophthalmologic evaluation in 2 to 3 days. It is important to have the suture ends closest to the cornea tucked under more distal sutures to avoid corneal irritation (see Fig. 230-12).

Blunt Trauma

After sustaining blunt trauma, the eyelids are frequently swollen shut and the globe is difficult to visualize. Trying to pry the eyelids open with your fingers can be frustrating; it increases the intraocular pressure and usually results in obtaining an unsatisfactory view of the globe. A wire or adjustable eyelid speculum can help tremendously. Insertion of the eyelid speculum provides a significantly improved view of the cornea and anterior chamber and allows your hands to remain free for examination of the globe at the slit lamp. If a speculum is not available, try your best to assess the patient's visual acuity and the integrity of the globe and anterior chamber. If the anterior chamber is flat, a ruptured globe is certain and no further attempts to assess the eye should be made. A metal shield should be placed and an ophthalmologist consulted. A hyphema is also evidence of significant ocular trauma and necessitates an ophthalmology consult. If the globe appears intact and vision is preserved, next check ocular motility. Restricted upgaze or lateral gaze suggests a blowout fracture with entrapment (see "Blowout Fractures," below). Feel the orbital rim above and below for step-off deformities. Test for cutaneous sensation along the distribution of the inferior orbital nerve (below the eye and ipsilateral side of the nose). Perform a slit-lamp examination with fluorescein staining to check for abrasions, lacerations, foreign bodies, hyphema, iritis, and lens dislocation. Traumatic iritis is common, causing cell and flare to be seen on slit-lamp examination. If no corneal epithelial defect is seen, iritis can be treated with one drop of Pred Forte four to five times a day. The pupil can be constricted or dilated after sustaining trauma. It is important to look for pupillary irregularity, because the pupil will often peak toward the site of a penetration or rupture. If the anterior chamber is of normal depth and not shallow, one drop of Mydriacyl 1% will dilate the pupil and allow an easier funduscopic view. Non-Caucasian brown-eyed individuals will frequently require an additional drop of phenylephrine 2.5% to achieve adequate dilation. If vision as well as ocular anatomy and function are preserved, outpatient follow-up by an ophthalmologist in the next 48 h should be planned. If a ruptured globe is suspected (blind eye, flat anterior chamber, obvious full-thickness laceration, intraocular foreign body), no attempts at eye manipulation or IOP measurements should take place and an ophthalmologist should be consulted.

Treatment:

1. Assess globe integrity and vision.
2. If ruptured globe is suspected, do not attempt to check IOP; place a protective metal eye shield, check tetanus status, administer intravenous cephalosporin, let the patient take nothing by mouth, and call ophthalmology.
3. If ruptured globe is not suspected, proceed with the following.
4. Check eye motility and cutaneous sensation.

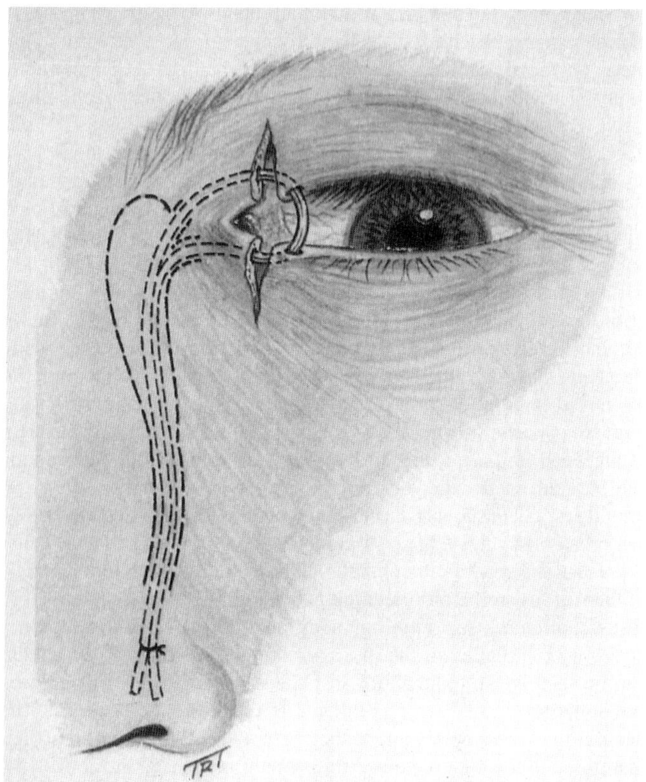

FIG. 230-13 (Plate 14). Traumatic canalicular laceration repair requires microsurgical stenting to reestablish patency.

5. Obtain Waters view and/or orbital CT if blowout fracture or orbital/intraocular foreign body is suspected. Treat accordingly.
6. Slit-lamp examination of corneal, conjunctival, scleral, and anterior chamber structures.
7. Dilate if anterior chamber depth is normal for funduscopic view.
   Caucasians: Mydriacyl 1%, one drop.
   All others: Mydriacyl 1%, one drop, plus phenylephrine 2.5%, one drop.
8. Ophthalmology referral within 48 h if no injuries are found.

HYPHEMA Blood in the anterior chamber is referred to as a hyphema (see Fig. 230-8). Hyphemas generally can be classified as either traumatic or spontaneous. Traumatic hyphemas are usually the result of bleeding from a ruptured iris root vessel. Both blunt and penetrating trauma can cause hyphemas. Spontaneous hyphemas are frequently associated with sickle cell disease. All hyphemas, regardless of etiology, should be seen by an ophthalmologist. ED management consists of assessing concomitant injury (ruptured globe, intraocular foreign body) and managing rises in intraocular pressure. The patient's head should be elevated to promote settling of suspended red blood cells inferiorly, so as not to clog the entire 360° of trabecular meshwork. The pupil should be dilated to avoid "pupillary play" (constriction and dilation movements of the iris in response to changing lighting conditions). Because an iris vessel is usually involved, pupillary activity can put the vessel on stretch, promoting additional bleeding. Pupillary dilation *does not* compromise the angle and aqueous outflow in normal individuals, and many ophthalmologists choose to dilate hyphemas for the above reasons. Intraocular pressure control is important and consists of topical β blockers, intravenous mannitol, topical α-adrenergic agonists (apraclonidine), and oral, topical, or intravenous carbonic anhydrase inhibitors (CAIs) such as Diamox, Trusopt, and Neptazane. In patients suspected of having sickle cell disease (either by history or if the hyphema was spontaneous), carbonic anhydrase inhibitors should be strictly avoided. CAIs will lower the aqueous pH in the anterior chamber, causing the red blood cells to sickle and become less flexible, thereby clogging outflow through the trabecular meshwork and increasing intraocular pressure. Rebleeding can occur 3 to 5 days later in up to 30 percent of cases, sometimes causing potentially blinding elevations of IOP and necessitating surgical anterior chamber "washouts." Because of this risk, some ophthalmologists believe in admitting all patients with hyphemas, while others will choose to follow them closely as outpatients. Generally those with hyphemas occupying one-third or less of the anterior chamber can be followed closely as outpatients. Because of the variance in treatment philosophy, the ED physician should not take the responsibility of deciding to discharge a patient with a hyphema. This decision should be made by the ophthalmologist on call after he or she has examined the patient.

Treatment:

1. Elevate the patient's head.
2. Administer atropine 1% one drop tid.
3. Administer prednisolone acetate 1% (Pred Forte) one drop qid.
4. If globe is intact, measure IOP.
5. If IOP is greater than 30 mmHg, administer topical β blocker (Timoptic 0.5%), one drop. Give PO or IV acetazolamide (Diamox) 500 mg and add mannitol 1 to 2 g/kg IV if there is no response to the above.
6. If IOP is greater than 24 mmHg and the patient is sickle cell trait–positive, treat as above *except avoid Diamox*.
7. Arrange for ophthalmology consult.

BLOWOUT FRACTURES The most frequent sites of orbital blowout fractures are the inferior wall (maxillary sinus) and medial wall (ethmoid sinus). A Waters view x-ray will frequently show a cloudy maxillary sinus on the side of the trauma. This represents blood and fluid in the maxillary sinus from fracture of the orbital floor. Fractures of the medial wall can be associated with subcutaneous emphysema, sometimes exacerbated by sneezing or blowing the nose. Fractures of the inferior wall with entrapment of the inferior rectus muscle can cause restriction of upgaze and diplopia (Fig. 230-14, Plate 15). Isolated blowout fractures with or without entrapment do not require immediate surgery and can be referred to ophthalmology, plastic surgery, oral maxillofacial (OMF) surgery or an ear/nose/throat specialist (depending on the local referral patterns) for repair within the next 3 to 10 days. CT scanning with 1.5-mm cuts of the orbit should take place, and oral antibiotics (Keflex 250 to 500 mg qid for 10 days) are often recommended because of the presence of sinus wall fractures. All blowout fractures with normal initial eye examination in the ED should be referred to an ophthalmologist for an outpatient full dilated

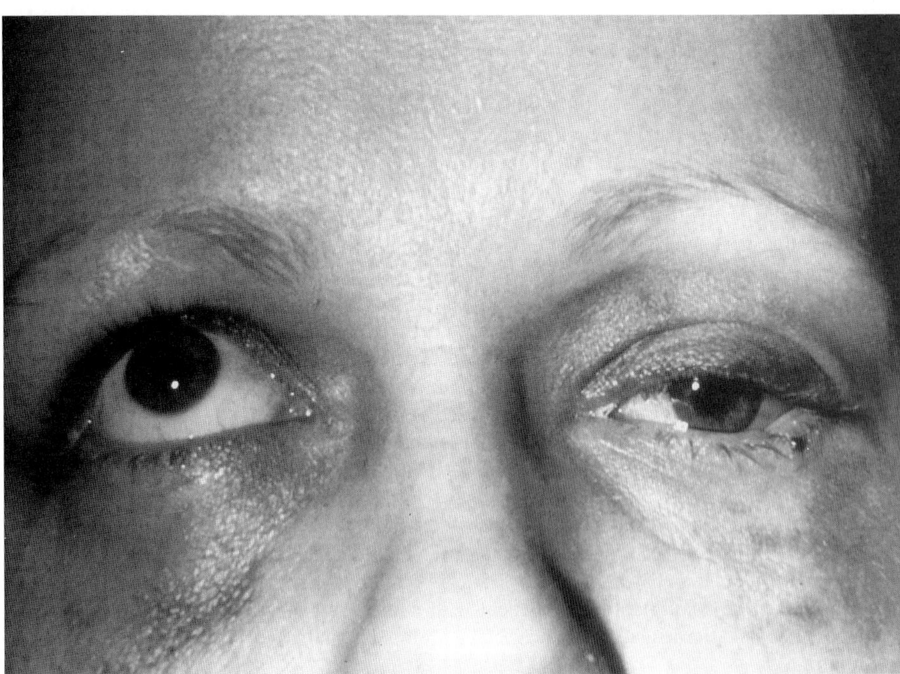

FIG. 230-14 (Plate 15). Inferior wall blowout fracture of the left eye with entrapment of the inferior rectus muscle. The patient's left eye is unable to look upward, causing diplopia on upgaze.

examination to rule out any unidentified retinal tears or detachments. Some 32 percent of blowout fractures are associated with ocular trauma (abrasion, traumatic iritis, hyphema, lens dislocation/subluxation, retinal tear or detachment); therefore a careful eye examination in the ED and referral to an ophthalmologist are essential.

Penetrating Trauma/Ruptured Globe

Penetrating ocular trauma can occur from numerous sources (BB pellets, lawn mower projectiles, hammering, knife and gunshot wounds). Any projectile injury has the potential for penetrating the eye. Any lid laceration from a sharp object, especially if it involves the upper and lower eyelid has the potential to have lacerated the globe and requires a slit-lamp examination. Clues to a ruptured globe or intraocular foreign body include shallow anterior chamber, hyphema, irregular pupil, significant reduction in preinjury visual acuity, and poor view of the optic nerve and posterior pole on direct ophthalmoscopy. It is not unreasonable to dilate the eye with Mydriacyl 1% and phenylephrine 2.5% to obtain a better view of the posterior segment of the eye, facilitating identification of an intraocular foreign body or retinal detachment. A modified Seidel test is helpful in identifying wound leaks (see Fig. 230-7). Any penetrating injury is considered a ruptured globe and mandates an eye shield and ophthalmology consultation. Tetanus status should be determined and intravenous cephalosporin administered. Do not attempt to measure IOP if a ruptured globe is suspected. A Waters view x-ray and orbital CT scans can be helpful in locating and confirming the presence of orbital and intraocular foreign bodies.

Treatment:

1. If ruptured globe suspected, do not attempt to check IOP, place a protective metal eye shield, check tetanus status, administer intravenous cephalosporin, caution the patient to take nothing by mouth, and call ophthalmology.
2. Obtain a Waters view x-ray and/or orbital CT scans if foreign bodies are suspected.

Chemical Trauma

CHEMICAL OCULAR INJURY A chemical injury to the eye is a true ocular emergency. The potential for chemical injury requires immediate recognition and treatment in the field and by the triage nurse. Immediate intervention consists of copious irrigation with at least 1 to 2 L of saline. Topical anesthesia and placement of a Morgan lens allows the irrigation to be delivered effectively and directly to the corneal surface. This is one situation where a delay even to assess visual acuity is inappropriate. Litmus paper or the pH portion of a urine dipstick can be used to assess the pH of the tears in the lower cul-de-sac. Irrigation should continue until pH testing improves to the range of 6 to 8. Both acid and alkali burns can be blinding; however, the majority of acid burns tend to coagulate proteins, thereby limiting the depth of penetration. Alkali burns (lye, ammonia) can rapidly penetrate the cornea, and aqueous pH can rise within minutes of exposure, causing damage to intraocular structures such as the iris and lens. After copious irrigation has been administered and the pH of the tears is close to normal, the eye should be inspected for any particulate matter and visual acuity should be assessed. A topical cycloplegic agent such as 0.25% scopolamine or 1% cyclopentolate should be used tid for pain reduction if an epithelial defect is present. Erythromycin ophthalmic ointment should be instilled qid if both eyes are affected. If only one eye is affected and an epithelial defect is present, adding a pressure patch for the first 12 to 24 h will sometimes make the eye more comfortable. Any patient with corneal clouding or epithelial defect after irrigation should receive prompt ophthalmology referral.

Patients with chemosis (edema of the bulbar conjunctiva overlying the white sclera) and no corneal or anterior chamber findings should be treated after irrigation with erythromycin ointment qid and referred for an ophthalmologic exam in the next 48 h. These patients are considered to have "chemical conjunctivitis."

Treatment:

1. Immediate copious irrigation with a minimum of 1 to 2 L of saline or until tear pH is 6 to 8.
2. If there is no corneal epithelial defect and the anterior segment is normal, administer erythromycin ointment qid.
3. If there is a corneal epithelial defect or there is clouding, administer erythromycin ointment, cycloplegia (cyclopentolate 1% or scopolamine 0.25%), and optional eye patching. Provide for ophthalmology referral within 24 h.

CYANOACRYLATE ("SUPER GLUE/CRAZY GLUE") Cyanoacrylate adhesives are commonplace and often easily accessible to children. Accidental instillation into the eye and adnexa can cause the lids to adhere and adhesive clumps to form on the cornea. Most of the time these accidental instillations are not permanently harmful to the eye. Medicinal-grade cyanoacrylates are used occasionally directly on the cornea to seal corneal perforations and are not considered toxic to the cornea. The only concern is the mechanical abrasive effect of hard, irregular glue aggregates rubbing against the cornea with eye movement and blinking. Erythromycin is instilled heavily into the eye and on the surface of the eyelids to moisten, lubricate, and provide antibiotic coverage. Initial debridement of the surface glue clump should be limited to easily removable pieces. The glue will loosen and become easier to remove in a few days. Referral to an ophthalmologist should take place within 24 to 48 h.

Treatment:

1. Moisten glue with erythromycin ointment and remove as much as can be removed easily without causing damage to underlying tissue.
2. Apply erythromycin ointment heavily into eye (if not glued completely shut) and eyelids five or six times a day.
3. Refer to ophthalmologist in next 24 to 48 h.

ULTRAVIOLET KERATITIS ("WELDER'S FLASH") Pain, tearing, photophobia, and foreign-body sensation typically occur 6 to 12 h after unprotected ocular exposure to welding or sun-tanning lights. The history is diagnostic in these cases. Slit-lamp examination with fluorescein staining shows superficial punctate keratitis (SPK); this appears as numerous small microdots of staining on the corneal surface seen under high magnification using the cobalt-blue light. Treatment consists of cycloplegia, erythromycin ointment, and pressure patching overnight. Oral narcotic analgesia is sometimes necessary.

Treatment:

1. Instill cycloplegic agent: 1% cyclopentolate or 0.25% scopolamine, one drop in each eye; this may be repeated by the patient q 6 to 8 h if needed for pain reduction.
2. Erythromycin ophthalmic ointment now, then qid once the patch is removed.
3. Pressure patching for comfort for the first 24 h; bilateral is preferable but seldom practical.
4. Consider oral narcotic analgesia if pain is severe.
5. Ophthalmology referral within 48 h (this condition is usually self-limited, with complete recovery).

ACUTE VISUAL REDUCTION/LOSS

Painful Visual Reduction/Loss

ACUTE ANGLE-CLOSURE GLAUCOMA Acute angle-closure glaucoma presents with cloudy vision, eye ache and/or headache, increased intraocular pressure, and frequently nausea and vomiting. Abdominal symptoms can sometimes be misleading and delay the diagnosis. Acute angle closure typically occurs in a patient with *no* previous history of glaucoma. These patients generally have narrow anterior chamber angles and suddenly develop "pupillary block" when the pupil becomes middilated and the iris leaflet touches the lens. This prevents circulation of the aqueous humor from the posterior chamber (where it is produced by the ciliary body) through the pupil and into the anterior chamber (where it is filtered out of the eye through the trabecular meshwork located in the angle). The continuous production of aqueous in the posterior chamber is trapped and the increasing hydrostatic pressure bows the iris forward, further compromising the angle and inhibiting outflow (Fig. 230-15). Intraocular pressure rises and eventually exceeds the capacity of the corneal pump mechanism, causing the cornea to become edematous and less transparent. This explains the foggy vision or halos patients complain of and the hazy appearance of the cornea on physical examination. The pupil is *middilated and nonreactive* (Fig. 230-16, Plate 16). Pressures of 50 mmHg and greater are not uncommon. Treatment, aimed at pressure reduction, consists of using suppressants of aqueous production such as topical β blockers, α-adrenergic agonists (apraclonidine), and oral or intravenous CAIs (Diamox). Because patients are frequently nauseated, intravenous CAIs are preferable to oral ones. Intravenous mannitol is very good at quickly lowering intraocular pressure and should be considered an adjunct to treatment if there are no contraindications. Pilocarpine frequently will not cause the iris to constrict during the acute attack until the pressure is reduced. This is due to pressure-induced ischemic paralysis of the iris. Pilocarpine 1 or 2% should be added once the pressure is reduced to make the pupil miotic, thereby pulling the peripheral iris away from the angle. This maneuver will help protect against recurrence until an ophthalmologist can perform the definitive treatment procedure of creating a peripheral laser iridectomy.

Treatment:

1. Identify middilated, nonreactive pupil with increased IOP.
2. Topical β blocker (Timoptic 0.5%), one drop.

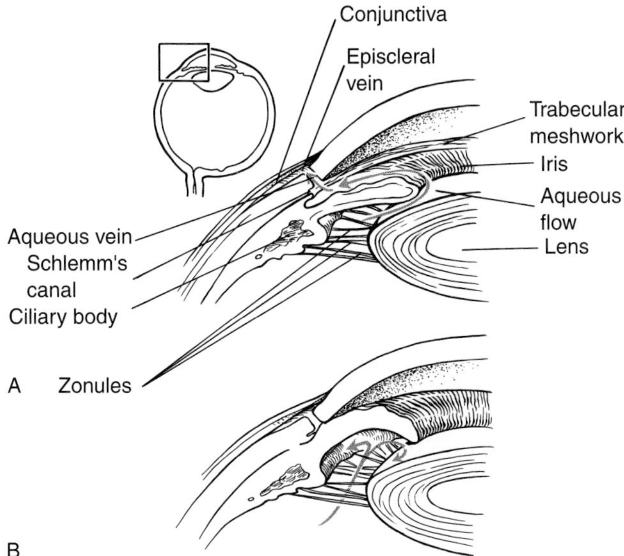

FIG. 230-15. A. Normal flow of aqueous from ciliary body, through the pupil and out through the trabecular meshwork and Schlemm's canal located in the anterior chamber angle. **B.** Angle-closure glaucoma with pupillary block. Iris leaflet bows forward, blocking the chamber angle and prohibiting aqueous outflow. Meanwhile aqueous production continues and IOP rises.

3. Topical α agonist (Iopidine 0.1%), one drop.
4. Topical steroid (Pred Forte 1%), one drop q 15 min for four doses, then hourly.
5. CAI (acetazolamide) 500 mg IV or PO.
6. Mannitol 1 to 2 g/kg IV.
7. Recheck IOP hourly.
8. Topical pilocarpine 1 to 2%, one drop qid once IOP is below 40 mmHg.
9. Consult ophthalmology.

OPTIC NEURITIS Optic neuritis is the most common cause of acute reduction of vision due to optic nerve dysfunction in patients 20 to 40 years of age. Women are more frequently affected. Reduction of vision is rapid and frequently painful (especially with eye movement). Color vision is commonly more affected than visual acuity. The red desaturation test is helpful in identifying optic neuropathies (have the patient look with one eye at a dark red object, then test the other eye to see if the object looks the same color. The affected eye will often see the red object as pink or lighter red). An afferent pupillary defect is commonly present. Visual acuity can range from mildly reduced to no light perception (NLP). If the optic disk is swollen and edematous on the affected side (papillitis), the patient is said to have anterior optic neuritis. If the head of the optic nerve is normal in appearance, the patient is said to have retrobulbar neuritis. The Optic Neuritis Treatment Trial (ONTT) showed that 1 year after an attack of optic neuritis, there was no difference in visual outcome between the patients treated with intravenous steroids and those given a placebo. Treatment with intravenous steroids, however, was associated with a slightly lower 2-year risk of subsequent development of multiple sclerosis, especially in patients whose MRI showed periventricular white matter lesions. For this reason, some physicians will consider intravenous steroids for any attack of optic neuritis, although no treatment is also acceptable. *Initial treatment with oral steroids is contraindicated* and, for unexplained reasons, had the least favorable outcome in the ONTT. Children can develop optic neuritis with similar initial findings except that the majority of them tend to have bilateral optic nerve swelling (simulating papilledema), and a viral illness is frequently associated with an attack. Subsequent development of multiple sclerosis occurs less frequently in children.

Treatment:

1. Check visual acuity, do red desaturation test, APD, eye pain with movement.
2. Check optic nerve head for papillitis (usually unilateral), may be bilateral in children or normal in retrobulbar neuritis.
3. Discuss with ophthalmologist or neurologist whether to treat with IV steroids* or discharge without treatment.

Painless Visual Reduction/Loss

CENTRAL RETINAL ARTERY OCCLUSION Sudden, profound, painless, monocular loss of vision is characteristic of a central retinal artery occlusion (CRAO). The event is often preceded by episodes of amaurosis fugax. The first branch off the internal carotid artery is the ophthalmic artery, which supplies the central retinal artery, which, in turn, provides the blood supply to the inner retina. If the central retinal artery becomes occluded, the retina will infarct and become pale, less transparent, and edematous. The macula is the thinnest portion of the retina and the intact underlying choroidal circulation remains visible through this section of retina, creating the illusion of a "cherry-red spot." In fact, the macular area tends to maintain its normal color while the surrounding ischemic retina turns pale, thus causing this

*Steroid regimen: methylprednisolone 250 mg IV qid for 3 days, followed by oral prednisone 1 mg/kg per day for 11 days.

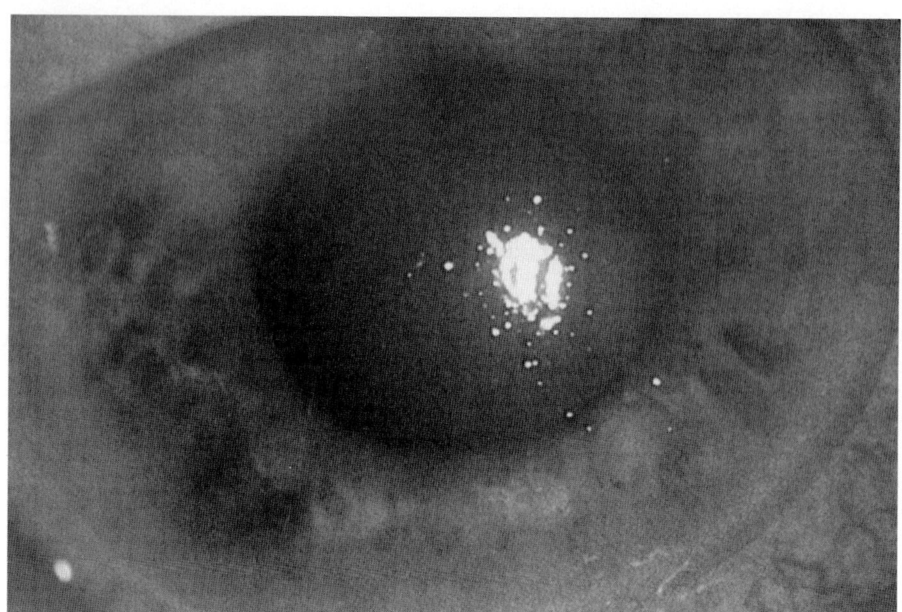

FIG. 230-16 (Plate 16). Acute angle-closure glaucoma. Pupil is middilated and nonreactive. The cornea is hazy due to stromal edema.

classic finding on funduscopy (Fig. 230-17, Plate 17). An APD is a common finding associated with a CRAO. Causes include embolus (carotid and cardiac), thrombosis, giant-cell arteritis, vasculitis (lupus), sickle cell disease, and trauma. Often the patient will have atrial fibrillation. The retina will sustain irreversible damage within 90 min of total occlusion, so treatment should begin immediately. Unfortunately these patients rarely respond to therapy, but because the visual loss is usually so profound, every attempt should be made to reestablish circulation to the retina. Treatment in embolic cases (the majority) is aimed at trying to convert a CRAO into a branch retinal artery occlusion (BRAO). In the attempt to dislodge the embolus from the central artery and into one of its retinal branches, the other retinal branches may become reperfused, thereby reducing the size of the infarct. Maneuvers include digital massage, IOP-lowering drugs, and vasodilation techniques (breathing into a paper bag to increase Pa_{CO_2}). An ophthalmologist should be consulted immediately to evaluate the patient and decide whether performing an IOP-lowering anterior chamber paracentesis is indicated.

Treatment:

1. Consult ophthalmology the moment the diagnosis is made.
2. Administer ocular massage: Firm, steady digital pressure on the globe through closed lids for about 15 s, followed by sudden release of pressure. This may be repeated several times.
3. Administer topical β blocker (Timoptic 0.5%), one drop.
4. Give Diamox 500 mg IV or PO.
5. Consider having the patient breathe into a paper bag for 5 to 10 min if there are no respiratory contraindications.

CENTRAL RETINAL VEIN OCCLUSION Thrombosis of the central retinal vein causes retinal venous stasis, edema, and hemorrhage. Loss

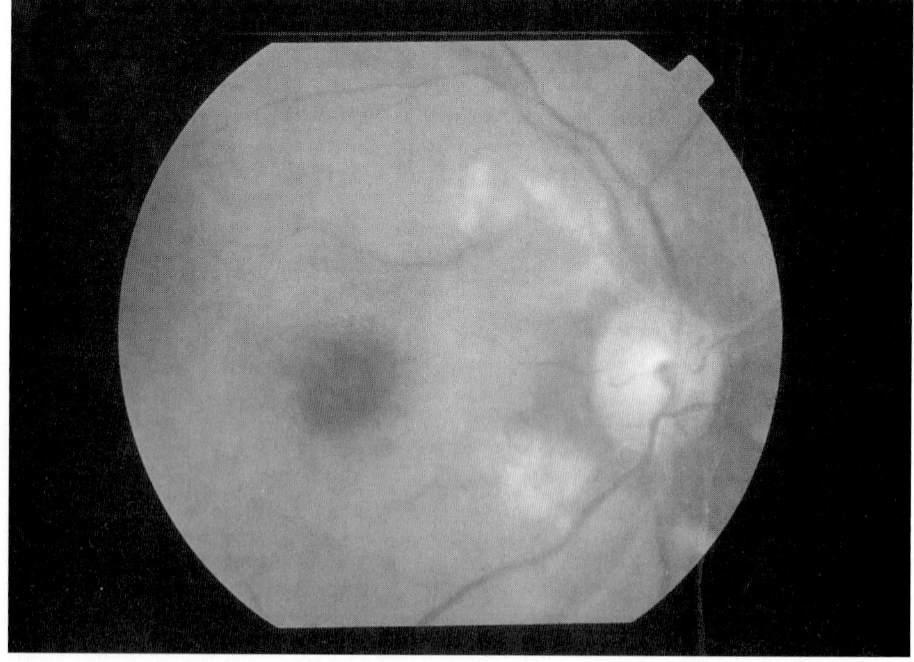

FIG. 230-17 (Plate 17). Central retinal artery occlusion. Note macular ''cherry-red spot'' and retinal pallor between macula and disk. The retinal veins appear normal size, but the arteries are barely visible and attenuated.

of vision is variable, painless, monocular, and rapid. Funduscopic examination typically reveals optic disk edema and diffuse retinal hemorrhages in all quadrants (''blood-and-thunder fundus,'' Fig. 230-18, Plate 18). The contralateral optic nerve and fundus are generally normal, which helps distinguish central retinal vein occlusion (CRVO) from papilledema, and the diffuse retinal hemorrhages help distinguish it from optic neuritis (the peripheral retina is normal in optic neuritis). Typically these patients have a history of hypertension, although hypercoagulable disorders, vasculitis, and glaucoma may also be associated. No specific treatment is available, although the addition of aspirin 60 to 325 mg daily is reasonable. These patients should be referred to an ophthalmologist for confirmation of the diagnosis and monitoring of ischemia-induced neovascularization.

Treatment:

1. Ophthalmology referral.
2. Consider aspirin 60 to 325 mg/day PO.

GIANT-CELL ARTERITIS (TEMPORAL ARTERITIS) Giant-cell arteritis (GCA) is a systemic vasculitis involving medium-sized arteries in the carotid circulation and can include the aorta and its primary branches. GCA can cause a painless ischemic optic neuropathy with devastating visual consequences and rapid contralateral involvement if not diagnosed and treated promptly. Patients are generally over 50 years of age and frequently have a history of polymyalgia rheumatica. Women are more commonly affected than men. Symptoms may include headache, jaw claudication, myalgias, fatigue, fever, anorexia, and temporal artery tenderness. Up to 33 percent may have associated neurologic symptoms such as transient ischemic attacks or stroke. The patient can develop rapid and profound visual loss, with the contralateral eye becoming involved within days to weeks. The physical examination will frequently reveal an APD if the optic nerve circulation is involved. An elevated Westergren sedimentation rate is usually present, with the majority of biopsy-proven cases in the range of 70 to 110. The added presence of an elevated C-reactive protein also suggests the diagnosis. Treatment consists of several doses of intravenous steroids, followed by oral steroids. Steroids should not be delayed while waiting for a temporal artery biopsy to be performed. Biopsies will still be positive a week after initiation of steroid therapy.

Treatment:

1. Order sedimentation rate and C-reactive protein.
2. Consult patient's personal physician.
3. If highly suspicious or any visual loss: Admit for methylprednisolone 250 mg q 6 h IV for 3 days and temporal artery biopsy.
4. If not suspicious and no visual involvement: prednisone 80 to 100 mg PO per day and close outpatient monitoring.

NEURO-OPHTHALMOLOGY

Approximately 38 percent of all the neurons in the brain have some association with the visual system; therefore an understanding of neuro-ophthalmology is essential.

Bell's Palsy

Bell's palsy is a dysfunction of peripheral cranial nerve (CN) VII commonly of viral origin. The orbicularis muscles are involved, frequently resulting in incomplete closure of the eyelids on the affected side. If the eye rolls up under the upper lid on attempted blinking (*Bell's phenomenon*), the cornea will be moistened and the risk of corneal exposure keratitis and subsequent ulceration will be less. These patients should still use viscous topical wetting agents, such as Celluvisc or Lacrilube, to keep the corneal epithelium from breaking down. Ophthalmology referral for outpatient monitoring of the cornea is warranted. The patient's medical doctor or neurologist should follow the patient for the dysfunction of CN VII and be involved in the decision to institute or forego oral steroid treatment, since this remains an area of controversy.

Treatment:

1. Test ipsilateral abduction [rule out genu VII Bell's palsy*]

*Genu VII Bell's palsy is a CVA masquerading as a peripheral seventh-nerve Bell's palsy. It is a stroke involving CN VI and the ipsilateral CN VII as it genuflects around the sixth-nerve nucleus. This results in a CN VII palsy identical to a typical Bell's palsy (affecting the upper and lower face ipsilaterally) but with the added finding of the patient's inability to abduct the ipsilateral eye (CN VI palsy). This underscores the importance of EOM testing in all Bell's palsy patients to avoid misdiagnosis of a CVA.].

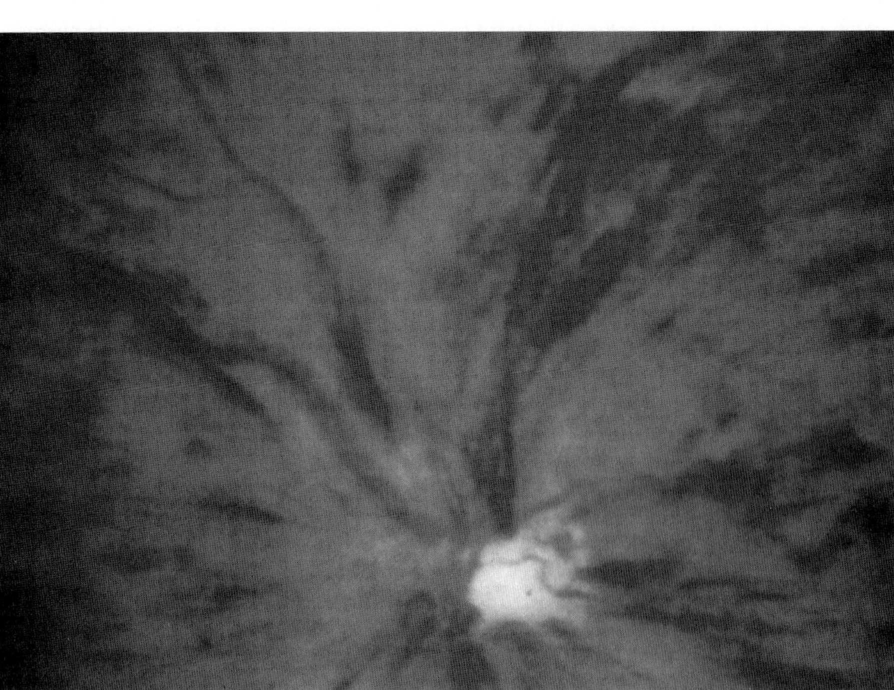

FIG. 230-18 (Plate 18). Central retinal vein occlusion ''blood and thunder fundus.'' Note diffuse retinal hemorrhages in all retina quadrants and blurred disk margins.

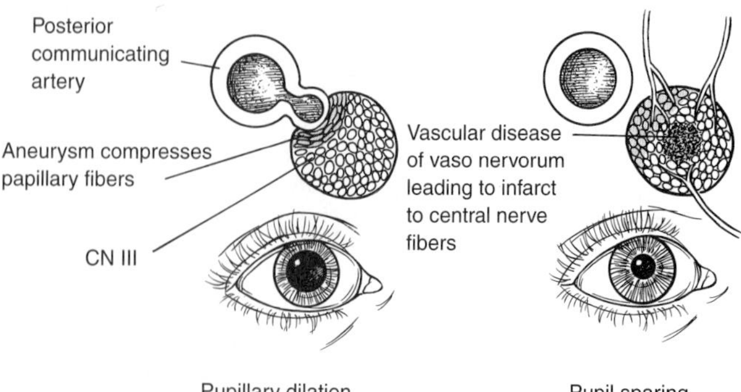

FIG. 230-19. PCA aneurysm compresses the peripherally located pupillomotor fibers of cranial nerve III, causing a nerve palsy and pupillary dilation. Diabetes and hypertension can cause microvascular compromise of the central nerve fibers causing a nerve palsy with pupil sparing.

2. Have patient use eye lubricants every 2 h (Celluvisc or artificial tears) and ointment at bedtime.
3. Consider oral steroids
4. Refer to ophthalmology for outpatient monitoring of cornea.

Diabetic/Hypertensive Cranial Nerve Palsies

Chronic diabetes and hypertension can eventually create vascular compromise to the vasa nervorum of any CN. Frequently the patient will present with new-onset diplopia and an isolated CN III or VI palsy will be found on physical examination. The CN palsy is often painful, but it can be painless. The *pupil is spared* in acute diabetic CN III palsy due to vascular compromise of the central nerve fibers (the efferent pupillomotor fibers run in the periphery of the nerve—see Fig. 230-19). Extraocular muscle testing will reveal an inhibition of ipsilateral medial gaze, upward gaze, and downward gaze as well as ptosis in an acute CN III palsy. Lateral gaze (abduction) will be preserved, and diplopia will be worse when the patient attempts to look toward the contralateral side due to inability to adduct the eye (medial rectus dysfunction). In an acute CN VI palsy, lateral gaze will be diminished (abduction) on the ipsilateral side and diplopia will be worse when the patient is trying to look to the affected side (lateral rectus dysfunction). If no other associated neurologic symptoms or findings are present and the blood sugar and blood pressure are under control, the patient can be discharged with ophthalmology and/or neurology follow-up. Many of these palsies will resolve or improve over the following 3 months. Imaging is indicated if the history or physical suggests an intracranial lesion or if the palsy fails to improve over the next 6 to 12 weeks.

Posterior Communicating Artery (PCA) Aneurysm

Acute cranial nerve III palsy with *ipsilateral pupillary dilation* is a PCA aneurysm until proven otherwise. Concomitant headache is a frequent but not absolute finding. Expansion of an aneurysm of the posterior communicating artery frequently causes compression of the outer fibers of CN III. The pupillomotor fibers are located in the outer portion of CN III; therefore the pupil becomes dilated on the affected side (see Fig. 230-19). These patients require emergent blood pressure reduction, neuroimaging, and neurosurgical consultation.

Internuclear Ophthalmoplegia (INO)

A stroke or demyelinating disease involving the medial longitudinal fasciculus (MLF) will cause the patient to experience diplopia, most noticeable when he or she attempts to look to the side opposite the lesion. EOM testing reveals an ipsilateral adduction weakness (medial rectus muscle only—not a CN III palsy).

EXAMPLE If a patient has experienced a right (MLF) stroke, the right medial rectus muscle will not function when he or she attempts a leftward gaze and the patient will not be able to adduct the right eye. The left eye will abduct but may experience some nystagmus on leftward gaze. The patient will be able to look to the right without difficulty unless there is bilateral involvement. The patient will also be able to look up and down, revealing that the superior and inferior rectus muscles are functioning and that this is not a CN III palsy.

Treatment:

1. Same as with any newly diagnosed CVA.
2. Consider demyelinating disease if the patient is young.

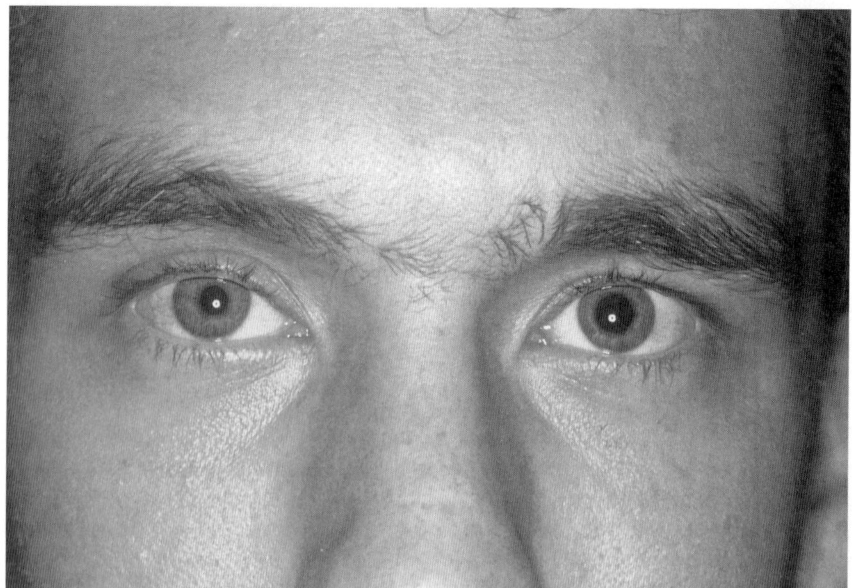

FIG. 230-20 (Plate 19). Horner's syndrome. Note ptosis and miosis of the right eye. This patient sustained an acute right carotid artery dissection after being hit in the neck with a football.

Horner's Syndrome

The physical findings of ipsilateral ptosis and miosis are characteristic of Horner's syndrome (Fig. 230-20, Plate 19). Interruption of the sympathetic nerve impulses controlling the Mueller muscle in the upper eyelid and the iris dilators cause these classic findings. Interruption can occur anywhere along the pathway from the brain stem to the sympathetic plexus surrounding the carotid artery (Fig. 230-21). It is very important to determine whether this syndrome is acute or chronic. Patients with chronic disease can be evaluated on an outpatient basis, but all cases of acute disease require a full emergent evaluation. Workup includes a chest x-ray, CT of the brain and cervical region, and a carotid angiogram if a carotid dissection is suspected (acute Horner's syndrome with neck pain).

Causes of Horner's syndrome include, in adults, CVA, tumors, internal carotid dissection, herpes zoster, and trauma. In children, the causes include neuroblastoma, lymphoma, and metastasis.

Treatment:

1. Determine whether the condition is chronic or acute.
2. Chronic: outpatient workup by personal physician.

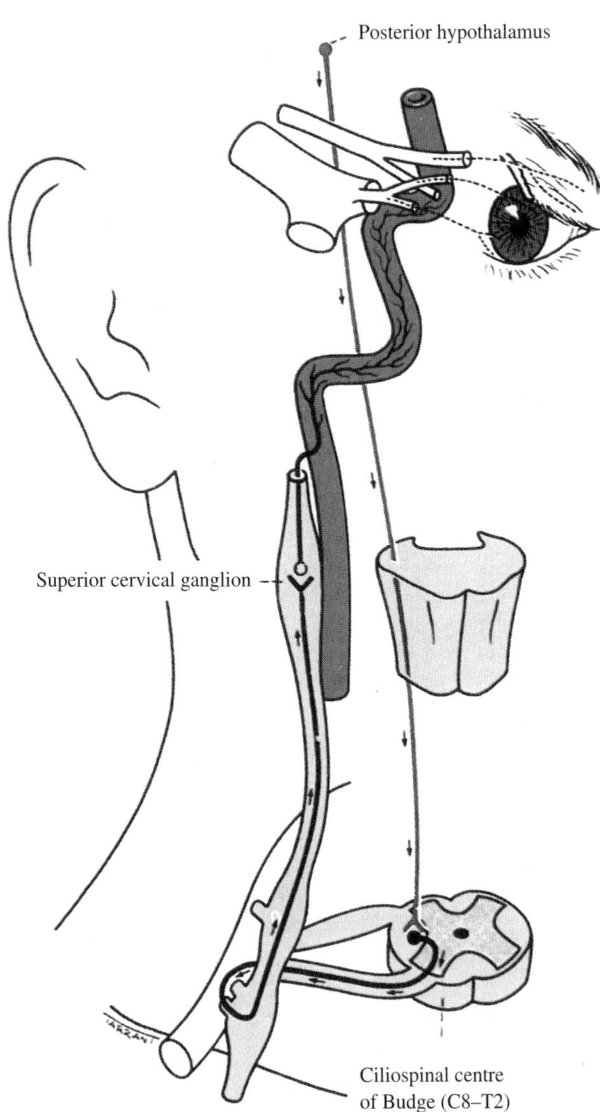

FIG. 230-21. Sympathetic nerve pathway of the eye. An interruption anywhere along this pathway can cause Horner's syndrome.

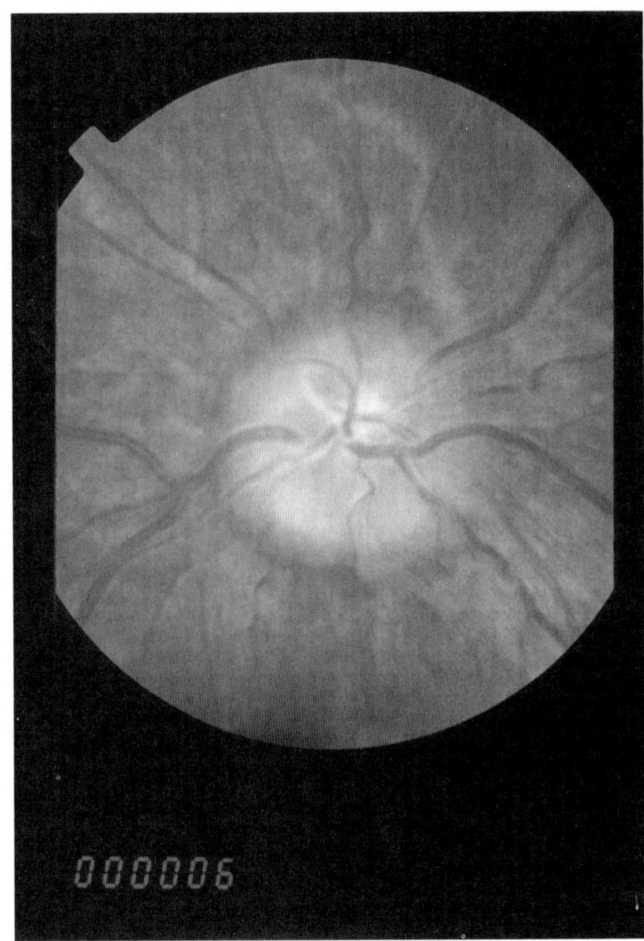

FIG. 230-22 (Plate 20). Optic nerve head edema. Vascular congestion, elevation of the nerve head, and blurred disk margins are characteristically seen in papilledema, papillitis, and compressive lesions of the optic nerve.

3. Acute: Evaluate for CVA, tumor, or carotid dissection.*

Papilledema

Papilledema is generally defined as bilateral edema of the head of the optic nerve due to increased intracranial pressure. It is a common finding in malignant hypertension, pseudotumor cerebri, intracranial tumors, and hydrocephalus. Any disease process that increases the ICP and thereby inhibits vascular or axoplasmic flow in the optic nerve causes congestion and edema of the nerve head. When only one nerve head is involved, it generally is not related to increased ICP. Monocular optic nerve edema or binocular involvement not associated with increased ICP is usually referred to as *optic nerve edema* or, if inflammatory in origin, *papillitis* (i.e., optic neuritis). Frequently the term *papilledema* has been used interchangeably in the literature to refer to monocular or binocular nerve head edema; however, most neuro-ophthalmologists reserve the term *papilledema* for bilateral nerve involvement due to increased ICP. Regardless of the etiology, the clinical findings on ophthalmoscopy of papilledema and papillitis are identical: the disk margins are blurred, the cup is diminished or absent, and the nerve head is elevated with vascular congestion (Fig. 230-22, Plate 20). Frequently flame-shaped hemorrhages are seen on

*Neck pain and acute Horner's syndrome suggests carotid dissection and can occur spontaneously (usually at above age 30) or traumatically (see Fig. 230-21).

or adjacent to the nerve head. A distinguishing feature of papilledema is prolonged preservation of visual acuity (frequently patients are visually asymptomatic). In this respect they differ markedly from patients with optic neuritis, who generally present with decreased visual acuity.

Pseudotumor Cerebri (Idiopathic Intracranial Hypertension)

Increased ICP, papilledema, normal cerebrospinal fluid, and normal CT/MRI characterize pseudotumor cerebri. Most patients are 20- to 30-year-old obese women, although this condition can occur at any age. Patients complain of nausea, vomiting, headaches, and transient visual obscurations. They can develop CN VI paresis, causing horizontal diplopia (double vision on lateral gaze). A variety of conditions (pregnancy) and exogenous agents (oral contraceptives, vitamin A, tetracycline, nalidixic acid, and corticosteroid withdrawal or prolonged use) have been associated with this poorly understood disease. It can be self-limited, but the recurrence rate can be as high as 40 percent and permanent loss of visual field can occur. Treatment is aimed at weight reduction and use of diuretics. Serial lumbar punctures are sometimes performed to reduce ICP.

Treatment:

1. Identify papilledema.
2. Perform neuroimaging of brain (CT/MRI).
3. If CT/MRI normal, perform lumbar puncture and record opening pressure, send CSF for routine diagnostics.
4. If ICP is elevated and scans and CSF are normal, discuss with ophthalmologist/neurologist institution of diuretics (Diamox 500 mg PO bid) and outpatient visual field monitoring.

BIBLIOGRAPHY

Chang B, Cullom R: *The Wills Eye Manual: Office and Emergency Room Diagnosis and Treatment of Eye Disease,* 2d ed. Philadelphia, Lippincott, 1994.

Kanski J: *Clinical Ophthalmology: A Systematic Approach,* 3d ed. London, Butterworth-Heinemann, 1994.

Kline L: *Optic Nerve Disorders: Ophthalmology Monographs,* no. 10. San Francisco, American Academy of Ophthalmology, 1996.

Spalton D, Hitchings R, Hunter P: *Atlas of Clinical Ophthalmology,* 2d ed. London, Mosby–Year Book Europe, 1994.

Trobe J: *The Physician's Guide to Eye Care.* San Francisco, American Academy of Ophthalmology, 1993.

Vaughan D, Asbury T, Riordan-Eva P: *General Ophthalmology,* 14th ed. Norwalk, Appleton & Lange, 1995.

Weingeist T, Liesegang T, Slamovits T: *Basic and Clinical Science Course, 1997–1998.* San Francisco, American Academy of Ophthalmology, 1997.

Wright K: *Textbook of Ophthalmology.* Baltimore, Williams & Wilkins, 1997.

231 COMMON DISORDERS OF THE EXTERNAL, MIDDLE, AND INNER EAR

Anne Urdaneta
Michael Lucchesi

NORMAL ANATOMY

External Ear

The auricle, or pinna, is the visibly external portion of the ear, whose trumpet shape enables it to collect air vibrations. It consists of a thin plate of elastic cartilage with a tightly adherent covering of skin. The external auditory canal (EAC) is an S-shaped skin-lined tube that extends from the auricle to the tympanic membrane. The outer one-third of the EAC is composed of an incomplete cartilaginous tube; its thick skin contains hair follicles and apocrine and sebaceous glands. The inner two-thirds of the canal is composed of bone covered by a thin layer of tightly adherent skin, which is easily torn by minimal trauma.

The blood supply to the external ear is derived from the posterior auricular, superficial temporal, and deep auricular arteries. Venous drainage of the external ear is into the superficial temporal and posterior auricular veins and then into the external jugular vein. The posterior auricular vein frequently connects to the sigmoid sinus, providing a route for extension of infection into the intracranial cavity.

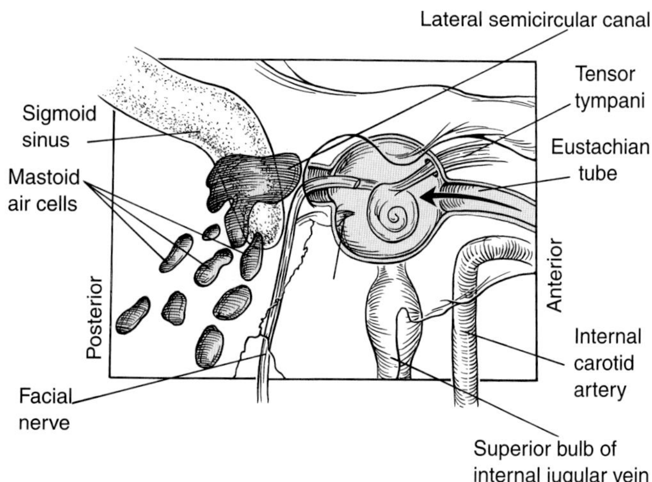

FIG. 231-1. Sagittal section of the middle ear and related structures.

Middle Ear

The middle ear is an air-containing cavity in the petrous temporal bone. It contains the auditory ossicles, which function to transmit vibrations of the tympanic membrane (TM) to the perilymph of the internal ear. It communicates with the nasopharynx anteriorly by the eustachian tube and with the mastoid air spaces posteriorly by the aditus ad antrum (Fig. 231-1).

The TM is a thin, pearly gray, fibrous membrane, which, when illuminated, produces a cone-shaped light reflex anteroinferiorly. Superiorly, the pars flaccida is a relatively slack portion of the membrane lying between the malleolar folds; the remainder of the membrane is tense and is called the pars tensa. The auditory ossicles are the malleus, incus, and stapes. Both the incus and the handle and lateral processes of the malleus are typically visible through the TM (Fig. 231-2). The

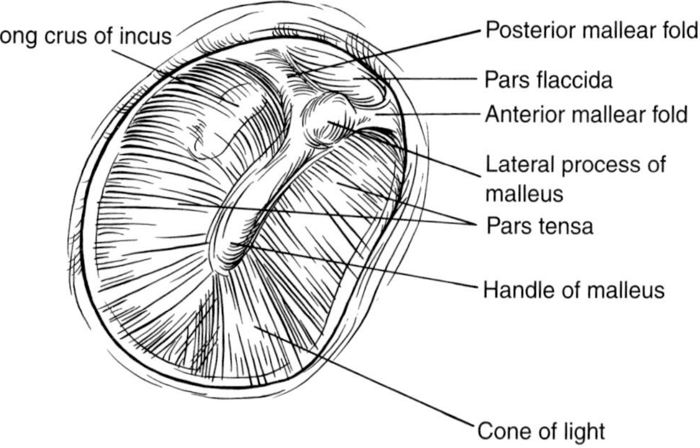

FIG. 231-2. Right tympanic membrane as seen through the otoscope.

relationships of the facial nerve, sigmoid sinus, and internal carotid artery to the tympanic cavity are shown in Fig. 231-1.

Inner Ear

The inner ear consists of the cochlea, which contains the auditory sensory receptors, and the vestibular labyrinth, which contains balance receptors. Cristae in the semicircular canals detect angular acceleration and macules detect linear acceleration. Afferent nerves from the vestibular labyrinth connect to brain stem nuclei to maintain smooth movement of the eyes during head movement and to the cerebellum to control oculomotor and postural functions. Blood supply is from the vertebrobasilar system. A branch of the anteroinferior cerebellar artery, the internal auditory artery, supplies the vestibular labyrinth. (See Fig. 231-3).

COMMON EAR COMPLAINTS

Otalgia

Primary otalgia is caused by auricular and periauricular disease, while referred otalgia is caused by disease originating from remote structures. Referred otalgia is common because of the multiple cranial nerves and branches of the cervical plexus that supply sensory innervation to both the ear and other structures of the head and neck. The sensory innervation of the ear is mediated by the fifth, seventh, ninth, and tenth cranial nerves as well as the cervical plexus, with much overlapping and variability. Common causes of primary and referred otalgia are listed in Table 231-1.

PRIMARY OTALGIA The mandibular division of the trigeminal nerve mediates sensory innervation from the anterior outer ear: the auricle, tragus, EAC, and external surface of the TM. The facial nerve carries sensory innervation from the EAC and the skin behind the auricle. The glossopharyngeal nerve and the auricular branch of the vagus nerve (the Arnold nerve) carry sensory input from the medial ear structures. Branches of the second and third cervical nerves form the greater auricular and lesser occipital nerves, which receive input from the skin over the parotid gland and behind the ear, respectively.

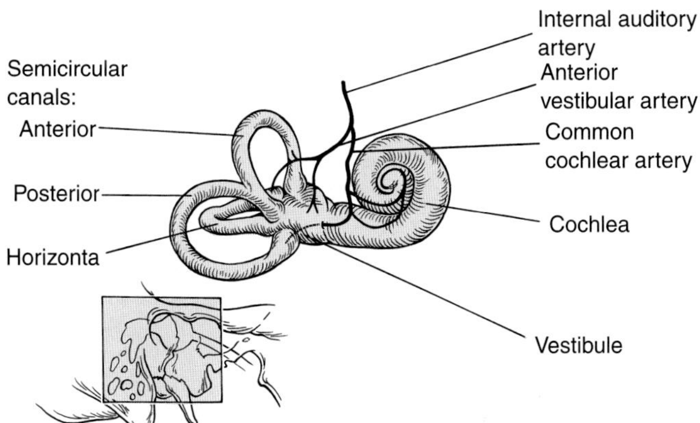

FIG. 231-3. Schematic drawing of the bony labyrinth containing the vestibular and auditory sensory organs. The otolithic organs (utricle and saccule) lie in the vestibule. The internal auditory artery divides into the common cochlear artery and the anterior vestibular artery. The anterior vestibular artery provides the blood supply to the anterior and horizontal semicircular canals but not to the cochlea. Isolated occlusion of the anterior vestibular artery may therefore cause acute vestibular syndrome without hearing loss.

TABLE 231-1 Causes of Otalgia

Primary	Referred	Neuralgias
Trauma	Dental	Trigeminal
Infection	TMJ disease	(Tic douloureux)
Otitis externa	Abscessed teeth	Herpetic geniculate
Otitis media	Malocclusion	(Ramsay Hunt)
Mastoiditis	Bruxism	
Bullous myringitis	Trauma	
Foreign bodies	Retro- and oropharyngeal	
Cerumen impaction	Tonsillitis	
Cholesteatoma	Abscess	
Neoplasms	Neoplasm	
	Nasal cavity	
	Sinusitis	
	Deviated septum	
	Throat and neck	
	Foreign body	
	Thyroid disease	
	Cervical strain	
	Neoplasm	

Disease from any portion of the ear or its surrounding skin and structures may result in primary otalgia. A history and physical examination of the external ear, EAC, and TM will usually identify the cause of primary otalgia, with specific therapy as appropriate.

REFERRED OTALGIA The maxillary and mandibular divisions of the trigeminal nerve receive sensory input from the nasopharynx, paranasal sinuses, teeth, parotid gland, and muscles of mastication. The facial nerve carries sensory innervation from the nasal mucosa and the ethmoid and sphenoid sinuses. The glossopharyngeal nerve carries sensory innervation from the nasopharynx, eustachian tube, soft palate, posterior pharynx, and tonsils. The vagus nerve mediates sensation from the valleculae and piriform sinuses, from the larynx via the superior laryngeal nerve, and from the cervical esophagus and trachea via the recurrent laryngeal nerve.

Abscessed and impacted teeth, usually mandibular molars, frequently cause ear pain. Malocclusion, bruxism, mandibular trauma, temporomandibular joint (TMJ) disorders, and ill-fitting dentures are frequent causes of otalgia.[1] Trigeminal neuralgia, or tic douloureux, causes severe unilateral facial pain. Herpetic geniculate neuralgia, or Ramsay Hunt syndrome, is herpes simplex of the EAC and auricle with facial palsy which may persist long after the disappearance of the vesicles (postherpetic neuralgia).

The diagnosis of the source of referred otalgia requires a history and physical examination that encompasses the nasal and oral cavities, nasopharynx, oropharynx, throat, and neck. Again, further evaluation and treatment depend upon diagnosis.

Tinnitus

Tinnitus is the perception of sound without external stimulation. It may be constant, pulsatile, high- or low-pitched, hissing, clicking, or ringing. It is most prevalent between the ages of 40 and 70 and has no gender predominance.[2]

Tinnitus is divided into two types: objective and subjective. Objective tinnitus may be heard by the examiner. Subjective tinnitus is more common. Its exact mechanism is unknown, although it is believed to result from damage to cochlear hair cells. Causes are outlined in Table 231-2.[2]

Pharmacologic side effects are the cause of tinnitus in at least 10 percent of cases.[2] The most commonly implicated drugs are aspirin (which may produce tinnitus in doses as low as 1.5 g/day) and aspirin-containing compounds, nonsteroidal anti-inflammatory drugs, and anti-

TABLE 231-2 Common Causes of Tinnitus

Objective	Subjective
Vascular	Sensorineural hearing loss
AV malformations	Hypertension
Arterial bruits	Conductive hearing loss
Mechanical	Head trauma
Enlarged eustachian tube	Medication
Palatomyoclonus	TMJ disorders
Stapedial muscle spasm	Depression, stress
	Neurologic
	Acoustic neuroma
	Multiple sclerosis
	Benign intracranial hypertension
	Meniere's disease
	Cogan syndrome

biotics, particularly aminoglycosides. (See Table 231-3 for a list of common ototoxic agents.)

Accurate diagnosis usually requires referral to an otolaryngologist. Many medications have been suggested as therapies, but antidepressants are currently the only class of drug found to be useful in alleviating tinnitus in which no correctable cause can be found.

Vertigo

Vertigo is the sensation of motion, either internal (''I feel myself turning'') or external (''things seem to spin around me''). It may also be a sensation of linear movement, such as tilting. A careful history and physical examination should distinguish vertigo from other symptoms that cause light-headedness, such as postural hypotension, leg weakness, or peripheral neuropathy.

The history should identify the onset, duration, and frequency of the symptom as well as the presence of crucial movements or positions that precipitate it. Ask about accompanying symptoms such as nausea, vomiting, otalgia, tinnitus, hearing loss, or a sensation of aural fullness. Finally, any clearly precipitating events such as head trauma or recent upper respiratory tract infections should be identified.

In addition to a general physical exam, the Dix-Hallpike maneuver[3] may be performed to check for benign positional vertigo. The maneuver is performed by starting with the patient sitting up, with the patient's head held firmly in the examiner's hands. The patient is quickly laid supine while turning his or her head to one side and extending the neck. After a latent period of about 2 s, a rotatory nystagmus may appear, generally toward the downward-facing ear (clockwise when the patient's head is to the left, counterclockwise when it is to the right). When the patient is again seated upright, a reverse rotatory nystagmus may be observed. The maneuver should be repeated in each direction a number of times to determine whether the nystagmus is extinguishable.

The differential diagnosis of vertigo is large and may be divided into central and peripheral types (Table 231-4).[3–5] Acoustic neuroma should be considered if there is a concomitant unilateral sensorineural hearing loss. Vertigo may be a symptom of a vertebrobasilar insufficiency or stroke. While classic teaching has stated that vertebrobasilar insufficiency should be accompanied by brain stem findings such as diplopia, dysarthria, dysphagia, or focal deficits, isolated vertigo in a patient with risk factors for stroke is becoming more commonly recognized.[6] Peripheral causes of vertigo, or vestibular vertigo, include benign positional vertigo (BPV), labyrinthitis, Meniere's disease, and perilymphatic fistula. Common causes of peripheral vertigo are discussed below. See Chap. 223 for further discussion.

BENIGN POSITIONAL VERTIGO BPV is the most common form of peripheral vertigo. Generally, the patient will complain that the vertigo occurs with head movement, typically while turning over in bed or quickly turning the head to one side; it usually lasts seconds to minutes. It is most often idiopathic in nature but is also common secondary to head trauma or viral infections. The peak age of onset is during the sixth decade in the idiopathic group, with a 2:1 female predominance, and in the fourth and fifth decades in the posttraumatic group, with no gender predominance. The pathophysiology of BPV is disputed, but it has been thought to result from lesions of the otolith organs of the inner ear or from deposits in the semicircular canals. BPV is by definition paroxysmal and positional and is reproducible using the Dix-Hallpike maneuver. The nystagmus elicited is usually but not always extinguishable.[3]

LABYRINTHITIS Labyrinthitis, or vestibular neuronitis, is characterized by the acute onset of a severe vertiginous episode, often accompanied by nausea or vomiting but usually without tinnitus or hearing loss. Typically the symptom develops over a period of hours and peaks the first day, with a gradual and complete recovery in days. It is usually caused by a viral infection from an upper respiratory tract pathogen.

MENIERE'S DISEASE Meniere's disease, or endolymphatic hydrops, is a diagnosis of exclusion. The classic presentation is of episodic vertigo, hearing loss, tinnitus, and a sensation of aural fullness, although not all symptoms may be present and they may not all occur simultaneously. The symptoms may last seconds to hours, and episodes typically occur in clusters followed by periods of remission. The pathophysiology is thought to be a dilatation of the endolymph-containing spaces of the inner ear, although the primary causative factor is unknown.

TABLE 231-3 Ototoxic Agents

Loop diuretics	Topical agents
Ethacrynic acid	Solvents
Furosemide	Propylene glycol
Bumetanide	Antiseptics
Salicylates	Ethanol
NSAIDs	Antibiotics
Quinine	Polymyxin B
Antibiotics	Neomycin
Aminoglycosides	
Erythromycin	
Vancomycin	
Chemotherapeutic agents	
Cisplatin	
Carboplatin	
Vinblastine	
Vincristine	

TABLE 231-4 Causes of Vertigo

Systemic	Central	Peripheral
Autoimmune disorders	Acoustic neuroma	Benign positional
Hypo- and hyperthyroidism	Multiple sclerosis	Labyrinthitis
Diabetes mellitus	Vascular insufficiency	Meniere's disease
Anemia	Vertebrobasilar stroke or insufficiency	Cogan syndrome
Leukemia		Perilymphatic fistula
Otosyphilis		

PERILYMPHATIC FISTULA Perilymphatic fistula is another cause of vestibular vertigo lasting minutes to hours and involves rupture of the cochlear membranes with leakage of perilymph from the middle to the inner ear. It may result from surgery, from strenuous physical activity such as weight lifting, or from excessive pressure changes such as may occur during scuba diving or flying.

Primary treatment of vestibular vertigo is often medical and aimed at suppression of the vestibular system. Antihistamines such as meclizine, phenothiazines such as prochlorperazine, and scopolamine have all been used in the treatment of peripheral vertigo. Specific treatment for Meniere's disease may also include salt restriction and diuretics. Surgery may be necessary for cases refractory to medical therapy.

For those patients in whom BPV may be diagnosed with reasonable certainty, an appropriate plan is a course of medical therapy with otolaryngologic follow-up if symptoms persist more than 1 week. All others should have prompt neurologic or otolaryngologic referral to rule out a central origin of the symptom.

Hearing Loss

Hearing loss may be divided into conductive and sensorineural types; the Weber and Rinne tests may be performed to differentiate between the two. The term *sudden hearing loss* refers only to the sensorineural type.

SUDDEN HEARING LOSS Sudden hearing loss (SHL) is a sensorineural hearing loss occurring over 3 days or less. The incidence increases with increasing age, and there is no gender predominance. Indicators of poor prognosis include more severe hearing loss on presentation and the presence of vertigo. Although most cases of SHL are idiopathic, implicated etiologies include infection, vascular causes, and trauma as well as metabolic disturbances and ototoxic drugs (Table 231-5).[7]

Viral infections, most typically mumps, have long been associated with SHL. Because of the terminal branches and interosseous location of the blood supply to the inner ear, the ear is uniquely vulnerable to a variety of vascular and hematologic diseases. Cogan syndrome is an autoimmune disorder that presents with a bilateral hearing loss classically associated with tinnitus and vertigo. SHL may also be caused by mechanical or traumatic rupture of the cochlear membranes.

Many common medications have been implicated in SHL (see Table 231-3).[8–14] Although a variety of mechanisms are responsible for medication-induced SHL, a general rule is that risk of hearing loss increases with increasing dosage and length of use and is further aggravated by factors that impair drug metabolism and excretion, such as renal insufficiency.

TABLE 231-5 Causes of Sudden Hearing Loss

Infection	Rheumatologic
Mumps	Temporal arteritis
Epstein-Barr virus	Polyarteritis nodosa
Herpes	Wegener granulomatosis
Cytomegalovirus	Other
Syphilis	Meniere's disease
Labyrinthitis	Cogan syndrome
Hematologic and vascular	Acoustic neuroma
Leukemia	Pharmacologic
Sickle cell anemia	Cochlear rupture
Polycythemia	Conductive
Berger disease	Otitis externa
Cerebral aneurysm	Otitis media
Metabolic	Ruptured tympanic membrane
Diabetes mellitus	Neoplasms
Hyperlipidemia	Otosclerosis

The evaluation of SHL begins with a complete history and physical examination. Sudden conductive hearing loss results from obstruction of the EAC or from disturbances of the TM or ossicles. An evaluation of all current medications for possible ototoxic agents is necessary. A history of trauma or recollection of a ''popping'' noise preceding the hearing loss is a helpful diagnostic clue. Coexistent tinnitus or vertigo may point to Meniere's disease. Systemic illness should be considered.

The differential diagnosis includes both potentially reversible and potentially ominous causes. If the physical examination does not identify the cause, emergency otolaryngologic consultation is necessary.

INFECTIONS

Otitis Externa

Otitis externa includes infections and inflammation of the external auditory canal (EAC) and auricle. It may be divided into acute diffuse and malignant types.

ACUTE DIFFUSE OTITIS EXTERNA **Definition and Diagnosis** Also known simply as otitis externa (OE) or swimmer's ear, this infection is characterized by pruritus, pain, and tenderness of the external ear. Physical signs include erythema and edema of the EAC, which may spread to the tragus and auricle. Other signs are clear or purulent otorrhea and crusting of the EAC. As the disease progresses, the pain becomes intolerable and is present with mastication or any movement of the periauricular skin. Increasing edema eventually narrows the EAC lumen and may cause hearing impairment. In severe cases, infection may spread to the periauricular soft tissues and lymph nodes, and there may be lateral protrusion of the auricle secondary to inflammation.

Pathophysiology Predisposing factors for the development of OE are trauma to the skin of the EAC and elevation of the local pH. Constant contact with water, from swimming, bathing, or a humid environment both elevate the pH of the EAC skin and may cause maceration. Trauma is most commonly caused by scratching or by overzealous disimpaction of cerumen. Cerumen is an acidic mixture of sebaceous and apocrine gland secretions and desquamated epithelial cells. It forms a physical barrier that protects the EAC skin from violation, while the acidic pH has antimicrobial properties.

Microbiology The most common organisms implicated in OE are *Pseudomonas aeruginosa* and *Staphylococcus aureus*,[15] although one study found a polymicrobial etiology in one-third of patients and an anaerobic bacterial etiology in one-quarter, with *Bacteroides* species predominating.[16]

Otomycosis, or fungal OE, accounts for approximately 10 percent of cases, with a high percentage found in tropical climates.[17] A history may reveal the presence of diabetes or other immunocompromised states or previous long-term therapy with antibiotics. Most (80 to 90 percent) of otomycosis is due to *Aspergillus* species, and physical examination may reveal a black, blue-green, or yellow discoloration of the EAC. The second most common fungal pathogen is *Candida*.[17]

Noninfectious causes include contact dermatitis from topical medications or resins in hearing aids, seborrhea, and psoriasis.

Treatment The treatment of OE involves analgesia, cleansing of the EAC, acidifying agents, topical antimicrobials, and sometimes steroids. Cleansing may be done with gentle irrigation using hydrogen peroxide, and gentle debridement by the physician with a suction aspirator such as a Frasier suction.

A variety of topical agents exist that combine an antimicrobial agent with either an acid and/or a steroid. Table 231-6 lists the components of many otic preparations. No single agent has been shown to be more effective than the others, although the lower-pH preparations are thought to be better.[15] The burning associated with the acidic preparations may reduce compliance, however, and patients unable to tolerate the low pH of otic preparations may instead use the slightly more alkaline ophthalmic drops. Also, if there is suspected TM perforation or the TM cannot be visualized, antibiotic drops should be prescribed. Cortisporin Otic *Suspension* should only be used; the solution is toxic to the middle ear. The medication should be instilled into a cleansed ear while it is facing up, with this position held for 3 min. This should be done four times daily for at least 10 days or until after the resolution of symptoms. If edema of the EAC obstructs the lumen, a commercial wick or piece of gauze may be inserted into the EAC and kept moist with the otic drops.

Bacterial and fungal cultures may guide treatment of nonresponsive cases. Oral antibiotic therapy should be reserved for febrile patients and those with periauricular extension. All patients with OE should be taught to avoid predisposing factors in order to eliminate recurrences. Strategies include ear plugs while swimming or bathing (cotton wool impregnated with Vaseline or commercial ear plugs), occasional, brief use of a hair dryer to remove EAC water, and avoidance of cotton-tipped applicators or other devices to remove cerumen.

Specific treatment of otomycosis consists of antifungal agents such as clotrimazole. *Aspergillus* is not sensitive to most oral antifungals with the exception of itraconazole.[17] With noninfectious OE, removal of the offending agent is the first step in treatment. Topical steroid drops may be used for seborrhea and psoriasis.

Finally, all patients should be instructed to follow up with their primary physician or an otolaryngologist if the condition worsens at any time or does not respond to treatment in 1 week; these patients must be evaluated for the more serious disease of malignant otitis externa.

MALIGNANT OTITIS EXTERNA **Definitions** Malignant otitis externa (MOE) is a potentially life-threatening infection of the EAC with variable extension to the skull base. It is almost always caused by *P. aeruginosa*. The term *MOE* actually refers to a spectrum of disease. When it is limited to the soft tissues and cartilage, it is called necrotizing otitis externa (NOE). When there is involvement of the temporal bone or skull base it is called skull-base osteomyelitis (SBO).

TABLE 231-6 Some Common Topical Otic Preparations

Preparation	Constituents	Comments
CiproHC Otic	Ciprofloxacin Hydrocortisone	Not safe with perforation
Cortisporin Otic	Neomycin Polymixin B Hydrocortisone	Use suspension* only Theoretic potential for ototoxicity; no longer widely used.
Floxin Otic	Ofloxacin	Safe with perforations; 5 drops bid
Otic Domeboro	2% Acetic acid solution	pH 4.5–6.0
VoSol HC Otic	Acetic acid Hydrocortisone	pH 3.0

*Solution is thinner and more easily absorbed through the round window or a perforation.

Pathophysiology MOE begins as a simple otitis externa that then spreads to the deeper tissues of the EAC and infects cartilage, periosteum, and bone, with the normal anatomy of the ear serving as the conduit for the spread of infection. The cartilaginous floor of the EAC has clefts, known as the fissures of Santorini, through which the infection may spread to deeper structures. The parotid gland and TMJ are anterior, the mastoid air cells are posterior, and the skull base, carotid artery, jugular bulb, and sigmoid sinus are inferomedial. Infection may spread to any of these structures as well as to the seventh cranial nerve as it exits the stylomastoid foramen and the ninth, tenth, and eleventh cranial nerves at the jugular foramen.

The typical patient with MOE is the elderly diabetic. The impaired immune response of the diabetic, which is further compromised in the elderly, may predispose to the onset of pseudomonal infection. Furthermore, the cerumen of diabetic patients has been found to have a higher pH than that of normal controls; this represents an additional breakdown in local defense mechanisms. Finally, the small blood vessel disease of diabetics may lead to cartilaginous degeneration, further promoting the spread of infection.

Microbiology The most common causative organism of MOE is *P. aeruginosa*. *Aspergillus* has been reported to cause SBO, usually in patients who are immunosupressed due to AIDS or other causes. *Aspergillus* SBO also has a different presentation than typical pseudomonal SBO in that the infection generally begins in the middle ear rather than in the EAC.

Diagnosis Any elderly, diabetic, or immunocompromised patient presenting with OE or any person with persistent OE despite 2 to 3 weeks of topical antimicrobial therapy should be suspected of having MOE. The typical presentation is similar to that of OE: otalgia and edema of the EAC with or without otorrhea. The otalgia may be out of proportion for routine OE. Granulation tissue may be evident on the floor of the EAC near the bone-cartilage junction.

The history and physical examination should also be directed toward determining the extent of progression of the disease by identifying involvement of nearby structures. Parotitis may be present, and trismus indicates involvement of the masseter muscle or TMJ. Cranial nerve involvement is a serious sign; the history and examination should specifically rule out facial palsy and hoarseness or dysphagia. The seventh cranial nerve is usually the first affected, and the presence of dysfunction of the ninth, tenth, or eleventh cranial nerve implies even more extensive disease. Lateral or sigmoid sinus thrombosis and meningitis are also possible complications.

Certain patients may have an atypical clinical presentation and require special mention. MOE in children tends to to be rapidly progressive; thus children may be more ill appearing upon presentation, with fever, leukocytosis, and even bacteremia. Also, the TM, middle ear, and facial nerve are more likely to be involved in children than in adults. AIDS patients with MOE tend to be younger, have etiologic organisms other than *Pseudomonas,* and tend to have a worse prognosis than patients without AIDS.

Diagnosing MOE depends first on having a high index of suspicion; emergent otolaryngologic consultation is necessary. The next step involves radiographic confirmation and staging of the disease with CT of the head, focusing on the EAC and temporal bone (Table 231-7).[17]

Treatment Once the diagnosis of MOE has been made, the patient must be admitted to the hospital for parenteral antibiotics. Therapy with an aminoglycoside and antipseudomonal penicillin, or cephalo-

TABLE 231-7 Staging of Malignant Otitis Externa

RADIOLOGRAPHIC STAGING	
Stage I	Soft tissue involvement only (NOE)
Stage II	Bony involvement limited to mastoid (Early SBO)
Stage III	Extensive SBO (May involve occipital, facial or contralateral temporal bone)
CLINICAL STAGING	
Stage I	Involvement limited to EAC and mastoid
Stage II	SBO with cranial nerve involvement
Stage III	Extension to brain and meninges

Key: NOE, necrotizing otitis externa; SBO, skull-base osteomyelitis; EAC, external auditory canal.

sporin, or quinolone is standard, and should be initiated in the emergency department. Selected cases may be managed with oral quinolones, depending on the otolaryngologist's preference.

The ultimate prognosis of MOE is primarily based on the stage of disease at presentation. Earlier stages are likely to completely resolve with a single course of antibiotic therapy, while more advanced stages may require surgical debridement and may ultimately prove fatal.

Otitis Media

EPIDEMIOLOGY Otitis media (OM) is primarily a disease of infancy and childhood. Although adults may present with OM, its incidence and prevalence peak in the preschool years and then decrease with increasing age. There is little or no literature to suggest that the diagnosis or management of OM in adults differs from that in children. The decrease in incidence of OM from childhood through adolescence is thought to be due to the changing anatomy of the eustachian tube; between infancy and adulthood the eustachian tube angle and length both increase, promoting drainage of the middle ear and offering a greater physical barrier to the migration of bacteria from the nasopharynx to the middle ear.

MICROBIOLOGY The most common bacterial pathogens in acute OM are *Streptococcus pneumoniae, Haemophilus influenzae,* and *Moraxella catarrhalis.* The predominant organisms involved in chronic OM are *Staphylococcus aureus, P. aeruginosa,* and anaerobic bacteria.[18] Viruses probably play a role in the pathogenesis of OM in that they may promote bacterial superinfection by impairing eustachian tube function and other host defense mechanisms; they may also interfere with host response to antimicrobial drugs.

DIAGNOSIS The patient with OM will present with otalgia with or without fever. Otorrhea and hearing loss are variably present, while tinnitus, vertigo, and nystagmus are uncommon. The TM may be retracted or bulging. It may be red in color, indicating inflammation, or it may be yellow or white, due to middle ear secretions. Pneumatic otoscopy demonstrates impaired mobility. The facial nerve should always be assessed because of its proximity to the middle ear.

TREATMENT Oral antimicrobial agents are the therapy of choice for acute OM. Initial treatment should be with one of the following, for 7 to 10 days: amoxicillin, trimethoprim-sulfamethoxazole, or erythromycin plus sulfamethoxazole. OM unresponsive to initial therapy should be treated with one of the alternate drugs for the same period of time; this method will generally eradicate organisms that are resistant to one of the drugs. Topical therapy should be avoided in cases with an associated TM rupture. Since pain usually continues for 8 to 24 h after the initiation of antibiotics, the addition of acetaminophen or ibuprofen analgesia is appropriate. OM with effusion requires treatment with the same antimicrobials, but for 3 weeks, and prednisone may be added.[18]

Adults with simple acute OM should receive follow-up to assess treatment efficacy and to ensure that there is no anatomic obstruction to the eustachian tube, as for example, from occult carcinoma. Any patient who presents with complications of OM or who appears septic should have urgent consultation for diagnostic and therapeutic tympanocentesis and possible admission for intravenous antibiotics.

Complications

Complications of OM can be divided into intratemporal and intracranial types. Perforation of the TM is a common intratemporal complication and most often occurs in the pars tensa from the increased pressure of middle ear secretions, with resultant otorrhea. Healing usually occurs in 1 week, although a chronic perforation may result. A temporary conductive hearing loss may occur with OM secondary to fluid in the middle ear; the hearing loss resolves as the fluid is resorbed. Acute serous labyrinthitis may occur when bacterial toxins enter the inner ear via the round window. Facial nerve paralysis is an uncommon complication but requires emergent otolaryngology consultation.

ACUTE MASTOIDITIS One of the most serious complications of acute OM is acute mastoiditis. This occurs as infection spreads from the middle ear to the mastoid air cells via the aditus ad antrum. When this opening becomes blocked, the mastoid cavity becomes a closed space, and the mastoid air cells become filled with fluid and inflamed. Spread through venous channels to the overlying periosteum is referred to as *acute mastoiditis with periostitis.* In addition to otalgia and fever, patients with mastoiditis will have postauricular erythema, swelling, and tenderness, with protrusion of the auricle and obliteration of the postauricular crease. Although the diagnosis can usually be made based on the history and physical examination, certain radiographic tests are indicated. Mastoid radiographs will demonstrate mastoid clouding due to fluid accumulation, and CT may delineate the extentof bony involvement. Mastoiditis requires admission for intravenous antibiotics, tympanocentesis, and myringotomy. Cefuroxime is frequently chosen as an initial empiric agent.[19] Incision and drainage of subperiosteal abscess or mastoidectomy may ultimately be indicated.

CHRONIC MASTOIDITIS Chronic mastoiditis presents with chronic otorrhea and has an increased incidence in patients with nasopharyngeal tumors, Down syndrome, or craniofacial abnormalities. Each of these predisposing factors can cause obstruction of the eustachian tube. *P. aeruginosa* is the most common cause of chronic mastoiditis. Tuberculosis may also present as chronic mastoiditis.[19]

INTRACRANIAL COMPLICATIONS Intracranial complications of OM are more likely with chronic than with acute OM and are, in general, decreasing with the widespread use of antibiotics in the treatment of OM. However, suppurative intracranial extension is a severe complication, and suggestive signs and symptoms should be investigated appropriately. Meningitis is the most common intracranial complication of OM; the most prevalent causative organisms are *Strep. pneumoniae* and *H. influenzae* type b. Extradural abscess and subdural empyema are also potential complications.

LATERAL SINUS THROMBOSIS Lateral sinus thrombosis (LST) is another ominous complication of acute OM. It arises from extension of infection and inflammation in the mastoid, with eventual inflammation of the adjacent lateral or sigmoid sinus. Reactive thrombophlebitis with mural clot formation, intraluminal empyema, or perforation of the venous wall may occur. A high index of suspicion is necessary to diagnose LST because the common clinical findings are similar to those found in acute OM or mastoiditis.

Headache is the most common symptom, with papilledema, sixth-nerve palsy, and vertigo being less frequently present.[20] Angiography with venous phase and magnetic resonance imaging (MRI) are more sensitive than computed tomography (CT) in diagnosing LST. Although in the majority of cases of LST no bacterial isolates are recovered, antibiotic therapy is the initial treatment of choice. The agent should cover *Staphylococcus, Streptococcus,* and upper respiratory anaerobes and have good penetration of the blood-brain barrier. A combination of intravenous penicillin or nafcillin, ceftriaxone, and metronidazole has been recommended as an initial empiric regimen.[20] Most patients will also require surgical intervention.

CHOLESTEATOMA A serious complication associated with chronic OM is cholesteatoma. Aural cholesteatoma is composed of epidermis and exfoliated keratin within pneumatized spaces of the temporal bone. It is an erosive, expanding lesion originating within the middle ear or mastoid air cells. As the cholesteatoma expands, it may erode the ossicular chain, bony labyrinth, or facial nerve canal. Cholesteatomas are often infected and their intracranial extensions may be life-threatening.

Bullous Myringitis

DEFINITION Bullous myringitis is a painful condition of the ear characterized by bulla formation on the TM and deep EAC. Its epidemiology, etiology, and pathology are poorly understood. It may occur at any age, frequently after an upper respiratory tract infection.

PATHOPHYSIOLOGY The blisters are believed to occur between the highly innervated outer epithelium and the inner fibrous layer of the TM, explaining the severe otalgia. The blisters may be blood-filled, serous, or serosanguinous. Middle ear effusions may be present, either sympathetic in origin or as a result of medial rupture of bullae. Otorrhea as a result of ruptured bullae is short-lived. A reversible hearing loss is commonly associated with the condition and may be conductive, sensorineural, or mixed.

MICROBIOLOGY Although bullous myringitis was originally associated with influenza epidemics, since then numerous pathogens have been implicated in its etiology, including *Mycoplasma pneumoniae, Chlamydia psittaci,* and numerous viral pathogens. Herpes simplex has not been implicated as a causative agent.[21]

DIAGNOSIS Patients with bullous myringitis typically present with severe, throbbing otalgia, often with hearing loss. Otoscopy reveals multiple fluid-filled blisters, which may be yellow to red in color. There may be bloody otorrhea or hemotympanum.

TREATMENT As the etiologic agent of bullous myringitis remains elusive, treatment of the condition consists of warm compresses and systemic analgesia with acetaminophen or nonsteroidal anti-inflammatory drugs (NSAIDs). Oral antibiotics may be added in cases with an associated middle ear effusion, since some of these may represent a concomitant otitis media.

TRAUMA TO THE EAR

Although trauma to the ear is rarely life-threatening, its associated morbidity is significant and includes hearing loss and poor cosmetic outcome.

Abrasions can cause partial loss of the covering epidermis. Abrasions that do not penetrate to the underlying perichondrium should be thoroughly irrigated with normal saline. If there are any embedded foreign bodies, they should be meticulously removed to prevent infection and ''tattooing'' of the wound. A topical antimicrobial ointment with a contoured nonpressure dressing should be applied. The wound should be reevaluated in 24 h. Lacerations of the auricle require delicate closure with careful realignment to maintain the natural contour. (See Chap. 38.) Prior to closure, a thorough examination is required to determine the magnitude of the injury, followed by cleansing and irrigation with normal saline. Further exploration can be done with a sterile cotton swab to determine the actual extent of the injury and explore for any remaining foreign bodies. In simple lacerations not involving the perichondrium or cartilage, the skin can be approximated with everting nylon sutures. In lacerations involving the cartilage, the perichondrium should be sutured using 5-0 or 6-0 absorbable sutures. If debridement is necessary, the otolaryngologist may be consulted. After skin closure, an antimicrobial ointment and a firm, contoured, nonpressure dressing should be applied. Complete or partial avulsion injuries, especially those involving tissue loss exposing large areas of cartilage, should be referred to an otolaryngologist or plastic surgeon.[22, 25]

Thermal Injuries

FROSTBITE With its position of prominence and large surface area, the auricle is extremely susceptible to extremes in temperature. The thin subcutaneous tissue makes the auricle particularly susceptible to cold-induced injury. In frostbite, the ear will initially appear pale. In superficial frostbite injuries, the underlying tissue remains soft and pliable. In deep injuries, the underlying tissue is very hard. With rewarming, the ear may become painful, with edema and blister formation. If blisters do form, they should be allowed to reabsorb spontaneously. The ear should be aseptically and quickly rewarmed with saline-soaked gauze that has been warmed to 38 to 40°C (100.4 to 104°F). The rewarming process may be very painful and conscious sedation may be necessary.

BURNS Burns of the upper body occur frequently, with burns of the face and neck representing about 30 percent of all burn injuries. In one study of patients sustaining significant facial burns, 42 percent suffered burns to the ears.[26] Direct thermal burns may be severe enough to cause necrosis and sloughing of the entire external ear. Even with lesser injury, disruption of the auricular skin can lead to damage of the underlying cartilage, which, once damaged, is particularly susceptible to infection. Factors that affect the healing of burn injuries include the depth of the burn, development of infection, and external pressure or friction on the burned auricle.[23] Otochondritis is a potentially disfiguring complication of otic burns. Chondritis may occur in up to 20 percent of significant otic burns and may appear anywhere from 2 to 5 weeks after the injury. The hallmarks of chondritis consist of helical dull pain followed by erythema, edema, exquisite tenderness to palpation, and an increase in the auriculocephalic angle (lateral protrusion of the ear from the head).[26] Once chondritis is present, treatment must be aggressive to preserve ear architecture; it usually consists of surgical debridement. Systemic antibiotics alone are generally considered ineffective.

First-degree burns involve only the superficial layers. Vascular congestion and dilation occur in the intradermal vessels. First-degree burns can be gently cleaned, and the patient can be discharged with mild analgesics as needed. Second-degree burns exhibit destruction of varying depths of epidermis, with coagulation necrosis. Third-degree burns involve destruction of all skin elements with coagulation of the subdermal plexus.

Burns more severe than first-degree should be seen in consultation with a burn unit or an otolaryngologist. If the burn is an isolated injury and a mild second-degree type, treatment in the emergency department should consist of meticulous cleaning and irrigation with normal saline, application of a non-sulfa-containing antimicrobial ointment, and a nonpressure dressing. Silvasulfadiazine ointment can cause skin pigmentation changes and should not be used above the clavicles. Referral should be made within 24 h. Substantial second-degree burns with blistering or any third-degree burns should be referred to a burn center for further management.

Hematoma

A hematoma can develop from almost any type of trauma to the ear. As a result of the lack of subcutaneous fat on the anterior surface of the auricle, blunt force applied to this area tends to shear the perichondrium from the underlying cartilage and tear the adjoining blood vessels. The cartilage depends on the perichondrial blood vessels for viability. Any separation can result in necrosis. In addition, a subperichondral collection can lead to stimulation of the overlying perichondrium, which can result in an asymmetrical formation of new cartilage and deformity of the auricle. The resultant deformed auricle has been referred to as ''cauliflower ear,'' which was fairly common in wrestlers and boxers of the past. The auricular hematoma itself presents as a painful swelling after trauma, which obscures the normal contour of the ear. The hematoma may accumulate immediately or several hours after the insult; if it is large enough, it may have an ecchymotic hue. In the past, the advised treatment was aspiration of the hematoma. More current literature suggests that aspiration alone does not completely evacuate the clot and therefore leads to deformity and increased morbidity. The goal of treatment is to remove the fluid collection and maintain pressure in the area for several days to prevent reaccumulation of fluid.[24,25] After local anesthesia, and using sterile technique, a circular incision should be made through the skin with caution not to violate the underlying perichondrium. The incision should be the minimal necessary to drain the underlying hematoma and positioned in an area with the least exposure (the inner curvature of the helix or anthelix). The hematoma can then be removed by gentle suction or curettage.[24–28]

A dental roll or a firm sterile pledget can then be placed over the resutured site with through-and-through sutures connected to a similar bolster on the opposite side.[22] A nonpressure dressing with antibiotic ointment should then be applied and the patient given instructions as to reevaluation within 24 h to assure there has been no reaccumulation. Prophylactic antibiotics can be reserved for immunocompromised patients and should cover *P. aeruginosa* and *Staphylococcus aureus*, the two likely participants in posttraumatic chondritis.

Foreign Bodies

Foreign bodies in the external canal are commonly seen in the emergency department. The variations can include anything from cotton, pencil erasers, or pieces of toys to illicit drugs and insects. Organic materials such as beans, seeds, and vegetable matter may conform to the contour of the canal or expand if moistened, complicating the dilemma of removal. Insects that crawl into the ear can actually survive for a long period of time, causing a local inflammation and a great deal of distress to the patient.

The evaluation of a patient with a foreign body in the ear should begin with calming the patient and placing him or her in the reclined position. Occasionally the complaint may be sudden pain while in the recumbent position, as in the case of an embedded insect. Most of the time, the history will reveal the type of material in the ear. A thorough examination and visualization of the complete tympanic membrane is mandatory. Inability to visualize the entire canal, contact of the foreign body with the tympanic membrane, or the presence of a perforation mandates the use of an operative microscope and speculum, with obvious consultation. Foreign bodies in children medial to the bony isthmus often require conscious sedation or even general anesthesia for safe extraction.[29] Cerumen loops, a right-angle hook, and alligator forceps are the instruments of choice for the removal. Live objects should be drowned with a 2% lidocaine solution or viscous lidocaine, which immediately paralyzes the bug and provides modest topical anesthesia to the cutaneous area. The liquid can then be suctioned out with butterfly tubing and the insect removed with gentle suction or forceps under direct visualization. Care must be taken to assure that no debris of the insect remains in the canal. Irrigation with room-temperature water is adequate for small particles such as hard sand or cerumen and can mobilize distally positioned objects. Irrigation should not be used unless the tympanic membrane is completely visualized and free of perforation, and it can be utilized only for nonorganic matter, which will not expand when moistened.

Complete inspection of the ear canal after removal of the foreign body is important to exclude more significant injury to the canal skin, tympanic membrane, and ossicles caused by the foreign body or its extraction. Small abrasions heal spontaneously. Topical antibiotics should be considered in cases where there was more serious cutaneous damage or where the foreign body consisted of organic material (see Table 231-6).[29]

Cerumen Impaction

Occasionally the diagnosis is made as patients present with unrelated complaints, but more often, patients complain of decreased hearing, a sensation of pressure or fullness in the ear, dizziness, tinnitus, or pain. The symptoms are often precipitated by the use of cotton-tipped applicators. Most of the time, cerumen loops can be used. In the particularly difficult cases or where cerumen is completely occluding the canal, softening of the cerumen can be accomplished with half-strength hydrogen peroxide, sodium bicarbonate drops, mineral oil, or over-the-counter preparations such as Debrox or Cerumenex for 30 min. If irrigation is the treatment of choice, it can usually be accomplished with a metal ear syringe, a flexible 18-gauge intravenous catheter, or a syringe attached to the tubing of a butterfly infusion catheter. Body-temperature irrigant is the solution of choice. The catheter should be inserted into the cartilaginous canal (distal third) and a pulsatile flow should be inserted along the superior portion of the external auditory canal. Irrigation of the canal when the middle ear is not infected often causes a temporary redness of the tympanic membrane; therefore, the subsequent diagnosis of otitis media should be made with caution.

Tympanic Membrane Perforation

Tympanic membrane perforations can occur as a result of blunt, penetrating, or noise trauma. When it is secondary to blunt or noise trauma, the perforation almost always occurs in the pars tensa, usually anteriorly or inferiorly. The pars tensa, the largest area of the tympanic membrane, is only a few cell layers thick.

The patient usually complains of an acute onset of pain and hearing loss, with or without bloody otorrhea. There may also be associated vertigo and tinnitus, but this is usually transient unless there has been injury to the inner ear or rupture of the round or oval windows.[30] In evaluating these injuries, the canal must be cleared of blood and debris. The tympanic membrane should be completely visualized. Greater than 90 percent of tympanic membrane perforations heal spontaneously. Those occurring secondary to blunt or noise trauma can be safely discharged and referred to a specialist for further evaluation and a formal audiogram as soon after the injury as possible. Patients should be instructed not to allow water to enter the canal of the ear. They do not need topical or systemic antibiotics. Perforations in the posterosuperior quadrant or those secondary to penetrating trauma have a greater likelihood of damaging the ossicular chain or, in the case of the latter, a retained foreign body and should be referred to an otolaryngologist within 24 h.[30,31]

Lightning fatally strikes approximately 600 persons annually in the United States and leaves thousands more survivors with permanent sequelae. Although the blast effect associated with a lightning strike plays a part in perforations, conducted electrical current from cutaneous sites via the external auditory canal and into the middle or inner ear structures is another hypothesized mechanism for lightning-induced otologic injuries.[29] Tympanic membrane perforation is the most common sequela.

Barotrauma

Barotrauma to the middle ear, also called barotitis media, is discussed in Chap. 192.

REFERENCES

1. Kreigsberg MK, Turner J: Dental causes of referred otalgia. *Ear Nose Throat J* 66:398, 1987.
2. Seidman JD, Jacobsen GP: Update on tinnitus. *Otolaryngol Clin North Am* 29:455, 1996.
3. Dix MR, Hallpike CS: Pathology, symptomatology and diagnosis of certain disorders of the vestibular system. *Proc R Soc Med* 45:341, 1952.
4. Weber PC, Warren YA: The differential diagnosis of Meniere's disease. *Otolaryngol Clin North Am* 30:977, 1997.
5. Hotson JR, Baloh RW: Current concepts: Acute vestibular syndrome. *N Engl J Med* 399:680, 1998.
6. Norrving B, Magnusson J, Holtas S: Isolated acute vertigo in the elderly: Vestibular or vascular disease? *Acta Neurol Scand* 91:43, 1995.
7. Hughes GB, Freedman MA, Haberkamp TJ, Guay ME: Sudden sensorineural hearing loss. *Otolaryngol Clin North Am* 29:393, 1996.
8. Rohn GN, Meyerhof WL, Wright GC: Ototoxity of topical agents. *Otolaryngol Clin North Am* 26:747, 1993.
9. Schweitzer VG: Ototoxicity of chemotherapeutic agents. *Otolaryngol Clin North Am* 26:759, 1993.
10. Jung TTK, Rhee C, Lee CS, et al: Ototoxicity of salicylate, nonsteroidal anti-inflammatory drugs, and quinine. *Otolaryngol Clin North Am* 26:791, 1993.
11. Brummett RE: Ototoxicity of vancomycin and analogues. *Otolaryngol Clin North Am* 26:821, 1993.
12. Brummett RE: Ototoxicity liability of erythromycin and analogues. *Otolaryngol Clin North Am* 26:811, 1993.
13. Matz GJ: Aminoglycoside cochlear ototoxicity. *Otolaryngol Clin North Am* 26:705, 1993.
14. Rybak LP: Ototoxicity of loop diuretics. *Otolaryngol Clin North Am* 26:829, 1993.
15. Selesnick SH: Otitis externa: Management of the recalcitrant case. *Am J Otol* 15:408, 1994.
16. Brook I, Frazier EH, Thompson DH: Aerobic and anaerobic microbiology of external otitis. *Clin Infect Dis* 16:955, 1992.
17. Bojrab DI, Bruderly T, Abdurazzak Y: Otitis externa. *Otolaryngol Clin North Am* 29:761, 1996.
18. Brook I: Otitis media: Microbiology and management. *J Otolaryngol* 23:269, 1994.
19. Myer CM III: The diagnosis and management of mastoiditis in children. *Pediatr Ann* 20:662, 1991.
20. Garcia RDJ, Baker AS, Cunningham MJ, Weber AL: Lateral sinus thrombosis associated with otitis media and mastoiditis in children. *Pediatr Infect Dis J* 14:617, 1995.
21. Marais J, Dale BAB: Bullous myringitis: A review. *Clin Otolaryngol* 22:497, 1997.
22. Lee D, Sperling N: Initial management of auricular trauma. *Am Fam Physician* 53:2339, 1996.
23. Lawson W: Management of acute trauma, in Lucente FE, Lawson W, Novick NL (eds): *The External Ear*. Philadelphia, Saunders, 1995, pp 174–188.
24. Ruder RO: Injuries of the pinna, in Gates GA (ed): *Current Therapy in Otolaryngology—Head Neck Surgery*, 5th ed. St Louis, Mosby, 1994, pp 127–131.
25. Gilmer PA: Trauma of the auricle, in Bailey BJ (ed): *Head Neck Surgery—Otolaryngology*. Philadelphia, Lippincott, 1993, pp 1557–1563.
26. Skedros D, Goldfarb LW, : Chondritis of the burned ear: A review. *Ear Nose Throat J* 71:359, 1990.
27. Starck WJ, Kaltman SI: Current concepts in the surgical management of traumatic auricular hematoma. *J Oral Maxillofac Surg* 50:800, 1992.
28. Templer J, Renner GJ: Injuries of the external ear. *Otolaryngol Clin North Am* 23:1003, 1990.
29. Backous DD, Minor LB, et al: Trauma to the external auditory canal and temporal bone. *Otolaryngol Clin North Am* 29: 1996.
30. Stiernberg CM, Strunk CL: Ear injuries in sports. *Texas Med J* 82: 1986.
31. Armstrong BW: Traumatic perforations of the tympanic membrane: Observe or repair? *Laryngoscope* 82:1882, 1972.

FACE AND JAW EMERGENCIES

W. F. Peacock IV

FACIAL CELLULITIS

Facial cellulitis represents a group of diseases requiring individualized diagnosis and treatment. Periorbital and orbital cellulitis are covered in Chap. 117.

Pathophysiology

A bacterial infection may enter the soft tissues from virtually any skin violation. Patient risk is increased by immunosuppression, alterations in vascularity (e.g., previous radiation treatment), underlying systemic disease (e.g., diabetes), and the presence of foreign bodies or appliances precluding normal host defenses. A remote history of silicone injections may predispose to recurrent episodes of cellulitis.[1]

The most likely pathogens causing facial cellulitis include *Haemophilus influenzae* type b, *Streptococcus pneumoniae*, *Strep. pyogenes*, *Strep. viridans*, *Staphylococcus aureus*, *Bacteroides fragilis*, *B. melaninogenicus*, and other pathogens found in deep neck abscesses.[2]

Clinical Features

The history should examine recent prodromal events (e.g., insect bites, trauma), allergen exposure, chronic dental caries, painful mastication, previous treatments with radiation, or silicone injections. The presence of dental or cosmetic appliances, nasal discharge, or vision changes should be ascertained. Systemic signs of infection should be excluded, such as fever and vomiting. A thorough head and neck exam is required. Occult infection, with extension from other head and neck structures, should be excluded.

Diagnosis

Cellulitis is classically defined by pain, erythema, edema, increased tactile temperature, and dysfunction of the involved structure. The diagnosis is usually based upon these clinical findings. When there is a focus with purulent drainage, such as an abscess, cultures may yield the organism.

The differential diagnosis includes insect envenomation or other traumatic event, dental caries with abscess formation, occult head and neck infection, orbital or periorbital cellulitis, sinusitis with erosion of the bony cortex, otitis externa, erysipelas, viral exanthems (e.g., erythema infectiosum), parotitis, impetigo, systemic lupus erythematosus, herpes zoster, dermatitides, angioneurotic edema, and allergy.[3,4]

Treatment

Analgesics and antipyretics should be administered as indicated. Broad-spectrum antibiotic therapy, ensuring coverage of staphylococcal and streptococcal species, is indicated. When possible, all foreign bodies and appliances should be removed. Initially recommended antibiotics are amoxicillin/clavulanate or ampicillin/sulbactam. Alternatives include vancomycin plus aztreonam.[2] If cellulitis is secondary to underlying abscess or osteomyelitis, diagnostic evaluation and treatment for the underlying source is necessary.

Disposition

Hospitalization, with antibiotic therapy initiated in the emergency department (ED), is required for patients with facial cellulitis and the following associated conditions:

1. Systemic signs of sepsis
2. Antibiotic intolerance for any reason (e.g., emesis)
3. Immunosuppressive therapies or illness
4. Extensive areas of erythema or induration
5. Unremovable head/neck appliances or foreign bodies
6. Inability to comply with outpatient therapy

Outpatient therapy is appropriate in selected cases. Patients should be instructed to return to the ED for fever, difficulty swallowing or breathing, inability to take their antibiotics for any reason, or if there is worsening of their condition. The patient should be seen the following day for evaluation. If there is continued progression, admission for inpatient antibiotics is warranted. Patients at the extremes of age should have a lower admission threshold.

TEMPOROMANDIBULAR JOINT DYSFUNCTION

The temporomandibular joint (TMJ) combines both a hinge and gliding action. The articular surfaces are separated by the articular disk (also known as the meniscus), which assists in the hinge action between the mandibular condyle and the disk and the gliding action between the disk and temporal bone. Part of the lateral pterygoid muscle inserts into the anterior portion of the disk. Closure of the mandible is by the powerful muscles of mastication, which include the masseter, temporalis, and medial pterygoid. The jaw is opened by forward traction on the mandibular neck by the lower portion of the lateral pterygoid, with assistance from the digastric, mylohyoid, and geniohyoid muscles. Lateral movement of the jaw is by unopposed contraction of one of the lateral pterygoids. Protrusion occurs by the combined action of the medial and lateral pterygoids, and retrusion occurs by contraction of the posterior temporalis with the suprahyoid muscles.

In population studies, TMJ dysfunction is estimated to have a prevalence of 6 to 12 percent, with a 2:1 female preponderance.[5] However, in most treatment samples, women of about age 38 constitute 85 to 90 percent of patients.[5]

Pathophysiology

There is no single clear explanation for all manifestations of TMJ pain. Chronic TMJ dysfunction probably results from a variety of causes, either singly or in combination, and includes neuromuscular disturbance, anatomic deviations as a result of trauma or congenital formation, dental abnormalities, TMJ manifestations of systemic disease, and psychic tension.

Classification[6] is initially based upon whether the primary pathologic event is intracapsular (e.g., disk pathology) or extracapsular (e.g., myositis). This may be difficult to determine.

Myofascial disorders are characterized by pain and spasm of the muscles around the joint; there may be inflammation, tendinitis, or trismus. The patient may report associated bruxism or jaw clenching. Dental malocclusion is felt to play only an indirect role. Most studies have found no significant correlation between occlusal parameters and signs or symptoms of temporomandibular disorders.[7]

Anatomic internal derangement may occur as the result of disk displacement. This may be the result of single major traumatic event (motor vehicle accident, whiplash, direct blow) or secondary to chronic microtrauma (bruxism, jaw hypermobility with chronic injury).

Degenerative joint disease may result from chronic internal derangement or secondarily as the result of systemic disease [e.g., rheumatoid arthritis, systemic lupus erythematosus (SLE)]. At the extreme end of the spectrum, joint ankylosis can occur.

Clinical Features

The patient's chief complaint is usually of pain localized to one of the muscles of mastication. The masseter is the most frequently identified painful area, followed by the temporalis, sternocleidomastoid, trapezius, splenius capitis, and cervical spine musculature.[5] One-third of patients complain of earache.[5] There may be unilateral headache, or pain about the TMJ. Discomfort may be exacerbated by yawning, chewing, jaw clenching, or bruxism. Eighty percent report their discomfort as unilateral.[5]

The onset of discomfort is insidious in 75 percent of patients, with the remainder attributing their onset to a trauma (injury, surgery, bruxism, stress event).[5] In the absence of an acute trauma (e.g., fracture), acuity of onset is not related to ultimate outcome.[5]

Physical findings may include limitation in the range of motion of the mandible, defined as restricted if the distance between the upper and lower incisors is less than 35 mm.[5] With clicking, there may be irregular jaw motion with opening of the mouth.[5] Because the pain is frequently unilateral, there may be jaw deviation. Clicking or popping at the TMJ may be audible or palpable by the physician.

Palpation should be performed at the muscles of mastication to assess for areas of sensitivity, induration, rigidity, size, and swelling. The condylar heads may be palpated just anterior to the tragus with the teeth together and then with the teeth apart.

A careful head and neck exam is warranted to exclude other more malignant causes of facial pain.

Diagnosis

The ED diagnosis of TMJ dysfunction is predominately based upon the history and physical findings. In the absence of acute trauma without the suggestion of an infectious or neoplastic lesion, there is little necessity for x-rays. It is rare to find abnormalities of the joint with plain radiography unless there is degenerative joint disease.

If acute trauma is the etiology, the initial radiographic evaluation of the TMJ is usually a panoramic view of the mandible. The principal advantage of the panoramic view is the ability to demonstrate pathology causing discomfort from sites other than the TMJ. Other imaging modalities include computed tomography (CT) scanning and magnetic resonance imaging (MRI), but these are not relevant in the ED setting.[6]

Since patients with TMJ are frequently women in their thirties, men of any age and older women presenting with their first onset of pain should prompt concern. An expanded differential, including other etiologies of facial pain, should be considered but can usually be excluded by history and physical exam. Jaw pain secondary to angina, sinusitis, toothache, otitis, septic TMJ, alternative diagnoses of headache (e.g., temporal arteritis), neoplastic lesions, and trigeminal neuralgia[5] may be considered.

Treatment

Recommendations to the patient may include the following:

1. Use ice or hot packs to the reduce pain and muscle spasm.
2. Eat soft foods to reduce chewing stress (no chewing gum or ice).
3. As much as possible, disengage the teeth by keeping them slightly apart.
4. Control body position: do not sit with the chin resting on the hand and do not sleep with the pillow pushing against the TMJ.

The physician may prescribe nonsteroidal anti-inflammatory drugs as indicated by the patient's discomfort. Muscle relaxants may be helpful. If narcotic use is necessary, it should be of limited duration.[8,9]

Many patients with chronic TMJ have been treated with oral appliances; however, controlled studies have shown no benefit for these over placebo.[5]

DISLOCATION OF THE MANDIBLE

Epidemiology

Mandibular dislocation is a common problem in emergency medicine.[10] Dislocations are usually preceded by a preexisting risk factor. These include general joint laxity, neurologic disease resulting in increased muscular activity, and extrapyramidal side effects of neuroleptic medication.[11] In a population study of 400 patients with symptomatic TMJ dysfunction, only 1.8 percent sustained recurrent mandibular dislocation.[11]

Pathophysiology

The mandible can be dislocated in an anterior, posterior, lateral, or superior plane. Anterior dislocation is most common and occurs when the mandibular condyle is forced in front of the articular eminence. The jaw is then kept in this position by muscular spasm. Anterior subluxation occurs in up to 70 percent of normal individuals but can be spontaneously reduced by the patient.[12] A predisposition to symptomatic anterior dislocation includes anatomic predilection (a shallow glenoid fossa), loss of joint capsule integrity (previous trauma), or increased muscle tone. Once the jaw is dislocated, muscular spasm, particularly from the temporalis and lateral pterygoid muscles, tends to prevent reduction. Dislocations are most frequently bilateral, but they also occur unilaterally.[12]

Anterior dislocations are classified as acute, chronic recurrent, or chronic.[12] Acute dislocations usually present shortly after their occurrence, owing to severe discomfort. In chronic recurrent dislocations, precipitating factors should be considered. This includes dystonic reactions and hypermobile syndromes (e.g., Marfan, Ehlers-Danlos).[12] Chronic dislocations, where the condyle is displaced from the fossa for an extended time, occur in patients unable or unwilling to obtain prompt medical treatment (e.g., severe mental illness, alcoholism, etc.).

Posterior dislocations are rare. They follow a direct blow to the chin that does not break the condylar neck. In this dislocation, the mandibular condyle is thrust against the mastoid. As a result, the condylar head may prolapse into the external auditory canal.[12]

Lateral dislocations are always associated with jaw fracture. With a lateral dislocation, the condylar head is forced laterally and then superiorly into the temporal space.

Superior dislocations occur from a blow to the partially open mouth that forces the condylar head upward. Associated injuries include cerebral contusions, facial nerve palsy, and deafness. Mandibular fractures are not always present.[12]

Clinical Features

Patients with acute dislocation usually present with severe pain, difficulty in speaking or swallowing, or malocclusion. There may be loose or missing teeth and areas of sensory deficit at the chin or mouth.

With anterior dislocation, pain is localized anterior to the tragus. The symptoms are frequently reported to have begun acutely following extreme mouth opening. Anterior dislocation has been reported to have occurred after laughing, yawning, vomiting, taking a large bite, trauma, oral sex, dental extraction, overstretching of the mouth during general anesthesia, or tonsillectomy.[11,12] As opposed to anterior dislocation, all other types of mandibular dislocation tend to require significant trauma.

All patients with a history of possible mandibular dislocation should have a good head, neck, and dental examination. With anterior dislocations, there is a visible and palpable preauricular depression from the displacement of the mandibular condyle. There will also be difficulty with jaw movement. If the dislocation is unilateral, there is deviation of the jaw away from the dislocation.

When a posterior dislocation is considered, the external auditory canal should be visualized. Baseline hearing function should be verified. With lateral dislocations, the condylar head is palpable in the temporal space and there are always signs of a jaw fracture (e.g., malocclusion). When a superior dislocation is suspected, a thorough exam is needed, especially focusing on the head, neck, and neurologic systems.

Diagnosis

In the cooperative patient with a spontaneous nontraumatic anterior dislocation, the diagnosis is based upon clinical grounds. In other dislocations, radiographs may be needed to confirm clinical suspicion. In the setting of significant trauma, radiographs should be obtained to exclude fracture. The panoramic view usually demonstrates the pathology and excludes other mandibular injury. Specific jaw or TMJ films may be helpful. In the patient with more serious trauma, where there may be a superior dislocation or intracranial injury, a CT scan will provide more information.

The differential diagnosis of jaw dislocation includes mandibular fracture, traumatic hemarthrosis, acute closed locking of the TMJ meniscus, and TMJ dysfunction.[12]

Treatment

Reduction may be attempted in closed anterior dislocations without fracture. Most attempts are made easier with analgesia. A short-acting intravenous muscle relaxant (e.g., midazolam) helps to decrease muscle spasm.[11] Appropriate airway and hemodynamic monitoring is required. A systemic analgesic (e.g., narcotic) may also be considered. Conscious sedation has also been used successfully.[10]

Alternatively, local anesthetic can be placed into the joint capsule.[11] Using aseptic technique, a 21-gauge needle is placed into the preauricular depression just anterior to the tragus and 2 mL of 2% lidocaine is injected.[12] (See Fig. 232-1.)

There are two methods for reducing an anterior mandibular dislocation.[12] The most commonly used technique requires the patient to be firmly seated, with the head against the wall or chair back, positioned

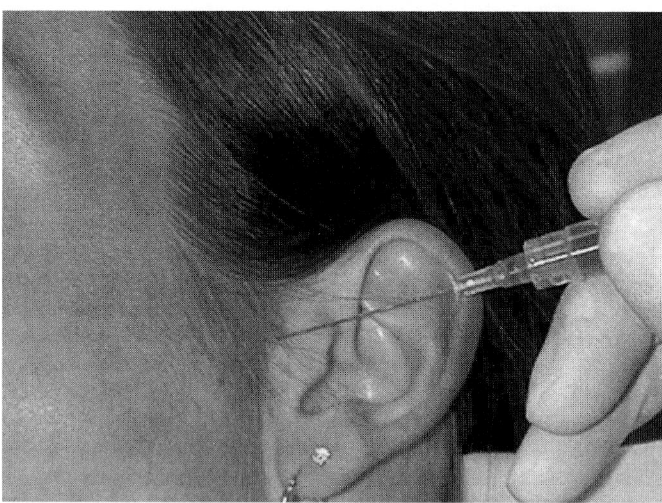

FIG. 232-1. Site of injection for dislocated mandible local anesthesia.

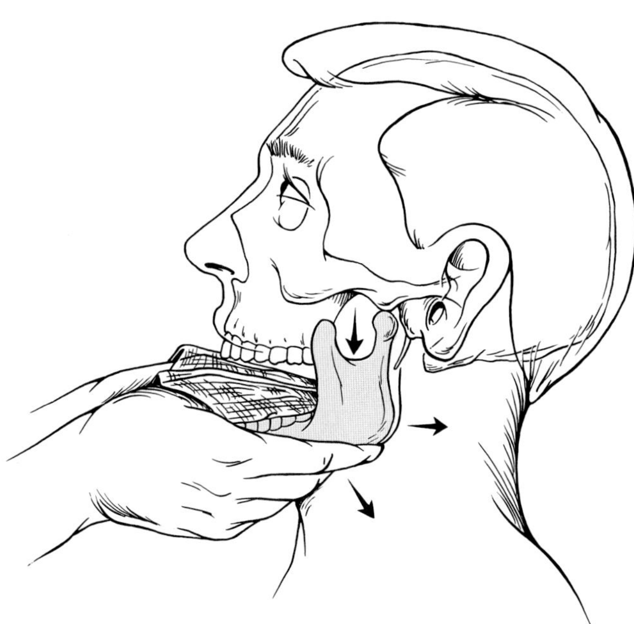

FIG. 232-2. The temporomandibular joints in normal and dislocated positions, and positioning for mandibular relocation in a seated patient. Positioning for mandibular relocation in a recumbent patient.

so that the examiner's flexed elbow is at the level of the patient's mandible. Facing the patient, the examiner places his or her gloved thumbs in the patient's mouth, over the occlusal surfaces of the mandibular molars, as far back as possible. The fingers should curve beneath the angle and body of the mandible. Using the thumbs, the examiner applies pressure downward and backward. Slightly opening the jaw may help disengage the condyle from the anterior eminence. (See Fig. 232-2). When the dislocation is bilateral, it may be easier to relocate one side at a time. Some suggest that the examiner may wish to wear gauze over the thumbs for protection, should the mandible snap closed after reduction.[12]

The second technique requires the examiner, standing behind the recumbent patient, to place the thumbs on the molars and apply downward and backward pressure.[12]

If the reduction is successful, the patient should be able to close his or her mouth immediately. Postreduction radiographs are not usually required unless the procedure was difficult or traumatic or there is significant discomfort postprocedure.

Complications from the reduction itself are unusual but can include iatrogenic fracture or avulsion of the articular cartilage.[10]

Disposition

Patients with dislocations that are open, superior, associated with fracture, that manifest any nerve injury, or that are unreducible by closed technique should be emergently referred to a head and neck or oral surgeon.

Following the successful reduction of an acute dislocation, patients are placed on a soft diet and cautioned against opening their mouths more than 2 cm for the following 2 weeks.[11] They should be instructed to support the mandible with a hand when they yawn. Nonsteroidal analgesics may be required to manage initial discomfort.

In all dislocations, follow-up is recommended. In severe cases, intermaxillary fixation may be required to control jaw motion during healing. Chronic dislocations may require operative intervention.

MASTICATOR SPACE ABSCESS

Pathophysiology

The masticator space consists of four potential spaces bounded by the muscles of mastication. (See Fig. 232-3.) These spaces include the masseteric, superficial temporal, deep temporal, and pterygomandibular spaces.[13] Since they are contiguous, it is rare for a single one to be infected. Secondary infection usually occurs by extension from one of the anterior spaces (buccal, sublingual, or submandibular).

Infection of the masseteric space most frequently arises via extension from soft tissue infection around the third molar. Rarely, it may follow as a complication to an inferior alveolar nerve block, an open fracture at the angle of the mandible, or as an extension from osteomyelitis of the zygoma or temporal bones.[14]

The temporal spaces are rarely involved. If this occurs, it is usually the result of a serious, overwhelming infection. The pterygomandibular space is usually infected secondarily by extension from the sublingual or submandibular spaces or from infection from around the third molar. Untreated, infection can spread to the adjacent spaces of the head and neck that are contiguous with the mediastinum, resulting in mediastinitis, pericarditis, and death.[15]

Soft tissue infections of the spaces in the perimandibular and parapharyngeal region are frequently caused by oral anaerobes. These include *Peptostreptococcus*, *Fusobacterium* sp., *Bacteroides* sp. (*oralis* and *melaninogenicus*), *Propionibacterium*, and *Clostridium* sp.[2] Masticator space infections are frequently mixed, with at least two organisms present.[15]

Clinical Features

The most frequent acute clinical findings are facial swelling, pain, erythema, and trismus.[15] In chronic infection the patient may be afebrile but may complain of progressive trismus.[15]

Constitutional signs include fever, malaise, dehydration, dysphagia, nausea, or vomiting. In more advanced cases, systemic signs of sepsis are present.

History and physical exam features are variable. When infection occurs in the masseteric space, there is posteroinferior facial swelling

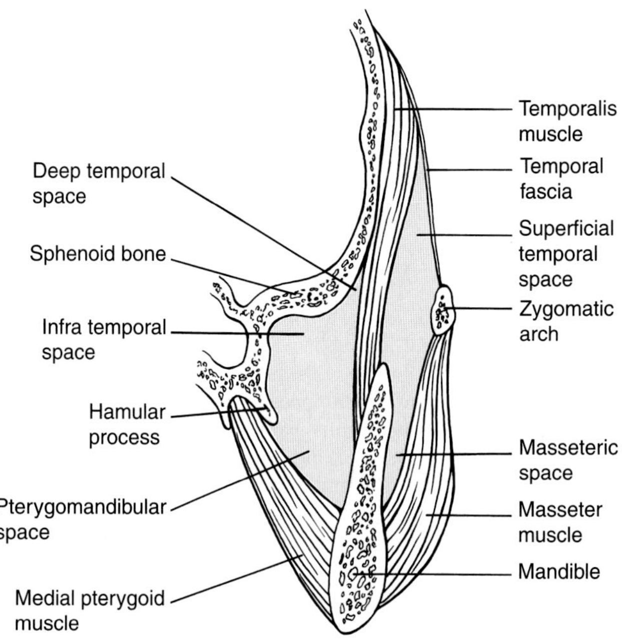

FIG. 232-3. Masticator space.

with mild to moderate trismus. If the temporal space is infected, there is soft tissue swelling over the temporalis and significant trismus. Trismus without swelling suggests pterygomandibular space abscess.

Diagnosis

The diagnosis of masticator space infection is clinical. Radiographs occasionally demonstrate osteomyelitis of the mandible. CT may define the extent of an abscess but is not required in the management of those well enough to be treated as outpatients. CT may be needed in more ill-appearing patients. Abscess culture usually yields *Streptococcus* and oral anaerobes but is unnecessary in uncomplicated immunocompetent patients.

Because the parotid gland overlies the masseter, diagnostic confusion with parotitis can result when there is swelling over these structures. Useful distinctions are that the symptoms of parotitis are cyclically related to eating, whereas the pain of an abscess is constant,[14] and parotitis is not associated with the significant trismus that accompanies infection of the masticator space.[15] Other diagnoses to consider with lateral jaw pain include jaw discomfort of angina, masticator space neoplasm, TMJ dysfunction, referred dental pain, pharyngeal infection, tonsillitis or peritonsillar abscess, and otitis media or externa. History and physical exam are usually sufficient to exclude these other considerations.

Treatment

Therapy is determined by the patient's condition. In unilateral masticator space infections, airway compromise is rare; however, the possibility should always be considered. Emergent ear, nose, and throat (ENT) consultation is required in patients with airway compromise, severe trismus, vomiting, palpable abscess, large or diffuse areas of cellulitis, large areas of induration, or systemic signs of sepsis.

For patients requiring hospitalization, intravenous antibiotics should be started in the ED. Large doses of penicillin, 20 million units daily, are appropriate. In penicillin-allergic patients, clindamycin is a good alternative.[2,16] Analgesics should be administered as needed.

In candidates for outpatient management, antibiotic selection is as follows: penicillin as a first choice, erythromycin, or clindamycin may be selected. Antibiotics should be continued for 10 to 14 days.

Disposition

Stable afebrile patients with minimal symptoms, only slight trismus, no palpable abscess or induration, and without vomiting or systemic signs of infection may be considered for discharge on oral antibiotics and analgesics. They should have follow-up in 24 h and should receive precise discharge instructions to return should they experience difficulty in swallowing or breathing, fever, vomiting, or inability to take their medication for any reason.

SALIVARY GLANDS

The salivary glands are generally considered as comprising two major groups: the parotid and the submandibular. The facial nerve passes through the superficial portion of the parotid gland. The parotid (Stenson) duct opens into the mouth opposite the upper second molar.

The submandibular and sublingual glands lie beneath the tongue. The submandibular ducts open into the mouth at either side of the frenulum of the tongue. The multiple sublingual ducts open into the sublingual fold or directly into the submandibular duct.

Disorders of the salivary glands may have inflammatory, neoplastic, immunologic, or traumatic causes. Only the most common disorders are discussed below. It is important to determine which glands are involved; whether single or multiple glands are affected; whether there is pain, tenderness, or a palpable mass; the acuity of symptoms and their precipitants, whether symptoms are persistent or recurrent; and whether associated problems such as dry mouth or eyes, joint symptoms, or diabetes are present.

MUMPS AND OTHER VIRAL PAROTITIS

Prior to the advent of the vaccine in 1968, mumps caused by the paramyxovirus was the most frequent cause of painful parotid swelling in children between the ages of 5 and 15.[2,17,18] The incubation period is 12 to 21 days.[17] Patients are infective from 3 days prior to 7 days after salivary gland swelling.[19] Repeat episodes of mumps occur but are rare. Viral parotitis can also be caused by influenza, enteroviruses, cytomegalovirus, and the human immunodeficiency virus (HIV).[18]

Symptoms progress from initial fever and malaise to increasing pain and stiffness with chewing.[18] Parotid swelling, bilateral in 70 percent of patients, follows.[17] The angle of the mandible may be obliterated.[18] There may be edema of the surrounding area, but there is no discharge from the Stenson duct. In 10 percent, the submandibular glands are involved.

Usually benign in children, mumps can be severe in adults. Although 25 percent of men suffer orchitis, only 5 percent of women manifest oophoritis.[19] Possible complications include mastitis, pancreatitis, myocarditis, meningoencephalitis, encephalomyelitis, and sensorineural deafness.[17,18]

The diagnosis of mumps can be made solely on clinical grounds.[17] Amylase levels may be elevated.[18] There is no specific therapy. Treatment is supportive. Children with mumps should be excluded from school or day care for 9 days following the onset of parotid swelling.[18]

SUPPURATIVE PAROTITIS

Parotitis can occur in any debilitated or dehydrated patient. About one-third of cases occur postoperatively.[20] Suppurative parotitis is believed to occur from the retrograde migration of oral bacteria.[19] Predisposing conditions are ductal abnormalities (e.g., stricture), drugs or therapies decreasing the flow of saliva (e.g., phenothiazines, antihistamines, parasympathetic inhibitors, radiation treatment), and poor oral hygiene.[17,20]

Suppurative parotitis presents clinically as a tender, erythematous, and swollen parotid gland. It is bilateral in up to 20 to 25 percent of cases.[19] Pain may extend from the ear to above the mandible. Swelling may progress over the face and neck. The angle of the mandible may be obliterated.[18] Fever and trismus may be present, and pus (which should be cultured) may be expressed from the Stenson duct.[20] Abscesses can occur, although the fluctuance may be difficult to appreciate on physical exam.

Suppurative sialoadenitis can occur in the other salivary glands, but the expected pathogens and recommended treatment are the same. Usual bacteria are *Staph. aureus* mixed with anaerobes.[17,20] In chronically ill, dehydrated, or hospitalized patients, *Pseudomonas*, *Enterobacter*, *Klebsiella*, enterococci, *Proteus*, and *Candida* spp. can be found.

The diagnosis is strictly clinical.[17] No specific testing is available. Examination will identify the parotid as the source of discomfort. In patients failing to improve after several days of treatment, CT or ultrasound should be considered to identify a possible abscess. Because it may aggravate the condition, sialography is contraindicated during the acute stage.[17]

It may be difficult to differentiate viral and suppurative parotitis. The differential is broad and includes sialolithiasis (Table 232-1). Bacterial parotitis is usually associated with higher fever, greater warmth, and more overlying erythema as compared with viral parotitis. Lymphadenitis can present with similar findings but usually involves an identifiable source of infection, is not localized to the parotid, and will not cause purulent discharge from the Stenson duct.

Hydration to ensure salivary flow, massage, local heat, and sialogogues (such as lemon drops) are the mainstays of therapy. The

TABLE 232-1 Causes of Salivary Gland Enlargement

Sialolithiasis
Metabolic
Malnutrition, anorexia/bulimia
Vitamin A, B, or niacin deficiency
Celiac disease, cystic fibrosis
Alcoholism, cirrhosis
Uremia
Hormonal
Diabetes, hyperlipidemia
Hypothyroidism
Testicular atrophy
Pregnancy, lactation
Menopause
Infectious
HIV
Cat-scratch disease
Tuberculosis, atypical mycobacteria
Histoplasmosis, actinomycosis
Viral (mumps, influenza, enteroviruses, cytomegalovirus)
Bacterial suppurative parotitis
Drugs/Toxins
Thiourea, methimazole, phenylbutazone
Oxyphenbutazone, phenothiazines
Thiocyanate, iodides and iodine-containing drugs
Heavy metal poisoning (Pb, Hg, Cu)
Others
Sjögren's syndrome, Mikulicz's syndrome, sarcoidosis
Collagen vascular diseases, obesity
Primary tumors, lymphoma
Congenital cysts
Pneumoparotitis (air insufflation)

patient should receive antibiotics effective against the expected pathogen. Initially recommended antibiotics are amoxicillin/clavulanate or ampicillin/sulbactam.[2] Alternative choices include clindamycin, antistaphylococcal penicillin, cefoxitin, or vancomycin plus metronidazole.[2] Antibiotics should be continued until culture results are known.

Patients who are clinically stable and able to complete their antibiotic regimen may be discharged for outpatient management. Those with hemodynamic instability, vomiting, severe complicating disease, or other factors precluding compliance with their antibiotic therapy should be admitted for intravenous antibiotics. When an abscess is identified, ENT consultation for consideration of surgical drainage is necessary.

SIALOLITHIASIS

Salivary calculi can be seen at any age, peak in the third to sixth decades, and have a male predominance. More than 80 percent of stones occur in the submandibular gland; most of the remainder are found in the parotid.[17,19] The sublingual glands are rarely involved. Submandibular sialoliths are more common because of more viscous and alkaline secretions as well as the anatomically ''uphill'' path of the Wharton (submandibular) duct.[20] Sialoliths are composed mostly of calcium phosphate and organic matrix.[19] Multiple stones are seen in approximately 25 percent of patients who present with an initial stone.[20]

The symptoms of pain, swelling, and tenderness are similar to those of parotitis and the two conditions may be difficult to differentiate. However, ductal obstructive symptoms (pain and swelling) are exacerbated by meals, when salivary secretion is stimulated.[17,20] Sialolithiasis usually presents with unilateral swelling and pain in the affected gland. The stone may be palpated within the duct. If there is superimposed infection, the diagnosis may be difficult.

Diagnosis is usually clinical. Although intraoral radiographs visualize more than 90 percent of calculi, extraoral radiographs demonstrate only about 50 percent. This is despite the fact that 80 percent of submandibular calculi are radiopaque.[19] Only 20 percent of parotid calculi are visualized by plain radiography.[17]

Sialography, diagnostically limited in the detection of small stones and extrinsic masses, is being replaced by ultrasound, CT, and MRI. These diagnostic procedures are rarely indicated emergently.

Diagnosis and therapy may be initiated on the basis of clinical findings. Conservative treatment is usually effective. Initial management consists of analgesics, antibiotics if there is concurrent infection, massage, and sialogogues (e.g., lemon drops).[17,19] Easily located distal calculi may be digitally ''milked'' from the duct.[19] Alternatively, they may be removed by the specialist by either dilation or incision of the ductal orifice. Most patients with sialolithiasis may be discharged for outpatient management. If there is a concurrent abscess, disposition should be guided by the recommendations for abscess management, as outlined above. Proximal or intraglandular sialoliths should be referred for outpatient ENT evaluation.

Complications of salivary duct obstruction include recurrent or persistent obstruction, sialectasia (irregular dilations of the ductal system resulting in stasis and further stone formation), and superimposed infection.[19]

SALIVARY GLAND ENLARGEMENT

The majority of causes of salivary gland enlargement do not require emergency intervention. However, the patient should be instructed to seek appropriate follow-up for definitive diagnosis and treatment.

Salivary gland enlargement can result from a large number of conditions. (See Table 232-1.) HIV may cause painless gradual enlargement.[17] Other infectious diseases, such as sarcoidosis, cat-scratch disease, tuberculosis, atypical mycobacterial infections, and actinomycoses may present as a chronic form of sialoadenitis.[17,19]

Neoplastic lesions may present with enlarged salivary glands. Less than 3 percent of all head and neck tumors are found in the salivary glands.[17] Although about 70 to 80 percent of salivary tumors arise in the parotid, 75 to 90 percent are benign.[17,20]

ED disposition and outpatient follow-up should be based upon the suspected underlying cause of salivary gland enlargement.

REFERENCES

1. Rapaport MJ, Vinnik C, Zarem H: Injectable silicone: Cause of facial nodules, cellulitis, ulceration, and migration. *Aesthet Plast Surg* 20:267, 1996.
2. Fairbanks DN: *Antimicrobial Therapy in Otolaryngology—Head and Neck Surgery,* 8th ed. American Academy of Otolaryngology—Head and Neck Surgery Foundation, 1996.
3. Middleton DB, Ferrante JA: Periorbital and facial cellulitis. *Am Fam Physician* 21:98, 1980.
4. Biederman GR, Dodson TB: Epidemiologic review of facial infections in hospitalized pediatric patients. *J Oral Maxillofac Surg* 52:1042, 1994.
5. Marbach JJ: Temporomandibular pain and dysfunction syndrome: History, physical examination, and treatment. *Rheum Dis Clin North Am* 22:477, 1996.
6. Talley RL, Murphy GJ, Smith SD, et al: Standards for the history, examination, diagnosis, and treatment of temporomandibular disorders (TMD): A position paper: American Academy of Head, Neck, and Facial Pain. *Craniology* 8:60, 1990.
7. Mitchell RJ: Etiology of temporomandibular disorders. *Curr Opin Dentistry* 1:471, 1991.
8. Westesson PL: Reliability and validity of imaging diagnosis of temporomandibular joint disorder. *Adv Dent Res* 7:137, 1993.
9. Tarro AW: The treatment of TMJ disorders: A current update. *J Mass Dent Soc* 40:125, 1991.

10. Totten VY, Zambito RF: Propofol bolus facilitates reduction of luxed temporomandibular joints. *J Emerg Med* 16:467, 1998.
11. Undt G, Kermer C, Piehslinger E, Rasse M: Treatment of recurrent mandibular dislocation, part I: Leclerc blocking procedure. *Int J Oral Maxillofac Surg* 26:92, 1997.
12. Luyk NH, Larsen PE: The diagnosis and treatment of the dislocated mandible. *Am J Emerg Med* 7:329, 1989.
13. Peterson LJ: Odontogenic infections, in Cummings CW (ed): *Otolaryngology—Head and Neck Surgery*, 2d ed. St. Louis: Mosby–Year Book, pp 1199–1215.
14. Mandel L: Submasseteric abscess caused by a dentigerous cyst mimicking a parotitis: Report of two cases (Review). *J Oral Maxillofac Surg* 55:996, 1997.
15. Doxey GP, Harnsberger HR, Hardin CW, Davis RK: The masticator space: The influence of CT scanning on therapy. *Laryngoscope* 95:1444, 1985.
16. Baker AS, Montgomery WW: Oropharyngeal space infections. *Curr Clin Top Infect Dis* 8:227, 1987.
17. Krause GE, Meyers AD: Management of parotid swelling. *Comp Ther* 22:256, 1996.
18. Peter JR, Haney HM: Infections of the oral cavity. *Pediatr Ann* 25:572, 1996.
19. Johnson A: Inflammatory conditions of the major salivary glands. *ENT J* 68:94, 1989.
20. Langlais RP, Benson BW, Barnett DA: Salivary gland dysfunction: Infections, sialoliths, and tumors. *ENT J* 68:758, 1989.

NASAL EMERGENCIES AND SINUSITIS

Thomas A. Waters
W. F. Peacock IV

EPISTAXIS

Because the blood supply of the nasal mucosa ultimately originates from the internal and external carotid arteries, acute epistaxis has the potential to be very serious, especially when the patient is frail or elderly. Still, most cases of epistaxis are self-limited and can be managed conservatively. Epistaxis has an increased incidence during the dry, cold winter months, due to abrupt temperature changes and exposure to dry heat.

Pathophysiology

The origin of epistaxis can be broadly divided into two categories: anterior and posterior. Anterior epistaxis is more common in young patients, while posterior is the most common in older patients. Determining the origin of bleeding will help guide treatment. Some common causes are listed in Table 233-1.

TABLE 233-1 Common Etiologies of Epistaxis

Infection
Rhinitis
Nasopharyngitis
Sinusitis
Trauma
Self-induced (i.e., nose-picking)
Facial bone fractures
Nasal foreign body
Iatrogenic
Nasal surgery
Local irritants
OTC nasal sprays
Cocaine abuse
Other chemical irritants
Dry nasal mucosa
Allergic rhinitis
Atrophic rhinitis
Hypertension and atherosclerotic cardiovascular disease
Tumors (benign or malignant)
Primary
Secondary
Acquired or hereditary coagulopathies
Hereditary hemorrhagic telangiectasia

Anatomy

The nose functions to warm and humidify air and therefore requires a vigorous blood supply (Fig. 233-1). Its blood supply originates from both the internal and external carotid arteries. The posterior and inferior aspects of the nasal cavity are supplied by the sphenopalatine artery, which is a branch of the maxillary artery. The internal carotid artery gives rise to the ophthalmic artery, which supplies the anterior-superior nasal cavity by the anterior and posterior ethmoidal arteries. The nasal septum receives its blood supply from multiple arteries. The superior labial branch of the facial artery supplies the vestibule and inferior-anterior septum. The posterior and superior septum is supplied by branches of the sphenopalatine, anterior ethmoidal, and posterior ethmoidal arteries. These all join to form Kiesselbach's plexus.

ANTERIOR EPISTAXIS

Anterior epistaxis represents 90 percent of nosebleeds, with the majority originating from Kiesselbach plexus. This area has been referred to as the "picking zone," and is also the area most prone to drying and cracking due to environmental effects. Anterior nose bleeds result from any process that causes mucosal hyperemia.

Hereditary hemorrhagic telangiectasia (HHT), or Osler-Weber-Rendu disease, is an unusual, but severe, cause of recurrent anterior nosebleeds. HHT is an autosomal-dominant disorder, characterized by mucosal telangiectasia throughout the airway and gastrointestinal tract.

Clinical Features

The history can provide valuable insight as to the location of the epistaxis. Questions that are important to ask include:

- Which side is bleeding?
- Do you have a sensation of blood in back of throat?
- Do you have a history of previous epistaxis, trauma, head/neck tumor, radiation therapy, or head/neck surgery?
- Is there a family history of bleeding disorders?
- Are you using anticoagulants, aspirin, or NSAIDs?

Typically, with anterior epistaxis, the bleeding is unilateral and the patient will not report the sensation of blood in the posterior oropharynx.

In anterior epistaxis one can often visualize the area of bleeding. However, proper lighting and suction are essential. Adequate lighting is best achieved by the use of an ENT head lamp or with a head mirror. Universal precautions must be observed by the examiner and the patient's clothing should be protected with a gown. The patient should be seated in a chair leaning forward with the head inclined anteriorly. This helps to visualize the nasal cavity, minimizes backward blood flow, and decreases gagging.[1] The assessment of the patient must include a complete set of vital signs, as well as a thorough exam of the oropharynx and nasopharynx. Additionally, a general physical overview is necessary to evaluate for signs of systemic coagulopathy.

Laboratory investigation is not routinely required. Exceptions to this are in the patient with multiple or prolonged episodes of hemor-

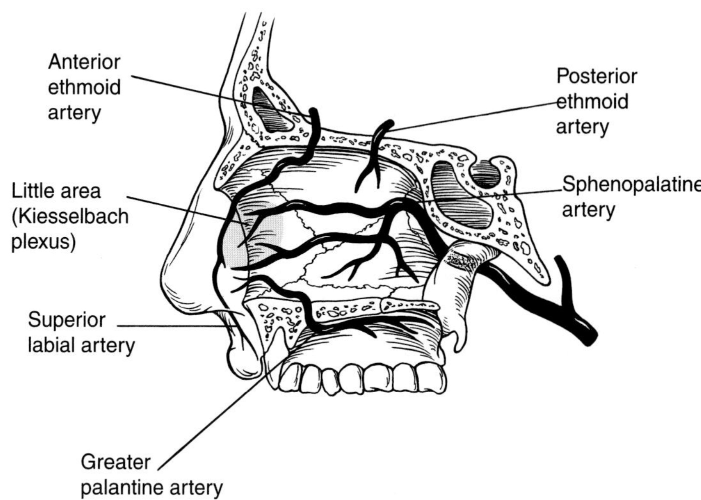

FIG. 233-1. Arterial blood supply to the nasal cavity. The most common site of nasal hemorrhage is at Little area, located on the nasal septum. The most common site of posterior epistaxis is at the lateral nasal branch of the sphenopalatine artery, which enters the nasal cavity behind the middle turbinate. AE, anterior ethmoid; GP, greater palatine; LA, Little area; PE, posterior ethmoid; SL, superior labial; SP, sphenopalatine (lateral nasal branch).

rhage when there is a clinical suspicion of coexisting anemia or if coagulopathy is suggested by either the history or physical exam.

Treatment

The treatment of anterior epistaxis includes direct pressure, vasoconstrictive agents, nasal packing, and cautery. Despite a frequently elevated blood pressure in the setting of acute epistaxis, initial efforts at stabilization should focus on direct control of hemorrhage. Once the bleeding has been stopped and patient anxiety regarding exsanguination resolved, elevated blood pressure usually spontaneously resolves. Persistent or extremely high elevations of blood pressure can then be addressed.

Most episodes of anterior epistaxis can be managed by direct pressure to the nose. This is achieved by compressing the elastic areas of the nose between the thumb and middle phalanx of the index finger. Pressure must be continuously maintained for 10 to 15 min, and confirmed with a clock, as patients frequently underestimate the amount of time that has elapsed. Release of pressure to see if the bleeding has stopped will not allow adequate clot formation and may result in continued bleeding.

Vasoconstrictive agents may be used in conjunction with all other treatment modalities. Table 233-2 lists common vasoconstrictive agents. These compounds can be instilled into the nasal cavity by a spray bottle, an atomizer, or cotton swab. If the area of bleeding can be visualized, cotton swabs or pledgets are preferred. This provides excellent contact with the mucosa and can provide direct pressure to the site.

If the source of bleeding is easily visualized anteriorly, cautery can be attempted with either silver nitrate or electrocautery. Cautery should not be performed indiscriminately. It can lead to septal perforation if used in an overzealous fashion. Silver nitrate sticks can be used as an aid in the management of well-visualized anterior nose bleeds. It should only be attempted after the bleeding has already been stopped and the offending area is well visualized. It is extremely difficult to cauterize an actively bleeding site by chemical means.

Electrical and thermal cautery are best left for the otolaryngologist. It is difficult to control or estimate the depth of cautery achieved with the battery-powered cautery devices available. Significant trauma can occur to the nasal mucosa, septal cartilage, and the skin surrounding the nares.

Anterior Nasal Packing

Anterior nasal packing should be performed on any patient in which direct pressure and vasoconstrictors are unsuccessful in controlling epistaxis. The use of nasal tampons, or sponges, is a very quick and effective method for controlling epistaxis. Nasal tampons, which are initially rigid, are inserted along the floor of the nasal cavity against the septum. They are made of synthetic, sponge-like material that expands to many times its original size after installation of saline or the absorption of blood (see Fig. 233-2). Insertion of the device can be facilitated by coating the tampon with water-soluble antibiotic ointment. This ointment will also help delay expansion until after the tampon is in place. Patients report such commercial devices to be significantly more comfortable than traditional gauze or balloon packing. This, coupled with the ease of insertion when compared to gauze packing, has made such devices very popular. Placement of a traditional anterior nasal pack may be considered when the bleeding is difficult to control, or other methods fail (see Fig. 233-3).

Any patient who has undergone nasal packing may be considered for prophylactic treatment against toxic shock syndrome (TSS) with

TABLE 233-2 Vasoconstrictive and Anesthetic Agents Used in Epistaxis

Phenylephrine (Neo-Synephrine) 0.5–1.0% concentration mixed with 4% lidocaine*
Oxymetozaline (Afrin) 0.05% concentration mixed with 4% lidocaine*
Epinephrine 0.25 mL of 1:1000 concentration mixed with 20 mL of 4% lidocaine*

* The maximum dose of lidocaine applied to the nasal mucosa should not exceed 4 mg/kg.

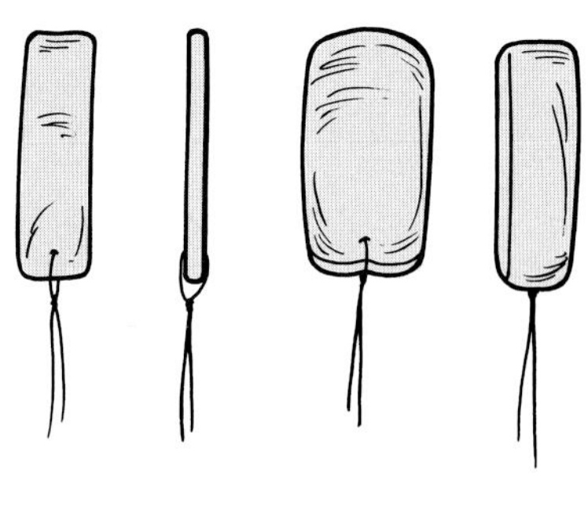

FIG. 233-2. The Merocel nasal sponge in its desiccated (left) and hydrated (right) forms.

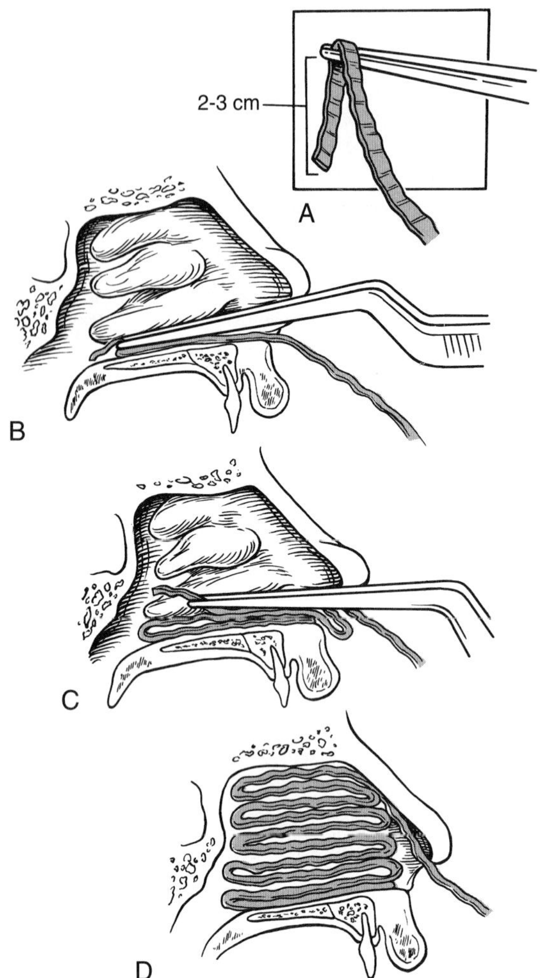

FIG. 233-3. The key to placement of an anterior nasal pack that will control epistaxis adequately and stay in place is to lay the packing into the nasal cavity in an "accordion" manner, so that part of each layer of packing lies anteriorly, preventing the gauze from falling posteriorly into the nasopharynx. **A.** The first layer of $\frac{1}{4}$-in. petrolatum-impregnated gauze strip is grasped approximately 2 to 3 cm from its end. **B.** The first layer is then placed on the floor of the nose through the nasal speculum (not pictured here). The beyonet forcepts and nasal speculum are then withdrawn. **C.** The nasal speculum is reintroduced on top of the first layer of packing, and a second layer is placed in an identical manner. After several layers have been placed, it is often useful to reintroduce the bayonet forceps to push the previously placed packing down onto the floor of the nose, making it tighter and more secure. **D.** A complete anterior nasal pack can tamponade a bleeding point anywhere in the anterior nasal cavities and will stay in place until removed by the physician or patient.

antistaphylococcal medications. Coating the pack with antibiotic ointment before placement helps decrease the amount of nasal bacteria, as well as decreases the number of episodes of bacteremia.[2] The recommended regimen is either cephalexin (250 or 500 mg qid) or amoxicillin/clavulanate (250 or 500 mg tid). In the patient who cannot tolerate these, clindamycin (150 to 300 mg qid) or trimethoprim/sulfamethoxazole DS (bid) can be used as a second choice.[2]

Approximately 25 percent of properly placed anterior nasal packs fail to control the hemorrhage.[1] In such a case, emergency ENT consultation should be obtained if replacing the pack does not control the bleeding. Patients may also experience reflux of blood through the ocular puncta and need to be warned about this. No specific therapy is indicated if this occurs.

Anterior packing alone is a relatively benign procedure. Complications associated with anterior nasal packing include: dislodgement of the pack, persistent bleeding, sinusitis, septal necrosis, and, rarely, TSS. Any patient presenting after nasal packing with fever, rash, nausea, or vomiting, should be considered suspicious for TSS.

Anterior Packs in Children

Anterior epistaxis is fairly common in children. In a study of 1218 children age 11 to 14, 6 percent had experienced epistaxis. The most common cause is idiopathic or related to upper respiratory infections. Treatment is by direct pressure. In the rare case when packing is required, conscious sedation may be needed.

Removal of Anterior Nasal Packs

Removal of nasal packing should be performed at follow-up, after 2 to 3 days. When nasal tampon removal is planned, the pack should be first rehydrated with 5 cc of normal saline. If a gelfoam packing has been placed, this can be left to be absorbed by the body. Recurrent epistaxis may accompany packing removal.

Disposition

Hospital admission is rarely required for patients when good control of anterior epistaxis has been obtained. If bleeding persists after placement of an anterior pack, the possibility of inadequate packing or a posterior bleed needs to be considered. If epistaxis cannot be controlled, or is posterior in origin, emergency ENT consultation should be requested.

At the time of discharge, patients should be given these instructions:

- Do not manipulate the external nares or insert any foreign object into the nasal cavity. If there is no packing, as an exception, the patient may apply petrolatum jelly or triple-antibiotic ointment to dry mucosa. This is performed gently with a sterile cotton-tipped applicator once or twice daily for 3 to 4 days.
- Do not use aspirin or nonsteroidal anti-inflammatory agents for 3 or 4 days.
- If bleeding recurs from simple anterior epistaxis, where no packing has been inserted, home measures may be tried before returning to the emergency department. Patients may be advised to use an over-the-counter vasoconstrictor nasal spray (such as phenylephrine or oxymetazoline) and pinch their nose, with proper technique, for 10 to 15 min. If the bleeding continues, compression may be repeated twice more. If after three unsuccessful attempts, the bleeding continues, they should return to the emergency department immediately. Patients who have had an anterior pack inserted should return if bleeding occurs around the packing or if there is a sensation of blood trickling down the back of the throat. They should be advised to leave the pack in place and not attempt to remove it themselves.
- The patient should follow-up with a primary care or ENT physician in 2 to 3 days.

POSTERIOR EPISTAXIS

Posterior epistaxis represents only 5 percent of nosebleeds presenting to the ED.[3] It is more common in elderly patients and is believed to be due to arteriosclerosis of the large posterior vessels of the nasal cavity. Hypertension is also a large contributor to posterior epistaxis. One study reported that 64 percent of patients with posterior epistaxis had a previous diagnosis of hypertension. Forty-eight percent were actually hypertensive with a systolic blood pressure (BP) greater than 180 or diastolic greater than 110 at the time of their epistaxis. The most common site of bleeding is posterior to the inferior turbinate, occurring 6 to 7.5 cm posterior to the vestibule, and emanates from branches of the sphenopalatine artery.[4] The actual bleeding site usually cannot be visualized.

Clinical Features

Bleeding is typically more profuse than with anterior epistaxis and may be more difficult to control. Blood can often be seen flowing down the posterior oropharynx, or from both nares. The latter is thought to be more common with posterior epistaxis because the site of hemorrhage is closer to the choanae and blood is more likely to reflux to the unaffected side. Direct visualization of the bleeding site may require use of a fiberoptic nasopharyngoscope. Anytime an anterior pack has been placed, and the patient continues to feel blood trickle down the posterior pharynx, a posterior bleed must be considered. A complete set of vital signs, and a thorough head, neck, and naso/oropharyngeal exam should be performed. A general physical overview, searching for evidence of systemic coagulopathy is warranted.

Because posterior epistaxis patients are at greater risk for morbidity and mortality, lab evaluation is often appropriate. This should include hemoglobin and hematocrit, blood type and screening for a possible transfusion, INR/PTT, and any other baseline lab as indicated by the patient's underlying comorbidities. Finally, an intravenous line should be established.

Posterior Nasal Packing

The treatment of posterior epistaxis is posterior nasal packing. Direct pressure is ineffective. The use of cautery in posterior epistaxis is best left to an otolaryngologist. Attempts at cauterizing a vigorously bleeding posterior hemorrhage is nearly impossible and often leads to increased bleeding. Severe damage to the posterior nasal cavity can be sustained with blind attempts at chemical, heat, or electrocautery. The use of vasoconstrictors and anesthetic agents in the treatment of posterior epistaxis is the same as for anterior bleeding.

In the past, physicians were taught to construct a posterior nasal pack using a gauze roll and silk ties. In actual practice, this is a time-consuming and difficult procedure. This practice has been superseded by the advent of commercial devices such as nasal sponges, the Nasostat epistaxis balloon (Sparta Surgical Corp., Hayward, CA), and the Storz epistaxis catheter (Storz Instrument., St. Louis, MO). These tools allow for rapid control of epistaxis with minimal preparation. The use and insertion of the nasal tampons in posterior epistaxis is the same as discussed for anterior epistaxis. A longer sponge is utilized to obtain both anterior and posterior tamponade.

The procedure for insertion of a commercial nasal catheter is as follows:

- The nasal cavity is prepared using vasoconstrictors and anesthetic agents.
- A test is performed for leakage by filling the anterior balloon with 25 mL of water and the posterior balloon with 8 mL of water. If no leak is detected, the water is removed.
- The device is lubricated with 4% lidocaine jelly and inserted into the nasopharynx. The patient opens his or her mouth, and the catheter is advanced until the distal balloon tip is visible in the posterior pharynx.
- The posterior balloon is slowly filled with 4 to 8 mL of water, and the device is pulled anteriorly so that it wedges in the posterior nasopharynx.
- While gentle traction is maintained, the anterior balloon is slowly inflated with 10 to 25 mL of water, providing anterior tamponade. Inflation should be stopped immediately if the patient complains of significant pain. However, some discomfort is usually present.
- Bilateral packing may be necessary to control hemorrhage.
- Analgesics are usually required.

If a commercial device is not available, a Foley catheter can be used to construct a posterior pack. The procedure for placement of the Foley catheter is identical to the procedure described above with only slight differences. The tip of the Foley catheter must be trimmed off to avoid stimulation of the posterior pharynx. The Foley catheter must be pulled anteriorly and held in the forward position by a transverse clamp across the catheter, external to the nasal septum. Ensure that alar necrosis does not result by inserting padding between the nasal alae and the clamp. After placement of a Foley catheter, the anterior nasal cavity is packed as previously described.

The procedure of inserting a posterior nasal pack is very uncomfortable and stressful to the patient. After placement, the patient often continues to have significant discomfort and may require sedation.

Posterior nasal packs carry a significant morbidity. Problems include difficulty swallowing; eustachian tube dysfunction; otitis media; sinusitis; nasal synechiae; hypoventilation with resultant hypoxia; cardiac dysrhythmias; cardiac arrest; accidental dislodgement into the airway; or aseptic necrosis of the nasal alae, columella, palate, and nasal mucosa. In patients with severe COPD or CHF, posterior nasal packing can result in hypoxia.

Embolization and Ligation

If epistaxis is refractory to the above treatments, more extensive and specialized techniques may be needed. These include arterial ligation or embolization. These options should only be performed by a specially trained physician.

Surgical ligation can be performed as treatment for posterior epistaxis. The external carotid artery can be ligated distal to the lingual branch. However, this is rarely successful in controlling epistaxis secondary to the extensive collateral circulation. Ligation of the ethmoidal vessels and the maxillary artery have been successful in controlling hemorrhage. Angiographic embolization of the vessels supplying the bleeding site is usually used when bleeding has failed to respond to packing or arterial ligation. A 96 percent success rate has been reported in patients with severe or intractable epistaxis.[5] The risks of embolization include neurologic and ocular complications from accidental embolization of the cerebral or ophthalmic arteries. Despite this, in experienced hands embolization results in low morbidity and negligible mortality.[5]

Disposition

All patients with posterior epistaxis should have emergent consultation with an otolaryngologist. Attempts at controlling bleeding with the appropriate balloon technique should not be delayed pending the arrival of a specialist physician. Because of the potential for serious morbidity and mortality associated with posterior packing, patients are usually admitted for observation. They may need sedation secondary to severe discomfort and require monitoring for hypoxia. Prophylactic antibiotics are generally given (see anterior packing).

NASAL FRACTURE

Pathophysiology

Any significant central midface trauma should be considered highly suspicious for the presence of a nasal bone fracture. A direct impact is most likely to cause a fracture because there is no soft tissue to dissipate the force of the blow. The pathomechanics of the resulting fracture vary according to the site, direction, and intensity of impact, as well as the characteristics of the bone that is struck. In younger patients, bones are denser and more elastic, whereas in older patients, bones are less dense and more brittle.

Clinical Features

A careful history can usually ascertain the severity of trauma incurred. In cases where the forces involved are severe, the physician must be suspicious of cervical spine injury or closed-head injury. These injuries take precedence over any concurrent nasal fracture. Epistaxis may be frequently associated with nasal trauma.

Findings suggestive of a nasal fracture include swelling, tenderness, crepitance, ecchymosis, or nasal deformity. Indirect evidence of nasal fracture include periorbital ecchymosis, epistaxis, and rhinorrhea. A general physical exam, specifically focused on the head, neck, and neurologic system, is necessary to exclude associated injury.

After spraying the nasal mucosa with a vasoconstricting agent, search for defects in the mucosa, septal hematoma, and bony displacement. Finally, palpate the injured nose checking for crepitance, step-offs, and instability. Severe edema often precludes immediate detection of nasal fractures.

The diagnosis of nasal fracture is predominately based upon historical and physical exam findings. Nasal radiographic studies are usually not required for diagnosis or management. Radiographic imaging selection depends upon suspicion of other associated facial fractures.

Treatment

A simple, minimally or nondisplaced nasal fracture does not require specific treatment other than analgesia, nasal decongestants, and protection from further injury. If significant epistaxis occurs, nasal packing can be placed as previously discussed, but is usually unnecessary. All patients with suspected nasal bone fractures should be given follow-up for reevaluation with either a plastic surgeon, otolaryngologist, or an oral and maxillofacial surgeon, once the swelling has subsided, usually in 2 to 5 days. Grossly displaced nasal fractures should receive consultation in the ED for correction.

Complications

The complications of a nasal fracture include nasal deformity, deviated nasal septum, septal hematoma, cribiform plate fracture, and associated facial, head, or spinal injuries.

A septal hematoma is a rare complication. It is a collection of blood beneath the septal perichondrium. Easily visualized using an otoscope, it appears as a bluish, fluid-filled sac overlying the septum. Such a hematoma is easily managed by making an incision for drainage, followed by packing the nasal cavity to prevent reaccumulation. If undiagnosed or left untreated, it may progress to an abscess or result in avascular necrosis (AVN) of the cartilaginous septum within three to four days. Septal AVN is associated with the cosmetic complications of saddle nose deformity, retraction, and changes in phonation.

Fracture through the cribiform plate of the ethmoid bone is associated with a cerebrospinal fluid (CSF) leak through torn meninges. It represents a violation in the integrity of the subarachnoid space. Cerebrospinal fluid rhinorrhea is suspected in any patient presenting with a clear nasal discharge following facial injury. CSF rhinorrhea is usually seen within the first week as cerebral edema resolves, but it may be delayed days to weeks following a traumatic event. If untreated, possible sequelae include meningoencephalitis or brain abscess. Fortunately, this is rare.

The identification of CSF rhinorrhea can be difficult in nasal injuries because it is not unusual for there to be a clear transudate from the traumatized nasal mucosa. One method of detecting CSF is to put a drop of the suspected liquid on a piece of filter paper and see if a clear area surrounds a central blood stain. An alternative is that CSF can be detected by using a glucose reagent strip. If the glucose content of suspected fluid is greater than 30 mg/dL, then the presence of CSF is suggested. These tests should not be used to definitively exclude the diagnosis. All patients with suspected CSF rhinorrhea should undergo a head CT and urgent neurosurgical consultation. If a fracture of the cribiform plate is clinically suspected, the patient should be placed in an upright position, intranasal packing avoided, and immediate neurosurgical consultation obtained. Coughing, sneezing, nose blowing, and straining by the patient should be avoided.

Other injuries often seen with nasal trauma are fractures of the orbital wall, sinuses, and zygoma. The emergency physician should also be suspicious of cervical spine damage or closed-head injury in any patient with significant facial trauma.

Disposition

An isolated nasal bone fracture does not itself warrant admission to the hospital. The patient should be advised to initiate measures to reduce swelling immediately. Discharge instructions should instruct intermittent ice application for 24 to 48 h, elevation of the head, even while sleeping, and over-the-counter decongestants as needed. They should also include head-injury instructions and advise the patient to be alert for CSF rhinorrhea. All patients should be given follow-up with an appropriate specialist at 2 to 5 days.[5] Although nondisplaced fractures rarely need further treatment, follow-up should be provided secondary to the cosmetic importance of the injury.

NASAL FOREIGN BODIES

Children frequently insert foreign bodies in their nares that may require removal by a physician. Items that may be found in the nasal cavity are limited only by the child's imagination. Among foreign bodies most often found in children's nostrils are food, paper, and pieces of toys.[6,7] Dried beans and vegetable matter are particularly concerning because they tend to absorb fluid and swell, increasing discomfort and making removal more difficult. Other common foreign bodies include rocks, buttons, and button batteries.

Clinical Features

When obtaining a history, interact with the child in a nonjudgmental manner. Many children are hesitant to admit placing a foreign body in their nose for fear they will elicit displeasure from their parents or the physician. In 73 percent of cases, the insertion of the foreign body is actually observed by the caregiver or the child reported the presence of a foreign body.[8] The treating physician should suspect a nasal foreign body in a child who presents with any of the following:

- Sensation of unilateral nasal obstruction
- Persistent, foul-smelling rhinorrhea despite proper antibiotic treatment
- Persistent unilateral epistaxis

In addition to a nasal examination, a complete head and neck physical exam should also be performed. The ears should be carefully checked for foreign bodies, and the lungs auscultated for wheezing.

Treatment

If the child is cooperative and the foreign body visible, it is possible to remove the object in the emergency department. In small or uncooperative children, a papoose board may be used for patient restraint. The nasal mucosal is generally prepared with vasoconstrictors and anesthetics (1 cc of phenylephrine mixed with 3 cc of 4% xylocaine). In uncooperative children, aerosolized adrenaline (racemic epinephrine) can be used to decongest the nasal mucosa and loosen the foreign body.[9] When administered in the aerosolized form by the parent, it causes little or no distress to the child. Following this, visualization with an appropriate-sized nasal speculum is attempted.

If the object appears loose after vasoconstriction, an attempt to remove it can be made using a number of different techniques including:

- Positive pressure technique.
- Removal by a suction catheter.
- Grasping the object with bayonet or alligator forceps.
- Passing any blunt-hooked instrument beyond the object, rotating the instrument, and pulling the foreign body out.
- Passing a Fogarty vascular catheter past the foreign body, inflating the balloon and removing the catheter and foreign body.

The latter four techniques are all acceptable but require a cooperative child, or conscious sedation, to prevent damage to the nasal mucosa.

Regardless of the technique utilized, the airway must be protected and appropriate material for managing airway obstruction should be immediately available. The examiner should be careful not to advance the foreign body any deeper into the nasopharynx.

Positive Pressure Technique

The successful use of this method is well documented.[9–11] It can be performed in both cooperative and uncooperative patients, and it is less invasive. After vasoconstrictors, positive pressure can be applied by the patient, if cooperative, or the caregiver. The caregiver is instructed to give a puff of air to the mouth of the child while occluding the unobstructed nare with a finger. The foreign body is usually expressed from the nose onto the cheek of the caregiver. Repeated attempts may be necessary.

Disposition

Despite anxiety generated in the mind of the parent, most patients with nasal foreign bodies can be discharged home even if removal attempts are unsuccessful. Admission need only be considered if the patient exhibits constitutional symptoms such as fever, malaise, or lethargy. If attempts to remove the foreign body are unsuccessful, the patient should follow-up with an otolaryngologist within one to two days. If foreign body removal was successful, no further follow-up or treatment is required.

SINUSITIS

Acute sinusitis is defined as acute inflammation of the paranasal sinuses of less than three weeks duration. It has been reported to affect 14 percent of the population.[12] In 1992, direct medical costs of sinusitis reached almost $2.4 billion.[12] Despite the frequency of the disease, it often goes unrecognized or misdiagnosed. Once an accurate diagnosis has been made, appropriate treatment is essential to avoid the complications associated with acute sinusitis. Mastoid sinus disease is covered in Chap. 231.

Pathophysiology

There are six distinct nasal sinuses: two maxillary, two frontal, one sphenoidal, and the ethmoidal air cells. The biologic function of the paranasal sinuses remains unknown. Various hypotheses as to their function have been suggested, including humidification of air, pressure equalization, reduction in the weight of the skull, provision of vocal resonance and sound projection, and assisting in olfaction.

Sinusitis occurs when there is an acute obstruction of the normal drainage mechanisms of the sinuses. Efficiency of sinus drainage consists of three elements: ostial patency, ciliary apparatus function, and the quality of the nasal secretions. Although an alteration in any of these components can result in sinusitis, obstruction of the mucociliary drainage at the osteomeatal complex is generally accepted as the major cause.

Viral upper respiratory tract infections and allergic rhinitis are the most common initiating factors in sinusitis.[13] Edema from rhinitis causes obstruction at the osteomeatal complex, followed by reabsorption of the air in the sinus, that results in negative pressure. Negative pressure causes a collection of transudate within the sinus cavity. If bacteria are present, multiplication leads to suppuration. It is most commonly caused by *Streptococcus pneumoniae* in 37 percent, and *Haemophilus influenzae* in 38 percent of cases.[14] Other organisms seen in acute sinusitis include, in decreasing order of frequency, other haemophilus species, *Streptococcus pyogenes, Moraxella catarrhalis,* alpha streptococci, and gram-negative bacilli with mixed anaerobes.[14]

Chronic sinusitis results from unresolved acute sinusitis of more than three weeks duration. In chronic sinusitis, polymicrobial anaerobic species are found in over 50 percent of cases. The anaerobic bacteria of chronic sinusitis consist of peptostreptococcus in 22 percent and prevotella species in 15 percent of cases.[14] Decreasing in order of frequency, other species include bacteroides, *Propionibacterium,* and *Fusobacterium.*[14] A number of aerobic species are found in chronic sinusitis, including streptococci, *Staphylococcus aureus,* haemophilus species, and *M. catarrhalis.*[14] In pediatric cases with chronic sinusitis, bacteria are most likely to represent the pathogens of acute sinusitis.[14]

Nosocomial sinusitis is associated with nasotracheal or nasogasric tubes. It is frequently due to gram-negative bacilli, and is commonly mixed. *Pseudomonas aeruginosa* is seen in 48 percent of cases, followed by *Klebsiella* (28 percent), enterobacter species (28 percent), *Proteus mirabilis* (20 percent), *Escherichia coli* (12 percent), β-hemolytic strep (12 percent), bacteroides species (8 percent), and *S. aureus* (4 percent).[14] Pseudomonas is the predominant pathogen in individuals with cystic fibrosis, and is common in patients with nasal polyps.[14]

As many as 70 percent of HIV patients develop sinusitis. In addition to the usual pathogens, they may be infected with opportunistic bacteria, viruses, or fungi.[14] Consequently, cultures are essential in this subgroup.

Clinical Features

The classic symptoms of acute sinusitis include pain overlying the affected area, decreased sense of smell, fever, headache, and purulent nasal discharge. These symptoms are often difficult to differentiate from upper respiratory infection or allergic rhinitis, and have been found to be poor indicators of sinus infection. The best indicators of bacterial sinusitis are, in decreasing order of predictive value, maxillary toothache, mucopurulent discharge, poor response to nasal decongestants, and abnormal transillumination.[15,16] Although maxillary toothache is a good predictor of acute sinusitis, it is only found in 11 percent of patients with the disease.[15]

The presence of ethmoidal sinusitis usually causes the patient to complain of a dull, aching sensation behind the eye. Infection of the frontal and maxillary sinuses generally causes pain over the affected sinus. Ethmoidal sinusitis can spread to orbit, retroorbital area, and central nervous system. The headache seen in sinusitis is usually aggravated by bending forward, coughing, or sneezing, although these findings have poor sensitivity and specificity.[15]

Typically the physician may find tenderness to palpation and percussion over the involved sinus. Direct visualization of the nasal cavity may show swollen, erythematous mucosa with purulent exudate draining from the ostia. Diminished transillumination of the affected sinus is also seen. However, results regarding the sensitivity of the various techniques is conflicting, and there is a significant amount of interobserver variability.[16] The physical should include comprehensive head, neck, and neurologic system examination. It should be directed to specifically exclude indications of infectious spread beyond the sinus cavity, as well as complications and confounders in the differential diagnosis.

In the emergency department, acute sinusitis is generally a clinical diagnosis based on history and physical exam. Standard radiography can visualize the paranasal sinuses, but there is no consensus role for their use in emergency diagnosis. The most reliable radiographic signs include sinus opacity, air fluid levels, or at least 6 mm of mucosal thickening.

The primary role of CT is to diagnose sinusitis when the differential diagnosis is unclear and to define anatomy before surgery.[17] Only 62 percent of patients with sinus-related symptoms will have CT evidence of abnormality.[18] Interestingly, 16 percent of patients without sinus-related symptoms will have abnormalities on CT scanning.[18] Therefore, CT is not routinely indicated in the emergency department setting. It should be considered in immunosuppressed or toxic patients.

Cultures are not routinely required. However, they should be considered in patients with HIV, chronic immunosuppression (e.g., transplant patients), those who demonstrate any signs of infectious spread external to the sinus cavity, or in those who are systemically toxic.

Differential Diagnosis

The most important points to consider are those diagnoses arising as complications from sinusitis. These include any evidence of infectious extension from the sinus cavity, such as periorbital cellulitis, brain abscess, subdural empyema, meningitis, or cavernous sinus thrombosis. Such patients are febrile, extremely ill, may have unstable vital signs, can demonstrate altered mental status, meningismus, or focal neurologic findings. None of these symptoms are compatible with diagnosis of sinusitis. The history and physical should be structured such as to exclude these diagnoses.

The differential diagnosis of patients with signs and symptoms of facial pain includes tension headache, migraines, and cluster headache. Headache syndromes can usually be excluded based upon limited and historical evidence of an infectious process. Cluster and migraine headache patients usually have a history of similar headache, and sinusitis is never preceded by aura or other prodromal neurologic symptoms. Tension headache may exhibit trigger points and its distribution does not suggest sinusitis. Occasionally, however, the above disorders can coexist with sinusitis, making diagnosis more difficult.

Other diagnoses to consider include nasal polyp or foreign body. While a foreign object or polyp may cause purulent rhinorrhea, a physical exam localizing either can exclude sinusitis as the primary etiology of the discharge. Dental pain is usually localized to a single tooth, exquisitely sensitive to percussion, with little other symptoms to support the diagnosis of sinusitis. Likewise, temporomandibular syndrome may result in facial pain, but it is usually localized to the region of the temporomandibular joint, exacerbated by jaw movements, and has no associated infectious findings. Trigeminal neuralgia may cause facial pain. However, there is no evidence of infection, the symptoms are intermittent, and the pain character does not suggest sinusitis.

Finally, other diagnoses may mimic bacterial sinusitis. These include viral infection of the upper respiratory tract, nasal congestion, allergic rhinitis, and mucosal engorgement due to rebound following excessive topical decongestant use.

Treatment

Antimicrobial therapy reduces or eliminates bacteria in the maxillary sinus and improves symptoms in acute bacterial sinusitis.[19] Empiric therapy against the typical pathogens seen in acute sinusitis is usually appropriate. Timely treatment helps prevent complications.

Antibiotics usually recommended for the treatment of acute sinusitis in the outpatient environment include amoxicillin, amoxicillin-clavulanate, or erythromycin plus sulfonamide. Alternatives include third-generation cephalosporins, clarithromycin, azithromycin, doxycycline, or trimethoprim sulfamethoxazole.[14] In chronic sinusitis, recommended antibiotics include amoxicillin-clavulanate or ampicillin sulbactam. Alternatives include clindamycin, a cephalosporin plus metronidazole, or doxycycline.[14] When HIV or cystic fibrosis complicates the presentation, the initial choice of antibiotics is clindamycin in addition to ciprofloxacin. Alternatives include augmented penicillin plus ciprofloxacin or gentamicin.[14] The recommended duration of therapy varies. Most authorities recommend either 10-, 14-, or 21-day regimens.[14,20]

Over-the-counter nasal spray decongestants or antihistamines, such as pseudoephedrine, phenylephrine, oxymetazoline, and phenylpropanolamine, are commonly used, but there is scant literature to support the practice.[21–23] While some authors feel that decongestants are important in treatment, [23] there are unproven theoretical concerns that vasoconstrictors may impede mucociliary transport.[22,24] If topical decongestants are prescribed they should be of limited duration due to rebound mucosal congestion and edema if their use exceeds five to seven days.[23] Oral antihistamines may be of use in allergic rhinosinusitis.[23] However, in suppurative sinusitis, they may result in thickening of secretions, with crust formation, at the osteomeatal complex.[23] No superior therapeutic benefit of the newer nonsedating antihistamines has been documented in comparison to older sedating antihistamines.[23] While soporific side effects can be avoided with newer nonsedating antihistamines, they have the drawback of increased cost, and some have significant drug interactions (e.g., terfenadine or astemizole with macrolides or ketoconazole may cause ventricular dysrhythmias).[23]

Topical steroids have been shown to reduce local inflammation, thus increasing ostial drainage. However, there is inadequate data to justify their use in all patients with acute sinusitis. If allergic rhinitis is a significant contributing factor, corticosteroids may be indicated.

Complications

Persistent sinusitis can result in extension of the infectious process into the surrounding tissues. Bony destruction, originating from the frontal sinus, can extend anteriorly. This leads to the development of a doughy edematous forehead called Potts puffy tumor. If a frontal bone osteomyelitis extends posteriorly, a frontal brain abscess, meningitis, subdural empyema, or epidural abscess can develop. Extension from the ethmoid sinus can result in orbital or periorbital cellulitis. Finally, direct extension from the paranasal sinus to the venous or lymphatic system can cause cavernous sinus thrombosis. All patients suspected of having any infection extension of infection beyond the paranasal sinuses should undergo immediate CT scanning, intravenous antibiotic therapy, and emergent consultation with the appropriate specialist.

Disposition

Most patients with acute sinusitis can be treated as outpatients. Any patient demonstrating evidence of infectious spread beyond the sinus cavity should be admitted to the hospital, including patients who appear toxic, are febrile with neurologic signs, or have orbital/periorbital cellulitis.

Patients who are candidates for discharge should be advised to follow-up with their primary care physician or an otolaryngologist if their symptoms persist longer than 5 to 7 days despite appropriate treatment. Patients with evidence of chronic sinusitis (symptoms greater than three weeks) should follow-up with an otolaryngologist within 5 to 7 days. At discharge, they should be instructed to see their doctor promptly, or return to the emergency department if they develop uncontrolled fever, severe or worsening headache, vision changes, or persistent vomiting.

REFERENCES

1. Monux A, Tomas M, Kaiser C, Gavilon J: Conservation management of epistaxis. *J Laryngol Otol* 104:868, 1990.

2. Rubin J, Rood S, Myers E, Johnson J: The Management of Epistaxis. Self-Instructional Package. Alexandria, VA: American Academy of Otolaryngology-Head and Neck Surgery, 1990.
3. Viducich RA, Blanda MP, Gerson LW: Posterior epistaxis: Clinical features and acute complications. *Ann Emerg Med* 25(5):592, 1995.
4. DeWeese DD, Saunders W, Schuller D, Schleuning A II (eds): *Otolaryngology–Head and Neck Surgery*, 7th ed. St. Louis: CV Mosby, pp 113–124, 1988.
5. Elahi MM, Parnes LS, Fox AJ, et al: Therapeutic embolization in the treatment of intractable epistaxis. *Arch Otolaryngol Head Neck Surg* 121(1):65, 1995.
6. Baker O: Foreign bodies of the ears and nose in childhood. *Pediatr Emerg Care* 3:67, 1987.
7. Nondapalan V, McIlwain JC: Removal of nasal foreign bodies with a Fogarty biliary balloon catheter. *J Laryngol Otol* 108:758, 1994.
8. Tong MCF, Ying SY, van Hasselt CA: Nasal foreign bodies in children. *Int J Pediatr Otorhinolaryngol* 35:207, 1996.
9. Douglas AR: Use of nebulized adrenaline to aid expulsion of intranasal foreign bodies in children. *J Laryngol Otol* 110:559, 1996.
10. Backlin SA: Positive pressure technique for nasal foreign body removal. *Ann Emerg Med* 25(4):554, 1995.
11. Finkelstein JA: Oral Ambu-bag insufflation to remove unilateral nasal foreign bodies. *Am J Emerg Med* 14:157, 1996.
12. Kaliner MA, Osguthorpe JD, Fireman P, et al: Sinusitis: Bench to bedside current findings, future direction. *Arch Otolaryngol Head Neck Surg* 116:51, 1997.
13. Gwaltney JM Jr: Sinusitis, in Mandell RG Jr, Bennett JE (eds): *Principles and Practice of Infectious Diseases*, 3rd ed. New York, Churchill Livingstone, 1990, pp 510–514.
14. Fairbanks DN: *Antimicrobial Therapy in Otolaryngology—Head and Neck Surgery*, 8th ed. American Academy of Otolaryngology—Head and Neck Surgery Foundation, 1996.
15. Williams JW Jr, Simel DL: Does this patient have sinusitis? Diagnosing acute sinusitis by history and physical examination. *JAMA* 270:1242, 1993.
16. Williams JW, Simel DL, Roberts LR, et al: Clinical evaluation of sinusitis. *Ann Intern Med* 117:705, 1992.
17. Diaz I, Bamberger DM: Acute sinusitis seminars. *Respir Infec* 10(7):14, 1995.
18. Calhoun KH, Waggenspack GA, Simpson CB, et al: CT evaluation of the paranasal sinuses in symptomatic and asymptomatic populations. *Arch Otolaryngol Head Neck Surg* 104:480, 1991.
19. Gwaltney JM Jr: State-of-the-art: Acute community-acquired sinusitis. *Clin Infect Dis* 23:1209, 1996.
20. Williams JW, Holleman OR Jr, Samsa GP, et al: Randomized controlled trial of 3 vs 10 days of trimethoprim/sulfamethoxzole for acute maxillary sinusitis. *JAMA* 273(13):1015, 1995.
21. Malm L: Pharmacological background to decongesting and anti-inflammatory treatment of rhinitis and sinusitis [Review]. *Acta Otolaryngol Suppl (Stockh)* 515:55, 1994.
22. McCormick DP, John SD, Swischuk LE, Uchida T: A double-blind, placebo-controlled trial of decongestant-antihistamine for the treatment of sinusitis in children. *Clin Pediatr (Phila)* 35(9):457, 1996.
23. Mabry RL: Therapeutic agents in the medical management of sinusitis [Review]. *Otolaryngol Clin North Am* 26(4):561, 1993.
24. Min YG, Kim HS, Suh SH, et al: Paranasal sinusitis after long-term use of topical nasal decongestants. *Acta Otolaryngol (Stockh)* 116(3):465, 1996.

ORAL AND DENTAL EMERGENCIES

Ronald W. Beaudreau

Although few life-threatening dental emergencies occur, oral and dental complaints commonly result in emergency department (ED) visits in the United States. Oral emergencies generally can be divided into three categories: (1) orofacial pain, (2) orofacial trauma, specifically dentoavleolar trauma, and (3) hemorrhage. Early manifestations of many systemic illnesses are evident in the oral environment and may provide clues to the diagnosis of systemic illnesses. Oral lesions may cause pain or anxiety, and it is important that the emergency physician be familiar with common oral pathology and its management. An understanding of dental anatomy and the attachment apparatus is essential for the recognition and management of oral disease.

ORAL AND DENTAL ANATOMY

The normal adult dentition consists of 32 permanent teeth. The adult dentition has four types of teeth: 8 incisors, 4 canines, 8 premolars, and 12 molars. The primary or deciduous dentition consists of 20 teeth of three types: 8 incisors, 4 canines, and 8 molars. Figure 234-1 shows the eruptive pattern of both the primary and permanent dentition. *Agenesis,* or lack of formation of a tooth or teeth, especially maxillary lateral incisors and third molars, is not uncommon. Likewise, extra or *supernumerary teeth* are not uncommon. Each tooth type is designed for a specific function in the process of mastication. Incisors are used for biting and cutting, canines and premolars for ripping, and molars for grinding. Figure 234-2 illustrates one commonly used tooth numbering system; however, description by the emergency physician of the tooth type and location is appropriate. Mastication is an important initial step in the digestive process and thus nutrition. The dentition is also important in the development of the mandible and maxilla and aesthetic development of the midface.

Anatomy of the Teeth

A basic understanding of dental anatomy is important in understanding dental disease. Table 234-1 lists commonly used dental nomenclature. A tooth consists largely of *dentin,* which surrounds the *pulp,* or neurovascular supply of the tooth (Fig. 234-3). Dentin is a homogeneous material produced by pulpal odontoblasts throughout life. It is deposited as a system of microtubules filled with odontoblastic processes and extracellular fluid. The *crown,* or portion of the tooth that is visible, consists of a thick *enamel* layer overlying the dentin. Enamel, the hardest substance in the human body, consists largely of hydroxyapatite and is produced by ameloblasts prior to eruption of the tooth into the mouth. The *root* portion of the tooth extends into the alveolar bone and is covered with a thin layer of *cementum.*

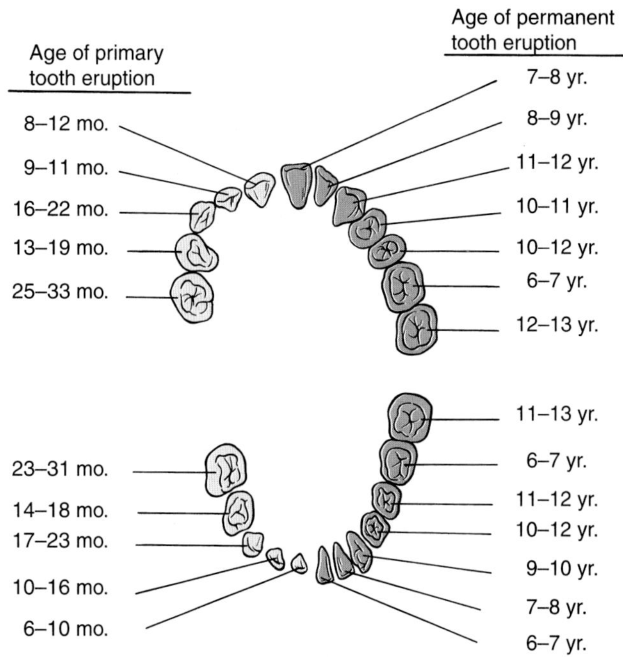

FIG. 234-1. Normal eruptive patterns of the primary and permanent dentition.

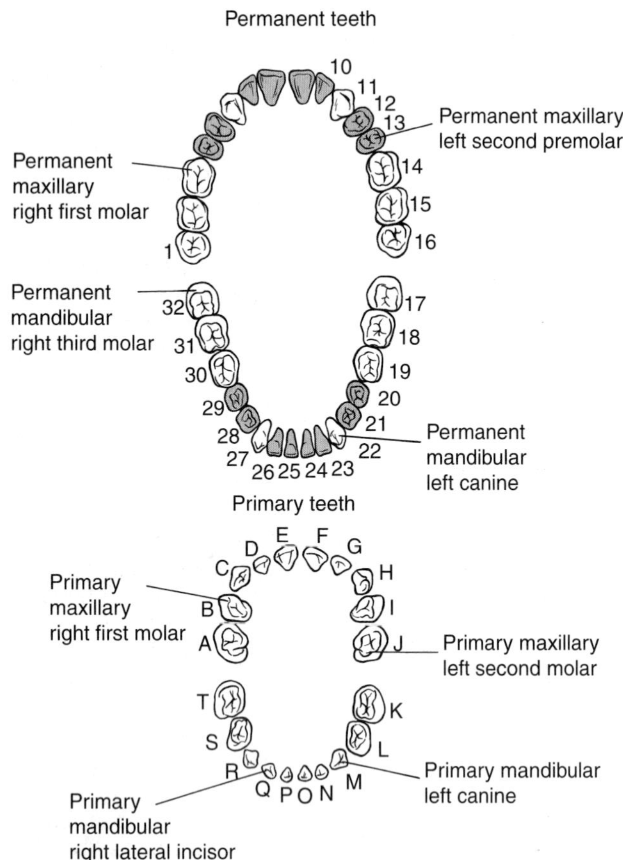

FIG. 234-2. Identification of teeth.

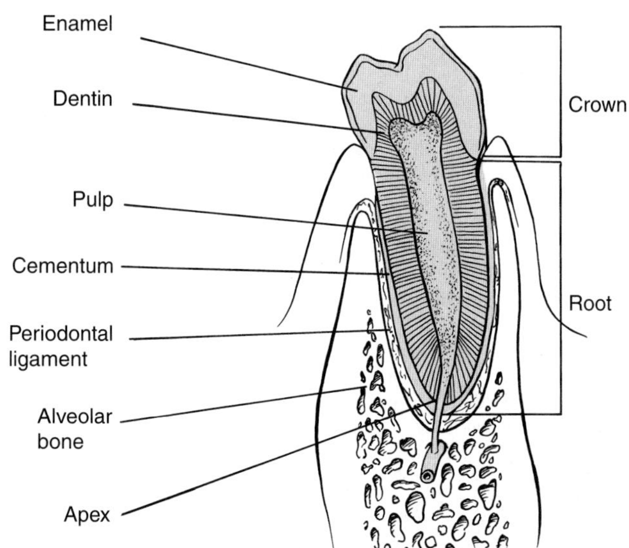

FIG. 234-3. The dental anatomic unit and attachment apparatus.

The Normal Periodontium

The periodontium, or attachment apparatus, is essential for maintaining the integrity of the dentoalveolar unit. The attachment apparatus consists of a gingival component and a periodontal component. The gingival component includes the junctional epithelium, gingival tissue, and gingival fibers. The periodontal component includes the periodontal ligament, alveolar bone, and cementum of the root of the tooth. The periodontal ligament consists of collagen fibers that extend from the alveolar bone to the root of the tooth, adhering to the cementum via a hemidesmosomal attachment. The latter component forms the majority of the attachment apparatus, and the former aids primarily in maintaining the integrity of the periodontal ligament. Disease states such as gingivitis and periodontal disease weaken and destroy the attachment apparatus, resulting in tooth mobility and tooth loss.[1]

Gingival tissue is keratinized stratified squamous epithelium. It can be divided into the free gingival margin and the attached gingiva. The free gingiva is the portion that forms the 2- to 3-mm-deep *gingival sulcus* in the disease-free state. The attached gingiva adheres firmly to the underlying alveolar bone and extends to the oral vestibule and floor of the mouth. There the tissue becomes nonkeratinized *alveolar mucosa.* This nonkeratinized tissue covers the mucosal surface of the cheeks, lips, and floor of the mouth.[1]

TABLE 234-1 Commonly Used Dental Terminology

Anatomically descriptive terms for tooth surfaces	
Interproximal	The surfaces between two adjacent teeth
Mesial	The interproximal surface facing anteriorly or toward the midline
Distal	The interproximal surface facing posteriorly or away from the midline
Occlusal	The chewing surface
Facial	Toward the face, a general term applicable to all teeth
Labial	Toward the lips, specific to anterior teeth
Buccal	Toward the cheek, specific to posterior teeth
Palatal	Toward the palate, specific to maxillary teeth
Lingual	Toward the tongue, specific to mandibular teeth
Apical	Toward the tip of the root of the tooth
Radicular	Associated with the root, especially the apical region
Coronal	Toward the crown of the tooth
Incisal	Toward the biting edge of incisors
Cervical	Related to the junction of the crown and root of the tooth

OROFACIAL PAIN

Pain of Odontogenic Origin

TOOTH ERUPTION Discomfort is commonly associated with the eruption of primary or deciduous teeth in infants. Irritability, drooling, and decreased intake are commonly associated findings. An associated low-grade fever (37.9°C) and diarrhea are more controversial findings. No scientific data support an association of teething, fever, and diarrhea. It is plausible that mild dehydration from excessive salivary production or a decrease in intake may result in a low-grade fever, and changes in feeding habits may result in diarrhea. One must be careful in attributing either to tooth eruption. Other sources for fever must be carefully sought.[2] Other common causes of orofacial pain are listed in Table 234-2.

As with the primary dentition, eruption of permanent teeth, especially third molars, or *wisdom teeth,* may result in significant pain. Gingival irritation and inflammation associated with tooth eruption are common and must be distinguished from *pericoronitis.* Pericoronitis, although usually associated with the eruption of third molars, can be associated with any tooth. Gingival tissue overlying the occlusal surface of an erupting tooth, or *operculum,* progressively becomes inflamed secondary to impaction of food and debris beneath the operculum. Direct trauma from opposing teeth during mastication compounds the inflammatory process. Normal gingival irritation associated with tooth eruption is replaced by a progressive inflammatory process re-

TABLE 234-2 The Differential Diagnosis of Orofacial Pain

Odontogenic origin	
Dental caries	Pericoronitis
Reversible pulpitis	Postrestorative pain
Irreversible pulpitis	Postextraction discomfort
Pulpal necrosis and abscess	Postextraction alveolar osteitis
Dentinal sensitivity	Bruxism
Tooth eruption	Cervical erosion
Periodontal pathology	
Gingivitis	Periodontal abscess
Periodontal disease	Acute necrotizing gingivostomatitis
Orofacial trauma	
Dental fractures:	Facial fractures
Subtle enamel cracks	Alveolar ridge fractures
Ellis fractures	Soft tissue lacerations
Dental luxation and avulsion	Traumatic ulcers
Infection	
Oral candidiasis	Hand, foot, and mouth disease
Herpes simplex types 1 and 2	Sexually transmitted diseases
Varicella-zoster, primary and secondary	Mycobacterial infections
Herpangina	Mumps
Malignancies	
Squamous cell carcinoma	Leukemia
Kaposi's sarcoma	Graft-versus-host disease
Lymphoma	Melanoma
Other etiologies	
Cranial neuralgias	Ulcerative disease:
Stomatitis and mucositis:	Lichen planus
Uremia	Cicatricial pemphigoid
Vitamin deficiency	Pemphigus vulgaris
Other	Erythema multiforme
Erythema migrans	Crohn's disease
Pyogenic granuloma	Behçet's syndrome

sulting in frank infection. Because of the close proximity of the masseteric space to third molars, associated trismus is common and portends the potential for extension into the communicating parapharyngeal spaces. Treatment consist of appropriate antibiotic therapy with penicillin VK 500 mg qid, erythromycin 250 mg qid, or clindamycin 300 mg qid, local irrigation of food and debri from underneath the operculum, saline mouth rinses, and analgesic therapy with nonsteroidal anti-inflammatory drugs (NSAIDs) and narcotic preparations as appropriate. Referral to a general dentist or an oral and maxillofacial surgeon within 24 to 48 h is essential. If pericoronitis is related to trauma from an opposing tooth, as is frequently the case with third molars, concomitant extraction of the opposing tooth and antibiotic therapy will bring marked relief within 24 h.[3] Definitive treatment is extraction of the associated tooth by a general dentist or oral and maxillofacial surgeon.

DENTAL CARIES AND PULPAL PATHOLOGY *Dental caries* represents the loss of integrity of the tooth enamel secondary to dissolution of hydroxyapatite from prolonged exposure to the acidic metabolic by-products of plaque bacteria. Caries most commonly occurs in areas where plaque accumulates such as pits and fissures of the occlussal surface, interproximally, and along the gingival margins. When a sufficient breach of enamel integrity has occurred, sensitivity to cold or sweet stimulus may result. With dentinal involvement, caries progression occurs more rapidly, spreading along dentinal microtubules. At this stage, direct communication between the oral environment and the vital dental pulp has been established, and inflammatory changes in the pulpal tissue are evident histologically.

The pulpal inflammatory process is initially reversible, but with continued stimuli, the pulp's ability to respond and repair is jeopardized. *Irreversible pulpitis* can be distinguished from *reversible pulpitis* by the duration of symptoms. Both require a stimulus to initiate a painful response; however, in reversible pulpitis, the duration of pain is short, lasting seconds, as compared with irreversible pulpitis, in which the pain may last for minutes to hours. The most common stimulus is thermal, although sweet or sour stimulus also can elicit a painful response. Spontaneous odontogenic pain most frequently represents pulpal death or necrosis. Pain elicited with heat stimulus is most commonly associated with pulpal necrosis, but some painful response to heat with irreversible or irreversible pulpitis may occur. Distinguishing where a particular tooth falls on the continuum is impractical for the emergency physician. Treatment focuses on providing adequate analgesia and referral to a general dentist. The definitive treatment for irreversible pulpitis and pulpal necrosis is root canal therapy or dental extraction.[4,5]

PERIRADICULAR PATHOLOGY The most common cause of severe odontogenic pain is periapical pathology. *Periapical granuloma,* more appropriately termed *periradicular periodontitis,* is the most common periapical lesion. This lesion is not a true granuloma but rather slowly expanding granulation tissue associated with the root apex. Most commonly, periradicular periodontitis is a result of pulpal inflammation or necrosis, but it can be associated with trauma. *Periapical* or *radicular cyst* and *periradicular abscess* are clinically and radiographically identical lesions to periradicular periodontitis. A periapical cyst has an epithelial lining originating embryologically from the rest of Malassez, and a periradicular abscess represents the accumulation of associated inflammatory cell. All three lesions are only associated with the apical region of teeth with severely inflammed or necrotic pulps and may cause significant pain. Radiographically, these periapical lesions appear as a slight widening of the periodontal ligament space, thinning of the lamina dura, or a frank radiolucent area associated with the apex on a periapical dental radiograph (Fig. 234-4). Radiographic evaluation with a panorex is rarely useful for identification of all but the most extensive periradicular lesions but can be important in identifying more significant painful osseous pathology. Erosion of a periradicular abscess through the cortical bone results in subperosteal extension with intraoral or facial swelling and fluctuance. A small swelling of the gingiva with a draining fistula adjacent to the affected tooth is known as a *parulis.*[4,5]

Pain of dental origin may be diffuse in nature, presenting as a headache, sinus pain, eye pain, or jaw or neck pain or may be localized to a single tooth. One must remember to consider myocardial infarction as an etiology of jaw pain. Identification of the offending tooth is best accomplished by eliciting pain with percussion of the suspected teeth with a dental mirror handle or similar metallic object. Definitive treatment of periradicular periodontitis, periapical cysts, and abscesses is root canal therapy or extraction of the affected tooth. This, however, is not prudent in the ED. Subperiosteal extension and the resulting fluctuant abscess should be incised and drained orally. The emergency physician should treat dental abscesses or other periapical lesions with oral antibiotics such as penicillin VK 500 mg qid, clindamycin 300 mg qid, or erythromycin 500 mg qid and provide adequate analgesia with an NSAID. Narcotic analgesia may be indicated in the first 24 to 48 h. Prompt referral to a dentist for definitive treatment such as root canal therapy or extraction is indicated.[4,5]

FACIAL CELLULITIS Spread of odontogenic infections into the various facial tissue spaces is relatively common. Buccal extension of a periapical infection of the mandibular teeth will involve the buccinator space. Maxillary labial extension of infection primarily will involve the infraorbital space. Perforation through the lingual cortical bone of mandibular molars, particularly the second and third molars, usually occurs below the mylohyoid ridge, affecting the submandibular space. Lingual

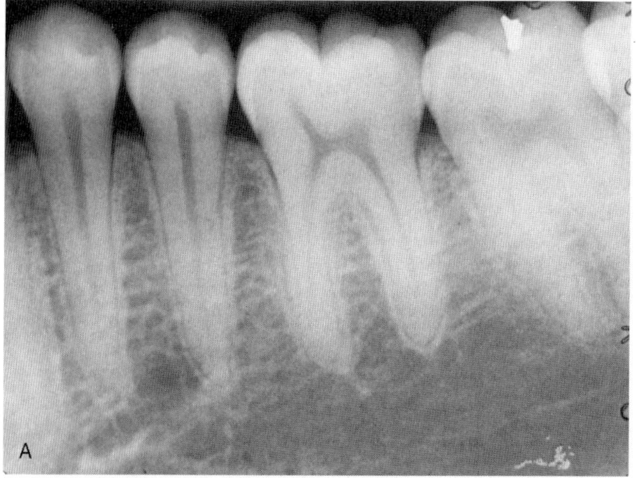

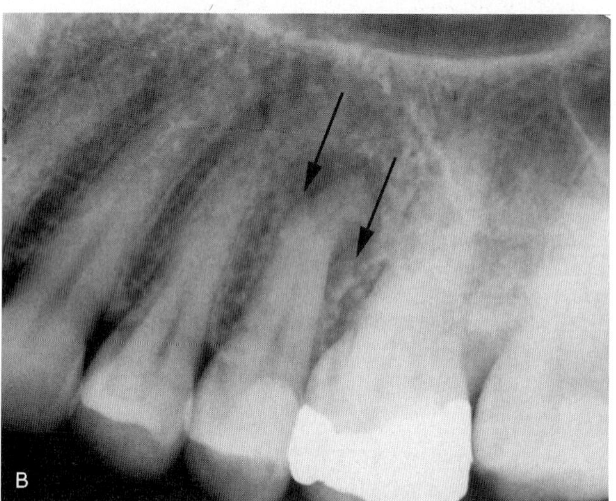

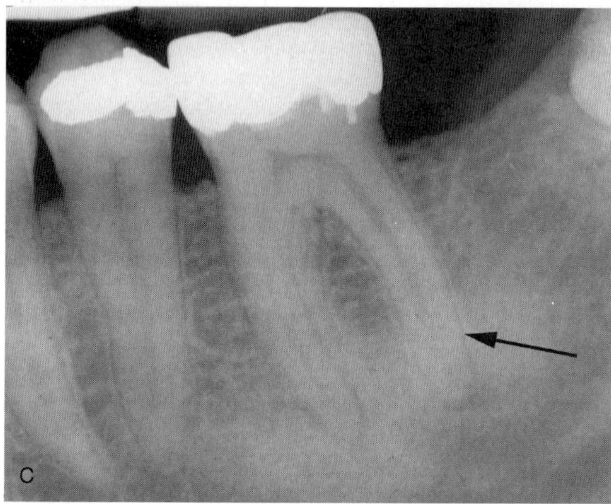

FIG. 234-4. A. The radiographic appearance of a healthy tooth with a normal periodontal ligament space and distinct lamina dura compared with the radiographic appearance of a periapical abscess, periradicular periodontis, and periradicular cyst. **B.** A frank periapical radiolucency. **C.** Subtle radiographic loss of the periapical lamina dura and widening of the periodontal ligament space. (*Courtesy of Gary M. Beaudreau, D.M.D.*)

spread of periapical infections associated with mandibular anterior teeth will affect the lingual space. The submandibular space and lingual space communicate with each other at the posterior border of the mylohyoid muscle.

Cellulitis of bilateral submandibular spaces and the lingual space is called *Ludwig's angina* and is potentially life threatening. Clinically, Ludwig's angina is a rapidly spreading cellulitis that results in brawny induration of the suprahyoid region and elevation of the tongue. Involvement of the floor of the mouth pushes the tongue posteriorly. Epiglottic involvement is not uncommon. As a result, airway compromise is the immediate primary concern. The primary focus of initial management is maintenance of a patent airway. Timely administration of high-dose penicillin and metronidazole or cefoxitin is essential. An aminoglycoside may be added to extend coverage, and in the penicillin-sensitive person, clindamycin may be substituted. Immediate oral and maxillofacial surgical consultation and hospitalization for incision and drainage and intubation as indicated are necessary.[6]

Infection of the infraorbital space may have a potentially devastating outcome if retrograde spread via the ophthalmic veins occurs, and the cavernous sinus becomes involved. *Cavernous sinus thrombosis* presents as an infraorbital or periorbital cellulitis with rapidly developing meningeal signs, sepsis, and coma. Early recognition and treatment with high-dose intravenous antibiotic as above are essential in decreasing morbidity and mortality.

POSTEXTRACTION ALVEOLAR OSTEITIS Pain in the initial 24 to 48 h after dental extraction, termed *periosteitis,* is common and responds well to analgesics. Depending on the tooth removed, density of the bone, and amount of associated trauma that occurred during extraction, significant discomfort can occur. *Postextraction alveolar osteitis,* or *dry socket,* usually occurs on the second or third postoperative day and is associated with exquisite oral pain. Dislodgment of the clot from the socket or fibrinolytic dissolution of the clot results in exposure of the alveolar bone to the oral environment. This initiates an inflammatory response resulting in a localized osteomyelitis of the exposed bone. A higher incidence of dry sockets has been identified in females on hormone replacement therapy probably secondary to increased plasmin fibrinolytic activity as a result of exogenous estrogens. Other risk factors for developing postextraction alveolar osteitis include smoking, preexisting pericoronitis or periodontal disease, traumatic extractions, and a prior history of alveolar osteitis.[7,8]

The incidence of postextraction alveolar osteitis is 2 to 5 percent of all extractions but is considerably higher (20–35 percent) among impacted third molar extractions. Many studies have shown that topical antibiotic placement such as tetracycline or clindamycin at the time of surgery or chlorhexidine mouth rinses after extraction reduce by nearly tenfold the incidence of dry sockets. Dental radiographs should be taken to ensure the absence of a retained root tip or other foreign body. Thorough irrigation of the dental socket with sterile normal saline and packing it with oil of cloves– or eugenol-impregnated gauze results in an almost immediate improvement in level of comfort. Dental anesthesia may be necessary to adequately irrigate and pack a dry socket. Antibiotic therapy is indicated in the most severe cases, and daily packing changes are important. Thus referral to a dentist within 24 h is indicated.[7,8]

Managing postoperative dentoalveolar sequelae is in the realm of emergency medicine. Postoperative pain is a common presentation. Pain immediately postoperative is most commonly related to the trauma of surgery. Providing adequate analgesia is important in these patients. Postoperative edema such as with extraction of third molars is best managed with ice packs and elevation of the head of the bed to 30°. Most oral and maxillofacial surgeons premedicate patients with Decadron in complex cases to minimize swelling. Swelling normally peaks in the first 24 to 48 h. Trismus is common postoperatively and can result from infection, direct injury to the temporomandibular joint, injury to the muscles of mastication during administration of the inferior alveolar nerve block or during the surgery, and most commonly, normal perioperative inflammation. Trismus peaks in the first 24 h and usually decreases thereafter unless an infective process is the etiology. Postoperative trismus should resolve entirely by 1 week. If trismus persists, stretching exercises usually are initiated by the oral and maxillofacial surgeon.[9]

DENTINAL SENSITIVITY Improper tooth brushing techniques may result in cervical erosion and abrasion, recession of the gingival tissue, and exposure of the root surface to the oral environment. In this setting, teeth may be very sensitive to cold stimulus. Microscopic or macroscopic fractures of the enamel also will result in pain on cold stimulus or mastication. Avoidance of the inciting stimulus is recommended. There are several therapies available to a dentist such as topical flouride application or restorative repair of areas of significant toothbrush abrasion that may be helpful.[3]

POSTRESTORATIVE PAIN Pain may occur after a dental restorative procedure. Trauma from mechanical instrumentation of the tooth or direct exposure of the pulpal tissue during instrumentation may result in pain. Pain associated primarily with mastication may be a result of improper occlusion of the new restoration. Analgesia and referral to the patient's general dentist are the treatment of choice. After endodontic therapy, patients may experience exquisite pain secondary to instrumentation or a buildup of gaseous pressure in the pulp chamber and may require a dentist to reopen the tooth because analgesics may be inaffective.

Periodontal Pathology

PERIODONTAL DISEASE Gingival inflammation and bleeding, or *gingivitis,* results from the accumulation of plaque along the gingival margins. Hormonal variations of puberty, adolescence, and pregnancy, as well as many medications such as phenytoin, also may result in gingival inflammation. As the inflammatory process progresses, destruction of the attachment apparatus occurs, and the gingival sulcus deepens, resulting in periodontal pockets and *periodontitis.* Periodontal pockets create a favorable environment for plaque accumulation, maturation, and mineralization into *calculus.* Further destruction of the periodontal attachment results. Eventually, sufficient bone loss causes tooth mobility and tooth loss.[1,10]

The pathogenesis of periodontal disease is uncertain, but there is a very strong association between adult periodontitis and *Bacteroides gingivalis.* Many other specific bacteria have been shown to have a role in periodontitis. Destruction of tissue collagens, proteoglycans, and the connective tissue matrix is a major feature of gingivitis and periodontitis. Three theories for the etiology of this destruction have been proposed. Tissue destruction may occur as a result of the direct effects of bacterial plaque and their metabolic products, an accelerated host immune response, or immune deficiencies involving neutrophil function or the autologous mixed lymphocyte response.[1,10]

Four distinctive types of periodontal disease have been identified. These include adult, rapidly progressing, juvenile, and prepubertal periodontitis.[10] Etiology, age and sex predilection, and clinical course of disease vary by type. A definite association between juvenile periodontitis and *Actinobacillus actinomycetemcomitans* exists. More severe and rapidly progressing periodontitis, especially those types affecting a younger population such as the prepubertal and juvenile periodontitis, appears to be associated with decreased neutrophil chemotaxis or phagocytosis. Systemic illnesses such as human immunodeficiency virus (HIV) infection, diabetes, lazy leukocyte syndrome, Down syndrome, and cyclic neutropenia are associated with severe periodontal disease.[1]

Periodontal disease is the most common cause of tooth loss today. It usually progresses painlessly but may present as gingival bleeding or tender, swollen ginigval tissue. Treatment is directed at slowing or arresting the progression of disease primarily by the removal of plaque and its by-products.[1] Antibiotics may play a role in treatment. Referral to a dentist for definitive treatment is indicated because the treatment involves extensive dental cleaning, instruction and improvement in oral hygiene, and periodontal surgery in some cases.

PERIODONTAL ABSCESS When plaque and debris are entrapped in the periodontal pocket, a periodontal abscess may form, resulting in severe pain. Small periodontal abscesses respond to local therapy with warm saline rinses and antibiotics such as penicillin VK 500 mg PO qid or erythromycin 250 mg PO qid. Larger periodontal abscesses require incision and drainage. Saline mouth rinses four times a day are useful. Analgesics are essential.

ACUTE NECROTIZING ULCERATIVE GINGIVITIS Acute necrotizing ulcerative gingivitis (ANUG) is an aggressively destructive process (Fig. 234-5). Also known as *Vincent's disease* or *trench mouth,* it is part of a spectrum of disease ranging from localized ulceration of the gingiva to often fatal noma, in which localized ulceration and necrosis spread to the adjacent tissues of the cheeks, lips, and underlying facial bones.[11,12] ANUG is also related to Vincent's angina or tonsilar ulceration and necrosis. The diagnostic triad includes pain, ulcerated or "punched out" interdental papillae, and gingival bleeding. Secondary signs include fetid breath, pseudomembrane formation, "wooden teeth" feeling, foul metallic taste, tooth mobility, lymphadenopathy, fever, and malaise.[12,13]

The differential diagnosis for ANUG is quite extensive, but herpes gingivostomatitis is most difficult to differentiate. Herpes gingivostomatitis usually has smaller vesicular eruptions, less bleeding, more systemic signs, and lack of interdental papilla involvement.[12,13]

The etiology of ANUG is still poorly understood, but three patterns of disease have been clearly identified: the malnourished child pattern, the young adult stress pattern, and the HIV-positive adult pattern. It appears to be an opportunistic infection in a host with lowered resistence. It is believed that suppression of the humoral and cell-mediated immune response in HIV infection, severe malnourishment, and perhaps stress are responsible for this lowered host resistence. Anaerobic bacteria such as *Treponema, Selenomonas, Fusobacterium,* and *Prevotella* are uniformly identified. These bacteria appear to invade otherwise healthy tissue, resulting in an aggressively destructive disease process.[12,13]

The most important predisposing factor is HIV infection. Previous necrotizing gingivitis infection is the second most important predisposer. Other contributing factors include poor oral hygiene, unusual emotional stress, poor diet, inadequate sleep, Caucasian heritage, age

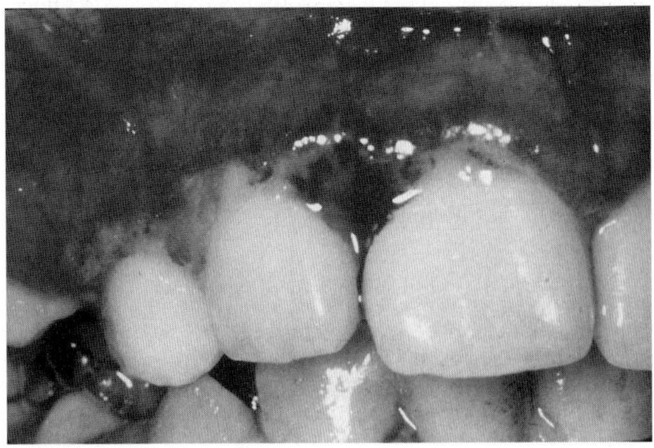

FIG. 234-5. Acute necrotizing ulcerative gingivitis. (*Courtesy of Philip J. Hanes, D.D.S.*)

less than 21 years, poor socioeconomic status, recent illness, alcohol use, tobacco use, acatalasia, and various infections such as malaria, measles, and intestinal parasites.[12,13]

The treatment is threefold. Primarily, identification and resolution of the predisposing factors are essential. Bacterial control using chlorhexidine oral rinses twice daily, professional debridement and scaling by a dentist, and adjunctive antibiotic therapy with metronidazole 250 mg tid are the mainstay of treatment.[12] A significant reduction in pain can be expected within 24 h of institution of this regimen.[3] Finally, supportive therapy with a soft diet rich in protein and vitamins and plenty of fluids is important in establishing and maintaining a disease-free state.[12]

Cranial Neuralgias

Trigeminal neuralgia is the most common of the cranial neuralgias. Others include postherpetic neuralgia, glossopharyngeal and vagal neuralgia, and superior laryngeal neuralgia. All these are far less common. Trigeminal neuralgia is undoubtedly one of the most painful presentations involving the face.[14]

Trigeminal neuralgia affects adults 30 to 60 years of age most commonly. Females constitute 60 percent of the patients. Patients report recurrent episodes of excruciating paroxysmal pain of short duration separated by pain-free periods. Painful episodes have been described as stabbing in nature resembling a severe electric shock. Contraction of the facial and masticatory muscles during an episode is characteristic, resulting in the term *tic douloureux*. Physical stimulation of a trigger point is the usual inciting event. Trigeminal neuralgia is almost always unilateral, following the anatomic distribution of the involved cranial nerve. The maxillary branch of the fifth cranial nerve is most commonly affected.[14]

The pathogenesis of trigeminal neuralgia is still unknown. The two prevailing theories include the vascular compression theory and the demyelination theory. Neither adequately explains the disease. Diagnosis is based on clinical presentation. Since 3 percent of patients with trigeminal neuralgia have multiple sclerosis, referral to a neurologist is essential. Comprehensive examination of the head and neck is required to eliminate organic pathology such as acoustic neuroma or a nasopharyngeal carcinoma.[14]

Trigeminal neuralgia may respond well to the administration of carbamazepine (100 mg/bid initially and gradually increasing as needed to a maximum dose of 1200 mg daily). Surgery is reserved for patients who do not respond to medications.[14]

Nonparoxysmal pain of neuropathic origin may develop (1) in patients who have had long-standing neuralgias, (2) secondary to surgical trauma along the distribution of the affected nerve branch, and (3) in association with viral infections, drugs, or heavy metal intoxication. Other neuropathies such as alcoholic and diabetic sensory neuropathies also may affect the oral cavity.

SOFT TISSUE LESIONS OF THE ORAL CAVITY

Lesions of the oral mucosa are common and, when symptomatic or noticed by patients, may require identification and treatment by the emergency physician. Treatment depends on the appropriate diagnosis. Thus familiarization with common oral pathology is important.

Oral Candidiasis

Candidiasis commonly affects the oral cavity. Nearly 60 percent of healthy adults harbor candidal microorganisms. Concurrent histologic evidence of tissue invasion and clinical manifestations of candidal infections are the primary means for diagnosing oral candidiasis. Many predisposing factors influence the development of oral candidiasis. These include the extremes of age, intraoral prosthetic devices such as dentures, malnourished states, associated mucosal disorders, concurrent infections, antibiotics, and immunocompromised conditions such as acquired immunodeficiency syndrome (AIDS), transplant recipients, radiation therapy, and chronic immunosuppressive therapy. Three oral clinical types have been described. The most common type is the psuedomembranous type with white, curdlike plaques. These plaques can be easily scraped off to reveal an underlying erythematous mucosal base. The second type is atrophic or erythematous and usually involves the dorsum of the tongue. Atrophy of the filiform papillae is seen. Finally, the lesions of hyperplastic candidiasis are raised white plaques that can only be partially removed with scraping due to deeper infiltration into the underlying tissue. Perioral candidiasis also may occur and is commonly seen as angular cheiltis or scaling patches of the perioral facial tissues. Treatment is with topical oral antifungal agents such as nystatin oral suspension 500,000 units qid or systemic agents such as fluconizole 200 mg bid.[11,15,16]

Aphthous Stomatitis

Aphthous stomatitis or ulceration is one of the most common oral lesions, affecting 20 percent of the normal population (Fig. 234-6). Although uncertain, significant evidence suggests that the etiology appears to be a cell-mediated immune response to a yet unidentified triggering agent. Three etiologic factors are known to predispose aphthous ulcer formation: an immune imbalance, a breach in the mucosal barrier, and an allergic response. Aphthous ulceration involves the nonkeratinized epithelium, especially the labial and buccal mucosa, and begins as an erythematous macule that ulcerates and forms a central fibropurulent eschar. Lesions measure from 2 to 3 mm to several centimeters in diameter, are painful, and frequently are multiple. They usually resolve spontaneously in 10 to 14 days. Aphthous stomatitis occurs in a major and minor form. The major form has larger, deeper ulcers that take up to 6 weeks to heal. A third form called *herpetiforme apthae* have up to 100 ulcers each 1 to 2 mm in diameter and take 7 to 10 days to heal. Treatment consist of topical corticosteroids such as betamethasone syrup or 0.01% dexamethasone elixir as a mouth rinse. Fluocinonide 0.05% gel applied topically to isolated lesions is acceptable. Resolution typically occurs 2 days after therapy. Aphthous major is more resistant to therapy and may require intralesional steroid injection or systemic steroid therapy.[16,17]

Herpes Simplex

Herpes simplex type 1 most commonly affects the oral cavity. Herpes simplex type 2 can occur orally and will be discussed later. The primary infection, herpes gingivostomatitis, causes acute painful ulcerations on the gingiva and mucosal surfaces. Fever and lymphadenopathy are commonly associated findings and may occur up to 3 days prior to

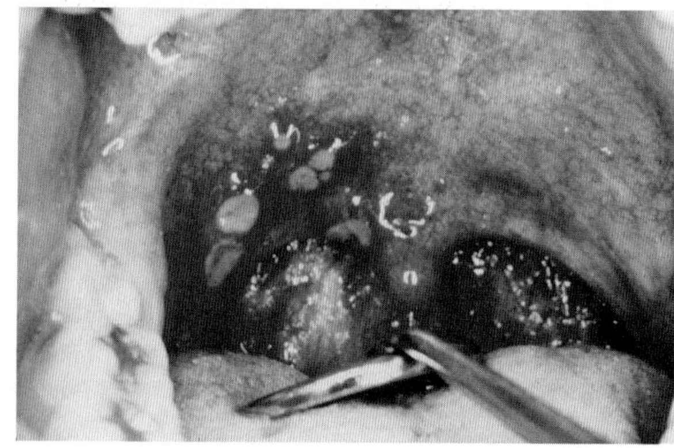

FIG. 234-6. Apthous stomatitis. (*Courtesy of Baldev Singh, B.D.S., Ph.D.*)

the appearance of oral lesions. Vesicular lesions appear and rupture after 1 to 2 days, leaving painful ulcers that heal gradually over 1 to 2 weeks. Secondary infection affects mostly the lips but may affect the hard palate and attached gingiva. By adulthood, most of the population has been exposed to herpes simplex type 1. The virus is harbored in sensory ganglion such as the gasserian ganglion of the trigeminal nerve. Periodic stresses activate the virus from its normally dormant state and allow for infection along the sensory distribution of the affected nerve. A prodrome of burning or tingling frequently occurs 1 to 2 days preceding outbreak of the characteristic vesicular lesion. Vesicles rupture within 2 to 3 days, forming small, shallow ulcers that heal in 6 to 10 days. Treatment is usually palliative; however, antiviral therapy with acyclovir 400 mg tid or valacyclovir 500 mg bid for 5 days initiated during the prodromal phase lessens the severity and duration of the ulceration.[11,16]

Varicella-Zoster

The varicella-zoster virus causes chickenpox in its primary infection, resulting in the typical vesicular eruption. It occurs most commonly in childhood but may affect patients at any age. The rash begins on the face and trunk, spreading to involve the entire body over the course of several days. Fever, malaise, pharyngitis, and rhinitis are associated. Vesicular involvement of the oropharynx is common and may precede skin involvement. Treatment is palliative, although special care in maintaining adequate hydration is important when oral lesions are present.

Herpes zoster, a latent infection of varicella, typically begins with a 1- to 4-day prodrome of exquisite pain in the area innvervated by the affected nerve. Although more commonly found on the trunk, herpes zoster may occur in the distribution of the trigeminal nerve 15 to 20 percent of the time. During it prodomal stage, herpes zoster may present only as oral or facial pain, a headache, or a toothache. Vesicular eruptions characteristically occur unilaterally, not crossing the midline, and last 7 to 10 days. Intraoral lesions are most commonly associated with a facial outbreak but can occur alone. Treatment is largely palliative, although early treatment with acyclovir 800 mg 5 times per day for 7 to 10 days or valacyclovir 1 g tid for 7 days reportedly will lessen the outbreak and the likelihood or severity of postherpetic neuropathy.[11,16]

Herpangina

Herpangina is caused by coxsackievirus group A, types 1–6, 8, 10, and 22 most commonly. Most commonly occurring in the summer and autumn, herpangina presents with a sudden onset of high fever, sore throat, headache, and malaise followed by eruption of oral vesicles 1 to 2 mm in size within 24 to 48 h. The vesicles quickly rupture, leaving numerous shallow, painful ulcers. The soft palate, uvula, posterior pharynx, and tonsilar pillars are usually affected, sparing the buccal mucosa, tongue, and gingiva. The disease lasts 7 to 10 days and can be distinguished from herpetic gingivostomatitis by the lack of gingival involvement.[11]

Hand, Foot, and Mouth Disease

Coxsackievirus type A16, and occasionally types A4, A5, A9, and A10, are associated with hand, foot, and mouth disease. This entity is characterized by the development of a few small vesicles on the tongue, gingiva, soft palate, and buccal mucosa. These vesicles rupture, resulting in painful, shallow ulcers with a surrounding red halo. The lateral and dorsal aspects of the fingers and toes are frequently involved and aid the diagnosis. The buttocks, palms, and plantar surfaces of the feet may be affected. Fever is usually of short duration, and the disease lasts 5 to 8 days. Treatment is palliative.[11]

Traumatic Ulceration

Traumatic ulcers are a result of direct trauma to epithelial tissue causing in a painful area of erythema with a central fibropurulent eschar. They most commonly occur on the tongue, lips, and buccal mucosa. Common sources of trauma include rough or jagged edges on teeth or restorations, ill-fitting dentures, or mishaps during oral hygiene. Trauma from dental injection may result in ulceration. Removal of persistent sources of trauma is essential; otherwise, treatment is palliative.[16]

Lesions of the Tongue

Many systemic conditions and local stimuli affect the appearance of the tongue. Asymptomatic deep fissuring of the dorsal surface is common and probably represents a developmental phenomenon. Many systemic conditions, various vitamins deficiencies, and iron-deficiency anemia cause atrophy of the filiform papillae, resulting in a smooth erythematous appearance. Excessive intake of hot, spicy foods also can result in a smooth appearance. Occurrence of ectopic thyroid tissue on the midline posterior portion of the tongue is called a *lingual thyroid* and is a common finding. Some of the common conditions affecting the tongue not discussed elsewhere will be mentioned here.

ERYTHEMA MIGRANS Erythema migrans, geographic tongue, or benign migratory glossitis is a common benign finding on oral examination, occurring in 1 to 3 percent of the population. Females are affected twice as often as males. The typically multiple, well-demarcated zones of erythema on the tongue are due to atrophy of the filiform papillae. The lesions concentrate on the tip and lateral borders of the tongue and heal in several days, only to quickly reappear in other areas. Lesions can occur on any oral mucosa site. These lesions usually are asymptomatic; however, a burning sensation or sensitivity to hot or spicy foods has been described. Etiology is yet unknown; however, fluctuations with stress and menstrual cycle occur. Generally, treatment is not indicated because this entity is benign. Reassurance of patients is usually sufficient. In patients in whom discomfort is a major factor, oral topical steroids such as fluocinonide gel applied several times daily may provide relief.[18–20]

MEDIAN RHOMBOID GLOSSITIS Median rhomboid glossitis is believed to be a developmental defect of the dorsal surface of the tongue. It appears as a small 1 by 2 cm ovoid erythematous area just anterior to the circumvallate papillae. The area is devoid of papillae and usually asymptomatic. Recently, it has been suggested that this lesion represents an area of erythematous candidiasis. No treatment is necessary.[20]

BLACK HAIRY TONGUE First reported by Lusitanus in 1557, black hairy tongue represents yellow to brown discoloration of elongated filiform papillae. This entity is rare, affecting 0.15 percent of the population. Normal papillae are 1 to 2 mm in length, but these elongate up to 12 to 18 mm, taking on the characteristic hairlike appearance. Only the dorum of the tongue anterior to the circumvallate papillae is affected. The condition is usually asymptomatic but of significant concern to the patient. The etiology remains obscure. Treatment consist of frequent brushing of the tongue and avoidance of predisposing factors such as tobacco, strong mouthwashes, and antibiotics. Resolution usually occurs spontaneously, and surgical clipping is rarely needed.[20]

STRAWBERRY TONGUE Strawberry tongue is associated with erythrogenic, toxin-producing *Streptococcus pyogenes*. Clinically, the tongue has prominent red spots on a white-coated background. Microscopically, the fungiform papillae are hyperemic with a smooth glossy surface. Treatment is with antibiotics directed at group A streptococci.[20]

Leukoplakia and Erythroplakia

Leukoplakia is defined by the World Health Organization as a white patch or plaque that cannot be scraped off or characterized clinically or histopathologically as any other disease.[21] Leukoplakia is the most common oral precancer; however, only 2 to 4 percent of leukoplakic lesions are carcinoma.[22] The prevalence is approximately 20 to 39 per 1000 persons, affecting males twice as frequently as females. Etiology is unknown, but tobacco, alcohol, ultraviolet radiation, candidiasis, human papillomavirus, tertiary syphilis, and trauma have all been implicated. The most common intraoral site involved is the buccal mucosa. Other sites of involvement include the hard and soft palates, maxillary gingiva, and lip mucosa. Biopsy is mandatory for all persistent leukoplakic lesions, yet most demonstrate no dysplastic changes histologically. Leukoplakic lesions of the floor of the mouth, tongue, and vermilion border are most likely associated with malignancy. Lesions demonstrating dysplastic changes warrant removal.[21]

Erythroplakia is defined as a red patch that similarly cannot be clinically or pathologically characterized as any other disease. Although erythroplakia is far less common than leukoplakia, it has a far greater potential for dysplastic findings histologically.[22]

Oral Cancer

Oral cancer accounts for 2 to 4 percent of the cancers in the United States.[23] More than 90 percent of all oral malignancies are squamous cell carcinoma.[22] Lymphomas (both Hodgkin's and non-Hodgkin's), Kaposi's sarcoma, and melanoma comprise most of the remainder. Several intrinsic and extrinsic etiologic factors for oral squamous cell carcinoma have been identified. Extrinsic factors include tobacco use, especially chewing tobacco or snuff; excessive alcohol consumption; and sunlight exposure (Fig. 234-7). Intrinsic factors include general malnutrition and iron-deficiency anemia, especially chronic forms such as Plummer-Vinson syndrome.

Specific etiologic factors play varying roles in oncogenesis. Oral candidiasis, especially in its hyperplastic form, promotes the development of oral squamous cell carcinoma. Immunosuppressive states such as HIV infection slightly increase one's risk of oral cancer, and oncogenic viruses such as human papillomavirus, herpes simplex virus, and various adenoviruses and retroviruses may play some role in the etiology of oral cancer.[19,22]

Oral squamous cell carcinoma has four common morphologic presentations. It can be exophytic, or mass-forming, with an irregular or papillary surface. Endophytic, or ulcerative, cancers usually present as depressed irregular ulcers with rolled borders. Leukoplakic and erythroplakic lesions, when malignant, are felt to represent squamous cell carcinomas that have yet to form a mass or ulcerate.[19]

The most common site involved in oral cancer is the tongue, particularly the posterolateral border, accounting for approximately 50 percent of oral cancers in the United States. Cancer of the floor of the mouth accounts for nearly 35 percent.[19] Cancer of the lips is common and usually secondary to sunlight exposure. Table 234-3 lists the common signs and symptoms of oral cancer; unfortunately, oral cancer is generally painless, and patients are often unaware of the presence of a mass until it is advanced. Early diagnosis is the key to successful treatment of oral squamous cell carcinoma. Careful oral screening by emergency physicians through methodical examination of the oral cavity should reveal most oral carcinomas. All ulcers, erythroplakic lesions, and leukoplakic lesions of the oral cavity that do not respond to palliative treatment in 10 to 14 days warrant biopsy.

Treatment depends on site of involvement and staging of disease. It consists primarily of wide radical excision, radiation therapy, or a combination of the two. Adjunctive chemotherapy has been used to aid in tumor debulking. The prognosis depends on site and tumor stage, but an overall 5-year survival rate for patients with lesions that have not metastasized is 76 percent, 41 percent when cervical nodes are involved, and 9 percent when metastasis below the clavicle has occurred.[19]

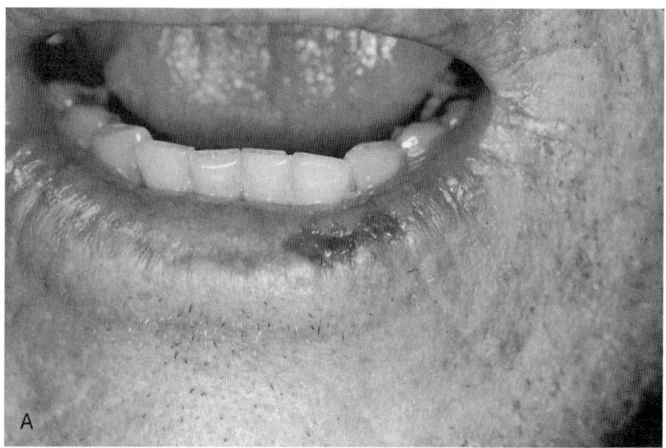

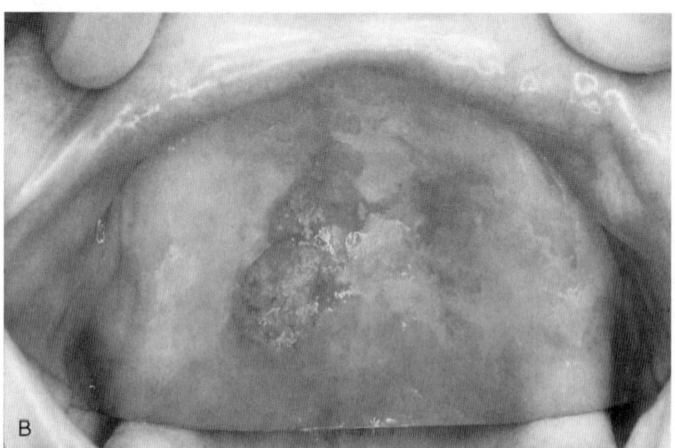

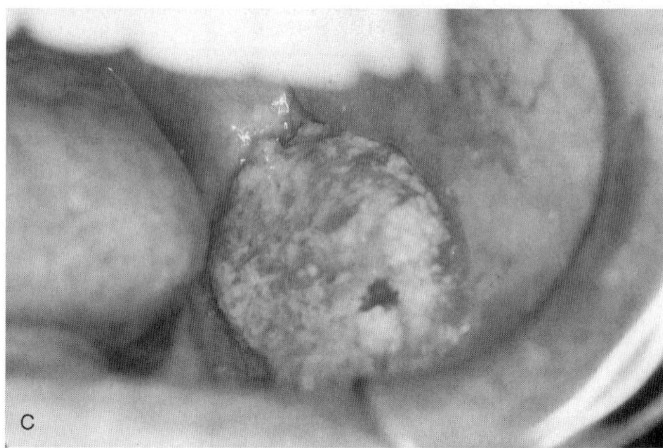

FIG. 234-7. Oral squamous cell carcinoma. **A.** Squamous cell carcinoma of the lip secondary to sun exposure. **B.** Squamous cell carcinoma of the hard palate. **C.** Verrucous carcinoma secondary to dipping snuff. (*Courtesy of H. Anthony Neil, D.D.S.*)

Other

Fordyce granules that are slightly elevated, cream-colored spots seen frequently on the vermilon border of the lips and buccal mucosa represent ectopic sebaceous glands.[25] *Linea alba* is a white line on the buccal mucosa at the level of the occlusal surface. It is caused by normal friction from the facial surfaces of the teeth during mastication. *Leukedema*, which is a normal variant, is a grayish white appearance

TABLE 234-3 Signs and Symptoms of Oral Cancer

Signs
- Nonhealing ulcer: can be in form of crater with elevated, indurated margins
- Bleeding: resulting from ulceration
- Lymphadenopathy
- Rigidity: lesion fixed to surrounding tissue
- Induration: hardness of the lesion
- Functional interference: such as speech and mastication

Symptoms
- Pain
  - Secondary to ulceration
  - Secondary to trauma related to functional interferences
- Parathesias
- Drooling: secondary to functional interferences

Source: From Marder.[24] Used with permission.

to the mucosal surfaces secondary to thickening of the mucosa and edema of the spinosal layer. It usually affects the buccal musosa bilaterally and can be diagnosed by its disappearance on eversion or stretching of the mucosal surface.[19] Firm exophytic enlargement along the lingual surface of the mandible (*torus mandibularis*) or of the hard palate (*torus palatinus*) represents benign exostoses of the associated bone. The etiology is unknown, but no therapeutic intervention is required.[26] Other entities that cause oral lesions such as pemphigoid, pemphigus, lichen planus, and erythema multiforme are discussed later as manifestations of systemic disease.

OROFACIAL TRAUMA

Dentoalveolar Trauma

Dentoalveolar trauma is a very common reason for ED visits. Approximately 20 percent of all school-age children will experience oral trauma. The most common mechanism of injury is falls. Sporting injuries, fights, and motor vehicle collisions account for most of the remainder. Injury to the maxillary central incisors accounts for 70 percent of dental injuries.[27] The management of dentoalveolar trauma depends on the extent of tooth and alveolar involvement, the degree of development of the apex of the tooth, and the age of the patient. In isolated fractures of a tooth, treatment decisions are based on the vitality of the tooth and, in a vital tooth, the proximity to the pulpal tissue. Involvement of the root of the tooth compromises the attachment apparatus and thus the ability of a dentist to adequately restore the tooth to function. Isolated alveolar bone trauma rarely occurs.

DENTAL FRACTURES A simple classification of dental fractures is the Ellis classification shown in Fig. 234-8. The goal of the emergency treatment of a fractured tooth is maintaining pulpal vitality. The proximity of the fracture to the pulp and the length of time before treatment are most important in determining outcome. Treatment is aimed at sealing the dentinal tubules and creating a barrier between the dental pulp and the oral environment. In properly treated uncomplicated dental fractures, 1 to 2 percent of the affected pulps undergoes necrosis. Since pulpal necrosis is a process, it can occur at any time after trauma, and serial follow-up with a dentist is recommended.[4,29]

Ellis class I fractures involve the enamel portion of the tooth only. Generally, no emergent treatment of these fractures is indicated, except to smooth sharp corners that may irritate the tongue or mucosa. An emory board or similar instrument is sufficient. Referral to a general dentist for aesthetic repair depends on the degree of cosmetic concern of the patient.[4,28,29]

Ellis class II fractures involve the dentin of the tooth and require intervention by the emergency physician. These fractures account for 70 percent of tooth fractures. Generally, patients express sensitivity to hot or cold stimuli as well as air passing over the expose surface during breathing. The Ellis class II fracture can be identified both by the patient's symptomatology and visualization of exposed dentin, which is a creamy yellow color compared with the whiter enamel. One may need to use gauze to wipe blood from the fractured tooth surface to determine the classification. Because dentin is microtubular in structure, communication between the oral environment and the dental pulp is established with exposure of the dentin. The thickness of remaining dentin determines the rate of pulpal contamination. Greater than 2 mm of remaining dentin is felt to offer some protection to the pulpal tissue. Microorganism contamination of the pulp, oral irritants, or desiccation from mouth breathing initiates an inflammatory process in the pulpal tissue. A delay in treatment increases the likelihood of pulpal necrosis. Thus it is the responsibility of the emergency physician not only to identify such a fracture but also to cover the exposed dentin to decrease pulpal contamination. This is best achieved using a glass ionomer cement that is easily mixed according to the manufacturer's instructions and carefully applied to the dried exposed dentin. A calcium hydroxide dental base such as Dycal historically has been recommended. It is now felt that this provides a less effective dentinal seal. Although calcium hydroxide is acceptable, glass ionomer is recommended in the recent literature because it is hydrophilic and fluid from the dentinal tubules does not weaken the seal. Referral to a dentist within 24 h is mandatory to best ensure tooth vitality.[4,28,29]

In Ellis class III fractures, exposure of the pulp has occurred. On wiping the fractured surface dry with sterile gauze, blood originating from the pulp of the tooth is easily identified. A class III fracture is a true dental emergency, and immediate attention by a dentist or oral and maxillofacial surgeon is indicated. One should attempt to cover the exposed dentin with a glass ionomer cement or calcium hydroxide base as in class II fractures until urgent dental evaluation can occur. If this is not possible because of the size of exposure, then maintaining a sterile environment by isolating the tooth with moist sterile gauze is important. If the pulpal exposure is extremely small, placing a glass ionomer or calcium hydroxide base is adequate until dental evaluation within 24 h. Prompt appropriate treatment lessens the likelihood of pulpal necrosis by minimizing pulpal contamination. For all but the most minuscule pulpal exposures, definitive treatment is endodontic

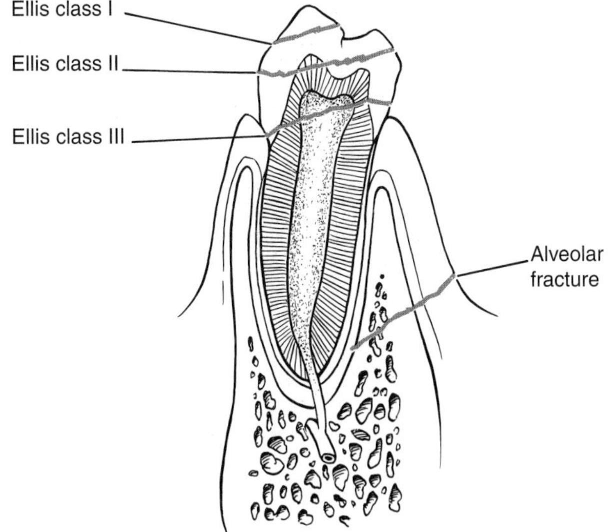

FIG. 234-8. Ellis classification for fractures of anterior teeth.

or root canal therapy. Oral analgesics should be prescribed and topical analgesics avoided.[4,28,29]

Crown root fractures account for 5 percent of all injuries of the permanent dentition. Extraction of the coronal segment is required. If less than one-third of the root is involved, root canal therapy can be performed by a dentist, and restoration of the tooth may be possible. Careful attention must be paid to identifying fractures of the root because they can be clinically obscure.[29]

The age of the patient becomes important in dental trauma for several reasons. As indicated earlier, dentin is formed throughout the life of a tooth. Thus, in younger patients, especially those less than 12 years of age, the pulp of anterior teeth is quite large and the dentinal layer is thin. Dental fractures in this age group more commonly involve the pulp of the tooth. Even when the pulp is not exposed directly, the dentinal layer separating the pulp from the oral environment is thin, so contamination is more likely. Fortunately, in this age group the apex of the root also is usually incompletely formed, allowing for a greater pulpal regenerative capability. In this age group, a blush of the pulp underneath a thin translucent dentinal layer in a class II fracture should be treated like a class III fracture. As one ages, more dentin is formed. Thus, in older patients, the pulpal chamber may be very small and pulpal exposure highly unlikely. Understanding the effects of age on the dentin layer is important for treatment of Ellis fractures.[28,29]

CONCUSSIONS, LUXATIONS AND AVULSIONS The same forces that cause dental fractures may result in loosening of a tooth from the attachment apparatus. Careful evaluation of the teeth for tenderness, malpositioning or mobility must be performed. Luxations account for nearly 50 percent of injuries to teeth.[27] Five distinct types of luxations have been described. (1) *Concussion* injuries are defined as injury to the supporting structures of a tooth with clinical tenderness to percussion but no mobility. (2) *Subluxation* is defined as an injury to the attachment apparatus resulting in mobility without clinical or radiographic evidence of dislodgment of the tooth. (3) *Extrusive luxation* is defined as partial avulsion or dislodgment of a tooth from the alveolar bone. (4) *Lateral luxation* is defined as dislodgment of a tooth laterally with concomitant fracture of the alveolar bone. (5) *Intrusive luxation* is defined as displacement of a tooth into its socket with associated alveolar fracture. Treatment of luxations depends on identifying and assessing tooth involvement, permanent or primary tooth involvement, and presence of root fracture and/or significant associated alveolar fracture.[4,27,28]

A concussive injury to a tooth represents a minor injury. The degree of tenderness to percussion determines the treatment. Stabilizing the tooth by splinting it to adjacent teeth is not indicated. Management of pain with NSAIDs, soft diet, and referral to a dentist to confirm the diagnosis and exclude more severe injury, are the most appropriate courses of action for the emergency physician. Removal of the occlusal forces from the tooth by a dentist may aid in comfort and healing. Similarly, a subluxed tooth generally does not require splinting. Again, removal from occlusion by a general dentist may be beneficial. Subluxation represents a more significant injury and is associated with a higher incidence of subsequent pulpal necrosis. Clinically, bleeding around the tooth is common.[4,27]

Extrusive luxation requires repositioning the tooth in its original position and splinting to stabilize the tooth during healing. Repositioning the tooth may require local anethesia. Firm, gentle pressure usually will reposition the tooth. If a clot has formed apical to the tooth, then more aggressive manipulation may be required. Stabilization is ideally obtained with a flexible wire splint place by a dentist. In the ED, a temporary splint with Coe-Pak (Fig. 234-9) as described by Medford[30] is acceptable until the patient can see a dentist or oral and maxillofacial surgeon within 24 h. Care must be taken to avoid excess material placement, especially on the occlusal surface, because interference in occlusion will place stresses on the tooth during mastication. Splinting

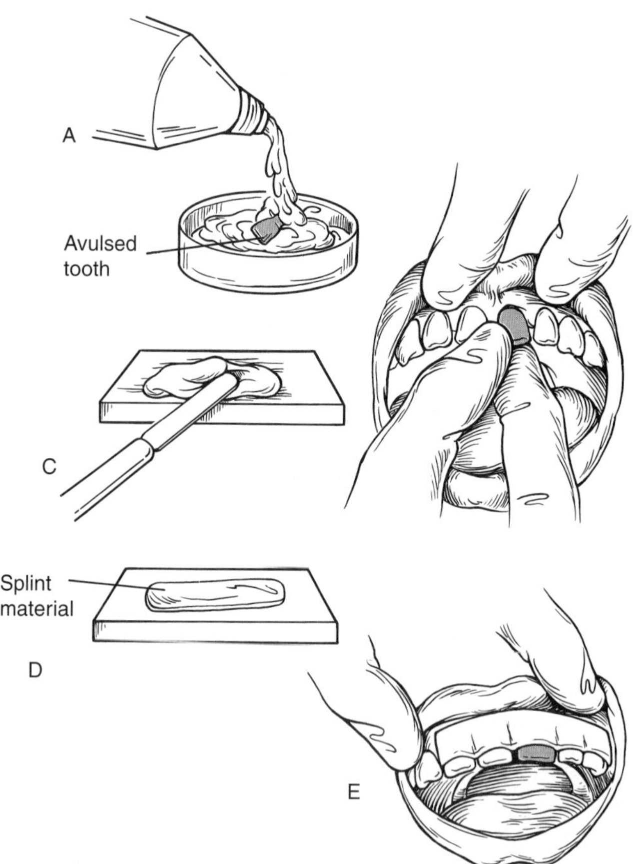

FIG. 234-9. Reimplantation and stabilization of an avulsed tooth. **A.** Tooth is rinsed. **B.** Tooth is placed back into socket. **C.** Splint material is ready for application. **D.** Packing is molded over reimplanted tooth and two adjacent teeth to each side.

should be maintained for 1 to 2 weeks. Close follow-up by a dentist is necessary to identify early occurrence of any of the potential postluxation sequelae such as internal and external root resorption, ankylosis, and pulpal necrosis.[4,27]

A lateral luxation represents a more extensive injury with associated crazing or fracture of the surrounding alveolar bone. Repositioning of the tooth is generally more difficult. It usually can be accomplished by manipulating the displaced tooth with thumb and forefinger. Once the apex has been dislodged from its locked-in position labially, apically directed axial pressure will reposition the tooth. Intraarch stabilization is necessary for a minimum of 2 weeks. Temporary splinting with Coe-Pak is acceptable if a minimal associated alveolar fractured occurred. Otherwise, splinting by an oral and maxillofacial surgeon or general dentist in the ED is mandatory.[4,27]

Intrusive luxations are the most serious because significant damage to the alveolar socket and periodontal ligament occurs. Root resorption is common as a result of damage to the periodontal ligament. Recommended treatment is allowing the tooth to reerupt on its own or to orthodontically extrude the tooth over 3 to 4 weeks.[27]

Total displacement of a tooth from its socket, or *avulsion,* accounts for up to 16 percent of all injuries to teeth. It is necessary to reimplant avulsed permanent teeth as soon as possible. Reimplantation is possible if performed within 2 to 3 h. Ideally, the tooth should be reimplanted by the patient or health care provider at the scene to minimize this time. The tooth should be rinsed with sterile normal saline or tap water to remove debris. Care should be taken to handle only the crown portion of the tooth, and it should be reimplanted immediately into the socket. If this is not possible, or if the risk of aspiration is high, such as in a young child or a patient with a decreased level of consciousness, then the tooth should be transported with the patient to the ED. Acceptable transport media include isotonic solutions such as Hank's solution, sterile saline, and milk. Commercial preparations of Hank's solution such as Save-A-Tooth (TPS, Biologic Rescue Products, Inc.) are available and come with a useful transport container as part of the system. If the avulsed tooth was not recovered, radiographs to ensure that the tooth was not aspirated are indicated.[31–33]

Survival of the periodontal ligament fibers that remain attached to the root of an avulsed tooth is key to successful reimplantation. Milk is an acceptable storage medium due to its osmolarity and essential concentration of calcium and magnesium ions. Hank's solution, a pH-balanced cell culture medium, is the best transport medium and has been found to maintain periodontal ligament cell viability for up to 4 to 6 h. It also has been found that Hank's solution can help to restore cell viability in a tooth that has been avulsed longer than 20 and 60 min.[32,33]

In the ED, prior to reimplantation, the tooth should be thoroughly rinsed clean of dirt and debris with sterile saline or preferably Hank's solution. The root of the tooth should not be scrubbed, and care should be taken not to disrupt existing periodontal fibers. If an avulsed tooth with an open apex has been dry for less than 20 min, then the prognosis for reestablishing a vital pulp is good. If the apex is completely closed, then revitalization is not possible. If the tooth has been dry from 20 to 60 min regardless of apices, it is recommended that the tooth be soaked in Hank's balanced salt solution for 30 min. This has been found to decrease the chance of ankylosis. For an avulsed tooth that has been dry for greater than 60 min, the periodontal cells are dead, and the goal is to reduce root resorption. It is recommended that the tooth be soaked in citric acid for 5 min, then 2% stannous flouride, and finally doxycycline for 5 min prior to reimplantation.[31]

Preparation of the dental socket plays little role in the success or failure of the reimplanted tooth. The socket is prepared by carefully removing the clot and irrigating gently with sterile normal saline. As little manipulation as possible of the socket should occur. Local anesthesia is usually required. Reimplantation is accomplished with firm pressure and having the patient bite on gauze until more permanent stabilization can be arranged. Anterior teeth are most commonly affected, and Fig. 234-10 illustrates the morphology of the maxillary central incisor to assist reimplantation in the proper orientation. Early improper reimplantation holds a higher success rate for tooth salvage than delayed reimplantation resulting from waiting for an oral and maxillofacial surgeon. Stabilization by an oral and maxillofacial surgeon or using a temporary method such as Coe-Pak is necessary.[31–33]

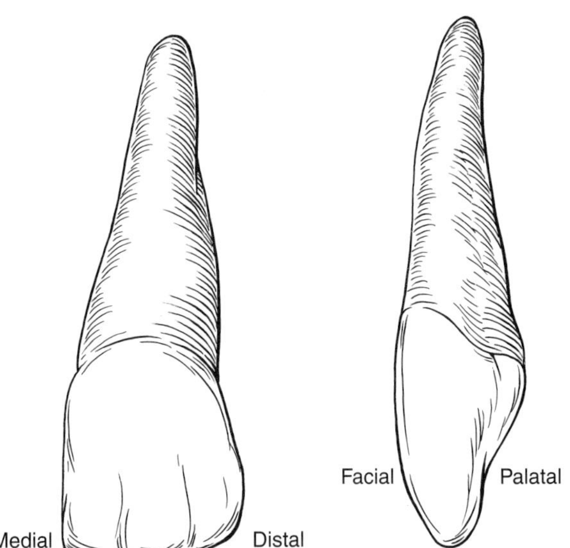

FIG. 234-10. Illustration of a maxillary left central incisor. Note that the part of the tooth facing medially comes to more of a right angle at the incisal edge than occurs distally. The facial portion of the tooth is more convex.

Avulsion or luxation of primary teeth is treated differently from that of permanent teeth. Thus identification of primary teeth in patients aged 6 to 12 years when the dentition is mixed is essential. Avulsed primary teeth are not reimplanted. More severe luxations in primary teeth generally require extraction of the tooth. Repositioning or reimplanting primary teeth risks injuring the underlying permanent teeth and thus is avoided. Intruded primary teeth are an exception and generally are left alone to reerupt into normal position. Primary teeth maintain space and allow for adequate growth of the mandible and maxilla to accommodate their permanent successors. Thus postavulsion orthodontic space maintenance may be important. Referral to a general dentist for follow-up is essential to ensure optimal long-term outcome.[28,31]

Posttraumatic sequelae are variable. Pulp canal obliteration, pulpal necrosis, internal resorption and external resorption of the root, and ankylosis may occur. The severity of luxation or avulsion is the most important determining factor in sequela occurrence. Transient apical breakdown occurs with all type of luxations but is especially common with extrusive and lateral luxations. More than 50 percent of extrusively luxated teeth undergo pulpal necrosis within 1.5 years or the traumatic event.[27]

Significant force must occur to dislodge or fracture teeth, and associated alveolar ridge fracture is common. Care to ensure the integrity of the maxilla and mandible is also important. Stabilization of repositioned or reimplanted teeth is essential for optimal results. This is best accomplished with semirigid fixation by a general dentist or oral surgeon. Stabilization is maintained for 1 to 2 weeks depending on the involvement of alveolar bone. Early placement back into function is felt to improve the success rate by decreasing ankylosis and resorption of the root. Decisions concerning when to remove the stabilization should be left to the consultant. With significant alveolar ridge fracture, segments may require intermaxillary stabilization. Oral and maxillofacial surgical consultation is necessary. Stabilization in these patients is usually maintained for up to 6 weeks in order to ensure adequate healing.[28,31]

Soft Tissue Trauma

Repair of associated injuries of gingival, lip, mucosal, and facial soft tissues should occur after stabilization of hard tissue in the oral cavity. Otherwise, intricate repairs may be damaged and torn during the manipulation required to reduce, reimplant, and stabilize subluxed or avulsed teeth or associated bony fractures.

Oral lacerations can involve any of the soft tissues of the mouth. Large intraoral lacerations (>1 cm) are susceptible to ulceration and secondary infection and tend to heal in a fibrotic mass. Intraoral lacerations should be inspected carefully for foreign material, including tooth fragments, and irrigated well with sterile normal saline. Retained foreign bodies serve as a nidus for infection and can result in need for later surgical removal and poor aesthetic outcome. Crushed and nonviable tissue should be debrided. Close approximation of the wound edges rather than a tissue seal is desired to allow drainage. Resorbable suture material such as 4-0 chromic is generally used. Black silk (4-0) is easier to use but requires removal in 7 to 10 days. When resorbable sutures are used, care should be taken to place the sutures so that the knots are buried. Prophylactic antibiotics generally are not indicated except with the most extensive lacerations. Forty-eight-hour follow-up is necessary to monitor healing.

Lacerations of the lips and tongue require special consideration. Care should be taken in wound-edge approximation of lacerations on the dorsum of the tongue because reepithelialization across the wound edge is important. If the edges are not well approximated, the epithelia will migrate downward and will result in an epithelial cleft and a bifid appearance. This is both a cosmetic and a functional problem requiring revision. Small tongue lacerations in children, where the edges remain approximated, need not be sutured. Bleeding can be controlled with pressure using gauzes or moistened tea bags (see below). Extensive tongue lacerations in children require conscious sedation and may be best referred for repair.

Lip lacerations are a potential cosmetic problem, so careful closure is essential. In lacerations involving the vermilion border, alignment of the border is important and should be completed first. The portion of the laceration extraoral to the wet-dry line of the lip and involving the skin of the face should be closed with 6-0 nylon monofilament or Prolene. The intraoral portion of the laceration is repaired in the same manner as any oral laceration. Because of the musculature of the lips, any deep laceration requires closure of the deep layers using a 4-0 resorbable suture material such as Polyvicryl to decrease the likelihood of the wound edges opening on removal of the suture. With any laceration involving the face or other aesthetic areas, sutures should be removed as early as possible, generally in 5 days, so as to decrease scarring from the suture material. Careful daily cleansing of the wound with dilute hydrogen peroxide and application of a triple-antibiotic ointment makes suture removal easier and improves the aesthetic results.

Controversy concerning closure of through-and-through lip laceration exists. Some advocate leaving the intraoral portion of the laceration open; however, it is my recommendation that mucosal lacerations larger than 1 cm be repaired. Generally, the intraoral component should be repaired first, and then, from an extraoral approach, the laceration should be cleansed and irrigated aggressively. A deep layer of sutures may be necessary in large lacerations. The skin then should be closed aesthetically. Prophylactic antibiotics such as penicillin VK or erythromycin 250 mg PO qid for about 5 days, are indicated.

Laceration of the maxillary labial frenulum, unless unusually large, does not require repair. These lacerations can be very painful, so adequate analgesia must be prescribed. Because of the vascularity of adjacent tissue, lacerations to the lingual frenulum usually do need to be repaired. Resorbable suture such as 4.0 chromic is appropriate.

Other soft tissue injuries commonly occur. Intraoral contusions and ecchymoses are prevalent with facial trauma. Ecchymoses and petechial hemorrhages to the soft palate, uvula, and pharynx from direct trauma or from the negative pressure created from suction are frequently associated with fellatio. Treatment is mainly palliative, with reassurance to the patient and NSAIDs for discomfort.

HEMORRHAGE

Spontaneous Hemorrhage

Spontaneous gingival hemorrhage is not uncommon. A history of recent dental therapy such as periodontal scaling or curettage is important because resulting hemorrhage after scaling is easily controlled with peroxide mouth rinses or direct gingival pressure A careful medical history must be obtained because systemic diseases such as clotting factor deficiencies, leukemia, and end-stage liver disease that result in a hypocoagulable state may first manifest as spontaneous gingival hemorrhage. Overanticoagulation with oral agents may present as spontaneous gingival bleeding. The need for laboratory evaluation depends on a careful history and physical examination. Treatment depends on the specific cause of bleeding in the event that local measures are unsuccessful.

Postoperative Bleeding

Postextraction bleeding is not uncommon. Dislodgment of the clot may result in recurrent or continued bleeding. Generally, firm pressure applied to the extraction site is adequate to control bleeding. This is best accomplished by neatly folding a 2 × 2 gauze pad and placing it over the extraction site, applying firm pressure by clenching firmly with the opposing teeth. This pressure must be held firmly, not a chewing action, for 20 min or until hemostasis is complete. Also, pressure with a used tea bag aids hemostasis because the tannic acid is a natural hemostatic agent. If direct pressure is not successful, then application of Gel-Foam, Avitene, or Instat to the socket may provide a matrix for clot formation. Sutures should be used for holding such agents in place or to close the gingiva over the socket. The gingiva should not be closed under pressure, especially along the suture line, since this may result in necrosis of the gingival flap. If these methods are unsuccessful, the vasoconstrictive effect of direct instillation of lidocaine with epinephrine may aid hemostasis. Finally, if hemostasis still cannot be obtained, then oral and maxillofacial surgical consultation becomes necessary.

Bleeding may occur after periodontal surgery secondary to underlying clotting abnormalities or from dislodgment or instability of the periodontal packing. It is important that the practitioner who performed the surgical procedure be contacted to direct care because positioning of the periodontal flap is critical for successful therapy.

ORAL MANIFESTATIONS OF SYSTEMIC DISEASE

Vitamin Deficiencies

In the developed world today, significant vitamin deficiency is uncommon. Patients with malabsorption syndrome and eating disorders, fad dieters, and alcoholics are notable exceptions. Most significant vitamin deficiencies have characteristic oral manifestations.

RIBOFLAVIN A diet deficient in riboflavin causes many abnormalities. Oral manifestations include glossitis and angular cheilitis, sore throat, and swelling and erythema of the oral mucosa. Seborrheic dermatitis is seen commonly in chronic riboflavin deficiency. A normocyctic normochromic anemia is also common.[19]

NIACIN Severe niacin deficiency results in a condition known as *pellagra*. Once common in the southeastern United States, it manifests as a dermatitis (especially on sun-exposed areas), dementia, and diarrhea. Oral manifestations include angular cheilitis, stomatitis, and glossitis. The tongue typically appears smooth and fiery red. Untreated severe deficiencies ultimately may result in death.[19]

PYRIDOXINE Pyridoxine deficiency is extremely uncommon because pyridoxine occurs almost universally in foods. Deficiency states occur not uncommonly in patients taking a number of drugs such as isoniazid that are pyridoxine antagonists. Deficiency states result in weakness, dizziness, and seizure activity. The oral manifestations are similar to those of pellagra, with glossitis and angular cheilitis.[19]

VITAMIN C A deficiency of vitamin C is known as *scurvy* and is limited to people with diets deficient in fresh fruits and vegetables such as inner-city infants and the edentulous elderly. The clinical symptoms are related to the vitamin's role in collagen synthesis. Typically, wound healing is impaired, and decreased vascular wall integrity results in widespread petechial hemorrhages or ecchymoses. Oral manifestations include the typical gingival lesion, or scorbutic gingivitis, with gingival swelling and ulceration. Spontaneous gingival hemorrhage, tooth mobility, and increased severity of periodontal disease are also common. Severe deficiency can result in death secondary to spontaneous intracranial hemorrhage.[19]

VITAMIN D A deficiency of vitamin D historically was quite common and in children is called *rickets* and in adults *osteomalacia*. Essential in the absorption of calcium from the small intestines and, in conjunction with parathyroid hormone, reabsorption from the distal tubule of the kidney, manifestations of a deficiency state are related to problems with calcium homeostasis. This is manifested primarily as inadequate calcification of the bones. Otherwise, there are no specific oral manifestation of vitamin D deficiency.[19,34]

VITAMIN K Seen most commonly in patients with a malabsorption syndrome or whose gastrointestinal flora have been irradicated by long-term antibiotic use, vitamin K deficiency results in coagulation abnormalities. A deficiency in vitamin K results in inadequate synthesis of prothrombin and other clotting factors. Spontaneous gingival hemorrhage is not uncommon in severe vitamin K deficiency.[19]

Anemia

IRON-DEFICIENCY ANEMIA Iron-deficiency anemia is the most common cause of anemia in the world today. In severe deficiencies, patients may complain of fatigue, palpitations, light-headedness, and lack of energy. Oral manifestations include angular cheilitis, diffuse or patchy atrophic glossitis, and mucosal atrophy. Associated oral candidiasis is common. Such oral changes are rarely seen in the developed world because iron-deficiency anemia is identified relatively early.[19]

MEGALOBLASTIC ANEMIA Dietary deficiency of cobalamin (vitamin B_{12}) or folate is uncommon. A deficiency state leads to megaloblastic anemia. Pernicious anemia is a result of poor absorption of cobalamin or extrinsic factor. Intrinsic factor is produced by the parietal cells of the stomach and combines with cobalamin in the duodenum, enabling its absorption in the small intestine. Pernicious anemia is a result of a lack of intrinsic factor secondary to an autoimmune destruction of the parietal cells of the stomach. Gastric bypass and severe gastrointestinal disease also may result in a decreased production of intrinsic factor and thus absorption of cobalamin. Cobalamin is essential for the production of nucleic acids. Consequently, rapidly dividing cells such as the hematopoetic cells and mucosal lining are affected most. The most common systemic complaints associated with pernicious anemia are fatigue, weakness, shortness of breath, headache, parathesias, and diminished vibratory and positional sense. Oral manifestations reportedly affect up to 50 percent of patients and include atrophic glossitis and erythematous mucositis. A frequent complaint is a painful or burning sensation of the tongue, lips, and buccal mucosa. Angular cheilitis and hyperkeratosis are also common. Biopsies of unaffected mucosal surfaces reveal atrophy, inflammatory changes, loss of melanin pigments, and glycogen depletion. Treatment involves parenteral supplementation of the deficient vitamin.[19,35]

Endocrine Abnormalities

THYROID HORMONE The most common findings of hypothyroidism include lethargy, fatigue, dry coarse skin, facial and extremity swelling, hoarseness, constipation, and weakness. Oral manifestations are related to the accumulation of glycosaminoglycans in the oral tissues, causing macroglossia and thickened lips. If hypothyroidism occurs in childhood, teeth may fail to erupt, although tooth formation is unimpaired.[19]

Grave's disease is the most common type of hyperthyroidism and is associated with an increased metabolic rate, tachycardia, nervousness, weight loss, heat intolerance, emotional lability, and muscle weakness. The most prominent feature of hyperthyroidism, however, is exopthalamus. No characteristic oral findings are associated with hyperthyroidism.[19]

PARATHYROID HORMONE Findings of hypoparathyroidism are related to the resulting serum hypocalcemia. Common oral findings include Chvostek's sign, or twitching of the upper lip secondary to tapping the facial nerve just below the zygomatic arch. This is indicative of latent tetany associated with hypocalcemia. If hypoparathyroidism occurs during childhood, odontogenesis may be affected, and pitting enamel hypoplasia, widened pulp chamber, short roots, hypodontia, and failure of teeth eruption may occur.[19,36]

Uncontrolled production of parathyroid hormone may result from a pituitary adenoma or primary hyperparathyroidism or from a chronically low serum calcium level secondary to the renal failure of secondary hyperparathyroidism. Primary hyperparathyrodism occurs most commonly over the age of 60 years and is four times more prevalent in females. The classic findings of hyperparathyroidism include ''stones, bones, and abdominal groans.'' Stones refer to an increased incidence of kidney stones. Abdominal groans refer to the tendency to develop duodenal ulcers. Bones refer to a variety of osseous lesions such as the radiographic subperiosteal resorption of the phalanges of the index and middle fingers. Generalized loss of the lamina dura surrounding the roots of teeth is an early finding. With disease progression, loss of trabeculation results in a ground glass radiographic appearance of the mandible and maxilla. Persistent disease results in the development of other osseous lesions such as the brown tumor of hyperparathyroidism. These lesions occur most commonly in the mandible, clavicle, ribs, and pelvis and appear radiographically as well-demarcated unilocular or multilocular radiolucencies.[19]

GROWTH HORMONE Pituitary dwarfism is caused by a lack of growth hormone production by the anterior pituitary gland. Characteristic features include the remarkably short stature of the patient with normal body proportions. The maxilla and mandible of affected persons are smaller than usual. Tooth eruption is typically delayed from 1 to 3 years. Root formation is often delayed, and third molars ageneisis is common. Also, tooth size is usually smaller.[19]

Gigantism is a result of overproduction of growth hormone prior to closure of the bony epiphyses and, if untreated, results in extreme heights. Acromegaly is a result of overproduction of growth hormone in an adult patient, resulting in renewed growth in the small bones of the hand as well as the membranous bones of the skull and mandible. Similar oral findings occur in both cases. True macrodontia is a characteristic finding of gigantism. Mandibular prognathia with an anterior open bite is seen characteristically in acromegaly. Abnormal growth of the mandible and maxilla may result in diastema formation between the teeth. Soft tissue growth may result in thickening of the soft palate and a uniform macroglossia.[19]

ADRENAL CORTICOSTEROIDS Addison's disease is due to insufficient production of adrenal corticosteroids and results in gastrointestinal upset, fatigue, anorexia and weight loss, and salt craving. A characteristic bronzing of the skin is evident, and orally, brown macular pigmented lesions are common. The hyperpigmentation of the oral mucosal is caused by excessive melanin production and may be the first manifestation of Addison's disease.[19]

Hypercortisolism results in slow weight gain, particularly in the central areas of the body. No characteristic oral findings are noted; however, ''moon facies'' from deposition of fat in the facial region is characteristic.[19]

INSULIN Most of the systemic complications of diabetes are related to the microangiopathy caused by the disease.[19] Oral manifestations are associated more commonly with insulin-dependent diabetes mellitus but may be associated with non-insulin-dependent diabetes mellitus. Periodontal disease is more common and more aggressive in the diabetic patient. Wound healing postoperatively is delayed, and diabetics are prone to infections secondary to impairment of neutrophil function. In the poorly controlled diabetic patient, gingival erythema and proliferation are common.[37] The poorly controlled diabetic patient is more susceptible to oral candidiasis. Erythematous candidiasis with its central papillary atrophy of the tongue is reported in up to 30 percent of diabetic patients. An increased incidence in benign migratory glossitis is seen in insulin-dependent diabetes. Diabetic sialadenosis, or diffuse nontender enlargement of the parotid salivary glands, is not uncommon. Xerostomia is a common complaint of diabetic patients, yet no conclusive studies demonstrating an actual decrease in saliva production exists. Oral complaints in diabetic patients are extremely common and may lead to a new diagnosis of diabetes.[19,37]

Renal Failure

Findings associated with chronic hypocalcemia and secondary hyperparathyroidism of renal failure are common. These findings were described previously. Uremic stomatitis is an uncommon finding of renal failure. When present, it is commonly associated with acute renal failure and a blood urea nitrogen level of greater than 30 mmol/L. The characteristic manifestation is an erythematous, pseudomembranous stomatitis. This presents as white mucoid plaques or crusts on the gingiva, buccal mucosa, tongue, and floor of thc mouth, possibly extending into the pharynx. Ulcerative lesions are less common. Patients usually complain of oral pain or a burning sensation. The etiology is uncertain, but it is felt that the urease in oral flora metabolizes salivary urea to ammonia. It is this free ammonia that damages the oral mucosa. An astute clinician may be able to detect an odor of ammonia.[38]

Medication-Related Soft Tissue Abnormalities

Gingival hyperplasia is associated with many commonly used medications (Fig. 234-11). Historically, phenytoin-related gingival hyperplasia has been described. Approximately 50 percent of patients on phenytoin will develop significant gingival hyperplasia. Many other medications are known to cause gingival hyperplasia, such as calcium channel blockers, especially nifedipine, and cyclosporine. Concomitant use of two agents known to cause gingival hyperplasia results in accelerated gingival proliferation. With phenytoin hyperplasia, enlargement begins in the interdental papillae. Characteristics of the gingival tissue depend on oral hygiene and secondary inflammation. In the absence of inflammation, gingival proliferation results in dense tissue, normal in coloration, with a smooth, stippled, or granular texture. Inflammation results in edematous changes and erythematous coloration. Inflamed tissue bleeds readily. Histologically, an increase in collagen fibers, in fibroblasts, and in glycosaminoglycans is seen. Epithelial acanthosis also occurs. The characteristics of gingival hyperplasia related to cyclosporine and calcium channel blockers appear to be identical to those of phenytoin hyperplasia. The etiology of drug-related gingival hyperplasia remains unclear, but clearly, poor oral hygiene increases its likelihood and severity. Treatment includes fastidious oral hygiene to slow the hyperplasia and gingivectomy in advance cases.[39]

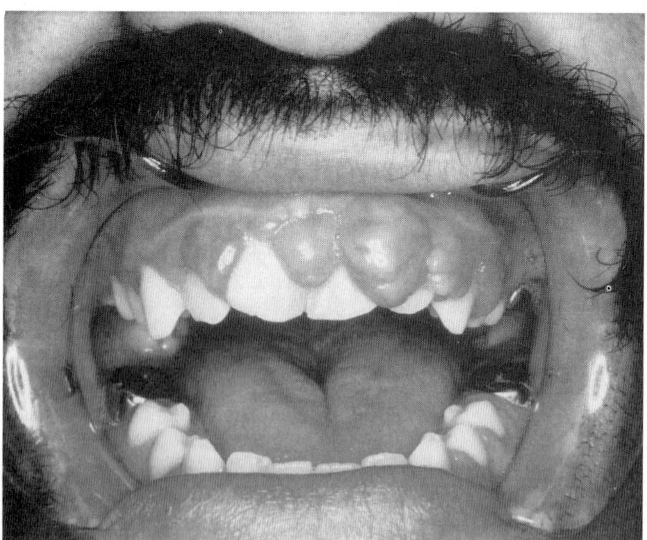

FIG. 234-11. Gingival hyperplasia secondary to cyclosporine. (*Courtesy of Philip J. Hanes, D.D.S., M.S.*)

Many other medications are known to cause abnormalities of the oral mucosa or dental structures. Allergic mucositis, erythema multiforme, and fixed drug type reactions are examples. Xerostomia and associated mucosal alterations are a side effect of many medications such as anticholinergics, antidepressants, and antihistamines.[1] Tetracycline taken systemically during tooth formation results in a characteristic gray-brown discloration of the dental enamel. Systemic flouride ingestion, although significantly reducing caries rates, in higher than the recommended 1 ppm may result in significant enamel defects called *flourosis.* Flourosis is dose-dependent and is primarily an aesthetic concern, with the most common abnormality being lusterless, opaque white discolored areas on the teeth.

Heavy Metal Intoxication

Ingestions of one of several heavy metals can lead to systemic manifestations. Lead poisoning, or *plumbism,* is the most common heavy metal poisoning. Systemic signs of lead poisoning are highly variable depending on the age of the patient and the amount of lead ingested. Symptoms range from colic, iritability, fatigue, and anemia to encephalopathy. Intraorally, lead poisoning presents as an ulcerative stomatitis or a bluish hue to the buccal mucosa. The classic bluish lead line on the ginigiva, secondary to subepithelial deposits of lead sulfide, also may be seen. In addition, a tremor on tongue thrusting, excessive saliva production, metallic taste, and severe periodontal disease may occur. Treatment is chelation therapy.[40]

Granulomatous Disease

SARCOIDOSIS Sarcoidosis is a multisystem granulomatous disease with an uncertain etiology. The lungs, lymph nodes, skin, and eyes are affected most commonly. Skin lesions are common and include classic painless erythematous nodules, erythema nodosum, on the extremities. Oral involvement is primarily limited to enlargement of major and minor salivary glands, and xerostomia is a common complaint. Mucoceles of the minor salivary glands are common, and biopsy of these lesions may result in the diagnosis of sarcoidosis.[19]

WEGENER'S GRANULOMATOSIS Wegener's granulomatosis causes necrotizing lesions of the upper and lower respiratory tracts, kidney, and small arteries and veins. Any organ system can be involved. Orally, a distinctive form of gingivitis called *strawberry gingivitis* is seen. Originating from the interdental gingiva, strawberry gingivitis is characterized by a hyperemic granular hypertrophy of the gingival tissue. Eventually involving the entire gingiva and periodontal tissue, tooth mobility and loss are common. Poor healing at the site of tooth loss also occurs. Oral ulceration, jaw claudication, and temporomandibular joint arthralgia also may occur. Oral lesions are frequently the first manifestation of Wegener's granulomatosis. Since the disease is uniformly fatal without early detection and treatment, familiarity with this entity is important.[19,41]

MYCOBACTERIAL INFECTIONS Most oral lesions of tuberculosis represent secondary infection from a primary pulmonary infection, but primary oral tubercular lesions can occur. Discovery of oral lesions prior to diagnosis of pulmonary tuberculosis is rare. Prior to effective antitubercular therapeutic regimens, oral lesions were considered a poor prognostic indicator. Secondary oral tubercular lesions are usually painful, irregular, nodular ulcers surrounded by an area of erythema affecting the tongue, lips, and palate most commonly. Lesions also may be leukoplakic. Primary lesions more commonly affect the gingiva. Tubercular osteomyelitis of the mandible is uncommon but has been reported.[19,42]

Oral lesions of lepromatous leprosy occur most commonly in the first 5 years of disease and are reported to affect up to 60 percent of patients. This is in contrast to tuberculoid leprosy, in which the oral cavity is rarely involved. The most commonly affected oral sites are the anterior maxillary gingiva, hard and soft palates, uvula, and tongue. In most patients, intranasal lesions precede oral involvement. Mucosal lesions may appear as yellowish sessile, enlarging nodules that may ulcerate and necrose with time. A pink or red discoloration of the maxillary incisors is the only specific dental finding. However, involvement of the maxilla in children can affect the development of teeth. Specific gingival involvement is limited to the premaxillary gingiva and is associated with underlying bony destruction and eventual loss of teeth.[43]

CROHN'S DISEASE Crohn's disease is an inflammatory disease that may affect the entire gastrointestinal tract from mouth to anus. A wide variety of oral lesions may be associated with Crohn's disease. The most common lesions are diffuse or nodular swelling of the oral and perioral tissue, a cobblestone appearance to the mucosa, and deep granulamatous ulcers surrounded by hyperplastic margins, fissuring on the midline of the lower lip. Oral lesions may be asymptomatic or painful. Additionally, angular cheilitis and submandibular lymphadenopathy can occur. Metallic dysguesia and gingival and buccal mucosal bleeding have been reported. Although these findings may be associated with any orofacial granulomatosis, it is important to note that the oral manifestations of Crohn's disease precede the gastrointestinal lesion in 30 percent of patients.[44]

PYOGENIC GRANULOMA A pyogenic granuloma is a common, benign proliferation of connective tissue in a sessile or pedunculated manner in response to local trauma or irritation. It occurs primarily on the gingiva. Despite its name, this lesion is not a true granuloma but rather an accumulation of granulation tissue. A specific pyogenic granuloma occurring in pregnancy is referred to as a *pregnancy tumor* (Fig. 234-12). This tumor is benign and usually recurs if removed during pregnancy. If the tumor does not regress 2 to 3 months postpartum, definitive removal is indicated.[45]

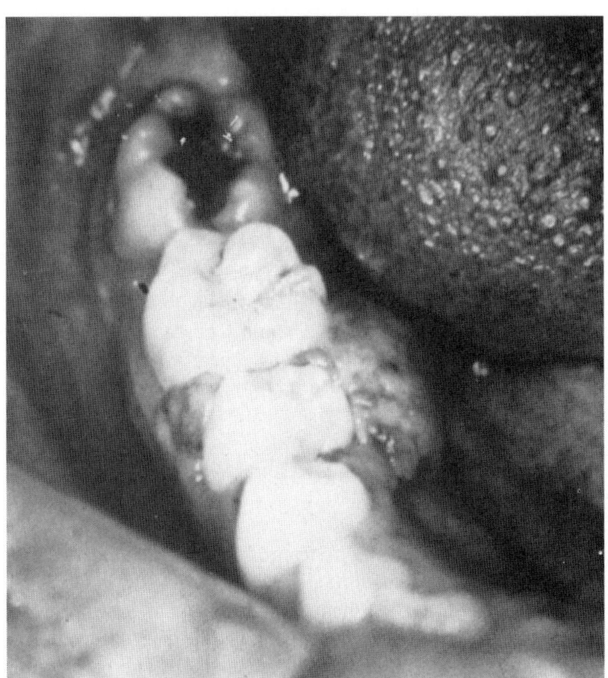

FIG. 234-12. Pyogenic granuloma.

Collagen Vascular Disease

Collagen vascular diseases are a group of disorders that includes systemic lupus erythematosus and systemic sclerosis or scleroderma. They are immunologically mediated. Nearly a quarter of systemic lupus patients develop oral lesion affecting the palate, buccal mucosa, or gingiva. These lesions may be lichenoid in appearance with associated ulceration, pain, erythema, and hyperkeratosis.

Systemic sclerosis patients characteristically have microstomia secondary to perioral contractures as a result of the deposition of collagen in the perioral tissue. Limited mobility of the tongue and crenations of the buccal mucosa are common in severe disease. Trigeminal paresthesias and hyperesthesia are found in 4 percent of systemic sclerosis patients. Dental radiographs reveal a diffuse widening of the periodontal ligament space, and a panorex view in up to 70 percent of patients shows varying degrees of resorption of the posterior ramus, coronoid process, and mandibular condyles.[46]

Leukemia

Patients with leukemia frequently experience easy bruising and spontaneous gingival hemorrhage secondary to thrombocytopenia. Common oral findings include petechial hemorrhage of the soft palate. Leukemic patients are more prone to oral candidiasis and oral herpetic infections. Ulceration of the oral mucosa as a result of severe neutropenia, or neutropenic ulcers, occurs in leukemia due to the host's inability to combat normal oral flora. These ulcers are typically deep, punched-out lesions with a gray-white necrotic base. They occur most commonly after mucosal trauma, herpes infection, or chemotherapeutics. Acute leukemias, particularly acute monocytic forms, cause infiltration of leukemic cells into oral soft tissue, especially gingival tissue, resulting in swollen, boggy hyperplastic gingivitis. Gingival lesions can be a result of direct infiltration, as shown in Fig. 234-13, due to drug toxicity, from graft-versus-host disease, or secondary to marrow or lymphoid tissue depression.[47] Infiltration of leukemic cells into the periapical tissue clinically and radiographically resembles periapical inflammatory disease.[48]

Chronic Vesiculoulcerative Disease

PEMPHIGUS VULGARIS Pemphigus vulgaris is a rare disease with an incidence of 0.5 to 3.2 per 100,000 persons annually. It is important,

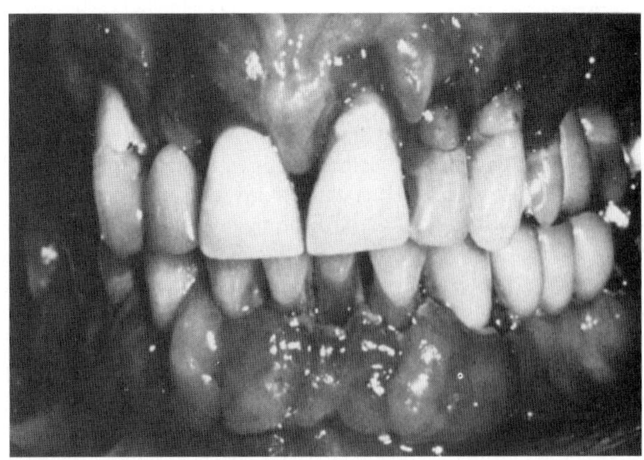

FIG. 234-13. Oral manifestations of leukemia.

though, because without treatment, its mortality rate is high. Oral manifestations occur in up to 70 percent of patients and are frequently the first sign of disease, preceding cutaneous lesions by up to a year. Oral lesions are also the most difficult to treat. Ulceration results from autoantibodies attacking the deeper layer of the stratum spinosum of the epidermis, resulting in an intraepithelial split. Females are affected slightly more commonly, with a female-to-male ratio of 2:3. Pemphigus vulgaris most commonly affects people in their sixth decade of life. Typical lesions are superficial erosions with ragged edges found on any oral mucosal surface. Involvement of the soft palate is most common, occurring 80 percent of the time. The buccal mucosa is the next most common site of involvement (46 percent), followed by the tongue (20 percent). Cutaneous lesions appear as fluid-filled vesicles and bullae. Lesions can be induced by firm lateral pressure on apparently normal skin (Nikolsky's sign). Treatment includes systemic corticosteroids as well as other immunosuppressive agents and is beyond the realm of emergency medicine. Referral to an appropriate consultant is necessary.[16,49]

CICATRICIAL PEMPHIGOID Cicatricial pemphigoid is a chronic vesiculobullous mucocutaneous disorder with an autoimmune etiology. Autoantibodies against the basement membrane result in subepithelial cleft formation. Cicatricial pemphigoid affects people in the seventh decade of life, with no race predilection. The ratio of males to females 1:2.27. Oral lesions are seen in approximately 85 percent of patients, but any mucosal or cutaneous site can be affected. Oral lesions may begin as a desquamative gingivitis or vesiculobullous lesions. Oral lesions eventually become denuded, leaving a painful, erythematous, irregularly bordered erosion or ulcer. Lesions may persist for weeks. Significantly, ocular involvement occurs in 65 percent of cicatricial pemphigoid patients and, if untreated, may lead to blindness. Referral to an ophthalmologist is essential. Diagnosis is by biopsy and immunofluorescent staining of perilesional mucosa. Histologically, the lesions show inflammatory infiltrates surrounding subepithelial bullae. Treatment must be individualized. Treatment of isolated oral lesions with topical steroids is acceptable. Intralesional steroid injections may be useful. Systemic involvement or persistent oral lesions require systemic steroid therapy.[16,50]

ERYTHEMA MULTIFORME Erythema multiforme most commonly affects men in the third or fourth decade of life. Early cutaneous lesions are concentric erythematous circular rings resembling a target (target lesion). Oral lesions are painful erythematous patches that undergo necrosis, forming large ulcerations with irregular borders. They occur most commonly on the lips, labial mucosa, buccal mucosa, tongue, floor of the mouth, and soft palate, sparing the hard palate and gingiva. Erythema multiforme is a spectrum of diseases that includes toxic epidermal necrosis in its most severe form. Stevens-Johnson syndrome includes ocular and genital involvement accompanying oral lesions. Treatment is with systemic steroids in all patients except those with isolated oral lesions. In such patients, topical steroids may be adequate.[16,51]

LICHEN PLANUS Lichen planus is one of a group of chronic cutaneous vesiculoerosive diseases affecting approximately 1 percent of the population. Females are affected three times as often as males. Certain drugs such as ACE inhibitors have been shown to cause lichenoid-type reactions, and these must be differentiated from lichen planus. Lichen planus is a result of T-lymphocyte attack on the basal cell layer. Approximately, 50 percent of patients with cutaneous lesions have oral lesions, but only 25 percent of patients have isolated oral lesions. Lichen planus can affect any mucosal surface; however, orally, the buccal mucosa is most common (Fig. 234-14). In its reticular form, lichen planus appears as multiple scattered white papules interconnected via white lines called *Wickham's striae*. Definitive diagnosis is via biopsy and immunofluorescent staining. The reticular and papular patterns are usually asymptomatic and require no treatment. Symptomatic erosive and atrophic forms of lichen planus, especially those involving the tongue, can be treated successfully with topical corticosteroids. Some question concerning the premalignant potential of lichen planus, especially the erosive form, exists, but less than 1 percent of oral lichen planus undergoes malignant transformation.[16,52]

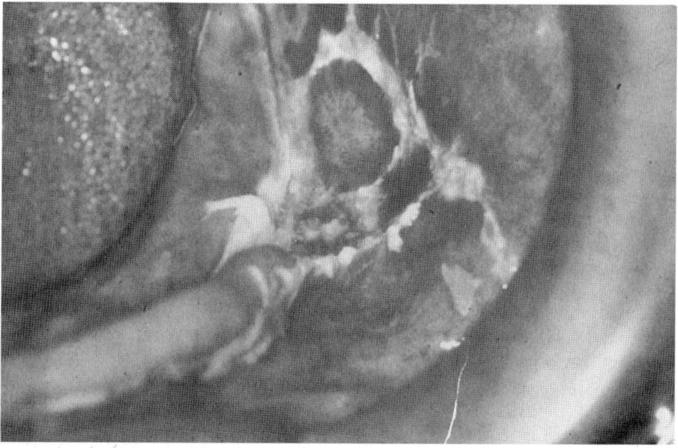

FIG. 234-14. Lichen planus. (*Courtesy of Baldev Singh, B.D.S., Ph.D.*)

Graft-versus-Host Disease

Graft-versus-host disease occurs in up to 50 percent of allogeneic bone marrow transplants despite HLA matching and immunosuppressive therapy. In graft-versus-host disease, the transplanted bone marrow cells recognize the host as foreign, and transplanted hematopoetic cells attack the host. Systemic manifestations of the disease vary by the severity of disease, organ system affected, and acute versus chronic disease. Oral manifestations include lesions in a fine white papular pattern, interlacing white striae in a lichenoid or reticular pattern, and a desquamative pattern occurring commonly on the tongue and labial and buccal mucosa. Posttransplant ulcerations related to the induced neutropenic state occur in the first 2 weeks. Ulcerations that persist longer must be attributed to graft-versus-host disease. Xerostomia and a burning oral sensation are common. The oral lesions and xerostomia as a result of chronic graft-versus-host disease may persist for years. An increased incidence of periodontal disease and dental caries is associated with decreased salivary flow. The principal approach to treatment is to prevent disease with the addition of other immunosuppressive agents. Oral topical steroids improve healing of oral ulceration and psoralen and ultraviolet A (PUVA) therapy may be used on cutaneous oral lesions.[47,53]

Sexually Transmitted Diseases

GONORRHEA Oral gonococcal infection with *Neisseria gonorrhoeae* is not uncommon. The most frequent mode of transmission is fellatio. Consequently, it is seen more commonly in females and homosexual males. A stomatitis may occur with fiery red and inflammed oral mucosa. More commonly, a pharyngitis involving the uvula and tonsils occurs. Gonococcal pharyngitis may present with or without pustules or exudate. In the carrier state, a normal pharyngeal appearance may be present. Treatment is the same as with genital involvement.[11,54]

SYPHILIS The primary chancre of syphillis can occur orally and may affect the lips, gingiva, hard and soft palates, buccal mucosa, pharynx, and tongue. Chancre of the lip is the most common oral site involved. Tongue involvement is next in frequency, followed closely by the tonsils. An oral chancre is similar in appearance to the genital counterpart. Initially, the lesion may be an erythematous papule that erodes into the classic painless, punched-out ulcer that becomes firm and indurated.[11,54]

Secondary syphilis follows the onset of the primary lesion by 9 to 90 days. Systemic symptoms such as fever, malaise, generalized lymphadenopathy, weight loss, and arthralgia are common during the secondary stage. Oral lesions are common and frequently accompany cutaneous lesions but may occur alone. They are usually multiple, oval-shaped, slightly raised ulcers or erosions covered with a gray membrane. They occur most commonly on the tip and sides of the tongue. Condyloma lata rarely occur intraorally.[11,54]

Tertiary syphilis can occur many years after the initial infection. Intraorally, the tongue is enlarged in a lobulated or irregular pattern with atrophic and hypertrophic areas. A single gumma is unusual. Chronic interstitial glossitis may result in fissuring of the tongue. In late syphilis, the tongue atrophies secondary to ischemia associated with chronic interstitial glossitis, resulting in balding of the tongue with thinning and wrinkling of the mucosal surface. Gummatous infiltration of the hard palate also may occur.[11,54]

Congenital syphilis affects the formation of both the anterior and posterior teeth. The permanent maxillary incisors are most affected. These *Hutchinson incisors* are usually shorter than the lateral incisors and barrel-shaped, resembling a screwdriver. The central portion of the incisal edge may be notched. The posterior molars, or *mulberry molars,* are narrower at the oclussal surface, and the normally occurring four cusps are replaced by many more, resulting in the characteristic mulberry appearance.[11,19,54]

Diagnosis of syphilis is with serology or dark-field examination of the primary and secondary lesions. Benzathine penicillin G 2.4 million units intramuscularly is used to treat primary, secondary, and latent syphilis of less than 1 year duration. VDRL at 3, 6, 12, and 24 months is necessary. Weekly injections for 3 weeks are necessary for the treatment of infections of greater than 1 year duration. Daily ceftriaxone injections for 10 days in the penicillin-allergic patient are an alternative.[11,54]

HERPES TYPE 2 Ninety percent of all herpes type 2 occurs in the anogenital region, but with oral-genital contact, oral lesions may occur. Oral herpes type 1 and type 2 infections are clinically indistinguishable, with primary infection frequently causing a gingivostomatitis and associated fever and malaise. Lesions may last up to 2 weeks. Secondary or recurrent lesions occur as a result of the same predisposing factors as type 1. Definitive diagnosis is made in the laboratory by viral cultures or DNA probe. Treatment of primary genital lesions with acyclovir 400 mg PO tid or Valtrex 1g PO/bid for 10 days is recommended. Acyclovir 400 mg PO tid or valacyclovir 500 mg PO bid for 5 days shortens the course of disease, and prophylactic therapy reduces recurrences and subclinical shedding of herpes simplex type 2.[11,16,54]

HUMAN PAPILLOMAVIRUS Human papillomavirus is probably the most common sexually transmitted disease today. HPV-6, -11, and -45 are most commonly associated with *condyloma acuminatum,* or *venereal warts.* Although most commonly affecting the anogenital region, oral lesions can occur. Intraorally, the labial and buccal mucosa, palate, tongue, and gingiva are most commonly affected, although any site can be involved. Lesions many be solitary or multiple and are sessile or pedunculated nodules. Treatment is with electrosurgical or laser therapy.[11,54]

Acquired Immunodeficiency Syndrome

There are numerous oral manifestations of HIV infection. Primary HIV infection, occurring from 1 to 6 weeks after contact, is an acute viral syndrome but may have associated intraoral findings such as a sore throat, mucosal erythema, and focal ulceration. Persistent generalized lymphadenopathy, particularly of the cervical lymph nodes, is present in 70 percent of otherwise asymptomatic HIV-infected patients. The presentation of acquired immunodeficiency syndrome (AIDS) is highly variable, and numerous oral manifestations can occur. Oropharyngeal candidiasis is the most common oral finding and may lead to the initial diagnosis of AIDS. HIV-related gingivitis is distinctive, presenting as a 2- to 3-mm linear band of erythema along the gingival free margin. Periodontitis among the HIV-infected population is common and usually more aggressive and painful in its presentation. Such necrotizing periodontitis is distinguished from acute necrotizing ulcerative gingivitis, which is also a common finding, by it distribution and microbiology. Viruses such as herpes simplex virus, varicella-zoster virus, and Epstein-Barr virus are fairly common and produce more significant disease when present in the immunocompromised patient. Hairy leukoplakia, somewhat distinctive hyperkeratotic and epithelial hyperplastic lesions on the lateral borders of the tongue, strongly suggests HIV infection. Kaposi's sarcoma is the most common malignancy associated with AIDS and appears orally as a nonblanching brown to purplish macule or papule affecting most commonly the gingiva or hard palate. Lymphoma, primarily non-Hodgkin's lymphoma, is the second most commonly associated cancer. Many less common findings occur such as aphthous-like ulcerations, mulloscum contagiosum, verruca vulgaris, thrombocytopenia, salivary gland enlargement, and mucosal hyperpigmentation. With the concurrent use of newer therapeutic agents such as the nonnucleoside inhibitors, protease inhibitors, and the nucleoside inhibitors, significantly fewer opportunistic infections are seen.[19,55]

Other

Many other diseases have intraoral manifestations. Of note, mucopolysaccharidosis and amyloidosis show some degree of magroglossia. Ectodermal dysplasia results in varying degrees of xerostomia and oligodontia. Several other diseases such as amelogenesis imperfecta, dentinogenesis imperfecta, and osteogenesis imperfecta cause significant defects of the enamel and dentin.

REFERENCES

1. Williams RC: Periodontal disease. *N Engl J Med* 322:373, 1990.
2. Jaber L, Cohen I, Mor A: Fever associated with teething. *Arch Dis Child* 67:234, 1992.
3. Matthews RW, Peak JD, Scully C: The efficacy of management of acute dental pain. *Br Dent J* 176:413, 1994.
4. Antrim DD, Bakland LK, Parker MW: Treatment of endodontic urgent care cases. *Dent Clin North Am* 30:549, 1986.
5. Montgomery S, Ferguson CD: Diagnostic, treatment planning, and prognostic considerations. *Dent Clin North Am* 30:533, 1986.
6. Iwu CO: Ludwig's angina: A report of seven cases and review of current concepts in management. *Br J Oral Maxillofac Surg* 28:189, 1990.
7. Sorenson DC, Preisch JW: The effect of tetracycline on the incidence of postextraction alveolar osteitis. *J Oral Maxillofac Surg* 45:1029, 1987.
8. Colby RC: The general practitioner's perspective of the etiology, prevention, and treatment of dry socket. *Gen Dent* 45:461, 1997.
9. Garibaldi JA: Dentoalveolar surgical sequelae. *Compend Contin Educ Dent* 19:407, 1998.
10. Suzuki JB: Diagnosis and classification of periodontal disease. *Dent Clin North Am* 32:195, 1988.
11. Laskaris G: Oral manifestations of infectious diseases. *Dent Clin North Am* 40:395, 1996.
12. Horning GM: Necrotizing gingivostomatitis: NUG to noma. *Compend Contin Educ Dent* 17:951, 1996.
13. Horning GM, Cohen ME: Necrotizing ulcerative gingivitis, periodontitis, and stomatitis: Clinical staging and predisposing factors. *J Periodontol* 66:990, 1995.
14. Donlon WC, Jacobson AL, Truta MP: Neuralgia. *Otolaryngol Clin North Am* 22:1145, 1989.

15. Fotos PG, Vincent SD, Hellstein MAJ: Oral candidiosis. *Oral Surg Oral Med Oral Pathol* 74:41, 1992.
16. Glass BJ, Kuhel RF, Langlais RP: Treatment of common orofacial conditions. *Dent Clin North Am* 30:421, 1986.
17. Vincent SD, Lilly GE: Clinical, historic, therapeutic features of apthous stomatitis: Literature review and open clinical trial employing steroids. *Oral Surg Oral Med Oral Pathol* 74:79, 1992.
18. Espelid M, Bang G, Johannessen AC, et al: Geographic stomatitis: Report of 6 cases. *J Oral Pathol Med* 20:425, 1991.
19. Neville BW, Damm DD, Allen CM, et al: *Oral and Maxillofacial Pathology.* Philadelphia: Saunders, 1995.
20. Sarti GM, Haddy RI, Schaffer D, et al: Black hairy tongue. *Am Fam Phys* 41:1751, 1990.
21. Bouquot JE, Gorlin RJ: Leukoplakia, lichen planus, and other oral keratoses in 23,616 white Americans over the age of 35 years. *Oral Surg Oral Med Oral Pathol* 61:373, 1986.
22. Mashberg A, Samit AM: Early detection, diagnosis, and management of oral and oropharyngeal cancer. *CA* 39:67, 1989.
23. Silverberg E, Lubera JA: Cancer statistics. *CA* 39:3, 1989.
24. Marder MZ: The standard of care for oral diagnosis as it relates to oral cancer. *Compend Contin Educ Dent* 19:569, 1998.
25. Halperin V, Jefferis KR, Huddleston SO, et al: The occurrence of fordyce spots, benign migratory glossitis, median rhomboid glossitis, and fissured tongue in 2478 dental patients. *Oral Surg Oral Med Oral Pathol* 6:1072, 1953.
26. Kolas S, et al: The occurrence of torus palatinus and torus mandibularis in 2478 dental patients. *Oral Surg Oral Med Oral Pathol* 6:1134, 1953.
27. Johnson R: Descriptive classification of trauma: The injuries to the teeth and suporting structures. *J Am Dent Assoc* 102:195, 1981.
28. Dumsha, TC: Luxation Injuries. *Dent Clin North Am* 39:79, 1995.
29. Rauschenberger CR, Hovland EJ: Clinical management of crown fractures. *Dent Clin North Am* 39:25, 1995.
30. Medford HM: Temporary stabilization of avulsed teeth. *Ann Emerg Med* 11:490, 1982.
31. Trope M: Clinical management of the avulsed tooth. *Dent Clin North Am* 39:93, 1995.
32. Blomlof L: Milk and saliva as possible storage media for traumatically exarticulated teeth prior to replantation. *Swed Dent J* 8:1, 1981.
33. Lindskog S, Blomlof L: Influence of osmolality and composition of some storage media on human periodontal ligament cells. *Acta Odontol Scand* 40:435, 1982.
34. Finkelman D, Butler WT: Vitamin D deficiency and skeletal tissues. *J Oral Pathol* 14:191, 1985.
35. Greenberg MS: Clinical and histological changes of the oral mucosa in pernicious anemia. *Oral Surg Oral Med Oral Pathol* 52:38, 1981.
36. Walls AWG, Soames JV: Dental manifestations of autoimmune hypoparathyroidism. *Oral Surg Oral Med Oral Pathol* 75:452, 1993.
37. Cianciola LJ, Park BH, Bruck E, et al: Prevalence of periodontal disease in insulin-dependent diabetes mellitus (juvenile diabetes). *J Am Dent Assoc* 104:653, 1982.
38. Hovinga J, Roodvoets AP, Gaillard J: Some findings in patients with ureamic stomatitis. *J Maxillofac Surg* 3:124, 1975.
39. Dongari A, McDonnell HT, Langlais RP: Drug-induced gingival overgrowth. *Oral Surg Oral Med Oral Pathol* 76:543, 1993.
40. Granstein RD, Sober AJ: Drug and heavy metal induced hyperpigmentation. *J Am Acad Dermatol* 5:1, 1981.
41. Handlers JP, Waterman J, Abrams AM, et al: Oral features of Wegener's granulomatosis. *Arch Otolaryngol* 111:267, 1985.
42. Brennan TF, Vrabec DP: Tuberculosis of the oral mucosa: Report of a case. *Ann Otol Rhinol Laryngol* 79:601, 1970.
43. Bucci F, et al: Oral lesions of lepromatous leprosy. *J Oral Med* 42:4, 1987.
44. Frankel DH, Mostofi RS, Lorincz AL: Oral Crohn's disease: Report of two cases in brothers with metallic dysgeusia and a review of the literature. *J Am Acad Dermatol* 12:260, 1985.
45. Daley TD, Nartey NO, Wysocki GP: Pregnancy tumor: An analysis. *Oral Surg Oral Med Oral Pathol* 72:196, 1991.
46. Eversole LR, Jacobsen PL, Stone CE: Oral and gingival changes in systemic sclerosis (scleroderma). *J Periodontol* 55:175, 1984.
47. Barrett AP: Gingival lesions in leukemia: A classification. *J Periodontol* 55:585, 1984.
48. Peterson DE, Gerar H, Williams LT: An unusual instance of leukemic infiltrate: Diagnosis and management of periapical tooth involvement. *Cancer* 51:1716, 1983.
49. Lamey P-J, Rees TD, Wright JM, et al: Oral presentation of pemphigus vulgaris and its response to systemic steroid response. *Oral Surg Oral Med Oral Pathol* 74:54, 1992.
50. Ahmed AR, Kurgis BS, Rogers RS: Cicatricial pemphigoid. *J Am Acad Dermatol* 24:987, 1991.
51. Bastuji-Garin S, Rzany B, Stern RS, et al: Clinical classification of cases of toxic epidermal necrolysis, Stevens-Johnson syndrome, and erythema multiforme. *Arch Dermatol* 129:92, 1993.
52. Jungell P: Oral lichen planus: A review. *Int J Oral Maxillofac Surg* 20:129, 1991.
53. Barrett AP, Bilous AM: Oral patterns of acute and chronic graft-v-host disease. *Arch Dermatol* 120:1461, 1984.
54. Fiumara NJ: Venereal disease of the oral cavity. *J Oral Med* 31:36, 1976.
55. Scully C, McCarthy G: Management of oral health in persons with HIV infection. *Oral Surg Oral Med Oral Pathol* 73:215, 1992.

DISORDERS OF THE NECK AND UPPER AIRWAY

Theresa A. Hackeling
Rudolph J. Triana, Jr.

This chapter discusses common infections and the most important conditions that can obstruct the upper airway. The upper airway infections are pharyngitis, epiglottitis, peritonsillar abscess, and retropharyngeal abscess. Noninfectious conditions that can obstruct the airway are posttonsillectomy bleeding, caustic ingestion, foreign bodies, and laryngeal trauma.

PHARYNGITIS

Pharyngitis is an infection or irritation of the pharynx and tonsils. It rarely occurs in infants younger than 1 year and is uncommon in infants younger than 2 years. It peaks between the ages of 4 to 7 years but recurs throughout life. Seasonal variation occurs, with a higher incidence in winter.[1]

Causal agents of pharyngitis include viruses, bacteria, fungi, and parasites (Table 235-1). Most often, viruses are the culprits. Rhinovirus and adenovirus are the most common, but Epstein-Barr virus, herpes simplex virus, influenzavirus, parainfluenzavirus, and coronavirus are responsible for about 5 percent of the infections.[2] Fungal and, very rarely, parasitic infection occurs in an immunocompromised host, but such infections are rarely found in immunocompetent patients. The most common bacteria causing pharyngitis include *Streptococcus pyogenes* [group A β-hemolytic streptococcus (GABHS)], *Mycoplasma, Chlamydia, Neisseria,* and *Corynebacterium.* GABHS is responsible for 15 percent of all pharyngitis and is associated with significant nonsuppurative sequelae in the form of acute rheumatic fever (ARF) or acute glomerulonephritis (AGN).[2] Because of the sequelae associated with GABHS, there is a greater emphasis placed on early diagnosis and treatment of this causal agent. This organism produces three extracellular pyrogenic exotoxins (A, B, and C) that facilitate tissue penetration. Almost every body tissue is subject to infection, but the skin and throat are favorite targets because of host-dependent surface receptor sites.[2]

Endemic year-round GABHS pharyngitis has its peak occurrence in the late winter and early spring.[1] After an incubation period of 2 to 5 days, patients develop the sudden onset of sore throat, painful swallowing, chills, and fever. Headache, nausea, vomiting, and abdominal pain are common associated symptoms.

On physical examination of patients with typical GABHS, there are erythematous tonsils, discrete tonsillar exudate; enlarged, tender

TABLE 235-1 Causes of Pharyngitis

VIRUSES
Rhinovirus
Adenovirus
Epstein-Barr virus
Herpes simplex virus
Influenzavirus
Parainfluenzavirus
Coronavirus
Varicella virus
BACTERIA
Streptococcus species
Staphylococcus species
Haemophilus influenzae
Bordetella pertussis
Mycoplasma pneumoniae
Chlamydia pneumoniae
Neisseria gonorrhoeae
Corynebacterium diptheriae, C. pyogenes, C. ulcerans
FUNGI
Candida albicans
Cryptococcus
Blastomycosis
Histoplasma
PARASITES
Leishmania brasiliensis
Toxoplasma gondii

anterior cervical lymph nodes; and uvula edema. Often, palatal petechiae accompany the marked erythema of the throat and tonsils. Viral and bacterial agents often present with a more vesicular and petechial pattern on the soft palate and tonsils of the pharynx and no exudate. Clinical differentiation between viral and bacterial infection can be difficult.

Throat culture remains the most effective method for diagnosis. A single throat swab cultured correctly on a blood agar plate has a sensitivity of 90 to 95 percent in detecting the presence of a GABHS.[3] A disadvantage of culturing a throat swab is the delay in obtaining the culture results. Rapid antigen detection tests (RADTs) have been developed for the identification of GABHS directly from throat swabs. Most of the RADTs currently available have an excellent specificity (>95 percent) compared to blood agar plate cultures.[4] Either a positive throat culture or RADT result provides adequate confirmation of the presence of GABHS in the pharynx, but a negative RADT result should be confirmed with a throat culture.

All patients with pharyngitis should receive symptomatic treatment. Gargling with warm saltwater, drinking warm liquids, and rest are important. Patients unable to tolerate oral fluids or who become dehydrated should be given intravenous fluids. Young children and geriatric patients should be carefully assessed for their ability to remain well hydrated.

A number of antibiotics are effective against GABHS. These agents include penicillin and its congeners (e.g., ampicillin and amoxicillin), as well as numerous cephalosporins, macrolides, and clindamycin. However, penicillin remains the drug of choice because of its proven efficacy, safety, narrow spectrum, and low cost. Erythromycin is a suitable alternative for patients allergic to penicillin. First- or second-generation cephalosporins are also acceptable for penicillin-allergic patients who do not manifest immediate hypersensitivity. Most oral antibiotics, except the newer macrolides, must be administered for 10 days to achieve maximal pharyngeal eradication of GABHS. It has been reported that azithromycin, cefuroxime, cefixime, and cefpodoxime can be used to achieve comparable bacteriologic and clinical cure rates among patients with streptococcal pharyngitis when given for less than 5 days.[3] Close contacts and family members should be cultured, and those whose results are positive should be treated.

All types of pharyngitis can lead to suppurative complications, including cervical lymphadenitis, peritonsillar abscess, retropharyngeal abscess, sinusitis, and otitis media.

EPIGLOTTITIS

Epiglottitis is a potentially life-threatening disease that can lead to rapid, unpredictable airway obstruction resulting in hypoxia and respiratory arrest. It is an inflammatory condition, usually infectious, primarily of the epiglottis but often including the aeryepiglottic folds and the loose connective tissue in the pre-epiglottic and paraglottic spaces. Some clinicians prefer the term *supraglottitis* because the process rarely involves just the epiglottis.

Epiglottitis is traditionally reported to affect children between the ages of 2 and 8 years.[5] Epiglottitis and meningitis are the most common life-threatening diseases caused by *Haemophilus influenzae* type b (Hib). With the introduction of the Hib vaccine, the incidence of epiglottitis in children has been reduced, while the incidence in adults appears to be increasing.[6] Epiglottitis is more common in African Americans than in whites or Hispanics.[7] Incidence peaks in the spring and the fall and in during the summer months.[8]

Epiglottitis can be caused by bacteria, viruses, and fungi (Table 235-2), but the commonest cause is Hib.[9,10] Other pathogens that have been isolated include *Streptococcus* species, *Staphylococcus* species, *Moraxella catarrhalis, Klebsiella, Mycobacterium tuberculosis, Candida* species, respiratory syncytial virus, varicella virus, adenovirus, and herpesvirus.

Patients with epiglottitis caused by Hib typically experience a 1- to 2-day prodrome that resembles a benign upper respiratory tract infection. The symptom constellation associated with epiglottitis is listed in Table 235-3.

Physical examination of a patient with epiglottitis may reveal an appearance of apprehension, drooling, and difficulty lying supine. Stridor and protrusion of the tongue are frequently noted. The stridor associated with epiglottitis is primarily inspiratory and is softer and lower pitched than in children with croup.[11] Fever is initially absent in 30 to 50 percent of cases and may develop later.[11] Patients often position themselves sitting up, leaning forward, mouth open, head extended, and panting. Thick oral pharyngeal secretions are commonly present, with little or no cough. Movement of the upper trachea or

TABLE 235-2 Causes of Epiglottitis

BACTERIA
Haemophilus influenzae
Streptococcus species
Staphylococcus species
Moraxella catarrhalis
Klebsiella pneumoniae
FUNGI
Mycobacterium tuberculosis
Candida albicans
VIRUSES
Varicella virus
Adenovirus
Herpesvirus
Respiratory syncytial virus

TABLE 235-3 Signs and Symptoms of Epiglottitis

Fever
Dysphagia
Stridor
Apprehension
Drooling
Pooling of secretions
Labored breathing
Protrusion of the tongue
Tender larynx
Erect position
Panting

thyroid cartilage is often quite painful and is a marker for supraglottic infection.

Diagnosis is made by history, clinical examination, radiographs, and laryngoscopy. Lateral cervical soft tissue radiographs demonstrate obliteration of the vallecula, swelling of the aryepiglottic folds, edema of the prevertebral and retropharyngeal soft tissues, and ballooning of the hypopharynx (Fig. 235-1).[12] The edematous epiglottis appears enlarged and thumb-shaped. Blood and surface cultures of the epiglottis are useful to confirm the presence of Hib but should be postponed until an artificial airway has been established.

Patients should be treated with extreme care because of the possibility of unpredictable sudden airway obstruction. While severe cases of epiglottitis are easily recognized, as many as 36 percent of less severe cases are initially misdiagnosed as pharyngitis.[9] Therefore, clinicians must maintain heightened suspicion for this disease. All patients with suspected epiglottitis require immediate otolaryngologic consultation, and the emergency physician must be prepared to establish a definitive airway at all times. Patients should never be left unattended. Initial treatment consists of supplemental humidified oxygen, intravenous hydration, monitoring, and intravenous antibiotics. Heliox can be given to temporarily decrease airway resistance. In cases of airway obstruction in the emergency department, endotracheal intubation must be attempted, but the physician should be prepared for a very difficult intubation secondary to the swollen, distorted anatomy. In the case of intubation failure, the last resorts for preserving the airway in adult and pediatric patients are cricothyrotomy and needle cricothyrotomy, respectively. Current antibiotic recommendations include cefuroxime, cefotaxime, or ceftriaxone as first-line drugs.[10] Alternative antibiotics include ampicillin-sulbactam and trimethoprim-sulfamethoxazole. The use of steroids to decrease inflammation and edema remains controversial, but they are used empirically by many otolaryngologists.

PERITONSILLAR ABSCESS

Peritonsillar abscess (PTA) is the most frequently occurring deep-space infection of the head and neck.[13,14] It is an acute, usually infectious, accumulation of purulent material between the tonsillar capsule and the superior constrictor muscle of the pharynx (Fig. 235-2). It is thought to be a complication of follicular tonsillitis that progresses from local cellulitis to abscess. A secondary mechanism of abscess development may occur through seeding of bacteria throughout the tonsil via the bloodstream or lymphatics.[15]

PTAs are more common during the second and third decades.[13] The incidence of PTAs corresponds to the incidence of streptococcal pharyngitis and tonsillitis, occurring with greatest frequency from November to December and from April to May.

Cultures of aspirates from PTAs characteristically produce a mixture of aerobic and anaerobic flora.[16] The most predominant infective organisms in PTAs are *S. pyogenes, Bacteroides, Peptostreptococcus,* and *Staphylococcus aureus.*[14,16] β-lactamase producing organisms are present in up to one half of all culture specimens.[14]

Symptoms of a PTA include fever, malaise, ''hot-potato voice,'' sore throat, odynophagia, dysphagia, and otalgia. Signs of a PTA include dehydration, unilateral tonsillar hypertrophy, palatal edema, contralateral deflection of the swollen uvula, inferior and medial displacement of the infected tonsil, tender cervical lymphadenopathy, drooling, rancid breadth, and trismus (Fig. 235-3).

The differential diagnosis of a PTA includes cellulitis, infectious mononucleosis, herpes simplex tonsillitis, retropharyngeal abscess, neoplasm, foreign body, and internal artery carotid aneurysm.

The diagnostic gold standard of a PTA is aspiration of pus through an 18-gauge needle. This should be done by individuals trained in the technique who can manage complications of the procedure. Prior to aspiration lidocaine spray or gel is used to anesthetize the overlying mucosa topically. Then, 1 to 2 mL lidocaine with epinephrine, using a 25-gauge needle, can be injected into the mucosa of the anterior tonsillar pillar. Once adequate anesthesia is achieved, an 18-gauge needle should be directed medially and superiorly within the abscess cavity. The needle should penetrate no more than 1 cm. A needle guard can be made by cutting the distal tip of a needle cover and

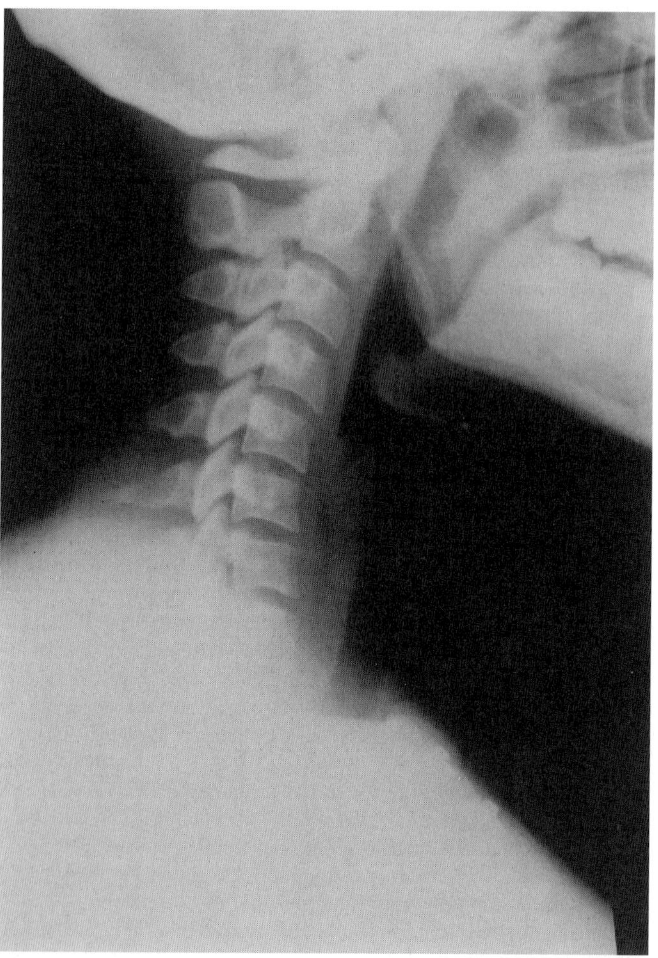

FIG. 235-1. Lateral radiograph demonstrating thumbprinting of the epiglottis and ballooning of the parapharyngeal space consistent with epiglottitis.

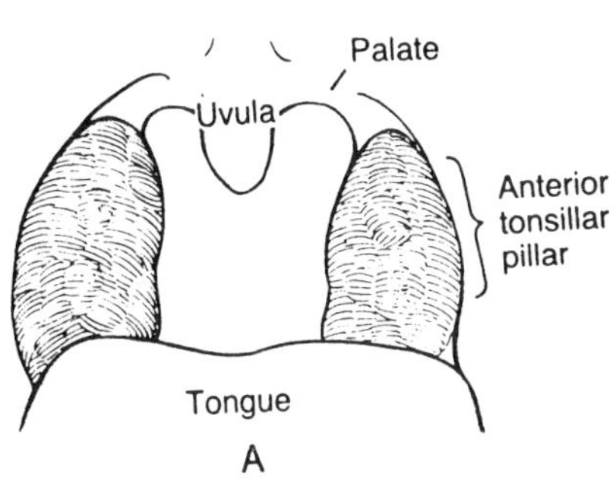

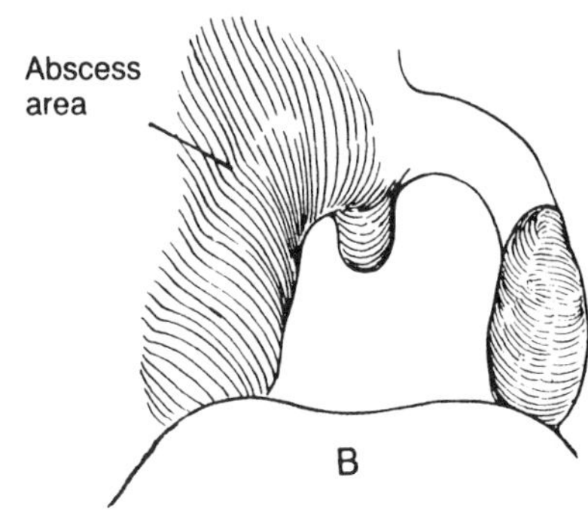

FIG. 235-2. **A.** In tonsillitis, the tonsils are enlarged. They may be covered by white exudate. The margin between the tonsil and the anterior tonsillar pillar is well defined. **B.** In peritonsillar abscess, the tonsil, palate, and anterior tonsillar pillar may be bulging medially in one unit. The margin between the tonsil, palate, and anterior tonsillar pillar is somewhat effaced. The uvula is usually edematous and may be pointing toward the opposite tonsil. The safest area to aspirate a peritonsillar abscess is usually just above the tonsil in the soft palate. This location will serve to guard the deep vessels of the neck from inadvertent injury. (From Abelson TI, Witt WJ, in Roberts JR, Hedges JR, eds: *Clinical Procedures in Emergency Medicine,* 2d ed. Philadelphia, Saunders, 1991, with permission.)

replacing it over the needle so that less than 1 cm of the needle is exposed. Note that the carotid artery lies laterally and inferiorly, and care should be taken to avoid this area. Often, multiple aspirations may be required to find the abscess. Attempts should first begin on the superior aspect of the anterior tonsillar pillar and then progress inferiorly. Any pus aspirated should be sent for Gram stain, aerobic cultures, and anaerobic cultures. Children with trismus in whom adequate examination is not possible should be brought to the operating room and examined under anesthesia. When the airway is not in jeopardy and either a complete examination or aspiration is not possible, a computed tomography (CT) scan of the neck may be required to better evaluate this area.

The majority of PTAs can be treated effectively with outpatient needle aspiration, antibiotics, and pain medication. Incision and drainage or tonsillectomy can be performed when needle aspiration fails. A contrast CT scan of the neck is recommended when the results of needle aspiration are negative and a parapharyngeal- or retropharyngeal-space process is suspected. A PTA in a child requires hospitalization, intravenous hydration, antibiotics, and removal of the abscessed tonsil under general anesthesia. High-dose penicillin is the drug of choice, although, in light of current microbiologic findings of penicillin-resistant organisms, treatment with penicillin alone may be ineffective. Ampicillin-sulbactam, clindamycin, cefotaxime, and metronidazole should be considered. Ten days of antibiotics after aspiration is usual. Previous antibiotic treatment does not always prevent the development of peritonsillar abscess. Many patients presenting with peritonsillar abscess have been treated with antibiotics at the time of presentation.

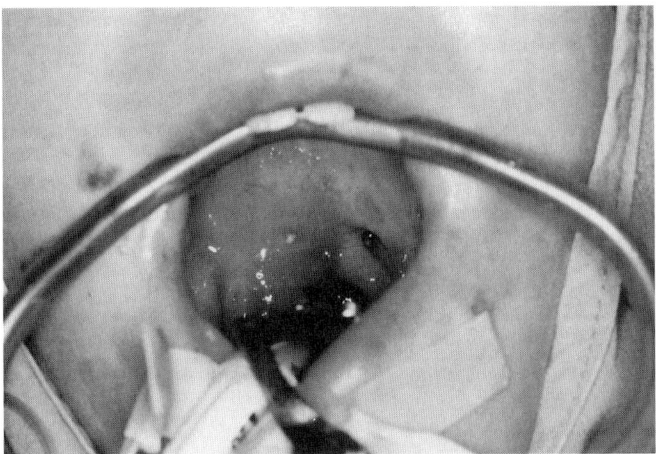

FIG. 235-3. Open-mouth view with mouthgag present in a patient demonstrating tonsillar hypertrophy, palatal edema, and uvula deviation consistent with a peritonsillar abscess.

Complications of a PTA include airway obstruction, rupture of the abscess with aspiration of the contents, thrombophlebitis, ulceration of the large submaxillary arteries, epiglottitis, septicemia, endocarditis, retropharyngeal abscess, and mediastinitis.

RETROPHARYNGEAL ABSCESS

A retropharyngeal abscess is an infection of the deep neck spaces resulting from suppuration and necrosis of the lymph nodes in those spaces. The retropharyngeal space is a connective tissue pocket that extends from the base of the skull to the level of the tracheal bifurcation. The two paramedial chains of lymph nodes (nodes of Rouvier), which drain the nasopharynx, adenoids, and posterior nasal sinuses, can be found within this space.

Although a retropharyngeal abscess is relatively uncommon, it occurs most frequently in very young children. The majority of children treated for this infection are younger than 12 months of age, and almost one-third of cases occur in children less than 6 months of age.[17] There is a higher incidence of retropharyngeal abscess in young children because of the prominence of several lymph nodes in the space between the posterior pharyngeal wall and the prevertebral fascia. By 3 to 4 years of age, these lymph nodes atrophy and are no longer functional.[17] Predisposing factors for the development of a retropharyngeal abscess include a penetrating foreign body, such as a nasogastric tube or nasotracheal tube; trauma; pharyngitis; tonsillitis; otitis media; nasal or dental procedures; and tonsillectomy or adenoidectomy.

Signs and symptoms include fever, dysphagia, neck pain, limitation of cervical motion, cervical lymphadenopathy, sore throat, poor feeding, muffled voice, and difficulty breathing. Symptoms in children less than 1 year of age are more likely to include stridor and neck swelling. The intense inflammation and swelling associated with a retropharyngeal abscess can lead to inflammatory torticollosis, which is unilateral spasm of the sternocleidomastoid muscle, causing posturing of the head with the occiput rotated toward the affected side.

Cultures from retropharyngeal abscesses have revealed a polymicrobial milieu including aerobes and anaerobes. The most common aerobic species isolated are *Streptococcus viridans* and *S. pyogenes.* Most of the staphylococcal species isolated are β-lactamase producing. *Bacteroides* and *Peptostreptococcus* are the most commonly isolated anaerobes.[18,19] Aerobes and anaerobes work synergistically to increase the severity of the disease.

Radiographs and CT scans are helpful diagnostic tools. A lateral soft-tissue radiograph of the neck taken during inspiration with moderate cervical extension demonstrates thickening and protrusion of the retropharyngeal wall. However, even a small degree of flexion in children normally causes a marked forward bulge of the posterior pharyngeal wall that can be misleading. In adults, the posterior pharyngeal tissue is more constant appearing in flexion and extension, and the width of the soft tissue should not exceed the width of the adjacent vertebral body. A CT scan from the skull base to the clavicles with intravenous contrast is the gold standard for diagnosing deep neck space infections if there is suspicion on radiographs because CT differentiates abscess formation from other causes of retropharyngeal thickening.

All patients suspected of having a retropharyngeal abscess should have immediate otolaryngologic consultation and be admitted to the hospital. Close observation for airway obstruction is the highest priority. Procedures to relieve acute airway obstruction include endotracheal intubation, tracheostomy, cricothyrotomy, and fiberoptic endotracheal intubation. Intravenous hydration and antibiotic treatment should be started in the emergency department until the patient can be brought to the operating room for transoral or transcervical incision and drainage. Antibiotics effective against normal oropharyngeal flora, penicillin-resistant *S. aureus,* and *Bacteroides* should be used. Clindamycin combined with an aminoglycoside, or penicillinase-resistant penicillin combined with a third-generation cephalosporin and metronidazole, is a reasonable antibiotic choice.[18,19]

Catastophic complications from retropharyngeal abscess include extension of the infection into the mediastinum, and upper airway asphyxia from direct pressure or sudden rupture of the abscess.[20]

POSTTONSILLECTOMY AND ADENOIDECTOMY BLEEDING

Tonsillectomy with and without adenoidectomy is one of the most common surgical procedures performed in the United States.[21] It is estimated that 750,000 tonsillectomies with or without adenoidectomies are performed annually.[22] Since this surgery has become an outpatient procedure, complications that were previously evident in the hospital are now presenting to the emergency department. Postoperative bleeding is a well-known complication that can lead to death from airway obstruction or hemorrhagic shock. Estimates of the incidence of posttonsillectomy hemorrhage range from 1 to 10 percent.[21,23]

Classically, hemorrhage occurs between 5 and 10 days postoperatively, but it has been seen as late as 6 weeks postoperatively.[24] There is a significantly higher of incidence of bleeding in the age group between 16 and 25 years of age, with males having a slightly higher predominance than females.[25,26] Hemhorrhage is rare in children under 3 years of age.[27]

Emergency management of posttonsillectomy bleeding consists of ensuring an adequate airway and controlling the bleeding. Otolaryngologic consultation is necessary. Massive bleeding is rare. However, when it occurs, intubation may be the only means of protecting the airway. Each patient should be placed on a monitor, intravenous access should be obtained, blood should be typed and crossmatched, and direct pressure should be applied to the bleeding tonsillar bed while otolaryngologic consultation is obtained. Significant bleeding typically comes from a specific vessel, while generalized oozing comes from the tonsillar bed. More commonly, patients present with bleeding that can be controlled by silver nitrate, electric cautery, or direct pressure with ringed forceps, oxidized cellulose, thrombin packs, or gauze moistened with an equivolume solution of 1:1000 epinephrine and 1% lidocaine. If direct pressure fails, local infiltration of 1 to 3 mL 1% lidocaine with 1:1000 epinephrine may be attempted until the otolaryngologist arrives.

CAUSTIC INGESTION

Esophageal, pharyngeal, and tracheolaryngeal injury can occur from ingestion of bases (alkalis or caustics), acids, and bleaches. Children represent the largest group of caustic injuries, resulting mostly from accidental ingestion. Most adult caustic injuries are suicide attempts.

Ingestion of base-containing substances produces the most significant injury because bases cause liquefactive necrosis, which allows deep penetration of the caustic material.[28] Such substances include lye (NaOH and KOH), ammonia (NH_4OH_4), hair relaxers, hair straighteners, and electric dishwasher soaps. Small amounts of caustic materials can cause significant injury.[28] The injury associated with alkaline substances is completed almost immediately on mucosal contact. Acidic substances cause less severe injury because they cause a coagulation necrosis, which tends to limit extension into the muscular layer.[28]

Patients presenting with caustic injuries of the upper aerodigestive tract display a wide variety of symptoms and physical findings, depending on the anatomic area of involvement (Table 235-4). Studies have failed to show a consistent relationship between symptoms and signs and the ability to predict the severity of injury.[28–30] Absence of oropharyngeal lesions does not exclude esophageal, gastric, or tracheal injury. Eight to 20 percent of patients without oropharyngeal lesions have esophageal burns.[30] Conversely, the presence of oropharyngeal lesions does not necessarily mean that the esophagus or trachea is involved.

The essence of the physical examination is to try to determine the extent of the injury. The examination begins with a careful history, including the type, amount, and brand name of the ingested product. The precise location and extent of the burn in the oropharynx and pharynx should be noted. Complete examination, including the extremities, groin, and chest, is necessary to detect caustic spills to those areas. Patients with oral mucosal burns and tongue edema should be monitored closely for developing airway obstruction, which may be heralded by dyspnea, hoarseness, and stridor. Because symptoms can develop as early as 1 h postingestion or as late as 5 h postingestion, emergency departments should observe children who have ingested caustic substances for at least 5 h.[28] The patient should be given nothing by mouth. Gastric lavage and emesis are contraindicated.

Fiberoptic laryngoscopy is a valuable adjunct in the assessment of the larynx and hypopharynx for injury. Blind nasotracheal or nasogastric intubation may lead to obstructive bleeding or esophageal or pharyngeal perforation, and should not be performed. In a patient with rapid airway deterioration and poor visualization of the larynx, emergency cricothyrotomy or tracheotomy may be necessary. Intravenous steroids are used by many otolaryngologists, but the issue remains very controversial.

Chest and neck radiographs may reveal airway edema, free air, aspiration, mediastinal air, or obstruction. Immediate esophagoscopy and laryngoscopy should be performed in any caustic or acidic inges-

TABLE 235-4 Symptoms of Caustic Ingestion

Pharynx, larynx	Pain, odynophagia, mucosal ulceration, tongue edema, drooling, stridor, hoarseness, refusal to eat or drink
Esophagus	Dysphagia, odynophagia, chest pain, back pain
Stomach	Thoracoabdominal pain, abdominal tenderness, vomiting, hematemesis

tion in a symptomatic patient.[31] Asymptomatic patients observed for 5 h may be safely discharged as long as home observation can be provided, the patient is close to medical care, and follow-up can be provided the next day.[31]

Bleach ingestion is the one exception to the general rule of performing immediate endoscopy and bronchcospy.[31] Bleaches are chlorides that are oxygenating compounds. Sodium hypochlorite is the most common component in such products as Clorox and Comet. In the United States, bleaches typically are only 2.5 percent acid, which produces a superficial ulceration that does not result in stricture or residual sequelae. Management of chlorine bleach ingestion includes careful oropharyngeal examination. If no burns are present and the patient is tolerating fluids by mouth, the patient may be safely discharged with follow-up scheduled in 12 h.[31]

FOREIGN BODIES OF THE AERODIGESTIVE TRACT

Foreign bodies in the aerodigestive tract can be life threatening if not detected early. It is estimated that approximately 1500 people die annually from complications related to foreign-body ingestion and aspiration, with children being the commonest victims.[32] Although a history of solid-particle ingestion is important, this information is often missing for children. The most common foreign body ingested by children is a coin, the second most common is food (e.g., peanuts and popcorn).[33] Because many of the symptoms may be subtle in children, a high index of suspicion is required to arrive at the correct diagnosis before several days have passed. In all children with choking, stridor, wheezing, or unexplained cough, foreign-body aspiration should be suspected. The symptoms in adults are more obvious because adults recognize the symptoms and seek help early. The most common foreign bodies in adults are fishbones, dentures, meat, and meat bones (Fig. 235-4).[34]

Symptoms of laryngeal or tracheal foreign-body aspiration classically follow sudden onset of choking or coughing. Symptoms are listed in Table 235-5. The stridor resembles croup, with a high-pitched inspiratory quality usually associated with a barking cough. Wheezing may be heard throughout the lung fields but is usually loudest over the involved area.[35] Chronic cough or wheezing that fails to respond to medical management, especially in a child without a history of previous reactive airway disease, should raise suspicions of an airway foreign body. In contrast to patients with foreign-body aspiration, patients with foreign-body ingestion usually complain of dysphagia, chest pain, or nausea, which may be accompanied by drooling and vomiting. Cough is uncommon, since most symptoms are related to the pharynx, esophagus, and stomach.

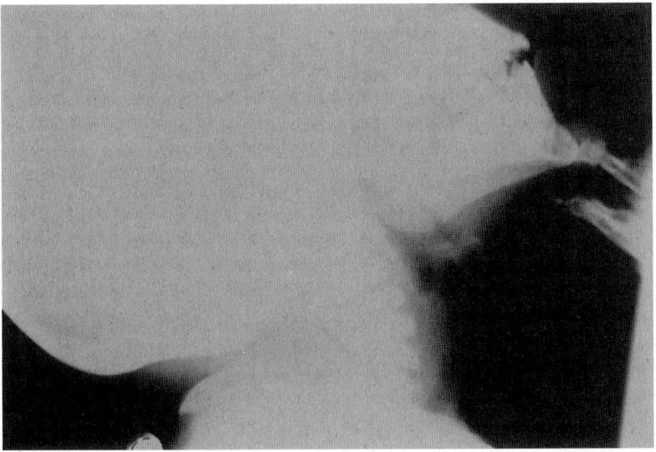

FIG. 235-4. Lateral radiograph demonstrating a fishbone in the soft tissues of the pharynx.

TABLE 235-5 Signs and Symptoms of Foreign-Body Aspiration versus Ingestion

FOREIGN BODY ASPIRATION
Cough
Shortness of breath
Wheezing
Stridor
Dysphonia
Recurrent pneumonia
FOREIGN BODY INGESTION
Dysphagia
Drooling
Vomiting
Chest pain

It is crucial to obtain a careful history and a precise description of the foreign body ingested or aspirated. Careful questioning of the parents may uncover an episode of choking or vomiting that was dismissed at the time as insignificant. Although they are not always diagnostic, routine chest radiographs should be obtained. Because some foreign bodies may be very thin and poorly seen in one dimension, both anteroposterior and lateral radiographs are essential. Both inspiratory and expiratory films should be obtained. Changes related to inspiration and expiration are the most common abnormal findings, consisting of differential inflation or a shift of the mediastinum toward the object with inspiration. Atelectasis, hyperinflation, and aerophagia are radiographic findings consistent with foreign-body aspiration.[35]

In contrast to foreign-body ingestions, all suspected foreign-body aspirations require bronchoscopic evaluation by a consulting otolaryngologist. See Chaps. 72 and 129 and for discussions of foreign-body ingestion and aspiration.

LARYNGEAL TRAUMA

External laryngeal trauma is reportedly rare, occurring in approximately 1 in every 30,000 emergency room visits.[36] However, the actual number of laryngeal injuries is probably underestimated, since many cases go unrecognized, and the victims of the most severe laryngeal trauma frequently die at the scene of the accident. Several authors suggest that an increase in the incidence of laryngotracheal injury patients reaching the emergency room alive is a result of improved prehospital care and the development of specialized regional trauma units.[36,37]

Blunt trauma to the larynx occurs primarily as the result of motor vehicle accidents (dashboard), personal assaults, or sports injuries. The basic mechanism for blunt external injury to the laryngotracheal skeleton is compression of the larynx on the anterior cervical bodies. The varying densities of the hard and soft tissues of the larynx and the rotation of these elements around fixed points cause tearing of the cartilage and mucosa. Injuries range from mucosal tears, to cartilaginous fractures of the hyoid, cricoid, or thyroid, to dislocation of the cricoarytenoid joints or vocal cords. The so-called clothesline injury is a form of blunt laryngeal trauma that deserves special attention due to its severity. This typically occurs when the victim is riding a motorcycle or snowmobile and the neck strikes a stationary object, such as a wire fence or tree limb. The transfer of such a large amount of force to the neck crushes the laryngeal cartilage and may cause laryngotracheal separation. Asphyxiation often occurs at the scene, and survivors of such injuries may have an airway held together precariously by mucous membranes bridging the cartilage.

The larynx of a child responds to blunt trauma differently than does that of an adult. The pediatric larynx is situated higher in the neck and is protected by the mandible. Although the larynx of a child has relatively smaller dimensions, fractures are less common due to the elasticity of the pediatric cartilaginous skeleton. However, the lack of fibrous tissue support and the loose attachments of the mucous membranes increase the likelihood of soft-tissue damage in children.[38]

An upper airway injury should be suspected in any patient with anterior neck trauma. The classic symptoms associated with laryngeal trauma are listed in Table 235-6. With the exception of a subtle change in voice, injuries may be initially asymptomatic. With more significant or worsening injury, the patient may become increasingly aware of pain. Dyspnea, cough, and hemoptysis are common symptoms of tracheobronchial injury. Subcutaneous emphysema of varying degrees is a common finding. When the laryngeal lumen is severely compromised, aphonia and apnea may occur, signaling the need for immediate establishment of an alternative airway.[36]

If the airway is stable, a thorough physical examination of the neck and larynx is required. Bleeding, expanding hematomas, bruits, and loss of pulses are signs associated with vascular injury.[37,38] Other signs of laryngeal trauma include stridor, hemoptysis, subcutaneous emphysema, and tenderness or deformity of the laryngeal skeleton. The type of stridor may suggest the location of the lesion. Inspiratory stridor is typically indicative of partial supraglottic airway obstruction, as might occur from edema, hematoma, foreign body, soft-tissue injury, or cartilaginous fractures. Expiratory stridor may portend lower airway pathologic conditions in the trachea. Inspiratory and expiratory stridor suggest partial obstruction at the level of the glottis.

Flexible fiberoptic nasopharyngolaryngoscopy is the examination of choice, since it allows immediate assessment of airway integrity while maintaining cervical spine immobilization. In stable patients, CT is helpful in defining the extent of injury and need for structural repair.[36] In cases of massive blunt trauma, CT scanning is not indicated, since patients require immediate tracheostomy, direct laryngoscopy, and open exploration. Cervical spine radiographs should be performed to rule out vertebral injury, and soft-tissue anteroposterior and lateral radiographs of the neck should be obtained. Deep cervical and prevertebral air is the most common finding on radiographs of the cervical spine and on CT (Figs. 235-5 and 235-6).

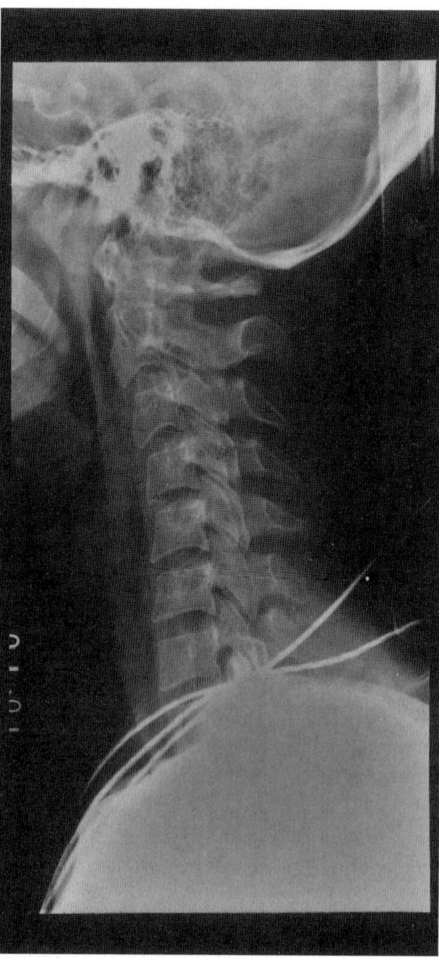

FIG. 235-5. Lateral radiograph demonstrating air in the retropharyngeal space after blunt laryngeal trauma.

The two primary goals in the management of acute laryngeal trauma are preservation of life by maintaining the airway and restoration of function. There is controversy regarding the best way to establish an alternative airway in blunt laryngeal trauma. Some authors believe that intubation following laryngeal trauma is hazardous, since the endotracheal intubation of a traumatized larynx may cause iatrogenic injury as well as the loss of an already precarious airway.[36,37,39] Other authors suggest that orotracheal intubation is a safe method of establishing an airway in this setting if it is done with a small tube under direct visualization.[40] If the lumen of the laryngeal airway is compromised by ecchymosis and edema but there is no gross disruption of the laryngeal mucosa or displacement of the arytenoids and the tracheal lumen can be identified, then the airway may be secured with an endotracheal tube advanced over the bronchscope.[40] When the laryngeal lumen cannot be visualized because of gross anatomic disruption or edema and hemorrhage, urgent tracheostomy is the preferred method of controlling the airway and avoiding further injury to the larynx.[41] An emergent tracheotomy is performed through a midline vertical skin incision, and the trachea should be entered at a level lower than usual (fourth or fifth tracheal ring.) Cricothyrotomy may be difficult because of cervical emphysema and swelling, and should be avoided if possible in suspected laryngeal trauma, since it may further injure the subglottis.[39] Retrograde intubation should not be attempted.

TABLE 235-6 Classic Signs and Symptoms of Blunt Laryngeal Trauma

Hoarseness
Laryngeal pain
Dyspnea
Dysphagia
Cough
Hemoptysis
Aphonia

NECK MASSES

Neck masses may be due to congenital disorders, infection, or neoplastic lesions. With careful attention to the history and physical examination and selected imaging tests, the physician can arrive at a correct diagnosis.

The patient's age may give a clue to the diagnosis (Table 235-7). Neck masses in children represent benign conditions in 90 percent of cases.[42] Neck masses in infants and children commonly include branchial cleft abnormalities, thyroglossal duct cysts, lymphangiomas, hemangiomas, or benign lymphadenopathy.[43] Branchial cysts are round, smooth, and movable, but they are not tender unless they

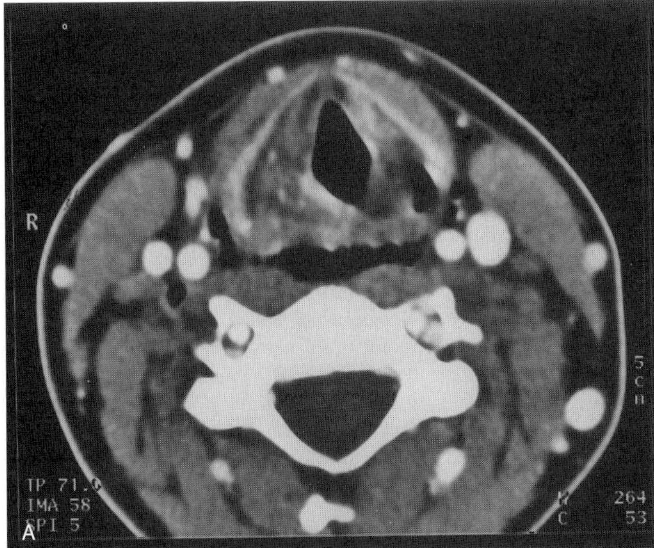

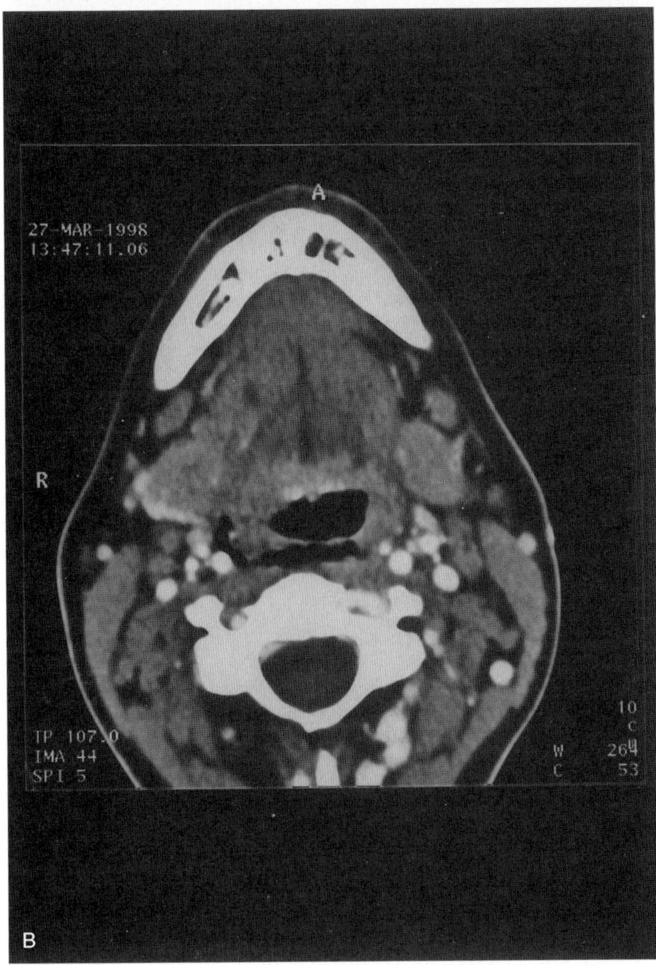

FIG. 235-6. Two axial computed tomographic (CT) cuts demonstrating air in the retropharynx after blunt laryngeal trauma.

TABLE 235-7 Neck Masses by Age

INFANT
Hemangioma
Lymphangioma
Branchial cleft cyst
Rhabdomyosarcoma
CHILD
Reactive lymphadenopathy
Branchial cleft cyst
Thyroglossal duct cyst
YOUNG ADULT
Reactive lymphadenopathy
Mononucleosis
Hodgkins disease
Branchial cleft cyst
Thyroglossal duct cyst
ADULT
Salivary gland or parotid infection or neoplasm
Oral cavity neoplasm
Metastatic carcinoma
Lymphoma
Thyroid disorder

become infected. They are located along the anterior border of the lower sternocleidomastoid muscle (Fig. 235-7). In contrast, thyroglossal duct cysts are found in a subhyoid position, either midline or just to the left of midline (Fig. 235-8). These cysts commonly enlarge after an upper respiratory illness. Lymphangiomas are most commonly found in the lateral cervical region along the jugular chain of lymphatics as a result of sequestration of lymphatic channels and failure to communicate with the internal jugular system. Sixty-five percent of these soft, painless, compressible lymphangiomas are present at birth, and 90 percent are clinically detectable by the end of the second year of life.[44] Large lesions may result in airway and feeding problems. Hemangiomas are congenital vascular malformations that on physical

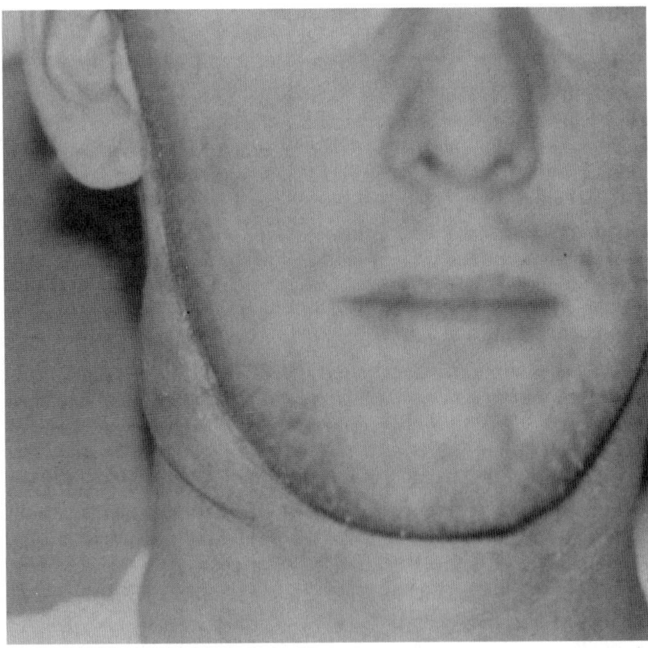

FIG. 235-7. Lateral neck mass in an adolescent demonstrates an infected branchial cleft cyst. It can be found anatomically along the sternocleidomastoid muscle.

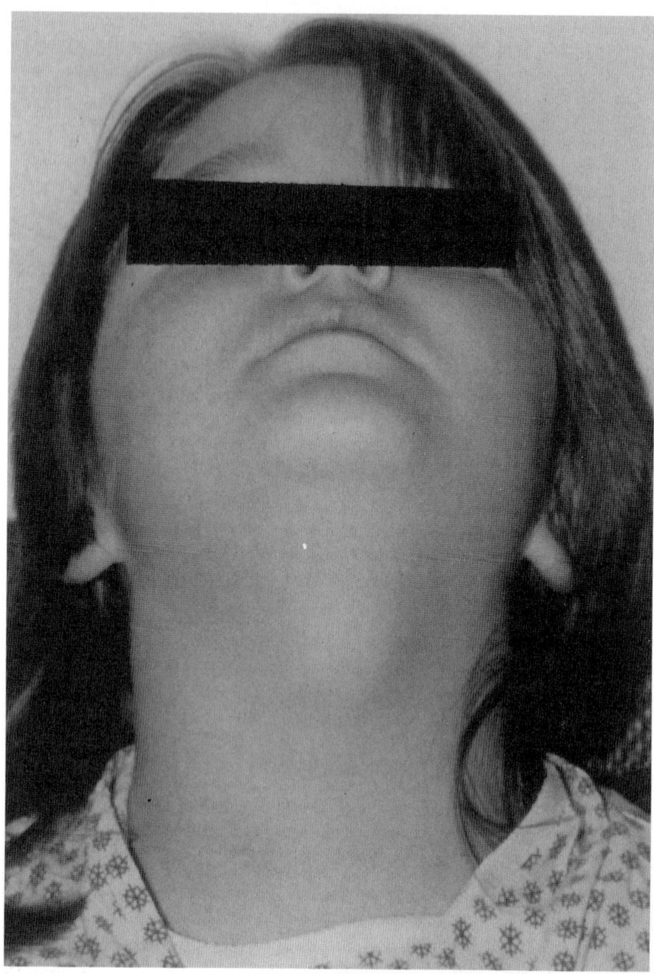

FIG. 235-8. Midline mass in an adolescent demonstrating a thyroglossal duct cyst.

examination are soft, mobile, and frequently have a bluish hue. They undergo a proliferative phase soon after birth, followed by an involutional phase, which is usually complete by age 2 to 3. Almost 90 percent of hemangiomas resolve spontaneously.[45] General lymphadenopathy is also common in infants and children and usually is infectious in origin.[46]

Neck masses in adolescents and young adults represent either infection or tumor. Significant cervical lymphadenopathy, malaise, and pharyngitis are the symptom complex for mononucleosis. A single, large, inflamed anterolateral neck mass in this age group that develops after an upper respiratory infection suggests a branchial cleft cyst. Young adults with multiple, rubbery low-neck masses, night sweats, fever, and malaise may have Hodgkin disease or lymphoma.

In adults, 80 percent of neck masses are neoplastic.[47] The most common cause of a unilateral neck mass in a middle-aged person with a history of tobacco use is squamous cell carcinoma of the upper aerodigestive tract metastatic to the cervical lymph nodes. Other common neoplasms that present in the neck include tumors of the parotid, submandibular, and minor salivary glands, and Hodgkin and non-Hodgkin lymphomas. Neoplastic lymph nodes usually feel firm, and, although initially mobile, they become fixed to surrounding structures as the cancer invades their capsules. Infectious neck masses can be seen in adults, but these nodes can be differentiated from their malignant counterparts by their soft and sometimes fluctuant appearance. Untreated suppurative lymphadenopathy can lead to deep neck infections and should be treated aggressively.

Other common neck masses seen in all age groups include prominent normal structures, such as the pulsatile carotid bulb or the hard transverse process of the first cervical vertebra.[45] Carotid aneurysm, while uncommon, should be suspected if a patient has an expanding neck mass or a history of cervical trauma. Thyroid masses are common. Diffuse nodular thyroid enlargement that is present for many years suggests a simple goiter, whereas a solitary thyroid nodule, although usually benign, may represent thyroid cancer. Epidermal and dermal inclusion cysts are very superficial and result from recurrent cutaneous inflammation.

In addition to age, the history often helps to limit the differential diagnosis. Infectious processes usually develop over hours to days and have associated pain, redness, warmth, and fever. Patients often have a preceding upper respiratory tract or dental infection. Infected congenital cysts may have enlarged on earlier occasions and resolved with antibiotics. Submandibular gland infections (sialadenitis) often wax and wane, are exacerbated by eating, and may cause a foul taste in the mouth as the gland decompresses. Hodgkin disease and lymphomas are associated with night sweats, malaise, itching, and/or fever. Neoplastic disease usually occurs in patients with a history of heavy smoking and alcohol abuse. Such patients often present with dysphagia, otalgia, dyspnea, voice change, or weight loss.

The head and neck examination should include thorough visualization of the ears, nose, oral cavity, oropharynx, nasopharynx, hypopharynx, and larynx. Factors critical in the neck examination include mass consistency and location, as described above. A variety of laboratory studies may prove useful. A heterophil antibody test may reveal mononucleosis in a young patient with pharyngitis and cervical lymphadenopathy. Serologic tests for HIV infection may help in the evaluation of an at-risk patient with multiple enlarged cervical lymph nodes. Intradermal antigen testing for tuberculosis and a control substance, thyroid function tests, and a complete blood cell count with differential counts can each provide useful data in appropriate situations. Several imaging studies can yield helpful information. Chest radiographs may show a primary lung carcinoma or findings consistent with tuberculosis or lymphoma. CT can delineate cervical anatomic relationships and reveal such pathologic conditions as primary aerodigestive tract cancer.

All patients with neck masses must be assessed for airway patency and protection. Patients with any airway concerns, such as stridor or difficulty breathing, or patients with signs of infection, should be evaluated immediately by an otolaryngologist. All other patients may be referred on an outpatient basis.

REFERENCES

1. Denny FW Jr: Tonsillopharyngitis. *Pediatr Rev* 15:185, 1994.
2. Middleton DB: Pharyngitis. *Primary Care* 23:719, 1996.
3. Bisno AL, Gerber MA, Gwaltneyy JM, et al: Diagnosis and management of group A streptococcal pharyngitis: A practice guideline. *Clinical Infect Dis* 25:574, 1997.
4. Gerber MA: Comparison of throat cultures and rapid strep tests for diagnosis of streptococcal pharyngitis. *Pediatr Infect Dis J* 8:820, 1989.
5. Dashefsky B: Life-threatening infections. *Pediatr Emerg Care* 7:244, 1991.
6. Ryan M, Hunt M, Snowberger T: A changing pattern of epiglottitis. *Clin Pediatr* 31:532, 1992.
7. Wurtele P: Acute epiglottitis in children and adults: A large-scale incidence study. *Otolaryngol Head Neck Surg* 103:902, 1980.
8. Senior B, Radkowski D, MacArthur C, et al: Changing patterns in pediatric suppraglottitis: A multi-institutional review, 1980–1992. *Laryngoscope* 104:1314, 1994.
9. Fonanarosa PB, Polsky SS, Goldman GE: Adult epiglottitis. *J Emerg Med* 7:223, 1989.
10. Carnfelt C: Etiology of acute infectious epiglottitis in adults: Septic versus local infection. *Scand J Infect Dis* 21:52, 1990.
11. Navarrete ML, Quesada P, Garcia M, et al: Acute epiglottitis in the adults. *J Laryngol Otol* 105:839, 1991.
12. Sarant G: Acute epiglottitis in adults. *Ann Emerg Med* 10:58, 1981.

13. Blokmanis A: Ultrasound in the diagnosis and management of peritonsillar abscesses. *J Otolaryngol* 23:260, 1994.
14. Ungkanont K, Yellon RF, Weissman JL, et al: Head and neck space infections in infants and children. *Otolaryngol Head Neck Surg* 112:375, 1995.
15. Childs W, Baugh RF, Diaz JA: Tonsillar abscess. *J Nat Med Assoc* 83:333, 1991.
16. Brook I, Frazier EH, Thompsom DH: Aerobic and anerobic microbiology of peritonsillar abcess. *Laryngoscope* 101:289, 1991.
17. Hartmann RW: Recognition of retropharyngeal abscess in children. *Am Fam Physician* 46:193, 1990.
18. Asmar BI: Bacteriology of retropharyngeal abscess in children. *Pediatr Infect Dis J* 9:595, 1990.
19. Coutlhard M, Isaacs D: Retropharyngeal abscess. *Arch Dis Child* 66:1227, 1991.
20. Barratt GE, Kipman CF, Coulthard WS: Retropharyngeal abscess: A 10-year experience. *Laryngoscope* 94:455, 1984.
21. Cressman WR, Meyer CM: Management of tonsillectomy hemorrhage: Results of a survery of pediateric otolaryngology fellowship programs. *Am J Otolaryngol* 16:29, 1995.
22. Segal C, Berger G, Baskar M, et al: Adenotonsillectomies on a surgical day-clinic basis. *Laryngoscope* 93:1205, 1983.
23. Steketee KE, Reisdorff EJ: Emergency care of post tonsillectomy and adenoidectomy hemorrhage. *Am J Emerg Med* 13:518, 1995.
24. Chowdhury K, Tewfik TL, Schloss MD: Post tonsillectomy and adenoidectomy hemorrhage. *J Otolaryngol* 17:46, 1988.
25. Kristensen S, Tveteras K: Post tonsillectomy hemorrhage: A retrospective study of 1150 operations. *Clin Otolaryngol* 9:347, 1984.
26. Roberts C, Jayarmachandran S, Raine CH: A prospective study of factors which may predispose to post-operative tonsillar fossa hemorrhage. *Clin Otolaryngol* 7:13, 1992.
27. Wiatrak BJ, Meyer CM III, Andrews TM: Complications of adenotonsillectomy in children under 3 years of age. *Am J Otolaryngol* 12:170, 1991.
28. Eihorn A, Horton L, Altieri M, et al: Serious respiratory consequences of detergent ingestion in children. *Pediatrics* 84:472, 1989.
29. Forsen JW, Muntz HR: Hair relaxer ingestion. *Ann Otol Rhinol Laryngol* 102:781, 1993.
30. Friedman EM: Caustic ingestions and foreign bodies in the aerodigestive tract of children. *Pediatr Clin North Am* 36:1403, 1989.
31. Christensen HBT: Prediction of complications following unintentional caustic ingestion in children: Is endoscopy necessary? *Acta Paediatr* 84:1177, 1995.
32. Webb WA: Management of foreign bodies of the upper gastrointestinal tract. *Gastroenterology* 94:204, 1988.
33. Crysdale WS, Sendi KS, Yoo J: Esophageal foreign bodies in children: Fifteen-year review of 484 cases. *Ann Otol Rhinol Laryngol* 100:320, 1991.
34. Friedman EM: Caustic ingestions and foreign bodies in the aerodigestive tract of children. *Pediatr Clin North Am* 36:1403, 1989.
35. Healy GB: Management of tracheobronchial foreign bodies in children: An update. *Ann Otol Rhinol Laryngol* 99:889, 1990.
36. Schafer SD, Close LG: The acute management of laryngeal trauma: An update. *Ann Otol Rhinol Laryngol* 98:98, 1989.
37. Burke JF: Early diagnosis of traumatic rupture of the bronchus. *JAMA* 181:682, 1962.
38. Meyer CM, Orobello P, Cotton RT, et al: Blunt laryngeal trauma in children. *Laryngoscope* 97:1043, 1987.
39. Chagnon FP, Mulder DS: Laryngotracheal trauma. *Chest Surg Clin North Am* 6:733, 1996.
40. Gussack GS, Jurkovich GJ, Luterman A: Laryngotracheal trauma: A protocol approach to a rare injury. *Laryngoscope* 96:660, 1986.
41. Furhman GM, Stieg FH, Buerk CA: Blunt laryngeal trauma: Classification and management. *J Trauma* 30:87, 1990.
42. Maisel RH: When your patient complains of a neck mass. *Geriatrics* 35:103, 1980.
43. Weissler MC: Evaluating the patient with a neck mass. *Hosp Med* Feb, 1994.
44. Radkowki D, Arnold J, Healy GB, et al: Thyroglossal duct remnants: Preoperative evaluation and management. *Arch Otolaryngol Head Neck Surg* 117:1378, 1991.
45. Weissler MC: The differential diagnosis of neck masses. *Hosp Med* March:39, 1994.
46. Bamji M, Stone RK, Kaul A, et al: Palpable lymph nodes in healthy newborns and infants. *Pediatrics* 78:573, 1986.
47. Youn WP: Evaluation of neck masses in children. *Am Fam Physician* 51:1904, 1995.

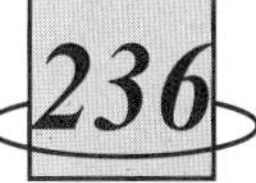

236 COMPLICATIONS OF AIRWAY DEVICES

Rudolph J. Triana, Jr.
Theresa A. Hackeling

Even with expertise and meticulous planning, complications of airway management are bound to occur. Most complications are due to many factors, including inadequate preparedness, inadequate assessment, failure to anticipate or recognize the complication, and inadequate skill during the airway crises.[1] This chapter focuses on complications of airway devices, including endotracheal tubes, tracheostomy tubes, laryngeal stents, and alternative speech devices.

ENDOTRACHEAL TUBES

Acute complications of endotracheal intubation range from minor to catastrophic. Minor complications, such as lip lacerations, corneal abrasions, tooth fractures, or tongue injuries, occur in 5 percent of patients with normal airways.[2] The blades of the laryngoscopes and the use of adjuvant airway devices and malleable stylets are well known to contribute to lip lacerations. Some patients present with dry lips, and merely opening their mouth or stretching their lips may lead to a lip laceration. Application of petroleum jelly or an antibiotic ointment to the lips before manipulating the oral cavity may reduce the extent of injury. In most cases, eye damage is an avoidable complication of securing an airway. The physician preparing to intubate the patient should remove any objects hanging from scrub clothes or gowns. Anesthesia masks, syringes hanging from endotracheal tubes, and stylets must be carefully watched, since they may also cause corneal abrasions. After the induction of anesthesia and before manipulation of the airway, a lubricant and tape or occlusive dressing should be applied to the eyes. Another relatively common complication of securing the airway is dental damage. Facial trauma increases the risk of damage. Proper techniques and avoidance of rocking the laryngoscope back can help to avoid tooth fracture. Tongue laceration, ischemia, or lingual nerve injury may occur as a result of oropharyngeal airway misplacement, use of an inappropriately sized airway device, pressure on the orotracheal tube, or injudicious use of a laryngoscope.[3]

More serious complications of endotracheal intubation include damage to the soft tissues of the pharynx, formation of a false passage, aspiration of particulate matter, and dislocation of the arytenoid cartilage or vocal cords.[4] Repetitive intubation or "blind stabs" are more likely to result in such problems.[5] Unfortunately, many such complications go unnoticed in the emergency department. Formation of a false passage is one injury that will become evident early in the emergency department because the patient will not be adequately oxygenated or ventilated (Fig. 236-1). In the case of placement of the endotracheal tube into a false passage, the tube should be removed immediately and replaced under fiberoptic guidance.

The emergency physician should be well prepared to deal with common complications of intubation, such as laryngospasm, endotracheal tube obstruction, and pnuemothorax. Laryngospasm is a serious complication of securing a difficult airway. In addition to the problem of hypoxia and its sequelae, acute pulmonary edema is a well documented phenomenon that often accompanies laryngospasm and makes the problem more difficult to handle.[1] The best approach to relieving laryngospasm is to try continuous positive-pressure bag-mask ventilation. If this technique is unsuccessful, more neuromuscular blockade should be administered to the patient. If the first two maneuvers fail, 1 to 2 mL lidocaine on a 25-gauge needle can be injected into the

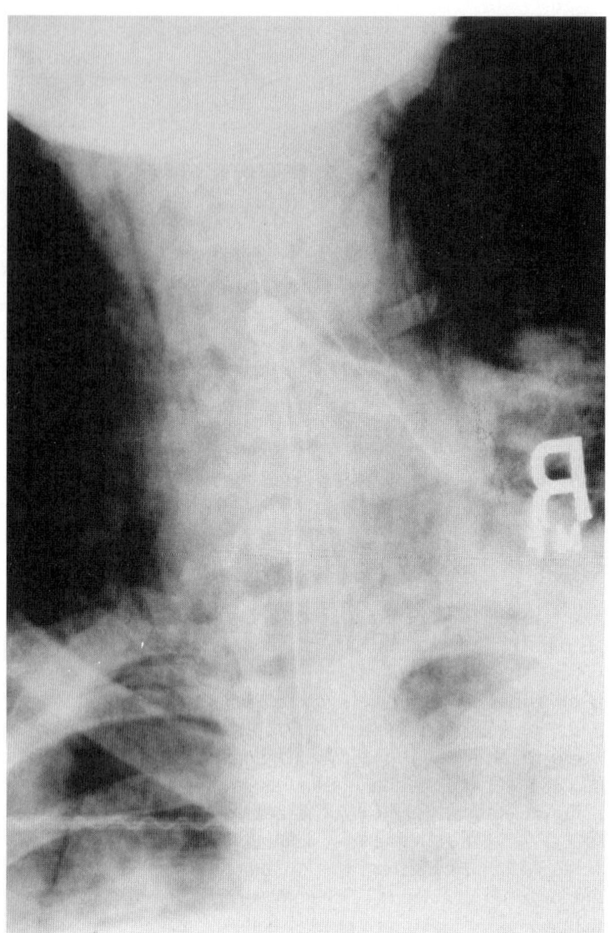

FIG. 236-1. Anteroposterior radiograph demonstrating creation of a false passage by the tracheostomy tube and subcutaneous air in the soft tissues of the neck.

cricothyroid membrane. The advantage of this technique is that it anesthetizes the vocal cords and immediately results in coughing and subsequent passage of air.

Endotracheal tube obstruction is a known complication that occurs frequently while the patient is in the emergency department. The tube is often plugged with friable tissue, thick mucous secretions, or granulation tissue. Options of treatment include suction techniques using saline solution or *N*-acetyl cysteine (Mucomyst), or removal and placement of a larger endotracheal tube.

Pneumothorax can also result when securing an airway by overzealous initial ventilation with high volumes and pressures. Clinical assessment and a chest radiograph should thus be performed after each endotracheal intubation to confirm tube placement and to look for evidence of a pneumothorax. All intubated patients with a pneumothorax require immediate chest tube placement and reassessment of the ventilation parameters.

TRACHEOSTOMY TUBES

The emergency department care of a patient with a tracheostomy tube can be problematic due to difficulty with patient communication, urgency of airway control, and unfamiliarity with tracheal equipment. An understanding of tracheal anatomy, tracheal equipment, and the complications and management of tracheostomies can assist the emergency physician in managing such patients.

A standard tracheostomy is a surgical procedure that creates an opening between cartilaginous rings in the airway by suturing the skin to the anterior tracheal wall (Fig. 236-2). Current indications for tracheostomy tube placement include the maintenance of airway patency in patients with functional or mechanical airway obstruction, the provision of airway access for suctioning retained airway secretions, the prevention of aspiration in a patient with glottic dysfunction, significant obstructive sleep apnea, and the management of patients who require long-term access for ventilatory support.

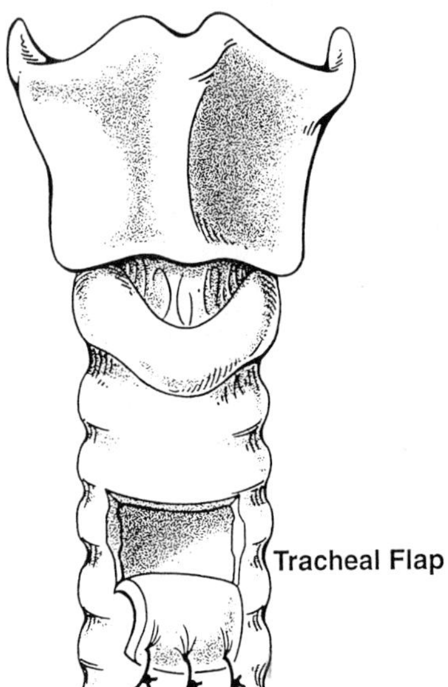

FIG. 236-2. Creation of a tracheal flap.

There are many tracheostomy tubes available, including those made of plastic, silicone, nylon, and metal. They vary in luminal diameter, length, angle of the curvature, presence of an inner cannula, obturators, locking mechanisms at the hub, cuffs, valves, and fenestrations (Fig. 236-3). The size of the tracheostomy tube is defined by the size of the inner diameter. Adult tracheostomy tubes range from 4.0 to 10.0 mm, and pediatric tracheostomy tubes range from 0.0 to 4.0 mm. Some tubes are designed to work with an artificial voice through an airport above the tracheostomy, with a tracheoesophageal prosthesis, and with other voice devices. Obturators fit through the tracheal tube to create a smooth surface during insertion. Inner cannulas provide a mechanism for clearing the artificial airway without losing patency. It should be noted that pediatric tracheostomy tubes never have an inner cannula due to the small size of the inner diameter. Most pediatric and adult tracheostomy tubes have a 15-mm standard respiratory connection that may be used with ventilator tubing and a bag-valve device.

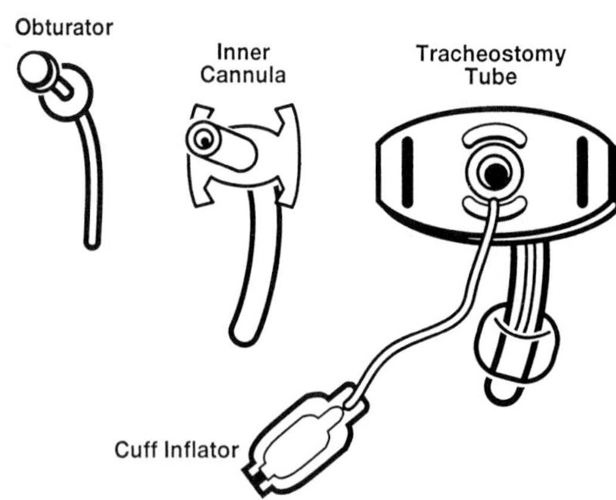

FIG. 236-3. Contents of a tracheostomy tube.

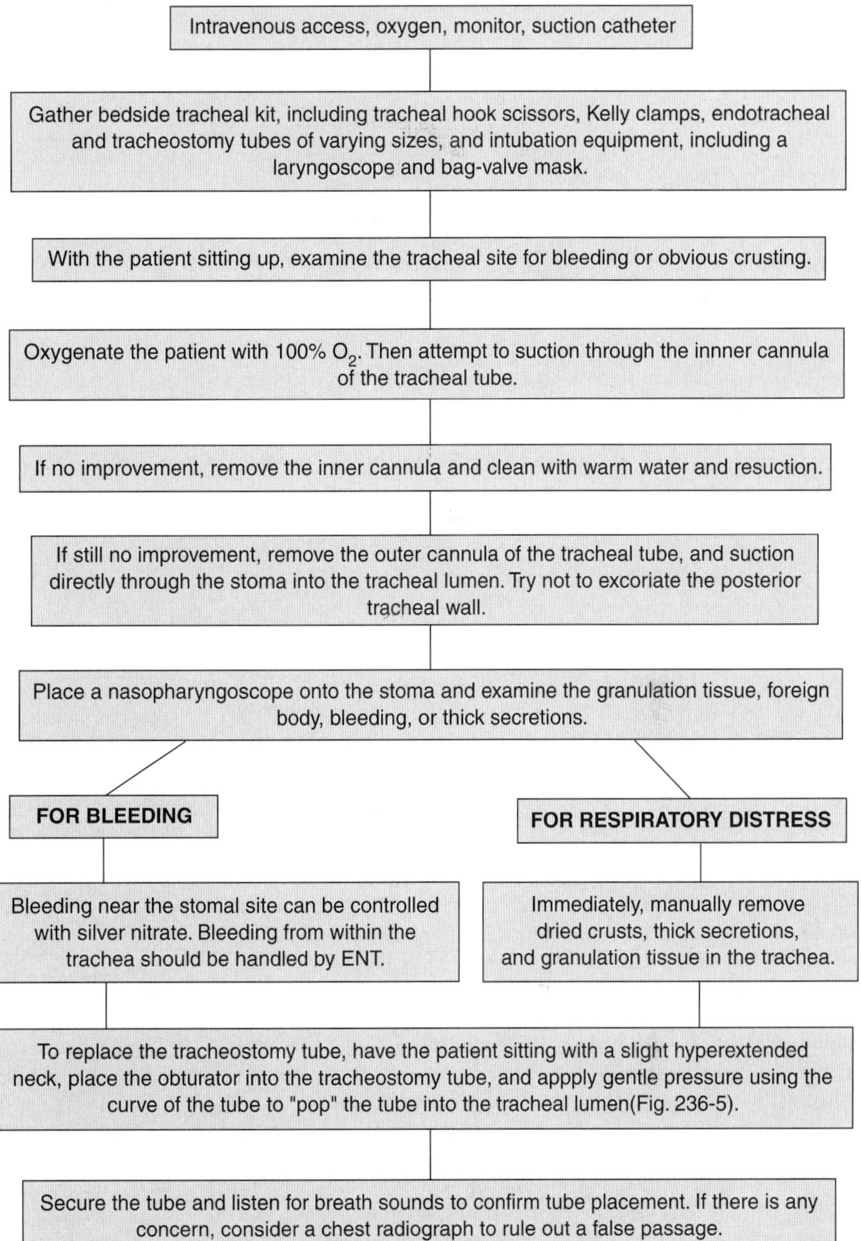

Intravenous access, oxygen, monitor, suction catheter
Gather bedside tracheal kit, including tracheal hook scissors, Kelly clamps, endotracheal and tracheostomy tubes of varying sizes, and intubation equipment, including a laryngoscope and bag-valve mask.
With the patient sitting up, examine the tracheal site for bleeding or obvious crusting.
Oxygenate the patient with 100% O_2. Then attempt to suction through the innner cannula of the tracheal tube.
If no improvement, remove the inner cannula and clean with warm water and resuction.
If still no improvement, remove the outer cannula of the tracheal tube, and suction directly through the stoma into the tracheal lumen. Try not to excoriate the posterior tracheal wall.
Place a nasopharyngoscope onto the stoma and examine the granulation tissue, foreign body, bleeding, or thick secretions.
FOR BLEEDING
FOR RESPIRATORY DISTRESS
Bleeding near the stomal site can be controlled with silver nitrate. Bleeding from within the trachea should be handled by ENT.
Immediately, manually remove dried crusts, thick secretions, and granulation tissue in the trachea.
To replace the tracheostomy tube, have the patient sitting with a slight hyperextended neck, place the obturator into the tracheostomy tube, and appply gentle pressure using the curve of the tube to "pop" the tube into the tracheal lumen(Fig. 236-5).
Secure the tube and listen for breath sounds to confirm tube placement. If there is any concern, consider a chest radiograph to rule out a false passage.

FIG. 236-4. Algorithm for evaluation of the tracheostomy patient.

Tracheostomy tubes with balloon cuffs are used in the first postoperative week to prevent aspiration of blood or secretions. To prevent tracheomalacia and stenosis, cuffless tracheostomy tubes are used after 1 week if the patient is not ventilator dependent.

The most common complications of tracheostomy tubes include accidental decannulation, tube obstruction, infection, development of a bleeding tracheoinnominate fistula, and tracheal stenosis (Fig. 236-4). Accidental decannulation can occur in the early or late period after tracheostomy tube placement, particularly when patients cough or extend their neck. To replace the tube, hyperextend the patient's neck and, using the curve of the tube, gently direct the tube into the opening (Fig. 236-5). Hyperextension of the neck places the larynx and trachea in a very anterior position, thereby facilitating placement of the tube. If a tracheostomy tube is not readily available, an endotracheal tube may be quickly inserted into the stoma in order to maintain airway security. In cases of extreme airway compromise, the patient may be endotracheally intubated from above in order to secure the airway and allow time to assess the tracheostomy site. The only time the patient

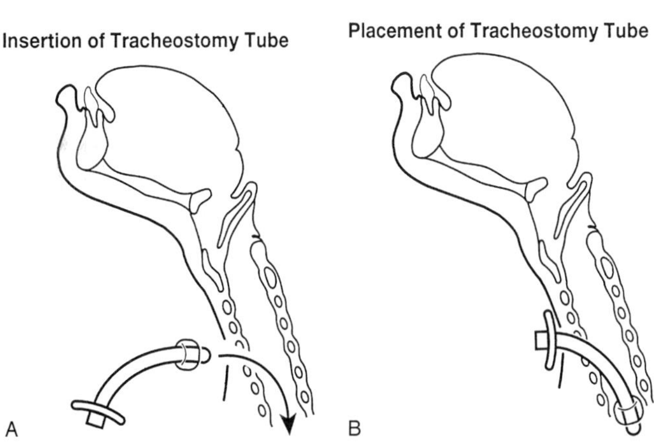

FIG. 236-5. Insertion and placement of the tracheostomy tube.

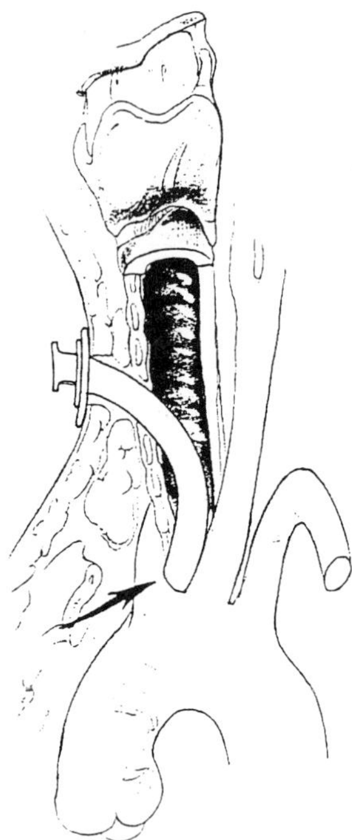

FIG. 236-6. The arrow points to the position of the tracheostomy tube in relation to the innominate artery. This close approximation facilitates creation of a tracheoinnominate fistula.

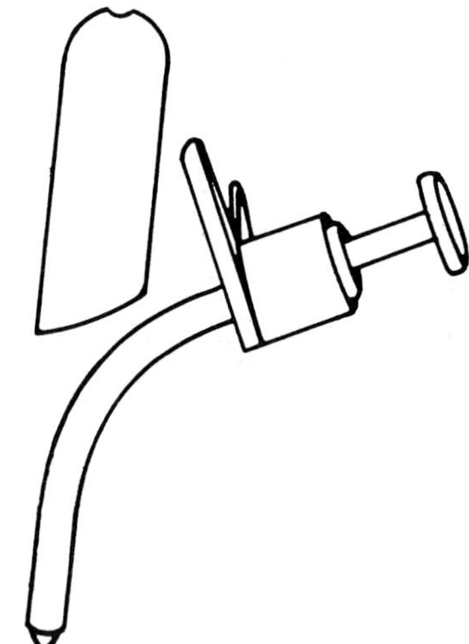

FIG. 236-7. Relation of the tracheostomy tube to the laryngeal stent. The stent lies superior within the lumen of the trachea.

may not be endotracheally intubated orally is in the case of a laryngectomy. Patients who have had a laryngectomy will have a tracheal stoma and sometimes a tracheostomy tube in place but will not have an accessible airway passage from their mouth. The only access to the tracheal bronchial tree in laryngectomy patients is through the neck.

Tracheostomy tube obstruction with mucous plugging is a common complication of this airway device. Secretions may act by a ball-valve mechanism, allowing air in but restricting outward ventilation. Dried crusts and secretions and other obstructing lesions should be manually removed. The inner cannula of the tracheostomy tube must be removed, and often the entire tracheostomy tube must be removed and cleaned with sterile saline water. If profuse, thick secretions are seen in the trachea, they should be suctioned after preoxygenation and placement of sterile saline solution to aid in loosening the secretions. Prolonged use of large suction catheters without preoxygenation will cause hypoxemia.

All indwelling tracheostomy tubes are contaminated with normal and sometimes pathogenic flora. Stomal skin infection, tracheitis, and bronchitis can be a recurring problem.[6] *Staphylococcus aureus, Pseudomonas,* and *Candida* are often identified.[6] Broad-spectrum antibiotics are indicated in the setting of clinical disease.

Bleeding is one of the most common complications in the early period after tracheostomy tube placement. Hemorrhage most commonly occurs between the first and third week postoperatively.[7] Sources of hemorrhage include granulation tissue, thyroid arteries, the thyroid gland, the tracheal wall, or the innominate artery.[7] If bleeding is slow, the tube may be removed, and the stoma and tracheal wall should be examined. Local bleeding can be controlled with silver nitrate or electrocautery. With more brisk bleeding, the tracheostomy tube should be kept in place until an airway is placed below the bleeding site. Maneuvers to control bleeding include local digital pressure, hyperinflation of the cuff, and mild traction of the tube with manual pressure. These maneuvers are particularly essential in cases of tracheoinnominate fistula. Tracheoinnominate artery fistula is a rare but life-threatening complication occurring in approximately less than 1 percent of all tracheostomies.[8] Bleeding results from direct pressure of the tip of the tracheal cannula against the innominate artery (Fig. 236-6). Some patients may present with premonitory tracheal stomal bleeding (a sentinel bleed) or hemoptysis. Such bleeding may be mild to severe and should not be taken lightly, since the potential exists for sudden massive hemorrhage. Immediate otolaryngologic consultation is required, and operative intervention is lifesaving.

Less commonly seen is the presentation of tracheal or stomal stenosis. Tracheal stenosis results from necrosis at the pressure points of the cuff that become scar and result in airway narrowing. Signs and symptoms include dyspnea, wheezing, stridor, or inability to clear secretions. Treatment includes humidified oxygen, nebulized racemic epinephrine, and early administration of steroids. Radiographs may be helpful in demonstrating narrowing of the trachea, but flexible bronchoscopy is the diagnostic modality of choice. Immediate otolaryngologic consultation is warranted.

LARYNGEAL STENTS

The surgical management of laryngotracheal stenosis often employs techniques that utilize tracheal stents for various periods of time. Placement of an endolaryngeal stent renders a patient tracheostomy dependent until the stent is removed, due to blockage of the airway at the laryngeal level by the solid stent (Fig. 236-7). There are many different endolaryngeal stent designs and materials, including silastic endolaryngeal molds secured by cutaneous buttons, a stent secured

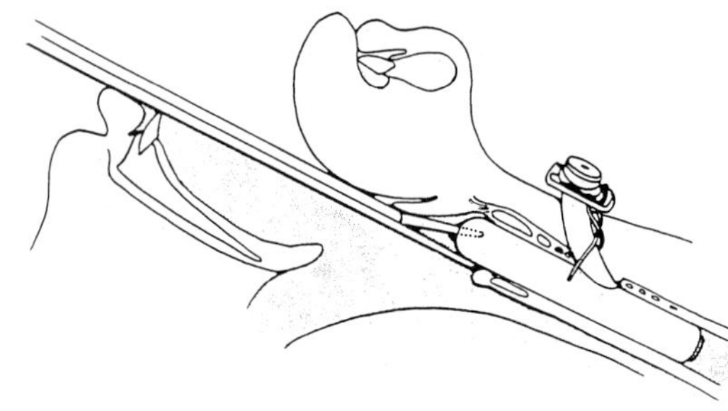

FIG. 236-8. The Abouker stent, which is commonly used in pediatric laryngotracheal reconstruction, involves a metal tracheostomy tube that is wired to a silastic stent that remains in the tracheal lumen.

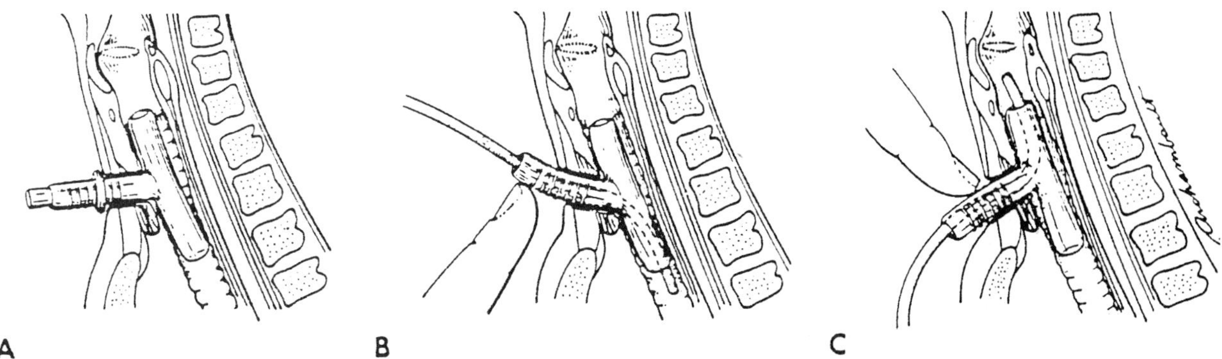

FIG. 236-9. Suctioning is required of both the upper and lower limbs of the Montgomery T tube. If necessary the entire T tube can be removed.

by a strap that comes out the tracheal stoma and is attached to the skin, the Abouker stent complex (used in pediatric airway surgery), and the Montgomery T-tube stent. Although endolaryngeal stents are secured by buttons or straps, a known complication of these devices is dislodgement. If a stent becomes dislodged but the tracheostomy tube remains in position, airway security is not an issue. The operating surgeon should be notified when extrusion or dislodgment of any stent occurs.

The Abouker stent, which is commonly used in pediatric laryngotracheal reconstruction, consists of a metal tracheostomy tube wired to a silastic stent that remains in the tracheal lumen (Fig. 236-8).[9] Removing the inner cannula of the trachesotomy tube should relieve airway obstruction in patients with Abouker stents. Only the inner cannula can be removed. The tracheostomy tube cannot be removed because it is wired to the stent.

The Montgomery T-tube configuration is commonly used in adult laryngotracheal reconstruction.[10] It is a modification of a tracheostomy tube that does not have an inner cannula. Humidification and suctioning of the T tube is essential to prevent mucous plugging. Airway obstruction should be addressed by first suctioning both the upper and lower limbs of the T tube (Fig. 236-9). If suctioning both limbs of the T tube does not relieve the obstruction, the T tube should be removed and the trachea should be cannulated with an appropriately sized tracheostomy tube or an endotracheal tube.

SPEECH DEVICES

Speech in patients who are tracheostomy-tube dependent was nonexistent prior to the late 1980s. The development of the Passy-Muir valve has enabled patients to produce lung-powered speech. The Passy-Muir valve is a one-way valve that fits directly over the opening of the tracheostomy tube. The patient may breathe freely through the tracheostomy tube. Speech is created when the patient exhales hard enough to close the Passy-Muir valve and the air is thus directed up through the vocal cords and out the mouth (Fig. 236-10).[11]

Complications with the Passy-Muir valve may initially present as airway obstruction or an inability to speak. In such cases, the speaking device should be removed from the tracheostomy tube so that air can pass freely during both inhalation and exhalation. If this does not improve the situation, the physician should assess the tracheostomy tube for evidence of obstruction.

Speech in postlaryngectomy patients has also improved dramatically with the use of the Blom-Singer voice prosthesis. This one-way valve is surgically placed between the posterior wall of the trachea

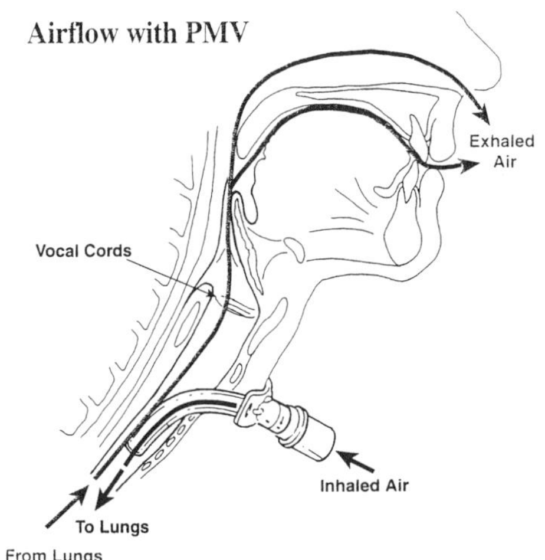

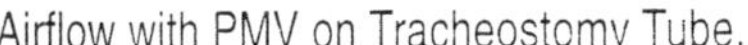

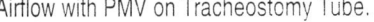

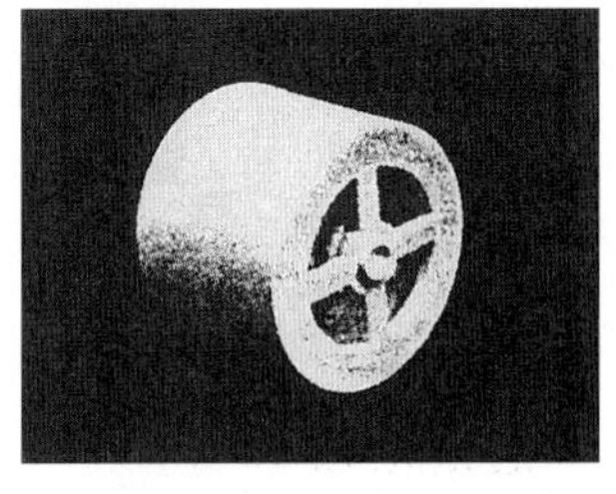

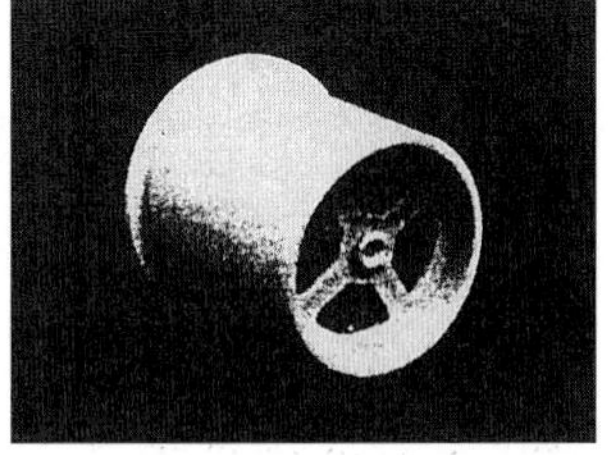

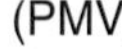

FIG. 236-10. The Passy-Muir valve is a one-way valve that fits directly on the opening of the tracheostomy tube. Speech is created when the patient exhales as air is passed up through the vocal cords and out the mouth.

through the anterior wall of the cervical esophagus. To speak, patients exhale while occluding the tracheal stoma with their thumb, thus forcing the exhaled air into the esophagus. The air vibrates the esophagus (as a belch does) and the resultant tone is used to provide speech.[11] Two common complications with the Blom-Singer speech devices are aspiration of the valve and dislodgment. Patients with aspiration are likely to present with persistent cough and respiratory distress. Initial evaluation may include passing a flexible scope into the tracheal stoma to see if the prosthesis has been dislodged. In addition, a chest radiograph may show the valve. If there is suspicion of aspiration, an otolaryngologic consultation is indicated for further bronchoscopic evaluation.

A more common problem is dislodgment or extrusion of the prosthesis. If the prosthesis has just fallen out, recannulate the tracheoesophageal fistula as soon as possible using a small Foley catheter (10 or 12 French). Many times, a stiffer tube, such as a red rubber catheter, facilitates cannulation of the fistula. Sterile surgical lubricant or lidocaine jelly may be applied to the tube or on a cotton swab applicator, which can identify the fistula prior to placement of the tube. If the fistula can be cannulated, the tube should be secured to the neck or chest, and the patient should follow up with a speech pathologist or otolaryngologist the next day. If recannulation is not easily achieved, repeated attempts are not recommended because they may result in formation of a false tract. If recannulation is unsuccessful, an otolaryngologist should be consulted immediately.

REFERENCES

1. Mallampati SR: Recognition of the difficult airway, in Benumof JL (ed): *Airway Management: Principles and Practice.* St. Louis, Mosby-Year Book, 1996, pp 126–142.
2. Anderson DA, Braun TW, Herlich A: Eye injury during general anesthesia for oral and maxillofacial surgery:etiology and prevention. *J Oral Maxillofac Surg* 53:312, 1995.
3. Brimacombe J: Bilateral lingual nerve injury following tracheal intubation. *Anaesthesia Intens Care* 21:107, 1993.
4. Lee TS, Jordan JS: Pyriform sinus perforation secondary to traumatic intubation in the difficult airway patient. *J Clin Anesth* 6:152, 1994.
5. Jensen NF: Arytenoid injury and subluxation in anesthetic practice. *Am J Anesth* 1:145, 1995.
6. Tayal VS: Tracheostomies. *Emerg Med Clin North Am* 12:707, 1994.
7. Jones JW, Reynolds M, Hewitt RL, et al: Tracheoinnominate artery erosion: Successful management of a devastating complication. *Ann Surg* 184:194, 1977.
8. Ross CB, Morris JA: Tracheoinnominate artery fistula: A potentially fatal complication of tracheostomy. *J Tenn Med Soc* 81:446, 1988.
9. Zalzal GH: Use of stents in laryngotracheal reconstruction in children: Indications, technical considerations, and complications. *Laryngoscope* 98:849, 1988.
10. Montgomery WW, Montgomery SK: Manual for the use of Montgomery laryngeal, tracheal, and esophageal prostheses. *Ann Otol Rhinol Laryngol* 99(suppl 150):2, 1990.
11. Singer MI, Blom ED: An endoscopic technique for voice restoration after total laryngectomy. *Ann Otol Rhinol Laryngol* 89:529, 1980.

APPROACH TO THE DERMATOLOGIC PATIENT IN THE EMERGENCY DEPARTMENT

William J. Brady
Marcus L. Martin

The chief complaint "rash" is encountered in approximately 5 percent of ED visits nationwide; additionally, cutaneous findings are felt to contribute significantly toward the correct diagnosis and management in another 5 percent. In children, rashes are encountered even more often. A medical record survey of pediatric patients presenting to an academic ED revealed that 31 percent of cases primarily involved a dermatologic aspect; an additional 9 percent of ED patients demonstrated various skin findings that did not relate to the chief complaint, yet may have contributed to the final diagnosis and management plan.[1] The dermatologic syndromes seen in the ED span the spectrum of cutaneous disease. The majority of skin lesions involve infections, irritants, and allergies.[2] Fortunately, few presentations represent life- or limb-threatening skin disorders. Visual diagnosis using pattern recognition is the key to cutaneous diagnosis. The recommended approach to the patient with skin disease in the ED is (assuming resuscitation or stabilization is not required):

- Determine the chief complaint.
- Obtain a brief history (duration, rate of progression, location of lesions).
- Perform the dermatologic examination (morphology, distribution).
- Formulate the differential diagnosis based upon lesion morphology and distribution.
- Elicit additional issues from the history (associated complaints, comorbidity, medications, exposures) and include/exclude syndromes in the differential based upon this information.
- Perform ancillary investigations, if necessary.
- Obtain dermatologic consultation if necessary and/or arrange for appropriate referral (primary care or dermatologic).

DIAGNOSTIC APPROACH

The History

The emergency physician should determine the chief complaint and obtain a brief history (discomfort, duration, rate of progression, and location of lesions). The secondary history should include issues relating to the lesion—morphology, evolutionary nature, rate of progression, and distribution. Associated systemic complaints and mucosal systems must be identified. Ask about exposures to medications (over-the-counter, prescription, and illicit), immunizations, toxins, chemicals, foods, animals, insects, plants, and ill contacts. Sexual history, if appropriate, as well as medical and family histories, should be reviewed. Asking about medication use, sun exposure, or particular food ingestion may also yield helpful information.

The Examination

The dermatologic physical examination must be performed on the disrobed patient in a room with adequate lighting. All skin and mucosal surfaces must be inspected, including hair, nails, scalp, and mucous membranes. Then, the specific skin lesions must be inspected. A magnifying lens and a portable lamp are helpful for conducting the examination.

The skin should be examined in a systematic, methodical, orderly process. The distribution, pattern, arrangement, morphology, extent, and evolutionary changes of the lesions must be determined. Distribution is the location of the skin findings while the pattern is the anatomic, functional, and physiologic arrangement of the lesions. For example, the patient with a unilateral band-like arrangement of lesions on the thorax suggest varicella-zoster infection (Fig. 241-5). Skin diseases often present with a predilection for certain body areas; as such, location will assist in narrowing the diagnostic possibilities (Table 237-1). From the anatomic perspective, the skin surfaces that are usually considered as separate areas of distribution include scalp, hair, face, eyelids, mouth, trunk, axilla, perineum, extremities, and nails; the extremities may be further subdivided into upper versus lower and proximal versus distal, as well as wrists/ankles and hands/feet (Fig. 239-5). Rashes on exposed portions of the skin should prompt inquiries about sun exposure, jewelry, or topical agents. Refer to Table 237-2 for a differential diagnosis of skin lesions as a function of location.

Lesion arrangement refers to both the symmetry and configuration. Bilateral symmetry suggests either a systemic internal event or symmetric external exposure, as seen in erythema multiforme, with plaque-like lesions on the flexor surfaces of the extremities (Fig. 241-1A) or in the patient with contact dermatitis related to a lotion application. An asymmetric arrangement supports a localized process. Configuration may apply to a single lesion with reference to its individual features or, alternatively, to multiple lesions and their relationship to one another. For instance, internal configuration is illustrated by the relationship between the central papule relative to the erythematous ring in the target lesion of erythema multiforme (Fig. 241-1B); on the total-body scale, configuration is demonstrated by clustering of lesions in a herpes virus infection (Fig. 241-5) or by a linear arrangement in poison ivy or oak. Other terms used to describe the lesion configuration are listed in Table 237-3.

Recognition of the primary lesion is vital in establishing the diagnosis. The primary lesion is the lesion which has not been altered by secondary issues, including healing, complicating infection, medication application, or scratching. Examples of primary skin lesions include macules, papules, nodules, tumors, cysts, plaques, wheals, vesicles, bullae, and pustules. Secondary lesions have had their appearance altered due to disease evolution or various external factors as noted above, and include crusts, scales, fissures, erosions, ulcerations, excoriations, atrophy, scarring, and lichenification. See Table 237-4 for a listing with description of the various morphologic descriptors of dermatologic lesions; refer to Tables 237-5 and 237-6 for a differential diagnosis of the various skin disorders relative to primary and secondary lesion morphologies that can use the "Burn rule of 9's" (Chap. 194, "Thermal Burns") to estimate the degree of skin involvement.

Diagnostic Techniques

The potassium hydroxide preparation is used in patients with suspected molluscum contagiosum and dermatophytic infections. The test is performed on loose skin scales, nail pairings, subungual debris, short residual hairs, or small pearly globules (from a molluscum body). The material is placed on the microscope slide, gently crushed, and mixed with two drops of a 20% KOH solution. The specimen is then warmed; boiling will produce artifactual change. Excess solution may be re-

TABLE 237-1 Distribution and Pattern Descriptors

DISTRIBUTION		
Scalp	Trunk	Further subdivision of Extremities:
Hair	Axilla	Upper *vs.* Lower
Face	Perineum	Proximal *vs.* Distal
Eyelids	Extremities	Wrists/Ankles
Mucosa (eyes, lips)	Nails	Hands/Feet
Mouth		
PATTERN		
Sun-, clothing-, jewelry-, or agent-exposed	Hair-bearing	Apocrine
Intertriginous	Palmar/plantar	Acneiform
Flexor/extensor	Pityriasis rosea	Acrodermatitis

moved by placing a paper towel at the corner of the slide. A coverslip may be applied for especially thick specimens; gentle pressure on the coverslip will compress the material adequately for viewing. Thick skin scrapings may also be allowed to set in the potassium hydroxide solution for 20 min, which should allow additional dissolving. The material is then viewed under a microscope at low power with the condenser and light at low levels. As the slide is scanned, rapidly focus up and down. True hyphae are long, branching, green rods of constant width that cross the borders of epithelial cells. Molluscum bodies are oval discs with homogeneous cytoplasm. In hair fragments, the organisms appear as small round spores packed closely within the hair shaft.

Scabies and lice preparations are useful in patients with possible infestation. In scabies infestations, the rash itself may resemble other dermatologic syndromes; microscopic analysis will confirm the diagnosis. The donor site for skin specimen selection is very important. The best sites include burrows (10-mm elongated papule with a pustule or vesicle) and papules located on the fingers, wrists, and elbows. Within the vesicle or pustule, a small black dot is noted, which is the mite. The point of the scalpel is scraped across the lesion while holding the skin taut; the mite is then removed. A single drop of mineral oil may be applied to the blade to ensure that the scrapings adhere to the

TABLE 237-2 Differential Diagnosis Relative to Lesion Distribution/Pattern

Pattern	Differential Diagnosis
Flexor areas of skin	Atopic dermatitis, candidiasis, eczema, ichthyosis
Sun-exposed (face, upper thorax, distal extremities)	Sunburn, photosensitive drug eruption, photosensitive dermatitis, systemic lupus erythematosus, viral exanthem, porphyria
Acrodermatitis (distal extremities)	Viral exanthem, atopic/contact dermatitides, eczema, Rocky Mountain spotted fever, gonococcemia
Pityriasis rosea (anterior and posterior thorax)	Pityriasis rosea, secondary syphilis, drug eruption, atopic/contact dermatitis, psoriasis
Clothing-covered (thorax and distal lower extremities)	Contact dermatitis, psoriasis, folliculitis
Acneiform (face and upper thorax)	Acne, drug-induced acne, irritant dermatitides

TABLE 237-3 Lesion Configuration Descriptors

Descriptor	Configuration
Annular	ring-like or pertaining to the outer edge
Arcuate	curved or pertaining to the curve
Circinate	circular
Confluent	blending together
Dermatomal	belt-like or limited to one side of body in anatomic dermatome
Discoid	solid, round, slightly raised or pertaining to a disk
Discrete	separate or individual
Grouped	clustered
Guttate	scattered or droplike
Gyrate	coiled or winding
Herpetiform	creeping
Iris	concentric circles
Linear	in a line
Polycyclic	overlapping circles or borders of irregular curves
Retiform	net-like
Serpiginous	snake-like

instrument. The material is then placed on the microscope slide with an additional drop of mineral oil; gentle pressure on the coverslip will flatten thick specimens. Using low power, the slide is scanned for presence of the mite, eggs, or feces. Mites are eight-legged creatures that are easily identified on thin smears; thick specimens may require additional viewing to look for the mite. Additional findings supportive of the diagnosis include eggs (smooth ovals) and feces (clusters of red-brown pellets). Lice are usually found on the scalp, eyelashes, and pubic areas, and may be visible to the unaided eye. Moving objects in the area should be grasped with forceps and placed on a slide and viewed under low power. Head lice are long and thin while pubic lice are shorter and broad.

The Tzanck smear, useful in blistering disorders, assists in establishing the diagnosis of a herpes infection—herpes simplex, herpes zoster, and varicella. The choice material for examination is obtained from the base of a recently unroofed lesion; purulent fluid at the base of the lesion is removed with a scalpel and placed on a microscope slide. The material is allowed to air dry and then is stained with either Giemsa or Wright's stain. Using low power, the slide is scanned for epithelial cells. Multinucleated giant cells, indicative of a herpes infection, are a syncytium of epidermal cells with multiple overlapping nuclei. The presence of the multinucleated giant cell does not distinguish herpes simplex, herpes zoster, and varicella syndromes. Wood's light examination is helpful in several different situations, including erythrasma (a superficial *Corynebacterium* infection of moist skin in the groin, axilla, and web spaces), tinea versicolor (a superficial fungal infection), certain pseudomonal skin infections, and porphyria cutanea tarda. Wood's light is an ultraviolet source that emits light at a wavelength of 365 nm. The following fluorescent findings are noted in these conditions: erythrasma—red or pink; tinea versicolor—green or yellow; pseudomonas—yellow or green; and porphyria cutanea—orange or yellow (urine only). Other laboratory investigations are of

TABLE 237-4 Lesion Morphology

Descriptor	Morphology	Lesion Nature (Primary/Secondary)	Height Relative to Adjacent Skin
Erosion	Ruptured vesicle/bulla with denuded epidermis	Secondary	Depressed
Excoriation	Linear erosion	Secondary	Flat
Fissure	Linear cracks in skin surface	Secondary	Flat
Ulcer	Epidermal/dermal tissue loss	Secondary	Depressed
Macule	Flat, circumscribed discoloration 1 cm or less in diameter; color varies	Primary	Flat
Petechiae	Nonblanching purple spots less than 2 mm in diameter	Primary	Flat
Sclerosis	Firm, indurated skin	Secondary	Flat/Elevated
Telangiectasia	Small, blanchable superficial capillaries	Primary	Flat
Purpura	Nonblanching purple discoloration of the skin	Primary	Flat
Abscess	Tender, erythematous, fluctuant nodule	Primary	Elevated
Cyst	Sack contining liquid or semisolid material	Primary	Elevated
Nodule	Palpable solid lesion less than 1 cm in diameter	Primary	Elevated
Tumor	Palpable solid lesion greater than 1 cm in diameter	Primary	Elevated
Scar	Sclerotic area of skin	Secondary	Flat/Elevated
Wheal	Transient, edematous papule or plaque with peripheral erythema	Primary	Flat/Elevated
Vesicle	Circumscribed, thin-walled, elevated blister less than 5 mm in diameter	Primary	Elevated
Bulla	Circumscribed, thin-walled, elevated blister greater than 5 mm in diameter	Primary	Elevated
Pustule	Vesicle containing purulent fluid	Primary	Elevated
Papule	Elevated, solid, palpable lesion less than 1 cm in diameter; color varies	Primary	Elevated
Plaque	Flat-topped elevation formed by confluence of papules greater than 0.5 cm in diameter	Primary	Elevated
Comedo	Papule with an impacted pilosebaceous unit	Primary	Elevated

limited value; selected tests are listed in Table 237-7 with the respective dermatologic disease.

TOPICAL THERAPIES

In general, the maxim ''if it's dry, wet it, and if it's wet, dry it'' applies to the initial therapy of many rashes. Water, protein, and lipid losses characterize dry skin diseases. Emollient creams and lotions restore water and lipids to the epidermis, hasten the healing process, and reduce pruritus and pain. Emollients are moisturizers that reduce skin dryness and decrease skin friction and the sensation of tightness. In patients with chronic drying dermatitides, ointments are best used, particularly in the winter months; in warm weather climates, less viscous, less oily preparations, such as a cream, are better tolerated by the patient. Open wet dressings using tap water or normal saline not only reduce discomfort due to the drying but also cleanses the skin by painlessly loosening crusts and exudates. The various wet cutaneous syndromes involve similar protein and lipid losses due to excessive flow of transudative or exudative fluid from the diseased skin with leaching of the complex macromolecules of the epithelial cells. Drying agents retard this flow of fluid and associated biologic materials from the body, assisting in the curative process.

Corticosteroids

Urticaria, angioedema, and toxicodendron and other contact/allergic dermatitides are potential indications for systemic corticosteroids. Other dermatologic syndromes, such as erythema multiforme, toxic epidermal necrolysis, and vasculitis, are best treated with systemic steroids only after consultation with a dermatologist. Eczema and psoriasis, both of which are chronic dermatologic conditions, are likely to rapidly improve after systemic steroid therapy. Both will also rebound as rapidly with discontinuation of treatment; further, such management increases the possibility of development of pustular psoriasis. Oral prednisone has been used successfully in urticaria patients. In a recent small study, the addition of prednisone burst therapy (40 mg

TABLE 237-5 Differential Diagnosis of Selected Skin Disorders Relative to Primary Lesion Morphology

Lesion Morphology	Differential Considerations
Macule	Drug eruption (fixed or photosensitive); nevus, tattoo (ink); lice infestation; rheumatic fever; syphilis (secondary); viral exanthem erythema multiforme; toxic-infectious erythemas; meningococcemia (early); external trauma (ecchymosis); vitiligo; tinea vesicolor; cellulitis (early)
Papule	Acne; basal cell carcinoma; melanoma; nevus; warts; molluscum contagiosum; skin tags; atopic dermatitis; urticaria; eczema; folliculitis; insect bites; vasculitis; psoriasis; scabies; toxicodendron dermatitis (poison ivy, oak, or sumac); erythema multiforme; varicella (early); gonococcemia
Plaque	Eczema; pityriasis rosea; tinea corporis and versicolor; psoriasis; seborrhcic dermatitis; urticaria; syphilis (secondary); erythema multiforme
Nodule	Basal cell, squamous cell, or metastatic carcinoma; melanoma; erythema nodosum; furuncle; lipoma; warts
Wheal	Urticaria; angioedema; insect bites; erythema multiforme
Pustule	Acne; folliculitis; gonococcemia; hidradenitis suppurativa; herpetic infection (herpes simplex, herpes zoster, varicella); impetigo; psoriasis; rosacea; pyoderma gangrenosum
Vesicle	Herpetic infection (herpes simplex, herpes zoster, varicella); impetigo; toxicodendron dermatitis (poison ivy, oak, or sumac); thermal burn; friction blister; toxic epidermal necrolysis; bullous pemphigoid; pemphigus vulgaris
Bulla	Bullous impetigo; toxicodendron dermatitis (poison ivy, oak, or sumac); thermal burn; friction blister; toxic epidermal necrolysis; bullous pemphigoid; pemphigus vulgaris

Please note that this list is not exhaustive; it represents the more common syndromes that are likely to be encountered in the ED.

daily for 4 days) markedly reduced the pruritus and hastened the clinical improvement. The authors of this study felt that the patients' conditions improved more rapidly and more completely, and without apparent adverse effects, when prednisone was administered.[3] Patients with poison ivy or oak who require systemic steroids should be treated with oral prednisone (1 mg/kg body weight) with a slow two- to three-week taper. Other contact or allergic dermatitides may benefit from an abbreviated course (four days) of oral prednisone.

Topical corticosteroids are a powerful tool in the management of dermatologic disease. Numerous agents are available for use. They differ in concentration, base components, and cost. Familiarity with a single agent in each potency class is sufficient to safely and effectively treat any steroid-responsive skin ailment. Corticosteroid potency or strength, i.e., the anti-inflammatory property, is measured by the agent's ability to induce vasoconstriction. Agents' strengths are rated using the vasoconstricting ability on a scale of one to seven with lower scale numbers correlating with more potent corticosteroids—group I agents are the most powerful corticosteroids while group VII medications are the least potent. Marked variation in potency is seen among various corticosteroids while much less difference in strength is encountered for individual agents at varying concentrations. Many corticosteroids are fluorinated. Fluorination greatly increases the potency

TABLE 237-6 Differential Diagnosis of Selected Skin Disorders Relative to Secondary Lesion Morphology

Lesion Morphology	Differential Considerations
Scales	Psoriasis; pityriasis rosea; toxic-infecious erythemas; secondary syphilis; dermatophytic infection (tineas); tinea versicolor; xerosis (dry skin); thermal burn (first degree)
Crusts	Eczema; dermatophytic infection (tineas); impetigo; contact dermatitis; insect bite
Erosions	Candidiasis; dermatophytic infection (tinea); eczema; toxic epidermal necrolysis; toxic-infectious erythemas; erythema multiforme; primary blistering disorders (bullous pemphigoid and pemphigus vulgaris); brown recluse spider bite
Ulcers	Aphthous lesions; chancroid; decubitus ulcer; thermal or friction injury; subacute/chronic ischemia; malignancy; chancre (primary syphilis); primary blistering disorders (bullous pemphigoid and pemphigus vulgaris); brown recluse spider bite; pyoderma gangrenosum; stasis ulcer; factitial

Please note that this list is not exhaustive; it represents the more common syndromes that are likely to be encountered in the ED.

but also increases the risk of adverse reactions and should not be used in pregnancy.

Use of the appropriate-strength steroid is strongly encouraged at the start of therapy. The use of a less powerful agent is not likely to either spare the patient from potential adverse effect or produce adequate control of the disease. Hydrocortisone, perhaps the most frequently used topical corticosteroid in the outpatient setting, is available over-the-counter in strengths up to 1% and by prescription to a maximum of 2.5%. Hydrocortisone is safe and may be used on most body surfaces, including the face, genitalia, flexure creases, and intertriginous zones; it also is safe for use in infants and children. For the treatment of diseases involving the palms and soles, hydrocortisone is a poor choice in that the thickened skin does not allow adequate penetration of this relatively low-potency steroid. Corticosteroids of moderate potency, including triamcinolone acetonide and fluocinoline acetonide, are useful in severely inflamed skin and on the thicker skin of the scalp, trunk, extensor surfaces, and palms/soles; these agents should not be applied to the face or genitals nor used in the infant. Fluorinated steroids should not be prescribed to pregnant women. See Table 237-8 for recommendations of corticosteroid potency relative to dermatologic disease.

Different skin surfaces respond differently to topical corticosteroid therapy; this different response rate varies relative to the absorption

TABLE 237-7 Selected Laboratory Investigations Useful in the Diagnosis of Dermatologic Disease

Laboratory Test	Dermatologic Disease
Sedimentation rate	Leukocytoclastic vasculitis
Urinalysis (active sediment)	Leukocytoclastic vasculitis
Microbiologic studies	Infectious syndromes (toxic-infections erythemas, tick-borne illnesses, STDs, etc.)
Platelet count/coagulation studies	Purpuric/petechial states

TABLE 237-8 Recommendations of Corticosteroid Potency Relative to Dermatologic Disease*

Groups I and II	Groups III, IV, and V	Groups VI and VII
Psoriasis	Atopic dermatitis	Nonspecific dermatitis, of face, eyelids, and perineum
Eczema, of hand (severe)	Stasis dermatitis	
Poison ivy (severe)	Seborrheic dermatitis	
Atopic dermatitis (severe)	Tinea	
	Scabies	
	Nonspecific dermatitis, of face (severe)	

*Group I, highest potency; Group VII, lowest potency.

of the steroid into the deeper tissues. The relatively thin skin surfaces of the face respond very rapidly to the use of group VII agents, whereas the thicker skin of the palms and soles requires a highly potent steroid. Issues that result in an effective higher potency application when using a low-potency agent include: raw, inflamed skin (such skin more rapidly and readily absorbs medication); treatment regions involving skin surfaces in frequent contact, such as intertriginous areas (the apposition of two skin surfaces produces enhanced absorption of drug similar to the effect to an occlusive dressing); and areas of skin surfaces enclosed under tight clothing, such as the diaper area (once again, enhanced absorption of the agent due to the occlusive effect of the garment). In general, lower potency agents are acceptable in these situations.

The application of creams, ointments, gels, and lotions is relatively straightforward. The medication, applied in thin layers, should be massaged into the skin as directed daily. Prewashing the skin prior to corticosteroid application is unnecessary. Patients should be advised to follow directions closely, both early and late in the treatment course. Early application with either extra medication per dose or more frequent medication administrations is not desired; likewise, both a reduced frequency of application or a decreased amount of medication as the disease process responds to therapy can cause relapse. Optimum application regimens have not been determined for topical corticosteroids in most dermatologic syndromes. The more potent agents are best applied two to three times daily for 1 to 2 weeks followed by a drug-free week; additional therapy may be required as determined by the disease as well as by the particular patient's response to the initial therapy. Agents from the less potent steroid groups may be applied three times daily for 2 to 4 weeks followed by a seven day steroid-free period.

The prescription of the correct amount of topical steroid is at times difficult. The burn rule of nines may be used to estimate the amount of topical corticosteroid to prescribe. Calculate the percentage of body surface area requiring therapy; then, multiply the percentage by a correction factor of 30. This calculation will provide the amount of topical corticosteroid in grams for a single application. Next, determine the number of administration required in the treatment course. For example, a tid regimen for a duration of 10 days ultimately requires 30 applications. The number of applications is multiplied by the amount required for a single use. In general, 9 g of topical steroid will cover 9 percent of the body surface area in a tid application for a single day.

Tachyphylaxis refers to the decrease in responsiveness to a drug as a result of enzyme-mediated events. The term is used in relation to topical corticosteroids in reference to acute tolerance to the vasoconstricting ability. In general, vasoconstriction has been demonstrated to decrease progressively over time when a topical steroid is applied. Such reductions in strength due to tolerance are encountered as early as four days into the treatment course in all potency groups yet are felt to be more important in groups I and II. A reasonable strategy to employ to counter the development of tachyphylaxis is the use of interrupted application schedules; such an interrupted treatment course might include an initial tid application for two weeks followed by a single week of drug holiday followed by a repeat of the cycle.

Antihistamine Agents

Antihistamines (H_1 antagonists) are frequently used in the management of dermatologic disease, particularly in the control of pruritus. These agents include diphenhydramine and hydroxyzine and are dosed using these guidelines: for diphenhydramine, adult: 25 to 50 mg po q6h; children: 4 to 6 mg/kg/24 h po given q6 to 8h not to exceed 200 mg in 24 h; and for hydroxyzine, adult: 25 to 100 milligrams po q8h; children: 2 to 4 mg/kg/24 h po q8 to 12h not to exceed 200 mg in 24 h. Parenteral H_1 antagonists may also be used intramuscularly or intravenously. H_2 antagonists (e.g., ranitidine or famotidine) have also demonstrated some benefit in the patient with an allergic-mediated event, particularly urticaria. The second-generation antihistamine agents, including astemizole, cetirizine, fexofenadine, and loratadine, are newer agents that may be used in certain circumstances. In general, the newer antihistamines offer the advantages of reduced dosing frequency and less sedative effect, but they are more costly. Comparisons of these new medications to hydroxyzine are generally favorable; comparisons among these second-generation agents do not demonstrate significant differences.[4,5] The use of topical antihistamine preparations is discouraged. Topical antihistamine agents are readily absorbed; dosing is therefore difficult to predict. Accidental overdosage may result in the patient who aggressively applies the preparation and/or is also using similar oral agents. Numerous other antipruritic therapies are recommended including Domeboro solution (diluted 1:10 aluminum sulfate) soaks, potassium permanganate baths, and oatmeal baths.

Antimicrobial Agents

Topical antibacterial agents are used primarily as adjuncts to wound dressings; these agents rarely are useful as primary therapy for superficial bacterial infections of the skin. The exception to this statement is topical mupirocin, which is reportedly as effective as oral antimicrobial agents in the management of impetigo. Concerning wound dressings, the agents commonly used include polymyxin B, bacitracin, neomycin, and silver sulfadiazine. Suggested benefits of these medications include reduced adherence of bandaging material to the wound, as well as less coagulum and decreased bacterial colonization. The impact on the rate of wound healing and the prevention of wound infection are less well characterized. Another use of topical antibacterial agents is the treatment of aphthous stomatitis with oral tetracycline rinses. Systemic antibiotic therapy is of use in certain dermatologic syndromes and is discussed in those areas.

Various topical antifungal agents are available for the treatment of candida and the dermatophytic infections. The imidazole and polyene classes of agents are the most commonly used in outpatient medicine. Members of the imidazole class include clotrimazole, miconazole, and ketoconazole, while the polyenes are represented by nystatin and amphotericin B. Generally, the imidazoles are effective against yeasts and dermatophytes, whereas the polyenes are useful only in the treatment of candidal infections. In that diagnostic confusion that may arise in the fungal etiology of the superficial infection, polyene agents are best avoided; imidazole agents will treat all such superficial fungal infections. Dermatophytic and yeast infections should be treated for prolonged periods to reduce the possibility of recurrence; in general, a two- to four-week period of therapy is advised. In cases involving significant discomfort, combination agents composed of imidazole and corticosteroid agents reduce discomfort and eradicate the organism.

Selenium sulfide shampoo is effective against tinea versicolor when applied for 30 min daily for 14 days.

Acyclovir has been used extensively in patients with various herpes virus infections, including acute varicella, varicella zoster virus infections (''shingles''), and herpes simplex infections. Valacyclovir[6] and famciclovir[7] are acceptable therapies.[8] In general, these agents do not offer significant advantage over acyclovir with the exception of reduced dosing frequency—perhaps increasing compliance and, therefore, the possibility of an improved outcome.

Infestations with lice are treated with topical lindane, permethrin 1%, or pyrethrins. These agents are reasonably effective against adult lice but are less useful against the unhatched eggs—the nit. Consequently, a second application 5 to 10 days after the initial treatment should clear the new generation of lice, which was not affected by the first use. Central nervous system toxicity has been reported in small infants treated with lindane; as such, permethrin or pyrethrins should be used in children less than one year of age. Scabies may also be treated with a single overnight application of lindane or permethrin 5% covering the entire nonhair-bearing skin surface.

Topical Agent Vehicle Considerations

The vehicle, or medication base, is the substance in which the active ingredient is dispersed. The base determines the rate at which the active ingredient is absorbed through the skin. Components of some bases may cause irritation or allergy. Creams, a mixture of oils, water, and preservative, are white in color and greasy in texture. Creams are the most versatile vehicle and can be applied to any body surface area; they are particularly useful in the intertriginous areas. Creams are best used for acute therapy only; chronic application may cause excessive drying. Ointments are composed of greases such as petroleum jelly and are preservative-free; little water is added to this vehicle. This vehicle is translucent and, when applied to the skin, remains greasy. This greasy consistency may aid in the lubrication in particularly dry lesions. In general, ointment vehicles allow deeper tissue penetration when compared to the cream base. Ointments are too occlusive, providing very thorough coverage with deep tissue penetration while allowing little movement in moisture and other material into and out of the skin. Acute exudative syndromes, as well as intertriginous areas of the body, should not be treated with topical steroids using the ointment vehicle. Gels are greaseless mixtures of propylene glycol and water at times with alcohol. Gels have a translucent appearance and are described as ''sticky.'' Alcohol-containing gels are best used for acute exudative lesions such as poison ivy dermatitis, whereas alcohol-free combinations should be applied to dry, scaling conditions. In denuded areas, the alcohol component may cause discomfort. Gels are of particular use in the scalp area; their presence does not alter the arrangement of the hair and therefore more tolerable for the patient from the cosmetic perspective. Solutions or lotions may contain water or alcohols in addition to other agents. They are clear or milky in appearance; with their liquid consistency, they are best applied to the scalp and other dense hair-bearing areas without leaving significant residue on the hair. In denuded areas, the alcohol component may cause discomfort. Guidelines for specialty consultation or hospital admission are similar. First, extensive skin involvement by erythroderma, bullae, or a palpable purpura suggests the need for rapid ED consultation followed by hospital admission. However, certain dermatologic syndromes typically present with generalized involvement and do not require specialty care; classic examples include urticaria and angioedema, acute varicella, and toxicodendron dermatitis. If the diagnosis is in question in the patient with a generalized rash consider the need for dermatologic consultation.

General medical concerns that might prompt consultation and admission include cardiorespiratory instability, the systemic signs and symptoms, multisystem involvement, significant comorbidity, patient age, poor home environment, or the need for the initiation of aggressive medical therapy.

REFERENCES

1. Shivaram V, Christoph RA, Hayden GF: Skin disorders encountered in a pediatric emergency department. *Pediatr Emerg Care* 9:202, 1993.
2. Feldman SR, Fleischer AB, McConnell RC: Most common dermatologic problems identified by internists, 1990–1994. *Arch Intern Med* 158:726, 1998.
3. Pollack CV, Romano TJ: Outpatient management of acute urticaria: The role of prednisone. *Ann Emerg Med* 26:547, 1995.
4. Tharp MD: Cetirizine: A new therapeutic alternative for chronic urticaria. *Cutis* 58:94, 1996.
5. Goldsmith P, Dowd PM: The new H1 antihistamines. *Dermatol Clin* 11:87, 1993.
6. Acosta EP, Fletcher CV: Valacyclovir. *Ann Pharmacother* 31:185, 1997.
7. Crumpacker C: The pharmacological profile of famciclovir. *Semin Dermatol* 15(suppl):14, 1996.
8. Stein GE: Pharmacology of new antiherpes agents: Famciclovir and valacyclovir. *J Am Pharm Assoc* NS37:157, 1997.

238 DISORDERS OF THE FACE AND SCALP

Lisa May

The list of cutaneous disorders affecting the face and scalp is quite long. This chapter focuses on those disorders that are more specific to this distribution and likely to be encountered in an acute care setting.

ACNEIFORM ERUPTIONS

Although acne vulgaris is a common chronic problem that likely would not be encountered as a chief complaint in the emergency department setting, several acneiform eruptions may develop with alarming clinical presentations prompting a patient to seek immediate attention. As these disorders are uncommon and require a dermatologic consultation, they are discussed only briefly. These disorders include acne fulminans, pyoderma faciale, dissecting cellulitis of the scalp, and acne keloidalis.

Acne fulminans is a severe form of cystic acne with ulcerating cysts. It most commonly affects the chest and back of young males. Severe scarring may result. It may have systemic associations including fever, myalgias, arthralgias, malaise, and anorexia. Treatment includes systemic corticosteroids and isotretinoin (Accutane). As isotretinoin has potentially severe side effects, including devastating teratogenicity in women who become pregnant while on this medication, it should be administered only by those familiar with the use of Accutane and able to follow the patient during the entire course of therapy.

Pyoderma faciale is an inflammatory cystic acneiform eruption on the central face of young women. Comedones are absent. Scarring is likely to result and thus treatment should be instituted rapidly. Treatment consists of systemic corticosteroids and isotretinoin (Accutane). Again, a dermatology consultation is recommended.

Dissecting cellulitis of the scalp is an inflammatory and scarring disease of the scalp and neck. It is most commonly seen in young African-American males. Clinically, the disease begins with boggy tender nodules on the scalp and neck. The nodules suppurate and develop sinus tracts. Hair loss develops over these nodules, and with time, a permanent scarring alopecia results. The etiology is unknown. It may be seen in association with acne conglobata and hidradenitis suppurativa, where together these three diseases are referred to as the follicular occlusion triad. Treatment is difficult and often unsuccessful. Therapy includes topical and systemic antibiotics; topical, intralesional, or oral corticosteroids; isotretinoin; and excision. Therapy is best managed by a dermatologist.

Acne keloidalis is a perifollicular inflammatory process of the scalp resulting in hypertrophic and keloid scarring. The exact etiology is unknown. It is most common in African-Americans, and it is more common in males than females. The primary lesions are follicular-based papules and pustules on the occipital scalp. The individual keloidal papules enlarge and coalesce to form keloidal plaques with an associated scarring alopecia. Treatment includes topical antibiotics such as clindamycin solution (Cleocin-T solution), topical corticosteroids such as flucinonide (Lidex) solution, and oral antibiotics such as tetracycline. Repeated intralesional corticosteroids may help relieve pruritus and pain, and soften keloidal plaques. Surgical excision and Laser excision are often unsatisfactory.

SEBORRHEIC DERMATITIS

Because seborrheic dermatitis is such a common disorder, its recognition and management are important in any clinical setting including the emergency department. Although the exact etiology is unclear, the yeast, *Piytrosporum ovale,* may play a role in the pathogenesis of this disease.

Clinical Features

Clinically, one sees erythema and waxy scale in the skin folds and hair-bearing areas of the face, scalp, chest, and groin. Common sites of involvement include the scalp, the pinna of the ear, the posterior auricular sulcus, the eyebrows, and the alar grooves of the nose. Itching is quite variable but usually mild. Any age may be affected but the elderly and debilitated are more likely to have extensive involvement. In newborns, seborrheic dermatitis is often referred to as cradle cap. Extensive seborrheic dermatitis that is poorly responsive to treatment may be seen in association with HIV.

Diagnosis

Diagnosis is based on clinical examination. A skin biopsy is rarely necessary. The differential diagnosis includes tinea capitis, psoriasis of the scalp, rosacea, and cutaneous lupus erythematosus. Seborrheic dermatitis is diffuse and rarely associated with hair loss; thus if hair loss is present or the eruption is focal, fungal cultures should be obtained to rule out tinea capitis. As seborrheic dermatitis is uncommon between infancy and puberty, tinea capitis should always be excluded in this age group. Rosacea and seborrheic dermatitis may overlap, but if the predominant features are inflammatory papules and pustules, the patient should be treated for rosacea.

Treatment

Therapy is aimed at controlling the disease; treatment is not curative. Initial treatment should consist of an antidandruff shampoo containing zinc pyrethrin (Head and Shoulders), selenium sulfide (Selsun Blue), salicylic acid (Neutrogena T-Sal), or tar (Polytar or Neutrogena T-Gel). Nizoral shampoo can also be used and is now available over the counter. The shampoo should be lathered into the scalp and left on for 5 to 10 min before rinsing. Shampooing should be performed three times a week. A topical corticosteroid such as flucinonide solution may be applied to the scalp in severe cases. For the face, hydrocortisone 1% or 2.5% applied bid should be the initial management. The use of higher-potency topical corticosteroids on the face can lead to the development of perioral dermatitis and should be avoided. Patients should treat the seborrheic dermatitis until clear and then on a prn basis.

ERYSIPELAS AND FACIAL CELLULITIS

Erysipelas and cellulitis are infections of the dermis and subcutis with erysipelas being more superficial than cellulitis. The distinction between the two is subtle and therapeutically irrelevant. Erysipelas is more likely to occur in the young and in the elderly.

Pathophysiology

Cellulitis may be a primary process or it may complicate another dermatosis. On the face, it may begin at a site of minor trauma that is often inapparent. A group A streptococcus is the most likely cause of erysipelas. *Haemophilus influenzae* may be a causative organism in children; although this is not as common because of the widespread use of the *H. influenzae* vaccine. *Staphylococcal spp* and *Streptococcal spp* are the most likely pathogens of cellulitis.

Clinical Features

Erysipelas and cellulitis of the face presents as a hot, bright red, tender, indurated plaque (Fig. 238-1). The area of involvement is sharply demarcated and expands peripherally. They do not clear centrally. Vesicles or bullae may be present. They may be unilateral or bilateral. When unilateral, erysipelas and cellulitis need to be distinguished from early herpes zoster infection. When bilateral, they may be mistaken for the malar eruption of systemic lupus erythematosus.

Fever and lymphadenopathy are often present. Periorbital cellulitis can be associated with orbital cellulitis and has the risk of developing an orbital abscess, cerebral abscess or meningitis.

Diagnosis

Diagnosis is based on clinical presentation. A biopsy is rarely necessary and often not helpful. Needle aspiration of the leading edge for culture has a low yield. A complete blood count and blood cultures should be performed to exclude bacteremia. An imaging study and an ophthalmologic consultation should evaluate periorbital cellulitis.

Treatment

Cellulitis or erysipelas of the face warrants parenteral therapy in an inpatient setting. Unless history is suggestive of an unusual organism, therapy should be directed toward *Staphylococcal spp* and *Streptococcal spp* in adults. Coverage should include these organisms and *H. influenzae* in children. Again, an immediate ophthalmology consultation should be obtained if there is any question of orbital involvement.

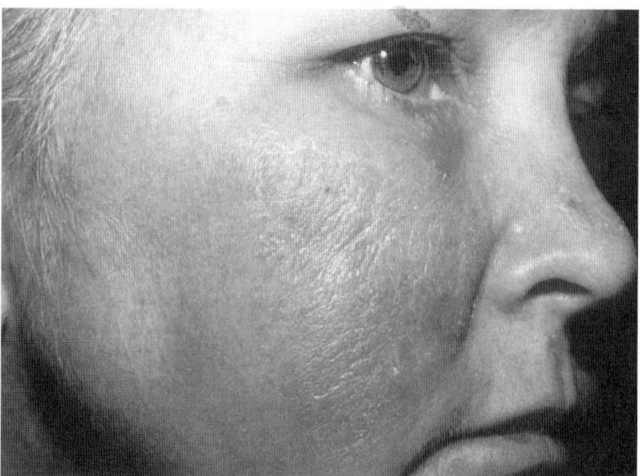

FIG. 238-1. Facial cellulitis. Erythema and edema involve the cheek, nasal bridge, and the upper and lower eyelids.

HERPES ZOSTER INFECTION

Herpes zoster infections (''shingles'') can occur anywhere on the body but most commonly involve the thoracic dermatomes. Involvement of the trigeminal nerve occurs in about 10 percent of herpes zoster infections. Involvement of the face and scalp has the most potentially serious sequelae and thus is discussed here.

Clinical Features

Herpes zoster results from reactivation of latent varicella-zoster virus (VZV). The initial eruption of varicella-zoster virus is chickenpox. Pain or dysesthesia precedes the eruption by 3 to 5 days. Erythematous papules progress to clusters of vesicles with an erythematous base. The vesicles crust in about 1 week. Generalized eruptions may occur in immunocompromised patients.

Any of three branches of the trigeminal nerve may be involved on the face. Involvement of the ophthalmic branch (V1), especially with vesicles on the tip of the nose indicative of involvement of the nasociliary branch, is of serious concern. Involvement of this area raises the possibility of developing keratitis. Therefore, an ophthalmology consult should be obtained.

The virus may spread to motor root ganglia, resulting in motor weakness or paralysis. Ramsay-Hunt syndrome results from facial and auditory nerve involvement. The cutaneous eruption consists of zoster lesions in the external auditory canal (Fig. 238-2) and on tympanic membrane. Bell's palsy and possible deafness or vertigo may result.

Diagnosis

The differential diagnosis includes herpes simplex infections, impetigo, and contact dermatitis. A Tzanck preparation and a viral culture can confirm the diagnosis. The yield is higher when the tests are performed on early intact vesicles. A Tzanck preparation allows for visualization of multinucleated giant cells. It is useful to determine if an eruption is viral in origin; however it is unable to distinguish between herpes simplex and varicella zoster viruses. Viral culture should be obtained by opening a vesicle and scraping the base of a vesicle onto a synthetic (not cotton) swab to be placed in viral culture media. Growth may take as long as one week.

Again, ophthalmic nerve involvement requires an ophthalmology consultation to rule out ocular complications.

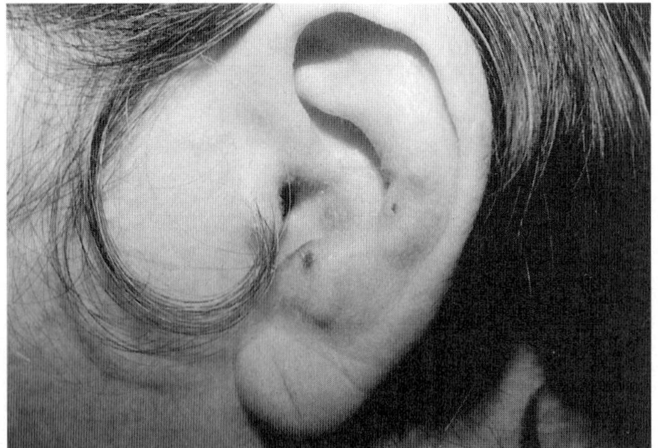

FIG. 238-2. Herpes zoster infection. This example demonstrates clustered intact vesicles and crusts of the pinna and external auditory canal. Patients with this distribution are at risk of developing Ramsay-Hunt syndrome with facial nerve involvement resulting in Bell's palsy.

Treatment

Antiviral medications are helpful if given within the first 72 h after the eruption begins. Antiviral therapy can shorten the time to healing, decrease new lesion formation, and possibly decrease the pain and duration of postherpetic neuralgia. Acyclovir (800 mg po five times per day for 7 days), famciclovir (500 mg po tid for 7 days), and valacyclovir (1 g po tid for seven days) are recommended outpatient regimens.

Symptomatic treatment includes Domeboro's solution compresses 1:40 dilution for 15 min qid followed by Polysporin ointment or Silvadene cream. Analgesics are often necessary as well.

HERPES SIMPLEX VIRUS INFECTIONS

Herpes simplex virus (HSV) type I most commonly occurs on the face. Initial infection occurs during childhood or adolescence and varies in its presentation. Many individuals experience mild symptoms while a few experience a debilitating eruption. Recurrences tend to be mild and occur primarily on the lips, in the nose, and in the oral cavity.

The typical lesions of HSV are painful, grouped vesicles with an erythematous base. The primary eruption may be preceded by constitutional symptoms. The characteristic primary eruption is a gingivostomatitis with herpetic lesions on the lips and in the oral cavity. It may persist for weeks. The differential diagnosis includes erythema multiforme, Coxsackie virus, varicella zoster virus, idiopathic aphthae, and, rarely, Behcçet's disease and pemphigus vulgaris.

Recurrent HSV is typically seen as herpes labialis (''fever blisters'' or ''cold sores''). The individual often experiences a prodrome of localized tingling or burning several hours before the onset of the eruption. The herpetic lesion usually occurs along the lip margin and completely heals within 10 days. Ultraviolet light, fever, or local trauma can induce these eruptions.

The diagnosis is established in the same manner as that for herpes zoster with a positive Tzanck preparation and viral culture.

Treatment for primary HSV gingivostomatitis includes symptomatic treatment, as mentioned previously for herpes zoster infections, including compresses and topical antibiotics. If mild, oral antiviral medications are not necessary; in more severe cases, use acyclovir (200 mg po five times per day for 5 days). Immunocompromised patients with severe involvement require hospitalization for intravenous acyclovir. Treatment can continue for up to 10 days if lesions have not crusted. Recurrent HSV does not require oral antiviral therapy. Patients with recurrent disease should be instructed to avoid triggers, especially the sun, by using sunscreen and a lip balm with ultraviolet light protection.

ECZEMA HERPETICUM

In individuals with cutaneous diseases, most commonly atopic dermatitis, HSV or VZV can infect the dermatitic skin. This disorder is referred to as eczema herpeticum or Kaposi's varicelliform eruption. Initially, the infection may be mistaken as an exacerbation or impetiginization of the dermatitis. Pustules or confluent areas of pus develop. Constitutional symptoms and adenopathy are usually present. Dissemination of the virus is possible; mortality reports in this disorder are as high as 10 percent. Furthermore, scarring may be extensive if the viral infection is not treated early and aggressively.

An immediate dermatology consultation is warranted if this diagnosis is entertained. Depending on the extent of involvement, oral or intravenous acyclovir should be used. The underlying cutaneous disease requires aggressive treatment as well.

OTHER INFECTIOUS DISEASES OF THE FACE

In addition to the infections mentioned above, numerous other infections can occur on the face. In children, impetigo on the face is common, as is dermatophyte infections (tinea faciei and tinea barbae). Staphylococcal folliculitis is also seen on the face. The face and scalp are also a common site of involvement in secondary syphilis in which individuals develop "moth-eaten" alopecia, scaly or moist papules around the nose and at the angles of the mouth. Flat warts are frequently seen in males as a result of spreading the virus by shaving. Numerous molluscum contagiosum on the face of an adolescent or adult are suggestive of HIV. Patients with this disorder should be tested for HIV.

Uncommon infectious diseases on the face include blastomycosis, histoplasmosis, leishmaniasis, leprosy, tuberculosis, sporotrichosis, actinomycosis, and atypical mycobacterium infections.

CUTANEOUS LUPUS ERYTHEMATOSUS

Lupus erythematosus is a connective tissue disease of uncertain etiology. It may be a systemic disease with many organ systems involved or confined exclusively to the skin. Cutaneous lupus erythematosus can be divided into three major types: acute cutaneous lupus, subacute cutaneous lupus, and chronic cutaneous lupus. All three types may occur on the face. This section focuses on the malar rash of acute cutaneous lupus and the discoid lesions of chronic cutaneous lupus erythematosus.

Acute Cutaneous Lupus Erythematosus

The classic eruption of acute cutaneous lupus is the malar or butterfly rash. In most cases, this eruption is associated with systemic disease. It usually occurs simultaneously with the onset or flare of SLE. This eruption is induced by ultraviolet radiation. The malar rash is more common in whites than in African-Americans.

Clinically, the malar rash consists of erythema on the medial cheeks and across the bridge of the nose. Induration, scale, or telangiectasias may be present. Occasionally, the eyelids may be involved which makes the eruption difficult to distinguish from heliotrope rash of dermatomyositis.

Diagnosis is based on clinical examination and the presence of other systemic symptoms suggestive of SLE. This eruption is by no means specific for lupus erythematosus. The differential diagnosis includes rosacea, erysipelas, dermatomyositis, seborrheic dermatitis, medication-induced photosensitivity, polymorphous light eruption, and allergic contact dermatitis. Skin biopsy may be helpful especially if the diagnosis is in question. Initial laboratory evaluation includes a complete blood count, chemistry profile to include BUN and creatinine, urinalysis with evaluation of urine sediment, antinuclear antibodies, double-stranded DNA, and complement.

If the diagnosis of SLE is likely, a rheumatology consultation should be obtained for further evaluation and management. The urgency of this consultation is dependent on the patient's systemic complaints. If other signs or symptoms of SLE are not present, the other entities in the differential diagnosis should be explored. A nonemergent consultation with a dermatologist is recommended.

Chronic Cutaneous Lupus Erythematosus

Chronic cutaneous lupus erythematosus is referred to as discoid lupus erythematosus (DLE). It is an eruption that results in scarring and pigmentary changes in the skin. DLE is most commonly seen in African-Americans. Only 10 percent of patients with this type of lupus develop systemic disease.

Clinically, the lesions of DLE occur in a photodistributed area, especially on the face, ears, scalp, and neck. The lesions begin as erythematous or hyperpigmented papules or plaques that enlarge leaving central depigmentation (Fig. 238-3). Follicular plugging may be visible, especially in ear lesions. On the scalp, a scarring alopecia with typical discoid lesions may occur. More extensive involvement of the trunk and extremities is more likely to be associated with systemic disease.

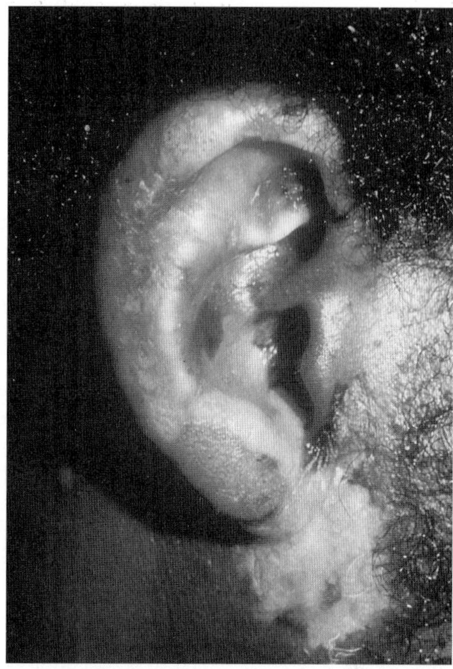

FIG. 238-3. Discoid lupus erythematosus. The external ear and preauricular cheek is a common site of involvement. Central depigmentation with surrounding erythema and hyperpigmentation is typical of discoid lupus erythematosus.

The lesions of DLE are quite characteristic and the diagnosis can often be made clinically. A skin biopsy is performed to confirm the diagnosis or to make a diagnosis in atypical clinical presentations. As DLE is a chronic disease and individuals suspected of having this disorder should be referred to a dermatologist for long-term management.

PHOTOSENSITIVITY

The types of reactions to ultraviolet light are varied. In many disorders, ultraviolet light aggravates, but does not cause, the disease. Examples of this type of reaction include lupus erythematosus, porphyria cutanea tarda, dermatitis associated with niacin deficiency (pellagra), and recurrence of HSV. Other disorders are caused primarily by the sun. The most common is a sunburn reaction. Sunburn reaction, exogenously induced photosensitivity, and polymorphous light eruption are discussed here.

Sunburn

A sunburn reaction is the inflammatory response to skin injury as a result of ultraviolet radiation. It may be minimal with little discomfort to the patient, or it may be severe with extensive blistering. Individuals with fair skin, light eyes, and naturally light hair color are more susceptible to sunburns; however, even darker pigmented skin can develop skin injury with large enough ultraviolet light exposure.

The sunburn reaction begins 2 to 6 hours after exposure and peaks in one to three days. Erythema and warmth in sun-exposed areas occurs. Vesiculation may result that is equivalent to a second-degree burn.

The most important part of treatment is to stress prevention. Education includes counseling the patient to avoid the midday sun, to apply liberally and frequently a broad-spectrum sunscreen (UVA and UVB protection with SPF 15 to 30), to wear protective clothing, and to seek shade. Sunburns can be treated symptomatically with NSAIDs, with tepid baths, and by applying topical antibiotics to areas of vesiculation. Emollients may be soothing but will not prevent eventual exfoliation. Individuals should also be advised to avoid the sun until the eruption resolves.

Exogenous Photosensitivity Disorders

These disorders result from topical application or ingestion of an agent that causes the skin to be more sensitive to ultraviolet light. Photosensitivity disorders may be phototoxic or photoallergic. The clinical differences are subtle and do not impact on acute management of a patient; therefore, the reader is referred to a reference or dermatology textbook for further information.

Topical photosensitizers usually result in a cutaneous eruption at their sites of application. Ultraviolet exposure is necessary for the eruption to occur. Furocoumarins are the most common group of agents causing topical photoeruptions. Lime juice applied to the skin, fragrances, figs, celery, and parsnips are examples of furocoumarins. Other topically applied agents causing photosensitivity include PABA esters, topical psoralens, musk ambrette, and salicylanilide antibacterials. The typical clinical eruption is a severe sunburn-like reaction, often with vesiculation. Often a linear appearance suggests that an externally applied substance is the culprit.

Numerous ingested substances can result in a photosensitivity eruption as well. Table 238-1 lists the most common offending agents. Because these agents are ingested and distributed throughout the body, the eruption involves all sun-exposed areas. The characteristic distribution of a photosensitivity eruption is the face, posterior neck, dorsal hands, and extensor arms. Certain areas including the creases of the eyelids, the upper lip, the V of the anterior neck, and the posterior auricular neck are spared.

The diagnosis is based on identifying the offending agent. If the diagnosis is unclear, other photosensitivity disorders, such as lupus erythematosus and polymorphous light eruption, should be excluded. Photopatch testing performed by a dermatologist or allergist may be helpful in identifying the photosensitizing agent.

The causative agent should be discontinued, if possible. Initial management includes topical corticosteroids and management similar to a sunburn reaction. The patient should avoid the sun until the eruption has cleared completely.

CONTACT DERMATITIS OF THE FACE

Two types of contact allergies are likely to result on the face. The first is the result of an aerosolized allergen. The second is direct physical contact that is most prominent on the sensitive skin of the face.

TABLE 238-1 Medications Commonly Causing Photosensitivity Eruptions

Aminodarone
Chlorpromazine
Chloroquine/hydroxychloroquine
Furosemide
NSAIDs
Psoralen
Sulfonamides
Sulfonylreas
Tetracyclines
Thiazides

TABLE 238-2 The Differential Diagnosis of Alopecia

Nonscarring	Scarring
Alopecia areata	Kerion tinea capitis
Secondary syphilis	Herpes zoster infection
Traumatic alopecia	Dissecting cellulitis of the scalp
Trichotillomania	Folliculitis decalvans
Traction alopecia	Acne keloidalis
Contact dermatitis	Discoid lupus erythematosus
Androgenic alopecia	Lichen planopilaris
Thyroid disorders	Morphea
Telogen effluvium	Sarcoidosis
Medications	Scleroderma
Hair shaft abnormalities	Turmors (squamous cell carcinoma, basal cell carcinoma, melanoma, metastatic disease, cylindroma, lymphoma)

Clinically, allergic contact dermatitis resulting from an aerosolized allergen presents as erythema or scale with or without vesiculation. The involvement is diffuse with upper and lower eyelids affected. This distribution is in contrast with photosensitive eruptions in which nonsun-exposed areas, such as the upper eyelids and the upper lip, are spared. Direct allergic contact dermatitis tends to be most prominent on the most sensitive skin, such as the eyelids. Examples of aerosolized contactants include rhus (poison ivy, oak) when the plant has been burned. Examples of common contactants affecting the face include nickel, nail polishes, toothpaste, preservatives in make-up, contact lens solutions, eyeglasses, and hair care products. Chemical-splash injuries are a common cause of facial-irritant contact dermatitis. A thorough history is necessary to uncover the offending agent. Referral to a dermatologist or allergist may be necessary if the history is unrevealing.

Avoiding the offending agent is the most crucial part of treatment. Medical treatment will be of little value if the offending agent is not removed from the patient's environment. Depending on the severity, topical or oral corticosteroids and oral antihistamines are used in medical management. Domeboro's compresses can be beneficial as well. Only low-potency topical corticosteroids should be used on the face. Hydrocortisone 2.5%; cream or ointment should be tried initially. Careful application around the eyes is important because topical corticosteroid use has been implicated in causing cataracts and glaucoma. Oftentimes, extensive and severe periocular involvement requires oral prednisone.

HAIR LOSS

Hair loss can be a very alarming event leading to visits to an emergency department. The causes of hair loss are numerous and are typically divided into scarring and nonscarring alopecia. Nonscarring alopecia may be reversible where as scarring alopecia is rarely reversible. The differential diagnoses for alopecia are listed in Table 238-2. Several of the more common types are discussed here.

Tinea Capitis

Tinea capitis is a dermatophyte infection of the scalp. It is most commonly seen in children, particularly African-American children.

CLINICAL FEATURES Clinically one sees areas of alopecia with broken-off hairs and scale at the periphery. The alopecia is patchy and usually nonscarring (Fig. 238-4). Occasionally, tinea capitis is associated with an intense inflammatory response. This is manifested as a boggy, tender, indurated plaque with superficial pustules and overlying alopecia. This is referred to as a kerion, and it may result in permanent scarring and alopecia.

DIAGNOSIS Diagnosis is based on a positive potassium hydroxide preparation or positive fungal culture. A potassium hydroxide preparation of the hair is necessary; scraping only the scalp rarely gives a positive KOH exam. Culture is often necessary to establish or confirm the diagnosis. Wood's light examination may be helpful as certain types of dermatophytes fluoresce under Wood's light examination.

TREATMENT After a diagnosis is established, the current first-line therapy is griseofulvin. Topical treatment alone is not affective. Ultramicrosized griseofulvin at doses of 15 mg/kg/day given bid with meals is recommended. Individuals should be treated for six weeks, at which time the patient should be reevaluated to determine whether therapy should be continued longer. Nizoral shampoo at least three times per week is recommended in addition to griseofulvin.

DISPOSITION Other family members, especially children, and other close contacts, such as classmates at school or day care, should be evaluated as well. Other affected members should be treated simultaneously to prevent reinfection. Follow-up is crucial and should be stressed as persistent infection may only manifest as scale and go unrecognized by caregivers. Follow-up should be with a primary care provider or a dermatologist.

Alopecia Areata

Alopecia areata (Fig. 238-5) is disease of unknown etiology that results in nonscarring alopecia. Clinically, one will loose round patches of hair leaving behind smooth bald skin. Inflammation or scale is not present. Any hair-bearing area may be affected, but the scalp is the most common site of involvement. Rarely, patients loose all of their scalp or body hair; these are referred to as alopecia totalis and alopecia universalis, respectively. Diagnosis is based on clinical examination. ''Exclamation point'' hairs may be noted at the periphery. Alopecia areata may be associated with hyperthyroidism; thus, checking a TSH is warranted. Secondary syphilis may result in patchy alopecia described as ''moth-eaten'' alopecia. Often, scale is present. If secondary syphilis is suspected by history, a screening test, such as an RPR or VDRL, should be performed.

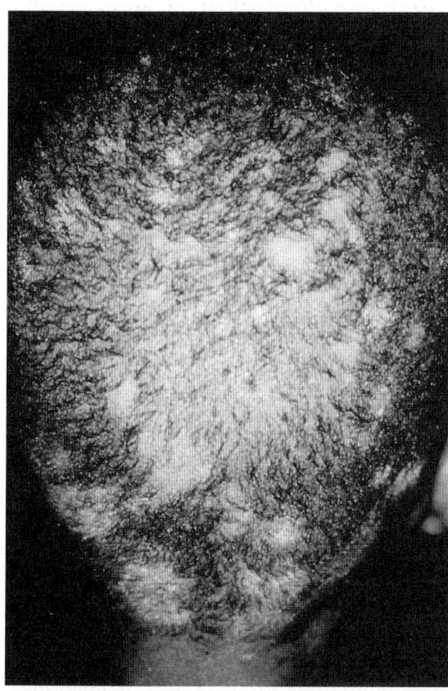

FIG. 238-4. Tinea capitis. Patchy areas of hair loss with broken-off hairs and scale is characteristic of tinea capitis.

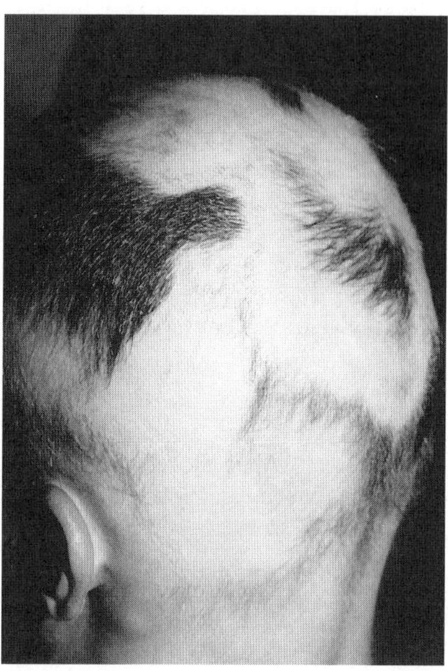

FIG. 238-5. Alopecia areata. This patient's hair loss results in areas of complete balding. The etiology is unknown.

Patients should be counseled that localized alopecia areata usually resolves spontaneously within two to six months. Extensive disease is less likely to resolve. If the disease is extensive, rapidly progressive, or of significant cosmetic concern, the patient should be referred to a dermatologist for treatment. Multiple therapies have been reported including topical, intralesional, and, rarely, systemic corticosteroids; anthralin; contact sensitizers such as dichloronitrobenzene; and photochemotherapy. None is universally successful, and all have potential complications; thus, only those health care providers who can follow the patient long-term to monitor for potential benefit and complications should administer therapy.

Telogen Effluvium

Telogen effluvium is hair loss resulting from a major stressful event. This may include pregnancy and delivery, major surgery, major illness usually requiring hospitalization, or crash diets. The event causes hair to arrest in the telogen growth phase of the hair. Two to three months after the event, when new hairs are growing, the telogen hairs are shed. The patient often notices hair clogging the shower drain or numerous hairs on the pillow upon rising in the morning. The patient and the patient's family notice appreciable thinning that is sudden and often quite alarming. Diagnosis is based on diffuse hair loss in the appropriate clinical setting. A related disorder is anagen effluvium, which is secondary to systemic chemotherapeutic agents. Patients should be reassured that complete hair loss is unlikely and actually heralds new hair growth.

BIBLIOGRAPHY

Gould JW, Mercurio MG, Elmets CA: Cutaneous photosensitivity diseases induced by exogenous agents. *J Am Acad Dermatol* 33(4):551, 1995.

Laman SD, Provost TT: Cutaneous manifestations of lupus erythematosus. *Rheum Dis Clin North Am* 20(1):195, 1994.

DISORDERS OF THE HANDS, FEET, AND EXTREMITIES

Lisa May

Dermatological conditions affecting the hands, feet, and extremities encompass a great majority of skin diseases. This chapter focuses on the disorders that are most likely encountered in an acute care setting. This is by no means a comprehensive review of the subject. The reader is referred to the suggested reading section at the end of this section for a more in-depth coverage of this topic.

ACUTE PARONYCHIA

Paronychia is inflammation of the nail folds. It may be acute or chronic in nature, is seen more often in women than in men, and is associated with frequent wetting of the hands.

Pathophysiology

Acute paronychia results from trauma to the cuticle or nail fold allowing bacteria or yeast to enter. Aggressive manicuring can contribute to this process in adults while nail biting and thumb sucking contribute in children. Excessive water exposure also softens the cuticle allowing for easier entry of organisms. Continued water exposure prevents the reforming of the cuticle, thus providing an environment for colonization of the area with bacteria or yeast. This process results in a chronic paronychia. The most common organisms found in acute paronychia include *Staphylococcal* and group A *Streptococcal* species. The organisms most likely involved in chronic cases are *Candida, Staphylococcus,* and *pseudomonas*.

Clinical Features

Acute paronychia presents as a rapid onset of swelling, tenderness, and redness of the nail fold. A pustule or abscess may develop and pus can often be expressed from the space between the nail fold and the nail. Erythematous streaks may extend proximally from this area and may be associated with fever. Chronic paronychia has a less abrupt onset, and swelling, tenderness, and redness will wax and wane. Retraction of the cuticle is prominent in chronic paronychia, and the nail plate usually has horizontal ridging [Fig. 239-1 (Plate 21)].

Other noninfectious causes of paronychia include psoriasis, dermatitis, and even certain medications including Accutane. Because of injury to the proximal nail fold and cuticles, these patients are at risk of developing secondary infection as well. A clue to the diagnosis is sudden exacerbation of the nail disease without exacerbation of other cutaneous disease.

Diagnosis

The diagnosis of paronychia is based primarily on clinical examination and history. In chronic cases, differentiating between bacterial and *Candida* paronychia may be difficult clinically. Therefore, a fungal culture should be obtained in addition to a bacterial culture.

Treatment

If an abscess or fluctuance is present, immediate treatment includes drainage of the affected area. To perform this procedure, a no. 15 scalpel blade is inserted between the nail plate and the cuticle. The nail fold is then gently massaged to aid in drainage. An incision does not need to be made through the nail fold. Cultures should be obtained in recurrent or chronic cases. Drainage should be followed with warm

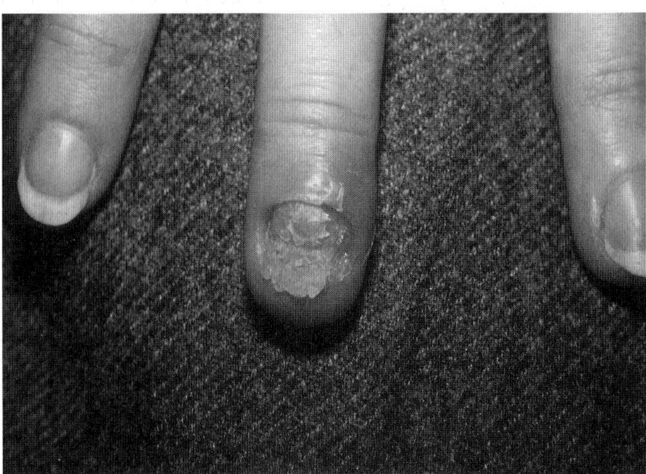

FIG. 239-1 (Plate 21). Chronic *candida paronychia.* The cuticle is absent. Erythema and edema are prominent at the proximal and lateral nail folds. The dystrophic ridged nail is a sign of chronic disease.

tap water soaks for 10 to 15 minutes three times a day for one to two days in acute cases. In chronic cases, the area should be kept as dry as possible. In mild acute cases, topical antibiotics like mupirocin (Bactroban) can be applied twice a day for seven days. In more severe acute cases, oral antibiotics such as cephalexin or dicloxacillin (250 mg po qid for 10 days) should be started until culture results and sensitivities have returned.

In chronic paronychia, the hands should be kept dry. Avoiding prolonged water exposure is imperative. In occupations where this is not feasible, such as bar tending, janitorial services, or dish washing, the patient should wear a pair of thin cotton gloves underneath rubber or vinyl gloves. The cotton gloves should be changed frequently as sweating can lead to maceration and further contribute to the problem. All manicuring should be stopped. Drying agents are the treatment of choice. A 2% to 4% thymol in absolute alcohol can be compounded by a pharmacist and applied to the area four times a day. Topical antifungal solutions, such as clotrimazole solution, can be used twice a day as well. Acute flares should be treated like acute paronychia with drainage and antibiotics. Occasionally, severe or recalcitrant candidal paronychia may require oral antifungal therapy with fluconazole or itraconazole. Such cases should be referred to a dermatologist.

Disposition

The patient should be told to avoid water exposure, wear gloves, and avoid manicuring nails as mentioned above. If the patient has not improved in 10 to 14 days in cases of acute paronychia, refer the patient to a dermatologist. Chronic paronychia may take weeks to months to improve; however, lack of response to the above-mentioned treatments or frequent relapses are indications for referral to a dermatologist.

TINEA PEDIS AND TINEA MANUUM

Tinea pedis is a fungal infection of the feet and is often referred to as athlete's foot. Tinea manuum is a dermatophyte infection of the hand. It is often unilateral and associated with tinea pedis. Tinea pedis is very common and usually begins in early adulthood. It is rare in children. Men are more often affected than women. Predisposing factors include hot, humid weather, excessive sweating, and occlusive footwear.

Pathophysiology

Dermatophyte infections result from invasion of the stratum corneum by dermatophytes. *Trichophyton rubrum, Trichophyton mentagrophytes,* and *Epidermophyton floccosum* are the most common organisms causing tinea pedis/manuum. *T. mentagrophytes* is most likely to cause inflammatory bullous tinea pedis. Dermatophyte infections are transmitted from person-to-person or from animal-to-person via fomites or direct contact.

Clinical Features

There are three main types of tinea pedis. The most common type of tinea pedis is the interdigital type. This type manifests as maceration and scale in the web spaces between the toes. Ulceration may even be present in severe cases with secondary bacterial and candidal infection (Fig. 239-2).

The second type, which is seen in tinea manuum as well, presents as chronic, dry scales with little, if any, inflammation on the palmar or plantar surfaces. It often extends to the medial and lateral aspects of the feet but not the dorsal surface. When present on the feet in this distribution, it is often described as a moccasin distribution. Polycyclic or annular patterns may be seen. Maceration between the toes is common. Onychomycosis may be present with numerous, but usually not all, nails having onycholysis (separation of the nail from the nail bed), and thick subungual debris. Oftentimes, if one hand is involved, both feet are involved as well. It is unclear why the other hand is spared in this ''two foot, one hand'' type of fungal infection (Fig. 239-3).

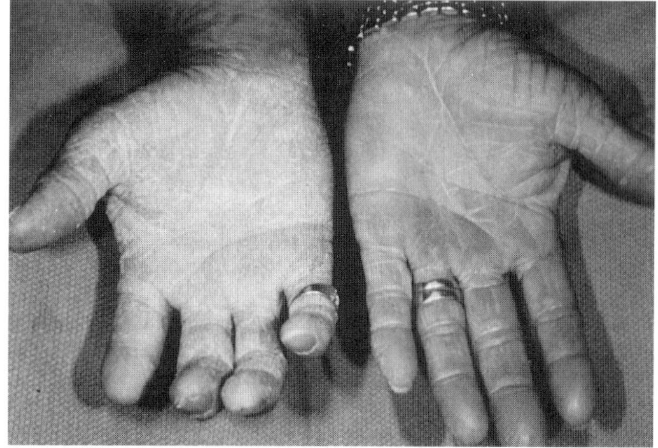

FIG. 239-3. Tinea manuum. The right hand has a markedly scaly palm while the left hand is uninvolved. This presentation is typical of tinea manuum. The feet would likely be involved as well.

The third type of fungal infection presents as an acute, painful, pruritic vesicular eruption on the palms or soles. Erythema is a prominent feature. Toenails and web spaces are usually not involved.

Diagnosis

Diagnosis is based on clinical examination and identification of fungal elements on a potassium hydroxide preparation or with fungal culture. Involvement between the toes and dystrophic toenails support the diagnosis of a fungal infection. Remember, however, that psoriasis, and even chronic hand and foot dermatitis, can involve the web spaces and can cause dystrophic nails.

Although a KOH examination appears to be a simple test, it is often difficult to perform and interpret by inexperienced clinicians. Even in experienced hands, the KOH exam may have a low yield in the noninflammatory type of tinea pedis/manuum. To perform a KOH exam, the area to be scraped (the peripheral scaling margin or vesicle roof) is cleaned with an alcohol swab. With a no. 15 scalpel blade, the scale is scraped onto a glass slide. A coverslip is then placed over the specimen and a drop of 10% potassium hydroxide solution is placed at the edge of the coverslip and allowed to diffuse under the coverslip. The specimen is then heated gently under an alcohol flame to aid in dissolving the keratin of the squamous cells. The specimen is then viewed under 10× magnification. Hyphae appear as light-green, thin strands that cross over cells and have branches (Fig. 239-4).

If a positive KOH exam cannot be obtained, scraping of scale can be sent to the laboratory for KOH exam and fungal culture.

Treatment

If a positive KOH exam is obtained, nonbullous tinea pedis and manuum can be treated with topical antifungal agents. Imidazole antifungal agents such as clotrimazole (Lotrimin and Mycelex), miconazole (Micatin and Monistat), ketoconazole (Nizoral), or econazole (Spectazole) cream should be used twice a day. Treatment should be continued

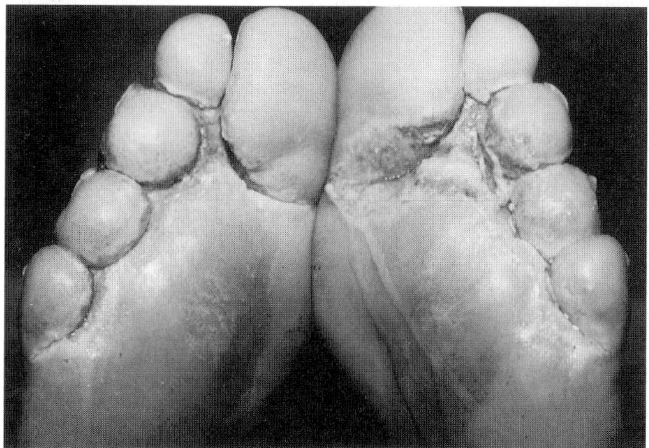

FIG. 239-2. Ulcerative interdigital tinea pedis. Secondary bacterial and/or *candida* infection complicate this case of interdigital tinea pedis. This eruption is quite painful and debilitating.

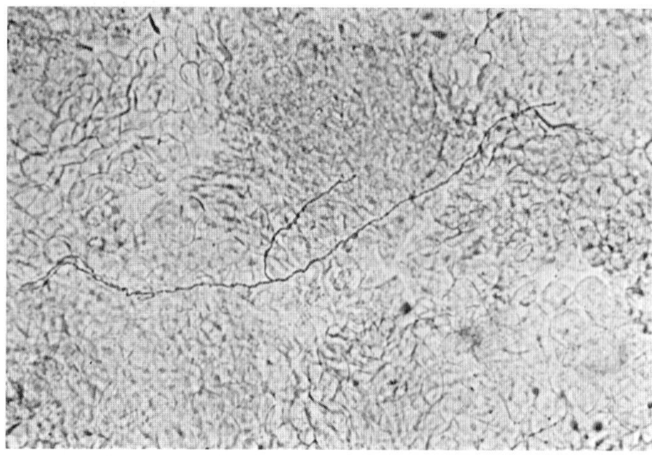

FIG. 239-4. Positive KOH exam. As viewed under 10× magnification, long, thin branching hyphae are seen.

for one week after clearing has occurred. Although econazole cream is more expensive, it is preferred for interdigital tinea pedis as it has antibacterial properties to treat secondary bacterial (often corynebacterium) infection. Topical terbinafine (Lamisil) cream is a fungicidal agent. It is nonprescription and is used once a day. It is currently used in cases that have not responded to other topical agents. Patients should be warned that tinea pedis is often a chronic disease and that recurrences are common. Recurrences or failure to clear with topical medications may warrant treatment with oral agents. Such patients should follow up with a primary care provider or dermatologist.

Furthermore, patients and physicians should be aware that these topical agents do not treat nail infections. Thus, if a patient desires treatment of onychomycosis as well, an oral agent such as itraconazole, fluconazole, or terbinafine is needed. Because onychomycosis does not require emergent attention, such patients should see their primary care provider or dermatologist should they wish to pursue treatment of onychomycosis.

If a positive KOH cannot be obtained, but the clinical examination is highly suspicious for a fungal infection, empiric therapy is not unreasonable. Prior to starting therapy, obtaining scrapings for fungal culture is suggested. As positive KOH exams are difficult to obtain after treatment has started, culture results (whether positive or negative) can help the follow-up physician choose the most appropriate therapy.

Bullous tinea pedis often does not respond to topical treatment. If the patient is experiencing minimal discomfort, a topical agent can be tried initially. In more severe cases, oral antifungal treatment is necessary. Itraconazole 200 mg qd for 14 days or terbinafine 250 mg po for 14 days are effective. The prescribing physician should be familiar with the potential drug interactions and the uncommon but serious side effects (hepatotoxicity and erythema multiforme/toxic epidermal necrolysis) prior to prescribing these medications.

Disposition

In addition to the specific treatment mentioned above, patients should be educated about aggravating or exacerbating factors. Patients should be told to keep their hands and feet as dry as possible. After bathing, web spaces should be thoroughly dried. A hair dryer may be helpful in achieving satisfactory drying. Socks should be changed anytime a patient notes that his or her socks are damp from sweating. Shoes and socks should be removed when possible.

The patient should also be instructed to follow up with a dermatologist if the eruption is not clear in four to six weeks.

HAND AND FOOT DERMATITIS

Hand and foot dermatitis simply means inflammation of the skin of the hands and/or feet. The term is used to encompass several more specific disorders. These include allergic contact dermatitis, irritant contact dermatitis, dyshidrosis, and atopic dermatitis of the hands.

Pathophysiology

As this term relates to several different diagnoses, the pathophysiology is based on the specific disorder. Allergic contact dermatitis is a delayed hypersensitivity reaction to one of many possible allergens. On the hands, allergens may include rhus (poison ivy/poison oak), nickel, chromate, and rubber components of gloves. Some of the more common agents that cause allergic contact dermatitis on the foot are rhus, rubber accelerators found in shoes, dyes in leather and socks, and dichromates used in tanning leather.

Irritant contact dermatitis is an immediate nonimmunological response from chemical damage to the skin. Strong irritants such as acids or phenol may cause severe immediate irritation (''chemical burn''). Weaker irritants including soaps, detergents, friction, and cold, dry air cause a more chronic dermatitis.

The cause of dyshidrosis is unknown. It tends to occur equally in men and women during early to mid-adulthood (ages 20 to 40).

Atopic dermatitis is more often a disease of infancy and childhood; however, persistence into adulthood is possible. Hand or foot involvement is usually not the only cutaneous finding.

Clinical Features

In acute allergic contact dermatitis, erythema with papules, vesicles, and/or bullae is present. It is intensely pruritic and excoriations are noted. Chronic allergic contact dermatitis has less prominent vesiculation and more scale, lichenification, and fissuring. Distribution is the most helpful clue to aid in diagnosis. When the hands or feet are involved in allergic contact dermatitis, the eruption tends to be present on the dorsal surfaces sparing the palms, soles, and web spaces. The thick stratum corneum of the palms and soles prevents penetration of potential allergens. Furthermore, distribution with linear streaks suggests a plant allergy such as rhus hypersensitivity (Fig. 239-5*A*). Sharp demarcation of footwear indicates a reaction to a component of the patient's shoes (Fig. 239-5*B*). An eruption also present behind

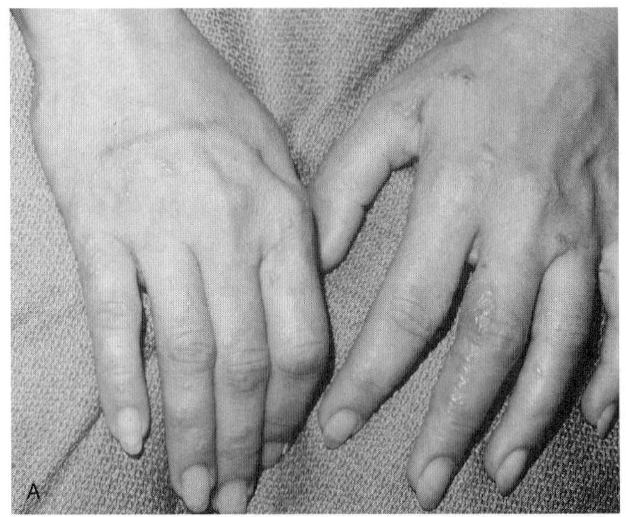

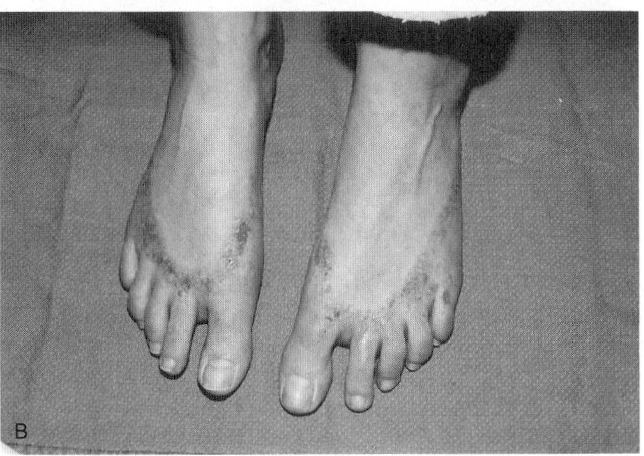

FIG. 239-5. Allergic contact dermatitis. **A.** Allergic contact dermatitis from exposure to poison ivy. Erythema, vesiculation and bullae are present on the fingers and the dorsal surfaces of the hands. Note the linear streak across the right hand. This finding is a diagnostic clue for rhus contact dermatitis (poison ivy). **B.** Allergic contact dermatitis to the straps of sandals. Erythema, scale and excoriations are noted in a symmetric patterned distribution matching to this patient's footwear.

the earlobes, around the neck or at the site of a pant snap suggests a possible nickel allergy.

Irritant dermatitis resulting from a strong irritant like an acid or alkali initially begins as immediate burning in the exposed area. Vesiculation and bullae formation with surrounding erythema follow. In severe reactions, necrosis and ulceration may even be present. These eruptions often occur as a result of accidental exposure. Irritant dermatitis from weaker irritants presents as erythema, scale, and fissuring. Vesiculation is less prominent, and often is not present. Irritant contact dermatitis is a common problem in occupations that require frequent handwashing or water exposure, such as health care workers, bartenders, and housewives.

Dyshidrosis initially begins as very small, deep-seated, pruritic vesicles on the lateral aspects and the volar surfaces of the palms and soles. The dorsal surface of the distal phalanges may also become involved. A key feature separating this disorder from other dermatitides is the lack of erythema at the onset. Over time, the vesicles may form pustules or desquamate to leave small collarettes of scales. In chronic cases, erythema and scales become more prominent and may be difficult to distinguish from other forms of hand and foot dermatitis.

Atopic dermatitis of the hands and feet often presents as erythematous, pruritic scaly patches with prominent involvement of the dorsal surfaces as well as the palms and soles. Chronic atopic dermatitis will also have hyperpigmentation and lichenification and fissuring. Oftentimes, other areas of the body are involved. Common areas of involvement include the antecubital and popliteal fossae, the posterior neck, and the wrists and ankles.

Diagnosis

The diagnosis is made on clinical grounds. Differentiation between the above-mentioned disorders, however, may be extremely difficult or impossible at times. More than one disorder may be present at a time, such as atopic dermatitis complicated by irritant dermatitis. One should try to elicit an occupational or hobby history that may indicate a specific causative agent. A history of an atopic diathesis (atopic dermatitis, allergic asthma, allergic rhinitis) in the patient or other family members should be sought as well. If an allergen is suspected, referral to a dermatologist for skin patch testing can help determine the exact agent responsible. A fungal infection should always be considered in the differential diagnosis. A potassium hydroxide preparation can exclude this possibility. A dermatophytid eruption is another possibility. In this disorder, the hands break out in a dermatitic eruption as a result of a dermatophyte infection of the feet. Checking the patient's feet should be part of the clinical examination. Finally, psoriasis, lichen planus, pityriasis rubra pilaris, keratodermas, and autoimmune bullous diseases should be considered in the differential diagnosis. Rarely is a biopsy indicated, as it cannot differentiate between the different types of dermatitis.

Treatment

If an offending agent is discovered, it should be removed from the patient's environment. All antihistamine, anesthetic, antibiotic, and anti-itch creams should be stopped as they may cause a second allergy. In addition, water, soaps, detergents, and lotions should be avoided, as they may be irritating. The hands or feet should be well protected when performing any potentially irritating activities such as housecleaning, gardening, or hobbies using glues or chemicals. Friction should be avoided as well. Lubrication with products such as Vaseline petroleum jelly, Eucerin cream, or Aquaphor ointment should be used frequently and liberally.

Acute eruptions with vesiculation can be treated with an astringent soak. The most commonly used astringent is aluminum acetate (Burow's solution). One Domeboro's powder packet or tablet is mixed with one pint of water then applied with a towel or gauze to the affected area for 15 to 20 min qid. A high-potency topical corticosteroid such as fluocinonide (Lidex) ointment is then applied two to three times a day. Weaker nonfluorinated topical corticosteroids, such as hydrocortisone 2.5% or desonide, should be used on the face, in skin folds, and on children. Antihistamines are also valuable, especially to relieve nighttime pruritus. Hydroxyzine (Atarax) 25 to 50 mg every 6 hours should be tried initially. In severe cases with debilitating eruptions, systemic glucocorticoids are indicated. In allergic contact dermatitis secondary to rhus, the eruption usually persists for three to four weeks, thus treatment should continue throughout this period to prevent return of the eruption once the prednisone is stopped. Prednisone beginning at 40 to 60 mg with a 2- to 3-week taper is recommended. Relative contraindications to prednisone use include diabetes, hypertension, active peptic ulcer disease, psychiatric disease, and immunodeficiency. If prednisone is prescribed to such patients, close follow-up is necessary.

Chronic eruptions should be treated with high-potency topical corticosteroids two to three times a day. Ointments are preferred as they help with lubrication. Hydroxyzine can provide symptomatic relief from itching. Systemic glucocorticoids should be avoided in chronic cases. Although they may provide temporary relief, rebound disease after cessation of the glucocorticoid is common. Furthermore, patients become overly dependent on this medication and the chronic effects of corticosteroid therapy then become an issue.

Severe irritant contact dermatitis with skin necrosis should be treated in a similar manner as a thermal burn. Debridement, and even skin grafting, may be necessary. Immediate referral to burn specialists or a burn center is warranted.

Disposition

Hospitalization is rarely indicated except in instances of severe chemical burns. Burn specialists (either plastic surgeons or dermatologists) should be consulted and the patient should be treated in a burn center if necessary. If the diagnosis is in question, consultation by a dermatologist should be sought. All acute dermatitis can be treated initially in the emergency department. The patient should be instructed to follow up with a primary care physician or dermatologist if the eruption does not clear in three to four weeks, if systemic glucocorticoids are begun in the emergency department, or if patch testing is necessary. Chronic dermatitis should be seen by a primary care physician or dermatologist in two to three weeks to assess the need for prolonged treatment and to follow for possible complications to topical corticosteroids.

PSORIASIS

The hands and feet are common sites of involvement in psoriasis. Two types of psoriasis are seen. The first is psoriasis vulgaris or plaque-type psoriasis. Often, these patients have disease involvement of other areas especially the elbows, knees, scalp, and gluteal cleft. Sometimes, however, the hands or the feet may be the only involved site. The second type of psoriasis involving the palms and soles is palmoplantar pustulosis. This is a rare form of pustular psoriasis confined to the palms and soles.

Pathophysiology

Psoriasis is an inherited disease in which the principal abnormality is a shortening of the keratinocyte cell cycle resulting in an overproduction of cells 28 times normal. The causes underlying this rapid cell cycle are not clear; however, immunological factors play a complex role in this process.

Clinical Features

In psoriasis vulgaris, erythema, scales, and fissures are seen in discrete plaques on the palms or soles (Fig. 239-6*A*). Extensive disease may

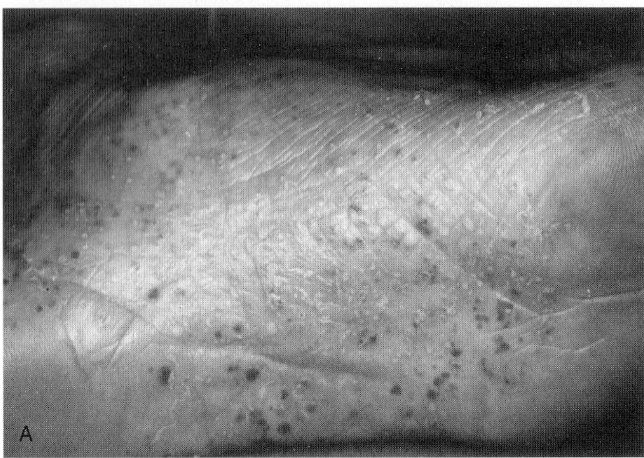

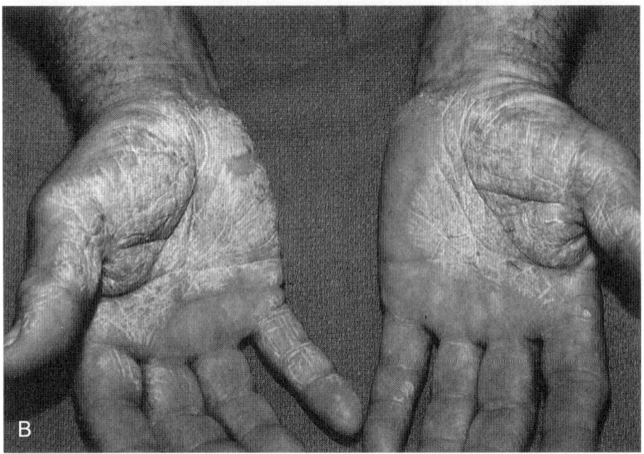

FIG. 239-6. Psoriasis. **A.** In plaque type psoriasis, erythematous plaques with thick scale are present on the palms. Hand dermatitis and lichen simplex chronicus may be difficult to differentiate clinically from this type of psoriasis. **B.** Pustules in various stages of evolution are seen in this typical example of palmoplantar pustulosis.

extend over the entire palms, soles and dorsal surfaces of the hands or feet. Onycholysis (separation of the nail plate from the nail bed), nail pits, and yellow discoloration of the nails help support the diagnosis of psoriasis. Hand and foot dermatitis, lichen simplex chronicus, and Reiter's syndrome should be included in the differential diagnosis.

In pustular psoriasis of the palms and soles, erythema, minimal scale, and numerous sterile pustules are seen. The pustules are in various stages of evolution from small pustules to larger confluent ''lakes of pus'' to crusts to rings of scale (Fig. 239-6*B*). It is most commonly seen bilaterally in the instep of the foot, the thenar, and hypothenar eminences of the hands. The differential diagnosis includes tinea pedis or manuum, *Staphylococcus aureus* infection, herpes simplex infection, and dyshidrosis.

Diagnosis

Complete examination of the skin focusing on the sites commonly affected by psoriasis including the elbows, knees, scalp, lower back, gluteal cleft, and nails may reveal other areas of involvement to aid in diagnosing psoriasis. If no other psoriatic plaques are noted, differentiation from hand and foot dermatitis can be difficult. A biopsy may be helpful in this instance. A KOH examination should be performed to rule out a dermatophyte infection. Bacterial and viral cultures should be obtained when disease is localized to one area.

Treatment

Initial treatment includes the use of topical corticosteroids, tar preparations, and lubrication. A tar solution containing 1 teaspoon of a tar emulsion such as Balnetar or Zetar in a quart of water, should be used to soak the palms and soles for 15 to 20 minutes twice a day. Application of a high- or ultra high-potency topical corticosteroid such as fluocinonide (Lidex) or clobetasol propionate 0.05% (Temovate) or betamethasone dipropionate (Diprolene) 0.05% ointment follows this soak. Liberal use of emollients such as Vaseline petroleum jelly, Aquaphor healing ointment, or Eucerin cream should be encouraged.

Disposition

The above-mentioned treatment should be discussed with the patient. The chronicity of this disease and the slow response to treatment should also be mentioned. Psoriasis of the palms and soles is exceedingly difficult to treat and the patient should be warned that complete clearing is unlikely and treatment is aimed at controlling symptoms. Because of the chronicity of this disorder, follow-up with a dermatologist in four to six weeks is recommended. The patient should be educated about other treatments, such as acitretin (Soriatane), psoralen-ultraviolet light A, or methotrexate, that are available should the above recommendations fail; however, referral to a dermatologist is recommended to commence such treatment. Immediate consultation with a dermatologist is usually not necessary, but follow-up in several days to four weeks is warranted, depending on the degree of involvement and severity of symptoms.

LICHEN SIMPLEX CHRONICUS

Epidemiology

Lichen simplex chronicus (LSC) is an extremely pruritic eruption that can involve any part of the body. Most commonly, the ankles, lower extremities, neck, scrotum, and vulva are involved. In LSC, the inciting event is often unknown. The pruritus is intense, thus leading to scratching. Scratching intensifies the itching, which then perpetuates the scratching.

Clinical Features

LSC presents as a one or several intensely pruritic well-demarcated plaques. As a result of chronic scratching and rubbing, lichenification is the prominent feature. Erythema, hyperpigmentation, and excoriations are also present. Scale is minimal. The ankles, shins, dorsal feet, and hands may be affected.

Diagnosis

The diagnosis is based on history and clinical examination. The differential diagnosis includes a dermatophyte infection (ringworm), nummular eczema, psoriasis, and squamous cell carcinoma. A KOH exam is helpful to rule out a dermatophyte infection. Psoriasis oftentimes involves numerous areas of the body, most commonly the elbows, knees, the lower back, the gluteal cleft, and the scalp. Psoriasis tends to have less pruritus, less lichenification, and more silvery scale. Nummular eczema is characterized by more lesions and less lichenification. If the diagnosis is in question, a skin biopsy is suggested.

Treatment

Interrupting the scratch-itch cycle is the most important aspect of treatment. High potency topical corticosteroids such as fluocinonide (Lidex) ointment should be applied to the plaque two to three times a day. Antihistamines should be used for pruritus and nighttime sedation. Benadryl or Atarax 25 to 100 mg every 6 hours is recommended.

Disposition

The chronicity of the disease and its slow response to treatment should be discussed with the patient. Furthermore, the sedating nature of antihistamines and their avoidance when driving or operating heavy machinery should also be discussed. Follow-up with a primary care provider or a dermatologist should be arranged in four to six weeks, especially if response to treatment has been minimal.

VENOUS STASIS DERMATITIS AND VENOUS LEG ULCERS

Epidemiology

Stasis dermatitis and venous leg ulcers result from chronic venous insufficiency. Stasis dermatitis and venous ulcers are seen in the middle-aged to elderly population. Approximately 80 percent of leg ulcers are venous stasis ulcers resulting from chronic venous insufficiency.

Pathophysiology

Chronic venous insufficiency is the cause of stasis dermatitis and venous leg ulcers. Chronic venous insufficiency is usually due to episodes of phlebitis or varicose veins. This results in poor venous return from the lower extremities leading to increased hydrostatic pressure and lower extremity edema. It is most common on the medial ankle where the inferior perforate connects the superior and deep venous systems and the hydrostatic pressures are the greatest.

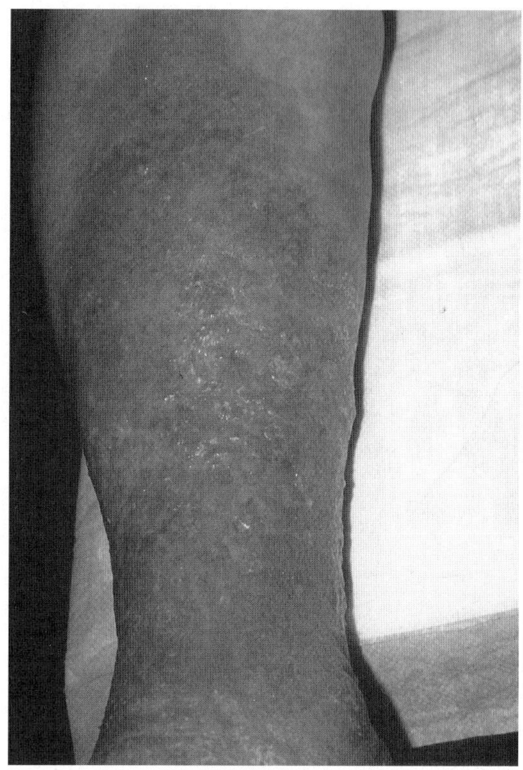

FIG. 239-7 (Plate 22). Stasis dermatitis. Note the surrounding red-brown pigmentation and the central weepy erythema on the pretibial leg.

Clinical Features

Dependent edema, erythema, and orange-brown hyperpigmentation characterize early stasis dermatitis. The medial distal legs and the pretibial leg are the areas most frequently affected. More chronic and severe cases may have bright weepy erythema and even ulceration [Fig. 239-7 (Plate 22)]. Like other dermatitic processes, pruritus is common. Bacterial infection may complicate stasis dermatitis. The presence of honey-colored crust and pustules suggest secondary bacterial infection. Cellulitis and lymphangitis may even be present.

Stasis ulcers often begin within areas of stasis dermatitis. The medial and lateral malleolus and the medial aspect of the calf are the most common sites of involvement. The ulcer often has an aching quality with dependency. The ulcer has a punched out appearance with orange-brown hyperpigmentation at the borders and a moist pink base. Peripheral pulses are usually present.

Diagnosis

Diagnosis of stasis dermatitis is based on the history and physical examination. Other disorders to consider include allergic contact dermatitis (especially to topical preparations used to treat underlying stasis changes), lichen simplex chronicus, and xerotic dermatitis. Especially in association with acute exacerbation, secondary infection with *Staphylococcus aureus* should be excluded with a bacterial culture.

Stasis ulcers are also diagnosed on the basis of a history and physical examination. Bacterial cultures should be obtained if secondary bacterial infection is suspected. The differential diagnosis of leg ulcers is quite long and broad (Table 239-1). If the ulcer does not have the clinical findings mentioned above, other diagnoses should be considered, and appropriate history sought and tests performed. This is particularly important for certain disorders, such as arterial ulcerations, pyoderma gangrenosum, and polyarteritis nodosa, that require immediate attention. For instance, if peripheral pulses are absent and the patient has a history of claudication, vascular blood flow studies should be performed to rule out arterial ulcers. If the patient reports a rapidly developing ulcer that began as a pustule or erythematous nodule and has violaceous overhanging borders, pyoderma gangrenosum should be suspected. If the diagnosis is in question, consultation with a dermatologist is indicated.

Treatment

Attempts should be made to determine and correct the underlying cause of dependent edema. Venous hypertension should be reduced by leg elevation and the use of support stockings. Weeping eruptions should be treated with an astringent compress like Domeboro's solution. A low- to midpotency topical steroid such as fluocinolone acetonide (Synalar) 0.025% cream or hydrocortisone 2.5% cream should be used twice a day. The patient should be told the medication is used to treat the erythema, scale, and pruritus. Hyperpigmentation will not respond to treatment; therefore, the medication should be discontinued when erythema, scale, and pruritus resolve. Oral antihistamines, such as Benadryl or Atarax, should be used for pruritus and for nighttime sedation. Secondary bacterial infection should be treated with cephalexin, dicloxacillin, or ciprofloxacin for 7 to 10 days. Evidence of cellulitis or lymphangitis may require hospitalization for intravenous antibiotics. Topical neomycin, antihistamine creams, and anesthetic creams should be avoided as they may cause allergic contact dermatitis when used in this setting.

Because venous leg ulcers are chronic and slow to heal, emergency department treatment should focus on treating underlying causes of edema, stasis dermatitis, secondarily infected ulcers, cellulitis, or lymphangitis. Follow-up should be arranged with a dermatologist, with a vascular surgeon, or at a leg ulcer clinic for further treatment.

TABLE 239-1 The Differential Diagnosis of Leg Ulcers

Venous stasis
Arteriosclerosis
Diabetes
Hypertensive ischemic ulcer

Embolic
  Cholesterol
  Atheromatous
  Septic

Vasculitis
  Polyarteritis nodosa
  Wegener's granulomatosis

Cryoglobulinemia
Pyoderma gangrenosum
Panniculitis
Sickle cell anemia

Deep fungal infections
  Blastomycosis
  Coccidioidomycosis
  Cryptococcus
  Mycetoma
  Histoplasmosis
  Sporotrichosis

Bactcrial
  Ecthyma
  Ecthyma gangrenosum
  Atypical mycobacterium
  Tuberculosis
  Nocardia
  Tertiary syphilis

Chronic herpes simplex virus
Leishmaniasis
Sarcoidosis
Bites

Burns
  Thermal
  Chemical
  Electrical

Factitial
Traumatic
Pressure

Neoplasia
  Basal cell carcinoma
  Squamous cell carcinoma
  Malignant melanoma
  Cutaneous T-cell lymphoma
  Leukemia cutis
  Cutaneous metastases

ERYTHEMA NODOSUM

Epidemiology

Erythema nodosum is an inflammatory eruption of the subcutaneous fat. It has numerous possible etiologies. As a result, all age groups can be affected [Fig. 239-8 (Plate 23)].

Pathophysiology

Erythema nodosum is classified as a panniculitis–inflammation of the subcutaneous fat. Table 239-2 lists many of the potential causes of erythema nodosum. In about 40 percent of cases, the etiology remains unknown.

Clinical Features

Tender, warm, ill-defined erythematous nodules characterize erythema nodosum. It is most commonly seen on the pretibial area of the lower extremities. The upper extremities and trunk can occasionally be involved. Numerous lesions are usually present. Ulceration is not a feature of erythema nodosum and suggests the possibility of another type of panniculitis.

Diagnosis

Clinical exam is characteristic of a panniculitis. Individual lesions may be mistaken for bacterial cellulitis; however, the nodular component supports the diagnosis of erythema nodosum. If a presumed bacterial cellulitis has no obvious portal of bacterial entry, erythema nodosum should be considered in the differential diagnosis. If the diagnosis

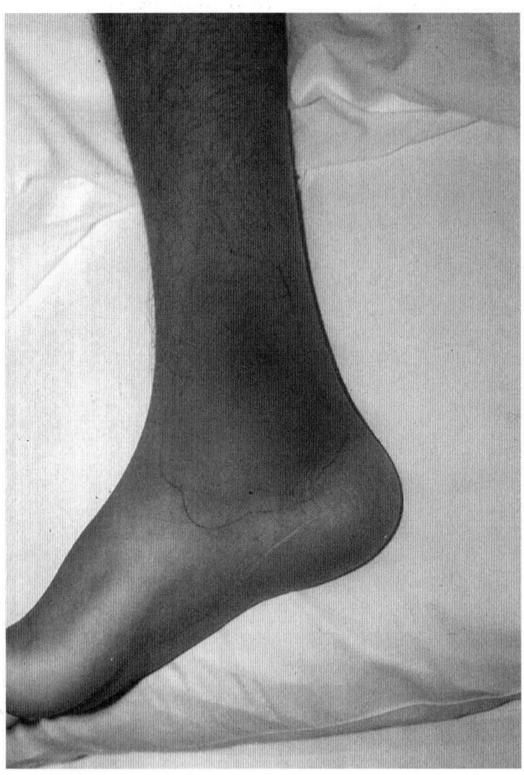

FIG. 239-8 (Plate 23). Erythema nodosum. An erythematous indurated nodule is seen. This patient's disease was initially diagnosed as cellulitis. However, after no response to antibiotics, a biopsy confirmed the diagnosis of erythema nodosum. Most patients with erythema nodosum will have multiple lesions.

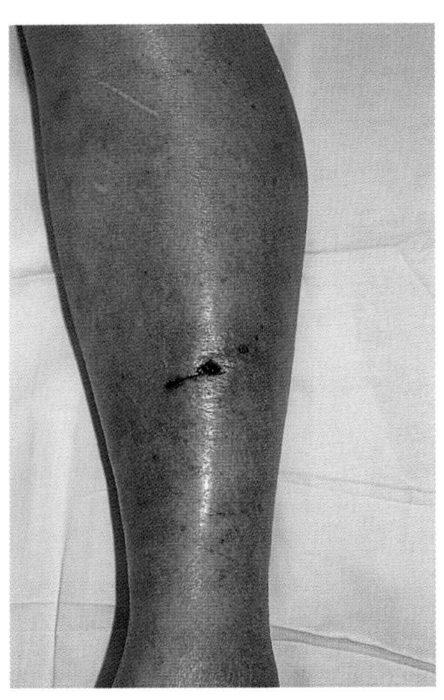

PLATE 1 (FIG. 42-1A). This patient's leg was punctured by a wooden stake 2 days prior to presentation. Surrounding cellulitis and

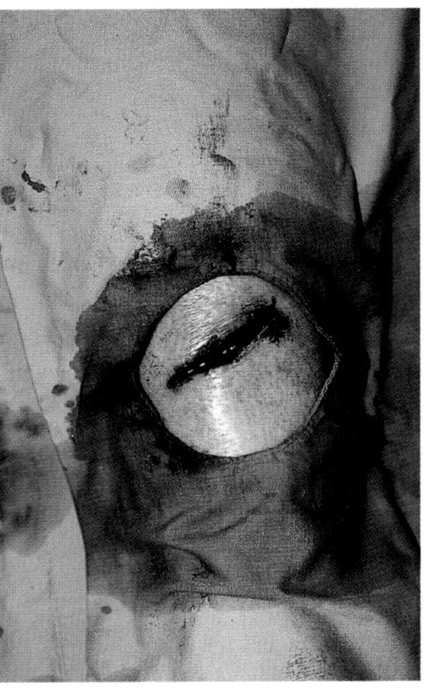

PLATE 2 (FIG. 42-1B) point tenderness lateral to the wound increased the probability of a retained foreign body.

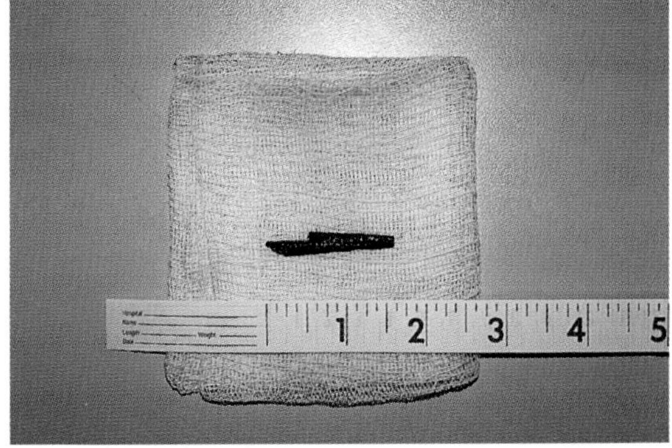

PLATE 3 (FIG. 42-1C). The entrance to the wound was extended, and 1.5-cm piece of wood was removed from a 3.5-cm-deep wound.

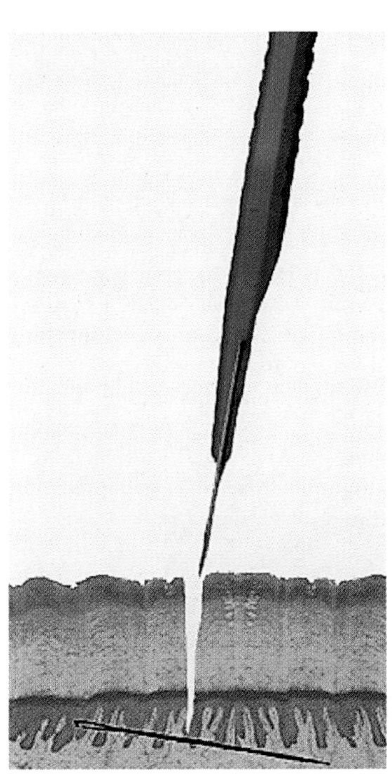

PLATE 4 (FIG. 42-2A). An incision is made perpendicular to the needle at its midpoint. The needle is grasped through the incision with a hemostat and backed out of the puncture wound. The entrance site is enlarged with a skin incision. If the incision passes to the side of the object, the skin is undermined.

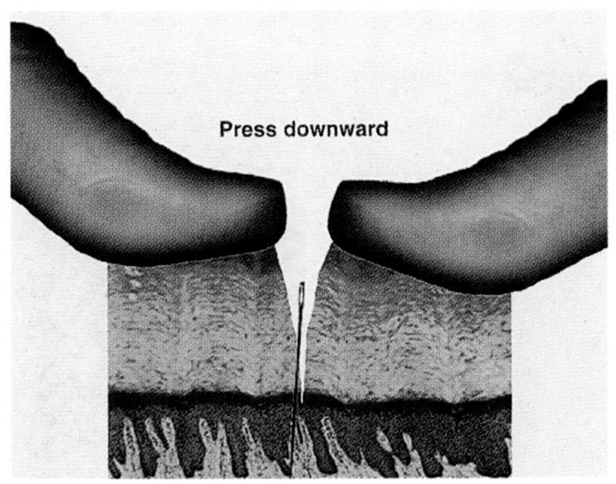

PLATE 5 (FIG. 42-3C). Pressure on the skin edges displaces the foreign body into the center of the wound.

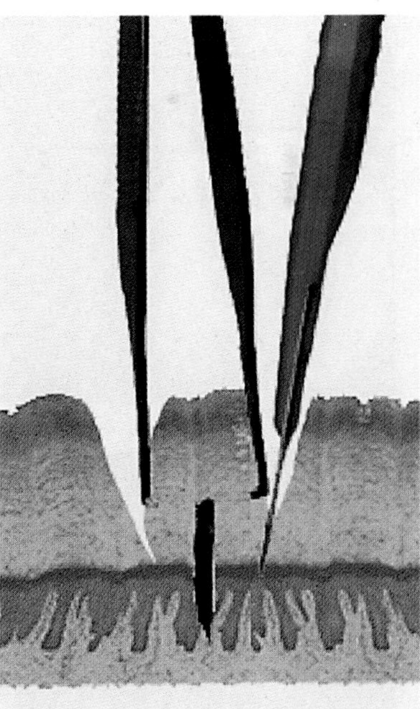

PLATE 6 (FIG. 42-5B). Block excision is effective for foreign bodies that are friable, difficult to find, buried in fatty tissue, or stain surrounding tissue. A small, elliptical incision is made around the original wound. The incision is undercut until contact is made with the foreign body. The block of tissue is grasped with a forceps, the foreign body is clamped with a hemostat, and both are removed.

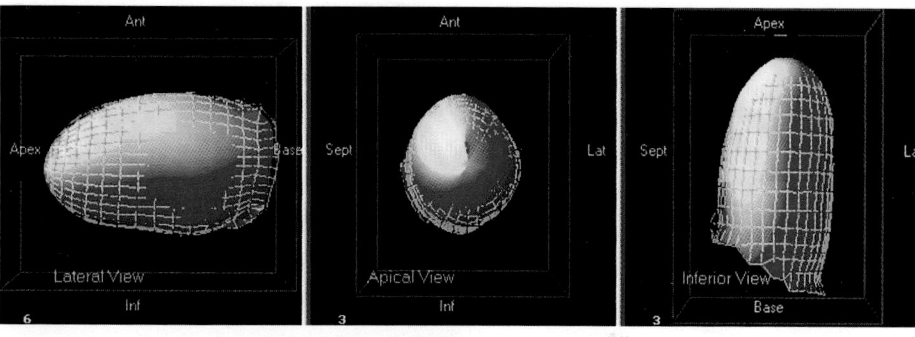

PLATE 7 (FIG. 57-7). Three-dimensional representation of gated SPECT data at end diastole.

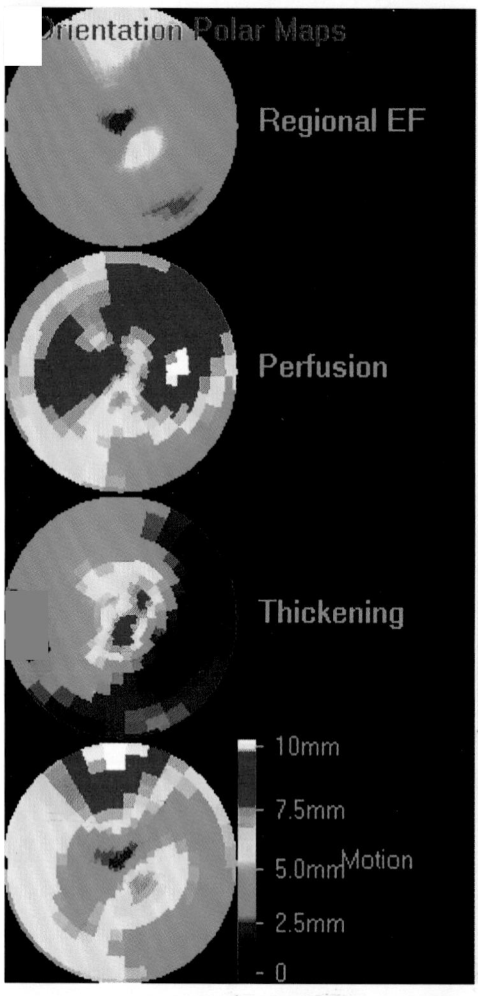

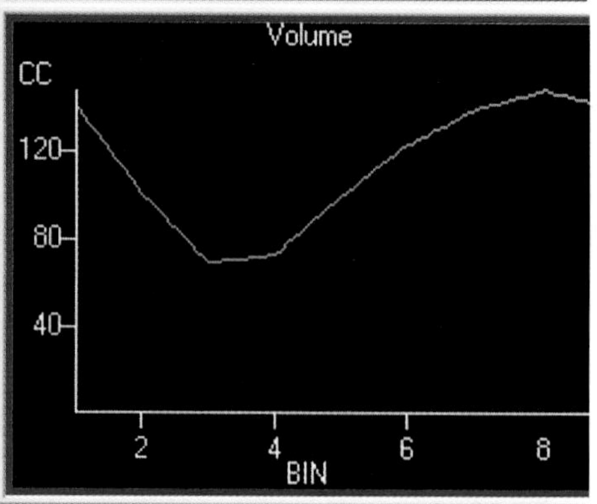

PLATE 8 (FIG. 57-8). Bull's-eye representation of gated SPECT data. Hypoperfusion of the proximal inferolateral wall as well as mild hypokinesis and diminished wall thickening. There is preserved global left ventricular function.

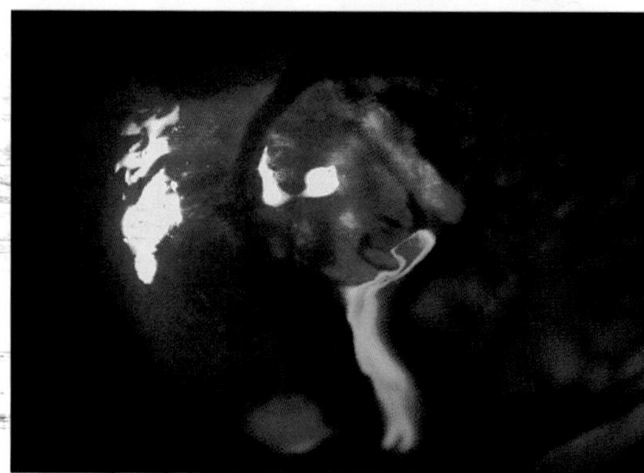

PLATE 9 (FIG. 230-7). Positive Seidel test showing aqueous leaking through a full-thickness corneal wound. Aqueous will turn fluorescein lime-green under a cobalt-blue light as it oozes through the wound while being observed at the slit lamp.

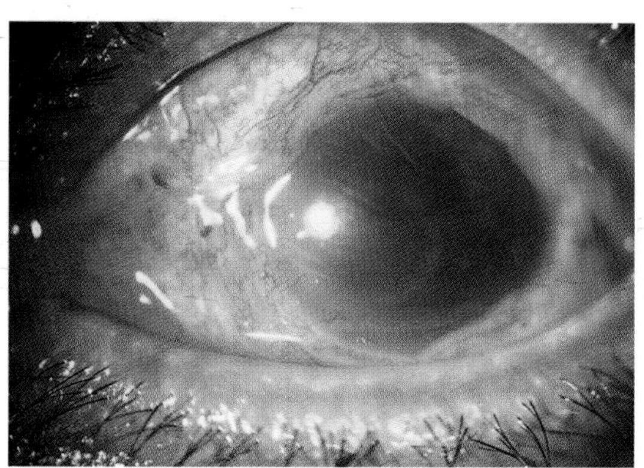

PLATE 10 (FIG. 230-8). Hyphema secondary to blunt trauma. Note the blood filling the lower half of the anterior chamber and hazy appearance of cornea suggesting increased IOP.

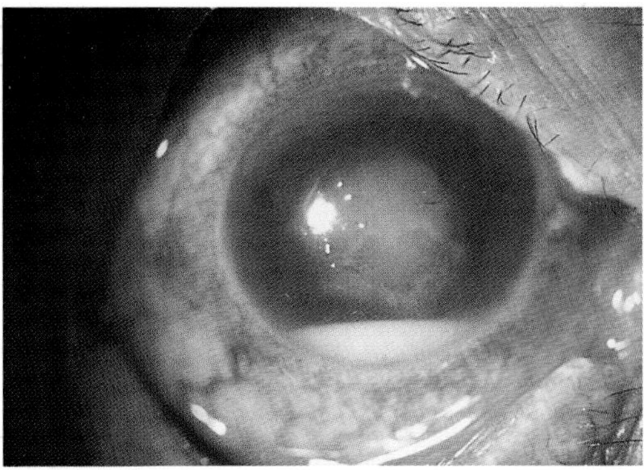

PLATE 11 (FIG. 230-9). Corneal ulcer with hypopyon. The ulcer is seen as a shaggy white corneal infiltrate surrounding the borders of the epithelial defect. The hypopyon represents the accumulation of white cells layering out in the lower one-sixth of the anterior chamber.

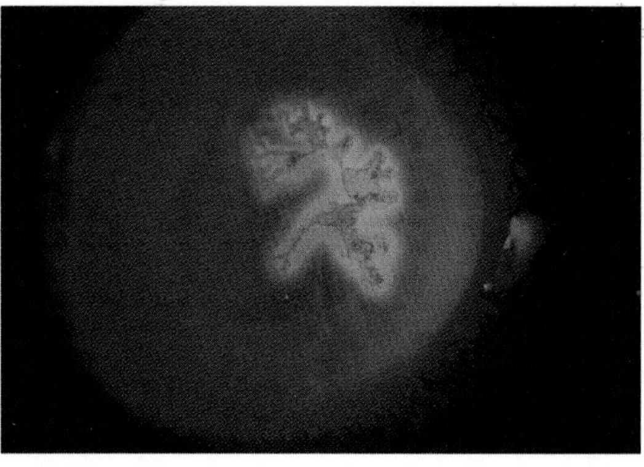

PLATE 12 (FIG. 230-10). Herpes simplex corneal dendrite seen with fluorescein staining and cobalt-blue light.

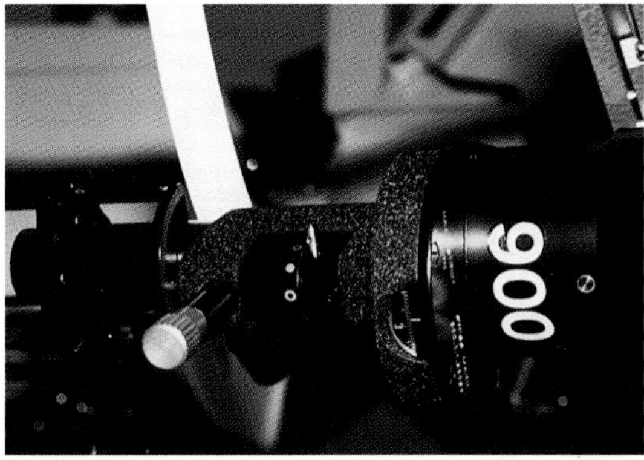

PLATE 13 (FIG. 230-11). Slit-lamp measuring wheel. The length of the light beam on the cornea can be varied and the reading on the dial represents the length in millimeters. Useful in measuring corneal abrasion dimensions.

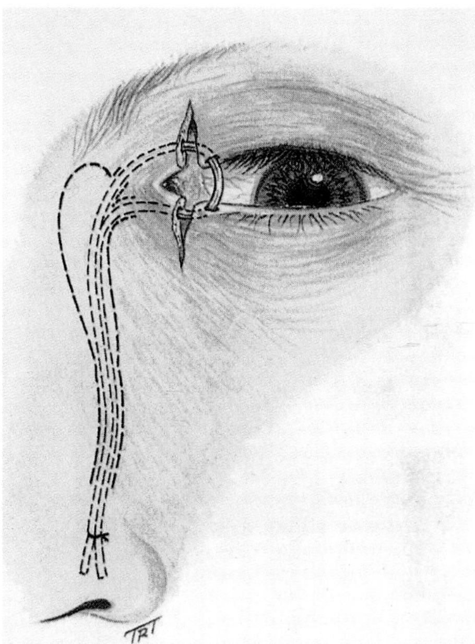

PLATE 14 (FIG. 230-13). Traumatic canalicular laceration repair requires microsurgical stenting to reestablish patency.

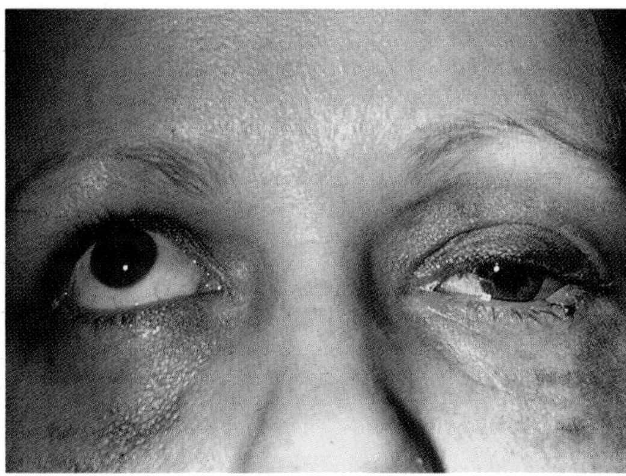

PLATE 15 (FIG. 230-14). Inferior wall blowout fracture of the left eye with entrapment of the inferior rectus muscle. The patient's left eye is unable to look upward, causing diplopia on upgaze.

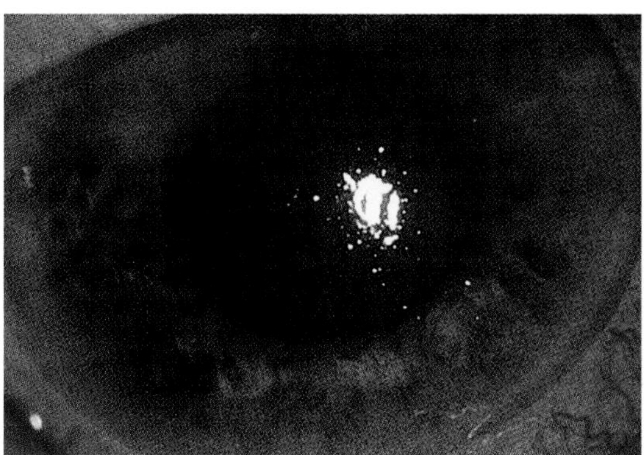

PLATE 16 (FIG. 230-16). Acute angle-closure glaucoma. Pupil is middilated and nonreactive. The cornea is hazy due to stromal edema.

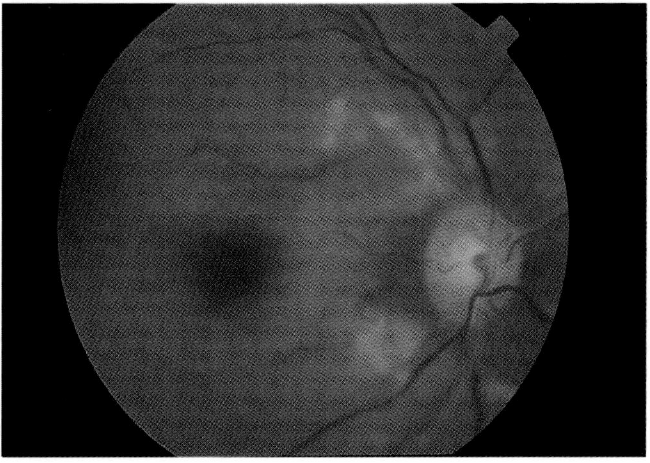

PLATE 17 (FIG. 230-17). Central retinal artery occlusion. Note macular "cherry-red spot" and retinal pallor between macula and disk. The retinal veins appear normal size, but the arteries are barely visible and attenuated.

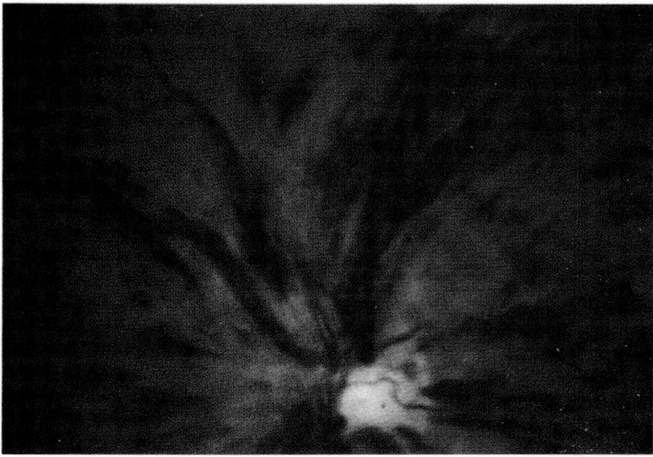

PLATE 18 (FIG. 230-18). Central retinal vein occlusion "blood and thunder fundus." Note diffuse retinal hemorrhages in all retina quadrants and blurred disk margins.

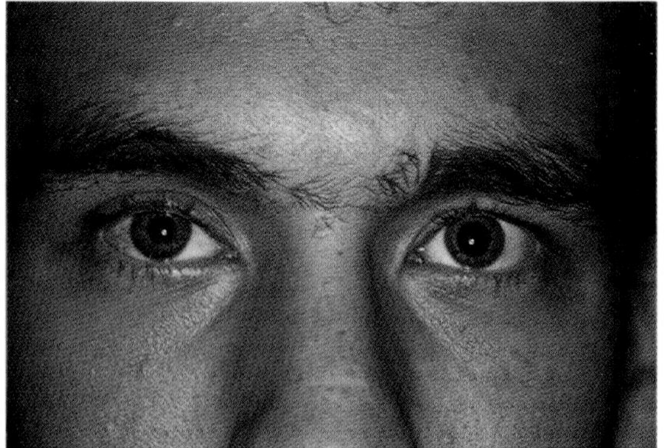

PLATE 19 (FIG. 230-20). Horner's syndrome. Note ptosis and miosis of the right eye. This patient sustained an acute right carotid artery dissection after being hit in the neck with a football.

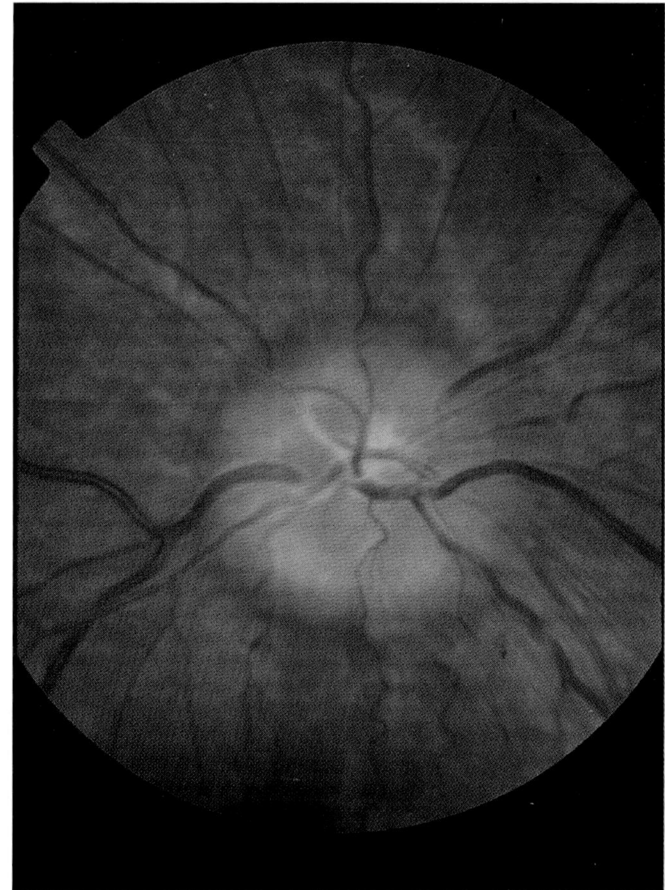

PLATE 20 (FIG. 230-22). Optic nerve head edema. Vascular congestion, elevation of the nerve head, and blurred disk margins are characteristically seen in papilledema, papillitis, and compressive lesions of the optic nerve.

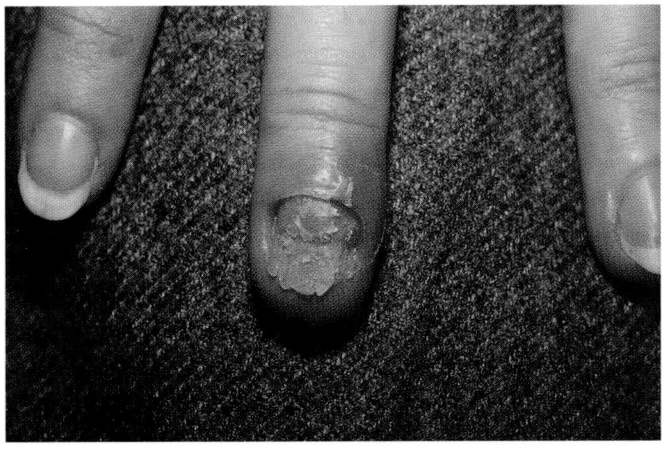

PLATE 21 (FIG. 239-1). Chronic *candida paronychia*. The cuticle is absent. Erythema and edema are prominent at the proximal and lateral nail folds. The dystrophic ridged nail is a sign of chronic disease.

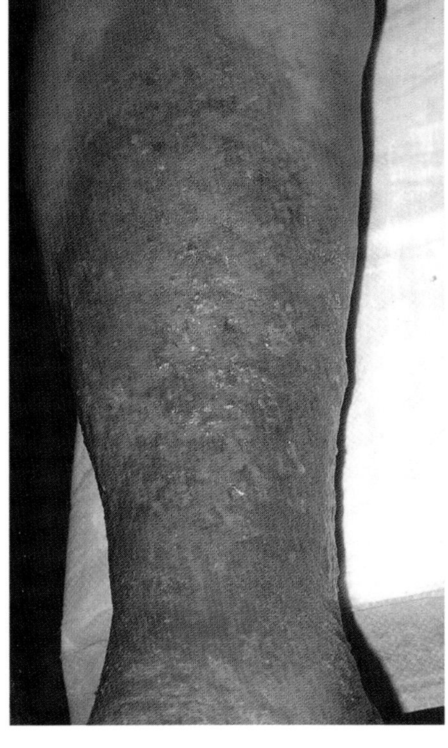

PLATE 22 (FIG. 239-7). Stasis dermatitis. Note the surrounding red-brown pigmentation, the central weepy erythema on the pretibial leg.

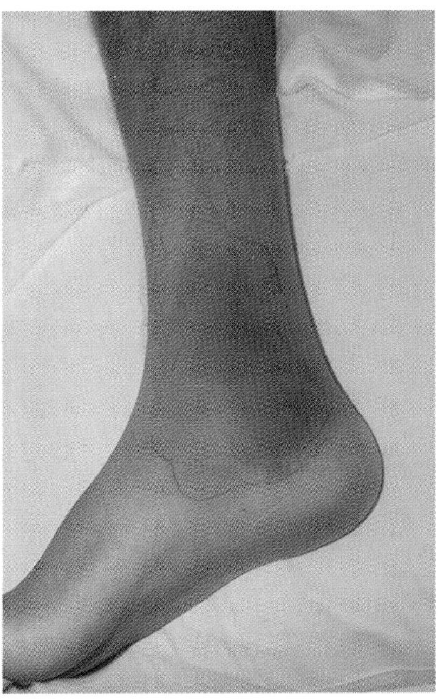

PLATE 23 (FIG. 239-8). Erythema nodosum. An erythematous indurated nodule is seen. This patient's disease was initially diagnosed as cellulitis. However, after no response to antibiotics, a biopsy confirmed the diagnosis of erythema nodosum. Most patients with erythema nodosum will have multiple lesions.

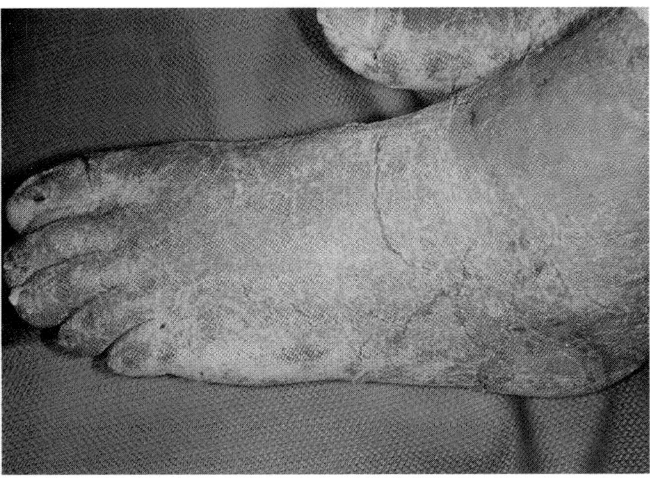

PLATE 24 (FIG. 239-9). Norwegian scabies. The thick scale, erythema, and exudate resemble a foot dermatitis. This disorder should not be forgotten when presented with a patient with extremely pruritic scaly eruption. Norwegian scabies is more common in immunocompromised and debilitated patients.

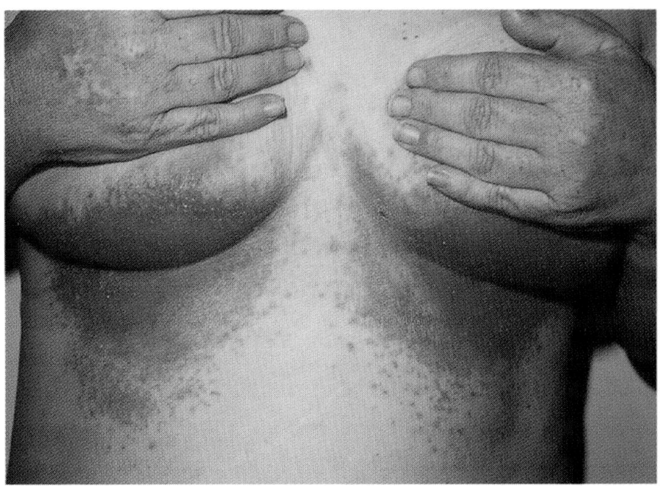

PLATE 25 (FIG. 240-2). Candida intertrigo. Note the bright-red erythema, erosions, and satellite papules and pustules in this striking example of inframammary candida intertrigo. A KOH examination will confirm the diagnosis.

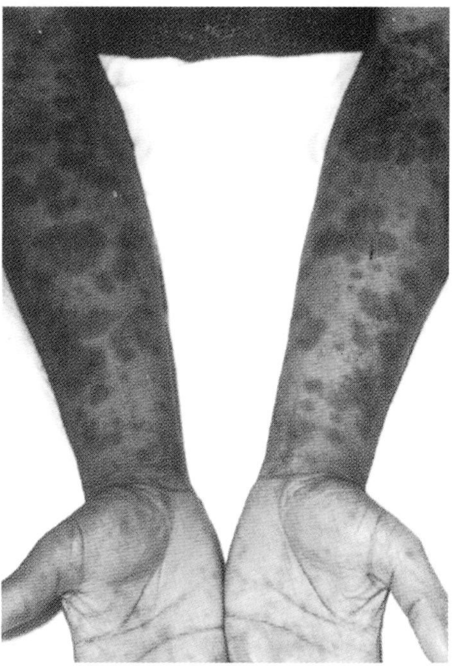

PLATE 26 (FIG. 241-1A). Erythema multiforme: Symmetrical, plaque-like lesions involving the flexor surface of the upper extremities—lesions which may be misdiagnosed as the IgG-mediated urticarial allergic reaction. Also note the erythematous macules on the palms. (Reprinted with permission from Brady W, DeBehnke D, Crosby D: Dermatologic emergencies. *Am J Emerg Med* 12:217, 1994.)

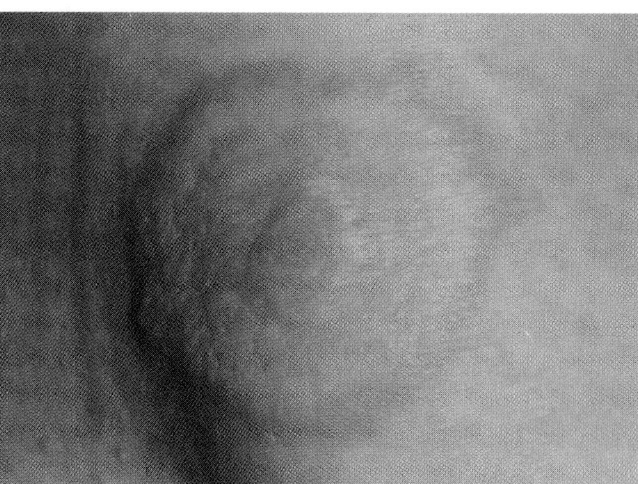

PLATE 27 (FIG. 241-1B). Iris or target lesion, a finding strongly suggestive of EM. This iris lesion is composed of a central bullous lesion with dusky, edematous center and erythematous halo. (Reprinted with permission from Brady W, DeBehnke D, Crosby D: Dermatologic emergencies. *Am J Emerg Med* 12:217, 1994.)

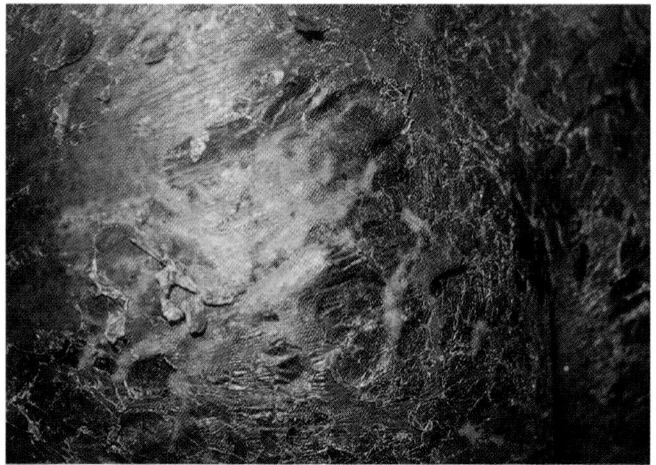

PLATE 28 (FIG. 241-2). Exfoliative dermatitis—generalized, warm erythema accompanied by scaling or flaking.

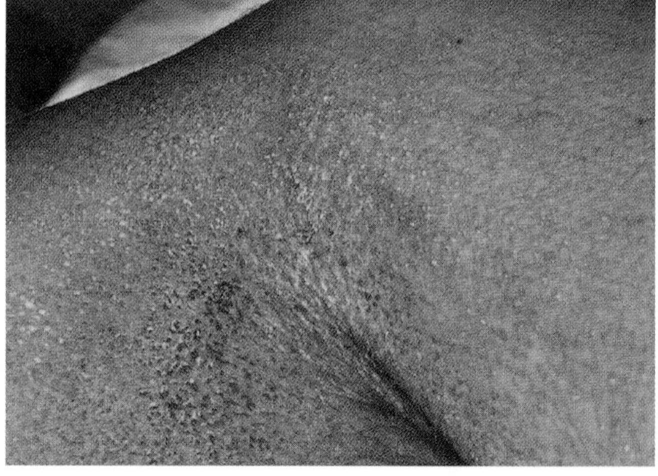

PLATE 29 (FIG. 241-3). Blanching, nonpruritic erythroderma with a ''rough'' texture in a patient with toxic shock syndrome. (Reprinted with permission from Brady W, DeBehnke D, Crosby D: Dermatologic emergencies. *Am J Emerg Med* 12:217, 1994.)

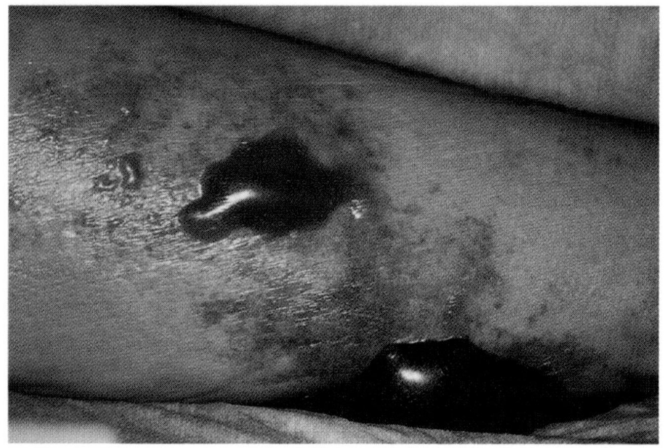

PLATE 30 (FIG. 241-4). Large bullous lesions on the lower extremity in a patient with streptococcal toxic shock.

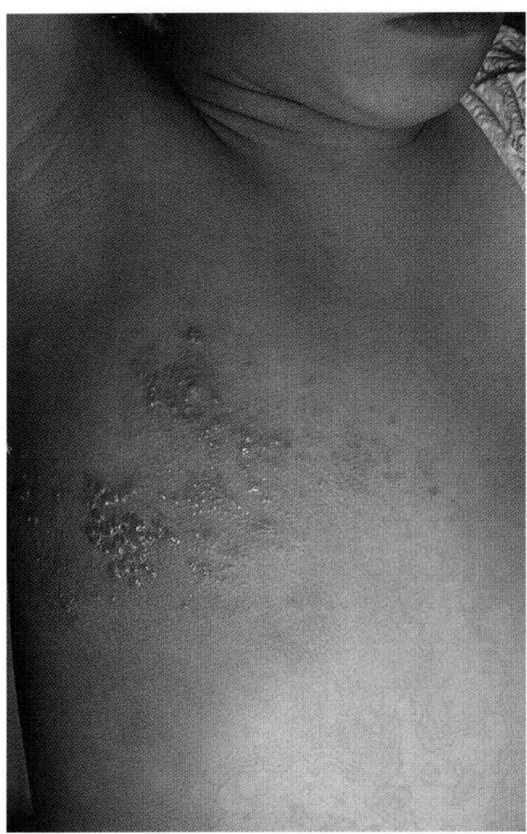

PLATE 31 (FIG. 241-5). A single dermatomal involvement in a patient with herpes zoster infection in a thoracic distribution.

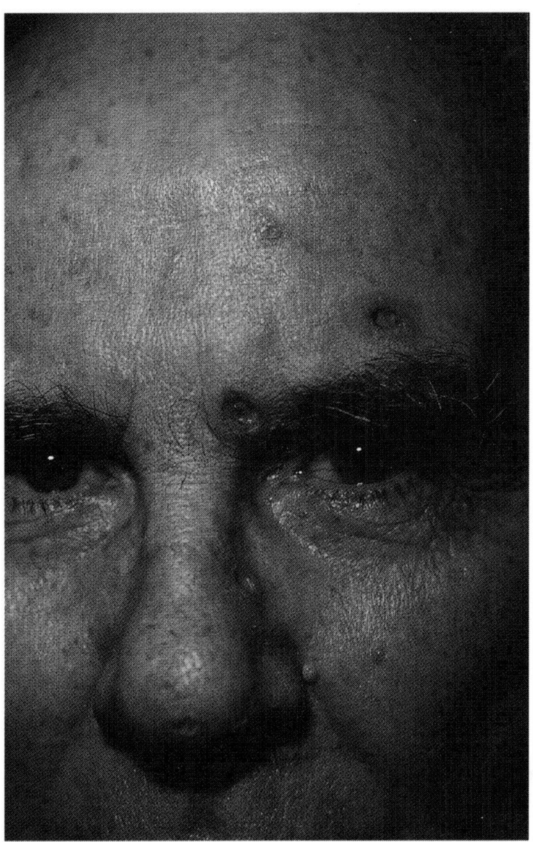

PLATE 32 (FIG. 241-6). Herpes zoster ophthalmic infection: Facial zoster involving the ophthalmic branch of the fifth cranial nerve with nasal lesions strongly suggestive of corneal infection.

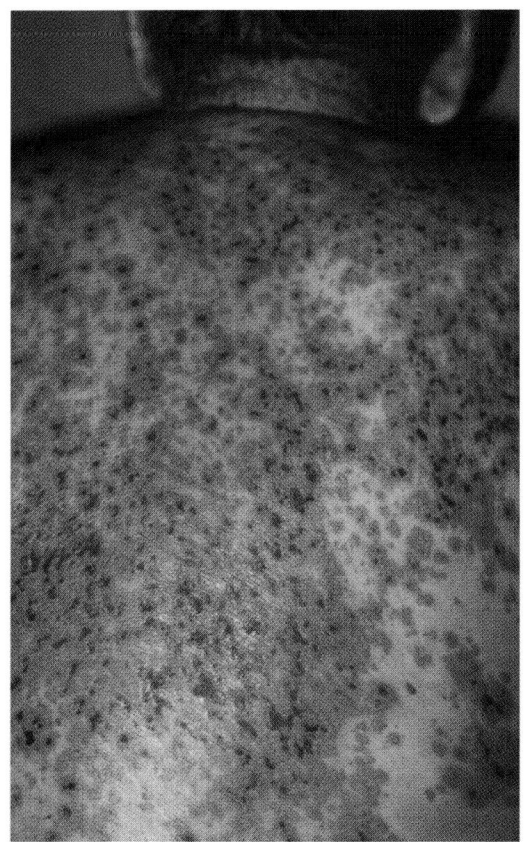

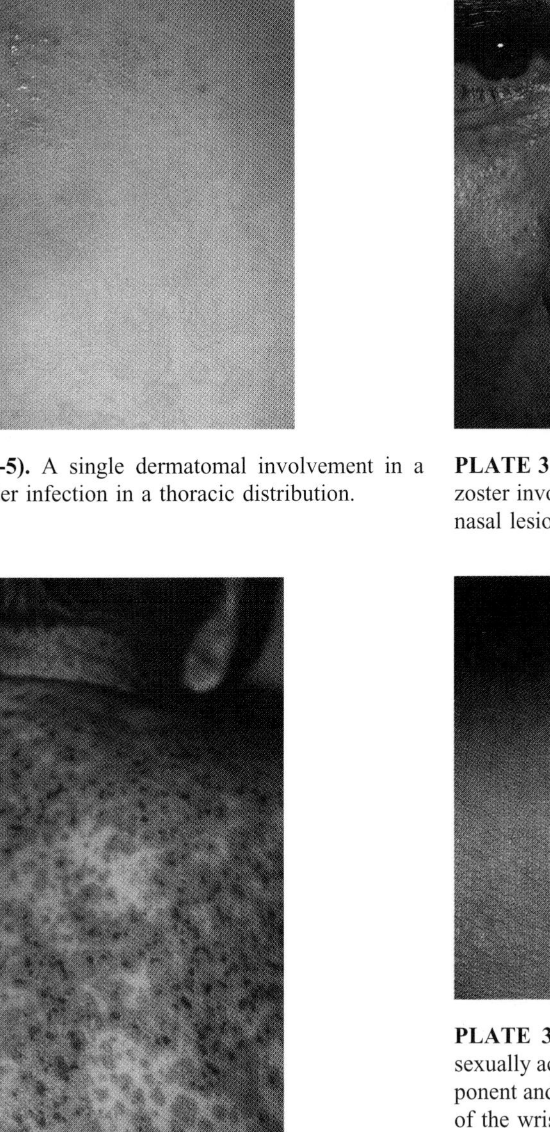

PLATE 33 (FIG. 241-7). Disseminated HSV infection in an immunocompromised adult patient; note the widespread distribution of vesicular lesions on an erythematous base.

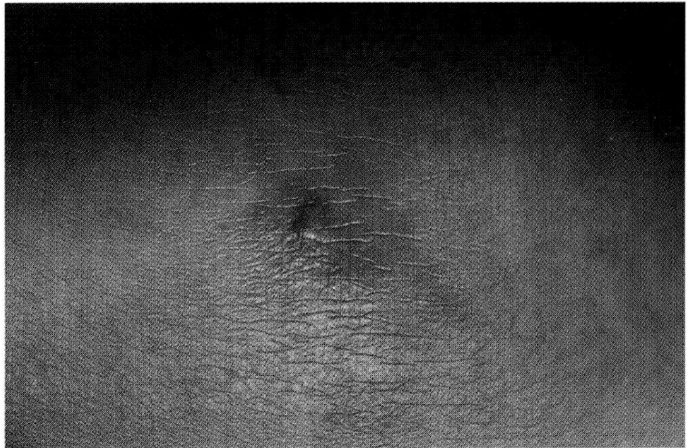

PLATE 34 (FIG. 241-8). Disseminated gonococcal infection in a sexually active adult female; note maculopapule with a petechial component and an erythematous periphery located on the extensor surface of the wrist.

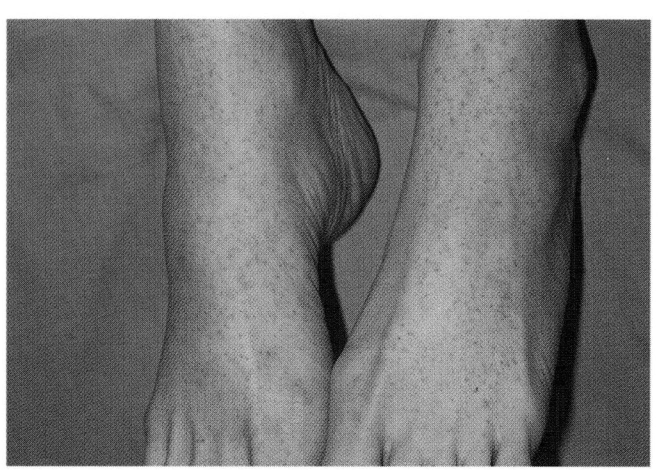

PLATE 35 (FIG. 241-9). A patient with Rocky Mountain spotted fever revealing petechiae on the ankles.

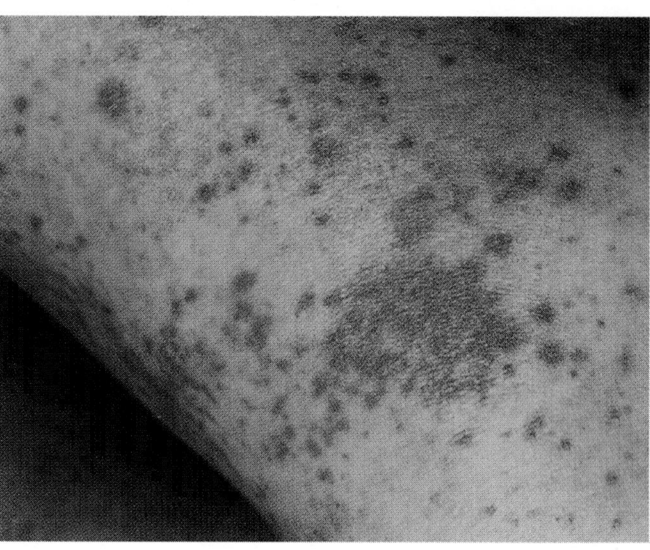

PLATE 36 (FIG. 241-10). Early findings of meningococcemia with petechiae evolving into purpuric lesions. (Reprinted with permission from Brady W, DeBehnke D, Crosby D: Dermatologic emergencies. *Am J Emerg Med* 12:217, 1994.)

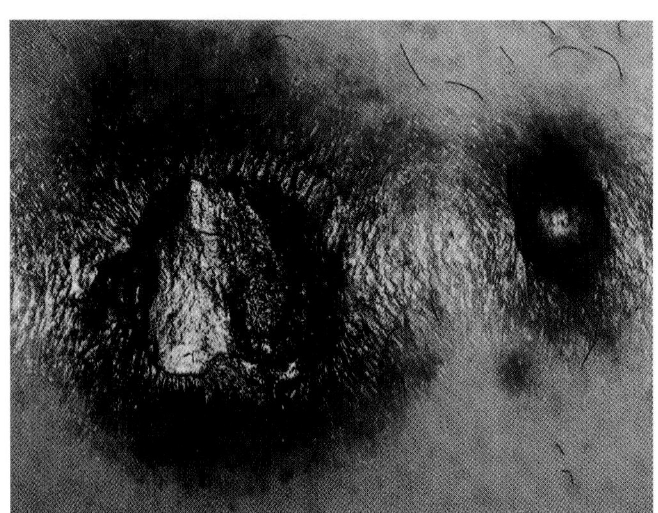

PLATE 37 (FIG. 241-11). Purpura fulminans with hemorrhagic bullae. (Reprinted with permission from Tangoren IA et al: Ecchymoses and epidermal necrosis in a 75-year-old man with bacteremia. *J Crit Illness* 13:108, 1998.)

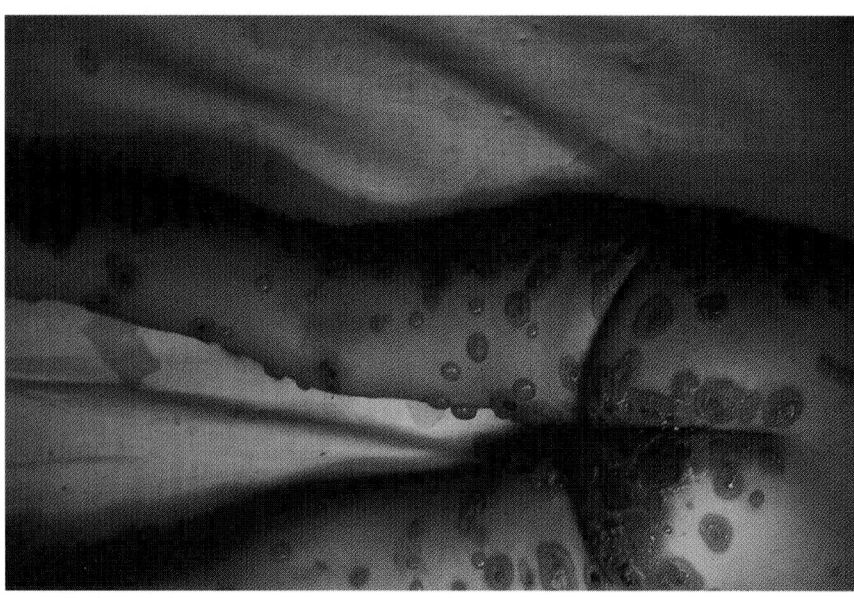

PLATE 38 (FIG. 241-12). Scattered bullous lesions intermixed with erosions and painful inflammatory plaques.

TABLE 239-2 The Causes of Erythema Nodosum

Infectious
- Fungal
  - Blastomycosis
  - Coccidioidomycosis
  - Histoplasmosis
  - Dermatophyte
- Bacterial
  - Streptococcal infections
  - Campylobacter
  - *Yersinia sp.*
  - Tuberculosis
  - Leprosy
- Parasitic
  - Leishmaniasis
  - Toxoplasmosis
- Viral
  - Herpes simplex
  - Infectious mononucleosis

Pharmacological
- Sulfonamides
- Oral contraceptive pills
- Penicillin
- Bromides
- Vaccines

Sarcoidosis

Inflammatory bowel disease

Pregnancy

Behcet's syndrome

Leukemia and lymphoma

Idiopathic

is unclear, a deep punch biopsy or an incisional biopsy including subcutaneous fat is indicated. After the diagnosis of erythema nodosum is established, one must search for possible etiologies. Work-up includes a thorough history and physical examination. Further evaluation, as directed by history and physical findings, may include a throat culture, a stool culture, a complete blood count, a chest radiograph to rule out sarcoidosis, and placement of a PPD.

Treatment

Therapy focuses on treatment of the underlying cause. If such a cause is not clearly established, symptomatic relief can be obtained with bedrest, leg elevation, and nonsteroidal anti-inflammatory agents. These measures can be instituted in the emergency department until the patient can be seen by dermatologist. Other treatments, including oral potassium iodide (SSKI) and systemic corticosteroids, may be required; however, they should not be started until the etiology is established.

PYOGENIC GRANULOMA

Epidemiology

Pyogenic granulomas most commonly occur in children and young adults. Pyogenic granuloma is also more common in pregnant women in whom it is referred to as granuloma gravidarum.

Pathophysiology

A pyogenic granuloma is a benign proliferation of immature capillaries occurring at the site of minor skin trauma. The name is a misnomer as it is neither an infection nor a granuloma.

Clinical Features

A pyogenic granuloma initially presents as a bright red, shiny papule with a thin collarette of hyperkeratosis. It may be ulcerated and tends to bleed profusely with minor injury. Later, the lesion reepithelializes and becomes a dull red to purple color. Although these lesions can occur anywhere on the body, the extremities, especially the hands, are the most common sites of involvement. The differential diagnosis includes amelanotic melanoma, squamous cell carcinoma, bacillary angiomatosis, and cutaneous metastasis.

Diagnosis

The diagnosis is often suspected on clinical grounds; however, a biopsy of the lesion should be performed to confirm the diagnosis and to rule out the above-mentioned disorders, especially an amelanotic melanoma. These two disorders can be indistinguishable by clinical examination alone.

Treatment

Referral to a dermatologist for biopsy is indicated. If the lesion is bleeding profusely in the acute setting, hemostasis can be obtained with pressure and electrocautery. Destruction of the lesion, excision, or a shave biopsy followed by electrodesiccation and curettage are the treatments of choice. These lesions will rarely resolve completely without treatment.

OTHER DISORDERS AFFECTING THE HANDS AND FEET

Several other generalized skin disorders have classic clinical findings on the palms and soles. These disorders are discussed in more detail in Chap. 241; however, they are mentioned briefly here so as to be reminded of these disorders when a patient presents with a complaint in one of these body regions.

Erythema multiforme has characteristic findings on the palms and soles. These lesions are erythematous macules with a violaceous, dusky or bullous center. They are commonly referred to as target or iris lesions. Discovering such lesions should incite a search for similar lesions on the rest of the body, hemorrhagic erosions on the mucosal surfaces, and conjunctival hemorrhage in the eyes.

Secondary syphilis also has characteristic palm and sole lesions. These lesions are red-brown to brown macules on the palms and soles. Although patients with darker pigmented skin may have several hyperpigmented macules as a normal finding, recent onset or failure of the patient to recall such lesions should increase the clinician's suspicion of secondary syphilis. These lesions are often asymptomatic and may be the only indication of secondary syphilis. A high index of suspicion is necessary, and appropriate further clinical examination and serology should be carried out.

Rocky Mountain spotted fever may also present initially with palm or sole lesions. These appear as blanching erythematous macules that later become nonblanching petechial lesions. These lesions start distally and spread proximally.

Kawasaki disease, scarlet fever, and toxic shock syndrome may all have palmar erythema as a prominent feature. The palms and soles will desquamate as these diseases progress.

Furthermore, when considering pruritic eruptions of the extremities, one must always think about scabies. The hands, feet, and elbows

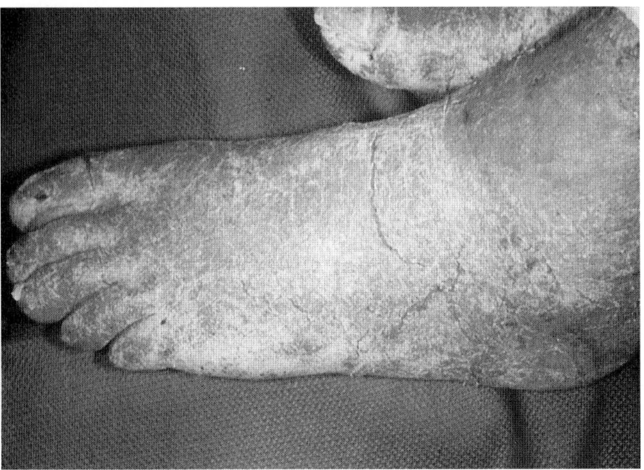

FIG. 239-9 (Plate 24). Norwegian scabies. The thick scale, erythema, and exudate resemble a foot dermatitis. This disorder should not be forgotten when presented with a patient with extremely pruritic scaly eruption. Norwegian scabies is more common in immunocompromised and debilitated patients.

along with the groin are the most common areas of involvement. Diagnostic burrows will most likely be found in the hyperkeratotic skin of the palms and soles particularly along the web spaces and the wrist. When the scabetic mite burden becomes quite high, Norwegian scabies results. Thick hyperkeratosis resembling dermatitis results [Fig. 239-9 (Plate 24)]. See Chap. 242 for further discussion.

Finally, all the major types of skin cancer including malignant melanoma, squamous cell carcinoma, and basal cell carcinoma can occur on the extremities.

BIBLIOGRAPHY

Omura EF, Rye B: Dermatologic disorders of the foot. *Clin Sports Med* 13(4):825, 1994.

Hochman LG: Paronychia: More than just an abscess. *Int J Dermatol* 34(6):385, 1995.

Epstein E: Hand dermatitis: Practical management and current concepts. *J Am Acad Dermatol* 10:395, 1984.

Epstein E, Maibach HI: Palms and soles, in Roenigk HH, Maibach HI (eds): *Psoriasis,* 2d ed. New York, Marcel Dekker, 1990, p 121.

Katz HI: Systemic antifungal agents used to treat onychomycosis. *J Am Acad Dermatol* 38:S48, 1998.

Ryan TJ, Burnand K: Diseases of the veins and arteries—Leg ulcers, in Champion, et al (eds): *Rook/Wilkinson/Ebling Textbook of Dermatology,* 5th ed. Oxford, Blackwell Scientific, 1992, pp 1963-2013.

Bondi EE, Lazarus GS: Panniculitis, in Fitzpatrick TB, et al (eds): *Dermatology in General Medicine,* 4th ed. New York, McGraw-Hill, 1993, pp 1392-1345.

240 DISORDERS OF THE GROIN AND SKIN FOLDS

Lisa May

When discussing the skin folds of the body, one is referring to the groin, intergluteal cleft, axilla, inframammary folds, and pannus folds. The skin folds have unique characteristics that set them apart from other regions of the body. For one, these areas are almost continuously occluded. As a result, scale does not develop; maceration and fissuring develop instead. This alters the appearance of papulosquamous diseases and inflammatory processes in this region. The occlusion also allows for the development of a warm, moist environment favorable to the growth of fungi, yeast, and bacteria. Finally, the skin folds—in particular, the groin, intergluteal cleft, and the axilla—are the major sites in the body of apocrine glands. Thus, certain disease processes of these structures such as hidradenitis suppurativa occur predominantly in this area. Although many skin diseases can affect the skin folds to some degree, this chapter focuses on common disorders where skin fold eruptions are the main cutaneous finding.

TINEA CRURIS

Tinea cruris is a fungal infection of the groin commonly called jock itch. Tinea cruris is very common in males. It is uncommon in females and exceedingly rare in children. Tinea cruris results from invasion of the stratum corneum by the dermatophyte types of fungi. It is transmitted from person-to-person via fomites and from animal (usually kittens or puppies)-to-person via direct contact or fomites.

Clinical Features

One sees erythema with a peripheral annular slightly scaly edge in the groin and extending onto the inner thighs (Fig. 240-1) and even the buttocks. The penis and scrotum are not affected. This feature is important in distinguishing tinea cruris from other eruptions in the groin as most other eruptions will affect the scrotum.

Other common disorders to be included in the differential diagnosis include candidiasis, erythrasma, lichen simplex chronicus, allergic and irritant contact dermatitis, and extramammary Paget's disease. A more extensive list of inflammatory processes of the intertriginous areas can be found in Table 240-1. See the description under intertrigo for a comparison of the features of these disorders.

Diagnosis

The diagnosis is established by a positive potassium hydroxide (KOH) examination. A KOH preparation will demonstrate branching hyphae (Fig. 239-4). If a KOH examination is negative, one of the other above-mentioned disorders should be considered.

Treatment

Antifungal creams such as clotrimazole (Lotrimin or Mycelex), ketoconazole (Nizoral), or econazole (Spectazole) twice a day is the initial treatment. Clotrimazole is suggested initially as it is of low cost and

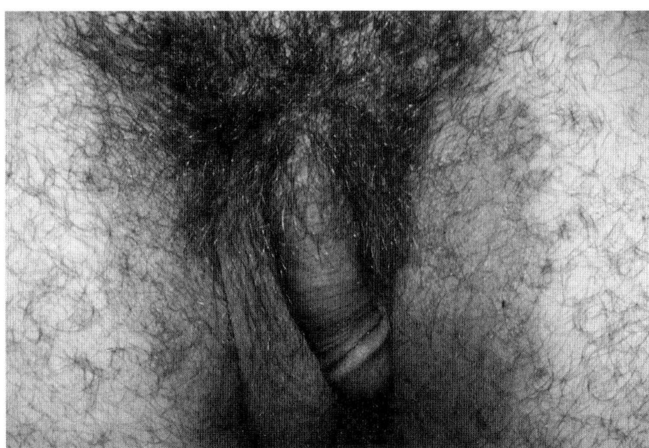

FIG. 240-1. Tinea cruris. Erythema with a more prominent, arciform leading edge on the inner thighs is typical of tinea cruris.

TABLE 240-1 Inflammatory Disorders of the Skin Folds

Infectious
Tinea cruris
Candida intertrigo
Erythrasma
Dermatitis
Seborrheic dermatitis
Intertrigo/irritant contact dermatitis
Allergic contact dermatitis
Atopic dermatitis
Lichen simplex chronicus
Psoriasis
Infestations
Scabies
Pediculosis pubis
Neoplasia
Bowen's disease (squamous cell carcinoma in situ)
Extramammary Paget's disease
Histiocytosis X (in diaper dermatitis)
Hidradenitis suppurativa
Cutaneous Crohn's disease
Hailey-Hailey disease (benign familial pemphigus)
Darier's disease
Lymphogranuloma venereum
Granuloma inguinale
Acrodermatitis enteropathica (zinc, biotin, or essential fatty acid deficiency)

is nonprescription. Spectazole also has antibacterial properties and is preferred if maceration is present. Treatment also includes keeping the affected area as cool and dry as possible. Wearing loose-fitting clothing is recommended. Antifungal powders such as Zeasorb AF should be used on a daily basis to prevent recurrences.

Disposition

The patient should follow up with a primary care provider or dermatologist if the eruption has not resolved in 4 to 6 weeks.

CANDIDA INTERTRIGO

Candidal infections of the skin favor moist, occluded areas of the body. Although any skin fold may be involved, superficial candida infections are commonly seen in the diaper area of infants, the vulva and groin of women, the glans penis (balanitis) in uncircumcised males, and the inframammary and pannus folds of obese patients. Antibiotic therapy, systemic corticosteroid therapy, urinary or fecal incontinence, immunocompromised states, and obesity are predisposing factors. Women with vulvar or inner thigh involvement will often have vaginal candidiasis as well. Frequently, intertrigo is multifactorial with candida complicating other inflammatory intertriginous disorders.

Clinical Features

The typical presentation is erythema and maceration with surrounding small erythematous papules or pustules [Fig. 240-2 (Plate 25)]. These satellite pustules are a characteristic finding differentiating candida intertrigo from other inflammatory disorders affecting the skin folds. Patients will complain of burning or itching. The other inflammatory disorders listed in Table 240-1 should be considered in the differential diagnosis.

Diagnosis

The rim of satellite pustules helps to distinguish candida intertrigo from other eruptions of the skin folds. A KOH preparation of the pustules or a leading edge scale may demonstrate short hyphae and spores; however, these may be difficult to find in cases with just erythema and maceration. If candida is suspected but not visualized on KOH preparation and the diagnosis is in question, a fungal culture should be obtained.

Even if the diagnosis of candida intertrigo is confirmed by a KOH preparation, it is important to obtain a thorough history to rule out an underlying disorder that may be secondarily infected with Candida.

Treatment

Keeping the affected area dry and cool is a very important part of treatment and should be stressed to the patient. After bathing, air drying or drying with a hair dryer should be encouraged. Clothing should be loose and lightweight. Astringent solutions such as aluminum acetate (Burow's solution) aid in drying weepy inflamed eruptions. One Domeboro's powder packet or tablet is mixed with 1 pint of water, then applied with a towel or gauze to the affected area for 15 to 20 min qid. A topical antifungal cream such as clotrimazole, ketoconazole (Nizoral), or econazole (Spectazole) should be applied bid. Spectazole has the advantage of antibacterial properties as well; however, it is more expensive. The addition of hydrocortisone 1% cream bid can speed symptomatic relief and healing. Furthermore, drying powders, such as Zeasorb AF, should be used on a daily basis.

Patients with vulvar candidiasis should be evaluated for candida vaginitis and treated appropriately if found. Patients with candida balanitis often have a female sexual partner with candida vaginitis, so this person should be evaluated and treated as well. In infants or in adults with urinary or fecal incontinence, diapers or sanitary pads should be changed frequently. Zinc oxide paste applied over the antifungal agent provides a barrier to the irritation of urine and feces.

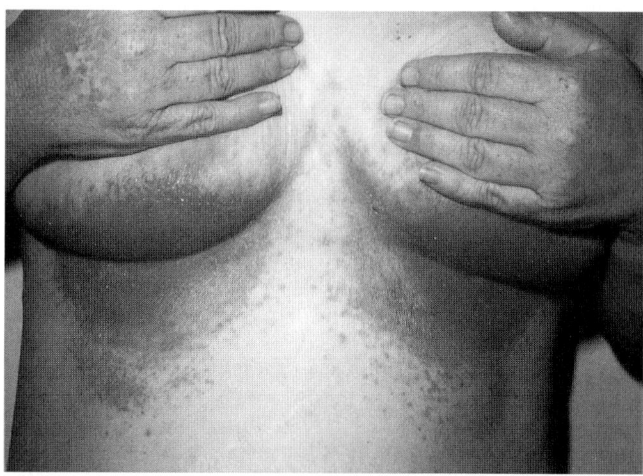

FIG. 240-2 (Plate 25). Candida intertrigo. Note the bright-red erythema, erosions, and satellite papules and pustules in this striking example of inframammary candida intertrigo. A KOH examination will confirm the diagnosis.

Disposition

Failure to respond to treatment may indicate another etiology of the eruption, and reevaluation by the patient's primary care provider or dermatologist should be sought.

INTERTRIGO AND DIAPER DERMATITIS

Intertrigo refers to inflammation of the skin folds. It is an irritant dermatitis resulting from moisture, heat, friction, and irritating substances like urine and feces. Intertrigo is common in the skin folds of obese patients where sweating and maceration occur. It is also a frequent occurrence in the diaper area of infants where it is referred to as diaper dermatitis.

Clinical Features

Intertrigo presents as erythema, maceration, and fissures in the occluded area of skin folds, especially the groin and inframammary fold. Satellite papules and pustules are absent. Burning and pruritus are present.

Diagnosis

Intertrigo is a diagnosis of exclusion. Other causes of skin fold erythema and fissuring such as candida intertrigo, erythrasma, tinea cruris, allergic contact dermatitis, seborrheic dermatitis, inverse psoriasis, and extramammary Paget's disease must be considered. Differentiating candida intertrigo from inflammatory intertrigo can be difficult. Candida intertrigo will have satellite pustules as a prominent feature. If positive, a KOH examination supports the diagnosis of candida intertrigo. A negative KOH examination, however, does not rule out this possibility, as yeast is difficult to obtain and visualize with this procedure. A scraping of peripheral scale or a pustule to send for fungal culture is suggested.

Erythrasma is a bacterial infection caused by *Corynebacterium minutissimum*. Its distribution is the same as tinea cruris in the groin, but other skin folds may be affected as well. The color is often an orange-red color without a prominent leading edge. The diagnosis of erythrasma is confirmed by the presence of coral-red fluorescence under Wood's light examination.

Clinically, irritant dermatitis cannot always be distinguished from allergic contact dermatitis. A history should be taken to uncover any possible contact allergens or irritants such as neomycin-containing ointments, anesthetic creams, Benadryl cream, deodorants, feminine hygiene sprays, or other lotions, solutions, or home remedies.

Complete skin examination will help to uncover other signs of seborrheic dermatitis or psoriasis. Furthermore, extramammary Paget's disease and Bowen's disease (squamous cell carcinoma in situ) may be clinically indistinguishable from intertrigo—they may even be secondarily infected with candida. Little or no response to therapy are indications to biopsy the affected area to exclude these diagnoses.

Treatment

As this eruption results from irritation by moisture, heat, and friction, these factors should be eliminated. Keeping the areas dry and cool is helpful. The patient should avoid tight-fitting clothing, especially undergarments. Weight loss can help as well. All potential irritants should be avoided. In diaper dermatitis, disposable diapers are preferred because of their highly absorbent properties. Diapers should be changed frequently, and periods free of diaper wear to dry and cool the affected skin is recommended. Zinc oxide paste provides an excellent barrier to urine and fecal material.

It is a common occurrence for the practitioner to be uncertain of the diagnosis. As a result, treatment is often aimed at both anticandidal and anti-inflammatory therapy. Several pitfalls of this approach exist. First, if used alone, topical corticosteroids can cause persistence or worsening of candida intertrigo. Second, the commonly prescribed combination medications, Lotrisone and Mycolog, contain a high-potency fluorinated corticosteroid. The occlusive nature of skin folds allows for better and deeper penetration of these high-potency corticosteroids, resulting in an increased risk of steroid-induced atrophy and striae. If combination therapy is warranted, Vytone-HC 1% (Vioform and 1% hydrocortisone) has anticandidal effects with a mild topical corticosteroid more appropriate for use in the intertriginous areas.

For moist weepy intertrigo, astringent compresses can be used. Domeboro's compresses, as described above for candida intertrigo, are recommended.

Secondary bacterial impetiginization can occur and should be treated with oral antibiotics with staphylococcal and streptococcal coverage.

SEBORRHEIC DERMATITIS

Seborrheic dermatitis is one of the most common skin disorders. It most notably affects the scalp ("dandruff") and creases of the face and ears; however, other skin folds such as the intergluteal cleft, groin, the axilla, inframammary folds, and the umbilicus can be affected. Severe and extensive seborrheic dermatitis is more common in debilitated patients, patients with HIV, and patients with Parkinson's disease.

The exact cause of seborrheic dermatitis is unknown. Overgrowth of *Pityrosporon ovale,* a yeast that normally inhabits hair follicles and sebaceous ducts, with resultant inflammatory response has been implicated.

Clinical Features

Seborrheic dermatitis of the scalp and skin folds of the face presents as erythema with a waxy yellow scale. When seborrheic dermatitis affects other skin folds, erythema and maceration are noted. Extension of the eruption onto the pubic area and central chest may be seen.

Diagnosis

The diagnosis is made on clinical examination of the skin folds with special attention to the scalp and creases of the face. Without examination of the face and scalp, the groin or other skin fold involvement is hard to differentiate from the other inflammatory disorders such as candida intertrigo, inverse psoriasis, allergic contact dermatitis, or erythrasma.

Treatment

Patients should be told that treatment is not expected to result in a cure. Treatment is aimed at relieving signs and symptoms of disease; the eruption will return after treatment ceases. Shampoos can be used on the scalp and other hair-bearing areas. These include shampoos containing zinc pyrithione (Head and Shoulders), selenium sulfide (Selsun or extra-strength Head and Shoulders), salicylic acid (Neutrogena T-Sal), or tar preparations (Neutrogena T-Gel). Nizoral shampoo can be effective as well and is now available over-the-counter. Seborrheic dermatitis is very responsive to low-potency corticosteroids. Hydrocortisone 1% cream can be used in mild cases, while hydrocortisone 2.5% cream or desonide (DesOwen) cream or lotion may be required initially in more severe cases. If these initial treatment options fail, the patient should be instructed to follow up with a dermatologist.

LICHEN SIMPLEX CHRONICUS

The scrotum, vulva, and perianal area are common sites of involvement with lichen simplex chronicus. Clinically, lichenification, hyperpigmentation, and excoriation are prominent features (Fig. 240-3). Treatment is the same as for LSC in other areas except low-potency corticosteroid (hydrocortisone 2.5% or desonide) ointments should be used. In cases of perianal LSC, patients should be instructed to cleanse the perianal area thoroughly to remove fecal debris and tissue paper that may be irritating. Witch hazel pads are recommended for cleansing.

HIDRADENITIS SUPPURATIVA

Hidradenitis suppurativa is a chronic scarring inflammatory disorder of the apocrine gland–bearing areas of the body. These glands are located predominantly in the groin, intergluteal cleft, vulva, and axilla. Hidradenitis suppurativa begins after puberty and is seen slightly more frequently in women. It is more likely seen in obese patients. Hidradenitis suppurativa may be seen in association with acne conglobata, dissecting cellulitis of the scalp, and pilonidal cysts (the follicular occlusion syndrome).

The initiating event in hidradenitis suppurativa is occlusion of the apocrine gland and pilosebaceous follicular unit. The exact mechanism resulting in this occlusion is unknown. This occlusion results in the development of inflammatory nodules and abscesses. Bacterial infection is only a secondary process and not the cause of this disorder.

Clinical Features

Initially, hidradenitis suppurativa begins as a painful deep erythematous nodule usually in the axilla or groin. The inflammatory nodule may resolve on its own or develop into a sterile abscess that may open to the surface and drain. Such a lesion may persist and periodically drain, develop a sinus tract and continually drain, or heal with scarring. New lesions may develop in the same area and interconnect. Open comedones, which normally are not present in these body regions, may be seen. Comedones with multiple openings are characteristic of hidradenitis suppurativa. Scarring may be pitted, bridging, or hypertrophic (Fig. 240-4). The extent of involvement is variable with some patients experiencing only localized intermittent lesions with minimal scarring and others with continuously active disease in the axilla, groin, intergluteal cleft, and buttocks.

Diagnosis

The diagnosis is made clinically. The location, types of lesions, comedones, and scarring are clues to diagnosing hidradenitis. Other disorders to include in the differential diagnosis of mild disease include

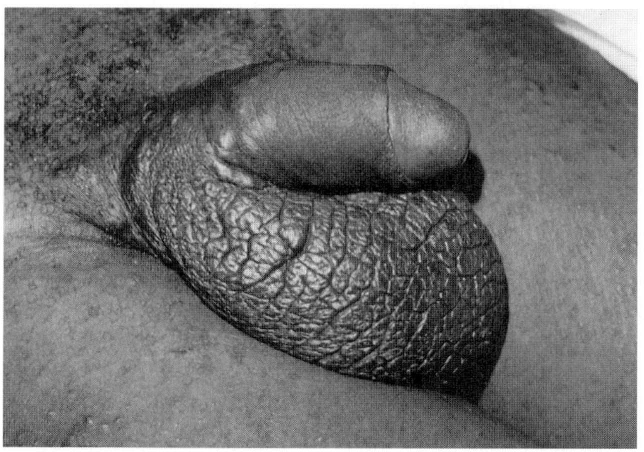

FIG. 240-3. Lichen simplex chronicus. Pronounced lichenification and hyperpigmentation is typical of lichen simplex chronicus. The scrotum is a common site of involvement.

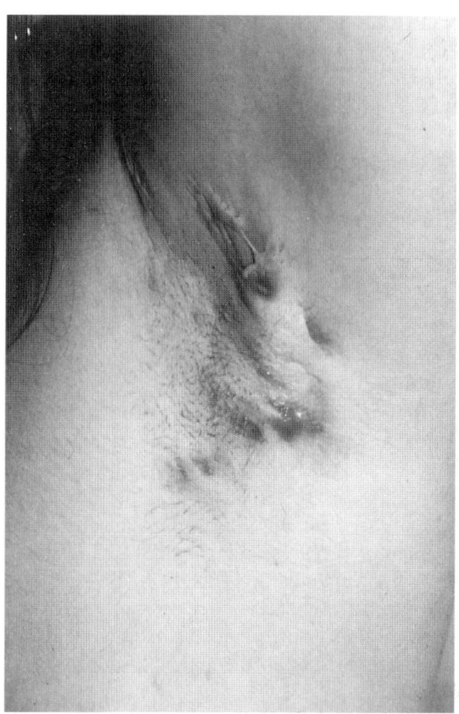

FIG. 240-4. Hidradenitis suppurativa. A typical example of hidradenitis suppurativa displaying active inflammatory nodules, sinus tracts, pitted scars, and double-headed comedones.

inflamed epidermal inclusion cysts, inflamed pilonidal cysts, and furuncles. Severe disease should be distinguished from cutaneous Crohn's disease, lymphogranuloma venereum, granuloma inguinale, and actinomyces. Epidermal inclusion cysts may be singular or multiple and usually have a distinct opening (punctum) to the surface. Usually, only one cyst is inflamed at a given time. Scarring is not a characteristic finding. The patient often gives a history of the presence of a nontender flesh-colored nodule from which cheesy, foul smelling material could be expressed. Pilonidal cysts are singular and located over the coccyx or sacrum in the midline. A furuncle is a staphylococcal abscess (''boils'') resulting from folliculitis. Perianal cutaneous Crohn's disease may have a very similar clinical appearance to hidradenitis with inflammatory nodules, sinus tracts, and fistulas. A thorough history and physical examination will help identify or exclude this disease. If uncertain, a skin biopsy for histopathology and culture will differentiate hidradenitis from cutaneous Crohn's disease, lymphogranuloma venereum, granuloma inguinale, and actinomyces.

As secondary bacterial infection can occur, cultures of draining lesions should be performed.

Treatment

Medical and surgical treatment options exist for hidradenitis suppurativa. The therapy chosen depends on the extent and severity of the disease. Acutely inflamed nodules should be treated with intralesional corticosteroids (triamcinolone 3 to 5 mg/mL). Acutely inflamed abscesses should be incised and drained. Mild-to-moderate chronic disease should be treated with oral antibiotics in a similar manner as treating acne. This includes using tetracycline 500 mg PO bid, minocycline 50 mg PO bid, or erythromycin 500 mg PO bid for at least 1 month. If bacterial infection is discovered from bacterial culture results, antibiotic treatment should be tailored to the specific organism and its drug sensitivities. Surgical excision may be necessary if lesions do not respond to the above mentioned treatments. Such patients should be referred to a plastic or dermatologic surgeon.

In addition to the previously mentioned therapy, severe disease may require oral prednisone or isotretinoin (Accutane). Such patients should be referred to a dermatologist for management. Patients should be told about the chronicity of this disease. Aggravating factors such as tight-fitting clothing should be avoided. Obese patients should be encouraged to loose weight. Antibacterial cleansers (Hibiclens) or a topical antibiotic solution (Cleocin T) should be prescribed to prevent secondary bacterial infection.

SEXUALLY TRANSMITTED DISEASES

Sexually transmitted diseases are mentioned briefly so as not to forget them when presented with a patient with an eruption in these areas. Sexually transmitted diseases can occur in the intergluteal cleft, the perianal area, and the groin with or without genital involvement. The chancre of primary syphilis and condyloma lata of secondary syphilis can occur in these areas. The perineum or perianal area is a common site for primary or recurrent herpes simplex virus. The sacrum is also a common site of recurrent HSV. Condyloma acuminatum frequently involves the inguinal creases and perianal area in addition to the genitalia. Furthermore, pediculosis pubis (''crabs'') and scabies should be considered in pruritic excoriated eruptions of the groin and axilla. Finally, the clinical findings in granuloma inguinale and lymphogranuloma venereum predominate in the inguinal folds.

BIBLIOGRAPHY

Guitart J, Woodley DT: Intertrigo: A practical approach. *Compr Ther* 28(7):402, 1994.

Parks RW, Parks TG: Pathogenesis, clinical features and management of Hidradenitis suppurativa. *Ann R Coll Surg Engl* 79(2):83, 1997.

GENERALIZED SKIN DISORDERS

William J. Brady
Daniel J. DeBehnke

This chapter describes selected generalized skin disorders in adults, and discusses their dermatologic diagnosis and treatment. Discussed below are erythema multiforme; toxic epidermal necrolysis (TEN); the toxic infectious erythemas; disseminated viral infections; Rocky Mountain spotted fever; meningococcemia; purpura fulminans; and the systemic bullous diseases.

ERYTHEMA MULTIFORME

Erythema multiforme (EM) is an acute inflammatory skin disease presenting across a spectrum. It ranges from a localized papular eruption of the skin (EM minor) to a severe, multisystem illness (EM major) with widespread vesiculobullous lesions and erosions of the mucous membranes, Stevens-Johnson syndrome (SJS). The disorder strikes all age groups with the highest incidence in young adults (age range 20 to 40 years), affects males twice as often as females, and occurs commonly in the spring and fall. Infection, especially mycoplasma and herpes simplex, drugs, especially antibiotics and anticonvulsants, and malignancies are common precipitating factors. However, there is no identifiable etiology in approximately 50 percent of cases.[1]

The pathogenesis of EM remains largely unknown. Most likely, it is the result of a hypersensitivity reaction with the demonstration of immunoglobulin and complement components in the cutaneous microvasculature on immunofluorescence studies of skin biopsy specimens, circulating immune complexes in the serum, and mononuclear cell infiltrate on histologic examination.[1,2]

Patients frequently experience malaise, fever, myalgias, and arthralgias. Diffuse pruritus or a generalized burning sensation can occur before the skin develops lesions. The morphologic configuration of the lesions is quite variable, hence the descriptor ''multiforme.'' Maculopapular [Fig. 241-1*A* (Plate 26)] and target [iris, Fig. 241-1*B* (Plate 27)] lesions are the most characteristic. Erythematous papules appear symmetrically on the dorsum of the hands and feet, and the extensor surfaces of the extremities. The maculopapule evolves into the classic target lesion during the next 24 to 48 h. As the maculopapule enlarges, the central area becomes cyanotic, occasionally accompanied by central purpura or a vesicle. Urticarial plaques may also occur with or without the iris lesion in a similar distribution. Vesiculobullous lesions, which may be pruritic and painful, develop within preexisting maculopapules or plaques, usually on the extensor surface of the arms and legs, less frequently involving the trunk. Vesiculobullous lesions are most often found on mucosal surfaces, including the mouth, eyes, vagina, urethra, and anus; they may also be seen on the trunk. Ocular involvement occurs in approximately 10 percent of patients with EM minor while the SJS variant experiences ophthalmologic lesions in almost 75 percent of cases.

The various lesions develop in successive crops during a 2- to 4-week period, and crops heal over 5 to 7 days. Scarring is rarely a problem except in cases of secondary infection or in heavily pigmented

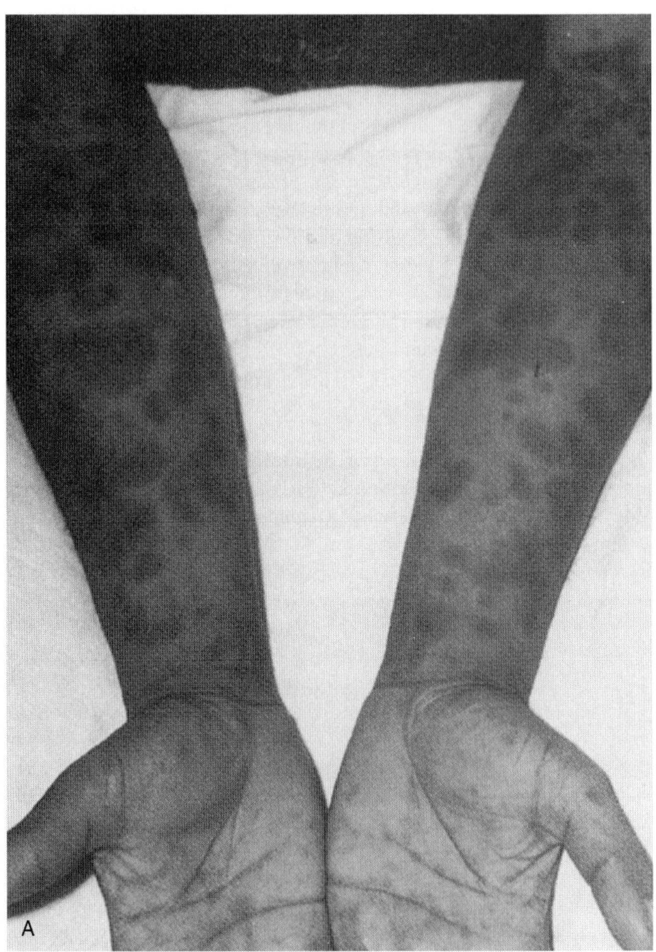

FIG. 241-1A (Plate 26). Erythema multiforme: Symmetrical, plaque-like lesions involving the flexor surface of the upper extremities—lesions which may be misdiagnosed as the IgG-mediated urticarial allergic reaction. Also note the erythematous macules on the palms. (Reprinted with permission from Brady W, DeBehnke D, Crosby D: Dermatologic emergencies. *Am J Emerg Med* 12:217, 1994.)

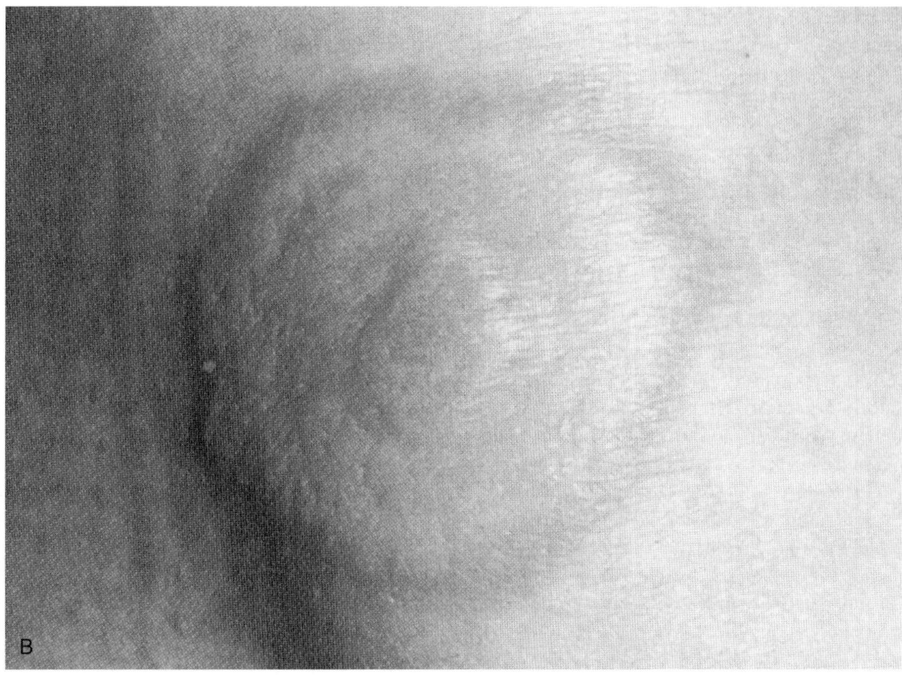

FIG. 241-1B (Plate 27). Iris or target lesion, a finding strongly suggestive of EM. This iris lesion is composed of a central bullous lesion with dusky, edematous center and erythematous halo. (Reprinted with permission from Brady W, DeBehnke D, Crosby D: Dermatologic emergencies. *Am J Emerg Med* 12:217, 1994.)

patients in whom hypopigmentation or hyperpigmentation may occur. Recurrence may be noted on repeat exposure to the etiologic agent, a special concern in cases associated with herpes simplex infection or medication use.[3] The rate of EM recurrence is very high in children with HSV infection. For example, 75 percent of children with a prior history of HSV-related EM experienced erythema multiforme recurrence after *herpes simplex* virus reactivation.[3] Fluid and electrolyte disorders, as well as secondary infection from cutaneous sites, represent the most frequent complications, as well as the most common causes of death in the EM patient. The differential diagnosis of EM includes herpetic (both *herpes simplex* virus and varicella zoster virus) infection; vasculitis; TEN; various primary blistering disorders (pemphigus and pemphigoid); urticaria; Kawasaki disease; and the toxic-infectious erythemas.

Outpatient treatment of EM minor with topical corticosteroids is possible, but steroids should not be applied to eroded areas of the skin. Dermatologic consultation and close follow-up are advised. Those patients with extensive disease, systemic toxicity, and/or mucous membrane involvement require hospitalization, optimally in the intensive care or burn unit setting.

Systemic steroids are commonly used and provide symptomatic relief, but are of unproven benefit in influencing the duration and outcome of EM.[4] Many authorities recommend a short, intensive steroid course, 60 to 80 mg/day of prednisone in divided doses, particularly in drug-related cases, with abrupt cessation in 3 to 5 days if no favorable response is noted. Systemic analgesic agents and antihistamines provide symptomatic relief. Stomatitis is treated with diphenhydramine and viscous lidocaine mouth rinses. Blisters are treated with cool, wet Burow's solution (aluminum sulfate/calcium acetate in aqueous solution) compresses. Ocular involvement should be monitored by an ophthalmologist; unfortunately, burst-steroid therapy does not appear to reduce either the chance of development or significance of existing ocular lesions. Acyclovir may reduce recurrence of HSV infection and, therefore, lessen the potential for another bout of EM; prolonged, prophylactic acyclovir therapy may reduce the chance of recurrent EM related to HSV.[3] EM, particularly SJS, has significant morbidity and a mortality of approximately 10 percent despite aggressive therapy.

TOXIC EPIDERMAL NECROLYSIS

Toxic epidermal necrolysis is an explosive dermatosis characterized by tender erythema, bullae formation, and subsequent exfoliation. Patients may be systemically ill on presentation. Many authorities consider the SJS variant of EM and TEN as the same process.[2] TEN is found in all age groups without predilection to gender. The syndrome has multiple possible etiologies with medications representing the most common cause.[1,2,5,6] Sulfa and penicillin antibiotics, anticonvulsants, and oxicam NSAIDs are the most frequent drug triggers for TEN.[7,8] Other causes include malignancy and human immunodeficiency virus (HIV).[6] In many cases, an etiology is not found.

The pathogenesis is poorly understood and may be partly an immunologic and partly a genetic predisposition. The tendency to develop TEN may be linked to a highly specific genetic defect in the detoxification of the culprit drug or its reactive metabolites.[9] Human lymphocyte antigen (HLA) typing has also suggested a possible genetic predisposition.

Patients with TEN often present with a one- to two-week prodrome of malaise, anorexia, arthralgias, fever, or upper respiratory infection symptoms. Skin tenderness, pruritus, tingling, or burning may be found at this time. Skin signs begin with a warm erythema, initially only involving the eyes, nose, mouth, and genitalia, but later becoming generalized. The erythematous areas become tender and confluent within hours. Flaccid, ill-defined bullae then appear within the areas of erythema. Lateral pressure with a finger on normal skin adjacent to a bullous lesion dislodges the epidermis producing denuded dermis, demonstrating Nikolsky's sign. The bullae form along the cleavage plane between the epidermis and the dermis. The epidermis is then shed in large sheets, leaving raw, denuded areas of exposed dermis. The average time of onset after exposure to the inciting agent is 2 weeks. Cutaneous extension follows an unpredictable time course, ranging from 24 h to 15 days with a minority of severe cases demonstrating rapid, extensive involvement within 24 h.

Prolabial blistering and erosive lesions are disfiguring and often impair adequate oral intake, contributing to hypovolemia. Ocular complications include purulent conjunctivitis, painful erosions, and potential blindness. Anogenital lesions are common. Additional mucous membrane involvement includes the gastrointestinal, urinary, and respiratory tracts. The two major complications and leading causes of death in TEN are infection and hypovolemia with electrolyte disorders. A broad range of pathogens is usually found, with staphylococcal and pseudomonal species predominating. The mortality rate has been reported as being between 25 and 30 percent. These clinical variables are associated with poor prognosis: advanced age; extensive disease; idiopathic nature; multiple medication use; steroid therapy; azotemia; hyperglycemia; leukopenia; and thrombocytopenia.[7] The differential diagnosis of TEN includes staphylococcal scalded skin syndrome (SSSS); EM, toxic shock syndrome (staphylococcal and streptococcal); exfoliative drug reactions; primary blistering disorders (pemphigus and pemphigoid); and Kawasaki syndrome.

Management of TEN requires hospitalization in a critical care setting or, optimally, a burn unit.[7] In most cases, therapy is similar to the approach for the burn patient. Immediate concerns center on the airway, because sloughing of airway and respiratory epithelium can occur. Hypovolemia and electrolyte abnormalities should be corrected. Prompt, aggressive antibiotic administration is necessary in suspected or documented infection; initial prophylactic antibiotics are not recommended by most. The advice of the burn center should be followed for any topical dressings that are applied before transfer.

EXFOLIATIVE DERMATITIS

Exfoliative dermatitis, a cutaneous reaction produced in response to a drug or a chemical agent or to an underlying systemic disease, is a condition in which most or all of the skin surface is involved with a scaly erythematous dermatitis. Males are affected twice as often as females, and most patients are over the age of 40.[10] The mechanisms responsible are not known although drug-induced exfoliative dermatitis may be mediated by an increased activity of sensitized suppressor-cytotoxic T lymphocytes.

Exfoliative dermatitis can have an abrupt onset, particularly when related to a drug, contact allergen, or malignancy, whereas exacerbations related to an underlying cutaneous disorder usually evolve more slowly. In many cases, exfoliative dermatitis tends to be a chronic condition with a mean duration of five years when related to a chronic illness; a shorter course often follows suppression of the underlying dermatosis, discontinuation of causative drugs, or avoidance of allergen. Both idiopathic and chronic disease-related exfoliative dermatitis can continue for 20 or more years; death is rare.

Generalized erythema and warmth are noted and are similar to that seen in the patient with TEN, but skin tenderness is usually lacking. Erythema is accompanied by scaling or flaking and the patient often complains of pruritus and skin tightness [Fig. 241-2 (Plate 28)]. The process usually begins on the face and upper trunk with progression to other skin surfaces. The patient usually has a low-grade fever. Excessive heat loss and hypothermia can complicate erythroderma. Widespread cutaneous vasodilation may result in high-output congestive heart failure. The disruption of the epidermis results in increased transepidermal water loss, and continued exfoliation can result in significant protein loss and negative nitrogen balance. Chronic inflammatory exfoliation produces many changes, such as dystrophic nails, thinning scalp and body hair, and patchy or diffuse pigmentation changes.

The differential diagnosis of exfoliative dermatitis includes staphylococcal scalded skin syndrome, EM, TEN, toxic shock syndrome (staphylococcal and streptococcal), and Kawasaki disease. Considerable effort must be made to determine the underlying etiology, including evaluation for underlying malignancy, and biopsy of involved skin. Patients generally require emergent dermatologic consultation and admission. Hypothermia and hypovolemia should be corrected, and systemic corticosteroids are often given after consultation.

TOXIC INFECTIOUS ERYTHEMAS

A number of infectious syndromes caused by toxigenic bacteria with toxin-mediated dermatologic manifestations have been described, including toxic shock syndrome (TSS), streptococcal toxic shock syndrome (STSS), SSSS, bullous impetigo, and scarlet fever. In certain cases, the bacteria are colonizers with the disease resulting only from the toxin (e.g., TSS); in other instances, the toxigenic organism produces infection with clinical manifestations developing from both the infectious process and the presence of the toxin (e.g., STSS, SSSS, bullous impetigo, and scarlet fever).

Toxic Shock Syndrome

Discussion of the general features and management of TSS are discussed in Chap. 138, while the dermatologic features are discussed below.[11]

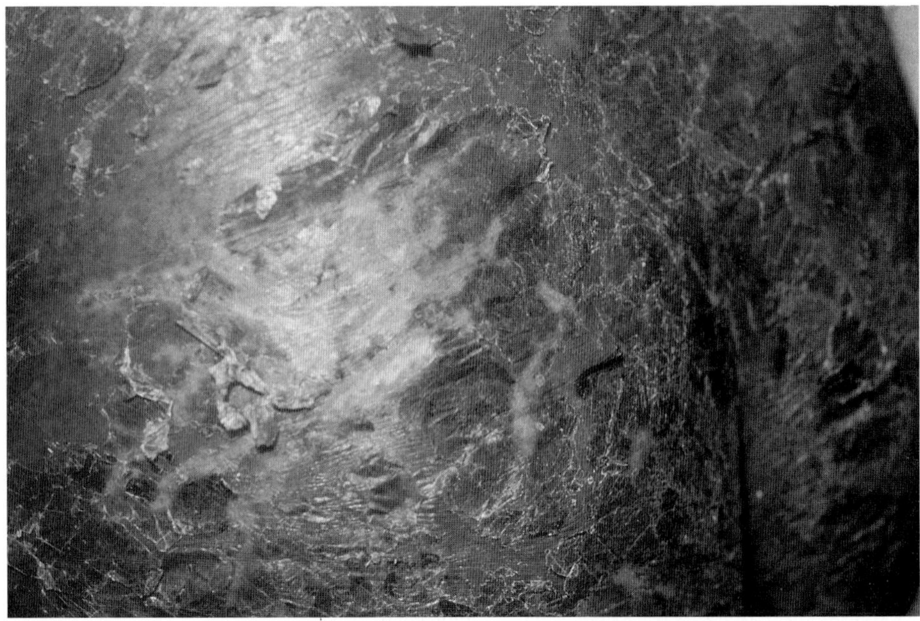

FIG. 241-2 (Plate 28). Exfoliative dermatitis—generalized, warm erythema accompanied by scaling or flaking.

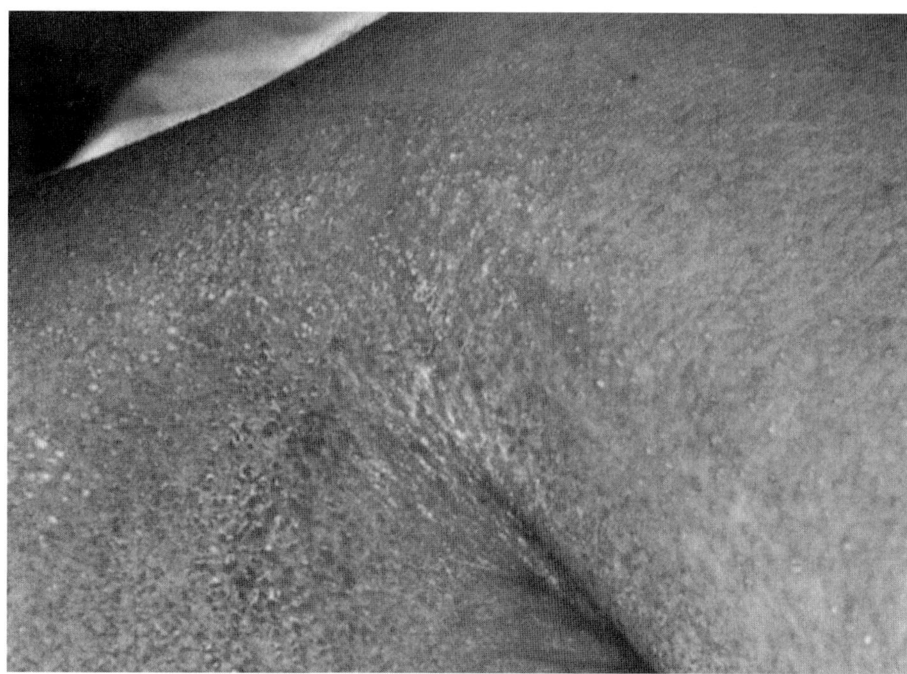

FIG. 241-3 (Plate 29). Blanching, nonpruritic erythroderma with a "rough" texture in a patient with toxic shock syndrome. (Reprinted with permission from Brady W, DeBehnke D, Crosby D: Dermatologic emergencies. *Am J Emerg Med* 12:217, 1994.)

The dermatologic hallmark of TSS is nonpruritic, blanching macular erythroderma, a characteristic feature and a major criterion for the diagnosis [Fig. 241-3 (Plate 29)]. The erythroderma is usually diffuse, although it may be confined to the extremities or trunk and may resemble sunburn. The rash may be subtle and is often missed in heavily pigmented patients or when the patient is examined in a poorly illuminated room. Erythroderma may resolve in 3 to 5 days, and a fine desquamation of the hands and feet follows in 5 to 14 days. Other dermatologic manifestations include conjunctival and mucosal hyperemia, petechiae, alopecia, and fingernail loss. The differential diagnosis is broad and includes scarlet fever; Rocky Mountain spotted fever; leptospirosis; rubeola; meningococcemia; streptococcal TSS; SSSS; Kawasaki syndrome; toxic epidermal necrolysis; SJS; gram-negative sepsis; and exfoliative drug eruptions.

Streptococcal Toxic Shock Syndrome

STSS is an uncommon clinical syndrome that involves multiple organ systems with fever, hypotension, and skin findings.[12] The causative agent of this clinical disorder is *Streptococcus pyogenes* (group A *Streptococcus*). Streptococcal species produce extracellular proteins called streptococcal pyrogenic exotoxins (SPEs). Invasive soft tissue streptococcal infection, such as cellulitis, myositis, or fasciitis, is a common factor in the etiology of STSS.

The clinical presentation of STSS includes fever, hypotension, skin edema, and erythema, or bullae [Fig. 241-4 (Plate 30)]. Subsequent desquamation occurs less commonly than during staphylococcal TSS. The same major and minor criteria used for the diagnosis of staphylococcal TSS can be helpful in identifying patients with STSS. According to a consensus document[13] clinical features must include isolation of group A streptococci (*S. pyogenes*) and hypoperfusion, as well as evidence of multisystem dysfunction. Because up to 75 percent of cases of STSS have associated soft-tissue infection, a thorough skin examination for the site of infection is warranted. Palpate muscle groups for tenderness, indicating possible myositis or fasciitis, and evaluate for secondary compartment syndrome. Treatment is oxygenation and fluid resuscitation. Because soft-tissue infection plays a large role in STSS, aggressive management of infection is essential. The site of infection should be identified, incised, and drained, and nonviable tissue debrided. Parenteral nafcillin, or oxacillin, or vancomycin, and a first-generation cephalosporin are often given as initial therapy.

Staphylococcal Scalded Skin Syndrome

Staphylococcal scalded skin syndrome develops in patients with clinically inapparent staph infections caused by an exotoxin produced by *Staphylococcus aureus*. It occurs primarily in infants and young children, and also in immunosuppressed adults or those with renal insufficiency. The exotoxins involved, collectively known as exfoliatin, are elaborated by the bacteria, released into the circulation, and cause acantholysis and intraepidermal cleavage of the skin.[14]

An episode of SSSS frequently begins as a clinically inapparent staphylococcal infection of the conjunctiva, nasopharynx, or umbilicus. The disease course can be divided into three phases: initial/erythroderma; exfoliative; and desquamation/recovery. Initially, the patient (or parent) notes the sudden appearance of a tender erythroderma, usually diffuse, although localized disease has been described. The involved skin may have a sandpaper texture. Tender erythema is prominent in the perioral, periorbital, and groin regions, as well as in the skin creases of the neck, axilla, popliteal, and antecubital areas. The mucous membranes are spared. The exfoliative stage begins on the second day of the illness. The erythematous skin wrinkles and peels off at sites of minor trauma or with minimal lateral pressure with the examiner's fingertip, illustrating the positive Nikolsky's sign (also found in TEN). Large, flaccid, fluid-filled bullae and vesicles then appear. These lesions easily rupture and are shed in large sheets; the underlying tissue resembles scalded skin and rapidly desiccates. After 3 to 5 days of illness, the involved skin desquamates, leaving normal skin in 7 to 10 days. The differential diagnosis for SSSS includes toxic epidermal necrolysis, TSS, exfoliative drug eruptions, and localized bullous impetigo.

Management includes fluid resuscitation and correction of electrolyte abnormalities, as well as identification and treatment of the source of the toxigenic staphylococcus with oxacillin or vancomycin. Corticosteroids are not recommended.

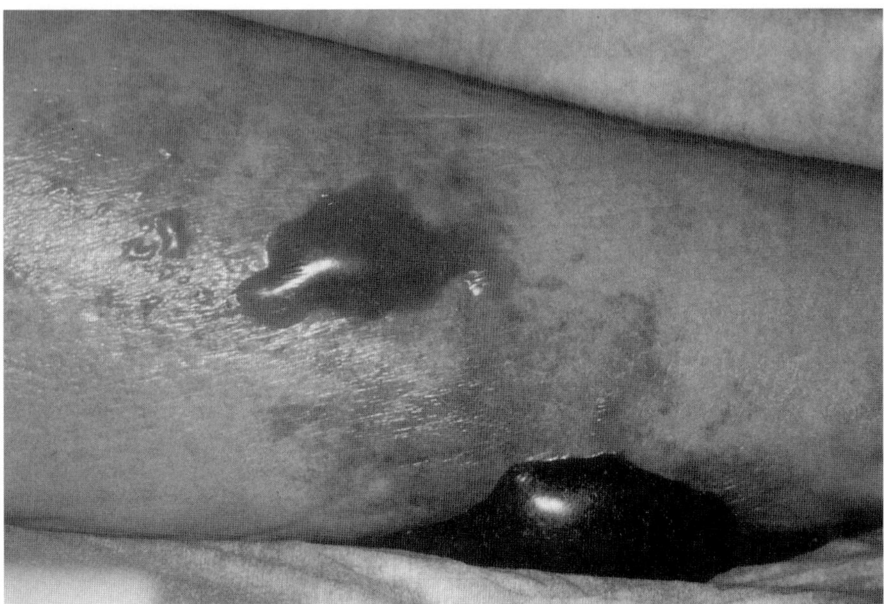

FIG. 241-4 (Plate 30). Large bullous lesions on the lower extremity in a patient with streptococcal toxic shock.

DISSEMINATED VIRAL INFECTIONS

Infectious Exanthems

Many viral infections are associated with generalized morbilliform cutaneous eruptions. The list is exhaustive, but the most common include adenoviruses; cytomegalovirus; coxsackie and echoviruses; Epstein-Barr virus; hepatitis B virus; human herpesvirus-6; paramyxovirus; respiratory syncytial virus; rotaviruses; rubella virus, and human immunodeficiency virus. Other agents associated with generalized eruptions include mycoplasma; *Borrelia* spp; *Legionella; Leptospira; Listeria;* meningococci; rickettsiae; and *Treponema pallidum.* Erythematous macules and papules, or, less often, vesicles and petechiae, usually develop centrally, sparing the palms and soles. Diagnosis and differential diagnosis are based upon history and physical examination. Drug eruption should always be considered in the differential. Skin lesions usually resolve in 7 to 10 days, and are treated symptomatically.

Herpes Zoster

Varicella zoster infections (VZI), also referred to as shingles or zoster, represent reactivation of the previously dormant virus, *Herpesvirus varicellae,* in a patient with an altered immune response. At reactivation, the virus travels down specific sensory nerves to the skin resulting in the skin manifestations of shingles. Patients with lymphoma, leukemia, or diabetes mellitus, and who are immunocompromised, are at risk for reactivated or disseminated infection.[15]

The rash of herpes zoster consists of clusters of vesicles and papules grouped on an erythematous base. Vesicles initially appear clear but become cloudy or purulent over several days. They eventually rupture and crust over. The lesions usually appear along an individual dermatome [Fig. 241-5 (Plate 31)]; less often, adjacent dermatomes are involved. The lesion clusters are usually discrete and separated by normal skin; in the severe case, the cluster may become confluent along the dermatome. Approximately 60 percent of all zoster infections involve the trunk, followed by the head, extremity, and perineal regions in decreasing incidence.[16] Unilateral involvement that abruptly halts at the midline is helpful in correctly identifying the rash; occasionally, a few lesions appear immediately beyond the midline. Involvement of the nose must prompt evaluation for corneal involvement [Fig. 241-6 (Plate 32)].

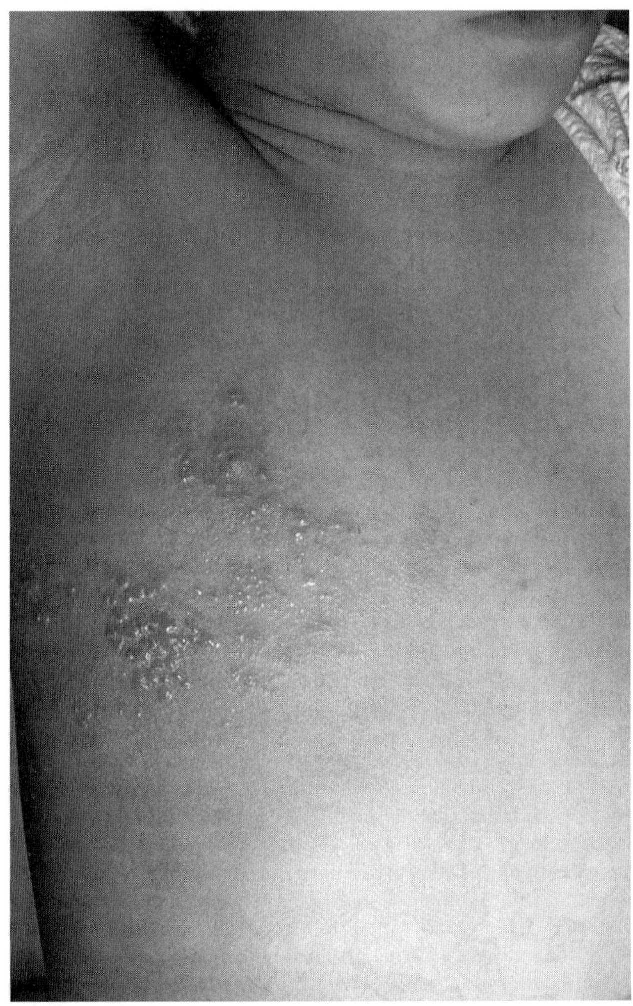

FIG. 241-5 (Plate 31). A single dermatomal involvement in a patient with herpes zoster infection in a thoracic distribution.

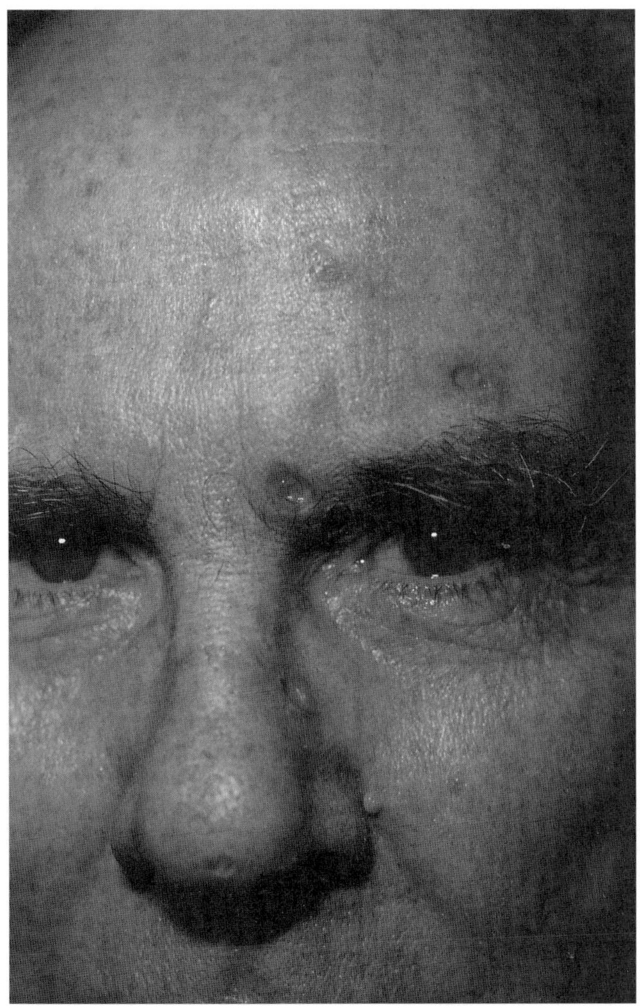

FIG. 241-6 (Plate 32). Herpes zoster ophthalmic infection: Facial zoster involving the ophthalmic branch of the fifth cranial nerve with nasal lesions strongly suggestive of corneal infection.

Approximately one-half of cases with VZI—particularly those patients with AIDS or reticuloendothelial malignancy—experience viremia and may exhibit solitary lesions totaling less than 30 scattered across the body. Patients with AIDS, using immunosuppressive medications, or with active reticuloendothelial malignancy more often demonstrate true dissemination in which widespread vesicular lesions are distributed evenly across the trunk, extremities, and head. In fact, patients with Hodgkin's disease are particularly prone to dissemination with 15 to 50 percent of cases demonstrating involvement of the skin, lungs, and central nervous system. Patients with disseminated herpes zoster infection require admission and treatment with parenteral antiviral therapy.

Herpes Simplex and Eczema Herpeticum

The vast majority of HSV type 1 or type 2 infections involve only localized areas of skin or mucous membranes. In neonates, and adults with atopic dermatitis, malignancy, immunosuppression, and the acquired immunodeficiency syndrome (AIDS), the HSV infection may disseminate, resulting in widespread vesicles, pustules, and ulcerations, and causing multisystem involvement. The neonate may acquire the infection either in utero due to maternal infection during pregnancy or during delivery. Adults undergoing chemotherapy or transplant recipients who are HSV seropositive may reactivate HSV and develop disseminated disease. Patients with atopic dermatitis are also at risk of disseminated disease, which is called eczema herpeticum.[17]

The vesicular rash, initially present in some form in up to 70 percent of patients, ranges from the scattered vesicle to full-body distribution. Lesions are vesicular, of similar size, 2 to 3 mm in diameter, clustered together in groups, and arrayed on an erythematous base [Fig. 241-7 (Plate 33)]. The lesions frequently umbilicate. Occasionally, the disseminated forms of HSV present cutaneously with different lesion morphology and appearance. Rather than grouped, the lesions may occur singularly with a widespread distribution; the lesions may also appear as pustules with purulent blister fluid. Bacterial superinfection is common. Regardless of their initial appearance, the lesions will ulcerate with crusting. A Tzanck preparation, in which fluid from an intact vesicle is applied to a microscope slide and stained with Wright's or Giemsa stain, often demonstrates multinucleated giant cells. If necessary, cultures of vesicle fluid can be obtained for confirmatory diagnosis. The patient's course may be complicated soon after by multiorgan failure. Treatment is admission to a critical care unit with parenteral antiviral therapy and antibiotics for bacterial superinfection.

Eczema herpeticum is an association of two common conditions—atopic dermatitis and HSV infection. The most severe forms of eczema herpeticum tend to occur in the young infant and the adult immunocompromised patient. Lesions appear initially in the area of the preexisting

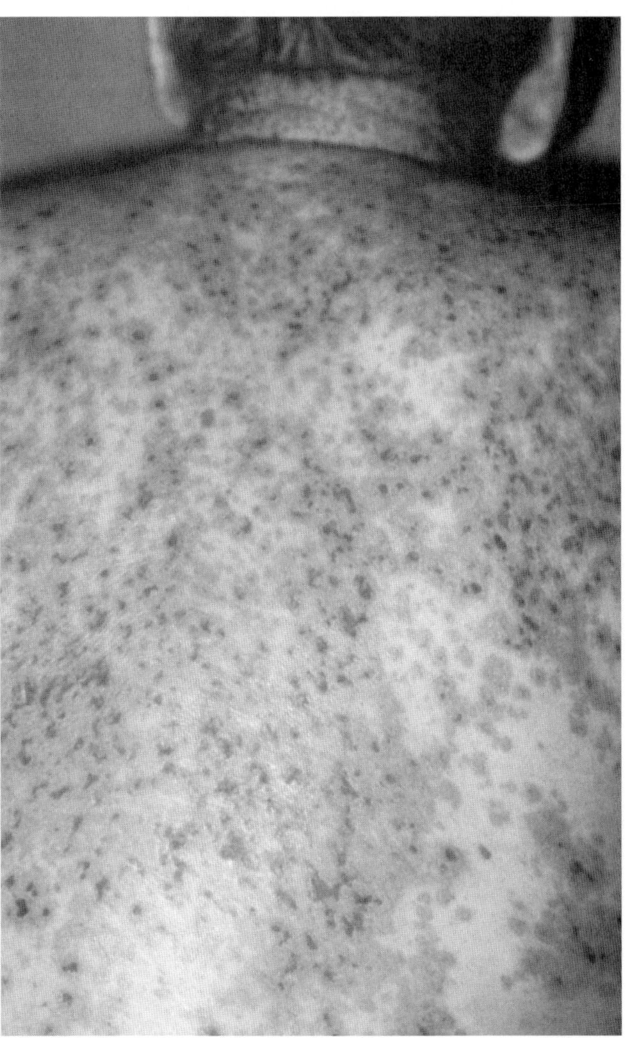

FIG. 241-7 (Plate 33). Disseminated HSV infection in an immunocompromised adult patient; note the widespread distribution of vesicular lesions on an erythematous base.

dermatitis, but eventually may disseminate. The underlying atopic dermatitis and bacterial superinfection may alter lesion appearance. Dermatologic consultation is usually necessary to aid in disposition decisions. Selected cases of local eczema herpeticum can be managed in the outpatient setting, with oral acyclovir and antibiotics. More severe or disseminated cases require admission.

DISSEMINATED GONOCOCCAL INFECTION

About 2 percent of patients with mucosal genitourinary (GU) infection will develop disseminated gonococcal infection (DGI). Risk factors for dissemination are not well known, but asymptomatic local disease and active menses seem to be somehow associated. Up to 75 percent of patients with DGI were diagnosed in either late pregnancy, the immediate postpartum period, or within one week of the onset of menses. Disseminated disease, once common in women, now is noted to occur with increased frequency in men. Disease manifestations result from both organism and immune complex dissemination. Fever, arthralgias, and multiple papular, vesicular, or pustular skin lesions characterize gonococcemia. The rash develops on the extensor surfaces of the wrists, palms, and hands and the dorsal aspects of the ankles and feet. The lesions, usually numbering less than 10 to 20, initially appear as small red papules or maculopapules [Fig. 241-8 (Plate 34)] with a petechial component and an erythematous periphery. Lesions either resolve rapidly or evolve into vesicles with purulent fluid, which develop gray necrotic centers. The necrotic center is theorized to be the embolic focus of the gonococcal organism. Ultimately, the lesions become hemorrhagic.

The differential diagnosis includes other petechial syndromes including Rocky Mountain spotted fever (RMSF); meningococcemia; staphylococcal acute endocarditis; vasculitides (particularly Henoch-Schönlein's purpura and leukocytoclastic vasculitis); enteroviral infections; bacterial sepsis (gram-positive and gram-negative) with disseminated intravascular coagulation; and typhus. The distribution of the rash is similar to that encountered in the RMSF patient, initially seen on the wrists and ankles. The number of lesions in the DGI arthritis-dermatitis patient, however, is markedly less compared to the total lesion count in both RMSF and meningococcemia cases. Further, the rash of DGI is pustular rather than obviously petechial and hemorrhagic, as are the lesions of RMSF and meningococcemia. Lastly, the DGI patient usually does not demonstrate systemic toxicity as commonly seen in RMSF and meningococcemia victims. Reiter's syndrome may be confused with the gonococcal arthritis-dermatitis syndrome. Patients with Reiter's syndrome present with urethritis, conjunctivitis, arthritis, and a psoriasis-like cutaneous eruption; patients with Reiter's syndrome do not demonstrate petechiae, macules, papules, or maculopapules.

The diagnosis of DGI is made in the sexually active patient with complaints of tenosynovitis, arthralgias, and the appropriate dermatologic findings. Gram's stain of fluid from unroofed lesions may demonstrate *Neisseria gonorrhoeae.* Blood cultures may be positive with an increased yield in the early phase of illness with active bacteremia, and urethral or cervical specimens can be obtained for culture or gonococcal antigen. Cultures of the various mucosal surfaces—i.e., cervical and vaginal—are frequently sterile in the patient with disseminated disease states. Antimicrobial agents of choice include ceftriaxone and ciprofloxacin; spectinomycin may be used in patients with intolerance to the initial treatment choices. Treatment regimens include ceftriaxone 1 g intravenously daily for seven doses or parenteral ciprofloxacin over a similar duration.

ROCKY MOUNTAIN SPOTTED FEVER

Rocky Mountain spotted fever, a potentially fatal multisystem illness caused by *Rickettsia rickettsii,* is introduced to humans via the tick vector. Without adequate, timely management, the mortality rate increases to 50 percent. After introduction of the organism to body tissues, it disseminates via the blood stream and invades vascular endothelium causing a necrotizing vasculitis. Constitutional symptoms of fever, headache, and myalgias develop about one week after exposure. The rash in classic RMSF is evident 4 days (range: 1 to 15 days) after the onset of fever and other symptoms. In a minority of patients, usually the adult, the rash is not noted during the entire disease course. This entity, Rocky Mountain ''spotless'' fever, occurs in approximately 15 percent of cases.

The rash first appears on the wrists and ankles, and rapidly spreads to the palms and soles [Fig. 241-9 (Plate 35)]. As the rash moves centrally, the proximal extremities, trunk, and face are involved. The skin lesions at onset are described as discrete macules or maculopapules that blanch with pressure. The initial lesions evolve into petechiae over two to four days, fade slowly over two to three weeks, and heal occasionally with resultant hyperpigmentation. Rarely, the petechiae may coalesce into ecchymotic areas with eventual gangrene of the distal extremities, nose, ear lobes, scrotum, and vulva—purpura fulmi-

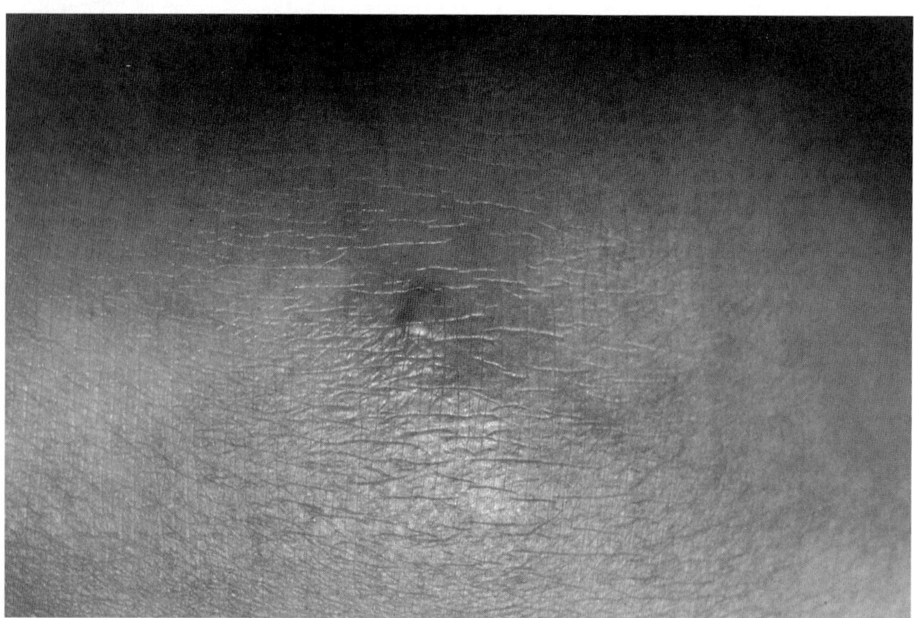

FIG. 241-8 (Plate 34). Disseminated gonococcal infection in a sexually active adult female; note maculopapule with a petechial component and an erythematous periphery located on the extensor surface of the wrist.

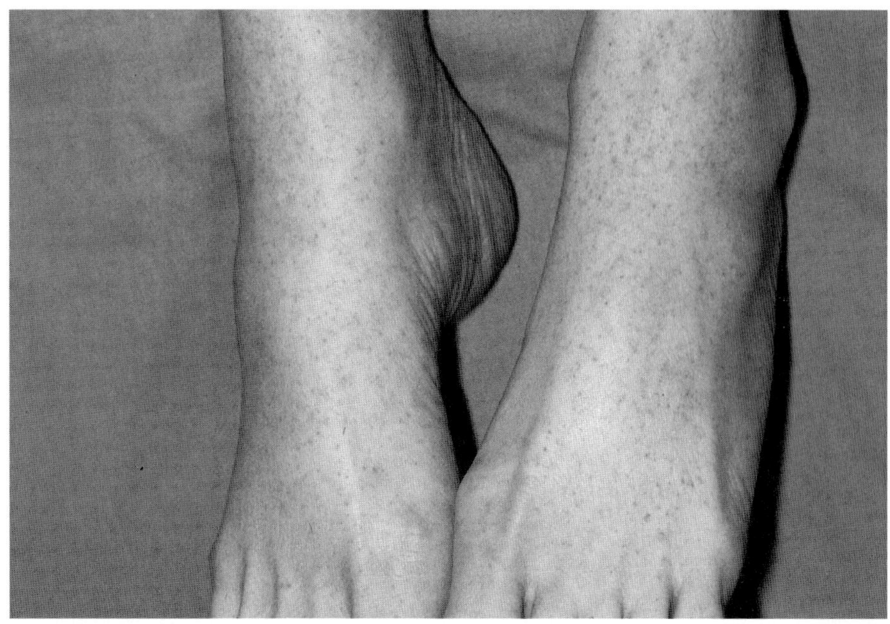

FIG. 241-9 (Plate 35). A patient with Rocky Mountain spotted fever revealing petechiae on the ankles.

nans. For further discussion of the treatment of this and other tick borne diseases, see Chap. 145.

MENINGOCOCCEMIA

Meningococcemia is a potentially fatal infectious illness caused by the gram-negative diplococcus *Neisseria meningitidis*. Meningococcal disease presents across a wide clinical spectrum in both acute and chronic forms. The acute entities include pharyngitis, meningitis, and bacteremia. Meningococci are present in the nasopharynx of 2 to 20 percent of the general population (the carrier state); during epidemics, the organism is found in up to 30 percent of people without evidence of active disease.

The illness usually strikes patients younger than 20 years of age with the vast majority of cases occurring in children and infants younger than 5 years of age. Epidemic outbreaks occur when a particularly virulent strain of the organism is introduced into a closed, confined population. The highest rates of infection are reported in the winter and spring months, although sporadic cases appear throughout the year. The organism is transmitted through aerosolized droplets of respiratory secretions from asymptomatic carriers and less frequently from actively infected patients. The mortality rate ranges from 5 to 28 percent, although most patients treated appropriately early in the disease course recover. Patients with acute meningococcal infection who exhibit signs of circulatory insufficiency, a peripheral white blood cell count of less than 10,000 cells/μL, or a coagulopathy have a high probability of developing organ system failure followed by death.[18,19]

After exposure to the organism, clinical infection develops usually within 3 to 4 days (range: 2 to 10 days) and progresses rapidly to severe illness. The patient may complain of severe headache, sudden

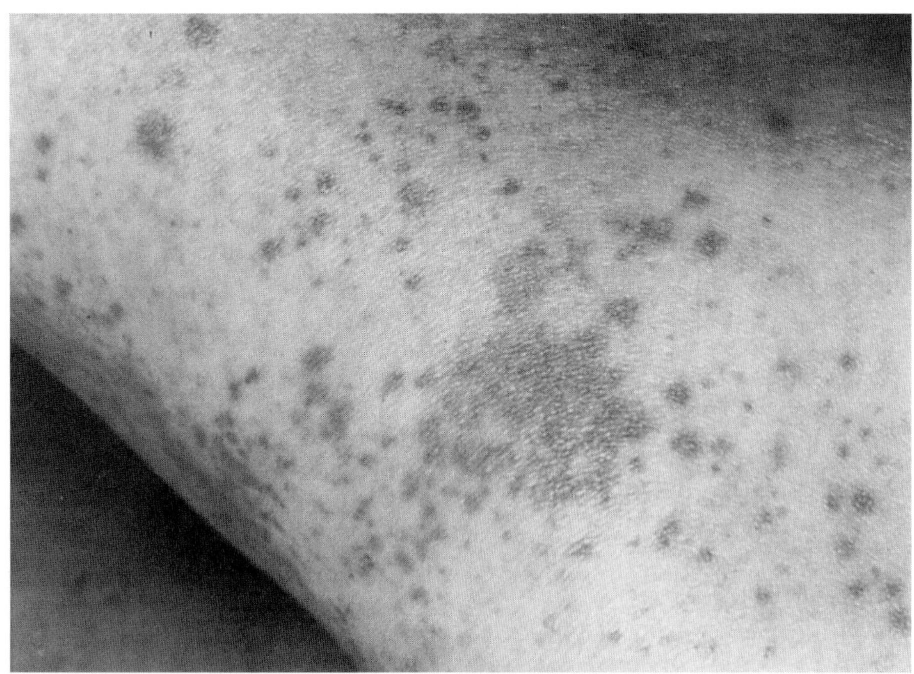

FIG. 241-10 (Plate 36). Early findings of meningococcemia with petechiae evolving into purpuric lesions. (Reprinted with permission from Brady W, DeBehnke D, Crosby D: Dermatologic emergencies. *Am J Emerg Med* 12:217, 1994.)

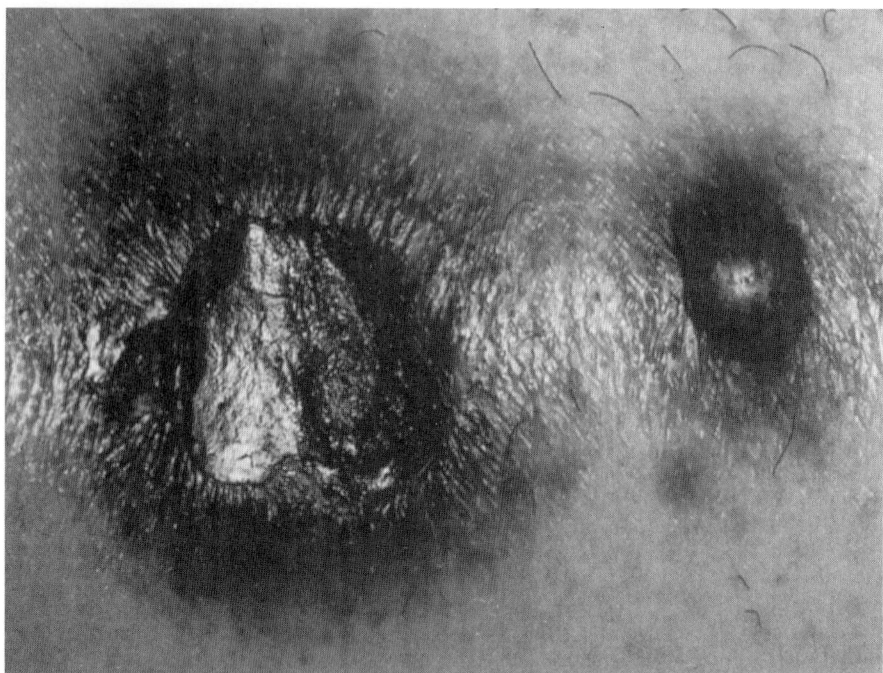

FIG. 241-11 (Plate 37). Purpura fulminans with hemorrhagic bullae. (Reprinted with permission from Tangoren IA et al: Ecchymoses and epidermal necrosis in a 75-year-old man with bacteremia. *J Crit Illness* 13:108, 1998.)

fever, altered mental status, nausea, vomiting, myalgias, arthralgia, and a stiff neck. A rash is frequently noted on presentation and is an invaluable clue to the correct diagnosis early in the disease course. The dermatological manifestations include petechia, urticaria, hemorrhagic vesicles, macules, and/or maculopapules [Fig. 241-10 (Plate 36)]. The classic petechial lesions are found on the extremities and trunk but also are noted on the palms, soles, head, and mucous membranes. The petechiae evolve into palpable purpura with gray necrotic centers, a pathognomic finding for meningococcal infection. The skin findings result from the organism's invasion and destruction of the endothelium. Histopathologic analysis shows an infectious vasculitis.

Fulminant meningococcal disease is found in less than 5 percent of patients, and presents with sudden prostration, petechiae with areas of ecchymosis, and distributive shock. This rapidly progressive version of meningococcemia is complicated by purpura fulminans, a severe form of disseminated intravascular coagulation. Large ecchymotic areas (usually the extremities, acral portions of the face, and genitalia) become necrotic or gangrenous.[18,19]

The diagnosis of acute meningococcal disease relies on recognition of an ill-appearing patient with an associated petechial rash and the nonspecific symptoms of fever, headache, altered sensorium, and body aches. Additional historical points, physical findings, and laboratory results supportive of the diagnosis include known exposure to active disease; rapid progression of nonspecific symptoms with the associated petechial rash; Gram's stain of skin lesions or cerebral spinal fluid demonstrating gram-negative intracellular diplococci; and latex agglu-

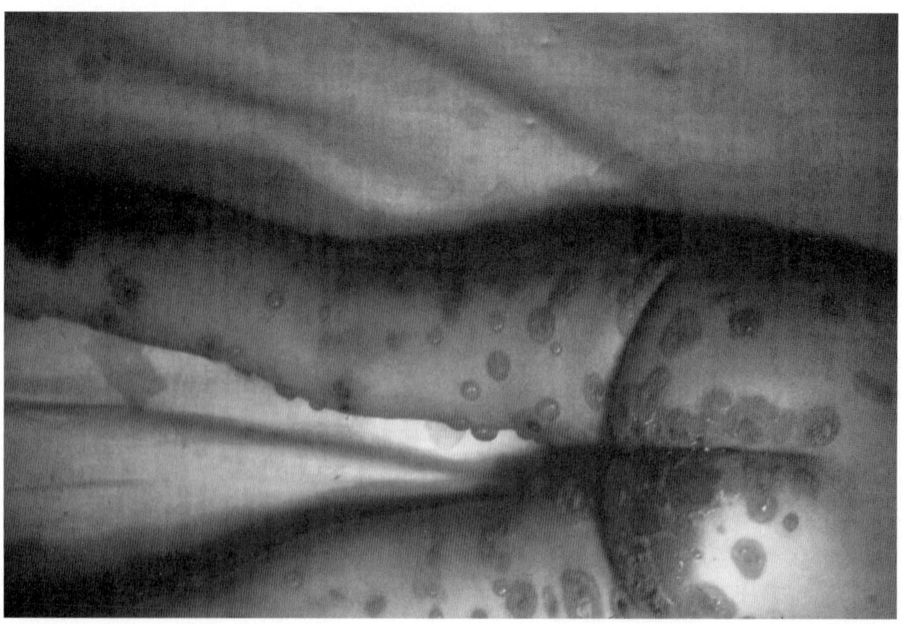

FIG. 241-12 (Plate 38). Scattered bullous lesions intermixed with erosions and painful inflammatory plaques.

tination of the cerebrospinal fluid. The differential diagnosis includes RMSF, TSS, acute gonococcemia, bacterial endocarditis, vasculitis (Henoch-Schönlein purpura or leukocytoclastic vasculitis), enteroviral infections, and bacterial sepsis (gram-positive and gram-negative) with disseminated intravascular coagulation.

Antibiotics must be given as soon as possible in a patient suspected of acute disease. In adults, an appropriate agent is ceftriaxone; due to the increased prevalence of cephalosporin-resistant pneumococcus, parenteral vancomycin is also often empirically given.

PURPURA FULMINANS

Purpura fulminans (PF) is a rare vascular disorder that is characterized by fever, shock, multiorgan failure, and the rapid development of hemorrhagic skin necrosis. It is associated with dermal vascular thrombosis resulting from vascular collapse and disseminated intravascular coagulation (DIC). Purpura fulminans can result from hereditary or acquired protein C deficiency, activated protein C resistance, or protein S deficiency. It may also result from any condition that causes DIC.

Purpura fulminans presents with the dermatologic triad of widespread ecchymoses, hemorrhagic bullae [Fig. 241-11 (Plate 37)], and epidermal necrosis. Commonly, cyanosis with initial ecchymoses and ultimate necrosis of the tip of the nose, ears, and genitalia frequently occur; in general, distal tissue areas with end-circulation are affected. Large confluent ecchymoses can develop, often on the extremities—from distal to proximal—as well as on the perineum, buttocks, and abdomen. The extremities are often involved symmetrically. Treatment is directed at the underlying cause.

BULLOUS DISEASES (Pemphigus Vulgaris and Bullous Pemphigoid)

Pemphigus vulgaris (PV) is a generalized, mucocutaneous, autoimmune, blistering eruption with a grave prognosis characterized by intraepidermal acantholytic blistering. Bullous pemphigoid (BP) is a generalized mucocutaneous blistering disease of the elderly, with an average age of 70 years at the time of initial diagnosis.[20,21] Although the blisters are deeper in the skin than in PV (below the epidermal basement membrane), the prognosis of BP is better with less associated comorbidity and a significantly more rapid response to therapy.[20,21]

The primary lesions of PV are vesicles or bullae [Fig. 241-12 (Plate 38)] that vary in diameter from less than 1 cm to several centimeters; they commonly first affect the head, trunk, and mucous membranes.[20,21] The blisters are usually clear and tense, originating from normal skin or atop an erythematous or urticarial plaque. Within two to three days, the bullae become turbid and flaccid. Rupture soon follows, producing painful, denuded areas. These erosions are slow to heal and prone to secondary infection. Nikolsky's sign is invariably positive in PV and absent in other autoimmune blistering diseases. Mucous membranes are affected in 95 percent of PV patients; in as many as 25 percent, the mucous membranes are the primary sites of involvement. Blisters on mucous membranes are more transitory than blisters on the skin in that they are more vulnerable to rupture; this is particularly true in the mouth, where ragged ulcerative lesions readily develop after inadvertent biting of the tissues.

BP is characterized by the presence of tense blisters (up to 10 cm in diameter) that arise from either normal skin or from erythematous or urticarial plaques; ulceration with tissue loss follows. Sites of predilection include the intertriginous and flexural areas. Pruritus, occasionally accompanied by a burning sensation, is noted with the appearance of the blistering. Lesions of the oral cavity occur in BP, but with less consistency and severity than in PV. Because the blisters in the oral cavity rupture very easily and heal without scarring, involvement in the mouth is often overlooked. Oral involvement may occur in as many as 40 percent of patients. It is unusual for oral mucosal lesions to precede the cutaneous eruption as in PV.

The differential diagnosis of PV and BP includes the vesiculobullous diseases; dermatologic consultation is required for diagnosis.

Limited oral intake and accelerated protein, fluid, and electrolyte losses through the involved skin can rapidly lead to hypoalbuminemia with significant hypovolemia and electrolyte disturbances in both PV and BP; therefore, dermatologic consultation is advised for treatment and disposition.

REFERENCES

1. Rzany B, Hering O, Mockenhaupt M, et al: Histopathological and epidemiological characteristics of patients with erythema exudativum multiforme major, Stevens-Johnson syndrome and toxic epidermal necrolysis. *Br J Dermatol* 135:6, 1996.
2. Paquet P, Pierard GE: Erythema multiforme and toxic epidermal necrolysis: A comparative study. *Am J Dermatopathol* 19:127, 1997.
3. Weston WL, Morelli JG: Herpes simplex virus-associated erythema multiforme in prepubertal children. *Arch Pediatr Adolesc Med* 151:1014, 1997.
4. Kakourou T, Klontza D, Soteropoulou F, Kattamis C: Corticosteroid treatment of erythema multiforme major (Stevens-Johnson syndrome) in children. *Eur J Pediatr* 156:90, 1997.
5. Guillaume JC, Roujeau JC, Revuz J, et al: The culprit drugs in 87 cases of toxic epidermal necrolysis (Lyell's syndrome). *Arch Dermatol* 123:1166, 1987.
6. Porteous DM, Berger TG: Severe cutaneous drug reactions (Stevens-Johnson syndrome and toxic epidermal necrolysis) in human immunodeficiency virus infection. *Arch Dermatol* 127:740, 1991.
7. Kelemen JJ, Cioffi WG, McManus WF, Mason AD, Pruitt BA: Burn center care for patients with toxic epidermal necrolysis. *J Am Col Surg* 180:273, 1995.
8. Roujeau JC, Kelly JP, Naldi L, et al: Medication use and the risk of Stevens-Johnson syndrome or toxic epidermal necrolysis. *N Engl J Med* 333:1600, 1995.
9. Wolkenstein P, Charue D, Laurent P, Revuz J, Roujeau JC, Bagot M: Metabolic predisposition to cutaneous adverse drug reactions: Role in toxic epidermal necrolysis caused by sulfonamides and anticonvulsants. *Arch Dermatol* 131:544, 1995.
10. Wong KS, Wong SM, Tham SM, et al: Generalized exfoliative dermatitis: A clinical study of 108 patients. *Ann Acad Med* 17:520, 1988.
11. Freedman JD, Beer DJ: Expanding perspectives on the toxic shock syndrome. *Adv Intern Med* 36:363, 1991.
12. Hoge CW, Schwartz B, Talkington DF, et al: National Centers for Disease Control and Prevention: The changing epidemiology of invasive group A streptococcal infections and the emergence of streptococcal toxic shock-like syndrome: A retrospective population-based study. *JAMA* 269:384, 1993.
13. The Working Group in Severe Streptococcal Infections: Defining the group A streptococcal toxic shock syndrome: Rationale and consensus definition. *JAMA* 269:390–391, 1993.
14. Resnick SD: Staphylococcal toxin-mediated syndromes in childhood. *Semin Dermatol* 11:11, 1992.
15. Friedman-Kein AE: Herpes zoster: A possible early clinical sign for the development of acquired immunodeficiency syndrome in high-risk individuals. *J Am Acad Dermatol* 14:1023, 1986.
16. Goh CL, Khoo L: A retrospective study of the clinical presentation and outcome of herpes zoster in a tertiary dermatology outpatient referral clinic. *Int J Dermatol* 36:667, 1997.
17. Novelli VM, Atherton DJ, Marshall WC: Eczema herpeticum: Clinical and laboratory features. *Ann Intern Med* 27:231, 1988.
18. Tesoro LJ, Selbst SM: Factors affecting outcome in meningococcal infection. *Am J Dis Child* 145:218, 1991.
19. Algren JT, Lal S, Cutliff SA, et al: Predictors of outcome in acute meningococcal infection in children. *Crit Care Med* 21:447, 1993.
20. Seidenbaum M, David M, Sandbank M: The course and prognosis of pemphigus: A review of 115 patients. *Int J Dermatol* 27:580, 1988.
21. Venning VA, Frith PA, Bron AJ, et al: Mucosal involvement in bullous and cicatricial pemphigoid. A clinical and immunopathological study. *Br J Dermatol* 118:7, 1988.

INFESTATIONS AND BUG BITES

Lisa May

HUMAN SCABIES

Human scabies is an infestation of the skin by *Sarcoptes scabiei.* Human scabies occurs worldwide and affects all races and social classes. It is a quite common disorder, accounting for approximately 2 percent of all dermatologic visits in the United States. The mite is transmitted from human to human by close physical contact. Although children and young adults are most commonly affected, infestation may occur at any age.

Pathophysiology

The scabetic mite resides in a burrow within the stratum corneum, the most superficial layer of the epidermis. Most individuals have an average of 12 mites at any given time. When the mite burden becomes high, numbering in the millions, a crusted form of scabies develops. This is called Norwegian scabies. It is most commonly seen in association with an immunocompromised state, particularly HIV; mental retardation; dementia; or physical disability. The time from infestation to clinical symptoms is about 3 to 4 weeks.

Clinical Features

Scabies tends to be an extremely pruritic eruption, often disturbing sleep (except Norwegian scabies, which tends to have minimal associated pruritus). The most common sites of involvement include the hands, feet, flexural surfaces of the elbows and knees, umbilicus, groin, and genitals. Facial involvement is usually seen only in infants. The pathognomonic lesion, or burrow, is a fine erythematous linear or curved lesion with central scale (Fig. 242-1). Burrows are most often visible in the web spaces of the fingers, the lateral aspects of the fingers, the volar surface of the wrists, the instep of the feet, and the shaft of the penis. Often, however, burrows are not present, especially in patients with excellent hygiene. Excoriations and pruritic papules may be the only visible cutaneous feature. Vesicles are often seen in infants and young children.

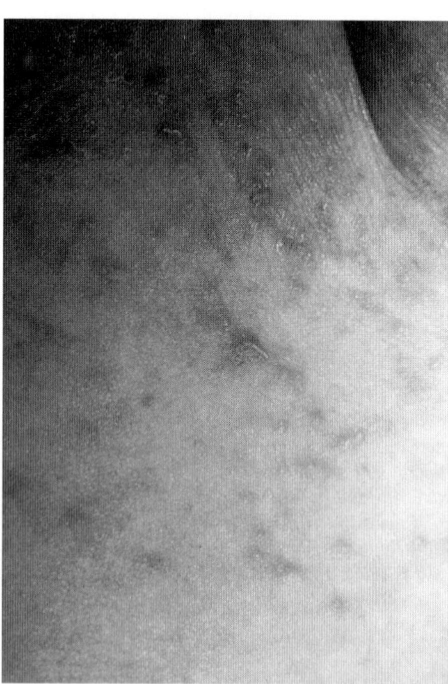

FIG. 242-1. Human scabies. Numerous scabetic burrows are visible near the axilla of this infant infested with scabies.

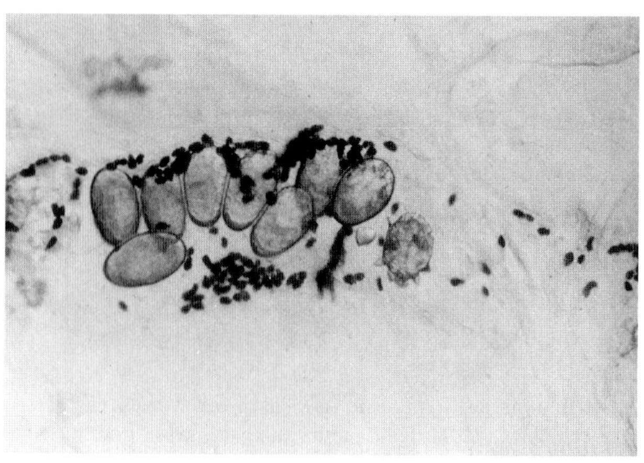

FIG. 242-2. Scabies preparation. The immature mite, ova, and scybala (fecal pellets) are present in this scraping of a burrow. The presence of any one of these elements is considered a positive scabies preparation result.

In Norwegian scabies (Fig. 239-9), one develops thick, dirty-appearing hyperkeratosis on the hands and feet. The nails are often affected as well. Because of the large mite burden, this form of scabies is highly contagious.

Diagnosis

The diagnosis is based on a high clinical suspicion and a positive scabies preparation. The diagnosis should be entertained when more than one family member itches. Other disorders to consider in the differential diagnosis include other bite reactions, body lice, atopic dermatitis, neurotic excoriations, and delusions of parasitosis. Suspected cases of scabies should be confirmed by performing a scabies preparation. To perform a scabies preparation, one scrapes or superficially shaves a lesion (preferably a burrow) with a 15 blade. The sample is placed on a glass slide, covered with immersion oil and a cover slip, and examined under the microscope. Mites, eggs, or scybala (feces) will be visible (Fig. 242-2). When possible, the diagnosis should be confirmed with a scraping prior to treatment.

Treatment

Topical scabicides are the treatments of choice. The topical preparation should be applied from the neck down to the feet, with special attention paid to applying the lotion around and under fingernails, in the web spaces of the fingers and toes, and in the umbilicus.

Permethrin 5% cream (Elimite) and lindane 1% lotion (Kwell) are equally effective. Either preparation should be left on overnight and rinsed off the following morning. Lindane is easier to apply and less expensive than permethrin, but lindane resistance has been reported. Furthermore, because of reports of neurotoxicity with the use of lindane in infants, this medication should not be used in children under 6 years of age or in pregnant women. Patients with extensive involvement should be treated again in 1 week.

All household members and sexual contacts at high risk of acquiring scabies should be treated concurrently even if they are asymptomatic, since a delay from the time of infestation to the development of symptoms exists. Nursing homes, institutions, hospital staff, and schools should be notified, and any symptomatic individuals should be treated. Bed linens, towels, and clothing should be washed and dried in a dryer on high heat.

Since pruritus is a common complaint, antihistamines, such as diphenhydramine hydrochloride (Benadryl) or hydroxyzine, should be prescribed as well. A mid-potency topical corticosteroid may also provide relief from itching. In addition, obvious secondary bacterial infection should be treated with an antistaphylococcal agent.

Disposition

Patients should be educated that itching may take weeks to subside. If they are still symptomatic in 2 weeks, they should seek follow-up for repeat evaluation and treatment.

PEDICULOSIS

Pediculosis capitis (head lice) is an infestation of the hair and scalp by the mite *Pediculus capitis. Pediculus corporis* is the body louse, and pubic lice is an infestation of the pubic hair by *Phthirus pubis.*

Head Lice

This disorder is most commonly seen in school-aged children or in children attending day-care centers. However, any age group can be affected. It is very uncommon in African Americans. The louse is passed from person to person via close contact. The organism may live away from a host on furniture, clothing, linens, hats, or hairbrushes for several weeks, and thus may be passed to another who comes in contact with these articles.

PATHOPHYSIOLOGY Head lice feed off human blood and therefore remain close to the scalp. When the louse lays its eggs, the ova, or nits, are cemented to the hair shaft. The ova hatch within 7 days. The ova encasement remains attached to the hair shaft and grows out with the hair. By the time the nits are a distance of 1 cm or more away from scalp, they have probably hatched.

CLINICAL FEATURES The patient usually experiences pruritus. This itching may be mild or quite intense. The occiput and posterior neck are common sites of pruritus, and excoriations on the neck may be noted.

DIAGNOSIS The diagnosis is made on clinical inspection of the scalp for lice and nits (Fig. 242-3). Unlike flakes of scale, which can easily be moved up and down the hair shaft, nits are firmly attached to the shaft. If the diagnosis is in question, suspected organisms or ova can be viewed underneath a microscope.

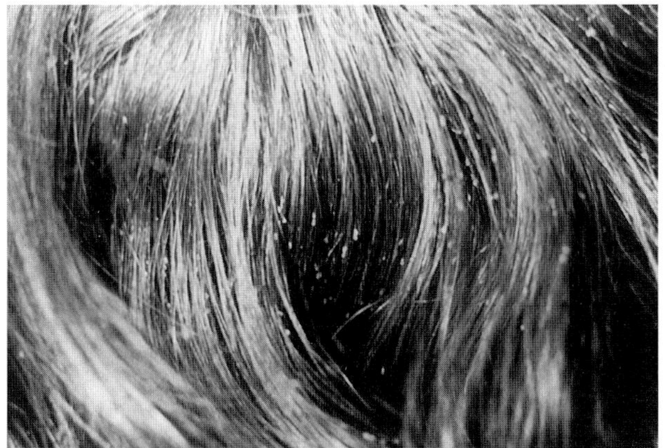

FIG. 242-3. Head lice. Nits are clearly visible, firmly attached to the hair shafts.

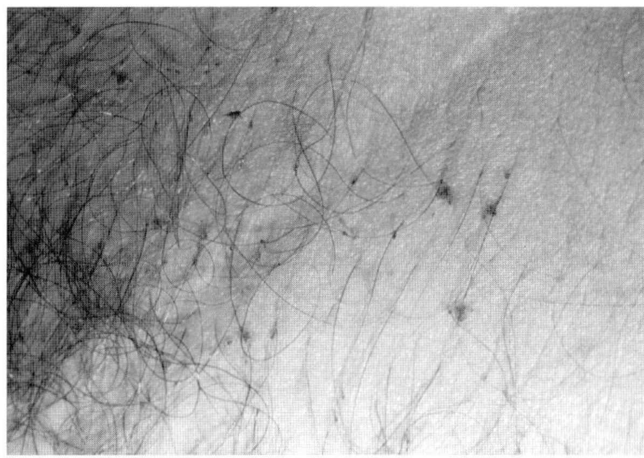

FIG. 242-4. Pubic lice. Pubic lice are seen on the skin surface, and nits are attached to the pubic hairs.

TREATMENT Two important aspects of treatment should be addressed: treating the current infection and preventing reinfestation. Several agents may be used to treat the infestation. Permethrin 1% (Nix) rinse should be used as first-line therapy. Unlike lindane and pyrethrins, permethrin is ovacidal as well as pediculicidal. After shampooing, the treatment should be applied to the scalp for 10 min. For cosmetic reasons, nits can be removed by rinsing the hair in a 50% vinegar solution and then combing the hair with a fine-toothed comb.

To prevent reinfestation, all close contacts should be examined and affected individuals treated, including family members, classmates at school or day care, roommates, or health care workers in an institutional setting. Schools and day-care centers should be notified so that appropriate measures can be undertaken to evaluate other individuals.

Clothing, hats, and bed linens should be washed with hot water and dried in a dryer on high heat for 20 to 30 min. Carpets and sofas should be thoroughly vacuumed. Hairbrushes should be washed in hot water with the pediculicide product.

Patients should be reexamined in 7 to 10 days.

Pediculosis Pubis

In general, pubic lice is a sexually transmitted disease. Rarely, it may be passed from person to person via infested clothing, bed linens, and so on. Affected individuals should be evaluated for other sexually transmitted diseases. One report indicated that as many as 30 percent of individuals with pubic lice have another sexually transmitted disease. In children, the possibility of sexual abuse should be considered.

As with head lice, the main complaint with pubic lice is itching, which may vary in intensity. Pubic hair of the groin is most commonly infested, but body hair and eyelashes may be affected as well. Close inspection reveals the lice and nits (Fig. 242-4).

Treatment involves the same medications as for head lice, listed above. Permethrin (Nix) is the preferred initial therapy and should be applied to the affected area for 10 min and then rinsed. Eyelash infestations should be treated by manually removing as many lice and nits as possible and then applying petrolatum to the lashes two to three times a day for 10 days.

Pediculosis Corporis

Body lice is currently uncommon in the United States. Infestation is more likely to occur in persons with poor hygiene or overcrowded living conditions. The lice reside on hair-bearing areas of the body but attach their nits to clothing. The lice and nits can survive as long as 30 days without contact with a human host. Clinically, the bite is often not perceived by an individual but leaves a pruritic red urticarial papule. This lesion is not distinguishable from other bite reactions. A clue to diagnosis is that areas not covered by clothing, such as the face and hands, are usually spared. A high index of suspicion is needed, especially in patients with poor hygiene. Close inspection of clothing reveals nits, especially along clothing seams.

The body louse is the vector for epidemic typhus fever (*Rickettsia prowazekii*), trench fever (*Rickettsia quintana*), and relapsing fever (*Borrelia recurrentis*).

Treatment is similar to that for head or pubic lice. Since the nits can survive long periods without human contact, infested clothing and linens should preferably be destroyed. If not, recommendations include washing and drying on hot cycles and ironing the seams of the textiles. Oral antihistamines and topical corticosteriods may be necessary when itching is severe. Secondary infection, if present, should be treated.

SPIDER BITES

Although spiders are ubiquitous and instill fear in many individuals, significant disease is very uncommon. Numerous spiders may bite, leaving an urticarial papule with two central puncture wounds. Only the bites of two types of spiders in the United States result in significant reactions: *Loxosceles reclusa* (the brown recluse spider) and *Latrodectus mactans* (the black widow spider).

Brown Recluse Spider Bites

As the name implies, the brown recluse spider is a reclusive organism. Humans encounter this spider in attics, storage sheds, crawl spaces, and woodpiles. Encounters with humans are uncommon.

PATHOPHYSIOLOGY Brown recluse spiders are not aggressive and bite humans in self-defense. The venom results in epidermal and subcutaneous necrosis. This reaction is a local process around the bite site.

CLINICAL FEATURES Because the bite itself is painless, patients cannot recall being bitten. Only a history of potential exposure can be elucidated. Rarely does a patient see the bite or capture the spider. About 6 to 8 h after the bite, pain associated with a red-to-violaceous discoloration develops. Two central puncture wounds are often visible on close inspection. Initially, the bite site may look like a bruise. It may even form a bulla. Over the next several hours to days, necrosis of the skin and subcutis will occur (Fig. 242-5). This reaction may remain localized or spread to 25 cm in diameter. The spread is in a gravitational direction. Healing is very slow and results in scarring. Secondary infection is common.

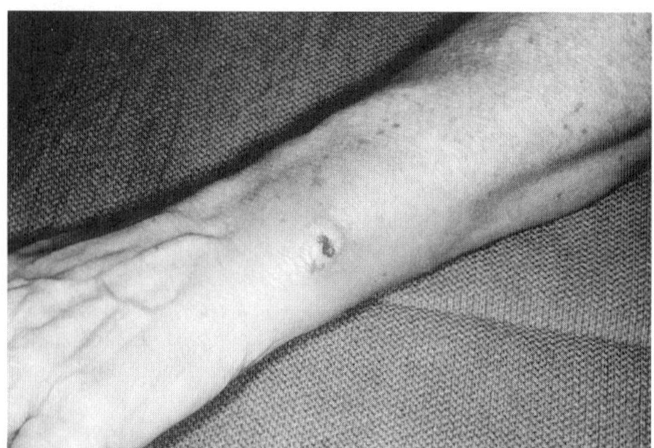

FIG. 242-5. Brown recluse spider bite. A central area of necrosis with surrounding erythema is noted.

Systemic symptoms are unlikely, but if they occur, the victim experiences fever, malaise, nausea, vomiting, hemolytic anemia, thrombocytopenia, disseminated intravascular coagulation, seizures, and coma.

DIAGNOSIS Diagnosis is based on history of potential exposure and clinical course. The spider varies from tan to dark brown and has a violin-shaped marking on its back. It ranges from 0.2 to 2.5 cm in length. Because of the distinct marking, the brown recluse spider is often known as the violin or fiddle-back spider.

The differential diagnosis includes necrotizing fasciitis, pyoderma gangrenosum, toxic reactions to other biting organisms, and infectious processes.

TREATMENT Initial treatment includes elevation of the affected area, inactivity, and ice compresses to decrease erythema and edema and prevent the spread of venom. Additional treatment for brown recluse spider bites is controversial and includes dapsone, débridement and skin grafting, and systemic corticosteroids. For small areas of involvement, observation and prevention of secondary infection are recommended. Dapsone, a leukocyte inhibitor, has been reported to prevent progression. Dapsone doses should begin at 25 mg twice daily. Patients should be monitored closely for side effects, including hemolysis and agranulocytosis. Dapsone should not be prescribed to individuals with glucose-6-phosphate dehydrogenase deficiency.

Débridement and skin grafting should be delayed until wounds have stabilized, since the venom may delay wound healing. The role of systemic corticosteriods is also controversial. They are recommended for systemic symptoms. Consultation by a dermatologist or other physician with experience in bite reactions should be sought to rule out other potential causes and determine the most appropriate course of therapy. Outpatient management with close follow-up is appropriate for mild-to-moderate cases. Extensive necrosis, rapid progression, or systemic symptoms may require close monitoring in a hospital setting.

Black Widow Spider Bites

Black widow spider bites are rare but serious. Black widow spiders live in webs close to the ground in secluded areas, such as under rocks or logs or in barns, sheds, or outhouses. Only female black widow spiders are capable of envenomation.

CLINICAL FEATURES The bite of a black widow spider may or may not be painful. Black widow spiders release a neurotoxic venom upon biting the victim. Local reaction is minimal, with mild erythema and edema. Within 20 to 40 min of the bite, the victim begins to develop muscle cramps locally and then generally. A painful, rigid abdomen, mimicking an acute abdomen, is seen. Other systemic symptoms include nausea, vomiting, anxiety, diaphoresis, respiratory distress, urinary retention, hypertension, shock, and coma. In less than 1 percent of cases, death results. Symptoms generally peak in 2 to 3 h and resolve over 2 to 3 days.

DIAGNOSIS Diagnosis is based on potential exposure, clinical history, or identification of the organism. The red hourglass marking on the undersurface of its abdomen readily identifies the spider.

TREATMENT In most cases, treatment is supportive. Muscle relaxants and intravenous calcium gluconate may be useful. Narcotics and benzodiazepines should be used judiciously for pain relief. Antivenin (Lyovac) is available but should be reserved for those at greatest risk of morbidity, including the very young, the elderly, pregnant women, and those with cardiovascular disease. Since the antivenin is a horse serum preparation, risks include anaphylaxis and serum sickness.

TICK BITES

Tick bites are common in the United States and are vectors for several serious systemic diseases, including Rocky Mountain spotted fever, Lyme disease, ehrlichiosis, and tularemia. These diseases are discussed elsewhere in this text.

The bite of a tick is usually painless. It may become pruritic over time. Through the mouth parts, the tick cements itself to the skin to obtain a blood meal. As a result, ticks are difficult to remove from the skin. A tick can be recognized as a dark-brown to black organism firmly adherent to the skin. It enlarges as its body becomes engorged with the host's blood. The best approach to removing a tick is to grasp it with tweezers as close to the skin as possible and gently pull with steady pressure. Methods such as burning the tick with a flame, pouring alcohol on it, or covering it with petroleum jelly will not dislodge the tick. If the entire tick is not removed, the patient may develop a foreign-body reaction, which is best treated by excision of the area.

OTHER BITES

Numerous other organisms bite and sting. Common bites include those of mosquitoes, chiggers, fleas, bedbugs, and flies. Some of these insects are disease vectors, and such diseases are discussed elsewhere in this text. The type and distribution of the lesion produced provide hints as to the causative insect.

For instance, mosquitoes and flies tend to bite exposed skin, producing urticarial pruritic papules. Chiggers (''red bugs'') are mites that dwell on the ground. They crawl up clothing and bite in high-temperature areas, usually around elastic bands of socks, shirts, and pants. Their bite produces an intensely itchy papule or vesicle. Fleas jump from the ground or furniture. Thus, their bites are seen on the exposed areas around the ankles. Flea bites may be papular or vesicular. Bedbugs reside within walls and mattresses of homes or hotels and tend to bite victims in rows of three (''breakfast, lunch, and dinner bites''). Insects that bite, but not those that sting, may be repelled by insect repellent, such as diethyltoluamide (DEET). Symptomatic treatment, if necessary, consists of topical corticosteriods and oral antihistamines.

HYMENOPTERA STINGS

Hymenoptera includes bees, wasps, hornets, and fire ants. When provoked, these insects inject their stinger into the victim. Bees can only sting once, but yellow jackets, other wasps, and hornets can sting repeatedly. The sting is initially very painful. Local erythema and swelling occur. Local and systemic hypersensitivity reactions can also occur. Local hypersensitivity reactions result in exaggerated swelling. If the sting occurs around the mouth or neck, airway compromise may result. Systemic hypersensitivity is an anaphylactic response, and its recognition and treatment are discussed elsewhere in this textbook.

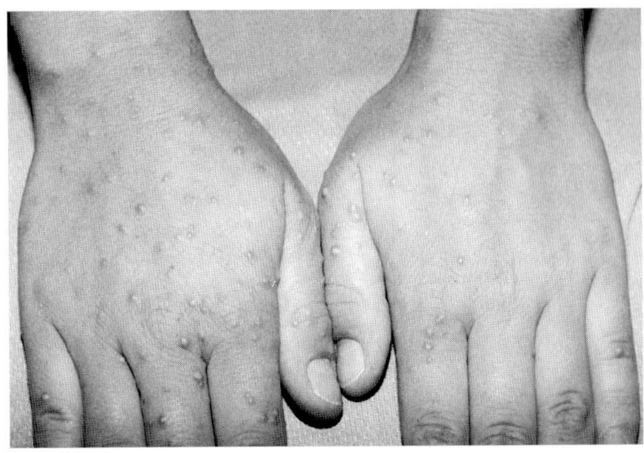

FIG. 242-6. Fire ant bites. This individual unknowingly disturbed a fire ant mound. She received numerous painful stings that developed into pustules with an erythematous base.

Fire ants are seen in the southern United States but continue to migrate northward. They dwell in mounds on the ground. When the mound is disturbed, numerous fire ants rapidly run out of the mound. As a result, the victim is usually stung by many fire ants simultaneously. Each ant can sting repeatedly. Anaphylaxis has been reported following fire ant bites. Their sting is very painful and results in a pustule with an erythematous base (Fig. 242-6).

Initial treatment of hymenoptera stings includes removing the stinger as quickly as possible, since the stinger continues to release venom. A lateral motion with a knife, fingernail, or credit card is preferred over trying to pull the stinger straight out. Elevation and ice compresses can prevent further swelling.

BIBLIOGRAPHY

Goddard J: *Physicians Guide to Arthropods of Medical Importance,* 2d ed. Boca Raton, FL, CRC Press, 1996.

INITIAL APPROACH TO TRAUMA

Edward E. Cornwell III

Trauma in America remains a major public health challenge, accounting for nearly 150,000 deaths each year and an enormous burden to both the health care system and the economy in general. Injury is the fourth leading killer of Americans and the single greatest cause of death before the age of 45. Trauma causes more deaths among children and adolescents (ages 1 to 19) than all diseases combined. Apart from the loss of life, the economic burden (>$100 billion annually) and the number of years of life lost before age 65 (>4.1 million) due to traumatic injury exceed those same measures due to cancer and heart disease combined.[1–3]

TRAUMA SYSTEMS

The importance of a systems approach to trauma care becomes clear when one considers the timing of death occurring secondary to traumatic injuries. The pattern of mortality takes on roughly a trimodal distribution where three peak occurrences are seen. The first peak occurs in the prehospital setting largely due to devastating head and major vascular injuries. Efforts to reduce deaths in this setting are largely societal, complex, and multidisciplinary and include such multifaceted activities as drunk driving laws; safe road construction; seat belt, helmet, and airbag laws; and violence-prevention activities such as counseling, education and outreach efforts, handgun control, and dissemination of conflict resolution skills.[4,5] A second peak incidence of deaths due to traumatic injuries occurs in the early minutes and hours after a patient's arrival at the hospital. Deaths in this peak are largely due to major head, chest, and abdominal injuries. Attempts to decrease deaths in this setting are largely aimed at rapid transport of patients to the most appropriate facility and prompt resuscitation and identification of injuries requiring surgical intervention. This is the most important function of a trauma system. The third peak in the trimodal distribution of deaths occurs in the intensive care unit where the sequelae of organ hypoperfusion experienced in the early postinjury period are seen. Specifically, patients who have survived the initial injury, transport, and operative resuscitation die in this setting as a result of the systemic inflammatory response syndrome and multisystem organ failure.

In recognition of the need to establish a system where injured patients are rapidly triaged to the most appropriate setting, Congress passed the Trauma Care Systems Planning and Development Act of 1990.[2] This act required each state to develop a Model Trauma Care System Plan to be used as the reference document. Since this act did not carry with it specific appropriated funds, the level of implementation has varied from state to state. Ultimately, each state must determine the appropriate facility for various types of injuries, and some states have come to rely on a verification process offered by the American College of Surgeons in order to designate certain hospitals as trauma centers.[6] An effective trauma system requires the teamwork of emergency medicine, trauma surgery, and trauma care subspecialists.

While each state ultimately has responsibility for designating trauma centers, some have come to rely on the guidelines of the American College of Surgeons.[7] Examples of requirements of various levels of trauma centers are listed in Table 243-1. In addition to the listed essentials, a trauma center must have all the required features of lower-level trauma centers.

In short, trauma centers are verified on the basis of commitment of personnel and resources needed to maintain a state of readiness to receive critically injured patients. A well-functioning trauma system ensures that *not only are there appropriately designated trauma centers but also specific triage criteria to designate which patients should be transported to these centers* (Table 243-2).

PRIMARY SURVEY

In accordance with the principles of advanced trauma life support, injured patients are assessed and treated in a fashion that establishes priorities based on their presenting vital signs, mental status, and injury mechanism.[8] A process that consists of an initial primary assessment, rapid resuscitation, and a more thorough secondary survey followed by diagnostic tests and ultimate triage constitutes the initial approach to trauma care (Table 243-3).

When available, a history obtained from a patient, witnesses, or prehospital provider may provide important information regarding circumstances of the injury (single-car accident, a fall, exposure, smoke inhalation), preexisting medical conditions (depression, cardiac disease, pregnancy), or medications (steroids, β blockers) that may suggest certain patterns of injury or the physiologic response to injury.

A *primary survey* is undertaken quickly with the goal of identifying and treating life-threatening conditions. Specific lethal problems (discussed in further detail below) that should be identified immediately are airway obstruction, tension pneumothorax, massive hemorrhage, open pneumothorax, flail chest, and cardiac tamponade. During the primary survey, the following are quickly assessed:

a. *A*irway maintenance with C-spine control
b. *B*reathing/ventilation
c. *C*irculation with hemorrhage control
d. Neurologic *d*isability
e. *E*xposure, where the patient is completely undressed

Some specific points are emphasized regarding the various components of the trauma evaluation.

Airway with C-Spine Control

Rapid assessment for airway patency includes inspecting for foreign bodies or maxillofacial fractures that may result in airway obstruction. The chin-lift or jaw-thrust maneuver or the insertion of an oral or nasal airway is a first response for the patient making inadequate respiratory effort. A two-person technique is suggested, where one devotes undivided attention to maintaining in-line immobilization and preventing excessive movement of the cervical spine. Comatose patients (Glasgow Coma Scale score 3–8; see "Disability" below) should be intubated tracheally to protect the airway and to prevent the secondary brain injury that occurs with hypoxemia. Log rolling and pharyngeal suction may be necessary to prevent aspiration if the patient vomits. A team approach, where surgeons and emergency medicine physicians work together, is utilized for patients whose anatomy or severe maxillofacial injury precludes endotracheal intubation. In such cases, a surgical airway by means of cricothyroidotomy may be necessary. Agitated trauma patients suffering from head injury, hypoxia, or drug- or alcohol-induced delirium may present a danger to themselves. In these circumstances, paralyzing agents such as succinylcholine or vecuronium, along with a small dose of diazepam or midazolam, may be necessary to enable safe airway management. See Chap. 15 for details, dosages, and techniques.

TABLE 243-1 Essential Characteristics of Levels I, II, and III Trauma Centers

Level I (not required of levels II, III, and IV trauma centers)
24 h availability of all surgical subspecialties (including cardiac surgery/bypass capability)
Neuroradiology, hemodialysis available 24 h
Program that establishes and monitors effect of injury prevention/education efforts
Organized trauma research program
Level II (not required of levels III and IV trauma centers)
Cardiology, ophthalmology, plastic surgery, gynecologic surgery available
Operating room ready 24 h a day
Neurosurgery department in hospital
Trauma multidisciplinary quality assurance committee
Level III (not required of level IV trauma centers)
Trauma and emergency medicine services
24 h x-ray capability
Pulse oximetry, central venous and arterial catheter monitoring capability
Thermal control equipment for blood fluids
Published on-call schedule for surgeons, subspecialists
Trauma registry

The issue of C-spine clearance is one that has received much attention in the recent past. Ultimately, "clearance" of a C-spine is both a radiologic and a clinical undertaking. This implies that patients who do not demonstrate evidence of bony fractures or subluxation on x-ray may still have significant injuries that are not appreciated if they cannot cooperate with a thorough physical examination. On the other hand, precious time should not be expended on multiple views in patients who have critical head, thoracic, and abdominal injuries that may require rapid intervention. In these patients, after a cross-table lateral view of the C-spine, the cervical collar should be left in place until the patient ultimately can cooperate with the clinical examination or undergo more sophisticated studies (e.g., CT scans or MRI of the spine).

TABLE 243-2 Maryland Criteria for Mandatory Transport to a Trauma Center

Abnormal vital signs (GCS < 14 or systolic BP < 90) (respiratory rate < 10 or > 29)
Multiple-system trauma
Penetrating wound to
Head, neck, or torso
Gunshot wound(s) to extremities proximal to elbow and knee
An extremity with neurovascular compromise
CNS injury (head, spine)
Suspected pelvic fracture
Mechanism of injury
Vehicular deformity
Intrusion into passenger compartment greater than 12 in
Major vehicular deformity greater than 20 in
Ejection
Entrapment
Falls greater than three times the patient's height
Fatality in same passenger compartment
Rapid deceleration
Auto-pedestrian/auto-bicycle injury with significant impact (>5 mi/h)
Vehicular rollover
Exposure to blast/explosion

Finally, the practice of obtaining multiple C-spine x-rays in awake, alert patients with normal examinations (no pain or tenderness with the neck in neutral position and rotated in all four directions) is excessive. A prospective study undertaken at a large level I trauma center evaluated nearly 2000 patients admitted with blunt trauma.[8] Five-hundred and forty-nine of these patients were alert, oriented, and clinically nonintoxicated and had a normal neck examination. These patients subsequently underwent anteroposterior, lateral, and odontoid views of the cervical spine at a minimum. Additional films were necessary for clearance in 59 percent of patients. The total resources used on these 549 patients were 2272 spine films, 78 CT scans, 1 MRI, and 17 additional hospital days just to clear the C-spine. There was not a single injury identified in this group of patients, suggesting that clinical examination alone is reliable to assess the neck in blunt trauma patients who are alert, nonintoxicated, and have no neck symptoms.

Breathing

With the patient breathing or now intubated and being ventilated with 100% oxygen, the thorax and neck should be inspected, auscultated, and palpated to detect abnormalities such as a deviated trachea, crepitus, flail chest, sucking chest wound, fractured sternum, and absence of breath sounds on either side of the chest. Possible interventions here include application of an occlusive dressing to a sucking chest wound, withdrawal of the endotracheal tube from the right mainstem bronchus; reintubation of the trachea if no breath sounds are heard, and insertion of large chest tubes (38Fr) to relieve hemopneumothorax. Evacuated blood should be collected in an autotransfusion device. The volume of blood that returns should be noted immediately, since 1500 cc of hemorrhage may require a thoracotomy.

Circulation with Hemorrhage Control

Hemorrhagic shock, a common cause of postinjury death, should be assumed to be present in any hypotensive trauma patient until proven otherwise. Direct pressure should be used to control obvious external bleeding, and a rapid assessment of hemodynamic status is essential during the primary survey. This includes evaluation of level of consciousness, skin color, and presence and magnitude of peripheral pulses. Attention should be paid to the specifics of heart rate and blood pulse pressure (systolic minus diastolic blood pressure), particularly in previously young, healthy trauma patients (Table 243-4).

Not all hemorrhage is hemorrhagic shock, and the unsuspecting clinician may fail to appreciate ongoing hemorrhage with blood loss of up to 30 percent of the circulating blood volume. While class I hemorrhage (loss of up to 15 percent of circulating blood volume) is associated with minimal symptoms and is clearly not shock, class III hemorrhage associated with gross hypotension is readily appreciated as a state of hypoperfusion. Yet, consider a young, healthy trauma victim who has lost 25 percent of his circulating blood volume (class II hemorrhage) and had a preinjury blood pressure of 130/70 mmHg and a pulse rate of 60. If this patient experiences a 50 percent increase in his pulse rate (to a rate of 90) and a greater than 50 percent decrement of his pulse pressure (from 130/70 mmHg pulse pressure of 60 to 116/90 mmHg pulse pressure of 26), the unsuspecting clinician may assume that the patient is "hemodynamically stable." A false sense of security may lead to delays in aggressively pursuing the source of bleeding (ultrasound, peritoneal lavage, operative exploration). From this example it should be clear that the practice of omitting diastolic

TABLE 243-3 A Step-by-Step Procedure for Trauma Resuscitation

1. *Notification by Prehospital Personnel:* The receiving emergency department should be informed about:
    - Airway patency
    - Pulse and respirations
    - Level of consciousness
    - Immobilization
    - Mechanism of injury and blood loss at the scene
    - Anatomic sites of apparent injury
2. *Preparation for Receiving the Trauma Victim*
    - Assign tasks to team members
    - Check and prepare vital equipment
    - Summon surgical consultant and other team members not present
3. *Primary Survey:* The most immediately lethal injuries are taken care of as they are identified.
    - Airway
        - Clear airway: chin lift, suction, finger sweep
        - Protect airway
            - Depressed level of consciousness or bleeding, tracheal intubation without neck movement
        - Surgical airway
    - Breathing
        - Ventilate with 100% oxygen
        - Check thorax and neck
            - Deviated trachea
            - Tension pneumothorax (intervention—needle decompression)
            - Chest wounds and chest wall motion
            - Sucking chest wound (intervention—occlusive dressing)
            - Neck and chest crepitation
            - Multiple broken ribs
            - Fractured sternum
            - Pneumothorax
        - Listen for breath sounds
            - Correct tracheal tube placement?
            - Hemopneumothorax?
                - Chest tube(s)—38-Fr
                - Collect blood for autotransfusion
    - Circulation
        - Apply pressure to sites of external exsanguination
        - Assure that two large-bore IVs established
            - Begin with rapid infusion of warm crystalloid solution
            - If arm sites unavailable, insert a large central line or perform a saphenous cutdown at the ankle
        - Assess for blood volume status
            - Radial and carotid pulse, BP determination
            - Jugular venous filling
            - Quality of heart tones
        - Beck triad present?
            - Pericardiocentesis or echocardiogram
            - Decompress tamponade
                - Pericardiocentesis
                - Thoracotomy with pericardiotomy
        - Hypovolemia
            - After 2 L of crystalloid begin blood infusion if still hypovolemic; in children use two 20 mL/kg boluses then 10 mL/kg blood boluses if still unstable
        - Near-term pregnant patient—place roll under right hip
    - Disability
        - Brief neurological examination
            - Pupil size and reactivity
            - Limb movement
            - Glasgow Coma Scale
    - Exposure
        - Completely disrobe the patient
        - Logroll to inspect back
    - Continuing resuscitation
        - Monitor fluid administration
            - Consider central line for CVP monitoring
            - Use fetal heart rate as indicator in pregnant women
            - Record all events
4. *Secondary Survey:* A thorough search for injuries is carried out in order to set further priorities.
    - Trauma series x-rays: lateral cervical spine, supine chest, AP pelvis
    - Head-to-toe examination looking and feeling; quickly bring problems under control as they are discovered
        - Scalp wound bleeding controlled with Raney clips
        - Hemotympanum?
        - Facial stability?
        - Epistaxis tamponaded with balloons if severe
        - Avulsed teeth, broken jaw?
        - Penetrating injuries?
        - Abdominal distension and tenderness?
        - Pelvic stability?
        - Perineal laceration/hematoma?
        - Urethral meatus blood?
        - Rectal examination for tone, blood, and prostate position
        - Bimanual vaginal examination
        - Peripheral pulses
        - Deformities, open fractures
        - Reflexes, sensation
    - Large gastric tube (32-Fr) inserted
    - Foley catheter inserted
        - Blood?
        - Pregnancy test
    - Logroll the patient to feel and see the back, flanks, and buttocks if not already done
    - Splint unstable fractures/dislocations
    - Assure that tetanus prophylaxis is given
    - Consult with surgeon regarding further tests or immediate need for surgery or preferred IV medications; consider:
        - Emergency thoracotomy to provide aortic compression of cross-clamping
        - Aortogram or upright chest x-ray to rule out ruptured aorta
        - Cystogram if pelvic fracture present or blood in urine
        - IVP or enhanced CT scan of the abdomen
        - FAST or diagnostic peritoneal lavage
        - Head CT scan
        - IV mannitol for neurologic decompensation
        - IV steroids for possible spinal cord injury
        - IV antibiotics for possible ruptured abdominal viscus
        - IV antibiotics for perineal, vaginal, or rectal lacerations
        - Pelvic arteriogram and embolization for pelvic hemorrhage

blood pressures (and reporting "116/palpable," thus omitting the pulse pressure) is potentially hazardous. The alert, suspicious clinician identifies hemorrhage before it reaches the class III category of obvious shock.

Two large intravenous lines should be established and blood obtained for laboratory studies. While there are varying preferences, I prefer a percutaneous large line in the groin for unstable patients in whom upper extremity veins are not available. This is so because subclavian lines are potentially dangerous in the hypovolemic patient, saphenous vein cutdown at the ankle may not be appropriate for the patient with an injured lower extremity, and complications encountered from the femoral venous line may be minimized if the line is removed quickly on completion of resuscitation in the early postoperative period. Unstable patients without an obvious indication for surgery should be assessed for their response to 2 L of rapid infusion of crystalloids. If there is not marked improvement, type O blood should be transfused (O-negative for females of childbearing age). Auscultation for breath sounds and heart sounds and inspection of neck veins

TABLE 243-4 Estimated Fluid and Blood Losses Based on Patient's Initial Presentation

	Class I	Class II	Class III	Class IV
Blood loss (mL)*	Up to 750	750–1500	1500–2000	>2000
Blood loss (percent blood volume)	Up to 15%	15–30%	30–40%	40%
Pulse rate	<100	100–120	120–140	>140
Blood pressure	Normal	Normal	Decreased	Decreased
Pulse pressure (mmHg)	Normal or increased	Decreased	Decreased	Decreased

*Assumes a 70 kg patient with a preinjury circulating blood volume of 5 L.
BV = blood volume.

are included in the assessment of circulation because two major causes of hypotension may be present in trauma patients with minimal blood loss: *cardiac tamponade* (hypotension, agitation, distended neck veins, muffled heart sounds) and *tension pneumothorax* (hypotension, distended neck veins, absent breath sounds).

Echocardiography and abdominal ultrasonography, now becoming available in many emergency departments, are rapid, noninvasive ways to assess for fluid in the pericardium and peritoneal cavity.

A discussion of the longstanding controversies involving *fluid resuscitation* is beyond the scope of this chapter. However, reference must be made to a landmark paper published by Bickell and associates.[9] In their prospective, randomized study of victims of penetrating torso injuries in Houston, patients were randomized to receiving immediate IV fluid resuscitation versus withholding fluid until operative intervention could be undertaken. A lower mortality was identified among the group with delayed fluid resuscitation, prompting the authors to speculate that giving fluids before operative control could be achieved is harmful. However one interprets this study, the fact that there were inordinate delays (sometimes >50 min) between hospital arrival and surgical intervention should help achieve consensus around at least one concept: the importance of rapid triage of critically injured patients, particularly those with penetrating trauma, to an appropriate trauma center. One is hard pressed to identify any beneficial interventions that would justify a delay in rapid transport.

The inability, after nearly three decades, to demonstrate an unequivocal advantage of colloid therapy (which is more expensive than crystalloids) has led to near-universal acceptance of a balanced salt crystalloid (normal saline or Ringer's lactate) as the fluid of choice for initial resuscitation.

Disability

An abbreviated neurologic evaluation should now be performed, including level of consciousness, pupil size and reactivity, and motor function. The Glasgow Coma Scale (Table 243-5) should be used to quantify the patient's level of consciousness: possible scores range from 3 (no response) to 15 (high response on all measures). Despite the common comorbid presence of drug and alcohol abuse in trauma patients, it is only safe to assume that patients presenting with a GCS score of less than 15 and an appropriate mechanism have a head injury until proven otherwise. The GCS can be utilized to determine the severity of injury (minor injury GCS 13 and 14, moderate injury GCS 9 to 12, severe injury–coma GCS 3 to 8) and therefore the urgency with which the CT scan is obtained. New head injury guidelines have been formulated by an evidence-based methodology performed by the Brain Trauma Foundation in conjunction with the American Association of Neurological Surgeons.[9,10] Among the updated recommendations are (1) a suggested guideline for the placement of devices for intracranial pressure (ICP) monitoring for head-injured patients with GCS scores of 3 to 8 and a traumatic intracranial lesion and (2) concerns about prolonged prophylactic hyperventilation in the absence of an identified increase in ICP. The result of these two recommendations produces a heightened emphasis on the importance of the head CT scan. Only a head CT would identify the intracranial lesion that would lead to placement of an ICP catheter, and it is only with identification of such an increase in ICP that prolonged hyperventilation (until recently a practice routinely taught) can be justified. Accordingly, patients who are comatose after head injury should be intubated with in-line neck immobilization and transported to the CT scanner with the same sense of urgency that a hypotensive patient with a gunshot wound to the abdomen would be rushed to the operating room.

Exposure

No primary survey is complete without thoroughly disrobing the patient and examining the total body surface area carefully for bruises, lacerations, impaled foreign bodies, and open fractures. If hemodynamically stable and if the airway is ensured, the patient should be logrolled, with one attendant assigned to maintain cervical stabilization. Check the back, and thoracic and lumbar spine for tenderness. Check the gluteal cleft and perineum for injury. When the exam is completed, the patient should be covered with warm blankets to prevent hypothermia.

When derangements in any of the components of the primary survey are identified, treatment is undertaken immediately. Once the primary survey is complete, securing of the airway, intravenous catheters as well as urinary and gastric catheters, and monitors should be

TABLE 243-5 The Glasgow Coma Scale Measure of Level of Consciousness

Measure	Response	Score
Eye opening	Opens:	
	Spontaneously	4
	To verbal command	3
	To pain	2
	No response	1
Verbal	Oriented and converses	5
	Disoriented and converses	4
	Inappropriate words	3
	Incomprehensible sounds	2
	No response	1
Motor	Obeys verbal command	6
	To painful stimulus:	
	Localizes pain	5
	Flexion-withdrawal	4
	Abnormal flexion (decorticate rigidity)	3
	Extension (decerebrate rigidity)	2
	No response	1

achieved. At this point a *secondary survey,* a more thorough head-to-toe evaluation, is undertaken. It should be stressed that the secondary survey is not initiated until the primary survey (ABCs) is assessed to be adequate and resuscitation has been initiated.

SPECIFIC INJURIES OF IMPORTANCE

Having discussed the initial assessment of the injured patient, emphasis is placed on specific injuries of importance. These injuries are critical in that they are identified during the primary survey, represent impending demise, and require an immediate response.

Traumatic arrests In most emergency medical systems, paramedics transport patients without vital signs to a hospital while cardiopulmonary resuscitation (CPR) is initiated (unless obvious signs of death are present). On arrival to the Emergency Department (ED), a critical decision must be made regarding the level of intervention. A recently published large series analyzing 862 patients undergoing ED thoracotomy at a regional trauma center yields interesting information.[12] There were 385 patients (45 percent) with blunt trauma, 147 (17 percent) with stab wounds, and 330 (38 percent) with gunshot wounds. The overall number of neurologically intact survivors was 34 (3.9 percent), and the series was large enough and sufficiently equally divided among mechanisms of injury to permit subgroup analysis. There were 259 patients with blunt trauma and no vital signs in the field. There were no survivors in this group. This is a consistent finding among other series, and clearly ED thoracotomy for this group of patients should be abandoned. The greatest proportion of neurologically intact survivors was among patients with stab wounds to the chest (20 of 109, 18 percent). Their survival rate improved to 23 percent among thoracic stab wound victims with vital signs in the field and to 38 percent among those who were moribund but had some vital signs on arrival to the ED. Therefore, the strongest recommendation for ED thoracotomy can be made for victims with penetrating chest trauma with witnessed signs of life in transport or the ED and at least cardiac electrical activity on arrival.[12–15] More liberal indications (although not with total consensus) would include victims with abdominal trauma with cardiac electrical activity, in whom thoracotomy is performed for resuscitation and aortic cross-clamping before operating room laparotomy rather than for hemorrhage control, and patients with blunt torso trauma who have some vital signs on arrival.

Severe Head Trauma Head trauma with coma (GCS 3 to 8) suggests that rapid assessment of the intracranial injury must be undertaken and the patient should be intubated for airway protection and to avoid secondary brain injury associated with hypoxemia. These patients present a dilemma, because ultimately they may be found to have anything ranging from a normal head CT scan to a devastating, nonsurvivable brain injury. The challenge is to quickly identify patients with intracranial injuries that may benefit from neurosurgical evacuation. In such cases, minutes may make a difference in the ultimate patient outcome. Accordingly, all nonessential procedures should be prioritized to a time after the head CT is performed. The patient is intubated with in-line neck immobilization, and the C-spine collar is reapplied. A rapid chest x-ray may be justifiable to rule out pneumothorax and to assess endotracheal tube placement, particularly if the film can be developed as the patient is being transported to the CT scan suite. This implies that in the well-run trauma center the critically multisystem-injured patient has ongoing diagnostic workup and therapeutic resuscitation occurring in a smooth transition between ED, x-ray suite, operating room, and postoperative intensive care setting.

Tension Pneumothorax, Open Pneumothorax, and Massive Hemothorax These are all diagnoses that should be made during the primary survey requiring rapid placement of a chest tube. Absent breath sounds on the side of a gunshot wound, stab wound, or chest wall ecchymosis (associated with tympany in the case of pneumothorax and percussion dullness in the case of hemothorax) in a patient with respiratory distress and tachycardia suggest the diagnosis.

Abdominal Gunshot Wounds with Hypotension This deserves special mention. Palpation tenderness elicited on ED admission identifies the need for surgery and should prompt *immediate transport to the operating room* without further workup. Placement of nasogastric, urinary, and intravenous catheters should proceed in the operating room as the patient is being prepared for general anesthesia. The importance of time is emphasized because of the large amount of hemorrhage necessary (>2 L in the 70-kg patient) to produce severe hypotension in a young, previously healthy patient. A false sense of security with these patients brought on by the absence of hypotension is hazardous.[16]

SECONDARY SURVEY

While resuscitation continues, a secondary survey should be undertaken. The secondary survey is a rapid but thorough physical examination for the purpose of identifying as many injuries as possible. With this information, the resuscitating physician and his or her surgical colleague can set logical priorities for evaluation and management. Frequent assessments of the patient's blood pressure, pulse rate, and central venous pressure should continue.

The examination is conducted in a head-to-toe fashion, beginning with the scalp. Scalp lacerations can bleed profusely. This bleeding can be controlled with plastic Raney clips that grasp the full thickness of the scalp and galea. The tympanic membranes should be visualized to detect hemotympanum, and the pupil examination should be repeated. if epistaxis is a problem, a Foley catheter or a nasal balloon should be inserted to provide posterior tamponade. The examination continues over the neck and thorax. A lateral cervical spine x-ray (if not already obtained), a chest x-ray, and an anteroposterior pelvic x-ray should be obtained while the secondary survey continues. A 32-Fr gastric tube should be inserted into the stomach and connected to suction. When there is facial trauma or basilar skull fracture, the gastric tube should be inserted through the mouth rather than the nose. The urinary meatus, scrotum, and perineum are inspected for the presence of blood, hematoma, or laceration.

A rectal examination is done, noting sphincter function and whether the prostate is boggy or displaced. Rectal blood should be noted. If the prostate is normal and there is no blood at the urethral meatus, a Foley catheter can be placed in the bladder. If a urethral injury is suspected (meatal blood present), a urethrogram should be obtained prior to passing the catheter. If the prostate is displaced, it should be assumed that the urethra is disrupted. Catheterization should not be attempted if the urethra is injured. The urine should be examined for blood. If the patient is a woman of childbearing age, a pregnancy test should be obtained. A bimanual vaginal examination should be performed. If blood is present, a speculum examination will be necessary to identify a possible vaginal laceration in the presence of a pelvic fracture. Palpate all peripheral pulses. The patient should be logrolled to either side while keeping the neck immobilized so that every inch of the patient's body is seen and felt. The extremities should be evaluated for fracture and soft tissue injury. Peripheral pulses should be felt. A more thorough neurologic examination can now be done, carefully checking motor and sensory function.

Radiographic Imaging

In patients who are not rapidly transported to the operating suite or the CT scanner after the initial assessment, standard radiographic imaging includes *lateral C-spine, chest, and pelvic radiographs.* The chest x-ray and pelvic films image the three regions (left hemithorax, right hemithorax, and extraperitoneal pelvis) outside the true peritoneal cavity that can accommodate volumes of hemorrhage sufficient to produce gross hypotension. X-rays in penetrating trauma are dictated by bullet entry site and include a chest x-ray for patients with torso penetrating trauma and appropriate extremity films to rule out fractures in patients with penetrating extremity injuries.

Echocardiography has become a useful diagnostic tool for emergency medicine physicians and trauma surgeons.[17] A focused abdominal sonographic examination for trauma (FAST) is a rapid diagnostic tool performed with a 3.5-MHz probe that assesses for fluid in (1) the pericardium, (2) the hepatorenal recess of Morrison (a common location for blood in patients with hemoperitoneum), (3) the pelvis around the bladder, and (4) the perisplenic region. Abdominal sonography in the trauma patient is rapidly supplanting *diagnostic peritoneal lavage* as the procedure of choice to detect hemoperitoneum in the unstable trauma patient for whom transport to the CT suite is unsafe.

DISPOSITION

Options include moving the patient to the operating room, admission to the hospital, or transfer to another facility. The primary and secondary survey must have been completed, and a gastric tube and a Foley catheter should be in place unless a urethral injury was detected. In most urban hospitals, the trauma surgeon should have been present for the secondary survey, and he or she should assume direction of the diagnostic workup and disposition of the case at that time. In rural hospitals that transfer severe trauma cases, the resuscitating physician should relate all the physical findings discovered during the primary and secondary surveys to the physician receiving the patient. Laboratory results, x-rays, and the flow sheet showing blood pressure, pulse, fluids infused, urine output, gastric output, and neurologic findings should accompany the patient. If a diagnostic peritoneal lavage was performed, a sample of the lavage fluid should accompany the patient. A patient who is being transported to another facility should be accompanied by personnel capable of administering fluids and monitoring vital signs and pupillary changes. Mannitol should be available if there is neurologic deterioration enroute.

The hallmark of trauma care in patients without obvious indications for surgery identified on the initial assessment is *serial examination.* An *observation area* is extremely useful for these patients. Such an area (typically with nursing care provisions analogous to those of an intermediate care unit in most hospitals) allows for serial observations of patients with (1) closed head trauma who have regained consciousness but require repeat neurologic examinations, (2) penetrating abdominal wounds (stab wounds or tangential gunshot wounds) who require repeat abdominal examinations, (3) patients receiving repeat chest x-rays for penetrating chest trauma without pneumothoraces, (4) blunt abdominal trauma with normal physical examination on initial evaluation, and (5) documented blunt injuries to the liver, spleen, or kidney who are clinically stable and are being managed nonoperatively. An observation area for these patients should allow for more rapid triage from the ED and for serial evaluations of multiple patients in a convenient setting and should provide for rapid transport to the operating room in patients whose clinical examination deteriorates.

REFERENCES

1. Baker SP, O'Neill B, Ginsburg MJ, Li G: *The Injury Fact Book,* 2d ed. New York, Oxford University Press, 1992.
2. General Accounting Office: *Trauma Care: Life-Saving System Threatened by Unreimbursed Costs and Other Factors.* Report to the Chairman, Subcommittee on Health for Families and the Uninsured, Committee on Finance, U.S. Senate. Washington, DC: GAO (HRD-91-57), 1991.
3. Committee on Trauma Research, Commission on Life Sciences, National Research Council and the Institute of Medicine: *Injury in America: A Continuing Public Health Problem.* Washington, DC: National Academy Press, 1985.
4. Cornwell EE III, Jacobs D, Walker M, et al: National Medical Association Surgical Section: Position paper on violence prevention: A resolution of trauma surgeons caring for victims of violence. *JAMA* 273:1788, 1995.
5. Cornwell EE III, Berne TV, Belzberg H, et al: Health care crisis from a trauma center perspective: The L.A. story. *JAMA* 276(12):940, 1996.
6. Committee on Trauma American College of Surgeons: *Resources for Optimal Care of the Injured Patient: 1999.* Chicago, American College of Surgeons, 1998.
7. American College of Surgeons Committee on Trauma: *Advanced Trauma Life Support for Doctors, Instructor Course Manual,* 6th ed. Chicago, American College of Surgeons, 1997.
8. Velmahos GC, Theodorou D, Tatevossian R, et al: Radiographic cervical spine evaluation in the alert asymptomatic blunt trauma victim: Much ado about nothing? *J Trauma* 40(5):768, 1996.
9. Bickell WH, Wall MJ Jr, Pepe PE, et al: Immediate versus delayed fluid resuscitation for hypotensive patients with penetrating torso injuries. *N Engl J Med* 331:1105, 1994.
10. Brain Trauma Foundation: Indications for intracranial pressure monitoring. *J Neurotrauma* 13:667, 1997.
11. Brain Trauma Foundation: The use of hyperventilation in the acute management of severe traumatic brain injury. *J Neurotrauma* 13:699, 1997.
12. Branney SW, Moore EE, Feldhaus KM, Wolfe RE: Critical analysis of two decades of experience with postinjury emergency department thoracotomy in a regional trauma center. *J Trauma* 45(1):87, 1998.
13. Esposito TJ, Jurkovich GJ, Rice CL, et al: Reappraisal of emergency room thoracotomy in a changing environment. *J Trauma* 31:881, 1991.
14. Velmahos GC, Degiannis E, Souter I, et al: Outcome of a strict policy on emergency department thoracotomies. *Arch Surg* 130:774, 1995.
15. Feliciano DV, Bitondo CG, Cruse PA, et al: Liberal use of emergency center thoracotomy. *Am J Surg* 152:654, 1986.
16. Cornwell EE III, Velmahos GC, Berne TV, et al: Lethal abdominal gunshot wounds at a level I trauma center: Analysis of "TRISS fallouts." *J Am Coll Surg* 187(2):123, 1998.
17. Rozycki GS, Ochsner MG, Frankel HL, et al: A prospective study of surgeon performed ultrasound as the initial diagnostic modality for injured patient assessment. *J Trauma* 39:492, 1995.

PEDIATRIC TRAUMA

William E. Hauda II

Trauma is the leading cause of death and disability in children over 1 year of age. The most common reason for injury is a motor vehicle crash. Because children have different anatomy and physiology, the management of injuries in children differs is some respects compared with adults. Knowledge of these differences is crucial for emergency physicians to provide expedient and effective care to injured children. Many injuries can be initially managed in a general hospital emergency department (ED), but care of the most seriously injured children requires prompt triage and transportation to a designated pediatric trauma center.

EPIDEMIOLOGY

Trauma is responsible for over 600,000 pediatric hospitalizations each year in the United States,[1] and is the second leading cause of ED visits after infections.[2] Head injury is the most frequent cause of death.[3] Motor vehicle injuries are the leading cause of death among children over the age of 1 year, accounting for 18 percent of all deaths and 37 percent of all deaths due to trauma.[4] Motor vehicle crashes are also the most frequent cause of injury.[1,3] Alcohol use by a driver is a factor in almost 25 percent of these crashes.[5] Under the age of 1 year, suffocation is the most common cause of death due to injury.[4] The other leading causes of death are drowning, fire/burn, and firearms. Death rates for boys over the age of 5 is twice the rate for girls.[4] Children who are economically disadvantaged are 2.6 times more likely to die from trauma.

Homicide accounts for about 25 percent of pediatric deaths. Infants are 10 times more likely to die from homicide than are children 5 to

9 years of age.[4] Rates of death from injury among children have declined over the past 10 years in the United States in all categories except for firearms, suffocation, and poisoning.

TRAUMA RESUSCITATION PRIORITIES

The priorities in managing children with traumatic injuries do not differ greatly from that of injured adults (see Chap. 243). However, as with nontraumatic resuscitation, emphasis is placed upon airway management and the recognition and treatment of shock. Injuries and conditions that require immediate lifesaving intervention are treated during the primary survey (Table 244-1). All other conditions are identified and managed during the secondary survey.

A team approach will help to minimize confusion during the initial resuscitation. Tasks for individual members of the team include airway management, cervical spine stabilization, intravascular line placement, assessment of the child by system, and preparation and administration of mediations and fluids. A team leader not directly involved in patient care can facilitate the overall management of the patient because that person is not dedicated to a particular task.

Airway

The most important step in trauma care for children is airway intervention. Many preventable traumatic deaths among children are due to loss of an adequate airway or due to hypoxia. Proficient training in airway skills and aggressive airway management leads to a reduction in the number of pediatric deaths. Often, only airway opening and support are needed to prevent death. However, because pediatric trauma patients infrequently require intubation, many health care providers have inexperience with more advanced methods.[6] Proficient management of a child's airway requires an understanding of the anatomy of children (see Chap. 11, "Pediatric Airway Management").

OXYGEN High-flow oxygen should be applied to all trauma patients. Patients who are not hypoxemic initially may become so as their condition changes if they are not given supplemental oxygen. A nonrebreathing mask is the usual method of delivery, but blow-by oxygen is acceptable in a child who fights having the face mask. Continuous-pulse oximetry should be monitored.

TABLE 244-1 Primary Survey Goals

Identify	Intervene
Airway	
Airway obstruction	Open airway, remove obstruction
Breathing	
Apnea	Positive pressure ventilation
Hypoxia	Supplemental oxygen administration
Tension pneumothorax	Needle thoracostomy, tube thoracostomy
Massive hemothorax	Tube thoracostomy
Open pneumothorax	Occlusive dressing, tube thoracostomy
Circulation	
Shock	Fluid bolus, blood products
Pericardial tamponade	Fluid bolus, pericardiocentesis, thoracotomy
Cardiac arrest	Thoracotomy if penetrating trauma
Disability	
Spinal cord injury	Immobilization, steroids
Cerebral herniation	Hyperventilation, mannitol
Exposure	
Hypothermia	Warmed fluids, external warming
Exsanguinating hemorrhage	Direct pressure, air splints

BASIC AIRWAY MANEUVERS Basic airway techniques are covered in detail in Chap. 11, "Pediatric Airway Management." In the trauma patient, care must also be taken to avoid injuries to the head or neck while managing the child's airway. The cervical spine should be protected by stabilization, not traction, with one provider dedicated to this task. The airway should be opened by using the jaw-thrust technique. This technique minimizes movement of the cervical spine, yet still easily opens the airway. Prolonged maintenance of the jaw-thrust can be tiring. Thus, in an unconscious child, placement of an oral airway can be considered, whereas, if the child is conscious or has an intact gag reflex, a nasopharyngeal airway should be used instead. Constant reassessment of the airway status is necessary, as airway adjuncts can become occluded by blood, vomit, or tissue swelling.

ENDOTRACHEAL INTUBATION If the airway cannot be maintained by basic maneuvers, the child requires hyperventilation, or access is needed for medication administration, then the child should be intubated by the oral route. The most experienced airway provider should perform the intubation. A trauma patient who is a child requires several considerations beyond the normal concerns. First, cervical spine stabilization must be maintained throughout the procedure. Excessive cervical spine movement can occur during endotracheal intubation. Thus, at least two persons will be needed to perform the intubation: one for cervical spine stabilization and one to intubate. Secondly, selection of the induction agents requires consideration of the patient's hemodynamic state, risks, and likelihood of cerebral injury. For example, the use of ketamine must be avoided in head-injured patients. The propensity for thiopental to cause hypotension minimizes its utility in trauma patients. Frequently used agents include fentanyl and etomidate. The choice of a paralytic agent is less dependent on a child's condition. Succinylcholine or vecuronium are commonly used. Third, some patients will require pretreatment with pharmacologic agents prior to intubation. Lidocaine should be considered in head-injured patients, although the importance of using it has not been firmly established. Atropine should be given to all patients younger than age 6, especially if succinylcholine will be used as the paralyzing agent.[7] These issues are covered in detail in Chap. 10, "Pediatric Cardiopulmonary Resuscitation" and in Chap. 11, "Pediatric Airway Management."

SURGICAL AIRWAY Rarely will the emergency physician or emergency medical service provider need to perform a surgical airway on a child. However, the difficulty with performing this technique has perpetuated the need for preparation and training. Because of the relative small size of a child's airway, needle cricothyroidotomy is the preferred first attempt at securing a surgical airway. A 14- to 16-gauge catheter is placed through the cricothyroid membrane and is attached to a jet insufflator. A bag-valve mask can be used for a short time, but high pressures are needed to ventilate through the small catheter. Although ventilation will be limited, oxygenation is achievable for up to 2 h, or until a more definitive airway can be established by additional oral attempts or more advanced techniques.[8] (See Chap. 11, "Pediatric Airway Management.")

Cervical Spine

The cervical spine must be immobilized in any patient with a suspected spinal injury until cervical spine injury can be excluded. Immobilization is performed at the same time that airway management is started. Cervical spine immobilization can be provided by the same individual that maintains the jaw thrust. Whenever possible, a hard cervical collar should be used. However, due to the limited number of sizes available, a properly fitting collar may not be possible. Omitting the application of a cervical collar is acceptable in children for whom no properly fitting rigid collar is available. The child should be placed on a spinal board or in a pediatric immobilizer designed for trauma immobilization. The head should be secured to the board by using towel rolls or commercially available head blocks and tape applied across the forehead and under the chin of the collar. If a collar is not used, tape should not be applied under the chin, because this may prevent the mouth from opening. The child's body is secured to the board by straps or wide cloth tape. Blanket rolls should be placed on either side of the child to prevent lateral movement of the child if logrolling becomes necessary to clear the airway. Clearance of the child's cervical spine by clinical or radiographic methods should wait until the primary survey is completed.

Breathing

All trauma patients should receive supplemental oxygen. Assessment of breathing entails identifying inadequate oxygenation or ventilation or the potential for deterioration. Children with respiratory failure should have positive pressure ventilation (PPV) started immediately. PPV may render an innocuous pneumothorax into a compromising injury, and such a possibility should be actively monitored. If the presence of a small pneumothorax is already known, a tube thoracostomy may be appropriate early in the resuscitation efforts. Children with respiratory distress may not have a striking presentation, but still require immediate attention to minimize complications. Cyanosis, poor end-organ function, and desaturation on pulse oximetry will identify a child with severe hypoxemia. A child with mild hypoxemia may manifest more subtle signs, such as agitation and poor capillary refill. Signs of inadequate ventilation in the young child include tachypnea, nasal flaring, grunting, retractions, and stridor or wheezing. Often, signs of inadequate oxygenation and ventilation will coexist in children. Auscultation of the chest can identify a large pneumothorax or hemothorax. Because breath sounds are easily transmitted across a small chest, breath sounds should be sought in both axilla. If signs of inadequate oxygenation do not improve rapidly with high-flow oxygen administration, then PPV must be started.

TENSION PNEUMOTHORAX The classic presentation of a tension pneumothorax is absent breath sounds, tympany, hypotension, and jugular venous distention due to high intrathoracic pressures. Children rarely have this complete presentation. If suspected during the primary survey, a catheter decompression should be performed, followed by tube thoracostomy.

MASSIVE HEMOTHORAX The classic presentation of a massive hemothorax is absent breath sounds, dullness to percussion on the affected side of the chest, and hypotension. Jugular venous distention is unlikely because the circulatory volume is low. Tube thoracostomy is needed for effective management. Operative thoracotomy should be considered if the initial drainage is greater than 15 mL/kg or the chest tube output exceeds 4 mL/kg/h.

OPEN PNEUMOTHORAX The skin wound of an open pneumothorax should be occluded on three sides with a dressing of petrolatum gauze or a plastic sheet. An open pneumothorax may be associated with a tension pneumothorax. An occlusive dressing is applied and air can no longer escape through the wound; leaving one side of the dressing open to act as a flutter valve will minimize the development of a tension pneumothorax. A tube thoracostomy need only be performed after completing the primary survey.

Circulation

Hypovolemic shock is the most common form of shock in children. Recognizing the subtle early signs of shock can be daunting even for experienced emergency physicians. Children can maintain an adequate blood pressure, even in the face of severe blood loss, but other signs of shock will be apparent. Monitoring blood pressure alone to diagnose shock is unreliable in pediatric patients. Signs of shock include tachycardia, cool extremities, capillary refill time longer than 3 s, altered level of consciousness, weak distal pulses, and low urine output. Hypothermia can be a confounding factor, because it also can affect skin perfusion.

The treatment of shock in trauma is based on the same principles as other forms of hypovolemic shock. Crystalloid fluid boluses of 20 mg/kg given over 20 min or less are used to resuscitate the child. If two boluses of crystalloid fail to correct signs of shock, then blood (packed red blood cells) should be given using 10 mL/kg boluses. In small children, the blood bank should hold several aliquots from a single donor unit to minimize the risk of a transfusion reaction.

CARDIAC ARREST Absent pulses in a child with traumatic injuries portends a poor outcome. In children with penetrating chest or abdominal trauma, a resuscitative thoracotomy can be lifesaving if vital signs were recently lost. In children with traumatic arrest from blunt trauma, the outcome is always death.[9] Standard advanced cardiac life-support algorithms are followed, but most commonly injured children will have asystole or pulseless electrical activity. Early administration of blood products should be used and any identified injuries treated.

CARDIAC TAMPONADE This condition is rare in children. Most commonly it results from penetrating trauma. Beck's triad consists of hypotension, muffled heart sounds, and jugular venous distention. Diagnosis can be confirmed by echocardiography prior to treatment. Initial fluid boluses may be temporizing, but pericardiocentesis and resuscitative thoracotomy can be lifesaving.

VASCULAR ACCESS Achieving vascular access is one of the most difficult tasks in an injured child. In an adult patient, ''two large bore'' intravenous lines are placed; in a child, placing a single functioning intravenous line is often considered a success. Ideally two lines are placed so that blood and medications or fluids can be given simultaneously. Practically, a functioning intravenous line is all that may be readily achieved, and is usually adequate. Consideration should be given to early intraosseous line placement in a severely injured child, because any fluids, medications, or blood products can be given through this line. The femoral vein is the next easiest site because of the identifiable landmarks and the relative ease of the procedure compared with other central venous lines in children (see Chap. 17, ''Vascular Access'').

Disability

The next goals in the primary survey are to identify neurologic abnormalities in the child. Level of consciousness is assessed by either the Glasgow Coma Score (GCS) or the AVPU system wherein the child's consciousness is rated as (present or absent): *A*lert, responds to *V*erbal stimuli, responds to *P*ainful stimuli, or *U*nresponsive. The GCS is commonly used in trauma databases, and lower scores have been associated with increased mortality rate. An arbitrary cutoff of 8 is often quoted as the score that should prompt endotracheal intubation in trauma patients. This point has been chosen because mortality rate is greatly increased with GCSs below this level. The AVPU system is recommended by the American Heart Association as an easier system to use.[7]

A pupillary exam is used to recognize early signs of increased intracranial pressure and herniation. Several case reports can be found of children with a high level of consciousness who had a dilated pupil and then rapidly developed a herniation syndrome.

Examination of the motor strength of each limb concludes the disability exam. Gross strength is all that is noted during the primary survey, so that paralysis from a spinal cord or central neurologic event is recognized. If a spinal cord injury is strongly suspected, then IV steroids are started immediately[10] (see discussion below).

Exposure

The final part of the primary survey serves to identify any important wounds and to detect or prevent hypothermia. Actively bleeding wounds or penetrating wounds will direct the priority of actions taken during the resuscitation and secondary survey. Bleeding is controlled by direct pressure, using air splints on the extremities if needed. A rectal temperature should be obtained for all pediatric trauma patients, but especially if the temperature outside is cool. Children become hypothermic much easier than adults due to their high body surface area. Hypothermia can develop in the emergency department despite a seemingly comfortable ambient temperature. Whenever possible, keep the child covered. Warm fluids to 40°C if large amounts of IV fluids or blood products are used.

Prehospital Considerations

Standards of care in the prehospital environment have been slow in developing. Many pediatric patients are being treated in systems which lack the experience and standards of care that are needed to manage children appropriately. IV access is the prehospital advanced life-support intervention that is most often performed,[6] although the beneficial effects may be rare.[11] IV success rates are as high as 93 percent.[6] Airway management, however, is often more difficult, with many studies showing success rates from 57 to 79 percent, far lower than the success rates with adult patients. Minimizing scene times is an important issue in pediatric trauma management. Placing IV lines en route to the hospital unless a prolonged extrication is required can shorten field times.[6]

POSTRESUSCITATION PRIORITIES

Secondary Survey

The goal of the secondary survey is to identify all other injuries to a trauma patient. It does not begin until the completion of the primary survey. All body areas are completely examined. Resuscitation priorities are established, and any life-threatening injuries should already have been managed. Any needed x-rays, laboratory studies, or diagnostic procedures in the ED are also performed during this phase.

The presence of family will often be helpful to calm and console frightened and injured children. Additionally, during this phase a complete history should be obtained using the AMPLE format (*A*llergies, *M*edications, *P*ast medical history, time of *L*ast meal, *E*vents leading up to the injury).

Stabilization

In this phase, all of the child's injuries are managed definitively, or the child is stabilized sufficiently to allow safe transfer to a facility that can provide a higher level of care. Continual reassessment is crucial, because some injuries may be only manifest over time and complications from therapeutic interventions can occur. Emphasis is placed on monitoring the airway and circulatory status of pediatric trauma patients. Endotracheal tube dislodgment, development of a pneumothorax, regurgitation of stomach contents, occult hemorrhage causing shock, and worsening neurologic function are all frequently seen in injured children. Careful monitoring of fluid administration will prevent inadvertent overhydration. Analgesia and sedation should be used judiciously; often these elements are neglected in injured pediatric patients.

Referral to Pediatric Center

Pediatric trauma centers are designed to provide optimal care to pediatric trauma patients by having all pediatric specialties immediately available to the children. This is a capability-oriented approach. Designation of the trauma center is done by the state government, and the requirements vary from state to state. Several capabilities would be ideal for the pediatric trauma center.[12] The hospital should have a dedicated pediatric trauma service directed by a pediatric trauma surgeon. Comprehensive pediatric services should be available from scene care to rehabilitation and reintegration into the family and society. The trauma team should be immediately available at all times and be capable of treating at least two patients simultaneously. Other pediatric specialists should be on site or immediately available including emergency medicine, anesthesiology, neurosurgery, radiology, orthopedics, pediatric intensive care, and nursing. A pediatric intensive care unit is essential.

Use of trauma triage scores can help identify a child who needs a more experienced team for care. However, not all systems are easy to use. Two common scores used are the pediatric trauma score (PTS) and revised trauma score (RTS) (Table 244-2). Advantages of these scores over other systems are that they include physiologic variables instead of relying only on anatomic variables. Higher numbers are associated with a higher likelihood of survival and, thus, a reduced need for trauma center care. A child with an RTS of less than 12 or a PTS of less than 8 should be taken to a trauma center.

Some indications for transfer to a pediatric trauma center are listed in Table 244-3.

The need to transfer a patient to a pediatric trauma center should be based on the need for treatment that the initial hospital cannot provide. Ideally, a seriously injured child would receive care from a pediatric trauma specialist. However, this is impractical and not always achievable. Additionally, adolescents (age 12 and over), whose anatomic and physiologic characteristics are essentially those of adults, account for up to 50 percent of injured children. Younger children

TABLE 244-2A Pediatric Trauma Score

	−1	+1	+2
Size (kg)	<10	10–20	>20
Airway	Unmaintained	Maintained	Normal
Systolic blood pressure (mmHg)	<50	50–90	>90
Level of consciousness	Comatose	Altered	Awake
Wounds	Major open	Minor open	None
Skeletal trauma	Open/multiple	Closed	None

TABLE 244-2B Revised Trauma Score

Number	Glasgow Coma Score	Systolic Blood Pressure	Respiratory Rate
4	13–15	>89	10–29
3	9–12	76–89	>29
2	6–8	50–75	6–9
1	4–5	1–49	1–5
0	3	0	0

TABLE 244-3 Indications for Transfer to a Pediatric Trauma Center

Mechanism of injury	Ejected from motor vehicle Fall greater than 3 times child's height Prolonged extrication Death of another occupant in motor vehicle
Anatomic injury	Multiple severe trauma More than three long bone fractures Spinal fractures or spinal cord injury Amputations Severe head or facial trauma Penetrating head, chest, or abdominal trauma

Source: Adapted from Harris et al,[12] with permission.

may do better with pediatric traumatologists. Children are more likely to have successful nonoperative management of blunt trauma injuries at a designated pediatric trauma center.[13] At least one study has shown that pediatric patients can be appropriately managed in ''adult'' trauma centers, but the data may be biased by not including children referred to a pediatric trauma center from the prehospital environment. There are no studies to date that have shown that children receive better care in an ''adult'' trauma center as compared with a designated pediatric trauma center.

Transportation

Because only 8 percent of hospitals have a pediatric intensive care unit, most critically injured children will need transportation to another facility. The first step is to assure that all identified injuries are treated to the best ability of the referring hospital and that the child is maximally stabilized. Few areas possess a dedicated pediatric critical care transport team to manage the patient during the transportation. The next best option is to have a critical care transport team with some pediatric experience (pediatric nurse or pediatrician) traveling with the child. Indications for pediatric critical care experience on the transport team are endotracheal intubation, potential airway compromise, spinal injury, hemodynamic instability, pressor infusions, skull fractures, pelvic fractures, or a child currently receiving blood products. Standard advanced life-support crews can be used for children without airway problems or hemodynamic instability. Increasingly, pediatric trauma centers have their own home-based interhospital transport systems and will arrange transportation from referring sites.

MANAGEMENT OF INJURIES

Head Trauma

Cerebral trauma is the leading cause of death due to injury in children.[14] Most of these deaths occur outside of the hospital. The most common mechanisms of injury differ by age. Falls are most frequent in children less than 2 years of age. Preschoolers also are most frequently injured in falls, but motor vehicle crashes account for 25 percent. In school-age children, falls and motor vehicle crashes occur with equal frequency. Lastly, in adolescents, sports injuries and motor vehicle crashes are about equal.

Children frequently have head injuries because of several factors. A child's head encompasses a relatively larger proportion of body mass and area. The bones of the neck are not fully developed, so the head is attached on a largely ligamentous connection. The incompletely myelinated brain is more susceptible to shear forces during trauma. Because of cartilage in the skull and the presence of open sutures, young children are better able to tolerate increased intracranial pressure than are adolescents and adults.

CLINICAL FINDINGS Most children will have suffered a mild head injury and present with no or few symptoms in the ED. Common symptoms associated with head injury include vomiting, headache, and lethargy.[15] For children with more significant cerebral injuries, the signs and symptoms are not markedly different from those for adults. The most difficult aspect of evaluation is often the neurologic exam. It is difficult to ascertain inappropriate behavior or mental status particularly in the very young. Level of consciousness can be rated by the AVPU system or the GCS. A pupillary exam can identify impending herniation even in a child without distress. Asymmetry of spontaneous movements is, of course, a telling clue. Older children can then be asked to move their fingers and toes. Sensory function should be assessed by withdrawal from pain or the ability to feel touch in older children. In young children, look for signs of fontanelle fullness (increased intracranial pressure ICP) or retinal hemorrhages (shaken baby syndrome).

INCREASED INTRACRANIAL PRESSURE Signs of increased ICP in children are most commonly vomiting, dizziness, headache, irritability, and decreased level of consciousness. Management is not remarkably different from adult management (see Chap. 11). Aggressive hyperventilation in children has been associated with worsened cerebral ischemia as compared with more moderate hyperventilation in head-injured children.[16] Children with suspected increased ICP should be mildly hyperventilated (P_{CO_2} 30 to 34 mmHg) and should have their hemodynamic status maximized with judicious use of fluids and blood. Fluid restriction should not be an acute consideration. The head of the bed should be elevated to 20° to 30°, and the neck should be straight, to optimize venous drainage. IV mannitol in a dose of 0.5 to 1.0 g/kg can be used to lower ICP. Although mannitol may acutely lower ICP by removal of free water and decreased blood viscosity, frequent administration will lead to increased serum osmolality. Further, it is felt that, initially following administration, ICP may in fact be transiently increased due to an initial increase in intravascular volume. Although concern has frequently been expressed, neither phenomenon has been shown to be detrimental clinically. Local preferences will dictate practice. Lasix (furosemide) (1.0 mg/kg) may decrease edema, as well. Currently, no studies have shown steroids to be helpful. Aggressive hyperventilation should be reserved for children with signs of impending herniation.

POSTTRAUMATIC SEIZURES Seizures following traumatic head injury are relatively uncommon, occurring in about 5 percent of hospitalized patients.[17] About half of these patients will never have a seizure again. Of the remaining half, 50 percent have rare seizures and 50 percent have frequent seizures. Children with loss of consciousness, lower GCS, longer duration of coma, and computed tomography (CT) scan abnormalities are at increased risk for seizures. Intracranial injuries most commonly seen are subdural hemorrhages, depressed skull fractures, and intracranial lacerations.[17] Only 50 percent of children with posttraumatic seizures will have abnormalities on CT scanning.[17] Use of anticonvulsant medication as prophylaxis in the absence of a seizure or following a single seizure is controversial. Children with two or more seizures, or seizures lasting more than a few minutes, should receive anticonvulsant therapy. Prophylactic anticonvulsant therapy should be strongly considered in a child with a GCS under 8, even if no seizures have yet occurred, because the risk of developing acute posttraumatic seizures is high and many of these children already have high ICPs that will increase further with a seizure.[17]

Although phenytoin has been the standard anticonvulsant studied, the improved safety profile of fosphenytoin will likely cause its replacement. Dosage is the same (17 mg/kg IV load) except that fosphenytoin is measured in phenytoin equivalents. Acute seizures should be managed with a benzodiazepine such as lorazepam, midazolam, or diazepam.

As with adults, proximity of seizure to the event predicts long-term likelihood of epilepsy. Immediate seizures are least likely to result in long-term problems.[17]

RADIOGRAPHY Since the primary goal of the evaluation is to identify increased ICP and to identify injuries that require surgical intervention, plain films are rarely appropriate. In suspected child abuse, skull films are essential to document current or past skull fractures. A child who will undergo a CT examination does not need plain films unless a skull fracture is strongly suspected (subgaleal hematoma may be a clue) and the CT does not show a fracture. A CT scan is indicated in children who fall into a moderate- or high-risk category (Table 244-4).[18] Children in the low-risk category generally do not need a CT scan unless other circumstances, such as lack of follow-up, dictate a need for a study.

Obtaining a CT scan in a young child will often require sedation and the inherent risks associated with it. Midazolam (0.1 mg/kg IV) is commonly used. Obviously, preparations must be made for the unexpected deterioration of a child's condition after sedatives are used.

MANAGEMENT Children in the low-risk category can be safely discharged home to follow up with the primary care provider by phone or in person. Discharge instructions should clearly state the need to return to the ED if any symptoms in the moderate-risk category occur. Children who have an intracranial injury or skull fracture should have an immediate neurosurgical consultation in the ED or shortly after being admitted. These patients must be managed in a pediatric intensive care unit.

SPECIFIC INJURIES **Scalp Injuries** Because the scalp is richly vascularized, some children have developed shock due to significant blood loss, violating the dogma that "head injuries do not cause shock." The area under a laceration should be palpated to determine if a skull fracture is present.

TABLE 244-4 Risk Groups for Head Computed Tomographic Evaluation

Low Risk	Moderate Risk	High Risk
No symptoms	Persistent vomiting	Penetrating injury
Dizziness	Altered level of consciousness after injury or at baseline	Depressed level of consciousness
Headache	Loss of consciousness >5 min	Focal neurologic findings
Vomited 1–2 times	Posttraumatic seizure	Signs of herniation
Loss of consciousness <5 min	Alcohol/drug intoxication	
Minor soft tissue injury	Age <2 years and symptoms	
	Multiple trauma	
	Serious facial injury	
	Suspected abuse	
	Basilar or other skull fracture	
	Vomiting >8 h from injury	

Source: Adapted from Masters et al,[18] with permission.

Concussion By definition, these are transient injuries with no demonstrable cerebral injury on CT scan. Other symptoms often coexist in children, such as dizziness, vomiting, and headache. Amnesia is frequent and may be antegrade or retrograde in relation to the event. No specific management is needed except analgesia and observation, often in the home setting if the parent is responsible. Most children will have no long-lasting effects from a concussion, but long-term cognitive and behavioral changes have been described after even apparently trivial trauma.

Contusion A contusion is a focal area of bruising or tearing of brain tissue. These are the most common injuries seen on CT scans of children following head injury. Management includes hospital observation and neurosurgical evaluation. Some patients will worsen and require supportive care for cerebral edema, but these children rarely require operative intervention. Most children with such injuries do well.

Epidural Hemorrhage These uncommon injuries are greatly feared because they can occur after seemingly minor trauma.[15] Falls from heights less than 5 ft (<2 m) are associated with epidural bleeds in children under 5 years of age.[15] Usually these injuries are due to a fall, with a direct blow to the side of the head. The classic description of a brief loss of consciousness followed by a lucid interval, with subsequent clinical deterioration is relatively uncommon, occurring in only about 25 percent of patients with epidural hemorrhage.[15] Patients will often have vomiting or a headache. As consciousness becomes altered, the ipsilateral pupil may dilate. Hemiparesis and seizures are late signs. Surgical drainage is often required, although some small epidural hemorrhages can be observed in the intensive care unit setting. Prognosis is excellent for a child whose results on neurologic examination are normal at the time of diagnosis, suggesting that early identification of epidural bleeds may improve outcome.[15]

Subdural Hemorrhage Often these injuries are caused by shearing of the bridging venous vessels to the brain. Either direct trauma or indirect shaking has been known to cause these injuries. Patients will present with signs of increased ICP. Although the presentation of syncope with the so-called lucid interval has traditionally been associated with epidural hematomas, the presentation is more likely to point to a subdural hematoma, not because of greater association, but because subdural hematomas are much more common. Subacute or chronic subdurals may require contrast-enhanced CT scanning to detect the isodense lesion. Hemorrhage size and altered mental status are the primary indicators for operative intervention.

Intraparenchymal Hemorrhage These injuries are associated with substantial force, a penetrating injury, or a predisposing factor such as a vascular malformation. Signs of increased intracranial pressure will usually be present. Management is determined by the extent and location of hemorrhage.

Skull Fractures Three basic types of skull fractures occur: linear, depressed, and basilar skull fractures.

LINEAR SKULL FRACTURES These are the most common of all pediatric skull fractures and usually occur at the point of impact. Associated intracranial hemorrhage occurs in up to 50 percent of parietal fractures and 75 percent of occipital fractures. Subgaleal hemorrhages are also commonly seen. The presence of a skull fracture mandates a CT scan and inpatient observation. Children with isolated linear skull fractures can be observed on a pediatric ward, but prompt neurosurgical intervention must be available.

DEPRESSED SKULL FRACTURES CT scanning occasionally misses these injuries, so plain skull films should be obtained in a child with a normal CT scan and a suspicion of a depressed fracture. Tangential views are often necessary. Neurosurgical management depends on the nature of the injury, but intensive care unit admission is required of all patients.

BASILAR SKULL FRACTURES Unlike the other skull fractures, basilar skull fractures are best seen on a CT scan. Signs that suggest the presence of a basilar skull fracture include periorbital bruising (raccoon eyes), hemotympanum, mastoid bruising (Battle sign), and cerebrospinal fluid atorrhea or rhinorrhea. Management is usually symptomatic and requires neurosurgical expertise.

Spinal Trauma

Spinal trauma is relatively uncommon in young children but is more commonly seen in adolescents.[19] Cervical spine injuries predominate, although thoracic and lumbar injuries also occur (see lap-belt syndrome, below). Fractures or dislocations not related to birth trauma are very rare in children less than 16 months of age, having yet to be reported in the literature. Motor vehicle crashes are the most common reason for spinal injury, followed by falls and sports events. In young children, falls predominate and, in older children, motor vehicle crashes predominate. Due to increased flexibility of the spine and spinal column in younger children, fractures and dislocations rarely occur with minor trauma, and spinal cord injury without radiographic abnormality (SCIWORA) can occur. Adolescents more commonly have fracture patterns similar to those of adults. Also, 50 percent of spinal injuries and 67 percent of cervical spinal injuries in children under the age of 12 occur between the occiput and C2. By comparison, adolescents and adults more commonly experience lower cervical spine injuries.[19] Younger children also less frequently have thoracic or lumbar injuries. Signs and symptoms of spinal cord injury are nearly always evident in the pediatric population when present following injury. Part of the reason for this pattern of injury is that an immature child's spine and an adult's spine have several differences (Table 244-5).

Children with incomplete spinal cord deficits have a better prognosis for improvement in neurologic condition than those children with complete spinal cord injuries. Spinal cord trauma is associated with a higher mortality rate in children than in adults.

CLINICAL FINDINGS Presentation is related to the presence or absence of a spinal cord injury. Children with fractures only will have pain, tenderness, or overlaying soft tissue injury. Children with spinal cord injuries with or without fracture will present based on the type of spinal cord injury.

Over 50 percent of children with SCIWORA have a delayed onset of paralysis, sometimes up to 4 days.[20] Many of these children have transient paresthesias, numbness, or weakness at the time of or shortly after the injury. Because most spinal injuries fail to improve substantially, even in children, the most important factor in prognosis is the initial neurologic status.[20] Children with fractures and neurologic symptoms do worse than children with SCIWORA alone.[20]

TABLE 244-5 Spinal Column Differences in Children

Ligamentous laxity
Underdevelopment of supporting muscles
Partially ossified vertebrae
Wedge-shaped vertebrae
Horizontal facet joints
Higher fulcrum of flexion
Instability of atlanto-occipital joint

RADIOGRAPHY Cervical spine radiographs should be obtained on any patient with neurologic symptoms including coma, or if any symptoms are referable to the neck. Up to 66 percent of spinal cord injuries in children have no radiographic abnormality and thus fall into the category of SCIWORA.[20] Widening of the prevertebral soft tissues to 8 mm or more in front of C2 or more than 75 percent of the adjacent vertebral body width is considered abnormal. In infants, however, this becomes less reliable.

In alert unintoxicated adult blunt trauma patients without neck symptoms, cervical spine radiographs can be forgone and cervical spine immobilization can be released. Because children have a much lower frequency of cervical spine fractures, following this algorithm in children is appropriate. Any child with neurologic complaints, neck pain, limited neck movement, neck tenderness, or evidence of neck trauma, must have plain films consisting of at least three views: lateral, anteroposterior, and odontoid. The single lateral cervical spine radiograph has been shown to miss fractures and result in a delay in diagnosis.[21] If the child has neck pain but no neurologic symptoms, plain radiography is generally all that is required to clear the cervical spine. Occult fractures and misinterpretation of plain films do occur, so if there is any doubt, a CT scan should be obtained. If the child had paresthesias, numbness, or weakness or currently has neurologic symptoms, a CT scan is also recommended.[20] If all plain film radiographs are negative, but the diagnosis of SCIWORA is being entertained, then a flexion and extension lateral cervical spine x-ray must be obtained to identify any ligamentous instability. This is not detectable on CT scan. These films should be done under close supervision and only in an awake and cooperative patient. Fluoroscopy may be helpful, as well. Anytime the diagnosis of SCIWORA is considered, the child requires a neurosurgical consultation from the ED and admission for observation.[20]

MANAGEMENT Treatment of spinal cord injuries in the prehospital and ED settings consists of immobilization, diagnosis of the specific injury, and steroid administration. Prehospital personnel must be instructed that an infant's relatively large head may cause the neck to flex in the standard supine position, so they require padding behind the shoulders to prevent this. Steroids should be started if there is evidence of a neurologic deficit with a loading dose of 30 mg/kg of methylprednisolone.[10] Steroids should be started within 8 h of the injury. Those who receive steroids within 3 h should be maintained on steroids for 24 h. Those who receive steroids 3 to 8 h after the injury require maintenance for 48 h. The maintenance dose is 5.4 mg/kg/h. The maintainance dose is initiated 45 min after the initial bolus. Children with a spinal cord injury require immediate neurosurgical consultation. If a spinal fracture is also present, a pediatric orthopedist should also be consulted.

Chest Trauma

Children, with their relatively compliant chest walls, may not show external evidence of serious intrathoracic trauma. Blunt trauma occurs more frequently than penetrating trauma and may be equally as serious. Isolated chest trauma in children carries a 4 to 12 percent mortality rate. Most children with chest trauma will have other significant injuries. In a multiply-injured child, death is 10 times more likely if chest trauma is present.[22] Penetrating chest injuries are becoming more frequent as the number of firearm injuries steadily increases in the United States. Children under the age of 12 are more likely to be injured in unintentional crossfire and require a longer hospitalization than do adolescents and adults.

Evaluation of a patient who has evidence of, or who has a good mechanism for, chest injury should include a thorough physical examination looking for bony defects, crepitus, paradoxical chest movement, and unequal breath sounds. A chest x-ray should be taken. To minimize interruption of the resuscitation, a supine chest x-ray can be initially obtained. A rib fracture is a sensitive indicator of serious underlying injury.[22] The most common injury is pulmonary contusion, but this may not be visible on the early ED chest x-ray.[22]

Most injuries requiring emergent treatment can be identified on the standard supine anteroposterior chest x-ray. Mediastinal widening is common on supine chest x-rays, but aortic injury is quite rare in children who survive to the ED. An upright chest x-ray, preferably using posteroanterior technique, will often obviate the need for additional studies. Aortography is still considered essential to exclude aortic injury, when suspected, although contrast-enhanced spiral CT scanning may also identify aortic injury. If an abdominal CT scan is obtained, additional occult chest injuries are often detected, but these rarely require emergent therapy.

Tube thoracostomy alone is usually sufficient management for pneumothorax or hemothorax, both of which are uncommonly associated with blunt trauma in children. Other specific injuries should be managed as outlined in the primary survey section. Emergent thoracotomy should be performed selectively as with adults. Survival from pulseless arrest at the scene or en route to the ED is rare in both blunt and penetrating trauma.[9] Only children who have sustained penetrating trauma and experience a loss of vital signs in the ED should have a resuscitative thoracotomy performed. In all other cases, the attempt is futile and the financial costs are high.[9]

Abdominal Trauma

DIAGNOSIS The physical examination of a child's abdomen is frequently misleading in the detection of intraabdominal injury. Children with severe injuries can have minimal physical findings, while other children may have occult serious injuries. Physical exams have been shown to be unreliable in up to 45 percent. In most children with abdominal symptoms or a mechanism of injury to the abdomen, an investigative study should be obtained.

Diagnostic peritoneal lavage (DPL) has been shown to be quite accurate in the identification of serious intraabdominal injury in children.[23]

False-negative DPLs are unusual. False-positive rates are in the range of 4.5 to 14 percent.[23] DPL criteria considered indicative of the need for laparotomy in children are listed in Table 244-6. Elevated amylase levels are associated with both pancreatic injury and bowel injury.[24] Because DPL is invasive and most children will not need an operation to manage their injuries (see below), abdominal CT scan is gaining popularity. A DPL is indicated, however, in children who have hemodynamic instability or other nonabdominal injuries that require immediate operative management. Some authors have also advocated use of DPL before CT scan in stable patients with an equivocal exam, because of its higher sensitivity; if the DPL is positive by red blood cell (RBC) criteria only, then a CT scan is performed to determine the need for laparotomy based on the extent of solid organ injury.[23]

Abdominal CT scanning has been recommended for management of hemodynamically stable children with potential intraabdominal injury. Advantages of CT scanning include its noninvasiveness and the ability to visualize the retroperitoneum. Disadvantages of CT scanning include time spent in radiology away from the trauma room, lower accuracy for hollow organ and pancreatic injury, and radiation exposure. Indications for obtaining a CT scan in children include abdominal tenderness, abdominal distention, abdominal bruising, hematuria, vomiting, neurologic obtundation, dropping or low hematocrit, and absent bowel sounds.[25] CT scan and operative findings correlate within splenic injury grade level in 86 percent of cases.[26] Normal CT findings in blunt trauma are strongly predictive of both no-future-deterioration and no-need-for-future operative intervention.[25] Normal CT findings virtually eliminate an intraabdominal injury; however, subtle signs such as unexplained peritoneal fluid, bowel wall enhancement, and bowel wall thickening are associated with bowel trauma.[25]

Ultrasound screening of the abdomen prior to CT has been shown to reduce the need for abdominal CT scans without missing significant injuries.[27] Currently, there is insufficient reported experience to recommend its routine use in the evaluation of pediatric trauma patients.

The general approach to evaluation of the abdomen in a child is outlined in Fig. 244-1.[28]

TABLE 244-6 Criteria for a Positive DPL

Study	Greater Than or Equal to
Red blood cells	
Blunt	100,000 RBCs/μL or gross blood
Penetrating—stab	100,000 RBCs μL or gross blood
Penetrating—gunshot	5,000 RBCs/μL or gross blood
White blood cells	
Blunt	500 WBCs/mm^3
Penetrating	500 WBCs/mm^3
Gastric contents	Any
Amylase	20 IU/L
Alkaline phosphatase	6 IU/L

SPLENIC TRAUMA The spleen is the most commonly injured abdominal organ in children. Children are more likely to be hemodynamically stable than adults even with the same degree of splenic injury.[26] Children with splenic injuries are more likely to be managed nonoperatively than adults.[26] Several reasons are thought to explain this difference. The spleen in children has a thicker capsule. There are larger amounts of elastin and smooth muscle in both the capsule and the splenic vessels. Children tend to have lower-velocity injuries and overall lower Injury Severity Scores.[26] Children who are more likely to require operative intervention include those with a higher Injury Severity Score, an injury sustained in a motor vehicle crash, or a greater amount of hemoperitoneum. Any child who requires a splenectomy should receive pneumococcal vaccine to prevent postsplenectomy sepsis.

HEPATIC TRAUMA The liver is the second most commonly injured abdominal organ in children. Similar to splenic trauma, these injuries can often be managed conservatively. The rate of fatal hemorrhage is higher with hepatic injury than with splenic injury. Diagnosis is often made by abdominal CT scanning in stable trauma patients. Unstable patients often require operative intervention to control hemorrhage.

PANCREATIC TRAUMA Although pancreatic trauma is uncommon in children, occurring in less than 10 percent of blunt trauma patients, trauma is the most common cause of acute pancreatitis. Handlebar injuries are the most common mechanism of injury and often cause isolated pancreatic trauma.[29] A high index of suspicion is required because symptoms are often delayed and morbidity is related to delay in diagnosis. Serum amylase levels are often elevated, but the degree of elevation does not correlate with the degree of pancreatic injury.[29] Serum lipase levels have not been studied in children. CT scanning has at best an 85 percent sensitivity to identify pancreatic injury in the acute setting.[29] Sensitivity is highest when both oral and IV contrast are used. Children with abdominal pain and an elevated serum amylase require an abdominal CT scan and should be hospitalized for observation even if the CT scan findings are normal.[29] Complications of pancreatic injury include pseudocyst formation, acute pancreatitis, and relapsing pancreatitis.

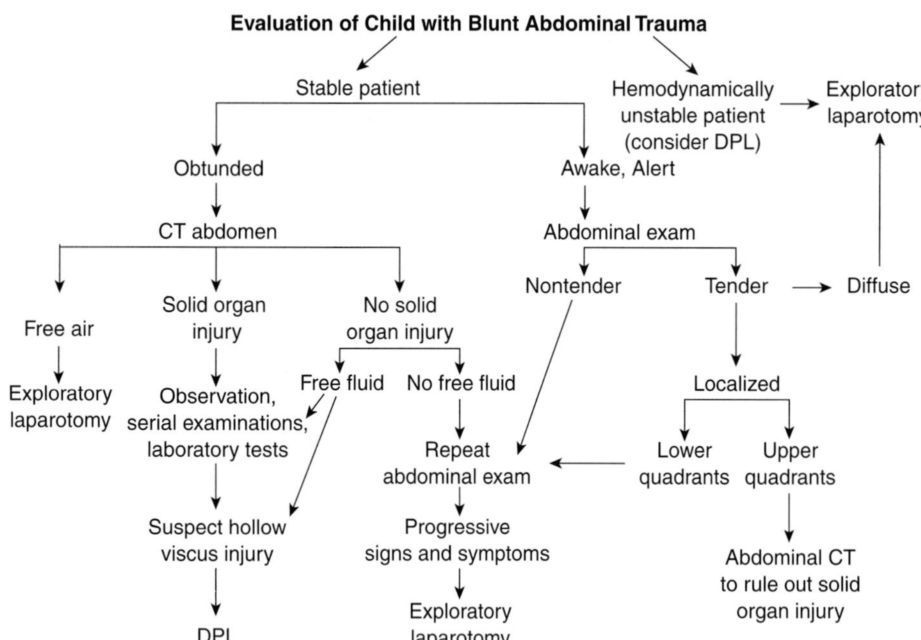

FIG. 244-1. Management algorithm for a child with suspected blunt abdominal injury. In an alert child, we heavily rely on the presence or absence of abdominal tenderness when making decisions for further evaluation. In a child with a closed head injury, an abdominal CT scan gives the most information but does not exclude hollow organ injury. *Abbreviations:* CT, computed tomography; DPL, diagnostic peritoneal lavage.

BOWEL TRAUMA Intestinal injuries occur in less than 5 percent of children with blunt abdominal trauma. The jejunum is most frequently injured, followed by the ileum and cecum. The duodenum is particularly prone to the development of hematomas in the wall, leading to obstruction. The physical examination is often quoted as being unreliable in diagnosing bowel injury following blunt trauma. Children with abdominal wall injuries (bruising or abrasions), tenderness on palpation, or a mechanism of a direct blow to the abdomen require further investigation to rule out bowel injury. In hemodynamically stable patients, a contrast-enhanced CT scan can often increase the suspicion of a bowel injury. CT scans are diagnostic for bowel injury in only 25 percent of cases. Pneumoperitoneum or extravasation of enteral contrast is considered diagnostic of bowel injury and requires immediate laparotomy. Nondiagnostic findings include free peritoneal fluid without solid organ injury and bowel wall enhancement or thickening. A child with a tender abdomen and these nondiagnostic but suggestive radiographic findings requires an exploratory laparotomy or DPL to rule out an intestinal perforation.[28] Complications of bowel injury include peritonitis, obstruction, and intestinal strictures.

Bowel injury is associated with seat-belt use in less than 5 percent of children admitted to trauma centers. A particular entity, the lap-belt complex, consists of intestinal or mesenteric injury with a concomitant lumbar spine injury due to a lap belt. It has also been shown to occur with three-point restraints (lap belt/shoulder-harness restraints) when the lap belt is incorrectly positioned over the abdomen. The intraabdominal injury often occurs at the midlumbar level. Most commonly, the jejunum is injured. Any child with a lumbar fracture or an anterior abdominal bruise from a seat belt must have a thorough search for intraabdominal injury. If a spinal injury is present, but the CT scan is negative, the child should be admitted for observation or a DPL should be performed.

Pelvic and Genitourinary Trauma

Trauma to the genitourinary (GU) tract should be considered in all children with multiple trauma, a pelvic fracture, or injury to the flank, back, or groin. GU injuries are uncommon in children, occurring in only 10 percent of trauma patients. Symptoms and physical findings are often nonspecific, including back pain, abdominal pain, hypotension, and abdominal wall trauma. Pelvic fractures, particularly anterior ring fractures, are associated with urethral and bladder injury. Children are less likely to die of hemorrhage from a pelvic fracture than are adults. Often, other coexisting injuries mask the signs and symptoms of GU trauma in a multiply-injured child.

Hematuria is considered the hallmark finding in GU trauma, although it is a nonspecific finding. The degree of hematuria does correlate with the severity of injury, although renal pedicle disruption can be associated with no hematuria.[30] The radiographic evaluation of an injured child with hematuria is based on clinical presentation. Children with gross hematuria or more than 20 RBCs/hpf and unstable vital signs or the emergent need for operative intervention for other injuries require an IVP in the ED. Children who have hematuria of more than 10 RBCs/hpf and stable vital signs should have CT of the abdomen performed. Asymptomatic microscopic hematuria in children with blunt trauma and no apparent injuries is a low-yield indication for emergent abdominal CT scanning. These cases can be followed as outpatients.

Cystourethrography is required on all patients with suspected lower urinary tract injuries (for example, blood at urethral meatus, high prostate, or anterior pelvic fracture). Straddle injuries account for 20 percent of the cases of urethral injury (motor vehicle crashes account for most of the other 80 percent). Straddle injuries are also associated with pubic fractures, testicular injuries, and labial or scrotal hematomas and lacerations. Sexual abuse should be considered in a girl with a straddle injury and a history that does not seem compatible with the injury.

Burns

Despite continuing improvement in burn care, many children continue to suffer death and significant morbidity from burns. Burns are the second most common cause of accidental death among children under the age of 4 years. Younger children are more commonly injured by scalding water, accidental spills being twice as frequent as intentional immersions. Older children are more commonly burned by flame.[31]

DIAGNOSIS Resuscitation principles are unchanged for pediatric burn patients.[32] Management of airway and circulation is paramount. Any traumatic injuries should be managed without regard to the burn itself. Aggressive airway management is crucial, as large burns may

TABLE 244-7 Criteria for Burn Center Referral

Second- and third-degree burns over 20 percent body surface area
Third-degree burns over 10 percent burn surface area
Second- and third-degree burns over 10 percent burn surface area in child under 10 years old
Second- and third-degree burns on face, hands, feet, genitals
Second- and third-degree circumferential burns
Electrical burns
Lightning burns
Chemical burns on face, hands, feet, genitals
Inhalation burns
Patients with burns and significant preexisting medical disorders that affect burn management
Inability or inexperience in pediatric burn management at referring facility

require high-volume fluid resuscitation, leading to airway edema and the inability to intubate the child later. Early intubation particularly with inhalational burns cannot be overemphasized. Burn surface area (BSA) cannot always be estimated by the "Rule of Nines" in children because the proportion of body surface area changes with growth. A Lund and Browder chart that is age-appropriate should be used (see Fig. 194-2). Alternately, the burn area can be estimated by using the child's palm as 1 percent. Fluid resuscitation can be estimated by the Parkland formula (4 mL/kg × %BSA), the modified Brooke formula (2 mL/kg × %BSA), or the Shriners formula (5000 ml × BSA in m^2 + 2000 mL × total surface area in m^2). All formulas call for one-half the estimated fluid to be given in the first 8 h after the burn, the second one-half in the following 16 h so that the total volume is given in 24 h. All resuscitation formulas are a guide only. Proper management requires that the response to fluid administration be carefully monitored and adjustments be made individually.[32]

CRITERIA FOR BURN CENTER REFERRAL Table 244-7 lists the criteria for referral to a burn center from the American Burn Association. Predictors for mortality rate in children by importance are burn size over 30 percent, age less than 4 years, and the presence of an inhalation burn.[31] Any questions regarding an individual patient should be directed to the regional burn center.

REFERENCES

1. Rosenberg ML, Rodriguez JR, Chorba TL: Childhood injuries: Where we are. *Pediatrics* 86:1084, 1990.
2. National Safety Council (NSC): *National Safety Council Accident Facts*, 1987 ed. Chicago, NSC, 1987.
3. Rhodes M, Smith S, Boorse D: Pediatric trauma patients in an "adult" trauma center. *J Trauma* 35:384, 1993.
4. Fingerhut LA, Warner M: *Injury Chartbook, Heath, United States*, 1996–97. Hyattsville, MD, National Center for Health Statistics, 1997.
5. Centers for Disease Control (CDC): Alcohol related traffic fatalities involving children: United States, 1985–1996. *MMWR* 46:1130, 1997.
6. Lavery RF, Tortella BJ, Griffin CC: The prehospital treatment of pediatric trauma. *Pediatr Emerg Care* 8:9, 1992.
7. Chameides L, Hazinski MF, eds: *Textbook of Pediatric Advanced Life Support*. Dallas, American Heart Association, 1994.
8. McCarty DL, Surpure JS: Pediatric trauma: Initial evaluation and stabilization. *Pediatr Ann* 19:584, 1990.
9. Sheikh AA, Culbertson CB: Emergency department thoracotomy in children: Rationale for selective application. *J Trauma* 34:322, 1993.
10. Bracken MD, Shepard MJ, Holford TR, et al: Administration of methylprednisolone for 24 or 48 hours in the treatment of acute spinal cord injury. *JAMA* 20:1597, 1997.
11. Teach SJ, Antosia RE, Lund DP, et al: Prehospital fluid therapy in pediatric trauma patients. *Pediatr Emerg Care* 11:5–8, 1995.
12. Harris BH, Barlow BA, Ballantine TV, et al: American Pediatric Surgical Association principles of pediatric trauma care. *J Pediatr Surg* 27:423, 1992.
13. Hall JR, Reyes HM, Meller JL, et al: The outcome for children with blunt trauma is best at a pediatric trauma center. *J Pediatr Surg* 31:72, 1996.
14. Kraus JF: Brain injuries among infants, children, adolescents, and young adults. *Am J Dis Child* 144:684, 1990.
15. Schutzman SA, Barnes PD, Mantello M, et al: Epidural hematomas in children. *Ann Emerg Med* 22:31, 1993.
16. Skippen P, Seear M, Poskitt K, et al: Effect of hyperventilation on regional cerebral blood flow in head-injured children. *Crit Care Med* 25:1402, 1997.
17. Lewis RJ, Lee L, Inkelis SH, et al: Clinical predictors of post-traumatic seizures in children with head trauma. *Ann Emerg Med* 22:1114, 1993.
18. Masters SJ, McClean PM, Arcarese JS, et al: Skull x-ray examinations after head trauma. *N Engl J Med* 316:84, 1987.
19. Hadley MN, Zabramski JM, Browner CM, et al: Pediatric spinal trauma: Review of 122 cases of spinal cord and vertebral column injuries. *J Neurosurg* 68:18, 1998.
20. Pang D, Wilberger JE: Spinal cord injury without radiographic abnormalities in children. *J Neurosurg* 57:114, 1982.
21. Dietrich AM, Ginn-Pease ME, Bartkowski HM, et al: Pediatric cervical spine fractures: Predominately subtle presentation. *J Pediatr Surg* 26:995, 1991.
22. Peclet MH, Newman KD, Eichelberger MR, et al: Thoracic trauma in children: An indicator of increased mortality. *J Pediatr Surg* 25:961, 1990.
23. Rothenberg S, Moore EE, Marx JA, et al: Selective management of blunt abdominal trauma in children: The role of peritoneal lavage. *J Trauma* 27:1101, 1987.
24. McAnena OJ, Marx JA, Moore EE: Peritoneal lavage enzyme determinations following blunt and penetrating abdominal trauma. *J Trauma* 31:1161, 1991.
25. Ruess L, Sivit CJ, Eichelberger MR, et al: Blunt abdominal trauma in children: Impact of CT on operative and nonoperative management. *AJR* 169:1011, 1997.
26. Powell M, Courcoulas A, Gardner M, et al: Management of blunt splenic trauma: Significant differences between adults and children. *Surgery* 122:654, 1997.
27. Katz S, Lazar L, Rathaus V, et al: Can ultrasonography replace computed tomography in the initial assessment of children with blunt abdominal trauma? *J Pediatr Surg* 31:649, 1996.
28. Jerby BL, Attorri RJ, Morton D Jr: Blunt intestinal injury in children: The role of the physical examination. *J Pediatr Surg* 32:580, 1997.
29. Arkovitz MS, Johnson N, Garcia VF: Pancreatic trauma in children: Mechanisms of injury. *J Trauma* 42:49, 1997.
30. Abou-Jaoude WA, Sugarman JM, Fallat ME, et al: Indicators of genitourinary tract injury or anomaly in cases of pediatric blunt trauma. *J Pediatr Surg* 31:86, 1996.
31. Morrow SE, Smith DL, Cairns BA, et al: Etiology and outcome of pediatric burns. *J Pediatr Surg* 31:329, 1996.
32. Mlcak R, Cortiella J, Desai MH, et al: Emergency management of pediatric burn victims. *Pediatr Emerg Care* 14:51, 1998.

GERIATRIC TRAUMA

O. John Ma
Daniel J. DeBehnke

With the rapid growth in the size of the elderly population, the incidence of geriatric trauma is expected to increase as well. Although the elderly experience the same types of injuries that younger individuals do, there are differences in the incidence and patterns of trauma. Emergency physicians need to be aware of many of these unique injury mechanisms and patterns associated with geriatric trauma. Elderly patients also respond differently to traumatic injuries because age-related changes may produce a diminished physiologic reserve.

Therefore, special management principles need to be applied in caring for geriatric trauma victims.

EPIDEMIOLOGY

Persons 65 years of age and older represent a large and growing segment of the population. According to the 1990 United States Census, 30.9 million people, representing 12.5 percent of the total population, were 65 years of age or older. This marked a 21.3 percent increase in this segment of the population from the 1980 Census figures. The U.S. Census Bureau projects that those over 65 years of age will increase to 52 million by the year 2020. The number of people over 85 years of age also is growing at an accelerated pace, with estimates that they will number 6.7 million by the year 2020.[1]

While persons over 65 years of age represent 12 percent of the population, they account for 36 percent of all ambulance transports, 25 percent of hospitalizations, and 25 percent of total trauma costs.[1] Although the elderly are less likely to be involved in trauma compared with other age groups, they are more likely to have fatal outcomes when they are injured. Approximately 28 percent of deaths due to accidental causes involve persons 65 years of age and older. Also, the elderly have the highest population-based mortality rate of any age group.[1]

Definitions

Defining the term *elderly* is a difficult task because it involves both chronologic and physiologic components. The literature has divided the elderly population into two groups: the *young old* (65 to 80 years of age) and the *old old* (80 years of age and older).[1] Although this is a somewhat arbitrary division, it is helpful in interpreting the literature on geriatric trauma.

One of the difficulties in describing the elderly population is the potential discrepancy between chronologic age and physiologic age. *Chronologic age* is the actual number of years the individual has lived. *Physiologic age* describes the actual functional capacity of the patients' organ systems in a physiologic sense. Comorbid disease states such as diabetes mellitus, coronary artery disease, renal disease, arthritis, and pulmonary disease can decrease the physiologic reserve of certain patients, which makes it more difficult for them to recover from a traumatic injury.[2,3] *Physiologic reserve* describes the various levels of functioning of the patients' organ systems that allows them to compensate for traumatic derangement. For example, a 65-year-old patient with diabetes, arthritis, and chronic obstructive pulmonary disease may have less physiologic reserve and hence an older physiologic age compared with an 80-year-old without any comorbid conditions.

CLINICAL FEATURES

Common Mechanisms of Injury

The elderly will experience similar types of injuries that younger individuals do. There are differences, however, in the incidence and patterns of injury for elderly patients compared with younger persons.

Falls

Falls are the most common accidental injury in patients over 75 years of age and the second most common injury in the 65 to 74 age group. Fifty percent of elderly persons who fall do so repeatedly. Most individuals who fall will do so on a level surface, and most will suffer an isolated orthopedic injury.[1,4] Falls are reported as the underlying cause of 9500 deaths each year in patients over the age of 65 years. Many falls in the elderly population occur in residential institutions such as nursing homes. In the over 85 age group, 20 percent of fatal falls occur in nursing homes.[4]

There are age-related changes in postural stability, balance, motor strength, and coordination that make the elderly more prone to tripping and falling and may explain the increased incidence of falls in this population. Also, decreased visual acuity and increased memory loss can cause the patient difficulty in recognizing and avoiding environmental hazards. Acute, preexisting, and chronic diseases also may lead to falls. Syncope has been implicated in many cases of elderly patients who fall, and this may be secondary to dysrhythmias, venous pooling, autonomic derangement, hypoxia, anemia, or hypoglycemia. Other contributing factors include alcohol and medications, most notably sedative, antihypertensive, antidepressant, diuretic, and hypoglycemic agents.[4]

Motor Vehicle Crashes

Motor vehicle–related injuries rank as the leading mechanism of injury that brings elderly patients to a trauma center in the United States. Motor vehicle crashes are the most common mechanism for fatal incidents in elderly persons through 80 years of age.[1] Emergency physicians should anticipate an increase in motor vehicle trauma involving the elderly due to the growth in this subset of the population and the increase in elderly drivers and occupants. Recent data by Li and colleagues[5] have shown that the crash fatality rate among the elderly is considerably higher than for younger age groups. As noted earlier, similar effects of acute and chronic medical conditions can influence the incidence of motor vehicle crashes. The patient may have decreased cerebral and motor skills and may have memory and judgment losses that can compound the difficulty in operating a motor vehicle. The patient also may have decreased auditory or visual acuity that makes it more difficult to recognize dangerous traffic situations. Furthermore, decreased strength and slower reaction times may hinder an individual's ability to respond to a hazardous traffic situation.[1] One study reported that the number of motor vehicle crashes per driver's license increased with age in elderly drivers. Elderly drivers typically collided in an intersection with a crossing vehicle, which they reported not noticing or seeing so late they did not have enough time to avoid it.[6]

Pedestrian-Automobile Accidents

When elderly patients are struck by automobiles, devastating injuries may result. The 65 and older age group accounts for 22 percent of pedestrian-automobile fatalities in the United States.[1] Elderly pedestrians struck by a motor vehicle are much more likely to die compared with younger pedestrians.[7] Postural changes due to musculoskeletal decline may lead to kyphosis, which results in difficulty in lifting the head to see and obey traffic signals. Traffic signals, which operate at a crossing rate of 4 ft/s, may not account for the elderly's slower walking speeds.[1] Thus elderly individuals may not have enough time to safely cross an intersection. Reduced peripheral vision and decreased hearing may limit access to information needed to make rational decisions about crossing the street. Again, cognitive, memory, and judgment skills may be diminished and could play a role in pedestrians being struck by automobiles.

Violence

The overall increase in violent crimes in the United States has not spared the elderly. Violent assaults account for 4 to 14 percent of trauma admissions in this age group. Elderly persons are seen as ideal targets for robberies because they may possess various age-related physical deficiencies.[1] Just as in the younger population, ethanol consumption by the assailant or victim has been found to be involved in the majority of fatal assaults. While blunt trauma, to date, has been the most frequent injury mechanism, penetrating injuries are on the rise.[1] Emergency physicians also should have a heightened suspicion for elder or parental abuse in the geriatric trauma patient (see Chap. 292, "Abuse in the Elderly and Impaired").

DIAGNOSIS AND ASSESSMENT

Primary and Secondary Surveys

As in all trauma patients, the primary survey should be conducted expeditiously. Special attention should be paid to anatomic variations that may make airway management more difficult. These include the presence of dentures (which may occlude the airway), cervical arthritis (which adds danger to extending the neck), or temporomandibular joint arthritis (which may hinder mouth opening). A thorough secondary survey is essential to uncover less serious injuries. These injuries, which include various orthopedic and "minor" head trauma, may not be severe enough to cause problems during the initial resuscitation but cumulatively may cause significant morbidity and mortality. An important point to note is that patients with no apparent life-threatening injuries actually can have potentially fatal injuries if there is some degree of limited physiologic reserve. Seemingly stable geriatric trauma patients can deteriorate rapidly and without warning.

History

Since elderly patients may have a significant past medical history that affects their trauma care, obtaining a precise history is vital. Often the time frame for obtaining information about the traumatic event, past medical history, medications, and allergies is quite short. Medical records and consultation with the patient's family physician may be helpful. Family members also may be able to provide information regarding the traumatic event and the patient's previous level of function.

Vital Signs

Early assessment and frequent monitoring of vital signs are essential in the geriatric trauma patient. The clinician, however, should not be led into a false sense of security by "normal" vital signs. In a study by Scalea and colleagues[8] of 15 patients initially considered to be hemodynamically "stable," 8 had cardiac outputs of less than 3.5 L/min and none had an adequate response to volume loading. Of 7 patients with a normal cardiac output, 5 had inadequate oxygen delivery.

There is progressive stiffening of the myocardium with age that results in a decreased effectiveness of the pumping mechanism. An 80-year-old will have approximately 50 percent of the cardiac output of a 20-year-old even without significant atherosclerotic coronary artery disease. The myocardium also becomes less sensitive to endogenous and exogenous catecholamines. Conduction defects may be exacerbated by the stress of illness or trauma. A normal tachycardic response to pain, hypovolemia, or anxiety may be absent or blunted in the elderly trauma patient.[9] Medications such as beta blockers may mask tachycardia and hinder evaluation of the elderly patient. Emergency physicians should be wary of a "normal" heart rate in the geriatric trauma victim.

RECOGNITION AND DIAGNOSIS OF COMMON INJURY PATTERNS

Head Injury

With aging, the brain undergoes progressive atrophy and decreases in size by about 10 percent between the ages of 30 and 70 years.[10] Subtle changes in cognition, memory, and data acquisition may confound the emergency physician's evaluation of the elderly patient's mental status. When evaluating the patient's mental status during the neurologic examination, it would be a grave error to assume that alterations in mental status are due solely to any underlying dementia or senility.

Elderly persons suffer a much lower incidence of epidural hematomas than the general population.[10] This has been attributed to the relatively more dense fibrous bond between the dura mater and the inner table of the skull in older individuals. There is, however, a higher incidence of subdural hematomas in elderly patients. As the brain mass decreases with advancing age, there is greater stretching and tension of the bridging veins that pass from the brain to the dural sinuses. The increased "dead space" within the skull may delay symptoms of intracranial bleeding.[9,10] More liberal indications for computed tomographic (CT) scanning are justified.

Cervical Spine Injuries

In one study[11] cervical spine injuries in patients 60 years of age and older accounted for 12 percent of the injuries. The pattern of cervical spine injuries in the elderly is very different than in younger patients. Ryan and associates[11] found that the incidence of C1 and C2 fractures rose as the population aged. This rise in upper-level fractures was due to a significant increase in the incidence of odontoid fractures in the elderly. When the elderly trauma patient presents with neck pain or a potential mechanism for spine injury (fall, mvc), emergency physicians need to place special emphasis on maintaining cervical immobilization until the cervical spine is properly assessed. Because underlying cervical arthritis may obscure fracture lines, the elderly patient with persistent neck pain and negative plain radiographs should undergo CT scanning of the neck, and flexion-extension views if imaging is negative but symptoms or suspicion for injury persists.

Chest Trauma

Chest trauma, both minor and severe, can compromise elderly individuals. In blunt trauma, there is an increased incidence of rib fractures due to osteoporotic changes. The pain associated with rib fractures, along with any decreased physiologic reserve, may predispose patients to respiratory complications.[12] More severe thoracic injuries, such as hemopneumothorax, pulmonary contusion, flail chest, and cardiac contusion, can quickly lead to decompensation in elderly individuals whose baseline oxygenation status may already be diminished.

Geriatric patients are more susceptible to developing hypoxia and respiratory infections following trauma. In the elderly, diminished elasticity of the lungs along with progressive changes in the chest wall can lead to a reduction in pulmonary compliance and in the ability to cough effectively. Total lung surface area decreases as alveolar and small airway support diminishes with advancing age. There also is reduced mucociliary clearance of foreign material and bacteria and increased colonization of the oropharynx with gram-negative organisms. All these factors result in an increased risk for elderly patients to develop nosocomial gram-negative pneumonia.[9,12]

Also, the great vessels tend to be more rigidly fixed, allowing for easier disruption from transmitted forces.

The main therapeutic goal is aggressively maintaining adequate oxygen delivery. Frequent arterial blood gas analysis may provide early insight into elderly patients' respiratory function and reserve. Prompt tracheal intubation and use of mechanical ventilation should be considered in patients with more severe injuries, respiratory rates greater than 40 breaths per minute, or when the Pa_{O_2} is less than 60 mmHg or the Pa_{CO_2} is greater than 50 mmHg. While nonventilatory therapy helps to prevent respiratory infections and is always desirable, early mechanical ventilation may avert the disastrous results associated with hypoxia.[12]

Emergency physicians should remember that chest trauma alone does not necessarily forecast a bleak outcome. In one series, most of the patients sustaining blunt chest injuries were discharged home to their preinjury level of independence.[12]

Abdominal Trauma

The abdominal examination in elderly patients is notoriously unreliable compared with younger patients, even in the absence of distracting pain, injuries, or altered sensorium. Even with an initially benign physical examination, emergency physicians must have a high index of suspicion for intraabdominal injuries in patients who have associated pelvic and lower rib cage fractures. For older patients, the adhesions associated with previous abdominal surgical procedures may increase the risk of performing diagnostic peritoneal lavage in the emergency department.[1] Therefore, CT scanning with contrast material is a valuable diagnostic test. It is important to ensure adequate hydration and baseline assessment of renal function prior to the contrast load for the CT scan. Some patients may be volume depleted due to medications such as diuretics. This hypovolemia coupled with contrast administration may exacerbate any underlying renal pathology.[1] For unstable patients, and especially those with multiple scars on the abdominal wall from previous procedures, the trauma ultrasound examination is the ideal diagnostic study to detect free intraperitoneal fluid. In prospective studies by emergency physicians and trauma surgeons, ultrasonography has been demonstrated to be highly sensitive and specific for the identification of free intraperitoneal fluid. It also is rapid, portable, noninvasive, and easily repeatable.[13]

Orthopedic Injuries

HIP FRACTURES Many elderly patients are predisposed to orthopedic injuries due to osteopenic and osteoporotic changes in their skeletal structure. Hip fracture is the single most common diagnosis that leads to hospitalization in all age groups in the United States. Hip fractures occur primarily in four areas: intertrochanteric, transcervical, subcapital, and subtrochanteric. Intertrochanteric fractures are the most common, followed by transcervical fractures.[9] Emergency physicians must be aware that pelvic and long bone fractures are not infrequently the sole etiology for hypovolemia in elderly patients. Timely orthopedic consultation, evaluation, and treatment with open reduction and internal fixation should be coordinated with the diagnosis and management of other injuries.

LONG BONE FRACTURES Long bone fractures of the femur, tibia, and humerus may produce a loss of mobility with a resulting decrease in the independent lifestyle of elderly patients.[9] Geriatric patients who present with femoral fractures have been found to have a significantly higher rate of preexisting medical conditions than patients with proximal humeral fractures.[14] Early orthopedic consultation for intramedullary rodding of these fractures may result in increased early mobilization.

UPPER EXTREMITY INJURIES Falls on the outstretched hand increase the elderly's risk for Colles's fractures. After the diagnosis is confirmed by radiographs, these fractures usually can be treated with closed reduction and immobilization. The incidence of humeral head and surgical neck fractures in elderly patients also is increased by falls on the outstretched hand or elbow.[9] Localized tenderness, swelling, and ecchymosis to the proximal humerus are characteristic of these injuries. Early orthopedic consultation and treatment with a shoulder immobilizer or surgical fixation should be arranged. Social services may need to be contacted to arrange for assistance with routine daily activities for some elderly patients being discharged home after an orthopedic injury.

TREATMENT

Special Management Principles

Emergency physicians often are faced with the challenging task of assessing elderly trauma patients' cardiovascular status and reserve. First, recent work by Ma and colleagues[15] has demonstrated that elderly trauma patients are less likely to be appropriately transported to trauma centers. Therefore, significantly injured older patients may have their injuries underappreciated yet present to nontrauma centers. The work by Scalea and colleagues[8] demonstrated that trauma physicians themselves frequently fail to recognize the severity of hemodynamic instability in geriatric patients. Therefore, early invasive monitoring has been advocated to help physicians assess the elderly's hemodynamic status. Scalea and coworkers showed that by reducing the time to invasive monitoring in elderly trauma patients from 5.5 to 2.2 h, and thus recognizing and appropriately treating occult shock, the survival rate of their patients increased from 7 to 53 percent. Survival was improved because of enhanced oxygen delivery through the use of adequate volume loading and inotropic support. These authors concluded that urgent invasive monitoring provides important hemodynamic information early, aids in identifying occult shock, limits hypoperfusion, helps prevent multiple organ failure, and improves survival.[8]

The insertion of invasive monitoring lines seldom occurs in some emergency departments because of institutional practice and availability of equipment. Given the clear empirical evidence for the value of rapid assessment and early intervention,[8] every effort should be made by emergency physicians to expedite emergency department (ED) care of elderly trauma patients and prevent unnecessary delays. In the ED evaluation of blunt trauma patients, the chest radiograph, cervical spine series, and pelvic radiographs are necessary diagnostic tests during the secondary survey. After ordering this set of plain radiographs, emergency physicians must resist the temptation of trying to appease consultants by immediately obtaining plain films of every other body region that may have sustained minor trauma. While it is vital to be thorough in the diagnosis of occult orthopedic injuries, expending a great deal of time in the radiology suite, especially if off-site, may compromise patient care. Only a few radiologic studies, such as emergent head and abdominal CT scans, can take precedence over obtaining vital information from invasive monitoring, depending on the situation. Elderly trauma patients will benefit most from an expeditious transfer to the intensive care unit so that their hemodynamic status can be further monitored. After ensuring that their hemodynamic status has been stabilized, patients can be transported back to the radiology suite for further plain radiographic studies. If in doubt, extremities can be temporarily splinted.

In the ED, emergency physicians must make critical management decisions regarding volume resuscitation without the benefit of sophisticated invasive monitoring devices. Geriatric trauma patients can decompensate with overresuscitation just as quickly as they can with inadequate resuscitation.[9] Elderly patients with underlying coronary artery disease and cerebrovascular disease are at a much greater risk of suffering the consequences of ischemia to vital organs when they become hypotensive after sustaining trauma. During the initial resuscitative phase, crystalloid, while the primary option, should be administered judiciously because elderly patients with diminished cardiac compliance are more susceptible to volume overload. Strong consideration should be given to early and more liberal use of red blood cell transfusion. This practice early in the resuscitation would enhance oxygen delivery and help minimize tissue ischemia.

DISPOSITION

Prevention, Prognosis, and Outcome

For elderly patients who are discharged home after sustaining an injury from a fall, it is appropriate for emergency physicians to encourage them to work with their primary care physician to arrange for a social worker to conduct a home safety assessment to help prevent future falls. Chronic medications that may adversely affect the vestibular system, cause profound sedation, or produce postural hypotension should be identified; patients can then discuss alternative therapies or dosages with their primary care physicians.[4] When discharging home a patient with a new medication prescription, emergency physicians should select drugs that are least centrally acting, least associated with postural hypotension, and have the shortest duration.

Among geriatric trauma patients who are hospitalized, the mortality rate has been reported to be between 15 and 30 percent. These figures far exceed the mortality rate of 4 to 8 percent found in younger patients.[1] In general, multiple organ failure and sepsis cause more deaths in elderly patients than in younger trauma victims.[16] Geriatric patients also are more likely to die following minor traumatic events.[17]

Several markers for poor outcome in elderly trauma victims have been determined. Age greater than 75 years, Glasgow Coma Scale score of 7 or less, presence of shock on admission, severe head injury, and the development of sepsis are associated with worse outcome and higher mortality figures.[18] The Injury Severity Score has been found by many investigators to have poor correlation with mortality rates.[19]

The ultimate goal in care of elderly trauma patients is to return them to their preinjury state of independent function. There are conflicting data on the ability of elderly patients to return to independent living. A study by Oreskovich and colleagues[20] showed a mortality rate of 15 percent among their geriatric trauma patients, and a dismal 12 percent of patients returning to their baseline independent state. Public debate has raised questions about the ethics and cost-benefits of trauma care for the elderly. However, DeMaria and colleagues[21,22] demonstrated that immediately after discharge, one-third of trauma survivors return to independent living, one-third return to dependent status but living at home, and one-third require nursing home facilities. Altogether, at long-term follow-up, 89 percent returned home after trauma and 57 percent returned to independent living. The findings of DeMaria and colleagues are supported by the investigation of van Aalst and colleagues,[18] who also showed that the majority of their elderly trauma patients regained an independent level of function.

Many questions regarding the ultimate outcome of geriatric trauma patients remain unanswered. In light of the investigations by DeMaria[21] and van Aalst[18] and their colleagues showing that elderly patients can return to independent living after trauma and the study by Scalea and colleagues[8] demonstrating the beneficial effect of early invasive monitoring, it appears that aggressive resuscitation efforts for geriatric trauma patients are warranted.

In summary, the acute management principles of geriatric trauma continue to evolve. Emergency physicians must remain familiar with the various mechanisms of injury unique to the elderly trauma patient. Special management and treatment axioms, outlined in Table 245-1, should be applied early when caring for the geriatric trauma patient.

TABLE 245-1 Geriatric Trauma Management Axioms

1. Assume that patients have limited physiologic reserve.
2. Seemingly minor injuries may actually be life-threatening in the face of limited physiologic reserve.
3. "Stable" patients may quickly become unstable, with little warning.
4. Low threshold for ordering of head and abdominal CT scanning is justified.
5. Early invasive hemodynamic monitoring often will provide valuable diagnostic and resuscitation information.
6. Early, aggressive oxygen use and mechanical ventilation may be necessary in some patients.
7. Blood transfusion for volume replacement early in the resuscitation phase will improve oxygen delivery in hypovolemic patients.
8. Overresuscitation is as detrimental as inadequate resuscitation.
9. The patient's environment and social situation need to be considered as potentially playing a major role in the trauma suffered and for convalescence, particularly if the patient is to be discharged from the ED.

REFERENCES

1. Schwab CW, Kauder DR: Trauma in the geriatric patient. *Arch Surg* 127:701, 1992
2. MacKenzie EJ, Morris JA, Edelstein SL: Effect of pre-existing disease on length of hospital stay in trauma patients. *J Trauma* 29:757, 1989.
3. Morris JA, MacKenzie EJ, Edelstein SL: The effect of pre-existing conditions on mortality in trauma patients. *JAMA* 263:1942, 1990.
4. Tinetti ME, Speechley M: Prevention of falls among the elderly. *N Engl J Med* 320:1055, 1989.
5. Li G, Baker SP, Longlois JA, Kelen GD: Are female drivers safer? An application of the decomposition method. *Epidemiology* 9:379, 1998.
6. Hakamies-Blomqvist LE: Fatal accidents of older drivers. *Accidents Anal Prevent* 25:19, 1993.
7. Sklar DP, Demarest GB, McFeeley P: Increased pedestrian mortality among the elderly. *Am J Emerg Med* 7:387, 1989.
8. Scalea TM, Simon HM, Duncan AO, et al: Geriatric blunt trauma: Improved survival with early invasive monitoring. *J Trauma* 30:129, 1990.
9. Demarest GB, Osler TM, Clevenger FW: Injuries in the elderly: Evaluation and initial response. *Geriatrics* 45:36, 1990.
10. Kirkpatrick JB, Pearson J: Fatal cerebral injury in the elderly. *J Am Geriatr Soc* 26:489, 1978.
11. Ryan MD, Henderson JJ: The epidemiology of fractures and fracture-dislocations of the cervical spine. *Injury* 23:38, 1992.
12. Allen JE, Schwab CW: Blunt chest trauma in the elderly. *Am Surg* 51:697, 1985.
13. Ma OJ, Mateer JR, Ogata M, et al: Prospective analysis of a rapid trauma ultrasound examination performed by emergency physicians. *J Trauma* 38:879, 1995.
14. Sartoretti C, Sartoretti-Schefer S, Ruckert R, et al: Comorbid conditions in old patients with femur fractures. *J Trauma* 43:570, 1997.
15. Ma MH-M, MacKenzie E, Alberta R, Kelen GD: Compliance with prehospital protocols for major trauma patients. *J Trauma* 46:168, 1999.
16. Horst HM, Obeid FN, Sorensen VJ, et al: Factors influencing survival of elderly trauma patients. *Crit Care Med* 14:681, 1986.
17. Smith DP, Enderson BL, Maull KI: Trauma in the elderly: Determinants of outcome. *South Med J* 83:171, 1990.
18. van Aalst JA, Morris JA, Yates HK, et al: Severely injured geriatric patients return to independent living: A study of factors influencing function and independence. *J Trauma* 31:1096, 1991.
19. Osler T, Hales K, Baack B, et al: Trauma in the elderly. *Am J Surg* 156:537, 1988.
20. Oreskovich MR, Howard JD, Copass MK, et al: Geriatric trauma: Injury patterns and outcome. *J Trauma* 24:565, 1984.
21. DeMaria EJ, Kenney PR, Merriam MA, et al: Survival after trauma in geriatric patients. *Ann Surg* 206:738, 1987.
22. DeMaria EJ, Kenney PR, Merriam MA, et al: Aggressive trauma care benefits the elderly. *J Trauma* 27:1200, 1987.

TRAUMA IN PREGNANCY

Nelson Tang

An injured pregnant woman presents two patients, simultaneously requiring timely and effective evaluation, stabilization, and definitive care. Furthermore, the inherent changes in maternal anatomy and physiology during pregnancy make effective diagnosis of serious injury more difficult and may result in delays in recognition and initiation of therapy. As in other aspects of trauma care, injuries in pregnancy require a thoughtful and consistent approach to diagnosis and treatment.

Trauma remains the leading cause of nonobstetric morbidity and mortality in pregnant women. The conventional paradigm that fetal survival depends wholly on maternal stabilization and well-being is fundamentally accurate. It has become increasingly apparent, however, that especially in relatively minor traumatic events the severity of maternal injuries may be a poor predictor of fetal distress and outcome.[1-3] Successful outcomes for both mother and fetus require a collaborative effort among the prehospital provider, emergency physician, trauma surgeon, obstetrician, and neonatologist.

EPIDEMIOLOGY

It has been consistently estimated that significant trauma complicates 6 to 7 percent of all pregnancies.[2] Trauma during pregnancy is associated with an increased risk of preterm labor, placental abruption, fetal-maternal hemorrhage, and pregnancy loss. Maternal trauma-related mortality rate does not appear to be different from that of nonpregnant women.[4,5]

The most common cause of blunt abdominal trauma is motor vehicle crash, accounting for up to 70 percent of acute injuries. This is followed by falls and direct assault in decreasing order of frequency.[1,2,6] The incidence of falls appears to increase with advancement of pregnancies, presumably due to alterations in maternal balance and coordination. Minor abdominal trauma may yet result in fetal demise. Up to 5 percent of patients with minor trauma may experience abruption. The role of domestic violence during pregnancy is of significant concern, with one large series describing more than 31 percent of trauma in pregnant women as intentional injuries and as many as 88 percent of those cases implicating the husband or boyfriend as perpetrator.[7] Whether this represents a change in epidemiology or reporting, the need for vigilance by emergency physicians for domestic or intimate violence during pregnancy is clear.

Penetrating injuries are less common than blunt trauma during pregnancy. Gunshot wounds are the most common form of penetrating trauma. Some of these injuries may be self-inflicted and represent attempts to terminate pregnancies.[6] Fetal mortality rates in penetrating injuries are as high as 70 percent. While the rate of maternal visceral injuries is 19 to 38 percent, there remains a 60 to 90 percent chance of fetal injury. This is presumably due to the protective effect of the gravid uterus on maternal viscera.

PHYSIOLOGIC CHANGES OF PREGNANCY

A normal pregnancy creates complex changes in maternal anatomy and physiology, many of which begin as early as the first trimester and continue throughout its term. Significant alterations to the maternal reproductive, cardiovascular, respiratory, and gastrointestinal systems as well as maternal anatomy make the evaluation of an acutely injured pregnant patient more difficult. An understanding of these physiologic changes is essential to the appropriate diagnosis and management in such cases. These are discussed in detail in Chap. 99, ''Normal Pregnancy,'' but will be noted here in brief.

Maternal blood volume begins to expand at approximately week 10 of gestation and peaks at 45 to 50 percent increase from baseline at week 28, resulting in a state of hypervolemia. Red cell mass increases to a lesser extent, leading to the relative physiologic anemia of pregnancy. Cardiac output is increased by 1.0 to 1.5 L/min at week 10 of pregnancy and remains elevated until the end of pregnancy. Heart rate in the mother is generally increased by 10 to 20 beats per minute in the second trimester, accompanied by decreases in systolic and diastolic blood pressures of 10 to 15 mmHg.

These changes can be frequently misleading during maternal resuscitation in trauma and make clinical findings difficult to interpret. A pregnant woman may lose 30 to 35 percent of circulating blood volume before manifesting hypotension or clinical signs of shock.[2] Uterine arteries vasoconstrict, resulting in diminished fetal blood flow and tissue oxygenation before significant evidence of maternal hypovolemia.

After week 12 of gestation, the uterus becomes an intraabdominal organ, removing it from the relative protection of the maternal pelvis and making it more susceptible to direct injuries. The bladder also moves anteriorly into the abdomen in the third trimester of pregnancy, increasing its susceptibility to injury. Uterine blood flow may increase to upward of 600 mL/min, making severe maternal hemorrhage from uterine injury possible. The gravid uterus also causes passive stretching of the abdominal wall and peritoneum as it enlarges and may lead to diminished sensitivity to injury and irritation from intraperitoneal blood.[4] At or about week 20 of gestation, the expanding mass of the gravid uterus may lead to the supine hypotension syndrome in which venous return and cardiac output are diminished by compression of the maternal inferior vena cava in the supine position. The enlarging uterus may additionally cause engorgement of lower extremity and lower abdominal vessels, predisposing the patient to severe retroperitoneal hemorrhages in acute injuries to these areas.

As pregnancy progresses, the diaphragm is raised by as much as 4 cm and tidal volume increases by 40 percent as residual volume diminishes by 25 percent. Functional residual capacity is similarly decreased, and the compensatory increase in ventilation results typically in respiratory alkalosis. Serum pH is usually maintained at normal values by renal compensation. These changes may significantly impair the ability of a pregnant trauma patient to compensate for respiratory compromise.

The gastrointestinal tract demonstrates diminished motility, and there is delayed gastric emptying during pregnancy. This increases the likelihood of gastroesophageal reflux and the potential for aspiration from acute injuries as well as from resuscitative interventions, including endotracheal intubation. The small bowel is moved upward in the abdomen by the enlarging uterus, protecting the small bowel to some degree from lower abdominal injuries. It does, however, increase the chance of complex bowel injuries in penetrating trauma of the upper abdomen.[4] The liver is typically unaffected by pregnancy, and the most common etiology of abdominal hemorrhage remains splenic injury, as in nonpregnant patients.

MATERNAL AND FETAL INJURIES

Until about week 12 of gestation, the uterus is protected to a large degree by the bony structure of the maternal pelvis. As a result, direct fetal injury is relatively infrequent in blunt abdominal trauma during pregnancy. When fetal injuries do occur, they are typically seen in later gestation and tend to involve the fetal skull and brain. These injuries are frequently sustained in association with fractures to the maternal pelvis when the fetal head is engaged. When the uterus is penetrated by a sharp object or projectile, the fetus has a high probability of sustaining injury.[6,8]

Uterine rupture is a relatively uncommon complication of blunt trauma sustained during pregnancy. Its incidence has been reported as 0.6 to 1.0 percent of injuries in pregnancy and is more likely to occur during the late second and third trimesters and when there is direct and forceful impact upon the uterus.[4,6] The fetal mortality rate in such cases is nearly 100 percent, whereas maternal mortality is less than 10 percent. The presentation of uterine rupture may be quite nonspecific, but loss of the palpable uterine contour, ease of palpation of fetal parts, or radiologic evidence of abnormal fetal location is suggestive of the diagnosis.

Uterine irritability and the onset of preterm labor may be precipitated by acute abdominal trauma during pregnancy. Numerous reports have noted the management of premature labor in pregnant trauma patients with tocolytic agents, but the use has not been generally recommended and requires individualization.[1,9] Tocolytic agents have numerous described adverse side effects, such as fetal and maternal tachycardia, which may complicate the evaluation of trauma patients. Additionally, their use may further impair the ability to diagnose other significant traumatic injuries, specifically placental abruption. If tocolytics are considered, an obstetrician should be consulted prior to administration.

Second only to maternal death, abruptio placentae is the most common cause of fetal death. Abruptio placentae complicates 1 to 5 percent of minor injuries during pregnancy and up to 40 to 50 percent of major traumas.[1,6] Placental abruption has been described as being caused by the deformation of the elastic uterus around the relatively inelastic placenta. Further exacerbated by increased intrauterine pressures, shear forces are applied to the placental base, leading to separation from the uterine wall. Findings consistent with abruptio placentae include abdominal pain, vaginal bleeding, and tetanic uterine contractions. Placental abruption may also lead to the introduction of placental products into the maternal circulation, stimulating disseminated intravascular coagulation (DIC). The correlation and predictive value of DIC with respect to fetal mortality remains unsettled.[7,10]

The fetal and maternal circulations are normally separate during pregnancy, and fetal red blood cells may enter the maternal bloodstream in cases of traumatic injury. The incidence of such fetal-maternal hemorrhage in trauma during pregnancy is four to five times that which occurs in pregnancies not complicated by injury.[4,6] Fetal-maternal hemorrhage occurs in over 30 percent of significant trauma in pregnant patients and is implicated in the sensitization and subsequent isoimmunization of Rh-negative patients. As little as 0.1 to 0.3 mL of fetal cells is sufficient to sensitize 70 percent of Rh-negative women.[11] The fetal hemorrhage itself poses the direct risks of fetal hypovolemia, anemia, distress, and death. Anterior placental location appears to be associated with increased risk of fetal-maternal hemorrhage.[1]

EMERGENCY TREATMENT

Prehospital Care

An effort to ascertain the possibility of pregnancy should be made during the initial evaluation of all acutely injured women of childbearing age. As in the care of all trauma victims, initial priorities remain the ABCs of resuscitation. All pregnant trauma patients should receive supplemental oxygen, as the gravida becomes less able to compensate for hypoxia. Similarly, early intubation must be considered when indicated by the nature or severity of injuries. Peripheral intravenous lines with crystalloid infusions should be initiated in the prehospital setting.

For pregnant patients beyond 20 weeks of gestation who must be transported in the supine position or in whom spinal immobilization is indicated, a wedge should be placed under the right hip area tilting the patient toward her left side to avoid hypotension from inferior vena cava compression by the gravid uterus. Alternatively, the uterus may be manually maneuvered to the left side of the abdomen by transport personnel. Pneumatic antishock trousers are rarely used now, but if considered in a pregnant patient, the abdominal compartment must not be inflated, because that may cause uteroplacental compression and impair venous return to the heart. An integral part of the prehospital role in trauma management is the appropriate triage to receiving facilities. If pregnancy in a trauma patient is identified or suspected, transport should be initiated to a designated trauma center with sufficient capabilities to manage such patients. Advanced notification of the receiving facility should be made to enable the assembly of the appropriate hospital personnel to continue the resuscitation and management efforts.

Emergency Department Management

Upon arrival in the emergency department, the prehospital resuscitative measures already undertaken should be reviewed and continued as appropriate. Since maternal stability and survival offer the best chance for fetal well-being, initial efforts must be directed toward the adequate resuscitation of the mother. No critical interventions or diagnostic procedures should be withheld from the treatment of pregnant trauma patients out of concerns for potential adverse fetal consequences. A trauma surgeon and obstetrician should be involved early in the evaluation and management of a significantly traumatized pregnant patient.

The initial sequence of trauma resuscitation is unchanged in the emergency treatment of an injured pregnant patient. The patient is kept in the left lateral decubitus position to the extent possible to minimize vena caval compression. Securing the airway and ensuring the adequacy of ventilation in addition to the administration of supplemental oxygenation are of primary concern. Gastric tube decompression must be performed early, since delayed stomach emptying makes the possibility of aspiration a particular concern during pregnancy. Sources of hemorrhage should be identified and controlled, because maternal blood loss and hypovolemia occur at the expense of fetal hypoperfusion. Adequate large-bore vascular access is essential, and crystalloid infusions may need to be adjusted upward by as much as 50 percent to account for the additional plasma volumes in pregnancy.[4,8] The use of vasopressor agents poses a risk of impaired uterine perfusion and should not be initiated until adequate volume replacement has been administered. Their use should not be restricted, however, if required for maternal resuscitation. Initial laboratory studies include complete blood counts, blood typing, and Rh status, as well as coagulation profiles to determine the possibility of DIC. Low serum bicarbonate levels have been shown to be associated with adverse fetal outcomes, and routine determination of the levels may be of predictive value.[2] After the primary trauma survey, an organized and methodical secondary system survey must be performed to ensure the identification of all potential injuries.

Attention should next be turned to the gravid abdomen. Gestational age can be assessed rapidly by palpating uterine fundal height. At week 20 of gestation, the fundus may be palpated at or about the level of the umbilicus. The abdomen and uterus should be examined for evidence of injury as well as palpated for uterine tenderness or contractions. If abdominal or pelvic trauma is suspected, a sterile pelvic examination is indicated to inspect for injuries of the lower genital tract, vaginal bleeding, or rupture of amniotic membranes. Fluid in the vaginal canal with pH of 7 is suggestive of amniotic fluid, whereas a pH of 5 is consistent with vaginal secretions. A branchlike pattern upon drying of vaginal fluid on a microscopy slide or "ferning" is also diagnostic of amniotic fluid.

The Kleihauer-Betke assay is an acid elution technique that differentially stains fetal and maternal red blood cells based on differences in hemoglobin and may be performed on maternal blood to quantify the degree of fetal-maternal hemorrhage in Rh-negative gravidas. The sensitivity of the typical laboratory Kleihauer-Betke test is generally incapable of detecting small quantities of transfused fetal blood. Thus, administration of one prophylactic dose of Rh immune globulin (Rho-

GAM) is indicated with all Rh-negative pregnant trauma patients beyond 12 weeks of gestation who are evaluated for abdominal injury. One 300-μg dose of RhoGAM protects against 30 mL of fetal blood. The use of the Kleihauer-Betke test may be helpful in identifying greater amounts of fetal-maternal inadvertent transfusion and determining the need for additional doses of immune globulin. Its utility, however, as a predictor of fetal morbidity or adverse pregnancy outcome has not been demonstrated.[1,9,12] Tetanus prophylaxis has no deleterious fetal effects and should be routinely administered as indicated following trauma.

The indications for emergent laparotomy remain unchanged in the evaluation of pregnant trauma patients. Similarly, diagnostic peritoneal lavage (DPL) and abdominopelvic computed tomography (CT) scan remain valid modalities for the evaluation of intraabdominal injuries from acute trauma. DPL should be performed with an open, supraumbilical technique in patients with evidence of a gravid uterus. The fetus appears to tolerate surgery and anesthesia well if adequate oxygenation and uterine perfusion are maintained.[6] The performance of emergent DPL and surgery have not been shown to have an association with fetal loss, and these procedures should not be withheld out of concern for fetal compromise when indicated in trauma.[2] Additionally, a recent large multi-institutional retrospective review has shown that emergent cesarean delivery results in a fetal survival rate as high as 75 percent when gestation is at or longer than 26 weeks, fetal heart tones are present on admission, and the procedure is performed at the earliest indication of fetal distress.[3]

Radiologic Evaluation

The use of diagnostic radiologic imaging in the emergency treatment of pregnant trauma patients adheres to the fundamental principles of trauma management. While the judicious acquisition of studies is indicated to minimize fetal exposure to the potential effects of ionizing radiation (Table 246-1), no tests should be withheld if necessary for appropriate maternal evaluation and treatment. The principal concerns regarding radiation exposure in utero are the possibilities of childhood neoplasia, fetal loss, congenital malformations, and microcephaly.[13] Thus, studies should be limited to those needed, as radiation exposure sequelae are cumulative. The greatest risk to fetal viability is within the first 2 weeks following conception, and the highest potential for malformation is during embryonic organogenesis from 2 to 8 weeks after conception.[13] Adverse fetal effects due to radiation exposure are negligible from doses of less than 10 rad. The standard trauma plain radiographs, such as cervical spine, chest, and pelvis films, deliver significantly less than 1 rad each.[4,13] Fetal exposure can be further decreased by appropriate shielding of the maternal abdomen and pelvis during many studies.

TABLE 246-1 Fetal Radiation Exposure from Common Radiologic Studies

Radiologic Study	Exposure (rad)
Cervical spine film	≤0.001
Chest film	0.001–0.005
Abdomen film	0.10–0.5
Pelvis film	0.15–0.5
Lumbar spine film	0.5–1.5
Head CT scan	0.05–0.1
Abdominopelvic CT scan	1.0–5.0

Abbreviation: CT, computed tomography.

Abdominopelvic CT scanning, pelvic angiography, and pelvic fluoroscopy result in the highest delivered doses of radiation. The amount is typically 2 to 5 rad, with some variation due to equipment quality, techniques used, and duration of study.[4,13] Radiation exposure in CT may be reduced by performing modified studies and the use of dose-reducing techniques, such as reducing the number of slices obtained.[13] Diagnostic evaluations with magnetic resonance imaging and ventilation-perfusion scanning have not been reported to cause adverse pregnancy outcomes. Potential effects of contrast agents have not been definitively studied, and their use requires individualization.

Fetal Assessment

A rapid assessment of fetal condition should be initiated with auscultation of fetal heart tones to determine fetal viability and identify fetal distress. Assessment of fetal heart tones may be augmented by use of a Doppler stethoscope or ultrasound. It has been suggested that fetal viability in the setting of trauma is directly related to the presence or absence of fetal heart tones on presentation, and that if these are confirmed absent, then the remainder of treatment efforts be directed solely at maternal resuscitation.[3] Normal fetal heart rates are in the range of 120 to 160 beats per minute. The most likely cause of fetal bradycardia is acute hypoxia. In acute injuries, maternal hypotension, hypothermia, respiratory compromise, or placental abruption are likely etiologies. Similarly, in the setting of acute trauma, the finding of fetal tachycardia may also represent a hypoxic or hypovolemic state.

The use of bedside ultrasound has become an increasingly valuable adjunct to initial trauma assessment and management. Portable ultrasound has been shown to be rapid, noninvasive, and facilitates serial examinations.[14] In cases of trauma during pregnancy, ultrasonography may also be of particular value in the evaluation of general fetal condition. Fetal size and estimated gestational age, the presence of fetal heart motion, fetal activity or demise, placental location, and amniotic fluid volume can be assessed.[4,15] The efficacy of ultrasound, however, for the diagnosis of specific trauma-related injuries remains unproven. Several recent reports have suggested the relative inability of ultrasound to diagnose uterine rupture or fetal-placental injuries, and its sensitivity is insufficient to exclude the diagnosis of placental abruption.[12,15] The intraabdominal anatomic distortions of late third-trimester pregnancy may further limit the diagnostic capability of ultrasound in acute trauma.

In the management of blunt trauma during pregnancy, external fetal monitoring is indicated for gestational age estimated beyond 20 weeks. The initiation of fetal tocodynamometry is recommended at the earliest possible stage of evaluation following maternal stabilization, preferably in the emergency department. Fetal monitoring is utilized to assess both uterine contractile activity as well as fetal heart rate. Beyond the viable gestational age of 23 weeks, the presence of fetal tachycardia, lack of beat-to-beat or long-term variability, or late decelerations on tocodynamometry are diagnostic of fetal distress and may be indications for emergent cesarean delivery.

The identification of frequent uterine activity on external fetal monitoring has been shown to be a sensitive predictor of abruptio placentae beyond 20 weeks of gestation. In a major prospective study, no cases of abruptio placentae were identified unless more than 8 contractions per hour were found during the first 4 h of tocodynamometry.[1] A minimum of 4 h of external tocodynamometric monitoring appears to be predictive of immediate adverse pregnancy outcomes and is indicated for all pregnant patients evaluated for trauma. Patients demonstrating 3 to 7 contractions per hour of persistent uterine irritability should have tocodynamometry extended to a minimum of 24 h. They may subsequently be safely discharged if uterine contractions abate and other reasons for further evaluation do not exist. Patients with fewer than 3 contractions per hour during an initial 4-h observation period can be safely discharged. This approach has been shown to have the same pregnancy outcomes among discharged patients when compared with uninjured controls.

TABLE 246-2 Estimated Neonatal Survival Rates by Gestational Age

Gestational Age (Weeks)	Survival (%)
22	0
23	15
24	55
25	60
26	≥75

PERIMORTEM CESAREAN DELIVERY

The need to perform perimortem cesarean delivery in cases of maternal cardiac arrest arises extremely infrequently. Nevertheless, it involves complex ethical, medical, and emotional considerations. The largest review of reported attempts to date in the literature revealed fewer than 200 successful fetal outcomes from the procedure.[16] The time to delivery from the onset of maternal arrest was found to be critical to fetal survival with good neurologic outcome. Excellent outcomes were reported when delivery took place within 5 min of maternal death. Survival was unlikely if delivery occurred after 20 min of maternal arrest. It has since been recommended that the procedure be performed after 4 min of maternal resuscitation. Recently, the first successful out-of-hospital perimortem cesarean delivery was reported and with a time interval of 34 min between maternal collapse and delivery, although with severe neurologic deficits in the infant.[17]

Consideration of perimortem cesarean delivery must be made only after immediate and optimal advanced maternal cardiopulmonary resuscitative measures have been instituted. The procedure may be attempted in gestations estimated at beyond 23 weeks[17] (Table 246-2). Full maternal resuscitation must continue unabated while preparing for and during the actual delivery. It is universally recommended that the procedure be performed rapidly with the most readily available materials and that a single vertical incision be made to enter the peritoneum, followed by a vertical uterine incision to deliver the fetus. Successful maternal revival following fetal delivery has been reported. Improved venous return to the central circulation, increased maternal oxygen delivery following removal of the high uterine demand, and decreased pooling of blood in the uteroplacental circulation have all been suggested explanations.

DISPOSITION

The decision to admit or discharge after the emergency assessment and management of a pregnant trauma patient is ultimately based on the nature and severity of presenting injuries. Patients suffering severe multisystem trauma will have their further management assumed by trauma surgeons and consultant obstetricians. Even in cases of seemingly minor but potentially significant injuries, admission to a trauma service capable of further observation and management is appropriate. Patients who demonstrate evidence of fetal distress or uterine irritability during the initial assessment require admission under the extended evaluation and care of an obstetrician capable of emergency delivery as necessary. Patients who must be transferred to other facilities for definitive trauma or obstetric care must be appropriately stabilized prior to transfer, with provisions for an appropriate level of care during transport. There must be strict adherence to transfer policies that comply with COBRA and EMTALA regulations. Clearly, the ongoing need for an interdisciplinary approach to patient management in such cases remains even after admission.

Although external fetal monitoring may be initiated in the emergency department, the monitoring is typically continued in the labor and delivery suite under the direction of an obstetrician. If the extended period of monitoring demonstrates no evidence to suggest fetal or maternal injury or distress, the patient may be discharged. Upon discharge, the patient must be carefully advised to seek medical attention immediately if she should develop abdominal pain or cramping, vaginal bleeding, leakage of fluid, or perception of diminished fetal activity. The decision to discharge an injured pregnant patient from the emergency department must be made carefully. A high index of suspicion should be maintained for occult injuries as well as a low threshold for obstetric consultation when indicated. To screen for the possibility of interpersonal violence, a thorough social services evaluation or referral should be made in all but the most obvious cases of accidental injury. Adequate obstetric follow-up care must be ensured for all pregnant trauma patients when discharged from the emergency department.

REFERENCES

1. Pearlman MD, Tintinalli JE, Lorenz RP: A prospective controlled study of outcome after trauma during pregnancy. *Am J Obstet Gynecol* 162:1502, 1990.
2. Scorpio RJ, Esposito TJ, Smith LG, et al: Blunt trauma during pregnancy: Factors affecting fetal outcome. *J Trauma* 32:213, 1992.
3. Morris JA, Rosenbower TJ, Jurkovich GJ, et al: Infant survival after cesarean section for trauma. *Ann Surg* 223:481, 1996.
4. Pearlman MD, Tintinalli JE: Evaluation and treatment of the gravida and fetus following trauma during pregnancy. *Obstet Gynecol Clin North Am* 18:371, 1991.
5. Esposito TJ, Gens DR, Smith LG, et al: Trauma during pregnancy: A review of 79 cases. *Arch Surg* 126:1073, 1991.
6. Trauma during pregnancy. *Am Coll Obstet Gynecol Tech Bull* 161, 1991.
7. Poole GV, Martin JN, Perry KG Jr, et al: Trauma in pregnancy: The role of interpersonal violence. *Am J Obstet Gynecol* 174:1873, 1996.
8. American College of Surgeons Committee on Trauma: *Advanced Trauma Life Support Student Course Manual.* Chicago, American College of Surgeons, 1997.
9. Dahmus MA, Sibai BM: Blunt abdominal trauma: Are there any predictive factors for abruptio placentae or maternal-fetal distress? *Am J Obstet Gynecol* 169:1054, 1993.
10. Ali J, Yeo A, Gana TJ, et al: Predictors of fetal mortality in pregnant trauma patients. *J Trauma* 42:782, 1997.
11. Mollison PL: Clinical aspects of Rh immunization. *Am J Clin Pathol* 60:287, 1973.
12. Towery R, English P, Wisner D: Evaluation of pregnant women after blunt injury. *J Trauma* 35:731, 1993.
13. Goldman SM, Wagner LK: Radiologic management of abdominal trauma in pregnancy. *Am J Radiol* 166:763, 1996.
14. Nordenholz KE, Rubin MA, Gularte GG, et al: Ultrasound in the evaluation and management of blunt abdominal trauma. *Ann Emerg Med* 29:357, 1997.
15. Ma OJ, Mateer JR, DeBehnke DJ: Use of ultrasonography for the evaluation of pregnant trauma patients. *J Trauma* 40:665, 1996.
16. Katz VL, Dotters DJ, Droegemueller W: Perimortem cesarean delivery. *Obstet Gynecol* 68:571, 1986.
17. Kupas DF, Harter SC, Vosk A: Out-of-hospital perimortem cesarean section. *Prehosp Emerg Care* 2:206, 1997.

HEAD INJURY

Thomas D. Kirsch
Salvatore Migliore
Teresita M. Hogan

EPIDEMIOLOGY

Injuries are the leading cause of death in persons less than 45 years old with up to 50 percent of these due to head trauma. This chapter discusses all aspects of head injuries, but focuses on the more severe category of injuries now referred to as traumatic brain injuries (TBI). According to national data, approximately 1.5 million people per year sustain a nonfatal TBI. More than 370,000 persons are hospitalized annually with TBI, and 52,000 per year sustain a fatal TBI.[1] In 1996, there were more than 750,000 ED visits for intracranial head injuries and 2.6 million visits for open wounds to the head.[2] TBI is also the major cause of traumatic disability in the United States, leading to 80,000 annual cases of residual neurologic disability. The costs for treatment of both acute and chronic TBI have been estimated to be $4 billion dollars annually.[3]

The most commonly affected groups are young male adults. The elderly and young children are also at greater risk because of underlying anatomic and physiologic factors. In addition, alcoholics are at an increased risk for TBI. Ethanol-intoxicated individuals have a 40 percent greater chance of sustaining a head injury than sober individuals.[4] The causal agent for TBI a mortality varies greatly by age and other demographic factors. For example, the leading cause of TBI-related deaths in the 15- to 24-year-old age group is gunshot wounds, while for those over 65 years it is falls.

ANATOMY

The scalp is composed of five layers; skin, subcutaneous tissue, galea, areolar tissue, and the pericranium. There is potential for severe blood loss due to the heavy blood supply in the subcutaneous tissue and the loose areolar connection to the pericranium.

The skull is a rigid container made up of eight major bones. The bones of the skull have two solid layers separated by cancellous bone, which adds further rigidity and strength. The inner surface of the skull is lined by the dura. While protecting the brain from external forces, the rigid skull does not allow for the expansion of the intracranial contents. Fractures of the skull, particularly of the temporal bone can disrupt the enclosed meningeal artery and lead to epidural hematoma.

The adult brain weighs between 1300 and 1500 g and occupies 80 percent of the total volume of the skull. The brain's three basic structures—the cerebral hemispheres, the cerebellum and the brainstem—are divided by two major fixed dura attachments. The *falx cerebri* vertically separates the two major halves of the cerebrum down to the level of the brainstem. The *tentorium cerebelli* separates the cerebellum and brainstem from the cerebrum at the base of the skull. The inner edge of the tentorium cerebelli is the site of the most common brain herniation syndrome, uncal herniation. The cerebrum is further anatomically divided into major lobes named after the bones overlying them: frontal, temporal, parietal, occipital.

The brain is covered with multiple anatomic layers and potential spaces. The outermost layer next to the skull is the *dura*. It is between the dura and the skull where bleeding from the meningeal arteries causes epidural hematomas. Underneath is a thinner fibrous material called the *arachnoid*. The *pia* is closely associated with the gray matter of the brain and is the inner most layer. Between the arachnoid and the pia is the *subarachnoid space* where cerebrospinal fluid (CSF) circulates. In the average adult, there is 150 mL of CSF surrounding the brain and spinal cord. Approximately 500 mL of CFS is produced in the choroid plexus of the lateral ventricles each day.

PATHOPHYSIOLOGY

Physiology

The brain accounts for only 2 percent of total body weight, but consumes 20 percent of the body's total oxygen requirement and 15 percent of total cardiac output. The volume of cerebral blood flow (CBF), the cerebral perfusion pressure (CPP), and the blood oxygen levels determine the amount of oxygen delivered to cerebral tissue. Under normal circumstances the major regulatory mechanisms of CBF are the P_{CO_2}, blood pressure, and pH. As hypotension or hypoventilation leads to increased P_{CO_2} and decreased pH, the cerebral vasculature dilates to increase CBF and deliver more oxygen. Vasoconstriction occurs with hypertension, hypocarbia and alkalosis. CBF is also responsive to P_{O_2}, with cerebral vasodilatation occurring as P_{O_2} decreases.

Because it is not possible to accurately measure the CBF in a clinical setting, the CPP is used as a surrogate indicator for monitoring. The CPP is the pressure gradient against which cerebral perfusion must work and is the result of the mean arterial pressure (MAP) minus the intracranial pressure.[5] This is summarized by the equation, CPP = MAP − ICP. Under normal conditions, the ICP is 0 to 10 mmHg. Therefore, CPP is closely related to the MAP. The brain has the ability to maintain a constant cerebral blood flow by vasodilatation or vasoconstriction to counter changes in the MAP in hypotensive or hypertensive settings. This self-maintenance is known as *autoregulation* and functions when the CPP is between 50 and 150 mmHg (Fig. 247-1). Outside this range autoregulation is disrupted, and CBF follows a more linear passive-pressure relationship to CPP. Patients with TBI often lose autoregulation and CBF follows a linear relationship directly proportional to the CPP. Under these conditions, normal cerebral blood flow may not be restored until the CPP is greater than 90 mmHg.[5] Below this value, cerebral blood flow may not be sufficient to support cerebral oxygenation, resulting in tissue ischemia. In 1996, the Brain Trauma Foundation made several recommendations regarding CPP, MAP, and ICP for patients with TBI.[6] CPP should be maintained at 70 mmHg or greater. To achieve this, two things must occur: the MAP must be 90 mmHg or greater (which would mean a SBP of 120 to 140 mmHg) and the ICP no greater than 20 to 25 mmHg.[6] Under these guidelines, any patient with severe TBI must have a MAP >90 mmHg maintained. If this is achieved and the patient exhibits progressive neurologic deterioration or evidence of herniation not attributable to extracranial sources, then the ICP is most likely elevated and CPP decreased. In this situation, CSF drainage by ventriculostomy is the best intervention, followed by mannitol given as a bolus. Hyperventilation should not be used prophylactically due to potentially serious side effects from decreased CBF. If it is used prophylactically, then a Pa_{CO_2} of 30 to 35 mmHg should be maintained. Hyperventilation should only be performed for treatment of documented intracranial hypertension. It is generally reserved for increased ICP that is refractory to treatment modalities such as adequate CPP, CSF drainage, sedation, neuromuscular blockade, mannitol.[6]

The calvarium is a closed space housing three components: the brain, blood, and CSF. Volume increase in one of these components leads to either a decrease in another component or an increase in intracranial pressure. Patients with a TBI-caused mass lesion or cerebral edema have an increase in brain volume. Initially, as pressure increases, the CSF is displaced into the spinal canal, a process called *CSF buffering*. The elastic properties of the brain provide further compensation by allowing tissue compression. As the volume increases beyond the regulatory capacity, the ICP increases, leading to decreased CBF, the loss of autoregulation, and tissue ischemia or herniation. Rapid rises in the ICP can lead the *Cushing reflex* of hypertension, bradycardia, and respiratory irregularities. This triad is classic for an acute rise in ICP, but is seen in only one-third of cases, and is more common in children than adults.

Traumatic Brain Injury

TBI results from either direct or indirect forces to the brain matter. Direct injury is caused immediately by the forces of an object striking the head or by penetrating injury. Indirect injuries are from acceleration/deceleration forces that result in the movement of the brain inside the skull. These injuries are caused by the shearing

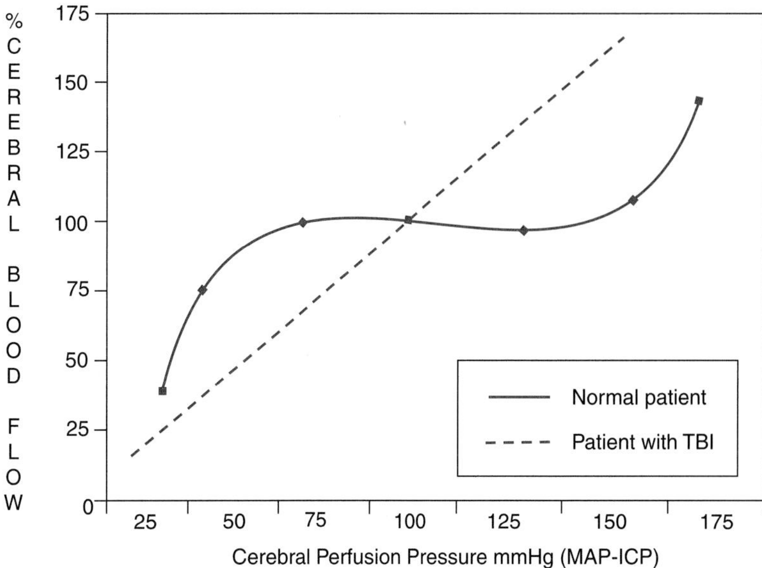

FIG. 247-1. Normal cerebral blood flow autoregulation curve and the abnormal relationship in TBI. In normal settings (solid line) the CBF remains relatively constant between a CPP of 50–150. Outside these ranges the relationship of CBF to CPP is more direct and linear. For patients with TBI, the relationship is direct through all CPP (dotted line).

forces generated by the variable movements of different areas of the brain against one another and by the impact of the brain against the skull.

PRIMARY INJURY TBI is further described as either primary or secondary injury. Primary neuronal damage occurs immediately at impact and is dependent upon the cause and severity of the inciting event. These injuries are irreversible and therefore prevention of the injury event and mitigation of the injury forces applied to the brain are the only means to reduce morbidity and mortality. Preventive measures include safer roads, barriers to prevent falls, and gun control legislation. In addition, bicycle and motorcycle helmets, seatbelts, airbags, and soft surfaces on playgrounds are effective in reducing the morbidity and mortality from TBI.

SECONDARY INJURY Secondary damage occurs from minutes to days after the event. Secondary injuries result from either intracranial or systemic causes. Secondary intracranial injuries are the result of neurophysiologic and anatomic changes at the cellular level. Besides the direct damage to cells, secondary injuries cause cerebral edema that, along with mass lesions such as epidural and subdural hematomas, increases the ICP.[7]

Systemic Causes Once an injury has occured, the greatest benefit for patients can be provided by preventing the systemic causes of secondary injury. These include correcting hypoxemia, hypotension, anemia, hyperglycemia, and hyperthermia, and evacuation of intracranial masses. Hypotension (SBP <90) and hypoxemia (Po_2 <60) have been associated with a doubling of TBI mortality.[8] Anemia (hematocrit <30 percent) also leads to increased mortality due to decreased oxygen-carrying capacity. Patients with acute subdural hematomas have a 30 percent mortality rate if operated on within four hours compared to a 90 percent mortality rate after four hours.[9]

BRAIN HERNIATION When intracranial pressure increases beyond the capability of physiologic and limited physical compensation, brain herniation can occur. There are four major brain herniation syndromes: uncal and central transtentorial, cerebellotonsillar and upward posterior fossa. The most common site of herniation occurs when the uncus of the temporal lobe is displaced inferiorly through the medial edge of the tentorium (Fig. 247-2). This is usually due to an expanding lesion in the temporal lobe or lateral middle fossa. Uncal transtentorial herniation leads to compression of the third (occulomotor) nerve, causing an ipsilateral fixed and dilated pupil. Further herniation compresses the pyramidal tract leading to contralateral motor paralysis. In 20 percent of cases, the pupillary changes are contralateral, or motor changes are ipsilateral, so decompressive trephination (''burr holes'') should be bilateral when trephination on the expected side does not yield expected results.

Central transtentorial herniation is less common and occurs with midline lesions in the frontal or occipital lobes, or in the vertex. The most prominent symptoms are initial bilateral pinpoint pupils, bilateral Babinski's signs and increased muscle tone. This is followed by fixed midpoint pupils, prolonged hyperventilation, and decorticate posturing.

Cerebellotonsillar herniation occurs when the cerebellar tonsils herniate through the foramen magnum. This causes pinpoint pupils, flaccid paralysis, and sudden death. Upward transtentorial herniation results from a posterior fossa lesion and leads to a conjugate downward gaze with absence of vertical eye movements, pinpoint pupils, and rapid death.

THE CLINICAL SPECTRUM OF TBI

The Glasgow Coma Scale (GCS) was developed as a standardized scoring system allowing reliable interobserver neurologic assessment of patients with head injuries.[10] An accurate GCS score can only be obtained after resuscitation. A GCS during the initial resuscitation phase has limitations and may be artificially low. The postresuscitation GCS is used to categorize the severity of traumatic brain injuries and is based upon three factors: eye opening, verbal function, and motor function (Table 247-1). The best response in a stabilized patient from each area is added for a score that ranges from 3 to 15. The GCS for intubated patients cannot be assessed for verbal response, and paralyzed patients cannot be assessed for any of the three categories. The following recommendations are based on nonintubated, nonsedated postresuscitation GCS. A GCS of less than 9 is considered a severe TBI, moderate is 9 to 13, and mild is 14 to 15.

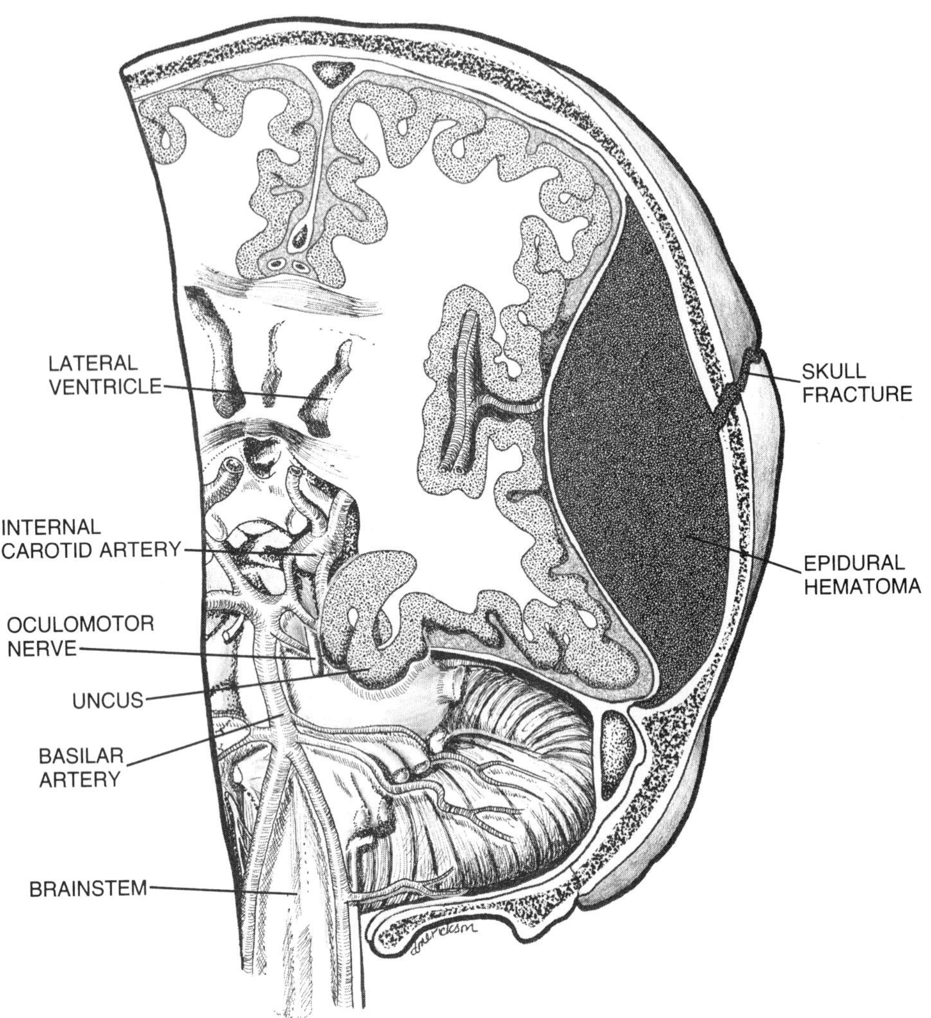

FIG. 247-2. Anterior view of transtentorial uncal herniation caused by a large hematoma. Note the skull fracture overlying the hematoma.

TABLE 247-1 The Glasgow Coma Scale for All Age Groups

	4 yrs to Adult	Child <4 yrs	Infant
EYE OPENING			
4	Spontaneous	Spontaneous	Spontaneous
3	To speech	To speech	To speech
2	To pain	To pain	To pain
1	No response	No response	No response
VERBAL RESPONSE			
5	Alert and oriented	Oriented, social, speaks, interacts	Coos, babbles
4	Disoriented conversation	Confused speech, disoriented, consolable, aware	Irritable cry
3	Speaking but nonsensical	Inappropriate words, inconsolable, unaware	Cries to pain
2	Moans or unintelligible sounds	Incomprehensible, agitated, restless, unaware	Moans to pain
1	No response	No response	No response
MOTOR RESPONSE			
6	Follows commands	Normal, spontaneous movements	Normal, spontaneous moves
5	Localizes pain	Localizes pain	Withdraws to touch
4	Movement or withdrawal to pain	Withdraws to pain	Withdraws to pain
3	Decorticate flexion	Decorticate flexion	Decorticate flexion
2	Decerebrate extension	Decerebrate extension	Decerebrate extension
1	No response	No response	No response
3–15			

GCS reporting should be modified for intubated and paralyzed patients.

Mild TBI

Mild TBI traditionally included patients with a GCS of 13. But studies have shown that 38 percent of patients with a GCS of 13 have findings on CT scan and 8 percent require neurosurgical intervention. Only 10 percent of patients with a GCS score of 15 will have positive CT scans, less than 1 percent will require surgery.[11] Therefore, most authors now include patients with a GCS of 13 in the moderate TBI group.

Mild TBI accounts for 70 to 80 percent of all patients with head injuries seen in the emergency department. These injuries have been increasingly recognized as a significant cause of long-term morbidity. Furthermore, approximately 3 percent of patients presenting with mild TBI may ''talk and deteriorate'' within 48 h postinjury.[12]

With a report of a blow to the head, mild TBI patient presentations range from asymptomatic to confusion or amnesia for the event. Brain CT scans are indicated for almost all patients with a GCS of 14 or less. For those with a GCS of 15, specific symptoms or physical findings indicate the need for a CT scan. These include a reported loss of consciousness or posttraumatic seizure, a history of a coagulopathy, vomiting or amnesia (Fig. 247-3). Physical findings indicating the need for a brain CT include a skull fracture, large subgaleal swelling, focal neurologic findings, unexplained asymmetric pupils, distracting injuries or intoxication.[13]

Patients with an initial GCS score of 15 that is maintained, and a normal CT scan may be discharged home. Those with a positive CT scan require neurosurgical consultation and admission. Admitting patients with mild TBI for observation without a CT scan should be done with caution, as patients may rapidly deteriorate requiring an emergent CT scan and neurosurgical intervention. This delay in identifying an intracranial mass may increase morbidity and mortality. It has been suggested that the most cost-effective and prudent approach is to CT scan these patients as part of the emergency department evaluation and to discharge those with negative scans and normal exams, rather than admitting them for observation.[14]

Patients with an initial GCS score of 14 and a normal CT scan should be observed in the emergency department for 6 to 12 h. This group can be discharged home if they remain neurologically intact and improve their GCS score to 15. Any patient discharged home should have a reliable home companion who can competently carry out appropriate head injury instructions.

Most mild TBI patients return to full recovery within weeks after the injury and by one year, 85 to 90 percent are effectively recovered. Unfortunately, 10 to 15 percent will continue having complaints such as impaired memory, inability to concentrate, headaches, and dizziness.[15]

Moderate TBI

Moderate TBI (GCS 9 to 13) accounts for approximately 10 percent of patients with head injuries. Mortality rates for patients with isolated moderate TBI is less than 20 percent, but long-term disability is as high as 50 percent. Overall, 40 percent of moderate TBI patients have a positive CT scan and 8 percent require neurosurgical intervention.[16] Approximately 10 percent of all moderate TBI patients will deteriorate due to secondary brain injury and progress to severe TBI.

Most patients with moderate TBI should be admitted because of the potential for deterioration (Fig. 247-4). Those with an initial GCS of 13 who return to normal, who remain intact after a 6-12h observation period, and who have a normal CT, can be discharged to family. Those with positive CT scans need neurosurgical consultation and admission to a monitored observation unit. If an institution has inadequate facilities to properly manage these patients, they should be transferred.

Severe TBI

Severe TBI (GCS <9) accounts for approximately 10 percent of all emergency department patients with TBI. The mortality of severe TBI approaches 40 percent with deaths usually occurring within 48 h. Long-term disability is common, with less than 10 percent of patients making even a moderate recovery. The management of patients with severe TBI has three primary goals: to identify other life-threatening injuries, to prevent further secondary brain injury, and to identify treatable mass lesions. Management decisions are delineated in the algorithm, (Fig. 247-5).

EVALUATION AND MANAGEMENT

Prehospital

The care of the head-injured patient begins in the pre-hospital setting with EMS personnel. Assessing the history of the event and the patient's condition and mental status immediately after the injury is important. Securing the patient's airway and cervical spine, establishing IV access, and controlling bleeding are the initial priorities. Hypoxia and hypotension need to be identified and corrected rapidly on the scene. As discussed earlier, hypotension (SBP <90 mmHg) has been associated with a significant increase in mortality. Patients with isolated severe head trauma resuscitated with 250 cc of hypertonic (7.5%) saline in the prehospital setting had a significantly higher SBP on arrival to the emergency department and significantly decreased mortality rate when compared to those resuscitated with lacerated ringers alone.[17] A retrospective review of 169 consecutive TBIs found that patients with more severe TBIs tended to have higher admission and postoperative glucose values, and patients with glucose levels greater than 150 mg/dL had worse neurologic outcomes.[18] In animal models, hyperglycemia may aggravate ischemic neurologic injury. However, ''separation of cause and effect is difficult because hyperglycemia constitutes a hormonally mediated response to more severe injury.''[19] Therefore, it is recommended that glucose should not be administered without first checking a blood glucose finger stick in the comatose trauma patient.

Emergency Department

The ED physician should follow ATLS protocols for the evaluation and stabilization of all trauma patients. Airway control with cervical spine stabilization, breathing, and circulation are the first priorities. Only after the ABCs are secure can a neurologic and mental status examination be conducted to evaluate disability. Exposure of the patient of identify other life-threatening abnormalities can then be completed. Early recognition and treatment of hypoxemia, hypotension, and anemia are the hallmark to reducing morbidity and mortality from TBI.

HISTORY A careful history is important for all patients with TBI. For the unconscious patient, the past medical history and the patient's baseline mental status must be obtained from the paramedics, bystanders, or the family. Important historical points include the mechanism of injury, the patient's condition before and after the trauma, the past medical history and the recent use of drugs or alcohol. Important information regarding the condition after the injury includes the length of the loss of consciousness, vomiting and if seizure activity occurred. A history of anticoagulant use or a coagulopathy must be determined for all patients. Potential for associated unidentified injuries conditions should be sought. These include entities such as hypothermia, inhalation injuries, and toxic exposures including carbon monoxide.

AIRWAY/BREATHING Hypoxia, defined as a Po_2 <60 mmHg, increases mortality from TBI. All patients with severe TBI require intubation and ventilation with 100 percent O_2. Because cervical fractures are seen in 3 to 4 percent of patients with TBI, in-line cervical spine stabilization is essential. Orotracheal rapid sequence intubation (RSI) is preferred because when performed properly using appropriate

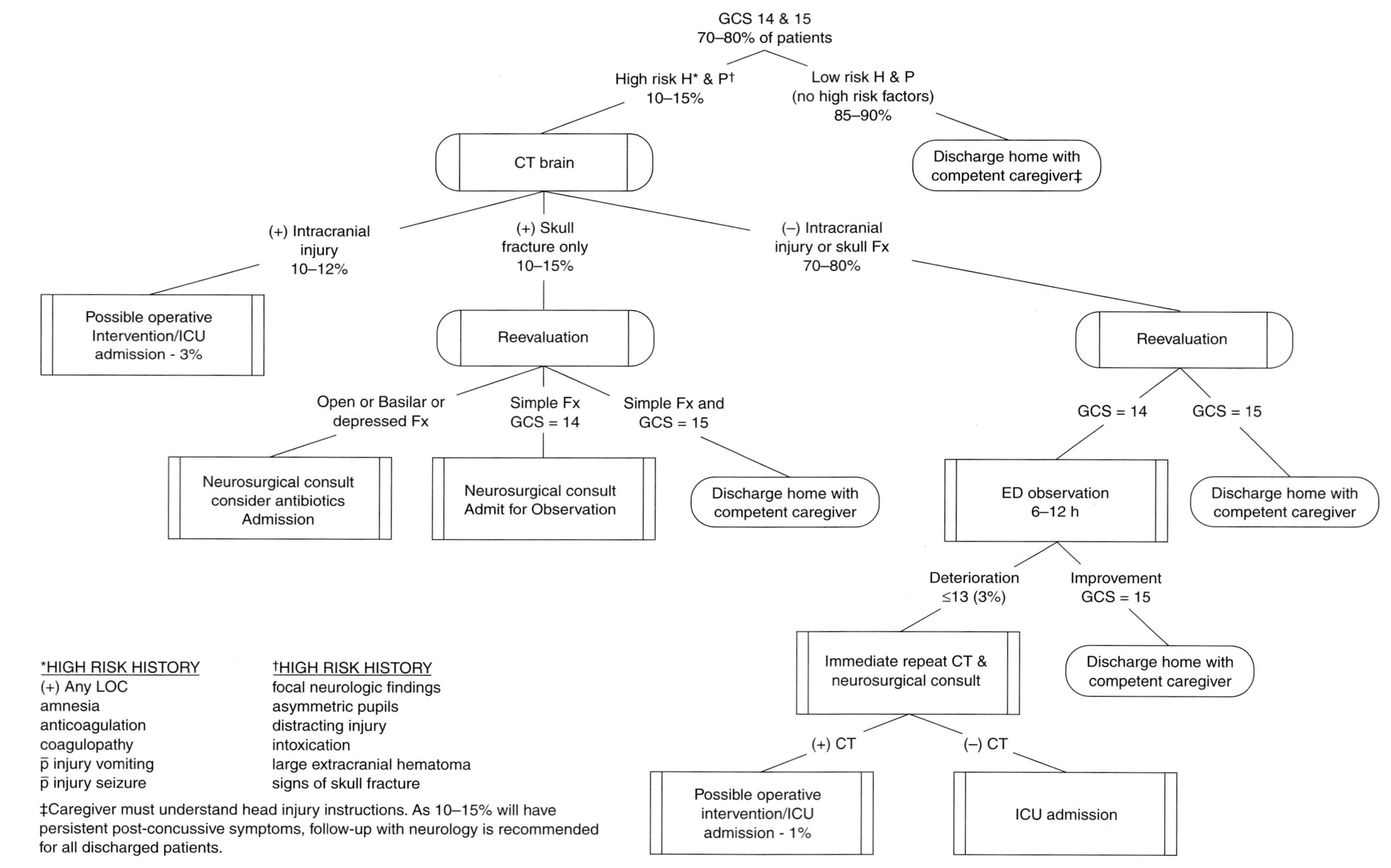
GCS 14 & 15
70–80% of patients
High risk H* & P†
10–15%
Low risk H & P
(no high risk factors)
85–90%
Discharge home with
competent caregiver‡
CT brain
(+) Intracranial
injury
10–12%
(+) Skull
fracture only
10–15%
(–) Intracranial
injury or skull Fx
70–80%
Possible operative
Intervention/ICU
admission - 3%
Reevaluation
Reevaluation
Open or Basilar or
depressed Fx
Simple Fx
GCS = 14
Simple Fx and
GCS = 15
GCS = 14
GCS = 15
Neurosurgical consult
consider antibiotics
Admission
Neurosurgical consult
Admit for Observation
Discharge home with
competent caregiver
ED observation
6–12 h
Discharge home with
competent caregiver
Deterioration
≤13 (3%)
Improvement
GCS = 15
Immediate repeat CT &
neurosurgical consult
Discharge home with
competent caregiver
(+) CT
(–) CT
Possible operative
intervention/ICU
admission - 1%
ICU admission
*HIGH RISK HISTORY
(+) Any LOC
amnesia
anticoagulation
coagulopathy
p̄ injury vomiting
p̄ injury seizure
†HIGH RISK HISTORY
focal neurologic findings
asymmetric pupils
distracting injury
intoxication
large extracranial hematoma
signs of skull fracture
‡Caregiver must understand head injury instructions. As 10–15% will have persistent post-concussive symptoms, follow-up with neurology is recommended for all discharged patients.

FIG. 247-3. Algorithm for the evaluation and treatment of mild brain trauma.

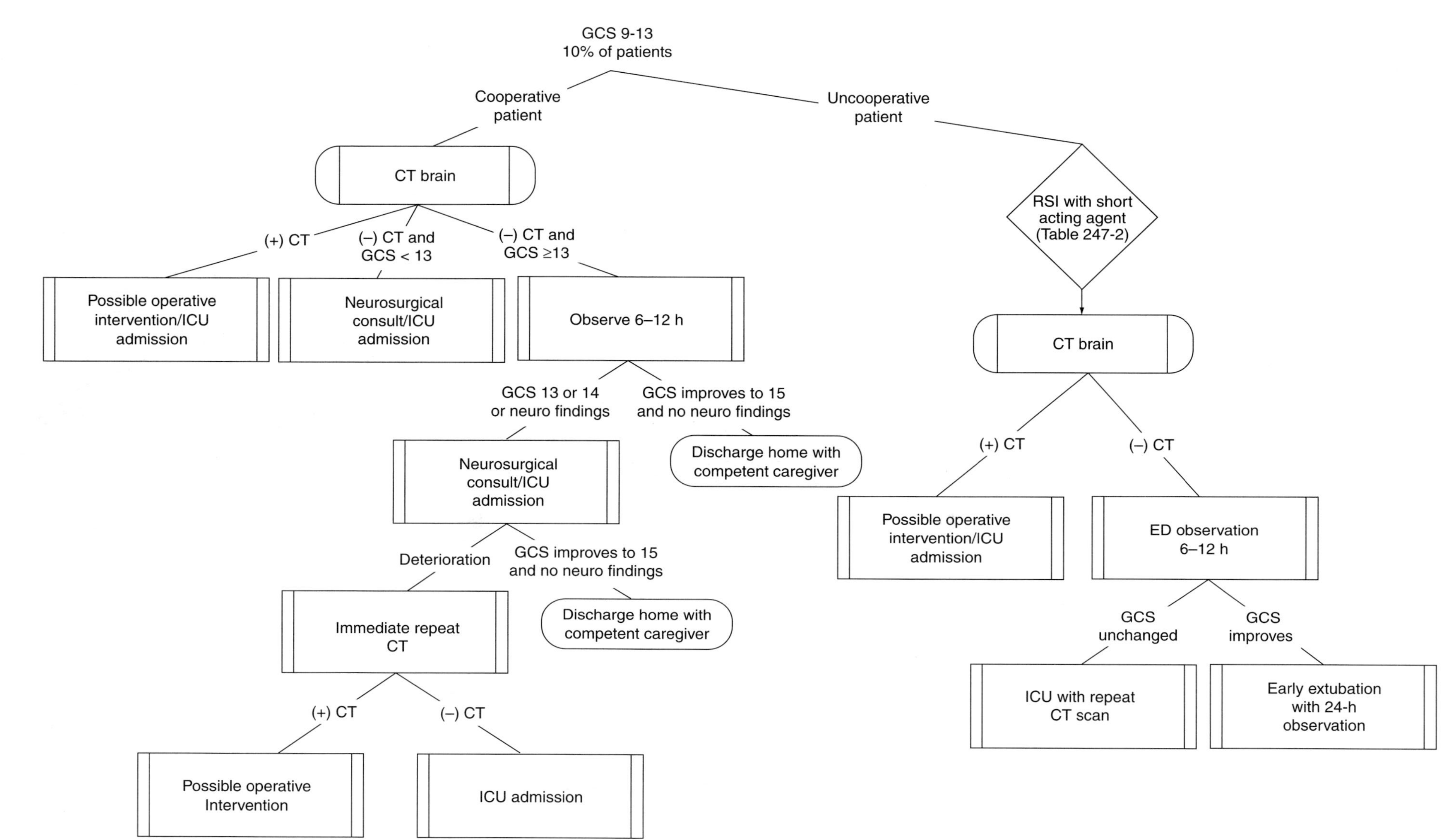

FIG. 247-4. Algorithm for the evaluation and treatment of moderate brain trauma.

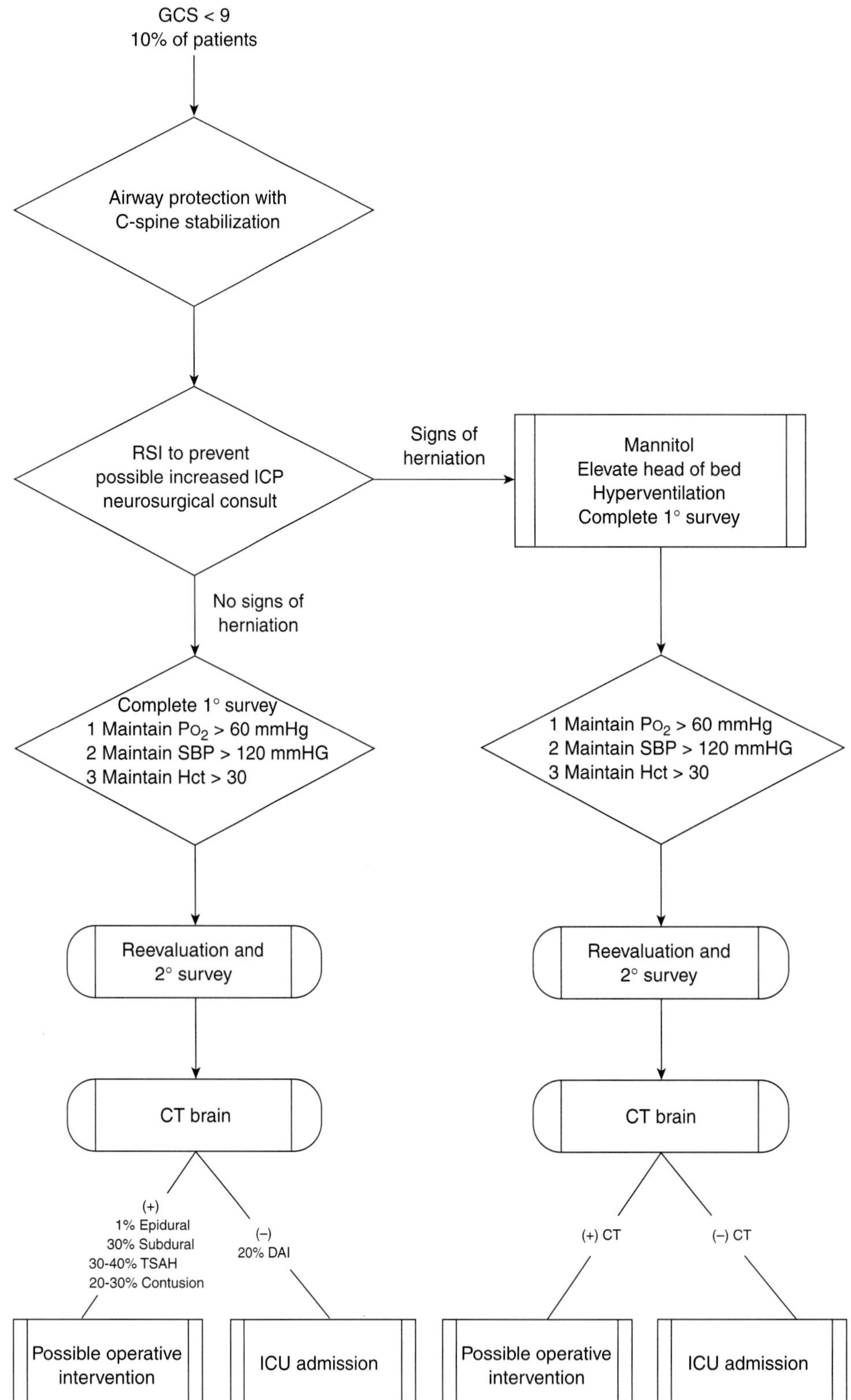

FIG. 247-5. Algorithm for the evaluation and treatment of severe brain trauma.

agents the patient's physiology is optimized, increased ICP is prevented and it has the lowest complication rate. The ideal induction agent should both blunt the increase in ICP and yet not decrease the MAP (Table 247-2). Barbiturates have been shown to decrease ICP and decrease cerebral metabolic oxygen demand. Therefore, the use of a short-acting barbiturate as an induction agent and not for long-term barbiturate coma may be considered. Thiopental in a dose of 3 to 5 mg/kg has advantages of being both rapid in onset of action and short-acting. Unfortunately, thiopental is a cardiovascular depressant. Patients who are hypotensive should either receive a lower dose, 0.5 to 1 mg/kg or another inducting agent, such as etomidate (0.3 mg/kg). Ketamine should be avoided because it increases ICP. Short-

TABLE 247-2 Agents for Rapid Sequence Intubation of Patients with Severe TBI

Pretreatment (given 2–3 min prior to paralysis)	
Agent	Purpose
Lidocaine 1.5 mg/kg IV	Hemodynamic stability
Fentanyl 3–5 mg/kg IV	Hemodynamic stability and analgesia
Vecuronium (0.01 mg/kg) or pancuronium (0.01 mg/kg) IV	Defasciculating
Paralysis and induction agents	
Thiopental 3–5 mg/kg (normotensive) or 0.5–1 mg/kg (hypotensive)	Sedation
Succinylcholine 1.5 mg/kg	Paralysis

Source: Walls RM: Rapid sequence intubation in head trauma. *Ann Emerg Med* 22(6):1008, 1993.

acting paralytic agents are preferred to facilitate serial neurologic exams that can identify worsening brain injury. Although succinylcholine (1.5 mg/kg) can cause a rise in the ICP, this may be blunted by administering a defasciculating dose of vecuronium (0.01 mg/kg) two to three minutes prior to succinylcholine. These same guidelines should be followed for comatose patients, who are also susceptible to increases in ICP with laryngoscopy and intubation. Lidocaine should also be used as a pretreatment agent because of its potential to prevent hemodynamic changes (Table 247-2). Although nasotracheal intubation is not contraindicated in TBI, it should rarely be used for patients with TBI due to its higher complication rate, lower success rate, and potential for marked increase in ICP if not carried out perfectly. In the presence of a basilar skull fracture, nasotracheal intubation also leads to an increased risk of meningitis.

CIRCULATION Once the airway is secured, aggressive fluid resuscitation may be required to prevent hypotension and the resulting secondary brain injury. Studies have shown an increase in mortality from 27 to 50 percent for patients with isolated TBI who had a single episode of systolic blood pressure of less than 90 mmHg. Adequate fluid resuscitation has not been shown to increase ICP. Guidelines recommend that the MAP be maintained at 90 mmHg (systolic blood pressure of 120 to 140 mmHg) to achieve adequate cerebral perfusion.[20] Hypotension in the setting of trauma should generally be addressed with vigorous fluid and blood replacement. The use of pressors is potentially dangerous and seldom indicated. However, in the absence of shock from volume loss, pressors may be used in an effort to maintain adequate cerebral perfusion. In these cases, monitoring should include cardiac output, continuous arterial blood pressure, and, optimally, intracranial pressure measurement. The pressors indicated for raising MAP to maintain cerebral perfusion are norepinephrine and phenylephrine. Norepinephrine dosages range from 2 to 80 μg/min and should be begun low and titrated slowly to the desired effect. Phenylephrine doses range from 40 to 180 μg/min and are similarly titrated.

Hypertension is a critical finding and must be taken as a Cushing's response in the setting of head injury. The finding of hypertension and bradycardia should initiate measures to decrease intracranial pressure. If hypertension exists independent of increased intracranial pressure, then the systemic pressure should be lowered by no more than 30 percent of the mean arterial blood pressure by using nipride. Pressor agents may be needed to maintain the MAP, although this has not been formally studied. Anemia is also associated with increased mortality. Therefore, external and internal bleeding need to be controlled quickly and the hematocrit should be kept above 30. Head injury alone rarely produces hypotension (except as a preterminal event). Exceptions to this include hypovolemic shock in infants due to epidural bleeding or subgaleal hematoma, or massive blood loss from scalp lacerations in any age group.

DISABILITY **The Glasgow Coma Scale** The initial neurologic examination of ATLS is to assess the level of consciousness using the AVPU system: *Alert*, responds to *Verbal* stimuli, responds to *Painful* stimuli or is *Unresponsive*. This same assessment provides most of the information needed to calculate the Glasgow Coma Scale. The GCS taken at any time does not replace an appropriate neurologic exam.

The Neurologic Exam Other important aspects of the neurologic examination in the initial trauma evaluation include assessing pupils for size, reactivity, and anisocoria. Motor function, cranial nerve function, deep tendon reflexes, and evaluation of sensory changes are also useful to indicate the presence of an intracranial injury. Brainstem function in the unresponsive patient is assessed by observing respiratory pattern and eye movements. Oculovestibular (cold calorics) and oculocephalic (doll's eyes) responses are not checked until the cervical spine has been fully cleared.

Pupils are assessed for size and reactivity. A fixed and dilated pupil is highly suggestive of an ipsilateral hematoma with uncal herniation that requires rapid operative intervention. Direct ocular trauma should also be assessed. Bilateral fixed and dilated pupils suggest poor tissue perfusion, (i.e., hypoxemia) bilateral uncal herniation or drug effect, whereas bilateral pinpoint pupils suggest either opiate use or a pontine lesion.

Altered motor function can indicate brain, spinal cord or peripheral nerve injuries. Careful attention is paid to signs of increasing ICP and herniation. Movement in unresponsive patients is assessed by the application of painful stimuli. Decorticate posturing (abnormal upper extremity flexion and lower extremity extension) is indicative of an injury above the midbrain. Decerebrate posturing (abnormal arm extension and internal rotation with wrist and finger flexion and internal rotation and extension of the lower extremities) is a result of a more caudal injury and a worse outcome.

After the primary survey a secondary survey is needed to identify other significant injuries. Up to 60 percent of patients with severe TBI will have other major injuries.

DIAGNOSTIC RADIOGRAPHY FOR TBI All patients with moderate to severe TBI require urgent head CT scan after stabilization. Delays in obtaining a CT scan can lead to a catastrophic delay in emergent neurosurgical interventions. Therefore, if the patient with moderate TBI is uncooperative or combative, intubation using RSI is often the best option. If this is undertaken, the best neurologic exam possible just prior should be performed, and may be valuable to subsequent neurosurgical consultation. Prior to the availability of CT scanning, skull films were the standard diagnostic test. Skull films will be positive in 5 percent of patients with mild TBI. Unfortunately, they often miss basilar skull fractures and do not reliably detect underlying intracranial pathology. CT scans are much more accurate and useful.

There is increasing agreement about the need to scan patients with a GCS of less than 14, but debate remains regarding the indicators for CT scanning for patients with a GCS of 15. Specific signs and symptoms can be indicative of intracranial lesions in these patients. These include a history of loss of consciousness, seizure, vomiting, alcohol use, or physical findings of large subgaleal swelling or amnesia. If any of these findings is present, patients shall have a less than 5 percent chance of having an intracranial lesion and a less than 1 percent chance of requiring neurosurgical intervention. Those with a GCS of 15 and none of these findings have not been shown to have adverse outcomes. Patients on anticoagulants or with coagulopathies are also at higher risk and should be scanned.

Control of the agitated patient with head injury is critical in the evaluation and stabilization of these cases. Haloperidol easily crosses the blood-brain barrier, has few adverse respiratory or cardiac effects, and does not interfere with the neurologic exam. However, contraindications to haloperidol include coma and severe toxic CNS depression. This limits its utility in severely inebriated patients and those patients whose mental status changes may deteriorate to coma. Haldol's slow onset of 10 to 30 min, even when given IV, diminishes it's utility in the more severely agitated patients.

Midazolam has sedative, hypnotic, anxiolytic, and amnestic effects. It easily crosses the blood brain barrier, reduces intracranial pressure and augments cerebral perfusion pressure.[22] Midazolam also causes skeletal muscle relaxation and is an effective anticonvulsant. However, it will not control psychotic symptoms. Its use is contraindicated in severe hypotension and may be limited by respiratory depression. Admission of a continuous infusion may allow maintenance of adequate sedation while preserving an intact airway. However, close monitoring is required for patients on midazolam infusion; airway protection by intubation is often indicated. Midazolam's rapid clearance allows for an adequate neurologic exam within minutes of discontinuation.

Propofol is an intravenous sedative hypnotic with onset of action less than 1 min with a duration of less than 10 min. Propofol decreases elevated intracranial pressure while not significantly decreasing cerebral perfusion pressure.[23] For conduction and maintenance of sedation, a variable rate infusion method is preferable over intermittent bolus doses. Patients will generally require maintenance rates of 20 to 75 μg/kg/h during the first 10 to 15 min. Dose may be decreased to 25 to 50 μg/kg/h and titrated to clinical response. Propofol is contraindicated with cardiovascular instability and hypotension. It is recommended for use in patients who are intubated and mechanically ventilated.

Treatment for Increased ICP

It is critical that intracranial pressure be maintained at less than 20 to 25 mmHg. Above this value results in a significant increase in morbidity and mortality. Several strategies may be used to achieve this goal. All patients with severe TBI and evidence of increased ICP should have the head of the bed elevated to 30 degrees, adequate volume resuscitation to a MAP of 90 mmHg, and maintenance of adequate arterial oxygenation. After these steps several other treatment modalities may be used to lower intracranial hypertension.

Hyperventilation has been widely used to reduce ICP but it is no longer recommended as a prophylactic intervention.[6] Because of the extreme sensitivity of the cerebral vasculature to CO_2 levels, hyperventilation leads to vasoconstriction that reduces ICP within 30 s. Unfortunately, hyperventilation and the resultant vasoconstriction can also cause cerebral ischemia. Hyperventilation should be reserved for head-injured patients with signs of increasing ICP (such as unilateral dilated pupil, motor posturing, and worsening mental status) despite other therapeutic measures (i.e., a last resort). If hyperventilation is used, it should be initiated as temporary measure and the P_{CO_2} should be monitored closely and returned to the 30 to 35 mmHg range as soon as possible.[6]

Osmotic agents such as mannitol reduce ICP by osmotic diuresis with an onset within 30 min and lasting approximately 6 to 8 h. Mannitol has the additional benefit of expanding volume, initially reducing hypotension, and improving the blood's oxygen-carrying capacity. The recommended dose is 0.25 g/kg to 1 g/kg. There is no dose-dependent effect seen with mannitol; therefore, some authors advocate the lower range of the suggested dose. However, due to the diuresis, over time there will be a net intravascular volume loss, requiring hemodynamic monitoring. The Brain Trauma Foundation recommends that CSF drainage is preferable to mannitol. In the ED, where an IC catheter may not be readily available, mannitol may be used.

In addition to the above measures, monitoring of ICP should be performed for all patients with evidence of increased ICP, herniation, and a GCS score of less than 8. A ventricular catheter offers the best method to directly monitor ICP and thus calculate CPP. Under this setting, any rise in ICP above 20 to 25 mm HG may be reduced by CSF drainage. This treatment has the most favorable risk-to-benefit ratio. If CSF drainage is not effective in reducing ICP, then mannitol should be administered, assuming adequate MAP. Barbiturates have been shown to reduce cerebral metabolic rate. However, the use of barbiturate coma is rarely indicated in the emergency department as its effect occurs relatively late. The recommended dose of pentobarital is 10 mg/kg over 30 min. Steroids have no proven role in treating patients with TBI. Studies addressing this issue have not demonstrated improved outcome with their use.

EMERGENCY DECOMPRESSION When other methods to control the ICP have failed, patients with signs of herniation may need emergency decompression by trephination (''burr holes''). CT scanning before attempting trephination is recommended to localize the lesion and direct the decompression site. If CT scan is unavailable, or the patient is unstable for CT due to signs of rapidly progressive neurologic deterioration and herniation, then trephination should be considered.

As a final premorbid action for rapidly increasing intracranial pressure from traumatic hematoma expansion uncontrolled by medical therapy, emergency cranial surgical decompression may be attempted. If the cervical spine is stable, then optimally the patient's head is rotated so that the side with the dilated pupil is superior. The head should be stabilized and supported to prevent movement. A temporal burr hole should be attempted first by making a 4-cm vertical skin incision two finger-breadths anterior and three finger-breadths superior to the anterior tragus of the ear. When skull is reached, then a handheld drill should be inserted and drilled until the inner skull table is reached. A thin rim of bone should be left and scooped out under direct visualization with a curette.

If the temporal burr hole fails to yield blood or reverse signs of herniation then a frontal burr hole three finger-breadths from the midline and three finger-breadths from the hairline may be made. Should the second burr hole fail to improve the patient's condition, a final parietal burr hole can be placed four finger-breadths behind the frontal hole. Rarely, in cases with a high frontal injury, false lateralizing signs can occur due to Kernihan's notch. In these cases, the entire procedure should be repeated on the opposite side of the skull.

MANAGEMENT OF SPECIFIC INJURIES

Scalp Laceration

Because of a rich blood supply, loose connective, tissue and relatively loose attachment to the pericranium, scalp lacerations can lead to massive blood loss. During the resuscitation phase of trauma care, scalp hemorrhages should be controlled as rapidly as possible. If direct pressure is not effective, lidocaine with epinephrine can be infiltrated locally, and vessels can be clamped or ligated if still necessary. Early closure with irrigation and debridement is the best method to control bleeding. Wounds should be carefully examined prior to closure. Blood clots and debris should be cleaned away to examine for underlying fractures and galeal lacerations. Large galeal disruptions should be repaired, but small one can be left alone.

Skull Fracture

Skull fractures are usually categorized by location (basilar vs. the skull convexity), pattern (linear, depressed, or comminuted) and whether they are open or closed. Up to 50 percent of patients with skull fractures, including depressed fractures will not have significant loss of consciousness or any neurologic findings. This is why a careful physical exam and wound exploration is essential. Complicated skull fractures include those that are open or depressed, those that involve a sinus, and those that cause intracranial air (pneumocephalus).

LINEAR AND COMMINUTED FRACTURES The management of linear and simple comminuted skull fractures is the same. Even open fractures (fractures with an overlying laceration) in and of themselves do not usually indicate admission or surgical exploration. However open fractures require careful cleaning and repair. Wounds should be explored gently so as not to drive bone fragments into the brain. A neurosurgeon should be consulted and a head CT scan performed to ensure that there is no underlying brain injury. Closure of these wounds should be undertaken only in consult with a neurosurgeon prior to CT scan. The use of prophylactic antibiotics following an open skull fracture is controversial.

Particular care should be taken in evaluating fractures that cross the middle meningeal artery or a major venous sinus. Occipital fractures also require aggressive evaluation, as they are associated with a 33 percent complication rate, including increased risk of subarachnoid hemorrhage. Fractures that are depressed beyond the thickness of the skull require operative repair. Depressed skull fractures are associated with an increased risk of intracranial injury, infections, and early seizures. CT scans are, therefore, indicated for all of these patients.

BASILAR SKULL FRACTURE Basilar skull fractures occur in 3.5 to 24 percent of all patients with head injuries. The most common type of basilar skull fracture is longitudinal through the petrous portion of the temporal bone. This usually involves the external auditory canal and the tympanic membrane. These fractures are commonly associated with a torn dura leading to CSF leakage and a risk of traumatic meningitis. Signs and symptoms associated with basilar skull fractures include CSF otorrhea or rhinorrhea, mastoid ecchymosis (Battle's sign), periorbital ecchymoses (raccoon eyes), hemotympanum, vertigo, decreased hearing or deafness and seventh nerve palsy. Periorbital and mastoid ecchymoses are often absent on presentation to the ED, but develop gradually over the first hours after an injury. A nasal discharge that leaves a large clear ring when dripped onto a paper towel, or that is positive for glucose, indicates a basilar skull fracture with CSF leak. In general, patients with a skull fracture should be hospitalized. Approximately 20 percent of patients with CSF fistulas develop meningitis. A recent meta-analysis supports the use of prophylactic antibiotics by demonstrating a significant reduction in meningitis for patients receiving prophylactic antibiotics.[24] Administration of antibiotics should only be done in consultation with either a neurosurgeon or head and neck surgeon. Common organisms responsible for meningitis in these patients are *Pneumococcus*, *Streptococcus*, and *Haemophilus influenzae*. If prophylactic antibiotics are instituted, they should have broad coverage with good penetration into the meninges. A third-generation cephalosporin such as ceftriaxone at 1 to 2 g per day is a reasonable choice. Most CSF leaks will resolve spontaneously within a week.

Cerebral Contusion/Intracerebral Hemorrhage

Contusions are one of the most frequent types of TBI (Fig. 247-6). Contusions most commonly occur in the subfrontal cortex, the frontal and temporal lobes, and occasionally in the occipital lobes. The are often associated with a subarachnoid hemorrhage. Contusions may occur at the site of the blunt trauma or the opposite site of the brain, known as a ''contrecoup'' injury.

Intracerebral hemorrhage can occur days after significant blunt trauma, often at the site of resolving contusions. This complication is more common with patients with a coagulopathy. CT scans in the immediate postinjury phase are often normal.

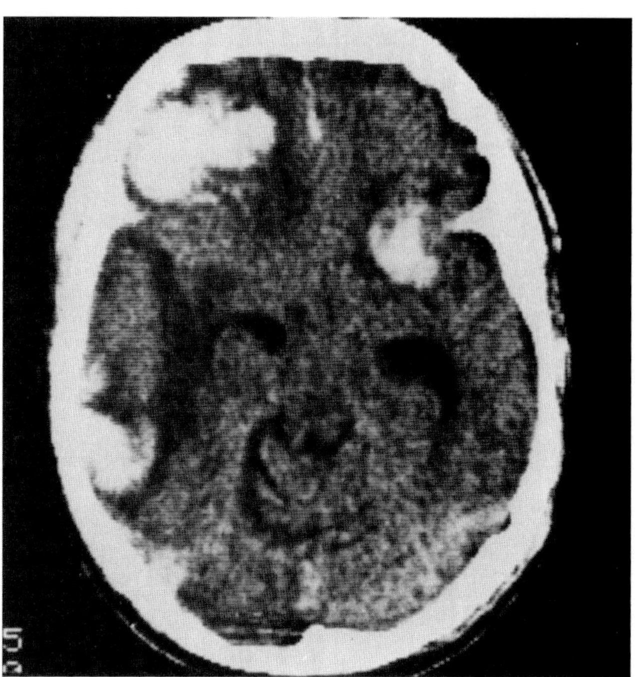

FIG. 247-6. Cerebral contusion with associated hemorrhage occurring subfromtally on the left, in the posterior temporal region.

Subarachnoid Hemorrhage

Traumatic subarachnoid hemorrhage (tSAH) results from the disruption of subarachnoid vessels and presents with blood in the CSF (Table 247-3). In one large European head-injury study, one-third of all patients with moderate to severe head injuries demonstrated traumatic subarachnoid hemorrhage on early CT scans,[25] making tSAH the most common CT abnormality finding in patients with moderate to severe TBI. The overall incidence of tSAH is as high 40 percent when including CT abnormalities. When the CT scan is positive for tSAH, the amount of blood seen on the CT scan is inversely related to the presenting GCS and percent of positive outcomes. The outcome of patients with tSAH was significantly worse than that of patients with no SAH on first CT scan. Overall, 60 percent of the former group resulted in an unfavorable outcome defined as death, persistent vegetative state, or severe disability compared to only 30 percent in the latter group. Mortality in the early tSAH group was 42 percent compared to 14 percent in the no SAH group.[25] Recent data have demonstrated the use of nimodipine at 2 mg/h for 7 to 10 days followed by 360 mg daily until day 21 to significantly lower this unfavorable outcome by 55 percent compared to the placebo group.[26]

Patients with tSAH can present with mild to severe TBI. Those with isolated tSAH often present with a headache and photophobia and mild meningeal signs. A CT scan is generally diagnostic but care must be taken on reports of delayed intracranial hematomas, especially subdural hematomas, exist in the literature for patients who exhibited nonfocal neurologic exams with negative initial CT scans.[27] Unfortunately, delayed findings may not be detected for one to two months after initial insult. Generally, scans performed six to eight hours or more after injury will demonstrate tSAH. However, delays can occur in 3 to 5 percent of patients. Careful instructions and discharge in the care of a competent adult are therefore necessary to detect these delayed injuries. Referral for reexamination by a physician in 24 to 48 h is usually required for all patients with an initial negative CT scan. The disposition of any patient with tSAH requires immediate neurosurgical consultation and admission to an intensive care unit.

TABLE 247-3 Intracranial Hematomas

	Type of Patient	% of TBI	Anatomic Location	CT Findings	Common Cause	Classic Symptoms
Epidural	Young, rare in the elderly and age <2	1	Potential space between skull and dura mater	Biconvex, football-shaped hematoma	Skull fracture with tear of the middle meningeal artery	Immediate LOC with a ''lucid'' period prior to deterioration (only occurs in 20%)
Subdural	More risk for the elderly and alcoholics	25–30	Space between dura mater and arachnoid	Crescent- or sickle-shaped hematoma	Acceleration-deceleration with tearing of the bridging veins	Acute: rapid LOC-lucid period possible Chronic: altered MS and behavior with gradual decrease in consciousness
Subarachnoid	Any age group following blunt trauma	30–40	Subarachnoid	Blood in the basilar cisterns and hemispheric sulci and fissures	Acceleration-deceleration with tearing of the subarachnoid vessels	Mild to moderate TBI with meningeal signs and symptoms
Contusion/ intracerebral hematoma	Any age group following blunt trauma	20–40	Usually anterior temporal or posterior frontal lobe	May be normal initially with delayed bleed	Severe or penetrating trauma; shaken baby syndrome	Symptoms range from normal to unconscious

Epidural Hematoma

Epidural hematomas are the result of blood collecting in the potential space between the skull and the dura mater. They occur in only 0.5 to 1 percent of all head-injured patients and in less than 10 percent of those with head injuries who are comatose. Most (80 to 90 percent) result from blunt trauma to the temporal or temporoparietal area with an associated skull fracture and middle meningeal arterial disruption (Fig. 247-7). Occasionally, trauma to the parietooccipital region or the posterior fossa causes tears of the venous sinuses with epidural hematomas. Almost all epidural hematomas are associated with skull fractures, and 80 percent will progress to uncal herniation. Additional cerebral lesions occur in 24 percent of patients, but they are usually not life-threatening. Epidural hematomas are rare in the elderly and children less than age two. In the elderly, the dura mater is firmly attached to the skull, which decreases the likelihood of dissection into the potential space. The less rigid skull of younger children protects against skull fractures and the resultant disruption of the middle meningeal artery.

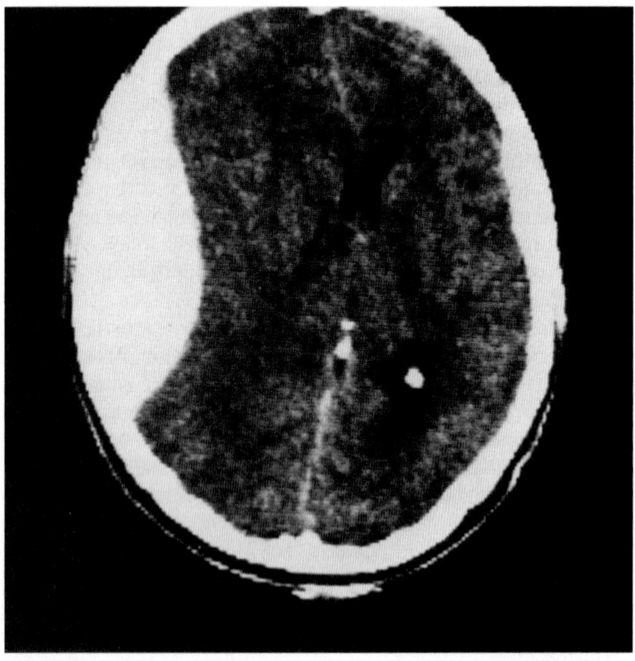

FIG. 247-7. A typical epidural hematoma with a lenticular-shaped configuration.

The classic history of an epidural hematoma is for the patient to experience immediate loss of consciousness after significant blunt head trauma. The patient then awakens and has a lucent period prior to again falling unconscious as the hematoma expands. Unfortunately, this ''classic'' syndrome occurs in only about 20 percent of cases. The majority of patients either never loose consciousness or never regain consciousness after the injury.

The diagnosis of an epidural hematoma is based on CT scan and physical findings. On CT scans, epidural hematomas appear biconvex (football shaped), typically in the temporal region.

The high-pressure arterial bleeding of an epidural hematoma can lead to herniation. The sequence of epidural bleeding and herniation usually occurs within hours. Therefore, early recognition and intervention is key to reduce morbidity and mortality. More than 90 percent of patients with recognized epidurals will have the hematoma operatively evacuated within 48 h. One-third of these will be evacuated within the first 12 h. Bilateral emergency department trephination (burr holes) are only indicated if definitive neurosurgical care is not available. Full recovery can be expected if the hematoma is evacuated prior to herniation or to the presence of neurologic deficits. Otherwise, irreversible brain injuries from increased ICP may insue, resulting in a less favorable outcome.

Subdural Hematoma

Subdural hematomas (SDH) are caused by sudden acceleration-deceleration of brain parenchyma with subsequent tearing of the bridging veins. These vessels are located beneath the dura mater and result in blood clots forming between the dura mater and the arachnoid (Fig. 247-8). SDHs occur in approximately 30 percent of all severe TBI.

Brains with extensive atrophy, such as the elderly and alcoholics, are more susceptible to subdural hematomas because of the relatively smaller brain volume in a larger cranial vault. Children under the age of two are also at increased risk of subdural hematomas. This is related to transfer of the force that limits the risk of sustaining epidural hematomas as discussed above. In addition, children have a larger

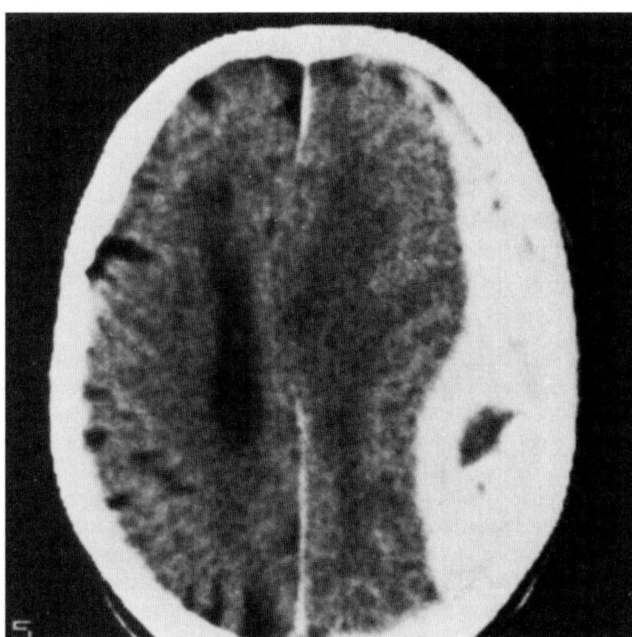

FIG. 247-8. A large acute subdural hematoma with a midline shift and ipsilateral ventricular effacement.

head to body ratio than adults, which increases the overall risk of head injury.

Blood tends to collect more slowly than epidural hematomas because of its venous origin. However, unlike the epidural hematomas, SDH have more associated brain parenchyma injury so outcome is less favorable. The mortality rate averages 60 percent for patients with acute SDH, but can be significantly lowered with early surgical intervention.[9]

Traditionally, subdural hematomas have been classified as acute, subacute, and chronic, depending on time of presenting signs and symptoms. In acute SDH patients present between 3 and 14 days. After 2 weeks, patients are defined as having a chronic SDH. There is no specific clinical syndrome associated with a subdural hematoma. Acute cases usually present immediately after severe trauma and often, the victim is unconscious. However, chronic subdurals may present in the elderly or alcoholic with vague complaints or mental status changes. These patients often do not recall an injury. On CT scan, acute SDH are hyperdense (white), crescent-shaped lesions. Subacute SDH are isodense and more difficult to identify. A CT scan with intravenous contrast can assist in identifying a subacute SDH. A chronic SDH appears hypodense as the iron in the blood is phagocytized.

The definitive treatment of subdurals depends on the type and on associated brain injuries. Mortality and the need for surgical repair are greater for acute and subacute SDH. Chronic subdurals can sometimes be managed without surgery depending of the severity of the symptoms.

Diffuse Axonal Injury

Diffuse axonal injury (DAI) is the disruption of axonal fibers in the white matter and brainstem. Shearing forces on the neurons generated by sudden deceleration cause DAI. A relationship exists between the force of sudden deceleration and the amount of DAI observed in all cases of TBI except for assaults and whiplash. The classic cause of DAI is an MVC. In infants, the ''shaken baby syndrome'' is a well-described tragic cause.

Injury occurs immediately and is essentially irreversible. There is a rapid or immediate increase in ICP. Patients present unresponsive. The state may be prolonged or permanent until death. A CT scan of a patient with DAI may be normal, but the classic triad demonstrates hemorrhagic injury to the corpus callosum, the midbrain or pons, and retraction of the Balls of Cajal. The treatment options for DAI are very limited, but attempt to prevent secondary damage by reducing cerebral edema.

Penetrating Injury

In the United States, gunshot wounds (GSW) are now the leading cause of death from TBI; GSW result in more than 33,000 deaths annually. Of these, slightly more than half are from homicide, with most of the remaining suicides. As a bullet passes through the brain, it creates a cavity 3 to 4 times greater than its diameter. The damage, however, is due to more than just the penetration of the bullet. Also involved in a major transfer of kinetic energy of the bullet to the brain matter. The amount of transferred kinetic energy is dependent on the mass of the missile and the velocity squared ($E = \frac{1}{2} mv^2$). The result is that a small increase in bullet velocity results in large increases in energy delivered and resultant damage. The resulting concussive force can damage tissue outside of the bullet's path. (Wound ballistics is discussed in detail in Chap. 256.)

The prognosis of a patient with a GSW to the brain can be predicted by the GCS if they are not intoxicated. Patients with a GCS of greater than 8, and reactive pupils have a 25 percent mortality risk. Those with a GCS of less than 5 approach 100 percent mortality. All patients with a penetrating GSW to the brain should be intubated and treated with prophylactic antibiotics and anticonvulsants.

Stab wounds have very low energy and impart only direct damage to the area contacted by the penetrating object. Therefore, the morbidity and mortality from these injuries is much less than from those with GSWs. Essentially all patients sustain penetrating injury require operative intervention. Impaled objects should be left in place until surgical removal. Patients should receive broad-spectrum antibiotics and be admitted.

COMPLICATIONS/LONG-TERM PROBLEMS

Seizures

There are three periods in which patients with TBI are susceptible to seizures: acute, early, and late. Acute seizures occur within minutes of the head injury; early seizures occur within one week of head injury; late seizures occur after one week of head injury. Acute seizures are associated with a high mortality from expanding hematomas. However, if the patient survives, the situation is the least likely to be associated with a long-term seizure disorder. Late seizures are most likely to result in a prolonged seizure disorder. Seizures are four times more common following penetrating trauma than blunt trauma.

Because seizures result in hypoxia, increased cerebral ischemia, and increased ICP, the use of anticonvulsants, such as phenytoin, is recommended for all patients with severe TBI for one week after the injury. Indications include patients with intracranial hemorrhage or hematoma, depressed skull fractures or penetrating injuries, a posttraumatic seizure or any patients who are paralyzed. Long-term use of anticonvulsants has not been shown to decrease incidence of seizures beyond one week.[28] If the patient is no longer paralyzed, and not had a breakthrough seizure for one week, the anticonvulsant can be discontinued.

Concussion

A concussion is any brief and temporary interruption of neurologic function following head trauma. Concussions may occur with or without loss of consciousness. Symptoms of amnesia and confusion are the hallmarks of concussion. Duration of amnesia is predictive of

TABLE 247-4 Evaluation and Management of Patients with Concussions

Concussion Grade	Symptoms	Action
Grade 1	No loss of consciousness Confusion without amnesia	Remove from event. Examine immediately and every 5 min for the development of amnesia or postconcussive symptoms at rest and with exertion. If asymptomatic at 20 min with rest/exertion, can return to event. If two grade 1 concussions, then no sports for the day. If three grade 1 concussions, then out for season and no contact sports for 3 months.
Grade 2	No loss of consciousness Confusion and amnesia	Remove from event for the day. Refer for exam the next day. May return to athletic activities after 1 week if asymptomatic with rest/exertion. If two grade concussions, no play for 1 season; if three grade 2 concussions, termination of season.
Grade 3	Loss of consciousness	Transport to ED for evaluation—evaluate per mild to moderate TBI protocols. Return to sport at 1 month if asymptomatic for a 2-week period. If two grade 3 concussions or positive imaging, then season is terminated.

Source: Adapted with permission, from, Sports Medicine Committee: *Guidelines for the Management of Concussion in Sports.* Denver, Colorado Medical Society, 1991.

injury severity. Other symptoms include dizziness, headaches, nausea, and vomiting. The patient with concussion may appear dazed with a blank stare while others may cry for no apparent reason. Most of these signs and symptoms may resolve prior to arrival in the emergency department and the patient's only complaint may be that of a headache. Most patients with brief loss of consciousness, GCS 15, and amnesia less than 1 h, recover within 6 to 12 weeks.[15]

SPORTS-RELATED CONCUSSION Sports-related concussions are common injuries, but their true incidence is greatly underreported. Sports most commonly associated with concussion are boxing, football, soccer, baseball, and basketball. The management of any patient with TBI or concussion is the same as described above. However, for the athlete with a concussion, special consideration must be made for their safe return to a sporting activity. Based on degree of signs and symptoms of the athlete, a grading scale of 1 to 3 is used. A higher grade is associated with greater risk of sustaining permanent brain damage or even death if an additional injury is sustained (Table 247-4).

POSTCONCUSSIVE SYNDROME Regardless of the cause of head injury, patients with TBI may experience persistent symptoms postinjury. Despite exhaustive work-ups, postconcussive syndrome (PCS) patients may continue to have very vague complaints such as headaches, dizziness, inability to concentrate, and memory changes. After one year, 85 to 90 percent of these patients effectively recover. The remaining 10 to 15 percent have persistent postconcussive syndrome (PPCS). Risk factors for patients developing PPCS from PCS are female sex, ongoing litigation, and low socioeconomic status. While all PCS and PPCS patients should be referred to their primary physicians or neurologist, amitriptyline at 25 to 50 mg/day has been shown to help patients with headaches, depression, and insomnia.[29] Regardless of treatment options, physicians need to relay two important messages to any patient with TBI. The symptoms usually clear, but the time needed is generally weeks to months.[15]

Infections

Patients with traumatic brain injuries are at increased risk for CNS infections. Several factors increase the risk. Skull fractures and CSF leaks, as discussed earlier, are risk factors for developing meningitis. In addition to CNS infections, patients intubated and on neuromuscular blockade are shown to have longer ICU stays, an increased risk for aspiration pneumonias, and, tend toward sepsis. Due to controversies regarding use of prophylactic antibiotics, consultation with the neurosurgeon or intensivist should be obtained prior to their administration.

Patients who present with a history of a skull fracture and fever or other symptoms of meningitis should be treated with antibiotics. The source of infection depends on the time since the injury. Within 72 hours, pneumococcus is generally the cause. After that, gram-negative organisms and *Staphylococcus aureus* become more common. Patients should given vancomycin and a third-generation cephalosporin, such as ceftazidime, until cultures confirm the cause.

REFERENCES

1. Sosin DM, Sniezek JE, Waxweiler RJ: Trends in deaths associated with traumatic brain injury, 1979–1992. *JAMA* 273(22):1778, 1995.
2. National Center for Health Statistics. National Hospital Ambulatory Medical Care Survey: 1996 emergency department summary. *Adv Data* 293:1, 1997.
3. Max W, McKenzie EJ, Rice DP: Head injuries: costs and consequences. *J Head Trauma Rehab* 6:76, 1991.
4. Honkanen R, Smith G: Impact of acute alcohol intoxication on patterns of non-fatal trauma: Cause-specific analysis of head injury effect. *Injury* 22:225, 1991.
5. Chestnut RM: The management of severe traumatic brain injury. *Emerg Med Clin North Am* 15:581, 1997.
6. Chestnut RM: Guidelines for the management of severe head injury: What we know and what we think we know. *J Trauma* 42:S19, 1997.
7. Doberstein CE, Hovda DA, Becker DP: Clinical considerations in the reduction of secondary brain injury. *Ann Emerg Med* 22:993, 1993.
8. Chestnut RM, Marshall LF, Klauber MR, et al: The role of secondary brain injury: Determining outcome from severe head injury. *J Trauma* 34:216, 1993.
9. Seelig JM, Becker DP, Miller JD, et al: Traumatic acute subdural hematoma: Major mortality reduction in comatose patients treated under four hours. *N Engl J Med* 304:1511, 1981.
10. Teasdale G, Jennett B: Assessment of coma and impaired consciousness: A practical scale. *Lancet* 2:81, 1974.
11. Stein SC, Ross SE: Mild head injury: A plea for routine early CT scanning. *J Trauma* 33:11, 1992.
12. Rockswold GL, Pheley PJ: Patients who talk and deteriorate. *Ann Emerg Med* 22:1004, 1993.
13. Arienta C, Caroli M, Balbi S: Management of head-injured patients in the emergency department: A practical protocol. *Surg Neurol* 48:213, 1997.
14. Shackford SR, Wald SL, Ross SE, et al: The clinical utility of computed tomographic scanning and the neurologic examination in the management of patients with minor head injuries. *J Trauma* 33:385, 1992.
15. Alexander MP: Mild traumatic brain injury: Pathophysiology, natural history, and clinical management. *Neurology* 45:1253, 1995.
16. Stein SC, Ross SE: Moderate head injury: A guide to initial management. *J Neurosurg* 77:562, 1992.
17. Vassar MJ, Fischer, RP, O'Brien PE, et al: A multicenter trial for resuscitation of injured patients with 7.5 percent sodium chloride: The effect of added dextrose 70. *Arch Surg* 128:1003, 1993.

18. Lam AM, Winn HR, Cullon BF, Sendling BS: Hypoglycemic and neurologic outcome in patients with head injury *J. Neurosurg* 75:545, 1991.
19. Prough DS, Lang J: Therapy of patients with head injuries: Key parameters for management. *J Trauma* 42:S10, 1997.
20. Bullock R, Chestnut R, Clifton G, et al: *Guidelines for the Management of Severe Head Injury*. New York, Brain Trauma Foundation, 1996.
21. Bullock R, Chestnut R: *Consensus Statement Guidelines for Management of Severe Head Injury*, New York: Brain Trauma Foundation, 1995.
22. Papazian L, Albanese J, Thirion X, et al: Effect of bolus doses of midazolam on intracranial pressure and cerebral perfusion pressure in patients with severe head trauma. *Brit J Anaesth* 71:267, 1993.
23. Fowler SB, Herizog J, Wagner BK: Pharmacological interventions for Agitation in head-injured patients in the acute care setting. *J Neurosci Nurs* 27(2):119, 1995.
24. Brodie HA: Prophylactic antibiotics for posttraumatic cerebrospinal fluid fistulae. *Arch Otolaryngol Head Neck Surg* 123:749, 1997.
25. Kakarieka A, Braakman R, Schakel EH: Clinical significance of the findings of subarachnoid blood on CT scan after head injury. *Acta Neurochir* 129(1-2):1, 1994.
26. Harders A, Kakarieka A, Braakman R: Traumatic subarachnoid hemorrhage and its treatment with nimodipine. *J Neurosurg* 85:82, 1996.
27. Snoey ER, Levitt MA: Delayed diagnosis of subdural hematoma following normal computed tomography scan. *Ann Emerg Med* 23:1127, 1994.
28. Temkin NR, Dikman SS, Wilensky AJ, et al: A randomized, double-blind study of phenytoin for the prevention of post-traumatic seizures. *N Engl J Med* 323:497, 1990.
29. Label LS: Treatment of post-traumatic headaches: Maprotiline or amitriptyline? *Neurology* 41(suppl):247, 1991.

SPINAL CORD INJURIES

Bonny J. Baron
Thomas M. Scalea

Spinal injuries are probably the most devastating of all trauma-related injuries. Treatment of multiple associated injuries often supersedes definitive management of spinal injuries. Emergency physicians must prioritize management yet not lose sight of the potential ramifications of spinal trauma. Stabilization of primary injury and prevention of secondary injury are the goals in order to optimize final outcome.

EPIDEMIOLOGY

The incidence of traumatic spinal cord injury (SCI) in the United States has been estimated at 30 cases per million population at risk. Thus, 8000 to 10,000 new cases can be expected annually. The actual incidence is probably higher. Minor injuries are often not reported, and those associated with trauma fatalities may go unnoticed. SCI is predominantly a disease of young men. The mean age has been reported as 33.5 years,[1] with a male-to-female predominance of 4 to 1. Spinal injury occurs more frequently on weekends and holidays and during summer months. The majority (90 percent) of cases are caused by blunt trauma with most of these from motor vehicle crashes.

FUNCTIONAL ANATOMY

The vertebral column serves as the central supporting structure for the head and trunk and provides bony protection for the spinal cord. It consists of 33 vertebrae: 7 cervical, 12 thoracic, 5 lumbar, 5 sacral (fused to form the sacrum), and 4 coccygeal, which are usually fused (Fig. 248-1).

Vertebrae

In accordance with their weight-bearing function, the vertebrae become larger toward the lower end of the column, but all are built on the same fundamental plan. A typical vertebra is composed of a body anteriorly and a vertebral arch posteriorly (Fig. 248-2). Between the body and arch is the vertebral foramen, through which the spinal cord runs. The vertebral arch is made up of two pedicles, two laminae, and seven processes (one spinous, two transverse, and four articular). The spine has the potential to move in flexion, extension, lateral flexion, rotation, or circumduction (combination of all movements). The articular processes form synovial joints that act as pivots of the spinal column. The orientation of these articular facet joints changes at different levels of the spine. Differences in orientation of the facet joints account for variations in motion of specific regions of the vertebral column. A series of ligaments serve to maintain the alignment of the spinal column. The anterior and posterior longitudinal ligaments run along the vertebral bodies. Surrounding the vertebral arch are the ligamentum flavum and the supraspinous, interspinous, intertransverse, and capsular ligaments. The intervertebral disks lie between adjacent vertebral bodies. Each disk consists of a peripheral annulus fibrosus and a central nucleus pulposus. The annulus fibrosus is composed of fibrocartilage. The nucleus pulposus is a semifluid, gelatinous structure

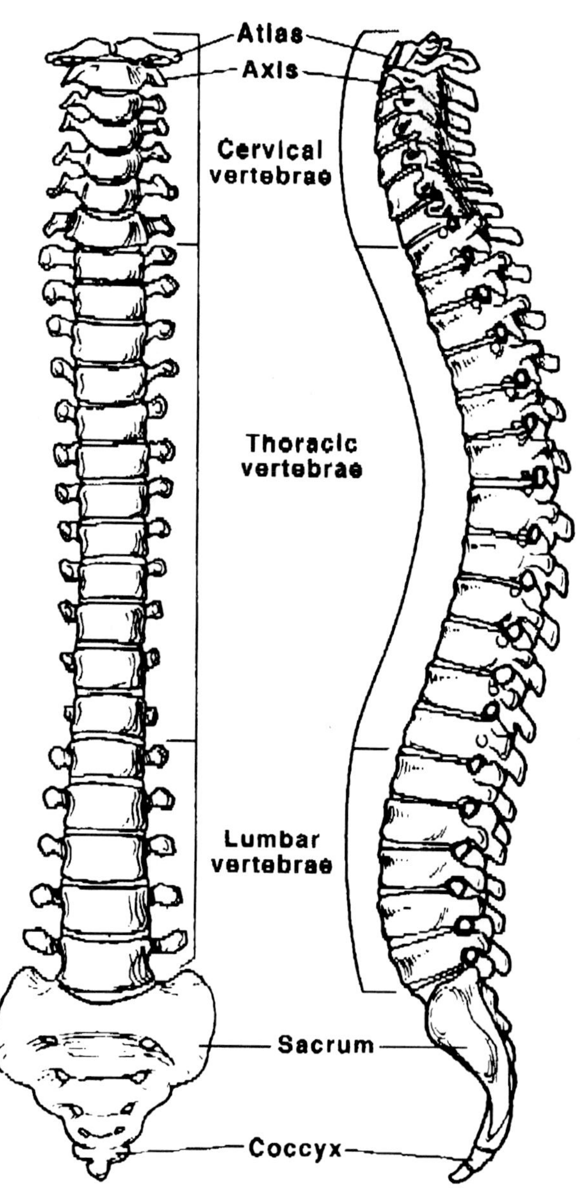

FIG. 248-1. The vertebral column. There are three vertebrae divided into cervical, thoracic, lumbar, sacral, and coccygial.

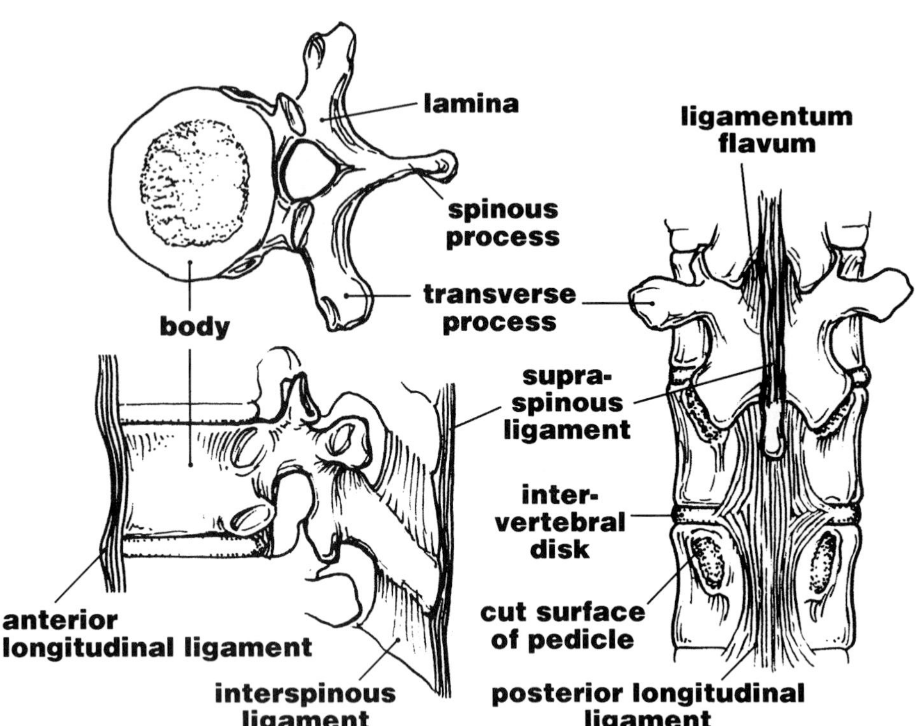

FIG. 248-2. Vertebra. Each vertebra consists of a vertebral body and posterior element. They are stabilized by an anterior longitudinal ligament, posterior ligament, and interspinous ligament.

made up of water and cartilage fibers. With advancing age, the proportion of water decreases and fibrocartilage increases. The disks act as shock absorbers to distribute axial load. When compressive forces exceed the absorptive capacity of the disk, the annulus fibrosus ruptures, allowing the nucleus pulposus to protrude into the vertebral canal. This may result in spinal nerve or spinal cord compression.

Spinal Stability

The determination of spinal stability is an important factor in the evaluation of the injured spine. White and Panjabi define stability as the ability of the spine to limit patterns of displacement under physiologic loads so as not to damage or irritate the spinal cord or nerve roots and to prevent incapacitating deformity or pain due to structural changes.[2] CT evaluation applied to Denis's three-column system for classification of thoracolumbar injuries can be used to assess spinal stability. According to Denis, the spine consists of three columns.[3] The anterior column is formed by the anterior part of the vertebral body, the anterior annulus fibrosus, and the anterior longitudinal ligament. The middle column is formed by the posterior wall of the vertebral body, the posterior annulus fibrosus, and the posterior longitudinal ligament. The posterior column includes the bony complex of the posterior vertebral arch and the posterior ligamentous complex. In order for an injury to be unstable, there must be disruption of at least two columns. In evaluating stability, it is also important to include the degree of compression of the vertebral body. Vertebral body compressions of more than 50 percent are generally considered unstable.

Thoracic and Lumbar Spine

The thoracic spine is a rigid segment. The additional support provided by its articulation with the rib cage imparts a stiffness to the thoracic spine 2.5 times that of the ligamentous spine alone. Relative to other regions of the vertebral column, a large force is necessary to overcome the intrinsic stability of the thoracic spine. While injury to the thoracic spine is less common than in other regions, when it does occur it is usually significant. The spinal canal is narrower than that found in either the cervical or lumbar spine. The large spinal cord diameter relative to canal diameter increases the risk of cord injury. When cord injuries occur, most are neurologically complete. Of additional importance is the association between fractures of the thoracic spine and severe pulmonary injuries, including mediastinal hemorrhage. Patients with blunt chest trauma and mediastinal widening should be evaluated for both aortic and thoracic spine injuries.[4]

The spine is divided into alternating mobile and fixed segments. The thoracolumbar junction (T11-L2) is considered a transitional zone between the fixed thoracic and mobile lumbar regions. This distinction is important because the transitional zones sustain the greatest amount of stress during motion. These areas are most vulnerable to traumatic injuries. In addition to this change in bony anatomy, the thoracolumbar junction serves as the level of transition from the end of the spinal cord (about L1) to the nerve roots of the cauda equina. Relative to the thoracic spine, the width of the spinal canal is greater. Despite a large number of vertebral injuries at the thoracolumbar junction, most are associated with normal neurologic exams or incomplete neurologic findings.

Relative to the thoracic and thoracolumbar regions, the lower lumbar spine is the most mobile. Isolated fractures of the lower lumbar spine rarely result in complete neurologic injuries. When neurologic injuries occur, they are usually complete cauda equina lesions or isolated nerve root injuries.

Sacrum and Coccyx

The sacrum supports the lumbar vertebral column and transmits loads from the trunk to the pelvic girdle and into the lower limbs. It consists of five rudimentary vertebrae fused to form a single wedge-shaped bone. The upper border articulates with the fifth lumbar vertebra. The inferior border articulates with the coccyx. Laterally, the sacrum articulates with the iliac bones to form the sacroiliac joints. The vertebral foramina together form the sacral canal. The sacral canal contains the nerve roots of the lumbar, sacral, and coccygeal spinal nerves and the filum terminale.

The coccyx consists of four vertebrae fused together to form a triangular bone, which articulates with the sacrum. Except for the first vertebra, the remaining coccygeal vertebrae consist of bodies only.

Injuries of the sacral spine and nerve roots are very unusual. When they occur, they are frequently associated with fractures of the pelvis. There are multiple different classification schemes of sacral fractures that help to predict neurologic deficits and establish treatment protocols. In general, transverse fractures through the body are most significant in that they cause injury to part or all of the cauda equina. Longitudinal fractures may cause radiculopathy. If there is involvement of the central sacral canal, however, bowel or bladder dysfunction may also occur.[5] Careful neurologic evaluation is essential. Motor and sensory evaluation of the sacral nerve roots should be performed. Rectal examination will assess anal sphincter tone and the bulbocavernosus reflex.

Coccygeal injuries are usually associated with direct falls onto the buttocks. Patients typically describe intense pain with sitting and straining. Diagnosis of fracture is made on rectal examination. Pain will be elicited with motion of the coccyx. X-rays are not needed. Treatment is symptomatic, and includes analgesics and use of a rubber doughnut pillow.

Spinal Cord

The spinal cord is a cylindrical structure that begins at the foramen magnum, where it is continuous with the medulla oblongata of the brain. Inferiorly, it terminates in the tapered conus medullaris at the lower border of the first lumbar vertebra. The conus is continued at its apex by a prolongation of the pia mater, the filum terminale, which extends to the base of the coccyx. The spinal cord gives rise to 31 pairs of spinal nerves: 8 cervical, 12 thoracic, 5 lumbar, 5 sacral, and 1 coccygeal. Each spinal nerve emerges through the intervertebral foramen corresponding to the appropriate spinal cord level. There is disproportionate growth in the length of the spinal cord and the vertebral column. As a result of this inequality, the length of the nerve roots increase and at lower levels, both progressively. The lower nerve roots, inferior to the conus medullaris, form an array of nerves around the filum terminale; this is called the *cauda equina*.

CLINICAL FEATURES

Damage to the spinal cord is the result of two types of injury. First is the direct mechanical injury from traumatic impact. This insult sets into motion a series of vascular and chemical processes that lead to secondary injury. The initial phase is characterized by hemorrhage into the cord and formation of edema at the injured site and surrounding region. Local spinal cord blood flow is diminished owing to vasospasm and thrombosis of the small arterioles within the gray and white matter. Extension of edema may further compromise blood flow and increase ischemia. A secondary tissue degeneration phase begins within hours of injury. This is associated with the release of membrane-destabilizing enzymes, mediators of inflammation, and disturbance of electrophysiologic coupling by disruption of calcium channel pathways. Lipid peroxidation and hydrolysis appear to play a major role in this secondary phase of spinal cord injury.[6]

Spinal Cord Lesions

It is important to distinguish between complete and incomplete spinal cord injuries. The severity of injury determines the prognosis for recovery of function. The American Spinal Injury Association defines a complete neurologic lesion as the absence of sensory and motor function below the level of injury. This includes loss of function to the level of the lowest sacral segment. In contrast, a lesion is incomplete if sensory, motor, or both functions are partially present below the neurologic level of injury. This may consist only of sacral sensation at the anal mucocutaneous junction or voluntary contraction of the external anal sphincter upon digital examination.[3] In assessing neurologic function, spinal shock must be considered. Patients in spinal shock lose all reflex activities. This generally resolves, with the return of the bulbocavernosus reflex occurring first. Lesions cannot be deemed complete until spinal shock has resolved. Complete lesions have a minimal chance of functional motor recovery. Patients with incomplete lesions are expected to have at least some degree of recovery.

Clinical syndromes classify incomplete spinal cord lesions. Damage to specific sections of the spinal cord results in predictable physical findings (Table 248-1).

A discussion of the anatomy may be helpful.

A large number of descending and ascending tracts have been identified in the spinal cord. The three most important of these in terms of neuroanatomic localization of cord lesions are the corticospinal tracts, spinothalamic tracts, and dorsal (posterior) columns.

The corticospinal tract is a descending motor pathway. Its fibers descend from the cerebral cortex through the internal capsule and the middle of the crus cerebri. The tract then breaks up into bundles in the pons and finally collects into a discrete bundle, forming the pyramid of the medulla. In the lower medulla, approximately 90% of the fibers cross (decussate) to the side opposite that of their origin and descend through the spinal cord as the lateral corticospinal tract. These fibers synapse on lower motor neurons in the spinal cord. The 10 percent of corticospinal fibers that do not decussate in the medulla descend in the anterior funiculus of the cervical and upper thoracic cord levels as the ventral corticospinal tract. Damage to the corticospinal tract neurons (upper motor neurons) in the spinal cord results in ipsilateral clinical findings such as muscle weakness, spasticity, increased deep tendon reflexes, and a Babinski sign.

The two major ascending pathways that transmit sensory information are the spinothalamic tracts and the dorsal columns. The first neurons of both of these afferent systems begin as sensory receptors situated in the skin and stretch receptors of muscles. Their cell bodies are located in the dorsal root ganglia of the spinal nerves. The spinothalamic tract transmits pain and temperature sensation. As the axons of the first neurons enter the spinal cord, most rise one or two levels before entering the dorsal gray of the spinal cord, where they synapse with the second neuron of the spinothalamic tract. The second neuron immediately crosses the midline in the anterior commissure of the spinal cord and ascends in the anterolateral funiculus as the lateral spinothalamic tract. When the spinothalamic tract is damaged in the spinal cord, the patient experiences loss of pain and temperature sensation in the contralateral half of the body. The sensory loss begins one or two segments below the level of the lesion. The dorsal columns transmit vibration and proprioceptive information. Neurons enter the spinal cord proximal to pain and temperature neurons. They differ from pain and temperature neurons in that they do not immediately synapse. Instead, these axons enter the ipsilateral dorsal column and do not synapse until they reach the gracile or cuneate nuclei of the medulla. From these nuclei, fibers cross the midline and ascend in the medial lemniscus to the thalamus. Injury to one side of the dorsal columns will result in ipsilateral loss of vibration and position sense. The sensory loss begins at the level of the lesion. Light touch is transmitted through both the spinothalamic tracts and the dorsal columns. Therefore, light touch is not completely lost unless there is damage to both the spinothalamic tracts and the dorsal columns.

Concerning the spinal nerves and their relationship to the vertebrae, each spinal nerve is named for its adjacent vertebral body. Because there is an additional pair of spinal nerve roots compared to the number of vertebral bodies, the first seven spinal nerves are named for the first seven cervical vertebrae, each exiting through the intervertebral foramen above its corresponding vertebral body. The spinal nerve exiting below C7, however, is referred to as the C8 spinal nerve, though no eighth cervical vertebra exists. All subsequent nerve roots,

TABLE 248-1 Spinal Cord Syndromes

Syndrome	Etiology	Symptoms	Prognosis
Anterior cord	Direct anterior cord compression Flexion of cervical spine Thrombosis of anterior spinal artery	Complete paralysis below the lesion with loss of pain and temperature sensation Preservation of proprioception and vibratory function	Poor
Central cord	Hyperextension injuries Disruption of blood flow to the spinal cord Cervical spinal stenosis	Quadriparesis—greater in the upper extremities than the lower extremities. Some loss of pain and temperature sensation, also greater in the upper extremities	Good
Brown-Séquard	Transverse hemisection of the spinal cord Unilateral cord compression	Ipsilateral spastic paresis, loss of proprioception and vibratory sensation and contralateral loss of pain and temperature sensation	Good
Cauda equina	Peripheral nerve injury	Variable motor and sensory loss in the lower extremities, sciatica, bowel/bladder dysfunction and ''saddle anesthesia''	Good
Spinal shock	Partial or complete injury at the T6 level and above	Areflexia, loss of sensation, and flaccid paralysis below the level of the lesion; a flaccid bladder and loss of rectal tone; bradycardia and hypotension	Complete lesions have a poor prognosis Incomplete lesions have some degree of recovery

beginning with T1, exit below the vertebral body for which they are named.

During fetal development, the downward growth of the vertebral column is greater than that of the spinal cord. Because the adult spinal cord ends as the conus medullaris at the level of the lower border of the first lumbar vertebra, the lumbar and sacral nerve roots must continue inferiorly below the termination of the spinal cord to exit from their respective intervertebral foramina. These nerve roots form the cauda equina. A potential consequence of this arrangement is that injury to a single lower vertebra can involve multiple nerve roots in the cauda equina. For example, an injury at the L3 vertebra can involve the L3 nerve root as well as the lower nerve roots that are progressing to a level caudal to the L3 vertebra.

Anterior Cord Syndrome

The anterior cord syndrome results from damage to the corticospinal and spinothalamic pathways with preservation of posterior column function. This is manifest by loss of motor function and pain and temperature sensation distal to the lesion. Only vibration, position, and crude touch are preserved. This syndrome may occur following direct injury to the anterior spinal cord. Flexion of the cervical spine may result in cord contusion or bone injury with secondary cord injury. Alternatively, thrombosis of the anterior spinal artery can cause ischemic injury to the anterior cord.[7,8] Immediate evaluation with computed tomography CT or magnetic resonance imaging MRI may reveal an extrinsic mass that is amenable to surgical decompression. The overall prognosis for recovery of function historically has been poor and remains so today.[5]

Central Cord Syndrome

The central cord syndrome is usually seen in older patients with preexisting cervical spondylosis who sustain a hyperextension injury. The injury preferentially involves the central portion of the cord more than the peripheral. The centrally located fibers of the corticospinal and spinothalamic tracts are affected. The neural tracts providing function to the upper extremities are most medial in position. The thoracic, lower extremity, and sacral fibers have a more lateral distribution. Clinically, patients present with decreased strength, and to a lesser degree, decreased pain and temperature sensation, more in the upper than the lower extremities. Spastic paraparesis or spastic quadraparesis can also be seen. The majority will have bowel and bladder control, although this may be impaired in the more severe cases. Prognosis for recovery of function is good; however, most patients do not regain fine motor use of their upper extremities.[7,9,10]

Brown-Séquard Syndrome

The Brown-Séquard syndrome results from hemisection of the cord. It is manifest by ipsilateral loss of motor function, proprioception, and vibratory sensation, and contralateral loss of pain and temperature sensation. The most common cause of this syndrome is penetrating injury. It can also be caused by lateral cord compression secondary to disk protrusion, hematomas, bone injury, or tumors. Of all of the incomplete cord lesions, this has the best prognosis for recovery.[7,9]

Cauda Equina Syndrome

The cauda equina is composed entirely of lumbar, sacral, and coccygeal nerve roots. An injury in this region produces a peripheral nerve injury rather than a direct injury to the spinal cord. Symptoms may include variable motor and sensory loss in the lower extremities, sciatica, bowel and bladder dysfunction, and ''saddle anesthesia'' (loss of pain sensation over the perineum).[7] Because peripheral nerves possess the ability to regenerate, the prognosis for recovery is better than that for spinal cord lesions.

MECHANISM OF INJURY

Accidents involving motor vehicles are the principal cause of traumatic injury to the spinal cord. Other etiologies, in descending order of frequency, include falls, gunshot wounds, and injuries secondary to sports or recreational activities.

Fractures of the spine can be divided into minor and major injuries. Minor injuries are those that are localized to part of a column and do not cause instability. These fractures often result from direct blunt trauma to the posterior elements of the spine. Minor injuries include isolated fractures of the transverse, spinous, and articular processes. Major spinal injuries can be classified into four categories: (1) compression (wedge) fractures, (2) burst fractures, (3) flexion-distraction (seat belt–type injuries) and (4) fracture/dislocations.[11]

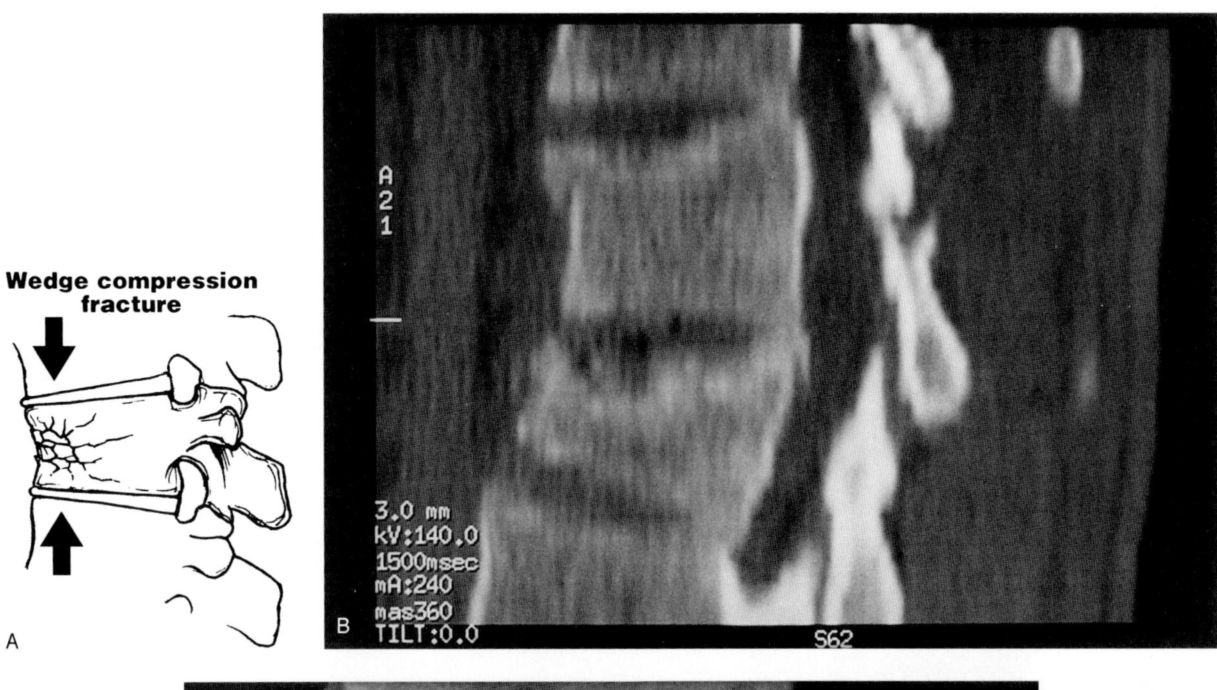

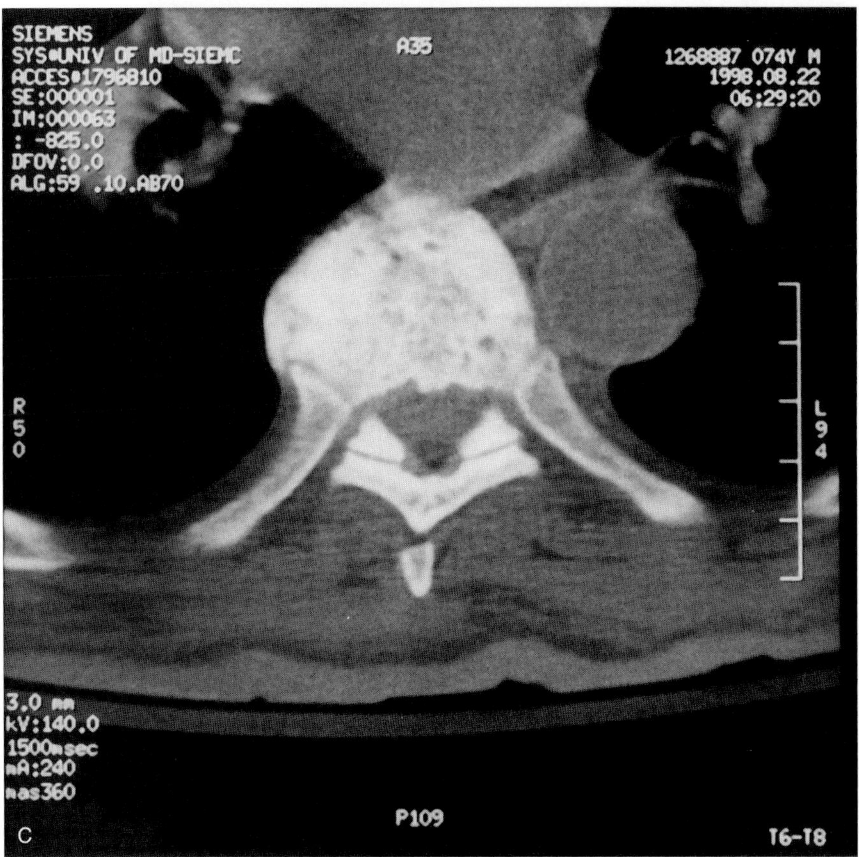

FIG. 248-3. Wedge compression fractures are often caused by axial unloading with failure of the anterior column. **A,** Schematic of a compression fracture. **B,** Lateral reconstruction of a CT demonstrating the anterior wedging. **C,** Demonstrates the anterior wedging and vertebral body fracture. Note the lack of retropulsion of elements into the spinal canal.

Compression fractures result from axial loading and flexion, with subsequent failure of the anterior column (Fig. 248-3). The middle column remains intact. These injuries are usually stable unless they are greater than 50 percent. They are unlikely to be directly responsible for neurologic damage.

Burst fractures occur following failure of the vertebral body under axial load (Fig. 248-4). In contrast to compression fractures, both the anterior and middle columns fail. There is retropulsion of bone and disk fragments into the canal. This may cause spinal cord compression.

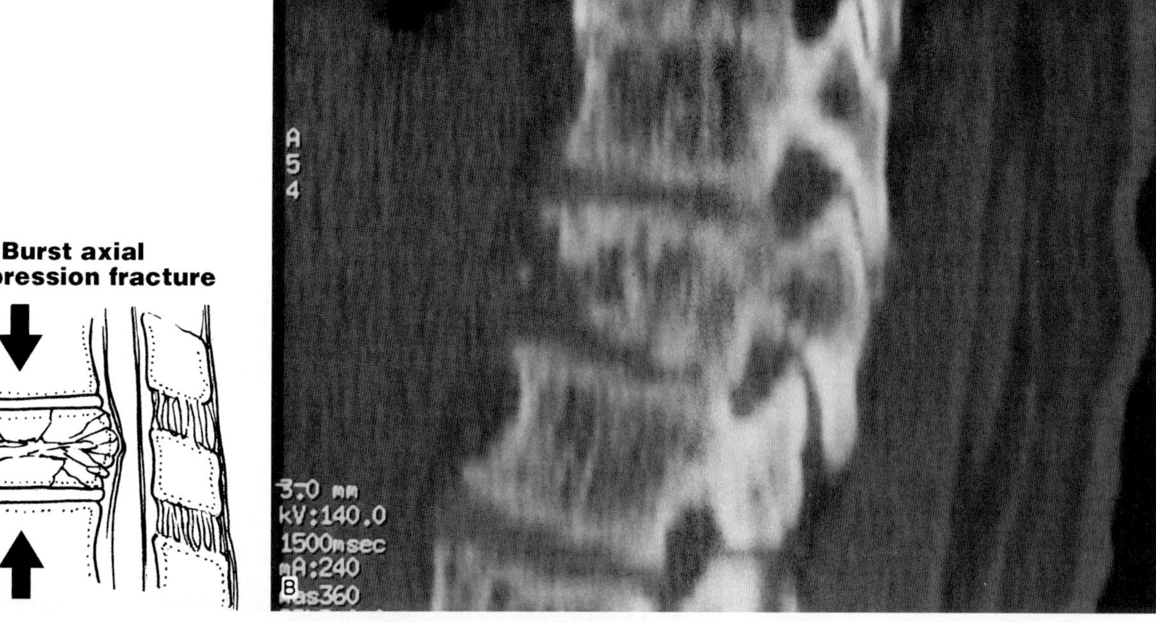

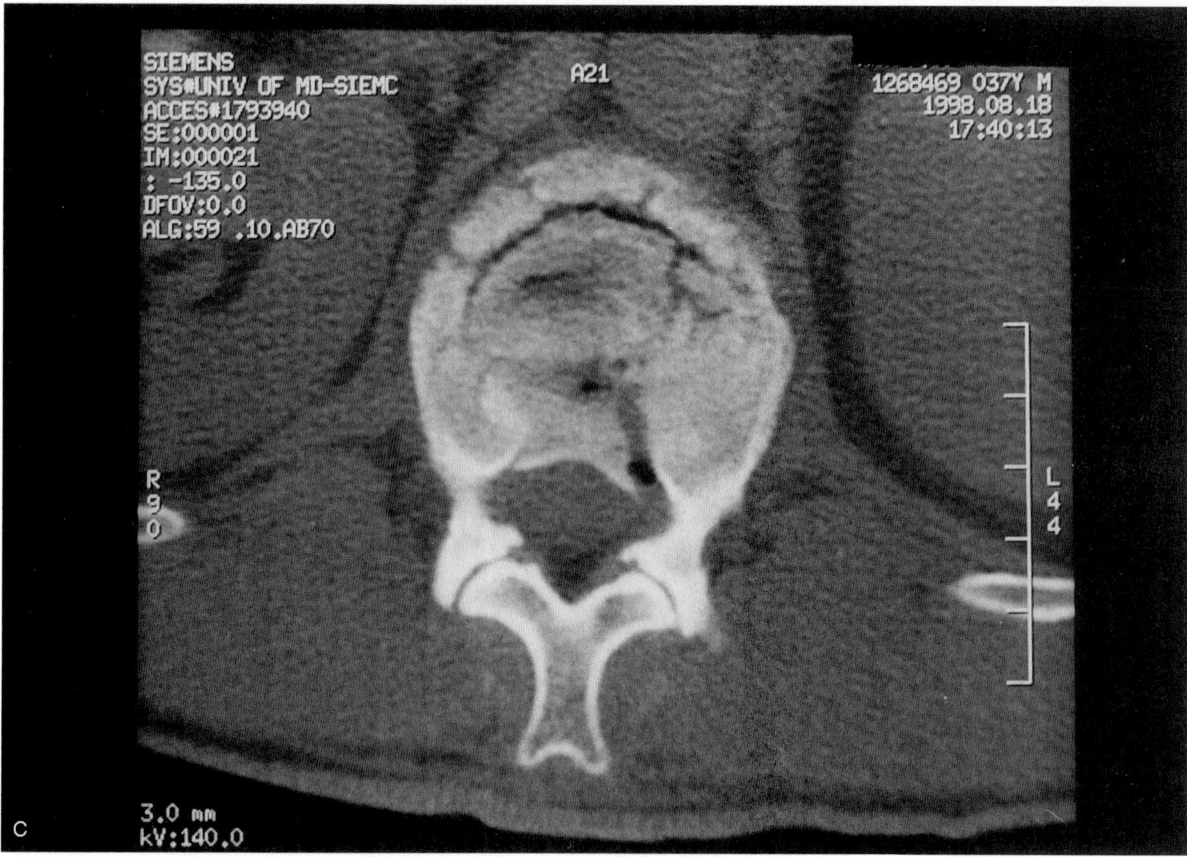

FIG. 248-4. Burst fractures are also caused by axial unloading. Both anterior and middle columns have failed. **A,** Schematic of the forces transmitted. **B,** Lateral reconstruction CT scan demonstrating failure of both the anterior and middle columns. **C,** Demonstrates the burst vertebral body. Note the retropulsion of elements into the spinal canal.

Flexion-distraction injuries are commonly seen following seat belt–type injuries, particularly where lap belts alone are used (Fig. 248-5). The seat belt serves as the axis of rotation during distraction, and there is failure of both the posterior and middle columns. The intact anterior column prevents subluxation. Typical radiographic findings reveal increased height of the posterior vertebral body, fracture of the posterior wall of the vertebral body, and posterior opening of the disk space.

Fracture-dislocations are the most damaging of injuries (Fig. 248-6). Compression, flexion, distraction, rotation, or shearing forces lead to failure of all three columns. The end result is subluxation or dislocation.

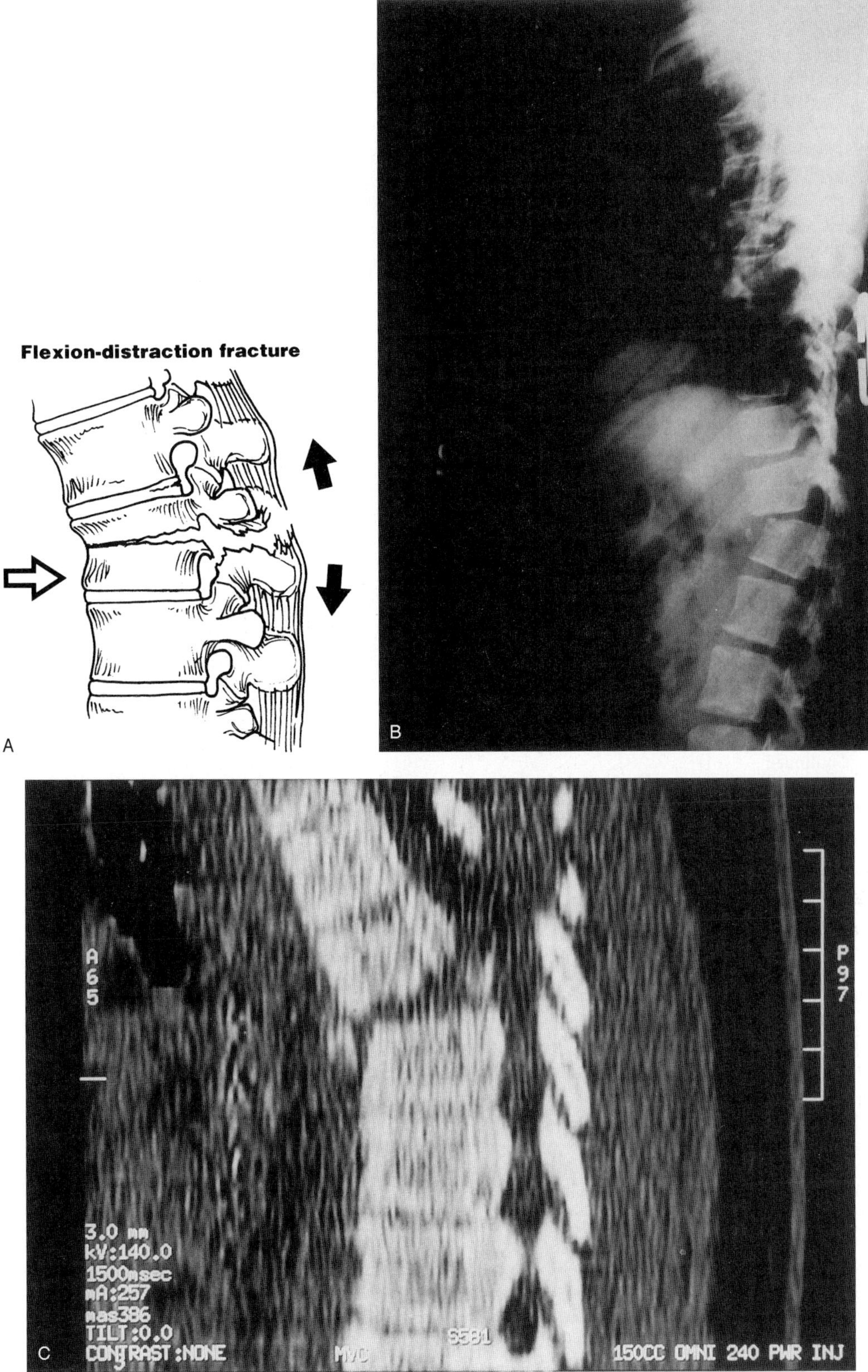

FIG. 248-5. Flexion-distraction injuries involve rotation of forces. This results in failure of both the posterior and middle columns. **A,** Schematic of the forces transmitted. **B,** Plain films demonstrating a flexion distraction injury. **C,** Lateral CT reconstruction confirming the pattern, also demonstrating posterior opening of the disc space. **D,** Shows loss of the middle column with fracture through the lateral elements.

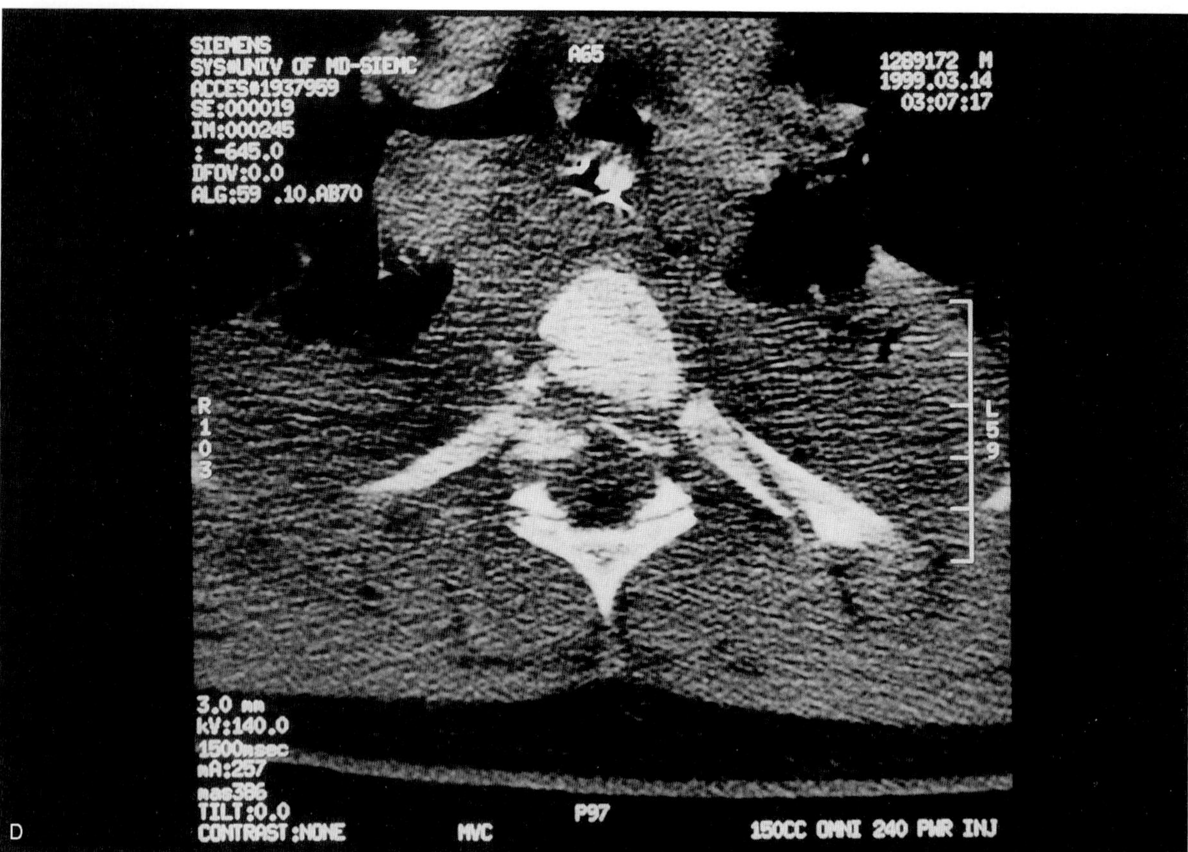

FIG. 248-5. Continued

Blunt Injury

MOTOR VEHICLE–RELATED INJURIES Motor vehicle crashes usually result in acceleration-deceleration injuries. Multiple vertebral structures are subjected to the forces involved, including the anterior and posterior bony elements, disks, interspinous ligaments, and musculature. The cervical spine is the most susceptible to injury by this mechanism, but the thoracic and lumbar regions are also at risk. The majority of victims are involved in low-impact crashes. Most commonly, the soft tissues are injured. Patients complain of pain in the posterior neck and back. High-speed, high-energy crashes are more likely to result in structural damage to the spine. Lap-only seatbelts have been associated with thoracolumbar injuries.

Pedestrians struck by vehicles and motorcyclists are at considerable risk for multiple skeletal injuries, including spinal injuries. These patients have no protective structure surrounding them and are therefore subject to forces applied directly to their bodies.

The challenge to the emergency physician is to distinguish between minor injury and an unstable spine. Obvious neurologic deficits mandate emergent treatment for an unstable injury. In the absence of deficits, the mechanism of injury with an understanding of the forces involved should guide management. When in doubt, it is best initially to overtreat and overstudy in order to avoid missing a significant injury.

Falls

Falls from a height are associated with fractures of the lower extremities, pelvis, and spine. Scalea et al. studied 161 patients who fell from a height of one or more stories, nearly one-fourth of whom suffered spine fractures.[12] Of the latter, 74 percent sustained a major compression or burst fracture. The most common site of injury was the thoracolumbar junction. A thorough neurologic evaluation must be part of the early assessment of patients with vertical deceleration injury. All patients must be presumed to have unstable spine fractures until proven otherwise.

Sports Injuries

Spinal injuries occur in both contact and noncontact sports. The specific injury is related to the mechanism, the force involved, and the point of application of the force rather than to the specific sport. Injuries can occur to the supporting tissue, the disk, or the bone. The majority of injuries are self-limiting soft tissue injuries. Injuries at the level of the disk result in disk herniation or degeneration. Those that occur at the level of the bone can range from minimal avulsion-type fractures to compressions or fracture dislocations. Most bony injuries are not associated with neurologic sequelae. Rarely, however, sports injuries do result in significant neurologic compromise. When neurologic impairment occurs, it is usually secondary to direct axial forces. Catastrophic injuries have been associated with football, water sports (especially diving), gymnastics, rugby, and ice hockey.[13]

Penetrating Injury

The majority of penetrating spinal cord lesions are caused by gunshot wounds. These wounds may be localized to the spine or may involve transperitoneal trajectories. The spinal cord may be injured by direct contact with the bullet, by bony fragments, or from concussive forces.[14] Most gunshot wounds result in stable vertebral injuries, although cord lesions are often complete. Stabbing injuries are much less common. These may be inflicted by a variety of implements including knives, axes, icepicks, screwdrivers, and glass fragments. The majority of stab

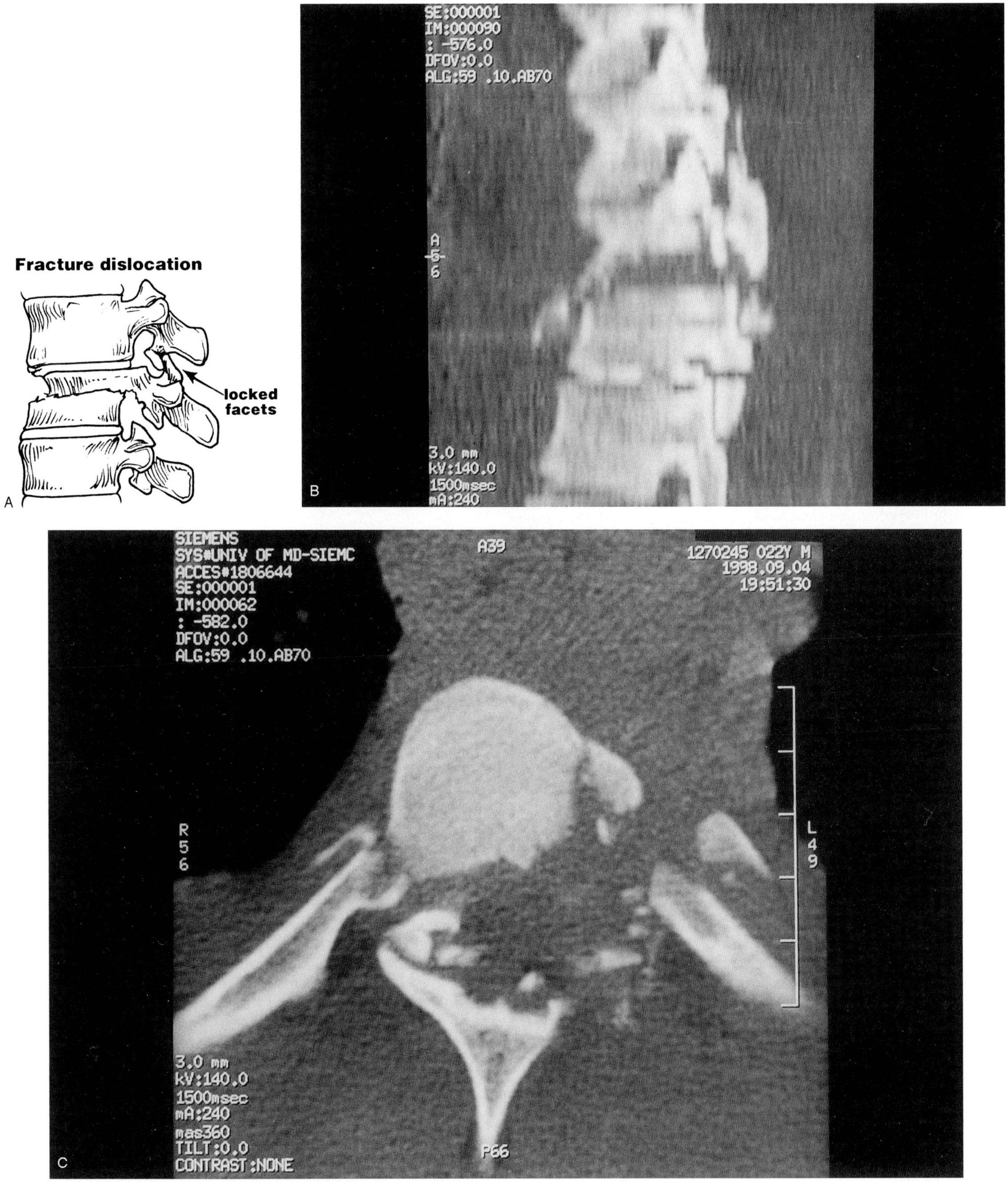

Fracture dislocation

locked facets

A

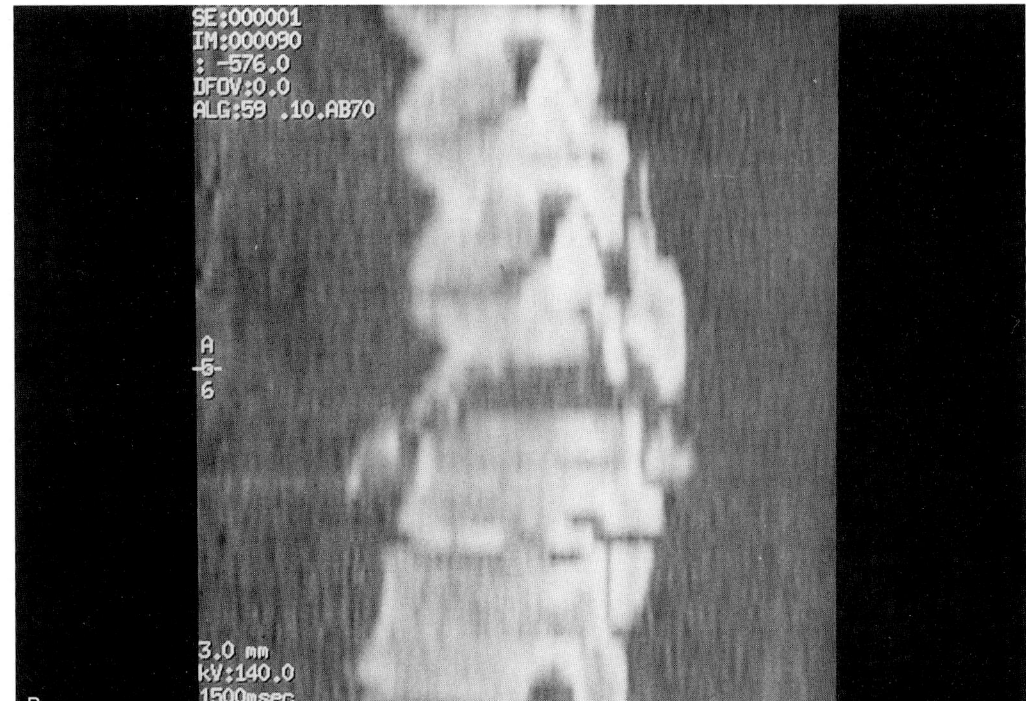

C

FIG. 248-6. Fracture dislocations are the most damaging of injuries leading to failure of all three columns. **A,** Demonstrates these injuries schematically. **B,** Lateral CT reconstruction demonstrating loss of all three columns. **C,** Demonstrates the dislocation and displacement of the vertebral body.

wounds involve incomplete Brown-Séquard lesions of the thoracic cord. These have the best prognosis of incomplete spinal injuries. The prognosis for patients with stab injuries to the spine and incomplete paralysis is significantly better than that for patients with gunshot wounds to the spine and a similar extent of paralysis.

TREATMENT

The initial care of a patient with a spinal cord injury must be performed in conjunction with the evaluation and treatment of coexisting injuries, both potential and diagnosed. As with all multiply injured patients, this involves prehospital evaluation and triage, which should be designed to deliver the patient to the most appropriate level of care for the compendium of injuries. In addition, prehospital therapy must include stabilization of the patient as well as control of the underlying problem if possible. Emergency department (ED) evaluation must be tailored to rapidly identify injuries and institute early therapy.

Prehospital Care

The prehospital treatment of patients with spinal cord injury involves recognition of patients at risk, proper triage, and early care. All patients who have complaints of neck or back pain or who have tenderness on prehospital assessment must be presumed to have a spine injury until proven otherwise. Traditionally, all patients with significant injury above the clavicle are also presumed to have cervical spine injury regardless of related complaints. All patients with neurologic complaints must be presumed to have a spinal cord injury. Sometimes this is obvious, as in a patient with flaccid paraplegia. More often, symptoms are much more subtle (numbness or tingling in an extremity). Appropriate triage is imperative, as the results of the treatment for spinal cord injury are somewhat time-related. Therefore, initial triage to a center that is capable of rapid diagnostics and therapeutics is essential to optimize outcome following spinal cord injury.

Triage can be difficult. Patients may be asymptomatic or may have suffered a concomitant head injury that makes them unable to describe their injuries and hence does not allow for neurologic assessment in the field. Other injuries may preclude accurate hospital assessment. The mechanism of injury is an important criterion on which prehospital providers can rely. High-speed or roll-over vehicular accidents are commonly associated with spinal injury. Even more commonly, axial loading injuries such as substantial falls from a height produce spinal cord injuries, generally in the area of the thoracolumbar junction. Diving and surfing accidents, where force is transmitted through the cranium and into the cervical spine, typically produce cervical spine injuries. Any patient at risk by mechanism of injury must be presumed to have a spinal cord injury. While this may result in a substantial rate of overtriage, the consequences of undertriage can be devastating.

Prehospital care for spinal injuries involves immobilization of the entire spine and initial fluid therapy as proposed by the American College of Surgeons.[15] The entire cervical spine can be immobilized with a rigid cervical collar supplemented with sandbags and tape. The thoracic and lumbar spine can be immobilized utilizing a long backboard. Patients are ''papoosed'' onto the boards to maintain spinal alignment. Patients should be transported completely immobilized. Fluid therapy is begun and tailored to avoid hypotension. While there is little scientific evidence to support any single target for systolic or mean arterial blood pressure in patients with spinal cord injuries, a mean arterial pressure of 65 to 70 mmHg seems a reasonable target. Optimal perfusion of the spinal cord is one of the therapies that can be implemented in the field to lessen the chances of secondary spinal injury.

Prehospital personnel must balance the issues of time of transport with the level of expertise of the various hospitals within their system. All efforts should be made to deliver patients with symptomatic spinal injuries to the areawide spine center. Delays engendered by transport to a different site can be costly. Clearly, patients who are not hemodynamically stable must be taken to the closest available hospital.

ED Stabilization

ED evaluation should not differ substantially from any patient with multiple injuries (see Chap. 243). It involves a stepwise search for immediately life-threatening injuries. Airway concerns are paramount. Real consideration should be given to immediate airway control in patients with cervical spine injuries no matter how stable they seem at the time of presentation. The higher the level of spinal injury, the more compelling the indication for early airway intervention. The roots of the phrenic nerve, which supplies the diaphragm, emerge at the third, fourth, and fifth cervical vertebral levels. Thus, any patient with an injury at C5 or above should be intubated. It may be prudent to intubate parents with cervical cord lesions even below this level. Significant spinal cord edema may progress rostrally to involve the roots of the phrenic nerve. Many patients can initially support ventilatory function utilizing intercostal muscles or abdominal breathing, but they eventually tire and then develop respiratory failure. As the evaluation process for these patients often involves transport outside of the ED, the authors feel strongly that early airway control is the safest route. Patients who develop respiratory failure in the CT scanner or the MRI suite may suffer respiratory arrest before it can be recognized and the airway secured. This risks anoxic brain damage and worsening spinal cord injury from hypoxia.

AIRWAY It is important to try to perform a complete neurologic assessment if possible before patients are intubated and sedated. The spine must be kept immobilized while the airway is managed. In general, this is accomplished using orotracheal intubation with in-line cervical stabilization (without distraction force) and cricoid pressure. Nasal intubation can be performed in patients while maintaining spine immobilization, though it is not our preferred method and presents considerable difficulties. Nasal intubation is generally a blind technique. Virtually all patients with potential cervical spine trauma require sedation before nasal intubation can be accomplished; but if respirations become substantially depressed, nasotracheal intubation may not be possible. If patients are inadequately prepared they may resist intubation. Motion of an unstable fracture can worsen spinal injury. If patients are over-sedated, they may become hypoxic and lose the ability to protect the airway. Also, nasal intubation is performed with a smaller endotracheal tube, which can compromise respiratory therapy later during the hospitalization. Fiberoptic bronchoscopy (FOB) may be required, particularly in those with pulmonary injuries or significant atelectasis. Bronchoscopy can be used for diagnostic purposes or to facilitate removal of inspissated mucous plugs or blood. A relatively large endotracheal tube (8.0 mm or greater in size) is needed during FOB in order to ensure that ventilation is not compromised during the procedure. An 8.0 mm endotracheal tube is often too large for nasotracheal intubation. In addition, the limiting factor in minimizing tube size is the increasing respiratory resistance to gas flow imposing increased work for the patient with each spontaneous breath. Thus, the work of breathing is greater with tubes of 6 to 7 mm internal diameter, sometimes used for nasal intubation, than with tubes of 8 mm or greater internal diameter. The most limiting aspect of nasal intubation is the inability to move the cervical spine to attain the ''sniff'' position, optimal for the procedure. Finally, nasal intubation increases the risk of sinusitis, which later becomes symptomatic.

Nasal intubation with fiberoptic guidance is a useful technique. It does carry many of the concerns of nasal intubation previously mentioned. It is, however, not a blind technique and can be directed, maximizing the chances of successful airway management.

Patients with spinal cord injuries often have concomitant chest injuries and/or abdominal injuries. A careful survey must be completed for each of these. Respiratory failure in a spinal cord–injured patient can certainly come from tension pneumothorax or blood loss into the chest.

HYPOTENSION Following airway stabilization, hemodynamic stability is the most pressing concern. Fluid therapy is generally the treatment of choice to support cardiovascular functioning. Patients with spinal cord injuries often present with hypotension, which must be differentiated as to its cause: spinal cord injury, blood loss, or both. Injury to the spinal cord at the level of the cervical or thoracic vertebrae causes sympathetic denervation. There is a loss of α-adrenergic tone and dilatation of the arterial and venous vessels. Elimination of sympathetic arterial tone results in hypotension. Systemic vascular resistance is reduced. Loss of sympathetic innervation to the heart (T1 through T4 cord levels) leaves the parasympathetic cardiac innervation via the vagus nerve unopposed, resulting in bradycardia. While it is true that neurogenic shock is associated with bradycardia, it should never be assumed that a patient with hypotension and bradycardia is suffering from isolated neurogenic shock. Vital signs are often nonspecific. Patients with neurogenic shock may have concomitant hemorrhagic shock and may not be able to mount a tachycardic response. Blood loss must be presumed to be the cause of hypotension until proven otherwise. In general, patients with neurogenic shock are warm, peripherally vasodilated, and bradycardic. They seem to tolerate hypotension relatively well. This makes some sense, as peripheral oxygen delivery is presumably normal. They have incurred mechanical sympathectomy, thus cardiovascular function is not impaired.

The mechanism of injury is important in determining whether hypotension is from spinal cord injury or blood loss. Soderstrom et al. have demonstrated that 70 percent of patients with blunt trauma have hypotension secondary to the spinal cord injury.[16] However, in almost one-third of the patients, blood loss at least partly explained the hemodynamic instability. Hypotension from spinal cord injury is highly unusual in patients with penetrating injury. Zipnick et al. have demonstrated that over 90 percent of hypotensive patients with penetrating spinal cord injury have blood loss to at least partly explain their hypotension.[17]

In all patients, a rapid search for potential blood loss should be undertaken. A chest x-ray will identify blood loss within the thorax. Retroperitoneal blood loss can come from concomitant pelvic fractures or may be secondary to lumbar arterial bleeding from spine fractures, especially in patients with substantial falls from a height. This can be a difficult diagnosis to make. Every patient with a spinal fracture should have an abdominal investigation. In hemodynamically unstable patients, CT scanning is too time-consuming; therefore ultrasound or diagnostic peritoneal lavage should be used (see Chap. 252). Retroperitoneal bleeding should be suspected in patients without evidence of intraabdominal blood loss who develop abdominal distention or tenderness.[12] Plain x-rays that demonstrate spinal fractures should help with the diagnosis. Angiography may be necessary for both diagnosis and treatment of ongoing bleeding.

NEUROLOGIC EXAMINATION Once patients are stabilized and other life-threatening injuries have been excluded or treated, a detailed neurologic examination should be performed if still possible. Details of history include whether the patient has had a loss of consciousness. Ask about the presence or absence of sensory or motor symptomatology in the field. A patient who was asymptomatic in the field and has neurologic deterioration in the ED requires emergent therapy. The presence of neck or back pain, or urinary or fecal incontinence clearly defines the patient at risk for spinal cord injury.

Physical examination should delineate the level of spinal cord injury, if any (Fig. 248-7). Document the initial neurologic performance. If patients deteriorate later, a complete initial neurologic examination must be documented for comparison purposes. The presence or absence of neck or back tenderness should be noted. A careful motor examination should be performed. Motor function for muscle groups should be tested and recorded on a scale of 0 to 5 (Table 248-2). The level of sensory loss should be determined. Gross proprioception or vibratory function must be investigated to examine posterior column function. Deep tendon reflexes should be tested. Anogenital reflexes should also be tested, because ''sacral sparing'' with preservation of the reflexes denotes an incomplete spinal cord level even if the patient has complete sensory and motor loss. The neurosurgeon must be notified emergently. To test the bulbocavernosus reflex, squeeze the penis to determine whether the anal sphincter simultaneously contracts, and assess rectal tone at the same time. Priapism implies a complete spinal cord injury. The cremasteric reflex is tested by running a pin or a blunt instrument up the medial aspect of the thigh. If the scrotum rises, there is some spinal cord integrity. The area around the anus should be tested with a pin. An ''anal wink'' (contraction of the anal musculature) indicates some sacral sparing.

DIAGNOSTIC IMAGING

Certainly one of the real dilemmas facing the clinician in the ED is which patient requires evaluation for a potential spinal cord injury (Fig. 248-8). A multiplicity of examinations exists. Blind application of expensive diagnostic testing risks inappropriately increasing the cost of medical care and potentially rendering resources unavailable to other patients. Diagnostic testing must evaluate the possibility of injury to both bone and spinal cord. While these often occur in concert, this is not always the case. While one would always like to limit diagnostic testing to those who require it, the consequences of a missed spinal cord injury can be devastating. Removing a collar or allowing a patient to walk with an unstable spine risks converting a patient with no spinal cord injury to one with a complete level. Thus, it is prudent to completely image and evaluate all patients with the possibility of spinal cord pathology.

In general, an x-ray of the cervical spine is part of the standard triage for blunt trauma. The utility of plain films of the cervical spine over the clinical examination to identify injury in patients who are alert, oriented, and have no neck or back pain is questionable.[18,19] Many centers have abandoned use of cervical spine x-rays in such patients. There is a substantial difference, however, in patients who are not alert and awake. The frequency of cervical spine injury in association with blunt head trauma is about 2 to 5 percent. However, it increases to almost 9 percent in patients with significant head injury, defined as a Glasgow Coma Scale score <10.[20]

Plain x-rays are clearly indicated in all patients with neck pain or cervical tenderness. The presence of pain or tenderness has over an 80 percent sensitivity for cervical spine injury. Cervical spine injury is very unusual in patients without pain or tenderness but may occur in approximately 1 percent.[19] Thus, the mechanism of injury should also be taken into account when the decision is made whether to image a patient's cervical spine. In a study of 233 patients, nine variables correlated significantly with cervical spine injury. They were: falls, symptoms of numbness, sensory loss, weakness, neck spasm, neck tenderness, objective sensory and motor loss, and weakness or loss

TABLE 248-2 Motor Grading System

0	No active contraction
1	Trace visible or palpable contraction
2	Movement with gravity eliminated
3	Movement against gravity
4	Movement against gravity plus resistance
5	Normal power

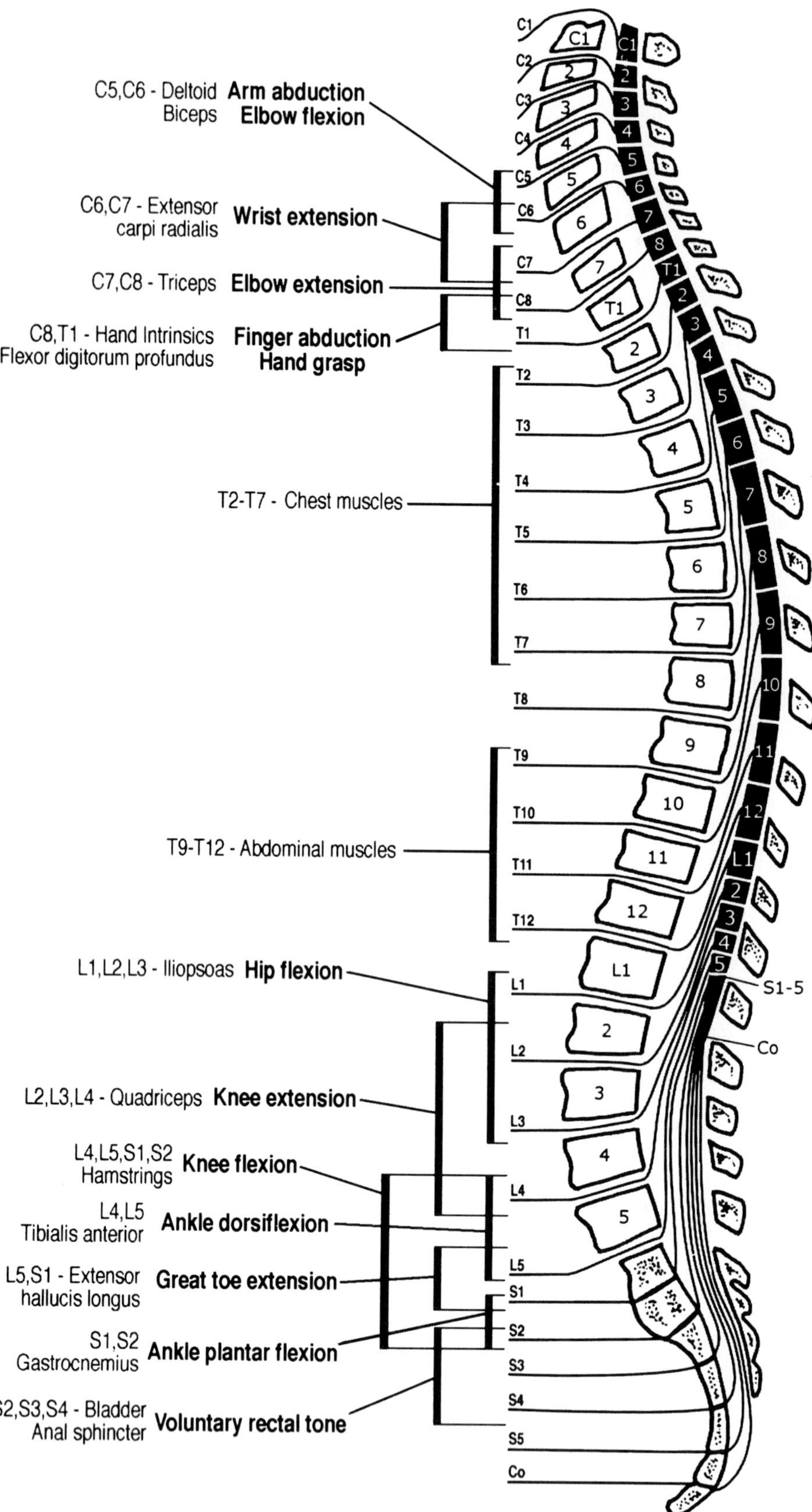

FIG. 248-7. Spinal cord level. This level can be delineated by physical examination, including a detailed neurologic examination.

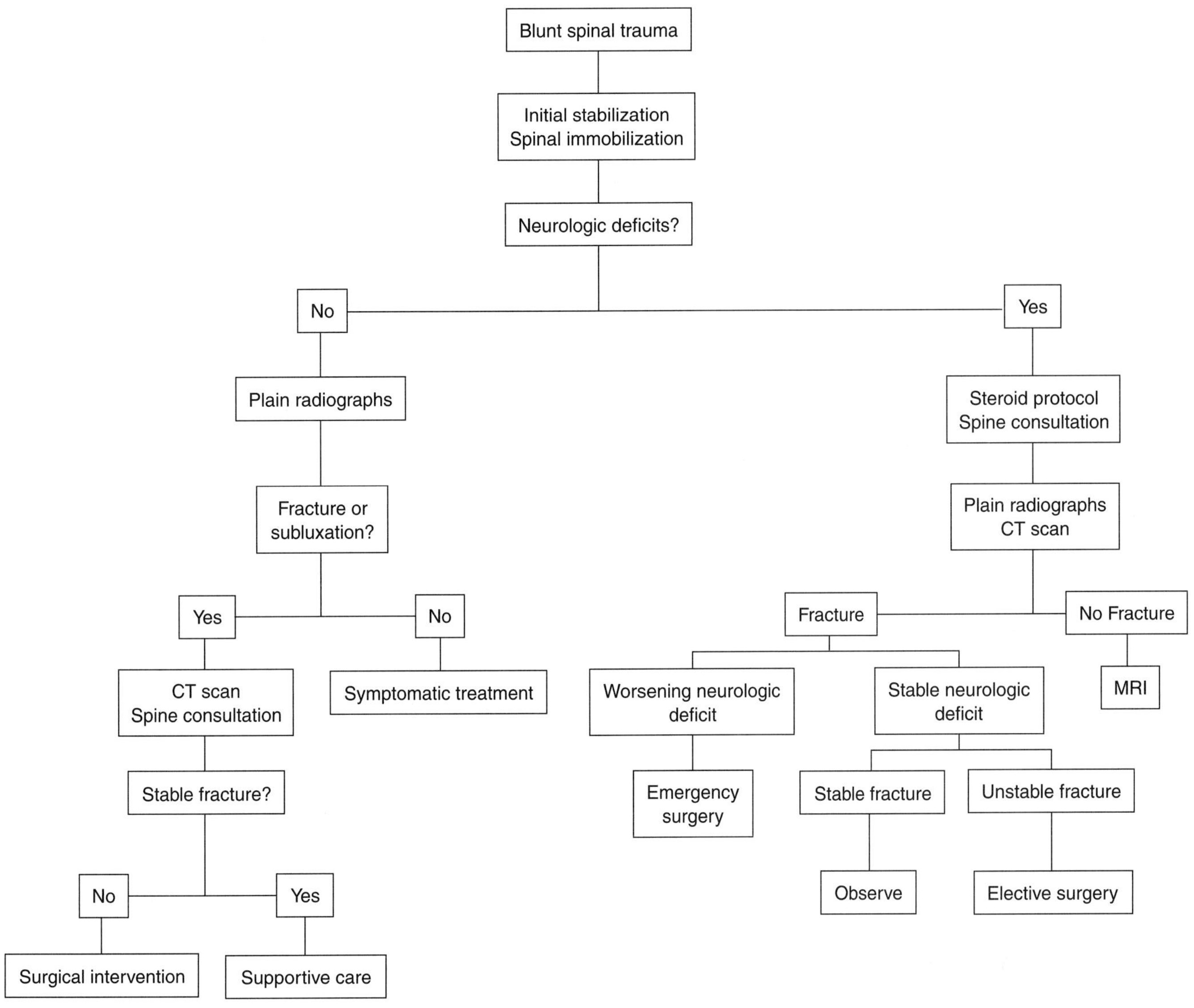

FIG. 248-8. Algorithm for blunt spinal trauma.

of anal sphincter tone. Correlation of cervical injury with involvement in a motor vehicle crash approached statistical significance.[21] Unfortunately, there are significant limitations to the study that do not allow accurate assessments. Apart from a paucity of patient-related information, the study appears to show that falls greater than 10 ft are not significantly associated with spine injury. The question of how much force is required before cervical spine injury is likely remains largely unanswered at this time, but studies are underway to develop decision guidelines.

The ''gold standard'' for the identification of bony cervical injury includes three views of the cervical spine: AP, lateral, and odontoid. They allow for imaging of the entire cervical spine. It is important that all seven cervical vertebrae be imaged, including the junction between the seventh cervical and the first thoracic vertebrae. A single lateral cervical spine film is important as an initial screening radiograph. It will identify 90 percent of injuries to bone and ligaments. Cervical immobilization must be maintained until the patient also has an AP and open-mouth odontoid view. If the initial lateral view is normal and the patient is neurologically intact, the AP and open-mouth views can be delayed until other injuries are adequately stabilized. The combination of lateral, AP, and odontoid views is generally adequate to identify or at least raise the suspicion of cervical spine injury.

Visualization of the entire cervical spine often can be problematic. Patients' body habitus or the presence of upper extremity injuries may limit the clinician's ability to pull on the arms, a maneuver necessary to visualize all seven vertebral bodies. An alternative is a swimmer's view, which is aimed through the axilla in an attempt to image the lower cervical spine. Oblique views (45°) can also be obtained. These views have the added advantage of showing the neural foramina well. They demonstrate the pedicles as well as the laminae, which should stack like shingles on a roof. A newer technique is CT scanning of the cervical spine which can visualize the entire cervical spine well but not the atlantooccipital junction.

Patients can have cervical spine injury even with normal plain films. In fact, a normal lateral cervical spine film may only identify 90 percent of significant bony and ligamentous injuries. The film must be examined for the presence or absence of prevertebral swelling. The prevertebral space anterior to C3 should be less than 5 mm. The predental space should be less than 3 mm. The open-mouth odontoid view will identify many of the remaining abnormalities.[22] Still, plain films of the neck may not identify patients with pure ligamentous injuries. In these patients, ligaments are disrupted but the spine spontaneously reduces to a normal position. Motion, however, risks neurologic injury.

Flexion and extension views demonstrate the degree of spinal column stability. In general, these views are obtained when patients have pain or tenderness but normal plain films.[23] They can only be obtained in a fully awake, unsedated cooperative patient. The patient carefully and slowly flexes and extends the neck. Motion should be limited by increasing pain or the appearance of any neurologic symptomatology. A stepoff of 3.7 mm or an angulation of greater than 11° denotes cervical spine instability.[24] It is possible to have ligamentous injury even with normal flexion/extension films, since muscle tone can splint the bones in a stable configuration. Most patients in this latter category note pain improvement with analgesics after a few days. Reliable patients without a substantial mechanism of injury with persistent pain but normal radiographs, including flexion/extension views, can be discharged in a hard collar with outpatient follow-up. Most patients' symptoms will resolve over a few days. A patient with persistent symptoms will require additional outpatient workup. Unreliable patients or those with a significant mechanism of injury or risk factors, such as advanced age, should undergo MRI.

Plain films of the thoracic and lumbar spine are the initial examinations generally utilized to image these spinal levels. Many of the same principles used for cervical spine imaging are important for thoracic and lumbar imaging. All patients with a mechanism of injury, those with complaints of back pain, and those who have tenderness on physical examination must be assumed to have a fracture of the thoracic or lumbar spine. They must be kept immobilized. AP and lateral films are generally obtained and examined for abnormality. In general, the lateral x-rays are much more easily obtained with patients still on a backboard. Skin breakdown and pressure sores can develop very quickly, particularly in obese patients. Our goal is to remove patients from the backboard in less than 2 h. Patients can then be nursed supine in a bed as long as they are logrolled. A standard hospital mattress provides adequate spinal support. However, patients must be carefully moved and care must be taken to keep spinal immobilization complete in transfers from bed to stretcher. It may be helpful to place patients back on a backboard for the transportation phases of their care. Alternatively, a scoop stretcher may be used for transport.

It can be difficult to image the upper thoracic spine adequately, even if maximal power of the x-ray beam is used. One alternative is to clear the reliable patient by physical examination. Unreliable or unexaminable patients with a concerning mechanism should be logrolled until they become examinable. Patients with point tenderness and normal films are a special subset. CT scanning can be useful in this subset, though the yield is low. The thoracic spine has inherent stability from the rib cage. Few fractures in these patients will be unstable. Alternatively, patients can be treated with analgesics and investigated selectively if symptoms persist.

More recently, CT has assumed a much more important role in the imaging of spine injuries. Plain films can be imperfect and may miss a number of such patients. Newer-generation helical scanning is rapid, and CT allows for a complete three-dimensional imaging of bony structures. CT scanning is indicated in almost all patients with proven bony spinal injury, as it allows for more precise anatomic description of the fractures. CT can reveal the exact anatomy of an osseous injury and the extent of spinal canal impingement by bone fragments. CT is vital in helping to determine the stability of an injury. CT scans are indicated for all patients with subluxations or fractures that can be seen on plain films. CT scans are also useful in patients with neurologic deficits but no apparent abnormalities on plain films, those with severe neck or back pain and normal plain films, and those in whom the thoracic and lumbar spine should be examined to define the anatomy of a fracture and the extent of impingement on the spinal canal. CT is especially useful when the lower cervical spine cannot be adequately visualized on plain films because of overlying soft tissues.

MRI is not as sensitive as CT for picturing bone injuries precisely. On the other hand, MRI is superb at defining neurologic, muscular, and soft tissue injury. It is the diagnostic test of choice for describing the anatomy of nerve injury. Entities such as herniated disks or spinal cord contusions are easily seen on MRI. Many of these require only supportive therapy. However, some require acute surgical intervention. Early identification helps plan therapy. MRI may also be used to identify ligamentous injury and it is indicated in all patients with neurologic symptoms or physical findings but no clear explanation on plain films and/or CT scanning.

MRI is indicated and should be part of the ED workup in patients with neurologic findings with no clear explanation following plain films and CT scanning. CT myelography is an alternative when MRI is unavailable and immediate diagnosis of a neurologic lesion is required. If the patient is neurologically stable and MRI is unavailable, delayed MRI and/or transfer to a tertiary care facility may be appropriate.

The determination of a spinal column injury at one level should prompt imaging of the remainder of the spine. Approximately 10 percent of patients with one spine fracture will have a second fracture. Often plain films will suffice, but multilevel CT scanning and/or MRI may be necessary to investigate such patients completely.

TREATMENT

The goals of treatment are to prevent secondary injury, alleviate cord compression, and establish spinal stability. Spinal immobilization must be maintained. Unnecessary movement of a potentially unstable spine must be avoided in order to prevent additional injury.

Once the patient is stabilized, it should be determined whether the patient has a neurologic deficit and/or the spinal column is unstable. If either of those conditions exists, subspecialty consultation should be requested emergently. The consultant, be it a neurosurgeon or orthopedic surgeon, must have the opportunity to perform a detailed neurologic examination early in the patient's course, so as to optimize outcome. Patients with progressive neurologic deterioration require urgent surgical intervention. The method of stabilization (collar or traction) must be determined, as must the need for further CT or MRI imaging.

Corticosteroids

High-dose methylprednisolone has been shown to be effective in the treatment of blunt spinal cord injury. The National Acute Spinal Cord Injury Study (NASCIS) group conducted a series of multi-institutional studies to evaluate the efficacy of methylprednisolone in spinal trauma.[2] Methylprednisolone infusion resulted in improvement of both motor and sensory function in patients with complete and incomplete neurologic lesions. This positive outcome was dependent upon dosage of steroids and time of administration. The current recommended steroid protocol for victims of spinal injury with neurologic deficits is as follows:

1. Treatment must be started within 8 h of injury.
2. Methylprednisolone (30 mg/kg) bolus administered intravenously over 15 min.
3. This is followed by a 45-min pause.
4. A maintenance infusion of methylprednisolone (5.4 mg/kg per hour) is continued for 23 h.

NASCIS evaluated only blunt spinal cord injury. Patients with penetrating injuries were excluded from the study. The role of steroids in the treatment of penetrating cord injury is currently unclear.

The major neuroprotective mechanism of high dose methylprednisolone is its inhibition of free radical-induced lipid peroxidation.[25] Other proposed beneficial actions of methylprednisolone include its ability to increase levels of spinal cord blood flow, increase extracellular calcium, and prevent loss of potassium from injured cord tissue. Methylprednisolone is advocated in preference to other steroids because it crosses cell membranes more rapidly and completely.

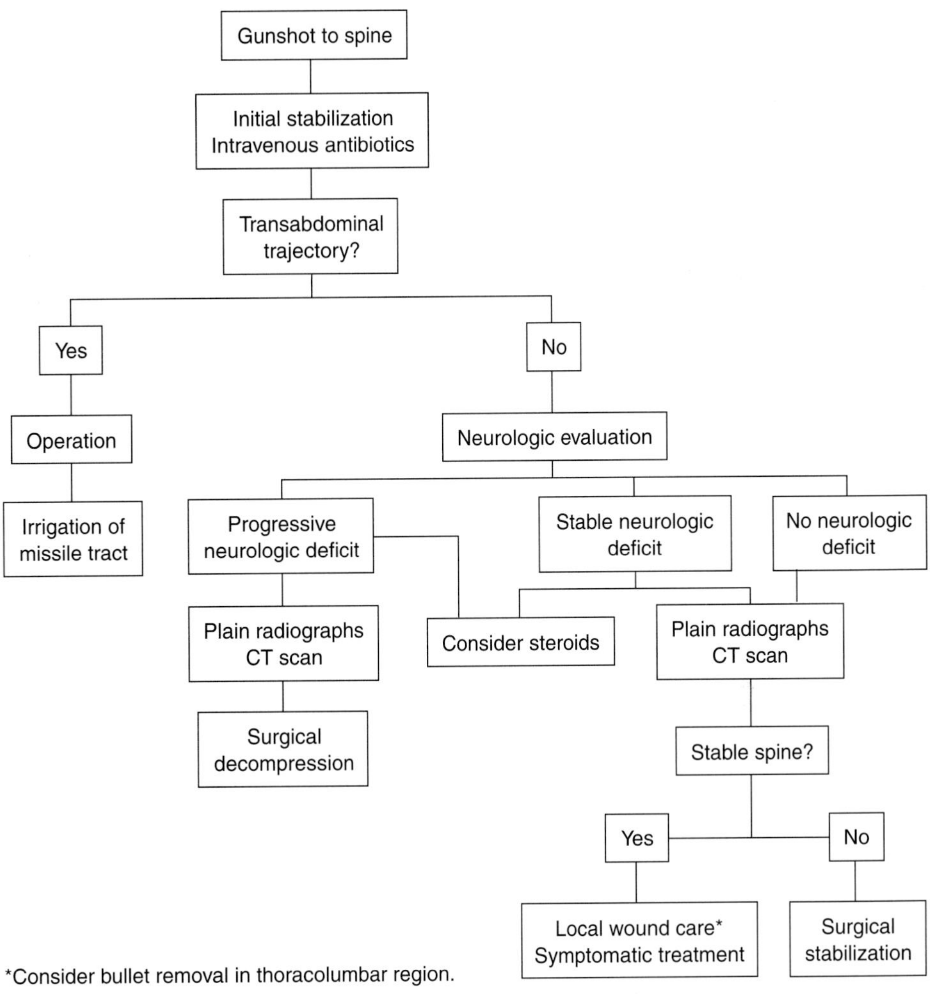

FIG. 248-9. Algorithm for gunshot to spine.

Penetrating Injury

Treatment goals are the same for penetrating and blunt spinal injury. There are, however, additional considerations in penetrating trauma (Fig. 248-9). Optimal treatment of these injuries has been the subject of debate. One concern is that of infectious complications related to the presence of foreign bodies. Additional contamination is associated with transperitoneal and transintestinal trajectories of gunshot wounds to the spine. Intravenous antibiotics should be given in the ED. Surgical debridement with laminectomy has not proven effective in reducing the incidence of infectious complications, as most are managed nonoperatively. If the patient requires laparotomy for abdominal trauma, irrigation and debridement of the spinal injury through the missile tract may be appropriate.[14]

As with blunt trauma, there is general agreement that progressive neurologic deficits warrant surgical decompression. The indication for removal of bullet and bone fragments in those patients with nonprogressive neurologic deficits is less clear. Wound location may determine the need for surgical intervention. Bullet removal has not been shown to significantly improve the neurologic status of patients with stable cervical and thoracic spinal cord lesions. In contrast, a collaborative study by the National Spinal Cord Injury Model Systems demonstrated that bullet removal from the thoracolumbar spine significantly improved motor recovery in both complete and incomplete injuries.[26] Most vertebral injuries to the spine following penetrating trauma are stable and require only symptomatic treatment with a supportive orthosis and analgesics.

Nonoperative Spinal Stabilization

The goal of stabilization is to reduce deformities and then restrict motion and maintain alignment. In the cervical spine, it is important to determine the adequacy of cervical bony reduction. Subluxations are generally reduced using Gardner-Wells tongs, which are placed into the soft tissue of the temples under local anesthesia. The location and type of injury determine the amount of weight applied. The upper cervical spine generally requires less weight for traction than the lower cervical spine. Depending upon location, initial weight should be started at 5 to 10 lb. Weight should be increased in 2.5-to 5-lb increments. Ideally, this should be done under fluoroscopic guidance. If fluoroscopy is unavailable, radiographs and neurologic examinations should be performed after each increment of weight. The radiographs should be evaluated for alignment of the spinal column and to ensure that overdistraction has not occurred. Neurologic performance can improve if reduction is achieved. Inability to achieve adequate reduction is an indication for early spinal decompression and fusion.

Spinal orthoses are used to immobilize well-reduced cervical fractures. The cervical spine is the region most effectively stabilized by external splinting devices. There is less soft tissue separating the brace from the spine at this level. In addition, some braces can be solidly secured by fixation points at the cranium and the thoracic cage. Cervical orthoses consist of cervical and cervicothoracic types. Cervical collars fit around the neck and contour to the mandible and occiput. They restrict flexion and extension in the middle and lower cervical spine. Lateral bending and rotational movements, however, are poorly controlled. Examples of cervical orthoses include the hard collar, the Philadelphia collar, and the Miami J collar. Cervicothoracic braces provide additional support. The ''gold standard'' is the halo cervical immobilizer, which provides the most rigid stabilization. Consisting of a halo ring pinned to the skull, a vest, and upright posts, it can be used for traction and reduction of unstable fractures as well as immobilization.

Immobilization of the upper thoracic spine by orthoses is difficult. Fortunately, an intact rib cage and sternum provide relative stability. Although brace immobilization is not always necessary in the treatment of these fractures, braces can provide additional comfort. Thoracic corsets provide minimal control of motion and are appropriate only for minor injuries. Jewett and Taylor braces provide intermediate control of spinal motion. Maximum limitation of motion is provided by the Risser jacket and the body cast.

The thoracolumbar junction and lower lumbar regions are also difficult to immobilize externally. The splints are limited by the lack of an adequate caudal fixation point. The functions of most thoracolumbosacral orthoses (TLSOs) are the following: to create an awareness and remind the patient to restrict movements, to support the abdomen and relieve some of the load on the lumbosacral spine, to provide some restriction of motion of the upper lumbar and thoracolumbar spine by three-point fixation, and to reduce lumbar lordosis in order to provide a straighter, more comfortable lower back.

Complications of external immobilization devices include pain, pressure, muscle weakness and disuse atrophy, venous compromise, psychological dependence, ineffective stabilization, and pin-site complications (halovest).[27]

Operative Management of Spine Injuries

The indication for operative stabilization is somewhat controversial and varies from institution to institution. Those favoring an aggressive approach stress the importance of early mobilization of the multiply injured patient as it helps decrease pulmonary problems, skin breakdown, deep venous thrombosis, and pulmonary embolus. Early stabilization allows for this early mobilization. Rigid fixation may also decrease time in hospital as well as long-term pain and deformities.

Those advocating a nonoperative approach point out the possibility of worsening neurologic performance by operative manipulation. In addition, the long-term results with operative intervention may not be substantially better than with nonoperative therapy.

All would agree that progressive neurologic deterioration is an indication for urgent surgery. In addition, spinal instability should most often be managed operatively even in the case of a complete spinal cord level. This helps prevent long-term deformity.

AGE CONSIDERATIONS

Elderly

Osteoporosis and degenerative bone changes predispose the elderly to injury from low-energy trauma. A significant number of injuries occur following falls. Central cord syndrome is the most common incomplete lesion. Compression fractures are the most common bone injuries in the thoracic and lumbar spine. In addition to decreased bone density, pathologic lesions may also be responsible for compression fractures. If a minor mechanism of injury results in a fracture, metastatic disease and multiple myeloma should be excluded as causes. The most important principle of therapy in the elderly is early mobilization and rehabilitation. Prolonged immobilization results in more systemic complications and higher mortality. Decisions involving operative versus nonoperative treatment should take this into account.

Children

Anatomic and biomechanical features unique to the immature spine account for differences in injury patterns between pediatric and adult patients. The pediatric spine has increased phyisologic mobility because of several factors. Laxity of the interspinous ligaments and joint capsules, the horizontal orientation of facet joints, incompletely ossified wedge-shaped vertebrae, and the underdeveloped neck and paraspinous musculature all contribute to increased flexibility, particularly of the cervical spine. This elasticity affords children some protection against spinal trauma. When spinal injury occurs in the pediatric population, however, it is generally secondary to mechanisms involving considerable force. The resulting injuries are associated with a high degree of neurologic compromise at presentation. In addition, there is an increased occurrence of spinal cord injury without radiographic evidence of abnormality (SCIWORA) in patients younger than 10 years.[28] Growth plate fractures are most common, but these are difficult to detect on plain radiographs. If spinal cord injury is suspected, based on history or results of the neurologic examination, normal spine radiographs cannot be used to exclude injury. Immobilization must be maintained. Neurologic deficits should be aggressively evaluated with CT scan and MRI.

An additional concern in the pediatric population is child abuse. Vigorous shaking of infants, termed ''shaken baby syndrome,'' may result in avulsion or compression fractures of the spine. A history that is inconsistent with the nature and extent of the injuries should raise the suspicion of child abuse. A thorough search for associated injuries should be undertaken, and appropriate governmental agencies notified.

REFERENCES

1. Burney RE, Maio RF, Maynard F, et al: Incidence, characteristics, and outcome of spinal cord injury at trauma centers in North America. *Arch Surg* 128:596, 1993.
2. White AA, Panjabi MM: *Clinical Biomechanics of the Spine*, 3rd ed. Philadelphia, Lippincott, 1990.
3. Denis F: The three column spine and its significance in the classification of acute thoracolumbar spinal injuries. *Spine* 8:817, 1983.
4. Woodring JH, Lee C, Jenkins K: Spinal fractures in blunt chest trauma. *J Trauma* 28:789, 1988.
5. Denis F, Davis S, Comfort T: Sacral fractures: An important problem. Retrospective analysis of 236 cases. *Clin Orthop* 227:67, 1988.
6. Bracken MB, Shepard MJ, Collins WF, et al: A randomized, controlled trial of methylprednisolone or naloxone in the treatment of acute spinal cord injury: Results of the second national acute spinal cord injury study. *N Engl J Med* 322:1405, 1990.
7. Ditunno JF, Young WS, Donovan WH, et al (eds): *American Spinal Injury Association: Standards for Neurological and Functional Classification of Spinal Cord Injury*, rev ed. Chicago, American Spinal Injury Association, 1992.
8. Schneider RC: The syndrome of acute anterior cervical spinal cord injury. *J Neurosurg* 12:95, 1995.
9. Bosch A, Stauffer ES, Nickel VL: Incomplete traumatic quadriplegia: A ten year review. *JAMA* 216:473, 1971.
10. Schneider RC, Cherry G. Pantek H: The syndrome of acute central cervical spinal cord injury with special reference to the mechanisms involved in hyperextension injuries of the cervical spine. *J Neurosurg* 11:546, 1954.
11. Denis F: Spinal instability as defined by the three-column spine concept in acute spinal trauma. *Clin Orthop Rel Res* 189:65, 1984.
12. Scalea T, Goldstein A, Phillips T, et al: An analysis of 161 falls from a height: The ''jumper syndrome''. *J Trauma* 26:706, 1986.
13. Tall RL, De Valut W: *Spinal injury in sport: Epidemiologic considerations.* Clinics in Sports Medicine. 12:441, 1993.
14. Kihtir T, Ivatury RR, Simon R, et al: Management of transperitoneal gunshot wounds of the spine. *J Trauma* 31:1579, 1991.
15. American College of Surgeons: The Advanced Trauma Life Support Course. Chicago, Illinois 1997.
16. Soderstrom C, McArdle DQ, Ducker TB, Militello PR: The diagnosis of intra-abdominal injury in patients with cervical cord trauma. *J Trauma* 23:1061–1065.

17. Zipnick R, Scalea TM, Trooskin SZ, et al: Hemodynamic responses to penetrating spinal cord injuries. *J Trauma* 35:578–583, 1993.
18. Bachulis BL, Long WB, Hynes GD, et al: Clinical indications for cervical spine radiographs in the traumatized patient. *Am J Surg* 153:473–477, 1987.
19. Roberge RJ, Wears RC, Kelly M, et al: Selective approach of cervical spine radiography in alert victims of blunt trauma: A prospective study. *J Trauma* 28:784–788, 1988.
20. Bayless P, Ray VG: Incidence of cervical spine injuries in association with blunt head trauma. *Am J Emer Med* 7:139–142, 1989.
21. Jacobs LM, Schwartz R: Prospective analysis of acute cervical spine injury: A methodology to predict injury. *Ann Emerg Med* 15:44, 1986.
22. Chiles BW III, Cooper PR: Acute spinal injury. Current concepts. *New Engl J Med* 334:514–520, 1996.
23. MacDonald RL, Schwartz ML, Mirich D, et al: Diagnosis of cervical spine injury in motor vehicle crash victims: How many x-rays are enough? *J Trauma* 30:392–397, 1990.
24. Panjabi MM, Tech D, White AA: Basic biomechanics of the spine. *Neurosurg* 7:76, 1980.
25. Hall ED: The neuroprotective pharmacology of methylprednisolone. *J Neurosurg* 76:13, 1992.
26. Waters RL, Adkins RH: The effects of removal of bullet fragments retained in the spinal canal. A collaborative study by the National Spinal Cord Injury Model Systems. *Spine.* 16:934, 1991.
27. Benzel EC (ed.): *Biomechanics of Spine Stabilization,* ed 1, New York, McGraw-Hill, pp. 247–262, 1995.
28. Hadley MN, Zabramski JM, Browner CM: Pediatric spinal trauma: Review of 122 cases of spinal cord and vertebral column injuries. *J Neurosurg* 68:18, 1988.

MAXILLOFACIAL TRAUMA

Stephen Colucciello

Up to 60 percent of patients with severe facial injuries have multisystem trauma and have potential for airway compromise. The alarming nature of facial injuries may divert attention from more occult life threats. Management requires a coordinated team approach, necessitating involvement of emergency physicians, and surgical specialists in ear-nose-throat (ENT), trauma, plastics, and oral surgery (Table 249-1).

TABLE 249-1 Pitfalls in the Management of Maxillofacial Injuries

1. *Poor airway management.* Be prepared. Remember that the sitting position may be lifesaving (after the cervical spine and associated injuries have been ruled out). The tongue becomes a dangerous ''foreign body'' in the flail mandible.
2. *Inappropriate focus on the face.* Gross injuries tend to distract. Initially focus on the airway, hemorrhage, and associated life-threatening injuries.
3. *Casual physical exam.* Observe, palpate, and ask the patient to move the face and jaw. The eye and mouth exam deserve special attention.
4. *Poor choice and timing of x-rays.* Get skull films if suspicious of frontal bone fractures. Periorbital fractures usually require computed tomography. The critically ill may have facial imaging deferred until they stabilize.
5. *Failure to consult.* Recognize high-risk patients, including those with decreased vision, periorbital fractures, tripod and naso-ethmoidal-orbital injuries, LeFort fractures, open mandibles, and pediatric injuries.
6. *Lack of documentation.* Litigation is common in facial fractures and involves criminal, civil, and malpractice issues. Document meticulously.

ETIOLOGY/INCIDENCE

The etiology of facial fractures varies between urban and rural environments. Penetrating trauma and assault-related injuries are more common in cities, whereas motor vehicle crashes (MVCs), sporting, and other recreational injuries are seen frequently in community hospitals. In community emergency departments (EDs), the nose and mandible are the most common facial fractures; in trauma centers, however, midface and zygomatic injuries are more frequent. Domestic violence and elder and child abuse are important causes of facial trauma. Facial injury accounts for the majority of ED visits related to domestic violence. As many as one-fourth of women with facial trauma are victims of domestic violence.[1] If a woman has an orbital fracture, the likelihood of sexual assault or domestic violence rises to more than 30 percent.[2] Falls are also an important cause of facial injury in the very young and the elderly.

Potential injuries associated with facial trauma are those of the head, cervical spine, and eye. As many as 20 to 50 percent of victims of facial trauma sustain concurrent brain injury, especially those with upper face and midface fractures.

Although most series show no increased incidence in cervical spine injury with facial trauma (1 to 4 percent), this is of statistical interest only. One must consider possible spinal injury in all patients with significant or suspected maxillofacial fractures, because it takes considerable force to shatter the midface or upper face. Always rule out cervical spine injury clinically or radiographically in such patients. One study has linked carotid artery injury to severe facial trauma.[3]

Periorbital fractures may be associated with globe disruption. The dangerous triad of limited extraocular movement, limited visual acuity, and limited visual fields should be checked in all those with facial injury.

Blindness occurs in 0.5 to 3 percent of patients with facial fractures and is most frequent in patients with LeFort III (2.2 percent), LeFort II (0.64 percent), and zygomatic fractures (0.45 percent).[4] MVCs and gunshot injuries are responsible for most cases of visual loss.

In addition to the physical consequences of facial trauma, there are psychological costs as well. More than one-quarter of patients with significant facial trauma may develop posttraumatic stress disorder.[5]

ANATOMY

The facial buttresses, bony arches joined by suture lines, provide vertical and horizontal support. Vertical stability depends on the zygomatic-maxillary buttress laterally and the frontal process of the maxilla medially. The zygomatic-maxillary arch and the hard palate bolster the horizontal face. Sutures linking these facial bones rupture in predictable fashion during trauma. Knowledge of their location enables one to palpate these sutures to detect diastasis or tenderness.

Sutures found at borders of the sphenoid wings, pterygoid plate, and the zygomatic arch anchor the face to the skull. These are the structures disrupted in LeFort injuries (Fig. 249-1).

The most complex aspect of facial anatomy is the orbit, an elaborate structure comprised of seven different bones: maxilla, zygoma, frontal, sphenoid, palatine, ethmoid, and lacrimal. Between these bones lie the orbital foramina, through which course cranial nerves II, III, and VI and branches of V. Rupture of orbital bones may compress these fissures and cause blindness through traction, rupture, or compression of the optic nerves.

PREHOSPITAL CARE

The major concern in prehospital care is control of the airway. The mouth should be cleared of any foreign body or debris and suctioned of blood. The tongue may block the airway, and a jaw thrust or modified chin lift without neck extension often relieves the obstruction. With severe mandible fractures, these maneuvers may not elevate the

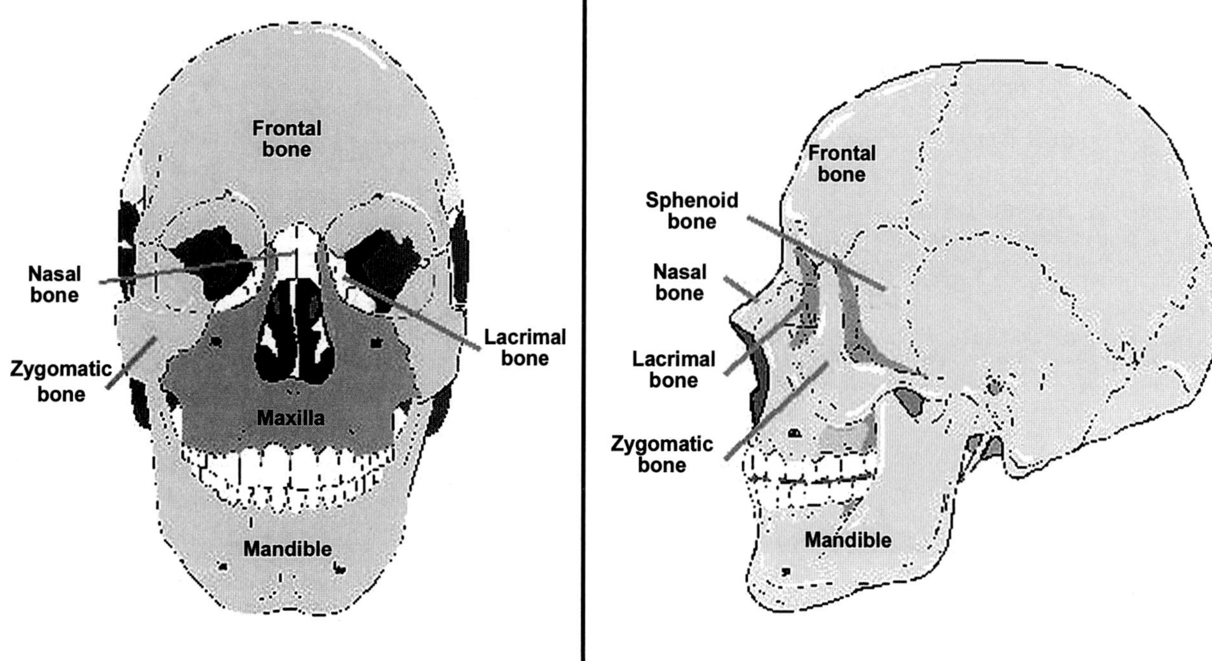

FIG. 249-1. Coronal and lateral facial bone anatomy. (Reprinted with permission from Isenhour J, Colucciello S: Maxillofacial trauma, in Ferrera P et al: *Trauma Management.* St. Louis, Mosby, 2000.)

tongue, necessitating manual extraction. As a rule, any patient with trauma above the clavicles should have the cervical spine immobilized.

If there is copious bleeding and massive facial injury, early notification allows the ED to prepare for a difficult airway.

EMERGENCY MANAGEMENT: RESUSCITATION

The compelling and sometimes grotesque nature of facial injuries must not distract physicians from following the routine, sequential trauma protocol. The most urgent complication of facial trauma is not shock, but airway compromise, particularly with midfacial and lower facial trauma.

Airway

Simple intervention, such as the chin lift without neck extension, jaw thrust, and oropharyngeal suctioning, often clears the airway. In mandibular fractures, however, loss of bony support may result in a *flail mandible,* leaving the tongue to obstruct the airway.[6] In this case, open the mouth and pull the tongue forward with a gauze pad, towel clip, or a large suture placed through the anterior tongue. When the cervical spine has been cleared, clinically or radiographically, allow the patient to sit up and lean forward, and give the patient a tonsil-tip suction. This position may be lifesaving in patients with significant mandible fractures. Patients who do not respond to simple maneuvers may require intubation.

Intubation Considerations

Because the cribriform plate may be disrupted, avoid nasotracheal intubation in patients with midface trauma. Nasotracheal intubation can result in nasocranial intubation or dramatic nasal hemorrhage. Admittedly, these complications are rare, and some patients have successfully intubated via the nasotracheal route.[7] Nonetheless, orotracheal intubation is often successful even with severely distorted facial anatomy.

Rapid-sequence intubation carries particular risk in facial trauma. These dangers include the failure to intubate and subsequent failure to ventilate with a bag-valve mask. Before paralyzing any patient, evaluate the degree of difficulty anticipated for mask ventilation. Patients with distortion of the maxilla or mandible may be impossible to bag, because the mask will not fit tightly on an unstable face.

In such cases, consider an awake intubation. Options include sedation with a benzodiazepine, droperidol, or other induction agent in a dose that minimizes respiratory depression. If a patient with severe maxillofacial trauma is given paralytics, prepare for immediate backup cricothyroidotomy. *Preparation* in this case implies more than locating a surgical tray: it extends to povidone-iodine on the neck, a ready blade, an opened cricothyroidotomy tray, and a tracheostomy tube at the bedside.

Some authors describe creative approaches to intubation in facial trauma. Fiberoptic intubation with patients in the semiprone position may be useful in penetrating injuries of the face.[8] The traditional supine intubating position may be impossible with a ruined maxilla that falls into the airway. Such airways may clear when a patient lies on his or her side (although this may be both awkward and disconcerting to the physician). The Bullard intubating blade and the laryngeal mask airway are all used to manage a difficult airway in patients with a crushed face.

Other alternatives include percutaneous transtracheal ventilation and retrograde intubation as a temporizing measure. Both require considerable preparation, and the most dependable alternative airway is surgical. Emergency cricothyroidotomy, being faster and associated with fewer complications, is preferable to emergency tracheostomy.

Hemorrhage Control

Patients rarely develop shock from facial bleeding. In hypotensive patients, look for other sources of blood loss, such as intrathoracic, intraabdominal, and retroperitoneal hemorrhage. Control maxillofacial bleeding with direct pressure, and avoid blind clamping in wounds, because important structures such as facial nerve or parotid duct may be injured. Severe pharyngeal bleeding may require packing of the pharynx and hypopharynx around a cuffed endotracheal tube. In patients with LeFort fractures, manual reduction of the face should stem bleeding. Grasp the anterior hard palate at the maxillary arch and realign the fragments.

Severe nasal bleeding requires direct pressure to the nares, or combined posterior and anterior packing, taking care not to pack the cranium. In the case of massive nasopharyngeal bleeding, a Foley catheter placed along the floor of the nose and inflated with saline may be lifesaving. Nasopharyngeal dual-lumen balloons are commercially available for this purpose.

Once the airway is secure and gross hemorrhage controlled, only then search for life threats in the chest, abdomen, and pelvis.

HISTORY

Obtain a history regarding the injury from the patient, witnesses, and prehospital care providers. It is important to determine the mechanism and time of injury and to assess for loss of consciousness. Allergies and tetanus status are standard inquires.

The following three ''face-oriented'' questions are essential: (1) ''How is your vision?'' (2) ''Is any part of your face numb?'' and (3) ''Are your teeth meeting normally?'' These questions target eye involvement, injury to facial nerves, and alignment of central and lower face.

Question the patient regarding vision, diplopia, and whether there is pain with eye movement. Monocular double vision occurs with lens dislocation or with corneal or retinal injury, whereas binocular double vision implies dysfunction of the extraocular muscles or nerves. Pain on eye movement suggests injury to the orbit or globe.

There should be a high index of suspicion for domestic violence. If the mechanism of injury is not an MVC, ask women about domestic violence. Although a victim of domestic violence may tell the triage nurse that they fell or ''ran into a door,'' most patients reveal the true etiology if directly questioned by a physician. Child abuse and elder abuse are important considerations when patients at the extremes of age present with facial trauma. More than half of all abused children are injured in the head, face, mouth, or neck.[9]

PHYSICAL EXAMINATION

Inspection

Begin the examination by viewing the patient from the front. Facial elongation occurs with high-grade LeFort fractures. Then view the face from above looking down (bird's-eye view) and from below up (worm's-eye view). These perspectives reveal subtle asymmetries. Because posttraumatic Bell palsy occurs with fractures of the temporal bone, test the muscles of facial expression. Ask patients to smile, frown, whistle, raise their brows, and close their eyes tightly. Look for ecchymosis around the eyes (raccoon eyes) and over the mastoid area (Battle sign) for associated basilar skull fracture. These findings usually develop over several hours and are often absent on admission, despite serious facial trauma.

Palpation

Palpation will disclose the majority of facial fractures. The entire face should be palpated carefully for tenderness, bony crepitus, and subcutaneous air. The presence of subcutaneous air is pathognomonic for fracture of a sinus or nose.

During palpation, target vulnerable sutures such as those on the infraorbital rim and the zygomatic-frontal suture located on the upper lateral aspect of the orbit. Simultaneous palpation of the zygomatic arches will reveal any asymmetry. The best way to distinguish tenderness of the soft tissues of the cheek from bony tenderness is by intraoral palpation. Place a gloved finger inside the patient's mouth and on the buccal surface of the upper molars (outside the teeth). In this position, locate the examining finger under the zygomatic arch. This method will identify displacement or collapse of the arch.

To assess facial stability, open the patient's mouth and grasp the maxillary arch (*not* the central incisors—which might pull out). LeFort fractures are best diagnosed by rocking the maxillary arch and simultaneously feeling the central face for movement with the opposite hand. This maneuver is more sensitive for maxillary fractures than are plain films.

Test sensation. Although anesthesia of the face may be secondary to nerve contusion, it often signifies a fracture. Damage to the infraorbital nerve (often due to blowout or rim fractures) results in anesthesia of the ipsilateral upper lip, nasal mucosa at the vestibule, lower eyelid, and maxillary teeth. Lower lip and lower dental anesthesia occurs with mandibular fractures.

Periorbital and Orbital Exam

The eye exam deserves particular attention, especially when there is periorbital injury. The exam should be performed early during the ED encounter, because, if not timely, progressive lid edema may prevent further examination. If lids are already swollen, lid retractors help visualize the globe. The bird's-eye and worm's-eye views help detect exophthalmos or enophthalmos.

The pupil exam includes reactivity, and whether the pupils line up in the horizontal plane. A teardrop-shaped pupil indicates a ruptured or otherwise penetrated globe in patients without preexisting iridectomy. Examine for hyphema, although this usually requires a patient to be sitting. The presence of a hyphema correlates with significant visual loss. The Snellen chart, either standard or hand held, if feasible to administer, should be used to document visual acuity. If the patient cannot see the chart, record finger counting or, barring that, the presence or absence of light perception. Early recognition of traumatic optic neuropathy should trigger an emergency consultation, because timely decompressive surgery may prevent blindness.

The best way to detect damage to the optic nerve or retina is the swinging-flashlight test. An abnormal pupil (Marcus Gunn) initially dilates (rather than constricts) when first exposed to a light that swings between both eyes.

Subconjunctival hemorrhage is often present with periorbital fractures, and lateral hemorrhage frequently accompanies zygomatic fractures. Soft tissue bruising provides other important clues. Periorbital ecchymosis (raccoon eyes) result from a variety of insults, including basilar skull fracture, as well as direct trauma to the periorbital area. Fractures of the orbit, nose, and midface also produce raccoon eyes.

In patients with severe periorbital trauma, measure the distance between the medial canthi. In average adults, the intercanthal distance should be 35 to 40 mm—or approximately the width of a patient's eye. Widening of this distance is called telecanthus and portends serious orbital injury. In patients with telecanthus, the bridge of the nose appears wide, but the distance between the pupils is unchanged. This is usually seen with naso-ethmoidal-orbital (NEO) trauma. A more serious condition known as hypertelorism occurs when the interpupillary distance increases. In this case, the orbits are dislocated and literally ''blown apart.'' This devastating injury usually results in blindness.

Extraocular motions must be evaluated for restriction. Fractures of the zygomatic and infraorbital floor frequently cause diplopia, especially on upward gaze. Significant pain with extraocular motions provides a clue to occult injury.

Palpate the entire orbit for tenderness, subcutaneous air, and deformity. Inexperienced physicians frequently neglect the superior and lateral rims.

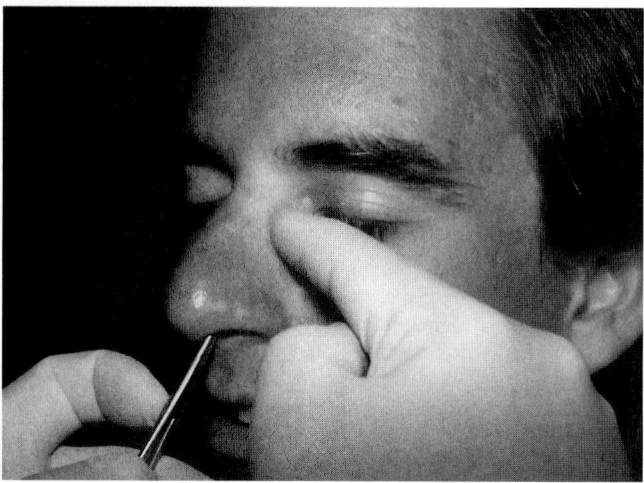

FIG. 249-2. Intranasal palpation test. (Reprinted with permission from Isenhour J, Colucciello S: Maxillofacial trauma, in Ferrera P et al: *Trauma Management.* St. Louis, Mosby, 2000.)

Bimanual Palpation Test

One of the most important concerns is the status of the medial orbital area (the NEO complex). Consider this injury if the medial canthus is tender, or if the patient has telecanthus. When an NEO injury is suspected, the bimanual nasal palpation test is a helpful adjunct (Fig. 249-2).

To perform this test, anesthetize the nose with either cocaine or lidocaine. Then insert a clamp or long cotton swab into nose. Use the clamp or swab to press intranasally against the medial orbital rim (just inside the medial canthus). Simultaneously use the other hand to press the medial canthus. If the bone moves, the NEO complex is fractured.

Penetrating Injuries

With periorbital penetrating injuries, consider occult globe penetration. When the orbital septum is violated, fat protrudes from the wound, signaling possible globe perforation. Injuries to the medial third of the eyelids often damage the lacrimal apparatus and should be considered high risk. Check all lid lacerations for disruption of levator palpebral muscle and tarsal plate.

Nose

Inspect the nose from various angles to detect any deformity. Posttraumatic edema often obscures nasal deviation. The patient can assist in the exam by identifying preexisting nasal deformity. Palpation will detect crepitus, subtle deformity, and subcutaneous air. The two most important potential findings are septal hematoma and cerebrospinal fluid (CSF) rhinorrhea. Septal hematoma appears as a bluish, bulging mass on a widened septum. If in doubt, palpate the septum with a cotton swab to appreciate the doughy swelling.

CSF mixed with blood forms a double ring or *halo sign* when dropped on a paper towel or a bed sheet. This occurs because blood and CSF have different diffusion properties. This finding is *not* specific for CSF and will occur with traumatized rhinorrhea. Unlike CSF, simple rhinorrhea (absent blood) does not contain glucose. Unfortunately, the bedside glucose tests cannot distinguish between spinal fluid and rhinorrhea. However, a standard laboratory glucose test can make the distinction.

Ears

Examine the pinna for subperichondral hematoma. The ear canals should be inspected for lacerations and CSF leak. Hemotympanum appears as a purple (not red), often bulging, eardrum. Tympanic membrane ruptures are also seen in conjunction with fractures of the mandibular condyle. In the presence of a basilar skull fracture, the mastoid area may be ecchymotic (Battle sign.)

Oral and Mandibular Exam

During inspection, determine whether the jaw is deviated. Deviation results from either a condylar fracture or dislocation. The chin will point away from a dislocation and toward a fracture. While the patient opens and closes the mouth, look for malocclusion. With LeFort fractures, patients may be unable to close the mouth due to premature occlusion of the molars. Zygomatic fractures also prevent jaw closure if the bone fragment either presses against the masseter or impinges on the coronoid process of the mandible. Test for anesthesia of the lips and gingiva, usually due to a fracture-associated nerve injury.

An intraoral exam may reveal significant pathology. The exam should include manipulation of each tooth, a search for intraoral lacerations, and stress of the mandible. Essentially all fractures can be detected or excluded by both palpating and stressing the jaw. By placing a finger in the external ear canal while a patient opens and closes the mouth, one can palpate the mandibular condyle during jaw motion.

Tongue-Blade Test

The tongue blade, or spatula, test is a useful technique to detect mandibular fractures (Fig. 249-3). Although unnecessary in patients with an obvious fracture, it enables physicians to determine the need for x-rays in patients with jaw pain and no obvious instability. The patient should be asked to bite down forcefully on a tongue blade. The physician then twists the tongue blade in an attempt to break the blade. Patients with a broken jaw will reflexively open their mouth, whereas those with an intact mandible will break the blade. In one study, this test was more than 95 percent sensitive and nearly 65 percent specific for mandibular fracture.[10]

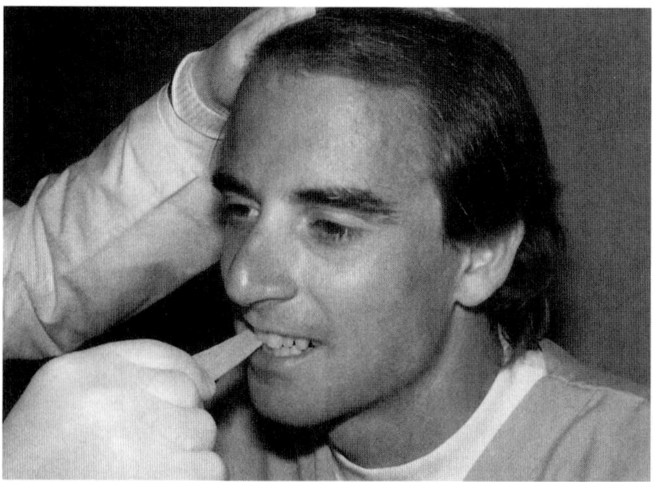

FIG. 249-3. Tongue blade test. (Reprinted with permission from Isenhour J, Colucciello S: Maxillofacial trauma, in Ferrera P et al: *Trauma Management.* St. Louis, Mosby, 2000.)

RADIOLOGY

The choice and timing of radiographic studies depends on the clinical stability of the patient. Management of head, chest, and abdominal trauma takes precedence over facial imaging. In the critically injured, diagnostic imaging of the face, including computed tomography (CT), may be deferred for days, until the patient's condition has stabilized.

It is not always clear which patients require facial imaging. In one study, physical examination alone detected 90 percent of clinically significant fractures.[11] However, management was altered in 17 percent of patients based on either CT or plain films.[11] CT scan is not always required before surgical repair. Some authorities consider scans expensive, time consuming, and labor intensive, adding little information to that gained from physical examination and plain films.

Because immediate surgical intervention is rarely indicated for patients with facial trauma, some argue that most x-rays or CTs may be deferred in the ED. If adequate follow-up is available, a facial surgeon could determine the need for imaging studies at the time of outpatient consultation. On the other hand, because many patients with facial fractures are noncompliant when it comes to follow-up, definitive ED diagnosis of an injury *theoretically* prompts patients to keep the consultative appointment.

Plain Films

Plain films are useful screens for maxillofacial injury and are available in all hospitals. For the uninitiated, the numerous overlapping lines and complex shadows make interpretation challenging.

One of the most useful approaches is to assess symmetry. Consider the right and left sides as mirror images. Are there lucencies or shadows that are unilateral? Are the sutures and sinuses symmetrical? Look for bony integrity and subcutaneous air. While air/fluid levels in the sinuses may occur with acute sinusitis, in the presence of trauma they are nearly pathognomonic for sinus fracture. Clouding of a sinus may be secondary to soft tissue swelling, or due to complete filling of the sinus with blood. When seen in the superior aspect of the maxillary sinus, a soft tissue density may represent herniation of orbital contents through the orbital floor (Fig. 249-4).

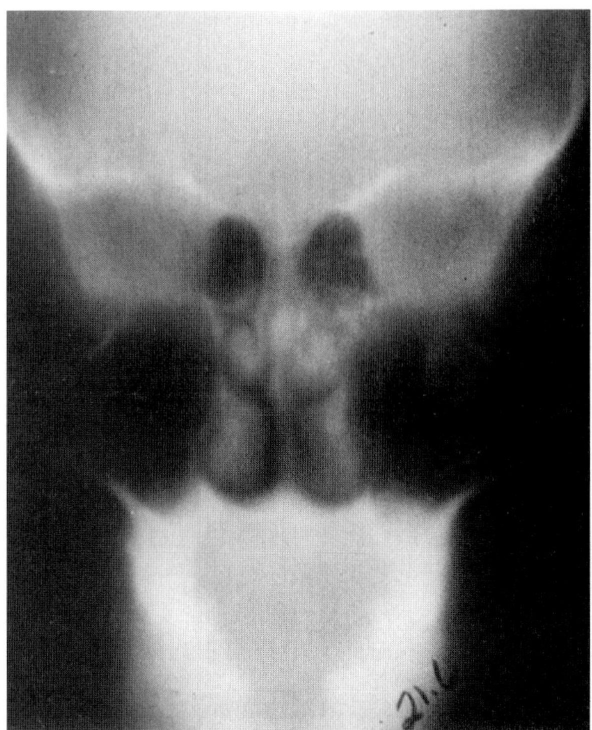

FIG. 249-4. Orbital tomogram showing classical ''teardrop'' herniation of orbital tissue into the maxillary sinus.

Radiographic Views of the Face

The Waters or occipital-mental view is the single most valuable study of the midface. It evaluates continuity of orbital rims, provides an initial diagnosis of blowout fractures, and will demonstrate air/fluid levels in maxillary sinus.

The posterior-anterior (PA or Caldwell) view, which best details the bones of the upper face, confirms ethmoidal and frontal sinus fractures, as well as lateral orbital injuries.

The cross-table or upright laterals are difficult to read and are not very helpful. On occasion, they suggest elongation of the face in LeFort injuries or disruption of the posterior sinus wall. Look for air/fluid levels in sphenoid or ethmoidal sinuses.

The submental-vertex view, known colloquially as the ''jug handle'' or zygomatic arch view, shows the base of the skull and the zygomatic arches. It may be the only film necessary for suspected arch fractures.

The Towne view is useful for evaluating the mandibular ramus and condyles, as well as the base of the skull.

Computed Tomography

CT provides a conclusive diagnosis of complex maxillofacial fractures. Opinions regarding the role of CT vary widely. Some authorities recommend routine CT scanning for every case of significant facial trauma, whereas others feel it is superfluous. Its greatest utility lies in evaluating patients with known or suspected periorbital and midface fractures. Scans are especially useful to evaluate the globe and orbital fissures. Specialized views—such coronal, sagittal, or parasagittal cuts, thin-slice scans, and three-dimensional reconstruction—are useful in particular circumstances. In general, the slices should be in a plane 90° to that of the suspected fracture—and not parallel to the fracture line. Three-dimensional CT is superior to two-dimensional CT for serious midface fractures, such as tripod and complex maxillary fractures.[12]

Multiply injured patients, who are intubated, unconscious, or sedated, frequently have significant and unsuspected facial fractures. If they require a CT of the head, consider adding a scan of the face for clinically stable patients. Slightly more than 10 percent of such patients may have unsuspected facial fractures needing surgical repair.[13] However, an unstable patient with severe concomitant injuries should not receive a facial scan if it delays emergency surgery.

CT with various manipulations, such as coronal and axial views, is essential for management of particular complex fractures. However, plain films still have an important role in screening for maxillofacial injury. In the case of clinically obvious, complex facial injuries (in particular, periorbital and midface fractures), plain films may be eliminated and CT performed directly. Coronal films should be ordered for periorbital fractures, and thin-slice scans may be appropriate in this area.

Cost

Although charges vary among institutions, a full CT of face with coronals results in a charge of approximately $900. This contrasts with the average charge of $100 to $200 for plain film of the face.

Magnetic Resonance Imaging

Magnetic resonance imaging (MRI) is useful to consultants who wish to visualize the soft tissues of the face, particularly the optic nerve or retrobulbar hemorrhage. MRI does *not* adequately delineate fractures, however.

SPECIFIC FACIAL FRACTURES

Frontal Sinus/Frontal Bone Fractures

This injury commonly results from a direct blow to the frontal bone with a blunt object—classically, a lead pipe or brick. This fracture is frequently associated with intracranial injury, secondary to disruption of the posterior table of the sinus. Dural tears are frequent, and patients may have associated injuries to the orbital roof (leading to blindness), as well as to the brain.[14] Late complications include cranial empyema or mucopyoceles. Mucopyoceles are collections of pus and mucus that occur when fractures block the nasal frontal duct, preventing sinus drainage.

Physical examination may reveal disruption or crepitance of the supraorbital rims or subcutaneous emphysema. Fractures are often overlooked because of traditional prohibitions against skull films for head trauma. Patients with a suggestive mechanism or examination benefit from skull films or a Caldwell view of the face. If a depressed or posterior wall fracture is seen on plain film, obtain CT. Patients with hard signs of a frontal bone fracture (subcutaneous air, bony step-off, etc.) require only a CT.

Consult with an ENT specialist or a neurosurgeon regarding antibiotic use in patients with frontal sinus fractures. Many specialists recommend antibiotics that cover common sinus pathogens, although the literature lacks definitive evidence on this issue. Frequently prescribed antibiotics include first-generation cephalosporins, amoxicillin-clavulanate, erythromycin, and trimethoprim-sulfamethoxazole. Patients with depressed fractures, or those who have posterior wall involvement, require intravenous antibiotics, admission, and consultation. Those with isolated fracture of the anterior wall may be treated as outpatients.

Naso-Ethmoidal-Orbital Injuries

Suspect NEO injuries in those with trauma to the bridge of the nose or medial orbital wall (Fig. 249-5). The mechanism of injury is usually dramatic, and these fractures are not likely due to fisticuffs. NEO fractures are frequently associated with lacrimal disruption and dural tears. Patients may complain of pain on eye movement, and physical examination may reveal traumatic telecanthus or epiphora (tears spilling over the lid).

If the medial canthus is tender, perform the intranasal palpation test and examine for CSF rhinorrhea. Plain radiographs are insensitive.[15] If the examination is suggestive, order a CT of the face to include coronal sections and thin axial slices through the medial orbital wall.

If an NEO fracture is present, consult a maxillofacial surgeon. As with many facial fractures, antibiotics are frequently prescribed for CSF leaks; however, no controlled studies have proven their efficacy. Some believe prophylactic antibiotics increase the risk of resistant organisms.

Orbital Fractures

Blowout fractures are the most common orbital fractures. These injuries occur when a blunt object strikes the globe, resulting in expansion of orbital contents and subsequent rupture through the bony floor. A direct blow to the orbital rim will also result in a blowout. Four clinical findings suggest the diagnosis. (1) Rare patients may have enophthalmos, or sunken globe, when a large section is ruptured. (2) Infraorbital anesthesia is a more common finding and develops when the infraorbital nerve is contused by the initial trauma or when compressed by bony fragments. Anesthesia of the maxillary teeth and

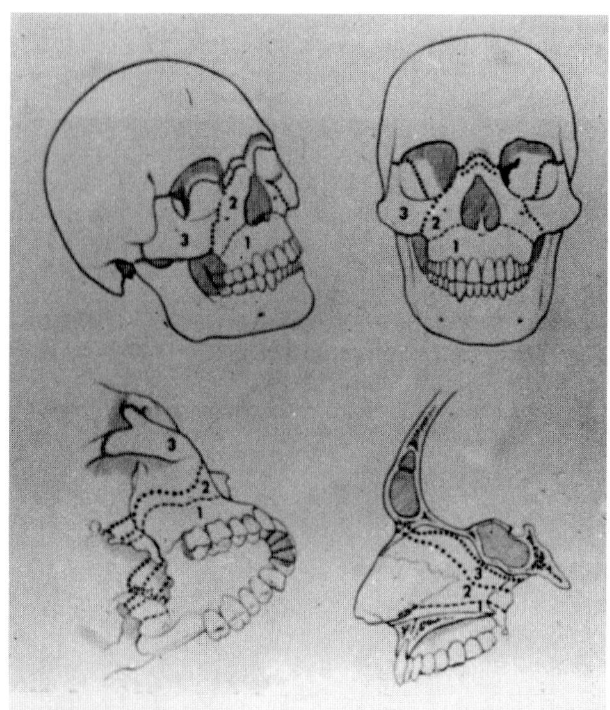

FIG. 249-5. Schematic of midfacial fracture lines: Le Fort I, II, and III. (Reprinted with permission from Dingman RO, Natvig P: *Surgery of Facial Fractures.* Philadelphia, Saunders, 1964, p 248.)

upper lip is more reliable than numbness over the cheek. (3) Diplopia, particularly on upward gaze that usually indicates inferior rectus muscle entrapment, is another important clinical finding. However, the etiology of diplopia may be multifactorial and does not necessarily imply entrapment of extraocular muscles. True entrapment occurs in only a small minority of patients with diplopia, and etiologies that are more common include direct muscle injury, damage to the third nerve, or entrapment of periorbital fat. Mechanical entrapment is readily diagnosed by the forced duction test. To perform this test, apply a few drops of ophthalmic anesthetic in the conjunctival sac, grasp the inferior sclera with a toothed forceps, and gently tug upward. In true entrapment, the eye remains fixed. It is not imperative that an emergency physician perform this test, because CT scanning and consultation are necessary for patients with posttraumatic diplopia. (4) Occasionally, a step-off deformity can be palpated over the intraorbital rim. Subcutaneous emphysema is pathognomonic for fracture into a sinus or nasal antrum.

Plain films are useful in the diagnosis of blowout fractures. The "hanging teardrop" sign is seen with herniation of orbital fat into the maxillary sinus, whereas the "open bomb-bay door" results from bone fragments that protrude into the sinus. Air/fluid levels in the maxillary sinus are frequently seen in association with these signs. At least one author suggests that only patients with well-defined indications for surgery (enophthalmos of more than 2 mm and/or persistent diplopia) require any imaging studies at all.[16] This is perhaps a minority view.

Once a blowout fracture is confirmed either radiographically or clinically (i.e., diplopia or subcutaneous air), obtain a CT scan with coronal sections to determine the surface area of the broken floor. This film could be done as an outpatient study, but it may be expedient to obtain it during the ED stay. Patients with orbital fractures tend to have low compliance with follow-up.[17] Some centers have used ultrasound to evaluate orbital floor fractures, but this is not as sensitive as CT.

There is significant controversy as to timing and necessity of orbital floor repair. Some specialists use CT to determine the need for surgery, whereas others repair the orbit only if there is enophthalmos or persistent diplopia. Although enophthalmos mandates surgical repair, most diplopia (up to 70 percent) resolves spontaneously within several months.

Many consultants recommend antibiotics active against sinus pathogens for patients with subcutaneous emphysema. Patients with fractures into the sinus should avoid blowing their nose to prevent accumulation of subcutaneous air.

In rare circumstances, malignant periorbital emphysema may jeopardize vision by injuring the retina or optic nerve. In such cases, emergency cantholysis may salvage the patient's vision. In patients with massive emphysema, and no evidence of an open globe, measure the intraocular pressure. If the pressure is significantly elevated, immediately consult an ophthalmologist and discuss the need for an emergency cantholysis.

Orbital Fissure Syndromes

The oculomotor and ophthalmic divisions of the trigeminal nerve course through the superior orbital fissure. A fracture of the orbit involving this canal compresses these nerves, leading to the superior orbital fissure syndrome. This condition is characterized by paralysis of extraocular motions, ptosis, and periorbital anesthesia.

A more serious variant is the orbital apex syndrome, which involves the optic nerve. Patients with the orbital apex syndrome have all the aspects of the superior orbital fissure syndrome, plus blindness or decrease in visual acuity. The swinging-flashlight test and visual acuity testing are crucial to the diagnosis. Patients with these syndromes need emergent ophthalmic intervention to save their vision. Although few emergency practioners have experience, cantholysis can be considered an ED procedure. It involves anesthetizing then crushing the lateral canthal fold to achieve hemostasis. The lateral canthal ligament is cut and the lids spring apart relieving intraocular pressure.

Nasal Fractures

Cosmesis and the ability to breathe through the nose are key issues in nasal fractures. Apart from management of a septal hematoma, a fractured nose is of little medical concern, unless deformity or airway obstruction is present. Ask the patient several key questions to evaluate nasal fractures: (1) "Have you ever broken your nose before?" (2) "How does your nose look to you?" (3) "Are you having trouble breathing through your nose?" Because nasal deformity may be due to either new or old trauma, solicit the patient's opinion. On physical examination, observe for deformity and palpate for crepitus. The intranasal exam is key to detect septal hematoma, as described earlier. Drain any septal hematomas in the ED after anesthetizing with a topical anesthetic such as cocaine or benzocaine. Use a no. 11 blade to incise the inferior portion of the hematoma and allow it to drain. Packing the nose with Vaseline (petroleum jelly) gauze will prevent reaccumulation of blood. After drainage, reevaluate the patient in 2 to 3 days or arrange for ear-nose-throat follow-up.

The need for nasal films remains controversial. Nasal films do not determine the need for intervention and do not affect surgical planning. Despite the presence of a fracture on x-ray, there is no need for intervention if there is no cosmetic deformity and no obstruction to airflow. Obvious nasal deformity (new or old) in the absence of radiographic findings may prompt rhinoplasty.

For these reasons, many physicians never, or only rarely, order nasal x-rays. Some might obtain nasal films because of patient insistence. Patients with obvious deformity or difficulty breathing through the nose should be referred to a consultant on an outpatient basis. Those with significant swelling or questionable deformity need reevaluation in 5 to 7 days, when edema has resolved. This follow-up is more valuable than radiographic imaging.

Zygomatic Fractures

Zygoma fractures occur in two major patterns: the most serious injury is the tripod fracture, whereas the most common is the arch fracture. The zygoma forms a tripod, which abuts the frontal, maxillary, and temporal bones. The classic tripod fracture involves the infraorbital rim, a diastasis of the zygomatic-frontal suture, and disruption of the zygomatic-temporal junction at the arch. The fragment may drop, and pull the lateral canthus, causing the eye to "tilt." Later, the cheek will flatten, but edema usually obscures this finding in the ED.

Look for lateral subconjunctival hemorrhage and infraorbital anesthesia. A significant percentage of patients with large lateral subconjunctival hematomas have associated zygomatic injury. Either trismus or an open bite will appear if the zygoma impinges on the masseter or coronoid process. Palpate the zygomatic arch from within the mouth to detect arch fractures.

Plain films, consisting of the jug-handle or arch view, are adequate for suspected arch fractures, and the Waters view can screen for tripod injury. Order CT scans for tripod fractures that are diagnosed or suggested by plain films. In those cases where tripod fractures are unmistakable on physical examination, plain films are superfluous and patients should go directly to CT. The scans delineate injury to the orbital floor and guide surgical planning.

Patients with tripod fractures require admission for open reduction and internal fixation of displaced fragments. Those with fractures of the arch may be scheduled for outpatient elevation and repair.

Maxillary Fractures

Fractures of the maxilla are high-energy injuries. An impact 100 times the force of gravity is required to break the midface. Accordingly, these patients often have significant multisystem trauma. Many require resuscitation and admission.

If the patient is conscious, inquire about malocclusion and visual symptoms. On physical examination, a patient may have an open bite, facial lengthening, CSF rhinorrhea, or periorbital ecchymosis. LeFort fractures are best diagnosed by grasping and rocking the hard palate. In most cases, parts of the midface will shift with this maneuver, but greenstick and impacted fractures may be immobile. Although the classic fracture patterns are diagrammed in this text (Fig. 249-5) they are more likely to be seen in print than in the ED. In clinical practice, fracture patterns are often mixed, with a low-grade LeFort on one side and a higher grade on the other.

In LeFort I, a transverse fracture separates the body of the maxilla from the lower portion of the pterygoid plate and nasal septum. With stress of the maxilla, only the hard palate and upper teeth move. A pyramidal fracture of the central maxilla and the palate defines a LeFort II injury. Facial tugging moves the nose but not the eyes. LeFort III, also called *cranial-facial disjunction,* occurs when the complete facial skeleton separates from the skull. The fracture extends through the frontozygomatic suture lines, across the orbit and through the base of the nose and ethmoid region. The entire face, including most of both orbits, shifts with mobilization. The LeFort IV fracture (not initially described by LeFort) involves the frontal bone as well as the midface.

These catastrophic injuries often require aggressive airway control and frequently intubation. Look for associated injuries, especially intracranial spinal thoracic, and abdominal. A test of visual acuity, if at all possible, is especially important for patients with LeFort III fractures, where the incidence of blindness is high. Plain films are unnecessary, and CT scans of the face may be ordered in conjunction with brain CT in clinically stable patients. Patients with complex maxillary fractures require admission for open reduction and internal fixation. Even if surgery is delayed, admission is prudent to monitor these often multiply injured victims.

Mandibular Fractures

After nasal bone injury, mandibular fractures are the second most common facial fracture. Assaults and falls on the chin are responsible for most injuries. Because of its ring shape, fractures are often multiple. Most injuries are to the body, angle, and the condylar process. An impact to the point of the jaw may transmit forces through the condyles that can fracture the temporal bone and rupture the eardrum.

History and physical examination will detect nearly all injuries. Ask patients whether their teeth approximate normally and whether they have pain on jaw movement. Evaluate jaw opening and search for intraoral lacerations to determine whether the fracture is open or closed. Gingival lacerations may be hidden between the teeth. Ecchymosis under the tongue is a sensitive finding for mandibular fracture, and fracture-induced injury to the mandibular nerve produces anesthesia of the lower lip.

Patients with normal occlusion and a negative tongue-blade test rarely require imaging studies. Radiography may include panorex, Towne, and lateral oblique views. If the symphysis is involved, consider occulusal films if other views are normal. Sometimes plain films are normal despite a condylar fracture. If films are normal but clinical suspicion remains high, consider a CT scan of the condyles.

Patients with open fractures require admission and intravenous antibiotics. Penicillin G (2 to 4 million units IV) or clindamycin (600 to 900 IV) is considered the drug of choice, but clindamycin and first-generation cephalosporins are good alternatives. Patients may be made more comfortable with a Barton bandage, which is an Ace bandage wrapped around the jaw and head. This prevents excessive jaw movement. Many patients with closed fractures may be managed as outpatients after consultation with an oral surgeon.

Temporomandibular Joint Dislocation

Dislocation of the temporomandibular joint (TMJ) may occur from blunt trauma to the jaw, seizures, or excessive mouth opening. Consider that patients who mumble after a seizure may not be postictal but instead be suffering from TMJ dislocation. Unlike condylar fractures, where the jaw points toward the side of injury, the chin deviates away from the side of the dislocation. In the less common bilateral dislocation, the chin juts forward. In a TMJ dislocation, the condyle becomes locked anterior to articular eminence and will not slide back secondary to muscle spasm. If a patient has jaw deviation and an open bite after a blow to the mandible, x-rays are indicated to detect fracture. However, films are not required to diagnose spontaneous or recurrent mandibular dislocations brought on by wide opening of the mouth.

Mandibular reduction is a simple ED procedure. The physician wraps his or her thumbs in gauze and stands behind the seated patient (Fig. 249-6). Standing on a footstool may increase the mechanical advantage if the physician is short or the patient is tall. Position the thumbs on either of the posterior molars or on the mandibular ridge. (The posterior molars are less slippery but will endanger the physician's digits when the jaw snaps into place.) To unlock the mandible, press downward and forward, and the joint should relocate. A rocking motion is helpful. If the patient has significant spasm or is difficult to reduce, inject the TMJ or lateral pterygoids with a local anesthetic, to facilitate relocation. Intravenous benzodiazepines are also helpful in this situation. Immediately after reduction, apply a Barton bandage to prevent repeat dislocation. Unless cautioned ahead of time, patients will test their jaw movement after reduction and re-dislocate the mandible. Patients must drink a liquid diet through a straw for several days and should follow up with an oral surgeon.

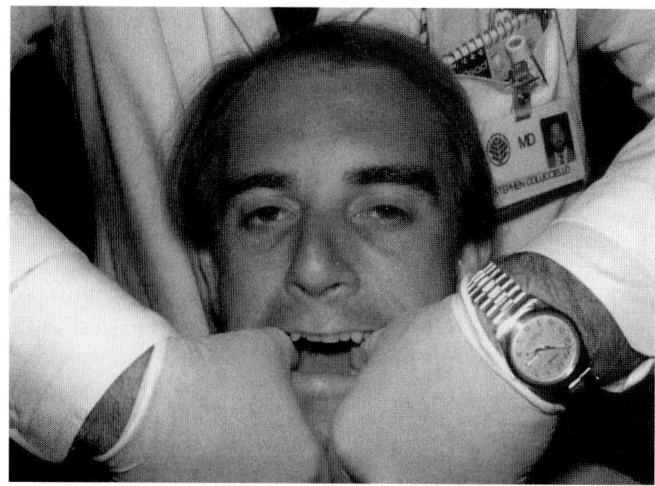

FIG. 249-6. Temporomandibular joint relocation technique. (Reprinted with permission from Isenhour J, Colucciello S: Maxillofacial trauma, in Ferrera P et al: *Trauma Management*. St. Louis, Mosby, 2000.)

SPECIAL CIRCUMSTANCES

Penetrating Trauma to the Face

Over a third of patients with penetrating trauma to the face have significant complications, including intracranial injury, blindness, or infection.[18] Shotgun blasts to the face are especially problematic, and globe injury is common.

The most immediate concern is airway management, which often requires emergency intubation or cricothyroidotomy. Not only is the risk of intracranial injury high, but there is also the possibility of cavernous sinus fistulas. The bullet's path may endanger the great vessels of the neck, and zone III injuries to the carotid are common. Patients at risk require angiography.

Infection is also a concern in patients with gunshot wounds to the face, especially if there is intraoral trajectory. In this situation, administer intravenous antibiotics effective against oral flora.[19]

Children versus Adults

Pediatric anatomy and developmental concerns influence the management of facial fractures in children.

ETIOLOGY Be suspicious of nonaccidental trauma in cases of pediatric maxillofacial injury. Associated skull fractures, a torn frenulum, and facial bruising may signify child abuse. Children with facial injuries should be completely undressed and examined for other stigmata of nonaccidental trauma. Some may require a radiographic skeletal survey to detect occult or prior trauma.

FRACTURE PATTERNS Fracture patterns relate to developmental anatomy. Young children have a higher incidence of frontal bone injury due to its prominence. Infants and toddlers almost never suffer midface fractures. The dearth of maxillary fractures under age 6 is due to the lack of sinuses in the midface. It is these sinuses that weaken the facial buttresses and predispose adults and adolescents to LeFort injury. As the child grows, the sinuses pneumatize, and fractures shift to the midface and lower face. By age 12 to 15, the fracture pattern resembles that in adults.

ASSOCIATED INJURIES Children with facial trauma also have dissimilar associated injuries than adults. Because the pediatric skull is more prominent, children have much higher incidence of intracranial injuries. Up to 60 percent of children with significant facial fractures have head injury. In addition, the dynamics of cervical injury vary between children and adults. Children are more likely to suffer an upper, rather than lower, cervical spine injury and are also prone to spinal cord injury without radiographic abnormality (SCIWORA).

AIRWAY MANAGEMENT A young child's airway is subject to subglottic stenosis and tracheomalacia. For this reason, avoid cricothyroidotomy in children younger than age 12. Intubation is the definitive airway of choice in children who need emergency airway management. If intubation is impossible, percutaneous transtracheal jet ventilation provides temporary airway control until a formal tracheotomy is feasible.

COMPLICATIONS AND TIMING OF FOLLOW-UP Because subsequent facial growth may be asymmetric, pediatric facial fractures can lead to serious cosmetic deformities. Subcondylar fractures of the jaw and displaced nasal fractures are of particular concern in children under age 5. Condylar fractures in this age group predispose children to facial deformity, micrognathia, and ankylosis of the TMJ. Consultation is essential.

Early follow-up is important in all pediatric facial fractures, because a child's facial skeleton heals faster than that of an adult. Within a week, early callous formation makes delayed reduction troublesome.

REFERENCES

1. Ochs HA, Neuenschwander MC, Dodson TB: Are head, neck and facial injuries markers of domestic violence? *J Am Dent Assoc* 127:757, 1996.
2. Hartzell KN, Botek AA, Goldberg SH: Orbital fractures in women due to sexual assault and domestic violence. *Ophthalmology* 103:953, 1996.
3. Marciani RD, Israel S: Diagnosis of blunt carotid injury in patients with facial trauma. *Oral Surg Oral Med Oral Pathol Oral Radiol Endod* 83:5, 1997.
4. Zachariades N, Papavassiliou D, Christopoulos P: Blindness after facial trauma. *Oral Surg Oral Med Oral Pathol Oral Radiol Endod* 81:34, 1996.
5. Bisson JI, Shepherd JP, Dhutia M: Psychological sequelae of facial trauma. *J Trauma* 43:496, 1997.
6. Bavitz JB, Collicott PE: Bilateral mandibular subcondylar fractures contributing to airway obstruction. *Int J Oral Maxillofac Surg* 24:273, 1998.
7. Rosen CL, Wolfe RE, Chew SE, et al: Blind nasotracheal intubation in the presence of facial trauma [see comments]. *J Emerg Med* 15:141, 1997.
8. Neal MR, Groves J, Gell IR: Awake fibreoptic intubation in the semi-prone position following facial trauma. *Anaesthesia* 51:1053, 1996.
9. Jessee SA: Physical manifestations of child abuse to the head, face and mouth: A hospital survey. *ASDC J Dent Child* 62:245, 1995.
10. Alonso LL, Purcell TB: Accuracy of the tongue blade test in patients with suspected mandibular fracture. *J Emerg Med* 13:297, 1995.
11. Thai KN, Hummel RP III, Kitzmiller WJ, Luchette FA: The role of computed tomographic scanning in the management of facial trauma. *J Trauma* 43:214, 1997.
12. Ohkawa M, Tanabe M, Toyama Y, et al: The role of three-dimensional computed tomography in the management of maxillofacial bone fractures. *Acta Med Okayama* 51:219, 1997.
13. Rehm CG, Ross SE: Diagnosis of unsuspected facial fractures on routine head computerized tomographic scans in the unconscious multiply injured patient. *J Oral Maxillofac Surg* 53:522, 1995.
14. Martello JY, Vasconez HC: Supraorbital roof fractures: A formidable entity with which to contend. *Ann Plast Surg* 38:223, 1997.
15. Nolasco FP, Mathog RH: Medial orbital wall fractures: Classification and clinical profile. *Otolaryngol Head Neck Surg* 112:549, 1995.
16. Bhattacharya J, Moseley IF, Fells P: The role of plain radiography in the management of suspected orbital blow-out fractures. *Br J Radiol* 70:29, 1997.
17. Stewart MG, Chen AY: Factors predictive of poor compliance with follow-up care after facial trauma: A prospective study. *Otolaryngol Head Neck Surg* 117:72, 1997.
18. Chen AY, Stewart MG, Raup G: Penetrating injuries of the face. *Otolaryngol Head Neck Surg* 115:464, 1996.
19. Wallick K IV, Davidson P, Shockley L: Traumatic carotid cavernous sinus fistula following a gunshot wound to the face [review]. *J Emerg Med* 15:23, 1997.

250 PENETRATING AND BLUNT NECK TRAUMA

Bonny J. Baron

The optimal management of patients with blunt or penetrating neck injuries is challenging. Seemingly minor injuries can quickly become life threatening. Missed injuries and delayed diagnosis can result in serious complications and death. While ultimate management goals are the same, each mechanism has its own special considerations.

EPIDEMIOLOGY

There is a paucity of data regarding the epidemiology of blunt and penetrating neck trauma. The demographics are expected to mirror those of other trauma victims, particularly in urban settings. There is a predominance of young males, especially those in the 21- to 30-year-old age groups. The incidence of gunshot versus stab wounds varies from study to study. Penetrating neck trauma is associated with a high incidence of simultaneous injuries to other systems. Multiple injuries occur 44 to 52 percent of the time.[1] Serious injuries following blunt trauma are not as common. The latter injuries are probably underreported because many are not recognized initially. About half of blunt neck trauma is related to motor vehicle crashes.

ANATOMY

The neck contains a high concentration of vascular, aerodigestive, and spinal structures in a relatively confined space. Other susceptible structures include the thyroid and parathyroid glands, lower cranial nerves, brachial plexus, and thoracic duct. Many of these structures are in close proximity to the skin, and therefore vulnerable to injury. Only the spinal cord has bony protection.

There are several anatomic classifications of the neck. Traditionally, anatomists have defined the neck in terms of anterior and posterior triangles, as divided by the sternocleidomastoid muscle (Fig. 250-1). The anterior triangle is bounded by the midline of the neck, the lower border of the mandible, and the anterior border of the sternocleidomastoid muscle. Within this triangle are most major vascular and aerodigestive structures. The carotid artery, internal jugular vein, vagus nerve, thyroid gland, larynx, trachea, and esophagus all lie in the anterior triangle. The boundaries of the posterior triangle are the middle third of the clavicle, the anterior border of the trapezius muscle, and the posterior border of the sternocleidomastoid muscle. The posterior

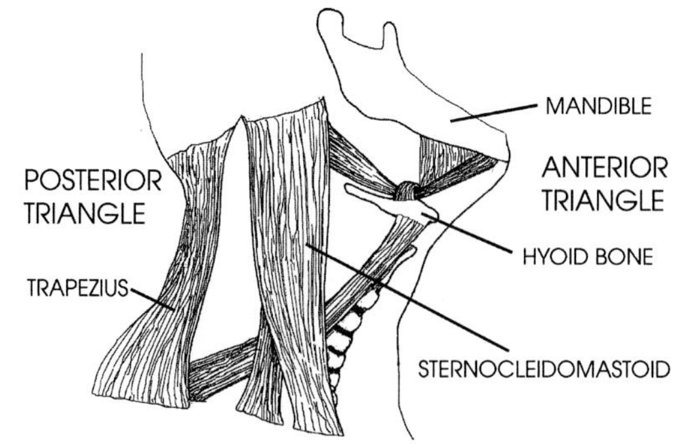

FIG. 250-1. Triangles of the neck.

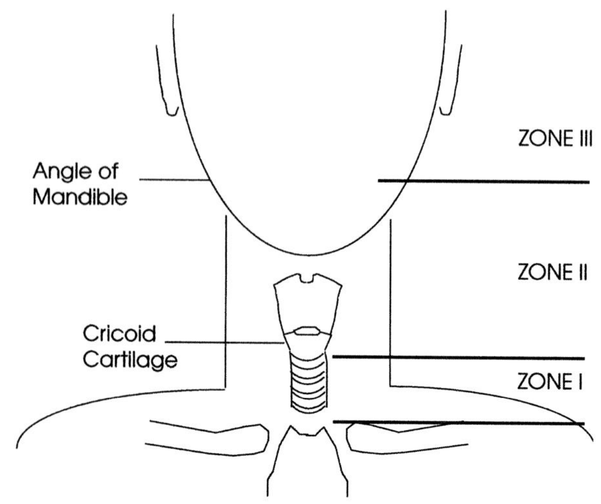

FIG. 250-2. Zones of the neck.

triangle has few vital structures, except at its base where the subclavian artery and brachial plexus are located.

An alternative anatomic classification divides the neck into three zones (Fig. 250-2). This classification was established to guide the clinician in the diagnostic and therapeutic management of penetrating injuries. Various authors have defined the zones differently. The most widely used classification is that of Roon and Christensen.[2] By their definition, zone I extends from the clavicles to the cricoid cartilage. Zone I includes the vertebral and proximal carotid arteries, major thoracic vessels, superior mediastinum, lungs, esophagus, trachea, thoracic duct, and spinal cord. Zone II extends from the inferior margin of the cricoid cartilage cephalad to the angle of the mandible. Injuries in zone II may involve the carotid and vertebral arteries, jugular veins, esophagus, trachea, larynx, and spinal cord. Zone III is located between the angle of the mandible and the base of the skull. The distal carotid and vertebral arteries, pharynx, and spinal cord are all at risk of injury in zone III.

The structures of the neck are supported by a series of fascial layers (Fig. 250-3). The superficial fascia surrounds the platysma muscle. This thin muscle covers the entire anterior triangle and the anteroinferior aspect of the posterior triangle. The platysma is the most superficial structure beneath the skin and subcutaneous tissue, and serves as an important planar landmark when evaluating penetrating neck injuries. Beneath the platysma is the deep cervical fascia, a series of fascial compartments that support the muscles, vessels, and viscera of the neck. The deep cervical fascia divides into the investing, pretracheal and prevertebral layers. The investing layer splits to enclose the sternocleidomastoid and trapezius muscles. The pretracheal layer attaches to the thyroid and cricoid cartilage and blends with the pericardium in the thoracic cavity. The prevertebral layer covers the prevertebral muscles and blends with the axillary sheath, which encloses the subclavian vessels. All three layers of the deep cervical fascia combine to form the carotid sheath. The tight facial compartments provide a tamponade effect, which limits potential for external bleeding from vascular injuries. Bleeding within these narrow compartments, however, can result in extrinsic compression and airway compromise.

INITIAL MANAGEMENT

The initial approach to patients with neck injury is performed according to Advanced Trauma Life Support (ATLS) protocols.[3] A directed primary survey, resuscitation, and secondary survey must all be performed expeditiously. Once the initial evaluation is completed, decisions concerning optimal diagnostic studies and definitive care are made.

Airway

Neck injuries can create some of the greatest challenges to airway management. All agree that any patient with acute respiratory distress, airway compromise from blood or secretions, massive subcutaneous emphysema, tracheal shift, or severe alteration in mental status must have early airway intervention. Controversy arises when presented with patients who have significant injury mechanisms without any immediate evidence of vascular injury or airway compromise. There are no published data that definitively outline the optimal approach in such patients. It is important to realize how quickly blood or air dissecting into fascial compartments can distort normal anatomy. Once this occurs, airway management becomes difficult, if not impossible. The risk of performing an unnecessary intubation is minimal compared

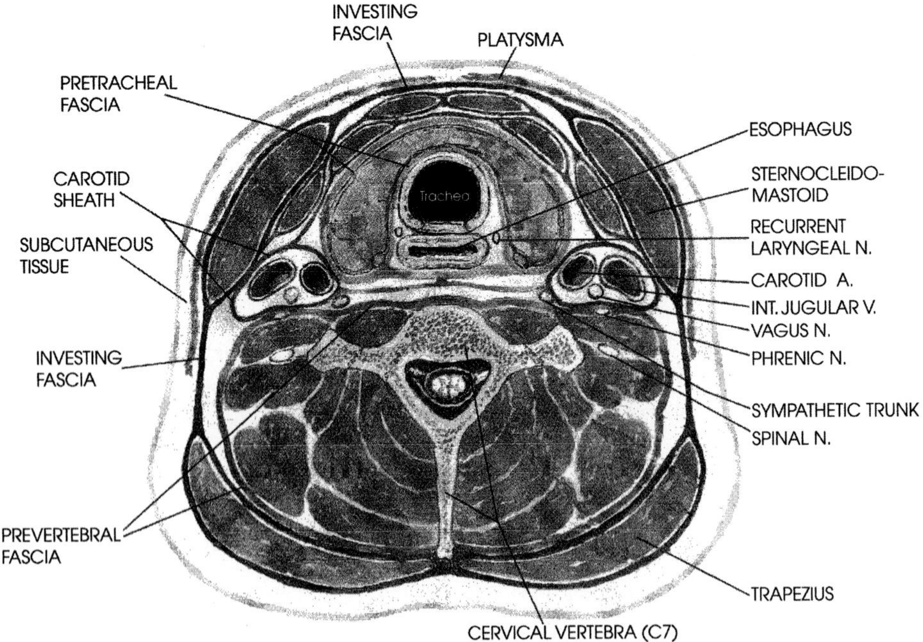

FIG. 250-3. Fascial layers of the neck. (Copyright 1989. Novartis. Modified with permission from *The Atlas of Human Anatomy,* p 30, illustrated by Frank H. Netter, M.D., Summit, NJ. All rights reserved.)

to the potential morbidity of a difficult intubation with respiratory distress and a distorted airway. It is particularly important to establish a definitive airway before a patient leaves the monitored setting of the Emergency Department for diagnostic studies. In most cases, orotracheal intubation with rapid sequence induction can be used.

If unsuccessful, the cricothyroidotomy is generally the next procedure of choice in adults. When performing a cricothyroidotomy care must be taken to avoid dislodging a contained hematoma. The integrity of the larynx should be evaluated prior to any intubation attempts, particularly in cases of blunt trauma. Intubation of a patient with a fractured larynx may result in complete transection or create a false passage, necessitating a tracheostomy. Occasionally, a tracheostomy site will be created by the injury itself. An existing tracheostomy may be intubated as a lifesaving means of securing the airway.[4] In all cases of blunt neck trauma, or in penetrating trauma in which a cervical spine fracture is suspected, immobilize the cervical spine in the neutral position.

Breathing

All patients should receive high-flow oxygen and be continuously monitored by pulse oximetry. Proximity of the base of the neck and the thorax predisposes both regions to injury. Difficulty ventilating a patient is indicative of either upper airway or thoracic injuries. Unequal breath sounds and asymmetric chest movement are signs of inadequate ventilation. These signs are associated with pneumo- or hemothoraces. Tracheal deviation may accompany a tension pneumothorax. Prompt recognition of these life-threatening complications and treatment with a tube thoracostomy will ensure adequate ventilation.

Circulation

Active bleeding is controlled by direct pressure at the site of injury. Do not clamp bleeding vessels, as additional damage to vascular or nervous structures may result. One should avoid placing intravenous access at a location where the IV fluid would flow toward the site of injury (for example, internal jugular or subclavian vein injury), and extravasate. Nasogastric tubes should be avoided during the initial resuscitation. Gagging and retching induced during NGT insertion could dislodge a clot and cause hemorrhage from a vascular injury.

Disability

A brief neurologic examination is mandatory. Neurologic deficits may indicate direct nerve or spinal cord injury, or they may result from cerebral ischemia caused by vascular injury. Early recognition of these deficits is important, particularly as patients are rapidly sedated and paralyzed for airway control.

Initial Radiographic Evaluation

The cervical spine must be imaged in all patients with a significant blunt trauma mechanism, particularly if they have an altered mental status. In cases of penetrating trauma, radiographs are evaluated for fractures and retained foreign bodies. Although the path of a missile is never known with certainty, localizing a bullet may determine or suggest a transcervical trajectory. In both blunt and penetrating trauma, the soft tissues should be examined for hematomas, air-column obstruction or deviation, subcutaneous emphysema, or retropharyngeal thickening. A chest radiograph must be obtained to evaluate for the presence of a pneumothorax, hemothorax, or air in the mediastinum.

Complete Evaluation

A complete history and thorough physical examination are performed. Information obtained from pre-hospital personnel should include mechanism of injury, symptoms, hemodynamic stability, and amount of blood loss at the scene. Once in the Emergency Department, if possible, the patient should be questioned about neck pain, difficulty breathing, dysphagia, odynophagia, hoarseness, hematemesis, hemoptysis, and any neurologic deficits. Examination of the neck requires a search for clinical signs of vascular, aerodigestive, and neurologic injuries. These include arterial bleeding, large or expanding hematomas, diminished pulses or bruits, lateralizing signs, tracheal deviation, air-bubbling through the wound, saliva in the wound, subcutaneous emphysema, and evidence of cranial nerve injuries. These clinical signs can be divided into hard and soft signs of injury (Table 250-1).[5] All signs require diagnostic investigation, but hard signs are more often associated with significant injury.

TABLE 250-1 Signs and Symptoms of Neck Injury

Hard Signs	Soft Signs
Hypotension in Emergency Department	Hypotension in field
Active arterial bleeding	History of arterial bleeding
Diminished carotid pulse	Tracheal deviation
Expanding hematoma	Nonexpanding large hematoma
Thrill/bruit	Apical capping on chest x-ray
Lateralizing signs	Stridor
Hemothorax >1000 cc	Hoarseness
Air or bubbling in wound	Vocal cord paralysis
Hemoptysis	Subcutaneous emphysema
Hematemesis	Seventh cranial nerve injury
	Unexplained bradycardia (without CNS injury)

PENETRATING INJURY

Mechanisms of penetrating injury can be categorized as stab, gunshot, shotgun, or miscellaneous sharp implements. All mechanisms have potential for causing serious injury. Seemingly innocuous wounds may involve multiple structures. Gunshot wounds cause damage both from the bullet itself and from the blast effect. In addition, the path of a bullet is unpredictable. Localizing a bullet will not delineate which structures it has traversed or disrupted. If the bullet has crossed the midline of the neck, however, there is a high probability of injury. Transcervical gunshot wounds are twice as likely to cause injuries to vital structures in the neck as are gunshot wounds that do not cross the midline.[6] Damage caused by shotguns depends largely on weapon-victim range, and type of weapon and shot used. Multiple pellets scattered across all three zones of the neck characterize these wounds.[7] Although the course of stab wounds is more limited than that of gunshot wounds, there is still clear potential for major injury.

Despite differences in mechanism, treatment principles are the same. Initial stabilization is always the primary concern. Once this is accomplished, attention is turned to examination of the wound itself. If the platysma muscle is clearly intact, local wound repair is all that is required. If the platysma has been violated it must be assumed that significant injury has occurred. Neck wounds must never be probed beneath the platysma in order to avoid disrupting hemostasis. The next priority is establishing wound location and determining which zones are involved. Vital structures at risk for injury can then be identified. Careful physical examination may reveal hard and soft signs of injury. A diagnostic plan, which will evaluate vulnerable structures, is then implemented.

Consultation

If the platysma is violated, immediate surgical consultation is indicated. Similarly, early involvement of radiologists will facilitate a nonoperative diagnostic work-up. A team approach will expedite stabilization, diagnosis, and definitive treatment. If the treating facility is unable to provide adequate diagnostic and surgical support, transfer should occur immediately after initial stabilization.

Diagnosis and Management

There is general agreement that patients who are hemodynamically unstable or have obvious aerodigestive injury require immediate surgical intervention. In those who are stable, the diagnostic approach is determined by the location of the wound. Nonoperative studies are used to identify injuries in zones I and III. Vascular control is often difficult to obtain in these zones. Zone I injuries require a thoracic surgical approach to gain proximal vascular control, important for arterial injuries. Both proximal and distal vascular control is easily obtained in zone II. For zone III, arterial injury proximal control is actually gained in zone II. More distal injury presents a difficult problem in zone III. Disarticulation of the mandible may be required for adequate exposure. Given these technical difficulties, routine exploration of zones I and III is not indicated. Both of these zones should be studied with angiography, as physical examination is not always reliable in identifying vascular injuries.[8] Zone I also requires diagnostic evaluation of the esophagus, as early injuries are often asymptomatic. The operative difficulties encountered in zones I and III are usually not a problem in zone II injuries.

Controversy surrounds the management of stable patients with zone II injuries. Literature supports both mandatory exploration of all injuries that penetrate the platysma as well as selective operation based on diagnostic studies. Mandatory exploration was popularized during World War II, as this intervention lead to markedly reduced morbidity and mortality. Advocates of mandatory exploration describe low complication rates following negative operations, as well as significant morbidity associated with missed injuries. There is also concern that diagnostic modalities that are used to detect aerodigestive injuries are inaccurate. Opponents of mandatory exploration cite its high negative exploration rate. In addition, an injury may be missed during surgical exploration. Alternatively, an injury may be discovered that is difficult to control surgically, such as a vertebral artery injury. Surgical exploration alone is often technically difficult with these injuries, particularly if the vascular anatomy and possible vertebral artery anomalies are not first identified by angiogram. Angiography helps clarify management. Complete occlusion of a vertebral artery in an asymptomatic patient with a normal contralateral vertebral artery and no evidence of a distal AV fistula is usually managed conservatively. The patient with active arterial bleeding, AV fistula, or pseudoaneurysm of the vertebral artery is preferably treated by percutaneous transcatheter embolization of the proximal and distal vertebral artery. On occasion, angiographic procedures are used during surgery to aid in obtaining vascular control. Obviously, if angiography is unavailable or unsuccessful, surgical exploration and repair is performed.[9] Selective management results in minimal nontherapeutic operations and spares the patient a surgical scar. No definitive evidence exists to establish one treatment paradigm as being more cost effective than the other.

Further controversy in the management of zone II injuries focuses on the diagnostic role of physical examination. Some advocate observation alone in asymptomatic patients with zone II injuries.[10,11] Studies supporting this management have been largely retrospective or had small sample sizes. Missed arterial and esophageal injuries have been demonstrated in asymptomatic patients.[5,8] Clinical signs and symptoms have low sensitivity, specificity, and predictive value.[5,8,12] In addition, multiple-injury patients may have associated injuries that make physical examination of the neck less reliable. Selective exploration based on the results of diagnostic studies should be done. This will decrease the rate of negative explorations, yet avoid missing injuries. Evaluation of zone II injuries should routinely include vascular and esophageal evaluation.

Angiography is currently the gold standard for evaluating vascular injury and can also be therapeutic. Duplex sonography is being used with increasing frequency. It is noninvasive, but it is operator-dependent and its sensitivity at detecting small lesions or intimal flaps is not yet established.

Esophageal evaluation must be performed in all patients because esophageal injuries with injuries in zones I and II are initially notoriously asymptomatic. Delayed treatment of esophageal perforations will result in neck space infections and mediastinitis. Ideally, evaluation should include both an esophagram and esophagoscopy. Using this combination of studies, the sensitivity of detecting injury is increased to nearly 100 percent.[13] Flexible, rather than rigid, esophagoscopy is the current procedure of choice.

Laryngotracheal injuries are of concern in zones I and II. Significant laryngotracheal injuries are rarely occult. Diagnosis is usually easy due to the anterior and superficial position of the trachea. Air-bubbling through the wound, dyspnea, stridor, hemoptysis, and subcutaneous emphysema are the most common signs and symptoms. Although optimal management is controversial, diagnostic evaluation with laryngoscopy and bronchoscopy is generally reserved for those who are symptomatic.

In summary, stable patients with zone I injuries should undergo angiography and esophagram, and/or esophagoscopy. Those with zone III injuries should undergo angiography. Patients with zone II injuries can undergo mandatory exploration or be evaluated with angiography and esophagram, and/or esophagoscopy. Patients with symptoms suggestive of laryngotracheal injury require laryngoscopy and bronchoscopy (Fig. 250-4). Despite the presence of a single wound, multiple zones may be involved. This happens most often when the injury is caused by a gunshot. Diagnostic evaluation should be liberal and account for all structures that may have been in the pathway of a trajectory.

It is important to recognize that to a large degree diagnostic evaluation is institution- and personnel-dependent. Available resources often determine the optimal diagnostic regimen.

Pediatric Considerations

Initial management of children is identical to that of adults. In children, however, certain predisposing factors may alter the diagnostic evaluation. The diagnostic process itself may be associated with significant morbidity. Young children must often be anesthetized to undergo diagnostic procedures. Angiography is technically more difficult due to the smaller vessel size. Hall et al. have suggested observation alone in asymptomatic children with zone II penetrating injuries.[14] The authors caution that this practice should only be followed if close, active observation by skilled consultants can be performed and operative facilities are immediately available.

BLUNT INJURY

Blunt neck trauma is rare. The head, shoulders, and chest offer protection to the neck when it is in the neutral position. Hyperextension,

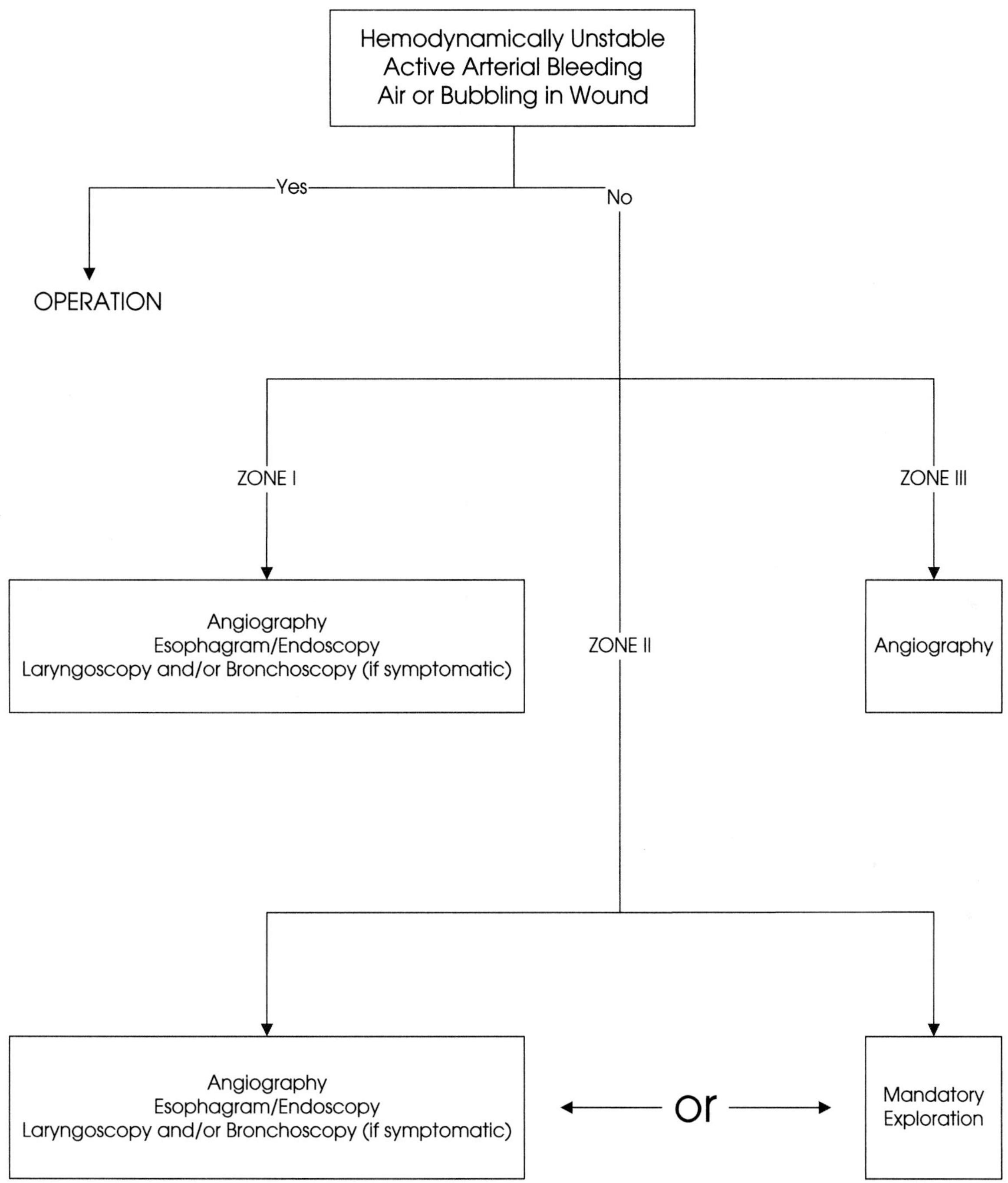

FIG. 250-4. Management of penetrating neck injury.

hyperflexion, rotation, and direct blows contribute to blunt injuries. Most commonly, injury results from motor vehicle crashes, when the extended neck strikes the steering wheel or dashboard.[15] Shearing forces from shoulder safety belts are also responsible for injury. Motorcycles, snowmobiles, and all-terrain vehicles have been implicated in ''clothesline'' injuries. These occur when the exposed neck strikes a stationary cord. They are associated with severe laryngotracheal and esophageal injuries. Other mechanisms include direct blows sustained during sports (football, karate, hockey), handlebar injuries from bicycles, assaults, and strangulation.[16]

Though uncommon, blunt cervical trauma can be lethal or can result in significant morbidity. Symptoms are often minimal, or delayed, and the diagnosis can be easily overlooked. Head, facial, and cervical spine injuries frequently accompany blunt neck trauma. Symptoms of vascular or aerodigestive injuries may be misinterpreted in the context of these associated injuries. A high index of suspicion must be maintained. Signs and symptoms or a significant injury mechanism mandate aggressive diagnostic evaluation, and admission for observation. As with penetrating trauma, surgical consultants should be involved in the initial assessment and management of all patients.

Laryngotracheal Injury

Laryngotracheal injury can range from soft tissue edema and ecchymosis to mucosal lacerations, vocal cord avulsion, fractures of the thyroid and cricoid cartilage, recurrent laryngeal nerve laceration, or complete laryngotracheal disruption. Classic symptoms include dysphonia, hoarseness, dysphagia, odynophagia, dyspnea, pain, hemoptysis, and stridor. Signs of injury include tenderness, subcutaneous emphysema, deformities, contusions, and tracheal deviation. Unfortunately, in contrast to penetrating tracheal trauma, which is frequently associated with signs and symptoms, blunt injury may present with few or no signs. Diagnosis requires a high index of suspicion.

Establishing an airway is the initial focus in management. Opinions vary as to the optimal method of achieving airway control. Some advocate endotracheal intubation by the most experienced personnel. Others recommend immediate tracheostomy. Those advocating tracheostomy believe that attempts at intubation may result in a false passage, adding further injury to an already compromised airway. Cricothyroidotomy should be avoided as this may worsen laryngeal injury. Any patient with suspected laryngotracheal injury should undergo chest, cervical spine, and soft tissue lateral neck radiographs. Subcutaneous emphysema, narrowing of the subglottic airway, and hyoid bone fractures may be seen on radiographs. Diagnostic work-up will then focus on identification of specific injuries. Laryngoscopy and bronchoscopy will evaluate vocal cord function, luminal integrity, and level of injury. CT is indicated in hemodynamically stable patients with secure airways. CT delineates the type and degree of injury, and is helpful in deciding which injuries can be managed conservatively and which require immediate operative intervention.

Pharyngoesophageal Injury

Blunt pharyngoesophageal injuries generally present with few or no symptoms. As with penetrating trauma, untreated, these perforations lead to life-threatening infections. Pharyngoesophageal injuries are usually associated with laryngotracheal injury. Laryngotracheal injury should prompt diagnostic evaluation of the esophagus with esophagram and esophagoscopy.

Vascular Injury

High suspicion of injury, coupled with early diagnosis and treatment of carotid injuries improves outcome. Injuries are often missed because there is a delay in the onset of signs and symptoms, and when these signs do develop they are often attributed to an associated head injury rather than a vascular injury. Any movement that distracts or compresses the artery can create injury. Five mechanisms of injury have been described: hyperextension with compression of the artery against the transverse process of the cervical spine; hyperflexion, with compression of the artery between the mandible and the spine; direct blows; intraoral trauma; and basal skull fracture causing tearing of the intracranial portion of the carotid artery.[17]

Two different lesions may occur following trauma. A pseudoaneurysm may form[18] or the vessel wall might dissect and cause secondary thrombosis, resulting in distal emboli or occlusion.[19] Clinical findings associated with closed carotid injury include neck hematomas, bruits, pulse deficits, ipsilateral Horner's syndrome, transient ischemic attacks, and contralateral motor or sensory deficits. Neurologic symptoms may develop immediately, or they may be delayed for several weeks. Outcome may be compromised once a deficit develops. The first step in diagnosis is a head CT to eliminate closed-head injury as the cause of symptoms. This should be followed by angiographic evaluation of the carotid arteries. Once the diagnosis of carotid injury is confirmed, the first line of treatment is anticoagulation. The rationale for systemic anticoagulation is to minimize clot formation at the site of intimal injury, decrease further propagation of the clot that has formed, and prevent embolization of clot from any pseudoaneurysm sac.[20] Medical management has been shown to provide good results in patients with minimal neurologic deficits. Patients with severe neurologic deficits on initial examination may benefit from surgical intervention.

There are several cases in the literature of vertebral injury following chiropractic neck manipulation. Cases of severe neurologic deficit following vertebral artery injury have also been reported with Yoga exercises, calisthenics, archery, and painting a ceiling.[21,22] All mechanisms of injury involve either cervical hyperextension, excessive contralateral rotation, or, most commonly, both. The vertebral arteries are susceptible to mechanical injury because of their relationship to neighboring bony structures and ligaments. Traumatic intimal disruption may lead to complete thrombotic occlusion, subintimal hematoma, dissection, or pseudoaneurysm formation. Distal branch occlusions may result from dissecting aneurysms, thrombus propagation from the neck, or thromboembolism. Patients may be asymptomatic, or they may have transitory or delayed neurologic symptoms. Symptoms vary from neck pain and occipital headache to Wallenberg's syndrome and lethal stroke. Wallenberg's syndrome (lateral medullary infarction syndrome) may include ipsilateral loss of cranial nerves V, IX, X, and XI, cerebellar ataxia, Horner's syndrome, and contralateral loss of pain and temperature sensation. Sudden death, quadriplegia, and "locked-in syndrome" (quadriplegia with loss of all lower cranial nerves) have also been described. Cerebral arteriography must be performed for any suspicion of vertebral artery injury. Anticoagulation and platelet aggregation inhibition are recommended, but the efficacy of this therapy has not been clearly established.

STRANGULATION

Significant external pressure applied to the neck results in strangulation. This is caused by hanging, ligature strangulation, manual strangulation, and postural strangulation. Circumstances surrounding strangulation injuries include homicides or assaults, suicides, accidents, and judicial executions. Depending on the method used, death from strangulation may occur by one of three mechanisms: injury to the spinal cord and brain stem; mechanical constriction of the neck structures; and cardiac arrest.[23] These are explained below.

Pathophysiology

Hanging occurs when pressure is exerted on the neck and then tightened by the weight of the victim's body. Hangings in which the body is suspended and the feet do not touch the ground are termed "complete." These generally occur with judicial hangings. All other positions of the body, when the feet are in contact with the ground, are referred to as "incomplete." The mechanism of death may differ depending on the method of hanging. If a victim drops a distance equal to his height, death usually results from fracture of the upper cervical spine and transection of the spinal cord. If a hanging is incomplete, or the victim drops a distance less than his height, the cervical spine is spared. Constriction causes jugular venous obstruction, stagnant cerebral blood flow and brain ischemia. Loss of consciousness results. Muscle tone decreases and compression of vital structures increases. Complete arterial occlusion and/or airway compromise result in death. Alternatively, cardiac arrest may occur due to carotid sinus stimulation and increased vagal tone.

In ligature and manual strangulation, the constricting force is external, but the weight of the body and head play no part. Postural strangulation is seen in infants. This results when the victim's neck is placed over an object and the weight of the body adds pressure to the neck. In all of these methods of strangulation, death probably results from airway obstruction (suffocation) or vascular occlusion, as previously described in incomplete hangings.

Fracture of the thyroid cartilage, hyoid, and larynx are associated with strangulation. Traumatic edema of the larynx and supraglottic tissue lead to airway compromise. Delayed mortality is often due to neurogenic pulmonary edema and aspiration pneumonia. Cerebral anoxia may cause neurologic damage. Neurologic deficits are not always immediately apparent, and may develop over time. Long-term psychiatric manifestations include psychosis, Korsakoff's syndrome, amnesia, and progressive dementia.

Clinical Presentation

Abrasions, ecchymosis, and a brownish compression groove may be apparent. A rise in venous pressure above the ligature can lead to the formation of Tardieu's spots. These petechial hemorrhages can best be seen in the skin and subconjunctival areas. Patients may complain of painful swallowing. Severe hoarseness and stridor are suggestive of an impending airway obstruction.

Treatment

Treatment is directed at airway, respiratory, cardiac, neurologic, and psychiatric complications. Endotracheal intubation should be performed if airway problems or severe blood gas abnormalities are evident. As noted above, C-spine fracture or instability is all but impossible except in judicial-style hangings, where a significant free-fall drop is designed to cause a death resulting in vertebral fracture. Thus, for most suicidal, and accidental hangings, cervical spine immobilization is unnecessary. Neurogenic pulmonary complications are best treated with controlled ventilation and positive end-expiratory pressure (PEEP). Cardiac monitoring is essential for the identification and management of dysrhythmias. Hyperventilation, fluid restriction, and diuretics will treat cerebral edema. Intracranial pressure monitoring may be useful in guiding therapy. Psychiatric support is often necessary in long-term survivors.

A high level of suspicion must be maintained in all patients who sustain compression injuries to the neck. Admission for 24 h is warranted to observe for delayed airway obstruction.

REFERENCES

1. Irish JC, Hekkenberg R, Gullane PJ, et al: Penetrating and blunt neck trauma: 10-year review of a Canadian experience. *Can J Surg* 40:33, 1997.
2. Roon AJ, Christensen N: Evaluation and treatment of penetrating cervical injuries. *J Trauma* 19:391, 1979.
3. American College of Surgeons, Committee on Trauma: *Advanced Trauma Life Support Course* (student manual), 6th ed. Chicago, ACS, 1997.
4. Shearer VE, Giesecke AH: Airway management for patients with penetrating neck trauma: A retrospective study. *Anesth Analg* 77:1135, 1993.
5. Baron BJ, Sinert RH, Kohl L, et al: The value of physical examination in penetrating neck trauma. *Acad Emerg Med* 4:347, 1997.
6. Demetriades D, Theodorou D, Cornwell E, et al: Transcervical gunshot injuries: Mandatory operation is not necessary. *J Trauma* 40:758, 1996.
7. Ordog GJ, Albin D, Wasserberger J, et al: Shotgun "birdshot" wounds to the neck. *J Trauma* 28:491, 1988.
8. Sclafani SJA, Cavaliere G, Atweh N, et al: The role of angiography in penetrating neck trauma. *J Trauma* 31:557, 1991.
9. Golueke P, Sclafani S, Phillips T, et al: Vertebral artery injury—Diagnosis and management. *J Trauma* 27:856, 1987.
10. Jurkovich GJ, Zingarelli W, Wallace J, et al: Penetrating neck trauma: Diagnostic studies in the asymptomatic patient. *J Trauma* 25:819, 1985.
11. Atteberry LR, Dennis JW, Menawat SS, et al: Physical examination alone is safe and accurate for evaluation of vascular injuries in penetrating zone II neck trauma. *J Am Coll Surg* 179:657, 1994.
12. Apffelstaedt JP, Muller R: Results of mandatory exploration for penetrating neck trauma. *World J Surg* 18:917, 1994.
13. Weigelt JA, Thal ER, Snyder WH, et al: Diagnosis of penetrating cervical esophageal injuries. *Am J Surg* 154:619, 1987.
14. Hall JR, Reyes HM, Meller JL: Penetrating zone-II neck injuries in children. *J Trauma* 31:1614, 1991.
15. Reece GP, Shatney CH: Blunt injuries of the cervical trachea: Review of 51 patients. *Southern Med J* 81:1542, 1988.
16. Fuhrman GM, Stieg FH, Buerk CA: Blunt laryngeal trauma: Classification and management protocol. *J Trauma* 30:87, 1990.
17. Li MS, Smith BM, Espinosa J, et al: Nonpenetrating trauma to the carotid artery: Seven cases and a literature review. *J Trauma* 36:265, 1994.
18. Sharma S, Rajani M, Mishra N, et al: Extracranial carotid artery aneurysms following accidental injury: ten years experience. *Clin Radiol* 43:162, 1991.
19. Watridge CB, Muhlbauer MS, Lowery RD: Traumatic carotid artery dissection: Diagnosis and treatment. *J Neurosurg* 71:854, 1989.
20. Fabian TC, Patton JH, Croce MA, et al: Blunt carotid injury, importance of early diagnosis and anticoagulant therapy. *Ann Surg* 223:513, 1996.
21. Schellhas KP, Latchaw RE, Wendling LR, et al: Vertebrobasilar injuries following cervical manipulation. *JAMA* 244:1450, 1980.
22. Raskind R, North CM: Vertebral artery injuries following chiropractic cervical spine manipulation—Case reports. *Angiology* 41:445, 1990.
23. Iserson KV: Strangulation: A review of ligature, manual, and postural neck compression injuries. *Ann Emerg Med* 13:179, 1984.

THORACIC TRAUMA

William M. Bowling
Robert F. Wilson
Gabor D. Kelen
Timothy G. Buchman

INTRODUCTION

Approximately 25 percent of nonmilitary trauma-related deaths are due to thoracic trauma. A majority of the deaths occur after the patient reaches the hospital. Mortality is relatively low (5 percent) for isolated chest injuries. With two or more organ systems involved, death will occur in about one-third. It is felt that as many as 10 percent of such deaths could have been prevented in the ED.[1]

Penetrating injuries have a different mechanism than blunt trauma. Nearly all penetrating injuries result in a pneumothorax, with hemothorax occurring in more than 75 percent. Blunt trauma causes injury by one or more of several mechanisms: compression (organ rupture), direct trauma (e.g., fracture), and acceleration/deceleration forces (vessel shear and tear). Penetrating trauma has the further distinction of being associated with abdominal injuries in about one-third of cases. Only 5 to 15 percent of patients with chest trauma will require a thoracotomy.

CHEST WALL, BRONCHI, LUNGS, AND DIAPHRAGM

Patients with chest trauma who develop acute, severe respiratory distress have a high mortality rate. About 10 percent of patients admitted with chest trauma required endotracheal intubation almost immediately upon entrance to the emergency department (ED). If shock is also present in addition to the respiratory distress, three-quarters will die. In patients with blunt chest trauma, the most frequent factors associated with acute respiratory distress included shock, coma, multiple rib fractures, and hemopneumothorax (Table 251-1). In patients with penetrating trauma, respiratory distress is usually associated with severe shock or hemopneumothorax (Table 251-2).

Initial Resuscitation, Airway Control, and Ventilation

Diagnosis of the cause of respiratory distress must be made promptly. If the patient is making little or no effort to breathe, central nervous system dysfunction due to head trauma, drugs, or spinal cord injury is the most likely problem. If the patient is attempting to breathe but is moving little or no air, upper airway obstruction should be suspected.

TABLE 251-1 Injuries in Patients with Respiratory Failure after Blunt Chest Trauma

Injury	Incidence, %	Mortality Rate, %
Flail chest/multiple rib fracture	75	52
Hemopneumothorax	55	39
Lung contusion	39	45
Extremity fracture	30	53
Intraabdominal	23	46
Intracranial	23	46
Myocardial contusion	13	57
Diaphragm	9	20
Paraplegia	4	100
Other	7	100

The most common cause of upper airway obstruction in comatose patients is prolapse of the tongue into the pharynx. Other causes of upper airway obstruction include dentures; vomitus; or blood clots in the pharynx, larynx, or upper trachea. Occasionally, direct trauma may cause fracture of the larynx or cricotracheal separation. Inspiratory stridor does not usually occur unless there is at least a 70 percent occlusion of the larynx or upper trachea. With any suspected laryngeal injury, cautious endoscopy should be performed in the operating room as soon as possible, but one must also be prepared to perform an emergency tracheostomy immediately if the airway occludes.

If the patient is attempting to breathe and the upper airway appears to be intact but the breath sounds are poor, thoracic problems such as flail chest, hemopneumothorax, diaphragmatic injury, or parenchymal lung damage should be considered. In all cases of respiratory distress, the airway must be secured. Following airway control, optimal oxygenation and ventilation should be provided.

CARDIAC ARREST DURING OR JUST AFTER ENDOTRACHEAL INTUBATION Although Rotondo et al[2] have pointed out that urgent paralysis and intubation of trauma patients who are combative or have complex injuries is relatively safe, one of the most frequent times for an emergency department patient to have a cardiac arrest is during or right after endotracheal intubation. Table 251-3 lists common causes for cardiac arrest during intubation. If the patient has poor venous return because of hypovolemia, ventilation with excessive pressures can further reduce venous return and cause cardiac arrest. Hypovolemic patients should probably be ventilated with tidal volumes of only 5 to 8 mL/kg at 10 to 14 times per minute until venous return is improved.

TABLE 251-2 Injuries in Patients with Respiratory Failure after Penetrating Chest Trauma

Injury	Incidence, %	Mortality Rate, %
Lung	55	69
Intraabdominal	36	83
Heart	29	63
Hemopneumothorax	18	42
Diaphragm	17	64
Chest wall	8	60
Extremity vessels	8	20
Other	41	63

TABLE 251-3 Causes of Cardiac Arrest with Endotracheal Intubation

Inadequate preintubation oxygenation and ventilation
Esophageal intubation
Intubation of the right (or left) main bronchus
Excess ventilation, further reducing venous return
Development of a tension pneumothorax
Systemic air embolism
Vasovagal response (rare)
Sudden development of severe alkalosis

If there is a lung injury or if there are fragile subpleural blebs, bagging the patient vigorously can also cause a tension pneumothorax to develop rapidly, further reducing venous return. Even if the lungs are normal, ventilatory pressure exceeding 70 to 80 cmH_2O can cause pulmonary damage. Excessive hyperventilation can also cause severe alkalosis, reducing ionized calcium levels and producing serious dysrhythmias.

Any patient with a lung injury, especially with hemoptysis, should be considered at risk for developing a systemic air embolus, particularly if high ventilatory pressures are used. Intrabronchial bleeding may also flood normal alveoli, causing severe hypoxemia.

Vasovagal responses are rare in injured patients, but they can occur during insertion of endotracheal, nasogastric, or chest tubes. One should be alert for the development of this problem in patients with nausea or inappropriate bradycardia that worsens as a procedure is being performed. Airway management techniques are discussed in Chaps. 14 to 16.

Initial Survey

Several life-threatening thoracic injuries should be recognized and treated during the initial survey. These are airway obstruction (noted above), tension pneumothorax, cardiac tamponade, massive hemothorax, open pneumothorax, and flail chest.

TENSION PNEUMOTHORAX The diagnosis of tension pneumothorax should be suspected based on clinical grounds alone. The presentation includes dyspnea, hypoperfusion, distended neck veins, diminished or absent breath sounds on the affected side, a hyperresonant percussion note on the affected side, and tracheal deviation to the opposite side. Not all elements of the presentation need be present to suspect the diagnosis. For example, the noise in the resuscitation area makes the percussion note difficult to hear. Also, distention of the neck veins may be absent in the face of hypovolemia.

If a tension pneumothorax is suspected, the next intervention must be the insertion of a small cannula (typically a 14-gauge intravenous catheter) through the chest wall into the pleural space. The purpose of this intervention is to convert the tension pneumothorax into an open pneumothorax. Although the classic description of this maneuver places the insertion point at the second interspace in the midclavicular line, any point in the superior, anterior, or lateral chest wall may be selected. Once the tension pneumothorax is decompressed (a hiss of gas exiting the pleural space may be audible) the patient's perfusion often improves within seconds. The initial survey should be completed and a chest tube (tube thoracostomy) inserted on the side of the tension pneumothorax as soon as practicable. Lack of improvement following decompression means that another cause of hypoperfusion should be sought immediately. If the neck veins remain distended, cardiac tamponade from pericardial blood (pericardial tamponade) must be suspected and treated immediately.

An x-ray of the chest should not be obtained in the patient with a suspected tension pneumothorax until after tube thoracostomy has been performed and the patient's perfusion improved.

PERICARDIAL TAMPONADE (CARDIAC TAMPONADE) Both blunt and penetrating thoracic injuries have the potential to cause blood to accumulate in the pericardium. Although stab wounds to the midchest are the most common cause, blunt compressive forces to the anterior heart can rupture the right atrium or its appendage while maintaining enough filling of the right ventricle to sustain life for a short interval. In either case, blood fills the poorly compliant pericardial sac, with pressure increasing sharply as each small increment of fluid accumulates.

The presentation of tamponade is similar to that of tension pneumothorax: both lesions cause obstruction of venous return to the heart. In addition to hypoperfusion and distended neck veins, the patient with tamponade may have ''muffled'' heart tones—muffling that is hard to hear in the busy environment of a trauma resuscitation. However, breath sounds should be audible bilaterally and the trachea should lie in the midline.

While the initial treatment of tamponade is emergency pericardiocentesis (described further on), immediate surgical intervention is required to control the bleeding. An intravenous bolus of fluid to transiently increase the pressure filling the right atrium may be helpful to increase cardiac output for a minute or two while preparations are being made for the pericardiocentesis and/or immediate surgical intervention.

Again, radiographs are conspicuous by their absence from this discussion. The poorly compliant pericardium, although full and under pressure from the blood within, casts a rather ordinary shadow on the chest x-ray. As little as 150 to 200 mL of blood may result in cardiac tamponade. Therefore, chest radiographs cannot be used to exclude this life-threatening diagnosis.

If surgery cannot be performed immediately, it may be wise to leave a cannula within the pericardial sac for serial aspirations as surgical preparations are being made. Aspiration of only 5 to 10 mL of fluid can substantially improve cardiac performance—again a consequence of the rigidity of the pericardium.

MASSIVE HEMOTHORAX Each hemithorax can potentially hold about 40 to 50 percent of the human circulating blood volume. While the hemithorax is ordinarily filled with air, a small amount of blood, and the tissues of the lung, blood can accumulate rapidly in the pleural space. A massive hemothorax in an adult is defined as 1500 mL or more—that is, about two-thirds of the available space in the hemithorax is occupied by blood.

Massive hemothorax is life-threatening by three mechanisms. First, the acute hypovolemia renders preload inadequate to sustain effective left ventricular function. Second, the collapsed lung induces hypoxia by disturbing ventilation-perfusion matching. Third, the pressure of the hemothorax compresses the vena cava (further impairing preload) and the pulmonary parenchyma, raising pulmonary vascular resistance.

If a radiograph of the chest has been obtained, the diagnosis of a massive hemothorax can be made if the aerated lung is completely surrounded by fluid (blood).

Immediate tube thoracostomy is required to initially manage the massive hemothorax. Surgical repair must be performed emergently. Common causes of massive hemothorax include injury to the lung parenchyma, to an intercostal artery, and to the internal mammary artery.

Patients with ''ordinary'' hemothorax will occasionally drain a moderate amount of blood but then rebleed or continue to bleed. If there is evidence of ongoing hemorrhage after initial drainage exceeding 600 mL/6 h (i.e., 100 mL/h for 6 h, 300 mL/h for 2 h, or 600 mL/h for 1 h), a ''massive hemothorax equivalent'' is diagnosed. In such cases of rebleeding/ongoing bleeding, conservative management requires thoracotomy, although occasional patients may be managed nonoperatively.

Since massive hemothorax is, by definition, associated with accumulation and subsequent drainage of large volumes of potentially ''clean'' blood, it is desirable to collect the effluent into an autotransfusion-prepared device. The decision to proceed with autotransfusion must be based on the patient's condition and the probability that the blood is free from contamination by enteral pathogens from an occult injury to the gastrointestinal tract.

OPEN PNEUMOTHORAX Open pneumothorax (discussed in detail further on) is an open communication between the outer chest wall and the pleural space. Respiratory distress is due to inability to ventilate the affected side. The injury is sometimes referred to as a ''sucking chest wound'' because of the sound produced as air moves through the wound. On examination, this injury is usually obvious. However, it may be obscured by the patient's position or clothing. Air entry is diminished on the affected side, and chest wall motion is less dynamic. The injury is very often associated with a hemothorax. The initial maneuver in the ED is to cover the wound with a three-sided dressing so that air can escape but not enter through the wound. Complete occlusion may convert the injury into a tension pneumothorax.

FLAIL CHEST The term *flail chest* refers to a free-floating segment of ribs that are no longer connected to the rest of the thorax. This entity is also described in detail further on. During the initial survey, the examiner must search for segmental paradoxical chest wall motion, which is easy to miss if not specifically sought. Air entry will be diminished on the affected side. Jugular venous pressure may be intermittently increased in rhythm with respirations due to pendelluft, as explained later in this chapter.

Ventilatory Support

In patients with chest trauma, impaired ventilation, in spite of measures to ensure an open airway, relief of chest wall pain, and drainage of hemopneumothorax, is an indication for ventilatory support. Respiratory failure associated with a flail chest is best treated by early endotracheal intubation and ventilatory assistance, particularly if there are associated injuries, and even if the patient's breathing intially seems adequate. Ventilatory assistance should also be strongly considered if the patient is in shock, has had multiple injuries, is comatose, requires multiple transfusions, is elderly, or has preexisting pulmonary disease. A respiratory rate greater than 30 to 35 breaths per minute, a vital capacity less than 10 to 15 mL/kg, and/or a negative inspiratory force (NIF) less than 25 to 30 cmH_2O can also be considered early indications for ventilatory support.

All trauma patients should be monitored by pulse oximetry. In patients with severe chest trauma, an arterial blood gas should be drawn soon after admission and at frequent intervals thereafter. If arterial P_{O_2} is less than 50 mmHg while the patient is breathing room air or less than 80 mmHg while the patient is breathing supplemental oxygen (equivalent to an F_{IO_2} of 0.4 or more), the patient should generally be given ventilatory assistance. Metabolic acidosis with an arterial P_{CO_2} insufficiently decreased to compensate for the decrease in $[HCO_3^-]$ is another indication for ventilatory support. Although there are several formulas relating the expected change in P_{CO_2} to the magnitude of the decrease in $[HCO_3^-]$, the simplest approach is to expect a 1:1 relationship. That is, for each milliequivalent per liter decrease in [HCO_3^-], ventilatory response should result in a decrease of Pco_2 of 1 mmHg. Thus, in the face of metabolic acidosis, Pco_2 less than 40 mmHg may still be inappropriately high. (See Chap. 21 for a detailed discussion.)

When used properly, pulse oximetry can also reduce the need for arterial blood gas (ABG) determinations; however, since the Sao_2 indicated by the pulse oximeter is often 2 to 3 percent higher than that seen with ABG, one should try to keep the saturation more than 92 to 93 percent.

Shock

At the same time that one is ensuring an adequate ventilation, efforts should be directed toward rapidly restoring a more than adequate tissue perfusion. After hemorrhagic shock, the cardiac output and oxygen delivery must be 25 to 50 percent greater than normal to adequately perfuse and oxygenate the intestinal mucosa and liver.[3]

Other preliminary studies indicate that capnometry to determine the end-tidal Pco_2 ($PETco_2$), particularly if combined with arterial Pco_2 determinations so that one can determine the arterial–end tidal CO_2 difference [P (a − ET)co_2] can also help monitor the adequacy of tissue perfusion ventilation. In general, a persistent $PETco_2 <$ 28 mmHg or P (a − ET)$co_2 >$ 10 mmHg is an indication of a poor prognosis.

If hypovolemic hypotension is present in patients with blunt chest trauma, it is most likely due to pelvic or extremity fractures, intraabdominal injuries, and/or intrathoracic bleeding.

In patients with penetrating chest trauma, the cause of shock will be intrathoracic injury in about three-quarters. The most frequent sources of intrathoracic bleeding are lung, heart, great vessels, and intercostal or internal mammary arteries. Up to one-half may have extrathoracic injuries contributing to the shock. When this occurs, it is most likely due to intraabdominal bleeding which often has a delayed diagnosis.

TREATMENT **Fluids** Failure to correct hypotension within 15 to 30 min greatly increases the mortality rate. In previously healthy patients requiring massive transfusions but having hypotension for less than 30 min, the mortality rate has averaged about 10 percent. However, if the hypotension is present for more than 30 min, the mortality rises to almost 50 percent. If the patient has preexisting disease or is over 65 years of age, the mortality with massive transfusions plus prolonged hypotension exceeds 90 percent.

To provide fluids rapidly in hypotensive patients, one usually needs at least two large intravenous catheters. If peripheral veins are not readily available, one may be forced to cannulate the subclavian or internal jugular veins. If a subclavian vein line is required, it should be inserted on the side of the injury. If one side of a chest is injured and the other lung is collapsed during insertion of a central intravenous line, impaired function of both lungs could be rapidly fatal.

Peripheral veins may be collapsed, unavailable, or inadequate. Especially in patients with thoracic trauma (and because of the activity required at the chest to deal with the direct consequence of that trauma) femoral venous cannulation is a preferred route of access for infusion of fluids. Seldinger technique is usually used (that is, "catheter over a guidewire") to insert a short, fat cannula, such as an "introducer" of the kind otherwise used in conjunction with pulmonary artery catheters. If percutaneous access to the femoral veins is difficult—as it often is when the patient has "bled out"—an experienced operator can place a cannula in the femoral vein via a saphenous vein cutdown in less than a minute. Such saphenous cutdowns are rare but can be lifesaving.

Irrespective of the route used to obtain vascular access, the goal is to stabilize the intravascular volume long enough to definitively manage the bleeding and only then to fully resuscitate the patient. Rapid resuscitation prior to control of the source can increase the rate and volume of blood loss, worsening hypothermia, immune suppression, and even mortality. Stopping the bleeding is the penultimate priority.

Chest Tube and Thoracotomy A large hemothorax or pneumothorax can seriously interfere with ventilation and venous return; consequently, it should be evacuated as rapidly as possible. If blood is being removed rapidly through the chest tube, the vital signs should be followed very closely. If the vital signs are improving, one can continue to evacuate the blood. However, if the vital signs deteriorate as the blood is being evacuated, in spite of the rapid infusion of intravenous fluids, the patient may be exsanguinating via the chest tube because the tamponading effect of the hemothorax has been removed. In such circumstances, the chest tube should be clamped and the patient taken directly to the operating room for an emergency thoracotomy.

If it is thought that the bleeding is from an internal mammary or intercostal artery, one can insert a 30-mL balloon Foley catheter into the chest at the injured site, inflate the balloon, and pull it back tightly against the inside of the chest wall. The Foley catheter can also be used to drain blood or air from the pleural cavity, and if adequate pressure is applied with the inflated balloon against the chest wall for 12 to 24 h by taping the stretched tube to the chest wall, the bleeding will usually remain controlled.

Cardiac Arrest

EXTERNAL MASSAGE In patients with cardiac arrest due to chest trauma, external cardiac massage is generally of no value and is in fact likely to be harmful. Since the trauma patient suffering cardiac arrest is generally hypovolemic, external massage is usually ineffective and may actually cause significant additional injury to the heart, liver, lungs, or great vessels. In addition, forced ventilation and external cardiac compression may result in air emboli in the coronary arteries.

INTERNAL (OPEN) MASSAGE Resuscitative thoracotomy can be helpful in selected patients, i.e. those with signs of life within 5 min of arrival in the ED and penetrating wounds of the chest. However, a resuscitative thoracotomy is seldom of benefit in (1) patients with blunt trauma, (2) patients with penetrating abdominal or head injuries, and (3) patients "dead at the scene."

Open cardiac massage is usually performed through an anterolateral incision in the fifth intercostal space on the side of the injury. The pericardium is opened vertically 1 to 2 cm anterior to the phrenic nerve. The thoracic incision allows direct inspection of the heart, control of bleeding sites in the chest, and complete evacuation of any pericardial tamponade or hemopneumothorax. In addition, a left thoracotomy allows the physician to compress or clamp the descending thoracic aorta.

Since about 60 percent of the cardiac output normally goes to the tissues below the diaphragm, clamping of the descending thoracic aorta can increase coronary and carotid blood flow almost threefold. If the arterial systolic blood pressure does not rise to 90 mmHg within 5 to 10 min of aortic cross-clamping, further resuscitation will probably be of no avail. On the other hand, if the proximal aortic pressure rises above 160 to 180 mmHg in a previously normotensive individual, it can damage the brain and/or left ventricle.

Diagnosis of Thoracic Injuries

SYMPTOMS The most frequent symptoms of thoracic trauma are chest pain and shortness of breath. The pain is usually well localized to the involved area of the chest wall, but not infrequently it is referred to the abdomen, neck, shoulder, or arms. Dyspnea and tachypnea are nonspecific and may also be caused by anxiety or pain from other injuries.

PHYSICAL EXAMINATION A thorough physical examination, directed toward detecting the potential presence of the six major conditions to be sought during the primary survey, can be performed rapidly. There should not be an excessive reliance on chest x-rays. Tension pneumothorax, in particular, should be diagnosed and treated before obtaining a chest x-ray.

Inspection CHEST WALL Without careful inspection of the chest wall, one can easily overlook contusions, flail chest, intrathoracic bleeding, and open ("sucking") chest wounds. The paradoxical motion of a flail chest may be minimal when the patient is first seen, especially if it involves the lateral or posterior thorax.

Although external bleeding is easily recognized, it may be difficult to determine whether the source is intrathoracic or from the chest wall itself. Most chest wounds that communicate with the pleural cavity are readily apparent because of the noise air makes as it passes through the tissue of the chest wall during ventilatory efforts. However, some wounds are open only intermittently and may not be discovered until or unless the patient makes increased ventilatory efforts.

NECK Distended neck veins, especially when the patient is sitting upright, may indicate the presence of pericardial tamponade, tension pneumothorax, cardiac failure, or air embolism. However, distended neck veins may not appear until hypovolemia has been at least partially corrected. If the face and neck are cyanotic and swollen, severe damage to the superior mediastinum with occlusion or compression of the superior vena cava should be suspected. Subcutaneous emphysema from a torn bronchus or laceration of the lung can cause severe swelling of the neck and face.

ABDOMEN A scaphoid abdomen may indicate a diaphragmatic injury with herniation of abdominal contents into the chest. Excessive abdominal movement during breathing may indicate chest wall damage that might not otherwise be apparent. A rocking-horse type of ventilation may indicate a high spinal cord injury with paralysis of intercostal muscles.

PALPATION Palpation of the chest should begin with determining whether the trachea is in its normal position, which is in the midline or slightly to the right. Palpation of the chest wall may reveal areas of localized tenderness or crepitus from fractured ribs or subcutaneous emphysema. Well-localized and consistent tenderness over ribs should be considered to be due to rib fractures, even if the initial x-rays appear to be normal.

Motion of a portion of the sternum or severe localized tenderness may be the only objective evidence of a fractured sternum. When a patient is coughing or straining, palpation can sometimes detect abnormal motion of an unstable portion of the chest wall better than visual inspection.

Percussion Percussion of the chest wall can be of some help in differentiating between a hemothorax and pneumothorax. Dullness to percussion over one side of the chest following trauma may be the first evidence that a hemothorax is present; hyperresonance, on the other hand, may indicate the presence of a pneumothorax. A fairly large hemothorax can be missed if the chest x-ray is taken while the patient is lying supine.

If the pericardial cavity is greatly distended by an effusion or tamponade, the area of cardiac dullness may extend beyond the midclavicular line on the left or the sternal border on the right. This sign is especially helpful if the point of maximal impulse is located more than an inch inside the left border of cardiac dullness.

Auscultation Whenever possible, the chest should be auscultated systematically and thoroughly, anteriorly, laterally, and posteriorly, and at both the bases and apices. If the breath sounds are equal bilaterally, the major bronchi are probably intact.

The presence of bowel sounds high in the chest may be the first indication of a diaphragmatic injury. Decreased breath sounds on one side usually indicate the presence of hemothorax or pneumothorax, but this may also occur if the endotracheal tube is in too far and only one lung is being ventilated. Before inserting a chest tube into a patient with an endotracheal tube and acute respiratory distress, with decreased breath sounds on one side, one should check the position of the endotracheal tube. Occasionally, persistently decreased breath sounds on one side are due to a bronchial foreign body or ruptured bronchus.

Injury to the Chest Wall

SOFT TISSUE INJURIES **Bleeding** Probing of a penetrating chest wound to determine its depth or direction can be dangerous because it can damage underlying structures and cause severe recurrent bleeding or a pneumothorax or air leak. Bleeding from chest wall muscles can be rather brisk at times and is best controlled initially by local pressure. Later, one can inspect the depths of the wound in the operating room and use ligatures to control the bleeding and carefully close the wound.

Open (Sucking) Chest Wounds Small open chest wounds can act as one-way valves, allowing air to enter during inspiration but none to leave during expiration, thereby causing an expanding pneumothorax. This not only reduces tidal volume but can also interfere with venous return. If the open chest wound exceeds two-thirds the area of the trachea, air will preferentially enter the pleural cavity through the chest wall opening rather than through the tracheobronchial tree into the lungs.

Sucking wounds of the chest should be covered immediately by a sterile, airtight dressing, such as a petrolatum gauze, and a chest tube should be inserted almost simultaneously at a separate site to relieve the pneumothorax. The chest tube is not inserted through the trauma wound because it is then likely to follow the missile or knife tract into the lung or diaphragm. The occlusive dressing itself has the potential to cause a tension pneumothorax. Sudden deterioration following placement of the occlusive dressing but prior to insertion of the chest tube should suggest the possibility of a tension pneumothorax. In this case, relief is obtained simply by removing the occlusive dressing. In the prehospital setting, the occlusive dressing is fastened to the skin on only three sides so as to allow air to escape during exhalation but none to enter during inhalation.

Tissue Loss Injuries caused by close-range shotgun blasts or high-powered rifles may destroy such large quantities of chest wall that it may be impossible to close the chest wall in the usual manner. Intubation and mechanical ventilation will be required until the defect is definitively closed. It is important, however, to cover the lungs and heart and close the diaphragm. For small defects, resection of adjacent ribs and a thoracoplasty may be adequate. With large defects, rotated muscle flaps and/or Marlex mesh may be required.

Subcutaneous Emphysema Subcutaneous emphysema usually develops because air from lung parenchyma or the tracheobronchial tree gains access to the chest wall through an opening in the parietal pleura. The air may also reach the chest wall from an interstitial lung injury by dissecting back along the bronchi into the hilum and mediastinum and then into the extrapleural spaces. Extensive subcutaneous emphysema should make one suspect an injury to the pharynx, larynx, or esophagus.

Patients with subcutaneous emphysema should be presumed to have an underlying pneumothorax, even if it is not visible on the chest x-ray. If the patient requires a general anesthetic or is to be placed on a ventilator, a chest tube should be inserted on the involved side(s), after inserting a finger to ensure that a pleural space is present. If subcutaneous emphysema is severe, a major bronchial injury should be suspected and sought by bronchoscopy.

If there appears to be any respiratory difficulty that may be due to mediastinal emphysema, a tracheostomy around which the skin and fascia are closed only loosely may serve to maintain adequate ventilation and also allow a route for air to escape from the mediastinum and subcutaneous tissue. Very rarely, linear incisions into the subcutaneous space of the chest wall may be required to relieve massive subcutaneous emphysema. Once the initiating cause is controlled, subcutaneous emphysema usually disappears gradually over a period of several days.

BONY INJURIES **Clavicular Fractures** Isolated clavicular fractures due to blunt trauma are usually relatively harmless. Occasionally, however, direct trauma produces sharp fragments that may injure the subclavian vein and produce a moderately large hematoma or venous thrombosis. Rarely, excess callus forming later at the site of a clavicular fracture may press against the subclavian artery or brachial plexus, producing a thoracic outlet syndrome.

Rib Fractures SIMPLE FRACTURES Rib fractures should be assumed to be present in any patient who has localized pain and tenderness over one or more ribs after chest trauma. Up to 50 percent of rib fractures (especially those involving the anterior and lateral portions of the first five ribs) may not be apparent on x-ray, particularly for the first few days after injury. Furthermore, injuries to the cartilaginous portions of the ribs may never be appreciated on x-ray.

The principal diagnostic goal with clinically suspected rib fractures is the detection of significant complications, especially hemopneumothorax, pulmonary contusion, or major vascular injury. If there is a suspicion of a pneumothorax that is not seen on the initial chest x-ray, the patient should also have inspiratory and expiratory films taken. As a general rule, a pneumothorax is seen better on expiratory chest films where the pneumothorax space takes up a larger percentage of the hemithorax. If the patient has severe trauma, if the rib fractures have sharp fragments, or if the patient has other injuries, serial chest roentgenograms (every 6 to 12 h for 24 to 48 h) should be obtained.

The pain of rib fractures can greatly interfere with ventilation. Strapping the chest with adhesive tape or a rib belt to relieve the pain may be effective in young, athletic individuals with only a few rib fractures; however, in less vigorous patients, strapping may significantly reduce ventilation and cause progressive atelectasis. Probably the best analgesic for mild to moderate chest wall pain is acetaminophen with codeine (Tylenol no. 3) or ibuprofen, 600 to 800 mg every 6 to 8 h as needed.

If the patient is admitted, an intercostal nerve block with bupivacaine (Marcaine) may dramatically relieve pain, muscle spasm, and ventilation for 6 to 12 h. Intrapleural catheters for administration of local anesthetics can also relieve chest wall pain quite well. Epidural analgesia usually works even better, but in many hospitals this requires admission to a step-down intensive care unit (ICU) for apnea monitoring.[4]

FIRST- AND SECOND-RIB FRACTURES Except with direct trauma, as from a hammer blow, it takes great force to fracture the first and second ribs. It is frequently associated with significant injuries such as blunt myocardial injury (formerly referred to as myocardial contusion), bronchial tears, or a major vascular injury. There is conflicting evidence in the literature as to whether first- or second-rib fractures are more likely to be associated with mortality. Nevertheless, 15 to 30 percent of either fracture type is associated with poor outcome, usually from head injury or rupture of a major vessel.

MULTIPLE RIB FRACTURES If a patient with fractured ribs, especially ribs 9, 10, and 11, becomes hypotensive and does not have a large hemothorax or tension pneumothorax, intraabdominal bleeding from the liver or spleen should be suspected.

In general, it is wise to hospitalize patients with fractured ribs for at least 24 to 48 h if they cannot cough and clear their secretions adequately, especially if they are elderly or have preexisting pulmonary disease. Admitting the patient also provides time to observe the patient for associated injuries that might not be apparent initially. Aspiration pneumonitis and fat embolism often do not become apparent clinically or on chest x-ray for at least 24 to 48 h.

Flail Chest PATHOPHYSIOLOGY Segmental fractures (i.e., fractures in two or more locations on the same rib) of three or more adjacent ribs anteriorly or laterally often result in an unstable chest wall and the phenomenon known as flail chest. This injury is characterized by a paradoxical inward movement of the involved portion of the chest wall during spontaneous inspiration and outward movement during expiration.

Although the paradoxical motion of the involved chest wall can greatly increase the work of breathing, the main cause of the hypoxemia of flail chest is the underlying lung contusion. In the past, pendelluft (a ventilatory phenomenon referring to movement of air back and forth between the injured and uninjured lungs with each breath) was considered to be an important cause of the hypoxemia seen with flail chest. However, pendulluft is probably significant only when the upper airway is partially obstructed.

Immediately after the injury, little flail may be apparent. Later, as fluid moves into the area of the pulmonary contusion, lung compliance falls, and more pressure is needed to inflate the lungs. The increasing pressure differential between intrathoracic and atmospheric pressure may then overcome the resistance of the muscles attached to the fractured ribs, thereby allowing the involved chest wall to develop increasing paradox. In addition, the patient may fatigue rapidly because of the decreased efficiency of ventilation and increased muscular effort. Thus, a vicious cycle of decreasing efficiency of ventilation, increasing fatigue, and hypoxemia may develop. In some instances, the increasing ventilatory fatigue can result in a sudden respiratory arrest.

TREATMENT **INITIAL THERAPY** Historically, belts and adhesive tape were applied to ''strap'' and stabilize the chest. These interventions actually inhibit expansion of the chest and thereby aggravate the atelectasis of the underlying lung. The preferred intervention is analgesia adequate to allow the patient to fully expand the underlying lung, with a goal of improving ventilation and pulmonary toilet.

NONVENTILATORY THERAPY Patients with mild to moderate flail chest and little or no underlying pulmonary contusion or associated injuries can often be managed without a ventilator, by (1) relief of pain by analgesics or intercostal nerve block, (2) frequent coughing and chest physiotherapy, and (3) restriction of intravenous fluids to prevent volume overload. However, ventilatory support should be provided if, in spite of this regimen, the arterial Po_2 remained less than 80 mmHg on supplemental oxygen.

VENTILATORY SUPPORT Indications for early ventilatory support of patients with flail chest include shock, three or more associated injuries, severe head injury, comorbid pulmonary disease, fracture of eight or more ribs, or age greater than 65 years. Early (prophylactic) ventilatory assistance in patients with flail chest and one or two additional injuries may reduce mortality to about 7 percent. This is in sharp contrast to a mortality rate of 69 percent in similar patients in whom ventilatory assistance is delayed until there is clinical evidence of respiratory failure. Ventilated patients seem to do better if intermittent mandatory ventilation (IMV), rather than controlled mandatory ventilation (CMV), is used.

One of the most controversial areas in the management of flail chest is the role of surgical fixation of the fractured ribs or the sternum. The aim of surgical fixation of the chest is to reduce the need for ventilatory assistance; however, this same objective can often be achieved with improved pain relief and ventilatory support. Although some European surgeons have claimed significant reductions in mortality and morbidity with surgical fixation of the flail chest, it is performed only infrequently in the United States.[5]

Sternal Fractures Fracture of the sternum has long been considered a serious and life-threatening injury. Sternal fractures occur most often in motor vehicle accidents and have been thought to be associated frequently with cardiovascular injury, particularly blunt cardiac trauma and especially in older women wearing seat belts. Some authors have reported mortality rates in patients with sternal fractures to be as high as 45 percent. However, in a large recent study of patients with sternal fractures collected over 6½ years, it was found that the incidence of sternal fracture as a result of motor vehicle collisions was 3 percent.[6] This series had a very low incidence of cardiac dysrhythmias requiring treatment [1.5 percent (4/272)], and mortality rate (0.7 percent).

The variability in the data likely reflect uneven definitions of blunt myocardial injury (BMI). Increasing evidence suggests that sternal fracture is not an indicator of significant blunt myocardial injury.[7,8] Authors of a small retrospective study have offered an algorithm approach to the consideration of BMI. Patients with blunt chest trauma without sternal fractures whose vital signs and ECG are normal require no further consideration of BMI. Patients with normal vital signs and ECG with sternal fractures should have repeat ECG alone in 6 h. If unchanged, then no further work up for BMI is required.[8] Institutional practices for the management of sternal fractures vary. Some admit for 24-h cardiac monitoring if the inner sternal cortex is disrupted.

TRAUMATIC ASPHYXIA Sudden, severe crushing of the chest may cause subconjunctival hemorrhage or petechiae together with vascular engorgement; edema; and cyanosis of the head, neck, and upper extremities. This clinical picture appears to be due to an abrupt sustained rise in superior vena caval pressure and concurrent closure of the airway after deep inspiration. Although these patients often look moribund initially, neurologic impairment is usually only temporary, and long-term morbidity is due primarily to associated injuries.[9]

Injury to the Lungs

PULMONARY CONTUSION Pulmonary contusions are a significant source of severe morbidity and mortality following penetrating and blunt trauma. While such trauma has long been recognized to be a source of deranged physiology, new diagnostic techniques, including computed tomography (CT), have made recognition of this common problem much more frequent. Prompt recognition and therapy can be lifesaving. Pulmonary contusion is defined as direct damage to the lung resulting in both hemorrhage and edema in the absence of a pulmonary laceration. The most typical cause of pulmonary contusion is a compression-decompression injury to the chest. In high-speed automobile crashes, airbags can attenuate but do not entirely prevent this injury. Consider the consequence of a rapid deceleration of the chest as causing a high-pressure wave that compresses the thoracic cavity. The force wave is transmitted directly to the lung because it is in contact with tissues of the chest wall. There is an instantaneous rise in intrathoracic pressure followed by a near instantaneous drop. The force wave coupled with the extraordinarily rapid changes in intrathoracic pressure are probably both necessary and sufficient to cause the injury.

Pathophysiology There appear to be two significant stages in the pathophysiology of pulmonary contusion. The first is related to the direct injury, while the second is related to the resuscitative measures directed at associated injuries that ultimately prove harmful to the lung, in particular, the administration of intravenous fluid. Administration of fluid in the setting of unilateral pulmonary contusion can cause an extravasation of fluid into the contralateral (uninjured) lung, probably in association with reflex attempts to increase blood flow through this uninjured lung. The mechanism appears to be a fall in pulmonary vascular resistance in the uninjured lung, causing pressures exerted by the right heart to increase hydrostatic pressure in the capillaries enough to force both blood and fluid out of those capillaries into the interstitium and alveoli. Unfortunately, the process is self-perpetuating in that, as each proximate segment of lung sees the full force of the right heart activity, it becomes functionally congested and contused and the process continues to the next uninjured segment of lung.

The pathologic changes associated with pulmonary contusion seem to be primarily the result of capillary damage. There is both interstitial and intraalveolar extravasation of red blood cells and accumulation of edema fluid in the interstitium. These two processes typically do not occur simultaneously, but rather in sequence. Initially, the problem is primarily intraalveolar hemorrhage. The edema follows, as would be expected from the usual course of injury followed by fluid resuscitation. This accumulation of debris and mucus secretions causes further atelectasis, which leads, in secondary fashion, to large areas of unventilated but still perfused lung. Intrapulmonary shunting is increased, resistance to airflow is increased, the elasticity of the lungs is reduced, and the amount of respiratory work to move gases in and out of the lungs is markedly increased. Thus the work of ventilation becomes prohibitive and the patient becomes hypoxic, hypercarbic, and acidotic. Adaptive increases in cardiac output are usually insufficient to overcome the hypoxic process and cardiopulmonary decompensation can occur very quickly. With a significant blow to the chest, there may be accompanying myocardial dysfunction (attributable to blunt force to the heart), which, in combination with a severe pulmonary contusion, can synergistically lead to a rapid downward spiral.

Diagnosis Areas of opacification of the lung seen on the chest x-ray within 6 h of blunt trauma are usually considered to be pulmonary contusions. The lung changes with aspiration pneumonia and fat embolism are not usually seen on chest x-rays for at least 12 to 24 h. The extent of the lung injury seen at thoracotomy or autopsy or on CT scan is usually much greater than suspected from chest x-rays.

Treatment Treatment of pulmonary contusions primarily involves maintenance of adequate ventilation. Chest physiotherapy, intercostal nerve blocks, epidural analgesia, and nasotracheal suction are used as needed to ensure that the patient takes deep breaths and coughs adequately. If ventilatory assistance is required, ventilation with IMV and positive end-expiratory pressure (PEEP) usually provides much better ventilation-perfusion matching, better venous returns, and quicker weaning than does standard controlled ventilation. An important determinant of the need for mechanical ventilation is the volume of contused lung. Patients with less than 18 percent of total lung volume (about one lobe) do not require such support, whereas patients with more than 28 percent of total lung volume involved in the contusion predictably require such support. Premorbid health status and associated injuries can, of course, affect the threshold for mechanical ventilation in either direction. The point is that the ''gray area'' is quite narrow—a reflection of the progressive nature of the injury.

Patients who have a severe unilateral lung injury and are responding poorly to conventional mechanical ventilation may benefit from synchronous independent lung ventilation (SILV) provided through a double-lumen endobronchial catheter. This technique helps prevent overinflation of the normal lung and underinflation of the damaged, poorly compliant lung.[10]

In severe pulmonary contusion, ordinary mechanical ventilation may be insufficient to reverse the hypoxemia. The first maneuver should be to place the good lung ''down'' by turning the patient to the decubitus position. This simple maneuver can improve ventilation/perfusion matching. While administration of nitric oxide gas is still considered experimental therapy at the time of this writing, it has proven to be a superb adjunct in many patients with contusion because the gas reaches only ventilated alveoli and exerts its vasodilator effects in precisely those ventilated alveoli. Failing these two maneuvers, consideration should be given to chemical paralysis and institution either of pressure-controlled inverse-ratio ventilation or high-frequency oscillation. Both modes cause hemodynamic changes that require experience and invasive monitoring to manage effectively.

HEMOTHORAX **Etiology** Hemothorax requiring a thoracotomy is most frequently caused by bleeding from lung injuries. However, the compressing effect of the shed blood, the high concentration of thromboplastin in the lungs, and the low pulmonary arterial pressure combine to help reduce bleeding from torn lung parenchyma, so that a thoracotomy is needed only in about 5 to 15 percent of patients admitted with chest trauma. The other causes of severe and/or continuing intrathoracic bleeding include damage to the great vessels of the chest or intercostal or internal mammary arteries.

Pathophysiology If there is more than 300 to 500 mL of blood in the pleural cavity, it should be removed as completely and rapidly as possible. Large clots can act as a local anticoagulant by releasing fibrinolysins and fibrinogenolysins from their surface. A large hemothorax also restricts ventilation and venous return. Bleeding from multiple small intrathoracic vessels often stops fairly rapidly after the hemothorax is completely evacuated.

Diagnosis A hemothorax should be suspected following trauma if the breath sounds are reduced and the chest is dull to percussion on the involved side. Fluid collections greater than 200 to 300 mL can usually be seen on good upright or decubitus roentgenograms of the chest. However, if the patient is supine, more than 1000 mL of blood may easily be missed because it may only produce a mild to moderate diffuse haziness on that side. Ultrasound use in trauma to detect hemothorax has not been well studied and techniques for such detection are currently being evaluated. Even so, plain chest x-rays give much more additional information.

Treatment THORACENTESIS A very small, stable hemothorax does not always have to be removed, but it should be carefully observed. If the hemothorax seems large enough to drain, we have avoided needle aspiration and have relied on chest tubes. Needle aspiration of a hemothorax is usually incomplete and may cause a pneumothorax or infection of the hemothorax.

CHEST TUBES **TECHNIQUE** Chest tubes for treatment of traumatic pneumothorax or hemothorax are usually inserted in the anterior axillary line just behind the lateral edge of the pectoralis major muscle. For a pneumothorax we tend to direct the tube as high and anteriorly as possible without the tip pressing on the mediastinum. For a hemothorax, the tube is usually inserted at the level of the nipple and directed posteriorly and laterally.

Once the insertion site is selected, the area around it is painted liberally with an iodophor preparation and then widely draped with a fenestrated sheet. A 22-gauge needle is used to liberally infiltrate the skin, subcutaneous tissue, and intercostal muscles down to the parietal pleura with 1% lidocaine (Xylocaine) with adrenalin, keeping the total amount of lidocaine used below 0.5 mL/kg (5 mg/kg).

A transverse incision 2 to 3 cm in length is then made and extended down to the intercostal muscles. The skin incision for the chest tube should be at least 1 to 2 cm below the interspace through which the tube will be placed. A large clamp is then inserted through the intercostal muscles in the next higher intercostal space, with care taken to prevent the tip of the clamp from penetrating the lung (Fig. 251-1*A*). The resulting oblique tunnel through the subcutaneous tissue and intercostal muscles usually closes promptly after the chest tube is removed, thereby reducing the chances of recurrent pneumothorax.

Once the clamp is pushed through the internal intercostal fascia, it is opened to enlarge the hole to approximately 1.5 to 2 cm. A finger is inserted along the top of the clamp through the hole to verify the position within the thorax and to make sure the lung is not stuck to the chest wall (Fig. 251-1*B*). This is particularly important if a chest x-ray has not been taken or if the x-ray does not clearly show that the lung is away from the chest wall.

For a simple pneumothorax, a 24F or 28F chest tube can be inserted. For a hemothorax, a 32F to 40F chest tube is preferred. When in doubt, the larger tube should be chosen for trauma situations. Smaller tubes may not drain blood adequately. The chest tube is grasped at its tip with the clamp and directed through the hole into the pleural space and advanced in the appropriate direction (Fig. 251-1*C*). The tube is advanced until the last side hole is 2.5 to 5 cm (1 to 2 in.) inside the chest wall. The tube is secured in place with a long, heavy suture (2–0 or 1–0) of nonabsorbable material placed in a U fashion around the tube. The suture is tied so as to pull the soft tissues snugly around the tube and provide an airtight seal. The tails of the suture can be wrapped around the tube in opposite directions approximately half a dozen times and then tied to secure the tube to the chest wall.

The open end of the tube is attached to a combination fluid-collection water-seal suction device, such as the Pleur-evac, with 20- to 30-cmH_2O suction (Fig. 251-2). If a significant hemothorax is known to be present or if a large amount of blood starts to drain immediately, consideration should be given to collection of blood in a heparinized autotransfusion device so that it can be returned to the patient either directly or after washing the red blood cells in saline.

After it appears that the chest tube is correctly situated and working properly, a sterile occlusive dressing is placed over the incision and additional layers of tape are used to secure the tube to the chest wall, so that it will not be accidentally pulled out.

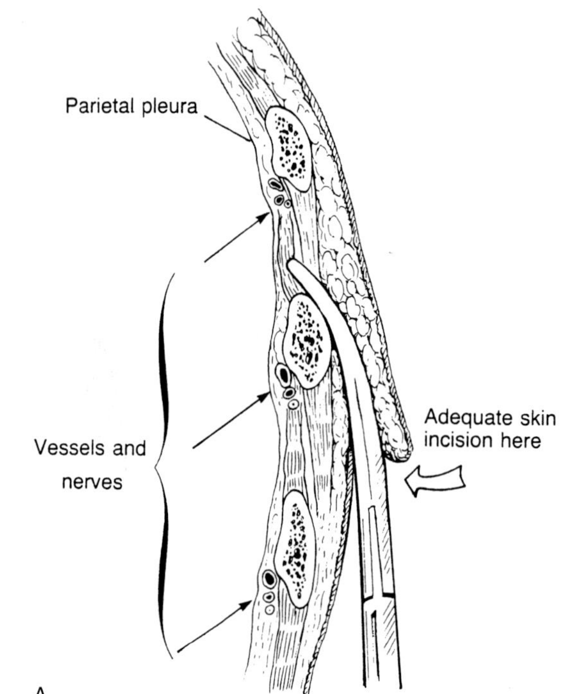

FIG. 251-1A. The clamp is inserted through the incision and is tunneled up to the next intercostal space. (From Roberts JR, Hedges JR: *Clinical Procedures in Emergency Medicine,* 2d ed. Philadelphia: Saunders, 1991, with permission.)

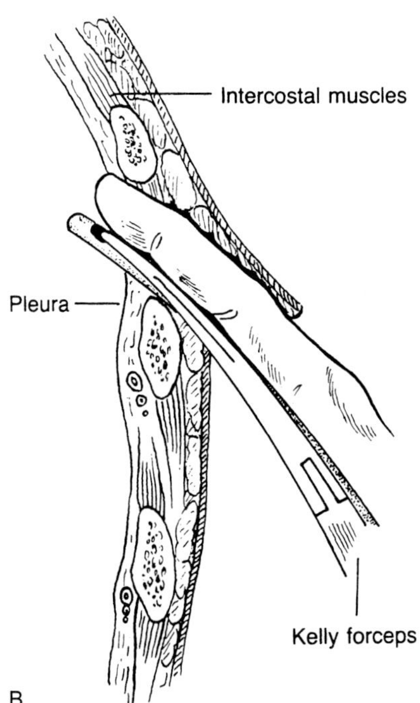

FIG. 251-1B. Using the finger as a guide, one places the tip into the pleural cavity. The pleura is punctured just above the rib to avoid intercostal vessels and nerves. (From Roberts JR, Hedges JR: *Clinical Procedures in Emergency Medicine,* 2d ed. Philadelphia: Saunders, 1991, with permission.)

The intrathoracic position of the chest tube and its last hole and the amount of air or fluid remaining in the pleural cavity should be checked with a chest x-ray as soon as possible after the tube is inserted. If there is a significant air leak, the chest films are best done as portables at the patient's bedside so as not to risk the development of a tension pneumothorax while the patient is off suction en route to the x-ray department.

If the patient is sent to the radiology department for x-rays, the chest tube should not be clamped because any continuing air leakage can rapidly collapse the lung and/or cause a tension pneumothorax. While the tube is unclamped, the water-seal bottle should be kept 1 to 2 ft lower than the patient's chest.

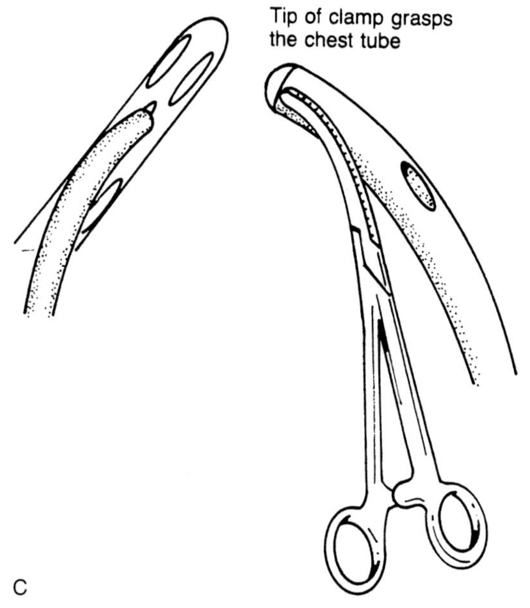

FIG. 251-1C. The tube is grasped with the curved clamp, with the tube tip protruding from the jaws. (From Roberts JR, Hedges JR: *Clinical Procedures in Emergency Medicine,* 2d ed. Philadelphia: Saunders, 1991, with permission.)

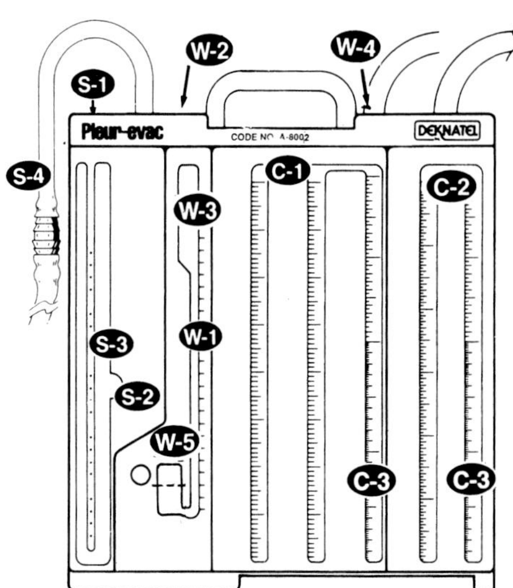

FIG. 251-2. Chest drainage. *A.* Suction control. S-1, atmospheric vent. Use this opening for filling the suction control chamber. This is also the vent to atmosphere. S-2, self-sealing diaphragm on face of unit. Use an 18- or higher-gauge needle, attached to a syringe, to remove fluid from this chamber. S-3, suction control pressure scale. When suction is applied and bubbling occurs, the approximate level of suction imposed is determined by the original fluid level. S-4, suction tubing for connection to suction source. If suction is not required, tubing should remain uncapped and unclamped, to allow air to exit and minimize possibility of tension pneumothorax. *B.* Water-seal chamber. The water-seal chamber serves three purposes: (1) acts as a one-way valve to allow air to exit from the pleural space; (2) serves as a manometer, measuring the amount of negativity in the patient's chest cavity; (3) allows for observation of the degree of air leak. W-1, water-seal pressure scale (to determine negativity in patient's chest cavity). Without suction, the pressure in the chest cavity is read directly by the fluid level in the calibrated water-seal pressure scale. With suction, add the reading from the suction control chamber setting to the reading of the water-seal pressure scale (e.g., -20 suction plus -10 water seal $= -30$ cmH_2O patient negativity). Patency of the patient's thoracic catheter can be observed as oscillation in the water-seal chamber. The water level rises and falls as the patient breathes. Oscillations may not be present when suction is operative, the lung is fully expanded, or the tubing is blocked or kinked. W-2, positive-pressure relief valve opens with increases in positive pressure, preventing pressure accumulation. W-3, high-negativity float valve preserves the water seal in the presence of high negativity. W-4, filtered high-negativity relief valve is provided to vent excessive negativity. W-5, self-sealing diaphragm is provided in the front of the unit to adjust the water level in the water-seal chamber. *C.* The major collection chamber is calibrated in 2-mL increments up to 200 mL. Over 200 mL, calibrations are in 5-mL increments. Fluids overflow from one section to the next. The capacity of the major collection chamber is 2000 mL. C-2, the minor collection chamber. Its collection capacity is 100 mL. C-3, self-sealing diaphragms are provided on the back of the unit for taking laboratory samples of patient drainage. (Adapted from instructions for use of the Pleur-evac, Deknatel, Inc., Fall River, MA.)

Serial chest auscultation, chest x-rays, and careful recording of the volume of blood loss and the amount of air leakage are important guides to the functioning of chest tubes. If a chest tube becomes blocked and a significant pneumothorax or hemothorax is still present, the tube should be replaced. This can often be done easily through the same incision. Irrigating an occluded chest tube or passing a Fogarty catheter through it in an effort to reestablish its patency seldom works well and almost certainly increases the risk of infection. If the chest tube is functional and well placed but a decubitus film shows a shift of some of the pleural fluid, the hemothorax is partially clotted; another chest tube placed with ultrasound guidance may be helpful. If a significant hemothorax persists, early evacuation of the clotted blood via thoracoscopy can prevent atelectasis.

If a chest tube is inserted because of a pneumothorax, it is left in place on suction for at least 24 h after all air leaks have stopped. If inserted for bleeding, it is left in place until the drainage is serous and less than 100 mL/24 h. However, if the patient is on a ventilator, many physicians would prefer to keep the chest tubes in case a new pneumothorax suddenly develops.

When the tube is to be removed, the patient is asked to take a deep breath and bear down, as in a Valsalva maneuver. While intrathoracic pressure and lung volume are at their maximum, the tube is quickly pulled out and petrolatum (Vaseline) gauze is immediately applied as an airtight dressing over the chest tube site. It is important that the patient be in full inspiration when the tube is pulled. The involuntary reflex while the tube is being pulled is a quick inspiratory effort because of the pleural pain. This may rapidly suck in several hundred milliliters of air just as the tube is being removed, necessitating reinsertion of another tube. Some surgeons put only one throw in their initial chest tube suture so that the ends can be unwound from the chest tube and then tied down to provide an airtight seal of the chest tube hole.

Following removal of the chest tube, a chest x-ray should be obtained to rule out a recurrent pneumothorax. Another chest x-ray should be obtained 12 to 24 h later to confirm continued complete expansion of the lungs.

Although there continues to be controversy about the need for prophylactic antibiotics in patients requiring a chest tube for a traumatic hemothorax and/or pneumothorax, a recent review by Wilson of the six available double-blind prospective studies showed a clear reduction in the incidence of pneumonia and/or empyema when antibiotics were given until the chest tubes were removed.[11] Studies suggest that giving antibiotics for just 24 h is adequate,[12] and one study suggests that only one dose of antibiotic need be given when thorecostomy tubes are required following penetrating trauma.[13]

AUTOTRANSFUSION In patients with massive bleeding into a body cavity, proper collection and autotransfusion of the shed blood may reduce the need for bank blood and its associated risks. Intrathoracic bleeding is generally ideal for this technique, because there is usually no contamination of the blood by bile or intestinal contents.

To use shed blood for autotransfusion, one adds citrate or heparin to it as it is removed (to keep it from clotting) and collects it in a special sterile container. The red blood cells are then usually washed with saline. Autotransfused blood can greatly reduce many of the risks of blood transfusion, but, in emergency situations, attempts at autotransfusion can be time-consuming and difficult. The suction used for collecting blood for autotransfusion is also not as efficient as the regular suction for keeping the operative field clear. As a consequence, if adequate type-specific blood is readily available, many centers make little effort to use autotransfusions. Furthermore, using more than five units of autotransfused blood may contribute to a tendency to a coagulopathy. If the cells are washed in a cell saver, more autotransfused blood can be given safely, but there is still some concern about the development of a coagulopathy. Generally it is easier and much faster to use bank blood unless (1) the bleeding is massive and not rapidly controllable by surgery, (2) the blood type is rare, and/or (3) there is difficulty with the cross-matching.

THORACOTOMY Most patients with intrathoracic bleeding can be treated adequately by intravenous administration of fluids and evacuation of the hemothorax with a chest tube. Fewer than 5 percent will require operative management. Massive hemothorax mandates operation. (See earlier discussion.) Selection of management approach must be made by a qualified surgeon in the context of available resources.

Occasionally, when the chest tube is initially inserted, blood emerges at an alarmingly rapid rate. If the patient's condition improves as the blood is being removed, continuing drainage of the blood and observation of the patient are in order. However, if the patient's vital signs deteriorate as the blood is being removed, loss of the tamponading effect of the hemothorax has probably allowed serious bleeding from the lung to recur. Consequently, the patient should be taken directly to surgery.

PNEUMOTHORAX **Pathophysiology** Collections of air or blood within the pleural cavity reduce vital capacity and increase intrathoracic pressure, thereby decreasing minute ventilation and venous return to the heart. During inspiration, the negative intrapleural pressure increases the tendency for air or blood to leak into the pleural cavity through any wound in the lung or chest wall. If there is any obstruction of the upper airway or if the patient has chronic obstructive lung disease, additional air may be forced into the pleural cavity during expiration, increasing the likelihood of tension pneumothorax with intrapleural pressures exceeding atmospheric pressure.

Diagnosis Failure to obtain a chest x-ray soon after admission and again in 4 to 8 h may result in missing significant intrathoracic injuries. The presence of a chest injury is usually readily apparent from the history and physical examination; however, accurate assessment of the damage, especially to intrathoracic organs, often requires serial chest x-rays and/or a CT scan.

A pneumothorax is not likely to cause severe symptoms unless it (1) is a tension pneumothorax, (2) occupies more than 40 percent of one hemithorax, or (3) occurs in a patient with shock or preexisting cardiopulmonary disease. If there is a suspicion of a pneumothorax but it is not clearly seen on the first chest roentgenogram, repeat films during expiration may be helpful. Apical-lordotic films may allow better visualization of an apical pneumothorax. Occasionally, a pneumothorax after a stab wound is delayed for more than 12 h. Consequently, serial chest x-rays every 6 h for 12 to 24 h are indicated in selected patients. In a recent study of 4106 patients with initially asymptomatic stab wounds of the chest, Ordog et al found that 12 percent of the patients required a tube thoracostomy for a delayed hemothorax or pneumothorax.[14] Current accepted practice is to observe the patient and repeat the film in 6 h. If no pneumothorax is noted on the repeat film, and there are no other concerns, the patient can be discharged.

One should assume that a tension pneumothorax is present and begin treatment without waiting for a chest x-ray if the patient has (1) severe respiratory distress, (2) decreased breath sounds and hyperresonance on one side of the chest, (3) distended neck veins, and (4) deviation of the trachea away from the involved side. Insertion of a large needle into the involved side through the second intercostal space in the midclavicular line may help confirm the diagnosis and provide temporary relief while a chest tube is inserted.

A small pneumothorax (less than 1.0 cm wide and confined to the upper one-third of the chest) that is unchanged on two chest roentgenograms taken 4 to 6 h apart in an otherwise healthy individual can usually be treated by observation alone. However, in most instances after trauma, a chest tube or small catheter should be inserted as a precautionary measure, especially if the patient cannot continue to be observed closely.

Occasionally a small pneumothorax is not apparent on chest x-rays but is seen on a CT scan of the chest or abdomen. This is referred to as an *occult pneumothorax.* Chest tube drainage of an occult pneumothorax is not required unless the patient is going to be on a ventilator.[15,16]

If only a pneumothorax is present, a small- to moderate-sized (24F to 28F) chest tube may be inserted anteriorly in the second intercostal space in the midclavicular line. However, a high midaxillary tube is generally preferable. Although some physicians insert chest tubes over trocars because it is less painful, especially if the lung is well away from the chest wall, we believe it is safer to avoid the trocar and insert chest tubes using a large hemostat. Catheter aspiration of a simple pneumothorax (CASP) is most suitable for the treatment of pneumothoraces caused by needles or catheters.

Complications In general, a small- or moderate-sized pneumothorax does not cause problems unless there is a continuing air leak or the patient has other trauma or preexisting cardiopulmonary disease. Also, a continuing air leak does not usually result in complications if the lung is completely expanded. However, if a combination of a pneumothorax and continued air leak is allowed to exist for more than 24 to 48 h, the incidence of empyema and bronchopleural fistula is greatly increased.

The most frequent reasons for failure to evacuate a pneumothorax rapidly and to completely expand the lungs are (1) improper connections or leaks in the external tubing or water-seal collection apparatus, (2) improper position of the chest tube(s), (3) occlusion of bronchi by secretions or a foreign body, (4) a tear of one of the large bronchi, or (5) a large tear of the lung parenchyma. If a pneumothorax persists in spite of one or two well-placed chest tubes and there is a large leak, emergency bronchoscopy should be performed to clear the bronchi and identify any damage to the tracheobronchial tree that may need repair. Continued large air leakage and failure of the lung to expand adequately in spite of these measures is an indication for early thoracotomy to control the air leak.

PNEUMOMEDIASTINUM Subcutaneous emphysema in the neck should make one look closely for a pneumomediastinum. The diagnosis of pneumomediastinum should also be suspected from the presence of a crunching sound (Hamman sign) over the heart during systole. The diagnosis is usually readily apparent on CT scans, but it can easily be missed on chest x-rays. Traumatic pneumomediastinum is of itself usually asymptomatic, but one must look closely for an injury to the larynx, trachea, major bronchi, pharynx, or esophagus.

PULMONARY HEMATOMAS Pulmonary hematomas are parenchymal tears filled with blood. These generally resolve spontaneously over a few weeks; however, if they become infected, they can form lung abscesses that may be very difficult to manage. These hematomas are more likely to become infected if a thoracotomy is performed, if there is prolonged chest tube drainage of the pleural cavity, and/or if prolonged ventilatory assistance is required.

PULMONARY LACERATIONS WITH HEMOPNEUMOTHORAX Major hemorrhage from lacerations of the lung following blunt trauma are usually caused by the sharp ends of fractured ribs. Occasionally, they may be caused by tearing of the lung at pleural adhesions during rapid deceleration injuries. Rarely, the adhesions themselves are quite vascular, and a torn adhesion will bleed enough to cause shock.

SYSTEMIC AIR EMBOLISM In patients with penetrating chest wounds, and particularly those with hemoptysis, positive-pressure ventilation must be used with great care. High ventilatory pressures, especially over 50 cmH_2O, may force air from an injured bronchus into an adjacent injured vessel, producing systemic air emboli. This probably accounts for many of the severe dysrhythmias or central nervous system (CNS) changes that occur when patients with penetrating chest wounds are intubated and ventilated. One should be particularly concerned about causing systemic air emboli if the patient has hemoptysis.

If systemic air embolism occurs, the head should be lowered, and an immediate thoracotomy should be performed to clamp the injured area of lung and then aspirate air from the heart and ascending aorta. Open cardiac massage with clamping of the ascending aorta may help push air through the coronary arteries. Cardiopulmonary bypass should be instituted promptly if available.

INTRABRONCHIAL BLEEDING Intrabronchial bleeding is poorly tolerated and can rapidly cause death from severe hypoxemia by flooding dependent alveoli. Patients with intrabronchial blood tend to die from ''drowning'' rather than from hypovolemia.

In patients with hemoptysis due to trauma, the uninvolved lung should be kept as free of blood as possible and nasotracheal suction and bronchoscopy used as often as necessary. If the bleeding is severe, a double-lumen endotracheal (Carlen) tube can sometimes be used to confine the bleeding to one lung. If a Carlen or similar split-function tube is not available or cannot be inserted, one may insert an endotracheal tube over a flexible bronchoscope into the bleeding main-stem bronchus. The balloon on the endotracheal tube can then be inflated as needed. If the bleeding is from the intubated lung, the endotracheal tube prevents blood from passing into the other lung, and ventilation of the other lung may then be maintained either spontaneously or via a mask or another endotracheal tube.

In some instances, the bleeding can only be controlled by occluding the involved bronchus with a Fogarty balloon catheter or by packing it with gauze until the bleeding site can be controlled surgically.

ASPIRATION Aspiration of gastric contents is quite common after severe trauma, especially if the patient is unconscious. If it is recognized promptly, immediate bronchoscopy should be performed to remove any residual food particles. Immediate irrigation of the tracheobronchial tree with buffered saline or a bicarbonate solution may also help reduce the severity of the chemical pneumonitis, but the value of such irrigation is controversial.

Radiologic changes are usually delayed for more than 12 to 24 h. If an opaque foreign body is aspirated into the tracheobronchial tree, it is usually readily diagnosed on x-ray. However, radiolucent foreign bodies are easily missed. Inspiratory and expiratory chest films may help diagnosis of a one-way valve effect due to a foreign body by demonstrating failure of one lung to empty properly during expiration. Occasionally, a foreign body can remain lodged in various bronchi, causing repeated pulmonary infections or hemoptysis for years before being discovered. Persistent or recurrent cough, atelectasis, or pneumonia after trauma should be indications for bronchoscopy and/or bronchography.

Tracheobronchial Injury

LOWER TRACHEA AND MAJOR BRONCHI Most injuries to major bronchi are due to rapid deceleration and shearing of more mobile bronchi from relatively fixed proximal structures. However, forced expiration against a closed glottis and/or compression against the vertebral column may cause bursting of these structures.

Numerous reports have emphasized that the most common presenting signs and symptoms are dyspnea, hemoptysis, subcutaneous emphysema, Hamman sign, and sternal tenderness. A large pneumothorax, pneumomediastinum, deep cervical emphysema, and an endotracheal tube balloon with a round appearance on chest roentgenograms may suggest tracheobronchial injury; however, approximately 10 percent are almost completely asymptomatic.

Most tracheobronchial injuries occur within 2 cm of the carina or at the origin of lobar bronchi. On bronchoscopy, the usual bronchial injury seen is a transverse tear in a main bronchus or a disruption at the origin of an upper lobe bronchus. The characteristic injury in the trachea is a vertical tear in the membranous portion near its attachment to the tracheal cartilages.

Even if the lung expands and the air leak stops, lacerations of the bronchi involving more than a third of the circumference should be repaired because they tend to eventually cause severe bronchial stenosis with repeated pulmonary infections or complete atelectasis. Untreated tracheal tears may result in severe mediastinitis.

The majority of airway injuries can be corrected using standard techniques. With complex ruptures, cardiopulmonary bypass can provide safety during correction of the lesion and may encourage repair of the involved lung rather than its resection.

Those patients who survive a tracheal transection generally have their injury in the cervical trachea and have no associated injuries. Intrathoracic tracheal transection is usually associated with two or more major injuries and is almost invariably fatal. Concurrent esophageal injuries occur in almost 25 percent of penetrating tracheobronchial injuries and are easily missed unless esophagoscopy or contrast studies are also performed.

CERVICAL TRACHEAL INJURIES Injuries to the cervical trachea from blunt trauma usually occur at the junction of the trachea and cricoid cartilage. This is most frequently caused when the anterior neck strikes the dashboard in an automobile accident. Evidence of trauma to the neck with subcutaneous emphysema should arouse suspicion of this injury. Inspiratory stridor usually indicates a 70 to 80 percent upper airway obstruction. However, cricotracheal separation is often only suspected when an endotracheal tube or bronchoscope cannot be inserted past the cricoid cartilage.

If the patient has a laceration of the trachea that is small and high, it may be managed simply by performing a tracheostomy below the injury. All lacerations of the trachea should be repaired.

Diaphragmatic Injury

ETIOLOGY In urban centers, diaphragmatic injuries are caused most frequently by penetrating trauma, particularly gunshot wounds of the lower chest or upper abdomen. Rupture due to blunt trauma is much less frequent and occurs in only 4 to 5 percent of patients hospitalized with chest trauma. If there is a fracture of the pelvis, the incidence increases to about 8 to 10 percent.

Because of the protective effect of the liver on the right and the possible increased weakness of the left posterolateral diaphragm, most series report that 80 to 90 percent of the diaphragmatic injuries following blunt trauma occur in that area. However, in the series of Brown and Richardson,[17] the incidence of right- and left-sided diaphragmatic rupture was almost equal.

NATURAL HISTORY Since 60 to 70 percent of normal ventilation depends on proper function of the diaphragm, trauma to this structure can cause serious ventilatory problems. However, the initial signs and symptoms are often masked by other injuries. Unless the diaphragmatic lesion is large, symptoms due to abdominal viscera in the thoracic cavity usually occur rather late. Over time, sometimes even years, a large amount of viscera can gradually work up into the chest through small diaphragmatic tears. The intrathoracic bowel may then become obstructed or strangulated or cause severe compression of the adjacent lung, a phenomenon we have referred to as *tension enterothorax.*

DIAGNOSIS With penetrating trauma, the diagnosis of diaphragmatic injury is often made only intraoperatively. However, if the entrance wound is in the abdomen and there is evidence of an intrathoracic injury or foreign body, one can assume that the missile or knife has traversed the diaphragm. In the series just mentioned, 59 percent of the patients with diaphragmatic injuries had diagnostic chest x-rays. However, eight of nine peritoneal lavages done in these patients were negative. In the only positive lavage, the lavage fluid drained out through a previously placed chest tube.

With blunt trauma, any abnormality of the diaphragm or lower lung fields on chest x-ray should arouse suspicion of a diaphragmatic tear. Occasionally a nasogastric tube is seen to go into the abdomen and then back up into the chest because the stomach has passed through a diaphragmatic tear.

Techniques for diagnosing the less obvious diaphragmatic injuries include (1) peritoneal lavage with a chest tube in place; (2) upper gastrointestinal (GI) series, looking for displacement of viscera into the chest; (3) pneumoperitoneum with carbon dioxide; (4) CT scan with contrast; and (5) intraperitoneal technetium sulfur colloid. However, up to 50 percent of diaphragmatic injuries are diagnosed only during a thoracotomy or laparotomy.

Subtle diaphragmetic injuries can be difficult to diagnose, particularly on the right. Axial CT scans that are virtually tangent to areas at risk are difficult to interpret unless there is herniation of abdominal contents through the defect. The advent of laparoscopy has provided a new, useful tool for identifying the smaller injuries, and this may well be the diagnostic mode of choice for patients who have no other indications for laparotomy. Caution should be exercised, since insufflated gas can leak from the abdomen across a violated diaphragm and cause acute cardiorespiratory embarassment.

THERAPY Laparotomy is necessary to repair the diaphragm. Thoracotomy may be necessary for associated chest injury, resuscitation, delayed repair of the diaphragm, or management of thoracic complications. Recently there have been several reports of repair using thoracoscopy techniques.

HEART

Penetrating Injury to the Heart

The many factors affecting survival from penetrating injury to the heart include the weapon used, the size of the myocardial injury, the injured cardiac chamber, coronary artery damage, the presence of tamponade, associated injuries, and the time taken to reach the hospital. Every patient with penetrating chest injury anywhere near the heart and shock on admission should be considered as having a cardiac injury until proven otherwise. The converse is not true, since about one-third of patients who arrive in an ED alive and are subsequently proven to have a penetrating cardiac wound have near-normal vital signs.

With early aggressive resuscitation and surgery, up to one-third of patients arriving in a trauma center in extremis with a cardiac injury can be saved. In patients brought to the operating room with signs of life and a recordable blood pressure, the survival rate should exceed 70 percent for gunshot wounds and 85 percent for stab wounds.

Prognosis in penetrating cardiac injury correlates with cardiovascular status on presentation. Those patients who reach the ED with near-normal vital signs typically have good outcomes, while few who lose signs of life during transport or on arrival to the ED survive with intact neurologic function. Patients who have no signs of life ''in the field'' are not candidates for resuscitative efforts.

PATHOPHYSIOLOGY Penetrating wounds of the heart are usually rapidly fatal, generally because of massive hemorrhage; fewer than one-fourth of the patients with this injury reach the hospital alive. Patients surviving more than 15 to 30 min usually have either a small wound or some component of pericardial tamponade. In a sense, pericardial tamponade is a two-edged sword; although it may prolong life by reducing the initial blood loss, the tamponade itself can be fatal by interfering with diastolic filling of the heart.

DIAGNOSIS **Clinical Features** All patients in shock with a penetrating wound of the chest between the midclavicular line on the right and the anterior axillary line on the left should be considered to have a cardiac injury until proven otherwise. If the only problem is tamponade and the patient is not hypovolemic, Beck's triad may be present. This consists of distended neck veins, hypotension, and muffled heart tones. The last is the least reliable sign; even with a large acute pericardial tamponade, which seldom is more than 200 mL, the heart tones are usually fairly clear.

Since patients with penetrating heart wounds are usually hypotensive, the neck veins will generally not distend until the blood volume is at least partially restored. On the other hand, chest injuries can cause the patient to breathe abnormally or strain, thereby causing neck vein distention even in the absence of tamponade. Other causes of Beck's triad include tension pneumothorax, myocardial dysfunction, and systemic air embolism.

Tamponade may also cause two Kussmaul signs. One is increased distention of neck veins during inspiration and the other is pulsus paradoxus. Paradoxical pulse is characterized by a drop in systolic blood pressure of more than 10 to 15 mmHg during normal spontaneous inspiration. The amount of paradox may be increased by hypovolemia.

Invasive Monitoring While the obstruction to cardiac venous return is usually evident on physical examination and by the finding of distended neck veins, occasionally a central venous catheter may be required to confirm the elevated central venous pressure in the setting of hypoperfusion. Patients in extremis should undergo diagnostic pericardiocentesis in lieu of central venous pressure following insertion of a central venous catheter.

X-Rays The pericardium is noncompliant. Whereas an obviously globular cardiac silhouette may suggest tamponade as the cause of hypoperfusion, the converse is not true: most patients with tamponade have very ordinary-appearing cardiac silhouettes.

Electrocardiography Electrocardiography (ECG) changes following cardiac injury are usually nonspecific. ST-T wave changes may indicate pericardial irritation or may reflect associated ischemia or hypoxia.

Echocardiography Transthoracic echocardiography (TTE) performed by both emergency physicians and trauma surgeons has been shown to be successful in the detection of pericardial fluid.[18–20] Accordingly, TTE is now frequently used in penetrating chest trauma for the evaluation of potential cardiac tamponade. It has been shown that TTE performed in the ED results in more rapid diagnosis, faster time to surgical intervention, as well as improved survival and neurologic outcome.[19] The presence of a hemothorax may limit the ability of TTE to detect occult cardiac injuries;[21] however, there are methods to distinguish hemothorax from pericardial fluid by using different views.

Echocardiography can identify pericardial fluid and may help localize missile fragments in the pericardium. While TTE remains a mainstay of rapid assessment and diagnosis, emergency physicians practicing in trauma centers will periodically encounter critically ill patients for whom the diagnosis of cardiac injury must be excluded while a series of other injuries are being addressed. In experienced hands, transesophageal echocardiography (TEE) is an efficient diagnostic tool, particularly if the patient is already intubated and ventilated and the probe can be inserted quickly.

Pericardiocentesis ACCURACY There is an increasing tendency to avoid the use of pericardiocentesis as a diagnostic procedure in acutely injured patients with possible tamponade. In Demetriades' series, the incidence of false-negative pericardiocentesis was 80 percent and the incidence of false-positives was 33 percent.[13] In addition to its inaccuracy, attempts at pericardiocentesis may injure the heart or cause dangerous delays in needed surgery.

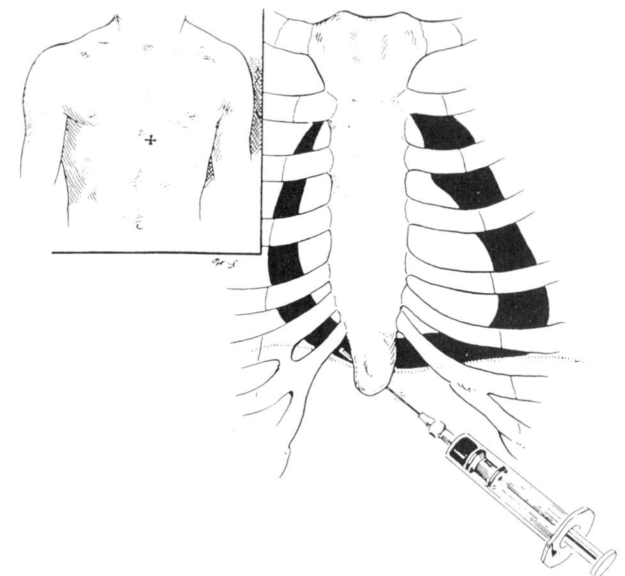

FIG. 251-3. The paraxiphoid technique for pericardiocentesis is usually performed with the needle directed toward the left shoulder or left scapula tip. *However,* if one aims toward the tip of the right scapula, the needle tends to go parallel to the lateral border of the right heart and is less apt to penetrate the coronary artery or myocardium. [From Wilson RF: Injury to the heart and great vessels, in Henning RS (ed): *Critical Care Cardiology.* New York: Churchill Livingstone, 1989, with permission.]

TECHNIQUE The paraxiphoid approach is commonly used. An 18-gauge, 10-cm spinal needle is attached to a stopcock and then to a 20-mL syringe. The pericardiocentesis should be done with continuous ECG monitoring if possible. The ECG monitoring is more sensitive if one attaches the V lead of the ECG to the metal pericardiocentesis needle using an insulated wire with alligator clips on both ends.

The needle is passed upward and backward at an angle of 45° for 4 to 5 cm and advanced slowly until the point seems to enter a cavity (Fig. 251-3). Most authors direct the needle toward the left scapula tip; however, directing the needle toward the right scapula is more likely to parallel the right border of the heart and is less likely to penetrate the right ventricle.

One should aspirate every 1 to 2 mm as the needle is advanced. One can insert a stylet or inject 0.5 to 1.0 mL of saline solution at intervals to be certain that the needle is not plugged. The needle is then carefully advanced until blood is obtained, cardiac pulsations are felt, or the ECG shows an abrupt change.

Generally, a large portion of the blood in the pericardial cavity is clotted. Consequently, one can usually remove only a few milliliters of blood without manipulating the needle. If 20 mL of blood can be drawn out easily and rapidly, it usually indicates that the blood is being aspirated from the right ventricle.

If an immediate thoracotomy is not possible in a patient with a positive pericardiocentesis, a plastic catheter (inserted over a needle or Seldinger wire) can be left in place for continuous drainage of intrapericardial blood until the cardiac wound can be surgically repaired.

COMPLICATIONS The pericardiocentesis needle can perforate the right ventricle as a coronary artery and cause tamponade as a consequence of the procedure itself. Dysrhythmias may also occur. A falsely negative pericardiocentesis may delay needed surgery.

Subxiphoid Pericardial Windows If the patient has been hemodynamically stable and echocardiography is either not available or equivocal, an alternative method for diagnosing pericardial tamponade is a subxiphoid pericardial window. Although this can occasionally be performed under local anesthesia in the ED in a cooperative patient, it is best done in the operating room under general anesthesia. If blood is found in the pericardium, the incision can be extended up as a median sternotomy to repair the cardiac wound.

TREATMENT **Fluid Replacement** It is essential that patients with penetrating wounds of the chest have two or more large intravenous lines in place, with at least one line in a leg vein in the event that the superior vena cava or one of its major branches is injured. It is particularly important to have an adequate or increased blood volume if hypovolemia or tamponade is present. If tamponade is present with an elevated central venous pressure, one should generally not be reluctant to administer further fluid and blood to improve venous return to the heart while moving the patient to an operating room.

Pericardiocentesis Pericardiocentesis can be both diagnostic and therapeutic. Patients who are in shock and may have a cardiac injury should have an emergency thoracotomy as soon as possible. If it is not possible to perform an emergency thoracotomy promptly, continuing pericardiocentesis to relieve the suspected tamponade should be attempted.

Removal of as little as 5 to 10 mL of blood from the pericardial sac may increase stroke volume by 25 to 50 percent, with a dramatic improvement in cardiac output and blood pressure. In patients who have small puncture wounds of the heart, pericardiocentesis may be curative, and thoracotomy may not be required as long as the vital signs remain stable for at least 24 to 48 h after the procedure.

Thoracotomy Occasionally, a highly selected, stable patient with a small penetrating cardiac injury, as by a needle or ice pick, may be successfully treated without surgery. However, all patients with hemodynamic instability and a suspected injury to the heart should have emergency thoracotomy.

INCISION For penetrating wounds over the precordium thought to involve the heart, an anterolateral thoracotomy is performed in the left fifth intercostal space, which is one interspace below the male nipple (Fig. 251-4). The incision should be as long as possible, extending from just lateral to the sternum to a point high in the axilla. In females, the breast is displaced upward, and the incision is made through the breast crease. The incision is extended through the intercostal muscle into the pleural cavity, with care taken not to injure the underlying lung or heart. A rib spreader is then inserted and opened widely so that two hands can fit inside the chest (Fig. 251-5). Cutting the intercostal cartilages above and below the incision may help increase the exposure. Not infrequently the internal mammary vessels, which lie about 0.5 to 1.0 cm lateral to the sternum, are cut; if so, they must be clamped and tied or suture-ligated.

When the injury is to the right of the sternum, a right thoracotomy is initially performed to control any bleeding sites, but strong consideration should be given to extending the incision across the sternum as a bilateral thoracotomy so as to be able to also control the descending aorta and, if needed, massage the heart directly. The sternum can be divided with a rib cutter. A bilateral anterolateral thoracotomy allows wide exposure of both sides of the heart and the proximal great vessels. In patients with a cardiac arrest, there is usually minimal bleeding from the thoracotomy incision until the circulation is restored. However, once circulation is restored, incisional bleeding may become quite severe, especially from the internal mammary arteries, which should be suture-ligated.

In hemodynamically stable patients with penetrating anterior chest trauma, a midsternotomy provides superior exposure for the organs most apt to be injured.[22] They feel that an anterolateral or lateral thoracotomy should be reserved for hemodynamically unstable pa-

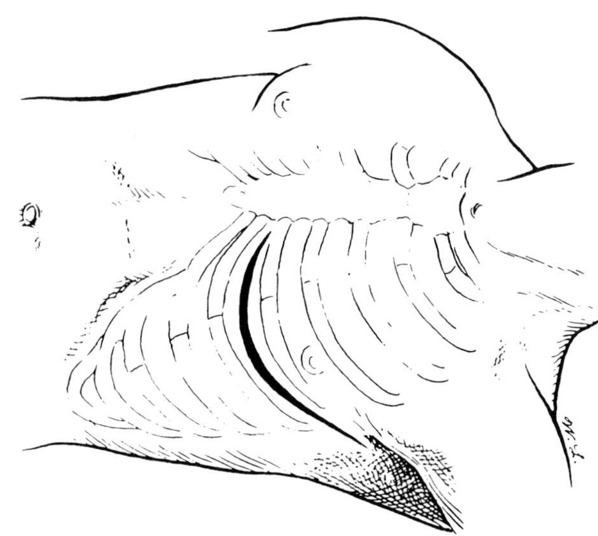

FIG. 251-4. Emergency thoracotomy to treat a stab wound of the heart or to perform open cardiac massage is usually done through an anterolateral thoracotomy approach. The incision extends along the fifth intercostal space with the skin incision placed in the inframammary crease. It extends from just lateral to the sternum to the midaxillary line. (From Geller ER: *Shock and Resuscitation.* New York: McGraw-Hill, 1993, with permission.)

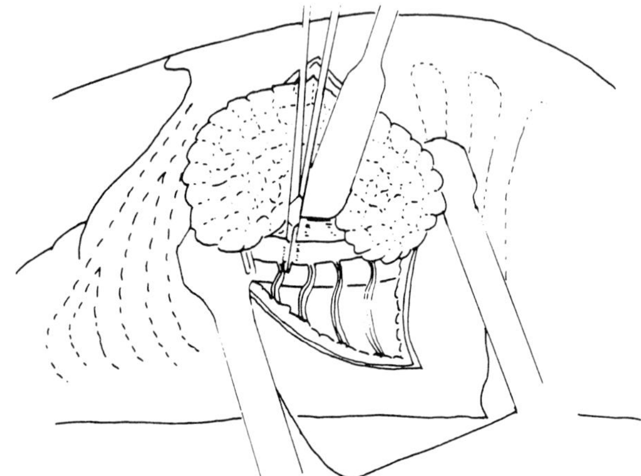

FIG. 251-5. If the descending thoracic aorta is to be cross-clamped, it is best done under direct vision. To accomplish this, the anterior thoracotomy must be large and the incision opened as widely as possible. The left lung is pulled up anteriorly as far as possible by an assistant standing at the right side of the table. The pleura and fascia anterior to the aorta are thin, but the tissue between the aorta and the vertebral column is often rather tough and must be incised to get around the aorta properly. A straight clamp is often easier to put around the aorta than a curved clamp and is less likely to rupture the intercostal vessels. (From Geller ER: *Shock and Resuscitation.* New York: McGraw-Hill, 1993, with permission.)

tients, or if posterior mediastinal injury is suspected or aortic cross-clamping is apt to be needed.

PERICARDIOTOMY Even when the pericardial sac is not distended with blood, it can be difficult to grasp the pericardium with a forceps. It may be necessary at times to ''hook'' the pericardium with one blade of a scissors and then grab it with a forceps or clamp. Another technique is to very carefully incise the pericardium near the apex of the heart with a small-bladed knife to produce a hole just big enough to allow the tip of one blade of a scissors. If a scalpel is used to open the pericardial sac, inadvertent injury to the underlying myocardium or left anterior descending coronary artery can easily occur.

The pericardial sac should then be opened from the diaphragm below to the great vessels above with a scissors in a longitudinal direction 1 to 2 cm anterior to the left (or right) phrenic nerve. If the pericardial sac is still tight around the heart, a transverse cut of the anterior pericardium just above the central diaphragm may greatly help with exposure. The liquid blood and clots in the pericardial sac should then be manually evacuated and cardiac massage initiated if needed.

CLAMPING THE DESCENDING AORTA The second maneuver in the patient with severe hypotension or a cardiac arrest is compression or clamping of the descending thoracic aorta to help improve coronary and cerebral arterial flow. Since more than 60 percent of the cardiac output goes through the descending thoracic aorta, cross-clamping of this vessel can increase blood flow to the coronary and cerebral arteries two- to threefold.

To expose the descending aorta, an assistant on the right side of the patient lifts the left lung anteriorly, almost out of the hemithorax, so that the aorta can be seen from the left side of the table. The pleura and fascia in front of the aorta are easily opened, but the tougher posterior tissue between the aorta and the vertebral bodies often has to be incised sharply.

After the aorta has been exposed, a finger or a vascular clamp can be hooked around it. In this way, clamping is performed under direct vision, and the chances of intercostal or esophageal injuries are reduced. To be sure that the clamp is applied properly, one should feel pulsations from the spontaneous heartbeat or cardiac massage above the clamp but none below. If a nasogastric tube is not in place and there is little or no blood pressure, it is possible that the esophagus was mistaken for the aorta. After the clamp is applied, the time is noted, and the left lung is allowed to drop back into the thorax.

CLAMPING INJURED LUNG If there is an obvious associated lung injury, it should be controlled with a vascular clamp or a lung clamp to prevent systemic air embolism and stop the bleeding and air leak until more definitive control can be accomplished. If there is a large central lung injury, one should put a clamp across the hilum. If the hilar clamp does not control the bleeding because the injury is too close to the heart, one may have to clamp the pulmonary vessels inside the pericardium.

EXAMINING THE HEART If the bleeding site(s) is (are) not obvious, one should first carefully examine the right ventricle and right atrium, which are the chambers most apt to be injured. If an injury is still not seen, the heart can be swung out laterally and anteriorly into the left hemithorax to allow better examination of the remainder of the heart. When examining the posterior heart, one should be very careful because lifting the heart straight up increases the possibility of entry of air into a left-sided or posterior cardiac perforation, and this could result in sudden fatal coronary or cerebral air embolism.

CONTROLLING CARDIAC WOUNDS Most atrial wounds can be controlled by the application of a Satinsky vascular clamp and then sewn with a running 3–0 or 4–0 polypropylene suture. Traditionally, wounds of the ventricles can generally be tamponaded by the operator's finger while pledgeted horizontal mattress sutures of 2–0 silk or Prolene are passed under the finger and tied by an assistant. However, given the uncontrolled setting and poor visualization, this procedure can only be considered of the highest risk for needle-stick injury and potential exposure to blood-borne infections. Thus, other techniques described below should be used. When a wound lies next to a major coronary artery, mattress sutures are placed beneath the artery so as to avoid ligation or compression of the vessel. Cardiac stapling can also be highly effective in the initial management of simple penetrating cardiac wounds.

For handling more difficult cardiac wounds, several other techniques are available. The insertion of a 5- or 30-mL balloon Foley catheter into a large or inaccessible (posterior) defect may allow for control of hemorrhage until a purse-string suture can be applied around the hole. Use of such a catheter also allows one to infuse fluids very rapidly, directly into the heart.

Wide horizontal mattress sutures placed on either side of a large defect and pulled together can also be used to control hemorrhage until cardiopulmonary bypass can be instituted. If cardiopulmonary bypass is not readily available, occlusion of the superior vena cava and inferior vena cava by vascular tapes or clamps can allow quick repair of large defects without causing exsanguinating hemorrhage. Before restarting the heart, if the caval occlusion technique is used, all air is evacuated from the various cardiac chambers by allowing bleeding through the injury prior to tying the final suture and then inserting large needles into the apex of the right and left ventricles while the heart is cautiously massaged.

CARDIAC MASSAGE Once cardiorrhaphy had been completed, internal cardiac massage can be performed as needed by compressing the heart between the palms of two hands or between one palm and the sternum. Warm—preferably 40 to 42.2°C (104 to 108°F)—saline solution poured over the heart may help prevent ventricular fibrillation. If ventricular fibrillation occurs, defibrillation with internal paddles, starting at 20 to 40 W/s should be performed. Lidocaine (1 mg/kg), correction of severe acidosis or alkalosis, and intravenous infusions of 1 to 2 g of $MgSO_4$ may help prevent recurrent ventricular fibrillation.

AIR EMBOLISM If severe dysrhythmia or cardiac arrest develops during endotracheal intubation or while the chest is being opened, aspiration of the cardiac chambers for air should be performed immediately. Systemic air embolism is most frequently diagnosed by seeing air bubbles in the coronary arteries. This serious complication is seldom mentioned in the literature but is seen in about 20 percent of patients with penetrating truncal trauma who have a cardiac arrest in the ED after endotracheal intubation. Patients rarely survive this complication.

CONTINUED CARE Once the heart develops a satisfactory rhythm, the descending thoracic aorta is gradually declamped as infusions of fluid and blood are administered, with care taken to keep the systolic blood pressure above 90 to 100 mmHg. One should also avoid systolic blood pressures greater than 160 to 180 mmHg because they may tear open cardiac repairs, excessively dilate the left ventricle, and/or cause intracerebral bleeding. The use of vigorous inotropes, such as epinephrine, should be particularly avoided at this point, as they may cause sudden, severe hypertension and can also increase the risk of recurrent ventricular fibrillation.

After the cardiac wounds and all bleeding vessels are controlled and an adequate cardiac output has been obtained, all clot is washed out of the pericardial and pleural cavities. One must look closely to make sure that the internal mammary arteries are intact or carefully suture-ligated. If the heart is edematous or dilated, the pericardium can be left open. Occasionally, the sternum cannot even be closed. In such instances, the skin can usually be stapled. The sternum can then be closed after several days when the cardiac edema and dilatation have resolved.

CORONARY ARTERY INJURIES Ligation of the cut ends is the treatment of choice for lacerations of small coronary vessels. Torn proximal coronary arteries may also be ligated if there is no evidence of cardiovascular dysfunction. However, such patients must be observed closely. If a large proximal coronary artery laceration results in dysrhythmias, myocardial infarction, or impaired hemodynamic function, an aortocoronary revascularization with a saphenous vein graft should be performed under cardiopulmonary bypass.

Blunt Injury to the Heart

ETIOLOGY AND MECHANISMS OF INJURY The most common cause of blunt cardiac trauma is a high-speed motor vehicle accident. However, myocardial injury has been documented in accidents involving vehicles going less than 20 mph. Other causes include direct blows to the chest, industrial crush injuries, falls from heights, blast injuries, and athletic trauma.

The heart is suspended relatively freely within the chest cavity from the great vessels, and this mobility plus its location between the sternum and the thoracic vertebrae make it susceptible to injury as a result of several mechanisms: (1) sudden horizontal acceleration and/or deceleration, causing the heart to impact against the sternum and vertebrae; (2) a compression between the sternum and vertebrae following a direct forceful blow to the chest; (3) a sudden increase in intrathoracic and intracardiac pressures, causing disruption of the myocardium or cardiac valves; (4) a ''hydraulic ram effect,'' with compression of the abdomen forcibly displacing abdominal viscera against the heart with sudden great force; and (5) strenuous or prolonged cardiac massage, particularly if done through the intact chest wall.

TYPES OF INJURIES Blunt trauma to the heart can cause a wide spectrum of injuries, including (1) rupture of an outer chamber wall, with resulting death from tamponade or bleeding; (2) septal rupture; (3) valvular injuries, of which injury to the aortic valve is the most common; (4) direct myocardial injury (contusion); (5) laceration or thrombosis of coronary arteries; and (6) pericardial injury.

Some authors have stressed the differences between myocardial concussion and myocardial contusion. With myocardial concussion, there is no anatomic cellular injury, but there is some dysfunction, as demonstrated by abnormal wall motion studies. With contusion, there is an anatomic injury, as demonstrated either by elevated CPK-MB isoenzymes or by direct visualization at surgery of autopsy. Because these are difficult to distinguish, the term *blunt myocardial injury* (BMI) is often used (see below).

DIAGNOSTIC PROBLEMS Blunt cardiac trauma can be very difficult to detect at times. The victim may have experienced severe multiple-system trauma, and the presence of a cardiac injury may be overshadowed by other, more obvious injuries. In addition, the forces that produce blunt cardiac trauma may cause little or no external evidence of injury. Therefore, a history of moderate to severe chest or upper abdominal injury, even without abnormalities on physical examination, should make one suspect cardiac injury (Table 251-4).

TABLE 251-4 Clues to Diagnosis of Blunt Cardiac Injury

History
High-speed motor vehicle accident
Crushed steering wheel
Angina-like chest pain
Physical examination
Tachycardia out of proportion to other findings
Any dysrhythmia
Any part of Beck triad
Evidence of severe anterior chest injury
Any evidence of heart failure
Radiography
Fractured sternum or first two ribs
Widened pericardial silhouette
Laboratory
Elevated CPK-MB levels
ECG
Dysrythmias or conduction disturbance
Elevated ST segments
Other studies
Impaired motion of anterior heart on two-dimensional echocardiogram or radionuclide angiography
PA catheter monitoring showing elevated PAWP, low cardiac output, and/or poor response to fluid

BLUNT MYOCARDIAL INJURY **Terminology** There has been great confusion regarding the appropriate appellation for cardiac injuries related to blunt trauma. The terms *cardiac* (or *myocardial*) *contusion, cardiac* (or *myocardial*) *concussion, blunt myocardial injury,* and *blunt cardiac injury* have all been proposed. Certainly there is a spectrum of injuries to the heart for which the term *blunt cardiac injury* would be appropriate, if not very specific. *Myocardial concussion,* sometimes referred to as *commotio cordis,* suggests no obvious gross or microscopic pathology to explain the phenomenon. However, sudden death from dysrhythmia can occur. The initiating mechanism is usually from a sudden direct force to the chest, while an individual is participating in certain sports (e.g., karate, hockey, etc.).[23] The term *myocardial contusion,* although somewhat out of favor currently, may in fact have a pathologic definition (see below). The term *blunt myocardial injury* (BMI), a more encompassing term although not universally accepted, has come into vogue, since *myocardial contusion* rarely exists in the strictest sense but is often associated with other injuries (e.g., coronary artery thrombosis, infarction related to hypotension). Also, the underlying pathologic definition is less important than determining the cardiac risk profile of patients with blunt chest trauma.

Pathologic Changes The pathologic changes seen in the myocardium typically include subendocardial hemorrhage and a much larger area of focal myocardial edema, interstitial hemorrhage, and myocytolysis with infiltrates of polymorphonuclear leukocytes. The areas most frequently involved are (1) the anterior right ventricular wall, (2) the anterior interventricular septum, and (3) the anterior-apical left ventricle.

Additional myocardial injury may occur if there are concomitant intimal tears or compression from adjacent hemorrhage and edema. Indeed, some feel that much of the myocardial injury seen is due to redistribution of coronary blood flow. Very occasionally, transient hypotension may cause complete occlusion of a previously diseased coronary artery.

Usually there is complete clinical recovery with minimal residual scarring within 3 to 6 weeks of a myocardial contusion. However, in rare cases with severe transmural injury, a ventricular aneurysm may develop.

Physiologic Changes In addition to rhythm and conduction disturbances, some reduction in cardiac output can be found in most victims studied. The degree of cardiac depression is directly related to the mass of contused myocardium. Screening tests, such as the ECG and

CPK-MB isoenzymes, usually do not accurately indicate the severity of the injury, nor are they predictive of major morbidity or mortality.

Although there seems to be a great concern about making the diagnosis, most patients with myocardial contusions have relatively little problem. However, occasionally there is a problem with an dysrhythmia, especially premature ventricular contractions (PVCs), atrial fibrillation, or a conduction defect, or there is clinical evidence of heart failure. Such problems are most apt to occur in patients with: (1) preexisting cardiac disease, (2) prolonged general anesthetics, or (3) hypotension because of other injuries.

Diagnosis Methods to diagnose myocardial injury have long been controversial. The variation in sensitivity reported for the various diagnostic tests has two origins. First, the tests require subjective interpretation. Second, there is no "gold standard" for comparison. Overall, significant BMI is an unlikely injury. A recent meta-analysis of studies of blunt cardiac trauma revealed that less than 3 percent of over 2200 patients in 25 prospective studies developed a cardiac complication (defined as requiring treatment or intervention). Most of these were ECG abnormalities (ventricular ectopy, superventricular dysrhythmias, symptomatic bradycardia). The most frequent cardiac rhythm finding, sinus tachycardia, was not considered, as it never required any specific treatment. ECG abnormalities requiring treatment were independently associated with a cardiac complications.[24]

Since diagnostic criteria (and even terminology) have not enjoyed universal or even general agreement, the focus has appropriately become predicting the likelihood of adverse events.

CLINICAL FEATURES Any patient involved in a motor vehicle accident involving speeds exceeding 35 mph and having any chest symptoms or signs should be suspected of having a BMI. Rarely, a patient with BMI will have angina-like pain that is not relieved by nitroglycerin.

Tachycardia that is out of proportion to the degree of trauma or blood loss may be the first sign of a BMI. Occasionally, an irregular rhythm due to atrial fibrillation or multiple premature atrial or ventricular contractions may be noted. Differentiation from an acute myocardial infarction in older individuals may be difficult in the ED.

RADIOLOGIC EXAMINATION The chest x-ray has its greatest value in the recognition of associated injuries. The closest x-ray correlates of BMI are pulmonary contusion or fractures of the first two ribs, the clavicles, or the sternum. Sternal fractures were thought to have been of importance, but, as noted above, when isolated, they are rarely associated with injury.[7,8]

Acute cardiac decompensation may be diagnosed by x-ray evidence of acute pulmonary edema (if the left ventricle is involved) associated with a normal-sized heart. Cardiac tamponade usually does not cause an enlarged cardiac silhouette, but a widened azygos vein is suggestive of this diagnosis.

ELECTROCARDIOGRAPHY As with other tests, the potential value of the ECG is controversial. Suggestions have ranged from a single ED-based ECG to 72 h of continuous ECG monitoring. A recent study of 71 patients with blunt chest trauma (not requiring admission to an intensive care unit) revealed that the initial ECG was predictive of subsequent clinically significant ECG events. Still, an initially normal ECG does not exclude the development of a clinically significant cardiac event, since, most abnormalities will develop within 24 h.[25] The most frequent ECG abnormality is sinus tachycardia, although this finding does not suggest increased risk in and of itself. Significant ECG findings include injury pattern, tachydysrhythmias, ST-T wave abnormalities, and ectopy—particularly premature ventricular contractions.

One reasonable approach is to obtain an initial 12-lead ECG. If it is normal, then the patient must be monitored for 4 to 6 h. If there are no untoward events, patients can be safely discharged.[26] (Some authorities advocate no further monitoring.) If the ECG is abnormal but there is no hemodynamic instability, the patient should be admitted to a monitored setting, with the 12-lead ECG repeated in 24 h. Some authorities suggest an intervening ECG at 6 and 12 h. Hemodynamic instability suggests an aggressive diagnostic approach (see below). If, at any time, the ECG is abnormal (or changed) or if there is ectopy or dysrhythmia, cardiac monitoring should be continued and a cardiology consult obtained.

CARDIAC ENZYMES Initially there was considerable controversy regarding the value of CPK-MB determination. Its certainly appeared that CPK-MB determinations were of questionable value and likely only to confuse, as they appeared to be of insufficient specificity and sensitivity.[27] Further, elevated MB fractions in this setting do not correlate with the clinical course.

Determination of cardiac troponins has shown promise[28] (Fig. 251-6), has been advocated as a laboratory criterion, and has even been proposed as the "gold standard" for the diagnosis of BMI. These determinations have been shown to have greater specificity for myocardial injury than CK-MB or myoglobin. However, the issue at this time appears no clearer than it was for CK-MB. A recent study found that troponin T (TT) had a specificity of 91 percent in predicting clinically significant ECG changes among those with blunt thoracic trauma, but the sensitivity was only 27 percent.[25] The authors concluded that TT determinations were useful. Using different criteria for the diagnosis of "myocardial contusion" (rather than untoward events), another study found very similar sensitivity (31 percent) and specificity (91 percent), minimally better than CK-MB.[29] The authors of the latter study conclude that TT has no important diagnostic value. More recent work suggests the sequential TT and troponin I (TI) may improve predictability for adverse events and need for intensive monitoring.

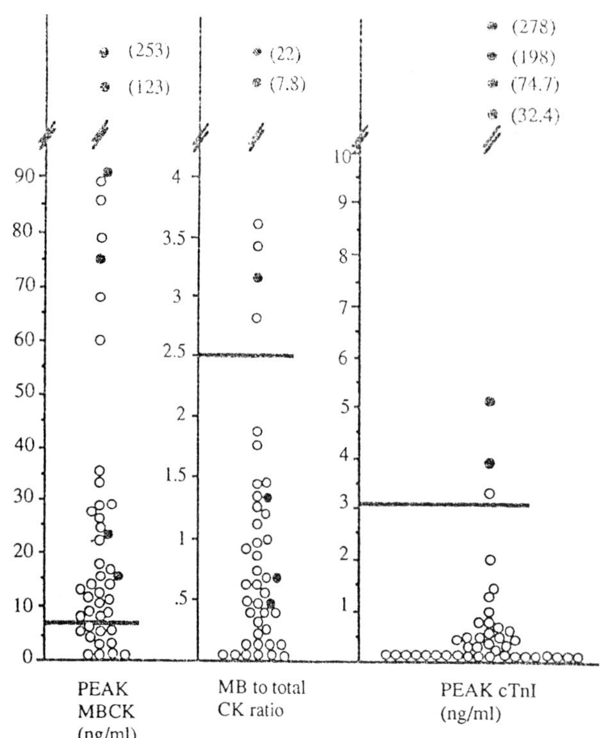

FIG. 251-6. Highest value of MBCK found *(peak)*, peak MBCK to total CK ratio, and highest value of cTnI. *Open circles* indicate patients without cardiac contusion; *solid circles* indicate those with contusion. *Heavy horizontal lines* indicate upper reference limits for each parameter. (From Adams et al,[28] reprinted with permission.)

There is intensive work in this area, but—as with other diagnostic tests—lack of agreement on definition or other end points; in the case of troponin, appropriate cutoff values and the type of assay used will continue to veil its potential usefulness.

ECHOCARDIOGRAPHY A recent detailed review concludes that echocardiography does not appear to be useful as a primary screening modality in the identification of patients likely to develop complications from myocardial injury.[30] It may well be the most sensitive test, but observed wall motion abnormalities often resolve and are usually clinically insignificant. However, patients who do develop cardiac complications may benefit from echocardiographic evaluation. Thus, the current recommendation is to use echocardiography in selected patients who demonstrate cardiac dysrhythmias or dysfunction.[31] While myocardial wall motion abnormalities may be present in stable patients with blunt chest trauma, this finding alone does not seem to predict the likelihood of a complication.

OTHER DIAGNOSTIC TESTS Technetium-labeled pyrophosphate scanning, thallium single-photon-emission computed tomography, and radionuclide angiography have all been controversially discussed in the literature. They do not appear to have any greater front-line diagnostic value than the diagnostic adjuncts already discussed.

Summary of Diagnostic Approach There is no consistent standard of care to advocate at this time. Certainly the trend toward identifying patients who require intensive monitoring or who are at higher risk for adverse events is better than trying to arrive at a diagnosis (BMI) that has poor clinical correlation. Certainly all patients should have a CXR. Any abnormalities found will help to stratify patients for risk and allow consideration of other diagnoses. All patients should have a 12-lead ECG and be initially monitored. A conservative practice would be to monitor all patients with significant chest wall trauma for up to 24 h, although, based on the current literature, 4- to 6-h of cardiac monitoring would be acceptable in patients who have been hemodynamically stable throughout. Patients with abnormal ECGs merit continued monitoring, serial 12-lead ECGs, and consideration for echocardiography. It is difficult to recommend outright the routine use of cardiac enzymes for screening purposes, although one cannot be faulted for considering cardiac troponin determination, particularly for delayed diagnosis. The reader is advised to stay abreast of this rapidly developing modality.

Patients with hemodynamic compromise at any time should not only be monitored in an intensive care unit setting, but also warrant echocardiography and a cardiac consultation for further diagnostic and therapeutic options.

Treatment Although some patients will require treatment of heart failure or rhythm or conduction disturbances, specific treatment interventions are seldom required. In general, blunt cardiac injuries cause death very rarely, as noted elsewhere,[24] and the incidence of clinically significant dysrhythmias or other cardiac complications is generally greatly overestimated.

Supplemental oxygen should be administered as needed to maintain the arterial P_{O_2} above 80 mmHg, and analgesics should be given as needed to reduce excessive pain. Coronary vasodilators should not be used unless the patient has suspected preexisting coronary artery disease. Cardiac dysrhythmias should be diagnosed early and treated appropriately. Prophylactic treatment of dysrhythmias is not indicated. Low cardiac output or hypotension should be treated with fluids or inotropic agents as indicated.

In the absence of dysrhythmias or hemodynamic instability, patients with BMI can safely undergo surgical procedures if the pulmonary artery wedge pressure and cardiac output are closely monitored.

If the patient remains in a low-output state despite adequate fluid resuscitation, inotropic support, and correction of any mechanical problems such as tamponade, use of an intraaortic balloon counterpulsation device should be considered.

There is some question as to whether patients with a myocardial contusion and an intramural thrombus seen on two-dimensional echocardiography should have prophylactic anticoagulation if not otherwise contraindicated. In limited studies, patients with echocardiographically proven right ventricular thrombi did not develop subsequent systemic or pulmonary embolization. Furthermore, anticoagulation is contraindicated in most cases of multiple trauma because of the potential for severe hemorrhage.

OTHER BLUNT CARDIAC INJURIES Cardiac rupture is the most frequent finding at autopsy in patients dying at the scene, and up to 90 percent with this injury die at the scene. Among those who reach the hospital, a few arrive seemingly stable. Most of these patients will deteriorate suddenly and resuscitation will most likely be unsuccessful. The diagnosis is suggested when shock is out of proportion to the degree of recognized injury despite attempts at hemorrhage control and volume repletion. Immediate thoracotomy and surgical repair is the only hope for a successful outcome.

Septal defects are rare but may be evident when a systolic murmur is heard and an infarct pattern is seen on the ECG. An ultrasound exam may also prove helpful. The diagnosis can be suspected when hypoxemia is severe with a normal CXR. Patients with atrial septal defects are unlikely to survive.

Rupture of the aortic valve is the most common valvular lesion found in patients who survive nonpenetrating cardiac injury. Patients with bioprosthetic heart valves are particularly likely to have traumatic valve injury. The next most frequent blunt valvular injury is laceration of a papillary muscle or the chordae tendineae of the mitral valve. The prognosis for rupture of a mitral papillary muscle or a mitral valve leaflet is grave, and death usually occurs within a few days after injury.

Direct injury to the coronary arteries from blunt chest trauma occurs very rarely, but if it causes pericardial tamponade or intrathoracic bleeding, immediate operation is required. Coronary artery thrombosis is also rare but has been reported. Coronary artery spasm does not appear to occur.

The incidence of major cardiac injury from blunt trauma resulting in cardiac tamponade or acute hemopericardium at autopsy has been reported to be about 6 percent. Hemopericardium or pericardial effusion with or without frank tamponade can occur without any evidence of blunt cardiac injury. This may develop acutely or may be delayed for more than a week. As with other causes of pericardial effusion, the rate of fluid accumulation is the main determinant of its hemodynamic consequences. In some instances, only echocardiography or autopsy provides the diagnosis. Small posttraumatic pericardial effusions can be seen with many cardiac injuries following blunt chest trauma but are usually of little or no consequence. They generally remain asymptomatic and resolve without any therapy. In rare instances, a patient may develop late constrictive pericarditis, occasionally with extensive calcification of the pericardium.

FOLLOW-UP It is important that patients with proven or suspected cardiac injury be closely observed, not only throughout their hospital stay but also later, for undiagnosed injuries or complications. One should look particularly for posttraumatic pericarditis, ventricular septal defect, valvular defects, and ventricular aneurysms.

POSTPERICARDIOTOMY SYNDROME **Etiology and Pathogenesis** The cause of the postpericardiotomy syndrome (PPCS) is still largely unknown, but it may be a delayed hypersensitivity reaction to the presence of damaged myocardium in the pericardial cavity. This damaged tissue can act as a foreign protein, inducing the production of autoantibodies against similar tissues. In fact, antimyocardial antibodies can be measured, and their serum concentration varies with the severity of the symptoms. Autogenous blood and lipids in the pericardium can also set up an inflammatory response that may be a contributing factor.

Diagnosis PPCS should be suspected in individuals who develop chest paint, fever, and pleural or pericardial effusions 2 to 4 weeks after cardiac trauma (or heart surgery). Patients may also have friction rubs, arthralgia, and pulmonary infiltrates. The blood count often shows a leukocytosis, and the ECG will often show ST-T wave changes consistent with pericarditis.

Treatment Treatment is primarily symptomatic. Salicylates and rest can often reduce symptoms dramatically within 12 to 24 h, but glucocorticoids are occasionally required. Rarely, drainage of pleural or pericardial fluid may be required to relieve symptoms or rule out other problems.

GREAT VESSELS OF THE CHEST

Penetrating Trauma

Of the patients who reach the hospital with penetrating chest wounds and require admission, only 5 to 15 percent require a thoracotomy, but up to 25 percent of the patients having such surgery have an injury to a great vessel. The survival rate with stab wounds is generally much higher than with gunshot wounds. Small knife wounds are often rapidly sealed off by surrounding tissue, especially vascular adventitia. This limits the amount of blood loss, particularly after hypotension develops. If the knife stays in place, it may temporarily seal the involved vessel.

The factors that determine the amount of tissue destruction caused by a bullet are discussed in Chap. 256.

TYPES OF VASCULAR INJURIES Simple lacerations of the great arteries of the chest can cause exsanguination, tamponade, hemothorax, or air embolism. Other vascular injuries include AV fistulas and false aneurysms, which may not be apparent for days or even months. As time goes on, AV fistulas tend to increase in size. Eventually, if more than 25 percent of the cardiac output goes through an AV fistula, high-output cardiac failure is likely to develop.

Pulmonary AV fistulas after penetrating chest trauma are said to be extremely rare because of the small pressure differential that usually exists between the pulmonary arteries and veins. However, if the patient develops hypoxemia out of proportion to the apparent lung injury and has a persisting pulmonary density, one should suspect this problem.

DIAGNOSIS **History** History is particularly important in establishing the goals of care when a patient arrives without signs of life. Unless the patient had signs of life "in the field" or in the ED, resuscitative efforts are not indicated. Witnessed traumatic arrest following penetrating thoracic injury requires immediate suspicion and intervention for tension pneumothorax and cardiac tamponade followed by emergent thoracotomy if the percutaneous maneuvers fail to substantially improve the perfusion. The contrast between declaring death and proceeding with truly emergent resuscitative maneuvers is obvious, and the decision is based on history alone.

The size of a knife, its depth, and the angle of penetration may indicate the vessels or organs most likely to be injured. If there are two skin wounds, it is helpful to know whether they represent two entrance wounds or an exit and an entrance wound. In some instances, a bullet that entered the chest without exiting is not evident on chest or abdominal x-rays because it is in lateral subcutaneous tissues or has entered a major vessel and has embolized. It is also extremely important to know, if possible, the caliber of the bullet and whether it was a high-velocity missile (>1000 ft/s).

Physical Examination Close inspection including lifting the skin edge with a forceps may be useful to determine the general trajectory. Under no circumstances should the wound be deeply probed to determine depth.

A large upper mediastinal hematoma may cause an acute superior vena caval syndrome, tracheal compression, and/or respiratory distress. Occasionally, a decreased upper extremity pulse may be noted. Unfortunately patients with injuries to major vessels at the thoracic inlet may have none of the usual diagnostic signs of significant vascular injury.

One should auscultate the entire chest for bruits after a penetrating injury. A systolic bruit, particularly over the back or upper chest, should make one suspect a false aneurysm involving one of the great vessels. A continuous bruit suggests an AV fistula. A millwheel murmur, thought to be due to the churning of air in the heart, may be diagnostic of air embolism. Loss of a peripheral pulse caused by an embolization of a bullet from a thoracic vascular injury is rarely but occasionally seen.

Radiography PLAIN RADIOGRAPHS Evidence of cervical or supraclavicular swelling or widening of the upper mediastinal silhouette or chest x-ray is often present in patients with injury to brachiocephalic vessels. A "fuzzy" foreign body (bullet) can be an important radiologic sign, and one should not assume that is is due to poor radiologic technique. Because foreign bodies tend to pulsate when they lie next to major vessels, their margins may appear indistinct on chest films. Therefore, a fuzzy foreign body contiguous with clear mediastinal structures on chest films can be an important x-ray clue to a vascular injury. Even if an angiogram is normal, a fuzzy foreign body should still be considered an indication for surgery.

COMPUTED TOMOGRAPHY SCAN CT scans are rarely performed immediately for penetrating wounds of the chest because of the usually precarious condition of the patient. However, in a stable patient, a CT scan can identify localized hematomas or collections of blood that may not be apparent on routine x-rays. If a persistent "mass" is adjacent to a great vessel and does not move with position changes by the patient, one should assume that a contained hematoma is present. Intravenous contrast provides additional help for demonstrating a vascular defect or false aneurysm on the CT scan. CT scans can be particularly helpful for suspected thoracic aorta trauma or dissection, and false-negative studies without an adjacent hematoma are very unusual if the CT scan has been performed and interpreted properly. Nevertheless, CT scans should be used primarily for screening for great vessel injuries rather than for definitive diagnosis.

ARTERIOGRAM Arteriograms may be particularly helpful in identifying major intrathoracic vascular injuries within contained hematomas, especially those resulting from penetrating wounds of the lower neck. Indeed, before exploring penetrating injuries of the thoracic inlet in hemodynamically stable patients, one should obtain a preoperative arteriogram to visualize the arch of the aorta and its major branches. Aortography is still considered by many to be the definitive study for examining injury to the aorta.

VENOGRAMS Venograms to identify major vascular injuries in the chest are seldom performed. A patient who is actively bleeding from a major venous injury is usually explored emergently because of unstable vital signs or continued blood loss through chest tubes. However, once a venous injury stops bleeding, the hemorrhage generally does not recur and does not require a thoracotomy.

CONTRAST SWALLOWS A contrast swallow may be performed on a stable patient if there is concern about an associated esophageal injury. Gastrogratin is used first but may miss up to half of esophageal leaks. Barium swallows have fewer false-negatives but can cause a worse mediastinitis if a perforation is present.

Endoscopy With penetrating wounds of the chest or lower neck in hemodynamically stable patients, it may be prudent to perform bronchoscopy and esophagoscopy to rule out an injury to the aerodigestive tract. In some patients with ''hemoptysis,'' the source may not be clear; such bleeding may result from injury to lung parenchyma, trachea, or a major bronchus. In other instances, it may be unclear whether mediastinal air is caused by an esophageal, pulmonary, or tracheobronchial injury.

Ultrasound There is much controversy on how to evaluate hemodynamically stable patients with transmediastinal gunshot wounds. Such injuries often result in either prompt surgical exploration or an extensive evaluation to rule out injury to the heart, great vessels, esophagus, or tracheobronchial tree. Recently, however, transesophageal echocardiography has been noted to be of great diagnostic help, particularly if the aortogram demonstrates an equivocal injury. (See discussion under ''Blunt Trauma to Great Vessels,'' below.)

TREATMENT **Initial Resuscitation** The standard ABCs (airway, breathing, circulation) of initial resuscitation should be followed aggressively if the patient is in shock. One of the problems occasionally seen with injuries to vessels in the thoracic outlet is massive mediastinal hematoma formation with resulting tracheal compression. Consequently, early endotracheal intubation should be performed. Tracheostomy should be avoided in patients with injuries at the thoracic inlet, at least initially, because of the possibility of precipitating massive bleeding from an otherwise controlled hematoma.

If the patient is in severe shock (systolic blood pressure <60 mmHg), surgery should be performed promptly and aggressive fluid replacement should not be employed until the major bleeding sites are controlled. With mild to moderate shock (systolic blood pressure = 60 to 88 mmHg), one should infuse 2000 to 3000 mL of balanced electrolyte solution in 10 to 15 min. If the shock is persistent, the patient is rushed to the operating room. If the patient is about to have a cardiac arrest in the ED, an immediate resuscitative thoracotomy should be performed there to control bleeding, provide internal cardiac massage, and cross-clamp the descending thoracic aorta as needed.

If rapid control of the bleeding sites and cross-clamping of the descending thoracic aortic arch do not raise the systolic blood pressure to at least 90 mmHg within 5 min, terminal cardiovascular failure is present; almost all of these patients will die in the operating room. Even if large doses of epinephrine or dopamine combined with aortic cross-clamping can raise the systolic blood pressure over 90 mmHg, death is still almost invariably the outcome.

Even if the patient's vital signs are relatively stable, one should probably perform a thoracotomy for continued bleeding if (1) a total of more than 1500 mL of blood is lost from the chest within the first 4 to 8 h and the patient is still bleeding, (2) the drainage of blood from the chest tubes continues to exceed 200 to 300 mL/h, or (3) the chest continues to be more than half full of blood on x-ray after the chest tubes are inserted and functioning well.

Bullets entering large systemic veins or the right heart can embolize to the lungs, whereas bullets entering the pulmonary veins or left heart can embolize to major systemic arteries. Some of these emboli cause no symptoms or signs and cannot be found except with multiple x-rays. Fluoroscopy in the operating room can be important in tracing these bullets, especially in the central veins or heart, because they can change position rapidly during the surgery itself.

Blunt Trauma to the Great Vessels of the Chest

INCIDENCE Approximately 80 to 90 percent of patients with blunt trauma to thoracic great vessels, particularly the aorta, die at the scene, and up to 50 percent of the remaining patients die within 24 h if not promptly treated. The frequency of these injuries appears to be increasing and is primarily related to the use of high-speed automobiles. Each year at least 5000 to 8000 individuals in the United States suffer traumatic rupture of the thoracic aorta or one of the other great arteries in the chest. Over 80 percent of the cases are due to automobile accidents.

MECHANISM OF INJURY The mechanical factors responsible for traumatic rupture of the thoracic aorta and its major branches are probably somewhat different for each anatomic area. For the descending aorta at the level of the isthmus, three mechanical factors thought to contribute to rupture are shearing stress, bending stress, and torsion stress. The difference in deceleration between the mobile aortic arch and the relatively immobile descending aorta puts the aortic isthmus under tension, and the resultant shearing stress can lead to rupture or tears opposite the site of fixation. Bending stress is produced as the heart exerts downward traction on the aortic arch, resulting in the hyperflexion of the blood-filled aortic arch on a transverse fulcrum created by the hilar structures of the left lung. Torsion stress occurs when anteroposterior compression of the chest with resultant displacement of the heart to the left is combined with an intravascular pressure wave transmitted to the aorta. These three forces can combine to produce maximum stress to the inner surface of the aorta at the ligamentum arteriosum, which is its point of greatest fixation.

The aortic injury tends to progress from the intima out toward the adventitia. The adventitia, which has the lowest elastic limit, seems to withstand these stresses better than the intima or media.

Rupture of the innominate or left subclavian artery at their origins probably results primarily from the interaction of two forces. One is a compression force that displaces the heart into the left chest and places the brachiocephalic vessels under tension at their attachment to the aortic arch. The other force occurs when hyperextension of the neck with rotation of the head to one side places the contralateral subclavian arteries under tension. Subclavian artery injuries can also occur just over the first rib, and injuries at that site are usually caused by direct trauma and/or excessive stretching.

PATHOLOGIC CHANGES Blunt aortic tears usually extend partially or completely around the vessel in a transverse or spiral direction. Preexisting disease, such as atherosclerosis or medial necrosis, does not appear to predispose to traumatic rupture. When the aortic tear involves all layers of the aortic wall, death by exsanguination is usually almost instantaneous. If the aortic tear does not involve the adventitia, and the parietal pleura and the surrounding mediastinal tissues remain intact, a false aneurysm often forms. The false aneurysm tends to expand, particularly if the patient is hypertensive, and about 50 percent of these, if untreated, will rupture within 24 h. However, some posttraumatic aortic false aneurysm remain intact and may not be detected for 20 years or longer. Although a lacerated subclavian artery occasionally forms a false aneurysm, it usually just occludes and does not require surgery.

It should be emphasized that the small hemothorax that is often present with blunt trauma to the aorta does not result from the aortic injury itself but rather from tears to adjacent small mediastinal vessels or other structures. In the same manner, although the widened mediastinum may be partly due to the aortic pseudoaneurysm, much of it is actually caused by bleeding from small mediastinal vessels.

NATURAL HISTORY Of the patients who reach a hospital and survive for 1 h, about half die within 24 h, and three-quarters die within 7 days. Of the remainder, most die within the next 1 to 3 months.

Many of the early deaths are caused by associated injuries, but even when the aortic injury is an isolated problem, diagnosis and repair should usually be accomplished on an urgent basis. All too often the patient dies of exsanguination before a definitive repair can

TABLE 251-5 Clinical Factors Suggesting Possible Traumatic Rupture of the Aorta

High-speed deceleration injury or side impact
Multiple rib fractures or flail chest
Pulse deficits
Hypertension
Systolic murmur over back
Hoarseness without laryngeal injury
Superior vena caval syndrome

be effected. Keeping the systolic blood pressure <120 mmHg and prevention of Valsalva maneuvers may avoid many of the early deaths.

LOCATION At least 90 percent of blunt aortic injuries in patients who reach the hospital alive occur in the isthmus of the aorta, between the left subclavian artery and the ligamentum arteriosum. The next most common sites involved are the innominate or left subclavian artery at their origin or a subclavian artery over the first rib. Patients do not usually survive injury to the ascending aorta, but this injury may be seen in up to one-third of the individuals who die at the scene of an accident, especially with vertical deceleration from falls from great heights or plane crashes. Tears in the lower aorta below the ligamentum arteriosum are quite uncommon but tend to occur adjacent to severely comminuted fractures of vertebral bodies.

DIAGNOSIS **History** The single most important factor in establishing the diagnosis of acute traumatic rupture of the aorta (TRA) is a high index of suspicion because of the nature of the trauma (Table 251-5). Even if there is no external evidence of chest injury, one should still be acutely aware of the possibility of this injury in anyone who has sustained an accident characterized by sudden severe deceleration or a high-speed impact from the side.

Patients with TRA usually complain primarily of their associated injuries and generally have no symptoms related to the aortic injury itself. The most common complaint that may be due to the aortic injury itself is retrosternal or interscapular pain from ''stretching'' or dissection of the adventitia of the aorta. Recurrence or exacerbation of the pain, particularly if associated with a rise in blood pressure (which may be due to excess fluid administration or inadequate pain control), may herald an impending rupture of the pseudoaneurysm. Less frequent symptoms, due primarily to pressure from the associated hematoma, include dysphagia, stridor, dyspnea, or hoarseness.

Physical Examination In many reports, at least one-third of the patients with blunt trauma to the aorta have no external evidence of thoracic injury at the time of the initial physical examination.

Physical findings that suggest aortic injury include (1) an acute onset of upper extremity hypertension, (2) difference in pulse amplitude between the upper and lower extremities, and (3) the presence of a harsh systolic murmur over the precordium or posterior interscapular area. Upper extremity hypertension has occurred in 31 to 43 percent of the patients reported in the literature and has been attributed to compression of the aortic lumen by a periaortic hematoma. However, the hypertension may also be secondary to stretching or stimulation of special receptors located in the vicinity of the aortic isthmus.

If the torn intima and media form a flap that acts as a ''ball valve,'' partial or complete aortic obstruction can occur. With partial obstruction, an ''acute coarctation syndrome'' can develop, with hypertension in the upper extremities and weak pulses or hypotension in the lower extremities. A systolic murmur, thought to be caused by turbulent blood flow across the area of transection, is found in fewer than 30 percent of the patients with acute aortic rupture. If complete aortic obstruction occurs, anuria and paraplegia can develop almost immediately. Other, less frequently encountered physical findings include hoarseness, voice change, superior vena cava syndrome, swelling at the base of the neck, and paraplegia.

Plain Chest X-Ray The results of a study by Gundry and colleagues[32] are shown in Table 251-6. These data confirm prior reports that a widened mediastinum visualized on an upright chest radiograph is the most sensitive and specific finding in patients subsequently shown to have traumatic rupture of the aorta (TRA). While secondary signs—including esophageal deviation, obscuration of the aortic knob, and loss of the paraspinal stripe—may suggest TRA or great vessel injury, these secondary signs are less predictive.

One of the main reasons that many unnecessary aortograms are preformed is a technically poor chest x-ray. The upper mediastinum tends to appear wider than normal if the chest x-ray is taken (1) anteroposteriorly (AP) rather than posteroanteriorly (PA), (2) with the patient less than 3¼ ft (100 cm) from the origin of the x-ray beam, (3) with the patient lying flat, or (4) with poor inspiration. The optimal chest x-ray is an upright PA chest x-ray taken at a distance of 6 ft (about 2 m) with the patient leaning forward about 10 to 15°.

The most accurate radiographic sign of TRA is usually deviation of the esophagus more than 1 to 2 cm to the right of the spinous

TABLE 251-6 Reliability of Selected Clinical and Radiographic Criteria in the Detection of Traumatic Rupture of the Aorta*†

Radiographic or Clinical Finding	Correlation with TRA	Sensitivity	Specificity	Accuracy
Widened mediastinum (under 65 years old)	$p = 0.001$	0.95	0.82	0.84
Widened mediastinum (all ages)	$p = 0.001$	0.80	0.82	0.82
Murmur	$p = 0.002$	0.32	0.93	0.84
Pneumothorax/pulmonary contusion	$p = 0.07$	0.22	0.67	0.51
Hemothorax	$p = 0.21$	0.25	0.88	0.81
1st/2nd rib fracture	$p = 0.39$	0.36	0.73	0.68

*All other clinical and radiographic criteria were less useful in detecting TRA.
†Sensitivity = TP/(TP + FN); Specificity = TN/(TN + F); Accuracy = (TP + TN)/All tests.
Source: From Gundry SR, Williams S, Burnes RE: Indications for aortography in blunt thoracic trauma: A reassessment. *J Trauma* 22:664, 1982, with permission.

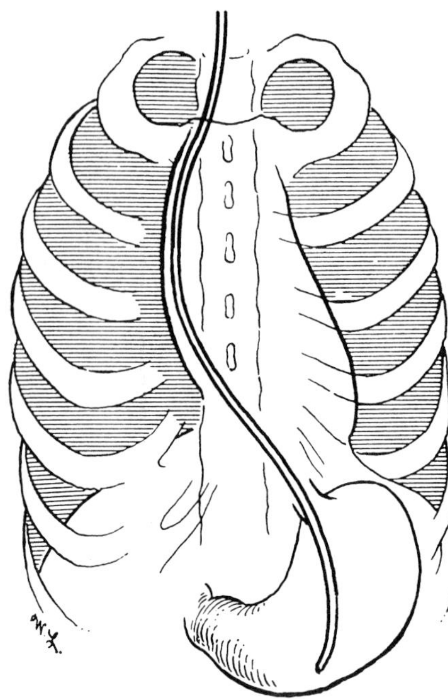

FIG. 251-7. Deviation of the esophagus (nasogastric tube) to the right is generally a very accurate sign of traumatic rupture of the aorta. If the distance from the nasogastric tube to the spinous process of the fourth thoracic vertebra is greater than 2.0 cm, it is almost 100 percent indicative of a torn descending thoracic aorta.

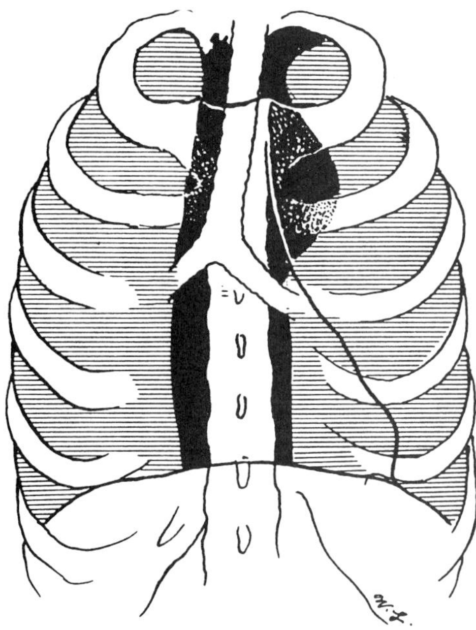

FIG. 251-8. Mediastinal hematomas, indicated by the blackened areas, may widen and displace the paratracheal stripe separating the right side of the tracheal air column from the medial border of the right lung by more than 5 mm. Mediastinal hematomas may also displace the right and left paraspinal lines in the lower thorax rather widely from the lateral edges of the thoracic spine. The paraspinal lines are not readily seen on most x-rays because of overlying structures.

process of T4 (Fig. 251-7). Patients in whom the esophagus is deviated less than 1.0 cm from the midline are unlikely to have a TRA. A nasogastric tube in a normal position virtually excludes TRA.

Blurring or obscuration of the aortic knob or descending aorta is almost as accurate an indication of TRA. Studies have shown that patients with a normal aortic contour and no evidence of deviation of the trachea or nasogastric tube to the right on the chest x-ray do not have TRA.

Other chest x-ray signs include displacement of the left main stem bronchus more than 40° below the horizontal, obliteration of the usual clear space between the aortic knob and the left pulmonary artery (apical cap), widening of the right paratracheal stripe, and displacement of the right paraspinous interface (Fig. 251-8).

The paratracheal stripe is a linear structure just to the right of the tracheal air column (Fig. 251-8). It extends from the thoracic inlet to the proximal right bronchus and normally measures less than 5 mm in thickness at a level 2 cm above the azygos vein. If the paratracheal stripe is more than 5 mm wide and/or is deviated to the right, this may be another sign of mediastinal hemorrhage.

The paraspinal lines lie between the pleura and the lung, projected away from the lateral margin of the thoracic spine. The right paraspinal line is usually not visible on routine chest x-rays, but if it is seen and if it is displaced to the right in the absence of spinal or sternal fractures, it may be of some diagnostic value.

The left paraspinal line may be distinguished from the image of the descending aorta by the fact that it is not continuous with the aortic knob. When displaced more than one-half the distance from the spine to the left margin of the descending aorta without spinal or sternal fractures, it is highly specific.

It often takes great force to fracture the first or second ribs or sternum, especially in young patients. Consequently, such fractures tend to be associated with an increased incidence of major intrathoracic injuries; however, it is now very controversial whether fractures of the first or second ribs are associated with a significantly increased incidence of TRA.

One should not assume that a TRA has been ruled out if the initial chest x-ray is normal. In up to one-third of patients with TRA, widening of the mediastinum and other characteristic changes may not be apparent on the chest x-ray until several hours after the injury. Two-thirds of patients above 65 years of age with TRA may not show mediastinal widening. Consequently, serial chest films should be taken in any patient with severe chest trauma at 6- to 12-h intervals during the first day and then daily for at least the next 3 days. Indeed, the circumstances of the trauma in such individuals should be the main indication for ordering an aortogram.

Transesophageal Ultrasound Although aortography is the ''gold standard'' for the diagnosis of traumatic disruption of aorta (TDA), it is positive in only about 10% of patients in whom injuries are suspected based on plain films. Further, it is an invasive procedure that requires 1 to 2 h. Unlike aortography, CT, or magnetic resonance imaging (MRI), transesophageal echocardiography (TEE) can be safely performed in hemodynamically unstable patients.[33]

The thoracic aorta is not readily imaged by TTE. However, with the advent of new-generation TEE transducers, the entire thoracic aorta can be imaged. TEE visualizes the aortic isthmus and descending aorta very well and allows assessment of the pericardial cavity (hemopericardium, tamponade), valve function (and potential rupture), pulmonary veins (potential avulsion), and regional wall motion abnormalities.

One study that examined the role of both aortography and TEE found 100 percent sensitivity and specificity, respectively, with higher accuracy for TEE than aortography.[34] In this study, there were no complications from TEE, which was performed in less than 30 min on average, as compared with aortography, which required over 75 min on average. Other studies have found the sensitivity and specificity of TEE (in the hands of cardiologists) to be as low as 63 and 84 percent respectively.[35] The differences in the various studies are likely attributable to local factors such as patient population, limited study enrollment, and operator experience. TEE in this setting may be performed by cardiologists, surgeons, and radiologists. Because of the variability of findings using this relatively new diagnostic modality, the exact role of TEE for aortic imaging in both blunt and penetrating chest injuries remains to be defined.

The complication rate from TEE is very low, with esophageal perforation (perhaps the most feared complication) being on the order of 2 to 3 per 10,000.

CT Scans CT scans, particularly helical (spiral) CT scans, are increasingly used as screening tools to evaluate patients with blunt chest trauma who are thought to be at risk for aortic and great vessel injury. Reports in the literature are contradictory regarding the sensitivity, specificity, and safety of this technique, which may well reflect the rapidly evolving technology as much as variation in technique and interpretation. The following comments apply to situations where technically adequate images can be obtained using a late-generation helical-capable CT scanner. Primitive CT scanners cannot be recommended for screening for aortic injury.

CT scanning is not a substitute for plain radiography or aortography. When a patient with an appropriate mechanism of injury (rapid deceleration) also has a chest radiograph suspicious for an aortic or great vessel injury, aortography should be the next step. However, there is a group of patients with an equivocal history and an equivocal radiograph. These patients may be screened to exclude an aortic injury using CT scans *provided that certain conditions are met.* The first and most important condition is that the patient is not thought to be at risk for great vessel injuries, since *injuries to the great vessels are commonly missed by axial CT.* The second condition is that the patient should be hemodynamically stable and capable of tolerating two dye loads, the first in CT and the second if aortography is required. We generally obtain a ''dry'' (noncontrast) view of the thoracic aorta first. If there is evidence of mediastinal hematoma on this initial study, we proceed to angiography. If the study appears normal, a CT ''angiogram'' is obtained using rapid infusion and helical scanning to collect images through the aortic arch and isthmus. If this study is entirely normal, we consider the aorta ''cleared.'' Abnormalities require an aortogram. This special use of CT has found its widest application in our practice with obese patients who cannot tolerate an erect chest x-ray owing to skeletal instability. We reiterate that CT scanning is not a substitute for the proven methods of chest x-ray and aortography, and the use of CT should probably be limited to screening under specific circumstances. Difficulties in demonstrating injuries near or involving the great vessels should allow information about a ''high-probability'' mechanism of injury to prevail and thus justify proceeding with aortography even in the face of a ''negative'' CT.

Magnetic Resonance Imaging MRI is a technically seductive method for investigating injuries to the aorta and great vessels. MRI has certainly emerged as the preferred tool for the evaluation of dissecting aneurysms of the thoracic aorta. However, even current-generation MRI instruments require long intervals in quiet patients who lie in an isolated room free of metallic objects to obtain satisfactory images—a requirement that is often difficult to meet in patients who are suspected of harboring major vascular injuries. For these reasons, the role of MRI in the evaluaton of blunt thoracic injuries remains indeterminate. As scan times become faster, the other limitations become less onerous.

Aortography If an aortic rupture is suspected on clinical or radiologic grounds, an aortogram should be performed. While waiting for the aortogram or surgery, it is important to ensure that the systolic blood pressure is kept below 120 mmHg. It is also important to protect the patient from excessive gagging or straining.

The most common finding on aortogram is a pseudoaneurysm of the isthmus of the aorta. A slight pouching out of the inferior or inner border of isthmus, sometimes referred to as a pseudodiverticulum, is normal but may be confused with a traumatic pseudoaneurysm. Bulging of the aorta laterally is a more reliable indicator of TRA. A linear filling defect caused by torn intima and media is the best evidence that a TRA is present.

A patient who is in shock from a suspected TRA or who has a rapidly expanding mediastinal hematoma should be taken directly to the operating room without undergoing aortography. It should be remembered that occasional false-negatives occur with aortography.

Although it is often thought that there is relatively little risk to angiography, local complications with conventional angiography may occur in up to 23 percent of cases, and systemic complications may occur in up to 9 percent.[36] Although the rates of amputation (0.1 percent) or death (0.3 percent) resulting from transfemoral studies is relatively low, if they occur in an individual with a negative study, the indications for the aortogram are apt to be questioned. Death has also occurred in at least two instances when the angiographic catheter was manipulated through the aorta at the level of a tear. If angiography is done in a hospital where relatively few cases are done each year, the incidence of complications can be increased up to 32-fold.

Intraarterial Digital Subtraction Angiography In an effort to improve the speed and accuracy of angiography and reduce the dose of contrast material, intraarterial digital subtraction angiography (IA-DSA) has been investigated. Studies have shown IA-DSA to be up to 100 percent accurate, as indicated by the results of surgery, conventional arteriography, serial chest x-rays, and clinical follow-up. The method is 50 percent faster than conventional aortography, and it can significantly reduce x-ray film costs. The use of smaller-caliber catheters for the intraaortic injection and a decrease in radiographic contrast media requirements also make this method safer than conventional arteriography.

TREATMENT Although it is essential to resuscitate severely injured patients aggressively and to correct hypotension and hypoxemia rapidly the patient with a TRA should not be allowed to develop a systolic blood pressure over 120 mmHg or to perform a Valsalva maneuver. Endotracheal intubation can likewise cause gagging and coughing. Therefore these patients should not be intubated ''awake.'' In addition to the standard paralytic and sedative drugs administered during rapid-sequence intubation, preemptive intravenous administration of lidocaine (1 mg/kg) to attenuate the vascular and bronchial responses prior to laryngoscopy may be advisable in patients with suspected or proven TRA. Fluid administration should be watched carefully, and administration of sedatives, analgesics, vasodilators, or even beta-adrenergic blockers may be required to keep the patient's systolic blood pressure at safe levels.

It is often important to insert a nasogastric tube in patients with multiple injuries, but it is essential that the patient with a suspected TRA not perform a vigorous Valsalva maneuver. Sudden gagging or bearing down can cause intraaortic pressure to rise abruptly to well over 200 mmHg and complete the rupture of a partially torn aorta. Similar precautions must be undertaken when inserting an endotracheal tube.

Since the initial report of a successful repair of an acute traumatic thoracic aortic disruption in 1958,[37] emergency operation has become the accepted standard for treatment. However, in selected cases, delays in surgical intervention may be warranted and safe. Such delay should be considered if (1) the patient is stable but the conditions for surgery are not ideal, or (2) the patient represents an extremely high operative risk because of associated injuries or preexisting medical conditions.

In a few centers with extensive experience with thoracic aortic surgery, the aortic repair may be preferentially performed by a rapid ''clamp and sew'' technique without an external shunt or cardiopulmonary bypass. Under these circumstances, an intravenous infusion of an alpha and beta blocker may be used to keep the systolic blood pressure in the upper portion of the body less than 150 mmHg so as to diminish the chances of intracerebral hemorrhage or left heart failure while the aorta is clamped. The operation must be rapid and precise, because clamping of the descending aorta for more than 30 min without perfusion of the distal aorta greatly increases the risk of damage to the spinal cord and abdominal viscera.

Because it allows increased time for a meticulous, unhurried repair and reduces the risk of ischemic damage to the spinal cord and abdominal viscera, repair of traumatic rupture of the thoracic aorta is often performed under partial cardiopulmonary bypass. If the patient's condition is stable, transfer to a hospital where cardiopulmonary bypass is available is wise, just in case problems develop during the repair.

Special Considerations in Less Frequent Great Vessel Injuries

ASCENDING AORTA **Incidence** Very few patients with ascending aortic injury survive long enough for the diagnosis to be established and repair to be carried out. These injuries are frequently associated with cardiac rupture or severe myocardial contusion, and the aortic tears are multiple in up to 15 to 20 percent. Most victims have been hit by or thrown from moving vehicles or have fallen from great heights.

Diagnosis Since most ascending aortic tears occur within the pericardium, if there is a small complete tear, there is often evidence of both shock and pericardial tamponade. The chest x-ray findings often show a widened superior mediastinum with or without obscuration of the aortic knob. Aortography is generally required for the diagnosis to be established. The aortogram usually shows a pseudoaneurysm with an intimal tear seen as an irregular filling defect within the lumen. If there is an associated valvular injury, aortic insufficiency of varying severity will usually also be seen.

Thoracic aortic injuries distal to the isthmus should be suspected with severe chest trauma in which a lower thoracic vertebra is severely crushed.

DESCENDING AORTA Injuries to the descending aorta are uncommon. The presentations include paraplegia (owing to injuries to vessels supplying the spinal cord), mesenteric ischemia, anuria, or lower extremity ischemia. Angiography is typically required for diagnosis, and cardiopulmonary bypass may be required for surgical management. The more distal the injury, the better the anticipated outcome—assuming that the patient does not exsanguinate prior to surgical repair. Immediate surgery is indicated.

OTHER GREAT VESSEL INJURIES **Innominate Artery** INCIDENCE In patients reaching the hospital alive, blunt injuries of the innominate artery are second in frequency only to rupture of the aorta at the isthmus. Associated injuries, such as rib fractures, flail chest, hemopneumothorax, fractured extremities, head injuries, facial fractures, and abdominal injuries, are found in more than 75 percent of these patients.

DIAGNOSIS Making a diagnosis of blunt injury to the innominate artery can be very difficult because there are no characteristic physical findings except for some diminution of the right radial or brachial pulse, which occurs in about 50 percent of the patients. Signs and symptoms of distal ischemia are uncommon. Occasionally, a systolic murmur may draw attention to a possible lesion in this area.

The chest x-ray findings are somewhat similar to those seen with TRA, but the mediastinal hematoma tends to be higher and the trachea and esophagus may be pushed to the left. Aortography must generally be performed for the diagnosis to be established. Associated injuries in other brachycephalic vessels or the aorta are found in about 10 percent of patients.

Subclavian Artery ETIOLOGY Although a subclavian artery is occasionally avulsed at its origin because of sudden deceleration, direct trauma to the distal artery with intimal damage and occlusion associated with fractures of the first rib or clavicle are more likely. Shoulder restraints that are loose may be a major factor in causing this injury.

DIAGNOSIS The most important sign of a subclavian occlusion is absence of a radial pulse. In the patient with only a partial laceration and no occlusion, the radial pulse may be preserved. Other physical findings that are highly suggestive of subclavian artery rupture are a pulsatile mass or a bruit in the root of the neck. Occasionally a patient may develop an acute subclavian steal syndrome if the subclavian artery occludes proximal to the origin of the vertebral artery.

Up to 60 percent of patients with blunt injury to the subclavian artery, especially from motor vehicle accidents, will also have some damage to the brachial plexus. Consequently, a complete neurologic examination preoperatively is important in these patients. A Horner's syndrome often indicates avulsion of nerve roots from the spinal cord.

The chest x-ray with subclavian artery injuries may show the presence of a widened superior mediastinum without obscuration of the aortic knob. The angiogram usually shows occlusion, but a pseudoaneurysm is occasionally found. Blunt subclavian artery injuries are associated with other major vascular injuries in about 10 percent of patients.

TREATMENT The treatment of acute subclavian artery injury is usually immediate repair. However, in certain high-risk patients who are doing poorly, occlusion by an interventional radiologist may be the treatment of choice. If the artery is already occluded, observation may be all that is required. The collateral circulation to the distal portions of the vessel is usually very good. However, if there has been severe blunt trauma to the shoulder girdle, many of the collateral vessels may be damaged, resulting in critical ischemia of the hand or upper extremity gangrene in about 30 percent.

ESOPHAGEAL AND THORACIC DUCT INJURIES

Esophageal Injuries

MECHANICAL TRAUMA Lacerations of the esophagus occur most frequently during endoscopic biopsy or dilatation of a narrowed or obstructed esophagus. The esophagus can also be injured by swallowed foreign bodies. Injury to the thoracic esophagus is seen only rarely in patients who reach the hospital alive.

If esophageal injury is suspected, an esophagogram should be obtained. The initial study should be performed using water-soluble contrast, since extravasation of barium into the mediastinum can complicate mediastinitis. However, a negative water-soluble contrast study should always be confirmed with a barium study owing to the former's relatively high false-negative rate.

Flexible esophagoscopy is being performed increasingly for diagnosis but may miss more than 20 percent of injuries, even if combined with an esophagogram. Some prefer rigid esophagoscopy in combination with bronchoscopy to rule out associated tracheobronchial injuries.

If treatment is delayed beyond 24 h, primary closure of a torn esophagus is usually not advisable because local edema, tissue necrosis, and infection make secure suturing and primary healing unlikely. If mediastinitis develops, it may be rapidly fatal unless the site is drained early and completely. Even if an esophageal repair is not attempted, continuous complete drainage of the stomach (preferably with a gastrostomy tube) and the adjacent mediastinum (with chest tubes) is important and may be necessary for up to several weeks.

In spite of all our technical and nutritional advances in recent years, the mortality rate for esophageal injuries ranges from 5 to 25 percent for those treated definitively within 12 h and 25 to 66 percent for those treated after 24 h.

Thoracic Duct Injuries

Most injuries to the thoracic duct in the chest result in a chylothorax. Because the thoracic duct in the chest tends to be slightly to the right of the midline, injuries to it usually cause a chylothorax on the right. Initially, the chyle may just accumulate in the mediastinum as a chyloma, but eventually, usually within 7 to 13 days, it will cause an increasing pleural effusion, especially after the patient begins to eat. Thoracic duct leakage in the chest can result in the loss of 1500 to 2500 mL/day of fluid with fat globules (demonstrated by Sudan III) and/or chylomicrons (demonstrated by lipoprotein electrophoresis) with minimal cholesterol.

Keeping the patient from eating and providing adequate drainage of the pleural cavity with a chest tube for several days usually results in spontaneous closure of the fistula. If the fistula persists and is large, nasogastric suction can help reduce the amount of chyle draining, and intravenous hyperalimentation can help prevent the protein malnutrition that can rapidly develop in these patients. If the patient is allowed to eat, a strict no-fat diet or a diet in which fat is given only as medium-chain triglycerides is preferred. If the drainage is greater than 1500 mL/day and leads to metabolic and nutritional problems or persists for more than 14 days, surgery to ligate the duct is generally indicated.

REFERENCES

1. Richardson JD: What's new in trauma and burns? *J Am Coll Surg* 184:210, 1997.
2. Rotondo MF, McGonigal MD, Schwab CW, et al: Urgent paralysis and intubation of trauma patients: Is it safe? *J Trauma* 34:242, 1993.
3. Diebel LN, Robinson RL, Wilson RF, Dulchavsky SA: Splanchnic mucosal perfusion effects of hypertonic versus isotonic resuscitation of hemorrhagic shock. *Am Surg* 59:495, 1993.
4. Luchette FA, Radfshar MR, Kaiser R, et al: Prospective evaluation of epidural versus intrapleural catheters for analgesia in chest wall trauma. *J Trauma* 35:165, 1993.
5. Galan G, Penalver JC, Paris E, et al: Blunt chest injuries in 1696 patients. *Eur J Cardiothorac Surg* 6:284, 1992.
6. Brookes JG, Dunn RJ, Rogers IR: Sternal fractures: A retrospective analysis of 272 cases. *J Trauma* 35: 46, 1993.
7. Wright SW: Myth of the dangerous sternal fracture. *Ann Emerg Med* 22:1589, 1993.
8. Chiu WC, D'amelio LF, Hammond JS: Sternal fractures in blunt chest trauma: A practical algorithm for management. *Am J Emerg Med* 15:252, 1997.
9. Jongewaard WR, Cogbill TH, Landercasper J: Neurologic consequences of traumatic asphyxia. *J Trauma* 32:28, 1992.
10. Inoue H, Suzuki I, Iwasaki M, et al: Selective exclusion of the injured lung. *J Trauma* 34:496, 1993.
11. Wilson RF: *Handbook of Antibiotic Therapy for Surgery Related Infections.* Philadelphia, Scientific Therapeutic Information, 1994, pp 294–331.
12. Cant PJ, Smyth S, Smart DO: Antibiotic prophylaxis is indicated for chest stab wounds requiring closed tube thoracostomy. *Br J Surg* 80:464, 1993.
13. Demetriades D, Breckon V, Breckon C, et al: Antibiotic prophylaxis in penetrating injuries of the chest. *Ann R Coll Surg Engl* 73:348, 1991.
14. Ordog GJ, Wasserberger J, Balasubramanium S, Shoemaker W: Asymptomatic stab wounds of the chest. *J Trauma* 36:680, 1994.
15. Collins JC, Levine G, Waxman K: Occult traumatic pneumothorax: Immediate tube thoracostomy versus expectant management. *Am Surg* 58:743, 1992.
16. Enderson BL, Abdalla R, Frame SB, et al: Tube thoracostomy for occult pneumothorax: A prospective randomized study of its use. *J Trauma* 35:726, 1993.
17. Brown GL, Richardson JD: Traumatic diaphragmatic hernia. *Ann Thorac Surg* 39:172, 1985.
18. Ma OJ, Mateer JR, Ogata M, et al: Prospective analysis of rapid trauma ultrasound examination performed by emergency physicians. *J Trauma* 38:879, 1995.
19. Plummer D, Brunette D, Asinger R, et al: Emergency department echocardiography improves outcome in penetrating cardiac injury. *Ann Emerg Med* 21:709, 1992.
20. Rozycki GS, Ochsner MG, Jaffin JH, Champion HR: Prospective evaluation of surgeons' use of ultrasound in the evaluation of trauma patients. *J Trauma* 34:516, 1993.
21. Meyer DM, Jessen ME, Grayburn PA: Use of echocardiography to detect occult cardiac injury after penetrating thoracic trauma: A prospective study. *J Trauma* 39:902, 1995.
22. Mitchell ME, Muakkassa FF, Poole GV, et al: Surgical approach of choice for penetrating cardiac wounds. *J Trauma* 34:17, 1993.
23. Maron BJ, Pollac LC, Kaplan JA, et al: Blunt impact to the chest leading to sudden death from cardiac arrest during sports activities. *N Eng J Med* 333:337, 1995.
24. Maenza RL, Seaberg D, D'Amico F: A meta-analysis of blunt cardiac trauma: Ending myocardial confusion. *Am J Emerg Med* 14:237, 1996.
25. Fulda GJ: An evaluation of serum troponin T and signal-averaged electrocardiography in predicting electrocardiographic abnormalities after blunt chest trauma. *J Trauma* 43:304, 1997.
26. Foil MB, Mackersie RC, Furst SR, et al: The asymptomatic patient with suspected myocardial contusion. *Am J Surg* 160:638, 1990.
27. Biffl WA, Moore FA, Moore EE, et al: Cardiac enzymes are irrelevant in the patient with suspected myocardial contusion. *Am J Surg* 169:523, 1994.
28. Adams JE, Davila-Roman VGH, Bessey PQ, et al: Improved detection of cardiac contusion with cardiac troponin-I. *Am Heart J* 131:308, 1996.
29. Ferjani M, Droc G, Dreux S, et al: Circulating cardiac troponin T in myocardial contusion. *Chest* 111:427, 1997.
30. Chan D: Echocardiography in thoracic trauma, in Eckstein M, Chan D (eds): *Contemporary Issues in Trauma.* Emerg Clin North Am 16:191, 1998.
31. Karalis DG, Victor MF, Davis GA, et al: The role of echocardiography in blunt chest trauma: A transthoracic and transesophageal echocardiographic study. *J Trauma* 36:53, 1994.
32. Gundry SR, Williams S, Burney RE: Indications for aortography in blunt thoracic trauma. A reassessment. *J Trauma* 22:664, 1982.
33. Sohn DW, Shin GJ, Oh JK, et al: Role of transesophageal echocardiography in hemodynamically stable patients. *Mayo Clin Proc* 70:925, 1995.
34. Kearney PA, Smith W, Johnson SB, et al: Use of transesophageal echocardiography in the evaluation of traumatic aortic injury. *J Trauma* 34:696, 1993.
35. Saletta S, Lederman E, Fein S, et al: Transesophageal echocardiography for the initial evaluation of the widened mediastinum in trauma patients. *J Trauma* 39:137, 1995.
36. Waugh JR, Sacharias N: Arteriographic complications in the DSA eras. *Radiology* 182:243, 1992.
37. Parmley LF, Mattingly TW, Manion WC: Nonpenetrating traumatic injury of the aorta. *Circulation* 17: 1086, 1958.

ABDOMINAL INJURIES

Thomas M. Scalea
Sharon A. Boswell

The evaluation of patients with abdominal injury cannot occur in a vacuum. It must be part of the systematic trauma evaluation designed to identify immediately life-threatening injuries and treat them first. Injuries that are potentially life-threatening can then be diagnosed in rank priority, allowing for the formation of a definitive plan of care.

Abdominal evaluation presents special challenges. There are five body cavities in which patients may be injured and sequester a significant volume of blood: the thorax, the abdomen, the retroperitoneum, muscle compartments, and "the street." A chest x-ray can easily diagnose intrathoracic blood loss. A pelvic film will diagnose pelvic fractures, the presence of which correlates strongly with retroperitoneal bleeding. External blood loss must be estimated based on prehospital provider information. The abdomen is a large body cavity, and patients can easily lose virtually their entire blood volume into it. There are no radiographic markers, and physical examination can be imprecise in the diagnosis of intraabdominal injury. Patients with missed injuries may not become symptomatic for 7 to 10 days postinjury, long after they are discharged home.

The management of intraabdominal injury continues to evolve. There are now many more injuries treated nonoperatively than there were 5 or 10 years ago. There continues to be debate as to which patients are safe for nonoperative management. Successful implementation of this strategy is contingent on accurate diagnostics and appropriate clinical follow-up.

The purpose of this chapter is to discuss the various issues concerning abdominal trauma. Clearly no one chapter can provide an indepth discussion of the multiplicity of issues concerning the evaluation and treatment of injury to the abdomen. It is our hope that we will be able to delineate these issues and provide the framework for clinical decision making when treating an injured patient.

PATHOPHYSIOLOGY OF INJURY

This year nearly 40 million people will be seen in this nation's emergency departments as a result of nonintentional injury. Over 2.5 million will remain hospitalized. In 1996 the number of deaths from nonintentional injury increased for the fourth consecutive year to 93,874. This trend is expected to continue.

The most common case of death and disability from nonintentional injury worldwide is the motor vehicle crash. In 1996 deaths from motor vehicle-related incidents in the United States alone rose to 43,300, and nearly 21 million people suffered disabling injury. Forty-one percent of these crashes were alcohol-related.

Falls, the second leading cause of accidental death in the United States, were responsible for 8,436,000 emergency department visits in 1994 and continue to account for more than 20 percent of all injury-related hospital admissions.

Increasing urban violence in the United States presumably has led to the continuously rising incidence of penetrating trauma. While penetrating trauma can be self-inflicted or accidental, more than 55 percent of these fatalities are caused by violence. In 1994 gunshot wounds and stabbing injuries accounted for 4,123,000 (10 percent) of all emergency department visits in the United States.

Abdominal trauma generally is divided into two types: blunt and penetrating. This is somewhat simplistic, and a skilled clinician must make more subtle differentiations within these injury patterns. Patients can suffer both blunt and penetrating trauma simultaneously. Patients involved in motor vehicle crashes may be impaled on objects at the time of impact. In addition, people who are shot or stabbed may be assaulted at the same time.

Blunt Trauma

Blunt trauma is the most common mechanism of injury seen in the United States. The injury pattern is often diffuse; thus all parts of the abdomen are at risk for injury. The biomechanics of blunt injury involve a compression or crushing by energy transmission directly to the patient. If the compressive, sheering, or stretching forces exceed the tolerance limits of the tissue or organ, the tissues are disrupted. This may result in injury to solid viscera such as the liver or spleen or rupture of hollow viscera such as the gastrointestinal tract.

Injury also can result from the movement of organs within the body. Some organs are rigidly fixed, whereas others are more motile. Injury is particularly common in areas of transition where one part is fixed and the other is free to move with some velocity. Typical examples in the abdomen include mesenteric or small bowel injuries, particularly at the ligament of Treitz or at the junction of the distal small bowel and right colon.

Falls from a height produce a unique pattern of injury. The degree of injury is a function of the distance, the surface on which the victim lands, and whether the fall has been broken by objects. Interestingly, intraabdominal injuries are very uncommon in patients who have fallen from a height. When they occur, they usually involve hollow visceral rupture and almost never cause hypotension.[1] Retroperitoneal injuries, however, are quite common because force is usually transmitted upward along the axial skeleton.

Pedestrians struck by cars may have unique patterns of injury because they are completely unprotected and all force is applied directly to the patient's body. Motorcyclists or bicyclists generally are poorly protected with the exception of a helmet. Their injuries are also compounded by the fact that motorcycles can travel at a great rate of speed.

Penetrating Trauma

Stab wounds are relatively straightforward. The wounding blade directly injures tissue as it passes through the body. Unfortunately, the penetrating object produces a hole no larger than the blade. External examination of the size of the wound may grossly underestimate the degree of internal damage. In addition, the trajectory of the blade is not apparent by external examination. Any stab wound located in the lower chest, pelvis, flank, or back must be presumed to have an abdominal injury until proven otherwise.

Gunshot wounds injure in several different ways. Bullets may directly injure organs. They also may do so secondarily from missiles such as bone or bullet fragments or from energy transmission from the bullet. Some bullets are designed to expand or break apart once they enter a victim. These tend to cause much more tissue destruction than a bullet that remains intact.

Entrance and exit wounds can approximate the missile trajectory. Plain radiographs help to localize the foreign body, allowing prediction of organs at risk. Unfortunately, bullets may not travel in a straight line. Thus all structures in any proximity to the presumed trajectory must be considered injured until proven otherwise (see Chap. 256, "Wound Ballistics").

DIAGNOSING ABDOMINAL INJURY

Solid Visceral Injuries

The organs of the abdomen involve a variety of both hollow and solid viscera that produce symptoms differently. Clearly, injuries to these viscera can, and often do, occur in concert with one another. Solid visceral injuries produce symptoms in a variety of ways. Substantial blood loss will produce alterations in vital signs, and patients often will present with or rapidly develop hypotension.[2] Some patients develop tachycardia, skin changes, and mental confusion with progressive blood loss.[2] These signs are tremendously nonspecific. Young patients may lose 60 percent of their total circulating blood volume and remain relatively asymptomatic.[3] Thus the assumption that a stable patient does not have an intraabdominal injury is hazardous. Abdominal tenderness, distension, and/or tympany may not be present until patients have nearly exsanguinated into their abdomen. In addition, it may be difficult to determine whether initial abdominal findings reflect hemoperitoneum or simply the patient's body habitus. Some patients develop exquisite abdominal tenderness early after development of hemoperitoneum. Others, however, remain asymptomatic for many hours or days. Thus, relying on physical examination to make the determination of hemoperitoneum will lead to an unacceptable rate of missed injuries.

Hollow Visceral Injuries

Hollow visceral injuries produce symptoms by the combination of blood loss and peritoneal contamination. Perforation of the stomach, small bowel, or colon is almost always accompanied by some blood loss such as from a concomitant mesenteric injury. Blood loss from the mesentery can be substantial. Gastrointestinal contamination will produce physical findings over a period of time. This assumes that the patient is awake and alert enough to complain of pain and demonstrate tenderness. Patients with closed head injuries or those who are significantly intoxicated may not demonstrate physical findings for hours or days after admission. In addition, patients with substantial injuries elsewhere may be distracted from their abdominal pain for a number of hours.

Gastrointestinal injuries may take as long as 6 to 8 h to manifest clear findings on physical examination. Gastric injuries produce abdominal symptomatology by chemical irritation when acidic contents are spilled into the abdominal cavity. This often occurs early in the treatment course but may take more time if patients are on H_2 blockers. The fluid within the small bowel and colon produce symptomatology by virtue of its bacterial content. Thus peritonitis is suppurative. Inflammation may take some hours to develop. The duodenum, on the other hand, is located within the retroperitoneum. If duodenal injuries are contained, there may be few early symptoms. Thus duodenal injuries represent a special subset of hollow visceral injuries that require more complete investigation, including the maintenance of a high index of suspicion.

The bladder is a hollow viscus whose fluid is not an irritant. Urine can be in the peritoneal cavity for days before producing symptoms. Retroperitoneal bladder injuries will produce virtually no symptoms. The bladder wall is tremendously well vascularized. Thus almost all patients with bladder injuries have significant hematuria. Intraperitoneal bladder rupture usually produces fluid in the abdomen. The amount of fluid will depend on the amount of urine in the bladder at the time of impact. If the bladder injury is contained within the retroperitoneum, there will be no free fluid. Physical examination will rarely diagnose a bladder injury. More sophisticated diagnostic testing is necessary to make this diagnosis.

Retroperitoneal Injuries

The diagnosis of retroperitoneal injuries can be extremely complicated. As with intraabdominal injuries, symptomatology and physical findings may be subtle or completely absent at the time of patient presentation. Occasionally, retroperitoneal injuries do produce symptomatology such as abdominal pain, even if they are relatively insignificant, such as a small retroperitoneal hematoma. Even computed tomography (CT) may miss retroperitoneal injuries initially.

Duodenal injuries also can be asymptomatic at the time of presentation. Duodenal wall hematomas can produce relative gastric outlet obstruction with abdominal pain, nausea, and vomiting (Fig. 252-1). Duodenal ruptures usually are contained within the retroperitoneum. They may present with abdominal pain, fever, and tenderness, although all of these may take hours or even days to become clinically obvious. Mechanism of injury should alert the clinician. Duodenal ruptures often occur from rapid increases in intraluminal pressure when both the pylorus and the proximal small bowel develop spasm. This is most often associated with high-speed vertical or horizontal decelerating trauma. Thus all such patients require some evaluation of the duodenum.

Pancreatic injuries also can be extremely subtle. They often accompany rapid decelerating injury. Pancreatic transection usually occurs in the midbody as the pancreas is displaced against the vertebral column. Thus unrestrained drivers who hit the steering column or bicyclists who hit the handlebars are at risk for pancreatic injury. Falls from height also can cause pancreatic injury.

The diagnosis of pancreatic injury can be elusive because many of these patients have very little in the way of symptoms at the time of presentation. Unfortunately, there are no biochemical or radiographic markers pathognomonic for the diagnosis. Elevations in serum amylase are nonspecific and not particularly useful. CT scanning may be normal initially. Relatively small pancreatic injuries can go on to become symptomatic days later. This is probably a result of leakage of pancreatic enzymes from the injured organ. Peripancreatic fluid develops and is activated, and a form of autodigestion occurs. Thus small pancreatic injuries ultimately may become larger and more symptomatic. These also can become superinfected with bacteria, producing a retroperitoneal abscess.

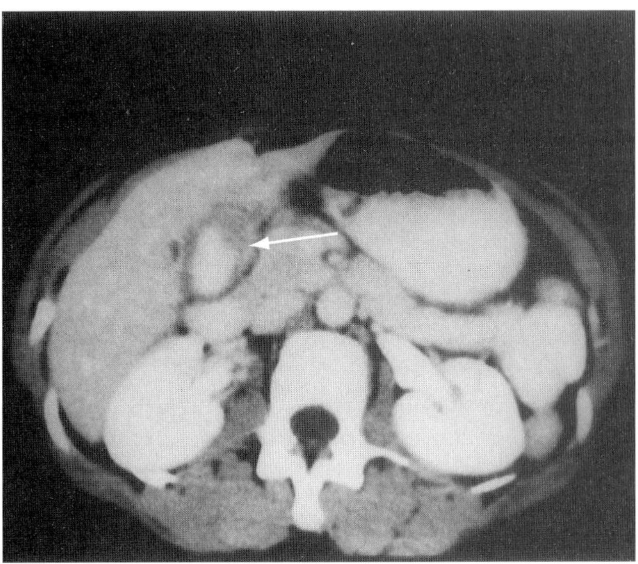

FIG. 252-1. Duodenal injury. CT scan demonstrating duodenal hematoma. Note the partial obstruction of the duodenum with an intramural hematoma. The injury resolved with nasogastric decompression and a short period of intravenous nutrition.

Urologic injuries often present with hematuria. Both the kidney and the bladder are well-vascularized organs, and even relatively minor injuries can produce an impressive amount of blood in the urine. Unfortunately, there are some injuries that may produce no hematuria. Ureteral injuries are common after penetrating trauma but also have been reported with blunt trauma, particularly vertical decelerating injuries. These injuries often present without hematuria. In addition, major renal hilar injuries such as vascular thrombosis and extraparenchymal vascular injury may have no hematuria at all (Fig. 252-2).

Diaphragmatic Injuries

Diaphragmatic injuries are particularly difficult to diagnose. A plain film of the chest demonstrating viscera in the chest or a nasogastric

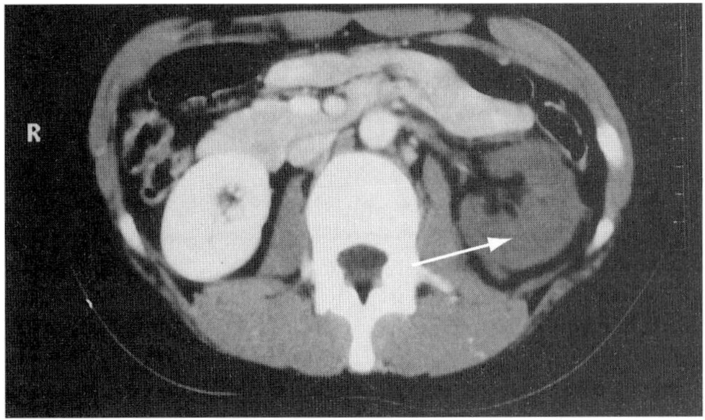

FIG. 252-2. Blunt renal artery injury. CT scan demonstrates lack of enhancement of the left kidney. There is no evidence of perinephric hematoma or other sources of retroperitoneal blood loss. The patient underwent renal artery revascularization with a successful outcome.

tube coiled in the thorax will definitively diagnose a diaphragm injury. More often, chest x-ray findings are far more subtle or completely absent. Diagnostic peritoneal lavage (DPL) can be helpful, particularly if the DPL fluid exits via a concomitantly placed chest tube or if follow-up chest x-ray demonstrates a new pleural effusion. Helical CT and magnetic resonance imaging (MRI) can both be helpful in determining the presence or absence of a diaphragmatic injury.[4] Occasionally, blind surgical exploration or a less invasive technique such as laparoscopy or thoracoscopy may be necessary to make the diagnosis of diaphragmatic injury.

ABDOMINAL EVALUATION AFTER BLUNT TRAUMA

A multiplicity of diagnostic modalities is available to evaluate the abdomen. These diagnostics are applied radically differently depending on whether the patient has sustained blunt or penetrating trauma. No test is foolproof, and each must be used in conjunction with an assessment of the patient's stability as well as associated injuries and physical findings. All too often the discussion surrounding evaluation of the abdomen centers on what diagnostic test should be used. Clinicians often fail to take into account several key issues such as the limitations of the diagnostic test and whether the patient needs abdominal evaluation at all.

Who Needs Evaluation?

All patients undergo physical examination as part of the primary and secondary surveys. Physical examination is often inadequate to make the diagnosis of intraabdominal injury. On the other hand, application of expensive diagnostic testing or prolonged observation in every patient is clearly not possible. Conversely, a missed injury may result in long-term disability or death. Clearly, any patient with abdominal pain or other physical findings requires further evaluation. The mechanism of injury and other prehospital details also provide important information to guide the clinician.

The abdomen extends through the pelvis and rises to approximately the fourth intercostal space during deep exhalation. Patients with evidence of lower chest or pelvic injury require abdominal evaluation. In addition, patients involved in high-speed collisions or collisions where there has been substantial deformity to the vehicle probably should undergo abdominal evaluation regardless of physiologic status or physical findings. This is particularly true if the patient was unrestrained. Motor vehicle crashes with fatalities or those in which there were other substantial injuries also should make the clinician suspicious of abdominal injury even in seemingly asymptomatic patients.

Abdominal evaluation is mandated in all patients who sustain unprotected injury. Patients who are unable tolerate a missed injury or delayed diagnosis should undergo early abdominal evaluation even if the indications seem somewhat soft. The elderly or those with chronic cardiovascular or pulmonary disease should undergo prompt evaluation, since a delayed diagnosis certainly will increase their morbidity and mortality. Lastly, patients with distracting injuries such as long bone injuries should undergo abdominal evaluation because such patients clearly have sustained sufficient force to produce injury, and a concomitant abdominal injury is certainly possible.

There is debate as to whether all patients with a decreased sensorium require abdominal evaluation. Closed head injury or the presence of alcohol and other intoxicants limits a patient's ability to complain of pain or demonstrate physical findings such as subtle tenderness. In addition, small injuries may progress while patients are under observation. Ethanol may reduce the amount of blood loss necessary to produce shock. In general, we prefer to be aggressive and evaluate the abdomen in most patients with head injuries and decreased levels of consciousness.

Techniques of Evaluation

In the past, abdominal diagnostics were designed merely to document that an abdominal injury existed. Organ-specific diagnosis was made at the time of surgery, since virtually all patients with intraabdominal injury underwent exploratory laparotomy. A large number of patients are now managed nonoperatively. Table 252-1 details the available diagnostic testing used for blunt abdominal trauma. Some specific comments, however, are important.

The vast majority of patients who undergo abdominal evaluation are found to have no injury. Thus it makes sense to use a rapid, inexpensive screening test that reliably excludes injury in most patients. More sophisticated and expensive testing can then be reserved for patients who are proven to have some intraabdominal injury. The choice of diagnostics largely depends on local interest and expertise. For instance, a community hospital that has a limited volume of injured patients may chose to observe patients. On the other hand, large municipal hospitals that are often inundated with injured patients cannot reliably provide serial examinations.

Exploratory laparotomy has the advantage of rapidly diagnosing intraabdominal injuries. While injuries certainly can be missed at the time of laparotomy, this is relatively rare. Blind exploration, however, is an inefficient way to make the diagnosis of abdominal injury most of the time with an excessive rate of nontherapeutic operations. On the other hand, it is occasionally appropriate.

Physical Examination

The abdomen should be examined for outward signs of injury such as abrasions or contusions to the abdominal wall. This should include the flank, back, and lower chest, as well as the anterior abdominal wall.

Physical examination is insensitive, as discussed earlier. In addition, injuries suspected on physical examination may be insignificant and require no therapy. Overall, if care depends on information gathered only by physical examination, care may be inappropriate up to 50 percent of the time.

Comprehensive serial physical examinations may be an acceptable method for identifying intraabdominal injury. These must be per-

TABLE 252-1 Diagnostic Testing

Techniques	Easy	Rapid	Sensitive	Specific	Retroperitoneum	Expensive	Repeatable	Invasive	Transport from ED
Physical Examination	Yes	Yes	No	No	No	No	Yes	No	No
DPL	Yes	Yes	Yes	Not at all	No	No	No	Yes	No
FAST	Yes	Yes	Yes	Not at all	No	No	Yes	No	No
CT	No	No	Yes	Yes	Yes	Yes	Yes	IV contrast	Yes

formed by the same senior-level clinician and should span a period of time of at least 16 to 24 h. The patient must be reliable and not have a condition where sensorium is altered. While there is little science describing this technique, we believe that physical examination must be performed at least every 30 minutes for the first 4 h and then hourly for an additional 4 to 6 h and every 2 to 4 h for the remainder of the 24-h observation period. This should be accompanied by frequent hematocrit determinations and measurement of serial vital signs. While this may be a rational technique in patients in a 23-h observation unit or in relatively quiet emergency departments that do not see a large volume of trauma, it is almost never applicable in high-volume centers that commonly see a multiplicity of injuries.

Plain Radiographs

Plain radiographs have an extremely limited use in the initial evaluation of patients with blunt abdominal trauma. They are incapable of making the diagnosis of hemoperitoneum. Even patients with hollow visceral injury often have normal radiographs. Occasionally, a chest x-ray will show free air under the diaphragm, and this will prompt laparotomy. However, universal use of plain films of the abdomen is not a cost-effective way of evaluating patients with blunt trauma.

Pelvic films, on the other hand, are standard in the evaluation process. Patients with pelvic fractures must be assumed to have high-energy injury mandating abdominal evaluation. Patients with pelvic fractures can have retroperitoneal blood loss. Thus abdominal evaluation must be rapid to avoid confusing retroperitoneal from intraabdominal blood loss. In addition, patients with thoracolumbar spine fractures have a mechanism that mandates abdominal evaluation. Thus any patient with pain or tenderness in the back must have radiographs to exclude a spine fracture. More sophisticated plain imaging such as intravenous pyelography (IVP) is occasionally useful. In patients who are hemodynamically stable, CT is far superior and has eliminated the use of IVPs. Retrograde urethrography is useful in males with pelvic fractures to exclude urethral injury.

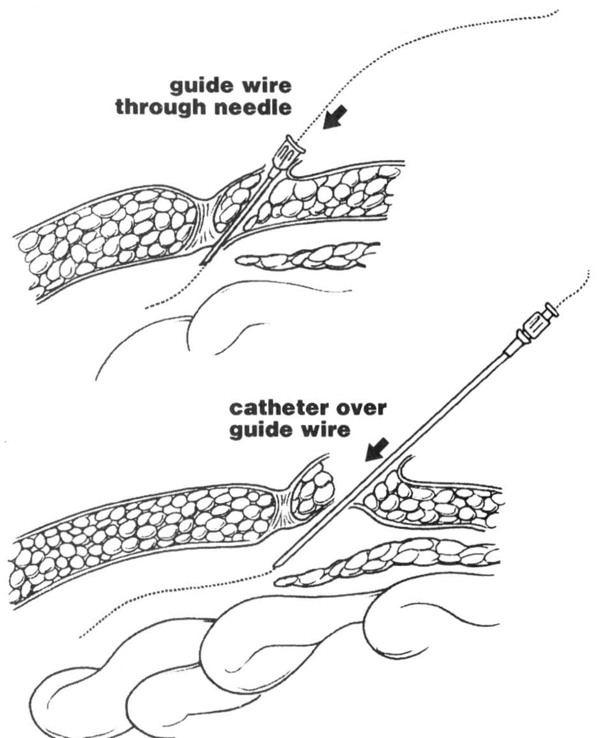

FIG. 252-3. Closed diagnostic peritoneal lavage (DPL). Closed percutaneous DPL is an effective manner of evaluating the abdomen for hemoperitoneum. A needle is inserted two finger breaths below the umbilicus after infiltration with local lidocaine with epinephrine. A guide wire can be then inserted into the abdomen and the peritoneal lavage catheter inserted over the guide wire. One liter of fluid is instilled and the abdomen is then drained.

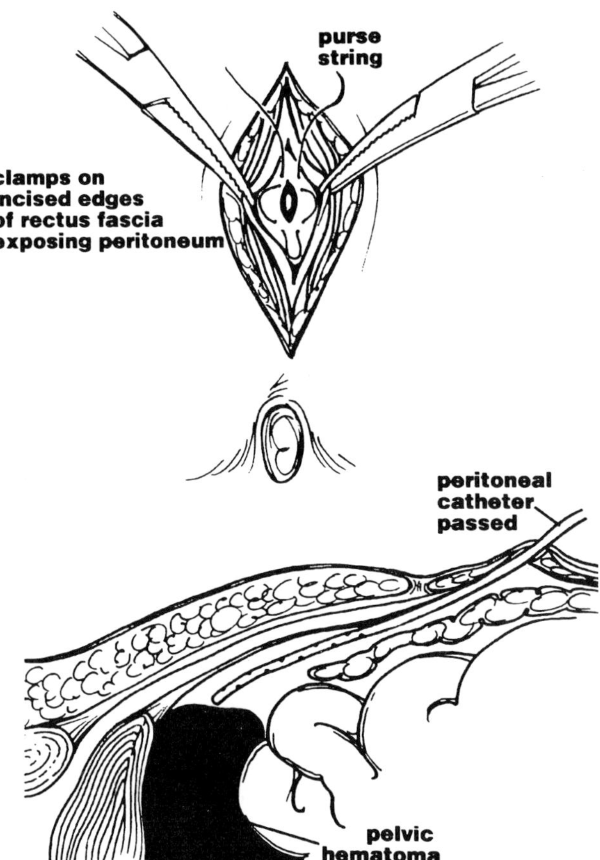

FIG. 252-4. Open diagnostic peritoneal lavage. Open diagnostic peritoneal lavage is a surgical procedure requiring some expertise. An incision is made under local anesthetic and can be performed in an infraumbilical or supraumbilical location. Patients with pelvic fractures must have their DPL performed open and above the umbilicus. An incision is made through the skin and subcutaneous tissue under local anesthesia. The fascia is opened and a purse-string suture placed in the peritoneum. The peritoneum is then opened within the purse-string suture and the catheter passed into the peritoneal cavity. Fluid is infused and returned as with a closed DPL.

Screening Examinations for Abdominal Injury

Both diagnostic peritoneal lavage (DPL) and ultrasonic abdominal evaluation are good screening tests for the presence of hemoperitoneum after blunt trauma. Both examinations are similar in that they identify the presence or absence of blood in the abdomen but can make no determination as to the etiology of the hemoperitoneum. DPL is rapid, safe, and inexpensive. There is approximately a 1 percent incidence of major complication. DPL can be performed using either an open or a closed technique (Figs. 252-3 and 252-4). We generally prefer closed percutaneous DPL because the complication rate is no different from the longer, more cumbersome open technique. A positive tap is defined as the aspiration of 10 cc of free-flowing blood. If the tap is negative, 1 L of saline is instilled into the abdomen and the abdomen is drained by gravity. It is not clear how much return is necessary to have the test be reliable. Some authors recommend that 250 cc of return is necessary.[5] One hundred thousand red blood cells per cubic centimeter is considered a positive lavage in blunt trauma. Thus only 25 cc of blood must accumulate in the abdomen (assuming complete mixing) for DPL to be positive.

Laparotomy based solely on a positive DPL for red blood cells results in a nontherapeutic procedure approximately 30 percent of the time.[6] Minimal injury to the liver or spleen or trivial mesenteric injuries can easily produce a hemoperitoneum sufficient to render DPL positive. Five hundred white cells per cubic centimeter had been suggested as another limit for positivity. More recently, white cell count DPL effluent has been criticized as being nonspecific.[7] We have abandoned the use of white cells as criteria for positive DPL. In addition, biochemical assays such as liver function tests or amylase determination are occasionally done in DPL effluent. None of these is an effective screen for intraabdominal or retroperitoneal injury. Decision on laparotomy should be made based on the patient's hemodynamic stability and associated injuries in concert with the results of the DPL. A patient with a positive DPL who is stable and does not exhibit signs of peritonitis is a candidate for nonoperative management.

Focused assessment with sonography for trauma (FAST) is a rapidly evolving technique to screen for intraabdominal injury. Like DPL, it can determine the presence or absence of hemoperitoneum. FAST is clearly operator-dependent, and considerable expertise is necessary to use FAST safely as a screening test for abdominal injury. FAST is extremely rapid and can be performed in under 1 minute by a skilled operator. Like DPL, FAST is nonspecific and is ineffective for imaging the retroperitoneum.

The number of cubic centimeters of intraabdominal fluid necessary for a positive FAST remains a subject of interest. Clearly, more skilled operators will be able to detect smaller amounts of fluid. Many people believe that several hundred cubic centimeters are necessary to be clearly visible using ultrasound.[8] Like DPL, FAST cannot determine the etiology of the fluid.

FAST is generally performed in four areas: perisplenic, perihepatic, pelvic, and pericardial, the so-called four P's. No matter which organ is injured, the perihepatic view is most commonly positive. Blood pools in Morison's pouch, the most dependent portion of the abdomen. FAST offers a view of the pericardium that can be extremely helpful. Pericardial tamponade is rare in patients with blunt injury.

The utility of FAST to determine the need for laparotomy is at best questionable. Several authors have described scoring systems for FAST. McKinney and colleagues have encouraging data that suggest that their scoring system is accurate in determining the need for laparotomy.[9] Unlike DPL, FAST can be done easily in a serial fashion.

Clearly, FAST has limitations. Its ability to detect small amounts of fluid is questionable even in very skilled hands. Thus a small bowel injury with a small amount of fluid may not be detected by the initial FAST. In addition, there are no data that suggest that a single FAST is capable of absolutely excluding intraabdominal injury. While the data on this are somewhat sketchy, a recent international consensus conference on the use of ultrasound for trauma concluded that prudent evaluation would involve a minimum of two ultrasound examinations performed at least 6 h apart.[10] This would need to be supplemented with serial physical examinations and laboratory evaluations to avoid missing an intraabdominal injury.

ORGAN-SPECIFIC DIAGNOSIS

At this juncture, only CT scanning can make the diagnosis of organ-specific injury in the abdomen. CT scanning images both the intraabdominal content and the retroperitoneum. Thus it is the diagnostic test of choice to investigate the duodenum and pancreas. In addition, it has almost completely supplanted use of the intravenous pyelogram (IVP) in the evaluation of urologic injuries. It is a more complete examination than IVP and assesses the status of the renal vasculature. It can diagnose urinary extravasation and images the ureters most of the time. It can quantitate the amount of blood in the abdomen and can image the individual organs with precision.

The disadvantages of CT are the expense and time required to perform the examination. In many centers, the CT scanner may be located some distance away from the emergency department, mandating transport of patients out of a monitored setting. This may limit the utility, particularly in critically ill patients. An additional disadvantage is the oral contrast material, which often produces nausea and vomiting or must be administered while the spine remains immobilized, and the intravenous contrast material, which has a small incidence of allergic reactions. Some have advocated that oral contrast is unnecessary for abdominal CT during the initial assessment.[11] While some institutions have adopted this practice or apply it only to selective patients, omission of oral contrast in the CT evaluation of blunt abdominal trauma requires further study before it is likely to gain widespread acceptance.

There are some patients who require CT scanning despite a normal ultrasound exam. Chiu and colleagues have demonstrated that up to 28 percent of all patients with specific physical findings or injury complexes may have intraabdominal solid visceral injury without hemoperitoneum.[12] These findings include abrasions or tenderness in the lower chest, abdomen, or pelvis. Other findings mandating CT are the presence of pelvic fractures or thoracolumbar spine fractures. Ultrasound may still have a role in the triage of these patients. Patients with a positive ultrasound should have CT scans performed urgently. Those with a normal ultrasound can have their CT scan performed in a less urgent fashion.

The increased resolution of helical CT allows for the identification of even very subtle injuries, although standard CT is almost always sufficient. CT scans should be performed with intravenous contrast agents in order to differentiate normal parenchyma from blood. Oral contrast agents are extremely helpful in detailing loops of bowel from the mesentery. Rectal contrast agents are virtually never needed for blunt trauma.

EVALUATION OF THE ABDOMEN AFTER PENETRATING TRAUMA

Stab Wounds

Mandatory exploration, a policy used in many trauma centers in the 1960s and early 1970s, has largely been abandoned. Mandatory exploration yields unacceptably high rates of nontherapeutic laparotomy. This is a particular concern because Feliciano and Renz have documented over 40 percent complication rates for nontherapeutic laparotomy in patients with penetrating abdominal injury.[13]

There are several diagnostic modalities available for the evaluation of patients with stab wounds to the anterior abdomen. Those most commonly employed are physical examination, DPL, and local wound exploration.

Physical examination may fail for all the reasons stated in the aforementioned discussion on use of physical examination in patients with blunt trauma. Accurate physical examination may be difficult if patients are intoxicated with either drugs or alcohol. Furthermore, retroperitoneal injury or tenderness from concomitant blunt trauma may produce abdominal tenderness in the absence of intraabdominal injury. Thus a single physical examination may be misleading much of the time. Serial physical examinations, on the other hand, have been shown to be accurate in the evaluation of patients with stab wounds to the abdomen.[14] This must be considered with all the provisos mentioned in the discussion on blunt trauma.

Closed percutaneous DPL, as described earlier, is an excellent technique to evaluate patients with anterior abdominal stab wounds. It is performed exactly as described previously for patients with blunt trauma. There is some controversy as to which level of red cells constitutes a positive DPL when used for stab wounds. There is a linear relationship between lavage count and rates of nontherapeutic laparotomy and missed injuries. Thus the lower the threshold for a positive lavage cell count, the higher is the rate of nontherapeutic laparotomy, but the lower is the rate of missed injury. If the threshold for a positive lavage count is set higher, there are fewer nontherapeutic laparotomies but more missed injuries. Most centers set between 10,000 and 20,000 red blood cells/μL as a threshold for laparotomy in patients with stab wounds. The accuracy increases from approximately 78 to 90 percent as the threshold for positivity decreases. Any patient who undergoes DPL must be observed in the hospital for at least 12 to 24 h.

Local wound exploration is a superb way to evaluate the abdomen after a stab wound (Fig. 252-5). It is important to remember that this is a surgical procedure and must be regarded as such. This requires good lighting, proper instruments, and an acceptable level of local anesthesia. Often this must be supplemented with intravenous conscious sedation. Digital probing of the wound or radiographic trajectograms with contrast material should be mentioned only to be condemned. These are completely inaccurate and lead to a very high rate of both nontherapeutic laparotomy and missed injuries.

If local wound exploration demonstrates no violation of the anterior fascia, the patient can be discharged home safely. If local wound exploration demonstrates clear violation of the fascia, several options are available. It is entirely reasonable to explore these patients because the rate of nontherapeutic laparotomy will be relatively low. On the other hand, if one wishes to absolutely limit the number of nontherapeutic laparotomies, positive local wound explorations can be followed by DPL. If DPL fluid exits the wound or is positive by cell count, the patient should then undergo laparotomy.

Perhaps it is most important to realize the limitations of local wound exploration. It is often difficult to follow the trajectory of a stab wound. If the clinician is not completely comfortable that this has been a technically satisfactory procedure, one must abandon the use of the local wound exploration in that patient and use another form of evaluation. Our preference would be to use DPL if the local wound exploration is not considered technically satisfactory.

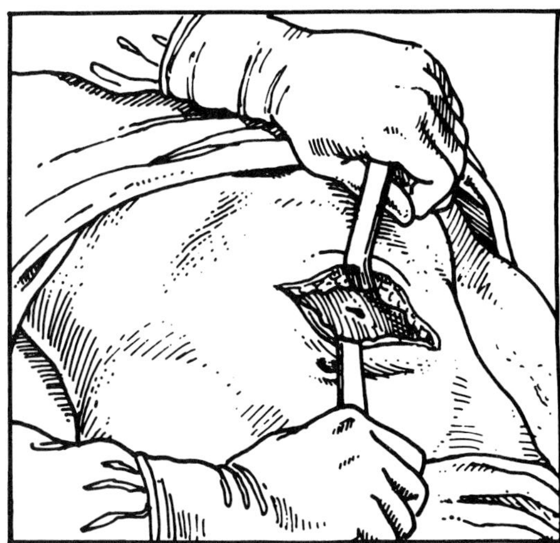

FIG. 252-5. Local wound exploration. Local wound exploration is the appropriate way to evaluate the abdomen after a stab wound. This is a surgical procedure requiring expertise, proper instrumentation, and lights. It is an appropriate diagnostic technique only for patients with anterior abdominal stab wounds. The stab wound is widened and explored down to the level of the fascia. A determination can be made whether the anterior fascia and/or posterior fascia has been violated.

Gunshot Wounds

A major concern with anterior abdominal gunshot wounds is to determine whether the missile traversed the peritoneal cavity. All patients with transabdominal gunshot wounds require exploration because virtually all of them will have intraabdominal pathology requiring surgery. Most often this can be determined by estimating trajectory. While it can be difficult to determine whether a hole is an exit wound or an entrance wound, a hole both in the anterior and posterior abdomen clearly defines a transabdominal trajectory. In the event of a single entrance, a plain film of the chest, pelvis, and/or abdomen often can determine trajectory. A lateral film may be necessary to help determine the trajectory precisely. A missile in a location that defines a transabdominal pathway mandates exploration.

Occasionally, in the case of tangential injuries or multiple gunshot wounds, it may be impossible to clearly estimate trajectory. Several options exist. It often may be safest to simply explore the patient. While the rate of nontherapeutic laparotomy may be relatively high, surgical exploration at least ensures that a potentially life-threatening injury will not be missed. The second option is to very carefully observe the patient with frequent physical examinations and laboratory values. The last option is to perform a peritoneal lavage. There are virtually no data that determine the correct threshold for red or white blood cell positivity in patients with gunshot wounds. The only purpose is to determine whether the missile traversed the abdominal cavity. Thus we generally set the threshold very low and explore patients if there is even a pink tinge to the effluent or the red blood cell count is 5000/cc.

THERAPY FOR ABDOMINAL INJURY

Laparotomy

Laparotomy is the ''gold standard'' therapy for intraabdominal injuries. As mentioned previously, it is definitive and rarely misses an injury. It allows for complete evaluation of virtually all structures within the abdomen and the retroperitoneum at a single point in time. Laparotomy may be exploratory in nature or may be performed to treat a diagnosed injury.

Indications for surgical abdominal exploration vary from institution to institution depending on location, expertise, and interest. Table 252-2 describes generally accepted indications for exploratory laparotomy. Certainly all patients with hypotension, abdominal wall disruption, or peritonitis mandate surgical exploration. In addition, the presence of extraluminal, intraabdominal, or retroperitoneal air either on plain film or CT should prompt surgical exploration. Finally, organ-specific diagnosis on CT often will mandate exploration. Examples include pancreatic injury, duodenal injury, renal injury with urinary extravasation outside Gerota's fascia, or a small bowel or colon injury.

Some patients have the diagnosis of injury made but are hemodynamically stable with a normal physical examination. This would include patients with a positive DPL or FAST or patients with a CT-diagnosed splenic or hepatic injury. Clearly, some of these patients may be managed nonoperatively. The ability to do so will involve readily available ancillary diagnostic testing such as CT scanning and angiography. This is discussed in more detail below. In smaller centers or community hospitals this may not be realistic. These patients are then best served by surgical exploration. In tertiary care centers some of these patients can be managed nonoperatively.

Special mention must be made of patients with fluid seen on CT scan without a clear source. Some will have hemoperitoneum from a trivial liver or splenic injury that is simply missed on CT. Unfortunately, others will have mesenteric injuries and/or small bowel injuries. Again, in many centers the safest course is to simply explore to avoid late diagnosis of gastrointestinal perforation or ischemia. In tertiary

TABLE 252-2 Indications for Laparotomy

	Blunt	Penetrating
Absolute	Anterior abdominal injury and hypotension Abdominal wall disruption Peritonitis Free air on chest x-ray CT diagnosed injury requiring surgery, i.e. pancreatic transection; duodenal rupture	Injury to abdomen, back and flank with hypotension Abdominal tenderness GI evisceration Positive DPL (GSW) High suspicion for transabdominal trajectory CT diagnosed injury requiring surgery, i.e., ureter or pancreas
Relative	Positive DPL or FAST in stable patient Solid visceral injury in stable patient Hemoperitoneum on CT without clear source	Positive local wound exploration (SW)

care centers some can be managed nonoperatively by means of careful observation and/or ancillary diagnostics.

The diagnostic dilemma is much less in patients with penetrating trauma. Diagnostic evaluation is undertaken only to infer the presence of abdominal injury. Specific organ injury is diagnosed at the time of surgical exploration. In stab wounds, the presence of hemoperitoneum or suspicion of gastrointestinal injury by physical examination should prompt exploratory laparotomy. A positive local wound exploration is a relative indication for operation. Any patient with a proven transabdominal trajectory following a gunshot wound requires laparotomy.

Some patients with penetrating trauma can be managed nonoperatively. For the most part, this involves patients with injury to the flank and back section. Only 9 percent of such patients who present hemodynamically stable have injuries mandating surgery.[15] Diagnostic adjuncts involve contrast-enhanced CT enema using oral, intravenous, and rectal contrast agents (Fig. 252-6). Perivascular hematomas can be investigated further with angiography. Endoscopy of the colon also may provide useful information.

NONOPERATIVE MANAGEMENT OF BLUNT TRAUMA

There is no question that many injuries previously thought to require surgery may now be managed nonoperatively. The evolution of this technique has been greatly advanced by the evolution of CT. CT makes the diagnosis of solid visceral injury and often can rule out other injuries requiring surgery. Solid visceral injuries can be graded as to severity.

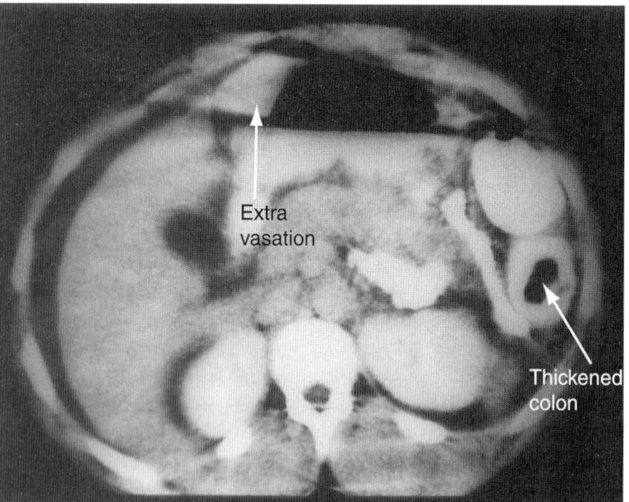

FIG. 252-6. Contrast enhanced CT enema. CT scan with oral, rectal, and intravenous contrast should be performed for asymptomatic patients with injury of flank and back. CT demonstrates a thickened left colon with contrast extravasation.

Unfortunately, CT grading may not agree with intraoperative observation.[16] In addition, CT grading does not always predict the success of nonoperative therapy.[17] This may be true for several reasons. CT provides a good description of the status of the internal parenchyma but does not provide three-dimensional injury anatomy. Operative grading, on the other hand, provides an excellent three-dimensional view of the organ but may underestimate internal damage. In addition, a traditional CT cannot provide information as to the integrity of the parenchymal vasculature. It is a single snapshot in time that cannot diagnose ongoing blood loss.

Organ-specific properties may affect the success or failure rate of nonoperative management. As patients age, the capsule of the spleen and liver weakens. Parenchymal changes may occur as well. Thus nonoperative management of even very severe injuries is the norm in children. Failure rates are much higher in adults. In addition, as patients age, the consequences of rebleeding become more substantial. Thus many tramatologists are less willing to attempt nonoperative management in elderly patients.

Over the last several years, several technologic advances have increased the sophistication of nonoperative management. The increased resolution of helical CT often identifies vascular injuries such as pseudoaneurysms or AV fistulas. Helical CT also can identify contrast material extravasation, indicating active bleeding. The role of angiography and nonoperative hemostasis has expanded greatly in nonoperative management of solid visceral injuries. Angiography has the ability to diagnose intraparenchymal vascular injury and evaluate the possibility of ongoing blood loss. Patients without vascular injury usually can be managed nonoperatively. In patients in whom vascular injury is diagnosed, percutaneous transcatheter embolization with either stainless steel coils or Gelfoam pledgets can arrest hemorrhage with a high degree of reliability.

Nonoperative Management of Hepatic Injury

Nonoperative management of hepatic injury has become the norm. Several recent large series have documented successful nonoperative treatment in 90 percent of patients who are hemodynamically stable at presentation.[18] Liver injuries are most commonly classified according to the system described by the American Association for the Surgery of Trauma (AAST) (Table 252-3). Unfortunately, most patients in these large series have had relatively low-grade injuries. Complications of nonoperative management of hepatic injuries include delayed bleeding, bile leak, intraabdominal sepsis, and missed intraabdominal injuries. These are relatively rare and occurred in only 5 percent of the largest series of nonoperative management of liver injuries.[18] However, the vast majority of complications occurred in higher-grade injuries.

TABLE 252-3 American Association for the Surgery of Trauma (AAST) Liver Injury Scale

Grade*		Injury Description
I.	Hematoma	Subcapsular, nonexpanding, <10 cm surface area
	Laceration	Capsular tear, nonbleeding, <1 cm parenchymal depth
II.	Hematoma	Subcapsular, nonexpanding, 10–50 percent surface area; intraparenchymal, nonexpanding, <10 cm in diameter
	Laceration	Capsular tear, active bleeding; 1–3 cm parenchymal depth, <10 cm in length
III.	Hematoma	Subcapsular, >50 percent surface area or expanding; ruptured subcapcular hematoma with active bleeding; intraparenchymal hematoma, >10 cm or expanding
	Laceration	>3 cm parenchymal depth
IV.	Hematoma	Ruptured intraparenchymal hematoma with active bleeding
	Laceration	Parenchymal disruption involving 25–75 percent of hepatic lobe or 1–3 Couinaud's segments within a single lobe
V.	Laceration	Parenchymal disruption involving >75 percent of hepatic lobe or >3 Couinaud's segments within a single lobe
	Vascular	Juxtahepatic venous injuries, i.e., retrohepatic vena cava/central major hepatic veins
VI.	Vascular	Hepatic avulsion

*Advance one grade for multiple injuries, up to grade III.

TABLE 252-4 American Association for the Surgery of Trauma (AAST) Spleen Injury Scale (1994 Revision)

Grade*		Injury Description
I.	Hematoma	Subcapsular, nonexpanding, <10 percent surface area
	Laceration	Capsular tear, nonbleeding, <1 cm parenchymal depth
II.	Hematoma	Subcapsular, nonexpanding, 10–50 percent surface area; intraparenchymal, nonexpanding, <5 cm in diameter
	Laceration	Capsular tear, active bleeding; 1–3 cm parenchymal depth, which does not involve a trabecular vessel
III.	Hematoma	Subcapsular, >50 percent surface area or expanding; ruptured subcapcular hematoma with active bleeding; intraparenchymal hematoma, >5 cm or expanding
	Laceration	>3 cm parenchymal depth or involving trabecular vessels
IV.	Hematoma	Ruptured intraparenchymal hematoma with active bleeding
	Laceration	Laceration involving segmental or hilar vessels producing major devascularization (>25 percent of spleen)
V.	Laceration	Completely shattered spleen
	Vascular	Hilar vascular injury that devascularizes spleen

*Advance one grade for multiple injuries up to grade III.

In the past, the failure of nonoperative management, either bleeding or bile leak, required operative management. More recently, it has become clear that many of these complications can be managed nonoperatively as well. Angiography with selective embolization is an effective means of treating even delayed blood loss from hepatic injuries. Percutaneous drainage can treat "bilomas" and can be used for hepatic abscesses. Endoscopic retrograde cholangiopancreatography (ERCP) with or without biliary stenting can be extremely helpful in decompressing clots from the biliary tree and definitively treating intraparenchymal hepatic ductal injury. Recently, Carrillo and colleagues reviewed 135 patients managed nonoperatively.[19] Thirty-two patients developed complications requiring intervention, with most of these patients having higher-grade injuries. A combination of the aforementioned techniques was successful in managing these complications nonoperatively 85 percent of the time.

Finally, nonoperative techniques can be combined with operation. Laparotomy and temporary packing to control hepatic injury ("damage control") are now commonplace. This can be followed by angiographic embolization to control arterial injuries deep within the substance of the liver. Other techniques can then be used once the patient has stabilized.

Nonoperative Management of Splenic Injury

Although nonoperative management of splenic injuries is the norm in children, its use in adults has been far less successful. Failure rates have been reported to be as high as 20 to 30 percent. This relatively high failure rate has prompted some authors to advocate limiting nonoperative management to patients under 55 years of age and those with a CT injury grade no higher than 3 (Table 252-4).

The addition of angiography to the treatment algorithm has radically changed the nature of nonoperative management for splenic injury. First reported by Sclafani and colleagues from Kings County Hospital, sequential DPL, CT, and angiography was used as a management algorithm in the care of patients with blunt trauma.[16] Stable patients with a positive DPL underwent CT. All patients with CT-diagnosed splenic injury were then treated angiographically. All vascular injuries identified at the time of angiography were treated with proximal coil embolization. Proximal embolization, similarly to splenic artery ligation, decreases the pressure head to the spleen, allowing for spontaneous hemostasis. Splenic viability and immune function are preserved by collateral vessels via the pancreatic branches of the splenic artery, the short gastric vessels, and collaterals from the superior mesenteric artery. In a series of approximately 150 patients, splenic salvage was 95 percent when this algorithm was used. Most important, a negative splenic arteriogram predicted successful nonoperative management 100 percent of the time.

The group from Memphis recently reported on 524 consecutive patients with blunt trauma.[20] Nonoperative management was attempted in 344 patients. Ninety-four percent were managed successfully nonoperatively, which represented 60 percent of the total splenic injuries. The indication for angiography was the presence of a pseudoaneurysm seen on helical CT. They used subselective embolization as opposed to proximal coil embolization. Only one patient developed clinically significant splenic infarction despite the subselective embolization. Importantly, nearly three-quarters of the patients had a pseudoaneurysm seen at the time of follow-up CT scan that was not seen at the time of initial scanning. The authors stressed the importance of follow-up CT even in asymptomatic patients.

It would seem that an initial helical CT scan, while valuable, is not definitive and that injuries evolve. In both series, higher-grade injuries had an increased likelihood of having a vascular injury identified. However, in the Brooklyn series, 12 percent of patients with grade 1 injuries had vascular injuries identified and embolized at the time of angiography.[16] Thus simple CT grading may not be sufficient to predict the success of nonoperative therapy. It would seem that careful follow-up is mandatory for all patients in whom nonoperative management is attempted. Follow-up CT scan has the potential to identify the progression, if any, of injury. In addition, it appears to reliably identify pseudoaneurysms not seen at the time of initial scanning. Alternatively, early, liberal use of angiography should help to identify patients with vascular injuries. Either of these techniques appears to radically decrease the incidence of delayed splenic rupture. This often presents at 7 to 10 days in patients who were stable initially following the diagnosis of splenic injury.

In fact, the term *delayed splenic rupture* is probably a misnomer. Instead, this more correctly is misdiagnosis of splenic vascular injury at the time of initial presentation, almost certainly small injuries such as pseudoaneurysms or AV fistulas. Over 7 to 10 days they expand and ultimately rupture, producing blood loss and corresponding symptoms. The term pulsating splenic hemorrhage more correctly describes this entity.

Neither of these series had a large proportion of high-grade splenic injuries contained within them. Recently, the group at the Shock Trauma Center prospectively evaluated a series of 73 patients.[21] All patients diagnosed with splenic injuries underwent early angiography. There was a large proportion of CT grade 3 and 4 injuries contained within this series. The presence of a vascular abnormality correlated with grading. The higher the grade, the more likely the patient was to have vascular injury at the time of angiography. Patients with high-grade injuries tended to have more severe injuries and often had multiple injuries. These were treated with a combination of proximal coil and subselective embolotechniques (Fig. 252-7). Nonoperative management was successful 88 percent of the time, and the splenic salvage rate was 94 percent in this series.

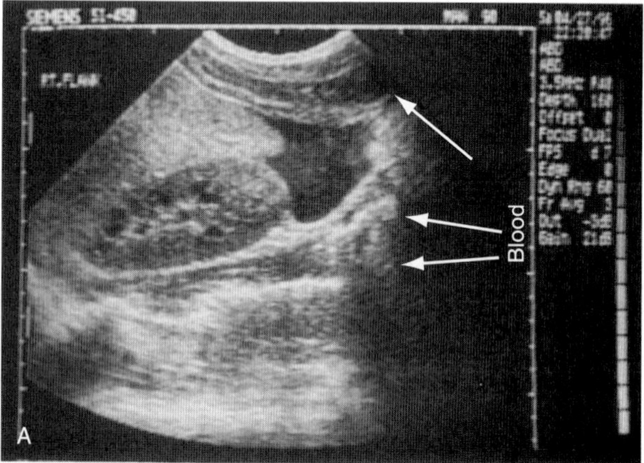

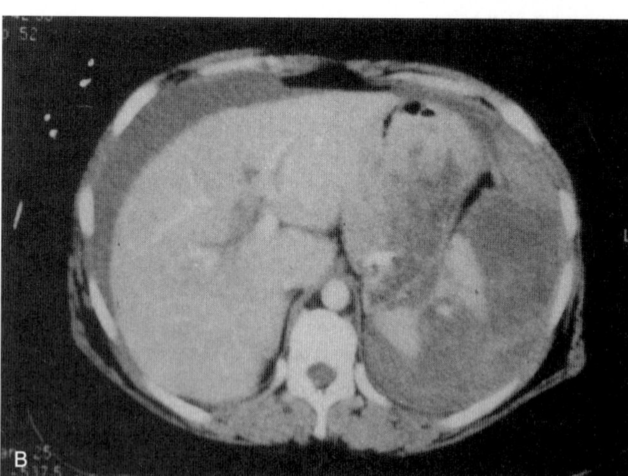

FIG. 252-7. Nonoperative management of splenic injuries. **A.** FAST in this 21-year-old female with blunt abdominal trauma clearly demonstrates hemoperitoneum. **B.** The patient remains hemodynamically stable and CT scan demonstrates a grade 4 splenic injury.

Nonoperative management for splenic injuries is certainly a safe and effective technique. However, this must involve a committed team of emergency physicians, surgeons, and invasive radiologists in order to safely manage patients with high-grade injuries nonoperatively. Coil embolization is a safe technique and an effective method of hemostasis. These innovative techniques should be performed in a tertiary care center under strict protocol in order to be managed safely.

REFERENCES

1. Scalea TM, Goldstein AS, Phillips TF, et al: An analysis of 161 falls from a height: The ''jumper syndrome.'' *J Trauma* 26:706, 1986
2. American College of Surgeons, Committee on Trauma: *Advanced Life Support Course, Student Manual.* ACS, 1993.
3. Scalea TM, Holman M, Fourtes M, et al: Central venous blood oxygen saturation: An early, accurate measurement of volume during hemorrhage. *J Trauma* 28:725, 1988.
4. Shanmuganathan K, Mirvis SE, White CS, Pomertanz SM: MR imaging evaluation of hemidiaphragms in acute blunt trauma: Experience with 16 patients. *AJR* 167:397, 1996.
5. Saunders CJ, Battistella FD, Whetzel TP, Stokes RB: Percutaneous diagnostic peritoneal lavage using a Veress needle versus an open technique: A prospective randomized trial. *J Trauma* 44:883, 1998.
6. Goldstein AS, Scalfani SJA, Kupterstein NH, et al: The diagnostic superiority of computed tomography. *J Trauma* 25:939, 1985.
7. Otomo Y, Henmi H, Mashiko K, et al: New diagnostic peritoneal lavage criteria for diagnosis of intestinal injury. *J Trauma* 44:991, 1998.
8. Branney SW, Wolfe RE, Moore EE, et al: Quantitative sensitivity of ultrasound in detecting free intraperitoneal fluid. *J Trauma* 39:375, 1995.
9. McKinney MG, Lentz K, Nunez D, et al: Can ultrasound replace diagnostic peritoneal lavage in the assessment of blunt trauma? *J Trauma* 37:439, 1994.
10. Glaser K, Ischmelitsch J, Kluiger P, et al: Ultrasonography in the management of blunt abdominal and thoracic trauma. *Arch Surg* 129:742, 1994.
11. Tsang BD, Panacek EA, Brant WE, Wisner DH: Effect of oral contrast administration for abdominal computed tomography in the evaluation of acute blunt trauma. *Ann Emerg Med* 30:7–13, 1997.
12. Chiu WC, Cushing BM, Rodriquez A, et al: Abdominal injuries without hemoperitoneum: A potential limitation of focused abdominal sonography for trauma (FAST). *J Trauma* 42:617, 1997.
13. Renz BM, Feliciano DV: Unnecessary laparotomies for trauma: A prospective study of morbidity. *J Trauma* 38:350, 1995.
14. Zubowski R, Nallathambi M, Ivatury R, Stahl W: Selective conservatism in abdominal stab wounds: The efficacy of serial physical examination. *J Trauma* 28:1665, 1988.
15. McCarthy MC, Lowdermilk GA, Canal DF, Broadie TA: Prediction of injury caused by penetrating wounds to the abdomen, flank, and back. *Arch Surg* 126:962, 1991.
16. Sclafani SJA, Shaftan GW, Scalea TM, et al: Nonoperative salvage of computer tomograph-diagnosed splenic injuries: Utilization of angiography for triage and embolization for hemostasis. *J Trauma* 39:818, 1995.
17. Mirvis SE, Whitley NO, Gens DR: Blunt splenic trauma in adults: CT-based classification and correlation with prognosis and treatment. *Radiology* 171:133, 1989.
18. Pachter HL, Knudson MM, Esrig B, et al: Status of nonoperative management of blunt hepatic injuries in 1995: A multicenter experience with 404 patients. *J Trauma* 40:31, 1996.
19. Carillo EH, Spain DA, Wohltmann CD, et al: Interventional treatment can improve the outcome of nonoperative management of hepatic injuries [abst]. *J Trauma* 45:202, 1998.
20. Davis KA, Fabian TC, Croce MA: Improved success in nonoperative management of blunt splenic injuries: Embolization of splenic artery pseudoaneurysms. *J Trauma* 44:1008, 1998.
21. Boyd-Kranis R, Hastings G, Fan CM, et al: Angiography and subselective artery embolization for nonoperative management of blunt splenic injury [abst]. *J Trauma* 45:199, 1998.

PENETRATING TRAUMA TO THE FLANK AND BUTTOCK

Alasdair K. T. Conn

Penetrating injuries to the flank and buttock challenge the physician because of the possibility of missed injuries to retroperitoneal structures. Gunshot and stab wounds in these areas must be carefully evaluated to determine whether there is retroperitoneal injury with intraperitoneal or vascular injury that might mandate immediate surgical intervention. Evaluation is difficult; the retroperitoneal structures are well protected by dense layers of musculature and the spine. There is significant risk of missed injury and delay in diagnosis. Fortunately, an increased armamentarium of diagnostic testing assists in timely diagnosis and allows for selective conservative management. The choice of management, conservative or operative, is determined based upon the emergency evaluation, making the emergency physician's input essential to a correct decision and a clinically successful outcome. Penetrating injuries to the buttock are relatively uncommon and some trauma centers report as few as three to five patients with this type of injury per year. Trauma centers in urban settings have reported 50 to 80 patients per year. With appropriate management the mortality is low, but case reports indicate that there is a potential for a missed injury to the bowel or major vessels, especially with shotgun or high velocity gunshot wounds, unless the clinician is vigilant in the emergency evaluation. This chapter outlines the evaluation of patients who present to the Emergency Department (ED) with penetrating trauma to the flank and to the buttock.

PENETRATING TRAUMA TO THE FLANK

Pathophysiology

The flank is the area between the anterior and posterior axillary lines, superiorly bordered by the sixth rib and inferiorly bordered by the iliac crest. Although a penetrating wound to the flank can produce intraperitoneal injury with the associated physical findings of peritonitis or hemoperitoneum with shock, it is possible that a penetrating flank wound only injures the retroperitoneal organs. A delay in diagnosis of duodenal, colonic, rectal, renal, pancreatic or major vascular injuries may result in the late appearance of septic or hemorrhagic shock.

The path of a gunshot or stab wound to the flank may track superiorly. Bullets may ricochet off the bony structures of the spine and produce a unique bullet path and injury pattern. Other intra-abdominal organs may be injured, such as the stomach or pancreas, the diaphragm, and intrathoracic organs. Inferior tracking will jeopardize the lower GI tract and colon. Treatment of these specific organ injuries is covered elsewhere in this text (see Chap. 251).

Clinical Features

Patients with penetrating trauma to the flank should be resuscitated and evaluated according to standard resuscitative protocols. Initial resuscitative efforts should be directed towards the primary survey (see Chap. 243). Information regarding the mechanism of injury, how much time has passed since the traumatic event, and the nature of the weapon should be obtained and recorded. In the case of a gunshot wound, the nature of the gun (shotgun, handgun, BB gun) and the range between the gun and the patient at time of the gun's discharge should be ascertained and noted in the emergency record. Following stabilization, an attempt should be made to find an exit wound, and a bullet path reconstructed. Baseline laboratory and radiologic data, including a hemogram, chest radiograph, urinalysis, and rectal exam with testing for occult blood, should be performed on all patients. In the presence of peritonitis, intravenous fluid and broad-spectrum antibiotics should be administered and urgent surgical consultation obtained. A suitable regime of antibiotics is ampicillin, gentamycin, and metronidazole initiated in the emergency department. Most patients are stable and will require additional diagnostic modalities.

Diagnosis

PORTABLE ULTRASOUND In a patient with a penetrating wound to the flank, portable ultrasonography can be utilized to determine if there is fluid in the abdominal cavity. In the absence of a preexisting medical condition (such as cirrhosis with ascites), such information may be invaluable. Although the sensitivity and specificity varies with the type of equipment used and the experience of the operator, fluid collections of 600 cc should easily be detected by the emergency physician.[1] For a patient with a gunshot wound this may be sufficient to recommend an operative approach. For a patient with a stab wound, even if hemodynamically stable, this indicates a significant intra-abdominal injury. Operative intervention is sometimes delayed pending further adjunctive diagnostic measures.

WOUND EXPLORATION Although local wound exploration under adequate local anesthesia using sterile technique is of value in anterior abdominal wounds, it is only of limited value in wounds of the flank. If local exploration demonstrates that the injury does not penetrate beyond fascia or muscle, the wound may be safely closed and the patient discharged from the ED with appropriate follow-up instructions. With deeper penetrating injuries, it is difficult to determine the extent of injury with local wound exploration. More information can usually be obtained by CT scanning. Deep wound exploration often leads to further hemorrhage and tissue damage and is of limited value. It is difficult, if not impossible, to ascertain the exact depth of a stab wound from deep wound exploration.

DIAGNOSTIC PERITONEAL LAVAGE Appropriately performed, diagnostic peritoneal lavage (DPL) is highly accurate in determining the presence of intraperitoneal injury; it does not detect the presence of a retroperitoneal injury. (For details of the technique, see Chap. 252.) The criteria of what constitutes a positive diagnostic lavage in penetrating trauma are different from the criteria for blunt trauma. The exact criteria vary from hospital to hospital, but a guide is a red cell count of $>10,000/mm^3$ as an indication to perform an exploratory laparotomy. Lavage fluid may also be analyzed for bowel content, white cells, or enzymes such as amylase; although criteria for what constitutes a positive lavage vary from center to center. In some hospitals, enzymatic assay and examination for bowel content have been abandoned. Others still advocate its use to ascertain if a bowel or pancreatic injury has occurred. In most institutions, the use of diagnostic peritoneal lavage for a stable patient has been replaced by CT scanning. In an unstable patient, DPL can be performed (especially if portable ultrasound is not immediately available) to rapidly detect the presence (or absence) of hemoperitoneum.

COMPUTED TOMOGRAPHY (CT) In many centers, computed tomography has become the diagnostic modality of choice in patients who present hemodynamically stable following a flank penetrating trauma.[2,3] Double (oral gastrografin and intravenous contrast) or triple (oral, intravenous, and rectal contrast) are used; rectal contrast should be used if there is even a remote likelihood of a rectal or sigmoid injury. Cooperation with the radiologist is essential as fine "cuts" through the site of injury may be required to delineate the injury tract. Particular attention should be paid to the presence of intraperitoneal fluid and any edema of the bowel wall. The latter may represent bowel perforation, although no leak is visible by leakage of the contrast.[4]

The majority of patients with identified injury will be found to have retroperitoneal hematoma, without bowel or solid organ damage. Rarely, a hematoma around one of the major blood vessels or the pancreas is evident, requiring further diagnostic testing such as angiography, venography, or endoscopic retrograde cholangiopancreatogram (ERCP). Occasionally, a gunshot wound may be observed to pass extraperitoneally, but concerns about blast effect may lead to the decision to perform laparoscopy.

Treatment

The treatment of penetrating trauma to the flank remains somewhat controversial, although there is a tendency toward more conservative management. Some patients present with signs and symptoms that mandate immediate exploratory celiotomy.

Although in the past, celiotomy was more liberally utilized, it should be reserved for those patients who present with these conditions:

- Hemorrhagic shock
- Peritonitis
- Evisceration
- Transabdominal missile path
- Intraperitoneal free air

At the time of surgery, all intraperitoneal and retroperitoneal organ structures should be evaluated according to standard operative procedures.

Although some surgeons still advocate mandatory exploratory laparotomy in an effort to detect all injuries early, most surgeons now advocate selective management with early CT scanning, which allows many injuries to be managed by close observation. Using this conservative approach, celiotomy rates have been decreasing from 100 percent to approximately 30 percent with the incidence of positive laparotomy rising from 15 percent to approximately 80 percent, without increases in untoward outcome.[5] Using this approach, the risks associated with the "negative laparotomy" (early: hemorrhage and infection; and late: complications small bowel obstruction) as well as added expense are avoided. Many recent reviews support this selective management approach.

Exploratory laparotomy is most commonly performed for flank gunshot wounds. Many flank stab wounds can be safely managed conservatively. In the case of high-velocity gunshot wounds, blast effect must be considered. Depending on the exact location and type of injury, consideration of the blast effect may lead to exploratory laparotomy if there is concern as to the bowel, bladder, or vascular integrity; or laparoscopy may be used to determine the extent of intraperitoneal injury. An experienced surgeon should perform laparoscopy, as bowel injuries may be difficult to detect.

With CT, the exact depth of a stab wound can often be determined. Decision algorithms based upon low-risk patients' flank stab wounds (penetration superficial to the deep fascia) or high-risk (penetration beyond the deep fascia) have been developed and appear to be clinically justified.[6] Hemodynamically stable patients with stab wounds to the flank can be risk-stratified based upon these contrast-enhanced computer tomography findings. Low-risk patients may be discharged immediately from the Emergency Department. High-risk patients require surgical consultation and should be admitted to the hospital, but in many cases a discharge decision can be made within 24 h.

PENETRATING BUTTOCK INJURIES

Pathophysiology

Penetrating trauma to the buttock may be either from gunshot wounds or stab wounds. Gunshot wounds have the greatest potential for injury; as the thick musculature and fat over the buttocks normally protects the gastrointestinal, genitourinary, and neurological systems from injury in all except the deepest penetrating trauma from stab wounds. With gunshot wounds, the risk of intraperitoneal injury is much higher and may necessitate immediate exploratory celiotomy. Injured systems requiring operative intervention are the lower GI tract, the lower GU tract, and, rarely, a vascular injury. A delay in diagnosis of colonic or rectal injury will contribute to increased mortality and morbidity. From the civilian trauma literature, approximately 30 percent of patients who present with gunshot wounds require surgery. Factors associated with surgical intervention include findings of peritonitis; a positive finding at sigmoidoscopy; gross blood in the urine; entrance wound above the level of the greater trochanters; and a transpelvic (as opposed to extrapelvic) bullet course.[7–9] Stab wounds to the buttock infrequently require laparotomy.

Clinical Features

Initial approaches to trauma resuscitation should be followed as noted earlier. Attention should be paid to the abdominal examination. If there is indication of peritonitis or of a gunshot with a transabdominal missile path, emergent surgical consultation should be obtained and preparations made for an exploratory laparotomy. Baseline hemogram, urinalysis, and rectal examination should be performed on all patients. If there is any concern of injury to the rectum because of blood being noted on rectal examination or because of the trajectory of the bullet, proctosigmoidoscopy should be performed.[10] Cystography should be performed on patients when there is blood on urinalysis or the proximity of the wound to the GI tract is a concern. Vascular injury to gluteal or internal iliac arteries has been reported from gluteal-penetrating wounds and may lead to exsanguinating external hemorrhage.[11] An intrapelvic injury may also cause injury to the internal iliac vessels with hypovolemic shock; this will require early operative intervention. In all patients, the peripheral pulses in lower extremity should be examined looking for decreased pulses or pallor as evidence of a proximal injury. Neurologic examination of the lower extremities to document any injury to the sciatic or femoral nerve should also be performed on all patients. Buttock wounds rarely cause damage to the sciatic plexus or femoral plexus. Injury could include transsection, partial transsection, or stretch injury secondary to the trauma. The presence of any symptomatic signs requires appropriate consultation.

Diagnosis

The signs of peritonitis, intrapelvic or transabdominal missile path, and intraperitoneal free air warrant immediate celiotomy. Proctosigmoidoscopy can be a great aid in the diagnosis of a rectal injury, and should be performed in the ED. To evaluate the lower GU tract, a cystourethrogram should be performed. This can be performed either as a separate study or in conjunction with CT scanning, with rectal and intravenous contrast and clamping the urethra catheter to obtain a CT cystogram. If the CT scan demonstrates a pelvic hematoma, angiography or venography may be indicated to document a significant vascular injury. Also, appropriate consultation should be obtained. Local wound exploration is of limited value in penetrating buttock injuries. For those patients who present with peritonitis, or if there is a concern of a rectal injury, broad spectrum intravenous antibiotics should be initiated in the ED. Operative therapy for rectal injuries should be directed at proximal colostomy, presacral drainage, and distal washout. Genitourinary tract injuries are repaired with appropriate drainage and often a suprapubic cystostomy.

REFERENCES

1. Branney SW, Wolfe RE, Moore EE, et al: Quantitative sensitivity of ultrasound in detecting free intraperitoneal fluid. *J Trauma* 39(2):375, 1995.
2. Easter DW, Shackford SR, Mattrey RF: A prospective, randomized comparison of computed tomography with conventional diagnostic methods in the evaluation of penetrating injuries to the back and flank. *Arch Surg* 126(9):1115, 1991.

3. Kirton OC, Wint D, Thrasher B, et al: Stab wounds to the back and flank in the hemodynamically stable patient: A decision algorithm based on contrast-enhanced computed tomography with colonic opacification. *Am J Surg* 173(3):189, 1997.
4. Himmelman RG, Martin M, Gilkey S, et al: Triple-contrast CT scans in penetrating back and flank trauma. *J Trauma* 31(6):852, 1991.
5. Boyle EM Jr, Maier RV, Salazar JD, et al: Diagnosis of injuries after stab wounds to the back and flank. *J Trauma* 42(2):260, 1997.
6. Velmahos GC, Demetriades D, Cornwell EE, et al: Gunshot wounds to the buttocks: Predicting the need for operation. *Dis Colon Rectum* 40(3):307, 1997.
7. Gilroy D, Saadia R, Hide G, et al: Penetrating injury to the gluteal region. *J Trauma* 32(3):294, 1992.
8. DiGiacomo JC, Schwab CW, Rotondo MF, et al: Gluteal gunshot wounds: Who warrants exploration? *J Trauma* 37(4):622, 1994.
9. Ferraro FJ, Livingston DH, Odom J, et al: The role of sigmoidoscopy in the management of gunshot wounds to the buttocks. *Am Surg* 59(6):350, 1997.
10. Mercer DW, Buckman RF Jr, Sood R, et al: Anatomic considerations in penetrating gluteal wounds. *Arch Surg* 127(4):407, 1992.
11. McCarthy MC, Lowdermilk GA, Canal DF, et al: Prediction of injury caused by penetrating wounds to the abdomen, flank and back. *Arch Surg* 126(8):962, 1991.

GENITOURINARY TRAUMA

Gabor D. Kelen

EPIDEMIOLOGY

Injuries to the genitourinary system occur in about 2 to 5 percent of adult trauma victims. The vast majority of these injuries are due to blunt trauma. Accurate overall estimates for children are not available, but it appears that about 10 percent of pediatric patients with blunt abdominal trauma have renal system injury.[1,2] More than 80 perecnt of those with injuries to the kidney have other concurrent injuries, about a third of them life threatening. Approximately 80 percent of the urogenital injuries involve the kidney, and about 10 percent involve the bladder. Significant ureteral injuries are relatively rare and are usually associated with penetrating trauma. Significant urethral injuries most often occur in males and are usually associated with pelvic fracture. Patients with anatomic anomalies, including tumor and hydronephrosis, appear more susceptible to injury.

CLINICAL APPROACH

The overall approach to trauma is discussed in Chap. 243. Only issues specific to genitourinary trauma are discussed here.

Renal system injuries rarely require immediate intervention. Investigation of renal injuries should not supercede evaluation of more life-threatening injuries. For example, with a pelvic fracture, determining the need for pelvic angiography is more important than determining whether a urethral injury exists. The patient may well die from a sheared major artery, whereas an injured urethra will never require immediate attention. The retrograde introduction of dye will render subsequent pelvic angiography very difficult, if not impossible.

During the detailed secondary survey, a concerted effort should be made to closely inspect the perineum. Blood on the underwear is an important finding. In both male and female patients, the folds of the buttocks should be spread in search of perineal lacerations, which often denote an open pelvic fracture. Such lacerations should not be probed lest a clot be disrupted and exsanguinating hemorrhage result. During the rectal examination, sphincter tone, the position of the prostate gland, and presence of any blood should be noted. If the prostate is riding high or feels boggy, there has been a disruption of the membranous urethra. Next, the scrotum is palpated and inspected for ecchymoses, laceration, and testicular disruption. Simultaneously, the length of the penis is palpated to inspect for blood at the meatus. In females, the labia are inspected for lacerations and hematomas. If there is any evidence of likelihood of trauma in this area, a bimanual vaginal examination is required. If there is blood in the vagina, a speculum examination is necessary to rule out vaginal laceration.

During the secondary survey, the trauma series x-rays are obtained and often include an anteroposterior view of the pelvis. The presence of a pelvic fracture has important implications in the workup of genitourinary injuries.

Generally, no urinary catheter should be introduced until the urine can be evaluated for hematuria. However, the placement of a urinary catheter for monitoring of urine output may be required in severely injured patients who cannot void. If there is doubt and placement of a catheter is urgent, a suprapubic approach may be the most prudent. In menstruating women, a specimen obtained with a catheter is likely to offer more accurate urinalysis than a spontaneously voided specimen.

The standard serologic and blood specimen results are generally not helpful in determining the presence or degree of renal injury in the acute setting.

BLUNT TRAUMA

Detection of Specific Injuries

The need to determine the existence of specific injuries is based on the clinical elements obtained in the history, physical examination, and plain films, and to some extent the age of the patient. Table 254-1 lists some key elements that should prompt the consideration of further evaluation of renal tract injury. The approach to evaluation is dependent on the following: blunt versus penetrating trauma, the presence of hematuria and whether it is gross or microscopic, associated injuries, mechanism of injury, hemodynamic stability, and age of the patient.[3] Each of these factors affects the approach somewhat. Renal injuries require staging for appropriate management (Table 254-2).[4] Staging is usually accomplished through use of an imaging modality, but sometimes exploration is required (see below).

MEATAL BLOOD Blood at the meatus is associated with urethral injuries. Urethral injuries are almost exclusively seen in males. Poste-

TABLE 254-1 Key Clinical Findings Associated with Renal System Injury

Acceleration or deceleration injury (renal pedical)
Lower rib fractures (kidney)
Fracture lower thoracic or upper lumbar spine
Pelvic fracture (urethra)
Abdominal trauma
Flank ecchymosis, tenderness, mass (kidney)
Straddle injuries (urethra)
Penetrating trauma (in vicinity of any part of the renal system)
Penile scrotal or perineal hematoma (urethra)
Gross hematuria
Microscopic hematuria in certain circumstances (see text)
Abnormally positioned prostate (posterior urethra)
Blood at penile meatus (urethra)

TABLE 254-2 Grading of Renal Injuries[4]

Grade	Injury
I	Contusion (microscopic or gross hematuria, with normal urologic study results) Subscapsular, nonexpanding hematoma without laceration
II	Parenchymal laceration <1.0 cm depth limited to cortex, no extravasation Nonexpanding hematoma, confined to retroperitoneum
III	Parenchymal laceration >1 cm depth with extravasation or collecting system rupture
IV	Laceration extending through to collecting system Vascular pedical injury, hemorrhage contained
V	Shattered kidney Avulsed hilum (devascularized kidney)

rior urethral injuries are commonly associated with pelvic fractures. A superiorly displaced prostate indicates disruption of the posterior urethra. Anterior urethral injuries are associated with straddle injuries and instrumentation.

When meatal blood is noted, a urinary catheter should not be placed in order to prevent the conversion of a partial urethral laceration into a complete transection. A retrograde urethrogram is virtually mandatory in this setting.

HEMATURIA For the purposes of trauma, microscopic hematuria is defined as more than five red blood cells (RBCs) per high-power field (hpf). A 10-mL specimen must be centrifuged for 5 min at 2000 revolutions for an accurate assessment. Gross hematuria is, of course, readily visible blood. Reddish urine does not necessarily indicate hematuria; several medications and toxic substances may cause discoloration (Table 254-3). Also, results of a dipstick evaluation may be erroneous, since myoglobin, a frequent finding in major trauma, reacts with the reagent.

TABLE 254-3 Substances and Medications Associated with Urinary Discoloration

Black	Brown	Red
Cresols	Benzene	Ampicillin
Levodopa	Carbon tetrachloride	Aniline
Methocarbamol	Chloroquine	Anthocyanin (beets, blackberries)
Phenazopyridine	Cresols	Betaine (fresh beets)
Phenol	Dinitrophenol	Deferoxamine
Quinine	Fava beans	Ibuprofen
	Hydroquinone	Lead (chronic)
	Lead	Lycopene (tomatoes, watermelon)
	Levodopa	Mercury
	Mercury	Myoglobin
	Methemoglobinemia	Napthalene
	Methocarbamol	Phenolphthalein (in laxatives)
	Metronidazole	Phenothiazines
	Naphthalene	Phenytoin
	Niridazole	Porphyrins
	Nitrofurantoin	Quinines
	Phenacetin	Rifampin
	Phenols	
	Phenothiazine	
	Phenytoin	
	Primaquine	
	Quinines	
	Sulfonamides	

The initially voided urine may provide clues as to the location of injury. When possible, at least two specimens (initial stream and terminal stream) should be obtained. Initial hematuria suggests injury to the distal system (i.e., urethra or prostate). Terminal hematuria suggests bladder neck injury. Continuous hematuria suggests upper renal system (bladder, ureter, or kidney) injury.

Many studies have demonstrated that, in adult patients with blunt trauma, the degree of hematuria does not correspond to the degree of injury. Gross hematuria may be seen with relatively minor renal contusions, whereas microscopic hematuria (or even no hematuria) may be seen in renovascular injuries. However, in the absence of significant hemodynamic compromise, isolated microscopic hematuria is unlikely to represent significant blunt injury. While there is no clinically validated or generally accepted upper limit of microscopic hematuria beyond which imaging is done, many physicians image patients where the degree of microscopic hematuria is ≥ 50 RBCs/hpf. A review of several major studies addressing this question concluded that isolated microscopic hematuria indicates significant injury in about 1 in 500 patients with such a finding.[3] Thus, the current consensus is that adult patients with isolated microscopic hematuria do not require further imaging studies. There are three exceptions. When the mechanism of trauma involves rapid deceleration, renal pedicle injuries may ensue but can present with minimal (or even no) hematuria. Also, hematuria in a patient with even transient hypotension should not be considered an isolated finding. Finally, microscopic hematuria may be a significant finding in children, as detailed later in the text.

All patients in whom microscopic hematuria is found with concurrent nonrenal injuires and those with hemodynamic instability should have a diagnostic imaging study, as discussed below. In such patients, computed tomography (CT) is often impractical. A ''one-shot'' intravenous pyelogram (IVP) can be obtained in the operating room.

Gross hematuria may occur from injury virtually anywhere in the renal tract. The finding of gross hematuria mandates a diagnostic imaging study that is chosen based on other findings (Table 254-4). For example, in the presence of pelvic fractures, gross hematuria should raise the possibility of bladder or urethral injury. Almost 95 percent of bladder injuries are associated with gross hematuria.

Special Considerations

RAPID DECELERATION FORCES Rapid deceleration injuries may result in renal pedicle and vascular injuries. Such injuries result in

TABLE 254-4 Selection of Diagnostic Imaging for Suspected Renal System Injury

Imaging Study	Suspected Injury
Retrograde urethrogram or cystogram	Urethral injury
CT (with IV contrast)	Renal injury (staging) Ureteral injury
Cystogram, plain film (retrograde)	Bladder injury
CT cystogram (retrograde)	Bladder injury
''One-shot'' IVP	Unstable patients taken to operating room
IVP	Alternative to CT in unstable patients Ureteral injury
Angiogram or venogram	Pedicle injuries, venous disruption
Retrograde pyelogram	Renal pelvis disruption

high mortality rates, but fortunately they are quite rare, occurring in less than 1 percent of blunt renal trauma. However, hematuria, the clue to renal injury, may not be present. Accordingly, patients whose mechanism of injury is from forces of rapid deceleration should have a renovascular imaging study. Since pedicle injuries virtually always occur in association with other significant injuries,[5] other indications for radiographic evaluation are likely. Many such patients have other indications for surgical exploration.

PEDIATRIC BLUNT TRAUMA Hematuria following blunt trauma may have different significance in the pediatric population.[6,7] Unlike the situation in adults, the degree of hematuria does seem to correlate with the degree of injury.[5] Many advocate that pediatric patients with any degree of hematuria, even if hemodynamically stable, should undergo imaging studies.[8,9] However, pediatric patients with less than 50 RBCs/hpf do not appear to have significant injuries.[5] Thus, it appears appropriate to perform imaging studies on only those patients with significant hematuria, as defined above.[3] Other standards for imaging studies for pediatric patients remain similar to those for adults.

Choice of Radiographic Study for Evaluation and Staging of Renal System Injury

The following should be considered when ordering studies in the trauma patient: (1) intravenous contrast agents can cause false-positive scan results for blood; (2) the total quantity of contrast required may limit the number of contrast studies, especially with shock; (3) hypotensive patients are at risk for developing contrast-induced acute renal failure; (4) abdominal CT reveals more information but requires a hemodynamically stable condition; and (5) an intraoperative IVP during an emergency laparotomy is needed to determine the status of the contralateral kidney.

A guideline for the selection of diagnostic imaging modalities is shown in Table 254-4.

PLAIN FILM Plain films are helpful in determining likelihood of renal trauma when abnormalities such as lower rib fractures, lower thoracic and upper lumbar spinal fractures, and pelvic fractures are seen. Loss of the psoas shadow or scoliosis may suggest injury. However, plain films are inappropriate for evaluating the renal tract.

COMPUTED TOMOGRAPHY Indications for imaging the kidneys following blunt trauma include gross hematuria, hematuria with multiple injuries or hemodynamic instability, and mechanisms that include rapid deceleration. When renal injury is suspected, CT is considered superior to other imaging modalities, including sonography, angiography, or IVP. CT is most likely to allow appropriate staging of renal injury (Table 254-2) and has several advantages. CT is a noninvasive modality with superior imaging detail that allows detection of even minor injuries and minimal extravasation, estimation of extent of hematoma, and simultaneous evaluation of other organs. The major disadvantage is that it can be performed only in a stable patient. Other disadvantages are cost and the difficulty in detecting vascular, particularly venous, injury. In children with hematuria, CT is the radiographic study of choice in evaluating renal injuries because a significant nonrenal intraabdominal injury is more likely than a renal injury.

Certain considerations should be kept in mind. Routine abdominal CT evaluation often stops at the iliac crests. In situations where renal system trauma is under consideration, the examination should be extended to the pelvis. Also, contrast enhancement is usually indicated for appropriate evaluation. Both oral and intravenous contrast material is often given when other intraabdominal trauma is under consideration. However, if enhanced CT is required to image the kidneys and collecting system appropriately, gastrointestinal contrast studies may need to be delayed to allow accurate interpretation.

MAGNETIC RESONANCE IMAGING Magnetic resonance imaging (MRI) is generally not a first-line imaging modality. However, its accuracy appears to be similar to that of CT. It may prove useful in stable patients who have dye allergy.

ANGIOGRAPHY Angiography has largely been replaced by CT. It still has a role when vascular injury is suspected and remains the gold standard for detecting renal venous injury. Arteriography may be indicated in selected patients when no renal function is evident on IVP or CT. Other indications include penetrating trauma where vascular injury is high, and when embolization is considered for persistent or delayed hemorrhage. It should be kept in mind that the kidney can tolerate only 4 to 6 h of warm ischemia. Arteriographic confirmation may cause an undue delay.

ULTRASOUND Ultrasound examination of the right upper quadrant (Morrison pouch) and the left upper quadrant (splenorenal recess) is part of the Focused Assessment for the Sonographic Examination of the Trauma Patient (FAST) examination (see Chaps. 243 and 295) but has little accepted role to date in the initial detection (or exclusion) of significant renal injury in the United States. Certain conditions, such as patient position and fractured ribs, make such examinations difficult to perform. Furthermore, sonography reveals nothing about renal function. In Europe, however, ultrasound is used as a technique of choice for the initial imaging modality in some centers.[10]

RADIONUCLIDE IMAGING Radionuclide imaging has a very limited role now, given the superiority of CT. It may still be useful in patients with iodinated dye allergy in whom technetium-99m glucoheptonate can be safely used.

INTRAVENOUS PYELOGRAM Formal IVP with or without tomograms can be used in stable patients if CT is unavailable. However, it is not the ideal study in the trauma setting, given the need for quality imaging. If used, the dose of contrast material needs to be greater than the standard 1 mL/kg to account for hemodilution for intravenous fluid administration and possible impaired renal perfusion. The recommendation is 2 mL/kg up to 150 mL of 60% iodinated contrast. In patients with a history of allergy, a nonionic agent, such as iohexol, can be used. Alternatively, noncontrast CT, radionuclide imaging, or MRI may offer satisfactory results.

IVP remains the mainstay of diagnosing ureteral injuries, although it is not infallable.[11] Extravasation of die is the classic finding, although on occasion there is absence or delay of contrast in the distal collecting system. However, many are now using spiral CT to diagnose ureteral injuries, since it offers the advantage of viewing the entire retroperitoneal space and has the ability to detect urinomas.

A ''one-shot'' IVP can be obtained in unstable patients in the emergency department or operating room. This technique entails injecting 2 mL/kg intravenous contrast material about 5 min before the film is taken. However, if the patient's blood pressure is 70 mmHg or less, the kidneys may not concentrate the contrast material and are more susceptible to injury by it.

CYSTOGRAPHY For suspected bladder injuries, plain-film cystogram is classically used. About 300 to 500 mL (5 mL/kg in children) of contrast media is instilled retrograde into the bladder under gravity from 2 ft (60 cm) above the patient. At a height of 2 ft, the intravesical pressure generated approximates the physiologic voiding pressure. Unless adequate bladder pressure is generated, the cystogram may be falsely negative. Ideally, the procedure is performed under fluoroscopy to avoid filling the peritoneal cavity with contrast material in the event of a tear. A film of the distended bladder is taken, and a postdrainage view is obtained to note any extravasation not evident on the initial film. Some authorities suggest that the bladder be ''washed out'' with saline solution prior to obtaining the post–''wash-out'' view.

Allowing intravenous contrast material to flow into the bladder following intravenous injection is not considered an appropriate technique,[12] although some continue to advocate clamping a urinary catheter to allow antegrade filling of the bladder.[13] A CT cystogram may be preferred in a patient who requires intravenous contrast-enhanced CT imaging for other indications.[14] However, contrast material must still be injected retrograde.[15] Postvoiding scans are generally not required, since CT allows full imaging of the retrovesicular space.

A prospective investigation studying indications for cystography in blunt trauma with hematuria or pelvic fracture concluded that it was appropriate and cost effective to restrict this procedure to patients with gross hematuria only.[16] The authors contend that patients with pelvic fracture and microscopic hematuria do not routinely require cystography.

Urethral injuries are also investigated by retrograde cystography. An unlubricated urinary catheter is placed about 2 to 3 cm into the navicular fossa of the distal urethra, and the balloon is inflated with 1 to 3 mL water. Approximately 20 to 30 mL of contrast material is injected. An oblique view is obtained. The entire length of the urethra is seen on the plain film when the x-ray is taken as the last 10 mL of the contrast solution is injected. Occasionally, a patient may be transferred from another facility with an indwelling urethral catheter in place. A retrograde urethrogram can still be performed without removing the catheter, by injecting contrast solution into the urethra through a small feeding tube placed adjacent to the urethral catheter.

Urethral injuries should not be investigated in cases of pelvic trauma until it is certain that pelvic angiography or embolization is not required. Also, if the prostate gland was grossly displaced on rectal examination, the urethra is transected, and a retrograde study is not needed, at least not during the initial evaluation.

CONTRAST STUDIES When both upper and lower tract injuries are suspected, imaging needs to be approached with particular attention to order. While the most serious potential injury should guide the order of obtaining images, oral contrast material should generally not be given before an IVP or cystogram because gastrointestinal contrast may obscure important findings. Patients with potential bladder injuries may require a retrograde urethrogram to evaluate possible urethral disruption first. If injury is noted, cystography can be accomplished by suprapubic puncture.

IMAGING CONSIDERATIONS FOR OTHER CONDITIONS A perinephric hematoma may initially be difficult to distinguish from a urinoma. A delayed CT image may demonstrate contrast, indicating a urinoma. Patients with such perinephric collections can be followed with ultrasound studies. A nuclear ^{99m}Tc renal scan can also detect a persistent urine leak.

Significant adrenal injuries are relatively rare. Adrenal hematomas may be found in up to 3 percent of patients with blunt abdominal trauma. They are usually associated with other significant thoracic and abdominal injuries. Adrenal hematomas can be followed by CT or sonography and usually resolve over a few months. Long-term sequelae are unlikely.

PENETRATING TRAUMA

About 10 percent of patients with renal injury related to stab wounds may not manifest hematuria. Thus, appropriate evaluation depends on clinical suspicion, the weapon involved, and patient characteristics. Generally, all stable patients with penetrating trauma with the potential of renal system injury should undergo imaging studies. Hematuria, microscopic or gross, does not correlate with injury from penetrating trauma.[17] The choice of imaging depends on the vicinity of the trauma. Thus, its presence alone mandates further evaluation.

Ureteral injuries are usually a result of bullet wounds. Again, hematuria is not a reliable finding in this setting. Imaging is required for penetrating injuries near ureters. Contusions from secondary energy forces related to bullets cannot be detected by imaging. They may come to light during surgical exploration.

Penetrating bladder injuries are usually accompanied by gross hematuria. As with other penetrating trauma, in the absence of hematuria, the need to perform imaging studies is driven by clinical concern.

Choice of Diagnostic Imaging for Penetrating Renal Trauma

CT with intravenous contrast material remains the primary imaging modality for penetrating trauma to the kidneys. It usually shows appropriate detail of injury to inform management decisions. At least one study has shown its utility for staging even penetrating injuries, allowing nonoperative management in selected patients (i.e., those with minor injury).[18] As with blunt trauma, sonography has no accepted role for detection or staging of renal injury in the United States at this time.

Ureteral injuries can be assessed by IVP or CT with contrast. Extravasation indicates injury. CT has the added advantage of being able to evaluate the extent of extravasation and other intraabdominal injuries. As with blunt trauma, cystography (plain film or CT) is required to evaluate penetrating injuries of the bladder. Unstable patients who require emergency laparotomy can undergo a "one-shot" IVP while in the operating room.

SPECIFIC INJURIES

Kidney Injuries

The kidneys are well protected in the retroperitoneal location surrounded by bulky musculature, fascia, and lower ribs. Considerable force is generally necessary to cause significant renal injury. Fractured ribs, vertebral transverse process fractures, flank bruises or hematomas, and hematuria may indicate injury. Contusions account for most (92 percent) renal injuries, with renal lacerations (5 percent), renal pedicle injuries (2 percent), and renal ruptures or shattered kidneys (1 percent) accounting for the rest.

RENAL CONTUSION Renal contusion accounts for over 90 percent of renal injuries. This relatively minor injury includes renal parenchymal ecchymosis, minor lacerations, and subcapsular hematomas with an intact renal capsule. Radiographically, results of the IVP are usually normal, and the CT may reveal edema with microextravasation of contrast material within the renal parenchyma. Subcapsular hematoma appears as a flattened portion of the renal cortex compressed by the hematoma under the renal capsule.

RENAL LACERATION Renal lacerations are classified as either minor cortical lacerations that do not involve the medulla or collecting system, or major renal lacerations that extend deep into the corticomedullary junction or collecting system (Table 254-2). The resulting perirenal hematoma may fill the perirenal space before it is tamponaded by the Gerota fascia. Renal lacerations account for approximately 5 percent of renal injuries. Radiographic studies demonstrate disruption of the renal outline, a perirenal hematoma, and possibly extravasation of contrast material adjacent to the kidney.

RENAL PEDICLE INJURY Renal pedicle injuries include lacerations and thrombosis of the renal artery, renal vein, and their branches. Renal pedicle injuries make up 2 percent of all renal injuries. These injuries result from high-velocity deceleration injuries and penetrating trauma. In blunt trauma, the most common renal pedicle injury is thrombosis of the renal artery, which follows tearing of the intima with intact adventitial and medial layers. There is bruising surrounding the renal artery, but no perirenal hematoma is found in renal pedicle lacerations. When the renal artery is occluded or divided, the IVP shows nonfunction, and the arteriogram reveals renal artery occlusion or bleeding. In such injuries, CT demonstrates a nonenhanced kidney with minimal peripheral enhancement from the renal capsular vessels (''rim sign''). Renal vein thrombosis results in delayed renal function and parenchymal swelling in the absence of ureteral obstruction.

RENAL RUPTURE Renal ruptures, or shattered kidneys, account for 1 percent of renal injuries. A large expanding perirenal hematoma accompanies renal rupture, and the patient becomes clinically unstable from continued bleeding. Radiographic studies reveal multiple deep lacerations, devitalized kidney fragments, and extravasation of contrast.

RENAL PELVIS RUPTURE Ruptures of the renal pelvis result in extravasation of urine into the perirenal space and along the psoas muscle. Renal pelvis ruptures are rare and are often associated with congenital renal anomalies. Radiographic studies reveal a normally functioning kidney, filling of the calyceal system, and extravasation of contrast without visualization of the ureter. Renal pelvis ruptures are often misdiagnosed as small renal lacerations. If the diagnosis is delayed, the patient may develop high fever, increased abdominal pain, and tenderness as the extravasation of urine continues into the retroperitoneal space. Sepsis may ensue. The diagnosis of renal pelvis rupture is confirmed by retrograde pyelogram.

Ureteral Injuries

Ureteral injuries are the rarest of all genitourinary injuries and are usually the result of penetrating trauma (Fig. 254-1). Blunt trauma, however, can induce a rupture at or just below the ureteropelvic junction as a result of hyperextension of the spine with the distal ureter fixed at the trigone of the bladder. Blast effects from gunshot wounds may cause microvascular thrombosis in the ureteral wall, delayed ureteral necrosis, and urinary fistula formation. Diagnosis is sometimes delayed. If the ureter is completely transected, hematuria may be absent.[11] IVP is likely to miss such injuries.[11] Enhanced CT or a retrograde pyelogram may be required for detection.

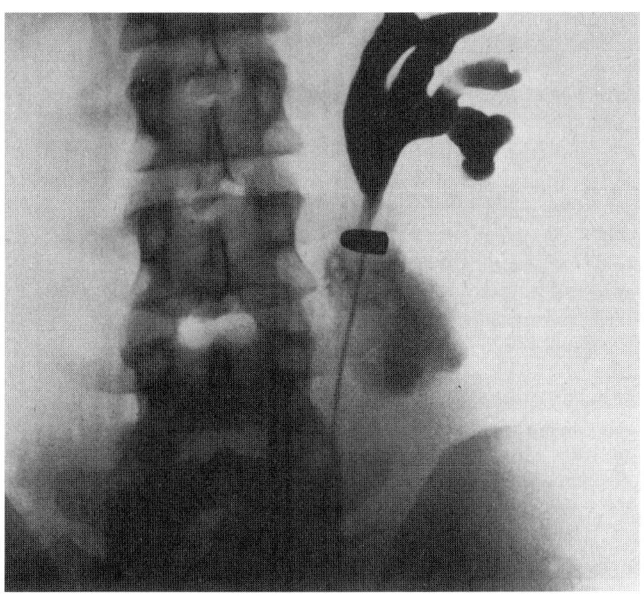

FIG. 254-1. Rare ureteral injury from a gunshot wound, with extravasation of contrast material on retrograde pyelogram.

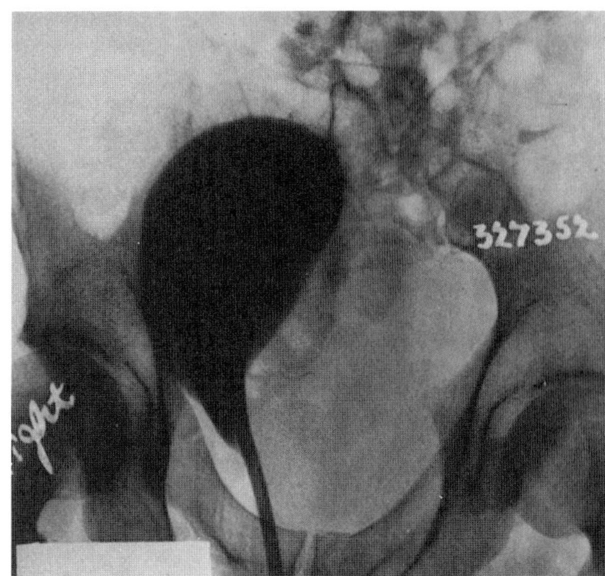

FIG. 254-2. Bladder contusion and displacement from pelvic hematoma.

Bladder Injuries

The bladder is an intraabdominal organ in children but is situated deep in the bony pelvis in adults. It is protected from all but the most severe injuries to the abdomen and pelvis. Bladder injuries are the second most common injury to the genitourinary tract after renal injuries and are usually associated with blunt trauma and pelvic fracture. Penetrating bladder injuries are often associated with injuries to other abdominal and pelvic organs.

BLADDER CONTUSION Bladder contusion is bruising of the bladder wall and resultant hematuria. A cystogram demonstrates an intact bladder outline. With a fractured pelvis, a large hematoma often results inside the bony pelvis, causing displacement of the bladder superiorly and laterally (Fig. 254-2). This finding can serve as an indicator of pelvic hemorrhage. Large bladder hematomas also alter the architecture of the bladder, which takes on the shape of an inverted pear, hence the term ''pear-shaped'' bladder. Hematomas are best detected by CT.

BLADDER RUPTURE There are two types of bladder injuries.[19] Intraperitoneal bladder rupture is usually a burst injury of a full bladder resulting in a 1-in laceration in the dome posteriorly, the only portion of the dome covered by the peritoneum. In this type of injury, urine is spilled into the peritoneal cavity. Extraperitoneal bladder rupture is more common. The rupture is usually located at the bladder neck. Associated pelvic ring fractures predominate. The classic triad includes abdominal pain and tenderness, hematuria (usually gross), and inability to void. If the rupture is intraperitoneal, there may be peritonitis. Kehr sign (pain referred to the shoulder), suggesting blood or urine irritating the diaphragm, may be a clue. Patients in whom bladder injury is suspected but who are unable to void spontaneously should have a retrograde or suprapubic catheter placed. Retrograde catheter placement should be avoided until urtheral disruption has been ruled out.

Bladder injuries are best diagnosed by cystogram or CT cystogram (see above). Gross extravasation indicates rupture. Intraperitoneal rupture is demonstrated by extravasation of contrast material in the cul-de-sac posterior to the bladder, along the paracolic gutters, and between the loops of intestine above the bladder. In extraperitoneal bladder rupture, the cystogram shows flamelike extravasation of contrast material streaking into the perivesical tissues. The washout film (not necessary with CT cystogram) is helpful when the extravasation is predomi-

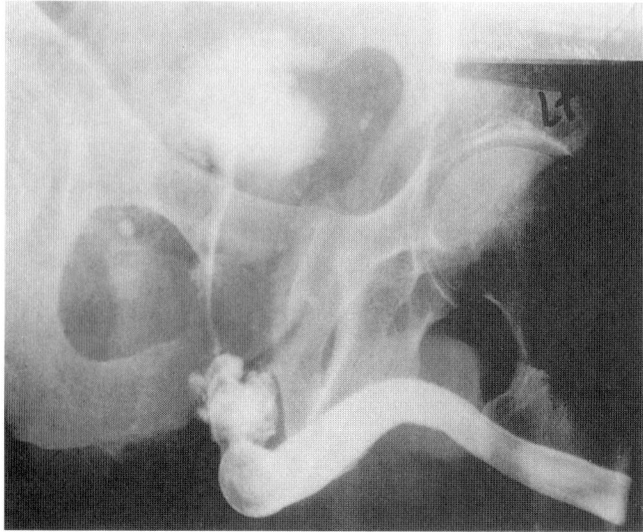

FIG. 254-3. Partial urethral laceration, with contrast extravasation at the site of injury and outlining the prostatic urethra and bladder.

nantly behind the bladder and obscured by contrast material in the full-bladder film of the cystogram. An irregular outline of an intact bladder may indicate contusion, hematoma, or an incomplete tear. Cystoscopy is not considered useful in this setting due to the gross hematuria and clot formation.[3]

Urethral Injuries

Urethral injuries in males occur in the posterior (prostatomembranous) urethra and in the anterior (bulbous and penile) urethra. Posterior urethral injuries are associated with pelvic fractures. Digital rectal and perineal examinations reveal the presence of a perineal hematoma or high-riding detached prostate, which is associated with complete posterior urethral disruption. Anterior urethral injuries result from direct blows to the urethra (e.g., fall-astride injuries, straddle injuries, or kicks) or from instrumentation, and in conjunction with a penile fracture. Examination reveals the classic ''butterfly'' perineal hematoma, limited by the attachments of the fascia lata.

In anterior urethral contusions, there is blood at the external urinary meatus, but the retrograde urethrogram findings are normal. In partial anterior urethral lacerations, the retrograde urethrogram reveals contrast extravasation at the site of injury and contrast material outlining the urethra proximal to the site of injury (Fig. 254-3). In complete anterior urethral lacerations, the retrograde urethrogram reveals contrast extravasation at the site of injury without contrast proximal to the site of injury.

Female urethral injuries should be suspected in extensive pelvic fractures. Eighty percent of female urethral injuries present with vaginal bleeding. Careful vaginal and endoscopic examination should be undertaken, even when the patient has menstrual bleeding or an indwelling tampon. Delayed diagnosis has resulted in labial edema, necrotizing fasciitis, and sepsis.

MANAGEMENT OF RENAL SYSTEM INJURIES

General management of trauma in the emergency department is discussed in Chapter 243. Only aspects specifically related to genitourinary system trauma are discussed here.

Patients with isolated microscopic hematuria (5 to 50 RBCs/hpf) in whom imaging was not indicated may be discharged from the emergency department. Strenuous activity should be proscribed. Follow-up urinalysis should be obtained in 1 to 2 weeks.

Kidney

Grade I and II renal injuries (Table 254-2) are usually managed nonoperatively. If there are no other medical considerations, such patients can be treated similarly to those with isolated hematuria. Renal contusions almost always resolve without sequelae unless there is a preexisting renal lesion, such as hydronephrosis, cyst, or tumor. Almost all minor lacerations heal without sequelae with conservative management.

Patients with grade III and IV injuries should be admitted to the hospital. Most of these patients will have other compelling reasons to be admitted or be taken to the operating room. Many stable adult patients with clearly delineated grade III and even grade IV injuries can still be managed nonoperatively.[20,21] Many centers attempt nonoperative management for all stable children unless the renal injury is particularly severe or the child fails conservative therapy.[8,22] Exploration itself is not without consequence, since it may accentuate considerable hemorrhage. Neither the volume of blood replacement nor the degree of extravasation is an indication for exploration in itself.[3] However, if exploration is undertaken for the evaluation of other injuries, repair of renal injuries is usually undertaken. If conservative management is attempted, frequent reassessment is required, and there should be a low threshold for ordering reimaging studies. Conservative management includes bed rest, hydration, serial hematocrit determinations, monitoring of vital signs, and serial urine specimens to assess the degree of hematuria. Patients with gross hematuria remain at bed rest until the gross hematuria resolves and remain at limited activity until microscopic hematuria resolves.

Indications for operative management are listed in Table 254-5.[3] Renal rupture is usually explored and nephrectomy usually required. Most, but not all, penetrating injuries are explored. The only widely accepted absolute indication for surgical exploration of a renal injury is persistent retroperitoneal bleeding with hemodynamic instability. As noted, CT may allow adequate staging even for penetrating injuries.[18] If the patient has other injuries warranting abdominal exploration, an intraoperative IVP may assist in determining the necessity for retroperitoneal exploration while also giving information regarding function of the contralateral kidney.

Renal pedicle injuries are usually associated with multiple life-threatening injuries, and the safest surgical option is nephrectomy. In a stable patient with an isolated renal pedicle injury, repair should be undertaken within 12 h of the injury if a viable kidney is to result. Thrombosis of segmental arteries is treated conservatively.

Surgical exploration consists of preliminary vascular control, debridement, and surgical repair. Early control of the renal vessels decreases the nephrectomy rate in potentially salvageable kidneys. Nephrectomy, however, may be necessary in unstable patients.

TABLE 254-5 Indications for Operative Exploration or Intervention in Renal Injury[3]

Uncontrolled renal hemorrhage
Penetrating injuries
Inadequate staging
Multiple kidney lacerations
Shattered (ruptured) kidney
Avulsed major renal vessel
Pulsatile or expanding hematoma found on abdominal exploration
Vascular injuries*
Extensive extravasation

*Only those found early (see the text).

Ureter

Ureteral injuries are managed intraoperatively. Unfortunately, not all ureteral injuries are found at the time of injury. Delayed presentations include infection, including sepsis, and urinoma formation. Contusions are missed by imaging studies, but, if noted at the time of exploration, can be managed expectantly or with placement of an internal stent.

Bladder

Incomplete bladder lacerations can be managed by catheter placement and observation. Contusions require no specific intervention. Intraperitoneal rupture and penetrating injuries require operative intervention. Extraperitoneal bladder ruptures are treated with urethral catheter drainage alone. In such cases, the catheter remains indwelling for 10 to 14 days, and the cystogram is repeated to verify healing before the urethral catheter is removed. Rarely, persistent urinary extravasation is seen, with a bony fragment remaining in the bladder wall or a pelvic fixation impinging upon the bladder.

Urethra

Anterior contusion heals with conservative management, with or without a urethral catheter, depending on whether the patient can void. Partial anterior urethral lacerations are managed with an indwelling urethral catheter (placed coaxially over a guide wire under fluoroscopic control) or with a suprapubic cystostomy. Complete lacerations of the anterior urethra are repaired surgically with debridement and end-to-end anastomosis over a urethral catheter.

Surgical repair is usually deferred for posterior urethral injuries. Suprapubic cystostomy is favored by most for bladder drainage. Partial posterior urethral lacerations are managed with a urethral catheter placed coaxially over a guide wire under fluoroscopic control or with a suprapubic catheter. In complete posterior urethral lacerations, the management remains controversial. The injury is managed with primary realignment of the lacerated urethra or with suprapubic cystostomy alone. Stricture formation occurs with both techniques. However, the subsequent urethral stricture in patients with primary realignment tends to be less extensive. The advantage of suprapubic cystostomy alone, especially in an unstable patient, is its simplicity. The impotence and incontinence rates are thought to be related to the extent of injury and are the same for both techniques.

In women, a layer repair of the urethral and associated vaginal injuries is performed over a urethral catheter. The voiding phase of the repeat cystogram is essential in confirming complete urethral healing.

The Full-Bladder Dilemma

Emergency physicians in nontrauma centers may encounter patients with a urethral injury precluding bladder catheterization but with a full urinary bladder. Such a patient may have to be transferred many miles to reach a center with a urologic service. Spontaneous or conscious bladder contraction may ensue, with spillage of urine into the perivesicle space, increasing the risk of infection. Guide-wire-aided placement of a temporary suprapubic catheter into the bladder can alleviate this problem. A large-bore Seldinger-technique central venous catheter or cavity drainage catheter may provide temporary relief. The exploring needle is inserted perpendicularly about two finger breadths above the symphysis pubis. The guide wire is inserted when urine returns. The catheter selected should be long enough to coil within the bladder so that it remains in the lumen of the bladder when it is empty. Because the bladder may be displaced by a large hematoma or extravasated urine, it is advisable to inject a few milliliters of contrast material into the bladder while obtaining an x-ray to confirm that the catheter is actually in the bladder.

GENITAL INJURIES

Testicular and Scrotal Injuries

The mobility of the testicle, cremaster muscle contraction, and the tough capsule of the testis (tunica albuginea) are responsible for the infrequent rate of injury to the testis. A direct blow to the testis impinging it against the symphysis pubis is the primary cause of blunt testicular injury. Blunt testicular injuries are either contusions or ruptures. Rarely, traumatic dislocation of the testicle to the inguinal canal has been reported. In testicular contusions or ruptures, the tunica vaginalis sac fills with blood (hematocele) and appears as a large, blue, tender scrotal mass. Penetrating injuries to the scrotum through the tunica vaginalis require exploration. Bilateral testicular injuries are often seen in penetrating trauma. Testicular ultrasound studies with colored Doppler studies can help delineate the extent of testicular trauma and are quite reliable in diagnosing ruptured testes.

Early exploration, evacuation of blood clots, and repair of testicular rupture tend to result in an earlier return to normal activity, decreased hematoma infection, and less testicular atrophy than does conservative management. Testicular salvage following penetrating trauma is on the order of 35 percent.[23]

Scrotal skin avulsion is managed by housing the testicle in the remaining scrotal skin even though the reconstruction places the skin under tension. Usually the scrotum returns to nearly normal size within a few months. In complete scrotal skin loss, the testicles are placed in pouches in the inner thighs.

Injuries to the Penis

Self-inflicted injuries of the penis include vacuum cleaner injuries and blade injuries. Vacuum cleaners cause extensive injury to the glans penis and some loss of the urethra, requiring debridement of devitalized tissue and reconstruction. Blade injuries range from superficial lacerations to complete amputation. Amputation of the penis is managed by reimplantation or local repair. Reimplantation is preferable if the distal penis is in satisfactory condition, and the ischemia time is less than 12 to 18 h. Loss of penile skin by avulsion injury or burns is managed by split-thickness skin grafts after the denuded penis is clean and uninfected. The avulsed skin should not be reapplied, for it invariably becomes necrotic and infected and must be subsequently removed.

Traumatic rupture of the corpus cavernosum of the penis or fracture of the penis occurs when the erect penis impacts forcibly on a hard object (sexual partner's pubis or the floor), receives a direct blow, or is subjected to abnormal bending. A cracking sound is heard, followed by penile pain, immediate detumescence, rapid swelling, discoloration, and distention. Urethral injuries may accompany penile ruptures. Penile ruptures are managed by immediate surgical evacuation of blood clot and repair of the torn tunica albuginea of the corpus cavernosum and urethra.

Zipper injury to the penis is caused when the penile skin is trapped in the trouser zipper. Mineral oil and lidocaine infiltration are useful in freeing the penile skin from the zipper. Otherwise, wire-cutting or bone-cutting pliers are used to divide the median bar (or diamond) of the zipper, which causes the zipper to fall apart, freeing the penile skin.

Contusions of the perineum or penis, which can result from straddle or toilet seat injuries, are treated conservatively with cold packs, rest, and elevation. If the patient is unable to void, catheter drainage is elected.

REFERENCES

1. Abdalati H, Bulas DI, Sivit CJ, et al: Blunt renal trauma in children: Healing of renal injuries and recommendations for imaging follow-up. *Pediatr Radiol* 24:573, 1994.
2. Stein JL, Bisset GS, Kirks DR, et al: Blunt renal trauma in the pediatric population: Indications for radiographic evaluation. *Urology* 44:406, 1994.

3. Ahn JH, Morey AF, McAninch JW: Workup and management of traumatic hematuria. *Emerg Med Clin North Am* 16:145, 1998.
4. Moore EE, Shackford SR, Pachter HL, et al: Organ injury scaling: Spleen, liver, kidney. *J Trauma* 29:1664, 1989.
5. Morey AF, Bruce JE, McAninch JW: Efficacy of radiographic imaging in pediatric blunt renal trauma. *J Urol* 156:2014, 1996.
6. Abou-Jaoude WA, Sugarman JM, Fallat ME, et al: Indicators of genitourinary tract injury or anomaly in cases of pediatric blunt trauma. *J Pediatr Surg* 31:86, 1996.
7. Quinlan DM, Gearhart JP: Blunt renal trauma in childhood: Features indicating severe injury. *Br J Urol* 66:526, 1990.
8. Levy JB, Baskin LS, Ewalt DH, et al: Nonoperative management of blunt pediatric major renal trauma. *Urology* 42:418, 1993.
9. Stein JP, Kari DM, Eastham J, et al: Blunt renal trauma in the pediatric population: Indications for radiographic evaluation. *Urology* 44:406, 1994.
10. Rosales A: The use of ultrasonography as the initial diagnostic exploration in blunt renal trauma. *Urol Int* 48:134, 1992.
11. Brandes SB, Chelsky MJ, Buckman RF, et al: Ureteral injuries from penetrating trauma. *J Trauma* 36:745, 1994.
12. Rehm CG, Mure AJ, O'Malley KF, et al: Blunt traumatic bladder rupture. The role of retrograde cystogram. *Ann Emerg Med* 20:845, 1991.
13. Sivit CJ, Cutting JP, Eichelberger MR, et al: CT diagnosis and localization of rupture of the bladder in children with blunt abdominal trauma: Significance of contrast material extravasation in the pelvis. *AJR* 164:1243, 1995.
14. Lis LE, Cohen AJ: CT cystography in the evaluation of bladder trauma. *J Comput Assist Tomogr* 14:386, 1990.
15. Mee SL, McAninch JW, Federle MP: Computerized tomography in bladder rupture: Diagnostic limitations. *J Urol* 137:207, 1987.
16. Fuhrman GM, Simmons GT, Davidson BS, Buerk CA: The single indication for cystography in blunt trauma. *Am Surg* 59:335, 1993.
17. Federle MP, Brown TR, McAninch JW: Penetrating renal trauma: CT evaluation. *J Comput Assist Tomogr* 11:1026, 1987.
18. Carroll PR, McAninch JW: Operative indications in penetrating renal trauma. *J Trauma* 24:587, 1985.
19. Cass AS, Luxenberg M: Features of 164 bladder ruptures. *J Urol* 138:743, 1987.
20. Cheng DL, Lazan D, Stone N: Conservative treatment of type II renal trauma. *J Trauma* 36:491, 1994.
21. Mansi MK, Alkhudar WK: Conservative management with percutaneous intervention of major blunt renal injuries. *Am J Emerg* Med 7:633, 1997.
22. Baumann L, Greenfield SP, Aker J, et al: Nonoperative management of major blunt renal trauma in children: In-hospital morbidity and long-term follow-up. *J Urol* 148:691, 1992.
23. Cline KJ: Penetrating trauma to the male external genitalia. *J Trauma* 44:492, 1998.

255 PENETRATING TRAUMA TO THE EXTREMITIES

Richard D. Zane
Allan Kumar

Emergent management of penetrating extremity injuries is an evolving and controversial subject. Recent advances in surgical technique enable arterial repair with an extremely low rate of postoperative thrombosis, making the recognition and rapid treatment of arterial injury of paramount importance. Associated injury to soft tissue, nerve, and bony structures are now the primary determinants of limb salvage. Emergency physicians play a crucial role in the management of penetrating extremity injuries by identifying injuries early and promptly initiating care crucial to limb rescue. Unnecessary delays in treatment can lead to irreversible limb ischemia and subsequent limb loss.

EPIDEMIOLOGY

In the past 10 years, there has been a surge in the number of violent crimes associated with firearm usage. Gun-related assaults, robberies, and murders have risen by 59 percent since 1987. Penetrating trauma accounts for up to 82 percent of all vascular injuries to the extremities. Gunshot and shotgun wounds account for nearly 65 percent of penetrating vascular extremity injuries, and stab wounds account for approximately 15 percent. Of patients presenting with gunshot wounds, 20 to 40 percent have extremity involvement, either isolated or in combination with other injuries. In 1950, a patient with a penetrating extremity injury with vascular involvement had a 50 percent chance of leaving the hospital with an amputated limb. With recent advances in emergency care, vascular surgery, invasive radiology, and the science of thrombosis, penetrating extremity injury results in amputation in fewer than 5 percent.[1] Despite this improved diagnosis, there is still a 15 to 40 percent long-term morbidity due to other complications, such as nerve damage, fractures, wound infections, open joint injuries, and compartment syndromes.[2]

PATHOPHYSIOLOGY

Gunshot and stab wounds account for the largest percentage of penetrating extremity injuries. Gunshot and blast injuries often present a diagnostic and management dilemma. A basic understanding of wound ballistics will enable astute clinicians to better plan the clinical management of patients who sustain a gunshot wound to the extremity. Diagnostic and treatment modalities as well as outcome differ with the type and severity of the injury. Although the damage from a stab wound can be relatively predictable with a good knowledge of clinical anatomy, the tissue damage inflicted by a missile or blast depends on a variety of factors (see Chap. 256, "Wound Ballistics"). The notion that projectile velocity alone determines the extent of damage is false. Wound profiles depend on variables that include the projectile's shape, construction, composition, angle of impact, flight characteristics in tissue (yawing, or turning sideways in relation to line of flight), velocity, and mass.[3] An example would be a shotgun blast. At close range, a shotgun creates a more severe wound than a high-velocity M-16 assault rifle would at the same range because of the increased total mass and fragmentation of the shotgun load. The impact of a missile on tissue also creates indirect damage due to pressure waves accelerating radially away from the point of penetration, thereby displacing tissue. This phenomenon, termed *temporary cavity,* can cause significant additional damage.[4] The severity of injury due to the temporary cavity varies inversely with the elasticity and density of the surrounding tissue. As an example, muscle and fat are relatively more elastic and therefore far less susceptible than bone or liver to this type of indirect damage. A third proposed mechanism of damage is termed shock wave: a sound wave traveling in front of the bullet is generated by the missile impact onto tissue. This theory has not been proven in multiple studies, and the nature of the subsequent damage is not well defined. Overall, tissue damage is usually proportional to the amount of fracture comminution and displacement, blood loss within the limb, and nerve or vascular injury. The wide variety of handguns available on the market and the availability of military-surplus weapons, as well as the inaccuracy of the information given to treating physicians about weapon and bullet type by the injured and their associates, make clinical findings and diagnostic modalities the best guides in determining management.

DIAGNOSIS AND MANAGEMENT

After the initial trauma resuscitation and primary and secondary surveys are complete, specific points of the victim's past medical history should be examined: preexisting vascular and neuromuscular deficits, and the events surrounding the injury, such as the type of gun and number of shots. An extremely careful and thorough physical examination is imperative to identify significant injuries rapidly and to determine whether immediate surgical intervention is necessary or which, if any, diagnostic studies are indicated. This may be challenging in the presence of other serious trauma or distracting injuries.

TABLE 255-1 Clinical Manifestations of Extremity Vascular Trauma

Hard signs
Absent or diminished distal pulses
Obvious arterial bleeding
Large expanding or pulsatile hematoma
Audible bruit
Palpable thrill
Distal ischemia (pain, pallor, paralysis, paresthesias, coolness)
Soft signs
Small, stable hematoma
Injury to anatomically related nerve
Unexplained hypotension
History of hemorrhage no longer present
Proximity of injury to major vascular structures
Complex fracture

The presentation of penetrating vascular injury varies widely. Prompt recognition of arterial injury is one of the fundamental goals of management. The presence and volume of the distal pulses in the affected extremity should be noted and compared with the unaffected limb. Ankle-brachial indices (ABIs) should be calculated on the affected and unaffected limbs (method described below). The color, temperature, and capillary refill time are important clinical indicators of more subtle injury to underlying vessels. Examination should also look for signs of compartment syndrome. Capillary refill alone is an unpredictable marker of vascular injury but may be useful in conjunction with other modalities. Only a small minority of patients (fewer than 6 percent) will present with classic "hard" signs of arterial injury (Table 255-1). These patients require expeditious operative management or, under certain circumstances, angiography (Fig. 255-1). A surgeon should be involved in the management of these patients as soon as possible. Patients with "soft" signs (Table 255-1) of arterial vascular trauma can usually be managed without surgical intervention on an inpatient surgical service.[5] Controversy surrounds the management of the patient with a wound in proximity to a major vascular structure but without clinical evidence of arterial injury. Historically, patients with these types of injuries were all surgically explored, which yielded a large number of negative exploratory surgeries, and thus angiography became popular. Angiography based on proximity alone yields abnormalities in 10 to 20 percent of the cases, with less than 2 percent requiring surgical intervention. Current practice regarding penetrating injuries in proximity to major vessels without any signs of vascular injury is to observe patients with clinically silent arterial injury. The natural course in these cases is likely benign, and these patients can be safely observed with serial examinations.

Duplex ultrasound has become a popular modality in the management of proximity injuries without evidence of arterial injury. Recent advances in duplex ultrasonography have shown highly accurate rates of detecting occult arterial injury (vide infra). Some clinicians use duplex ultrasound to distinguish between patients who require observation and those who can safely be discharged home.

Although venous trauma can bleed profusely, management by either ligation or reanastomosis often yields similar results.[6] Asymptomatic venous injury rarely results in long-term morbidity. During the initial trauma resuscitation, attempts should not be made to clamp or ligate bleeding vessels in an attempt to control bleeding. Nerves are bundled with vascular structures and can be easily damaged by blind clamping or ligation. Profuse bleeding should be initially controlled with direct pressure.

Although arterial injury is the most dramatic result of penetrating extremity injury and represents the most immediate life threat, injuries to major nerves are the most likely to lead long-term disability. Fortunately, 70 percent of peripheral nerve injuries noted during the initial examination recover completely within 6 months of the initial injury. A neuromuscular exam of the extremities should indicate both muscu-

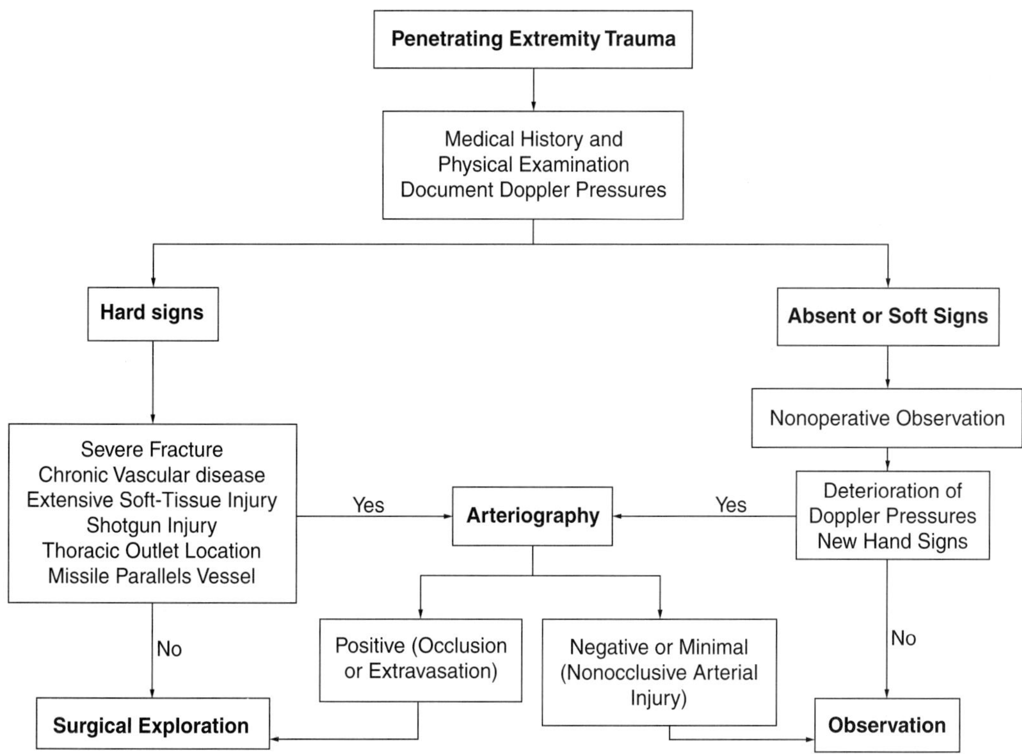

FIG. 255-1. Algorithm for the evaluation of an injured extremity for vascular trauma. (Adapted from Frykberg: Advances in diagnosis and treatment of extremity trauma. *Surg Clin North Am* 75:207, 1995.

TABLE 255-2 Clinical Examination of the Nerves of the Extremities

Nerve	Text of Motor Function	Test for Sensation
Axillary (C5–6)	Arm abduction Arm internal, external rotation	Lateral aspect of shoulder
Musculocutaneous (C5–6)	Forearm flexion	Lateral forearm
Radial (C5–8)	Forearm, wrist, and finger extension	Dorsoradial hand, thumb
Median (C6–T1)	Wrist flexion, finger adduction	Volar aspect of thumb and index finger
Ulnar (C7–T1)	Finger abduction	Volar aspect of little finger
Femoral (L1–L4)	Knee extension	
Obturator (L2–L4)	Hip adduction	
Superior gluteal (L4–S1)	Hip abduction	
Sciatic (L4–S3)	Knee flexion	
Deep peroneal (L4–S1)	Ankle and great toe dorsi flexion	
Superficial peroneal (L5–S1)	Foot eversion	
Tibial (L5–S2)	Ankle plantar flexion	
Posterior tibial (L5–S2)	Great toe plantar flexion	
Spinal L4		Medial calf
Spinal L5		Dorsal foot
Spinal S1		Lateral plantar foot

lar and sensory function (Table 255-2) and check for evidence of compartment syndrome. Patients with suspected nerve, orthopedic, or vascular injury or compartment syndrome should be immediately evaluated by surgical subspecialists.

The size and shape of the wounds, and soft tissue and obvious bony deformities, should be noted and thoroughly examined. Pain on palpation or movement of an extremity is suspicious for an underlying fracture. Penetrating trauma near a joint should be evaluated thoroughly for damage to the joint capsule, as associated long-term morbidity is significant. Radiologic evidence of air in a joint is evidence of joint penetration. Patients with obvious bony or joint capsule injury should be evaluated by an orthopedic surgeon. The majority of orthopedic surgeons will undertake arthroscopic exploration and ''wash out'' an involved major joint. Joint sepsis and destruction, rapid chondrolysis, and loss of anatomic contours can lead to long-term morbidity in the form of posttraumatic degenerative arthritis and decreased or total loss of flexibility. Metal fragments left in the joint space may dissolve in the synovial fluid, resulting in lead toxicity. Patients with penetrating injury proximal to, or overlying, a major joint without obvious joint penetration and without fracture can be splinted and discharged with 24-h orthopedic follow-up. Most orthopedic authors recommend discharging these patients on oral antibiotics, although the rationale has not been clearly established. Bony fractures as a result of penetrating injury are treated as open fractures. The injury is surgically debrided and the patient admitted for intravenous antibiotics.

DIAGNOSTIC MODALITIES

Radiographic Studies

Plain films, including anteroposterior and lateral views, of the involved extremities should be obtained in all cases. Oblique views may also offer additional information. It is important that the joints above and below the suspected injury site are imaged. Five general types of fracture patterns are created from bullets (Fig. 255-2). A drill hole pattern from penetration of cancellous bone is often seen in sites such as the proximal humerus, pelvis, and distal femur. These fractures have less comminution than those in cortical bone, because cancellous bone is more porous and less dense. Unicortical fractures of the metaphysis on long bones are often seen with bullet impact on a tangential plane. The majority of gunshot fractures of the diaphysis are comminuted, and the degree of comminution depends on the amount of energy transfer from the penetrating missile. Spiral fractures distant from the site of impact on the bone can occur if the bone is under a degree of torsional stress. There have also been reports of simple fractures of long bones caused by indirect damage from the temporary cavity. It is also important to note whether a joint has been penetrated, because this complication changes patient management. In the case of shotgun or blast injury, it is important to image the extremity distal to the injury in order to detect any pellets that may have embolized (Figs. 255-3 and 255-4).

Computed tomography, although rarely useful in the acute diagnosis and treatment of extremity trauma, is considered helpful in selected cases before definitive orthopedic care. It can help diagnose bony pathology and determine if intraarticular fractures, fragments, or foreign bodies are present. Magnetic resonance imaging, once thought to be a promising tool in the assessment of extremity trauma, is not readily available in many institutions, is time consuming, and often is of low yield.

Angiography can be used to delineate the extent, nature, and location of vascular injuries with special situations such as shotgun wounds, multiple or severe fractures, chronic vascular disease, thoracic outlet wounds, or extensive soft tissue injury. The widespread availability and accuracy of angiography led to it become the gold standard in the evaluation of patients with wounds in proximity to major neurovascular bundles. Arteriography for the evaluation of proximity injuries in

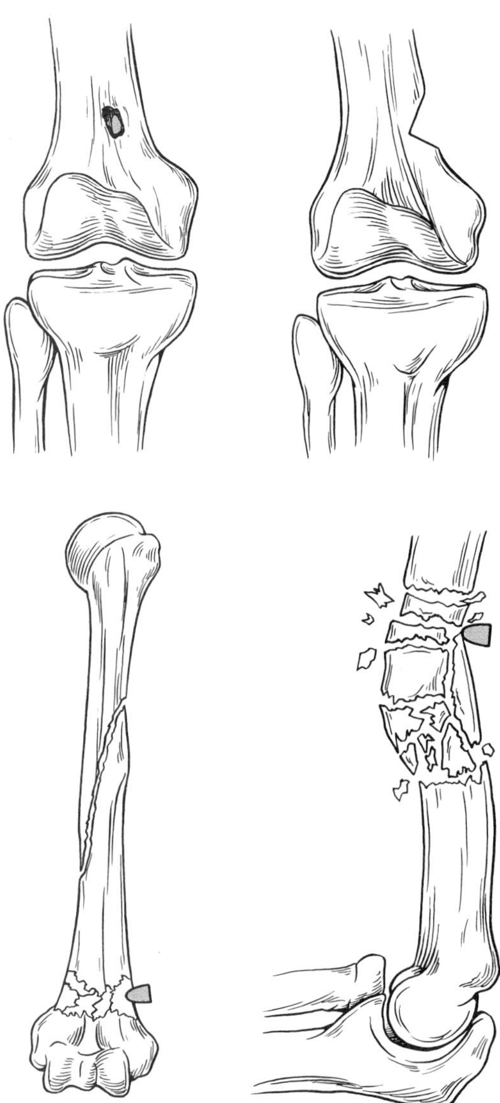

FIG. 255-2. Types of fracture patterns created with bullets: drill hole, unicortical, distant spiral, comminuted. The fifth type seen is a simple fracture.

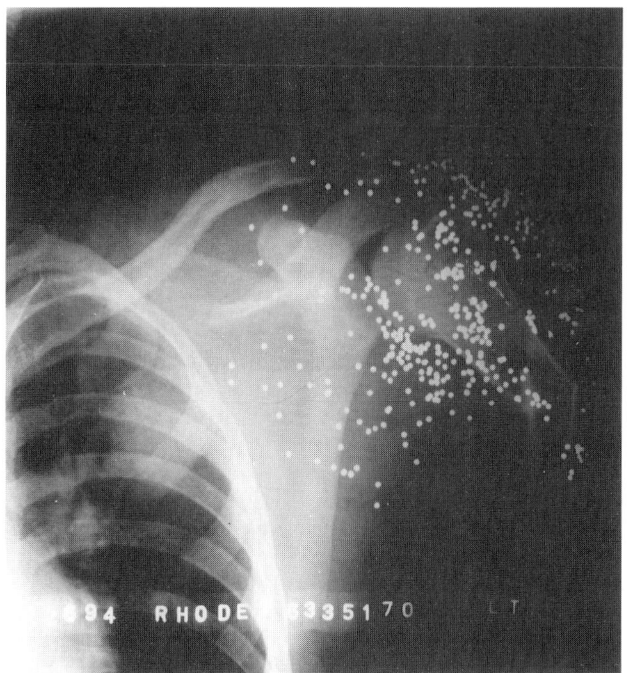

FIG. 255-3. Gunshot wound to the shoulder and axilla.

patients without hard signs of injury reveals normal results in 80 to 90 percent, with a complication rate of 1 to 2 percent from the procedure. Recent studies have shown that occult vascular injuries can exist, without hard clinical findings, in up to 23 percent of patients. Among these, however, fewer than 2 percent have surgically important lesions. Still, with observation and a careful examination, positive findings will eventually be more evident and the wounds subsequently repaired without increased morbidity.[7–10] The algorithm presented in Figure 255-1 outlines the approach to vascular injuries. In the presence of hard signs of vascular injury on clinical examination, immediate surgery is indicated in some conditions, without a preoperative angiogram. However, certain injuries are still best evaluated by angiography prior to surgical intervention. The need for angiography in patients with soft signs of vascular injury is still a matter of some debate among surgeons and radiologists. However, current practice in most centers is to observe patients with soft signs and conduct serial examinations. Angiography and surgery are delayed until there is clinical evidence of arterial injury.

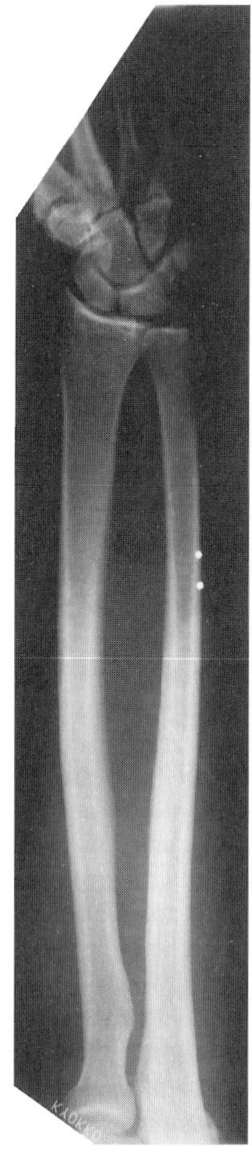

FIG. 255-4. Actual embolization of shotgun pellet, illustrating importance of obtaining images of the extremity distal to such injuries.

Digital subtraction angiography has also been used in evaluation of vascular trauma with accuracy similar to standard techniques but is less reliable in detecting intimal disruption. The test requires a cooperative patient, because it is extremely sensitive to motion artifact.[5]

Ankle Brachial Indices

Doppler devices are used to determine ABIs or wrist brachial indices. Diagnostic accuracy has been reported to be as high as 95 percent, but sensitivity and specificity vary depending on whether the classification of abnormal is set at a ratio of 1.0 or 0.9.[10,11] This test does not reliably detect nonocclusive arterial disease, such as intimal flaps and pseudoaneurysms. It can augment the clinical examination by objectively confirming the subjective impression of a diminished pulse in a patient under observation. To perform accurate ABIs, it is important to place the patient in supine position and measure the systolic blood pressure in all four extremities. To measure an ankle systolic pressure, a standard adult blood pressure cuff should be snugly wrapped around the ankle just above the malleoli. While using the Doppler flowmeter to monitor the signal from the posterior of the anterior tibial artery, distal to the cuff, inflate the cuff to a pressure approximately 30 mmHg above the systolic pressure to occlude flow temporarily. As the cuff is slowly deflated (2 to 5 mmHg/s), the pressure at which the Doppler flow signal is heard should be noted and recorded as the ankle systolic pressure. To assure accuracy, the upper extremity systolic blood pressure should be measured by using a Doppler flowmeter, as well. An ABI is then calculated by dividing the ankle systolic blood pressure by the greater of the two systolic upper extremity blood pressures. An ABI of greater than 1.0 is normal. An ABI of 0.5 to 0.9 is indicative of injury to a single arterial segment. An ABI of less than 0.5 is indicative of severe arterial injury or injury to multiple arterial segments. A difference of greater than 20 mmHg between the upper extremity blood pressures is indicative of upper extremity arterial injury. Underlying conditions, such as preexisting peripheral vascular disease or severe hypothermia, can also affect the accuracy of the ABI.

Duplex Ultrasonography

Duplex ultrasonography has a diagnostic accuracy of 96 to 98 percent and can image extremity vessels with as much resolution as contrast angiography. Advantages over angiography include an increased safety profile and rapid results. However, it is highly operator dependent and has not been tested in patients with severely injured extremities with open wounds or fractures, large hematomas, bulky dressings, or traction devices.[1,5,12]

DISPOSITION

Patients with hard signs of arterial injury are not a diagnostic dilemma. These patients require surgical intervention or, at the very least, expedient surgical evaluation and angiography. Patients with soft signs of arterial injury require inpatient observation. Patients with penetrating extremity injury, no signs of arterial injury, no bony or nervous injury, minimal soft tissue defect, and no signs of developing compartment syndrome can be safely discharged home with close follow-up after a period of observation and serial examinations. There is no consensus on the ideal observation time, but the current literature describes times from 3 to 12 h. Wound exploration in the emergency department should be reserved for those patients with suspected foreign bodies in the wound, for ligamentous involvement, or for control of minor venous bleeding. Wound exploration to control arterial or major venous bleeding should be done in the operating room. The general principles of wound management, including tetanus prophylaxis, apply here. Although controversial, there is no proven role for prophylactic antibiotics unless a wound is contaminated or patients have an underlying preexisting condition that would predispose them to infection.

REFERENCES

1. Frykberg ER: Advances in the diagnosis and treatment of extremity vascular trauma. *Surg Clin North Am* 75:207, 1995.
2. McAndrew MP, Johnson KD: Penetrating orthopedic injuries. *Surg Clin North Am* 71:297, 1991.
3. Hull JB: Management of gunshot fractures of the extremities. *J Trauma* 40(suppl):193, 1996.
4. Fackler ML: Gunshot wound review. *Ann Emerg Med* 28:194, 1996.
5. Modrall JG, Weaver FA, Yellin AE: Diagnosis and management of penetrating vascular trauma and the injured extremity. *Emerg Med Clin North Am* 16:129, 1998.
6. Yelon JA, Scalea TM: Venous injuries of the lower extremities and pelvis: Repair versus ligation. *J Trauma* 33:532, 1992.
7. Dennis JW, Frykberg ER, Crump JM, et al: New perspectives on the management of penetrating trauma in proximity to major limb arteries. *J Vasc Surg* 11:84, 1990.
8. Dennis JW, Frykberg ER, Veldenz HC, et al: Validation of nonoperative management of occult vascular injuries and accuracy of physical examination alone in penetrating extremity trauma: 5- to 10-year follow-up. *J Trauma* 44:243, 1998.
9. Feliciano DV, Herskowitz K, O'Gorman RB, et al: Management of vascular injuries in the lower extremities. *J Trauma* 28:319, 1988.
10. Gates JD: Penetrating wounds of the extremities: Methods of identifying arterial injury. *Orthop Rev* 10(suppl):2, 1994.
11. Nassoura ZE, Ivatury RR, Simon RJ, et al: A reassessment of Doppler pressure indices in the detection of arterial lesions in proximity penetrating injuries of extremities: A prospective study. *Am J Emerg Med* 14:151, 1996.
12. Bergstein JM, Blair JF, Edwards J, et al: Pitfalls in the use of color-flow duplex ultrasound for screening of suspected arterial injuries in penetrating extremities. *J Trauma* 33:395, 1992.

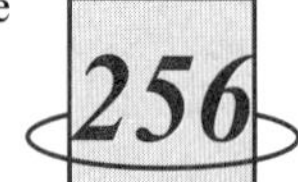

WOUND BALLISTICS

Jeremy J. Hollerman
Martin L. Fackler

EPIDEMIOLOGY

Violence involving firearms is a significant problem in the United States. Handguns are used in the overwhelming majority of cases because they are easy to carry and conceal. Many criminals now use semiautomatic handguns that carry up to 15 cartridges in their clips. Funds produced in the lucrative illegal drug trade enable drug traffickers to switch from cheap revolvers (Saturday night specials) to expensive modern high-technology semiautomatic pistols. Law enforcement has followed suit in this ''arms race.'' It is not surprising that multiple gunshot wounds are becoming more common.[1] A higher percentage of patients wounded by semiautomatic pistols are dead at the scene, increasing from 5 percent in 1985 to 34 percent in 1990 in Philadelphia County.[1] In that study, the percentage of firearm homicide victims with criminal records increased from 43 percent in 1985 to 67 percent in 1990. Of all the 1990 Philadelphia firearm homicide victims, 61 percent were intoxicated at the time they were killed, and 39 percent were using cocaine at the time of death compared with 9 percent in 1985.

Between 1983 and 1992, a total of 37 million handguns, rifles, and shotguns were produced in the United States. These were added to the pool of existing firearms. This figure does not include guns imported into the United States during the same period. In 1992, a total of 3 million handguns, rifles, and shotguns were produced in the United States, and 2.85 million more were imported.[2]

When tracing the ownership history of a firearm for a crime investigation, the record often stops at the point of the gun's first private sale. Except where expressly outlawed by individual states, anyone who owns a firearm is free to sell it without demanding identification and without keeping any record of the sale. The Brady law does not apply. Like most federal gun-sale laws it regulates only the transactions of federally licensed gun dealers.

Each day in the United States, there are 65 murders.[3] At least 68 percent of these are committed with firearms. Many of these murders and much of the urban gun violence result from disputes between criminals, so criminals are often the victims. The medical literature regarding the epidemiology of firearm-involved trauma is often misleading and sometimes outright false.[4,5]

GENERAL CONCEPTS

The medical literature is full of erroneous articles classifying gunshot wounds based on bullet velocity. Other bullet and tissue characteristics are at least as important as velocity.[6–8] Bullet *mass,* which is related to diameter and length, is a major determinant of how deeply the bullet will penetrate tissue. Bullet *construction* (such as whether the bullet is solid lead with no bullet jacket, is partially jacketed, or has a full metal jacket) is a primary determinant of whether the bullet will deform or fragment. Bullet shape and center of mass (which determine how soon it will yaw in its path through tissue), the *thickness of the body part wounded* (determining whether the bullet has a long enough path through tissue to deform or yaw) (Fig. 256-1), *tissue type* struck (e.g., femur versus lung), tissue elasticity, density, specific gravity, and internal cohesiveness [which determine how well the tissue will withstand tissue stretch (temporary cavitation) forces] are all important, in addition to bullet *velocity,* in determining the nature of the wound produced. The amount of kinetic energy ''deposited" or "retained'' in a victim wounded by a projectile is not a reliable predictor of wound severity,[9] and muzzle energy is not a reliable indicator of bullet performance.

An understanding of wound ballistics enables physicians to evaluate and treat missile wounds without repeating the errors of conventional ''wisdom.'' Based on common misconceptions about wound ballistics, many papers have suggested harmful and unnecessary treatment for gunshot wounds. An example of such an unnecessary and harmful recommendation is that for mandatory surgical excision of the tissue surrounding the bullet track (the path of the projectile through tissue) whenever an extremity wound is caused by a high-velocity bullet. This is based on the belief that these tissues will become necrotic. Clinical experience and research show this to be false.[10]

WOUNDING POTENTIAL

Every moving bullet has a maximum wounding potential determined by its mass and velocity. Bullets of equal wounding potential may produce wounds of very different severity, depending on bullet shape, internal and external construction, and which tissues they traverse.

Bullets with equal wounding potential often do not produce similar wounds. A heavier, slower bullet crushes more tissue but induces less temporary cavitation; most of the wounding potential of a lighter, faster bullet is likely to be used up forming a larger temporary cavity, but this bullet leaves a smaller permanent cavity (crushes less tissue).[9,12] The heavier, slower bullet causes a more severe wound in elastic tissue than the lighter, faster bullet, which uses up much of its wounding potential producing tissue stretch (temporary cavitation). This tissue stretch may be absorbed with little or no ill effect by elastic tissue such as lung or muscle. In less elastic tissue such as liver or brain, the temporary cavity produced by the lighter, faster bullet can produce a more severe wound. Penetration depth will be less with the lighter, faster bullet, and critical structures such as the heart may not be reached.

MECHANISMS OF WOUNDING

Both missile and tissue characteristics determine the nature of the wound. Missile characteristics are partly inherent (mass, shape, and construction) and are partly conferred by the weapon (longitudinal and rotational velocity). Tissue characteristics (elasticity, density, and anatomic relationships) also strongly affect the nature of the wound. The severity of a bullet wound is influenced by the bullet's orientation during its flight through tissue and by whether the bullet fragments[9] deform (into the typical mushroom shape of expanding hollow-point or soft-point bullets).

Two major mechanisms of wounding occur: the *crushing* of the tissue struck by the projectile (forming the permanent cavity), and the radial *stretching* of the projectile path walls (forming a temporary cavity) (Fig. 256-1). In addition, a sonic pressure wave precedes the projectile through tissue. The sonic pressure wave plays no part in wounding.[11]

Crushing of Tissue

A missile crushes the tissue it strikes, thereby creating a permanent wound channel (permanent cavity). If the bullet is traveling with its pointed end forward and its long axis parallel to the longitudinal axis of flight (0° of yaw, the angle between the long axis of the bullet and its path of flight), it crushes a tube of tissue no greater than its approximate diameter. When the bullet yaws to 90°, the entire long axis of the bullet strikes tissue. The amount of tissue crushed may be three times greater than at 0° of yaw.

When striking soft tissue with sufficient velocity, soft-point and hollow-point bullets deform into a mushroom shape. This increases surface area and the amount of tissue crushed. For most big-game hunting, such bullets are mandated by law. This is to increase the probability of prompt lethality, rather than the creation of a disabling but nonlethal wound causing an animal prolonged suffering. If the mushroomed diameter is 2.5 times greater than the initial diameter of the bullet, the area of tissue crushed by the bullet is 6.25 times greater than the amount that would have been crushed by the undeformed bullet.

Bullet fragmentation also increases the volume of tissue crushed.[8] After bullet fragmentation, bullet surface area is increased and much more tissue is crushed. For large handgun (e.g., .44 magnum) and rifle bullets, the striking of bone is one of the causes of early bullet fragmentation.

Comminuted fracture may be created by rifle and large handgun bullets striking bone. Bone fragments can become secondary missiles, crushing tissue. Many handgun bullets are unable to fragment bone significantly. When a large bone is struck, it is likely that the bullet will expend its wounding potential in the victim and will not exit.

Bullet fragments and secondary missiles, such as bone fragments, teeth, or coins, propelled by contact with the bullet are likely to increase the severity of the wound. Multiple perforations weaken tissue and create focal points for stress (stress risers). Tissue tears are particularly likely to occur at stress risers during temporary cavitation stretch.[9]

Unjacketed lead bullets cannot be driven faster than about 2000 ft/sec (610 m/s) without some of the lead stripping off in the barrel. This is avoided if a jacket made of a harder metal (such as copper or a copper alloy) is used to surround the lead. The jacket of a military bullet completely covers the bullet tip (a full metal jacket). Civilians often use hollow-point or soft-point bullets. Hollow-point bullets have a hole in the jacket at the bullet tip, and soft-point bullets have some of the lead core of the bullet exposed at the bullet tip. These constructions weaken the bullet tip, causing it to flatten on impact. This flattening often greatly exceeds bullet diameter, resulting in a mushroom-shaped projectile.

The hollow-point and soft-point bullets used by civilians are often more damaging to tissue than are military bullets fired from rounds

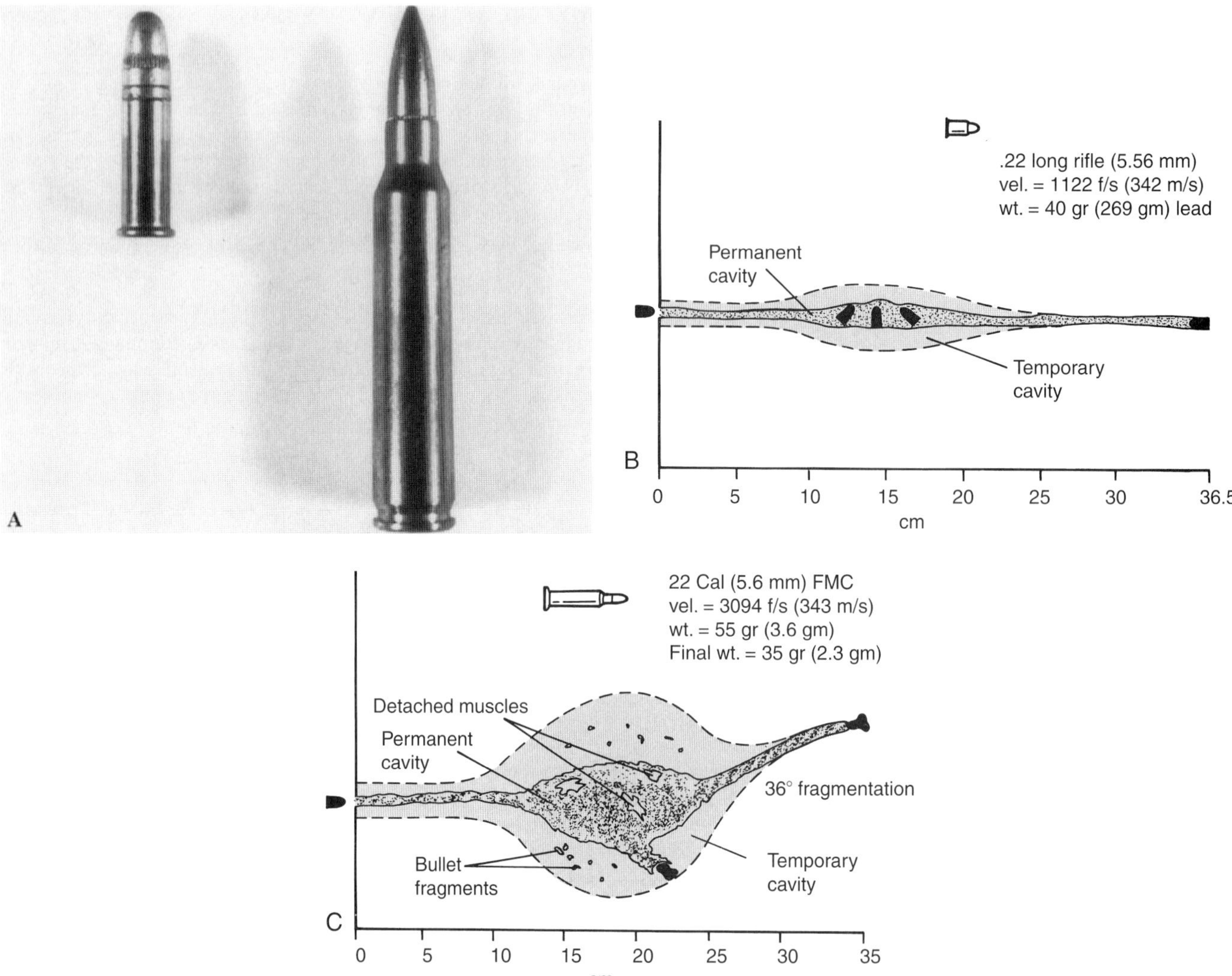

FIG. 256-1. A. The photograph shows a .22 long rifle round (*left*) and an M16 round (*right*). **B** and **C.** These are the wound profiles of the same .22 long rifle (B) and .224 caliber M-193 round of the M16A1 rifle (C). [Full metal case (FMC) is a synonym of full metal jacket (FMJ), the type of bullet used in the military.] This figure shows that caliber (bullet diameter in decimals of an inch or in millimeters) is only one indicator of wounding potential and not a very good one. Because of much higher velocity [3094 ft/s (943 m/s), as opposed to 1122 ft/s (342 m/s) for the .22 long rifle bullet], because it fragments in tissue, and because of greater bullet mass, the M16 bullet has the potential to cause a much more severe wound if the anatomic part struck is sufficiently thick. Note that, in the gelatin block, both the permanent cavity and the temporary cavity caused by the M16 bullet are much larger than those of the .22 long rifle bullet. As is usual for a non-deforming bullet, the temporary and permanent cavities caused by the .22 long rifle bullet are largest when the bullet has a 90° yaw. (From Hollerman et al (p 686),[4] with permission.)

otherwise configured identically.[6,9,13] Because of this, wounds produced by civilian hunting rifles, shotguns, and large-caliber handguns are usually more severe than wounds produced by military-rifle bullets of the same mass and velocity.[13]

Hollow-point and soft-point bullets either deform into a mushroom shape or stay undeformed. Up to one-third of hollow-point and soft-point handgun bullets fail to deform into a mushroom shape, usually due to insufficient bullet velocity or an excessively stiff or thick bullet jacket that prevents deformation.

When the tip of a hollow-point bullet is plugged with material such as clothing or drywall, bullet expansion into a mushroom shape in tissue is usually delayed and sometimes prevented. This causes deeper penetration of tissue, sometimes causing a perforating wound (having both and entrance and an exit). This may result in the injury of bystanders. Some recent handgun bullets have designs attempting to overcome this problem.

Projectiles penetrate more deeply as projectile velocity is increased, but only up to the point where velocity becomes sufficiently high to deform the projectile. Penetration decreases markedly from that point on. The greater the bullet diameter expansion from mushrooming, the less is the depth of penetration.[14]

There is a critical range of velocity for each handgun hollow-point and soft-point bullet, within which the bullet may perform as expected. Below this velocity range the bullet will have insufficient velocity to mushroom on impact, and at velocities above this range the bullet may fragment after impact, resulting in many light bullet pieces crushing tissue at a superficial depth.

Military full metal jacket bullets do not flatten at the bullet tip, i.e., they do not mushroom. Sometimes they can break and fragment as a result of yawing to 90°. The stress on the bullet as its long axis strikes tissue causes the sides of the bullet to flatten as if it had been squeezed in a vise. If the bullet breaks, it will usually do so at the cannelure, a circular groove around the bullet where it is crimped into the cartridge case. Although the M-193 military bullet of the M16 rifle fragments in soft tissue wounds with a characteristic pattern depending on range,[15] most other full metal jacket military bullets, such as those fired from the AK-47, AK-74, and the NATO 7.62-mm rifle (US version), do not fragment unless they strike a large bone.

If a bullet is jacketed, the bullet jacket usually cannot be distinguished from the lead core on standard radiographs, because the entire bullet is metallic density. Occasionally, as the bullet deforms or fragments, the bullet jacket separates from the bullet and is visible on a radiograph.

In extremity wounds, when a radiograph reveals an undeformed bullet lying in the soft tissues and no fracture is present, tissue disruption is usually minor. If a major vessel or nerve is divided, however, even a simple wound can have a severe effect.

Wounding is like real estate: location is the most important factor. A bullet of low wounding potential can cause a severe wound if it passes through a vital structure such as the spinal cord.

Temporary Cavitation (Tissue Stretch)

Fired from an appropriate and well-designed weapon, a bullet flies in air with its nose pointed forward; it yaws only 1° to 3°. Yaw occurs around the bullet's center of mass. In pointed rifle bullets, the center of mass is behind the midpoint of the bullet's long axis. Although the bullet's most naturally stable in-flight orientation would be with its heaviest part (its base) forward, for aerodynamically efficient flight it must fly point forward.

During flight, a bullet is stabilized against yaw by the spin imparted to it by the spiral grooves (rifling) in the gun barrel. The longer (and heavier) the bullet in relation to its diameter, the more rapidly it must be rotated to avoid significant yaw in flight. A gun barrel intended to fire a heavier bullet has rifling that makes a full turn in fewer inches of barrel length than the rifling in a barrel intended for a shorter, lighter bullet of the same caliber. This will cause a faster rate of bullet spin.

A gun with a shorter barrel will generally produce a bullet of lower velocity than would a weapon with a longer barrel when firing the same round. With shorter barrel length, the expanding gasses of the burning gunpowder have less time to accelerate the bullet before they are discharged into the atmosphere. A .22 long rifle round fired in a rifle will produce a bullet with up to 300 ft/s more velocity than would the same round fired in a handgun.

Although the bullet's spin is adequate to stabilize it against yaw in its flight through air, it is not adequate to stabilize it in its path through tissue, because of the higher density of the medium. If it does not deform, a pointed bullet eventually yaws to a base-forward position (180° of yaw). Expanding bullets lose the physical stimulus to yaw because, after mushrooming, their heaviest part is forward.

As a bullet passes through 90° of yaw or after it deforms into a mushroom shape, it is crushing its maximal amount of tissue (unless it fragments, which will crush more). It is slowed down rapidly, as its wounding potential is used up. The bullet creates a splash-type force in tissue, which spreads out radially. This force creates the temporary cavity. This aspect of the wounding process is analogous to the splash of a diver entering the water.

If a diver enters the water very straight and point forward (similar to a bullet at 0° of yaw), the splash may be minimal. If the diver does a belly flop (similar to a bullet at 90° of yaw), a large splash is induced. In tissue, this splash, the temporary cavity, produces localized blunt trauma.[9]

The maximal size of the temporary cavity occurs several milliseconds after the bullet has passed through the tissue. Because forces follow paths of least resistance, temporary cavitation is likely to be asymmetric and spread out through tissue planes.

The temporary cavity caused by common handgun bullets is generally too small to be a significant wounding factor in all but the most sensitive tissues (brain and liver). Center-fire rifle bullets and large handgun bullets (e.g., .44 magnum), often induce a large temporary cavity [10- to 25-cm (4- to 10-in) diameter] in tissue. This can be a significant wounding factor, depending on the characteristics of the tissue in which it forms.

Near-water-density, less elastic tissue (such as brain, liver, or spleen), fluid-filled organs (including the heart, bladder, and gastrointestinal tract), and dense tissue (such as bone) may be damaged severely when a large temporary cavity displaces them or forms within them. More elastic tissue (such as skeletal muscle) and lower-density elastic tissue (such as lung) are less affected by the formation of a temporary cavity.[16,17] Because of these tissue differences, transmitted blunt trauma from temporary cavitation caused by a bullet traveling 800 to 950 m/s can cause a more severe pulmonary contusion when the bullet traverses the chest wall musculature than the pulmonary contusion it would have caused if passing through the lung.[17]

Although the formation of a large temporary cavity often has devastating effects in the brain or liver, its effect in wounds of the extremities has frequently been exaggerated.[18] Fracture of large bones not hit by the bullet and tearing of major vessels or nerves by the temporary cavity are often mentioned in the literature but are rare in clinical experience. This includes a systematic review of 1400 rifle wounds sustained in the Vietnam conflict and analyzed in the Wound Data and Munitions Effectiveness Team (WDMET) study (R.F. Bellamy, personal communication). Most of the permanent damage done in wounds of the extremities is the result of structures being hit by the intact bullet, bullet fragments, or secondary missiles. As in all blunt trauma, shear forces develop and tear structures at points where one side is fixed and the other side is free to move. The temporary cavity is no exception. In the unlikely event that the blunt trauma caused by the temporary cavity tears a vessel wall, this is particularly likely to occur at the vessel origin.

BALLISTIC PROPERTIES AND THE WOUND PRODUCED

Animal experiments using military-rifle bullets[9] have clearly disproved the assertion that all tissue exposed to temporary cavitation is destroyed. Not only does the 14-cm diameter temporary cavity produced by the AK-74 not destroy a great amount of muscle, but the sizable stellate exit wound it causes in the uncomplicated thigh wound ensures excellent wound drainage, which assists healing.[9,16] A history that the wound was caused by a high-velocity bullet does not mandate radical excision of the wound path.[16,18]

The characteristics of the wounded tissue, the thickness of the body part, the point in the path of the bullet at which deformation into a mushroom shape, yaw or fragmentation occurs, and other factors strongly influence the wound produced.

Experiments with ballistic gelatin (which reproduces the projectile deformation and penetration depth of living animal muscle) have shown that most full metal jacketed rifle bullets yaw significantly only at tissue depths greater than the diameter of human extremities.

In the first 12 cm (the average thickness of an adult human thigh) of a soft tissue wound path, there is often little or no difference between the wounding effect of low- and high-velocity bullets when the high-velocity bullet is of the military full metal jacket type. This is particularly true of the relatively heavier military-rifle bullets such as those fired by the AK-47 and NATO 7.62-mm (USA version) rifle. A wound of an extremity caused by an AK-47 bullet that does not hit bone is often similar to a handgun bullet wound. No matter how high its velocity, if a non-deforming, heavy bullet does not break, fragment, or hit a large bone, it may exit an extremity with much of its wounding potential unspent. These same bullets are often lethal in chest or abdominal wounds because the trunk is thicker than an extremity and allows the bullet a sufficiently long path through tissue to yaw. Maximal temporary cavitation induced by the AK-47 bullet usually occurs at a tissue depth of 28 cm, much greater than the diameter of a human extremity.

A soft-point or hollow-point bullet fired from a civilian center-fire rifle deforms soon after entering tissue and produces a much more severe extremity wound than will a military full metal jacket bullet that does not break and fragment.

The more recently developed, smaller-caliber, AK-74 fires a bullet that is lighter than the AK-47 bullet and yaws earlier.[19] Its maximal temporary cavity occurs at a tissue depth of 11 cm. Extremity wounds from the AK-74 can be expected to be more severe than those from the AK-47.[19] The lighter, smaller AK-74 round allows a soldier to carry many more rounds of ammunition. This was the primary motivation for development of the M16 and the AK-74.

Caliber

Caliber (bullet diameter in decimals of an inch or in millimeters) is only one indicator of wounding potential but not a very good one (Fig. 256-1). Caliber indicates bullet diameter, but not bullet length, and therefore does not disclose bullet mass. Caliber also is independent of bullet velocity and bullet construction.

Unfortunately, commonly used weapon and bullet designations are often misleading. As an example, the .38 special and the .357 magnum use bullets that have the same diameter [.357 in. (9.07 mm)] (Table 256-1). The longer cartridge case of the magnum can hold more powder, giving the bullet higher velocity and greater wounding potential.

Gunshot Fractures

Handgun wounds of the extremities yield characteristic fracture patterns. Frequently seen are divot fractures of cortical bone, drill-hole fractures, butterfly fractures, and double butterfly fractures.[8] Nondisplaced fracture lines sometimes radiate from these defects. These usually heal well. The bullet hole itself can act as a stress riser. Spiral fractures extending proximally or distally from the bullet hole may result from the dissipation of stress forces at the bullet hole. Occasionally, remote spiral fractures at some distance proximal or distal to the bony gunshot wound also occur, probably because of the presence of stress risers, such as vascular channels in the bone, and the fact that the bone was under load and often torsional stress at the time of impact.[20]

In gunshot fractures from rifles and large handguns, a greater extent of comminution may be seen. These fractures often have complications because of the soft tissue damage these bullets cause.[8] The vascular compromise associated with these comminuted gunshot fractures increases the likelihood of delayed union or nonunion of the fracture. Wound infections are more common in this group. Early fasciotomy to prevent compartment syndrome is important, when needed.

At some hospitals, outpatient treatment is being used successfully for extremity fractures caused by handguns, if no significant neurologic or vascular compromise has occurred.[21]

Trunk Wounds

Bullets are not sterilized by the heat of firing. They can carry bacteria from the body surface or body organs, such as a perforated colon, deep into the wound.

In trunk wounds, an analysis of the bullet path is mandatory to determine whether a laparotomy is needed. Two radiographs in planes separated by 90°, computed tomography (CT), clinical examination, and peritoneal lavage are all useful. Abdominal CT is more accurate if performed before peritoneal lavage. If peritoneal penetration by a bullet is suspected, laparotomy is indicated.[22] The morbidity and mortality rates of an exploratory laparotomy that shows no significant

TABLE 256-1 Cartridge Case Name and Actual Bullet Diameter Used

Cartridge Cases	Actual Bullet Diameter (Inches)
Of common interest:	
32 Auto (ACP)	.312
380 Auto (ACP)	.355
9-mm Luger (9-mm Parabellum)	.355
38 Super	.355 or .357
38 Special	.357
357 Magnum	.357
44 Special	.4295
44 Magnum	.4295
444 Marlin	.4295
Others of interest:	
22 Hornet	.223 and .224
218 Bee	.224
219 Donaldson Wasp	.224
219 Zipper	.224
221 Remington Fireball	.224
222 Remington	.224
222 Remington Magnum	.224
223 Remington	.224
224 Weatherby Magnum	.224
225 Winchester	.224
22-250 Remington	.224
220 Swift	.224
243 Winchester	.243
244 Remington/6-mm Remington	.243
240 Weatherby Magnum	.243
256 Winchester Magnum	.257
250/3000 Savage	.257
257 Roberts	.257
25/06 Remington	.257
257 Weatherby Magnum	.257
30-06	.308
30-30 Winchester	.308
30 M1 Carbine	.308
7.62-mm × 39-mm (AK-47)	.308
30/40 Krag	.308
7.5-mm × 55-mm Swiss (Schmidt-Rubin)	.308
300 Savage	.308
7.62-mm Russian	.308
308 Winchester	.308
7.62-mm NATO	.308
30-06 Springfield	.308
300 H & H Magnum	.308
30-338	.308
300 Winchester Magnum	.308
308 Norma Magnum	.308
300 Weatherby Magnum	.308
303 British	.311
7.65-mm Mauser	.311
7.7-mm Japanese	.311

Often, both the numerical designation associated with the bullet and the cartridge case do not reflect exact measurements. As an example, the 44 Remington Magnum Pistol cartridge is 0.456 in in diameter at its distal end and uses a bullet with a 0.43-in diameter.[34] Both the .38 special and the .357 magnum use bullets that have the same diameter [0.357 in (9.07 mm)]. These bullets are often exactly the same weight. When trying to determine bullet type from a radiograph, in addition to correcting for magnification or deformation, one must look up actual bullet diameter rather than relying on the bullet name for its size.

Abbreviation: ACP, Automatic Colt Pistol.

Sources: Adapted from references 33 and 34.

intraabdominal injury are low compared with those of missed intestinal injury. CT is useful, especially when an exclusively body wall or retroperitoneal path is suspected. CT has largely replaced excretory urography as the preferred means of evaluating the urinary tract after penetrating trauma.

Any bullet wound below the nipple line should raise the question of whether the diaphragm or abdomen has been penetrated. CT sometimes can be used to make this determination. Laparotomy is required if peritoneal penetration cannot be excluded.[22]

Whenever a gunshot wound traverses the midline of the neck or the width of the mediastinum, perforation of the esophagus should be suspected. Esophageal evaluation should not be overlooked after angiographic evaluation of the neck or chest.

Head Wounds

In skull wounds, as elsewhere in bone gunshot fractures, inward beveling of the calvarial defect at the bullet entrance and outward beveling of the skull at the exit wound are typical.[23] This is due partly to the geometry of the skull and partly to the bullet-bone interaction. Characteristic fracture patterns of the skull can be used to identify entrance and exit wounds.[23] When there is a cranial exit wound, skull fractures propagate across the calvarium faster than the bullet travels through the brain, producing characteristic patterns of fracture. These fracture patterns sometimes allow differentiation of entrance and exit wounds.[23] Radial fractures often spread out in a star pattern from the entrance and to a lesser extent from the exit holes in the skull. Concentric heaving fractures may occur, connecting the arcs of the radial fractures around both the entrance and exit holes, if sufficient temporary cavitation forces are generated inside the brain to cause significant outwardly directed tissue splash forces inside the skull, pushing out the calvarium.[23] Because a fracture will not cross a preexisting fracture line, the temporal sequence of the occurrence of the fractures can sometimes be determined from the pattern of the fractures.

Brain, whose tissue properties include near-water density, very little elasticity, and poor tissue cohesiveness, is extremely sensitive to temporary cavitation forces. When disrupted by such forces, severe brain injury often results. In addition to the relative lack of elasticity of brain tissue, its enclosure in the rigid cranial vault magnifies brain disruption by temporary cavitation forces.

Pellet Wounds

Compared with a pointed rifle bullet, spherical pellets slow rapidly in its flight through air or tissue. In tissue, the entire wounding potential of a shot pellet at its entrance velocity is likely to be delivered to the target, often with no exit wound. At close range (less than 3 m), shotgun pellets remain tightly clustered. Therefore, shot pellet size makes little difference, as the entire load of the pellets functions as a unit, with a velocity virtually equal to muzzle velocity. Shotgun wounds at ranges of less than 5 m consist of multiple parallel wound channels. This grossly disrupts the blood supply to tissue between the wound channels.

The most severe civilian firearm wounds typically seen are those inflicted by a shotgun from close range. After a close-range or contact shotgun wound to the trunk, external examination of the patient, particularly after adequate volume resuscitation, often does not disclose the severity of the internal injuries present.

Major neural injury after shotgun wounding of the extremities may be more important than fracture or major vascular injury in determining the final outcome.[24]

During surgical exploration of a close-range shotgun wound, it is important to search for wadding, casing debris, plastic shot cup, and surface materials carried into the wound (e.g., clothing, glass, or wood). Many of these are radiolucent.[8]

Diagnosing long-range injury on the basis of the pattern of pellet spread is sometimes problematic. When shotgun pellets are tightly clustered or widely spread out, close-range injury or long-range injury (respectively) is usually suspected. However, in close-range injuries, the *''billiard ball'' effect* may cause considerable pellet spread.[25] When the tightly clustered group of shot at close range contacts the skin, the pellets at the front of the group are slowed. The pellets behind them in the group strike the pellets in front with an effect like a billiard ball break. This causes much more pellet spread in tissue than would be expected at close range. On radiographs, particularly in trunk wounds, this effect can simulate the pellet spread of a longer-range injury.[25] This pitfall can be avoided if the skin physical examination is correlated with the radiologic findings. If there is only one entrance wound hole, it is a close-range injury. If the distribution of the multiple skin entrance wounds is the same as the pellet spread on the radiograph, the injury occurred at longer range.

Recently manufactured BB guns and air guns that fire small pellets have considerably higher muzzle velocity [600 ft/s (183 m/s) or more] than older guns of this type. Penetrating injuries from these weapons are sometimes fatal. These air guns should not be considered toys. It is possible for someone to have been shot with a BB pellet that has penetrated the scalp, skull, and brain and think only a scalp wound is present.[26]

ASSESSMENT OF MISSILE TYPE AND LOCATION IN THE BODY

As in all of radiology, localization requires two views at 90°, or a tomographic image. CT of the head and body is often useful for analysis of bullet path.[8]

The CT digital scout radiograph, which can be used for missile localization, usually can be taken in anteroposterior and lateral projections without moving the patient. The ability to manipulate the display window and center enables visualization of bullets seen through dense structures, such as the shoulders and pelvis.

Assessment of Missile Type

On a radiograph, assessment of missile caliber is difficult because of magnification and missile deformation. If an undeformed bullet is seen in two views at 90°, and its degree of magnification is known, the approximate caliber of the bullet can be determined. Some bullets are difficult to distinguish because the diameter is similar to others (Table 256-1). Sometimes deformed bullets can be accurately characterized radiologically for intact bullet caliber and weight.[27]

Many radiographs show only fragments of the bullet and do not enable determination of the type of weapon and projectile that caused the wound. However, certain bullets deform or fragment in a characteristic pattern (such as the M16 military bullet, the Winchester Black Talon or SXT handgun bullets, and the .357 magnum 125-grain Remington semijacketed soft-point bullet) that can be used to identify them. Deformation of large lead shotgun pellets (e.g., 00 buckshot) after contact with bone can cause these to be confused with deformed bullet fragments.

MISSILE EMBOLIZATION

It always must be ascertained that the path from the entrance wound is consistent with the bullet's current location, because a bullet may have reached its present location by embolization. Arterial and venous embolization of bullets and shotgun pellets, as well as bullet movement within the subarachnoid space in the head and spine, have been reported. It is generally accepted that a missile freely floating within a cardiac chamber should be removed to prevent embolization.[28] Missiles clearly embedded in chamber walls are relatively safe.[28] Missile size does not seem to be especially important, as all sizes can produce morbidity after embolization. Two-dimensional echocardiography is useful in determining whether a missile is embedded in a chamber wall.[28] CT (particularly high-speed CT) and magnetic resonance imaging for nonmagnetic missiles also have a role. On chest radiographs, blurring of the margins of a pericardiac missile or fragment is a reason to suspect that the missile is in or next to the heart.[28]

Whenever a bullet is not found on radiographs of the body part predicted based on the entrance wound, the bullet's location is not known, and there is no exit wound, additional radiographs or fluoroscopy to find the bullet are mandatory. Immediately before surgery for missile removal, repeat radiographic confirmation of the exact location of the missile is usually indicated.

Interventional radiologic techniques are useful in bullet removal, including the removal of intravascular and intrarenal bullets. Significant deformation of an intravascular bullet is a relative contraindication to retrieval using a transarterial catheter because of potential damage to the intima. Arthroscopy sometimes can be used for removing bullets from joints, especially the knee.

Most bullets follow straight paths through the body, but sometimes, even in the absence of embolization, a bullet, particularly a handgun bullet, will not. It may ricochet off body structures, especially bone, or may follow fascial or tissue planes. Bullets traveling less than 1100 ft/s (335 m/s) are the ones most likely to be deflected by anatomic structures or to follow tissue planes. Bullet shape also influences the tendency to be deflected.

Far more common than bullet displacement by embolization from where it came to rest in the body at the end of its path is bullet movement due to the effect of gravity on a bullet that ends up free in the pleural space or peritoneal cavity.

LEAD FRAGMENTS AND LEAD POISONING

Lead fragments in soft tissue usually become encapsulated with fibrous tissue and do not cause problems. Bullet-induced lead poisoning is most common with intraarticular, disk space, and bursal locations of bullet fragments because of the solubility of lead is synovial fluid.[29,30] Lead fragments in the brain are usually relatively benign unless they are copper plated (as are many civilian .22 caliber bullets).[31] Copper-plated lead pellets produced a sterile abscess or granuloma in the brain of cats surgically implanted with missiles of this type.[31] This can be associated with downward migration of the missile, resorption of copper from the surface of the missile, progressive neurologic deficit, and sometimes the death of the cat. These findings were absent in cats whose brains were implanted with uncoated lead pellets.

Intraarticular fragments should be removed to avoid both the mechanical trauma and the destructive synovitis lead can cause.[29] Significant damage to the articular cartilage visible at surgery may be present as a result of lead synovitis, when radiographs remain normal except for bullet fragments.[29] If large fragments are present in the joint, they can cause severe mechanical trauma during motion. This motion can lead to further lead fragmentation.

Whether lead poisoning occurs depends largely on the surface area of the retained lead particles and their location in the body.[30] Sometimes the onset of clinical lead poisoning can be quite rapid, but usually it takes years.

Patients with retained lead pellets or lead bullet fragments should be advised that, on rare occasions, a fragment might erode into a bursa or joint space and cause lead poisoning. They should be assured that lead poisoning poses a threat *only if unrecognized and untreated.* They should be cautioned to inform their physician of the retained lead any time they seek treatment for problems such as headache, abdominal pain, personality change, or bizarre neurologic symptoms. Once the possibility of lead poisoning is considered, it can be easily confirmed or ruled out simply by determining the blood lead level.

EVIDENTIARY CONCERNS

Physicians must be aware of the importance of preserving evidence in patients being resuscitated after penetrating trauma. Do not cut through bullet holes or knife holes in clothing when removing it. Do not incise through skin wounds unless absolutely necessary. To preserve powder marks, do not scrub wounds unless necessary. Emergency departments must have a protocol for collecting clothing and other evidence so that it can be documented that it was always under surveillance or otherwise kept in such a way that tampering could not occur. Do not describe wounds as entry or exit wounds; instead, describe the appearance of wounds in detail, without interpretation. Describe the location, size, and shape of all gunshot wounds. Include the presence or absence of a soot ring, or skin or subcutaneous tissue tattooing with gunpowder, or the presence of subcutaneous gas (such as from a contact wound with injection into the subcutaneous tissues of gases from burning gunpowder). When a bullet or fragment is encountered, do not pick it up with a metallic clamp, so ballistic markings can be interpreted without the possibility that marks were made later with a surgical instrument. Prehospital personnel should receive similar instruction relative to preserving evidence at the scene. The history of the episode can be useful if the number of shots fired or the position of the victim relative to the assailant was observed.

The sharp bullet jacket edges that some soft-point and hollow-point handgun bullets have when they are deformed into a mushroom shape should be avoided. Infectious diseases such as hepatitis and HIV can pass from the victim to the health-care provider as a result of skin punctures from these sharp edges.

Some emergency medicine residency programs now include a course in forensic medicine.[32]

REFERENCES

1. McGonigal MD, Cole J, Schwab CW, et al: Urban firearm deaths: A five-year perspective. *J Trauma* 35:532, 1993.
2. United States Department of the Treasury Bureau of Alcohol Tobacco and Firearms Public Affairs Branch: Civilian firearms—Domestic manufacturing, exportation, importation, and availability for sale 1980–1992, in ATF Ready Reference 1993. Washington, DC, US Government Printing Office, 1993, pp 14–19.
3. Federal Bureau of Investigation: *Crime in the United States 1992: Uniform Crime Reports.* Washington, DC, US Department of Justice, 1993.
4. Suter EA: Guns in the medical literature: A failure of peer review. *J Med Assoc Ga* 83:133, 1994.
5. Kates DB, Schaffer HE, Lattimer JK, et al: Guns and public health: Epidemic of violence or pandemic of propaganda? *Tenn Law Rev* 62:513, 1955.
6. Hollerman JJ, Fackler ML, Coldwell DM, Ben-Menachem Y: Gunshot wounds: 1. Bullets, ballistics and mechanisms of injury. *AJR* 155:685, 1990.
7. Hollerman JJ, Fackler ML: Gunshot wounds: Radiology and wound ballistics. *Emerg Radiol* 2:171, 1995.
8. Hollerman JJ, Fackler ML, Coldwell DM, Ben-Menachem Y: Gunshot wounds: 2. Radiology. *AJR* 155:691, 1990.
9. Fackler ML, Surinchak JS, Malinowski JA, Bowen RE: Bullet fragmentation: A major cause of tissue disruption. *J Trauma* 24:35, 1984.
10. Fackler ML, Breteau JPL, Courbil LJ, et al: Open wound drainage versus wound excision in treating the modern assault rifle wound. *Surgery* 105:576, 1989.
11. Harvey EN, Korr IM, Oster G, McMillen JH: Secondary damage in wounding due to pressure changes accompanying the passage of high velocity missiles. *Surgery* 21:218, 1947.
12. Hollerman JJ: Wound ballistics is a model of the pathophysiology of all blunt and penetrating trauma. *Emerg Radiol* 5:279, 1998.
13. DeMuth WE Jr: Bullet velocity and design as determinants of wounding capability: An experimental study. *J Trauma* 6:222, 1966.
14. Wolberg EJ: Performance of the Winchester 9mm 147 grain subsonic jacketed hollow point bullet in human tissue and tissue simulant. *J Int Wound Ballistics Assoc* 1:10, 1991.
15. Fackler ML: Wounding patterns of military rifle bullets. *Int Defense Rev* 22:59, 1989.

16. Hampton OP Jr: The indications for debridement of gunshot (bullet) wounds of the extremities in civilian practice. *J Trauma* 1:368, 1961.
17. Daniel RA Jr: Bullet wounds of the lungs. *Surgery* 15:774, 1944.
18. Fackler ML: Wound ballistics: A review of common misconceptions. *JAMA* 259:2730, 1988.
19. Fackler ML, Surinchak JS, Malinowski JA, Bowen RE: Wounding potential of the Russian AK-74 assault rifle. *J Trauma* 24:263, 1984.
20. Smith HW, Wheatley KK Jr: Biomechanics of femur fractures secondary to gunshot wounds. *J Trauma* 24:970, 1984.
21. Woloszyn JT, Uitvlugt GM, Castle ME: Management of civilian gunshot fractures of the extremities. *Clin Orthop* 226:247, 1988.
22. Feliciano DV, Burch JM, Spjut-Patrinely V, et al: Abdominal gunshot wounds: An urban trauma center's experience with 300 consecutive patients. *Ann Surg* 208:362, 1988.
23. Smith OC, Berryman HE, Lahren CH: Cranial fracture patterns and estimate of direction from low velocity gunshot wounds. *J Forensic Sci* 32:1416, 1987.
24. Deitch EA, Grimes WR: Experience with 112 shotgun wounds of the extremities. *J Trauma* 24:600, 1984.
25. Messmer JM, Fierro MF: Radiologic forensic investigation of fatal gunshot wounds. *Radiographics* 6:457, 1986.
26. Lucas RM, Mitterer D: Pneumatic firearm injuries: Trivial trauma or perilous pitfalls? *J Emerg Med* 8:433, 1990.
27. Bixler RP, Ahrens CR, Rossi RP, Thickman D: Bullet identification with radiography. *Radiology* 178:563, 1991.
28. Robison RJ, Brown JW, Caldwell R, et al: Management of asymptomatic intracardiac missiles using echocardiography. *J Trauma* 28:1402, 1988.
29. Sclafani SJA, Vuletin JC, Twersky J: Lead arthropathy: Arthritis caused by retained intra-articular bullets. *Radiology* 156:299, 1985.
30. Linden MA, Manton WI, Stewart RM, et al: Lead poisoning from retained bullets: Pathogenesis, diagnosis, and management. *Ann Surg* 195:305, 1982.
31. Sights WP, Bye RJ: The fate of retained intracerebral shotgun pellets: An experimental study. *J Neurosurg* 33:646, 1970.
32. Smock WS: Development of a clinical forensic medicine curriculum for emergency physicians in the USA. *J Clin Forensic Med* 1:27, 1994.
33. *Sierra Rifle Reloading Manual,* 3d ed. Santa Fe Springs, CA: Sierra Bullets, 1989.
34. *Sierra Handgun Reloading Manual,* 3d ed. Santa Fe Springs, CA: Sierra Bullets, 1989.

FORENSICS

John E. Smialek

State laws and standard medical practices obligate physician/health care providers in the emergency departments (EDs) to serve as an interface between patients and the state within the context of the legal and justice systems. To comply with these additional responsibilities, physicians must be aware of legal obligations and must be able to recognize patterns of injury. Observations must be appropriately documented and evidence must be processed in a manner consistent with legal standards.

Each ED should provide its physicians with a standard protocol for responding to state-imposed legal responsibilities such as reporting requirements. As an example, all states impose an obligation to report certain types of injuries to state social services or law enforcement agencies. Generally, these reporting requirements are centered around the vulnerable patients such as children, the elderly, and other victims of domestic violence. Reporting laws for other types of injuries vary from state to state. There may be obligations to report gunshot wounds, knife wounds, assaults and burns.

The physician must also take a proper history from the patient and other reporting witnesses, which must include a statement regarding the origin of the injury. These statements must be documented verbatim for several reasons. Firstly, they may be self-serving and the explanation may change upon subsequent reflection. Secondly, such statements are of legal significance and are admissible in subsequent legal proceedings where they will be analyzed in minute detail.

In addition to obtaining this initial history, the physician must also provide a physical examination of the injury and documentation of that examination before the injury is altered by healing or medical treatment. The physical examination should be supplemented by other diagnostic and documentary tools, such as x-ray. The legal significance of injury assessment also warrants documentation of the injury by photograph. Therefore, an autofocus, Polaroid, or digital camera should be standard equipment in every ED. The newer digital cameras may also suffice but may be more prone to accusations of computer alteration.

PATTERNS OF INJURY

Classification

Injuries may be classified in a variety of ways. Mode of production is one method that includes blunt force, sharp force, missile, heat, electricity, and chemicals. Injuries may also be categorized according to the circumstances in which they were inflicted. Such circumstances are accidental, suicidal or homicidal. Wounds may also be characterized as surgical or ritual, depending on the setting in which these wounds are sustained. However, the most useful classification is based on the components of the injury pattern. Injuries consist of one or a combination of several of the following types of tissue damage:

1. Abrasion
2. Bruise (ecchymosis)
3. Contusion
4. Laceration/tear
5. Stab/cut
6. Bite
7. Burn
8. Missile penetration
9. Strangulation

Abrasion

An *abrasion* is the damage inflicted on the superficial layers of the skin (epidermis) by friction or pressure. An abrasion may be sustained by sliding on a rough carpet, producing what is commonly called a *rug burn.* A much more extreme version of an abrasion is the injury produced when a pedestrian is knocked to the pavement by an automobile, sustaining extensive friction injuries to the skin on various parts of the body. These injuries are commonly called *road burn* or *road rash.* While abrasions may be lacking in specific detail to allow an instrument of causation to be identified, some abrasion patterns may be very specific. These may include the abrasions resulting from a rope used as a ligature around the neck or extremities and rubbed against the skin, called *ligature marks.* Abrasions can also be caused by the irregular surface of the shoe sole or by an electrical cord used as a whip (Fig. 257-1).

BRUISE (ECCHYMOSIS) An *external bruise* represents bleeding beneath the skin. If sufficient bleeding occurs to create a lump, this is called a *hematoma.* Such injuries result from direct force applied to the skin surface, resulting in the tearing of subcutaneous blood vessels. The pattern of bleeding may be circular, surrounding a central bleeding point where the blow has stretched and torn a blood vessel wall. When multiple blood vessels are torn because of the use of a specific instrument, the bleeding pattern may conform to the outline of that instrument. For example, a blow inflicted with a human fist can produce multiple circular bruises in a pattern that conforms to the tips of the knuckles (Fig. 257-2). Similarly, pressure from fingertips such as occurs when someone grabs another by the arm may produce around

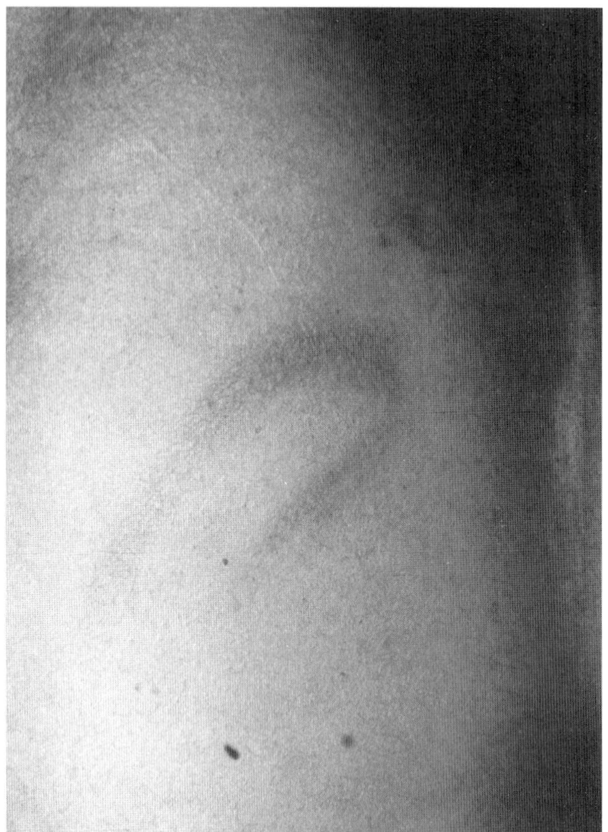

FIG. 257-1. Abrasion caused by electric cord.

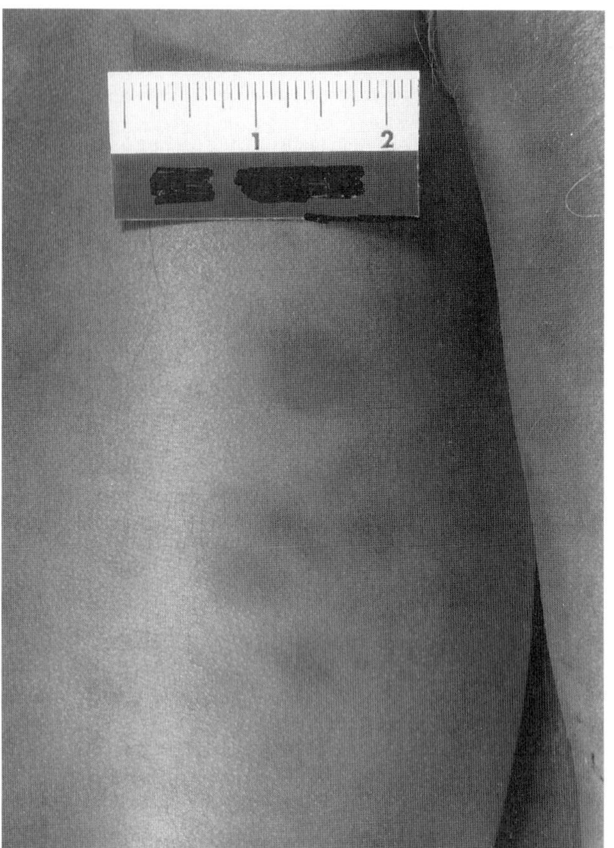

FIG. 257-2. Bruise pattern from knuckles.

of circular oval bruises. In contrast, a strike with a police baton can produce parallel linear bruises conforming to the diameter of the baton (Fig. 257-3).

Contusion

When sufficient force is applied to the surface of the body, the combination of friction or pressure and tearing of underlying blood vessels produces a bruise with an overlying abrasion. The term commonly used for this injury pattern is *contusion*, although some individuals use it interchangeably with bruise. Contusions as well as bruises have different appearances, depending on the pigmentation of the person's skin and the age of the injury. A bruise or contusion that is dark red or purple with well-defined margins is consistent with having been inflicted less than 48 h prior to examination. In contrast, a bruise or contusion that is yellow or brown or whose margins have begun to fade is certainly older than 48 h.

Laceration/Tear

A *laceration* is a tear of the skin. Depending on the amount of force used, the tear may be confined to the dermis or may extend through the full thickness of the skin. An example of an injury confined to the dermis is overstretching (Fig. 257-4). A full-thickness laceration extends into the subcutaneous tissue. When the injury is examined, *bridging* by intact blood vessels may be evident (Fig. 257-5). The resilience of elastic walled structures, such as arteries, allows them to maintain their integrity despite a blunt-force impact that tears the adjacent skin.

Because a laceration is usually the result of a crushing force, the margins of the laceration will show the effects of the pressure crushing the epidermal layer or skin surface. Depending on the instrument

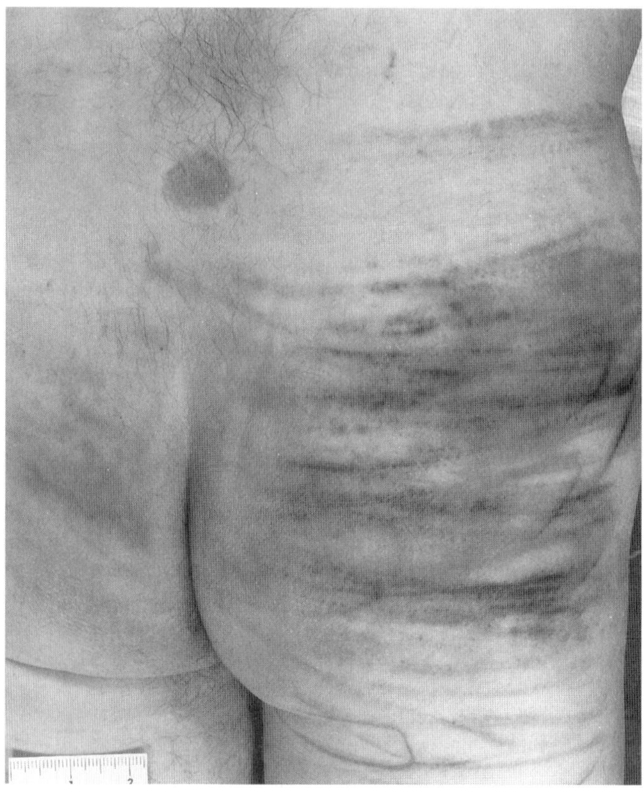

FIG. 257-3. Parallel linear bruises from police baton.

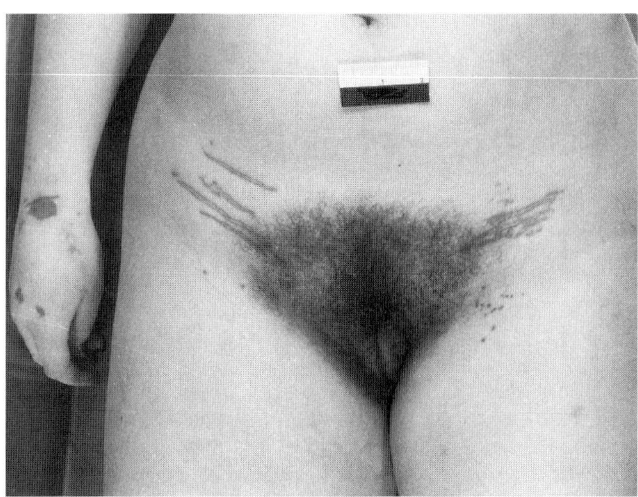

FIG. 257-4. "Overstretching" type laceration confined to the dermis.

causing the injury, a specific imprint may be evident when the margins of the laceration are reapposed. A laceration can also be called a tear but should never be called a cut, which implies the application of something other than blunt force. A common type of laceration occurs in protuberant areas of the body such as the elbow, knee, or eyebrow, where a fall against a hard surface such as a floor or pavement may result in the crushing of the skin against the underlying bone. Because the crushed skin margins may be nonviable, simple suturing of such a laceration without debridement will not result in healing by first intention.

Since lacerations often result from contact with a foreign object, residue from this object may be left within the wound. Recognition and recovery of particles of concrete, brick, or sand may be very helpful in the determination of whether an injury resulted from impact with an object such as a rock or the butt of a handgun (Fig. 257-6). This information should be included in the description of the injury.

Stab/Cut

A *stab* or *cut* is an injury inflicted on the skin by contact with a sharp object. Knife blades, shards of glass, and fragments of metal can penetrate the skin and leave a cutting pattern that will vary depending on the movement of the injured party and the object causing the injury. The sharp edge of these objects severs structures in the skin, leaving no evidence of bridging such as that seen in lacerations. Depending on the shape of the sharp object, the cut edges will be abraded accordingly while the ends of the wound may be squared or pointed (Fig. 257-7). Unique abrasions found around a stab wound may represent the effect of the hilt of a knife blade striking the skin (Fig. 257-7). Examination of the stab-wound track may reveal particles of the offending weapon, and such particles should be retained as evidence to assist in the identification of a weapon. The location of specific stabs or cutting wounds may suggest the manner in which they were inflicted. For example, cuts or stabs on the inner (volar) side of the wrist or forearm are consistent with efforts of individuals trying to

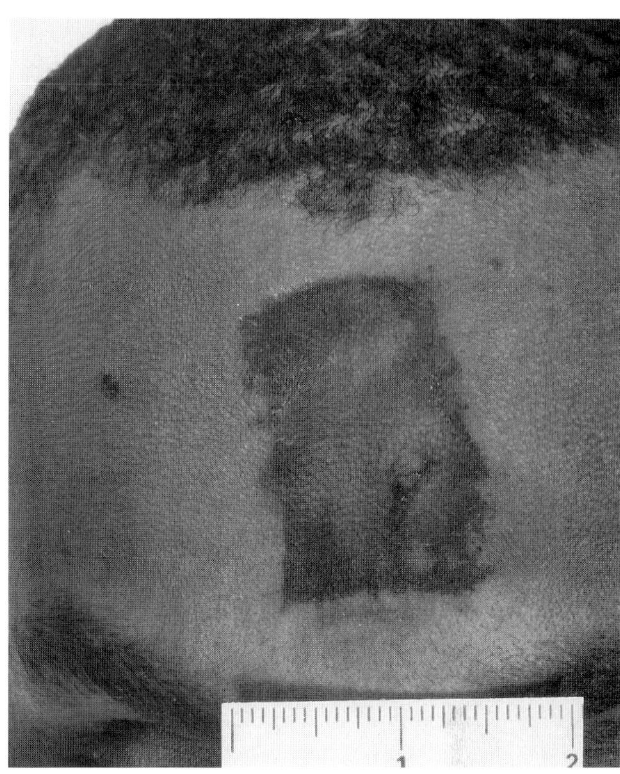

FIG. 257-6. Revealing pattern suggesting that injury was caused by butt of a handgun.

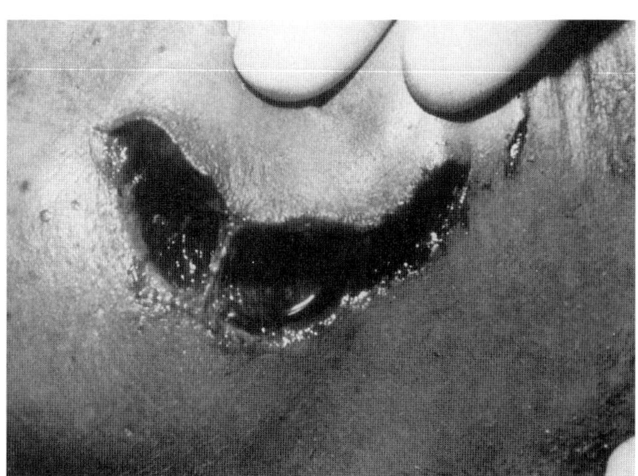

FIG. 257-5. Full thickness laceration with "bridging by intact blood vessels.

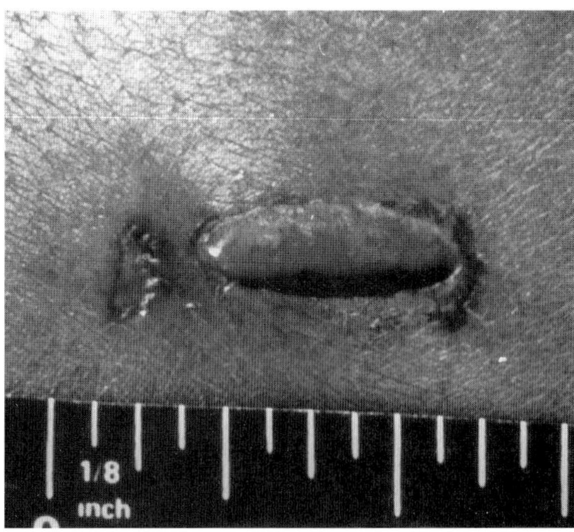

FIG. 257-7. Abrasion and bruise around periphery of stab wound suggesting cause is blunt trauma from hilt of a knife blade.

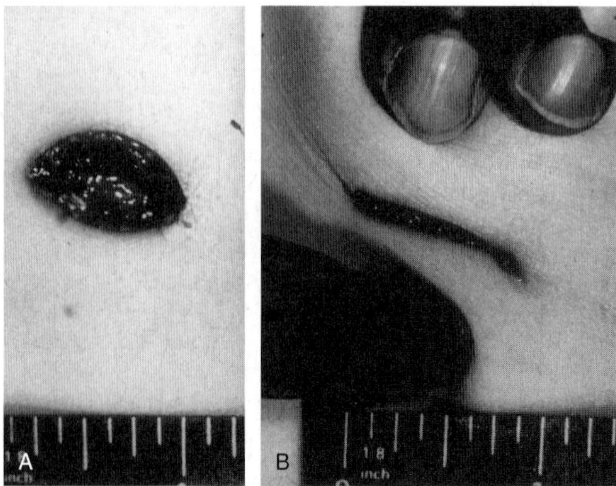

FIG. 257-8. Transparent tape applied over wound may aid in reconstruction and identification or verification of weapon.

protect themselves from an assailant by raising their arm in front of their body in a defensive posture. These are called *defense wounds* by forensic pathologists.

To properly evaluate the wound characteristics of cutting or stabbing wounds, the wound edges must be reapposed. The reapposition counteracts the effect of elastofibroretraction and allows the physician to observe the wound as it occurred. It also enables the physician to identify abraded margins as well as patterns of squared ends or pointed ends. A *squared end* results from the noncutting or blunt edge of a knife blade, whereas a *pointed end* results from contact with the sharp edge of a blade. The physician should use transparent tape to hold the edges of the wound together while the wound is photographed. This practice can be extremely valuable in the comparison of the wound with a suspected weapon (Fig. 257-8).

Another example of a patterned abrasion injury is the one caused by fragments of automobile glass. These characteristic wound patterns in human skin can enable the physician to identify whether the glass causing the injury is from a windshield or side auto window. The side window consists of tempered glass that breaks into 5-mm cubes, causing right-angle cuts to the left side of the face of the driver of the vehicle sustaining a driver-side impact. They may also be found on the right side of the face of passenger of a vehicle sustaining a passenger-side impact (Fig. 257-9*A*). Recognizing these patterns and their location can be useful in establishing who was driving the vehicle at the time of the collision. Cuts from windshield glass are distinguishable from side impact injuries. Windshield glass, which consists of thin layers of laminated glass, breaks into tiny splinters that produce superficial, parallel, linear cuts (Fig. 257-9*B*).

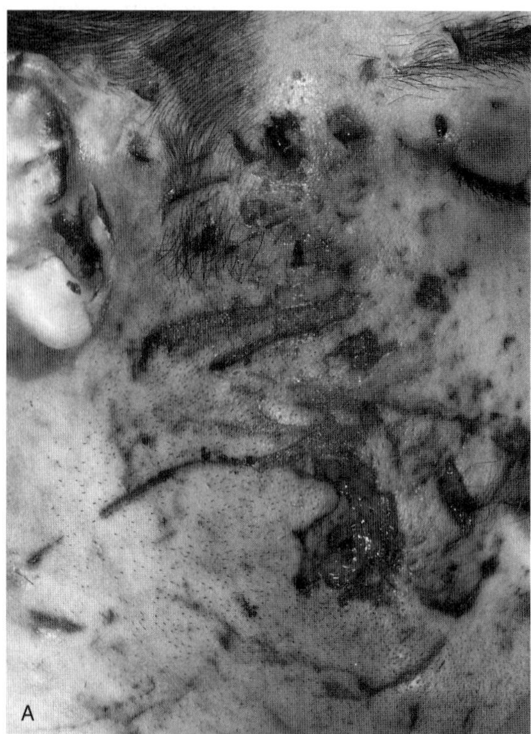

FIG. 257-9A. Right angle lacerations from side window glass of car made of tempered glass that brakes into 5 mm cubes.

Bite

Contact between human mouth and/or teeth and skin will leave evidence of the amount of force used in the contact as well as material (saliva) and/or teeth marks that can lead to the identification of the biter. Love bites or hickeys (suction injuries) result when there is extended oral contact with the skin of a partner involving sucking or biting. Hickeys are typically seen on the neck but may occur on any part of the body and usually exhibit no evidence of damage to the subepidermal layers, although discoloration from tissue fluid leakage may occur. On the other hand, *love bites*, and bites inflicted during a struggle, usually damage the dermis, leaving a partial or complete pattern of the dentition of the biter (Fig. 257-10). Not only can this bite pattern be used for comparison with the dental pattern of the suspect, but the recognition of the bite mark sustained during an attack should alert a physician to protect the skin surrounded by the bite pattern so that it can be swabbed to obtain saliva containing DNA material. A DNA profile can be compared with that of a suspect, providing almost 100 percent accuracy of identification. The most severe form of human bite is one that extends through the dermis into the subcutaneous tissue and results in the loss of blood. Thus, one can grade bite marks as first degree (mild), second degree (moderate), or third degree (severe). Using this grading system, a love bite would be considered in the mild category, whereas one similar to that occurring during a recent notorious boxing match as third degree (severe).

Burn

Injuries of the skin resulting from contact with electrical energy, extreme heat, heated objects, or certain chemicals often exhibit charac-

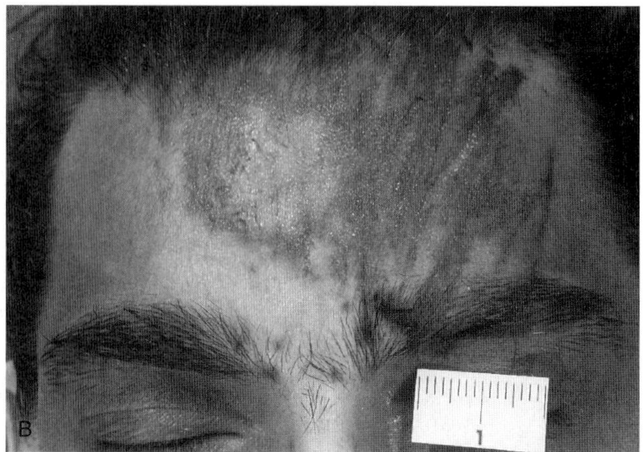

FIG. 257-9B. Linear lacerations and abrasions from windshield glass that brakes into tiny splinters.

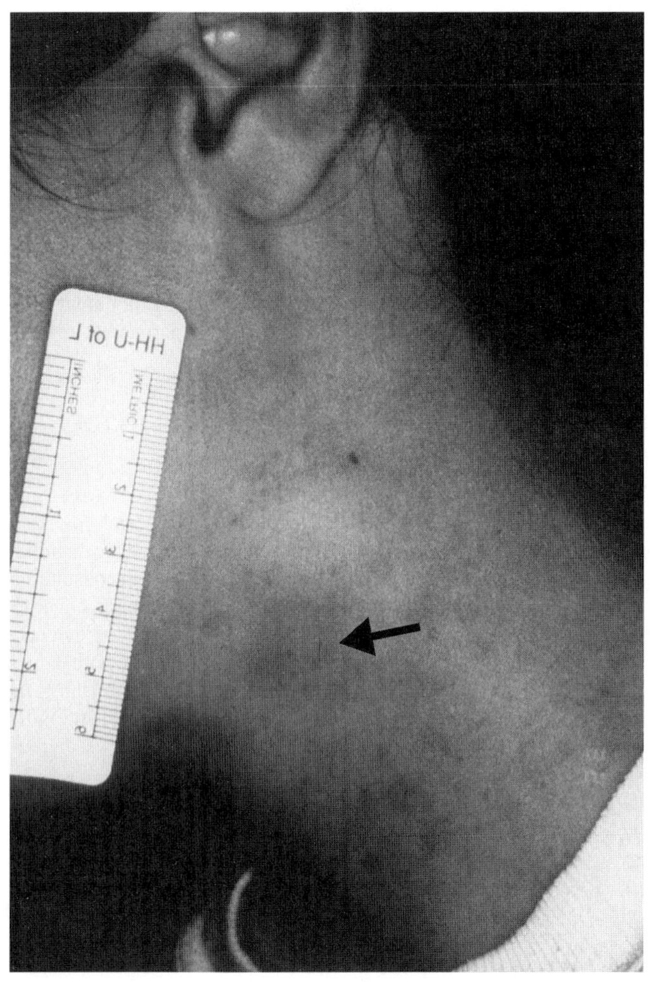

FIG. 257-10. Human bite revealing pattern of dentition.

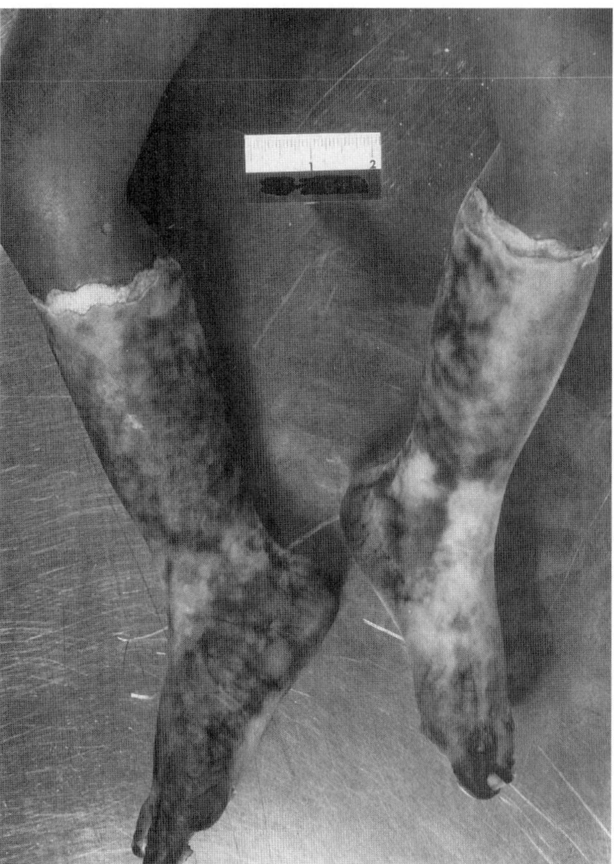

FIG. 257-11. Characteristic line of demarcation secondary immersion burn injury seen in abuse.

teristic patterns. For example, immersion of a child's buttock in 140°F (60°C) water will result in second-degree burns to the immersed skin. The resulting burn pattern will show a characteristic line of demarcation that represents the amount of skin immersed in the hot water (Fig. 257-11). Similarly, contact of the skin with electrical current can result in a central area of necrosis characteristically seen as black, charred tissue surrounded by a pale zone with a bright red peripheral margin.

Tremendous electrical force contained in a lightning strike may produce relatively little in the way of external evidence and may include only singeing of hair or slight charring of skin where contact occurs. An arborization or fernlike pattern of redness may be seen on the skin of fatally injured victims. A possible result of contact with a lightning strike is magnetization of certain metal articles on the victim's body.

Missile Penetration

The entrance wound of a skin penetration caused by a high-speed missile (such as a bullet) or a low-speed missile (such as an arrow) is circular, oval, or triangular, with a circumferential rim of abrasion. This abrasion pattern, produced by the friction sustained by the skin margins in contact with the missile, enables a physician to identify which hole is the exit and which is the entrance in a through-and-through gunshot wound. The outer skin edges of an exit wound do not come in contact with the missile and therefore do not sustain friction damage and do not exhibit this rim of abrasion. However, if a person is wearing tight clothing or the skin is resting against a hard, firm surface when the missile exits, the skin around the exit wound may be abraded from contact with this material. This produces a pattern called a *shored exit wound* (Fig. 257-12).

The presence of gunpowder residue surrounding a gunshot wound of the skin is a critical finding that needs to be described and documented with photographs before cleansing. The description of the distribution of the gunpowder residue, whether it consists of black smudging (soot) or stippling by particles of gunpowder, should include measurements with photographs. Wound photographs should always have a measurement scale in the field (Fig. 257-2). Clothing soiled with gunpowder residue must be protected and retained for collection by law-enforcement agencies for analysis in the crime lab. This type of evidence is used for determining the distance between the muzzle of the weapon firing the bullet and the injured party. Establishing this distance provides one parameter for evaluating the validity of accounts given by each of the parties as to the circumstances of the shooting. For example, one person may allege that there was a struggle and the gun was fired in self-defense, while the other person may say he or she was shot without threatening the shooter in any way.

Identification of the site of the entrance and exit of a gunshot wound path is an important step in the reconstruction of the shooting incident. When these incidents are not fatal, legal action often results, leading to a dispute over the accuracy of accounts given by each of the two parties: the injured party and the shooter.

Physicians without forensic training should avoid giving any opinion regarding a wound being an entrance or exit, or whether it was caused by firing at close range or a distance, or whether any type of activity or movement occurred during the shooting or what type of ammunition was used. Rather, physicians should document in as much

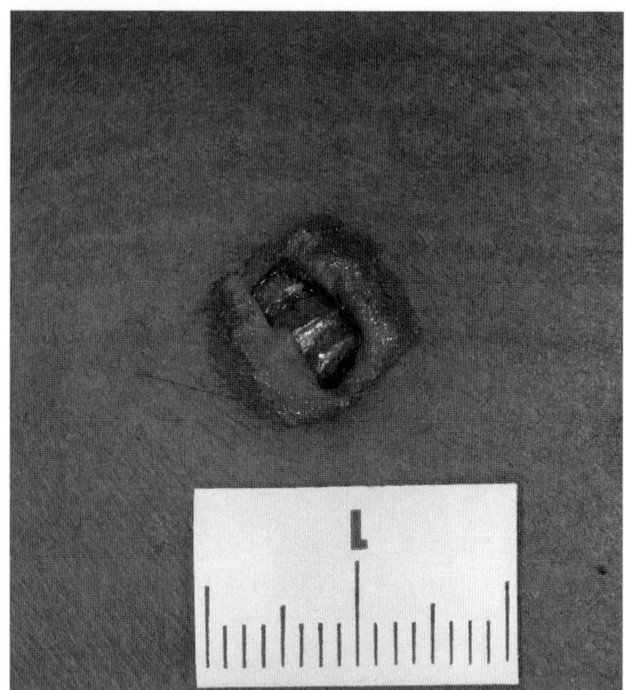

FIG. 257-12. Characteristic ''shored exit wound,'' an abrasion pattern resulting from missile exit when skin is resting against a hard surface.

detail as possible the information set out above for evaluation by those expert in this area.

Strangulation

Attempts to injure or kill a person by strangulation using one's hands, a ligature, or forearm, in a choke hold, may result in skin damage to the neck. For example, in manual strangulation, multiple bruises and scratches typical of contact with hands and fingernails will be seen on a victim's neck. On the other hand, if a ligature is forcefully wrapped around a victim's neck, a band of abrasion approximating the diameter of the ligature will be seen on the skin. Pinpoint hemorrhages, or petechiae, which are dramatically evident in the translucent conjunctival lining of the eyes, are important evidence of strangulation. These hemorrhages, which are the result of ruptured capillaries, occur when the buildup in pressure occurring when venous return from the head and face is obstructed. Since a period of 4 min is required for compression of the blood supply of the brain to result in irreversible neuronal damage and death, it is not surprising that so many attackers let go of their victim before death has occurred. If other force such as shooting, stabbing, or beating is not used, a victim may survive strangulation and appear in the ED, with evidence of neck injury and petechial hemorrhages in the eyes. Such victims should be examined for evidence of sexual assault, and vaginal swabs should be taken for identification with semen and DNA analysis.

The foregoing categories of injuries represent those most commonly seen in a trauma unit or a medical examiner office. However, readers who wish to become more familiar with the variety and details of injury are referred to several informative forensic medicine texts available in the medical library.

MEDICAL RECORDS

When an injury becomes the subject of a legal proceeding, the medical record documenting that injury and its subsequent treatment becomes a central part of the court deliberations, which may include obtaining testimony from the physician that created that record. The defendant or the accused is entitled to cross-examine that physician to establish or refute the validity of the medical information presented to the court. Physicians must recognize the legal responsibility that society places on them and be prepared to provide competent, professional testimony when required. The proper documentation of injuries includes the description of the details previously specified under *wound pattern*. The use of anatomic diagrams, together with photographs, makes the record more representative of the injuries as a physician saw them and more understandable by the lay members of a court. These items (charts, diagrams, and cameras) should be essential equipment in an ED, and photographs should become part of the permanent medical record.

PRESERVATION AND COLLECTION OF EVIDENCE

Preservation of blood samples, missiles, and debris found in wounds may be extremely valuable in identifying a particular weapon and tying this weapon to an assailant. However, this evidence is useful only if a proper chain of custody has been established. In handling such evidence, EDs should follow a protocol developed in consultation with the local law-enforcement agency. The use of a simple envelope that enables a physician to identify the patient, the date the evidence was recovered, where it was recovered from, and to whom it was given, and signed by the physician is adequate for establishing the chain of custody. Use of an appropriate receipt form documenting the transfer of this evidence should be an essential part of the medical record.

REPORT OF DEATH

This chapter has been confined to those issues relevant to the assessment of living patients. However, another important responsibility of the emergency physicians is that of notifying the local law-enforcement agency or medical examiner or coroner of a death that constitutes a medical examiner or coroner case.

Statutory language identifies those deaths that require an investigation by a medical examiner/coroner of the circumstances of the death. This enables one to determine whether an autopsy is necessary, which can then be carried out under the same statutory authority. Such deaths are generally those of individuals who die suddenly while not under the immediate care of a physician and any death associated with some type of injury, and usually include a category of any suspicious or unusual death. It should be emphasized that the length of time a patient has been in hospital, or the age of an injury associated with the underlying cause of death, is not a factor in determining whether the death should be reported to the medical examiner/coroner.

For example, the death of a person who sustained paraplegia from a gunshot wound of the back remains a medical examiner case despite the many medical procedures and complications that result from such an injury—even when many years have passed and the victim has died of a complication of paraplegia, such as a chronic urinary tract infection. The evidence of gunshot injury together wtih the medical treatment and any other intervening events leading up to the eventual death need to be assessed by the medical examiner/coroner. If a chain of events exists, leading from the gunshot wound to the immediate cause of death, then the manner of death would be determined to be homicide.

BIBLIOGRAPHY

Carmona R, Prince K: Trauma and forensic medicine. *J Trauma* 29:1222, 1989.
DiMaio DJ, DiMaio VJM: *Forensic Pathology.* New York, Elsevier, 1989.
DiMaio VJM: *Gunshot Wounds: Practical Aspects of Firearms, Ballistics and Forensic Techniques.* New York, Elsevier, 1985.
Goldsmith MF: U.S. forensic pathologists on a new case: Examination of living persons. *JAMA* 256:1685, 1986.

Jones NL: *Atlas of Forensic Pathology*. Igaku-Shoin, 1996.

Maryland Statute Health—General §5-704. Child Abuse and Neglect—Reporting of Abuse or Neglect—By Health Practitioner, Police Officer, Educator or Human Service Worker.

Mason JK: *Forensic Medicine: An Illustrated Reference*. Chapman and Hall, 1993.

Mittleman RE, Goldberg HS, Waksman DM: Preserving evidence in the emergency department. *Am J Nurs* 83:1652, 1983.

Mittleman RE, Stevens EC, Sorouon R: Obtaining saliva samples from bitemark evidence. *Law Enforcement Bull* November, 1980.

Parrish RF, Ing R: *Medical Examiner and Coroner Jurisdictions in the United States*. American Academy of Forensic Sciences, 1988.

Smialek JE: Forensic aspects of penetrating trauma, in *12th National Trauma Symposium, March, 1990*.

Spitz WU, Fisher RS: *Medicolegal Investigations of Death Investigation*, 3d ed. Charles C Thomas, 1993.

Wetli C, Rao V, Ivatury R, Cayten CC: *Gene: The Textbook of Penetrating Trauma*. Baltimore, Williams and Wilkins, 1995, pp 1084–1097.

INJURY CONTROL

Arthur L. Kellermann
Knox H. Todd

INTRODUCTION

Injuries account for about one-fourth of emergency department (ED) visits and they are the most common cause of death for Americans ages 1 to 44.[1] Because injuries disproportionately affect the young, they account for more years of potential life lost before age 65 than all causes of cancer and heart disease *combined*.

Epidemiological research shows that injuries, like diseases, tend to affect identifiable groups, follow an often predictable chain of events, and therefore are preventable. After an injury occurs, morbidity can be minimized by providing optimal acute care and subsequent rehabilitation. This combination of strategies—prevention, acute care, and rehabilitation—is called *injury control*.

A PUBLIC HEALTH APPROACH

William Haddon developed the classic approach to injury control by identifying the three principal factors of injury (host, vehicle, and environment) and subdividing each factor by the three temporal phases of an injury event: pre-event; the event itself; and the postevent phase. This resulted in a "phase-factor" matrix of nine discrete cells.[2] Examining these cells can suggest various strategies to prevent or control injuries. Since its introduction in 1972, the Haddon matrix has proven to be an invaluable tool for injury control.

Haddon outlined 10 generic injury-control strategies that can be utilized to break the chain of injury causation (Table 258-1).[3] Examining this list to identify promising approaches to injury control is known as *options analysis*. Certain options lend themselves more easily to one class of injuries than others. The best injury control option is not always the most obvious. Often a combination of approaches is superior to any single strategy.

The Injury Control Model

More than a century after yellow fever was controlled by targeting the vector of transmission, Haddon's work demonstrated that many injuries can be controlled by broadening our traditional emphasis on acute care and rehabilitation to include *preventive* efforts. Injury control draws on the expertise of many disciplines, including epidemiology, prevention, biomechanics, acute care, rehabilitation, law, and public administration. Prevention is attempted whenever practical. When prevention is not enough, acute care can minimize further damage from major trauma. After the victim is stabilized, long-term outcomes can be enhanced by optimal rehabilitation.

Haddon's approach was first applied to great effect in the control of deaths and injuries due to car crashes. Prior to his work, the Federal government poured millions of dollars into costly and largely ineffective media campaigns directed to the driver. Little progress occurred until the National Highway Traffic Safety Administration mandated changes in the design of motor vehicles, as well as the creation of safer roadways and driving environment. (See "Engineering" below.)[4]

These efforts produced one of the greatest public health achievements of this century. While the number of vehicle miles traveled in the United States has risen annually, today's crash fatality rate is less than one-third that of 1950. If the United States had not launched and maintained its highway traffic safety initiative, the annual toll of motor vehicle crash-related deaths, injuries, and costs would be thousands of lives and billions of dollars higher than it is today.

PREVENTION STRATEGIES

Active and Passive Countermeasures

Active countermeasures require the conscious cooperation of the individual. Examples include manual safety belts, motorcycle helmets, and child safety seats. *Passive* countermeasures, on the other hand, require little or no cooperation. Examples include air bags, automatic sprinkler systems, and spring-loaded kill switches on lawn mowers. In general, the less a countermeasure relies on user initiative, the more likely it will provide protection when needed. When used, manual safety belts reduce the risk of death in a car crash by 45 to 55 percent. However, they are effective only when buckled by the user. In contrast, air bags deploy in serious crashes virtually 100 percent of the time.

TABLE 258-1 Options Analysis: Strategies with Examples, for Injury Control

1. Prevent creation of the hazard. Ban production and sale of assault weapons to civilians.
2. Reduce the amount of hazard. Limit water heater temperature to 125° F (47.25° C).
3. Prevent the release of a hazard that already exists. Put dangerous medications in "child proof" containers.
4. Modify the rate of distribution of the release of the hazard from its source. Require fire-safe cigarettes that cannot easily ignite furniture or bedding.
5. Separate, by time or space, the hazard from that which is to be protected. Construct overpasses or underpasses to eliminate crossing streams of traffic.
6. Physically separate, by barriers, the hazard from that which is to be protected. Equip cabs with bullet- and knife-proof partitions.
7. Modify surfaces and basic structures to minimize injury. Equip all new cars with driver- and passenger-side air bags.
8. Make that which is to be protected more resistant to damage. Issue bulletproof vests to law enforcement officers and security guards.
9. Begin to counter damage already done. Promote citizen training in first aid and CPR.
10. Stabilize, repair, and rehabilitate the injured person. Implement trauma care systems throughout the United States.

Source: From Haddon.[2]

Education

Education is generally the first approach taken to encourage the public to accept an active countermeasure of proven efficacy. Implicit in its approach is the belief that once people are taught what to do, they will change their behavior and reduce their risk of injury. Driver's education programs, child pedestrian training, and bicycle helmet campaigns are examples of this strategy.

Although these campaigns are popular and attract large numbers of volunteers, they rarely result in sustained behavior change. One study evaluated the impact of a $78 million federal "alcohol safety action program." Although it was launched in dozens of communities around the United States, subsequent evaluation revealed that the program did not reduce the rate of alcohol-related fatalities in the target population.[5]

Robertson and colleagues evaluated a saturation advertising campaign promoting safety belts in one city served by two cable systems. One system aired over 1000 high-quality promotional spots; the other aired none. Subsequent observation revealed no difference in rates of safety belt use among subscribers of either system.[6]

Not all public education efforts have yielded such discouraging results. A large-scale community action campaign promoting bicycle helmet use in Seattle, Washington produced sharp increases in helmet sales. Observed rates of helmet use among school-aged children increased from 5.5 percent in 1986 to 40.2 percent in 1992. More importantly, head injuries that came to medical attention decreased by approximately two-thirds in this age group.[7]

The impact of many public education campaigns is blunted by *attenuation of effect.* No matter how powerful, pervasive, and repetitive a safety message may be, there are always some who never encounter it. Among those who see or hear the message, some actively reject it. Some are not sufficiently motivated to change their behavior. Among those changing their behavior, some relapse into old habits over time. Others fail to follow the message on a consistent basis. Finally, not everyone who adopts a protective strategy escapes injury.

Educational interventions may be enhanced by incorporating theoretical models that include important determinants of individual behavior.[8] These include a number of personal, community, and political factors. The PRECEDE health promotion model has been used with some success in planning injury prevention programs.[9] PRECEDE is an acronym for *predisposing, reinforcing,* and *enabling causes* in *educational diagnosis* and *evaluation.* Predisposing factors are characteristics of a patient, consumer, or community that motivate behavior. Reinforcing factors are rewards or punishments that are anticipated or follow as a consequence of these behaviors. Enabling factors are environmental characteristics that facilitate or hinder injury-prevention behaviors. This framework has been successfully used to assess educational needs and select appropriate strategies to encourage car seatbelt use and prevent motor vehicle injuries.[10]

Enforcement

Unfortunately, young males (the group that experiences the highest rates of serious injury) often resist behavioral change. When voluntary acceptance of a countermeasure of proven effectiveness is poor, compliance can be increased by making the countermeasure compulsory. The impact of "mandatory use" laws can be impressive. A study of Michigan's child safety seat law revealed that injuries declined 25 percent after passage of the law.[11] The 55-mph speed limit was estimated to have saved 2000 to 4000 lives annually. Raising the minimum age to purchase alcohol in 26 states decreased nighttime fatal crashes by an average of 13 percent.[12] After Victoria, Australia enacted legislation to make bicycle helmet use compulsory for all cyclists, rates of helmet use rose from 31 to 75 percent. During the same period, the number of insurance claims from bicyclists killed or injured after sustaining a head injury decreased by 70 percent.[13]

Community education and visible enforcement are needed to obtain maximal benefit from mandatory use laws. In Elmira, New York, an enforcement and publicity campaign promoting the state's seat belt law boosted compliance rates from 49 to 77 percent. Four months later, the rate of use sagged to 66 percent, but rebounded to 80 percent during a reminder campaign.[14]

Mandatory use laws are effective, but they are difficult to enact. People are quite willing to support measures limiting the ability of others to injure them but resist measures intended to protect them from their own actions. Speed limits, drunk driving laws, and measures to ban the carrying of weapons on commercial aircraft enjoy broad-based support, but mandatory seat belt laws, motorcycle helmet laws, and gun control are less popular. Mandatory use laws often engender spirited resistance from a vocal minority that view these laws as an infringement of "personal freedom."

Political backlash can block legislation or lead to the repeal of a successful law. Despite overwhelming evidence that motorcycle helmet laws save lives, 26 states repealed their statutes when federal incentives were relaxed in 1976. In these states, motorcycle crash fatality rates increased 40 percent.[15]

Opponents of mandatory use laws argue that individuals should be permitted to ignore sound safety policies if the level of risk is acceptable to them. Unfortunately, the circle of harm extends far beyond the victim. Motorcyclists and bicyclists who ride without a helmet face an increased risk of serious head injury or death. When such individuals are killed or disabled in a crash, families and loved ones lose companionship, dependents lose their principal source of financial support, employers lose productivity, and society is required to cover the expense of care. All of us, either directly or indirectly, bear the costs of preventable injury.

Engineering

Many injuries can be prevented by building safer vehicles and modifying the physical environment in which injuries occur. The cost to develop and implement passive countermeasures usually exceeds the cost of education campaigns. However, engineering is usually more effective because it does not require millions of users to permanently and consistently change their behavior.

Consider these examples. In contrast to the disappointing results of driver's education, federal standards for motor vehicle construction saved an estimated 37,000 lives between 1975 and 1978 alone. These standards addressed such issues as passenger restraint systems, windshields, fuel tank integrity, and the flammability of interior fabric. Introduction of air bags cut the nation's toll of deaths and injuries due to car crashes still further.

Construction of the interstate highway system saved lives as well. Modifications to the driving environment, such as banked curves, divided lanes of traffic, controlled ramps for ingress and egress, elimination of crossing streams of traffic, and the positioning of energy-absorbing pilings in front of fixed obstructions, cut the interstate highway death rate to less than half that for other roads.

These lessons can be applied to other hazardous products. Cigarettes cause more than half of U.S. fatalities due to house fires. Most occur when the smoker falls asleep in bed or leaves a burning cigarette on the arm of a sofa or chair. Television, radio, and print advertisements warning of the dangers of smoking in bed have had little no impact on this problem. Smoke detectors save lives by warning of an impending catastrophe in time to permit the occupants to evacuate the house, but they require a concerted effort to encourage people to install and maintain them.

Passive engineering of the home environment by installing sprinkler systems could be a very effective strategy. Unfortunately, residential sprinkler systems are expensive and often cannot be retrofitted into older homes. However, the cigarette itself could be modified to diminish its potential to ignite furniture or bedding.

Laws requiring products to be designed to diminish their potential to cause harm can be highly effective. Unfortunately, such laws are difficult to enact. Manufacturers often oppose such regulations because they fear it will raise the price of the products and discourage sales. In addition to the issue of personal freedom, concerns are often raised about cost, government interference, and reduced competitiveness with nonregulated manufacturers. If efforts to regulate a hazardous product fail, product liability lawsuits may force a needed change in product design.

PRACTICE OF INJURY CONTROL

Step 1: Define the Problem

Population-based data on the incidence and impact of injury are essential to define the scope of the problem and mobilize the resources necessary to achieve change. Public health surveillance is needed to monitor patterns and trends, and to evaluate the impact of countermeasures.

Several sources of information can be used for this purpose. Vital records or death certificates are useful to document the impact of injuries on overall rates of mortality, but they do not provide information about nonfatal injuries. Hospital discharge data and trauma registries can provide essential information about cases of major trauma, but population-based data are needed to calculate rates of injury. Furthermore, hospital admission statistics and trauma registry data do not capture patients who are treated and released from the ED.

Although injuries that are managed on an outpatient basis are generally assumed to be minor, they can result in significant long-term disability. This is particularly true of head, back, and hand injuries. Patients visiting an ED for injury have an increased risk for recurrent injury, especially if their index visit is related to alcohol abuse or violence.

Assignment of external cause of injury codes (''E-codes'') to every injury-related emergency department visit can substantially enhance community-based surveillance efforts. Several states mandate E-coding of all hospital admissions, but only one requires hospitals to E-code ED visits.

Step 2: Identify Causes and Risk Factors

Descriptive studies are usually conducted to determine *who* is injured, *what* kinds of injuries are involved, and *where, when,* and, *why* those injuries occur. These data provide essential clues to injury causation, and often generate hypotheses that can be investigated with analytical methods.

In some cases, the link between a risk factor and injury is so strong that no additional research is needed. For example, studies of automobile injury show that 50 percent of all fatal crashes and 60 percent of all fatal single-vehicle crashes involve alcohol.[16] In most cases, however, it is necessary to compare the rate of injury among those *with* a risk factor to the rate of injury in an otherwise similar group *without* a risk factor. Cohort, quasiexperimental, or experimental designs may be needed to reach a definitive conclusion. When the outcome of interest is rare, and exposure to the risk factor(s) of interest can be shown to precede the injury, case-control studies may be employed. Meticulous attention to methodology is essential to generate valid results and control for the effects of confounding variables.

Step 3: Develop and Test Interventions

Once the magnitude of the problem and its associated risk factors are identified, a variety of countermeasures may be considered for implementation. Careful attention must be given to the characteristics of the target population, the feasibility of the countermeasure(s), their acceptability to the target population, and cost. Pilot intervention programs are often helpful to test various strategies. The most promising program can then be selected for more widespread implementation.

Community education programs are often tried first because they are relatively easy to initiate, attract motivated volunteers, and are invaluable for raising public awareness. They can also help build public support for legislative changes at a later time. It is essential to take the views and values of the community into consideration at every step of the process. Citizen involvement is crucial to any program's success.

Most programs set milestones and predefined measures of success. For example, a campaign to prevent deaths and injuries in residential fires may identify selected measures of *structure* (staff hired, office space, cooperative agreements reached), *process* (number of pamphlets distributed, number of home visits made, total smoke detectors installed), or *outcome* (reductions in the rate of fire deaths, or a decline in hospital admissions due to burns and smoke inhalation).

It is not always feasible to demonstrate major impacts on rates of morbidity or mortality with small-scale demonstration projects. When this is the case, surrogate measures may be used to demonstrate program impact. For example, preintervention rates of smoke detector use in a target neighborhood can be compared with rates noted after an educational campaign. Telephone surveys can seek evidence of changes in knowledge, attitudes, and self-reported behavior. Self-reports do not guarantee long-term behavior change, but they confirm that a program is reaching the target group.

Step 4: Implement Effective Interventions and Evaluate Their Impact

Once a program is initiated on a large-scale basis, evaluation data should be collected to demonstrate its impact. Measures of cost-effectiveness (e.g., dollars spent per life saved or injury prevented) are particularly important. It is easy to tabulate the cost of a prevention program, but it is harder to document the savings from ''tragedies that didn't happen.'' Program support tends to wane over time, especially when no group or organization has an economic interest in seeing it continued. During more difficult economic times, prevention programs are often the first to go. Without documented evidence of impact, worthy programs can wither and die.

THE ROLE OF THE EMERGENCY PHYSICIAN IN INJURY CONTROL

Patient Education

Injury-control measures need not be implemented on a grand scale to make a difference. Emergency physicians can incorporate injury prevention into their clinical practice.[17] The impact of these bedside interventions can be substantial.

Special efforts should be made to correct factors that precipitated the injury or contributed to its severity. Otherwise, a patient is likely to return with a more serious injury in the future. A child sustaining a minor head injury while bike riding should be told to wear his bicycle helmet. The unbelted adult who sustained minor injuries in a low-velocity motor vehicle crash deserves a short lecture on the importance of safety belts.

However, any ED encounter is a ''teachable moment.''[18] Because emergency physicians are more likely to provide acute care to injured patients than any other physician group, they should have a special stake in preventing and controlling injuries. The mother who brings her child to the ED for evaluation of a severe otitis can leave the department with information about the importance of child safety seats, bicycle helmets, and four-sided fencing around her swimming pool. Emergency physicians have the opportunity to motivate patients to change high-risk behaviors and modify their home environment to decrease injury risk. Unfortunately, the ability to influence behavior from these brief emergency setting encounters have not been well studied.

Data Collection and Program Evaluation

If current trends towards capitated care continue, the ED will become a pivotal arena for prevention efforts and health resource utilization. Until now, the financial incentives of health care have encouraged hospitalization and provision of services. The move towards capitated payment will substantially increase the incentive to prevent, rather than treat illness and injuries. As the portal of entry for 40 percent of U.S. inpatients and virtually all admissions, the emergency department can play a key role in monitoring system performance, identifying high-risk groups, reducing the need for expensive inpatient care, and evaluating the impact of prevention programs.

Research

Emergency physicians are ideally positioned to conduct injury surveillance and evaluate countermeasures and should take the lead in community-based epidemiologic research. Research on pediatric injuries, alcohol-related trauma, drunk driving enforcement, firearm-related injuries, intimate violence, residential fires, and the biomechanics of trauma are important areas for emerging research.

Advocacy

Sometimes, evaluation data indicate that a countermeasure is effective but rarely used. When education is not enough to motivate behavioral change, legislation may have a major impact, particularly when coupled with ongoing education efforts and visible enforcement. For example, states with mandatory motorcycle helmet laws report compliance rates as high as 98 percent.

Coalition building is essential to assemble a broad base of support. Physician leadership is essential to the success of these efforts. The testimonies of health care providers, surviving family members, and disabled individuals are needed to give the statistics an emotional context. Information on the economic impact of injuries and the cost-effectiveness of countermeasures is also helpful.

It is also important to train the next generation of injury control experts. Research suggests that many medical students lack a fundamental understanding of the principles and practice of injury control.[19] Academic emergency physicians can play an important role by emphasizing the importance of injury control to their students and trainees.

REFERENCES

1. Ventura SJ, Peters KD, Martin JA, Maurer JD: *Births and deaths: United States, 1996. Monthly Vital Statistics Report,* Hyattsville, MD, National Center for Health Statistics, 1997. Vol. 46, No. 1, supp 2, pp 32–33.
2. Haddon W: A logical framework for categorizing highway safety phenomenon and activity. *J Trauma* 12:193, 1972.
3. Haddon W: Energy damage and the ten countermeasure strategies. *J Trauma* 13:321, 1973.
4. Waller JA: Reflections on a half century of injury control. *Am J Public Health* 84:664, 1994.
5. Zador P: Statistical evaluation of the effectiveness of "Alcohol Safety Action Projects—Part I." *Accid Anal Prev* 8:51,1976.
6. Robertson LX, Kelley AB, O'Neill B, et al: A controlled study of the effect of television messages on safety belt use. *Am J Public Health* 64:1071,1974.
7. Rivara FP, Thompson DC, Thompson RS, et al: The Seattle children's bicycle helmet campaign: Changes in helmet use and head injury admissions. *Pediatrics* 92:567, 1994.
8. Gielen AC: Health education and injury control: Integrating approaches. *Health Educ Q* 19:203, 1992.
9. Green LW, Kreuter MW: *Health Promotion Planning: An Educational and Environmental Approach,* 2d ed. Mountain View, CA: Mayfield Publishing, 1991.
10. Sleet DA: Health education approaches to motor vehicle injury prevention. *Public Health Rep* 102:606,1987.
11. Wagenaar AC, Webster DW: Preventing injuries to children through compulsory automobile safety seat use. *Pediatrics* 78:662, 1986.
12. Du Mouchel W, Williams AF, Zador PL: Raising the alcohol purchase age: Its effects on fatal motor vehicle crashes in twenty-six states. *J Legal Stud* 16:249, 1987.
13. Finch CF, Newstead SV, Cameron MH, Vulcan AP: *Head Injury Reductions in Victoria Two Years After Introduction of Mandatory Bicycle Helmet Use.* Melbourne, Australia, Monash University Accident Research Centre, 1993. Report No. 51.
14. Williams AF, Preusser DF, Blomberg RD, Lund AD: Seat belt use law enforcement and publicity in Elmira, New York: A reminder campaign. *Am J Public Health* 77:1450, 1987.
15. Watson GS, Zador PL, Wilks A: The repeal of helmet use laws and increased motorcyclist mortality in the United States, 1975–1978. *Am J Public Health* 70:579, 1980.
16. Polen MR, Friendam GD: Automobile injury: Selected risk factors and prevention in the health care setting. *JAMA* 259:76, 1988.
17. Dunn KA, Cline DM, Grant T, et al: Injury prevention instruction in the emergency department. *Ann Emerg Med* 22:1280, 1993.
18. Todd KH: Air bags and the teachable moment. *Ann Emerg Med* 28:242, 1996.
19. Butler RN, Todd KH, Kellermann AL, et al: Injury-control education in six U.S. medical schools. *Acad Med* 73:524, 1998.

INJURIES TO BONES, JOINTS, AND SOFT TISSUES

INITIAL EVALUATION AND MANAGEMENT OF ORTHOPEDIC INJURIES

Jeffrey S. Menkes

CLINICAL PHYSIOLOGY OF FRACTURES

The ability to properly assess and treat acutely injured patients in the emergency department depends largely on an understanding of the way fractures are created and how they heal. Practical knowledge of fracture physiology may provide the index of suspicion needed to diagnose an injury that might otherwise be missed. It may also help prevent or minimize complications and may form the basis for advising the patient regarding the outlook for ultimate recovery of function.

How Fractures Occur

Although fractures are sometimes described in terms of the external mechanism by which they are created, they may also be thought of simply in terms of the physiologic processes involved.

"TYPICAL" FRACTURES Most fractures are the result of significant trauma to healthy bone. The bony cortex may be disrupted by a variety of forces, including a direct blow, axial loading, angular (bending) forces, torque (twisting) stress, or a combination of these.

PATHOLOGIC FRACTURES Fractures that occur from relatively minor trauma to diseased or otherwise abnormal bone are termed pathologic fractures. This implies that a preexisting pathologic process has weakened the bone and rendered it susceptible to fracture by forces that, under normal circumstances, would not disrupt the cortex. Common examples of such injuries are fractures through metastatic lytic lesions, fractures through benign bone cysts (as in the humerus of Little League pitchers), and—perhaps most common—vertebral compression fractures in patients with advanced osteoporosis. Numerous other disease processes may render patients susceptible to pathologic fracture.

Because these injuries are often not associated with a history of significant trauma, pathologic fractures may go undetected unless there is a preexisting index of suspicion based on the knowledge that such injuries can occur.

STRESS FRACTURES In some cases, bone may undergo a "fatigue" fracture from repetitive forces applied before the bone and its supporting tissues have had adequate time to accommodate to such forces. An example is the insidious occurrence of a metatarsal shaft fracture in unconditioned foot soldiers (the so-called march fracture). The physiologic principle of stress fracture can be easily envisioned by anyone who has "cut" an aluminum finger splint to the desired length by bending it back and forth. The pliable metal—too hard to cut with an ordinary scissors—ultimately gives way in the face of repeated stresses requiring relatively little force.

The processes that render bone susceptible to stress fracture are not generally agreed upon. The important point is that diagnosis depends on a familiarity with the entity, because *x-rays are typically negative* early in the patient's course. Early diagnosis may be purely clinical, based on the history and physical findings. Days or weeks may pass before the fracture line or new bone formation becomes visible on x-ray, ultimately confirming the suspicions of the physician who, having made the correct presumptive diagnosis, will have treated the patient appropriately from the outset.

SALTER (EPIPHYSEAL) FRACTURES Fractures involving the physis—the cartilaginous epiphyseal plate near the ends of the long bones of growing children—are called Salter fractures after Salter and Harris, the physicians who devised the most popular method of classifying these injuries.[1] The supply of new bone material needed for the elongation of bones during growth is provided by specialized cells within the physis. When growth is completed, the physis is transformed into bone, ultimately fusing with the surrounding bone and disappearing as a distinct entity. By definition, Salter fractures cannot occur in fully grown adults.

Any damage to the epiphyseal plate during a child's growth may destroy part or all of its ability to produce new bone substance, resulting in aborted or deformed growth of the bone thereafter. The potential for growth disturbance from an epiphyseal injury is related to the number of years the child has yet to grow (the older the child, the less time remains for deformity to develop) and to the pattern of the fracture line through the epiphyseal area. Classification of Salter fractures and their clinical implications are discussed later in this chapter.

Fracture Healing

The physiology of fracture healing constitutes the basis for many decisions in the emergency department. The judgment as to whether an angulated fracture requires reduction or can be left to heal as is, the choice of treatment modality in relation to the patient's age, and the prognosis for regaining function or being left with residual deformity all require familiarity with the short- and long-term aspects of the healing process.

Fracture healing can be described in terms of three phases—the inflammatory, reparative, and remodeling— each of which gradually blends into the next.[2]

When a fracture occurs, the microscopic vessels crossing the fracture line are severed, depriving the damaged bone ends of their blood supply. In the ensuing hours and days, the bone ends necrose, triggering a classic inflammatory response. This early phase is brief but creates the tissue environment for the most predominant aspect of fracture healing: the reparative phase.

Soon, granulation tissue begins to infiltrate the area. Within this tissue are specialized cells capable of forming collagen, cartilage, and bone, the ingredients of callus, which gradually surrounds the fractured ends and stabilizes them. With time, the callus becomes more densely mineralized.

Meanwhile, the necrotic edges of the fragments are removed by osteoclasts, cells whose specific function is to resorb bone. That is why some "hairline" fractures do not appear on x-ray until days after injury. Initially invisible, the diagnostic fracture line appears only after necrotic bone has been resorbed from the area.

The final phase of bone healing, the remodeling phase, is the longest, often lasting years. Remodeling is the tendency of bone to gradually regain its original shape and contour. During this phase, the superfluous portions of callus are resorbed, and new bone is laid down along natural lines of stress. These internal layers, easily visible in x-rays of normal bone, are the bony trabeculae. Formation of trabecular bone is a physiologically efficient process, providing maximum strength relative to the amount of bone material used.

The anticipated success of remodeling is related to a number of factors. Young children have a greater capacity for remodeling than adults do. Accordingly, their potential for residual deformity is less, other circumstances being equal. Remodeling is also related to the magnitude and direction of unreduced angulation and to the fracture's location along the bone. Specific predictors of satisfactory remodeling include youth, proximity of the fracture to the end of the bone (but not involving the epiphyseal plate), and direction of angulation coinciding with the plane of natural joint motion.

Clinical decisions regarding the aggressiveness of fracture reduction are directly linked to a knowledge of this physiology. Angulation near the end of a long bone, for example, is more acceptable than angulation near the midshaft. Dorsal or volar angulation at the wrist has a better prognosis than ulnar or radial angulation because the natural plane of wrist motion is dorsal-volar. Mild angulation in a 2-year-old may be left to remodel on its own, whereas the same angulation in an adult may require correction.

ORTHOPEDIC EMERGENCIES

Some types of musculoskeletal trauma deserve special mention because a delay in their diagnosis or treatment can increase the chance of significant complications or a negative outcome.

Open Fracture

An open fracture (compound in older terminology) is a fracture associated with overlying soft tissue injury, creating communication between the fracture site and the external surface of the body. Although open fracture may initially convey the image of grossly exposed bone, the term is equally applicable to a simple puncture wound extending to the depth of an underlying fracture. Such puncture wounds may be created by external forces or by a sharp bone fragment transiently protruding through the skin before receding back beneath the surface.

The most dreaded complication of open fracture is osteomyelitis. Once established, osteomyelitis may result in months or years of pain, disability, medical therapy, surgical procedures, and ultimately amputation. Although osteomyelitis may be unavoidable in some cases, it becomes less likely when treatment is prompt and meticulous.

Open fractures are sometimes classified by severity, based on the length of the overlying laceration, extent of tissue damage, kinetic energy of the injuring force, and evidence or likelihood of significant contamination. Irrespective of these factors, any open fracture should be promptly and carefully treated. Elements in the care of open fractures are described later in this chapter.

Dislocation and Subluxation

A joint is dislocated when the articular surfaces of the bones that normally meet at the joint are completely out of contact with one another. This is distinct from subluxation, a condition in which the articular surfaces are only partially out of contact.

The urgency of treating dislocated joints is based on several factors. One is the potential for neurologic or circulatory compromise. The neurovascular bundle passing close to the affected joint is typically "kinked" around the deformity associated with the dislocation. Persistence of this condition can result in a neurologic or vascular deficit that may be temporary if the deformity is reduced promptly but irreversible if treatment is delayed.

Another consideration is that, the longer a joint has been dislocated, the more difficult it may be to reduce and the more likely it is to be unstable after reduction. This is probably due at least in part to edema, muscle spasm, and other tissue changes that increase over time.

Dislocation of the hip carries its own particular urgency in addition to those mentioned above: the danger of avascular necrosis of the femoral head. Avascular necrosis occurs because much of the blood supply to the femoral head is delivered through vessels that emerge from the acetabulum. When the joint is dislocated, circulation to the femoral head is disrupted. At some point, the vascular insult becomes irreversible, and bony necrosis is the ultimate result. Although aseptic necrosis may occur despite the physician's best efforts, its likelihood increases with the time delay until reduction.

Neurovascular Deficit

Naturally, any injury associated with neurologic or vascular compromise—such as may result from a severely deformed fracture—should be addressed as soon as possible. The longer a deficit goes untreated, the longer it is likely to persist and the greater the possibility that it will be irreversible. In some cases, simply reducing a deformity by means of longitudinal traction may restore circulation or nerve function, allowing the remainder of the patient's evaluation and treatment to proceed at a calmer pace.

PREHOSPITAL CARE

With the growing sophistication of emergency medical service (EMS) programs in many areas of the United States, important aspects of early care are no longer overlooked.

Preliminary Splinting

Effective splinting of the injured extremity is crucial for several reasons: (1) it reduces the patient's pain; (2) it reduces damage to nerves and vessels by preventing them from being repeatedly ground between the fragments or being stretched by increased angulation at the fracture site; (3) it reduces the chance of inadvertently converting a closed fracture to an open one as a sharp bone fragment pokes its way through the skin (considered a mishap of severe consequence, because of the potential for the disastrous complication of osteomyelitis), and (4) it facilitates patient transport and the taking of x-rays, by reducing the pain and manipulation associated with moving the patient from ground to ambulance to emergency department stretcher to x-ray table.

PREHOSPITAL SPLINTING DEVICES Many splinting devices are available to EMS systems. For injuries of the wrist or forearm, a foam-padded intravenous board can be wrapped in place, supplemented by a sling. The sling is important because optimal immobilization includes the joint above and the joint below the fracture. The sling keeps the elbow (the joint above) at rest.

For suspected injuries to the elbow or humerus, a sling-and-swathe arrangement works well. This involves applying a sling and then binding the affected arm to the thorax with a gauze wrap. An exception to this principle is immobilization of patients with suspected anterior dislocation of the shoulder. Such patients are unable to adduct the forearm against the thorax, and forcibly binding it there is painful and not recommended. A simple sling is adequate. (Anterior dislocation is unlikely if the patient prefers to keep the arm tightly bound against the thorax and abdomen.)

Injuries to the ankle can be immobilized in a pillow or well-padded cardboard splint. If fracture of the tibial shaft or knee is suspected, the device should extend well above the knee (to immobilize the joint above as well as the joint below).

Some injuries warrant specialized splints, such as winch-mechanism traction devices for femoral shaft fractures. Although such devices do not immobilize the hip (the joint above), the added element of traction makes this unnecessary. If a traction device is unavailable, the hip needs to be immobilized. This can be accomplished with military antishock trousers (MAST) with all compartments inflated or, less elegantly, by binding the legs together, then binding the patient to a backboard from ankles to thorax.

Other types of splints exist, but their use is controversial. Inflatable plastic splints, for example, are acceptable for injuries to the ankle or wrist, but are often used inappropriately for fractures of the humerus or femur. Because these devices normally do not extend above the elbow or knee, they provide inadequate immobilization for such injuries. Also, overinflation of plastic splints can seriously impair circulation. (If the splint cannot be dented by moderate thumb pressure, it is probably overinflated.) Inflatable splints should not be applied over clothing because underlying wrinkles in the clothing may cause pressure sores in swollen and vulnerable tissue.

Also controversial are nonmalleable aluminum splints because they are based on the "one size fits all" principle, which some physicians regard as "this size fits none." If used, aluminum splints should be very well padded because their hard surface may cause pressure sores. Like any splint, they should immobilize the joint above and the joint below the fracture if they are used for long-bone injuries. For example, an above-knee splint is needed for fracture of the tibial shaft. Aluminum splints should be removed as soon as possible, once a fracture is diagnosed or ruled out. If a fracture is confirmed, the splint should be replaced with another type of immobilization dressing before the patient leaves the emergency department.

Reducing Deformity in the Field

Many EMS programs do not recommend prehospital reduction of deformity of an injured extremity. If the deformity is near a joint (suggesting the possibility of dislocation), this is certainly good advice. Injudicious manipulation may convert a pure dislocation to a fracture-dislocation. Even if a fracture already exists, there will be no way to prove it was not caused by the manipulation.

A circumstance in which prehospital reduction of obvious fractures along the shaft of a long bone can be justified is the absence of a distal pulse. Minutes count in such cases. If reduction is attempted, it should be performed by means of longitudinal traction.

In the absence of a common standard, the indications for reduction of deformity by prehospital personnel ultimately remain at the discretion of the supervising EMS program.

EMERGENCY DEPARTMENT EVALUATION AND DIFFERENTIAL DIAGNOSIS

The importance of a careful history and physical examination cannot be overstated. Orthopedic diagnosis is sometimes thought of as being as simple as taking an x-ray where the patient says the pain is. This philosophy is probably responsible more than any other factor for physicians' missing significant injuries.

Although x-ray is of course an important adjunct, it is not the ultimate diagnostic resource, for the following reasons. The pain of a fracture or even a dislocation may be referred to another area. For example, patients with disruption of the sternoclavicular joint or fracture of the humeral shaft may present complaining of shoulder pain. If the x-ray is based solely on where the patient reports subjective discomfort, then the injury might not even be included on the film. The area x-rayed should be determined not only by the patient's chief complaint, but also by systematic palpation, looking for subtle deformity or significant point tenderness.

Some fractures or dislocations are apparent only on special x-ray views, which are not part of the standard series for that body part. Such special views will never be ordered unless the physician has already formulated a presumptive differential diagnosis before x-ray, based on the history and physical findings.

Some injuries may not be radiologically apparent on the first day regardless of what views are taken. Common examples of such injuries are fracture of the scaphoid (carpal navicular), nondisplaced fracture of the radial head, and stress fracture of a metatarsal. The classic radiologic signs accompanying such injuries, such as the fat-pad sign of the elbow, are not always conveniently present, but suggestive history and findings commonly are. In such cases, the diagnosis of fracture may have to be purely clinical until 7 to 10 days after injury, when enough bony resorption has occurred at the fracture site to reveal a lucency on x-ray. A bone scan may suggest the fracture even sooner, but on the day of injury, there may be no readily available test capable of demonstrating the pathology. Only the physician's clinical impression, arrived at through a systematic history and physical examination, will result in proper and timely treatment of a radiologically undemonstrable fracture.

History

The value of history taking in the case of orthopedic injuries is often underestimated. In fact, knowing the precise mechanism of injury or listening carefully to the patient's symptoms can be the key to diagnosing fractures or dislocations. For example, a history of shoulder injury combined with the complaint of dysphagia may be the only clue to the existence of posterior sternoclavicular dislocation. This entity, which causes pressure on the mediastinal structures, can often be demonstrated only by computed tomography (CT) scan and is associated with severe complications if treatment is delayed. Another example is a history of landing flat on the feet from a significant height, which should prompt the physician to consider fracture of one or both calcanei, as well as lumbar vertebral compression fracture.

History is often the only means of correctly assessing and treating young children who "just won't use the arm." Such children, who present with a seemingly paralyzed arm ("pseudoparalysis") after being pulled or yanked, may be incorrectly diagnosed as having a brachial plexus injury, when in fact the history and presentation are classic for subluxed radial head, an entity *not discernible on x-ray* and easily and quickly remedied by a proper reduction maneuver.

A careful history may enable the physician to diagnose posterior dislocation of the shoulder, another entity commonly missed on routine films. If the patient has (1) experienced a direct blow to the front of the shoulder, (2) landed forward on an outstretched arm, or (3) had a seizure or undergone violent muscle contraction for any other reason (e.g., contact with high-voltage current) and now complains of excruciating shoulder pain and severely limited motion, the diagnosis of posterior dislocation should be entertained. If the implications of the history are not appreciated, then the specific x-ray views needed to demonstrate the injury may never be ordered.

Table 259-1 provides further examples of mechanisms that might lead the clinician to suspect, or presumptively treat for, specific injuries. This is by no means a definitive or exhaustive list. Some of the mechanisms described may produce injuries other than those mentioned. Conversely, the injuries may be produced by mechanisms besides those listed.

Some musculoskeletal injuries or conditions may not necessarily be associated with a history of trauma. Occult fracture of the hip in an osteoporotic individual, occult stress fracture of a metatarsal in someone who has recently done an unusual amount of walking, and slipped capital femoral epiphysis in a preteenager or young adolescent, are all examples of injuries whose symptoms may be gradual and insidious in onset, unrelated to an isolated traumatic event. Tenderness to palpation or pain on weight-bearing or range-of-motion suggests the possibility of an occult or easily missed fracture. Depending on the index of suspicion, further studies, such as bone scan or magnetic resonance imaging (MRI), may be indicated to rule out significant pathologic conditions before the patient is allowed to resume weight-bearing.

History taking should not necessarily be limited to orthopedic issues. Depending on the situation, a general medical history should be obtained, since it may have implications for further workup, the potential for complications, or ultimate prognosis for recovery of function. For example, relevant items may include a history of heart

TABLE 259-1 Mechanisms Associated with Particular Orthopedic Injuries

Mechanism	Possible Injury
Bilateral compression of shoulders	Anterior or posterior sternoclavicular dislocation
Direct blow to medial clavicle	Posterior sternoclavicular dislocation
Fall, landing on point of shoulder	Acromioclavicular separation
Direct blow to anterior shoulder, fall on outstretched arm, seizure or electroconvulsive muscular activity	Posterior dislocation of shoulder
Yanking of infant's or toddler's arm	Subluxed radial head (sometimes misdiagnosed as brachial plexus injury because of pseudoparalysis of arm)
Fall, landing on outstretched arm or with elbow beneath the body	Fracture of radial head (may be occult on initial x-rays)
Wrist hyperextension (forced dorsiflexion)	Fracture of scaphoid (carpal navicular), lunate or perilunar dislocation, Colles fracture
Striking knee against dashboard in high-speed collision	Posterior dislocation of hip
Landing flat on feet from height	Calcaneus fracture (one or both); tibial plateau fracture (one or more); acetabular fracture (one or both); vertebral compression fracture, usually lumbar (one or more)
Ankle inversion force	Fracture of any of the malleoli, fracture of base of fifth metatarsal
Rotatory ankle force	Fracture of any of the malleoli, disruption of the anterior tibiofibular ligament with proximal fibular fracture (Maisonneuve injury)
Inversion, medial or lateral stress to forefoot; axial load on metatarsal heads with ankle plantarflexed	Midfoot dislocation

disease, anticoagulant medication, falling due to syncope or transient hemiparesis rather than simply stumbling, or an unsteady baseline gait that cannot withstand further impairment.

Physical Examination

Essential components of the examination for musculoskeletal trauma are (1) inspection for swelling, discoloration, or deformity; (2) assessment of active and passive range of motion of the joints proximal and distal to the injury; (3) palpation for tenderness or subtle deformity; and (4) verification of neurovascular status.

INSPECTION AND RANGE OF MOTION Gross deformity along the shaft of a long bone is of course pathognomonic for fracture. The presence of most dislocations or fractures near a joint can be inferred by deformity at the joint, loss of range of motion, and severe pain at rest. An exception is posterior dislocation of the shoulder, which, while intensely painful, may not be accompanied by obvious deformity. Chapter 263 has a more complete discussion of this entity.

PALPATION When gross deformity is not present, presumptive orthopedic diagnosis depends strongly on the findings noted on palpation. Palpation will disclose areas of bony step-off, as well as the precise location of point tenderness. If films are ordered before performing this phase of the examination, the wrong area may be x-rayed, because pain is commonly referred to a location distant from the injury site.

The palpation examination should be done systematically and consistently from one patient to the next. The area palpated should extend well beyond the location of the patient's subjective pain. For example, when an injured patient complains of shoulder pain, palpation should begin at the sternoclavicular joint and then proceed along the extent of the clavicle, onto the acromioclavicular joint, onto the humeral head, and along the entire humeral shaft. In addition, the scapula should be palpated for tenderness and the posterior aspect of the shoulder palpated for any unnatural prominence that might suggest a posterior dislocation. Injury to any of these areas may be reported by the patient as pain in the shoulder. Only a meticulous palpation examination may protect the physician from being misled by referred pain and missing a crucial diagnosis.

NEUROVASCULAR ASSESSMENT When injury involves an extremity, as opposed to the vertebral column, sensorimotor testing should be performed on the basis of *peripheral nerve* function, rather than nerve root and dermatomal distribution. In the upper extremity, the radial, median, and ulnar nerves should be tested. When the shoulder is anteriorly dislocated, two additional nerves—the axillary (supplying sensation to the lateral aspect of the shoulder) and the musculocutaneous (supplying sensation to the extensor aspect of the forearm)—should be checked as well. In the lower extremity, examination of the saphenous (sensory only), peroneal, and tibial nerves should be performed. Neurologic deficit, although not necessarily immediately reversible, is important to document early, particularly before the patient has undergone any significant manipulation or reduction maneuvers.

Assessment of vascular status should also be performed early. The sooner circulatory compromise is identified and addressed, the greater the chance of avoiding tissue infarction and necrosis. Such injuries as dislocation of the knee (tibiofemoral joint), fracture-dislocation of the ankle, and displaced supracondylar fracture of the elbow in children are commonly associated with vascular occlusion or disruption, with resulting circulatory impairment.

RADIOLOGIC EVALUATION

The area x-rayed and the particular views ordered should be based on the history and physical examination, rather than simply on where the patient reports subjective pain. The joint above and the joint below a fracture should be included on the films because injury at the proximal or distal joint may coexist with long-bone fractures.

Injuries that may require special views to be visualized include acromioclavicular separation, fracture of the scaphoid, posterior shoulder dislocation, and sternoclavicular dislocation. That is why formulation of a presumptive diagnosis *prior to* x-ray is crucial. The physician may never order the specialized views needed to demonstrate a particular injury unless he or she has already anticipated the injury by virtue of the history and physical examination.

Children who have sustained trauma at or near a joint may need comparison studies of the opposite extremity to differentiate fracture lines from normal epiphyseal plates or ossifying growth centers. This is particularly true for the pediatric elbow, which typically exhibits six separate ossification centers sequentially as the child grows.

Although the physician may be tempted to base diagnostic and treatment decisions on the radiologist's written report, this is not advisable for at least two reasons. First, a report of negative findings does not rule out significant injury. Fractures of the radial head, scaphoid, or metatarsal shaft, for example, may initially be undetectable on x-ray, even when special views are taken. Second, the terminology used by radiologists to describe malposition of fracture fragments or disrupted joints is often different from the terminology used by orthopedists. Because the emergency physician will often be conferring with an orthopedist regarding the initial management of a patient, and because this interaction commonly involves describing the radiologic appearance of a patient's injury, it is important that the two physicians ''speak the same language.'' This might not be achieved by simply relaying the radiologist's written description.

Describing Radiographs

When orthopedic consultation is indicated, proper management of the patient may rest on the emergency physician's accurate description of the x-ray. Often the narrative will influence the orthopedist's decision regarding the need for hospital admission and whether surgical versus nonsurgical management is warranted. In essence, the emergency physician should be able to transmit a virtual copy of the x-ray by means of verbal description.

There are various ways of classifying or categorizing fractures. The method presented here is intended to be the most practical from the standpoint of effective communication with a consultant who is not physically present.[3]

OPEN VERSUS CLOSED Although not a radiologic finding per se, this aspect of an injury is among the most important and should be conveyed to the orthopedist before any other. The implications of open fracture are of such significance that this factor alone may determine the patient's immediate care or ultimate disposition.

LOCATION OF THE FRACTURE Typical reference points used by orthopedists to describe the location of a fracture along the shaft of a long bone are the midshaft, the junction of the proximal and middle thirds, and the junction of the middle and distal thirds. Any fracture more proximal or distal than this may be localized in terms of its distance, in centimeters, from the bone end.

When a proximal or distal fracture extends into the adjacent joint, it is termed intraarticular. Intraarticular fractures have special significance because disruption of the joint surface may warrant surgery to restore the joint's contour and prevent subsequent traumatic arthritis. This feature of a fracture line, if present, constitutes important information.

Anatomic bony reference points should be cited when applicable. A fracture just above the condyles of the distal humerus or femur, for example, is most precisely called a *supracondylar* fracture. A fracture running from the greater to the lesser trochanter of the proximal femur is an *intertrochanteric* hip fracture, whereas a fracture just below the trochanters is *subtrochanteric,* and a fracture just above is said to involve the femoral *neck.* The area at or proximal to the coronoid process of the ulna is the *olecranon* and should be referred to as such, rather than simply the proximal ulna. Other bony landmarks include the radial head (proximal), radial styloid (distal), and greater tuberosity of the humerus. Numerous additional examples exist.

ORIENTATION OF THE FRACTURE LINE The most common orientations of fracture lines are illustrated in Fig. 259-1. Torus and greenstick fractures are seen almost exclusively in young children, whose bones are more pliable than those of adults. Note the segmental fracture, which is commonly described incorrectly as a comminuted fracture. To an orthopedist, the term *comminuted* implies splintering or shattering. A single large free-floating segment of bone between two well-defined fracture lines is a *segmental fracture.*

DISPLACEMENT AND SEPARATION *Displacement* refers to the position of the fracture fragments as nonconcentric or offset from each other. It is expressed in terms of direct measurement (4-mm displacement) or in terms of the percent of the width of the bone (e.g., 50 percent displacement or complete displacement). The direction of displacement is based on the position of the distal fragment in relation to the proximal.

Displacement should not be confused with separation, which is the distance two fragments have been pulled apart. Figure 259-2 illustrates principles of displacement and separation.

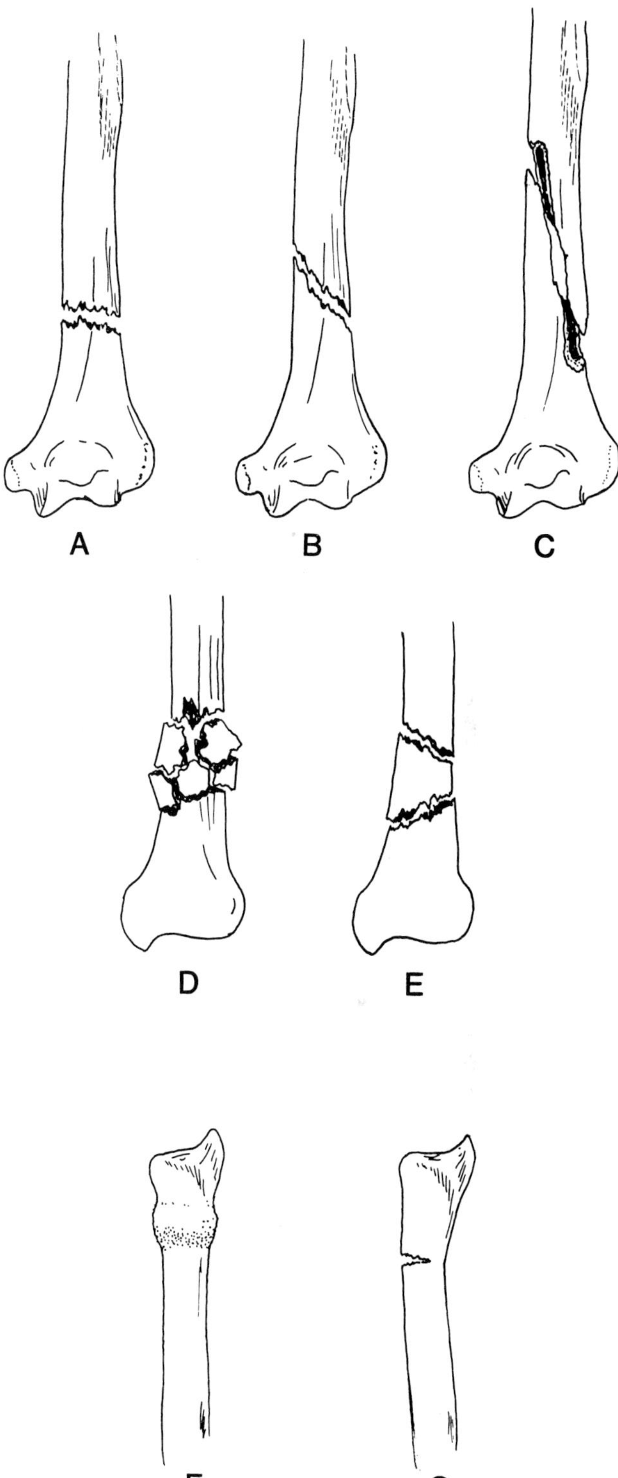

FIG. 259-1. Fracture line orientation. **A.** Transverse. **B.** Oblique. **C.** Spiral. **D.** Comminuted. **E.** Segmental. **F.** Torus. **G.** Greenstick.

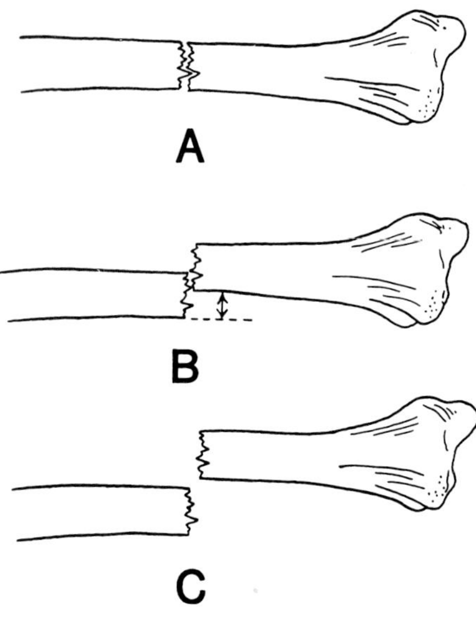

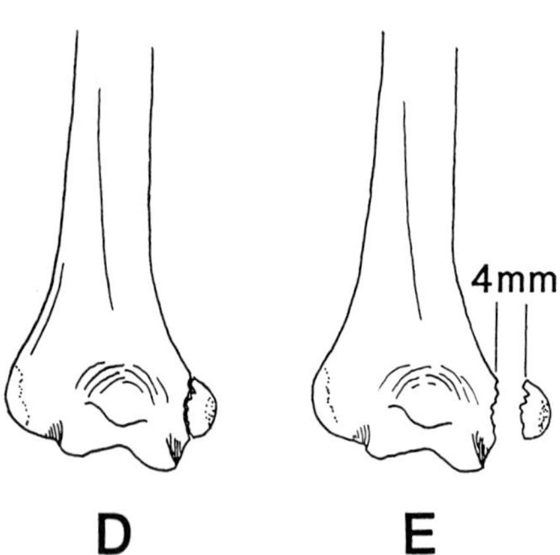

FIG. 259-2. Fracture displacement and separation. **A.** No displacement, slight separation. **B.** Fifty percent dorsal displacement. **C.** Complete dorsal displacement. **D.** Nondisplaced, no separation. **E.** A 4-mm separation.

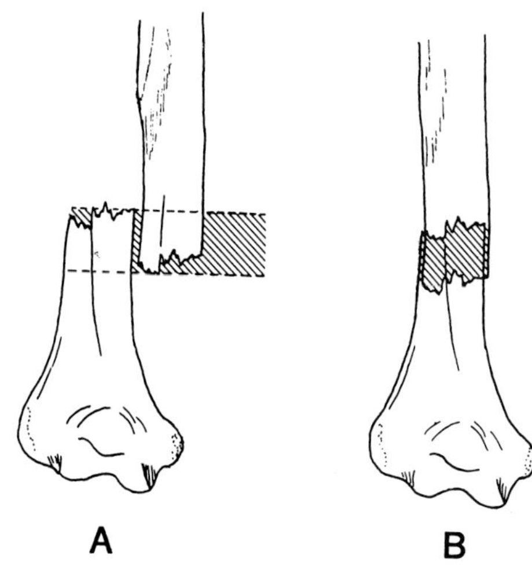

FIG. 259-3. Shortening at fracture site. **A.** Complete displacement with overriding. **B.** Impaction. In both cases, the width of the shaded area represents the amount of shortening.

SHORTENING Shortening is the amount by which the bone's length has been reduced and is expressed in millimeters or centimeters. Shortening can occur by impaction (telescoping of the fragments into one another) or by the overlap of two completely displaced fragments (Fig. 259-3). The latter is referred to by some orthopedists as overriding. Because an x-ray affords no depth perception, a fracture that appears impacted on one view must also be visualized at an angle 90° from the first to differentiate it from a fracture whose ends are completely displaced and overriding.

Depending on the location of the fracture and the age of the patient, shortening may have long-range functional implications and may have to be corrected by closed manipulation or by surgery.

ANGULATION Angulation is expressed in terms of two parameters: direction and amount (Fig. 259-4). Quantifying the angulation is relatively simple. The physician need only estimate the amount of ''unbending'' (expressed in degrees) that would be required to make the fragments parallel.

Describing the direction of angulation is more difficult because the terminology is less consistent among clinicians. Generally, when a fracture is near the midshaft of a long bone, the direction of angulation is the direction of the *apex* of the angle formed by the two fragments. Figures 259-4A and B both represent 30° of dorsal angulation. When a fracture is located near the end of a bone, however, angulation is described in terms of the direction the *terminal fragment* is deviated. Figure 259-4C also represents 30° of dorsal angulation, even though the apex of the angle formed by the fragments is pointing in the

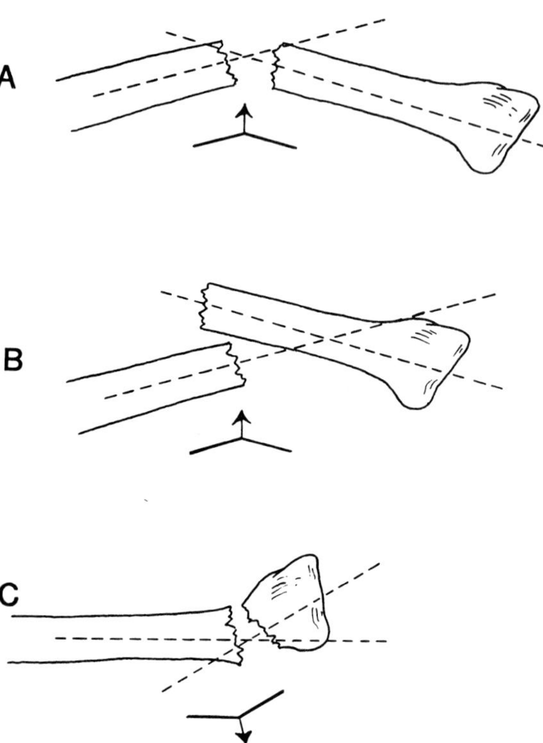

FIG. 259-4. Fracture angulation. All figures depict 30° dorsal angulation. **A.** and **B.** Direction is based on the apex of the angle drawn below the figures. **C.** Direction is based on the direction of the terminal fragment.

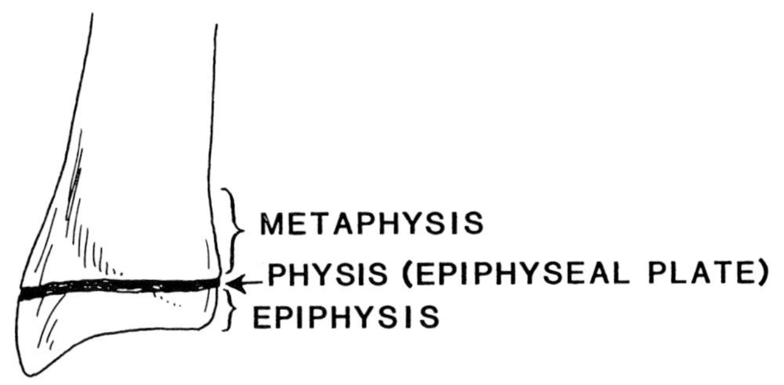

FIG. 259-5. Epiphyseal anatomy.

TABLE 259-2 Description of Salter Fractures

Salter Type	What Is Broken Off
I	The entire epiphysis
II	The entire epiphysis *with* a portion of the metaphysis
III	A portion of the epiphysis
IV	A portion of the epiphysis *with* a portion of the metaphysis
V	Nothing "broken off;" compression injury of the epiphyseal plate

opposite direction from that in the preceding figures. If there is a possibility of ambiguity in the description, specifying the *direction of deviation of the distal fragment* can usually resolve it.

Depending on the anatomic area involved, direction of angulation may be expressed as radial or ulnar, dorsal or volar, anterior or posterior, or lateral or medial.

ROTATIONAL DEFORMITY Rotational deformity—the extent to which the distal fracture fragment is twisted on its own axis relative to the proximal fragment—is generally not measurable on x-ray and sometimes not even radiologically apparent. This element of fracture description depends on physical examination. Its detection is particularly important in the phalanges of the fingers, where, if rotational deformity goes unrecognized and uncorrected, the affected finger will always be malaligned when the hand is closed.

FRACTURE COMBINED WITH DISLOCATION OR SUBLUXATION Injuries near a joint may involve dislocation or subluxation in combination with a proximate fracture. An example is fracture of one or more ankle malleoli, together with partial or complete displacement of the talus from beneath the tibia. Fracture-dislocations are significant injuries, often requiring surgical intervention. If, in describing the injury, the physician emphasizes the fracture component but expresses the dislocation or subluxation component as mere displacement, then the full severity may not be appreciated by the orthopedist. Such injuries should be described as fracture-dislocations or fracture-subluxations.

SALTER FRACTURES The physiology of Salter fractures—fractures involving the epiphyseal plate at the end of the long bone of a growing child—has already been discussed. Salter fractures are classified into five types, based on the pattern of the fracture line. Because the type generally correlates with the potential for future growth disturbance (and, consequently, with the aggressiveness of treatment required), the ability to classify such injuries based on their x-ray appearance is important.

Perhaps the easiest way to remember the Salter classification system is to think of these injuries not in terms of where the fracture line runs, but in terms of what has been broken off. Figure 259-5 illustrates the anatomy involved. Table 252-2 describes the five types of Salter fractures, which are illustrated in Fig. 259-6. The potential for growth disturbance is least for type I and increases with the classification number, the worst prognosis being associated with type V injuries.

Type I and type V Salter fractures may be radiologically undetectable. Type I injuries usually involve little or no separation of the epiphysis from the rest of the bone, and the lucent fracture line is not visible along the equally lucent epiphyseal plate. If the epiphysis and plate slip transversely along the end of the shaft, the abnormal position will be seen on x-ray, but slippage does not always occur. Diagnosis of acute Salter I fractures is usually clinical, based on the presence of swelling and tenderness in the region of the physis.

Type V injuries may be evident only retrospectively, when growth disturbance first begins to appear. At time of initial presentation, however, a history of a significant axial loading force, coupled with significant tenderness in the area of the epiphyseal plate, should suggest the possibility of a type V injury. Such children should be immobilized and referred for orthopedic follow-up.

TREATMENT IN THE EMERGENCY DEPARTMENT

Control of Pain and Swelling

Measures to reduce swelling should be initiated early. Severe swelling not only intensifies the patient's discomfort but may also delay the application of a long-term definitive immobilization dressing and may make the skin more susceptible to pressure sores. Although sometimes regarded as trivial modalities, the application of cold and elevation are both effective in keeping swelling to a minimum or at least preventing its progression. When cold is applied, the skin should be protected from direct contact with ice-cold temperatures.

Parenteral analgesics should be administered as necessary. If the patient is relatively comfortable at rest, medication may not be re-

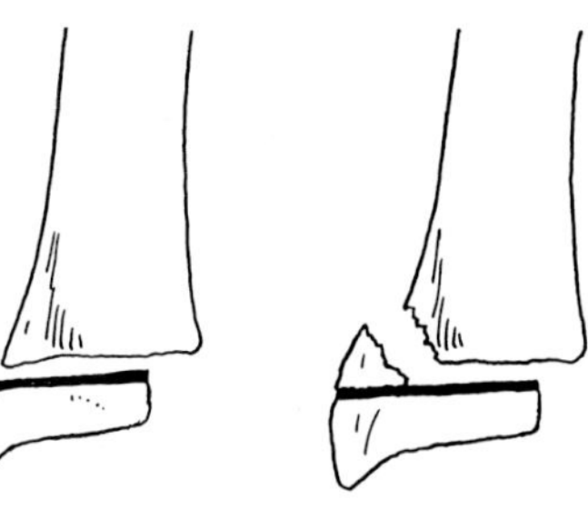

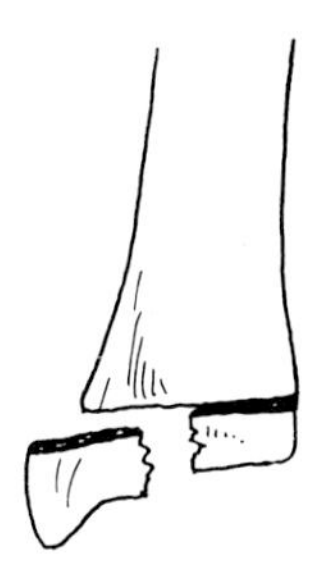

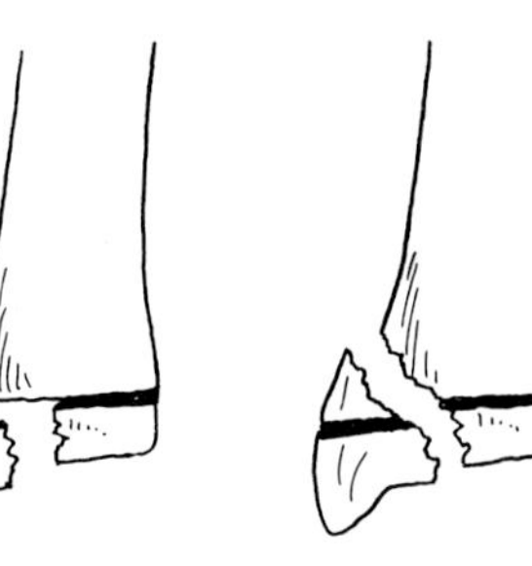

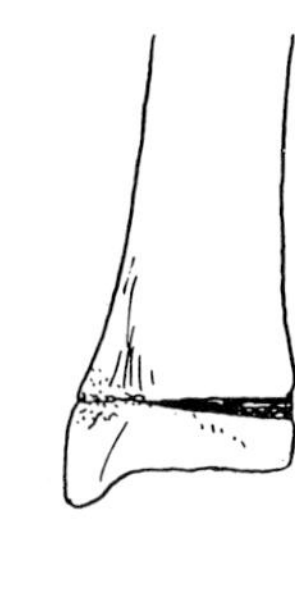

FIG. 259-6. Epiphyseal fractures based on Salter-Harris classification.

quired. Analgesics have virtually no effect on the pain of movement or manipulation unless combined with hypnotics or other central nervous system active agents. Jewelry, watches, or rings that can cause compression as an extremity swells should be removed if there is suspicion or confirmation of proximal injury.

Keeping the Patient NPO

Any patient who may be a candidate for prompt surgical fixation, manipulation, or any other procedure under general anesthesia or conscious sedation should be kept NPO from the moment of arrival until the need for, and timing of, such a procedure has been ascertained. This seemingly obvious point is commonly overlooked, particularly in a busy emergency department, where the process of clinical evaluation may be prolonged and hunger may develop in the interim.

Reducing Fracture Deformity

The long-term purpose of reducing significant deformity associated with fractures is, of course, restoration of normal appearance and function of the extremity. However, there are also short-term reasons for reducing deformity early in the patient's course, including (1) alleviating pain, (2) relieving the tension on nerves or vessels that may be stretched as they pass over the deformity, (3) eliminating or significantly minimizing the possibility of inadvertently converting a closed fracture to an open one when the skin is tented by a sharp bony fragment, and (4) restoring circulation to a pulseless distal extremity.

After the patient has been sedated, deformity at or near the midshaft of a long bone is usually easy to reduce with gradual, steady longitudinal traction. Any rotational deformity should be corrected only after the angular component has been addressed and should be performed while traction is maintained. If reduction is performed as a definitive procedure prior to immobilization, attention to rotational deformity is particularly important because of its profound effect on ultimate function. As discussed earlier, rotational deformity is much easier to appreciate by examining the patient than by examining the x-ray.

The nearer the deformity is to a joint, the more difficult it may be to correct and the more specialized the reduction maneuver may have to be. Who performs the procedure, the emergency physician or the orthopedist, is determined by a variety of circumstances, some of which may be specific to the particular practice environment. When deformity is associated with circulatory deficit, a true emergency exists, and the anticipated delay until reduction should be considered.

Reducing Dislocations

The techniques used to reduce specific dislocations are discussed in subsequent chapters. In general, prereduction x-rays are advisable unless circulation is threatened and prompt radiologic evaluation is not available. X-rays are needed because dislocations and fracture-dislocations may have the same clinical appearance on physical examination, but the techniques used to treat them may be markedly different. An example is simple anterior dislocation of the shoulder, as opposed to the same injury associated with complete fracture through the humeral neck. If the fracture is identified at the outset, the patient will be spared the pain of prolonged unsuccessful reduction attempts, and no question will arise as to exactly when the fracture might have occurred. Even ''pure'' dislocations may be associated with minute fracture fragments. A prereduction film will usually furnish proof of the preexistence of such fragments.

Of course, there are circumstances in which the potential benefits of a prereduction film may be outweighed by the associated expenditure of time and money. For example, a prereduction film may be omitted in a patient with a history of multiple recurrent dislocations of the shoulder, who presents with history, signs, and symptoms typical of another recurrence.

The importance of postreduction films is another consideration. Occasionally a joint may feel as though it has been reduced, when in fact it has not. Even when a maneuver is successful, the joint may redislocate after the patient leaves the emergency department. There is no way to prove that the joint was in anatomic position at the time of discharge, without a postreduction film. The obtaining of postreduction films is, of course, a matter of judgment and ultimately at the clinician's discretion.

Initial Management of Open Fractures

Open fractures, which may be complicated by subsequent osteomyelitis, warrant prompt and meticulous attention. The most important elements in the treatment of open fractures, aside from tetanus prophylaxis that applies generally to any wound, are irrigation, débridement, and antibiotics provided as soon as is practical. Although irrigation and debridement are commonly performed in the operating room, antibiotics may be administered in the emergency department.

Early administration of antibiotics can help reduce the incidence of infection in open fractures.[4,5] The longer the interval between the time of injury and the initiation of antibiotic therapy, the less likely that such therapy will be of benefit. Exactly what constitutes the ideal antibiotic is controversial. An accepted combination is a first-generation cephalosporin plus an aminoglycoside, but this is by no means the only regimen in use. Aerobic and anaerobic wound cultures can be obtained before antibiotics are administered.

Antibiotics by themselves are no substitute for irrigation and debridement, both of which have been well demonstrated to be crucial to reducing the incidence of osteomyelitis in open fractures by reducing bacterial contamination and the potential for bacterial colonization.[6,7] Irrigation should be extensive to (1) make the area more visible for inspection for foreign material, (2) float out nonviable tissue or at least float it into the field of vision so it can be removed, and (3) float out contaminated blood clots and bits of tissue. Pulsatile pumps may increase the effectiveness of irrigation, provided the stream is not too forceful. Excessive force will simply pack debris farther into the recesses of the wound.

Debridement of minor wounds that overlie a fracture may sometimes be performed in the emergency department. When tissue damage is moderate or severe, formal debridement and irrigation are commonly performed in the operating room.

ORTHOPEDIC CONSULTATION IN THE EMERGENCY DEPARTMENT

In many cases, such as hip fracture or both-bone fracture of the forearm, the need for hospital admission and/or orthopedic consultation in the emergency department is obvious. In some situations, however, differences of opinion may exist among emergency physicians, as well as among orthopedists, as to whether the patient needs to be seen by an orthopedist in the emergency department, or whether the patient may be treated in preliminary fashion and referred for subsequent definitive orthopedic management. Even patients with injuries that may ultimately require surgical repair, such as an unstable ankle fracture, may sometimes be immobilized and discharged for prompt orthopedic follow-up.

Some entities or situations that may warrant orthopedic consultation while the patient is still in the emergency department are discussed below.

Compartment Syndrome

The physiology and potentially catastrophic consequences of compartment syndrome are described later in this chapter. In cases of known or suspected compartment syndrome, orthopedic consultation should be obtained promptly. Emergency surgical intervention may be required to try to avert permanent tissue damage and muscle contracture.

Irreducible Dislocation

The emergency physician may sometimes be unable to reduce a dislocation, even with the aid of nerve block or pharmacologic sedation. While technique is certainly a factor, there may be other reasons closed reduction cannot be accomplished, such as the interposition of soft tissues or the presence of associated fractures. Orthopedic consultation should be sought in such cases. Timely reduction, which may sometimes only be achieved surgically, can help minimize the complications (and shorten the pain) resulting from a dislocated joint.

Circulatory Compromise

Circulatory deficit resulting from musculoskeletal injury warrants prompt orthopedic consulation. Even if circulation has been restored by the emergency physician through the correction of deformity, the orthopedist may wish to investigate the integrity of the involved vessels, and should at least be contacted in order to discuss the case.

Open Fracture

As mentioned earlier, some open fractures need to be treated aggressively in the operating room. Other types, such as those involving the phalanges, may often be irrigated in the emergency department and referred for follow-up. If there is any question, a discussion with an orthopedist can result in a mutually agreeable plan of care.

Injuries Requiring Surgical Repair

While some musculoskeletal injuries require operative intervention as soon as possible, others may be treated on a delayed basis. In many cases, orthopedists differ in their preferred approach to the timing of surgery. Orthopedic consultation, at least by telephone, is indicated in cases of musculoskeletal injury that the emergency physician believes may need operative fixation or repair. The orthopedist may then exercise his or her choice to admit the patient right away, or to see the patient in timely follow-up and schedule surgery at that time.

IMMOBILIZATION TECHNIQUES

Immobilization is indicated not only for fractures but also for dislocated joints that have been reduced. When a joint becomes dislocated, the ligaments that had provided it with stability are disrupted, and the joint is susceptible to redislocation until healing has occurred.

Whether plaster or fiberglass is used in the dressing depends on a number of factors, including the emergency physician's preference, the philosophy of the orthopedic community, the needs of the patient, and the hospital's resources. Fiberglass has the advantages of being lightweight, fast setting, and resistant to damage by moisture (although most splint dressings contain additional bandaging materials that need to be kept dry). Ultimately, the physician should use the material he or she is most comfortable with and can use most skillfully with best results.

Principles of Splinting

With the exception of the specific chemical substance involved, references to plaster in the following description are equally applicable to fiberglass.

The chemical reaction that causes plaster of paris (calcium sulfate) to crystallize, or set, is initiated by contact with water. The higher the water temperature, the faster the hardening process. However, the setting of plaster is an exothermic chemical reaction, which liberates heat. The faster plaster sets, the more heat it generates. This means, the maximum temperature to which the patient's skin is exposed will be the *additive* result of the water temperature plus the heat released by the plaster. For this reason, severe burns can result when plaster has been immersed in hot water, even though the temperature of the water itself was not sufficient to cause such burns. Although there is no universally prescribed ideal water temperature, a safe practice is to make the water slightly warmer than room temperature. If steam is visible, the water is almost certainly too hot.

To avoid irritation and minimize the potential for pressure sores, plaster dressings need to include several layers of padding between the plaster and the skin. When longitudinal splints are used, the padding need not be circumferential. Longitudinal padding will effectively protect the skin as long as it slightly exceeds the width and length of the splint. The best way to ensure this is to fashion the dry splint first and then measure the padding over it.

The length of a splint should be sufficient to provide ample leverage to immobilize the injured joint. To immobilize the elbow, for example, a splint should begin distal to the wrist and extend high up the lateral arm, to the level of the humeral neck. To effectively immobilize the ankle, a splint should extend from beneath the metatarsal heads to high calf. If the fracture is located along the midshaft of the distal extremity rather than at a joint, the splint should be long enough to immobilize the joint above and the joint below the fracture.

Splints may be fashioned from the plaster rolls normally used for casting or from prepadded material supplied on a continuous roll, which can be cut to length. When using common plaster rolls, determine the necessary length of the splint by measuring out a single layer along the extremity. Then, on a flat surface, unroll the plaster back and forth over itself to make a multilayered splint. For an adult, the splint should be at least 12 layers thick. Even more layers should be used for children, who typically remain as active as possible and have little regard for protecting the dressing.

When the dry splint has been prepared, measure out several layers of padding over it, making the padding longer and wider than the plaster. After setting the padding aside, grip each end of the splint and immerse it in water, keeping it submerged until bubbling stops (indicating the water has been fully absorbed into the interstices of the material). Then withdraw the splint and strip out the excess water by sliding the thumb and index finger along the length of the plaster on each side. (Be sure to use a stripping motion, rather than crumpling the dressing to wring out the excess water, or much of the plaster will be wrung out as well.)

The next step, frequently overlooked, is to lay the splint on a flat surface and massage the layers into one another so that they fuse. This creates a strong dressing that is solid on cross section. A splint whose separate layers are still visible on cross section is much weaker.

The padding should now be laid over the plaster and the dressing applied to the extremity, with the padded surface against the skin. An assistant can hold the splint against the extremity while it is wrapped in place with gauze bandage. Make sure the assistant uses the palms, rather than fingertips, when holding the plaster. Hardened finger dents can cause irritation or even pressure sores. If a compressive effect is desired, an elastic bandage may be wrapped over the gauze. (If an elastic bandage is wrapped directly onto plaster without an intervening layer of gauze, it will set into the plaster and lose its compressive function.)

While the plaster is setting, the physician may need to maintain the affected joint in a particular position. Again, the palms, rather than the fingers, should be used. Once the setting process is well underway, if the position of a joint is changed, the dressing will crack and become functionally useless. If the joint has gradually migrated from the desired position, the physician must decide either to accept the current position or remove the dressing and start over. There is no need to feel self-conscious about the latter course. Patients generally appreciate a desire for perfection by their physician.

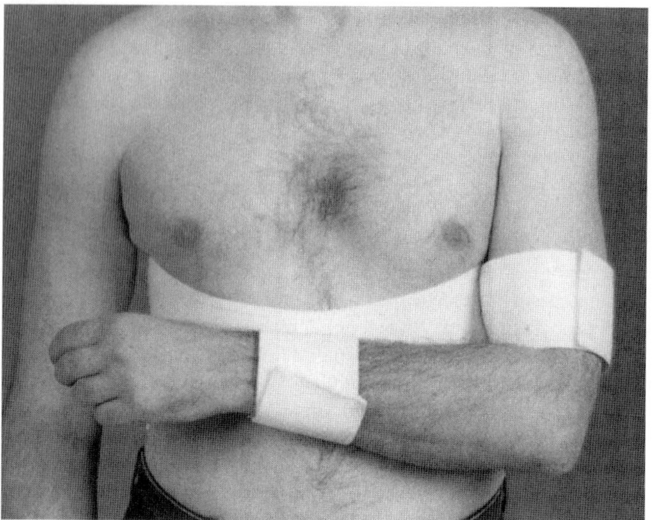

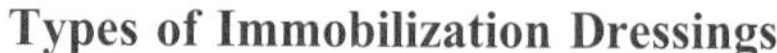

FIG. 259-7. Shoulder immobilizer.

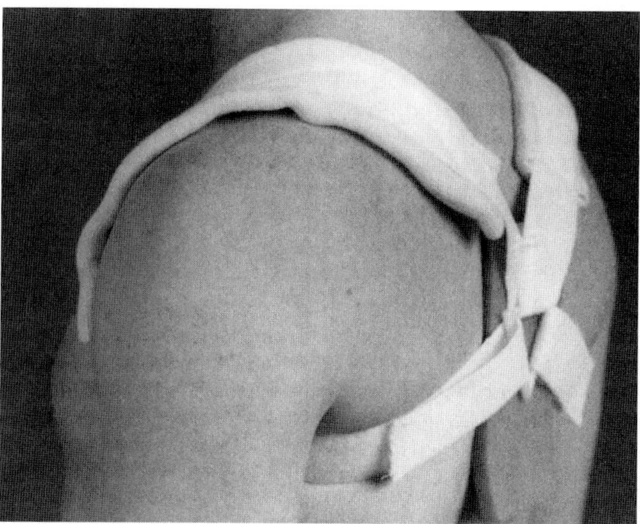

FIG. 259-8. Clavicle strap.

Types of Immobilization Dressings

The more common immobilization dressings used in the emergency department are discussed below.

SHOULDER IMMOBILIZER This is a removable, Velcro-fastened device that keeps the arm in "sling position" but allows less mobility than a sling (Fig. 259-7). A wide band wraps around the thorax. Two cuffs are attached to the thoracic piece, one on the lateral side, which grasps the upper arm, keeping it adducted against the thorax, and one anterior, which grasps the wrist, keeping the forearm against the abdomen. This dressing is suitable for fractures about the shoulder girdle, including clavicle and well-positioned humeral neck fractures, as well as for reduced anterior shoulder dislocations.

The shoulder immobilizer is also commonly used for acromioclavicular separations, although the ideal dressing for this injury is one that exerts upward pressure on the elbow and downward pressure on the clavicle. Commercial versions of such dressings exist, but they are cumbersome to apply and uncomfortable to wear, leading to noncompliance. A shoulder immobilizer (or sling and swathe) is an acceptable alternative dressing.

CLAVICLE STRAP (FIGURE-OF-EIGHT BANDAGE) The purpose of an immobilization dressing for clavicular fractures is to maintain support and minimize pain. The figure-of-eight bandage or strap (Fig. 259-8) has long been considered the "appropriate" immobilization device, but more recent studies have shown it to be no more effective than a simple sling or shoulder immobilizer in terms of providing comfort and achieving alignment of the fragments.[8] Generally, anatomic alignment can be maintained only by surgical fixation, but this is a controversial modality because of its association with a significant frequency of non-union and other complications. In any event, manipulation and realignment of the fragments are usually unnecessary unless there is compromise to the subclavian neurovascular structures, entrapment of tissue, or the likelihood of penetration of the skin by a sharp fragment. While untreated malalignment may result in a permanent "bump" at the fracture site after healing (of which the patient should be forewarned at the initial visit), this should not prevent the ultimate return of normal function.

Another consideration is that, in contrast to a simple sling, a clavicle strap may be awkward to apply, may require frequent readjustment, may cause problems related to pressure on the brachial plexus, and is often uncomfortable. Finally, some studies suggest that, depending on the location of the fracture, a figure-of-eight may actually *increase* the displacement of the fragments. Nevertheless, for the sake of completeness, a description of this still-common dressing is included here.

The clavicle strap (figure-of-eight dressing) consists of padded straps that pass down the anterior aspect of both shoulders and under the axillae. The right and left halves of the dressing meet in back, where they are attached to clips centered between the scapulae. The straps, whose tension is adjustable, exert backward pressure on each shoulder.

Patients or their parents should be cautioned to watch for paresthesias or swelling in the hands or fingers. Such symptoms suggest that the dressing is too tight, and it should be removed until symptoms disappear. The strap may then be reapplied more loosely.

LONG-ARM ULNAR GUTTER SPLINT This is a plaster splint that maintains the elbow in flexion, usually at 90° (Fig. 259-9). The upper extremity is placed in sling position (elbow flexed and palm facing the abdomen). The splint begins on the ulnar surface of the hand at the metacarpal heads and extends along the ulnar surface of the forearm, past the apex of the elbow, to a spot high on the lateral surface of the upper arm just opposite and below the axillary crease. It should be supplemented with a sling.

The most common error associated with fashioning this dressing is insufficient length. If the splint is not carried far enough above the

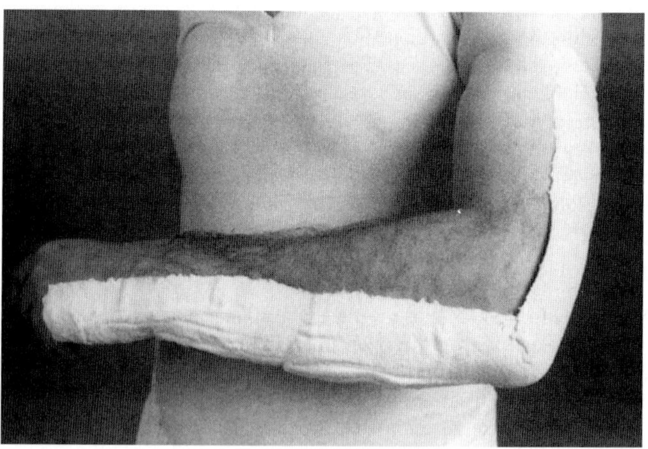

FIG. 259-9. Long-arm ulnar gutter splint.

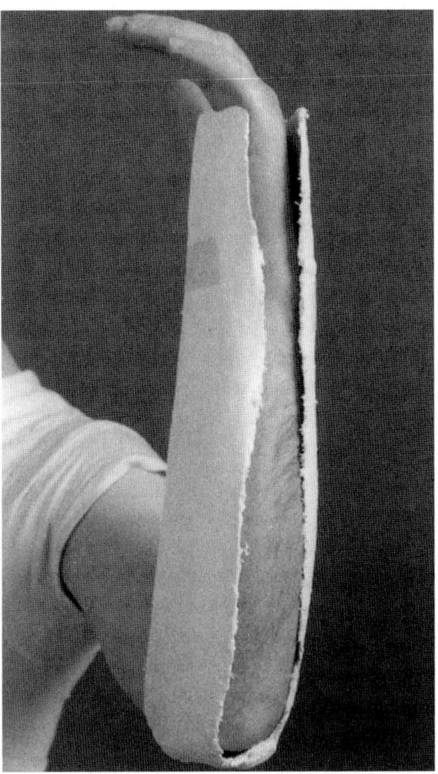

FIG. 259-10. Sugar-tong splint.

elbow, it will not be able to exert enough leverage to prevent motion of the joint.

The long-arm ulnar gutter is useful for injuries about the elbow, including radial head fractures, nondisplaced supracondylar humeral fractures, and reduced dislocation of the elbow.

SUGAR-TONG SPLINT This is a plaster splint that prevents motion of the wrist and elbow, including pronation-supination (Fig. 259-10). The upper extremity is placed in sling position, as described above. The splint begins on the extensor aspect of the hand at the level of the metacarpal heads and extends along the extensor aspect of the forearm, around the elbow and humeral condyles onto the flexor aspect of the forearm, and ultimately to the palmar aspect of the hand, ending at the level of the metacarpal heads. It is wrapped in place with gauze and often topped off with a compression bandage. It should be supplemented with a sling.

Proper length of the sugar-tong dressing is important. Too short a splint will fail to immobilize the wrist. If the dressing is too long, it will impair motion of the metacarpophalangeal joints, leaving them stiff and making the fingers more susceptible to swelling due to immobility.

The sugar-tong splint is appropriate for fractures about the wrist or distal forearm. Some orthopedists use it as a definitive dressing after reduction of wrist fractures.

"COCK-UP" WRIST SPLINT (TO BE AVOIDED) The "cock-up" splint is a removable device that encloses the forearm and hand, maintaining the wrist in a dorsiflexed position. The splint is fastened with Velcro straps. *Cock-up splints should not be used for fractures of the wrist or carpals* because such injuries are usually caused by forceful dorsiflexion and the splint only reproduces the position of injury, imposing considerable pain in the process. Fractures about the wrist are generally immobilized in neutral position with plaster dressings. Colles fractures may even be immobilized in slight palmar flexion after reduction.

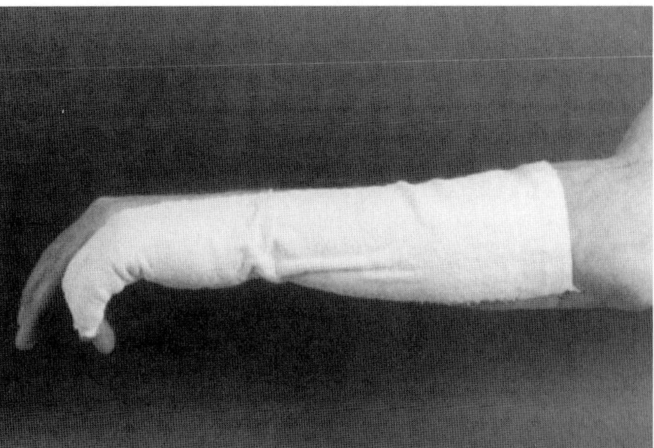

FIG. 259-11. Short-arm ulnar gutter splint.

"Cock-up" splints may be useful in some situations, such as to immobilize the wrist for tendinitis or to support it in the case of wrist drop due to radial nerve palsy. In such instances, dorsiflexion of the wrist will preserve the patient's grip strength.

SHORT-ARM ULNAR GUTTER SPLINT This plaster splint immobilizes the wrist and ulnar half of the hand (Fig. 259-11). It extends along the ulnar surface of the hand and forearm, beginning just proximal to the tip of the fifth finger and ending high onto the forearm. The splint should be wide enough to encompass the fourth and fifth rays (fingers and metacarpals) on both the extensor and palmar aspects of the hand. The splint is wrapped in place with the fourth and fifth fingers bound together, separated by a thin layer of padding to prevent maceration of the skin. The metacarpophalangeal joints and interphalangeal joints should be positioned in gentle flexion. The dressing should be supplemented with a sling.

The short-arm ulnar gutter is useful for fractures of the proximal phalanx of the ring or little finger, or for fractures of the fourth or fifth metacarpal (including the common "boxer's fracture"). The counterpart of this splint, the short-arm radial gutter, is designed in similar fashion but extends along the radial surface of the hand and forearm and is used for comparable injuries of the index or middle rays. It is fashioned with a hole that allows the thumb to pass through.

THUMB SPICA This plaster dressing immobilizes the wrist and thumb (Fig. 259-12). The term *spica* applies to any dressing that encompasses a main trunk plus one or more of its branches, in this

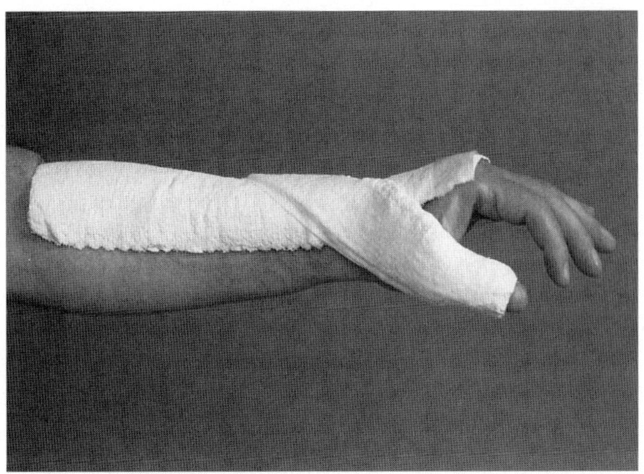

FIG. 259-12. Thumb spica splint.

case, the forearm plus the thumb. It is used for fractures of the scaphoid or for fractures of the thumb metacarpal or proximal phalanx.

A thumb spica can be fashioned from a single wide plaster splint, but a more effective and better-looking dressing can be made from two separate splints. The wrist piece runs along the extensor aspect of the hand and forearm beginning at the metacarpal heads and ending just short of the elbow. The more narrow thumb piece, approximately 2 in wide, extends from the tip of the thumb (which has been padded separately), along the outer aspect of the thumb metacarpal, and onto the extensor aspect of the forearm, well overlapping the first splint. Along their area of contact, the two splints are molded into each other, with no padding between them, to form a sturdy dressing. The plaster is wrapped in place with gauze, and a compression wrap may be added at the physician's discretion. The dressing is supplemented with a sling.

While the plaster is setting, optimal position can be achieved by keeping the wrist in *neutral* position and having the patient oppose the tips of the thumb and index fingers in the form of an "OK" sign. This preserves thumb-index pinch function, minimizing the patient's incapacitation. It also avoids reproducing the position of injury in the case of scaphoid fractures, which are typically caused by forced dorsiflexion of the wrist.

KNEE IMMOBILIZER This is a removable device that wraps around the upper and lower leg and maintains the knee in a fully or almost fully extended position (Fig. 259-13). The splint contains longitudinal metal struts and is fastened with Velcro straps.

The knee immobilizer is useful for a variety of injuries, including fracture of the lateral or medial tibial plateau, fracture or subluxation of the patella, meniscal injuries (provided the patient's knee is not locked in partial flexion), and ligamentous strains or tears.

POSTERIOR ANKLE MOLD This is a plaster splint that immobilizes the ankle (Fig. 259-14). It begins beneath the metatarsal heads, runs along the plantar aspect of the foot, and continues up the back of the lower leg, ending at high calf. The splint is used for severe ankle sprains or for stable ankle fractures, such as minimally displaced fractures of the distal fibula. Unstable fractures, such as those involving more than one malleolus or widening of the medial joint space (disruption of the deltoid ligament), may be supplemented by a sugar-tong component running down one side of the leg, beneath the heel, and up the other side. Where the two components overlap, they are molded together. The additional component helps minimize inversion-eversion of the ankle. Even more stability is provided by continuing the posterior splint past the back of the knee to high posterior thigh, using wider plaster for this area. With the knee slightly flexed, rotational motion at the ankle will be prevented as well.

While the plaster is setting, the ankle should be maintained in a position as close as possible to neutral, that is, at 90° to the leg. This maintains the width of the ankle joint and may allow the patient to regain range of motion more quickly after the dressing is removed. Because most patients with ankle injuries tend to keep the ankle plantar flexed, the physician will usually have to maintain passive dorsiflexion by exerting gentle pressure with a palm beneath the sole of the foot.

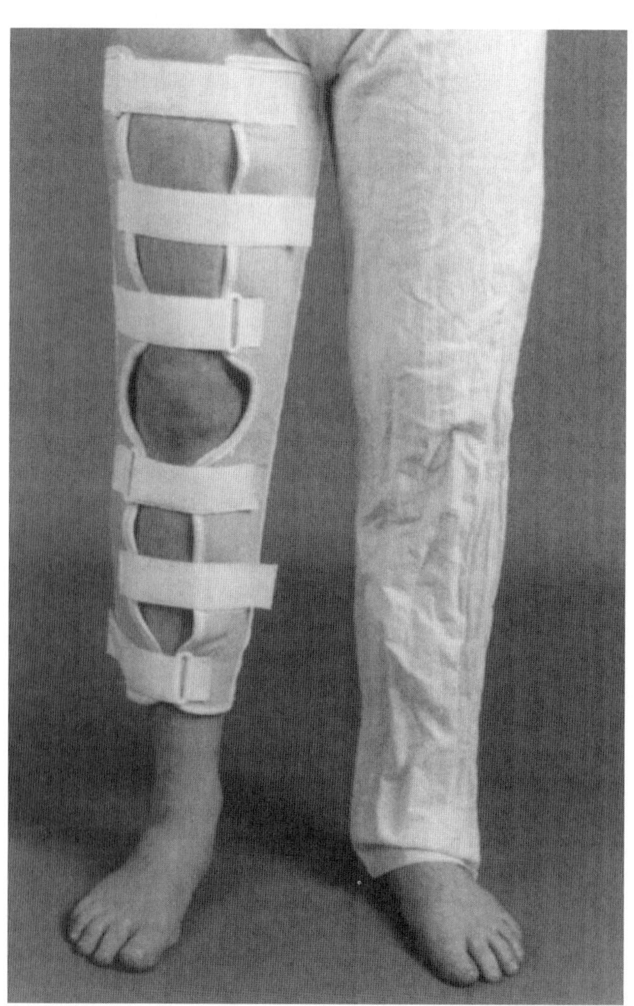

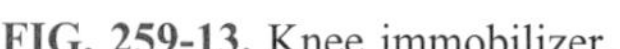

FIG. 259-13. Knee immobilizer.

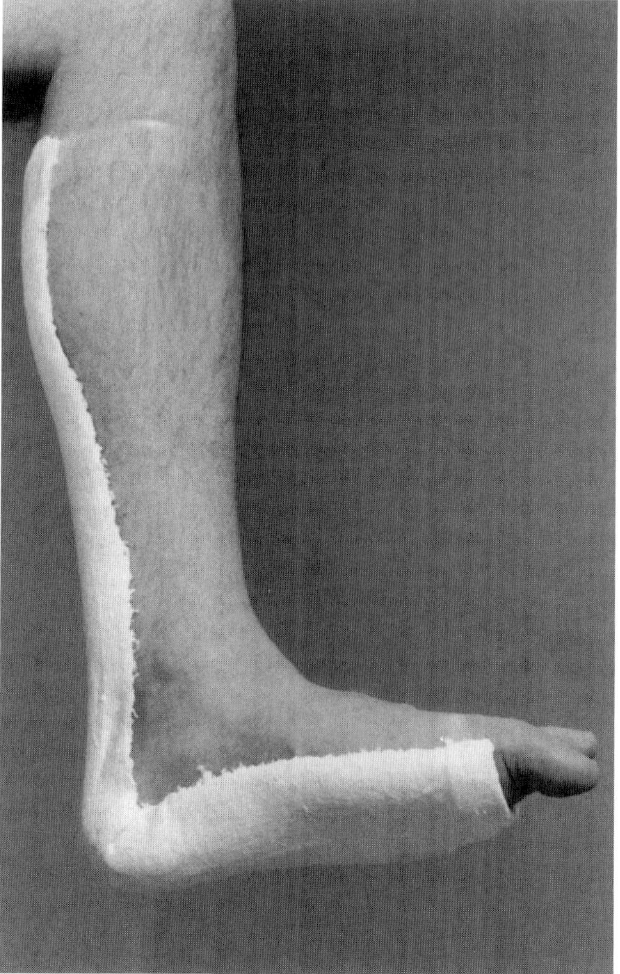

FIG. 259-14. Posterior ankle mold.

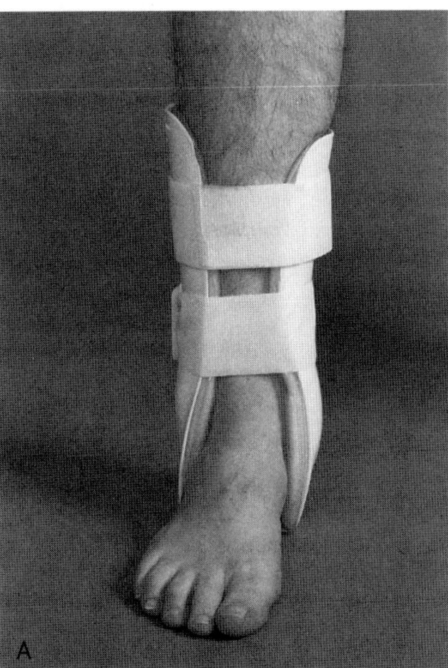

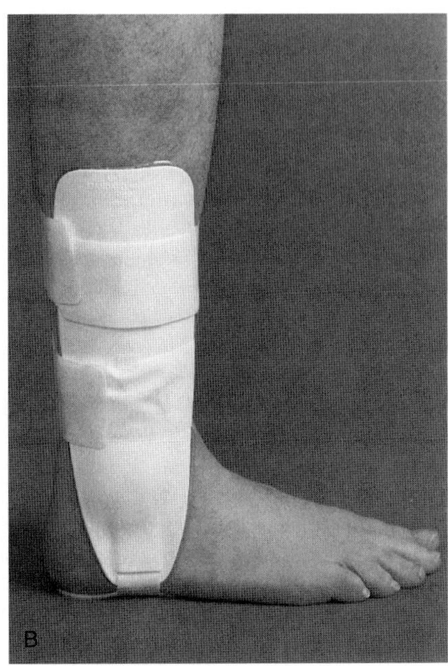

FIG. 259-15. **A** and **B.** Inflatable ankle stirrup.

An exception to the 90° principle is immobilization for rupture of the Achilles tendon. Patients with this injury should be immobilized in plantar flexion to reduce tension on the tendon.

ANKLE STIRRUP Like the posterior mold, the commercially available inflatable ankle splint (Fig. 259-15A and Fig. 259-15B) is useful for ankle sprains and minor avulsion fractures. It is equipped with valves and tubes to allow the addition or removal of air, although it usually comes optimally pre-inflated. Printed instructions are typically included, describing the method of determining and creating the proper degree of inflation and also describing rehabilitation exercises for the patient.

The ankle stirrup is essentially a ''sugar-tong'' splint held in place by Velcro straps. It prevents eversion and inversion but does not limit ankle plantarflexion or dorsiflexion. It is removable by the patient for purposes of bathing or when not bearing weight.

If the patient does remove the splint temporarily, a common error when re-applying it is to fail to unwrap the Velcro straps completely, specifically, to leave the straps attached posteriorly, so that the splint is ''hinged'' along its posterior aspect, like a ''book.'' This may result in the foot's persistently slipping forward and out of the splint. The clinician may wish to instruct the patient that the proper way to re-apply the splint is to unwrap the straps *all the way around*, so that the sides fall apart bilaterally, with the foot pad acting as the ''hinge'' on the plantar aspect (Fig. 259-16). The foot can then be positioned on the lower pad, and the sides brought together to adequately grasp the medial and lateral aspects of the ankle and lower leg. The final step is to wrap the straps about the posterior and anterior aspects of the dressing.

ADJUNCTS TO AMBULATION

Crutches

Crutches should be used by patients who can bear no weight at all on an injured lower extremity. Ideal crutch height is one hand width below the axillae. The grip bar should be adjusted to a height at which the elbows are still mildly flexed while supporting the body weight. The patient should be instructed to bear the pressure of the pads against the sides of the thorax rather than in the axillae, or brachial plexus injury might result (crutch palsy).

Any of several crutch gaits may be prescribed. With a two-point gait, the patient advances the crutches first, and then brings the well leg up to the crutches (''swing-to'' gait) or just past the crutches (''swing-through'' gait). With a three-point gait, the crutches and the injured extremity are all advanced together, and then the well extremity is advanced to meet them. The three-point gait results in slower forward progression than does the two-point gait, but requires less energy. Partial weight-bearing or no weight-bearing may be prescribed for the injured extremity, regardless of the gait used.

The method for negotiating stairs is similar for the two- and three-point gaits. Ascending stairs, the patient advances the well extremity up to the next step, followed by the crutches and the injured extremity. Descending stairs, the crutches are lowered first.

Walkers and Canes

Most elderly or infirm patients do not have the strength to use crutches safely. For them, a walker or cane is more suitable. Unfortunately, these devices are more appropriate for partial weight-bearing than for full non–weight-bearing conditions. Elderly patients who can bear no weight at all on an injured extremity may require initial bed rest and subsequent rehabilitation.

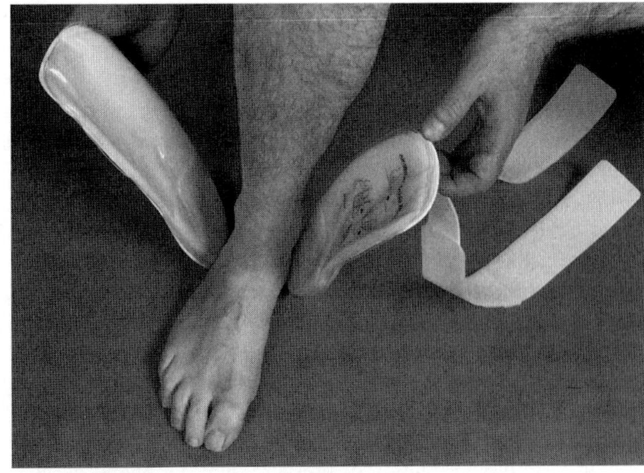

FIG. 259-16. Technique for applying ankle stirrup.

The technique for using a walker is essentially intuitive, with the patient simply lifting it and placing it a short distance ahead, then advancing up to it. By contrast, the technique for using a cane tends to be counterintuitive. Most patients instinctively hold a cane on the same side as the injured extremity. In fact, when the cane is held in the hand on the *well* side, much less strength is required to maintain balance, resulting in an easier and less awkward gait. The patient should be instructed to advance the cane (held on the well side) and the injured extremity simultaneously, then advance the noninjured extremity to meet them.

DISCHARGE INSTRUCTIONS

Continuous elevation of the injured part usually helps minimize swelling and pain. However, most individuals do not share the physician's knowledge that, to be effective, elevation must be above the level of the heart. Patients with an injured lower extremity often sit at home or at work with the leg resting on a chair, thinking they are complying with instructions. The patient should understand that the benefits of elevating a lower extremity can only be achieved in a recumbent or near-recumbent position, with the leg supported higher than the rest of the body.

Patients discharged in a lower-extremity plaster dressing should be cautioned not to rest the heel on the floor or any other hard surface. Plaster takes about 24 h to fully set. During this time, prolonged pressure on the heel can gradually create an indentation that may cause significant discomfort or even a pressure sore. This is not a consideration with fiberglass, which sets immediately.

If an upper-extremity sugar-tong dressing has been applied, the patient should be instructed to work the fingers (wiggle or wave) as much as possible to minimize stiffness and swelling. The sugar-tong splint should allow full flexion of the metacarpophalangeal joints.

Patients should be advised to watch the fingers or toes for excessive swelling, decreased sensation, or cyanosis, and to be alert for a significant increase in pain. Any of these signs or symptoms warrant a return to the emergency department or prompt evaluation by the follow-up physician.

When crutches, a cane, or a walker is supplied, instruction for use should be provided, and the patient's ability to navigate with such aids should be verified.

FOLLOW-UP

There is no universally prescribed follow-up interval for specific injuries. Physicians differ as to how soon patients should be seen. Generally, patients with unreduced fractures or injuries that require future surgical intervention should be seen within a few days.

Sometimes the situation may be discussed with the follow-up physician and an appointment arranged while the patient is still in the emergency department. Alternatively, the emergency physician may instruct the patient to contact the follow-up physician or clinic as soon as possible. If the name of the injury is written on the discharge instruction sheet, the patient can convey it at the time of the call. Based on this information, the follow-up physician can decide when the patient should be seen.

COMPLICATIONS

Complications associated with musculoskeletal injury may be early or delayed, and may occur minutes, days, weeks, or even months later.

Neurologic Deficit

Neurologic injury resulting from long-bone fractures or joint dislocations is usually due to traction or pressure on a peripheral nerve or a nerve plexus. Such complications usually manifest themselves early. Recovery may take hours, days, or weeks. Sometimes they are irreversible. Prompt reduction of deformity can often prevent, eliminate, or mitigate the effects of neurologic involvement, but is not a guarantee against permanent deficit.

Vascular Injury

Peripheral vessels that run close to a joint may sometimes be compressed or disrupted when that joint becomes dislocated, as, for example, with dislocation of the ankle or knee (tibiofemoral joint). Loss of peripheral pulse, or poor-to-absent capillary refill, calls for expeditious reduction of deformity. Even after reduction, evidence of significant vascular injury may be delayed. Patients who experience tibiofemoral dislocation, for example, may undergo routine post-reduction angiography to verify the integrity and patency of the popliteal vessels, regardless of whether a circulatory deficit was noted on initial examination.

Compartment Syndrome

The limbs are divided into ''compartments'' by longitudinal partitions of fascia. Each compartment is a closed space, whose fascial borders are firm and relatively unyielding. With musculoskeletal injury, either a direct blow or a fracture, there may be extravasation of blood, swelling of muscle tissues, and impairment of venous flow within a given compartment. Eventually, this leads to increased pressure, which can compromise circulatory perfusion of the muscles and nerves in that compartment. If the tissues remain ischemic for a sufficient period of time, irreversible necrosis and permanent neurologic damage and muscle contracture can occur.[9]

Clinical evidence of ongoing compartment syndrome is a true emergency, requiring expeditious diagnosis and aggressive treatment, sometimes surgical fasciotomy, to try to prevent permanent disability.

Early diagnosis of compartment syndrome is typically presumptive, based on index of suspicion. Classic signs of compartment syndrome, the five ''P's,'' have been described: pain, pallor, paralysis, pulselessness, and paresthesias. The problem is that, by the time all these signs are present, irreversible damage has almost always occurred. The emergency physician should be alert for the *earliest* sign of impending compartment syndrome, which is pain. Although some degree of pain is normally associated with fractures, it can usually be relieved by reduction, immobilization, and customary doses of oral or parenteral analgesics. Contrary to this is the pain associated with compartment syndrome, which is due to ischemia. It is perceived by the patient as deep, continuous, and poorly localized, and, unlike typical fracture pain, is extremely difficult to control, even with large and frequent doses of parenteral analgesics. In the upper extremity, the pain is typically exacerbated by passive extension of the patient's fingers. In the lower extremity, the usual exacerbating maneuver is passive flexion of the toes.

Other early signs of still-reversible compartment syndrome are tight swelling and tenseness along one aspect of an extremity, and paresthesias or hypesthesia in the area of skin served by the cutaneous nerve contained within the affected compartment. Unfortunately, none of these signs occurs consistently. However, they are sufficiently common that, when any of them is present (most commonly uncontrollable pain), the possibility of an evolving compartment syndrome should be considered and surgical consultation obtained. Patients with altered mental status, in whom pain and paresthesias cannot be relied upon as early indicators of compartment syndrome, need to be monitored for physical signs such as tenseness of the affected area, skin cyanosis (early) or pallor (late), and impaired circulatory status.

In some emergency departments, a percutaneous manometer is available to measure intracompartmental pressure. Under normal circumstances, the pressure should be close to zero. Pressures of 30–40 mm Hg usually indicate the need for fasciotomy. Once the pressure equals or exceeds the patient's diastolic blood pressure, perfusion of the tissues within the compartment is physiologically impossible, and fasciotomy may be indicated even in the presence of a palpable peripheral pulse.

Delayed and Late Complications

Patients who have sustained a fracture may be at risk for pulmonary fat embolus, usually originating from the marrow of a large bone, such as the femur. If fat embolism occurs, it usually does so within the first few days after injury, rather than in the first hours. This event may have a variable effect on pulmonary function, ranging from mild distress to severe or even fatal respiratory failure.

The most delayed complications of fractures include nonunion, malunion (healing with deformity), joint stiffness, traumatic arthritis of an involved joint, avascular necrosis of one of the bone fragments, and, in the case of open fractures, osteomyelitis.

ACKNOWLEDGMENTS

Original artwork: is by Eleanore Denton Rhodes, AMI.
Photography: is by Joy Miller, BPA., and Joe Driscoll.

REFERENCES

1. Salter RB, Harris WR: Injuries involving the epiphyseal plate. *J Bone Joint Surg* 45A:587, 1963.
2. Buckwalter JA, Einhorn TA, Bolander ME, Cruess RL: Healing of the musculoskeletal tissues, in Rockwood CA Jr, Green DP, Bucholz RW, Heckman JD (eds.): *Fractures in Adults*, vol 1, 4th ed. Philadelphia, Lippincott-Raven, 1996, pp. 261–304.
3. Schultz RJ: *The Language of Fractures.* Baltimore, Williams & Wilkins, 1972.
4. Antrum RM, Solomkin JS: A Review of antibiotic prophylaxis for open fractures. *Orthop Rev* 16:246, 1987.
5. Worlock P, Slack R, Harvey L, Mawhinney R: The prevention of infection in open fractures: An experimental study of the effects of antibiotic therapy. *J Bone Joint Surg* 70A:1341, 1988.
6. Chapman MW, Olson SA: Open fractures, in Rockwood CA Jr, Green DP, Bucholz RW, Heckman JD (eds.): *Fractures in Adults,* vol 1, 4th ed. Philadelphia, Lippincott-Raven, 1996, pp. 305–352.
7. Gustillo RB, Merkow RL, Templeman D: Current concepts review: The management of open fractures. *J Bone Joint Surg* 72A:229, 1990.
8. Anderson K, Jensen PO, Lauritzen J: Treatment of clavicular fractures: Figure of eight bandage vs. a simple sling. *Acta Orthop Scand* 57:71, 1987.
9. Whitesides TE Jr, Haney TC, Morimoto K, Harado H: Tissue pressure measurements as a determinant for the need of fasciotomy. *Clin Orthop* 113:43, 1975.

INJURIES TO THE HAND AND DIGITS

Robert L. Muelleman

Hand injuries are commonly encountered in the ED. The best outcome often depends on an accurate initial evaluation and treatment. This chapter covers soft tissue injuries distal to the volar wrist crease and fractures distal to the carpal bones.

EPIDEMIOLOGY

Each year in the United States, nearly 1.4 million patients present to the ED with hand and finger symptoms. A recent series of 1000 consecutive hand problems indicated that 42 percent had lacerations, 27 percent had contusions, 17 percent had fractures, and 5 percent had infections. Two-thirds of presenters were male and one-third were under 18 years old; one-third of the injuries occurred at home. The most common mechanism was blunt trauma (50 percent) followed by sharp object (25 percent).

ANATOMY

The hand consists of 27 bones: 14 phalangeal bones, 5 metacarpal bones, and 8 carpal bones arranged in 5 rays of metacarpals and phalanxes having its base at the carpometacarpal (CMC) articulation (Fig. 260-1).

The carpal bones are made up of two rows of four bones. They are concave on the volar surface and bridged by flexor retinaculum. This forms the carpal tunnel through which pass the median nerve and the nine long flexor tendons of the fingers. The bases of the second and third CMC articulation are fixed. The thumb, ring, and little finger have mobility at the CMC joint and provide movement that allows for grasp and adaptive movement of the hand.

The soft tissue supporting these bones and joints are the capsular ligamentous structures that give stability, the intrinsic muscles of the hand, and the tendinous structures that generate mobility. The collateral ligaments of the MP joints are tightest in flexion (Fig. 260-2). The IP collaterals are tight throughout the entire range of motion (Fig. 260-2). The intrinsic muscles of the hand are those that have their origins and insertions within the hand. They consist of the muscle of the thenar and hypothenar eminences, adductor pollicis, the interossei, and the lumbricals.

The thenar muscles cover the thumb metacarpal, originate in the flexor retinaculum and carpal bones, and insert at the base of the first metacarpal and first proximal phalanx. The thenar muscles consist of abductor pollicis brevis, opponens pollicis, and flexor pollicis brevis. The median nerve innervates all three. Adductor pollicis is innervated by the ulnar nerve and originates from the second and third metacarpals and inserts in the first proximal phalanx.

The hypothenar group includes opponens digiti minimi, the flexor digiti minimi, and the abductor digiti minimi. These muscles originate in the flexor retinaculum and carpal bones and insert at the proximal phalanx and metacarpal of the little finger. They are innervated by the ulnar nerve (Fig. 260-3).

There are seven interossei. The three palmar and four dorsal interossei lie between the metacarpal bones and originate from them. The palmar interosseus and the palmar portion of the dorsal interosseus have an insertion into the extensor hood. The palmar interosseus adducts the index, ring, and small finger. The dorsal portion of the dorsal interosseus inserts by tendons into the base of the proximal phalanx. The dorsal interosseous muscles abduct the fingers away from the midline. The interossei are innervated by the ulnar nerve (Fig. 260-4).

The lumbricals arise from the flexor digitorum profundus tendons in the palm and course radially to the metacarpophalangeal (MP) joints and reinforce the interosseous lateral band on the radial side of the digit. The lumbricals contribute little to the flexion of the MP joint; however, they contribute to the extension of the interphalangeal (IP) joints. The lumbricals play a critical role coordinating the flexor and extensor system of the digits. The median nerve innervates the radial two lumbricals, and the ulnar nerve innervates the ulnar two.

The extensor tendons course over the dorsal side of the forearm, wrist, and hand. Nine extensor tendons pass under the extensor retinaculum and separate into six compartments. In the dorsum of the hand, the extensores digitorum communis are connected by junctura. Because of this, a complete tendon laceration proximal to the junctura may still result in normal extensor function. In the finger, the extensor expansion divides into a central slip that attaches to the middle phalanx and into two lateral bands that join with the tendons of the lumbricals and interosseous muscles and that attach to the base of the distal phalanx (Fig. 260-5).

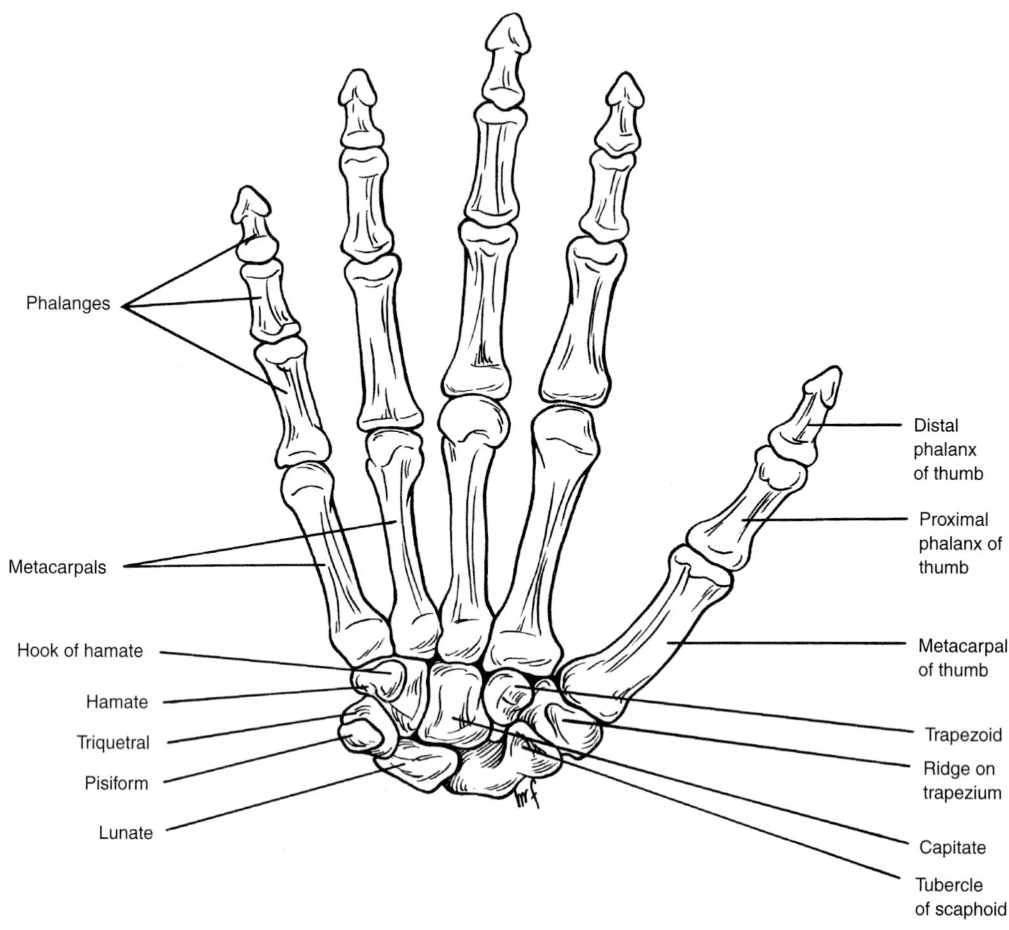

FIG. 260-1. Bones of the hand.

The flexor tendons course over the volar side of the forearm, wrist, and hand. Flexor carpi radialis, flexor carpi ulnaris, and palmaris longus primarily flex the wrist. The remaining nine tendons pass through the carpal tunnel. One tendon goes to the base of the distal phalanx of the thumb. The other four digits have two tendons each. The flexor digitorum superficialis (FDS) inserts into the middle phalanx and flexes all the joints it crosses. The flexor digitorum profundus (FDP) runs deep to FDS until the level of the MP joint where FDS bifurcates. FDP inserts at the base of the distal phalanx and acts primarily to flex the distal interphalangeal (DIP) joint as well as all other joints flexed by FDS (Fig. 260-6). Unlike the extensor tendons, the flexor tendons are enclosed in synovial sheaths, making them prone to deep space infections.

The hand and digits have dual blood supplies with contributions from the radial and ulnar arteries. The blood supply of the proximal portion of the hand is composed of a series of deep and superficial arches on the palmar and dorsal side. The blood supply of the fingers is distributed by the digital arteries that arise from the superficial palmar arch (Figs. 260-3 and 260-7).

The radial, ulnar, and median nerves innervate the hand. In the hand, the median and ulnar nerves have mixed motor and sensory function. The radial nerve (C5–T1) just has sensory function to the dorsal radial aspect of the hand. The ulnar nerve (C7–T1) supplies sensory function to the ulnar one and one-half fingers and motor function to the hypothenar muscles, ulnar two lumbricals, interossei, adductor pollicis, and the deep head of the flexor pollicis longus. The median nerve (C5–T1) supplies sensory function to the thumb and radial two and one-half fingers and motor function to abductor pollicis brevis, superficial head of flexor pollicis brevis, and opponens pollicis (Fig. 260-8). As the digital nerves course through the palm, they are superficial structures and are the structures most often injured, so that digital nerve sensation and two-point discrimination should be routinely assessed when evaluating lacerations of the palm (Fig. 260-9). The palm is often called "no man's land" because penetrating injuries in this area are so difficult to evaluate and treat. Careful neurovascular testing of the hand and digits is necessary for all palmar injuries that involve more than the skin, and hand consultation is advised if the extent of injury is uncertain. In the digits, digital nerves divide into volar and dorsal branches to supply sensation to the fingers. Knowing their location is important to properly perform a digital block (see Fig. 260-3).

PRINCIPLES OF EVALUATION

It is important not to let a visually striking hand injury delay the identification and treatment of other potentially life-threatening injuries. After hemorrhage control, assessment involves a detailed history, general hand examination, testing of nerves and tendons, anesthesia, and direct wound inspection. Comparison with the uninjured hand is helpful, especially to identify partial motor or sensory deficits.

History

The history should include the time and cause of injury as well as the possibility of associated crush, burn, or chemical exposure. The posi-

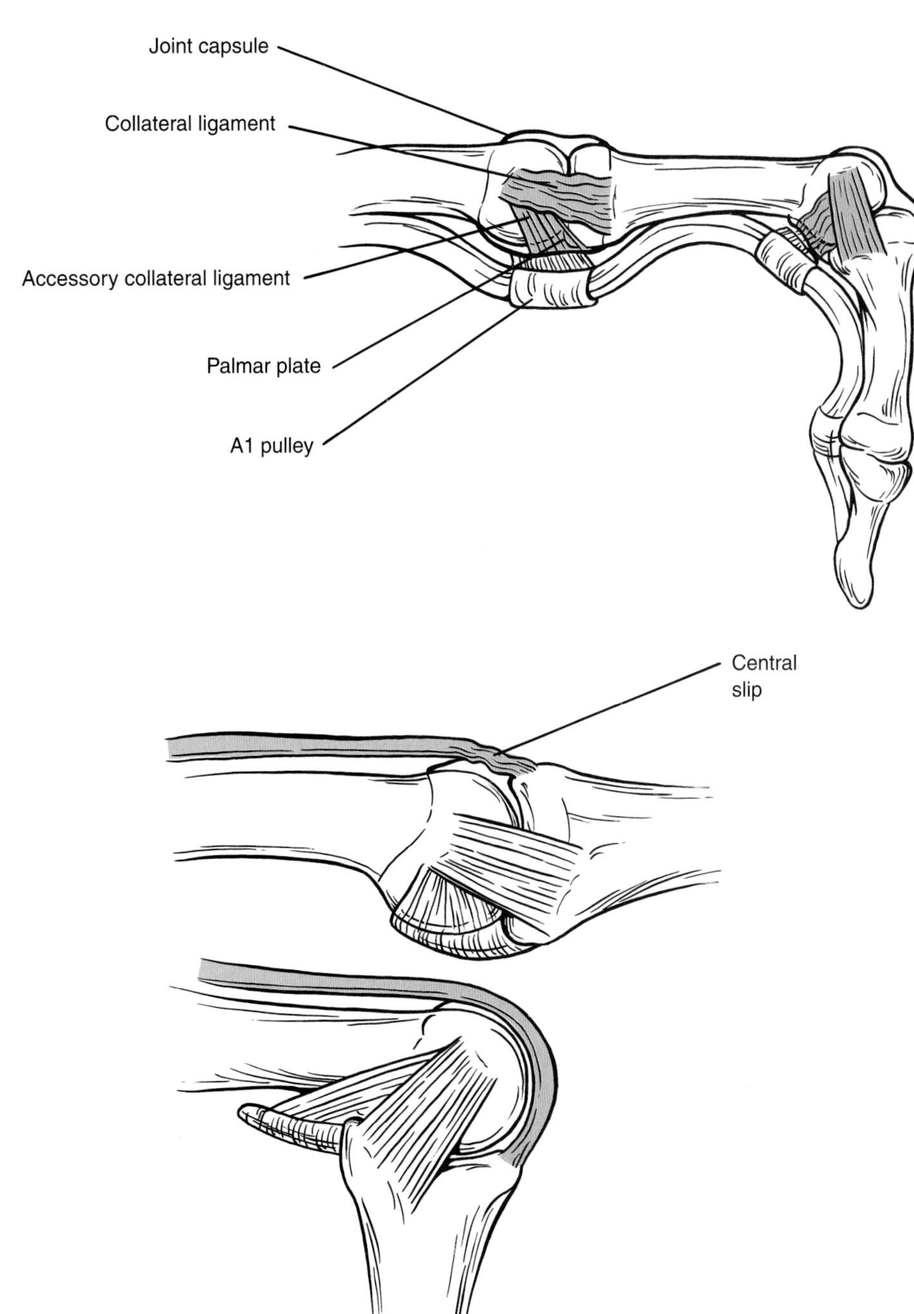

FIG. 260-2. Ligament attachments of the metacarpophalangeal and interphalangeal joints.

tion of the hand at the time of injury should be determined. Injuries with the digits in flexion may result in retraction of the cut end of the tendon when the digit is examined in neutral position. The patient's occupation, avocations, prior hand injuries, and handedness should be documented because they are important indicators of the functional impact of the injury.

General Hand Examination

The general examination should detail the extent of injury by documenting the amount of devascularization, status of the skin, posture of the fingers, and presence of deformity or active bleeding. Bilateral grip strength should be checked. Have the patient make a clenched fist to observe the orientation of the middle and distal phalanxes. They should be oriented parallel to each other with the nails positioned in the same plane when the fist is clenched. Then, starting with the fingers extended, the patient should draw the fingertips together, so that the tip of the thumb contacts the tips of the other four digits. This is a gross estimation of intact median, ulnar, and radial nerve motor function. Pincer function should also be routinely tested. Have the patient tightly grasp a piece of paper between the thumb and index finger. Weakness suggests median nerve or ulnar collateral ligament disruption, depending on the mechanism of injury being evaluated. Circulation is assessed by regional pulses and capillary refill.

NERVE TESTING To test the median nerve, have the patient flex the distal phalanx of the thumb against resistance. Test opposition by touching the tip of the thumb to the tip of the little finger. The patient may be able to accomplish this range of motion with loss of median

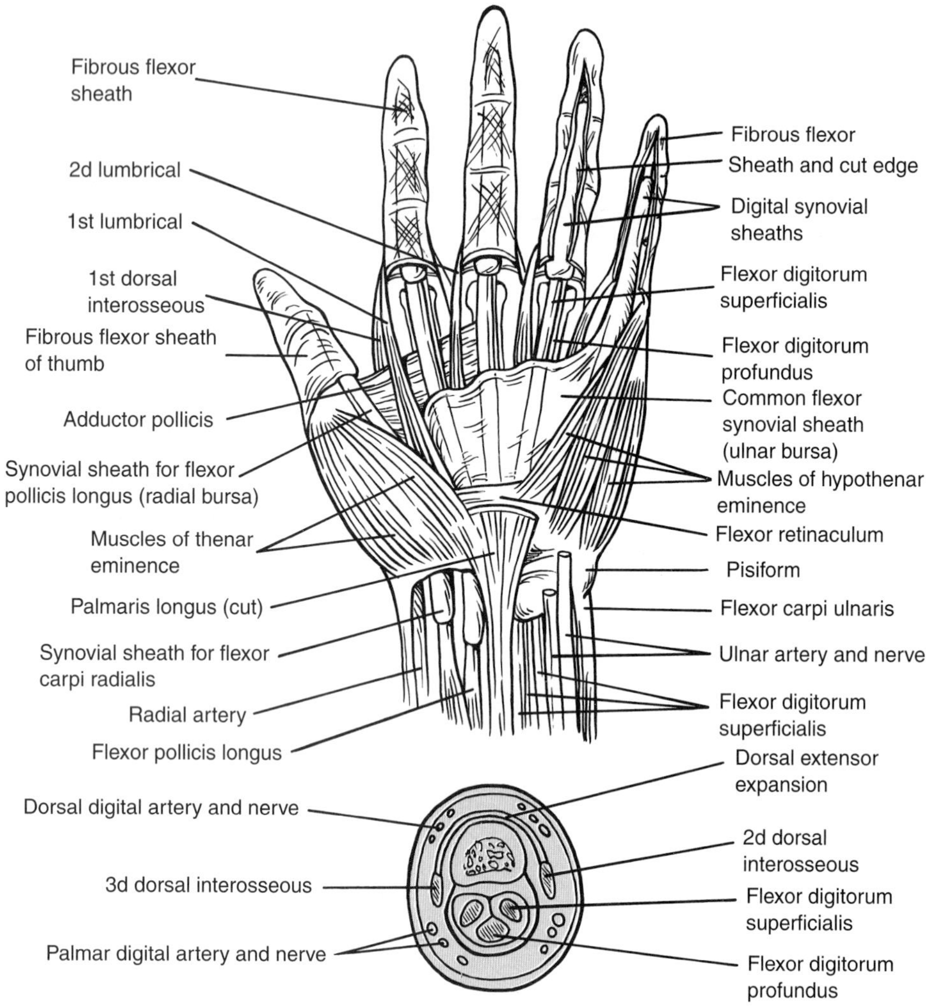

FIG. 260-3. Anterior view of the hand showing relationship of muscles and tendon sheaths.

nerve function due to compensation with muscle groups innervated by the ulnar nerve, but the patient will be unable to oppose against resistance if median nerve function is lost. Finally, test thumb abduction by placing the hand palm up and raising the thumb to the perpendicular while palpating the belly of the abductor pollicis muscle to insure it is contracting.

To test the ulnar nerve, spread the fingers apart against resistance and then push them together against resistance. To test the hypothenar muscles (ulnar innervation), extend the fingers and then move the fifth finger away from the others. To test thumb adduction (the ulnar nerve innervates the adductor pollicis muscles), bring the thumb tightly against the side of the index finger. Adductor strength can be further tested by interposing a piece of paper between the thumb and the side of the index finger and then trying to pull the paper away. To test the radial nerve, extend the fingers and wrist. With the thumb in the hitchhiking position, test its resistance to further extension.

Sensation is determined by two-point discrimination. Normal two-point discrimination is <6 mm at the fingertips and is often <2 mm. Both injured and noninjured fingers must be compared. Because patients are likely to guess correctly by chance, hand specialists recommend repeating two-point discrimination testing two to four times on each side of the digit. At least 80 percent accuracy is considered acceptable. Less than 80 percent or indeterminate accuracy suggests the possibility of digital nerve injury. A sensory deficit implies a potential digital artery laceration because of the close proximity of the two.

TESTING OF TENDONS In assessing tendon function, full range of motion of each tendon against resistance should be assessed and compared with the uninjured side. It is important to test resistance because up to 90 percent of a tendon can be lacerated with preservation of range of motion without resistance. In addition, pain along the course of the tendon during resistance testing suggests a partial laceration even if strength appears adequate. Patients can distinguish deep pain of tendon laceration from the superficial pain of lacerated skin. FDP is tested by flexing the DIP against resistance while the MP and proximal interphalangeal (PIP) are held in extension. Flexing the PIP against resistance while the remaining fingers are held in full extension tests FDS. Each finger must be tested separately.

Anesthesia and Direct Wound Examination

Anesthesia and direct wound inspection is necessary because partial tendon lacerations or intraarticular injuries are not always readily apparent. Sensation and range of motion should be tested before anesthesia. In general, if a laceration needs to be extended in order to properly view the wound, hand consultation is in order. A bloodless field can be facilitated by milking the digit proximally and then applying a local tourniquet or Penrose drain around the base of the digit. The tourniquet should not be stretched to more than 150 percent of its length, and it can be held in place with a hemostat. The digit can be milked by wrapping another Penrose drain circumferentially

FIG. 260-4. Origins, insertions, and actions of the palmar and dorsal interossei.

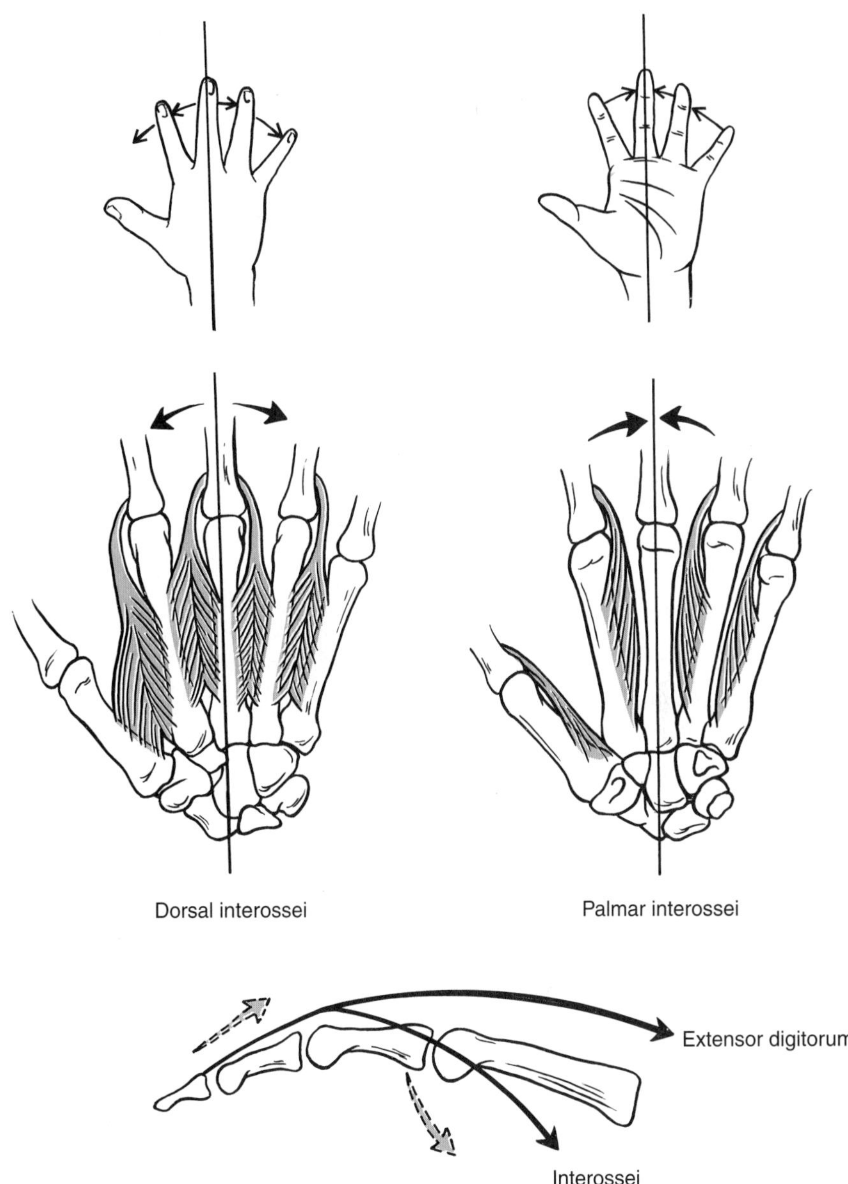

around the entire digit, going from distal to proximal or by reconfiguring a 4 × 4 gauze dressing into a narrow band and wrapping that circumferentially around the entire digit. Only moderate compression should be used to avoid compression injury to the digit. The tourniquet should not be left in place for more than 20 min. Contaminated wounds should be copiously irrigated with normal saline and antibiotics administered. Tetanus toxoid should be administered as needed.

Radiographs, Consultation, and Disposition

Radiologic evaluation should include at a minimum a posteroanterior (PA), lateral, and oblique projection. Similar projections are used for the digits, except that the x-ray beam is centered over the digits. Actual or suspected injuries of tendons and nerves should be referred to a hand specialist. Whether consultation is provided in the emergency department or in follow-up (1 to 3 days) depends on local resources. Often the skin can be closed, the hand splinted in the position of function, and at follow-up the wound can be extended, explored, and definitive repair performed by the hand specialist. Most hand specialists prefer to do definitive repair within a 3- to 5-day window after acute injury. While most tendon injuries <20 percent may not be surgically repaired, hand specialist follow-up and rehabilitation are still necessary to accurately determine the extent of injury, minimize scarring and tendon contraction, and minimize neuroma formation.

For patients with hand or digit lacerations that are sutured in the emergency department, and where there is no suspicion of neurovascular or tendon injury, follow-up evaluation and suture removal in the emergency department should always include repeat hand examination to make sure that significant injuries have not been missed.

TENDON INJURIES

Flexor Tendons

The most common cause of flexor tendon injury is a laceration. Flexor tendon lacerations can be subtle; however, the careful examiner will identify these injuries. A classification system for flexor tendon injuries

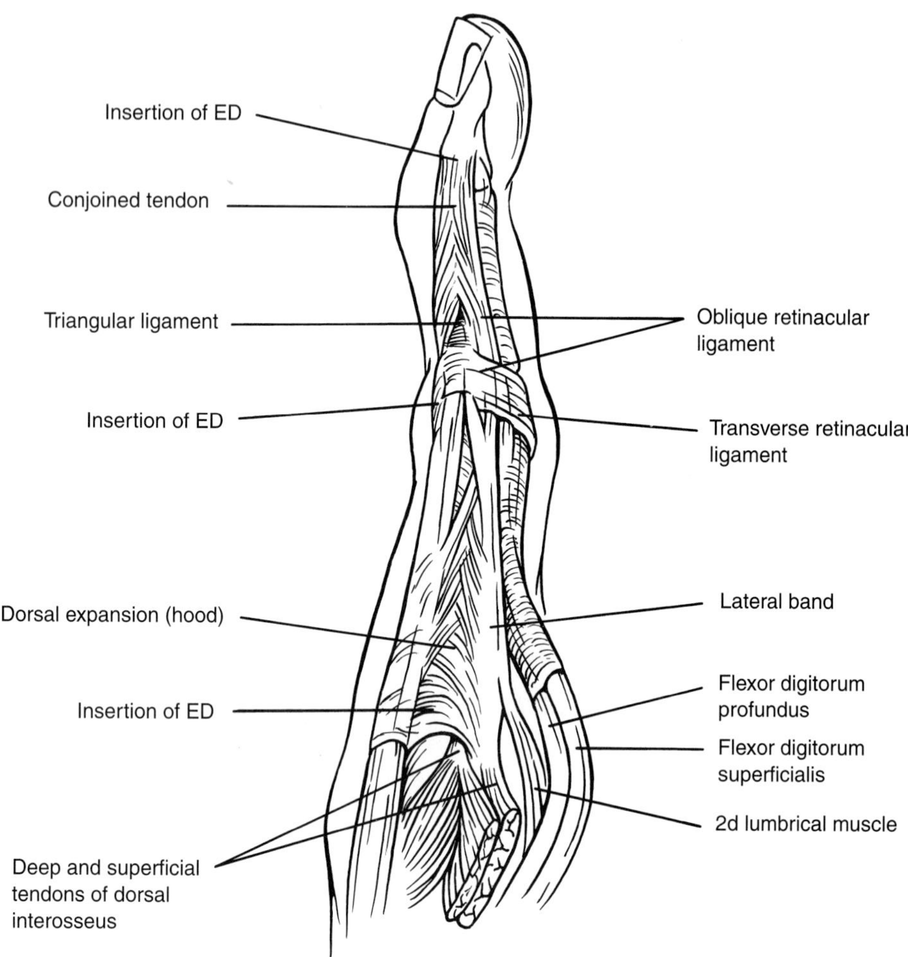

FIG. 260-5. The extensor mechanism in the finger.

has been developed based on location, treatment considerations, and prognosis.

ZONE I Extends from the insertion of FDS to the profundus tendon. Patients with these injuries lose flexion at the DIP. Retrieval of the proximal tendon is often difficult.

ZONE II Involves the portion of the digital canal occupied by both FDS and FDP. The close proximity of these tendons makes it essential for exact repair with minimal operative trauma. This region is often referred to as ''no man's land'' because of the frequent poor outcomes prior to the 1960s when improved repair techniques were developed. Lacerations in this zone are common, and partial lacerations are more common then complete.

ZONE III Extends from the distal edge of the carpal tunnel to the proximal edge of the flexor sheath. The lumbrical muscles originate from FDP in this region. Outcomes are generally favorable.

ZONE IV Involves the carpal tunnel and related structures. The area must be explored carefully because so many vital structures go through the carpal tunnel. Isolated injuries are the exception.

ZONE V Involves injuries to tendons proximal to the carpal tunnel. Injuries here tend to be severe and often involve multiple tendons as well as the median or ulnar nerve. It is essential to search for all major structures.

A hand surgeon should repair flexor tendon lacerations. Primary repair should occur within 12 h. Secondary repair can occur up to 4 weeks after the injury.

Another type of flexor tendon injury is the avulsion of FDP from its insertion in the distal phalanx. This can occur from a grasping motion against high-speed resistance. The patient will be unable to flex the distal phalanx. Prognosis depends on the size of the bony fragment, the length of time from injury to repair, and the blood supply to the tendon.

Extensor Tendon

The extensor tendons are the most common site of tendon injuries because of the superficial nature of the tendons on the dorsum of the hand. A classification system has been developed for assessing injury patterns, repair techniques, and rehabilitation.

ZONE I Involves the area over the distal phalanx and DIP. Injury can occur from blunt or sharp trauma. Complete laceration or rupture of the tendon at this level will result in the DIP joint flexed 40°. This injury after blunt trauma is often referred to as ''mallet finger,'' and it is the most common tendon injury in athletes. This injury has been classified as type I if there is tendon only rupture, type II if there is a small avulsion fracture, and type III if greater than 25 percent of the articular surface is involved. Types I and II can be treated with the DIP joint immobilized in slight hyperextension continuously for 6 to 10 weeks. Some hand surgeons may prefer operative treatment. Controversy exists whether treatment of type III injuries should be

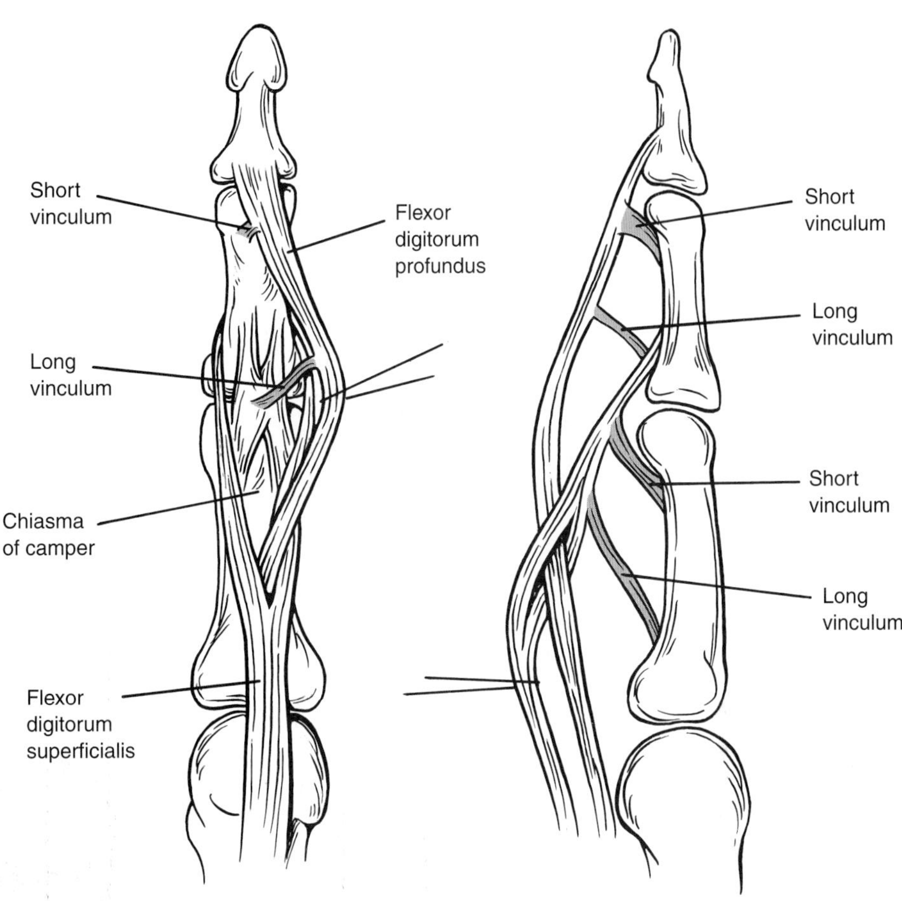

FIG. 260-6. Anatomy of flexor digitorum superficialis (FDS) and profundus (FDP).

conservative or operative. Chronic untreated mallet finger may develop a swan-neck deformity (Fig. 260-10). This is caused when the lateral bands are displaced proximally and dorsally, resulting in increased extension forces on the PIP joint.

ZONE II Involves the area over the middle phalanx. Injuries are usually due to laceration. Treatment is similar to zone I injuries.

ZONE III Involves the area over the PIP. The central tendon is the most commonly injured structure. Complete disruption of the central tendon may result in the volar displacement of the lateral bands, causing them to be flexors, along with the unopposed FDP. Additionally, the extensor hood retracts, causing extension of the MP and the DIP joints resulting in the boutonnière deformity (Fig. 260-11). Closed injuries are treated with the petrosal interphalangeal (PIP) joint immobilized in extension for 5 to 6 weeks.

ZONE IV Involves the area over the proximal phalanx. These injuries have clinical findings similar to zone III injuries. Often these injuries are less problematic because the joint is not involved and the tendon at this level is broad and flat.

ZONE V Involves the area over the MP. Open injuries to this area should be considered human bites until proven otherwise. Wounds from human bites should have delayed repair when free from infection. Clean wounds can be repaired primarily.

ZONE VI Involves the area over the dorsum of the hand. Because the tendons in this area are so superficial, even minor-appearing lacerations may be associated with one or more tendon injuries. If the laceration is proximal to the junctura tendineae, the patient may be able to extend the involved MP joint, because weak extensor forces are transmitted to the junctura from adjacent extensor tendons.

ZONE VII Involves the area over the wrist. Repair here can be difficult because of the presence of the extensor retinaculum. This thick, fibrous structure on the dorsum of the wrist contains 12 extensor tendons and 6 retinacular compartments that are lined with synovium.

ZONE VIII Involves the area of the distal forearm. Injuries to this area require a thorough exploration to identify all injured structures. The tendons frequently retract into the forearm and must be retrieved and repaired. As a general principle, lacerations of less than 25 percent don't require repair; 25 to 50 percent need simple suture repair, and greater than 50 percent need repair with a modified Kessler or similar technique. After repairs in zones V through VII, splinting should occur with the wrist in 15° extension, the MP joint in 15° flexion, and the IP in 15° flexion in the involved and adjacent digit.

LIGAMENT AND DISLOCATION INJURIES

Soft tissue injuries to the hand are extremely common. Accurate diagnosis and treatment are important to avoid complications such as joint luxatio, loss of motion, chronic pain, and deformity.

DIP

Dislocations of the DIP joint are uncommon because of the firm attachments of the skin and subcutaneous tissue to the underlying bone by osteocutaneous fibers. There is additional stability of the flexor and extensor tendons. When they do occur, they are usually dorsal. Longitudinal traction and hyperextension, followed by direct

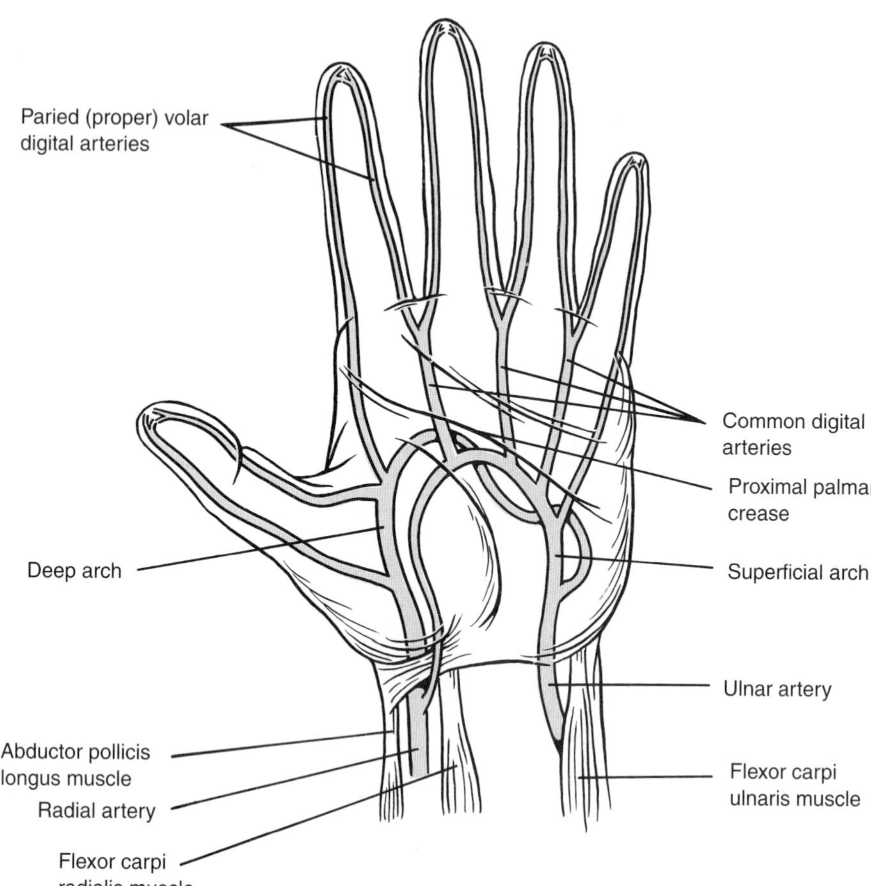

FIG. 260-7. The dual blood supply to the hands and digits.

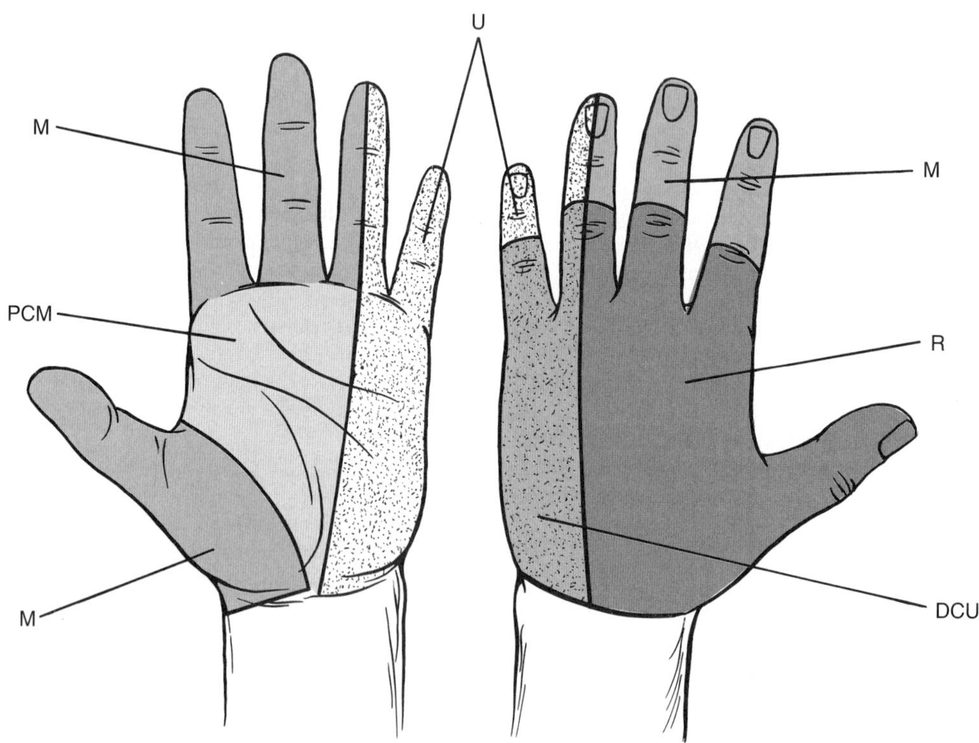

FIG. 260-8. The cutaneous nerve supply in the hand. M = median, R = radial, U = ulnar, PCM = palmar branch of median nerve, DCU = dorsal branch of ulnar nerve.

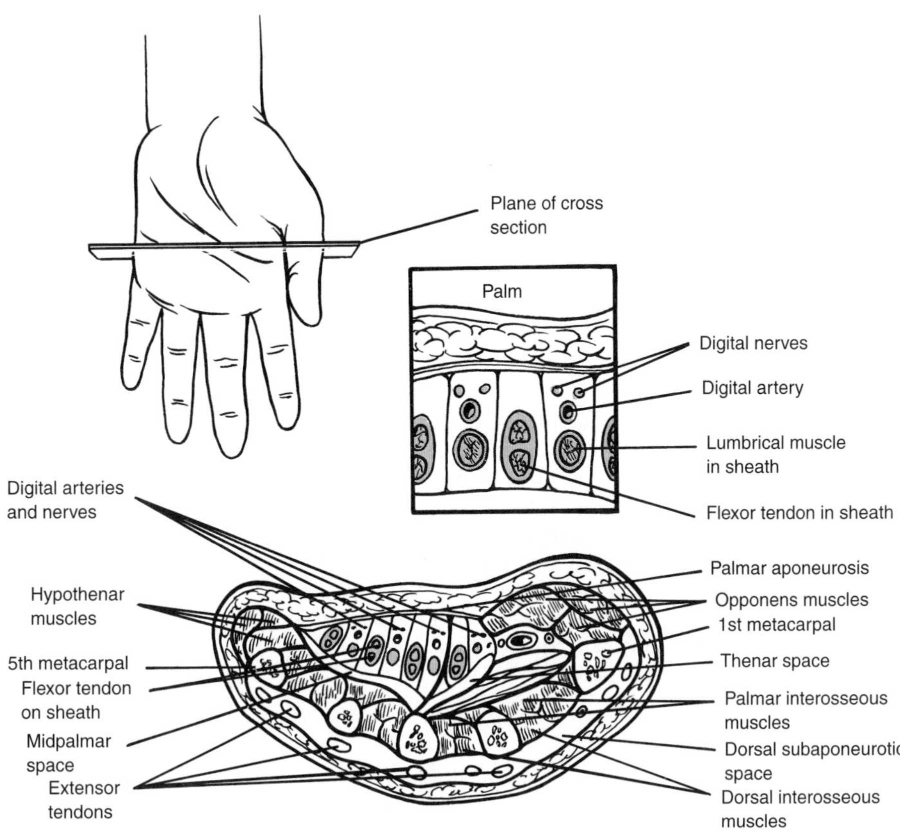

FIG. 260-9. Relationship of nerves, arteries, tendons, and muscles in the hand.

dorsal pressure to the base of the distal phalanx, accomplish reduction after digital nerve block. Irreducible cases may be due to the entrapment of an avulsion fracture, profundus tendon, or volar plate.

PIP

Dislocations of the PIP joint are one of the most common ligamentous injuries of the hand. The mechanism is usually due to axial load and hyperextension. Dorsal dislocation occurs when the volar plate ruptures. Lateral dislocations occur when one of the collateral ligaments ruptures with at least a partial avulsion of the volar plate from the middle phalanx. The digit is usually ulnarly deviated because the radial collateral ligament is six times more likely than the ulnar collateral ligament to rupture. Volar dislocations are rare. Dorsal dislocations are reduced similarly to DIP dorsal dislocations. After reduction, active motion and strength is tested. If testing is normal, the joint should be splinted at 30° flexion for 3 weeks. If the joint is irreducible or there is evidence of complete ligamentous disruption, operative repair is required.

MP

Dislocations of the MP joint are less common than at the PIP joint. The mechanism is usually due to hyperextension forces that rupture the volar plate causing dorsal dislocation. In simple dislocations (subluxation), the joint appears to be hyperextended 60 to 90° and the articular surfaces are still in contact. Reduction here does not involve hyperextension because it might convert a simple dislocation into a complex one. Reduction is performed with the wrist flexed to relax the flexor tendon and applying pressure over the dorsum of the proximal phalanx in a distal and volar direction. After reduction, the MP joint should be splinted in flexion. Complex dislocations appear less deformed. Because the volar plate is interposed in the MP joint space, closed reduction is usually not possible. Volar dislocations are rare and usually require operative reduction.

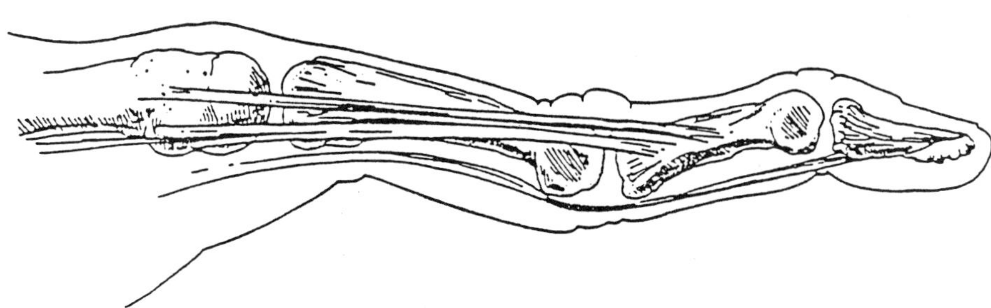

FIG. 260-10. Swan-neck deformity.

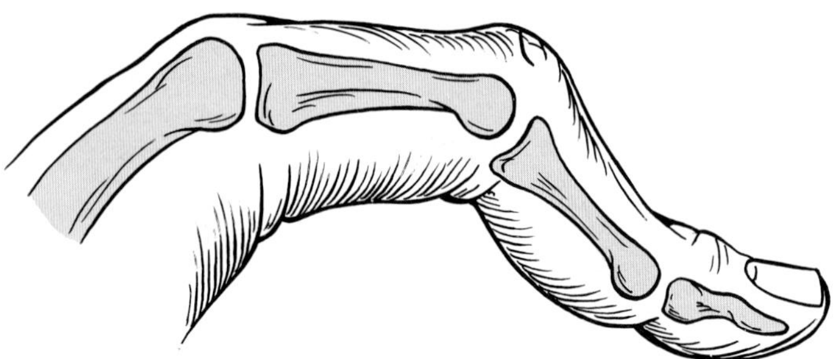

FIG. 260-11. Boutonnière deformity.

CMC

Dislocations of the carpometacarpal joint are uncommon because the joint is supported by strong dorsal, volar, and interosseous ligaments and are reinforced by the broad insertions of the wrist flexions and extensors. The cause is usually due to high-speed mechanisms such as motor vehicle crashes, falls, crushes, or clenched fist trauma. If a dislocation occurs, it is usually dorsal with associated fracture. Reduction of dorsal CMC dislocations can be attempted after regional anesthesia with traction and flexion with simultaneous longitudinal pressure on the metacarpal base. Early referral after reduction is needed to determine if further fixation is needed.

Thumb IP

Dislocations of the thumb IP are rare but, if present, usually open. The mechanism is usually hyperextension with rupture of the volar plate. Reduction is similar to the IP joints of the other digits. After reduction, the joint should be immobilized 3 weeks in mild flexion.

Thumb MP

Dislocations of the MP joint of the thumb are usually dorsal from a hyperextension force causing rupture of the volar plate. The dislocation may be simple or complex. Reduction, after radial nerve block, is accomplished with pressure directed distally on the base of the proximal phalanx with the metacarpal flexed and abducted.

Thumb MP Collateral Ligament Rupture

Rupture of the ulnar collateral ligament (gamekeeper's thumb; skier's thumb) occurs when the mechanism causes radial deviation (abduction) of the MP joint. The tear usually occurs at the insertion into the proximal phalanx. Often significant injury to the dorsal capsule and volar plate occurs. Stress testing of the ulnar collateral ligament is required and should be performed both in full extension and in 30° flexion. More than 40° of radial angulation indicates complete rupture and requires surgical consultation. Repair is best accomplished within 1 week. Radial collateral ligament rupture is not as common, and the mechanism is forced adduction.

Thumb CMC

Isolated thumb CMC dislocation is rare compared to the more common Bennett fracture dislocation. These are easy to reduce but unstable after reduction. After reduction, a thumb spica splint should be applied. These injuries should have a surgical referral for a decision on operative repair.

FRACTURES

Distal Phalanx

Fractures of the distal phalanx account for 15 to 30 percent of all hand fractures. Mechanisms are usually from crush or shearing forces. The fractures can be classified as tuft, shaft, or intraarticular. Tuft fractures can be associated with nail bed lacerations. Fractures at the base may be associated with flexor or extensor tendon involvement. Generally, these fractures are treated as soft tissue injuries with protective splinting.

Proximal and Middle Phalanx

The proximal phalanx has no tendinous attachments, therefore fractures frequently have volar angulation from the forces of the extensor and interosseous muscles. The middle phalanx has the FDS insert on the entire volar surface and the extensor tendon insert at the proximal base; therefore, fractures at the base have dorsal angulation and fractures at the neck result in volar angulation. A direct blow mechanism usually causes a transverse or comminuted fracture, while a twisting mechanism will more often result in a spiral fracture. Most often these fractures are stable and nondisplaced and can be treated with early protected motion by buddy taping. Unstable fractures amenable to closed reduction can be splinted from the elbow to the DIP with the wrist at 20° extension and the MP joint in 90° flexion. Midshaft transverse fractures, spiral fractures, and intraarticular fractures often require internal fixation.

Metacarpal (II-V) Fractures

The second and third metacarpals are relatively immobile, and fractures require anatomic reduction. The fourth and fifth metacarpals have 15 to 20° AP motion, which allows for some compensation. Metacarpal fractures are categorized as head, neck, shaft, or base fractures.

HEAD Fractures of the metacarpal head are usually due to a direct blow, crush, or missile. These fractures are distal to the insertion of the collateral ligaments and are often comminuted. If a laceration is present, a human bite must be considered. Treatment consists of ice, elevation, and immobilization with referral to a hand surgeon.

NECK Fractures of the metacarpal neck are usually due to a direct impaction force. A fracture of the fifth metacarpal neck is often referred to as a boxer's fracture. These fractures are usually unstable with volar angulation. Angulation of less than 20° in the fourth and 40° in the fifth metacarpal will not result in functional impairment. If greater angulation in these metacarpals occur, reduction should be attempted. In the second and third metacarpal, angulation of $<15°$ is acceptable. These fractures should be splinted with the wrist in 20° extension and the MP flexed at 90°. Fractures of the second or third metacarpal that are significantly displaced or angulated require anatomic reduction and surgical fixation.

SHAFT A direct blow usually injures fractures in this region. Rotational deformity and shortening are more likely in shaft fractures than in neck fractures. If manipulative reduction is necessary, operative fixation is usually indicated.

BASE Fractures at the base of the metacarpal are usually due to a direct blow or axial force. They are often associated with carpal bone fractures. Fractures at the base of the fourth and fifth metacarpal can result in paralysis of the motor branch of the ulnar nerve.

Thumb Metacarpal

Because of the mobility of the thumb metacarpal, shaft fractures are uncommon. Fractures usually involve the base.

EXTRAARTICULAR Extraarticular fractures are due to a direct blow or impaction mechanism. The mobility of the CMC joint can allow for 20° angular deformity. Angulation greater than this requires reduction and thumb spica splint for 4 weeks. Spiral fractures often require fixation.

INTRAARTICULAR Intraarticular fractures are due to impaction from striking a fixed object. Two fracture types have been described.

BENNETT FRACTURE A Bennett fracture is an intraarticular fracture with associated subluxation or dislocation at the CMC joint. The ulnar portion of the metacarpal usually remains in place. The distal portion usually subluxes radially and dorsally from the pull of abduction pollicis longus and the adductor pollicis. Treatment includes thumb spica splint and surgical referral.

ROLANDO FRACTURE A Rolando fracture is an intraarticular comminuted fracture at the base of the metacarpal. The mechanism of injury is similar to the Bennett fracture, but less common. Treatment includes thumb spica splint and surgical consultation.

BIBLIOGRAPHY

Belliappa PP, Scheker LR: Functional anatomy of the hand. *Emerg Med Clin North Am* 11:557, 1993.
Bowers WH: Sprains and joint injuries in the hand. *Hand Clin* 2:93, 1986.
Gaine WJ, Braidwood AS: Hand problems presenting to a district general hospital accident and emergency department. *J R Coll Surg Edinb* 41:401, 1996.
Gupta A, Kleinerl HE: Evaluating the injured hand. *Hand Clin* 9:195, 1993.
Weeks PM: Hand injuries. *Curr Probl Surg* 30:725, 1993.

261 INJURIES TO THE ELBOW AND FOREARM

Dennis T. Uehara
Harold W. Chin

ELBOW

Elbow Dislocation

The elbow is one of the most stable joints in the body. This stability is due to the adjacent muscular attachments, collateral ligaments, and inherent stability afforded by the hingelike articulation. Because of this stability, surgical repair for acute instability is usually not required, and chronic dislocations are unusual. Despite this, however, dislocations of the elbow are commonly seen, being third in large-joint dislocations, after glenohumeral and patellofemoral dislocations.

There are five general types of elbow dislocations: (1) posterior, (2) anterior, (3) medial, (4) lateral, and (5) divergent. The vast majority of elbow dislocations are posterior, all the others being uncommon. The mechanism of injury is usually a fall on the outstretched hand.

Clinically the patient presents with the elbow in 45° of flexion. The olecranon is prominent posteriorly, and the deformity resembles a displaced supracondylar fracture. If the patient is seen immediately after the injury, the bony landmarks can be identified. Later, however, the swelling may be quite severe, with no possibility of evaluating the injury topographically. A careful assessment of the neurovascular status is performed, with specific attention to the brachial artery and the ulnar, radial, and median nerves. The examination must be performed before and after manipulation, since neurovascular complications occur in 8 to 21 percent of patients, the most frequent being injury to the ulnar nerve. Vascular complications occur in 5 to 13 percent of elbow dislocations, with brachial artery injury the most common. Endean and coworkers found absence of a radial pulse before reduction, open dislocation, and other systemic injuries (head, chest, and abdomen) to be significantly associated with an arterial injury.

Radiographically, on the lateral view, both the ulna and radius are displaced posteriorly (Fig. 261-1). In the anteroposterior view, there may be lateral or medial displacement, with the ulna and radius in their normal relationship to each other. A search for associated fractures should be performed. In the child, a fracture of the medial epicondyle is most commonly seen. In adults, fractures of the coronoid process, radial head, capitellum, or olecranon may occur. Initially, these fractures should only be noted, with primary attention focused on the dislocation.

After adequate sedation, reduction is accomplished by gentle traction on the wrist and forearm in the direction in which it lies (Fig. 261-2). An assistant applies countertraction on the arm. Any medial or lateral displacement is corrected with the other hand. Downward pressure on the proximal forearm helps to disengage the coronoid process from the olecranon fossa. Distal traction is continued, and the elbow is flexed. With reduction, a palpable "clunk" is felt as the olecranon is seated in the humeral articular surface. The elbow is then moved through its full range of motion (ROM) to assess stability. If full smooth passive ROM is not possible, the postreduction radiograph should be examined for entrapment of the medial epicondyle, especially common in children (Fig. 261-3). Instability in extension suggests associated fractures or disruption of the capsule.

After reduction, the elbow is placed in a plaster splint from the axilla to the base of the fingers with the elbow in at least 90° of flexion. Because of the soft-tissue trauma and subsequent edema, cylinder casts should not be placed. A neurovascular follow-up examination should be obtained the following day.

Appropriate treatment of elbow dislocations requires adequate reduction and recognition of neurovascular complications, associated fractures, and postreduction instability. If there is any question of neurovascular compromise, the patient should be admitted for observation. Immediate orthopedic consultation should be sought if the dislocation is irreducible, if there is neurovascular compromise, for disruption of the joint capsule, if there are associated fractures, and for open dislocations.

Subluxation of the Radial Head (Nursemaid's Elbow)

Subluxation of the radial head is common among preschool children. The peak age is between 1 and 4 years, and it is usually not seen in children older than 7 years. The mechanism of injury is sudden traction on the hand with the elbow extended and the forearm pronated. Anatomically, during forceful traction, some fibers of the annular ligament, which encircles the radial neck, slip and become trapped between the radial head and capitellum. In the child up to age 5, the radial head is about the same size as the neck. After age 7, the size of the radial head is larger than the neck and subluxation does not occur.

Clinically the child sits comfortably with the parent, may even be playful, but does not use the injured arm. The arm is held in slight flexion and pronation. Supination is painful, and any effort to move the arm is resisted, although movement is free. The neurovascular examination is normal.

It is important to elicit the history of traction on the hand; the act may have been unrecognized by the parent or playmate or the history withheld because of a feeling of guilt or fear. Recently, an atypical history has been reported to occur in as many as 49 percent of radial

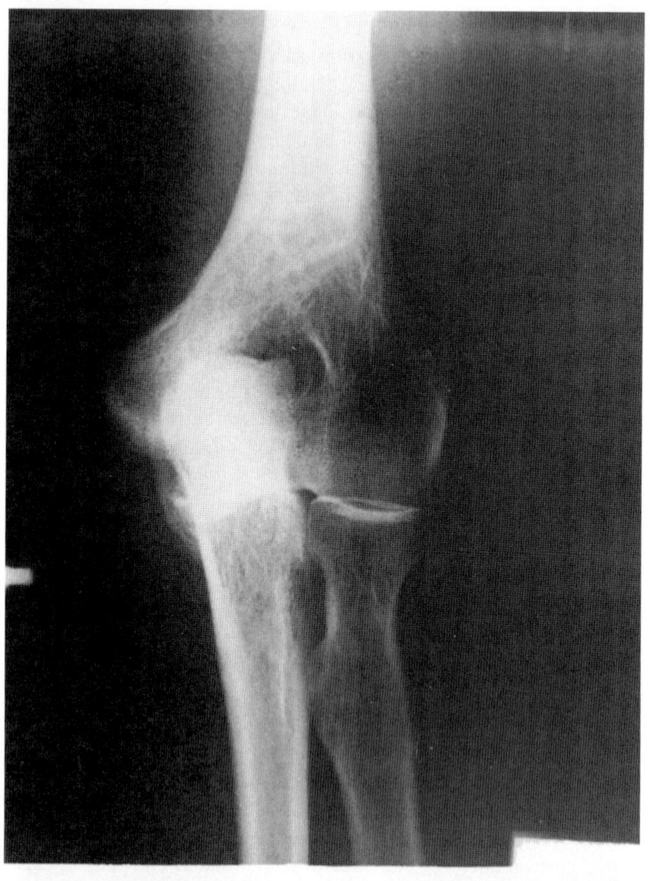

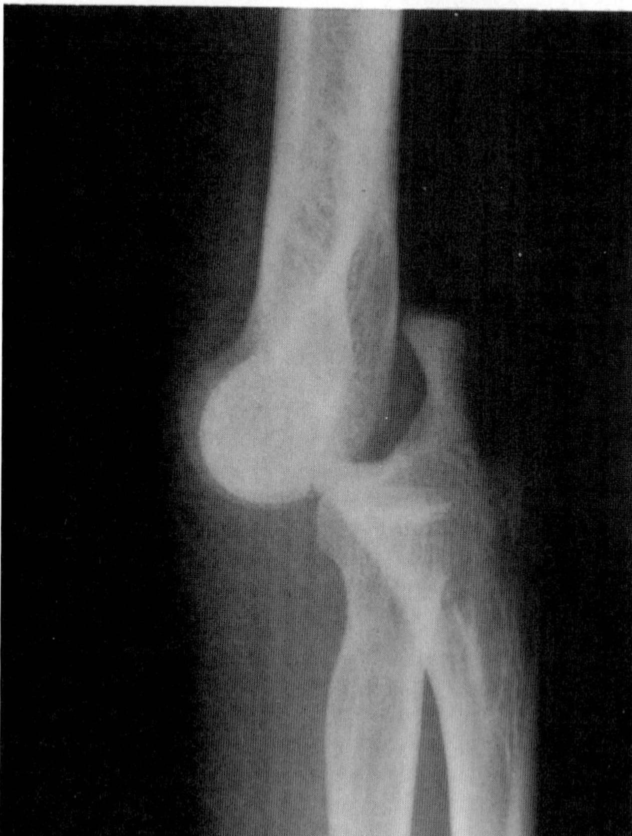

FIG. 261-1. Posterior dislocation of the elbow.

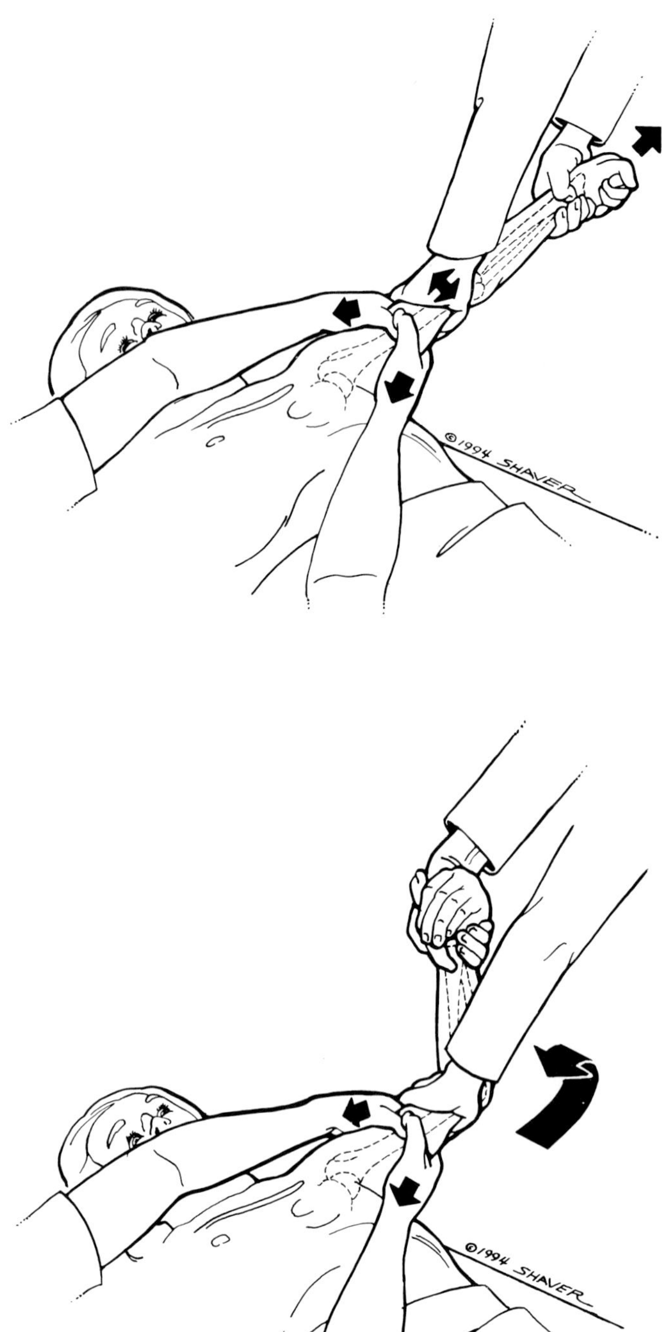

FIG. 261-2. Reduction of posterior elbow dislocation. **A.** Operator applies gentle traction as assistant applies countertraction. Displacement is corrected with the other hand. Downward pressure on the proximal forearm disengages the coronoid process from the olecranon fossa. **B.** Distal traction is continued as the elbow is flexed.

head subluxations. Any child not using an arm that is flexed and pronated and without signs of trauma should be considered to have a radial head subluxation unless the history strongly suggests another diagnosis. Radiographs are unnecessary unless another diagnosis is being considered or if reduction is not accomplished.

Reduction is carried out by firmly placing the thumb over the radial head while the other hand is placed on the wrist. The forearm is fully

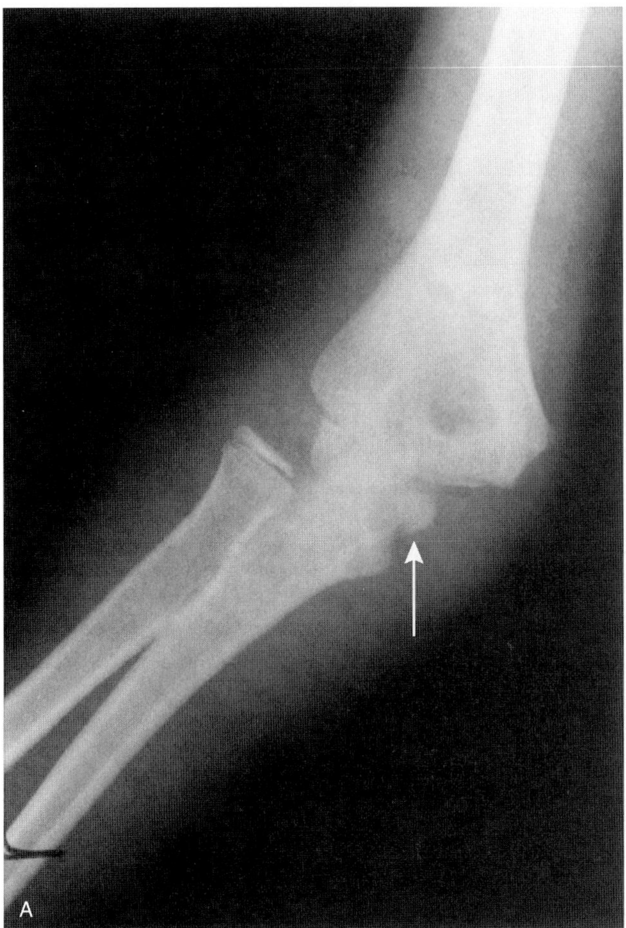

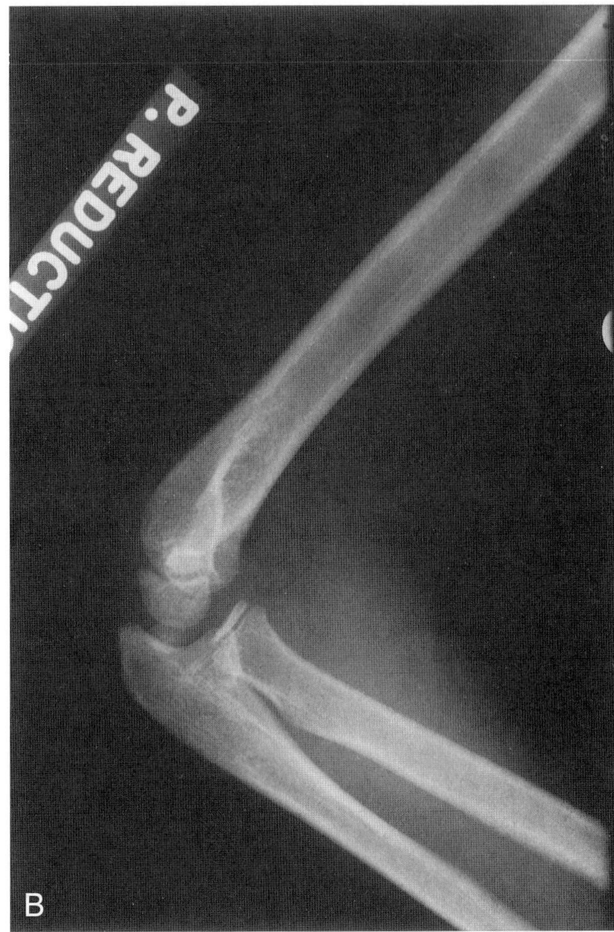

FIG. 261-3. Postreduction radiograph of a posterior elbow dislocation. The medial epicondyle is fragmented in the joint space and is seen in the anteroposterior and lateral radiographs (*arrow*).

supinated, and if a "click" is not felt, the elbow is flexed. This maneuver may be repeated if the initial attempt does not reduce the subluxation. Alternatively, the elbow may be extended. Both maneuvers are reported to be equally effective. Reduction as evidenced by a click is highly predictive and will result in relief from pain and, shortly thereafter, use of the affected arm.

After the first subluxation, no immobilization is required. For recurrent subluxations, however, orthopedic referral is needed. The patient's arm should be immobilized in a sling; some recommend a long-arm cast. Teach et al found a recurrence rate of 23.7 percent in either arm and 19.4 percent in the ipsilateral arm. Children 24 months or younger had a relative risk of 2.6 for recurrence when compared to children older than 24 months.

Intercondylar T or Y Fractures

Intercondylar fractures are much more common in adults than in children. Any distal humerus fracture in an adult should initially be assumed to be intercondylar rather than supracondylar (Fig. 261-4). A careful search should be made for a fracture line separating the condyles from each other and from the humerus. This distinguishes intercondylar T or Y fractures from other fractures of the distal humerus.

The mechanism of injury is a force directed against the elbow, driving the olecranon against the humeral articular surface separating the condyles and producing the typical fracture. These fractures are associated with severe soft-tissue injuries. Treatment in the young is directed at anatomic reduction. In older patients with severe injuries, treatment is often directed at joint motion through nonoperative means. As in supracondylar fractures, patients with severe swelling or displaced fractures should be admitted.

Supracondylar Fractures

These extraarticular fractures occur most commonly in children. Ninety-five percent are displaced posteriorly as a result of an extension force. When the mechanism of injury is due to a flexion force, the much less common anterior displacement occurs. There can also be various degrees of abduction, adduction, and rotation of the distal fragment.

EXTENSION-TYPE FRACTURES In an extension-type fracture, the patient will have significant swelling and tenderness at the elbow. The olecranon is prominent, and there is a depression proximally over the area of the triceps muscle. This appearance may be easily mistaken for a posterior elbow dislocation.

Radiographs may reveal a fat-pad sign in undisplaced fractures (Fig. 261-5). This is due to visualization of fat from the olecranon fossa (posterior fat pad) as it is displaced by the hemarthrosis. This may also occur anteriorly (anterior fat pad), although this is a less reliable sign. In some undisplaced fractures, the fracture line may not be seen, with the fat-pad sign being the only evidence of injury. Treatment should be initiated as though a fracture were identified, with splint immobilization and orthopedic consultation. In displaced fractures, the anteroposterior radiograph usually reveals a transverse

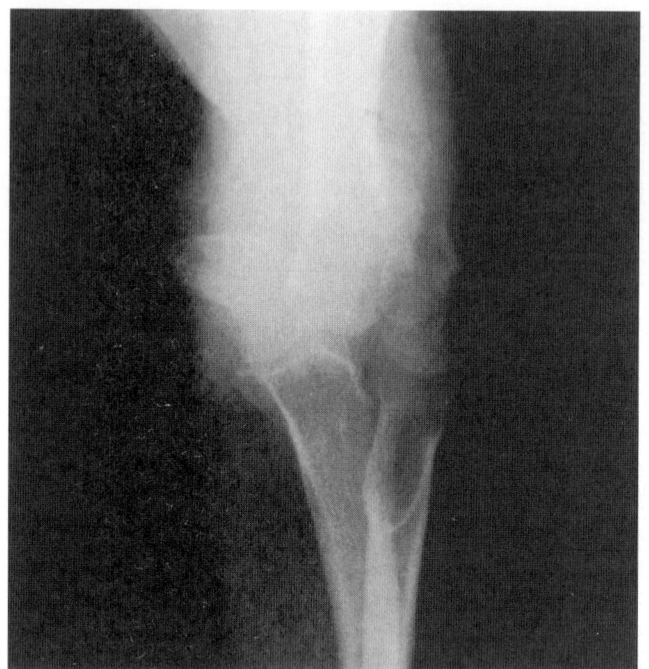

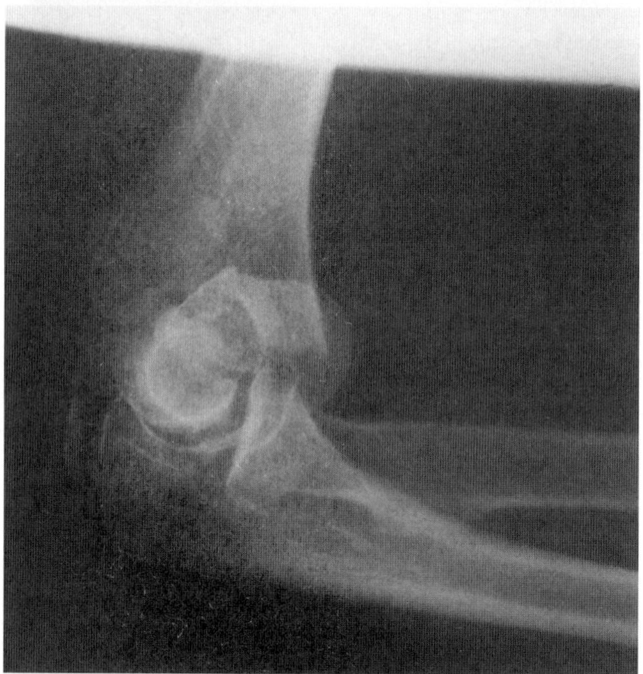

FIG. 261-4. Comminuted displaced and rotated intercondylar fracture (type IV).

fracture line. More severely displaced fractures may show medial or lateral displacement or rotation along the axis of the humerus (Fig. 261-6). The lateral radiograph will reveal the fracture line extending obliquely from posterior proximal to anterior distal. The distal fragment will be displaced proximally and posteriorly.

Treatment of undisplaced fractures consists of plaster immobilization. Displaced fractures have the best results when reduced by closed methods followed by traction or pin fixation. Patients with displaced fractures or severe swelling should be admitted for observation of neurovascular status.

FLEXION-TYPE FRACTURES Flexion-type fractures occur in fewer than 5 percent of supracondylar fractures. The mechanism is direct anterior force against a flexed elbow. This results in anterior displacement of the distal fragment. Since the mechanism is direct force, these fractures are often open.

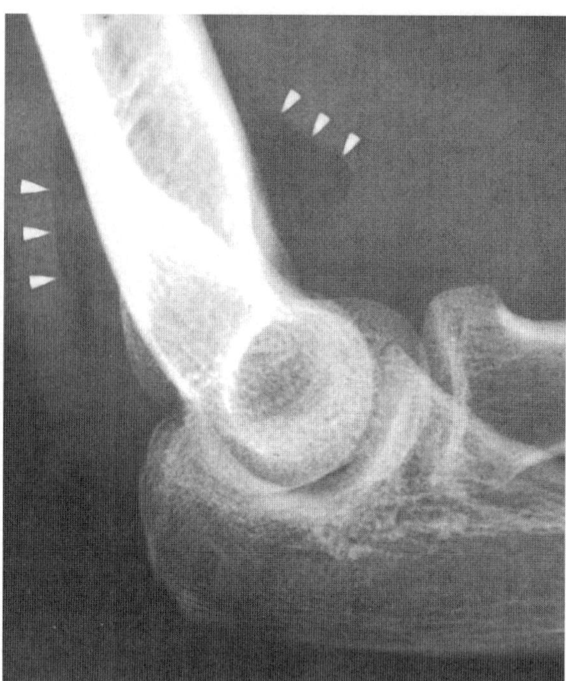

FIG. 261-5. Anterior and posterior fat pad signs.

Radiographs reveal an oblique fracture from anterior proximal to posterior distal. The distal fragment is anterior to the humerus.

Management consists of closed reduction and plaster immobilization or surgery if reduction cannot be maintained by closed methods.

COMPLICATIONS There are numerous complications of supracondylar fractures, including nerve and vascular injuries and those occurring late, such as nonunion, malunion, myositis ossificans, and loss of motion.

Associated injuries to the median, ulnar, and radial nerves have been well documented and have an incidence of 7 percent. Recently, Cramer and coworkers found a high incidence of anterior interosseus nerve injuries in their patients with supracondylar fractures. This nerve arises from the median nerve and innervates the flexor pollicis longus, the radial part of the flexor digitorum profundus, and the pronator quadratus. Since there is no sensory component to the anterior interosseous nerve, identification of the injury can be made only by specific muscle testing. Testing consists of flexion at the index finger distal interphalangeal and thumb interphalangeal joints. The mechanism of injury is usually traction, contusion, or a combination. Complete transection is rare, and entrapment within the fracture occurs only occasionally. Prognosis is excellent, with complete recovery in 2 to 6 weeks.

Acute vascular injuries must always be suspected in patients with supracondylar fractures. Absence of a radial pulse is common in children. This is most frequently due to transient arterial spasm. Rarely, there is a partial or complete transection of the brachial artery, an intimal tear and thrombosis, or entrapment within the fracture fragment.

The most serious complication is Volkmann's ischemic contracture. This classically occurs after a supracondylar fracture, when edema reduces venous outflow and arterial inflow. This results in ischemia, which, if unrelieved, will lead to muscle and nerve necrosis and eventual replacement by fibrotic tissue. Refusal to open the hand in children, pain with passive extension of the fingers, and forearm tenderness are signs of impending Volkmann's ischemia. It is now well understood

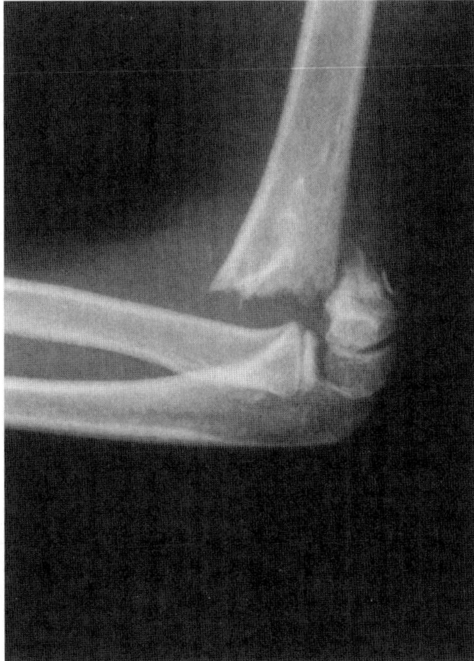

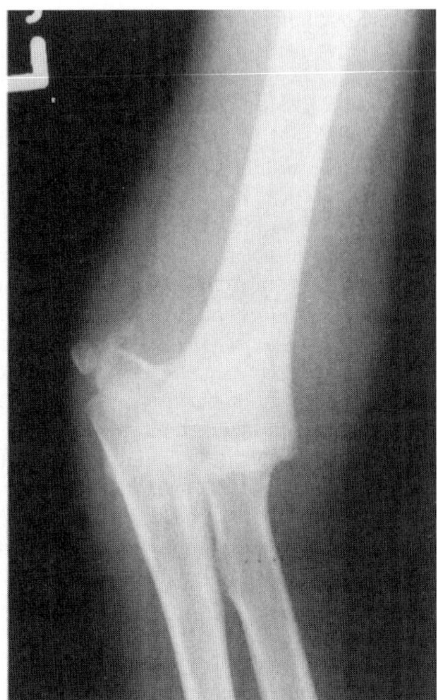

FIG. 261-6. Displaced supracondylar fracture. The distal fragment is displaced posteriorly, proximally, and medially. The proximal fragment is displaced anteriorly and distally.

that the mere lack of a radial pulse does not indicate ischemia unless accompanied by these signs.

Treatment of supracondylar fractures with absent radial pulse begins with fracture reduction and pinning. Extremities still without a pulse and with signs of ischemia are taken to the operating room for fasciotomy and/or brachial artery exploration. Extremities without a pulse and no signs of ischemia may be treated in one of 3 ways: (1) close observation, (2) observation for 24 to 36 h followed by arteriography and surgery if indicated, or (3) immediate surgical exploration.

Humeral Condyle Fractures

Although rare, lateral condyle fractures occur more frequently than medial condyle fractures. The mechanism is usually a fall on the outstretched arm or direct force applied to the posterior aspect of the flexed elbow. Examination reveals swelling and tenderness laterally, crepitus, and limitation of movement. Radiographs show a fracture line extending from the supracondylar ridge through the intertrochanteric articular surface. There may be displacement of the distal fragment posteriorly and distally from the pull of the extensor muscles.

Treatment for undisplaced and minimally displaced fractures (< 2 mm) is immobilization in a long-arm splint with the elbow flexed, the forearm supinated, and the wrist dorsiflexed to decrease the tension from the extensor muscles. The patient should be referred in 2 to 3 days to an orthopedist. Surgery is indicated for displaced fractures.

Medial condyle fractures usually occur as a result of a fall on the outstretched arm or a direct force applied to the olecranon. Pain and swelling medially are prominent findings. There is also pain with flexion of the wrist through action of the flexors. The proximity of the ulnar nerve requires a careful neurovascular examination. The fracture line is oblique from the supracondylar ridge through the trochlear groove.

Treatment of undisplaced and minimally displaced fractures is immobilization in a long-arm posterior splint with the forearm pronated and the wrist flexed to relieve tension of the flexors originating from the medial epicondyle. Referral to an orthopedist is made in 2 to 3 days and active ROM may be started in 2 to 3 weeks. Displaced fractures require open reduction and internal fixation, usually with screws.

Epicondyle Fractures

Lateral epicondyle fractures almost never occur, since the anatomic position of the condyle reduces the exposure to direct blows resulting instead in fractures of the lateral condyle. When they do occur, these fractures are usually avulsion fractures and may be treated by immobilization with the elbow flexed to 90° and the forearm in supination. The patient is referred to an orthopedist within 1 week.

Medial epicondyle fractures are more common and tend to occur in the pediatric and adolescent populations. The mechanism of injury is usually a posterior elbow dislocation with avulsion of a fragment of the medial epicondyle. In adults, the mechanism is from a direct blow to the prominent medial epicondyle. Examination reveals swelling and tenderness medially, and pain with flexion of the elbow or wrist from the forearm flexors. A careful search must be made of the radiographs to determine whether the fracture fragment is carried into the joint space after reduction of an elbow dislocation (Fig. 261-3).

Undisplaced and minimally displaced fractures are treated with a long-arm posterior splint with the forearm pronated and elbow and wrist flexed. The patient is referred to an orthopedist within 1 week, and early active ROM is begun. Fracture fragments entrapped within the joint require surgical removal if closed attempts are unsuccessful. Displaced fractures may be treated either surgically or by closed manipulation. These patients are splinted as described, and an acute referral is made to an orthopedist. Since the trochlea does not appear as an ossification center until after age 10 to 12 years, one must be mindful that a displaced medial condyle fracture may be associated with a significant trochlear fracture.

Trochlea Fractures

Owing to the anatomy and location of the trochlea, fractures are rarely seen. They are often the result of an elbow dislocation. Clinical findings include swelling, tenderness, and limitation of movement. Undisplaced fractures are treated with a posterior splint and referral in 2 to 3 days. Displaced fractures are treated by open reduction and internal fixation.

Capitellum Fractures

Like fractures of the trochlea, fractures of the capitellum are quite rare. The mechanism of injury occurs as a result of breaking a fall with the outstretched hand with the elbow in flexion or direct trauma to the elbow that is in full flexion. Three types of fractures are recognized: type I is a shearing of the capitellum from the lateral column, type II an osteochondral fracture of the anterior capitellum, and type III a comminuted or impacted fracture. Physical findings include tenderness and swelling laterally and limitation of ROM. Limitation of movement is due to mechanical obstruction from the fracture fragment in flexion or extension. Clinical as well as radiographic evaluation is also directed at determining associated injuries, especially a radial head fracture. Standard radiographs are generally sufficient to evaluate the injury. Special attention must be directed at the radiographs, since the fracture fragment consists largely of cartilage that will not be easily recognized, especially against the background of the humerus. The lateral radiograph may reveal the fragment anterior and proximal to its usual anatomic position.

Undisplaced fractures are initially treated in a long-arm splint with the elbow flexed to 90° and the forearm neutral. Although a recent paper described closed reduction for displaced fractures, most authors recommend open reduction and fixation with screws or Kirschner (K) wires.

Coronoid Fractures

Coronoid fractures are rare and often associated with elbow dislocations. Some classify these fractures according to the size of the fracture fragment and the stability of the joint. Type I fractures involve an avulsion the tip of the coronoid process, type II fractures involve 50 percent or less of the coronoid process, and type III fractures involve greater than 50 percent of the coronoid process and are unstable. Type I fractures may be treated with early immobilization. Types II and III fractures are generally unstable and are treated by open reduction and internal fixation. Emergency treatment consists of immobilization, ice, elevation, and early orthopedic consultation.

Olecranon Fractures

Fractures of the olecranon are common because of its subcutaneous location. The mechanism of injury is usually direct trauma to the tip of the elbow. Olecranon fractures may be avulsions, oblique or transverse intraarticular, or comminuted. Clinical findings include swelling and tenderness over the olecranon, limitation of movement, a palpable fracture line, and inability to fully extend the elbow. Because of its proximity, examination is especially directed at evaluation of ulnar nerve function. Ulnar nerve injuries are usually transient neuropathies. Standard anteroposterior and lateral radiographs will identify the fracture, the extent of comminution, and the articular surface involved. As many as 32 percent of olecranon fractures may be associated with other fractures, the commonest being fractures of the radial head or neck.

Undisplaced fractures (< 2 mm displacement) in both flexion and extension are treated with splint immobilization with the elbow placed in 45° of flexion. Follow-up is within 1 week. Displaced fractures (> 2 mm displacement) are treated by open reduction and excision of the proximal olecranon fragments or internal fixation with screws, plates, or tension-band wiring. Complications include loss of ROM, nonunion, ulnar nerve compression, and posttraumatic arthritis.

Radial Head Fractures

Radial head fracture is the most commonly encountered fracture about the elbow. The mechanism of injury is a fall on the outstretched hand with the force transmitted along the radius to the radial head, where it impacts on the capitellum. The result is a fracture of the weaker radial head or neck. An alternative mechanism is direct trauma to the lateral aspect of the elbow directly over the radial head. The patient complains of pain in the elbow, and examination reveals swelling and tenderness laterally. Rotation of the forearm with firm pressure over the radial head will elicit pain. Careful examination of the wrist and forearm for tenderness must be performed to determine whether there has been injury to the distal radioulnar ligaments or to the interosseus membrane. The latter injuries result in radioulnar dissociation (Essex-Lopresti) and proximal migration of the radius if the radial head is excised. Anteroposterior and lateral radiographs are generally sufficient, but occasionally radiocapitellar views are required. A fat-pad sign in a patient with an appropriate mechanism of injury is sufficient to make a presumptive diagnosis of a radial head fracture regardless of whether or not the fracture is visualized (Fig. 261-5).

Undisplaced and minimally displaced fractures are treated with sling immobilization and early ROM. Such patients have excellent results with little morbidity. All other fractures should be referred acutely to an orthopedist, since treatment varies from early motion to radial head excision and prosthetic radial head implantation.

ULNAR NEURITIS

Ulnar neuritis may be a compressive neuropathy or can be simply a result of direct repetitive stretching or friction. The two most common problem sites are at the elbow (cubital tunnel) and at the wrist (Guyon's canal). In cubital tunnel syndrome, the nerve may experience trauma or compression against the medial epicondyle, such as from pitching or playing golf. In Guyon's canal, damage may result from direct pressure, such as in holding bicycle handlebars.

Numbness or weakness in the ring and small fingers or medial elbow pain indicate ulnar nerve pathology. Tapping along the nerve may reveal the site of involvement. Signs and symptoms of cervical spine disease or thoracic outlet syndrome should also be sought.

To test for cubital tunnel syndrome, hold the elbow in maximum flexion for 1 min. This may reproduce or exacerbate symptoms due to peripheral ulnar nerve pathology. Cubital tunnel syndrome may in addition cause numbness over the dorsoulnar hand because of inclusion of the superficial branch. Thumb adduction is also weak because of the ulnar innervation of the adductor pollicis muscle. This can be tested by having the patient tightly hold a piece of paper between the thumb and the proximal phalanx of the index finger. If the phalanx must flex more than a few degrees, then the muscle is weak (Froment's sign).

Pathology in Guyon's canal spares this deep branch so that numbness of only the ring and small fingers, not of the hand, occurs. Similarly, Froment's sign is absent because the adductor pollicis is innervated by the deep branch.

Cubital tunnel syndrome in its milder form can initially be treated with rest. Failing this, orthopedic surgery to decompress or anteriorly transpose the nerve may be needed.

Guyon's canal syndrome is first treated with the wrist splinted in mild dorsiflexion and nonsteroidal anti-inflammatory drugs (NSAIDs). While resistant cases may respond to steroid injection into the canal, the majority will require surgical decompression.

EPICONDYLITIS

Lateral Epicondylitis

In this condition, also known as tennis elbow, pain is noted at the origin of extensors of the distal arm. While it occurs from racquet sports and repetitive manual labor, it may also occur spontaneously. When it is from racquet sports, a faulty backhand stroke is usually to blame. The extensor mass, especially the deep extensor carpi radialis brevis, rubs and rolls over the lateral epicondyle and radial head. In addition, there is pulling on the extensor origin, resulting in microtears.

Pain is increased over the lateral epicondyle with pronation of the forearm and concomitant dorsiflexion of the wrist against resistance. Lifting a chair with the affected hand in pronation should also exacerbate symptoms. Picking up a full cup of liquid also reproduces the pain.

Treatment includes avoidance of the painful activity and use of NSAIDs. Utilizing supination in daily grasping activities will aid in rest of the area. In the case of racquet sports, instruction in a quality backhand should be sought after the acute injury heals. Those who use a two-handed backhand are rarely afflicted. Orthopedic referral is advised for further evaluation and treatment.

Medial Epicondylitis

Although also known as golfer's elbow, this syndrome often occurs from racquet sports and pitching. Overuse of the flexor forearm muscles stresses and inflames the tendinous insertion at the medial epicondyle.

Pain will be noted over the medial epicondyle, and grip may be suboptimal secondary to pain. Pronation or wrist flexion against resistance will increase the pain over the medial epicondyle. About two-thirds of these patients have concomitant ulnar neuritis (cubital tunnel syndrome).

Treatment is conservative, with rest and NSAIDs. Play is gradually resumed after 6 weeks.

BICEPS RUPTURE

Functional Anatomy

The biceps muscle originates on the coracoid process (short head) and the superior glenoid labrum (long head) and inserts on the bicipital tuberosity of the radius. The long tendon runs over the head of the humerus in the bicipital groove and courses to its insertion inside the shoulder joint. This makes it susceptible to repetitive microtrauma and degenerative changes from repetitive overuse.

The biceps functions to flex the elbow and supinate the forearm. Ninety-seven percent of ruptures are proximal, occurring in the long head of the biceps. Distal rupture is rare, with fewer than 200 cases reported in the literature. Tendon rupture is usually the end result of repetitive microtrauma with degenerative changes and so is seen most frequently in patients between the fourth and sixth decades of life. Chronic glucocorticoid use and/or injection are also etiologic. The injury is unusual in young athletes. Rupture is precipitated by sudden or prolonged muscle contracture against resistance, such as with heavy lifting or a checked baseball swing.

Proximal Biceps Rupture (Long Head)

CLINICAL FEATURES Patients with acute ruptures usually relate a long history of tendinitis. Symptoms include anterior shoulder pain and an audible ''pop'' or ''snap'' during strenuous activity. Examination demonstrates tenderness, swelling, and crepitus over the bicipital groove. Flexion of the elbow elicits pain. Weakness in flexion and supination is minimal (10 to 20 percent) because of the function of the short head of the biceps. Ecchymoses and a visible gap in the muscle, caused by distal migration of the muscle mass with resulting egg-shaped swelling, are usually obvious. Slow contraction of the biceps makes this deformity more prominent. Rupture usually occurs in the proximal one-third of the tendon at the top of the bicipital groove. Occasionally this injury involves an avulsed fragment of bone. Radiographs are necessary to rule out an avulsion fracture.

DIFFERENTIAL DIAGNOSIS The differential diagnosis includes biceps tendinitis, subluxation-dislocation, rotator cuff disease, impingement syndrome, partial rupture, and osteochondral fracture.

TREATMENT Treatment is surgical repair of the tendon in the young athletic patient. The older patient can be treated conservatively with immobilization, followed by early and progressive mobilization and strengthening exercises as soon as pain subsides. Orthopedic consultation should be obtained in the emergency department. Admission is required only for surgical repair. Emergency department treatment consists of ice and analgesia. Outpatient treatment requires immobilization in a sling, analgesia, and intermittent application of ice for 48 to 72 h.

Distal Biceps Avulsion

CLINICAL FEATURES Almost all cases of distal biceps rupture occur in males, and 80 percent occur in the dominant extremity. A single traumatic event causes acute rupture, resulting in symptoms of pain in the antecubital fossa accompanied by a tearing or popping sensation. Examination will demonstrate tenderness, swelling, ecchymosis, and inability to palpate the biceps tendon in the antecubital fossa. Comparison with the uninjured extremity for asymmetry will aid in making the diagnosis. Deformity in the muscle is palpable as the biceps retract proximally during contraction. The patient can still flex the elbow and supinate the forearm because of intact brachialis and supinator muscles, but strength loss will be much more prominent (40 to 50 percent) than with proximal biceps ruptures. The rupture usually occurs at the tendon-osseous insertion and leaves no distal tendon fragment at the tuberosity. Avulsion fractures are unusual but should be ruled out by radiographs.

DIFFERENTIAL DIAGNOSIS The differential diagnosis includes biceps tendinitis, partial tear, bursitis, anterior capsulitis of the elbow, and annular ligament sprain.

TREATMENT Treatment is surgical tendon repair, and thus orthopedic consultation to plan for timing of repair is warranted. Emergency department treatment consists of ice and analgesia. If the patient is discharged home with plans for later surgical repair, immobilization in a sling and analgesia are standard.

TRICEPS RUPTURES

Functional Anatomy

The triceps muscle acts as both an extensor of the shoulder through its attachment to the scapula and as a powerful extensor of the elbow. All three heads form a common tendon attached to the olecranon.

Clinical Features

The triceps muscle is extraordinarily injury free, but rupture of the common tendon can occur. This is the least common of all tendon ruptures. Rupture most frequently occurs in young males (mean age, 26 years) secondary to trauma. There is an equal distribution between dominant and nondominant extremities. The site of rupture is usually the tendon-osseus junction, resulting in a high percentage of avulsion fractures of the olecranon. Musculotendinous junction and muscle belly ruptures are rare. The injury usually occurs as a result of indirect trauma from a fall on the outstretched extremity. Ruptures from direct blows and spontaneous ruptures from systemic illness have been reported.

Symptoms of acute rupture include pain and soft tissue swelling at the posterior elbow. The ability to extend the elbow is lost. Examination often shows a palpable defect proximal to the olecranon, along with localized tenderness and swelling. Radiographs of the elbow must be obtained, since olecranon avulsion fractures are present in greater than 80 percent of cases.

Differential Diagnosis

Differential diagnostic possibilities include olecranon bursitis, partial rupture or strain, degenerative joint disease, and olecranon fracture.

Associated fractures are common. Thus, a thorough upper-extremity examination must be carried out, and the posterior aspect of the elbow must be examined when other injuries are detected initially.

Treatment

Treatment is surgical repair of the tendon to restore extension strength. Orthopedic consultation should be obtained. Emergency department treatment consists of ice and analgesia. If the patient is discharged, a sling and analgesia, along with intermittent ice application, are usually prescribed.

FOREARM

Anatomy

The radius and ulna are joined together along their entire length by a fibrous interosseous membrane and touch only at their ends to form the complex proximal and distal radioulnar joints. The ulna is a comparatively straight bone, whereas the radius has an important outward bowing. During the motions of supination and pronation, the ulna holds a relatively fixed position, while the radius rotates around it. Because these bones have such a close relationship to one another, injury to either will have a direct impact on the other. A displaced or angulated fracture of one bone typically disrupts the other or causes a dislocation at the proximal or distal radioulnar joint, such as in the Monteggia and Galeazzi fracture-dislocations.

The radius and ulna are also under the influence of numerous muscle groups, such as those that supinate and pronate. The biceps brachii and the supinator insert on the proximal radius and are the powerful supinators of the forearm. The pronator teres inserts just distal to them and onto the midsection of the radius. As its name suggests, it is responsible for pronation. Radius fractures that are located between these muscle groups will result in marked displacement of the bone, with supination of the proximal segment and pronation of the distal portion. However, if the fracture is distal to the insertion of the pronator teres, these forces tend to neutralize one another and result in less rotational deformity.

The neuroanatomy is most easily understood by appreciating the neural control of the most basic components of wrist and finger movement (Fig. 261-7). The radial nerve travels over the lateral epicondyle and supplies the muscles involved in wrist extension before it gives

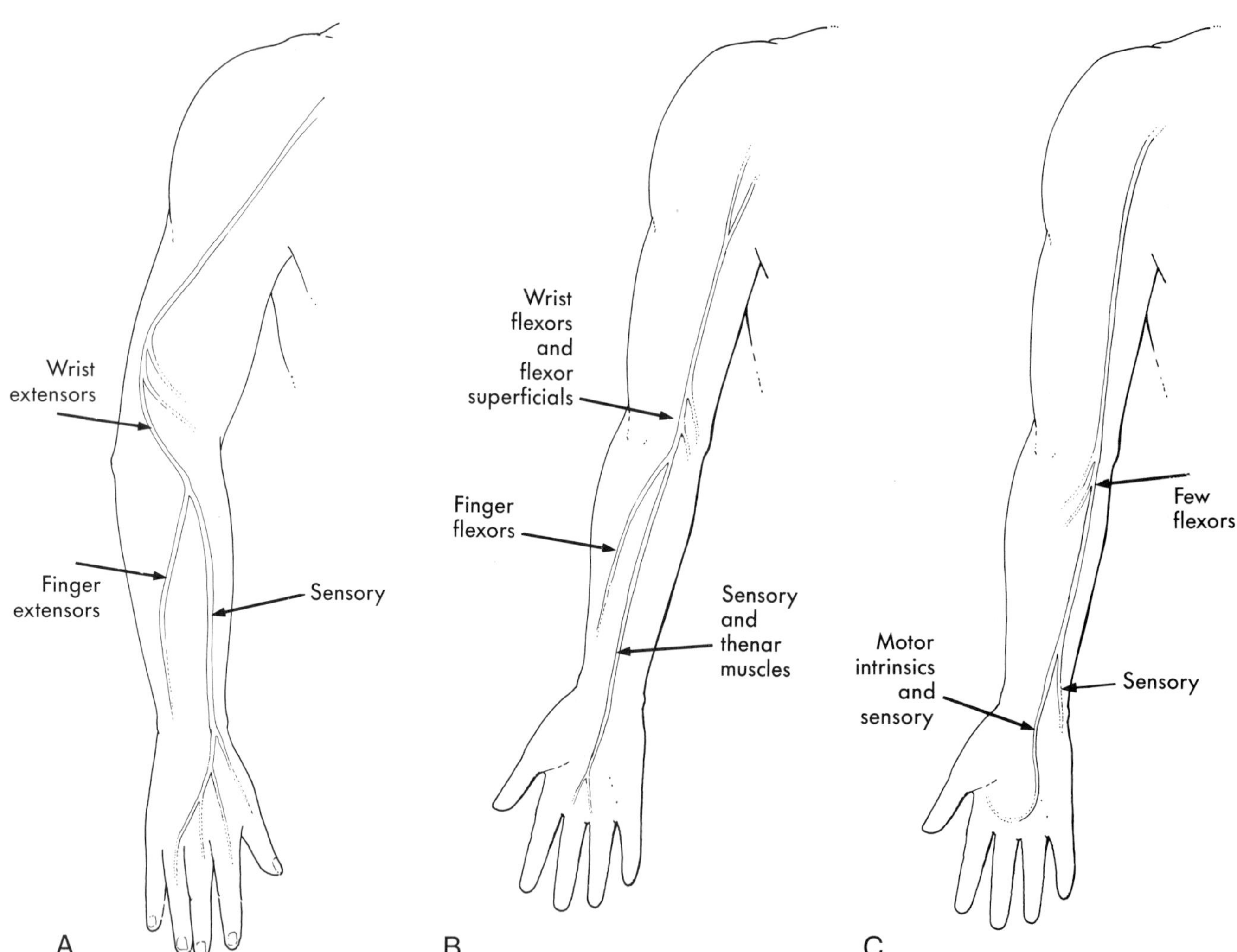

FIG. 261-7. **A.** The radial nerve controls wrist extension before branching into the posterior interosseous nerve. **B.** The median nerve controls wrist flexion and the flexor digitorum superficialis before branching into the anterior interosseous nerve (controls the deep finger flexors in the forearm) and a branch that innervates the thenar muscles and provides sensation to most of the palm. **C.** The ulnar nerve controls the intrinsic muscles and sensation to the ulnar side of the hand. [From Chin HW, Propp DA, Orban DJ: Forearm and wrist, in Rosen P, Barkin RM, et al (eds): *Emergency Medicine Concepts and Clinical Practice,* 3d ed, vol 1. St. Louis, Mosby Year Book, 1992.]

off a branch, the posterior interosseous nerve. This branch travels around the proximal radius and controls the muscles that extend the fingers and thumb. The remainder of the radial nerve is purely sensory and innervates the posterior aspect of the hand from the thumb to radial half of the ring finger. Quite simply, the proximal portion of the radial nerve controls the more proximal function of wrist extension, while the distal branch (posterior interosseus nerve) controls the more distal function of finger extension and another branch that is purely sensory. So an isolated injury (e.g., to the posterior interosseous branch) would affect finger extension but spare wrist extension and sensation to the dorsum of the hand. The single best test of radial nerve function is to have the patient extend both the wrist and fingers against resistance, and check the sensation over the dorsum of the hand.

The median nerve controls the basic movements of wrist and finger flexion and sensation on the volar surface of the hand from the thumb to the radial half of the ring finger. The proximal portion of the median nerve innervates the muscles that control wrist flexion and the flexor digitorum superficialis before it gives off the anterior interosseous nerve. This branch controls portions of the remaining deep finger flexors: flexor digitorum profundus, flexor pollicus longus, and pronator quadratus. The remaining portion of the median nerve provides sensation to most of the volar surface of the hand plus a motor branch to the thenar muscles of the thumb (recurrent branch of the median nerve). The median nerve is evaluated by assessing each of these distal branches. A simple test of the anterior interosseous nerve is the ability to make a circle, or ''OK'' sign, with the thumb and index finger; if so, this nerve is likewise ''OK.'' Abduction of the thumb (recurrent branch of the median nerve) and intact sensation on the radial side of the palm complete the evaluation of the median nerve.

The ulnar nerve provides innervation to a few forearm muscles but, more important, controls the intrinsic muscles of the hand and provides sensation to the little finger and the ulnar half of the ring finger. The ability to abduct the index finger against resistance and normal sensation on the ulnar side of the hand is an easy test of ulnar function.

Fractures of Both Radius and Ulna

A great amount of force is necessary to fracture both the radius and ulna. This injury occurs most often from vehicular trauma, falls from a height, or a direct blow to the forearm. The magnitude of the force determines the type of injury. A moderate force produces transverse or mildly oblique fractures. Comminuted and segmental fractures are produced by a high-impact force. As one might expect, these fractures are often displaced. Open fractures of the radius and ulna are second only to tibia fractures because of the subcutaneous location of the entire ulna and the distal portion of the radius.

Nondisplaced fractures of both bones are exceedingly rare because the force necessary to produce the injury is also sufficient to displace it. However, in this event, a long-arm cast is applied, and frequent reevaluation for potential displacement is necessary.

Displacement of both bones is generally the rule. Examination reveals swelling, deformity, and tenderness of the forearm. Careful assessment of the neurovascular status is imperative. Nerve injuries can be seen with severe open fractures but fortunately are uncommon with most closed injuries. Because of the excellent collateral circulation of the forearm, vascular compromise is generally not a major problem if either the radial or ulnar circulation is intact.

The fractures are clearly visible on the radiographs. Angulation and longitudinal alignment are easily evaluated, but changes in rotational alignment may be subtle. A rough estimate of rotational alignment can be made by noting the normal orientation of various bony prominences of these bones. On the anteroposterior radiograph, the radial styloid and radial (bicipital) tuberosity normally point in opposite directions, whereas the ulnar styloid and coronoid process do so on the lateral view. A change in this arrangement suggests rotation malalignment. Since these bones are also oblong rather than circular in their cross-sectional appearance, a sudden change in the bone's width at the fracture site is another clue to a rotational deformity.

Although there are some reports of adequate reduction using closed techniques, the potential for these injuries to subsequently displace, in spite of cast immobilization, makes this alternative unpredictable. An exception is the injury in a child. A child's ability to remodel bone and compensate for some malalignment makes closed reduction possible. Otherwise, these injuries invariably require open reduction and internal fixation, most commonly with compression plating and screws. The use of external fixation may be necessary in situations where infection is possible, such as severe open fractures, comminution, or bone loss. Internal fixation is delayed until the risk of infection is diminished.

Potential complications include reduced ability to supinate and pronate, osteomyelitis, nonunion, malunion, neurovascular injury, and compartment syndrome. Recognizing the development of a compartment syndrome is particularly important to prevent debilitating ischemic contractures of the forearm. The diagnostic findings are palpable induration of the area, pain with passive movement of the fingers, and pain that appears to be disproportionate to the physical findings. The presence of a palpable pulse does not exclude the diagnosis of compartment syndrome. Alterations in sensation and the pulse are late findings. Direct measurements of elevated compartment pressures confirm the diagnosis.

Ulna Fractures

Isolated fractures of the ulna most often result from direct blows to the forearm. The natural response to raise the forearm in defense of a blow from a club is why it is often referred to as a *nightstick fracture*. Undisplaced fractures are immobilized in a long-arm cast and closely followed for subsequent displacement of the fracture.

Displaced fractures are those with greater than 10° of angulation or displacement of more than 50 percent of the width of the bone at the site of the fracture. Open reduction and internal fixation with a compression plate and screws are necessary to prevent angulation, loss of length, and rotational deformity. These injuries should be closely scrutinized for any possible radius fracture or dislocation.

Fracture of the ulnar shaft with a radial head dislocation is often referred to as *Monteggia fracture-dislocation* (Fig. 261-8). It is typically a diaphyseal fracture in the proximal third of the ulna with an anterior dislocation of the radial head (60 percent of cases). Anterolateral and posterolateral dislocation of the radial head or a metaphyseal ulna fracture are other possibilities. Clinically, there are considerable pain and swelling at the elbow. The radial head may be palpable in an anterolateral or posterolateral location. The forearm may appear shortened and angulated. The ulnar fracture is clearly visible and may overshadow the less obvious radial head dislocation. As a rule, the radial head normally points to the capitellum in all radiographic views of the elbow. In a Monteggia fracture, the apex of the ulna fracture points in the direction of the radial head dislocation.

Monteggia fracture-dislocations are treated with open reduction and internal fixation of the ulna and closed reduction of the radial head dislocation. Children may be treated adequately by closed reduction of both bones and long-arm cast immobilization. Complications include nonunion, redislocation, infection, and paralysis of the posterior interosseus nerve. Remember that the nerve wraps around the proximal radius.

Radius Fractures

Radius fractures can be divided into those that are proximal and those that are distal to the junction of the middle and distal thirds of the bone. Excluding radial head fractures, isolated fractures of the proximal two-thirds of the radius are not common because it is relatively well

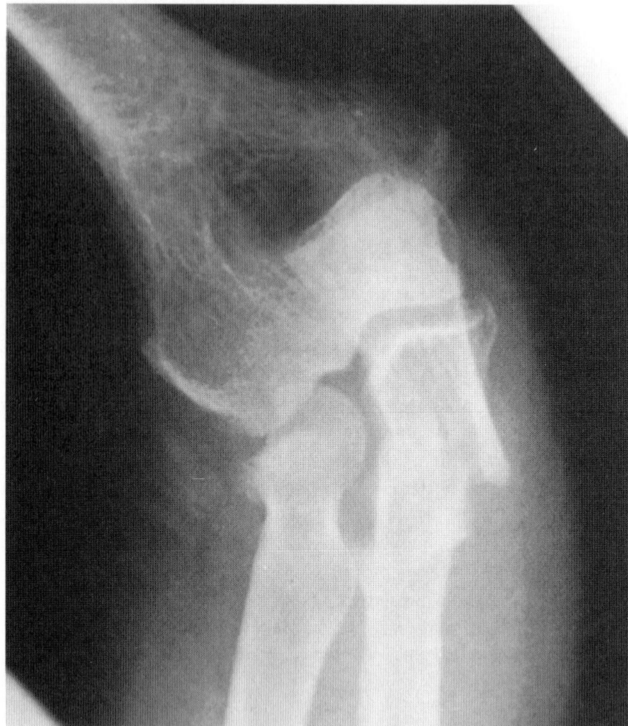

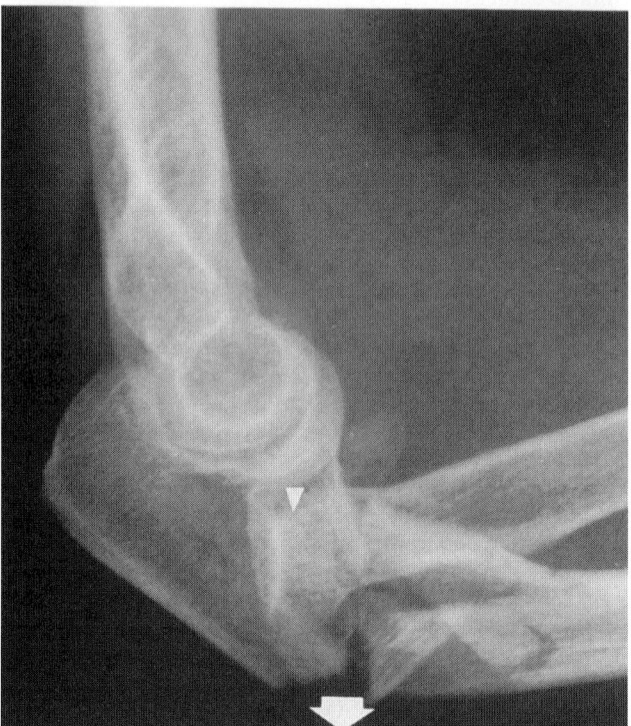

FIG. 261-8. Monteggia fracture-dislocation. The angulation of the comminuted fracture of the proximal ulna (*arrow*) points in the direction of the radial head dislocation (*arrowhead*).

protected from direct blows by the ulna and also by the surrounding musculature of the forearm. Undisplaced fractures are rare; these are treated with cast immobilization. Fractures of the proximal two-thirds of the radius are often displaced by both the force of the injury and the action of the supinators and pronators on the radius. They require internal fixation with plating and screws to maintain the reduction and to prevent rotational deformity.

Fractures of the distal third of the radial shaft are produced by falls on the outstretched hand in forced pronation or by a direct blow. Much like the Monteggia fracture-dislocation, the distal radial shaft fracture is often associated with a distal radioulnar joint dislocation, hence the name *reverse Monteggia fracture* or, more commonly, *Galeazzi fracture*. There are localized tenderness and swelling over the distal radius and wrist. The radius fracture is usually short oblique or transverse with dorsal lateral angulation. The distal radioulnar joint injury can be subtle. Radiographs may show only a slightly increased distal radioulnar joint space on the anteroposterior view. On the lateral view, the ulna is displaced dorsally. This injury is treated by open reduction and internal fixation of the radius fracture with compression plating and screws. The distal radioulnar joint reduction is held with immobilization of the forearm in supination or with K-wire fixation for 6 weeks.

BIBLIOGRAPHY

Cohen MS, Hastings H: Acute elbow dislocation: Evaluation and management. *J Am Acad Orthop Surg* 6:15, 1998.

Cramer KE, Green NE, Devito DP: Incidence of anterior interosseous nerve palsy in supracondylar humerus fractures in children. *J Ped Pediatr Orthop* 13:502, 1993.

Endean ED, Veldenz HC, Schwarcz TH, et al: Recognition of arterial injury in elbow dislocation. *J Vasc Surg* 16:402, 1992.

Harris IE: Supracondylar fractures of the humerus in children. *Orthopedics* 15:811, 1992.

Kuntz DG Jr, Baratz ME: Fractures of the elbow. *Orthop Clin North Am* 30(1):37, 1999.

Kurer MH, Regan MW: Completely displaced supracondylar fracture of the humerus in children. *Clin Orthop Rel Res* 256:205, 1990.

Letts M, Rumball K, Bauermeister S, et al: Fractures of the capitellum in adolescents. *J Pediatr Orthop* 17:315, 1997.

Malone CP: Open treatment for displaced articular fractures of the distal radius. *Clin Orthop* 202:104, 1986.

Ochner RS, Bloom H, Palumbo RC, et al: Closed reduction of coronal fractures of the capitellum. *J Trauma* 40:199, 1996.

Olney BW, Menelaus MB: Monteggia and equivalent lesions in childhood. *J Pediatr Orthop* 9:219, 1989.

Propp DA, Chin HW: Forearm and wrist radiology. *J Emerg Med* 7:393, 1989.

Royle SG: Posterior dislocation of the elbow. *Clin Orthop* 269:201, 1991.

Sacchetti A, Ramoska EE, Glascow C: Nonclassic history in children with radial head subluxations. *J Emerg Med* 8:151, 1990.

Schunk JE: Radial head subluxation: Epidemiology and treatment of 87 episodes. *Ann Emerg Med* 19:1019, 1990.

Skaggs D, Pershad J: Pediatric elbow trauma. *Pediatr Emerg Care* 13:425, 1997.

Teach SJ, Schutzman SA: Prospective study of recurrent radial head subluxation. *Arch Pediatr Adolesc Med* 150:164, 1996.

Wilkins KE: Supracondylar fractures: What's new? *J Pediatr Orthop* 6(part B):110, 1997.

WRIST INJURIES

Harold W. Chin
Dennis T. Uehara

The wrist comprises the area from the distal radius and ulna to the carpometacarpal joints. It is a complex unit with articulations among eight carpal bones and the distal radius and ulna. Injuries to this area are common and diagnosis is often difficult. An understanding of the functional anatomy, mechanics of injury, and clinical assessment is needed for proper diagnosis and treatment.

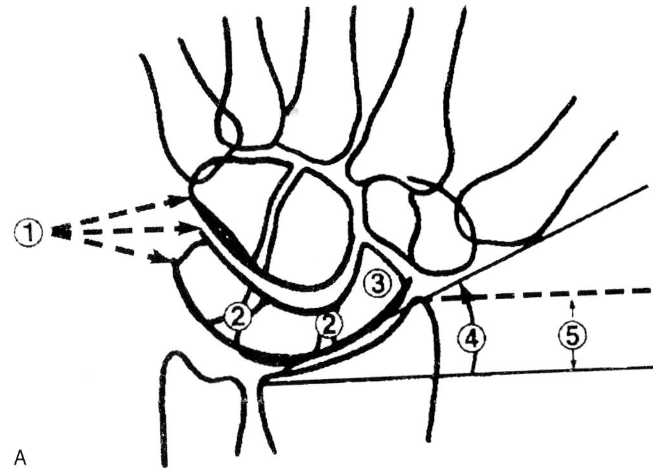

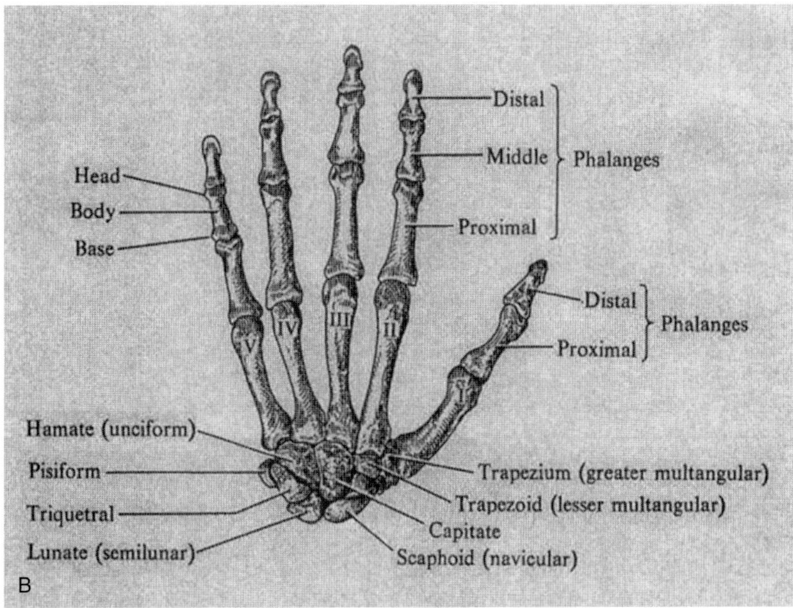

FIG. 262-1. A. Key elements on a normal PA view. (1) The carpal bones form three smooth arcs; (2) carpal bones are separated by a 1- to 2-mm space; (3) scaphoid has an elongated shape; (4) radius has an ulnar inclination of 15 to 25 degrees; (5) radial styloid projects 8 to 18 mm (average 13 mm). Half the lunate articulates with the radius, and the ulna and adjacent radial surface are equal in length (neutral ulnar variance). **B.** Bony anatomy. (With permission from Chin HW: Injuries of the wrist, in Hart RG, Rittenberry JJ, Uehara DT (eds): *Handbook of Orthopaedic Emergencies.* Philadelphia, Lippincott-Raven, 1998.)

ANATOMY

The distal radius is the only forearm bone that articulates directly with the bones of the carpus (scaphoid and lunate). The distal radius has three articular surfaces: radiocarpal, distal radioulnar, and the triangular fibrocartilage. The radiocarpal surface of the radius is concave and tilted in two planes. The radius has an ulnar inclination or tilt of 15 to 25 degrees in the frontal plane and a volar tilt of 10 to 15 degrees in the sagittal plane. The ulna is separated from the carpal bones by a cartilage complex on its distal end, the triangular fibrocartilage complex (TFCC). This cartilage complex forms a smooth continuous ulnarly directed extension of the distal radial surface and supports the lunate and triquetrum, on the distal ulna. The triangular fibrocartilage complex is also the main stabilizer of the distal radioulnar joint. The distal radius has a concave sigmoid notch on its ulnar aspect that articulates with the curvature of the ulnar head permitting rotation of the wrist. The distal radioulnar joint is also supported by dorsal and volar radioulnar ligaments that merge with the triangular fibrocartilage complex.

The eight carpal bones are arranged in two rows (Fig. 262-1*A*, *B*). The distal row (trapezium, trapezoid, capitate, and hamate) is quite stable. These carpal bones are joined tightly together and to their adjoining metacarpals. The distal carpal row and metacarpals move together as a unit forming a relatively rigid stable arch. The proximal row (scaphoid, lunate, triquetrum, and pisiform) is also arranged in an arch in the frontal plane located between the distal radius and distal carpal row. The proximal carpal row functions as a mobile middle link or "intercalated segment" in this arrangement. By virtue of its position, the proximal carpal row is potentially unstable. The scaphoid holds a unique position, acting as a stabilizing strut and linking the proximal and distal carpal rows on the radial aspect of the wrist. This explains the scaphoid's greater propensity for injury.

The forearm muscles that insert onto the base of the metacarpals produce wrist motion. There are no direct tendon insertions on the carpal bones (except for the pisiform that is a sesamoid bone of the flexor carpi ulnaris). The carpal bones move passively in response to hand position. Although the radiocarpal joint is often referred to as the "wrist joint," it is important to realize that wrist motion is nearly equally divided between the radiocarpal and midcarpal joint. This is best appreciated when viewing carpal movement from the sagittal view. During flexion and extension each row moves in the same direction and with similar degrees of angulation.

The carpal bones are stabilized to one another by intrinsic ligaments and to the bones of the forearm by the extrinsic ligaments. The key extrinsic ligaments are arranged in three arcades; two are volar and one dorsal. The two volar ligaments are arranged in two inverted V-shaped arches. The apex of one arch inserts on the lunate supporting the proximal carpal row, while the other arch reaches out to the distal carpal row with its apex inserting onto the capitate. There is an inherently weak area (space of Poirier) between these two palmar arches. This area lies at the junction of the lunate and capitate and also widens with dorsiflexion of the wrist. Forceful dorsiflexion of the wrist could tear the capsule here and produce a perilunate or lunate dislocation. There is a single dorsal arcade that acts as a sling across the back of the wrist. These arcades have origins on the rim and styloid of the radius on one side, and distal ulna and triangular fibrocartilage complex on the other side; injuries to either insertion point are therefore potentially unstable.

The intrinsic ligaments are largely responsible for holding the carpal bones together as a kinematic unit in their respective carpal rows. Because the proximal carpal row is a mobile middle link in this three-link system, the intrinsic ligaments within this segment are particularly important because of their greater propensity for injury. The intrinsic ligaments of the proximal carpal row are named after the respective carpal bones they connect: the scapholunate and triquetrolunate. The proximal carpal row is also under important internal dynamic forces. The palmar flexed posture of the scaphoid produces a flexion torque on the lunate that is counterbalanced by an extension torque from the triquetrum. Unfortunately, this delicate balance is lost if either ligament is disrupted, and produces a volar or dorsal tilt of the proximal carpal row and carpal instability.

CLINICAL ASSESSMENT

An individual's age affects the maturity of the bones and influences the type of injury. Children are more likely to sustain injuries to the immature, weaker epiphyseal plate or metaphysis of the radius. Their carpus is mostly cartilage that helps cushion them from injury. Carpal injuries are rare in children. Young adults, particularly those with active lifestyles, are more likely to be injured with greater force and disrupt either the carpus or distal radial metaphysis that often involves the articular surface. In the elderly, the weak point is the brittle distal radial metaphysis.

Injuries most often occur from falls on the outstretched hand. Impact on the thenar eminence is more likely to injure the scaphoid and its supporting ligaments. An impact on the hypothenar eminence is likely to cause injury to the triquetrum and the pisiform, and to their supporting ligaments.

Pinpointing areas of tenderness and correlating it to anatomical landmarks on the wrist will help determine what structure may be injured and the best way to evaluate it with a radiograph. The most noteworthy landmark on the dorsum of the wrist is the anatomical snuffbox. The scaphoid is palpable at the base of this triangle and the radial styloid forms its proximal base. The extensor pollicis longus creates the ulnar border of the snuffbox, as it wraps around Lister's tubercle, a palpable small bony prominence on the distal radius. The scapholunate joint is located just distal to Lister's tubercle. Immediately ulnar to the scapholunate junction is a palpable indentation in the middle of the wrist that is the location of the lunate and capitate. When the wrist is flexed, the lunate is palpable as it rises out of this fossa. The ulnar styloid is the bony prominence on the ulnar aspect of the wrist. The triquetrum and triangular fibrocartilage complex are located just distal to it.

A clearly visible landmark on the volar aspect of the wrist is the wrist crease that marks the location of the proximal carpal row. The scaphotrapezium joint is palpable at the base of the thenar eminence. The pisiform is the visible bony prominence at the base the hypothenar eminence. The hook of the hamate is palpable within the soft tissue of the hypothenar eminence a centimeter away, at a 45-degree angle radial from the pisiform.

RADIOGRAPHY

The clinical examination should determine which radiographs are necessary to support the diagnosis. Standard views of the wrist include posteroanterior, lateral, and oblique views. Although these views are sufficient in the majority of cases, other projections may be necessary to profile specific carpal injuries.

The key to interpreting the radiograph is to first assure proper positioning, then identify specific features on each projection. On a properly positioned posteroanterior view, the distal radius and ulna should not overlap at their distal articulation and the axis of the third metacarpal should parallel that of the radius. Besides looking for disruption of the bony cortex, key elements on the PA view are illustrated on Fig. 262-1.

On the PA view, three smooth arcs outline the articular surfaces at the radiocarpal and midcarpal joints. Two of these arcs are formed by the proximal and distal articular surfaces of the scaphoid, lunate, and triquetrum. The third arc is formed by the proximal articular surface of the capitate and hamate in the midcarpal joint. Any distortion of these lines implies a possible fracture, dislocation, or subluxation at the site.

The carpal bones fit together like a jigsaw puzzle, the pieces are separated by a narrow 1 to 2 mm joint space. This space is increased or obliterated with ligament disruption, carpal instability patterns, or fractures/dislocations. This occurs most often around the lunate at the scapholunate and capitolunate joints. Unfortunately, incorrect positioning can produce overlap patterns that could be misinterpreted as pathological. For example, radial deviation of the wrist causes normal physiological palmar rotation of the proximal carpal row. The dorsal rim of the lunate will overlap the capitate and obliterate the capitolunate joint space. The scaphoid that should appear elongated on the PA view appears shorter as it rotates palmar and can be confused with a rotatory subluxation of the scaphoid.

The radial styloid should project 8 to 18 mm beyond the distal radioulnar joint and create an ulnar inclination to the distal radius of 15 to 25 degrees on the PA view. Distal radius fractures can alter these measurements. At the distal radioulnar joint, the ulna and adjacent portion of the radius should be of equal length, and the distal radius should articulate with at least half the lunate. The extrinsic ligaments, along with the triangular fibrocartilage complex, prevent ulnar translocation (the migration of the carpals down the ulnar tilt of the radiocarpal surface). The lunate would have less contact and support from the radius if ulnar migration were present. A shorter ulna (negative ulnar variance) also provides less support to the lunate and increases the potential shear stress to the lunate. Although negative ulnar variance is a normal variant, its presence predisposes the lunate to injury.

The lateral radiograph is important for determining carpal alignment and degree of fracture angulation. The first step, again, is assuring that the wrist is properly positioned on the radiograph. The radius and ulna should completely overlap one another, and the radial styloid should be centered over the distal radial articular surface. The key features on this view are illustrated on Fig. 262-2.

The axis of the radius, lunate, and capitate is colinear on the lateral view. If the articular surfaces of these bones were highlighted, they would appear as three consecutive Cs in a row. This provides a simple radiographic assessment of wrist dislocation. Measurement of the capitolunate and scapholunate angles is a more precise assessment of carpal alignment. The axis of the capitate, lunate, and scaphoid runs through the center of their proximal and distal articular surfaces. The axis of the lunate and capitate should nearly overlap and form an angle that is less than 10 to 20 degrees. The scaphoid is normally palmar flexed on the lateral view; its axis should form an angle that is between 30 to 60 degrees with the lunate. Deviation from either of these angles suggests ligament disruption and carpal instability patterns Fig. 262-3.

Fractures of the distal radius are the most common fracture in the wrist. While a displaced fracture is the obvious deformity, the alteration

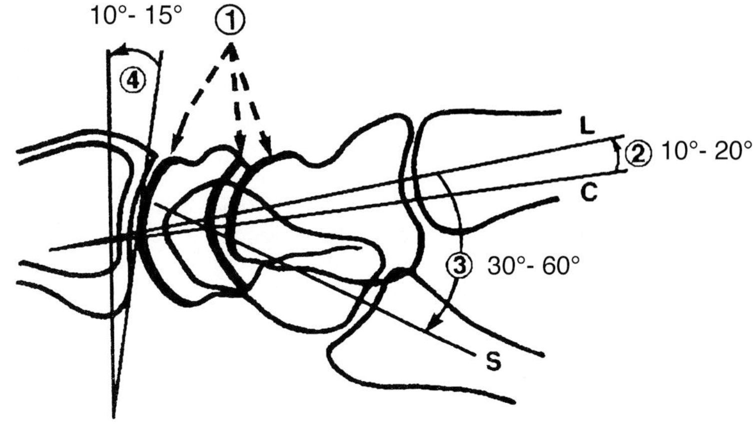

FIG. 262-2. Key elements on a normal lateral view. (1) three Cs sign; (2) capitolunate angle is <10 to 20 degrees; (3) scapholunate angle is <60 degrees; (4) radial volar tilt of 10 to 15 degrees. (With permission from Chin HW: Injuries of the wrist, in Hart RG, Rittenberry JJ, Uehara DT (eds): *Handbook of Orthopaedic Emergencies.* Philadelphia, Lippincott-Raven, 1998.)

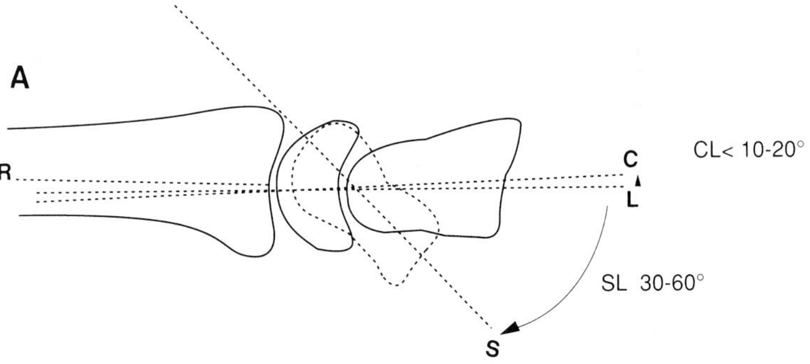

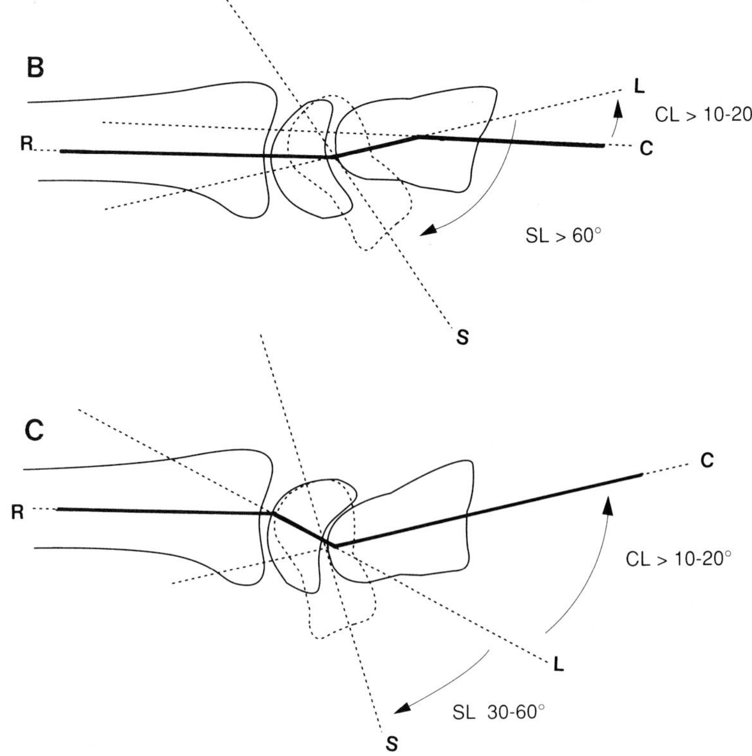

FIG. 262-3. A. Normal wrist. Axis of the radius (R), lunate (L), and capitate (C) are colinear. The capitolunate angle (CL) is less than 20 degrees and the scapholunate angle (SL) is between 30 and 60 degrees. **B.** Dorsal intercalated segment instability (DISI). The lunate tilts dorsal and slides palmar, increasing the capitolunate angle. The scaphoid tilts more palmar and increases the scapholunate angle. The axes of the radius, lunate, and capitate take on a zigzag pattern (dark line). **C.** Volar intercalated segment instability (VISI). The lunate tilts palmar and the capitolunate increases, but the scapholunate angle is maintained. The zigzag pattern is in the opposite direction.

of the normal volar tilt of 10 to 15 degrees of the distal articular radial surface has greater long-term consequences. The shape of the distal radius, distal ulna, and triangular fibrocartilage has a significant influence on carpal alignment and movement.

Other radiographic views profile specific areas of the wrist. Oblique views are performed in either partial pronation or supination. They project the scaphotrapezium joint or pisiform away from the overlapping adjacent carpal bones. The scaphoid view is a coned-down PA view of the scaphoid in ulnar deviation. This position extends the normal flexed posture of the scaphoid so that the bone is profiled lengthwise. This may assist in detecting subtle fractures. The carpal tunnel view is a tangential view through the carpal tunnel and is helpful in visualizing the pisiform and hook of the hamate. Motion studies are dynamic views in flexion, extension, and radial and ulnar deviation. They examine relative carpal movement to one another and stress the intercarpal ligaments for laxity characterized by widening of the intercarpal space. Likewise, the grip compression or fist view is a stress view in the PA projection of a tightly clenched fist. The capitate is pushed into the proximal carpal row and forces the carpal bones apart if the intrinsic intercarpal ligaments are torn.

LIGAMENTOUS INJURIES

The lunate is located in the middle of the wrist, so it is not surprising that the majority of ligamentous injuries are centered on the lunate. These injuries usually result from forceful dorsiflexion of the wrist, most often from a fall on the outstretched hand. The various injuries occur sequentially depending on the degree of force, and range from isolated tears to perilunate and lunate dislocations.

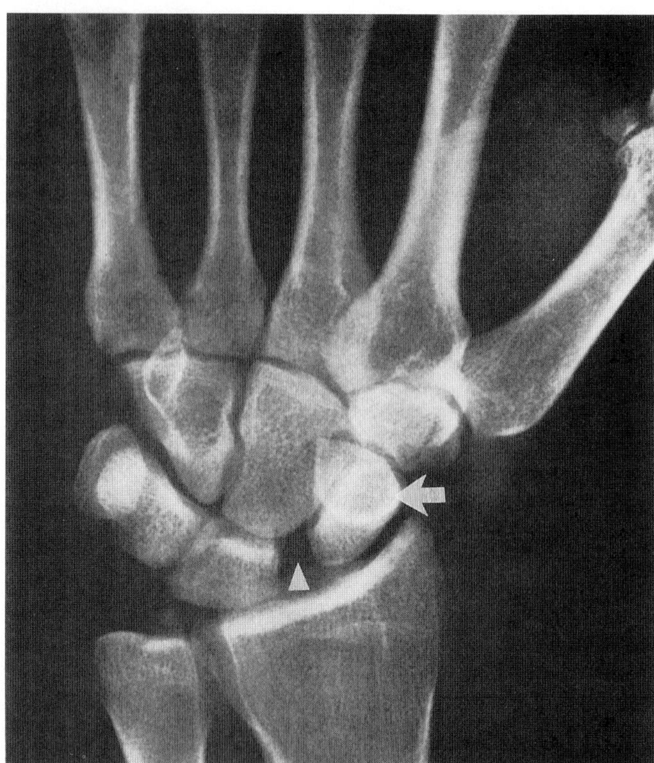

FIG. 262-4. Scapholunate dissociation with accompanying rotatory subluxation of the scaphoid. The scaphoid and lunate are separated by a gap of more than 3 mm (arrowhead) and the scaphoid appears shorter from rotation with a dense ring (cortical ring sign, arrow).

Scapholunate Ligament Instability

The scapholunate ligament is the intrinsic ligament that binds the scaphoid and lunate. Because the scaphoid bridges the proximal and distal carpal rows, it is not surprising that the scapholunate ligament also has a greater propensity for injury. It is the most common ligament injury of the wrist. Injury most often is from a fall on the outstretched hand with impact on the thenar eminence. These individuals will complain of pain and swelling on the radial side of the wrist and sometimes a clicking sensation with wrist movement. Examination reveals localized tenderness on the dorsum of the wrist in the area immediately distal to Lister's tubercle. Ballottement of the scaphoid may also produce pain in this area.

This injury is often referenced to the various radiographic appearances it may take. There are three different radiographic signs that may occur separately or in combination with one another. Scapholunate dissociation is a widening of the scapholunate joint space on the PA projection of more than 3 mm (Fig. 262-4). This has been called the ''Terry Thomas'' sign, named after a British comedian with notable dental diastema between his upper front incisors. If it is not apparent on routine views, a grip-compression stress view or motion study may be necessary to demonstrate the abnormal gap. These maneuvers are particularly helpful in identifying an incomplete tear of the ligament. Rotatory subluxation of the scaphoid is another abnormality that often accompanies scapholunate dissociation. A torn scapholunate ligament can cause the scaphoid to tilt more palmar and increase the scapholunate angle to greater than 60 degrees on the lateral view (normal angle is 30 to 60 degrees). On the PA view, the scaphoid tilts toward the observer. The scaphoid appears shorter as it is viewed more on its end and the circular cortex of the bone becomes visible like a ring (cortical ring sign; see Fig. 262-4). A third possible radiographic abnormality is a carpal instability pattern, dorsal intercalated segment instability (DISI). The normal flexed posture of the scaphoid produces a flexion torque on the lunate that is counterbalanced by an extension torque from the triquetrum. When the scapholunate ligament is torn, this balance is disrupted. The lunate tilts dorsal from the unopposed extension torque from the triquetrum, while the scaphoid tilts more palmar (rotatory subluxation of the scaphoid) because it has lost support from the lunate. The dorsal tilt of the lunate also causes a slight flexion tilt of the capitate. In the lateral view, the normal colinear arrangement of the axes of the radius, lunate, and capitate are replaced by a characteristic zigzag pattern. Both the scapholunate and capitolunate angles are increased. The concept of the proximal carpal row being the middle-link or ''intercalated segment'' in this system, combined with the lunate's pathological dorsal tilt and zigzag pattern, is how this abnormality came to be named dorsal intercalated segment instability, DISI (see Fig. 262-3*B*).

These injuries are treated acutely with a radial gutter splint or posterior mold. Appropriate orthopedic referral is necessary because these injuries require either closed reduction and pinning or, more often, open reduction and surgical repair of the ligament. Early severe degenerative arthritis is a possible sequelae if left untreated.

Triquetrolunate Ligament Instability

The triquetrolunate ligament binds the triquetrum and lunate on the ulnar aspect of the wrist. Injury to this ligament is the ulnar equivalent of the scapholunate ligament injury. Triquetrolunate ligament injury, however, occurs less often and is more stable. This injury most often results from falls on the outstretched dorsiflexed hand with impact on the hypothenar eminence. There will be localized tenderness on the ulnar aspect of the wrist just distal to the ulna. Ballottement of the triquetrum may produce a painful clicking sensation.

A complete tear of this ligament removes the influence of the triquetrum to counterbalance the flexion torque from the palmar-flexed scaphoid. The lunate hence tilts palmar, and the capitate extends slightly in response. A zigzag pattern in the opposite direction of scapholunate injury is produced. The capitolunate angle is increased greater than 10 to 20 degrees; however, the scapholunate angle is unaffected because the scapholunate ligament is still intact. The lateral radiograph reveals the volar intercalated segment instability (VISI) pattern (see Fig. 262-3*C*). The PA radiograph may reveal a widening of the triquetrolunate joint space and obliteration of the capitolunate joint space because of the volar tilt of the lunate.

These injuries are treated acutely with an ulnar gutter splint or posterior mold and referred to an orthopedist. Immobilization in a cast for six to eight weeks followed by a protective splint is sufficient in most cases. Open reduction and internal fixation is generally reserved for chronic injuries. Unrecognized injuries can result in early degenerative arthritis and a chronically painful wrist.

Perilunate and Lunate Dislocations

Perilunate and lunate dislocations represent the final stages of midcarpal ligament disruption. Much like the scapholunate and triquetrolunate injuries, these injuries are also the result of forceful dorsiflexion and impact on the outstretched hand, but usually with much greater force, such as a fall from a height or impact from a motor vehicle accident. The injury can begin on either side of the lunate, but typically starts on the radial side, tearing the scapholunate ligament. It progresses around the lunate in a semicircular fashion, tearing the volar ligament arcade at the radiocapitate ligament. Remember that the extrinsic ligaments form two strong volar arcades with an inherently weak area between them that widens with dorsiflexion of the wrist. This space of Poirier lies at the junction of the lunate and capitate. The space of Poirier is opened further as additional loading disrupts the triquetrolunate ligament. Besides ligament disruption, any number of the surrounding carpal bones can fracture along an arc around the lunate (see Fig. 262-5). If a sufficient force is applied, the ligaments and carpal bones surrounding the lunate are stripped away. The capitate is displaced posterior to the lunate, producing a perilunate dislocation. If the capitate rebounds with sufficient force, it can push the lunate off the radius and into the palm, creating a lunate dislocation. These injuries are all part of a continuous spectrum of ligamentous disruption.

On clinical examination, there is often generalized swelling, pain, and tenderness. However, a gross deformity, typical of many other joint dislocations, is often absent and can be misleading. Radiographic interpretation is the key to diagnosis. The perilunate dislocation is best appreciated on the lateral view. The linear arrangement of the three Cs sign is disrupted with the capitate, represented by the third C, displaced posterior to the lunate. The lunate still maintains its contact with the radius. The scapholunate and capitolunate angles are increased. On the PA view, the three smooth arcs are disrupted and the capitolunate joint space is obliterated as the bones overlap one another. The scapholunate and triquetrolunate joint space may either be increased because of torn ligaments, or obliterated by rotation of fractured carpal fragments. The scaphoid will appear shortened from rotatory subluxation or fracture. A perilunate dislocation may, unfortunately, overshadow any associated carpal bone fracture. The scaphoid

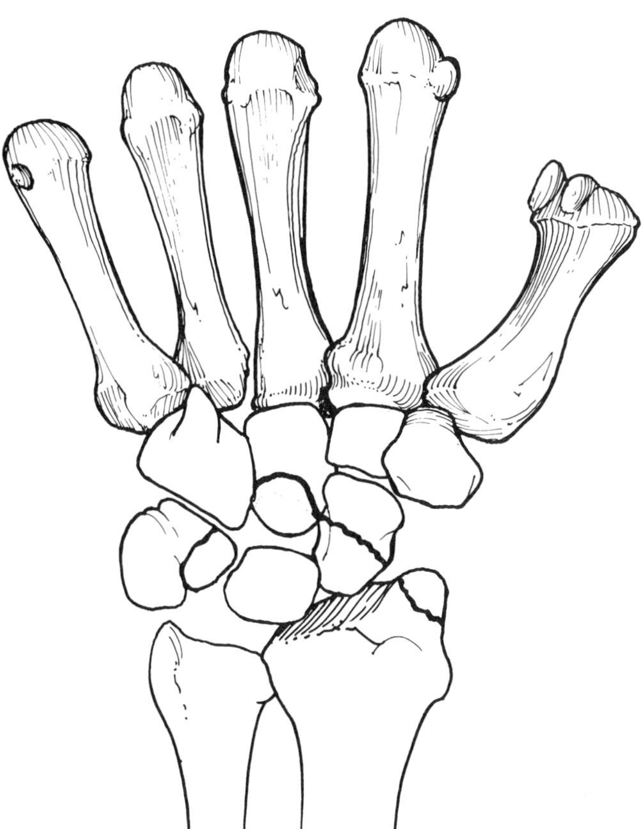

FIG. 262-5. Perilunate and lunate dislocations can fracture any of the carpal bones that surround the lunate in an arc pattern.

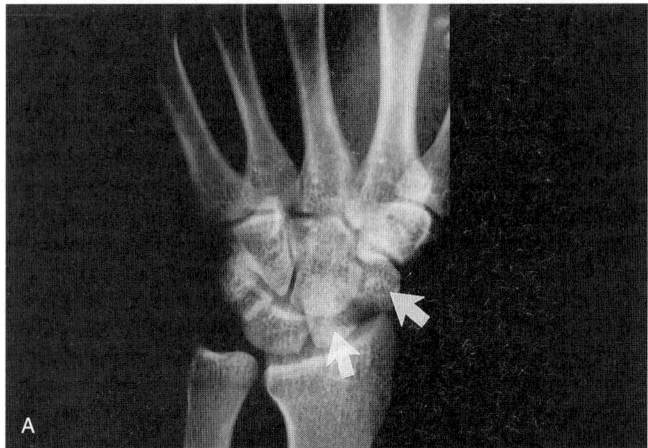

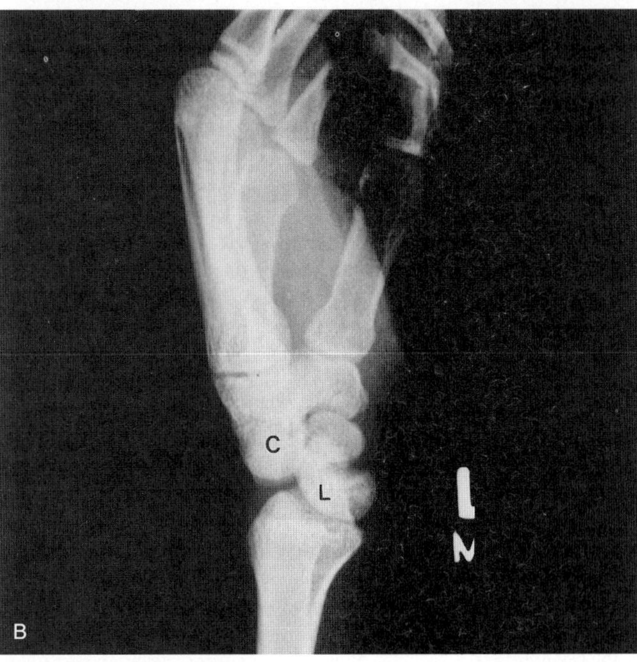

FIG. 262-6. Transscaphoid perilunate dislocation. **A.** PA view shows subtle overlap of the lunate and capitate. A displaced scaphoid fracture is present (arrows). **B.** Lateral view shows the lunate (L) maintaining contact with the radius while the capitate (C) is positioned posterior to the lunate. (With permission from Chin HW, Visotsky J: Ligamentous wrist injuries. *Em Med Clin North Am* 11:3, 1993.)

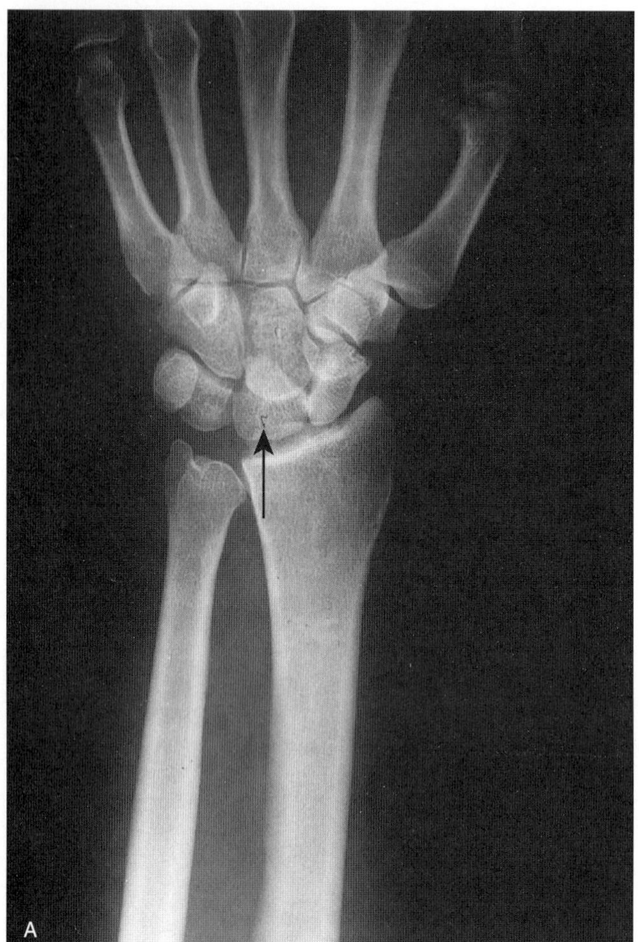

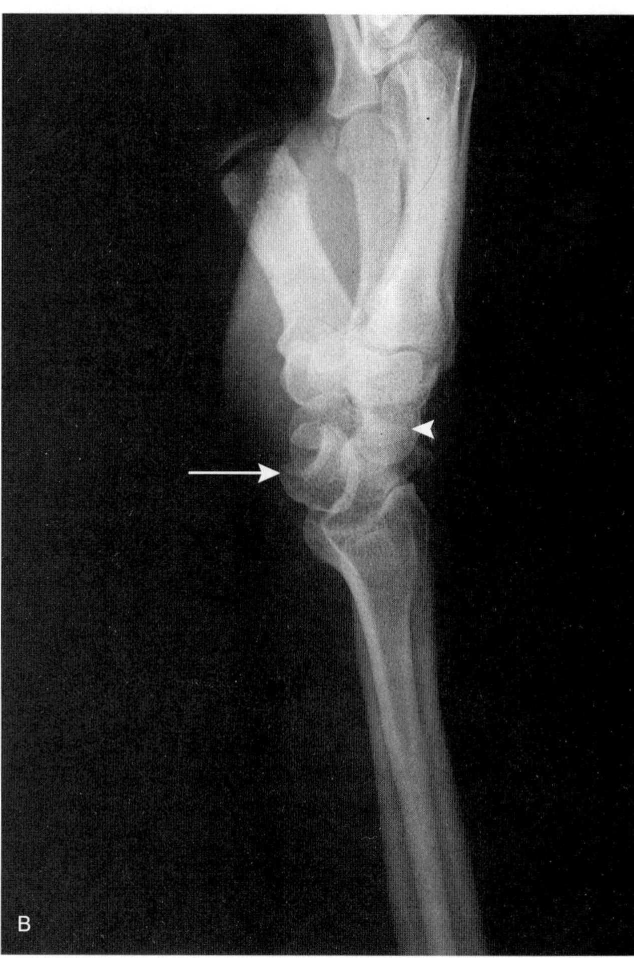

FIG. 262-7. Lunate dislocation. **A.** PA view reveals pathognomonic triangular shape of lunate (piece of pie sign, arrow). **B.** Lateral view shows lunate tilting into the palm (spilled teacup sign, arrow) and the capitate positioned posterior to the lunate (arrowhead). Note the associated scaphoid and triquetrum fractures. (With permission from Chin HW, Visotsky J: Ligamentous wrist injuries. *Em Med Clin North Am* 11:3, 1993.)

and capitate are most often involved, so it is prudent to carefully inspect these bones for fractures. These fractures are designated by adding the prefix ''trans'' to the carpal's name; e.g., transscaphoid perilunate dislocation (see Fig. 262-6*A*, *B*).

A lunate dislocation has many similar and several distinct features when compared to a perilunate dislocation. On the lateral view, it also disrupts the three Cs sign. The lunate (represented by the middle C) is pushed off the radius and into the palm. This has been called the ''spilled teacup'' sign because it resembles a cup spilling in the direction of the palm. The capitate may rebound back and even rest on the radius. On the PA view, the lunate has a triangular shape (''piece-of-pie'' sign) that is pathognomonic for lunate dislocation (see Fig. 262-7*A*, *B*). The signs of ligament disruption and the associated carpal fractures described with perilunate injuries may also be present.

All patients with perilunate or lunate dislocations require emergency orthopedic consultation. Treatment is determined by the extent of injury. Closed reduction and long-arm splint immobilization is appropriate for reducible dislocations. Open, unstable, and irreducible dislocations require open reduction and internal fixation, with repair of the ligaments and fractures. Some clinicians operate on all perilunate and lunate dislocations. The complications are development of carpal instability patterns that lead to early degenerative arthritis, delayed union, malunion, nonunion, avascular necrosis, and, occasionally, median nerve compression from the volar dislocation of the lunate into the carpal tunnel.

CARPAL BONE FRACTURES

Carpal bone fractures account for 7 to 10 percent of all hand injuries. Unfortunately, they are among the most commonly missed wrist injuries. It is important that a high index of suspicion is maintained and a focused examination is used to recognize these injuries. The following carpal fractures are listed in descending order of occurrence.

Scaphoid Fracture

The scaphoid is an oblong bone that has the unique role of linking and stabilizing the two rows of carpal bones. This, unfortunately, increases its propensity to injury, making it the most common carpal fracture. The injuries usually result from a fall on an outstretched dorsiflexed hand or by an axial load directed along the thumb's metacarpal. There is pain along the radial side of the wrist and localized tenderness in the anatomical snuffbox. Examining the wrist in ulnar deviation exposes more of the scaphoid to direct palpation in the anatomical snuffbox. Eliciting pain in this area, when the patient resists supination or pronation of their hand, or pain with axial pressure directed along the thumb's metacarpal is also suggestive of injury.

Standard and scaphoid views should be carefully examined for any cortical disruption (see Fig. 262-8). The scaphoid view profiles the bone lengthwise and may assist in detecting subtle fractures. Distortion

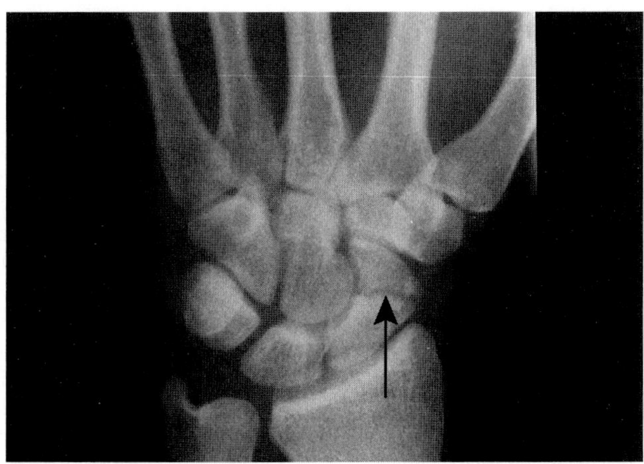

FIG. 262-8. Scaphoid fracture in the middle third or waist (arrow).

of a soft tissue fat stripe that lies adjacent to the radial side of the scaphoid is also suggestive of injury. Two-thirds of the fractures occur at the waist or middle third of the bone, 16 to 28 percent in the proximal third, and 10 percent in the distal third. A scaphoid fracture may also have an associated injury in 12 percent of cases involving either the radius, neighboring carpals, a carpal instability pattern, or dislocation.

A scaphoid fracture can develop avascular necrosis of the proximal fracture segment that can lead to disabling arthritis. There are several reasons that this occurs. The vascular supply to the scaphoid enters the distal portion of the bone through small branches off the radial artery and the palmar and superficial arteries. A fracture could therefore disrupt the blood supply to the proximal segment. In general, the more proximal, oblique, or displaced the fracture, the greater the risk of developing avascular necrosis. A scaphoid fracture is considered unstable if there is even as little as 1 mm of displacement, rotation, angulation, shortening, or if a carpal instability pattern is present. Two thirds of the scaphoid's surface is also articular. This only adds to the scaphoid's problems, because articular fractures are more difficult to heal.

Because 10 percent of initial radiographs fail to detect a fracture, it is imperative that initial treatment also be directed by clinical suspicion until follow up studies can exclude the diagnosis. Nondisplaced fractures and those that are only clinically suspected can be treated in a short-arm thumb spica splint or cast. Displaced or unstable fractures should be placed in a long-arm thumb spica splint or cast, and should be seen promptly by the orthopedic surgeon for definitive treatment. The main complications are avascular necrosis, delayed union, nonunion, malunion, and subsequent early degenerative arthritis.

Triquetrum Fractures

Triquetrum fractures are either dorsal avulsion fractures or fractures through the body. Avulsion fractures are produced when a twisting motion of the hand is suddenly resisted, or a hyperextension shear stress pushes the hamate or ulnar styloid against the triquetrum. Fractures of the body occur from direct trauma and are seen in association with perilunate and lunate dislocations (part of the arc fractures). There will be localized tenderness over the dorsum of the wrist in the area immediately distal to the ulnar styloid. The dorsal avulsion fracture is best seen on the lateral view or an oblique view in partial pronation (see Fig. 262-9). It appears as a tiny flake of bone on the dorsum of the triquetrum. Triquetral body fractures are usually nondisplaced because numerous ligaments encase the bone. These are best seen on the PA view.The dorsal avulsion fractures are treated with a wrist splint for six weeks and have an excellent prognosis for full recovery.

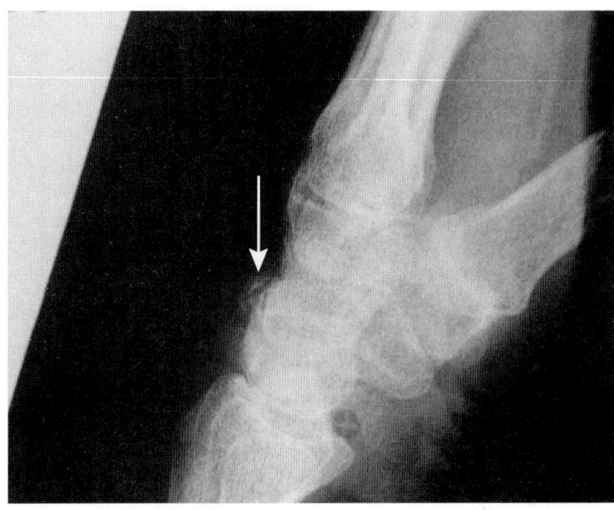

FIG. 262-9. Dorsal avulsion fracture of the triquetrum (arrow).

Fractures though the body are treated with a cast for six weeks. Those associated with perilunate/lunate dislocations may require internal fixation. Nonunion is possible, but avascular necrosis has not been reported.

Lunate Fracture

Lunate fractures generally occur in association with other carpal injuries. It is rare to have an isolated lunate injury. Like many other carpal injuries, it usually is the result of a fall on the outstretched hand. There will be localized tenderness in the middle of the wrist. The lunate is present in the shallow indentation on the mid-dorsum of the wrist. If the wrist is flexed the lunate is easily palpable as it rises out of the floor of this indentation. Axial pressure applied along the third metacarpal ray may also elicit pain in this same area and is suggestive of injury. Like the scaphoid, the lunate's blood supply enters through the distal end. A fracture risks producing avascular necrosis to the proximal portion. Because the lunate is nestled in the middle of the wrist, overlap with other carpal bones may make it difficult to identify an injury on a plain radiograph. Clinical suspicion should dictate the acute treatment. A thumb spica splint should be applied until further evaluation by the orthopedist. MRI and CT to identify occult fractures have replaced tomography and bone scans. The major complication is avascular necrosis (Kienböck's disease) that can lead to lunate collapse, osteoarthritis, chronic pain and decreased grip strength. Repetitive trauma to the lunate can also produce microfractures of the bone and subsequent osteonecrosis (see Fig. 262-10). Individuals with ulnar negative variance are at increased risk of developing Kienböck's disease, because a shorter ulna provides less support to the lunate.

Trapezium Fracture

The trapezium is a saddle-shaped bone that is adjacent to the thumb metacarpal. Injuries are produced by a direct blow to the thumb or from a dorsiflexion and radial deviation force. Vertical fractures are rare and are an analog of a Bennett's fracture (an intra-articular proximal thumb metacarpal fracture). Thumb movement is painful. There is tenderness at the apex of the anatomical snuffbox and at the base of the thenar eminence. This injury is best profiled on a 20-degree pronated oblique view. Nondisplaced fractures are treated in a thumb spica cast or splint for six weeks. Displaced fractures require open reduction and internal fixation. The major complication is nonunion.

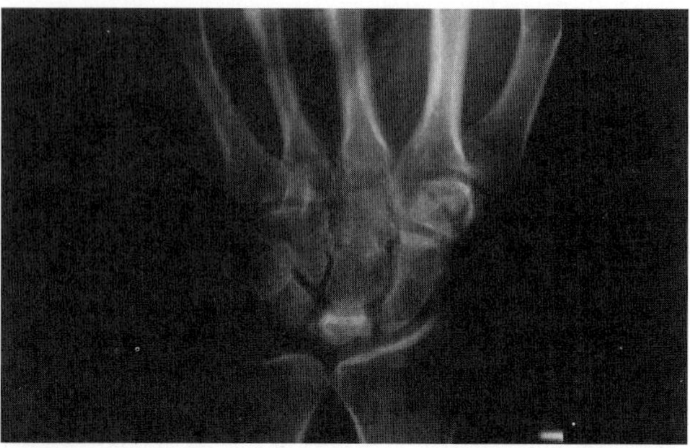

FIG. 262-10. Kienböck's disease, osteonecrosis, and collapse of the lunate. (With permission from Chin HW, Visotsky J: Wrist fractures. *Em Med Clin North Am* 11:3, 1993.)

Pisiform Fracture

The pisiform is a sesamoid bone within the flexor carpi ulnaris tendon. It is positioned immediately volar to the triquetrum and is the palpable bony prominence at the base of the hypothenar eminence. Injuries usually result from a fall directed on the hypothenar eminence. There will be localized tenderness on the pisiform itself. If the wrist is flexed, the pisiform can be grasped and ballotted between the examiner's fingers. This should elicit pain. Because the pisiform and hook of the hamate form the bony walls of Guyon's canal that contains the ulnar nerve and artery, it is important to exclude injury to them. Radiographs in partial supination or the carpal tunnel view are the optimal views because they remove the overlap with the triquetrum present on standard views (see Fig. 262-11). Multiple ossification centers in the pisiform may be confused with a fracture; however, these will have smoother margins and lack the perfect jigsaw puzzle fit seen with fracture fragments. Pisiform fractures are treated either in a compression dressing or a splint in 30 degrees of flexion and ulnar deviation that relaxes the tension from the flexor carpi ulnaris. These fractures have an excellent prognosis.

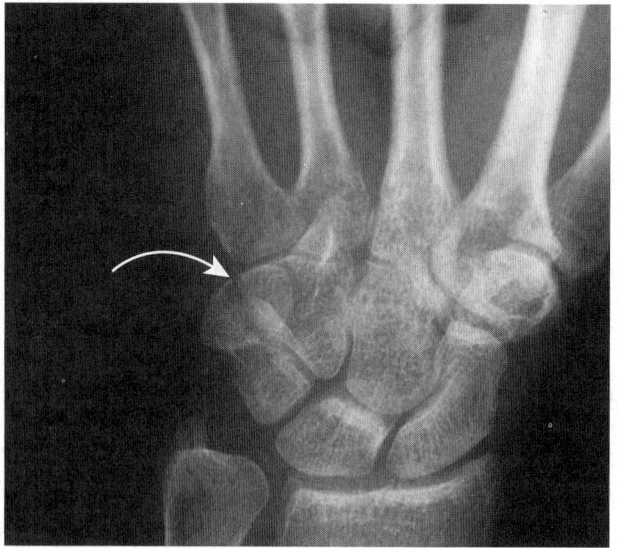

FIG. 262-11. Pisiform fracture PA view with a thin lucency in the center of the bone (arrow). (With permission from Chin HW, Visotsky J: Wrist fractures. *Em Med Clin North Am* 11:3, 1993.)

Hamate Fracture

Hamate fractures may involve the body of the hamate, the hook of the hamate, or any of its articular surfaces. Body fractures are rare and are generally associated with fracture/dislocations of the fourth or fifth metacarpals. Most hamate fractures involve the hamate hook, which is a small bony prominence on its volar side. The classic mechanism is an interrupted swing with golf club, bat, or racquet. The handle impacts against the hypothenar eminence and compresses the bone. The hook of the hamate is palpable in the soft tissues of the hypothenar eminence, just 1 cm distal and at a 45-degree radial angle from the pisiform. There will be localized tenderness here. Standard and carpal tunnel views are necessary to visualize the fracture. Occult fractures may be visualized by bone scan or computed tomography. These injuries are treated with compression dressing or splint. Nonunion is common and excision of the bone may be necessary. Injury to Guyon's canal and the ulnar nerve or artery are potential complications.

Capitate Fracture

The capitate is an elongated carpal bone that has a large proximal articular head that contacts the lunate; the midportion is the neck and the distal end is the body. Capitate fractures most often occur in the neck, and usually occur in conjunction with a scaphoid fracture. This association of scaphoid and capitate fractures is called the ''scaphocapitate syndrome.'' Isolated capitate fractures are rare. These injuries result from forceful dorsiflexion of the hand with impact on the radial side. The scaphoid is fractured first, followed by the capitate through its neck. This can continue around the lunate creating other so-called arc fractures, and eventually a perilunate or lunate dislocation. Capitate fractures also share the same legacy of potential avascular necrosis of the proximal fracture segment. Like the scaphoid and lunate, the capitate's blood supply enters through the distal end.

Physical examination will reveal diffuse swelling and tenderness over the capitate. The capitate neck fractures are best seen on the lateral radiograph. The head of the capitate should be carefully noted because it can rotate as much as 180 degrees. Unfortunately, capitate fractures are most often overlooked because the accompanying scaphoid fracture or perilunate/lunate dislocation overshadows it. Most of these fractures are displaced, and require closed or open reduction with internal fixation. Avascular necrosis, delayed union, nonunion, and malunion may complicate them.

Trapezoid Fracture

This is an extremely rare fracture accounting for only 1 percent of all carpal fractures. The injury results from an axial load onto the index metacarpal. There will be tenderness on the radial side that is augmented by applying pressure along the index metacarpal ray. These injuries are difficult to see on standard radiographs, and CT or MRI may be necessary to visualize it. These fractures are treated with a thumb spica cast or splint.

DISTAL RADIUS AND ULNA FRACTURES

Fractures of the distal metaphysis of the radius and ulna are among the most common injuries affecting the wrist. Among the factors that influence the type and amount of displacement of the fracture are the point and direction of impact, the degree of force, and the patient's age. In general, the thinner cortices of the elderly make them more likely to sustain extraarticular fractures, whereas younger adults often sustain more complicated intraarticular fractures.

Colles' Fracture

Colles' fracture results most often from falls on the outstretched hand. This mechanism produces a distal radial metaphysis fracture that is dorsally angulated and displaced. Compression forces on the dorsal side often produce dorsal comminution of bone. The fracture line may also comminute and extend into the radioulnar or radiocarpal joint (''die-punch'' fracture). A fracture of the ulnar styloid is often present and may be suggestive of injury to the triangular fibrocartilage complex (Fig. 262-12).

The wrist has the characteristic dorsiflexion, or ''silver-fork,'' deformity. These individuals may complain of palmar paresthesias from tension or pressure on the median nerve. Anteroposterior radiographs reveal a distal metaphyseal fracture of the radius that often appears shortened from the angulation or comminution of the bone. The lateral view provides the best view of the dorsal angulation and comminution. In general, potentially unstable fractures have more than 20 degrees of angulation, intra-articular involvement, marked comminution, or more than a centimeter of shortening. These injuries are more likely to develop loss of reduction, distal radioulnar joint instability, radiocarpal instability patterns, and subsequent arthritis.

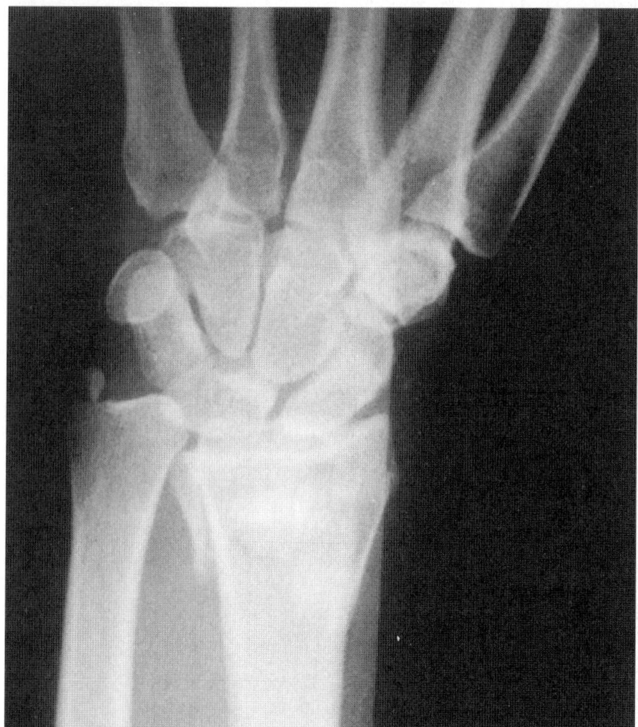

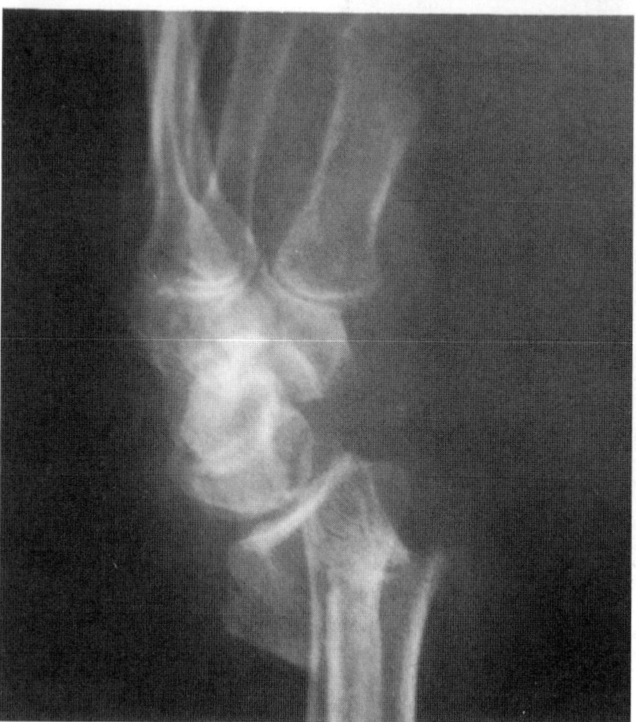

FIG. 262-12. Colles' fracture. (With permission from Chin HW, Visotsky J: Wrist fractures. *Em Med Clin North Am* 11:3, 1993.)

Stable fractures may be treated with a compression dressing and splint until they can be evaluated by an orthopedic surgeon. Otherwise, closed reduction is performed, with traction provided by finger traps while the fracture fragment is pushed distal and palmar while the patient's forearm is firmly held. The goal is to restore the volar tilt, radial inclination, and proper length to the radius. This is particularly important in younger patients. The volar tilt ideally should be restored to its normal position, but a minimum of neutral or zero degrees of angulation may be acceptable. Although most Colles' fractures can be treated with closed reduction and cast immobilization, those that are unstable, severely comminuted, or intra-articular may require casting with pinning, external fixation with possible bone grafting, or open reduction and internal fixation. Good to excellent results are achieved in 56 to 81 percent of patients with these more aggressive treatment alternatives. All open and neurovascularly compromised fractures require prompt evaluation by the orthopedic surgeon.

Complications include malunion, median nerve injuries, triangular fibrocartilage complex injuries, secondary radioulnar and radiocarpal instability patterns, and arthritis. These can produce a weak, stiff, and painful wrist.

Smith's Fracture

Smith's fracture, or ''reverse Colles' fracture,'' is a volar angulated fracture of the distal radius. These injuries result from a fall or direct blow on the dorsum of the hand and wrist or from falls on the outstretched hand in supination that then shifts into a pronated position. The hand is displaced palmar in a ''garden-spade deformity.'' The anteroposterior radiograph looks much like the Colles' fracture, with a distal metaphyseal radius fracture that may be shortened and comminuted. The lateral radiograph shows the volar angulated and displaced fracture (Fig. 262-13).

The treatment objectives and complications are much like those seen with Colles' fracture. In this case, however, the angulation is in the opposite direction.

Barton's Fracture

Barton's fractures are dorsal or volar rim fractures of the distal radius. The dorsal rim fractures result from a dorsiflexion and pronation force, whereas the less common volar rim fracture is produced by a fall on the outstretched hand in supination. These injuries are often fracture dislocations or subluxations, because the carpus or hand is frequently displaced in the direction of the fracture. Accompanying ligamentous injuries create radiocarpal instability. This is often not fully appreciated in the acute setting but can lead to various secondary carpal instability patterns and premature degenerative arthritis.

The anteroposterior radiograph often shows a comminuted fracture of the distal radial metaphysis. The lateral view reveals an intra-articular fracture of the volar or dorsal rim of the radius, which may be accompanied by carpal subluxation in the same direction (Fig. 262-14*A*, *B*).

Minimally displaced fractures can be treated acutely with closed reduction and a splint or cast until they can be reevaluated by the orthopedist. Unstable fractures involve more than 50 percent of the radial articular surface or have accompanying carpal subluxation and

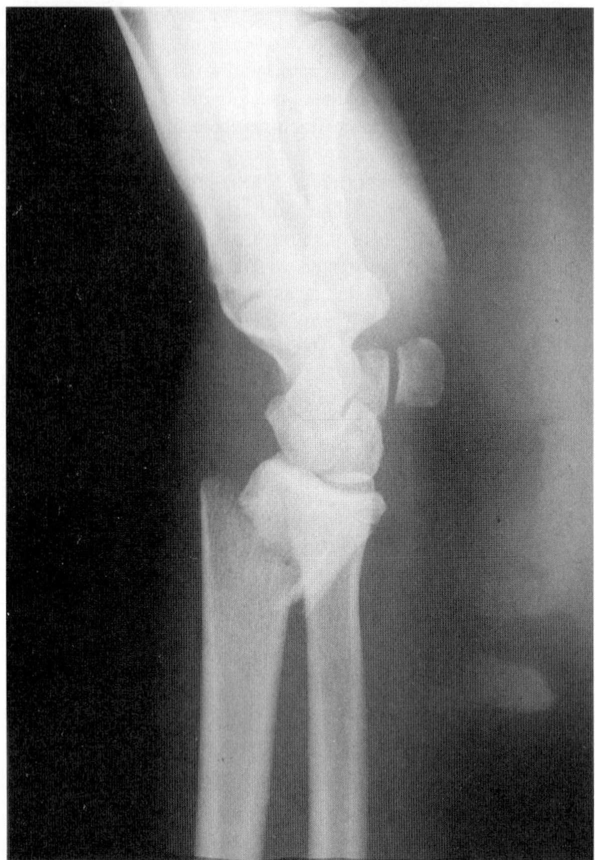

FIG. 262-13. Smith's fracture.

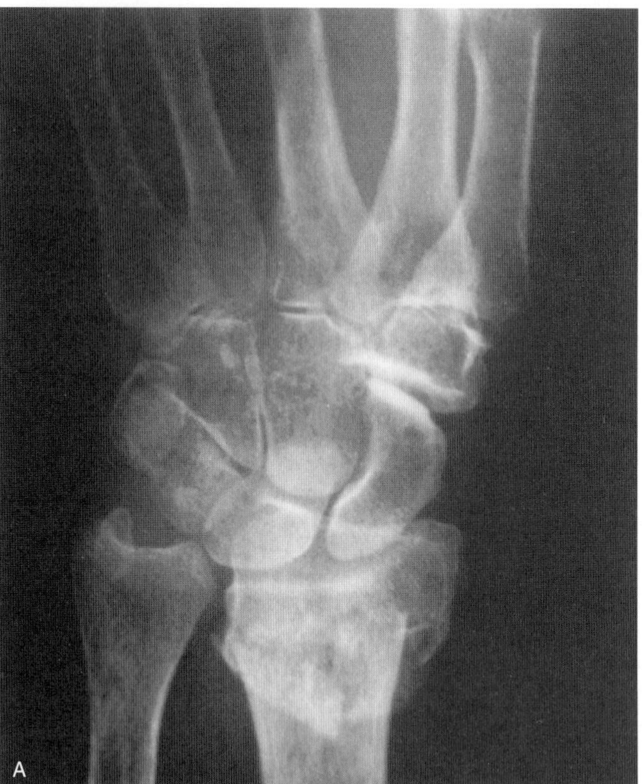

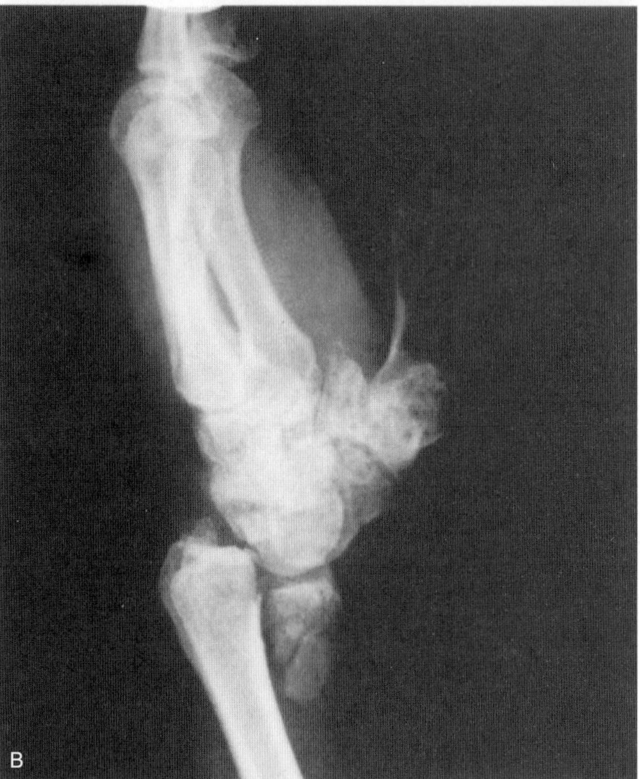

FIG. 262-14. Volar Barton's fracture. **A.** AP view. **B.** Lateral view. (With permission from Chin HW, Visotsky J: Wrist fractures. *Em Med Clin North Am* 11:3, 1993.)

require reduction and immobilization by the orthopedist. These injuries often require open reduction and fixation with pins or a buttress plate.

Radial Styloid Fracture

A force directed along the radial side of the hand can produce a transverse or oblique fracture that runs from the scaphoid fossa to the metaphysis of the radius. It is best seen on the anteroposterior radiograph as a thin, lucent line beneath the radial styloid. Because the major carpal ligaments along the radial side of the wrist insert on the radial styloid, displacement of this fracture can produce carpal instability. Displaced fractures often require open reduction and internal fixation. Displacement of as little as 3 mm is often associated with accompanying scapholunate dissociation. Failure to recognize these intercarpal ligament tears adds to the potential for subsequent posttraumatic arthritis.

Ulnar Styloid Fracture

Forced radial deviation, dorsiflexion, and rotatory stress fracture the ulnar styloid. The ulnar styloid fracture may be isolated or may accompany other injuries, such as Colles' fracture. Displaced fractures can be associated with tears of the triangular fibrocartilage complex, which is the main stabilizer of the distal radioulnar joint. These individuals complain of a painful clicking or locking sensation in the wrist.

Ulnar styloid fractures are treated acutely with a splint or cast in slight ulnar deviation and neutral positioning of the wrist. Arthrograms or MRI imaging may be necessary to delineate the full extent of these injuries.

Radioulnar Disruption

Radioulnar joint disruption is generally seen with intra-articular or distal radial shaft fractures (Galeazzi's fracture-dislocation), or with fractures of both bones of the forearm. These more apparent injuries often overshadow radioulnar joint disruption and, unfortunately, cause these injuries to be unrecognized until subsequent pain and diminished wrist movement are appreciated.

Isolated radioulnar joint dislocations are uncommon and are unrecognized acutely in as many as 50 percent of cases. Dorsal dislocation of the ulna results most often from falls on the wrist in hyperpronation. The rare volar dislocation results from forced hypersupination of the wrist. These individuals present with a painful wrist that has restricted range of motion. There may be a palpable prominence of the ulnar head, but this can be quite subtle and easily overlooked.

The anteroposterior radiograph reveals narrowing and overlap of the distal radioulnar joint. The lateral radiograph demonstrates either volar or dorsal displacement of the ulna, which is normally centered and overlapping the radius. Because slight oblique positioning of the wrist can produce a misleading appearance of ulnar displacement, it is crucial that a properly positioned lateral view be obtained. A true lateral view should have superimposition of the four-ulnar metacarpals, superimposition of the proximal pole of the scaphoid with the lunate and triquetrum, and the radial styloid centered over its distal articular surface. CT scanning may be necessary to establish the diagnosis if plain films are inconclusive. Immobilizing the wrist in supination reduces dorsal dislocations, whereas volar dislocations are placed in pronation. These injuries unfortunately have a high recurrence rate, particularly if there are delays in diagnosis, and may require reconstructive surgery.

BIBLIOGRAPHY

Altissimi M, Antenucci R, Fiacca C, Mancini GB: Long-term results of conservative treatment of fractures of the distal radius. *Clin Orthop* 206:202, 1986.

Bradway JK, Amadio PC, Cooney WP: Open reduction and internal fixation of displaced, comminuted intra-articular fractures of the distal end of the radius. *J Bone Joint Surg Am* 71A:839, 1989.

Breckenbaugh RD: Accurate evaluation and management of the painful wrist following injury. *Orthop Clin North Am* 15:289, 1984.

Bryan RS, Dobyns JH: Fractures of the carpal bones other than the navicular. *Clin Orthop* 149:107, 1980.

Chernin MM, Pitt MJ: Radiologic disease patterns at the carpus. *Clin Orthop* 187:72, 1984.

Cooney WP, Bussey R, Dobyns JH: Difficult wrist fractures. *Clin Orthop* 214:136, 1987.

Cooney WP, Dobyns JH, Linscheid RL: Fractures of the scaphoid: A rational approach to management. *Clin Orthop* 149:90, 1980.

Dunn AW: Fractures and dislocations of the carpus. *Surg Clin North Am* 52:1513, 1972.

Frykman G: Fractures of the distal radius: A clinical and experimental study. *Acta Orthop Scand* 108:1, 1967.

Green DP: The sprained wrist. *Am J Fam Pract* 19:114, 1979.

Green DP, O'Brien ET: Classification and management of carpal dislocations. *Clin Orthop* 149:55, 1980.

Johnson R: The acutely injured wrist and its residuals. *Clin Orthop* 149:33, 1980.

Linscheid RL: Kinematic considerations of the wrist. *Clin Orthop* 202:27,1986.

Linscheid RL, Dobyns JH, Beabout JW: Traumatic instability of the wrist. *J Bone Joint Surg Am* 54:1612, 1972.

Malone CP: Open treatment for displaced articular fractures of the distal radius. *Clin Orthop* 202:104, 1986.

Mayfield JK: Wrist ligamentous anatomy and pathogenesis of carpal instability. *Orthop Clin North Am* 15:209, 1984.

O'Brien ET: Acute fractures and dislocations of the carpus. *Orthop Clin North Am* 15:237, 1984.

Propp DA, Chin HW: Forearm and wrist radiology. *J Emerg Med* 7(4):393, 1989.

Rand JA, Linscheid RL, Dobyns JH: Capitate fractures. *Clin Orthop Rel Res* 165:205, 1982.

Waeckerle JF: A prospective study identifying the sensitivity of radiographic findings and the clinical efficacy of clinical findings in carpal navicular fractures. *Ann Emerg Med* 16:733, 1987.

263 INJURIES TO THE SHOULDER COMPLEX AND HUMERUS

Dennis T. Uehara
John P. Rudzinski

Function of the upper extremity is intimately dependent on the shoulder complex. Movement is effected through an intricate mechanism with integration of muscles, ligaments, osseous components, and a system of joints all working in harmony. Through its joint system, which consists of four joints, the sternoclavicular, glenohumeral, acromioclavicular, and scapulothoracic, the upper extremity is able to move through a complex and wide range of motion. The following discussion focuses on the major soft tissue and osseous components of the shoulder complex and humerus and those injuries that create loss of motion, instability, and pain.

STERNOCLAVICULAR DISLOCATIONS

The sternoclavicular joint is the most frequently moved nonaxial joint of the body because almost any movement of the upper extremity is transferred proximally to this joint. It also has the least amount of bony stability of any major joint because less than half of the medial end of the clavicle actually articulates with the upper sternum. Joint stability therefore depends on the integrity of the surrounding ligaments, which give the sternoclavicular joint surprising strength. As a result, the majority of injuries to this area are simple sprains, dislocations being uncommon.

A sprain of the sternoclavicular joint can result from the shoulder being forced forward suddenly or from a medially directed force applied to the shoulder. Pain and swelling are localized to the joint, and treatment is symptomatic with ice, sling, and analgesics. Differential diagnosis should include consideration of septic arthritis, especially in intravenous drug abusers.

Sternoclavicular dislocations are uncommon, accounting for only 3 percent of a series of 1603 shoulder girdle injuries. Dislocations usually result from motor vehicle accidents or sports injuries, but spontaneous dislocations have been reported. Posterior sternoclavicular joint dislocations are much less common than anterior dislocations. A posterior dislocation may result from a direct blow or from an indirect force to the shoulder if the shoulder is rolled forward at the time of impact. An anterior sternoclavicular joint dislocation may result from the same indirect force if the shoulder is rolled backward at the time of impact. Of note is that the medial clavicular epiphysis is the last epiphysis of the body to appear radiographically (age 18) and the last to close (age 22 to 25). As a result, physeal injuries in this age group can easily be misdiagnosed as a dislocation.

Patients with a sternoclavicular joint dislocation have severe pain that is exacerbated by arm motion and when in the supine position. The shoulder appears shortened and rolled forward. On examination, anterior dislocations have a prominent medial clavicle end that is visible and palpable anterior to the sternum. In posterior dislocations, the medial clavicle end is less visible and not palpable, and the patient may have signs and symptoms of impingement of the superior mediastinal contents (Fig. 263-1). Routine radiographs may not be diagnostic although specialized views or tomograms may be helpful. Computed tomography (CT) is the imaging procedure of choice.

Closed reduction of anterior sternoclavicular joint dislocations is usually attempted with the patient supine and with a sandbag or pad between the shoulders. Direct pressure over the clavicle may reduce

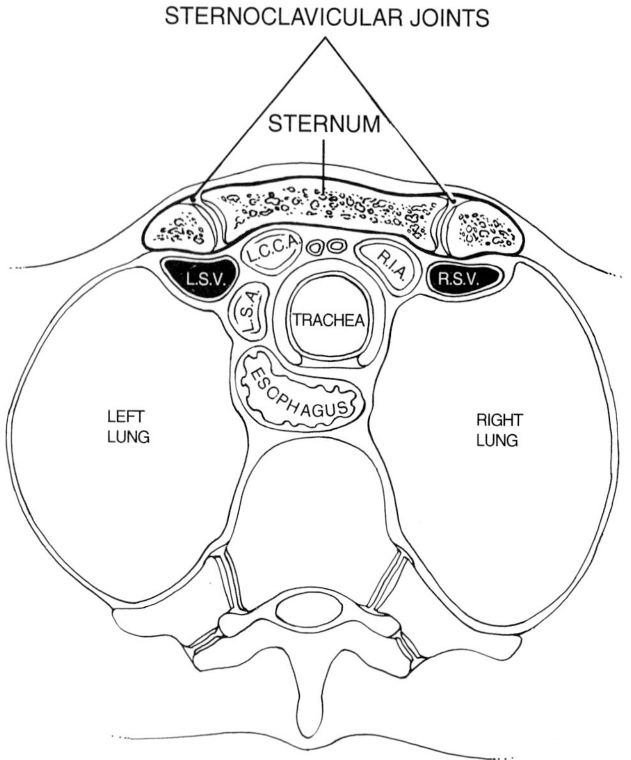

FIG. 263-1. The relationship of the sternoclavicular joint to adjacent structures. RSV, right subclavian vein; RIA, right innominate artery; LCCA, left common carotid artery; LSA, left subclavian artery; LSV, left subclavian vein.

the dislocation.The patient is usually discharged in a figure-of-eight clavicle harness. Unfortunately, many anterior dislocations prove unstable and recur as soon as direct pressure is released. Patients may subsequently undergo open reduction, or the position of the deformity may be accepted and no further treatment rendered.

In posterior dislocations, life-threatening injuries to adjacent structures may result in a pneumothorax or in compression or laceration of the great vessels, trachea, or esophagus. Local swelling may obscure any deformity, and routine radiographs are often not conclusive, making diagnosis difficult. Additional injuries should be aggressively sought and addressed. Orthopedic consultation for stabilized patients may attempt closed reduction, with thoracic surgical backup. A towel clip is often used to grasp and pull the medial clavicle forward and back into place. Open reduction may be necessary.

CLAVICLE

Clavicle fractures account for 5 percent of all fractures seen in the emergency department and for 44 percent of significant injuries to the shoulder girdle. This is the most common fracture of childhood, with almost half of these injuries occurring by the age of 7. The clavicle functions as a strut, connecting the shoulder girdle to the trunk, and provides support and mobility for upper-extremity function. The clavicle also protects the adjacent lung, brachial plexus, and subclavian and brachial blood vessels.

The most common mechanism of injury is a blow to the shoulder. Transmission of the compressive force results in a buckling of the clavicle, which fractures once a critical force is achieved. Children will often have a greenstick or buckle-type fracture or a bowing deformity without a definite fracture. Open fractures, due to extreme tenting of the overlying skin, may occasionally be seen.

Eighty percent of clavicle fractures involve the middle third, 15 percent the distal third, and 5 percent the medial third. Patients typically present with swelling, deformity, and tenderness localized to the clavicle. The arm is slumped inward and downward and is supported by the other extremity. Routine clavicle radiographs may miss fractures due to overlap of surrounding structures, particularly with fractures at either end of the bone. Diagnosis of these may require special views or specialized techniques, such as tomography or computed tomography (CT) scan.

Numerous forms of treatment have been described for this common injury. Simple immobilization with a sling is often successful, with displaced fractures often treated with a figure-of-eight brace. A shoulder spica or open reduction may be required for severely displaced fractures, poor patient compliance, or for complications. Healing may occur as rapidly as 2 weeks for infants, with most adults healing in a 4- to 6-week period.

Although the vast majority of these fractures have a benign course, serious associated injuries and complications may occasionally occur. Penetrating or blunt trauma may result in associated lung, neurovascular, or first-rib injuries. Injury to the adjacent vascular structures, usually the subclavian artery, subclavian vein, internal jugular vein, or axillary artery, may be life-threatening. Distal clavicle fractures with displacement typically are associated with rupture of the coracoclavicular ligament and may require operative intervention to avoid nonunion. Medial clavicle fractures may be associated with intrathoracic injuries or develop late complications, such as arthritis. Significant callus formation may result in subsequent compression of adjacent neurovascular structures and is cosmetically deforming.

SCAPULA

The scapula links the axial skeleton to the upper extremity and serves as a stabilizing platform for motion of the arm. Fracture of the scapula is an infrequent occurrence, accounting for less than 1 percent of all fractures. Due to the high energy typically required to fracture this protected bone, there is a greater than 80 percent association of injuries to the ipsilateral lung, thoracic cage, and shoulder girdle.

Significant scapular injury occurs most frequently in men between 25 and 40 years of age, usually as a result of motor vehicle accidents, falls, or other severe trauma. The mechanism of injury is from a direct blow, trauma to the shoulder sometimes with injury of the acromion or coracoid, or a fall on the outstretched arm. An indirect axial load transmitted via the outstretched arm may result in a scapular neck fracture, while the indirect force of a shoulder dislocation may result in fracture of the glenoid. Scapular fractures may be classified by their anatomic location: body, glenoid neck, intraarticular glenoid, spine, coracoid, and acromion (Fig. 263-2). Fractures of the body and glenoid neck are the most common.

A patient with an isolated scapular fracture typically will present with localized tenderness over the scapula and the ipsilateral arm held in adduction. The shoulder may have a flattened appearance. Radiographs consisting of an anteroposterior shoulder, lateral scapula, and axillary will identify most fractures. However, scapula fractures are often associated with other significant injuries, and hence diagnosis may be delayed or initially missed entirely. In Ada and Miller's series, 96 percent of scapular fractures had associated injuries, of which rib fractures were the most common, followed by pulmonary, humeral head, and shoulder girdle injuries. Other injuries may include neurovascular, abdominal, and spine trauma.

Rarely, significant trauma may result in scapulothoracic dissociation. This syndrome consists of lateral scapular displacement, clavicular disruption, and severe soft-tissue injury. This injury is sometimes associated with brachial plexus avulsion, subclavian artery disruption, or both. Its presence may be suspected by neurovascular findings or by lateral displacement of the scapula visualized on a nonrotated chest radiograph.

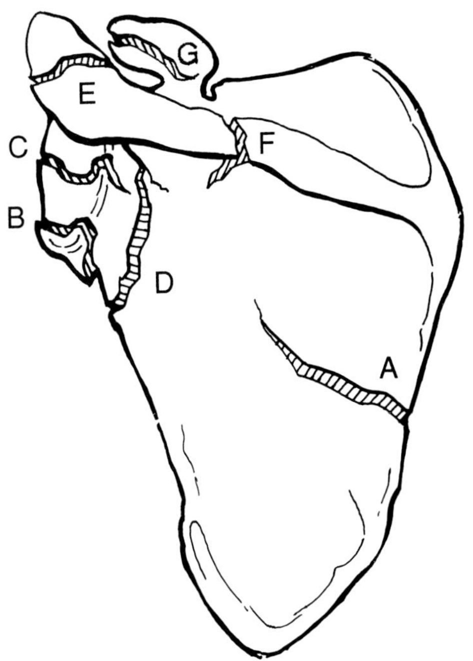

FIG. 263-2. Sites of scapula fractures. **A.** Body. **B.** Glenoid rim. **C.** Intraarticular glenoid. **D.** Neck. **E.** Acromion. **F.** Spine. **G.** Coracoid.

The vast majority of scapular fractures are treated nonsurgically, with a sling for immobilization, ice, analgesics, and early range-of-motion exercises. Surgical intervention may be necessary for significant or displaced articular fractures of the glenoid, angulated glenoid neck fractures, acromial fractures associated with a rotator cuff tear, and some coracoid fractures. Fractures of the glenoid, acromion, or coracoid are more likely to be associated with long-term disability.

Complications of scapular fractures themselves are uncommon. Although many of these fractures heal with some degree of malunion, typically this does not result in significant disability. Most long-term disability is a result of other, associated injuries.

ROTATOR CUFF INJURIES

The rotator cuff consists of the tendons of the supraspinatus, infraspinatus, subscapularis, and teres minor muscles (see also Chap. 275). These tendons coalesce with the capsule of the glenohumeral joint and attach to the greater and lesser tuberosities of the humerus. The main function of the rotator cuff is to provide dynamic stability to the glenohumeral joint. This is accomplished by contraction of muscles that compress the humeral head in the glenoid and by selective contraction resist the actions of major shoulder girdle muscles. The end result is a stable scapulohumeral articulation with the ability to perform smooth, coordinated motion. Injuries to the rotator cuff occur as a result of acute trauma, such as from a dislocation of the glenohumeral joint and as a result of chronic injuries.

Tears of the rotator cuff after glenohumeral dislocation are common but unfortunately often missed. They should be suspected in all patients over the age of 40 years, in patients with luxatio erecta, and in patients who are unable to abduct or externally rotate the arm after a glenohumeral dislocation.

Chronic injuries occur as a result of impingement and decreased vascularity, both common with advancing age. Impingement is explained by the anatomic relationship of the rotator cuff to osseus and soft-tissue structures. It is ''sandwiched'' among the humeral head, acromion, coracoid, and the coracoacromial ligament. Compression of the rotator cuff between the humeral head and the coracoacromial arch (acromion, coracoid, and coracoacromial ligament) leads to tendon attrition and degeneration. Disease of the rotator cuff is a continuum of injury from mild inflammation to rupture. The initial stage is characterized by inflammation and edema, resulting in mild pain with activity. There is no limitation of motion or weakness. There may be mild tenderness over the greater tuberosity. This stage of disease is most common in patients less than 25 years of age and is completely reversible.

In the second stage there is increased tendinitis, and the pain is more intense and seems to be worse at night. Tenderness is more diffuse. Overhead motion is painful, and there is some limitation of abduction and external rotation.

The third stage of disease is characterized by significant rotator cuff degeneration and tears. Most patients are over the age of 40 with a long history of symptoms. They have more pain, limitation of motion, and weakness. Patients with complete rotator cuff tears have tenderness over the greater tuberosity and acromioclavicular joint. They also have limitation of motion and weakness, especially to abduction and external rotation. Disease at this stage is considered irreversible.

Treatment in the early stages consists of rest, with sling immobilization, nonsteroidal anti-inflammatory drugs, ice, and local injections. Treatment of rotator cuff tears is initially symptomatic, followed by consideration for surgery either arthroscopically or open. (See Chap. 275 for more detailed discussion of shoulder pain.)

ACROMIOCLAVICULAR JOINT INJURIES

Injuries to the acromioclavicular joint are commonly seen in emergency practice. Although they may occur in any age group, the majority occur in young, active males. Emergency management consists of identifying the severity of injury, recognizing associated injuries, and managing selected patients as outpatients.

Anatomy

The acromioclavicular joint is a diarthrodial joint that, together with the sternoclavicular joint, connects the upper extremity to the axial skeleton. The support of the acromioclavicular joint is through the acromioclavicular and coracoclavicular ligaments and the strong attachment of the trapezius and deltoid muscles (Fig. 263-3). The acromioclavicular joint is surrounded by a thin capsule, which is reinforced by the acromioclavicular ligaments. The superior fibers of this ligament blend with the fascia of the trapezius and deltoid, which attach to the clavicle and acromion. The acromioclavicular ligaments provide horizontal stability to the joint. The tough coracoclavicular ligaments consist of two parts, the more lateral trapezoid and the medial conoid. They attach the distal inferior clavicle to the coracoid process of the scapula. The coracoclavicular ligament is the major suspensory ligament of the upper extremity and provides vertical stability to the acromioclavicular joint.

Mechanism of Injury

The mechanism of injury is usually direct trauma to the acromioclavicular joint from a fall with the arm adducted, as typically may occur in a sporting activity. An indirect mechanism is a fall on the outstretched hand with transmission of force to the acromioclavicular joint. The result is that the scapula and shoulder girdle are driven inferiorly while the clavicle remains in its normal position. This is confirmed by observing the opposite clavicle, which is at the same level as the injured one.

Clinical Features

The diagnosis of acromioclavicular joint injuries is made clinically. The typical mechanism of injury, as well as tenderness and deformity

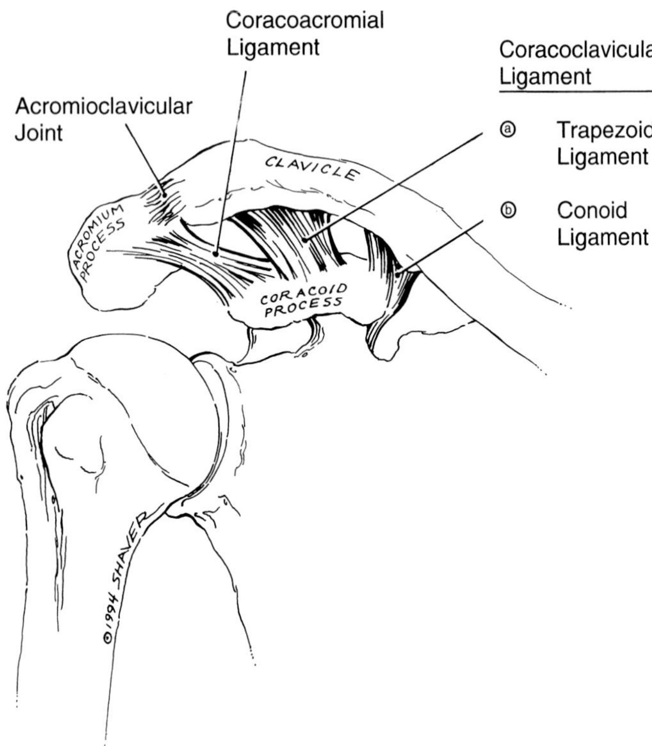

FIG. 263-3. Anatomy of the acromioclavicular joint.

at the acromioclavicular joint, is confirmatory. Radiographs are useful for identifying other fractures and determining the severity of injury. Acromioclavicular radiographs should specifically be ordered because they require only one-third to one-half the penetration of standard shoulder films. Shoulder technique will overpenetrate the acromioclavicular joint, and small fractures may be missed. Although standard acromioclavicular radiographs are generally sufficient, an axillary view is required to identify posterior clavicular dislocation (type IV, see below). Routine use of stress radiographs has been standard practice. Recently, however, Bossart and colleagues have called this practice into question. Their study suggests that stress radiographs are of low yield and that their routine use should be abandoned. Although some agree, others disagree, citing occult type III (see below) injuries that can be unmasked only with stress radiographs.

Classification of Injury

The classification of acromioclavicular joint injuries classically describes three types of injuries. Rockwood describes three others (Fig. 263-4). Types I, II, and III are common; types IV, V, and VI are rare. The anatomic injury, radiographic findings, and physical findings are summarized in Table 263-1.

Treatment

Treatment of type I injuries consists of rest, ice, analgesics, and immobilization, followed by early range-of-motion exercises. Most agree that type II injuries should be similarly treated. Various straps and braces have been used to reduce the dislocation, but none has proven successful. A simple sling remains the most convenient and effective. Prognosis for type I and II injuries is excellent, with only a small percentage who develop late symptoms requiring excision of the distal clavicle. Treatment of type III injuries (Fig. 263-5) is controversial, with proponents for both conservative and operative philosophies. A recent trend among directors of orthopedic residency programs, however, reveals a shift to conservative treatment with sling immobilization. Both strategies have yielded good results in selected patients, with the specific management operator dependent. Treatment decisions are based on such factors as age, occupation, and activity level. Types IV, V, and VI are severe injuries, and most authors recommend surgical repair. Because other injuries are associated with these more severe forms of acromioclavicular joint injuries (especially type VI), a careful clinical and radiographic examination must be performed.

TABLE 263-1 Classification and Physical Findings in Acromioclavicular Joint Injuries

Type	Injury	Radiograph	Examination
I	Sprained acromioclavicular ligaments	Normal	Tenderness over acromioclavicular joint
II	Acromioclavicular ligaments ruptured; coracoclavicular ligaments sprained	Slight widening of acromioclavicular joint; clavicle elevated 25–50% above acromion; may be slight widening of the coracoclavicular interspace	Tenderness and mild step-off deformity of acromioclavicular joint
III	Acromioclavicular ligaments ruptured; coracoclavicular ligaments ruptured; deltoid and trapezius detached	Acromioclavicular joint dislocated 100%; coracoclavicular interspace widened 25–100%	Distal end of clavicle prominent; shoulder droops
IV	Rupture of all supporting structures; clavicle displaced posteriorly in or through the trapezius	May appear similar to type II and III; axillary radiograph required to visualize posterior dislocation	Possible posterior displacement of clavicle
V	Rupture of all supporting structures (more severe form of type III injury)	Acromioclavicular joint dislocated; generally 200–300% disparity of coracoclavicular interspace compared to normal shoulder	More pain; gross deformity of clavicle
VI	Acromioclavicular ligaments disrupted; coracoclavicular ligaments, deltoid, and trapezius may be disrupted	Acromioclavicular joint dislocated; clavicle displaced inferiorly	Severe swelling; multiple associated injuries

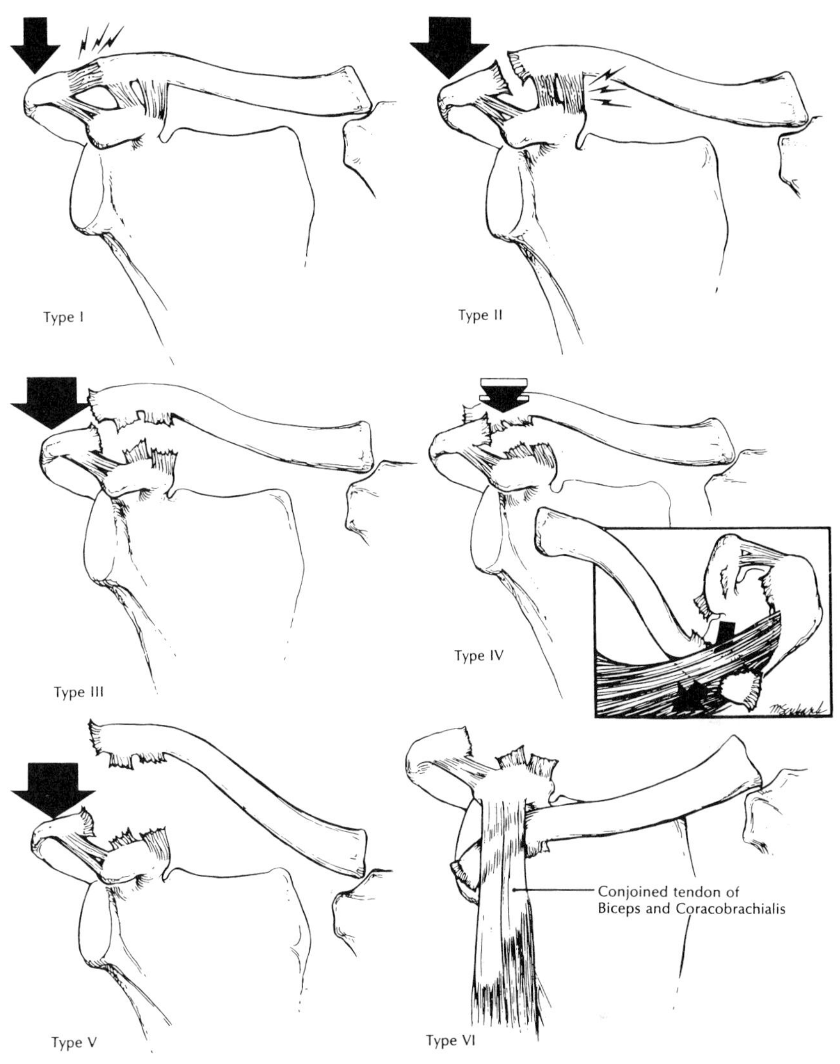

FIG. 263-4. Classification of acromioclavicular joint injuries. (From Rockwood CA, Green DP, Bucholz RW: *Rockwood & Green's Fractures in Adults,* 3d ed. Philadelphia, Lippincott, 1991, with permission.)

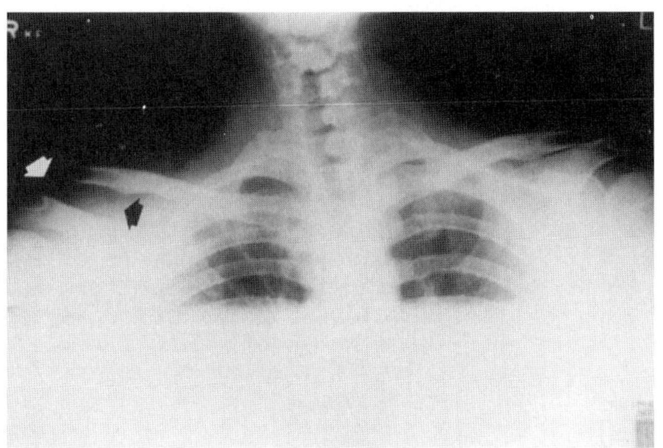

FIG. 263-5. Type III acromioclavicular dislocation. Note the dislocation of the acromioclavicular joint (*white arrow*) and increased coracoclavicular interspace (*black arrow*).

DISLOCATION OF THE GLENOHUMERAL JOINT

Dislocation of the glenohumeral joint is the most common major joint dislocation. Anterior dislocations are by far the most common. Posterior dislocations are described but occur in less than 2 percent of cases. Other dislocations include inferior (luxatio erecta) and superior (very rare).

Anterior Glenohumeral Dislocations

There are four types of anterior dislocations. In subcoracoid dislocation, the commonest type, the humeral head is displaced anterior to the glenoid and inferior to the coracoid. In a subglenoid dislocation, the humeral head lies inferior and anterior to the glenoid fossa. In a subclavicular dislocation, the head of the humerus is displaced medial to the coracoid below the clavicle. In the very rare intrathoracic dislocation, the head of the humerus lies between the ribs and thoracic cavity.

The mechanism of injury may be direct force, but an indirect force is commoner. The combination of abduction, extension, and external rotation with sufficient force will cause an anterior dislocation.

The patient is usually in severe pain. The arm is in slight abduction and external rotation. The shoulder is "squared off," lacking the normal rounded contour. The patient resists abduction and internal rotation. The humeral head can often be palpated anteriorly. Because neurovascular injuries occur, a careful examination must be performed. The axillary nerve is most commonly injured. This nerve may be tested by pinprick sensation over the skin of the deltoid muscle.

Anteroposterior and scapular lateral or Y radiographs should be obtained before reduction is attempted. Although the anteroposterior radiograph will reveal the dislocation, the scapular Y radiograph will indicate the direction of dislocation: anterior or posterior. Bony injuries reported in the literature include fractures of the anterior glenoid lip, greater tuberosity, coracoid, and acromion, and compression fractures of the humeral head (Hill-Sachs lesion).

Many reduction techniques have been described. The three main categories are traction, leverage, and scapular manipulation. Success rates are between 70 and 90 percent regardless of technique. The use of conscious sedation is recommended, but any reduction technique may be attempted without medication when performed slowly and atraumatically. It is important for the physician to be comfortable with two or three techniques in case of a failed first attempt. Considerations in selection of a technique include ease of performance, effectiveness, as little trauma and pain as possible, requirement for medication, number of assistants, and time for procedure.

HIPPOCRATIC (MODIFIED) A modification of the Hippocratic method uses traction-countertraction (Fig. 263-6). The patient is supine with the arm abducted and elbow flexed at 90°. A sheet is tied and placed across the thorax of the patient and then around the waist of the assistant. Another sheet is tied and placed around the forearm of the patient at the elbow and the waist of the physician. The physician gradually applies traction as the assistant provides countertraction. Gentle internal and external rotation or outward pressure on the proximal humerus may aid reduction.

STIMSON The patient is placed prone on a gurney with the dislocated extremity hanging over the side and a 10-pound weight attached to the wrist. Complete muscle relaxation is required. Twenty to 30 min is required to allow reduction to occur.

Although safe, effective, and easy to learn, the time involved and constant monitoring by a nurse are drawbacks to this technique.

MILCH The patient is supine. The physician slowly abducts and externally rotates the arm to the overhead position (Fig. 263-7). With the elbow fully extended, traction is applied. With the other hand, pressure may be placed on the humeral head to manipulate it over the lip of the glenoid.

This technique is well tolerated by the patient, effective, and atraumatic. It is the technique of choice for many physicians

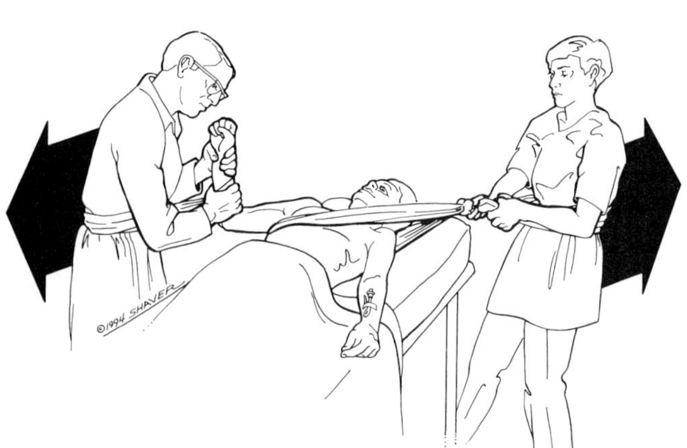

FIG. 263-6. Modified Hippocratic technique.

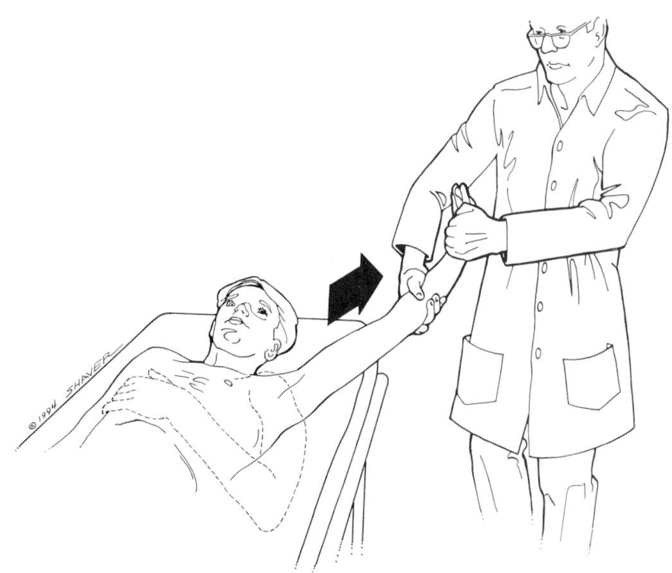

FIG. 263-7. Milch technique.

SCAPULAR MANIPULATION The patient is positioned with weights in the same manner as the Stimson technique (Fig. 263-8). After adequate sedation, the physician pushes the tip of the scapula medially using the thumbs, while stabilizing the superior aspect with the cephalad hand.

Several reports have recently been published. Physicians have found this technique relatively painless, fast, and in one study 90 percent successful.

EXTERNAL ROTATION The patient is supine with the arm adducted to the patient's side. With the elbow at 90° of flexion, the arm is slowly externally rotated. No longitudinal traction is applied. It is important to perform the movement slowly to allow time for spasm and pain to resolve. Reduction is usually complete prior to reaching the coronal plane and is often not noted either by the patient or physician.

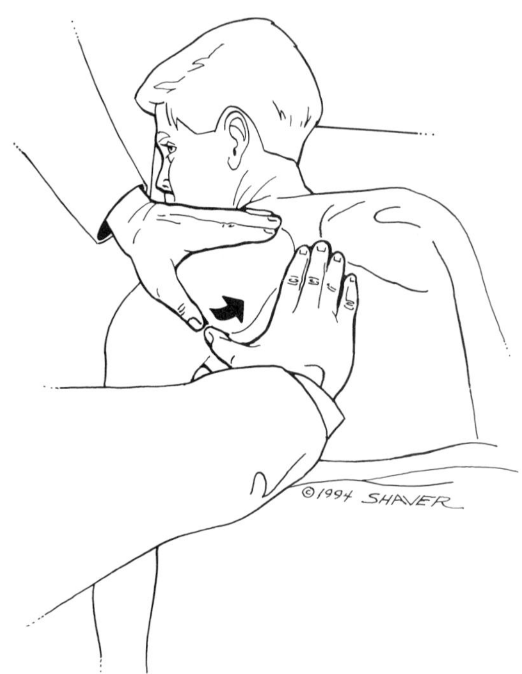

FIG. 263-8. Scapular manipulation technique.

This method has been reported to be 78 percent successful, relatively atraumatic, safe, and easily learned.

COMPLICATIONS Complications are frequently encountered in patients with anterior glenohumeral dislocations. The most common complication is recurrent dislocation, which is age dependent. Those patients less than 20 years of age have a greater than 90 percent recurrence; those older than 40 years have a 14 percent recurrence. Other complications include fractures and injuries to nerves and the rotator cuff. Vascular injuries are rare but when they occur tend to involve the axillary artery in elderly patients. Clinical findings of vascular injury include absent radial pulse, axillary hematoma, bruising of the lateral chest wall, and an axillary bruit.

Bony injuries are common and include fractures of the humeral head (Hill-Sachs lesion), anterior glenoid lip, and greater tuberosity. Neural injuries occur in 10 to 25 percent of acute dislocations. Of these injuries, which are the result of traction neuropraxia, most occur in the axillary nerve. This injury is temporary and resolves spontaneously. The common test of sensation over the skin of the deltoid muscle may not be reliable, with only an electromyogram providing an accurate evaluation. Other nerves injured are the radial, ulnar, median, musculocutaneous, and brachial plexus.

A frequent but often missed injury is a tear of the rotator cuff. This injury, which increases with age, has a greater than 80 percent occurrence in patients older than 60 years. Treatment is surgical.

Posterior Glenohumeral Dislocations

Posterior dislocation may occur with the humeral head in the subacromial (most commonly with the humeral head behind the glenoid and beneath the acromion), subglenoid, or subspinous. The latter two are rare.

The usual mechanism is an indirect force that produces forceful internal rotation and adduction. This mechanism may occur during a fall or from violent muscle contraction from a seizure or electric shock. Direct force to the anterior shoulder can also produce a posterior dislocation.

Posterior dislocations are reported to be commonly missed. Thus, a careful examination and radiographic evaluation are essential. Clinical findings include the following:

1. The arm is adducted and internally rotated.
2. The anterior shoulder is flat and the posterior aspect full.
3. The coracoid process is prominent.
4. The patient will not allow external rotation or abduction because of severe pain.

Although the anteroposterior radiograph is helpful, the scapular Y radiograph is diagnostic. In this radiograph, the humeral head is seen in a posterior position.

Since severe pain and muscle spasms are the norm, muscle relaxation and analgesia are paramount. The reduction is performed with the patient supine. Traction is applied to the adducted arm in the long axis of the humerus. An assistant gently pushes the humeral head anteriorly into the glenoid fossa.

Most complications are fractures, including fractures of the posterior glenoid rim, humeral head (reversed Hill-Sachs deformity), humeral shaft, and lesser tuberosity. Neurovascular and rotator cuff tears are less common than in anterior dislocations.

Inferior Dislocations (Luxatio Erecta)

Although inferior dislocation is a rare injury, it is one that will be seen in a busy emergency practice. It is always a severe injury and is associated with significant soft-tissue trauma or fracture. The mechanism of injury is a hyperabduction force, which levers the neck of the humerus against the acromion. As the force continues the inferior capsule tears, and the humeral head is forced out inferiorly.

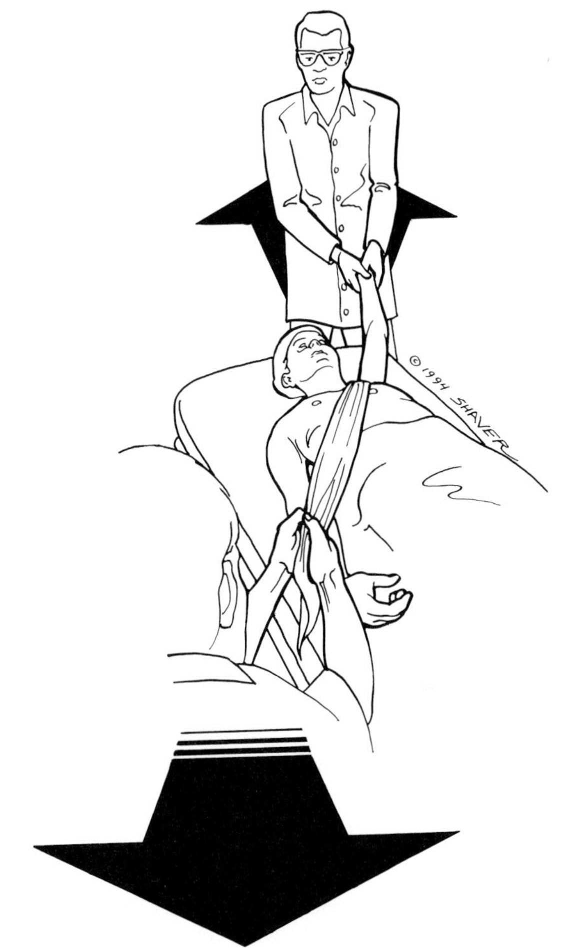

FIG. 263-9. Reduction of luxatio erecta.

The patient is in severe pain. The humerus is fully abducted, the elbow is flexed, and the patient's hand is on or behind the head. The humeral head can be palpated on the lateral chest wall. This clinical presentation is difficult to mistake for another condition.

Reduction consists of traction in an upward and outward direction in line with the humerus (Fig. 263-9). The assistant applies countertraction. Reduction is signaled by a ''clunk.'' The arm is then brought to the patient's side and immobilized in a shoulder immobilizer.

Complications include severe soft-tissue injuries and fractures of the proximal humerus. The rotator cuff, which is always detached, requires orthopedic follow-up. Neurovascular compression injuries are usually found but almost always resolve following reduction. When the humeral head is buttonholed through the inferior capsule, the dislocation is irreducible, and operative reduction is required.

HUMERUS FRACTURES

Proximal Humerus

Fractures of the proximal humerus are a relatively common problem in the emergency department, representing 5 percent of all fractures. They typically occur in elderly osteoporotic patients via an indirect mechanism, such as a fall on an outstretched hand with the elbow extended. Eighty percent of such fractures can be easily managed by the emergency physician, but the remainder have significant displacement and are a challenge to correctly diagnose and treat. Fortunately, the shoulder joint has an intrinsic reserve of range of motion, which can often provide a surprisingly functional outcome despite seemingly crippling injuries.

The proximal humerus is composed of the articular segment, the greater and lesser tuberosities, and the proximal humeral shaft. Muscles of the rotator cuff insert on the humeral tuberosities, and the biceps tendon travels between them. The humeral circumflex arteries enter in the area of the bicipital groove and the tuberosities to supply blood flow to the articular segment.

Patients with fractures typically present with pain, swelling, and tenderness about the shoulder. Crepitus and ecchymosis may be present, and the arm is generally held closely against the chest wall. A neurovascular examination should be performed, since the brachial plexus and axillary arteries are near the coracoid process and not uncommonly injured. The axillary nerve is the most commonly injured nerve, and sensation over the skin of the deltoid muscle should be tested routinely. Injury to the axillary artery is the commonest vascular injury and may be suggested by paresthesias, pallor, pulselessness, or an expanding hematoma. Vascular injuries may occur with even trivial trauma in atherosclerotic elderly patients.

Radiographs consisting of anteroposterior, lateral shoulder, and axillary views will correctly diagnose most proximal humerus fractures. Fractures of the articular surface may be suggested by a fat fluid level or by a superior joint hematoma that appears to push the humerus downward in the joint as a ''pseudosubluxation.'' A transthoracic lateral radiograph, tomograms, CT scan, and magnetic resonance imaging scan may also be of value.

The Neer classification system uses the relationship of the proximal humerus segments (greater and lesser tuberosities, anatomic neck, and surgical neck) to guide the management of these fractures. Significant fragment displacement is defined as greater than 1-cm separation or greater than 45° of angulation between fragments. The number of fracture fragments significantly displaced determines the classification in the Neer system (Fig. 263-10).

A one-part fracture may have any number of fracture lines, but no major segment is significantly displaced. The surrounding soft tissue and periosteum hold fracture fragments together. One-part fractures comprise over 80 percent of all proximal humerus fractures. Treatment generally consists of immobilization with a sling and swathe or collar and cuff, ice, analgesics, and referral. Early exercise is important to avoid adhesive capsulitis. The overall prognosis is generally good.

Two-part fractures account for 10 percent of proximal humerus fractures, with the remaining 10 percent evenly split between three-part and four-part fractures. Such displaced fractures are more frequently associated with complications and are often difficult to manage. Treatment considerations include integrity of the blood supply, integrity of the rotator cuff, likelihood of union, associated dislocations and neurovascular injuries, and the functionality of the patient. Closed reduction, intraoperative treatment, or a combination of the two may be necessary. Emergent orthopedic consultation for multipart fractures facilitates subsequent reduction and referral.

Any fracture involving the anatomic neck or the articular surface may result in compromise of the blood supply to the articular segment. Ischemic necrosis of the articular segment may ultimately require insertion of a humeral head prosthesis for these relatively uncommon fractures. Greater tuberosity fractures accompany up to 15 percent of anterior shoulder dislocations. Significant displacement of a greater tuberosity fragment implies a concomitant rotator cuff tear, with surgical repair often necessary for the active patient. Fracture of the lesser tuberosity should alert the examiner to a potential posterior shoulder dislocation. Significantly angulated surgical neck fractures are at risk for neurovascular damage (axillary neurovascular structures and brachial plexus) and should be immediately immobilized and radiographed in the position of presentation. Children may have significant displacement or separation of the proximal humeral epiphysis and may require exact reduction if near skeletal maturity. A shoulder spica is often used after reduction.

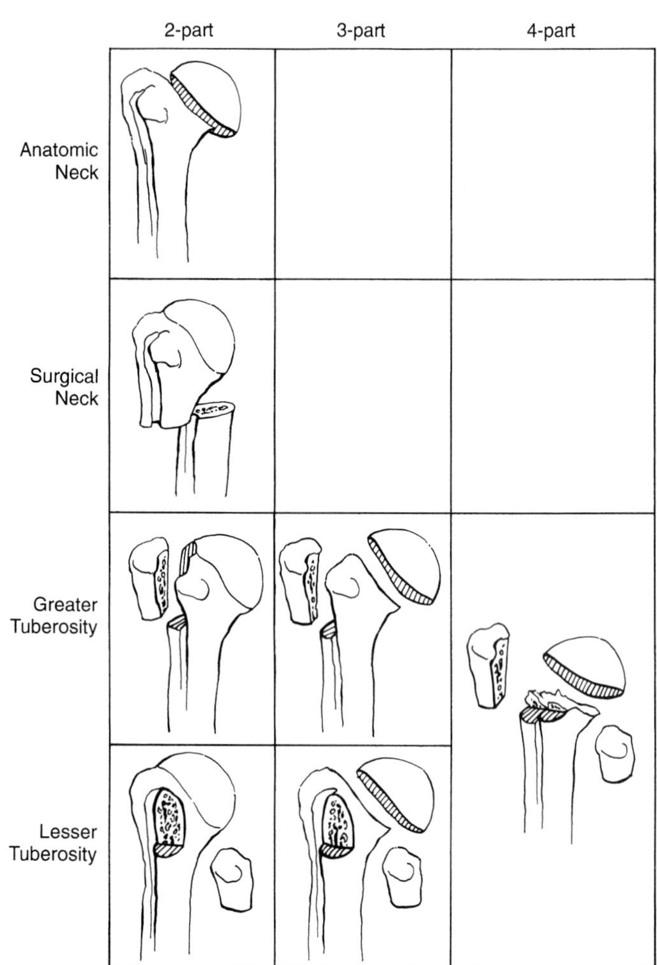

FIG. 263-10. The Neer classification system for proximal humerus fractures.

Humeral Shaft

Fractures of the humeral shaft occur in a bimodal age distribution, with peaks in the third and seventh decades of life, representing active young men and osteoporotic elderly women, respectively. The most common site of fracture is the middle third. Neurovascular injuries are a common complication of these fractures and are a direct result of the anatomy of the upper extremity. Displacement of fracture fragments is common as a result of the insertions and actions of the various muscles (deltoid, biceps, triceps, supraspinatus, and pectoralis major) that act on the upper arm (Fig. 263-11).

Humeral shaft fractures may be caused by a direct blow that produces a bending force, which results in a transverse fracture. It may also be caused by an indirect mechanism, such as a fall on the outstretched hand that produces a torsion force, resulting in a spiral fracture. A combination of bending and torsion forces results in an oblique fracture, sometimes with comminution, producing the ''butterfly'' fragment. The humerus is also a common site of pathologic fractures, especially from metastatic breast cancer.

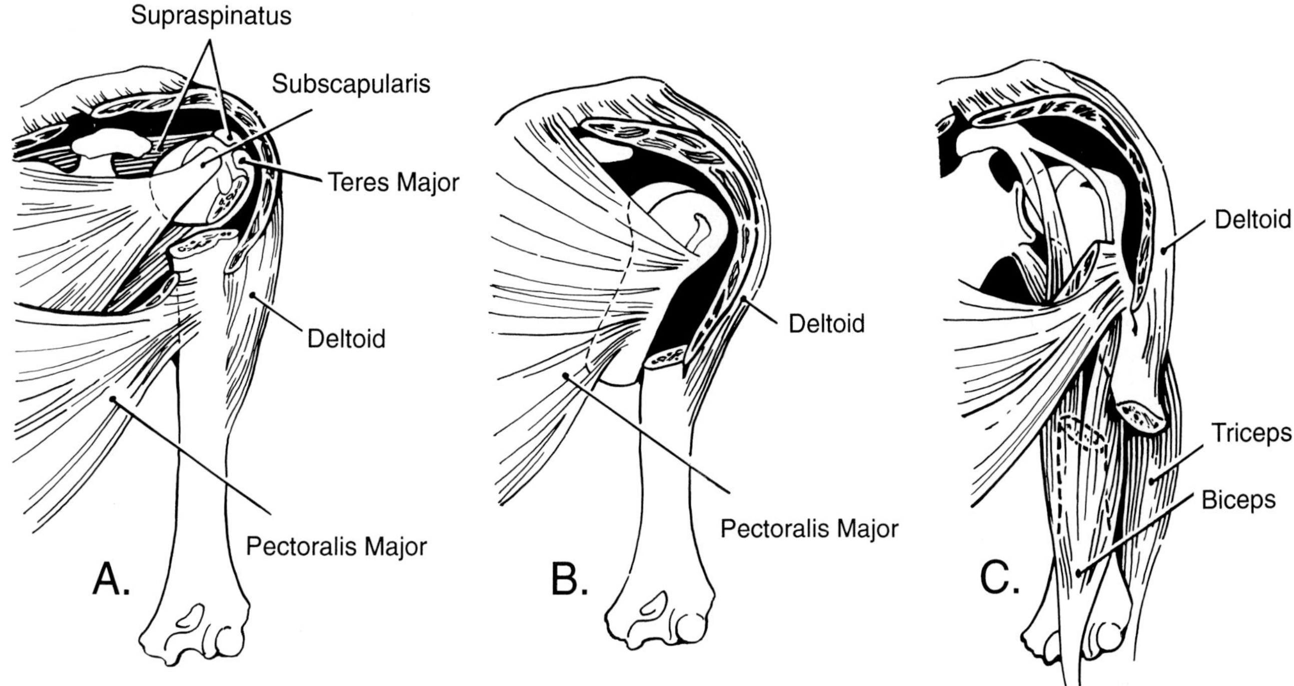

FIG. 263-11. The actions of the muscles inserting on the humeral shaft determine fracture angulation and displacement. Humeral fractures anterior view: **A.** Angulation of fragments with fracture line distal to rotator cuff insertion. **B.** Angulation of fragments with fracture line distal to pectoralis major insertion. **C.** Angulation of fragments with fracture line distal to deltoid insertion.

Clinical examination reveals localized tenderness, swelling, pain, and abnormal mobility or crepitus on palpation. Displaced fractures are associated with shortening of the upper extremity. Attention must be given to the initial neurovascular status, and reevaluation must be performed, especially after manipulation. Radiographs should include two views of the humerus, and consideration should be given to radiographic examination of the shoulder and elbow as well.

The vast majority of closed fractures of the shaft of the humerus are managed nonoperatively. The treatment of uncomplicated fractures includes immobilization, ice, analgesia, and referral. Closed treatment options include the coaptation splint (sugar tong), a hanging cast, functional bracing, and external fixation. A simple sling and swathe are adequate for most emergency management. Some surgeons favor internal fixation for patients with transverse fracture lines, very proximal or very distal humerus fractures, pathologic fractures, multiple trauma, and fractures associated with neurovascular injuries.

Complications include injury to the brachial artery or vein, or the radial, ulnar, or median nerves. A radial nerve injury, which is the most common, may be manifested by a wrist drop and altered sensation at the dorsal first web space. The incidence of radial nerve palsy ranges from 10 to 20 percent. Fractures of the distal third are particularly prone to entrapment of the radial nerve either as a result of the initial injury or after closed reduction. The majority of patients have eventual return of nerve function without operative intervention.

BIBLIOGRAPHY

Ada JR, Miller ME: Scapular fractures. *Clin Orthop* 269:174, 1991.

Beach WR, Caspari RB: Arthroscopic management of rotator cuff disease. *Orthopedics* 16:1007, 1993.

Bossart PJ, Joyce SM, Manaster BJ, et al: Lack of efficacy of ''weighted'' radiographs in diagnosing acute acromioclavicular separation. *Ann Emerg Med* 17:20, 1988.

Breazeale NM, Craig EV: Partial-thickness rotator cuff tears. *Orthop Clin North Am* 28:145, 1997.

Camden P, Nade S: Fracture bracing the humerus. *Injury* 23:45, 1992.

Cook DA, Peiner JP: Acromioclavicular joint injuries. *Orthop Rev* 19:510, 1990.

Cox JS: Current method of treatment of acromioclavicular joint dislocations. *Orthopedics* 15:1041, 1992.

Damschen DD, Cogbill TH, Siegel MJ: Scapulothoracic dissociation caused by blunt trauma. *J Trauma Injury Infect Crit Care* 42:537, 1997.

Gallay SH, Hupel TM, Beaton DE, et al: Functional outcome of acromioclavicular joint injury in polytrauma patients. *J Orthop Trauma* 12:159, 1998.

Gartsman GM, Brinker MR, Khan M: Early effectiveness of arthroscopic repair for full-thickness tears of the rotator cuff. *J Bone Joint Surg* 80:33, 1998.

Golden RH, Chow AW, Edwards JE, et al: Sternoarticular septic arthritis in heroin users. *N Engl J Med* 289:616, 1973.

Heim D, Herkert F, Hess P, et al: Surgical treatment of humeral shaft fractures: The Basel experience. *J Trauma* 35:226, 1993.

Kothari RU, Dronen SC: Prospective evaluation of the scapular manipulation technique in reducing anterior shoulder dislocation. *Ann Emerg Med* 21:1349, 1992.

Meister K, Andrews JR: Classification and treatment of rotator cuff injuries in the overhand athlete. *J Orthop Sports Phys Ther* 18:413, 1993.

Ono K, Inagawa H, Kiyota K, et al: Posterior dislocation of the sternoclavicular joint with obstruction of the innominate vein: Case report. *J Trauma Injury Infect Crit Care* 44:381, 1998.

Press J, Zuckerman JD, Gallagher M: Treatment of grade III acromioclavicular separations: Operative vs nonoperative management. *Bull Hosp Joint Dis* 56:77, 1997.

Rawes ML, Dias JJ: Long-term results of conservative treatment for acromioclavicular dislocation. *J Bone Joint Surg* 78-B: 410, 1996.

Riebel GD, McCabe JB: Anterior shoulder dislocation: A review of reduction techniques. *Am J Emerg Med* 9:180, 1991.

SooHoo NF, Rosen P: Diagnosis and treatment of rotator cuff tears in the emergency department. *J Emerg Med* 14:309, 1996.

Zahiri CA, Zahiri H, Tehrany F: Anterior shoulder dislocation reduction. *Orthopedics* 20:515, 1997.

INJURIES TO THE SPINE

James L. Larson, Jr

EPIDEMIOLOGY

The most important sequela of injuries to the spinal column is damage to the spinal cord. There are an estimated 10,000 new cases of spinal cord injury each year, rendering approximately 5000 people quadriplegic.[1] In addition to the personal tragedy, tremendous financial costs are involved in the care of the spinal cord-injured patient. In 1996, the costs during the first year after a spinal cord injury located from C1 through C4 averaged $417,000. Lifetime medical costs were estimated at $1,350,000 for the same patients.[1] The estimated annual cost of medical, rehabilitative, and vocational care for all spinal cord-injured patients in the United States is $2 to 4 billion.[2]

Injuries to the spinal cord are due to blunt trauma in about 90 percent of cases. The most common injury mechanism is a motor vehicle accident, followed by assaults—mostly gunshot wounds, falls, and sporting accidents.[1] The cervical spine is the most common site for injury to the spinal cord (61 percent), followed by the thoracolumbar junction (19 percent), the thoracic spine (16 percent), and the lumbosacral spine (4 percent).[3]

EVALUATION

Resuscitation

Injuries to the spine and spinal cord are frequently associated with other injuries. Initial resuscitation of the patient with multiple injuries from trauma focuses on airway, breathing, and circulation (the ABCs). The patient with a potential spine injury should undergo immobilization to prevent deterioration during resuscitation. Patients who are at risk for spine injury include those who have had automobile and motorcycle accidents, falls, and diving accidents. Any patients complaining of neck pain, weakness, parethesias, or paralysis should be considered to have a spinal cord injury. A patient with a history of trauma and an altered level of consciousness should always be treated as if a spinal cord injury were present.

Spinal immobilization is important to prevent secondary injury. The components of spinal immobilization include a long spine board, a semirigid cervical spine collar, and ''sandbags'' or other devices to limit head and neck motion. Cervical spine collars alone are ineffective at limiting spine motion.[4] The process for moving a patient onto a spine board or for examination of the back involves a ''log-roll.'' One person is required to maintain the head and neck in neutral position while a minimum of two other people gently roll the patient. The person holding the head directs the team to avoid nonsynchronous motion.

The patient with a spinal cord injury may also present with hypotension due to a loss of sympathetic function and vasodilation below the level of the injury. In a multiply injured patient, other causes of hypotension should be vigorously pursued. Hypotension due purely to a spinal cord injury will be associated with a bradycardia. Hypotension from acute hemorrhage and hypovolemia will be associated with a tachycardia. The initial treatment of hypotension is intravenous fluid. Atropine may be used for significant bradycardia, and vasopressors such as dopamine can be employed if the patient does not respond to fluid boluses.

Airway Management

Patients with multiple trauma are frequently intubated without knowledge of the condition of the cervical spine. Regardless of the airway management technique selected, movement of the spine should be minimized. Intubation techniques for patients with possible spinal injury include nasotracheal intubation with and without bronchoscopic guidance, orotracheal intubation, transtracheal intubation, and cricothyrotomy.[5] Methods for protecting the spinal cord during orotracheal intubation to prevent further injury have been studied in cadavers. These studies have shown that manual in-line stabilization using a dedicated person to hold the head and neck in a neutral position is superior to the use of a Philadelphia collar alone.[6–8] During proper in-line stabilization, no traction is applied to the head and spine. Axial traction is discouraged because it can cause distraction of cervical spine fractures.[9]

Physical Examination

After the primary survey has been performed and any immediately life-threatening conditions have been addressed, a complete neurologic examination should be performed. The motor exam should assess the strength of all extremities. Any deficits should be localized to a nerve root level (Table 264-1). The sensory exam should ensure that sensation is present in all extremities. Sensory innervation follows the dermatome pattern. The loss of sensation at and below a given dermatome can localize the level of the injury (Fig. 264-1). Priapism should be considered as evidence of a spinal cord injury. Rectal examination may reveal decreased tone due to spinal cord injury. Prognosis can be difficult to determine in the early stages of a spinal cord injury owing to the temporary condition of spinal shock. Spinal shock as defined here is different than the spinal neurogenic shock discussed in Chap. 31. Spinal shock, a condition seen frequently in the first 24 h after injury, is defined by a complete loss of segmental cord reflexes in addition to paralysis. Only after the spinal shock has remitted can any definitive prognosis be given. Resolution of spinal shock is heralded by return of segmental reflexes (bulbocarvernosus in males).

RADIOGRAPHIC EVALUATION

The Asymptomatic Patient

The use of clinical criteria to ''clear'' the cervical spine and avoid unnecessary radiographs in selected trauma patients has been suggested

TABLE 264-1 Motor Examination

Loss of Function	Level of Spinal Cord Lesion
Spontaneous breathing	C4
Shrugging of shoulders	C5
Flexion at elbow	C6
Extension at elbow	C7
Flexion of fingers	C8, T1
Intercostal, abdominal muscles	T1 to T12*
Flexion at hip	L1, L2
Adduction at hip	L3
Abduction at hip	L4
Dorsiflexion of foot	L5
Plantarflexion of foot	S1, S2
Rectal sphincter tone	S2–S4

*Localization of lesions in this area is best accomplished with the sensory examination.
Source: From Galli et al,[29] with permission.

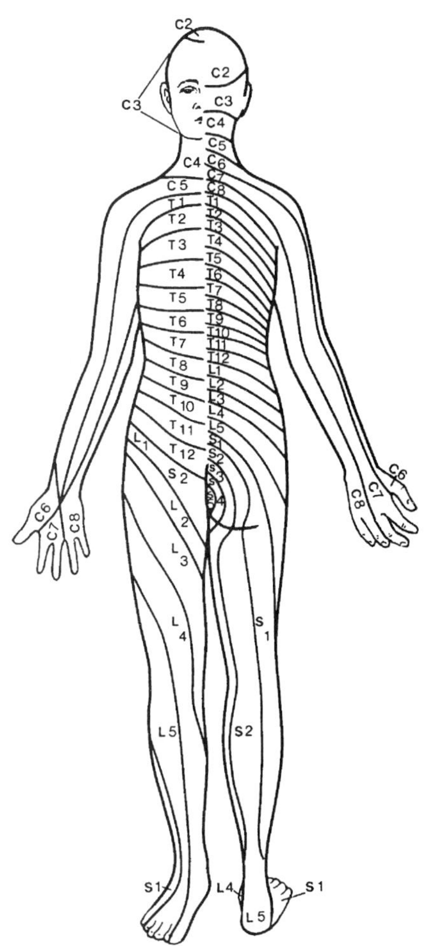

FIG. 264-1. Dermatomes.

by authors of several studies.[10–12] The criteria examined were a combination of relevant historical and physical examination features. Patients meeting the criteria did not have significant cervical spine injury requiring radiographs.[13] The criteria that excluded cervical spine injury in these blunt trauma patients were:

1. Alertness, absence of intoxication
2. Absence of neck pain
3. Absence of neck tenderness
4. Absence of painful distracting injuries
5. Absence of sensory or motor deficit

Trauma patients who do not meet all of these criteria should have plain radiographs to evaluate the cervical spine. These should include lateral, anteroposterior, and odontoid views. If these views are normal and the patient is cooperative and has no neurologic signs or symptoms, active range of motion and/or flexion-extension views can be used to further evaluate the cervical spine.

Cervical Spine Radiographs

LATERAL VIEW The lateral view radiograph detects 70 to 80 percent of traumatic cervical spine injuries.[14] The lateral view should include the cervothoracic junction, as 10 percent of cervical spine fractures will occur at this level.[15] Gentle traction on the upper extremities may move the shoulders out of the way and increase the yield of the interval view. Another radiographic technique for defining the bony anatomy of the cervicothoracic junction is the ''swimmer's'' view. This can be difficult to perform because of the positioning of the patient and film and difficult to interpret owing to overlying bone shadows and obliteration of the posterior spine. If plain radiographs do not define the cervicothoracic junction in a patient with suspected cervical spine injury, the patient should remain in cervical immobilization and alternate methods such as computed tomography (CT) should be employed.[16]

The lateral view should be inspected methodically to detect abnormalities (Table 264-2). Alignment should be evaluated by following anatomic lines (Fig. 264-2). There should be no stepoffs or breaks in the lines. The anterior longitudinal ligament line follows along the anterior surface of the vertebral bodies. This line should follow the normal lordotic curve of the spine. The line of the posterior longitudinal ligament runs along the posterior bodies of the vertebrae and is immediately anterior to the spinal cord. A change of 11° or more in the angle of this line at an interspace should be considered evidence of ligamentous injury (Fig. 264-3). The spinolaminal line is formed by the junction of the lamina with the spinous process at each vertebra. Fractures of the odontoid or C2 pedicles can be detected by examining the spinolaminal line. The spinolaminal line connecting C1 with C3 should pass within 1 mm of the spinolaminal junction of C2. Displacement of more than 1 mm suggests anterior or posterior displacement of the odontoid or a hangman's fracture[5] (Fig. 264-4). The last line is the line connecting the tips of the spinous processes.

Examination of the soft tissues of the neck may be helpful in defining injury. The upper limits of normal dimensions of the prevertebral tissue are 6 mm at C2 and 22 mm at C6.[17] Injury to the cervical spine can cause hematomas and edema that increase the size of the prevertebral space as seen on the lateral view radiograph. Abnormal width of the prevertebral tissues occurs in 33 to 60 percent of cervical spine injuries.[17]

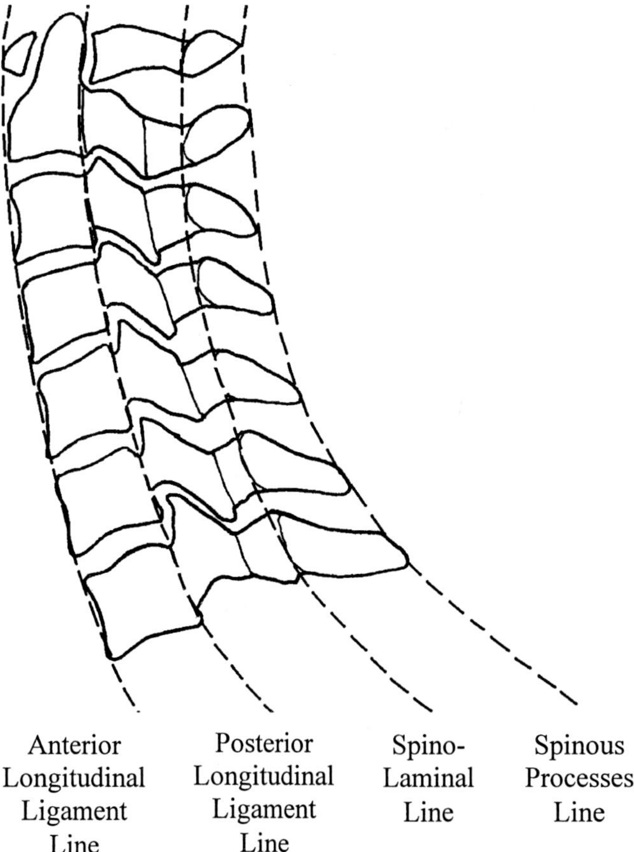

FIG. 264-2. Alignment of the lateral cervical spine.

TABLE 264-2 Criteria for Clearing the Cervical Spine Cross-Table Lateral View

All seven vertebral bodies must be clearly seen, including the C7–T1 junction.
Evaluate proper alignment of the posterior cervical line and the four lordotic curves: anterior longitudinal ligament line, posterior longitudinal ligament line, spinolaminal line, and tips of spinous processes.
Evaluate the predental space (3 mm in adults, 4–5 mm in children)
Evaluate each vertebra for fracture and increased or decreased density (e.g., suggestive of a compression fracture, metastatic lesion, osteoporosis).
Evaluate the intervertebral and interspinous processes. (Abrupt angulation of more than 11° at a single interspace is abnormal).
Evaluate if there is fanning of the spinous processes, suggestive of posterior ligament disruption.
Evaluate the prevertebral soft tissue distance. Less than 7 mm at C2 or less than 5 mm at C3–C4 is considered normal. Note that in children less than 2 years old, the prevertebral space may appear widened if the film is not an inspiratory one.
Evaluate the atlantooccipital region for possible dislocation.

Source: From Van Hare,[30] with permission.

ANTEROPOSTERIOR (AP) VIEW The AP view is ineffective in evaluating the upper cervical spine because the structures of the face and mandible obscure the bony anatomy. The lateral cortex of the articular masses can show evidence of fracture or dislocation if they are angled as compared with superior or inferior neighbors. The spinous processes can be seen on end, and abnormal widening may indicate a hyperflexion sprain or interfacetal dislocation.

ODONTOID VIEW The odontoid or open-mouth view shows the odontoid and its relationship to the lateral masses of C1. The dens should be centered between the lateral masses, and the lateral masses of C1 should be directly over the lateral portions of C2. Rotation of the head may cause some displacement of the lateral masses and asymmetry of the relationship of the dens and C1. Rotation can be detected by using the space between the central incisors, which should be in the midline in an unrotated view. Displacement of the lateral masses due to rotation will cause one side to be displaced medially and the opposite side displaced laterally.[5]

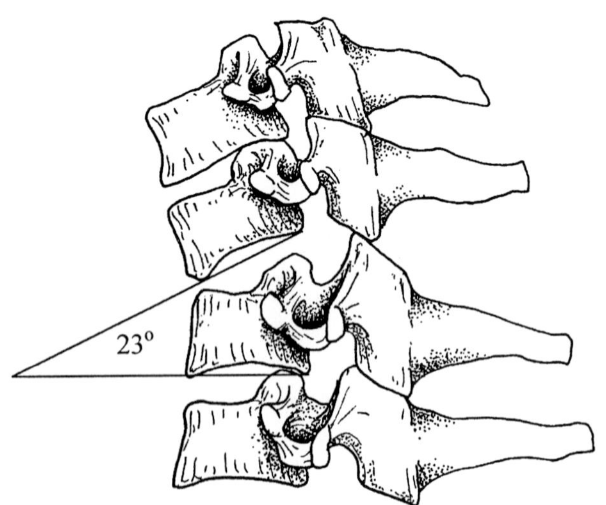

FIG. 264-3. Angulation.

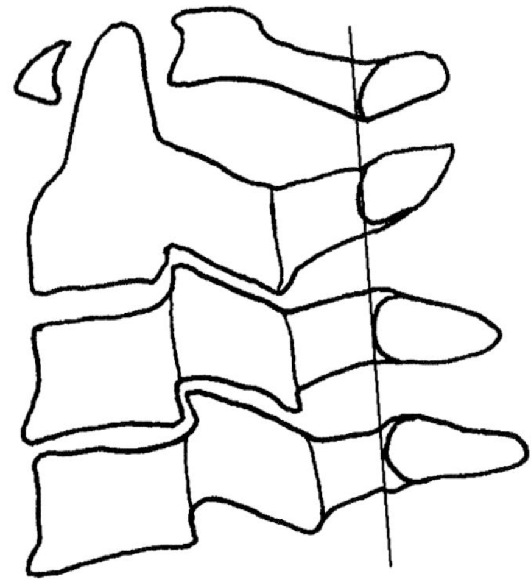

FIG. 264-4. Spinolaminal alignment.

FLEXION-EXTENSION VIEWS An injury to the ligamentous structures of the spine may occur without a bone fracture. If the initial radiographs show no evidence of fracture but are suggestive of subluxation or if suspicion of a ligamentous injury exists, flexion and extension views may be performed. Anterior subluxation injuries are exacerbated in flexion and reduced in extension. This should only be performed in awake, cooperative patients. The flexion and extension should be halted at the point where they cause the patient pain.[16]

Computed Tomography Scanning

CT scanning is indicated in any major fracture or fracture/dislocation of the spine. CT scanning can improve the detection of fractures in areas poorly visualized by plain radiography; these areas comprise the C1, C2, C6 and C7 vertebrae. CT scanning is less useful for purely soft tissue injuries seen with ligamentous disruption.

CT scanning can miss fractures oriented in the axial plane.[18] Subluxations and dislocations are also sometimes missed with CT scanning.[19] When plain radiography is combined with CT for difficult-to-visualize vertebrae, almost all abnormalities will be identified.[19]

Magnetic Resonance Imaging (MRI)

MRI is better than CT for defining the soft tissue injury seen with spine fractures and is indicated in all patients who have neurologic deficits from a spinal cord injury. MRI can evaluate the epidural space for herniated intervertebral disks, hematoma, and bone fragments and can image the spinal cord for edema, hemorrhage, or laceration.[20] MRI is more time-consuming than CT scanning and should be used only for patients who are hemodynamically stable.

CERVICAL SPINE INJURIES

Anatomy

The forces that lead to cervical spine injury have been studied in laboratory settings. These experiments have revealed that specific patterns of injury are associated with the initial dominant force present at the time of injury. A classification system for describing cervical spine injuries based on the biomechanical force responsible for the

TABLE 264-3 Cervical Spine Injuries: Mechanism of Injury

Flexion
Anterior subluxation (hyperflexion sprain)
Bilateral interfacetal dislocation
Simple wedge (compression) fracture
Clay-shoveler's (coal-shoveler's) fracture
Flexion teardrop fracture
Flexion-rotation
Unilateral interfacetal dislocation
Pillar fracture
Fracture/separation (pedicolaminar fracture)
Vertical compression
Jefferson burst fracture of atlas
Burst (bursting, dispersion, axial-loading) fracture
Hyperextension
Hyperextension dislocation
Avulsion fracture of anterior arch of atlas
Extension teardrop fracture
Fracture of posterior arch of atlas
Laminar fracture
Traumatic spondylolisthesis (''hangman's'' fracture)
Lateral flexion
Uncinate process fracture
Injuries caused by diverse or poorly understood mechanisms
Occipitoatlantal dissociation
Occipital condylar fractures
Dens fractures

Source: From Harris,[16] with permission.

injury has been proposed by Harris Table 264-3. A description of selected cervical spine fractures based on this classification follows.

An understanding of the anatomy of the cervical spine is essential to the classification of injuries. For the purpose of understanding how mechanisms of injury affect the spine, consider the spine as consisting of two columns. The anterior column is composed of those structures anterior to the posterior longitudinal ligament. The ligamentous structures in the anterior column are the intervetebral disk, the annulus, and the anterior and posterior longitudinal ligaments. The posterior column is made up of the vertebral arch, the ligamentum flavum, the capsular ligaments and the interspinous and supraspinous ligaments. The posterior ligamentous elements resist flexion forces and the anterior ligamentous elements resist extension forces.

Mechanism: Hyperflexion

ANTERIOR SUBLUXATION Anterior subluxation is also known as *hyperflexion sprain*. The posterior ligamentous structures fail because of the hyperflexion of the cervical spine. A pure subluxation injury has no associated fractures. Radiographic findings can include a ''fanning'' or widening of the spinous processes at the level of injury. The disc space may be widened posteriorly and narrowed anteriorly. Abrupt angulation change of more than 11 degrees at a single interspace may also signal an injury[21] (Fig. 264-3).

Cervical spine radiographs may be normal if the hyperflexion sprain has not caused a fracture and the subluxation has been reduced. Flexion and extension views should be obtained in awake and cooperative patients to further evaluate for injury. Flexion views will exaggerate the radiographic abnormalities and extension views will reduce them. Anterior subluxation is a stable injury but mandates consultation to institute proper treatment, ensure absence of any associated spinal injuries, and prevent the development of delayed instability and pain syndromes.

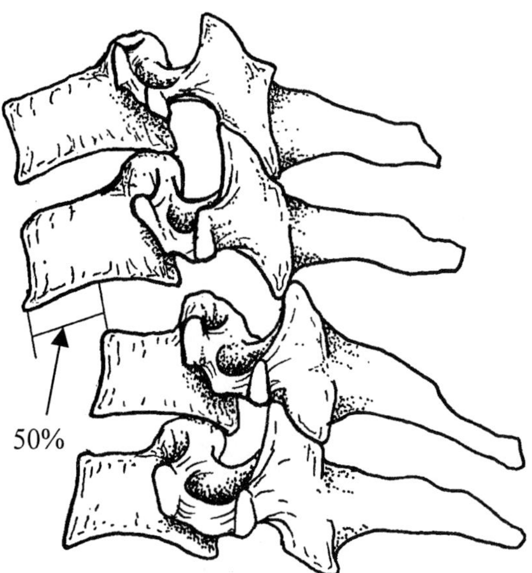

FIG. 264-5. Bilateral intrafacetal dislocation.

BILATERAL INTERFACETAL DISLOCATION (BID) BID occurs when disruption to all ligamentous structures due to hyperflexion allows the articular masses of the involved vertebra to dislocate superiorly and anteriorly over into the intervertebral foramen inferior to the involved vertebra (Fig. 264-5). Radiographically, the vertebra can be seen dislocated anteriorly to at least 50 percent its width. The injury is mechanically unstable and usually presents with neurologic findings.[16] A ''perched'' vertebra is seen in partial BID, when the articular masses of the involved vertebra are perched on the superior articular processes of the subjacent vertebra. This configuration is also mechanically unstable but may not present with neurologic compromise.[16] Using the term *locked facets* to describe a BID is misleading because the injury is unstable. Immediate specialist referral is necessary to reduce the dislocation.

SIMPLE WEDGE FRACTURE A wedge fracture of a vertebra is caused by compression between two other vertebrae. The superior end plate fractures while the inferior surface of the vertebra remains intact (Fig. 264-6). The posterior ligaments may be disrupted, leading to an in-

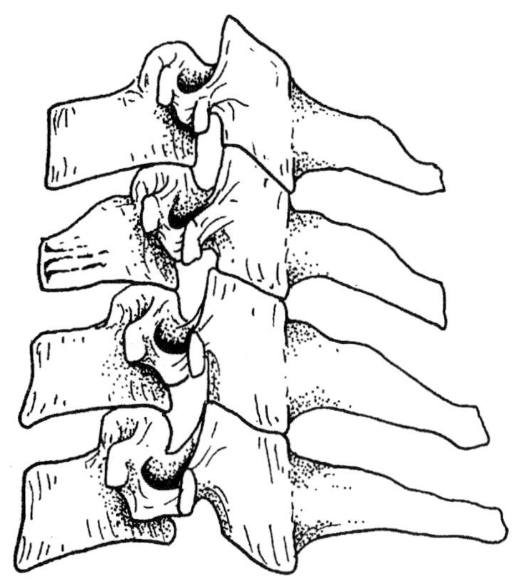

FIG. 264-6. Wedge fracture.

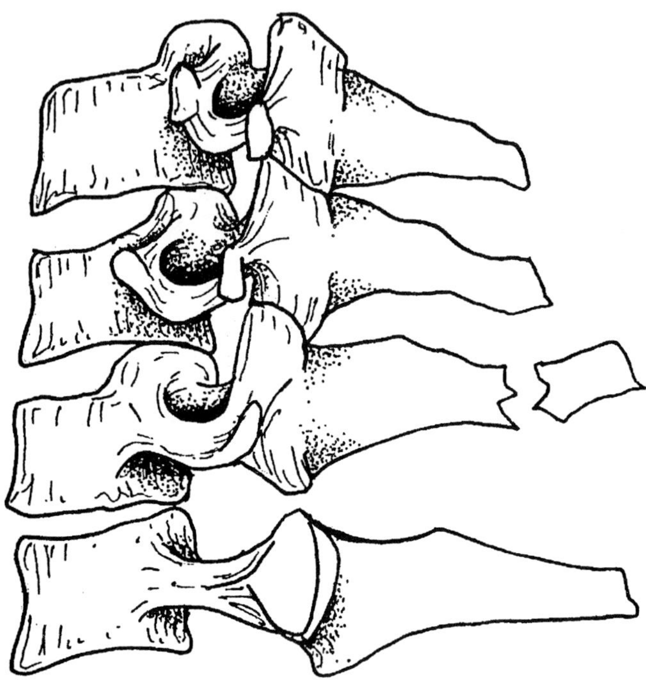

FIG. 264-7. Clay-shoveler's fracture.

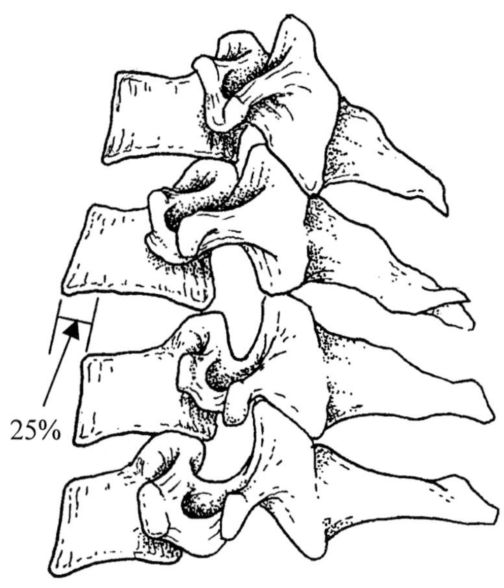

FIG. 264-9. Unilateral facet dislocation.

crease in the distance between spinous processes. Posterior element disruption makes the injury unstable. The simple wedge fracture is differentiated from a burst fracture by the absence of a vertical fracture of the vertebral body. Immediate specialist consultation is necessary if stability of the posterior ligament is not assured.[16]

CLAY-SHOVELER'S FRACTURE An avulsion of the spinous process of the lower cervical vertebrae, classically C7, is known as a clay-shoveler's fracture (Fig. 264-7). Intense flexion against contracted posterior erector spinal muscles causes avulsion of the spinous process. An isolated clay shoveler's fracture is mechanically stable. Conservative treatment with ice, analgesia, rest, and early referral is indicated.[16]

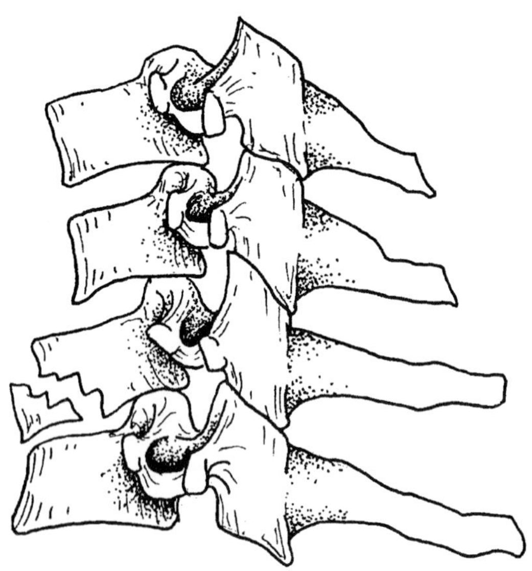

FIG. 264-8. Flexion teardrop fracture.

FLEXION TEARDROP FRACTURE Extreme flexion can cause the flexion teardrop fracture (Fig. 264-8). The associated anterior cord syndrome is due to impingement of the spinal cord by the fracture hyperkyphosis. There is complete disruption of all ligamentous structures at the level of the injury. The ''teardrop'' is the anteroinferior portion of the vertebral body, which is separated and displaced from the remaining portion of the vertebra. This injury is mechanically unstable and requires immediate attention from a spine specialist.[16]

Mechanism: Flexion and Rotation

UNILATERAL INTERFACETAL DISLOCATION Simultaneous forces of flexion and rotation can produce a unilateral facet dislocation. The articular mass and inferior facet on one side of the vertebra are anteriorly dislocated (Fig. 264-9). Radiographically, the AP view will reveal the rotation, because the spinous processes will not be projected directly over one another. The affected spinous process will point toward the side of the vertebra that is dislocated. The involved vertebra will be displaced anteriorly less than 50 percent of the width of a vertebra on the lateral view. The dislocation is mechanically stable unless there is a fracture at the base of the inferior articular mass of the dislocated vertebra or a fracture of the superior articular mass of the inferior vertebra. Immediate consultation of a specialist is recommended because of the long-term complications of an unreduced injury.[16]

Mechanism: Extension and Rotation

PILLAR FRACTURE Extension and rotation can cause impaction of a superior vertebra on the articular mass of its inferior neighbor. The resultant vertical or oblique fracture of the articular mass is called a *pillar fracture* (Fig. 264-10). The adjacent lamina and pedicle remain intact. The lateral view may show a ''double-outline'' sign at the level of the injury. This can be differentiated from the normal lateral radiograph, in which the articular masses are imposed on one another and only a single radiographic density is seen. The double outline occurs when the fractured articular mass is displaced posteriorly and causes two radiographic shadows. The AP projection will show an

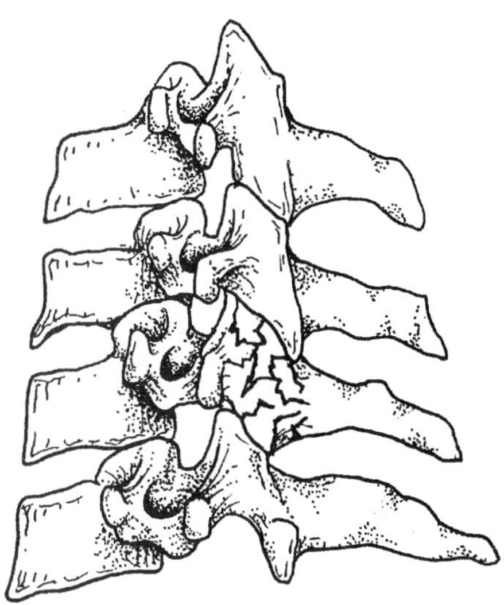

FIG. 264-10. Pillar fracture.

abnormality of the lateral column and a fracture at the level of the injury. The fracture is considered stable. Immediate specialist consultation is indicated.[16]

FRACTURE SEPARATION Harris has described the fracture/separation as a pedicolaminar fracture because it involves fractures of the pedicle and lamina. There are varying degrees of fracture, ranging from fractures without displacement to disruption of the anterior longitudinal ligament and disk rupture. The lateral radiograph may show rotation of the involved articular mass as compared with the uninvolved lateral mass at the level of the injury. Anterior listhesis may be seen in more severe mechanisms. The AP view may show disruption of the lateral column. Immediate consultation is recommended.

Mechanism: Vertical Compression Injuries

BURST FRACTURE OF THE LOWER CERVICAL SPINE A direct axial load causes a burst fracture of the lower cervical spine. The axial force causes the vertebra to burst with fragments displacing in all directions (Fig. 264-11). The spinal cord may be injured if a fragment enters the spinal canal. The lateral radiograph may show a fracture of the superior and inferior vertebral end plate and retropulsion of the posterior segment of the vertebra into the spinal canal. The AP view will show a vertical fracture and widening of the interpedicular distance. This injury is unstable. Immediate consultation is recommended.[16]

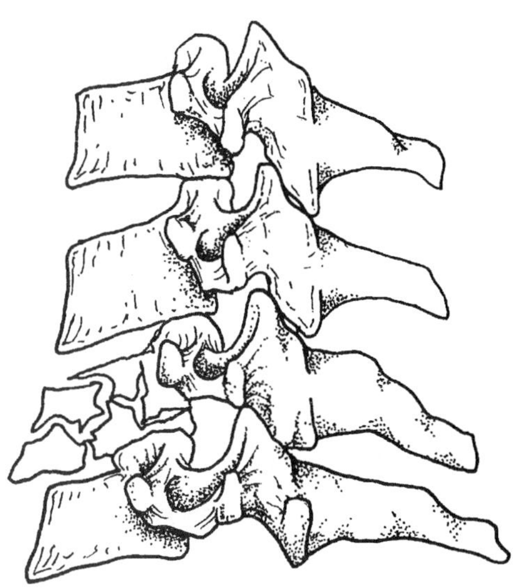

FIG. 264-11. Burst fracture.

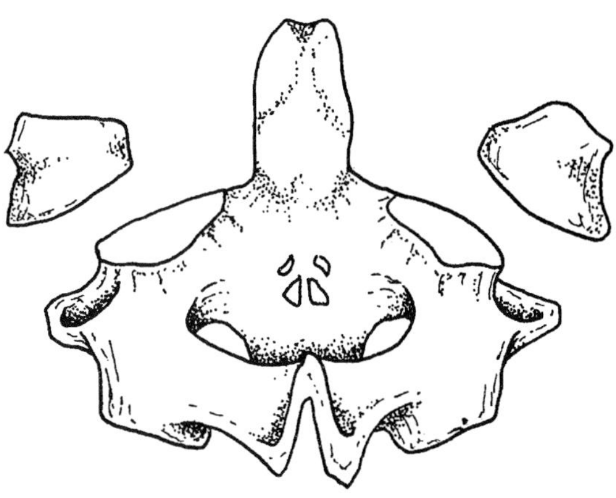

FIG. 264-12. Jefferson fracture.

JEFFERSON FRACTURE The Jefferson fracture is usually produced when the cervical spine is subjected to an axial load due to a direct blow to the top of the head. The occipital condyles are displaced downward and produce a burst fracture by driving the lateral masses of C1 apart (Fig. 264-12). The lateral masses will be displaced laterally on the open-mouth odontoid radiograph. A fracture through only one lateral mass will cause unilateral displacement on the open-mouth view. Instability is likely if the lateral masses are displaced significantly. If the displacement of the lateral masses on each side added together is greater than 7 mm, rupture of the transverse ligament is likely. Immediate specialist consultation is necessary for all Jefferson fractures.

Mechanism: Hyperextension Injuries

HYPEREXTENSION DISLOCATION A hyperextension injury involves a complete tear of the anterior longitudinal ligament and intervertebral disk with disruption of the posterior ligamentous complex. Facial trauma with a central cord syndrome is the most common clinical presentation. Radiographically the vertebrae are normally aligned because the dislocation will be reduced. Diffuse prevertebral soft tissue swelling is usually present. Other signs include a disk-space widening anteriorly or a fracture of the anteroinferior end plate of the vertebrae.[16] If the patient has no neurologic deficit and no evidence of fracture, flexion-extension films may be used to help define ligamentous instability. Any evidence of instability requires immediate specialist consultation.

AVULSION FRACTURE OF THE ANTERIOR ARCH OF ATLAS A hyperextension may avulse the inferior pole of the anterior tubercle of C1. This is most readily detected on the lateral view (Fig. 264-13). The presence of perivertebral soft tissue swelling and absence of cortication distinguish it from the ununited secondary ossification center of the inferior pole of the tubercle. A fracture involving the entire anterior arch is unstable. Immediate specialist consultation is recommended.[16]

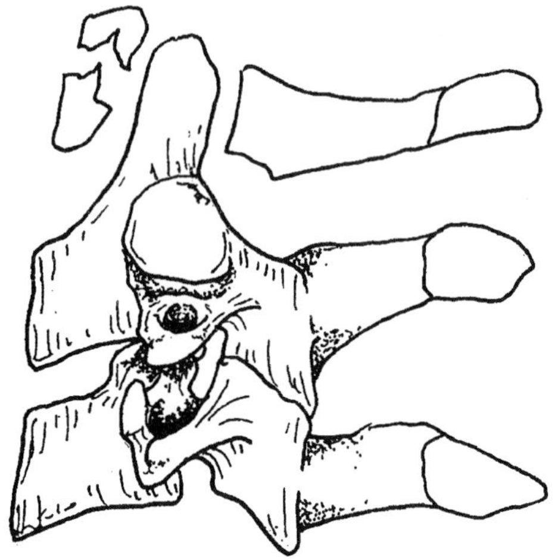

FIG. 264-13. Avulsion fracture of the anterior arch of the atlas.

EXTENSION TEARDROP FRACTURE A hyperextension mechanism may cause the anterior longitudinal ligament to avulse the inferior portion of the anterior vertebral body at its insertion (Fig. 264-14). The most common location is at C2. The height of the fragment usually exceeds its width. This fracture is more common in older patients with osteoporosis. The extension teardrop fracture is unstable in extension and immediate specialist consultation is necessary.[16]

FRACTURE OF POSTERIOR ARCH OF THE ATLAS Hyperflexion of the cervical spine may compress the posterior arch of the atlas between the occipital bone and the spinous process of the axis. This is to be differentiated from the Jefferson fracture of C2. Prevertebral soft tissue swelling is much more prevalent with the more extensive Jefferson fractures. CT scanning will ultimately define which fracture is present. This fracture is frequently associated with other cervical spine fractures, and specialist consultation is recommended.

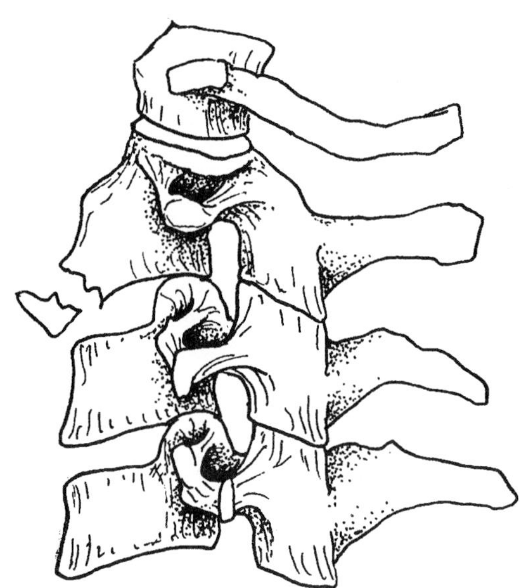

FIG. 264-14. Extension teardrop fracture.

LAMINAR FRACTURE Isolated laminar fractures are caused by hyperextension and may be subtle on plain radiographs. Associated spinous process fractures may be present. CT scanning is required to define the extent of spinal cord involvement. This injury is considered stable; immediate specialist consultation is recommended.

HANGMAN'S FRACTURE The hangman's fracture is located in the pedicles of C2, with C2 displacing anteriorly on C3 (Fig. 264-15). The fracture is caused by an extension mechanism and is seen in judicial hangings. Suicidal hangings do not usually cause the extreme hyperextension seen in judicial hangings and do not cause a hangman's fracture. The same fracture is seen in motor vehicle and diving accidents where sudden hyperextension forces are applied in deceleration. Owing to the large diameter of the spinal canal at the level of C2, even displacement of C2 on C3 may not cause neurologic injury, and these patients may be neurologically intact. This injury is unstable and mandates immediate consultation.

Mechanism: Lateral Flexion

UNCINATE PROCESS FRACTURE Pure lateral flexion is rare in most mechanisms of injury. Lateral flexion can cause a transverse fracture at the base of the uncinate process as the lateral aspect of the superior vertebral body fractures the inferior uncinate process. During the initial injury, the degree of lateral neck flexion is limited because the head strikes the shoulder. This fracture may be seen in the AP or lateral view. Immediate consultation is recommended.

Poorly Understood Mechanisms

OCCIPITOATLANTAL DISSOCIATION (OAD) In occipitoatlantal dissociation, the skull may be displaced anteriorly or posteriorly or distracted from the cervical spine. OAD frequently results in death. Severe OAD is easily detected on the lateral radiograph. Occipitoatlantal subluxation is more difficult to detect on radiographs. Harris has described a method for detecting occipitoatlantal injury. The basion-axial interval (BAI) can be measured in most lateral radiographs. This is the distance between the basion and a line extending from the posterior cortex of C2. The BAI should not exceed 12

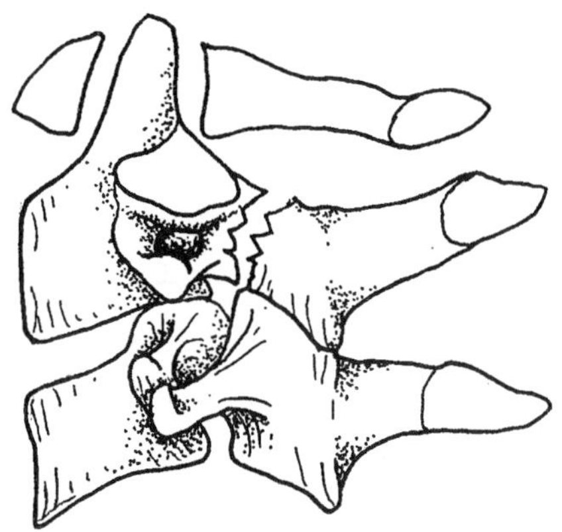

FIG. 264-15. ''Hangman's'' fracture.

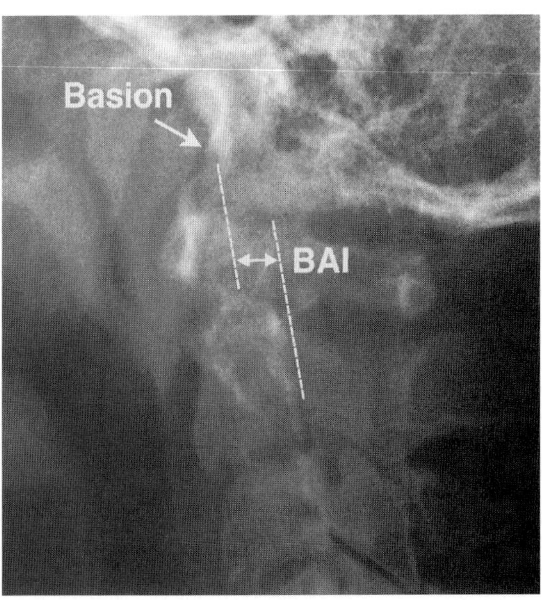

FIG. 264-16. Basion-axial interval (BAI).

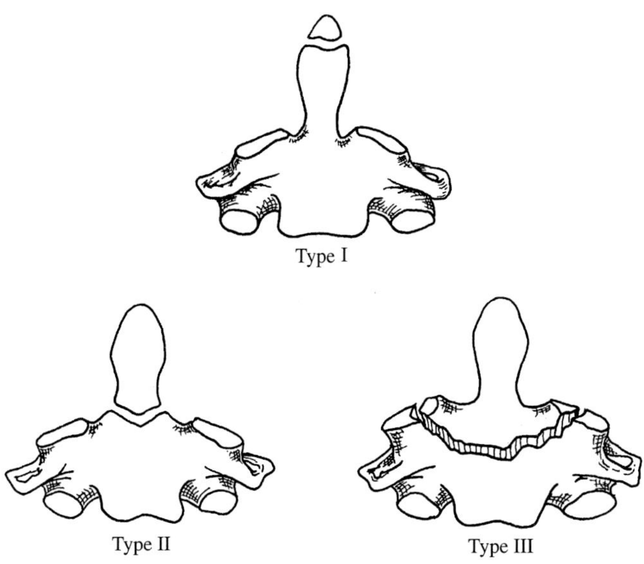

FIG. 264-18. Odontoid fractures.

mm (Fig. 264-16). The basion-dental interval (BDI) is the distance between the basion and the superior cortex of the dens. This distance should also be less than 12 mm (Fig. 264-17). Atlantooccipital injuries are extremely unstable and mandate immediate specialist consultation.

TRANSVERSE LIGAMENT DISRUPTION The transverse ligament is located anterior on the inside of the ring of C1 and runs along the posterior surface of the dens. The transverse ligament is crucial to maintaining the stability of the first and second vertebrae. Pure ligamentous rupture without an associated fracture can occur in older patients with a direct blow to the occiput, as would occur in a fall. Without a fracture present, radiographic diagnosis relies on identifying the atlanto-dens interval, also known as the *predental space*, which is viewed on the lateral x-ray. The space is between the posterior aspect of the anterior arch of C1 and the anterior border of the odontoid. The space should be 3 mm or less in adults. More than 3 mm of space implies damage to the transverse ligament; more than 5 mm implies rupture of the transverse ligament. Immediate specialist consultation is necessary for these injuries.

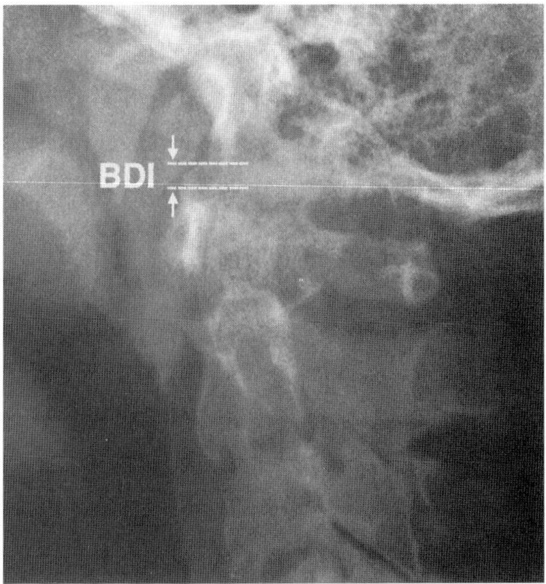

FIG. 264-17. Basion-dental interval (BDI).

ODONTOID FRACTURES One-third of all fractures of the ring of C1 occur in combination with fractures of the odontoid.[22] Odontoid fractures make up 7 to 14 percent of cervical spine fractures.[23] Fractures of the odontoid are usually due to major forces and frequently involve other injuries to the cervical spine as well as multisystem trauma.[24] Awake patients will usually complain of immediate and severe high cervical pain with muscle spasm aggravated by movement. The pain may not be severe and can radiate to the occiput of the head. Neurologic injury presents in 18 to 25 percent of cases. This can range from minimal sensory or motor loss to quadriplegia.[25] Classification of odontoid fractures relies on identifying the level of injury. Type I fractures are avulsions of the tip. The transverse ligament remains attached to the dens, the fracture is stable, and the injury carries a good prognosis. Type II fractures occur at the junction of the odontoid and the body of C2. This is the most common odontoid fracture. Type III odontoid fractures occur through the superior portion of C2 at the base of the dens (Fig. 264-18). Immediate specialist consultation is recommended.

THORACOLUMBAR SPINE INJURIES

Anatomy

The thoracolumbar spine (TLS) is relatively more protected and stable than the cervical spine. Vertebrae T1 through T10 are fixed, owing to their articulation with the thoracic cage. Large forces are required to fracture thoracic vertebrae and neurologic abnormalities are common. The mobility of the thoracolumbar junction predisposes it to injury. The thoracolumbar junction is second only to the cervical spine in frequency of injury. The spinal cord ends at

TABLE 264-4 Classification of Thoracolumbar Spine Injury

Major Injuries*	Minor Injuries†
Wedge compression fractures	Transverse process fracture
Chance fractures	Spinous process fracture
Burst fractures	Pars interarticularis fracture
Flexion distraction injuries	
Translational injuries	

*Assume to be unstable; should be cared for at a center with either orthopedic or neurosurgical spine specialists.
†Implies isolated fracture with no neurologic deficits, generally are stable.
Source: From Savitsky and Voley,[28] with permission.

approximately L1 at the conus medullaris. The individual nerve roots extending from the conus medullaris constitute the cauda equina. These nerve roots are less susceptible to damage and neurologic injury, as trauma to the lower lumbar and sacral segments occurs less often and is less severe.

Mechanism of Injury and Classification

McAfee et al.[26] have classified TLS injuries into major and minor fractures (Table 264-4). A discussion of the classification follows. Wedge compression fractures are the result of flexion causing compression of the anterior body of the vertebra. Plain radiographs demonstrate loss of anterior height in the traumatized vertebra. The posterior height and cortex are intact. CT scanning should be performed to define the stability of the posterior elements and sparing of the neural canal. These fractures are not usually associated with neurologic compromise but should be treated as unstable until evaluation is complete. A flexion mechanism causing anterior vertebral compression with involvement of the posterior cortex defines the burst fracture. Lateral plain radiography will show the loss of anterior and posterior height; AP views will show and increase in the interpedicular distance; and a CT scan will define the extent of the injury. The burst fracture should be considered unstable. A Chance fracture is caused by a flexion around an axis anterior to the anterior spinal longitudinal ligament. A high-speed motor vehicle accident with the occupant in a lap belt will produce this mechanism. The Chance fracture involves the spinous process, lamina, transverse processes, pedicles, and vertebral body.[27] The lateral radiograph will show the fracture through the posterior elements and vertebral body. A CT scan may help to define the injury but can miss it if the fracture is in the same plane as the scan. The Chance fracture should be considered unstable.

A flexion-distraction mechanism places the anterior portions of the spine under compression while distracting the posterior elements. The lateral radiograph shows loss of height in the anterior portion of the vertebra with increased interspinous spaces posteriorly (''fanning''). This injury is unstable.

Translational injuries are the result of large shear forces that cause complete disruption of spine stability. The lateral radiograph will show translation of one or more vertebral segments on subsequent segments. Associated neurologic injury is common. Specific injuries include slice fractures, rotational fracture/dislocations, and pure dislocations.[28] Minor fractures include spinous process fractures, transverse process fractures, and pars interarticularis fractures. Minor fractures have no associated neurologic compromise and are considered stable.

REFERENCES

1. National Spinal Cord Injury Statistical Center (NSCISC): *Spinal Cord Injury: Facts and Figures at a Glance.* Birmingham, AL: NSCISC, 1998.
2. Woolsey RM: Modern concepts of therapy and management of spinal cord injuries. *Crit Rev Neurobiol* 4:137, 1988.
3. Fife D, Kraus J: Anatomic location of spinal cord injury relationship to the cause of injury. *Spine* 11:2–5, 1986.
4. Kaufman WA, Lunsford TR, Lunsford BR, Lance LL: Comparison of three prefabricated cervical collars. *Orthop Prosthet* 39:4:21, 1986.
5. Mahoney B: Cervical spine injuries, in Ruiz E, Cicero JJ (eds): *Emergency Management of Skeletal Injuries.* St Louis: Mosby, 1995, pp 71–94.
6. Majernick TG, Bieniek R, Houston JB, et al: Cervical spine movement during orotracheal intubation. *Ann Emerg Med* 15:417, 1986.
7. Aprahamian C, Thompson BM, Finger WA, et al: Experimental cervical spine injury model: Evaluation of airway management and splinting techniques. *Ann Emerg Med* 13:584, 1984.
8. Holley J, Jorden R: Airway management in patients with unstable cervical spine fractures. *Ann Emerg Med* 18:1237, 1989.
9. Bivins HG, Ford S, Bezmalinovic Z, et al: The effect of axial traction during orotracheal intubation of the trauma victim with an unstable cervical spine. *Ann Emerg Med* 17:25, 1988.
10. Hoffman JR, Schriger DL, Mower W, et al: Low risk criteria for cervical spine radiography in blunt trauma: A prospective study. *Ann Emerg Med* 21:1454, 1992.
11. Velmahos GC, Theodorou D, Tatevossian R, et al: Radiographic cervical spine evaluation in the alert blunt trauma victim: Much ado about nothing? *J Trauma* 40:768, 1996.
12. Roberge RJ, Wears RC, Kelly M, et al: Selective application of cervical spine radiography in alert victims of blunt trauma: A prospective study. *J Trauma* 28:784, 1988.
13. Kreipke DL, Gillespie KR, McCarthy MC, et al: Reliability of indications for cervical spine films in trauma patients. *J Trauma* 29:1438, 1989.
14. Blahd WH, Iserson KV, Bjelland JC, et al: Efficacy of the post-traumatic cross table lateral view of the cervical spine. *J Emerg Med* 2:243, 1985.
15. Ross SE, Schwab CW, David ET, et al: Clearing the cervical spine: Initial radiologic evaluation. *J Trauma* 27:1055, 1987.
16. Harris J: Spine, including soft tissues of the pharynx and neck, in Harris J, Harris W, Novelline R (eds): *The Radiology of Emergency Medicine,* 3d ed. Baltimore: Williams & Wilkins, 1993, pp 127–282.
17. Paakkala T: Prevertebral soft tissue changes in cervical spine injury. *CRC Crit Rev Diagn Imaging* 24:201, 1985.
18. Acheson MB, Livingston RR, Richardson ML, et al: High-resolution CT scanning in the evaluation of cervical spine fractures: Comparison with plain film examinations. *AJR* 148:1179, 1987.
19. Woodring JH, Lee CL: The role and limitations of computed tomographic scanning in the evaluation of cervical trauma. *J Trauma* 33:698, 1992.
20. Mirvis SE, NessAiver M: Magnetic resonance imaging of acute cervical spine trauma, in Harris JH, Mirvis SE (eds): *The Radiology of Acute Cervical Spine Trauma.* Baltimore: Williams & Wilkins, 1996, pp 114–179.
21. White AA III, Punjabi MM: *Clinical Biomechanics of the Spine,* 2d ed. Philadelphia: Lippincott, 1990.
22. Bauer RD, Errico TJ, Waugh TR, Cohen W: Evaluation and diagnosis of cervical spine injuries: A review of the literature. *Cent Nerv Syst Trauma* 4:71, 1987.
23. Mouradian WH, Fietti VG, Cochran GVB: Fractures of the odontoid: A laboratory and clinical study of mechanisms. *Orthop North Am Clin* 9:985, 1978.
24. Schatzker J, Rorabeck CH, Waddel JW: Fractures of the dens 1971. *J Bone Joint Surg* 53B:392, 1971.
25. Stauffer ES: Management of spine fractures C3–C7. *Orthop Clin North Am* 17:45, 1986.
26. McAfee PC, Hansen YA, Fredrickson BE, et al: The value of computed tomography in thoracolumbar fractures. *J Bone Joint Surg* 65A:461, 1983.
27. Smith WS, Kaufer H: Patterns and mechanisms of lumbar injuries associated with lap seat belts. *J Bone Joint Surg* 51A:239, 1969.
28. Savitsky E, Votey S: Emergency department approach to acute thoracolumbar spine injury. *J Emerg Med* 15:49, 1997.
29. Galli RL, Spaite DW, Simon RR: *Emergency Orthopedics: The Spine.* Norwalk, CT: Appleton & Lange, 1989, p 9.
30. Van Hare RS: The ring of C2 and evaluation of the cross-table lateral view of the cervical spine. *Ann Emerg Med* 21:733, 1992.

TRAUMA TO THE PELVIS, HIP, AND FEMUR

Mark T. Steele

TRAUMA TO THE PELVIS

Pelvic fractures constitute 3 percent of all skeletal fractures and about 5 percent of patients admitted to hospitals because of trauma have pelvic fractures.[1] These fractures and concomitant injuries are a frequent cause of death from blunt trauma sustained in automobile accidents. Fortunately, the mortality has decreased. Most pelvic fractures are secondary to automobile passenger or pedestrian accidents, but about one-third are the result of minor falls in older persons and from major falls or industrial accidents.[2] This chapter discusses the most common fractures of the pelvis, femur, and hip, the mechanisms of injury, radiologic evaluation, and treatment.

Anatomy and Biomechanics

The major functions of the pelvis are protection, support, and hematopoiesis. The pelvis consists of the two innominate bones, which are made up of the ilium, ischium, and pubis; the sacrum; and the coccyx. The two innominate bones and sacrum form a ring structure, which is the basis of pelvic stability. This stability is dependent on the strong posterior sacroiliac, sacrotuberous, and sacrospinous ligaments (Fig. 265-1).[3] Any single break in the ring will yield a stable injury without significant risk of displacement. An injury with two breaks in the ring is unstable with the risk of displacement. The iliopectineal, or arcuate, line divides the pelvis into the upper, or false, pelvis, which is part of the abdomen, and the lower, true pelvis. In addition, this line constitutes the major portion of the femorosacral arch, which, along with the subsidiary tie arch (bodies of pubic bones and superior rami), supports the body in the erect position. In the sitting position, the weight-bearing forces are transmitted by the ischiosacral arch augmented by its tie arch, the pubic bones, inferior pubic rami, and ischial rami. When traumatized, the tie arches fracture first, especially at the symphysis pubis, pubic rami, and just lateral to the sacroiliac (SI) joints. Incorporated in the pelvic structure are five joints that allow some movement in the bony ring. The lumbosacral, SI, and sacrococcygeal joints, and the symphysis pubis allow little movement. The acetabulum is a ball-and-socket joint that is divided into three portions: the iliac portion, or superior dome, is the chief weight-bearing surface; the inner wall consists of the pubis, and is thin and easily fractured; and the posterior acetabulum is derived from the thick ischium.

The pelvis is extremely vascular, a fact that is significant in pelvic fractures. The nerve supply through the pelvis is derived from the lumbar and sacral plexuses. Injury to the pelvis may produce deficits at any level from the nerve root to small peripheral branches.

The lower urinary tract is contained in the pelvis (Fig. 265-2). In the adult, the bladder lies behind the symphysis and pubic bones, and the peritoneum covers the dome and base posteriorly. The location of the bladder and the degree of peritoneal reflection are determined by urine content. The lower gastrointestinal tract housed in the pelvis includes a small portion of the descending colon, the pelvic, or sigmoid, colon, the rectum, and the anus. In women, the uterus and vagina are also housed in the bony pelvis.

Clinical Evaluation

HISTORY Assume that all victims of serious or multiple trauma have fractures of the pelvis. A patient with a suspected pelvic fracture should be questioned about details of the accident to determine the mechanism of injury and about prehospital evaluation and treatment. The patient should be specifically questioned to determine areas of pain, last urination or defecation, present bladder sensation, and the last solid and fluid intake. In addition, the time of the last menses or the presence of pregnancy, current medications, and allergies should be ascertained.

PHYSICAL EXAMINATION Symptoms and signs of pelvic injuries vary from local pain and tenderness, especially with walking, to pelvic instability and severe shock. The physician must maintain alertness, perception, and concern in evaluating these patients. On inspection look for perineal and pelvic edema, ecchymoses, lacerations, and deformities. Look for hematomas above the inguinal ligament or over the scrotum (Destot's sign). Roll the patient over if appropriate and examine the areas over-lying the sacrum and coccyx. On palpation feel for irregularities, crepitance, or movement at the iliac crests, pubic rami, and ischial rami. Palpation of a bony prominence or large hematoma or tenderness along the fracture line is possible by rectal examination (Earle's sign). Compress the pelvis lateral to medial through the iliac crests, anterior to posterior through the symphysis pubis, and anterior to posterior through the iliac crests. Compress the greater trochanters and determine the range of motion of the hips. On rectal examination, superior or posterior displacement of the prostate, or rectal injuries are indicative of intraperitoneal and urologic injury. Proctoscopic examination may be required to fully assess for the presence of rectal tears.[4] Decrease in anal sphincter tone may suggest neurologic injury and blood at the urethral meatus, urologic injury. Pelvic examination should be carefully performed in women to detect the presence of blood or lacerations suggesting the possibility of open fracture. Carefully evaluate neurovascular function. If a pelvic fracture

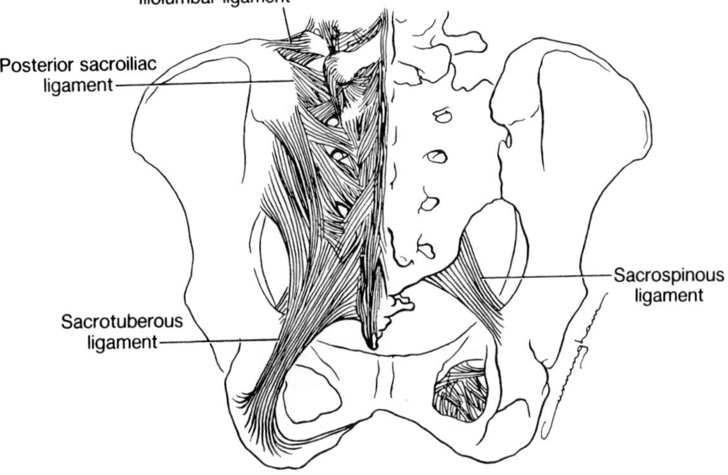

FIG. 265-1. The major posterior stabilizing structures of the pelvic ring, that is, the posterior tension band of the pelvis, include the iliolumbar ligament, the posterior sacroiliac ligaments, the sacrospinous ligaments, and the sacrotuberous ligaments. (From Tile M. Anatomy. In: *Fractures of the Pelvis and Acetabulum.* Baltimore: Williams & Wilkins, 1984, p 11. Used with permission.)

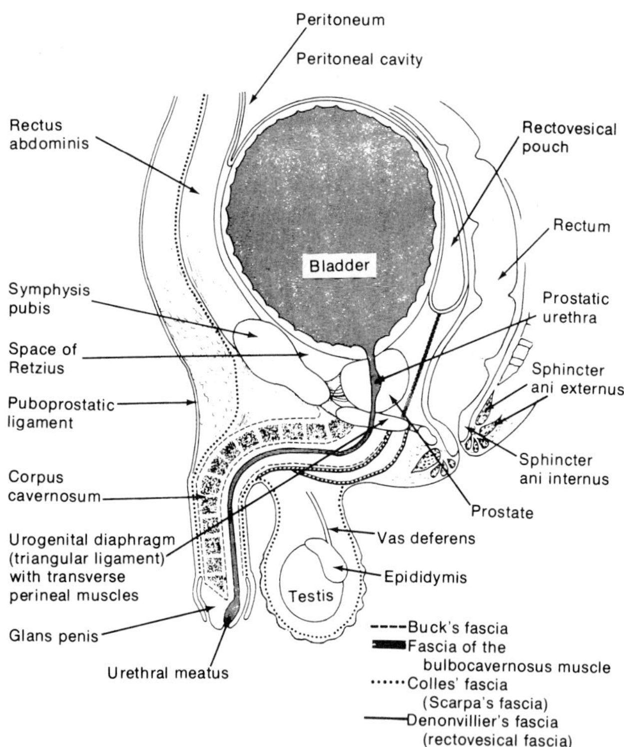

FIG. 265-2. Sagittal section of the male pelvis showing the relation of the full bladder. [From Kane WJ: Fractures of the pelvis, in Rockwood CA Jr, Green DP (eds): *Fractures,* Vol. 2. Philadelphia, Lippincott, 1975, pp 916, 917. Used with permission.]

is found, assume intra-abdominal, retroperitoneal, gynecologic, and urologic injuries until proved otherwise.

RADIOLOGIC EVALUATION Stabilization of the patient takes priority over obtaining x-ray films. Unnecessary movement may produce further injury or cause more blood loss. After stabilization, roentgenographic evaluation of the pelvis is a must in all unconscious patients who have sustained multiple injuries. Lower extremity long bone fractures as well as pelvic symptoms or signs are also indications for roentgenograms. A standard anteroposterior (AP) view of the pelvis is indicated in the presence of multisystem blunt trauma or if pelvic fracture is suspected. If additional studies are needed, lateral views, AP views of either hemipelvis, internal and external oblique views of the hemipelvis, or inlet and outlet views of the pelvis may be done. An inlet view shows anterior-posterior displacement of ring fractures (Figs. 265-3 and 265-4). An outlet view shows superior-inferior displacement. Oblique views of the hemipelvis are true AP and lateral views of the acetabulum. Tomography, computed tomography (CT) scans, and special studies may be needed to fully evaluate and manage patients, particularly for acetabular and sacral fractures. CT is superior to plain radiography in assessing the posterior pelvic arch and acetabulum[5] and has the added advantage of being able to identify the presence or absence of ongoing pelvic hemorrhage.[6] Angiography or venography may be necessary to determine a source of bleeding. The patient's condition must dictate what is done and when.

Classification and Treatment of Pelvic Fractures

BREAK IN THE PELVIC RING Pelvic fractures include those that involve a break in the pelvic ring, fractures of a single bone without a break in the pelvic ring, and acetabulor fractures. Pelvic fractures involving a break in the pelvic ring can be complex and therefore difficult to classify. These injuries range from low-energy stable fractures to high-energy unstable patterns. The most clinically useful classification by Young (Table 265-1), is presented.[7] It differentiates fracture patterns based on mechanism of injury and direction of causative force. Incidence of complications (i.e., urogenital and vascular) is correlated with the fracture pattern, making identification of the type more clinically significant and useful.

Three main types of patterns have been identified. The first and most common mechanism, lateral compression (LC) (Figs. 265-5 through 265-9), accounts for close to half the injuries. Motor vehicle accidents in which a car is broadsided or a pedestrian struck from the side are examples. Anteroposterior compression (APC) (Figs. 265-10, 265-11, and 265-12) is the second type, accounting for about 25 percent of injuries. Head-on motor vehicle accidents are the classic example. The least common mechanism is vertical shear (VS) (Fig. 265-13) typified by a fall or jump from a height, accounting for about 5 percent of fractures. A combination (CM) of other injury patterns make up the other 20 to 25 percent of injuries.

The different injury types may be suggested by history, but can also be differentiated radiographically. The alignment of pubic rami fractures is one such clue to the mechanism and direction of force. Horizontal fractures suggest lateral compression injury, whereas vertical ones point to an anteroposterior direction of force. If there is sacroiliac joint diastasis and an associated crush fracture of the sacrum, then the injury is due to lateral compression. Central hip dislocations suggest a lateral compression mechanism whereas posterior dislocation suggests an anteroposterior force. With vertical shear patterns, fractures are vertical in alignment with vertical displacement of fragments. Based on the recognition of the fracture pattern, one can then predict the likelihood of severe hemorrhage or urogenital injury (Table 265-2).

Mortality usually is due to associated injuries, although pelvic hemorrhage is also a contributor. Mortality rates approach 25 percent for severe APC and VS injuries, whereas it is about 13 percent with

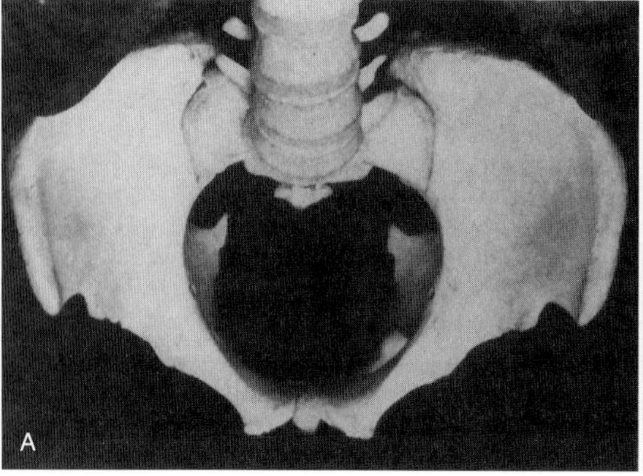

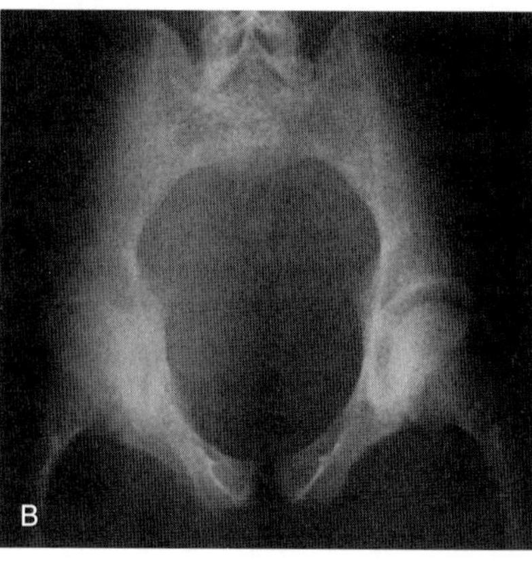

FIG. 265-3. A. Anatomic appearance in the inlet projection. **B.** Radiologic appearance in the inlet projection. (From Tile M. Assessment. In: *Fractures of the Pelvis and Acetabulum.* Baltimore: Williams & Wilkins, 1984, p 63. Used with permission.)

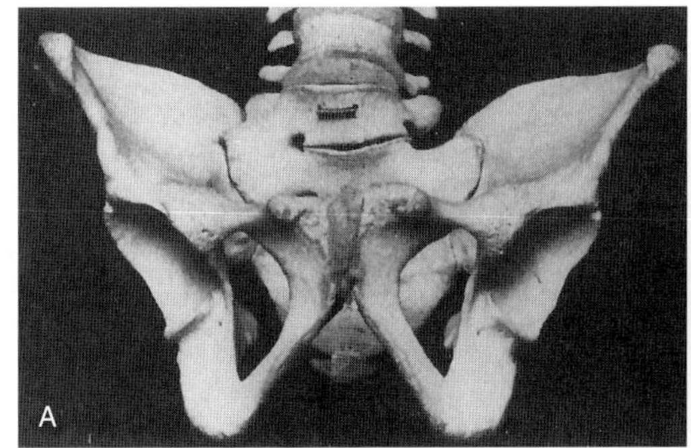

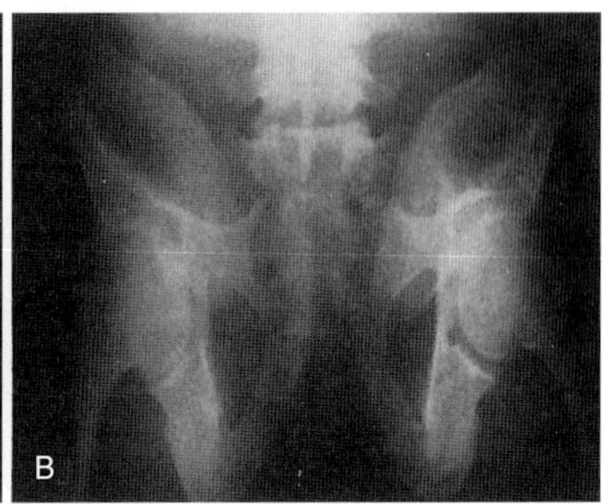

FIG. 265-4. A. Anatomic appearance in the outlet projection. **B.** Radiologic appearance in the outlet projection. (From Tile M. Assessment. In: *Fractures of the Pelvis and Acetabulum.* Baltimore: Williams & Wilkins, 1984, p 64. Used with permission.)

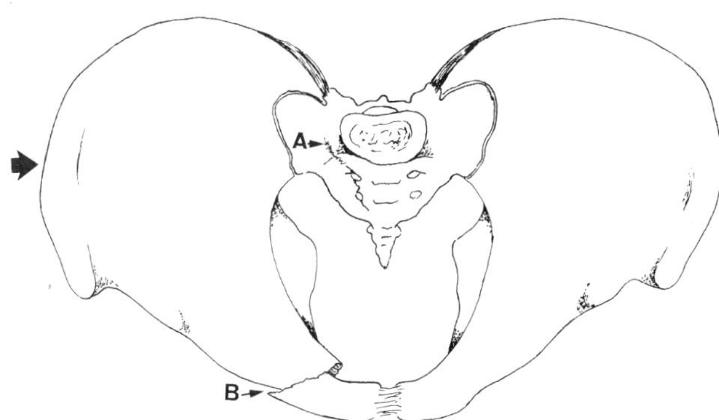

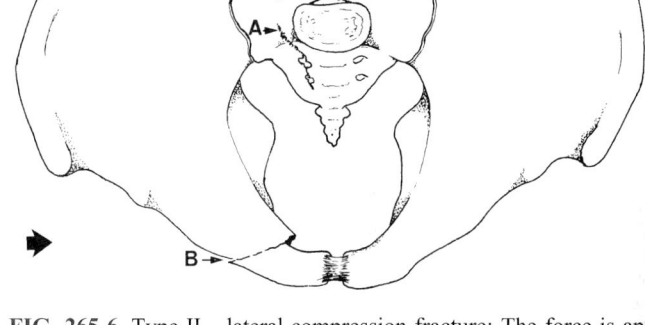

FIG. 265-5. Type I—lateral compression fracture: The lateral force is applied posteriorly (*arrow*). This causes a crush effect on the SIJ: this may be visible radiographically as a sacral fracture (**A**). The characteristic fracture pattern of the pubic rami will be seen (**B**). No ligamentous injury is seen.

FIG. 265-6. Type II—lateral compression fracture: The force is applied anteriorly (*arrow*), causing the typical anterior public rami fractures (**B**). In this case, however, rotation of the pelvis around the anterior sacral margin may occur, causing rupture of the posterior sacroiliac ligaments (*R*). A crush fracture of the sacrum may also be seen (**A**).

TABLE 265-1 Injury Classification Keys According to the Young System

Category	Distinguishing Characteristics
LC	Transverse fracture of pubic rami, ipsilateral or contralateral to posterior injury I—Sacral compression on side of impact II—Crescent (iliac wing) fracture on side of impact III—LC-1 or LC-II injury on side of impact; contralateral open-book (APC) injury
APC	Symphyseal diastasis and/or longitudinal rami fractures I—*Slight* widening of pubic symphysis and/or anterior SI joint; stretched but intact anterior SI, sacrotuberous, and sacrospinous ligaments; intact posterior SI ligaments II—Widened anterior SI joint; disrupted anterior SI, sacrotuberous, and sacrospinous ligaments; intact posterior SI ligaments III—Complete SI joint disruption with lateral displacement; disrupted anterior SI, sacrotuberous, and sacrospinous ligaments; disrupted posterior SI ligaments
VS	Symphyseal diastasis or vertical displacement anteriorly and posteriorly, usually through the SI joint, occasionally through the iliac wing and/or sacrum
CM	Combination of other injury patterns, LC/VS being the most common

Abbreviations: APC, anteroposterior compression; CM, combination; LC, lateral compression; VS, vertical shear.

LC injuries.[8] Mortality has been shown to be reduced with early fracture fixation and patient mobilization.[9] In addition to mortality, the fracture type and severity can also predict the organ injury pattern and resuscitation needs. The treatment of LC-I and APC-I injuries consists of a few days of bedrest followed by protected weight-bearing. The treatment of LC-II injuries generally requires three to six weeks of bedrest followed by progressive weight-bearing or open reduction and internal fixation. LC-III, APC II and III, and VS injuries typically require open reduction and internal fixation within 5 to 14 days of

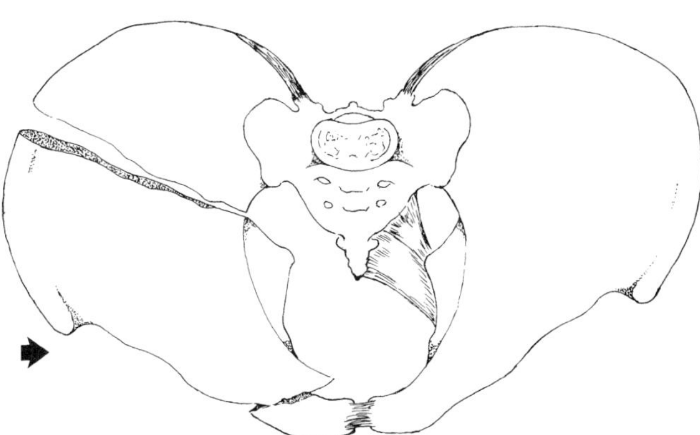

FIG. 265-7. Alternatively (compared to Fig. 265-6), a fracture of the iliac wing may occur which dissipates the rotational forces and thus leaves the posterior ligaments intact.

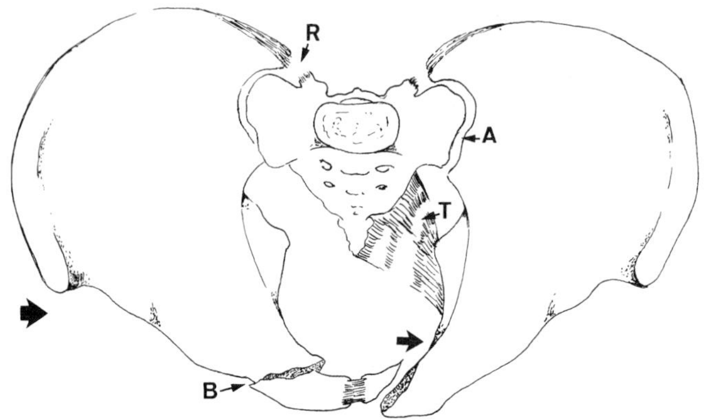

FIG. 265-8. Type III—lateral compression fracture: The force is applied anteriorly (*arrow*), causing internal rotation of the anterior hemipelvis. Continuing through to the contralateral hemipelvis (*arrow*), the force causes it to rotate externally. The result is a pattern of lateral compression on the ipsilateral side, with apparent AP compression on the contralateral side. This results in rupture of the posterior sacroiliac ligaments on the ipsilateral side (*R*) and sacrospinous/sacrotuberous complex (*T*) and anterior ligaments (**A**) on the contralateral side. Typical public rami fractures (**B**) are to be expected.

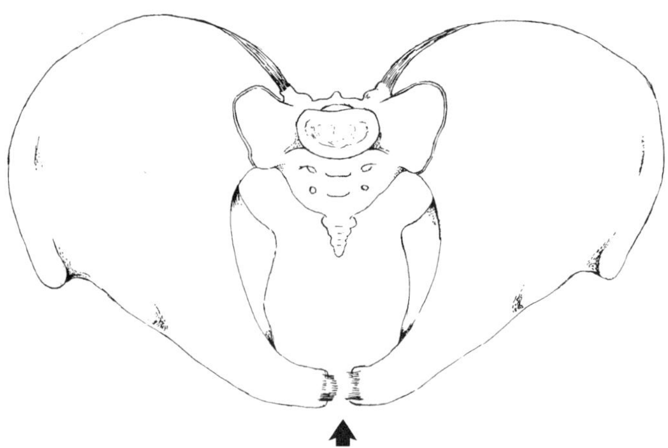

FIG. 265-10. Type I—AP compression fracture: The force is delivered in an AP direction (*large arrow*), tending to "open" the pelvis. This gives rise to mild splaying of the symphysis, due to rupture of the anterior sacroiliac ligaments.

injury.[10] The long-term outcome/disability following open reduction and internal fixation of unstable pelvic fractures is generally fair with three-quarters having some mild disability and about 75 percent of those employed preinjury returning to their preinjury occupations.[11]

True open-book type fractures with an intact posterior ring have the greatest potential benefit from anterior external fixator placement. Stabilization decreases the volume of the pelvis with resultant tamponade of hemorrhage.[5] The tamponade effect is less if the posterior arch of the pelvis has been disrupted. Anterior stabilization should be considered in hemodynamically unstable patients with unstable pelvic fractures.[12] Fracture patterns potentially amenable to external fixator placement include LC-III, APC II or III, and VS fractures. There is evidence that external fixation improves clinical outcome, but there is no prospective randomized trial to prove that acute external fixation decreases morbidity and mortality in those patients.[13] The risk of fixator placement is higher in obese patients due to the development of skin breakdown and infection.

AVULSION AND SINGLE BONE FRACTURES **Anterior Superior Iliac Spine (Fig. 265-14)** This fracture typically occurs in adolescents because of forceful contraction of the sartorius muscle. Symptoms and signs are local pain, tenderness, and swelling and pain with flexion or abduction of the thigh. There is minimal displacement of the anterior superior iliac spine visible on the AP film of the pelvis.

Anterior Inferior Iliac Spine This fracture occurs because of forceful contraction of the rectus femoris muscle. Symptoms and signs are sharp pain in the groin, difficulty with ambulation, and inability to flex the hip. The AP film shows downward displacement of the fragment, but this must be differentiated from the epiphyseal line of the os acetabuli.

Ischial Tuberosity This fracture results from forceful contraction of the hamstrings (such as with kicking), and the fracture is seen in youths whose apophyses are not united. Symptoms and signs include acute or chronic pain with sitting or on flexing the thigh with the knee extended. Rectal examination reveals tuberosity tenderness. The roentgenogram shows detachment of the apophysis from the ischium with minimal displacement. The apophysis closes between ages 20 and 25 years.

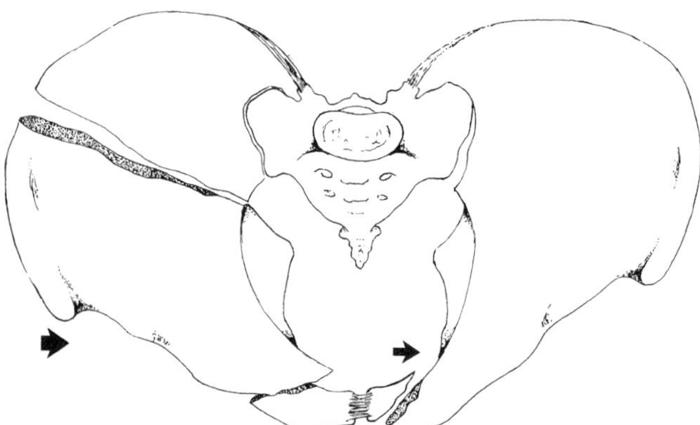

FIG. 265-9. Alternatively (compared to Fig. 265-8), as in type II B fractures (Fig. 265-7) there may be an iliac wing fracture sparing the posterior SIJ on the ipsilateral side.

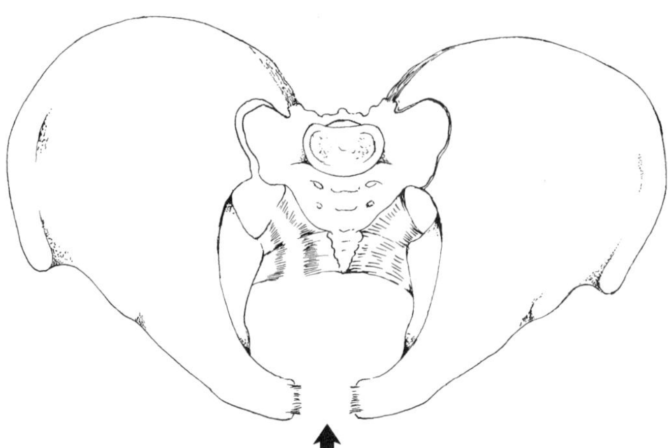

FIG. 265-11. Type II—AP compression fracture: The AP force vector (*large arrow*) has caused further "opening" of the anterior pelvis, with additional rupture of the anterior sacroiliac, sacrotuberous, and sacrospinous ligaments.

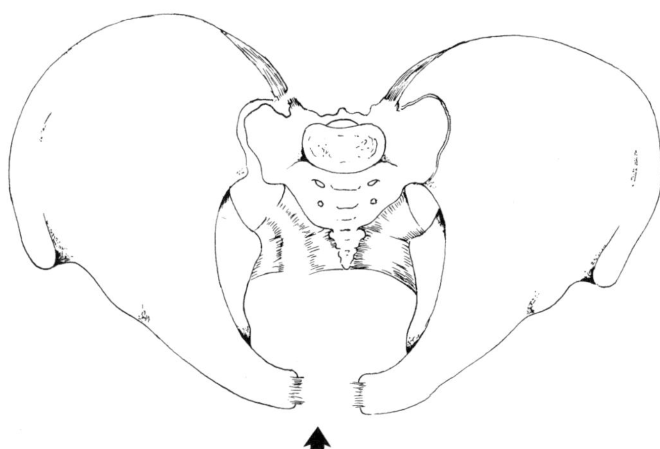

FIG. 265-12. Type III—AP compression fracture: There is total disruption of the SIJ due to wide ''opening'' of the pelvis. All supporting ligament groups, including the posterior sacroiliac ligaments, may be disrupted.

TABLE 265-2 Local Associated Injuries

	% OCCURRENCE		
	Severe Hemorrhage	Bladder Rupture	Urethra
Lateral compression fractures			
Type I	0.5	4.0	2.0
Type II	36.0	7.0	0.0
Type III	60.0	20.0	20.0
AP compression fractures			
Type I	1.0	8.0	12.0
Type II	28.0	11.0	23.0
Type III	53.0	14.0	36.0
Vertical shear fractures	75.0	15.0	25.0
Mixed patterns	58.0	16.0	21.0

Source: From Young JWR, Burgess AR: *Radiologic Management of Pelvic Ring Fractures: Systematic Radiologic Diagnosis.* Baltimore, Urban & Schwarzenberg, 1987. (Used with permission.)

Treatment of avulsion fractures is conservative including the use of nonsteroidal antiinflammatory drugs (NSAIDs), rest in a position of comfort, and the use of crutches with partial weight bearing initially followed by full weight bearing.[11] Follow-up with the patient's primary care physician or orthopedist within 1 to 2 weeks is recommended. Patients generally resume normal activities within 3 to 4 weeks of those injuries.

Single Ramus of Pubis or Ischium (Fig. 265-14) These injuries are commonly seen in the elderly, and the mechanism of injury is usually a fall with direct trauma.[10] Symptoms and signs include local pain and tenderness and inability to ambulate. Examination of the pubic bones will usually distinguish a fracture of the pubis from a femoral neck fracture. The AP roentgenogram of the pelvis typically shows a nondisplaced fracture of the ramus. Treatment is symptomatic including the use of NSAIDs or opioid analgesics and crutches as needed. Orthopedic or primary care follow-up within one to two weeks is recommended.

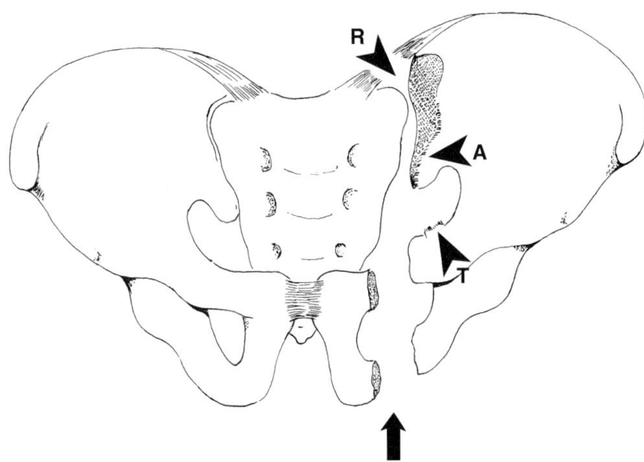

FIG. 265-13. Vertical shear vector: The injury force vector is delivered in a vertical plane (*large arrow*), causing disruption along this line. Fractures of the pubic rami are usually seen anteriorly, while fractures of the sacrum, SIJ, or iliac wing are usually seen posteriorly. The fractures are vertical and are associated with vertical displacement of fragments. Ligamentous injury to the posterior (*R*) and anterior (*A*) sacroiliac ligaments may be seen, as well to sacrospinous/sacrotuberous (*T*), and (possibly) symphysis ligaments.

Ischium Body Fractures The incidence of ischial body injury is very low. The mechanism of injury is violent, external trauma, such as a fall in a sitting position. Symptoms and signs include local pain and tenderness, and pain with hamstring movement. The x-ray film shows fracture of the body or tuberosity of the ischium. A large fragment with comminution or a butterfly pattern may be seen on the AP film of the pelvis. Treatment consists of rest, analgesics, the use of a donut-ring cushion for sitting and crutches as needed. Outpatient primary care or orthopedic follow-up within one to two weeks is recommended.

Iliac Wing (Duverney) Fractures (Fig. 265-14) The mechanism of injury in an iliac wing fracture is direct trauma, usually lateral to medial.[10] Symptoms and signs include pain, swelling, and tenderness over the iliac wing. There is severe pain on ambulation, and Trendelenburg's sign (waddling gait) is present. Although accompanying abdominal injuries are infrequent, abdominal rigidity, lower quadrant tenderness, and ileus are common findings. The AP film of the pelvis typically shows minimal displacement of fragments. Treatment is conservative[5] including analgesics and outpatient primary care or orthopedic follow-up. Hospital admission is not necessary unless the fracture is open or there is significant abdominal muscle spasm associated with the fracture making abdominal exam difficult.

Sacral Fractures These fractures account for approximately 4 to 5 percent of all pelvic fractures. Transverse fractures of the sacrum (Fig. 265-14) are more common with massive pelvic injuries. The mechanism of injury of lower transverse sacral fractures is direct trauma by a posterior-to-anterior force. Upper transverse fractures are typically the result of a flexion injury such as associated with a fall from a height or being struck in the lower back with a heavy load. A rectal examination with the other hand on the sacrum causes pain and movement at the fracture site. Roentgenogram interpretation may be difficult, and exactly aligned AP views are necessary to show the fracture. Look for a transverse fracture line at the level of the lower SI joint, and irregularity, buckling, or sharp angulation of the foramina. Examine the body and wings closely. A lateral view may show displacement anteriorly. Neurologic injury does not occur with fractures

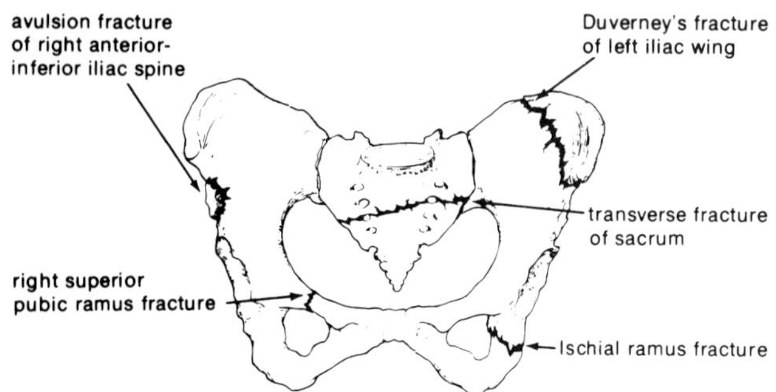

Type I: Fracture of individual bones without break in pelvic ring. Examples shown above.

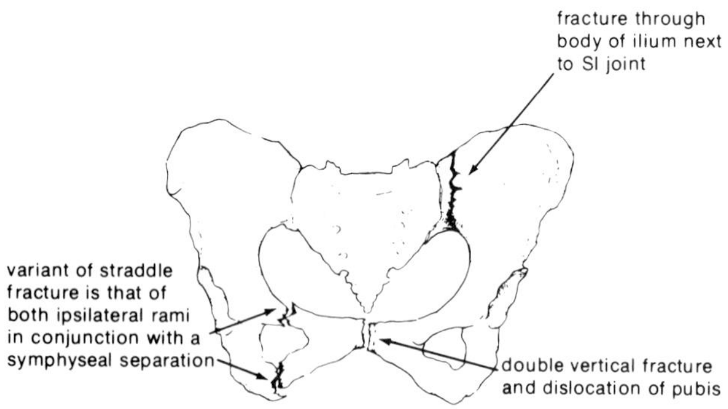

Type II: Single break in the pelvic ring. See examples above.

Malgaigne fracture consisting of symphyseal dislocation and fracture of the ilium.

Type III: Double break in pelvic ring.

FIG. 265-14. Pelvic fractures (type I, II, and III) according to classification by Key JA, Conwell HE: *The Management of Fractures, Dislocations, and Sprains,* 4th ed. St. Louis, Mosby, 1946, p 857, as adapted by Kane WJ: Fractures of the pelvis, in Rockwood CA Jr, Green DP (eds): *Fractures,* 4th ed. Philadelphia, JB Lippincott, 1996. vol. 2, pp 1119–1142.

below the S4 level. Sacral root injury may be present in up to one-third of patients with upper transverse fractures.[15,16] Treatment of simple transverse fractures without neurologic deficit consist of bedrest, analgesics, and orthopedic follow-up. Early orthopedic consultation and surgery is generally indicated for fractures associated with neurologic disability. Lengthy disability may occur with these latter injuries.

Coccyx Fractures Coccygeal fractures are more frequent in women and are generally caused by direct violence or a fall in the sitting position. Symptoms and signs include pain, tenderness, and swelling and ecchymoses over the lower sacral region. There may be pain on getting up from a sitting position or straining at stool. The rectal examination reveals pain with movement of the coccyx. A roentgenogram is not needed if physical examination verifies that this is the only fracture, but AP and lateral views with sharp flexion of the thighs may demonstrate the fracture. Treatment consists of bedrest, sitz baths, stool softeners, and sitting on a donut-ring cushion. Primary care or orthopedic follow-up within 2–3 weeks is recommended. Surgical excision of the distal fracture fragment is rarely indicated if symptoms become chronic.

ACETABULAR FRACTURES Acetabular fractures account for 20 percent of pelvic fractures and are usually secondary to automobile accidents.[17] The fracture force is either transmitted laterally through the hip or through the femur as with a knee-versus-dashboard mechanism. Acetabular fractures are seen commonly with other injuries including femur, hip fractures and dislocations, and knee injuries. The roentgenographic anatomy of acetabular fractures is shown in Fig. 265-15. There are four anatomic types of fractures, and all are associated with hip dislocations: posterior, ilioischial column, transverse, and iliopubic column. In addition, combinations of any of these fractures can occur.

Posterior Fracture The mechanism of injury in a posterior fracture is direct trauma to a flexed knee and hip. Anteroposterior and lateral radiologic views easily demonstrate the posterior acetabular fracture with the posterior hip dislocation. Complications are sciatic nerve injury, which may occur in up to 40 percent of this fracture type, and femoral fractures.

Ilioischial Column Fracture The mechanism of injury is posteriorly directed force to a knee with the thigh abducted and flexed. The AP x-ray film demonstrates a large, medially displaced fragment with

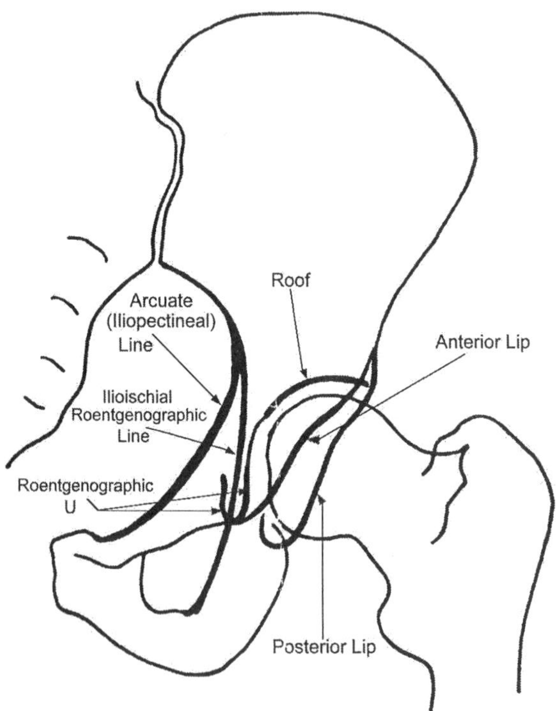

FIG. 265-15. Roentgenographic anatomy of type IV acetabular fractures.

central dislocation of the femoral head. The most common complication is sciatic nerve injury.

Transverse Fracture of Acetabulum The mechanism is force lateral to medial over the greater trochanter, or force posterior to anterior on the posterior pelvis with the hip flexed. An AP x-ray film clearly demonstrates the fracture with a central hip dislocation.

Iliopubic Column Fracture The mechanism of injury is a lateral force to the greater trochanter with the hip externally rotated. On roentgenography, there is marked external rotation of the hip. The ilioischial line is disrupted, and the anterior lip is fractured. Further discussion on acetabular fractures appears below under "Trauma to the Hip and Femur."

Early orthopedic consultation and hospital admission is indicated for patients with acetabular fractures. Nondisplaced fractures may be treated with bedrest and analgesics. Early reduction and internal fixation is indicated for displaced fractures. Significant long-term disability is associated with acetabular fractures.

Complications of Pelvic Fractures

It is imperative to recognize associated injuries. Acute complications include hemorrhage, urogynecologic injury, rectal injury, ruptured diaphragm, and nerve root injury.

HEMORRHAGE Hemorrhage is estimated to be the cause of death in about 50 percent of total pelvic injuries.[18] Retroperitoneal bleeding is an inevitable complication, and up to 4 L of blood can be accommodated in this space until vascular pressure is overcome and tamponade occurs. It is thought that approximately 90 percent of pelvic bleeding is from the fractures and low pressure venous plexus. Both small and large vessels, especially the superior gluteal and internal pudendal branches of the internal iliac artery, can also be disrupted, with hemorrhage dissecting from the back to the buttocks.

General resuscitative measures include massive crystalloid, colloid, and blood replacement. In one series of high-energy pelvic fractures, patients on average required about six units of blood transfused.[19] The average transfusion requirement for APC injuries was about 15 units, VS injuries 9 units, and LC injuries about 3.5 units. Aggressive resuscitation of these patients along with treatment of extrapelvic injuries and early or delayed open reduction and internal fixation of the fractures may reduce mortality.[20]

The use of the antishock garment is controversial. It may be helpful in controlling bleeding sites by immobilizing fractures and compressing the pelvis. Disadvantages include decreased visibility and access to the abdomen and lower extremities and the risk of compartment syndrome with prolonged application. This garment is generally only recommended for pelvic stabilization in the pre-hospital and ED setting. Early orthopedic consultation should be considered for placement of external fixator device to help control hemorrhage in patients with persistent hemodynamic instability.

If the patient is exsanguinating, angiography can be done and small arterial bleeding sites controlled by transarterial embolization. Most authorities agree that aggressive fluid and blood replacement is the best initial therapy along with correction of hypothermia and coagulopathy. Placement of an external fixator and laparotomy should also be considered prior to angiography.[21] Overall, only about two percent of patients with pelvic fracture require embolization and efficacy approaches 100 percent when utilized.[22] Younger age, shorter time from injury to embolization, and hemodynamic stability are associated with improved survival.

UROGYNECOLOGIC INJURY Urinary tract injuries are discussed in Chap. 254. Gynecologic injuries are uncommonly associated with pelvic trauma. Vaginal laceration is the most common injury seen with anterior pelvic fractures. A bimanual pelvic examination should be performed on all women with pelvic fractures. If blood is found in a woman of childbearing age, a speculum examination must be carried out to distinguish menses from laceration. Treatment is irrigation and debridement in the operating room with repair of wounds and antibiotic therapy.

A high fetal death rate is associated with pelvic trauma in pregnancy if the mother is in shock; if there is placental, uterine, or direct fetal injury; or if the mother dies. Immediate caesarean section must be considered (see Chap. 246, "Trauma in Pregnancy").

RECTAL INJURIES Rectal injuries are uncommon and are usually associated with urinary injuries and ischial fractures. Diagnosis is by rectal examination or by protoscopy, whereupon blood is found in the rectum. Treatment includes a diverting colostomy with washout of the distal colon, and presacral space drainage. Antibiotics should be given as soon as the injury is discovered.

RUPTURED DIAPHRAGM Ruptured diaphragm associated with fracture of the pelvis may be more common than previously thought. It may be associated with rib injuries. Suspect the diagnosis with physical findings such as displacement of the heart toward the right, absent breath sounds, or presence of bowel sounds in the chest. Confirmation is by x-ray and CT scan. Diagnosis is difficult if the defect is small.

NERVE ROOT INJURY Nerve root or peripheral nerve injuries can occur because of traction, pressure from hemorrhage, callus or fibrous tissue, and impingement-laceration by bone fragments. The onset of symptoms and signs may be delayed, but deficits usually follow a nerve root pattern. Lumbar nerve root injuries are associated with SI joint dislocation or fracture. Sacral root injuries are associated with sacral fractures, especially fractures of S1 and S2.

Pelvic Fractures in Children

Commonly caused by automobile-pedestrian accidents, pelvic fractures in children have a high incidence of concomitant injuries because of the smaller protection afforded by the developing pelvis and the significant trauma incurred.[14] Hemorrhage determines mortality. Children in shock who respond poorly to fluid replacement have the highest mortality. Frequent concomitant injuries include head and neck injuries, intra-abdominal injuries, and long bone fractures. The incidence of genitourinary injuries is similar to that of adults. Major thoracic injuries are rare but particularly dangerous because they are often overlooked.

Postponement of surgery until stabilization of circulation is recommended unless the patient is exsanguinating despite treatment. If the child does not respond to transfusions equal to the estimated total blood volume (TBV) (88 mL/kg × wt [kg] = TBV) within 1 h, suspect major vascular injury and operate. Both arterial and venous injuries are associated with significant SI joint injury.

Except for pelvic avulsion fractures, early orthopedic consultation and hospitalization is indicated. Surgical treatment for pelvic fractures is indicated less frequently in children than in adolescents or adults because of children's ability to remodel pelvic fractures and because early ambulation is not critical.[14] Nondisplaced fractures can generally be treated with bedrest alone. Displaced fractures can be treated with distal femoral skeletal traction on the displaced side of the hemipelvis. Severely malaligned Malgaigne fractures may occasionally require open reduction and internal fixation.

TRAUMA TO THE HIP AND FEMUR

Anatomy

The hip is a ball-and-socket joint made up of the acetabulum and the femur. The hip includes the acetabulum and the proximal femur two to three inches below the lesser trochanter. The functions of the hip are weight-bearing and movement. The fibrous capsule that surrounds the joint on all sides is exceedingly strong. It attaches around the acetabulum proximally and runs to the intertrochanteric line distally on the anterior surface. Posteriorly, it falls short of the intertrochanteric crest and inserts on the neck of the femur. It is weakest posteriorly.

The blood supply of the femoral head is derived from nutrient branches of the obturator, medial femoral circumflex, lateral femoral circumflex, and superior and inferior gluteal arteries. These course beneath the reflection of the capsule on the neck of the femur and also along the ligamentum teres. The capsular vessels are much more important than those of the ligamentum teres.

Clinical Evaluation

PHYSICAL EXAMINATION The examination of the hip begins with a detailed history and complete examination of the patient. The pelvis and hip are then carefully evaluated. The unclothed, erect patient is inspected for a list, injuries, scars, or asymmetry of the muscles. Gait should be tested, if possible.

If the patient is a trauma victim, after primary survey and initial stabilization observe the position of the extremities, looking for deformities, shortening, rotation, lacerations, or bruises, and test for stability and range of motion. On palpation, feel for irregularities in movement at the iliac crest, pubic rami, and ischial rami. Compress the pelvis lateral to medial through the iliac crest; anterior to posterior through the symphysis pubis; and anterior to posterior through the iliac crest, seeking pain and tenderness. Also, compress the greater trochanters of the hips.

If no significant abnormalities are found, range of motion of the hips should then be studied. If rotation of the hip with the leg in extension is painful all other maneuvers should be done cautiously. If a hip or pelvic fracture or dislocation is identified in a trauma victim, *assume* that intra-abdominal, retroperitoneal, and urologic injuries have occurred as well, until it has been proved otherwise. Always perform a detailed neurovascular examination and a rectal examination, looking for displacement of the prostate in male patients. Associated femoral shaft fractures should be ruled out.

RADIOLOGIC EVALUATION Roentgenographic evaluation of the pelvis and hips is a must in all unconscious patients who have sustained multiple injuries. The threshold for obtaining radiographs in demented elderly patients who have sustained minor falls should also be relatively low because those patients may be particularly difficult to evaluate.[23] Lower extremity long bone fractures, as well as pelvic symptoms or signs, are also indications for these x-ray examinations. The x-ray evaluation should include a standard AP and a lateral view of the pelvis. If further studies are needed, AP views of either hemipelvis, internal and external oblique views of the hemipelvis as described by Judet and colleagues, or "inlet" and "tilt" views may be done. In certain instances, such views allow better identification and detail of the acetabulum and femoral head and neck. Always inspect not only the hip joint but also the femur and knee when evaluating hip disorders on x-ray films. Disorders to the knee and the femoral shaft often occur with hip injuries. Significant hip pain with weight-bearing following trauma and normal radiographs suggest the possibility of occult fracture, especially at the femoral neck or acetabulum.[24] The patient should be prescribed protected weight-bearing and the emergency physician should communicate with the patient's primary care provider or orthopedist regarding close follow-up for possible CT or MR hip imaging to rule out occult fracture.[25,26] MR is reliable in detecting occult fractures within 24 h of injury.

Classification/Epidemiology of Hip Fractures

The estimated incidence of hip fractures in the United States is about 80 per 100,000 population.[27] The incidence increases with age and doubles for each decade past the age of 50. The incidence is about two to three times higher in women than men and fractures are more common in white than nonwhite women.

The possibility of elder abuse should be considered in all elderly patients with falls and fractures. Evidence of physical abuse such as bruises and burns, especially if they are unexplained, and of various ages and certain patterns should raise the physician's clinical suspicion of abuse. Patterns or well-defined shapes, such as an emersion pattern or rope or restraint marks on the wrists or ankles, should also raise suspicion. Signs of neglect, such as dehydration, malnutrition, poor hygiene, extensive bed sores, urine burns or excoriations, and fecal impactions, should also increase suspicion for elder neglect. Interactions between family or caregivers and the patient should be observed and Social Services should be consulted and abuse reported as required by law when appropriate.[28]

Hip fractures are classified as femoral head and neck (intracapsular) and trochanteric, intertrochanteric, and subtrochanteric (extracapsular) (Fig. 265-16). The prognosis for successful union and restoration of normal function varies considerably with the fracture.

In intracapsular fractures with displacement, the femoral neck vessels are compromised due to a tear or compression secondary to an intracapsular hemarthrosis. The blood supply through the ligamentum teres may not be sufficient to nourish the entire femoral head. Therefore, avascular necrosis inevitably results (15 to 35 percent overall) unless some of the capsular vessels remain intact. Basilar neck and intertrochanteric fractures below the capsule rarely sever important arteries. Morbidity and mortality associated with hip fractures is primarily due to patient immobilization and the development of deep venous thrombosis and pulmonary embolus. Even with modern treatment modalities, mortality following hip fracture ranges from 15 to 35 percent within one year of surgery and 25 to 50 percent of the survivors will not regain their ability to ambulate.[29] Factors predictive of increased mortality include male sex, increased age, dementia, institutionalization, poorly controlled systemic disease, and the development of postoperative complications. There is some evidence that early (<72 h) hip fracture fixation of low impact hip fractures in the elderly reduces morbidity and mortality.[30–32]

FEMORAL HEAD FRACTURES Isolated femoral head fractures occur infrequently. They are usually associated with dislocations of the hip. Shear fractures of the superior aspect of the femoral head are associated with anterior dislocations, and shear fractures of the inferior femoral head are associated with posterior dislocations.

In most instances, the symptoms and signs are those of the associated dislocation rather than of the fracture itself. The standard AP and lateral x-ray views usually demonstrate the fragment adequately. When there is an associated dislocation, the postreduction films offer a better view of the fracture fragment.

Orthopedic consultation should be obtained in the ED for these fractures. Treatment is to reduce the associated dislocation and then attain anatomic reduction of the fracture fragment. Complications are associated with the high-energy trauma that produces the fracture-dislocation, that is, the more comminuted the fracture, the more severe the dislocation and the greater the severity of trauma to the patient. Life-threatening injuries must then be ruled out.

The prognosis is related to the severity of the initial trauma resulting in the dislocation. Poor prognostic indicators include delay between hip dislocation and reduction, repetitive unsuccessful relocation at-

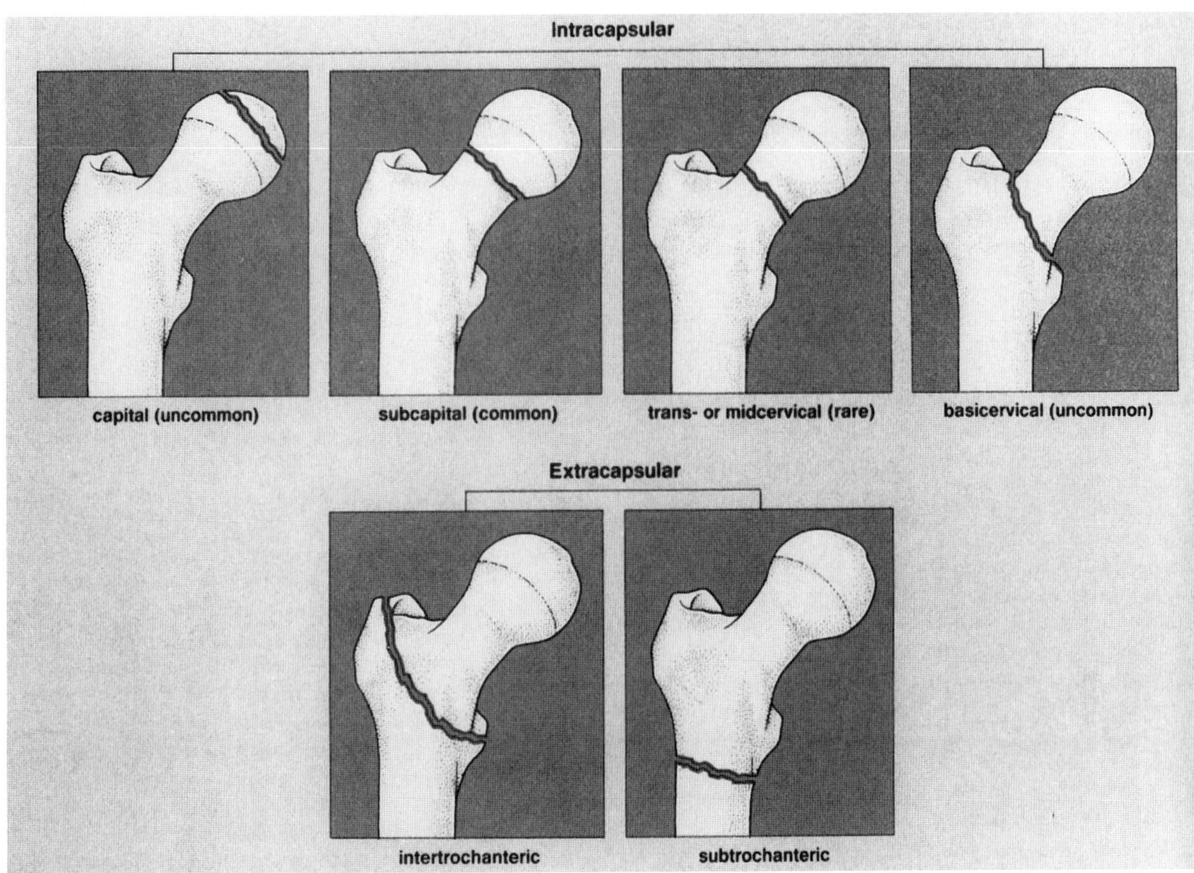

FIG. 265-16. Fractures of the proximal femur are traditionally classified as intracapsular and extracapsular. (From Greenspan A. *Orthopedic Radiology*. Philadelphia: JB Lippincott, 1988, p 5.17. Used with permission.)

tempts and associated injuries. Posttraumatic arthritis occurs in one-third to two-thirds of patients, avascular necrosis in 10 to 20 percent and myositis ossificans in approximately 1 to 2 percent.[33]

FEMORAL NECK FRACTURES Femoral neck fractures are commonly seen among older adults, due to osteoporosis, and occur more frequently in women than in men. These fractures are rare among the younger population. The cause of such fractures is usually minor trauma secondary to falls (90 percent) or torsion in the patient with osteoporosis or osteomalacia. In younger patients, the high kinetic energy sustained in the major trauma causes a fracture through normal bone with marked soft tissue disruption and comminution.

The classification of femoral neck fractures is by fragment displacement. The symptoms seen with femoral neck fractures range from complaints of mild pain in the groin or inner thigh in patients with an incomplete fracture to moderate to severe pain in patients with displaced fractures.

Patients who have sustained a fracture without displacement may walk with some limping rather than being completely unable to bear weight. Their only physical findings are minor pain with movement and minimal muscle spasm limiting range of motion. In contrast, displaced fractures cause severe pain, inability to ambulate, limited range of motion, and no palpable movement of the extracapsular head. The patient lies with the extremity in *slight* external rotation, abduction, and shortening.

Radiographic evaluation is essential in any patient suspected of having a femoral neck fracture. Stress fractures, however, may not show up on x-ray for days or weeks, so repeat films or bone scans in symptomatic patients are necessary. The standard AP view should have the patient maximally internally rotated to best demonstrate the femoral neck. The AP view should be inspected for a fracture line starting on the superior surface of the neck. These fracture lines routinely become complete within 10 to 14 days. Also, disruption of Shenton's line may be appreciated on the AP view in some instances. If there is any concern that the patient has sustained a fracture that is not visible on the initial x-ray examination, the patient should be conservatively treated and x-ray films should be made again in 10 to 14 days; or the physician may order a CT or MRI, which demonstrates the fracture in most instances. In contrast, displaced fractures are obvious on the AP film, but a lateral view should also be done to ascertain the exact position.

Orthopedic consultation should be obtained in the emergency department for these fractures. The orthopedic surgeon's goal of treatment for femoral neck fractures is anatomic reduction and stability. Treatment for nondisplaced or impacted fractures is somewhat controversial but usually involves a form of internal fixation. This is due in part because up to 15 percent of impacted fractures can develop secondary displacement without surgery. Conservative treatment is generally only considered if the patient is medically unfit for surgery or the fracture is several weeks old and the patient is walking without pain.[22] Displaced fractures definitely require emergency surgery for fixation. Prosthetic hip replacements may be required in certain instances, particularly in those patients over age 70.[27] The timing of surgery remains controversial. Early surgery (<72 h) is indicated in fit patients, whereas surgery should be delayed if correctable comorbidities are present. Special note should be made of stress fractures because some are treated in a conservative manner and others are treated with internal fixation, depending on the type of fracture and the patient's cooperation. Skeletal traction is contraindicated with femoral neck fractures because it may further compromise femoral head blood flow.

The complications of femoral neck fractures are significant. They include infections, emboli, and avascular necrosis, which is the most feared early complication. Avascular necrosis has an incidence of 15 percent in nondisplaced fractures and rises to near 90 percent with untreated, completely displaced fractures. A higher incidence is also associated with more severe fractures or fractures that are not surgically reduced to anatomic position within 48 h. Nonunion in nondisplaced fractures is rare but occurs in approximately 20 to 30 percent of patients with displaced fractures.[22]

TROCHANTERIC FRACTURES Greater trochanteric fractures are usually due to avulsions at the insertion of the gluteus medius. In the younger population (7 to 17 years of age), this is a true epiphyseal separation, in contrast to the adult population, in which this is due to direct trauma.[22] The patient presents with pain, especially with abduction and extension, and a limp. Also, there is tenderness to palpation over the greater trochanter.

Standard AP and lateral x-ray views reveal displacement in the superior-posterior area, or comminution. The treatment is generally conservative with protected weight-bearing recommended until the patient is asymptomatic. Outpatient orthopedic referral is indicated. Orthopedic consultation for possible surgical fixation may be indicated for fracture displacement of greater than 1 cm.[22]

Lesser trochanteric fractures due to an avulsion secondary to a forceful contraction of the iliopsoas are commonly seen in children and young athletic adults, particularly gymnasts and dancers. These patients present with pain during flexion and internal rotation maneuvers. In most instances, the treatment is bedrest and then gradual weight-bearing to regain full activity. Outpatient followup by primary care or orthopedics is advised. Full recovery generally occurs within three weeks.

If greater than 2-cm displacement is seen on the standard AP and lateral views, then screw fixation by the consulting orthopedic surgeon may be indicated.

INTERTROCHANTERIC FRACTURES These fractures are defined as extracapsular fractures occurring in a line between the greater and lesser trochanters. Intertrochanteric fractures generally occur in the elderly and are more common in women, again due to the high incidence of osteoporosis. The mechanism of injury is usually a fall or occasionally an automobile accident. It is postulated that a rotational component along with the direct trauma is involved in some instances as well.

Symptoms and signs include pain, swelling of the hip, local ecchymosis, and pain with any hip movement or weight-bearing. Moreover, the extremity is markedly externally rotated and shortened, in contrast to the minimal deformities associated with femoral neck fractures. These fractures are classified as stable or unstable. Stable fractures are defined as ones in which the medial cortices of the neck and femoral fragments abut. X-ray evaluation should include AP and lateral views, with the AP view having as much internal rotation as possible to adequately visualize the neck.

Severe life-threatening injuries must be excluded. The consulting orthopedic physician can then admit the patient to the hospital and perform surgical fixation to attain a stable reduction as soon as possible, although this is not an emergency. Buck's traction (Fig. 265-17) may temporarily help reduce pain.

The complications and prognosis are related to other associated injuries and prior disease. The overall mortality is approximately 10 to 30 percent. Infection can be a major problem, with an incidence of up to 17 percent.[34] Thromboembolic disease is especially a problem if postoperative mobilization does not occur quickly. Avascular necrosis is rare in these patients, and nonunion is also uncommon. Morbidity is due to the patient's inability to return to prefracture activity.

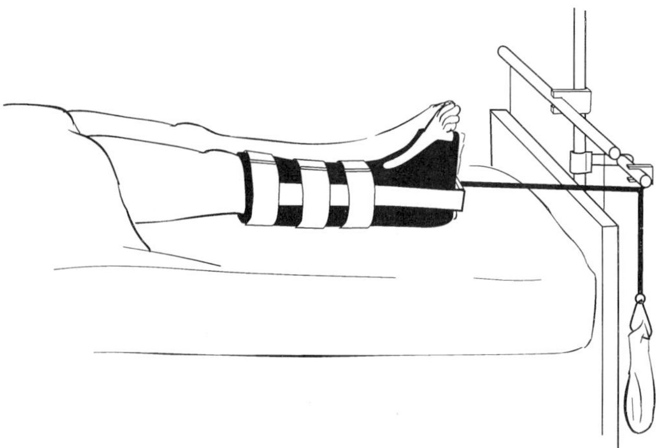

FIG. 265-17. Buck's traction.

SUBTROCHANTERIC FRACTURES Subtrochanteric fractures may be seen in two different populations. They usually occur secondary to falling in the 40- to 60-year-old patient with osteoporotic or weakened bone. The second population is young persons who have suffered major trauma with significant kinetic energies directed into the femur. These fractures may be an extension of an intertrochanteric or other isolated fracture and are usually classified as stable or unstable, with stable defined as bony contact of the medial and posterior femoral cortices.

The symptoms and signs are similar to those of trochanteric or femoral fractures, with local pain, deformity, swelling, crepitance, etc. These patients can lose a large amount of blood into the thigh area and may present in hypovolemic shock. Because this injury is due to significant trauma, other, more life-threatening injuries must be excluded prior to treatment of this specific fracture.

Standard AP and lateral x-ray views of the hip are necessary to properly assess the fracture. Moreover, x-ray studies of the pelvis, femur, and knee are indicated to rule out associated fractures.

Treatment consists of immobilization with a traction apparatus. Hare (Dyna-Med, Carlsbad, CA) or Sager (Minto Research & Development, Redding, CA) splints (Figs. 265-18 and 265-19) may be employed in the prehospital setting. Proper evaluation of the entire patient to rule out associated severe injuries should be conducted. After the patient has stabilized and secondary evaluation has occurred, orthopedics should be consulted. Open reduction and internal fixation is generally indicated for fracture management.[34]

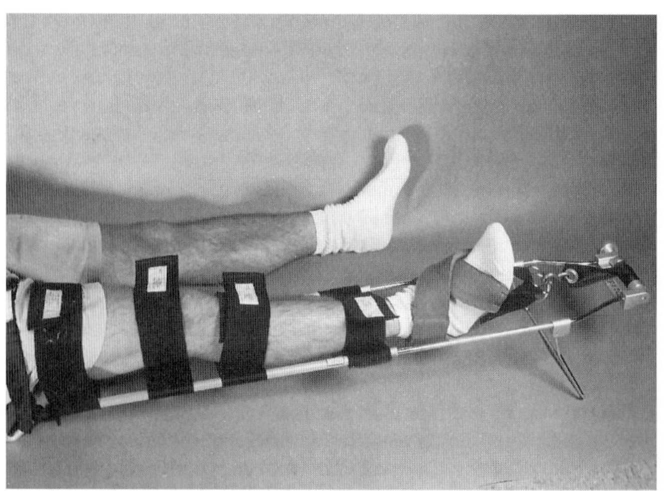

FIG. 265-18. Hare traction splint.

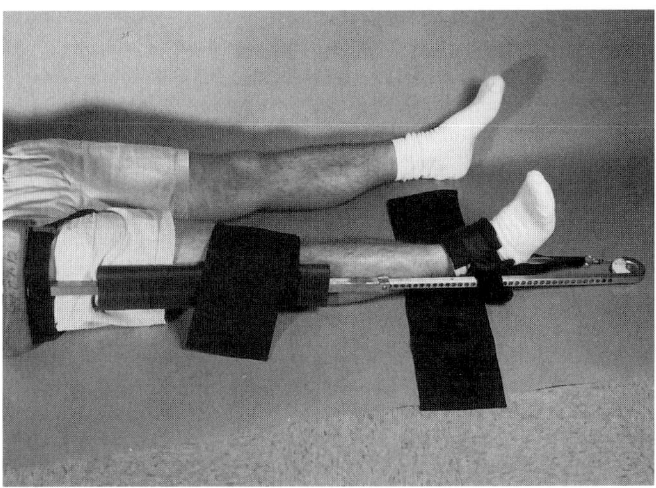

FIG. 265-19. Sager traction splint.

The complications are similar to those of intertrochanteric fractures, except that there is a higher incidence of nonunion. Malunion and delayed union occur as well in this population. Prognosis is better for proximal fractures that are not comminuted.

Hip Dislocations

Hip dislocations can be classified as anterior, posterior, and central. Acetabular fracture with central hip dislocation has been discussed under acetabular fractures.

ANTERIOR DISLOCATIONS About 10 percent of hip dislocations are anterior (Fig. 265-20*A* and *B*), and the majority are secondary to automobile accidents, but they may also result from a fall, or a blow to the back while squatting. In anterior dislocations, the femoral head rests anterior to the coronal plane of the acetabulum. Anterior dislocations can be superior or inferior (obturator, thyroid, perineal) depending on the degree of hip flexion present at the time of injury. If the hip is abducted, externally rotated, and flexed at the time of injury, inferior dislocation occurs. If the hip is abducted, externally rotated, and extended, superior dislocation occurs. The mechanism of injury is forced abduction that causes the femoral head to be levered out through an anterior capsular tear. The affected extremity is in abduction and external rotation. However, the clinical appearance of superior versus inferior dislocations is dramatically different (Fig. 265-20*C* and *D*). Neurovascular compromise is an unusual, but possible complication.

An AP film of the pelvis easily demonstrates the femoral head to be anterior to the acetabulum. A lateral view illustrates the anterior dislocation more clearly, although it may be difficult to obtain because of the patient's pain.

Treatment for the dislocation is early closed reduction, usually under conscious sedation. Strong, in-line traction is done with simultaneous flexion and internal rotation. Finally, the hip is abducted once the head clears the rim of the acetabulum. The dislocation should be reduced quickly, within a few hours, because the longer the delay in reduction, the higher the incidence of avascular necrosis. Postreduction radiographs should be specifically examined for acetabular or femoral head fractures and the possibility of small fragments in the joint not appreciated on the initial films.

POSTERIOR DISLOCATIONS Posterior dislocations (Fig. 265-21*A*) constitute 80 to 90 percent of hip dislocations. They are caused by force applied to a flexed knee, directed posteriorly. Acetabular fractures may result as well. On examination, the extremity is found to be shortened, internally rotated, and adducted (Fig. 265-21*B*). Concomitant life-threatening injuries must be ruled out.

Anteroposterior and lateral x-ray films of the pelvis and hip will reveal the dislocation, but further assessment of the acetabulum and femur must be done to rule out fractures. The oblique views of Judet and colleagues will reveal an acetabular fracture. Also, inferior femoral head fracture will be seen on the AP or oblique view. Hip dislocations are difficult to recognize if there is an associated femoral shaft fracture, so roentgenograms of the pelvis and hips should be routinely obtained in such cases.

The treatment of posterior dislocation without fracture is closed reduction under conscious sedation or general anesthesia, as quickly as possible and always within six hours. In-line traction, gentle flexion to 90°, and then gentle internal-to-external rotation is done (Allis maneuver, Fig. 265-22). The Stimson maneuver (Fig. 265-23) may prove useful in certain situations.

Complications include sciatic nerve injury in about 10 percent of the patients and avascular necrosis that increases in direct proportion to the delay in adequate reduction.

Hip Injuries in Children

FRACTURES AND DISLOCATIONS Fractures of the proximal end of the femur are extremely rare in children and are usually due to severe trauma. Trauma may produce a displaced epiphysis or a fracture of the neck, trochanteric, or subtrochanteric region. Traumatic epiphyseal separation is probably less common than the previously mentioned fractures, but is more common than dislocation. The treatment of displaced fractures is anatomic reduction, followed by internal fixation surgically. Nondisplaced fractures of the intertrochanteric and subtrochanteric regions may be treated with skin or skeletal traction followed by abduction spica casting.[35] There is a significant complication rate, especially avascular necrosis with transepiphyseal and transcervical (femoral neck) fractures.

Traumatic dislocations in children are rare, but are more common than hip fractures. They are more common in boys and more common between ages 2 and 5, and 11 and 15. The frequency of left versus right is equal, and bilateral dislocations are reportable. Posterior dislocations occur with an 80 to 85 percent frequency. The mechanism of injury and the clinical picture are similar to those seen in traumatic dislocation in the adult. The presence of an associated fracture is rare.

The treatment is closed reduction. Dislocation is an orthopedic emergency, and reductions should be done within six hours. Delay in reduction past 24 h is associated with a much higher incidence of complications.

Bursitis

Approximately 18 bursae surround the hip joint. These are derived developmentally from and are physiologically similar to synovium and tendon sheaths. As a result, they suffer from the same inflammatory afflictions which cause problems to the joint itself. Conditions that affect the bursae include traumatic inflammation, which is usually secondary to overuse or excessive pressure; infections; metabolic disorders such as gout; and benign and malignant growths.

Treatment consists of rest, ice, anti-inflammatory medications orally and, occasionally, intrabursal injections. Ultrasound physical therapy may help as well. The prognosis is good as long as associated problems such as infection and low-back disk disease are ruled out. Mechanical problems, especially leg length discrepancies, must be sought and, if found, properly treated so that further trochanteric bursitis does not occur.

Femoral Shaft Fractures

Fractures of the shaft of the femur most often occur in men during their most active period in life. Falls, industrial and automobile acci-

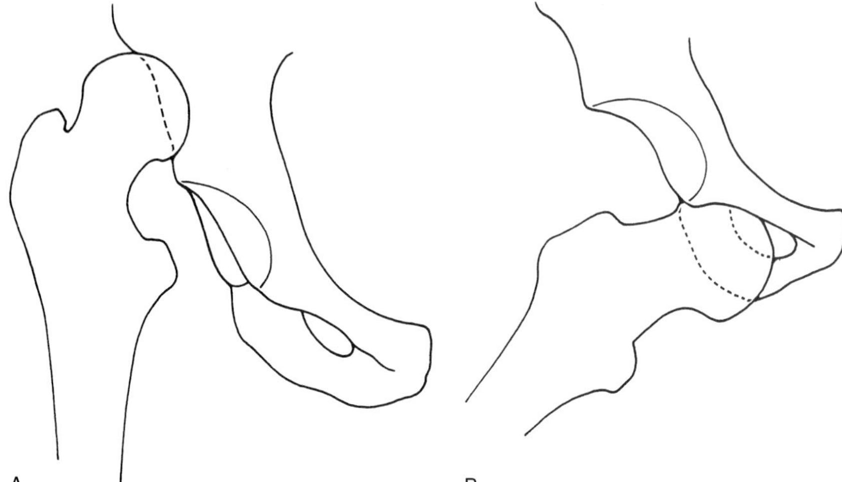

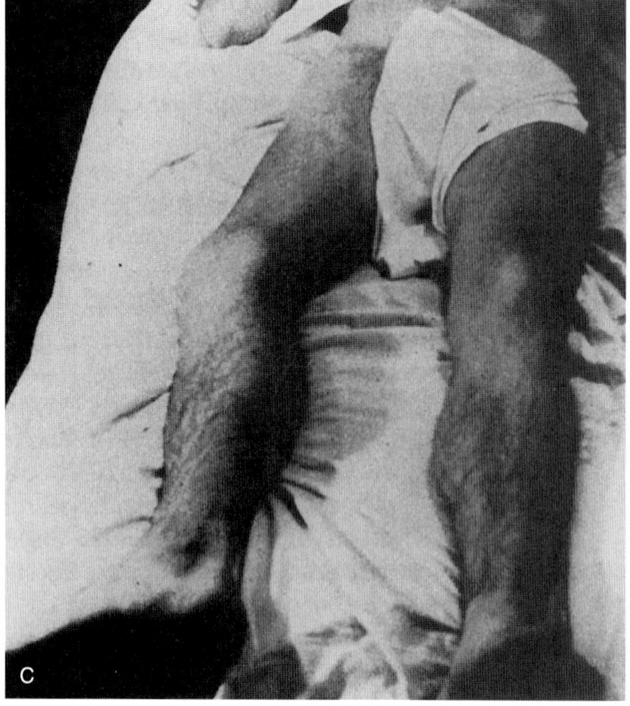

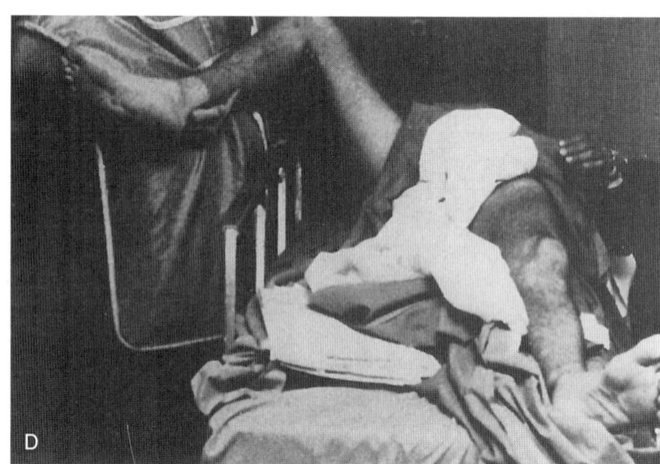

FIG. 265-20. A. Anterior superior dislocation of the hip. **B.** Inferior dislocations (obturator, thyroid, or perineal). **C.** Clinical appearance of a superior-type anterior dislocation of the hip. **D.** Clinical appearance of an inferior-type dislocation of the hip. (From Rockwood CA Jr, Green DP, Bucholz RW (eds). *Fractures in Adults,* 3rd ed, vol. 2. Philadelphia: JB Lippincott, 1991, pp 1576, 1578, 1587, 1588. Used with permission).

dents, and gunshot wounds account for the majority of these fractures.[36] Severe, direct trauma may result in transverse fractures (most common) with displacement, oblique or spiral oblique fractures, or badly comminuted segments. Pathologic fractures are uncommon but can occur secondary to metastases (breast, lung, or prostate most common) or rarely secondary to primary bone tumors such as osteogenic sarcoma.

Spiral midshaft femur fractures can occur in toddlers who are running and trip with a twisting motion.[37] Midshaft femur fractures in children are often the result of neglect or abuse; however, up to 80 percent of fractures during the first year of life are possibly due to abuse.[38] The suspicion of abuse should be greater if the fracture occurs in an infant, child with preexisting brain damage, child with bilateral femur fractures, subtrochanteric femur fractures, or fractures occurring in children with other concomitant trauma. Distal metaphyseal chip fractures and delays in the family seeking medical care for the child should also raise the clinical suspicion for abuse. A femoral fracture in a young child with no history suggestive of abuse or significant trauma should suggest the possibility of osteogenesis imperfecta.

The femur is surrounded by large muscle groups with a rich vascular supply. Therefore, femoral fractures may result in a loss of 1 L or more of blood into the soft tissue of the thigh, producing clinical shock. The initial evaluation should always include careful neurovascular examination of the extremity. Vascular occlusion or disruption can occur, but nerve damage is rare.

Femoral shaft fractures are generally evident in the field to prehospital personnel because of the shortening, deformity and associated swelling. Initially, basic stabilization of the patient should take place in the field, along with spinal assessment and immobilization. External hemorrhage should be controlled by direct pressure, open wounds covered with a sterile dressing and then neurovascular examination of the extremities performed. It is best to splint the affected extremity with a traction splint at the time of injury. Hare (Dyna-Med, Carlsbad, CA) or Sager (Minto Research & Development, Redding, CA) traction splints can be placed over the trousers, applying traction to a sling around the ankle and forefoot. Traction splints are relatively contraindicated in cases of open fracture with grossly contaminated exposed

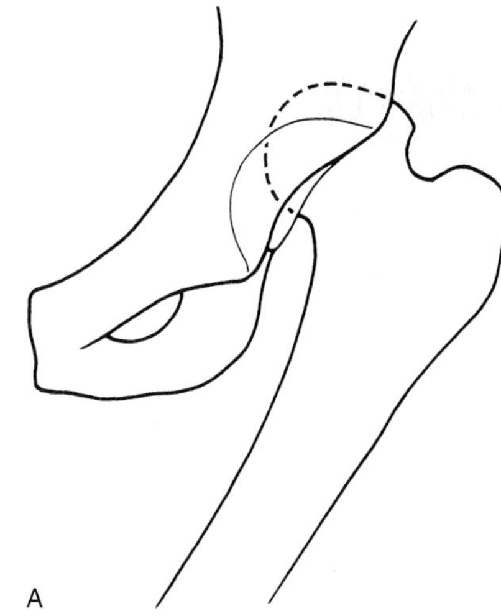

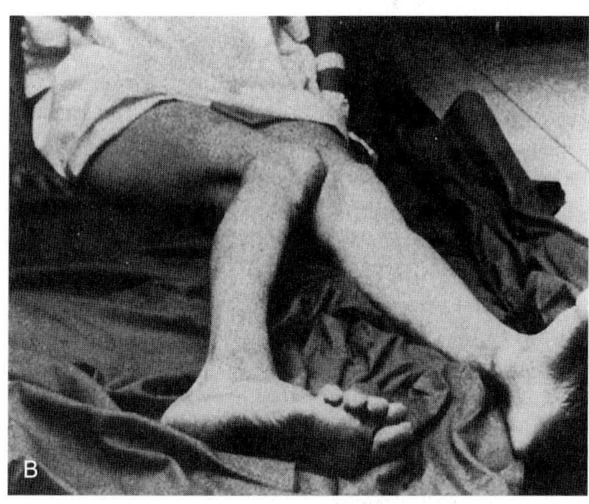

FIG. 265-21. **A.** Posterior dislocation of the hip. **B.** The clinical appearance of a posterior dislocation of the right hip. (From Rockwood CA Jr, Green DP, Bucholz RW (eds). *Fractures in Adults,* 3rd ed, vol. 2. Philadelphia: JB Lippincott, 1991, pp 1580, 1591. Used with permission.)

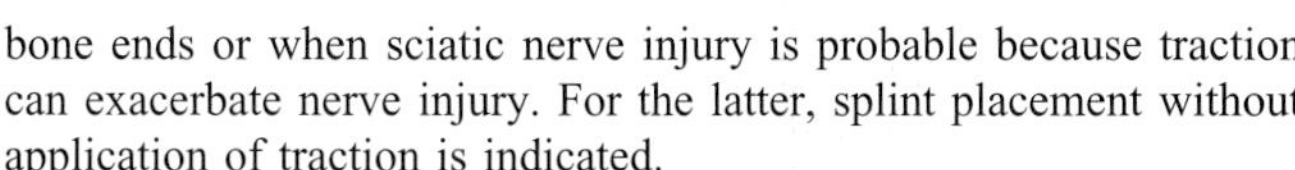

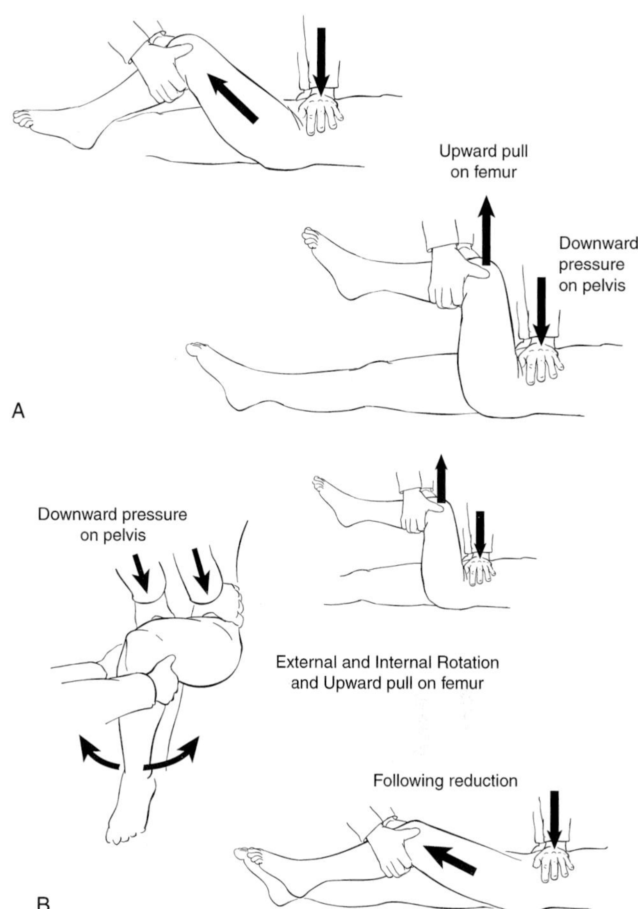

FIG. 265-22. **A** and **B.** Allis maneuver.

bone ends or when sciatic nerve injury is probable because traction can exacerbate nerve injury. For the latter, splint placement without application of traction is indicated.

Emergency Department management includes basic stabilization of the patient followed by careful neurovascular examination of the affected extremity. Open fractures require broad spectrum antibiotics, debridement, and copious irrigation, generally in the operating room. Radiographs of the femur are generally lower priority in the acute resuscitation phase and parenteral analgesics are generally required if there is no contraindication to their use. Orthopedic consultation should be obtained early and most patients require hospitalization and surgical intervention.

Definitive management options include traction, external fixation, pins and plaster, and internal fixation. In infants and in children up to 2 years of age or 30 pounds, fractures of the shaft of the femur are treated by direct overhead traction applied to both legs (Bryant's traction) followed by spica casting. Spica casting is also used for children up to age six. In an older child or young adult, the Fisk-type of traction by means of a half-Thomas ring and Pearson attachment, to allow flexion of the knee, is satisfactory for unstable fractures followed by spica casting or cast bracing. External fixation and flexible intramedullary rod fixation are being employed more frequently in this age group.[39] The intermedullary interlocking nailing is the method

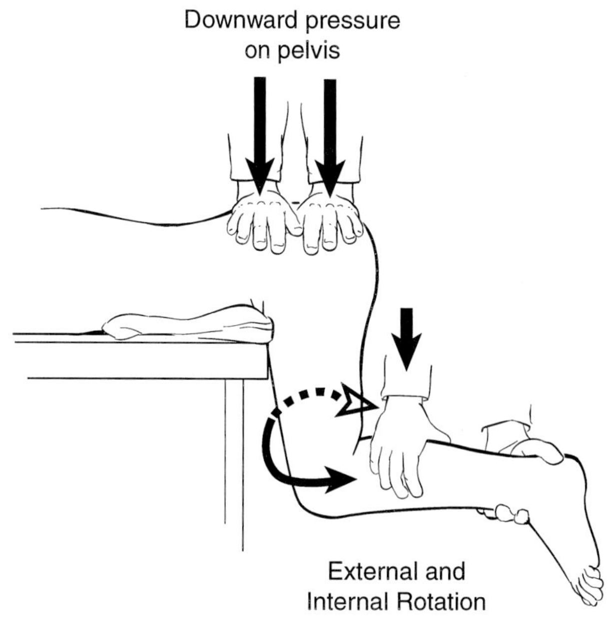

FIG. 265-23. Stimson maneuver.

of choice for the treatment of uncomplicated fractures of the mid shaft and junction of the upper and middle third of the femur in adults, except where comminution is so extensive that stability with the rod cannot be maintained. In cases where comminution is severe, either dual-plating or the use of a compression plate device can result in excellent fixation. Open femur fractures require early orthopedic consultation for copious irrigation and debridement in the operating room. These injuries can generally be nailed immediately.[40] In severely contaminated open fractures, external fixation may be the preferred method of treatment.

The overall prognosis of midshaft femur fractures is very good, with most patients being able to return to work within six months. Union rates approach 100 percent, with non-union being very uncommon. Mild degrees of limb shortening or malalignment can result in limp and posttraumatic arthritis.

Patients with preexisting internal hardware may suffer recurrent fractures with trauma. These fractures tend to be very severe and comminuted because the bone is weaker than the hardware. Evaluation and treatment principles are the same as without hardware. Hardware migration, loosening and rarely breakage can occur. Pain at the site and radiographic changes compared to old films are present. Infection, suggested by pain at the fracture site and fever, may also occur, but is uncommon with closed procedures.

REFERENCES

1. Mucha P Jr, Farnell MB: Analysis of pelvic fracture management. *J Trauma* 24:379, 1984.
2. Moreno C, et al: Hemorrhage associated with major pelvic fracture: A multispecialty challenge. *J Trauma* 26:987, 1986.
3. Tile M: Anatomy, in: *Fractures of the Pelvis and Acetabulum.* Baltimore: Williams & Wilkins, 1984, pp 11, 63–64.
4. Strate RG, Grieco JG: Blunt injury to the colon and rectum. *J Trauma* 23:384, 1983.
5. Yang AP, Iannacone WM: External fixation for pelvic ring disruptions. *Orthop Clin North Am* 28:331, 1997.
6. Cerva DS Jr, Mirvic SE, Shanmuganathan K, et al: Detection of bleeding in patients with major pelvic fractures: Value of contrast-enhanced CT. *Am J Roentgenology* 166:131, 1996.
7. Young JWR, Burgess AR: *Radiologic Management of Pelvic Ring Fractures: Systematic Radiologic Diagnosis.* Baltimore: Urban & Schwarzenberg, 1987.
8. Dalal SA, Burgess AR, Siegel JH, et al: Pelvic fracture in multiple trauma: Classification by mechanism is key to problem of organ injury, resuscitation requirements and outcome. *J Trauma* 29:981, 1989.
9. Riemer BL, Butterfield SL, Diamond DL, et al: Acute mortality associated with injuries to the pelvic ring: the role of early patient mobilization and external fixation. *J Trauma* 35:671, 1993.
10. Burgess AR, Jones AL: Fractures of the pelvic ring, in Rockwood CA Jr, Green DP, Bucholz RW, Heckman JD (eds): *Fractures in Adults*, 4th ed. Philadelphia, JB Lippincott, 1996, pp 1575–1615.
11. Gruen GS, Leit ME, Gruen RJ, et al: Functional outcome of patients with unstable pelvic ring fractures stabilized with open reduction and internal fixation. *J Trauma* 39:838, 1995.
12. Routt ML Jr, Simonian PT, Swiontkowski MF: Stabilization of pelvic ring fractures. *Orthop Clin North Am* 28:369, 1997.
13. Wolinsky PR:Assessment and management of pelvic fracture in the hemodynamically unstable patient. *Orthop Clin North Am* 28:321, 1997.
14. Canale ST, Beaty JH: Part I—Fractures of the pelvis, in Rockwood CA Jr, Wilkins KE, Beaty JH (eds): *Fractures in Children*, 4th ed. Philadelphia, JB Lippincott, 1996, pp 1109–1193.
15. Denis F, Davis S, Comfort T: Sacral fractures: An important problem. *Clin Orthop* 227:67, 1988.
16. Gibbons KJ, Solonick DS, Razazk N: Neurologic injury and patterns of sacral fractures. *J Neurosurg* 72:889, 1990.
17. Tile M: Fractures of the acetabulum; in Rockwood CA Jr, Green DP, Bucholz RW, Heckman JD (eds): *Fractures in Adults*, 4th ed. Philadelphia, JB Lippincott, 1996, pp 1617–1658.
18. Cryer HM, Miller FB, Evers BM, Rouben LR: Pelvic fracture classification: correlation with hemorrhage. *J Trauma* 28:973, 1988.
19. Burgess AR, Eastridge BJ, Young JW, Ellison TS: Pelvic ring disruptions: Effective classification system and treatment protocols. *J Trauma* 30:848, 1990.
20. Gruen GS, Leit ME, Gruen RJ, et al: The acute management of hemodynamically unstable multiple trauma patients with pelvic ring fractures. *J Trauma* 36:706, 1994.
21. Ben-Menachem Y: Exploratory angiography and transcatheter embolization for control of arterial hemorrhage in patients with pelvic ring disruption. *Tech Orthop* 9:271, 1995.
22 Agolini SF, Shah K, Jaffe J, et al: Arterial embolization is a rapid and effective technique for controlling pelvic fracture hemorrhage. *J Trauma* 43:395, 1997.
23. Lindberg EF, Macias D, Gipe BT: Clinically occult presentation of comminuted intertrochanteric hip fractures. *Ann Emerg Med* 21:1511, 1992.
24. Alba E, Youngberg R: Occult fractures of the femoral neck. *Am J Emerg Med* 10:64, 1992.
25. Conway WF, Totty WG, McEnery KW: CT and MR imaging of the hip. *Radiology* 198:297, 1996.
26. Pandey R, McNally E, Ali A, Bulstrode C: The role of MRI in the diagnosis of occult hip fractures. *Injury* 29:61, 1998.
27. Zuckerman JD: Hip fracture. *N Engl J Med* 334:1519, 1996.
28. Kleinschmidt KC: Elder abuse: A review. *Ann Emerg Med* 30:463, 1997.
29. Ahmad LA, Eckhoff DG, Kramer AM: Outcome studies of hip fractures: A functional viewpoint. *Orthop Rev* 23:19, 1994.
30. Rogers FB, Shackford SR, Keller MS: Early fixation reduces morbidity and mortality in elderly patients with hip fractures from low-impact falls. *J Trauma* 39:261, 1995.
31. Bredahl C, Nyholm B, Hindsholm KB: Mortality after hip fracture: Results of operation within 12 hours of admission. *Injury* 23:83, 1992.
32. Fox HJ, Pooler J, Prothero D, et al: Factors affecting the outcome after proximal femoral fractures. *Injury* 25:2977, 1994.
33. Rosenthal RE, Coker WL: Posterior fracture dislocation of the hip. *J Trauma* 19:572, 1979.
34. Lyons AR: Clinical outcomes and treatment of hip fractures. *Am J Med* 103:51S, 1997.
35. Levy J, Ward WT: Pediatric femur fractures: An overview of treatment. *Orthopedics* 16:183, 1993.
36. Bucholz RW, Brumback RJ: Fractures of the shaft of the femur, in Rockwood CA Jr, Green DP, Bucholz RW, Heckman JD (eds): *Fractures in Adults*, 4th ed. Philadelphia, JB Lippincott, 1996, pp 1827–1918.
37. Thomas SA, Rosenfield NS, Leventhal JM, et al: Long-bone fractures in children: Distinguishing accidental injuries from child abuse. *Pediatrics* 88:471, 1991.
38. Kasser JR: Femoral shaft fractures, in Rockwood CA Jr, Wilkins KE, Beaty JH (eds): *Fractures in Children*, 4th ed. Philadelphia, JB Lippincott, 1996, pp 1195–1230.
39. Buckley SL: Current trends in the treatment of femoral shaft fractures in children and adolescents. *Clin Ortho Rel Res* 338:60, 1997.
40. Bucholz RW, Jones A: Current concepts review: Fractures of the shaft of the femur. *J Bone Joint Surg* 73A:1561, 1991.

KNEE INJURIES

Mark T. Steele

Injuries to the knee are common in our exercise and sports-oriented society. Because the knee is essential for ambulation, one must be familiar with the examination of the normal and abnormal knee to be able to recognize, treat, and appropriately refer specific injuries. This chapter deals with examination of the knee and with recognition of fractures and dislocations of the patella; fractures of femoral condyles; fractures of the tibial spines, tuberosity, and plateaus; ligamentous and meniscal injuries of the knee joint; knee dislocation; quadriceps and patellar tendon ruptures; patellar tendinitis and chondromalacia patellae; penetrating injuries and foreign bodies; total knee replacement and postarthroscopy problems; and osteochondritis dissecans.

An accurate diagnosis of the injured knee is required before proper treatment can be instituted. The first examination is usually the easiest to perform and may be the most valid because the patient does not anticipate pain and therefore does not guard, and involuntary muscular spasm, inflammation and effusion causing further limitation of the examination may not yet have occurred.

EXAMINATION

The examination of the knee is divided into five phases: history, observation, inspection, palpation, and stress testing.

The current mechanism of injury as well as any prior serious injuries or surgical procedures frequently clarifies subtleties in the examination, allowing a more accurate diagnosis and appropriate treatment.

The patient should be examined while walking, if possible, and in both the sitting and lying positions. Take note of the gait, muscular development, functional range of motion, and the ability of the patient to extend the flexed knee against minimal resistance.

The knee should be inspected for swelling, ecchymoses, effusion, masses, patella location and size, muscle mass, erythema, and evidence of local trauma. With the patient supine, note whether leg lengths are equal or unequal. Lastly, ask the patient to perform the best possible active range of motion.

Initially the neurovascular status of the leg should be noted. As with all orthopedic examinations, the noninjured or normal knee should be compared with the injured knee during all aspects of the examination but especially during palpation and stress testing. When palpating the knee, begin in the nontender areas and work lastly toward the tender area so that the patient does not guard or become apprehensive. The patella and patellar facets, as well as the femoral and tibial condyles, should be palpated for pain and crepitance. Effusion, tenderness, increased temperature, strength, sensation, and location of pulses should be noted.

Examine the patella for size, shape, and location with the knee in flexion; check mobility with the knee in extension. The patella should be compressed to check for pain as well as moved laterally and medially to ascertain possible subluxation. The popliteal space should be palpated for masses, swelling, and pulses. Both the medial and lateral joint lines should be palpated because tenderness at those locations suggests the possibility of meniscal injury. Palpation of the medial and lateral collateral ligaments should also be performed with tenderness once again suggesting the possibility of injury.

The final phase of the examination of the knee is stress testing (also see section on Ligamentous and Meniscal Injuries). This is the most difficult aspect of the examination although potentially the most informative. The patient must be reassured and relaxed and made as comfortable as possible. This may require allowing the leg to hang over the side of the bed with the bed supporting the posterior thigh rather than the physician holding the leg, as is usually done during stress testing. The uninjured, hopefully normal, opposite knee should be examined first to determine the patient's normal laxity. A brief summary of the instabilities and tests to demonstrate them are presented in the section on ligamentous and meniscal injuries.

RADIOGRAPHIC EVALUATION

The Ottawa Knee Rules (Table 266-1) for determining the need for x-rays have proven sensitive for fracture[1] and have resulted in reduced emergency department waiting times and costs. The Pittsburgh Knee Rules (Table 266-2) are similar and recently were prospectively shown to be as sensitive, but more specific than the Ottawa Rules.[2] They also have the added advantage of being applicable to both children and adults. A recent evaluation[3] suggested that point tenderness is not a good predictor of knee fracture in children. This study suggested that applying a rule of an inability to bear weight and inability to flex the knee to 90° would decrease x-rays ordered by 75 percent without any missed fractures.

TABLE 266-1 Ottawa Knee Rules: Guidelines for X-Ray

1. Patient older than 55 years
2. Tenderness at the head of the fibula
3. Isolated tenderness of the patella
4. Inability to flex knee to 90 degrees
5. Inability to transfer weight for four steps both immediately after the injury and in the ED

Anteroposterior, lateral, and oblique radiographs are typically obtained if x-rays are determined to be necessary.[4] Fat fluid levels (lipohemarthrosis) may be identified on a lateral view of the knee which is suggestive of intra-articular fracture.[5] Oblique views are particularly helpful at detecting subtle tibial plateau fractures (internal oblique view is best to visualize lateral plateau, external oblique film best to visualize medial plateau). A tunnel or intercondylar view provides a clear view of the intercondylar region and is particularly useful in identifying tibial spine fractures. The sunrise (skyline, axial, or tangential) view is most useful in detecting nondisplaced vertical or marginal fractures of the patella which may be missed with the conventional three views. The sunrise view is indicated if patellar subluxation or fracture is suspected. CT scanning may be necessary to fully delineate the extent of tibial plateau fractures.[6] MRI is also helpful in this regard, having the added benefit of being able to assess soft tissue injury (i.e., ligamentous and meniscal).

FRACTURES

Fractures of the Patella

Fractures of the patella occur from a direct blow such as with the knee striking a car dashboard in an MVA, a fall on the flexed knee, or forceful contraction of the quadriceps muscles, which can occur with falling or stumbling. Fractures may be transverse, comminuted,

TABLE 266-2 Pittsburgh Knee Rules

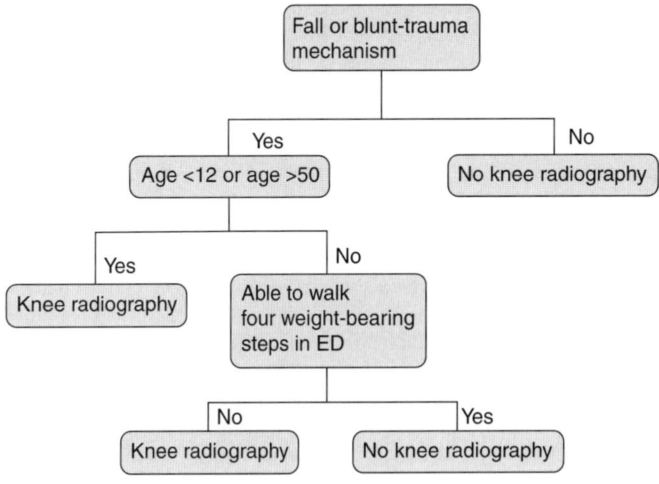

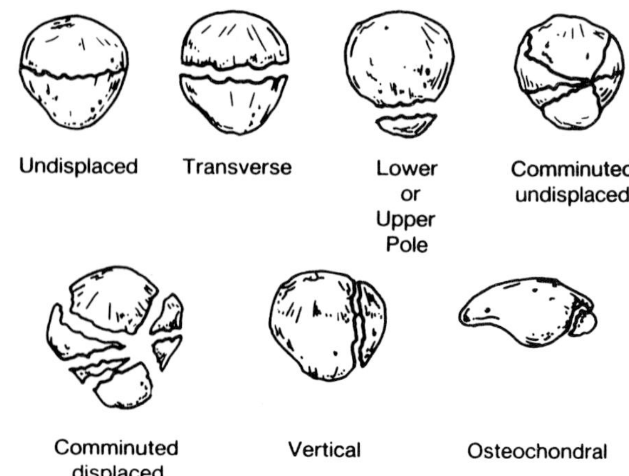

FIG. 266-1. Classification of patellar fractures. (From Hohl M, Johnson EE, Wiss DA. Fractures of the knee, in Rockwood CA Jr, Green DP, Bucholz RW (eds): *Fractures in Adults,* 3d ed, vol. 2. Philadelphia, Lippincott, 1991, p. 1765. Used with permission.)

or of the avulsion type, when the quadriceps or patellar tendon pulls off a small portion of the patella (Fig. 266-1).

Transverse fractures of the patella are most common, followed by stellate and comminuted fractures.[7] Patients with nondisplaced fractures may be ambulatory. Physical examination reveals focal patellar tenderness, swelling, and effusion. It is imperative that the integrity of the extensor mechanism of the knee be checked by having the patient perform a straight-leg raise against gravity. Transverse fractures are more likely to be displaced and have a disrupted extensor mechanism. Differential diagnosis of patellar fractures radiographically includes bipartite patella. This condition involves the superior lateral corner of the patella, is typically bilateral, and is differentiated from fracture by its smooth cortical margins.

A nondisplaced fracture of the patella with an intact extensor mechanism is initially treated in the emergency department with a knee immobilizer, ice, elevation, and nonsteroidal anti-inflammatory drugs and/or opioid analgesics. Such fractures are generally treated in a long leg cast for a total of six weeks of immobilization.[7] During this period the patient should be encouraged to walk on crutches initially, with partial weight-bearing progressing to full weight-bearing as tolerated. Fractures that are displaced greater than 3 mm, or that are associated with the disruption of the extensor mechanism, require early referral to orthopedics for open reduction and internal fixation.[7] This generally consists of tension-band wiring of the patella and suturing of the retinaculum. Severely comminuted fractures may be treated surgically by removal of smaller fragments (or all fragments if they are small) and suturing of the quadriceps and patellar tendons. All open fractures must be debrided and irrigated by orthopedics in the operating room and antistaphylococcal antibiotics should be administered. The overall prognosis for patellar fractures is good.[7]

Fractures of Femoral Condyles

Fractures of the femoral condyles account for 4 percent of femur fractures and include supracondylar, intercondylar, condylar, and distal femoral epiphyseal fractures (Fig. 266-2). Most often, these injuries are secondary to direct trauma from a fall with axial loading or a blow to the distal femur. Examination reveals pain, swelling, deformity, rotation, shortening, and an inability to ambulate. Although neurovascular injuries are uncommon, the potential for popliteal artery injury exists so the status of distal sensation and pulses must be checked. The space between the first and second toe, innervated by the deep peroneal nerve, should be tested for sensation. In addition, a search for ipsilateral hip dislocation or fractures, and damage to the quadriceps apparatus must be made. Incomplete or nondisplaced fractures in any age group and stable impacted fractures in the elderly can be treated with cast immobilization.[7] Open reduction and internal fixation is generally required for displaced fractures or if there is any degree of joint incongruity present.[8] Therefore, leg splinting and orthopedic consultation is essential. The overall progress of these injuries is fair. Complications include deep venous thrombosis, fat embolus syndrome, delayed or malunion, and the subsequent development of osteoarthritis.

Fractures of the Tibial Spines and Tuberosity

Although isolated injuries of the tibial spine are uncommon, they usually result in cruciate ligament insufficiency. The injury is most often caused by a force directed against the flexed proximal tibia in an anterior or posterior direction, resulting in incomplete avulsion of the tibial spine, with or without displacement, or complete fracture of the spine. Vehicular and sporting accidents are the most common causes of these injuries.[7] Fracture of the anterior tibial spine is about tenfold more common than fracture of the posterior spine. Examination shows a painful, swollen knee, secondary to hemarthrosis, inability to extend fully, and a positive Lachman's sign (see section on Ligamentous and Meniscal Injuries). If the fracture is incomplete or nondisplaced, it should be immobilized in full extension in a knee immobilizer. Protected weight bearing and outpatient orthopedic follow-up within a few days to a week is advised. Complete, displaced fractures require early orthopedic consultation and often need open reduction, and internal fixation.

The quadriceps mechanism inserts on the tibial tubercle. A sudden force to the flexed knee with the quadriceps muscle contracted may result in a complete or incomplete avulsion of the tibial tubercle. The fracture line may extend into the joint. Examination reveals pain and tenderness over the proximal anterior tibia with pain on passive or active extension. If the avulsion is small or nondisplaced, the fragment may be maintained in position by immobilization; otherwise, open

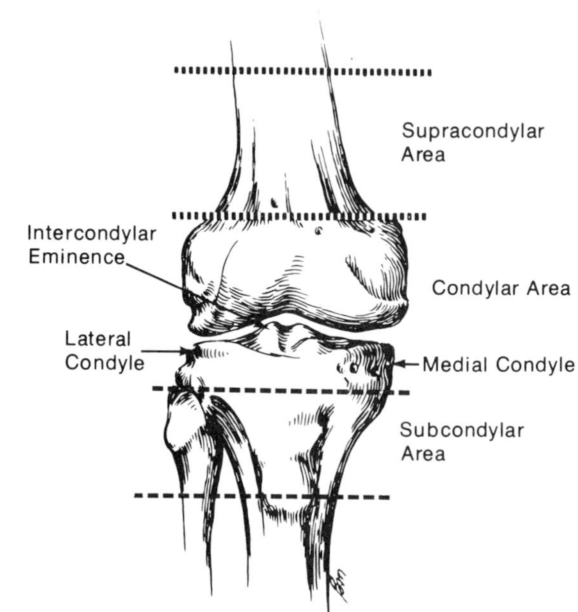

FIG. 266-2. The supracondylar and condylar areas of the femur, and the medial and subcondylar areas of the tibia. [Modified from Hohl M, Larson RL: Fractures and dislocations of the knee, in Rockwood CA Jr, Green DP (eds): *Fractures,* vol 2. Philadelphia, Lippincott, 1975, pp 1132, 1147. Used by permission.]

reduction and internal fixation are necessary.[7] (See also section on Injuries to Tibial Tubercle.)

Fractures of the Tibial Plateaus

Fractures of the tibial plateaus are seen more commonly in the older population and can be very difficult to detect. They are produced by valgus or varus forces combined with axial loading, which drives the femoral condyles into the articulating surface of the tibia. A fall from a height or the leg being struck by the bumper of a car are common causes of these fractures.[9] Both medial and lateral plateaus may be fractured simultaneously although the lateral plateau is more often fractured.[7] Direct trauma to the lateral aspect of the knee may account for the preponderance of lateral tibial plateau fractures. The patient presents with painful swelling of the knee and limitation of motion. Radiographs may demonstrate a fracture but often only show a lipohemarthrosis on the lateral view. Careful review of the x-rays is essential. Ligamentous instability may be present in up to one-third of those injuries. Anterior cruciate and medial collateral ligament injuries are associated with lateral plateau fractures whereas posterior cruciate and lateral collateral ligament injuries occur with medial plateau fractures.[7] If one plateau is fractured but not displaced, treatment in a knee immobilizer, without weight-bearing, is indicated with outpatient orthopedic follow-up scheduled within a few days to a week. Long-term treatment of these nondisplaced fractures consists of a long leg cast and prolonged non weight-bearing. Depression of the articular surface necessitates early orthopedic consultation and open reduction and elevation of the bony fragment. The treatment goal is precise reconstruction of the articular surfaces to allow for early range of motion so as to minimize the development of osteoarthritis.[7] Potential complications of those fractures include popliteal artery injury with high energy displaced fractures, the development of deep venous thrombosis and osteoarthritis. The prognosis for these injuries is fair.

LIGAMENTOUS AND MENISCAL INJURIES

The knee joint depends on ligaments and muscles for support (Fig. 266-3). It is frequently subjected to injuries from traumatic forces while extended or in various stages of flexion. These traumatic forces include abduction, flexion, and internal rotation of the femur on the tibia; adduction, flexion, and external rotation of the femur on the tibia; hyperextension; and anteroposterior displacement. By far the most common are abduction, flexion, and internal rotation of the femur on the tibia, which produce injuries to the medial side of the knee. Injuries to the lateral side of the knee are produced by adduction, flexion, and external rotation. Such forces may result in a strain or rupture of the medial or lateral collateral ligaments, the anterior or posterior cruciate ligaments, the capsular structures, or a tear in the medial or lateral meniscus, singularly or in combination. Functional instability of the knee is determined by stress testing, which will demonstrate abnormal laxity when properly done.

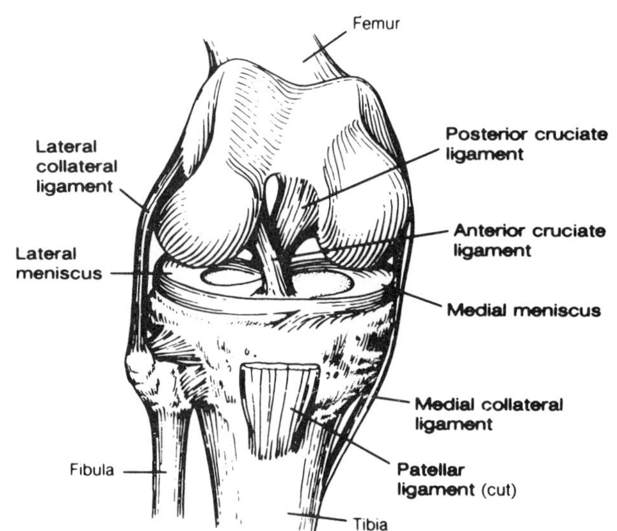

FIG. 266-3. Ligaments of the right knee joint. The articular capsule and the patella have been removed. (From Spencer AP, Mason EB: *Human Anatomy and Physiology.* Menlo Park, Benjamin/Cummings, 1979, p 174. Used by permission.)

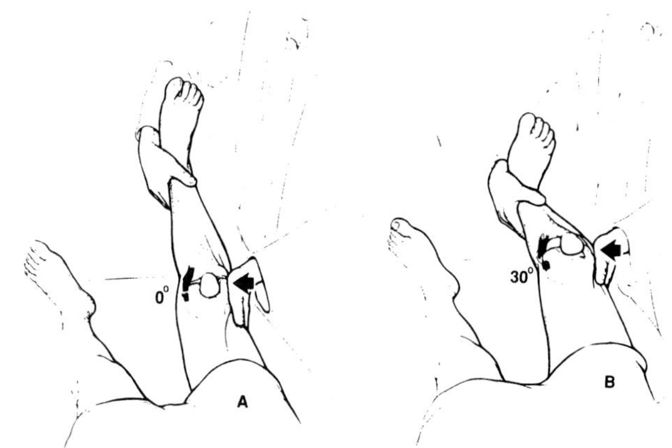

FIG. 266-4. Valgus stress in full extension **(A)** and in 30° of flexion **(B).** (From Scott WN. *Ligament and Extensor Mechanism Injuries of the Knee: Diagnosis and Treatment.* St. Louis, Mosby-Year Book, 1991, p 91. Used with permission.)

Initial stress testing is an abduction or valgus deformity (Fig. 266-4) applied to the knee, which is in approximately 30° of flexion, to determine the integrity of the medial capsular and ligamentous structures. The medial collateral ligament supplies the majority of restraint to valgus deformities of the knee in all stages of flexion. A varus or adduction force is then applied to the lateral aspect of the knee, again with approximately 30° of flexion, to ascertain the integrity of the lateral structures. The lateral collateral ligament, similar to the medial collateral ligament, is the major restraint to varus laxity on the knee at all positions of flexion. If there is a demonstrated laxity of greater than 1 cm without a firm end-point as compared to the other knee, there is a complete rupture of the medial or lateral collateral ligament.[10] If there is laxity with a firm end-point or a laxity of less than 1 cm, an incomplete or partial tear is present. If there is no demonstrated instability but there is pain, the patient has suffered a strain in the ligamentous structures tested. The patient who is unstable with the varus or valgus test performed with 30° of flexion should be brought into full extension, if possible, and similar maneuvers carried out. Medial instability in full extension indicates a severe lesion involving the cruciate ligaments and posterior capsule along with the medial ligaments. Lateral instability in extension likewise indicates a severe injury that may involve the posterolateral corner of the knee as well as the cruciate ligaments. Peroneal nerve injuries may also occur in lateral injuries.

Injury to the anterior cruciate ligament may be the most common ligamentous injury today.[10] The mechanism of injury is usually noncontact; a deceleration, hyperextension, or marked internal rotation of the tibia on the femur results in an injury to the cruciate. This injury is often associated with a ''pop'' and swelling that develops within hours. This pop is considered pathognomonic for anterior cruciate injury.[11] There may be an associated medial meniscal tear as well. Such a

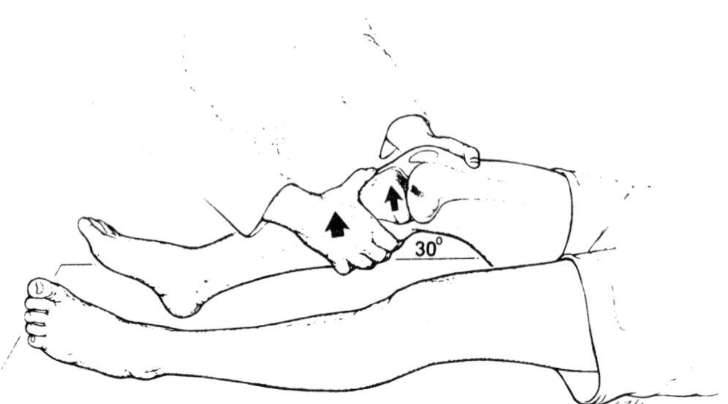

FIG. 266-5. The Lachman test is performed with the knee flexed between 15° and 30°. (From Scott WN. *Ligament and Extensor Mechanism Injuries of the Knee: Diagnosis and Treatment.* St. Louis, Mosby-Year Book, 1991, p 94. Used with permission.)

mechanism of injury combined with the presence of a traumatic effusion is very suggestive of a disruption of the anterior cruciate ligament.

The diagnosis of the anterior cruciate ligament injury is ascertained by using the Lachman test (Fig. 266-5), the anterior drawer sign, (Fig. 266-6) and the pivot shift (Fig. 266-7).[12] Although the anterior drawer sign has been used for a long time, it is not very sensitive. The maneuver is done with 45° flexion at the hip and 90° flexion at the knee. The physician then attempts to forwardly displace the tibia from the femur. A displacement of greater than 6 mm as compared to the normal, opposite knee indicates that there has been an injury to the anterior cruciate ligament. There are false-negatives associated with this maneuver. The Lachman test is a much more sensitive test.[10] The examiner places the knee in 20° of flexion by resting it on a pillow and stabilizes the femur above the knee with his or her nondominant hand. The dominant hand is placed behind the leg at the level of the tibial tubercle, and the examiner introduces an anterior force, attempting to displace the tibia forward. If a displacement of greater than 5 mm as compared to the opposite knee occurs, or if there is a soft, mushy end-point, then a tear in the anterior cruciate ligament has occurred. Although this examination is more sensitive than the anterior drawer and able to identify partial tears in the anterior cruciate ligament when the examiner is skilled, it is difficult on patients who have large legs. The pivot shift is the third maneuver by which the examiner can determine the integrity of the anterior cruciate ligament. The pivot shift is easily performed once the examiner is familiar with it, but it may be somewhat painful to the patient. While the patient is supine and relaxed, the examiner lifts the heel of the foot to approximately 45° of hip flexion with the knee fully extended. The opposite hand grasps the knee with the thumb behind the fibular head. The

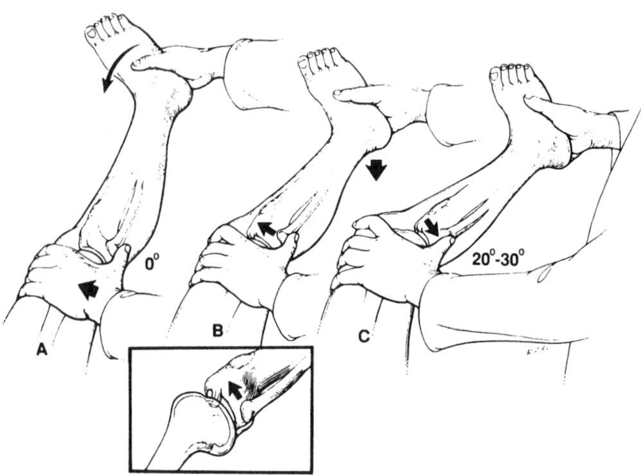

FIG. 266-7. In the pivot shift of Galway and MacIntosh, the test is done with the knee in full extension with application of a valgus and internal rotation stress. The ''clunk'' of reduction is felt in the first 20° to 30° of flexion. (From Scott WN. *Ligament and Extensor Mechanism Injuries of the Knee: Diagnosis and Treatment.* St. Louis, Mosby-Year Book, 1991, p 95. Used with permission.)

examiner then internally rotates the ankle and knee, applies a valgus force to the knee, and flexes the knee. If an anterior subluxation of the tibia is present, a sudden visible, audible, and palpable reduction of the subluxation occurs at about 20 to 40° of flexion. This indicates a deficit in the anterior cruciate ligament, which is required to stabilize the knee in this position. There are other tests described in the literature to determine the integrity of the anterior cruciate ligament, including the jerk test and dynamic extension testing.

The posterior cruciate ligament can also suffer an isolated injury or be injured in combination with other ligamentous structures of the knee. In contrast to anterior cruciate injuries, isolated posterior cruciate injuries are seen much less frequently. The posterior cruciate ligament provides initial resistance to posterior translation at all angles of flexion of the knee. The mechanism of injury then is usually an anterior to posterior force applied to the tibia or lower leg. Posterior cruciate injuries are seen in association with other ligamentous injuries when a serious injury has occurred to the knee. A deficit in this ligament is determined by the posterior drawer test (Fig. 266-8). The knee is examined with flexion at the hip and at the knee as described for the anterior drawer sign. The physician applies a posterior force to the tibial tubercle. If there is displacement posteriorly, then the examiner

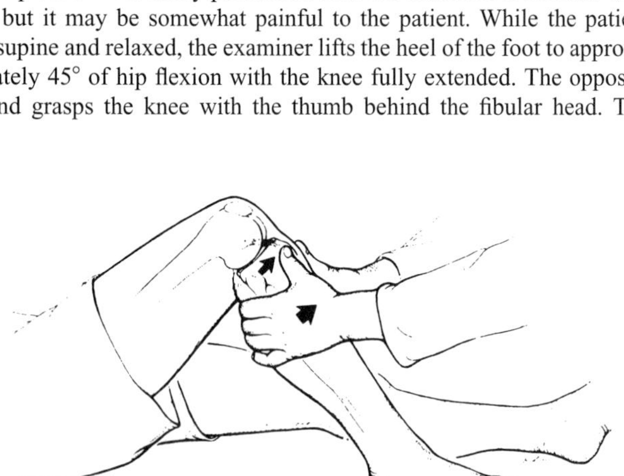

FIG. 266-6. Anterior drawer test. (From Scott WN. *Ligament and Extensor Mechanism Injuries of the Knee: Diagnosis and Treatment.* St. Louis, Mosby-Year Book, 1991, p 95. Used with permission.)

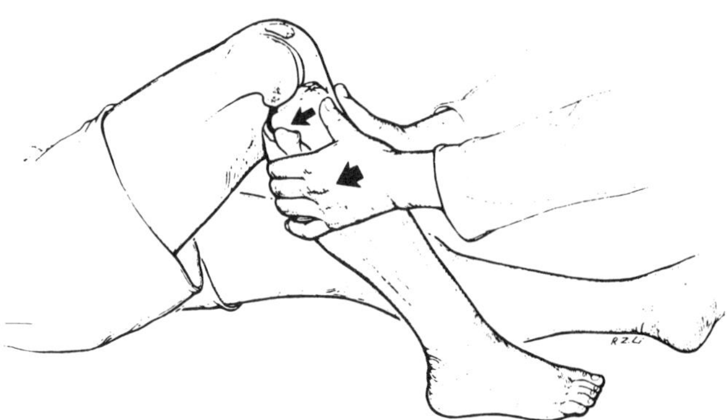

FIG. 266-8. Posterior drawer test. (From Scott WN. *Ligament and Extensor Mechanism Injuries of the Knee: Diagnosis and Treatment.* St. Louis, Mosby-Year Book, 1991, p 97. Used with permission.)

can diagnose an injury to this ligament. The physician might also notice a posterior sag or drop back of the tibial tubercle due to loss of integrity of the posterior cruciate when observing the knee with 45° flexion at the hip and 90° flexion at the knee. This test can be misleading, however, if there is a straight anterior instability resulting in a subluxation of the knee forward. This abnormal position would give the physician the false impression of too much posterior play when performing the posterior drawer test because the knee would be reduced to its normal anatomic alignment from the forwardly subluxed position.

Combined instabilities of the knee are often seen, especially in athletes. Anteromedial and anterolateral instability are the two that occur most frequently. They result from external rotation and abduction or adduction forces placed on the knee. Virtually any combination of medial and lateral instabilities of the knee can occur, however.

One knee injury that is especially difficult to detect is injury to the posterolateral structures. Posterolateral instability usually involves a tear of the popliteus-arcuate complex, which may occur in combination with lateral ligament injury and possible anterior or posterior cruciate ligament injury. Isolated injuries to the popliteus-arcuate complex can occur themselves but are rare. Isolated posterolateral instability is demonstrated by testing at 0 to 30° of flexion for maximal posterior translation, and at 90° of flexion for maximal external rotation as compared to the normal opposite knee. Further testing to determine the integrity of the lateral collateral ligament and anterior or posterior cruciates must be done as well.

Most ligamentous injuries of the knee present with hemarthroses. In fact, approximately 75 percent of all hemarthroses are due to disruption of the anterior cruciate ligament.[10] Serious ligament injuries, however, may present with minimal pain and no hemarthrosis due to complete disruption of the ligamentous and capsular fibers, allowing leakage of the blood into the soft tissue spaces. Hemarthrosis can also be due to osteochondral fractures or fractures that extend into the joint line or peripheral meniscal tears. Traumatic hemarthroses usually occur within minutes to hours of injury, in contrast to chronic effusions of the knee due to synovial inflammation, which occur one to two days after strenuous use of the joint.

Plain radiographs in ligamentous injuries are typically normal or only reveal an effusion. An avulsion fracture at the site of attachment of the lateral capsular ligament on the laterial tibial condyle (Segond fracture) is a marker for anterior cruciate ligament rupture.[13] Cortical avulsion of the medial tibial plateau (very uncommon) is associated with tears of the posterior cruciate ligament and medial meniscus.[14] Continued refinements in MRI have resulted in high-quality images of the ligamentous and meniscal structures of the knee resulting in an accuracy rate of close to 90 percent for meniscal and cruciate ligament disruption.[7] The ordering of this examination, however, is typically done by the patient's primary care provider or orthopedist in follow-up.

Stable injuries involving a single ligament with minor strain can be managed with a knee immobilizer, ice packs, elevation, nonsteroidal anti-inflammatory agents, and ambulation as soon as is comfortable for the patient.[15] When knee immobilizers are placed, the patient must be instructed to perform daily range of motion exercises to avoid contracture and maintain mobility. These complications are more common in the elderly and can occur after only a few days of immobilization. While there is no universally accepted regimen for range of motion exercise, one regimen is to apply ice first to relieve pain, and then perform 10–20 knee flexion-extensions (no weights should be added) three or four times a day. These injuries should be referred to an orthopedic surgeon or the patient's primary care provider within the next few days to a week for follow-up examination. Complete rupture of an isolated ligament can generally be treated conservatively in the same fashion with quadriceps strengthening, range of motion exercises, and functional bracing being part of the follow-up care.[11] Professional athletes with single ligament ruptures or patients with more than one ligament torn and an unstable knee necessitate immediate orthopedic consultation so that definitive surgical management can be planned.

Arthrocentesis may be of therapeutic benefit in patients with large, tense effusions of the knee. Recurrence of the effusion following aspiration, however, is common. Arthrocentesis may also be of assistance diagnostically if the etiology of the effusion is not clearly due to trauma. The presence of blood and glistening fat globules is pathognomonic of lipohemarthrosis, which indicates intra-articular knee fracture. The major complication of arthrocentesis is septic arthritis.

Meniscal Injuries

Meniscal injuries of the knee occur by themselves or in combination with ligamentous injuries. For example, anterior cruciate injuries are commonly associated with meniscal injuries. Cutting, squatting, or twisting maneuvers may cause injury to the meniscus. The medial meniscus is approximately twice as likely as the lateral meniscus to be injured. Four-fifths of the tears involve the peripheral posterior aspect of the meniscus.[16] Many maneuvers have been described in the literature to determine whether a meniscus has been injured. Most of these tests, however, have an unacceptable specificity and sensitivity. Although the diagnosis of a meniscal tear is difficult to make in certain patients, a combination of a suggestive history and physical findings on examination should lead the emergency physician to consider the diagnosis. On questioning the patient, the physician should ask if the patient experiences locking of the knee joint on either flexion or extension that is painful and limits further activity. This sign clearly points to the diagnosis of a torn meniscus. Effusions that occur after activity; a sensation of popping, clicking, or snapping; a feeling of an unstable joint, especially with activity; or tenderness in the anterior joint space after excessive activity suggests the diagnosis of a meniscal tear. When performing a physical examination, a physician should attempt to identify atrophy of the quadriceps muscle due to disuse, and joint line tenderness, which is very suggestive. Various maneuvers, such as McMurray's test or the grind test, are useful but, as mentioned earlier, are positive only about 50 percent of the time.[17] If a tentative diagnosis of a meniscal tear is considered, referral to an orthopedic surgeon or the patient's primary care provider is warranted. Nonsteroidal anti-inflammatory agents and partial weight-bearing are advised pending follow-up. Definitive diagnosis can be made by MRI or arthroscopy with the latter having the advantage of allowing for definitive surgical treatment (usually partial meniscectomy or meniscal repair).

The patient who presents to the emergency department with a locked knee can experience a great deal of pain along with loss of mobility. Following conscious sedation, one can attempt to unlock the knee by positioning the patient with the leg hanging over the edge of the table with the knee in 90° or greater of flexion. After a period of relaxation, the physician can apply longitudinal traction to the knee with internal and external rotation in an attempt to unlock the joint. If this maneuver is unsuccessful, consultation with the orthopedic surgeon is recommended.

Knee Dislocation

Knee dislocation (Fig. 266-9) is a result of tremendous ligamentous disruption due to hyperextension, direct posterior force applied to the anterior tibia, force to the fibula or medial femur, force to the tibia or lateral femur, or rotatory force resulting in anterior, posterior lateral, medial, or rotatory dislocation. This injury typically occurs following sporting accidents and falls and posterior dislocation is most common. With posterior dislocation, there is complete disruption of the anterior and posterior cruciate ligaments and the posterior joint capsule. The extensor mechanism of the knee may also be disrupted and should be checked postreduction. Because of knee instability reduction very often occurs spontaneously. A severely unstable knee in multiple

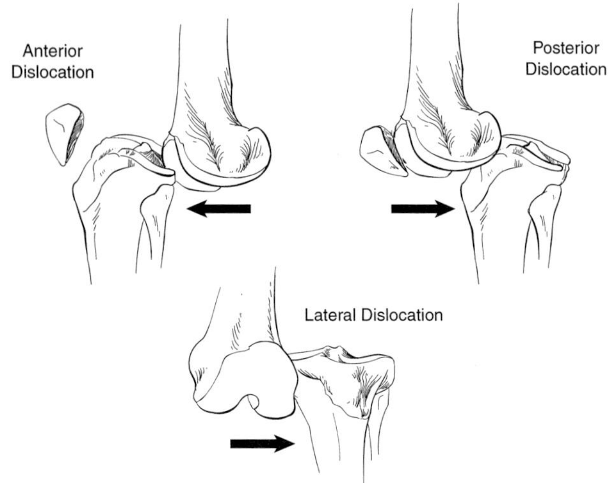

FIG. 266-9. Types of dislocations. 1. Anterior; 2. posterior; and 3. lateral. (From DePalma AF. *Management of Fractures and Dislocations: An Atlas.* Philadelphia, WB Saunders, 1970, p 1621. Used by permission.)

directions is suspicious for a spontaneously reduced knee dislocation. Suspicion of the injury is important because of the high incidence of associated complications, including popliteal artery injury (50 percent incidence) and peroneal nerve injury (mostly with posterolateral dislocations), in addition to ligamentous and meniscal injury.

Early reduction of the dislocation employing longitudinal traction is essential. Neurovascular status of the extremity should be documented pre- and postreduction. Hospitalization is required and orthopedic consultation should be obtained immediately.

Controversy exists regarding when to obtain arteriography in patients with knee dislocation. Because of the high incidence of popliteal artery injury (up to one-third of patients) and poor outcomes related to delays in vascular reconstruction, some authors recommend arteriography for all confirmed knee dislocations.[18] Others have suggested clinical examination alone is reliable in identifying patients requiring arteriography and/or surgical intervention.[19] Patients with an absent pulse or other signs of vascular injury (i.e., bruit, distal ischemia) require immediate vascular surgical consultation for surgical exploration. Patients with an absent pulse prereduction with return of a pulse postreduction probably necessitate arteriography.[20] Patients with normal pulses pre- and postreduction along with normal Doppler pressure indices (Ankle-Brachial Index) (see Chap. 55) can probably be safely observed in the hospital with serial vascular examinations. Presence of normal distal pulses, however, does not preclude occult popliteal artery injury.[21] As a result, if any doubt exists, arteriography should be performed.

Patella Dislocation

Dislocation of the patella usually occurs from a twisting injury on the extended knee and is more common in women. The patella is displaced laterally over the lateral condyle, resulting in pain and deformity of the knee (Fig. 266-10). Tearing of the medial knee joint capsule often occurs. Reduction is accomplished following conscious sedation by flexing the hip, hyperextending the knee, and sliding the patella back into place. This results in immediate relief of pain, but further soreness from capsular injury persists for a period of time. The patella and knee should be x-rayed to rule out a fracture, and the knee should be immobilized after reduction. Follow-up with a primary care provider or orthopedist within one to two weeks is suggested. Partial weight-bearing progressing to full weight-bearing, nonsteroidal anti-inflammatory agents, and isometric quadriceps strengthening exercises are also indicated. Recurrent lateral dislocation of the patella occurs in about 15 percent of patients, and superior, horizontal, and intercondylar dislocations require referral to an orthopedic surgeon for possible surgical intervention.

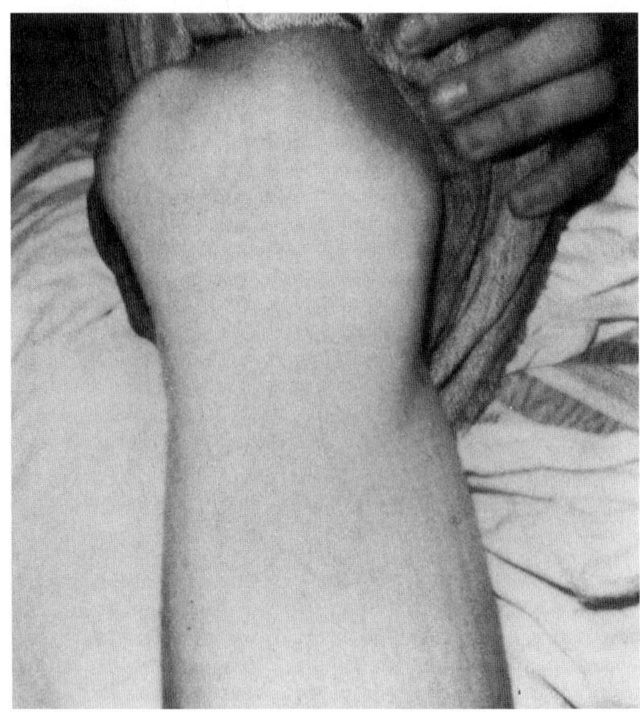

FIG. 266-10. Lateral dislocation of the patella. (From Lyman JI, Ervin ME. Management of common dislocations, in Roberts JR, Hedges JR (eds). *Clinical Procedures in Emergency Medicine.* Philadelphia, WB Saunders, 1985, p 634. Used with permission.)

Quadriceps/Patellar Tendon Rupture

Rupture of the quadriceps or patellar tendons can occur from forceful contraction of the quadriceps muscle or falling on a flexed knee. Patellar tendon rupture occurs most commonly in individuals under age 40 with a history of tendinitis or past steroid injections. Quadriceps tendon rupture is most frequent in the over 40 age group.[7] There is significant pain, diffuse swelling, and the patient is unable to extend a flexed knee against mild resistance in both instances. Depending on the tendon ruptured, a defect may be palpable above or below the patella. A ''high-riding patella'' may be seen on the lateral x-ray of the knee with patellar tendon rupture (Fig. 266-11). The treatment is surgical repair of the involved tendon[22] within the first 7 to 10 days following rupture to achieve the best results. Orthopedic consultation in the emergency department is indicated.

Osteochondritis Dissecans

Osteochondritis dissecans is a disorder in which a segment of articular cartilage and subchondral bone become partially or totally separated from the underlying bone. It is a rare condition of unknown etiology that has been thought to result from acute or chronic trauma. It typically is found in adolescents, is generally unilateral, and most often involves the nonweight-bearing lateral aspect of the medial femoral condyle. Patients generally complain of pain and swelling but typically do not recall any specific incident of trauma. The condition can be diagnosed on routine radiographs with tunnel views being particularly helpful. Treatment is conservative with protective weight-bearing if the epiphy-

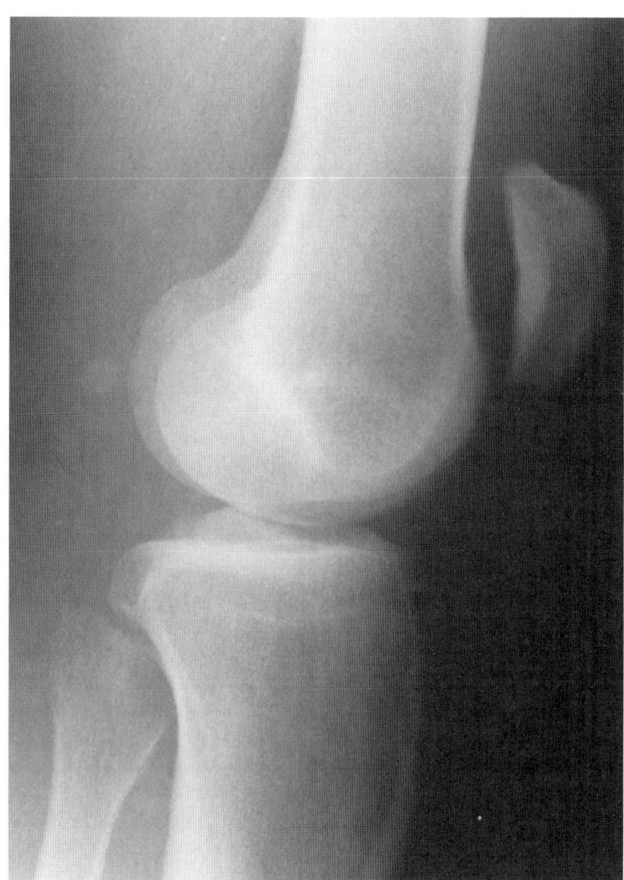

FIG. 266-11. Patella alta.

ses are still open. If the epiphyses are closed and the fragments are detached, the prognosis for healing is poor. Arthroscopy for the retrieval of loose bodies or arthrotomy for pinning or bone grafting of the detached lesions is suggested in this instance.[23]

Osteonecrosis

Osteonecrosis is a bony infarction caused by disruption of blood supply to the bone. Osteonecrosis is divided into two main categories, primary (spontaneous, idiopathic) and secondary. The etiology of primary osteonecrosis remains unknown. Secondary causes include steroid therapy, systemic lupus erythematosus, alcoholism, sickle cell disease, and renal transplantation. Patients with osteonecrosis are typically elderly women who present with acute knee pain. The weight-bearing surface of the medial femoral condyle of the knee is the most common site of involvement. Physical exam generally reveals tenderness over the involved femoral condyle or tibial compartment. Secondary osteonecrosis occurs in a younger age group. Plain radiographs are typically normal early in the course of the disease but MR scanning is diagnostic. Initial treatment is nonoperative and consists of protected weight-bearing and the use of nonsteroidal anti-inflammatory drugs. The outcome of the disease depends on the percentage of the weight-bearing surface of the joint involved. Treatment options for advanced stages of the disease include arthroscopic debridement, curettage or drilling of the lesion, bone grafting, high tibial osteotomy, use of osteochondral allografts, and total knee arthroplasty.[24]

Patellar Tendinitis

Also known as ''jumpers knee,'' patellar tendinitis is primarily seen in runners, basketball and volleyball players, and high jumpers. Pain is referred to the area of the patellar tendon and is worsened when going from sitting to standing or when running up hills. Point tenderness can be found at the distal aspect of the patella or proximal part of the patellar tendon. Treatment consists of heat, nonsteroidal anti-inflammatory agents, and quadriceps strengthening exercises. Steroid injections predispose to tendon rupture so should be avoided.

Chondromalacia Patellae

Chondromalacia patellae is an overuse syndrome of the articular cartilage of the patella. The condition is caused by patellofemoral malalignment, which leads to a tracking abnormality of the patella, placing excessive lateral pressure on the articular cartilage. It is most common in young, active women and the pain is generally localized to the region of the anterior knee. Stair climbing and rising from a chair exacerbate the pain.

Two tests may aid in the diagnosis. The patellar compression test is performed by pushing the patella distal in the trochlear groove with the knee extended and quadriceps muscles tightened. This maneuver illicits pain. The apprehension test is performed on a relaxed leg. When the patella is pushed laterally, the quadriceps muscles contract in anticipation of pain. Treatment of this condition consists of rest, nonsteroidal anti-inflammatory medication, and quadriceps strengthening exercises.[25]

Post Arthroscopy Presentations

Patients may rarely present to the emergency department following arthroscopy secondary to pain and swelling. Effusions are common following arthroscopy, but joint infection is very uncommon. Diagnostic arthrocentesis should be performed if joint infection is suspected. Arthrocentesis may be helpful therapeutically for large tense effusions. Intra-articular injection of bupivacaine and morphine after traumatic knee injuries and arthroscopy reduces the need for systemic analgesia, but morphine is more effective and can provide relief longer.[26]

Penetrating Knee Injury/Joint Foreign Bodies

If the knee joint has clearly been violated due to penetrating injury, orthopedic consultation should be obtained for joint irrigation in the operating room. If penetration is suspected, but is in doubt, injection of the joint with sterile methylene blue can help to confirm the diagnosis. Extravasation of dye indicates penetration and the need for irrigation. Remember that the history obtained must recreate the position of the knee when the penetrating injury occurred. Many occupational injuries occur with the knee flexed, but the joint is examined with the knee resting in extension. Failure to anticipate the trajectory of injury with the knee flexed could lead to misdiagnosis and failure to anticipate joint penetration.

Radiopaque foreign bodies (i.e., metal, glass) will visualize on conventional radiographs. In general, foreign bodies in the knee joint need to be removed. A bullet in the joint can destroy the cartilage and lead poisoning can occur.[27] A bullet lodged in the bone only, however, does not necessitate removal. Antibiotics to cover streptococci and staphylococci are generally indicated for both penetrating knee wounds and foreign bodies. Tetanus prophylaxis should be administered if indicated.

KNEE INJURIES IN CHILDREN

Although knee injuries do occur in children, they are usually the result of fractures of the bone rather than significant ligamentous injuries. Ligamentous injuries can occur in children but are not common. Careful examination and radiographic evaluation usually reveal that the ligaments are intact and there has been an epiphyseal injury. Meniscal tears also occur in children with a much lower incidence than in adults.

The characteristic finding of meniscal tears in children is that they have a more insidious history than in the adult. Patellar fractures are also infrequent in children. They can be difficult to diagnose because of the difficulty in evaluating the radiographs. The opposite knee should be x-rayed for comparison views to help the physician in the diagnosis of a fracture. Lastly, dislocations are, fortunately, an extremely rare condition in children. If they occur, however, they have the same ominous complications as in the adult.

Separation of Distal Femoral Epiphysis

This is a common epiphyseal injury in adolescents that can occur in the anterior plane or coronal plane. The anterior separation is usually the result of a hyperextension injury. The more common coronal separation is a result of abduction and adduction forces, most often occurring during sports activities or play. The patient complains of acute injury with inability to bear weight with displaced fractures and presents with a flexion deformity. As with most epiphyseal injuries, the examiner finds circumferential tenderness around the entire epiphyseal plate, and effusion and swelling are typically present. The standard radiographic views for evaluating the knee are required. The Salter-Harris classification is used to classify these fractures, with type II being the most common. Stress films may be necessary to diagnose Salter-Harris I injuries. The treatment of nondisplaced fractures is above the knee cast immobilization with the knee in 20° of flexion for four to six weeks. Displaced Salter-Harris I or II fractures require reduction with gentle traction followed by cast immobilization. Displaced Salter-Harris III and IV fractures typically require open reduction and internal fixation. The prognosis of these fractures is generally good, with return to normal activities expected within four to six months. Complications include popliteal artery injury with markedly displaced fractures and peroneal nerve injury.[28]

Separation of Proximal Tibial Epiphysis

The separation of the proximal tibial epiphysis is a rare phenomenon because the tibia is well protected. The mechanism of injury is usually indirect forces of abduction or hyperextension against a fixed knee. Occasionally this injury is due to a direct force such as encountered in an automobile-pedestrian accident. Again, the classification is the Salter-Harris method. The symptoms and signs are similar to those of all other knee injuries, with pain, swelling, effusion, and a limited range of motion, especially extension-flexion. As with all epiphyseal injuries, there is circumferential tenderness over the injured growth plate. Stress examination reveals instability to the various maneuvers. Standard radiographs to evaluate the knee are recommended, with stress films required if no injury is seen, but one is suspected. Careful evaluation looking for an occult fracture line is important. The treatment for nondisplaced fractures is a long-leg cast with the knee flexed approximately 30° for six to eight weeks. Displaced injuries require closed reduction followed by casting. If reduction is not anatomic, which is commonly the case with types III and IV, closed or open reduction followed by external or internal fixation is indicated. Vascular compromise is the primary complication occurring in up to 10 percent of cases. Knee instability, joint disease, and growth disturbances can occur in up to 10 to 20 percent of these injuries. The overall prognosis is fairly good for these injuries.[28]

Injuries to the Tibial Tubercle

Two problems can occur at the tibial tubercle. The first is the acute avulsion of the tibial tubercle; the second is the classic Osgood-Schlatter lesion. Avulsion injuries are usually incurred as an acute event during sports and play. The patient presents with the inability to walk, because of the injury, as well as with localized tenderness and swelling. The lateral radiographic view is most important because it demonstrates both the size of the fracture fragment and the degree of displacement. A minimally displaced, small avulsion fragment can be treated in a long-leg cast. Larger fragments are treated by open reduction and internal fixation. The overall prognosis is good. In contrast, Osgood-Schlatter lesions present with a vague history in adolescent boys. The pain is mild and intermittent, allowing the child to continue to participate in sports and play but not at a full level of involvement. Pain is aggravated by running, jumping, kneeling, squatting, and climbing or ascending stairs. Osgood-Schlatter disease is seen bilaterally in approximately 25 percent of the cases. In contrast to patients with avulsion injuries, patients with Osgood-Schlatter lesions experience pain with range of motion, especially range of motion against resistance, and not at rest. The treatment is symptomatic and supportive. There are minimal complications, and the prognosis is excellent.[28]

Fracture of the Intercondylar Eminence of the Tibia

This fracture is usually encountered in 8- to 15-year-old youths, who most often relate a history of a fall from a bicycle. This causes the intercondylar eminence to be avulsed from the tibia, resulting in a painful and acutely swollen knee. The patient has a positive Lachman's test and a drawer sign, and may have concomitant medial collateral ligamentous instability to valgus stress testing. Radiographs usually reveal evidence of a fracture on the lateral view with the knee slightly flexed. The treatment is immobilization in full extension in most instances, as this can reduce the fracture fragment to its anatomic state. Persistent displacement of the fracture should be treated surgically. The concomitant injuries to the medial collateral ligaments do not often require surgical intervention and can be treated while the patient is recovering from the fracture. The prognosis with proper treatment is good.[28]

Osteochondral Fractures

Osteochondral fractures occur infrequently in children and adolescents. If they do occur, they occur most often in adolescent boys and are usually fracture fragments from the femoral condyles or the patella. The mechanism of injury is a direct blow to the knee, flexion-rotation of the knee, or patellar dislocation. The history is typically one of an acute injury with a pop or snap, causing severe pain and an acute effusion. The fracture is difficult to see on radiographs, so careful attention should be paid to the femoral condyles as well as to the patella. Treatment is surgical removal of the fracture fragment or surgical fixation of the fragment. Prognosis is good for small fragments not involving the weight-bearing surface of the joint. Prognosis is less favorable for larger fragments involving the weight-bearing surface.[28]

REFERENCES

1. Stiell IG, Wells GA, Hoag RH, Sivilotti ML, et al: Implementation of the Ottawa Knee Rules for the use of radiography in acute knee injuries. *JAMA* 278:2075, 1997.
2. Seaberg DC, Yealy DM, Lukens T, Auble T, Mathias S: Multicenter comparison of two clinical decision rules for the use of radiography in acute, high-risk knee injuries. *Ann Emerg Med* 32:8, 1998.
3. Cohen DM, Jasser JW, Kean JR, Smith GA: Clinical criteria for using radiography for children with acute knee injuries. *Pediatr Emerg Care* 14:185, 1998.
4. Gray SD, Kaplan PA, Dussault RG, Omary RA, et al: Acute knee trauma: How many plain films are necessary for the initial examination? *Skeletal Radiol* 26:298, 1997.
5. Lugo-Olivieri CH, Scott WW Jr, Zehovni EA: Fluid-fluid levels in injured knees: Do they always represent lipohemarthrosis? *Radiology* 198:499, 1996.
6. Walker CW, Moore TE: Imaging of skeletal and soft tissue injuries in and around the knee. *Radiol Clin North Am* 35:631, 1997.

7. Wiss DA, Watson JT, Johnson EE: Fractures of the knee, in Rockwood CA Jr, Green DP, Bucholz RW, Heckman JD (eds): *Fractures in Adults,* 4th ed. Philadelphia, JB Lippincott, 1996, pp 1919–1999.
8. Schatzker J: Fractures of the distal femur revisited. *Clin Ortho* 347:43, 1998.
9. Watson JT: High-energy fractures of the tibial plateau. *Orthop Clin North Am* 25:723, 1994.
10. Swenson TM, Harrer CD: Knee ligament injuries: current concepts. *Orthop Clin North Am* 26:529, 1995.
11. Scuderi GR, Scott WN, Install JN: Injuries of the knee, in Rockwood CA Jr, Green DP, Bucholz RW, Heckman JD (eds): *Fractures in Adults,* 4th ed. Philadelphia, JB Lippincott, 1996, pp 2001–2126.
12. Scott WN: *Ligament and Extensor Mechanism Injuries of the Knee: Diagnosis and Treatment.* St. Louis, Mosby-Year Book, 1991, pp 87–99.
13. Kerr HD: Segond fracture, hemarthrosis, and anterior ligament disruption. *J Emerg Med* 8:29, 1990.
14. Hall FM, Hochman MG: Medial segond-type fracture: Cortical avulsion off the medial tibial plateau associated with tears of the posterior cruciate ligament and medial meniscus. *Skeletal Radiol* 26:553, 1997.
15. Hughston JC: Knee Ligaments: Injury and Repair. St. Louis, Mosby-Year Book, 1993.
16. Hardin GT, Farr J, Bach BR Jr: Meniscal tears: Diagnosis, evaluation, and treatment. *Orthop Rev* 21:1311, 1992.
17. Evans PJ, Bell GD, Frank C: Prospective evaluation of the McMurray test. *Am J Sports Med* 21:604, 1993.
18. Dennis JW, Jagger C, Butcher JL, Menawatt SS, et al: Reassessing the role of arteriograms in the management of posterior knee dislocations. *J Trauma* 35:692, 1993.
19. Kendall RW, Taylor DC, Salvian AJ, O'Brien PJ: The role of arteriography in assessing vascular injuries associated with dislocations of the knee. *J Trauma* 35:875, 1993.
20. Merrill KD: Knee dislocation with vascular injuries. *Orthop Clinic North Am* 25:707, 1994.
21. Gable DR, Allen JW, Richardson JD: Blunt popliteal artery injury: Is physical examination enough for evaluation? *J Trauma* 43:541, 1997.
22. Haas SB, Callaway H: Disruptions of the extensor mechanism. *Orthop Clin North Am* 23:687, 1992.
23. Garrett JC: Osteochondritis dissecans. *Clin Sports Med* 10:569, 1991.
24. Patel DV, Breazeale NM, Behr CT, Warren RF, et al: Osteonecrosis of the knee: Current clinical concepts. *Knee Surg Sports Traumatol Arthrosc* 6:2, 1998.
25. Zappala FG, Taffel CB, Senderi GR: Rehabilitation of patellofemoral joint disorders. *Orthop Clin North Am* 23:555, 1992.
26. VanNess SA, Gittiris ME: Comparison of intra-articular morphine and bupivicaine following knee arthroscopy. *Orthop Rev* 23:743, 1994.
27. Bolanos AA, Demizio JP Jr, Vigorita VJ, Bryk E: Lead poisoning from an intra-articular shotgun pellet in the knee treated with arthroscopic extraction and chelation therapy. A case report. *J Bone Joint Surg* 78:422, 1996.
28. Sponseller PD, Beaty JH: Fractures and dislocations about the knee, in Rockwood CA Jr, Wilkins KE, Beaty JH (eds): *Fractures in Children,* 4th ed. Philadelphia, JB Lippincott, 1996, pp 1231–1329.

LEG INJURIES

Paul R. Haller
Ernest Ruiz

Lower leg injuries are common. The tibia is the most common long bone fractured. Significant soft tissue injuries to the leg can also occur. Documentation of the history and the physical examination are crucial to the proper evaluation of lower leg injuries. A knowledge of the anatomy aids in the interpretation of findings.

ANATOMY

Bone

Support for weight bearing is provided primarily by the tibia, a bone triangular in cross section that lies subcutaneously in the anterior aspect of the leg. Although it is in harm's way, it has a thick cortex and significant force is required to fracture it. Proximally, the tibia is splayed out to form the medial and lateral plateaus that articulate with the femoral condyles. The lateral plateau is higher and smaller than the medial and is more susceptible to fracture. The distal tibia articulates with the fibula laterally and the talus inferiorly. This articulation is supported by the ankle syndesmosis, a series of ligaments that lie inferior to the interosseous membrane. The fibula lies lateral and posterior to the tibia. Its smaller diameter allows it to be broken with less force than the tibia. Patients can remain ambulatory after a fibula fracture, because it bears little weight. The tibia and fibula are connected by a dense interosseous membrane.

Compartments

The cylinder of the lower leg is divided into four chambers or compartments by bone and dense layers of fascia. It is useful to describe the neurovascular and muscular anatomy in terms of the position of the nerves and muscles in these four compartments: (1) The anterior compartment is bordered by the tibia medially, the interosseous ligament posteriorly, and the anterior crural septum on its lateral aspect. It contains the muscles that dorsiflex the ankles and toes. The anterior tibial artery runs through this compartment before becoming the dorsal pedal artery of the foot. The deep peroneal nerve that also traverses this compartment supplies motor function to the dorsal flexors of the foot and toes. It provides sensory innervation to the web space of the first and second toes. (2) The lateral compartment is circumscribed by the anterior peroneal septum, the fibula, and the posterior peroneal septum. It houses the superficial peroneal nerve, which is sensory to the lateral dorsum of the foot, and motor control for the muscles within the compartment that evert the foot. The peroneal nerve runs just lateral to the fibular head, where it is exposed to direct trauma. (3) The superficial posterior compartment contains muscles that plantar flex the ankle (gastrocnemius, soleus, and plantaris). The sural nerve runs through it before providing sensory innervation to the lateral heel. No major arteries traverse this compartment. (4) The deep posterior compartment contains muscle groups that plantar flex the toes. The tibial nerve provides motor control to these muscles and sensation for the sole of the foot. This compartment also contains the posterior tibial artery, whose pulse can be felt posterior to the medial malleolus of the ankle. The physical findings produced by increased pressure within each compartment are tabulated in Chap. 270.

EVALUATION

Leg injuries are initially evaluated with a directed history, including the amount and type of violence that occurred. The history may also give clues about nontraumatic soft tissue injuries. On examination, nerves should be evaluated by checking sensation in the web space, lateral heel, and sole of the foot. Motor tests should include the ability to plantar and dorsal flex the foot, as well as to evert the foot. The extent of soft tissue injury is evaluated visually and by palpating the muscle groups. The tibia and fibula should be palpated along their entire lengths. The popliteal, dorsal pedal, and posterior tibial pulses should be palpated. An absent or decreased pulse may indicate the need for urgent fracture reduction and vascular evaluation. Patients with tibial shaft fractures are unable to bear weight or lift their foot off of the cart. Patients with fibular fractures alone are often able to bear weight.

Simple anteroposterior and lateral x-rays of the leg that include the knee and ankle are sufficient to evaluate leg injuries. If ankle or knee injuries are suspected, then further x-ray evaluation is needed. If a tibial shaft fracture is suspected, the leg should be splinted with a radiolucent device to control pain and prevent further soft tissue damage prior to obtaining films. Check pulses, movement, and sensation before and after moving the leg.

TREATMENT

Detailed attention to soft tissue injuries is critical to treating lower leg injuries properly. Often it is the extent of such injury, rather than the fracture itself, that determines the outcome. Wounds should be cleansed and debrided of loose tissue and foreign material. Tetanus immunization should be given, if indicated. Splinting of fractures will prevent further damage to soft tissue caused by movement of the sharp bone fragments. Carefully palpate the compartments to detect any possible compartment syndrome. If such is suspected, inform the consulting surgeon so that appropriate priorities can be set in the management of the injury. Parenteral antibiotics should be administered in open-fracture cases.

COMPLICATIONS

Wounds that are not adequately cleansed and debrided are very prone to infection, an event not preventable by the use of antibiotics alone. Patients with compartment syndromes may develop permanent disability if the syndromes are not suspected or diagnosed. Fractures that are not adequately aligned or immobilized heal poorly or not at all. If a vascular injury is not urgently repaired, amputation can result.

SPECIFIC INJURIES

Fibula Fractures

Isolated fibula fractures usually result from a direct blow. They are relatively uncommon. Since this bone only bears 15 percent of the body weight, patients are often able to walk despite the fracture. Proximal fibular fractures are often the result of external rotation, whereas distal fractures usually result from internal rotation. Repetitive trauma, particularly in runners beginning their training, may result in stress fracture of the distal fibula. A mild soreness caused by a low-velocity injury and a fibula fracture can be treated with immobilization using an elastic wrap (distal fibula) or a knee immobilizer (proximal fibula). More impressive pain and disability can be treated with crutches and casting or Robert Jones splinting. Nonunion is uncommon. Pain medication, cessation of the activity that caused the activity, and the use of ice and elevation are also recommended.

Tibia Fractures

A low-energy event such as a skier falling down and suffering a boot-top "tib/fib" fracture will have a more benign course than a motorcyclist who shatters a tibial shaft. In the setting of a tibial fracture, an intact fibula is a welcome finding in that this suggests that less energy was involved. The fibula may also help support or splint the fractured tibia. The extent and type of soft tissue damage incurred may determine the method used to immobilize the tibia. The majority of fractures of the tibia will require a prompt evaluation by an orthopedist while the patient is in the emergency department. Information that will assist the orthopedist includes (1) the general health of the patient and the presence of other injuries, (2) location of the fracture, (3) the pattern of the fracture lines, (4) the number of fracture fragments, (5) whether the fibular shaft is also fractured, and (6) the extent of soft tissue damage, including vascular compromise, soilage, and the possible presence of compartment syndromes.

Achilles Tendon Rupture

When the soleus and gastrocnemius muscles contract, the Achilles tendon pulls up the calcaneous, plantar flexing the foot. Rupture often occurs in sports settings, especially in poorly conditioned players. Forceful plantar flexion results in rupture of the tendon. A popping sound is heard by the patient, who then has difficulty ambulating. This injury is also likely to occur in individuals who have rheumatoid arthritis, lupus erythematosus, or prior steroid injection of the tendon. It frequently ruptures 2 to 6 cm above its attachment to the calcaneous, where it has its poorest vascular supply. A gap may be palpated at this point, and a dent may be visible. The Thompson-Doherty test is performed by squeezing the midportion of the calf of the patient lying in the prone position. An intact Achilles tendon is demonstrated by a plantar flexion of the foot. Another test is to have the patient walk on his or her toes. The diagnosis does not usually require imaging, but computed tomography or magnetic resonance imaging can be helpful in ambiguous cases. In the emergency department, the patient should be splinted in neutral position with a Robert Jones splint, with prompt referral to an orthopedist. Crutches will be needed for ambulation.

Gastrocnemius Rupture

The medial head of the gastrocnemius is frequently injured during athletic events. A forceful plantar flexion of the foot, often with an extended knee, results in partial tear or rupture of the medial head of the gastrocnemius near its origin on the distal femur. This may be the result of a fall on a plantar-flexed foot or the sudden plantar flexion that occurs in the back leg of an athlete serving a tennis ball. Predisposing factors include inadequate stretching, prior muscle injury, and advanced age.

The athlete feels a sudden sharp pain on the medial aspect of the proximal gastrocnemius. It is painful to ambulate and plantar flexion is uncomfortable. On exam, the proximal medial calf is tender, and may be swollen and bruised. Walking on tiptoes is possible, but uncomfortable. The history is similar to that of Achilles tendon rupture, but the pain and tenderness are more proximal, and the Thompson test is negative in patients with gastrocnemius muscle rupture. Rupture of a Baker cyst should also be considered in the diagnosis, along with deep vein thrombosis.

Treatment typically consists of immobilization with a posterior splint, crutches for ambulation, ice, and pain medications. A mild rupture may be treated simply with rest and non-weight bearing.

Shin Splints

The term *shin splints* describes pain over the lateral and anterior tibia that occurs with exertion and is relieved by rest. Athletes may suffer this early in their training, particularly when running on a hard surface. The only physical finding may be tenderness to the anterior or lateral tibia. Radiographs may be useful to detect a stress fracture of the tibia, but a bone scan is more sensitive. Treatment consists of cessation of the offending activity, usually for several weeks.

Osgood-Schlatter Disease

This lesion is typically seen in athletic teenagers. Girl and boy athletes are both affected. Football, soccer, basketball, gymnastics, and ballet can cause this injury. The anatomic lesion is the partial separation of the tibial tuberosity at the insertion of the patellar tendon. In about one-fourth of cases, it is a bilateral process. Palpation of the tibial tuberosity reveals tenderness and induration. A lateral x-ray of the proximal tibia with the knee flexed 30 degrees reveals an elevation of the distal portion of the tubercle off of the tibia. Alternatively, ultrasound can be used. Cold compresses, anti-inflammatory drugs, and stopping the offending activity is standard treatment. Follow-up with an orthopedist is advisable for this sometimes chronic condition.

Tibial Tuberosity Fractures in Children

Acute fracture of the tibial tuberosity is the result of contraction of the quadriceps, resulting in a strong pull on the infrapatellar ligament in a young athlete. Usually a leaping motion is involved. On examination,

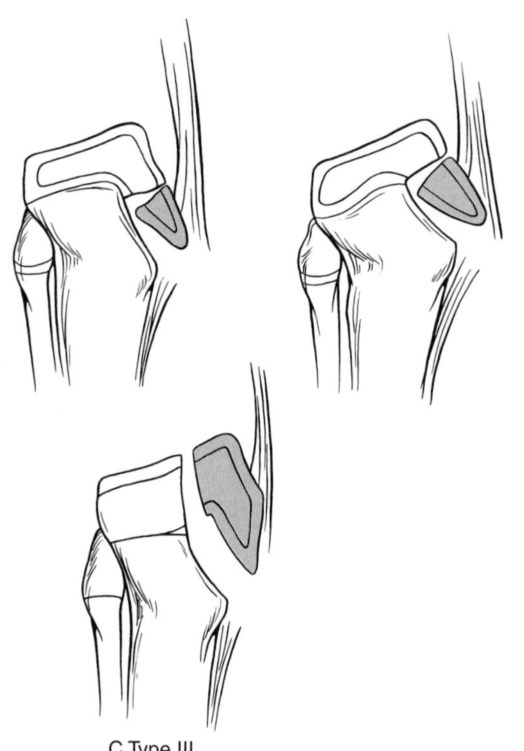

FIG. 267-1. Ogden's classification of tibial tuberosity fractures: **A.** type I (fracture between secondary ossification centers), **B.** type II (fracture splitting secondary ossification centers from primary ossification center), and **C.** type III (fracture into the articular surface of the knee). From Ruiz and Cicero (1995), with permission.

there is pain and tenderness at the tibial tuberosity. There may be a knee joint effusion if the fracture extends into the knee (Salter III). Anteroposterior and lateral x-rays are used to define the fracture. The fracture may be in the plane of the growth plate (Ogden type II) or the fracture plane may be distal to the growth plate (Ogden type I) (Fig. 267-1). A type III Ogden fracture extends into the knee joint. Orthopedic consultation should be obtained for these fractures, because operative reduction and fixation are often needed. Some Ogden type I injuries can be managed with a knee immobilizer and crutches. However, orthopedic follow-up is needed within 1 to 2 days.

Toddler Fractures

A twisting of the lower leg caused by a fall can result in this spiral fracture of the distal third of the tibia. Although it is most often seen in children just learning to walk, it may occur up to age 6. Examination of a frightened child may be difficult. Tenderness and swelling may be palpated at the fracture site. More often, the presentation is one of a limping child with no clear history of injury. In this setting, an x-ray of both the tibia and the femur should be obtained. The fracture may be subtle and visible on only one view. Sometimes the fracture is only seen during resorption and callus formation. Treatment involves a long leg cast for 2 to 4 weeks, with weight bearing as tolerated. Orthopedic consultation should be obtained.

BIBLIOGRAPHY

Dunn JF Jr: Osgood-Schlatter disease. *Am Fam Physician* 41:173, 1990.
Krause BL, Williams JP, Catterall A: Natural history of Osgood-Schlatter disease. *J Pediatr Orthop* 10:65, 1990.
Leach RE: Fractures of the tibia and fibula, in Rockwood CA, Green DP, Bucholz RW (eds): *Fractures in Adults,* 3d ed. Philadelphia, JB Lippincott, 1991, p 1915.
Ogden JA, Tross RB, Murphy MG: Fractures of the tibial tuberosity in adolescents, *J Bone Joint Surg [Am]* 62:205, 1980.
Ruiz E, Cicero JJ (eds): Emergency Management of Skeletal Injuries. St Louis, CV Mosby, 1995.

ANKLE INJURIES

John A. Michael
Ian G. Stiell

EPIDEMIOLOGY

Injuries to the ankle are a common presenting complaint in emergency departments (EDs). The majority of patients are younger than age 40 and are equally distributed between males and females. Fractures, most commonly of the lateral malleolus, are seen in 15 percent of these patients.[1,2] Below the age of 50, fractures are more common in men and, above this age, fractures are more common in women. Fracture-dislocations are more common in women.

ANATOMY

The ankle joint bears the weight of the body. An understanding of ankle injuries depends on not only a thorough knowledge of the anatomy of the joint but also on the mechanism of force that caused the injury.

The proximal part of the joint, or mortise, is comprised of distal fibula and tibia. This fits on top of the talus, or plafond, the distal part of the joint. These three bones are bound together by three groups of ligaments. Bony stability is provided by the medial and lateral malleoli extending over the plafond. Ligamentous stability is provided by the lateral ligament complex, the medial deltoid ligament, and the syndesmosis. The lateral malleolus is attached to the anterior and posterior aspects of the talus and to the calcaneus, respectively, by the anterior talofibular, posterior talofibular, and the calcaneofibular ligaments. The medial collateral or deltoid ligament is a thick triangular band of tissue that originates on the medial malleolus. The superficial fibers insert on the navicular, the sustentaculum of the calcaneus, and the talus, while a deep set of fibers insert on the medial aspect of the talus. The syndesmosis is a group of four distinct ligaments that attach the distal fibula to the tibia just above the plafond (Fig. 268-1).

The ankle joint is sometimes described as having a range of motion in only the plantar-dorsiflexion plane, however, a small degree of medial-lateral movement does occur. The four groups of muscles that serve the ankle joint are supplied by branches of the sciatic nerve. Dorsiflexion is accomplished by tibialis anterior, extensor digitorum longus, and extensor hallucis longus muscles that run over the anterior aspect of the joint. On the medial side of the joint, the tibialas posterior, flexor digitorum longus, and flexor hallucis longus run behind the medial malleolus and contribute to inversion of the joint. Laterally, running behind the distal fibula, the peroneous and brevis muscles contribute to eversion and plantar flexion. These two peroneal tendons share a common synovial sheath that is held in place by a groove on the posterior aspect of the lateral malleolus and the superior retinaculum. Plantar flexion is provided by the soleus and gastrocnemius muscles. The blood supply of the foot is served by branches of the popliteal artery.

Almost all injuries of the ankle joint are due to an abnormal motion of the talus within the mortise. Motion of the talus causes a stress on the malleoli and the ligaments, causing injury. If the injury allows shifting of the position of the talar dome within the mortise, then the injury has the potential to be unstable. Fractures above the plafond may be unstable, and injuries that cause disruption on both sides of

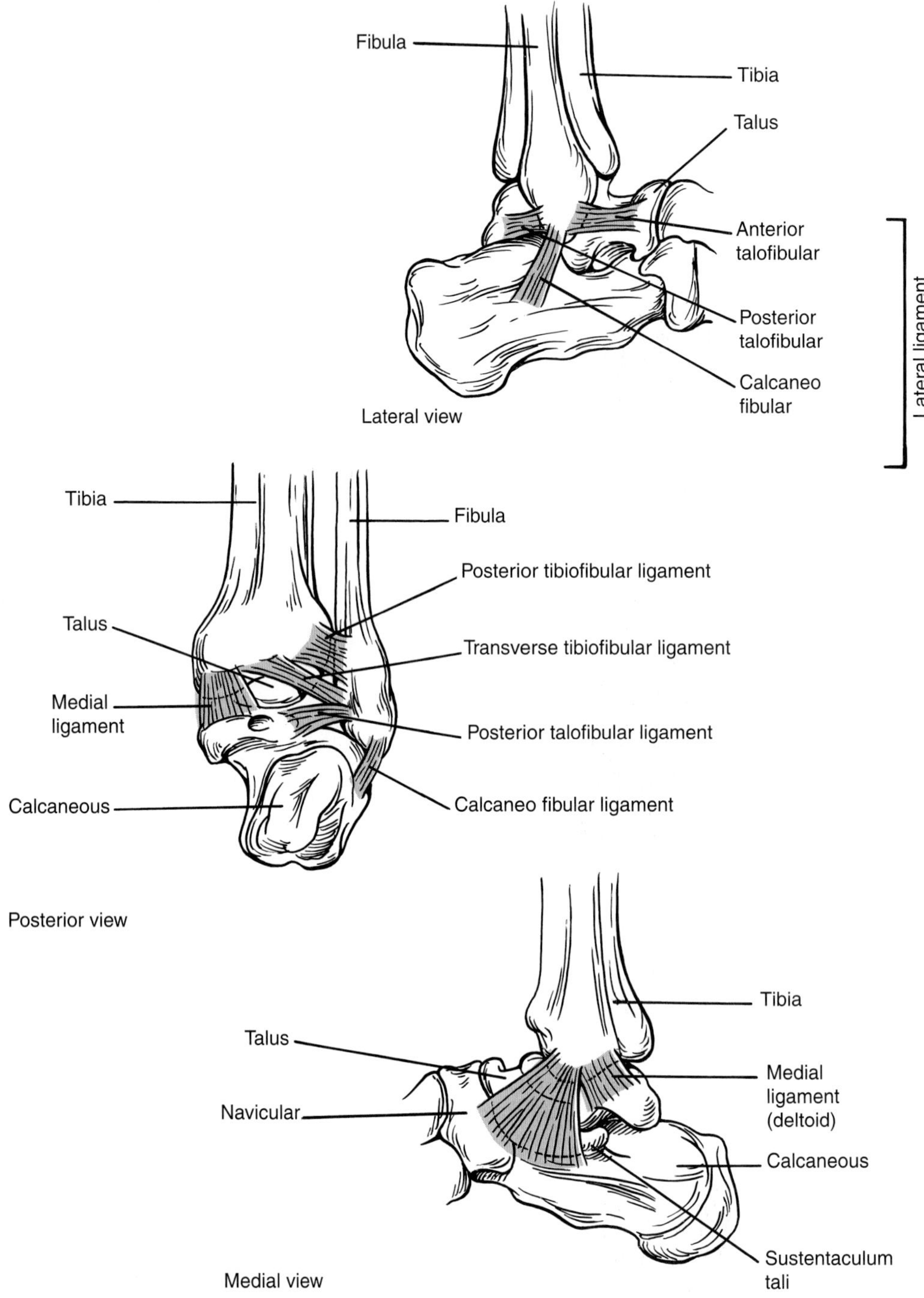

FIG. 268-1. Anatomy of the ankle joint.

the joint are unstable. Instability can result from a fracture of a malleolus and rupture of a ligament, fracture of both malleoli, or rupture of both ligaments.

EVALUATION

History

Although knowledge of the mechanism of the injury is important, many patients can not recollect the exact movement that caused the injury. The classification systems used to describe ankle injuries utilize the direction of the deforming force to describe the potential injury. This information is useful, but, to emergency physicians, the circumstances surrounding the injury are of greater importance in consideration of other injuries. The potential for associated injuries is greater in an individual who has jumped from a 12-foot fence than in a basketball player who came down on one foot from a hoop jump. Likewise, an elderly woman is more likely to have a second injury when she trips on a curbstone and falls to the pavement on an outstretched hand. The treatment of patients who have chronic medical conditions like diabetes or peripheral vascular disease, which can cause sensory deficits, or who are on chronic immunosuppressive therapy has to be approached with caution. A normal-appearing ankle or minimal tenderness on examination does not exclude the necessity of further evaluation. The ability to bear weight immediately after an injury, with subsequent increase in pain and swelling as the patient continues to ambulate, suggests a sprain rather than a fracture. Finally, the time of the injury, as well as previous bony or soft tissue injuries to the ankle, need to be documented.

Physical Examination

Once significant swelling has taken place, the examination of the ankle becomes more difficult. This may be temporized in the busy ED by the application of ice at triage and getting the patient to elevate the foot. Although tempting, the patient should not be examined in a wheelchair, but on a stretcher. It is critical to examine the joint above and below the injury. Note the position, swelling, and skin integrity of the injured ankle. Ask the patient to plantar and dorsiflex the ankle actively, then put the ankle through a passive range of motion. Soft tissue injuries are more likely when there is a significant difference between the passive and active range of motion. Increased pain with dorsiflexion is suggestive of a syndesmosis injury. Palpate the area of obvious injury last: Hurt the patient initially and their cooperation will rapidly diminish. Compare the injured ankle to the normal ankle. Tenderness of the knee, the fibular head, or the proximal fibular shaft suggests a fibulotibial ligament tear or a Maisonneuve fracture. Compress the fibula toward the tibia just above the midpoint of the calf in order to exclude clinically an isolated syndesmotic sprain. Starting at least 6 cm proximal, palpate the posterior aspects of lateral and medial malleoli to the distal tips of the shaft. Examine the Achilles tendon. If there is tenderness or a defect, perform the Thompson test. With the patient prone on a stretcher, squeeze the calf: loss of plantar flexion indicates a complete rupture of the tendon. Palpate the midfoot and hindfoot over the calcaneus, the tarsals, and the base of the fifth metacarpal. Patients can complain of an ankle injury when they have actually injured the foot or the Achilles tendon. Injuries to these structures are not excluded with the three-view ankle series.

Many acutely injured ankles are too painful or swollen for tests of ligamentous stability to be performed accurately. In these circumstances, the tests can be deferred to the physician who is going to follow the case. If the circumstances allow an examination, perform the following: With the foot hanging freely, grasp the posterior calcaneus with one hand and stabilize the distal leg with the other hand. With the foot in a few degrees of plantar flexion, test the anteroposterior stability of the joint by moving the foot while holding the tibia in a stable position. A positive anterior drawer test is greater than 5 mm of movement in comparison to the normal ankle. Evert and invert the foot. More than a 10° movement in comparison to the other foot is a positive talar tilt test. Inversion instability or anteriposterior laxity suggests the disruption of two or more of the lateral collateral ligaments. Eversion instability suggests a disruption of the deltoid complex. Some orthopedists feel that the anterior drawer test and the talar tilt test should be performed as stress radiographs, with comparison films of the other ankle before any conclusions are made. This is not practical in the ED, and these tests can be done in follow-up or consultation.

Perform a neurovascular examination. This includes palpation of the dorsalis pedis and posterior tibial pulse and capillary refill. Check the foot for motor and sensory impairment. Ask the patient to walk four steps: if the patient can transfer weight from one foot to another and the findings on physical examination as outlined above are normal, the likelihood of a significant fracture is nil.

IMAGING

The Ottawa Ankle Rules have provided a significant advance in the evaluation of ankle injuries in the ED. Previous studies suggested that not all patients who presented to the ED needed radiographs.[3] The Ottawa Ankle Rules were derived from an initial series of studies[4–6] and then were prospectively validated.[1,7,8] These studies involved over 9000 patient encounters and 200 emergency physicians. Two further studies by the same group found the implementation of the rules to be cost effective and that, once taught, emergency physicians continued to use them.[9,10] Although these studies were carried out in eight academic and community emergency departments in Canada, other studies at independent sites in the United States,[11,12] the United Kingdom,[13] and France[2] have further validated their use. Additionally, it has been demonstrated that nurses at triage can apply the rules successfully.[11,13] Only two studies have failed to replicate these results,[14,15] but these studies were found to have either a flawed methodology or did not accurately assess the rules as developed.

The rules are simple to apply and are illustrated in Fig. 268-2. The rules can be used on patients with an injury to the ankle, which is clinically broadly defined as the area of the distal leg and the midfoot subject to twisting injuries. Mechanisms of injury include twisting, direct blunt trauma, and falls. The rules were not developed for patients under the age of 18. Clinical judgment should prevail if the examination is unreliable due to lack of cooperation, intoxication, distracting injuries, or a diminished sensation in the leg. To assess the ability to bear weight, ask the patient to take four steps. If the patient can complete two transfers to the injured ankle, the patient passes the test.

Various objections that have been raised in the United States to applying these rules include, but are not limited to, the malpractice potential of missing any fracture, however insignificant; the patient's expectation of a radiograph and perception of a full assessment; and the physician's perception that the proportion of patients with fractures who present with ankle injuries is higher in the United States. Communication with the patient, such as an explanation of the thoroughness of the clinical examination, and the fact that a chip fracture, if missed, is treated like a sprain, is often effective. The saving of time and money for the patients should help them to accept the completeness of the evaluation. Additionally, studies done in the United States show a similar 15 percent fracture rate as demonstrated in Canada, the United Kingdom, France, and Scandinavia.

An excellent review of radiologic subtleties in the diagnosis of extremity injuries is found in Weissman.[16] Utilization of computed tomography and magnetic resonance imaging in the assessment of ankle injuries, although useful, is not appropriate for the ED.

INJURIES, TREATMENT, AND PROGNOSIS

Soft Tissue

LIGAMENTOUS SPRAINS **Lateral Ligament Complex** Sprains of the lateral ankle are the most common ankle injury, and the great majority are minor. The classification systems for ligamentous injuries to the lateral ankle are quite confusing. Older texts describe a purely anatomic classification scheme: A grade 1 injury is described as a complete rupture of one ligament and a grade 3 injury is a complete disruption of the three-ligament complex. More recent articles describe a more functional system: In this scheme, patients with grade 1 injuries have microscopic tears of the ligament, minimal swelling, normal findings on stress testing, and the ability to bear weight. Grade 2 injuries have a partial disruption of the ligament, significant swelling, indeterminant results on stress testing, and difficulty bearing weight. The ankle with a grade 3 injury has a ruptured ligament, swelling and ecchymosis, abnormal results on stress testing, and the inability to bear weight. These two classification systems are probably of little value to emergency physicians. A much more useful approach divides the injuries into two groups: stable, and potentially unstable or unstable.[17] If stress testing can be accomplished in the ED and the findings are normal, then the patient has a stable lateral ankle sprain and can be so treated. If results on stress testing are clearly abnormal or are

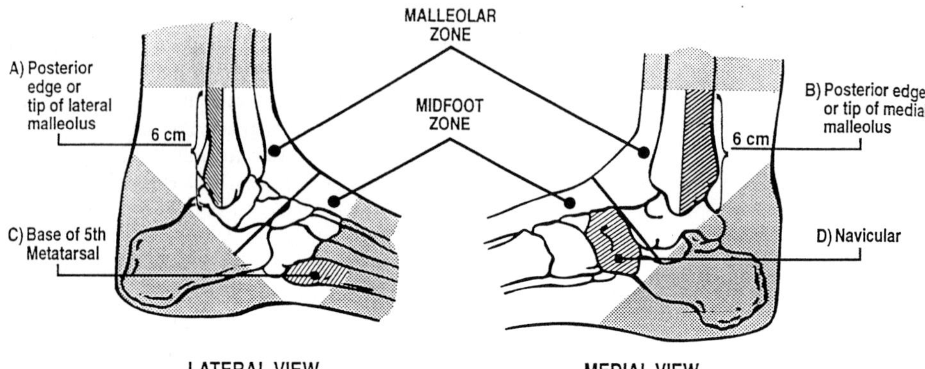

a) An ankle x-ray series is only required if:

There is any pain in malleolar zone and any of these findings:

i) bone tenderness at A
OR
ii) bone tenderness at B
OR
iii) inability to bear weight both immediately and in ED

b) A foot x-ray series is only required if:

There is any pain in midfoot zone and any of these findings:

i) bone tenderness at C
OR
ii) bone tenderness at D
OR
iii) inability to bear weight both immediately and in ED

FIG. 268-2. The Ottawa Ankle Rules for ankle and midfoot injuries.

indeterminate because of excessive swelling or pain, then the sprain should be treated as unstable.

Treatment of lateral ankle sprains has been equally controversial. A recent review of the English-language medical literature yielded 84 articles dealing primarily with soft tissue injuries of the ankle for a 30-year period.[18] The authors categorized the data to compare pharmacotherapy, surgical repair, active immobilization, cryotherapy, and diathermy. Although the average quality of the studies on a 10-point scale was 4 and no statistical analysis was performed, they made the following conclusions. Nonsteroidal anti-inflammatory drugs (NSAIDs) were associated with quicker recovery and less pain, active mobilization was the treatment of choice, and cryotherapy was useful. Unfortunately, only seven of the studies classified the degree of injury, and NSAIDs were compared with placebo rather than to acetaminophen. A review of more recent literature includes some fairly well performed prospective studies.[19–21] Most of these studies treated patients with grade 2 or 3 ankle sprains with compression, rest, and cryotherapy for 24 to 72 h. They then usually compared two treatment groups: (1) weight bearing with an ankle brace that allows plantar-dorsiflexion while resisting inversion and (2) eversion and plaster immobilization for up to 6 weeks. Patients in the early-mobilization groups returned to work or sport earlier than the immobilization groups, but at late follow-up there were no differences in outcomes. Additionally, direct comparisons of operative repair with cast, cast alone, and early controlled mobilization of acute grade 3 ankle sprains suggest that there is no difference in long-term outcome.[22]

The data indicate that individuals with stable and unstable ankle sprains, who are unable to bear weight easily, should be treated with rest, ice, compression, and elevation (RICE) for 24 to 72 h, depending on the amount of swelling and degree of pain. Individuals who can easily bear weight and have a stable joint probably need no more than simple analgesics and an elastic bandage, near normal activity with no sports involvement or prolonged walking, and follow-up in 1 week if they still have discomfort. Patients who are unable to bear weight in the ED but appear to have a stable joint can be given an ankle brace and be told to apply it in 24 to 72 h and to follow with their primary care physician or orthopedist within 1 week for a repeat evaluation. Patients who clearly have an unstable joint should be referred to an orthopedic surgeon, with consideration of a posterior mold. Timing of consultation depends on local preferences, but it would be prudent to establish communication early, as the ultimate decision on the method of treatment lies with the orthopedic surgeon.

Medial Ligament Complex An isolated sprain of the deltoid ligament is rare and is usually associated with a fibular fracture or significant tear of the tibial-fibular syndesmosis resulting from an eversion stress. When there is significant medial malleolus tenderness and swelling, Maisonneuve fracture is suspected and careful attention should be paid to the proximal fibula and fibular shaft. If the radiographs of the ankle and the fibula are negative, then a significant syndesmosis tear should be suspected. Patients with these type of injuries should be treated with RICE and early referral to an orthopedist.

Tibiofibular Syndesmotic Complex These injuries are usually associated with a hyperdorsiflexion injury. The talus moves in a superior direction and separates the fibula and tibia resulting in a partial or complete rupture of the syndesmosis. Patients usually complain of pain just above the plafond. These are significant injuries with prolonged recovery and should be treated with RICE and early consultation.

An excellent review of deltoid ligament, syndesmosis, and other "atypical ankle sprains" can be found in the work by Clanton and Porter.[17]

PROGNOSIS OF LIGAMENTOUS INJURIES The long-term complications of ankle sprains include functional instability (a subjective sensation of giving way without mechanical instability), mechanical instability (a demonstrable laxity), chronic pain, stiffness, and recurrent swelling. The documented incidence of complications is highly variable, and varies from 6 to 40 percent.[19,22] The long-term sequelae can be reduced with early rehabilitation. Physical therapy should be directed initially at active and passive range of motion exercises followed by early mobilization, strengthening exercises, proprioceptive training and, finally, restoration of normal activity.

STRAINS AND CONTUSIONS Strains are injuries to muscles or tendons and usually are not associated with a specific injury but rather are due to repetitive stress. The stress can be due to overuse secondary to athletic activity or to poorly fitting footwear. Treatment includes simple analgesics (anti-inflammatory medications may be of benefit), rest, identification and correction of provocative factors, and specific rehabilitative exercises. Contusions are usually caused by direct trauma, typically from a baseball or a hockey puck. Fractures are rare and usually are of the bone cortex only. Treatment is symptomatic with simple analgesics and ice.

PERONEAL TENDON SUBLUXATIONS AND DISLOCATIONS These injuries can be easily misdiagnosed as lateral ankle sprains. The mechanism is described by a sudden hyperdorsiflexion of the foot while the peroneal tendons are taut in eversion. This injury is most often associated with skiing. The superior retinaculum holding the peroneal tendons in place is stripped off the posterolateral malleolus. In more severe injuries, a small avulsion fracture will be noted on a radiograph, and the peroneal tendons dislocate or more often sublux anteriorly over the distal tip of the fibula. Consider this injury when tenderness and ecchymosis over the posterior edge of the lateral malleolus is noted in the absence of tenderness over the anterior talofibular ligament. It is important to consider this diagnosis in the acute setting: the treatment is frequently operative repair of the retinaculum.[17]

Fractures and Dislocations

CLASSIFICATION SCHEMES There are multiple classifications of ankle fractures. The more complex utilize both the position of the foot at the time of injury and the deforming force. These classifications are useful in predicting associated injuries. In the Lauge-Hansen classification system, the first word refers to the position and the second word refers to the force. The Danis-Weber classification is based on the level of the fracture of the fibula. Proximal fractures of the fibula are associated with damage to the syndesmosis and the increased likelihood of an unstable fracture. There are three types of injury in this classification scheme: The type A (fracture of fibula below the syndesmosis) is a supination injury and corresponds to the Lauge-Hansen-type suppination-adduction injury. The type B injury (fibular fracture at level of syndesmosis) is associated with external rotation force and corresponds with the suppination-eversion injury of Lauge-Hansen. The type C injury (fibular fracture above the syndesmosis) is associated with an external rotation-abduction force and corresponds with the pronation-eversion or abduction Lauge-Hansen injuries. The AO classification system amplifies the Danis-Weber system by subdividing each classification type into three subtypes to better describe associated medial injuries (Fig. 268-3).

Henderson described the simplest classification system based on radiographic appearance. This scheme is commonly utilized and uses the terms unimallelolar, bimalleolar, and trimallelolar to describe fractures of the ankle.

Although it is important to have a basic understanding of these classification systems, the most essential aspects of ankle injuries to appreciate is the stability of the injury and the exclusion of associated injuries (Table 268-1).

TREATMENT All fractures of the ankle, with the exception of fibular avulsion fractures, require immobilization by cast alone or surgical reduction with subsequent casting. Avulsion fractures are treated as stable ankle sprains if they are minimally displaced, less than 3 mm in diameter, and there is no indication of a medial ligamentous injury. The treatment goal with all other ankle fractures is to restore the anatomic relationship of the ankle, maintain reduction during the healing process, and institute early mobilization of the ankle. To ensure this, the talus has to be anatomically positioned in the mortise, the joint line has to be parallel to the ground, and the articular surface has to be smooth. The means to attain this goal is not only dependent on the type of fracture but also on the age and athletic expectations of the patient. Local preferences may also play a role in this decision. Most fractures, with the exception of unimalleolar injuries, require open reduction and fixation. The Maisonneuve fracture (AO type C2-3), although considered an unstable injury, can generally be treated with cast immobilization for 6 to 8 weeks, depending on the stability of the syndesmosis.[15] The Bosworth fracture, a rare variation of the Maisonneuve fracture where the proximal fibula gets trapped behind the tibia, usually requires operative reduction. The debate over the necessity of operative treatment for unimalleolar fractures with associated syndesmosis and deltoid ligamentous injuries is complex and beyond the scope of this text. Stable fibular fractures are treated with a short leg-walking cast for 6 weeks.

The timing of consultation is discussed below. In the interim, fractures should be splinted with a posterior mold and kept non-weight-bearing in all cases and elevated with application of ice in many. The analgesic need of the patient should be addressed. There is absolutely no basis for the practice of withholding analgesics until operative consent is obtained.

OSTEOCHONDRAL FRACTURES Osteochondral fractures are due to acute trauma or repetitive stress. These injuries vary from a deformation of the cartilage overlying the talar dome to a free-floating avulsion fracture. The staging and treatment of these lesions are complex, and orthopedic consultation is required. Treatment can involve excision or cast immobilization for up to 6 weeks.[17]

PROGNOSIS OF ANKLE FRACTURES Early complications and sequelae of ankle fractures are several and include skin necrosis and osteomyelitis in the short term and chronic pain, osteoarthritis, malunion, nonunion, and reflex sympathetic dystrophy in the long term. Although most of these problems are rare, postreduction arthritis can complicate up to 30 percent of fractures.

FRACTURE-DISLOCATIONS AND OPEN FRACTURES Dislocations of the ankle joint can occur in one of four planes and are frequently associated with a fracture. The posterior dislocation is most common and happens usually when the foot is plantar flexed and a backward force is applied. The injury is usually associated with rupture of the tibiofibular ligaments or fracture of the lateral malleolus. The anterior dislocation occurs with a dorsiflexed foot and fracture of the anterior aspect of the tibia. Lateral displacement is accompanied by ligamen-

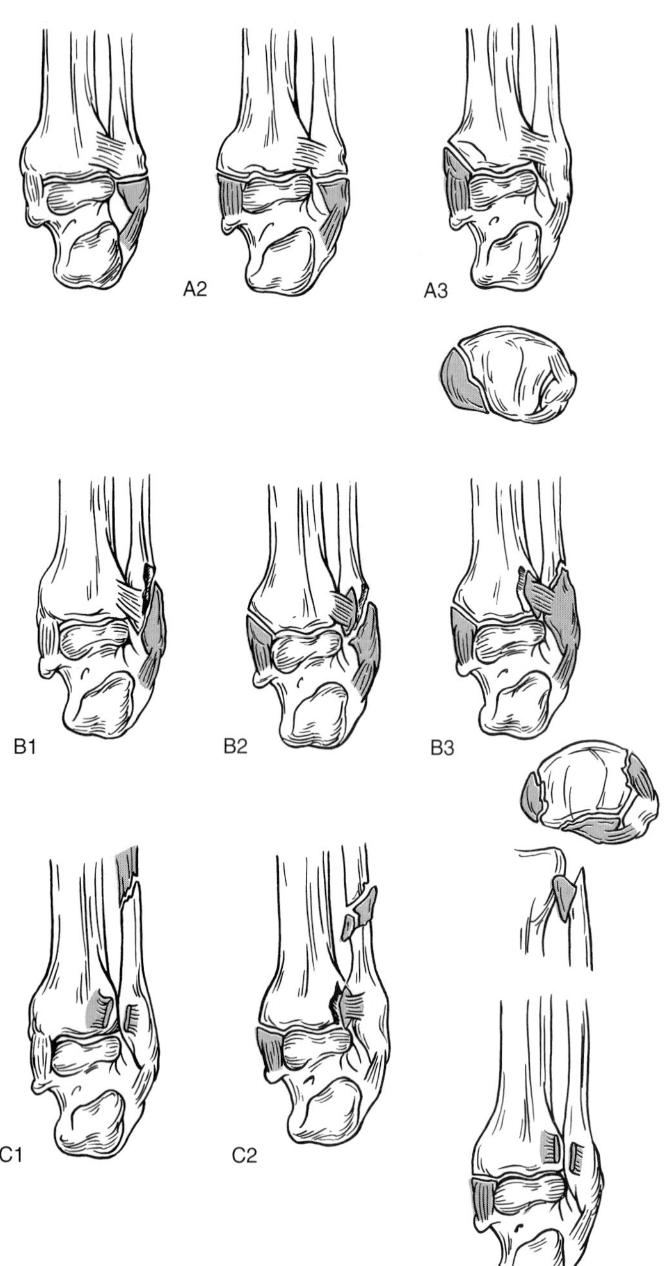

FIG. 268-3. The AO amplification of the Danis-Weber classification of ankle fractures.

TABLE 268-1 Associated and Occult Injuries of the Ankle

Injury	Clinical Suspicion	Confirmatory Test
Important to identify in the emergency department		
Fracture of base of fifth metatarsal	Examine lateral foot, tenderness to palpation	Anteroposterior foot radiograph
Maisonneuve fracture	Examine proximal fibula and shaft, tenderness to palpation	Fibula radiograph
Peroneal tendon dislocation	Palpable anterior tendon dislocation or subluxation	Clinical examination
Usually identified in follow-up of ankle sprains		
Osteochondral injuries	Diffuse ankle swelling, passive plantar flexion	Ankle mortise view/CT scan
Syndesmosis tear	Significant ankle pain, positive squeeze test	Widened mortise with weight bearing
Anterior calcaneal process fracture	Tenderness more inferioanterior than a typical ankle sprain	Lateral ankle radiograph/CT scan
Lateral talar process fracture	Tenderness just distal to the tip of fibula	Ankle mortise view/CT scan
Os trigonum	Tenderness anterior to Achilles tendon	Lateral ankle radiograph

tous disruption and fracture of either or both malleoli. Finally, the talus can be displaced upward with a significant impaction. There will be an associated fracture of the talar dome or tibial plafond and disruption of the syndesmosis.

Patients with fracture-dislocations of the ankle are at considerable risk of neurovascular compromise and conversion of a closed fracture to an open one. Under most circumstances, the reduction of fracture-dislocations is left to an orthopedic surgeon. However, if there is vascular compromise indicated by absent pulses and a cool dusky foot or tenting of the skin caused by fractured bone, the emergency physician should perform the reduction. Do not delay reduction in order to obtain radiographs. If possible, place the patient on the stretcher, with the affected foot hanging over the side with a flexed knee. This forces the leg into external rotation and the foot into internal rotation. It also gives the physician the advantage of gravity. Administer adequate intravenous analgesia with the appropriate cardiorespiratory monitoring. The heel and foot should be grasped with both hands (with an assistant stabilizing the proximal leg), and downward traction and rotation applied in the opposite direction of the mechanism of the injury. Little force is required. A splint is applied once distal perfusion is restored and the foot is again elevated. Irreducible fractures are quite rare and, of course, require open reduction.

Protect open fractures from further contamination by applying a wet, sterile dressing over the wound with a gauze roll. No studies substantiate the application of betadine-soaked gauze to the laceration site. Splint the injury until radiographs and definitive treatment are available. Tetanus-diphtheria toxoid is given as necessary, and tetanus immunglobulin considered if the wound is grossly contaminated. The antibiotic of choice is cephalexin, and an aminoglycoside is added if the wound is grossly contaminated. Consider clindamycin for patients with penicillin allergy.

PEDIATRIC INJURIES

A different injury pattern has to be considered in the pediatric population. Patients with immature bones are more likely to have fractured the growth plate than to have sprained a ligament. The distal fibular and tibial growth plates are usually closed by the age of 16 and then the pattern of injury mimics that in adult patients. The Salter-Harris classification system describes the pattern of injury in skeletally immature individuals (Fig. 268-4).

Soft tissue injuries are rare in the pediatric population. Look for an anterior dislocation of the pernoneal tendon in young athletes who complain of lateral ankle pain. If the tendon is palpated anterior to the lateral malleolus, it can be relocated by pronating the foot while in dorsiflexion. A patient with a normal radiograph and tenderness over the growth plate of the lateral malleolus has a Salter I fracture.

The Salter type I and II fibular fractures are usually associated with an inversion injury and are treated with closed reduction and a walking cast for 4 weeks. Closed reduction with a short or long leg cast for 6 weeks is the treatment for a Salter type II tibial fracture (pronation-eversion force) with an associated greenstick fibular fracture. Salter type III and IV fractures (significant adduction force) of the distal tibia with an associated fibular shaft fracture often require open reduction and fixation. Type V fractures (axial force) are rare and are treated with closed reduction and non-weight-bearing. Unfortunately, type V fractures can result in bone growth retardation. The prognosis of other pediatric fractures, however, is excellent.

TIMING OF CONSULTATION

No set of rigid rules for the timing of orthopedic consultation exists to guide emergency physicians for each specific ankle injury. Although it may be reasonable to request an in-person orthopedic consultation in an academic center at 3 o'clock in the morning for a stable ankle fracture, this will not endear a community-based emergency physician to his orthopedic colleagues. Although it may be perfectly acceptable for an emergency physician in some countries to apply a circular short leg cast to an AO type A1 or a Salter type I or II fibular fracture and arrange follow-up, this approach would not be common practice in other locales (Table 268-2).

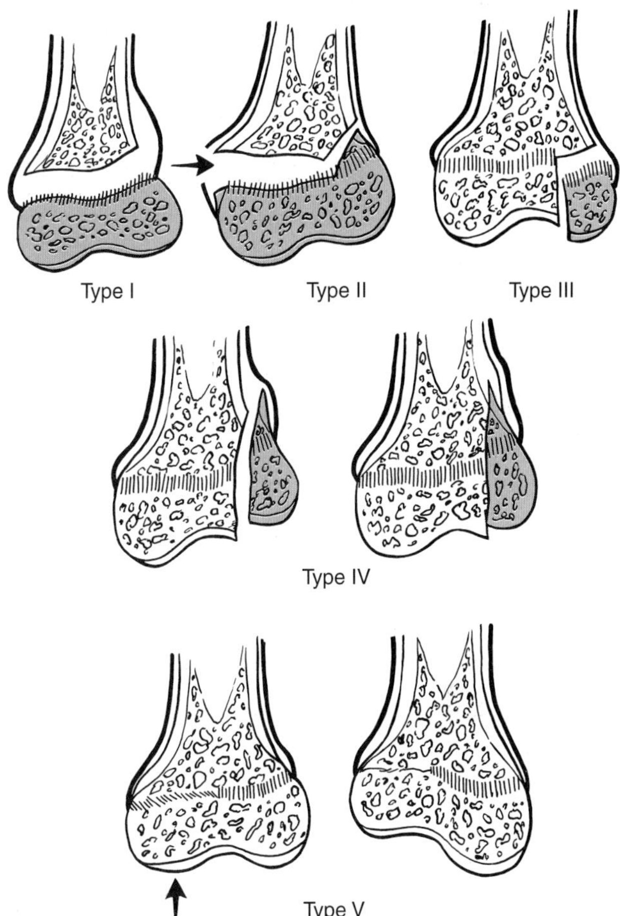

FIG. 268-4. Salter-Harris classification of pediatric fractures.

EMERGENCY DEPARTMENT TREATMENT ISSUES

Pharmacotherapy

The need for analgesia should always be addressed. As individual perception of pain varies, a simple ankle sprain may only require an elastic bandage or acetaminophen in most patients, while some will require oral narcotics. Although some studies suggest that the anti-inflammatory effect of NSAIDs is useful in treating ligamentous injuries,[18] other studies suggest that there is no benefit.[23] Patients who are in significant distress or who should be kept NPO because of anticipated surgery require parenteral analgesia.

Immobilization

Noncircular cast immobilization can be accomplished with a Jones bandage or a posterior mold. A Jones bandage has more padding and probably is more comfortable for patients with severe bruising and swelling, but may not accomplish the same degree of immobilization as a posterior mold. The patient should be supine on a stretcher. Apply two to three layers of abdominal pads, extending from the distal foot to just below the knee, and hold them in place with 4-inch elastic

TABLE 268-2 Timing of Consultation

Immediate Consultation in Emergency Department	Deferred Consultation*	Within 1 Week
All open fractures	Stable unimalleolar fractures	Potentially unstable sprains
All fracture dislocations	Unstable ligamentous injuries	
All dislocations	Acute peroneal dislocations	
All trimalleolar fractures†	Pediatric Salter I, II	
All bimalleolar fractures†		
Unstable unimalleolar fractures†		
Pediatric Salter III, IV, V†		
Maisonneuve fractures†		

*Implies that communication is established at time of diagnosis and specific time of consultation has been set.
†Consultation can be delayed in the emergency department in fractures without neurovascular compromise and appropriate splinting.

bandages. A four-inch cotton cast padding can be applied, in place of the abdominal pads, in a circular fashion overlapping by at least 50 percent with a minimum of three complete layers. The Jones bandage should not be used for more than a couple of days.

A posterior mold is most easily applied if the patient is prone on a stretcher with the knee flexed to 90°. Most emergency departments have a prepackaged padded splint material available. For extra padding, apply a single layer of 4-inch cotton cast padding from the toes to the knee, followed by a 4-inch plaster or fiberglass splint. The wet splint should extend along the plantar surface of the foot and the calf from just distal of the first metatarsal-phalangeal joint to the fibular head (Fig. 268-5). Hold the splint in place with 4-inch elastic bandages. As the splint hardens, keep the ankle at a 90° angle and mold the splint about the instep and malleoli. Use three or four layers of cotton cast padding, if prepackaged splints are not available, followed by 15 to 20 layers of 4-inch plaster fashioned into a slab of appropriate length. If more support is required, especially in the setting of an unstable joint, another slab can be added to give additional medial-lateral support. Size the patient, if necessary, for crutches and instruct in their appropriate use. For a weight-bearing patient, a cast shoe can be applied.

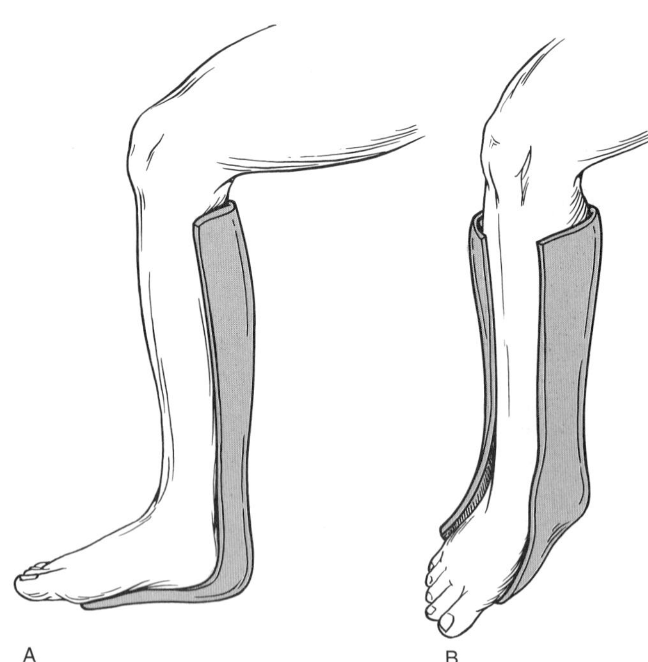

FIG. 268-5. Short leg posterior splint with and without a stirrup splint.

Ankle Braces

Several different ankle braces (which allow dorsiplantar flexion but do not allow inversion or eversion of the ankle) are available. These devices vary from complex applications of athletic tape, to lace-up splints and inflatable plastic stirrup-type braces. Although few studies exist that compare these braces, it is clear that any device that speeds mobilization and weight bearing will promote early return to full function.[19,21]

Cryotherapy and Other Modalities

Ice packs have been shown to limit swelling and decrease pain.[18] The pack is applied directly to the ankle or the splint and is left on for 20 min at a time. It can be repeated every few hours. Ultrasound has not been shown to promote healing.[18,24]

REFERENCES

1. Stiell IG, McKnight RD, Greenberg GH, et al: Interobserver agreement in the examination of acute injury patients. *Am J Emerg Med* 10:14, 1992.
2. Auleley G-R, Ravaud P, Giraudeau B, et al: Implementation of the Ottawa Ankle Rules in France. *JAMA* 277:1935, 1997.
3. Auletta AG, Conway WF, Hayes CW, et al: Indications for radiography in patients with acute ankle injuries: Role of the physical examination. *AJR* 157:789, 1991.
4. Stiell I, Wells G, Laupacis A, et al: Multicentre trial to introduce the Ottawa Ankle Rules for use of radiography in acute ankle injuries. *BMJ* 311:594, 1995.
5. Stiell IG, McDowell I, Nair RC, et al: Use of radiography in acute ankle injuries: Physicians attitudes and practice. *Can Med Assoc J* 147: 1671, 1992.
6. Stiell IG, Greenberg GH, McKnight RD, et al: Decision rules for the use of radiography in acute ankle injuries. *JAMA* 269:1127, 1993.
7. Stiell IG, McKnight RD, Greenberg GH, et al: Implementation of the Ottawa Ankle Rules. *JAMA* 271:827, 1994.
8. Stiell IG, Greenberg GH, McKnight RD, et al: A study to develop clinical decision rules for the use of radiography in acute ankle injuries. *Ann Emerg Med* 21:384, 1992.

9. Anis AH, Stiell IG, Stewart DG, et al: Cost-effectiveness analysis of the Ottawa Ankle Rules. *Ann Emerg Med* 26:422, 1995.
10. Verbeek PR, Stiell IG, Hebert G, et al: Ankle radiograph utilization after learning a decision rule; A 12 month follow-up. *Acad Emerg Med* 4:776, 1997.
11. Pigman EC, Klug RK, Sanford S, et al: Evaluation of the Ottawa clinical decision rules for the use of radiography in acute ankle and midfoot injuries in the emergency department: An independent site assessment. *Ann Emerg Med* 24:41, 1994.
12. Verma S, Hamilton K, Hawkins HH, et al: Clinical application of the Ottawa Ankle Rules for the use of radiography in acute ankle injuries: An independent site assessment. *AJR* 169:825, 1997.
13. Salt P, Clancy M: Implementation of the Ottawa Ankle Rules by nurses working in an accident and emergency department. *J Accid Emerg Med* 14:363, 1997.
14. Lucchesi GM, Cerasani C, Jackson RE, et al: Sensitivity of Ottawa Ankle Rules. *Ann Emerg Med* 26:1, 1995.
15. Kerr L, Kelly AM, Grant J, et al: Failed validation of a clinical decision rule for the use of radiography in acute ankle injury. *NZ Med J* 107:294, 1994.
16. Weissman BN: The radiologic diagnosis of subtle extremity injuries. *Emerg Med Clin North Am* 3:600, 1985.
17. Clanton TO, Porter DA: Primary care of foot and ankle injuries in the athlete. *Clin Sports Med* 16:435, 1997.
18. Ogilvie-Harris DJ, Gilbart M: Treatment modalities for soft tissue injuries of the ankle: A critical review. *Clin J Sport Med* 5:175, 1995.
19. Konradsen L, Holmer P, Sondergaard L: Early mobilizing treatment for grade III ankle ligament injuries. *Foot Ankle* 12:69, 1991.
20. Karlsson J, Eriksson BI, Sward L: Early functional treatment for acute ligament injuries of the ankle. *Scand J Med Sci Sports* 6:341, 1996.
21. Eiff MP, Smith AT, Smith GE: Early mobilization versus immobilization in the treatment of lateral ankle sprains. *Am J Sports Med* 22:83, 1994.
22. Munk B, Holm-Christensen K, Lind T: Long term outcome after ruptured lateral ankle ligaments. *Acta Orthop Scand* 66:452, 1995
23. Dupont M, Beliveau P, Theiriault G: The efficacy of antiinflammatory medication in the treatment of the acutely sprained ankle. *Am J Sports Med* 15:41, 1987.
24. Williamson JB, George TK, Simpson DC, et al: Ultrasound in the treatment of ankle sprains. *Injury* 17:176, 1986.

FOOT INJURIES

John A. Michael
Ian G. Stiell

The foot is a complex, highly evolved structure that bears the weight of the body and acts as a lever to propel the body forward while walking or running. It is designed to carry the body over varied terrain with little apparent difficulty. Although most injuries are minor and heal with time, undertreated and unrecognized injuries can result in significant long-term pain and disability. Radiographs are sometimes difficult to interpret, and seemingly minor abnormalities can be associated with a significant injury.

ANATOMY

Chopart and Lisfranc joints divide the foot into three regions. The talus and the calcaneum comprise the hindfoot. The midfoot contains the cuneiforms, the cuboid, and the navicular. The metatarsals and the phalanges make up the forefoot (Fig. 269-1). There are a total of 28 bones and 57 articular surfaces. Numerous intrinsic muscles and ligaments contribute to the integrity of the foot's structure. The biomechanical specifics of the foot involved in ambulation are extremely complex. In general, eversion and inversion occur about the subtalar and calcaneotarsal joints, whereas adduction-abduction and flexion-extension occur about the metatarsophalangeal and interphalangeal joints.

The body weight when standing is distributed about the heel to the rear and the five metatarsal heads to the front. The curved shape of the foot is held in position by three arches. The shape of the bones, the arrangement of the ligaments, and the tone of the muscles maintain the position of the arches. The plantar aponeurosis covers the sole of the foot and is a strong band of fascia that originates on the medial side of the calcaneum and fuses with the fibrous sheaths of the phalanges.

The blood supply of the foot comes from branches of the popliteal artery. The anterior tibial artery serves the dorsum of the foot, and its branch, the dorsalis pedis, can be palpated over the dorsum of the midfoot. Branches of the posterior tibial and the peroneal arteries serve the sole. The motor and sensory nerves of the foot include branches of both the femoral and sciatic nerves and include branches of the saphenous, sural (sensory), and deep and superficial peroneal nerves (both sensory and motor).

The essential parts of the anatomy of concern include, but are not limited to, the following. The first metatarsal bears twice the weight as any other metatarsal, and injuries to this bone require a more conservative approach. The blood supply to the foot is tenuous, and major fractures of the talus and subtalar dislocations are complicated by avascular necrosis. The base of the second metatarsal is the ''keystone'' of the Lisfranc complex, and any injury to this area has to be treated with caution.

EVALUATION

History

As with all injuries, it is important to obtain an adequate history. Many injuries to the foot are associated with significant forces or falls from a height, and other injuries have to be sought. Generally, most foot injuries are caused by direct or twisting forces. Twisting forces are associated with avulsion-type injuries and are generally more minor than the injuries caused by direct trauma. Previous injuries, general medical condition, and repetitive mechanisms are all important to

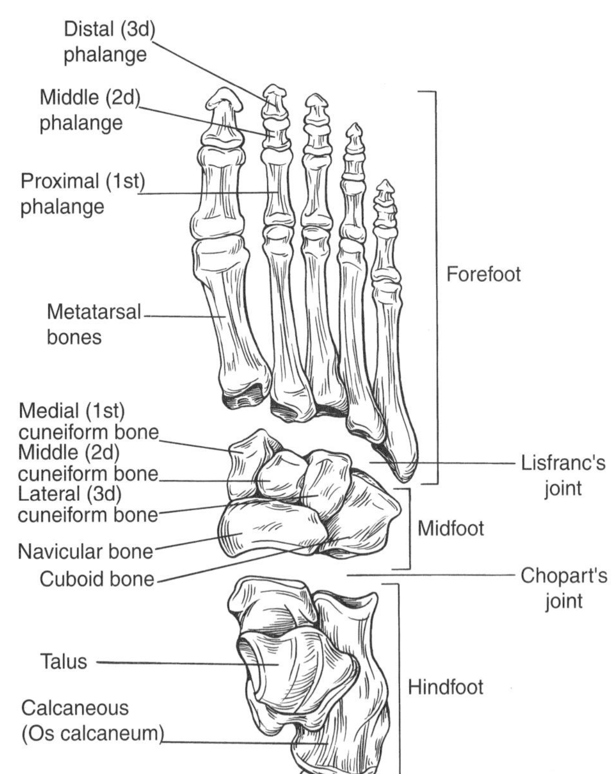

FIG. 269-1. Bony anatomy of the foot.

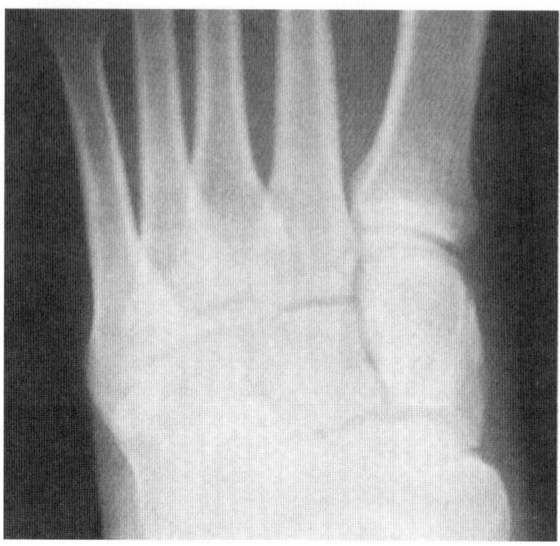

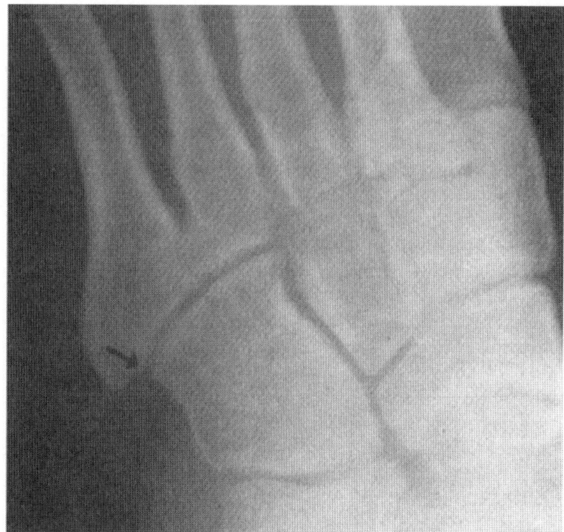

FIG. 269-2. Normal radiographic anatomy of the Lisfranc joint.

elicit from the patient. Increasing inability to ambulate after an injury and increasing pain may be suggestive of a minor sprain or of an impending vascular catastrophe. Special care should be paid to puncture wounds. Consider the type of shoes worn, the possibility of a foreign body, and the potential of tetanus.

Physical Examination

Elevation of the foot and the application of ice at triage will facilitate the physical examination. The patient should be examined on a stretcher. Examination of the foot includes an ankle examination (see Chap. 268, ''Ankle Injuries''). The foot should be inspected for any loss of skin integrity, for deformity, and finally for swelling and ecchymosis. Passive range of motion should be assessed and compared with the uninjured foot. Palpate the achilles tendon, the calcaneum, the dorsum of the midfoot, and then the metatarsals and phalanges. Pay special attention to the base of the fifth metatarsal and the area over the base of the second metatarsal. Actively move the various joints of the foot through their range of motion. Next, grasp two adjacent metatarsal heads and move them in opposite dorsiplantar directions. Finally, if the foregoing exam does not suggest a specific injury, observe the patient ambulating. Normal findings on examination and the ability to complete several weight transfers to the injured foot essentially excludes a significant injury.

IMAGING

Patients with normal findings on examination of the hindfoot and forefoot and on examination of the ankle and midfoot (see Fig. 268-2, the Ottawa Ankle Rules, from the previous chapter) probably do not need radiographs. Clinical judgment should always prevail in the decision-making process. Abnormal findings on examination mandate a complete, three-view, standard foot series. If there is pain about the heel, an axial view of the calcaneum should be added. The lateral view of the foot and the axial view of the calcaneum are important in excluding hindfoot injuries, while the anteroposterior (AP) and oblique projections are more useful in delineating midfoot and forefoot injuries.

Other plain radiographic views, bone scans, and computed tomographic (CT) scans are seldom utilized by emergency physicians in the evaluation of foot injuries. Emergency physicians, however, should occasionally order comparison weight-bearing AP radiographs of the foot to exclude a subtle diastasis (greater than 1 mm) at the Lisfranc joint. The criteria for a normal radiograph are detailed in Fig. 269-2.[1]

INJURIES AND TREATMENT

Acute Soft Tissue Injuries

Puncture Wounds are discussed in Chap. 43. Complicated foot infections, gunshot wounds to the foot, and many lawn mower injuries require consultation and/or operative debridement.[3,4] The latter two open injuries require a careful search for associated vascular and tendon injuries, radiographs to document foreign-body presence and bony involvement, consideration of tetanus vaccine and immunoglobulin administration, aggressive wound irrigation, analgesics, and antibiotics in most cases. Do not rely on the presence of fever, abnormal radiographs, or elevated white cell counts and erythrocyte sedimentation rates to exclude the diagnosis of osteomyelitis.[2,5]

TURF TOE Forced hyperextension of the the first metatarsophalangeal causes a sprain or tear of the joint capsule. The injury is usually associated with a push-off mechanism from a hard surface. The treatment is conservative, with analgesics and with a supportive shoe to prevent further dorsiflexion.

PLANTAR FASCIA RUPTURE This is a tear in the plantar fascia at the point of insertion on the calcaneum. Patients describe a sudden pop and pain that is usually associated with sudden plantar flexion of the foot. Treatment is nonoperative.

TENDON RUPTURES Acute ruptures of the tendons of the foot are rare and are usually associated with penetrating or lacerating injuries. Extensor and flexor hallucis tendon injuries are repaired primarily. The treatment of other tendon transections is controversial.

CRUSH INJURIES AND COMPARTMENT SYNDROME Injuries caused by crush-type mechanisms without associated skin or bone injuries may appear innocuous. These injuries, however, place the foot at risk for the development of compartment syndrome. Compartment syndrome should be suspected when there is pain out of proportion to the injury. Typically, the foot is tensely swollen, and the pain is not relieved by elevation and is increased by passive dorsiflexion of the big toe. Paresthesias may be present, but pedal pulses and capillary

TABLE 269-1 Differential Diagnosis of Subacute and Chronic Foot Pain

Condition	Diagnosis	Etiology/Pathology	Treatment
Diagnosis on inspection			
Bunions	Swelling and pain, medial 1st MTP	Friction from poorly fitted shoewear	Special pads, rarely surgery
Corns	Callus formation, sole or dorsal toes	Friction from poorly fitted shoewear	Special pads
Ingrown toenails	Overgrowth of nail into adjacent tissue	Improper nail trimming	Surgical excision
Paronychia	Purulent infection between cuticle and nail	Poor toenail care	Incision and debridement
Hammertoe	DIP/IP plantar flexor deformity	Compression from poorly fitted shoewear	Special pads
Fallen arches	Loss of medial arch	Stretched ligaments from poorly fitted shoewear	Orthotics
Hindfoot pain			
Plantar fasciitis	Tenderness over plantar fascia of medial foot, increased with dorsiflexion of toes	Inflammation caused by prolonged standing or overuse	Rest, NSAIDs, orthotics
Subcalcaneal bursitis	Tenderness over the base of calcaneum	Overuse syndrome	Rest, NSAIDs, special pads
Achilles tendon bursitis	Tenderness lateral to the Achilles tendon	Friction caused by back of shoe	Special pads
Tarsal tunnel syndrome	Tenderness medial and inferior to medial malleolus, diagnosis confirmed by nerve conduction studies	Repetitive subtalar pronation leading to entrapment of tibial nerve	Rest, NSAIDs, steroid injection, surgical release
Os trigonum syndrome	Tenderness anterior to Achilles tendon	Chronic impingement from prolonged plantar flexion	NSAIDs, surgical excision
Forefoot pain			
Morton neuroma	Episodes of lancinating pain in the 3rd or 4th MT interspace, relieved by shoe removal; reproduced by compression of interspace or MT heads	Impingement of the interdigital nerve, caused by perineural fibrosis	NSAIDs, nerve block, surgical release
Metatarsal stress fractures	Insidious onset of aching pain, with tenderness over the affected MT shaft; confirmed by bone scan	Repetitive stress in runners, usually affecting MT 2 or 3	Analgesics, rest, reevaluation of training method

Abbreviations: DIP/IP, distal interphalangeal/interphalangeal joint; MT, metatarsal; MTP, metatarsophalangeal; NSAIDs, nonsteroidal anti-inflammatory drugs.

refill are often preserved. If compartment syndrome is suspected, intracompartmental pressures must be measured. There are multiple compartments in the foot. The measure of pressure in these small compartments is technically difficult, and orthopedic consultation may be necessary to exclude this diagnosis. Immediate fasciotomy is required once the diagnosis is confirmed.

DIFFERENTIAL DIAGNOSIS OF SUBACUTE AND CHRONIC FOOT PAIN Patients frequently present to the ED with the complaint of foot pain of varying duration. Although several disorders that cause pain are obvious on inspection, including bunions, ingrown toenails, corns, hammertoes and blisters, other problems require a directed physical examination of the foot. The diagnosis and treatment of these disorders is described in Table 269-1.

Fractures and Dislocations

HINDFOOT Talar fractures are uncommon. Minor avulsion fractures of the neck, body, and lateral process are usually treated with a posterior slab, crutches, and orthopedic follow-up. Os trigonum and transchondral talar dome fractures are difficult to identify in the ED and are sometimes diagnosed in the follow-up of "ankle sprains." Major fractures of the talar neck and body are associated with severe dorsiflexion and axial forces. These injuries often require open reduction and merit immediate orthopedic consultation. These fractures are frequently complicated by avascular necrosis.

Peritalar or subtalar dislocations are rare. In this injury, the calcaneotalar and talonavicular joints are disrupted while the tibiotalar joint remains intact. Although the dislocation can occur in any direction, medial dislocation is by far the most common and is the result of a severe rotational-inversion force. These injuries require immediate orthopedic consultation and emergent reduction. Closed reduction can sometimes be accomplished using conscious sedation in the ED, although frequently a general or regional anaesthetic in the operating room is required.

An axial load to the heel, caused by a fall from a height, is the mechanism associated with most fractures of the calcaneum. These injuries are frequently associated with other injuries, most commonly vertebral column, forearm, and other lower extremity fractures. Fractures should be categorized as intraarticular or extraarticular.

Although the more common subtalar, intraarticular fractures are usually obvious on the lateral foot radiograph, some compression fractures may be subtle. When this injury is suspected by mechanism or examination, carefully examine the radiograph utilizing the measurement of Boehler's angle. If the angle is less than 20°, suspect a fracture (Fig. 269-3). The criterion for open reduction of these fractures is controversial, with CT scanning playing an important diagnostic and preoperative planning role. Seek immediate orthopedic consultation. In the interim, apply a well-padded posterior splint, elevate the foot, and address analgesic needs. Comminuted fractures of the calcaneum can be extremely painful. The incidence of compartment syndrome with these fractures is high.

Extraarticular fractures are less common and usually are associated with a rotational mechanism as well as an axial load. Included are fractures of the tuberosity, the sustentaculum tali, anterior process avulsion, and extraarticular oblique body fractures. Most nondisplaced fractures can be treated conservatively with a posterior slab, crutches, and early orthopedic consultation.

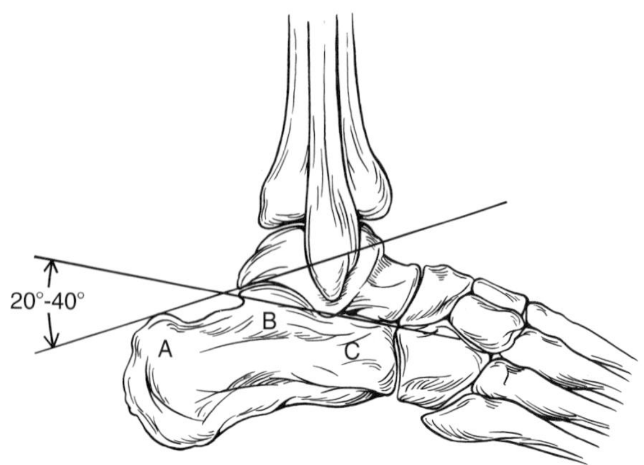

FIG. 269-3. Boehler's angle is formed by two lines, one between the posterior tuberosity **(A)** and the apex of the posterior facet **(B)**, and the other between the apex of the posterior facet **(B)** and the apex of the anterior process **(C)**. An angle less than 20 degrees suggests a calcaneal compression fracture.

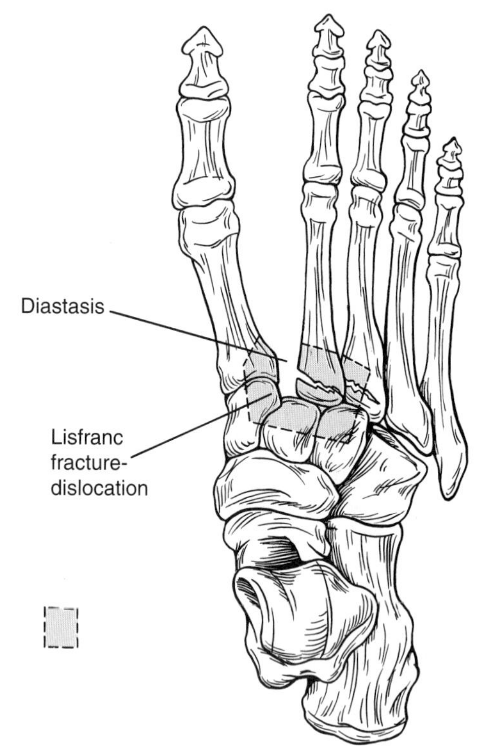

FIG. 269-4. Fracture of the base of the second metatarsal.

MIDFOOT Isolated fractures of the navicular, cuboid, and cuneiforms are uncommon and are difficult to identify on radiograph. Fractures of the navicular are most common and can involve the tuberosity, the dorsal surface, and the body. Isolated fractures of the cuboid and cuneiforms are extremely rare, and an associated injury to the Lisfranc joint should be sought. Most isolated injuries of the tarsal bones are treated conservatively.

The six-bone tarsometatarsal complex is known as the Lisfranc joint. Injuries to this joint are not uncommon, and unfortunately up to 20 percent of these injuries are missed in the ED.[6] The force required and the mechanism of injury are varied and can range from a seemingly minor rotational force to severe axial load as seen in an automobile accident. The great majority of injuries to the Lisfranc joint are associated with fractures, usually of the metatarsals, the cuboid, or the cuneiforms. A fracture of the base of the second metatarsal is pathognomonic of a disruption of the ligamentous complex (Fig. 269-4). The Lisfranc injury is classified by the direction of the dislocation. A divergent dislocation describes metatarsals splayed in both medial and lateral directions, usually between the first and second metatarsals. In isolated dislocations, one or more metatarsals are displaced from the rest. In homolateral dislocations, all five metatarsals are displaced in the same direction, either laterally or medially. Suspect this injury if there is point tenderness over the midfoot or when there is laxity between the first and second metatarsals in a dorsal-plantar direction. Diagnosis is made radiographically on the AP view when there is more then a 1-mm gap between the bases of the first and second metatarsals. Weight-bearing radiographs may be required to make the diagnosis. Injuries to the Lisfranc joint frequently require open reduction and fixation or percutaneous placement of Kirschner wires and non-weight-bearing for several weeks. These injuries are complicated by pedal artery damage in the short term and degenerative arthritis and chronic pain in the long term.

FOREFOOT Metatarsal fractures are most often associated with a crush or more occasionally with a twisting injury. Metatarsal fractures are divided into shaft and neck fractures. Nondisplaced shaft injuries are usually treated conservatively with either a walking cast or an

TABLE 269-2 Timing of Consultation for Foot Injuries

Immediate Consultation in Emergency Department	Deferred Consultation*	Within 1 Week	Pro Re Nata
All open fractures	Extraarticular calcaneous fractures	Avulsion fractures calcaneous	Pseudo-Jones fracture
All fracture dislocations	First metatarsal fractures	Avulsion fractures tarsal	Phalangeal fractures
Major talar neck and body fractures†	Displaced metatarsal shaft	Metatarsal fractures	Phalangeal dislocations
Intraarticular calcaneous fractures†	True Jones fractures	Pediatric metatarsal fractures	Soft tissue injuries
All Lisfranc injuries†	Tendon ruptures and lacerations	Ruptured plantar fascia	
Most gunshot wounds	Retained foreign bodies		
Suspected compartment syndrome			

* Implies that communication is established at time of diagnosis and that the specific time of consultation has been set.
† Consultation can be delayed in the emergency department in fractures without neurovascular compromise and with appropriate splinting.

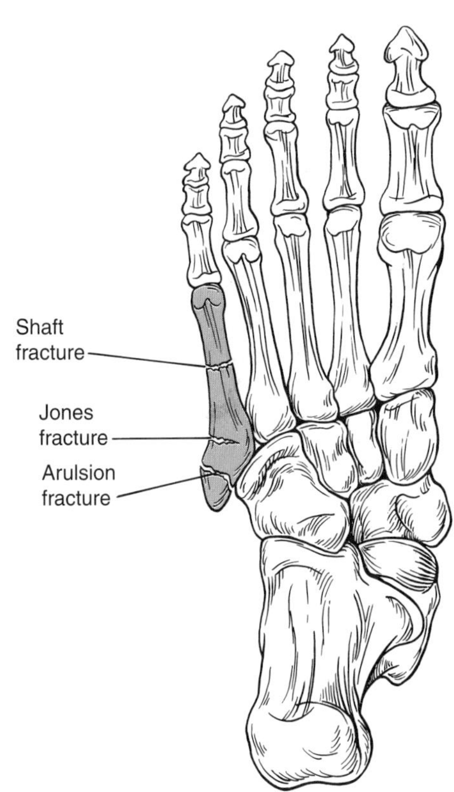

FIG. 269-5. Fractures of the fifth metatarsal.

orthopedic shoe. An exception is a fracture of the first metatarsal shaft. Keep this injury non-weight-bearing. Likewise, displaced shaft fractures of the middle metatarsals can be treated with closed reduction, followed by immobilization in a cast and non-weight-bearing for 6 weeks. A displaced first metatarsal fracture will often require an open reduction and fixation. Metatarsal neck fractures generally follow the treatment of shaft fractures, but postreduction instability of displaced neck fractures is not uncommon and open fixation is sometimes required.

Fifth metatarsal fractures are the most common of the metatarsal fractures. Shaft fractures usually can be treated conservatively, as above. The Jones fracture is described as a transverse fracture through the base of the fifth metatarsal 15 to 31 mm distal to the proximal part of the metatarsal. This fracture is frequently complicated by nonunion or malunion and should be treated with a non-weight-bearing cast for 6 weeks. The ''pseudo-Jones'' is an avulsion fracture of the tuberosity of the base and can be treated with a cast shoe. (Fig. 269-5).

Most nondisplaced phalangeal fractures can be treated conservatively with ''buddy taping'' and, occasionally, a cast shoe. Address the patient's analgesic need and arrange orthopedic consultation on a prn basis. Advise against prolonged ambulation or standing in the first week. Displaced fractures can be manipulated into position by using a digital block and manual traction. Some authors advocate open reduction of some displaced fractures, especially of the big toe.

Most dislocations of the forefoot involve the the distal interphalangeal and posterior interphalangeal joints of the second through fifth toes. These injuries can be easily reduced by manual traction and treated with buddy taping as needed. Dislocations of the big toe are rare, occasionally difficult to reduce, and require walking-cast immobilization for 3 weeks.

OPEN FRACTURES Open fractures of the foot require immediate orthopedic consultation. In the interim, protect open fractures from further contamination by applying a wet, sterile dressing over the wound with a gauze roll. Splint the injury until definitive treatment is available. Consider tetanus immunoglobulin if the wound is grossly contaminated. The antibiotic of choice is cephalexin, and add an aminoglycoside if the wound is grossly contaminated. Consider clindamycin for patients with a penicillin allergy. If there is going to be a significant delay to operative management, the wound should be irrigated.

PEDIATRIC INJURIES

Fractures of the foot are rare in children, presumably due to the flexibility of the immature bone and cartilage. Comparison radiographs may be of some benefit in the evaluation of these injuries. Generally, most fractures occur in the metatarsals, and these injuries are usually treated conservatively. Orthopedic consultation can be deferred, with the exception of injuries to the first metatarsal, and complications are usually minimal. Fractures of the calcaneum, talus, tarsals, and phalanges are rare. Injuries to the base of the second metatarsal suggest that a significant injury has occurred, and immediate orthopedic consultation is required. Crush injuries of the pediatric foot should be treated with care; compartment syndrome is more common in children than adults, even without fracture.[7]

TIMING OF CONSULTATION

Like ankle injuries, no set of rigid rules for the timing of orthopedic consultation exists to guide emergency physicians for each specific foot injury. In Table 269-2 a general guideline is set forth. Timing of consultation will vary with local preferences.

EMERGENCY DEPARTMENT TREATMENT ISSUES

Analgesia

The need for analgesia should always be addressed by the emergency physician. As individual perception of pain varies, a fifth metatarsal tuberosity fracture may require acetaminophen and a cast shoe in most patients, whereas others will require hydrocodone or oxycodone with acetominophen. Patients who are in significant distress, or who should be kept NPO because of anticipated surgery, require parenteral analgesia.

Immobilization

Most fractures of the foot can be splinted by a posterior slab or a Jones bandage (the appropriate method of application is discussed in Chapter 268, ''Ankle Injuries''). Cast shoes, variably called orthopedic, Reece, or post-op shoes, are useful in splinting minor foot fractures when the patient is allowed to bear weight on the injured extremity. Cast shoes can also be applied over a posterior splint to allow weight bearing. Apply an appropriately sized piece of felt or cotton padding between the two phalanges when they are being buddy taped.

Cryotherapy

Ice packs have been shown to limit swelling and decrease pain.[8]

REFERENCES

1. Stein RE: Radiological aspects of the tarsometatarsal joints. *Foot Ankle* 3:286, 1983.
2. Laughlin TJ, Armstrong DG, Caporusso J, et al: Soft tissue and bone infections from puncture wounds in children. *West J Med* 166:126, 1997.
3. Boucree JB, Gabriel RA, Lezine-Hanna JT: Gunshot wounds to the foot. *Orthop Clin North Am* 26:191, 1995.
4. Anger DM, Ledbetter BR, Stasikelis PJ, et al: Injuries of the foot related to the use of lawn mowers. *J Bone Joint Surg* [*Am*] 77:719, 1995.

5. Lavery LA, Harkless LB, Ashry HR, et al: Puncture wounds: Normal laboratory values in the face of severe infection in diabetics and non-diabetics. *Am J Med* 101:521, 1996.
6. Englanoff G, Anglin D, Hutson HR: Lisfranc fracture-dislocation: A frequently missed diagnosis in the emergency department. *Ann Emerg Med* 26:229, 1995.
7. Silas SI, Herzenberg JE, Meyerson MS, et al: Compartment syndrome of the foot in children. *J Bone Joint Surg* [*Am*] 77:356, 1995.
8. Ogilvie-Harris DJ, Gilbart M: Treatment modalities for soft tissue injuries of the ankle: A critical review. *Clin J Sport Med* 5:175, 1995.

COMPARTMENT SYNDROMES

Ernest Ruiz

Compartment syndromes are serious and often insidious problems that must be considered in the emergency department (ED) on a frequent basis. The incidence of compartment syndromes overall is unknown, but the conditions that can cause it are myriad and common. Early diagnosis and treatment are curative, whereas delay results in permanent and severe disability. An understanding of the pathophysiology and the early signs of the process is crucial if an emergency physician is to intercede appropriately. Compartment syndromes occurring in the limbs are the subject of this chapter.

PATHOPHYSIOLOGY

Compartment syndromes are due to increased pressure within closed tissue spaces that compromises the flow of blood through nutrient capillaries in muscles and nerves. The complex relationships between time, Starling forces, systemic and venous pressure, and reperfusion injury are not completely understood. The clinical variables of each case make a definitive explanation of how capillary blood flow is compromised a difficult exercise. However, a common factor is elevated tissue pressure. Normal tissue pressure is about zero and usually less than 10 mmHg. Capillary blood flow within the compartment is compromised at pressures greater than about 20 mmHg, and muscle and nerves are at risk for ischemic necrosis at pressures greater than about 30 to 40 mmHg. Of the tissues within the compartments, nerve is most sensitive, followed by muscle tissue. Blood flow through arteries, arterioles, and collaterals is not compromised significantly at these pressures. Nevertheless, tissues within the compartment that are dependent on the nutrient capillaries become ischemic and then necrotic if the compartment pressure is not reduced promptly. By the time that distal pulses are reduced, muscle necrosis has occurred. Ischemic muscles hurt, and this pain is exacerbated by active muscle contraction and by passive stretching of the muscle.

An increase in compartmental pressure can be caused by (1) compression of the compartment, for example, by burn eschar, a circumferential cast, or a pneumatic pressure garment; and (2) by a volume increase within the compartment due to hematoma and edema. Direct trauma with resulting bleeding and edema is probably the most common cause, but overexertion (shin splints) and limb compression during recumbency as a result of alcohol or drug overdose are also common causes. Mubarak and Hargens[1] developed a classification of the acute compartment syndromes (Table 270-1) listing the myriad of possible causes. Their text is highly recommended for readers wishing to learn more about this topic.

COMPARTMENTS AT RISK

Virtually any muscle mass invested in fascia is at risk, given the right conditions.

TABLE 270-1 Classification of Acute Compartment Syndromes

Decreased compartment size
Constrictive dressings and casts
Closure of fascial defects
Thermal injuries and frostbite
Increased compartment contents
Primarily edematous accumulation
Postischemic swelling
Arterial injuries
Arterial thrombosis or embolism
Reconstructive vascular and bypass surgery
Replantation
Prolonged tourniquet time
Arterial spasm
Cardiac catheterization and angiography
Ergotamine ingestion
Prolonged immobilization with limb compression
Drug overdose with limb compression
General anesthesia with knee-chest position
Thermal injuries and frostbite
Exertion
Venous disease
Venomous snakebite
Primarily hemorrhagic accumulation
Hereditary bleeding disorders (e.g., hemophilia)
Anticoagulant therapy
Vessel laceration
Combination of edematous and hemorrhagic accumulation
Fractures
Tibia
Forearm
Elbow (e.g., supracondylar)
Femur
Soft tissue injury
Osteotomies (e.g., tibia)
Miscellaneous
Intravenous infiltration (e.g., blood or saline)
Popliteal cyst
Long leg brace

Source: From Mubarak and Hargens,[1] with permission.

Upper Extremity

The upper arm has an anterior and a posterior compartment. The anterior compartment contains the biceps-brachialis muscle and the ulnar, median, and radial nerves (Fig. 270-1). The posterior compartment contains the triceps muscle. Fortunately, the compartments of the upper arm are relatively roomy, and compartment syndromes are uncommon in this location. The forearm has volar and dorsal compartments that are further subdivided into smaller compartments by investing fascia at mid-forearm (Fig. 270-2). The volar compartment contains wrist and finger flexors, and the dorsal compartment contains wrist and finger extenders. The hand has thenar and hypothenar compartments, containing the intrinsic muscles of the thumb and little finger, respectively. The interosseous muscles of the hand are contained in their own compartments (Fig. 270-3).

Lower Extremity

There are three gluteal compartments of the buttocks. One contains the tensor muscle of the fascia lata, another the gluteus medius and minimus, and the third the gluteus maximus. The sciatic nerve lies adjacent to the gluteus maximus and can be compressed by it.

The thigh has three compartments: the anterior, medial, and posterior. The anterior compartment contains the vastus lateralis, the vastus

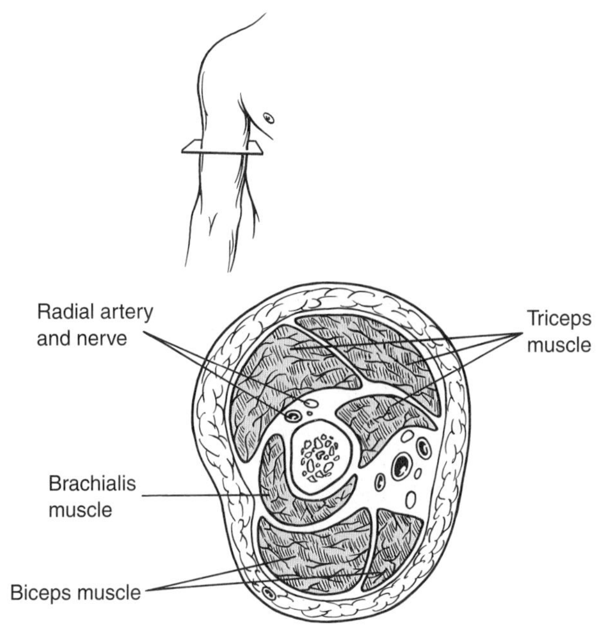

FIG. 270-1. The biceps-brachialis (anterior) and triceps (posterior) compartments of the right arm.

intermedius, and the vastus medialis muscles, as well as the sartorius and rectus femoris muscles. The femoral artery and nerve also traverse the anterior thigh compartment. The medial compartment contains the adductor longus, the adductor brevis, and the adductor magnus muscles, plus the gracilis muscle. The posterior compartment contains the semimembranosus, the semitendinosus, and the biceps femoris muscles. The sciatic nerve also traverses the posterior compartment.

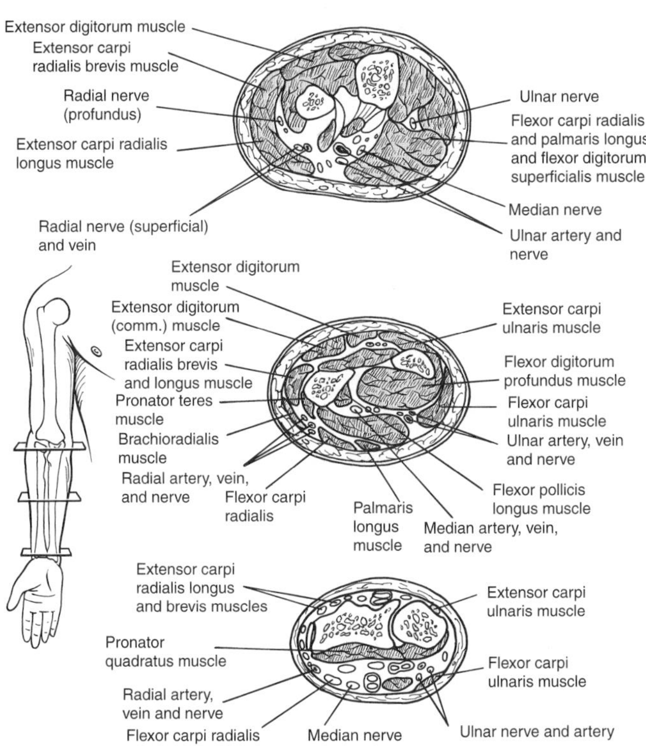

FIG. 270-2. Forearm compartments: transverse sections through the right forearm at various levels.

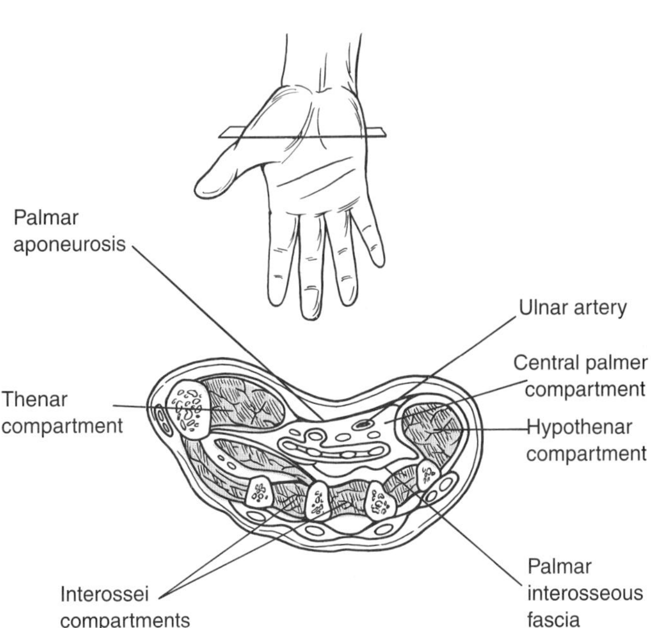

FIG. 270-3. Hand compartments: transverse section through the right hand.

The leg has four compartments (Fig. 270-4). The anterior compartment, the compartment most frequently involved by this syndrome, contains the tibialis anterior muscle and the extensor muscles of the toes—the extensor hallucis longus and the extensor digitorum longus muscles. The anterior tibial artery and the deep peroneal nerve are also located in this compartment. The lateral compartment, which is frequently involved when the anterior compartment is involved, contains the peroneous longus and brevis muscles, as well as the superficial peroneal nerve. The deep posterior compartment contains the tibialis posterior muscle, the flexor digitorum longus muscle, and the flexor hallucis longus muscle. It also contains the posterior tibial artery and the tibial nerve. The superficial posterior compartment contains the gastrocnemius muscle, the soleus muscle, and the sural nerve.

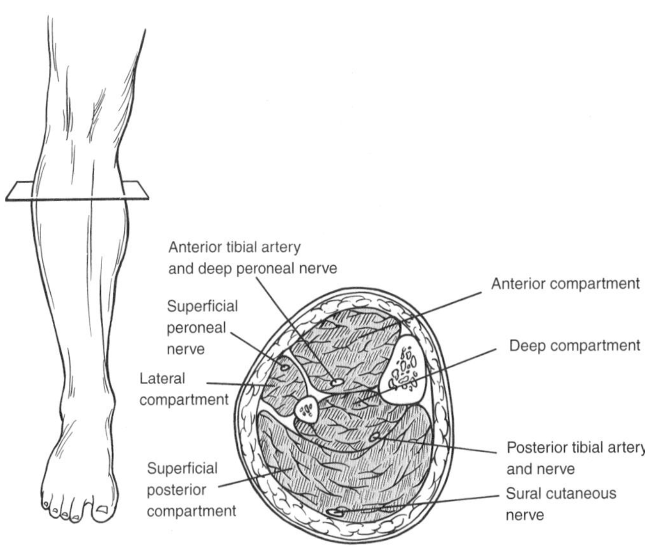

FIG. 270-4. The four compartments of the leg.

TABLE 270-2 Symptomatology of Acute Compartment Syndromes

Upper extremity	
Upper arm	
Anterior compartment	Pain on active and passive flexion and extension of the elbow Hypoesthesia in the distribution of the median, ulnar, and radial nerves
Posterior compartment	Pain on active and passive flexion and extension of the elbow Hypoesthesia over the dorsum of the hand
Forearm	
Volar compartment	Pain on active and passive flexion and extension of the fingers Hypoesthesia over the palm of the hand
Dorsal compartment	Pain on active and passive flexion and extension of the fingers
Hand	
Thenar and hypothenar compartments	Pain on thumb and little finger opposition
Interosseous compartments	Pain on abduction and adduction of the fingers
Lower extremity	
Gluteal compartments	Pain on active and passive flexion and extension of the hip Sciatic nerve paresthesias
Thigh compartments	Pain on active and passive flexion and extension of the knee Sciatic nerve paresthesias with posterior compartment involvement
Leg	
Anterior compartment	Pain on active and passive dorsiflexion and plantar flexion of the foot Hypoesthesia of the first web space
Lateral compartment	Pain on active and passive eversion and inversion of the foot Hypoesthesia of the first web space
Superficial posterior compartment	Pain on active and passive plantar flexion and dorsiflexion of the foot Hypoesthesia of the lateral foot
Deep posterior compartment	Pain on dorsiflexing the toes and everting the foot Hypoesthesia of the plantar surface of the foot

DIAGNOSIS

The history, including mechanism of injury, is very important, since many patients at risk for the syndrome are severely ill or injured and cannot relate whether they are experiencing pain. Palpation of the compartments in question may or may not reveal tenseness and swelling; when in doubt, the resuscitating physician should measure tissue pressure.

Alert and intact patients will virtually always relate that they are experiencing severe and constant pain over the involved compartment. Palpation of the compartment will also elicit pain. Active contraction of the involved muscles will increase the pain, as will passive stretching of the muscles (Table 270-2). Hypoesthesia resulting from compromise of nerves traversing the involved compartment appears at about the same time as muscle weakness and pain.

Possible compartment syndromes associated with injuries such as fractures or penetrating wounds should prompt an immediate surgical consultation, since the presence of a compartment syndrome may influence subsequent treatment choices.

Pressure Measurement

In patients without a clear need for surgical consultation, measuring the compartment pressures in the ED assures safe patient disposition and management. Compartment pressure can be quickly and easily measured using a commercially available battery-powered monitor [Stryker STIC Monitor (Stryker Instruments, Kalamazoo, MI) or Ace Intracompartmental Pressure Monitor (Ace Medical Company, Los Angeles, CA)] that has a self-contained pressure transducer and readout. Compartment pressure is measured after careful aseptic preparation, insertion of the side-ported 18-guage needle into the compartment, and injection of a small volume of sterile saline while keeping the apparatus level. There is a brief overshoot as resistance to flow and inertia is overcome, but within a second of time a plateau of pressure will be reached that is the compartment pressure in mmHg. Always check the accuracy of the transducer by filling the needle and transducer with saline and holding it level and open to the atmosphere. It should read zero. Measure the pressure twice, whether normal or high, to assure that the needle had not become lodged in fibrous tissue.

When an electronic pressure transducer and monitor, as is used for vascular pressure measurement, are available, they can be used as follows: (1) Attach a short length of intravenous (IV) extension tubing to a stopcock and then to a pressure transducer. (2) Fill the transducer and tubing with sterile saline. Adjust the height of the transducer to the level of the compartment in question. Zero the transducer with the tubing open to the atmosphere at the level of the compartment. (3) After antiseptic skin preparation, fill a 16-gauge catheter over needle with sterile saline. Insert it into the compartment and remove the metallic needle. Attach the IV tubing to the catheter. (4) Inject a small quantity (less than 1 mL) of saline through the transducer and into the compartment while observing the monitor. A small overshoot will be seen and then the pressure will plateau at true compartment pressure. Wilson and colleagues[2] found this system as accurate as the Stryker device. Uppal and coworkers[3] describe a system that uses the Intravenous Alarm Control (IVAC) pump as a monitor. EDs that use the IVAC pump may wish to study his report.

The technique of Whitesides and colleagues[4] for compartment pressure measurement had the advantage of requiring only basic materials available in every ED. Unfortunately, the required three-way stopcock is now hard to find, having been replaced by two-way stopcocks for most applications. Electronic pressure transducers have become standard pieces of equipment in the ED and are easier to use. However, those anticipating situations lacking electronic monitoring should obtain the supplies and be familiar with the Whitesides method. This requires a 20-mL syringe, a three-way stopcock, two IV extension tubes, a Luer male blood pressure cuff adaptor, a bedside mercury manometer, a small bottle of sterile saline, and an 18-gauge needle. Assemble the apparatus as shown in Fig. 270-5. The bottle of saline is vented with an 18-gauge needle, and the needle on the apparatus is then inserted into the saline and saline withdrawn until the IV extension is half-filled. When removing the needle from the saline bottle, it is important to avoid getting any air in the needle. The needle is then placed in the compartment and the apparatus kept at the level of the needle and the stopcock turned so that it is open in all three directions. Two people are required for this test. One watches the manometer while the other slowly and gently depresses the plunger in the syringe while watching the saline meniscus. When the meniscus moves toward the patient, the operator notifies the manometer watcher, who notes the reading at that instant. In this way, only a minute amount of saline is injected into the compartment. As with the other methods, measure the pressure twice.

Measure the patient's systolic and diastolic systemic pressure during the time that compartment pressure is measured, as some surgeons use the mean arterial pressure[5] or diastolic pressure[4] in combination with compartment pressure to decide when emergency fasciotomy is needed. Other surgeons prefer to operate on clinical grounds only. In

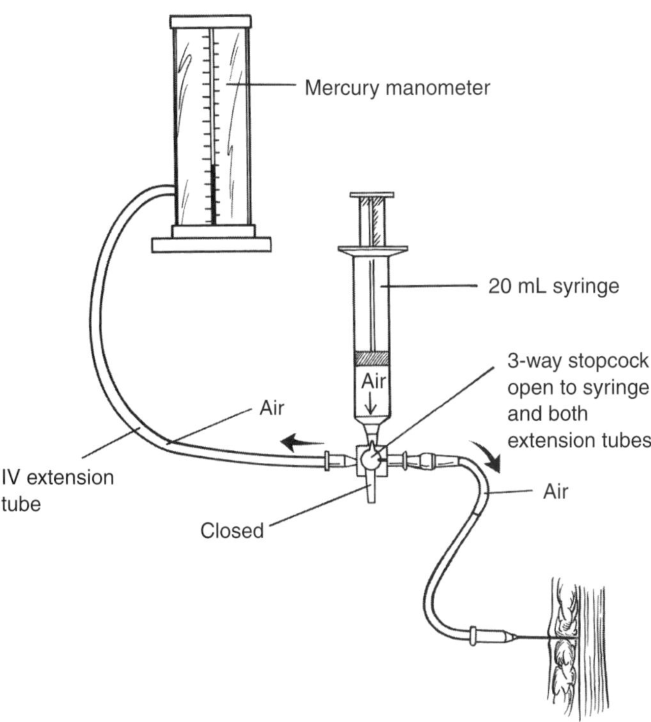

FIG. 270-5. The Whitesides method. Tissue pressure is measured by determining the amount of pressure with this closed system that is required to overcome the pressure within the closed compartment while injecting only a minute quantity of saline.

general, a compartment pressure of 35 to 40 mmHg is considered grounds for emergency fasciotomy.

Needle Placement

In general, the needle is placed where the patient describes the most pain or in the location that is most tense to palpation on examination. If the compartment in question is in a deep position or is small, as in the intrinsic muscle compartments of the hand, many surgeons will opt to operate on purely clinical grounds. The forearm is another region that can be difficult because of nervous and vascular structures in the midst of muscle bellys and numerous fascial septa. An accepted technique when the patient has a forearm fracture is to make volar and dorsal punctures adjacent to the fracture, at the carpal tunnel, and a volar puncture proximal to the fracture.[6] Of course, surgical consultation would be in order. The deep posterior compartment of the leg is reached by inserting the needle behind the medial surface of the tibia and directing it horizontally to the center of the leg.

Complications

Injecting too much saline into the compartment can result in false high readings. Inserting the needle into an artery or vein in a hypocoagulable patient can result in the development of a compartment syndrome. Injecting air into the tissues can confuse x-ray interpretation, adding open fracture and gas-forming organism infection to the differential diagnosis.

MANAGEMENT

Compartment pressures between 15 and 20 mmHg are problematic. If the problem is acute and the patient is reliable, the patient can be told to return for repeat measurement if symptoms do not improve. A pressure of 20 mmHg can be damaging if it persists for several hours; therefore, admission or surgical consultation will be needed for unreliable patients. Pressures greater than 20 mmHg demand admission and surgical consultation. A pressure of 30 to 40 mmHg is generally considered grounds for emergent fasciotomy in the operating room. Fasciotomy is accomplished by making a longitudinal skin incision over the compartment. The underlying fascia is then split the length of the compartment, allowing the contained muscle to expand. Do not recommend ice cooling, because muscle perfusion may be decreased by it. Do not recommend elevation of the limb, because the resulting decrease in arterial perfusion pressure may also decrease muscle perfusion. Bed rest would provide the best chances for improvement when conservative management seems to be in order.

REFERENCES

1. Mubarak SJ, Hargens AR: *Compartment Syndromes and Volkman's Contracture*. Philadelphia, WB Saunders, 1981.
2. Wilson SC, Vrahas MS, Berson L, Paul EM: A simple method to measure compartment pressures using an intravenous catheter. *Orthopedics* 20:403, 1997.
3. Uppal GS, Smith RC, Sherk HH, Mooar P: Accurate compartment pressure measurement using the Intravenous Alarm Control (IVAC) pump. *J Orthop Trauma* 6:87, 1992.
4. Whitesides TE, Haney TC, Morimoto K, Harada H: Tissue pressure measurements as a determinant for the need of fasciotomy. *Clin Orthop* 113:43, 1975.
5. Heppenstall RB, Sapega AA, Scott R, et al: The compartment syndrome: An experimental and clinical study of muscular energy metabolism using phosphorous nuclear magnetic resonance spectroscopy. *Clin Orthop* 226:138, 1988.
6. Royle SG: The role of tissue pressure recording in forearm fractures in children. *Injury* 23:549, 1992.

RHABDOMYOLYSIS

Francis L. Counselman

Rhabdomyolysis was first described in the Book of Numbers in the Old Testament. During the flight from Egypt, a number of Israelites experienced symptoms of rhabdomyolysis after eating hemlock-seed-fed quail.[1] In the early 1900s, the clinical syndrome of muscle pain, weakness, and dark urine became known as Meyer-Betz disease.[2] In the 1940s, Bywaters and Beall described acute renal failure as a complication of rhabdomyolysis observed in Londoners suffering from crush injuries during the German blitz.[3] Today, we realize rhabdomyolysis is a complication of a variety of disease processes and injury.

PATHOPHYSIOLOGY

Rhabdomyolysis is a syndrome characterized by injury to skeletal muscle with subsequent release of intracellular contents. These contents include myoglobin, creatine phosphokinase (CPK), aldolase, lactate dehydrogenase (LDH), serum glutamic-oxaloacetic transaminase, and potassium. Although numerous causes of rhabdomyolysis have been described, the common terminal event appears to involve the disruption of the Na^+,K^+-ATPase pump and calcium transport, resulting in increased intracellular calcium and subsequent muscle cell necrosis.

Several classifications systems have been developed to characterize the numerous causes of rhabdomyolysis. None of these systems are universally recognized, and each has its own limitations. In addition, many patients have multiple causes of rhabdomyolysis (e.g., alcohol abuse and hypokalemia). Table 271-1 lists the various causes. In general, the most common causes of rhabdomyolysis appear to be

TABLE 271-1 Causes of Rhabdomyolysis

Direct muscle injury
Crush
Electrical injury
Lightning injury

Drugs of abuse
Amphetamines
Caffeine
Cocaine
Ethanol
Gasoline (sniffing)
Heroin
LSD
Marijuana
Mescaline
Methamphetamines
Opiates
Phencyclidine (PCP)
Polyweed
Toluene

Excessive muscular activity
Acute dystonia
Contact sports
Delirium tremens
Isometric exercise
Lethal catatonia
Psychosis
Seizures
Sports/basic training
Status asthmaticus

Genetic disorders
Involving carbohydrate metabolism
- Adenine diaminose deficiency
- α-Glucosidase deficiency
- Amylo-1,6-glucosidase deficiency
- Cytochrome disturbances
- Myophosphorylase deficiency
- Phosphofructokinase deficiency
- Phosphoglycerate kinase deficiency
- Phosphoglycerate mutase deficiency

Involving lipid metabolism
- Carnitine deficiency
- Carnitine palmitoyltransferase deficiency

Immunologic diseases
Dermatomyositis
Polymyositis

Infection
Bacterial
- Gas gangrene
- Group A β-hemolytic strep
- Legionnaires' disease
- *Salmonella*
- Septic shock
- *Shigella*
- *Staphylococcus aureus*
- *Streptococcus pneumoniae*

Viral
- Coxsackie virus
- Cytomegalovirus
- Echovirus
- Epstein-Barr virus
- Hepatitis
- Herpes simplex virus
- HIV
- Influenza A and B
- Rotavirus

Rickettsial
- Rocky Mountain spotted fever

Parasites
- Trichinosis

Miscellaneous

Ischemic injury
Compartment syndrome
Compression
Sickle cell disease
Vascular occlusion (embolism, thrombus)
Vasculitis

Medications
Amphotericin B
Antihistamines
Azathioprine
Barbiturates
Benzodiazepines
Butyrophenones
Chlorpromazine
Cimetidine
Clofibrate
Codeine
Colchicine
Corticosteroids
Cotrimoxazole
Epsilon aminocaproic acid
Inhalation anesthetics
Isoniazid
Lindane
Lithium
Lovastatin
Methadone
Monoamine oxidase inhibitors
Narcotics
Neuroleptic agents
Organic solvents
Pentamidine
Phenothiazines
Phenylpropanolamine
Phenytoin
Procainamide
Quinine
Salicylates
Serotonergic agents
Succinylcholine
Theophylline
Tricyclic antidepressants
Trimethoprim-sulfamethoxazole
Vasopressin

Metabolic Disorders
Diabetic ketoacidosis
Hyperaldosteronism
Hypernatremia
Hypokalemia
Hyponatremia
Hypophosphatemia
Hypothyroidism
Nonketotic hyperosmolar coma
Thyroid storm

Temperature related
Heatstroke
Hyperthermia
Hypothermia
Malignant hyperthermia
Neuroleptic malignant syndrome

Toxins

Brown spider bite	Isopropyl alcohol
Carbon monoxide	Mercuric chloride
Centipede bite	Methanol
Cyanide	Snake venom
Ethylene glycol	Tetanus toxin
Haff disease	Typhoid toxin
Hymenoptera sting	Water hemlock

alcohol and drug abuse, toxin ingestion, trauma, infection, strenuous physical activity, and heat-related illness.

Consider hereditary causes in patients with a history of recurrent rhabdomyolysis and exercise intolerance. Patients in coma are at risk for development of rhabdomyolysis due to immobility from unrelieved pressure upon gravity-dependent body parts. In one study, the most common positions leading to rhabdomyolysis were the lateral decubitus, lithotomy, sitting, knee-chest, and prone positions.[4] Alcohol consumption can result in rhabdomyolysis secondary to coma-induced muscle compression and a direct toxic effect. Nutritional compromise and hypophosphatemia, both common in alcoholics, increase the risk of rhabdomyolysis. Alcohol is considered to be a causative or contributory factor in approximately 20 percent of all cases of rhabdomyolysis.[5] Drugs of abuse that have commonly been implicated in acute rhabomyolysis include cocaine, amphetamines, LSD, heroin, and phencyclidine (PCP). Common medications associated with the development of rhabdomyolysis include diuretics, narcotics, theophylline, corticosteroids, benzodiazepines, phenothiazines, and tricyclic antidepressants.

Viral and bacterial infections have been known to cause rhabdomyolysis. Strenuous physical activity, as seen in athletes, military recruits, and outdoor laborers, is a common cause of rhabdomyolysis. Factors that further increase the risk in this group of patients include poor physical conditioning, inadequate fluid intake, high ambient temperatures, and high humidity levels.[6]

CLINICAL FEATURES

The presenting symptoms of rhabdomyolysis are usually acute in onset and include myalgias, stiffness, weakness, malaise, low-grade fever, and dark (usually brown) urine. Symptoms relating to the musculoskeletal system, however, may be present in only 271 percent of cases.[7] Nausea, vomiting, abdominal pain, and tachycardia can occur in severe rhabdomyolysis. On occasion, mental-status changes are present secondary to urea induced encephalopathy. Swelling and tenderness of the involved muscle groups and hemorrhagic discoloration of overlying skin may be observed, but only in a minority of cases. Muscle swelling may not become apparent until after rehydration with intravenous (IV) fluids. The muscle groups involved may be localized or diffuse, depending on the etiology. Commonly, the postural muscles of the thighs, calves, and the lower back are involved. An important point to remember is that acute rhabdomyolysis may be present without any of these signs or symptoms, and the patient may have essentially normal findings on physical examination. For this reason, the diagnosis is often made only after soliciting a historical clue (e.g., recent cocaine use) or finding an elevated serum CPK or the presence of myoglobinuria on routine laboratory testing.

DIAGNOSIS

An elevated serum CPK level is the most sensitive and reliable indicator of muscle injury. The degree of CPK elevation correlates with the amount of muscle injury and the severity of illness, but not the development of renal failure or other morbidity. Most authors require a fivefold or greater increase in serum CPK, without cardiac or brain injury, as the requirement for making the diagnosis of rhabdomyolysis. In general, serum CPK begins to rise approximately 2 to 12 h after the onset of muscle injury, peaks in 24 to 72 h, and then declines at the relatively constant rate of 39 percent of the previous day's value. Ongoing muscle necrosis should be suspected in patients with elevated CPK values that fail to decrease in this manner. The isoenzyme CPK-MM (found in skeletal and cardiac muscle) is responsible for the majority of the elevation in serum CPK. The CPK-MB fraction (found primarily in cardiac, but also skeletal, muscle) may also be elevated, but should not exceed 5 percent of the total CPK level.

Myoglobin is an oxygen-binding protein found in skeletal and cardiac muscle and involved in oxidative metabolism. Myoglobin elevation occurs before CPK elevation following muscle injury and then is rapidly cleared from the plasma through renal excretion and metabolism to bilirubin. Myoglobin enters the urine when the plasma concentration exceeds 1.5 mg/dL and causes the typical reddish brown discoloration when urine myoglobin exceeds 100 mg/dL.[7] Since myoglobin contains heme, qualitative tests such as the dipstick (utilizing the orthotoluidine reaction) does not differentiate between hemoglobin and myoglobin. Therefore, suspect myoglobinuria when the urine dipstick is positive for blood, but no red blood cells are present on microscopic examination. Radioimmunoassay is only slightly more sensitive than the dipstick technique in identifying myoglobinuria, but usually not necessary. Since myoglobin levels may return to normal within 1 to 6 h after the onset of muscle necrosis, the absence of an elevated serum myoglobin or the absence of myoglobinuria does not exclude the diagnosis. In one study, 26 percent of patients with rhabdomyolysis did not have myoglobinuria.[7]

Other laboratory studies may be useful to identify the common complications of rhabdomyolysis, as well as the underlying etiology. Electrolytes, calcium, phosphorus, and uric acid levels should be determined in order to identify hyperkalemia, abnormal calcium and phosphorus levels, and hyperuricemia. A urinalysis should be performed on all patients. Serum creatinine and blood urea nitrogen (BUN) are useful as a baseline and to identify acute renal failure. Since disseminated intravascular coagulation (DIC) is a complication, all patients suspected of rhabdomyolysis should have a baseline CBC and DIC screen (e.g., prothrombin time, partial thromboplastin time, fibrin split products, and fibrinogen). Other common laboratory findings in rhabdomyolysis include elevated levels of aldolase, LDH, urea, creatine, and aminotransferases. Magnetic resonance imaging (MRI) has recently been shown to be highly effective in localizing rhabdomyolysis and is more sensitive than computed tomography or ultrasound in detecting abnormal muscle.[8] The high intensity lesions on T2-weighted MRI are most likely due to edema and inflammation of the muscles, rather than to permanent histologic changes.[9] Further laboratory testing to identify the underlying cause(s) of rhabdomyolysis should be based on the medical history and clinical presentation.

COMPLICATIONS

The complications of rhabdomyolysis include acute renal failure (ARF), metabolic derangements, DIC, and mechanical complications (e.g., compartment syndrome or peripheral neuropathy) (see Table 271-2). ARF is the most serious complication of rhabdomyolysis. Although rhabdomyolysis is thought to account for 5 to 8 percent of all cases of ARF,[10] the incidence of this complication in rhabdomyolysis is less clear. It is estimated that between 0[11] and 271 percent[12] of patients with rhabdomyolysis develop ARF, with 33 percent the most often quoted figure.[7] This wide range probably reflects the multifactorial

TABLE 271-2 Complications of Rhabdomyolysis

Acute renal failure
Metabolic derangements
Hypercalcemia (late)
Hyperkalemia
Hyperphosphatemia
Hyperuricemia
Hypocalcemia
Hypophosphatemia (late)
Disseminated intravascular coagulation
Mechanical complications
Compartment syndrome
Peripheral neuropathy

etiology necessary for the development of ARF. Factors known to contribute to rhabdomyolysis-induced ARF include hypovolemia, acidosis/aciduria, tubular obstruction, and the nephrotoxic effects of myoglobin. Renal tubular obstruction occurs secondary to precipitation of uric acid and myoglobin. Ferrihemate, the breakdown product of myoglobin, is responsible for the direct toxic effect on the kidneys. This effect, however, appears to occur only in the presence of hypovolemia and aciduria (pH < 5.6). The ARF may be oliguric (most common) or nonoliguric. The need for dialysis, serum potassium and calcium levels, and mortality rates appear to be similar for both rhabdomyolysis-induced ARF and non-rhabdomyolysis-induced ARF. Patients with rhabdomyolysis-induced ARF, however, do have higher serum uric acid and anion gap levels.[7] Neither the presence of myoglobinuria nor the degree of CPK elevation is predictive of which patients are at risk for developing ARF.

The serum potassium level is elevated in 10 to 40 percent of cases, due to release of potassium from injured skeletal muscle.[7,13] Renal function, however, appears to be the most important determinant of the degree of elevation. Hyperkalemia can be a significant complication of rhabdomyolysis if acute renal failure occurs.

Elevated uric acid levels can occur, especially in crush injures, due to release of muscle adenosine nucleotides and subsequent conversion to uric acid by the liver. Uric acid levels usually correlate with serum CPK levels.

Initially in rhabdomyolysis, serum phosphorus levels may be elevated, due its leakage from injured muscle. Later in the disease course, mild hypophosphatemia may be seen, but rarely requires treatment. Hypocalcemia, the most common metabolic complication, occurs early in rhabdomyolysis and is usually asymptomatic. It has been attributed to the deposition of calcium salts in necrotic muscle, due to the hyperphosphatemia and decreased levels of 1,25-dihydroxycholecalciferol. These soft tissue calcifications can sometimes be observed on x-ray of the involved limb muscles. The hypocalcemia can occur, however, without elevated levels of phosphorus. Later, as calcium is mobilized from damaged muscle, serum calcium levels rise and symptomatic hypercalcemia may be observed.

Disseminated intravascular coagulation occurs in severe rhabdomyolysis and can result in hemorrhagic complications. The DIC usually resolves spontaneously within several days.

The mechanical complications of rhabdomyolysis consist of compartment syndrome and peripheral nerve injury. Compartment syndrome occurs secondary to marked swelling and edema of the involved muscle groups. This swelling will often not occur until after IV hydration. Characteristic signs and symptoms include pain, parasthesias, paralysis, pallor, and pulselessness. Of these, a sensory deficit is the most reliable physical finding.[14] If the intracompartmental pressures exceed 30 to 35 mmHg, fasciotomy is recommended. The associated muscle swelling may also cause pressure on peripheral nerves, resulting in neuronal ischemia and causing parasthesias or paralysis. Nerve injury is often proximal, and multiple nerves may be involved in the same extremity.[15] These peripheral neuropathies usually resolve within a few days or weeks, though, in a minority of patients, they can be permanent.

TREATMENT

Prehospital Care

For victims of crush injury, or patients strongly suspected of having rhabdomyolysis and prolonged extrication/transport times, IV rehydration with normal saline should be initiated as soon as possible. In one small series, aggressive infusion of crystalloids at a rate of approximately 1.5 L/h helped prevent the development of ARF in seven crush-injury victims.[16] The addition of sodium bicarbonate to each liter of crystalloid may be considered, but there are no controlled studies in the preshospital setting to confirm its benefit.

Emergency Department

Once in the emergency department, aggressive IV rehydration remains the mainstay of therapy. This should be continued for the first 24 to 72 h. Curry and colleagues recommend rapid correction of the fluid deficit with IV crystalloids followed by infusion of 2.5 (mL/kg)/h, with the goal of maintaining a minimum urine output of 2 (mL/kg)/h.[10] Others recommend a goal of 200 to 300 mL of urine output each hour. Sodium bicarbonate, 44 to 271 meq added to each liter of normal saline, or 1 mmol/kg administered as an IV bolus, has been recommended to maintain a urine pH of 6.5 or above to prevent the development of ARF.[10,16] Alkalinization is not without risks, however, since it can exacerbate the hypocalcemia observed in rhabdomyolysis.

To assist in diuresis, 20% mannitol is commonly recommended, although there are no prospective studies on its benefit. This may given as a single 1g/kg IV dose over 30 min,[10] or as 25 g IV initially, followed by 5 g/h IV, for a total of 120 g/day. Mannitol should only be given after volume replacement and avoided in patients with oliguria or with other causes of potential hypertension. Intravenous furosemide (40 to 200 mg) has also been used to assist in maintaining an adequate urine output following IV hydration.[13] Despite appropriate treatment however, dialysis may be necessary to treat rhabdomyolysis-induced ARF.

All patients should have a Foley catheter placed to monitor urine output. Patients should be placed on a cardiac monitor because of the risk of dysrhythmias secondary to metabolic complications. For patients with heart disease, comorbid conditions, or preexisting renal disease, or for elderly patients, hemodynamic monitoring may be necessary to avoid fluid overload. Serial measurements of urine pH, arterial pH, electrolytes, CPK, calcium, phosphorus, BUN, and creatinine should be performed.

Hypocalcemia observed early in rhabdomyolysis usually requires no treatment. Calcium should only be given to treat hyperkalemia-induced cardiotoxicity or profound signs and symptoms of hypocalcemia. Hypercalcemia, on the other hand, is frequently symptomatic and normally responds to saline diuresis and IV furosemide. Hyperphosphatemia should be treated with oral phosphate binders when serum levels exceed 7 mg/dL. Similarly, the hypophosphatemia, which may occur late in rhabdomyolysis, only requires treatment when the serum level is less than 1 mg/dL. Hyperkalemia, which is usually most severe in the first 12 to 36 h following muscle injury, can be significant when associated with ARF. Treatment should be initiated to prevent cardiac complications. Traditional insulin and glucose therapy, though recommended, may not be as effective in rhabdomyolysis-induced hyperkalemia. The use of ion-exchange resins (e.g., sodium polystyrene sulfonate) is effective, as is dialysis.

Finally, avoid the use of prostaglandin inhibitors such as nonsteroidal anti-inflammatory agents because of their vasoconstrictive effects on the kidney. Most importantly, treat the underlying etiology of the rhabdomyolysis.

DISPOSITION

All patients with suspected rhabdomyolysis require admission for IV hydration, diuresis, management of complications, and treatment of the underlying etiology. For at least the initial 24 to 48 h, these patients should probably be admitted to a monitored bed to identify dysrhythmias secondary to the metabolic complications. The nephrology service should be consulted to evaluate the need for dialysis for all patients presenting with ARF or symptomatic hyperkalemia unresponsive to therapy.

REFERENCES

1. Poels PJE, Gabreels FJM: Rhabdomyolysis: A review of the literature. *Clin Neurol Neurosurg* 95:175, 1993.

2. Meyer-Betz F: Beobachtungen an einem Eigenartigen mit Muskellahmungen verbunden Fall von Hamoglobinurie. *Dtsch Arch Klin Med* 101:85, 1911.
3. Bywaters EGL, Beall D: Crush injuries with impairment of renal function. *BMJ* 1:427, 1941.
4. Szewczyk D, Ovadia P, Abdullah F, Rabinovici R: Pressure-induced rhabdomyolysis and acute renal failure. *J Trauma* 44:384, 1998.
5. Haller RG, Knochel JP: Skeletal muscle disease in alcoholism. *Med Clin North Am* 68:91, 1984.
6. Line RL, Rust GS: Acute exertional rhabdomyolysis. *Am Fam Physician* 52:2712, 1995.
7. Gabow PA, Kaehny WD, Kelleher SP: The spectrum of rhabdomyolysis. *Medicine (Baltimore)* 61:141, 1982.
8. Lamminen AE, Hekali PE, Tinla E, et al: Acute rhabdomyolysis: Evaluation with magnetic resonance imaging compared with computed tomography and ultrasonography. *Br J Radiol* 62:326, 1989.
9. Shintani S, Shiigai T: Repeat MRI in acute rhabdomyolysis: Correlation with clinicopathological findings. *J Comput Assist Tomogr* 17:786, 1993.
10. Curry SC, Chang D, Connor D: Drug- and toxin-induced rhabdomyolysis. *Ann Emerg Med* 18:1068, 1989.
11. Sinert R, Kohl L, Rainone T, Scalea T: Exercise-induced rhabdomyolysis. *Ann Emerg Med* 23:1301, 1994.
12. Feinfeld DA, Cheng JT, Beysolow TD, Briscoe AM: A prospective study of urine and serum myoglobin levels in patients with acute rhabdomyolysis. *Clin Nephrol* 38:193, 1992.
13. Knochel JP: Rhabdomyolysis and myoglobinuria. *Annu Rev Med* 33:435, 1982.
14. Moore RE, Friedman RJ: Current concepts and pathophysiology in diagnosis of compartment syndromes. *J Emerg Med* 7:657, 1989.
15. Shields RW, Root RE, Wilbourn AJ: Compartment syndromes and compression neuropathies in coma. *Neurology* 36:1370, 1986.
16. Ron D, Taitelman U, Michaelson M, et al: Prevention of acute renal failure in traumatic rhabdomyolysis. *Arch Intern Med* 144:277, 1984.

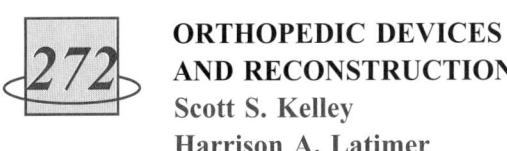

ORTHOPEDIC DEVICES AND RECONSTRUCTIONS

Scott S. Kelley
Harrison A. Latimer

Orthopedic surgery is unique in its abundant use of implants to reconstruct the musculoskeletal system. Implants may be used to replace a degenerated structure or simply to stabilize a bone or ligament while it heals. The goal is a painless, functioning spine or extremity. Implants are used in fractures, arthrodesis, arthroplasty, and ligament fixation.

This chapter reviews the common types of orthopedic implants. Postoperative complications that may be seen in an emergency department following implant use, including breakage, migration, and infection, are discussed.

COMMON ORTHOPEDIC IMPLANTS STABILIZING BONE TO BONE

Plates and Screws

Plates and their accompanying screws are commonly used to add stability while fractures, osteotomies, or arthrodeses fuse. They come in many different shapes and sizes because they have been designed to fit different areas of the skeleton. They all share the common function of stabilizing bone in an anatomically acceptable position while it heals to itself. To perform this function, the plate must be securely attached to bone with multiple screws to each fragment. When this method is used to manage fractures, the bones are placed in direct contact, and healing occurs without the large amount of callus formation seen with casting or intramedullary nailing (Fig. 272-1). Therefore, it is often difficult to determine when fracture union is complete, and it is not uncommon for the fracture line to be visible more than 1 year after surgery (Fig. 272-2).

COMPLICATIONS Early complications include wound infections, either superficial and amenable to antibiotics or deep and requiring surgical débridement. Later complications include nonunion of the fracture. Plate-screw constructs are simply temporizing measures. If the bone does not heal, the plate will eventually bend or break or the screws will pull out of the bone (Fig. 272-3). Plates and screws are sometimes removed, and the bone is then at risk for refracture (often through a screw hole) for approximately 7 months.

Intramedullary Rods

Since their popularization during World War II, solid, single intramedullary rods have become the most common method of treating femoral and tibial fractures and, more recently, some humeral fractures (Fig. 272-4). They have also been used to stabilize osteotomies or arthrodeses. Over the last decade their application to fractures has been extended by the addition of proximal and distal interlocking screws that add rotational stability. Over the past 5 years open fractures have been treated with intramedullary nails that are placed with minimal reaming of the bones. All these advances have led to the greater number of emergency patients who have intramedullary rods or nails.

Intramedullary rods are placed through an incision at the end of the bone, avoiding the joint surface. The intramedullary canal is then mechanically reamed to a slightly larger size than the nail. The nail is then inserted, and interlocking screws are added if needed for stability at the fracture or osteotomy. The immobilization of the fracture is less than that gained with plates and screws, and therefore the healing process involves visible callus formation at the fracture site (Fig. 272-5). In open fractures, minimal or no reaming, which retains the maximum blood supply to the injury, may be performed and requires a smaller-diameter rod. Although less popular today than single, solid rods, multiple, small, flexible rods are still sometimes used to gain fracture stability (see Fig. 272-6).

COMPLICATIONS As with all surgery, infection is the most worrisome early complication and still occurs with a 1 to 2 percent incidence in closed fractures despite the use of perioperative antibiotics. Unreamed nails are commonly used for open fractures and have up to a 25 percent infection rate. The number of emergency department encounters for postoperative infectious complications will increase. Due to their central location, rods have a greater mechanical strength than plates and screws. They, however, will also fail (usually after 1 year) by breaking at an unhealed facture site (Fig. 272-7). With weight bearing, the interlocking screws may break, often without loss of fracture stability. Any noninterlocked nail may work its way back out of the bone and irritate surrounding soft tissue. Femoral rods may then cause trochanteric bursitis. The multiple, small, flexible rods are notorious for this problem and often become palpable under the skin (Fig. 272-8). Nonunion of the fracture occurs more frequently with open fractures, and therefore the small unreamed nails used for these fractures are at risk for breakage.

External Fixators

External fixators have been widely used to stabilize open fractures. A fixator is preferred over cast immobilization because it allows the physician access to the soft-tissue injury. External fixators also may be used to temporarily stabilize an extremity while life- or limb-threatening surgery is performed. Certain types of closed fractures, such as distal radius fractures, may require an external fixator to maintain an adequate reduction of the fracture.

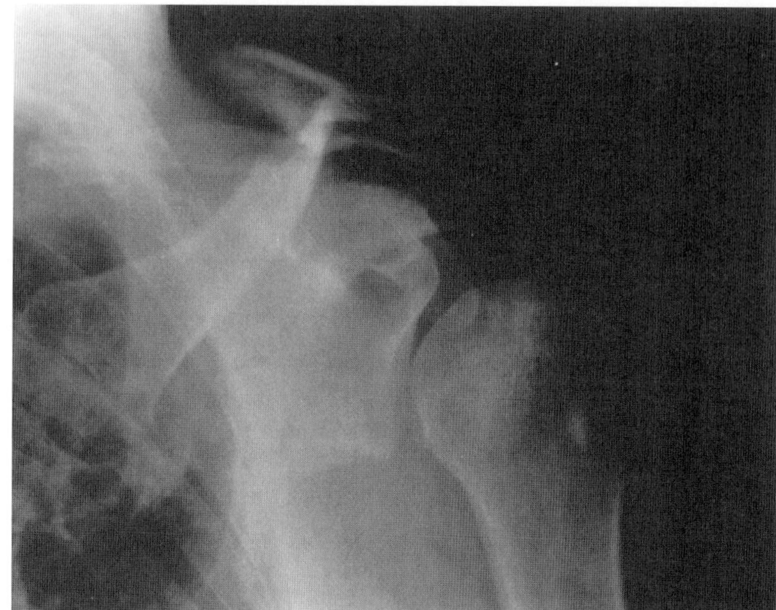

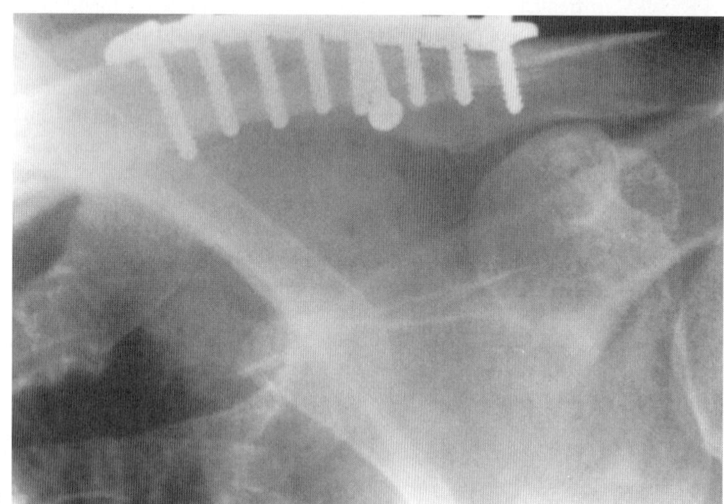

FIG. 272-1. A. This clavicle fracture was rigidly fixed with a plate and screws. **B.** Note that the fracture is healing without significant callus formation.

Nontraumatic uses of external fixators include stabilization of arthrodeses; special clamps may be used to add compression that enhances union. More recently, complex wire and ring (Ilizarov) fixators have been used to lengthen bones and correct deformities.

The external fixator is divided into two components: the fixation pins or wires and the external frame. The threaded pins or wires are inserted into each fragment at a distance from the fracture site. When connected to the frame, they are able to rigidly hold the bone so that union occurs (Fig. 272-9).

COMPLICATIONS Because external fixation is usually chosen for severe open fractures, which have a higher rate of infection, emergency department visits are not uncommon. Patients present with increased redness, swelling, or drainage at the previous open wound site. The skin should be prepared and deep cultures obtained by aspiration or swab. The fixation pins and wires very commonly sustain pin tract infections, which may easily be treated by releasing the skin around the pin site with a no. 11 blade after adequate local anesthesia. Oral antibiotics may be given empirically. With time, the fixator pins may loosen in the bone. The clamps connecting the pins to the frame may also loosen. This may result in instability or loss of reduction at the fracture site. This will usually be detectable clinically (unstable fractures are painful when stressed) or by radiographs.

Fixation Wires and Pins

Small smooth or threaded percutaneous pins (Fig. 272-10) are often used in the small bones of the hand or foot to add stability while fracture union occurs. The hand and foot possess an excellent blood supply, which usually results in early union. The pins are cut off outside the skin so that they may be removed between 3 and 9 weeks postoperatively.

Internal cerclage wires are often used to hold structures that have fractured under tension. Examples are tuberosity fractures of the proximal humerus (Fig. 272-11) or patella fractures. Cerclage wires may also be used with or without a plate to stabilize a fracture around a prosthetic joint implant (Fig. 272-12). They serve the same role as a screw, which cannot be placed through the implant.

COMPLICATIONS As with external fixation pins, the most common complication of using percutaneous pins is pin-tract infection. Such infections can be treated by removing the pin, but this should only

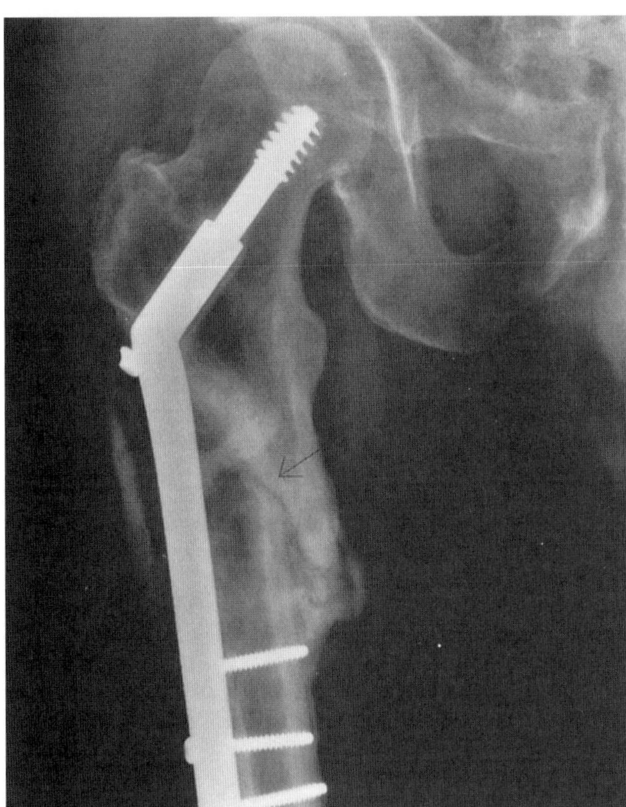

FIG. 272-2. This femur fracture is rigidly healed at 1 year, but the fracture line (*arrow*) is still present.

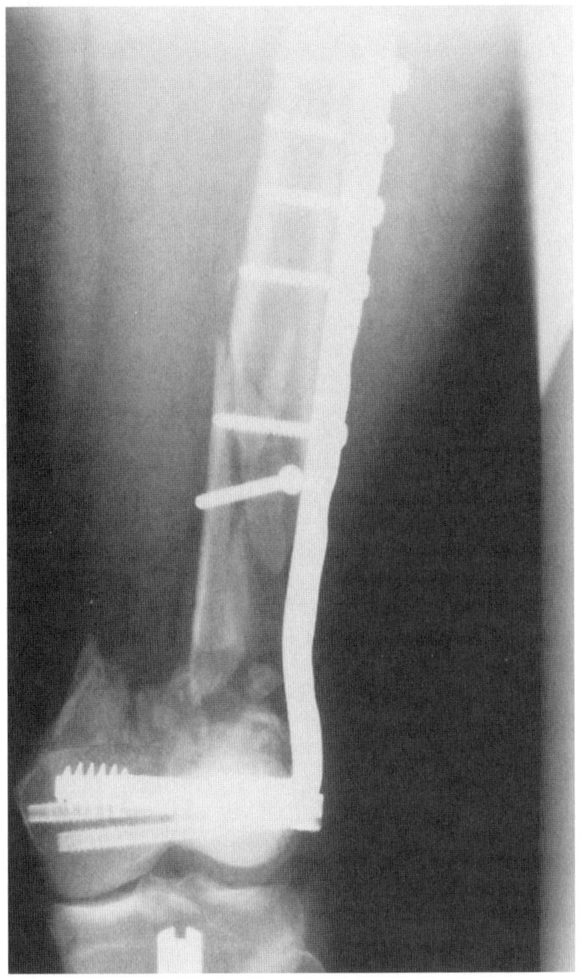

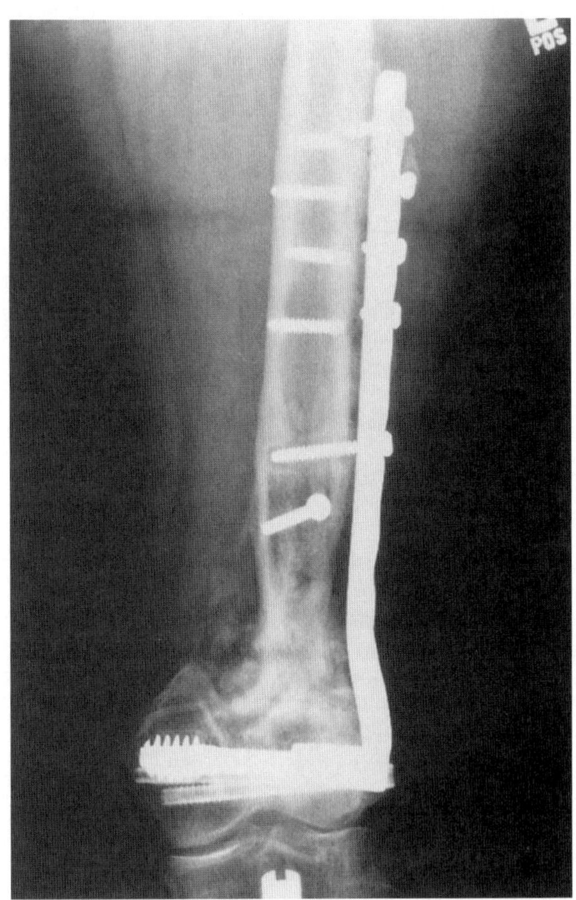

FIG. 272-3. **A.** This severely comminuted, open distal femur fracture was fixed with a plate and screws. **B.** Despite bone grafting, the screws broke before the fracture healed.

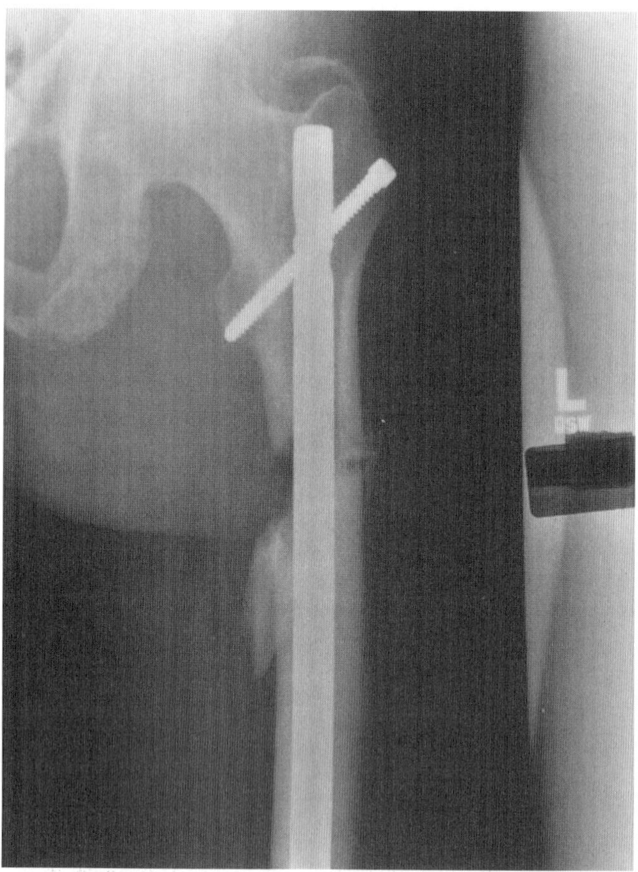

FIG. 272-4. This femur fracture was stabilized with an intramedullary rod.

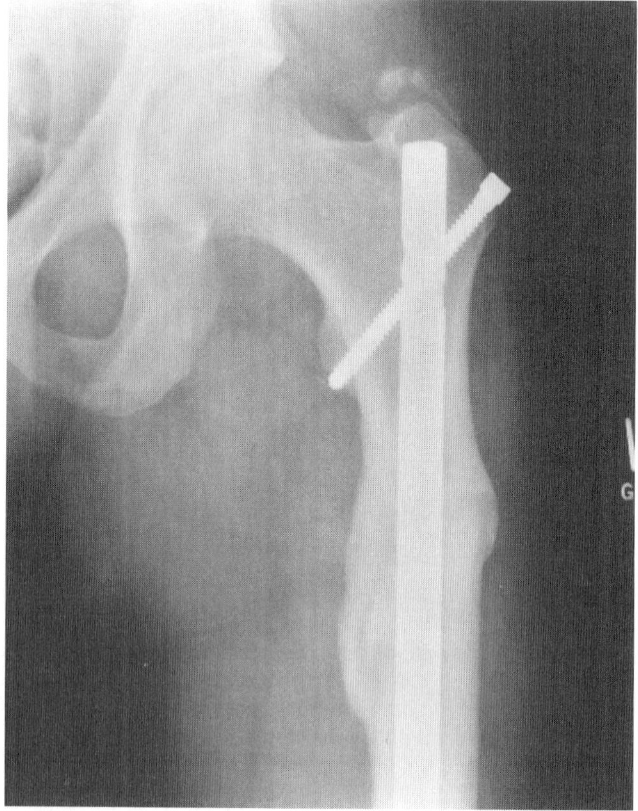

FIG. 272-5. Note the large callus formation at the fracture site.

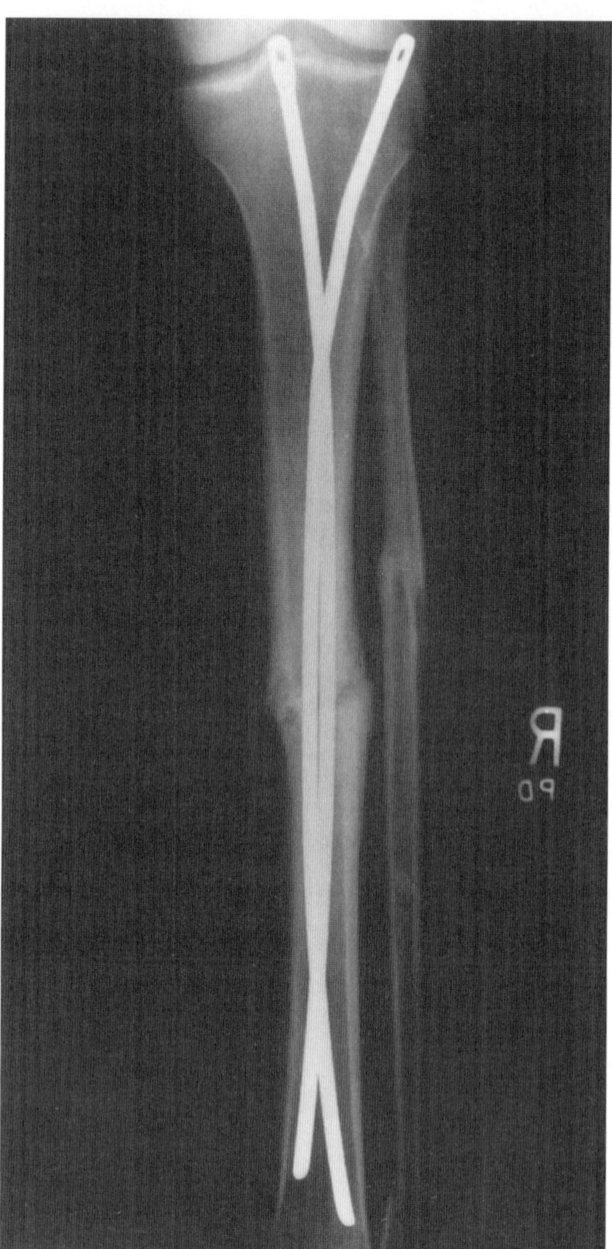

FIG. 272-6. These Ender rods were chosen to stabilize this open tibia fracture.

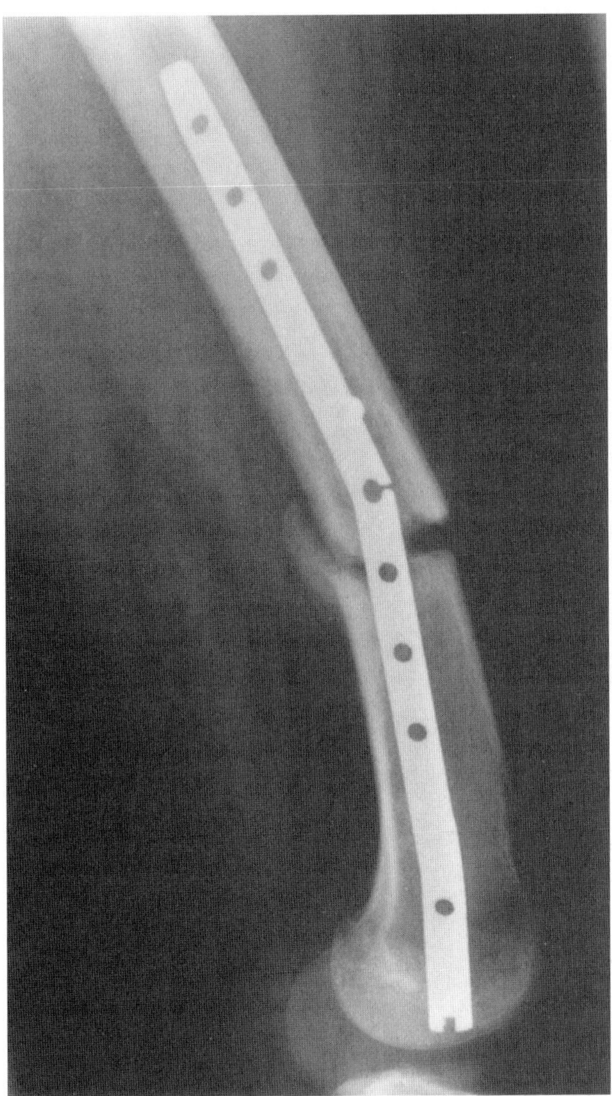

FIG. 272-7. This distal femoral intramedullary nail broke before fracture union occurred.

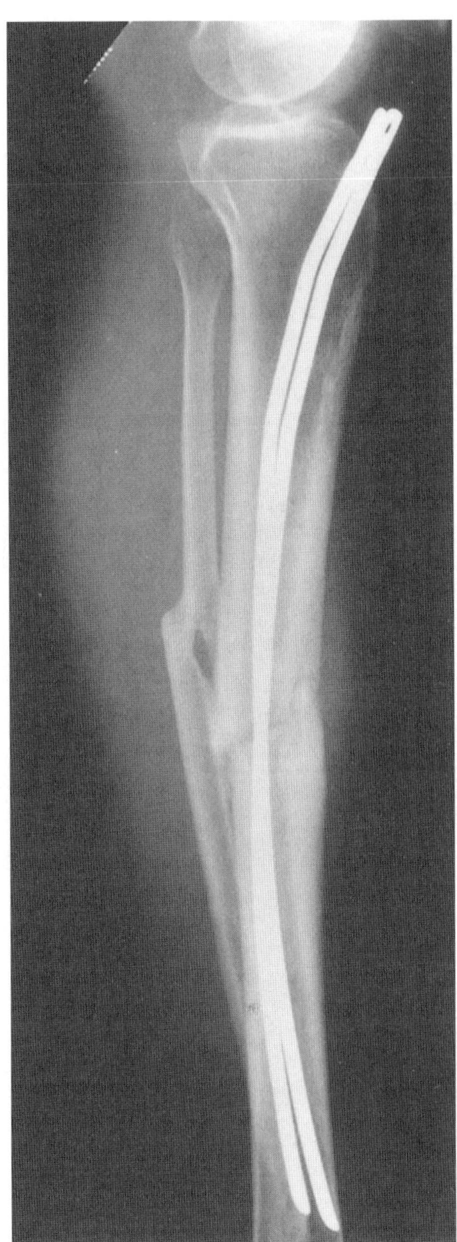

FIG. 272-8. The Ender rods have "backed out" of the bone and were prominent just under the skin.

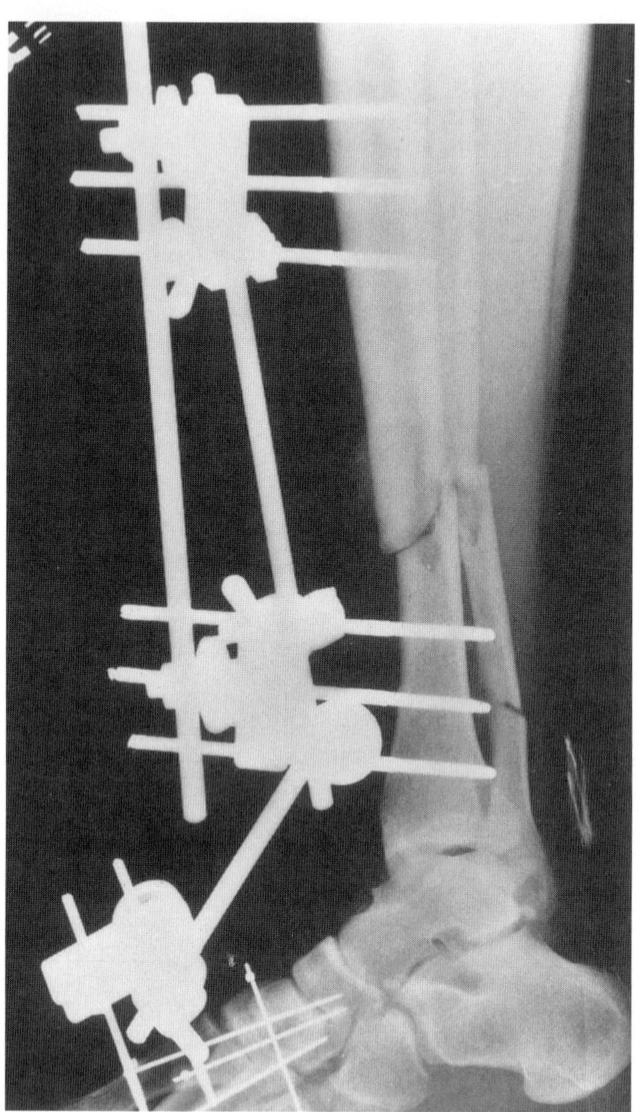

FIG. 272-9. This external fixator is used to stabilize the open tibia fracture while still allowing access to the soft tissue wound.

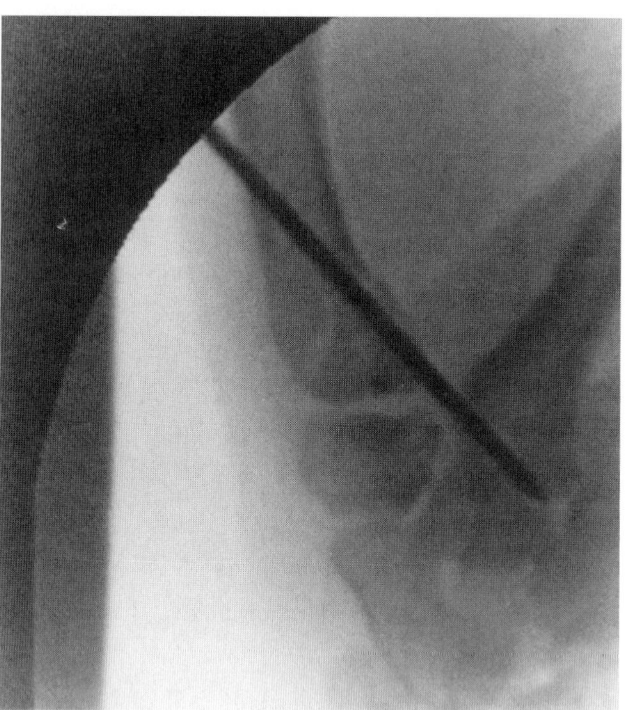

FIG. 272-10. This smooth pin was used to stabilize the fracture at the base of the thumb metacarpal.

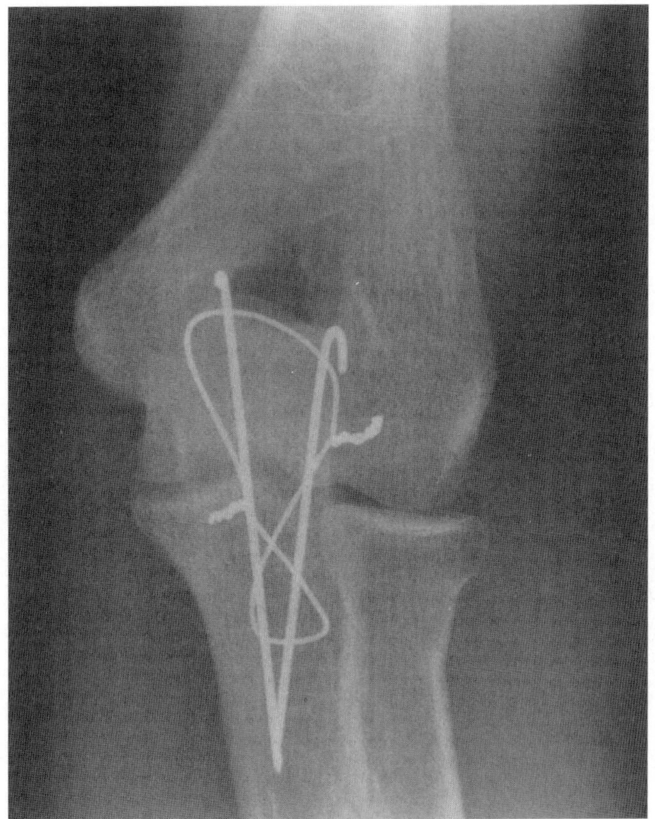

A

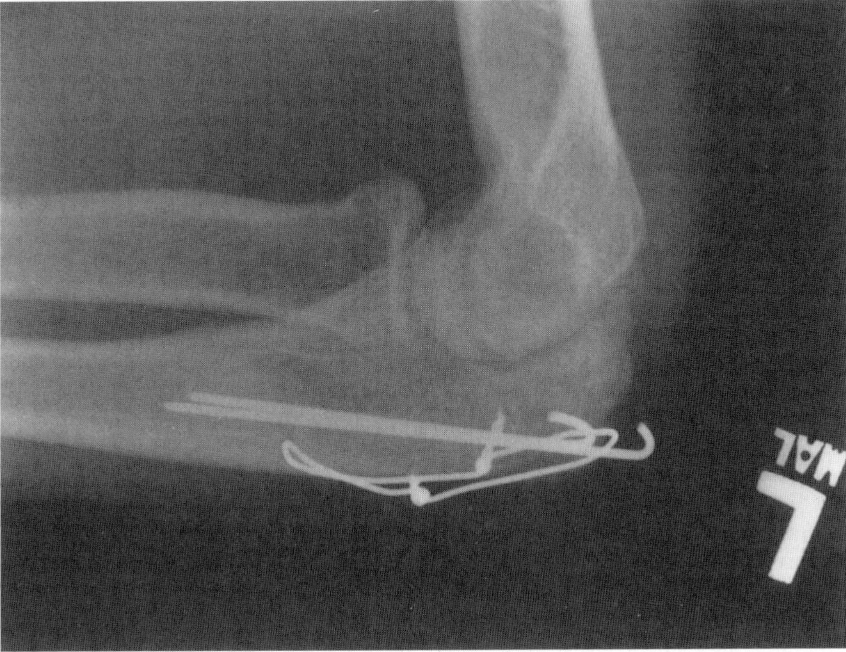

B

FIG. 272-11. A. and **B.** This olecranon fracture was stabilized with two smooth pins and a cerclage wire, which allowed joint motion during healing.

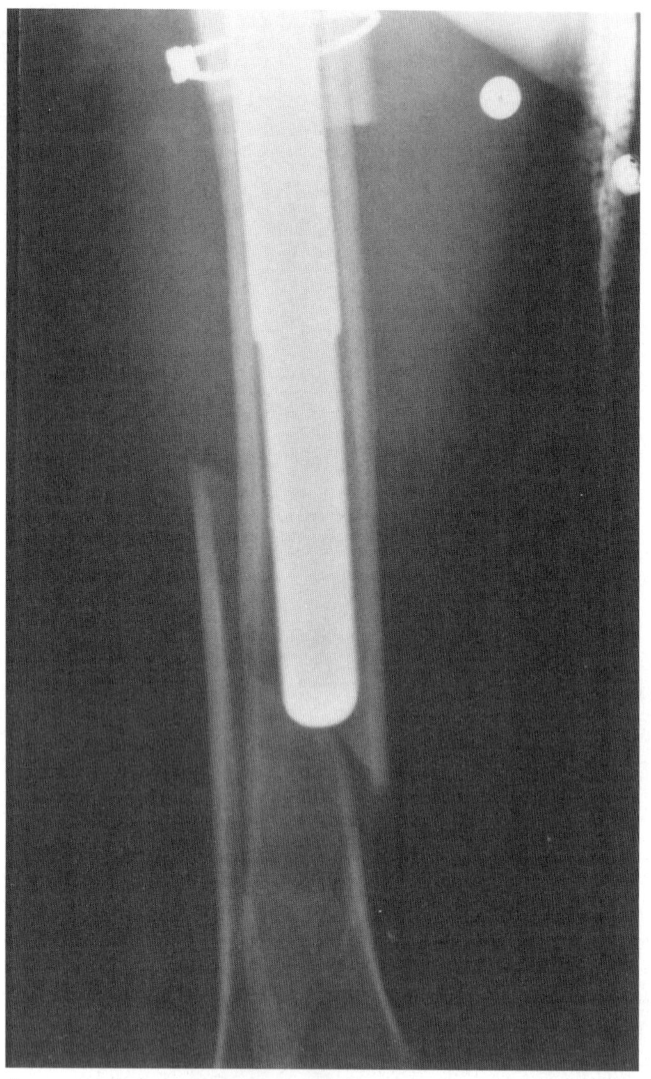
A

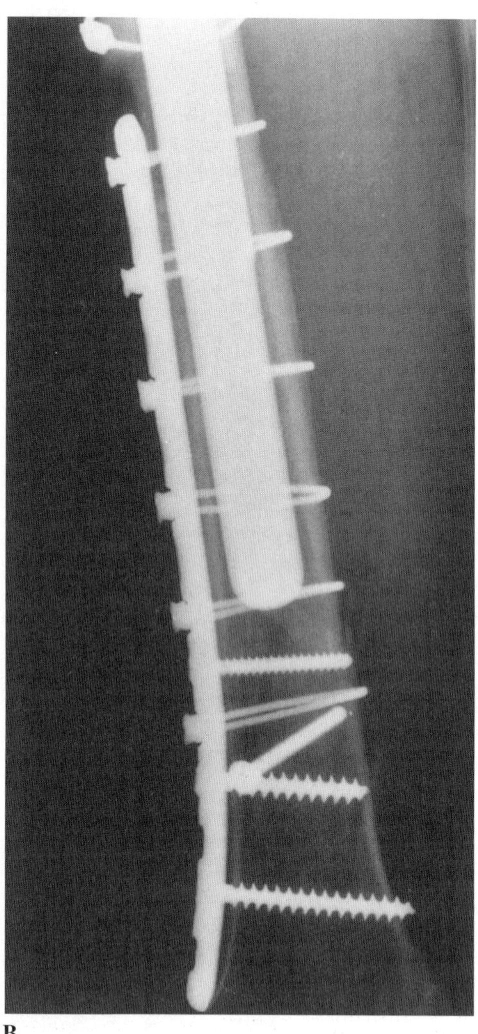
B

FIG. 272-12. A. and **B.** This periprosthetic fracture is stabilized by a special plate designed for use with wires or screws.

be done after consultation with an orthopedist. A course of oral antibiotics may also be indicated. Complications of cerclage wires include wire breakage prior to union or perforation of a wire through thin overlying skin.

Cervical Spine Implants

The cervical spine is unique from the rest of the vertebral column due to the common use of halo fixation. A halo is simply a ring external fixator that is rigidly attached to the outer skull table with pins. Usually, four rods are used to connect this ring to a well-molded plastic or plaster body jacket. The halo limits the motion of the cervical spine, allowing fractures to heal or arthrodesis to unite.

The most common cervical implant is a posterior cerclage wire (Fig. 272-13), which limits motion between adjacent vertebrae while fusion occurs. A bone block taken from the iliac crest is often used as a biologic implant in the anterior cervical spine to gain fusion. Special plates and screws have been developed for the anterior cervical spine. Their use is likely to accelerate in the future.

COMPLICATIONS As with other external fixators, the most common complication of halo fixation is pin-tract infection. Infected pins are usually removed and a new pin placed in an alternative site. Loose, noninfected pins should never be tightened because this risks penetration of the inner skull table and resultant meningitis. The internal implants will fail if the vertebrae fail to unite.

Anterior and Posterior Thoracolumbar Spine Implants

Although the number of spinal instrumentation systems is overwhelming, the basic concepts are simple. A rigid plate or rod is connected to the spine to limit motion between vertebral segments and allow healing or fusion to occur. There are three ways of connecting the rod or plate to the vertebrae: with a hook, a wire, or a screw. When reduced to these terms, the instrumentation is much simpler.

Most advances in spinal instrumentation arose from the treatment of childhood scoliosis. The first was the Harrington rod-hook system (Fig. 272-14), introduced in 1960 and still in use today. Two major lessons were learned in the development of this system: (1) extremely durable materials were needed to avoid breakage; and (2) no matter how rigid the instrumentation, failure was inevitable if fusion did not occur (Fig. 272-15). Over the years, many instrumentation systems have been developed with special hook designs that allow the basic Harrington rod concept to be used for a multitude of spinal problems.

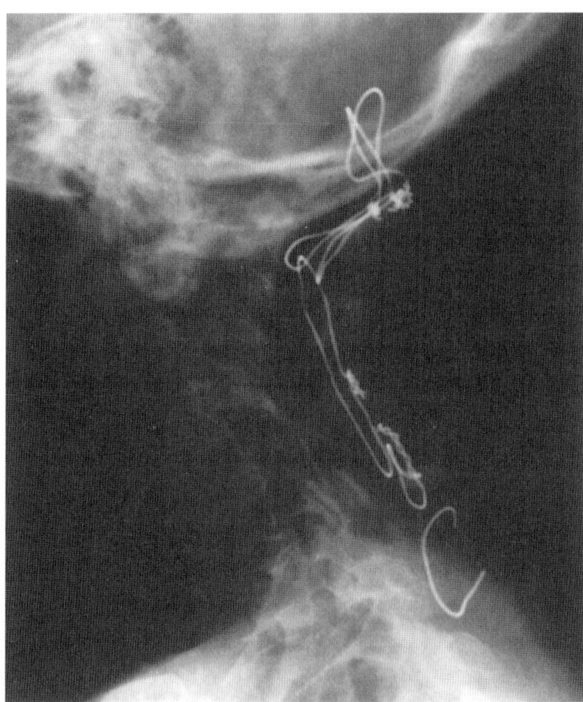

FIG. 272-13. This patient underwent posterior fusion of the entire cervical spine, with internal cerclage fixation supplemented by an external halo for 6 months.

In the 1970s, Eduardo Luque developed a system in which smooth metal rods were laid along the spine and wired to each segment. This created an extremely rigid construct that did not require postoperative bracing. This system is still in use today with only slight modifications (Fig. 272-14). Current systems may use combinations of hooks, screws, and wire for improved fixation and correction of deformity.

The drawback of rod-hook and rod-wire systems is the need for the implant to immobilize over a large number of vertebral levels. This problem has been addressed by pedicle screws placed directly into the vertebral body. This technique dates back to 1949. Because the screw passes through both the posterior and anterior spinal elements, excellent fixation is obtained (Fig. 272-16). This allows the surgeon to greatly reduce the number of segments immobilized. The pedicle screws are then connected to a rigid rod or plate.

Posterior spinal instruments are more commonly used than anterior instrumentation, due in part to the ease and safety of the posterior approach. Numerous types of anterior instrumentation have been developed (Fig. 272-17) using same principal of connecting to the vertebrae with a screw that in turn connects to a bridging plate, rod, or cable system.

COMPLICATIONS Early emergency visits usually involve wound problems. Diagnosis of an infection is supported by the presence of severe pain and an elevated temperature, white blood cell count, and erythrocyte sedimentation rate. Painful acute implant failure is not common, but Harrington-type hook implants may disengage. The patient usually notes an acute ''pop'' and an immediate increase in pain. This is usually best demonstrated on the lateral radiograph because the hook will no longer be under the vertebral lamina (Fig. 272-18). Rod breakage is usually a late occurrence due to failure of the fusion to prevent motion. Patients greater than 3 months postoperative usually will not have instability. Rod breakage should be easily detectable on standard anteroposterior and lateral radiograph views. Pain complaints from spine surgery patients are commonly encountered in the emergency department. Narcotics should be given sparingly, and communication with the orthopedic surgeon is often helpful in the management of patients with chronic pain.

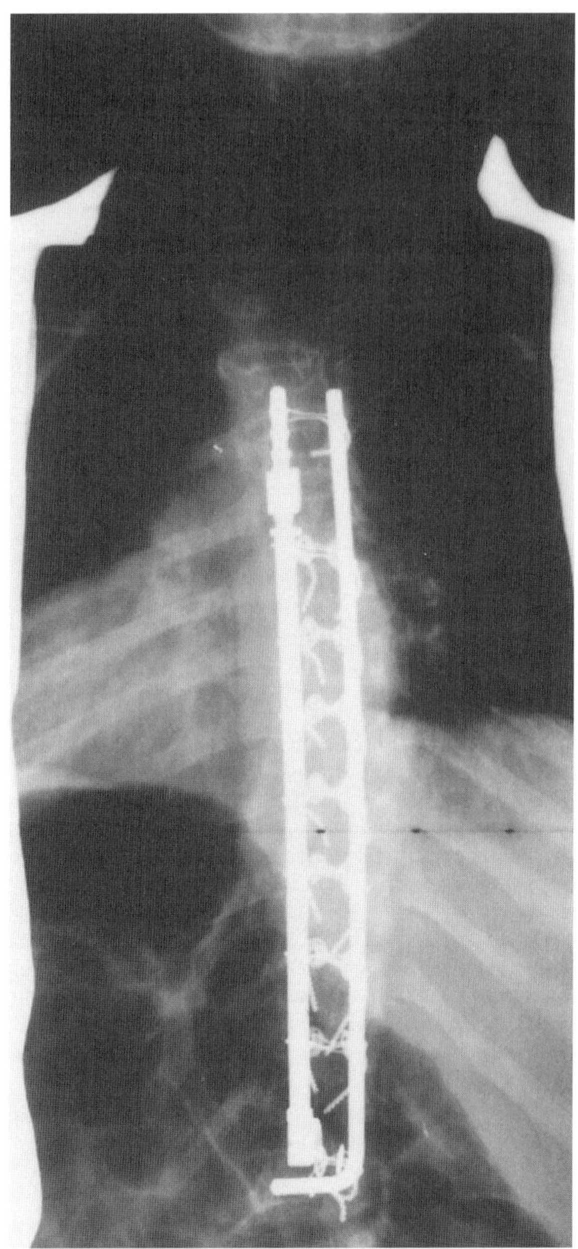

FIG. 272-14. This patient's posterior spine fusion was stabilized by a Harrington rod on the left and a Luque rod on the right.

COMMON ORTHOPEDIC IMPLANTS STABILIZING SOFT TISSUE TO BONE

The fitness craze of the last 15 years has led to a greater number of sports-related injuries. This has also resulted in greater need for reliable methods of stabilizing avulsed ligaments or tendons to bone. Graft implants are also more commonly used and must be stabilized while they heal to the host bone. These type of implants are most commonly used in the knee.

Thousands of anterior cruciate reconstructions are performed each year in the United States. The ruptured cruciate ligament may be replaced with harvested hamstring tendons or one-third of the patella tendon still connected at each end to a bone block from the patella

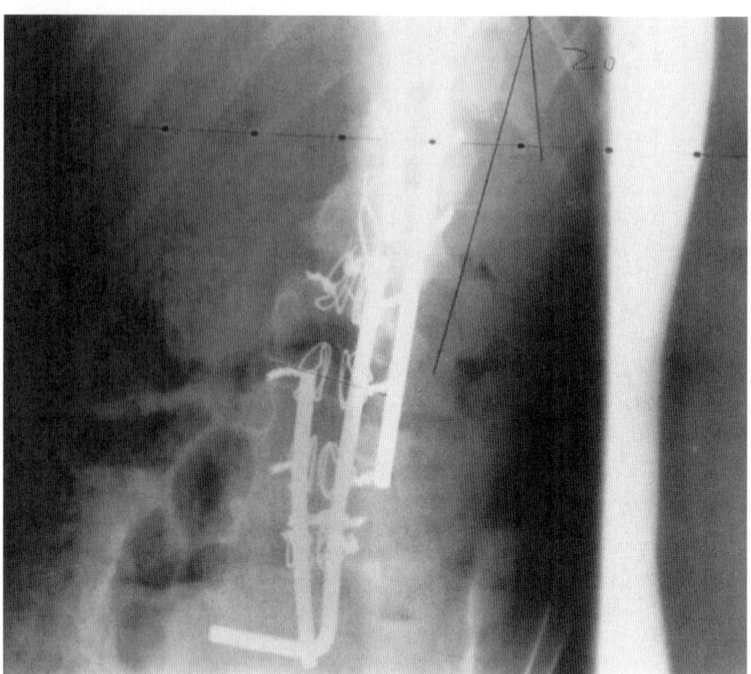

FIG. 272-15. This double Luque rod construct broke prior to fusion.

and the tibia. It may also be replaced by a cadaveric patella tendon graft. These reconstructions not only increase the knee's stability but also lower the risk of future meniscal injuries.

The graft may be stabilized by heavy sutures or directly stabilized to bone with a metalic implant. Hamstring tendon grafts have no bone; therefore, they are usually left attached to the tibia, threaded through the knee, and then stabilized by heavy permanent suture ties to a screw or staple. The free bone-patella-bone grafts may also be stabilized in this fashion but are more commonly held by ''interference'' screws that are placed parallel to the graft bone in the tunnel. The threads then engage and stabilize the graft bone to the host bone (Fig. 272-19).

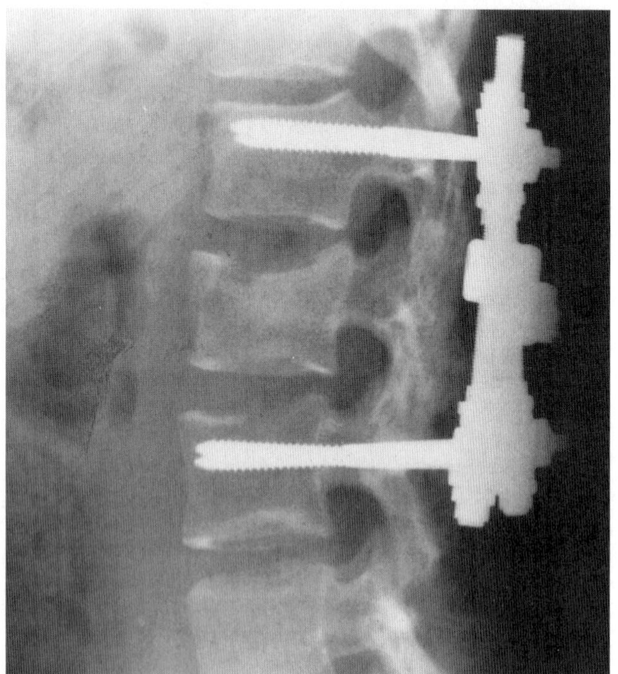

FIG. 272-16. The fracture has been reduced and stabilized with pedicle screws attached to posterior bars.

It is difficult to suture directly to bone. Previously this was performed by drilling small holes through which the suture could be threaded. More recently, special sutures that are coupled to metallic implants that can be drilled into the bone have been developed. These are often seen around the shoulder and have greatly simplified surgical techniques (Fig. 272-20).

COMPLICATIONS Although rare, postoperative infection (presenting as increased pain and fever) is a catastrophic early complication of knee reconstructions. Immediate surgical débridement is usually indicated. The most common complication of soft-tissue-stabilizing implants is loss of fixation. This may occur through failure of the suture or the bone-implant interface. Migration of anterior cruciate ligament metallic implants into the joint has not been a problem.

Often an athlete will present to an emergency department with an injury to a previously reconstructed knee. The reconstructed anterior cruciate ligament may be injured in the same manner as the original ligament, or the patient may simply have sustained a meniscal injury. Great psychological stress may accompany reinjury, and this diagnosis should therefore be deferred to an orthopedist. If surgery was performed less than 8 weeks previously, the knee examination should also be deferred to the treating orthopedist, since the graft itself may not have healed fully to bone. Placement of a knee immobilizer is usually a simple temporizing measure. The orthopedist is often unable to perform an optimal examination until 7 to 10 days after the injury, when inflammation has subsided. Patients will often not accept this long an interval, and earlier referral is probably indicated if the patient's anxiety is obvious. During the interim, cold therapy, gentle active range-of-motion exercises, and nonsteroidal anti-inflammatory drugs are beneficial.

TOTAL JOINT ARTHROPLASTY

Prosthetic replacement of joints is extremely common in the United States. The indication for arthroplasty is a painful degenerated joint that severely impairs the quality of life of the patient. Almost every joint of the upper and lower extremity has had prosthetic replacements designed for it. The weight-bearing joints of the lower extremity must tolerate much higher forces than the joints of the upper extremity.

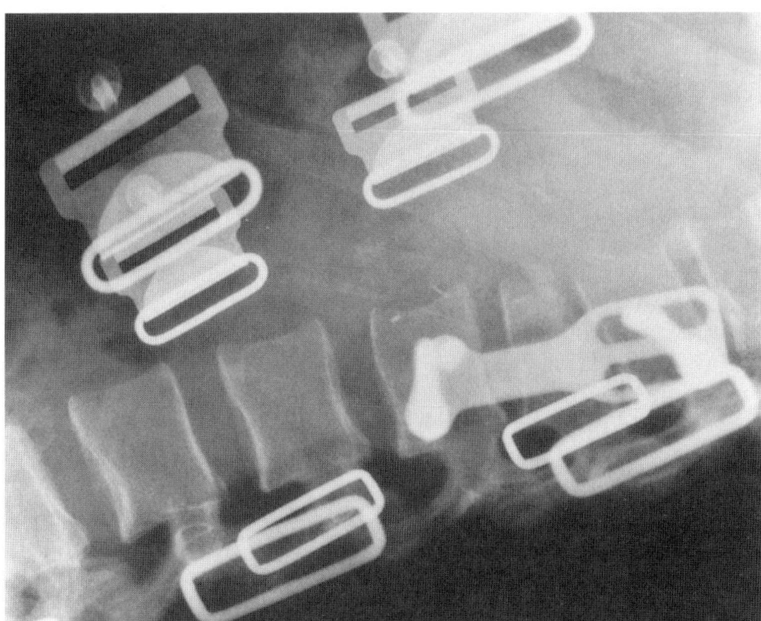

FIG. 272-17. An anterior spine plate and screws are used to stabilize this lumbar burst fracture. The numerous buckles are from the molded plastic jacket, which adds additional support.

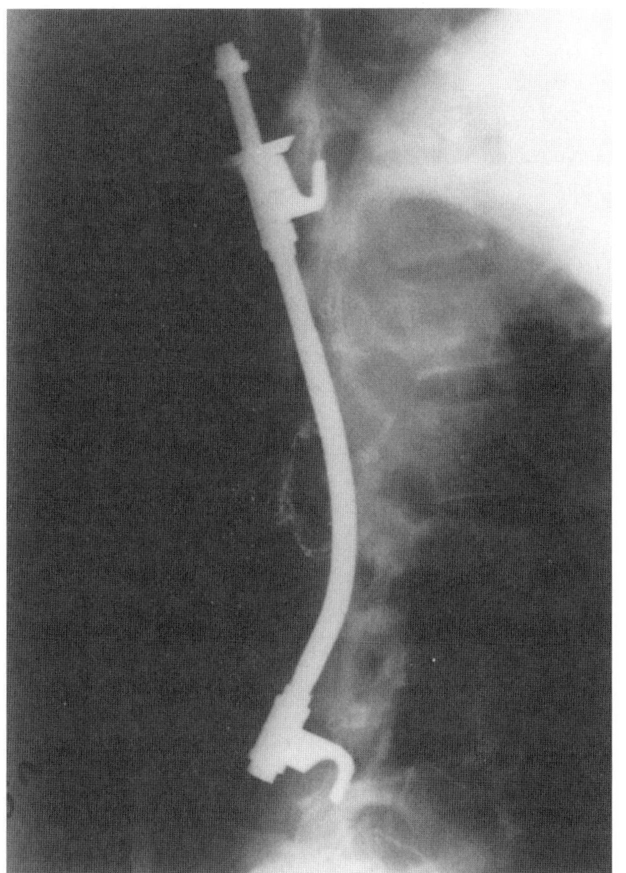

A

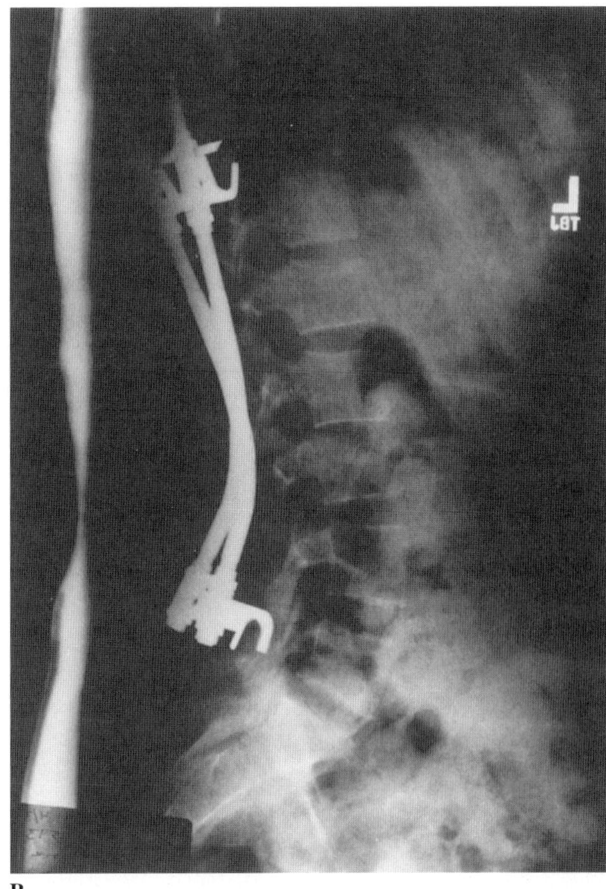

B

FIG. 272-18. A. This hook-and-rod system was used to stabilize a lumbar burst fracture. B. The patient noted a ''pop'' with forward bending, and the lateral radiograph confirms that the top hook was disengaged.

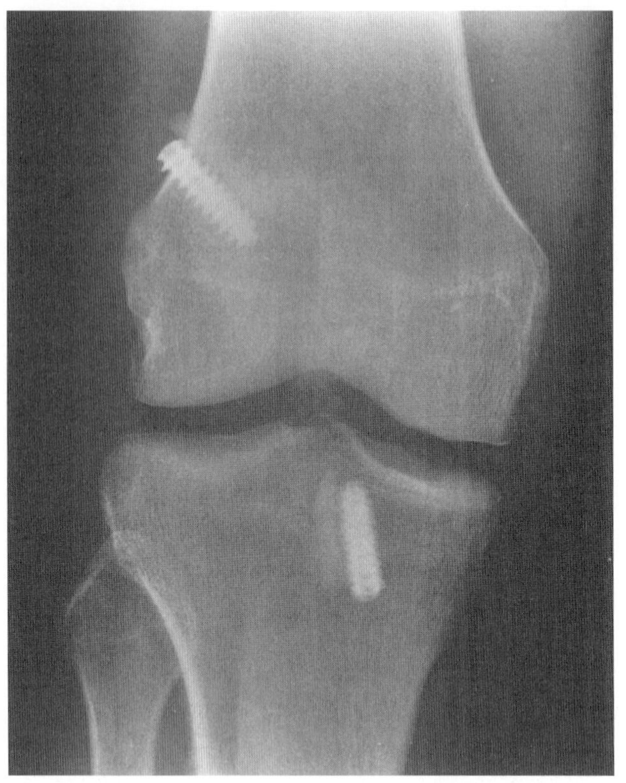

A

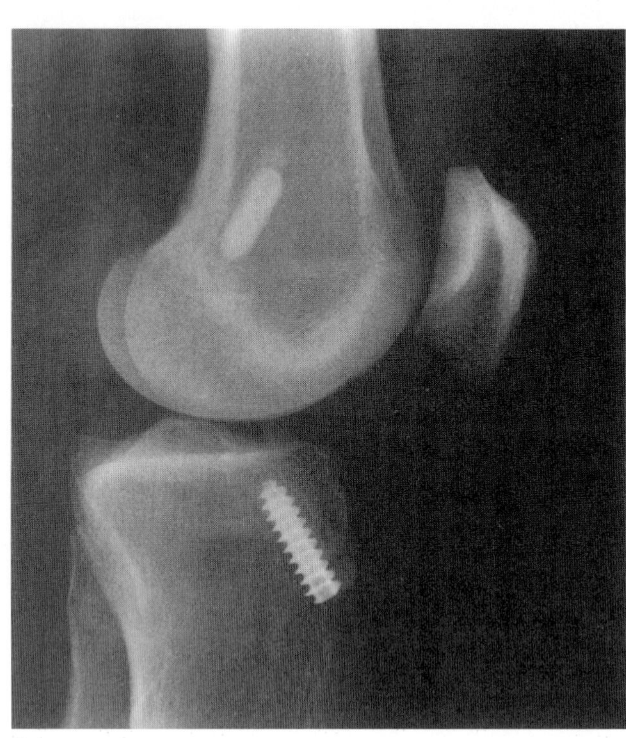

B

FIG. 272-19. A. and **B.** These interference screws rigidly fix the anterior cruciate ligament graft.

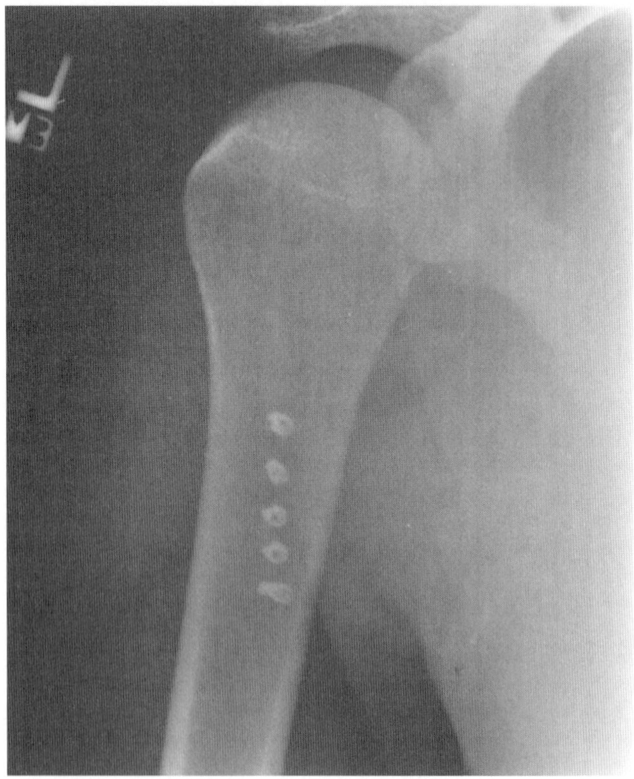

FIG. 272-20. These metal-anchored sutures were used to repair a ruptured pectoralis major insertion to the proximal humerus.

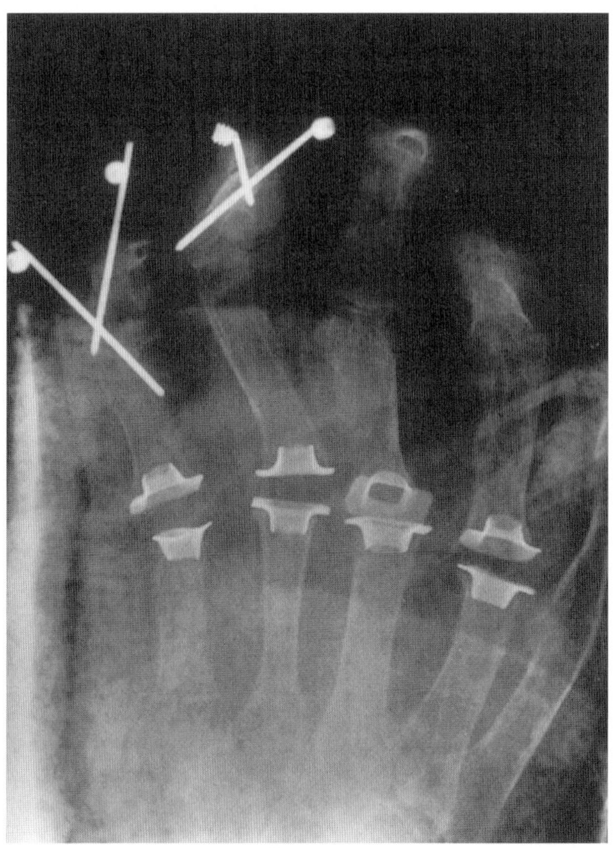

FIG. 272-21. This patient with rheumatoid arthritis underwent MCP silastic implants with metal grommets.

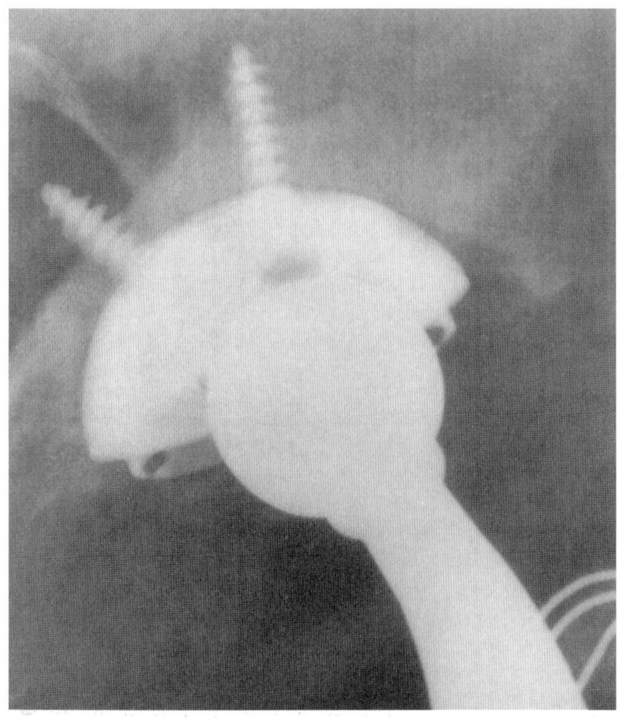

A

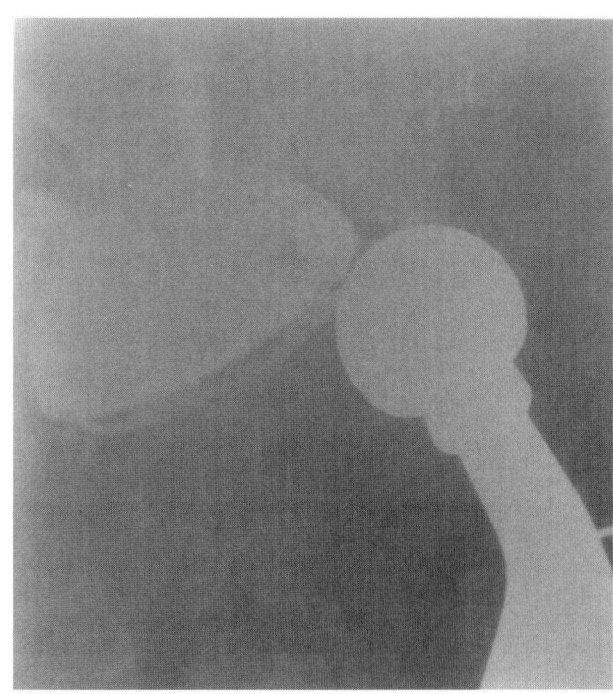

B

FIG. 272-22. A. and **B.** This patient's total hip arthroplasty is dislocated. The slight asymmetry on the first view was not detected, and further radiographs were needed to diagnose the dislocation.

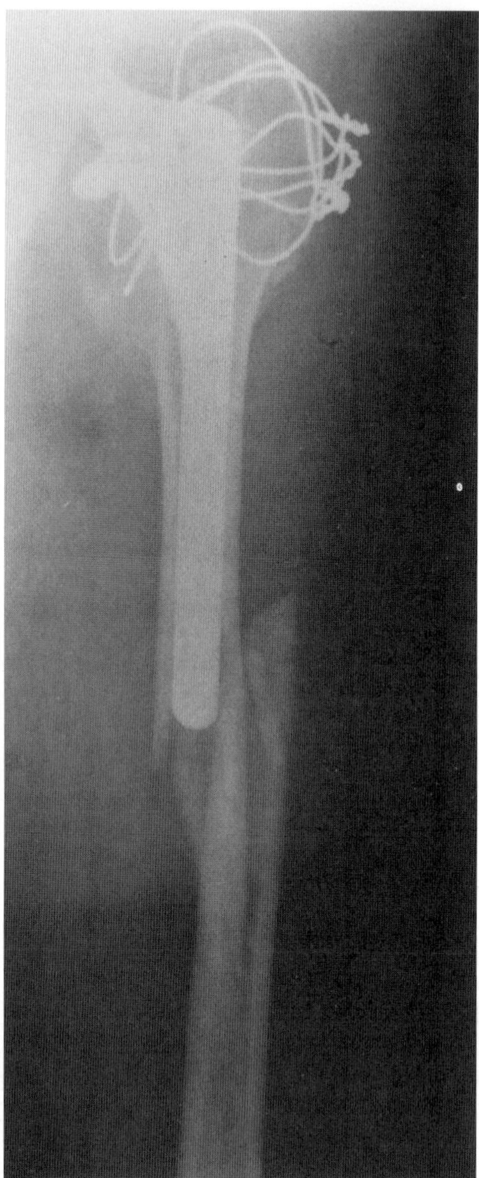

FIG. 272-23. This patient sustained a periprosthetic femur fracture during a fall.

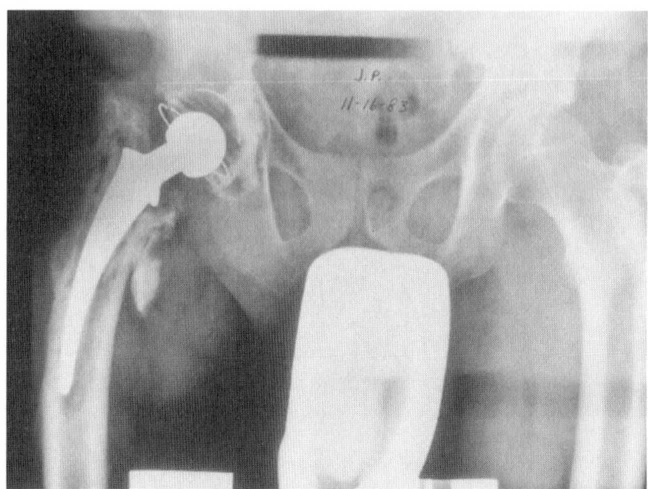

FIG. 272-24. This right cemented total hip arthroplasty is obviously loose, with associated proximal femoral bone loss.

Fortunately, the bones of the lower extremity are much larger, which allows for better fixation of the prosthetic devices.

The elbow and knee arthroplasties function in a similar manner, in that they both control the length of the extremity. As they bend, the extremity shortens. The hip and shoulder also function similarly because they position the extremity in space and have free motion in three planes.

Prosthetic Types

There is a great deal of variation between the design of prostheses for different joints. The small joints of the hand and foot are often replaced with silicone interpositional arthroplasties. The joint surfaces are excised and a silicone spacer is inserted. A metal grommet may be placed in the bone first to allow for improved wear properties (Fig. 272-21). These implants will survive if the forces across them remain low. Silicone implants are also used for wrist arthroplasty.

Large-joint arthroplasties may be subdivided into total joint arthroplasty in which both sides of the joint are addressed and hemiarthroplasty in which only one side is replaced. Hemiarthroplasties are most often used in the ball and socket joints of the shoulder and hip with only the ball portion being replaced. It is attached to a stem that is inserted in the intramedullary canal. Hemiarthroplasty is most commonly used for fractures involving the proximal humerus and proximal femur.

Total joint arthroplasty was first popularized by Sir John Charnley for the hip. A metal femoral prosthesis articulates with a plastic pelvic cup. Often a metal backing is added to the cup. These metal-on-plastic

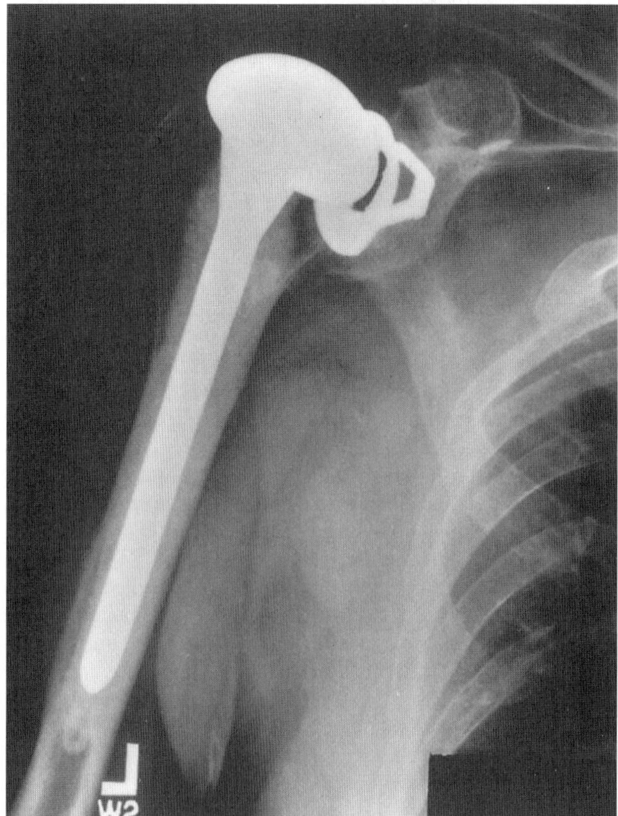

FIG. 272-25. This total shoulder arthroplasty has a well-fixed cemented humeral component.

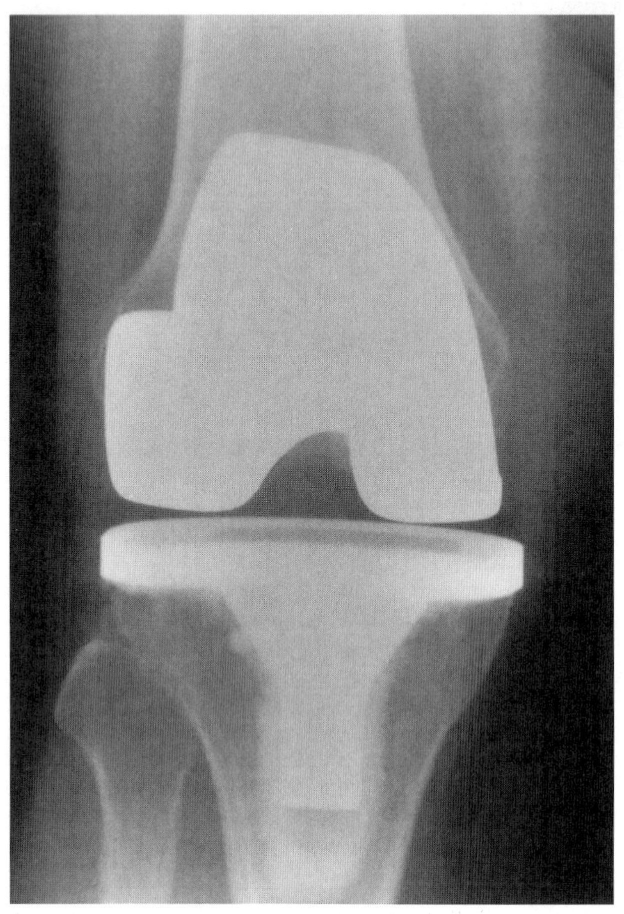
A

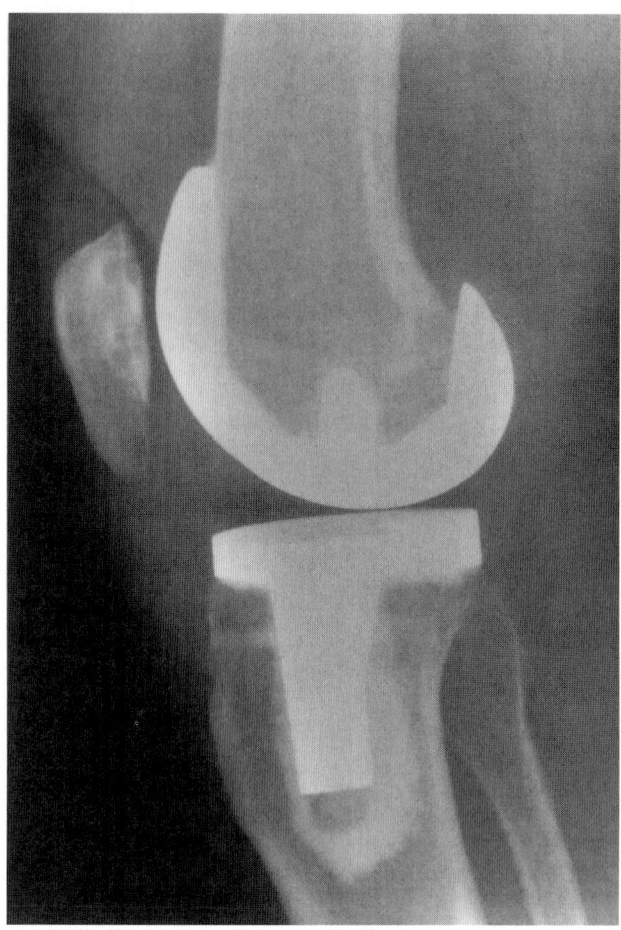
B

FIG. 272-26. A. and **B.** This patient with osteoarthritis underwent a total knee arthroplasty, with all components cemented.

total joints have been adapted to almost every other joint but are most commonly used in the knee followed by the hip, shoulder, elbow, wrist, ankle, and infrequently the small bones of the hand.

Total joints may also be divided into constrained or nonconstrained implants. The rate of loosening from the bone is much higher with constrained implants, which are designed with the two components locked together in a hingelike fashion that prevents dislocation. Constrained designs are used mostly with revision work where the amount of soft tissue loss leads to an unstable joint. The exception is the elbow, where primary (first time) constrained prostheses are often used, because this joint has very little inherent soft tissue stability.

Motion between the implant and the host bone will cause pain. Three methods of fixing the prosthesis to the bone may be used. The implant may be press-fit, allowing the gross bone structure to stabilize the implant. The implant may be seated in polymethylmethacrylate cement that bonds to both the bone and the implant in much the same manner mortar stabilizes a post in a hole or a tile on the floor. Implants with special coatings and surfaces that allow bone to grow directly into the implant were introduced in the 1980s.

The results of modern joint arthroplasty are excellent. The results are much better where the forces are low or the bones are large. Currently, total hip and total knee arthroplasty has a greater than 90 percent success rate at 15 to 20 years.

Complications

All of the joints are prone to similar complications such as dislocation, prosthetic breakage, periprosthetic fractures, infection, and loosening. It is possible for any nonconstrained implant to dislocate. The diagnosis is usually obvious, but should be confirmed by biplane radiographs, because one view may not clearly show the dislocation (Fig. 272-22). Because many of today's implants are modular (snap together in the operating room), relocation should not be attempted without discussion with an orthopedic surgeon. Disassembly of the prosthesis during attempted closed reduction has been reported. Consent for reduction under anesthesia should be obtained prior to any heavy sedation. It is safest to relocate modular implants under fluoroscopy.

Modern alloys have greatly reduced the incidence of prosthetic breakage. More commonly the bone around the prosthesis fractures (Fig. 272-23). Other than making the diagnosis of a periprosthetic or prosthetic fracture the emergency medicine physician will generally not be involved in the treatment of these problems.

Total joint arthroplasty should not be painful. Any time a patient presents with new onset of pain around a prosthesis, loosening of the prosthesis must be suspected. Loosening occurs in two ways: from infection or from the loss of implant fixation. Late loosening is usually characterized by insidious onset of pain and rarely presents to the emergency department. Many criteria for radiographic evidence of loosening have been presented in the orthopedic literature. Radiographic loosening is usually detected as migration of the implant over time with lytic destruction of bone around the prosthesis (Fig. 272-24).

Infection of a total joint arthroplasty is a catastrophic event. In the first few weeks postoperatively the prosthesis may sometimes be salvaged by immediate surgical débridement and intravenous antibiotics. The most sensitive emergency screening tests are an erythrocyte sedimentation rate or C-reactive protein. Aspiration of any joint should

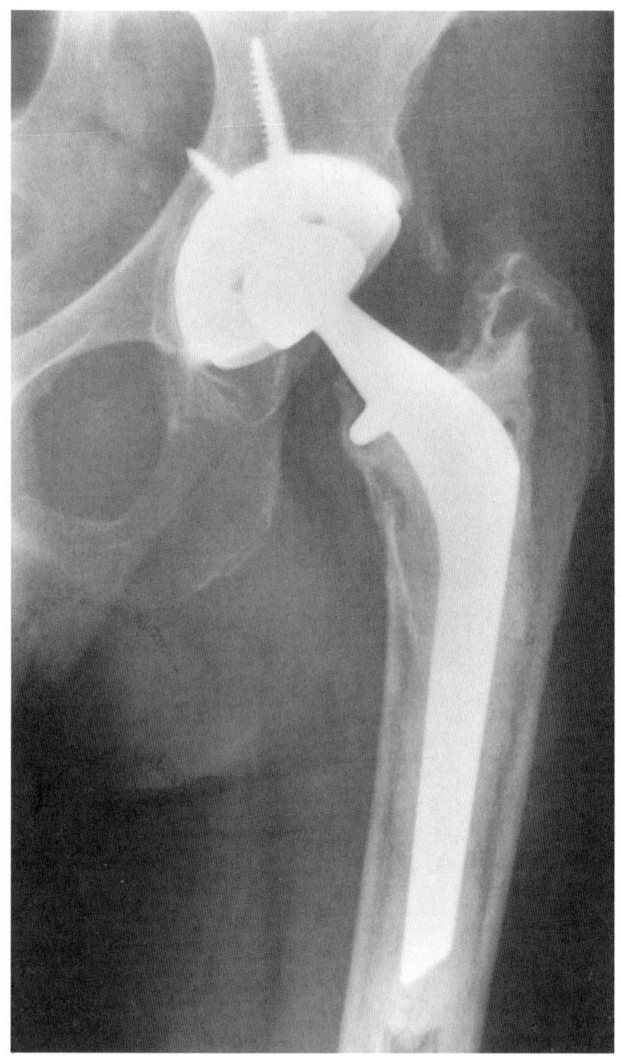

FIG. 272-27. This "hybrid" total hip arthroplasty has a cemented femoral component and a noncemented acetabular component that is additionally fixed with screws.

be performed prior to administration of any antibiotics but should never be performed without a surgeon's approval. It is possible for an uninfected implant to be infected by a needle aspiration. Late infections of a prosthesis require removal of a prosthesis to clear the infection.

Some of the most serious complications involving total joint arthroplasties involve the soft tissue structures around the joint. Ligaments holding the joint together can disrupt causing instability of the joint. Tendons that pass around the joint can rupture leading to loss of function of the joint. If diagnosed early they can often be repaired with an excellent result.

COMPLICATIONS OF UPPER EXTREMITY ARTHROPLASTIES The silicone interpositional arthroplasties may fail and create particles that cause an inflammatory response. This is differentiated from an infection by radiographs showing the radiolucent silicone "spacers" and aspiration of fluid for cell count, Gram stain, and culture.

The elbow joint has greater complications than any other commonly replaced joint. Even in the best centers infection rates of 10 percent or greater are not uncommon. This may be due to the thin soft tissue over the posterior elbow. Loosening rates at the elbow are also high due to the need for a constrained prosthesis and limited bone for fixation.

The shoulder's humeral component is extremely durable (Fig. 272-25). The glenoid component with its small bone surface area for fixation is prone to failure. Dislocation of the shoulder can only be diagnosed with a true anteroposterior and either axillary or transcapular lateral radiograph. Acute loss of motor power may be the result of a rotator cuff tear.

COMPLICATIONS OF LOWER EXTREMITY ARTHROPLASTY Silicone interpositional arthroplasty is also used in the feet, but the failure rates are much higher due to the higher forces. Ankle arthroplasty has had limited success because the small bones of the hind foot do not allow adequate fixation to withstand the high forces placed across the ankle joint.

The knee has excellent inherent ligamentous stability and therefore unconstrained implants (Fig. 272-26) are usually used today. It is possible for these implants to dislocate; however, it is not as common as in the shoulder or hip. Instability can develop in knee arthroplasties if a ligament is disrupted such as the medial collateral ligament or the posterior cruciate ligament. Diagnosis is by the same examination methods used on nonreplaced knees. Disruption of the quadriceps mechanism is a disastrous complication and must be considered if the patient is unable to straight leg raise. When the patella tendon ruptures, repair rates are extremely poor if not diagnosed and treated early.

The hip, like the shoulder, may be addressed by hemi- or total arthroplasty. The acetabulum is usually not replaced in fracture management, but almost always replaced for arthritis. The acetabulum is replaced by a plastic shell that accepts the head of the femoral component. This plastic liner may also be metal backed which allows for bone ingrowth or more even stress transfer when cemented (Fig. 272-27). The hip is the most common joint to dislocate. This is confirmed by biplane radiographs and because these prostheses are often modular, great care and often fluoroscopy should be used during relocation. Reattachment of the trochanter after the transtrochanteric approach is usually performed with wire. These wires commonly break during the healing process but are not usually a problem.

BIBLIOGRAPHY

Browner BD, Jupiter JB, Levine AM, Trafton PG: *Skeletal Trauma,* 2d ed. Philadelphia, Saunders, 1998.

Chapman MW: *Operative Orthopaedics,* 2d ed. Philadelphia, Lippincott, 1993.

Delee J, Drez D: *Orthopaedic Sports Medicine.* Philadelphia, Saunders, 1994.

Green DP: *Operative Hand Surgery,* 3d ed. New York, Churchill Livingstone, 1993.

Harrington PR, Dickson JH: An eleven-year clinical investigation of Harrington instrumentation: A preliminary report on 578 cases. *Clin Orthop* 117:157, 1976.

Morrey BF: *Joint Replacement Arthroplasty.* New York, Churchill Livingstone, 1991.

Muller ME, Allgower M, Schneider R, Willenger H: *Manual of Internal Fixation,* 3d ed. Berlin, Springer-Verlag, 1991.

Rockwood CA Jr, Green DP, Bucholz RW, Heckman JD: *Fractures in Adults,* 4th ed. Philadelphia, Lippincott-Raven, 1996.

Rothman RH, Simeone FA: *The Spine,* 3d ed. Philadelphia, Saunders, 1992.

NONTRAUMATIC MUSCULOSKELETAL DISORDERS

NECK PAIN

Myron M. LaBan

Neck pain has an encyclopedic list of causes, including trauma, degenerative disease, infections, neoplasms, congenital variations, inflammatory arthritis, and psychic tension. An evaluation of neck pain requires an understanding of the anatomy of the cervical spine. The cervical spine consists of seven vertebrae; the fifth through the seventh are alike in shape and size, whereas the first cervical vertebra (atlas) and the second (axis) differ in structure. The lower third through seventh vertebral bodies articulate with each other via their superior and inferior articular processes, enabling limited rotation and lateral flexion. The atlas (C1) supports the occipital condyles and the axis (C2). Its inferior articulations resemble the other inferior vertebral articulations. The dens and its stabilizing horizontal ligament enable rotation between C1 and C2. The transverse processes of each of the cervical vertebrae are perforated by a foramen through which the vertebral vessels pass. Topographically, the first cervical vertebra is located immediately behind the angle of the mandible, the transverse process of the atlas is positioned between the angle of the mandible and the mastoid process, the hyoid bone is anterior to the level of C3, the thyroid cartilage is anterior to C4, and the cricoid cartilage is at the level of the sixth cervical vertebra.

The muscles of the neck are compartmentalized into seven fascial planes. These planes normally enable pain-free movement of one muscle group on the other. Following acute neck trauma, petechial hemorrhages and edema within these same fascial planes may produce limited motion associated with complaints of stiffness, pain, and swelling.

The stable but flexible cervical spine is linked by both ligaments and disks. Because of major structural differences, the cervical disks are less likely than lumbar disks to prolapse. The cervical spine is more mobile, the superincumbent weight is less, the nucleus pulposus is more anteriorly displaced and, unlike the lumbar spine, the annulus is reinforced posteriorly in its entire width by the posterior longitudinal ligament.

The eight paired cervical spinal roots exit the intervertebral foramina between the superior and inferior pedicles, except for the upper two cervical roots. Unique to the cervical spinal roots, in over half the cases the ventral and dorsal roots are separate at the neural foramina. In these cases, isolated irritation of the dorsal (sensory) root posteriorly by an osteophyte may produce only sensory complaints. Similarly, ventral root (motor) compromise by a degenerative or herniated disk may produce only painless, progressive weakness. Segmental motor or sensory signs associated with a root disorder are called *radiculopathies.* Signs and symptoms of spinal cord disease are called *myelopathies.*

The sinuvertebral nerves from the dorsal root reenter the intervertebral foramina supplying sensory innervation to the ligaments of the spinal canal. Anteriorly, they supply the posterior longitudinal ligament and posteriorly the ligamentum flavum, meninges, and associated vessels. Ascending and descending branches also supply the zygoapophyseal joints, providing position sense.

The cervical portion of the spinal cord surrounded by spinal fluid is suspended laterally to the enveloping dura by 20 dentate ligaments. The dura in turn is attached cephalad to the rim of the foramen magnum and within the vertebral spinal canal is cushioned from trauma by epidural fat.

CLINICAL FEATURES

The source of neck pain can often be determined by a thorough and searching history. In most cases, patients can identify the inciting event or an exacerbating maneuver or position that causes pain. Following trauma, note the exact nature of the impact with reference to positioning; accompanying lacerations of the head, neck, or face; the use of restraints; the use of protective sports equipment; associated limb or trunk fractures or contusions; and loss of consciousness or seizures. The date of injury, the patient's age and occupation, preexisting medical conditions, and other contributing factors should also be identified. Determine the character of pain and its distribution. Ask about specific neurogenic symptoms, including extremity weakness, incoordination, numbness or paresthesias, and sphincter and sexual dysfunction. Patients with visual, auditory-vestibular, and pharyngeal-laryngeal symptoms often require direct questioning to elicit complaints. The results of previous imaging studies and prior response to medication or physical treatment may be diagnostic.

The physical examination begins with an observation of a loss of neck flexibility, unless a mechanism of injury is present for possible cervical fracture or spinal cord injury. In such cases, the neck should remain immobilized until radiographs are obtained and reviewed by the emergency physician. Pain may cause splinting of the head on the shoulders during position change. Active and passive movement should be assessed, including rotation (chin to shoulder) and lateral flexion (ear to shoulder). When localized ipsilateral neck pain is experienced toward the side of head movement, zygoapophyseal joint irritability is suspected. When ipsilateral pain radiates to shoulder or arm (Spurling sign), a radicular component may be present. Contralateral neck pain suggests either a primary ligamentous or a muscular source of discomfort as these structures are stretched.

Palpate the posterior cervical triangle, the supraclavicular fossa, and carotid sheaths, and the anterior neck. Auscultation of the carotid and the subclavian arteries may demonstrate bruits, in the former associated with potential cerebral insufficiency and in the latter instance with a thoracic outlet or vascular steal syndrome. Symptomatic occipital neuralgia can be replicated by firm pressure over the occipital notch, producing scalp numbness or burning dysesthesias in the occipital nerve distribution. Various compression and distraction maneuvers of the cervical spine are also diagnostically useful. They include vertical skull compression or lateral flexion positions that replicate radicular symptoms and manual vertical distraction, a reverse Spurling maneuver, which "unloads" the spinal roots and adjacent cervical vertebral joints, thereby reducing pain.

An evaluation of neck discomfort is incomplete without shoulder, arm, and neurologic examination (Table 273-1), since cervical spinal radiculopathies can cause upper extremity pain, paresthesias, and weakness. Knowledge of the dermatome, sclerotome, and myotome referral distribution of spinal root irritation is also essential to diagnosis. Look for muscle atrophy or fasciculations. A loss of triceps reflex suggests C7 root pathology, whereas a loss of biceps reflex suggests a C5-C6 root syndrome. Motor strength is tested by the "break" maneuver, whereby the patient is given a maximal advantage of position and strength and the examiner "breaks" the muscle, comparing one side with the other. The triceps is tested by having the patient extend the elbow and maximally resist the examiner's efforts to flex the elbow. A smooth, asymmetric "give" rather than a "ratchety" break suggests C7-C8, posterior cord, or radial nerve involvement. Similarly, other muscle groups are tested and patterns of weakness are correlated with the clinical history and symptoms. Local nerve

TABLE 273-1 Signs and Symptoms of Cervical Radiculopathy

Disk Space	Cervical Root	Pain Complaint	Sensory Abnormality	Motor Weakness	Altered Reflex
C1-C2	C1-C2	Neck, scalp	Scalp		
C4-C5	C5	Neck, shoulder, upper arm	Shoulder, thumb	Spinati, deltoid, biceps	Reduced biceps reflex
C5-C6	C6	Neck, shoulder, upper medial, scapular area, proximal forearm, thumb	Thumb and index finger, lateral forearm	Deltoid, biceps, pronator teres, wrist extensors	Reduced biceps and brachioradialis reflex
C6-C7	C7	Neck, posterior arm, dorsum proximal forearm, chest, medial $\frac{1}{3}$ scapula, middle finger	Middle finger, forearm	Triceps, pronator teres	Reduced triceps reflex
C7-T1	C8	Neck, posterior arm, medial proximal forearm, median inferior scapular border, medial hand, ring and little fingers	Ring and little fingers	Triceps, flexor carpi ulnaris, hand intrinsics	Reduced triceps reflex

palpation also is a useful adjunct to the examination. C5-C6 root lesions often elicit tenderness over the brachial plexus at Erb's point in the supraclavicular fossa, whereas a C8-T1 root lesion can cause tenderness over the distal ulnar nerve at the elbow.

Sensory symptoms of pain or dysesthesias are difficult to evaluate, particularly when motor signs are absent. This is all too often the case in cervical spinal radiculopathies. The discrete separation of the motor and sensory roots at the cervical neural foramina is the explanation for motor sparing despite severe sensory symptoms. Marked C7 root irritability without motor weakness of the triceps (radial nerve C7-C8) or the pronator teres (median nerve C6-C7) can present only with aching at the medial, middle scapular border, or aching in the myotome distribution to the chest, axilla, or triceps. Numbness or tingling in the C7 dermatome distribution to the middle finger may be the only symptom of spinal root irritation.

Early cervical spinal myelopathies can only be recognized if the examiner looks for them, so a full neurologic examination that includes the lower extremities is needed to evaluate neck pain. Common signs and symptoms include hyperreflexia, a positive Babinski sign, gait disturbance, lower extremity weakness, impaired fine hand movement, or upper and lower extremity spasticity.

The need for radiographs depends on the clinical condition suspected. If degenerative disease is suspected, oblique views of the cervical spine can identify foraminal narrowing. Both the dens and the lowest cervical and upper thoracic vertebrae should also be visualized. Flexion-extension films are useful if instability is suspected. Magnetic resonance imaging is now the preferred test to evaluate the cervical cord.

Electromyographic (EMG) studies can diagnose neural structural abnormality, assess the level and the degree of severity, and provide a prognostic baseline and an objective means of reassessment. Both EMG and nerve conduction velocity testing are needed if there is progressive motor impairment or when confusion exists as to the level of neural compromise. Unfortunately, EMG findings lag 2 weeks behind a patient's actual clinical state. EMG is a test of motor dysfunction. If the sensory root is solely compromised and the motor root spared, the EMG findings may be normal.

CERVICAL SOFT TISSUE INJURIES

Hyperflexion-hyperextension injuries to the cervical spine result in stretching of soft tissues, intervertebral joints, nerve roots, and adjacent peripheral nerves. The most common precipitating events are motor vehicle accidents, falls, and sport injuries. Staged automobile accidents using cadavers have demonstrated injuries ranging from petechial hemorrhage and edema, muscle and ligament distraction, vertebral dislocations and fractures, to herniations of the intervertebral disk. The forces applied during motor vehicle crashes are multiple and depend on the position of the head and neck as well as the type of accident. Forces applied include flexion, extension, rotation, and vertical compression. A rear-end collision propels the trunk forward on the pelvis, throwing the head into hyperextension and stretching the anterior structures of the neck. Hyperextension injuries include hyperextension dislocation; atlas fractures including avulsions of the anterior arch, extension teardrop fractures, or fractures of the posterior arch; laminar fracture; traumatic spondylolisthesis; and other fracture dislocations. A head-on impact initially produces acute flexion, compressing the anterior neck structures. Hyperflexion injuries include anterior subluxation; unilateral or bilateral interfacet dislocations; vertebral compression fractures; avulsion fractures of the spinous processes; and complete subluxation with disruption of the posterior ligaments, facet capsule, and annular disk fibers. Both hyperextension and hyperflexion injuries are also associated with rebound flexion and extension, respectively. To compound the mechanism of injury further, a vertical component may be added as the cervical spine is compressed when the individual's trunk is lifted by the force of impact.

Passengers forewarned of an impending rear collision can potentially protect themselves by flexing the neck and tucking the chin against the chest. An extended head potentiates the risk of ligamentous rupture and articular dislocation. Areas of preexisting degenerative disease are most susceptible to injury.

Postinjury complaints are highly variable and, besides neck pain, may include headache, vertigo, dysesthesias, visual symptoms, dizziness, tinnitus, dysphagia, and hoarseness. Typically, pain is delayed for a number of hours following an accident. Restricted cervical range of motion can be associated with radicular patterns of myotome weakness suggesting cervical root compromise. Headache can occur from stretching and tearing of occipital muscles and the occipital nerve. The cause of vertigo is unknown but could be due to brainstem contusion, trauma to sympathetic fibers that accompany vertebral arteries, vertebral artery insufficiency secondary to atherosclerosis, or osteophytic compression of the vertebral arteries. Spatial instability affecting balance is not uncommon, and patients describe a feeling of "sliding" or "veering" with changes of direction rather than true vertigo. This rather unique description of spatial instability may be due to injury to the zygoapophyseal joints of the neck rather than the inner ear. Dysphagia can occur as a result of pharyngeal edema or a retropharyngeal hematoma. Vocal hoarseness can be attributed to stretching of the recurrent laryngeal nerve, often associated with marked edema of the sternocleidomastoid muscles and carotid sheaths, potentially increasing neck circumference by one collar size. In such a case, however, blunt neck or laryngeal injury should always be suspected and evaluated with computed tomography of the neck. The most devastating complication of hyperflexion-hyperextension injury is the central cord syndrome, which may occur in the presence of cervical spondylosis, spinal stenosis, ankylosing spondylitis, or disk herniation. There may be no radiographic evidence of spinal trauma. Findings of central cord syndrome include weakness of both upper and lower extremities with predominance of weakness in the former; or upper and lower extremity spasticity. (See Chap. 264, ''Injuries to the Spine,'' for further discussion.)

Cervical spine x-ray films are of value to exclude fracture or subluxation, and flexion-extension views can demonstrate vertebral instability. Initial roentgenograms may reveal only an initial loss of the normal cervical lordosis, with subsequent studies possibly demonstrating evidence of new ligamentous ossification. Extension views of the cervical spine can demonstrate vacuum clefts in the anterior surface of the cervical disks, suggesting the presence of an avulsed disk.

Treatment initially consists of splinting of the neck with a fitted soft cervical collar fastened in slight flexion, and the use of topical ice packs for the first 24 h. Heat should be applied after 24 h. Early mobilization exercises starting at 72 h to restore flexibility should be combined with superficial moist heat and a gradual reduction in the use of the soft collar. Early in recovery, diathermy and/or cervical traction may aggravate symptoms. However, later these modalities are useful when ligamentous or articular pain persists or for treatment of radicular symptoms. In both instances treatment must be based on a specific diagnosis. Oral analgesics, including narcotics, initially are appropriate for pain relief. Muscle relaxants are not very effective. With chronic discomfort, oral nonsteroidal anti-inflammatory drugs are useful. Where occipital neuralgia or myofascial symptoms are sources of continuing pain, local injections of a mixture of long-acting steroid and 1% lidocaine followed by ice massage and ultrasound are useful.

CERVICAL DISK PATHOLOGY

Cervical disk herniations occur as the nucleus pulposus protrudes through the posterior annulus fibrosis, producing either an acute radiculopathy or occasionally a myelopathy. Cervical spondylosis and stenosis are associated with a subtle progression of symptoms, including neck stiffness or localized pain, occipital neuralgia, extremity-referred radicular pain, and occasionally clinical manifestations of a progressive myelopathy.

Acute Cervical Disk Herniations

Evidence of degeneration of the nucleus pulposus and the annulus fibrosis usually antecedes cervical disk herniation. These protrusions are usually confined by the posterior longitudinal ligament but can occasionally extrude through this ligament as free fragments. Direct posterior ruptures, although infrequent, can produce progressive myelopathy, whereas the more common posterolateral herniations precipitate the symptoms and signs of an acute cervical radiculopathy. Disk prolapse is $1\frac{1}{2}$ times more common in males, occurring most often in the fourth decade. The levels of most frequent involvement are C6-C7 (C7 root), usually left sided, and C5-C6 (C6 root), usually right sided.

The symptoms of an acute cervical disk prolapse include neck pain, headache, sclerotomal referral to the shoulder and along the medial scapular border, myotome pain in the spinal root distribution to the shoulder and arm, and dermatomal sensory dysesthesias of the appropriate finger. Motor signs include fasciculations, atrophy and weakness in the myotome distribution of the spinal root, loss of deep tendon reflexes; and, with cervical myelopathy, lower extremity hyperreflexia, Babinski sign and, rarely, loss of sphincter control. Cervical hyperextension and lateral flexion to the symptomatic side can replicate the symptoms, as can a Valsalva maneuver, whereas manual cervical distraction in flexion alleviates them. A thorough and searching examination, including muscle testing, easily delineates the level of root involvement (see Table 273-1).

Electroneuromyography can be complementary in diagnosis and will exclude occult peripheral mononeuropathies and acute brachial plexopathies. Cervical spine x-ray films are often more useful in these syndromes for what they fail to reveal rather than what they demonstrate. The presence of degenerative disease may mask a soft cervical disk protrusion. In younger adults, x-ray films may be normal, failing to reveal even a large herniation. In this instance, magnetic resonance imaging is necessary for diagnosis.

Treatment consists of analgesics sufficient to control pain, a cervical soft collar and, without evidence of carotid bruits or myelopathy, a trial of intermittent cervical traction. If the symptoms and signs of acute cervical root compression fail to respond to conservative treatment or reoccur, surgery may be recommended if imaging demonstrates a prolapsed cervical disk with root compression. Indications for hospital admission include:

1. Intractable radicular pain unresponsive to treatment.
2. Progressive upper extremity weakness, especially in the C7 distribution.
3. Progressive lower extremity myelopathic signs, such as positive Babinski sign, hyperreflexia, motor weakness, and bladder or bowel dysfunction.

Cervical Spondylosis and Stenosis

Cervical spondylosis is a progressive condition that can present either as a loss of cervical flexibility or as neck pain. Neck pain is due to local zygoapophyseal joint degeneration. Degenerative disk disease predisposes individuals to progressive osteoarthrosis of the cervical zygoapophyseal joints. A loss of disk height associated with annulus bulging produces cervical segment instability, excessive facet weight bearing, and incongruous joint motion during neck movement, accelerating articular degeneration. Altered mechanical stresses produce traction osteogenesis with subsequent spur formation. Spurs can encroach posteriorly on the spinal canal, producing cervical myelopathy; laterally on the intervertebral foramen, producing cervical radiculopathy; and anteriorly on the esophagus, producing dysphagia.

The combination of a congenitally narrowed spinal canal further compromised by a vertebral osteophytic bar anteriorly, and a buckling ligamentum flavum posteriorly, increases the risk of myelopathy secondary to cervical spinal stenosis as the diameter of the spinal canal is reduced to less than 12 mm. Cervical spinal stenosis can also occur in about 20 percent of patients with lumbar spinal stenosis. Selective impingement of the dorsal spinal root by an osteophyte arising from the zygoapophyseal joint can present with complaints of digital numbness or vague myalgias, which on subsequent appraisal can be related to the known myotome distribution of a spinal root. The C6 nerve root emerges between the C5 and C6 vertebrae and is the earliest and most frequent site of a degenerative disk. Since the C6 myotome encompasses most of the major proximal shoulder muscles, a complaint of bilateral shoulder pain should raise suspicion of C6 radiculopathy. Spurious osteophytes can produce Horner syndrome, vertebral-basilar symptoms, severe radicular symptoms without associated neck pain, painless upper extremity myotome weakness, and chest pain mimicking angina. Radiographic studies demonstrating typical segmental degenerative changes may in fact bear no relation to the actual spinal root level of the presenting complaint. For example, foraminal encroachment visible on x-ray views may be more severe at C5-C6, with the patient presenting with both clinical and EMG evidence of a progressive C7 radiculopathy arising from the C6-C7 level.

Localized neck pain and stiffness attributable to arthritis at the zygoapophyseal joint can be treated with cervical collar support, superficial ice massage, ultrasound, flexibility exercises, and nonsteroidal anti-inflammatory drugs. Cervical traction therapy may aggravate pain due to arthritis. For cervical radicular pain, though, intermittent cervical traction initially in the formal setting of an outpatient physical therapy facility, followed by ongoing home cervical traction, is an effective approach. Myofascial pain can often be managed with topical ice, deep kneading massage, stretching exercises, and local injections of steroids and lidocaine. The prompt recognition and correction of aggravating factors, such as emotional stress or prolonged postural neck hyperextension related to overly soft seating or to the use of bifocal glasses during reading, may in itself be curative.

BIBLIOGRAPHY

Caillet R: *Neck and Arm Pain,* 3d ed. Philadelphia, FA Davis, 1991.

DeLisa JA (ed): *Rehabilitation Medicine: Principles and Practice,* 2d ed. Philadelphia, JB Lippincott, 1993.

Ellenberg M, Honet JC: Clinical pearls in cervical radiculopathy, in LaBan MM (ed): *Physiatric Pearls.* Philadelphia, WB Saunders, 1996, p 47.

Saruhashi Y, Hukuda S, Katsuura A, et al: Clinical outcomes of cervical spinal cord injuries without radiographic evidence of trauma. *Spinal Cord* 36:567, 1998.

THORACIC AND LUMBAR PAIN SYNDROMES

Paul J.W. Tawney
Cara B. Siegel
Myron M. LaBan

THORACIC SPINE

Although spine pain complaints are more common at cervical and lumbar levels, thoracic complaints can be as disabling. This region of the spine is comparatively stable and protected both by the rib cage and the orientation of the facet joints. In this region, the spinal cord and paired segmental nerves traverse the narrowest of bony canals and any compromise of the available space can result in rapid and profound neurologic deficits.

Thoracic spine fractures occur most commonly at the T10–L2 levels and can occur from direct trauma as well as forced hyperflexion of the trunk, as in lap-belt injuries. Vertebral fractures resulting from spinal osteoporosis occur in 8 percent of women over 80 years of age. Such compression fractures are usually wedge-shaped and stable. The presenting symptom is usually severe pain, and accompanying myelopathy is rare. However, when long tract signs, such as hyperreflexia, Babinski's sign, and urinary incontinence are present, a malignancy metastatic to the spine must be suspected. An epidural metastasis may present similarly as an acute myelopathy with or without pain or abnormal x-rays. Myelography, computed tomography (CT), or magnetic resonance imaging (MRI) is needed to differentiate the relatively rare thoracic disk protrusion (1 percent of all disk herniations) from a spinal cord tumor. Pain from thoracic root lesions is usually worse while reclining at night and is relieved by assuming an erect position. Patients may sleep sitting up in a chair. They may on initial examination demonstrate Babinski reflexes that disappear after a brief period of rest. Slowed lumbar spinal evoked potentials can also be diagnostic in confirming thoracic spinal myelopathy.[1,2]

Localized paravertebral pain can be associated with an acute facet syndrome. Plica entrapped within the thoracic zygapophyseal joints can produce severe and disabling pain. Radicular pain and localized stiffness associated with osteoarthrosis of these same vertebral joints cause chronic pain and can result in narrowing of the neural and spinal canals. The latter can lead to signs and symptoms of thoracic spinal stenosis.

Rheumatoid spondylitis primarily affecting young men may initially present as thoracic spinal pain or stiffness. A loss of chest expansion to less than 1 in. at nipple line is suggestive and, with x-rays of the sacroiliac joints, is often diagnostic.

Herpes zoster neuralgia can also be associated with acute thoracic radiculopathy. It is difficult to diagnose before vesicles and bullae are evident.

Diabetic thoracic radiculopathy may present as abdominal pain. When this condition is suspected, electromyography (EMG) demonstrating thoracic paraspinal and abdominal muscle segmental denervation (T7–T12) can be diagnostic.

LUMBAR SPINE

Epidemiology

Low back pain is second only to the common cold as a cause of industrial absenteeism and is the primary cause of reduced working capacity. Sixty to 90 percent of the population will experience back pain in their lifetime. Fifty percent of people will have a recurrent episode. It is one of the most common reasons for a physician office visit. The yearly prevalence in working age adults is 50 percent. Over 5 million individuals are disabled with low back pain, making it the number one disability in workers less than 45 years old.[3,4] In 85 percent of cases, no definitive diagnosis or source of the pain can be given. The natural history of low back pain is that 90 to 95 percent of patients, even if they have sciatica, will be better within 2 months,[5] regardless of the type of treatment rendered.[6] Economic and psychosocial costs for this common disorder are substantial.[7]

Pathophysiology and Clinical Features

The causes of lumbosacral pain are as diverse and as complex as are the interrelated anatomic structures of the lumbar spine itself. Any innervated structure in the region can be a pain generator. The specific pain generator is rarely identified. Deep somatic pain due to mechanical irritation, inflammation, or even increased vascular pressure can emanate from the vertebral column, surrounding muscles, tendons, ligaments, or fascia. Discomfort of articular origin, either lumbar zygapophyseal or sacroiliac joints, can also be recognized by known sclerotome patterns of pain referral.[8] Pain due to nerve irritation can be perceived locally and distally. Nonspinal causes of low back pain must also be considered.

One rational approach to the diagnosis and treatment of low back pain or sciatica is predicated on an understanding of the process of spinal degeneration as described by Kirkaldy-Willis and Farfan.[9] Initially beginning with an alteration in the hydroscopic quality of the nucleus pulposus, it can progress from annular degeneration of a single disk to multilevel involvement. Sequential disk degeneration with associated zygapophyseal joint compromise can be associated with relatively infrequent disk prolapses. More often, progressive posterior facet disease is associated with foraminal or spinal canal encroachment, producing symptoms associated with lateral or central spinal stenosis.

Spinal Stenosis

Spinal stenosis can be a cause of back and lower extremity pain. It is defined as any narrowing of the lumbar spinal canal, nerve root canal, or intervertebral foramina, the predominant etiology being degenerative changes. Diagnosis is usually by CT or MRI. Incidence and prevalence as the primary source of pain is difficult to establish as it can also be found in asymptomatic individuals. The clinical presentation is usually that of an older individual with a long history of back pain. Ninety percent also have leg pain, as the key sign is lower extremity pain exacerbated with walking and relieved with sitting (neurogenic claudication). However, this still has a broad differential, including osteoarthritis of the hip and vascular claudication due to peripheral vascular disease. Ambulation producing lumbar, gluteal, or calf pain may be a manifestation of peripheral vascular disease, but it is also indistinguishable from that of lumbar spinal stenosis. Both vascular insufficiency and spinal stenosis are aggravated by activity and relieved by rest. Vascular signs in the former case or neurologic abnormality in the latter instance can lead to the diagnosis, but arteriography or MRI or CT scan may be necessary for confirmation. Most helpful associations with spinal stenosis are age older than 65, absence of pain when seated, wide-based gait, and production of thigh pain with sustained lumbar extension of 30 s. Physical examination findings are not particularly helpful in ruling in or ruling out spinal stenosis.[10]

Three-Joint Complex Degeneration

The combined retrogressive and proliferative changes in the disk anteriorly and in the posterior joints present with both clinical symptoms and roentgenographic changes referred to as combined three-joint complex degeneration. The vertebra-disk-vertebra joint and the paired facet joints comprise the three-joint complex. Three distinct stages in the evolution of this process can be recognized clinically. The *stage of dysfunction* is associated with complaints of pain and stiffness, often without radiographic or clinical abnormality. The *stage of instability* is associated with evidence of spinal segment movement best exemplified by radiographic evidence of the presence of pseudospondylolisthesis, usually at the L4–L5 level, secondary to advanced degenerative disk disease with preservation of the stabilizing pars interarticularis. This phase of degeneration can be clinically recognized by the presence of limited spinal flexibility, reactive scoliosis, reduction in the lumbar lordosis, and, on occasion, the presence of neurologic abnormality, including alterations in deep tendon reflexes, reductions in muscle strength, and restricted straight leg raise (SLR) signs.

The final stage of stabilization is clinically associated with a marked loss of lumbar flexibility. ''Stiffness'' is a primary complaint that may supersede pain, particularly following periods of immobility. Prolonged standing or walking may precipitate symptoms of localized radicular pain, paresthetic complaints of numbness or tingling, and motor symptoms of ''weakness'' or ''instability'' with or without corroborative motor signs. Articular facet, laminar, and vertebral enlargement associated with osteophytic formation progressing to vertebral fusion are characteristic x-ray features of this stage.

The zygapophyseal (facet) joints are true synovial joints innervated by the medial branches of the dorsal rami. It has been estimated that 15 to 40 percent of chronic back pain is due to the zygapophyseal joints. The clinical presentation overlaps considerably with low back pain of other etiologies. The diagnosis remains one of exclusion and confirmation by analgesic injection.[11]

Sacroiliac Joint Disease

Mechanical dysfunction can occur within the sacroiliac (SI) joints. Sacroiliac joint pain is commonly referred to the inguinal and anterolateral thigh, as well as the lower abdominal quadrants, often simulating an acute appendicitis or ovarian cyst. Inflammatory processes can involve the SI joints, as in the seronegative spondyloarthropathies. Early in this process there may be little or no correlation between symptom severity and radiographic evidence of joint involvement. The pain is usually experienced over the joints themselves, radiating to the anterior lateral or posterior thighs. Usually worse at night, the pain may be bilateral, alternating from side to side. Prolonged standing or sitting, especially on long car trips, exacerbates the discomfort. ''Weakness'' or stiffness, primarily in the morning, is also a predominant symptom of sacroiliitis. When in young men, stiffness may be associated with new-onset rheumatoid spondylitis; the earliest complaint may be that of chest pain and stiffness rather than that of low back pain. The earliest sign may be that of restricted chest expansion of less than 1 in. at the nipple line. Unfortunately, chest expansion measurement, Schober test of lumbar range, and other sacroiliac tests are poor for following disease progression.[12]

Radiculopathy

Radicular pain derives from irritation of the proximal portion of the spinal nerve as a result of ischemia, chemical irritation by contents of the nucleus pulposus, or mechanical compression. Kuslich,[13] performing progressive local anesthesia during spinal surgery, has observed that compressed or chemically irritated nerve roots are perceived as painful when stretched, while normal nerve roots do not reproduce pain. The outer annulus and posterior longitudinal ligament also could be stimulated to produce pain.[13] Ninety-five percent of disk herniations occur at L4–L5 or L5–S1. Without complaint of sciatica, or pain below the knee in a dermatomal distribution, the chance of a herniated nucleus pulposus is 1 in 1000. Complaints of muscular pain in the myotome and sensory dysesthesias in the dermatome distribution of a spinal root may be accompanied by referred pain in the sclerotome distribution. Compromise of L5 and S1 roots can be experienced, respectively, as muscular pain in the anterior tibial compartment simulating ''shin splints,'' and muscular pain in the calf mimicking a thrombophlebitis. Proximal L5 and S1 root compression is suggested distally by the presence of pain to palpation over the peroneal nerve (L5) at the fibular head and the tibial nerve (S1) in the tarsal tunnel. Sensory complaints in the presence of radicular syndromes may be useful in localizing root levels of involvement. Paresthesias in the great toe suggest L5 root involvement, and in the little toe S1 radiculopathy.

Other Causes of Lumbar Pain

Neurogenic pain in the low back region can be associated with herpes zoster as manifest in shingles or in femoral nerve mononeuropathy that is often associated with diabetes. Pain is due to loss of the pain inhibitory system in the central or peripheral nervous system. It is described as burning, tingling, or skin crawling. It is intensified by what would otherwise be nonpainful sensory stimulation, such as light touch (allodynia). It may persist after cessation of the provoking stimulus (hyperpathia).

Additionally, pain of remote origin, even outside the spine itself, can present as lumbar pain. Lesions within the central nervous system, and in the spinal cord at or above the lumbar area, can also produce both low back pain and radicular leg discomfort. Parasagittal brain tumors and thoracic root lesions, including neurofibromata, can simulate lumbar root syndromes.

Distal nerve entrapment syndromes also can present with primary complaints of lumbosacral pain. The most notable example of this situation is tibial nerve entrapment (S1) in the tarsal tunnel behind the medial ankle malleolus.

Pain to direct palpation over the ischial tuberosities, greater trochanters, or sciatic notches may suggest localized abnormality, including a bursitis at the tuberosity or trochanter or an enthesitis; that is, inflammation at the tendinous attachment of muscle to bone, at the insertion of the hip abductor and extensor muscle groups. Trochanteric bursitis itself can mimic lumbar radiculopathy with distal pain referral along the iliotibial band to the lateral knee. Excessive lateral trunk sway to the stance leg during ambulation, a compensated Trendelenburg gait, suggests primary intraarticular hip abnormality. On examination, corroborative evidence of an initial loss of hip internal rotation may be associated with medial groin pain and a positive Patrick sign, which may radiate to the knee. Attempting to "walk around," primary hip disease produces excessive stress at both the ipsilateral sacroiliac joint and the greater trochanter. Each, singly or together, may initially appear to be the salient problem until the loss of hip mobility is identified as the progenitor of the other complaints.

Based on their shared segmental innervation, pain from visceral disorders, including those of kidney, pancreas, and gallbladder; duodenal ulcers; colonic diverticulitis; expanding abdominal aortic aneurysm; epidural hematoma or abscess; and endometriosis, can all mimic primary low back disorders. Pain from a leaking abdominal aortic aneurysm is constant and aching and may be referred to the lower abdomen and inguinal areas as well as the low back. In the evaluation of low back pain in the elderly, an abdominal aortic aneurysm must always be considered in the differential diagnosis. Costovertebral angle percussion pain is invariably associated with retroperitoneal pathology, most often kidney. Spinal cord compression can develop as a first sign of malignancy or as a complication. It is usually associated with back pain and should always be suspected if there are any neurologic signs or sphincter dysfunction. A history of associated systemic symptoms and a lack of therapeutic response to a trial of initial bedrest, combined with an abnormal abdominal, pelvic, neurologic, or rectal examination, are usually sufficient to redirect the examination to the appropriate extraspinal problem.[12]

Diagnosis

Due to the prevalence, cost, concern for suboptimal care, and a growing body of evidence on low back pain, the Agency for Health Care Policy and Research (AHCPR) commissioned guideline development for evaluation and treatment of acute low back pain.[14] The *Quick Reference Guide for Clinicians* is a distilled version of the *Clinical Practice Guideline,* with summary points for ready reference on a day-to-day basis.[15] Text, figures, and tables from the *Quick Reference* are referenced throughout this chapter.

The AHCPR guideline defines acute low back problems as activity intolerance due to lower back or back-related leg symptoms of less than 3 months' duration. This includes new episodes in patients with recurrent low back problems. A focused medical history and physical examination are sufficient to assess the patient with an acute or recurrent limitation due to low back symptoms of less than 4 weeks' duration. Patient responses and findings on the history and physical examination, referred to as "red flags" (Table 274-1), raise suspicion of serious underlying spinal conditions. The medical history and physical examination can also alert the clinician to nonspinal pathology (abdominal, pelvic, and thoracic) that can present as low back symptoms.[15]

AHCPR classifies low back problems into working categories:

Potentially serious spinal condition—tumor, infection, spinal fracture, or a major neurologic compromise, such as cauda equina syndrome, suggested by a red flag.

Sciatica—back-related lower limb symptoms suggesting lumbosacral nerve root compromise.

Nonspecific back symptoms—occurring primarily in the back and suggesting neither nerve root compromise nor a serious spinal condition.

Objectives of the diagnostic process are to rule out a serious systemic disease and neurologic compromise by searching for "red flags" for spine fracture, tumor, infection, cauda equina syndrome, or nonspinal pathology. Given the many variables impacting onset and persistence of back problems, one must also assess social or psychological distress (nonphysical factors) that may amplify or prolong pain.[16]

If a potentially dangerous problem is not present, diagnostic testing in the first 4 weeks of symptoms is not helpful. Ultimately, the treatment goal is to improve activity tolerance rather than focus on pain.

TABLE 274-1 Red Flags for Potentially Serious Conditions

From Medical History		
Fracture	Tumor	Cauda Equina
Major trauma, such as vehicle accident or fall from height. Minor trauma or even strenuous lifting (in older or potentially osteoporotic patient).	Age over 50 or under 20. History of cancer. Constitutional symptoms, such as recent fever or chills or unexplained weight loss. Risk factors for spinal infection: recent bacterial infection (e.g., urinary tract infection); IV drug abuse; or immune suppression (from steroids, transplant, or HIV). Pain that worsens when supine; severe nighttime pain.	Saddle anesthesia. Recent onset of bladder dysfunction, such as urinary retention, increased frequency, or overflow incontinence. Severe or progressive neurologic deficit in the lower extremity.
From Physical Examination for any Potentially Serious Conditions		
	Unexpected laxity of the anal sphincter. Perianal/perineal sensory loss. Major motor weakness: quadriceps (knee extension weakness); ankle plantar flexors, evertors, and dorsiflexors (footdrop).	

Evaluation and treatment algorithms and tables are provided within the guideline to assist in initial and follow-up assessment of patients. A patient's estimate of personal activity intolerance due to low back symptoms contributes to the clinical assessment of the severity of the back problem, guides treatment, and establishes a baseline for recommending daily activities and evaluating progress.[15]

Spinal fracture may be suspected in major trauma, such as motor vehicle accident or fall from height, or minor trauma, or even strenous lifting in an older or potentially osteoporotic patient. The examiner must give credence to the history, age, and circumstances of onset in establishing a diagnosis. For example, an elderly woman with acute onset, severe midthoracic pain, without a history of trauma, can be presumed to have an osteoporotic vertebral compression fracture until proved otherwise. Sacral insufficiency fractures may also be considered in elderly women.[17] Compression fracture is increasingly likely in patients over age 50 and more so for those over 70 years old. History of trauma or steroid use also supports this in the differential diagnosis (see Table 274-1).

Less than 1 percent of patients presenting to a general medical clinic with low back pain (LBP) had cancer.[16] All patients with cancer-related LBP had at least one of the following: age ≥50 (80 percent); previous history of breast, lung, or prostate cancer (33 percent); unexplained weight loss, fever, chills; failure of conservative therapy; no relief with bedrest or supine position; and pain duration >1 month. Percussion pain over the bony spine itself supports the presence of an osseous abnormality, such as compression fracture, metastasis, or disk or vertebral infection.[18]

In patients found to have a spinal infection, fever was only associated 27 percent of the time. Other factors that raise the suspicion of infection are IV drug use, urinary tract infection, skin infection, and immune suppression due to steroids, transplant, or HIV. Disk space infections are relatively uncommon and are most often associated with recent disk surgery. However, they can also occur in association with a remote infection, that is, kidney, skin, distal trauma to a bursa, or in the drug addicted, or can also arise spontaneously in rare cases.[18]

The onset of lumbosacral pain associated with bilateral leg pain radiation and a sudden loss of bladder control should be presumed to be a midline herniated disk with the threat of paraparesis (cauda equina syndrome). This demands careful neurologic exam including rectal examination for sensory changes (''saddle anesthesia''), examination for motor and reflex function, and examination for possible immediate consultation for emergent imaging and possibly surgical intervention.

Physical Examination

Guided by the medical history, the physical examination includes: general observation of the patient; a regional back examination; neurologic screening; and testing for sciatic nerve root tension. The examination is mostly subjective because patient response or interpretation is required for all parts except reflex testing and circumferential measurements for atrophy.

Addressing Red Flags

Physical examination evidence of severe neurologic compromise that correlates with the medical history may indicate a need for immediate consultation. The examination may further modify suspicions of tumor, infection, or significant trauma.[15] If it does, then the physical examination must include abdominal, vascular, neurologic, and lower extremity evaluation. Abdominal visceral palpation and auscultation over the aorta and renal arteries, as well as an assessment of peripheral pulses, color, and temperature, should be routine.

Observation and Regional Back Examination

With the patient disrobed, the spine and pelvis should be observed for abnormal spinal curves, pelvic tilts, or the presence of spinal-pelvic lists, all suggesting splinting or guarding in response to pain. Each vertebra should be palpated to identify point tenderness that suggests bony involvement. The gait should be observed for a loss of normal, symmetric spinal-pelvic rhythm. Asymmetric posturing suggests pain or weakness to which the patient is biomechanically accommodating. Guarding or splinting can best be demonstrated at slower cadences and can be dramatically accentuated by spinal extension and flexion maneuvers.

Extension and lateral flexion toward the painful side of the lumbar spine on the pelvis narrows the neural foramina and loads the zygapophyseal joints on the ipsilateral side and aggravates local articular pain. Similarly, extension and lateral flexion to the opposite side reduce the load on the symptomatic joints and open the neural foramina, reducing pain. Flexion maneuvers can demonstrate painful limitations of spinal-pelvic range of motion as measured from fingertips to toes; adjacent spinal segments may be visualized to move as a singular unit in response to localized guarding.

Palpation of the paraspinal muscles and the spinal vertebral processes in relation to their relative excursion to each other vividly dramatizes this loss of spinal segment mobility.

The presence of an acute lumbar radiculopathy associated with a ''tethered'' root or prefixed spinal root syndrome initiates a precipitous sequence of maneuvers on the painful side in an effort to unload the root, which includes a lateral thrust of the spine, elevation, and forward thrust of the pelvis, as well as acute flexion of the hip and knee to reduce tension on the inflamed nerve root.

With mechanical dysfunction of posture or the presence of neurologic signs such as alteration of deep tendon reflexes, weakness, atrophy, restricted or crossed straight leg–raising (CSLR) signs, and the presence of long tract signs or sphincter dysfunction, the diagnosis of primary spinal-neural pathology becomes self-evident.

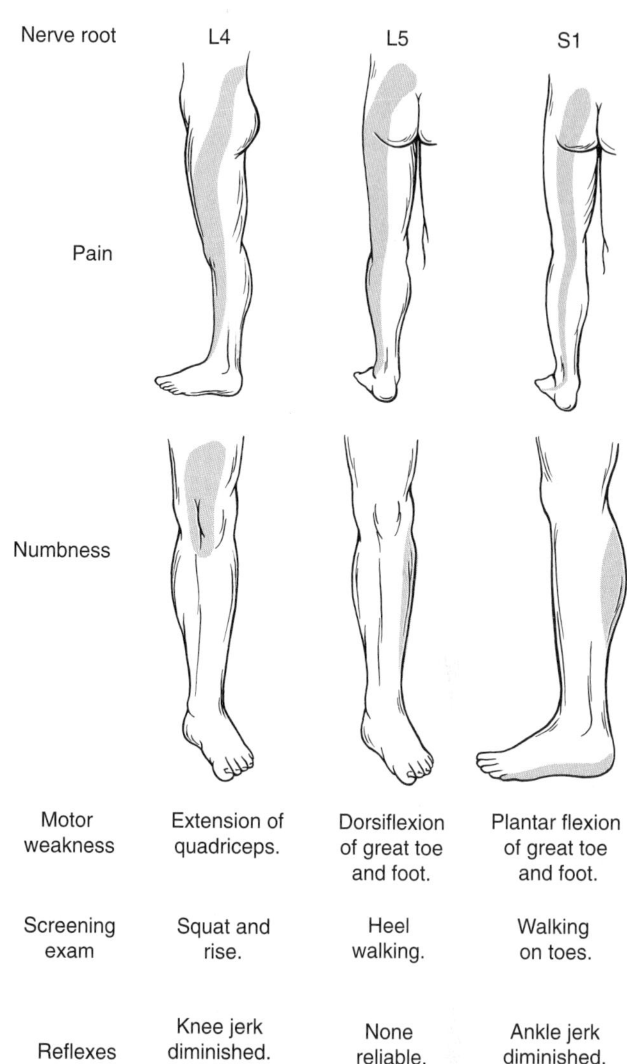

Nerve root
L4
L5
S1
Pain
Numbness
Motor weakness
Extension of quadriceps.
Dorsiflexion of great toe and foot.
Plantar flexion of great toe and foot.
Screening exam
Squat and rise.
Heel walking.
Walking on toes.
Reflexes
Knee jerk diminished.
None reliable.
Ankle jerk diminished.

FIG. 274-1. Testing for lumbar nerve root compromise.

Establishing a diagnosis in the absence of neurologic signs is more difficult. The examiner must rely to a greater extent on the details of the history and the ability to replicate and alleviate symptoms by anatomic maneuvers.[19]

Neurologic Screening

The neurologic examination can focus on a few tests that seek evidence of nerve root impairment, peripheral neuropathy, or spinal cord dysfunction. As noted, over 90 percent of all clinically significant lower extremity radiculopathy due to disk herniation involves the L5 or S1 nerve root at the L4–L5 or L5–S1 disc level. The clinical features of nerve root compression are summarized in Fig. 274-1.

Testing for Muscle Strength

An inability to walk on either the heels or the toes because of weakness in the foot dorsiflexors or plantar flexors, respectively, suggests an L5 radiculopathy in the former case and S1 root involvement in the latter instance. Similarly, difficulty in assuming or arising from a squatting position may indicate quadriceps weakness associated with

L4 root compromise. Muscle atrophy can be detected by circumferential measurements of the calf and thigh bilaterally. Differences of less than 2 cm in measurements of the two limbs at the same level may be a normal variation.[15] Weakness of the hip flexors suggests L3 compromise, of the quadriceps L4, the foot dorsiflexors and great toe extensors L5, and the calf S1 radiculopathy. Deep tendon reflexes are tested and compared one side with the other. An absent or reduced knee jerk suggests an L4 radiculopathy, biceps femoris jerk L5, and an asymmetric Achilles reflex an S1 root compression syndrome.[19] Up-going toes in response to stroking the plantar footpad (Babinski or plantar response) may indicate upper motor neuron abnormalities (such as myelopathy or demyelinating disease), rather than a common low back problem. Testing light touch or pressure in the medial (L4), dorsal (L5), and lateral (S1) aspects of the foot (see Fig. 274-1) is usually sufficient for sensory screening.[15]

Clinical Tests for Sciatic Tension

Straight leg–raising testing can be both confusing and diagnostic. The SLR test (Fig. 274-2) can detect tension on the L5 and/or S1 nerve root. SLR may reproduce leg pain by stretching nerve roots irritated by a disk herniation. Pain below the knee at less than 70° of straight leg raising, aggravated by dorsiflexion of the ankle and relieved by ankle plantar flexion or external limb rotation, is most suggestive of tension on the L5 or S1 nerve root related to disk herniation. Reproducing back pain alone with SLR testing does not indicate significant nerve root tension.[15] A CSLR sign occurs when contralateral leg elevation produces sciatic pain in the symptomatic leg. Crossover pain is a stronger indication of nerve root compression than pain elicited from raising the straight painful limb. A markedly positive SLR in the younger patient is more likely associated with a prolapsed intervertebral disk than in an older patient, particularly when it is associated with a positive CSLR.

Additional confirmatory maneuvers include an exacerbation of pain with foot dorsiflexion or with the addition of head flexion with the SLR maneuver held at the symptomatic limit of sciatic pain tolerance. In the older patient, positive SLR or CSLR tests are less specific as to pain etiology but do suggest a radicular component of involvement.[19] Sitting knee extension (Fig. 274-3) can also test sciatic tension. The patient with significant nerve root irritation tends to complain or lean backward to reduce tension on the nerve.[15]

Inconsistent Findings and Pain Behavior

The patient who embellishes a medical history, exaggerates pain perception, or provides responses on physical examination inconsistent with known physiology can be particularly challenging.[15] This condition can be objectified in the physical exam with the use of Waddell's nonorganic physical signs.[20] Tests can be included in the flow of the general physical exam for the back. Testing includes tenderness to superficial skin rolling; report of low back pain with axial loading or when the whole body is rotated as one; the "flip test," in which the patient does not report pain with seated straight leg raise (often using distraction of manual muscle testing the quadriceps or ankle dorsiflexors) but reports pain at a low angle on the supine SLR; weakness or sensory loss in a nonanatomic distribution; and overreaction with "pain behaviors." If three or more of these signs are present, it represents increased psychological distress on the part of the patient to their condition. While it can be frustrating to the clinician, it is usually not purposeful, nor is it evidence of malingering or a mental disorder. Considering it a "cry for help" on the part of the patient allows the clinician to offer appropriate support and psychological intervention as follow-up. In patients with recurrent back problems, inconsistencies and amplifications may simply be habits learned during previous medical evaluations. In working with these patients, the clinician should attempt to identify any psychological or socioeconomic pressures that might be influenced in a positive manner. The overall goal should always be to facilitate the patient's recovery and avoid the development of chronic low back disability.[15] In the emergency department, one must also be aware of the patient demonstrating drug-seeking behavior.

In patients with pain, further diagnostic studies are often considered, especially given the difficulty of establishing a definitive anatomic structure to account for the patient's condition.

Diagnostic Studies

Prior to ordering imaging studies the clinician should have noted either the emergence of a red flag or physiologic evidence of tissue insult or neurologic dysfunction.[15]

Plain x-rays of the lumbar spine are recommended for ruling out fractures in patients with acute low back problems when any of these

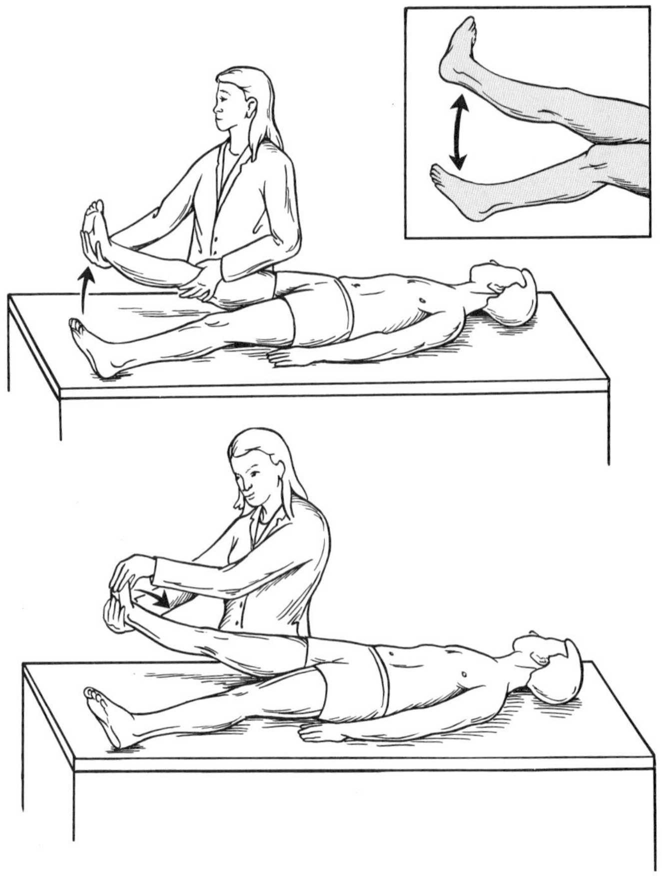

FIG. 274-2. Instructions for the straight leg–raising (SLR) test. 1. Ask the patient to lie as straight as possible on a table in the supine position. 2. With one hand placed above the knee of the leg being examined, exert enough firm pressure to keep the knee fully extended. Ask the patient to relax. 3. With the other hand cupped under the heel, slowly raise the straight limb. Tell the patient, "If this bothers you, let me know, and I will stop." 4. Monitor for any movement of the pelvis before complaints are elicited. True sciatic tension should elicit complaints before the hamstrings are stretched enough to move the pelvis. 5. Estimate the degree of leg elevation that elicits complaint from the patient. Then determine the most distal area of discomfort: back, hip, thigh, knee, or below the knee. 6. While holding the leg at the limit of straight leg raising, dorsiflex the ankle. Note whether this aggravates the pain. Internal rotation of the limb can also increase the tension on the sciatic nerve roots.

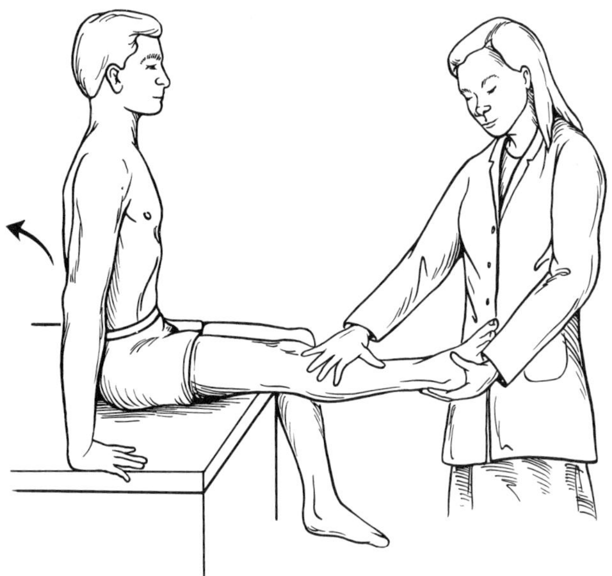

FIG. 274-3. Instructions for sitting knee extension test. With the patient sitting on a table, both hip and knees flexed at 90 degrees, slowly extend the knee as if evaluating the patella or bottom of the foot. This maneuver stretches nerve roots as much as a moderate degree of supine SLR.

red flags are present: recent significant trauma (any age), recent mild trauma (patient age over 50), history of prolonged steroid use, osteoporosis, or patient age over 70. Oblique views are not necessary.[14] Laboratory tests such as erythrocyte sedimentation rate (ESR), complete blood count (CBC), and urinalysis (UA) can be useful to screen for nonspecific medical diseases (especially infection and tumor) of the low back.[15] Plain x-rays in combination with CBC and ESR may be useful for ruling out tumor or infection in patients with acute low back problems when any of these red flags are present: prior cancer or recent infection, fever over 100°F, IV drug abuse, prolonged steroid use, low back pain worse with rest, or unexplained weight loss. If tumor or infection is suspected, CT or MRI may be considered in the presence of red flags, even if plain films are negative. In the presence of red flags suggesting cauda equina syndrome or progressive major motor weakness, prompt use of CT, MRI, myelography, or CT-myelography is recommended. Because these conditions may require timely surgical intervention, planning and choice of study is best carried out in consultation with a surgeon. In patients with acute back problems who have had prior back surgery, MRI with contrast is the imaging test of choice because it can help distinguish disk herniation from scar tissue from previous surgery.[14] A bone scan can detect physiologic reactions to suspected spinal tumor, infection, or occult fracture.[15]

When the neurologic examination is less clear, however, further physiologic evidence of nerve root dysfunction should be considered before ordering an imaging study. Electromyography (EMG), including H-reflex tests, may be useful to identify subtle focal neurologic dysfunction in patients with leg symptoms lasting longer than 3 to 4 weeks. Sensory evoked potentials (SEPs) may be added to the assessment if spinal stenosis or spinal cord myelopathy is suspected.[15]

There is a 20 to 40 percent false-positive rate with plain films, CT, MRI, and myelogram. The altered anatomic structures identified may not be responsible for the patient's pain. Most findings on these studies are consistent with normal degenerative changes and are also found in asymptomatic individuals. Any imaging abnormalities must correlate with the patient's symptoms and signs to be of value in guiding treatment.

Treatment

In the evaluation of back syndromes, the examiner's goal is to discriminate between pain of neurogenic origin and pain of musculoskeletal origin, as well as to rule out nonspinal pathology. Although the potential for surgical intervention is by far greater with neurologic than with musculoskeletal involvement, in both instances surgery is indicated in less than 1 percent of all cases. If no red flags are identified that would require diagnostic imaging or immediate consultation, symptomatic treatment may be initiated. Fortunately, the majority of all lumbosacral syndromes respond to routine symptomatic treatment, including relative rest, progressive activity, simple comfort measures such as superficial heat, and oral analgesics.[19]

Patient Education

If the initial assessment detects no serious condition, assure the patient that there is "no hint of a dangerous problem" and that "a rapid recovery can be expected." The need for education varies among patients and during various stages of care. An obviously apprehensive patient may require a more detailed explanation. Patients with sciatica may have a longer expected recovery time than patients with nonspecific back symptoms and thus may need more education and reassurance. Any patient who does not recover within a few weeks may need more extensive education about back problems and the reassurance that special studies may be considered if recovery is slow.[15] This points out the necessity of follow-up referral in this patient population.[19]

Medication

Comfort is often a patient's first concern. Nonprescription analgesics will provide sufficient pain relief for most patients with acute low back symptoms. If treatment response is inadequate, as evidenced by continued symptoms and activity limitations, prescribed pharmaceuticals or physical methods may be added. Table 274-2 summarizes comfort options.[15] Muscle relaxants seem no more effective than NSAIDs for treating patients with low back symptoms, and using them in combination with NSAIDs seems to have no demonstrated benefit. Side effects including drowsiness have been reported in up to 30 percent of patients taking muscle relaxants.[15]

Opioids appear no more effective than safer analgesics for managing low back symptoms. Opioids should be avoided if possible and, when chosen, used only for a short time. Poor patient tolerance and risks of drowsiness, decreased reaction time, clouded judgment, and potential misuse/dependence have been reported in up to 35 percent of patients. Patients should be warned of these potentially debilitating problems.[15]

Physical Methods

Manipulation, which is defined as manual loading of the spine using short- or long-leverage methods, is safe and effective for patients in the first month of acute low back symptoms without radiculopathy. For patients with symptoms lasting longer than 1 month, manipulation is probably safe, but its efficacy is unproved. If manipulation has not resulted in symptomatic and functional improvement after 4 weeks, it should be stopped and the patient reevaluated.[15,16]

Other interventions, including traction, massage, diathermy, ultrasound, cutaneous laser application, biofeedback, application of shoe lifts, and transcutaneous electrical nerve stimulation (TENS), have not yet been found to provide any lasting benefit. Instruction in self-application of heat or cold may be provided for temporary symptom relief. Additionally, invasive techniques such as needle acupuncture and injection procedures (injection of trigger points in the back; injection of facet joints; injection of steroids, lidocaine, or opioids in the epidural space) have no proven benefit.[15]

AHCPR Guidelines for Activity Limitations

To avoid both undue back irritation and debilitation from inactivity, recommendations for alternate activity can be helpful. Bedrest is reserved for patients with the most severe limitations (due primarily to leg pain).[15] This should not exceed 2 days. In general, especially if no red flags have arisen, patients should be instructed to return to their usual daily activities including work as soon as able. The AHCPR guidelines outline the approach described below to activity limitations.

AVOIDING UNDUE BACK IRRITATION Activities and postures that increase stress on the back also tend to aggravate back symptoms. Patients limited by back symptoms can minimize the stress of lifting by keeping any lifted object close to the body at the level of the navel. Twisting, bending, and reaching while lifting also increase stress on the back. Sitting, although safe, may aggravate symptoms for some patients. Advise these patients to avoid prolonged sitting and to change position often. A soft support placed at the small of the back, armrests to support some body weight, and a slight recline of the chair back may make required sitting more comfortable.[15]

AVOIDING DEBILITATION Until the patient returns to normal activity, aerobic (endurance) conditioning exercise such as walking, stationary biking, swimming, and even light jogging may be recommended to help avoid debilitation from inactivity. An incremental, gradually increasing regimen of aerobic exercise (up to 20 to 30 minutes daily) can usually be started within the first 2 weeks of symptoms. Such conditioning activities have been found to stress the back no more than sitting for an equal time period on the side of the bed. Patients should be informed that exercise may increase pain slightly at first. If intolerable, some exercise alteration is usually helpful.[15]

Conditioning exercises for trunk muscles are more mechanically stressful to the back than aerobic exercise. Such exercises are not recommended during the first few weeks of symptoms, although they may later help patients regain and maintain activity tolerance.[15]

There is no evidence to indicate that back-specific exercise machines are effective for treating acute low back problems. Neither is there evidence that stretching of the back helps patients with acute symptoms.[15]

WORK ACTIVITIES When requested, clinicians may choose to offer specific instructions about activity at work for patients with acute limitations due to low back symptoms. The patient's age, general health, and perceptions of safe limits of sitting, standing, walking, or lifting (noted on initial history) can provide reasonable starting points for activity recommendations. Table 274-3 provides a guide for recommendations about sitting and lifting. The clinician should make clear to patients and employers that even moderately heavy unassisted lifting may aggravate back symptoms. Any restrictions are intended to allow for spontaneous recovery or time to build activity tolerance through exercise. Activity restrictions are prescribed for a short time period only, depending upon work requirements (no benefits are apparent beyond 3 months' restriction).[15]

TABLE 274-2 Symptom Control Methods

Prescribed Pharmaceutical Methods	Prescribed Physical Methods	
Recommended		
Nonprescription analgesics Acetaminophen (safest) NSAIDs (Aspirin,* Ibuprofen*)		
Nonspecific low back symptoms and/or sciatica Other NSAIDs*	Nonspecific low back symptoms Manipulation (in place of medication or a shorter trial if combined with NSAIDs)	
Options		
Nonspecific low back symptoms and/or sciatica Muscle relaxants†,‡,§ Opioids†,‡,§	Nonspecific low back symptoms Physical agents and modalities† (heat or cold modalities for home programs only) Shoe insoles†	Sciatica Manipulation (in place of medication or a shorter trial if combined with NSAIDs) Physical agents and modalities† (heat or cold modalities for home programs only) Few days' rest§ Shoe insoles†

*Aspirin and other NSAIDs are not recommended for use in combination with one another due to the risk of GI complications.
†Equivocal efficacy.
‡Significant potential for producing drowsiness and debilitation; potential for dependency.
§Short course (few days only) for severe symptoms.

TABLE 274-3 Guidelines for Sitting and Unassisted Lifting

Symptoms	Severe	→	Moderate	→	Mild	→	None
Sitting*	20 min	→	→	→	→	→	50 min
Unassisted lifting†							
Men	20 lb	→	20 lb	→	60 lb	→	80 lb
Women	20 lb	→	20 lb	→	35 lb	→	40 lb

*Without getting up and moving around.
†Modification of NIOSH Lifting Guidelines, 1981, 1993. Gradually increase unassisted lifting limits to 60 lbs (men) and 35 lbs (women) by 3 months, even with continued symptoms. Instruct patient to limit twisting, bending, reaching while lifting and to hold lifted object as close to umbilicus as possible.

REFERRAL

Referral for continuing outpatient care is absolutely critical. When seen on a one-time basis in the emergency center, each patient should be provided with an opportunity for follow-up in the event that the problem fails to respond to initial treatment. No matter how searching the physical examination, and notwithstanding the experience of the examiner, clinical manifestations can change rapidly, often dramatically, for example, the blossoming of the skin manifestations of herpes zoster 2 days after pain onset, to be recognized only by subsequent evaluations and further diagnostic studies such as MRI or EMG. Also, if the patient is given activity limitations and work restrictions, the limitations and restrictions require reevaluation to further substantiate need for these limits and to instruct patients in progressive return to activity. Referral to a specialist in physical medicine and rehabilitation for conservative spine care, a spine surgeon, or a multidisciplinary spine center offers the patient comprehensive management that would hopefully reduce future emergency department visits, especially as the patient's condition becomes more complex and perhaps less acute.

REFERENCES

1. Bauer RD, Errico TJ: Thoracolumbar spine injuries, in Errico TJ, Bauer RD, Waugh T (eds): *Spinal Trauma*. Philadelphia, JB Lippincott, 1991, pp 195–270.

2. Bruckner FE, Greco A, Leung AWL: "Benign thoracic pain" syndrome: Role of magnetic resonance imaging in the detection and localization of thoracic disc disease. *J R Soc Med* 82:81, 1989.
3. Frymoyer JW: Back pain and sciatica. *N Engl J Med* 328:291, 1988.
4. Deyo RA, Tsui-Wu YJ: Descriptive epidemiology of low back pain and its related medical care in the United States. *Spine* 12:264, 1987.
5. Andersson GBJ, Svensson H-O, Oden A: The intensity of work recovery in low back pain. *Spine* 8:880, 1983.
6. Carey TS, Garrett J, Jackman A, et al: The outcomes and costs of care for acute low back pain among patients seen by primary care practitioners, chiropractors, and orthopedic surgeons. *Spine* 14:913, 1995.
7. Nachemson AL: Newest knowledge of low back pain: A critical look. *Clin Orthop* 279:8, 1992.
8. LaBan MM: "Vesper's curse" night pain—the bane of Hypnos. *Arch Phys Med Rehabil* 65:501, 1984.
9. Kirkaldy-Willis WH, Farfan HF: Instability of the lumbar spine. *Clin Orthop* 165:110, 1982.
10. Fritz JM, Delitto A, Welch WC, Erhard RE: Lumbar spinal stenosis: A review of current concepts in evaluation, management, and outcome measurements. *Arch Phys Med Rehabil* 79:700, 1998.
11. Dreyer SJ, Dreyfuss PH: Low back pain and the zygapophysial (facet) joints. *Arch Phys Med Rehabil* 77:290, 1996.
12. LaBan MM: The lumbosacral pain syndrome, in Kaplan PE (ed): *The Practice of Physical Medicine.* Springfield, IL, Charles C Thomas, 1984, pp 107–160.
13. Kuslich SD, Ulstrom CL, Michael CJ: The tissue origin of low back pain and sciatica: A report of pain response to tissue stimulation during operations on the lumbar spine using local anesthesia. *Orthop Clin North Am* 22(2):181, 1991.
14. Bigos S, Bowyer O, Braen G, et al: *Acute Low Back Problems in Adults. Clinical Practice Guideline No. 14.* Rockville, MD: Agency for Health Care Policy and Research, Public Health Service, US Department of Health and Human Services, December 1994. AHCPR Publication No. 95-0642.
15. Bigos S, Bowyer O, Braen G, et al: *Acute Low Back Pain Problems in Adults. Clinical Practice Guideline, Quick Reference Guide No. 14.* Rockville, MD, Agency for Health Care Policy and Research, Public Health Service, US Department of Health and Human Services, December 1994. AHCPR Publication No. 95-0643.
16. Deyo RA, Rainville J, Kent DL: What can the history and physical examination tell us about low back pain? *JAMA* 268(6):760, 1992.
17. Grasland A, Pouchot J, Mathieu A, et al: Sacral insufficiency fractures: An easily overlooked cause of back pain in elderly women. *Arch Intern Med* 156(6):668, 1996.
18. Honan W, White GW, Eisenberg GM: Spontaneous infectious discitis in adults. *Am J Med* 1001:85, 1996.
19. LaBan MM: Low back pain-lumbosacral strain-lumbar disc disease, in Leek JC, Gershwin ME, Fowler WM (eds): *Principles of Physical Medicine and Rehabilitation in Musculoskeletal Diseases.* Orlando, FL, Grune & Stratton, 1986, pp 309–333.
20. Waddell G, McCullogh JA, Kummel E, Venner RM: Nonorganic physical signs in low back pain. *Spine* 5:117, 1980.

Agency for Health Care Policy and Research (AHCPR) clinical practice guidelines are available at: AHCPR Publications Clearninghouse toll-free at 800-358-9295 or write to: AHCPR Publications Clearinghouse, PO Box 8547, Silver Spring, MD 20907.

275 SHOULDER PAIN

D. Monte Hunter

Shoulder pain is one of the most common musculoskeletal complaints of patients over age 40. Work, recreation, and normal daily activities all place great demands on the shoulder. Of all adult patients presenting for evaluation of shoulder pain, one-third related their pain to work, one-third related their pain to athletic activity, and one-third could not identify any one specific precipitating event or factor.

Injuries involving the rotator cuff are the most common cause of shoulder pain. While these injuries can be acute, they more commonly occur from chronic overuse. Overuse can produce pathologic changes in the rotator cuff structures that progress along the continuum starting with subacromial bursitis from mechanical irritation, progressing to rotator cuff tendinitis, and eventually leading to partial and full thickness rotator cuff tears. Laborers who work with their arms above the horizontal and athletes of all ages, especially throwers, swimmers, and racquet sports enthusiasts, are the most susceptible to chronic overuse injuries. Acute injuries to the rotator cuff usually require significant trauma such as extreme forced hyperabduction or hyperextension of the upper extremity.

While disorders of the rotator cuff are the most common cause of shoulder pain, conditions affecting other intrinsic structures of the shoulder complex also can cause pain. Additionally, extrinsic disorders can refer pain to the shoulder and must be considered in the differential diagnosis. A focused history and physical examination carried out with an understanding of the complex anatomy and function of the shoulder are essential in determining the source of shoulder pain. Establishing the proper diagnosis, initiating the appropriate treatment, and making timely referrals for follow-up are critical in preserving the function and mobility of the shoulder.

FUNCTIONAL ANATOMY

The shoulder is the most versatile and yet the most vulnerable joint in the body. With range of motion greater than any other joint in the body, the shoulder is designed for mobility rather than stability. The ultimate function of the shoulder is to help position the hand and upper extremity for accurate and efficient use. The shoulder is also designed to provide strength and power to upper extremity movements. To meet the many demands placed on it, the shoulder uses three bones, four joints, and a specialized set of soft tissues consisting of muscles, tendons, ligaments, and bursae.

Bones and Joints

The humerus, clavicle, and scapula make up the bony structures of the shoulder complex. The scapula has two bony extensions, the coracoid and the acromion, which help protect the rotator cuff and play important roles in shoulder function.

The four joints of the shoulder include the glenohumeral, acromioclavicular, sternoclavicular, and scapulothoracic. All of these must work together to provide full shoulder motion and function. The *glenohumeral joint* is the most prominent and complex joint of the shoulder. This ball-and-socket joint is the central axis of motion of the shoulder. While the glenohumeral joint enjoys great freedom of motion, it is also recognized as the least stable joint in the body. To help improve its stability, this joint relies on three components. The first is the labrum, a fibrous band of tissue lining the glenoid cavity, analogous to the meniscus of the knee. The labrum increases the surface contact area of the humeral head within the glenoid. The second component consists of three glenohumeral ligaments, which aid stability by reinforcing the joint capsule. Finally, four specialized muscles known as the rotator cuff encompass the glenohumeral joint and provide stability during motion.

The *sternoclavicular* and *acromioclavicular joints* work together to contribute to glenohumeral motion. Rotation at the acromioclavicular joint and elevation at the sternoclavicular allow complete arm elevation. The *scapulothoracic joint* represents the articulation of the scapula on the posterior wall of the thorax. Scapular motion is essential for overall shoulder motion: every degree of scapulothoracic motion allows two degrees of glenohumeral motion.

Muscles

The muscles of the shoulder complex not only generate motion and power for the upper extremity but also provide significant stability for the glenohumeral joint. The deltoid, which drapes the shoulder complex and forms its contour, acts as a powerful and independent elevator of the arm. Along with the pectoralis, the deltoid is the major mover of the upper extremity.

The rotator cuff consists of four muscles: the supraspinatus, the infraspinatus, the teres minor, and the subscapularis. All originate on the scapula, traverse the glenohumeral joint, and insert on the proximal humerus. The rotator cuff functions primarily as a dynamic stabilizer of the glenohumeral joint. The rotator cuff muscles also contribute significantly to the power of the upper extremity, providing 30 to 50 percent of the power in abduction and 90 percent in external rotation (Figs. 275-1, 275-2).

The *supraspinatus* originates on the posterior and superior aspect of the scapula, passes beneath the acromion, and inserts on the great tuberosity of the humerus. It initiates arm elevation and abducts the shoulder. It also balances the power of the deltoid, keeping the humerus centered in the glenoid during deltoid contraction.

The *infraspinatus* originates on the posterior scapula just inferior to the scapular spine. It inserts on the posterior aspect of the greater tuberosity and acts primarily as an external rotator of the arm (Fig. 275-1).

The *teres minor* originates on the lateral border of the scapula just inferior to the infraspinatus and inserts on the posterior aspect of the humerus. It works with the infraspinatus to provide external rotation (Fig. 275-1).

The *subscapularis* is the only rotator cuff muscle that arises from the anterior aspect of the scapula. It attaches to the lesser tuberosity of the humerus and provides internal rotation of the arm (Fig. 275-2).

The *long head of the biceps tendon*, although not formally considered part of the rotator cuff, assists in rotator cuff function. This tendon courses superiorly in the bicipital groove of the humerus between the greater and lesser tuberosities, passes between the subscapularis and supraspinatus tendons, and penetrates the glenohumeral joint to insert on the labrum (Fig. 275-2). During arm elevation, the tendon of the long head of the biceps depresses the humeral head, helping it remain centered in the glenoid.

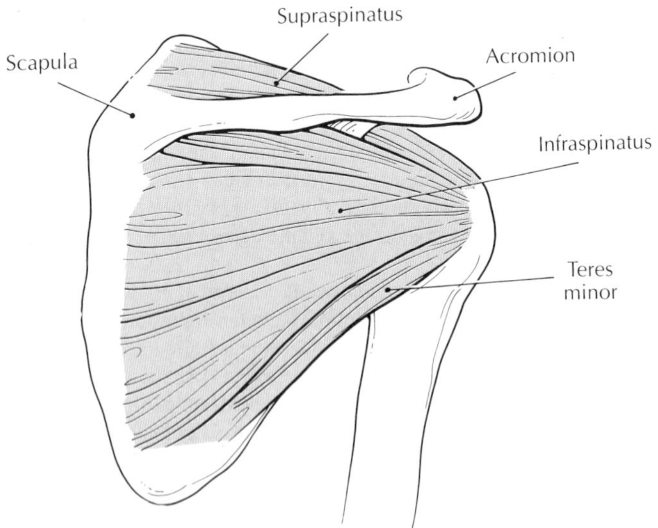

FIG. 275-1. Posterior view of shoulder illustrating rotator cuff muscles.

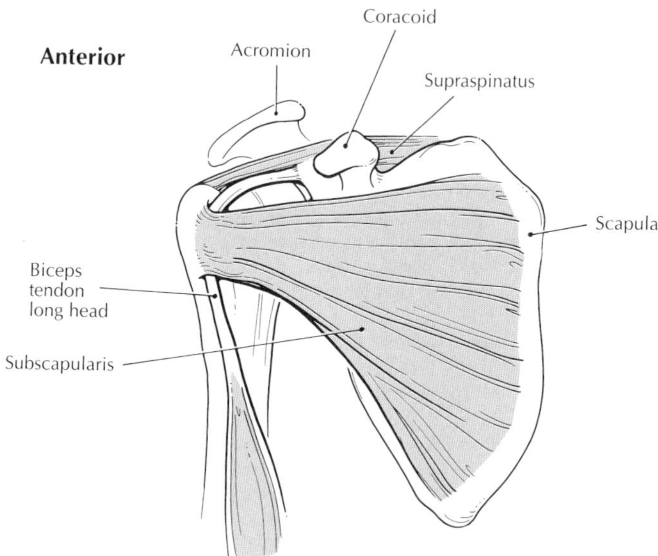

FIG. 275-2. Anterior view of shoulder illustrating supraspinatus and long head of biceps.

Bursae

The bursae facilitate motion between the components of the shoulder. There are eight identifiable bursae in the shoulder complex. However, only one, the large subacromial bursa, also known as the subdeltoid bursa, is clinically significant. The subacromial bursa is extraarticular; its roof adheres to the undersurface of the deltoid, and its floor to the underlying rotator cuff. A thick layer of synovial fluid between the roof and the floor normally allows smooth frictionless motion between the rotator cuff and adjacent structures.

Coracoacromial Arch

The coracoacromial arch is an important anatomic concept in understanding shoulder pathology. The arch is formed by the coracoid posteriorly, by the acromion anteriorly, and by the coracoacromial ligament, which forms the anterior roof of the arch (Fig. 275-3). The humeral head provides the floor of the arch. This arch defines the space within which the muscles of the rotator cuff, the tendon of the long head of the biceps, and the subacromial bursa must fit and function. The coracoacromial ligament is considered vestigial; however, by virtue of its position it can contribute to compression or impingement of the rotator cuff.

IMPINGEMENT SYNDROME

Repetitive use of the arm overhead or above the horizontal compresses the rotator cuff and related structures between the humeral head and coracoacromial arch (Fig. 275-4). The *impingement syndrome* refers to the pathologic changes that occur in the structures of the rotator cuff due to this repetitive compression. Also referred to as *painful arc syndrome*, *cuffitis*, *supraspinatus syndrome*, and *bursitis*, impingement syndrome is the leading cause of shoulder pain and dysfunction. A basic understanding of this concept is essential for the proper evaluation and treatment of the patient with shoulder pain.

Pathophysiology

Repetitive impingement of the bursa, rotator cuff, and biceps tendon produces pathologic changes in these structures that progress in a predictable pattern. Early on, repetitive motion produces mechanical

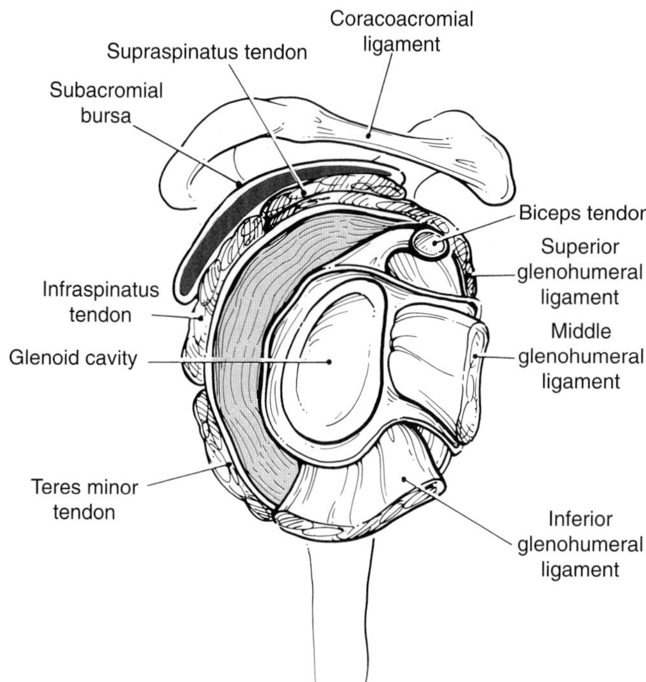

FIG. 275-3. Lateral view of shoulder illustrating coracoacromial arch with rotator cuff and subacromial bursa.

inflammation of the subacromial bursa and underlying rotator cuff. As activities that cause impingement continue, inflammation of the rotator cuff tendons worsens. Chronic inflammation in time leads to degeneration and eventual tearing of the rotator cuff. Degeneration of the rotator cuff exposes the biceps tendon, making it susceptible to degeneration and rupture. As the soft tissue restraints of the shoulder wear out, degenerative disease sets in and is typical of the advanced stages of the impingement syndrome.

Most of the pathologic changes in the rotator cuff due to impingement occur near the humeral insertion of the tendon. This area is referred to as the *critical zone* and has been identified as relatively avascular. Repetitive compression causes relative ischemia in this area. Over time this area degenerates and ultimately fails. The critical zone is the most common site of all rotator cuff abnormalities. The supraspinatus, due to its location in the coracoacromial arch, is the most commonly affected muscle of the rotator cuff.

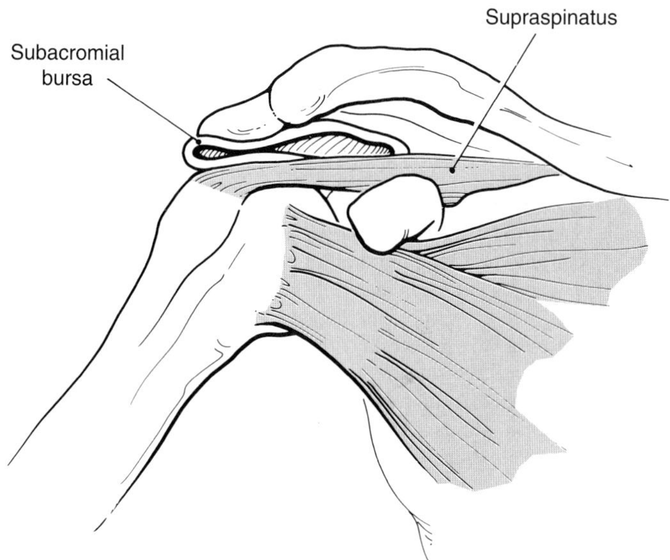

FIG. 275-4. Impingement of subacromial bursa and rotator cuff.

Three stages of impingement are identifiable. Stage 1 is characterized by local inflammation, edema, and hemorrhage and is most commonly associated with subacromial bursitis and early rotator cuff tendinitis. These changes are considered reversible. Stage 2 is characterized by inflammation, thickening, and fibrosis of the rotator cuff tendons. Stage 3 is characterized by degeneration and rupture of the rotator cuff tendon. Degenerative changes in the bony structures of the shoulder usually accompany stage 3. Stages 2 and 3 are considered to be irreversible.

Clinical Features

Specific maneuvers on physical examination test for signs of impingement by compressing the rotator cuff and bursa between the humeral head and coracoacromial arch. Neer's impingement test requires the examiner to move the patient's straightened arm smoothly but forcibly to full abduction. This compresses the cuff and bursa against the undersurface of the acromion. A second test, Hawkins' impingement test, requires the examiner to position the patient's arm in 90° of abduction and 90° of elbow flexion. Rotation of the arm inwardly across the front of the patient's body compresses the cuff and bursa between the humeral head and coracoacromial ligament. These tests are considered positive if they reproduce pain.

Emergency Department Treatment

The goals of treatment of impingement lesions are twofold: to reduce pain and inflammation and, more importantly, to prevent progression of the process. Regardless of the stage of impingement identified, a conservative treatment program initiated by the emergency physician should include the following:

1. *Relative rest and modification of activities.* However, immobilization should be avoided whenever possible. Brief periods of support with a sling may be prescribed.
2. *Medication to reduce pain and inflammation.* Often analgesics are required to control pain during stage 2 and 3 impingement. Nonsteroidal anti-inflammatory agents can be prescribed for a 7- to 10-day course.
3. *Cryotherapy.* The application of ice to the affected shoulder for 10 to 15 min two to three times per day can have analgesic effects and is thought to reduce local inflammation and edema.
4. *Gentle range of motion.* Two simple exercises can help the patient maintain glenohumeral motion. Pendulum swings are done with the patient slightly bent at the waist with the arm hanging freely in front of the body. Gentle arcs of motion to the level of pain tolerance can be carried out for 5 to 10 min daily. The size of the arcs should increase daily as symptoms allow. Also, having the patient walk his or her fingers up the wall to the level of pain tolerance can also help preserve glenohumeral motion.
5. *Stretching and strengthening.* During stage 1 impingement, stretching and strengthening may be initiated early on. Entering stage 2 and 3 impingement, stretching and strengthening are most effectively carried out under the supervision of a physical therapist. This is an important part of the treatment of impingement and is usually prescribed by the primary care physician or orthopaedist, who can monitor the patient's response to therapy.
6. *Corticosteroid injections.* While local corticosteroid injections into the subacromial space can be effective for pain relief, their deleterious effects on soft tissues have been well documented. These include muscular atrophy, weakness, and further tissue degeneration. Injec-

tion directly into the substance of the tendon can lead to necrosis and rupture. Even in the primary clinician's office setting, the judicious use of corticosteroids is advised, with no more than two to three injections being recommended in one specific area. While a single injection is not believed to be harmful, caution is still advised for use in the emergency department because of the potential harmful effects of repeated injections and difficulty in ensuring reliable follow-up.

Follow-up

Timely referral for all stages of impingement is crucial to help preserve function and mobility in the shoulder. Clinical follow-up is usually recommended after 7 to 14 days for stage 1 and 2 lesions. For stage 3 lesions, associated with chronic disability or other concern for rotator cuff tears, more acute follow-up is recommended.

If symptoms have diminished at the time of follow-up, a supervised course of therapy with emphasis on rotator cuff stretching and strengthening may be prescribed. If the symptoms persist or have worsened, the clinical physician may attempt a subacromial injection of glucocorticoid to help arrest the inflammatory response. If symptoms persist despite full conservative measures after 6 to 12 weeks of treatment, further workup with arthrography, magnetic resonance imaging (MRI), or arthroscopy to rule out rotator cuff tearing may be carried out at the discretion of the primary clinical provider.

SUBACROMIAL BURSITIS

Pathophysiology

Subacromial bursitis is associated with stage 1 impingement and is typically characterized by localized edema and inflammation in the subacromial bursa. More importantly, an early inflammation of the rotator cuff tendon usually coexists. Subacromial bursitis typically is seen in patients under 25 years of age and usually results from mechanical irritation from repetitive overhand activities. It is important that this condition be recognized because it is reversible. If left unrecognized and untreated, it progresses to the irreversible conditions associated with stage 2 and stage 3 impingement.

Primary subacromial bursitis is rare but should be considered in patients with shoulder pain who have rheumatoid arthritis, tuberculosis, gout, or pyogenic infections.

Clinical Features

Patients usually describe the pain of subacromial bursitis as a dull aching sensation deep within the shoulder, frequently following activity and usually improving with rest. Patients usually seek medical attention only when the symptoms affect their work, performance, or ability to compete. On physical examination, no muscular atrophy or asymmetry is present unless the symptoms have been chronic. Little if any tenderness is elicited on palpation; however, when tenderness is present it typically will be found on the lateral aspect of the proximal humerus or on deep palpation in the subacromial space. Full range of motion in the shoulder is usually preserved but may be painful, especially between 60° and 100° of abduction. The pain is worse when resistance is applied to the arm in 90° of abduction. Muscle strength in the deltoid and rotator cuff muscles is usually not affected. Impingement signs and impingement injection tests are usually positive.

Radiographic Findings

Most often radiographs are normal in the early stages of impingement associated with bursitis.

Emergency Department Treatment

The goals of treatment of subacromial bursitis and early rotator cuff tendinitis are twofold: to reduce pain and inflammation and, more importantly, to prevent progression of this reversible process to the irreversible stages of rotator cuff tendinitis and degeneration.

More than 90 percent of patients with subacromial bursitis respond to conservative measures. An effective conservative treatment plan has been outlined previously in this section. Since inflammation of the bursa is typically due to overuse, a short period of relative rest is indicated. Immobilization is not indicated and, in fact, can be detrimental, leading to adhesions and loss of motion. Total inactivity usually is not necessary. *Relative rest* implies avoidance of those activities that reproduce symptoms; e.g., a tennis player should avoid serving but can continue to hit ground strokes, and a laborer should avoid working with his or her arms over the head. Nonsteroidal anti-inflammatory agents are effective in reducing pain and inflammation. Analgesics are rarely needed to control pain. Localized ice treatment for 10 to 15 min two to three times per day will help reduce pain and inflammation. As pain diminishes, the patient should begin gentle range of motion, stretching, and strengthening exercises.

Follow-up

Clinical follow-up is recommended in 7 to 14 days. To simply diagnose ''bursitis'' and treat the symptoms does the patient a disservice and places the patient's shoulder at risk for future dysfunction. At the time of follow-up, if the patient's symptoms have diminished, a supervised course of therapy with emphasis on rotator cuff strengthening may be prescribed. If symptoms persist or have worsened, a subacromial injection of a glucocorticoid may help arrest the inflammatory response. If symptoms persist despite full conservative measures after 6 to 12 weeks of treatment, further workup with arthrography or MRI to rule out rotator cuff disease may be initiated at the discretion of the patient's primary clinician.

ROTATOR CUFF TENDINITIS

Pathophysiology

Inflammation of the rotator cuff tendons occurs initially in stage 1 of impingement. Continued repetitive mechanical impingement leads to irreversible fibrosis and thickening of the tendons of the rotator cuff, the hallmark of rotator cuff tendinitis. These findings are thought to represent the second stage of impingement. The supraspinatus is the tendon most commonly affected; however, any of the rotator cuff tendons may be involved.

Clinical Features

Patients with rotator cuff tendinitis are typically between the ages of 25 and 40 years, but the duration of the symptoms is more useful than age in making this diagnosis. The patient will report prior episodes of shoulder pain or a long duration of pain before seeking treatment. Since the lesion is not reversible, time and activity modification alone will not improve the symptoms. Patient describe the pain as a deep, aching discomfort that interferes with work and normal daily activities. Night pain, especially sleeping on the affected arm or with the arms above the head, will interfere with sleep. On examination, disuse atrophy of the shoulder musculature may be present if symptoms have been chronic. Palpation of the rotator cuff insertion at the lateral aspect of the proximal humerus will usually produce pain and tenderness. During range-of-motion maneuvers, fibrosis and scarring within the tendon can cause crepitus. A sensation of catching also may be present if scar tissue is trapped beneath the acromion. Both active and passive motion may be limited due to the scarring. Rotator cuff strength testing will reveal mild to moderate weakness. Pain will usually be present when resistance is applied. The individual muscles of the rotator cuff can be isolated and tested individually. To test the supraspinatus, abduct the arm to 90° and place it forward 30° with the thumb pointed down in the so-called empty beer can position. Pain or weakness against resistance in this position suggests injury to the supraspinatus. External rotation tests the infraspinatus and the teres minor. To test external rotation, place the patient's arm against the body with the elbow bent to 90° and the forearm in neutral position. Stabilize the elbow against the patient's waist and instruct the patient to rotate the arm outward. In this same position, with the elbow flexed and fixed against the patient's body, have the patient rotate the arm inward around the front of the body against resistance. This internal rotation tests subscapularis function.

The impingement sign is usually positive because the inflamed tendons are compressed beneath the coracoacromial arch. Injection of subacromial anesthetic may diminish pain but generally does not improve motion or strength significantly.

Radiographic Findings

Radiographs are most often normal but may yield helpful diagnostic clues. The presence of osteophytes off the inferior clavicle or acromion represents a long-standing process. These osteophytes can contribute to further injury to the underlying tendons. The soft tissues of the subacromial space should be inspected for evidence of calcification.

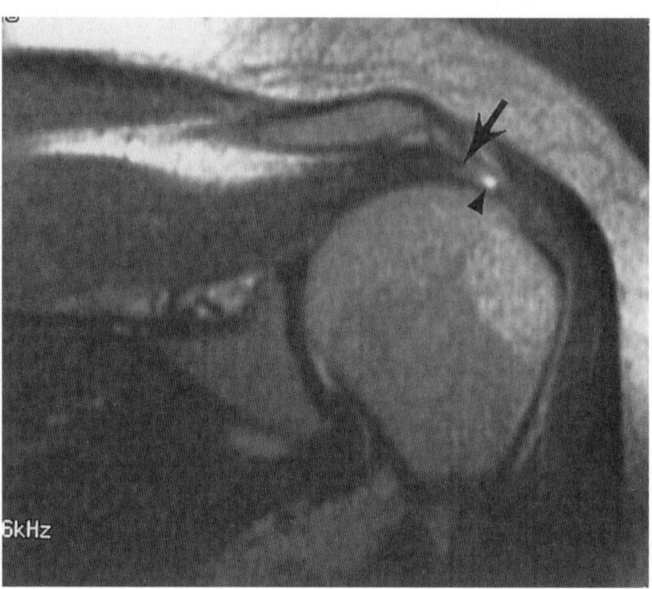

FIG. 275-5. Rotator cuff tear. MRI coronal image of shoulder reveals tear in supraspinatus tendon at the critical zone (arrow) with edema (point).

Emergency Department Treatment

Treatment of tendinitis emphasizes controlling symptoms, preserving motion, and improving strength and flexibility. Immobilization should be avoided, although an arm sling may be provided for comfort and support during acute symptoms. Nonsteroidal anti-inflammatory agents can help reduce pain and inflammation, and occasionally analgesics are necessary. Gentle range-of-motion exercises are recommended as early as symptoms allow to prevent further contraction and scarring.

Follow-up

Referral for follow-up is recommended in 7 to 14 days. Early physical therapy with treatment to reduce inflammation along with a supervised stretching and strengthening program are an integral part of treatment. Most patients with tendinitis respond to conservative management, experiencing no significant dysfunction. However, if symptoms persist despite conservative measures, further investigation for a possible degenerative rotator cuff tear may be pursued by the patient's primary physician.

ROTATOR CUFF TEARS

Tears in the rotator cuff muscles can occur from acute trauma, chronic overuse, or a combination of the two. Acute rotator cuff tears account for approximately 10 percent of all rotator cuff tears and usually occur as a result of significant trauma. Traumatic causes typically involve a fall on an outstretched arm, causing extreme hyperabduction or hyperextension. Lifting a heavy object or catching a heavy object as it falls can also cause acute rotator cuff tears. Chronic rotator cuff tears account for 90 percent of all rotator cuff tears and are usually due to progressive degeneration. Stage 3 impingement is associated with 95 percent of all chronic tears. If a degenerative tear is present, it is prone to extension with acute trauma.

Rotator cuff tears can be further classified as full thickness or partial thickness. Full thickness tears, as the name implies, involve the full extent of the tendon. Partial thickness tears, on the other hand, can exist on either the superior or inferior surface of the tendon or in the mid substance of the tendon. Partial thickness tears are twice as common as full thickness tears and most commonly occur on the inferior aspect of the tendon. Acute full thickness rotator cuff tears from a single injury are rare. Partial thickness rotator cuff tears are more likely to occur from an acute injury, especially in younger patients.

The type and extent of the tear have significant implications for the ultimate treatment and prognosis. Full thickness tears usually require surgical treatment, whereas partial thickness tears often respond to conservative management. In the emergency department it may be impossible to distinguish a full thickness tear from a partial thickness tear or even from an acute flare-up of rotator cuff tendinitis. However, it is important for the emergency physician to understand the pathophysiology of these conditions and their implications to shoulder function. Proper recognition, early intervention, and proper referral can preserve shoulder motion and function.

Pathophysiology

The critical zone of the rotator cuff is an area of relative avascularity near the humeral insertion of the tendon. Repetitive compression and impingement cause ischemia in this area. With time this area degenerates and ultimately tears. The critical zone is the most common site of all rotator cuff tears. The supraspinatus, due to its location within the coracoacromial arch, is the most commonly injured rotator cuff muscle (Fig. 275-5).

The bony structures of the shoulder can also contribute to rotator cuff tears. The acromion, which forms part of the roof of the coracoacromial arch, may be described as flat, curved, or hooked (Fig. 275-6). One clinical study associated a hooked acromion with 80 percent of rotator cuff tears, whereas a flat acromion was associated with fewer than 3 percent of tears.

Acute traumatic rotator cuff tears, which account for 10 percent of all rotator cuff tears, require a significant force. For a single traumatic event to cause a rotator cuff tear, the force must overcome the tensile strength of the tendon. However, the tensile strength of the tendon is greater than that of bone; therefore, a bony avulsion injury of the humerus is much more common than an isolated rotator cuff tear following acute trauma (Fig. 275-7).

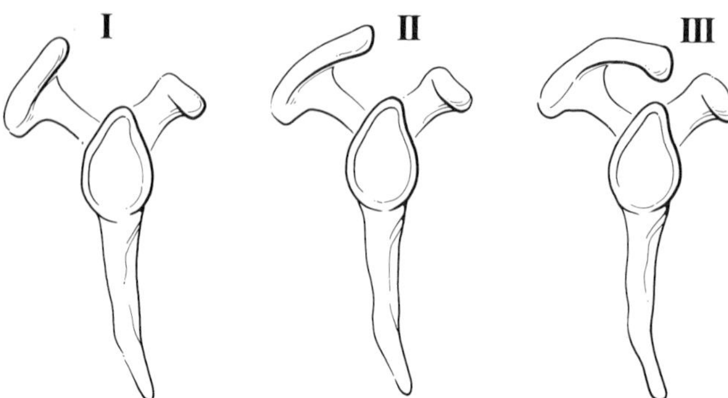

FIG. 275-6. Acromial morphology. I. Flat. II. Curved. III. Hooked.

Clinical Features

Patients with rotator cuff tears are almost always more than 40 years of age; rotator cuff tears in the young are rare. In general, the older the patient with shoulder pain, the more likely the presence of a rotator cuff tear. The clinical features of a chronic rotator cuff tear differ from those of an acute tear. Approximately one-half of all patients with chronic rotator cuff tears recall a specific trauma or an event associated with the onset of pain; however, the trauma is usually not significant. Patients more commonly report a history of gradual and progressive pain, which initially is described as worse at night. The pain eventually becomes persistent. The pain may be described as diffuse but is commonly localized to the lateral aspect of the upper arm. The patient typically reports flares of bursitis and tendinitis that initially responded to rest, anti-inflammatory agents, and glucocorticoid injections. However, as the rotator cuff weakens, the frequency, intensity, and duration of the symptoms increase and are less responsive to the usual treatments. Shoulder dysfunction progressively worsens and interferes with work, recreation, and normal daily activities. Arm elevation, external rotation, and lifting even light objects worsen the symptoms.

On examination, disuse atrophy may be present in patients with chronic rotator cuff tears. Palpation may produce discomfort at the lateral aspect of the upper arm or in the subacromial region. Active motion is variably limited by pain and weakness. Muscle strength is compromised, especially in abduction and external rotation. In fact, one study directly correlated the size of a rotator cuff tear with the strength of external rotation. The ''drop arm test'' is positive if the patient is unable to hold or lower a fully extended arm without dropping it. Crepitus and pain are usually present on range-of-motion testing. Injection of anesthetic into the subacromial space may diminish pain but will not improve motion or strength.

With acute injuries, such as a fall or catching a heavy object as it falls, the patient may report a sensation of ''tearing in the shoulder'' followed by severe pain and inability to raise the arm. An acute rotator cuff tear will produce immediate significant pain and disability. Asymmetry may be noted due to significant local swelling. A rotator cuff defect from the tear may be palpable overlying the humeral head. Active motion will be limited, with inability to abduct or externally rotate the arm against even minimal resistance. The drop arm test is positive and impingement signs are typically positive, but testing for them may not be practical after an acute injury. Injection of anesthetic into the subacromial space will not improve motion or strength.

Radiographic Findings

Radiographic findings may be supportive but are rarely diagnostic, yielding few specific clues unique to rotator cuff tears. With a large tear, the humeral head can ''button hole'' through the defect of the rotator cuff and assume a superior position to the glenoid. However, this is rarely appreciated. More often, radiographs will reveal findings associated with chronic rotator cuff pathology: sclerosis of the humeral head, degenerative joint disease at the acromioclavicular joint, osteophytes off the undersurface of the acromion and/or clavicle, and a hooked acromion.

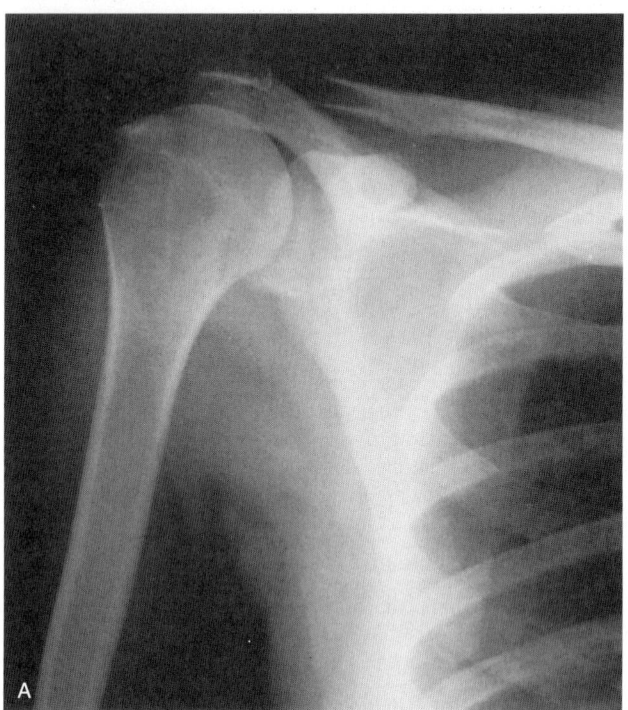

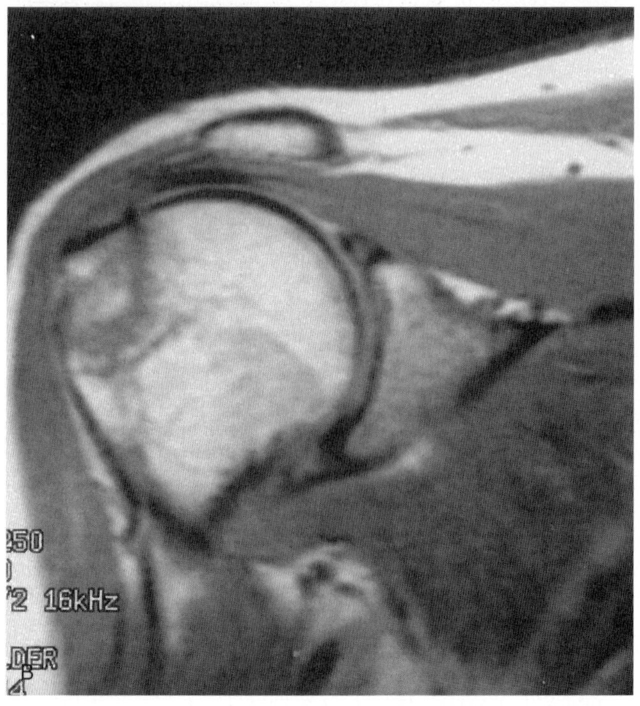

FIG. 275-7. Tensile strength of rotator cuff tendon is greater than bone. The patient suffered acute hyperabduction injury to arm causing extreme shoulder pain and dysfunction. Initially, radiographs (*A*) were interpreted as normal. MRI (*B*) of shoulder revealed avulsion fracture of humerus at site of supraspinatus tendon insertion.

Emergency Department Care

It may be clinically impossible to differentiate an acute rotator cuff strain from a partial-thickness or full-thickness rotator cuff tear. The immediate goal of emergency care for suspected rotator cuff injuries is to provide support, protection, pain relief, and most important, to help prevent further dysfunction and disability. An arm sling can be provided for support and comfort until acute symptoms subside. However, the perils of prolonged immobilization—stiffness, weakness, and loss of motion—should be emphasized to the patient. Appropriate analgesia should be provided, as should instruction in the proper use of ice two to three times per day to reduce pain and inflammation. When symptoms allow, gentle range-of-motion exercises such as pendulum swings and walking the fingers up the wall should be started.

Follow-up

Any patient with a suspected acute rotator cuff tear or with significant disability should receive prompt referral to an orthopaedist within 7 days. Young patients with full-thickness rotator cuff tears usually require surgical repair. Functional results are better if repair is carried out within 3 weeks of injury, before retraction, fibrosis, tendon degeneration, and muscular atrophy have occurred. Partial thickness or chronic tears may respond to conservative measures; however, early referral is warranted. If symptoms are improving at follow-up, conservative measures with physical therapy may be initiated. If significant symptoms and dysfunction persist, additional evaluation by MRI or CT arthrography may be pursued to determine the full extent of injury.

Following acute injuries, any evidence or suspicion of neurovascular compromise requires immediate orthopaedic consultation.

CALCIFIC TENDINITIS

Pathophysiology

Calcific tendinitis is considered a unique and still poorly understood disease process. It is characterized by the deposition of calcium hydroxyapatite crystals within one or more tendons of the rotator cuff. In time, the calcium deposition undergoes spontaneous resorption, with subsequent healing of the tendon. Calcific tendinitis does not appear to be related to any generalized disease process nor does its presence correlate with episodes of trauma or incidence of rotator cuff tears.

Primary tendon degeneration as a result of chronic repetitive microtrauma, age, or tissue hypoxia is considered to be the primary cause of this disorder. The supraspinatus is by far the most commonly affected tendon, with calcium deposition usually occurring 1 to 2 cm proximal to the insertion on the humerus; however, any of the rotator cuff tendons as well as the tendon of the long head of the biceps may be affected. After a variable period following the deposition of the calcium, spontaneous resorption occurs. The factors triggering resorption are unclear. With resorption of the calcium, the defect in the tendon remodels and heals.

The initial formation of the deposit is associated with few, if any, symptoms and little dysfunction. However, significant pain is associated with the resorption of the calcium deposit. This pain is thought to be due to the relative increase in pressure and volume within the tendon caused by vascular proliferation and the formation of granulation tissue.

Clinical Features

Patients in their thirties and forties are most commonly affected. This process is rarely seen in patients over 70. Of patients older than age 30 with shoulder pain, calcification in the rotator cuff tendons is found in approximately 7 percent. However, in asymptomatic patients between 31 and 40, 10 to 20 percent demonstrate rotator cuff calcification on routine radiographs. Of these patients, 35 to 45 percent will eventually become symptomatic. Females are affected more commonly than males, and calcification is often present bilaterally.

The onset of pain typically coincides with the resorption of the calcium deposit rather than the formation of it. Symptomatic patients experience sudden onset of shoulder pain, usually at rest. Any shoulder motion reproduces significant pain. The pain is often worse at night and interferes with sleep. The symptoms are usually self-limited, lasting 1 to 2 weeks in most cases. However, occasionally symptoms may be more indolent, producing less acute pain but lasting several weeks.

During an acute attack with intense pain, patients hold their arm across their body and often are reluctant to move it. Often a point of maximum tenderness can be palpated, usually over the proximal humerus near the tendinous insertion of the rotator cuff. Active and passive motion both are limited due to pain. Patients often report a sensation of catching when they move their shoulder through an arc of motion. Crepitus is frequently present with motion.

Radiographic Findings

Routine shoulder radiographs will reveal the calcific deposits. Deposits in the supraspinatus are readily visible on films in neutral rotation. Internal rotation of the humeral head best reveals deposits in the infraspinatus and teres minor. In patients with acute pain where resorption is actively occurring, calacium deposition may be ill defined or barely visible. However, during the formative phase, the deposit is usually dense, well defined, and easily visualized.

Emergency Department Treatment

The emergency department management of calcific tendinitis should be tailored to reduce the patient's symptoms and help protect shoulder function. During an acute attack, analgesics are usually necessary to calm the intense pain. A sling for brief periods of immobilization may be provided, but prolonged immobilization should be avoided to prevent loss of motion. The patient should be instructed to rest the shoulder in abduction on the back of a chair as often as is tolerable. Sleeping with a pillow beneath the axilla can also help prevent restricted motion. Gentle and progressive range-of-motion exercises should be emphasized and encouraged. In the acute phase, local application of ice for 10 to 15 min, two to three times per day, may provide analgesia and help control inflammation and edema. Local heat application may be used once acute symptoms have diminished.

Local needling of the calcific deposits in the emergency department has been described for the patient in acute pain. A point of maximum tenderness on palpation can be isolated, and the presence of calcification can be confirmed with radiographs. A local anesthetic, such as 2 percent xylocaine or bupivacaine without epinephrine, is used to anesthetize subcutaneous tissues corresponding to the anticipated site of needle placement. An 18-gauge needle can then be placed at the site of calcification. This may decompress the tendon and ease the pain acutely and may speed ultimate resorption of the deposit. Following this procedure, analgesics should be prescribed. Nonsteroidal anti-inflammatory agents for 7 to 10 days may also be helpful.

Follow-up

The patient should follow up with an orthopaedist within a week, regardless of whether he or she has undergone acute needling of the calcium deposit in the emergency department. Conservative measures such as physical therapy, local needling, and injection of local anesthetics at the site of the deposit may be prescribed. Surgical removal of the calcium deposit is usually considered only after all conservative measures have been exhausted.

ADHESIVE CAPSULITIS

Adhesive capsulitis, commonly referred to as the *frozen shoulder syndrome*, causes significant discomfort and dysfunction. It is characterized by markedly restricted joint motion and pain. This condition usually occurs in middle-aged patients and is uncommon in patients younger than 40 years of age and in those older than 70 years. It is more common in women, particularly postmenopausal women. The incidence in the general population is 2 to 5 percent; this increases to 10 to 20 percent in patients with diabetes. An increased incidence is also associated with patients with a history of trauma, cervical disc disease, thyroid disease, intracranial lesions, and personality disorders. It is rarely associated with the presence of rotator cuff tears.

Pathophysiology

The exact etiology of adhesive capsulitis remains unclear, and the pathophysiology remains poorly understood. Following injury or with chronic inflammation, the shoulder joint capsule becomes thickened and contracted. Pain initially limits motion. Decresed motion allows additional inflammation. Fibrosis and scarring between the capsule, rotator cuff, subacromial bursa, and deltoid progress, further restrict motion. The joint capsule normally has an inferior pouch or ''axillary fold,'' which stretches to accomodate the humeral head during progressive elevation and external rotation of the shoulder. With fibrosis and thickening, the capsule is drawn tightly around the humeral head and the axillary fold is obliterated, restricting shoulder motion.

Autoimmune mechanisms as well as autonomic nerve dysfunction also have been implicated as causes of adhesive capsulitis, but the mechanism remains unclear.

Clinical Features

A period of shoulder immobilization following an injury or failure to mobilize the shoulder following a stroke are considered predisposing factors in the development of adhesive capsulitis. Frequently, however, no precipitating cause can be identified. Symptoms may develop insidiously over several months. Pain is described typically as diffuse and aching, is poorly localized, and often extends down the upper arm. The pain is often described as worse at night.

A painful stiffened shoulder is the hallmark finding on examination. Active and passive range of motion are limited, especially in abduction and in internal and external rotation. Disuse atrophy may be present. Pain is not usually reproducible by palpation but is present at the limits of motion as the fibrosed capsule is stretched. Impingement testing is difficult due to restricted motion. Posterior glenohumeral dislocation must always be considered in the patient with restricted motion of the shoulder.

Radiographic Findings

X-rays should be obtained to rule out a posterior glenohumeral dislocation. These should include three views at right angles to each other, typically an anteroposterior view of the humerus in internal and external rotation and an axillary or ''y'' view of the scapula. Adhesive capsulitis yields few specific diagnostic radiographic clues. Glenohumeral joint volume is described, but may be difficult to appreciate.

Emergency Department Treatment

The goal of treatment is to reduce pain and initiate restoration of motion and function. In the emergency department, this treatment consists of administering analgesics and anti-inflammatory agents and instructing the patient in the proper use of heat and ice to reduce discomfort. The patient should be instructed in general progressive range-of-motion exercises, such as pendulum swings and walking the fingers up the wall using the affected arm. A sling may be provided for comfort, but its long-term use should be discouraged to prevent further loss of motion.

Follow-up

Prompt orthopedic referral, at least within 1 to 2 weeks, is warranted. If conservative measures fail, arthroscopy and manipulation of the shoulder under general anesthesia to break up adhesions may be considered by the orthopaedist.

Prevention is the best treatment, and the emergency physician plays a vital role. Prolonged immobilization of the shoulder or upper extremity following injury should be avoided. Prompt referral to the patient's primary care provider or orthopaedist following shoulder injuries is indicated. It allows the patient to begin early progressive motion and physical therapy, where indicated.

DISORDERS OF THE BICEPS TENDON

Pathophysiology

The tendon of the long head of the biceps, by virtue of its position, can be a common cause of shoulder pain. Disorders of the biceps tendon can result from progressive impingement or may occur due to isolated inflammation or injury. The tendon of the long head of the biceps courses through the bicipital groove on the anterior aspect of the proximal humerus and inserts on the superior aspect of the labrum in the glenohumeral joint. The tendon may become inflamed or partially dislocated, sublux out of the bicipital groove, or rupture altogether.

Clinical Features

Patients with bicipital tendinitis present with acute, intense, localized pain at the anterior aspect of the shoulder. Palpation of the tendon within the bicipital groove reproduces the intense pain. Forearm supination, one of the main actions of the biceps, will also reproduce pain, especially when resistance is applied.

The tendon may sublux or momentarily dislocate from the bicipital groove if the transhumeral ligament, which forms the roof of the groove, tears from degeneration or acute trauma. Resisted forearm supination may cause subluxation that is palpable and accompanied by a painful popping sensation as the tendon subluxes.

In younger patients, mild trauma may cause complete rupture of the biceps tendon. In older patients, chronic impingement and degeneration may lead to rupture. On examination, the classic finding is described as a ''popeye'' deformity caused by contraction of the muscle from the side of the tear proximally.

Emergency Department Treatment

Supportive care and pain relief are the mainstays of emergency department care. Tendinitis and subluxation are managed conservatively. The emergency physician may provide a sling for brief use as needed for support and comfort. Analgesics and anti-inflammatory agents may be used in conjunction with prescription of relative rest, use of ice for 10 to 15 min two to three times per day, and elevation to reduce swelling.

Follow-up

For complete tears, referral to an orthopedist is recommended for surgical consideration, although frequently complete tears of the proximal biceps are managed conservatively. Conservative treatment will usually result in a 10 to 15 percent loss of strength in the muscle and will leave a cosmetic deformity.

OSTEOARTHRITIS

Since the glenohumeral joint is non-weight-bearing, primary osteoarthritis is rare. When it does occur, presentation is similar to that of degenerative disease in other joints; the patient experiences gradual and progressive onset of pain, which is worse with motion and better with rest. This usually occurs concurrently with degenerative disease of the acromioclavicular joint.

Secondary osteoarthritis is usually more common and usually associated with a previous fracture, recurrent dislocations, or with an underlying rheumatologic, metabolic, or endocrinologic disorder. Emergency department care of both primary and secondary arthritis includes analgesics, anti-inflammatory agents, and gentle exercises to preserve range of motion. Prompt referral should be made for further evaluation of possible underlying rheumatologic or inflammatory conditions.

DIFFERENTIAL DIAGNOSIS

Aches and pains in the shoulder are not always due to bursitis or tendinitis. Although disorders of the rotator cuff and other intrinsic structures of the shoulder are the most common cause of pain, extrinsic conditions outside the shoulder complex can refer pain to the shoulder. It is critical and can be life preserving to distinguish extrinsic causes from intrinsic causes of shoulder pain.

The Neck

The neck is the most common source of pain referred to the shoulder. Degenerative disease of the cervical spine, degenerative disc disease, and herniated nucleus pulposus can all refer pain to the shoulder. These symptoms may occur acutely or gradually. The pain is usually worse during daytime activities and better at night when activities cease. The patient with a C5–C6 herniated disk may present with pain very similar to that due to rotator cuff disease. Careful and thorough examination of the cervical spine and a complete neurovascular examination should be included in the evaluation of any patient with shoulder pain. On examination, range of motion in the neck may be restricted and may reproduce symptoms in the shoulder. Axial loading may especially cause referred pain. If a cervical condition is considered to be the source of pain, cervical radiographs including oblique views should be obtained. In the absence of neurologic findings, conservative measures may be inititiated. In the emergency department, the patient may be fitted with a soft cervical collar and provided with analgesics and anti-inflammatory agents as needed for comfort.

The Brachial Plexus

An injury to the brachial plexus can cause pain referred to the shoulder and can produce weakness and atrophy in the muscles of the shoulder within weeks of injury. Radiographic evaluation of the cervical spine should be included in the emergency department evaluation of patients with suspected brachial plexus injury or involvement.

Brachial plexus neuritis is uncommon but can be very painful. It is usually determined to be of viral origin. The inflammation of the brachial plexus can lead to weakness and atrophy of the muscles of the shoulder complex within weeks following the onset of pain. Cervical spine radiographs should be included in the workup. Brachial plexus neuritis is usually self-limiting. Referral to a neurologist should be arranged if a patient is suspected of having this disorder.

Vascular Injuries

Injuries to the blood vessels also can cause shoulder pain. The most serious recognized vascular injury is acute thrombosis of the axillary artery. Repetitive mechanical trauma or explosive stress from lifting heavy objects can compress and contuse the intimal lining of the axillary artery. This predisposes the artery to thrombosis. Acute thrombosis requires primary thrombolytic therapy.

Neurologic Injury

The most common neurologic injury about the shoulder involves compression of the suprascapular nerve. This nerve originates from the brachial plexus distal C5–C6 nerve roots and courses posteriorly to the suprascapular notch. Not uncommonly, this nerve becomes entrapped beneath the transverse ligament at the level of the notch. Traction injuries from explosive movements can also injure the nerve. On examination, infraspinatus atrophy and associated weakness and external rotation will typically be found. The initial treatment is conservative. Electromyographic and nerve conduction velocity studies will reveal the extent and location of nerve injury. Surgery for decompression is considered if conservative measures fail.

Thoracic Outlet Syndrome

Compression of the brachial plexus and blood vessels proximal to the shoulder can cause shoulder pain. Women in the child-bearing years are affected three times more commonly than men. The medial trunk of the brachial plexus is most commonly affected, and the symptoms usually involve pain that radiates through the shoulder to the medial forearm and occasionally to the small and ring ringers. Patients can usually identify motions that reproduce the symptoms. Fatigue often prevents the use of the arms above shoulder level.

Radiographic evaluation may reveal evidence of a prior clavicle fracture with malunion or the presence of a cervical rib band, which are associated with compression of the brachial plexus. Treatment is generally conservative, although surgical decompression may be considered if the symptoms become debilitating or refractory to conservative measures.

Pancoast's Tumor

This tumor, when present in the superior sulcus of the lung, may compress the brachial plexus against the chest wall and cause shoulder pain. The patient may experience local or radicular shoulder pain or sense a fullness in the supraclavicular fossa.

Thoraco-Abdominal Disorders

Finally, a large number of cardiothoracic disorders can cause shoulder pain. These include myocardial ischemia and infarction, pneumonia, and pulmonary embolism and infarction. Any thoracic or abdominal disorder that irritates the diaphragm can also cause referred shoulder pain. Finally, abdominal disorders that can cause shoulder pain include biliary tract disease, splenic injury or inflammation, perforated viscus, or ruptured ectopic pregnancy.

BIBLIOGRAPHY

Blevins FT: Rotator cuff pathology in athletes. *SportsMed* 24(3):205, 1997.

Delee JC, Drez D, Jr (eds): *Orthopaedic Sports Medicine: Principles and Practice*. Philadelphia: Saunders, 1994.

Green S, Buchbinder R, Glazier R, Forbes A: Systematic review of randomised controlled trials of interventions for painful shoulder: Selection criteria, outcome assessment, and efficacy. *Br Med J* 316(7128):354, 1998.

Ionnotti JP (ed): *Rotator Cuff Disorders: Evaluation and Treatment*. American Academy of Orthopaedic Surgeons Monograph Series, 1991.

Rockwood CA, Matsen FA (eds): *Orthopedics*. Philadelphia: Saunders, 1990.

EMERGENCIES IN SYSTEMIC RHEUMATIC DISEASES

Mary Chester Morgan Wasko

Complaints related to the musculoskeletal system account for 1 of 7 visits to the primary care provider and an abundance of emergency room visits. Evaluating the patient with musculoskeletal problems requires a thorough, thoughtful history and examination to determine whether the symptom is a local problem or a manifestation of a systemic disease, and whether a local problem is potentially catastrophic, as in the case of an unrecognized septic joint in a rheumatoid arthritis patient.

Life-threatening manifestations of rheumatic disease are infrequent. They most often result directly from internal organ involvement from systemic conditions such as systemic lupus erythematosus (SLE) or other vasculitides; examples include alveolar hemorrhage in SLE and aortic arch dissection in temporal arteritis. Alternatively, they may be a complication of treatment itself, such as infection in the setting of immunosuppression, or gastrointestinal hemorrhage complicating nonsteroidal anti-inflammatory drug (NSAID) use. Either can lead to serious morbidity and increased mortality if not recognized and managed promptly.

Table 276-1 highlights common presenting musculoskeletal complaints that warrant prompt evaluation and a fundamental differential diagnosis for each. Before diagnostic tests are obtained, an accurate clinical assessment is imperative.

TABLE 276-1 Emergent Musculoskeletal Clinical Signs and Symptoms

Feature	Differential Diagnosis
History of significant trauma	Soft tissue injury, internal derangement, or fracture
Hot, swollen joint	Infection, systemic rheumatic disease, gout, pseudogout
Constitutional signs and symptoms (e.g., fever, weight loss, malaise)	Infection, sepsis, systemic rheumatic disease, malignancy
Weakness:	
Focal	Focal nerve lesion (compartment syndrome, entrapment neuropathy, mononeuritis multiplex, motor neuron disease, radiculopathy*)
Diffuse	Myositis, metabolic myopathy, toxin, paraneoplastic syndrome, degenerative neuromuscular disorder, myelopathy,* transverse myelitis
Neurogenic pain (burning, numbness, paresthesia):	
Asymmetric	Radiculopathy,* reflex sympathetic dystrophy, entrapment neuropathy
Symmetric	Myelopathy,* peripheral neuropathy
Claudication pain pattern	Peripheral vascular disease, giant cell arteritis (jaw pain), lumbar spinal stenosis

*Radiculopathy and myelopathy may be due to infectious, neoplastic, or mechanical processes.

Source: From American College of Rheumatology Ad Hoc Committee on Clinical Guidelines: Guidelines for the Initial Evaluation of the Adult Patient with Acute Musculoskeletal Symptoms. *Arthritis Rheum* 39(1): 2, 1996. Reproduced with permission.

This chapter provides an overview of emergencies in rheumatology, with a focus on systemic rheumatic disease.

RHEUMATIC EMERGENCIES ASSOCIATED WITH RISK OF MORTALITY

The Airway and Respiratory System

Life-threatening respiratory compromise occurs by two major mechanisms in rheumatic diseases: difficulty ventilating due to airway obstruction and impaired ventilation due to weakness (Table 276-2). Relapsing polychondritis is an inflammatory disease affecting cartilage and usually begins with the abrupt onset of pain, redness, and swelling of the ears or the nose. The airway is affected in roughly 50 percent of patients, causing inflammation, destruction, and ultimate collapse of tracheobronchial cartilage. Patients report throat tenderness over cartilaginous structures and hoarseness. Less commonly they experience shortness of breath, cough, or stridor. Repeated exacerbations ultimately may cause asphyxiation. Pulmonary function studies with flow-volume loops detect airway obstruction more reliably than bronchoscopy. Emergency tracheostomy may be helpful, depending on the level and extent of airway compromise. Hospitalization for careful observation and high dose corticosteroids is necessary during acute exacerbations.

Rheumatoid arthritis (RA) may cause cricoarytenoid dysfunction. RA patients with cricoarytenoid arthritis may complain of pain with speaking or swallowing, hoarseness, or stridor. If the joints become fixed in a closed position, airway compromise mandates emergency tracheostomy. Presentation with the above signs is an urgent indication for fiberoptic laryngoscopy.

The respiratory muscles may be impaired by inflammatory muscle disease. In dermatomyositis and polymyositis, respiratory insufficiency is uncommon at presentation but complicates poorly controlled or chronic disease. Patients should be observed for nasal flaring, as they may be too weak to generate intercostal retractions. Chest x-rays are normal or show "high-riding" diaphragms unless pulmonary involvement or an aspiration pneumonitis coexists. Admission for disease control and stabilization is indicated in any patient with inflammatory muscle disease and respiratory impairment. Patients with active or advanced disease may require intubation and ventilation for respiratory support. The clinical course can be followed at bedside with measurements of peak inspiratory and expiratory forces. Respiratory failure is predictable with peak inspiratory effort of less than 30 percent of predicted or vital capacity of less than 50 percent of predicted.

Pleurisy is common in RA and systemic lupus erythematosus (SLE). It may be asymptomatic in RA, but roughly half of lupus patients have signs and symptoms of pleurisy during the course of their disease. All effusions in rheumatic disease patients should be aspirated for diagnosis. Rheumatoid pulmonary effusions characteristically have very low glucose levels, but so do effusions associated with indolent infections such as tuberculosis. Rheumatic, infectious, and malignant effusions are often exudative and either polymorphonuclear or mononuclear cells may predominate. In the patient without lupus nephritis, nonsteroidal anti-inflammatory drugs (NSAIDs) (e.g., indomethacin, 25 to 50 mg tid) usually suffice. Prednisone in moderate doses 10 mg po tid is reserved for patients failing this regimen.

Pulmonary hemorrhage can complicate Goodpasture's disease, SLE, hypersensitivity vasculitis, and Wegener's granulomatosis due to vasculopathic or vasculitic lung involvement. Ankylosing spondylitis (upper lobes), scleroderma, and, rarely, RA and other rheumatic diseases can lead to pulmonary fibrosis. Patients may present with abrupt decompensation with a history of a well-tolerated slow decline. In myositis, however, interstitial pneumonitis may become apparent with quiescent muscle disease, progress rapidly, and result in fulminant respiratory failure; these patients should be hospitalized to rule out infection and be treated with aggressive immunosuppression.

TABLE 276-2 Respiratory Manifestations of Rheumatic Diseases

Disease	Common	Infrequent	Rare
SLE	Serositis, effusion	Infiltrate	Hemorrhage, effusion, "shrinking lungs," fibrosis
RA	Nodules, effusion	Pulmonary fibrosis	Cricoarytenoid obstruction
Spondyloarthropathies		Pulmonary fibrosis	Pulmonary infiltrates, ARDS
Relapsing polychondritis	Airway obstruction	Tracheobronchial collapse	
Polymyositis and dermatomyositis		Hypoventilation with hypoxemia, respiratory failure Interstitial pneumonitis	
Scleroderma	Pulmonary fibrosis	Pulmonary hypertension	
Vasculitides			
Wegener's	Sinusitis, nasal ulcers, pulmonary nodules, infiltrate, bronchospasm, hemoptysis	Hemorrhage	

Cardiac Diseases

The heart is affected in many rheumatic diseases, with potential involvement extending from the pericardium to the endocardium. Of the rheumatic diseases, RA and juvenile rheumatoid arthritis (JRA) are most often associated with pericarditis. Pericarditis is usually asymptomatic, but occasional patients with chest pain attributed to costochondritis may have symptomatic pericarditis. Chest pain is characteristically positional, and a pericardial rub is usually heard. SLE often causes symptomatic pericarditis, particularly in the elderly. Patients also report symptoms typical of a flare, such as rash, oral ulcers, or joint pain. Symptoms tend to be consistent from one flare to the next, and therefore a thorough review of systems is key. When symptomatic pericarditis is diagnosed, malignancy and infection must be considered and excluded if clinically indicated. Treatment is similar to that for pleurisy above. Pericardial tamponade and constrictive pericarditis from either RA or SLE are uncommon.

While therapy has greatly improved long-term survival in SLE, late mortality from premature atherosclerotic disease is being recognized. Precordial chest pain in SLE is not always due to serositis or costochondritis, particularly with long-standing disease, and angina should be considered. Other causes of precordial pain are listed in Table 276-3.

Myocardial infarction (MI) in rheumatic diseases is not usually related to underlying disease. The noteworthy exceptions are Kawasaki disease (see Chap. 132, "Musculoskeletal Disorders in Children") and polyarteritis nodosa (PAN). PAN is a form of vasculitis affecting small- and medium-caliber arteries of the skin (nodular, urticarial, or multiform rashes), gut (abdominal angina), and kidneys (hypertension, hematuria). Coronary arteries are commonly involved. MI and PAN are usually clinically silent, but when MI occurs it can occur at any age.

Mortality in SLE from premature atherosclerosis is well recognized. Angina always should be considered in SLE patients with chest complaints, especially with long-standing disease and in those on steroids.

Acute rheumatic fever (ARF) remains an important cause of pancarditis. ARF follows streptococcal pharyngitis within a few weeks. It is heralded by rapid development of fever and acute polyarthritis (in adults) or migratory arthritis (in children). A few patients have a more insidious onset. Supportive clinical clues are the presence of subcutaneous nodules, chorea, or erythema marginatum, but only a third of patients will have one of the latter major manifestations. Diagnosis is based on documenting the clinical involvement and antecedent streptococcal infection. The throat should be cultured and antistreptolysin O (ASO) or streptozyme titers determined at intervals to document a fourfold change in titer over a month. Other baseline tests include serial chest x-rays, echocardiography and ECGs to monitor the carditis; and acute phase reactants (erythrocyte sedimentation rate, C-reactive protein). The fever and arthritis respond rapidly and completely to salicylate therapy, but salicylates should be held until the diagnosis is clear. Patients should be placed at bedrest until clinical and laboratory parameters begin to normalize.

Rheumatic fever is only one disease associated with migratory arthritis (Table 276-4). Bacterial endocarditis or septicemia due to common bacterial pathogens and the prodromal phase of pulmonary mycoplasma or fungal infections must be considered. Children with Henoch-Schoenlein purpura and cefaclor (Ceclor) serum sickness often have migratory articular and periarticular involvement. Stage II Lyme disease can be manifested by migratory articular involvement, with

TABLE 276-3 Precordial Chest Pain in Rheumatic Diseases

Pericarditis, pancarditis
Angina, myocardial infarction
Dermatomal herpes zoster
Costochondritis
Vertebral compression fracture (thoracic radiculopathy)
Rib fracture
Pulmonary embolus
Gastroesophageal reflux

TABLE 276-4 Conditions Associated with Migratory Arthritis

Rheumatic fever
Subacute bacterial endocarditis
Henoch-Schönlein purpura
Cefaclor hypersensitivity (children)
Septicemia: staphylococcal, streptococcal, meningococcal, gonococcal
Pulmonary infection: *Mycoplasma,* histoplasmosis, coccidioidomycosis
Lyme disease

TABLE 276-5 Cardiac Manifestations of Rheumatic Diseases

Disease	Common	Infrequent	Rare
SLE	Pericarditis	Angina, myocarditis	Tamponade, constrictive pericarditis
Ankylosing spondylitis		Aortic stenosis/ insufficiency, dissection	Drop attacks
Relapsing polychondritis		Aortic insufficiency, dissection	
Polymyositis and dermatomyositis		Arrhythmias, myocarditis	
Scleroderma		Myocardial fibrosis, arrhythmias	Cor pulmonale
Vasculitides		Angina, myocardial infarction	

individual joints resolving over hours to days. Often young adults with polyarthritis are empirically treated with intravenous penicillin for disseminated gonococcus (GC) until a streptococcal infection is confirmed. The arthritis of ARF does not respond to antibiotic therapy; therefore prompt improvement suggests the diagnosis of GC.

Valvular heart disease is a recognized extraarticular manifestation of the seronegative spondyloarthropathies, particularly ankylosing spondylitis. Fibrotic changes of the aortic valve are usually asymptomatic, with dysfunction occurring more often in patients with long-standing, severe disease. Scar tissue also may impair cardiac conduction, leading to drop attacks. Relapsing polychondritis can affect the valves, causing aortic insufficiency and aneurysm. This may develop early after diagnosis and is a grave development. Table 276-5 summarizes cardiac involvement in rheumatic diseases.

ADRENAL INSUFFICIENCY

Rheumatic disease patients on glucocorticoids are usually instructed to seek medical care urgently if an illness like gastroenteritis prevents taking or absorption of prednisone. In general, the course of a rheumatic disease is not worsened by administration of stress glucocorticoids for a day during an acute illness, even if the dose is much larger than the usual daily dose. A large dose of glucocorticoid may cause labile hyperglycemia in diabetic patients, but no more so than the underlying acute condition. Other medications used to treat rheumatic diseases can be held safely for a brief bout of gastroenteritis. These include NSAIDs, cyclophosphamide or chlorambucil, methotrexate, hydroxychloroquine (Plaquenil), and calcium channel blockers, if they are only used to treat Raynaud phenomenon.

Rarely, patients treated with steroids in the past 18 months develop adrenal insufficiency. They may have early symptoms of weakness, depression, fatigue, and postural dizziness, or late life-threatening vomiting. The serum chemistries usually do not reveal hyponatremia or hyperkalemia in patients with adrenal insufficiency after prednisone withdrawal because that steroid has no mineralocorticoid activity. If adrenal insufficiency is a remote possibility, stress steroids should be administered. Dexamethasone is preferable, as that steroid will not interfere with assays of other adrenal steroids during subsequent diagnostic testing. Prior to the administration of stress steroids, a cortisol level should be drawn in the emergency room. Under stress, normally functioning adrenal glands generate a level in excess of 20 μg/dL.

RHEUMATIC PRESENTATIONS WITH HIGH RISK OF MORBIDITY

The Cervical Spine and Spinal Cord

Cervical spine disease and its neurologic risk is well recognized in rheumatoid arthritis and ankylosing spondylitis. In RA, pannus formation and destruction of ligamentous supporting structures may lead to atlantoaxial subluxation; an atlantodental distance in excess of the normal 3.5 mm seen in a lateral flexion view suggests instability (in children under 12, 4 mm of widening is normal). Cord compression may occur acutely following a trivial injury or be more insidious. Subtle clues include a change in bowel or bladder function, new weakness, numbness, or paresthesias. Instability may lead to cranial migration of the odontoid. Complaints relating to vertebral insufficiency (e.g., vertigo) may be reported. Lhermitte sign, an electric shock sensation radiating down the back on neck flexion, is a classic indication of cervical spine instability. Strength may be difficult to assess in an RA patient, so subtle differences in reflexes are particularly informative. Lateral cervical spine films in flexion are essential for evaluation. Neck flexion should not be forced, but rather studied at a degree considered comfortable by the patient.

The ankylosed, inflexible cervical spine in a patient with a seronegative spondyloarthropathy (e.g., ankylosing spondylitis) is susceptible to fracture with minor trauma. A whiplash-type injury or a blow from behind may result in new neck pain in an ankylosed area. The complaint of new neck pain requires a careful history and examination, with attention to possible trauma to the neck and evidence of peripheral nerve damage. Fractures are most commonly transverse through a disc space, leading to greater risk of dislocation and cord compression.

Intubation of patients with rheumatic cervical spine disease is best addressed in an elective, controlled situation after the cervical spine has been assessed. In an emergency, a patient with a stiff or arthritic neck should be intubated by the most experienced operator available. Atlantoaxial instability should be assumed, and extremes of head manipulation avoided.

The spinal cord can be affected by transverse myelitis in SLE, or a number of factors can induce an anterior spinal artery syndrome in patients with rheumatic diseases. The anterior spinal artery is a direct branch of the aorta; dissection of the aorta, vasculitis, or embolism can impair blood supply to the anterior cord and produce a clinical picture distinct from transverse myelitis or metastatic tumor by sparing of posterior column function (position sense and vibration).

The Eye

Temporal arteritis (TA) often causes sudden blindness, usually before the condition is diagnosed. Blindness can be prevented, however, if prodromal visual changes and coexistent symptomatology are recognized. Prodromal changes in vision almost always precede blindness.

TA is a granulomatous arteritis of the thoracic aorta and its branches; the vasculitis and ischemia in this distribution induce characteristic signs and symptoms: new headache, tender scalp, fluctuating vision, diminution or loss of a brachial pulse, pain in the jaw or tongue while chewing or talking, and constitutional symptoms. An elevated Westergren sedimentation rate (>50 mm/h), elevated liver function studies (particularly the alkaline phosphatase), and unexplained anemia are common laboratory abnormalities.

TA affects the middle-aged and elderly. Polymyalgia rheumatica (PMR), with proximal shoulder and hip girdle morning stiffness and aching, coexists in 10 to 30 percent of these patients. Prodromal changes in vision almost always precede blindness. A high index of suspicion is critical when evaluating anyone older than 50 with a new headache, fluctuating vision, or jaw, tongue, or upper extremity claudication. Diagnosis is established on temporal artery biopsy. If the clinical diagnosis is reasonably certain, steroid therapy should be initiated at a prednisone dosage of 60 mg/day to prevent blindness; this will not obscure pathologic findings if the biopsy is obtained within a week. Symptoms of PMR are easily controlled with prednisone, 5 to 7.5 mg po tid, and those patients without signs and symptoms of TA should not be unnecessarily treated with high-dose steroids.

Sjögren's syndrome, a lymphocytic infiltration of the lacrimal and salivary glands causing dry eyes and dry mouth, may complicate many rheumatic diseases or occur independently. It predisposes the patient to corneal irritation, ulceration, and superimposed infection.

In RA, a red eye requires careful evaluation. Under bright natural light, examination can reveal the difference between episcleritis, which is self-limiting, and scleritis, which is an emergency. Episcleritis is a painless injection of the episcleral vessels giving the eye a pink-red appearance; it rarely impairs vision. As it is self-limiting, no therapy is indicated. Scleritis causes exquisite ocular tenderness. The eye has a deep purplish discoloration. Visual impairment and scleral thinning with rupture are feared outcomes. High-dose steroids and intensive ophthalmologic management are required.

Hypertension

While hypertension can complicate PAN or SLE with renal involvement or RA with drug-induced renal toxicity (fluid retention, nephritis, or renal papillary necrosis), hypertension is a feared complication of systemic sclerosis (scleroderma). Hypertensive renal crisis was the leading cause of death in scleroderma until the advent of angiotensin-converting enzyme (ACE) inhibitors. The most susceptible patients have rapidly progressive skin changes and present within the first few years of diagnosis with complaints related to hypertension. Laboratory studies reveal rapidly progressive renal insufficiency and frequently a microangiopathic hemolytic anemia and thrombocytopenia. The hypertension results from sclerosis and impaired renal glomerular perfusion causing hyperreninemia. Dehydration from gastroenteritis or diuretics may precipitate the crisis. These patients should be hospitalized and promptly treated with captopril. Any intervention such as diuretics that might exacerbate volume contraction and the underlying pathophysiology should be avoided.

Other rheumatic diseases may affect the kidneys but are not acutely life-threatening. Renal involvement in SLE, PAN, or Wegener's granulomatosis may result in hypertension. Drug-induced nephrotoxicity (hypertension, fluid retention, nephritis, or renal papillary necrosis) is seen in rheumatic disease patients using nonsteroidal anti-inflammatory agents, usually with preexisting hypertension or renal disease.

The Kidney

Most systemic rheumatic diseases may affect kidney function. Glomerulonephritis is a major determinant of morbidity in patients with lupus and Wegener's granulomatosis. Urinalysis abnormalities (hematuria, proteinuria) and hypertension are apparent before serum creatinine rises. Patients with lupus and nephrotic syndrome can develop renal vein thrombosis due to urinary loss of antithrombin III; they present with flank pain and proteinuria. In diffuse scleroderma, renal dysfunction secondary to hypertension and microangiopathy typically develops rapidly over days to a few weeks.

Occasionally, a patient with active polymyositis or metabolic muscle disease develops acute renal insufficiency due to rhabdomyolysis. In metabolic muscle disease, myalgias and muscle breakdown can be triggered by exercise. Myoglobinuria should be suspected when the urine is brown and the dipstick shows blood but no red blood cells. In contrast to a hemolytic state, the serum is clear, creative phosphokinase is elevated, and haptoglobin is normal. Patients should be hydrated with normal saline to restore intravascular loss that accompanies muscle necrosis. Lasix and mannitol also are indicated to preserve urinary output.

A final consideration is medication nephrotoxicity. Patients, particularly the elderly, treated with nonsteroidal anti-inflammatory drugs can develop renal insufficiency and fluid retention on the basis of alteration in renal blood flow; this is mediated by prostaglandin inhibition. A decline in renal function in any rheumatic disease patient should prompt a search for remediable causes of renal dysfunction, either related to drug therapy or to the rheumatic disease itself. See Chap. 271, ''Rhabdomyolysis.''

BIBLIOGRAPHY

Ad Hoc Committee on Clinical Guidelines: Guidelines for the initial evaluation of the adult patient with acute musculoskeletal symptoms. *Arthritis Rheum* 39:1, 1996.

Anderson BC: Diagnosing bursitis of the hip. *IM Intern Med* 19:12, 1998.

Bailey JP Jr, Rahn DW: Acute monarthritis. *Bull Rheum Dis* 46:1, 1997.

Bennett DA, Bleck TP: Recognizing impending respiratory failure from neuromuscular causes. *J Crit Ill* 3:46, 1988.

Halla J: Rheumatology emergencies. *Bull Rheum Dis* 46:4, 1997.

Kelley WN, Harris ED Jr, Ruddy S, Sledge CB: *Textbook of Rheumatology*. Philadelphia: Saunders, 1997.

Killion MJ: Recognizing acute adrenal insufficiency in the perioperative patient. *IM Intern Med* 19:30, 1998.

Klippel JH (ed): *Primer on the Rheumatic Diseases,* 11th ed. Atlanta, GA: Arthritis Foundation, 1997.

Mandell BF: *Acute Rheumatic and Immunological Diseases*. New York: Marcel Dekker, 1994.

HAND INFECTIONS

Mark W. Fourre

Patients with hand infections routinely use the emergency department (ED) as their initial site of care. It is important for the emergency physician to accurately diagnose and treat the infection because failure to do so will likely cause long-term morbidity and disability. The hand is one of the most elegant and complex features of the human body, and the emergency physician must understand the basic anatomy and functions of the hand in order to appropriately manage the patient.

Infection is most commonly introduced by an injury to the dermis. The infection initially may remain superficial, as a cellulitis, or localized, as a paronychia or felon. Left untreated, these infections ultimately will spread along anatomic planes or to adjacent compartments in the hand. Deeper injuries may directly seed underlying structures, giving rise to rapidly spreading infections such as seen with closed-fist injuries or cat bites. Rarely, hematogenous spread may be the source of hand infections.[1]

A directed history must be obtained to delineate a likely cause of the infection. Patients who present with systemic symptoms secondary to a hand infection are seriously ill, and parenteral antibiotics with inpatient management is indicated. A history of chronic illness or immunodeficiency must alert the physician to the possibility of atypical pathogens.[2,3]

Since hand infections tend to disseminate along anatomic compartments and planes, the physical examination should be directed at defining the anatomic limits of the infection. The examiner should document if the process involves the skin, subcutaneous tissues, fascial spaces, tendon, joint, or bone.[4] If deep structures of the hand are involved, emergent consultation with a hand specialist is indicated because treatment likely will involve inpatient care and drainage in the operating room.

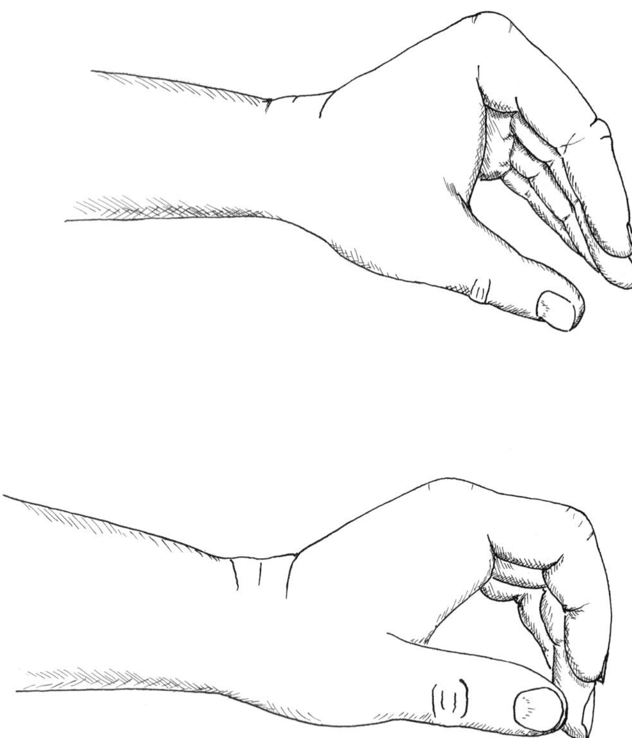

FIG. 277-1. Positioning the hand during immobilization. Top position is used when splints are applied in fractures or severe sprains. Bottom position is position of function used when applying a soft bond dressing.

With the exception of superficial cellulitis, hand infections are surgical problems that must be managed using accepted surgical principles.[5] First, if there is pus, drain it. Superficial and discrete infections, such as paronychia and felons, can be drained in the ED. All other infections involving deep structures in the hand should be treated in the operating room by a hand surgeon. Second, immobilize and elevate the extremity. This will rest the hand, reduce inflammation, avoid secondary injury, and limit anatomic extension of the infection. Immobilization is accomplished by applying a bulky hand dressing and splinting the hand in a position of function: the wrist at 15 to 30° of extension, the metacarpophalangeal (MCP) joints at 50 to 90° of flexion, and the interphalangeal (IP) joints at 5 to 15° of flexion (Fig. 277-1). The hand may be elevated on pillows or suspended using stockinet. Third, broad-spectrum antibiotics should be initiated (Table 277-1). Finally, serial examinations should be performed to ensure that an effective management plan has been instituted. If the patient is not admitted to the hospital, timely and appropriate follow-up must be arranged by the emergency physician.

MICROBIOLOGY

The bacterial etiology of hand infections depends on the source of the offending inoculum. Since *Staphylococcus* and *Streptococcus* species routinely colonize the skin, they are the bacteria most frequently isolated from hand infections.[1,6] Polymicrobial infections, including anaerobes, are the rule rather than the exception, and antibiotic coverage must be chosen accordingly.

Intravenous drug abusers typically present with abscesses or deep space infections secondary to *Staphylococcus aureus*. Although most commonly caused by direct introduction of a contaminated needle through inadequately cleaned skin, the infection may have spread hematoginously from a previously established bacterial endocarditis.[1] Paronychia and felons are commonly caused by minor trauma associated with chewing fingernails or exposing minor injuries to saliva. Most of these infections are polymicrobial in origin, with most harboring anaerobic bacteria.[7]

Bacteria found in infections caused by animal bites reflect the oral flora of the involved species. This encompasses a broad range of bacteria, including gram-positive, anaerobic, and gram-negative organisms. In human bites, *Eikenella corrodens* is a common pathogen. Although sensitive to penicillin and ampicillin, *Eikenella* is relatively resistant to numerous antibiotics, including first-generation cephalosporins, nafcillin, and clindamycin. Therefore, a β-lactamase inhibitor drug alone or a first-generation cephalosporin in combination with penicillin is required for prophylactic antibiotic coverage for human bites and for treatment of hand infections caused by human bites. Cat and dog bites may harbor *Pasteurella multicida*,[5,8] which typically produces an aggressive, rapidly spreading cellulitis that quickly becomes suppurative. *Pasteurella* is also sensitive to penicillin and ampicillin, and antibiotic coverage is the same as is indicated in human bites. Initial antibiotic coverage is reviewed in Table 277-1. For a complete discussion on animal bites, see Chap. 43, ''Puncture Wounds and Animal Bites.''

Care must be exercised when managing patients with diabetes or acquired immunodeficiency syndrome (AIDS) because they may harbor atypical infections caused by *Mycobacterium* or *Candida albicans*.[2,3] Patients who are immunocompromised or asplenic may be at risk for rapidly progressive and fatal infections. Aggressive intervention is indicated in these settings.

CELLULITIS

Cellulitis is the most superficial of hand infections and may be treated definitively with antibiotics if diagnosed early enough in its course. Diagnosis is made by documenting erythema, warmth, and edema to the affected portion of the hand. The examiner must document lack of involvement of any deeper structures in the hand. Specifically, range of motion of the digits, hand, or wrist should not be uncomfortable for the patient, and palpation of the deeper structures of the hand should not produce any tenderness.

The most common offending organism is *Streptococcus pyogenes*, although *S. aureus* and other pathogens are identified occasionally. An antistaphylococcal penicillin or first-generation cephalosporin is recommended for initial treatment.[4] For more extensive involvement, parenteral antibiotics should be instituted. Inpatient management should be reserved for patients who are immunocompromised or systemically ill and for rapidly spreading infections.

The hand should be immobilized in a position of function, and the patient should keep the hand elevated at all times. Finally, close follow-up should be arranged, with reexamination occurring within the next 24 h.

FLEXOR TENOSYNOVITIS

Flexor tenosynovitis is a surgical emergency that must be diagnosed promptly by the examining physician and managed aggressively by both the emergency physician and the hand surgeon. Failure to accurately diagnose and manage a flexor tenosynovitis will lead to loss of function of the digit and eventually loss of function of the entire hand. Diagnosis is made by recognizing the classic clinical findings described by Kanavel. The four cardinal signs are tenderness over the flexor tendon sheath, symmetric swelling of the finger, pain with passive extension, and a flexed posture of the involved digit at rest.[9,10]

The infection usually is associated with penetrating trauma of the affected area, although the patient may be unaware of this injury. *Staphylococcus* is the most common bacteria isolated; however, infec-

TABLE 277-1 Initial Antibiotic Coverage for Common Hand Infections

Infection	Initial Antibiotic	Likely Organisms	Comments
Cellulitis	First-generation cephalosporin (cephalexin) *or* antistaphylococcal penicillin (amoxicillin-clavulanate, dicloxacillin)	*S. pyogenes, S. aureus*	Consider vancomycin for intravenous drug abusers
Felon/paronychia	First-generation cephalosporin (cephalexin) *or* antistaphylococcal penicillin (amoxicillin-clavulanate, dicloxacillin)	Polymicrobial, *S. aureus,* anaerobes	Antibiotics indicated for infections with associated localized cellulitis
Flexor tenosynovitis	β-Lactamase inhibitor (ampicillin/sulbactam) *or* first-generation cephalosporin (cefazolin) and penicillin	*S. aureus,* streptococci, anaerobes, gram-negatives	Parenteral antibiotics are indicated; consider ceftriaxone for *N. gonorrhoeae*
Deep space infection	β-Lactamase inhibitor (ampicillin/sulbactam) *or* first-generation cephalosporin (cefazolin) and penicillin	*S. aureus,* streptococci, anaerobes, gram-negatives	Inpatient management
Animal bites (including human)	β-Lactamase inhibitor *or* first-generation cephalosporin and penicillin	*S. aureus,* streptococci, *E. corrodens* (human), *Pasteurella multocida* (cat), anerobes and gram negatives	All animal bite wounds should receive prophylactic oral antibiotics
Herpetic whitlow	None, unless secondary bacterial contamination is present	Herpes simplex	Consider acyclovir; no surgical drainage is indicated

tions often harbor anaerobes and are routinely polymicrobial in origin.[5,6,11] One should suspect disseminated *Neisseria gonorrhoeae* in any patient who has a recent history consistent with a sexually transmitted disease.

The emergency physician should initiate treatment with parenteral antibiotics. This should include a β-lactamase inhibitor or first-generation cephalosporin and penicillin. Vancomycin should be considered for patients who abuse drugs intravenously because they may harbor methicillin-resistant *S. aureus* (MRSA).[1] Any spontaneous exudate from the infection should be sent for Gram stain and culture with sensitivities.

The hand should be immobilized and elevated, and a hand surgeon should be consulted on an emergent basis. If the infection is identified early in its course, conservative therapy may be indicated initially. The patient would then be treated with parenteral antibiotics, immobilization, elevation, and reevaluation within 24 h. The decision to manage the patient without operative intervention must be made with involvement of the hand surgeon.

DEEP SPACE INFECTIONS

The hand offers numerous compartments in which infections may propagate and migrate. The volar surface of the hand encompasses many potential spaces that may become infected by direct inoculation or spread from surrounding structures. These include the thenar space, the midpalmer space, the radial bursa, and the ulna bursar (Figs. 277-2 and 277-3).

The volar aspect of the hand is covered by the tough and relatively fixed tissues of the palm; the veins and lymphatics course through the softer tissues on the dorsum of the hand; thus, regardless of the precise anatomic site of infection or inflammation, the dorsum of the hand always will swell whenever there is an inflammatory process. For this reason, a deep space infection initially may be misdiagnosed as a cellulitis over the dorsum of the hand if the practitioner does not obtain a thorough history and conduct a complete examination including palpation of the volar surface of the hand to elicit tenderness, induration, or fluctuance. Since these compartments are contiguous with the flexor tendons of the hand, range of motion of the digits often produces significant pain for the patient.

Occasionally, infections will arise in the web space. These ''collar button'' abscesses present with pain and swelling of the web space causing separation of the affected digits. Examination reveals induration or fluctuance in the dorsal and/or volar web space along with erythema, warmth, and tenderness. *S. aureus* and *Streptococcus* species are the most common organisms isolated.[9,10]

The emergency physician should initiate parenteral antibiotics (see Table 277-1), and the hand should be immobilized and elevated. The patient likely will require analgesia while in the ED. Emergent evalua-

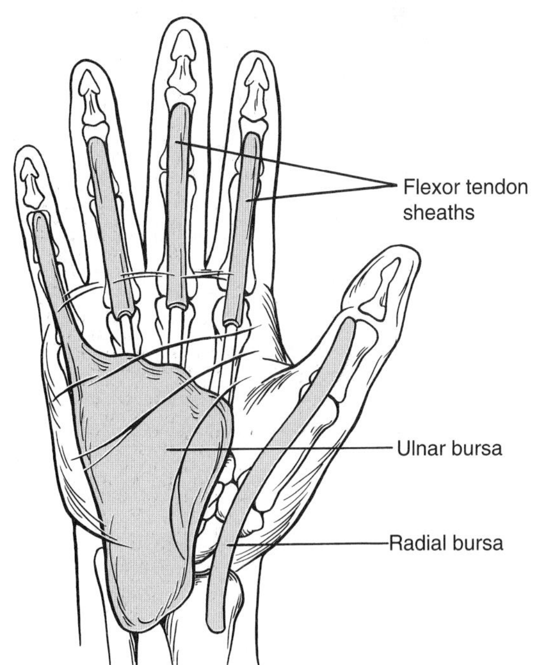

FIG. 277-2. Anatomy. Flexor tendon infections may travel quickly along established anatomic planes and spread quickly to the ulnar and radial bursae.

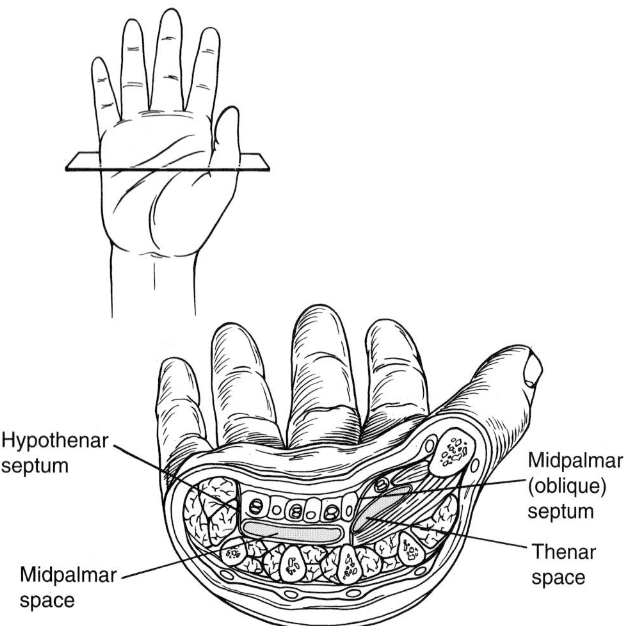

FIG. 277-3. Deep palmar spaces. The midpalmar and thenar spaces are deep in the structures of the hand. The proximity to vital structures necessitates an aggressive management course including parenteral antibiotics and referral to a hand surgeon for drainage.

tion by a hand surgeon is required because drainage of the infection should be undertaken in the operating room.

INFECTIONS FROM CLOSED-FIST INJURIES

The most common "human bite" infection of the hand is actually the result of a patient striking another individual's teeth with a clenched fist. Because of the force associated with the contact and the penetrating nature of the human incisor, these infections tend to occur on multiple planes, and infection spreads rapidly to adjacent compartments. Skin, extensor tendons, joint space, bone, and surrounding deep spaces often are involved because the inoculum of saliva may traverse all these structures.

The physical examination should document the extent of the infection. Hand x-rays are indicated because closed-fist injuries are often associated with fractures. Since most of these wounds are open, a Gram stain and culture with sensitivities should be obtained for both aerobic and anaerobic bacteria.

The most common organisms reflect the natural flora of the mouth and include *Streptococcus* species, *S. aureus*, anaerobes, *E. corrodens,* and *Neisseria* species.[5,8] Antibiotics should be initiated immediately (see Table 277-1). The wound should be cleansed, irrigated, and left open. The hand should be immobilized in the position of function and elevated. Disposition should be arranged in consultation with the hand surgeon.

PARONYCHIA

A paronychia is an infection of the lateral nail fold or paronychium (Greek: *para,* "beside" + Greek: *onyx,* "nail"). Occasionally this may extend to the cuticle or eponychium (Greek: *epi,* "upon" + *onyx*). These common conditions are usually caused by minor trauma such as nail biting, manicures, or hang nails. The infection starts as a small area of induration that may be erythematous and tender.[4]

Most paronychia contain both aerobic and anaerobic bacteria. *S. aureus* and *Streptococcus* species are the most common aerobic bacteria cultured from these abscesses.[7] Chronic peronychium may occur, particularly in patients who are immunocompromised. Atypical bacterial or fungal infections such as *C. albicans* have been identified in these cases.

If no fluctuance is identified, the paronychia may be treated with warm soaks, elevation, and antibiotics (see Table 277-1). Early intervention may prevent the need for surgical drainage. After suppuration has occurred, the infection will exhibit either fluctuance or identifiable pus that will necessitate drainage. Minor infections can be treated with elevation of the paronychium or epionychium with a flat probe or no. 11 blade (Fig. 277-4). This procedure sometimes can be performed without placing a digital block or providing analgesia.

More extensive infections that do not communicate directly with the nail fold may require incision directly into the area of greatest fluctuance. A digital block should be performed using lidocaine or bupivicaine prior to these more invasive procedures. Severe infections with pus beneath the nail require removal of a portion of the lateral or proximal nail to ensure adequate drainage.[9] Rarely, a free-floating nail will be encountered on a bed of pus, necessitating removal of the entire nail.

Following incision and drainage, the patient should be instructed to keep the hand elevated and immobilized. Warm soaks may be initiated to keep the wound open and clean. The patient should be scheduled for reevaluation in 24 to 48 h. If significant cellulitis is present, a short course of antibiotics should be prescribed.

FELON

A felon is a subcutaneous pyogenic infection of the pulp space of the distal finger or thumb. The septa of the finger pad produce multiple individual compartments and confine the infection under pressure. The patient presents with marked throbbing pain and a red, tense distal pulp space. Infection typically begins with minor trauma to the dermis overlying the finger pad. With time, the bacterial infection gradually spreads between septa forming multiple compartmentalized abscesses.

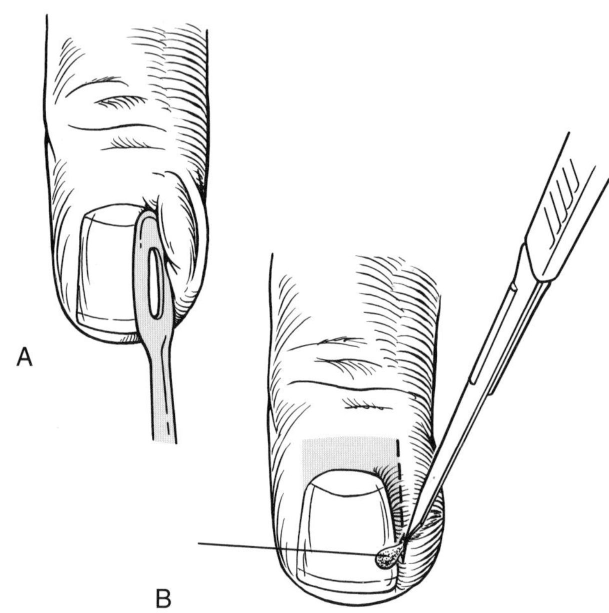

FIG. 277-4. Paronychia. **A.** The eponychial fold is elevated using a flat probe or no. 11 blade in order to allow the wound to drain. **B.** Alternately, a no. 11 blade may be used to incise the area of greatest fluctuation directly into the epionychium. The wound may then be gently probed with a small clamp to ensure drainage.

Left untreated, the infection may spread to the flexor tendon sheath and the interphalangeal joints, or eventually, osteomyelitis may develop.

S. aureus is the most common organism; however, *Streptococcus* species, anaerobes, and gram-negative organisms are encountered frequently. A Gram stain and culture should be obtained because these infections may be difficult to eradicate, and chronic infections may be caused by atypical organisms.[1,4] If osteomyelitis has developed, positive identification of the offending organism is necessary because long-term antibiotic therapy will be indicated.

If the finger pad is swollen and tense, or if there is any palpable fluctuance, drainage must be undertaken for healing to begin. A digital block must be performed because the procedure would be extremely painful without adequate anesthesia. A long-acting anesthetic such as bupivacaine should be used because postoperative discomfort is considerable. Most felons can be drained adequately with a limited incision and drainage procedure. A unilateral longitudinal approach is the most frequently used technique because it spares the sensate volar pad and achieves adequate drainage (see Fig. 277-5*A*).

A no. 11 blade is introduced lateral to the paronychium and is directed in a volar direction until pus is encountered. The incision should be extended to ensure adequate drainage, although it should not extend to the distal interphalangeal (DIP) flexor crease. Likewise, the incision should not carry through the distal end of the finger pad because this would likely cause instability and loss of sensation to the distal fingertip. A small clamp may be used to bluntly dissect septa to ensure complete drainage. If the wound is large enough, a small wick may be placed to encourage continued drainage.[9,10]

If the felon is pointing toward the volar fat pad, a longitudinal volar approach may be used, as depicted in Fig. 277-5*B*. Care should be exercised to avoid extending the incision to the flexor crease of the DIP joint. More extensive incisions such as the fishmouth, hockey stick, and through-and-through incisions are rarely, if ever, indicated. These incisions are routinely associated with loss of sensation to the fingertip and instability of the finger pad.[9,10]

Following drainage, the wound should be irrigated and then dressed with a dry, sterile dressing. The patient should be instructed to keep the extremity elevated, and the wound should be reevaluated in 24 to 48 h. Warm soaks may be initiated to keep the wound clean and promote continued drainage.

Most felons have significant associated cellulitis that should be treated with oral antibiotics.[12] A first-generation cephalosporin or antistaphylococcal penicillin should be prescribed for 7 to 10 days or until the infection has abated. Felons not responding to treatments outlined earlier should be referred to a hand specialist for more definitive management and long-term follow-up.

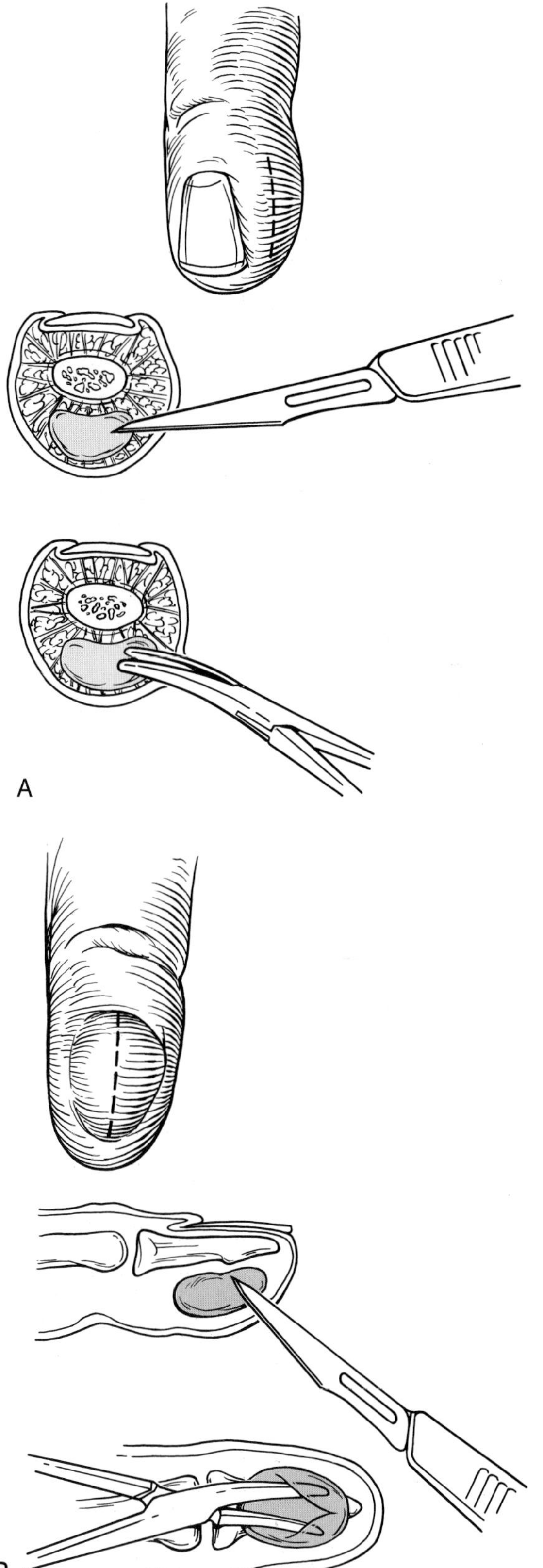

FIG. 277-5. Felon. **A.** The unilateral longitudinal approach is the most frequently used method for draining felons. This approach minimizes interference with sensate areas of the finger pad. **B.** If the felon is pointing on the volar surface of the finger pad, the longitudinal volar approach may be used.

HERPETIC WHITLOW

Herpetic whitlow is a viral infection of the distal finger caused by the herpes simplex virus. Infection typically occurs when the dermis has come in contact with oral herpetic infections. Herpetic whitlow in children tends to be associated with gingivostomatitis and herpes simplex type 1 (HSV-1), whereas adults most commonly harbor herpes simplex type 2 (HSV-2).[13] Health care professionals historically have been at risk for this infection, although the incidence appears to have diminished with the advent of latex gloves.

The patient will present with a burning, pruritic sensation similar to all herpes simplex infections. On examination, the lesion is erythematous and tender, with vesicular bullae being the hallmark of herpetic whitlow (Fig. 277-6). Although indurated, the infection is not tense, as is seen in a felon. It is important that a herpetic whitlow not be misidentified as a felon because incision and drainage may result in increased morbidity and prolonged failure to heal. If there is any question concerning the diagnosis of herpetic whitlow, a vesicle may be unroofed, and the drainage may be used for a Tzanck smear to confirm the diagnosis.

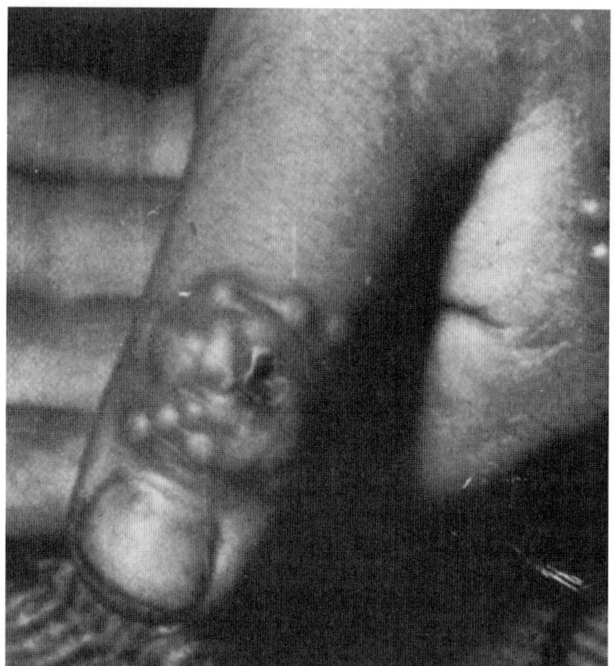

FIG. 277-6. Herpetic whitlow is shown. (From Domonkos AN: Clinical dermatology, in *Andrews' Diseases of the Skin*. Philadelphia: Saunders, 1971).

Treatment consists of immobilization, elevation, and pain medication. Antiviral agents such as acyclovir may shorten the course of duration and have been shown to prevent recurrent infections.[14,15] The patient must be instructed in the management of the infection, and the finger should be kept in a clean dressing to prevent autoinoculation or spread of the herpes infection to other individuals.

NONINFECTIOUS INFLAMMATORY STATES OF THE HAND

General Principles

Patients with noninfectious inflammatory states of the hand often present to the ED for diagnosis and relief of their symptoms. Most often the patient has experienced an acute exacerbation of the symptoms related to recent overuse, either in the workplace or at home. Chronic conditions are also frequently encountered in the ED when patients are unable to access a primary care provider or when their symptoms persist despite previous evaluations.

Inflammatory states of joints and tendons can be markedly painful, with classic signs of inflammation being present. It is critical that the emergency physician not mistake an acute bacterial infection for an inflammatory condition. In severe cases of inflammatory tendinitis or arthritis, the physical examination may be identical to that found in conditions caused by acute septic arthritis or suppurative tenosynovitis. If there is any question concerning the diagnosis, the patient must be managed aggressively for infection, and an appropriate hand specialist should be consulted.

If an inflammatory state is confidently diagnosed, the patient initially should be treated with conservative measures. These include rest, immobilization, elevation, and initiation of anti-inflammatory agents.

Tendinitis and Tenosynovitis

Inflammatory tendinitis may involve the flexor or extensor tendons of the hand. Most commonly the patient is able to relay a history of repetitive motion directly affecting the inflamed tendon. Palpation of the tendon produces tenderness. Active or passive movement of the tendon produces significant pain.

Treatment involves placing the patient in a splint in the position of function with instructions for rest and elevation of the affected area. Effective doses of anti-inflammatory agents should be prescribed on a scheduled basis. In patients with simple synovitis, injection of a depot steroid (such as 40 mg/mL triamcinolone mixed with 0.5% bupivacaine) into the synovial sheath is useful but should be done only when one is absolutely certain there is not infection. Accurate injection is important and may be challenging. One technique is to impale the tendon, as confirmed by distal motion on manipulation of the needle, and then to withdraw the needle while applying very gentle pressure to the plunger. When loss of resistance is felt, the needle is in the tendon sheath.

Patients should be referred to their primary care physician or a qualified hand surgeon for prompt follow-up. The patient also should be directed to return to the ED for worsening pain, increased swelling, or any signs of infection, including fever and erythema.

Trigger Finger

Tenosynovitis can develop in the flexor sheaths of the fingers and thumb. Scarring or inflammation may cause the tendon to become nodular which results in friction and catching between the tendon and its sheath, usually in the vicinity of the A1 pulley. This is referred to as *stenosing tenosynovitis*, or *trigger finger*. The patient experiences binding of the tendon, usually as the finger extends, relieved by a painful ''snap'' as the tendon clears the obstruction. Occasionally, this condition may progress to the point that the finger locks, usually in flexion. Early stages of trigger finger have been treated successfully with depot steroid injection into the tendon sheath, although there may be recurrence. Surgical division of the A1 pulley is usually curative.

DeQuervain's Stenosing Tenosynovitis

DeQueirvain's tenosynovitis is a common condition that occurs in patients who have experienced excessive use of the thumb. Often no good cause can be found. This is a tenosynovitis of the extensor pollicis brevis and abductor pollicis tendons, where they lie in the groove of the radial styloid.

The patient presents with pain along the radial aspect of the wrist that extends into the forearm. The definitive examination that confirms the diagnosis is Finkelstein's test (Fig. 277-7), in which the patient grasps the thumb in the palm of the hand and the examiner ulnar

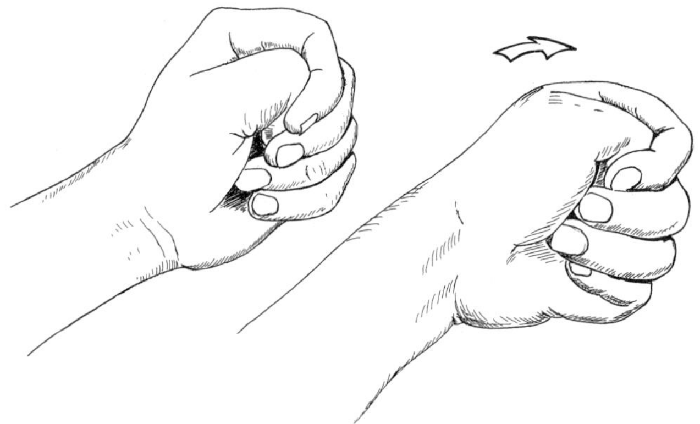

FIG. 277-7. The Finkelstein test is shown. The thumb is cupped in the closed fist and ulnar deviation reproduces pain along the extensor pollicis and abductor pollicis.

deviates the thumb and hand. This produces sharp pain along the involved tendons.

DeQuervain's tenosynovitis can be treated with injection into the tendon sheath of 1 mL of 0.5% bupivacaine mixed with 40 mg (1 mL) triamcinolone. This is accomplished by palpating the tendon with the thumb in hyperextension, and injecting 1 cm proximal to the tip of the radial styloid. Distention of the tendon sheath should be seen distal to the retinacular ligament. The tendon itself must not be injected, and care must be taken to avoid subcutaneous or intradermal injection of steroid because this may cause cutaneous thinning and depigmentation. A thumb spica splint should be applied to keep the thumb in a neutral position for 3 weeks. Instruct the patient to remove the splint briefly each day and perform range of motion exercises to prevent joint stiffness. Anti-inflammatory medication should be prescribed for 10 to 14 days. Recurrence of this condition is not uncommon, particularly when related to occupational stress. Persistent cases should be referred to a hand surgeon.

Carpal Tunnel Syndrome

Carpal tunnel syndrome is a peripheral mononeuropathy that involves entrapment of the median nerve in the carpal canal or tunnel, which is covered by the tense transverse carpal ligament. Whenever a condition causes swelling in the carpal tunnel, the median nerve is compressed, causing parasthesias that extend into the index and long fingers and the radial aspect of the ring finger and along the palmar aspect of the thumb.[16] The patient often complains of awakening at night with pain in the hand. In addition, patients often complain of numbness when driving a car or maintaining the hand in an extended position for a prolonged period of time.

Direct trauma to the wrist may exacerbate symptoms; however, a more common scenario involves overuse syndromes where the patient relays a history of repeated flexion and extension of the wrist that results in edema in the carpal tunnel. Other edematous conditions such as pregnancy and congestive heart failure may acutely exacerbate symptoms in patients with a predisposition for carpal tunnel syndrome.[17] It is also more common in diabetes and rheumatoid arthritis.[16]

Tinel's sign may support the diagnosis and involves tapping the volar aspect of the wrist over the median nerve. A positive sign produces paresthesias that extend into the index and long finger. Phalen's sign is more sensitive (50 percent) and specific (75 percent) and involves flexing the wrist maximally and holding it in this position for at least 1 min. The patient complains of tingling and numbness along the median nerve distribution. Both signs are subject to false-positive and false-negative results and electrodiagnostic techniques may be required to confirm the diagnosis.[18]

Initial treatment of carpal tunnel syndrome involves placing a volar splint to maintain the wrist in neutral position and giving the patient anti-inflammatory agents. Infiltration of the carpal tunnel with a mixture of 1 mL of 0.5% bupivacaine and 40 mg (1 mL) of triamcinolone may be beneficial, if the physician is experienced in the procedure. Unfortunately, this technique often provides only temporary relief. If this does not improve the condition, or if symptoms recur, surgical intervention is necessary to release the entrapment.

This condition may have a relapsing course, and permanent deficits of the median nerve occasionally are seen. Carpal tunnel syndrome should be diagnosed early, and the patient should be referred to a hand surgeon in a timely fashion.

Dupuytren's Contracture

Dupuytren's contracture is a poorly understood disorder resulting in fibroplastic changes of the subcutaneous tissues of the palm and volar aspect of the fingers. There appears to be a genetic component, and the condition is found most commonly in men of northern European descent.[19] This process eventually may lead to tethering and joint contracture. Firm longitudinal thickening and nodularity of the superficial tissues usually are readily appreciated. The diagnosis is made by identifying a nodule in the palm, usually at the distal palmar crease of the ring or small finger, which is held in the classic flexion contracture.[20] This condition should be referred to a skilled hand specialist because surgical excision of the fibrotic bands is usually palliative.

REFERENCES

1. Hausman MR, Lisser SP: Hand infections. *Orthop Clin North Am* 5:171, 1992.
2. Kour AK, Looi KP, Phone MH, et al: Hand infections in patients with diabetes. *Clin Orthop* 331:238, 1996.
3. Mann RJ, Peacock JM: Hand infections in patients with diabetes mellitus. *J Trauma* 17:376, 1977.
4. Moran GJ, Talan DA: Hand infections. *Emerg Med Clin North Am* 11:601, 1993.
5. Spiegel JD, Szabo RM: A protocol for the treatment of severe infections of the hand. *J Hand Surg* 13A(2):254, 1988.
6. Phipps AR, Blanshard J: A review of in-patient hand infections. *Arch Emerg Med* 9:299, 1992.
7. Brook I: Aerobic and anaerobic microbiology of paronychia. *Ann Emerg Med* 19(9):994, 1990.
8. Callaham M: Controversies in antibiotic choices for bite wounds. *Ann Emerg Med* 17(12):2321, 1988.
9. Green DP (ed): *Operative Hand Surg*, 3d ed. New York: Churchill-Livingstone, 1993.
10. Dahir K (ed): *The Hand: Primary Care of Common Problems*, 2d ed. New York: Churchill-Livingstone, 1990.
11. Zellweger G, Simmen HP, Meyer VE, et al: Infection in the upper body: Hand and burn-sound microbiology and considerations for antimicrobial therapy. *J Burn Care Rehabil* 13(2):298, 1992.
12. Mack GR: Superficial anatomy and cutaneous surgery of the hand. *Adv Dermatol* 7:315, 1992.
13. Gill MJ, Arlette J: Herpes simplex virus infection of the hand. *Am J Med* 84:89, 1988.
14. Laskin OL: Acyclovir and suppression of frequently recurring herpetic whitlow. *Ann Emerg Med* 102(4):494, 1985.
15. Hurst LC, Gluck R, Sampson SP, et al: Herpetic whitlow with bacerial abscess. *J Hand Surg* 16A(2):311, 1991.
16. Atroshi I, Gummesson MS, Johnsson R, et al: Prevalence of carpal tunnel syndrome in a general population. *JAMA* 282:153, 1999.
17. Hales TR, Bernard BP: Epidemiology of work-related musculoskeletal disorders. *Orthop Clin North Am* 27(4):679, 1996.
18. Kuhlman KA, Hennessey WJ: Sensitivity and specificity of carpal tunnel syndrome signs. *Am J Phys Med Rehabil* 76(6):451, 1997.
19. McFarlane R: Invitational lecture: American Society of Hand Therapists Nineteenth Annual Meeting, Dupuytren's disease. *J Hand Ther* 8:13, 1997.
20. Riolo J, Young L, Pidgeon L: Dupuytren's contracture. *South Med J* 84(8):983, 1991.

ACUTE DISORDERS OF THE JOINTS AND BURSAE

John H. Burton

EPIDEMIOLOGY

Acute disorders of the joints affect a collection of patients with diseases that span a vast spectrum of age, acuity, and etiologies. A young child with an acute septic arthropathy may reside at one end of this spectrum, whereas an elderly patient with an acute exacerbation of osteoarthritis may lie at the other, both patients unified by an acutely painful hip. Emergency physicians must differentiate conditions that require immediate attention from those that require less urgent therapy. A careful, methodical process utilizing certain unifying approaches within the clinical history, physical examination, laboratory evaluation, and ra-

TABLE 278-1 Examination of Synovial Fluid

	Normal	Noninflammatory	Inflammatory	Septic
Clarity	Transparent	Transparent	Cloudy	Cloudy
Color	Clear	Yellow	Yellow	Yellow
WBC/μL	<200	<200–2000	200–50,000	>50,000
PMNs (%)*	<25	<25	>50%	>50%
Culture	Negative	Negative	Negative	>50% positive
Crystals	None	None	Multiple or none	None
Associated conditions		Osteoarthritis, trauma, rheumatic fever	Gout, pseudogout, spondyloarthropathies, RA, Lyme disease, SLE	Nongonococcal or gonococcal septic arthritis

*The white blood cell count (WBC) and percent polymorphonuclear leucocytes (%PMNs) are affected by a number of factors, including disease progression, affecting organism, and host immune status. The joint aspirate WBC and %PMNs should be considered part of a continuum for each disease, particularly septic arthritis, and should be correlated with other clinical information. SLE, systemic lupus erythematosus; RA, rheumatoid arthritis.

diographic assessment will lead to appropriate diagnosis, treatment, and disposition.

CLINICAL FEATURES

Many pathways provoke acute joint complaints: degradation and degeneration of articular cartilage (osteoarthritis), deposition of immune complexes or immune-system-related phenomena (rheumatoid arthritis, rheumatic fever, and gonococcal arthritis), crystal-induced inflammation (gout and pseudogout), seronegative spondylarthropathies (ankylosing spondylitis and Reiter's syndrome), and bacterial invasion (septic or Lyme arthritis) or viral invasion (viral arthritis). These processes impact joint capsules and surfaces, resulting in a cascade of reactive and inflammatory events.

The most useful tool for evaluation of joint disorders is evaluation of synovial fluid. Table 278-1 lists the diagnostic characteristics of synovial fluid. However, joint aspiration may be difficult or impossible in smaller joints or those with minimal effusions. Identifying the distribution and number of affected joints is also necessary for diagnosis (Table 278-2). A migratory pattern of joint involvement may be helpful as well (Table 278-3).[1,2]

TABLE 278-2 Classification of Arthritis by Number of Affected Joints

Number of Joints	Differential Considerations
1 = Monoarthritis	Trauma-induced arthritis Infection/septic arthritis Crystal-induced (gout, pseudogout) Osteoarthritis (acute) Lyme disease Avascular necrosis Tumor
2–3 = Oligoarthritis	Lyme disease Reiter's syndrome Ankylosing spondylitis Gonococcal arthritis Rheumatic fever
>3 = Polyarthritis	Rheumatoid arthritis Systemic lupus erythematosus Viral arthritis Osteoarthritis (chronic)

Age and gender are also aids to diagnosis. Although no clinical pattern is diagnostic, certain general observations are helpful. Septic arthritis is important in infants and children,[3] with typical affecting organisms characteristic of age and development (Table 278-4). Additionally, a number of infectious and inflammatory processes are unique to childhood (Table 278-5).[3] In teen and adult years, sexual activity results in an increase in prevalence of gonococcal arthritis and Reiter syndrome associated with chlamydial urethritis.[4]

Crystal-induced arthritides commonly affect middle-aged adults. Gout is the commonest inflammatory joint disease in men over age 40.[5] The classic gout patient is a middle-aged man with an acute monoarthritis. Women, however, are generally spared the onset of gout until later middle age and can develop polyarticular involvement.[5]

As age progresses, the incidence of rheumatoid and osteoarthritis increases. Whereas osteoarthritis is a disease of older adults (over age 60), rheumatoid arthritis tends to strike earlier with a predilection for women three to four times that of men.[1] Additionally, rheumatoid arthritis classically demonstrates a progressive course with additive, polyarticular involvement of symmetric joints.[6]

DIAGNOSIS

Examination of Synovial Fluid

Joint fluid should routinely be analyzed for culture, Gram stain, leukocyte count with differential, and a wet preparation for crystals.[7] Glucose and lactate levels may be assessed as well. Cultures should include those for gonococci and anaerobes, when appropriate. Certain disease mechanisms are associated with classic joint aspirate findings (Table 278-1).

TABLE 278-3 Common Joint Disorders Displaying a Migratory Distribution Pattern

Gonococcal arthritis
Acute rheumatic fever
Lyme disease
Viral arthritis
Systemic lupus erythematosus

TABLE 278-4 Commonly Encountered Organisms in the Septic Arthritis Patient

Patient/ Condition	Expected Organisms	Antibiotic Considerations
Neonates and infants	Staphylococcus, gram-negative bacteria, group B Streptococcus, Candida	Nafcillin* plus aminoglycoside or third-generation cephalosporin, ampicillin-sulbactam
Children <5 years	Staphylococcus, *Haemophilus influenzae*	Nafcillin* plus cefuroxime, ampicillin-sulbactam
Older children and healthy adults	Staphylococcus, Gonococcus, Streptococcus	Nafcillin* plus third-generation cephalosporin, ampicillin-sulbactam
Involvement of the foot	Staphylococcus, Pseudomonas	Nafcillin* plus ceftazidime or aminoglycoside
Intravenous drug users	Staphylococcus, gram-negative bacilli	Nafcillin* plus aminoglycoside, ampicillin-sulbactam
Sickle-cell patients	Salmonella	Ciprofloxacin, ofloxacin, or ceftriaxone

*First-generation cephalosporin may be substituted for penicillinase-resistant penicillin. Vancomycin should be employed for treatment of suspected methicillin-resistant staphylococci.

Laboratory Tests

In the acute setting, few tests other than the joint aspirate contribute meaningfully to the diagnostic evaluation. Although the erythrocyte sedimentation rate (ESR) is frequently elevated in a number of acute inflammatory and reactive arthritides (septic, gonococcal, crystal-induced, spondyloarthropathies, and rheumatoid and Lyme arthritis),[8] the ESR is neither specific nor sufficiently sensitive for disease or as a marker for disease progression. The most promising and applicable levels of ESR sensitivity have been reported as 90 percent in children and young infants with septic arthritis.[2,9]

The white blood cell count (WBC) also has poor sensitivity and specificity. Notably, in pediatric septic arthritis, the total WBC is reported as 30 to 60 percent sensitive, with a left shift of the differential approaching 66 percent sensitivity.[2,9] Similar findings have been described in the adult population as well.[10]

Although routine (as in the case of WBC and ESR) in the consideration of a potentially infected joint, blood cultures have limited utility as well. Cultures should be drawn prior to antibiotic therapy. Blood cultures, in the setting of acute septic arthritis in adult and pediatric patients, have demonstrated sensitivities of 23 and 40 percent, respectively.[10,11]

Additional laboratory assessment may be required for follow-up, including rheumatoid factor, antinuclear antibodies, antineutrophil cytoplasmic antibodies, HLA-B27 tissue typing, lupus anticoagulant, and repeat synovial fluid analysis.[12]

TABLE 278-5 Differential Considerations for the Acutely Inflamed Pediatric Joint

Trauma
Septic arthritis
Rheumatic fever
Gonococcal arthritis
Lyme disease
Sickle-cell crisis
Henoch-Schönlein purpura
Calvé-Perthes disease
Slipped capital femoral epiphysis
Reactive/toxic synovitis
Osteomyelitis
Juvenile rheumatoid arthritis
Transient synovitis
Hemophilia

Radiology

Radiographs of an inflamed joint should be obtained when trauma, tumor, ankylosing spondylitis, avascular necrosis, or osteomyelitis are in the differential diagnosis. Radiographic evidence of osteomyelitis has been noted to follow infection by 7 to 14 days.[1,2] Radioisotope scanning is not usually required for emergency department diagnosis[3] but can be useful to detect osteomyelitis, occult fracture, avascular necrosis, or tumor.

ARTHROCENTESIS

Accurate diagnosis of articular problems often depends on aspiration and examination of synovial fluid from the affected joint(s) (Table 278-1).

Technique for Preparation of Selected Arthrocentesis Site

The skin overlying the affected joint should be free of cellulitis or impetigo in order to avoid contamination of the joint space during arthrocentesis. Other relative contraindications to joint aspiration are coagulopathy, hemarthrosis in hemophiliac patients, and the presence of a prosthetic joint. However, if the concern for septic arthritis is high, arthrocentesis may be performed in these settings after consultation.

The technique for preparation of any selected joint begins with overlying skin preparation and proper anesthesia. A large area overlying and adjacent to the affected joint is cleansed with povidone-iodine solution. After air drying, the skin is cleaned with an alcohol wipe to remove the povidone-iodine solution from the skin surface. This prevents the introduction of the povidone-iodine antiseptic into the joint, which can result in chemical irritation, or sterilization of the aspiration sample. Sterile drapes are then placed over the site.

Anesthesia is accomplished with infiltration of a local anesthetic by using a 25- to 30-gauge needle. Intraarticular injection of anesthetic should be avoided, because it can inhibit bacterial growth and may result in a spuriously negative culture in an early septic joint.[10]

A large-bore needle (18 or 19 gauge) should be used for aspiration of the joint. Smaller joints may require a smaller-bore needle to enter the joint space. The anticipated volume of fluid within the joint space should direct the selection of syringe size. As much synovial fluid should be removed as possible to optimize diagnosis and relieve pain from joint capsule distention. Aspirated fluid should promptly be sent for appropriate studies, including culture, Gram stain, leukocyte count with differential, and crystal analysis.

Shoulder

ANTERIOR APPROACH Insert the needle just lateral to the coracoid process. This technique is performed with the patient sitting in an

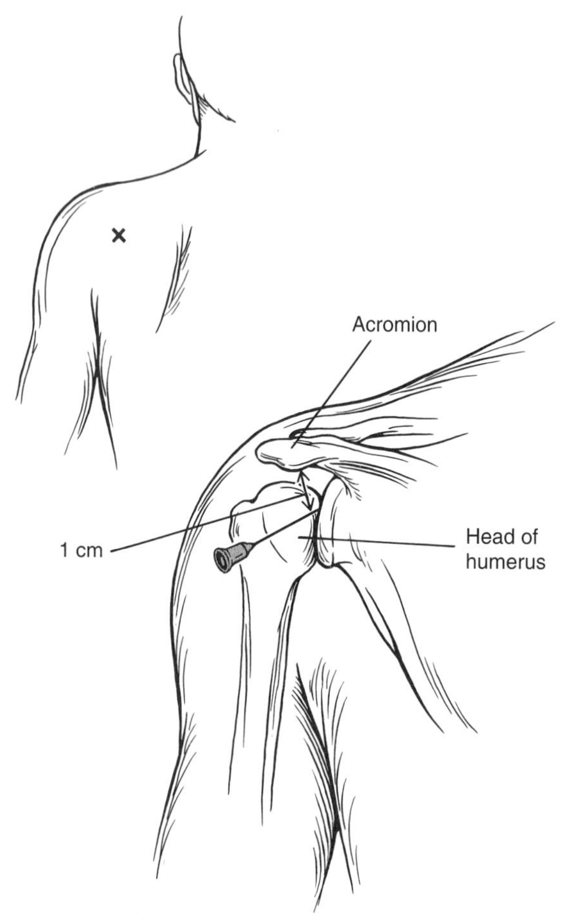

FIG. 278-1. Arthrocentesis of the shoulder, posterior approach.

upright position, facing the examiner. The needle is directed posteriorly between the coracoid process and the humeral head. Because of the difficulty in locating the coracoid process, a posterior approach to the glenohumeral joint may be preferable in some patients.

POSTERIOR APPROACH Sit the patient upright with his or her back toward you. The spine of the scapula is palpated to its lateral limit: the acromion. The posterolateral corner of the acromion is located. The point for needle insertion lies 1 cm inferior and 1 cm medial to the posterolateral corner of the acromion (Fig. 278-1). A $1\frac{1}{2}$-in needle is directed anterior and medial toward the presumed position of the coracoid process. The glenohumeral joint is located at a depth of approximately 1 to $1\frac{1}{2}$ in.

Elbow

A lateral approach to the elbow is used. Place the elbow in 90 degree flexion, resting on a table, with the hand prone. Locate the radial head, lateral epicondyle of the distal humerus, and the lateral aspect of the olecranon tip. These three landmarks form the anconeus triangle. The center of this triangle is the site for needle entry into the skin. The needle should be directed medial and perpendicular to the radius (Fig. 278-2).

Wrist

Landmarks for wrist arthrocentesis are palpable with the wrist in a neutral position. Noted landmarks are the radial tubercle of the distal radius, the anatomic snuff-box, the extensor pollicis longus tendon, and the common extensor tendon of the index finger (Fig. 278-3). The needle should be inserted perpendicular to the skin slightly ulnar to the radial tubercle and the anatomic snuff-box between the extensor pollicis longus and the common extensor tendons.

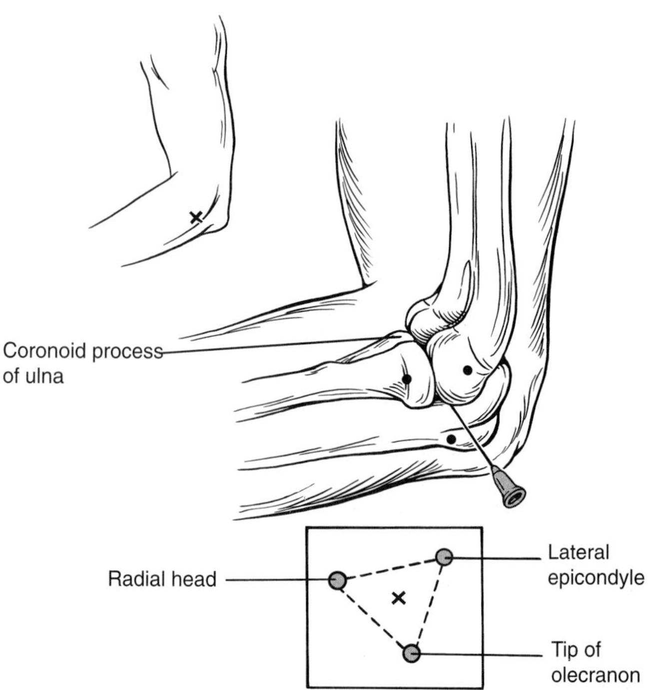

FIG. 278-2. Arthrocentesis of the elbow.

Hip

Hip arthrocentesis may be performed by either an anterior or a medial approach. Due to the belief that patients, particularly children, with a septic hip should undergo open surgical assessment and drainage, an orthopedic consultant performs this procedure.[3] Controversy exists regarding the utility of ultrasound, bone scan, or magnetic resonance

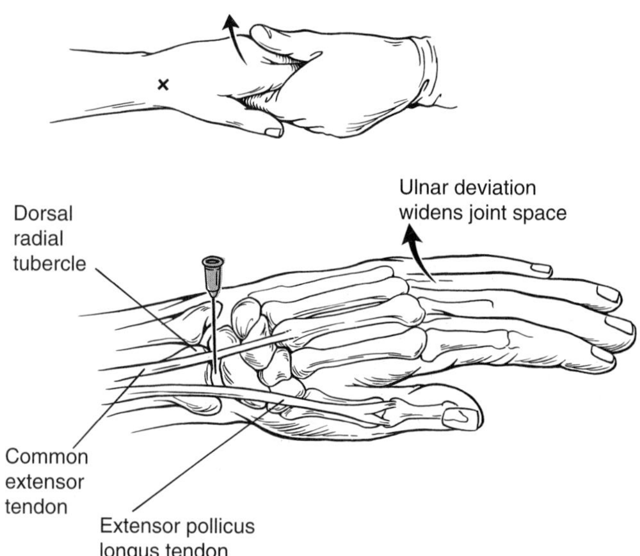

FIG. 278-3. Arthrocentesis of the wrist.

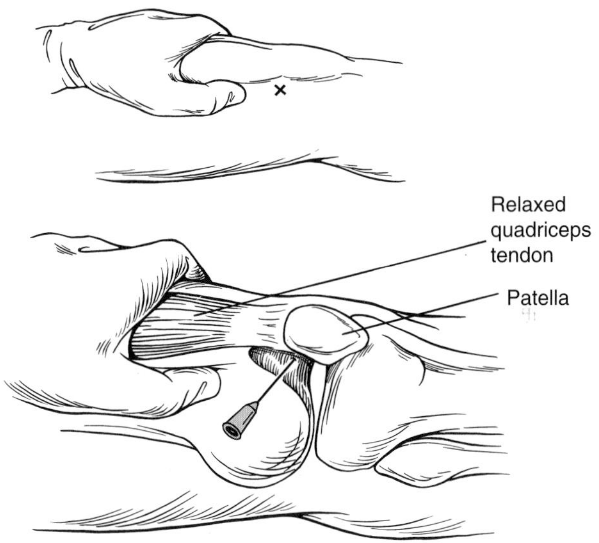

FIG. 278-4. Arthrocentesis of the knee, lateral approach.

imaging as a screening test prior to open surgical evaluation.[13,14] Immediate consultation with orthopedics is therefore desirable when a diagnosis of septic hip is considered.

Knee

The knee joint can be entered either medial or lateral to the patella. With the patient supine, the knee should be fully extended and the quadriceps muscle relaxed. The midpoint of the patella is identified. The insertion point of the needle is located approximately 1 cm inferior to the patellar edge, either lateral (Fig. 278-4) or medial (Fig. 278-5) to the middle of the patella. The needle should be directed posterior to the patella and horizontally toward the joint space. Compression applied over the joint space or ''milking'' of the bursae, on the patellar side opposite of the needle insertion site, may facilitate aspiration.

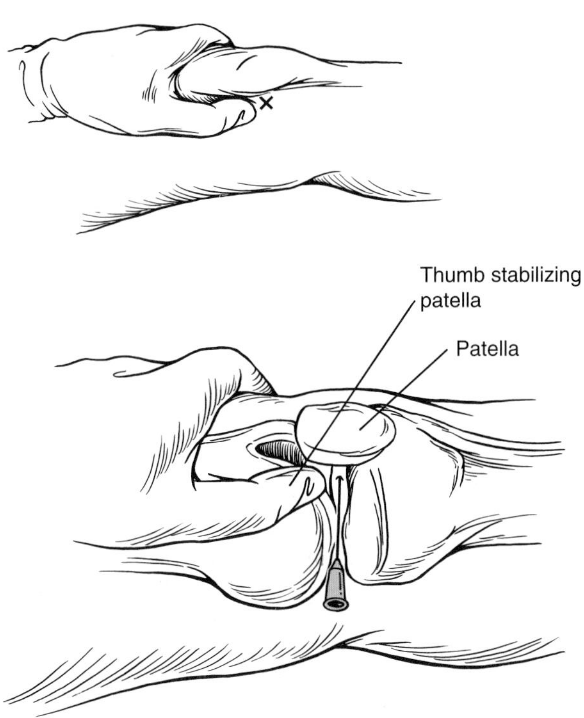

FIG. 278-5. Arthrocentesis of the knee, medial approach.

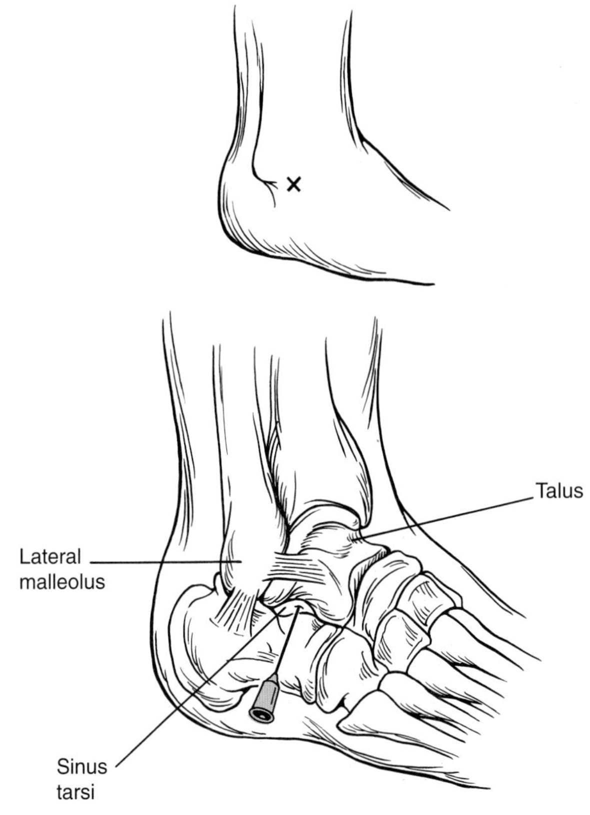

FIG. 278-6. Arthrocentesis of the ankle, lateral approach.

Ankle

Ankle arthrocentesis may be performed at either the subtalar joint (lateral approach) or the tibiotalar joint (medial approach). The subtalar joint is entered just below the tip of the lateral malleolus with the foot perpendicular to the leg (Fig. 278-6). The needle should be directed medially toward the joint space.

The tibiotalar joint is approached with the patient supine and the foot initially perpendicular to the leg. This position facilitates the location of a sulcus lateral to the medial malleolus and medial to the tibialis anterior and extensor hallucis longus tendons (Fig. 278-7). The foot is then plantar flexed with the needle entering the skin overlying the sulcus. The needle should be angled slightly cephalad as it passes between the medial malleolus and the tibialis anterior tendon.

SPECIFIC CONDITIONS

Traumatic Arthritis

Traumatic hemarthrosis has a high association with ligamentous injury or an intraarticular fracture. Effusions following trauma may range from small to large painful ones that impede range of motion. Aspiration of very large traumatic effusions will provide pain relief and increase range of motion. Treatment of traumatic hemarthrosis consists of immobilization, ice, and elevation of the affected joint. In the absence of a fracture or significantly unstable joint requiring immediate orthopedic evaluation, follow-up is needed for possible ligamentous and articular injuries.

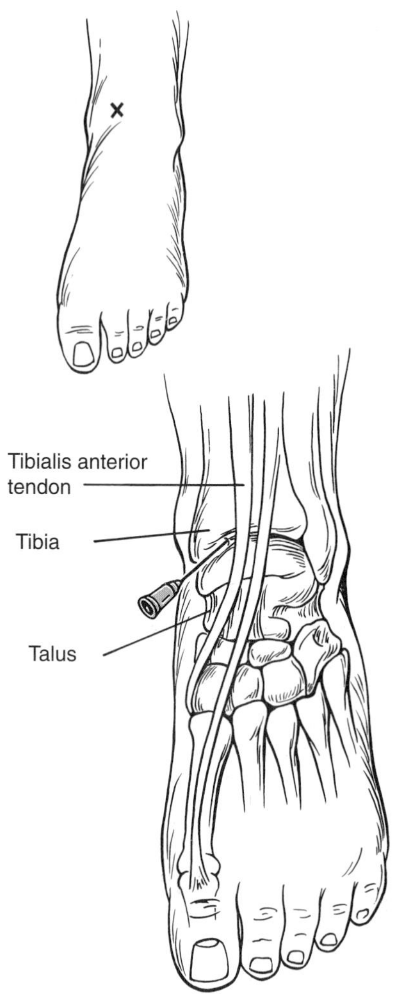

FIG. 278-7. Arthrocentesis of the ankle, medial approach.

Spontaneous hemarthrosis usually indicates underlying systemic illness and should trigger a search for primary or secondary coagulopathies. Hemophiliacs should receive specific clotting factor replacement (see Chap. 212), and their joints should generally not be aspirated. Follow-up should be provided with hematology and orthopedics.

Nongonococcal Septic Arthritis

Three mechanisms can lead to septic arthritis: (1) hematogenous spread of bacteria, (2) migration of bacteria from a focus contiguous to a joint, and (3) direct inoculation of bacteria into the joint.

Septic arthritis is a medical emergency. A rampant bacterial infection with a normal inflammatory response can destroy a joint within hours to days. The involved joint can become exquisitely painful over a few hours. On examination, effusions may be scant, with significant splinting and resistance to movement.

Although the classic bacterial arthritis patient is described as febrile with chills and rigors, a 10-year retrospective review of 43 adult patients noted presence of fever or rigors in only 40 and 21 percent of patients, respectively.[10] Thus, the absence of constitutional symptoms should not preclude a septic arthritis diagnosis. A suspicion for a bacterial infection should always guide clinical decision making when approaching patients with monoarthritis.

After joint aspiration, if septic arthritis cannot be excluded, the patient should be admitted for pain control and parenteral antibiotics until synovial culture results are available. Consultation with the orthopedics or infectious disease departments is desirable. Repeat closed needle aspiration, arthroscopy, or open surgical drainage may be required, depending on a number of factors, including consultant preference, patient age, affected joint, and likelihood of septic source.

Gonococcal Arthritis

Gonococcal arthritis is the most common cause of septic arthritis in adolescents and young adults.[3] Joint infection will typically have a prodromal phase where migratory arthritis and tenosynovitis predominate before pain and swelling settle on one or more septic joints. Vesiculopustular lesions, especially on the fingers, may be found.

Synovial fluid cultures are often negative in gonococcal arthritis, with only 25 to 50 percent of cases yielding positive identification of the organism. Cultures of the posterior pharynx, urethra, cervix, and rectum, prior to antibiotic treatment, may increase the culture yield.[3]

Treatment for gonococcal arthritis follows the same principles as treatment for nongonococcal septic arthritis. *Neisseria gonorrhoeae,* in the setting of arthritis, remains sensitive to penicillin, and extended antibiotic coverage is typically not required following identification of the organism.

Crystal-Induced Synovitis (Gout and Pseudogout)

Crystal-induced synovitis is primarily an illness of middle-aged and elderly adults. Uric acid (gout) and calcium pyrophosphate (pseudogout) are the two most common crystalline agents, with gout representing the most common form of inflammatory joint disease in men older than age 40.[5] Patients typically present with joint pain that acutely evolves over hours, as in acute gout attack, or over a single day, as in pseudogout. An acute gout or pseudogout attack often follows trauma, surgery, a significant illness, or change in medications that results in an abrupt change in uric acid levels. Crystalline involvement of joints has a predilection for the lower extremities. Although the first metatarsophalangeal joint is a classic focus for acute gout, no joint is the exclusive site of involvement for either crystal.

The diagnosis of a crystal-induced synovitis is by joint aspiration and identification of crystals through a polarizing microscope. Uric acid crystals appear needle shaped and blue when the source of light is perpendicular to the crystal. Calcium pyrophosphate is yellow in this alignment, with a rhomboid shape. Crystals should be located within phagocytes from aspirates of synovial fluid or inflamed tissues adjacent to the affected joint.

Serum uric acid levels have limited utility in diagnosis, as up to 30 percent of patients will have normal uric acid levels during an acute attack.[5] The joint aspirate WBC is often high with gout, approaching 100,000/mm^3 in some cases.[5] However, the presence of crystals, absence of findings on Gram stain/culture and, frequently, the dramatic response to nonsteroidal anti-inflammatory drugs (NSAIDs) will clarify the diagnosis. When the diagnosis of a septic joint cannot be excluded, hospital admission until cultures and/or clinical response clarify the diagnosis is the safest course of action.

When the diagnosis of gout or pseudogout is established, a NSAID, such as indomethacin, is standard first-line therapy. All NSAID dosing should be adjusted for renal function and continue for approximately 1 week. For patients with normal renal function, the initial dose of indomethacin is 50 mg. Therapy is continued three times a day for 3 to 5 days. Substantial pain relief typically occurs within 2 h of NSAID administration.[15] Additional treatment for pseudogout is typically not required.

Colchicine, although uncommonly necessary, may also be employed as an alternative in the treatment of acute gout. Oral colchicine is typically administered at a dose of 0.6 mg/h until intolerable side effects (vomiting or diarrhea) or efficacy ensue. Intravenous administration of colchicine, particularly at toxic levels, can be associated with serious side effects, with risks such as bone marrow suppression, neuropathy, myopathy, and death. Consequently, intravenous colchicine is rarely used.

Patient disposition is determined by consideration of effective analgesia and the inclusion or elimination of septic arthritis as a diagnosis in the patient evaluation. Once the symptoms of an acute crystal-induced synovitis episode have resolved, long-term control may be achieved with reduction or elimination of gout-inducing agents (diuretics, aspirin, or cyclosporine) and treatment with prophylactic drugs, such as allopurinol or probenecid.

Lyme Disease

The arthritic manifestations associated with Lyme disease occur in the weeks, months, or years following the primary, stage I infection. Typically, a monoarticular or oligoarticular, asymmetric involvement of joints is noted, with brief exacerbations followed by complete remission. Large joints are most often affected. A migratory pattern of oligoarthritis may be noted, in addition to brief attacks of bursitis and tendonitis.

Arthrocentesis yields an inflammatory synovial fluid with cultures uncommonly positive. The diagnosis of Lyme arthritis is initially suspected in patients residing in, or with a recent visit to, an endemic area. A history of tick bite or erythema chronicum migrans (ECM) rash is helpful but often absent. In patients with no history of rash, tick bite, or endemic location, a constellation of characteristic stage II and stage III findings—such as fatigue, neurologic abnormalities, and/or cardiac conduction disturbances—may be helpful in establishing the diagnosis. Ultimately, definitive diagnosis requires the history or presence of the ECM rash, multiorgan system involvement, or laboratory confirmation through enzyme-linked immunosorbent assay, immunofluorescent antibody titer, or isolation of the *Borrelia burgdorferi* spirochete from a clinical specimen.

Given the difficulty of making a definitive diagnosis in many patients, treatment of suspected Lyme arthritis is often initiated on the grounds of high clinical suspicion. Treatment is administered for 3 to 4 weeks with a number of antibiotics recognized as effective, including doxycycline, penicillin G, amoxicillin, or ceftriaxone. Intravenous antibiotic therapy is reserved for those patients with more severe presentations.

Rheumatoid Arthritis

Rheumatoid arthritis is distinguished by its symmetric, polyarticular involvement, with noted sparing of the distal interphalangeal (DIP) joints. Patients will describe stiffness of the joints occurring after prolonged periods of inactivity (morning stiffness). Multisystem involvement is characteristic, and depression, fatigue, and generalized myalgias are also common. Extraarticular symptoms and signs include pericarditis, myocarditis, pleural effusion, pneumonitis, and mononeuritis multiplex syndrome.

Articular involvement is noted for symmetric, painful, tender joints. A "boggy," slightly edematous synovium may be palpated. Sparing of the DIP joints is the rule, with an additive involvement of affected joints during the course of the illness. Arthrocentesis of synovial fluid is typically noted for an inflammatory profile.

Treatment during an acute exacerbation is directed at reducing pain and inflammation. Salicylates or other NSAIDs are the cornerstone of treatment, with immobilization providing added relief from joint movement pain. Corticosteroids may be utilized for brief periods with long-term therapy using agents such as antimalarials, gold, and methotrexate.

Osteoarthritis

Osteoarthritis is distinguished from rheumatoid arthritis by a lack of constitutional symptoms and/or multisystem involvement. Destruction of joints in osteoarthritis may involve the DIP joints, with less dramatic symmetric, polyarticular exacerbations. Although osteoarthritis is a chronic, polyarticular disease, patients may present with an acute monoarthritis exacerbation, typically of the knee. Effusions are small and difficult to aspirate. When analyzed, however, synovial fluid is noted to be noninflammatory.

Radiographs contribute to the diagnosis of osteoarthritis, demonstrating characteristic joint space narrowing due to destruction of articular cartilage. Treatment, as in rheumatoid arthritis, involves rest of affected joints and the use of salicylates or NSAIDs. Because of the noninflammatory and destructive nature of osteoarthritis, corticosteroids are not used in the disease. Disease progression often necessitates total joint replacement.

Reiter's Syndrome

Reiter's syndrome, or reactive arthritis, is a seronegative spondyloarthropathy characterized by an acute, asymmetric oligoarthritis preceded 2 to 6 weeks by an infectious illness. The classic triad of Reiter's syndrome is arthritis, urethritis, and conjunctivitis. A history of all three components is not necessary for diagnosis. *Chlamydia* or ureaplasma are common inciting infectious agents, particularly with regard to a precipitating urethritis. Diarrhea has also become recognized as an entity that may precipitate a reactive arthritis. A history of recent diarrhea or enteric infection while traveling abroad may suggest a recent *Salmonella* or *Shigella* infection as an inciting factor for the disease.[4]

Joint involvement is typically found in the lower extremities, particularly the heels of the feet. A diffuse swelling of an entire digit (sausage digit) may be found as well but is not specific to Reiter's syndrome alone.[1] Synovial fluid aspirates demonstrate an inflammatory profile. Treatment is supportive with emphasis on pain control and NSAID therapy. Antibiotics have not been found to contribute to treatment of Reiter's syndrome patients.

Ankylosing Spondylitis

Another of the seronegative spondyloarthropathies—ankylosing spondylitis—demonstrates an arthritic predilection for the spine and pelvis. Ankylosing spondylitis is similar to rheumatoid arthritis in its association with morning stiffness and multisystem involvement with constitutional symptoms such as malaise, weakness, and fatigue. However, ankylosing spondylitis is clearly differentiated in its association with hereditary factors, particularly the HLA-B27 antigen and negative rheumatoid factor.

Ankylosing spondylitis is suspected in individuals younger than age 40 who note insidious onset of symptoms that improve with exercise, are associated with morning stiffness, and last longer than 3 months.[16] Radiographic findings, in addition to genetic predisposition, are helpful in the diagnosis of ankylosing spondylitis. Squaring of the vertebral bodies (bamboo spine) and sacroiliitis are some of the more classic findings. Treatment consists of pain control with short-term and long-term management with NSAIDs.

BURSITIS

The term *bursitis* refers to any acute or chronic inflammatory process involving one of the more than 150 bursae identified throughout the human body.[17] Bursitis is classified by etiology, body location, and presence of infection. Etiologic entities include trauma, crystal-induced, rheumatoid, and idiopathic forms. Presence of infection is noted by classification as septic or nonseptic. *Staphylococcus aureus* accounts for the majority of identified infectious agents, but *Staphylococcus epidermis* and *Streptococcus* species are also encountered.

Bursitis is a relatively common condition, due to the number of bursae and the minimal trauma required to initiate a clinically evident process. The affected site is determined by the activity precipitating the event and/or the relatively superficial location of many bursae. Certain entities are frequently associated with occupations or activities that precipitate their occurrence: "carpet layer's knee" (prepatellar bursitis) or "student's elbow" (olecranon bursitis).

General principles of management include restraint from further trauma/injury, elevation, and a compressive dressing. Drug therapy with NSAIDs is the primary pharmacotherapeutic intervention. Injection of the affected bursa with steroids is controversial and should be avoided when septic bursitis cannot be excluded. Specifically, olecranon and prepatellar bursitis are not uncommonly complicated by infection.

Septic bursitis generally responds well to oral antibiotics, with emphasis on coverage of *Staphylococcus* and *Streptococcus* species. Selected patients will require more aggressive interventions, including admission to hospital, administration of parenteral antibiotics, incision and debridement, and open irrigation. These patients typically have more advanced, purulent infection within the bursa, extensive spread of infection/cellulitis to surrounding soft tissues, suspected joint involvement, or failure to respond to oral antibiotics and outpatient interventions.

Specific Conditions

OLECRANON BURSITIS The olecranon bursa overlies the olecranon process on the extensor surface of the elbow. Patients with olecranon bursitis present with a tense, edematous bursa that is often tender to palpation. Pain elicited with range of motion at the elbow is minor until the motion tightens and compresses the distended overlying bursa. The bursa is frequently erythematous and warm.

Distinguishing nonseptic bursitis from the septic and crystal-induced forms is a clinical challenge. Patients with crystal-induced bursitis will often demonstrate gouty tophi overlying the elbow extensor surface. Presence of crystals in bursal fluid analysis is diagnostic.

Septic bursitis and nonseptic bursitis are difficult to distinguish. No definitive conclusion can be reached solely on the basis of physical exam findings or history, although one report has noted the utility of a comparison of surface temperature of the affected bursa with the unaffected side.[17] These authors reported a temperature difference exceeding 2.1°C to be highly predictive of a septic bursal fluid aspirate.

Most authors advocate the importance of aspirating bursal fluid,[17–20] which is performed both for diagnostic and therapeutic purposes. Bursal fluid, like joint aspirates, demonstrates characteristic findings (Table 278-6). The utility of any one finding is limited, however, and the culture represents the definitive test for presence or absence of infection.

Aspiration of olecranon bursitis fluid is undertaken by means of a lateral approach to the affected bursa. As in joint aspirates, a sterile technique should be utilized, with evacuation of as large amount of fluid as possible.

Management of patients with olecranon bursitis follows the aforementioned general bursitis management principles. When a septic bursitis is definitively excluded, a steroid injected into the bursa may expedite resolution of inflammation.[20] However, a septic process usually cannot be excluded during the initial evaluation of an acute olecranon bursitis. As a consequence, utilization of steroid injection should be approached with caution.

Antibiotic treatment is usually effective with a 14-day course of oral antibiotic therapy.[17,19] Selected patients who may require parenteral therapy or operative management are generally distinguished by their toxic appearance, systemic signs of infection, extensive cellulitis to surrounding tissues, failure of outpatient interventions, or immunocompromised host status.

PREPATELLAR BURSITIS Prepatellar bursitis may affect any of the four bursae surrounding the extensor aspect of the knee. As in other bursitis conditions, a history of overuse or trauma to the prepatellar area is often elicited. Clinical findings are consistent with those of olecranon bursitis.

Aspiration of prepatellar bursal fluid should be approached by either a medial or lateral approach to the affected bursa. The incidence of prepatellar septic bursitis is much less than that of olecranon bursitis (approximately 75 percent less).[17] Treatment emphasizes conservative management and occasionally requires antibiotic therapy or admission following the same approach as already outlined for patients with septic olecranon bursitis.

TABLE 278-6 Characteristics of Bursal Fluid in Patients with Septic and Nonseptic Olecranon and Prepatellar Bursitis

	Septic	Traumatic and Idiopathic	Crystal Induced
Appearance	Purulent; may be straw colored or serosanguineous	Straw colored, serosanguineous, or bloody	Straw colored to bloody
Leukocytes/μL	1500–300,000; mean 75,000	50–11,000; mean 1100	1000–6000; mean 2900
Differential count	Predominantly PMNs	Predominantly mononuclear	Highly variable
Ratio bursal fluid to serum glucose	<50%	>50%	Unknown
Gram stain	Positive in 70%	Negative	Negative
Crystals present	No	No	Yes
Culture results	Positive	Negative	Negative

Source: From McAfee and Smith,[17] with permission.

REFERENCES

1. Barth WF: Office evaluation of the patient with musculoskeletal complaints. *Am J Med* 102(suppl 1A):3S, 1997.
2. Schemata HR: Arthritis of recent onset. *Postgrad Med* 97:52, 1995.
3. Shaw BA, Kasser JR: Acute septic arthritis in infancy and childhood. *Clin Orthop* 257:212, 1990.
4. Pinals RS: Polyarthritis and fever. *N Engl J Med* 330:769, 1994.
5. Joseph J, McGrath H: Gout or "pseudogout": How to differentiate crystal-induced arthropathies. *Geriatrics* 50:33, 1995.
6. Harris ED Jr: Rheumatoid arthritis. Pathophysiology and implications for therapy. *N Engl J Med* 322:1277, 1990.
7. Schmerling RH, Delbanco TL, Tosteson ANA, Trentham DE: Synovial fluid tests: What should be ordered? *JAMA* 264:1009, 1990.
8. Malleson PN: Management of childhood arthritis: Part 1. Acute arthritis. *Arch Dis Child* 76:460, 1997.
9. Del Beccaro MA, Champoux AN, Bockers T, Mendelman PM: Septic arthritis versus transient synovitis of the hip: The value of screening laboratory tests. *Ann Emerg Med* 21:1418, 1992.
10. Schlapbach P: Bacterial arthritis: Are fever, rigors, leucocytosis and blood cultures of diagnostic value? *Clin Rheumatol* 9:69, 1990.
11. Wilson NIL, DiPaola M: Acute septic arthritis in infancy and childhood. *J Bone Joint Surg [Br]* 68:584, 1986.
12. Callegari PE, Williams WV: Laboratory tests for rheumatic diseases: When are they useful? *Postgrad Med* 97:65, 1995.
13. Fink AM, Berman L, Edwards D, Jacobson SK: Immediate ultrasound guided aspiration and prevention of hospital admission. *Arch Dis Child* 72:110, 1995.
14. Alexander JE, Seibert JJ, Aronson J, et al: A protocol of plain radiographs, hip ultrasound, and triple phase bone scans in the evaluation of the painful pediatric hip. *Clin Pediatr (Phila)* 27:175,1988.

15. Shrestha M, Morgan DL, Moreden JM, et al: Randomized double-blind comparison of the analgesic efficacy of intramuscular ketorolac and oral indomethacin in the treatment of acute gouty arthritis. *Ann Emerg Med* 26:682, 1995.
16. Calin A: Seronegative spondyloarthritides. *Med Clin North Am* 70:323, 1986.
17. McAfee JH, Smith DL: Olecranon and prepatellar bursitis: Diagnosis and treatment. *West J Med* 149:607, 1988.
18. Smith DL, McAfee JH, Lucas LM, et al: Septic and nonseptic olecranon bursitis: Utility of the surface temperature probe in the early differentiation of septic and nonseptic cases. *Arch Intern Med* 149:1581, 1989.
19. Ho G, Tice AD, Kaplan SR: Septic bursitis in the prepatellar and olecranon bursae: An analysis of 25 cases. *Ann Intern Med* 89:21, 1978.
20. Smith DL, McAfee JH, Lucas LM, et al: Treatment of nonseptic olecranon bursitis: A controlled, blinded prospective trial. *Arch Intern Med* 149:2527, 1989.

SOFT TISSUE PROBLEMS OF THE FOOT

Frantz R. Melio

In 1990 the National Center for Health Statistics conducted a National Health Interview Survey that included a list of the three most common podiatric problems: bunions, corns and calluses, and ingrown toenails. In response, 13.2 out of 1000 people reported being afflicted by bunions, 24.5 per 1000 with ingrown toenails, and 20 per 1000 with corns or calluses. Advanced age, poverty, and female gender were associated with increased risk for these diseases. It is thus apparent that chronic foot problems play an important role in U.S. health care.[1] Patients with chronic or complicated foot problems generally should be referred to a dermatolgist, orthopedist, general surgeon, or podiatrist, depending on disease and local resources.

CORNS AND CALLUSES

Pressure or irritation causes focal hyperkeratotic lesions of the skin of the foot. The cause of these lesions can be external (poorly fitted shoe) or internal (bunion). These areas of epidermal accumulation are defined as *calluses.* Calluses serve a protective function and should not be treated if they are not painful. Calluses grow outward but are soon pushed inward by continued pressure and become corns. Corns also develop in areas of scarring and between toes. Corns are classified as hard or soft. Hard corns are seen over bony protuberances where the skin is dry. Soft corns are seen between toes where the skin is moist. Corns may be painful or painless, but pressure on the corn usually produces pain. Corns interrupt the normal dermal lines and can thus be differentiated from calluses. Hard corns may resemble warts; however, when pared, warts bleed and corns do not. Soft corns resemble tinea, which often leads to misdiagnosis and mistreatment.[2–4]

Treatment of symptomatic lesions consists of paring with a no. 15 blade scalpel and application of a pad on or around the lesion to relieve pressure. Avoiding constrictive footwear is also important. Keratolytic agents are advocated by some authors but are thought to be too toxic and better avoided by others. Patients should be referred to a podiatrist, since therapy includes repeated paring and possibly surgery to correct any underlying source of pressure.[2–4]

Keratotic lesions may be an indication of more severe underlying disease, deformity, local foot disorder, or mechanical problem. Other causes of keratotic lesions include syphilis, psoriasis, arsenic poisoning, rosacea, lichen planus, basal cell nevus syndrome, and, rarely, malignancies.[3]

PLANTAR WARTS

Plantar warts are caused by the human papillomavirus. These warts are fairly common and contagious. They may be painful and are usually found over bony prominences. Single lesions are endophytic and hyperkeratotic. A mother-daughter wart is similar to a single lesion except for a small vesicular satellite lesion. Mosaic warts are often painless, closely grouped, and may coalesce. Diagnosis is usually made clinically. There are many therapeutic options. Treatment is complicated by the fact that many of these lesions will resorb spontaneously within 2 years. These patients may require prolonged treatment in resistant cases and should be referred.[3,5]

TINEA PEDIS

The incidence of tinea pedis in industrialized countries has been estimated at 10 percent of the population. It has been estimated that in high-risk patients as many as 70 percent are affected. In the United States, $240 million per year is spent on products used to treat tinea pedis. Factors that predispose to infection include hot and humid climate, occlusive footwear, infrequent changes of socks or shoes, hyperhidrosis of the feet, conditions that lead to maceration of the feet, and repeated exposure of the feet to fungi combined with some form of minimal trauma. In high-risk groups, such as the elderly and immunocompromised patients, infections can become chronic and resistant to treatment and can disseminate. Tinea pedis can usually be prevented with proper hygiene. These measures include daily bathing and drying of feet, wearing absorbent socks and changing them daily, wearing shoes that "breathe" and changing them daily, wearing different footwear for sporting activities, and using drying agents and antifungals for prophylaxis in high-risk groups.[6]

The causative fungal organisms of tinea pedis usually belong to the dermatophytes, with *Trichophyton rubrum* being the most frequently responsible, accounting for approximately 60 percent of cases. The *Microsporum* species, *Candida,* and saprophytic fungi also account for many occurrences.[6]

Clinically, tinea pedis appears in a variety of forms, ranging from mild scaling to acute inflammation. The most common form is interdigital infection. Interdigital presentation may be as benign as a fissure in the toe web, usually between the fourth and fifth toes. More commonly, the affected interspaces appear white, macerated, and soggy as a result of multiple simultaneous infections (dermatophyte and bacteria). These complex infections usually begin with dermatophyte infection of the toe web. The fungi produce antibiotics that select for an antibiotic-resistant bacterial population (both gram-positive and gram-negative). These bacteria induce further inflammation and damage to the epithelium. The bacteria also produce anifungal by-products and quickly predominate. It has now been recognized that these bacteria alone are also etiologic agents of tinea pedis. The more severe the infection, the more likely that other organisms such as yeast and saprophytic fungi are also involved. These lesions are pruritic and may become painful when the patient wears a closed shoe or exercises.[6,7]

A second form of tinea pedis is the hyperkeratotic or moccasin-type infection. This is a chronic form of tinea that is characterized by scaly eruptions, fissuring, pruritus, erythema, and the absence of vesicles and pustules. It is usually limited to the weight-bearing surfaces of the feet and spares the intertriginous areas. *T. rubrum* is the most frequent causative organism.[6,7]

The vesicular form is another common presentation of tinea pedis. This infection is characterized by vesicles and vesicopustules and is most commonly caused by *T. mentagrophytes, Epidermophyton floccosum,* and rarely, *Microsporum.* The lesions usually begin on the non-weight-bearing areas of the soles and can extend along the entire plantar surface, to the intertriginous areas, up over the toes, and onto the dorsum of the foot. Patients experience a burning pain and pruritus. An ulcerative form of tinea may be the result of secondary pyogenic bacterial infection involving these vesicles.[6,7]

Tinea infections must be differentiated from other lesions that affect the foot. Juvenile plantar dermatosis is a lesion frequently confused with tinea. Affected children have dry, cracked, red scaly patches on the toe pads and anterior plantar surface of the feet; the toe webs and insteps are spared. Treatment consists of lubricants and occlusion, with socks at night. Contact dermatitis is characterized by involvement of the dorsal surface of the feet, with well-demarcated, red patches that may contain tiny vesicles. Psoriasis presents as thick scaly lesions that spare the web spaces and affect the heel. Erythrasma is a low-grade chronic infection that may involve the web spaces. Symmetric patches are also present in the groin and axillae. These lesions fluoresce bright "coral red" under Wood's lamp examination. Pitted keratolysis is a diphtheroid bacterial infection which produces marked hyperkeratosis with multiple 1- to 3-mm punched-out pits on the plantar surface of the foot. Id reactions, which are immunologic reactions to antigenic products of fungal infections, may present as sterile vesicles.[3,6,7]

Diagnosis of tinea pedis is made clinically. Fungal cultures, due to bacterial overgrowth and fungal suppression, are usually very low yield.[6]

Due to the complexity of these infections, the ideal medication must be antifungal, antibacterial, and have local drying as well as anti-inflammatory properties. The imidazole group of antifungals (miconazole, clotrimazole, econazole, ketoconazole, oxiconazole, sulconazole and thoconazole) meet all these criteria and are also effective against *Candida.* Remember to avoid simultaneous treatment with erythromycins. These agents are an excellent choice for initial, empiric treatment of tinea pedis. Some of these medications are available in over-the-counter preparations. These topical antifungals generally should be applied for 2 to 3 weeks. Topical terbinafine and butenafine, applied for 1 to 2 weeks, may be used as an alternative.[8]

Creams and solutions are most often appropriate when treating tinea. Ointments hold the active ingredient at the site longer but should not be used on oozing or moist lesions. Sprays may also be helpful; they evaporate quickly, leaving the medication on the surface for absorption.[6]

Oral therapy with itraconazole, fluconazole, or terbinafine has recently been advocated. These medications are generally well tolerated, have been shown to be as effective as topical therapy, and require only a one week duration of treatment.[9,10]

The role of topical glucocorticoids is controversial. While the anti-inflammatory properties are advocated, the inhibition of cellular defenses may prolong the duration of infection. More important, the low level of anti-inflammatory action that the imidazoles possess is usually sufficient.[6]

Other aspects of therapy include proper hygiene such as daily foot cleaning, drying, and changes in socks and footwear. Application of drying agents such as aluminum chloride (Drysol) or aluminum acetate (Burow's solution and Domeboro) may assist in preventing hyperhidrosis and help control infection. Tight occlusive shoes should be avoided, and soft absorbent socks should be worn. High-risk patients should be told not to walk barefoot.[3,6,7]

Most patients respond to the measures outlined above. However, some infections are resistant to conservative therapy and require prolonged oral antifungal medication. These patients would benefit from appropriate referral.[3,6,7]

ONYCHOMYCOSIS

Dermatophyte fungi are the most frequent cause of nail plate invasion, with *T. rubrum* being the most common organism. Other organisms that can lead to nail infection include *Scopulariopsis brevicaulis, Scytalidium* species, *Aspergillus* species, *Acremonium* species, and *Candida.* The elderly, patients with psoriasis, diabetics, and immunocompromised individuals are more prone to developing onychomycosis.[11–14] Nail infections usually spread from surrounding infected skin. The infection can be either under or within the nail plate. If allowed to progress, these infections lead to severe disturbances in nail growth. The affected toenails appear opaque, discolored, and, at times, hyperkeratotic. Treatment of this disease process is complicated by the fact that topical antifungals are poorly absorbed through the nail. Newer oral antifungals (itraconazole, terbinafine, and fluconazole) have become the preferred first-line agents used in the treatment of onychomycosis. Continuous (daily for 12 weeks) and pulse (daily therapy for 1 week a month for 3 to 4 months) therapies have been studied. Pulse therapy appears to be as effective and have fewer side effects than continuous therapy. Oral terbinafine appears to be the most cost-effective of these agents.[11,15–19]

Surgical or chemical debridement of the nail matrix may play a role as adjunctive therapy to the preceding oral antifungals. Patients should be referred to a podiatrist or other appropriate practitioner for continued care because these lesions often require prolonged care. Even with optimal treatment there is a very high recurrence rate. Autoavulsion and traumatic avulsion of involved toenails is common.[4,11,19]

ONYCHOCRYPTOSIS (INGROWN TOENAIL)

Ingrown toenails occur when a segment of the nail plate penetrates the nail sulcus and subcutaneous tissue. Curvature of the nail plate is the most common predisposing factor. The lesion usually occurs as a result of external trauma or self-treatment. Onychocryptosis is characterized by inflammation, swelling, and infection of the medial or lateral aspect of the toenail. The great toe is the most commonly affected. Protracted infection may result in periungual ulcerative granulation. In patients with underlying diabetes or arterial insufficiency, cellulitis, ulceration, and necrosis may lead to amputation if treatment is delayed. If infection is not present at the time of presentation, simple elevation of the nail with placement of a wisp of cotton between the nail plate and the skin, daily foot soaks, and avoidance of pressure on the nail is usually sufficient treatment. Another option, if no infection is present, is to remove a small spicule of the offending nail. A digital block is placed as described below. The area is cleaned, and the skin is prepared for surgical procedure. An oblique portion of the affected nail is trimmed about one- to two-thirds of the way back to the posterior nail fold. The nail groove should then be debrided, and a nonadherent dressing placed[3,4,20] (Fig. 279-1).

If granulation or infection is present, then partial removal of the nail plate is indicated. This is performed by placing a digital block and preparing the area for a surgical procedure. The entire affected area, one-quarter or less of the nail plate, is cut longitudinally (anterior

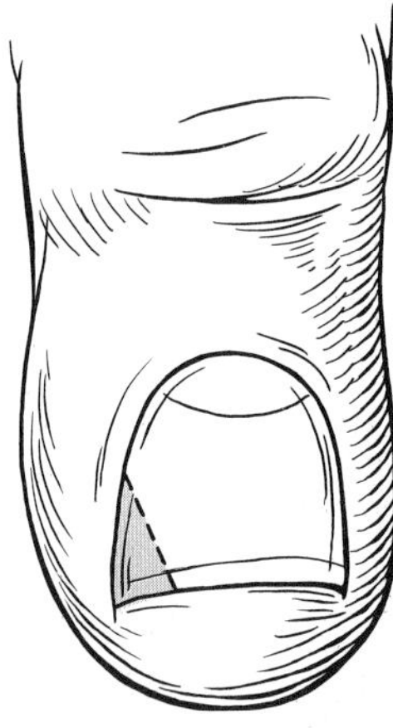

FIG. 279-1. Partial toenail removal.

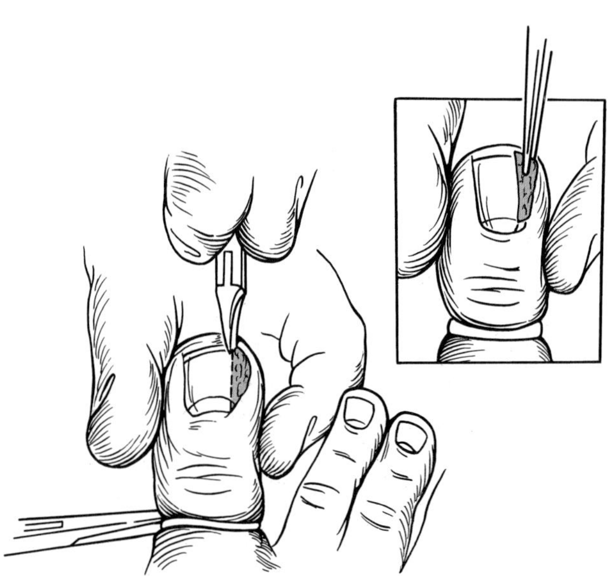

FIG. 279-2. Partial toenail removal (infection present).

to posterior), including the portion of the nail beneath the cuticle. English anvil scissors or a nail splitter are the optimal instruments for cutting the nail. The affected cut portion of the nail is then grasped with a hemostat and, using a rocking motion, removed from the nail groove. The nail groove is then debrided and a dressing is placed[20] (Fig. 279-2).

One may also cauterize the exposed nail plate. However, cauterization should only be performed by those with appropriate experience with this procedure.[20] An 88% phenol mixture can be applied for 30 s with a cotton-tipped applicator. The phenol is then rinsed with an alcohol solution. Any phenol that comes in contact with healthy tissues must be removed immediately. Silver nitrate also may be used to cauterize the area and should be left on the nail matrix for 1 min. Cauterization is not without risk, as these chemicals may cause extensive tissue destruction. Hemostasis is also extremely important in order to avoid inadvertent absorption of these toxins.

Once the procedure is completed, a nonadherent gauze or antibiotic ointment should be placed on the wound. A bulky dressing should then be placed on the toe. The wound should be checked in 24 to 48 h.[20]

OTHER NAIL LESIONS

Other common toenail afflictions include paronychia and subungual hematoma, which are treated similarly to when they occur in the fingers. Hyperkeratotic toenails can be a problem in the elderly. These may become so severe as to affect gait and cause ulcerations and infections. Patients with these lesions require referral for repeated trimming or nail plate removal.[3,4]

BURSITIS

There are many bursae in the foot, all of which may become a source of pain. Pathologic bursae can be divided into noninflammatory, inflammatory, suppurative, and calcified. Noninflammatory bursae are usually pressure-induced and are found over bony prominences. Inflammatory bursae are commonly due to gout, syphilis, or rheumatoid arthritis. Suppurative bursitis is due to the invasion of the bursae, usually from adjacent wounds, by pyogenic organisms (primarily staphylococcal species). Acute bursitis can lead to the formation of a hygroma or calcified bursae. In severe cases, pressure on bursae can lead to fistula and ulcer formation. Diagnosis of these lesions is dependent on analysis of bursal fluid, which can be obtained by large-bore needle aspiration. Fluid should be sent for cell count; protein, glucose, and lactate (elevated in septic bursitis) levels; crystal analysis; and Gram stain as well as culture (since initial Gram stains are often negative). Treatment of the bursitis depends on its cause. In all cases one should avoid further pressure to the area by instructing the patients to be non-weight-bearing. Septic bursitis should be initially treated with a penicillinase-resistant semisynthetic penicillin while awaiting culture results. Repeated aspiration or incision and drainage may become necessary.[21–23]

PLANTAR FASCIITIS

Plantar fasciitis is an inflammation of the plantar aponeurosis. The plantar fascia's main function is to anchor the plantar skin to the bone, thus protecting the longitudinal arch of the foot. The cause of plantar fasciitis is usually overuse in the physically active patient or in the patient unaccustomed to activity. Other causes include abnormal joint mechanics, tightness of the Achilles tendon, shoes with poor cushioning, abnormal foot position and anatomy, and obesity. In the younger patient, collagen vascular diseases and rheumatic diseases can lead to this entity. Patients present with pain on the plantar surface of the foot that is worse on arising and after physical activity. Examination usually reveals a point of deep tenderness at the anterior medial aspect of the calcaneus, the point of attachment of the plantar fascia. Plantar fasciitis is generally a self-limiting disease. Short-term treatment consists of rest, ice, nonsteroidal anti-inflammatory agents, heel and arch support shoe inserts, and dorsiflexion night splints (molded ankle-foot orthosis that holds the plantar fascia and Achilles tendon stretched.) Patients should be taught Achilles tendon stretching exercises and be told to avoid walking barefoot on hard surfaces. In severe cases, a short-leg walking cast may be applied to unload and rest the plantar fascia. Glucocorticoid and local anesthetic injections may be helpful. Glucocorticoid injections are associated with plantar fascia rupture and potentially serious sequelae. Only those with appropriate experience should perform this procedure.[24–27]

Long-term therapy consists of proper foot support, stretching, and strengthening exercises. Surgical intervention may be required in refractory cases. Patients should be referred to a podiatrist, orthopedist, or other appropriate practitioner.[25]

TARSAL TUNNEL SYNDROME

This compression neuropathy of the posterior tibial nerve has recently received greater recognition as a cause of foot and heel pain. After coursing inferiorly to the medial malleolus, the posterior tibial nerve enters the tarsal tunnel. The plantar aspect of the tarsal tunnel is bound by the talus and calcaneus bones and by the tibialis posterior, flexor hallucis longus, and flexor digitorum longus. The dorsal aspect is bound by the inelastic flexor retinaculum, which extends from the medial malleolus to the calcaneus to the abductor hallucis muscle.

In the setting of overuse, running and activities requiring restrictive footwear (e.g., ski boots, skates) have been implicated. The edema of pregnancy may also be a precipitant. Hyperpronation while running makes the nerve more vulnerable both to direct trauma from stretch and to indirect trauma from inflammation of the surrounding structures resulting in compression.

Pain is noted at the medial malleolus, the heel (calcaneal branch), and sole (medial or lateral plantar branch), depending on the site and severity of compression. Distal calf pain may result due to retrograde radiation (Valleix phenomenon). Similiar to carpal tunnel syndrome, the pain is often worse at night. More advanced compression may result in weak toe flexion. Tinel's sign is positive inferior to the medial malleolus. Simultaneous dorsiflexion and eversion of the ankle exacerbates symptoms.

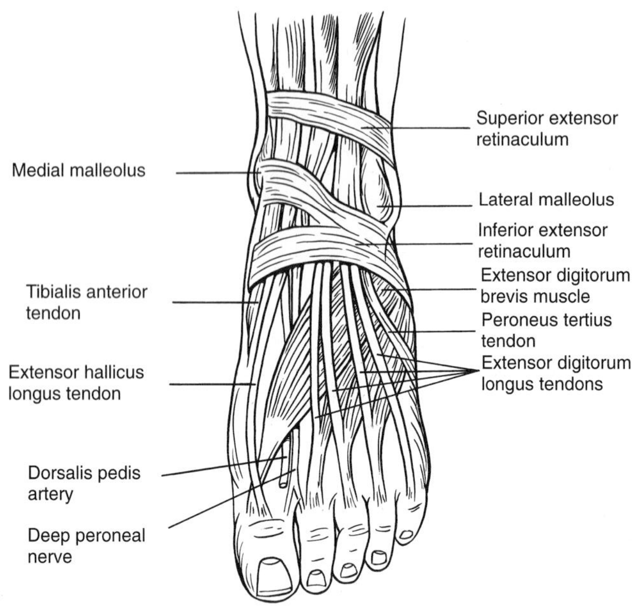

FIG. 279-3. Tendons of the foot.

The differential diagnosis includes plantar fasciitis and, if limited to the heel, Achilles tendinitis. Plantar fasciitis will cause point tenderness over the plantar heel and worse pain upon morning standing. Tarsal tunnel syndrome causes greater medial heel and arch pain due to involvement of the abductor hallucis muscle. Fasciitis pain may improve with gradual ambulation throughout the day, whereas tarsal tunnel worsens. In addition, tarsal tunnel syndrome may produce distal calf pain, whereas fasciitis does not.

Initial treatment includes avoidance of the exacerbating activities and use of NSAIDs. If there is no improvement or symptoms recur after a few weeks, then orthopaedic evaluation and treatment, which include electromyographic studies, steriod injection, orthotic devices, or surgery, are recommended.

GANGLIONS

A ganglion is a common benign synovial cyst. Ganglia are 1.5 to 2.5 cm in diameter and are often attached to a joint capsule or tendon sheath. Although ganglions typically occur in the wrist, they may also occur in the foot. These lesions typically arise in the anterolateral aspect of the ankle but can occur in many areas of the foot. The pathogenesis of these lesions is unknown. The two most popular theories are (1) that they are produced by herniation of the tendon sheath, and (2) that they arise from focal myxomatous degeneration of collagenous tissues caused by trauma. Ganglions may appear suddenly or gradually, may enlarge and diminish in size, and may be painful or asymptomatic. On examination one notes a firm, usually nontender, cystic lesion. Diagnosis is usually made clinically, although ultrasound and MRI are useful if there is any question of the diagnosis. Aspiration and instillation of glucocorticoids leads to the complete resolution of ganglions in some cases. Most ganglions require complete surgical excision.[28,29]

TENDON LESIONS

Tendon lesions usually require referral and/or consultation with a podiatrist or orthopedist to aid in treatment decisions (Figs. 279-3 and 279-4). Tenosynovitis and tendinitis may occur in the foot, usually due to overuse. Patients present with pain over the involved tendon. The flexor hallucis longus, posterior tibialis, and Achilles tendon are most commonly involved. Treatment consists of rest, ice, and oral anti-inflammatory agents.[30,31]

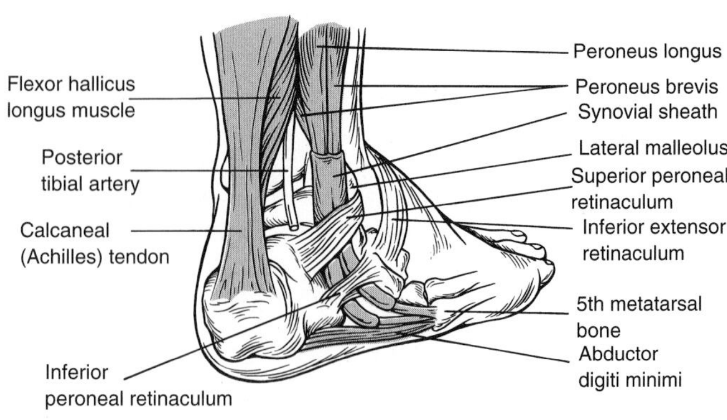

FIG. 279-4. Tendons of the foot.

Tendon lacerations are usually traumatic. The usual mechanism of injury is a cut to the dorsal or plantar aspect of the foot. Tendon lacerations should be explored and repaired if the ends of the tendon are visible in the wound. The foot should be casted in dorsiflexion after the repair of extensor tendons, and in equinus after repair of flexor tendons. Unfortunately, tendon repairs in the foot have a relatively high complication and disability rate. Specialty consultation is appropriate.[30,31]

Spontaneous rupture of the Achilles, tibialis anterior, and posterior tibialis tendons is fairly common. Diagnosis and proper treatment of tendon ruptures is aided by ultrasound, CT scanning, and MRI studies. Orthopedic consultation should be obtained to aid in proper therapeutic decisions. Achilles tendon ruptures are usually due to forceful dorsiflexion and occur more commonly in males. Patients present with pain, a palpable defect in the area of the tendon, and inability to stand on tiptoes. Squeezing the calf of the prone patient whose knee is flexed at 90° will normally cause the foot to plantar flex. This response will be absent in patients with Achilles tendon ruptures. Treatment is generally surgical in younger patients and conservative (casting in equinus) in older patients.[30,31]

Ruptures of the anterior tibialis tendon are rare. These usually occur after the fourth decade and are not excessively painful. Patients present with varying degrees of foot drop and a palpable defect distal to the ankle joint in the area of the tendon. In most cases, disability is minimal and surgery is not necessary.[30,31]

Spontaneous ruptures of the posterior tibialis tendon also occur after the fourth decade. Two-thirds of these cases occur in women. The presentation is usually chronic and insidious. Patients notice a gradual flattening of their arch, with modest discomfort and swelling over the medial ankle. Examination reveals absence of the tendon's normal prominence and weakness on inversion of the foot. Patients find it impossible to stand on tiptoes. Treatment may be conservative or surgical, depending on the duration of the tear and activity of the patient.[30,31]

Another tendon rupture of note is rupture of the flexor hallucis longus, which presents as a loss of plantar flexion of the great toe. This lesion must be repaired in ballet dancers but not in the nonathlete.[30,31]

Disruption of the peroneal retinaculum can occur as a result of a blow during dorsiflexion of the foot. Besides pain localized to the peroneal tendon behind the lateral maleoles, the patient complains of a clicking when walking as the tendon subluxes. Treatment is generally surgical repair.

PLANTAR INTERDIGITAL NEUROMA (MORTON'S NEUROMA)

Neuromas may form in a plantar digital nerve, usually proximal to its bifurcation. These neuromas may occur in any of the digital nerves but are most common in the third interspace. The cause of these lesions is thought to be local irritation of the nerve due to entrapment, usually from tight-fitting shoes. Women between the ages of 25 and 50 years are the most commonly affected group. Patients present with pain located in the area of the metatarsal head. The pain is described as burning, cramping, or aching. Pain is worsened by ambulation and resolved by rest and removal of shoes. The pain may radiate to the affected toes, and patients may note numbness in the toes. Pain is usually easily reproduced upon palpation of the area, and at times a mass is felt. Diagnosis is usually made clinically, but nerve conduction studies, electromyograms, ultrasound studies, and MRI may be helpful at times. Conservative treatment consists of wearing wide shoes with good metatarsal head supports and metatarsal head off-loading inserts. Local glucocorticoid injections can be curative. Conservative therapy is often unsuccessful, and patients may ultimately require neurolysis or surgical intervention.[24,32]

COMPARTMENT SYNDROME

Compartment syndromes have been more commonly described to affect the arms and legs. Nine compartments have been identified in the foot. Compartment syndrome occurs when an elevation of tissue pressure within one of these nonyielding fascial compartments impedes vascular flow. In the foot, the cause of compartment syndrome is usually a high-energy injury associated with multiple fractures. Crush injuries are more likely to cause compartment syndrome. Compartment syndromes have been reported in association with midfoot fractures and rearfoot fractures, burns, contusions, bleeding disorders, postischemic swelling after arterial injury or thrombosis, venous obstruction, exercise, and prolonged pressure to the affected area. There have also been reports of chronic compartment syndromes due to overuse. Patients typically present with severe acute pain that is worsened on active or passive movement, swelling, paresthesias, and neurovascular deficits. The only reliable method to diagnose compartment syndrome is by obtaining intracompartmental pressures. Once the diagnosis is made, fasciotomy should be performed emergently. The sequelae of compartment syndrome range from transient neurologic compromise to complete myoneural necrosis, fibrosis, and ischemic contractures. The prognosis of compartment syndrome is directly related to the time delay in diagnosis and treatment.[33,34]

IMMERSION FOOT (TRENCH FOOT)

Immersion foot is the result of prolonged exposure of the foot to a moist, nonfreezing (but below 60°F, 15.56°C), occlusive environment. Immersion foot is classically seen in military operations, but the homeless civilian population is also particularly at risk. Prolonged cooling of the extremities produces direct soft tissue injury, with the peripheral nerves being most affected. Wet conditions accelerate the injury, as do factors that reduce circulation to the extremities. These factors include constrictive footwear, prolonged immobilization, hypothermia, smoking, dehydration, nutritional deficiencies, trauma, and underlying disease. When first seen, the injured area is pale, anesthetic, pulseless, immobile, but not frozen. After several hours of rewarming, a vigorous hypermia develops associated with severe burning pain and reappearance of proximal sensation. Edema and bullae, at times sanguinous, may develop as perfusion increases. This hyperemic phase may last weeks, and hyperhidrosis is a prominent late feature. Patients may develop fever and lymphadenopathy. The injury evolves slowly, and anesthesia may be permanent. Differential diagnosis includes cellulitis and fungal infections. Treatment is conservative and includes admission for bedrest, leg elevation, and air drying of feet at room temperature. Antibiotics play little or no role in the recovery process but should be given if superinfection is present.[35,36]

PLANTAR FIBROMATOSIS

Plantar fibromatosis, or Dupuytren's contracture of the plantar fascia, does not occur as commonly as in the hand. Plantar fibromatosis is a disorder of fibrous tissue proliferation, which slowly invades the skin and soft tissues. Presentation is generally in adolescence or young adulthood. Patients present with small (0.5 to 1.0 cm), asymptomatic, palpable, slowly enlarging, fixed, firm masses on the plantar aspect of one or both feet. These lesions tend to be in the non-weight-bearing areas of the foot. Toe contractures do not occur. These lesions have a tendency to reabsorb spontaneously. Treatment is conservative, and only rarely is surgery indicated. These patients should be referred to the appropriate consultant for continued care.[23,29,37]

FOOT ULCERS

Foot ulcers can generally be classified as neuropathic or ischemic by the predominant etiologic factor and clinical features. Infection can be a complicating factor in either type of ulcer. Diabetics are prone to both types of ulcers and in addition are more apt to develop infections. It has been estimated that proper foot care in diabetics (including prophylaxis and treatment of foot ulcers) could reduce the number of lower limb amputations by 44 to 80 percent.[38,39]

Ischemic ulcers are secondary to vascular compromise, usually due to atherosclerosis of larger vessels. Ulcers rarely develop due to problems with the microcirculation in an area. These ulcers are seen in the setting of a cool foot, dependent rubor, pallor on elevation, atrophic shiny skin, and diminished pulses. Patients may complain of symptoms of intermittent claudication and leg pain in the supine position, relieved by dependency. If the underlying vascular disease is corrected, these ulcers usually heal quickly. Without reconstructive surgery, the prognosis is poor and amputation is often inevitable.[40–42]

Neuropathic ulcers are essentially pressure ulcers. Patients at risk are those with absent or distorted foot sensation. These include patients with diabetes, leprosy, tabes dorsalis, and other congenital or acquired neuropathies. Their feet are prone to ischemia from pressure by ill-fitting shoes, foreign bodies, abnormal bony prominences, and most commonly from the daily stresses of walking. The ulcers are usually well circumscribed with surrounding white calluslike material. The

TABLE 279-1 Selected Empirical Antimicrobial Regimens for Foot Infections in Patients with Diabetes Mellitus*

Non-limb-threatening infection:
Oral regimen
  Cephalexin
  Clindamycin
  Dicloxacillin
  Amoxicillin-clavulanate
Parenteral regimen
  Cefazolin
  Oxacillin or nafcillin
  Clindamycin

Limb-threatening infection:
Oral regimen
  Fluoroquinolone and clindamycin
Parenteral regimen
  Ampicillin-sulbactam
  Ticarcillin-clavulanate
  Cefoxitin or cefotetan
  Fluoroquinolone and clindamycin

Life-threatening infection:
Parenteral regimen
  Imipenem-cilastatin
  Vancomycin, metronidazole, and aztreonam
  Ampicillin-sulbactam and an aminoglycoside

*These regimens may require adjustment if the patient has a history of allergies or if there are clinical or epidemiologic factors suggesting unusual pathogens. Doses should be commensurate with the severity of infection, with adjustment for renal dysfunction when indicated.
Source: From Caputo GM, Cavanaugh PR, Ulbrecht JS, et al: Assessment and management of foot disease in patients with diabetes. *N Engl J Med* 331:859, 1994.

foot (if there is no underlying vascular disease) has normal temperature, color, and pulses. Defects in touch, pressure, or proprioception are noted on examination. Motor weakness and muscular atrophy may also be present. These changes can lead to abnormal gait and foot anatomy.[38–40]

Once an ulcer becomes infected, two aspects of therapy are essential for healing: thorough debridement and complete pressure relief. Debridement must be aggressive; wet-to-dry dressing changes are not sufficient. Once debridement is completed, the role of wet-to-dry dressing is controversial. These dressings may prevent drying of the ulcer and eschar formation. To date, no topical agents or foot soak has been conclusively found to be beneficial for the healing of diabetic ulcers. Relief of pressure is accomplished by either complete bed rest or by total contact casting.[38–40]

Antibiotics and often admission are warranted for the treatment of infected ulcers. Infections are usually polymicrobial. The most common organisms are *Staphylococcus aureus* and beta-hemolytic streptococci. Other organisms found in diabetic foot ulcers are various species of Enterobacteriaceae and anaerobes, enterococci, and *P. aeruginosa.* Superficial cultures of infected ulcers are unreliable. Cultures should be obtained of any purulent drainage and of aspirates from fluctuant areas. Antibiotics should initially be broad spectrum to cover the wide variety of possible infective organisms. Choices depend on the severity of infection (Table 279-1). Cellulitis and signs of deep soft tissue infection require hospitalization for antibiotics and strict bed rest. Abscesses should be incised and drained. X-rays should be considered if there is any suspicion of subcutaneous gas, foreign body, osteomyelitis, and Charcot foot. MRI and bone scan may be indicated to determine the presence of osteomyelitis. Palpation of bone in the depths of infected pedal ulcers has been shown to strongly correlate with osteomyelitis. With diabetics, a serum glucose level should be obtained, as it is often elevated. Patients with nonhealing foot ulcers should undergo evaluation to determine the underlying etiology of the ulcer (vascular, diabetic, or other systemic disease, including malignancies). Hyperbaric oxygen has been advocated by some as beneficial in the treatment of both infected and noninfected foot ulcers.[38–40,43–47]

MALIGNANT MELANOMA

The incidence of malignant melanoma is increasing, thus making consideration of this disease process important. Malignant melanoma of the foot accounts for up to 15 percent of all cutaneous melanomas. Melanomas can present as an atypical, pigmented, or nonhealing lesion of the foot, including the nail. These malignancies often imitate more common foot disorders such as fungal infections and plantar warts. Since prognosis is directly related to early diagnosis, a high index of suspicion must be maintained. All skin lesions that are either atypical or not healing despite treatment should be referred for biopsy.[29,48]

FOOT LESIONS INDICATIVE OF DISSEMINATED DISEASE

Many disease processes may be manifest by foot lesions. Acquired immunodeficiency syndrome may present with a variety of foot lesions, including Kaposi's sarcoma and nonhealing ulcers and those caused by bacterial and fungal infections such as histoplasmosis (which can present as maculopapular eruptions or depressed pits of the soles).[49] These patients may develop neuropathies presenting as both paresthesias and dysesthesias. Secondary syphilis presents as a nonitching polymorphic rash that affects both the soles and palms. The rash of Rocky Mountain spotted fever, which is initially discrete, macular, and later petechial, is also found on the palms and soles. Cutaneous forms of tuberculosis have also been described that affect the feet. Hand-foot-and-mouth disease causes small vesicular lesions on the soles, palms, buttocks, and in the mouth. This entity is caused by coxsackievirus and occurs in the late summer and fall.

REFERENCES

1. Levy LA: Prevalence of chronic podiatric conditions in the U.S.: National Health Survey 1990. *J Am Podiatr Med Assoc* 82:221, 1992.
2. Silfverskiold JP: Common foot problems: Relieving the pain of bunions, keratoses, corns and calluses. *Postgrad Med* 89:183, 1991.
3. Birrer RB, Dellacorte MP: Skin and nail disorders of the foot. *Emerg Med* 25:27, 1993.
4. Helfand AE: Nail and hyperkeratotic problems in the elderly foot. *Am Fam Phys* 39:101, 1989.
5. Glover MG: Plantar warts. *Foot Ankle* 11:172, 1990.
6. Page JC, Abramson C, Wei-Li L, et al: Diagnosis and treatment of tinea pedis: A review and update: *J Am Podiatr Med Assoc* 81:304, 1991.
7. McBride A, Cohen BA: Tinea pedis in children. *Am J Dis Child* 146:844, 1992.
8. Evans EG: Tinea pedis: Clinical experience and efficacy of short treatment. *Dermatology* 194 (suppl 1):3, 1997.
9. DelRosso JQ: Advances in the treatment of superficial fungal infections: Focus on onychomycosis and dry tinea pedis. *J Am Osteopath Assoc* 97:339, 1997.
10. Tausch I, Decrois J, Gwiezdzinski Z, et al: Short-term itraconazole versus terbinafine in the treatment of tinea pedis or manus. *Int J Dermatol* 37:140, 1998.
11. Hoffman AF, Driver VR: Onychomycosis. *Clin Podiatr Med Surg* 13:13, 1996.
12. Midgley G, Moore MK: Nail infections. *Dermatol Clin* 14:41, 1996.
13. Levy LA: Epidemiology of onychomycosis in special risk populations. *J Am Podiatr Med Assoc* 87:546, 1997.
14. Gupta AK, Lynde CW, Jain HC, et al: A higher prevalence of onychomycosis in psoriatics compared with non-psoriatics: A multicentre study. *Br J Dermatol* 136:786, 1997.
15. Gupta AK, De Doncker P, Scher RK, et al: Itraconazole for the treatment of onychomycosis. *Int J Dermatol* 37:303, 1998.

16. Drake LA, Shear NH, Arlette JP, et al: Oral terbinafine in the treatment of toenail onychomycosis: North American multicenter trial. *J Am Acad Dermatol* 37:740, 1997.
17. Brautigam M: Terbinafine versus itraconazole: A controlled clinical comparison in onychomycosis of the toenails. *J Am Acad Dermatol* 38:S53, 1998.
18. Bootman JL: Cost-effectiveness of two new treatments for onychomycosis: An analysis of two comparative clinical trials. *J Am Acad Dermatol* 38:S69, 1998.
19. Gupta AK, Scher RK, De Doncker P: Current management of onychomycosis: An overview. *Dermatol Clin* 15:121, 1997.
20. Malusky LP: Podiatric procedures, in Roberts JR, Hedges JR (eds): *Clinical Procedures in Emergency Medicine,* 3d ed. Philadelphia: Saunders, 1998.
21. Hernandez PA, Hernandez WA, Hernandez A: Clinical aspects of bursae and tendon sheaths of the foot. *J Am Podiatr Med Assoc* 81:366, 1991.
22. Lawson KS, Schwarian JS, Awbrey BJ: Septic bursitis of the foot: Diagnosis, management and end-result. *J Foot Surg* 29:379, 1990.
23. Jahss MH: Miscellaneous soft-tissue lesions, in Jahss MH (ed) *Disorders of the Foot and Ankle: Medical and Surgical Management,* 2d ed. Philadelphia: Saunders, 1991. p 1514.
24. Jones FK, Masear VR: Painful syndromes of the foot: Diagnosis and management. *Clin Plast Surg* 18:639, 1991.
25. Singh D, Angel J, Bentley G, et al: Fortnightly review: Plantar fasciitis. *Br Med J* 315:172, 1997.
26. Powell M, Post WR, Keener J, et al: Effective treatment of chronic plantar fasciitis with dorsiflexion night splints: A crossover prospective randomized outcome study. *Foot Ankle Int* 19:10, 1998.
27. Acevedo JI, Beskin JL: Complications of plantar fascia rupture associated with corticosteroid injection. *Foot Ankle Int* 19:91, 1998.
28. Wu KK: Ganglions of the foot. *J Foot Ankle Surg* 32:343, 1993.
29. Potter GK, Ward KA: Tumors, in McGlamry ED, Banks AS, Downey MS (eds): *Comprehensive Textbook of Foot Surgery,* 2d ed. Baltimore: Williams & Wilkins, 1992, p 1136.
30. Jahss MH: Tendon disorders of the foot and ankle, in Jahss MH (ed): *Disorders of the Foot and Ankle: Medical and Surgical Management,* 2d ed. Philadelphia: Saunders, 1991, p 1461.
31. Silvani S: Management of acute tendon trauma, in McGlamry ED, Banks AS, Downey MS (eds): *Comprehensive Textbook of Foot Surgery,* 2d ed. Baltimore: Williams & Wilkins, 1992, p 1450.
32. Wu KK: Morton's interdigital neuroma: A clinical review of its etiology, treatment, and results. *J Foot Ankle Surg* 35:112, 1996.
33. Myerson M, Manoli A: Compartment syndromes of the foot after calcaneal fractures. *Clin Orthop* 290:142, 1993.
34. Whitesides TE: Compartment syndromes of the lower extremity, in Jahss MH (ed): *Disorders of the Foot and Ankle: Medical and Surgical Management,* 2d ed. Philadelphia: Saunders, 1991, p 2584.
35. Wrenn K: Immersion foot: A problem of the homeless in the 1990s. *Arch Intern Med* 151:785, 1990.
36. Frey CC, Shereff MJ: Chemical, environmental, and foreign-body injuries to the foot and ankle, in Jahss MH (ed): *Disorders of the Foot and Ankle: Medical and Surgical Management,* 2d ed. Philadelphia: Saunders, 1991, p 2564.
37. Lee TH, Wapner KL, Hecht PJ: Plantar Fibromatosis. *J Bone Joint Surg* 75A:1080, 1993.
38. American Diabetic Association: Foot care in patients with diabetes mellitus. *Diabetes Care* 16(suppl 2):19, 1993.
39. Caputo GM, Cavanagh PR, Ulbrecht JS, et al: Assessment and management of foot disease in patients with diabetes. *N Engl J Med* 331:854, 1994.
40. Miller OF: Essentials of pressure ulcer treatment: The diabetic experience: *J Dermatol Surg Oncol* 19:759, 1993.
41. Tam M, Moschella SL: Vascular skin ulcers of limbs. *Cardiol Clin* 9:555, 1991.
42. Kaufman JL, Leather RP: Vascular diseases of the foot, in Jahss MH (ed): *Disorders of the Foot and Ankle: Medical and Surgical Management,* 2d ed. Philadelphias Saunders, 1991, p 1787.
43. Lipman BT, Collier BD, Timinis ME, et al: Detection of osteomyelitis in the neuropathic foot: Nuclear medicine, MRI and conventional radiography. *Clin Nucl Med* 23:77, 1998.
44. Grayson ML, Gibbons GW, Balogh K, et al: Probing to bone in infected pedal ulcers: A clinical sign of underlying osteomyelitis in diabetic patients. *JAMA* 273:721, 1995.
45. Yang D, Morrison BD, Vandongen YK, et al: Malignancy in chronic leg ulcers. *Med J Aust* 164:718, 1996.
46. Zamboni WA, Wong HP, Stephenson LL, et al: Evaluation of hyperbaric oxygen for diabetic wounds: A prospective study. *Undersea Hyperb Med* 24:175, 1997.
47. Faglia E, Favales F, Aldeghi A, et al: Adjunctive systemic hyperbaric oxygen therapy in treatment of severe prevalently ischemic diabetic foot ulcers: A randomized study. *Diabetes Care* 19:1338, 1996.
48. Miller G, James JH: Malignant melanoma of the foot. *Practitioner* 234:647, 1990.
49. Burns S: Podiatric manifestations of AIDS. *J Am Podiatr Med Assoc* 80:15, 1990.

BEHAVIORAL DISORDERS: CLINICAL FEATURES

Douglas A. Rund

Psychiatric disorders are common in the emergency department patient population. Estimates of the proportion of emergency department patients who present with a psychiatric disorder range from a few percent to more than a third. This variability is partly due to differences in patient population and utilization of alternatives for psychiatric crisis intervention. When patients are screened for mental disorders including substance abuse, many patients have unrecognized psychopathology that is relevant to their assessment and treatment in the emergency setting. Subgroups of the emergency patient population at higher risk for psychiatric disorders include those who are self-referred for nonurgent problems, patients with chest pain, and the "after midnight" group of emergency department patients, who had more psychiatric illness (56 percent) than the daytime group (20 percent). Sometimes, psychiatric disorders clearly make up the primary reason for an individual's presentation to an emergency department. In other cases, psychiatric disorders lead to injury and illness. Such conditions create the need for emergency care. As screening studies have shown, psychiatric disorders may form part of the current or past medical history of a patient, yet possess little importance for the immediate clinical condition.

In studies that report categories of psychiatric illness seen in the emergency department, the most prominent diagnoses are substance abuse, affective disorders, anxiety disorders, antisocial personality disorder, and severe cognitive impairment. Among repeat users of the emergency department, persons with schizophrenia are overrepresented.

Psychiatric disorders can cause substantial impairment in social or occupational functioning or marked distress. Patients or their families are often unwilling to seek psychiatric care because of the stigma of mental illness. Their evaluation in the emergency department is their point of entry into the health care system. Also, due to poor judgment, financial considerations, or cognitive impairment, many psychiatric patients do not regularly seek medical attention until an emergency intervenes. They then seek emergency treatment for their medical needs. The most serious manifestations of mental illness (suicide, psychosis, and violent behavior) are medical emergencies and consequently are appropriately dealt with in the emergency department. Emergency physicians require substantial knowledge and skill to be able to recognize psychiatric disorders, perform crisis intervention and stabilization, and refer the patient for psychiatric hospitalization or outpatient care as needed.

DIAGNOSIS

In the assessment of patients presenting with psychiatric symptoms, as with other medical conditions encountered in the emergency department, it is crucial to promptly stabilize the patient's acute condition and evaluate the major complaint immediately. Formulating a specific diagnosis must necessarily follow initial stabilization procedures in this clinical process. The determination that an individual is suicidal and in need of hospitalization, for instance, is more important than deciding whether that person suffers from schizophrenia or psychotic depression.

Nevertheless, provisional psychiatric diagnoses can be made in the emergency department. Recognition of specific behavioral syndromes can assist in evaluating the presenting complaint, pursuing associated symptoms, and determining treatment and disposition. Emergency physicians should be sufficiently familiar with commonly seen psychiatric illnesses to describe their predominant clinical features.

Structured Diagnostic Criteria

Over the past 15 years, awareness of the earlier unreliability of psychiatric diagnosis guided the development of operational criteria for separate and distinct mental disorders. These rules allow researchers and clinicians to agree on the presence or absence of a particular disorder. In addition, the criteria are based on observable signs and the patient's report of symptoms, not on unconscious psychic mechanisms. This simplifies the task of diagnosis for emergency physicians and other nonpsychiatrists because extensive knowledge of pathophysiology and unconscious mental processes is not essential.

The current official diagnostic nomenclature, published in 1994 by the American Psychiatric Association, is the *Diagnostic and Statistical Manual of Mental Disorders,* fourth edition, commonly known as DSM-IV. A copy of DSM-IV should be available for reference in the emergency department because it contains both the list of criteria for each disorder, and additional material on demographics, associated symptoms and syndromes, and differential diagnosis. Future revisions of DSM-IV will likely be based to a greater degree on biologic criteria as more is learned about biochemical, structural, and genetic features of various psychiatric illnesses.

Multiaxial Diagnostic System

The DSM-IV diagnoses are made on a multiaxial system in which each axis refers to a different domain of information. This system aids in making a comprehensive assessment, organizing complex clinical information, and communicating between professionals. Axis I disorders comprise the clinical syndromes of mental disorders. Conditions listed on Axis II are the personality disorders and developmental disorders, including mental retardation, which may underlie the more florid Axis I syndrome. Axis III notes general medical conditions. Axes IV and V record psychosocial stressors and adaptive functioning. It is generally unnecessary for the emergency physician to make a complete multiaxial diagnosis, but knowledge of this system may facilitate an understanding of medical records and psychiatric consultants' notes. For instance, a patient with previous medical records containing DSM-IV diagnoses of Axis I: alcohol intoxication; Axis II: antisocial personality disorder; and Axis III: scalp laceration, should be recognized as likely to display features of the Axis II personality disorder, although the patient's chief complaint may be a new problem.

PSYCHIATRIC SYNDROMES (AXIS I DISORDERS)

The organization and major categories of Axis I disorders covered here are listed in Table 280-1. A useful strategy for making a DSM-IV diagnosis is to classify the primary feature into a major category, consider possible nonpsychiatric etiologies for the complaint, and then use the decision trees in Appendix B of DSM-IV to identify the appropriate diagnosis. The decision trees guide the clinician who is unfamiliar with the intricacies of the criteria within a category to identify the features that distinguish closely related conditions.

TABLE 280-1 Axis I Disorders

Delirium, dementia, and amnestic and other cognitive disorders
Substance induced disorders
Mental disorders due to a general medical condition
Schizophrenia and other psychotic disorders
Mood disorders
Anxiety disorders
Somatoform disorders
Factitious disorders
Dissociative disorders
Eating disorders
Adjustment disorders

Delirium, Dementia, Amnestic, and Other Cognitive Disorders

This group of syndromes is characterized by a clinically significant deficit in cognitive or memory function due to a general medical condition. There are several distinct and common causes of organic brain syndromes in which the causative factor is known; for example, vascular dementia and alcohol withdrawal delirium. In these cases, the specific diagnosis is listed in DSM-IV. In other cases, the etiologic factor should be specified using the descriptor "due to [general medical disorder or substance]" for example, "delirium due to hepatic encephalopathy."

DEMENTIA The essential clinical feature of *dementia* is a pervasive disturbance of cognitive functioning in several areas including memory, abstract thinking, judgment, personality, and other higher cortical functions such as language. If clouding of consciousness is present, then the patient does not have solely a dementing illness, but has *delirium* or intoxication. The presence of global cognitive impairment may be detected by a bedside cognitive examination, such as the Mini Mental State Examination, and additional confirmatory history should be gathered from an informant, such as a family member. Memory disturbance is usually the earliest sign to be apparent to others, and unless it is very mild, it can be easily identified by examination.

Patients with dementia may be brought to the emergency department after having been found wandering away from home or an institution. Because the onset of most forms of dementia is slow and gradual, presentation to the emergency department often occurs only when some acute worsening of mental status occurs, which may be the result of a superimposed medical illness, adverse drug effect, or environmental change. The demented patient's diminished intellectual and physiologic resources allow abrupt worsening of function with the addition of such stressors.

Early in the course of dementia, anxiety, depression, or psychosis may dominate the clinical picture and obscure cognitive dysfunction. For this reason, a high degree of clinical suspicion of dementia should be maintained when evaluating an elderly patient with no prior psychiatric history who presents with new psychiatric problems. Demented persons are also prone to unrecognized physical illness because of inability to perceive or describe symptoms. Careful examination and appropriate laboratory testing are always indicated in the initial and ongoing evaluation of such patients.

It must be noted that dementia is not synonymous with the older designation of "chronic organic brain syndrome," which implies irreversiblity. Common causes of potentially reversible dementia include metabolic and endocrine disorders, polypharmacy, and depression. Often, especially in elderly patients, depression may present with prominent cognitive impairment, a condition erroneously labeled "pseudodementia," but more accurately called *dementia of depression.* The presence of a relatively acute onset, prominent mood changes, and vegetative disturbances such as loss of appetite and weight, sleep disturbance, or expressions of guilt or suicidal ideation all point to depression as the cause. In these situations, treatment of the mood disorder may lead to resolution of the cognitive impairment, although recent studies indicate that many such patients have evidence of brain dysfunction and only partial treatment response.

DELIRIUM Like dementia, *delirium* is characterized by global impairment in cognitive function, but is distinguished from it in two major ways. In delirium, the patient has clouding of consciousness, a reduction in the awareness of the external environment (manifest as difficulty sustaining attention), varying degrees of alertness ranging from drowsiness to stupor, and sensory misperception.

The primary distinguishing feature of delirium is the course that is typically acute, with rapid deterioration in hours or days, rather than months as with dementia. Also, the severity of delirium fluctuates over the course of hours; the patient may appear normal at one time and wildly agitated a few hours later. Extreme changes in psychomotor activity, ranging from restlessness and hyperactivity to stupor, are frequent in delirium, but uncommon in dementia except in the later stages when a delirious state may be superimposed. Finally, hallucinations, often visual, are common in delirium. They typically have a vivid quality to which the patient reacts strongly. The hallucinations contrast with the visual hallucinations seen by psychotic patients, which are often described and experienced indifferently.

Substance-Induced Disorders

INTOXICATION When recent ingestion of a specific exogenous substance produces maladaptive behavior and impairment of judgment, perception, attention, emotional control, or psychomotor activity, and the patient does not display features of delirium, hallucinosis, or other organic brain syndromes, a diagnosis of *intoxication* is made. When the offending substance is known, it should be specified (e.g., alcohol intoxication or amphetamine intoxication). The specific features of intoxication syndromes commonly seen in the emergency department are described in greater detail in the section on toxicology.

As a general rule, the diagnosis of intoxication can be rather easy when laboratory analysis reveals the type and amount of intoxicant circulating in the system. The clinical features of alcohol intoxication are familiar to experienced emergency physicians and range from impaired judgment and coordination through ataxia, lethargy, and coma. When repeated episodes of intoxication occur in a brief period of time, the individual by definition has a substance abuse disorder, and the additional diagnosis is made.

WITHDRAWAL *Withdrawal* can follow cessation or reduction in use of a substance of abuse. The category signifies a syndrome characteristic of withdrawal from that particular drug, when the clinical syndrome does not satisfy the criteria for delirium or another organic brain syndrome. For example, mild forms of alcohol withdrawal would be classified here, but if the patient is confused, hallucinating, and agitated, a diagnosis of alcohol withdrawal delirium is indicated. The diagnosis is made by identification of the withdrawal syndrome along with evidence of recent use of the substance in a pattern sufficient to produce withdrawal when the amount ingested is decreased. Specific withdrawal patterns depend on the agent customarily used.

Alcohol withdrawal, for instance, includes up to four stages: autonomic hyperactivity (6 to 8 h after cessation of drinking); hallucinations (24 h after withdrawal); major motor seizures (1 to 2 days); and global confusion (3 to 5 days after last use of alcohol). Some withdrawal syndromes, particularly from alcohol or barbiturates, can be life threatening.

Mental Disorders Due to a General Medical Condition

DSM-IV has implemented a major change in the classification of psychiatric symptoms caused by medical conditions. The previous terminology of "organic brain syndrome" and the subtypes organic mood disorder, organic delusional disorder, for example, have been eliminated because of the implication that the "functional" mental disorders were unrelated to biologic changes in brain function. Using DSM-IV, where there is evidence that a psychiatric disturbance is a direct physiologic consequence of a general medical condition or substance, the mental disorder is specified as ". . . due to" the medical problem; for example, "major depression due to hypothyroidism." Common medical causes of psychotic and mood disorders are covered in Chap. 281.

Schizophrenia and Other Psychotic Disorders

Schizophrenia and related disorders are marked by the presence of psychotic symptoms, primarily delusions and hallucinations. *Delusions* are defined as fixed false beliefs that are not amenable to arguments or facts to the contrary and that are not shared by others of similar cultural background. Common delusions are of several types. *Persecutory delusions* are those in which one believes that one is being attacked, followed, harassed, or conspired against. *Grandiose delusions* are those that involve themes of special powers or abilities. *Bizarre delusions* are those with patently absurd content, such as believing that one's thoughts are controlled by extraterrestrial beings. *Hallucinations* are false perceptions experienced in a sensory modality and occurring in clear consciousness. Auditory hallucinations are the most common, followed in order of prevalence by visual, tactile, olfactory, and gustatory. The most prevalent psychosis is *schizophrenia,* described in detail in the next section. The other psychotic disorders, discussed briefly, are less common. A decision tree helpful in evaluating psychotic symptoms is presented in Fig. 280-1.

SCHIZOPHRENIA Schizophrenia is one of the most serious public health problems in the world and accounts for 25 percent of all hospitalized patients. The essential features are a deterioration in functioning, the presence of active-phase symptoms (hallucinations, delusions, disorganized speech or behavior, catatonic behavior, or negative symptoms) for at least one month, and the relative absence of a mood syndrome. Research has established the importance of genetic factors in its cause, and schizophrenia is most likely a group of disorders of varying etiology that share a final common pathway, much as is the case with mental retardation. It is a brain disease, and there is no evidence that psychosocial stressors or poor parenting are responsible for the cause of the illness, although these may have a profound effect on the patient's adaptation to this usually chronic disorder.

Schizophrenia usually starts in late adolescence or early adulthood, although the onset can occur at any age. The childhood history of schizophrenics often is marked by shyness, oddness or eccentric behavior, school difficulties, or paranoid behaviors, but such features are not always present. A prodromal phase, in which a gradual deterioration of function is noted, usually precedes the development of active delusions or hallucinations. Such deterioration usually includes the worsening of social withdrawal or the new onset of social withdrawal, odd behavior or speech, and difficulty in functioning in school or work. Patients or their families rarely seek care until the onset of the active phase of psychosis. Schizophrenics seldom seek care at all because they lack insight; they do not realize that their perception, thoughts, and behavior are abnormal.

Antipsychotic drugs usually reduce the severity of delusions and hallucinations. Other manifestations of schizophrenia less responsive to antipsychotics include negative symptoms (lack of volition, blunting of emotion, anhedonia, and inattention). Such symptoms result in lasting impairment in self-care, work, and social relations.

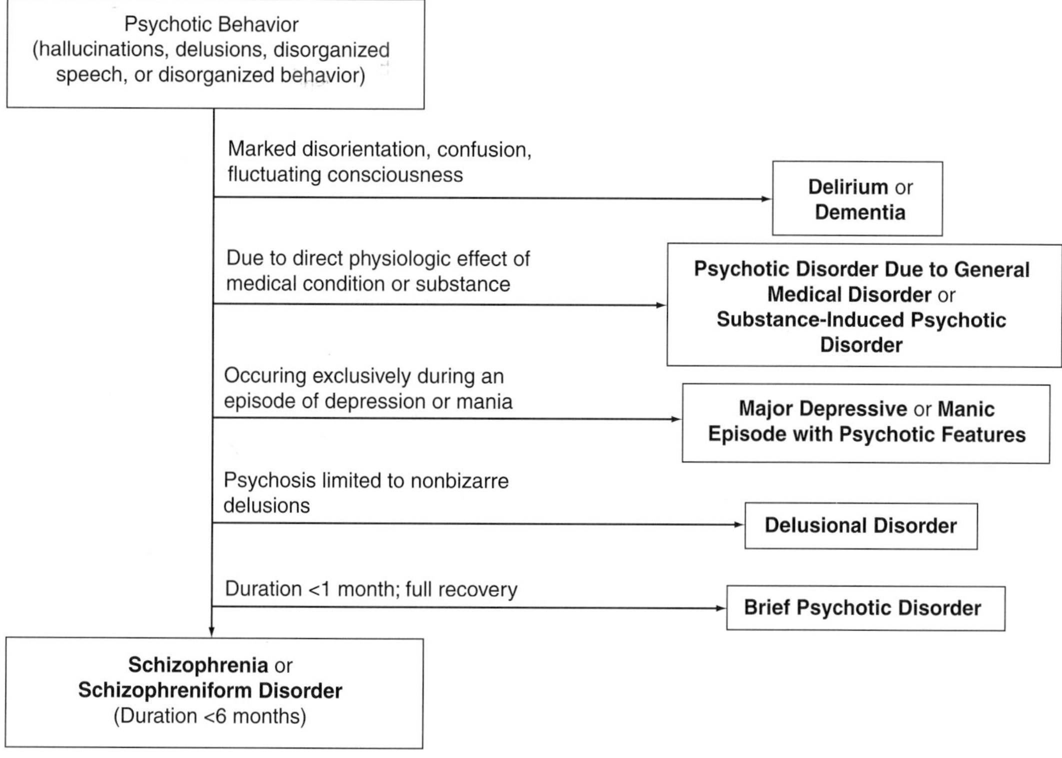

FIG. 280-1. Decision tree for evaluating psychosis.

Disorganization of thinking and behavior characterizes schizophrenia. Disheveled appearance and grooming, bizarre behavior, poor judgment, and loosening of associations indicate such disorganization. *Loosening of associations* refers to a loss of the normal logical connections between one thought and the next; the schizophrenic's speech is often vague, rambling, disjointed, or nonsensical. Fantastic experiences and bizarre ideas are described in an indifferent manner and unchanging facial expression.

Common reasons for persons with schizophrenia to come to the emergency department include worsening of psychosis resulting from stress or noncompliance with medication, suicidal behavior, assaultiveness (often as a result of paranoid thinking), and extrapyramidal side effects of neuroleptic drugs. Schizophrenics constitute a large share of the chronic homeless population and may be brought in, by authorities, in a confused state, obviously unable to attend to their basic needs. Their poor judgment and disorganization may lead to disregard for medical problems, so attention must be given to their physical status as well as the psychiatric problem.

SCHIZOPHRENIFORM DISORDER *Schizophreniform disorder* is diagnosed when the patient meets the criteria for schizophrenia but the symptoms have been continuously present for less than six months. A rapid onset over a few days and good premorbid functioning are more common than in schizophrenia.

BRIEF PSYCHOTIC DISORDER Some individuals may become acutely psychotic after exposure to an extremely traumatic life experience. If such a pyschosis lasts for less than four weeks, it is termed a *brief psychotic disorder*. Precipitants of the psychosis include the death of a loved one or a life-threatening situation such as combat or a natural disaster. Emotional turmoil, confusion, and extremely bizarre behavior and speech are common.

DELUSIONAL DISORDER *Delusional disorder* is a syndrome distinct from schizophrenia characterized by persistent nonbizarre delusions. Unlike schizophrenia, delusional disorder is rarely characterized by impairment in daily functioning, and the patient may appear outwardly normal aside from the strange ideas expressed. The onset is in middle or late adulthood, and the delusions develop over months or years. Several subtypes have been identified, the most common of which is the persecutory type, in which the delusions follow themes of being conspired against, cheated, followed, poisoned, or harassed. Other types of delusional disorder include delusional jealousy, in which the patient has an unsubstantiated conviction that one's partner is unfaithful, and the somatic type, in which patients believe they emit a foul odor or are infected with parasites.

Emergency medical evaluation may be occasioned by threats or acts of violence directed at the alleged persecutors, by suicidal behavior, or by involuntary commitment. Delusional disorders are uncommon, and more likely causes of this syndrome are psychotic depression or chronic stimulant abuse.

Mood Disorders

The mood disorders are the most prevalent of the major psychiatric disorders, affecting about 10 to 15 percent of the general population at some time in their lives. Depressive disorders are the major cause of completed suicide. An unsuccessful attempt may bring the patient to the emergency department. Mood disorders, substance abuse, and anxiety disorders are the most common psychiatric diagnoses in emergency patients.

Mood, or *affective,* disorders differ from the normal extremes of sadness and happiness in that characteristic clusters of psychological and vegetative symptoms (depressive or manic syndrome) are present, and functioning is impaired. Any of the features of schizophrenia such as delusions, hallucinations, or disorganization may be present, but if a full depressive or manic syndrome exists, a diagnosis of a psychotic mood disorder is required. Another important characteristic of affective disorders is that they tend to be episodic, with periods of remission and normal function.

In	Interest
S	Sleep
A	Appetite
D	Depressed mood
C	Concentration
A	Activity
G	Guilt
E	Energy
S	Suicide

FIG. 280-2. *In SAD CAGES.* A screening mnemonic for major depression. (From Rund DA, Hutzler JC: *Emergency Psychiatry.* St. Louis: Mosby, 1983, with permission.)

MAJOR DEPRESSION The essential features of *major depression* are a persistent dysphoric (sad) mood or pervasive loss of interest in usual activities, lasting for at least two weeks. Associated psychologic symptoms include guilt over past deeds, self-reproach, feelings of worthlessness or hopelessness, inability to experience pleasure, and recurrent thought of death or suicide. ''Vegetative symptoms'' involve physiologic functioning and include loss of appetite and weight, sleep disturbance, fatigue, inability to concentrate, and psychomotor agitation or retardation. The depression may begin gradually or rapidly but usually will have been present for several weeks before the patient comes for treatment.

When the patient complains of the full spectrum of depression symptoms, the diagnosis of major depression is easy to make, but when the chief complaint is a single symptom such as insomnia or fatigue, it will be necessary to elicit the other symptoms of major depression to make the diagnosis. Somatic complaints such as vague pain or weakness may be part of major depression, as may generalized anxiety. A useful screening mnemonic is presented in Fig. 280-2.

Major depression is more common in women, persons with a family history of depression or suicide, and individuals with medical or other psychiatric illnesses. When a medical disorder or drug produces a depressive syndrome through a presumed biologic effect on the brain, the diagnosis should be ''depression due to (the offending condition).'' Major depression is often superimposed on other mental disorders such as substance abuse, personality disorders, and anxiety disorders. Depression in the elderly may go unrecognized by the emergency physician. Screening tools for depression recognition in the geriatric population can be helpful in diagnosis.

Primary mood disorders tend to display more biologic features, are more familial, and respond better to somatic antidepressant treatment than do mood disorders due to medical disorders. The lifetime risk of suicide is 15 percent, so prompt and aggressive treatment is strongly indicated. Major depression is often recurrent, so certain patients must be maintained on long-term treatment to prevent relapse.

BIPOLAR DISORDER Bipolar disorder, previously termed *manic-depressive illness,* is characterized by the ocurrence of mania. A full manic syndrome is one of the most striking and distinctive conditions in clinical practice. The essential disturbance in mood is one of elation or irritability. Manics feel ''on top of the world,'' expansive, energetic, and precarious but may quickly become argumentative, hostile, and sarcastic, especially when their plans are thwarted.

The vegetative signs of mania are a decreased need for sleep, increased activity, rapid pressured speech, and racing thoughts. Manics may have grandiose ideas, such as unrealistic plans to start a business or run for public office, and if the grandiosity reaches delusional proportions, such patients may believe themselves to be famous, fabulously wealthy, or blessed with special powers and abilities. Poor judgment in spending money and sexual behavior may lead to problems that prompt manics' families to seek treatment for them, because manics usually lack insight into their abnormal condition and deny that anything is wrong. For this reason, reports from informants such as relatives often reveal important information to substantiate the diagnosis. Because patients who have had a manic episode almost invariably have depressions at some time (the other ''pole'' of bipolar disorder), a past history of depression may also help in diagnosis.

The disorder is equally common in men and women, and the onset is usually in the third and fourth decades. Complications include suicide, substance abuse (excessive alcohol use is common during the manic phase), and marital and occupational disruption. The course of bipolar disorder is episodic, with the duration, frequency, and regularity of the episodes varying greatly. Depressive episodes are more frequent than manic episodes.

DYSTHYMIC DISORDER *Dysthymic disorder* is a more chronic and less severe form of depressive illness and was previously termed depressive neurosis. Depressed mood must have been present most of the day, more days than not, for at least two years. Psychotic features are not seen, and these patients often have a life-long gloomy, pessimistic outlook. Women are more often affected, and the onset is in childhood, adolescence, or early adulthood. Associated personality disorders and substance abuse are common. When vegetative symptoms are present, they are usually less severe than with major depression. Major depression may be superimposed on dysthymia, often in association with stressful life events. When major depression complicates dysthymia, the patient may be brought in for evaluation because of the severity of symptoms or treatment following a suicide attempt.

Anxiety Disorders

The anxiety disorders are mental disorders in which apprehension, fears, and excessive worry dominate the psychological life of the individual. Pathologic degrees of anxiety are accompanied by varying degrees of autonomic activity out of proportion to any real danger or threat. Because anxiety is a ubiquitous condition and frequently is associated with medical illness, depression, neurologic syndromes, and psychoses, a diagnosis of a primary anxiety disorder should be made by exclusion of other causes.

Anxiety disorders are diagnosed in 4 to 8 percent of the general population, and are more often diagnosed in women than men. Because of the physical nature of certain symptoms associated with anxiety disorders, patients often seek treatment and evaluation in medical rather than psychiatric settings.

PANIC DISORDER Patients who experience recurrent attacks of severe anxiety are said to suffer from *panic disorder*. A panic attack consists of a sudden extreme surge of anxiety and dread accompanied by autonomic signs, including palpitations, tachycardia, shortness of breath, chest tightness, dizziness, sweating, and tremulousness. The symptoms develop over a few minutes at most and may either be unprovoked or occur with a phobic stimulus, such as a crowded store. After the attacks begin, some patients start to avoid situations that seem to precipitate the panic (phobic avoidance). Such behavior can severely impair their functioning. When activities are severely limited, the complication of *agoraphobia* is diagnosed. In agoraphobia, the patient tends to avoid situations where ready escape or assistance during an attack are not possible. The frequency and severity of panic attacks wax and wane, but the illness is generally chronic. Unless agoraphobia is severe, most patients are married, employed, and seldom require psychiatric hospitalization unless depression is superimposed on the anxiety disorder.

Because of the very real and frightening nature of the panic attack and its unexpected occurrence, the emergency department is a frequent initial source of medical attention. The presenting complaints may mimic a variety of medical emergencies and careful exclusion of an organic etiology is mandatory. History-taking should include questions about domestic violence and sexual abuse or assault because sometimes these experiences are the source of panic attacks.

GENERALIZED ANXIETY DISORDER When anxiety attacks are absent, yet the patient complains of persistent worry, tension, or free-floating anxiety, a diagnosis of generalized anxiety disorder should be considered. This condition lasts at least six months and is characterized by apprehensive worrying, muscle tension, insomnia, irritability, restlessness, jumpiness, or distractibility. Muscle tension may be so severe that the patient actually experiences diffuse muscular pain. Associated autonomic symptoms include the cardiopulmonary, gastrointestinal, and neurologic symptoms seen in panic attacks. In generalized anxiety disorder, such symptoms occur more continuously and chronically than in panic disorder.

PHOBIC DISORDERS Phobic disorders, other than agoraphobia, are an unusual cause of self-referral to the emergency department. In phobias, the anxiety symptoms are recognized as excessive and occur when the patient is exposed to, or anticipates exposure to, a specific situation, which then leads to avoidance of the stimulus to a degree that interferes with the patient's life. In social phobia, the situation involves having the attention of others drawn to the patient. Such activities as public speaking or meeting strangers create a fear that the patient will be embarrassed in some way. Specific phobia are quite common; they involve fear of a very specific stimulus such as animals, heights, dark, or flying.

OTHER ANXIETY DISORDERS *Posttraumatic stress disorder* is an anxiety reaction to a severe psychosocial stressor, usually life-threatening, such as military combat, fire, rape, or natural disaster. Symptoms involve repetitive and intrusive memories of the event, nightmares, emotional numbing, survivor guilt, and varying degrees of depression and anxiety. Substance abuse appears to be a frequent complication.

Obsessive-compulsive disorder is a mental disorder in which the patient experiences intrusive thoughts or images that cannot be eliminated from the mind. Typical thoughts involve images of graphic violence to self or others, contamination, or perverse sexual behavior that the patient would not carry out but nevertheless obsessively fantasizes about. To control the obsessive thoughts, the individual may engage in compulsive behavior or rituals such as excessive washing, repetitive checking, or counting. When the obsessions and compulsions occupy a great deal of time, the patient may become significantly disabled and seek psychiatric attention. The sense of helplessness and the impairment can lead to the development of depression, which also leads the patient to seek help.

Somatoform Disorders

Many patients have particular complaints or symptoms for which no medical explanation can be identified. When a physical cause has been clearly eliminated, and the complaint is not delusional or occurring in the context of a depression or anxiety disorder, somatoform disorders may be considered. When the complaint involves a loss of function, usually in the neurologic system (e.g., paralysis, blindness, numbness) and psychological factors are deemed etiologic, a *conversion disorder* may be present. The term conversion reflects Freud's hypothesis that unexpressed emotion associated with a traumatic event or situation could be ''converted'' into physical symptoms and signs. Conversion disorders are much more common in culturally and psychologically unsophisticated persons. This diagnosis should be made with extreme caution, if at all, in the emergency department because studies indicate that many patients diagnosed with conversion disorder eventually develop signs of a physical disorder explaining the symptom. Erroneous attribution to a mental disorder obviously deprives the patient of appropriate medical treatment.

Some patients have a wide variety of complaints and long complicated histories of medical problems that have no apparent medical cause. Such individuals may have *somatization disorder,* a disorder beginning in the teens and twenties, usually in women, and leading to considerable unnecessary diagnostic and surgical intervention. The prototypical patient is a middle-aged woman who describes a ''positive review of systems'' in a dramatic and confusing way. Conversion symptoms, menstrual complaints, multifocal pain, sexual and gastrointestinal symptoms, dizziness, and diverse psychiatric symptoms are common findings. The diagnosis is made when the patient has a history of a variety of medically unexplained symptoms involving multiple organ systems. As with conversion disorder, a firm diagnosis of somatization disorder should not be made on the basis of a single visit to the emergency department, but the identification of somatizing behavior is useful for future reference, because these patients frequently make repeated contacts.

Hypochondriasis may be diagnosed when the patient is preoccupied with fears of serious illness, fears that persist despite appropriate medical evaluation and reassurance.

Finally, when pain is the sole complaint and the intensity and secondary disability are unexplained by a known physical ailment, a diagnosis of *pain disorder* may be considered.

Identification of a somatoform disorder in the emergency department has such profound implications on future management that it is advisable to avoid making a firm diagnosis of these disorders unless a long history of prior similar complaints is documented and no organic disease has become apparent. This wisdom is tempered additionally because well-established conversion or other ''psychogenic'' complaints provide absolutely no protection against the development of a treatable medical disorder; new complaints always warrant careful examination for objective findings. When the physician is quite sure that no organic disease exists, the patient may be reassured that no serious physical illness is present. Avoid telling the patient that it is ''all in your head'' because this is not likely to be believed. Regular follow-up with a general internist or family physician is the best management for somatization disorder. Patients with this disorder notoriously resist psychiatric referral and treatment.

Dissociative Disorders

The dissociative disorders are a group of uncommon and poorly understood conditions where the central feature is a sudden alteration in the normal integration of identity and consciousness. The dissociation often occurs under severe stress and may or may not be recurrent, although it is rarely permanent. The forms of dissociative state relevant to emergency practice are *psychogenic amnesia,* a temporary loss of memory for important personal details that is not due to an organic cause, and *psychogenic fugue,* in which a similar loss of memory and assumption of new identity are accompanied by travel away from home. Dissociative disorders are difficult to distinguish from malingering, in which the individual in pursuit of a clear goal, such as avoiding incarceration or military duty, may consciously feign amnesia. As always, organic causes such as drug intoxication or loss of memory such as that resulting from transient global amnesia must be ruled out.

Other conditions in this category include *multiple personality disorder* and *depersonalization disorder.*

PERSONALITY (AXIS II) DISORDERS

Personality refers to an enduring pattern of perceiving, relating to, and reacting to one's environment and interpersonal relations. When a pattern of behavior is lifelong, not limited to periods of illness, and causes significant impairment in social and occupational functioning or considerable distress, a *personality disorder* is present. Some individuals are painfully aware of the consequences of their behavior but are unable to alter these fundamental ways of dealing with their world. Most of the patients who are seen clinically in medical and psychiatric settings who are diagnosed with a personality disorder lack a clear awareness of how their behavior alienates others or aggravates their own stress. Even when such insight is possible, actual personality change is unlikely.

TABLE 280-2 Behavioral Characteristics that Suggest Various Clusters of Personality Disorders

Behavior	Personality Disorder Group
Eccentric, odd, isolated, withdrawn, suspicious, inhibited, no friends, overly sensitive	Paranoid, schizoid, schizotypal
Emotional, dramatic, angry, seductive, impulsive, erratic	Antisocial, histrionic, borderline, narcissistic
Anxious, fearful, nervous, cautious	Dependent, avoidant, obsessive-compulsive

Source: Rund DA, Hutzler JC: *Emergency Psychiatry.* St. Louis: CV Mosby, 1983; DSM-IV, with permission.

The patient presenting with a personality disorder may often be recognized by the characteristic effect the interaction has on the physician and medical staff. Antisocial patients, for instance, are disliked immediately; they seem to be in control of their behavior unlike psychotic or depressed patients, but nonetheless have repeatedly engaged in maladaptive behavior. The patient may be seen as using the emergency department for some vague, or obvious, goal. These disorders are the most common secondary diagnosis in the malingerer.

The emergency physician seldom needs to decide which of the personality disorders relates appropriately to the patient. General categories of personality disorders are grouped in Table 280-2. When such features are present and seem to be interfering with some important aspect of the patient's life, personality disorder can be suspected. The presenting complaint should be evaluated appropriately, because patients with well-established character disorders still develop bona fide medical illnesses.

The personality disorder that constitutes a disproportionate share of emergency visits is *antisocial personality disorder.* The patient shows a continuous pattern of maladaptive behavior displaying disregard for the rights of others in a variety of ways: criminal behavior, fighting, lying, abuse and neglect of dependents and spouses, financial irresponsibility, recklessness, and inability to sustain enduring attachments to others.

The sociopathic behavior begins before the age of 15, but the diagnosis may not be made until after the age of 18. Sociopathy is much more frequent in males, in lower socioeconomic classes, and in relatives of alcoholics and sociopaths. Alcohol and drug abuse, imprisonment, multiple divorces, traumatic injury, accidental and violent deaths, and poor medical compliance are common complications.

Management of the antisocial patient in the emergency department is often frustrating, but anger toward the patient can be minimized and the interaction hastened along by setting firm limits on behavior, focusing on the chief complaint, and providing the patient with necessary information about the medical problem at hand. No effective psychiatric intervention can be forced on the patient, although certain patients may benefit from substance abuse treatment, psychotherapy, or organized religion when motivated to make changes in their lives. Fortunately, the most violent and disruptive behavior of many antisocials seems to ''burn out'' in the late twenties or after, although their adjustment to society often continues to be marginal.

BIBLIOGRAPHY

American Psychiatric Association. *Diagnostic and Statistical Manual of Mental Disorders,* 4th ed. Washington, DC: American Psychiatric Association, 1994.

Cannon M, Jones P, et al: Premorbid social functioning in schizophrenia and bipolar disorder: Similarities and differences. *Am J Psychiatry* 154:11, 1997.

Kandel ER: A new intellectual framework for psychiatry. *Am J Psychiatry* 155:4, 1998.

Lamarre CJ, Patten SB: Evaluation of the modified mini-mental state examination in a general psychiatric population. *Can J Psychiatry* 36:507, 1991.

Meldon SW, Emerman CL, Schubert D: Recognition of depression in geriatric ED patients by emergency physicians. *Ann Emerg Med* 30:4, 1997.

Munizza C, Furlan PM, d'Elia A, et al: Emergency psychiatry: A review of the literature. *Acta Psychiatr Scand Suppl* 374:1, 1993.

Tintinalli JE, Peacock FW, Wright MA: Emergency medical evaluation of psychiatric patients. *Ann Emerg Med* 23:859, 1994.

281 BEHAVIORAL DISORDERS: EMERGENCY ASSESSMENT AND STABILIZATION

Jeffery C. Hutzler
Douglas A. Rund

This chapter presents the principles of medical and psychiatric evaluation of patients with behavior disorders and reviews the management of suicidal and violent patients. The majority of psychiatric patient visits to emergency departments occur at night when psychiatric services are limited; therefore, the hospital must be staffed at off-hours with adequate personnel adept at handling patients who are suicidal, violent, or otherwise distraught or psychotic.

EMERGENCY APPROACH TO PSYCHIATRIC ASSESSMENT

Decision Making

A decision strategy for emergency psychiatric assessment should follow this sequence of questions: (1) Is the patient stable or unstable? (2) Does the patient have a serious medical condition that is causing abnormal behavior or thought processes? (3) If the cause of changes in behavior is not due to an underlying medical condition, it will be primarily *psychiatric* or *functional.* What is the diagnosis and severity? (4) Is a psychiatric consultation necessary? (5) When should the patient be forcibly detained for emergency evaluation?

Physical Restraint

Situations that require emergency stabilization, sometimes against a patient's wishes, involve a patient stating that he or she is potentially or actually violent, suicidal, or developing rapidly progressive medical conditions causing disturbed behavior (e.g., hypoglycemia, meningitis, or other causes of delirium). Disturbances involving actual or threatened violence are the most difficult for emergency department staff. The staff, of course, fear injury or that such patients will escape and hurt themselves or others. There are always limitations in security personnel and immediately available staff. There are often limitations in the physical facility itself in regard to restraining such patients.

Violent behavior demands immediate restraint. Hospital security forces and police are best equipped and best trained to subdue such patients with the least chance of staff or patient injury. Staff in the emergency department should not attempt to subdue a patient unless they are fully trained to do so. An initial show of force (four or five male attendants) may be sufficient to induce the patient to accept physical or chemical restraint without further resistance. Under ideal circumstances, the emergency department staff should organize themselves to be able to subdue a violent person if security personnel are not immediately available. This requires training and practice. The approach to the patient usually requires five team members with one member assigned to each limb and the leader assigned to the head. When approached from different directions and grabbed simultaneously, the violent person can usually be immobilized and restrained.

Potentially violent behavior requires the summoning of adequate force and the adoption of a nonthreatening attitude by a physician and staff. A physician should never have his or her hands out when approaching a patient or make other gestures that might be interpreted as an attack. The physician should also stay distant from the patient, avoid excessive eye contact, and maintain a somewhat submissive posture and tone of voice. Ideally, the physician should stand in a location that neither threatens the patient nor blocks his or her own retreat from the room. Allowing the patient to ventilate feelings verbally is important. Setting limits on acceptable behavior and making neutral comments may diffuse a potentially violent situation. Adequate force nearby should be visible to the patient, and the patient should clearly be told that certain kinds of behavior will result in restraint.

The decision to release a patient from physical restraints should be made jointly by medical and nursing personnel on the basis of a judgment regarding the patient's condition and behavior and not as a result of the patient's bargains or threats. Restraints should be removed in a stepwise fashion, from four limbs to two, to none.

Stabilization of an actively suicidal patient requires adequate suicide precautions. All dangerous objects are removed from the patient in the treatment room. Staff members should watch the patient closely and not allow the patient to leave the examining room unaccompanied by a staff member. Some institutions have members of the security staff available to provide supervision.

Patients who are threatening or demonstrate actual or potential violent behavior should be disrobed, gowned, and searched for weapons. Seemingly innocuous objects such as belts or belt buckles can be used by a patient to inflict self-injury or injury to others. Some emergency departments have installed metal detectors to prevent highly lethal weapons from entering the department. It has been determined that other patients do not resent the use of metal detectors because they feel safer themselves.

Initial Evaluation

The most effective tool available for the evaluation of behavioral disorders, particularly where ''organic'' mental disorders may be involved, is an excellent record of a patient's medical-psychiatric history. The history (including the use of medication, alcohol, or other drugs), physical examination, neurologic examination, and mental status examination should be incorporated into the early stages of evaluation of a person with disturbed behavior.

The changed behavior is a good starting point for inquiry. Sudden onset of major changes in behavior, mood, or thought in an individual who previously had functioned normally may be the result of an urgent medical disorder. Few ''functional'' or purely psychiatric behavioral disorders begin as abruptly as those caused by a medical condition. Behavioral disorders have resulted from all of the following life-threatening conditions:

Central nervous system (CNS) infection: meningitis or encephalitis
Intoxication
Alcohol or drug withdrawal
Hypoglycemia

Hypertensive encephalopathy
Hypoxia
Intracranial hemorrhage
Poisoning
CNS trauma
Seizure disorder
Acute organ system failure

A sudden change in behavior, especially in a patient over the age of 40, is a potentially important indicator of a new and correctable process. Neurologic symptoms associated with the behavioral changes should be explored. Such symptoms include fainting, dizziness, brief periods of disorientation, impairment of speech, confusion, loss of consciousness, headaches, and difficulty performing previous routine tasks.

The most important information about such behavioral changes will come from the patient's family. If the family is unavailable, friends or coworkers should be contacted and questioned. Third-party information may be the only source of information on a patient unable to give a cogent history. The source may be able to report substance abuse and can describe the level of previous functioning. Of course, it is important to get a history of any previous psychiatric illness or treatment. Similar previous change in behavior over past years weighs against the onset of a new "organic" process. However, it is important to weigh present information carefully to avoid a quick assumption that a patient's presentation is due to repeated occurrences of a preexisting disorder. In other words, psychiatric patients also develop medical illnesses producing change in behavior.

A medical history and review of systems is particularly important. The necessary questions can be addressed to the patient, or if he or she cannot answer these questions, a family member. Recent medical illnesses or symptoms such as infections, head trauma, fever, human immunodeficiency virus risk factors, difficulty in breathing, and dizziness should be investigated. A history of neurologic symptoms is particularly important. Any recent changes such as periods of confusion, speech difficulties, or syncope are suggestive of an organic disorder. A history of exposure to toxic substances such as heavy metals, organic solvents, or other occupational hazards may suggest a cause for newly disturbed behavior. To complete the investigation, family and social history may identify stressors in the patient's environment that are either a direct cause of changes in behavior or accentuate any responses to underlying disease.

Prescribed drugs, over-the-counter medications, illicit drugs, and alcohol can all create disturbed behavior. It is difficult to ask questions about drug use with certain patients such as the elderly,[1] the "important" patient, or those known personally by the emergency department personnel, but it is necessary. In particular, it is important to ask about the use of sedative-hypnotics, stimulants, psychotropic agents, anticonvulsants, anticholinergic agents, antiparkinsonian agents, cardiovascular drugs, diuretics, hormones, analgesics, anti-inflammatory drugs, anti-infective agents, and other categories of prescription drugs. Many of these medications cause changes in behavior when taken even in therapeutic doses. Ask specifically about over-the-counter drugs because patients rarely consider these "medications." Over-the-counter analgesics containing salicylates, anticholinergics, antihistamines, or bromides may produce delirium or toxic psychosis. Alcohol and street drugs such as phencyclidine, LSD, mescaline, amphetamines, or cocaine can produce a toxic psychosis similar to acute schizophrenia or mania. Hypnosedatives such as barbiturates or benzodiazepines may produce a confusional state or delirium both with intoxication and withdrawal.

Many emergency department patients meet diagnostic criteria for alcohol abuse, and patients with chronic mental illness have an even higher incidence of alcohol abuse than the general population. The many syndromes associated with alcohol abuse should be recognized by emergency physicians. These include intoxication, withdrawal, delirium, hallucinosis, alcohol amnestic disorder, paranoid behavior, and dementia. Alcohol screening tests are useful in disturbed patients even when the odor of ethanol is not present.

TABLE 281-1 Mental Status in the Emergency Department: An Outline

Behavior	What is the patient doing?
Affect	What feelings is the patient displaying?
Orientation	Does the patient know what is happening, where, and when?
Language	Is the patient understanding and being understood?
Memory	Can the patient recall historical details, recent and remote?
Thought content	Is the patient reporting beliefs that make little sense?
Perceptual abnormalities	Is the patient experiencing unusual sensory phenomena?
Judgment	Is the patient able to make rational decisions?

Detecting partner violence in the emergency department is an important aspect of the initial evaluation. In one study,[2] nearly 14 percent of emergency visits by women were associated with acute partner violence. Three brief questions will detect the majority of women with a history of physical or nonphysical violence in the past year. These three questions are

1. "Have you been hit, kicked, punched, or otherwise hurt by someone within the past year? If so, by whom?"
2. "Do you feel safe in your current relationship?"
3. "Is there a partner from a previous relationship who is making you feel unsafe now?"

Patients with positive screens should have this history documented in the medical record, and they should be offered counseling and referral to a safe shelter.

Mental Status Examination

The objective of the mental status examination is to distinguish functional from organic disorders. A great deal of the information obtained in mental status examinations becomes evident through patient observation and the initial patient interview (Table 281-1). Abnormal mental status examination findings suggest an organic basis for abnormal thought or behavior. Lability of affect, the necessity to repeat simple questions, irritability, disorientation, and lack of cooperation are some signs of organic dysfunction.

Important components of the mental status examination include level of consciousness, spontaneous speech, behavioral observation, physical appearance, the relaying of history information, attention, and language comprehension. This information is usually easily obtained during history taking. The more traditional mental status examination relies on specific assessment of orientation, memory, intellect, judgment, and affect.

The physician should compare his or her own direct observations of the patient's behavior with reports from the patient's family and friends. Documentation of the patient's orientation should include an assessment of attention, ability to concentrate on a specific task, and the traditional evaluation of person, place, and time. The patient should be asked the day, month, and year and place where he or she is presently being examined. Impaired language performance, including difficulty with speech, reading, writing, and word finding, may indicate a neurologic disorder. Memory is often divided into three categories: immediate, recent, and remote. Immediate memory is tested by asking a patient to repeat a series of digits (usually five) forward and backward. Recent memory can be tested by asking the patient to repeat three unrelated words immediately and then again after 3 to 5 min. The patient should be able to restate these after 3 to 5 min. The patient may also be asked about events that have occurred in the last few hours. Remote memory can be tested by asking about previous addresses, occupations, or historical events from an early period in the patient's life. Tests of memory should include details of significant personal, national, and international historical events. All history should be corroborated.

Investigation of higher cognitive functions includes assessment of a patient's general command of information; mental calculation, especially subtraction, such as serial sevens; and spelling of words forward and backward (such as world). Patients with organic disease often have difficulty spelling backward or performing serial calculation. The patient's affect or outward display of emotion should be evaluated for sadness, euphoria, and anxiety. This may help distinguish between cognitive disturbance induced by depressive disorders and dementia due to significant cerebral pathology. An examiner can draw some conclusions regarding a patient's thought processes during the patient's own telling of his or her history.

Disordered thought processes include paranoid or grandiose delusions, fixed false beliefs, and delusional denial of illness. Such beliefs should be compared with reports from family and friends.

Visual hallucinations do occur in functional psychotic illnesses (schizophrenia or affective disorder), but most often result from organic disease. A patient with visual hallucinations should always be assumed to have organic pathology until proven otherwise.

Judgment may be impaired in organic disease, and historical evidence of faulty judgment should be elicited. Insight about judgment can be gained by asking a patient how he or she would deal with day-to-day problems, such as finding the way home from the hospital.

Finally, the examiner should test for specific focal neurologic deficits, including apraxias, agnosias, right-left disorientation, aphasias, and inability to follow complex spoken and written commands. Such signs may or may not occur in association with other localizing neurologic signs, such as asymmetric reflexes, paresthesia, or hemiparesis.

Ask the patient to "draw a clock face." The physician can draw a circle on a piece of paper and ask the patient to fill in the numbers on the paper to look like a clock face. If the patient can put in the numbers correctly in a clock face, he or she should then be asked to put the hands at the position to read a specific time. If the patient cannot do these tasks, organic disease is present.

Accurately diagnosing and understanding behavioral emergencies in the elderly is difficult but important. Syndromes include confusion, agitation, psychosis, and behavioral regression. Diagnoses that cause emergency syndromes such as this in the elderly are listed in Table 281-2.

TABLE 281-2 Diagnoses That Cause Emergency Behavioral Syndromes in the Elderly[1]

Delirium
Medications (especially anticholinergic agents), physical illness (especially infections and metabolic diseases), and drug withdrawal states (especially alcohol).

Dementia
Alzheimer's disease and multi-infarct dementia account for 75 percent. However, treatable causes include drugs, depression, endocrine diseases, normal pressure hydrocephalus, subdural hematomas, and alcohol dependency.

Medications
Psychotropic drugs, digitalis, cimetidine, and anticonvulsant medications.

Physical illnesses
Renal and hepatic failure, chronic obstructive pulmonary disease, cardiovascular illnesses, and electrolyte imbalance.

Depression
Bipolar disorder, major depression, melancholia, psychotic depression.

Alcohol intoxication/dependency
Alcoholism, alcohol abuse secondary to chronic depression, decreased tolerance/increased sensitivity to alcohol.

Physical Examination

The objectives of physical examination are to identify disorders that may cause or have an impact on the behavior disorder and identify the presence of medical problems that may need special care in, or are inappropriate for, management in a psychiatric setting.

A physical examination should be conducted on every patient. Vital signs are a simple physical screening test of patients with altered behavior. Abnormal vital signs, when observed, must not automatically be dismissed as secondary to anxiety or stress. Bradycardia can be seen in patients with hypothyroidism, Stokes-Adams syndrome, or elevated intracranial pressure. Tachycardia may be apparent in patients suffering from hyperthyroidism, infection, heart failure, pulmonary embolus, or alcohol withdrawal. Fever is often associated with extreme hyperthyroidism or thyroid storm, vasculitis, alcohol withdrawal, sedative-hypnotic withdrawal, meningitis, or various inflammatory processes. Hypothermia is observed in sepsis, dermal disease, hypoendocrine status, CNS dysfunction, and intoxication. Hypotension may be an indicator of shock, Addison's disease, hypothyroidism, or medication side effects. Hypertension may be associated with hypertensive encephalopathy or stimulant abuse. Tachypnea is seen in patients with metabolic acidosis, pulmonary embolism, pneumonia, cardiac failure, or fever. Any such disorders may result in a secondary behavioral disturbance. The limited expense of, and useful information provided by, vital signs justifies their use in all patients.

A general physical examination should ideally be conducted with the patient completely disrobed and gowned. The patient should be carefully checked for signs of trauma. Contusions or abrasions of the head, face, and neck may be common if the patient is bellicose and may suggest the possibility of otherwise unsuspected head injuries. Extremities should be checked for frostbite or other evidence of exposure-related injury. If trauma is demonstrated or suggested by history, the mechanism of injury should be carefully reconstructed. For a variety of reasons, patients may omit or underreport the extent and cause of trauma.

Chest, cardiac, and abdominal examinations should be carefully performed and a careful neurologic examination should be specific for features that suggest organic disease. Other neurologic signs, such as bilateral asterixis or multifocal myoclonus, are often associated with delirium.

Laboratory Evaluation

The selection of particular laboratory tests emerges from diagnostic needs suggested by the history and by the findings of mental status examination and physical examination. Fluid and electrolyte disorders are common in elderly patients. Hypoglycemia can precipitate aggressive or agitated behavior, and an elevated white blood cell count may signify infection in patients with acute changes in mental status. Tests

TABLE 281-3 Laboratory Tests to Help Identify Causes of Agitation

Test	Cause of Agitation
White blood cell count	Infection
Serum electrolytes, calcium, magnesium	Hypo- or hypernatremia, hypo- or hypercalcemia, hypomagnesemia (delirium tremens)
Blood glucose	Hypoglycemia
Liver function	Alcoholic hepatitis, hepatic encephalopathy
Serum amylase	Pancreatitis
Blood urea nitrogen	Renal failure, uremic encephalopathy
Serum creatinine	Renal failure, uremic encephalopathy
Creatine phosphokinase	Rhabdomyolysis, myocardial infarction
Electrocardiogram	Myocardial infarction
Chest x-ray	Pneumonia, pneumothorax
Arterial blood gases	Hypoxemia, pulmonary embolus
Toxicologic analysis	Toxic effects of anticholinergics, cimetidine, alcohol and sedative hypnotic drugs, dopamine agonists (L-dopa, amantadine, bromocriptine), lidocaine, pentazocine, corticosteroids, stimulants, cocaine, phencyclidine, opiates (such as meperidine)
Cerebrospinal fluid	Central nervous system infection, intracranial bleeding
Computerized axial tomography	Mass lesion, stroke, atrophy
Magnetic resonance imaging	Stroke, demyelination
Electroencephalogram	Seizure (generalized, complex partial, nonconvulsive status)

that can be helpful when a patient presents with agitation are listed in Table 281-3.

EMERGENCY SITUATIONS REQUIRING EMERGENCY INTERVENTION

Suicide

The annual rate of suicide in the United States is about 11/100,000 accounting for at least 31,000 deaths annually.[3] There seem to be epidemiologic differences between suicide attempters and suicide completers. Suicide completers, for instance, are more likely than attempters to be older, male, living alone, or physically ill. These are high-risk patients who need to be carefully assessed. The ratio of attempted suicides to completed suicide is estimated to be about 40:1.

A suicide attempt is not a common accompaniment of the ''downward'' portion of the normal mood swings occasionally experienced by everyone. Only about 2 percent of the general population have seriously considered taking their lives and only about 1 percent have actually attempted suicide. Therefore, suicide attempters must be taken seriously. The attitude of the staff should be empathic; suicide precautions should be instituted; and, following medical management, the assessment of suicide risk should be carefully evaluated and documented. The decision to hold and hospitalize such patients should be given serious consideration.

Suicidal thinking is more frequent among women than among men and is associated with a clinical depression, social isolation, undesirable life events, and early parental loss. Suicidal thinking may precede an actual attempt by many months and may persist long after improvement in mental status and personal relationships.

Negative attitudes toward the suicide attempter have been documented among all types of emergency personnel: paramedics, nurses, and emergency physicians. A negative attitude intensifies a patient's already low self-esteem, thus increasing the risk of subsequent suicide and making it difficult to establish a therapeutic relationship.

Schizophrenia, substance abuse, and depression are psychiatric diagnoses that place a suicidal patient at relatively high risk.[3] Personality disorder and adjustment disorder implying a transient situational disturbance are frequent diagnoses in suicide attempters and are generally associated with relatively lower completion risk than the major psychiatric illnesses noted previously. Patients with these disorders still show a higher risk of completed suicide than the general population.

Drug overdose accounts for the overwhelming majority of all contemporary suicide attempts. Drugs used for suicide attempts tend to parallel prevailing prescribing patterns. Toxicity of the agent and the lethal intent of the patient help assess the relative risk. A patient taking a large dose of amitriptyline would be considered at greater risk than someone taking a few antihistamine tablets. Some patients may be relatively unaware of a drug's potential toxicity, however, and such knowledge and their continuing intent to die must be assessed by questions such as ''Were you surprised to find yourself alive after taking the overdose?''

Violent attempts (shooting, jumping, hanging) are generally considered serious and a high-risk factor for a future attempt. A number of reports have described a ''wrist-cutting syndrome'' in young, unmarried women whose self-mutilation, although repetitive, has seldom been thought to be serious in intent. These acts usually have been carried out in a state of mounting tension with depersonalization followed by relief after self-mutilation. A significant number of ''wrist slashers,'' or self-mutilators, however, whose cases have been followed for 5 to 6 years, have committed suicide.

In determining suicide risk, a general rule is that the risk of a successful suicide rises with advancing age. Men are two to three times more likely than women to complete suicide, whereas women are two or three times more likely than men to attempt suicide. Patients who are single, divorced, separated, widowed, or unemployed are at higher risk than those who are married and employed.

A psychotic patient who attempts suicide requires careful observation, whatever restraint necessary, and evaluation by a psychiatrist. A psychotic patient may respond unpredictably to distorted perceptions in a fearful or driven manner.

Secondary gain is a term that indicates that while the primary motive for a suicide attempt appears to be death, the attempt may meet another need such as attention or a plea for emotional help. When such needs are met by the attempt, a secondary gain is achieved and the risk of subsequent suicide attempt is lessened momentarily. It is dangerous, however, to assume that secondary gain is the cause of a suicide attempt with an initial evaluation in an emergency department. All suicide behaviors should be taken seriously.

Perhaps the most important part of the assessment of the suicide attempter is a determination of the patient's feelings and thoughts at the time of the interview. The patient who experiences helplessness, exhaustion, overwhelming depression, and a clear expression of intent to die certainly remains at high risk. If a patient expresses continuation of such feelings at the time of the interview, the physician has sufficient evidence that the patient needs psychiatric consultation immediately. Some patients, however, seem to equate self-injury with other forms of emotional discharge such as crying, talking to a friend, or becoming inebriated. They do not perceive the event as an attempt to end their life. When asked about their feeling at the time of the attempt, such patients may indicate that they were angry or vengeful. Attitudes and affect that generally indicate a good prognosis at the time of the interview are anger, remorse, or embarrassment. A patient who sits quietly, refusing to provide additional information to an examiner, should be considered at high risk. Feelings of hopelessness, helplessness, or exhaustion seem to be among the clearest indicators of long-term suicidal risk in patients hospitalized at one time for depression.

Patient disposition can be aided by estimating the lethality of the attempt and the likelihood of rescue. When there is a high likelihood of rescue and low lethality, a patient is considered at lower risk than in the reverse situation. A patient who makes a hanging attempt in a desolate wooded area is at greater risk than a person who takes a handful of relatively nontoxic pills in front of witnesses.

Patients who have made previous suicide attempts have traditionally been considered to be at greater risk for future suicide. Prior attempts seem a particularly ominous sign, particularly if the intensity and apparent lethality of the suicide attempts escalate with each subsequent attempt.

A "No Harm Contract"[4] is very useful in the emergency department in evaluating suicidal risk. The "No Harm Contract"[4] is a verbal or written agreement, initiated by the emergency room physician or psychiatrist, in which the suicidal patient is asked to agree not to harm or kill himself or herself for a particular period of time. This can be therapeutic, helping to reveal the intent of the patient and reduce it. It can also be diagnostic in assessing the nature and severity of a patient's suicidality. It can uncover specific issues precipitating suicidal thoughts and the ability of the patient to contract for safety.

A very difficult decision in the emergency department is when to discharge a child or adolescent patient who has expressed suicidal thoughts or behavior. Consideration of the following criteria is suggested before discharging a child or adolescent patient with suicidal ideation or behavior from the emergency department:[5]

1. The patient must not be imminently suicidal.
2. The patient must be medically stable.
3. The patient and the parents agree to return to the emergency department if suicidal intent recurs.
4. The patient must not be intoxicated, delirious, or demented.
5. Potentially lethal means of self-harm have been removed.
6. Treatment of underlying psychiatric diagnoses has been arranged.
7. Acute precipitants to the crisis have been addressed and attempts been undertaken to resolve them.
8. The physician believes that the patient and family will follow through on treatment recommendations.
9. The patient's caregivers and social supports are in agreement with the discharge plans.

Adolescents who complete suicide are more likely to have had histories of substance or drug abuse, disruptive disorders, anxiety, mood disorder, or schizophrenia. Precipitating events are usually stressors such as disciplinary crises, being in trouble with the law or at school, or the loss of a relationship.[6]

A summary of high-risk and low-risk suicide profiles is presented in Table 281-4.

TABLE 281-4 Evaluation of Suicide Risk in Adults and Adolescents

Demographic and Social Profile	High Risk	Lower Risk
Sex	Male	Female
Marital status	Separated, divorced or widowed	Married
Family history	Chaotic, conflictual Family history of suicide	Stable
Job	Unemployed	Employed
Relationships	Recent conflict or loss of a relationship	Stable relationships
School	In disciplinary trouble	No disciplinary problems
Religion	Weak or no suicide taboo	Strong taboo against suicide
Health		
Physical	Acute or chronic illness Excessive drug or alcohol use	Good health Little or no drug or alcohol
Mental	Depression (Sig ECAPS) Schizophrenia or bipolar history Panic disorder Disruptive behavior Feelings of helplessness or hoplessness	No depression No psychosis Minimal anxiety Directable, oriented Has hope
Suicide ideation	Frequent, intense, prolonged	Infrequent, low intensity, transient
Suicide attempts	Repeated attempts Realistic plan High risk Guilt Continuing wish to die	No prior attempts No plan High likelihood of rescue Embarrassment about suicide ideation No continuing wish to die
Other	Lack of concern Unsupportive family Socially isolated	Good insight Concerned family Socially integrated

Clinical Management

High-risk patients whose suicide intent is strong and immediate require immediate psychiatric hospitalization. Moderate-risk patients are those who present in a serious suicidal crisis, but who, because of a positive response to initial intervention and favorable social support, are not judged to be in immediate danger. Hospitalization can often be avoided with such patients, provided practical outpatient treatment can be established immediately. Such determinations are most often made in concert with a psychiatric consultant. Available means of suicide, such as firearms or drug caches, should be removed, and any psychotropic medication should be used judiciously and prescribed conservatively. It is important to have a family member take charge of a patient's medications.

Before discharging a patient, the physician must be certain that the patient has a good social support system and there is an absence of clearly pathologic features that predispose the patient to subsequent suicide. The support system usually includes a place to live and family or friends who will support the patient emotionally.

Low-risk patients frequently present with suicidal threats or minor attempts that occur in the context of a clearly definable external crisis. Social support is usually available and responsive. However, because many attempts that appear trivial on first glance are found to have more serious implications on closer examination, all patients presenting following a suicide attempt should be carefully assessed. If there is any question about the safety of discharging a suicidal patient, and psychiatric consultation is not immediately available, the patient should be hospitalized.

Chemical Restraint

Chemical restraint should be administered after gathering as much information as possible to enable provisional diagnostic assessment. Once initial medical history, physical examination, and laboratory information have been obtained, if a patient continues to chafe against restraints and to show uncontrolled behavior, the use of a pharmacologic intervention to assist in behavioral control might be considered. Although a variety of medications can be used, the only one with a clear advantage over the rest is lorazepam (Ativan), a potent benzodiazepine that has the advantages of the wide therapeutic index of the class, rapid onset of action, and the ease of administration by parenteral or oral routes. Lorazepam is the only benzodiazepine that can be reliably administered intramuscularly (IM), and its oral and parenteral potencies do not greatly differ, allowing for ease in dosage calculation. Alternative medications such as short-acting barbiturates have a much narrower therapeutic index, and sedating neuroleptic medications such as the phenothiazines have the disadvantage that those which are most sedating also cause the greatest difficulty with orthostatic hypotension. Useful dosage levels of lorazepam would be 1 to 2 mg orally (PO) or IM every half-hour until an adequate level of sedation is achieved. If this is insufficient, haloperidol can be used. The dose is 5 mg IM in younger adults and 1 to 2 mg IM in the elderly. However, haloperidol should not be given to those with Parkinson's disease or other movement disorder. The combination of haloperidol (5 mg) and lorazepam (2 mg) is sometimes given initially to calm agitated behavior, especially if psychotic features are present. Droperidol (Inapsine), 2.5 to 5 mg intravenously (IV), ensures rapid onset of tranquilization. Hypotension from droperidol occurs in a number of patients and is generally treated with a 250 to 500 mL crystalloid infusion.

Consultation and Referral

In the ideal setting, all emergency departments would have psychiatric consultation available at all times. However, in many instances, the physician in the emergency department will be forced to rely on more limited resources. Many psychiatric problems leading to emergency department presentation do not require immediate definitive treatment. In many instances, disposition following initial screening can be made to a variety of secondary sources of evaluation and treatment. Judgments regarding referral depend on assessment of a patient's likelihood of becoming violent toward self or others. Clues that suggest potential violence include hostile behavior, verbal aggressiveness, or statements about violent intent. Such patients need immediate hospitalization. Marked disorientation and confusion require evaluation for organic components. In the absence of such indications, referral can be made to a psychiatrist or a psychiatric facility. Results of the emergency department medical and psychiatric evaluation should be summarized in writing and provided to the consultant. The patient should receive clear discharge instructions and should have a follow-up interval for any medical or surgical disorders that were identified.

REFERENCES

1. Tueth MJ: Diagnosing psychiatric emergencies in the elderly [review]. *Am J Emerg Med* 12:364, 1994.
2. Feldhaus KL, Koziol-McLain J, Amsbury HL, et al: Accuracy of 3 brief screening questions for detecting partner violence in the emergency department. *JAMA* 277:1357, 1997.
3. Jamison UR, Baldessarini RJ: Effects of medical interventions on suicidal behavior. *J Clin Psychiatry* 60(suppl 2):3, 1999.
4. Stanford EJ, Goetz RR, Bloom JD: The No Harm Contract in the emergency assessment of suicidal risk. *J Clin Psychiatry* 55:344, 1994.
5. Press BR, Khan SA: Management of the suicidal child or adolescent in the emergency department [review]. *Curr Opin Pediatr* 9:237, 1997.
6. Schaffer D, Craft L: Methods of adolescent suicide prevention. *J Clin Psychiatry* 60(suppl 2):70, 1999.

PSYCHOTROPIC MEDICATIONS

Richard A. Nockowitz
Douglas A. Rund

The emergency physician must be able to administer certain selected psychotropic medications appropriately and recognize and manage side effects, toxicities, and adverse interactions with other medications.

There are four major classes of psychotropic medications dealt with here: antipsychotics, anxiolytics/sedative-hypnotics, antidepressants, and mood stabilizers such as lithium and anticonvulsants. There are multiple indications for several of these medications, particularly the antidepressants and anticonvulsants. However, only the antipsychotic and anxiolytic classes have undisputed utility on an emergency basis. Antidepressants and lithium are rarely prescribed by the emergency physician, primarily because they have long latencies of action and multiple side effects and require careful long-term monitoring. Only in exceptional circumstances, in consultation with a psychiatrist who agrees to provide follow-up care, might the emergency physician elect to initiate antidepressant or lithium therapy. Extensive pretreatment evaluation and detailed patient education weigh heavily against prescribing lithium, MAOIs, or heterocyclic antidepressants in the emergency department.

The emergency physician should be familiar with the emergency indications, common side effects, toxic reactions, and common interactions of the psychotropic medications. Caution in prescribing is the rule. Certain cases are bound to be complex, requiring detailed psychiatric evaluation, and serious medical disorders may coexist with psychiatric disorders. Patients with medical disorders, a history of serious side effects with psychotropic medication, or apparent need for more than one psychoactive medication usually require psychiatric consultation.

ANTIPSYCHOTICS (NEUROLEPTICS)

Indications

Because antipsychotic medications are symptom-specific (not disease-specific), they are useful in nearly all psychoses, whether primary (due to psychiatric illness) or secondary (substance-induced or due to a general medical condition). In the emergency setting, they are most often indicated to control agitated or psychotic behavior that constitutes an imminent danger to the patient or others.

A known allergy to a specific antipsychotic medication is a contraindication to its use and to use of other antipsychotic medications of the same class. Most patients who claim to be allergic to antipsychotic medications, however, actually describe a history of acute dystonic reactions when questioned more carefully.

Guidelines

Low-potency antipsychotics (Table 282-1) such as chlorpromazine (Thorazine) and thioridazine (Mellaril) may cause significant hypotension and thus are rarely used in emergency medicine. High-potency antipsychotics such as haloperidol (Haldol) and fluphenazine (Prolixin) have relatively few anticholinergic and alpha-blocking effects and are remarkably safe, even at high doses. They are the emergency antipsychotic agents of choice.

Optimal pharmacologic management of acute agitation or psychosis is to use a high-potency neuroleptic such as haloperidol intravenously. Oral or intramuscular dosing is also acceptable if intravenous administration is not possible. In most patients, the initial drug is haloperidol. The initial dosage of 2 mg is doubled every 45 min until the symptoms are controlled, the patient is calmed, or the behavior is stabilized. The best approach is not to think of the dosages as cumulative but rather to find the one single dosage that effectively treats the symptoms. Once this is accomplished, use this particular effective dose on an ''as needed'' basis each time the patient's symptoms reappear. Some clinicians augment this strategy with a dose or two of a benzodiazepine (e.g., 1 or 2 mg lorazepam) to control the symptoms. This proves useful in certain circumstances, such as with an agitated psychotic or manic patient, because there is a synergistic effect between the two medications. Additionally, the benzodiazepine may prevent potential extrapyramidal problems that occasionally occur with neuroleptic use. These are easily managed if they do occur, however, as discussed in the following section. One advantage to using haloperidol intravenously is an exceptionally low incidence of extrapyramidal side effects compared with the incidence seen with intramuscular or oral routes of administration. Dosages may need to be half those described or less if the patient is elderly, debilitated, brain-injured, or has AIDS.

TABLE 282-1 Commonly Used Antipsychotic Agents

Generic Name	Brand Name	Approximate Equivalent Dose, mg	Relative Potency
Phenothiazines			
Aliphatic			
Chlorpromazine	Thorazine	100	Low
Triflupromazine	Vesprine	30	Low
Piperidines			
Mesoridazine	Serentil	50	Intermediate
Thioridazine	Mellaril	100	Intermediate
Piperazines			
Acetophenazine	Tindal	15	Intermediate
Perphenazine	Trilafon	10	Intermediate
Trifluoperazine	Stelazine	5	High
Fluphenazine	Prolixin, Permitil	2	High
Thioxanthines			
Aliphatic			
Chlorprothixene	Taractan	100	Low
Piperazine			
Thiothixene	Navane	4	High
Dibenzapine			
Loxapine	Loxitane, Daxolin	15	Intermediate
Dihydroindolones			
Molindone	Moban	10	Intermediate
Butyrophenones			
Haloperidol	Haldol	2	High
Droperidol	Inapsine (for injection)	2	High

Side Effects

Antipsychotics block dopamine receptors throughout the central nervous system (CNS). Dopamine receptor blockade in the mesolimbic areas accounts for their antipsychotic properties. Dopamine blockade in the nigrostriatal tract is responsible for the majority of motor side effects, including acute dystonias, akathisia, and Parkinson's syndrome.

Acute dystonias, which usually occur in young males during the trial phase of antipsychotic treatment, are probably the most common side effect of antipsychotic medications seen in the emergency department. Muscle spasms of the neck, face, and back are the most common dystonias, but oculogyric crisis and even laryngospasm may also occur. When a drug history is not carefully obtained, dystonias are often misdiagnosed as primary neurologic illnesses (seizures, meningitis, tetanus, etc.). Treatment with either 1 to 2 mg of benztropine IV or 50 to 100 mg of diphenhydramine IV rapidly corrects the dystonia. Dystonias often recur, even if the antipsychotic is decreased or discontinued, however, unless an antiparkinsonian drug such as benztropine, 1 mg PO two to four times daily, is administered over the next several days.

Akathisia, a sensation of motor restlessness with a subjective desire to move, can begin several days to several weeks after initiation of antipsychotic treatment. Often misdiagnosed as anxiety or exacerbation of psychiatric illness, akathisia is aggravated by subsequent increases in antipsychotic dosage. Other coexisting extrapyramidal effects, such as cogwheel rigidity and shuffling gait, suggest antipsychotic effect, but these signs are not invariably present. Management can be difficult, but some useful strategies are known. If possible, the dosage of the antipsychotic should be decreased. The best treatment is probably administration of beta blockers. Propanolol 30 to 60 mg per day is a good starting dose. Some patients need 90 to 180 mg per day as blood pressure and heart rate allow. Antiparkinsonian or anticholinergic drugs such as benztropine, 1 mg PO two to four times daily, may also afford some relief. In refractory cases, the antipsychotic may need to be changed to an atypical agent, as discussed below.

Antipsychotic-induced *Parkinson's syndrome* is particularly common in the elderly and usually begins in the first month of treatment. A complete Parkinson's syndrome, including bradykinesia, resting tremor, cogwheel rigidity, shuffling gait, masked facies, and drooling can occur, but often only one or two features of the syndrome are obvious. Antipsychotic dosage reduction and/or anticholinergic medication is usually effective.

Whereas antidopaminergic extrapyramidal side effects (EPS) such as acute dystonia, akathisia, and Parkinsonism occur more often with high-potency neuroleptics, anticholinergic and anti-adrenergic effects are more commonly seen with low-potency neuroleptics. Both anticholinergic and alpha-blocking effects are dose-related and much more common in the elderly.

Anticholinergic effects range from mild sedation to delirium. Peripheral manifestations may include dry mouth and skin, blurred vision, urinary retention, constipation, paralytic ileus, cardiac dysrhythmias, and exacerbation of narrow-angle glaucoma. The central anticholinergic syndrome is characterized by dilated pupils, dysarthria, and an agitated delirium. Discontinuation of the antipsychotic and institution of supportive measures is the most prudent therapy. Physostigmine, 1 to 2 mg administered slowly IV may temporarily reverse the syndrome but may be very toxic and should be reserved for life-threatening situations.

Cardiovascular side effects are seen almost exclusively with low-potency antipsychotics. The exception to this is the rare occurrence of torsades de pointes caused by high dosages of high-potency neuroleptics such as haloperidol and droperidol. Alpha-adrenergic blockade and a negative inotropic effect on the myocardium may cause pronounced orthostatic hypotension and, rarely, cardiovascular collapse. Usually the hypotension can be easily managed with IV fluid. In severe cases, agonists, such as metaraminol (Aramine) or norepinephrine (Levophed), may be required.

Neuroleptic malignant syndrome (NMS) is an uncommon idiosyncratic reaction to neuroleptic drugs manifested by rigidity, fever, autonomic instability (tachycardia, diaphoresis, and blood pressure abnormalities), and a confusional state. Elevation of muscle enzymes, such as creatinine phosphokinase (CPK) and aldolase, the white blood cell count, and liver function tests are often seen. While high-potency antipsychotics may be more likely to cause the disorder, all antipsychotics are potential offenders. NMS is a medical emergency and has a mortality rate as high as 20 percent. Management includes immediate discontinuation of the antipsychotic medication, hydration, and meticulous supportive treatment in an intensive care setting. Anticholinergic medications are not helpful and may worsen the condition by further impairing centrally mediated temperature regulation. Medications such as dantrolene sodium or bromocriptine are sometimes used to relieve the rigidity. See Chap. 153 for a detailed discussion.

Overdose

While antipsychotics are rarely fatal when taken alone, overdose can present some unique management problems. With the exception of thioridazine (Mellaril), antipsychotics are potent antiemetics. The antiemetic effect may interfere with pharmacologic induction of emesis, and gastric lavage is often required. Agents with beta-agonist activity such as isoproterenol are contraindicated for cardiovascular support because beta-stimulated vasodilatation may worsen hypotension. Extrapyramidal effects may also be prominent in antipsychotic overdosage and are best treated with 50 to 100 mg IV of diphenhydramine (Benadryl).

ATYPICAL AGENTS

Clozapine

Clozapine (Clozaril) is an ''atypical'' antipsychotic medication in that it is preferentially more active at limbic than at striatal dopamine receptors and causes few or no EPS. Unfortunately, it may produce agranulocytosis, so its use is reserved for patients with schizophrenia unresponsive to standard agents and for those suffering from severe EPS or tardive dyskinesia with the standard agents. Use of clozapine requires weekly complete blood counts (CBC) the first 6 months of use and then every 2 weeks after that. Any white blood cell count less than 3500 requires closer monitoring, whereas a white blood cell count less than 2000 or absolute granulocyte count less than 1000 mandates immediate discontinuation of the drug and consultation with a hematologist. Fever may be a side effect during the first few weeks of therapy and should prompt an immediate CBC. If the CBC is normal, the fever will typically reverse. Clozapine is strongly sedating, strongly anticholinergic, and has considerable hypotensive effects. It also poses a substantial risk for inducing seizures, particularly when higher doses are used. Respiratory depression and arrest have been reported rarely, and there is a suggestion that coprescription of a benzodiazepine may increase the risk for this side effect.

Commonly reported features of overdose include altered sensorium (drowsiness, delirium, and coma), tachycardia, hypotension, respiratory depression and failure, hypersalivation, and seizures. Management, in addition to administration of activated charcoal, is symptomatic and supportive. Epinephrine and its derivatives should be avoided, as should antidysrythymics such as procainamide and quinidine. Close surveillance, including cardiac and vital sign monitoring, should continue for several days because of risk of delayed toxic effects. Fatal overdosages have been reported, usually at dosages over 2500 mg.

Risperidone

Risperidone is another ''atypical'' antipsychotic medication whose pharmacologic profile of potent serotonin (5-HT_2) antagonism and moderate dopamine (D_2) antagonism probably accounts for its relatively lower risk of EPS. Unlike clozapine, it does not have increased risk of agranulocytosis. Common side effects include sedation, insomnia, constipation, and weight gain. Cardiovascular effects may include small, short-term increases in heart rate, accompanied by reduced systolic/diastolic blood pressure, orthostatic hypotension, and QT-interval prolongation. Seizures have been reported in 0.3 percent of patients.

Features of overdose generally reflect exaggerated pharmacologic effects: drowsiness, sedation, tachycardia, hypotension, EPS, prolonged QT, widened QRS and, in several instances, seizure. Management is basically supportive. Cardiovascular monitoring is imperative. Should antidysrhythmic therapy be required, agents such as disopyramide, procainamide, and quinidine, which have the potential for QT-prolonging effects, should be avoided. As with more traditional antipsychotics, agents that may worsen effects of β-adrenergic blockade, such as bretylium, epinephrine, and dopamine, should also be avoided.

Olanzapine

Olanzapine (Zyprexa) has a chemical profile very similar to that of clozapine and thus causes little or no EPS. It also has the advantage of not being known to cause agranulocytosis and thus does not require monitoring of the white blood count. Its main adverse effects can include considerable weight gain, sedation, and mild anticholinergic activity. Little is known at this time about effects of overdose, but exacerbation of brain side effects such as somnolence and anticholinergic signs would be expected.

Quetiapine

Quetiapine (Seroquel) is the newest atypical antipsychotic agent and, like the others, is characterized by a high $5\text{-HT}/D_2$ binding ratio, responsible for its low incidence of EPS, while maintaining its antipsychotic effect. It has a high affinity for histaminic and α-adrenergic receptors, however, causing prominent adverse effects of sedation, orthostatic hypotension, and some dizziness. Little is known about effects of quetiapine in overdose.

ANXIOLYTICS

Indications

Severe emotional distress may indicate a need for psychotropic medication, even if the patient is not psychotic or an imminent threat to him- or herself or others. While not a substitute for psychotherapy, short-term anxiolytic therapy may be particularly beneficial in the anxious, agitated patient during a psychosocial crisis. Anxiolytics are also indicated for acute panic reactions unresponsive to reassurance.

Anxiolytics have utility in medical and surgical emergencies as well. Nonpsychiatric uses include facilitation of cooperation and mus-

TABLE 282-2 Commonly Used Benzodiazepines

Generic Name	Brand Name	Approximate Half-life, h	Usual Total Oral Dose, mg
	ANXIOLYTICS*		
Alprazolam	Xanax	12	1–6
Chlorazepate	Tranxene	48	15–60
Chlordiazepoxide	Librium	20	15–60
Diazepam	Valium	35	15–60
Lorazepam	Ativan	16	2–6
Midazolam	Versed	2	—‡
Oxazepam	Serax	15	20–60
Prazepam	Centrax	15†, 100†	20–60
	HYPNOTICS		
Flurazepam	Dalmane	2†, 72†	15–30 qhs
Temazepam	Restoril	15	15–30 qhs
Trizolam	Halcion	2	0.125–0.5 qhs

*Anxiolytics are administered in divided doses, usually three or four times daily.
†Flurazepam and prazepam have active metabolites with long half-lives.
‡Midazolam is available for parenteral use only.

cle relaxation during painful procedures; controlling seizures; treating alcohol, sedative, or hypnotic withdrawal; and allaying anxiety when a painful procedure such as surgery has been delayed.

Benzodiazepines are contraindicated in patients with known hypersensitivity to benzodiazepines and in acute, narrow-angle glaucoma. Pregnancy, particularly in the first trimester, is a relative contraindication.

Guidelines

Before prescribing anxiolytics, the emergency physician should try to rule out any serious underlying psychiatric illness. Because agitation and anxiety may indicate incipient psychosis or major affective disorder, anxiolytics should be used with extreme caution in patients with a history of major psychiatric illness. The possibility that a patient may be feigning illness to procure controlled substances should also be considered.

Benzodiazepines are very effective anxiolytics with a high therapeutic index. Nonbenzodiazepine anxiolytics (e.g., barbiturates and propanediols) have low therapeutic indices and high addiction potential. Except in the rare case of an allergy to benzodiazepines, nonbenzodiazepine anxiolytics have little use in modern psychopharmacology. Buspirone hydrochloride (BuSpar), an atypical anxiolytic medication that does not interact with the benzodiazepine-GABA receptor complex, has a delayed onset of action of days to weeks, which makes it impractical for use in emergent situations. Since it does not have cross-tolerance with other sedative/hypnotics or alcohol, it is not useful in treatment of sedative/hypnotic or alcohol withdrawal.

Certain benzodiazepines have relatively long half-lives (Table 282-2), including diazepam (Valium), chlordiazepoxide (Librium), flurazepam (Dalmane), and prazepam (Centrax). Agents with long half-lives gradually accumulate in the body and thus have a greater potential for causing sedation and confusion, particularly in the elderly. For short-term use, these agents may benefit the young, healthy person in crisis who complains of insomnia but is also anxious during the day. A single bedtime dose both induces sleep and has a mild anxiolytic effect the following day. For the most part, however, with the exception of the use of diazepam in seizures, short-acting benzodiazepines such as lorazepam (Ativan), oxazepam (Serax), and alprazolam (Xanax) are the preferred agents in emergency medicine. Alprazolam (Xanax), 0.25 to 0.50 mg PO, is a particularly effective treatment in acute panic attack. Lorazepam, an agent with very low cardiopulmonary toxicity, is particularly well suited for emergency use. Dosages of 1 to 2 mg PO or IM are usually effective. Only midazolam (Versed), a very short-acting agent, and lorazepam (Ativan) have reliable intramuscular absorption. As with all benzodiazepines, dosage adjustments may be necessary: higher dosages may be required in patients with histories of alcohol or sedative/hypnotic abuse; lower dosages in patients with hepatic disease or severe debilitation. Because they potentiate other CNS depressants, benzodiazepines should be used with extreme caution in intoxicated patients. Benzodiazepines particularly suppress hypoxic respiratory drive and should be used with caution in patients with hypercarbia, especially if the patient is also receiving supplemental oxygen.

Side Effects

Benzodiazepine side effects are usually mild and easily treated. Drowsiness, decreased mental alertness, sedation, and ataxia are the most common side effects. Such effects can usually be managed conservatively by decreasing the dose and advising the patient to avoid potentially hazardous activities, such as driving or operating dangerous machinery. Excessive sedation and overdose can be reversed with flumazenil by giving 0.2 mg IV over 15 to 30 s and then 0.2 to 0.4 mg every 30 to 60 s up to 1 to 3 mg total dose depending on the circumstances. This is contraindicated, however, in mixed overdoses and chronic benzodiazepine use. Infrequent paradoxical responses to benzodiazepines of insomnia and agitation are more common in the elderly and require discontinuation of the medication. Because benzodiazepines have abuse potential and high street value, the emergency physician should never prescribe more than a week's supply.

HETEROCYCLIC ANTIDEPRESSANTS (HCAs)

Although tricyclic antidepressants (named for their three-ring structure) were first synthesized in the nineteenth century, their antidepressant properties were not recognized until the late 1950s. Since that time, other "cyclic" antidepressant agents have been formulated thus creating need for the more general term *heterocyclic* (Table 282-3). The therapeutic effect of HCAs is believed to be related to secondary downregulation of norepinephrine and serotonin postsynaptic receptors after initial blockade of presynaptic reuptake of norepinephrine and serotonin. HCAs are primarily indicated for major depression but may also be effective for dysthymic disorder, panic disorder, agoraphobia, obsessive compulsive disorder, enuresis, and school phobia. As pre-

TABLE 282-3 Commonly Used Heterocyclic Antidepressants

Generic Name	Brand Name	Usual Dose mg/day
	TRICYCLICS	
Amitriptyline	Amitril, Elavil, Endep	75–200
Amoxapine	Asendin	100–300
Desipramine	Norpramin, Pertofrane	75–200
Doxepin	Adapin, Curetin, Sinequan	75–200
Imipramine	Janimine, Presamine, SK-Pramine, Trofranil	75–200
Nortriptyline	Aventyl, Pamelor	40–150
Pritriptyline	Vivactil	15–40
Trimipramine	Surmontil	75–200
	OTHERS	
Maprotiline	Ludiomil	100–150
Trazodone	Desyrel	100–200

viously advised, initiation of HCA therapy in the emergency department is not routinely recommended.

Side Effects

HCAs have low therapeutic indices. Side effects are common and often occur with customary dosages, even though serum levels may be within the designated therapeutic range. The majority of side effects are either anticholinergic or cardiotoxic.

Anticholinergic side effects are the most common. They are particularly likely to occur with concomitant use of other drugs with anticholinergic properties, such as low-potency antipsychotics, antiparkinsonian agents, antihistamines, and over-the-counter sleeping remedies. Both peripheral and central effects may occur. Peripheral effects include dry mouth, metallic taste, blurred vision, constipation, paralytic ileus, urinary retention, tachycardia, and exacerbation of narrow-angle glaucoma. Central effects include sedation, mydriasis, agitation, and delirium. Mild to moderately severe anticholinergic effects may be managed by dosage reduction, change to a medication with fewer anticholinergic properties, or addition of urecoline, 10 to 25 mg PO three times daily. For acute urinary retention, urecoline, 2.5 to 5 mg may be given subcutaneously. When anticholinergic effects become life-threatening, physostigmine, 1 to 2 mg administered *very slowly* IV, may be used. If physostigmine toxicities ensue, the effects can be reversed with IV atropine sulfate, 0.5 mg for each 1.0 mg of physostigmine administered.

Cardiac side effects of HCAs may include nonspecific T-wave changes, prolonged QT interval, varying degrees of AV block, and atrial and ventricular dysrhythmias. Orthostatic hypotension from α-adrenergic blockade may be significant, particularly in the elderly.

HCA therapy may also be complicated by allergic obstructive jaundice; decreased seizure threshold (especially with maprotiline, clomipramine, and amoxapine); and, very rarely, agranulocytosis.

Trazodone has little in common with other HCAs. It lacks significant anticholinergic or cardiac conduction effects but may be associated with marked sedation, ventricular dysrhythmias, and significant orthostatic hypotension. It may also cause priapism, a urologic emergency.

MONOAMINE OXIDASE INHIBITORS (MAOIs)

MAO catalyzes the oxidation of biogenic amines (tyramine, serotonin, dopamine, and norepinephrine) throughout the body. The therapeutic effect of MAOIs is probably related to their ability to increase norepinephrine and serotonin in the CNS. They are recommended for atypical major depressive episodes, characterized by hyperphagia, hypersomnolence, reversed diurnal variation (worse in the evening), emotional lability, so-called leaden paralysis (heavy leaden feelings in arms or legs), and rejection hypersensitivity. They are also occasionally useful in selected cases of HCA-refractory major depression and panic disorder. Only two agents in this class, phenelzine (Nardil) and tranylcypromine (Parnate), are commonly used in the United States. As with HCAs, initiation of therapy in the emergency department is not recommended. The physician who initiates MAOI therapy must have firmly established an appropriate indication for use and provided the patient with extensive counseling about toxic interactions with numerous medications and foods.

Side Effects

In general, MAOIs have fewer side effects than do HCAs. *Orthostatic hypotension,* although occasionally severe, usually responds to supportive therapy. *CNS irritability,* including agitation, motor restlessness, and insomnia, is managed by dosage reduction or addition of a benzodiazepine. Occasionally, MAOIs, like other antidepressant medications, actually precipitate a manic episode. *Autonomic side effects,* such as dry mouth, constipation, urinary retention, and delayed ejaculation, sometimes occur but are usually mild.

MAOIs block oxidative deamination of tyramine and may precipitate a *hypertensive crisis* when certain drugs, such as sympathomimetic amines, L-dopa, narcotics, or HCAs, or tyramine-containing foods are ingested. Common tyramine-containing foods include aged cheese, beer, wine, pickled herring, yeast extracts, chopped liver, yogurt, sour cream, and fava beans. The onset of the crisis is usually heralded by a severe headache. While hypertension is potentially the most serious effect, cardiac dysrhythmias, restlessness, diaphoresis, mydriasis, and vomiting may also occur. Beta-blocking agents are contraindicated, since they may intensify vasoconstriction and worsen hypertension. Although death may occur from hypertensive intracranial hemorrhage, the vast majority of patients recover completely from the hypertensive episode within a few hours. The MAOI can be restarted the following day after dietary counseling is reinforced.

Drug-drug interactions often complicate MAOI therapy. MAOIs potentiate the actions of sympathomimetics, anticholinergics, and oral hypoglycemics. They also inhibit metabolic degradation of alcohol, barbiturates, and narcotics. When combined with meperidine (Demerol), MAOIs may cause a variety of adverse effects, including hypotension, hypertension, fever, and neuromuscular irritability. While the interactions listed are among the most common, the list is far from exhaustive. More comprehensive accounts may be found in standard references.

SELECTIVE SEROTONIN REUPTAKE INHIBITORS (SSRIs)

Since the introduction of fluoxetine (Prozac) in 1988, the SSRIs have become the most commonly prescribed antidepressants in the United States. Other SSRIs currently available include sertraline (Zoloft), paroxetine (Paxil), fluvoxamine (Luvox), and citalopram (Celexa). SSRIs are primarily indicated for treatment of major depressive episodes but also have utility in dysrhythmia and anxiety disorders including generalized anxiety disorder, panic disorder, and obsessive compulsive disorder. Because of their favorable side effect profile and relative safety in overdose, some have argued that institution of an SSRI by an emergency department physician may occasionally be appropriate if (1) the patient can be assessed to rule out general medical causes for the depression, (2) ongoing substance abuse can be ruled out, and (3) the patient can be followed in the emergency setting until picked up by another health care provider. However, this rationale has rightly been questioned because of the concern over SSRIs and other antidepressants precipitating mania. The detection of bipolar disorder, because of its many variations and subtle forms, requires evaluation by an experienced psychiatrist. All antidepressants carry some degree of risk for precipitating a manic or mixed episode in a patient predisposed to bipolar illness.

Side Effects

SSRIs lack the anticholinergic and cardiac effects typical of the HCAs, although there have been several reports of symptomatic bradycardia with fluoxetine. The side effect profile of SSRIs reflect their potent serotonin antagonism. Among the most common side effects are headaches, dizziness, sexual dysfunction, nausea, diarrhea, insomnia, and agitation. Less common side effects are akithisia and apathy syndrome. A significant advantage of SSRIs is their high therapeutic index and associated low lethality, even when large quantities are ingested acutely.

An SSRI discontinuation syndrome has become apparent, more commonly with agents having a shorter half-life (e.g., sertralene, paroxetelene). It typically presents several days after cessation of one drug and is characterized by a flulike syndrome including nausea, vomiting, fatigue, myalgias, vertigo, headache, insomnia, and sometimes parathesias. Treatment is to reinstate SSRI therapy and taper more gradually.

A serotonin syndrome with SSRIs can occur when SSRIs are combined with other serotonergic medications such as the MAOIs. The syndrome is manifest by both CNS (restlessness, tremor, myoclonus, hyperreflexia, and seizures) and gastrointestinal (nausea, vomiting, diarrhea) irritability. Consequently, SSRIs or any medication that enhances serotonin levels should not be combined with MAOIs. Treatment of the serotonin syndrome consists of discontinuing the serotonergic agents and providing supportive care.

NEWER "COMBINATION" ANTIDEPRESSANTS

Whereas most tricyclic antidepressants enhance norepinephrine levels, SSRIs enhance serotonin levels, and psychostimulants (a category not discussed here) enhance dopamine levels. The newer antidepressants evidence "combinations" of these effects through various mechanisms. Examples of this include venlafaxine, bupropion, nefazodone, and mirtazapine.

Venlafaxine (Effexor)

Venlafaxine, which is structurally distinct from other antidepressants, is conceptually a combination of a tricyclic and an SSRI in that it enhances both serotonin and norepinephrine (as well as dopamine slightly) through reuptake blockade. It's advantages are relative freedom from medication interactions and no significant affinity for muscarinic, histaminic, and α-adrenergic receptors. Although lack of blockade for various receptors improves its side-effect profile somewhat, common complaints include agitation and insomnia, nausea, occasional dizziness, constipation, and sweating. Potential problems associated with venlafaxine include dose-related, sustained hypertension and the growing awareness of a significant discontinuation syndrome requiring very slow tapering of the drug. The hypertension needs to be monitored and may require lowering of the medication. The discontinuation syndrome can be significant. It usually occurs within days to 2 weeks after lowering or stopping the drug and is similar to SSRI discontinuation symptoms. It can be treated with an SSRI or by increasing the venlafaxine and tapering it more slowly. Venlafaxine should not be used in combination with an MAOI.

Bupropion (Wellbutrin)

Bupropion is also structurally unique and works by initiating reuptake inhibition of both norepinephrine and dopamine, the former more than the latter. It also interacts with few other medications and has a favorable side-effect profile due to its minimal anticholinergic and antihistaminic effects. It is being used also to aid in smoking cessation.

Common side effects include some initial restlessness and insomnia that typically resolves within 2 weeks. It is noted for having the lowest incidence of sexual side effects, which are common with other antidepressants, including SSRIs. In fact, when bupropion is added for SSRI-induced sexual dysfunction, sexual functioning improves in many patients. One concern with this drug had been a dose-related increase in the incidence of seizures. However, further study has shown no higher incidence at usual therapeutic dosages compared with other antidepressants. Caution should be taken when using this drug in patients with bulimia or metabolic disturbances predisposing to seizures. Likewise, individual doses greater than 200 mg and daily dosages greater than 400 mg should be avoided. Combination with an MAOI is to be avoided as well. Bupropion may be the least likely of all antidepressants to precipitate a switch into mania.

Nefazodone (Serzone)

Nefazodone inhibits serotonin reuptake inhibitors and blocks postsynaptic serotonin receptors (5-HT_2) at the same time. It is similar chemically to trazodone but possesses less α-adrenergic blockade. Common side effects are dizziness, headache, dry mouth, and nausea. Some patients also have problems with orthostatic hypotension and drowsiness. Anxiety is less of a problem with this drug compared with SSRIs, and sexual side effects are less common. It may be particularly useful for depression-associated insomnia.

Mirtazapine (Remeron)

Mirtazapine antagonizes inhibitory norepinephrine autoreceptors and heteroreceptors, causing increased release of norepinephrine and serotonin. The main side effects are somnolence, increased appetite, weight gain, and dizziness. Although serotonin enhancement is one of this drug's end results, it is via a very different mechanism, and the typical SSRI side effects are usually minimal. Given the limited clinical experience with this relatively new medication, effects of overdose are not well known.

MOOD STABILIZERS

Although lithium has been the mainstay of bipolar disorder (manic-depression) treatment for years, anticonvulsants such as carbamazepine, valproic acid, and now gabapentin and lamotrigine have come to play an increasingly important role in the management of this and other neuropsychiatric disturbances.

Lithium

Lithium carbonate is indicated for both acute mania and maintenance therapy in bipolar disorder. It also has utility in some cases of major depression (both unipolar and bipolar) and in some disorders characterized by episodic explosive outbursts or self-mutilation. Its mechanism of action is not exactly known, although it may relate to reducing dopaminergic function, enhancing serotonergic function, or reducing "excessive signaling" by the phosphytidylinositol system. The extensive pretreatment evaluation and long latency of action preclude the use of lithium as an emergency psychotropic medication. The emergency physician should be aware, however, of its side effects and signs of toxicity.

Side Effects

Patients vary widely in susceptibility to lithium side effects. While most of the serious adverse effects are associated with toxic serum levels, mild side effects such as gastrointestinal distress, dry mouth, excessive thirst, fine tremors, mild polyuria, and peripheral edema are often seen even when serum levels lie within the designated therapeutic range. This is particularly common during the first few weeks of therapy. Many of the more chronic side effects, including polyuria, nephrogenic diabetes insipidus, benign diffuse goiter, hypothyroidism, skin rashes and ulcerations, psoriasis, and leukocytosis without a left shift, appear unrelated to serum lithium levels. Underlying neurologic illness, dehydration, salt-restricted diets, and childbirth predispose to both minor and major side effects.

Toxicity and Overdose

The severity of lithium toxicity is related to both the serum lithium level and the duration of the elevated level. Even in acute overdose, symptoms may not be fully apparent for up to 48 h. As a general rule, lithium toxicity is rare at serum levels of less than 2 mEq/L. Early signs of toxicity include nausea and vomiting, dysarthria, lethargy, and a coarse hand tremor. As toxicity worsens, neurologic symptoms increase. Ataxia, myasthenia, incoordination, hyperreflexia, muscle fasciculation, blurred vision, and scotomas may develop. Eventually, confusion, choreoathetosis, myoclonus, and seizures occur, and the patient may finally become comatose. Cardiovascular toxicity is unusual at serum levels of less than 4 mEq/L. In addition to nonspecific

T-wave changes, high lithium levels may be associated with hypotension, AV conduction defects, ventricular tachydysrhythmias, and eventually complete cardiovascular collapse.

Because lithium toxicity may result in permanent neurologic sequelae, it should be considered a medical emergency. General supportive care, with particular attention to fluid and electrolyte balance, is the foundation of therapy. Lithium excretion may be facilitated by forced saline diuresis and alkalinization of the urine with IV sodium lactate. Mannitol, 50 to 100 mg IV, may also be added to promote osmotic diuresis. Aminophylline, 500 mg given slowly IV, also promotes lithium clearance by both suppressing renal tubular reabsorption of lithium and increasing renal blood flow. If the serum level exceeds a 4 mEq/L, the patient should be dialyzed immediately. Dialysis may also be required for serum levels in the range of 2 to 4 mEq/L if the patient's clinical condition is poor.

Anticonvulsants

These drugs all act through different mechanisms to cause either enhanced GABA inhibitory function or decreased glutamate and aspartate excitatory release, both of which ultimately result in neuronial relaxation or stabilization. They have come to be used for mood stabilization in rapid-cycling, cyclothymic, and mixed states of bipolar illness. Recent studies have demonstrated their superiority over lithium for such indications. Other uses are for impulsive aggression, behavioral disturbances in head-injured patients and patients exhibiting self-injurious behavior, and even for the irritability commonly seen in severe personality disorders. The side effects of carbamazepine and valproic acid are well known from their use as anticonvulsants.

Gabapentin is well tolerated, has few drug interactions, and does not need blood level monitoring. It may be titrated quickly and may be useful for patients already on multiple medications or with hepatic impairment. The main disadvantages are drowsiness, ataxia, and nausea at high dosages.

Lamotrigine is also well tolerated, with few adverse behavioral or cognitive effects. It does have some drug interactions (carbamazepine, valproate) and risk of potentially severe and fatal rash such as Stevens-Johnson and toxic epidermal necrolysis. The rash is more common in children and seems to be related to starting at too high a dosage, titrating too rapidly, and concomitant valproate therapy. Such a rash dictates immediate cessation of the medication in almost all circumstances. There may be additive toxicity with carbamazepine as well, causing more ataxia and dizziness than when used alone.

BIBLIOGRAPHY

Andersson C, Chankos M, Mailman R, et al: Emerging roles for novel antipsychotic medications in the treatment of schizophrenia. *Psychiatr Clin North Am* 21(1): 151–179, 1998.

Brown ES, Dilsaver SC, Bowers TC, et al: Droperidol in the interim management of severe mania: Case reports and literature review. *Clin Neuropharmacol* 21(5): 316–318, 1998.

Chan BS, Graudins A, Whyte IM, et al: Serotonin syndrome resulting from drug interaction. *Med J Aus* 169(10): 523–525, 1998.

Gultmacher B: *Concise Guide to Psychopharmacology and Electroconvulsive Therapy*. Washington: American Psychiatric Association, 1994.

Hassan E, Fontaine DK, Nearman HS: Therapeutic consideration in the management of agitated or delirious critically ill patients. *Pharmacotherapy* 18(1): 113–129, 1998.

Hughes JR, Goldstein MG, Hurt RD: Recent advances in the pharmacotherapy of smoking. *JAMA* 281(1): 72–76, 1999.

Hyman SE (ed): *Manual of Psychiatric Emergencies*, 3d ed. Boston: Little, Brown, 1994.

Janick PT, et al: *Principles and Practice of Psychopharmacotherapy*. Baltimore: Williams & Wilkins, 1997.

Seetle EC, Jr: Antidepressant drugs: Disturbing and potentially dangerous adverse effects. *J Clin Psychiatry* 16(595): 25–30, 40–42, 1998.

Trzepacz PT: Delirium. advances in diagnosis, pathophysiology, and treatment. *Psychiatr Clin North Am* 19(3): 429–448, 1996.

283 ANOREXIA NERVOSA AND BULIMIA NERVOSA

Alexander H. Sackeyfio
Susan J. Gottlieb

Anorexia nervosa and bulimia nervosa have reached epidemic proportions in the last 15 years. These diseases were once viewed as purely psychological in nature. However, increasing evidence has confirmed that both disorders involve physical complications, and knowledge of and ability to treat the medical complications of eating disorders are crucial for the patient's well-being.

Eating disorders affect between 5 and 10 percent of adolescent girls and young women, and up to 0.10 percent of males. Originally regarded as rich girls' diseases, they are now recognized across all socioeconomic and racial groups and in patients between the ages of 8 and 80. The onset of anorexia is usually between 12 years of age and the mid-thirties, with a bimodal distribution at ages 13 to 14 and 17 to 18. Bulimia usually begins between the ages of 17 and 25. The onset of both disorders has been reported in older persons.[1,2]

Anorexia, with its resulting starvation syndrome, is more likely to be recognized than is the commoner bulimia, which is frequently concealed from both family and physician. Table 283-1 lists the signs and symptoms that suggest a diagnosis of anorexia, and Table 283-2 lists the signs and symptoms of bulimia.

Anorexic patients[3] may present with one or all of the following:

1. Refusal to maintain body weight over a minimum normal weight for age and height; for example, weight loss or failure to make expected weight gain during a period of growth, leading to body weight 15 percent below normal
2. Intense fear of becoming obese even when underweight
3. Disturbance in the way in which body weight, shape, or size is perceived; for example, an obviously underweight or even emaciated patient's complaining of being fat or believing that one area of the body is "too fat"
4. Absence of at least three consecutive expected menstrual cycles (primary or secondary amenorrhea)

A diagnosis of bulimia[3] is suggested by the following:

1. A minimum average of two episodes of binge eating (rapid consumption of a large amount of food in a short period of time) per week for at least 3 months
2. A feeling of lack of control over the eating behavior during the eating binges
3. Regular engagement in self-induced vomiting, use of laxatives, strict dieting, fasting, or vigorous exercising in order to prevent weight gain
4. Persistent overconcern with body shape and weight

TABLE 283-1 Clues to Undiagnosed Anorexia Nervosa

Unexplained growth retardation
Unexplained primary amenorrhea
Weight loss of unknown origin
Unexplained hypercholesterolemia or carotenemia in a thin person
Exercise abuse
Membership in a vulnerable vocational group (see last item in Table 283-2)

TABLE 283-2 Signs and Symptoms of Bulimia in Adolescents and Young Adults

Hypokalemia of unknown cause or complications of hypokalemia (cardiac, renal, central nervous system)
Metabolic acidosis related to laxative abuse or excessive exercise
Parotid gland or submandibular gland enlargement, esophagitis, esophageal bleeding or rupture
Large unexplained weight fluctuations or weight loss
Unexplained elevations of serum amylase level
Unexplained secondary amenorrhea
Extensive loss of dental enamel or onset of many new caries
Scars on the knuckles of the hand (from induced vomiting)
Presence of juvenile diabetes mellitus
Other disorders of impulse control (alcoholism, drug abuse, borderline personality disorder)
Member of predisposed vocational group (models, ballet students or professionals, wrestlers, jockeys)

A third diagnosis[3] to be considered is eating disorder not otherwise specified. It is characterized by

1. For females, all criteria for anorexia except still menstruating
2. All criteria for anorexia except normal weight
3. All criteria for bulimia but lower frequency or duration
4. Regular use of compensatory weight control measures after small amount of food
5. Chewing and spitting out but not swallowing large amounts of food
6. Binge-eating disorder

The diagnosis of an eating disorder should be considered in a premenarchal patient who engages in potentially unhealthy weight-control practices and/or demonstrates obsessive thinking about food, weight, and height, especially if there is a delay in the maturation for gender and age. Families of patients with eating disorders tend to be outwardly orderly, respectable, and conventional. However, the inner dynamics of the family involve a rigid adherence to secret obligations and stifling prohibitions. Honesty and spontaneity are discouraged, and true autonomy and self-gratification are submerged beneath the adolescent's desire to please and gain approval from other family members.

ETIOLOGY

The onset of anorexia most often occurs during adolescence.[1] Normal physiologic changes that are preparation for the reproductive function, namely, an increase in total body fat (up to 200 percent in adolescent females) as well as the accumulation of fat around the chest and hips, are perceived as "fatness," and the adolescent begins to diet to lose the unwanted weight. Various reasons have been proposed for the progression of "normal" dieting into an eating disorder. Some feel that, for the anorexic, restriction of eating serves as a part of a general need to control impulses and disturbing feelings. Others have suggested that the central problems might be an avoidance of adulthood, an emergent panic related to the challenge of late adolescence, and the loss of the security enjoyed by the child and early adolescent.[1,2]

Bulimics have an intense need for approval, a high self-expectation, and a poor body image. Bingeing provides escape from boredom, anger, and loneliness and is sometimes a preferred social experience, especially when interpersonal intimacy has been elusive. Purging adds to an already negative self-image. Binge eating in bulimics almost always begins as a response to hunger from dieting and weight loss. Late in the syndrome, binge eating becomes generalized to deal with emotional distress.[1,2]

DIAGNOSIS

The differential diagnosis includes both psychiatric and medical disorders. Schizophrenics can present with an aversion to eating and sometimes with eating and purging. In depressive illness, anorexia and hyperphagia can be part of the presenting symptoms. Hysterics, patients with inadequate personality disorders, and patients with borderline personality disorders may also exhibit eating disorders.

A number of medical disorders should be considered, including superior mesenteric artery syndrome, inflammatory bowel disease, chronic hepatitis, Addison disease, diabetes, hyperthyroidism, hyperemesis gravidarum, tuberculosis, and malignancy. About 20 percent of teenage diabetics also have an eating disorder.[1] Extremely thin people in professions requiring low weight (e.g., ballet dancers, models, and jockeys) and runners may or may not have an eating disorder.[2]

PATHOPHYSIOLOGY

Eating disorders are associated with a number of physiologic changes (Table 283-3). Cachectic patients are relatively well adapted to their chronically deprived, mildly catabolic state. The hypothalamus is affected by low fat intake, which disturbs the reproductive, metabolic, growth, and neurohypophyseal hormones. There is an associated fall in metabolic rate, protein levels are preserved, and cell-mediated immunity tends to be normal.[4]

TABLE 283-3 Physiologic Changes Associated with Eating Disorders

HEMATOLOGIC
Normochromic and normocytic anemia
Leukopenia with relative lymphocytosis
Low sedimentation rate
Reduced C3 complement level
ELECTROLYTE
Hypokalemia
Hyponatremia
Hypomagnesemia
Hypocalcemia
Hypophosphatemia
CARBOHYDRATE METABOLISM
Low serum insulin levels
High serum glucagon levels
Starvation ketosis and hypoglycemia
Abnormal glucose tolerance due to fasting
Hypercholesterolemia
ENDOCRINE
Normal T4 and low T3 levels
High serum cortisol level without diurnal variation
Low serum luteinizing hormone, follicle-stimulating hormone, and estradiol levels
Low total urinary estrogen level
Increased growth hormone level
Pseudo-Bartter's syndrome (laxative and diuretic abusers)
Decreased antidiuretic hormone secretion (diabetes insipidus)
Decreased peripheral adrenergic activity with normal adrenomedullary function

Self-induced vomiting results in various disorders. Dental problems are caused by gastric acid regurgitation into the oral cavity. In addition, the oral hygiene of most anorexics is poor, and the vigorous brushing often done by bulimics aggravates dental problems. This poor oral hygiene, together with dietary deficiencies and dehydration of the soft tissue of the mouth, can cause gingivitis and dental erosion.

Parotid and submandibular gland enlargement is often seen. Oral lacerations and contusions, and callus formations on knuckles from stimulating the gag reflex, are common. Dysphagia, hematemesis, and, rarely, rupture of the esophagus, subcutaneous emphysema, or pneumomediastinum can occur following excessive purging. Easy bruising due to loss of bile salts and poor absorption of vitamin K is another complication. Severe hypokalemia and hypovolemia often accompany recurrent vomiting. Ipecac abuse can cause a dermatomyositis-like syndrome and cardiomyopathy. Hyperamylasemia, probably of salivary gland origin, is associated with purging episodes.

Laxative abuse produces weight loss mainly by dehydration and hypokalemia. Common nonspecific complaints of laxative abuse include constipation, diarrhea, abdominal cramping, and bloating. Severe potassium depletion due to chronic laxative abuse and intense physical exercise may contribute to myonecrosis. Specific effects include melanosis coli and cathartic colon. In carthartic colon, the colon is converted into an inert tube incapable of propelling the fecal stream without large doses of laxatives. This condition is not entirely reversible and may require colectomy. Brownish gray hyperpigmented areas on the skin are reported as complications of phenolphthalein-containing laxatives (e.g., Correctol and Ex-Lax).

Diuretic abuse results in dehydration and multiple serum abnormalities, including hypokalemia, hypercalcemia, hyperuricemia, hypomagnesemia, and hyponatremia.

Binge eating after a period of starvation can result in acute gastric distention and/or pancreatitis. Postbinge pancreatitis has a reported 10 percent mortality rate.

Periods of starvation result in hypoglycemia, which is a poor prognostic indicator. Hypoglycemia is often associated with hypothermia, coma, and infections, and may be fatal. Starvation leads to low insulin levels that are insensitive to both glucose and amino acid infusion. Gastric distention and reduced gastric emptying produce enhanced satiation and prolonged intermeal intervals. Food has been demonstrated to remain in the stomachs of anorexics for up to 24 h.

Starvation causes decreased hypoxic ventilatory drive, vital capacity, tidal volume, and minute ventilation. In addition, the surfactant pool is reduced, resulting in ''stiffer'' lungs with a greater tendency to collapse. The muscles of ventilation are affected by starvation, causing reduced diaphragm mass and respiratory muscle weakness.

Cardiovascular changes include brady- and tachyarrhythmias due to cardiomyopathy or electrolyte abnormalities. ST-T wave changes and Q-T-interval prolongation may be evident. Decreased peripheral adrenergic activity with normal adrenomedullary function results in bradycardia and orthostatic hypotension.

Dermatologic changes include pedal or pretibial edema with or without hypoalbuminemia, excessive loss of subcutaneous fat, brittle hair and nails, pellagra or scurvy, and petechiae or purpura.

Peripheral neuropathy, most likely a product of chronic malnutrition, is a notable complication.[5] Localized compression neuropathies secondary to subcutaneous tissue loss can also develop. Some patients experience paresthesias of the fingers and toes. Deep tendon reflexes may be diminished, and gross motor coordination may be impaired.

Anorexics are especially likely to be compulsive exercisers. Stress fractures[6] in the feet, march hemoglobinuria, and various musculoskeletal overuse syndromes have been identified as complications of compulsive exercise.

Osteoporosis is common in anorexics. It usually affects the femur, radius, and spine, in order of decreasing frequency. Estrogen deficiency is not a major causative factor. Any patient with an eating disorder who has been amenorrheic and low in weight for more than a year should undergo bone-density studies. A femur fracture has been reported in a young anorexic who tripped on a rug.[6]

Adolescent diabetics induce ketosis by skipping insulin for a day or two to lose weight; sometimes they overeat and increase insulin in compensation. The abuse of insulin and food can lead to severe metabolic consequences. Young diabetics with frequent hospitalizations should be evaluated for a coexisting eating disorder.

PSYCHOLOGICAL PRESENTATIONS

In addition to the presenting physical symptoms, psychological manifestations may be detected on emergency evaluation. Depression, including suicidal ideation, is the primary psychological complication of eating disorders. Other psychological manifestations include obsessive-compulsive personality traits, with rumination about food, calories, and weight. Ritualistic eating and exercising behavior are also evident. Perfectionistic striving often results in deterioration of friendships and leisure activities.

Impulse-control disorder is a psychological complication of eating disorders more commonly seen in bulimics than in anorexics. Other behavioral manifestations include shoplifting and stealing, sexual promiscuity, drug and alcohol abuse, and self-mutilation.

PROGNOSIS

As with most mental illnesses, the earlier the onset, detection, and treatment, the better the prognosis. Eating disorders can have potentially irreversible effects on the physical and emotional growth of adolescents. There is evidence suggesting improved outcome with early treatment, and therefore the threshold for intervention should be lower than with adults. The prognosis for individuals who have engaged in maladaptive eating patterns for years is guarded. Behaviors may remain constant, or the patient may improve briefly and return to the eating disorder during stressful times. Psychological immaturity persists in about 50 percent of the patients, with difficulties in social adjustment, and one-third continue to have problems with eating. Chronicity increases the risk of morbidity.

Despite advances in the understanding of anorexia and bulimia nervosa, eating disorders are still associated with significant long-term rates of morbidity and mortality. Mortality figures range from 2 to 5 percent to a high of 18 percent. Abnormally low albumin levels and low body weight (<60 percent ideal body weight) best predict a lethal course. High creatinine and uric acid levels predict chronicity in anorexics.[7] Death may result from suicide, starvation, metabolic catastrophe, infection, and cardiac insufficiency. Agents used to induce weight loss may lead to fatal complications.

TREATMENT

Emergency management of patients with eating disorders involves consideration of the complications and effects of the disorder. Nutritional rehabilitation should be the primary goal of treatment in both anorexia and bulimia. Anorexics tend to need a very gradual introduction of macronutrients. Bulimics tend to need fewer calories initially, and it is important to normalize the eating pattern.

Normotensive, hypokalemic, hypochloremic metabolic alkalosis is typical of purging eating-disorder patients. They appear to adapt to these metabolic states, and treatment should consider the whole metabolic state. Automatic replacement of individual deficiencies should be discouraged, since this could be dangerous, with fluid overload and overcorrection as common complications.

Medications have been used in eating disorders. The most helpful in anorexia is cyproheptadine hydrochloride (Periactin). Antidepressants have proved useful in bulimics. Fluoxetine (Prozac), imipramine or desipramine, and phenelzine sulfate (Nardil) have been extensively evaluated and found to be useful.[8]

Emergency management is best accomplished using total parenteral nutrition and slowly correcting the metabolic derangement. Cachectic patients do not need or secrete inducible enzymes, such as lipase or lactase. They have reduced gastric emptying and atrophy of the villi of the small intestines. The use of tube feeding can lead to hypertonic dehydration, hypernatremia, prerenal azotemia, and refeeding pancreatitis. Circulatory volume and caloric requirements should be advanced slowly. The refeeding syndrome, with severe cardiopulmonary and neurologic complications, has been described in anorexics and is associated with rapid electrolyte shifts, hypophosphatemia, hypokalemia, and hypomagnesemia.[9] Anorexics usually present with bradycardia, and monitoring the pulse rate may be the simplest, noninvasive way of monitoring fluid replacement. Serum and urine electrolyte, phosphorous, and magnesium levels should be closely monitored.

A period of 48 h in an inpatient setting is essential to determine the extent and severity of the illness and its complications. Eating disorders units are specifically designed for such evaluations, but they can also be performed in a regular medical unit with involvement of a multidisciplinary psychiatric and internal medicine team.

Hospitalization is suggested for the following:

1. Weight loss greater than 30 percent over 3 months
2. Severe metabolic disturbance
3. Depression severe enough to be at risk for suicide
4. Severe binge eating and purging
5. Failure to maintain outpatient weight contract
6. Psychosis
7. Family crisis
8. Need to confront the patient's and family's denial
9. Need for initiation of therapy (individual, family, and/or pharmacotherapy)
10. Complex differential diagnosis

Treatment algorithms for anorexia nervosa and bulimia nervosa appear in Figs. 283-1 and 283-2.

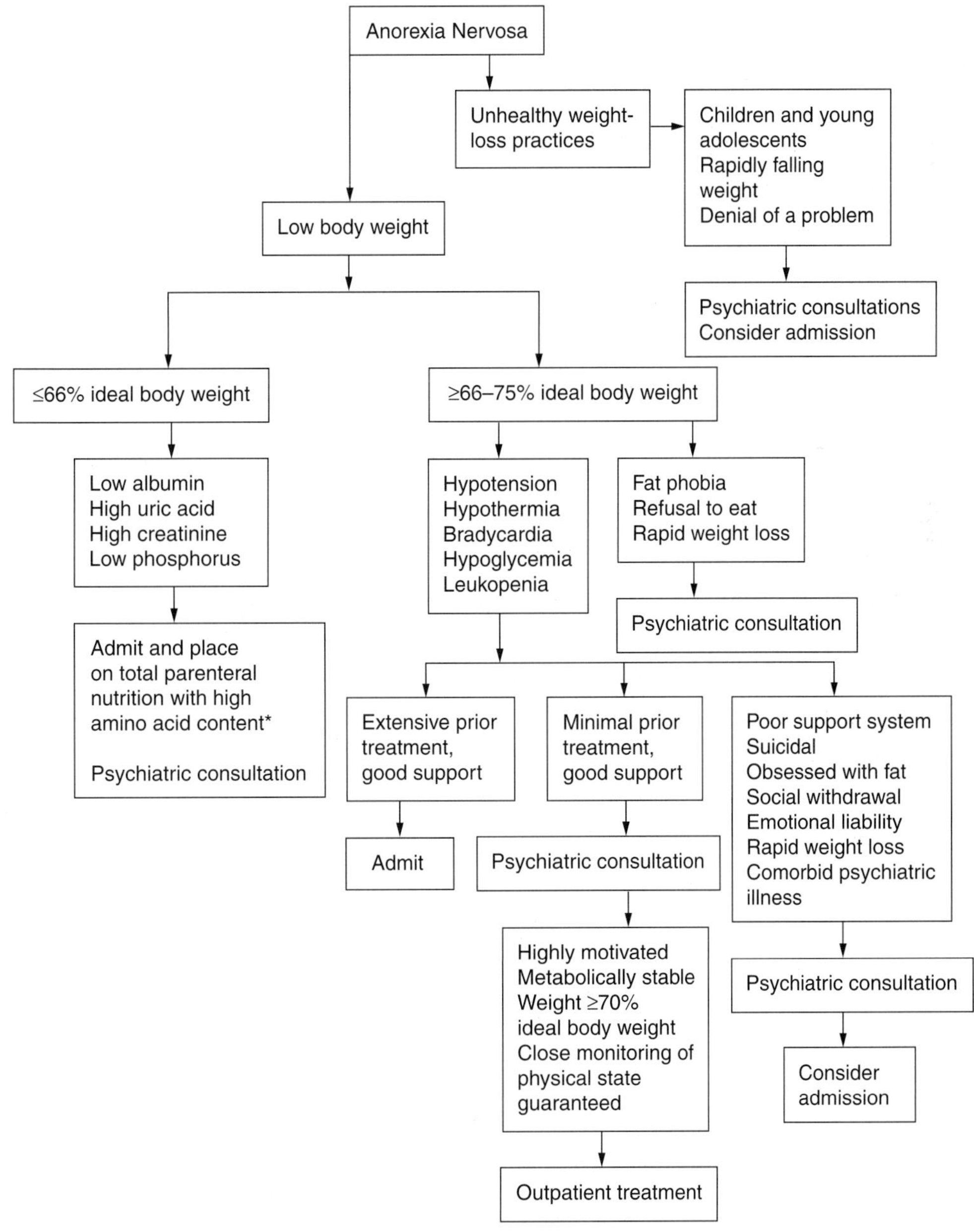

* A little nutritional support is good. Too much is *LETHAL.*

FIG. 283-1. Treatment algorithm for anorexia nervosa.

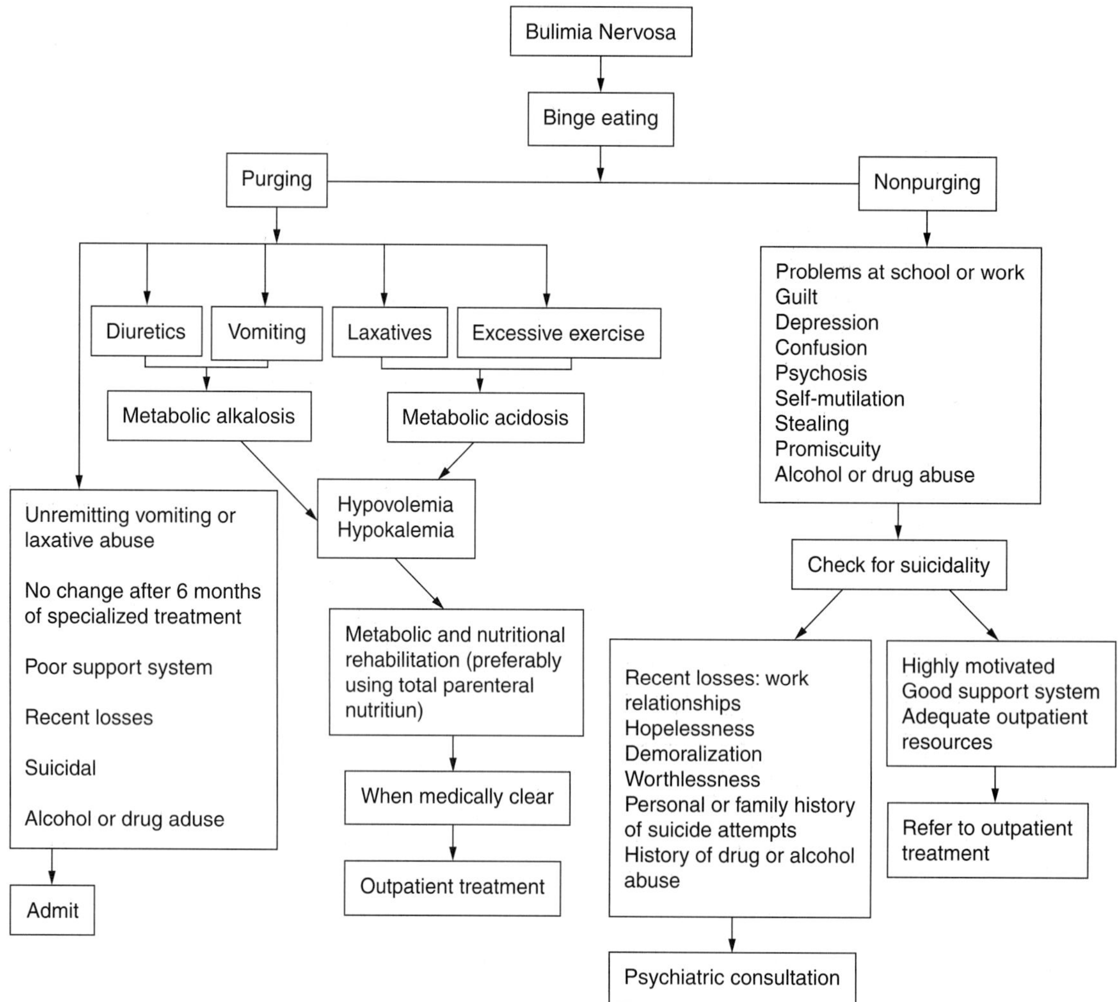

FIG. 283-2. Treatment algorithm for bulimia nervosa.

A trial of outpatient psychological treatment can be attempted if food restriction and weight loss are of less than 3 months' duration and if there is a very positive family support system. Referral to a local health professional who specializes in the treatment of eating disorders or to a self-help group can be obtained by contacting the following national organizations:

National Association of Anorexia Nervosa and Associated Disorders (ANAD)
PO Box 7
Highland Park, IL 60035
847-831-3438
www.healthtouch.com/level1/leaflets/anad/anad001.htm

Anorexia Nervosa and Related Eating Disorders, Inc. (ANRED)
PO Box 5102
Eugene, OR 97405
541-344-1144
www.anred.com

American Anorexia/Bulimia Association, Inc. (AABA)
165 W. 46th St. #1108
New York, NY 07666
212-575-6200
http://members.aol.com/AmanBu

National Eating Disorders Organization (NEDO)
6655 S. Yale Ave.
Tulsa, OK 74136
918-481-4044
www.laureate.com

Academy for Eating Disorders, Montefiore Medical Center (AED)
111 E. 210th St.
Bronx, NY 10467
718-920-6782
www.acadeatdis.org

REFERENCES

1. Comerci GD: Eating disorders in adolescents. *Pediatr Rev* 10(2):37, 1988.
2. Garner DM, Garfinkel PE: *Anorexia Nervosa: A Multidimension Perspective.* New York, Bruner/Mazel, 1982.
3. American Psychiatric Association: *Diagnostic and Statistical Manual of Mental Disorders,* 4th ed. Washington, 1994.
4. Garner DM, Garfinkel PE (eds): *Handbook of Treatment for Eating Disorders,* 2d ed. New York, Guilford Press, 1997.
5. Mackenzie JR, LaBan MM, Sackeyfio AH: Prevalence of peripheral neuropathy in patients with anorexia nervosa. *Arch Phys Med Rehabil* 70:827, 1989.
6. LaBan MM, Wilkins JC, Sackeyfio AH, Taylor RS: Osteoporotic stress fractures in anorexia nervosa. *Arch Phys Med Rehabil* 76:884, 1996.

7. Herzog W, Deter HC, Fiehn W, Petzold E: Medical findings and predictors of long-term physical outcome in anorexia nervosa: A prospective, 12-year follow-up study. *Psychol Med* 27:269, 1997.
8. Hoffman L, Halmi K: Psychopharmacology in the treatment of anorexia nervosa and bulimia nervosa. *Psychiatr Clin North Am* 16:767, 1993.
9. Solomon SM, Kirby DF: The refeeding syndrome: A review. *J Parenteral Nutrition* 14:90, 1990.

PANIC DISORDER

Susan L. Siegfreid
Linda Meredith Nicholas

Panic attacks are short-lived episodes of anxiety or intense fear, accompanied by a range of somatic symptoms, which may include tachycardia, tachypnea, dyspnea, chest tightness, weakness, nausea, dizziness, and paresthesias. *Panic disorder* is characterized by recurrent, spontaneous panic attacks. Panic disorder may occur with or without agoraphobia, a condition typified by avoidance of places or situations associated with anxiety. Panic disorder with agoraphobia may be severely disabling, as patients may be incapable of functioning socially or occupationally.

Since many of the symptoms of panic overlap with those of acute medical illness, the first point of contact for patients with panic disorder is often the emergency department. Data from the Epidemiologic Catchment Area study found that, when compared with patients who had either other psychiatric or medical problems, patients with panic disorder had the highest rates of use of emergency room services.[1] A study by Simpson and colleagues reported that this increased utilization preceded the diagnosis of panic disorder by up to 10 years.[2] Therefore, it is important for emergency clinicians to understand panic disorder, its common presentations, and its treatment.

EPIDEMIOLOGY

Panic disorder is relatively common, with a national lifetime and 12-month prevalence of 3.5 and 2.5 percent,[3] respectively, and a cross-national lifetime prevalence of 1.6 to 2.2 percent.[4] The age of onset is usually from late adolescence to mid-30s. The incidence may have a bimodal distribution with the first peak in late adolescence, followed by a second, smaller peak in the mid-30s.[5]

Women are two to three times more likely to develop panic disorder than men. There is some evidence that panic attacks may remit during pregnancy, only to be exacerbated in the postpartum period.[6,7] Cultural factors may play a role in the presentation of panic disorder. A study by Bell and coworkers found that sleep paralysis and hypertension are common symptoms of panic disorder in the African American population.[8] *Ataque de nervios* is an anxiety syndrome in Hispanic cultures that, at times, has a similar presentation to panic disorder.[9]

PATHOPHYSIOLOGY

The etiologic basis of panic disorder is not known. It is most likely multifactorial in origin, with genetic, behavioral, and biologic underpinnings.

Family and twin studies suggest a genetic etiology. First-degree relatives of patients with panic disorder have a four- to sevenfold increased risk of developing the disorder,[10] and monozygotic twins have a higher concordance for panic disorder than dizygotic twins.[11]

Cognitive-behavioral theorists propose that panic disorder is a learned response to interoceptive cues. Heightened awareness of body functions and/or cognitive misinterpretation of these cues are postulated to trigger a conditioned fear response.[12] Anticipatory anxiety and agoraphobia develop as a person begins to associate panic attacks with a particular place or situation.

Neurobiologic research into the etiology of panic disorder utilizes two main approaches: studies that use provocative (''panicogenic'') substances and studies that use known pharmacologic treatments. These approaches have implicated multiple neurotransmitters or neuropeptides, including norepinephrine, serotonin (5-hydroxytryptamine or 5-HT), γ-aminobutyric acid (GABA), and cholecystokinin (CCK) among others.

Panic disorder patients are generally hypersensitive to carbon dioxide inhalation.[13] One model proposes that carbon dioxide stimulates the locus ceruleus, which contains noradrenergic neurons, and induces panic by stimulating norepinephrine release.[14] In addition, there is also some evidence for impaired receptor sensitivity in panic disorder.[13]

Two agents have been reported to provoke panic attacks by effects on serotonergic receptors. Fenfluramine and *m*-chlorophenylpiperazine (m-CPP) both cause panic in challenge tests.[13] Theories that attempt to explain the results of these tests, as well as to incorporate the known efficacy of serotonergic agents in treating panic disorder, include the following: increased sensitivity of postsynaptic receptors, decreased or increased central nervous system serotonin activity, or interactions between serotonin and norepinephrine, GABA or CCK.[13]

Recently, much attention has been given to the neuropeptide, CCK, as an important mediator in panic disorder. It is present in many of the neuroanatomic areas thought to be involved in panic disorder, including the cerebral cortex, hippocampus, and brainstem. A tetrapeptide form of CCK causes panic when administered to panic disorder patients, and its effects are attenuated by imipramine, a tricyclic antidepressant with efficacy in treating panic.[15] There are also close interactions between CCK and GABA, serotonin and dopamine, as well as endogenous opioids and the excitatory amino acid, glutamate.[15]

The provocative agents sodium lactate, yohimbine, and caffeine, which reproducibly induce panic in patients with panic disorder, have not as yet implicated clear mechanisms by which panic attacks occur.

CLINICAL FEATURES

The cardinal features of panic disorder are recurrent, unexpected panic attacks and persistent worry about having another attack and its potential implications, such as heralding a serious medical illness. Panic attacks are of sudden onset and include feelings of apprehension, fear, and discomfort; they are relatively brief, with a peak in about 10 min and resolution within 1 h. The attacks are accompanied by characteristic somatic and/or cognitive symptoms.[5]

Somatic symptoms are referable to the major organ systems in the body. Cardiovascular complaints include palpitations/tachycardia or chest pain/discomfort. Respiratory symptoms of shortness of breath or the sensation of being smothered are common. A choking sensation and nausea or gastric distress comprise the majority of gastrointestinal complaints. Neurologic symptoms include dizziness, unsteadiness, light-headedness, trembling, shaking, or paresthesias. Sweating, hot flushes, or chills are also common. Cognitive symptoms include feelings of unreality about or being detached from one's environment (derealization) or one's self (depersonalization), as well as the fear of going crazy, losing control, or dying.[5] Some patients alter their behavior to minimize their risk of having more panic attacks, even to the point of becoming fearful of leaving their home and being in places or situations where escape or finding help would be difficult if a panic attack occurred (agoraphobia).[5]

DIAGNOSIS

The panic attacks must not be better accounted for by another psychiatric or medical disorder (Table 284-1). The patient's age, presenting symptoms, time course of symptom development and resolution, and lack of other identifiable medical causes are often helpful in considering the differential diagnosis of a panic attack.[16] For a diagnosis of panic disorder, a patient must have recurrent, unexpected panic attacks

TABLE 284-1 Medical Differential Diagnosis of Panic

Cardiovascular
Angina
Myocardial infarction
Congestive heart failure
Mitral valve prolapse
Pulmonary
Asthma
Pulmonary embolus
Hyperventilation
Endocrine
Hyperthyroidism
Hypoglycemia
Pheochromocytoma
Carcinoid syndrome
Cushing's syndrome
Neurologic
Migraines
Complex partial seizures
Transient ischemic attacks
Meniere's disease
Drug-induced
Sympathomimetics
Caffeine
Theophylline
Thyroid preparations
Selective serotonin reuptake inhibitors
Yohimbine
Anticholergics
Nicotine
Marijuana
Hallucinogens
Cocaine
Corticosteroids
β-Agonists
Drug withdrawal
Alcohol
Barbiturates
Benzodiazepines
Opiates
β-Antagonists
Psychosocial
Partner violence
Sexual abuse or assault
Other situational stressors

followed by at least a month of persistent fear of having additional attacks, worry about the implications or consequence (e.g., going crazy or having a heart attack), or a significant change in behavior.[5]

Psychiatric Differential Diagnosis

A panic attack is an episode of intense fear that develops abruptly and reaches a peak within 10 min. During a panic attack, at least four of 13 characteristic symptoms must be present, as listed in Table 284-2. Panic attacks are characterized in the *Diagnostic and Statistical Manual of Mental Disorders,* 4th edition (DSM-IV), as (1) *unexpected* (uncued), (2) *situationally bound* or cued (i.e., always occurring with exposure to a specific trigger), or (3) *situationally predisposed* (i.e., likely to occur in exposure to a given situation). Situationally bound or predisposed panic attacks may occur in association with a wide range of psychiatric disorders, including social phobia, specific phobia, acute or posttraumatic stress disorder, separation anxiety disorder, obsessive-compulsive disorder, and depressive disorders. The occurrence of spontaneous or unexpected panic attacks is necessary for a diagnosis of panic disorder. Patients should always be questioned regarding what situation triggered the attacks. It is often useful to ask if their panic attacks occur "out of the blue" or to inquire if they are ever awakened by panic attacks, in order to determine if the panic attacks are spontaneous versus triggered.

Medical Differential Diagnosis

Patients presenting with multiple somatic complaints consistent with a panic attack, even if they are known to have panic disorder, should have a thorough medical history documentation, physical examination and, when indicated, other specific tests performed to rule out medical causes. The differential diagnosis is quite extensive, as listed in Table 284-1, and panic disorder is a diagnosis of exclusion.

The psychosocial history should include questions regarding substance use, situational psychosocial stressors, partner violence, and sexual abuse or assault that may be exacerbating or precipitating panic attacks. The clinician should carefully review the patient's concurrent medical problems, as well as prescribed and over-the-counter medications. Substance intoxication and withdrawal states may also induce panic. A history of caffeine use is important, as panic patients are often exquisitely sensitive to methylxanthines.

Physical exam findings in panic patients most commonly are transient tachycardia and mildly elevated systolic blood pressure. Laboratory findings, when present, are most consistent with hyperventilation with low levels of sodium bicarbonate. The presence of any medical abnormalities suggests a diagnosis other than panic disorder.

ASSOCIATIONS

Panic disorder is closely associated with other psychiatric and medical conditions. Comorbid psychiatric disorders include depression in up to 50 to 65 percent, other mood disorders, substance abuse and dependence, posttraumatic stress disorder, other anxiety disorders, and personality disorders.[5] Certain medical conditions have been associated with panic disorder but are unrelated to its etiology. Panic disorder has well-documented associations with mitral valve prolapse and asthma.[5]

TABLE 284-2 Symptoms of a Panic Attack

Somatic Symptoms	Cognitive Symptoms
Palpitations, pounding heart, or tachycardia	Fear of losing control
Sweating	Fear of dying
Sensations of shortness of breath or smothering	Derealization (feeling of unreality) or depersonalization (feeling detached from oneself)
Trembling or shaking	
Feeling of choking	
Chest pain or discomfort	
Nausea or abdominal distress	
Feeling dizzy, unsteady, light-headed, or faint	
Paresthesias	
Chills or hot flushes	

Other medical conditions such as idiopathic cardiomyopathy, hypertension, atypical chest pain without evidence of coronary artery disease, irritable bowel syndrome, chronic obstructive pulmonary disease, Parkinson's disease, and migraine headaches have also been associated with panic attacks.[17]

COURSE

The course of panic disorder is variable in frequency and severity. Some patients suffer only intermittent attacks, whereas others have attacks almost continuously. In general, the course of the illness is chronic, with a waxing and waning pattern. Panic disorder patients also can have situationally predisposed attacks when exposed to certain cues or triggers, limited symptom panic attacks in which fewer than four of the 13 recognized diagnostic somatic or cognitive symptoms occur, and nocturnal panic attacks. A 4- to 6-year follow-up study of patients from a tertiary care setting after treatment showed that 30 percent were asymptomatic, 40 to 50 percent were improved, and 20 to 30 percent remained the same or were worse.[18] Lifetime rates of suicide attempts are similar for patients with uncomplicated panic disorder and uncomplicated major depression (7 and 7.9 percent, respectively), whereas rates for patients with comorbid panic disorder and depression are 19.5 percent.[19] Thus, panic disorder should be diagnosed and appropriately treated in order to prevent significant morbidity and mortality.

TREATMENT

Treatment of panic disorder starts with recognition of the illness. Ballenger[20] has proposed that the following screening question be asked of patients for rapid identification: ''Have you experienced brief periods for seconds or minutes of an overwhelming panic or terror which was accompanied by racing heart, shortness of breath or dizziness?''[20] Once panic disorder is diagnosed, the next step is to educate the patient about the disorder, providing reassurance that they are not dying or going crazy, and emphasizing that it is an illness that can be effectively treated. A study by Swinson and colleagues found that, in addition to education and reassurance, instruction on exposure to the situation that triggered the panic attack was potentially helpful in reducing the long-term sequelae of panic disorder.[21]

Both cognitive-behavioral therapy (CBT) and pharmacotherapy are effective treatment modalities for panic disorder.[22] Choice of treatment is based on an individual assessment of risks, benefits, efficacy, availability, acuity, and patient preference. Both CBT and pharmacologic treatment, with the exception of benzodiazepines, take at least 4 weeks for most patients to notice significant benefit. If there is no improvement within 6 to 8 weeks of a particular treatment, often a different treatment is required or combined CBT and medication is used.

TABLE 284-4 Tricyclic Antidepressants

Advantages	Concerns
Single daily dose	Delayed onset
Treats comorbid depression	Anticholinergic effects
Demonstrated efficacy	Postural hypotension
Generics available	Sexual side effects
No abuse potential	Weight gain
	Initial stimulation
	Dangerous in overdose

Cognitive Behavioral Treatment

CBT involves education about the disorder, symptom and thought records, learning anxiety management skills (e.g., breathing retraining), changing cognitions associated with panic attacks (cognitive restructuring), and exposure to feared situations, usually utilizing a hierarchy created by the patient and therapist.[22]

Medications

Four classes of drugs have been found to be effective in treating panic disorder: selective serotonin reuptake inhibitors (SSRIs), tricyclic antidepressants (TCAs), monoamine oxidase inhibitors (MAOIs), and benzodiazepines. Tables 284-3 to 284-6 list some of the advantages and disadvantages of each class.

ANTIDEPRESSANTS Treatment with antidepressants is considered by many clinicians to be the mainstay of treatment for panic disorder, since the potential complications of abuse, dependence, and withdrawal are not associated with their use. Additionally, antidepressants may be beneficial in treating comorbid depression disorders. Due to safety considerations and side-effect profiles, SSRIs are considered the drugs of choice. Although sexual side effects may be problematic with all three antidepressant classes, SSRIs lack the anticholinergic side effects, cardiovascular effects, and toxicity in overdose associated with TCAs or MAOIs. However, SSRIs are likely to be more expensive than generic TCAs or benzodiazepines.

When initiating treatment with SSRIs and TCAs, the starting dose should be lower than that used to treat depression, because panic disorder patients often are extremely sensitive to side effects. It is helpful to advise patients that they may temporarily notice some increased anxiety or activation when initiating treatment or increasing the dose. Patients should also be told that it might take several weeks before there are noticeable benefits.

TABLE 284-3 Selective Serotonin Reuptake Inhibitors

Advantages	Concerns
Single daily dose	Delayed onset
Treats comorbid depression	Initial stimulation
Safety	Sexual side effects
Well tolerated	Requires dose titration
No abuse potential	
Demonstrated efficacy	

TABLE 284-5 Monoamine Oxidase Inhibitors

Advantages	Concerns
Single daily dose	Delayed onset
Treats comorbid depression	Drug interactions
Effective	Dietary restrictions
No abuse potential	Sexual side effects
	Weight gain
	Dangerous in overdose

TABLE 284-6 Benodiazepines

Advantages	Concerns
Rapid onset	Discontinuation reactions
Demonstrated efficacy	Sedation
Well tolerated	Multiple daily dosing
General antianxiety effects	Abuse potential
Relatively safe in overdose	Dependence
Generics available	Inter-dose rebound
Tolerance rare for antipanic effects	

MAOIs are usually reserved as second-line treatment due to the dietary restrictions and risk of hypertensive crisis. Interestingly, controlled studies with MAOIs were done prior to the introduction of the panic disorder diagnosis in the 1980 DSM-III and examined the use of phenelzine for treatment of "phobic neurosis."[22] Studies of the use of reversible monoamine oxidase inhibitors (RIMAs), which do not require adherence to a tyramine-free diet, have showed effectiveness in treating panic and phobic symptoms.[23,24] Currently, RIMAs are not approved for use in the United States.

BENZODIAZEPINES For patients in whom more rapid control of panic symptoms is necessary, such as those who are unable to fulfill expected major psychosocial obligations (work, school, etc.), benzodiazepines may be the drug of choice. Alprazolam has been the most extensively studied benzodiazepine and is currently the only one approved by the Food and Drug Administration for treatment of panic disorder. It may be initiated at a dose of 0.5 mg four times daily. In double-blind studies, alprazolam, in the 5- to 6-mg/day dosage range, reduces panic attack frequency, anticipatory anxiety, phobic avoidance, and disability.[22] Studies suggest that diazepam, lorazepam, and clonazepam in equivalent doses may also be effective in treating panic disorder.

Benzodiazepines may also be administered acutely for a patient who is having a panic attack, regardless of the etiology of the panic. They should be used with caution in patients with a respiratory disorder or in those who have a history of substance abuse or dependence.

It may be beneficial to initiate treatment with both an antidepressant and a benzodiazepine, with the goal to later taper or minimize the benzodiazepine dose as the antidepressant begins to control symptoms. A controlled trial of alprazolam as an adjunct to imipramine during the first 4 to 6 weeks of treatment demonstrated that patients receiving both drugs had a more rapid therapeutic response.[25] However, 10 of 17 patients were unable to discontinue the alprazolam in 2 weeks following the treatment period. Thus, the benefits of a rapid response must be weighed with the risk of difficulty in discontinuing the benzodiazepine.

Both CBT and pharmacologic treatment, with the exception of benzodiazepines, take at least 4 weeks for most patients to notice significant benefit. If there is no improvement within 6 to 8 weeks of a particular treatment, often a different treatment is required or combined CBT and medication are used. Acute treatment usually lasts at least 12 weeks. If medication is being used, often a taper and discontinuation are attempted after 1 year of maintenance treatment. It is unclear whether further CBT sessions ("booster sessions") are beneficial in prevention of relapse. Relapse is treated with CBT and/or medication.

DISPOSITION

Usually, treatment for panic disorder can be initiated in an outpatient setting. If a patient is already being treated for panic disorder, consult with the treating physician before initiating or changing medication. Psychiatric consultation in the emergency department is an option, if consultation is available. The patient should be referred to his or her primary care physician or a psychiatrist for follow-up care.

Patients who are suicidal or who are so incapacitated that they are unable to care for themselves require psychiatric hospitalization. In such cases, a psychiatric evaluation is necessary to determine the extent of dangerousness and need for inpatient treatment.

REFERENCES

1. Klerman GL, Weissman MM, Ouellette R, et al: Panic attacks in the community: Social morbidity and health care utilization. *JAMA* 265:742, 1991.
2. Simpson RJ, Kazmierczak T, Power KG, et al: Controlled comparison of the characteristics of patients with panic disorder. *Br J Gen Pract* 44:352, 1994.
3. Kessler RC, McGonagle KA, Zhao S, et al: Lifetime and 12-month prevalence of DSM-III-R psychiatric disorders in the United States: Results from the National Comorbidity Survey. *Arch Gen Psychiatry* 51:8, 1994.
4. Weissman MM, Bland RC, Canino GJ, et al: The cross-national epidemiology of panic disorder. *Arch Gen Psychiatry* 54:305, 1997.
5. American Psychiatric Association: *Diagnostic and Statistical Manual of Mental Disorders,* 4th ed [DSM-IV]. Washington, DC, American Psychiatric Association, 1994.
6. George DT, Landenheim JA, Nutt D: Effect of pregnancy on panic attacks. *Am J Psychiatry* 44:1078, 1987.
7. Cohen LS, Sichel DA, Dimmock JA, et al: Postpartum course in women with preexisting panic disorder. *J Clin Psychiatry* 55:289, 1994.
8. Bell CC, Hildreth CJ, Jenkins EJ, et al: The relationship of isolated sleep paralysis and panic disorder to hypertension. *J Natl Med Assoc* 80:289, 1988.
9. Liebowitz MR, Salman E, Justino CM, et al: Ataque de nervios and panic disorder. *Am J Psychiatry* 151:871, 1994.
10. Knowles JA, Weissman MM: Panic disorder and agoraphobia, in Oldham JM, Riba MB (eds): *American Psychiatric Press Review of Psychiatry,* vol 14. Washington, DC, American Psychiatric Press, 1995, p 383.
11. Perna G, Caldirola D, Arancio C, et al: Panic attacks: A twin study. *Psychiatry Res* 15:69, 1997.
12. Barlow DH, Cohen AS, Waddell MT, et al: Panic and generalized anxiety disorder: nature and treatment. *Behav Ther* 15:431, 1984.
13. Bourin M, Baker GB, Bradwejn J: Neurobiology of panic disorder. *J Psychosom Res* 44:163, 1998.
14. Klein DF, Gorman JM: A model of panic and agoraphobic development. *Acta Psychiatr Scand* 335:87, 1987.
15. Bradwejn J, Koszycki D: Imipramine antagonizes the panicogenic effects of CCK-4 in panic disorder patients. *Am J Psychiatry* 15:261, 1994.
16. Zun LS: Panic disorder: Diagnosis and treatment in emergency medicine. *Ann Emerg Med* 30:92, 1997.
17. Zaubler TS, Katon W: Panic disorder in the medical setting. *J Psychosom Res* 44:25, 1998.
18. Katschnig H, Amering M, Stolk JM, et al: Predictors of quality of life in a long-term follow-up study of panic disorder patients after a clinical drug trial. *Psychopharmacol Bull* 32:149, 1996.
19. Johnson J, Weissman MM, Klerman GL: Panic disorder, comorbidity, and suicide attempts. *Arch Gen Psychiatry* 47:805, 1990.
20. Ballenger JC: Treatment of panic disorder in the general medical setting. *J Psychosom Res* 44:5, 1998.
21. Swinson RP, Soulios C, Cox BJ, et al: Brief treatment of emergency room patients with panic attacks. *Am J Psychiatry* 149:944, 1992.
22. American Psychiatric Association: Practice guideline for the treatment of patients with panic disorder. *Am J Psychiatry* 155(suppl):1, 1998.
23. Bakish D, Saxena BM, Bowen R, et al: Reversible monoamine oxidase inhibitors in panic disorder. *Clin Neuropsychopharmacol* 16(suppl 2):S77, 1993.
24. Garcia-Borreguero D, Lauer CJ, et al: Brofaromine in panic disorder: A pilot study with a new reversible inhibitor of monoamine oxidase-A. *Pharmacopsychiatry* 25:261, 1992.
25. Woods S, Nagy LM, Koleszar AS, et al: Controlled trial of alprazolam supplementation during imipramine treatment of panic disorder. *J Clin Psychopharmacol* 12:32, 1991.

CONVERSION DISORDER

Gregory P. Moore
Kenneth C. Jackimczyk

For a diagnosis of conversion disorder to be made, the following five criteria must be met:[1]

1. A symptom is expressed in which there is a change or loss of physical function suggesting a physical disorder.
2. The patient has experienced a recent psychological stressor or conflict.
3. The patient unconsciously produces the symptom.
4. The symptom cannot be explained by a known organic etiology or culturally sanctioned response pattern.
5. The symptom is not limited to pain or sexual dysfunction.

PATHOPHYSIOLOGY

An illustrative example involves the case of a young wife who is scheduled to visit her debilitated father in the hospital. His recent diagnosis of cancer has left her distraught, and the sight of him depresses her greatly. On the morning of her visit, she suddenly becomes blind.

This example typifies a conversion disorder in which conflict is caused by the patient's intense, but psychically unacceptable, urge to avoid a required action (in this case, visiting her father). The physical symptom (blindness) allows expression of the urge (how can she drive there if she is blind?) without consciously confronting the feelings that led to the wish. At the same time, the symptom imposes morbidity as a punishment for the wish. Often, the presenting symptom will have a symbolic relationship to the conflict, but this is not always the case. In this case, the sight of her father is distressing and therefore loss of sight is the chief complaint. Conversion disorders are often thought of as nonverbal exertion of control on the environment. Two mechanisms are responsible for the symptoms. The first is *primary gain,* in which the symptom allows patients to avoid confronting their uncomfortable feelings. The second is *secondary gain,* in which uncomfortable situations are avoided and support is given that might not normally be available. In the aforementioned case, secondary gain would occur if the patient's husband then stayed home from work to tend to his "blind" wife.

Conversion disorders are described as rare, with an annual incidence in outpatient psychiatric settings of 0.01 to 0.02 percent. An incidence of 5 to 16 percent among inpatients with psychiatric consultations has been noted. Most agree that the incidence is declining. Cases predominantly involve neurologic and orthopedic manifestations, and are seen in the military during times of war, in victims of industrial accidents, and in victims of violence. Conversion disorders are much more frequent in women than men, accounting in the former for up to 80 percent of cases in some series. The most common ages of presentation are adolescence or early childhood, although other age groups are also affected. Conversion disorders are more prevalent in rural, lower socioeconomic, and less educated populations. Other predisposing factors include medical illness, depression, anxiety, schizophrenia, somatization disorder, dependent personality disorder (5 to 21 percent of patients), borderline personality disorder, and passive aggressive personality disorder.[2,3]

CLINICAL FEATURES

Conversion disorders usually present as a single symptom with a sudden onset related to a severe stress. Precise history taking is imperative for making the diagnosis, focusing both on how the problem affects the patient and the surrounding events at time of onset. It may be necessary to interview the patient and family separately to confirm diagnostic suspicions. The most reliable diagnostic criterion for conversion disorder is either a previous history of it or a somatization disorder (each found in one-third of cases). Symptoms may vary in cases of recurrence.[2–4]

Motor complaints, usually involving voluntary muscles, are more common than sensory complaints.[2–4]

Rarely, the autonomic and endocrine systems are involved. Vomiting can be a psychogenic manifestation of disgust, and pseudocyesis (false pregnancy) can represent either a wish for or fear of pregnancy.

Classic symptoms of conversion disorders include paralysis, aphonia, seizures, coordination disturbances, akinesia, dyskinesia, blindness, tunnel vision, anosmia, anesthesia, and paresthesia. Pseudoseizures represent 10 to 40 percent of conversion disorders referred to psychiatrists. Patients may describe their condition with surprising lack of concern, considering the severity of the symptom (*la belle indifférence*). This was previously thought to be a hallmark of the disorder, but it is absent in about half of the cases and is found just as often in patients with organic disease. It is no longer considered diagnostic.[2,5]

Diagnosis is made first and foremost by ruling out organic pathology. Absence of a medical condition does not solely support the diagnosis of conversion disorder because the appropriate psychological criteria must also be met. Suspicion for the disorder should arise when no physical findings related to the symptom are found or the examination is not consistent with known anatomic or pathophysiologic states. Several techniques that can be used in the physical examination are helpful in testing for true neurologic deficits (Table 285-1). Appropriate laboratory and ancillary studies should be ordered to confirm suspected organic disease. It is important to remember, however, that organic disease may be present concurrently with conversion disorder.[6]

DIFFERENTIAL DIAGNOSIS

Careful history taking and physical examination should be used to rule out neurologic disease. A high index of suspicion should be maintained for physical disorders that have a vague onset, such as systemic lupus erythematosus, multiple sclerosis, polymyositis, Lyme disease, and drug toxicity or poisoning. Schizophrenia and depression may have associated conversion disorders. In somatization disorders, the symptoms are more chronic and involve multiple organ systems. With hypochondriasis, patients are usually without loss of function and display the conviction that some terrible undiscovered illness is present. Hypochondriacal patients will be overly concerned with symptoms. In cases of factitious symptoms, usually associated with malingering, patients will consciously complain about symptoms to get out of undesirable duty or to receive sympathy or undeserved compensation. These patients rarely have neurologic complaints.[7] Amobarbital interviews have been used to diagnose both conversion disorder and/or coexisting diagnoses. They may be therapeutic as well.[8]

TREATMENT AND PROGNOSIS

The patient does not have the insight that the symptoms have no organic cause. Confronting the patient and insisting that nothing "real" is wrong is not helpful in alleviating symptoms and may worsen the patient's condition. The symptoms should be neither trivialized nor reinforced. If the precipitating factor is identified, correction of the situation should be attempted. Meanwhile, the patient should receive reassurance that no serious medical problem has been identified. If both the results of initial testing and exam are negative, it should be suggested to the patient that the symptoms will resolve. Nonspecific supportive therapy should be prescribed. For instance, in the example cited at the beginning of this chapter, it could be suggested that the patient visit her father less often, call daily instead, and have her husband accompany her to the hospital. She should expect the blindness to resolve if she follows this course.[2,9]

TABLE 285-1 Physical Examination Techniques Used to Distinguish True Neurologic Deficits and Conversion Disorder

Function	Technique
Sensation	
Yes–no test	Patient closes eyes and responds "yes" or "no" to touch stimulus. "No" response in numb area favors conversion disorder.
Bowlus and Currier test	Patient extends crossed arms with thumbs pointed down and palms facing together. Fingers (but no thumbs) are interlocked, and then hands are rotated inward toward chest. The distortion of body position makes false responses to sensory stimuli difficult.
Strength test	Patient closes eyes. Test "strength" by touching finger to be moved. True lack of sensation would not allow patient to ascertain finger to be moved.
Pain	
Gray test	With abdominal pain due to psychological factors, patient will close eyes during palpation. In pain of organic basis, patient is more likely to watch examiner's hand in order to anticipate pain.
Motor	
Drop test	When patient with paralysis of nonorganic etiology lifts thumb, affected limb will drop more slowly or fall with exaggerated speed as compared with unaffected limb. Additionally, an extremity dropped from above the face will miss it.
Stretch reflex test	Patient contracts a muscle at maximum strength while counteraction is provided. Examiner suddenly jerks the muscle into extension. This will produce a stretch reflex that reveals patient's true muscle strength.
Thigh adductor test	Examiner places hands against inner thighs of patient. Patient is told to adduct normal leg against resistance. With pseudoparalysis, other leg will adduct.
Hoover test	Examiner's hands cup both heels of patient, and patient is asked to elevate normal leg. With pseudoparalysis, other leg will push downward. Absence of downward pressure of normal leg when patient is instructed to lift weak leg indicates noncompliance.
Sternomastoid test	Patient with conversion hemiplegia cannot turn head to weak side.
Coma	
Corneal reflex	Corneal reflexes remain intact in awake patient.
Bell's phenomenon	Eyes divert upward when lids opened, whereas eyes remain in neutral position in true coma.
Lid closing	In true coma, lids when opened close rapidly initially then more slowly as lids descend. Awake patients will have lids stay open, snap shut, or flutter.
Seizures	
Corneal reflex	Usually intact in pseudoseizure.
Abdominal musculature	Palpation of abdominal musculature reveals lack of contractions with pseudoseizure.
Blindness	
Opticokinetic drum	Rotating drum with alternating black and white stripes or piece of tape with alternating black and white sections pulled laterally in front of patient's open eyes will produce nystagmus in patient with intact vision.

Source: Adapted from Purcell.[6]

Referral is mandatory. Patients with conversion disorders may need repetitive reassurance and suggestion that symptoms will resolve before returning to full function. Periodic follow-up is also important to monitor for subtle organic disease. Between 25 and 50 percent of patients diagnosed with conversion disorders later develop serious organic conditions.[2,10]

Most conversion disorders are brief and quickly resolve. Favorable prognostic factors are (1) lack of other psychiatric disorders, (2) sudden severe stress as a precipitating cause, and (3) absence of medical problems. Some cases are resistant and require hypnosis or amobarbital interview for resolution. This should be coordinated by the primary care provider. Lorazepam has also been found helpful in management of this condition. Approximately 25 percent of patients will have another episode over the ensuing 1 to 6 years, which may involve the same or a new symptom complex.[2,10]

Some patients develop a chronic form of the disorder with complications including contractures and atrophy of muscle groups. In addition, unnecessary diagnostic tests may lead to iatrogenic complications.

REFERENCES

1. American Psychiatric Association: *Diagnostic and Statistical Manual of Mental Disorders,* 4th ed, rev. Washington, DC, 1994.
2. Kaplan HI, Sadock BJ (eds): Conversion disorder, in *Comprehensive Textbook of Psychiatry,* vol 1, 6th ed. Baltimore, Williams and Wilkins, 1995, pp 1252–1255.
3. Binzer M, Andersen PM, Kullgren G: Clinical characteristics of patients with motor disability due to conversion disorder: A prospective control group study. *J. Neurol Neurosurg Psychiatry* 63:83, 1997.
4. Dula DJ, DeNaples L: Emergency department presentation of patients with conversion disorder. *Acad Emerg Med* 2:120, 1995.
5. Lazare A: Conversion symptoms. *N Engl J Med* 305:745, 1981.
6. Purcell TB: The somatic patient. *Emerg Clin North Am* 9:137, 1991.
7. Dubovsky SL, Weissberg MP (eds): Hypochondriasis, in *Clinical Psychiatry in Primary Care,* 3d ed. Baltimore, Williams and Wilkins, 1986, pp 1–22.
8. Fackler SM, Anfinson TJ, Rand JA: Serial sodium Amytal interviews in the clinical setting. *Psychosomatics* 38:558, 1997.
9. Silver FW: Management of conversion disorder. *Am J Phys Med Rehabil* 75:134, 1996.
10. Hafeiz HV: Hysterical conversion: A prognostic study. *Br J Psychiatry* 136:548, 1980.

BREAKING BAD NEWS: NOTIFYING THE LIVING OF DEATH

James Brown
Glenn Hamilton

INTRODUCTION

Of the 90+ million emergency department (ED) visits in 1995, 339,000 (0.4 percent) deaths occurred in the department.[1] The timing and nature of death is often unexpected and traumatic to the survivors. In one study, 65 percent of ED deaths were considered unexpected versus 7 percent of inpatient deaths.[2] Compounding this difficult, acute situation the ED staff generally have no prior relationship with the patient or the family.[3]

Death notification training is deficient throughout medical education. Medical students question how well they are prepared to tell a family about death.[4] One-half of emergency physicians report training in death notification during medical school, and only one-third during residency. Seventy percent of ED physicians find death notification to be emotionally draining. Without proper training, this role is even more difficult.[5] Educational programs involving videotaping of death notifications and role playing can assist physicians in developing the necessary skills.[6–8] The ED staff can become desensitized, or preoccu-

TABLE 286-1 Sequence of Events

Preparation—Private area/room set aside. Family gathered. Family advised of ongoing efforts if any. Social services/chaplain contacted. Physician mentally and physically prepares.
Notification—Introduce yourself and identify family members. Sit down. Give brief synopsis of events to date. Express sympathy and tell the family that the patient has died.
Grief Response—Give physical comfort if able. Do not move away. After initial response, ask one of group a question about the patient. Reassure family that no suffering was involved, if appropriate. Support other physicians/EMS where possible. Stand up. Advise family that you will contact family physician and coroner. Leave the room.
Viewing the body—Allow the family to view the deceased. Don't force a viewing. Body is prepared prior to viewing. Member of staff accompanies family.
Concluding process—Express condolences. Ask if family has further questions. Inquire about autopsy/organ donation. Sign papers. Identify those at risk for pathological grief. Avoid prescribing sedatives. Arrange follow-up as appropriate. Tell the family when to leave.

Source: Modified from Hamilton[12] and Walters.[3]

pied with moving on to the living patients who are waiting. One-quarter of families describe the ED staff as cold, unsympathetic, and not reassuring.[9]

PREPARING FOR NOTIFICATION

An organized approach is essential (Table 286-1). A secluded area close to the ED is available for the family and friends. This area includes a telephone to allow the contact of relatives, friends, and other supporters. Ideally, a member of the clergy or a social worker is present during the discussions. If the family arrives while resuscitation efforts are continuing, a physician or trained member of the hospital staff informs them of the resuscitation and its progress. Updates are given frequently (every 5 to 10 min) until the effort concludes.[10] Sharing information and empathy during this time allows family members to become knowledgeably prepared for the potential outcome.

The emergency physician must prepare prior to speaking with the family. After leaving the resuscitation room, the physician must mentally ''change gears'' over 15 to 30 s. Knowing what to do and what to anticipate can be reassuring. A calm demeanor is essential for effective communication with the family. It is important to collect one's thoughts and organize the presentation. If clothing is soiled, it is changed before the notification. An appropriate amount of time is allotted. Other tasks in the department are delegated to others, or families are informed of the reason for delay. Advance information about which family members are present and their preparation is obtained when possible. This information can be gathered from the clergy, nurse, or physician who has served as intermediary. It is best not to go alone. If clergy or social services support is not yet present, or will not be available in a timely fashion, nursing staff can be enlisted.

TELLING THE SURVIVORS

It is the physician's responsibility to inform family members of the death.[11] As soon as the physician enters the room, the physician should introduce the team to the patient's family. The leading family member is identified and all parties, including the physician, are seated, if possible. Sitting minimizes the chance of trauma occurring from fainting or falling, and signals the family that the physician will remain as long as is needed. The deceased should be addressed by name. The family is then given a very brief summary of the patient's response to treatment, if any. This should be done in plain language, avoiding medical jargon. After these few brief phrases, the family is told that the patient has died and sympathy is expressed. To avoid confusion, terms such as ''passed on'' or ''no longer with us'' should not be used. Providing unnecessary detail before announcing the death can rouse false hopes, and can cause extreme anxiety in family members.

Once the initial statement is made, allow a brief period for the initial grief response (30 to 60 s). The physician may give physical comfort to the family if the physician is comfortable doing so. After the initial delay, asking the most stable survivor for their perception of the event allows the initial presentation of information to conclude. Families may receive some comfort from statements that the patient suffered no pain (if appropriate) and that everything possible was done. They are told that the coroner/medical examiner and their private physician will be contacted. They are also told that the physician will return to answer any questions they may have.[12]

GRIEF REACTION

Individual responses to the death of a loved one vary greatly. The initial response has been described as a ''psychic pain spike.'' Although it lasts only a brief amount of time, usually 5 to 15 min, it occurs. During this period, the family can make no decisions. Once this period of acute grief has ended, the family members will progress through other reactions: denial, anger, and/or guilt.[13]

Denial is one of the more frequent reactions to the news of death. The bereaved family may express disbelief, or insist that the information provided cannot be true. The family may insist upon viewing the deceased, and this should be done when possible.[13] Denial may be a protective mechanism, giving the mind time to absorb the situation. It is accepted and tolerated patiently, allowing the bereaved some time to adjust.[3]

Family who find difficulty accepting death may find an outlet in anger. This may be directed at the physician or staff. Accusations of negligence or statements about what should have been done may be often made. Although difficult to accept, the physician must see these as expressions of grief. This anger is often misplaced guilt at causing or failing to prevent the death. Unconscious frustration with the deceased for abandoning the bereaved can find its outlet in anger directed at others. A defensive posture on the part of the physician is counterproductive. Reflecting the family members' feelings back to them, and not accepting them personally, is the best response. Eventually the anger will dissipate, allowing the family to move on with the grieving process. The physician's handling of this immediate response is an important step in facilitating grief.

Guilt is a nearly universal emotion in the grieving process. There may be issues between the deceased and the bereaved that can no longer be resolved. It is important to intercept survivor's self-accusations and to address the components of survivor's guilt where possible. Exoneration by the physician can be very comforting.[3]

The emotional response to the news of death is dependent upon the cultural background of the bereaved. Responses vary from hysterical crying to cold distraction. Regardless of the initial response, the bereaved must be allowed to express their feelings. The physician's response to these expressions is one of calm and silence. If possible, gently touching the bereaved can be more important than any words. Clichés such as ''It's God's will'' or ''Life must go on,'' should be avoided.[13]

Normal grieving lasts six to eight months. Physical symptoms include headache, irritability, fatigue, insomnia, restlessness, dyspnea, or anorexia. Emotional symptoms include guilt, denial, anger, depression, difficulty concentrating, lack of organization, and preoccupation with the deceased. These symptoms become pathological grief if persistent over a prolonged period of time or with heightened intensity. Other manifestations of pathological grief may include an exacerbating or remitting pattern of grief or signs of physical disability. Pathological grief can be seen with multiple symptoms including apathy, panic attacks, overactivity, hostility with paranoia, suppression of hostility with resultant flat affect, depression, or symptoms resembling those of the deceased.[3]

Recognition of survivors at risk for or manifesting pathological grief allows for early intervention. Risk factors for pathological grief include sudden or unexpected death, death of an infant or child, death involving suicide or homicide, or death where guilt may be appropriate (i.e., survivor contributed to the death). The death of a spouse is a particularly significant risk factor for pathological grief. A surviving spouse with children may not have time to mourn appropriately. Those spouses with a high-conflict relationship, long duration of marriage, or a dependent relationship upon the deceased are particularly at risk. In the 2 years after losing a spouse over 50, the risk of the survivor dying is increased over fourfold.[3,14]

Physicians may be asked to provide sedatives, tranquilizers, or sleeping medications for the bereaved. The grieving process requires active work on the part of the bereaved. The survivors must learn to adjust to the absence of the deceased, form new relationships, and learn to live in their environment without their loved one. This process is delayed by tranquilizing medications. Their use is to be avoided except in cases of pathological grief and then only as part of a comprehensive psychotherapy plan. Requests for medication should be met with empathy and reassurance.

VIEWING THE BODY

After the family has undergone the initial grief reaction, they should be offered an opportunity to view the body of the deceased, without pressuring them to do so. Failure to view the body may prolong the process by not permitting the survivors to believe the person is really dead.[3,9,15,16] While most find viewing the body to be a helpful experience, those who do not view the body express no regret about their decision.[17]

The body is prepared prior to viewing. Blood and body secretions are cleaned off. The eyes are closed and the body is covered except for the hands and face. If permitted by the circumstances and local protocol, tubes and catheters are removed. If disfigurement has occurred, these areas are bandaged. The family is warned about the temperature and color changes of the deceased. The body is placed in a smaller room away from the treatment area to give the mourners more privacy. The physician, clergy, or nursing staff accompanies the family to provide support or answer questions. The family is encouraged to speak to and touch the deceased if they wish. A family member may wish to be alone with the deceased. This is permitted in appropriate circumstances; a staff member should remain close by for support. The deceased should be referred to by name or "him" or "her" and never by "it" or "the body."[3,11,13]

CONCLUDING PROCESS

Even after the family has an opportunity to view the body, there are several important processes left. Now is the time to make requests for autopsy and organ donation. Any signing of papers is done at this time and copies are given to the family. Any further questions are addressed at this time. Arrangements for funeral home and release of the body are made. The family is told that the patient's private physician will be contacted.[11] The physician and staff should be sympathetic but not apologetic. Families may misinterpret such expressions as an admission of guilt. Expressions such as, "You have my sympathy," or "I know this is very hard for you," are superior to, "I'm sorry."[3,11]

As in any other emergency encounter, follow-up arrangements conclude the visit. The survivors are educated about common grief symptoms. They are told to expect these as a normal part of grieving. At the minimum, the family should have the name and number of a staff member who can provide further information or answer questions that may arise.[11] Most authors recommend a follow-up phone call or letter within one week and again in two months.[3] One facility has established a program in which the staff sends a sympathy card, phone calls are made periodically during the year following the death, and the attending physician sends a letter explaining the autopsy findings.[5]

Finally, the family is told that it is time to leave. Survivors are frequently so overwhelmed with events that they do not know when to leave. They are escorted to the door and given reassurance again. Suggestions are made about contacting other friends or family for notification and funeral preparations.

SPECIAL CONSIDERATIONS

Long Distance Notification

If the survivors have not been notified of their family member's arrival in the ED, then initiate telephone contact. The caller should identify him- or herself and establish the identity of the survivor. Ideally, death notification is not made over the phone. The survivor is told that their relative or friend is severely injured or ill and that they need to come to the hospital immediately. Instruct them to drive carefully.[18]

There are times when distance, environmental, or other factors make physical notification inadvisable. One study showed that many survivors preferred to be notified by telephone if the driving time exceeded one hour.[19] Notification should not be rushed but should proceed in the same fashion as if done in person. The notification should not be forced; if the family member seems unprepared, offer to speak with another family member in the home or another relative. After the notification is made, if the survivor is alone, offer to contact some supporting person. If pathological grief is present, ensure the safety of the survivor by contacting other supporters to attend them. If the survivor appears suicidal, local police may need to be contacted. If no adult is present, ask the oldest child how to contact an adult relative. Assure the child that an adult will be contacting them shortly. Depending on the circumstances (distance, time of day, weather), the survivor should be instructed to come to the hospital driven by some supporter.[18,19]

Coroner's Cases

In most states, the coroner and/or medical examiner has the responsibility to investigate the cause of death within their jurisdictions. Cases the medical examiner may choose for further investigation include those of a sudden, mysterious, unusual, or unnatural nature. Deaths with a possible public health danger, deaths in police custody or in prison, or violent death (including those resulting from motor vehicle crashes) are also medical examiner cases. Autopsy is usually performed in these cases and the family is informed. Organ donation may still be possible, in consultation with the medical examiner.[11] Prior to viewing of the body by the family, resuscitative lines and tubes must be left in place. Except in very unusual circumstances, such as homicide, the viewing of the deceased is still able to take place.

Autopsy

Despite the clinical advantages of the information gained, autopsy rates have continued to decline in the United States. This decline is primarily the responsibility of physicians. Physicians may believe they already know everything about the case, and not want to stress the family further. Medical students are not taught the importance of the autopsy. Finally, the Joint Commission on Accreditation of Hospitals eliminated its minimum autopsy rate of 20 percent in 1971.[20]

Advantages of the autopsy include improvement in medical care nearly half the time, frequently by clarifying the diagnosis.[21] Diagnosis of new diseases is aided by the autopsy. Autopsies can assist in the grieving process by demonstrating to the family that they did not contribute to the death. Despite physicians' fear that the autopsy will lead to increased liability exposure, postmortem examinations are more often used as a defense.[22]

Public misperceptions concerning autopsy abound. Some of the misperceptions are that diagnostic tests are infallible; autopsy disturbs the patient's "peace"; bodily mutilation occurs; funeral arrangements will be delayed; it's too late to accomplish anything positive; religious prohibitions are present; the family never gets the results; and if an autopsy is necessary, one will be requested.[23]

The most senior physician involved with the case should approach the family with the request for autopsy. Specific points to be discussed include that the autopsy is done by specialists in pathology (an analogy to surgery may be helpful); specific determination of cause of death may help to dispel any doubt the family has; funeral arrangements will not be disturbed; and no mutilation occurs.[11] If the family is concerned about religious prohibitions, they can be reassured that autopsy is not prohibited by most of the major religions,[24] and can be encouraged to consult with the chaplain. The physician requesting the autopsy must be aware of local and institutional policies regarding billing and payment for autopsies. Many teaching institutions consider the autopsy as part of comprehensive care and do not submit a charge. However, there is great variation on policies in community, state, and municipal hospitals, and the patient's family should be so informed when they make their decision about an autopsy.

Organ Donation

Despite a growing need for transplantable organs, health care professionals are uncomfortable approaching families for organ donation.[25] While actually harvesting organs in the ED would be a rare event, many organs can be harvested up to 24 h after death if the body is refrigerated within 4 h of death. These harvestable organs include such tissues as cornea, bone, skin, tendon, fascia, cartilage, saphenous vein, and heart valves.[26] Contraindications to donation include age greater than 80, death from infectious disease, cancer (although corneas may still be donated), or toxic exposure.[26,27] Patients with fatal exposures to cocaine, ethanol, carbon monoxide, lead, and barbiturates have donated successfully. Consultation with a toxicologist is recommended in these circumstances.[28]

There are several barriers to tissue procurement in the ED. One study showed that only 43 percent of families were approached, with a successful donation rate of 12 percent. Reasons given for not approaching families included coroner's case (35 percent), family not available (20 percent), family too upset (18 percent), deceased medically unsuitable (14 percent), and no patient identification (12 percent). Time constraints are an additional barrier to successfully obtaining donation. Limited time to both develop rapport with families and to allow them to come to terms with the death, along with a busy staff, have been cited as reasons for unsuccessful donation efforts.[26]

The appropriate time to make a request for organ donation is after the family has viewed the body. At this point an interval has occurred from the actual notification and the bereaved have had time to come to accept the death as real. A premature request for organ donation may leave the family with doubts about the resuscitative efforts. The family is informed that they are not charged for any procedures related to the donation and that no alteration in appearance of the deceased occurs.[19]

Pediatric Concerns

Regardless of the etiology of the child's death, survivors are at increased risk of pathological grief.[3] Divorce is common after the death of a child.[29] Parents of deceased children display a wide range of emotional responses, but anger and guilt with associated despair predominate.[30] These emotions may be related to a sense of failure of the parent's protective role.[31] Both parents are equally devastated and unable to support each other adequately.[19] The need to care for surviving children may not allow time for proper grieving to occur. In particular, a perinatal death with either a surviving twin or subsequent pregnancy within five months places families at higher risk for pathological grief responses.[32]

Surviving children are also deeply affected by the death of a sibling. Feelings of abandonment, fear of death, and guilt predominate. If the child wished their sibling dead at a time near the death, they may believe that their "magical" thinking was causative.[19] Parents, unable to deal with their own grief, may explain the death in misleading or vague terms.[3]

The autopsy is particularly helpful in cases of pediatric death. It gives an organic, identifiable cause of death, helping to alleviate guilt. It can offer a source of comfort to the family that the knowledge gained may be useful in helping other children. Organ donation is also useful in this fashion.[3,15,33]

REFERENCES

1. McCaig LF: *Advance Data: National Hospital Ambulatory Medical Care Survey: 1996 Emergency Department Summary.* Hyattsville, MD, National Center for Health Statistics, 1997, p 20.
2. Tolle S: Communication between physicians and surviving spouses following patient deaths. *J Gen Intern Med* 1:309, 1986.
3. Walters DT: Family grief in the emergency department. *Emerg Med Clin North Am* 9:189, 1991.
4. Sykes N: Medical student's fears about breaking bad news. *Lancet* 1089:564, 1989.
5. Schmidt TA: Emergency physician's responses to families following patient death. *Ann Emerg Med* 19:125, 1990.
6. Schmidt TA: Sudden death in the ED: Educating residents to compassionately inform families. *J Emerg Med* 10:643, 1992.
7. Tolle SW: A program to teach residents humanistic skills for notifying survivors of a patient's death. *Acad Med* 64:505, 1989.
8. Wolraich ML: Training physicians in communication skills. *Dev Med Child Neurol* 21:773, 1979.
9. Parrish GA: Emergency department experience with sudden death: A survey of survivors. *Ann Emerg Med* 16:792, 1987.
10. Jones WH: Sudden death: Survivors' perceptions of their emergency department experience. *J Emerg Nursing* 7:14, 1981.
11. Olsen JC: Death in the emergency department. *Ann Emerg Med* 31:758, 1998.
12. Hamilton GC: Sudden death in the ED: Telling the living. *Ann Emerg Med* 17:382, 1988.
13. Edlich RF: On death and dying in the emergency department. *J Emerg Med* 10:225, 1992.
14. Jacob S: An epidemiological review of the mortality of bereavement. *Psychosom Med* 39:344, 1977.
15. Finlay I: Your child is dead. *BMJ* 302:1524, 1991.
16. Soreff SM: Sudden death in the emergency department: A comprehensive approach for families, emergency medical technicians, and emergency department staff. *Crit Care Med* 7:321, 1979.
17. Jones WH: Emergency room sudden death: What can be done for the survivors? *Death Educ* 2:231, 1978.
18. Dubin WR: Sudden unexpected death: Intervention with the survivors. *Ann Emerg Med* 15:54, 1986.
19. Leash RM: *Death Notification: A Practical Guide to the Process.* Hinesburg, VT, Upper Access, 1994.
20. McPhee SJ: To redeem them from death: Reactions of family members to autopsy. *Am J Med* 80:665, 1986.
21. Gambino SR: The autopsy: The ultimate audit. *Arch Pathol Lab Med* 108:444, 1984.
22. Webster JR: Obtaining permission for an autopsy: Its importance for patients and physicians. *Am J Med* 86:325, 1989.
23. Brown HG: Perceptions of the autopsy: Views from the lay public. *Hum Pathol* 21:154, 1990.
24. Geller SA: Religious attitudes and the autopsy. *Arch Pathol Lab Med* 108:494, 1984.
25. Prottas J: Health professionals and hospital administrators in organ procurement: Attitudes, reservations, and their resolutions. *Am J Public Health* 78:642, 1988.

26. Lewis LM: Tissue and organ procurement in the emergency department setting. *Am J Emerg Med* 11:347, 1993.
27. Rivers EP: Organ and tissue procurement in the acute care setting: Principles and practice—Part 2. *Ann Emerg Med* 19:193, 1990.
28. Leikin JB: The toxic patient as a potential organ donor. *Am J Emerg Med* 12:151, 1994.
29. Baumer J: Family recovery after the death of a child. *Arch Dis Child* 63:942, 1988.
30. Sanders CM: A comparison of adult bereavement in the death of a spouse, child, and parent. *Omega* 10:303, 1980.
31. Rando T: Bereaved parents: Particular difficulties, unique factors, and treatment issues. *Social Work* 30:19, 1985.
32. Rowe J: Follow-up of families who experience a perinatal death. *Pediatrics* 62:166, 1978.
33. Beckwith J: The value of the pediatric post mortem examination. *Pediatr Clin North Am* 36:29, 1989.

PATIENTS WHO ABUSE ALCOHOL AND OTHER DRUGS: EMERGENCY DEPARTMENT IDENTIFICATION, INTERVENTION, AND REFERRAL

Edward Bernstein
Judith A. Bernstein
Gail D'Onofrio

BACKGROUND AND RATIONALE

Epidemiology

Alcohol is implicated in more than 100,000 deaths annually in the United States, including 30,000 from unintentional injury and 17,700 from intentional injury.[1] Illicit drug use is associated with over 20,000 deaths,[1] more than 500,000 emergency department (ED) visits,[2] and one-third of the newly diagnosed cases of AIDS each year.[3] The economic cost of alcohol and other drug abuse in the United States was estimated at $276 billion for 1995. Alcohol abuse and alcoholism accounted for 60 percent of this figure, while illicit drug abuse and dependence (controlled substances used for nonmedical purposes) accounted for the remaining 40 percent.[4]

Substance abuse not only affects the individual user but has far-reaching implications for families, communities, the workplace, and the health care system. One out of four Americans experiences family problems related to alcohol, and an estimated 28 million children of alcoholics are at risk because of family dysfunction associated with alcoholism.[5] At the end of 1996, 1.4 million incarcerated adults were seriously involved with alcohol and drugs, and these individuals were parents to 2.4 million children.[6] Substance abuse is also a serious problem in American industry, with daily alcohol use by 8 percent of the work force and illicit drug use in the past year by 15 percent. Approximately 70 percent of the illicit drug users are employed.[5] Despite the proven effectiveness of treatment in breaking the cycle of addiction and reducing recidivism, clinical medicine has until recently lacked the social mandate, resources, will, and training necessary to treat alcohol and drug addiction adequately, and has deferred to the criminal justice system.[7]

Emergency Department Recognition of Substance Abuse

The percentage of ED patients who test positive for blood alcohol at the time of the visit ranges from 6 to 34 percent for injured patients and 1 to 19 percent for the noninjured.[8] At the time of an urban ED visit, 17 percent of patients were found to meet stringent criteria for alcohol abuse and 19 percent for alcohol dependency, while only 9 percent of the study group were breath alcohol positive, and only 14 percent reported a drinking problem. Among a 1-year sample of more than 7100 patients presenting to another urban ED, 41 percent (n = 2931) screened positive for alcohol or drug abuse on a health-needs history.[9] Rates of substance abuse as high as 50 percent have been reported among trauma patients,[10] and alcohol is a major risk factor for virtually all categories of injury.[11]

Although emergency physicians are experts in the stabilization, diagnosis, and treatment of acute alcohol and drug emergencies and their secondary complications, they often fail to detect and refer patients for treatment of addiction. In one study, for example, while ED physicians documented past or current alcohol use on the ED chart for 69 percent of patients with an elevated saliva alcohol level (reflecting acute intoxication), they documented alcohol use in only 46 percent of those with positive results on a screening test for at-risk behavior or dependence.[12] Referral rates as low as 13[11] and 23 percent[12] have been reported among ED patients with documented substance abuse problems. As a result, many ED patients who could be assisted in breaking the cycle of addiction continue to visit the ED with trauma and medical problems.

Time constraints, insufficient education, lack of role models in training programs, inadequate treatment resources, and the misperception that the patient's substance abuse is not an appropriate concern for a health-care provider all act as barriers to systematic detection and referral.[11] Provider attitudes of disinterest, avoidance, disdain, and pessimism are also common, especially when physicians are confronted with hostile, manipulative, or combative patients. Negative stereotypes of patients with substance abuse problems may reflect a physician's prior personal or family issues with substance abuse.

Patients with alcohol and drug problems are primarily encountered in the medical, rather than the treatment, system. According to the Institute of Medicine, more than 5 million Americans currently need treatment for drug abuse.[7] In a recent study, only 3 percent of weekly drug users were in contact with the drug treatment system, but 43 percent had encounters with primary health agencies, 39 percent with the criminal justice system, and 10 percent with the welfare system.[13] In addition, the ED is the usual source of extraprison care for many detainees and prisoners, and most of the 5.5 million individuals currently in the criminal justice system either are or will be returned to their communities to become ED patients again.

Emergency physicians have both an opportunity and an imperative to link patients presenting to the ED with the substance abuse treatment system. The ED, with its high prevalence rate, is an excellent site for taking advantage of a teachable moment in order to increase detection and referral rates and reduce harm associated with substance abuse.

Effectiveness of Brief Intervention

The effectiveness of screening, detection, and brief intervention was established four decades ago in an urban hospital ED study by Chavetz and associates.[14] A randomized, controlled trial among a population consisting primarily of homeless men demonstrated that it was possible to enhance the system of care even in such a hard-to-reach group by "establishing emotionally meaningful communication with these patients." As a result of this intervention, 65 percent completed a referral to an alcohol clinic, compared to 1 percent of the control group. Forty percent completed five or more voluntary visits, compared to 0 percent of the control subjects, who were managed by the ED staff in the routine manner.

That ED intervention represented a paradigm shift from the legacy of prohibition, the Harrison narcotics laws, and their underlying perspective of substance abuse as a moral weakness requiring criminal sanctions for individuals with substance abuse problems and penalties for physicians who tried to intervene. Shortly before the Chafetz study was published, the American Medical Association recognized alcoholism as a disease for the first time and encouraged physicians to care for patients with this problem as they would other sick individuals.

Many models for brief intervention have now been tested. A review of 32 controlled trials of brief counseling, primarily in the alcohol field, found that not only was brief counseling more effective than no treatment, but it compared favorably with more traditional treatments in 11 of 13 randomized trials.[15] The elements common to these trials were feedback, responsibility, advice, menu or choice, empathy, and self-efficacy (FRAMES). A World Health Organization study evaluating heavy problem drinkers across 12 nations with very different cultural orientations and social circumstances confirmed these results.[16] A randomized, controlled trial of brief intervention in 17 community-based primary care practices involving 64 physicians and 723 subjects in 10 Wisconsin counties demonstrated significant reductions in alcohol consumption.[17]

Treatment successes have also been associated with significant cost savings. The California Drug and Alcohol Treatment Assessment Study, for example, demonstrated a gain of $7 for every dollar invested in treatment; overall, the $200 million spent on treatment resulted in a $1.5 billion savings for California taxpayers.[18]

Changing Role of Emergency Department Physicians

In light of the enormous impact of alcohol and other drug abuse on society and individuals, it is no longer sufficient to treat only the emergency condition and the medical complications of substance abuse without providing proper screening, brief counseling, and referral to further treatment when appropriate. Connecticut State Law 472 mandates universal screening in the health care setting and requires documentation of training in intervention for all personnel working in health care institutions and clinical settings licensed by that state.

In the current managed-care environment where hospitals and physicians are competing intensely for market share and beginning to share economic risks with payers of health care, the desire to contain costs has given impetus to efforts to provide a more consistent approach to the needs of the patient with substance abuse. There is a growing recognition of the importance of a public health approach and the need for early identification, intervention, and access to treatment.

Research is currently under way at a number of EDs to discover best practices. A growing number of emergency physicians and nurses are engaged in helping patients with alcohol and drug problems to change negative behaviors. In some EDs, social workers, addiction specialists, volunteers from Alcoholics Anonymous or Narcotics Anonymous, or health promotion advocates (peer educators) are part of a team approach to providing identification, counseling, referrals to the treatment system, and access to primary health care and other needed services (e.g., housing, food, clothing, and jobs). Alcohol and injury studies in Rhode Island, Connecticut, and Georgia use an intervention conducted by social workers. Project Neighborhood in Missouri employs certified substance abuse counselors in an urban ED. A New York State hospital–based intervention program employs nurses who screen patients at the bedside and perform an interview. At Kaiser in Oregon, a health maintenance organization that has a broad series of prevention and intervention programs, patients are screened with a standardized instrument and referred to a health counselor for interview. Harborview Trauma Center employs social workers to intervene at the trauma center.

One of the first of these models to report ED data is Project ASSERT at Boston Medical Center,[9] in which trained community outreach workers from cultural backgrounds similar to those of the patients use a health-needs history to screen for substance abuse and other preventable conditions, and implement a brief negotiated interview (BNI) when substance abuse is identified. Patients are approached in the ED examining rooms in order to evaluate their overall health and safety needs and provide health education and referral. Among 7118 adult ED patients screened for alcohol and drug problems during the first study year, 2931 problem situations were detected and 1096 ED patients enrolled. Among 245 enrollees who participated in a 90-day follow-up, there was a significant reduction in harm at posttest in self-reported behavior, including a 45 percent decrease in drug-abuse severity scores, a 67 percent reduction in the number of enrollees using cocaine or crack, 62 percent reduction in the number using marijuana, a 56 percent reduction in alcohol use, and a 64 percent reduction in binge drinking. Over 50 percent reported following up with a treatment referral. Patients were also linked to primary care and other preventive services. Treatment options were negotiated with patients, and potential treatment slots were explored. Once placement was secured, taxicab vouchers were provided as needed for transportation to the selected facility.

TECHNIQUES FOR IDENTIFICATION AND BRIEF INTERVENTION

Early Identification and Screening in the Emergency Department

CRITERIA It is important for emergency physicians to distinguish between *at-risk* alcohol and drug abuse and *dependent* use. Any illicit drug use poses potential risk to the user, such as a criminal arrest, cocaine chest pain, seizures, heroin overdose, asthma exacerbation as a result of smoking drugs, and intentional or unintentional injury under the influence of drugs.

For alcohol risk, the National Institute on Alcohol Abuse and Alcoholism (NIAAA) has developed the following definitions for at-risk drinking among individuals between the ages of 21 and 65: for men, 14 drinks per week or 4 drinks per occasion; and for women, 7 drinks per week and 3 drinks per occasion.[19]

According to the American Psychiatric Association criteria,[20] the diagnosis of alcohol or substance *dependence* requires that at least three of the following criteria be present during a 12-month period:

1. Tolerance manifested by the need for markedly increased amounts of substance over time to achieve intoxication or the desired effect or by a markedly diminished effect with continued use of the same amount of the substance
2. Withdrawal manifested by a characteristic withdrawal syndrome or substance (or closely related substitute) taken to relieve or avoid withdrawal symptoms
3. Consuming larger amounts of substance over a longer period of time than intended
4. Persistent desire or unsuccessful attempts to cut down on or control use
5. A great deal of time spent in substance-related activities, such as obtaining the substance, consuming the substance, or recovering from the its effects
6. Important social, occupational, or recreational activities given up or reduced because of substance use
7. Continued substance use despite knowledge of a recurrent psychological or physical problem that is likely to have been caused by or exacerbated by use

HISTORY Universal screening in the ED would require that the past medical history include such questions as, Has your partner or any one you live with harmed you? Do you smoke? Do you drink beer, wine, liquor, or distilled spirits? Do you use drugs now and then?

An initial history should include questions about smoking first, then use of alcohol, and finally use of illegal substances in order to normalize the questions; create a nonjudgmental, matter-of-fact atmosphere; and thus enhance the likelihood of obtaining accurate information. If the initial response to drinking is positive, NIAAA guidelines recommend using the CAGE instrument, described below, and following up with quantity and frequency questions, such as, How many drinks containing alcohol do you consume in a typical week? and What is the maximum number of drinks you have had on any given occasion during the last month?

Similar questions can be asked for use of illegal substances. Questions about drugs should elicit the type of substance used, the frequency, the quantity (hits for crack and bags for heroin), the route, and whether drugs are used in combination with each other or with alcohol. It is also important to include an inquiry about nonmedical use of prescription drugs, since this is a common source of problems among women. If concerns about drugs and alcohol arise based on these data, it is recommended that brief intervention and referral be delayed to attend to acute medical issues before negotiating behavior change with the patient. Addressing the secondary diagnosis of alcohol and drug abuse dependency should be an integral part of an appropriate and safe discharge and follow-up plan.

SCREENING TESTS Although the initial history is important, the limitations of making a clinical diagnosis of an alcohol problem based only on blood, saliva, or breath alcohol testing; smell on breath; self-report; or presenting complaint have been described. A brief screening instrument, such as the CAGE test, is easy to administer, assists in identifying dependent drinkers who would benefit from entry into treatment, and may facilitate the process of matching an individual to the most appropriate treatment resource. In one study, 31 percent of patients presenting to an urban ED had positive results on the screening test, while only 13 percent were biochemically positive for alcohol using a saliva alcohol test.[12]

The CAGE, a mnemonic for the following questions, has been studied extensively, is easy to remember, and is easy to use:

C: Have you ever felt that you should *c*ut down on your drinking?
A: Have people ever *a*nnoyed you by criticizing your drinking?
G: Have you ever felt bad or *g*uilty about your drinking?
E: Have you ever had a drink first thing in the morning to steady your nerves or get rid of a hangover (*e*ye-opener)?

A score of 1 or more is positive for females, and a score of 2 or more is positive for males. Although the CAGE test is designed for assessing lifetime dependency, it should be prefaced with the phrase "in the last 12 months" in order to detect current problems. Patients tend to reveal less when the test is preceded by direct, closed-ended questions about quantity and frequency of drinking. Under such circumstances, the ability of the instrument to detect alcoholism is reduced by a third compared to when the test is preceded by an open-ended question, such as, "Do you drink beer, wine, or liquor now and then?"[21] Because of these findings, the CAGE test and other screening instruments should be employed as part of the history of present illness or past medical history, and not be used later in the physician-patient interaction as part of an intervention to change behavior.

The CAGE test has been specifically studied for its applicability to the ED.[8] The *sensitivity* (the proportion of individuals with a condition who have a positive test) was reported as 75 percent for at-risk drinkers, and 76 percent for dependent drinkers. The *specificity* (the proportion of individuals without the condition who have a negative test) was 88 percent for at-risk drinkers and 90 percent for dependent drinkers.

Intervention

VALUE OF BRIEF INTERVENTION IN THE EMERGENCY DEPARTMENT The best site for intervention is wherever the individuals who need help can be found. The first principle of intervention is that it comes *to* people, instead of people having to seek it out. The second is that it be timely, and the best time for early intervention is the crisis that brings the person with an alcohol or drug problem into the system for a medical, social, or criminal justice problem. An ED visit, for example, appears to be a teachable moment. Brief interventions have been shown to be effective for the at-risk user to negotiate behavior change, and for the dependent drinker and drug user to negotiate referral to treatment. The entire interaction can be accomplished in less than 10 min, and the dialogue can take place either at discharge or while suturing or casting.

INTERVENTION METHODS The BNI is a dialogue format developed in a busy urban ED for negotiating change in substance-related behaviors. In this method, the practitioner is the facilitator rather than the agent of change. The BNI may result in behavior change for the individual who is at risk and facilitates contact with the treatment system for the individual who is dependent. Through negotiation, patients' needs are tailored to solutions, and patients are matched with treatment modalities they are able to accept.

The BNI is based on the principles of brief motivational interviewing developed by Miller and Rollnick,[22] which are encapsulated in the FRAMES acronym (feedback, responsibility, advice, menu or choice, empathy, and self-efficacy). Brief cognitive motivational intervention also incorporates elements of a stages-of-change model,[23] in which five stages of change with highly predictable patterns are identified: precontemplation, contemplation, preparation, action, and maintenance, with the possibility of setbacks along the spiral pathway. Substance abusers are thought to cycle through these five stages in the course of changing their addiction behavior. Intervention techniques have been developed to suit each of these stages and explore with individuals the pros and cons of their behavior. In this process, the interventionist assists the addicted person to (1) define the problem, (2) identify his or her present stage, and (3) move through the stages of change toward recovery.

The BNI is used to assist patients to recognize and change behaviors that pose significant health risks. The goal of the interaction is to facilitate resolution of ambivalence through exploration of conflicting motivations (the pros and cons of drug use) and negotiate possible strategies for change, depending on the patient's readiness to change. The patient is seen to possess a unique store of knowledge—his or her own life history—that is essential for behavioral change to occur and just as important for achieving the goal as the interviewer's expertise. The BNI is used to increase intrinsic motivation so that change arises from within, rather than being imposed from without. The patient identifies both the problem and the solutions in order to own them. The general principles for successfully negotiating behavior change include (1) respect for the autonomy of patients and their choices; (2) negotiation based on readiness to change, and tailoring of interventions to level of readiness; (3) appreciation that ambivalence is expected, and exploitation of ambivalence is an important tool for facilitating change; (4) selection of targets for change by the patient, not the expert; (5) definition of the expert as a provider of information and support; and (6) reliance on the patient as the active decision maker.[24] "A patient's motivation to change can be enhanced by using a negotiation method in which the patient, not the practitioner, articulates the benefits and costs involved."[25] This theoretical understanding is the basis of the assertion that the BNI is more productive than simple advice.

The BNI protocol is based on mnemonics familiar to all emergency medical specialists, ABC and CPR:

A: Assessment
B: Brief intervention
C: Call back

C: Cultural competence
P: Patient choice
R: Readiness

The BNI consists of the following steps:

1. *Establish rapport with the patient* throughout the clinical encounter. Establish an atmosphere of positive regard in which the patient is not a problem but a person who has a problem.
2. *Ask the patient's permission to discuss the pros and cons of drug use.* Use open-ended questions and empathic and reflective listening. Explore the importance to the patient of the issues that emerge, and establish which of the pros and cons has the greatest salience in order to concentrate on those with the highest priority.
3. *Summarize what the patient says* to indicate that you understand what has been said (and to be sure you are correct in your interpretation). This summary technique can also elicit more information as trust develops.
4. *Ask the patient to describe his or her readiness to change.* A drawing of a ruler with a scale of 1 to 10 is used to elicit readiness to change use of drugs and or alcohol, as well as readiness to enter treatment. The patient points to the location on the scale that describes the current state of readiness for each score.
5. *Negotiate with the patient based on his or her perception of readiness* (not ready, unsure, or ready). Find out where the patient finds him or herself on the readiness ruler on a scale of 1 to 10 (a score of 1 is least ready and a score of 10 is most ready). If the patient is (a) *ready (a score of 8 to 10),* then the interviewer will solicit previous experience in attempting to quit, and brainstorm alternatives; (b) *unsure (a score of 5 to 7),* then the pros and cons of drugs or alcohol use and the pros and cons of change or treatment need to be explored, further assessment may be proposed, and the question posed, What will it take to help you take a few steps toward being more ready, say, going from 6 to 8?; (c) *not ready (a score of 1 to 4),* then the interviewer expresses concern, offers information about the affects of drugs and alcohol, provides a list of resources for further reference, and suggests the possibility of further contact (Table 287-1).

THE REFERRAL PROCESS

If a patient is ready to accept referral, a staff member who is familiar with treatment resources can assist the patient in making an appointment or plans to enter a treatment program. Each ED should provide a resource list for staff and a printed handout or brochure for patients with names, addresses, and phone numbers of treatment programs. The following resources should be available: inpatient detoxification; outpatient detoxification; acupuncture; methadone maintenance; outpatient individual and group counseling; residential communities; self-help groups, such as Alcoholics Anonymous, Narcotics Anonymous, or Alanon; programs focused on the needs of women; and programs that are culture specific.

TABLE 287-1 Sample Brief Negotiated Interview Dialogue

Speaker	Dialogue	Procedure
Physician	"Hello, Mr. Smith, I'm Dr. B. You had a pretty bad fall, but the x-ray doesn't show any fracture."	Establish atmosphere of respect; start with patient's own concerns.
Patient	"That's good news. I really took quite a fall. I couldn't use the arm to drive, and I thought I had broken it."	
Physician	"How did the fall happen?" (examining the shoulder)	
Patient	"I had just gotten home from a party. I was going up the stairs, lost my balance, and fell backwards on my shoulder."	
Physician	"That must have been upsetting! Were you drinking a lot?"	Establish empathy; unite with patient's feeling without condoning the behavior.
Patient	"I must have lost count."	
Physician	"Do you mind talking a little bit about the drinking?"	Ask permission to discuss substance use.
Patient	"What about my drinking?"	
Physician	"Well, would you help me to understand what it is that you like about your drinking?"	Begin discussion of pros and cons of drinking with open-ended question.
Patient	"I really like the taste of beer, and I like drinking with my friends after work. It helps me to loosen up."	
Physician	"Anything else?"	Ask open-ended question; explore pros.
Patient	"I like meeting new people at the bar."	
Physician	"Is there anything less enjoyable about your drinking?"	Explore cons.
Patient	"The fall that I took tonight and the fact that I lost count of my drinks concerns me."	
Physician	"Anything else, any other injuries?"	
Patient	"Last month I wrecked my car, and I got in a fight with my girlfriend tonight about flirting. I guess I can really be a jerk sometimes."	
Physician	"Let's see if I got this right. On the one hand, drinking is a way of relaxing with friends, loosening up and meeting new friends; while on the other hand, you may get too loose and lose count, get argumentative, and do things you wish you hadn't and even injure yourself."	Provide summary (reflective listening).

TABLE 287-1 *Continued*

Speaker	Dialogue	Procedure
Patient	"You got it."	
Physician	"Do you think you may be losing control of your drinking and drinking more than usual?"	
Patient	"I haven't thought about it that way, but you have a point."	
Physician	"On a scale of 1 to 10, like this ruler, how ready are you to cut back on your drinking?"	Assess readiness to change behavior.
Patient	"Oh, I think I'm about a 6. I'm pretty fed up with the problems I've been having. I don't know if I can do it, though."	Patient is unsure.
Physician	"What would it take to get you more ready?"	Keep negotiating.
Patient	"I suppose if I have another accident like tonight. But that's pretty stupid, to wait for something else to happen."	
Physician	"Well, if you were ready to make some changes, what are your options? What could you do to get more control over your drinking?"	Assist in generating options; return control and responsibility to patient.
Patient	"I could drink less and maybe socialize in a different setting where I don't feel the pressure to show off about how much I can handle."	
Physician	"That sounds like a great idea. Studies show that drinking 14 or more drinks in a week or 4 or more drinks on any occasion puts you at risk for injury and illness."	Offer feedback; reinforce positive movement.
Patient	"My friends and I drink a lot more than that."	
Physician	"Would you consider getting a further assessment of your drinking or talking with a good counselor about possible strategies to help you to get your drinking under control? Are you ready for some help?"	Assess readiness to accept referral for treatment.
Patient	"To tell you the truth, I would prefer to do it on my own. But maybe you can give me a phone number of this person in case I just can't."	
Physician	"I would be glad to. You are not alone. There are a lot of people who have succeeded in making these changes and would give you support, and there are formal support groups like Alcoholics Anonymous. Good luck, and feel free to give me a call to let me know how you are doing. Here's a prescription for the pain. Be sure to apply ice for the next 12 h to reduce the swelling. A discharge nurse will be in to give you instructions and a list of numbers you can call."	For unsure patients, offer a concrete support system, something written to take home, and a chance to talk to you again if needed (call back).
Patient	"Thank you, doc."	

If, for example, a patient who is injecting drugs is not ready to accept an ED referral, it may be possible to negotiate contact with a harm-reduction program, such as a community-based needle-exchange program that provides sterile needles in exchange for potentially contaminated needles. Such programs have documented effectiveness in reducing the spread of HIV[24–28] and hepatitis B and C[29] among injection drug users and are effective in facilitating entry into the drug treatment system.[3]

MEDICAL CLEARANCE FOR DETOXIFICATION

Medical clearance for transfer to a detoxification or other treatment facility should include the following components:

1. *Past history.* Inquire about past history of hospitalization for delirium tremens, alcohol-related seizures, hepatitis, and pancreatitis; screen for severity of alcohol withdrawal signs and symptoms; review past medical illness and medications; and rule out underlying medical conditions related to substance abuse.
2. *Recent history.* Inquire about and document recent falls, assaults, pedestrian or motor vehicle injuries, head injuries, tuberculosis status, and productive cough; and review notes made by the registered nurse, emergency medical technician, or referring facility.
3. *Examination.* Undress the patient completely; perform a careful evaluation for trauma, hypovolemia, and gastrointestinal bleeding, including a rectal examination for stool guaiac if orthostatic vital signs are abnormal or gastrointestinal bleeding is reported; assess and document a set of orthostatic vital signs, including temperature and O_2 saturation by pulse oximetric analysis for patients with history of lung disease or respiratory symptoms; and evaluate the level of withdrawal (e.g., gait, tremulousness, and change in mental status).
4. *Laboratory testing.* Determine the serum glucose level for diabetics and for patients with altered sensorium; obtain serum levels of lithium and anticonvulsants as appropriate; and obtain serum potassium levels for patients on diuretics.
5. *Mental health status.* Assess for psychiatric issues and obtain a consultation if the patient is dangerous to him- or herself or others.
6. *Specific risk factors.* Assess routinely; for example, think twice about transferring older people with comorbid conditions.
7. *Specific conditions.* Screen and treat for seizure disorder or alcohol-related seizure.
8. *Medications.* Assure that a reasonable supply of medications is sent with the patient until prescriptions can be filled.
9. *Discharge.* Clear only when the patient is ambulatory, alert, oriented, and able to take fluids orally; if pulse is less than 100 beats per minute and body temperature is less than 38.3°C (101°F); and if there is no significant change in mental status.

10. *Document.* Chart a clear plan for safe discharge, including the method of patient transfer to the detoxification facility.

REFERENCES

1. McGinnis JM, Foege WH: Actual causes of death in the United States. *JAMA* 270:2207, 1993.
2. Update: Syringe-exchange programs: United States, 1996. *MMWR* 46:565 1997.
3. Substance Abuse and Mental Health Services Administration, Office of Applied Studies: *Mid-Year Preliminary Estimates from the 1996 Drug Abuse Warning Network.* Rockville, MD, US Department of Health and Human Services, 1997.
4. Harwood H: *Economic Costs of Alcohol and Drug Abuse.* Fairfax, VA, Lewin Group, 1998.
5. Institute for Health Policy, Brandeis University: *Substance Abuse, The Nation's Number One Health Problem: Key Indicators for Policy.* Princeton, Robert Wood Johnson Foundation, 1993.
6. National Center on Addictions and Substance Abuse at Columbia University (CASA): *Behind Bars: Substance Abuse and America's Prison Population, Executive Summary.* http://www.casacolumbia.org/pubs/jan98/summary.htm.
7. Institute of Medicine: *Pathways of Addiction: Opportunities in Drug Abuse Research.* Washington, National Academy Press, 1996.
8. Cherpital CJ: Screening for alcohol problems in the emergency department. *Ann Emerg Med* 26:158, 1995.
9. Bernstein E, Bernstein J, Levenson S: Project ASSERT: An ED-based intervention to increase access to primary care, preventive services, and the substance abuse treatment system. *Ann Emerg Med* 30:181, 1997.
10. Dunn CW, Donovan DM, Gentilello L: Practical guidelines for performing alcohol intervention in trauma centers. *J Trauma* 42:299, 1997.
11. Lowenstein SR, Weissberg MP, Terry D: Alcohol intoxication, injuries and dangerous behaviors and the revolving emergency department door. *J Trauma* 30:1252, 1990.
12. Bernstein E, Tracey A, Bernstein J, Williams C: Emergency department detection and referral rate for patients with problem drinking. *Substance Abuse* 17:69, 1996.
13. Weisner C, Schmidt L: Expanding the frame of health services research in the drug abuse field. *HSR* 30:707, 1995.
14. Chavetz ME, Blane HT, Abrams HS, et al: Establishing treatment relations with alcoholics. *J Nerv Ment Dis* 134:395, 1962.
15. Bien TH, Miller WR, Tonigan JS: Brief interventions for alcohol problems: A review. *Br J Addict* 83:315, 1993.
16. WHO Brief Intervention Study Group: A cross-national trial of brief interventions with heavy drinkers. *Am J Public Health* 86:948, 1996.
17. Fleming MF, Barry KL, Manwill LB, et al: Brief physician advice for problem drinkers: A randomized controlled trial in community based primary care practice. *JAMA* 277:1039, 1997.
18. Gerstein DR, Harwood HJ, Sutter N, et al: *Evaluating Recovery Services: The California Drug and Alcohol Treatment Assessment.* Sacramento, State of California Department of Alcohol and Drug Programs, 1994.
19. National Institute of Alcohol Abuse and Alcoholism: *The Physician's Guide to Helping Patients with Alcohol Problems.* Washington, US Department of Health and Human Services, Public Health Service, National Institutes of Health publication 95-3769, 1995.
20. American Psychiatric Association: *Diagnostic and Statistical Manual of Mental Disorders,* 4th ed. Washington, DC, 1994.
21. Steinweg DL, Worth H: Alcoholism: The keys to the CAGE. *Am J Med* 94:520, 1993.
22. Miller WR, Rollnick S: *Motivational Interviewing: Preparing People to Change Addictive Behaviors.* New York, Guilford, 1991.
23. Prochaska JO, Velicer WF, Rossi JS, et al: Stages of change and decisional balance for 12 problem behaviors. *Health Psychol* 13:39, 1994.
24. Rollnick S, Heather N, Bell A: Negotiating behavior change in medical settings: The development of brief motivational interviewing. *J Ment Health* 1:25, 1992.
25. Rollnick S, Kinnersley P, Stott N: Methods of helping patients with behavior change. *Br Med J* 307:188, 1993.
26. Des Jarlais DC, Paone D, Friedman SR, et al: Regulating controversial programs for unpopular people: Methadone maintenance and syringe exchange programs. *Am J Public Health* 85:1577, 1995.
27. Lurie P, Drucker E: An opportunity lost: HIV infections associated with lack of a national needle-exchange programme in the USA. *Lancet* 349:604, 1997.
28. Hurley SF, Jolley DJ, Kaldor JM: Effectiveness of needle-exchange programmes for prevention of HIV infection. *Lancet* 349:1797, 1997.
29. Hagan H, Jarlais DC, Friedman SR, et al: Reduced risk of hepatitis B and hepatitis C among injection drug users in the Tacoma syringe exchange program. *Am J Public Health* 85:1531, 1995.

288 PHYSICIAN WELL-BEING

Sanford H. Koltonow

Physician well-being is an important personal and professional issue. Career satisfaction correlates with the following issues: (1) control over working conditions, (2) hospital administrative support, (3) having time for family and personal life, and (4) departmental security. The practice of emergency medicine requires a large knowledge base and advanced cognitive and interpersonal skills. Not quite as obvious is the need for excellent *intrapersonal* skills. Situations arise that conflict with one's personal values and produce intense feelings of uneasiness. To remain effective, coping methods need to be used that are adaptive and resolve conflict. The thought that one can meet *all* of a patient's needs ignores one's own needs for supports and limits.

Stress is necessary as a force that motivates. When excess stress becomes detrimental, it is more appropriately called distress. Much like Starling's law, each individual has his or her own curve with a point beyond which further stress causes less, rather than more, output.

Burnout is a state of physical, emotional, and mental exhaustion that occurs as a result of intense involvement with people over long periods in emotionally demanding situations. Burnout symptoms are characterized, in their extreme form, by physical depletion and chronic fatigue, feelings of helplessness and hopelessness, and the development of negative attitudes toward self, work, life. and others. Among physicians, symptoms of burnout are thought to be potential precursors of more severe manifestations of impairment, including alcoholism, drug abuse, and suicidal ideation.

Emergency physicians practice in an environment that can foster burnout. Critical decisions must be made with incomplete information. Noises, smells, crowding, children, families, terminal illnesses, substance abusers, psychiatric patients, police, and criminals are part of every day. It is easy to become overwhelmed.

The American Medical Association defines an impaired physician as "one who is unable to practice medicine with reasonable skill and safety because of physical or mental illness, including deterioration though the aging process, loss of motor skill, or excessive use . . . of drugs, including alcohol." Various estimates of impairment range from 7 to 13 percent. Well before attrition occurs, there are warning signs that, with awareness, can be identified and remedied before a patient's care and a physician's status are threatened.

Suicide, the ultimate manifestation of impairment, accounts for one-third of the premature deaths among physicians. The percentage is higher for women, particularly young women. Annually, over 100 physicians complete suicide.

BURNOUT

This is a condition born of good intentions. Doctors who fall prey to it are, for the most part, individuals who have striven for perfection in their careers. It grows from unrealistic goal setting. Burnout is fostered by common personality characteristics of those that choose and succeed in emergency medicine. Near-compulsive overachievement, denial of one's limits, a low level of trust, distant interpersonal relationships, and independent self-sufficiency are common. An effect is that the processing of deep feelings is repressed. Instead of addressing their own symptoms of personal stress, *physicians tend to project feelings* of irritability, anger, and frustration on others: patients, nurses, and their families.

The ability to dissociate feelings from one's work is an adaptive coping mechanism for working with contagious disease and dangerous situations, but it can also help physicians ignore their own vulnerabilities. They may not recognize the toll that a lifestyle of little sleep, poor diet, and little time for recreation or reflection may be having on themselves and their families. Dissociation becomes deadly when the ''it can't happen to me'' philosophy is used to justify increasing alcohol and drug consumption or other self-destructive behaviors.

Fear of incompetence is nearly universal among physicians and is the source of many of the stressors related to medical decision making. When dealing with other people's lives, mistakes can have life-threatening ramifications. If one cannot accept his or her limits and the possibility of making a mistake, one must (at least hope to) be perfect and all-knowing, a situation that promotes arrogance and a strong need to defend against perceived criticism. Even symbolic challenges, perhaps by someone asking a question about care or interjecting a different opinion, can strike deep at defense mechanisms, frequently resulting in inappropriate physician behavior.

PROFESSIONAL ENVIRONMENT STRESSORS

Stressors arising from nonmedical issues within the professional environment as well as from a physician's personal environment can also compound the difficulties in providing quality emergency care.

In urban areas, anywhere from 30 to 50 percent of patients receive *all* of their medical care from the emergency department. Their needs can be immense, including such basic needs as food, shelter, heat, and transportation, which makes assisting these patients much more difficult. Additionally, a physician may be drawn into a patient's dependency needs, creating interpersonal conflict.

Emergency departments and physicians are commonly required to become agents of the police and courts. Laws exist that compel emergency physicians' involvement with intoxicated, violent, and psychotic patients. This also may include victims of personal crimes, such as sexual assault and abuse, where physicians must collect evidence for legal proceedings.

Victims of major trauma are frequently victims of crime, and physicians are frequently subpoenaed to provided testimony in legal proceedings, which are inconvenient. In addition, in such settings, it is not unusual to be cross-examined with hostility.

Death and Dying

Death and dying involve physicians in sharing one of a family's most personal and powerful times. Emergency physicians need to become comfortable exploring patient's wishes and informing families of unexpected death and morbidity, for they will be called on to do so often. Empathy requires emotional energy. Speaking with a grieving family forces a physician to face both system and personal conflicts.

The need of the patient and family for compassion is a difficult process to rush. Their wishes and belief systems deserve exploration. There are questions from loved ones about the events leading up to a death that must be dealt with empathically to facilitate the grieving process. Offering understanding, comfort, compassion, and solace can be important source of satisfaction for physicians. Often, deaths resurrect powerful feelings in physicians, based on prior personal experiences.

Some difficulties of physicians may stem from the belief that a physician's career represents the battle against death and disease. Facing a surviving family or counseling a dying patient may symbolize ''failure'' in that battle. In addition, a physician can become a target for misplaced anger and denial.

Malpractice Litigation

Universally, physicians feel the need to expend significant resources to prevent malpractice litigation (as opposed to the resources used to prevent malpractice). For those unfamiliar with the process, a medical malpractice lawsuit can be frightening. It seems to strike at one's very being and self-worth. Many physicians will respond with disbelief, then anger, and finally depression. The process of meetings, testimony, and eventually the trial can be dehumanizing. Physicians who succumb to the emotional trauma of a lawsuit respond in such a consistent manner that it has become known as malpractice stress syndrome (MSS).

The single factor most predictive of a dysfunctional response is the experience of isolation. Embarrassment and self-doubt can cause avoidance of one's very sources of support. Colleagues' responses may reinforce a physician's feeling of shame. Knowing the physician is busy preparing a defense, colleagues may change their referral and social patterns, which can be interpreted as judgment about the facts of the case.

Self-doubt frequently carries over to personal life. Either for reasons of not wanting to bring home the pain or from feelings of shame for getting named in a lawsuit, many physicians withdraw from their spouses and families, furthering their isolation.

PERSONAL ENVIRONMENTAL STRESSORS

Sleep Deprivation

Shift work and scheduling difficulties are the most common sources of stress, career dissatisfaction, and attrition in emergency medicine. People who work swing shifts have a shortened life expectancy. Circadian principles acknowledge the body's natural rhythms and can help in integrating one's work schedule with one's personal life and promote quality sleep and, thus, health.

SLEEP PHYSIOLOGY Sleep occurs in discrete stages. The bulk of delta sleep or *slow wave sleep* (SWS) occurs early in the sleep period. There is an increase in SWS in subjects who perform challenging intellectual tasks. SWS is thought to be vital for *physical* recuperation. Those deprived of SWS often complain of fatigue and muscle aches.

Rapid eye movement (REM) *sleep* is characterized by rapid conjugate eye movements, a change in electroencephalogram to a pattern similar to wakefulness, the occurrence of dreams, increase in oxygen consumption, and increased cerebral blood flow. Those with shorter sleep periods will likely have REM deprivation, which is difficult to make up. REM sleep is thought to be vital for *psychological* well-being. Those deprived of it complain of irritability and moodiness. They also score higher on testing of aggressive behavior. REM sleep may also be important in the consolidation of complex learning. Experimental subjects deprived only of REM sleep but allowed the other phases begin displaying a thought disorder reminiscent of psychosis within 3 to 4 days.

Humans have a 25 h circadian clock. Many physiologic functions follow circadian patterns and can be transposed by keeping experimental subjects awake at night and sleeping during the day. This process is known as *entrainment* of the circadian rhythm. Many circadian patterns have been demonstrated to be sensitive to entrainment, including alertness and basal body temperature. The *primary* stimulus for spontaneous awakening is a rise in body temperature; thus, the duration of the sleep period depends more on the phase of the circadian rhythm than on the prior period of wakefulness. This partly explains why those working short stretches of nights sleep fewer hours during the

TABLE 288-1 Strategies and Recommendations to Assist in the Health of Shift Workers

Given the right set of circumstances, the best strategy is to work the same shift all of the time and keep the same sleep pattern.
For those unable to maintain consistent sleep patterns, use compromise strategies such as anchor sleep and napping to mitigate circadian disruptions.
Rotate all shifts in a clockwise direction, with at least 1-month minimum time per rotation.
One or two night shifts in a row causes minimal circadian disruption.
Sleep in a quiet, darkened room, minimizing disruptions. When working nights, give the work schedule to likely daytime callers.
Start the awake period with a high-protein meal and switch to complex carbohydrates toward bedtime. Avoid caffeine and high-calorie, high-fat snack food before sleep. Eat meals regularly.
Use bright light (more than 10,000 lux) for 2 h after rising, as an adjunct for entraining to new shifts.
Get regular exercise. Vigorous aerobic exercise after rising may diminish the time needed to adjust to new shifts. Avoid heavy exertion before attempting to sleep.
Work with family and friends to plan regular quality time together.
Do not try to live a day-shift lifestyle while working night shifts. Hold administrative meetings early in the morning or late in the afternoon when working night shifts. Respect the circadian rights of those working nights by excusing them from meetings held during the day.

Source: Adapted from Whitehead et al, with permission.

daytime than those working night shifts regularly, leading to REM sleep deprivation.

Many physicians attempt to use pharmaceuticals to assist them in falling asleep. Essentially all decrease the proportion of REM sleep. Stimulants, including nicotine and caffeine, impede onset of sleep and normal sleep stage progression.

Studies on sleep deprivation show that the ability to perform challenging intellectual tasks is slowed but otherwise relatively unchanged; however, motivation to perform routine tasks is diminished. Because the quality of emergency medical practice often depends on properly performing routine tasks that may follow prolonged periods of intellectual exertion, it is imperative for physicians who work different shifts to schedule themselves in ways that minimize risk to patients.

SUPPORTIVE STRATEGIES When planning shift rotations, it is healthier to rotate forward (days to afternoons to midnights), since the human circadian rhythm is 25 h long. Many physicians favor 12 h shifts to increase the number of days off. When rotating shifts, however, it takes longer to reset the biologic clock across a 12 h change than it does for an 8 h change (see Table 288-1).

The circadian "gold standard" is not to change shifts at all, but those working only night shifts must maintain a daytime sleep pattern, even during days off, to avoid reentrainment to a daytime pattern. Working nights for long periods is difficult due to pressures to participate in daytime family and social activities or to be involved regularly in administrative activities.

There is a compromise known as *anchor sleep*, which minimizes circadian disruption. By sleeping a block of at least 4 h at the same time every day, one tends to anchor the circadian rhythm. It can be useful for permanent night-shift workers during their days off or during short periods of irregular shift work, making it easier to return to "normal" sleep patterns.

Social life is important for shift workers. Maintaining close ties with family and friends helps to relieve stress and mitigates the sense of temporal isolation that shift workers face. Planning for quality social time is as vital as planning for work.

Family

The personality characteristics chosen by and supported in medicine often conflict with family and self-care priorities. With the increasing complexity of a physician's clinical and administrative schedule, social and community obligations, as well as the spouse's and children's interests. are most likely to suffer. A family deserves planned blocks of time that are sacrosanct.

Specific hardships are associated with being in a relationship with a physician. Two-physician families are becoming more common, with their own specific pressures. Living with the persistent demands of medicine, most physician couples live for the future, convinced that eventually there will be time for each other. The couple unconsciously assumes that the delay will not endanger the quality of the relationship, and it will remain as fresh and intense as the day it was postponed.

Complex defense mechanisms, learned in the milieu of the emotional and physical fatigue of training and practice, frequently lead to a blunting of one's ability to respond to deep personal feelings. The most common complaint from physician families entering counseling is that the physician member is emotionally unreachable, if not physically absent.

Physicians become professionally comfortable being decisive and responsible. Rarely are the feelings or opinions of others welcomed—physicians merely give "orders." As experts, they know what is best for the patients. It becomes a common scenario to translate this to the home, expecting that problems will be solved by directive. The physician is tired, communication falters, and compromise is one sided as the family member decides to "let it go; at least he's [or she's] finally home." Arrogance is enabled. Conflict is postponed until crisis develops.

Spouses can benefit from a support organization. The aim is to assist in understanding medical stress, share coping mechanisms, reduce isolation, and understand their own role in the patterns that shape their intimate relationships. Serious consideration should be given to using a trained communication facilitator and formal group structure for spouses' groups.

Finally, if a physician provides medical treatment to his or her family, the care given can be unsuitable—either excessive or inadequate. A physician can not remain objective in assessing loved ones, and it is most often inappropriate to try. Both the physician and his or her family deserve as complete and thorough an evaluation as would be provided to patients arriving at their emergency department.

Aging

Aging sometimes makes it physically difficult to do all that is required. Changes in the shift rotations are harder. Visual and hearing acuity may suffer. It may be difficult to accommodate medical problems; for example, at what time do you take your morning and evening doses of medications when you are working midnights? What if your diuretic takes effect during trauma resuscitation? How does a professional group deal with the inevitable increase in sick time needed by an aging group of physicians? When does the slowing of reflexes exceed acceptable tolerances?

Career transitions are available in many specialties, but, as a new specialty, emergency medicine does not have as much experience in tailoring the practice to accommodate older physicians, and options other than leaving the field need to be developed.

STRATEGIES FOR WELL-BEING

Table 288-2 lists the author's principles for promoting personal well-being. The overriding tenets are self-awareness and self-responsibility.

TABLE 288-2 Principles for Promotion of Physician Well-Being

Commit to being aware of your stresses and anxieties. Relate to stress as a challenge to overcome, not as something intolerable with power over your life.
Maintain perspective. Don't take yourself too seriously. Develop a separate identity, one not dependent on your role as a physician.
Allow yourself space to be human. Realize medicine is not the cause of your problems or unhappiness—you are free to choose the lifestyle and work environment. Confront the options.
Be here now. If your family, religion, community, or other activity is actually a priority, spend time with it. Your family deserves planned blocks of time that are sacrosanct.
Focus on the intrinsic rewards of medicine: altruism, interest in the science, the challenge of the patients who need your skills, and stimulation by the broad range of people with whom you work. There are rewards in medicine you find motivating. If these are not apparent, then this is an area in need of exploration.
Develop networks with your peers. Don't allow yourself to become isolated.
Support systems need to be acceptable to all concerned and not threaten professional status. You must have personal and professional confidants and accurate feedback. Learn to recognize maladaptive coping mechanisms in yourself and colleagues.
Expose students and residents to psychotherapists, who can establish scientific and interpersonal credibility. This exposure can facilitate their personal use during times of crisis.
Be certain there is adequate staffing provided to afford relief, time off, and backup in times of crisis.
Care for yourself by attending to your physical health: Make necessary provisions to assure adequate, quality sleep. Get regular exercise, control your weight, and pay attention to your diet. Provide for your relaxation. This is different from leisure. See your doctor(s) and follow *their* instructions.

No individual or institution created your conflicts or can resolve them. One can, however, mold the environment until it best suits one's needs. Choices and alternatives always exist.

Self-Assessment

During a particularly difficult period, most people know they feel stressed and may not be functioning as efficiently as they usually do. Frequently, this is attributed to a difficult patient, a busy shift, or a particular personal stressor outside of one's control. Self-awareness enables individuals to begin to appreciate their patterns of response from a wider perspective. Paradoxically, some physicians, when faced with the disillusionment of a lifestyle not realized, cling harder to their original motives—in denial. This process feeds upon itself, resulting in frustration.

Table 288-3 lists some questions to be used as a starting point to assess one's own emotional fatigue. If several of the answers are affirmative, perhaps this is evidence of divergence between personal values and career activities. This may motivate you to seek feedback from a trusted source.

Principles of Management

Common methods for overcoming professional fatigue use time management, support systems, debriefing/relaxation, administrative training, and physical self-care. Regardless of the validity of the need, one can not say yes to one commitment without saying no to something else. A process of *value clarification* helps identify those concepts one is willing to commit to and provides a starting point for determining personal priorities. One then should set life's major goals in all areas—physical, mental, financial, spiritual, social—according to the individual's most meaningful objectives.

Develop relationships with peers that go beyond the immediate clinical issues. Listen, and provide emotional support and challenge. Be the one to take the risk of talking about the things that are felt but ignored. Share the social reality of what living and practicing in current society is like, sharing thoughts, feelings, and strategies. The fear that someone may discover one's vulnerabilities needs to be resisted. This encourages low levels of trust in peers and tends to isolate one from the social supports needed in times of crisis.

Concern for the well-being of medical trainees must be constantly modeled in training. Many trainees do not have the advantage of *mentors* who share with them their mistakes, let down their guard, and demonstrate that a lack of perfection does not mean incompetence. Such mentors demonstrate that a mistake is compatible with excellence and compassionate care. Errors in problem solving can be used to improve learned behavior. A faculty that can mentor on personal/professional humility is the best prevention against medical arrogance.

Well-being committees within hospital or medical societies can provide education along with referral to other resources. Lines of communication are opened as physicians learn coping techniques that others have found effective. Topics to present to the medical staff include value clarification, goal setting, time management, grieving, and reframing. A well-being committee is different from professional assistance programs for impaired, disabled, or ''troubled'' physicians, though their work should complement one another.

The *critical incident stress debriefing* (CISD) team is an approach that attempts to reduce the severity of poststress disorders at the time of occurrence. Personnel who have experienced a critical or anxiety-provoking situation are debriefed as a group. The group is facilitated by experienced group leaders of similar professional background in conjunction with mental health professionals. This occurs within 72 h following the event. The goal is to intercede before unhealthy reactions have time to be fully incorporated. Each individual is asked to describe what he or she saw, heard, and felt. The incident becomes the setting to share feelings. Participants are given the message that the discomfort they are encountering is a normal reaction to an abnormal experience. It also allows the opportunity to identify those individuals who may need further assistance.

TABLE 288-3 Questions for Self-Assessment

Do you find the old ways of coping are not as reliable as they once were?
Do you find yourself becoming cynical about your colleagues or the ''system''?
Do you waste time at work, dreading to see patients or slowed by indecision?
Are you drinking, eating, or smoking more than is normal for you?
Is your self-esteem unduly affected by criticism?
Have you lost the intrigue with medicine?
Do you feel helpless over the loss of control in the direction that medicine is taking?
Do you have continuous problems with insomnia, fatigue, or depression?
Do you feel lonely or isolated? Do you avoid others so they don't see how unhappy you are?

Rapport

In emergency situations, one often does not have the benefit of an ongoing doctor-patient relationship. There are some easy things that emergency physicians can do to build rapport and trust. Most revolve around communicating the perception of listening and caring. Physicians should greet patients by name and introduce themselves, shaking hands when appropriate. Physicians should sit down whenever possible—regardless of how long physicians actually remain in the room, patients perceive it as much longer. When touching patients, do so gently with an air of caring. Respect a patient's privacy by closing curtains and exposing only that which is necessary. When clinically appropriate, listen to a patient's overall agenda—it may save time. Do not use complex language. If a patient is lying down, sit or bend down and put your eyes at the patient's level. Set expectations for a patient with the first encounter, i.e., "results will be back in 2 h, and I'll be back to discuss them then," or "I have a critical patient to care for but you'll be next." Finding a small need that you can fulfill (e.g., a glass of water, a pillow, a phone call) will help establish rapport.

Conflict Resolution

Conflict resolution skills are important in emergency medicine for interactions with patients, peers, physicians in other specialties, and other hospital staff. The issues of conflict differ; the dynamics, however, are similar.

Some people believe intrinsically that their concerns, no matter how minor, are more important than anyone else's. Demanding patients or families are best handled by acknowledging their expectations and attempting compromise. Sometimes, it is effective to acknowledge that the patient has been heard and his or her perspective considered, yet the physician has a different perspective and position. Although firmness may be necessary, rarely will anything be gained by hostility or by confrontation.

Administrators, nurses, and consultants may be other sources of conflict; often, ongoing personality conflicts exist, provoked by the intensity of the work environment. One needs to focus on finding the "common ground," which is the patient's needs.

Not every conflict is a battle that must be won. Healthy conflict resolution requires physicians to know when to stand up and when to negotiate or retreat.

Malpractice Litigation Support

Those concerned with physician well-being are beginning to explore malpractice litigation stress support groups. Several common attributes exist in the various models that have been proposed.

The group is educational. Risk management personnel describe what to expect at each step and clarify the meaning of legal terms. Physicians who have contended with lawsuits provide support by sharing their experiences. Hearing that others have felt similarly can be the initial crack in the wall of isolation built by the physician-defendant. Family members can provide insight into the process their family is experiencing and their emotional responses. This will often improve communication at home.

Information is available on how to establish litigation stress support groups, and many state medical societies already have such groups in place.

Physical Health

Most physicians do not get regular preventive health care. This may be due both to the tremendous time constraints of practice and to denial of one's vulnerability to illness. Either way, a physician can wind up caring less for self than for the patients.

Exercise helps maintain physical health and relieves emotional tension. In addition, setting aside the time for one's own health, within one's busy schedule and conflicting priorities, confirms with action the belief that caring for oneself is an important use of time.

The diets of many emergency physicians contribute to both poor health and fatigue: high in fat, sugar and caffeine, usually eaten quickly, without time to sit. Anticipating an urgent interruption also prevents one from relaxing.

Relaxation Techniques

Relaxation is different from leisure. Leisure activity is an important way to achieve balance. Physicians will find the stressors of leisure enjoyable in part because they are so different from the common stressors of professional life. Leisure activity will also usually involve family and friends. However, leisure activity frequently contains stressors of its own that tend to arouse and fatigue, rather then renew.

Relaxation is different from doing nothing. Relaxation actually increases awareness and focuses the mind while resting the body. It is a time to be present, to reflect, and to process experiences and feelings. Systematic relaxation requires concentration and deliberate mental activity. It will lead to lower arousal and release of strain. It can be particularly helpful if the relaxation does not require physically leaving the home, e.g., pleasure reading, gardening, hobbies, and crafts.

For those finding it difficult to achieve this level of relaxation, many techniques are available. Physicians will frequently respond to meditation, progressive muscle relaxation, selective awareness, self-hypnosis, somatics, yoga, breath control, and biofeedback. Many techniques have audiotapes available to help guide one conveniently through the learning process. For some, religious beliefs and activities may fulfill the need for relaxation. The important common denominator is quiet time that allows for personal reflection, integration, and planning.

IDENTIFICATION OF IMPAIRMENT

Emergency physicians frequently feel emotionally overwhelmed temporarily. When does this become maladaptive? Table 288-4 lists behaviors and thoughts, which when seen as a change in established behavior, are suggestive of problems.

Detecting impairment in others is much more difficult. Psychologically and chemically impaired professionals are often able to delay notice by protecting their job performance at the expense of every other dimension of their lives. The common signs of uncharacteristic behavior are frequently ignored. The phenomenon of family, neighbors, friends, and coworkers becoming involved in an exhaustive conspiracy *enabling* an impaired physician to appear to be functioning at his or her job is both common and tragic. Training in pharmaceutical use, functional psychiatric problems, and in the medical problems of addicted and abusing patients, helps physicians feel that they are experts capable of treating their own problems.

Intervention is almost always required with impaired physicians, because of the massive denial and other defense mechanisms they employ. Shame, embarrassment, fear, and guilt keep many health care workers from consciously accepting that they are not in control until confronted by either trusted colleagues or, more commonly, authorities. Intervention is a delicate task, requiring sensitivity, clear motives, and *specialized training*. Members of the physician's support system are consulted, and some are asked to be present at the intervention to deconstruct this "conspiracy of enabling." This will be the critical moment where a firm attitude of concern, without hostility or punitive overtones, has the opportunity to break through the defenses and enable the individual, for maybe the first time, to acknowledge the problem. At this point, the individual is very vulnerable and must be offered options.

The seriousness of the emotional impact of confrontation on the sick physician must be appreciated; it is critical to anticipate and prevent the possibility of a suicide or bodily harm by accident or

TABLE 288-4 Possible Signs and Symptoms of Burnout

Using home time only as time to rest, with withdrawal from family activities.
''Acting out'' behavior on spouse, family members, nurses, and staff.
Chronic complaining, cynicism, blaming others
Dreading to see patients.
Writing short, ambiguous charts; Quality Assurance or Utilization Review notice of inappropriate or unintelligible comments.
Requesting frequent consultations.
Inappropriate anger toward medicine, patients, staff, authority.
Over prescribing to a patient's symptoms.
Sharing personal problems with patients, blurring of boundaries.
Degrading of peers, backbiting, questioning motives of others.
Frequent illness, unexplained absence, and patterns of late arrival or early departures.
Frequent job changes.
Excessive ''toys'' that become time-consuming obsessions, such as computers, boats, and planes.
Spending nonwork time at the practice without apparent reason.
Unusual number of patient complaints.
Passive-aggressive response to change.

trauma. These possibilities are not uncommon, particularly among impaired health professionals.

RESOURCES

1. The Society and Center for Professional Well-Being of Durham, North Carolina, is a professional educational and consultative organization that produces programs on behalf of state and county medical societies, hospitals, and group practices. It offers unique programs in value clarification, practice assessment, mediation, and conflict resolution and is a source of manuals on developing litigation, spousal, and other support groups, as well as a speakers' bureau. Several active emergency physicians participate as speakers and contributors. (Contact: Dr. John-Henry Pfifferling, telephone 919-489-9167.)
2. The Talbot-Marsh recovery program for substance abuse and psychiatric disabilities in Atlanta, Georgia, specializes in treating health care professionals and is nationally recognized as a model for extended outpatient treatment of substance-abusing physicians. (Telephone 800-445-4232.)
3. The Menninger Clinic of Topeka, Kansas, provides individual, marital, and family therapy, and is a major psychoanalytic training program, as well. It also sponsors educational workshops in a retreat setting in Estes Park, Colorado, for a week each July. Designed specifically for physician couples, it focuses on the problem of balancing the demands of medical practice with the needs of self and family. (Contact: PO Box 829, Topeka, KS, 66601; telephone 800-288-7377.)
4. The Institute for the Study of Health and Illness is a nonprofit educational and research foundation focused on, among other things, the professional development of physicians who serve people who have life-threatening illnesses. Directed by Rachel Remen, MD, it offers books, tapes, and category I CME credit at small retreats that focus on topics such as loss, grief, personal limitation, impotence, isolation, and the examination of goals, values, and meanings. (Contact: ISHI, PO Box 316, Bolinas, CA 94924.)
5. ACEP, SAEM, and other medical societies provide state-of-the-art educational resources. Most of the topics in this chapter have been included in their presentations. ACEP has a membership section on well-being, which you may join for the informational newsletters of articles by other members, as well as to become active in supporting such issues with the college. (Contact: Well-Being Section, ACEP, PO Box 619911, Dallas, TX 75261-9911.)
6. The American Medical Association's Department of Mental Health has established the Physician's Health Foundation. Its purpose is to provide financial assistance for physicians disabled from any cause, including psychological or chemical impairment and HIV. Identification is through the state medical societies' physician's assistance programs. The foundation also supports research, focused education and retraining programs, job placement, and the International Conference on Physician Health. (Contact: Elaine Tejeck, telephone 312-464-5073.)

BIBLIOGRAPHY

Charles SC: Sued and nonsued physicians' self-reported reactions to malpractice litigation. *Am J Psychiatry* 142:437, 1985.

Gabbard G, Menninger RW, (eds): *Medical Marriages*. Washington, DC, American Psychiatric Press, 1988.

Gabbard G, Menninger RW: The psychology of postponement in the medical marriage. *JAMA* 261:2378, 1989.

Howell JB, Schroeder DP: *Physician Stress: A Handbook for Coping*. Baltimore, University Park Press, 1984.

Marshall AA, Smith RC: Physician's emotional reactions to patients. *Am J Gastroenterol* 90:4, 1995.

McCranie EW, Brandsma JM: Personality antecedents of burnout among middle-aged physicians. *Behav Med* Spring 1988.

Mitchell JT, Bray GP: *Emergency Services Stress*. Englewood Cliffs, NJ, Prentice Hall, 1990.

Pfifferling JH, in Scott CD, Hawk J: *Heal Thyself: The Health of Health Care Professionals*, New York, Brunner/Mazel, 1986.

Remen RN: *Kitchen Table Wisdom: Stories that Heal*. New York, Riverhead, 1996.

Sonneck G, Wagner R: Suicide and burnout of physicians. *Omega* 33:255, 1996.

Sulmasy DP: *The Healer's Calling: A Spirituality for Physicians*. New York, Paulist, 1997.

Whitehead DC, Thomas HR, Slapper DR: A rational approach to shift work in emergency medicine. *Ann Emerg Med* 21:1250, 1992.

CHILD ABUSE AND NEGLECT

Carol D. Berkowitz

SPECTRUM OF CHILD ABUSE AND NEGLECT

The concept of child maltreatment, defined as harm to a child because of abnormal child-rearing practices, is a broadening of the initial description of the battered child syndrome. Child maltreatment is an all-inclusive term covering physical abuse; sexual abuse; emotional abuse; parental substance abuse; physical, nutritional, and emotional neglect; supervisional neglect; and Munchausen syndrome by proxy.[1]

The ease with which physicians are able to recognize these disorders in part depends on their knowledge of normal children and normal development. The physical stigmata of maltreatment are characteristic, although the findings of neglect and sexual abuse are more subtle than those of gross physical trauma.

CHILD NEGLECT

Child neglect includes both physical and emotional neglect. Nearly 1 million cases of neglect occur annually in the United States. Neglect results from failure of the child's caregiver to provide adequate clothing, shelter, food, health care, and/or schooling. Children who are the victims of neglect may appear in the emergency department dirty, improperly clothed, and unimmunized. Their medical problems may not have been attended to in a timely manner. They may have suffered from burns or fractures because of inadequate supervision. Child neglect from early infancy can also result in the syndrome of failure to thrive (FTT). This syndrome usually affects children younger than age 3, although older children who remain in a nonnurturing environment show similar manifestations.

The FTT patient is often brought to the emergency department because of other medical problems, such as intercurrent infections; skin rashes, particularly severe monilial diaper dermatitis; or acute gastroenteritis.

The history of the acute illness may not alert the physician to the chronic nature of the underlying problem. The physical examination provides the clue to the diagnosis of long-standing malnutrition. Overall physical care and hygiene are frequently poor. Infants have very little subcutaneous tissue. The ribs protrude prominently through the skin, and the skin of the buttocks hangs in loose folds. There may be alopecia over a flattened occiput, reflecting that the baby has been allowed to lie on his or her back all day. Muscle tone is usually increased (although sometimes these babies are hypotonic). This increased tone is most notable in the lower extremities, and infants may manifest scissoring, similar to infants with cerebral palsy.[2]

FTT infants also show distinct behavioral characteristics.[3] They are wide-eyed and wary. If brought in close proximity to the examiner's face, they may purposely turn away to avoid eye contact. They become irritable if interpersonal interaction is pursued. They are difficult to console and are not cuddly. They prefer inanimate over animate objects and spend much time with their hands in their mouths. When left alone, they assume a ''straphanger's position,'' with their arms flexed at the elbows and extended over their shoulders.

Weights and lengths should be plotted on the appropriate growth curves. In general, weight is more adversely affected than length, although this depends on the duration of the neglect. This may be reflected in a body mass index [BMI = weight (kg)/height (m^2)] below the fifth percentile.[4] Likewise, long-standing neglect results in a diminution in the rate of growth of the head.

In addition to observing for these physical signs, physicians should obtain certain historical information, including the birth weight (to assess the rate of growth); any maternal use of cigarettes, alcohol, and/or drugs during pregnancy; previous hospitalizations; and the parental stature. A full social service assessment should also be obtained, although this is usually done by a medical social worker.

Infants suspected of suffering from significant environmental FTT should be admitted to the hospital. Weight gain in the hospital is felt to be the sine qua non of environmental FTT. Most infants gain weight within 1 to 2 weeks following admission; in addition, the hospitalization enables a more extensive social service assessment while the infant is in a protected environment. A skeletal survey of the long bones should be carried out to detect any evidence of physical abuse.[5]

Children over the age of 2 to 3 years with environmental neglect are termed psychosocial dwarfs. Their short stature is a more prominent finding than their low weight. These children manifest a classic triad of short stature, bizarre voracious appetite (eating from trash cans), and a disturbed home situation. They are frequently hyperactive and have delayed or unintelligible speech.[6] Psychosocial dwarfs have been studied endocrinologically and have been found to have a low to normal level of growth hormone that fails to increase with stimulation of insulin or arginine.[7] These children should also be admitted for evaluation and initiation of appropriate social intervention. The endocrinologic disturbances rapidly reverse following hospitalization or placement in a foster home.

MUNCHAUSEN SYNDROME BY PROXY

Munchausen syndrome by proxy (MSBP) is a relatively uncommon form of child abuse in which a parent either induces or fabricates an illness in a child in order to secure for himself or herself prolonged contact with health care providers.[8] Children with MSBP may arrive at the emergency department with reported symptoms such as bleeding, seizures, altered mental status, apnea, diarrhea, vomiting, fever, rash, or multiple organ system involvement. These symptoms may result from administration of agents such as warfarin or ipecac.[9] Often the cases are medically perplexing, and families frequently move from hospital to hospital, seemingly in search of diagnosis. Children with MSBP are often subject to multiple unnecessary tests as physicians seek to uncover the etiology of the disorder. The parent (biologic mother in 98 percent of cases) encourages the staff to do more diagnostic procedures and often seems uncharacteristically happy if a test is positive.

Social service and psychologic evaluation is mandatory in the evaluation and management of these children, who should be admitted to the hospital both to assure their safety and to institute needed therapy. Covert video surveillance has been used in some centers to document a parent's invasive actions.[10]

SEXUAL ABUSE

Victims of prior child sexual abuse are frequently difficult for inexperienced physicians to assess because of an unfamiliarity with the normal prepubertal genital examination.[11] Children who have been sexually abused are brought to the emergency department because of a disclosure about the abuse or because of other symptoms such as those referrable to the genitourinary tract, including vaginal discharge, vaginal bleeding, dysuria, urinary tract infections, or urethral discharge; behavior disturbances, including excessive masturbation, genital fondling, or other sexually oriented or provocative behavior; encopresis; regression; nightmares; and unrelated complaints.[12] Approximately 15 percent of children diagnosed in an emergency department as victims of sexual abuse in one report had unrelated complaints such as abdominal pain, asthma, and sore throat.

Children who are sexually abused rarely disclose their abuse until time has elapsed from the acute episode. Children who are seen immediately after an assault should be evaluated for evidence of acute injuries and for the presence of forensic material, such as semen.[13]

More often, several years have elapsed since the abuse was initiated, although it may be ongoing. Children 8 to 11 years of age frequently disclose that they have been victims of sexual abuse for a significant period of time. The assailant is known to the child in over 90 percent of cases.

A medical hsitory should be obtained from all children being evaluated for sexual abuse. Because evidence of the abuse may not be apparent until the child is examined, the physician may have to obtain additional medical history information after the physical assessment. The record of the medical history should include pertinent statements about whether the child has any underlying condition or has undergone any previous procedures that might cause changes in the anogenital area. Genitourinary surgery or trauma would be particularly important to note.

The child should be questioned directly about what happened. The child's name for genitalia and other body parts should be recorded, and all statements that the child makes concerning the abuse should be recorded verbatim. The demands of a busy emergency department may make it difficult for physicians to conduct a detailed and sensitive interview. In such cases, a hospital social worker should be consulted.[14]

Examining physicians must maintain a high index of suspicion of sexual abuse when evaluating children who have anogenital or behavioral complaints. The physical assessment should include an evaluation of the child's overall well-being and a general physical examination. The skin should be examined for bruises. Nongenital physical injuries are unusual, even following acute abuse. Rarely, there may be grip marks on the forearms or puncture wounds on the inner aspects of the lips caused by a slap to the face. The age of the child and the degree of sexual development should be noted.[15]

The genital examination should be confined to a careful inspection of the genitalia and perianal area. Generally, there is no need for a speculum examination unless the victim is an older adolescent or unless perforating vaginal trauma is suspected. Likewise, sedation is rarely needed, and most children can be reassured verbally if they are at all apprehensive. Careful inspection of the external genitalia is sufficient to establish physical evidence of genital injury. The examination is sometimes augmented by the use of a colposcope, to enable detection of subtle changes in the hymen.[16] The colposcope also facilitates photographing the external genital area. However, most emergency departments are not equipped with a colposcope, and this instrument is, in fact, not critical to an adequate assessment of the anogenital area. Magnification can easily be achieved with the use of hand-held lenses. Toluidine blue dye applied to the genital area may also detect subtle acute injuries.[17]

A number of different positions have been used to facilitate the examination. Infants may be seated on their parents' laps. Children are easily examined supine on the examining table with their legs in a frog-leg position. Some physicians also place all children in a prone knee-chest position to help fully assess the contour and homogeneity of the hymen. Placing a child in "stirrups" is usually unnecessary unless she is obese or has achieved adult stature.[18]

The normal prepubescent girl has full labia majora and small thin labia minora. The vaginal opening is covered by the hymen, a fine reddish-orange, thin-edged membrane. The thickness and color of the hymen varies as a function of age.[19,20] It is normally thick during infancy and again with the onset of puberty. In between, it is thinner, most often annular or crescentic, and smooth edged. The hymenal orifice can be measured, although there is a range of variation depending on the child's age, size, position, and degree of relaxation. Trauma may result in changes such as hymenal notches, also referred to as *concavities* or *clefts*.[21] Concavities at the 6:00 position are associated with prior penetrating trauma. Attenuation or reduction in the amount of hymenal tissue may lead to a gaping opening. Irregularities in the contour, particularly deep notches, are also associated with prior injury. Scarring, as evidenced by marked alteration in the vascular pattern (white areas or swirling vascularity), is an additional sign of healed injury. Erythema, on the other hand, may be secondary to irritation, inflammation, and/or chronic manipulation and is not specific for abuse.[22]

Physical findings indicative of a sexually transmitted disease should also be noted, including a vaginal discharge, warts consistent with condylomata acuminata or condylomata lata, and vesicles or ulcers consistent with herpes genitalia.

It is critically important for emergency physicians to be aware that the absence of physical findings does not preclude abuse. There are many sexually abusive activities (such as orogenital contact) that would not be expected to produce scarring trauma. In addition, as is true elsewhere in the body, injuries can heal without residual scarring.[23]

The genital examination in the sexually victimized young boy is less revealing. Rarely, there may be bite marks on the penis or scrotum. There may be a urethral discharge; the penis may become erect without tactile stimulation and remain erect.

The perianal examination is often more revealing, although it too may be completely normal in the case of either acute or chronic sodomy.[24] Acute penetration may produce no changes or may be associated with fissures; abrasions; hematomas; and changes in tone, including both dilatation and anal spasm. In the young female patient, anal penetration is easier than vaginal penetration, and changes in this area may be seen. Anal fissures or tags may be noted. The perianal folds, or rugae, may be thickened in some areas, thinned out in others, and distorted. The perianal skin may be lichenified and thickened secondary to frictional rubbing. Anal tone may be reduced when there has been repeated prior anal penetration. However, stool in the rectal ampulla may lead to similar dilatation, and one should be careful to note the presence or absence of stool.[25]

The laboratory evaluation of sexually abused children should include cultures of the throat, vagina (or urethra), and rectum for gonorrhea; and a culture from the vagina (or urethra) for *Chlamydia*. Rapid antigen assays are not considered reliable in prepubescent children.[26] A serologic test for syphilis is indicated if there is clinical evidence of syphilis, a history of syphilis in the assailant, or the presence of another sexually transmitted disease. HIV testing should only be done after appropriate counseling and if there is reason to suspect infection.[27]

A suspicion of child sexual abuse mandates that a report be filed with child protective services or law enforcement agencies. These agencies will pursue an investigation and attempt to ensure that the child is placed in a protected environment.

Although there is the likelihood that the child may be removed from the home, a return appointment for follow-up of cultures for sexually transmitted diseases and a referral for psychologic counseling should be given.

PHYSICAL ABUSE

The spectrum of injuries in children who have been intentionally traumatized is wide. Familiarity with this spectrum enables physicians in the emergency department to arrive at the correct diagnosis in a timely manner. Two-thirds of the victims of physical abuse are under the age of 3 years, and one-third are under 6 months. The physical vulnerability of such small children is easy to understand.

Historical data may raise suspicions of inflicted trauma. A history that is inconsistent with the nature or the extent of the injuries (e.g., a fractured femur in an infant from a fall off a bed), a history that keeps changing as to the circumstances surrounding the injury, a discrepancy between the story the child gives and the story the caretaker gives, a history of previous trauma in the patient or siblings, or a delay in seeking medical attention should raise one's index of suspicion of physical abuse.[28] Knowledge of normal motor development assists physicians in determining the likelihood that an injury happened in the stated manner. Children under the age of 6 months are incapable of inducing accidents or accidentally ingesting any drugs or poisons. The evaluating physician should record the developmental milestones the child has achieved, e.g., the age of sitting unsupported, walking, etc. A recent study showed that developmental milestones were recorded in none of the emergency department visits in which physical abuse was suspected.[29] Parental behavior in the emergency department should be observed, and it should be noted if the parents appear intoxicated or under the influence of drugs. The level of parental concern about the injury should also be noted.

Toddlers and older children should be questioned about the circumstances of the injury, and the comments should be recorded verbatim on the record. These statements are frequently admissible in court under exceptions to the hearsay rule and may help establish the diagnosis of child abuse.

The physical examination should note the child's overall hygiene and well-being. Normal children, especially toddlers who are just learning how to walk, may have multiple ecchymoses over the anterior shins, the forehead, and other bony prominences. Most falls result in bruises on only one body surface. Bruises over multiple areas, especially the low back, buttocks, thighs, cheeks, ear pinnae, neck, ankles, wrists, corners of the mouth, and lips suggest physical abuse. Handprints may be observed, or there may be uniform but bizarre bruises caused by belts, buckles, cords, or blunt instruments.[30] Bites produce bruising in a characteristic oval pattern, with teeth indentations along the periphery. Lacerations of the frenulum or oral mucosa may be present, especially in infants who have been force fed. Lacerations and abrasions in the genital area are seen in toddlers who are "punished" because of toilet-training accidents.

The duration of a bruise can be estimated by the color of the lesion. No discoloration is noted initially, although the bruised area may be swollen and tender. Within a day or two, the lesion becomes reddish-blue, and this lasts for about 5 days. This changes to green (days 5 to 7), then to yellow (days 7 to 10), and finally to brown (days 10 to 14) before resolving.[31] For instance, reddish-blue lesions are inconsistent with a 2-week-old injury. However, variability does exist and depends on the size and depth of the hematoma.[32]

Children with multiple bruises should be evaluated with a complete blood cell count, a differential blood count, and coagulation studies including a platelet count, a prothrombin time, and a partial thromboplastin time. Occasionally, a child with leukemia, aplastic anemia, or thrombocytopenia is brought for evaluation because of multiple bruises.

Burns constitute another form of inflicted injuries.[33] These may be scald burns caused by immersion in hot water. Such burns do not conform to a splash configuration; rather, an entire hand or foot ("glove-and-stocking" pattern) may be involved. There is sharp demarcation of the burn margin. The buttocks may be burned during toilet-training "punishment" by immersion in a bathtub filled with hot water. Knees, anterior thighs, feet, and portions of the abdomen are spared, and the buttocks and genitalia are scalded. Cigarette burns leave small (approximately 5 mm) circumferential scab-covered injuries. These lesions may resemble impetigo, as do scald injuries, which may resemble bullous impetigo. A culture of material from these lesions differentiates the burn from the infection. Other inflicted burns can result from forced contact with metal objects, such as an iron, curling iron, or heater grid.

Skeletal injuries may be detected when a child presents with unexplained swelling of an extremity or refusal to walk or to use an extremity. These fractures may take any form, but spiral fractures caused by torsion (twisting) of a long bone, and metaphyseal chip fractures, suggest inflicted injury, especially when present in infants under 6 months of age. Skeletal surveys referred to as a trauma series (or trauma x) should be obtained. These include films of all long bones, the ribs, the clavicles, the fingers, the toes, the pelvis, and the skull. They may reveal periosteal elevation secondary to new bone formation at sites of previous microfractures or periosteal injury; multiple fractures at different stages of healing; fractures at unusual sites such as the ribs, the lateral clavicle, the sternum, or the scapula; or repeated fractures to the same site. Such x-ray findings support the diagnosis of child abuse. Sometimes, bone scans will reveal fractures not readily apparent on x-rays.[34]

Head injuries are a serious and potentially lethal form of child abuse.[35] Infants with significant intracranial hemorrhage may have no apparent external injuries. Intracranial hemorrhages may result from vigorous shaking of the infant or from thrusting the infant down onto a surface, such as a mattress. This is referred to as shaken baby or shaken impact syndrome.[36] Older children may have been beaten about the head or face. Changes in mental status should therefore be evaluated by head computed tomography if there is any suspicion of abuse. Bruises around the ears, eyes, and cheeks, as well as swelling of the scalp secondary to subgaleal hematomas or underlying skull fractures, may be noted. Funduscopic examination may reveal retinal hemorrhages, which are usually associated with subdural hematomas. Such hemorrhages may result from direct trauma to the skull or severe shaking of the child.[37] These children should be evaluated with computed tomography, and coagulation studies should be performed to rule out underlying coagulopathies. Magnetic resonance imaging studies are also being used to help differentiate recent from older intracranial bleeding episodes. Additional eye injuries caused by trauma may include hyphema, lens dislocation, and retinal detachment.

Injuries to the abdomen are equally serious and are a common cause of death from child abuse.[38] Symptoms include recurrent vomiting, abdominal pain and tenderness, diminished bowel sounds, and/or abdominal distention. A history of injury as well as bruising of the overlying skin may be absent. Abdominal x-ray films may reveal a distended stomach with a "double-bubble sign" secondary to a duodenal hematoma. Diffuse distention may also be noted. Laboratory studies may reveal anemia, an elevated amylase level from traumatic pancreatitis, or hematuria from kidney trauma. Other abdominal injuries caused by trauma may include hepatic or splenic rupture, intestinal perforation, or rupture of intraabdominal blood vessels.

Any serious injury in a child under the age of 5 years should be viewed with suspicion. Other injuries that may be viewed as suggestive of child abuse include those which the child states were inflicted by another, were self-inflicted, or were inflicted by an unknown assailant.

The behavioral interaction between the child, the parent, and the physician may provide supportive evidence of the diagnosis of abuse. These children are often very compliant and submissive. They do not resist the medical examiner and readily submit to painful procedures such as blood drawing. They are overly affectionate to the medical staff, frequently preferring the nurse or the physician over the parent. Sometimes they are protective of the abusing parent, try to foster to his or her needs, and lie to cover up the true nature of the injury.

Parental behavior is less uniform, but certain distinct characteristics may be noted. The parents may not interact with the child in a comforting or supportive manner during the examination. They may become angry at the physician early in the course of the evaluation and may refuse diagnostic studies. They may appear to be intoxicated or under the influence of drugs. They may have brought the child in for seemingly minor complaints and ignored the major injuries or lesions. They may insist on hospital admission of the child for these minor problems and may readily confess they can no longer cope with the child. They may express fears of losing control.

The social service assessment may reveal an unstable home situation with frequent moves, poor parental support systems, low parental self-esteem (often caused by battering during their own childhood), parental substance abuse, and/or domestic violence. This adds further supportive evidence of a high-risk situation.

MANAGEMENT

Once the medical assessment has been completed, the physician must initiate the appropriate treatment. The medical management should be guided by the physical findings. Frequently, these children require hospitalization.

Although the specifics of the laws surrounding child abuse and neglect vary from state to state, every state does require that suspected cases be reported.[39] A verbal report is made initially to the police department and/or the child protection agency of the locality in which the abuse occurred. Law enforcement officers often appear in the emergency department, especially if the child does not require hospitalization. The child may be removed from the home and placed in protective custody, taken to a juvenile facility, placed temporarily with other relatives, or placed in a foster shelter home. The final disposition is dependent on a court hearing. The physician is also required to complete an official report detailing the specifics of the evaluation and giving his or her diagnostic opinion as to why the injuries or neglect are nonaccidental. The report should use nontechnical terms, e.g., *bruise* instead of *ecchymosis*, so the law enforcement and social service workers can understand the extent of the injuries.

Physicians are sometimes hesitant to report suspected cases. They are not "100 percent" certain. They are fearful of the parental response to the report. They are concerned about removing a child from the natural home. It is important to remember that physicians are required by law to report all suspected cases of abuse and neglect. Failure to report suspected cases can result in misdemeaner charges and lead to a fine or imprisonment. Additionally, physicians are protected by the law from legal retaliation by the parents.

Parental anger is a natural response to the filing of a report of suspected child abuse. The physician should refrain from being accusatory. Instead, the physician should note his or her concern about the child's well-being and advise the family that a physician is required by law to report any suspicions. The physician should verbally acknowledge the anger but persist in the role of child advocate. This job is facilitated in hospitals that have child abuse teams available to assist physicians in the emergency department.

REFERENCES

1. Reece RM: *Child Abuse: Medical Diagnosis and Management.* Philadelphia, Lea and Febiger, 1994.
2. Berkowitz CD: Failure to thrive, in Berkowitz CD (ed): *Pediatrics: A Primary Care Approach.* Philadelphia, WB Saunders, 1996, p 415.
3. Powell GF, Low JF, Speers MA: Behavior as a diagnostic aid in failure-to-thrive. *J Dev Behav Pediatr* 8:18, 1987.
4. Hammer LD, Kraemer HC, Wilson DM, et al: Standardized percentile curves of body-mass index for children and adolescents. *Am J Dis Child* 145:260, 1991.
5. Merten DF, Carpenter BLM: Radiologic imaging of inflicted injury in the child abuse syndrome. *Pediatr Clin North Am* 37:815, 1990.
6. Silver HK, Finkelstein M: Deprivation dwarfism. *J Pediatr* 70:317, 1967.
7. Powell GF, Brasel JA, Blizzard RM: Emotional deprivation and growth retardation simulating idiopathic hypopituitarism: I. Clinical evaluation of the syndrome. *N Engl J Med* 276:1271, 1967.
8. Meadow R: Munchausen syndrome by proxy. *BMJ* 299:248, 1989.
9. Rosenberg DA: Web of deceit: A literature review of Munchausen syndrome by proxy. *Child Abuse Negl* 11:547, 1987.
10. Southall DP, Plunkett MCB, Banks MW, et al: Covert video recordings of life-threatening child abuse: Lessons for child protection. *Pediatrics* 100:735, 1997.
11. Chadwick DL, Berkowitz CD, Kerns D, et al: *Color Atlas of Child Sexual Abuse* Chicago, Year Book Medical, 1989.
12. Seidel JS, Elvik SL, Berkowitz CD, et al: Presentation and evaluation of sexual misuse in the emergency department. *Pediatr Emerg Care* 2:157, 1986.
13. Berkowitz CD: Child sexual abuse. *Pediatr Rev* 12:443, 1992.
14. Levitt CJ: The medical interview, in Heger A, Emans SJ (eds): *Evaluation of the Sexually Abused Child: A Medical Textbook and Photographic Atlas.* New York: Oxford University Press, 1992, pp 31–38.
15. Woodling BA, Kossoris PD: Sexual misuse: Rape, molestation and incest. *Pediatr Clin North Am* 28:481, 1981.
16. Woodling BA, Heger A: The use of the colposcope in the diagnosis of sexual abuse in the pediatric age group. *Child Abuse Negl* 10:111, 1986.
17. Lauber AA, Souma ML: Use of toluidine blue for documentation of traumatic intercourse. *Obstet Gynecol* 61:644, 1982.
18. McCann L, Voris J, Simon M, et al: Comparison of genital examination techniques in prepubertal children. *Pediatrics* 85:182, 1990.
19. Berenson A, Heger A, Andrews S: Appearance of the hymen in newborns. *Pediatrics* 87:458, 1991.
20. Berenson A: Appearance of the hymen at birth and one year of age: A longitudinal study. *Pediatrics* 91:820, 1993.
21. Kerns DL, Ritter ML, Thomas RG: Concave hymenal variations in suspected child sexual abuse victims. *Pediatrics* 90:265, 1992.
22. McCann J, Wells R, Simon M, et al: Genital findings in prepubescent girls selected for non-abuse: A descriptive study. *Pediatrics* 86:428, 1990.
23. Finkel MA: Anogenital trauma in sexually abused children. *Pediatrics* 13:258, 1989.
24. Reinhart M: Sexually abused boys. *Child Abuse Negl* 11:229, 1987.
25. McCann J: Perianal findings in prepubertal children selected for non abuse: A descriptive study. *Child Abuse Negl* 13:179, 1989.
26. Hammerschlag MR, Doraiswarmy B, Alexander ER, et al: Are rectogenital chlamydial infections a marker of sexual abuse in children? *Pediatr Infect Dis J* 3:100, 1984.
27. Gellert G, Durfee M, Berkowitz CD: Developing guidelines for HIV antibody testing among victims of pediatric sexual abuse. *Child Abuse Negl* 14:9, 1990.
28. Newberger EH: Pediatric interview assessment of child abuse. *Pediatr Clin North Am* 37:943, 1990.
29. Limbos MA, Berkowitz CD: Documentation of child physical abuse: How far have we come? *Pediatrics* 102:53, 1998.
30. Berkowitz CD: Pediatric abuse: New patterns of injury. *Emerg Med Clin North Am* 13:321, 1995.
31. Wilson EF: Estimation of the age of cutaneous contusions in child abuse. *Pediatrics* 60:750, 1977.
32. Stephenson T, Bialas Y: Estimation of the age of bruising. *Arch Dis Child* 74:53, 1996.
33. Purdue GF, Hunt JL, Prescott PR: Child abuse by burning: An index of suspicion. *J Trauma* 28:221, 1988.
34. Kleinman PK (ed): *Diagnostic Imaging of Child Abuse*, 2d ed. Baltimore, Williams and Wilkins, 1998.
35. Alexander, R, Sato Y, Smith W, Bennett T: Incidence of impact trauma with cranial injuries ascribed to shaking. *Am J Dis Child* 144:724, 1990.
36. American Academy of Pediatrics, Committee on Child Abuse and Neglect: Shaken baby syndrome: Inflicted cerebral trauma. *Pediatrics* 92:872, 1993.
37. Budenz DL, Faber MG, Mirchandani HG, et al: Ocular and optic nerve hemorrhages in abused infants with intracranial injuries. *Ophthalmology* 101:559, 1994.
38. Cooper A, Floyd T, Barlow B, et al: Major blunt abdominal trauma due to child abuse. *J Trauma* 28:1483, 1988.
39. Forman DL: *Every Parent's Guide to the Law.* San Diego, Harcourt, Brace, 1998.

FEMALE AND MALE SEXUAL ASSAULT

Kim M. Feldhaus

EPIDEMIOLOGY

Sexual assault accounts for 5 percent of all violent crimes reported in the 1995 U.S. Uniform Crimes Report. An estimated one in five women will be raped during their lifetimes.[1] Prevalence studies suggest that at least 20 percent of all adult women and 12 percent of adolescent women have experienced some form of sexual abuse or assault during their lifetimes.[2] Most rape victims feel there is a stigma attached to being a victim of sexual assault. As a result, sexual assault is the most underreported violent crime. Authorities believe that as few as one in three cases are reported;[3] some estimates are as low as 10 percent.[4] The vast majority of information and statistics relate to female rape victims. Only recently has male sexual assault been recognized and reported. The estimated incidence is 2 to 4 percent of reported rapes.[5,6]

Many misconceptions are perpetuated about sexual assault. The most common is the assumption that rape is motivated by sexual desire. Rape is a violent crime, motivated by the need for power and control or by anger.[5] Recent literature detailing the injuries sustained by rape victims supports rape as a violent crime. Tintinalli and Hoelzer's study of 372 rape victims reported that facial or extremity injuries were most common, and gynecologic injuries accounted for only 7 percent of all injuries.[7] Genital injuries are not an inevitable consequence of rape, and lack of genital injuries does not imply consensual intercourse. Many victims are threatened with a weapon, the majority of victims suffer minor injuries, and only 1 to 2 percent require hospitalization.[5]

The physician's responsibility is to provide for the patient's physical and psychological well-being first; then, if the patient wishes to prosecute, to provide police with corroborative medical evidence. Victims should be encouraged to undergo an evidentiary examination; critical evidence may be lost if this exam is delayed. The victim may later choose not to proceed through the criminal justice system, as collection of forensic evidence does not commit her to seek prosecution.

CLINICAL FEATURES

The Female Rape Examination

HISTORY The purpose of the history is to obtain data tactfully about the assault, along with pertinent past medical history, in order to provide proper medical care. The victims should not have to relive every minute detail of the assault and, in fact, an extensively detailed history may hinder subsequent prosecution.[8,9] A professional, caring manner should be conveyed, and the history should be obtained in private; law enforcement personnel should not be present. Beginning with a general past medical history establishes the victim's trust in the physician.[4,8,10,11]

ASSAULT HISTORY[4,8,10,11]

1. *Who?* Did the victim know the assailant? Was it a single assailant or multiple? How many? Ask about their identity and race.
2. *What happened?* Was the victim physically assaulted? With what (e.g., gun, bat, or fist) and where? Determine the type and location of physical injuries and appropriately evaluate these injuries. Delineate actual or attempted vaginal, anal, or oral penetration. Did ejaculation occur? If so, where? Was a foreign object used? Was a condom used? This information will direct the physical examination to areas of potential injury.
3. *When?* When did the assault occur? This will determine the probability of detecting sperm (within 72 h) or acid phosphatase.
4. *Where?* Where did the assault occur? Corroborating evidence may be found based on the location of the assault.
5. *Douche, shower, or change of clothing?* Any of these activities performed prior to seeking medical attention may decrease the probability of sperm or acid phosphatase recovery.

MEDICAL HISTORY[4,8,10,11]

1. *Last menstrual period?* This will help to determine pregnancy risk.
2. *Birth control method?* This will also help to determine pregnancy risk.
3. *Last consensual intercourse?* If the patient has had recent intercourse (less than 3 days) prior to the attack, it may confuse laboratory analysis of sperm, acid phosphatase, and genetic typing.
4. *Allergies and prior medical history?* This information is necessary before prescribing antibiotics or pregnancy prophylaxis.
5. *Prior sexual assault?* Has this ever happened to the victim before?

PHYSICAL EXAMINATION[4,8,10,11] The physical exam should be performed thoroughly and compassionately. A female chaperone should be present if the examining physician is a man. Document a general medical examination, including vital signs and level of consciousness. Bruises, lacerations, or other signs of trauma should be described in detail; a body map may be useful. As many as 290 percent of rape survivors will have nongenital injuries.[2,5,12,13] The examiner should carefully inspect the victim's face, oral cavity, neck, breasts, wrist, thighs, and buttocks. Areas of tenderness should also be recorded. A pelvic examination should be performed, noting any vaginal discharge or genital lacerations or abrasions. Toluidine blue can be used to detect small vulvar lacerations.[4] Lacerations expose the deeper dermis, containing nuclei that absorb this stain. Prior to inserting the speculum, the dye is applied to the posterior fourchette with gauze and wiped away with lubricating jelly. A linear blue stain will highlight the vulvar lacerations. This simple procedure has doubled the reporting of genital lacerations. Colposcopic photographs may reveal other genital injuries, especially to the posterior fourchette.[14]

EVIDENTIARY EXAMINATION[4,10,11] Informed consent is required prior to evidence collection, and a system to maintain ''chain of evidence'' should be established. Most hospitals have a prepackaged rape kit with equipment and directions. The least invasive procedures should be performed first, and unnecessary duplication of procedures should be avoided. Any particulate matter should be collected. Examination with a Wood's lamp will reveal semen stains on a patient's body; these areas should be swabbed with a moistened cotton-tipped applicator. Saliva is obtained for secretor status during the oral cavity examination. Fingernail scrapings and hair samples are collected. During the pelvic examination, vaginal swabbings should be collected, along with gonorrhea and chlamydia cultures. Some physicians prefer to treat prophylactically and consider cultures irrelevant. If indicated by history, rectal or buccal swabs for sperm are collected. A rectal examination is performed if anal assault occurred. Emergency physicians should not examine wet mounts for the presence of sperm; this determination should be left to forensic scientists.[9,10] If blood is present, anoscopy or sigmoidoscopy should be performed. Blood samples are drawn for DNA testing, blood typing, and pregnancy testing. If photographs are used, they should be carefully labeled and given to the police.

The Male Rape Examination

History taking is similar to that in the female rape examination. The physical examination must be tailored to the particulars of the assault. For example, because the anus is penetrated and the victim is lying prone in the majority of cases, one should search for abrasions on the thorax or abdomen.

Victims of oral penetration require a careful examination of the oral cavity; pharyngeal edema or mucosal lacerations may be found. Swabs should be taken of buccal and gingival areas if indicated by history, and gonorrhea and chlamydia cultures of the pharynx can be taken.[6] In cases of anal assault, inspect the anus externally for signs of trauma. Up to half of victims will have minor genital injuries such as perineal contusions, anal fissures, or rectal mucosal tears.[5] Swabs from the victim's penis should be collected and may be examined for saliva if there is a history of oral copulation. If there is evidence of bleeding on rectal exam, the source should be sought via anoscopy or sigmoidoscopy. Obtain a rectal swabbing or a rectal aspirate in cases of anal assault for evidentiary purposes.[6] Sterile saline can be injected into the rectum, allowed to equilibrate, and then aspirated.

DIAGNOSIS

Rape is not a medical diagnosis but rather a legal determination. The definition of rape is based on legal, not medical, facts and contains three elements: (1) any degree of carnal knowledge; (2) nonconsent—unless the victim is a minor, intoxicated, or mentally incompetent; and (3) compulsion or fear of great harm.[4,58,10,11]

FORENSIC LABORATORY EVALUATION

Sperm Survivability

Historically, the courts and legal professions have placed a high significance on sperm detection as confirmatory evidence for rape.[9] The presence of sperm or seminal constituents in the vagina is evidence of recent sexual intercourse. The detection of sperm depends on several factors, including time lapse between the rape and the physical examination, whether the assailant is azoospermic, whether the victim douched prior to examination, and whether the assailant ejaculated.[4,10,11] Previous studies suggest that one-third to one-half of sexual assault victims will have sperm detected as part of the evidentiary examination.[7,12]

There is general agreement in the literature that 2 to 3 h is the average time for loss of sperm motility in a majority of patients.[4,11] Nonmotile sperm may persist for up to 24 h in the vagina and rectum and for up to several days in the cervical mucus.[8,11] In the mouth, seminal fluid is usually destroyed within hours by salivary enzymes. Semen stains found on the patient's body, clothing, or at the site of the assault (e.g., on bedding) often are useful in obtaining biologic specimens for forensic analysis.

Acid Phosphatase

Acid phosphatase detection in vaginal washings is helpful in cases of azoospermic ejaculations. Acid phosphatase is derived from cytoplasmic sources (erythrocytes, leukocytes, and thrombocytes) or tissue sources (bone, kidney, and liver). Various chemical means are used to differentiate the source of the acid phosphatase. However, a qualitative distinction between seminal and vaginal acid phosphatase cannot be made, because they are identical biochemically and immunologically. The only reliable distinction may be made quantitatively based on the high levels of acid phosphatase in seminal fluid.[11] The acid phosphatase determinations are most helpful when no sperm are found and acid phosphatase levels are markedly elevated, consistent with the presence of semen.[4,11]

Glycoprotein p30

The plasma glycoprotein p30 is unique to males and is produced in large quantities by the prostate. It is found in semen and follows a predictable pattern of degradation after intercourse. A positive glycoprotein p30 test indicates that coitus occurred within the past 48 h.[11]

Genetic Typing

Genetic typing helps to narrow the field of suspects but cannot specify an individual. Forensic analysis of evidence is used to determine genetic markers for the victim, the evidence, and the possible assailants. Four genetic markers are available in semen, blood, and vaginal fluid: ABO blood group antigens, peptidase A, phosphoglucomutase (PGM) and deoxyribonucleic acid (DNA).[4,11]

Of the general population, 80 percent secretes ABO antigens into other body fluids such as saliva. Secretor status is determined by testing for ABO blood type and then testing saliva for the presence of these antigens. Foreign antigens found on a victim may be from the assailant. Peptidase A and PGM are present in semen regardless of secretor status.[11] Peptidase A subtypes are common in black populations; typing of peptidase A is done when the assailant may have been black.[4] Peptidase A activity decreases rapidly after intercourse and can rarely be detected after 3 h. PGM has a number of subtypes. By combining ABO type and PGM subtypes, two individuals can be differentiated from each other 90 percent of the time.[11] PGM is rarely detected beyond 6 h. Semen stains found on a victim can be analyzed for these enzymes as well.

Deoxyribonucleic acid typing can be used to characterize an individual's unique genetic material and distinguish two individuals statistically. There is a 1 in 30 billion chance that two unrelated individuals will have the same DNA fingerprint.[9] This typing can be performed on very small samples of evidence, as well as on old or decomposing samples.

All evidence collected from a victim should be carefully labeled with the victim's name, the type and source of the evidence, the date and time of collection, and the name of the person who collected the evidence. Following instructions for proper collection and storage of evidence is critical to producing optimal laboratory results.[4,11]

TREATMENT

Treatment of the rape victim includes, first and foremost, management of any physical injuries according to standards of care, while attending to the psychological needs of the patient. Tetanus prophylaxis should be given if needed, lacerations sutured, and fractures casted. A pregnancy test should be obtained in order to identify any preexisting pregnancy; a negative pregnancy test should be documented before providing postcoital contraception. Routine drug screens or determination of alcohol levels are not recommended; they may be obtained if medically indicated and if the results will influence treatment.

Pregnancy Prophylaxis

When treating postmenarcheal female rape victims, physicians must consider pregnancy prophylaxis. Although the risk of pregnancy after an isolated sexual encounter during nonfertile periods of the menstrual cycle is thought to be less than 1 percent, it may rise to as high as 25 percent at midcycle.[15] Although the Food and Drug Administration has no approved medication for postcoital contraception, various regimens of high-dose estrogens are often used. Pregnancy prophylaxis must be initiated within 72 h of the sexual assault in order to be most effective.[16] Currently accepted therapy is the birth control pill Ovral (norgestrel plus ethinyl estradiol) 2 tablets orally initially and 2 tablets 12 h later.[17] Many women will experience nausea as a side effect of this regimen; prescribing an antiemetic is advised.[16] This regimen replaces the older 5-day diethylstilbestrol regimen, which had more side effects, lower compliance, and an increased risk of carcinogenesis.

Sexually Transmitted Disease Prophylaxis

Most of the literature demonstrates poor compliance of sexual assault patients with follow-up.[7,12,18] Therefore, prophylaxis for sexually transmitted diseases (STDs) should be given to all sexual assault victims. At a minimum, treatment for gonorrhea and chlamydia should be offered. The current guidelines from the Centers for Disease Control and Prevention (CDC) also recommend prophylaxis against *Trichomonas* and bacterial vaginosis.[19] Table 290-1 presents the current CDC guidelines for antibiotic choices. A negative pregnancy test should be documented on the chart prior to administering antibiotics; a positive pregnancy test will alter the choice of antibiotics. See Chapter 137 for further information on treatment of STDs. Hepatitis B prophylaxis should be considered if the assailant is felt to belong to high-risk

TABLE 290-1 Treatment of Sexually Transmitted Diseases Following Sexual Assault

Recommended regimens for gonorrhea prophylaxis:
Ceftriaxone 125 mg IM in a single dose
Alternative regimens:
Cefixime 400 mg orally in a single dose
or
Ciprofloxacin 500 mg orally in a single dose
or
Ofloxacin 400 mg orally

If pregnant:
Ceftriaxone 125 mg IM in a single dose (avoid quinolones and tetracyclines)

plus

Recommended regimens for chlamydia prophylaxis:
Azithromycin 1 g orally in a single dose or **doxycycline** 100 mg orally twice a day for 7 days
Alternative regimens:
Ofloxacin 300 mg twice a day for 7 days
or
Erythromycin base 500 mg four times daily for 7 days
or
Erythromycin ethylsuccinate 800 mg four times daily for 7 days

If pregnant:
Erythromycin base 500 mg four times daily for 7 days
or
Amoxicillin 500 mg orally three times a day for 7 days

plus

If coverage for trichomonas and bacterial vaginosis is desired:
Metronidazole 2 g orally in a single dose

Source: From the U.S. Department of Health and Human Services.[19]

group for the disease. The CDC recommends postexposure vaccination with the first dose administered at the time of the initial exam.[19] Administration of hepatitis B immune globin (HBIG) may also be considered. For those who have been vaccinated, a booster and HBIG should be given only if antibody titers are inadequate.

Counseling and Testing for Human Immunodeficiency Virus

The true risk of contracting human immunodeficiency virus (HIV) from a single sexual encounter is unknown but believed to be rare. Estimated rates are felt to be highest with receptive, unprotected anal intercourse (0.008 to 0.032 infections per episode with an HIV positive partner). The risk with receptive vaginal intercourse is 0.005–0.0015, and with insertive vaginal intercourse is 0.0003–0.0009 per episode. Local inflammation, bleeding, or trauma can affect the risk of transmission also.[20] Victims should be counseled regarding HIV testing and the need for repeat testing. Besides the uncertainty of risk of exposure after sexual assault, other factors complicating decision making about PEP for HIV include potential inability to identify or test the assailant for HIV; expense of PEP (about $700); side effects of medication (nausea, vomiting, anorexia in up to 50 percent of patients); the need for laboratory testing; and the need to provide follow-up with physicians informed about PEP for HIV. No specific guidelines for PEP in cases of sexual assault are available as of this writing. Physicians who consider offering postexposure therapy with antiretroviral agents should consider the likelihood of exposure to HIV, the risks and benefits of such therapy, the interval between exposure and therapy, the local epidemiology of HIV/AIDS, the nature of the assault, and any high HIV-risk behaviors exhibited by the assailant. Victims should be informed of the risks and benefits of antiretroviral therapy. If a patient decides to take postexposure therapy, the guidelines for occupational mucous membrane exposure would be followed with treatment begun within 72 h.[19] See Chap. 148 regarding occupational exposure guidelines.

ADMISSION INDICATIONS

The indication for admission is based on the nature of injuries sustained from the attack. Only 1 to 2 percent of victims sustain severe-enough injuries to require hospitalization.[5] The majority of injuries can be handled with outpatient follow-up.

FOLLOW-UP CARE

Ideally, counseling for sexual assault patients should be available 24 h a day in the emergency department. Often, a rape counselor will precede the physician in assessing a victim, preparing her for the examination, and providing moral support. Multidisciplinary *sexual assault response teams* are common in some areas of the country and work to provide coordinated, sensitive care of the sexual assault victim, including medical, legal, and psychological needs.[21] If no social worker or rape counselor is available when a sexual assault victim arrives, the physician should provide information on local rape counseling centers where the patient may seek further care.

Follow-up medical care is needed to ensure that any injuries have healed properly. In addition, follow-up at 7 to 14 days is necessary to ensure the effectiveness of the pregnancy prophylaxis and STD treatment. A male rape victim should be referred to an urologist or a proctologist. Young children should be referred to a pediatrician for evaluation. These follow-up instructions should be clearly explained in a written aftercare information sheet, as victims often recall very little of their emergency department encounter.[10]

REFERENCES

1. United States Department of Justice, Federal Bureau of Investigation: *Uniform Crime Reports.* Washington, DC, US Government Printing Office, 1993.
2. Council on Scientific Affairs, American Medical Association: Violence against women: Relevance for medical practitioners. *JAMA* 267:3184, 1992.
3. United States Department of Justice, Bureau of Justice Statistics: *Criminal Victimization in the United States 1994.* Washington, DC, US Government Printing Office, April 1996.
4. Dupre AR, Hampton HL, Morrison H, et al: Sexual assault. *Obstet Gynecol Surv* 48:640, 1993.
5. Geist RF: Sexually related trauma. *Emerg Med Clin North Am* 6:439, 1988.
6. Braen GR: The male rape victim: examination and management, in Warner CG (ed): *Rape and Sexual Assault.* Germantown, MD, Aspen Systems, 1980.
7. Tintinalli JE, Hoelzer M: Clinical findings and legal resolution in sexual assault. *Ann Emerg Med* 14:447, 1985.
8. Hampton HL: Care of the woman who has been raped. *N Engl J Med* 332:234, 1995.
9. Young WW, Bracken AC, Goddard MA, et al: Sexual assault: Review of a national model protocol for forensic and medical evaluation. *Obstet Gynecol* 80:878, 1992.
10. DeLahunta EA, Baram DA: Sexual assault. *Clin Obstet Gynecol* 40:648, 1997.
11. Hochbaum SR: The evaluation and treatment of the sexually assaulted patient. *Emerg Med Clin North Am* 5:601, 1987.
12. Rambow B, Adkinson C, Frost TH, et al: Female sexual assault: Medical and legal implications. *Annals Emerg Med* 21:727, 1992.
13. Ramin SM, Stain AJ, Stone IC, et al: Sexual assault in postmenopausal women. *Obstet Gynecol* 80:860, 1992.
14. Slaughter L, Brown CRV: Colposcopy to establish physical findings in rape victims. *Am J Obstet Gynecol* 166:83, 1992.

15. Ovral as a "morning after" contraceptive. *Med Lett Drugs Ther* 31:93, 1989.
16. American College of Obstetricians and Gynecologists (ACOG): *Practice Patterns: Emergency Oral Contraception.* Washington, DC, ACOG, 1996.
17. Trussell J, Ellertson C, Rodriguez G: The Yuzpe regimen of emergency contraception: How long after the morning after? *Obstet Gynecol* 88:1290, 1996.
18. Jenny C, Hooton TM, Bowers A, et al: Sexually transmitted diseases in victims of rape. *N Engl J Med* 322:713, 1990.
19. US Department of Health and Human Services: 1998 guidelines for treatment of sexually transmitted diseases. *MMWR* 47(RR-1):1, 1998.
20. Katz MH, Gerberding JL: The care of persons with recent sexual exposure to HIV. *Ann Int Med* 128(4):306–312, 1998.
21. American Medical Association: Experts hope team approach will improve the quality of rape exams. *JAMA* 275:973, 1996.

291 DOMESTIC VIOLENCE

Patricia R. Salber
Ellen H. Taliaferro

It has only been in the last 15 to 20 years that domestic violence has been acknowledged as a social problem with disastrous health consequences. In 1985, at a workshop, the Surgeon General of the United States identified domestic violence as one of the nation's most important health problems. In January 1992, the Joint Commission on the Accreditation of Healthcare Organizations mandated that all emergency departments and ambulatory care facilities establish written guidelines for the identification, evaluation, management, and referral of adult victims of domestic violence. In June 1992, the American Medical Association published guidelines for identification and intervention of domestic violence victims.[1]

In September 1994, the American College of Emergency Physicians approved a policy on emergency medicine and domestic violence that states:

- The identification and assessment for domestic violence is an important, specialized part of the evaluation of the emergency patient;
- Emergency medical services, medical school, and emergency medicine residency training programs incorporate training for identification, assessment, and intervention in domestic violence in their curricula;
- A collaborative, interdisciplinary approach with emergency physician leadership should be used to
    - Collect data on the incidence and extent of domestic violence
    - Develop clinical and academic research on domestic violence, and
    - Use this information to detect, diagnose, and intervene with these patients;
- Hospitals develop multidisciplinary approaches including policies and protocols for emergency department identification, treatment, and referral of domestic violence patients;
- The special nature of and the necessary resources for the domestic violence screening evaluation and examination should be recognized.[2]

Domestic violence is defined as the use of a pattern of assaultive and coercive behaviors, including physical, sexual, and psychological attacks, as well as economic coercion, which adults or adolescents use against their intimate partners. The behaviors used include emotional abuse, psychological abuse, intimidation, deprivation, isolation, economic abuse, stalking, and physical and sexual assault. There are multiple, sometimes daily events. Some are criminal acts and some are not; some are physically injurious and some are not; but all are psychologically and emotionally damaging. Domestic violence, then, is about the use of power by one partner to control the other.

EPIDEMIOLOGY

It is estimated that between 2 and 4 million women are battered each year in the United States.[3–5] Data from anonymous telephone surveys suggest that 20 to 25 percent of all adult women in the United States have been physically assaulted by an intimate partner at least once over their lifetime.[6] Furthermore, 32 percent of women who have been assaulted once will be battered again within 6 months of the initial incident,[7] and 34 percent of adults in the United States reported having witnessed a man beating his wife or girlfriend.[8]

Approximately 2000 battered women die as a result of partner abuse (homicide and suicide) each year, and 31 percent of female homicide victims were killed by an intimate (spouse, ex-spouse, boy/girlfriend) compared with only 4 percent of male victims.[9] Men and women seem to kill their partners for very different reasons. Men often kill in response to the woman's attempt to leave the abusive relationship, whereas women kill in self-defense or in retribution for prior acts of violence.[10–12]

Statistics from the Bureau of Justice show that, in greater than 90 percent of reported intimate assaults, victims are women.[4] Although some studies show that female-to-male aggression and male-to-female aggression occur at close to equal rates, the chance of the aggression ending in moderate to severe injury or injuries requiring medical treatment is much higher for female victims.[13] Controlling-type behaviors that are a key component of male-on-female domestic violence are rarely described in the context of female-on-male aggression.

Domestic violence is common among women who present to emergency departments for treatment, including in community hospital as well as urban teaching hospitals. Of all women seen in emergency departments, 2 to 3 percent are there because of acute trauma from physical abuse.[14–16] In one study, the incidence of acute domestic violence among women with a current male partner was 12 percent; however, only 23 percent of these women subjected to acute domestic violence presented for care because of trauma.[14] Of women seeking care in EDs, 14 percent have a history of having been physically or sexually abused within the past year, and 30 to 54 percent have a history of intimate partner abuse at sometime in their life.[14,16] Of women with a history of suicide attempts, 81 percent had experienced domestic violence at some time in their lives, compared with 19 percent of those with no history of suicide attempts.[17]

EMERGENCY DEPARTMENT PRESENTATIONS

In addition to being a direct cause of traumatic injury, domestic violence also contributes to other conditions frequently seen in emergency departments, such as depression, anxiety, hyperventilation, substance abuse, suicide attempts, sexually transmitted diseases (including HIV), complications of pregnancy, and headaches and other chronic pain syndromes.[18] Both batterers and their victims may abuse alcohol and drugs. Abused individuals with chronic medical conditions may present with exacerbations of their illnesses because the batterer withholds their medications or because they are not allowed to keep appointments with their office-based physician. A history of exposure to violence in the home during childhood has recently been associated with an increase in health risks and health-risk behaviors in adults (such as depression, substance abuse, and high-risk sexual behaviors).[19] It should be considered, therefore, a contributing factor to many conditions commonly treated in emergency departments.

BARRIERS TO DIAGNOSIS

Even though emergency physicians provide care for large numbers of battered women, a recent study documented that only domestic violence is documented in only a small percentage of cases.[14]

Physicians fail to make the diagnosis for many reasons. Until recently, it was distinctly unusual for medical students or residents to receive training about domestic violence. Instruction on how to recognize domestic violence is now part of the core curriculum for emergency medicine residencies. Physicians aware of domestic violence often have misconceptions that contribute to underdiagnosis. Some of these misconceptions are listed in Table 291-1.

Other barriers to diagnosing domestic violence were revealed in a 1993 study of California emergency department physician directors and nurse managers.[20] Respondents were asked to rank a list of possible obstacles to the identification of adult patients who had been abused as a "major problem," a "minor problem," or "not a problem." Almost half of the respondents listed patient factors such as fear of repercussion, denial, and failure to mention battering as the most significant obstacles to diagnosis. Conversely, staff factors, such as lack of training or awareness or staff busyness, were most frequently listed as "not a problem."

Another important reason for failure to diagnose is the failure to consider domestic violence in cases with nontrauma chief complaints. Battered women seek care in emergency departments for a wide variety of medical complaints, including anxiety, hyperventilation, depression, drug and alcohol intoxication, chronic pain syndromes, and symptoms suggestive of posttraumatic stress disorder (PTSD).

ROUTINE SCREENING FOR DOMESTIC VIOLENCE

Perhaps the most significant reason for missing the diagnosis of domestic violence is the failure to ask. Asking patients directly whether domestic violence is affecting their lives has the potential of overcoming many of these barriers to diagnosis as well as establishing the expectation that the physician believes that domestic violence is not acceptable. Research shows that patients will respond to direct questioning.[21] It has been reported that approximately 45 percent of battered women will speak to an emergency physician about the violence in their lives if direct inquiry is made, although fewer (24 percent) were willing to disclose if asked during a triage encounter.[21]

CONSEQUENCES OF FAILURE TO DIAGNOSE DOMESTIC VIOLENCE

Consequences of failure to diagnose may result in multiple visits to the ED and other provider settings. One study documented that 23 percent of battered women presented to clinicians between 6 and 10 times, and another 20 percent at least 11 times before the abuse was diagnosed.[22] In addition, misdiagnosis of battering-related symptoms such as mental illness can lead to misleading at best and inappropriate use of psychoactive medications or psychiatric hospitalization at worst. It has been estimated that many women hospitalized in psychiatric institutions are, in fact, battered women.[23]

Other consequences of failure to diagnose include an increase in the patient's feelings of hopelessness, despair, isolation, and entrapment. Battered women may resort to substance abuse or develop depression with and without suicide attempts. Continuing or escalating domestic violence can lead to permanent disability or death. Domestic violence has adverse consequences for the children of victims as well. Perpetrators of domestic violence abuse the children in the home in approximately 30 percent of cases.[24] Even if the children are not physically or sexually assaulted, experiencing or witnessing violence in the home as children has both short-term and long-term health consequences, including an increased incidence of adverse health-risk behaviors as adults.[19,25] Finally, failure to interrupt the cycle of violence can lead to repetition of violence in the next generation.[26]

TABLE 291-1 Common Reasons Why Physicians May Not Diagnose Domestic Violence in the Emergency Department

Patient withholds information
Fear of opening "Pandora's box"
Lack of physician training
Fear of offending patient
Time constraints
Does not know what to do about it
Believe intervention will not work

THE BATTERED WOMAN

Who Is She?

Any woman can become a victim of domestic violence. Although it is more commonly reported by women of color and poor women, domestic violence occurs in all socioeconomic classes, races, and cultural groups. It can occur regardless of age, educational background, or profession.

Why Does She Stay?

Many women stay in violent relationships because they are afraid of the consequences of escalating the violence. The highest number of fatalities from domestic violence occur when a woman leaves or tries to leave the relationship.[27] In addition to fearing for their own lives, battered women may fear for the safety of their children, pets, or others whom the batterer has threatened to harm if she leaves.

Some women stay because they have been systematically cut off from family and friends; they believe they have nowhere else to go. The batterer's control of information and giving of "disinformation" may make them think that no one will believe their story. They may also stay because of cultural or religious beliefs about the sanctity of the family.

For many battered women, especially women with small children, the lack of money or skills to obtain gainful employment can be a serious impediment to leaving the relationship. Their concern for their children's well-being may hold them in the relationship.

Finally, battered women may stay because they still love their partner; they don't want to end the relationship, they just want the violence to stop.

Why Doesn't She Tell?

A significant obstacle to identification is the battered women's reluctance to talk about, or outright denial of, battering. Many women do not tell physicians about the violence because the women fear that the information may not be confidential. They fear retribution if the batterer learns of the "betrayal." Some women do not tell because they are embarrassed or ashamed; they believe that their situation is unique and somehow related to their own failures in the relationship. Finally, they may not talk about it because they believe the physician does not care, cannot or will not help, or is too busy for this type of problem.

MEN WHO BATTER

Men who batter are of all ages and come from all socioeconomic, educational, racial, cultural, and religious backgrounds. One study that compared violent with nonviolent men found no statistically significant difference in demographic characteristics. Batterers were heterogeneous, failing to conform to a "batterer profile." Although batterers show higher levels of personality dysfunction than do nonviolent men, no particular personality disorder diagnosis has been identified that consistently discriminates between batterers and nonbatterers. The one thing batterers do have in common is the use of power to control the behavior of their partners and their children. Other common themes are the use of denial and minimalization as well as blaming others as justifications for their actions.

About 60 percent of men who batter grew up in violent homes where they either witnessed the battering of their mothers or they themselves were emotionally or physically abused. However, 40 percent of men who grow up in similarly violent homes do not go on to batter, and not all men who do batter experienced violence while growing up.

Both batterers and victims of battering may abuse alcohol and other drugs. Although use of alcohol is associated with the intensity of violent behaviors, there is no established link between the use of these substances and the *cause* of violence.

THE EFFECT OF DOMESTIC VIOLENCE ON CHILDREN

As many as 70 percent of children from violent homes witness their fathers beating their mothers. In addition, about 30 to 54 percent of reported cases of spousal abuse also report child abuse. One-quarter to one-half of children in violent homes are hurt incidentally during the violence or are injured when they try to intervene in the struggle. Several studies have documented that children exposed to violence in their homes have significant behavioral difficulties, including depression or PTSD, during childhood and later life. Several studies have documented a link between growing up in a violent home and later high-risk behaviors such as drug use, promiscuity, and criminal behaviors.

MAKING THE DIAGNOSIS OF DOMESTIC VIOLENCE

History and Physical Examination

The following findings are clues to battering that can be gleaned from the clinical history and physical examination:

Pregnancy. Pregnant women are high risk for battering; 40 percent of battering begins during the first pregnancy. Among all pregnant women, 17 percent have a history of domestic abuse, and 8 to 9 percent are battered during the index pregnancy; for pregnant teens, the figure is even higher. Any evidence of injury during pregnancy should prompt direct questioning about domestic violence.

Central pattern of injury. Battered patients are more likely to experience injuries to the head, neck, face, thorax, and abdomen than patients injured by other mechanisms.

Injuries suggesting a defensive posture. Forearm bruises or fractures may be sustained when women try to fend off blows to the face or chest.

Certain characteristic injuries. Fingernail scratches, bite marks, cigarette burns, and rope burns strongly suggest domestic violence.

An extent or type of injury inconsistent with the patient's explanation. Multiple abrasions and contusions to different anatomic sites, which are inconsistent with the history, should raise the possibility of abuse. An example of such an inconsistency would be a woman with a blowout fracture who says she injured herself falling off a bar stool.

Multiple injuries in various stages of healing. Just as x-rays that reveal old fractures help support a diagnosis of child abuse, evidence of new and old injuries help diagnose partner abuse.

Substantial delay between the time of injury and the presentation for treatment. Battered women may wait several days before seeking medical care. They may see their physician at inappropriate times for seemingly minor or resolving injuries. This may occur because they were prevented from leaving the house, or it might reflect their ambivalence about revealing the nature of their home life.

Frequent visits for vague complaints without evidence of physiologic abnormality. A woman who presents frequently with a variety of psychosomatic complaints previously ascribed to depression might actually be a victim of domestic violence.

Suicide attempts. Up to 25 percent of suicide attempts by women may be related to spousal abuse; 20 percent of pregnant battered women will attempt suicide. When asked what precipitated a suicide attempt, a battered woman may respond "I had a fight with my husband." The emergency physician can make the diagnosis by asking specifically if the fight was a physical fight and exploring whether there is a history of physical and psychological abuse suggestive of domestic violence.

Multiple prior visits. Review of the medical record may reveal frequent emergency department visits for a variety of complaints, including both trauma and nontrauma presentations. Extensive workups for chronic pelvic pain or other chronic pain syndromes may also suggest a history of domestic violence.

Partner's behavior. Partners accompanying victims of domestic violence may provide clues to the diagnosis by exhibiting controlling or abusive behavior. Furthermore, the victim may appear frightened of her partner or refuse to answer questions, instead deferring all responses to him.

Routine Screening for Domestic Violence

Although there are certain clues to abuse, the presentations of battered women in the emergency department are so varied that the diagnosis may be missed if the physician fails to ask directly about the presence of violence in the patient's life. As discussed earlier, many battered women will respond truthfully if questioned, in private (not at the triage desk) and in a sensitive, nonjudgmental way. Screening may be verbal or by a written questionnaire. The American Medical Association[1] suggests asking the following questions:

- Are you in a relationship in which you have been physically hurt or threatened by your partner? Have you ever been in such a relationship?
- Are you (have you ever been) in a relationship in which you felt you were treated badly? In what ways?
- Has your partner ever destroyed things that you cared about?
- Has your partner ever threatened or abused your children?
- Has your partner ever forced you to have sex when you did not want to? Does he ever force you to engage in sex that makes you feel uncomfortable?
- We all fight at home. What happens when you and your partner fight or disagree?

It is sometimes helpful to use framing clauses when verbally inquiring about domestic violence. Examples of this type of questioning are as follows:

- Violence in the home is very common and can be very serious. Therefore, I routinely ask all of my patients whether they are experiencing domestic violence, because no one should have to live in fear and because there is help available.
- Whenever I see injuries of this type, it is often because someone hit them with a fist. Is that what happened to you?
- Many women experience some type of physical abuse in their lives. Has this ever happened to you?

TREATMENT GOALS

If physicians have "getting her to a shelter" or "having him arrested" as the goal of the patient encounter, they are bound to become frustrated when dealing with cases of domestic violence. Leaving the relationship may not be the immediate goal of the patient, and she may be loathe to have her husband and the father of their children arrested. The safety of the woman and her children should be the first and foremost goal of every patient encounter. It is the woman, however, who must make the ultimate determination of whether it is safe to return home. By providing women with information about battering, risks, and options, the physician will help the woman to decide what is best for her and her family.

Assess Potential for Suicide or Homicide

The patient should be asked if she is contemplating suicide. Does she have a plan? Does she have a weapon or has she stockpiled medications in anticipation of a suicide attempt? Is she considering homicide as a means to ensure the safety of herself and her children? Does she have a plan or weapon? Psychiatric consultation should be obtained if suicidal or homicidal ideation are present; hospitalization may be indicated.

Safety Assessment

If considering discharge from the emergency department, it is imperative to assess the safety of the woman and her dependents. Although the safety assessment may be delegated to a domestic violence expert, such as a hospital-based social worker or a community-based advocate, the physician is responsible for assuring this assessment has been completed prior to discharge from the emergency department. Safety assessments include the following:

- Ask in detail about the nature of the abuse.
- Is there a pattern of escalating violence?
- Were the police called? Was the batterer arrested? If not, does she know where he is now?
- Does the batterer have a weapon, especially firearms, which can easily turn an abuse situation into a lethal situation?
- Is the woman afraid to go home? If so, does she have somewhere safe to go? Can she stay with friends or relatives? Is she afraid that the batterer would find her if she went to the home of someone he knows?
- Would she feel safer in a battered women's shelter? Emphasize that the location of these shelters is kept secret—the batterer would not be able to find her in a shelter.
- If she feels it is safe and she wants to go home, this choice should be respected. It is appropriate, however, to discuss with her the need to have a safety plan in case violence erupts again.

ESSENTIAL INFORMATION FOR BATTERED WOMEN

Although a battered woman may choose to return to the battering relationship at the end of the physician-patient encounter, important therapeutic interventions can help her begin the process of extricating herself and her children from the violence:

- She needs to know that she is not alone,
- She needs to know that there is help available for her and,
- She does not deserve to be beaten.

All battered women should be referred to hospital-based or community-based domestic violence experts, such as social workers or domestic violence advocates, for further evaluation and continuing intervention.

PREPARING THE EMERGENCY DEPARTMENT FOR OPTIMAL RESPONSE

The optimal response to battered women will require services beyond the confines of the emergency department or hospital. Battered women's shelters, police, and the legal community all provide necessary services. To be maximally effective, there must be coordination between the medical and legal communities.

Every emergency department should develop and maintain close relationships with hospital and community domestic violence experts who can assist in the management of cases of domestic violence. Emergency physicians should ensure that their hospital has a domestic violence committee that meets regularly and includes broad representation from the various hospital departments as well as community-based domestic violence experts. This committee can assume the responsibility for developing a uniform, institution-wide response to domestic violence as well continuing education of hospital staff and, if confidentiality can be assured, complex case review and management.

The emergency department must have current lists of resources available in the community to assist battered women. Battered women's shelters, legal aid, and other legal assistance, and appropriate social service agencies should be included on the list. Community coordinating councils on family violence can be an effective way of improving a community's response to domestic violence.

Protocols

The Family Violence Prevention Fund has analyzed protocols from emergency departments across the country. Sample protocols that can be used to help guide development of an institution's protocol can be obtained by calling the fund's special interest resource center at 415-252-8900. More important than written protocols, however, is the institutionalization of an optimal response to domestic violence victims as described in this chapter.

MEDICOLEGAL CONSIDERATIONS

Careful documentation in the medical record is crucial in domestic violence cases. Such documentation can assist the victim who seeks legal remedies such at temporary or permanent restraining orders, child custody, separation, or divorce. It is recommended that photographs of visible injuries be included. Be sure to obtain consent and to document the date and time of the photographs. A hand-drawn body map detailing areas of tenderness or hematomas should be included to document nonvisible injuries. *Physicians for a Violence-free Society,* which has developed materials to help physicians incorporate forensic documentation into their practices, can be contacted at 415-821-8209. Emergency physicians must be aware of their state's reporting requirements. Some states have mandatory reporting of known or suspected domestic violence; others have mandatory arrest, in addition to mandatory reporting. If the police are called, either at the woman's request or because of a reporting requirement, it is important to discuss a safety plan with the woman. Violence may escalate when the batterer discovers he has been reported, especially if he is not arrested, or if he is arrested but held for only a short period. Physicians must warn potential victims if serious homicidal intent is expressed. Failure to report domestic violence and reporting suspected domestic violence that is not substantiated are both potential sources of physician liability. States in which mandatory reporting exist should have liability protections similar to those for reporting suspected child abuse.

REFERENCES

1. American Medical Association (AMA): *Diagnostic and Treatment Guidelines on Domestic Violence.* Chicago, AMA, 1992.
2. American College of Emergency Physicians (ACEP): *Policy Statement: Emergency Medicine and Domestic Violence.* Dallas, ACEP, 1994.
3. Straus MA, Gelles RJ: Societal change and change in family violence from 1975 to 1985 as revealed by two national surveys. *J Marriage Fam* 48:465, 1986.
4. Bachman R: *Violence Against Women: A National Crime Victimization Survey Report.* Washington, DC, Government Printing Office; 1994; US Department of Justice, Office of Justice Programs, Bureau of Justice Statistics, NCJ-145325.
5. Bachman R, Saltzman LE: *Violence Against Women: Estimates from the Redesigned Survey.* Washington, DC, Government Printing Office, 1995; US Department of Justice, Office of Justice Programs, Bureau of Justice Statistics, NCJ-154348.

6. Freund KM: Domestic violence, in Carr PL, Freund KM, Soman S (eds): *The Medical Care of Women.* Philadelphia, WB Saunders, 1995, p 722.
7. El-Bayoumi G, Borum ML, Haywood Y: Domestic violence in women: Women's health issues, Part II. *Med Clin North Am* 82:391, 1998.
8. EDK Associates: *Men Beating Women: Ending Domestic Violence—A Qualitative and Quantitative Study of Public Attitudes on Violence Against Women.* New York, EDK Associates, 1993.
9. Craven D: *Sex Differences in Violent Victimization, 1994: Bureau of Justice Statistics Special Report.* Washington, DC, Government Printing Office, 1997; US Department of Justice, Office of Justice Programs, Bureau of Justice Statistics, NCJ-164508.
10. Abbott J: Injuries and illnesses of domestic violence. *Ann Emerg Med* 29(6):781, 1997.
11. Browne A: Assault and homicide in the home: When battered women kill, in Saks MJ, Sale L (eds): *Advances in Social Psychology,* vol 3. Hillsdale, NJ, Lawrence Erlbaum Associates, 1987.
12. Wilson MI, Daly M: Who kills whom in spouse killings? On the exceptional sex ratio of spousal homicides in the United States. *Criminology* 30:189, 1992.
13. Cascardi M, Langhinrichsen J, Vivian D: Marital aggression: Impact, injury and health correlates for husbands and wives. *Archiv Internal Med* 152:1178, 1992.
14. Abbott J, Johnson R, Koziol-McLain J, Lowenstein SR: Domestic violence against women: Incidence and prevalence in an emergency department population. *JAMA* 273:1763, 1995.
15. Muelleman RA, Lenaghan PA, Pakieser RA: Battered women: Injury locations and types.*Ann Emerg Med* 28:486, 1996.
16. Dearwater SR, Coben JH, Campbell JC, et al: Prevalence of intimate partner abuse in women treated at community Hospital emergency departments. *JAMA* 280:433, 1998.
17. Abbott J, Johnson R, Koziol-McLain J, Lowenstein S: Domestic violence against women: Incidence and prevalence in an emergency department population. *JAMA* 273(22):1763, 1995.
18. Salber PR: Introduction, in *Improving Health Care Response to Domestic Violence: A Resource Manual for Health Care Providers.* San Francisco, Family Violence Prevention Fund, 1998.
19. Felitti VJ, Anda RF, Nordenberg D, et al: Relationship of childhood abuse and household dysfunction to many of the leading causes of death in adults. The Adverse Childhood Experiences (ACE) Study. *Am J Prev Med* 14(4):245, 1998.
20. Lee D, Letellier P, McLoughlin E, Salber P: California Hospital Emergency Departments Response of Domestic Violence—Survey Report. Family Violence Prevention Fund, Aug. 1993, San Francisco (available by contacting the Fund 415-252-8900).
21. Hayden SR, Barton ED, Hayden M: Domestic violence in the emergency department: How do women prefer to disclose and discuss the issues? *J Emerg Med* 15:447, 1997.
22. Stark E, Flitcraft A: Medicine and patriarchal violence: The social construction of a "private" event. *Int J Health Serv* 9:461, 1979.
23. Jacobsen A, Richardson B: Assault experiences of 100 psychiatric inpatients: Evidence of the need for routine inquiry. *Am J Psychiatry* 144:908, 1987.
24. Jaffee P, Wolfe DA, Wilson SL: *Children of Battered Women.* Thousand Oaks, CA, Sage, 1990.
25. Knapp J: The impact of children witnessing violence. *Pediatr Clin North Am* 45(2):355, 1998.
26. Doumas D, Margolin GS, John RS: The intergenerational transmission of aggression across three generations. *J Fam Violence* 9(2):157, 1994.
27. Browne A: When Battered Women Kill. New York: The Free Press, 1987.

ABUSE IN THE ELDERLY AND IMPAIRED

Ellen H. Taliaferro
Patricia R. Salber

Although not a new problem, elder abuse continues to be an underrecognized and underreported cause of morbidity and mortality in the elderly for many reasons. Historical information often remains undetected during the medical evaluation process. Social stigmata surround the problem and, like all forms of domestic violence, it is the "disease that is lied about." Finally, detection of elder abuse and neglect is contingent upon physicians' awareness of the problem as well as their ability to recognize and understand the risk factors that often appear before a crisis occurs.

INCIDENCE AND PREVALENCE

General estimates of elder abuse in the United States indicate that it may affect nearly 10 percent of the elderly population. Research suggests that between 3 and 4 percent of the elderly population is affected.[1]

DEFINITIONS

Violence is any harm resulting from intentional action by oneself or others. A very narrow and concise definition of family violence was included in the Family Violence Prevention and Services Act of 1984 of the US Congress: "The term 'family violence' means any act or threatened act of violence, including any forceful detention of an individual, which (a) results or threatens to result in physical injury; and (b) is committed by a person against another individual (including an elderly person) to whom such person is or was related by blood or marriage, or otherwise legally related, or with whom such person is or was lawfully residing." Included in the broadest sense of this definition is psychological battery (e.g., humiliating, rejecting, corrupting acts, and psychosocial injury).

Practical working definitions that permit measurement of elder abuse employ three forms of maltreatment: physical abuse, neglect, and chronic verbal aggression. These definitions do not include material abuse (theft or misuse of an elder's money or other assets) or self-inflicted abuse or neglect (which is sometimes included in definitions of elder maltreatment).

SOCIAL AND ENVIRONMENTAL ETIOLOGIC FACTORS

While in general elderly victims are socially isolated from family and friends, many of them live with their abuser. When abuse occurs, it has been found that the abuser is often dependent upon the victim for housing, and financial and emotional support. Caretakers usually attempt to provide acceptable and appropriate care. However, when the caregiver is overwhelmed, frustrated, or resentful of the responsibilities involved in the task of caring for a less than fully independent elder, abuse and/or neglect may occur.

Certain conditions tend to set the stage for abuse or neglect. A 9-year prospective study of community-dwelling elders recently elucidated risk factors of elders likely to be abused.[2] Functional disability and worsening cognitive impairment, especially an acute decline, was significantly associated with elder mistreatment. Although poverty and minority status were also identified as risk factors, reporting bias was believed to have significantly overestimated their influence.

Risk factors for abuse also reside in the characteristics of the abuser. In one study,[3] elderly abuse victims and a nonabused control group were compared to explore the relationship of caretaker stress to caretaker psychopathology. The authors found that abuse is associated more with personality problems of the caretaker than with stress. Earlier studies substantiated financial dependency of the caretaker as a major risk factor. A more recent study concluded that in general abusers are heavily dependent individuals. That study included family caretakers who were disabled, cognitively impaired, or mentally ill. Other studies have uncovered substantial psychological impairment on the part of the abusers, as well as higher rates of alcoholism, arrest, and other deviant behavior. These deviant characteristics and behaviors appear to be related to the abusers' dependence on elderly relatives for financial assistance, housing, social support, and other help.

Because elder abuse is such a widespread public health problem in the United States and because physicians are in an ideal position to serve as professional advocates of the elderly who are abused, many medical specialty societies are addressing elder abuse through organizational policy statements. The American College of Emergency Physicians adopted a policy statement on the Management of Elder Abuse and Neglect in October 1997.[4] This statement contains the following recommendations:

1. Emergency departments should have written protocols on recognition and treatment of elder abuse.
2. Hospitals should have appropriate ancillary staff and other resources readily available to help in the assessment and disposition of those individuals who may be abused or neglected. The hospital staff should be educated in local laws governing the reporting of such incidents and in defusing potentially hostile situations.
3. Hospitals and emergency departments should establish relationships with agencies that oversee the management and investigation of elder abuse. In jurisdictions that have mandatory reporting requirements, persons reporting in good faith should be immune from liability for compliance.
4. Further research should be conducted in epidemiology, detection, prevention, and management of elder abuse and neglect; standardized definitions of elder abuse developed by the National Center on Elder Abuse should facilitate research in this area.

CLINICAL FEATURES

Mistreatment and/or neglect of elderly patients may be difficult to recognize. The problem is complicated by the fact that when abuse is suspected, it may be difficult to secure confirmation from the patient. The patient may welcome and be relieved by the physician's concern and identification. However, embarrassment, fear of abandonment, fear of retaliation, and fear of nursing home placement can prompt the patient to deny the physician's concerns.

Historical information should focus on the following: (1) detecting the presence of caretaker mental illness, mental retardation, dementia, or drug or alcohol abuse: (2) family history of violence; (3) caretaker dependence on the elder patient for housing, finances, or emotional support; (4) patient isolation, as reflected by the fact that the patient does not have the opportunity to relate with people or to pursue activities and interests in a manner that the patient chooses; (5) whether the patient and suspected abuser are living together; and (6) recent occurrence of stressful life events, such as loss of job, moving, or death of a loved one for the caretaker.[5]

Important historical information concerning the patient should include dependency needs. Problems such as mental confusion, immobility, and need for assistance with hygiene are most often associated with neglect, a common form of maltreatment of the elderly. Eliciting a history of cognitive impairment is essential, since abused victims have been found to have significantly greater cognitive impairment than nonabused elderly patients. Abused patients also have a greater history of problematic behavior such as incontinence, nocturnal shouting, wandering, or paranoia.[1]

An important direct question to put to the patient is, "Are you happy at home, or have you experienced any recent changes in mood or sleeping or eating patterns?" Look also for the sudden onset of behavioral signs and symptoms that suggest victimization: depression, fear, withdrawal, confusion, anxiety, low self-esteem, or helplessness.

Other historical indicators of abuse or neglect include a pattern of "physician hopping," unexplained delay in seeking treatment, lack of medical care, a series of missed medical appointments, previous unexplained injuries, explanation of past injuries inconsistent with medical findings, and previous reports of similar injuries.

The physical examination begins with an observation of the interaction between the patient and accompanying caretakers. The following are findings suggestive of abuse:

1. The patient appears fearful of his or her companion.
2. There are conflicting accounts of the injury or illness between the patient and caretaker.
3. There is an absence of assistance from the caretaker.
4. The caretaker displays an attitude of indifference or anger toward the patient.
5. The caretaker is overly concerned with the costs of treatment needed by the patient.
6. The caretaker denies the patient the chance to interact privately with the physician.

The mental status examination should try to elicit signs and symptoms of confusion or disorientation. These signs and symptoms are risk factors for elder abuse or neglect. If they are present, it is important to seek an underlying cause, especially if they are new, since they may represent underlying medical disorders or may be reflective of intentional or unintentional medication abuse or misuse resulting from abuse or neglect.

The general physical examination should focus on detecting signs and symptoms of poor personal hygiene, inappropriate or soiled clothing, dehydration, malnutrition, and worsening decubiti. Specific injuries suggestive of abuse are unexplained fractures or dislocations, unexplained lacerations or abrasions, burns in unusual locations or of unusual shapes, unexplained injuries to the head or face, the presence of sexually transmitted diseases, and unexplained bruises.

For example, bilateral bruises on the upper arms may indicate holding or shaking. Bruises may be similar to the shape of an object or be clustered on the trunk, indicating striking injuries. The presence of bruises in various stages of healing is suggestive of repeated abuse. Bruises around the wrists or ankles may occur secondary to being tied down. Bruises on the inside part of the thighs or arms are highly suggestive of intentional injury, since bruises obtained from falling are usually located on the outside surfaces of the extremities.

DIAGNOSIS

Detection and diagnosis of elder abuse is dependent on being open to what is reported by the patient or others. Without such openess, reported abuse may be dismissed as paranoia, dementia, or patient noncompliance. A high index of suspicion is necessary. When it is lacking, signs of abuse and neglect may be erroneously ascribed to frequent falls, accidental medication errors, failure to thrive, or the normal decline with aging.

There is no substitute for direct questioning when inquiring about abuse. In one report,[6] 33 percent of abused victims stated on initial presentation to the emergency department that they were involved in an abusive relationship. Another 6 percent of abuse cases were detected by eliciting information from other informants. The remaining cases were elicited by physical examination (43 percent) or by social service evaluation during hospitalization (19 percent).

TREATMENT

Elder abuse treatment is twofold. First, emergency department treatment of the injuries and illnesses resulting from abuse or neglect must be specific for the injuries and illnesses detected. Second, detection of elder abuse or neglect must be aimed at intervention. Therefore, all treatment, whether delivered in the emergency department or the hospital, for both victim and the victim's caregiver, should be on the basis of multidisciplinary assessment and may result in admission of the elderly patient to an extended-care facility.

Intervention includes the resolution of disposition problems brought about through caregiver exhaustion, the inability of patients to care for themselves in the community, and abandonment by individuals and institutions. Intervention requires a complex array of skills. For example, the serious problem of drug and alcohol abuse among the elderly must be recognized and addressed by emergency department staff. Physical problems often disguise the existence of a problem of substance abuse.

In cases of proven or strongly suspected elder abuse or neglect, intervention must include the involvement or adult protective services.[7] All 50 states have passed legislation aimed at protecting elderly victims of domestic abuse and neglect and establishing adult protective services programs. In 1997, it was reported that 42 states had mandatory reporting laws directed toward health care and social-service professionals. These laws require disclosure of suspected elder mistreatment despite the adult victims' wishes.

ADMISSION INDICATIONS

Elderly patients with problems requiring hospital admission should be admitted to the appropriate medical service, and the department of social services should be consulted for evaluation. Patients who do not medically require admission may need to be admitted for protective placement if they cannot be safely discharged to their caretakers or returned to their institutional setting.

DISPOSITION

Safety is a key issue. Patients must not be returned to their living situations if there is any doubt about their safety. A formal safety assessment may dictate consultation with domestic violence experts, such as a hospital-based social worker or an on-call community-based elder abuse professional. It is important to remember that abuse or neglect may occur when a caregiver is overwhelmed, frustrated, or resentful of the responsibilities involved in taking care of the patient. If indicated, caregivers should be provided with intervention options, such as arranging for home care, respite, or counseling, or should be given advice as to the appropriate care for their family member.

The serious problem of drug and alcohol abuse among the elderly must be recognized by emergency department staff and addressed through appropriate referrals. Communities with geriatric treatment centers provide a valuable resource for patients identified through emergency department visits. Identification of such centers and the referral opportunities they represent should be readily available to emergency department staff.

When discharge is safe and appropriate, aftercare instructions should include appropriate treatment and referral for identified injuries and illness. Referrals should include specific available services, such as ''Meals on Wheels,'' home health aides, visiting nurses, transportation, emergency shelter, legal aid, and medical and mental health services.

REFERENCES

1. Jones JS, Holstege C, Holstege H: Elder abuse and neglect: Understanding the causes and potential risk factors. *Am J Emerg Med* 15:579, 1997.
2. Lachs MS, Williams C, O'Brien S, et al: Risk factors for reported elder abuse and neglect: A nine-year observational cohort study. *Gerontologist* 37:469, 1997.
3. Pillemer K, Finkelhor D: Causes of elder abuse: Caregiver stress versus problem relatives. *Am J Orthopsychiatry* 59:179, 1989.
4. American College of Emergency Physicians: Policy statement: Management of elder abuse and neglect. *Ann Emerg Med* 31:149, 1998.
5. Kleinschmidt K: Elder abuse: A review. *Ann Emerg Med* 30:463, 1997.
6. Jones J, Dougherty J, Schelble D, et al: Emergency department protocol for the diagnosis and evaluation of geriatric abuse. *Ann Emerg Med* 17:1006, 1988.
7. Capezuti E, Brush BL, Lawson WT III: Reporting elder mistreatment. *J Gerontol Nurs* 23:24, 1997.

293 VIOLENCE IN THE EMERGENCY DEPARTMENT

Marshall C. McCoy

Violence once threatened only law enforcement personnel among those dealing with the public. Now it has spread into the health care arena. Violence has become a more frequent resolution of conflict and often with more devastating brutality. No health care providers are more at risk for violence than those involved with the first-line care of patients. Prehospital care providers have shown an increasing fear of violent calls and admit that violent encounters contribute to high levels of burnout.[1] Mock and coworkers found that violence occurs in 5 percent of emergency medical services runs, and an additional 14 percent of calls are precipitated by violence.[2] Recent surveys of emergency department residents have shown that one of their primary concerns is for their safety while working in the emergency department.[3] Although comprehensive data addressing the problem are still being collected from emergency department personnel, urban and rural hospitals are reporting a higher incidence of potential and actual violent episodes in their emergency departments.

By its nature, the emergency department has an atmosphere of controlled chaos. Emergency departments are open 24 h a day, provide generally unlimited and unrestricted access, and have readily available drugs. They are frequented by those who are fatigued or hungry, and they accommodate family and friends of critically ill patients and those for whom daily life stresses have heightened frustration and anxiety. Furthermore, emergency departments are frequented by substance abusers who are often violent. Other factors that may predispose the emergency department to violence are increasing waiting times, staff shortages, overcrowding, patients' financial problems, and the high expectations of the patients. These are just some of the predisposing factors that have escalated violent events in the emergency department.

It has been estimated that 50 percent of all health services providers will be involved in a violent episode in their career. In a 1988 survey of 127 teaching hospitals, 32 percent of the respondents had at least one verbal threat daily, 25 percent reported using restraints at least once daily, and 18 percent had at least one threat from a weapon monthly. Unfortunately, 7 percent reported a death related to emergency department violence in the past 5 years. Of the institutions responding, 35 percent lacked 24-h emergency department security, and of the nine respondents who reported a death, 55 percent lacked 24-h security.[4]

The prevalence of weapons has also led to more violence with increasing severity. It has been reported that close to 5 percent of all psychiatric patients who present to the emergency department for acute care have weapons. One study using metal detectors to screen all emergency department patients over a 6-month period found 33 hand guns, 1324 knives, 97 mace-type canisters, and various other items considered dangerous to the patient and staff.[5] Unfortunately, the escalating problem of violence in the emergency department is often not approached until after a violent event.

RECOGNIZING THE VIOLENT PATIENT

The only agreed upon predictors of violence are gender and alcohol abuse. Most perpetrators of violence are males with a history of substance abuse. The amount of education, ethnic background, marital status, or diagnosis are not reliable predictors, but they may be barriers to patient-staff interaction, which in itself may lead to frustration and anxiety for both the staff and patient. In turn, this subconscious conflict may precipitate a violent encounter.

The most obvious predictor of potential violence is the patient's history. Any patient with a history of being violent in the past must be taken seriously and handled cautiously. Trivializing a patient's threat, no matter how subtle, may be the cause of unrecognized violence escalation in its early stages.

Every patient exhibiting violent or threatening behavior should have a thorough physical and mental-status examination. This may require some form of control (restraints or sedation) before an examination can be completed. Using family members, friends, therapists, and/or medical records as a source of history may be valuable. It is the duty of the examining physician to differentiate between an organic and a functional cause of the behavior (Table 293-1). The treatment of an underlying disorder may completely remove any threat, such as the administration of intravenous glucose to a disoriented, aggressive hypoglycemic patient. The organic diseases most likely involved in a violent episode are those related to drugs and withdrawal syndrome(s), especially delirium tremors. According to the American Psychiatric Association, the presence of any one of the following indicators should prompt a search for an organic etiology: a patient older than 40 years of age with no previous psychiatric history; disorientation, lethargy or stupor; abnormal vital signs; visual hallucinations; or illusions.[6] A thorough evaluation should include laboratory work, toxicology screening, electrocardiograms, and, in some cases, computed tomography scans and lumbar puncture.

The most common functional disorder related to violent behavior is schizophrenia, especially in patients in paranoid subgroups or with personality disorders. The most dangerous functional disorder is manic behavior.

PRODROMES OF VIOLENCE

In most cases, violent behavior is not one of the presenting signs of the patient. Therefore, recognition of the prodromes of violence is necessary. The phases of escalation are generally agreed upon. The first is the anxiety phase, followed by defensiveness, and then physical aggression.[7] Each phase evokes a response that is proportionate to the patient's behavior. In general, verbal abuse is best handled by verbal response. Physical aggression is best handled by physical means. It is important to remember that, although these levels may be discrete, they also may overlap.

TABLE 293-1 Problems Associated with Violence

Psychiatric	Vascular malformation
Schizophrenia	Hypoglycemia
Paranoid ideation	Hypoxia
Catatonic excitement	AIDS
Mania	Electrolyte abnormality
Personality disorder	Hypothermia or hyperthermia
Borderline	Anemia
Antisocial	Vitamin deficiency
Delusional depression	Endocrine disorder
Posttraumatic stress disorder	Drugs
Decompensating obsessive-compulsive disorder	Unanticipated reaction to prescribed medication (especially sedatives in brain-injured or elderly patients)
Homosexual panic	Alcohol (intoxication and withdrawal)
Situational frustration	Amphetamines
Mutual hostility	Cocaine
Miscommunication	Sedative-hypnotic (intoxication or withdrawal)
Fear of dependency or rejection	PCP
Fear of illness	LSD
Guilt over role in disease process	Anticholinergics
Organic diseases	Aromatic hydrocarbons (e.g., glue, paint, gasoline)
Delirium	Steroids
Dementia	Antisocial behavior
Trauma	Violence with no associated medical or psychiatric explanation (these patients may be managed by the police or security)
CNS infection	
Seizures	
Neoplasm	
Cerebrovascular accident	

Abbreviations: AIDS, acquired immunodeficiency syndrome; CNS, central nervous system; LSD, lysergic acid diethylamide; PCP, phencyclidine.
Source: From Rice and Moore,[8] with permission.

Phase 1: Anxiety

The first level of behavior seen in a potentially violent patient is anxiety. This may not only occur with the patient. Family and visitors waiting long periods in the emergency department waiting room may also exhibit anxiety and should be dealt with before visiting the patient so as not to intensify the patient's behavior. In general, the signs of increasing anxiety are indicated by body language. Movements that seem to have no purpose other than to expend energy may be the first clue. These may include pacing, wringing of hands, clenching of fists, unwillingness to stay in the treatment area, or a disheveled appearance. Speech may be pressured and loud. Questions such as "Why am I here?" or "How long is this going to take?" may be asked. It is not necessarily what is said, but the manner of speech that gives a clue to the presence of anxiety. One of the most common reasons that a patient's condition may evolve beyond anxiety is that the staff ignores these signals, rather than acknowledging the potential for violence. Underestimating these gestures as a signal of potential violence is inviting a potential threat.

The appropriate response to the anxiety phase should be developing some type of rapport with the potentially violent patient. Time (a precious commodity to emergency staff and physicians) is usually all that is needed to establish this rapport. Listening to the patient's concerns and addressing him or her appropriately may be all that is required to diffuse the situation. To take an attitude of "I can't be bothered with such a matter" will only cause more anxiety in a person who may be feeling a loss of control. Most patients are fearful of this loss of control and usually welcome the opportunity to politely vent their feelings. This requires sympathy and empathy regarding their concerns. The patient must be treated honestly and with respect. This courtesy will go a long way in gaining rapport and ultimately avoiding future problems. Be supportive with responses that acknowledge the patient's feelings, such as "I understand why you are angry." A peace offering of food or drink may also help. Do not be judgmental. Concentrate on what the patient is saying and do not feign attention. Restating what the patient has just said may help clarify the patient's complaints and allow the patient to continue venting. Remain on the topic and, above all, remain calm. This will help the patient feel more in control.

Phase 2: Defensiveness

The next level in the continuum of violent behavior is characterized by defensiveness. At this point, the patient's behavior is volatile and becomes verbally abusive and profane. These verbal attacks may be directed to staff members or others in the department and may include statements about age, gender, weight, or heritage. The patient's behaviors are irrational and often have nothing to do with why the patient presented to the emergency department. The patient is losing control and may feel helpless. A patient may present to the emergency department in this stage, having passed the anxiety stage outside the hospital. If the patient is restrained, such as a patient in police custody, feelings of helplessness may be further magnified.

Such patients will challenge emergency department personnel and their authority and will respond to staff with body posturing and movements. Emergency department personnel must remain professional and avoid power struggles and loss of patience. Appropriate responses to this phase are preventing total loss of control by the patient and thus deflecting physical aggression. One must be firm in tone and action. The patient must have reasonable limits set and be made aware of the consequences of such continued behavior. Limits must be simple, clear, enforceable, and consistent among all emergency department personnel. Giving the patient reasonable choices may help diffuse the situation and make him or her feel rewarded for good behavior. Emergency staff must not overreact or make counterthreats or false promises. If others are present, the patient and the situation must be isolated. A show of force by uniformed security personnel may be in order, keeping in mind that such a presence may cause further escalation; however, this is the exception, not the rule. It is important that no consequence be stated that is not readily enforceable. Let the patient make the choice.

Phase 3: Physical Aggression

The third level of behavior that may be encountered is that of true physical aggression and assertive behavior. The patient is totally out of control, and no amount of verbal intervention is effective. The physically aggressive patient must be confronted and controlled physically, not only for the safety of the emergency department personnel, but for the safety of the violent patient, other patients, and visitors in the department. Only when all other interventions have failed and once the decision has been made to restrain, no further negotiation is warranted. Physical control of a patient may require personnel skilled in overcoming a person without injury to self or others. Physical control should never be attempted single-handedly and should preferably be deferred to a trained individual. It is important to remember that a health care provider has a *duty* to evaluate a patient's needs. Restraint, in some situations, is only fulfilling that duty. Using appropriate and nonharmful restraint enables the physician to provide necessary care for a violent patient. Physical control is implemented, not for punitive reasons, but in the interest of patient care and safety for others.

TABLE 293-2 Guidelines for Using Restraints

1. At least four persons should assist with restraining the patient, while a fifth staff member controls the patient's head and prevents biting. At no time should only one or two persons try to restrain a patient. Leather restraints are the safest and surest type of restraint.
2. Explain to the patient why he or she is being restrained. Give the patient a few seconds to comply, but do not negotiate. At a prearranged signal, the team grabs the patient and brings him or her to the floor in a backward motion without injuring him or her. The team applies restraints, then moves the patient to the seclusion room.
3. A staff member should always be visible to reassure the patient who is being restrained.
4. Restrain the patient with legs spread-eagled and one arm restrained to the side and the other arm restrained over the patient's head.
5. Remove all dangerous objects from the patient, including rings, shoes, matches, pens, and pencils.
6. Place restraints so that intravenous fluids can be given if necessary.
7. Raise the patient's head slightly to decrease feelings of vulnerability and to reduce the possibility of aspiration.
8. After the patient is in restraints, begin treatment using verbal intervention or rapid tranquilization.
9. Remove one restraint at a time at 5-min intervals until the patient has only two restraints on. Remove both of these restraints at the same time. Never leave only one limb in restraints.

Source: Adapted from Dubin WR, Weiss KJ in Michels R et al (eds): *Psychiatry,* vol 2. Philadelphia, Lippincott, 1985, with permission.

PHYSICAL RESTRAINTS

Restraints are used not only to control a patient when verbal interventions have failed but also to facilitate the appropriate evaluations of patients with underlying organic disorders who are too agitated or lack the mental capacity to be reasoned with and control themselves. When used properly and appropriately, restraints are more humane than allowing patients to injure themselves or others. Restraints should be used to prevent harm, to allow for further evaluation of a violent patient, or in response to a patient's request for them. Restraints should never be used with orthopedic problems or certain medical problems, such as myocardial infarction, when a worsening of symptoms may result from using the restraints and sensory deprivations may be more harmful than helpful (Table 293-2).

Once the decision to restrain a patient is made, appropriate personnel must be assembled. At least four to five people with a single team leader should be present. On the command of this leader, the procedure is carried out without undue force or harm to the patient or staff. Soft restraints should never be used on a truly violent patient, and once the patient is restrained the devices should not be removed except under the order of the treating physician, with the assent of the other health care providers, and with security personnel present. It is important that one explain the reason for restraint to the patient. Once restrained, the patient should not be abandoned.

Strict protocols for the use of restraints should be available in every emergency department. They should incorporate input not only from emergency department staff but from security, law enforcement, hospital legal departments, and, if possible, psychiatric services in order to present a consistent, lawful approach to the use of restraints. Once the protocol is developed, in-service meetings should be arranged to familiarize and train all emergency department personnel in the use of restraints.

Medicolegal issues are part of any restraining procedure. It is law that the minimal use of force be used to hold a violent patient.[8] The presence of security may be the only restraint needed. Anytime a person is placed in restraints, the medical chart should reflect the reason the patient was restrained. The chart should state clearly that a direct physician order is required to remove a restraint. No patient for whom restraints are needed should be allowed to leave the emergency department against medical advice. If necessary, contacting hospital legal authorities may be helpful. In general, restraining a patient against his or her will is preferable to facing the legal issues that arise when patients harm themselves or someone else in the emergency department and the threat of violence was clearly evident.

Restraining also allows the patient to be searched for weapons or drugs, although that is never the primary motivation. Searching can often be accomplished by simply asking the patient to allow such a search or by deferring to security personnel. The best search is done by undressing the patient. Emergency department staff should not attempt to take weapons from a patient without assistance; if weapons are obtained, they should never be returned, despite the patient's insistence.

Those who come to the emergency department in restraints should be left in restraints. Yet law enforcement officials often bring patients in handcuffs to the emergency department only to give them a summons and release them once treatment has begun. No person should be released from law enforcement personnel in the emergency department. If initial plans were to release the patients (the perpetrators), they should not have been brought to the emergency department, especially those refusing any type of care. Law enforcement officers should not be allowed to leave a patient unattended in the emergency department if physical restraint was needed earlier. Furthermore, prisoners in the emergency department should never be released from restraints; many an escape has taken place from a hospital setting.

CHEMICAL RESTRAINTS

At times a patient may be too violent, even while physically restrained, for an adequate evaluation to be performed. The use of pharmacologic agents can be a safe and effective means of controlling such patients, provided the drugs are used appropriately and that physicians are aware of their adverse affects (Table 293-3). The term *rapid tranquilization* has been used to describe delivery of medications in a titrated fashion to gain control of patients with psychiatric illness, substance abuse, dementia, or withdrawal symptoms.[9] Standard doses of neuroleptic agents or benzodiazepines are given at 30- to 60-min intervals until the desired effect is reached. In general, doses for elderly patients should be half of those used on younger patients.

Physicians who use any of these medications should become familiar with their adverse effects and the treatment of these effects, which include anticholinergic effects, hypotension, and extrapyramidal symptoms. Haloperidol is generally considered the neuroleptic of choice, since the adverse effects are usually less common. Short-acting benzodiazepines, such as lorazepam, are also recommended for intoxicated states and withdrawal syndromes. With the advent of flumazenil, a benzodiazepine antagonist, respiratory depression or oversedation with these agents can be reversed.

PREVENTION

The single best way to handle a violent patient or curtail the potential for violence in the emergency department is by prevention. Careful planning of the work area, cooperation with security, and training of all emergency department personnel to recognize violent patients are critical.

The physical plan of an emergency department should be one of controlled access. Visitation policies should be reasonable yet enforced. Some hospitals use visitor identification badges to monitor visitors in the department. A busy emergency department, packed full of visitors, only increases anxiety and tension. It is also the perfect place for a weapons-carrying violent patient to take hostages. Although a history from family and friends can be important in the evaluation of any potentially violent patient, interviews should be conducted in a safe, calm environment.

Seclusion rooms for interviewing patients should be safe for both the patient and the interviewer. Solid walls with sturdy, heavy furniture that would be awkward to lift should be used. Lighting should be able to be dimmed or brightened, depending on the circumstance. No free-standing objects, such as ashtrays, pictures, or pencils, should be allowed, since they all could become potential weapons. Exits should be clear of obstruction and readily available to the interviewer. Panic buttons may be installed or signals developed to be used in the event of threatening behavior on the part of the patient. If violent aggression does develop, the room should be large enough for a team of security personnel to safely overcome the patient without undue harm.

Deterrence is also a preventive technique. Signs outside the emergency department should clearly state that weapons of any type are not permitted, and trained hospital security personnel should be visible to everyone entering the emergency department. Not only does this set a tone of behavior, but security measures can be invaluable in preventing as well as curtailing any violence. The use of metal detectors and x-ray machines for personal articles, such as handbags, may allow for easy screening of those entering the treatment area. Once believed a luxury, metal detectors are now reasonably priced. Carefully placed monitors and alarm buttons may also be warranted. However, metal detectors, monitors, and alarms are only a part of an overall security system and complement personnel training in the management of potential and actual violent situations.[10,11]

Seclusion rooms and deterrent measures are needed, yet the education of the emergency department personnel is the most important factor in curbing violence in the emergency department. Several national programs, such as that offered by the National Crisis Prevention Institute, are invaluable in teaching a basic understanding of violent behavior, its recognition and management, and basic self-defense against violent patients. In-services by security personnel and law enforcement officials may also be of benefit. Physicians should learn how to examine a patient while still protecting their personal space in order to prevent injury should the patient lash out.

Common sense and a heightened awareness of the potential for violence is the first step in this education. Being aware of the position of one's body, clothing, and equipment in relation to the patient can save one from assault. The physician should never let a violent patient

TABLE 293-3 Rapid Tranquilization of Violent Patients

Cause of Violent Behavior	Drug Intervention*
Schizophrenia, mania, other psychoses	Lorazepam (Ativan) 2–4 mg IM combined with haloperidol (Haldol) 5 mg IM or thiothixene (Navane) 10 mg IM *or* An antipsychotic alone: Thiothixene (Navane) 10 mg IM Haloperidol (Haldol) 5 mg IM or droperidol 5 mg IM Loxapine (Loxitane) 10 mg IM
Personality disorder	Lorazepam (Ativan) 1–2 mg PO q1–2 h or 2 mg IM (0.05 mg/kg) q1–2 h
Alcohol withdrawal states†	For agitation, tremors, or change in vital signs: chlordiazepoxide (Librium) 25–50 mg PO q4–6 h For elderly patients or patients with liver disease: lorazepam 2 mg PO q2h For extreme agitation or patients not controlled with benzodiazepines: lorazepam 2–4 mg IM qh
Cocaine and amphetamine intoxication	For mild to moderate agitation: diazepam (Valium) 10 mg PO q8h For severe agitation: thiothixene 10 mg IM; haloperidol 5 mg IM; or droperidol 5 mg IM
Phencyclidine intoxication	For hyperactivity, mild agitation, tension, anxiety, excitement: diazepam 10–30 mg PO or lorazepam 2–4 mg IM (0.05 mg/kg) For severe agitation and excitement with hallucinations, delusions, bizarre behavior: haloperidol 5–10 mg IM or droperidol 5 mg IM

*All doses given at 30- to 60-min intervals; one-half dose for medically ill or older patients.
†Rapid tranquilization in alcohol withdrawal states is for severe agitation and behavioral control. The actual treatment of withdrawal is with a cross-tolerant medication.
Source: From Dubin and Weiss,[9] with permission.

get between him or her and the exit. Physicians should defer to trained security personnel if a patient needs to be searched or disarmed. Incidents and reasons for restraint must always be properly documented.

Violence in emergency departments is not uncommon. Both rural and urban hospitals are plagued by increasing episodes of violence. Careful preparation and a heightened awareness of the potential for violence are basic. Education is important in understanding the dynamics of violent behavior and will help to detect and manage the violent patient. Training should be reviewed periodically. Management strategies should involve a team of emergency department staff and security, law enforcement, and hospital legal departments. Strict policies should be established for visitation. Making the work environment safe will make all involved more comfortable. Health care providers should feel as safe at work as they do at home. Physicians should trust their intuition. If the physician is afraid, then the potential for violence probably exists.

REFERENCES

1. Tintinalli JE, McCoy M: Violent patients and the prehospital provider. *Ann Emerg Med* 22:1276, 1993.
2. Mock EF, Wrenn KD, Wright SW, et al: Prospective field study of violence in emergency medical service calls. *Ann Emerg Med* 32:33, 1998.
3. Anglin D, Kyriacou DN, Hudson HR: Resident's perspective on violence and personal safety in the emergency department. *Ann Emerg Med* 23:1082, 1994.
4. Lavoie FW, Carter GL, Danzel DF, Berg RL: Emergency department violence in United States' teaching hospitals. *Ann Emerg Med* 17:1227, 1988.
5. Dubin WR, Tarduff K, Maler G: Overcoming danger with violent patients: Guidelines for safe and effective management. *Emergency Medicine Reports,* vol 13, no 14, 1992.
6. *Seclusion and Restraint: The Psychiatric Uses.* Task Force Report 22. Washington, American Psychiatric Association, 1985.
7. *Nonviolent Crisis Intervention Workbook.* Brookfield, WI, National Crisis Prevention Institute, 1987.
8. Rice M, Moore G: Management of the violent patient, therapeutic and legal considerations. *Emerg Med Clin North Am* 9:13, 1991.
9. Dubin WR, Weiss KJ: *Handbook of Psychiatric Emergencies.* Springhouse, PA, Springhouse Corporation, 1991.
10. Thompson B, Nunn J, Kramer I, et al: Disarming the department: Weapon screening and improved security to create a safer emergency department environment. *Ann Emerg Med* 17:419, 1988.
11. Rankins RC, Hendey GW: Effect of a security system on violent incidents and hidden weapons in the emergency department. *Ann E Med* 33:6, 676, 1999.

CONTRAST STUDIES

John Eng

Iodinated intravascular contrast agents significantly improve the visualization of structures in many radiologic examinations, and millions of doses are administered each year in the United States for this purpose. As with any pharmaceutical product, appropriate use of intravascular contrast agents requires knowledge of the risks and benefits of their use. Unlike most drugs, however, contrast agents provide the potential benefit, not of a therapeutic effect, but of an improvement in diagnostic information.

This chapter begins with an introduction to the pharmaceutical properties of iodinated intravascular contrast agents, followed by clinical points to consider prior to their administration. While it is always advisable to discuss the need for iodinated contrast with a radiologist on a case-by-case basis, some general indications are offered. Iodinated contrast for visualization of the gastrointestinal tract is also briefly discussed. Finally, the diagnosis and treatment of contrast reactions are outlined. Throughout this chapter, *contrast agent* refers to iodinated intravascular contrast material unless otherwise indicated.

IODINATED INTRAVASCULAR CONTRAST AGENTS

Mechanism of Action

Iodinated intravascular contrast agents are water-soluble molecules that contain several radiodense iodine atoms per molecule. Following injection, contrast agents remain in the vascular space for only a short time and are rapidly distributed into the extracellular space. Contrast agents do not enter the intracellular space or cross an intact blood-brain barrier. They are rapidly excreted by the kidney via glomerular filtration without tubular resorption.

Since the radiodense iodine atoms absorb more x-rays than do biological tissues, contrast agents appear white (like the bones) if they are present in high enough concentration during examinations made with x-rays (radiographs). Contrast agents are visible on arteriography during the short time they are in high concentration in the vascular space. They are visible in the urinary tract during intravenous urography (IVU), after excretion by the kidney. Because of its ability to discriminate subtle differences in radiodensity, computed tomography (CT) shows the presence of contrast agents in all tissue compartments even though they may be present in relatively low concentration (compared to arteriography or radiography).

Types of Agents

Contrast agents are classified according to osmolality (Table 294-1). High-osmolality agents have been in clinical use since the 1950s, and they are often called ionic contrast agents because they are all organic salts (Fig. 294-1). Low-osmolality agents have been in use since 1986, and they are commonly called nonionic agents because all but one are organic molecules without electronic charge (Fig. 294-2). A number of studies have demonstrated that low-osmolality contrast agents are associated with at least a 50 percent reduction in the incidence of both minor and severe reactions (Table 294-1). Anecdotally, injection of low-osmolality agents is associated with less subjective effects, such as flushing, heat, chemical taste, and osmotic diuresis. Currently in the United States, low-osmolality contrast agents cost on average 8 to 10 times more than an equivalent dose of a high-osmolality agent. The use of low-osmolality contrast agents is surrounded by some controversy due to the significant cost differential for a relatively modest difference in the incidence of severe reactions, which are rare.

Types of Contrast Reactions

Contrast reactions can be divided into three categories: anaphylactoid, chemotoxic, and vasovagal (Table 294-2). Anaphylactoid reactions occur idiosyncratically, and they mimic allergic or anaphylactic reactions and shock. Anaphylactoid contrast reactions are not true anaphylactic reactions because they have no known consistent pathophysiologic mechanism. They may involve one or more of the following mechanisms: histamine release, complement activation, hapten formation, contact sensitivity, endovascular reactions, and central nervous system factors. However, unlike true immunoallergic or anaphylactic reactions, they do not involve IgE mediation. An increased risk of anaphylactoid contrast reaction is associated with a history of asthma, food or drug allergy, or a previous contrast reaction. Low-osmolality agents are associated with a lower risk of anaphylactoid contrast reaction.

Chemotoxic reactions are related to osmotoxic and other chemical effects of contrast agents. The pathophysiologic mechanisms for chemotoxicity are not well understood, but its occurrence is less idiosyncratic. Since many of the chemotoxic cardiovascular reactions, such as dysrhythmia and pulmonary edema, occur primarily with coronary artery injections, their occurrence in the emergency department setting is probably of less concern than in the cardiac catheterization suite.

Contrast agents can also cause vasovagal reactions, a result of increased vagal tone of the heart and blood vessels of unknown etiology but thought to be related to the central nervous system. In addition to being caused by contrast agents, vasovagal reactions may also be caused by the circumstances surrounding their administration, such as fear, anxiety, or discomfort from needle puncture.

RISK ASSESSMENT AND PATIENT PREPARATION

There are no absolute contraindications for receiving intravascular contrast agents. Certain clinical conditions either increase the risk of developing a contrast reaction or increase the severity of the reaction should one develop. Risk assessment and, in some cases, preventive measures should be performed prior to contrast administration. Considerations for patient preparation are summarized in Table 294-3, and additional comments are offered below.

History of Allergy

A history of asthma or severe allergy (e.g., anaphylaxis) to one or more allergens is associated with an increased risk of a contrast reaction. Patients with a history of asthma may have a fivefold greater risk of an adverse reaction than in the general population, and a history of allergy may double the risk.[1] A history of reaction during a previous contrast administration is associated with a three- to eightfold greater risk of a subsequent adverse reaction than in the general population.[1]

Renal Disease

Classically, the risk factors for developing renal insufficiency from contrast agents are preexisting renal insufficiency (creatinine level >

TABLE 294-1 Comparison of High- and Low-Osmolality Contrast Agents

Characteristic	High-Osmolality Agent (Ionic)	Low-Osmolality Agent (Nonionic)
Approximate osmolality relative to serum	5	2
Overall incidence of adverse reaction	5–8%	1–2%
Incidence of severe reaction	1–2 per 1000	1–2 per 10,000
Incidence of fatal reaction	1/40,000–1/170,000	1/200,000–1/300,000
Relative cost	1	8–10

1.5 mg/mL), diabetes mellitus, volume depletion, use of diuretics in cardiovascular disease, advanced age (>70 years), multiple myeloma, hypertension, and hyperuricemia.[2,3] More recent studies have shown that the most important risk is associated with the coexistence of diabetes *and* renal insufficiency.[4]

As a preventive measure, patients with preexisting renal insufficiency, diabetes, or volume depletion should receive hydration in the form of 0.45% sodium chloride at 100 mL/h beginning 12 h before and continuing 12 h after contrast administration. In patients with end-stage renal failure receiving chronic dialysis, contrast agent and extra fluid must be removed by dialysis, but the dialysis does not need to be performed emergently[5] unless there is significant underlying cardiac dysfunction (and thus increased risk of direct cardiac chemotoxicity).

Cardiac Disease

Patients with significant cardiac disease appear to be at increased risk for contrast reactions. Significant cardiac disease includes severe angina pectoris, congestive heart failure, severe valvular disease, primary pulmonary hypertension, or cardiomyopathy.

Metformin Therapy

Metformin (Glucophage) is an oral antihyperglycemic agent used to treat non-insulin-dependent diabetes mellitus. Development of potentially fatal lactic acidosis is a rare adverse effect of metformin and may occur if contrast-induced renal insufficiency (itself a rare event) develops. Therefore, metformin should be discontinued 48 h prior to contrast administration and withheld for 48 h afterward. The drug may be restarted after the patient's renal function is rechecked and found to be normal.

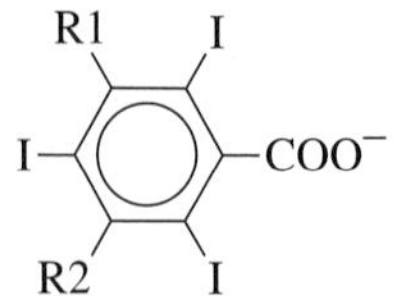

R1 I
I— —COO⁻
R2 I

FIG. 294-1. The general chemical structure of the anion of a high-osmolality contrast agent. The R groups are either diatrizoate or iothalamate, depending on the manufacturer. The corresponding cation is either sodium or meglumine.

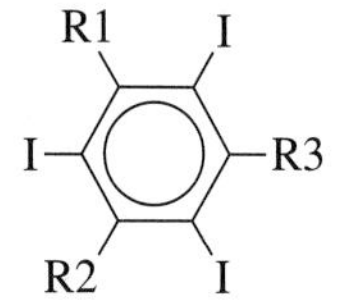

R1 I
I— —R3
R2 I

FIG. 294-2. The general chemical structure of a nonionic, low-osmolality contrast agent. There are four such agents currently on the market, each with a different R group: iohexol (Omnipaque), iopamidol (Isovue), iopromide (Ultravist), and ioversol (Optiray). All of the R groups contain multiple hydroxyl groups for solubility. A fifth low-osmolality agent, ioxaglate (Hexabrix), has a different chemical structure (not shown) that is unique because it is both ionic and low osmolality.

Anxiety

There is some evidence that severe contrast reactions may be partially mediated by anxiety. Therefore, an anxious patient should be reassured and calmed prior to contrast injection.

Other Diseases

In patients with pheochromocytoma, pretreatment with phentolamine, an α-adrenergic antagonist, is recommended prior to contrast administration. In a nonstabilized patient with recent seizures, pretreatment with diazepam may be advisable.[1] Convulsions or seizures following contrast administration may be due to a lowering of the seizure threshold, or they may be a final result of a severe hypotensive or vasovagal reaction.[4]

As mentioned above, hyperuricemia and dysproteinemias, such as multiple myeloma, are associated with an increased risk of contrast-induced renal insufficiency, but there is conflicting evidence regarding the strength of this relationship. Similarly, some studies suggest that sickle cell trait and disease are also associated with an increased risk of contrast reaction, but the significance of the relationship is unclear.

Premedication

Premedication with a steroid regimen has been shown in some studies to reduce the overall incidence of contrast reactions to both high- and low-osmolality agents. However, no controlled studies have been performed to determine whether premedication reduces the incidence

TABLE 294-2 Classification of Contrast Reactions

Reaction Type	Signs and Symptoms
Anaphylactoid	
Generalized urticaria	Hives (generalized)
Laryngeal or facial edema	Stridor, facial swelling
Bronchospasm	Wheezing, dyspnea
Cardiovascular collapse (shock)	Hypotension, sinus tachycardia
Chemotoxic	
Renal tubular injury	Rising creatinine
Cardiac dysrhythmia	Electrocardiographic changes
Cardiac impairment	Pulmonary edema
Neurotoxicity	Seizure
Mild reactions	Nausea, emesis, warmth, dizziness, headache, pallor, flushing, shaking, chills, diaphoresis, hives (localized), altered taste, pruritus
Vasovagal	Hypotension, sinus bradycardia

TABLE 294-3 Summary of Patient Preparation Prior to Intravascular Administration of Iodinated Contrast Agents

Item for Consideration	Action
Clinical history	Elicit any history of allergy, asthma, previous use of contrast material, renal insufficiency, diabetes, cardiac disease, seizures, metformin therapy
Creatinine level	Obtain in patients with suspected renal dysfunction (see Table 294-5)
Hydration	Consider in patients with renal insufficiency, diabetes, volume depletion
Premedication	Prescribe for patients with history of contrast allergy and possibly patients with history of severe allergy to a substance other than contrast material
Selection of low-osmolality agent	Refer to American College of Radiology guidelines (see Table 294-6)

of *severe* reactions. Most institutions prescribe premedication if there is a history of a significant (more than nausea, vomiting, or a few hives) reaction to a previous contrast injection.[6] Some institutions also premedicate if there is a history of severe allergy to any substance. There are no standard indications or protocols for premedication. Two commonly prescribed premedication regimens are listed in Table 294-4.[7,8]

Serum Creatinine

A baseline serum creatinine level should be determined prior to contrast injection for patients with suspected renal dysfunction or considered at increased risk for contrast-induced nephrotoxicity (Table 294-5).[4] Determination of the serum creatinine level is *not* necessary in patients without suspected renal dysfunction. Furthermore, in cases of suspected renal dysfunction, clinical judgment may determine that an urgently needed contrast-enhanced examination should not be delayed by determination of the serum creatinine level.

Selective Use of Low-Osmolality Agents

Because of their lower incidence of reactions, low-osmolality agents are used by many institutions with selected patients at higher risk for developing a contrast reaction. The American College of Radiology has suggested guidelines for the selective use of low-osmolality agents (Table 294-6).[4] These guidelines are the result of a consensus and are not evidence-based because it is difficult to study severe contrast reactions due to their rarity. Some practices have elected to use low-osmolality agents exclusively, especially since they are generally better tolerated by patients (e.g., less nausea, vomiting, flushing, and heat sensation).

TABLE 294-4 Commonly Prescribed Regimens for Premedication Prior to Contrast Administration

Regimen	Dosage
1	Methylprednisolone (Medrol) 32 mg PO 12 h and 2 h before contrast injection
2	Prednisone 50 mg PO 13 h, 7 h, and 1 h before contrast injection, *and* Diphenhydramine (Benadryl) 50 mg PO 1 h before contrast injection

Abbreviation: PO, oral.
Source: Regimen 1 from Lasser et al[7] and regimen 2 from Greenberger and Patterson,[8] with permission.

TABLE 294-5 Recommendations for Obtaining Serum Creatinine Level Prior to Administration of Intravascular Iodinated Contrast Agents

History of "kidney disease" as an adult, including tumor and transplant
Family history of kidney failure
Insulin-dependent diabetes mellitus of 2 years' duration or greater
Non-insulin-dependent diabetes mellitus of over 5 years' duration (if on diabetic medication for that period)
Paraproteinemia syndromes or diseases (e.g., myeloma)
Collagen vascular disease
Patients taking certain medications: metformin (Glucophage), nonsteroidal anti-inflammatory drugs, or nephrotoxic antibiotics (e.g., aminoglycosides)

Source: American College of Radiology,[4] with permission.

INDICATIONS FOR INTRAVASCULAR CONTRAST AGENTS

An intravascular contrast agent is required to visualize vascular structures in arteriography, venography, and vascular CT (e.g., aorta and

TABLE 294-6 American College of Radiology Suggested Guidelines for the Selective Use of Iodinated Intravascular Low-Osmolality Contrast Agents

Patients with a history of any previous adverse reaction to intravascular iodinated contrast material, with the exception of a sensation of heat, flushing, or a single episode of nausea or vomiting
Patients with asthma
Patients with a previous serious allergic reaction to materials other than contrast agents
Patients with known cardiac dysfunction, including recent or potentially imminent cardiac decompensation, severe dysrhythmias, unstable angina pectoris, recent myocardial infarction, and pulmonary hypertension
Patients with renal insufficiency (particularly those with diabetes)
Patients with generalized severe debilitation, as determined by a physician
Patients at high risk for contrast extravasation
Any other circumstances where, after due consideration, the radiologist believes there is a specific indication for the use of low-osmolality contrast material, examples of which include but are not restricted to (1) sickle cell disease, (2) patients at increased risk for aspiration, (3) patients who are very anxious about the contrast procedure or who request or demand the use of low-osmolality contrast material, and (4) patients in whom the risk factors cannot be satisfactorily established

Source: American College of Radiology,[4] with permission.

TABLE 294-7 Indications for Iodinated Intravascular Contrast Agents

Required
Arteriography
Venography
Intravenous urography
Vascular CT (CT aortography for injury, dissection, aneurysm; CT pulmonary arteriography for embolism)
Highly desirable but *not absolutely* required
CT for trauma to abdominal or pelvic organs
CT for abdominal or pelvic abscess
CT for appendicitis or diverticulitis
CT for bowel obstruction
CT for orbital infection
Not indicated
Musculoskeletal CT for trauma (e.g., face, spine, pelvis)
Cranial CT for trauma or acute neurologic symptoms
Abdominal CT for urolithiasis

pulmonary arteries). Intravascular contrast agent is also required to visualize the urinary tract in an IVU. In such situations, decisions regarding the use of intravascular contrast agents are concerned with whether to perform the examination. Aside from these indications, decisions regarding the use of contrast usually arise in the context of nonvascular CT. Although highly desirable in many situations, contrast enhancement is not *absolutely* required for nonvascular CT, and may not add much to the ED evaluation in many situations. While the potential imaging benefits versus the risks of contrast-enhanced CT should always be discussed with a radiologist on a case-by-case basis, some general guidelines are offered below (Table 294-7).

Vascular Computed Tomography

As with conventional angiography, intravascular contrast is required for CT evaluation of vascular structures. In the emergency department, such an examination is most commonly done to evaluate the aorta for trauma, dissection, or aneurysm. If the clinical suspicion is high, initial evaluation with conventional aortography should be considered instead of CT because, in such cases, aortography (requiring additional doses of contrast) would probably be performed whether or not the CT findings are positive.

Helical CT (a form of high-speed CT) has been used in conjunction with rapid contrast injection to perform CT pulmonary arteriography as an alternative to conventional arteriography for the detection of pulmonary embolism. A scintigraphic ventilation-perfusion scan is usually performed as a screening study prior to either type of pulmonary arteriography. If results of the ventilation-perfusion scan are normal or near normal, pulmonary embolism is ruled out and in most cases further evaluation with a contrast study is unnecessary.

Intravenous Urography and Urolithiasis

The IVU, or intravenous pyelogram, is the classic study for the evaluation of ureteral obstruction due to urolithiasis. During an IVU, contrast excreted by the kidney visibly flows in the urinary tract up to the level of obstruction. If the obstruction is partial, its severity may be estimated. However, the obstructing calculus is not always visualized. More recently, noncontrast helical CT has been applied to detect ureteral calculi directly in the setting of suspected obstruction.[9,10] The size and location of the calculus, which indicate the likelihood of spontaneous passage, can be accurately determined. However, the degree of functional obstruction cannot be evaluated without contrast administration. Therefore, noncontrast CT is not helpful in evaluating a patient with known calculi who presents with new symptoms.

Renal ultrasound is often requested in the evaluation of suspected acute ureteral obstruction. In such a setting, ultrasound is usually *not* helpful because (1) hydronephrosis may be absent in early acute ureteral obstruction, (2) a dilated renal collecting system may be due to causes other than acute ureteral obstruction, and (3) the detection of calculi within the kidney does not necessarily imply obstruction by a more distal calculus.

Abdominal Trauma

Intravenous contrast is indicated in all CT examinations performed to detect intraabdominal injuries from blunt trauma, including liver laceration, splenic laceration, renal trauma, bowel hematoma, pancreatic fracture, ureteral injury, and bladder perforation. Intravenous contrast agents differentiate normal organ parenchyma from hematoma within an area of injury. In patients for whom the risk of administering intravenous contrast is thought to be too great, noncontrast CT is probably still of benefit, but small-to-moderate intraabdominal injuries may be missed, especially if there is no associated intraperitoneal fluid from hemorrhage. Because of the importance of intravenous contrast, some institutions proceed with contrast injection (using a low-osmolality agent) in all patients undergoing emergent abdominal CT, regardless of past medical history. With such a policy, it is felt that the imaging benefits of contrast enhancement combined with an emergency situation outweigh any possible risk of adverse reaction.

In the setting of penetrating trauma to the back or flank, intravenous contrast material is administered as part of the "triple-contrast" CT, the other two types of contrast being orally and rectally administered. Triple-contrast CT should be reserved for patients who have a wound that penetrates the muscular fascia, are clinically stable, and have no obvious signs of intraperitoneal or other internal injury.[11] In such patients, intravascular contrast imaging is required to detect renal and vascular injuries, and rectal administration of contrast material is particularly important for detecting subtle colonic injury.

Acute Abdomen

Intravenous contrast enhancement is indicated for all CT examinations performed for the evaluation of acute abdomen. Acute abdominal conditions for which CT is commonly performed include appendicitis, diverticulitis, intraabdominal abscess, and bowel obstruction. While intravenous contrast material enhances the visualization of all of these conditions, its role is not as great as in CT for abdominal trauma. For example, mesenteric inflammation is detectable in the absence of intravenous contrast enhancement in the case of appendicitis or diverticulitis. Furthermore, intravenous contrast enhancement is not involved in the detection of the complications of acute gastrointestinal inflammation, such as bowel obstruction, abscess formation, and bowel perforation. One cause of an acute abdomen, bowel ischemia, is an exception, in that intravenous contrast enhancement plays a major role in its detection, especially when strangulation is present.

The role of intravenous contrast enhancement in the detection of intraabdominal abscess is somewhat controversial, and good opacification of bowel loops by an oral contrast agent is arguably more important than the use of intravenous contrast agents in optimal CT evaluation for the diagnosis of intraabdominal abscess. As in other pathologic processes in the female pelvis, radiologic evaluation of intrapelvic abscess in a female should usually begin with transabdominal and endovaginal ultrasound rather than CT. The uterus and ovaries are almost always better visualized by endovaginal ultrasound.

For the diagnosis of appendicitis, ultrasound with graded compression is an accurate alternative to contrast-enhanced CT.[12] The technique is rapid and requires no intravascular contrast material. Its main disadvantage is the requirement of a sonographer skilled in the specific technique of examining the appendix.

Focused helical CT of the appendix without intravenous contrast enhancement has been shown to be a cost-effective method of evaluating patients with clinically suspected appendicitis.[13] This examination is performed with both oral and rectal contrast material but without intravenous contrast agents, and images of only the axial levels surrounding the appendix are obtained.[14] A focused CT examination of the appendix should be considered only if the primary clinical question is the presence or absence of appendicitis. Evaluation for other intraabdominal pathologic conditions may be limited in this type of focused CT examination.

Cranial Computed Tomography

Contrast-enhanced cranial CT is rarely indicated in the emergency setting. Abnormalities detected only on contrast-enhanced cranial CT, such as meningitis, some subacute infarcts, and small metastases, rarely change the immediate diagnostic workup and treatment and are more appropriately evaluated with magnetic resonance imaging (MRI). In the case of infarction, administration of a contrast agent may exacerbate the patient's clinical condition. Furthermore, intravenous contrast material may obscure intracranial hemorrhage, especially in the subarachnoid space.

Skeletal Trauma

Since bone appears much denser on CT than does even intravascular contrast, imaging of the skeletal system does not require contrast injection. Emergent skeletal CT is most often performed to evaluate fracture of the axial skeleton. Intravenous contrast enhancement may be necessary to detect concomitant injury of the abdominal or pelvic organs.

CT of the spine, particularly of the lumbar spine, following administration of *intrathecal* contrast material is occasionally performed for the evaluation of back pain. This procedure, CT myelography, has been essentially replaced by MRI, which provides significantly better visualization of the spinal cord, nerve roots, and intervertebral disks. CT myelography should only be performed in special cases, such as preoperative evaluation and planning.

IODINATED GASTROINTESTINAL CONTRAST AGENTS

In most nonemergent fluoroscopic studies of the gastrointestinal tract, oral or rectal barium sulfate contrast material is preferred over iodinated contrast material (e.g., Gastrografin, Gastroview, Hypaque) be-

TABLE 294-8 Guidelines for the Diagnosis and Treatment of Contrast Reactions

Signs and Symptoms	Treatment	Treatment Interval	Treatment Precautions
Nausea and/or vomiting			
Transient	Supportive observation		
Severe, protracted	Prochlorperazine 5–10 mg IV or IM	Every 3–4 h	Give slowly; drowsiness
Urticaria			
Scattered, transient	Supportive observation		
Scattered, protracted	Diphenhydramine 25–50 mg PO/IV/IM	Every 2–3 h	Drowsiness, hypotension
Severe	Cimetidine 300 mg IV *or* Ranitidine 50 mg IV	Every 6–8 h	Give slowly; drowsiness
Profound, diffuse edema	See anaphylactoid reaction		
Bronchospasm (wheezing)	O_2 6 L/min by mask; pulse oximeter		
Isolated wheezing	Metaproterenol inhaler 2 puffs *or* Terbutaline inhaler 2 puffs *or* Albuterol inhaler 2 puffs	Every 4–6 h	Proper inhalation technique (use of spacer)
Moderate or severe	See anaphylactoid reaction		
Hypotension, isolated	O_2 6 L/min by mask; Trendelenburg		
Sinus tachycardia (shock)	Normal saline 1–2 L IV bolus *or* Lactated Ringer's 1–2 L IV bolus *and* If poorly responsive, see anaphylactoid reaction	Per blood pressure and urine output	Fluid overload
Sinus bradycardia (vagal)	Atropine 0.6–1.0 mg IV *and* IV fluids as for sinus tachycardia	Every 3–5 min up to 3 mg total	Monitor pulse rate; fluid overload
Laryngeal or facial edema (stridor)	See anaphylactoid reaction		
Anaphylactoid reaction	O_2 6 L/min by mask; pulse oximeter		
Moderate	Epinephrine 1:1000 0.1–0.3 ml SC (0.1–0.3 mg)	Every 10–15 min up to 1 ml	Noncardioselective β-blockers
Accelerating or severe	Epinephrine 1:10,000 1 ml IV (0.1 mg)	Every 5–10 min up to 10 ml	Give slowly; β-blockers (especially noncardioselective)

Abbreviations: IM, intramuscular; IV, intravenous; PO, oral; SC, subcutaneous.
Source: Modified from Bush and Swanson[1] and American College of Radiology,[4] with permission.

cause barium demonstrates the mucosa in greater detail and is less susceptible to dilution. However, iodinated contrast agents are indicated in many emergent situations in which barium contrast is contraindicated: (1) suspected or potential bowel perforation (including trauma or abscess), (2) administration before gastrointestinal surgery or endoscopy, and (3) evaluation of the position of percutaneously placed bowel catheters. Iodinated contrast agents are appropriate in these situations because they are rapidly reabsorbed from the peritoneal and interstitial spaces.[4] If a fluoroscopic study with iodinated contrast material does not demonstrate a suspected perforation, many radiologists repeat the study using barium to look for small leaks, which are often more apparent with barium than with iodinated contrast agents.

For gastrointestinal studies involving iodinated contrast material, low-osmolality agents are indicated in the following situations: (1) oral administration in patients who are at risk for aspiration, because contrast-induced pulmonary edema is less with low-osmolality agents; and (2) patients with fluid or electrolyte imbalances, because low-osmolality agents cause less dilution and fluid shifts into the bowel lumen.[4]

Following oral or rectal administration, a small amount of iodinated contrast agent (approximately 1 to 2 percent) is absorbed by the bowel and excreted into the urine.[4] Therefore, the risk of developing an anaphylactoid contrast reaction is theoretically the same as it is for intravascular administration, and the same preprocedural evaluation and precautions apply. However, moderate or severe contrast reactions are only very rarely reported following oral or rectal administration of iodinated contrast agents. Therefore, the actual risk may be lower than that for intravascular administration. These comments are also applicable to administration of iodinated contrast material into the bladder or male urethra for the evaluation of trauma. In such examinations, it is likely that absorption of the contrast agent is even less than in the gastrointestinal tract.

The administration of oral or rectal contrast material is important in a number of indications for abdominal CT. Unlike fluoroscopic studies, gastrointestinal CT studies entail no significant difference in diagnostic quality between barium and iodinated contrast agents because only very dilute gastrointestinal contrast material is required. Therefore, high-osmolality iodinated contrast agents may be routinely used for emergent CT evaluation of the gastrointestinal tract.

DIAGNOSIS AND TREATMENT OF CONTRAST REACTIONS

The great majority of adverse effects from contrast agents are mild or moderate events that are not life-threatening and require only observation, reassurance, and general supportive measures. However, vigilance must be maintained because most severe contrast reactions begin with mild-to-moderate symptoms and signs. The vigilance need not be prolonged because essentially all life-threatening contrast reactions occur immediately or within 15 min of injection.[15]

From a clinical perspective, acute reactions to contrast agents can be classified in the following types: (1) nausea and/or vomiting, (2) urticaria (hives) without respiratory symptoms, (3) bronchospasm (wheezing) without cutaneous or cardiovascular manifestations, (4) isolated hypotension, (5) vagal reaction, (6) isolated laryngeal edema, and (7) generalized anaphylactoid reaction.[1,4] Clinically, an anaphylactoid reaction is characterized by a severe or rapidly accelerating combination of one or more of the following: bronchospasm, generalized urticaria, angioedema, laryngeal spasm or edema, and hypotension with tachycardia (shock). Table 294-8 presents one approach to the treatment of acute contrast reactions. Contrast reactions may also have nonspecific manifestations, such as pulmonary edema, angina, seizure, or hypertensive urgency. Such reactions should be treated with standard therapies and protocols (see Chap. 30).

REFERENCES

1. Bush WH, Swanson DP: Acute reactions to intravascular contrast media: types, risk factors, recognition, and specific treatment. *AJR* 157:1153, 1991.
2. Byrd L, Sherman RL: Radiocontrast-induced acute renal failure: A clinical and pathophysiologic review. *Medicine* 58:270, 1979.
3. Katzberg RW: Urography into the twenty-first century: New contrast media, renal handling, imaging characteristics, and nephrotoxicity. *Radiology* 204:297, 1997.
4. American College of Radiology: *Iodinated Contrast Media,* 4th ed. Reston, VA, American College of Radiology, 1998.
5. Younathan CM, Kande JV, Cook MD, et al: Dialysis is not indicated immediately after administration of nonionic contrast agents in patients with end-stage renal disease treated by maintenance dialysis. *AJR* 163:969, 1994.
6. Cohan RH, Ellis JH, Dunnick NR: Use of low-osmolar agents and premedication to reduce the frequency of adverse reactions to radiographic contrast media: A survey of the Society of Uroradiology. *Radiology* 194:357, 1995.
7. Lasser EC, Berry CC, Tainer LB, et al: Pretreatment with corticosteroids to alleviate reactions to intravenous contrast material. *N Engl J Med* 317:845, 1987.
8. Greenberger PA, Patterson R: The prevention of immediate generalized reactions to radiocontrast media in high-risk patients. *J Allergy Clin Immunol* 87:867, 1991.
9. Smith RC, Verga M, McCarthy S, et al: Diagnosis of acute flank pain: Value of unenhanced helical CT. *AJR* 166:97, 1996.
10. Sommer FG, Jeffrey RB, Rubin GD, et al: Detection of ureteral calculi in patients with suspected renal colic: Value of reformatted noncontrast helical CT. *AJR* 165:509, 1995.
11. Boyle EM, Maier RV, Salazar JD, et al: Diagnosis of injuries after stab wounds to the back and flank. *J Trauma* 42:260, 1997.
12. Yacoe ME, Jeffrey RB: Sonography of appendicitis and diverticulitis. *Radiol Clin North Am* 32:899, 1994.
13. Rao PM, Rhea JT, Novelline RA, et al: Effect of computed tomography of the appendix on treatment of patients and use of hospital resources. *N Engl J Med* 338:141, 1998.
14. Rao PM, Rhea JT, Novelline RA, et al: Helical CT technique for the diagnosis of appendicitis: Prospective evaluation of a focused appendix CT examination. *Radiology* 202:139, 1997.
15. Shehadi WH: Death following intravascular administration of contrast media. *Acta Radiol Diagn* 26:457, 1985.

295 PRINCIPLES OF EMERGENCY DEPARTMENT SONOGRAPHY

Scott W. Melanson
Michael B. Heller

Emergency ultrasound examinations should usually be restricted to those areas that are amenable to the type of limited, goal-directed examinations described in this chapter and textbooks on emergency ultrasonography. Any abnormality noted on a bedside examination that the examiner cannot explain should be evaluated with further testing with formal ultrasound or another imaging modality. Many potential applications have been proposed, but only a half-dozen emergency department (ED) applications are firmly established as a major contribution to daily ED practice (Table 295-1). The first four of these are life-threatening, time-sensitive conditions for which the bedside ultrasound examination provides rapid, easily interpreted information that is often unavailable in a timely manner by any other means. The other two applications, for suspected obstructive renal disease and acute gallbladder pathology, are ordinarily not acutely life-threatening but are so common and so amenable to ultrasound studies that they have gained widespread acceptance as primary indications. Other potential applications, which are not reviewed in detail in this chapter, include determination of urinary bladder postvoid residual volume, soft-tissue foreign-body of deep venous thrombosis (DVT) evaluation, detection, soft-tissue abscess evaluation, and vascular access.

TABLE 295-1 Primary Indications for Emergency Department Ultrasound

Indication	Key Sonographic Finding
Abdominal aortic aneurysms	Aortic diameter >3 cm
Trauma evaluation	Hemoperitoneum
First-trimester pregnancy	Intrauterine pregnancy
Cardiac evaluation	Cardiac activity, pericardial fluid
Obstructive uropathy	Hydronephrosis
Gallbladder disease	Gallstones, sonographic Murphy sign*

*See the text for full details of sonographic findings.

FUNDAMENTALS

The basic principles and terminology employed in emergency ultrasonography are straightforward but differ in important respects from that of other imaging techniques. The ultrasound image is created electronically from high-frequency sound waves generated by the transducer (or probe), which also receives the reflected waves. The time required for the reflection of each structure determines its depth on the image, and the intensity of the reflection determines its shade on a black-to-white scale. A perfect reflector of ultrasound waves appears white and is referred to as *hyperechoic*. A perfect transmitter of ultrasound waves has no reflection and appears black, or *anechoic*. A great advantage of ultrasound is that most structures, particularly those not well visualized by standard x-ray, have intermediate echogenicity that is quite characteristic and allows for identification of normal and abnormal organs and tissues.

An important factor in determining the quality of the image is the frequency of the transducer employed: the lower the frequency, the greater the depth of penetration but the lower the resolution. For all the primary ED indications (except endovaginal ultrasound), a general-purpose probe of approximately 3.5 MHz is appropriate and will allow visualization even in obese patients. A 5 MHz probe can be used in thin adults or pediatric patients, providing better resolution. Some of the specialized applications, including many vascular and procedural uses (Table 295-2), require higher-frequency probes for adequate sonographic examination.

Color Doppler technology provides information on blood-flow characteristics of vascular structures by superimposing colors over the normal gray-scale image. The displayed colors, which range from red to blue, indicate the direction of blood flow relative to the transducer. While this technology is helpful in identifying vascular structures, it is not necessary for any of the primary ED applications of ultrasound.

TABLE 295-2 Examples of Specialized Applications for Emergency Department Ultrasound

Appendicitis
Ascites evaluation
Cardiac wall motion abnormalities
Deep venous thrombosis
Pelvic masses
Pleural fluid visualization
Procedural applications Abscess drainage Foreign-body removal Suprapubic aspiration Vascular access

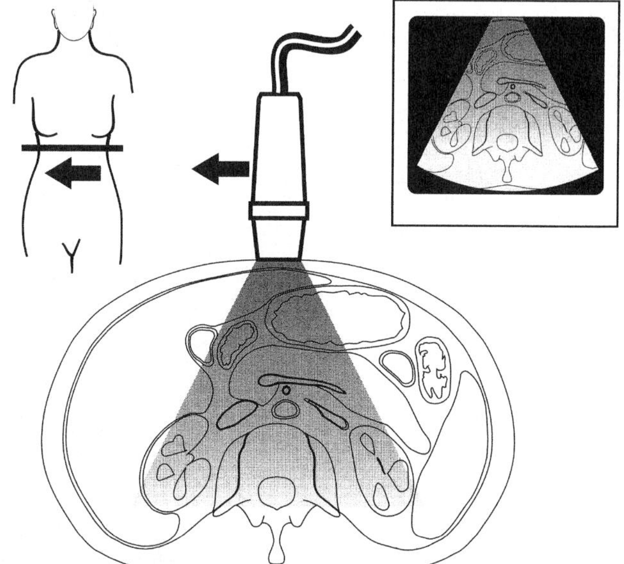

FIG. 295-1. Transverse ultrasound image. This is obtained by directing the marker dot on the probe toward the patient's right side. (From Heller M, Jehle D, eds: *Ultrasound in Emergency Medicine.* Philadelphia, Saunders, 1995, with permission.)

An important limitation of ultrasound is that even small amounts of air (e.g., in bowel loops and pneumoperitoneum) preclude effective visualization distal to the gas. Bone, too, is poorly imaged by ultrasound (compared to plain x-ray), and finding appropriate acoustic windows that avoid these problems is one of the skills required of the emergency sonologist.

Orientation

Certain arbitrary but generally accepted conventions are utilized for creating and displaying ultrasound images. The skin-transducer interface is placed at the top of the image. Each transducer has a mark of some sort, which is used for left-right orientation. The *marker always points to the left side of the screen, as viewed from in front.* When scanning in the transverse plane, the physician points the marker groove to the patient's right side, and the image is displayed as a cross section from the patient's feet (Fig. 295-1). For longitudinal or sagittal views, the *marker points to the patient's head*. The image then appears with the most cephalad portion on the left (Fig. 295-2).

The transmission of ultrasound waves is blocked by highly echogenic structures (e.g., gallstones), resulting in a relatively anechoic area distal to the echogenic structure. This effect is known as *acoustic shadowing. Acoustic enhancement* occurs distal to an anechoic, fluid-filled structure, such as the gallbladder. The area distal to the anechoic structure has increased echogenicity due to the greater number of ultrasound waves reaching this area through the anechoic structure. Examples of these phenomena are present in almost every ultrasound image. However, the many other technical factors that influence the creation of ultrasound images and artifacts are beyond the scope of this discussion. Two of the most common and useful are illustrated in Fig. 295-3.

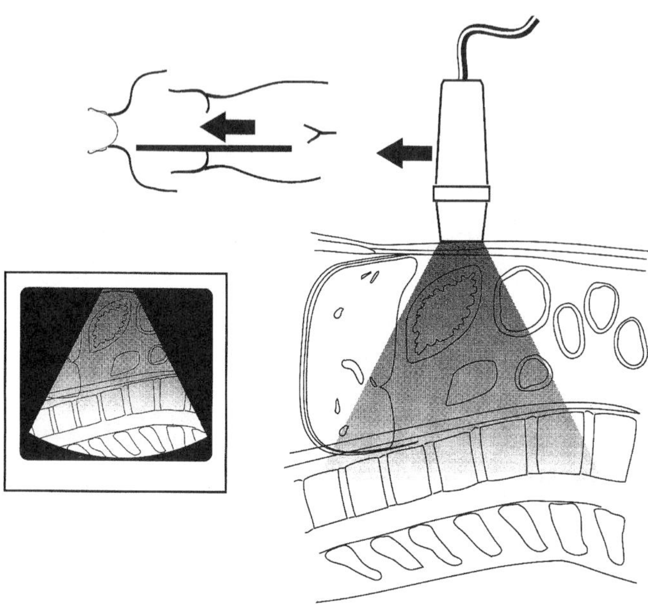

FIG. 295-2. Longitudinal ultrasound image. The marker dot on the probe is directed toward the patient's head. (From Heller M, Jehle D, eds: *Ultrasound in Emergency Medicine.* Philadelphia, Saunders, 1995, with permission.)

Characteristics of the Emergency Department Ultrasound Examination

The ED ultrasound examination is significantly different from the formal sonography that is performed in the radiology suite. The most important distinction is that the ED examination is very focused. Five of the six examinations seek only one primary finding: a yes-or-no answer (Table 295-1). This generally allows the examination to be performed in a single position (supine) and within only a few minutes. Also, the ED examination can be more interactive. The physician can use the patient's response and clinical findings together with the ultrasound image to aid in interpretation.

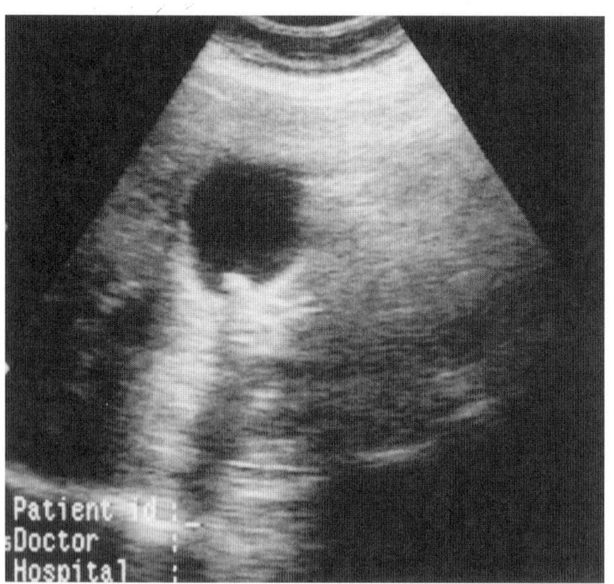

FIG. 295-3. Acoustic shadow created by solitary gallstone. Note increased echogenicity distal to gallstone (acoustic enhancement).

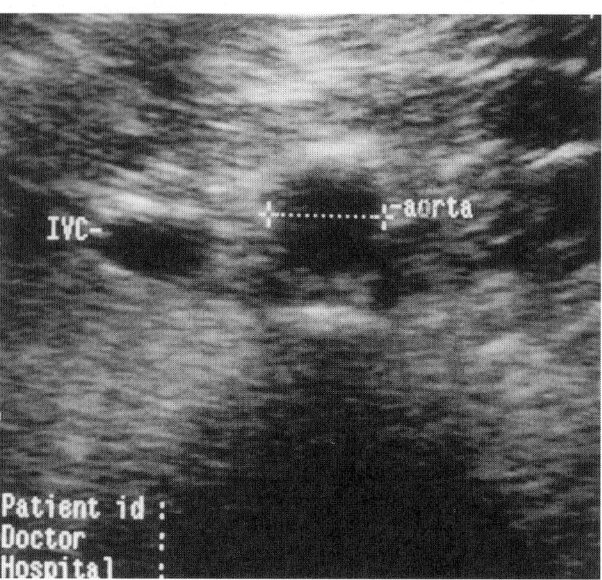

FIG. 295-4. Transverse view of a normal abdominal aorta and inferior vena cava (IVC). Note vertebral body is represented by the large hypoechoic area in the far field.

The ED applications described are usually performed with relatively modest, very portable, non-Doppler units. The addition of Doppler technology, which allows for evaluation of function (flow) as well as form (anatomy), can be expected to significantly expand the utility of bedside emergency ultrasound during the next decade.

PRIMARY INDICATIONS

Primary applications are those examinations that are critically time-dependent and/or of such nature that the information gained is likely to be of major benefit to the patient and physician (Table 295-1). These examinations each involve looking for only a few easily recognized findings. The straightforward, limited nature of these examinations allows emergency physicians to perform them with less formal training than the imaging specialist, occasionally under severe time constraints.

Abdominal Aortic Aneurysm

Ultrasound is as accurate as computed tomography (CT) and more accurate than angiography in measuring aneurysmal diameter. Specific indications for ultrasound evaluation of the aorta include abdominal pain in hypotensive patients and elderly patients with unexplained back, flank, or abdominal pain.

SONOGRAPHIC CONSIDERATIONS The aorta is located in the midline of the abdomen, to the left of the inferior vena cava (IVC), just anterior to the spine and posterior to all other abdominal contents (Fig. 295-4). The aorta normally tapers as it progresses distally, and any diameter greater than 3 cm is abnormal. An ultrasound examination that images the aorta from the diaphragm to its distal bifurcation is extremely accurate at confirming or refuting the diagnosis of abdominal aortic aneurysm (AAA). Although pressure on the transducer usually displaces intervening bowel gas, complete visualization is sometimes impossible. Such examinations are considerated indeterminate.

With experience, it is generally not difficult to differentiate the aorta from the IVC/Fog. The IVC, usually to the right of the aorta, has thinner walls and changes remarkably in size with probe pressure and the Valsalva maneuver. Both the aorta and the IVC are pulsatile, although the gentle, undulating pulsation of the IVC can, with experience, be differentiated from the forceful, centripetal aortic pulsation.

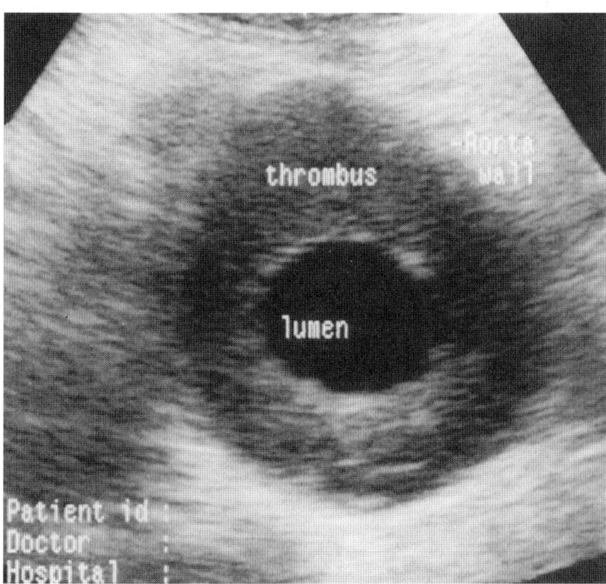

FIG. 295-5. Abdominal aortic aneurysm with intraluminal thrombus.

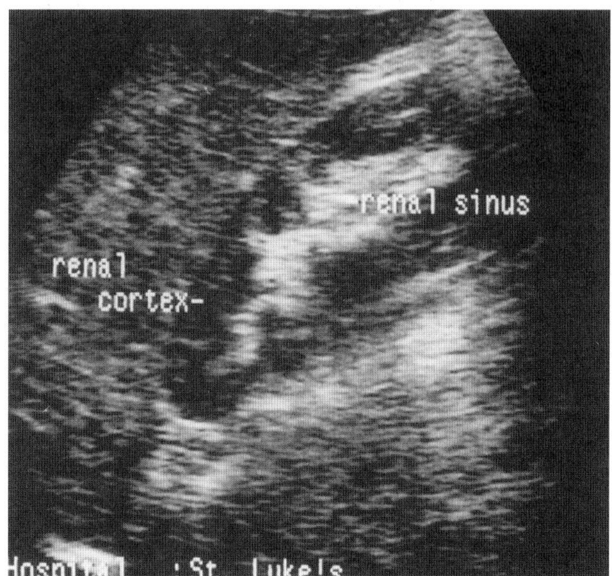

FIG. 295-6. Normal appearance of the right kidney.

The primary sonographic finding of AAA is an aortic diameter greater than 3 cm. When AAA is suspected, the aorta should be imaged in the transverse and sagittal planes from the diaphragm to its bifurcation at the level of the umbilicus. Transverse images measured horizontally from outside wall to outside wall are the most reliable in accurately determining true aortic size. Echogenic thrombus within the outer margins of AAAs is very common, and care must be taken to identify the outer limits of the aortic wall (Fig. 295-5). While ultrasound is very accurate in measuring AAA size, it is often impossible to determine sonographically whether the AAA has ruptured, since rupture most often occurs into the retroperitoneal space. A hypoechoic retroperitoneal hematoma may be seen but is often very difficult to identify. AAA rupture into the peritoneal space is usually fatal.

Renal Colic

Intravenous pyelogram (IVP), spiral CT, and ultrasound are all used in evaluating patients thought to have renal colic. Bedside ultrasound often allows a much more rapid diagnosis and disposition of ED patients than either IVP or spiral CT, and there are situations where the use of contrast material or iodizing radiation is unwise (e.g., pregnancy, renal insufficiency, and volume depletion). False-negative ultrasound results occur, but the sonographic appearance of hydronephrosis in the appropriate clinical setting aids in diagnosis, and negative findings on examination should lead to an alternative diagnosis.

SONOGRAPHIC CONSIDERATIONS A standard 3.5-MHz probe is generally used for renal scanning, but a 5-MHz transducer can be used with better resolution in thin adults and children. The right kidney is best visualized in the anterior to midaxially line over the lower ribs, but a subcostal approach can at times be successful in imaging the kidneys, avoiding the distraction of rib shadows. The left kidney is more difficult to see due to overlying bowel and stomach and the absence of the liver, which acts as an acoustic window, but is perfectly amenable to ED visualization as well. The best initial approach to the left kidney is somewhat more dorsally, in the posterior axillary line over the lower ribs. Occasionally, a posterior thoracic approach is necessary to adequately visualize the kidneys. Deep inspiration lowers the diaphragm and may move the kidneys caudally into a more easily visualized location. To fully evaluate the kidneys for hydronephrosis, both longitudinal and transverse images should be obtained, and both kidneys should be scanned with each examination.

The kidneys are retroperitoneal organs measuring approximately 12 cm in length and 5 cm in width and are divided into two sonographically distinct areas: the renal cortex and the renal sinus. The renal cortex occupies the periphery of the kidney and has an echogenicity similar to that of the liver or spleen. The renal sinus appears as a central echogenic stripe within the kidney and includes the collecting system as well as major vessels of the hilum (Fig. 295-6). Renal medullary pyramids appear hypoechoic relative to the cortex and are triangular in shape, occurring at the junction of the cortex and the more echogenic renal sinus. When the urine produced in a kidney flows freely into the bladder, there is no appreciable urine within the renal sinus and therefore no significant anechoic space within the hilum. Obstruction of urine outflow from a calculus results in the development of hydronephrosis, which appears as an anechoic fluid collection within the echogenic renal sinus (Fig. 295-7). Hydronephrosis can be graded

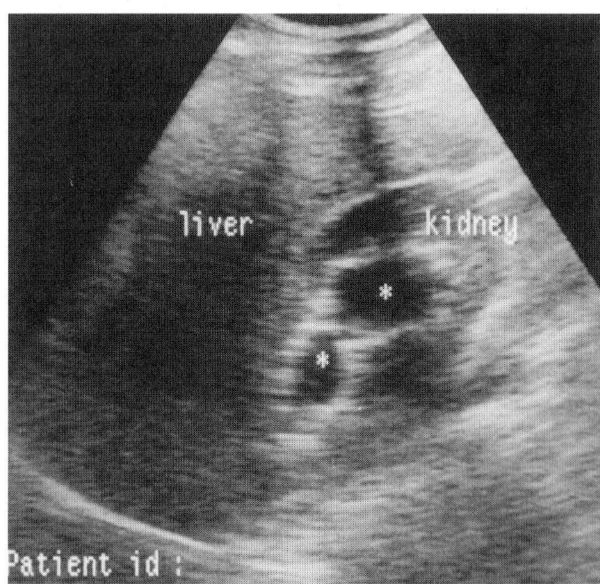

FIG. 295-7. Hydronephrosis of the right kidney with distended renal collecting system (*).

from mild, with minimal separation of the sinus echoes, to severe, manifested by extensive separation of the central echoes, with renal parerchymal thinning.

Renal cysts occur commonly and can be confused with hydronephrosis. Renal cysts are thin-walled, round, anechoic structures with distal acoustic enhancement that typically occur in the periphery of the kidney and lack the more echogenic border typical of the collecting system, as seen with hydronephrosis.

The urolith (calculus) causing the obstruction most often lodges at the ureterovesicular junction, the ureteropelvic junction, or the pelvic brim. While stones at the ureterovesicular junction can occasionally be seen sonographically through the bladder window, calculi are usually not identified on ultrasound examinations. One study found that the ureteral calculi were identified on ultrasound in only 19 percent of patients with documented stones, whereas spiral CT and IVP were able to identify 94 and 52 percent, respectively. Hydronephrosis was identified sonographically in 73 percent of the patients with ureteral calculi.[2] In another study, emergency physicians performed bedside renal ultrasound after a 500-mL bolus of normal saline solution in 108 patients suspected of having renal colic. When used in conjunction with the history and a kidney-ureter-bladder film, the emergency physicians were able to diagnose renal colic with a sensitivity of 97 percent. The specificity and accuracy were 59 and 83 percent, respectively.[3] It is possible that the fluid loading the patients received prior to the ultrasound studies resulted in a number of the false-positive results that contributed to the low specificity.

Hydronephrosis occurs in over 65 percent of pregnant women, peaking between 24 and 28 weeks of gestation. This is believed to be due to mechanical pressure of the enlarged uterus on the ureters and is usually more pronounced in the right kidney. This condition resolves within several weeks of delivery. False-positive scan results are also seen with overly vigorous hydration or a very full bladder. Peripelvic cysts and extrarenal pelvis are two fairly common conditions that may also cause confusion.

Gallbladder Disease

Ultrasound is generally accepted to be the modality of choice in the evaluation of biliary disease.[4] Greater than 90 percent of biliary disease is calculous in origin, and, regardless of composition, even the smallest of gallstones are visible sonographically. Conversely, only 15 percent of gallstones are visible with standard radiographs.

SONOGRAPHIC CONSIDERATIONS The gallbladder is an ideal organ for sonographic evaluation. This cystic structure is typically filled with anechoic bile and can be imaged through the liver, an excellent acoustic window. The gallbladder can be imaged in the right upper quadrant over the lower ribs or just below the costal margin. Deep inspiration moves the gallbladder caudally, often facilitating its visualization. The gallbladder varies in size, being smallest after fatty meals and largest after fasting, but it is typically 7 to 10 cm in length and 2 to 3 cm in width. The absence of reflective surfaces within the gallbladder results in distal acoustic enhancement. With experience and high-quality equipment, it is possible to visualize the common bile duct, especially when dilated, and this finding may be of considerable clinical import.

The primary sonographic finding in biliary disease is gallstones. Gallstones appear as bright, echogenic foci within the gallbladder and move with changes in position unless impacted (Fig. 295-8). A minority of gallstones float within the bile. Symptomatic gallstones may be very small in relation to the volume of the gallbladder, and a thorough search of the organ is mandatory. In order to ensure this, the patient should be instructed to halt inspiration when the gallbladder is well visualized. During this breath holding, the entire gallbladder should be visualized in one axis, sweeping from one side of the gallbladder to the other. This should be repeated with scanning done 90° to the axis of the first scanning plane, thus obtaining both sagittal and transverse images. *Acoustic shadows* appear as anechoic lines distal to the echogenic stones. These shadows are due to the blockage of ultrasound wave transmission distal to the stone and are helpful in identifying stones, often being more readily identified than the gallstone itself. Gallbladder polyps can mimic the appearance of gallstones but do not change position upon moving the patient and do not create acoustic shadows.

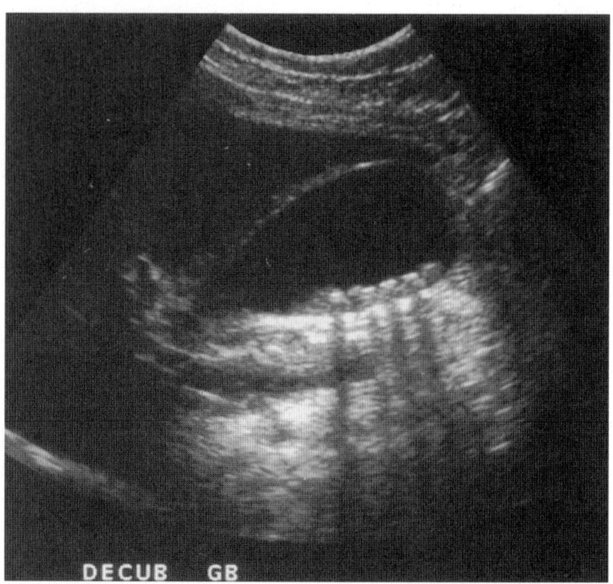

FIG. 295-8. Multiple dependent gallstones with acoustic shadowing.

A second extremely important sonographic finding of biliary disease is a positive sonographic Murphy sign. The sonographic Murphy sign is considered positive when the point of maximal tenderness to transducer pressure is directly over the sonographically located gallbladder. A positive sonographic Murphy's sign in the presence of cholelithiasis is reported to have a 92 percent positive predictive value for symptomatic gallbladder disease. Gallbladder wall thickening, defined as proximal gallbladder wall thickness greater than 3 mm, occurs in 50 to 75 percent of patients with acute cholecystitis, but this finding is not specific for cholecystitis. Edematous states, as well as such conditions as liver disease, AIDS, ascites, renal disease, and the postprandial state, can also result in gallbladder wall thickening. Gallbladder sludge is nearly always abnormal in the ambulatory patient, suggesting biliary disease. Sludge is composed of calcium bilirubinate and cholesterol granules, and generally form a bile-sludge layer within the gallbladder and does not create acoustic shadows (Fig. 295-9). Finally, a fluid collection around the gallbladder, or pericholecystitic fluid, is evidence of marked inflammation and often of perforation. This is usually seen in patients with other clinical and sonographic evidence of cholecystitis.

In summary, the sonographic signs of biliary disease are gallstones, sonographic Murphy sign, gallbladder wall thickening, gallbladder sludge, and pericholecystic fluid. The combination of a positive sonographic Murphy sign and any of the other sonographic findings described is highly reliable in diagnosing acute gallbladder disease. In fact, the presence of any two of the sonographic signs in the appropriate clinical setting is highly suggestive of the disease. Completely normal examination findings, including a negative sonographic Murphy sign, are reliable in excluding symptomatic gallbladder disease.

Focused Abdominal Sonography for Trauma

Abdominal CT scanning remains an important tool in evaluating trauma, with an accuracy of more than 90 percent in detecting intraab-

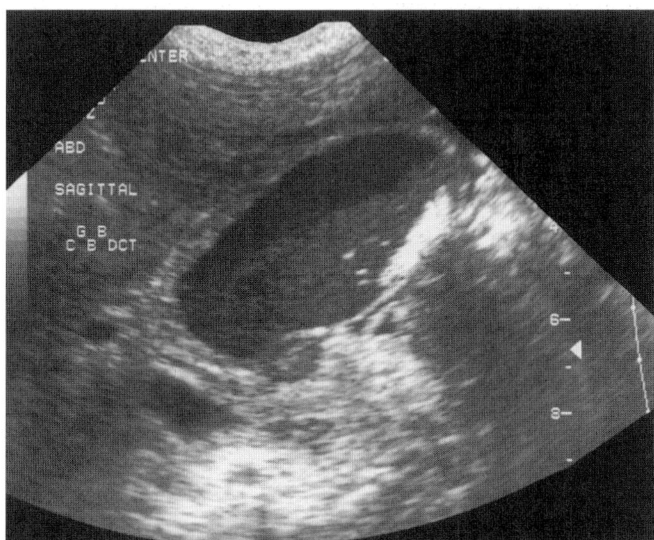

FIG. 295-9. Gallbladder sludge. The sludge is seen to layer out in the gallbladder. Multiple gallstones are also present. (From Heller M, Jehle D, eds: *Ultrasound in Emergency Medicine*. Philadelphia, Saunders, 1995, with permission.)

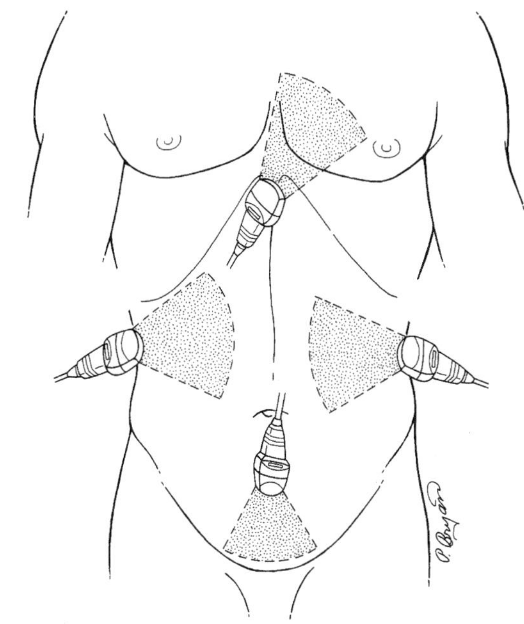

FIG. 295-10. Standard four views of the FAST examination. (From Sisley AC et al,[7] with permission.)

dominal injuries. However, CT is expensive and requires a hemodynamically stable, cooperative patient. It also involves contrast-medium administration and ionizing radiation. Diagnostic peritoneal lavage (DPL) has sensitivities greater than 90 percent for hemoperitoneum. However, up to one-third of laparotomies performed on the basis of positive DPL findings are unnecessary. As little as 20 mL of blood mixed with the standard liter of peritoneal lavage fluid will result in a positive DPL (100,000 red blood cells per cubic millimeter). In addition, this invasive procedure requires significant time and causes complications in up to 5 percent of patients.

Focused abdominal sonography for trauma (FAST) has proven to be a valuable tool in the evaluation of trauma victims. More than two dozen studies in European and North American centers have demonstrated that ED sonography has an accuracy similar to that of DPL for the detection of hemoperitoneum but has several advantages: it is more rapid (generally completed in under 5 min), requires no preparations (e.g., nasogastric tube and Foley catheter), has no contraindications, and is noninvasive. While ultrasound cannot reliably identify intraabdominal organ injuries (as can CT), it is accurate in predicting the need for laparotomy in trauma patients. Large studies have found the sensitivity of ultrasound to be 85 percent or higher with specificities of 96 percent or higher,[5] depending on the gold standards employed. Some studies have used the need for a therapeutic laparotomy as the gold standard, whereas others have used the presence of any intraabdominal injury or blood on CT as the gold standard, regardless of need for laparotomy (see Chap. 252 for further discussion.) Subcutaneous emphysema and marked obesity can impair the ability of ultrasound to image the abdomen, but it is uncommon that they prevent an adequate FAST examination. Training for as little as 2 to 8 has been sufficient for emergency physicians and surgeons to learn the FAST examination[6] and in many centers it has completely replaced DPL.

SONOGRAPHIC CONSIDERATIONS The primary finding in the FAST examination is anechoic fluid collections (blood) within the peritoneal cavity. The four standard views of the trauma ultrasound examination are depicted in Fig. 295-10. The right upper quadrant view, the easiest of the FAST examination views to visualize, is obtained by imaging over the lower rib cage in the area of the anterior to midaxillary line with the marker dot pointed cephalad. The liver, kidney, and Morison pouch are examined (Fig. 295-11). The Morison pouch is a potential space between the Gerota fascia of the kidney and the Glisson capsule of the liver and is usually devoid of fluid. Because the Morison pouch is one of the most posterior compartments of the supine abdomen, blood tends to accumulate in this space, creating an easily identified anechoic stripe (Fig. 295-12). Organ lesions, while not reliably identified on ultrasound, may appear as anechoic areas within the organ or as echogenic foci. The left upper quadrant view examines the potential space between the spleen and the kidney, the splenorenal space (Fig. 295-13). This view is obtained by placing the transducer in the mid to posterior axillary line over the lower left costal margin. Here again, blood will appear as an anechoic stripe

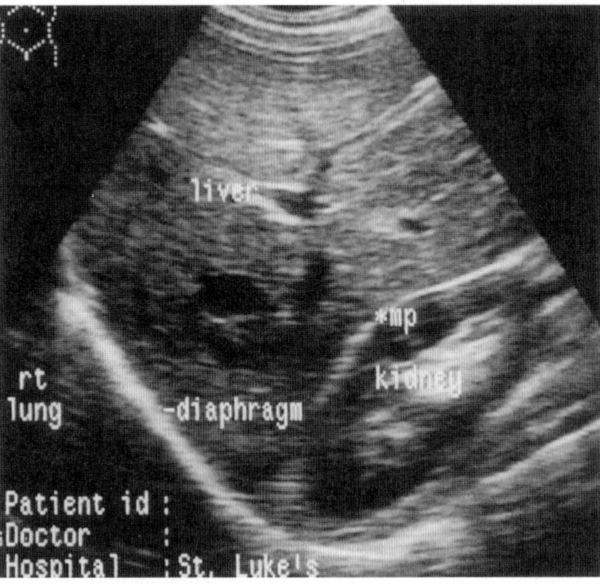

FIG. 295-11. Normal ultrasound image of the right upper quadrant demonstrating an absence of fluid in Morison's pouch (mp).

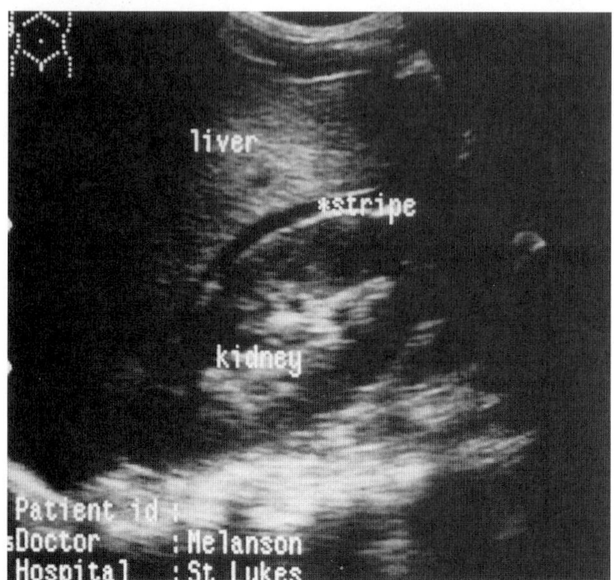

FIG. 295-12. Positive right upper quadrant FAST examination findings. Note "stripe" of fluid in Morison's pouch.

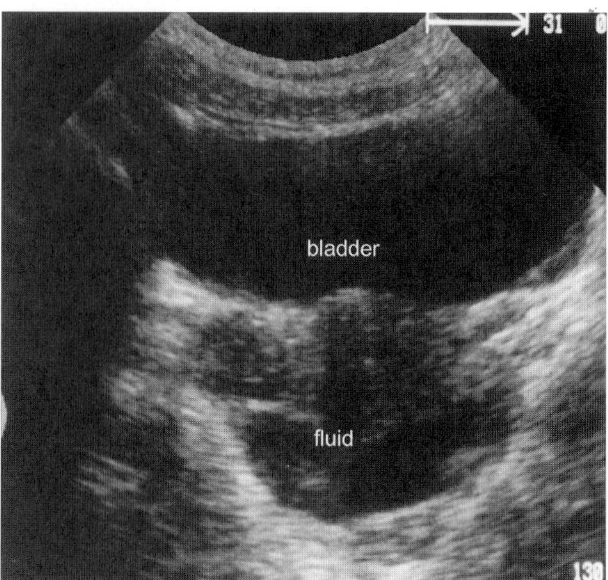

FIG. 295-14. Positive pelvic FAST examination findings. An anechoic fluid collection is seen distal to the large fluid-filled bladder.

between the spleen and kidney. While not routine, placing the patient into a Trendelenburg position may increase the amount of blood in the upper abdomen, facilitating sonographic identification of blood in both the right and left upper quadrant. Both upper abdominal views are also capable of identifying hemothorax, where the anechoic fluid collection appears above the diaphragm. Studies have found ultrasound to be at least as accurate as chest x-ray in identifying hemothorax.[7,8] The pelvis is the most dependent location within the intraperitoneal cavity in a supine patient, explaining why hemoperitoneum commonly collects in this location. The pelvic view seeks to identify intraperitoneal blood in the potential space between the rectum and uterus (pouch of Douglas) or its homologue in the male, the rectovesicular space. As with the other views, blood here appears as a fluid collection between two adjacent soft-tissue structures (Fig. 295-14). Unclotted intraperitoneal blood is anechoic, with sharp borders against the peritoneal confines. The pelvic view is facilitated by a full bladder, which can be produced by instilling 250 mL of normal saline solution via a Foley catheter. The full bladder acts as an acoustic window, optimizing the view of the pelvic structures. As little as 250 mL of intraperitoneal blood should be routinely noted with ultrasound; even smaller collections can often be identified.

The last view, that of the subcostal area, examines the heart for evidence of pericardial fluid collections, which would suggest cardiac injury (Fig. 295-15). Rapid ultrasound evaluation of the heart has resulted in faster times to diagnosis and to surgical intervention, as well as improved survival rates and neurologic outcomes in patients with penetrating cardiac injuries.[9] It is occasionally necessary to differ-

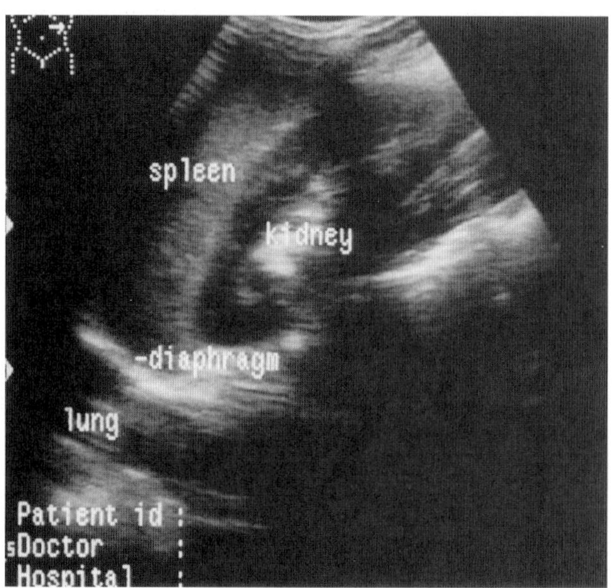

FIG. 295-13. Normal findings on left upper quadrant ultrasound. The potential space between the kidney and spleen is devoid of anechoic fluid.

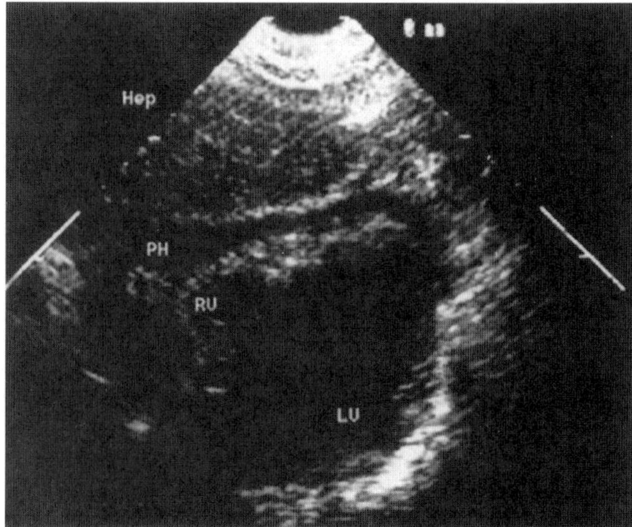

FIG. 295-15. Subcostal echocardiogram demonstrating pericardial hemorrhage (PH). Hep, hepatic parenchyma; RV, right ventricle; LV, left ventricle. (From Heller M, Jehle D, eds: *Ultrasound in Emergency Medicine.* Philadelphia, Saunders, 1995, with permission.)

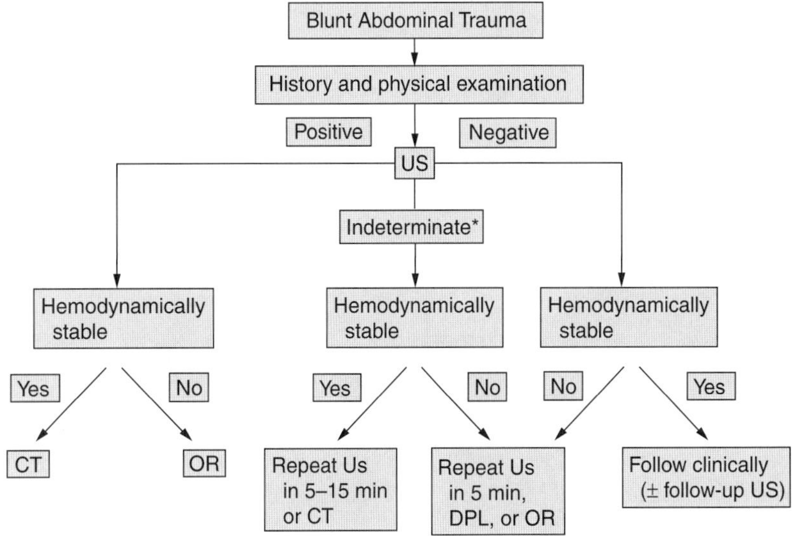

FIG. 295-16. Ultrasound utilization in a blunt abdominal trauma patient.

entiate pleural from pericardial fluid. Any fluid collection that follows the contours of the heart and is surrounded by the echogenic pericardium is pericardial fluid. There is no pleural reflection between the liver and heart; the subcostal view will therefore demonstrate pericardial, but not pleural, fluid. Blood within the pericardial space can appear anechoic but may be partially echogenic, depending on the degree of clotting and defibrination that occurs.

The great majority of research in the use of trauma sonography has focused on blunt abdominal trauma. The studies that have utilized ultrasound in penetrating abdominal trauma have found that sonography has a sensitivity and specificity for predicting need for laparotomy similar to those found for blunt trauma. Several studies have examined trauma sonography in blunt pediatric trauma and have demonstrated it to be as accurate in detecting hemoperitoneum in this setting as in the adult population.

A number of centers routinely repeat the ultrasound examination in all patients not taken immediately to surgery. The fact that ultrasound is inexpensive, rapid, and noninvasive makes this a practical approach to minimizing the chance of missing intraabdominal injuries that develop more slowly. Repeat scans are performed within 30 min to 6 h, depending on the stability of the patient.

Ultrasound can be easily incorporated into routine trauma care. Sonography is often performed at the completion of the primary survey, allowing rapid identification of hemoperitoneum. Figure 295-16 illustrates an algorithm depicting how ultrasound can be used in a clinical setting. A hemodynamically unstable patient with positive trauma ultrasound findings should be taken immediately to laparotomy. A stable patient with positive sonogram findings can be evaluated with CT to identify the specific organ lesion and to determine the feasibility of nonoperative intervention.

First-Trimester Pregnancy Evaluation

No set of historical factors, signs, or symptoms can accurately identify patients with ectopic pregnancy, and no laboratory tests are diagnostic of this condition. Sonographically identifying an intrauterine pregnancy can markedly reduce the possibility of ectopic pregnancy, since heterotopic pregnancies (concurrent intrauterine and ectopic pregnancies) occur with an incidence of less than 1:30,000 pregnancies, except for infertility or in vitro fertilization patients, who must be managed in concert with their obstetrician.

The incidence of ectopic pregnancy has been increasing for several decades. Stovall et al found that 7.5 percent of all ED patients with a positive pregnancy test, regardless of history, symptoms, or physical examination had an ectopic pregnancy.[10] Studies that evaluate ED patients with any abdominal pain, vaginal bleeding, risk factors for ectopic pregnancy, adnexal masses, or tenderness have found the incidence of ectopic pregnancy to be more than 10 percent. When ultrasound is used only in selected first-trimester ED patients (rather than all patients), 40 to 50 percent of the ectopic pregnancies are not identified. Approximately one-half of these ectopic pregnancies are ruptured at the time of diagnosis, which increases the risk of morbidity and mortality while decreasing the likelihood of subsequent normal pregnancy. Ultrasound evaluation of *all* first-trimester pregnant patients presenting to the ED with any abdominal or pelvic pain, vaginal bleeding, or risk factors for ectopic pregnancy has been recommended. Such an approach has been found to markedly decrease the frequency of delayed diagnoses and ectopic rupture at the time of diagnosis.[11] Emergency physicians have been proven capable of performing pelvic sonography in the evaluation of women at risk for ectopic pregnancy with an accuracy similar to that of obstetrics-gynecology consultants. Further, when an emergency physician performed the sonography, the patients were dispositioned much more quickly than when the ultrasound was performed by an obstetrics-gynecology consultant (60 versus 180 min).[12]

SONOGRAPHIC CONSIDERATIONS The pelvic organs can be imaged transabdominally or endovaginally. The transabdominal approach is best accomplished with a full bladder. The patient can avoid emptying the bladder, or 250 mL of normal saline solution can be instilled via a Foley catheter. The full bladder displaces bowel gas from the pelvis and functions as an acoustic window for the pelvic structures. The 3.5-MHz probe, or 5-MHz probe in thin patients, is used for this examination. Endovaginal scanning is performed with a 5- to 7.5-MHz probe designed for this purpose and is best performed with an empty bladder. A condom or sheath is placed over the transducer, which is then introduced several centimeters into the vagina. The endovaginal approach is not uncomfortable, and most patients prefer it to transabdominal probe pressure on a distended bladder. With the transducer tip in close proximity to the structures of interest, high-frequency, high-resolution probes can be utilized, resulting in much greater sonographic detail and allowing for earlier identification of an intrauterine pregnancy. While endovaginal scanning can identify a gestational sac as early as 4.5 weeks after the last menstrual period (LMP), transabdominal scanning is often not able to visualize it until 5.5 to 6 weeks after the LMP. In fact, all the landmarks of pregnancy are visualized approximately 1 week earlier with the endovaginal approach (Table 295-3). Transabdominal scanning provides a view of

TABLE 295-3 Earliest Sonographic Visualization of Embryonic Structures

Structure	Transabdominal, Weeks	Endovaginal, Weeks
Gestational sac	6	4.5
Yolk sac	6–6.5	5–5.5
Fetal pole	6.5–7	5.5–6
Cardiac activity	7	6

the entire pelvic contents, but with less resolution than the endovaginal approach. Endovaginal scanning can miss masses in the upper pelvis and lower abdomen due to the shallow depth of acoustic penetration of the higher-frequency transducer. These two approaches should, therefore, be thought of as complementary; one may yield the diagnosis if the first does not.

The primary ultrasound finding to be evaluated in first-trimester patients is evidence of an intrauterine pregnancy. The earliest sonographic finding of pregnancy is the gestational sac. This appears as a round or oval anechoic area within the uterus (Fig. 295-17). Care should be exercised in identifying gestational sacs, since up to 20 percent of ectopic pregnancies have a ''pseudogestational sac,'' which looks sonographically similar to a true gestational sac but is caused by intracavitary blood surrounded by a decidual reaction. True gestational sacs have two concentric echogenic rings surrounding the gestational sac (*double decidual sign*), representing the decidua parietalis and the decidua capsularis, and tend to appear to be adjacent to, not within, the echogenic endometrial complex (*intradecidual sign*). The first true embryonic structure that can be seen sonographically is the yolk sac (Fig. 295-9). This echogenic ringlike structure can be seen with endovaginal scanning at approximately 5 weeks after the LMP. As the pregnancy progresses, the fetus is seen at 5.5 to 6 weeks, with fetal parts being visible at 8 weeks endovaginally. Fetal cardiac activity can generally be seen from the time the fetal pole is identified but should always be present when the embryo is greater than 10 mm if the fetus is viable. The presence of fetal cardiac activity is very helpful

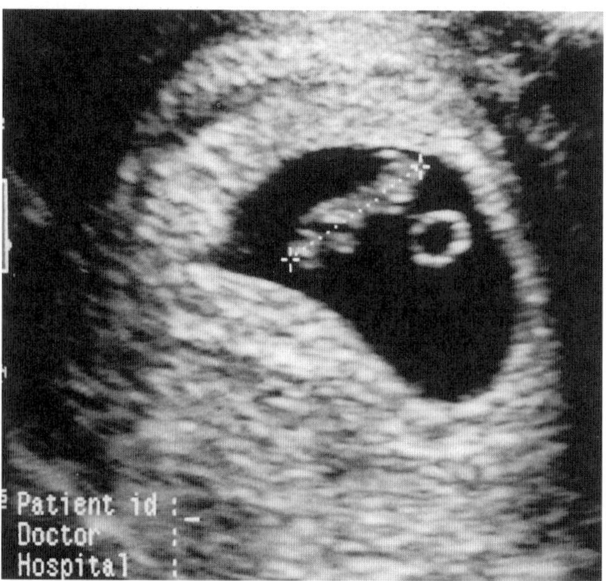

FIG. 295-17. Normal intrauterine pregnancy. The fetal pole (within calipers) and the round, echogenic yolk sac are seen within the anechoic gestational sac.

prognostically. The rate of spontaneous abortion is less than 5 percent when normal cardiac activity is seen at 8 to 12 weeks of gestation.

Although the primary goal of bedside US is to identify an intrauterine pregnancy, ectopic pregnancies can result in a number of sonographic findings. First, a living extrauterine pregnancy may be seen, obviously securing the diagnosis of ectopic pregnancy. This occurs in approximately 20 percent of ectopic pregnancies. The sonogram may also demonstrate abnormal structures suggestive of an ectopic pregnancy, such as an echogenic ringlike mass in the adnexae. The most common finding seen with ectopic pregnancies is that of an empty uterus with either no other findings or nonspecific findings (e.g., fluid in the cul-de-sac).

The quantitative β human chorionic gonadotropin (β-HCG) level is extremely helpful in evaluating pregnant patients with an empty uterus on ultrasound. A number of authors have suggested ''discriminatory zones,'' β-HCG levels above which an intrauterine pregnancy should be visualized if present. The value utilized in clinical practice depends on the skill of the sonographer, the quality of the ultrasound machine, and individual patient factors. Based on the work of several authors, it is expected that intrauterine pregnancy is detectable on endovaginal scanning if the β-HCG level is greater than 2000 MIU/mL.[11] In some institutions, the discriminatory zone could be as low as 1000 MIU/mL. Patients with β-HCG levels greater than this (the discriminatory zone) who do not have evidence of an intrauterine pregnancy on ultrasound are at very high risk for an ectopic pregnancy, and obstetrical consultation is needed. Such patients may undergo observation with repeat β-HCG level determinations, and ultrasound, laparoscopy, or surgical intervention, depending on the individual patient and the preferences of the obstetrician. For hemodynamically stable patient's with a β-HCG level less than 2000 MIU/mL and no intrauterine pregnancy on ultrasound, disposition is usually arranged in concert with the obstetrician. If the patient is discharged, obstetric follow-up is needed in 48 to 72 h, whereupon repeat β-HCG and ultrasound examinations are performed. Mateer and colleagues followed such a protocol and were able to decrease the number of delayed diagnoses of ectopic pregnancy from 43 to 28 percent, and the incidence of ectopic rupture at diagnosis decreased from 50 to 9 percent.[11]

Cardiac Ultrasonography

Two-dimensional echocardiography has become an invaluable tool in the evaluation of cardiac anatomy and function. Echocardiography is capable of evaluating myocardial wall motion, valve function, the great vessels, and pericardial fluid collections. The examination of these structures can be technically demanding, requiring specialized transducers and specialized training. Applications of bedside ultrasound by emergency physicians is therefore limited to critically time-dependent diagnoses that can be recognized by emergency physicians with a modicum of training and the standard ultrasound equipment available in the ED. The evaluation of cardiac trauma, pulseless electrical activity (PEA), and pericardial tamponade are such applications. The sonographic findings of interest in such settings are pericardial fluid collections and myocardial wall activity.

The use of ultrasound in the evaluation of potential cardiac trauma is discussed earlier, in the section on the FAST examination. Both blunt and penetrating trauma can result in hemopericardium, which can be rapidly diagnosed with ultrasound (Fig. 295-7). Electromechanical dissociation is a cause of PEA that has an extremely poor prognosis. An echocardiogram demonstrating a flaccid, inactive heart in a patient with PEA suggests very little chance of survival. In contrast, a hyperdynamic heart with small right-heart dimensions suggests hypovolemia, a readily treatable condition. Cardiac tamponade can be very difficult to diagnose at the bedside without the assistance of ultrasound. Echocardiography provides a means of rapidly determining whether a pericardial fluid collection is present, without which there can be no tamponade.

A number of windows used to sonographically evaluate the cardiac structures have been described. The *subcostal view* is the most useful to emergency physicians. This view can be obtained while other procedures are being performed with a 3.5-MHz transducer. Other views are best obtained using specialized transducer heads with small footprints (the surface area of the portion of the transducer that comes into contact with the patient) in order to image between the ribs. The subcostal view, obtained by placing the transducer in the area of the xiphoid process aiming toward the left shoulder, provides visualization of all four cardiac chambers. As always, structures that are closest to the transducer appear at the top of the image monitor; the liver, therefore, appears uppermost on the monitor, with the right atrium adjacent to it. The left atrium and ventricle appear closest to the bottom of the screen.

Other views used to evaluate cardiac structure include the left parasternal short-axis (LPSA), the left parasternal long-axis (LPLA), and the apical views. The *parasternal window* is obtained by placing the transducer between the second and fourth intercostal spaces adjacent to the sternum. In the LPLA, the ultrasound beam is directed in a plane parallel to a line drawn from the right shoulder to the left hip. This view images the aortic valve, proximal ascending aorta, and left ventricle well. The short-axis view (LPSA) is obtained by rotating the transducer 90°, so that the beam is parallel to a line drawn from the left shoulder to the right hip. Here the left ventricle appears as a round, thick-walled chamber, and the right ventricle appears more anteriorly in a crescent shape. The LPSA view is best used to image the mitral valve, papillary muscles, and aortic valve. The *apical view* is obtained by placing the transducer over the point of maximal cardiac impulse on the precordium (the apex) with the beam directed to the right shoulder. This view allows for the assessment of chamber size and the identification of aneurysms and intracardiac masses. The emergency physician can generally obtain the information necessary for the bedside indications mentioned above using only the subcostal view. The other views described may provide added information if the examiner has the appropriate equipment and training.

SONOGRAPHIC CONSIDERATIONS The echocardiographic evaluation of cardiac tamponade requires little training and can be rapidly performed at the bedside. The subcostal view should visualize any pericardial fluid collection large enough to result in tamponade. The pericardium is a dense, fibrous, echogenic sac that surrounds the heart. The pericardial space contains less than 50 mL of pericardial fluid under normal circumstances. Pericardial effusions appear as echo-free areas within the pericardial space. Small pericardial effusions (<100 mL) usually occupy a dependent position in the pericardial sac, while large effusions (>300 mL) are present both anteriorly and posteriorly. Whether a pericardial fluid collection affects cardiac function depends on such variables as the amount of fluid present, the rate of formation, and the underlying condition of the pericardium (diseased or not). Intrapericardial pressure rises abruptly after 80 to 200 mL of fluid has collected rapidly in the previously normal pericardial space. Early sonographic signs of increased intrapericardial pressure include right atrial and right ventricular collapse in diastole, but these findings are not always appreciable during the ED sonographic examination.

The interpretation of an echocardiographic finding of pericardial fluid collection must incorporate the clinical status of the patient. While the absence of a pericardial fluid collection excludes the diagnosis of cardiac tamponade, the mere presence of a pericardial fluid collection in an unstable patient is not diagnostic of pericardial tamponade. When pericardiocentesis is deemed necessary, sonographic localization of the heart will assist in determining the best approach for the procedure.

The patient with PEA (i.e., electrical cardiac activity without a palpable pulse) can be suffering from a wide variety of conditions, some fatal, some easily treated. Ultrasound greatly assists in the rapid diagnosis and treatment of such patients. The sonographic examination is straightforward. Cardiopulmonary resuscitation should be stopped briefly during the ultrasound examination. Any of the standard cardiac windows can be utilized, but the subcostal view has the advantages of easy imaging with standard ultrasound transducers and lack of interference with other procedures. Once visualized, the ventricles and valves are examined for evidence of activity. A patient in true electromechanical dissociation has no demonstrable cardiac activity. Several treatable causes of PEA can be diagnosed with a sonogram and appropriate treatment instituted. The ventricles of a hypovolemic patient contract vigorously, while the right-heart dimensions are diminished. Cardiac tamponade, another treatable cause of PEA, can also be easily diagnosed with echocardiography, as discussed above.

MISCELLANEOUS EMERGENCY DEPARTMENT APPLICATIONS

Formal radiology department ultrasound studies have been helpful in a great number of conditions beyond those already discussed. Emergency physicians, given the appropriate time, training, and equipment could technically perform any of these examinations at the bedside. This section discusses some applications that have been used by emergency physicians but are not now considered primary indications.

Deep Venous Thrombosis

Compression ultrasound has been performed by emergency physicians to evaluate ED patients suspected of having lower-extremity DVT.[13] Such studies detect venous thrombosis based on the fact that a vein filled with thrombus is not compressible whereas normal veins can be easily compressed. An examination of the lower extremity for DVTs, therefore, consists of sonographically identifying the common femoral vein and artery and proceeding distally to the trifurcation of the popliteal vein, imaging the veins at 3- to 5-cm intervals. The inability to compress a vein by transducer pressure is diagnostic of DVT in the portion of the vein being imaged. Echogenic thrombus is occasionally visualized within the vein, but slow-flowing blood may have a similar appearance, making this finding nonspecific. Compression ultrasound has been found to have both a sensitivity and a specificity of approximately 95 percent in venographically proven proximal leg DVTs, but the test is not accurate in identifying calf DVTs. Since approximately 20 percent of calf DVTs propagate to the proximal leg, repeat studies of the lower extremity are recommended in patients suspected of having a DVT found to have negative findings on compression ultrasound study. (See Chap. 55 for a detailed discussion.)

Visualization of Bladder and Fluid Collections

Ultrasound excels at identifying fluid collections, and a number of possible ED applications utilize this property. Unless devoid of urine, the bladder is very easy to identify on ultrasound, and most ultrasound machines have the ability to estimate bladder volume based on easily performed measurements. The invasive and painful procedure of catheterizing the bladder to determine postvoid residual volume can often be obviated by ultrasound. Furthermore, suprapubic bladder catheterizations and aspirations are easier and more likely to be successful when guided by ultrasound. Identifying abscesses is another area where ultrasound can be of assistance. With the use of high-frequency transducers (7.5 to 10 MHz), the presence or absence of fluid collections within subcutaneous masses can be determined. If an abscess is present, the depth of the abscess and surrounding structures (e.g., vessels) can be identified. The fluid within the abscess appears anechoic or has scattered echoes within a hypoechoic collection, representing necrotic debris. Just as ultrasound can identify hemothoraces, it can identify even small pleural effusions and guide aspiration attempts.

Procedural Uses

In addition to the bladder aspiration, mentioned above, there are several other procedural applications for ultrasound in the ED. While plain-film radiography or fluoroscopy is very accurate at identifying radio-paque foreign bodies, other objects, such as wood, can be very difficult to identify in a wound. Ultrasound is capable of identifying wooden objects as small as 2.5 by 1.0 mm in soft tissue and is also capable of identifying metal, plastic, glass, and vegetable matter.[14] With high-frequency probes (7.5 to 10 MHz), foreign bodies appear echogenic, often with acoustic shadowing.[15] With a small wound that is not amenable to exploration, it is acceptable to image directly over the potential entry site with the transducer and gel.

Sonography may also be used to assist in the percutaneous placement of central venous catheters.[16] Studies have found that the use of ultrasound to guide this procedure results in a decreased failure rate and lowers the overall incidence of complications.[17] Here, a 7.5- to 10-MHz probe identifies the location of the vein to be cannulated (e.g., internal jugular vein), and then the percutaneous puncture can be performed with accurate knowledge of the location of the vein. The vein is seen to compress considerably before puncture occurs.

Appendicitis

The sonographic evaluation of patients suspected of harboring acute appendicitis is mentioned here primarily as a cautionary note. The finding of a noncompressible appendix greater than 6 mm in diameter has been found to be helpful in making the diagnosis of appendicitis in the appropriate clinical setting.[18] However, several aspects of this examination make it particularly unsuited for performance by emergency physicians. This examination is generally quite time consuming, requires specialized training and experience, and can be very difficult technically. The diagnosis of appendicitis is also not as critically time dependent, as are such entities as ruptured AAA or hemoperitoneum in a trauma patient, and generally is best left in the hands of sonologists trained in this technique. Other potential uses for bedside ultrasound in the ED can be found in standard emergency ultrasound texts.

REFERENCES

1. Akkersdijk GJ, Puylaert JB, Coerkamp EG, de Vries AC: Accuracy of ultrasonographic measurement of infrarenal abdominal aortic aneurysm. *Br J Surg* 81:376, 1994.
2. Yilmaz S, Sindel T, Arslan G, et al: Renal colic: Comparison of spiral CT, US and IVU in the detection of ureteral calculi. *Eur Radiol* 8:212, 1998.
3. Henderson SO, Hoffner RJ, Aragona JL, et al: Bedside emergency department ultrasonography plus radiography of the kidneys, ureters, and bladder vs intravenous pyelography in the evaluation of suspected ureteral colic. *Acad Emerg Med* 5:666, 1998.
4. Simmons MZ: Pitfalls in ultrasound of the gallbladder and biliary tract. *Ultrasound Q* 14:2, 1998.
5. Porter RS, Nester BA, Dalsey WC, et al: Use of ultrasound to determine need for laparotomy in trauma patients. *Ann Emerg Med* 29:323, 1997.
6. Thomas B, Falcone RE, Vasquez D, et al: Ultrasound evaluation of blunt abdominal trauma: Program implementation, initial experience, and learning curve. *J Trauma* 42:384, 1997.
7. Sisley AC, Rozycki GS, Ballard RB, et al: Rapid detection of traumatic effusion using surgeon-performed ultrasonography. *J Trauma* 44:291, 1998.
8. Ma OJ, Mateer JR: Trauma ultrasound examination versus chest radiograph in the detection of hemothorax. *Ann Emerg Med* 29:312, 1997.
9. Rozycki GS, Feliciano DV, Schmidt JA: The role of surgeon-performed ultrasound in patients with possible cardiac wounds. *Ann Surg* 223:737, 1996.
10. Stovall TG, Kellerman AL, Ling FW, Buster JE: Emergency department diagnosis of ectopic pregnancy. *Ann Emerg Med* 19:1098, 1990.
11. Mateer JR, Valley VT, Aiman EJ, et al: Outcome analysis of a protocol including bedside endovaginal sonography in patients at risk for ectopic pregnancy. *Ann Emerg Med* 27:283, 1996.
12. Shih C: Effect of emergency physician-performed pelvic sonography on length of stay in the emergency department. *Ann Emerg Med* 29:348, 1997.
13. Jolly BT, Massarin CVT, Pigman EC: Color doppler ultrasonography by emergency physicians for the diagnosis of acute deep venous thrombosis. *Acad Emerg Med* 4:129, 1997.
14. Jacobson JA, Powell A, Craig JG, et al: Wooden foreign bodies in soft tissue: Detection at US. *Radiology* 206:45, 1998.
15. Hill R, Conron R, Greissinger P, Heller M: Ultrasound for the detection of foreign bodies in human tissue. *Ann Emerg Med* 29:353, 1997.
16. Hilty WH, Hudson PA, Levitt MA, Hall JB: Real-time ultrasound-guided femoral vein catheterization during cardiopulmonary resuscitation. *Ann Emerg Med* 29:331, 1997.
17. Randolph AG, Cook DJ, Gonzales CA, Pribble CG: Ultrasound guidance for placement of central venous catheters: A meta-analysis of the literature. *Crit Care Med* 24:2053, 1996.
18. Orr RK, Porter D, Hartman D: Ultrasonography to evaluate adults for appendicitis: Decision making based on meta-analysis and probabilistic reasoning. *Acad Emerg Med* 2:644, 1995.

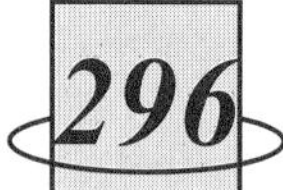

296 PRINCIPLES OF EMERGENCY DEPARTMENT USE OF COMPUTED TOMOGRAPHY

Stephanie Abbuhl
Patti J. Herling

BASIC PHYSICS AND TERMINOLOGY

Computed tomography (CT) is a technique that creates cross-sectional images with the use of x-rays and computerized image reconstruction. The patient passes through a gantry that contains an x-ray tube on one side and a set of detectors on the other. The gantry rotates around the patient, obtaining information from the detectors that is then analyzed by computer and displayed as an image. The image information can be manipulated by the computer to display a greater spectrum of densities than can be displayed on conventional x-ray film.

Image Formation and CT Numbers

The various shades of gray that make up a CT image are determined by the density of a structure and the amount of x-ray energy that passes through it. This phenomenon is referred to as the attenuation of the x-ray. The degree of beam attenuation on a CT image is quantified and expressed in Hounsfield units (HU), which are also referred to as CT numbers. Attenuation values span a range of 4000 CT numbers, from air at −1000 HU, to cortical bone at +3000 HU, and water is assigned the density of approximately 0 HU.

In conventional CT, each cross-sectional slice through a patient's body has a thickness, referred to as its *z* axis. The data are then further divided into tiny cubes of equal volume called *voxels* (volume elements). Each voxel is assigned a CT number that is determined by the degree to which the material in that voxel absorbed the x-ray beam. The two-dimensional CT image is formed by displaying the front face of each voxel, termed a *pixel* (picture element), in a composite matrix. The most common matrix size of CT scanners is 512 rows of pixels by 512 columns, or a total of 262,144 pixels[1] (Fig. 296-1).

Volume Averaging

Certain factors affect the accuracy of the Hounsfield units and the accuracy of the image. The degree of linear attenuation and the resultant CT number are determined by the average density of the material within that voxel. Therefore, when a voxel is filled with several structures (or the structure of interest is smaller than the voxel), the voxel will be assigned a CT number or HU that is subject to *volume averaging*

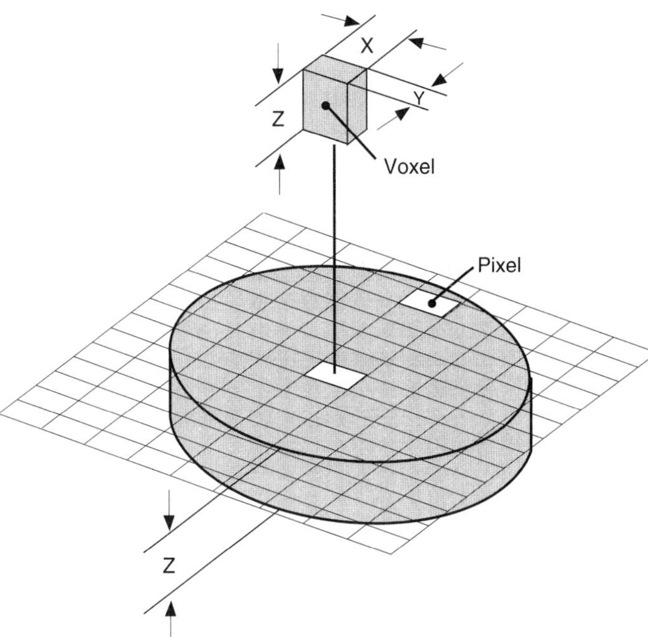

FIG. 296-1. The gray disc represents a cross-sectional slice corresponding to the patient. To create an image, the patient's data are segmented. A pixel is a two-dimensional square. A voxel incorporates the thickness of the slice and is a three-dimensional cube.

artifact. If the resolution of a very small structure is important, decreasing the scan thickness will improve accuracy. However, the benefits of thinner sections must be considered along with the risk of a higher radiation dose to the patient with the increased number of slices. Scanning protocols are designed to balance image resolution with acceptable radiation dose.

Image Noise

Although thinner sections increase image resolution, some of the advantages are lost due to increased image *noise,* also known as *quantum mottle.* Image noise is due to an insufficient number of x-ray photons reaching the detectors, resulting in a grainy image. Image noise can be reduced by increasing the radiation dose, but, again, a compromise between radiation exposure and image noise determines the quantitative x-ray dose.

Window and Level

Window width and *window level* are display settings that can be manipulated to optimize the appearance of the image. Selecting a window width determines the range of CT numbers that will be represented on a specific image. The computer assigns different shades of gray to CT numbers that fall within the selected range. CT numbers that are above the chosen range will appear white, while numbers below the chosen range will appear black. By increasing the window width, a greater range of CT numbers are each assigned to a shade of gray. This technique is used when it is desirable to view a variety of tissues that vary greatly in density (e.g., lung). The disadvantage to wider windows (400 to 2000 HU) is that subtle differences in density will not be visualized.

When the goal is to visualize a section of anatomy with minor discrepancies in tissue density, narrow window width is chosen (50 to 400 HU). A good example of the use of narrow window width is in the brain, where there is little difference in tissue densities; yet, with the higher contrast achieved with a narrow window, white and gray matter can be differentiated.

Window level determines the CT number that will be the center of the gray scale. The window level is generally set at the same value as the average attenuation number of the tissue of interest.

The image from a single data set can be displayed at different window widths and levels to highlight various tissues of interest. For example, in chest CT, settings that optimize the image of the soft tissue mediastinal structures use a moderate window width (e.g., 350) centered at a level just above water (e.g., +30). However, this setting does not allow visualization of the details of the lungs (Fig. 296-2*A*). On the other hand, lung settings use a wide window (e.g., 1400) and a low level (e.g., −600) to center the gray scale so it includes air densities (Fig. 296-2*B*). To optimize the image of a bony structure, a wide window (e.g., 1500) and a higher level (e.g., +305) would be used to center the gray scale toward higher-density tissues (Fig. 296-3).

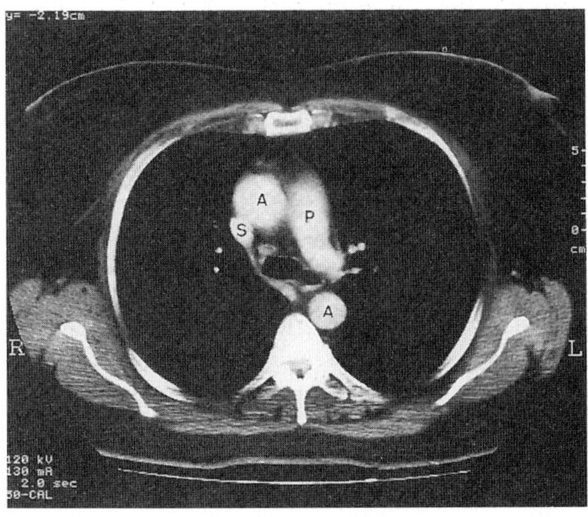

(a)

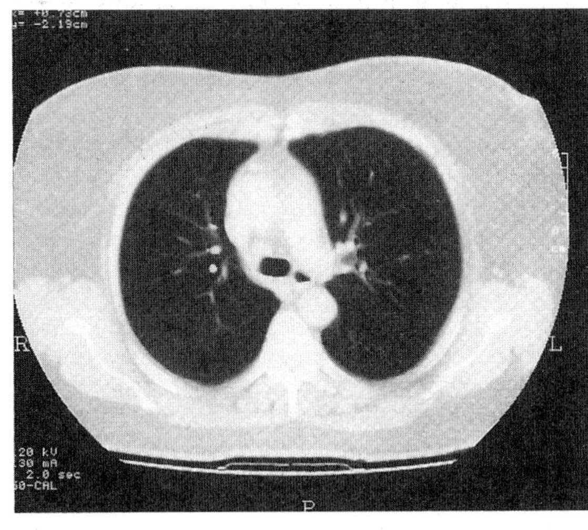

(b)

FIG. 296-2. CT windows. **A.** Mediastinal window. Note that the mediastinal anatomy is well shown; no lung detail can be seen. Note also the following structures: A, aorta; S, superior vena cava; and P, pulmonary artery. **B.** Lung window. Note that the vascular anatomy of the lungs is now well seen.

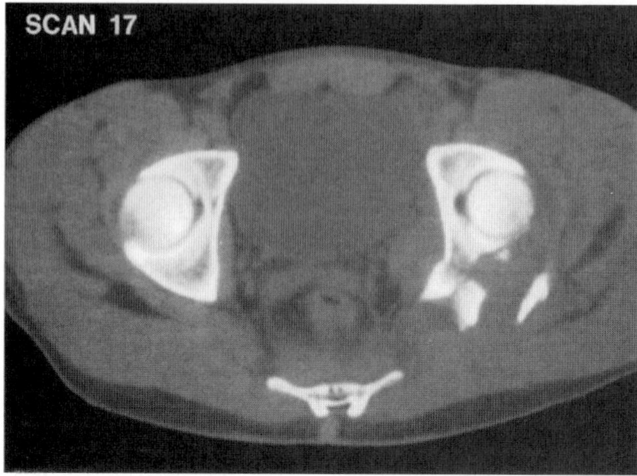

A

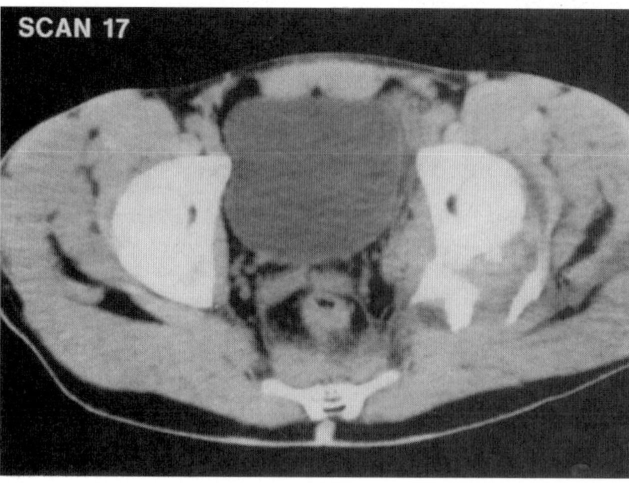

B

FIG. 296-3. **A and B.** The same CT scan at different window and level settings. A posterior wall fracture of the left acetabulum is shown at settings for bone **(A)** and at settings for soft tissue **(B)**. The wider window and higher level of the bone settings enable better visualization of bone detail but make all soft tissue structures nearly the same shade of gray. Soft tissue settings allow examination for hemarthrosis and adjacent soft tissue hematoma.

SCANNER GENERATION

The terms *first-generation through fourth-generation scanners* are used to represent the developments in technology that relate the configuration of the x-ray tube to the detectors. The first-generation scanners, which are no longer in use, had a thin x-ray beam pass linearly over the patient in a 180° arc, followed by a single detector on the opposite side.[2] Scanning time was very lengthy. Second-generation scanners used multiple detectors and a fan-shaped x-ray beam that continued to pass linearly across the patient before rotating. Scan times improved but were still very long.

Third-generation scanners represented a significant advance in technology, and scan times were greatly reduced. This design incorporates a fan-shaped beam and a detector array, and both move in a circle within the gantry. With the use of a rotating detector, all of the readings that make up a view can be recorded at the same time.[1] Third-generation scanners are the most common conventional models in use today.

Fourth-generation scanners have a detector array that is fixed and positioned in a complete circle within the gantry. The x-ray tube produces a fan-shaped beam that rotates around the patient. Scan times are theoretically shorter than with third-generation scanners, but few fourth-generation scanners have been installed.[2]

SPIRAL COMPUTED TOMOGRAPHY

The biggest technological advance came with the advent of spiral or helical scanning. Rather than scanning with the traditional axial method where the slices lie parallel to one another, spiral scanning obtains data continually in a spiral fashion. There is a continually rotating x-ray gantry and continuous table movement. This was achieved by a critical advance in hardware technology with the introduction of slip-ring interfaces in gantry construction, allowing for continuous rotation of the source detector assembly.[3] With conventional CT, a patient is required to hold his or her breath for each additional slice. When a patient breathes to varying depths with each slice, lesions as large as 1 cm can be missed as a result of slice *misregistration* (Fig. 296-4). In a typical spiral scanner, 60 images can be acquired in 1 min, therefore there is less breath holding, which decreases slice misregistration.

Because spiral scans are acquired at a slight slant, computer software must adjust for the angle by averaging the data. This statistical method of processing the data is referred to as *interpolation* (linear and nonlinear). The evolution of mathematical software processes enabling missing data to be estimated in helical data sets has also been critical to the advancement and success of spiral CT.[3] There is, however, a small decrease in resolution inherent to interpolation (Fig. 296-5).

The term *pitch* refers to the relation of table speed to slice thickness. If pitch is set at 1:1, the table will move at a speed that allows the gantry to rotate once for every slice thickness chosen. For example, with slice thickness at 5 mm, the table moves at a speed that allows the gantry to rotate once every 5 mm of table travel. If the pitch is adjusted to 2:1 and the slice thickness is maintained at 5 mm, the tube rotates only once for every 10 mm of table motion. Pitch is sometimes adjusted toward 2:1, which, in essence, "stretches the spring" and less data are acquired.[1] Pitch is usually set at close to 1:1 but may be increased when it is important to cover a long anatomic area in a very short time, as with CT angiography.

Spiral CT scanning has optimized the delivery of intravenous (IV) contrast. The rapid speed of the scanning technique allows for much finer control over which phase of IV contrast enhancement is imaged and allows for the possibility of obtaining more information from a single bolus of contrast. For example, in the abdomen, images can be obtained during the hepatic arterial, portal venous, and equilibrium phases. Delayed images are also easily and rapidly obtained when enhancement characteristics of certain lesions need to be visualized or when the urinary excretory phase must be imaged. This capability is widely utilized in trauma where major organ lacerations and active bleeding sites are best visualized during early phases of contrast enhancement, while bladder perforation may be better imaged on delayed contrast imaging.

The major advantages of helical scanning over conventional scanning are

1. Volumetric data acquisition is acquired rapidly.
2. Less contrast material is needed because of increased scanning speed.
3. Images can be retrospectively reconstructed at any desired interval or thickness or may be overlapping without rescanning the patient.
4. Respiratory, cardiac, and other motion artifacts are reduced.
5. The continuous nature of the data allows high-quality three-dimensional and multiplanar reconstruction.

Although the advantages of spiral CT predominate, there are some disadvantages:

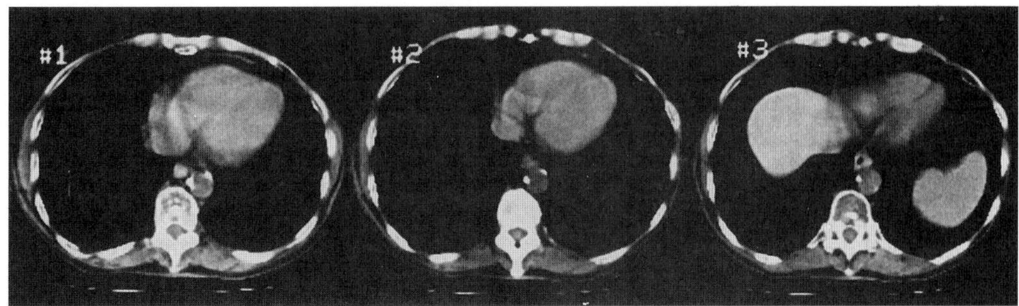
#1
#2
#3

FIG. 296-4. Slice misregistration caused by a patient's breathing. Each consecutive slice was 10 mm or more inferior, yet the second image appears the most superior. Lesions as large as 1 cm can be missed as a result of slice misregistration.

1. If pitch (relation of table speed to slice thickness) is increased from 1:1 toward 2:1, image resolution can be lost.
2. When scanning very large patients, there will be increased image noise if the milliampere setting cannot be maintained. Scanners vary regarding weight limitations, although the average maximum patient weight is approximately 350 lb.
3. Some image resolution may be lost due to the interpolation required to process spiral data.
4. Contrast material injection must be timed precisely, although this problem has been minimized with the use of established contrast protocols and power injectors.
5. Children and uncooperative adults need sedation and thus, close monitoring.

METHODS OF DAT

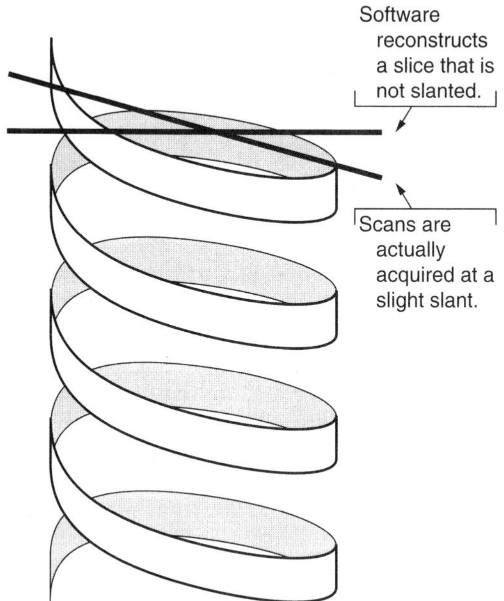
Software reconstructs a slice that is not slanted.
Scans are actually acquired at a slight slant.

FIG. 296-5. Spiral scans are acquired at a slight slant because of the continuous motion of the x-ray tube and table. By interpolating the data, the computer then creates an image that is not slanted. This process increases the effective slice thickness and causes some loss of image resolution. The more pronounced the slant, the more interpolation is required. The slant is affected by selected slice thickness and pitch.

Spiral CT scanners continue to have the capability of acquiring axial images. For example, at some institutions, CT protocols for cervical spine trauma use a spiral CT scanner to obtain axial images because of the potential improvement in image resolution in this anatomic area.

An important issue raised by the advent of spiral CT is what constitutes an appropriate examination archive. At this point, because of the enormous space required to store all the information, most CT scanners delete the raw data soon after the scan is acquired. Thus, it is important to select the reconstruction interval quickly and appropriately so that the opportunity is not lost to request additional reformatted images before the raw data is deleted.

GENERAL USES AND LIMITATIONS

As CT technology has advanced, the role of CT in the emergency department (ED) has also increased enormously. A CT scanner is in, or adjacent to, many EDs today in the United States, in recognition of its fundamental utility and to minimize necessity for patient transport. The only real disadvantages of CT are its relatively high cost and the use of ionizing radiation. Standard charges for conventional and spiral CT are the same. Head CT continues to be the primary imaging study for screening ED patients acutely, particularly for detection of acute hemorrhage, trauma, and cerebrovascular accident. Magnetic resonance imaging (MRI), however, may have an additional role when posterior fossa pathology or subtle parenchymal abnormalities are suspected. In general, CT is the imaging study of choice for the examination of the retroperitoneum and for many disorders of the abdomen and pelvis. At many institutions, spiral CT has become the primary imaging modality for detection of acute appendicitis[4] and ureteral calculi. It is also the modality of choice for many disorders of the mediastinum and lungs. Fractures and other bone pathology are often best visualized with CT, and it is excellent for detecting cervical spine, pelvic, and facial bone fractures.

Only a few areas of the body are poorly imaged with CT. The pituitary fossa and the posterior intracranial fossa are difficult to visualize because the adjacent bony structures cause significant streak artifact. MRI is the preferred study in these anatomic areas. CT is not sensitive in differentiating spinal cord or nerve roots from cerebrospinal fluid (CSF) unless contrast has been injected into the CSF space. MRI is the imaging study of choice to evaluate the spinal cord.

Although spiral scanning data can be reformatted into high-quality sagittal and coronal plane images, conventional CT is usually limited to the axial (transverse) plane. There are anatomic areas (such as the head and ankles) that can be positioned in the gantry of conventional CT scanners to obtain direct coronal images.

The role of CT in the evaluation of all potential ED presentations is beyond the scope of this chapter. The reader is referred to specific chapters of chief complaints or diagnoses for a discussion of the potential value of CT for each topic.

THE USE OF CONTRAST

Contrast materials for CT examinations can be administered via oral, rectal, intravenous, intraarterial, intraarticular, or intrathecal routes, and usage varies according to the examination desired. In general, contrast usage in the ED is limited to the oral and/or IV routes.

Oral Contrast

Oral contrast agents are used for most CT examinations of the abdomen and pelvis to ensure adequate contrast opacification and distention of the bowel. This is necessary to enhance the appearance of the bowel wall to detect hematoma, edema, mass, or laceration. This is usually achieved with *positive* contrast agents, such as iodine-based and barium-based agents. At times, however, *negative* contrast is optimal in the upper gastrointestinal tract and is achieved by using an oral water preparation. This is helpful, for example, when the indication for the abdominal CT is to evaluate the pancreas in a patient with jaundice. Occasionally, distention of the upper gastrointestinal tract can also be achieved by the additional administration of effervescent granules that cause gas formation within the bowel lumen. It is important that the radiologist and/or technologist know the purpose of the study so that the correct oral preparation is ordered. It is much more common to administer water-soluble iodinated oral agents to ED and trauma patients to avoid complications from extravasation of barium agents.

The iodine-based oral contrast used for CT is very dilute compared with the full-strength iodine-based contrast used for conventional radiography (upper gastrointestinal and barium enema series). Full-strength solutions may cause artifacts on CT because of their high density. Whereas full-strength iodine-based contrast aspiration may cause life-threatening pneumonitis, the dilute contrast used for CT poses much less risk. Nonetheless, use of this agent should either be avoided, or it should be used with caution in patients at risk for aspiration. If oral contrast is necessary in a patient with a known iodine allergy and a known gastrointestinal tract disorder, a dilute barium sulfate suspension should be administered instead.

Administering oral contrast takes approximately 2 h in a patient with a normal transit time if the entire bowel needs to be opacified. For example, intraluminal contrast must be present in the right colon to evaluate a patient adequately for possible appendicitis. For evaluating certain upper abdominal conditions, an additional 200 mL of oral contrast should be given just before scanning, to opacify the stomach and proximal small bowel. Not infrequently, an ED patient has nausea

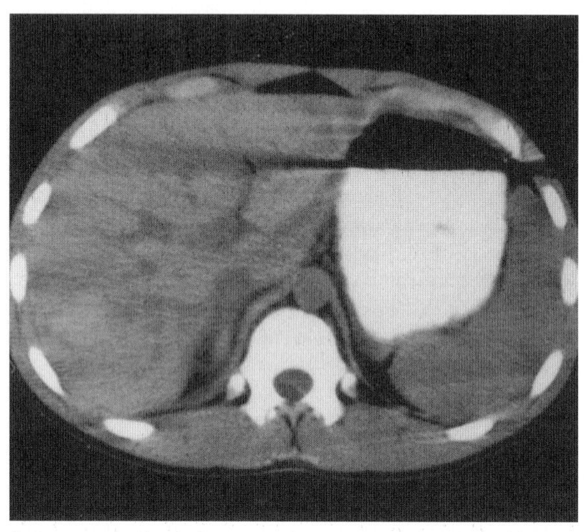

A

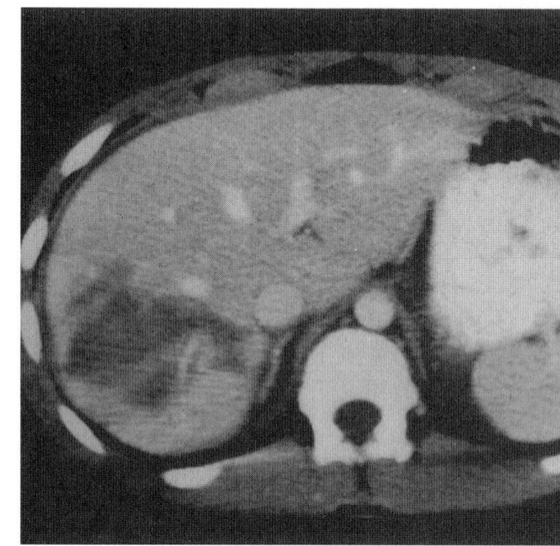

B

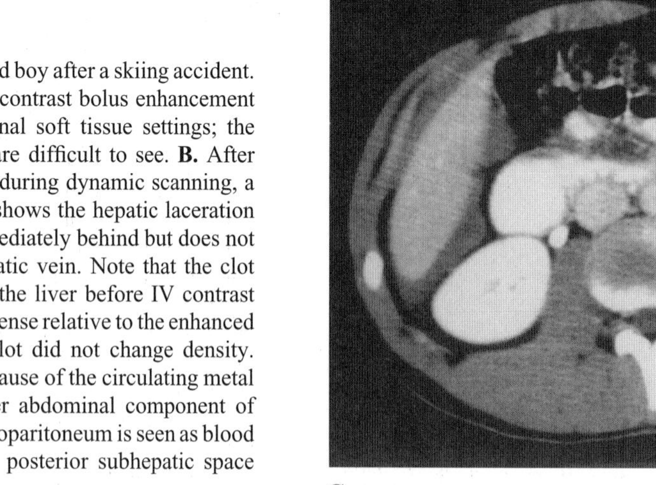

C

FIG. 296-6. Scans of a 16-year-old boy after a skiing accident. **A.** Scan before intravenous (IV) contrast bolus enhancement is displayed at standard abdominal soft tissue settings; the intrahepatic clot and laceration are difficult to see. **B.** After bolus IV contrast administration during dynamic scanning, a scan at the same level as in **(A)** shows the hepatic laceration well. The laceration extends immediately behind but does not apparently involve the right hepatic vein. Note that the clot appeared hyperdense relative to the liver before IV contrast administration and appears hypodense relative to the enhanced liver after bolus contrast. The clot did not change density. The liver increased in density because of the circulating metal in the IV contrast. **C.** The upper abdominal component of this patient's relatively small hemoparitoneum is seen as blood in the Morison pouch (the right posterior subhepatic space between the liver and kidney).

and vomiting, and a nasogastric tube and antiemetics are required in order to facilitate the oral contrast administration. Some contrast protocols use rectally administered contrast. The terms *double contrast* and *triple contrast* usually refer to the possible combined routes (oral, rectal, or vascular), but in some situations may refer to the concentration.

Intravenous Contrast

IV contrast is frequently utilized for emergency CT studies, because it creates a more detailed image of many structures, particularly abdominal, pelvic, and retroperitoneal organs. The contrast material causes beam attenuation that is directly related to the iodine concentration achieved by the vascular supply to that tissue. Abnormal tissue, whether due to a malignant, inflammatory, or infectious etiology, has different contrast enhancement patterns than normal tissue and may appear avascular, hypovascular, isodense, or hypervascular. Images can be obtained at various phases following contrast administration. Depending on the diagnosis in question, the study should be tailored to acquire data at the appropriate time (Fig. 296-6).

In certain circumstances, it may be necessary to perform both a noncontrast CT scan and a contrast CT scan. CT scans to evaluate patients with potential urinary tract calculi must initially be performed without IV contrast, because the presence of contrast can easily obscure any renal stones present. In addition, an obstructing ureteral calculus may often be detected on an unenhanced CT study. However, IV contrast can be useful to determine the exact level of ureteral obstruction or to determine whether a pelvic calcification lies within the ureter. It may also provide information on the function of the kidneys. In general, the best way to optimize any study is to discuss the purpose of the CT adequately with the radiologist and/or technologist performing the study.

REFERENCES

1. Romans LE: *Introduction to Computed Tomography.* Media, PA, Williams & Wilkins, 1995.
2. Napel SA: Basic principles of spiral CT, in Fishman EK, Jeffrey RB Jr (eds): *Spiral CT: Principles, Techniques and Clinical Applications.* New York, Raven, 1995, pp 1–9.
3. Brink JA: Technical aspects of helical (spiral) CT. *Radiol Clin North Am* 33:825, 1995.
4. Rao PM, Rhea JT, Novelline RA, et al: Effect of computed tomography of the appendix on treatment of patients and the use of hospital resources. *N Engl J Med* 338:141, 1998.

MAGNETIC RESONANCE IMAGING: PRINCIPLES AND SOME APPLICATIONS

Irwin D. Weisman

The significant advances in imaging technology of recent years have dramatically expedited diagnosis and improved outcomes in emergency department patients. Magnetic resonance imaging (MRI) has been at the forefront. In just a short time, it has become a major adjunct for neurologic and musculoskeletal evaluation. This chapter briefly describes MRI and elucidates its role in emergency medicine:

Magnetic resonance imaging has the following major advantages:

1. Like ultrasound, it does not use ionizing radiation and no short-term or long-term side effects have been demonstrated. This is in contrast to the high-energy ionizing radiation of computed tomography (CT) and other x-ray methods, which produce small but finite biologic damage that may have long-term carcinogenesis implications. Because of this consideration, where applicable, MRI should be preferred over CT and tomography in the pediatric and childlbearing female populations.
2. It produces variable-thickness, two-dimensional slices in any orientation through the body part of interest, thus optimizing visualization of tissues and their interfaces. With few exceptions, CT is restricted to a scan plane that is transverse to the long axis of the body.
3. Because of the different physical principles underlying magnetic resonance (as opposed to x-rays), it provides better contrast resolution and tissue discrimination in many areas compared with x-rays or ultrasound. For example, spinal cord, bone marrow, muscles, and tendons are better visualized with MRI than with CT. As a result, MRI is replacing invasive methods such as myelography, arthrography and, in limited situations, angiography.

MRI is a specific application of nuclear magnetic resonance to medical imaging.[1,2] Nuclear magnetic resonance was discovered simultaneously in 1946 by Bloch and colleagues at Stanford University[3] and by Purcell and colleagues at Harvard University.[4] Bloch and Purcell shared the Nobel Prize in 1952 for their outstanding contribution to the physical sciences.

PHYSICAL BASIS

The nuclei of hydrogen in water and fat molecules behave like small spinning bar magnets. When placed in a strong uniform magnetic field (greater than 0.01 tesla or 100 gauss), they execute a circular motion, or precession, weakly aligning to form a net nuclear polarization nearly parallel to the external magnet field. If a short pulse of radio frequency (rf) energy (radio wave), precisely tuned to the precession frequency of the water and fat proton nuclear magnets, is applied, the nuclei absorb a small amount of energy, change their alignment, and then gradually return to their previous equilibrium positions. In responding to the radio wave, the net nuclear magnetization generates a small voltage: the nuclear magnetic resonance signal. This can be detected and recorded electronically.

Two parameters T1 and T2, also known as respectively longitudinal and transverse relaxation times, govern the behavior of the electronic signal detected. The relaxation times are a function of the immediate environment of the resonating protons and vary in the different biologic tissues. For example, free water exhibits long T1 and T2 values and fat exhibits short T1 and relatively short T2 values. Image generation requires a large number of repetitions of the sequence that produces the nuclear resonance signal. The time between repetitions is called TR. For technical reasons, a two-pulse sequence is used to generate a particular type of signal called a spin echo. The spacing between pulses is labeled TE/2, and an echo occurs at a time TE. There are important relationships between the intensity of the nuclear magnetic resonance echo and TR, T1, TE, and T2. Based on the effects of the different relaxation times (T1 and T2), two types of imaging are carried out. Short repetition times (TR) between successive cycles of rf excitation pulses and short echo times (TE) produce stronger signals from tissues with relatively short T1 times, such as fat, especially bone marrow. Hence, weighting favoring short T1 results from pulse sequences using short TR and short TE. On the other hand, longer TRs eliminate much of the T1 signal difference between fat and water so that further manipulation of the rf pulse spacing (longer TE) will enhance signals from tissues with long T2 times, such as edema fluid. Long TR, TE pulse sequences preferentially weight long T2 tissues. Thus, the two basic methods of MRI scanning are labeled T1-weighted and T2-weighted imaging.

To construct an image from the tissue-specific signals of an object (for example, a patient), it is necessary to apply small, spatially inhomogeneous, three-dimensional magnetic fields called gradients. They modify the signal decay of the nuclear magnetization and spatially tag the hydrogen nuclear magnets in the object for mapping the image.

The actual reconstruction of an image is complex, just as in CT scanning, and requires a relatively fast computer with a large memory. The ultimate result is a two-dimensional, medically diagnostic, cross-sectional body image that is displayed on a video monitor and recorded on film or digitally stored on a hard disk or magnetic tape as a permanent record. In most gray-scale imaging formats, the strongest signal corresponds to maximum brightness on the black-and-white monitor. Therefore, in heavily T2-weighted images, water appears bright, whereas fat appears intermediate gray. On the other hand, on T1-weighted images, fat appears bright and water appears dark (Fig. 297-1). Table 297-1 lists the expected signal intensities for several biologic tissues in these two cases. Many newer and more sophisticated imaging pulse sequences have evolved from this imaging framework, such as chemical fat suppression, inversion recovery, short T1 inversion recovery (STIR), fluid attentuation inversion recovery (FLAIR), gradient echo recall, magnetization transfer, rapid acquisition with relaxation enhancement (RARE), echo planar, and diffusion gradient. For a more complete discussion of the technical aspects and clinical applications of MRI, readers are referred to more specialized texts.[5,6]

TABLE 297-1 Tissue Appearance in Magnetic Resonance Imaging

Tissue	T1 Image	T2 Image
Fat	Bright	Intermediate
Water	Dark	Bright
Muscle	Intermediate	Intermediate
Ligaments	Dark	Dark
Bone cortex	Dark	Dark

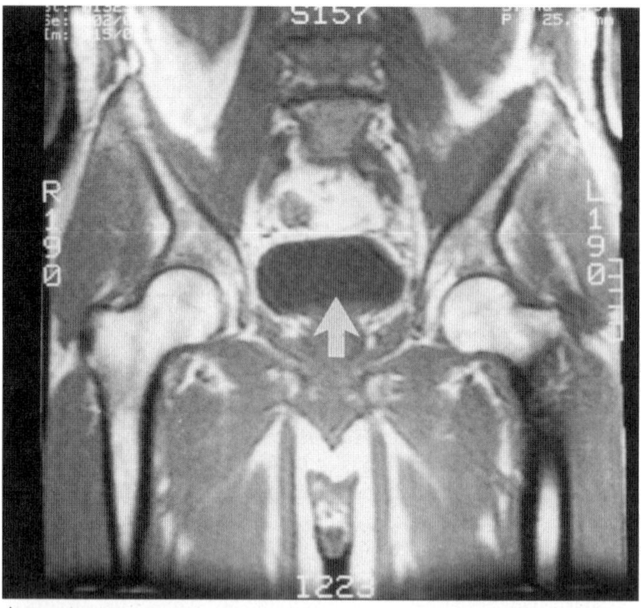

A

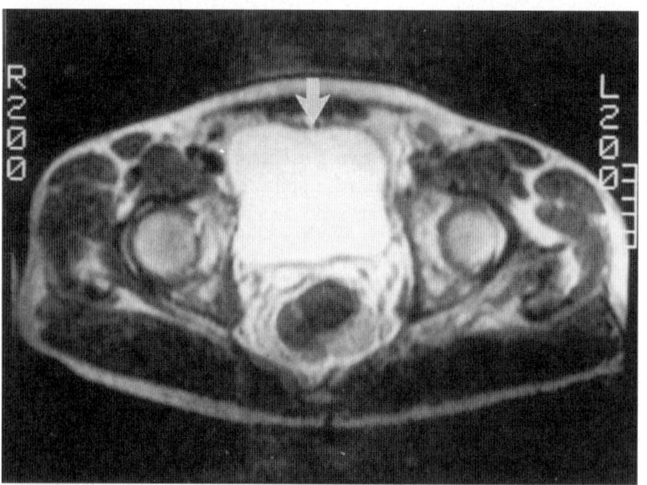

B

FIG. 297-1. Examples of T1-weighted and T2-weighted magnetic resonance images. **A.** T1-weighted coronal image: note that the urine in the bladder (*arrow*), which is essentially water with a long T1, appears dark, whereas the femoral bone marrow, subcutaneous, and perivesical fat (short T1) appear bright. **B.** T2-weighted axial image of the same patient as in **A:** note that the urine, which has a long T2, now appears bright, whereas the surrounding fat with its shorter T2 is intermediate in brightness.

The physical basis of image formation using MRI is quite different from CT, which is based on differential x-ray absorption coefficients. Even though both are tomographic imaging techniques, the meaning of bright and dark signals in MRI is relative to the pulse sequence eliciting them and has very little resemblance to the contrast in CT.

The core of an MRI system is the large magnet needed to generate the strong, constant, and uniform magnetic field, as well as the magnetic gradients. The magnet is composed of coils of a special superconducting wire that loses all resistance to electrical current when submerged in liquid helium. At this temperature, −450°F (−269°C), the coils can handle the relatively large currents of electricity required to produce the magnetic field. A specially designed, thermally insulated container encloses the magnet coils and the liquid helium. The liquid slowly boils away and must be replaced at regular intervals. The magnet is housed in a special room containing steel sheets and copper screen, which shield the system against interference by steel and radio waves on the outside and vice versa. The other components of the system, consisting of a radio transmitter, a sophisticated rf receiver, and a high-speed large-memory computer, are located near the operator's console just outside the room.

SAFETY

In a few cases, the large magnetic field could be a health hazard to the patient,[7,8] necessitating the use of alternative diagnostic methods such as ultrasound or CT. Internal cardiac pacemakers may be converted to an abnormal asynchronous mode by the magnetic field. Certain types of steel cerebral aneurysm clips (ferromagnetic as opposed to nonmagnetic stainless steel) may experience strong forces, with the potential of harming the brain. Small steel slivers imbedded in the eye (occasionally seen in asymptomatic sheet metal workers or welders) could injure the retina and cause blindness. Life-support equipment containing magnetic steel will be strongly attracted into the magnetic field, threatening both the patient and the system. Cochlear implants may be damaged or cause unacceptable injury due to eddy current heating effects. Patients in any of the aforementioned categories cannot be scanned with MRI. There are other devices, such as implantable cardiac defibrillators, neurostimulators, and bone growth stimulators, that may malfunction in the presence of high magnetic fields. Certain prosthetic heart valves contain nearly magnetic stainless-steel components that are subject to strong forces when placed in powerful magnetic fields. However, it has been pointed out that the forces on the valve from the heart exceed those generated by even high-field magnets, and hence this is a relative contraindication for MRI scanning.

The pulsed radio waves are a source of heat energy deposited within the body. Software programs built into the computers restrict the frequency of pulsing so that the maximum allowable power deposition averaged over the whole patient is never exceeded. Occasionally, skin burns have been reported when a patient's skin has come into direct contact with uninsulated rf leads, but proper precautions prevent this from happening.

The complete examination takes from 30 to 60 min, is painless, and is well tolerated by most patients. It does require suspension of all motion, except for breathing, for periods ranging from a few seconds to 15 min at a time, depending on the particular pulse sequence. Some patients are claustrophobic and have difficulty with the examination. Most problems of this nature are satisfactorily treated with minor tranquilizers administered orally. Infants, younger pediatric patients, and agitated adults need to be sedated, as in CT, because any motion degrades the MRI scan.

Some minor precautions are necessary. Magnetically encoded plastic cards, such as credit, cash, and parking cards, may be damaged when they come within a certain range of the magnetic field. Some watches with steel parts and hearing aids (and their batteries) are vulnerable to damage. Any ferromagnetic steel objects are potentially lethal missiles if carried into the magnet room. Patients need to leave such objects outside the scanning room.

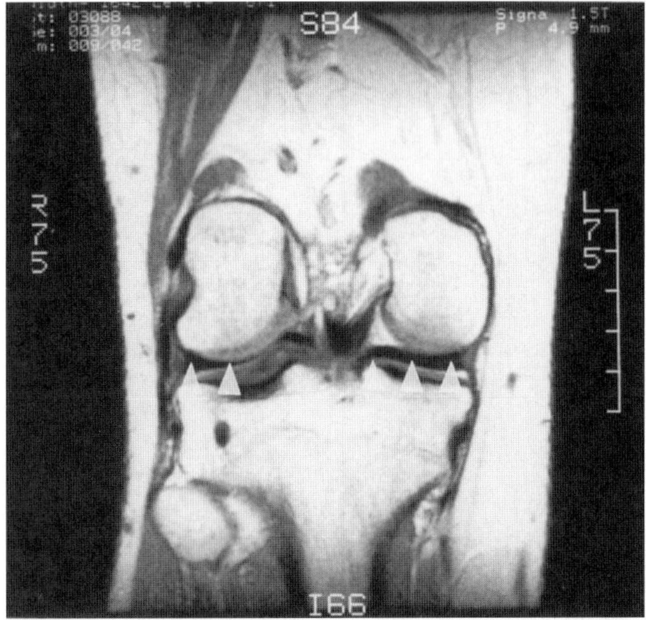

A

B

FIG. 297-2. Meniscal tear: **A.** Normal medial and lateral menisci as demonstrated on a magnetic resonance proton-density coronal image (partial T2 weighting). The menisci are the dark triangular structures marked with *arrowheads*. **B.** Proton-density coronal scan showing a large complex tear involving the posterior horn of the medial meniscus (*arrowheads*).

APPLICATIONS

MRI has been widely applied to the brain and spinal cord,[9] where it provides images that are superior in diagnostic quality to those obtained with CT. Furthermore, this information can be obtained with less risk to patients because CT myelography requires intrathecal contrast agents for a specific diagnosis. Although special intravenous contrast agents are frequently required to improve the sensitivity of MRI, they have been associated with much less toxicity and reactions as compared with the intravenous CT contrast agents.[10] Except in the cases of acute intracerebral hemorrhage, skull fracture, and some calcified brain lesions, MRI may completely replace CT of the head. The exact role of MRI versus CT in trauma and degenerative disease of the spine is still evolving. CT visualizes fracture fragment relationships and bone detail more optimally, but MRI visualizes the soft tissues with better resolution. Some spine surgeons still prefer CT myelography to MRI.

MRI has been useful in examining the chest and abdomen (especially the chest wall, mediastinum, liver, spleen, adrenals, and aorta), but has played a lesser role compared with CT, because of respiratory motion and heart pulsation artifacts that degrade anatomic delineation of critical structures. They can be compensated for, to some degree, with electrocardiograph and respiratory gating and associated electronic manipulation, but the methods are cumbersome and difficult to implement with an acutely ill patient. A recent innovation is the introduction of breath-hold MR cholangiography for the noninvasive evaluation of the biliary and pancreatic ducts.[11] It has had limited application to cooperative patients with biliary or pancreatic disease not amenable to ultrasound, CT, or other conventional methods. There has also been progress in cardiac MRI,[5,12] but introduction of these methods into the emergency practice are currently limited due to cost and availability.

MRI has a major role in other areas of the musculoskeletal system[6] especially the knee, shoulder, hip, and temporomandibular joints. Although MRI is not indicated for most acute fractures, it may be preferred in the diagnosis of rotator cuff tear of the shoulder, internal derangement of the knee (meniscus, tendon, and ligament tears), tendon or soft tissue injury to any of the small joints, soft tissue injury in the spine, and posttraumatic avascular necrosis of any bone. In addition, carpal tunnel syndrome has been evaluated using MRI. Figure 297-2 demonstrates a meniscus tear in the knee. Before MRI, arthrography, which involves injection of contrast agents into the joint, was used to detect cartilage injuries. This type of examination is not only painful but carries a small but measurable risk of infection and contrast reaction. MRI of these joints is painless and only requires that the patient be able to hold still for a moderate length of time. The information obtained in the knee and hips exceeds what can be obtained using other methods. In the hips, MRI has proven to be the most reliable method for detecting avascular necrosis.

In problematic cases, MRI has detected stress fractures and occult fractures in the small bones of the hand. Even though it does not visualize cortex, any break in the medullary cancellous bone can be readily detected.

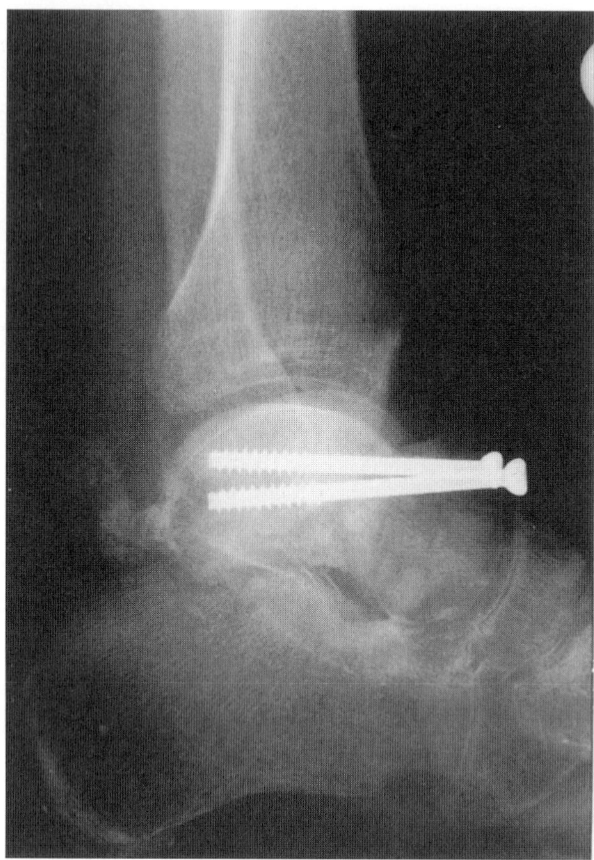

A

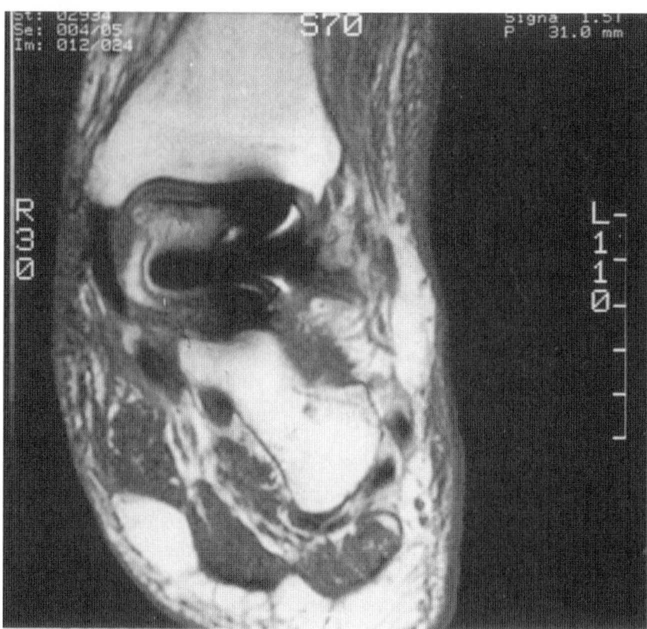

B

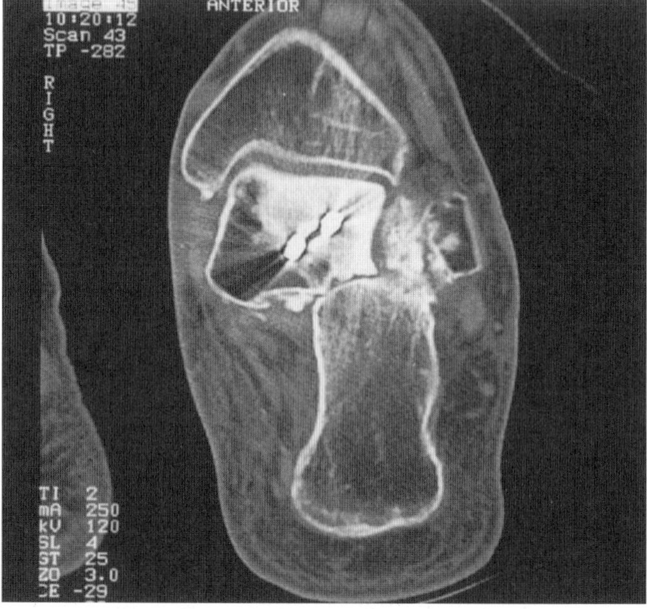

C

FIG. 297-3. Magnetic artifacts: **A.** Lateral radiograph of a foot of a patient with a talar fracture reduced with two cold-worked stainless-steel screws. **B.** Proton-density-weighted coronal magnetic resonance imaging: ferromagnetic artifacts almost completely obliterate the talar marrow signal, rendering it diagnostically useless. **C.** Ultra-high-resolution coronal computed tomographic (CT) scan on the same foot yields useful information on the condition of the talar fragments (nonunion and avascular necrosis). This is unusual in that the ferromagnetic properties of the screws are responsible for a disproportionate deleterious effect on the MRI compared with the CT. Note that both show a lateral calcaneal dislocation.

The sequelae of soft tissue musculoskeletal trauma, such as complete muscular or tendon tears, hemorrhage, and edema, are very easily diagnosed with MRI. Even injuries to the medium-sized nerves and brachial plexus can be demonstrated.[13,14]

MRI has also been used to study infection in bone and soft tissues, where in many cases it has been superior to modalities such as nuclear medicine and CT.[15–17] However, if the patient has a metallic prostheses in the region of abnormality, rf currents or magnetic field inhomogeneities due to the metal induce artifacts in the MRI scan that reduce the sensitivity (Fig. 297-3). This is even more of a problem in CT, where x-ray scattering from the prosthesis may completely obliterate the scan. Then, only nuclear medicine studies may be useful, in particular indium 111 tagged to white blood cells.

MRI is extremely sensitive and specific in detecting metastatic disease in bone when questions arise after a positive bone scan. MRI is neither practical nor cost effective to use for whole body surveys, but when applied to specific lesions the anatomic information expedites diagnosis.

CT continues to be the modality of choice for suspected head, spine, and abdominal injuries, because it is quick, more widely available, and more compatible with life-support equipment. Although MRI-compatible respirators and pulsed oxymeters are now available, most standard life-support equipment either contains magnetic steel components or sensitive electronics that will not operate properly in the presence of rf or large static or dynamic magnetic fields. MRI is used in an elective setting after a patient has been stabilized and there is time to address the less acute problems.

MRI IN THE EMERGENT SETTING

At present, there are two areas where MRI is the procedure of choice in the acute setting: (1) evaluation of suspected spinal cord compression

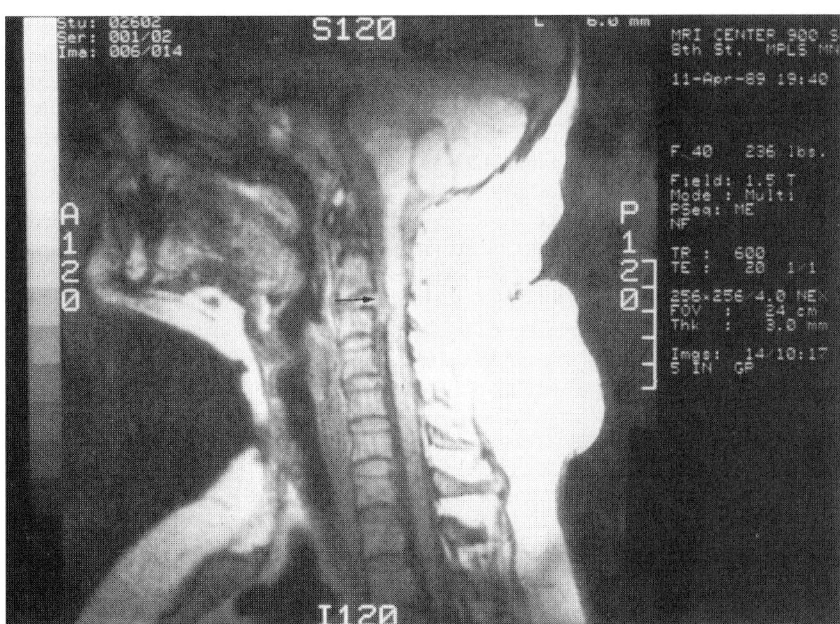

FIG. 297-4. Cervical spinal cord compression: T1-weighted sagittal magnetic resonance imaging demonstrates moderate spinal cord compression by an acute traumatically herniated disc at the C2–3 level (*arrow*). The patient was in a motor vehicle accident and also suffered associated bilateral C2 pedicle fractures.

from any cause and (2) radiographically occult femoral intertrochanteric and neck fractures. In both cases, the unique ability to form images in axial, coronal, or sagittal planes gives MRI a distinct advantage. Another major factor is the superb contrast resolution of MRI that facilitates detection of spinal cord injury or fracture through cancellous bone of the hip. Figure 297-4 demonstrates an example of cervical cord compression resulting from a traumatically herniated disc. Figure 297-5 is an example of an occult femoral intertrochanteric fracture best demonstrated on MRI. Small studies[18,19] have confirmed higher sensitivity and specificity for MRI as compared with radionuclide

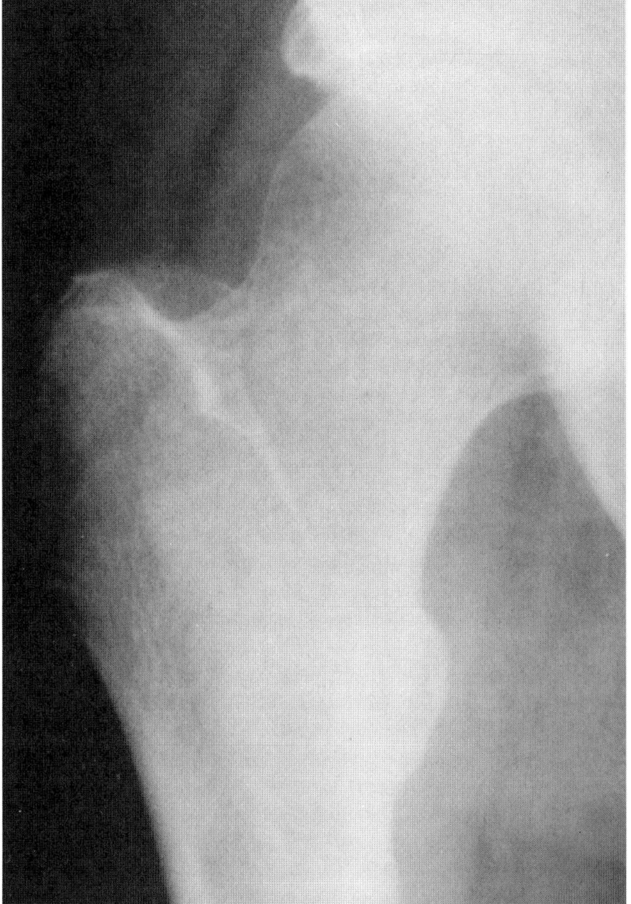

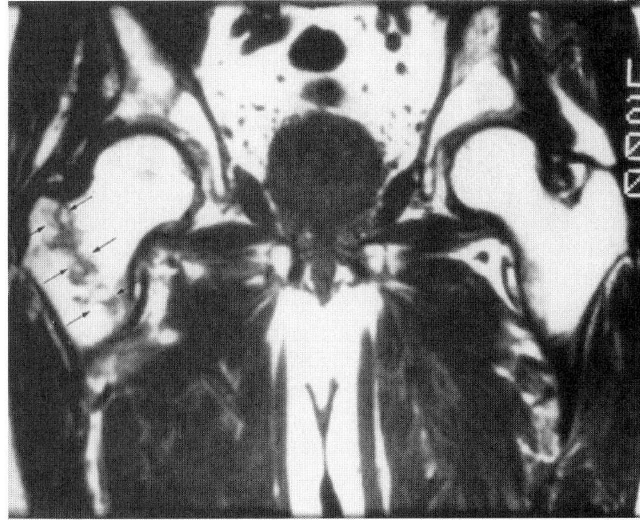

FIG. 297-5. Occult hip fracture: **A.** Anteroposterior radiograph of a 55-year-old patient on steroids who had right hip pain after a fall. No fracture is evident. **B.** T1-weighted coronal magnetic resonance scan of the same hip clearly demonstrates a non-displaced intertrochanteric femoral shaft fracture (*arrows*).

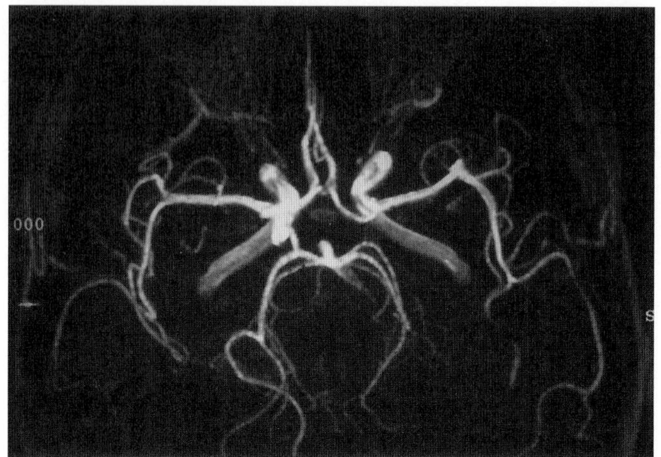

FIG. 297-6. Normal magnetic resonance angiogram of the circle of Willis in the brain. Summation image of maximum-intensity projection data from computer reconstructions after a three-dimensional time-of-flight acquisition in the axial plane. The examination required about 9 min, and no intravenous contrast was necessary.

bone scanning, tomography, and CT in the detection of occult fractures, especially in femoral head and neck fractures.

Another potential area for MRI evaluation in the acute setting is aortic dissection. MRI is superior to contrast-enhanced CT and possibly transesophageal ultrasound in delineating the intimal aortic flap. Unfortunately, many of these patients are unstable hemodynamically and are agitated, requiring life support and sedation. Thus, few, if any, good candidates for MRI. As more MRI-compatible life-support and monitoring equipment becomes available, this situation will change.

Finally, a second potential application is in pediatric fractures[20] when there may be significant injury to unossified cartilage around open growth plates. Fractures through cartilage are not seen on plane films but are easily identified on MRI.

One innovation—the development of low and very low magnetic field imaging systems—may have some impact on emergency departments. Most of the hazards previously delineated apply to high-field systems. In low-field systems where the magnetic flux density is less in magnitude and more restricted in spatial extent, it is easier to accommodate life-support equipment. The design of these units allows more access to the patient and reduces the chances of interference with the proper operation of the life-support electronics. Thus, installation of a low-field MRI scanner in the emergency department becomes more feasible. However, because of theoretical considerations, signal to noise is much less (i.e., less signal) at low field. Therefore, there may be trade-off in diagnostic quality of the scans. Some signal can be recovered with optimal design of the software and hardware, but this remains a controversial area. There may be a place for low-field MRI in the emergent setting in the evaluation of subacute intracerebral hemorrhage and brain edema.

MR angiography, which (except for innocuous intravenous contrast) is noninvasive, has been evolving slowly and improving steadily.[5,21,22] It may eventually be the method of choice in the emergent evaluation of suspected subarachnoid hemorrhage or in leaking aortic aneurysms. An example of a normal noncontrast MR angiogram is shown in Fig. 297-6.

Recent developments in echo planar and diffusion imaging make it possible to diagnose cytotoxic cerebral edema almost immediately after an acute ischemic event, even earlier than with CT or conventional MRI.[23] This has obvious implications with the advent of more aggressive lytic therapy aimed at early salvage of brain tissue after strokes.

MRI continues to evolve with more potential applications to emergency medicine in addition to its role in spinal cord compression, radiographically occult fractures, and acute aortic dissection. The new areas are diffusion imaging (to detect early strokes), noninvasive cerebral and body MRI angiography, and in the future cardiac and pulmonary MRI angiography. Taking advantage of its compatibility with life support equipment, further development of a low magnetic field system with improved signal to noise might accelerate introduction of the above applications into emergency medicine practice.

REFERENCES

1. Lauterbur PC: Image formation by induced local interactions: Example employing nuclear magnetic resonance. *Nature* 242:190, 1973.
2. Kumar A, Welti D, Ernst RR: NMR fourier zeugmatography. *J Mag Res* 18:69, 1975.
3. Bloch F, Hansen WW, Packard M: Nuclear induction. *Phys Rev* 69:127, 1946.
4. Purcell EM, Torrey HC, Pound RV: Resonance absorption by nuclear magnetic moments in a solid. *Phys Rev* 69:37, 1946.
5. Stark DD, Bradley WG Jr (eds): *Magnetic Resonance Imaging,* 3d ed. St. Louis, Mosby, 1999.
6. Stoller DW (ed): *Magnetic Resonance Imaging in Orthopaedics and Sports Medicine.* Philadelphia, Lippincott-Raven, 1997.
7. Shellock FG, Kanal E: *Magnetic Resonance: Bioeffects, Safety, and Patient Management.* New York, Raven Press, 1994.
8. Shellock FG, Kanal E: Magnetic resonance: Bioeffects and safety, in Stoller DW (ed): *Magnetic Resonance Imaging in Orthopaedics and Sports Medicine.* Philadelphia, Lippincott-Raven, 1997, pp 23–56.
9. Atlas SW (ed): *Magnetic Resonance of the Brain and Spine,* 2d ed. Philadelphia, Lippincott-Raven, 1996.
10. Murphy KJ, Brunberg JA, Cohan RH: Adverse reactions to Gadolinium contrast media: A review of 36 cases. *AJR* 167:847, 1996.
11. Fulcher AS, Turner MA, Capps GW, et al: Half-fourier RARE MR cholangiopancreatography: Experience in 300 subjects. *Radiology* 207:21, 1998.
12. Boxt LM (ed): Cardiac MR imaging. *MRI Clin North Am* 4:191, 1996.
13. Kellman GM, Kneeland JB, Middleton WD, et al: MR imaging of the supraclavicular region: Normal anatomy. *AJR* 148:77, 1987.
14. Kneeland JB, Kellman GM, Middleton WD, et al: Diagnosis of diseases of the supraclavicular region by use of MR imaging. *AJR* 148:1149, 1987.
15. Erdman WA, Tamburro F, Jayson HT, et al: Osteomyelitis: Characteristics and pitfalls of diagnosis with MR imaging. *Radiology* 180:533, 1991.
16. Morrison WB, Schweitzer ME: Diagnosis of osteomyelitis: Utility of fat-suppressed contrast-enhanced MR imaging. *Radiology* 189:251, 1993.
17. Ma LD, et al: CT and MRI evaluation of musculoskeletal infection. *Crit Rev Diagn Imaging* 38:535, 1997.
18. Deutsch AL, Mink JH, Waxman AD: Occult fractures of the proximal femur: MR imaging. *Radiology* 170:113, 1989.
19. Quinn SF, McCarthy JL: Prospective evaluation of patients with suspected hip fracture and indeterminate radiographs: Use of T1-weighted MR images. *Radiology* 187:469, 1993.
20. Jaramillo D, Shapiro F: Musculoskeletal Trauma in Children. *MRI Clin North Am* 6(3):521, 1998.
21. Krinsky G (ed): Magnetic resonance angiography of the body. *MRI Clin North Am* 6(2):223, 1998.
22. Litt A (ed): Magnetic resonance angiography of the central nervous system. *MRI Clin North Am* 3(3):375, 1995.
23. Gray L, MacFall J: Overview of diffusion imaging. *MRI Clin North Am* 6:125, 1998.

INTRAVENOUS DRUG USERS

Sarah A. Stahmer
Suzanne M. Shepherd

The practice of intravenous injection and the lifestyle of the intravenous drug user (IVDU), place the individual at risk for a wide variety of infectious and noninfectious complications.[1–3] In addition to those entities typically associated with IV drug use, such as endocarditis and hepatitis, IV drug use remains one of the greatest risk factors for acquiring the human immunodeficiency virus (HIV). The lifestyle associated with IV drug use increases the risk of trauma and sexually transmitted diseases. This population is also is placed at risk by a high incidence of homelessness, nutritional deficiencies, smoking and alcohol use, and mental illness.

Complications of the IVDU may be obvious from the start, such as a painful swelling due to a skin abscess. However, constitutional symptoms such as weakness, anorexia, body pains, weight loss, and fever are common and may be the only subtle sign(s) of serious underlying disease (Table 298-1).

It is estimated that over 2.5 million individuals have used IV drugs in the United States alone,[4] and the emergency department (ED) is a common the point of entry to health care.[5] Health care providers should be aware of drugs used in their catchment area and the street names and preparation and use rituals for those drugs. IVDUs should be asked about drug type(s) and amount, preparation of materials for injection (e.g., spitting on needles or use of saliva for drug reconstitution, reuse of needles), needle sharing, use of antibiotics, and coincident illness. Socioeconomic issues such as the IVDU's ability to purchase medications and return for follow-up also must be addressed when making dispositions. The IVDU patient should receive nonjudgmental instruction in measures to reduce their risk of complications and infections.

PATHOPHYSIOLOGY

A number of markers of immune dysfunction have been described in IVDUs separate from those produced by coincident HIV infection, other viral infections, or liver disease:

1. Exaggerated lymphocytosis and atypical lymphocytosis
2. Diminished lymphocyte responsiveness to mitogenic stimulation
3. Immunoglobulin G (IgG) and IgM hypergammaglobulinemia and increased opsonin production
4. A higher incidence of false-positive complement fixation tests for syphilis and febrile agglutinins

The use of IV drugs continues to play a major role in the acquisition and spread of HIV. In the United States, the proportion of AIDS cases directly attributable to IV drug use is estimated to exceed 30 percent, and HIV seroprevalence rates in IVDUs are as high as 10 to 50 percent.[6] In addition to transmission among IVDUs, HIV also can be spread to their sex partners and offspring. Transmission of HIV infection in IVDUs accelerated dramatically in the 1980s, largely due to the widespread use of injectable cocaine. Cocaine, by virtue of its highly addictive properties and short duration of effect, encourages frequent injections and widespread sharing of injection paraphernalia.

The prevalence of HIV in IVDUs has expanded the spectrum of diseases associated with IV drug use to include those typically associated with HIV infection.[7] HIV infection dramatically increases the probability of activation of latent *Mycobacterium tuberculosis* infection in IV drug users.[8] In addition, new tuberculosis infection is more likely to progress to active disease in HIV-infected drug users. AIDS-defining illnesses that present in IV drug users are similar in spectrum to those in non-IV drug users, but the distribution of such diseases appears to be different. IVDUs have proportionally more cryptococcal disease, *Pneumocystis carinii* pneumonia, tuberculosis, and wasting syndrome, and significantly less cytomegalovirus (CMV) infection, non-Hodgkin's lymphoma and Kaposi's sarcoma.[9] HIV-positive IVDUs also appear to be at increased risk of acquiring bacterial infections, such as skin abscesses, pneumonia, and endocarditis.[10–12] It has been hypothesized that HIV infection, even in the early stages, leads to early loss of regulation of immunoglobulin production, resulting in an ineffective response to bacterial infections. Greater immunosuppression, as defined by lower CD4 counts, is associated with both an increased risk of developing and dying from endocarditis. In those studies specifically comparing endocarditis in HIV- and non-HIV-infected IV drug users, there was no detectable differences in types of infecting organisms, frequency of right- and left-sided valve involvement, and duration of fever.

CLINICAL FEATURES

Fever

Fever is part of the presenting complaint in the majority of ED visits by IVDUs.[5,13–16] Fever is associated with infection in over two-thirds of patients. Prospective studies of febrile IVDUs have found bacteremia in up to 42 percent, pneumonia in 26 to 38 percent, and endocarditis in 6 to 13 percent.[13–16] These studies found that neither clinical judgment nor derived predictive rules were reliable in identifying those with serious underlying causes of fever.[13–16] While an elevated erythrocyte sedimentation rate (ESR) of greater that 100 mm/h is associated with serious infections in febrile IVDUs, a normal ESR does not reliably exclude serious disease.[17]

Noninfectious causes of fever in the IVDU include acute toxic reactions to substances of abuse, reactions to injected adulterants, and withdrawal syndromes. Cocaine and amphetamines can cause fevers acutely, occasionally in excess of 40°C (104°F). Adulterants used to dilute active substances can cause dramatic febrile reactions accompanied by alteration in mental status and leukocytosis.[18] One syndrome, associated with the use of cotton balls as filters for drug suspensions, is called *cotton fever.*[19] Patients with cotton fever develop high fever, chills, headache, dyspnea, myalgias, arthralgias, nausea, and vomiting within hours after injection. Physical findings may include tachypnea, tachycardia, abdominal pain, and inflammatory retinal nodules. Chest radiography may reveal inflammatory pulmonary granulomata. This is a self-limited syndrome that resolves completely within 24 h. While the cause of this syndrome remains unclear, it has been proposed that the acute symptoms are due to either endotoxin from gram-negative rods introduced by injection or the pyrogenic effect of injected cotton particulate matter. Patients withdrawing from barbiturates or heroin also may appear acutely ill, with chest and abdominal pain, diaphoresis, tachycardia, and fever.

Since there are no reliable markers excluding serious underlying disease in the febrile IVDU, common practice has been to obtain blood cultures and admit such patients for observation, awaiting culture results. In those patients for whom follow-up can be ensured and who

TABLE 298-1 Evaluation of IVDUs in the ED

Presenting Symptom	Other Findings	Possible Diagnosis	Ancillary Tests
Fever alone	Needle and track marks Heart murmur Rales and rhonchi Hypoxia	Pneumonia Endocarditis Occult bacteremia	Chest radiograph Blood cultures Urinalysis Erythrocyte sedimentation rate Echocardiogram
Fever and nausea/vomiting Rigors Abdominal pain	Diaphoresis Recent injection	Drug withdrawal "Cotton fever"	CBC Blood cultures
Fever and dyspnea/cough	Rales/rhonchi Purulent sputum Hypoxia	Bacterial pneumonia Atypical pneumonia Opportunistic pneumonia	Chest radiograph Blood cultures Sputum culture and gram-stain
Fever and weakness Weight loss Anorexia Night sweats Diarrhea	Cachexia Oral thrush	HIV infection Tuberculosis Hepatitis B and C	HIV serology Blood cultures Chest radiograph Sputum for AFB stain and culture Hepatitis serology
Fever and back pain	Heart murmur Focal neurologic signs Flank tenderness	Osteomyelitis Epidural abscess Endocarditis Renal abscess	Blood cultures Erythrocyte sedimentation rate Bone radiographs CT or MRI Urinalysis
Dyspnea/cough	Expiratory wheezes Rales/rhonchi Fever Pleuritic chest pain	Hypersensitivity reaction Non-cardiogenic pulmonary edema Pneumonia Septic pulmonary emboli Talc reaction	Chest radiograph Spirometry Echocardiogram Consider blood cultures
Painful limb	Localized erythema Tenderness Localized bruit Muscle pain/swelling Fever	Cellulitis Abscess Pseudoaneurysm Myositis Fasciitis Retained foreign body	Wound cultures Soft tissue radiographs CT Doppler ultrasound Consider blood cultures
Altered mental status	Obtundation Focal neurologic signs Meningismus Seizure	Drug overdose/intoxication Drug withdrawal CNS lesion Meningitis Tetanus	CT scan Drug screen Lumbar puncture Consider blood cultures
Eye pain/vision loss	Periorbital vesicles Subconjunctival lesions Keratitis Iridocyclitis Retinitis	Herpes zoster Kaposi's sarcoma Keratoconjunctivitis sicca Herpes simplex CMV Varicella-Zoster Toxoplasmosis Syphilis Fungal infection	

appear clinically well, outpatient evaluation is reasonable as long as an adequate number of cultures are obtained.[14]

Dyspnea

A wide range of both infectious and noninfectious causes may produce dyspnea and cough. The febrile IVDU with dyspnea and/or cough should be assumed to have tuberculosis until an alternative diagnosis is found, particularly those with known or suspected HIV.[20] Other common causes of dyspnea include both community-acquired and opportunistic pneumonia and septic pulmonary emboli from right-sided endocarditis. Opportunistic infections, such as *P. carinii* pneumonia, reflect the prevalence of HIV disease in this patient group.

Noninfectious causes of dyspnea include pneumothorax, hemothorax, and toxic reactions to injected substances.[21] Pneumo- and hemothorax are seen most commonly with the practice of "pocket shooting." As drug users run out of easily accessible veins, they will inject into veins in the supraclavicular fossa to access the subclavian, jugular, or brachiocephalic vein. When talc is injected, it can cause a syndrome of progressive respiratory distress and diffuse interstitial infiltrates known as *talc lung.*[22] Hypersensitivity reactions, associated with both heroin and cocaine injection, present with cough and wheezing and usually respond to inhaled beta-agonist therapy. Noncardiogenic pulmonary edema also has been described in association with heroin and cocaine use. Patients complain of dyspnea, and chest radiographs reveal diffuse alveolar infiltrates. Needles breaking off in the peripheral circulation can embolize into the lungs.[23] Pericarditis also has been reported secondary to central migration of a needle fragment.

Altered Mental Status

Causes of altered mental status include drug intoxication or withdrawal, stroke syndromes, hypoxia, delayed leukoencephalopathy, infectious diseases, mycotic aneurysms, and secondary trauma from either loss of consciousness and fall or drug-related violence.[24] CNS infections occur as primary infections, as embolic complications of distant infections (e.g., endocarditis), and as extensions of local vertebral osteomyelitis. Infections commonly seen in this population include epidural abscess, bacterial meningitis, fungal meningitis, and brain abscess. Bacterial meningitis is usually caused by meningococcus, pneumococcus, or *Staphylococcus aureus* spreading from a primary endocarditis. Patients also may develop mycotic aneurysms or meningitis due to coincident brain or epidural abscess or as an inflammatory response to microemboli and bacteremia from endocarditis. In addition, CNS infection may occur from opportunistic organisms in the patient with coincident HIV infection.

Stroke syndromes have been well-reported complications secondary to low-flow states during heroin intoxication, hypertensive hemorrhage from amphetamines, phencyclidine, or cocaine, and embolized vegetations from infectious endocarditis. Delayed leukoencephalopathies, both hypoxia-related and unrelated to hypoxia, have been reported in IVDUs but are rare.[25]

Back Pain

Epidural abscess is characterized by a chronic course of 1 to 15 months in most patients. However, a more acute course with pain, paraplegia, and urinary incontinence developing over several hours to days can occur. The earliest and most prominent symptom is localized pain, which may develop a radicular component. Cerebrospinal fluid (CSF) analysis often demonstrates a mononuclear pleocytosis and increased protein. Myelography, computed tomography (CT), and magnetic resonance imaging (MRI) can help to define the extent of infection. *S. aureus* and *Pseudomonas aeruginosa* are the most commonly reported bacterial isolates. *M. tuberculosis* also has been reported in those concurrently infected with HIV. Emergent neurosurgical evaluation should be obtained for adequate drainage and decompression of these lesions.

SPECIFIC INFECTIONS

Endocarditis

The incidence of endocarditis in the IVDU has been estimated to be 30 times that of the general population, or approximately 1.4 cases per 10,000 patients per year. Patients with IVDU-related endocarditis usually have no evidence of prior valve damage. Several mechanisms have been proposed by which IVDU contributes to endocardial injury. Talc, a common contaminant of injected material, has been recovered from subendothelial granulations during autopsy of IVDUs. In animal studies, valvular inflammation has been seen after repeated injection with horse serum or dead streptococci, suggesting that frequent antigenic exposure may produce valvular damage. Lastly, IV cocaine use has been associated with increased risk of endocarditis compared with other drugs. A likely basis for this increased risk is the fact that cocaine users inject more frequently, exposing the valves to frequent bacteremia and showers of particulate matter. Cocaine users are less likely to sterilize needles because cocaine does not need to be heated to go into solution. Furthermore, cocaine users are more likely to share needles and be injected by communal needles in "shooting galleries." An alternative explanation is that the vasoconstrictive properties of cocaine may cause interstitial or endothelial damage, predisposing to infection.

The cardinal sign of endocarditis in the IVDU is fever. There may be foci of infection, such as dental abscess, cellulitis, or septic pulmonary emboli. A cardiac murmur is present in over one-half of patients with endocarditis.[27] Right-sided murmurs, which vary with respiration, are usually pathologic and more specific for the diagnosis. Cough, pleuritic chest pain, and hemoptysis are common presenting complaints, particularly in patients with right-sided cardiac infection and septic pulmonary emboli. Pulmonary infiltrates on chest radiographs, associated with moderate hypoxia, have been described in over one-third of patients with IVDU-related endocarditis. Pulmonary findings may falsely lead the clinician to identify the lung as the primary source of infection. Pyuria and hematuria are ascribed to glomerulonephritis, embolic renal infarction, and perinephric abscess.

Blood cultures will be positive in over 98 percent of cases of IVDU-related endocarditis if three to five sets are obtained. True culture-negative endocarditis in the setting of high clinical suspicion and careful laboratory procedure is rare. *S. aureus* has been isolated from blood cultures in over half of patients. Up to one-third of *S. aureus* isolates, particularly those reported from large urban areas, are methicillin-resistant. *Streptococcus* is the second most frequently reported isolate, particularly *S. viridens. S. aureus* has a predilection for the tricuspid valve, whereas streptococci are more likely to involve left-sided structures.

Other less commonly isolated organisms include enterococci and gram-negative bacteria, particularly *P. aeruginosa, Serratia marcescens,* and *Klebsiella pneumoniae.* Other organisms, less frequently identified as causative agents, usually reflect local environmental pathogens or drug-injecting habits. For example, licking the needles prior to injection has been implicated in infections that result from oral pathogens such as *Eikinella corrodens, Hemophilus parainfluenzae, Bacterioides* spp. and *Neisseria* spp. Up to 20 percent of IVDU-related endocarditis is polymicrobial in nature. Although rare, fungal endocarditis has been reported increasingly. Most fungal infections are due to *Candida* spp., in particular *C. parapsilosis,* which accounts for over half of all isolates.

Although right-sided cardiac structures have been associated with IVDU-related endocarditis, any valve potentially can be involved. The tricuspid valve is infected in 40 to 50 percent, the mitral valve in 30 to 40 percent, the aortic valve in 10 to 20 percent, and multiple locations in 10 to 20 percent. Four types of valvular lesions have been described, vegetations, ring abscesses, cuspal tears or perforations, and ruptured chordae tendineae.

Diagnosis generally requires microbial isolation from a blood culture, which typically takes at least 24 h, and/or the ability to demonstrate typical lesions on echocardiography.[16] The classic findings of embolic phenomena, Janeway lesions and Roth spots, are usually not observed until the infection is advanced.

A complete blood count (CBC), chest x-ray, and urinalysis are useful screens, although no single abnormality is specific for endocarditis. Chest radiographs will be abnormal in over 50 percent of patients, and typical findings include infiltrates consistent with septic emboli, pneumonia, or congestive heart failure.

Transthoracic echocardiography (TTE) will reveal diagnostic cardiac lesions up to 80 percent of the time in patients (both IVDU and non-IVDU) in whom the diagnosis is strongly suspected. Transesophageal echocardiography (TEE) is the most sensitive imaging modality for demonstrating vegetations, myocardial and ring abscesses, and tricuspid valve involvement in IVDU-related endocarditis. The timing of echocardiography is debatable. Some echocardiographers advocate early imaging to confirm the diagnosis of endocarditis. Others have suggested that imaging should be performed only on those patients who have positive blood cultures, to assist in determining disease response to therapy and length of treatment.

Attempts to develop criteria that would prospectively identify endocarditis in the IVDU in the ED. with reasonable certainty have failed.[13–16] Generally, patients with suspected endocarditis should be cultured and admitted to the hospital. The need for empirical antibiotic therapy should be determined by the patient's clinical stability and ability to wait 24 h for the initial results of blood cultures. Treatment should be directed to *S. aureus* and *Streptococcus* spp., with consideration of local sensitivities and pathogens. Vancomycin or nafcillin and gentamicin are often initial therapy. The addition of an aminoglycoside has been shown to shorten the duration of bacteremia and duration of treatment in patients with *S. aureus* infections. Although 4 to 6 weeks of antibiotic therapy is standard, excellent cure rates have been achieved with only 2 weeks of treatment for patients with right-sided endocarditis caused by sensitive *S. aureus.*

Complications of endocarditis range from pump failure secondary to valve insufficiency, dysrhythmias due to myocardial infiltration, and pulmonary and systemic emboli. Mortality is related to the side of the heart involved, vegetation size, response to antibiotics, and compliance with treatment. Left-sided endocarditis is more likely to be complicated by left-sided congestive heart failure, septic cerebral emboli, and the need for surgery. Overall mortality for IVDU-related left-sided endocarditis is 14 to 21 percent, compared with 2 to 7 percent for IVDUs with right-sided endocarditis. Emboli can travel to the extremities, pulmonary bed, spleen, kidney, or brain. With right-sided endocarditis, septic pulmonary emboli occur in 30 to 60 percent of patients. Most complications related to right-sided endocarditis can be managed medically, and the prognosis is excellent. Valve replacement should be considered for those patients with congestive heart failure, failure to respond to antibiotics, myocardial abscess, or recurrent embolization. Early echocardiography can be instrumental in identifying those patients at risk for embolic events by identifying large (>2.0 cm) vegetations on valve leaflets.

Pulmonary Infections

S. pneumoniae and *H. influenzae* are frequent causes, and in those with septic emboli or endocarditis, *S. aureus* should be considered. Aspiration may result in infection with *S. pneumoniae*, polymicrobial oral flora, *S. aureus,* or *Pseudomonas* spp. *P. carinii,* cytomegalovirus, or atypical mycobacteria should be considered in HIV-positive patients. Drug-resistant tuberculosis also should be strongly considered. IVDU patients are also more likely to have extrapulmonary tuberculosis, including infection in cervical lymph nodes, CNS, bone, abdomen, genitourinary system, pericardium, skin, and the eyes.[28]

Because of the risk of atypical infection, coincident bacteremia, and endocarditis, admission to the hospital is recommended in all patients with pneumonia or other pulmonary infection. Patients should be placed on respiratory isolation until tuberculosis has been excluded.

Skin and Soft Tissue Infections

Unique features of skin infections in the IVDU[29,30] are (1) a high rate of skin and pharyngeal colonization with *S. aureus* and streptococcal species, (2) the high frequency with which cutaneous abscesses are due to oral flora,[31] and (3) the fact that infection with HIV also confers an additional risk for the development of skin abscesses.[10] The IVDU will self-inject, often multiple times a day, with unsterile needles, which may be licked prior to injection. Tap or toilet water or saliva often is used to dissolve narcotics, and each has been implicated as harboring the causative agent in both skin and blood-borne infections. Female gender is associated with increased incidence of skin infections, due to a relatively high rate of skin injection (skin popping).

Local infections of the skin and soft tissue include cellulitis, subcutaneous abscesses, septic phlebitis, necrotizing fasciitis, Fournier's gangrene, gas gangrene, and pyomyositis. Cellulitis is typically due to *S. aureus* and *Streptococcus* spp. Cultures from cutaneous abscesses are often polymicrobial, with aerobic gram-negative rods, anaerobic cocci, and bacilli.[31] Quinine, which is often used to ''cut'' heroin, can increase the risk of abscess formation. The extensive interconnected abscesses produced by skin popping provide ideal growth conditions for *Clostridium botulinum* and *C. tetani.* Broken needles lodged in the skin are foreign bodies that stimulate infection.[32] Groin injection has been associated with local gangrene and also the development of rapidly progressive and fatal Fournier's gangrene. Cutaneous abscesses in the neck may involve the carotid triangle and produce airway obstruction, vocal cord paralysis, and laryngeal edema.

Presenting signs and symptoms of cutaneous infections, including pyomyositis, are fever, pain, localized erythema, and edema. The painful area should be carefully inspected for fluctuance, crepitance, and lymphangitis. Infections over venipuncture sites suggest infected pseudoaneurysms. Pulsatile masses should be imaged with ultrasonography prior to incision and drainage, as attempts to aspirate or incise and drain an infected pseudoaneurysm can result in significant hemorrhage. Angiography may be required to identify vasospasm, thrombosis, emboli, mycotic aneurysms, or septic hematomas. Plain radiographs can demonstrate air in the soft tissues, which may be present even when localized tenderness and erythema are the only findings. CT is useful to clearly delineate the involvement of other structures and the extent of deep abscesses, especially in complex areas such as the neck. Whenever crepitus or subcutaneous air is detected or deep tissue or muscle involvement is suspected clinically, a prompt surgical consultation for possible exploration or debridement is appropriate. Wound botulism and tetanus have been reported in IVDUs.[33,34]

IVDUs with superficial cellulitis and no evidence of systemic involvement can be managed as outpatients. Empirical antibiotic choices should cover streptococci and staphylococci, and tetanus immunization should be updated. Febrile or toxic-appearing patients or those not responding to outpatient treatment should be admitted to the hospital. Blood and wound cultures should be obtained, and broad-spectrum intravenous antibiotics should be initiated pending culture results. For such patients, coverage should include a penicillinase-resistant synthetic penicillin or vancomycin plus an antipseudomonal aminoglycoside, antipseudomonal penicillin, or cephalosporin.Surgical consultation is needed for deep tissue and necrotizing soft tissue infections.

Vascular Infections

Vascular injury associated with IVDU includes inadvertent arterial injection with resultant vasospasm or thrombosis, septic thrombophlebitis, venous and arterial pseudoaneurysms and infected hematomas. Arterial injection rarely results in major vessel occlusion; instead, a commonly observed effect is pain, edema, and patchy mottling of the affected limb due to ischemia.[35] Peripheral pulses are usually preserved. Tissue necrosis and gangrene are the consequence of persistent focal ischemia. The etiology is thought to be a combination of vasospasm of distal vessels, embolization of particulate matter, and endothelial injury leading to thrombosis and vasculitis.[36]

For limb ischemia, the vascular surgeon should be involved early to decide if surgical intervention or intraarterial thrombolysis is indicated. However, the majority of cases involve distal vessels, and treatment is primarily supportive medical management with heparinization. Limb edema can progress to compartment syndrome or rhabdomyolysis. Fasciotomy may be required for compartment syndrome. For patients who develop rhabdomyolysis, careful monitoring of fluid balance and renal function is required.

Infected pseudoaneurysm is one of the most common vascular complications reported in IVDUs.[37,38] Although pseudoaneurysms can form in any artery, they are most often reported in the femoral, followed by the radial and brachial arteries. Venous pseudoaneurysms are relatively rare and are usually secondary to septic phlebitis. The femoral vein is the vessel most often involved. Patients with either infected arterial or venous pseudoaneurysms usually present with fever and a painful mass, typically in the groin. Although similar in gross appearance to an abscess, the presence of pulsations and often a bruit should suggest this diagnosis. Because of the disastrous hemorrhagic consequences of attempted incision and drainage or medical management with a course of antibiotics, all painful masses, particularly in the groin, should be imaged, usually with duplex ultrasonography. Treatment for infected pseudoaneurysm usually involves resection of the infected vessel. Broad-spectrum antibiotics should be initiated in the ED and should cover the most likely organisms. Early revascularization at the time of resection of the pseudoaneurysm may be necessary.[39]

Bone and Joint Infections

Bone and joint infections usually occur from (1) contiguous spread from an overlying skin or soft tissue infection or (2) hematogenous spread from a distant site. Infecting microorganisms tend to be unusual compared with the general population, with *Candida* and gram-negative organisms the most common examples. In IVDUs, osteomyelitic lesions are seen more frequently in the axial skeleton than in the bones of the extremities.[40]

Pyogenic infections are the predominant type seen involving bones and joints. In contrast to the general population, in which approximately two-thirds of bony infections are caused by *S. aureus,* the infecting organisms in an IVDU with osteomyelitis or septic arthritis is more likely to be polymicrobial and involve uncommon organisms, although recent studies have demonstrated an increasing frequency of *S. aureus* and groups A and G streptococcal bone infections in IVDUs. One also must consider gonococcal arthritis and tenosynovitis because of the high incidence of sexually transmitted diseases in this population. *E. corrodens* osteomyelitis also has been reported in IVDUs who lick their needles prior to injection. Nonpyogenic organisms may cause osteomyelitis and septic arthritis in IVDUs. Mycobacterial infections usually involve the ribs and vertebral column (Pott's disease). Symptoms include night sweats, fevers, weight loss, and localized pain. These are often associated with systemic involvement of the lungs, CNS, pelvic organs, and adrenal glands. *Candida* spp. have been reported with incidences as high as 20 percent in osteomyelitis in these patients.[41] Candidal infections are postulated to spread hematogenously. Some patients report an initial syndrome of high fever, headache, and myalgia lasting 3 to 4 days, followed by the appearance of metastatic lesions involving the skin, eye (choreoretinitis and endophthalmitis), and the bones and joints several days to weeks later. Rarely, *Aspergillus* spp. may cause osteomyelitis of the sternum in these patients.[40]

IVDU-related osteomyelitis is more likely to involve the vertebral column, particularly the lumbar segments.[42] Collected series have tabulated that 53 percent of all bony infections involved the vertebral column, 18 percent involved the sternoclavicular joint, and 17 percent involved the extremities, particularly the hip and knee joints.

Vertebral osteomyelitis usually presents with localized pain and tenderness to palpation over the involved bone. A soft tissue mass may be palpable, which in the case of *Candida* may not exhibit evidence of inflammation. Symptoms may be present for days in the case of bacterial infections to weeks in the case of fungal or mycobacterial infections. Many patients will exhibit neither fever nor leukocytosis. An elevated ESR is helpful if present, but its absence does not exclude these infections. If present, drainage from contiguous abscesses should be cultured. Biopsy or needle aspiration may be necessary for joint space and bony infections, especially in the case of unusual or fastidious organisms, such as *Mycobacterium, Candida,* or *Eikenella.* Appropriate imaging for osteomyelitis will vary with institution; however, MRI and CT are both useful. Patients with osteomyelitis warrant admission. Unless the patient appears septic or coincident endocarditis is a concern, antibiotic administration should be based on culture results. Antibiotic treatment will usually continue for 4 to 6 weeks.

Septic arthritis in the IVDU usually involves the knee or hip. Sternoclavicular infectious arthritis is also well described in this population and, if found, should strongly suggest IVDU. Patients often will note a recent history of trauma to the area, but causality has yet to be proven. Patients will note pain, localized tenderness, and swelling at the sites. The ESR is usually elevated, and fever and leukocytosis are usually present. Up to 80 percent will have normal plain radiographs; however, joint space widening, articular surface erosion, and surrounding soft tissue infection may be noted. Bone scans are often positive early in the process, and these infections also may be delineated with CT or MRI. The most sensitive but nonspecific finding on synovial fluid analysis is a white blood cell count greater than 20,000/mL with a predominance of neutrophils. Gram stain of the synovial fluid may aid in antibiotic selection. Immobilization, physical therapy, therapeutic arthrocentesis, and occasionally open drainage of a septic hip may be warranted.

Hepatic Disease

The IVDU may develop liver disease, including cirrhosis, from both parenterally and sexually transmitted hepatitis A, B, C, and G virus as well as the delta virus.[43–45] It is estimated that over 80 percent of IVDUs have had hepatitis, with the majority of reported cases due to hepatitis B and C. These patients frequently progress to chronic active hepatitis with a high mortality. When an IVDU patient presents with the clinical syndrome of acute hepatitis, appropriate laboratory testing includes serum transaminases, bilirubin levels, alkaline phosphatase, prothrombin time, and serologic testing. If other significant disease can be excluded, most can be managed as outpatients. Admission criteria include inability to tolerate oral intake, toxicity, and prolonged prothrombin time with bleeding. Patients should be counseled on both sexual contact and needle exposure and should be encouraged to inform all sexual and needle partners and household contacts of exposure. Seronegative patients should receive hepatitis B and A immunization.[43,44]

Ophthalmologic Infections

Ophthalmologic infections in the IVDU are usually the result of hematogenous seeding from a primary source of infection, such as endocarditis, or of opportunistic infections associated with coincident HIV disease. Bacterial endophthlamitis often presents acutely, with rapid progression of pain, redness, lid swelling, and decrease in visual acuity.[46] Inflammation is usually present in the anterior and posterior chambers. White-centered, flame-shaped hemorrhages (Roth spots), cotton wool exudates, and macular holes may be present. *S. aureus* is the most commonly isolated organism, followed by *Streptococcus* sp. A rare but rapidly destructive infection has been reported with *Bacillus cereus.* Treatment involves subconjunctival and systemic antibiotic therapy; surgical intervention may be needed. Fungal endophthalmitis, usually due to *Candida,* is more common than bacterial endophthalmitis. The clinical picture is often indolent, progressing over days to weeks. Symptoms include blurred vision, pain, and decreased visual acuity. White cotton-like lesions are seen on the choroid retina, with vitreous haziness. Uveitis, papillitis, and vitritis also have been reported.

Since 1980, a marked increase in *Candida* sp. infections has been reported in those individuals who use brown heroin. *Candida* chorioretinitis or endophthalmitis in these individuals is characterized by the appearance of a high fever, followed in 3 to 4 days by the appearance of ocular symptoms, cutaneous lesions, and costochondral involvement. Aspergillosis is the second most common fungal cause of endophthalmitis in IVDUs. Initial complaints often include decreased visual acuity, pain, and conjunctival injection. The physical examination may reveal iritis, vitritis, vitreal mass, or hyphema. The treatment is similar to that for *Candida.* The prognosis for both infections depends on prompt diagnosis and treatment. Fungal endophthalmitis secondary to *Torulopsis, Helminthosporium,* and *Penicillium* sp. also has been reported. As the incidence of HIV in these patients has increased, an increased frequency of cytomegalovirus, toxoplasmosis retinitis, and choroidal *Cryptococcus* and *Mycobacterium avium intracellulare* infections have been reported.

REFERENCES

1. Stein MD: Medical complications of intravenous drug use. *J Gen Intern Med* 5:249, 1990.
2. Cherubin CE, Sapira JD: The medical complications of drug addiction and the medical assessment of the intravenous drug user: 25 years later. *Ann Intern Med* 119:1017, 1993.
3. O'Connor PG, Samet JH, Stein MD: Management of hospitalized intravenous drug users: Role of the internist. *Am J Med* 96:551, 1994.
4. National Institute on Drug Abuse: *National Household Survey on Drug Abuse: Population Estimates 1990.* Washington, DC, US Department of Health and Human Services, publication no (ADM) 91-1732, 1991.
5. Makower RM, Pennycook AG, Moulton C: Intravenous drug abusers attending an inner city accident and emergency department. *Arch Emerg Med* 9:346, 1992.
6. Centers for Disease Control and Prevention: *HIV/AIDS Surveillance Report,* no 2. Atlanta, Centers for Disease Control and Prevention, 1995, p 7.
7. O'Connor PG, Selwyn PA, Schottenfeld RS: Medical care for injection-drug users with human immunodeficiency virus infection. *N Engl J Med* 331:450, 1994.
8. Selwyn PA, Hartel D, Lewis Va, et al: A prospective study of the risk of tuberculosis among intravenous drug users with human immunodeficiency virus infection. *New Engl J Med* 320:545, 1989.
9. Greenberg AE, Thomas PA, Landesman SH, et al: The spectrum of HIV-1 related disease among outpatients in New York City. *AIDS* 6:849, 1992.
10. Spijkerman IJ, van Ameijden EJ, Mientjes GH, et al: Human immunodeficiency virus infection and other risk factors for skin abscesses and endocarditis among injection drug users. *J Clin Epidemiol* 49:1149, 1996.
11. Pulvirenti JJ, Kerns E, Benson C, et al: Infective endocarditis in injection drug users: Importance of human immunodeficiency virus serostatus and degree of immunosuppression. *Clin Infect Dis* 22:40, 1996.
12. Selwyn PA, Feingolf AR, Hartel D, et al: Increased risk of bacterial pneumonia in HIV-infected intravenous drug users without AIDS. *AIDS* 2:267, 1988.
13. Marantz PR, Linzer M, Feiner CJ, et al: Inability to predict diagnosis in febrile intravenous drug abusers. *Ann Intern Med* 106:823, 1987.
14. Samet JH, Shevitz A, Fowle J, Singer DE: Hospitalization decision in febrile intravenous drug users. *Am J Med* 89:53, 1990.
15. Young GP, Hedges JR, Dixon L, Reeves J: Inability to validate a predictive score for infective endocarditis in intravenous drug users. *J Emerg Med* 11:1, 1993.
16. Weisse AB, Heller DR, Schimentoi RJ, et al: The febrile parenteral drug user: A prospective study in 121 patients. *Am J Med* 94:274, 1993.
17. Gallagher EJ, Gennis P, Brroks F: Clinical use of the erythrocyte sedimentation rate in the evaluation of febrile intravenous drug users. *Ann Emerg Med* 22:776, 1993.
18. Shannon M: Clinical toxicity of cocaine adulterants. *Ann Emerg Med* 17:1243, 1988.
19. Harrison DW, Walls RM: "Cotton fever": A benign febrile syndrome in intravenous drug abusers. *J Emerg Med* 8:135, 1990.
20. Selwyn PA, Sckell B, Alcabes P, et al: High risk of active tuberculosis in HIV-infected drug users with cutaneous anergy. *JAMA* 268:504, 1992.
21. Hind CR: Pulmonary complications of intravenous drug misuse: 1. Epidemiology and non-infective complications. *Thorax* 45:891, 1990.
22. Pare JP, Gilles C, Fraser RS: Long-term follow-up of drug abusers with intravenous talcosis. *Am Rev Respir Dis* 139:233, 1989.
23. Brunette DD, Plummer DW: Pulmonary embolization of needle fragments resulting from intravenous drug abuse. *Am J Emerg Med* 6:124, 1988.
24. Hestad K, Updike M, Selnes OA, Royal W: Cognitive sequelae of repeated head injury in a population of intravenous drug abusers. *Scand J Psychol* 36:246, 1995.
25. Rizzuto N, Morbin M, Ferrari S, et al: Delayed spongiform leukoencephalopathy after heroin use. *Acta Neuropathol* 94:87, 1997.
26. Prendergast H, Jerrard D, O'Connell J: Atypical presentations of epidural abscess in intravenous drug abusers. *Am J Emerg Med* 15:158, 1997.
27. Mathew J, Addai T, Anand A, et al: Clinical features, site of involvement, bacteriologic findings, and outcome of infective endocarditis in intravenous drug users. *Arch Intern Med* 155:1641, 1995.
28. Hind CR: Pulmonary complications of intravenous drug misuse: 2. Infective and HIV related complications. *Thorax* 45:957, 1990.
29. Beaufoy A: Infections in intravenous drug users: A two-year review. *Can J Infect Control* 8:7, 1993.
30. Stone MH, Stone DH, MacGregor HA: Anatomical distribution of soft tissue sepsis sites in intravenous drug misusers attending an accident and emergency department. *Br J Addict* 85:1495, 1990.
31. Summanen PH, Talan DA, Strong C, et al: Bacteriology of skin and soft-tissue infections: Comparison of infections in intravenous drug users and individuals with no history of intravénous drug use. *Clin Infect Dis* 20(suppl 2):S279, 1995.
32. Williams MF, Eisele DW, Wyatt SH: Neck needle foreign bodies in intravenous drug abusers. *Laryngoscope* 103(1 part 1):59, 1993.
33. Passaro DJ, Benson WS, McGee J, et al: Wound botulism associated with black tar heroin among injecting drug users. *JAMA* 279:859, 1998.
34. Centers for Disease Control and Prevention: Tetanus among injecting-drug users—California, 1997. *Morb Mortal Wkly Rep* 47:149, 1998.
35. Charney MA, Stern PJ: Digital ischemia in clandestine intravenous drug users. *J Hand Surg* 16A:308, 1991.
36. Woodburn KR, Murie JA: Vascular complications of injecting drug misuse. *Br J Surg* 83:1329, 1996.
37. Welch GH, Reid DB, Pollock JG: Infected false aneurysms in the groin of intravenous drug abusers. *Br J Surg* 77:330, 1990.
38. Cheng SW, Fok M, Wong J: Infected femoral pseudoaneurysm in intravenous drug abusers. *Br J Surg* 79:510, 1992.
39. Levi N, Rordam P, Jensen LP, Schroeder TV: Femoral pseudoaneurysms in drug addicts. *Eur J Vasc Endovasc Surg* 13:361, 1997.
40. Chadrasekar PH, Narula AP: Bone and joint infections in intravenous drug abusers. *Rev Infect Dis* 8:904, 1986.
41. Bisbe J, Miro JM, Latorre X, et al: Disseminated candidiasis in addicts who use brown heroin: Report of 83 cases and review. *Clin Infect Dis* 15:910, 1992.
42. Sapico FL, Montgomerie JZ: Vertebral osteomyelitis in intravenous drug abusers: Report of three cases and review of the literature. *Rev Infect Dis* 2:196, 1980.
43. Lee WM: Hepatitis B virus infection. *N Engl J Med* 337:1733, 1997.
44. Villano SA, Nelson KE, Vlahov D, et al: Hepatitis A among homosexual men and injection drug users: More evidence for vaccination. *Clin Infect Dis* 25:726, 1997.
45. Fong TL, Lee SR, Kim JP, et al: Prevalence of hepatitis G virus among intravenous drug abusers in Los Angeles. *Clin Infect Dis* 25:165, 1997.
46. Schlossberg D, Jan AM: Endopthalmitis in intravenous drug abuse. *Ann Ophthalmol* 25:77, 1993.

THE ALCOHOL-ABUSING PATIENT

William A. Berk

Alcoholism is a ubiquitous medical and social problem that crosses social and economic boundaries. Ethanol dependence, defined as regular use resulting in tolerance to the drug and the likelihood of withdrawal symptoms if intake is suspended, is experienced at one time in their lives by 4.4 percent of Americans.[1] Ethanol abuse, affecting another 3 percent of the population,[1] is a separate problem marked by social or medical problems that result from inappropriate use of ethanol but without the presence of dependence.[1] Examples of ethanol abuse include intermittent bouts of drinking resulting in aggressive or antisocial behavior or driving while intoxicated.[1]

Although alcoholism by itself is not a medical emergency, alcohol abuse and dependence are common threads in the presentation of many conditions in the emergency department. Such presentations include trauma, infections, acute alcohol intoxication and withdrawal, hepatitis, and pancreatitis. Alcohol is often used with other drugs, including cocaine, benzodiazepines, and marijuana. Emergency physicians should recognize alcoholism as both a contributor to a patient's presenting problems and as an underlying problem requiring care itself.

Alcoholism is a "primary, chronic disease with genetic, psychosocial, and environmental factors influencing its development and manifestations. . . [and] is characterized by impaired control over drinking, preoccupation with the drug ethanol, use of ethanol despite adverse consequences, and distortions in thinking, most notably denial. Each of these symptoms may be continuous or periodic."[2] Male gender, age of 25 to 34 years, poor education, preexistent psychiatric disorder, and homelessness are common associated factors. However, alcoholism is a disorder that crosses all socioeconomic boundaries and involves all age groups. Among the homeless, estimated at 250,000 on any given night and 3 million people per year in the United States, 20 to 45 percent are alcoholics.[1] Secondary psychiatric diagnoses, including antisocial personality, mania, and schizophrenia, are more common in alcoholics than in the general population. Suicide attempts and problems with drugs other than ethanol are also common among alcoholics.

The fact that almost 10 percent of the population experience at some time ethanol-related problems means that alcoholism touches most Americans' lives at some time, whether at home, on the road, or in the workplace.

The pathogenesis of alcoholism is multifactorial, with both genetic and environmental inputs. Studies of isolated twins, adopted children, and families in general have confirmed a heritable component to alcoholism. Similarly, twin research has shown that the risk of alcoholism for an identical twin of an alcoholic is much greater than that of a fraternal twin. Close relatives of alcoholics have a fourfold risk of alcoholism over control subjects, even when they are adopted children raised away from their genetic family from birth.

DIAGNOSIS

The diagnosis of alcoholism can be self-evident or exceedingly difficult (e.g., an executive who develops confusion when hospitalized for an unrelated medical condition and is abstinent for a few days).[3] Researchers utilizing sophisticated, comprehensive, and time-consuming diagnostic instruments have found that specialty physicians, including emergency physicians, miss the diagnosis in over half of all cases. Emergency physicians can maximize their success by consistently taking a social history, by asking repeatedly and pointedly about alcohol intake in patients who present with potentially associated conditions, by consulting medical records when available, and by conferring with patients' family members and associates.

EFFECTS OF ALCOHOL ON HEALTH

Ethanol abuse and its association with trauma represent a major public health issue. Forty percent of Americans will be involved in an ethanol-related motor vehicle collision in their lifetime, and over 40 percent of fatal motor vehicle accidents are associated with use of ethanol.[1] Those who drink are also at increased risk for accidents within the home and for injuries from assault.

Alcoholics have been estimated on average to have a life span 10 to 15 years shorter than that of moderate drinkers or nondrinkers.[4] Increased mortality rates result chiefly from heart and liver disease, cancer, and accidents. Although the occurrence of coronary artery disease is decreased among alcoholics, heavy ethanol use increases the likelihood of hypertension and can cause alcoholic cardiomyopathy. Ethanol is the most common cause of liver failure both in the United States and worldwide. Fatty liver is present in virtually all alcoholics, while 10 to 35 percent develop alcoholic hepatitis. Heavy ethanol use is also associated with increased risk of cancer of the esophagus, stomach, pancreas, liver, and breast.

TABLE 299-1 Some Adverse Health Effects Associated with Ethanol Abuse and Dependence

CENTRAL NERVOUS SYSTEM
Acute intoxication
Ethanol withdrawal
Seizures
Hallucinations
Wernicke's encephalopathy
Korsakoff's psychosis
Dementia
Depression, antisocial personality, suicidal ideation
GASTROINTESTINAL
Esophageal varices
Erosive gastritis
Alcoholic hepatitis or liver failure
Peptic ulcer disease
Pancreatitis
Oropharyngeal, esophageal, gastric, hepatic and pancreatic malignancies
CARDIOVASCULAR
Hypertension
Cardiomyopathy
Stroke
Dysrhythmias associated with intoxication or withdrawal
MUSCULOSKELETAL
Fractures secondary to ethanol-associated trauma
Myopathy
ENDOCRINE OR METABOLIC
Testicular atrophy
Alcoholic ketoacidosis
Folic acid and thiamine deficiencies
HEMATOPOIETIC
Thrombocytopenia secondary to marrow suppression, folate deficiency, splenic sequestration
Anemia secondary to marrow suppression, folate deficiency, gastrointestinal bleeding, splenic sequestration
Leukopenia secondary to marrow suppression, splenic sequestration
OTHER
Fetal alcohol syndrome
Breast cancer in women

Chronic toxicity from ethanol abuse may have serious health consequences for nearly every major organ system (Table 299-1).

There is good evidence that moderate ethanol use may actually promote health. A large population-based study found that subjects who consumed between one drink per month and one drink per day had a lower mortality rate than did those who drank either more or less.[5] This is the basis for the "U-shaped" curve of mortality in relation to alcohol consumption, with mortality greatest at the lowest and highest levels of consumption and lowest in the middle, at moderate levels of consumption. Decreased mortality rates may result from diminished coronary risk among users of ethanol, apparently mediated through increased blood high-density lipoprotein levels. While this effect persists at higher levels of ethanol use, the other deleterious effects of excessive chronic use outweigh the benefits.[5]

INJURED ETHANOL-INTOXICATED PATIENTS

Alcohol is an important predisposing factor for trauma of all types, but most important as far as morbidity and mortality rates are concerned

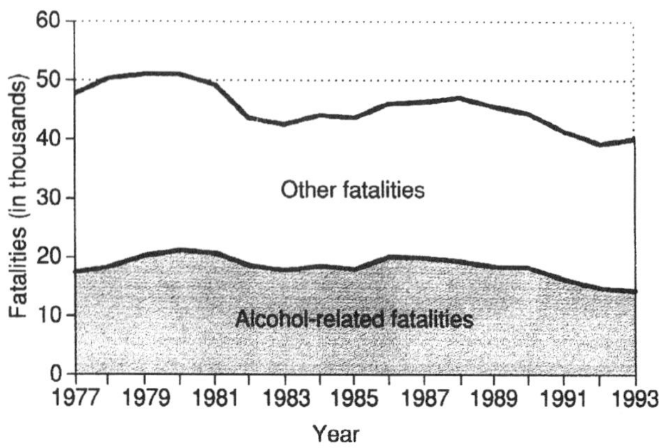

FIG. 299-1. Traffic fatalities 1977 to 1993: all versus those associated with use of alcohol. (From Campbell KE, Zobeck TS, Bertolucci D: Trends in Alcohol-Related Fatal Traffic Crashes, United States 1977–1993. Rockville, MD, National Institute on Alcohol Abuse and Alcoholism, 1995.)

is its association with motor-vehicle collisions. The proportion of fatal collisions involving a driver with a blood alcohol level greater than 10 mg/dL dropped from 51 to 41 percent between 1987 and 1996, when alcohol-related fatalities totaled 17,126 (Fig. 299-1). Nevertheless, alcohol-related motor-vehicle accidents continue to represent a significant public health problem with a large impact on emergency medicine practice.

Injured intoxicated patients present particular challenges for the clinician. In particular, the effect of ethanol on the sensorium complicates efforts at cost-effective diagnosis and treatment, since physical examination findings may be unreliable. Also, obtaining studies that require the patient's cooperation can be problematic, with the physician compelled to administer a second central nervous system depressant in order to satisfactorily evaluate injuries.

Evaluation of intoxicated head-injured patients is particularly difficult. Serious head injuries are easily overlooked in intoxicated patients, some of whom, especially in inner-city locales, may arrive at the emergency department with no definite history and no external signs of head trauma. In fact, the most common serious error made in management of intoxicated patients may be to assume for too long that a depressed or abnormal mental status is secondary to intoxication. Intoxicated patients should undergo computed tomography (CT) evaluation if there is a history of head injury and the rating on the Glasgow coma scale is less than 15; for any worsening of mental status while under observation; or if there is no improvement in mental status by 3 h after admission. Once the decision to perform CT has been made, no delay should be allowed due to lack of cooperation by the patient, which may be the result of ethanol, concomitant drug use, or head injury. Sedation may be required, with careful attention to airway protection and paralysis and intubation if necessary.

The general recognition that ethanol intoxication may also delay diagnosis of operatively remediable abdominal injuries makes it more likely that intoxicated injured patients will undergo such procedures and studies as intubation, diagnostic peritoneal lavage, and abdominal CT.[6] Such procedures and studies may not be necessary in all intoxicated patients. The results of one small study suggested that intoxicated trauma victims with a Glasgow coma scale rating of 15 and no abdominal complaints or physical findings suggestive of abdominal injury are candidates for careful observation.[7]

It is uncertain whether ethanol intoxication itself worsens the prognosis of injured patients. A study of over a million motor-vehicle accidents that attempted to control for safety-belt use, vehicle deformation, vehicle speed, and other factors found that drivers who drank were more likely to suffer a serious injury or death,[8] but other studies have found no difference in outcome for intoxicated injured patients.[9] Recent observations suggest that chronic alcoholism—but not acute alcohol intoxication—adversely affects the prognosis of injured patients.[10] These findings most likely reflect the comorbidity of underlying organ system dysfunction.

HYPOTHERMIA AND ETHANOL INTOXICATION

Most cases of hypothermia during winter months in urban settings are associated with ethanol use. Many homeless persons are heavy users of ethanol and on cold nights may employ ethanol to inure themselves to the effects of low temperature. While the sedative effects of ethanol may result in exposure predisposing to hypothermia, ethanol also directly contributes to body cooling by depressing central thermoregulatory mechanisms, decreasing shivering, and enhancing heat loss through vasodilatation. Management of the hypothermic intoxicated patient is similar to that of hypothermia in other patients. Prognosis is related to severity of hypothermia and the presence of underlying diseases, but does not appear to be adversely affected by ethanol intoxication.

ETHANOL WITHDRAWAL

Some alcoholics exhibit one or more symptoms of withdrawal upon discontinuation of ethanol intake. Symptoms and signs include tremor, anxiety, agitation, and signs of autonomic hyperactivity, including cardiac dysrhythmias, most frequently sinus tachycardia or atrial fibrillation. Seizures may occur, while hallucinations, usually visual, reflect moderate-to-severe withdrawal. Signs and symptoms of withdrawal are most likely to reach peak intensity at 48 h after the patient's last drink. There is wide variation in the timing of onset and peak severity of alcohol withdrawal, which reflects differences in patterns of ethanol intake, individual susceptibility to withdrawal, and concomitant illness. For example, significant withdrawal may occur while alcoholics still have detectable blood ethanol levels or within a short time after the last drink. Such situations probably reflect a recent pattern of decreased but continued intake of ethanol, or alcoholics' common practice of self-treatment with ethanol when symptoms first appear, followed by presentation for medical care if those symptoms fail to resolve.

Since ethanol withdrawal is a syndrome complex, more than one sign is present in most cases. When alcoholic patients present with a single sign typical of ethanol withdrawal, other causes should be considered. Seizures, in particular, can be due to other causes, most notably recent or remote head trauma, whether the patient recounts a history of head injury or not. Hallucinations may be secondary to a psychiatric disorder (although alcohol withdrawal hallucinations are more likely to be auditory, not visual) or concomitant drug use.

After the diagnosis of alcohol withdrawal is established, an examination for complicating medical conditions or injury should be performed. Patients with alcohol withdrawal may be volume depleted and require crystalloid infusion. If possible, patients should be placed in a quiet area with a minimum of stimulation. For patients who have experienced seizures, CT examination is indicated for focal seizures, when a focal neurologic finding is elicited, or when the patient has a persistent postictal defect in consciousness.[11]

Benzodiazepines are indicated for treatment of withdrawal, with most studies suggesting that lorazepam is the drug of choice, particularly in the elderly and those with significant liver disease.[12] The initial dose is 2 mg IV, followed by doses of 2 to 4 mg IV every 15 to 30 min until light sedation is attained. At the same time, 1 L of 5% dextrose in normal saline solution with 100 mg of thiamine and 4 g of magnesium sulfate is given IV over 1 to 2 h. Although magnesium has not been shown to be effective against ethanol withdrawal in general, hypomagnesemia has been closely associated with tremor in alcoholics and may play a role in the genesis of seizures. An alternative primary drug is phenobarbital, starting with a dose of 260 mg administered intravenously over 15 min, followed by doses of 130 mg every 30 to 45 min as needed. Phenobarbital has a relatively long half-life, 24 to 96 h, obviating the need for outpatient prescriptions if the patient is discharged.[13] Clinicians should approach treatment of alcohol withdrawal prepared to administer lorazepam (or phenobarbital) repeatedly and in cumulatively large doses. There is no evidence that prophylactic phenytoin prevents ethanol withdrawal seizures.[14]

Patients with alcohol withdrawal and complicating medical problems, such as infections or congestive heart failure, should be admitted to the hospital. Patients who fail to respond to one or two doses of sedative medications should also be admitted. Administration of more than 8 mg of lorazepam or 500 mg of phenobarbital is in most cases an indication for admission to a nursing unit where the patient can receive close observation by both nursing and physician staff, in many hospitals, an intensive care unit. Patients with mild alcohol withdrawal that respond to treatment may be discharged. If they have been given phenobarbital, no outpatient prescription is necessary. In any case, the benefit of prescribing outpatient benzodiazepines is doubtful if a patient is likely to resume drinking after discharge from the emergency department.

ELDERLY PATIENTS AND ALCOHOL

Fewer older people drink regularly, and intake among older drinkers is less than among younger people. Nevertheless, alcohol is still a significant problem among the elderly, and alcohol-related problems are by far the most common drug-related problem in this age group. Moreover, since many physicians are even less likely to consider the possibility of alcohol abuse or alcoholism in older than in younger patients, the diagnosis is often missed. Even so, the prevalence of alcohol-related hospitalizations during a recent year for people over 65 years of age was 54.7 per 10,000 population for men and 14.8 per 10,000 for women.[1] Alcohol plays a significant role in motor-vehicle collisions and other trauma involving the elderly and has a greater impact on the health of the elderly than on that of younger persons. Mortality and morbidity rates due to all types of trauma are higher for older patients.[15]

WOMEN AND ALCOHOL

Women are less likely than men to abuse alcohol but are more prone to experiencing alcohol-associated health problems, especially cirrhosis.[1] A population-based study found that, among those averaging six or more drinks per day, the relative risk for mortality for women was five times that of men. The reason for this is unclear but may be related to the fact that women have virtually no first-pass metabolism of alcohol by gastric alcohol dehydrogenase and a smaller volume of distribution than men, resulting in considerably higher blood alcohol levels following ingestion of a given dose of alcohol.[16]

Women who drink during pregnancy predispose their children to growth retardation in utero and to the fetal alcohol syndrome, characterized by facial dysmorphology and mental and growth retardation after birth. Even women who report intake of less than one drink a day are at increased risk of having a child in the bottom 10 percent for birth weight.[17] Since emergency physicians frequently diagnose pregnancy and patients with alcohol problems are often seen in emergency departments, emergency physicians are likely to have the opportunity to advise pregnant patients about the risks inherent in using alcohol during pregnancy.

LONG-TERM OUTLOOK FOR ALCOHOLICS

Alcoholic patients should be referred for counseling when possible. A fifth or more may achieve permanent abstinence with the aid of Alcoholics Anonymous or other self-help groups. Unfortunately, the rate of recidivism is related to socioeconomic status and availability of family and social support systems. Thus, while 60 percent of middle-class alcoholics remain ethanol free for at least 1 year after completing a rehabilitation program, the outlook is considerably bleaker for those who are less advantaged.

REFERENCES

1. Secretary of Health and Human Services: *Ninth Special Report to the US Congress on Alcohol and Health.* Washington, US Government Printing Office, 1997.
2. Morse RM, Flavin DK</AU>, for the Joint Committee of the National Council on Alcoholism and Drug Dependence and the American Society of Addiction Medicine to Study the Definition and Criteria for the Diagnosis of Alcoholism: The definition of alcoholism. *JAMA* 268:1012, 1992.
3. Moore RD, Bone LR, Geller G, et al: Prevalence, detection, and treatment of alcoholism in hospitalized patients. *JAMA* 261:403, 1989.
4. Ojesjo L, Hagnell O, Otterbeck L: Mortality in alcoholism among men in the Lundby community cohort, Sweden: A forty-year follow-up. *J Stud Alcohol* 59:140, 1998.
5. Klatsky AL, Armstrong MA, Friedman GD: Alcohol and mortality. *Ann Intern Med* 117:646, 1992.
6. Jurkovich GJ, Rivara FP, Gurney JG, et al: Effects of alcohol intoxication on the initial assessment of trauma patients. *Ann Emerg Med* 21:704, 1992.
7. Perez FG, O'Malley KF, Ross SE: Evaluation of the abdomen in intoxicated patients: Is computed tomography scan or peritoneal lavage always indicated? *Ann Emerg Med* 20:500, 1991.
8. Waller PF, Stewart JR, Hansen AR, et al: The potentiating effects of alcohol on driver injury. *JAMA* 256:1461, 1986.
9. Jurkovich GJ, Rivara FP, Gurney JG, et al: The effect of acute alcohol intoxication and chronic alcohol abuse on outcome from trauma. *JAMA* 1993:270:51, 1993.
10. Spies CD, Neuner B, Neumann T, et al: Intercurrent complications in chronic alcoholic men admitted to the intensive care unit following trauma. *Intensive Care Med* 22:286, 1996.
11. Feussner JR, Linfors EW, Blessing CL, Starmer CF: Computed tomography brain scanning in alcohol withdrawal seizures. *Ann Intern Med* 94:519, 1981.
12. Bird RD, Makela EH: Alcohol withdrawal: What is the benzodiazepine of choice? *Ann Pharmacother* 28:67, 1994.
13. Young GP, Rores C, Murphy C, Dailey RH: Intravenous phenobarbital for alcohol withdrawal and convulsions. *Ann Emerg Med* 16:847, 1987.
14. Chance JF: Emergency department treatment of alcohol withdrawal seizures with phenytoin. *Ann Emerg Med* 20:520, 1991.
15. Higgins JP, Wright SW, Wrenn KD: Alcohol, the elderly, and motor vehicle crashes. *Am J Emerg Med* 14:265, 1996.
16. Frezza M, Di Padova C, Pozzato G, et al: The role of decreased gastric alcohol dehydrogenase activity and first-pass metabolism. *N Engl J Med* 322:95, 1990.
17. Mills JL, Graubard BI, Harley EE, et al: Maternal alcohol consumption and birth weight: How much drinking during pregnancy is safe? *JAMA* 252:1875, 1984.

THE ELDER PATIENT

Arthur B. Sanders

Older patients represent a special population for emergency medicine. The approach that focuses on one chief complaint, and develops a differential diagnosis based on life-threatening and common diseases, may miss significant conditions in older persons. Older patients are more time consuming, more difficult to evaluate, and take more resources compared with younger adult patients. The complexity of their presentations and dispositions, as well as communication problems with the patients, their families, and primary care providers, all make the emergency department (ED) evaluation of elderly persons more difficult compared with younger adult patients.[1] The physiology of aging results in altered disease presentations, altered pharmacodynamics, and decreased functional reserve, as well as social problems, which must be dealt with in the setting of a busy ED.

EPIDEMIOLOGY

The demographics of the population in the United States demonstrate the importance of older persons in our society, the rapid growth of the elderly from 1920 projected to 2050, and the potential effects of these demographic changes on our health care system (Fig. 300-1). About 12 percent of the population was 65 years of age or older in 1990, whereas 20 percent of the population (or 55 million persons) will be 65 years of age or older by the year 2030.[2] The oldest elderly, those 85 years and above, are the most rapidly increasing segment of the population. This is also the population with the most health problems and in greatest need for health care. There is great variability in the physiologic age of individual patients. A 55-year-old with multiple chronic diseases and poor physiologic reserve may have a physiologic age much older than a healthy 80-year-old.

In 1990, about 15 percent of ED visits were made by patients 65 and older, and over 30 percent of older patients use ambulances to come to the ED.[3] The rate of ambulance use increases with age: more than half of those 85 years of age and older are transported by ambulances. Older patients require comprehensive emergency department services, and more than 40 percent are admitted to the hospital.[3] Older patients spend more time in the ED, require more ancillary tests, and are more likely to be admitted to critical care units.[4] A survey by the National Center for Health Statistics (NCHS) found that persons aged 65 to 74 years had an estimated 31.4 ED visits per 100 persons per year, and persons aged 75 years and older had 55.8 visits per 100 persons per year, twice the rate for younger persons.[5]

PATHOPHYSIOLOGY

To meet the needs of older persons in the emergency medical care system, principles of geriatric emergency medicine have been defined and are listed in Table 300-1.[6] Patients may present with vague or ambiguous symptoms, such as not feeling right, feeling weak, or not doing usual activities. Vague complaints, such as general weakness or functional decline, may indicate important diseases, such as sepsis, subdural hematoma, or myocardial infarction. Tools such as an assessment of functional status can be used for classifying and evaluating these complaints.

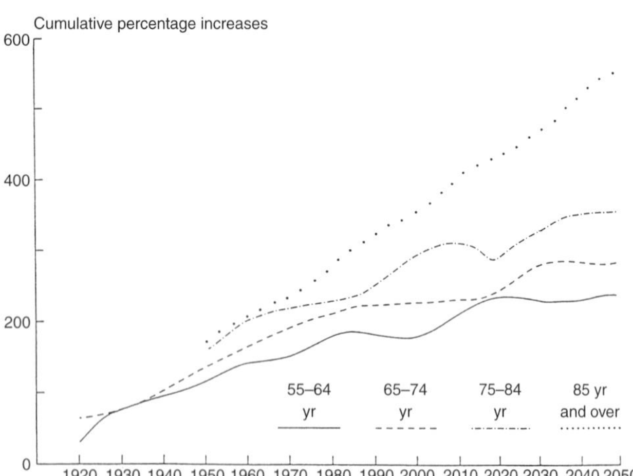

FIG. 300-1. Percentage increase of elderly population from 1920 projected to 2050. (From Eliastam M: Elderly patients in the emergency department. *Ann Emerg Med* 18:1222, 1989.)

TABLE 300-1 Principles of Geriatric Emergency Medicine

1. The patient's presentation is frequently complex.
2. Common diseases present atypically in this age group.
3. The confounding effects of comorbid diseases must be considered.
4. Polypharmacy is common and may be a factor in presentation, diagnosis, and management.
5. Recognition of the possibility for cognitive impairment is important.
6. Some diagnostic tests may have different normal values.
7. The likelihood of decreased functional reserve must be anticipated.
8. Social support systems may not be adequate, and patients may need to rely on caregivers.
9. A knowledge of baseline functional status is essential for evaluating new complaints.
10. Health problems must be evaluated for associated psychosocial adjustment.
11. The emergency department encounter is an opportunity to assess important conditions in a patient's personal life.

Source: From Sanders,[6] with permission.

Common diseases often present atypically in older persons,[7] resulting in missed diagnoses unless physicians understand and suspect the atypical presentations in this population. For example, fewer than half of patients 85 years of age and older will present with chest pain as a symptom of acute myocardial infarction. Instead, patients present atypically with dyspnea, syncope, weakness, or dizziness.[8] Acute abdominal catastrophes are often missed in older persons because of the atypical disease presentations. Abdominal guarding or even rigidity may be lacking with significant abdominal pathology. Fever or leukocytosis may not be present. Only about half the older patients with acute appendicitis have that diagnosed upon admission to the hospital. A large percent of patients with appendicitis present more than 48 h after the onset of symptoms, with up to 20 percent presenting after 3 days. The abdominal pain is vague, and the symptoms may be poorly localized. Classic patterns of pain and accompanying symptoms, such as nausea and vomiting, are present in only a minority of older patients with acute appendicitis.[9]

Older patients frequently will have confounding comorbid diseases, and emergency physicians must evaluate whether the presenting complaint reflects an exacerbation of one of the comorbid diseases or a new disease process. Comorbid diseases, especially those treated with multiple medications, may also affect the management and disposition of patients. Older adults take an average of 4.5 prescription drugs and 2.1 over-the-counter drugs each day.[10] About 30 percent of older persons will develop adverse medication effects, and they are twice as likely as younger adults to have adverse effects. Adverse medication effects account for approximately 5 percent of hospital admissions.[10] The number of medications that a patient takes is directly related to the chance of adverse drug effects. Normal aging results in a loss of cardiac, pulmonary, hepatic, and renal functional reserve. Thus, the margin of error decreases for many medications, such as nonsteroidal anti-inflammatory drugs. The distribution of drugs changes with age, lean body mass decreases, and the larger proportion of adipose tissue increases the volume of distribution of drugs, such as benzodiazepines, phenytoin, barbiturates, and phenothiazines, and prolongs their duration of action. Drug clearance depends primarily on hepatic and renal function. The decreased renal function with age may effect drugs such as digoxin and the aminoglycoside antibiotics. Drug receptor interactions also play a role in pharmacodynamics. Older persons have an increased sensitivity to warfarin and benzodiazepines. Common complications of medications or drug interactions include delirium, depression, functional decline, worsening dementia, orthostatic hypotension, weakness, dizziness, falls, and incontinence. The impact of new medications prescribed in emergency departments, such as anticholinergics, sedatives, and diuretics, as well as adverse interactions with current medicines, must be anticipated.[10]

Older persons will frequently have cognitive impairment that may not be recognized by health care providers. Cognitive impairment includes both acute confusional states (delirium) and dementia. Abnormal cognitive states in older patients affect the reliability of the history and impact disposition planning. Acute cognitive impairment can be an important symptom of sepsis, congestive heart failure, metabolic abnormality, adverse drug effect, or subdural hematoma. When older emergency department patients are screened for cognitive impairment, 30 to 40 percent of those who have no previous history of impairment will have abnormal cognition based on formal mental status exams.[11,12] About 10 percent of patients will meet formal criteria for delirium, which should be considered a symptom of a medical emergency. Formal tools for evaluation of cognition are recommended later in this chapter.

Accurate test interpretation requires a knowledge of which ''normal'' values are altered with aging. Although many laboratories control for age variations in neonates and children, few list control values for older patients. For example, laboratory parameters such as the sedimentation rate, glucose and creatinine levels, and arterial blood oxygen tension change with physiologic aging.

The likelihood of decreased functional reserve must be anticipated in older persons. Most patients are asymptomatic until they are stressed or reach a critical threshold in which symptoms are manifested. Most organ functions decline with age. Resting cardiac output decreases at approximately 1 percent per year after age 30. Pulmonary, renal, neurologic, and immunologic functions also decrease with age. Chronologic and biologic age, however, may vary considerably, depending on genetics, environment, health behaviors, diet, tobacco use, alcohol use, exercise, or stress. When older persons are stressed, for example, by extreme heat or cold, their regulatory mechanisms are not as effective.

Older persons must be viewed in the context of their home environment and social support network. Simply addressing an injury or illness may not be adequate. Over 20 percent reported a change in their ability to care for themselves following their emergency department visit.[13] An independent-living 80-year-old woman who sprains her ankle may become incapacitated. Enlisting the help of a social service network, home health providers, etc., will ensure that such patients are able to carry on the functions of daily living. In addition, many older persons need to rely on caretakers, so an assessment of the caretaker's ability to help the patient is important. Is the caretaker an elderly spouse who will predictably injure himself or herself in trying to lift a patient who is incapacitated by a new injury? Elder abuse and neglect is a significant issue[14] (see Chap. 292, ''Abuse in the Elderly and Impaired'') that should be assessed by questioning the patient and caretaker separately.

The emergency health care professional can play a key role in screening for such important conditions such as elder abuse, depression, alcoholism, malnutrition and incontinence, falls, and immunizations. In a multicenter study in which patients were screened, almost 80 percent of older patients demonstrated a problem in one or more of these areas.[15]

SPECIFIC ISSUES

This section reviews how the principles of geriatric emergency medicine (Table 300-1) can be applied to the specific medical conditions of altered mental status, functional decline, trauma, falls, and infections.

Altered Mental Status

Of emergency department older patients with no prior history of cognitive problems, 30 to 40 percent will meet the criteria for either delirium

I. ACUTE ONSET OR FLUCTUATING COURSE — BOX 1

Is there evidence of an acute change in mental status from the patient's baseline?

or

Did the (abnormal) behavior fluctuate during the day (i.e., tend to come and go or increase and decrease in severity)? No Yes

II. INATTENTION

Did the patient have difficulty focusing attention (e.g., being easily distractible or having difficulty keeping track of what was being said)? No Yes

III. DISORGANIZED THINKING — BOX 2

Was the patient's thinking disorganized or incoherent (e.g., rambling or irrelevant conversation, unclear or illogical flow of ideas, or unpredictable switching from subject to subject)? No Yes

IV. ALTERED LEVEL OF CONSCIOUSNESS

Overall, how would you rate the patient's level of consciousness?

—Alter (normal)

—Vigilant (hyperalert)
—Lethargic (drowsy, easily aroused)
—Stupor (difficult to arouse)
—Coma (unarousable)

Do any checks appear in this box? No Yes

FIG. 300-2. Confusion Assessment Method (CAM) worksheet. The diagnosis of delirium is suggested with the presence of the first two criteria and either the third or fourth criteria. From Inouye et al,[16] with permission.

or cognitive dysfunction, and this is often unsuspected by the physician.[11,12] Consequently, older patients should be routinely screened for cognitive dysfunction. The simplest screening tool is evaluation for orientation and three-item recall. If no problem is detected, no further testing needs to be done. If the screen is failed, further testing can be done. The Confusion Assessment Method (CAM) scale (Fig. 300-2)[16] is a useful tool for the emergency physician. Using the CAM scale, the patient is evaluated for (1) acute onset, (2) fluctuating course, (3) inattention, (4) disorganized thinking, and (5) altered level of consciousness. These factors are assessed through the emergency department history and observation, as well as structured questions such as three-item recall, stating the days of the week or months of the year backward. Patients who present with inattention—either acute onset or fluctuating course—and disorganized thinking or altered level of consciousness should be considered to have delirium and evaluated for acute medical problems as the cause. Cognitive function can be further assessed with formal mental status tools such as the Mini-Mental Status Exam (MMSE).[17] These scales are useful because they are widely accepted as indicative of cognitive dysfunction and can be followed by different clinicians over time (Fig. 300-3).

Delirium, dementia, or decreased level of consciousness are usually obvious on history and physical examination. The Glasgow Coma Scale (see Chap. 221) is useful for classifying a decreased level of consciousness. Acute mental status changes in older patients represent a medical emergency of presumed organic cause requiring extensive diagnostic tests to determine the etiology. The differential diagnosis is more difficult because a large number of disorders such as pneumonia, urosepsis, electrolyte imbalance, medication reaction, or congestive heart failure can cause a decrease in mental status.

Add points for each correct response.		Score	Points
Orientation			
1. What is the:	Year?	____	1
	Season?	____	1
	Date?	____	1
	Day?	____	1
	Month?	____	1
2. Where are we?	State?	____	1
	County	____	1
	Town or city?	____	1
	Hospital?	____	1
	Floor?	____	1
Registration			
3. Name three objects, taking one second to say each. Then ask the patient to repeat all three after you have said them. Give one point for each correct answer. Repeat the answers until patient learns all three.		____	3
Attention and calculation			
4. Serial sevens. Give one point for each correct answer. Stop after five answers. Alternate: Spell WORLD backwards.		____	5
Recall			
5. Ask for names of three objects learned in question 3. Give one point for each correct answer.		____	3
Language			
6. Point to a pencil and a watch. Have the patient name them as you point.		____	2
7. Have the patient repeat "No ifs, ands, or buts."		____	1
8. Have the patient follow a three-stage command: "Take a paper in your right hand. Fold the paper in half. Put the paper on the floor."		____	3
9. Have the patient read and obey the following: 'CLOSE YOUR EYES.' (Write it in large letters.)		____	1
10. Have the patient write a sentence of his or her choice. (The sentence should contain a subject and an object and should make sense. Ignore spelling errors when scoring.)		____	1
11. Have the patient copy the design. (Give one point if all sides and angles are preserved and if the intersecting sides form a quadrangle.)		____	1
		____ = Total	30

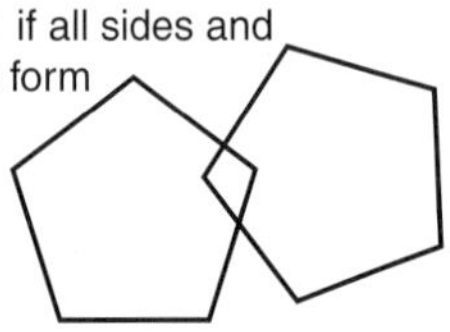

In validation studies using a cutoff score of 23 or below, the MMSE has a sensitivity of 87%, a specificity of 82%, a false-positive ratio of 39.4%, and a false-negative ratio of 4.7%. These ratios refer to the MMSE's capacity to accurately distinguish patients with clinically diagnosed dementia or delirium from patients without these syndromes.

FIG. 300-3. Mini-Mental State Examination (MMSE). Courtesy of Marshall Folstein. Reprinted from Folstein et al,[17] with permission.

Functional Decline

Functional decline represents a change in a patient's ability to perform tasks of independent living and is not a part of normal aging. This can be assessed with the use of a standard scale for Activities of Daily Living (ADL), which evaluates a patient's ability for bathing, dressing, toileting, transferring (in or out of a bed or chair), continence, and feeding (Table 300-2).[18] The patient is asked whether he or she can perform each of these functions with no assistance, with partial assistance, or cannot perform these functions. If a patient cannot perform these basic activities of daily living, then a caregiver is necessary. Deterioration in ADL generally follows an orderly progressive pattern of bathing, dressing, toileting (including continence), transferring, and feeding. When this pattern is not seen, such as a deterioration in feeding before the others, organ disease should be suspected. Another scale, the Instrumental Activities of Daily Living (IADL), assesses more sophisticated skills, such as telephone use, walking, shopping, preparing meals, housework, handiwork, laundry, taking medicines, and handling finances (Table 300-3).[19] It is best to use these formal scales in evaluating older patients and assessing changes over time. Acute functional decline represents an acute medical syndrome that needs

TABLE 300-2 Activities of Daily Living (ADL) Scale

- Bathing
- Dressing
- Toileting
- Transfer
- Continence
- Feeding

Source: From Katz et al,[18] with permission.

TABLE 300-3 Instrumental Activities of Daily Living (IADL) Scale

- Telephone use
- Walking
- Shopping
- Preparing meals
- Housework
- Handywork
- Laundry
- Take medicines
- Manage finances

Source: From Lawton and Brody,[19] with permission. © The Gerontological Society of America.

appropriate workup and treatment. An algorithm for the ED evaluation of functional decline is presented in Fig. 300-4.[20] The differential diagnosis for functional decline includes serious diseases such as myocardial infarction, sepsis, and subdural hematoma, as well as adverse drug reactions. Patients will often present with a vague symptom, such as weakness, that on further questioning and use of the scale is noted to be functional decline.

Trauma

Trauma is a major cause of morbidity and mortality among older persons. Although fewer than 20 percent of trauma patients are 65 years of age or older, older patients represent 28 percent of trauma deaths.[21,22] They are more likely to have significant complications and prolonged hospitalizations because of their decreased functional reserve.[21] Falls are the most common mechanism of injury for older persons, followed by motor vehicle crashes and pedestrian accidents. Regardless of injury severity or mechanism of injury, mortality increases for patients at 50 years of age and continues to increase with increasing age. The major challenge for emergency physicians who treat older patients who have multisystem trauma is that the standard physiologic indices, such as blood pressure and pulse, often remain within normal limits until the patient deteriorates acutely. Occult shock must be strongly suspected in all older patients who experience significant trauma. Early hemodynamic monitoring of older trauma patients

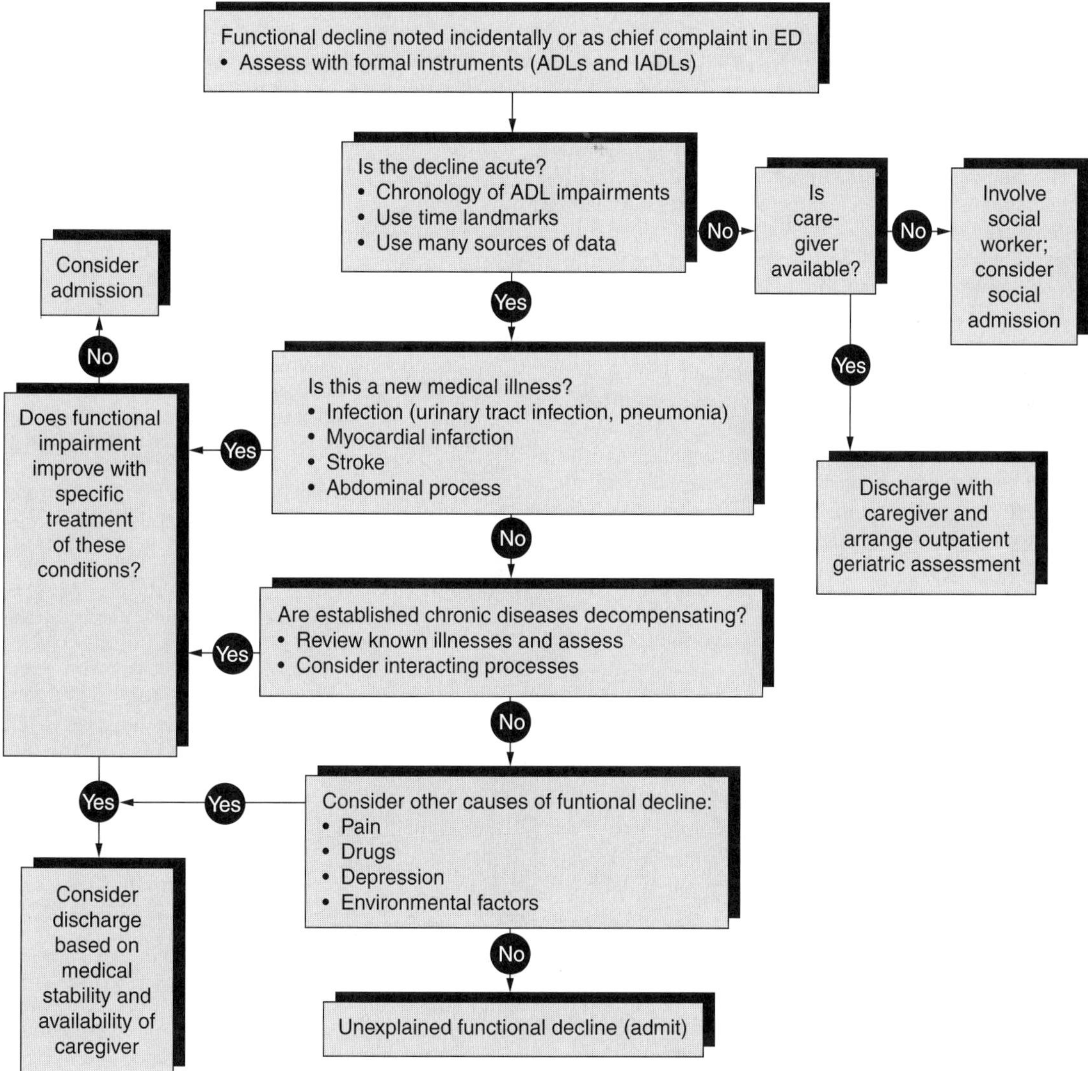

FIG. 300-4. Algorithm for the evaluation and management of functional decline in elderly patients. ADL, Activities of Daily Living scale; ED, emergency department; IADL, Instrumental Activities of Daily Living scale. From Lachs,[20] with permission.

can detect occult shock early in the course and improve the chance of survival.[21,22] (See Chap. 245, ''Geriatric Trauma.'')

Falls

Falls are not a normal part of aging. A fall is a symptom, and emergency physicians need to assess both the cause and the consequences of the fall. The causes of a fall may include acute or chronic diseases, medications, and environmental factors.[22] Consequences of a fall include injury and fear of falling, resulting in a decrease in activities. A fall can represent a sentinel event in an older person's life and result in a downward spiral of decreased activities, leading to death. As many as 50 percent of older patients admitted to the hospital after a fall die within 1 year. An emergency physician obtains the history of what caused the fall and determines whether further emergency department screening tests (electrocardiography, computed tomography, laboratory tests, social service consultation, etc.) will be done to evaluate the cause.[22] The patient should then be informed about fall assessment programs that decrease the incidence and morbidity from falls.

Infections

Multiple factors as well as changes in the immune system with age are responsible for the increased susceptibility to infection in the elderly.[23] In addition, older persons will have atypical disease presentations of sepsis. Focal symptoms or signs of infection may be lacking. Instead, patients may present with isolated fever or nonspecific symptoms of anorexia, weakness, fatigue, and functional decline as the only evidence of infection. Hypothermia may be evident instead of fever. The most common sites of infection include the lungs, urinary tract, abdomen, and skin.

Bacteremia and occult bacterial infection are common in the febrile elderly. Mellors and coworkers identified the following multivariate predictors of bacteremia and occult bacterial infection in febrile adults without localizing symptoms or signs: (1) age older than 50, (2) diabetes, (3) white blood cell count (WBC) more than 15,000, (4) neutrophil band count more than 1500, and (5) erythrocyte sedimentation rate more than 30 mm/h.[24] Patients with one or two of these factors had a seven- to eightfold relative risk for bacteremia or focal bacterial infection. Other studies in the febrile elderly have also found that leukocytosis and ''left shift'' on the WBC differential was also associated with a two- to threefold greater likelihood of bacterial infection.[25]

DISPOSITION

For all the foregoing reasons, elderly patients in EDs are more likely to require hospital admission for their illness or injury compared with younger patients. When discharged from an ED, elderly patients may not fully understand the instructions, may not be able to obtain and take prescribed medications, may not be able to access appropriate follow-up, or may not be able to care for their personal needs during the period of illness. An elderly patient's family, friends, and social support system should be informed and involved before the patient leaves the ED.

REFERENCES

1. McNamara RM, Rousseau E, Sanders AB: Geriatric emergency medicine: A survey of practicing emergency physicians. *Ann Emerg Med* 21:796, 1992.
2. Eliastam M: Elderly patients in the emergency department. *Ann Emerg Med* 18:1222, 1989.
3. Strange GR, Chen EH, Sanders AB: Use of emergency departments by elderly patients: Projections from a multicenter database. *Ann Emerg Med* 21:819, 1992.
4. Singal BM, Hedges JR, Rousseau EW, et al: Geriatric patient emergency visits: I. Comparison of visits by geriatric and younger patients. *Ann Emerg Med* 21:802, 1992.
5. McCraig LF: *National Hospital Ambulatory Medical Care Survey: 1992 Emergency Department Summary.* Washington, DC, National Center for Health Statistics, Centers for Disease Control and Prevention, US Department of Health and Human Services, 1994.
6. Sanders AB (ed): *Emergency Care of the Elder Person.* St Louis, Beverly Cracom, 1996.
7. Freedman ML: Detecting acute disease, in Bosker G, Schwartz GR, Jones JS, Sequeria M (eds): *Geriatric Emergency Medicine.* St Louis, CV Mosby Year Book, 1990, pp 9–15.
8. Bayer AJ, Chadha JS, Farag RB, et al: Changing presentation of myocardial infarction with increasing old age. *J Am Geriatr Soc* 34:263, 1986.
9. Horattas MC, Guyton DP, Wu D: A reappraisal of appendicitis in elderly. *Am J Surg* 160:291, 1990.
10. Evans R, Ireland G, Morley JE, et al: Pharmacology and aging, in Sanders AB (ed): *Emergency Care of the Elder Person.* St Louis, Beverly Cracom, 1996, pp 29–41.
11. Lewis LM, Miller DK, Morley JE, et al: Unrecognized delirium in ED geriatric patients. *Am J Emerg Med* 13:142, 1995.
12. Naughton BJ, Moran MB, Kadah H, et al: Delirium and other cognitive impairment in older adults in an emergency department. *Ann Emerg Med* 250:751, 1995.
13. Hedges JR, Singal BM, Rousseau EW, et al: Geriatric patient emergency visits: II. Perceptions of visits by geriatric and younger patients. *Ann Emerg Med* 21:808, 1992.
14. Kleinschmidt KC: Elder abuse: A review. *Ann Emerg Med* 30:463, 1997.
15. Gerson LW, Rousseau E, Hogan J, et al: A multicenter study of case findings in elderly emergency department patients. *Acad Emerg Med* 2:729, 1995.
16. Inouye SK, Van Dyck CH, Alessi CA, et al: Clarifying confusion: The confusion assessment method—A new method for detection of delirium. *Ann Intern Med* 113:941, 1990.
17. Folstein MF, Folstein S, McHugh PR: Mini-Mental State exam: A practical method for grading the cognitive state of patients for the clinician. *J Psychiatr Res* 12:189, 1975.
18. Katz S, Ford AB, Moskowitz RW, et al: Studies in illness in the aged: The index for ADL—Standardized measure of biologic and psychosocial function. *JAMA* 185:914, 1962.
19. Lawton MP, Brody EM: Assessment of older people: Self-maintaining and instrumental activities of daily living. *Gerontologist* 9:179, 1969.
20. Lachs MS: Functional decline, in Sanders AB (ed): *Emergency Care of the Elder Person.* St Louis, Beverly Cracom, 1996, pp 143–151.
21. Mandavia D, Newton K: Geriatric trauma. *Emerg Med Clin North Am* 16:257, 1998.
22. Evans R: Trauma and falls, in Sanders AB (ed): *Emergency Care of the Elder Person.* St Louis, Beverly Cracom, 1996, pp 153–170.
23. Crossley KB, Peterson PK: Infections in the elderly. *Clin Infect Dis* 22:209, 1996.
24. Mellors JW, Horwitz RI, Harvey MR, Horwitz SM: A simple index to identify occult bacterial infection in adults with unexplained fever. *Arch Intern Med* 47:666, 1987.
25. Wasserman M, Levinstein M, Keller E, et al: Utility of fever, white blood cells, and differential count in predicting bacterial infections in the elderly. *J Am Geriatr Soc* 37:537, 1989.

ADULTS WITH PHYSICAL DISABILITIES

Cara B. Siegel
Paul J.W. Tawney

Advances in medicine and surgery have prevented the deaths of many injured and sick patients. Although they survived, many such individuals live with significant impairments and disabilities. Some estimates are that 5 to 10 percent of the total population of the United States has major disabilities. Persons with disabilities seeking medical care in an emergency department (ED) may present with problems that are specific to their impairment or with signs and symptoms different from those that would occur in a nondisabled patient. The individual who is disabled is not unable, and every effort should be made to obtain the history directly from the patient. Do not automatically direct questions to persons with the disabled individual without first finding out whether the patient is capable of giving accurate responses. It is helpful to sit down and speak to a patient in a wheelchair at eye level, and to make an effort to use a dysphasic or dysarthric patient's communication system so that they may tell their story.

SPINAL CORD INJURY

Autonomic Dysreflexia

Patients with spinal cord injuries at or above the T6 level are at risk for developing autonomic dysreflexia (also called autonomic hyperreflexia).[1] This reflex is initiated by a noxious stimulus from below the level of the patient's spinal cord lesion. Intact sensory neurons below the level of the lesion transmit a message up the spinal thalamic tract and posterior columns, where interconnections stimulate the intermediolateral gray matter neurons, producing sympathetic outflow from spinal cord levels between T6 and L2, releasing norepinephrine, β-hydroxylase, and dopamine. This sympathetic reflex is relatively unopposed because the normal inhibitory impulses that would prevent it originate above T6 and are blocked at the level of injury.[1]

The sympathetic response produces a rise in blood pressure, vasoconstriction, skin pallor, and piloerection below the level of the lesion. Intact carotid and aortic arch baroreceptors detect the hypertension, producing increased parasympathetic activity in the vagus nerve and bradycardia. Sympathetic outflow above the lesion is inhibited, which causes profuse sweating, vasodilation, and skin flushing.[1,2]

Common symptoms and signs of autonomic dysreflexia are a pounding headache, profuse sweating and flushing above the level of the lesion with pallor below the level of the lesion, nasal congestion, feeling of apprehension or anxiety, visual changes, and, most significant, a marked increase in systolic and diastolic blood pressure above baseline.[1,2] Patients with spinal cord injury at or above the T6 level often have lower baseline systolic blood pressures, in the 90- to 110-mmHg range. Therefore, blood pressure elevations of 20 to 40 mmHg or systolic pressures of 130 to 150 mmHg are significant. Acute elevation in blood pressure is the most worrisome and potentially life-threatening manifestation of this syndrome.

A variety of stimuli can produce an acute episode of autonomic dysreflexia. The commonest causes usually involve the urinary system: bladder distention, urinary tract infection, and kidney stones. The second commonest reasons involve the colon: fecal impaction or bowel distention. However, any noxious stimulus below the level of injury can lead to autonomic dysreflexia, including other abdominal problems, such as ulcers, appendicitis, and gallstones. Other causes may be fractures, deep venous thrombosis (DVT), pressure ulcers, ingrown toenails, tight-fitting clothing, sunburns, blisters, heterotopic ossification, sexual intercourse, pregnancy, and labor and delivery.

Treatment starts with monitoring and controlling the patient's blood pressure. If possible, the patient should be sat up to lower blood pressure.[2–4] If the systolic blood pressure is above 150 mmHg, an antihypertensive agent with a rapid onset and short duration should be used to lower the blood pressure.[5] Nifedipine and nitrates are the most commonly used agents. More aggressive treatment should be undertaken if these agents do not adequately correct the elevated blood pressure.

After assessment of the blood pressure, the bladder should be checked for distention and infection.[3,4] If the patient does not already have a urinary catheter, one should be placed immediately. The stimulus of catheterization may add to the autonomic reflex, and lidocaine jelly should be used if it is readily available, but its lack should not delay the placement of the catheter. If the patient already has an indwelling Foley or suprapubic catheter, it should be checked for obstruction and correct placement. The bladder can be gently irrigated through either catheter with body-temperature normal saline solution to check for obstruction and improper placement.[4] Urine should be obtained for urinalysis and culture (see below).

If the problem does not appear to be bladder related, the physician should suspect fecal impaction.[3,4] Prior to the rectal examination, the patient's blood pressure should be managed, and the anal opening should be anesthetized with lidocaine jelly placed into the rectum for 5 min before beginning the examination.[4] The patient's blood pressure should be monitored to ensure that the hypertension is not aggravated during this procedure, since rectal examination can exacerbate autonomic dysreflexia. If the blood pressure increases, stop the examination, instill more anesthetic agent, and wait additional time. If the bladder or bowel does not appear to be the cause of the patient's symptoms, a search for other causes should be undertaken.

Following relief of an acute episode, patients should be monitored for at least 2 h after resolution to make sure that there is no recurrence. Patients with bladder distention do not routinely require discharge with an indwelling urinary catheter. It is best to discuss that option with the patient's physician. If the patient responds poorly or the cause has not been identified, the patient may need to be admitted for more aggressive pharmacologic control of blood pressure and a more thorough investigation of the cause.[2–5]

Urinary Tract Infection

A urinary tract infection should be suspected when a spinal-cord-injured patient presents with fever, discomfort over the kidney or bladder, change in spasticity, development of urinary incontinence, an episode of autonomic dysreflexia, cloudy or foul-smelling urine, a change in energy level, or a feeling of apprehension.[6,7] Unless there are confounding factors, the urinalysis shows pyuria and significant bacteruria. In a patient with the abovementioned symptoms and signs and pyuria, empiric treatment for urinary tract infection should be started. Absence of pyuria makes the diagnosis less likely but does not completely exclude it. Conversely, pyuria in an asymptomatic patient with spinal cord injury does not warrant treatment. Pyuria without infection can occur from irritation of the bladder wall in patients with indwelling catheters and in those who use intermittent catheterization.[8]

Significant bacteriuria for the spinal-cord-injured population is defined according to the method used for bladder emptying. For women who can spontaneously void, significant bacteriuria is defined as greater than 100,000 colony-forming units (CFUs) of bacteria per milliliter. For men who spontaneously void or use condom catheters, greater than 10,000 CFUs/mL is considered significant. For both women and men who use intermittent catheterization, greater than 100 CFUs/mL indicates significant bacteriuria. For patients with indwelling urethral or suprapubic catheters, any detectable level of bacteriuria is significant.[6]

Urinary tract infections in the spinal-cord-injured population are considered complicated urinary tract infections.[9] Antibiotics with broader-spectrum coverage should be used, since such organisms as *Proteus, Klebsiella, Pseudomonas, Serratia, Providencia,* enterococci, and *Staphylococcus* are more common. Because of the higher risk of upper-tract infection, 7 to 14 days of treatment should be considered.[10,11]

Asymptomatic bacteriuria is very common in patients with a neurogenic bladder that requires periodic or indwelling catheterization. Asymptomatic bacteriuria should not be routinely treated.[6] Because signs and symptoms of urinary tract infections may be less obvious in spinal-cord-injured individuals, the physician should be aware of subtle clues to the presence of infection and have a low threshold for urinalysis as the best method of diagnosis.[9]

Acute Abdomen

Classic signs of acute abdomen are often missing in patients with spinal cord injury. The diagnosis of perforated peptic ulcer, intestinal obstruction, appendicitis, peritonitis, cholecystitis, and renal abscess is often delayed because the classic findings of abdominal muscle rigidity, rebound, abdominal tenderness, fever, and leukocytosis may not be present.[12] In patients with spinal cord injury, other signs and symptoms suggestive of an acute abdomen are autonomic dysreflexia, referred shoulder tip pain, abdominal pain, abdominal distention, change in muscle spasticity, nausea and vomiting, and a sense of apprehension.[12–14] A high index of suspicion, along with laboratory and imaging tests, is necessary to avoid missing the diagnosis. One confounding factor is that urinary tract infections may present with similar signs and symptoms. Thus, the finding of pyuria or bacteruria alone should not be used to exclude the diagnosis of an acute abdomen.[13] Unexplained leukocytosis is a helpful, but not diagnostic, clue to the presence of an acute abdomen. While abdominal radiographs are also useful in the diagnosis of intestinal obstruction, many spinal-cord-injury patients have chronic dysmotility problems and have baseline increased bowel gas and air-fluid levels that may mimic a mechanical obstruction. Ultrasound, contrast, and computed tomography (CT) imaging studies are often required for correct diagnosis in such patients.[14]

Syringomyelia

Posttraumatic syringomyelia may present months to years after a spinal cord injury.[15] This process produces a cystic cavitation of the central cord that may extend over several levels. Ascending sensory level (i.e., a decrease or loss of sensation above the preexisting sensory level) and pain are the most common presenting symptoms. Motor weakness, a change in spasticity, and a change in deep-tendon reflexes may also be seen. Magnetic resonance imaging is the imaging study of choice for making the diagnosis of syringomyelia. Surgery is indicated in progressive neurologic deterioration.

Immobilization Hypercalcemia

Most cases of immobilization hypercalcemia are seen in adolescent boys following recent spinal cord injuries.[16] Risk factors include age less than 21 years, complete neurologic injuries, cervical injuries, prolonged immobilization, and dehydration.[16] Presenting symptoms include anorexia, nausea, headache, malaise, and depression in mild cases. In more severe cases, patients may have persistent nausea and vomiting, gastric dilatation, fecal impaction, and abdominal pain. Microscopic calcium deposition in the kidney may impair its ability to concentrate urine, leading to polyuria and polydipsia. Patients may also develop cardiac dysrhythmias and seizures.[16]

The pathophysiology of immobilization hypercalcemia is thought to be due to the combination of increased bone resorption and the inability of the kidneys to excrete the excess calcium. Compared to other age groups, an adolescent has a higher than normal bone turnover rate and more total bone mineral.[16] Immobilization causes a decrease in osteoblastic activity in the weight-bearing bones and an increased rate of bone resorption. Together, these factors lead to a higher-than-normal serum calcium level when subjected to a prolonged period of immobilization. In most cases, the kidneys can usually excrete the calcium, but in some patients this ability breaks down.

Treating immobilization hypercalcemia starts with hydration and diuresis with normal saline solution 2 to 3 L/day with the addition of furosemide. Calcitonin in doses of 1 to 4 IU/kg subcutaneously every 12 h can also effectively reduce the serum calcium level.[16]

Heterotopic Ossification

Heterotopic ossification (HO) is the formation of bone in the soft tissues.[17] The mechanisms of the formation of heterotopic bone are not precisely known. In spinal-cord-injured patients, it is more common among those with spasticity. Symptoms may present as early as 1 month after injury. Pain is prominent in other patients with HO but is often absent in spinal-cord-injured patients. For spinal-cord-injured patients, the commonest symptom of HO is a decreased range of motion. Other findings are a change in spasticity, fever, erythema, joint effusion, and swelling.[17] The differential diagnosis includes DVT, infection, and tumor. Sometimes HO and DVT are seen together.

The incidence of HO in spinal-cord-injured patients has been reported to be 16 to 53 percent. The most common sites are the hip, knee, femur, and shoulder.[18] Plain radiograph findings are often negative in the early stages of HO. The gold standard for diagnosis is the three-phase bone scan.[19,20] Serum alkaline phosphatase (ALP) levels have been used as a screening test for HO, since developing bone produces ALP.[21] However, this is a nonspecific test indicating increased bone metabolic activity, which may occur in fractures or tumors.[19]

Treatment for HO is usually disodium etidronate (20 mg/kg/day for 2 weeks followed by 10 mg/kg/day for 10 weeks) along with gentle physical therapy.[21] Referral to a physiatrist (a physician specializing in the care of patients with disabilities) or other spinal-cord-injury specialist is recommended to institute and monitor treatment.

BRAIN INJURY

Posttraumatic Hydrocephalus

Patients with a history of traumatic brain injury may present to the emergency department with the complaint of changing functional status, including psychomotor slowing, cognitive decline, change in gait, and loss of continence. An evaluation for possible infectious or metabolic causes must be undertaken, but a CT scan of the head is critical to exclude posttraumatic hydrocephalus.[22,23] A CT scan revealing periventricular lucency, diminishing sulci, and dilatation of the ventricles suggests posttraumatic hydrocephalus.[23] Consultation with a neurosurgeon for appropriate treatment options, such as shunting, should be undertaken.

Cerebrovascular Accident

Medical complications occur in up to 40 percent of stroke patients. Common complications include DVT, pulmonary embolism, skin breakdown, shoulder dysfunction, pneumonia, and increased risk of falls and injuries. Patients with strokes often have coexisting atherosclerotic heart disease. Heart disease is the second commonest cause of death during the first month after a stroke and the commonest cause after that.[24]

Leg Pain

In a brain-injured patient who presents with a swollen and painful leg, the differential diagnosis includes trauma (e.g., contusion, sprain, or fracture), DVT, heterotopic ossification, and reflex sympathetic dystrophy.[25] Especially with individuals whose impaired language or cognition hinder the history and physical examination, a high index of suspicion and liberal use of ancillary studies are critical. Plain radiographs are usually adequate for evaluating trauma. Noninvasive venous studies (duplex Doppler) are usually adequate for evaluating DVT. Once fracture and DVT have been ruled out, referral to a physiatrist or other specialist in the care of patients with brain injury should be arranged.

REFERENCES

1. Erickson RP: Autonomic hyperreflexia: Pathophysiology and medical management. *Arch Phys Med Rehabil* 61:431, 1980.

2. Colachis SC III : Autonomic hyperreflexia with spinal cord injury. *J Am Parapleg Soc* 15:171, 1992.
3. Kuric J, Hixon AK: *Clinical Practice Guidelines: Autonomic Dysreflexia.* Jackson Heights, NY, Eastern Paralyzed Veterans Association, 1996.
4. Consortium for Spinal Cord Medicine Clinical Practice Guidelines: *Acute Management of Autonomic Dysreflexia: Adults with Spinal Cord Injury Presenting to Healthcare Facilities.* Washington, Paralyzed Veterans of America, 1997.
5. Braddom RL, Rocco JF: Autonomic dysreflexia: A survey of current treatment. *Am J Phys Med Rehabil* 70:234, 1991.
6. The prevention and management of urinary tract infections among people with spinal cord injuries: National Institute on Disability and Rehabilitation Research consensus statement. *J Am Parapleg Soc* 15:194, 1992.
7. Stover SL, Lloyd LK, Waites KB, Jackson AB: Urinary tract infections in spinal cord injury. *Arch Phys Med Rehabil* 70:47, 1989.
8. Gribble MJ, Puterman ML, McCallum NM: Pyuria: Its relationship to bacteruria in spinal cord injured patients on intermittent catheterization. *Arch Phys Med Rehabil* 70:376, 1989.
9. Cardenas DD, Hooten TM: Urinary tract infections in persons with spinal cord injury. *Arch Phys Med Rehabil* 76:272, 1995.
10. Donovan WH, Stolov WC, Clowers DE, Clowers MR: Bacteruria during intermittent catheterization following spinal cord injury. *Arch Phys Med Rehabil* 59:351, 1978.
11. Stamm WE, Hooten TM: Management of urinary tract infections in adults. *N Engl J Med* 329:1328, 1993.
12. Juler GL, Eltorai IM: The acute abdomen in spinal cord injury patients. *Paraplegia* 23:118, 1985.
13. Bar-On Z, Ohry A: The acute abdomen in spinal cord injury individuals. *Paraplegia* 33:704, 1995.
14. Neumayer LA, Bull DA, Mohr JD, Putnam CW: The acutely affected abdomen in paraplegic spinal cord injury patients. *Ann Surg* 212:561, 1990.
15. Schurch B, Wichmann W, Rossier AB: Posttraumatic syringomyelia (cystic myelopathy): A prospective study of 449 patients with spinal cord injury. *J Neurol Neurosurg Psychiatry* 60:61, 1996.
16. Maynard FM: Immobilization hypercalcemia following spinal cord injury. *Arch Phys Med Rehabil* 67:41, 1986.
17. Garland DE: A clinical perspective on common forms of acquired heterotopic ossification. *Clini Orthop* 263:13, 1991.
18. Garland DE: Clinical observations in fractures and heterotopic ossification in spinal cord and traumatic brain injured populations. *Clin Orthop* 233:86, 1988.
19. Buschbacher R: Heterotopic ossifications: A review. *Crit Rev Phys Med Rehabil* 4:199, 1992.
20. Orzel JA, Rudd TG: Heterotopic bone formation: Clinical, laboratory, and imaging correlation. *J Nucl Med* 26:126, 1985.
21. Garland DE, Orwin JF: Resection of heterotopic ossification in patients with spinal cord injuries. *Clin Orthop* 242:169, 1989.
22. Long DF: Diagnosis and management of intercranial complications in traumatic brain injury rehabilitation, in Hors LJ, Zasler ND (eds): *Medical Rehabilitation of Traumatic Brain Injury,* Philadelphia, Hanley and Belfus, 1996, pp 333–362.
23. Doherty D: Posttraumatic hydrocephalus. *Phys Med Rehabil Clin North Am* 3:289, 1992.
24. Roth EJ, Nulls SF: Stroke rehabilitation secondary to comorbidities and complications. *Arch Phys Med Rehabil* 75:542, 1994.
25. Bontke CF: Medical complications related to traumatic brain injury. *Phys Med Rehabil* 3:43, 1989.

302 THE MENTALLY RETARDED ADULT

Linmarie Sikich
L. Jarrett Barnhill

Evaluating a developmentally disabled adult in the ED poses a number of challenges, including accurately assessing the ability of the individual to communicate his or her complaints, the ability to make an accurate diagnosis in the absence of sufficient historical information, and the recognition of unusual presentations of common disorders. In addition, 25 percent of individuals with developmental disabilities appear to have significantly increased pain thresholds that result in reduced responses to illnesses and to physical examinations.[1] Such pain insensitivity may limit recognition of medical problems (e.g., intestinal obstruction) until late in the disease process with potentially catastrophic consequences.[2] Treatment of developmentally disabled individuals is also complicated by questions about guardianship, decreased ability of the patient to understand the treatment recommendations and, often, inadequate preventative and routine medical care. However, it is essential that health care providers overcome these obstacles to provide care to this special population that has difficulty advocating for itself. This has become a growing issue over the past 20 years as large numbers of developmentally disabled adults have moved from specialized institutional settings where a small number of physicians were familiar with their special needs to individual and group homes in the community.

EPIDEMIOLOGY

The primary developmental disability is mental retardation. Mental retardation is defined as significant cognitive (IQ less than 70) and functional delays with onset before adulthood. Over 40 percent of individuals with mental retardation have associated medical conditions. Typically the lower the patient's IQ, the more likely a specific etiology of the mental retardation can be identified. Etiologic factors implicated in mental retardation may be prenatal, perinatal, postnatal, or traumatic. Genetic factors account for 7 to 15 percent of all mental retardation; there are 500 genetic syndromes known to be associated with mental retardation. Most of these genetic syndromes are multisystem disorders with a large number of associated medical problems. Cardiac, orthopedic, connective tissue, and neurologic disorders are particularly common.[3] Down syndrome (trisomy 21) is the most common genetic cause of mental retardation, accounting for 4 to 12 percent of all mental retardation, with an incidence of 1/1000 live births.[4] Fragile X is the most common single-gene disorder and accounts for 1 to 6 percent of all mental retardation. The incidence of fragile X syndrome in males is 1/1000 with almost all affected individuals having mental retardation. In females the incidence of fragile X syndrome is 1/2000, but less than half of females with fragile X syndrome have mental retardation. Other common genetic etiologies include Prader-Willi syndrome and Williams syndrome, each with a prevalence in live births of 0.1/1000, Lesch-Nyhan syndrome, with an estimated prevalence of 0.02/1000, and phenylketonuria (PKU), with a prevalence of 0.08/1000.[5] Exposures to toxins may cause as much as 15 percent of mental retardation with fetal alcohol syndrome (FAS) responsible for about 10 percent of all mental retardation.[6] Depending on the etiology, some medical problems are associated with specific mental retardation syndromes (Table 302-1).

It is estimated that between 1 and 2.5 percent of the population has mental retardation; thus 3 to 6 million individuals in the United States and 61 to 150 million in the world are affected. In recent decades, the reduction in the number of children born with mental retardation, coupled with the markedly improved survival of mentally retarded adults, has shifted the age distribution of persons with mental retardation. The largest age group with mental retardation is the 10- to 20-year-old group. Most studies have demonstrated increased medical problems in mentally retarded adults as compared with developmentally normal adults. These are particularly seizures and cardiovascular disorders.

Other developmental disorders important for health care providers to recognize are the autistic spectrum disorders and developmental language disabilities. Autism is defined by the presence of qualitative differences in social reciprocity, communication, and the ability to purposefully shift attention. About 50 to 70 percent of individuals with autism are also mentally retarded. The remainder, despite normal or superior cognitive abilities, has difficulty communicating their

TABLE 302-1 Medical Problems Associated with Specific Mental Retardation Syndromes

Syndrome	Incidence	%MR	Common Medical Problems
Down's	1/1000	4–12	Atlantoaxial instability; obesity; leukemia; dementia; sleep apnea; hypothyroidism; diabetes; cataracts; hearing loss; congenital heart disease
Fragile X	0.67/1000	1–6	Seizures; mitral valve prolapse; dilated great arteries; otitis
Fetal alcohol	2/1000	10	Seizures; congenital heart disease; eye problems; hearing loss
Prader-Willi	0.1/1000	0.4	Obesity; sleep apnea; hypoventilation; diabetes; inability to vomit; hypertension; ischemic heart disease
Williams	0.1/1000	0.4	Hypertension; supravalvular aortic stenosis; ulcers; renal artery stenosis; urethral stenosis; diverticulitis; vesicoureteral reflux; hypercalcemia
Lesch-Nyhan	0.02/1000	0.08	Severe self-injurious behavior; sudden death; gout; renal calculi; renal failure
Tuberous sclerosis	0.1/1000	0.4	Brain and skin tubers; seizures; rhabdomyomas of heart; angiomyolipomas of kidney; renal failure
Cerebral palsy	3/1000	12–30	Pain; contractures; seizures; respiratory and urinary tract infections

symptoms and understanding, appropriately generalizing, and responding to information about suggested medical treatments. A large number of autistic individuals have tactile defensiveness and become very agitated when they are touched, which complicates physical examination. Autism is estimated to have a prevalence of 1 to 2/1000 individuals, with as many as 5 to 7/1000 affected with milder forms of the disorder. Individuals with language disorders are also likely to have difficulty describing their medical history and understanding treatment recommendations. In both cases, the individuals' limitations may not be immediately obvious.

Over the past 20 to 30 years there has been a movement in the United States to remove mentally retarded individuals from institutional settings and care for them in the community. Consequently more than 60 percent of those institutionalized in the 1970s have been released into the community.[7] The push for deinstitutionalization has come from desires to improve the quality of life of affected individuals and to reduce societal costs. It is estimated that only 11 percent of American working-aged adults with mental retardation currently reside in institutions.[8] However, Strauss and colleagues found that adults with mental retardation who had been moved from an institutional setting to the community had a 51 percent greater mortality rate than those who remained in the state facility.[9] This difference rose to 67 percent when cancer deaths were excluded. The greatest increase in mortality was found in the two months following the move from the institution. Mortality was greater in those individuals who moved in 1995 as compared to 1993. Several hypotheses were proposed to explain the observed increase in mortality, but the most important was that the deinstitutionalized patients had relatively poor access to health care. For example, the caretakers of recent movers may have lacked adequate knowledge of the movers' baseline and thus did not recognize important changes, or the caretakers may not have been able to provide doctors with adequate past medical history. When these patients are evaluated by a physician, the greatest obstacle to patient care may be an inadequate past medical history.[10] Finally, physicians in institutions may be more familiar with the unusual presentations of common illnesses within the mentally retarded population or more experienced with the specialized evaluations these individuals require. These factors highlight the critical need for physicians, particularly those in emergency settings, to be familiar with the special needs of developmentally disabled patients.

GENERAL APPROACH

Assess the Individual's Developmental Level

Developmentally disabled individuals have a broad range of cognitive abilities. It is essential to approach patients in a manner consistent with their abilities and to be sensitive to and respectful of their thoughts and feelings. About 85 percent of mentally retarded individuals are mildly impaired; they typically function at about a fifth to sixth grade level, although under the stress of illness and the emergency department, this may be reduced. Once their anxiety is alleviated, they can generally provide some relevant history and describe many of their symptoms. They are also likely to understand simple written directions provided jargon is avoided. About 10 percent of mentally retarded adults are moderately affected; they function at the level of a preschool child, are likely to be able to follow commands, and may be able to answer simple questions. The remaining 5 percent are likely to have no expressive language although they sometimes can follow simple commands.

When assessing any verbal developmentally disabled individual, it is important to ask open-ended rather than yes/no questions to verify the patient's understanding of your question. It is also helpful to ask higher functioning individuals to repeat back information to make sure they have sufficient understanding. Many mentally retarded individuals have particular difficulties with time and causality concepts. Nonverbal patients may be able to point in response to simple questions; however, the bulk of information they provide is nonverbal. Painful regions of the body often become targets for self-injurious behaviors. Similarly, the patient may be splinting or mouthing a painful area. Finally, the mentally retarded often have reduced pain sensitivity that may lead to unusual illness presentations.

Collateral Informants

The evaluation of developmentally disabled patient usually requires collateral information from others, including parents or other family members, group home staff, or social service agency staff. The extent and importance of such information increases as the developmentally disabled patient's ability to communicate decreases. Unfortunately, the person with the patient may have relatively little information about the patient's current problems and/or past history. For example, 55 percent of caregivers in a community setting could not supply basic medical information about the patient. It is important to ask the collateral source explicitly how much information they have and whether there are others who can be contacted by phone who can provide additional information. It is also important to ask if they brought any written information with them. Frequently, lower functioning individuals will be living in group settings where a medical chart with a complete medical history, current medications, sleep logs, and longitudinal vital signs are available. Lack of sufficient information is likely to be the primary obstacle to care of the adult developmentally disabled individual.

TABLE 302-2 Frequently Used Medications and Side Effects

Medications	Frequency of Use[23]	Important Side Effects
Psychotropics	44%	
Antipsychotics		Extrapyramidal symptoms; neuroleptic malignant syndrome; dystonia can affect swallowing and breathing; sedation; orthostatic hypotension; weight gain; constipation
SSRIs		GI distress; agitation; insomnia; sedation
Benzodiazepines		Sedation; disinhibition; agitation; delirium
Anticholinergics		Blurry vision; urinary retention; constipation
Lithium		Hypothyroidism; delirium; cardiac arrhythmias
Anticonvulsants		Sedation; delirium; ataxia
Carbamazepine		Blood dyscrasias; rashes; constipation; lowers other drug levels
Lamotrigine		Severe rashes
Cardiovascular	25%	Overdosage may lead to cardiotoxicity
Laxatives	20%	Vitamin deficiencies
Bronchodilators	14%	Agitation; decreased bone mineralization
Analgesics	12%	Renal problems; anemia
Histamine blockers	10%	Psychosis
Thyroid supplement	8%	Psychosis; agitation; hot flashes; odd skin sensations

Essential Information

Because individuals with mental retardation have a broad range of function, it is essential to determine the patient's specific baseline in a number of areas.

1. How the patient normally communicates.
2. How aware they typically are of their environment.
3. What are their usual motor skills and level of activity.
4. What is the patient's elimination pattern? Constipation and urinary tract infections are common in the mentally retarded and often present with increased agitation or self-injurious behavior.
5. What are the patient's usual sleep pattern and appetite? Both may be disrupted with infectious and psychiatric disorders.

Many mentally retarded patients have multiple medical problems that, either directly or as a consequence of medication side effects, contribute to their acute problem. Therefore, it is essential to get a complete past medical history, an accurate list of medications and doses, and history of prior adverse reactions including allergies. Frequently used medications and associated side effects are shown in Table 302-2. Often increasing use of prn medications is associated with changes in mental status. Finally, one should ask about the patient's visual and hearing status and the use of assistive devices such as glasses, hearing aids, dentures, and walkers. Nearly 60 percent of mentally retarded adults have significant visual impairments, and they are twice as likely to have severe hearing impairments as nonmentally retarded individuals.[11,12] It is not unusual for someone with hearing or visual impairments to become agitated or withdrawn if an assistive device is lost or malfunctioning.

Next it is important to determine the patient's living situation. Even relatively minor changes in routine or caretakers can have a dramatic impact on the functioning of some developmentally disabled individuals, particularly those with autism. It is also essential to determine the patient's resources for appropriate follow-up care within the community. The provision of routine and preventative care is particularly important in the developmentally disabled population because of the higher incidence of medical problems. Finally, determine whether the patient has a guardian or, if not, whether they are capable of making their own decisions about medical care.

Physical Examination

A careful and thorough physical examination is essential because sufficient history is often not available to focus the examination. Often, developmentally disabled individuals will be very agitated or have extreme tactile defensiveness, making a thorough examination and detection of physical signs difficult. Special attention should be given to all body orifices (ears, nares, mouth, anus, vagina, and urethra) because foreign objects are often inserted into these areas without the caretakers' knowledge. A dental examination is also important because a large number of individuals with mental retardation have significant periodontal disease.

Vital signs should be obtained when the patient is calm, if possible. If not medically contraindicated, it may be helpful to offer the patient food or distractions (toys, magazines) so that they feel less threatened. It also is essential to carefully explain what you are doing and periodically check to see if the patient understands. It is usually very helpful to have a familiar person present during the examination and procedures, particularly if the patient is nonverbal. If none of these approaches decreases the patient's anxiety sufficiently to allow an evaluation, assistance is required to briefly hold the patient.

Ancillary Studies

Given the difficulties with communication and high frequency of medical problems observed in developmentally disabled adults, it is often useful to obtain ancillary studies that would ordinarily not be required in nondisabled adults. Although the results of some laboratory examinations (e.g., thyroid function tests) will not be available while the patient is in the ED, it is often important nonetheless to obtain them, particularly if there are any difficulties with phlebotomy or concerns about the adequacy of outpatient care. Most ancillary studies are chosen based on the complaints elicited or behavior observed. If the presentation does not suggest localizing symptoms or have helpful physical signs, generalized "screening" studies may be necessary. For most developmentally disabled patients, these screening studies include a complete blood count, electrolytes, liver function tests, urinalysis, and serum drug levels if the patient is on anticonvulsants or lithium[13,14] (Table 302-3). When obtaining these studies, it is essential that all procedures are carefully explained at the patient's developmental level. It may also be helpful to use topical anesthetic cream for phlebotomy.

Some presentations suggest the need for specific studies:

1. If agitation is the primary complaint, vitamin B_{12} levels, thyroid abnormalities, and the level of oxygenation as measured by pulse oximetry should be assessed, and impaction should be excluded with an abdominal radiograph.
2. If the agitation is cyclic, consider the possibility of a psychomotor seizure and the need for an EEG.
3. If "spells" are reported, an EEG, ECG, and pulse oximetry are appropriate.

TABLE 302-3 Suggested Ancillary Studies in Developmentally Disabled Adults

Situation	Diagnostic Evaluations
ED Screening	CBC; electrolytes; BUN; creatinine; liver function tests; serum drug levels (anticonvulsants; lithium); UA
If agitated	Add B_{12}; thyroid function (T4 and TSH); pulse oximetry; abdominal radiograph; consider EEG
"Spells"	Add EEG; ECG; pulse oximetry
Delirium	Add thyroid function tests (T4 and TSH); pulse oximetry; carnitine
GI Bleeding	Endoscopy; abdominal radiograph for foreign bodies
Ataxia	CK; cervical spine radiographs to evaluate atlantoaxial instability
Fatigue	Glucose; calcium; lactate; pyruvate; parathyroid hormone; prostate specific antigen; serum protein electrophoresis
Initial outpatient screening	ED screening plus chest radiograph; ECG; thyroid function tests (T4 and TSH); antinuclear antibody; erythrocyte sedimentation rate; B_{12}; folate

4. If a change in mental status or delirium has precipitated the evaluation, consider infections, seizures, and drug interactions or toxicities. Check thyroid function, carnitine levels (especially if patient is on valproic acid), and serum drug levels. Anticholinergics, antihistamines, and benzodiazepines are frequently associated with delirium and agitation.
5. If the patient presents with ataxia, consider drug toxicities, neuroleptic malignant syndrome (NMS), and atlantoaxial instability.
6. If fatigue is the primary complaint, consider viral illnesses, diabetes, and metabolic disturbances (including calcium, lactate, pyruvate, carnitine, and parathyroid).
7. If movement disorders are observed, withdrawal dyskinesias caused by reduction in antipsychotics and tardive dyskinesia should be considered.

FREQUENTLY ENCOUNTERED PROBLEMS

The incidence of medical problems is greater in the developmentally delayed population than in the general population. However, these problems often manifest in unusual ways. A recent study of elderly mentally retarded individuals found that 24 percent had arthritis; 23 percent had gastrointestinal problems (including 7.5 percent with ulcer disease); 23 percent had vascular disease; 16 percent had hypertension; 20 percent had respiratory disorders; and 19 percent had epilepsy.[15] Thirty-five percent of emergency department visits were precipitated by infections (usually respiratory); 33 percent by trauma; 15 percent by seizures; and 5 percent by gastrointestinal concerns.[15] In addition, agitation or aggression frequently leads to ED evaluations. In the study of recently deinstitutionalized adults with mental retardation, deaths were caused by respiratory problems (particularly pneumonia) in 24 percent; cardiovascular events in 22 percent; gastrointestinal illnesses in 15 percent; seizures in 15 percent; sudden asphyxiation in 9 percent; nonrespiratory infections in 4 percent; and trauma in 4 percent.[9]

Injuries

Injuries may be self-inflicted, accidental, or sustained by assault from others. Developmentally disabled individuals are quite vulnerable to assault, and it is important that health care providers be aware of the risk of abuse and their duty to report suspicious injuries. However, the majority of injuries that mentally retarded individuals experience are the result of self-injurious behaviors. Although self-injurious behaviors may be self-stimulating or compulsive, it is essential to rule out medical and environmental precipitants. This is particularly true if the self-injurious behaviors are of sudden onset. Bosch and colleagues found that in 28 percent of their patients, treatment of previously undiagnosed, painful medical conditions resulted in significant reductions in self-injurious behaviors.[16] Constipation, gastrointestinal reflux, and peptic ulcer disease were the most common disorders. In these cases, there had often been a cyclic pattern to the self-injurious behaviors or a recent exacerbation. Similarly, increased self-injurious behaviors are often observed with anxiety which frequently results from environmental changes. If no medical or environmental precipitants can be identified it may be useful to treat individuals with selective serotonin reuptake inhibitors (SSRI). However, mentally retarded individuals often respond to lower doses of these agents than individuals with obsessive compulsive disorder. Because these agents may take three to six weeks to act, it is essential that behavioral measures be taken to avoid further injury to traumatized tissues, such as covering affected areas (e.g., a helmet to prevent head-banging damage; mittens or splints to limit the ability to scratch or hit; or a helmet with a face mask to prevent biting). Very close supervision can also prevent a great deal of self-injurious behaviors. Other pharmacologic interventions being examined include the use of naltrexone or atypical antipsychotics.

Infections

Infections, which are often quite fulminant at the time of diagnosis, are frequent in the developmentally disabled population. Mentally retarded individuals frequently have oral-motor dyspraxias that result in frequent tracheal aspirations. Aspiration is also more common in individuals with esophageal reflux and with tube feedings. Urinary tract infections are common. An increased incidence of neurogenic bladder, limited mobility, and poor hygiene all contribute to this increase. Because individuals may initially not recognize or describe dysuria, they are at greater risk for pyelonephritis. With a history of repeated urinary tract infections, it is important to exclude congenital malformations of the urinary system. Skin infections are also frequent. In low functioning individuals, these most commonly occur over pressure points or in the skin folds of the genital and anal regions. Poor mobility and hygiene contribute significantly. In higher functioning individuals, skin infections may be a consequence of repeated biting or scratching or the insertion of foreign objects under the skin. Finally, 16 percent of mentally retarded individuals had severe periodontal disease as compared to 3 percent of controls.[17] It is likely that both poor hygiene and anticonvulsant use contribute to this finding.

Neurologic Problems

SEIZURES Thirty to 50 percent of all developmentally delayed individuals have seizure disorders. Often, an individual experiences several different types of seizures, which may have complicated presentations such as Lennox-Gastaut seizures. Occasionally, patients, particularly those who are verbal, also have pseudoseizures. As with any other patient, the priorities are to insure adequate oxygenation and to stop the seizure. Subsequently, one must determine the precipitants for the seizure, specifically whether the precipitant is medication or infection. Seizures are commonly precipitated by a change in medications. Frequently, in an effort to reduce side effects and potential drug interactions, efforts are made to reduce the number of anticonvulsants or to switch from an older agent such as phenobarbital even though the patient's seizures are under good control. Occasionally, unintentional medication changes occur when the developmentally disabled individual moves to new living situations because a medication has been forgotten or given incorrectly. Addition of new concurrent medications may also have altered the seizure threshold. For example, theophylline decreases seizure threshold. Infections, especially UTI may also precipitate seizures in individuals whose seizures had been previously well controlled.

DELIRIUM Developmentally disabled individuals appear to be particularly vulnerable to delirium. Typically caretakers will describe a relatively acute change in mental status. However, this change may be relatively subtle if the individual is inactive or nonverbal at baseline. Visual and tactile hallucinations and agitation are not uncommon. Most often the change in mental status is related to infection or to drug toxicity. Drug toxicity may occur at lower medication doses than observed in other populations. Toxicity may also be precipitated by interactions with other medications. For instance, erythromycin and fluoxetine both slow the metabolism of several anticonvulsants and may result in toxic levels. Anticonvulsants and anticholinergics frequently cause delirium. Less often, delirium results from metabolic disturbances including hyperglycemia, hypothyroidism, hypoxia, or vitamin or cofactor deficiencies (e.g., vitamin B_{12} in individuals with limited diets or carnitine in individuals treated chronically with valproic acid). In addition, changes in mental status are often seen in sleep apneas, which is common in Prader-Willi and Down syndromes.

DEMENTIA Dementia leads to many of the same symptoms as delirium but does so more gradually. Some subgroups of mentally retarded individuals appear especially likely to develop dementia. For instance, over 80 percent of individuals with Down syndrome who are older than 40 years, have symptoms of dementia. The differential diagnosis of dementia should include depression and chronic overmedication.

SPINAL CORD COMPRESSION DUE TO ATLANTOAXIAL INSTABILITY Individuals with Down syndrome are particularly vulnerable to spinal cord damage resulting from instability between the atlas and the axis of the cervical spine. This instability is a consequence of two factors. First, there is a general laxity of the connective tissue in Down syndrome. Second, congenital anomalies of the atlas and axis (particularly the odontoid process or hypoplasia of the posterior arch of the atlas) are common with an incidence of 26 percent in Down syndrome.[18] Although atlantoaxial instability is described primarily in Down syndrome, individuals with a number of other mental retardation syndromes associated with prominent hypotonia, connective tissue problems and bony malformation are also likely to develop atlantoaxial instability.

With atlantoaxial instability, the spinal cord is vulnerable to compression between the odontoid process anteriorly and the arch of the atlas posteriorly when the neck is flexed. Spinal cord compression may also occur during neck extension when there is atlantoaxial subluxation and/or dislocation. Intubation, cardiac catheterization, laryngoscopy, bronchoscopy, tracheal suctioning, sedation for neuroimaging, auditory- and visual-evoked potential studies, and dental work all involve positions with extreme neck extension and may be dangerous. The neurologic manifestations of atlantoaxial instability may be relatively subtle and include easy fatigability, difficulties in walking, neck pain, limited neck mobility, torticollis, incoordination and clumsiness, sensory deficits, problems with incontinence, and spasticity. These symptoms may progress to paraplegia, hemiplegia, quadriplegia or even death. Most individuals have had symptoms for more than a month prior to their diagnosis and many will have had symptoms for a year or more. Rarely, sudden subluxation has occurred when there is a sudden change in momentum (e.g., when a motor vehicle crashes and on carnival rides such as bumper cars and roller coasters).

Radiographic screening for atlantoaxial instability consists of measuring the atlantodens interval with intervals of greater than 4.5 mm considered suggestive of atlantoaxial instability. However, there has been a great deal of controversy about the reliability and stability of atlantodens interval measurements. Relatively few individuals with radiographic evidence of atlantoaxial instability are symptomatic and some symptomatic individuals have normal radiographs. Recently, some have argued that screening radiographs for atlantoaxial instability should be abandoned and careful neurologic exams should be substituted.[19]

Treatment of atlantoaxial instability typically involves surgical stabilization. There are frequent medical complications with procedures, but it is not clear that these are any greater in the developmentally disabled population than in the general population.

Psychiatric Disorders

Psychiatric disorders are estimated to afflict up to 50 percent of the developmentally disabled population. Although mood disorders, particularly depression, are most frequent, they are relatively unlikely to precipitate ED evaluations. Instead, emergency visits are usually precipitated by aggression or extreme agitation. In such cases, benzodiazepines or low-dose, low-potency antipsychotics, such as chlorpromazine, may be acutely helpful in controlling the patient's behavior sufficiently to proceed with an evaluation. However, it is essential to try to identify the underlying etiology of these behaviors and changes in their frequency or intensity. Undiagnosed, painful medical problems, including severe constipation, often lead to exacerbation.[16] Sleep apnea can also be manifest as increased irritability. In addition, anxiety may be manifest primarily as agitation. Often environmental factors can be identified that are increasing the patient's anxiety. Such factors may include changes in caretakers or recent onset of sensory deficits that have not yet been corrected. Sometimes the anxiety is the result of posttraumatic stress disorder. At other times, it may occur in the context of "panic attacks," which are manifested atypically due to language limitations. Akathisia, a dose-related side-effect syndrome caused by both typical and atypical antipsychotics, is manifest as agitation and hyperactivity. It should be considered anytime there is a history of worsening agitation with increased antipsychotic medications. Similarly, large doses of some of the newer anticonvulsants (e.g., gabapentin and lamotrigine) have been associated with agitation. Rarely, the agitation may occur in response to psychotic symptoms such as hallucinations or paranoid delusions.

If the patient appears to be psychotic, it is important to distinguish between true responses to internal stimuli, motor and verbal tics, and self-stimulating behaviors characteristic of autism. Catatonic behavior may reflect delirium, depression, or status epilepticus with absence or partial-complex seizures. Psychosis is probably the most common misdiagnosis in this population. Mood disorders typically present with changes in the patient's sleep, appetite, and activity level. Treatment with antidepressants is indicated and effective. Appropriate treatment for any underlying medical or psychiatric disorder should be undertaken. Remember that developmentally disabled individuals often require smaller doses of psychotropic medications and may be more sensitive to adverse effects.

Gastrointestinal Disorders

Mentally retarded individuals frequently present to the ED with gastrointestinal bleeding and it is the most common reason for hospital admission. In 70 percent of cases studied, erosive esophagitis was the diagnosis.[20] A large number of developmentally disabled individuals also have ulcers, usually duodenal. Such conditions respond well to aggressive treatment with proton pump inhibitors and H_2 blockers. In addition, perhaps as many as 40 percent of mentally retarded individuals have a neurogenic bowel with resulting constipation, overflow diarrhea, and infrequent rectal tears. It is important to carefully evaluate for constipation. Treatment must include both acute and long-term measures, including establishment of a regular stool pattern and provision of adequate fluid and fiber intake. It is also important to determine whether the patient has pica and may have developed bezoars. About 10 percent of individuals with pica will develop intestinal obstruction.[21] While surgery is often necessary for obstruction, it is also important to develop a treatment program to deal with the patient's pica. Behavioral measures are the cornerstone of such work, but pharmacologic interventions with SSRI may also be useful. It is also essential to determine whether a nutritional deficiency is related to pica. About 10 percent of mentally retarded individuals have parasitic infections. *Enterobius vermicularis* and *Strongyloides stercoralis* are common. Finally, there is a high prevalence of hepatitis within the mentally retarded population, particularly those individuals in group care.

Orthopedic Problems

As many as 50 percent of severely retarded individuals suffer from orthopedic problems. The problems are often multiple, with congenital abnormalities, limited mobility, obesity, and age-associated changes all contributing. Often these problems are painful and result in increased agitation. Treatment is generally symptomatic. However, efforts to increase mobility and reduce weight are also important.

Malignancies

Overall, the rates of malignancy in the developmentally disabled population do not differ from the general population.[22] However, malignancies are often much more advanced when diagnosed. Difficulties in communicating early, less-specific symptoms, markedly decreased self-monitoring (e.g., monthly breast self-examination), and a relative absence of preventative care, all contribute to this problem. Some mental retardation syndromes have an increased risk of malignancy. Adults with Down syndrome have a 10-fold increased risk for leukemia. Individuals with tuberous sclerosis are prone to brain tumors, particularly subependymal giant cell astrocytomas (SEGAs), rhabdomyomas of the heart, and angiomyolipomas of the kidney. Giant cell astrocytomas often present with an increase in seizure frequency.

REFERENCES

1. Biersdorff KK: Incidence of significantly altered pain experience among individuals with developmental disabilities. *Am J Ment Retard* 98:619, 1994.
2. Biersdorff KK: Pain insensitivity and indifference: Alternative explanations for some medical catastrophes. *Ment Retard* 29:359,1991.
3. Murphy CC, Boyle C, Schendel D, Decoufle P, Yeargin-Allsopp M: Epidemiology of mental retardation in children. *Ment Retard Develop Disabil Res Rev* 4:6, 1998.
4. Yeargin-Allsopp M, Murphy CC, Cordero JF, et al: Reported biomedical causes and associated medical conditions for mental retardation among 10-year-old children, metropolitan Atlanta, 1985 to 1987. *Develop Med Child Neurol* 39:142, 1997.
5. Gilberg C: *Clinical Child Neuropsychiatry*. Cambridge, England, Cambridge University Press, 1995.
6. Abel EL, Sokol RJ: Fetal alcohol syndrome is now the leading cause of mental retardation. *Lancet* ii:1222, 1986.
7. Braddock D, Hemp R, Bachedleder L, Fujiura G: *The State of the States in Developmental Disabilities,* 4th ed. Washington, DC, American Association of Mental Retardation, 1995.
8. Schoenman JA: Description of the U.S. working age disabled populations living in institutions and in the community. *Disabil Rehabil* 17:231, 1995.
9. Strauss D, Shavelle R, Baumeister A, Anderson TW: Mortality in persons with developmental disabilities after transfer into community care. *Am J Ment Retard* 102:569, 1998.
10. Minihan PM, Dean DH, Lyons CM: Managing the care of patients with mental retardation: A survey of physicians. *Ment Retard* 31:239, 1993.
11. Evenhuis HM: Medical aspects of aging in a population with intellectual disability. I. Visual impairment. *J Intellect Disabil Research* 39:19, 1995.
12. Evenhuis HM: Medical aspects of aging in a population with intellectual disability. II. Hearing impairment. *J Intellect Disabil Research* 39:27,1995.
13. Martin BA: Primary care of adults with mental retardation living in the community. *Am Fam Physician* 56:485, 1997.
14. Ryan R, Sunada K: Medical evaluation of persons with mental retardation referred for psychiatric assessment. *Gen Hosp Psychiatry* 19:274, 1997.
15. Tyler CV, Bourguet C: Primary care of adults with mental retardation. *J Fam Pract* 44:487, 1997.
16. Bosch J, Van Dyke DC, Smith SM, Poulton S: Role of medical conditions in the exacerbation of self-injurious behavior: An exploratory study. *Ment Retard* 35:124, 1997.
17. Scott A, March L, Stokes ML: A survey of oral health in a population of adults with developmental disabilities—comparisons with a national oral health survey of the general population. *Aust Dent J* 43:257, 1998.
18. Fenderson CB: Down syndrome and aging: Implications for rehabilitation. *Topics Geriatr Rehabil* 13:39, 1998.
19. American Academy of Pediatrics Committee on Sports Medicine and Fitness: Atlantoaxial instability in Down syndrome: Subject review. *Pediatrics* 96:151, 1995.
20. Orchard JL, Stramat J, Wolfgang M, Trimpey A: Upper gastrointestinal tract bleeding in institutionalized mentally retarded adults: Primary role of esophagitis. *Arch Fam Med* 4:30, 1995.
21. Danford DE, Huber AM: Pica among mentally retarded adults. *Am J Ment Deficiency* 87:141, 1982.
22. Evenhuis HM: Medical aspects of aging in a population with intellectual disability. III. Mobility, internal conditions and cancer. *J Intellect Disabil Res* 41:8, 1997.
23. Cooper SA: Clinical study of the effects of age on the physical health of adults with mental retardation. *Am J Ment Retard* 102:582, 1998.

THE HOMELESS PATIENT

Rama B. Rao
Lewis R. Goldfrank

Homelessness is a social problem of epidemic proportions worldwide.[1] In the United States alone, estimates of the homeless population range between 3 to 13.5 million. As much as 7.4 percent of the general population will experience homelessness in their lifetime.[2] Homelessness affects a diverse population of all ethnic groups and includes both urban and rural families, the elderly, children, veterans, migrant farm workers, mentally ill persons, and persons with substance abuse disorders. Minority groups are overrepresented in this population, most likely due to disparities in economic opportunities. Causes of homelessness are related to divorce or separation, domestic violence, pregnancy, adolescent runaways, substance abuse, eviction, acute or chronic unemployment, and the deinstitutionalization of persons with mental illness. A disparity between the need for low-income housing and its availability has also contributed to the epidemic of homelessness.

Homelessness has been defined in a variety of ways, including living on the "street," in shelters that provide temporary residence, or in single-room occupancy hotels with shared bathrooms. The consequences of homelessness are profound. A study of homeless adults in Philadelphia found that their age-adjusted mortality rate was nearly four times higher than that of the general population.[3] The median age of death of homeless adults in Atlanta was 44.[4] Infant mortality rates are more than twice those for nonpoor, domiciled mothers and 50 percent higher than those for poor domiciled mothers. The effects of homelessness on children may be profound and are discussed below. Other risks important to homeless populations include communicable diseases, environmental exposures to extreme heat or cold, and traumatic injury due to violent encounters, foraging for food, and seeking shelter.[5] These factors contribute greatly to acute medical illness in the homeless. Some of the increased risks are associated with poverty, and others are specific to undomiciled patients. Chronic illnesses, such as hypertension and diabetes, are neglected or poorly managed due to desperate living circumstances. Homeless individuals often delay care of minor medical problems until they become severe or unbearable.

The ED is often used as a primary source of medical care for acute and nonacute illnesses of the homeless.[6,7] Outpatient community- and shelter-based clinics provide medical care in a limited fashion and can lead to ED referral for more extensive evaluation and management. In some cities, homeless patients may arrive by police or emergency medical services because of extreme weather emergencies or other health and safety mandates. All of these factors make knowledge of this population important to emergency physicians. The management of the homeless patient is complex, and similarities to the domiciled layperson are limited. Medical evaluation and care, homeless health issues, and special conditions and populations are reviewed in this chapter.

CARE AND EVALUATION

Homeless patients may have both specific and nonspecific medical complaints.[8] Once the primary reason for the visit is addressed, a thorough examination of the entire body, including the skin and particularly the feet, should be considered. This is especially necessary for the homeless patient who presents disheveled, intoxicated, or with a significant psychosis. A valuable medical history may include the last evaluation for tuberculosis exposure, tetanus immunization status, vaccination status in children, psychiatric history, history of chemical dependence, and potential for substance withdrawal while receiving care in the emergency department. A social history may include family support, precipitants of homelessness, and prior contact with a social worker.

SPECIAL MEDICAL CONSIDERATIONS

Lower Extremity Diseases

Homeless patients have a variety of lower extremity disorders.[9] Such patients may spend a disproportionate amount of time with their legs in a dependent position while sleeping upright or ambulating for extended periods. The poverty associated with homelessness may prevent some patients from obtaining adequate or appropriately fitting socks and shoes that are seasonally appropriate. Ulcers and wounds from lack of foot protection, blisters from poorly fitting shoes, or bites from rats or insects may occur.

Some homeless patients may not have an available change of footwear or a place to change and bathe. Socks and shoes may not be removed for days to weeks for reasons such as warmth, fear that footwear may be stolen, embarrassment, or coexisting mental illness. These factors, along with limitations in hygiene, predispose to fungal infections, which can be treated with topical or oral therapy. Also of concern in this population is the condition known as trench foot.[10] Protracted exposure to moisture around the foot (usually from wet or sweaty socks) leads to absorption of water into the stratum corneum. Over 1 to 2 days, such exposure causes inflammatory changes that result in foot pain and skin breakdown. Bacterial superinfection with *Corynebacterium* species and *Pseudomonas* species can ensue. In the absence of superinfection, analgesia, leg elevation, and drying are adequate to treat trench foot. In colder climates, frostbite from formation of ice crystals in the tissues is a serious threat to limbs, ears, and nose. Careful in-hospital management is warranted, since the environmental risks persist as long as the patient remains homeless, and compliance with treatment may be difficult if not impossible.

Patients predisposed to peripheral vascular disease can have exacerbation of their illness due to inadequate nutrition, poor protein stores, alcoholism and substance use, use of tobacco, and inability to elevate the legs while sleeping upright. The resulting edema can lead to chronic venous stasis ulcers. The ulcers can become infected with common skin flora or even maggots (fly larvae). For uninfected ulcers, the use of venous support garments, such as Una boots, is a valuable management tool. Una boots are impregnated with antibiotic ointment and require less frequent changes. Infected ulcers require admission. The erythema associated with cellulitis may be difficult to distinguish from deep venous thrombosis or venous stasis changes. When the diagnosis is unclear, an evaluation of venous flow should be undertaken. For lesions infected with maggots, chloroform is a traditional therapy for deinfestation. Chloroform may not be available due to safety issues of combustibility. Ethyl chloride is an alternative. Ironically, maggots survive by ingesting necrotic tissue, keeping ulcers clean and well débrided. Once deinfestation is completed, close follow-up is mandatory, since natural débridement via fly larvae is terminated. Maggot infestation is a grave sign of serious neglect and suggests the inability to manage a clinical plan outside a supervised setting.

All homeless patients need education to minimize the risk of trench foot and fungal infections. Patients should be told to change or remove all footwear when environmental conditions allow, examine the feet, and attempt to find rest with the legs elevated. Intravenous drug abusers should be warned about the risk of skin infection from drug administration into the extremities. Community resources, which can provide clean, dry socks and well-fitting shoes, should be identified. Such preventive measures are especially important for diabetic patients and those who suffer from peripheral neuropathy.

Infections

Homeless patients develop common community-acquired respiratory infections, but tuberculosis is also a threat. The incidence of tuberculosis increases dramatically when people live under crowded conditions and when patients are immunosupressed from diseases such as AIDS, malnutrition, or alcoholism.[11] Multiple studies of various homeless populations confirm the high incidence and prevalence of tuberculosis in homeless patients. For homeless patients, compliance with a treatment regimen for an exposure to tuberculosis may be limited. Daily, directly observed therapy programs have been very successful by using incentives to organize therapy and decrease the risk of respiratory tuberculosis.

Homeless patients in shelters or other group living arrangement are also at higher risk than are domiciled patients for communicable skin diseases, such as pediculosis (lice), scabies, and impetigo. Deinfestation of lice and scabies is problematic for patients, since bathing facilities and the ability to wash and change clothing are limited. Patients may return to the environment where infestation originally occurred, and they are at high risk for reinfestation. A dermatologic disease known as bacillary angiomatosis-peliosis has been identified in homeless patients exposed to lice.[12] The causative organism is *Bartonella quintana,* and the condition can be treated effectively with macrolide antibiotics.

The living conditions of the impoverished can place them at risk for other infections. Diarrheal illness from the ingestion of improperly preserved or discarded food has been poorly studied but has been described by homeless patients and is particularly problematic when access to toilet facilities is limited. Fecal-oral transmission of illness is also increased.

Sexually transmitted diseases are prevalent in homeless individuals who engage in sexual activity voluntarily or by coercion to obtain food, shelter, cash, or other goods. Money for prophylactic condoms or other forms of contraception is limited, unavailable, or a low priority for survival. These problems, in addition to injected drug use, have lead to epidemic rates of HIV among the homeless. Discrimination and disability from HIV disease are also implicated as a cause of homelessness.

The management of HIV disease is complicated for both patients and medical practitioners even under ideal circumstances. Newer drug regimens, which include multiple medications, are expensive and depend on a reliable dosing schedule and follow-up. CD4+ counts and exposure to tuberculosis should be checked, and prophylaxis for *Pneumocystis carinii* pneumonia and tuberculosis should be offered accordingly. The use of reverse transcriptase and protease inhibitors may depend on the ability of patients to comply with therapy.[13]

Compliance

Prioritization of other life-sustaining activities, such as finding food or shelter, may interfere with compliance with medical regimens or follow-up despite the intention to do so.[14] Money may be unavailable for prescriptions. Even hospital-dispensed medications may be traded for cash or other items perceived as more essential, depending on the patient's level of despair and how well the patient understands the consequences of forgoing treatment. Some items necessary for treatment, such as insulin syringes or other medications, are valuable for illicit use and are at risk of theft. Agents such as insulin may lose their efficacy and safety when stored improperly. It may be impossible to refrigerate medications. A regular dosing medication schedule is complicated by a lifestyle devoid of daily routines.

Lack of medical insurance may cause patients to be turned away from medical care or follow-up. Negotiating eligibility for various types of state and federal medical coverage is usually complicated but may be of tremendous benefit to patients with chronic illnesses, for which poverty potentially thwarts adequate management. Patients should be referred to social workers familiar with eligibility requirements and processing. Unfortunately, even eligible patients may require several visits to social-services agencies to establish medical coverage, and this process alone may be too complex to complete.

Other barriers to care include lack of transportation or mental illness. The precarious existence of such patients must be considered with compassion, and they should be treated with a medical regimen that accommodates the limitations of their situation. For example, patients dependent on soup kitchens should have follow-up that does not compete with mealtimes. Shelter-based clinic systems may be more realistic than tightly scheduled appointments.

SPECIAL POPULATIONS

Women and Children

Women and children comprise a rapidly increasing proportion of the homeless population. Women may present for routine medical problems or as a result of domestic violence or rape, for which they are at particularly high risk.[15] Some women may resort to prostitution to support themselves or their children. Preventive gynecologic care is often inadequate and extends from inadequate screening for cervical cancer and venereal diseases to insufficient or absent prenatal care. The consequences are devastating. Children born to homeless mothers often have lower birth weights, higher rates of prematurity, and higher rates of infant mortality. Iron-deficiency anemia, malnutrition, elevated blood lead concentrations, and a higher rate of asthma are found in homeless children, as in other impoverished children.[16] Unlike impoverished domiciled children, homeless children are more likely to be inadequately immunized and suffer disproportionately from developmental delay or a lack of progression in school. The long-term psychological, social, and educational consequences of homelessness have yet to be evaluated.

Homeless adolescents, especially runaways, have high rates of alcoholism, illicit substance use, violent encounters, and psychiatric illness. Engaging in sex for survival has resulted in high rates of unplanned pregnancy, sexually transmitted disease, and HIV infection. Patients should be offered a variety of resources, including education regarding safe-sex practices, counseling, and the location and availability of drop-in centers. Social workers, psychiatrists, and adolescent specialists can cooperatively provide support for homeless runaways regardless of their chief medical complaint.

The Elderly

There are few studies of the homeless elderly.[17] Limited, fixed incomes with progressively increasing housing costs account for the displacement of many elderly people from their homes. Another factor may be gradual changes in cognitive and psychosocial performance, which may not be realized on a brief medical examination. For all people at risk, reassessment for organicity, dementia, and depression is essential to ensure an appropriate care plan.

Substance Use

Patients who are dependent on alcohol or illicit substances should be identified in order to facilitate appropriate disposition. For homeless patients who present intoxicated and sedated, close monitoring of body temperature, blood glucose monitoring, and serial evaluations for arousability should be performed in addition to a thorough physical examination. Whenever possible, a specific history of substance use should be obtained. A specific history of withdrawal from any sedative-hypnotic agent or ethanol should alert the clinician to the need for careful observation while primary evaluation of the chief complaint is undertaken. The patient should be asked whether he or she has a past history of participating in detoxification programs and whether that is a current desire. Accordingly, psychiatric evaluation can be undertaken.

Psychiatric Evaluation

Some homeless patients without documented history of chronic psychiatric illness or substance dependence may present to the emergency department with psychiatric complaints. The stresses of sustaining life without a home are associated with a variety of diagnoses, including adjustment disorders, substance use, and major depression.[18] Alternatively, some homeless patients have a chronic history of psychiatric illness, including schizophrenia or bipolar disorder, that may be partially responsible for precipitating homelessness.[19] The psychiatric assessment of homeless patients is important to providing adequate disposition of medical problems whose management may be compromised by mental illness. In addition, primary pharmacologic therapy can be evaluated or instituted in patients with chronic psychiatric disorders.

EMERGENCY DEPARTMENT TREATMENT

ED management includes the history and physical examination, as reviewed. Adjuncts to care include use of vitamin supplements and food, dispensation of medications, updating of immunizations, and reviewing documentation of past medical care. Pregnancy status and potential for sexually transmitted diseases should be investigated in homeless women of childbearing age. Appropriate gynecologic care, prenatal care, or family planning services can thus be arranged. Once a diagnosis and treatment plan are defined, patients should be assessed for language barriers, literacy, and capacity to comply with routine care instructions, medical regimens, or follow-up. An old chart may indicate immunization status, forgotten or disregarded health problems, and the ability of homeless patients to follow up. A lower threshold for admission should be maintained for patients with an impaired ability to manage their own care. This decision is easily acceptable if one appreciates how the patient arrived at the condition in question and how difficult, if not impossible, outpatient care may be in certain circumstances. A multidisciplinary approach to care, including social workers and nursing, medical, and psychiatric staff, may offer the most supportive environment for homeless patients. Such compassionate care in the ED, using trained and motivated individuals, will ensure that patients receive the care they need, increase patients' satisfaction, and reduce the rate of return emergency department visits among frequent users.[20]

REFERENCES

1. Institute of Medicine: *Homelessness, Health, and Human Needs.* Washington, National Academy Press, 1988.
2. Link BG, Susser E, Stueve A, et al: Lifetime and five-year prevalence of homelessness in the United States. *Am J Public Health* 84:1907, 1994.
3. Hibbs JR, Benner L, Klugman L, et al: Mortality in a cohort of homeless adults in Philadelphia. *N Engl J Med* 331:303, 1994.
4. Hanzlick R: Deaths among the homeless: Atlanta, Georgia. *MMWR* 36:297, 1997.
5. Hwang SW, Orav EJ, O'Connell JJ: Causes of death in homeless adults in Boston. *Ann Intern Med* 126:625, 1997.
6. Little GF, Watson DP: The homeless in the emergency department: A patient profile. *J Accid Emerg Med* 13:415, 1996.
7. Padgett DK, Struening EL, Andrews H, Pittman J: Predictors of emergency room use by homeless adults in New York City: The influence of predisposing, enabling and need factors. *Soc Sci Med* 41:547, 1995.
8. Brickner PW, Scharer LK, Conanan B, et al (eds): *Healthcare of Homeless People.* New York, Springer, 1985.
9. Wrenn K: Foot problems in homeless persons. *Ann Intern Med* 113:567, 1990.
10. Wrenn K: Immersion foot: A problem of the homeless in the 1990s. *Arch Intern Med* 151:785, 1991.
11. VonVille P, Holtzhauer F, Long T: Tuberculosis among homeless shelter residents. *MMWR* 40:869, 1991.
12. Koehler JE, Sanchez MA, Garrido CS, et al: Molecular epidemiology of Bartonella infections in patients with bacillary angiomatosis-peliosis. *N Engl J Med* 337:1876, 1997.
13. Bangsberg D, Tulsky JP, Hacht FM, Moss AR: Protease inhibitors in the homeless. *JAMA* 278:63, 1997.
14. Gelberg L, Gallagher TC, Andersen RM, Koegel P: Competing priorities as a barrier to medical care among homeless adults in Los Angeles. *Am J Public Health* 87:217, 1997.
15. Menke EM, Wagner JD: The experience of homeless female-headed families. *Issues Mental Health Nurs* 18:315, 1997.
16. Murata JE, Mace P, Strehlow A: Disease patterns in homeless children. *J Pediatr Nurs* 7:196, 1992.
17. Damrosch S, Strassner JA: The homeless eldery in America. *J Gerontol Nurs* 14:26, 1988.
18. Padgett DK, Struening EL: Influence of substance abuse and mental disorders on emergency room use by homeless adults. *Hosp Community Psychiatry* 42:834, 1991.
19. Bachrach LL, Santiago JM, Berren MR: Homeless mentally ill patients in the community: Results of a general hospital emergency room study. *Community Ment Health J* 26:415, 1990.
20. Redelmeier DA, Molin JP, Tibshirani RJ: A randomized trial of compassionate care for the homeless in an emergency department. *Lancet* 345:1131, 1995.

THE MORBIDLY OBESE PATIENT

Robert J. Vissers
Kathleen A. Raftery

Obesity is the condition of an excessive proportion of adipose tissue to total body weight. It is a common problem in the industrialized world, with approximately one-third of all adults in the United States estimated to be overweight.[1] Since body fat is difficult to measure in the clinical setting, body mass index (BMI) is frequently utilized. BMI is calculated by dividing the weight in kilograms by the square of the height in meters. A BMI greater than 28 kg/m^2 defines obesity in both sexes, and morbid obesity is associated with a BMI of 40 kg/m^2 or greater.

Morbidly obese patients pose a number of challenges for emergency health care providers. Prehospital care may be delayed due to problems in moving and transporting these patients. Appropriate-sized gurneys may not be readily available. Even providing common amenities, such as hospital gowns or bedpans of adequate size, can be difficult. In addition, the emergency department (ED) staff must anticipate and be prepared for challenges in performing technical procedures. Excess tissue makes access to body fluids and body cavities a formidable task, while performing imaging procedures can be difficult or impossible. Morbidly obese patients may also evince changes in cardiopulmonary physiology and patterns of traumatic injury, which add to the complexity of their care.[2] This chapter discusses these problems and suggests strategies and techniques that will facilitate the diagnosis and management of acute illness and injury in this unique group of patients.

PATHOPHYSIOLOGY

Cardiopulmonary Disease

Morbidity and mortality are considerably greater among the obese than in normal-weight patients, and many of the health risks associated with obesity increase progressively and disproportionately with increasing weight.[3] The most significant physiologic disturbances pertain to the cardiopulmonary system.[4]

Coronary artery disease, hypertension, and congestive heart failure are highly correlated with obesity. Both left- and right-sided heart failures are often observed in patients with obesity-hypoventilation syndrome. Obesity has also been linked to depressed left ventricular function even in young, asymptomatic patients.

Obesity is associated with an increased risk of venous thromboembolism, especially after surgery.[5] This is due to several factors found in the obese patient, including decreased levels of circulating antithrombin III, preexisting venous disease, and increased immobility.[6] The obesity-hypoventilation syndrome, also known as the *pickwickian syndrome,* occurs in 5 percent of the morbidly obese. Disturbances in the ventilation-perfusion relationship are prevalent.[7] Pulmonary hypertension is a common finding, resulting from chronic hypoxemia, hypoxic pulmonary vasoconstriction, and the added contribution of compromised cardiac function.[7]

Recognition of the increased risk of cardiorespiratory compromise in the morbidly obese patient is crucial, even when the patient presents to the ED with a problem unrelated to the cardiovascular system. The morbidly obese patient who states that he or she can only sleep in the upright position should be maintained in an upright position as much as possible or in a lateral position with the head up while performing procedures. Pulse oximetry should be used for monitoring, particularly if the patient needs to be supine. Elevate the head of a patient who is on a backboard by placing towels under the board.

Pregnancy

Obesity will also complicate pregnancy. Body weight before pregnancy and weight gain during pregnancy both influence labor, and obese women are more likely to require cesarean sections and to experience abnormal labor.[8] In addition, these infants tend to be heavier than those born to nonobese women, increasing the potential for difficult labor and delivery. Other complications such as hypertension, diabetes, preeclampsia, and eclampsia occur with increased frequency in pregnant obese women.

Trauma

The obese trauma patient is the product of two modern epidemics: the increasing prevalence of obesity and the increasing incidence of trauma.[2] Differences in the mechanisms of injury and associated injury patterns have been described, and obesity has been identified as an independent premorbid risk factor in trauma.[6]

TABLE 304-1 Procedural Problems and Solutions in the Morbidly Obese

Procedure	Problem	Solution
Bag-mask ventilation	Reduced pulmonary compliance	Occlude pop-off valve
Oral intubation	Access to airway Potentially difficult airway	Adjustable angle laryngoscope Objective predictors of difficulty Esophageal tracheal Combitube Surgical airway
Sphygnomanometry	Falsely elevated readings	Use larger cuff size
Pulse oximetry	Poor signal	Earlobe probe
Vascular access	Inability to locate vein/artery	Use 3- to 4-in. catheter Patient positioning Ultrasound-facilitated cannulation
Lumbar puncture	Difficulty in palpating landmarks Difficult to obtain cerebrospinal fluid	Upright patient positioning Increase needle length to 5 in.
Diagnostic peritoneal lavage	Accessing peritoneal cavity	Modified Seldinger technique

Excessive weight interferes with activities of daily living, therefore increasing the risk of injury. Moreover, the presence of obesity-related diseases such as diabetes, heart disease, and somnolence secondary to sleep apnea may contribute to accidents. Obese patients have also been noted to be less likely to wear seat belts because of poor fit or discomfort.

Obesity appears to protect the blunt trauma victim from head injury but is associated with a significantly higher incidence of injuries to the chest, primarily rib fractures and pulmonary contusions. It is hypothesized that the larger torso serves as a physiologic airbag, and although this offers some protection from head injury, there is an associated increase in thoracic injury. This may explain the dramatically higher mortality rate due to respiratory causes in morbidly obese trauma patients. A study that specifically examined the impact of obesity on mortality in blunt trauma found a 42.1 percent mortality rate in severely overweight patients, compared with 5.0 and 8.0 percent in the average and overweight groups.[9]

Despite the logistical difficulties the obese patient presents, the principles of trauma management must still be adhered to, with necessary spinal precautions maintained and full exposure obtained. The presence of subcutaneous fat obscures physical findings in thoracic and abdominal injuries.[6] The limitations of physical findings are further compounded by poor quality, portable chest radiographs in this population. A more aggressive approach to airway management with early intubation and assisted ventilation may be indicated.

The incidence of pelvic fractures is higher in the obese trauma victim. Portable films are often of a poorer quality in the obese patient, therefore any clinical suspicion of a pelvic fracture should be pursued by repeat views or computed tomography, despite a negative portable pelvic radiograph. A higher incidence of displaced ankle and elbow fractures has been described in obese patients sustaining minimal trauma (stumbling, low-energy falls).[10]

A higher frequency of postoperative morbidity and mortality has been recognized in obese patients undergoing elective surgery and is often attributed to their predisposition for pulmonary compromise and significant hypoxemia noted prior to, during, and after surgery. It is unclear if this is the primary cause of increased posttraumatic mortality in the obese patient or whether it is related to delayed diagnosis or intervention.

PROCEDURES

Procedures are more difficult to perform on the obese emergency patient (Table 304-1). Landmarks are obscured or nonpalpable, access is often impaired by excessive tissue, and positioning problems are common. Airway management may be difficult, intravenous access delayed, and investigations cumbersome or impossible to obtain in the obese patient. These factors all contribute to inevitable obstructions to rapid assessment and resuscitation. Having alternative approaches readily available is the ideal strategy. The appropriate equipment, such as the right blood pressure cuff, must be easy to access. Extra personnel are often required, and a minimum of six people is usually necessary to transfer the patient, particularly when cervical spine precautions must be maintained.

Airway Management

Obesity has not been shown to be an independent predictor of a difficult intubation.[11] Although a short thick neck seems to be more common in obese individuals, other objective predictors of a difficult intubation must be recognized and assessed. Use of the Mallampati scale,[12] a test based upon the pharyngeal structure visible when the patient's mouth is wide open, can be helpful. Another method is to measure the distance between the mentum of the chin and the hyoid bone or thyroid prominence. Less than three finger-breadths or less than 6 cm, respectively, when the head is extended, suggests a potentially difficult intubation. Atlantooccipital extension, maxillary overgrowth, temporomandibular joint mobility, nostril patency, and micrognathia are other anatomic features known to influence ease of intubation.

As with nonobese patients, the procedure of choice in the ED setting for the morbidly obese is tracheal intubation using rapid sequence induction (RSI) unless contraindications are present. Patients should be kept sitting upright or semirecumbent as long as possible prior to intubation.

Preoxygenation is critical, since morbidly obese patients will desaturate more quickly than normal adults.[13] If bag-mask ventilation is required, the obese patient often has reduced pulmonary compliance, which necessitates higher ventilatory pressures. The pop-off valve on the ventilation bag may have to be occluded in order to provide adequate ventilation.

Once the process of intubation is begun, access to the airway is enhanced by elevating both the head and shoulders with towels or by placing a rolled blanket between the scapulae and under the occiput. Elevation of the shoulders allows displacement of the breasts away from the midline. The greater elevation of the head places it in the sniffing position, and creates more space, as the chest wall of the morbidly obese patient may actually obstruct the handle of the laryngoscope. A shorter than average handle for the laryngoscope or an adjustable-angle laryngoscope is useful in this situation.

There are several other methods of securing a patent airway, including nasotracheal intubation, oral intubation, transtracheal jet ventilation (TTJV), the laryngeal mask airway (LMA), or the esophageal tracheal Combitube (ETC). Nasotracheal intubation is technically more difficult than orotracheal intubation but may be relatively advantageous if used by an experienced physician to intubate a spontaneously breathing patient with a short thick neck. Oral intubation should be used in the apneic trauma patient. TTJV requires higher ventilatory pressures and therefore may be less useful in the obese patient with decreased pulmonary compliance. The LMA may not provide adequate ventilation and may not protect against aspiration. Thus, it is not a first choice owing to the obese patient's tendency for rapid desaturation and aspiration. The ETC appears to be a reasonable alternative, providing ventilation as well as protection against aspiration, and its utility in the morbidly obese patient has been documented.[14] A fiberoptic bronchoscope can also be used to aid intubation, although visualization may be impaired by circumpharyngeal fat.

Finally, a cricothyrotomy may be indicated if other maneuvers fail. Needle cricothyrotomy is difficult given the anatomy of a morbidly obese patient's neck.

Electrocardiogram Analysis

Host factors such as body mass influence the ease of obtaining and interpreting an electrocardiogram (ECG). Landmarks for lead placement may be difficult to determine, and optimal lead placement and patient positioning may not be possible. Breast size and fat deposits in the chest wall can result in inaccurate lead placement. Variation in fat deposits in the chest wall and fat deposits surrounding the heart can lead to inconsistent voltage changes, although in general obese patients demonstrate loss of voltage.[15] Flattening or inversion of the T wave in the inferior or lateral leads is one consistent change. None of these ECG changes is pathognomonic for obesity, and such abnormalities should not be attributed to obesity alone.

Sphygmomanometry

Inadequate cuff width and circumference will artificially elevate pressure readings.[16] However, many morbidly obese patients are hypertensive, and a high pressure reading cannot always be blamed on inappropriate equipment. In order to minimize errors in blood pressure recording, a correct ratio of cuff width to arm circumference, approximately 2:5, should be chosen. The bladder length should be 80 percent of the arm circumference. The ED should stock a variety of sizes of blood pressure cuffs specifically for use in the obese population.

Pulse Oximetry

Tissue thickness can make the transmission of light waves more difficult in the extremely obese and thus make pulse oximetry readings unreliable. However, pulse oximetry in the moderately obese is generally accurate. In morbidly obese patients, the earlobe should be used instead of the finger for probe placement, as the earlobe is usually thinner than the digit, with higher perfusion, and the probe stays in place more easily. If use of an earlobe probe is not possible, use of the fifth digit of the hand or foot can be tried. Other areas of placement include the nose, lip, or temporal artery.[17]

Venous Access

Morbidly obese patients are notoriously difficult candidates for intravenous catheterization, venipuncture, or arterial puncture. Anatomy is distorted by subcutaneous fat, and landmark vessels are often not visible or palpable. This leads to multiple attempts, delay in access, and an increased incidence of central line placement with delays in changing a line after admission. All these factors contribute to a higher rate of complications, such as wound infection, pneumothorax, phlebitis, and thrombosis. In addition, standard 1.5-in. needles or catheters may not be long enough to penetrate the subcutaneous tissue and reach the target vessel; 3- or 4-in. needles and catheters are preferred. Locating the radial or femoral artery in order to obtain a sample for arterial blood gas analysis can also be extremely difficult. It may be necessary to change needle lengths on the prepackaged arterial blood gas syringes.

Various techniques can be employed to improve access to the vessel. Application of heat, light tapping over the vessel, active or passive pumping of the extremity, and application of topical nitroglycerin are commonly used to encourage vasodilation. Reactive hyperemia can be created by occluding the circulation for 3 to 4 min, then releasing the sphygmomanometer to 10 to 15 mmHg below the diastolic pressure.

The medial cubital and basilic veins are the first choice in the morbidly obese, since they are large, the antecubital crease is visible, and the skin and subcutaneous tissues are thinner in this area. Branches of the median and basilic veins on the volar surface of the forearm may be too deep to the adipose tissue to be easily accessed. The cephalic vein on the radial aspect of the wrist is a good second choice if it is not also obscured by fat. Another option is the vessels of the dorsum of the hand. The veins of the fingers may be accessible, especially those over the dorsal aspect of the thumb and forefinger. The veins of the feet are usually not good candidates, since they tend to be obscured by fat or the ravages of peripheral vascular disease. However, no vein should be excluded if it is accessible.

If peripheral veins are not available, a cutdown at the forearm veins or an attempt at cannulation of the external jugular vein should be the next choice. Cannulation of the femoral vein is another option, and will be facilitated by placing a towel under the ipsilateral buttock and having an assistant retract the panniculus. Venisection at the saphenous vein, a common alternative in patients of normal weight, will be challenging because of excess adipose tissue. Femoral catheterization is preferred over saphenous venisection in the obese patient with a palpable femoral pulse.

Because of the difficulty of peripheral access in the obese patient, a central line is more frequently required. Unfortunately, central line placement is also challenging.[18] Subclavian vein cannulation may be preferable to the internal jugular, since the bony landmarks are more easily palpable and the complication rate is lower than with other central venous access methods. The patient is usually placed in the Trendelenburg position. Change positions gradually while continuing to monitor the ECG and oxygen saturation. In some cases, as when the patient reports the need to sleep upright, the Trendelenburg position may be relatively contraindicated.[19] During subclavian line placement, abduction of the arm (as opposed to the standard recommendation of arm adduction) and retraction of chest tissue away from the clavicle may reduce excessive tissue layers at the site. It is common practice to insert a roll under the shoulders or a pillow lengthwise along the spine to improve access.

Ultrasound can facilitate venous cannulation and arterial puncture, allowing a higher success rate with fewer attempts because it is performed independent of landmarks.[20]

Lumbar Puncture

A lumbar puncture is difficult because landmarks tend to be obscured and depth is difficult to estimate. The procedure is most successfully performed with the patient sitting and bent forward. With the patient upright, the midline is easier to estimate and both iliac crests are usually palpable. Bone encountered after only a few centimeters usually represents spinous process and suggests an adjustment in the vertical plane above or below this point. A deeper bony encounter is likely lamina and requires a medial adjustment. Ultrasonography can be used as an aid to locating the vertebra.[21] Despite the excessive tissue, the standard 3-in. needle is adequate for many obese patients, although this may require pushing the needle hub to the point of dimpling the skin. The 5-in. needle is sometimes needed. It is best to have both sizes readily available. Tight intervertebral disk spaces are common in this population and may not allow passage of a 16- or 18-gauge needle. It may be necessary to use a much smaller gauge (albeit more flexible) needle as a guide for locating the disk, then a larger-gauge needle to puncture the space. The best choice is a 22- or 24-gauge needle, which allows adequate flow and decreases the likelihood of postpuncture headache.

Diagnostic Peritoneal Lavage

Diagnostic peritoneal lavage (DPL) is used for the early recognition of intraabdominal injury requiring celiotomy. In many centers, the use of DPL has been supplanted by imaging techniques because of increased accessibility to improved computed tomography (CT) and ultrasonography. However, size and weight restrictions and transport difficulties may preclude the use of CT scanning in the obese trauma victim. Abdominal ultrasonography is also less reliable in the morbidly obese patient. Therefore DPL may be the preferable diagnostic approach in these patients.

There are three general DPL techniques: the open, semiopen, and closed. In the open technique, a catheter is passed into the abdominal cavity through a large incision that exposes the peritoneum. This technique requires two people and in a normal-weight person may take more than 25 min.[22] Because of the larger incision required, the technical difficulties presented by the panniculus, and a potentially higher rate of wound infection and herniation, morbid obesity has been described as a relative contraindication to this procedure.

The traditional closed technique uses a larger trochar and is associated with an unacceptable rate of complications. A blind Seldinger technique using a smaller 18-gauge needle has been shown to be as efficient as the open technique. We recommend this as the method of choice in the obese patient. In patients whose abdominal wall thickness exceeds the reach of the needle, a modified Seldinger technique has been described in which 2- to 4-cm incision is carried down to the midline fascia and an 18-gauge needle is then inserted at that point. This procedure was used successfully in six morbidly obese patients whose weight exceeded the weight limit of the CT scanner.[22]

Imaging

Radiographs have limited utility in the morbidly obese. Standard film cassettes are too small to accommodate the entire chest or abdomen, and two or more films may be required. Excessive soft tissue can result in extremely underpenetrated films. Since transport is invariably problematic, morbidly obese patients may need to undergo portable radiography, resulting in lower-quality images.

CT and magnetic resonance imaging (MRI) scans are clearly superior to radiographs, offering better resolution and greater penetration. However, many CT scanners have a weight limit of 400 to 450 lb and a girth limit of 30 in. Most standard MRI scanners have a maximum shoulder-to-shoulder width of 52 in. and a weight limit of 350 lb. Thus many morbidly obese patients will be excluded from undergoing these studies. There are, however, private companies, veterinary schools, and zoos that have scanners with a larger capacity.

EQUIPMENT PROBLEMS SPECIFIC TO ED CARE

From the time the obese patient enters the waiting area to the time he or she leaves the ED, issues related to the patient's size challenge both personnel and equipment. Waiting-room chairs may be too small. Most wheelchairs also have weight limits and are not designed to safely accommodate patients weighing over 200 kg. Gurneys are often too small for the patient if the protective side rails are in place, and without the side rails the patient is not safe. In addition, collapsible gurneys are not designed to hold the weight of the morbidly obese patient, leading to instability and concomitant patient and staff danger. We recommend that EDs stock one heavy-duty stretcher (one with additional cross-brace supports) and at least one wheelchair designed to hold patients weighing more than 200 kg.

The comfort and modesty of morbidly obese patients should be thoughtfully considered during his or her ED stay.[23] The ED should stock oversized hospital gowns. Patients should also be allowed to wear their own night clothing as long as it does not obstruct care.

Any care that requires lifting or turning of the obese patient is difficult, as techniques used for average-sized patients cannot be used. In general, more than two providers should always be utilized to move the patient. Provision of an overhead trapeze will greatly facilitate patient-assisted transfers and should be available in the ED.

REFERENCES

1. Kuczmarski RJ, Flegal KM, Campbell SM, Johnson CL: Increasing prevalence of overweight among US adults. *JAMA* 272:205-11, 1994.
2. Boulanger B, Milzman D, Mitchell K, Rodriguez A: Body habitus as a predictor of injury pattern following blunt trauma. *J Trauma* 33:228, 1992.
3. Garrison RJ, Castelli WP: Weight and thirty-year mortality of men in the Framingham Study. *Ann Intern Med* 103:1006, 1985.
4. Ernst ND, Obarzanek E, Clark MB, et al: Cardiovascular health risks related to overweight. *J Am Diet Assoc* 97:S47, 1997.
5. Goldhaber S, Goldstein E, Stampfer M, et al: A prospective study of risk factors for pulmonary embolism in women. *JAMA* 277:642, 1997.
6. Boulanger BR, Milzman DP, Rodriguez A: Obesity. *Crit Care Clin* 10:613, 1994.
7. Lazarus R, Sparrow D, Weiss S: Effects of obesity and fat distribution on ventilatory function: The normative aging study. *Chest* 111:891, 1997.
8. Maeder EC Jr, Barno A, Mecklenburg F: Obesity: a maternal high-risk factor. *Obstet Gynecol* 45:669, 1975.
9. Smith-Choban P, Weireter L, Maynes C: Obesity and increased mortality in blunt trauma. *J Trauma* 31:1253, 1991.
10. Bostman A: BMI of patients with elbow and ankle fractures. *J Trauma* 37:62, 1994.
11. Rocke DA, Murray WB, Rout CC, Gouws E: Relative risk analysis of factors associated with difficult intubation in obstetric anesthesia. *Anesthesiology* 77:67, 1992.
12. Mallampati SR, Gatt SP, Gugino LD, et al: A clinical sign to predict difficult tracheal intubation: A prospective study. *Can Anaesth Soc J* 32:429, 1985.
13. Berthoud MC, Peacock JE, Reilly CS: Effectiveness of preoxygenation in morbidly obese patients. *Br J Anaesth* 67:464, 1991.
14. Banyai M, Falger S, Roggla M, et al: Emergency intubation with the Combitube in a grossly obese patient with bull neck. *Resuscitation* 26:271, 1993.
15. Eisenstein I, Edelstein J, Sarma R, et al: The electrocardiogram in obesity. *J Electrocardiol* 15:115, 1982.
16. Maxwell MH, Waks AU, Schroth PC, et al: Error in blood-pressure measurement due to incorrect cuff size in obese patients. *Lancet* 2:33, 1982.
17. Severinghaus J, Kelleher J: Recent developments in pulse oximetry. *Anesthesiology* 76:1018, 1992.
18. Dronen S, Younger J: Central venous catheterization and central venous pressure monitoring. In: Roberts JR, Hedges JR (eds): *Clinical Procedures in Emergency Medicine,* 3d ed. Philadelphia, Saunders, 1998, pp 358–385.
19. Burns S, Egloff M, Ryan B, et al: Effect of body position on spontaneous respiratory rate and tidal volume in patients with obesity, abdominal distension and ascites. *Am J Crit Care* 3:102, 1994.
20. Gilbert T, Seneff M, Becker R: Facilitation of internal jugular venous cannulation using an audio-guided Doppler ultrasound vascular access device: Results from a prospective dual-center, randomized, crossover clinical study. *Crit Care Med* 23:60, 1995.
21. Wallace DH, Currie JM, Gilstrap LC, Santos R: Indirect sonographic guidance for epidural anesthesia in obese pregnant patients. *Reg Anesth* 17:233, 1992.
22. Ochsner MG, Herr D, Drucker W, Champion HR: A modified Seldinger technique for peritoneal lavage in trauma patients who are obese. *Surg Gynecol Obstet* 173:158, 1991.
23. Wadden TA, Stunkard AJ: Social and psychological consequences of obesity. *Ann Intern Med* 103:1062, 1985.

INDEX

NOTE: Bold number indicates the start of the chapter that contains the main discussion of the topic; numbers followed with *f* and *t* refer to figure and table pages.

B

C

D

G

I

J

M

O

Q

R

S

W

X

Y

Z

ISBN 0-07-065351-8
90000
9 780070 653511
TINTINALLI/EMER. MED.

TABLE 247-1 The Glasgow Coma Scale for All Age Groups

	4 yrs to Adult	Child <4 yrs	Infant
EYE OPENING			
4	Spontaneous	Spontaneous	Spontaneous
3	To speech	To speech	To speech
2	To pain	To pain	To pain
1	No response	No response	No response
VERBAL RESPONSE			
5	Alert and oriented	Oriented, social, speaks, interacts	Coos, babbles
4	Disoriented conversation	Confused speech, disoriented, consolable, aware	Irritable cry
3	Speaking but nonsensical	Inappropriate words, inconsolable, unaware	Cries to pain
2	Moans or unintelligible sounds	Incomprehensible, agitated, restless, unaware	Moans to pain
1	No response	No response	No response
MOTOR RESPONSE			
6	Follows commands	Normal, spontaneous movements	Normal, spontaneous moves
5	Localizes pain	Localizes pain	Withdraws to touch
4	Movement or withdrawal to pain	Withdraws to pain	Withdraws to pain
3	Decorticate flexion	Decorticate flexion	Decorticate flexion
2	Decerebrate extension	Decerebrate extension	Decerebrate extension
1	No response	No response	No response
3–15			

GCS reporting should be modified for intubated and paralyzed patients.

TABLE 266-2 Pittsburgh Knee Rules

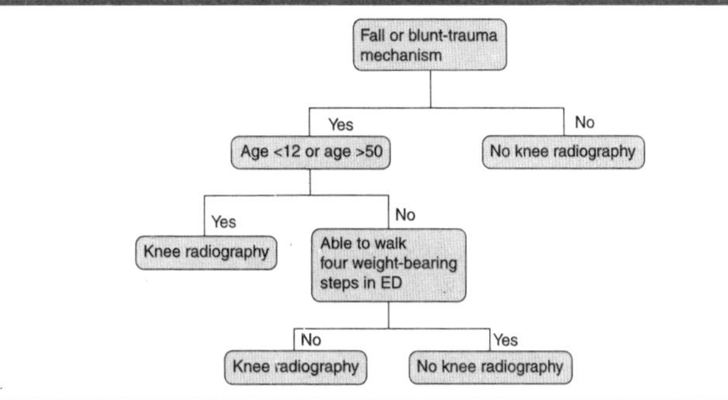

TABLE 266-1 Ottawa Knee Rules: Guidelines for X-Ray

1. Patient older than 55 years
2. Tenderness at the head of the fibula
3. Isolated tenderness of the patella
4. Inability to flex knee to 90 degrees
5. Inability to transfer weight for four steps both immediately after the injury and in the ED

TABLE 10-5 Length-Based Equipment Chart (Length, cm)

Item	54–70	70–85	85–95	95–107	107–124	124–138	138–155
Endotracheal tube size (mm)	3.5	4.0	4.5	5.0	5.5	6.0	6.5
Lip-tip length (mm)	10.5	12.0	13.5	15.0	16.5	18.0	19.5
Laryngoscope	1 Straight	1 Straight	2 Straight	2 Straight or curved	2 Straight or curved	2–3 Straight or curved	3 Straight or curved
Suction catheter	8F	8–10F	10F	10F	10F	10F	12F
Stylet	6F	6F	6F	6F	14F	14F	14F
Oral airway	Infant/small child	Small child	Child	Child	Child/small adult	Child/adult	Medium adult
Bag-valve mask	Infant	Child	Child	Child	Child	Child/adult	Adult
Oxygen mask	Newborn	Pediatric	Pediatric	Pediatric	Pediatric	Adult	Adult
Vascular access	22–24/23–25	20–22/ 23–25	18–22/ 21–23	18–22/ 21–23	18–20/ 21–23	18–20/ 21–22	16–20/ 18–21
Catheter/butterfly	Intraosseous		Intraosseous		Intraosseous		Intraosseous
Nasogastric tube	5–8F	8–10F	10F	10–12F	12–14F	14–18F	18F
Urinary catheter	5–8F	8–10F	10F	10–12F	10–12F	12F	12F
Chest tube	10–12F	16–20F	20–24F	20–24F	24–32F	28–32F	32–40F
Blood pressure cuff	Newborn/infant	Infant/child	Child	Child	Child	Child/adult	Adult

Directions for use:
1. Measure patient length with centimeter tape.
2. Using measured length in centimeters, access appropriate equipment column.

Source: Adapted from Luten et al,[9] with permission.